I. ATLAS OF DERMATOLOGY
Stephen F. Templeton / Thomas J. Lawley

A. Common Skin Diseases and Lesions

IA-1 Acne vulgaris **IA-2** Acne rosacea **IA-3** Psoriasis **IA-4** Atopic dermatitis **IA-5** Dyshidrotic eczema **IA-6** Seborrheic dermatitis **IA-7** Statis dermatitis **IA-8** Allergic contact dermatitis **IA-9** Lichen planus **IA-10** Pityriasis rosea **IA-11** Vitiligo **IA-12** Alopecia areata **IA-13** Urticaria **IA-14** Epidermoid cysts **IA-15** Seborrheic keratoses **IA-16** Keloids **IA-17** Cherry hemangiomas

B. Cutaneous Neoplasms

IB-18 Actinic keratoses **IB-19** Keratoacanthoma **IB-20** Basal cell carcinoma **IB-21** Squamous cell carcinoma **IB-22** Kaposi's sarcoma **IB-23** Mycosis fungoides **IB-24** Non-Hodgkin's lymphoma **IB-25** Metastatic carcinoma

C. Pigmented Lesions—Benign and Malignant

IC-26 Nevus **IC-27** Dysplastic nevi **IC-28** Superficial spreading melanoma **IC-29** Lentigo maligna melanoma **IC-30** Nodular melanoma **IC-31** Acral letiginous melanoma

D. Infectious Disease and the Skin

ID-32 Impetigo contagiosa **ID-33** Folliculitis **ID-34** Erysipelas **ID-35** Herpes simplex **ID-36** Varicella **ID-37** Herpes zoster **ID-38** Spread of herpes zoster with chemotherapy **ID-39** Verrucae **ID-40** Molluscum contagiosum **ID-41** Oral hairy leukoplakia **ID-42** Pseudomembranous oral candidiasis **ID-43** Tinea corporis **ID-44** Tinea cruris **ID-45** Tinea versicolor **ID-46** Scabies **ID-47** Erythema chronicum migrans **ID-48** Rocky Mountain spotted fever **ID-49** Disseminated gonococcemia **ID-50** Fulminant meningococcemia **ID-51** Primary syphilis **ID-52** Secondary syphilis **ID-53** Secondary syphilis **ID-54** Condylomata lata **ID-55** Chancroid **ID-56** Condylomata acuminata **ID-57** Skin lesions of neutropenic patients

E. Immunologically Mediated Skin Disease

IE-58 Systemic lupus erythematosus **IE-59** Discoid lupus erythematosus **IE-60** Dermatomyositis **IE-61** Dermatomyositis **IE-62** Scleroderma **IE-63** Scleroderma **IE-64** Erythema multiforme **IE-65** Erythema nodosum **IE-66** Vasculitis **IE-67** Pemphigus vulgaris **IE-68** Dermatitis herpetiformis **IE-69** Bullous pemphigoid

F. Skin Manifestations of Internal Disease

IF-70 Acanthosis nigricans **IF-71** Pretibial myxedema **IF-72** Sarcoid **IF-73** Neurofibromatosis **IF-74** Coumarin necrosis **IF-75** Pyoderma gangrenosum

II. ATLAS OF ENDOSCOPIC FINDINGS

II-1 Normal esophagus **II-2** Peptic regurgitant esophagitis **II-3** Ulcerated squamous cell carcinoma **II-4** Moniliasis of the esophagus **II-5** Barrett's metaplasia of the esophagus with an adenocarcinoma **II-6** Normal body of the stomach with rugal folds **II-7** Large, benign, lesser curve gastric ulcer **II-8** Gastric polyp **II-9** Arteriovenous malformation of the gastric mucosa **II-10** Normal pylorus **II-11** Normal duodenal bulb **II-12** Duodenal ulcer **II-13** Normal papilla of Vater **II-14** Periampullary carcinoma **II-15** Endoscopic papillotomy **II-16** Normal colon **II-17** Colonic adenomatous polyp **II-18** Multiple, small, colonic adenomatous polyps **II-19** Colon adenocarcinoma **II-20** Crohn's colitis **II-21** Severe ulcerative colitis **II-22** Kaposi's sarcoma involving the colon **II-23** Colonic varices **II-24** Ileal pouch

III. ATLAS OF FUNDUSCOPIC EXAMINATION

III-1 Cytomegalovirus **III-2** Hollenhorst plaque **III-3** Hypertensive retinopathy **III-4** Central retinal vein occlusion **III-5** Anterior ischemic optic neuropathy **III-6** Retrobulbar optic neuritis **III-7** Optic atrophy **III-8** Papilledema **III-9** Optic disc drusen **III-10** Retinal detachment **III-11** Glaucoma **III-12** Age-related macular degeneration **III-13** Diabetic retinopathy **III-14** Retinitis pigmentosa **III-15** Melanoma **III-16** Kayser-Fleischer ring

IV. ATLAS OF HEMATOLOGY

IV-1 Normal blood smear **IV-2** Megaloblastic anemia **IV-3** Liver disease **IV-4** Iron-deficiency anemia **IV-5** β Thalassemia intermedia **IV-6** Sickle cell anemia **IV-7** Traumatic hemolysis **IV-8** Spur cell anemia **IV-9** Uremia **IV-10** Hereditary spherocytosis **IV-11** Immunohemolytic anemia **IV-12** Leukoerythroblastic smear **IV-13A.** Normal granulocyte **IV-13B.** Normal monocyte and lymphocyte **IV-14A.** Normal eosinophil **IV-14B.** Basophil **IV-15** Normal granulocyte precursors in marrow **IV-16** Neutrophils with toxic granulation **IV-17** Band with Döhle body **IV-18** Hypersegmentation **IV-19A** Chédiak-Higashi anomaly **IV-19B** Pelger-Hüet anomaly **IV-20** Reactive lymphocytes **IV-21** Chronic granulocytic leukemia **IV-22** Promyelocytic leukemia **IV-23** Chronic lymphocytic leukemia **IV-24** Leukemia cells in acute lymphoblastic leukemia **IV-25** Hodgkin's disease, mixed cellularity **IV-26** Follicular lymphoma **IV-27** Multiple myeloma **IV-28** Diffuse large B cell lymphoma **IV-29** Burkitt's lymphoma **IV-30** Acute myelocytic leukemia **IV-31** Auer rod **IV-32** Normal bone marrow biopsy **IV-33** Aplastic anemia **IV-34** Marrow fibrosis **IV-35** Erythroid hyperplasia **IV-36** Granulocytic hyperplasia **IV-37** Megaloblastic erythropoiesis **IV-38** Marrow iron stores **IV-39** Ringed sideroblast

14TH EDITION

Harrison's

PRINCIPLES of INTERNAL MEDICINE

14TH EDITION

VOLUME 1

Harrison's

PRINCIPLES of INTERNAL MEDICINE

EDITORS

Anthony S. Fauci, MD
Chief, Laboratory of Immunoregulation; Director,
National Institute of Allergy and Infectious
Diseases, National Institutes of Health, Bethesda

Eugene Braunwald, AB, MD,
MA (Hon), MD (Hon), ScD (Hon)
Distinguished Hersey Professor of Medicine,
Faculty Dean for Academic Programs at Brigham
and Women's Hospital and Massachusetts General
Hospital, Harvard Medical School; Vice-President
for Academic Programs, Partners HealthCare
System, Boston

Kurt J. Isselbacher, AB, MD
Mallinckrodt Professor of Medicine, Harvard
Medical School; Physician and Director,
Massachusetts General Hospital Cancer Center,
Boston

Jean D. Wilson, MD
Charles Cameron Sprague Distinguished Chair
and Clinical Professor of Internal Medicine, The
University of Texas Southwestern Medical Center,
Dallas

Joseph B. Martin, MD, PhD,
FRCP (C), MA (Hon)
Dean of the Faculty of Medicine;
Caroline Shields Walker Professor of
Neurobiology and Clinical Neuroscience,
Harvard Medical School, Boston

Dennis L. Kasper, MD, MA (Hon)
William Ellery Channing Professor of
Medicine, Harvard Medical School;
Director, Channing Laboratory; Co-Director,
Division of Infectious Diseases; Executive
Vice-Chairman, Department of Medicine,
Brigham and Women's Hospital, Boston

Stephen L. Hauser, MD
Chairman and Betty Anker Fife Professor,
Department of Neurology, University of
California San Francisco, San Francisco

Dan L. Longo, AB, MD, FACP
Scientific Director, National Institute on
Aging, National Institutes of Health,
Gerontology Research Center,
Bethesda and Baltimore

McGraw-Hill
HEALTH PROFESSIONS DIVISION

New York   St. Louis   San Francisco   Auckland   Bogotá   Caracas   Lisbon   London   Madrid
Mexico City   Milan   Montreal   New Delhi   San Juan   Singapore   Sydney   Tokyo   Toronto

A Division of The McGraw·Hill Companies

Harrison's
PRINCIPLES OF INTERNAL MEDICINE
Fourteenth Edition

4567890 DOWDOW 0403020100

ISBN 0-07-020291-5 (COMBO)
0-07-020292-3 (VOL 1)
0-07-020293-1 (VOL 2)
0-07-912013-X (SET)

FOREIGN LANGUAGE EDITIONS
Arabic (Thirteenth Edition)—McGraw-Hill Libri Italia srl (est. 1996)
Chinese (Twelfth Edition)—McGraw-Hill Book Company–Singapore © 1994
Croatian (Thirteenth Edition)—McGraw-Hill Libri Italia srl (est. 1996)
French (Thirteenth Edition)—McGraw-Hill Libri Italia srl © 1995
German (Thirteenth Edition)—McGraw-Hill Libri Italia srl © 1995
Greek (Twelfth Edition)—Parissianos © 1994
Italian (Thirteenth Edition)—McGraw-Hill Libri Italia srl © 1995
Japanese (Eleventh Edition)—Hirokawa © 1991
Portuguese (Thirteenth Edition)—McGraw-Hill/Nueva Editorial Interamericana © 1995
Spanish (Thirteenth Edition)—McGraw-Hill Interamericana de España © 1994
Turkish (Thirteenth Edition)—McGraw-Hill Libri Italia srl (est. 1996)

This book was set in Times Roman by Monotype Composition Company. The editors were J. Dereck Jeffers, Martin J. Wonsiewicz, and Mariapaz Ramos Englis; editorial assistants were Rose Derario and Daniel J. Green. The production director was Robert Laffler. The index was prepared by Irving Tullar. The text and cover designer was Marsha Cohen/Parallelogram Graphics.

R.R. Donnelley and Sons, Inc., was the printer and binder.

Library of Congress Cataloging-in-Publication Data

Harrison's principles of internal medicine.—14th. ed./editors,
  Anthony S. Fauci . . . [et al.]
      p.   cm.
  Includes bibliographical references and index.
    ISBN 0-07-020291-5 (1 vol. ed.).—ISBN 0-07-912013-X (2 vol. ed.
: set).—ISBN 0-07-020292-3 (2 vol. ed. : bk 1).—ISBN
0-07-020293-1 (2 vol. ed. : bk 2)
    1. Internal medicine.   I. Harrison, Tinsley Randolph.
  II. Fauci, Anthony S.
    [DNLM: 1. Internal Medicine.   WB 115 H322 1998]
RC46.H333   1998
616—dc21
DNLM/DLC
for Library of Congress   97-14184

CONTENTS

SECTION 2
SPECIFIC ENVIRONMENTAL AND OCCUPATIONAL HAZARDS

APPENDICES

CONTRIBUTORS

Numbers in brackets refer to chapters written or co-written by the contributor.

ELIAS ABRUTYN, MD
Professor of Medicine and Public Health and Vice-Chairman, Medicine, Allegheny University of the Health Sciences, MCP Hahnemann School of Medicine, Philadelphia [146, 147]

MICHAEL J. AMINOFF, MD, FRCP
Professor of Neurology, University of California San Francisco, San Francisco [21, 361, 368]

KENNETH C. ANDERSON, MD
Associate Professor of Medicine, Harvard Medical School; Medical Director, Blood Component Laboratory, Dana-Farber Cancer Institute, Boston [115]

ELLIOTT M. ANTMAN, MD
Associate Professor of Medicine, Harvard Medical School; Director, Coronary Care Unit, Brigham and Women's Hospital, Boston [243]

GORDON LEE ARCHER, MD
Professor of Medicine and Microbiology/Immunology; Chairman, Division of Infectious Diseases, Department of Medicine, Medical College of Virginia, Virginia Commonwealth University, Richmond [140]

JAMES O. ARMITAGE, MD
Professor and Chairperson, Department of Internal Medicine, University of Nebraska Medical Center, Omaha [116]

ARTHUR K. ASBURY, MD
Van Meter Professor of Neurology; Vice-Dean for Faculty Affairs, University of Pennsylvania School of Medicine, Philadelphia [23, 381]

JOHN R. ASPLIN, MD
Assistant Professor of Medicine, Section of Nephrology, University of Chicago Pritzker School of Medicine, Chicago [278, 279]

JOHN C. ATHERTON, MRCP
Lecturer, Department of Medicine, Division of Gastroenterology and Institute of Infections and Immunity, University of Nottingham, Nottingham, England [156]

PAUL S. AUERBACH, MD, MS
Chief Executive Officer, American Medical Partners; Clinical Professor of Emergency Medicine, Stanford University School of Medicine, Stanford [392]

K. FRANK AUSTEN, MD
Theodore B. Bayles Professor of Medicine, Harvard Medical School; Director, Inflammation & Allergic Diseases Research Section, Division of Rheumatology and Immunology, Department of Medicine, Brigham and Women's Hospital, Boston [310]

BERNARD M. BABIOR, MD, PhD
Head, Division of Biochemistry, Department of Molecular and Experimental Medicine, The Scripps Research Institute; Professor and Staff Physician, Division of Hematology and Oncology, Department of Medicine, Scripps Clinic and Research Foundation, La Jolla [108]

KAMAL F. BADR, MD
Professor of Medicine and Director, Center for Glomerulonephritis, Renal Division, Emory University; Chief, Renal Section, Atlanta VA Medical Center; Attending Physician, Emory University Hospital, Atlanta [277]

DONALD S. BAIM, MD
Professor of Medicine, Harvard Medical School; Chief, Interventional Cardiology Section, Beth Israel Deaconess Medical Center, Boston [229, 245]

ANN SULLIVAN BAKER, MD*
Associate Professor of Medicine (Ophthalmology), Harvard Medical School; Director, Infectious Disease Service, Massachusetts Eye and Ear Infirmary; Physician, Massachusetts General Hospital, Boston [30]

KENNETH J. BART, MD, MPH, MSHPM
Associate Director, Office of International and Refugee Health, Department of Health and Human Services, Rockville [122]

M. FLINT BEAL, MD
Professor of Neurology, Harvard Medical School, Boston [372, 380]

* Deceased

ARTHUR L. BEAUDET, MD
Investigator, Howard Hughes Medical Institute; Professor, Departments of Molecular and Human Genetics, Pediatrics and Cell Biology, Institute for Molecular Genetics, Baylor College of Medicine, Houston [65]

ROBERT S. BENJAMIN, MD
Internist and Professor of Medicine, Chairman, Department of Melanoma/ Sarcoma Medical Oncology; Medical Director, Multidisciplinary Sarcoma Center, The University of Texas M.D. Anderson Cancer Center, Houston [100]

JOHN E. BENNETT, MD
Head, Clinical Mycology Section, Laboratory of Clinical Investigation, Division of Intramural Research, National Institute of Allergy and Infectious Diseases, National Institutes of Health; Director, Infectious Diseases Training Program, NIAID, NIH, Bethesda [202–210]

ERNEST BEUTLER, MD
Member and Chairman, Department of Molecular and Experiment Medicine, The Scripps Research Institute; Clinical Professor of Medicine, University of California, San Diego, San Diego [107]

DAVID R. BICKERS, MD
Carl Truman Nelson Professor, Chairman, Department of Dermatology, College of Physicians and Surgeons, Columbia University, New York [58]

BEVERLY M.K. BILLER, MD
Assistant Professor of Medicine, Harvard Medical School, Massachusetts General Hospital, Boston [328]

THOMAS D. BIRD, MD
Professor of Neurology, University of Washington; Chief of Neurology, Veterans Affairs Medical Center, Seattle [26, 367]

NEIL R. BLACKLOW, MD
Richard M. Haidack Distinguished Professor of Medicine, Molecular Genetics and Microbiology, and Chairman, Department of Medicine, University of Massachusetts Medical School, Worcester [189]

MARTIN J. BLASER, MD
The Addison B. Scoville Professor of Medicine; Director, Division of Infectious Diseases and Professor of Microbiology and Immunology, Vanderbilt University School of Medicine and VA Medical Center, Nashville [156, 160]

CLARA D. BLOOMFIELD, MD
Professor and Director, Division of Hematology and Oncology, Department of Internal Medicine; Director, Comprehensive Cancer Center, Ohio State University, Columbus [112]

JEAN L. BOLOGNIA, MD
Associate Professor of Dermatology, Yale University School of Medicine, New Haven [57]

GEORGE J. BOSL, MD
Chairman, Department of Medicine, Memorial Sloan-Kettering Cancer Center; Professor of Medicine, Cornell University Medical College, New York [98]

RICHARD C. BOUCHER, JR., MD
Professor of Medicine and Director, CF/Pulmonary Research and Treatment Center and Chief, Division of Pulmonary Disease/Critical Care Medicine, University of North Carolina at Chapel Hill; University of North Carolina Hospitals, Chapel Hill [257]

DAVID S. BRADFORD, MD
Chairman and Professor, Department of Orthopaedic Surgery, University of California San Francisco, San Francisco [16]

KAREN D. BRADSHAW, MD
Associate Professor of Obstetrics and Gynecology, The University of Texas Southwestern Medical Center, Dallas [52, 337]

HUGH R. BRADY, MD, PhD, FRCPI
Professor of Medicine and Therapeutics, University College Dublin; Mater Misericordiae Hospital, Dublin, Ireland [270, 273–275]

KENNETH D. BRANDT, MD
Professor of Medicine; Head, Rheumatology Division; Director, Multipurpose Arthritis and Musculoskeletal Diseases Center, Indiana University School of Medicine, Indianapolis [322]

EUGENE BRAUNWALD, AB, MD, MA (Hon), MD (Hon),
ScD (Hon), FRCP
Distinguished Hersey Professor of Medicine; Faculty Dean for Academic Programs at Brigham and Women's Hospital and Massachusetts General Hospital, Harvard Medical School; Vice-President for Academic Programs, Partners HealthCare System, Boston [1, 32–34, 36, 37, 226, 227, 232, 233, 237–241, 243, 244]

IRWIN M. BRAVERMAN, MD
Professor of Dermatology, Yale University School of Medicine, New Haven [57]

OTIS W. BRAWLEY, MD
Director, Office of Special Populations, Office of the Director, National Cancer Institute, National Institutes of Health, Bethesda [82]

GEORGE A. BRAY, MD
Professor of Medicine/Executive Director, Pennington Biomedical Research Center, Louisiana State University, Baton Rouge [75]

JOEL G. BREMAN, MD, DTPH
Deputy Director, Division of International Training and Research, Fogarty International Center, National Institutes of Health, Bethesda [216]

BARRY M. BRENNER, MD, AM (Hon), DSc (Hon), DMSc (Hon)
Samuel A. Levine Professor of Medicine, Harvard Medical School; Senior Physician and Director, Renal Division, Brigham and Women's Hospital, Boston [47, 49, 268–271, 273–277, 280]

CLAIRE V. BROOME, MD
Deputy Director, Centers for Disease Control and Prevention, Atlanta [145]

PHILIPPE BROUQUI, MD, PhD
Professor of Medicine, Faculté de Médecine, Marseilles, France [179]

ROBERT H. BROWN, JR., DPhil, MD
Associate Neurologist, Massachusetts General Hospital; Associate Professor of Neurology, Harvard Medical School, Boston [103, 370]

H. FRANKLIN BUNN, MD
Professor of Medicine, Harvard Medical School; Physician, Brigham and Women's Hospital, Boston [108, 109]

JOAN R. BUTTERTON, MD, MPhil, DTMH
Instructor in Medicine, Harvard Medical School; Clinical Assistant, Infectious Disease Division, Massachusetts General Hospital, Boston [128]

ALFRED E. BUXTON, MD
Professor of Medicine and Cardiology; Associate Chief of Cardiology, Temple University School of Medicine, Philadelphia [230, 231]

STEPHEN B. CALDERWOOD, MD
Associate Professor of Medicine (Microbiology and Molecular Genetics); Physician and Chief, Infectious Disease Division, Massachusetts General Hospital, Boston [128]

GRANT L. CAMPBELL, MD, PhD
Chief, Epidemiology Section, Bacterial Zoonoses Branch, Division of Vector-Borne Infectious Diseases, National Center for Infectious Diseases, Centers for Disease Control and Prevention, Fort Collins [164, 177]

CHARLES B. CARPENTER, MD
Professor of Medicine, Harvard Medical School; Director, Laboratory of Immunogenetics and Transplantation, Brigham and Women's Hospital, Boston [272, 306]

BRUCE R. CARR, MD
Professor of Obstetrics and Gynecology and Director, Division of Reproductive Endocrinology, The University of Texas Southwestern Medical Center, Dallas [52, 337]

GAIL H. CASSELL, PhD
Charles H. McCauley Professor and Chairman, Department of Microbiology; Professor, Departments of Pediatrics and Comparative Medicine, University of Alabama at Birmingham, Birmingham [180]

AGUSTIN CASTELLANOS, MD
Professor of Medicine and Director, Clinical Electrophysiology, University of Miami School of Medicine, Miami [39]

HUGO CASTRO-MALASPINA, MD
Associate Professor of Medicine; Associate Member, Memorial Sloan-Kettering Cancer Center, New York [110]

YUAN-TSONG CHEN, MD, PhD
Professor of Pediatrics and Chief, Division of Medical Genetics, Department of Pediatrics, Duke University Medical Center, Durham [347]

JOHN S. CHILD, MD
Professor of Medicine, University of California, Los Angeles; Co-Chief, Clinical Cardiology, UCLA Medical Center, Los Angeles [235]

L. CHINSOO CHO, MD
Assistant Professor, Department of Radiation Oncology, University of Texas Southwestern Medical Center, Harold C. Simmons Comprehensive Cancer Center, Dallas [396]

FREDRIC L. COE, MD
Professor of Medicine and Physiology and Chief, Nephrology Program, University of Chicago Pritzker School of Medicine, Chicago [268, 278, 279]

ALAN S. COHEN, MD
Distinguished Professor of Medicine in Rheumatology, Boston University School of Medicine, Boston [309]

JEFFREY I. COHEN, MD
Head, Medical Virology Section, National Institute of Allergy and Infectious Diseases, National Institutes of Health, Bethesda [186, 195]

JOHN M. COLFORD, JR., MD, MPH
Adjunct Assistant Professor, Department of Epidemiology and Biostatistics, University of California San Francisco, San Francisco [4]

FRANCIS S. COLLINS, MD, PhD
Director, National Human Genome Research Institute, National Institutes of Health, Bethesda [84]

WILSON S. COLUCCI, MD, FACC
Professor of Medicine and Physiology, Boston University School of Medicine; Chief, Cardiovascular Division, Boston Medical Center, Boston [241]

MAUREEN T. CONNELLY, MD, MPH
Instructor in Medicine, Harvard Medical School; Harvard Pilgrim Health Care, Boston [10]

MAX D. COOPER, MD
Professor of Medicine, Pediatrics, and Microbiology; Howard Hughes Medical Institute Investigator, University of Alabama at Birmingham, Birmingham [307]

LAWRENCE COREY, MD
Professor of Laboratory Medicine and Medicine and Head, Virology Division, University of Washington; Head, Program in Infectious Diseases, Fred Hutchinson Cancer Research Center, Seattle [184, 199, 201]

ANN M. COULSTON, MS, RD
Senior Research Dietitian, Stanford University Medical Center, Stanford [77]

MARK A. CREAGER, MD
Associate Professor of Medicine, Harvard Medical School; Director, Vascular Center, Brigham and Women's Hospital, Boston [247, 248]

RONALD G. CRYSTAL, MD
Bruce Webster Professor of Internal Medicine, Professor of Physiology and Biophysics; Chief, Division of Pulmonary and Critical Care Medicine, Department of Medicine, The New York Hospital–Cornell Medical Center, New York [320]

JOHN J. CUSH, MD
Medical Director, Arthritis Consultation Center, Presbyterian Hospital of Dallas, Dallas [321]

CHARLES A. CZEISLER, PhD, MD
Director, Sleep Disorders and Circadian Medicine, Associate Professor of Medicine, Harvard Medical School; Brigham and Women's Hospital, Boston [27]

GILBERT H. DANIELS, MD
Associate Professor of Medicine, Harvard Medical School; Co-Director, Thyroid Associates, Massachusetts General Hospital, Boston [328]

ROBERT B. DAROFF, MD
Professor of Neurology and Associate Dean, Case Western Reserve University; Chief of Staff and Senior Vice-President of Medical Affairs, University Hospitals of Cleveland, Cleveland [20]

CHARLES E. DAVIS, MD
Professor of Pathology and Medicine, University of California, San Diego School of Medicine; Director Emeritus, Microbiology Laboratory, UCSD Medical Center, San Diego [213]

MARGO DENKE, MD
Associate Professor of Internal Medicine, Center for Human Nutrition, The University of Texas Southwestern Medical Center, Dallas [72–74]

BRADLEY M. DENKER, MD
Assistant Professor of Medicine, Harvard Medical School; Associate Physician, Brigham and Women's Hospital, Boston [47]

DAVID T. DENNIS, MD, MPH
Chief, Bacterial Zoonoses Branch, Division of Vector-Borne Infectious Diseases, National Center for Infectious Diseases, Centers for Disease Control and Prevention, Fort Collins [164, 177]

ROBERT L. DERESIEWICZ, MD
Assistant Professor of Medicine, Harvard Medical School; Associate Physician, Channing Laboratory and the Division of Infectious Diseases, Brigham and Women's Hospital, Boston [142, 161]

ROBERT J. DESNICK, PhD, MD
Arthur J and Nellie Z Cohen Professor of Pediatrics and Genetics; Chairman, Department of Human Genetics, Mount Sinai School of Medicine, New York [343]

JULES L. DIENSTAG, MD
Associate Professor of Medicine, Harvard Medical School; Physician, Massachusetts General Hospital, Boston [93, 295–297, 301]

WILLIAM P. DILLON, MD
Professor of Radiology, Neurology, and Neurosurgery; Chief, Diagnostic Neuroradiology, University of California San Francisco, San Francisco [362]

ALAN R. DIMICK, MD
Professor of Surgery, University of Alabama at Birmingham; Director, Burn Center, University of Alabama Hospital, Birmingham [395]

CHARLES A. DINARELLO, MD
Professor of Medicine, University of Colorado Health Sciences Center, Denver [17, 125]

ROBERT G. DLUHY, MD
Associate Professor of Medicine, Harvard Medical School, Brigham and Women's Hospital, Boston [332]

RAPHAEL DOLIN, MD
Charles A. Dewey Professor and Chair, Department of Medicine, University of Rochester School of Medicine and Dentistry, Rochester [183, 191, 193]

DANIEL B. DRACHMAN, MD
Professor of Neurology and Neurosciences; Director, Neuromuscular Unit, The Johns Hopkins University School of Medicine, Baltimore [382]

JEFFREY M. DRAZEN, MD
Parker B. Francis Professor of Medicine, Harvard Medical School; Chief, Pulmonary Division, Brigham and Women's Hospital, Boston [249–251, 266]

THOMAS D. DUBOSE, JR., MD
Professor of Medicine and Integrative Biology; Director, Division of Renal Diseases and Hypertension; Vice-Chairman, Department of Internal Medicine, The University of Texas–Houston Medical School; Medical Director, Nephrology Section, Herman Hospital; Medical Director, University Kidney Center, Houston [50]

MARLENE DURAND, MD
Instructor, Harvard Medical School; Assistant in Medicine, Massachusetts General Hospital, Boston [30]

JANICE P. DUTCHER, MD
Professor of Medicine, Albert Einstein College of Medicine, Albert Einstein Cancer Center, Montefiore Medical Center, New York [104]

VICTOR J. DZAU, MD
Hersey Professor of the Theory and Practice of Medicine, Harvard Medical School; Chairman, Department of Medicine and Director of Research, Brigham and Women's Hospital, Boston [247, 248]

JEFFERY S. DZIECZKOWSKI, MD
Assistant Professor, Departments of Pathology and Internal Medicine, Wayne State University School of Medicine, Detroit [115]

J. DONALD EASTON, MD
Professor and Chair, Department of Clinical Neurosciences, Brown University School of Medicine; Neurologist-in-Chief, Rhode Island Hospital, Providence [366]

BARRY I. EISENSTEIN, MD
Vice-President, Science and Technology, Beth Israel Deaconess Medical Center, Boston [155]

LOUIS J. ELSAS II, MD
Professor of Pediatrics and Director of the Division of Medical Genetics, Emory University School of Medicine, Atlanta [349, 350]

JOHN W. ENGSTROM, MD
Associate Professor of Clinical Neurology, University of California San Francisco, San Francisco [16, 371]

ALAN EPSTEIN, MD
Assistant Professor of Medicine, Brown University, Providence [44, 288]

VIRGINIA L. ERNSTER, PhD
Professor of Epidemiology and Biostatistics, Department of Epidemiology and Biostatistics, University of California San Francisco, San Francisco [4]

KENNETH H. FALCHUK, MD
Associate Professor of Medicine, Harvard Medical School, Brigham and Women's Hospital, Boston [80]

ANTHONY S. FAUCI, MD
Chief, Laboratory of Immunoregulation; Director, National Institute of Allergy and Infectious Diseases, National Institutes of Health, Bethesda [1, 192, 305, 308, 319]

MURRAY J. FAVUS, MD
Professor of Medicine, Sections of Endocrinology and Nephrology, Department of Medicine, University of Chicago Pritzker School of Medicine, Chicago [279]

ROBERT G. FENTON, MD, PhD
Senior Investigator, Medicine Branch, Division of Clinical Sciences, National Cancer Institute, National Institutes of Health, Frederick [83]

THOMAS F. FERRIS, MD
Nesbitt Professor and Chairman, Department of Medicine, University of Minnesota; University of Minnesota Hospital and Clinics, Minneapolis [7]

HOWARD FIELDS, MD, PhD
Professor of Neurology and Physiology, University of California San Francisco, San Francisco [12]

GREGORY A. FILICE, MD
Associate Professor of Medicine, University of Minnesota; Chief, Infectious Disease Section, Veterans Affairs Medical Center, Minneapolis [167]

ROBERT W. FINBERG, MD
Professor of Medicine, Harvard Medical School; Chief, Division of Infectious Diseases, Dana-Farber Cancer Institute, Boston [87, 136]

JOYCE D. FINGEROTH, MD
Assistant Professor of Medicine, Harvard Medical School; Physician, Dana-Farber Cancer Institute, Boston [136]

DANIEL W. FOSTER, MD
Chairman and Professor of Internal Medicine, The University of Texas Southwestern Medical Center, Dallas [43, 76, 334, 335, 352]

ARNOLD S. FREEDMAN, MD
Associate Professor of Medicine, Harvard Medical School; Associate Professor of Medicine, Dana-Farber Cancer Institute, Boston [113]

GERALD H. FRIEDLAND, MD
Professor of Medicine and Epidemiology and Public Health, and Director, AIDS Program, Yale University School of Medicine, Yale-New Haven Hospital, New Haven [134]

LAWRENCE S. FRIEDMAN, MD
Associate Professor of Medicine, Harvard Medical School; Associate Physician, Massachusetts General Hospital, Boston [41, 42, 284, 287]

WILLIAM F. FRIEDMAN, MD
J.H. Nicholson Professor of Pediatrics (Cardiology); Senior Advisor, Clinical Affairs, to the Provost and Dean, University of California, Los Angeles School of Medicine and UCLA Medical Center, Los Angeles [235]

ROBERT F. GAGEL, MD
Professor of Medicine and Chief of the Section of Endocrinology, University of Texas M.D. Anderson Cancer Center, Houston [340]

JOHN I. GALLIN, MD
Director, NIH Warren Grant Magnuson Clinical Center; Associate Director for Clinical Research, Chief, Laboratory of Host Defenses, National Institute of Allergy and Infectious Diseases, National Institutes of Health, Bethesda [62]

JEFFREY A. GELFAND, MD
Sheldon M. Wolff Professor and Chairman, Department of Medicine, Tufts University School of Medicine; Physician-in-Chief, New England Medical Center, Boston [17, 125]

JAMES L. GERMAN III, MD
Member, New York Blood Center, Laboratory of Human Genetics, New York [66]

ANNE A. GERSHON, MD
Professor of Pediatrics, Columbia University College of Physicians and Surgeons; Attending Physician, Presbyterian Hospital, New York [196–198]

BRUCE C. GILLILAND, MD
Professor of Medicine and Laboratory Medicine, Associate Dean for Clinical Affairs, University of Washington School of Medicine, Seattle [314, 326]

HENRY N. GINSBERG, MD
Herbert and Florence Irving Professor of Medicine; Head, Division of Preventive Medicine and Nutrition, Department of Medicine, Columbia University College of Physicians and Surgeons, New York [341]

ELI GLATSTEIN, MD
Vice-Chairman and Clinical Director, Radiation Oncology, University of Pennsylvania Medical Center, Philadelphia [396]

ROBERT M. GLICKMAN, MD
Herrman L. Blumgart Professor of Medicine, Harvard Medical School; Chairman, Department of Medicine, Beth Israel Hospital, Boston [46, 286]

IRA J. GOLDBERG, MD
Professor of Medicine, Division of Preventive Medicine and Nutrition, Department of Medicine, Columbia University College of Physicians and Surgeons, New York [341]

ARY L. GOLDBERGER, MD
Associate Professor of Medicine, Harvard Medical School; Director of Electrocardiography and Arrhythmia Monitoring Laboratories, Beth Israel Deaconess Medical Center, Boston [228]

SAMUEL Z. GOLDHABER, MD
Associate Professor of Medicine, Harvard Medical School; Physician, Brigham and Women's Hospital, Boston [261]

LEE GOLDMAN, MD
Julius R. Krevans Distinguished Professor and Chairman, Department of Medicine and Associate Dean for Clinical Affairs, University of California, San Francisco School of Medicine, San Francisco [3, 11, 13]

DONALD E. GOODKIN, MD
Associate Professor, Department of Neurology; Medical Director, UCSF/Mt. Zion Multiple Sclerosis Center, San Francisco [376]

RAJ K. GOYAL, MD
Mallinckrodt Professor of Medicine, Harvard Medical School; Associate Chief of Staff for Research and Development, Brockton/West Roxbury VA Medical Center, West Roxbury [40, 283]

GREGORY C. GRAY, MD, MPH
Naval Health Research Center, Clinical Epidemiology Division, San Diego [180]

HARRY B. GREENBERG, MD
Professor of Medicine, Microbiology and Immunology, Stanford University School of Medicine and the VA Palo Alto Health Care System, Stanford [194]

NORTON J. GREENBERGER, MD, MACP
Professor and Chairman, Department of Medicine, University of Kansas Medical Center, Kansas City [285, 302–304]

JOHN S. GREENSPAN, BSc, BDS, PhD, FRCPath
Professor and Chair, Department of Stomatology and Director, Oral AIDS Center, School of Dentistry; Professor, Department of Pathology, and Director, AIDS Clinical Research Center, School of Medicine, University of California San Francisco, San Francisco [31]

JAMES E. GRIFFIN III, MD
Professor of Internal Medicine, The University of Texas Southwestern Medical Center, Dallas [336, 339]

ROBERT C. GRIGGS, MD
Professor of Neurology, Medicine, Pathology, Laboratory Medicine, and Pediatrics; Edward A. and Alma Vollertsen Professor of Neurophysiology; Chair, Department of Neurology, University of Rochester School of Medicine & Dentistry, Rochester [22, 383]

WILLIAM GROSSMAN, MD
Professor of Medicine, University of California San Francisco; Chief of Cardiology, University of California San Francisco Medical Center, San Francisco [229, 245]

RASIM GUCALP, MD, FACP
Associate Professor of Medicine, Department of Oncology, Montefiore Medical Center, Albert Einstein College of Medicine, New York [104]

BEVRA HANNAHS HAHN, MD, FACP
Professor of Medicine, Chief of Rheumatology, University of California, Los Angeles, Los Angeles [312]

ROBERT I. HANDIN, MD
Professor of Medicine, Harvard Medical School; Director, Hematology Division, Brigham and Women's Hospital, Boston [60, 117–119]

H. HUNTER HANDSFIELD, MD
Professor of Medicine, University of Washington School of Medicine; Director, STD Control Program, Seattle-King County Department of Public Health, Seattle [129]

STEPHEN L. HAUSER, MD
Chairman and Betty Anker Fife Professor, Department of Neurology, University of California San Francisco, San Francisco [1, 360, 366, 373, 376]

BARTON FORD HAYNES, MD
Frederic M. Hanes Professor and Chair, Department of Medicine; Professor, Department of Immunology, Director, Duke University Arthritis Center, Durham [305]

PATRICK H. HENRY, MD
Chairman, Department of Medicine, St. John's Mercy Medical Center, St. Louis [61]

BARBARA L. HERWALDT, MD, MPH
Medical Epidemiologist, Centers for Disease Control and Prevention, Division of Parasitic Diseases, Atlanta [217]

ROBERT S. HILLMAN, MD
Professor of Medicine, University of Vermont College of Medicine; Chairman of Medicine, Maine Medical Center, Portland [59, 106]

RAYMOND L. HINTZ, MD
Professor of Pediatrics, Head of the Division of Pediatric Endocrinology, Stanford University School of Medicine, Stanford [329]

MARTIN S. HIRSCH, MD
Professor of Medicine, Harvard Medical School; Physician, Massachusetts General Hospital, Boston [187]

BERNARD HIRSCHEL, MD
Associate Professor of Medicine; Head, HIV/AIDS Section, Division of Infectious Diseases, University Hospital, Geneva [173]

GARY S. HOFFMAN, MD, MS
Chairman, Department of Rheumatic and Immunologic Diseases, Cleveland Clinic Foundation; Professor of Medicine, Ohio State University, Columbus [323]

JOHN H. HOLBROOK, MD
Professor of Medicine and Chief, Division of General Internal Medicine, University of Utah School of Medicine, Salt Lake City [389]

MICHAEL F. HOLICK, PhD, MD
Professor of Medicine, Physiology and Dermatology, Boston University School of Medicine, Boston [353, 355]

STEVEN M. HOLLAND, MD
NIAID Investigator, Laboratory of Host Defenses, National Institute of Allergy and Infectious Diseases, National Institutes of Health, Bethesda [62]

STEVEN M. HOLLENBERG, MD
Assistant Professor of Medicine, Sections of Cardiology and Critical Care Medicine, Rush Medical College, Chicago [38]

KING K. HOLMES, MD, PhD
Professor of Medicine and Director, Center for AIDS and STD, University of Washington, Seattle [129, 130, 150, 166, 174]

RANDALL K. HOLMES, MD, PhD
Professor and Chair, Department of Microbiology, University of Colorado Health Sciences Center, Denver [144]

ERIC G. HONIG, MD
Associate Professor of Medicine, Emory University School of Medicine, Atlanta [258, 265]

JONATHAN C. HORTON, MD, PhD
Associate Professor of Ophthalmology, Neurology, and Physiology, University of California San Francisco, San Francisco [28]

THOMAS H. HOSTETTER, MD
Professor of Medicine, University of Minnesota School of Medicine; Director, Division of Renal Disease, University Hospital, Minneapolis [276]

LYN HOWARD, MB, DCh, FRCP, FACP
Head, Division of Clinical Nutrition, Professor of Medicine and Associate Professor of Pediatrics, The Albany Medical College, Albany [78]

HOWARD HU, MD, MPH, ScD
Associate Professor of Occupational Medicine, Harvard School of Public Health; Assistant Professor of Medicine, Harvard Medical School; Associate Physician, Channing Laboratory, Brigham and Women's Hospital, Boston [5, 390, 397]

GARY W. HUNNINGHAKE, MD
Professor of Internal Medicine and Director, Pulmonary, Critical Care and Occupational Medicine, University of Iowa College of Medicine, Iowa City [253]

DANIEL C. IHDE, MD
Professor of Medicine and Chief, Medical Oncology, Washington University School of Medicine, St. Louis [63]

EDWARD P. INGENITO, MD, PhD
Assistant Professor of Medicine, Harvard Medical School; Director, Pulmonary Function Laboratory, Brigham and Women's Hospital, Boston [266]

ROLAND H. INGRAM, JR, MD
Martha West Looney Professor, Emory University School of Medicine; Director, Pulmonary and Critical Care Medicine, Chief of Medicine, Emory-Crawford Long Hospital, Atlanta [32, 258, 265]

THOMAS S. INUI, ScM, MD
Professor and Chairman, Department of Ambulatory Care and Prevention, Harvard Medical School; Harvard Pilgrim Health Care, Boston [10]

CHARLES E. IRWIN, JR, MD
Professor of Pediatrics, Director of the Division of Adolescent Medicine, University of California San Francisco, San Francisco [8]

MARK A. ISRAEL, MD
Professor, Departments of Neurological Surgery and Pediatrics; Director, Preuss Laboratory of Molecular Neuro-Oncology, University of California San Francisco, San Francisco [375]

KURT J. ISSELBACHER, MD
Mallinckrodt Professor of Medicine, Harvard Medical School; Physician and Director, Massachusetts General Hospital Cancer Center, Boston [1, 41, 42, 44–46, 93, 281, 285, 288, 291–300, 302, 304, 342, 351]

RICHARD F. JACOBS, MD
Horace C. Cabe Professor of Pediatrics and Chief, Pediatric Infectious Diseases, Arkansas Children's Hospital and the University of Arkansas for Medical Sciences, Little Rock [163]

BRUCE E. JOHNSON, MD
Head, Lung Cancer Biology Section, Medicine Branch, National Cancer Institute, National Institutes of Health, Bethesda [102]

MICHAEL P. JOSEPH, MD
Physician, Weber Medical Clinic, Ltd., Olney [30]

MARK E. JOSEPHSON, MD
Professor of Medicine, Harvard Medical School; Director, Harvard-Thorndike Electrophysiology Institute and Arrhythmia Service, Beth Israel Deaconess Medical Center, Boston [230, 231]

EDWARD L. KAPLAN, MD
Professor, Department of Pediatrics, University of Minnesota Medical School, Minneapolis [236]

LEE M. KAPLAN, MD, PhD
Assistant Professor of Medicine, Harvard Medical School; Associate Chief for Research, Gastrointestinal Unit, Massachusetts General Hospital, Boston [45, 95]

DENNIS L. KASPER, MD, MA (Hon)
William Ellery Channing Professor of Medicine, Harvard Medical School; Director, Channing Laboratory; Co-Director, Division of Infectious Diseases; Executive Vice-Chairman, Department of Medicine, Brigham and Women's Hospital, Boston [1, 120, 127, 148, 152, 169]

LLOYD H. KASPER, MD
Professor of Medicine (Neurology) and Microbiology, Dartmouth Medical School, Hanover [219]

DONALD KAYE, MD
Klinghoffer Professor of Medicine, MCP Hahnemann School of Medicine, Allegheny University of the Health Sciences; Executive Vice-President for Health Affairs, Allegheny University of the Health Sciences; President and CEO, Allegheny University Hospitals, Philadelphia [126]

ELAINE T. KAYE, MD
Clinical Instructor in Dermatology, Harvard Medical School; Assistant in Medicine, Department of Medicine, Children's Hospital Medical Center, Boston [18]

KENNETH M. KAYE, MD
Assistant Professor of Medicine, Harvard Medical School; Associate Physician, Division of Infectious Diseases, Brigham and Women's Hospital, Boston [18]

JONATHAN R. KELLER, PhD
Head, Hematology and Gene Therapy Section, SAIC, Inc.; Intramural Research and Support Program, National Cancer Institute-Frederick Cancer Research and Development Center, Frederick [105]

GERALD T. KEUSCH, MD
Professor of Medicine and Chief, Division of Geographic Medicine and Infectious Diseases, New England Medical Center Hospitals, Boston [122, 158, 159, 161]

JAY S. KEYSTONE, MD, FRCPC
Professor of Medicine, University of Toronto; Tropical Disease Unit, Division of Infectious Disease, The Toronto Hospital, Toronto [123]

ELLIOTT D. KIEFF, MD, PhD
Harriet Ryan Albee Professor of Medicine; Professor of Microbiology and Molecular Genetics; Chairman, Virology Program, Harvard Medical School; Co-Director, Division of Infectious Diseases, Brigham and Women's Hospital, Boston [182]

LOUIS V. KIRCHHOFF, MD, MPH
Professor, Department of Internal Medicine, University of Iowa; Staff Physician, Department of Veterans Affairs Medical Center, Iowa City [218]

JAMES P. KNOCHEL, MD
Clinical Professor of Internal Medicine, University of Texas Southwestern Medical Center; Chairman, Department of Internal Medicine, Presbyterian Hospital, Dallas [356, 357]

HOWARD K. KOH, MD, PhD
Professor of Dermatology, Medicine and Public Health, Boston University Schools of Medicine and Public Health; Co-Director, Skin Oncology Program, Director, Cancer Prevention and Control Center, Boston [88]

ELISE C. KOHN, MD
Senior Investigator, Chief, Signal Transduction and Prevention Unit, Laboratory of Pathology, National Cancer Institute, National Institutes of Health, Bethesda [85]

ANTHONY L. KOMAROFF, MD
Professor of Medicine, Harvard Medical School, Boston [6]

WALTER J. KOROSHETZ, MD
Associate Professor of Neurology and Medicine; Associate Director, Stroke and Clinical Neurology Services, Massachusetts General Hospital, Harvard Medical School, Boston [378]

WILLIAM J. KOVACS, MD
Associate Professor of Medicine, Division of Endocrinology, Vanderbilt University School of Medicine, Nashville [53]

PHYLLIS E. KOZARSKY, MD
Associate Professor of Medicine, Emory University School of Medicine; Chief of Infectious Diseases, Emory Crawford Long Hospital, Atlanta [123]

BARNETT S. KRAMER, MD, MPH
Associate Director, Early Detection and Community Oncology Program, Division of Cancer Prevention and Control, National Cancer Institute, National Institutes of Health, Bethesda [82]

STEPHEN M. KRANE, MD
Persis, Cyrus, and Marlow B. Harrison Professor of Medicine, Harvard Medical School, Massachusetts General Hospital, Boston [353, 355, 358, 359]

DONALD W. KUFE, MD
Professor of Medicine, Harvard Medical School; Chief, Division of Cancer Pharmacology, Department of Medicine, Dana-Farber Cancer Institute, Boston [86]

HELENA KUIVANIEMI, MD, PhD
Associate Professor, Center for Molecular Medicine and Genetics, and Department of Surgery, Wayne State University School of Medicine, Detroit [348]

LEWIS LANDSBERG, MD
Irving S. Cutter Professor and Chairman, Department of Medicine, Northwestern University Medical School; Physician-in-Chief, Northwestern Memorial Hospital, Chicago [70, 333]

H. CLIFFORD LANE, MD
Head, Clinical and Molecular Retrovirology Section, Laboratory of Immunoregulation; Clinical Director, National Institute of Allergy and Infectious Diseases, National Institutes of Health, Bethesda [308]

THOMAS J. LAWLEY, MD
Professor and Chairman, Department of Dermatology, Emory University School of Medicine, Atlanta [54, 55, 311]

ALEXANDER R. LAWTON III, MD
Edward C. Stahlman Professor in Pediatric, Physiology and Cell Metabolism; Professor of Pediatrics and Microbiology, Head, Division of Pediatric Immunology and Rheumatology, Vanderbilt University School of Medicine, Nashville [307]

J. MICHAEL LAZARUS, MD
Associate Professor of Medicine, Harvard Medical School; Director of Clinical Services, Nephrology Division, Brigham and Women's Hospital, Boston [271, 272]

MATTHEW E. LEVISON, MD
Professor of Medicine and Chief, Division of Infectious Diseases, Allegheny University of the Health Sciences, Philadelphia [255]

ELLIOTT LEVY, MD
Instructor in Medicine, Harvard Medical School; Associate Physician, Brigham and Women's Hospital, Boston [276]

PETER LIBBY, MD
Professor of Medicine, Harvard Medical School; Director, Vascular Medicine and Atherosclerosis Unit, Brigham and Women's Hospital, Boston [242]

RICHARD W. LIGHT, MD
Professor of Medicine, Vanderbilt University; Director, Pulmonary Diseases Program, Saint Thomas Hospital, Nashville [262]

CHRISTOPHER LINDEN, MD
Associate Professor of Emergency Medicine, Division of Toxicology, University of Massachusetts Medical Center, Worcester [391]

LANCE A. LIOTTA, MD, PhD
Chief, Laboratory of Pathology, National Cancer Institute, National Institutes of Health, Bethesda [85]

MARC E. LIPPMAN, MD
Director, Lombardi Cancer Center; Professor of Medicine and Pharmacology, Georgetown University Medical School, Washington, DC [64, 91]

PETER LIPSKY, MD
Professor of Internal Medicine and Microbiology; Director, Harold C. Simmons Arthritis Research Center, Department of Internal Medicine, University of Texas Southwestern Medical Center at Dallas, Dallas [313, 317, 321]

LEO X. LIU, MD, DTMH
Assistant Professor of Medicine, Harvard Medical School; Division of Infectious Diseases, Department of Medicine, Beth Israel Deaconess Medical Center, Boston [214, 221, 222]

BERNARD LO, MD
Professor of Medicine and Director, Program in Medical Ethics, University of California San Francisco, San Francisco [2]

DAN L. LONGO, MD, FACP
Scientific Director, National Institute on Aging, National Institutes of Health, Gerontology Research Center, Bethesda and Baltimore [1, 61, 63, 81, 83, 105, 114, 192]

FRANK M. LONGO, MD, PhD
Associate Professor of Neurology, University of California San Francisco; Chief of Neurology, Veterans Affairs Medical Center, Department of Neurology, San Francisco [363]

NICOLA LONGO, MD, PhD
Assistant Professor of Pediatrics, Emory University School of Medicine, Atlanta [349, 350]

JOSEPH LOSCALZO, MD, PhD
Wade Professor and Chairman, Department of Medicine, Boston University School of Medicine; Physician-in-Chief, Boston Medical Center; Director, Whitaker Cardiovascular Institute, Boston [71]

FREDERICK H. LOVEJOY, JR, MD
William Berenberg Professor of Pediatrics, Harvard Medical School; Chief and Vice-Chairman, Department of Pediatrics, Children's Hospital, Boston [391]

DANIEL H. LOWENSTEIN, MD
Associate Professor of Neurology, Anatomy, and Neurosurgery, Robert B. and Ellinor Aird Chair in Neurology; Director, Epilepsy Research Laboratory, University of California San Francisco, San Francisco [365]

SHEILA A. LUKEHART, PhD
Research Professor of Medicine and Infectious Diseases, University of Washington, Seattle [174]

RICHARD B. LYNN, MD
Assistant Professor of Medicine, Jefferson Medical College, Thomas Jefferson University, Philadelphia [287]

HARALD S. MACKENZIE, MB, ChB, MRCP (UK)
Assistant Professor of Medicine, Harvard Medical School; Associate Physician, Brigham and Women's Hospital, Boston [269]

M. MONIR MADKOUR, DM (Cairo), FRCP (London)
Consultant Physician, Military Hospital, Riyadh [162]

LAWRENCE C. MADOFF, MD
Assistant Professor of Medicine, Harvard Medical School; Channing Laboratory, Brigham and Women's Hospital; Division of Infectious Diseases, Beth Israel Deaconess Medical Center, Boston [120, 135]

JAMES H. MAGUIRE, MD
Associate Professor of Medicine, Harvard Medical School; Associate Professor in Tropical Public Health, Harvard School of Public Health, Boston [132, 324, 393]

FRANCIS E. MARCHLINSKI, MD
Professor of Medicine, Allegheny University of the Health Sciences; Section Chief, Electrophysiology, Allegheny University Hospitals, Philadelphia [230, 231]

THOMAS J. MARRIE, MD, FRCPC
Professor of Medicine, Dalhousie University, Halifax [179]

JOSEPH B. MARTIN, MD, PhD, FRCP (C), MA (Hon)
Dean of the Faculty of Medicine; Caroline Shields Walker Professor of Neurobiology and Clinical Neuroscience, Harvard Medical School, Boston; formerly Professor of Neurology and Chancellor, University of California San Francisco, San Francisco [1, 12, 20, 24, 29, 360, 363, 366, 371, 372, 380]

JANET MAURER, MD
Head, Section of Lung Transplantation, Department of Pulmonary and Critical Care Medicine, The Cleveland Clinic Foundation, Cleveland [267]

ROBERT J. MAYER, MD
Professor of Medicine, Harvard Medical School; Clinical Director, Department of Medicine, Dana-Farber Cancer Institute, Boston [92, 94]

JOHN D. MCCONNELL, MD
Professor and Chairman, Department of Urology, The University of Texas Southwestern Medical Center, Dallas [48, 51]

EDWARD REGIS MCFADDEN, JR., MD
Argyl J. Beams Professor of Medicine and Director, Pulmonary and Critical Care Medicine, Case Western Reserve University School of Medicine, Cleveland [252]

MARGARET MCGOVERN, MD
Assistant Professor of Human Genetics and Pediatrics, Mount Sinai School of Medicine, New York [346]

NANCY K. MELLO, PhD
Professor of Psychology (Neuroscience), Alcohol and Drug Abuse Research Center, McLean Hospital, Belmont [388]

JERRY R. MENDELL, MD
Chairman and Professor of Neurology; Director, Neuromuscular Disease Center, The Ohio State University, Columbus [383]

JACK H. MENDELSON, MD
Professor of Psychiatry (Neuroscience), Alcohol and Drug Abuse Research Center, McLean Hospital, Belmont [388]

M.-MARSEL MESULAM, MD
Ruth and Evelyn Dunbar Professor of Neurology and Psychiatry; Director, Center for Behavioral and Cognitive Neurology; Director, Alzheimer's Program, Northwestern University Medical School, Chicago [25]

RICHARD A. MILLER, MD
Associate Professor of Medicine, University of Washington School of Medicine; Chief, Infectious Diseases Section, Veterans Affairs Puget Sound Health Care System, Seattle [172]

JOHN D. MINNA, MD
Professor, Internal Medicine and Pharmacology; Director, Hamon Center for Therapeutic Oncology Research, University of Texas Southwestern Medical Center, Dallas [90]

JEROME H. MODELL, MD
Professor of Anesthesiology; Executive Associate Dean, University of Florida College of Medicine, Gainesville [394]

STEPHEN A. MORSE, MSPH, PhD
Associate Director, Science Division AIDS/STDs and Tuberculosis Laboratory Research, National Center for Infectious Diseases, Centers for Disease Control and Prevention, Atlanta; Adjunct Professor of Microbiology and Immunology, Emory School of Medicine, Atlanta, and University of Alabama at Birmingham, Birmingham [150]

ARNOLD M. MOSES, MD, FACP
Professor of Medicine, State University of New York Health Science Center, Syracuse [330]

ROBERT J. MOTZER, MD
Associate Attending Physician, Memorial Sloan-Kettering Cancer Center; Associate Professor of Medicine, Cornell University Medical College, New York [96, 98]

HARALAMPOS M. MOUTSOPOULOS, MD
Professor and Director, Department of Pathophysiology, National University of Athens School of Medicine; Corresponding member, Academy of Athens; Athens, Greece [316, 318]

LÜTFIYE MÜLAZIMOGLU, MD
Associate Professor of Infectious Diseases and Clinical Microbiology, Section of Infectious Diseases, Marmara University, School of Medicine, Istanbul [153]

ROBERT S. MUNFORD, MD
Jan and Henri Bromberg Professor of Internal Medicine; Professor of Microbiology, The University of Texas Southwestern Medical Center, Dallas [124]

TIMOTHY F. MURPHY, MD
Professor of Medicine and Microbiology; Director, Division of Infectious Diseases, State University of New York at Buffalo, Buffalo [152]

DANIEL M. MUSHER, MD
Professor of Medicine and Professor of Microbiology and Immunology, Baylor College of Medicine; Chief, Infectious Diseases Section, Veterans Affairs Medical Center, Houston [141, 151]

ROBERT J. MYERBURG, MD
Professor of Medicine and Physiology and Director, Division of Cardiology, University of Miami School of Medicine, Miami [39]

LEE M. NADLER, MD
Chair, Department of Adult Oncology, Dana-Farber Cancer Institute; Chief, Division of Oncology, Brigham and Women's Hospital; Professor of Medicine, Harvard Medical School, Boston [113]

THEODORE ELLIOTT NASH, MD
Senior Scientist; Head, Gastrointestinal Parasite Section, Laboratory of Parasitic Disease, National Institute of Allergy and Infectious Diseases, National Institutes of Health, Bethesda [220, 224]

ROBERT L. NORRIS, MD, FACEP
Assistant Professor of Surgery, Department of Surgery, Division of Emergency Medicine, Stanford University, Stanford [392]

THOMAS B. NUTMAN, MD
Head, Helminth Immunology Section, Laboratory of Parasitic Diseases, National Institute of Allergy and Infectious Diseases, National Institutes of Health, Bethesda [223, 225]

RICHARD J. O'BRIEN, MD
Chief, Research and Evaluation Branch, Division of Tuberculosis Elimination, National Center for HIV, STD, and TB Prevention, Centers for Disease Control and Prevention, Atlanta [171]

PATRICK T. O'GARA, MD
Assistant Professor of Medicine, Harvard Medical School; Director, Clinical Cardiology, and Vice-Chairman for Clinical Programs, Department of Medicine, Brigham and Women's Hospital, Boston [34]

YVONNE M. O'MEARA, MD, MRCPI
College Lecturer, Department of Medicine and Therapeutics, University College Dublin; Consultant Physician, Mater Misericordiae Hospital, Dublin, Ireland [274, 275]

RICHARD J. O'REILLY, MD
Chairman, Department of Pediatrics; Chief, Bone Marrow Transplantation, Memorial Sloan-Kettering Cancer Center, New York [110]

ROBERT A. O'ROURKE, MD
Charles Conrad Brown Distinguished Professor in Cardiovascular Disease, The University of Texas Health Science Center at San Antonio, San Antonio [227]

JOHN A. OATES, MD
Professor and Chairman, Department of Medicine, Vanderbilt University School of Medicine; Physician-in-Chief, Vanderbilt University Hospital, Nashville [68]

RICHARD K. OLNEY, MD
Professor of Clinical Neurology, School of Medicine, University of California San Francisco, San Francisco [21]

ANDREW B. ONDERDONK, PhD
Associate Professor of Pathology, Harvard Medical School; Director, Clinical Microbiology Laboratory, Brigham and Women's Hospital, Boston [121]

SCOTT OSLUND, MD
Attending Physician, St. Francis Medical Center, Lynwood [392]

JOSEPH E. PARRILLO, MD
James B. Herrick Professor of Medicine, Rush Medical College; Chief, Sections of Cardiology and Critical Care Medicine; Medical Director, Rush Heart Institute, Rush–Presbyterian–St. Luke's Medical Center, Chicago [38]

JEFFREY PARSONNET, MD
Associate Professor of Medicine and of Microbiology, Dartmouth Medical School; Staff Physician, Infectious Disease Section, Dartmouth-Hitchcock Medical Center, Hanover [142]

SHREYASKUMAR R. PATEL, MD
Associate Professor of Medicine, Department of Melanoma/Sarcoma Medical Oncology, The University of Texas MD Anderson Cancer Center, Houston [100]

PETER L. PERINE, MD
Professor of Epidemiology, University of Washington, Seattle; Professor of Tropical Public Health and Medicine Emeritus, Uniformed Services University of the Health Sciences, Bethesda [175]

C.J. PETERS, MD
Chief, Special Pathogens Branch, Division of Viral and Rickettsial Diseases, National Center for Infectious Diseases, Centers for Disease Control and Prevention, Atlanta [200]

WALTER L. PETERSON, MD
Professor of Medicine, University of Texas Southwestern Medical School; Staff Physician, Dallas VA Medical Center, Dallas [284]

KEVIN J. PETTY, MD, PhD
Associate Director, Clinical Development, US Human Health, Merck & Company, Inc, Westpoint, Pennsylvania [19]

ELIOT A. PHILLIPSON, MD
Sir John and Lady Eaton Professor of Medicine and Chair, Department of Medicine, University of Toronto; Physician-in-Chief, Mount Sinai Hospital, Toronto [263, 264]

GERALD B. PIER, PhD
Associate Professor of Medicine, Harvard Medical School; Channing Laboratory, Brigham and Women's Hospital, Boston [139]

DANIEL K. PODOLSKY, MD
Professor of Medicine, Harvard Medical School; Chief, Gastrointestinal Unit, Massachusetts General Hospital, Boston [281, 291–293, 298–300]

RONALD E. POLK, PharmD
Professor of Pharmacy and Medicine, School of Pharmacy, Medical College of Virginia, Virginia Commonwealth University, Richmond [140]

MATTHEW POLLACK, MD
Professor of Medicine, Uniformed Services University of the Health Sciences, F. Edward Hébert School of Medicine, Bethesda [157]

JOHN T. POTTS, JR., MD
The Jackson Professor of Clinical Medicine, Massachusetts General Hospital, Harvard Medical School, Boston [353, 354]

LAWRIE W. POWELL, MD, PhD
Professor of Medicine, The University of Queensland; Director, Queensland Institute of Medical Research, The Bancroft Centre, Brisbane, Queensland, Australia [342]

DARWIN J. PROCKOP, MD, PhD
Professor and Director, Center for Gene Therapy MCP Hahnemann School of Medicine, Allegheny University of the Health Sciences, Philadelphia [348]

LOUIS J. PTÁČEK, MD
Associate Professor of Neurology and Human Genetics, The University of Utah School of Medicine, Salt Lake City [383]

DIDIER RAOULT, MD, PhD
Professor of Medicine and President of the University of Aix, Marseilles, France [179]

NEIL H. RASKIN, MD
Professor of Neurology, School of Medicine, University of California San Francisco, San Francisco [15, 364]

MARIO C. RAVIGLIONE, MD
Medical Officer, Tuberculosis Research and Surveillance Unit, Global Tuberculosis Programme, World Health Organization, Geneva [171]

SHARON L. REED, MD
Associate Professor of Medicine and Pathology and Director, Microbiology and Virology Laboratories, University of California, San Diego Medical Center, San Diego [215]

ANTONIO J. REGINATO, MD
Head, Division of Rheumatology; Professor of Medicine, Cooper Hospital/ University Medical Center, University of Medicine and Dentistry of New Jersey/Robert Wood Johnson Medical School at Camden, Camden [323]

RICHARD C. REICHMAN, MD
Professor of Medicine, Microbiology and Immunology and Head, Infectious Disease Unit, University of Rochester School of Medicine and Dentistry, Rochester [190]

NEIL M. RESNICK, MD
Associate Professor of Medicine, Harvard Medical School; Chief, Division of Gerontology, Brigham and Women's Hospital; Geriatric Research Education and Clinical Center, Brockton-West Roxbury Veterans Administration Medical Center, Boston [9]

VICTOR I. REUS, MD
Professor of Psychiatry, University of California San Francisco; Medical Director, Langley Porter Hospital, San Francisco [385]

HERBERT Y. REYNOLDS, MD
J. Lloyd Huck Professor of Medicine, The Pennsylvania State University; Chairman, Department of Medicine, University Hospital, The Milton S. Hershey Medical Center, Hershey [259]

STUART RICH, MD
Professor of Medicine, Rush Medical College; Director, Rush Heart Institute Center for Pulmonary Heart Disease, Chicago [260]

GARY S. RICHARDSON, MD
Instructor in Medicine, Harvard Medical School; Director, Sleep Disorders Service, Brigham and Women's Hospital, Boston [27]

HAL B. RICHERSON, MD
Professor of Internal Medicine, Allergy-Immunology Division, University of Iowa College of Medicine; University of Iowa Hospitals and Clinics, Iowa City [253]

CELESTE ROBB-NICHOLSON, MD, MPH
Assistant Professor of Medicine, Harvard Medical School; Assistant Physician, Massachusetts General Hospital, Boston [6]

CHERYL L. ROCK, PhD, RD
Associate Professor of Family and Preventive Medicine, University of California, San Diego, San Diego [77]

ALLAN H. ROPPER, MD
Chief of Neurology, St. Elizabeth's Medical Center; Professor of Neurology, Tufts University School of Medicine, Boston [24, 374]

LEON E. ROSENBERG, MD
Senior Vice-President, Scientific Affairs, Bristol-Myers Squibb Pharmaceutical Research Institute, Princeton [349, 350]

ROGER N. ROSENBERG, MD
Zale Distinguished Chair in Neurology; Professor of Neurology and Physiology, University of Texas Southwestern Medical Center; Attending Neurologist, Parkland Hospital and Zale-Lipsky University Hospital, Dallas [369]

WENDELL F. ROSSE, MD
Florence Reynaud McAlister Professor of Medicine and Medical Research, Department of Medicine, Duke University Medical School, Durham [109]

ARTHUR H. RUBENSTEIN, MD
Lowell T. Coggeshall Professor and Chairman of Medicine, University of Chicago Pritzker School of Medicine, Chicago [335]

MACK T. RUFFIN IV, MD, MPH
Assistant Professor, Department of Family Practice, Assistant Research Scientist, Department of Epidemiology, University of Michigan, Ann Arbor [77]

FRANCIS W. RUSCETTI, PhD
Chief, Laboratory of Leukocyte Biology, Division of Basic Sciences, National Cancer Institute–Frederick Cancer Research and Development Center, National Institutes of Health, Frederick [105]

THOMAS A. RUSSO, MD, CM
Assistant Professor of Medicine, Division of Infectious Diseases, Department of Medicine, State University of New York at Buffalo, Buffalo [168]

ARTHUR I. SAGALOWSKY, MD
Professor of Urology and Chief of Urologic Oncology, Department of Urology, The University of Texas Southwestern Medical Center, Dallas [97]

STEPHEN M. SAGAR, MD
Professor of Neurology, Case Western Reserve School of Medicine, Cleveland [375]

MATTHEW H. SAMORE, MD
Assistant Professor of Medicine, Harvard Medical School; Division of Infectious Diseases, Beth Israel Deaconess Medical Center, Boston [154]

I. HERBERT SCHEINBERG, MD
Senior Lecturer in Medicine, College of Physicians and Surgeons, Columbia University, New York [345]

W. MICHAEL SCHELD, MD
Professor of Internal Medicine and Neurosurgery; Associate Chair for Residency Programs, University of Virginia School of Medicine, Charlottesville [377]

HOWARD I. SCHER, MD
Chief, Genitourinary Oncology Service, Associate Attending Physician, Division of Solid Tumor Oncology, Department of Medicine, Memorial Sloan-Kettering Cancer Center; Associate Professor Medicine, Cornell University Medical College, New York [96]

ALAN L. SCHILLER, MD
Irene Heinz Given and John LaPorte Given Professor and Chairman of Pathology, Mount Sinai School of Medicine; Chairman of Pathology, The Mount Sinai Hospital, New York [359]

JOHN SPEER SCHROEDER, MD
Professor of Medicine, Stanford University School of Medicine; Division of Cardiovascular Medicine, Stanford Hospital, Stanford [234]

ANNE SCHUCHAT, MD
Medical Epidemiologist, Division of Bacterial and Mycotic Diseases, National Center for Infectious Diseases, Centers for Disease Control and Prevention, Atlanta [145]

MARC A. SCHUCKIT, MD
Professor of Psychiatry, University of California, San Diego, and Veterans Affairs Medical Center, San Diego [386, 387]

PETER H. SCHUR, MD
Professor of Medicine, Harvard Medical School; Senior Physician, Brigham and Women's Hospital, Boston [325]

DAVID S. SEGAL, PhD
Professor of Psychiatry, University of California, San Diego, La Jolla [387]

JULIAN L. SEIFTER, MD
Associate Professor of Medicine, Harvard Medical School; Physician, Brigham and Women's Hospital, Boston [280]

ANDREW P. SELWYN, MD, MA (Hon), FRCP, FACC
Professor of Medicine, Harvard Medical School; Director of Cardiac Catheterization, Brigham and Women's Hospital, Boston [244]

PETER A. SELWYN, MD, MPH
Associate Professor of Medicine, Epidemiology, and Public Health and Associate Director, AIDS Program, Yale University School of Medicine, Yale–New Haven Hospital, New Haven [134]

MARY-ANN SHAFER, MD
Professor of Pediatrics, Associate Director of the Division of Adolescent Medicine, University of California San Francisco, San Francisco [8]

STEVEN I. SHERMAN, MD
Assistant Professor of Medicine, University of Texas MD Anderson Cancer Center, Houston [340]

GEORGE R. SIBER, MD
Associate Professor of Medicine, Harvard Medical School, Boston; Vice-President and Chief Scientific Officer, Wyeth Lederle Vaccines and Pediatrics, Pearl River [154]

WILLIAM SILEN, MD
Johnson & Johnson Distinguished Professor of Surgery, Harvard Medical School; Surgeon-in-Chief Emeritus, Department of Surgery, Beth Israel Hospital, Boston [14, 289, 290]

FRED E. SILVERSTEIN, MD
Clinical Professor of Medicine, University of Washington; Partner, Frazier and Company, Seattle [282]

GARY G. SINGER, MD
Assistant Professor of Medicine, Washington University School of Medicine; Associate Director, Transplant Nephrology, Barnes-Jewish Hospital, St. Louis [49]

JEAN D. SIPE, PhD
Professor, Department of Biochemistry, Boston University School of Medicine, Boston [309]

CHRISTOPHER A. SLAPAK, MD
Assistant Professor of Medicine, Harvard Medical School; Division of Cancer Pharmacology, Dana-Farber Cancer Institute, Boston [86]

JAMES B. SNOW, JR., MD
Director, National Institute on Deafness and Other Communication Disorders, National Institutes of Health, Gaithersburg [29]

ARTHUR J. SOBER, MD
Associate Professor of Dermatology, Harvard Medical School; Associate Chief of Dermatology, Massachusetts General Hospital, Boston [88]

CLAUS O. SOLBERG, MD, PhD
Professor of Medicine and Chairman, Medical Department, University of Bergen, Bergen, Norway [149]

PETER SPEELMAN, MD
Chief, Division of Infectious Diseases, Tropical Medicine and AIDS, Department of Medicine, Academic Medical Center, University of Amsterdam, Amsterdam [176]

FRANK E. SPEIZER, MD
Edward H. Kass Professor of Medicine, Harvard Medical School; Co-Director, Channing Laboratory, Brigham and Women's Hospital, Boston [5, 254, 390]

ANDREW SPIELMAN, ScD
Professor of Tropical Public Health, Harvard School of Public Health, Boston [393]

JERRY L. SPIVAK, MD
Professor of Medicine and Oncology, The Johns Hopkins University School of Medicine, Baltimore [111]

WALTER E. STAMM, MD
Professor of Medicine and Head, Division of Allergy and Infectious Diseases, University of Washington, Seattle [131, 181]

ALLEN C. STEERE, MD
Professor of Medicine and Chief, Rheumatology/Immunology, New England Medical Center and Tufts University School of Medicine, Boston [178]

ROBERT S. STERN, MD
Professor, Department of Dermatology, Beth Israel Hospital, Boston [56]

DENNIS L. STEVENS, MD, PhD
Professor of Medicine, University of Washington School of Medicine, Seattle; Chief, Infectious Diseases, VA Medical Center, Boise [133]

RICHARD M. STONE, MD
Assistant Professor of Medicine, Harvard Medical School, Boston [101]

STEPHEN E. STRAUS, MD
Chief, Laboratory of Clinical Investigation, National Institute of Allergy and Infectious Diseases, National Institutes of Health, Bethesda [384]

DAVID H. P. STREETEN, MB, DPhil, FRCP
Professor of Medicine Emeritus, Department of Medicine, State University of New York, Health Science Center, Syracuse [330]

MORTON N. SWARTZ, MD
Professor, Department of Medicine, Harvard Medical School; Chief, James Jackson Firm Medical Services, Massachusetts General Hospital, Boston [378]

ROBERT A. SWERLICK, MD
Associate Professor, Department of Dermatology, Emory University School of Medicine, Atlanta [55]

RUP TANDAN, MD, MRCP
Associate Professor of Neurology; Director, Neuromuscular Disorders Section; Attending Neurologist, Medical Center Hospital of Vermont, Fletcher Allen Health Care, University of Vermont College of Medicine, Burlington [315]

JOEL D. TAUROG, MD
Professor of Internal Medicine, Department of Internal Medicine, University of Texas Southwestern Medical Center at Dallas, Dallas [317]

SCOTT J. THALER, MD
Instructor in Medicine, Harvard Medical School; Infectious Disease Division, Brigham and Women's Hospital, Boston [324]

LUCY STUART TOMPKINS, MD, PhD
Professor, Departments of Medicine (Division of Infectious Diseases and Geographic Medicine) and Microbiology and Immunology, Stanford University School of Medicine; Director, Clinical Microbiology Laboratory; Director, Hospital Epidemiology, Stanford University Medical Center, Stanford [165]

PHILLIP P. TOSKES, MD
Professor of Medicine and Director, Division of Gastroenterology, Hepatology and Nutrition; Associate Chairman for Clinical Affairs, Department of Medicine, University of Florida, Gainesville [303, 304]

NHU-LINH T. TRAN, MD
Fellow, Department of Dermatology, Emory University School of Medicine, Atlanta [88]

JEFFREY M. TRENT, PhD
Chief, Laboratory of Cancer Genetics; Director, Division of Intramural Research, National Human Genome Research Institute, National Institutes of Health, Bethesda [84]

GERARD TROMP, PhD
Assistant Professor, Center for Molecular Medicine and Genetics, Wayne State University School of Medicine, Detroit [348]

KENNETH L. TYLER, MD
Professor of Neurology, Medicine and Microbiology and Immunology, University of Colorado Health Sciences Center; Chief, Neurology Service, Denver Veterans Affairs Medical Center, Denver [379]

DAVID L. VALLE, MD
Professor of Pediatrics and Molecular Biology and Genetics, The Johns Hopkins Hospital School of Medicine, Baltimore [67]

EVERETT E. VOKES, MD
Professor of Medicine and Radiation and Cellular Oncology, University of Chicago, Chicago [89]

K. B. WAITES, MD
Associate Professor, Departments of Pathology, Microbiology, and Rehabilitation Medicine; Director of Clinical Microbiology, University of Alabama Hospitals and Clinics, Birmingham [180]

DAVID H. WALKER, MD
Professor and Chairman, Department of Pathology; Director, WHO Collaborating Center for Tropical Diseases, University of Texas Medical Branch, Galveston [179]

RICHARD J. WALLACE, JR., MD
Chairman, Department of Microbiology; Acting Director of Center for Pulmonary Infectious Disease Control; Professor of Medicine; John Chapman Professorship in Microbiology, University of Texas Health Center, Tyler [170]

PETER D. WALZER, MD
Professor of Medicine, University of Cincinnati College of Medicine; Associate Chief of Staff for Research, Cincinnati VA Medical Center, Cincinnati [211]

FREDERICK C.S. WANG, MD
Assistant Professor of Medicine, Harvard Medical School, Boston [182, 188]

LEONARD WARTOFSKY, MD
Professor of Medicine and Physiology, Uniformed Services University; Clinical Professor of Medicine, Georgetown, George Washington, and Howard University Schools of Medicine; Chairman of Medicine Washington Hospital Center, Washington DC [331]

CARL V. WASHINGTON, JR, MD
Assistant Professor of Dermatology, Emory University School of Medicine; Director, Mohs Surgery Unit, The Emory Clinic, Atlanta [88]

VISH WATKINS, MD
Clinical Research Physician, Lilly Research Laboratories, Eli Lilly and Company, Indianapolis [155]

STEVEN E. WEINBERGER, MD
Professor of Medicine, Harvard Medical School; Chief, Pulmonary and Critical Care Division, Beth Israel Deaconess Medical Center, Boston [33, 249–251, 256]

ROBERT A. WEINSTEIN, MD
Professor of Medicine, Rush Medical College; Chairman, Division of Infectious Diseases, Cook County Hospital, Chicago [138]

PETER F. WELLER, MD
Professor of Medicine, Harvard Medical School; Co-Chief, Division of Infectious Diseases and Chief, Allergy and Inflammation Division, Department of Medicine, Beth Israel Deaconess Medical Center, Boston [212, 214, 220–223, 225]

MICHAEL R. WESSELS, MD
Associate Professor of Medicine, Harvard Medical School; Channing Laboratory, Brigham and Women's Hospital; Division of Infectious Diseases, Beth Israel Deaconess Medical Center, Boston [143]

MEIR WETZLER, MD
Assistant Professor of Medicine, State University of New York at Buffalo, Buffalo [112]

NICHOLAS J. WHITE, DSc, MD, FRCP
Director, Wellcome-Mahidol University, Oxford Tropical Medicine Research Programme, Faculty of Tropical Medicine, Mahidol University, Bangkok; Wellcome Trust Clinical Research Unit, Centre for Tropical Diseases, Cho Quan Hospital, Ho Chi Minh City [216]

RICHARD J. WHITLEY, MD
Loeb Eminent Scholar in Pediatrics and Professor of Pediatrics, Microbiology and Medicine, University of Alabama at Birmingham, Birmingham [185]

GRANT R. WILKINSON, PhD
Professor of Pharmacology, Vanderbilt University School of Medicine, Nashville [68]

GORDON H. WILLIAMS, MD
Professor of Medicine, Harvard Medical School; Chief, Endocrine-Hypertension Division, Brigham and Women's Hospital, Boston [35, 246, 332]

JEAN D. WILSON, MD
Charles Cameron Sprague Distinguished Chair and Clinical Professor of Internal Medicine, The University of Texas Southwestern Medical Center, Dallas [1, 51, 53, 72–74, 79, 97, 327, 336, 338, 339]

BRUCE U. WINTROUB, MD
Professor of Dermatology, Executive Vice-Dean, School of Medicine, University of California San Francisco, San Francisco [56]

BEVERLY WOO, MD
Assistant Professor of Medicine, Harvard Medical School; Physician, Brigham and Women's Hospital, Boston [6]

ALASTAIR J.J. WOOD, MBChB, FRCP (Edin), FRCP (Lond)
Professor of Medicine and Professor of Pharmacology, Vanderbilt University School of Medicine; Attending Physician, Vanderbilt University Hospital, Nashville [69]

ROBERT L. WORTMANN, MD
Professor and Chairman of Medicine, East Carolina University School of Medicine, Greenville [344]

PAUL W. WRIGHT, MD
Director of Predoctoral Education and Professor of Family Practice, University of Texas Health Center, Tyler [170]

JOSHUA WYNNE, MD
Professor of Medicine and Chief, Division of Cardiology, Wayne State University; Chief, Section of Cardiology, Harper Hospital, Detroit [239]

KIM B. YANCEY, MD
Senior Investigator, Dermatology Branch, National Cancer Institute, National Institutes of Health, Bethesda [54, 311]

JAMES B. YOUNG, MD
Professor of Medicine, Northwestern University Medical School; Attending Physician, Northwestern Memorial Hospital, Chicago [70, 333]

ROBERT C. YOUNG, MD
President, Fox Chase Cancer Center, Philadelphia [99]

VICTOR L. YU, MD
Professor of Medicine, University of Pittsburgh; Chief, Infectious Disease Section, Veterans Affairs Medical Center, Pittsburgh [153]

DORI F. ZALEZNIK, MD
Assistant Professor of Medicine, Harvard Medical School; Physician, Beth Israel Deaconess Medical Center; Channing Laboratory, Brigham and Women's Hospital, Boston [127, 137, 148]

PETER J. ZIMETBAUM, MD
Instructor in Medicine, Harvard Medical School; Cardiovascular Division, Beth Israel Deaconess Medical Center, Boston [230, 231]

PHILIPPE E. ZIMMERN
Associate Professor of Urology, The University of Texas Southwestern Medical School, Dallas [48]

The first edition of *Harrison's Principles of Internal Medicine* was published nearly 50 years ago, and subsequent editions have incorporated advances that have occurred in biomedical research and clinical practice in the interim. In the 14th edition, the text has been revised to reflect further understanding of the biology and pathophysiology of disease and at the same time to retain those facts that, while not new, remain clinically useful and important. Virtually every chapter in the 14th edition has been completely or substantially rewritten, and major new chapters have been added. In this preface, we cannot describe all of these changes; however, we would like to call to the reader's attention those that are particularly noteworthy.

Part One, "Introduction to Clinical Medicine," contains new chapters dealing with the influence of environmental and occupational hazards on health. Disease prevention is becoming more important in the current era, and both general principles of prevention and specific guidelines for primary care physicians are presented in a new chapter on preventive medicine. Chapters on medical ethics, women's and adolescent health, geriatric medicine, medical complications of pregnancy, and cost awareness and quantitative aspects of medicine have been revised and updated.

Part Two, "Cardinal Manifestations and Presentation of Diseases," serves as a comprehensive introduction to clinical medicine. Major symptoms are reviewed by organ system and are correlated with specific disease states—the basis of differential diagnosis. New chapters have been added on fever and rash; hypothermia; faintness, syncope, and dizziness; weakness, abnormal movements, and imbalance; coma and acute confusional states; aphasia and other focal cerebral disorders; memory loss and dementia; heart murmur; hypertension; voiding dysfunction, incontinence, and other common urologic complaints; manifestations of cancer; and breast masses in women and men. For the first time in *Harrison's*, a comprehensive approach to the diagnosis and treatment of common eye disorders is presented. The chapter on diarrhea and constipation has been extensively revised, with a focus not only on etiology but also on acute and chronic treatment. The chapter on gastrointestinal bleeding has been rewritten to focus on early diagnosis and the latest approaches to treatment.

Part Three, "Genetics and Disease," has been extensively updated and includes a new formulation of the role of classic and molecular genetics in health and disease and a major revision of the chapter on cytogenetics.

Part Four, "Clinical Pharmacology," contains a new chapter on nitric oxide. Nitric oxide or its inhibition may be important in the management of coronary insufficiency, septic shock, erectile impotence, primary pulmonary hypertension, and the adult respiratory distress syndrome.

Part Five, "Nutrition," covers nutritional considerations related to clinical medicine, including nutritional requirements, assessment of nutritional status, protein-energy malnutrition, and diet therapy.

The core of *Harrison's* encompasses the disorders of the organ systems and is contained in Parts Six through Fifteen. These sections include succinct accounts of the pathophysiology of the major systems and emphasize disease manifestations, diagnostic procedures, differential diagnosis, and treatment strategies. The treatment sections of virtually every chapter have been amplified, supplemented by the liberal use of algorithms, and clearly highlighted.

Part Six, "Oncology and Hematology," has been completely reorganized and extensively rewritten under the direction of our newest editor, Dr. Dan L. Longo, who brings to the textbook a wealth of experience at the bench and bedside in both hematology and oncology. He has called upon a distinguished group of contributors to reorganize this section. The oncology chapters that were distributed among several sections in previous editions have been brought together in a single section on neoplastic disorders (with the exception

of tumors of the thyroid, central nervous system, and heart). There are eight new chapters, including those on the approach to the patient with cancer, cancer prevention and early detection, cancer cell biology, invasion and metastasis, sarcomas and bone tumors, and oncologic emergencies. Twenty-seven additional chapters have new authors. An effort was made to organize the chapters in a more uniform fashion and to include molecular and genetic mechanisms involved in tumors (and their clinical correlations) where that information is known. The chapter on lymphoid malignancies includes the novel classification scheme of the International Lymphoma Working Group. Where appropriate, diagnostic and management algorithms have been incorporated.

Changes in Part Seven, "Infectious Diseases," include a greater emphasis on the treatment of infections and infestations. Specific, current recommendations for therapy are made against a background of up-to-date information on the etiology, epidemiology, diagnosis, and prevention of infectious diseases. Special care has been taken to update and expand the information presented on the biology of microorganisms, microbial resistance to therapeutic agents, and emerging and reemerging infections, including mycobacterial infections, recently identified viral infections, and infections due to other newly recognized pathogens such as *Helicobacter pylori*. The revised chapter on the laboratory diagnosis of infectious diseases is complemented in this edition by the inclusion (as Appendix B) of comprehensive instructions for the collection and transport of specimens for culture. New and expanded chapters cover the health risks to travelers, the approach to patients with parasitic infections, and recommendations for the administration of standard and special-use vaccines. The chapter on the human retroviruses has been revised and expanded, as have the chapters on the biology of viruses and antiviral therapy. This edition's chapter on *Pneumocystis carinii* infection appears in Section 15, "Fungal Infections," reflecting the change in the classification of this pathogen from a protozoan to a fungus.

In Part Eight, "Disorders of the Cardiovascular System," a new chapter on atherosclerosis focuses not only on the importance of traditional risk factors but also on factors that influence plaque stability and instability. The current approach to the prevention of atherosclerosis is clearly delineated. An understanding of prevention of plaque instability is of critical importance, since it is now clear that plaque rupture can cause acute coronary syndromes (unstable angina and acute myocardial infarction) and sudden death.

Despite major advances in its diagnosis and therapy, acute myocardial infarction is the most common cause of death in industrialized nations. The new chapter on acute myocardial infarction provides important information on myocardial reperfusion therapy—thrombolysis and primary coronary angioplasty—and summarizes guidelines for acute coronary care and for risk stratification in the postinfarct patient.

Pulmonary thromboembolism is a major complication of the postoperative state and of a variety of illnesses. In Part Nine, "Disorders of the Respiratory System," major advances in prevention and therapy are presented in a new chapter that includes a useful algorithm for the work-up of patients with suspected pulmonary embolic disease. Enormous strides have been made in the use of lung transplantation for selected patients with end-stage, irreversible, pulmonary parenchymal and vascular disease, and a new chapter on this topic focuses on patient selection for this therapy.

In Part Ten, "Disorders of the Kidney and Urinary Tract," there has been considerable revision. In Part Eleven, "Disorders of the Gastrointestinal System," the new chapter on peptic ulcer and gastritis focuses on the role of *Helicobacter pylori*, with particular attention to its diagnosis and treatment. This chapter can be viewed as *the* definitive chapter on peptic ulcer and gastritis. The chapters on irritable bowel syndrome and diverticular diseases are also new, and the chapters on acute hepatitis and complications of cirrhosis have been extensively revised, the latter with a specific focus on the treatment of hepatic coma, ascites, and portal hypertension.

In Part Twelve, "Disorders of the Immune System, Connective Tissue, and Joints," the updating focuses on therapy. The chapter on "Introduction to the Immune System" has been completely rewritten and provides a comprehensive review of the human immune system. The chapter on HIV disease and AIDS is comprehensive and up-to-date and includes coverage of the natural history, epidemiology, and immunopathogenic mechanisms of HIV disease. In addition, the chapter contains both an organ system by organ system approach and a delineation of the major complications of HIV disease. The sections on therapy include a state-of-the-art discussion of the treatment of HIV infection with combinations of antiretroviral agents.

In Part Thirteen, "Endocrinology and Metabolism," there are new chapters on the hyperlipoproteinemias, lysosomal storage diseases, and glycogen storage disease. The chapter on diabetes mellitus includes a discussion of the impact of tight control on the development of diabetic complications.

As a new editor, Dr. Stephen L. Hauser, Chairman of the Department of Neurology at the University of California San Francisco, joins Dr. Joseph Martin in providing a comprehensive neurology section applicable to general internal medicine. Dr. Hauser's contributions to Part Fourteen, "Neurologic Disorders," have been substantial, including chapters on multiple sclerosis, disorders of the spinal cord, and stroke. The entire section on neurology has been extensively revised and updated. New or extensively rewritten chapters on neuroimaging, epilepsy, stroke, Alzheimer's disease, Parkinson's disease, ataxia, spinal cord disease, tumors, and chronic meningitis provide an up-to-date summary of this rapidly changing field. The traditional focus of *Harrison's* textbook—providing an in-depth review of the pathophysiologic basis of each neurologic disorder—has been retained, and important advances in molecular pathogenesis and treatment have been included. When possible, diagnostic and therapeutic algorithms have been prepared that standardize and simplify the approach to different neurologic problems. A major effort has been made to expand the neuroimaging figures throughout the section. The anatomic figures have also been expanded and improved.

Finally, Part Fifteen, "Environmental and Occupational Hazards," has been expanded and reorganized.

Beginning with the 12th edition of *Harrison's,* the editors decided to provide laboratory values expressed in two ways: according to the International System (SI) and according to the conventional laboratory terminology used by hospitals in the United States. We felt that this was important because, although the SI units are used in many scientific and medical journals in the United States and elsewhere and in hospitals in many parts of the world, there remains considerable resistance to their adoption from some hospitals and some medical journals. Thus, it is apparent that physicians in many parts of the world will have to live indefinitely with two systems of laboratory values—one for the practice of medicine and another for access to large parts of biomedical science. Consequently, in this edition we continue to list the SI units first and the conventional units in parentheses for all measurements except blood pressure,

which is given only in millimeters of mercury, and for those measurements in which the values are the same in both systems, as in the case of serum sodium measurements (expressed in meq/L and mmol/L). In most instances, the interconversion between SI and conventional units is straightforward. However, it is imperative that readers consult their own laboratory for normal values. Perhaps the greatest potential danger inherent in the existence of the two systems is in the interpretation of plasma glucose and plasma calcium levels, but caution should be observed in the interpretation of all laboratory values.

In view of the requirements for continuing education for licensure and relicensure, as well as the emphasis on certification and recertification, a revision of the *Pre-Test Self-Assessment and Review* will be published with this edition. It consists of several hundred questions based on *Harrison's,* along with answers and explanations for the answers. The *Companion Handbook* that was pioneered as a supplement to the 11th edition of *Harrison's* has been updated and will appear shortly after the publication of this edition. The 13th edition of *Harrison's* has been available in a CD-ROM version. An expanded CD-ROM version of the 14th edition will be available and will be regularly updated.

We wish to express our appreciation to our many associates and colleagues, who, as experts in their fields, have helped us with constructive criticism and helpful suggestions. We acknowledge especially the contributions of Gary Abrams, David Acker, Robert Alpern, Donna Ambrosino, Joseph Antin, Karen Antman, James Armitage, Cameron Ashbaugh, Tamar Barlam, Arthur L. Beaudet, Richard Blumberg, Timothy Brewer, Bruce Chabner, Paul Choi, Hal Churchill, Jeffrey Cohen, Oren Cohen, George Curlin, Richard T. Davey, Jr., Margo A. Denke, Judith Falloon, Christopher Fanta, Mark Feinberg, Paul Fitzgerald, Lawrence Friedman, Joseph L. Goldstein, Daryl Gress, Rachel Haft, Helen H. Hobbs, Stephanie James, Clay Johnston, Keith Joiner, Stephen Kohl, Catherine Lachenauer, John LaMontagne, H. Clifford Lane, James Maguire, James Mastrianni, Carol Mendelsohn, Kirk Miller, James Murtagh, Thomas Nutman, Mario Ostrowski, David Ozonoff, Jeffrey Parsonnet, John Reilly, Elizabeth Robbins, David Rosenthal, John Rutherford, Richard Schwartzstein, Robert Seder, Ellen Seely, Julian Seifter, John Spengler, Ray Swanson, Jorge Tavel, Scott Thaler, Kenneth Tyler, Mark Udey, Sasha Vinogradov, C. Fordham von Reyn, Ronald Walls, Fred Wang, Arnold Weinberg, Michael Weinblatt, Scott Weiss, Peter Weller, Michael Wessels, and Stephen Zucker.

This book could not have been edited without the dedicated help of our co-workers in the editorial offices of the individual editors. We are especially indebted to Pat Duffey, Caroline Figoni, Christy K. Gonzales, Terry Jones, Leslie LaPiana, Julie McCoy, Pamela Oliver, Jaylyn Olivo, Kathryn Saxon, Marie Scurti, and Elin Woodger.

Finally, we continue to be indebted to three outstanding members of the McGraw-Hill organization: Mariapaz Ramos Englis, Managing Editor; J. Dereck Jeffers, Editor-in-Chief; and Martin J. Wonsiewicz, Editorial Director. They are an effective team who have given the editors constant encouragement and sage advice and have been of enormous help in bringing this edition to fruition in a timely manner.

The Editors

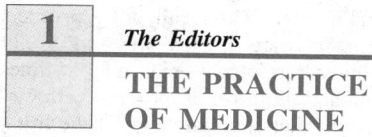

1 The Editors

THE PRACTICE OF MEDICINE

WHAT IS EXPECTED OF THE PHYSICIAN The practice of medicine combines both science and art. The role of science in medicine is clear. Science-based technology is the foundation for the solution to many clinical problems; the dazzling advances in biochemical methodology and in biophysical imaging techniques that allow access to the remotest recesses of the body are the products of science. So too are the therapeutic maneuvers that increasingly are a major part of medical practice. Yet skill in the most sophisticated application of laboratory technology and in the use of the latest therapeutic modality alone does not make a good physician. The ability to extract from a mass of contradictory physical signs and from the crowded computer printouts of laboratory data those items that are of crucial significance, to know in a difficult case whether to "treat" or to "watch," to determine when a clinical clue is worth pursuing or when to dismiss it as a "red herring," and to estimate in any given patient whether a proposed treatment entails a greater risk than the disease are all involved in the decisions that the clinician, skilled in the practice of medicine, must make many times each day. This combination of medical knowledge, intuition, and judgment defines the *art of medicine*. It is as necessary to the practice of medicine as is a sound scientific base.

The editors of the first edition of this book articulated what is expected of the physician in words that, although they reflect the gender bias of that era, still ring true as a universal principle:

> No greater opportunity, responsibility, or obligation can fall to the lot of a human being than to become a physician. In the care of the suffering he needs technical skill, scientific knowledge, and human understanding. He who uses these with courage, with humility, and with wisdom will provide a unique service for his fellow man, and will build an enduring edifice of character within himself. The physician should ask of his destiny no more than this; he should be content with no less.

Tact, sympathy and understanding are expected of the physician, for the patient is no mere collection of symptoms, signs, disordered functions, damaged organs, and disturbed emotions. He is human, fearful, and hopeful, seeking relief, help and reassurance. To the physician, as to the anthropologist, nothing human is strange or repulsive. The misanthrope may become a smart diagnostician of organic disease, but he can scarcely hope to succeed as a physician. The true physician has a Shakespearean breadth of interest in the wise and the foolish, the proud and the humble, the stoic hero and the whining rogue. He cares for people.

THE PATIENT-PHYSICIAN RELATIONSHIP It may be trite to emphasize that physicians need to approach patients not as "cases" or "diseases" but as individuals whose problems all too often transcend the complaints that bring them to the doctor. Most patients are anxious and frightened. Often they go to great ends to convince themselves that illness does not exist, or unconsciously they set up elaborate defenses to divert attention from the real problem that they perceive to be serious or life-threatening. Some patients use illness to gain attention or to serve as a crutch to extricate themselves from a stressful situation; some even feign physical illness. Whatever the patient's attitude, the physician needs to consider the setting in which an illness occurs—in terms not only of the patients themselves but also of their families and social backgrounds. Medical workups and records often fail to include essential information about the patient's origins, schooling, job, home and family, hopes and fears. Without

this knowledge, it is difficult for the physician to gain rapport with the patient or to develop insight into the illness. The ideal physician-patient relationship is based on thorough knowledge of the patient, on mutual trust, and on the ability to communicate with one another.

The direct, one-to-one physician-patient relationship, which traditionally characterized the practice of medicine, is in jeopardy, primarily because of the changing setting in which medicine is being practiced. Often the management of the individual patient requires the participation of a variety of trained professional personnel and of several physicians and indeed may be a team effort. The patient can benefit greatly from such collaboration, but *it is the duty of the primary physician to guide the patient through an illness*. To carry out this difficult task, the physician must have some familiarity with the techniques, skills, and objectives of specialist physicians and of colleagues in the fields allied to medicine. In giving the patient an opportunity to receive all the benefits of the important advances of science, the primary physician must, in the last analysis, retain responsibility for the major decisions concerning diagnosis and treatment.

Furthermore, patients are increasingly cared for by groups of physicians, clinics, hospitals, or health-maintenance organizations (HMOs) rather than by individual, independent practitioners. Whatever the potential advantages of such organized medical groups, there are also drawbacks, the chief of which is the *loss of the concept of the physician who is primarily and continuously responsible*. Even in the group setting, it is essential that each patient have a physician who has an overview of the problems and who is familiar with the patient's reaction to the illness, to the drugs given, and to the challenges that the patient faces. Moreover, because a number of physicians may, at any one time, contribute to the care of a particular patient, accurate and detailed medical records are essential to patient care.

The practice of medicine in a "managed care" setting puts additional stress on the classic paradigm of the physician-patient relationship. Many physicians find themselves in an environment where they must deal with a patient within a restricted time frame, with limited access to specialists, and under organizational guidelines that may at times compromise their ability to exercise their optimal clinical judgment. These circumstances provide a unique challenge to the physician to deliver excellent medical care while complying with the guidelines of the organization within which he or she practices. As difficult as these restrictions may be, it is the ultimate responsibility of the physician to determine what is best for the patient; this responsibility cannot be relinquished in the name of compliance with organizational guidelines.

Satisfactory physician-patient relationships in the tertiary care setting require that the physician be well versed in etiquette and ethics as well as in medicine. The diagnostic and treatment dilemmas of referring physicians must be respected, although the treatment provided prior to admission may not have been up to the standards of the current hospital or care setting. Differences of opinion that arise about patient management are best resolved in private discussions away from the bedside. When students or residents are involved in the care of a patient, they must be supervised by a senior physician. On the other hand, physicians must never misuse their position of authority in any manner that potentially exploits patients, staff, or trainees.

The modern hospital constitutes an intimidating environment for most patients. Lying in a bed surrounded by air jets, buttons, and lights; invaded by tubes and wires; beset by the numerous members of the health care team—nurses, nurses' aides, physicians' assistants, social workers, technologists, physical therapists, medical students, house officers, attending and consulting physicians, and many others; transported to special laboratories and x-ray chambers replete with blinking lights and strange sounds, it is little wonder that patients lose their sense of reality. In fact, the physician is often the only tenuous link between the patient and the real world, and a strong personal relationship with the physician helps to sustain the patient in such a stressful situation.

Many trends in contemporary society tend to make medical care impersonal. Some of these have been mentioned already and include (1) vigorous efforts to reduce the escalating costs of health care; (2) the increasing reliance on technologic advances and computerization for many aspects of diagnosis and treatment; (3) the increased geographic mobility of both patients and physicians; (4) the growing number of HMOs, in which the patient may have little choice in selecting a physician; (5) the need for more than a single physician to be involved in the care of most patients who are seriously ill; and (6) an increasing tendency on the part of patients to express their disappointments with the health care system by legal means (i.e., by malpractice litigation). Given these changes in the medical care system, maintaining the humane aspects of medical care and the empathetic qualities of the physician is a major challenge. It is now more important than ever that the physician consider each patient to be a unique individual deserving of humane treatment, regardless of personal or financial circumstances.

The American Board of Internal Medicine has defined humanistic qualities as encompassing integrity, respect, and compassion. Availability, the expression of sincere concern, the willingness to take the time to explain all aspects of the illness, and an attitude of being nonjudgmental with patients who have lifestyles, attitudes, and values different from those of the physician and which he or she may in some instances even find repugnant are just a few of the characteristics of the humane physician. Every physician will, at times, be challenged by patients who evoke strongly negative (and occasionally strongly positive) emotional responses. Physicians should be alert to their own reactions to such patients and situations and should consciously monitor and control their behavior so that the patients' best interests remain the principal motivation for their actions at all times.

The famous statement of Dr. Francis Peabody is even more relevant today than when delivered more than a half century ago:

The significance of the intimate personal relationship between physician and patient cannot be too strongly emphasized, for in an extraordinarily large number of cases both the diagnosis and treatment are directly dependent on it. One of the essential qualities of the clinician is interest in humanity, for the secret of the care of the patient is in caring for the patient.

CLINICAL SKILLS **History Taking** The written history of an illness should embody all the facts of medical significance in the life of the patient. If the history is recorded in chronologic order, recent events should be given the most attention. Likewise, if a problem-oriented approach is used, the problems that are clinically dominant should be listed first. Ideally, the narration of symptoms or problems should be in the patient's own words. However, few patients have sufficient powers of observation or recall to give a history without some guidance from the physician, who must be careful not to suggest the answers to the questions being posed. Often a symptom of concern to a patient has little significance, while a seemingly minor complaint may be of importance. Therefore, the physician must be alert to the possibility that any event related by the patient, however trivial or apparently remote, may be the key to the solution of the medical problem.

An informative history is more than an orderly listing of symptoms. Something is always gained by listening to patients and noting the way in which they describe their symptoms. Inflections of voice, facial expression, and attitude may betray important clues to the meaning of the symptoms to the patient. In listening to the history, the physician discovers not only something about the disease but also something about the patient.

With experience, the pitfalls of history taking become apparent. What patients relate for the most part consists of subjective phenomena colored by past experience; they differ widely in their responses to the same stimuli and in their coping mechanisms. Their attitudes are variably influenced by fear of disability and death and by concern over the consequences of their illness to their families. Sometimes the accuracy of the history is affected by language or sociologic barriers, by failing intellectual powers that interfere with recall, or by disorders of consciousness that make them unaware of their illness. It is not surprising, then, that even the most careful physician may at times despair of collecting factual data and be forced to proceed with evidence that represents little more than an approximation of the truth. It is in obtaining the history that the physician's skill, knowledge, and experience are most clearly in evidence.

The family history serves several functions. First, in rare single-gene defects a positive family history of a similarly affected individual or a history of consanguinity may have important diagnostic implications. Second, in diseases of multifactorial etiology with a familial aggregation, it may be possible to identify patients at risk for disease and to intervene before the development of overt manifestations. For example, recent weight gain may be a more ominous development in a woman who has a family history of diabetes than in one who does not. In certain situations the family history has major implications for preventive medicine. When a diagnosis of a hereditary condition known to predispose to cancer is made, it is the physician's obligation to follow up this possibility carefully in the patient, to survey the family, and to educate them about the need for long-term follow-up.

However accurate and complete, the medical history does much more than provide facts of critical importance. The very act of taking the history provides the physician with the opportunity to establish or enhance the unique bond that is the basis for the physician-patient relationship. An effort should be made to place the patient at ease, regardless of the circumstances. The patient should, at some point, have the opportunity to tell his or her own story of the illness without frequent interruption and, when appropriate, receive expressions of interest, encouragement, and empathy from the physician. It is helpful to develop an appreciation of the patient's perception of the illness, the patient's expectations of the physician and the medical care system, and the financial and social implications of the illness to the patient. The confidentiality of the physician-patient relationship should be emphasized, and the patient should be given the opportunity to identify any aspects of the history that should not be disclosed.

Physical Examination Physical signs are the objective indications of disease and represent solid, indisputable facts. Their significance is enhanced when they confirm a functional or structural change already suggested by the patient's history. At times, the physical signs may be the only evidence of disease, especially when the history is inconsistent, confused, or lacking altogether.

The physical examination should be performed methodically and thoroughly, with consideration for the patient's comfort and modesty. Although attention is often directed by the history to the diseased organ or part of the body, the examination of a new patient must extend from head to toe in an objective search for abnormalities. Unless the physical examination is systematic, important parts may be omitted, a common error even among skilled clinicians. The results of the examination, like the details of the history, should be recorded at the time they are elicited, not hours later when they are subject to the distortions of memory. Many inaccuracies stem from writing or dictating notes long after the examination has been concluded. Skill in physical diagnosis is acquired with experience, but it is not merely technique that determines success in eliciting signs. The detection of a few scattered petechiae, a faint diastolic murmur, or a small mass in the abdomen is not a question of keener eyes and ears or more sensitive fingers but of a mind alert to these findings. Skill in physical diagnosis reflects a way of thinking more than a way of doing. Physical findings are subject to change. Just because the examination is normal on one occasion does not guarantee that it will be normal on subsequent examinations. Likewise, abnormal findings may disappear during the course of illness. The physical examination should be repeated as frequently as the clinical situation warrants.

Laboratory Tests The increase in the number and availability of laboratory tests has increased our reliance on these studies for the solution of clinical problems. It is essential, however, to bear in mind the limitations of such procedures, which by virtue of their impersonal quality and complexity often gain an aura of authority regardless of the fallibility of the tests themselves, the instruments used in the tests, and the individuals performing or interpreting them. Moreover, the accumulation of laboratory data does not relieve the physician from the responsibility of careful observation and study of the patient. Physicians also must weigh the hazards and expense involved in the laboratory procedures they order. Moreover, laboratory tests are rarely ordered and reported singly. Rather, they are produced as "batteries" of multiple tests. The various combinations of laboratory tests are often useful. For example, they may provide the clue to such nonspecific symptoms as generalized weakness and increased fatigability by revealing abnormalities of hepatic function, suggesting the diagnosis of chronic liver disease. Sometimes a single abnormality, such as an elevated serum calcium level, points to a specific disease, such as hyperparathyroidism.

The thoughtful use of screening tests should not be confused with indiscriminate laboratory testing. The use of screening tests is based on the fact that a group of laboratory determinations can be carried out conveniently on a single specimen of blood at relatively low cost. Biochemical measurements, together with simple laboratory examinations such as blood count, urinalysis, and sedimentation rate, often provide the major clue to the presence of a pathologic process. At the same time, the physician must learn to evaluate occasional abnormalities among the screening tests that may not necessarily connote significant disease. An in-depth workup following a report of an isolated laboratory abnormality in a patient who is otherwise well is almost invariably wasteful and unproductive. Among the more than 40 tests that are performed on many patients, one or two are often slightly abnormal. If there is no suspicion of an underlying illness, these tests are ordinarily repeated to ensure that the abnormality does not represent a laboratory error. If an abnormality is confirmed, it is important to distinguish a minor one (less than two standard deviations) from a major one (more than two standard deviations). Even in the latter case, the decision of whether to proceed with further workup is left to the physician's clinical judgment.

Imaging Techniques The availability of ultrasonography, a variety of scans that employ isotopes to visualize organs heretofore inaccessible, computed tomography with its varying permutations, magnetic resonance imaging, and positron emission tomography has opened new diagnostic vistas, and has benefited patients because these new techniques have largely supplanted more invasive ones. While the enthusiasm for noninvasive technology is understandably justified, the expense entailed in performing these imaging tests is often substantial and is not always considered when ordering them. These examinations should be used judiciously.

Continued Learning The conscientious physician must be a perpetual student since the body of medical knowledge is constantly expanding and being refined. The profession of medicine should be inherently linked to a career-long thirst for new knowledge that can be used for the good of the patient. It is the responsibility of a physician to pursue continually the acquisition of new knowledge by reading, attending conferences and courses, and consulting with colleagues. This is often a difficult task under the circumstances of a busy practice; however, such a commitment to continued learning is such an integral part of being a physician that it should be given the highest priority.

Medicine on the Internet The explosion in use of the World-Wide Web, or Internet, through personal computers has had an important impact on many practicing physicians. The "Net" provides almost instantaneous availability of a wide range of information directly to the desk of a physician at any time of day or night and from anywhere in the world. It holds enormous potential for providing useful up-to-date practice guidelines, information on state-of-the-art conferences, journal contents, textbook chapters, and direct communication with other physicians and specialists, thereby expanding the depth and breadth of information available to the physician about the

diagnosis and care of patients. The potential benefit of this medium for the practicing physician is enormous, and it behooves physicians to become familiar with the use of the Internet. It is likely that most medical journals will ultimately be on-line. Yet, there is one important caveat. Certain authors post prepublication manuscripts on the Internet, and others supply unpublished data. In this regard, it is relatively easy to publish virtually anything on the Internet by using either a home page or a file server, thus circumventing the peer review process that is an essential feature of quality publication. Therefore, physicians who search the Internet for medical information must be aware of this potential for misinformation. Notwithstanding this limitation, appropriate use of the Internet is revolutionizing information access for physicians and will be a positive force in the practice of medicine.

THE DIAGNOSIS OF DISEASE Clinical diagnosis requires both aspects of logic—analysis and synthesis—and the more difficult the clinical problem, the more important is a logical approach to it. Such an approach requires that the physician list carefully each problem suggested by the symptoms and physical and laboratory findings and seek answers to each. Most physicians attempt consciously or unconsciously to fit a given problem into one of a series of syndromes. *The syndrome is a group of symptoms and signs of disordered function related to one another by means of some anatomic, physiologic, or biochemical peculiarity.* It embodies a hypothesis concerning the deranged function of an organ, organ system, or tissue. Congestive heart failure, Cushing's syndrome, and dementia are examples. In congestive heart failure, dyspnea, orthopnea, cyanosis, dependent edema, engorged neck veins, pleural effusion, rales, and hepatomegaly are connected by a single pathophysiologic mechanism—insufficiency of the cardiac pump mechanism. In Cushing's syndrome, moon facies, hypertension, diabetes mellitus, and osteoporosis are the consequence of excess glucocorticoids. In dementia, deterioration of memory, incoherent thinking, impaired language functions, visual-spatial disorientation, and faulty judgment are related to destruction of the association areas of the cerebrum.

A syndrome usually does not identify the precise cause of an illness, but it narrows the possibilities and may suggest certain special clinical and laboratory studies. The diagnosis is simplified greatly if a clinical problem conforms neatly to a well-defined syndrome, because only a few diseases need to be considered in the differential diagnosis. In contrast, the search for the cause of an illness that does not conform to a syndrome is more difficult because more diseases have to be considered. Even here an orderly approach that proceeds from symptom to sign to laboratory findings will usually result in the diagnosis.

CARING FOR THE PATIENT Patient care begins with the development of a personal relationship between the patient and the physician. In the absence of trust and confidence on the part of the patient, the effectiveness of most therapeutic measures is diminished. When there is confidence in the physician, reassurance may be the best treatment and all that is needed. Likewise, in those cases that do not lend themselves to easy solutions, a feeling by the patient that the physician is doing all that is possible is one of the most important benefits that can be provided. An important aspect of clinical decision making and patient care involves the "quality of life," a subjective assessment of what each patient values most. Such an assessment requires detailed, sometimes intimate knowledge of the patient, which can usually be obtained only through deliberate, unhurried, and often repeated conversation. As mentioned above, it is in these situations that the time constraints of a managed care setting may prove problematic. In situations where cure is impossible, enhancement of the quality of life is the major goal of therapy.

Assessing the Outcome of Treatments Clinicians generally use *objective* and readily measurable parameters to judge the outcomes of a therapeutic intervention. For example, findings on physical or laboratory examination—such as the level of blood pressure, the patency of a coronary artery on an angiogram, the size of a mass on a radiologic examination, or the titer of an antibody—can provide information of critical importance. However, patients usually seek medical attention for *subjective* reasons; they wish relief from pain, to preserve or regain function, and to enjoy life. Although these goals are often nebulous and differ among individuals, a patient's health status or quality of life can be separated into categories, such as bodily comfort, physical activity, social activity, personal and professional function, sexual function, cognitive function, sleep, vitality, and overall perception of health. Function in each of these important areas can be assessed by means of structured interviews or specially designed questionnaires. In a less formal way such assessments also provide useful parameters by which the physician can judge the patient's view of his or her disability and the response to treatment, particularly of chronic illness. The humane practice of medicine requires consideration and integration of both objective and subjective outcomes.

Drug Therapy Many new drugs have only a marginal advantage over the agents they are aimed to replace. The barrage of new information with which practitioners are deluged does little to provide a clear picture of clinical pharmacology; on the contrary, to most physicians new drugs are confusing. With some exceptions, however, the approach to a new drug should be one of caution. Unless the new agent is established beyond doubt to be a real advance, it is wiser to use agents whose efficacy and safety are well established.

Care of the Elderly Over the next several decades, the practice of medicine will be greatly influenced by the health care needs of the increasing numbers of the elderly. In the United States the population over age 65 will almost triple over the next 30 years, and it is essential that we understand and appreciate the physiologic processes associated with aging; the different responses of the elderly to common diseases; and disorders that occur commonly with aging such as depression, dementia, frailty, urinary incontinence, and fractures. The elderly have more adverse reactions to medications, in large part due to altered pharmacokinetics and pharmacodynamics. Commonly used drugs such as digoxin have prolonged half-lives, and tissues such as the central nervous system become more sensitive to certain drugs, such as the benzodiazepines and narcotics.

Diseases in Men versus Women There are significant gender differences in diseases that afflict both men and women. These have not been clearly evident because in the past many epidemiologic and clinical studies were carried out only in adult men. In ischemic heart disease, mortality rates may be higher in women. Hypertension is more prevalent in African-American women than in their male counterparts; diseases involving the immune system such as lupus erythematosus, multiple sclerosis, and primary biliary cirrhosis occur more frequently in women; and women have a greater longevity than men. Recently, considerable attention has been paid to women's health issues, a subject that has regrettably not received sufficient attention in the past. Such consideration should enhance our understanding of the mechanisms of gender differences in the course and outcome of certain diseases.

Iatrogenic Disorders An *iatrogenic disorder* occurs when the deleterious effects of a therapeutic or diagnostic regimen cause pathology independent of the condition for which the regimen is given. No matter what the clinical situation, it is the responsibility of the physician to use powerful therapeutic measures wisely, with due regard to their action, potential dangers, and cost. Every medical procedure, whether diagnostic or therapeutic, has the potential for harm, but it would be impossible to provide the benefits of modern scientific medicine if reasonable steps in diagnosis and therapy were withheld because of possible risks. *Reasonable* implies that the physician has weighed the pros and cons of a procedure and has concluded that it is advisable or essential for the relief of discomfort or the cure or amelioration of disease. For example, the use of glucocorticoids to arrest progressive systemic lupus erythematosus may produce Cushing's syndrome. In this instance, the benefits usually exceed the untoward side effects. However, much harm can result when the deleterious effects of a procedure or a drug exceed any possible advantages that might have been anticipated. Examples include the harmful and even fatal drug reactions that occasionally follow the use of antibiotics given for minor respiratory infections, the gastric hemorrhage or perforation caused by the administration of glucocorticoids for mild arthritis, and the development of fatal liver disease after needless transfusions of virus-contaminated blood or plasma.

However, the harm that a physician can do is not limited to the imprudent use of medication or procedures. Equally important are ill-considered or unjustified remarks. Many a patient has developed a cardiac neurosis because the physician ventured a grave prognosis on the basis of a misinterpreted finding of a heart murmur on auscultation. Not only the treatment itself but the physician's words and behavior are capable of causing injury.

The physician must never become so absorbed in the disease as to forget the patient who is its victim. As the science of medicine advances, it is all too easy to become so fascinated by the manifestations of disease that one disregards the ailing person's fears and concerns about suffering and death, job and family, the cost of medical care, and the specter of economic insecurity. Treatment of a patient consists of more than the dispassionate confrontation of a disease. It embodies also the expression of warmth, compassion, and understanding.

Informed Consent Patients often require diagnostic and therapeutic procedures that are painful and that pose some risk, such as surgical procedures, including biopsies, endoscopy, radiographic maneuvers involving the insertion of catheters, and many others. In most hospitals and clinics, patients undergoing such procedures are required to sign a form consenting to them. More important, however, the patient must understand clearly the risk entailed in these procedures; this is the definition of *informed consent*. It is incumbent on the physician to explain to the patient, in a clearly understandable manner, the procedures he or she faces, and to ascertain that the patient understands both the procedure and the attendant risks. By doing this conscientiously, much of the dread of the unknown that is inherent in hospitalization will be mitigated.

Accountability Throughout the world, physicians, once licensed to practice medicine, have not had to account for their actions except to their peers. In the United States, however, there have been increasing demands for physicians to account for the way in which they practice medicine by meeting certain standards prescribed by federal and state governments. The hospitalization of patients whose health care is reimbursed by the government (Medicare and Medicaid) and other third parties is subjected to utilization review. This means that the physician must defend the cause for and duration of a patient's hospitalization if it falls outside certain "average" standards. In some instances, a second opinion is necessary before a patient can have elective surgery. The purpose of these regulations is both to improve standards of health care and to contain spiraling health care costs. It is likely that this type of review will be extended to all phases of medical practice and will alter the practice of medicine profoundly.

Physicians also may be expected to give account of their continuing competence by mandatory continuing education, patient-record audit, recertification by examination (time-limited certification), or relicensing. While these measures probably enhance the physician's factual knowledge, there is no evidence that they have a similar effect on the quality of practice.

Practice Guidelines Physicians are faced with a large, often bewildering array of potentially useful diagnostic techniques and therapeutic measures from which to choose as they deal with individual patients. The intelligent and cost-effective practice of medicine consists of selecting those most appropriate to a particular patient and clinical situation. To aid physicians and other care-givers in making these selections, professional organizations and government agencies are developing formal clinical practice guidelines. These guidelines may be viewed as double-edged swords. On the one hand, when they are current and properly applied, they can provide a useful framework for managing patients with particular diagnoses or symptoms. They also offer guidelines that protect patients—particularly those with inadequate health care benefits—from receiving substandard care. They can also protect conscientious caregivers from inappropriate charges of malpractice, and they can protect society from the excessive costs associated with the overuse of medical resources. However, clinical guidelines tend to oversimplify the complexities of medicine. Different groups with differing perspectives may develop divergent recommendations regarding issues as basic as the need for a periodic sigmoidoscopy in middle-aged persons. Furthermore, guidelines do not—and cannot be expected to—take into account the uniqueness of each individual and of his or her illness. The practice of medicine strictly according to guidelines carries with it the danger of transforming medicine from a learned profession rooted in the biologic and behavioral sciences to a technical vocation. The challenge for the physician is to accept and incorporate into clinical practice the useful recommendations offered by the experts who prepare clinical practice guidelines without accepting them blindly or being inappropriately constrained.

Evidence-Based Medicine   The concept of evidence-based medicine means that clinical decisions are formally supported by data, particularly data derived from randomized, controlled clinical trials. There is a perception that many therapeutic decisions are made in the absence of a formal clinical trial that establishes efficacy. However, in a 1995 study at a university-affiliated hospital, it was concluded that 82 percent of primary treatments administered at that hospital were, in fact, evidence based. Evidence-based medicine was defined in the study as an intervention whose value had been established in one or more randomized controlled clinical trials or an intervention whose validity was so clear that randomized trials were unanimously judged to be unnecessary and would have been unethical if a placebo were involved. Eighteen percent of patients received symptomatic and supportive care without substantial evidence that it was superior to some other intervention, including no therapy. Nonetheless, there is a trend to require that therapy be scientifically validated. This approach will obviously have an impact on resource utilization.

Cost-Effectiveness in Medical Care   As the cost of medical care continues to rise, it is necessary to establish priorities in the expenditure of money for health care. In some instances, preventive measures offer the greatest return for the expenditure; outstanding examples include vaccination, immunization, reduction in accidents and occupational hazards, improved environmental control, and biochemical and molecular biologic screening of newborns. For example, the detection of phenylketonuria by newborn screening may result in a net saving of many thousands of dollars.

As resources become increasingly constrained, it is necessary to weigh the justification of performing costly procedures that provide only a limited life expectancy against the pressing need for more primary care for those persons who do not have adequate access to medical services. At the level of the individual patient, it is important to reduce costly hospital admissions as much as possible if total health care is to be provided at a cost that most can afford. This, of course, implies and depends on a close cooperative effort between patients, their physicians, their employers, third-party carriers, and government. It is equally important for individual physicians to know the cost of medicines that they prescribe and to monitor both the cost and effectiveness of those drugs. In the last analysis, the medical profession should provide leadership and guidance to the public in matters of cost control, and physicians must take this responsibility seriously without being or seeming to be self-serving. It is important, however, that the socioeconomic aspects of health care delivery not interfere with the welfare of patients. The patient must be able to rely on the individual physician as his or her principal advocate in matters of health care.

Research and Teaching   The title *doctor* is derived from the Latin *docere*, "to teach," and the physician should share information and medical knowledge with colleagues and with students of medicine and related professions. The practice of medicine is dependent on the sum total of medical knowledge, which in turn is based on an unending chain of scientific discovery, clinical observation, analysis, and interpretation. Advances in medicine depend on the acquisition of new information, i.e., on research, which must often involve patients; improved medical care requires the transmission of this information. As part of broader societal responsibilities, the physician should encourage patients to participate in ethical and properly approved clinical investigations if they do not impose undue hazard, discomfort, or inconvenience.

Incurability and Death   No problem is more distressing than that presented by the patient with an incurable disease, particularly when premature death is inevitable. What should the patient and family be told, what measures should be taken to maintain life, and how is death to be defined?

Although some would argue otherwise, there is no ironclad rule that the patient must immediately be told "everything," even if the patient is an adult and the head of a family. How much the patient is told should depend on the individual's ability and capacity to deal with the possibility of imminent death; often this capacity grows with time, and whenever possible, gradual rather than abrupt disclosure is the best strategy. A wise and insightful physician is often guided by an understanding of what a patient wants to know and when he or she wants to know it. This decision also may take into consideration the patient's religious beliefs, financial and business status, and to some extent the wishes of the family. The patient must be given an opportunity to talk with the physician and ask questions. Patients may find it easier to share their feelings about death with their physician, who is likely to be more objective and less emotional than family members.

One thing is certain; it is not for you to don the black cap and, assuming the judicial function, take hope away from any patient . . . hope that comes to us all.

William Osler

Even when the patient directly inquires, "Doctor, am I dying?" the physician must attempt to determine whether this is a request for information, a demand for reassurance, or even an expression of hostility. Most would agree that only open communication between the patient and the physician can resolve these questions and guide the physician in what to say and how to say it.

The physician should provide or arrange for emotional, physical, and spiritual support and must be compassionate, unhurried, and open. There is much to be gained by the laying on of hands. Pain should be adequately controlled, human dignity maintained, and isolation from family avoided. The last two in particular tend to be overlooked in hospitals, where the intrusion of life-sustaining apparatuses can so easily detract from attention to the whole person and encourage concentration instead on the life-threatening disease. The physician also must prepare to deal with guilt feelings on the part of the family when a member becomes gravely or hopelessly ill. It is important for the doctor to be able to assure the family that everything possible has been done.

The President's Committee for the Study of Ethical Problems in Medicine defined death as (1) irreversible cessation of circulatory and respiratory function or (2) irreversible cessation of all functions of the entire brain, including the brainstem. Clinical and electroencephalographic criteria permit the reliable diagnosis of cerebral death. According to the criteria adopted by the staff of the Massachusetts General Hospital and the Harvard Committee on Brain Death, death occurs when all signs of receptivity and responsivity are absent, including all brainstem reflexes (pupillary reactions, ocular movement, blinking, swallowing, breathing), and the electroencephalogram is isoelectric. Occasionally, intoxications and metabolic disorders may simulate this state; hence the diagnosis requires expert evaluation. Under the aforementioned circumstances, to continue with heroic, highly costly supportive measures merely for the purpose of preserving cardiac function is against the best interests of patient, family, and society. In such instances, the dilemma of continuing care could be avoided if the medical profession, in accord with social sanction, can be brought to redefine life and death by these criteria.

The following guidelines are deserving of consideration:

1. The diagnosis of brain death, based on the preceding criteria, should be corroborated by another physician and confirmed by clinical examination and EEG, repeated one or more times.

2. The family should be informed of the irreversibility of loss of brain function but should not be requested to ratify the decision whether the medical treatment should be discontinued. An exception to this limited decision-making power of the family might apply where the patient has directed the family that he or she wishes them to make the decision.
3. The physician, after consultation with a professional colleague, may withdraw supportive measures, assuming that nothing more can be offered.
4. The possibility that such patients may become sources of organs for grafting should not enter into the aforementioned decisions, although prior to the cessation of heart action the family may be asked whether this would be their wish, or the family may suggest that organs be used for this purpose. In many states, laws now require physicians to request organ donations. A question arises when the patient has indicated in advance a wish to be an organ or tissue donor whether the family must be approached, since many believe the patient's prior wishes carry overriding weight. This issue is controversial.

"Do Not Resuscitate" Orders and Cessation of Therapy
When carried out in a timely and expert manner, cardiopulmonary resuscitation is often useful in the prevention of sudden, unexpected death. However, unless there are reasons to the contrary, it should not be carried out when it merely prolongs life in a patient with terminal, incurable disease. The decision not to resuscitate a patient and decisions about the intensity of therapy and, indeed, whether or not treatment is to be delivered or continued to patients who are incurably and terminally ill must be reviewed frequently and must take into consideration any unexpected changes in the patient's condition. In this context the administration of fluids and food are considered therapies that may be withdrawn or withheld. These decisions also must take into account both the underlying medical condition and the wishes of the patient or, if these cannot be or have not been ascertained directly, those of a close relative or other surrogate who can be relied on to transmit the patient's feelings and to be guided by the patient's best interests and wishes. The patient's autonomy—whether the choice is to continue or discontinue treatment or to be resuscitated in the event of a cardiopulmonary arrest—is paramount. The courts have ruled that competent patients may be able to refuse therapy and that an incompetent patient's previously stated wishes regarding life support should be respected. The issues involving death and dying are among the most difficult in medicine. In approaching them rationally and consistently, the physician must combine both the art and the science of medicine.

BIBLIOGRAPHY

ELLIS J et al: Inpatient general medicine is evidence based. Lancet 346:407, 1996
LEWIN DI, SHURKIN JN: Scientific publishers rush journals into virtual print. J NIH Res 7:23, 1995
TAUBES G: Looking for the evidence in medicine. Science 272:22, 1996

2	*Bernard Lo*

ETHICAL ISSUES IN CLINICAL MEDICINE

Physicians frequently confront ethical issues in clinical practice that are perplexing, time-consuming, and emotionally draining. Experience, common sense, and simply being a good person do not guarantee that physicians can identify or resolve ethical dilemmas. Knowledge about common ethical dilemmas is also essential.

FUNDAMENTAL ETHICAL GUIDELINES

In patient care, physicians should follow two fundamental but frequently conflicting ethical guidelines: respecting patient autonomy and acting in the patient's best interests.

RESPECTING PATIENT AUTONOMY Competent, informed patients may exercise their self-determination and liberty by refusing recommended interventions and choosing among the available alternatives.

Informed Consent Informed consent requires physicians to discuss with the patient the nature of the proposed care, the alternatives, the risks and benefits of each, and the likely consequences and to obtain the patient's agreement to care. Informed consent involves more than obtaining patients' signatures on consent forms. Physicians need to educate patients, discuss options with them, answer questions, make recommendations, and help them deliberate. Patients can be overwhelmed with medical jargon, needlessly complicated explanations, or too much information at once.

Nondisclosure of Information Physicians may consider withholding a serious diagnosis, misrepresenting it, or limiting discussions of prognosis or risks out of fear that a patient will develop severe anxiety or depression or refuse needed care. Patients should not be forced to receive information against their will. Most people, however, want to know their diagnosis and prognosis, even if they are terminally ill. Generally, physicians should provide relevant information, while offering empathy and hope and helping patients cope with bad news.

Emergency Care Informed consent is not required when patients cannot give consent and delaying treatment would place their life or health in peril. People are presumed to want such emergency care, unless they have indicated otherwise.

Futile Interventions Autonomy does not entitle patients to insist on whatever care they want. Physicians are not obligated to provide futile interventions that have no physiologic rationale or when maximal treatment is failing. For example, cardiopulmonary resuscitation would be futile in a patient with multisystem failure that is worsening despite maximal therapy. But physicians should be wary of using the term "futile" in looser senses to justify withholding interventions when they believe that the probability of success is too low, no worthwhile goals can be achieved, the patient's quality of life is unacceptable, or the costs are too high. Such looser usages of the term are problematic because they may be inconsistent and mask hidden value judgments.

ACTING IN THE BEST INTERESTS OF PATIENTS The guideline of *beneficence* requires physicians to take actions for patients' benefit. Laypeople do not possess medical expertise and may be vulnerable because of their illness. They justifiably rely on physicians to provide sound advice and to promote their well-being. Physicians encourage such trust. For these reasons, physicians have a fiduciary duty to act in the best interests of their patients. Furthermore, the interests of the patient should take priority over physicians' self-interest or the interests of third parties, such as hospitals or insurers. These fiduciary obligations contrast sharply with the business world, where the goal is to maximize profits, not to act in the best interests of customers. The guideline of *"do no harm"* forbids physicians from providing ineffective interventions or acting without due care. This precept, while often cited, provides only limited guidance, because many beneficial interventions also have serious risks.

CONFLICTS BETWEEN BENEFICENCE AND AUTONOMY Patients' refusals of care may thwart their own goals or cause them serious harm. For example, a young man with asthma may refuse mechanical ventilation for reversible respiratory failure. Simply to accept such refusals, in the name of respecting autonomy, would fail to show caring. Physicians can elicit patients' expectations and concerns, correct misunderstandings, and try to persuade them to accept beneficial therapies. If disagreements persist after discussions, the patient's informed choices and view of his or her best interests should prevail. While refusing recommended care does not render a patient incompetent, it may lead the physician to probe further to ensure that the patient is able to make informed decisions.

Patients may not be able to make informed decisions because of unconsciousness, dementia, delirium, or other conditions. Physicians need to ask two questions regarding such patients: Who is the appropriate surrogate? What would the patient want done?

ASSESSING CAPACITY TO MAKE MEDICAL DECISIONS All adults are considered legally competent unless declared incompetent by a court. In practice, physicians usually determine that patients lack the capacity to make health care decisions and arrange for surrogates to make them, without involving the courts. By definition, competent patients can express a choice and appreciate the medical situation, the nature of the proposed care, the alternatives, and the risks, benefits, and consequences of each. Their choices should be consistent with their values and should not result from delusions or hallucinations. Psychiatrists may help in difficult cases because they are skilled at interviewing mentally impaired patients and can identify treatable depression or psychosis. When impairments are fluctuating or reversible, decisions should be postponed if possible until the patient recovers decision-making capacity.

CHOICE OF SURROGATE Physicians routinely ask family members to serve as surrogates for patients who lack decision-making capacity. Most patients want their family members to be surrogates, and family members generally know the patient's preferences and have the patient's best interests at heart. Patients may designate a particular individual to serve as proxy; such choices should be respected. Some states have established a prioritized list of which relative may serve as surrogate if the patient has not designated a proxy.

STANDARDS FOR SURROGATE DECISION MAKING
Advance Directives These are statements by competent patients to direct care if they lose decision-making capacity. They may indicate (1) what interventions they would refuse or accept or (2) who should serve as surrogate. Following the patient's advance directives respects his or her autonomy.

Oral conversations are the most frequent form of advance directives. While such conversations are customarily followed in clinical practice, casual or vague comments may not be trustworthy.

Living wills direct physicians to forego or provide life-sustaining interventions if the patient develops a terminal condition or persistent vegetative state. Generally patients may refuse only interventions that "merely prolong the process of dying."

A health care power of attorney allows patients to appoint a proxy to make health care decisions if they lose decision-making capacity. It is more flexible and comprehensive than the living will, applying whenever the patient is unable to make decisions.

Physicians can encourage patients to provide advance directives, to indicate both what they would want and who should be surrogate, and to discuss their preferences with surrogates. In discussions with patients, physicians can ensure that advance directives are informed, up-to-date, and address likely clinical scenarios. The federal Patient Self-Determination Act requires hospitals and health maintenance organizations to inform patients of their right to make health care decisions and to provide advance directives.

Substituted Judgment In the absence of clear advance directives, surrogates and physicians should try to decide as the patient would under the circumstances, using all information that they know about the patient. While such substituted judgments try to respect the patient's values, they may be speculative or inaccurate. A surrogate may be mistaken about the patient's preferences, particularly when they have not been discussed explicitly.

Best Interests When the patient's preferences are unclear or unknown, decisions should be based on the patient's best interests. Patients generally take into account the quality of life as well as the duration of life when making decisions for themselves. It is understandable that surrogates would also consider quality of life of patients who lack decision-making capacity. Judgments about quality of life are appropriate if they reflect the patient's own values. Bias or discrimination may occur, however, if others project their values onto the patient

or weigh the perceived social worth of the patient. Most patients with chronic illness rate their quality of life higher than their family members and physicians do.

Legal Issues Physicians need to know pertinent state laws regarding patients who lack decision-making capacity. A few state courts allow life-sustaining treatments to be withheld only if patients have provided written advance directives or very specific oral ones.

Disagreements Disagreements may occur among potential surrogates or between the physician and surrogate. Physicians can remind everyone to base decisions on what the patient would want, not what they would want for themselves. Consultation with the hospital ethics committee or with another physician often helps resolve disputes. Such consultation is also helpful when patients have no surrogate and no advance directives. The courts should be used only as a last resort when disagreements cannot be resolved in the clinical setting.

DECISIONS ABOUT
LIFE-SUSTAINING INTERVENTIONS

Although medical technology can save lives, it can also prolong the process of dying. Competent, informed patients may refuse life-sustaining interventions. Such interventions also may be withheld from patients who lack decision-making capacity on the basis of advance directives or decisions by appropriate surrogates. Courts have ruled that foregoing life-sustaining interventions is neither suicide nor murder.

MISLEADING DISTINCTIONS People commonly draw distinctions that are intuitively plausible but prove untenable on closer analysis.

Extraordinary and Ordinary Care Some physicians are willing to forego "extraordinary" or "heroic" interventions, such as surgery, mechanical ventilation or renal dialysis, but insist on providing "ordinary" ones, such as antibiotics, intravenous fluids, or feeding tubes. However, this is not a logical distinction because all medical interventions have both risks and benefits. Any intervention may be withheld, if the burdens for the individual patient outweigh the benefits.

Withdrawing and Withholding Interventions Many health care providers find it more difficult to discontinue interventions than to withhold them in the first place. Although such emotions need to be acknowledged, there is no logical distinction between the two acts. Justifications for withholding interventions, such as refusal by patients or surrogates, also are justifications for withdrawing them. In addition, an intervention may prove unsuccessful, or new information about the patient's preferences or condition may become available after the intervention is started. If interventions could not be discontinued, patients and surrogates might not even attempt treatments that might prove beneficial.

DO NOT RESUSCITATE (DNR) ORDERS When a patient suffers a cardiopulmonary arrest, cardiopulmonary resuscitation (CPR) is initiated unless a DNR order has been made. Although CPR can restore people to vigorous health, it can also disrupt a peaceful death. After CPR is attempted on a general hospital service, only 14 percent of patients survive to discharge, and even fewer in certain subgroups. DNR orders are appropriate if the patient or surrogate requests them or if CPR would be futile. To prevent misunderstandings, physicians should write DNR orders and the reasons for them in the medical record. "Slow" or "show" codes that merely appear to provide CPR are deceptive and therefore unacceptable. Although a DNR order signifies only that CPR will be withheld, DNR orders may lead to a reconsideration of the plans for care.

ASSISTED SUICIDE AND ACTIVE EUTHANASIA Proponents of these controversial acts believe that competent, terminally ill patients should have control over the end of life and that physicians should help them end their suffering. Opponents assert that such actions violate the sanctity of life, that suffering can generally be relieved, that abuses are inevitable, and that such actions are outside the physician's proper role. Whatever their personal views regarding these illegal acts, physicians need to respond to patients' inquiries with compassion and concern. Physicians need to elicit and address any underlying problems, such as unrelieved suffering, loss of control, or depression. Distress usually can be relieved more effectively, and after this is done patients generally withdraw their requests for these acts.

CARE OF DYING PATIENTS Patients often suffer unrelieved pain during their final days of life. Physicians may hesitate to order high doses of narcotics and sedatives, fearing they will hasten death. Relieving pain in terminal illness and alleviating dyspnea when patients forego mechanical ventilation enhances patient comfort and dignity. If lower doses of narcotics and sedatives have failed to relieve suffering, increasing the dose to levels that may suppress respiratory drive and hasten death is different from active euthanasia and is ethically appropriate. Physicians can also relieve suffering by spending time with dying patients, listening to them, and attending to their psychological distress.

CONFLICTS OF INTEREST

Acting in the patient's best interests may conflict with the physician's self-interest or the interests of third parties such as insurers or hospitals. The ethical ideal is to keep the patient's interests paramount. Even the appearance of a conflict of interest may undermine trust in the profession.

FINANCIAL INCENTIVES In managed care systems, physicians may serve as gatekeepers or bear financial risk for expenditures. Although such incentives are intended to reduce inefficiency and waste, the concern is that physicians may withhold beneficial care in order to control costs. In contrast, physicians have incentives to provide more care than indicated when they receive fee-for-service reimbursement or when they refer patients to medical facilities in which they have invested. Regardless of financial incentives, physicians should recommend available care that is in the patient's best interests—no more and no less.

DENIALS OF COVERAGE Utilization review programs designed to reduce unnecessary services may also deny coverage for care that the physician believes will benefit the patient. Physicians should inform patients when a plan is not covering standard care and act as patient advocates by appealing such denials of coverage. Patients may ask physicians to misrepresent their condition to help them obtain insurance coverage or disability. While physicians understandably want to help patients, such misrepresentation undermines physicians' credibility and violates their integrity.

GIFTS FROM PHARMACEUTICAL COMPANIES Physicians may be offered gifts ranging from pens and notepads to lavish entertainment. Critics worry that any gift from drug companies may impair objectivity, increase the cost of health care, and give the appearance of conflict of interest. A helpful rule of thumb is to consider whether patients would approve if they knew physicians had accepted such gifts.

OCCUPATIONAL RISKS Some health care workers, fearing fatal occupational infections, refuse to care for persons with human immunodeficiency virus (HIV) infection or multidrug-resistant tuberculosis. Such fears about personal safety need to be acknowledged, and institutions need to reduce occupational risk by providing proper training, equipment, and supervision. Physicians should provide appropriate care within their clinical expertise, despite personal risk.

MISTAKES Mistakes are inevitable in clinical medicine. They may cause serious harm to patients or require substantial changes in management. Physicians and students may fear that disclosing such mistakes could damage their careers. Without disclosure, however, patients cannot understand their clinical situation or make informed choices about subsequent care. Similarly, unless attending physicians are informed of trainees' mistakes, they cannot provide optimal care and help trainees learn from mistakes.

LEARNING CLINICAL SKILLS Learning clinical medicine, particularly how to perform invasive procedures, may present inconvenience or risk to patients. To ensure patient cooperation, students may be introduced as physicians, or patients may not be told that trainees will be performing procedures. Such misrepresentation undermines trust, may lead to more elaborate deception, and makes it difficult for patients to make informed choices about their care. Patients should be told who is providing care, what benefits and burdens can be attributed to trainees, and how trainees are supervised. Most patients, when informed, allow trainees to play an active role in their care.

IMPAIRED PHYSICIANS Physicians may hesitate to intervene when colleagues impaired by alcohol abuse, drug abuse, or psychiatric or medical illness place patients at risk. However, society relies on physicians to regulate themselves. If colleagues of an impaired physician do not take steps to protect patients, no one else may be in a position to do so.

CONFLICTS FOR TRAINEES Medical students and residents may fear that they will receive poor grades or evaluations if they act on the patient's behalf by disclosing mistakes, avoiding misrepresentation of their role, and reporting impaired colleagues. Discussing such dilemmas with more senior physicians can help trainees check their interpretation of the situation and obtain advice and assistance.

ADDITIONAL ETHICAL ISSUES

MAINTAINING CONFIDENTIALITY Maintaining the confidentiality of medical information respects patients' autonomy and privacy, encourages them to seek treatment and to discuss their problems candidly, and prevents discrimination. Physicians need to guard against inadvertent breaches of confidentiality, as when talking about patients in elevators. Maintaining confidentiality is not an absolute rule. The law may require physicians to override confidentiality in order to protect third parties, for example, reporting to government officials persons with specified infectious conditions, such as tuberculosis and syphilis, persons with gunshot wounds, and victims of elder abuse and domestic violence.

ALLOCATING RESOURCES JUSTLY Allocation of limited health care resources is unavoidable. Ideally, allocation decisions should be made as public policy, with physician input. At the bedside, physicians generally should act as patient advocates within constraints set by society and sound practice. *Ad hoc* rationing by the individual physician at the bedside may be inconsistent, discriminatory, and ineffective. In some cases, however, two patients may compete for the same limited resources, such as physician time or a bed in intensive care. When this occurs, physicians should ration their time and resources according to patients' medical needs and the probability of benefit.

ASSISTANCE WITH ETHICAL ISSUES Discussing perplexing ethical issues with other members of the health care team, colleagues, or the hospital ethics committee often clarifies ethical issues and suggests ways to improve communication and to deal with strong emotions. When struggling with difficult ethical issues, physicians may need to reevaluate their basic convictions, tolerate uncertainty, and maintain their integrity while respecting the opinions of others.

BIBLIOGRAPHY

AMERICAN COLLEGE OF PHYSICIANS: *American College of Physicians Ethics Manual.* Ann Intern Med, 117:947,1992

BEAUCHAMP TL, CHILDRESS JF: *Principles of Biomedical Ethics*, 4th ed. New York, Oxford University Press, 1994

DUNN PM et al: Medical ethics: An annotated bibliography. Ann Intern Med 121:627, 1994

EMANUEL LL: A professional response to demands for accountability: Practical recommendations regarding ethical aspects of patient care. Ann Intern Med 124:240, 1996

JONSEN AR et al: *Clinical Ethics*, 3d ed. New York, Macmillan, 1991

KASSIRER JP: Managed care and the morality of the marketplace. N Engl J Med 333:50, 1995

LO B: *Resolving Ethical Dilemmas: A Guide for Clinicians.* Baltimore, Williams & Wilkins, 1995

MEISEL A: *The Right to Die*, 2d ed. New York, Wiley, 1995

PELLOGRINO ED: The metamorphosis of medical ethics—a 30-year retrospective. JAMA 269:1158, 1993

QUANTITATIVE ASPECTS OF CLINICAL REASONING

The process of clinical reasoning is poorly understood but is based on factors such as experience and learning, inductive and deductive reasoning, interpretation of evidence that itself varies in reproducibility and validity, and intuition that often is difficult to define. In an effort to improve clinical reasoning, a number of attempts have been made to analyze quantitatively the many factors involved, including defining the cognitive approaches that clinicians apply to difficult problems, devising computerized decision support systems that are designed to emulate certain features of decision making, and applying decision theory to understand how judgments should be reached. While each of these approaches has advanced the understanding of the diagnostic process, all have practical and/or theoretical problems that limit their direct applicability to the care of the individual patient.

Nevertheless, these preliminary attempts to apply the rigor and logic inherent in the quantitative method have provided significant insights into the process by which clinical reasoning is accomplished, have identified ways in which the process may be improved, and have made it possible to minimize certain features of the workup that are not cost-effective.

In a simplified model, quantitative clinical reasoning includes five phases. The *first* consists of an investigation of the chief complaint through key questions that are included in the history of the present illness (Table 3-1). These questions are supplemented by the past medical history and by a physical examination that emphasizes detailed investigation of potential key organ systems. In the *second* phase, the physician may select from an array of diagnostic tests, each with its own accuracy and usefulness for investigating the possibilities raised in the differential diagnosis. Since each test has its costs, and some entail risk and discomfort as well, the physician must ask whether the history and physical examination are sufficiently diagnostic before ordering tests. *Third*, the clinical data must be integrated with test results to estimate the likelihood of conditions in the differential diagnosis. *Fourth*, the comparative risks and benefits of further diagnostic and therapeutic options must be weighed to reach a recommendation for the patient. In the *fifth* and final phase, this recommendation is presented to the patient, and after appropriate discussion of the options, a therapeutic plan is initiated. Each of the five steps in this simplified model of the clinical reasoning process can be analyzed individually.

HISTORY AND PHYSICAL EXAMINATION It originally had been assumed that physicians begin investigating a patient's chief complaint by obtaining a comprehensive history, which includes many, if not most, of the questions included in a full review of systems, and by performing an all-inclusive physical examination. However, experienced clinicians begin to form hypotheses based on the chief complaint and on the responses to initial questioning, and they ask further questions in a sequence that allows them to evaluate the initial hypotheses and, if necessary, shorten or amend the list of possibilities. In such a way, high-priority questions are selected from the almost limitless number that might be asked, and these specific questions are incorporated into the history of the present illness. Often, a key re-

Table 3-1

Phases of Clinical Reasoning and Decision Making

1. Investigation of the complaint by means of clinical examination (history and physical examination)
2. Ordering of diagnostic tests, each with its own intrinsic accuracy and usefulness
3. Integration of clinical findings with test results to assess diagnostic probabilities
4. Weighing of comparative risks and benefits of alternative courses of action
5. Determination of patient's preferences and development of a therapeutic plan

sponse, such as a history of melena, will be selected, a list of potential explanations for it will be formulated, and this list will then be trimmed, based on the response to more probing questions, so that a principal diagnosis can be selected and then tested. This process, termed *iterative hypothesis testing*, is an efficient approach to diagnosis and is preferable to attempts to gather every conceivable piece of information prior to formulating a differential diagnosis.

Advocacy of iterative hypothesis testing does not argue against the need for a systematic, thorough, and complete history of the present illness, past medical history, review of systems, family history, social history, and physical examination. For example, if a patient presents with abdominal pain, the physician should gather information regarding its location and quality as well as the factors that precipitate and/or relieve it. The physician then asks questions relating to the diagnoses that may be suspected based on the response to the initial questions. If the pain is suggestive of pancreatitis, the clinician would ask about alcohol intake, the use of thiazide diuretics or glucocorticoids, symptoms suggestive of concomitant gallbladder disease, a family history of pancreatitis, and questions aimed at uncovering the possibility of a posterior penetrating ulcer. Alternatively, if the discomfort seems more typical of reflux esophagitis, a different sequence of questions would be triggered. The use of iterative hypothesis testing encourages the physician to elicit detailed information in high-yield areas, without forgoing a systematic and thorough approach to the patient. The careful use of clear and, when possible, precise questions can increase the reproducibility and validity of the medical history but still cannot eliminate all variability. Findings on the history and physical examination should influence each other. The history focuses the physical examination on certain organs, and findings on physical examination should encourage more detailed review of certain systems.

Despite limitations in the reproducibility and validity of the medical history and physical examination, their critical importance in clinical reasoning should not be undervalued. Rather, they emphasize that care and diligence are critical in the application of these skills, and that physicians must recognize their limitations. For example, the history and physical examination are of limited value in predicting whether back pain is caused by a serious underlying disease, but careful auscultation of the heart during various bedside maneuvers (see Chap. 227) has been shown to be remarkably accurate in determining the cause of systolic murmurs. Even in the latter case, however, confirmation echocardiography will often be helpful.

When physicians use the history and the physical examination to arrive at a diagnosis, they are rarely certain of it. Therefore, it would be better to assess the likelihood of the diagnosis in terms of probabilities. All too frequently this probability is not expressed as an actual percentage but rather in such terms as "nearly always," "commonly," "sometimes," or "rarely." Since different physicians may assign different probabilities to the same terms, these imprecise words can lead to major misunderstandings among physicians or between the physician and the patient. Physicians should be as rigorous and quantitative as possible in their assessments, and when feasible, a quantitative expression of probability should be used. For example, rather than saying that it is unlikely that a radiographic pattern is indicative of a carcinoma of the colon, it would be preferable, if possible, to provide a more precise indication of the probability of carcinoma with this radiographic pattern. A 10 to 15 percent probability of carcinoma may be interpreted as "unlikely" but from a clinical perspective usually warrants further evaluation because of the serious consequences of missing a potentially resectable tumor.

Although such quantitative estimates would be desirable, they usually are not available in practice. Even experienced physicians often are unable to estimate accurately the likelihood of particular conditions. There is a tendency to overestimate the likelihood of relatively uncommon conditions, and physicians are especially poor at quantifying probabilities that are very high or very low. For example, a physician may not know whether the probability of bacterial meningitis or of another disease that could be diagnosed by a lumbar puncture in a patient with a severe headache is 1 in 20 or 1 in 2000. In both situations, the probability is low, but the decision as to whether a lumbar puncture should be performed may depend on this estimate.

As was emphasized in Chap. 1, the history and physical examination have other important purposes. They allow the physician to evaluate the emotional status of the patient and to understand how the present problems fit into the context of the patient's social and family life, and they encourage the development in the patient of confidence in the physician, which is so necessary for reaching an agreement on the coming plan of action.

DIAGNOSTIC TESTS: INDICATIONS, ACCURACY, AND USEFULNESS A diagnostic test should be ordered for specified clinical indications, be sufficiently accurate to be efficacious for such indications, and be the least expensive and/or risky of the available efficacious tests. No diagnostic test is totally accurate, and physicians often have difficulty interpreting test results. It is therefore critical to understand several commonly used terms in test analysis and epidemiology, including prevalence, sensitivity, specificity, positive predictive value, and negative predictive value (Table 3-2).

Although reports of the accuracies of diagnostic tests are commonly expressed in terms of positive and negative predictive values, these calculated values are dependent on the prevalence of the disease in the population being studied (Table 3-3). A test with a particular sensitivity and specificity has different positive and negative predictive values when used in groups of patients that have different prevalences of disease. For example, a mildly abnormal alkaline phosphatase level in a young adult with a known lymphoma suggests hepatic involvement by the tumor (i.e., it is likely to be a *true positive*), while the same alkaline phosphatase level as part of a routine screening battery of blood tests in an asymptomatic person of the same age is unlikely to be due to tumor (i.e., in this setting it is more likely to be a *false positive*).

Although the sensitivity and specificity of a test do not depend on the prevalence (or percentage of patients being tested who have the disease), they do depend on the spectrum of patients in whom the test is being evaluated. For example, measurement of a prostate-specific antigen for diagnosing carcinoma of the prostate (see Chap. 97) will appear to have a nearly perfect sensitivity and specificity if the diseased population has a palpable prostate nodule and an elevated serum acid phosphatase level while the nondiseased population is composed of normal medical students. If, however, without changing the prevalence of disease in the population being tested, the spectrum of the diseased and nondiseased patients is altered by including patients with other characteristics (i.e., if the population of patients with carcinoma of the prostate were composed principally of those without palpable nodules and with stage 1 disease, while the population without carcinoma of the prostate included elderly men with marked benign

Table 3-2

Definitions of Commonly Used Terms in Epidemiology and Decision Making

Test Result	Disease State Present	Disease State Absent
Positive	a (true positive)	b (false positive)
Negative	c (false negative)	d (true negative)
Prevalence (prior probability)	$= (a + c)/(a + b + c + d)$	$=$ all patients with the disease/all patients tested
Sensitivity	$= a/(a + c)$	$=$ true-positive test results/all patients with the disease
Specificity	$= d/(b + d)$	$=$ true-negative test results/all patients without the disease
False-negative rate	$= c/(a + c)$	$=$ false-negative test result/all patients with the disease
False-positive rate	$= b/(b + d)$	$=$ false-positive test results/all patients without the disease
Positive predictive value	$= a/(a + b)$	$=$ true-positive test results/all patients with positive test results
Negative predictive	$= d/(c + d)$	$=$ true-negative test results/all patients with negative results
Overall accuracy	$= (a + d)/(a + b + c + d)$	$=$ true-positive + true-negative test results/all tests

Table 3-3

How the Positive and Negative Predictive Values of the Same Test Vary Depending on the Prior Probability of Disease

INTERPRETATION OF TEST RESULT WHEN 10% OF PATIENTS TESTED HAVE THE DISEASE (PRIOR PROBABILITY = 10%)

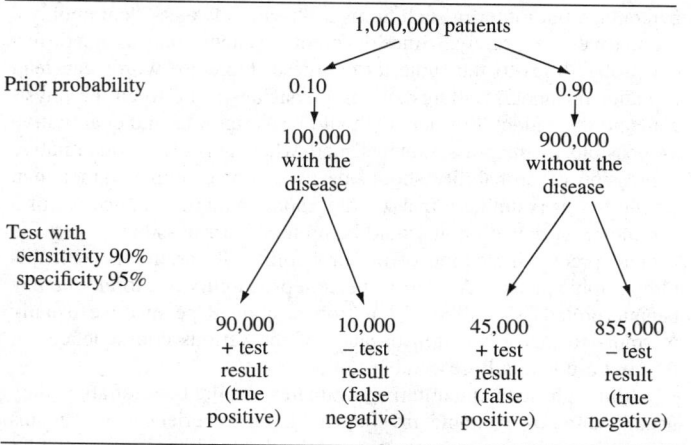

INTERPRETATION OF TEST RESULT WHEN 50% OF PATIENTS TESTED HAVE THE DISEASE (PRIOR PROBABILITY = 50%)

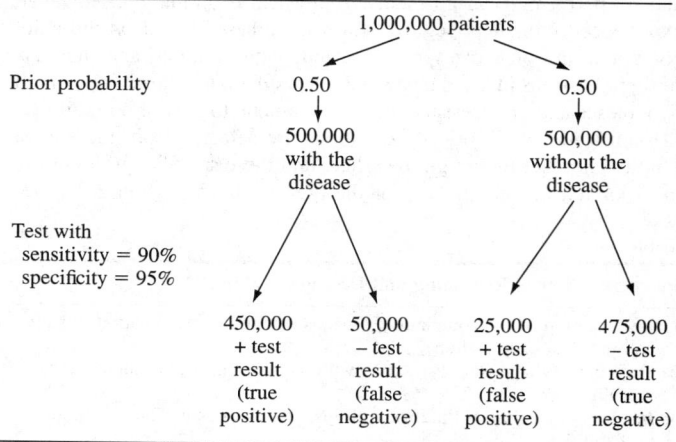

The probability of disease in a patient with a positive test result (positive predictive value) = 90,000/135,000 = 67%
The probability of no disease in a patient with a negative test result (negative predictive value) = 855,000/865,000 = 99%

The probability of disease in a patient with a positive test result (positive predictive value) = 450,000/475,000 = 95%
The probability of no disease in a patient with a negative test result (negative predictive value) = 475,000/525,000 = 90%

prostate hypertrophy), the sensitivity and specificity of the test would change dramatically. In the latter situation, the sensitivity and specificity of the prostate-specific antigen are not only lower than in the first example, because the spectrum of diseased and nondiseased patients has been changed, but more important, they may not be high enough for even this relatively accurate test to be recommended as a routine screening procedure. This example also demonstrates the methodologic problems encountered when applying data from one study to a different type of patient or when pooling data from studies of different subsets of patients.

In some situations, uncertainty about the sensitivity and specificity of the test in the type of patient being assessed may limit its clinical value. Since the physician rarely knows (or can know) the population on which every test that is ordered has been standardized, the results provide information that is far less decisive than usually thought. Furthermore, it may be quite difficult to distinguish random laboratory errors from test results that might be falsely positive or negative because of coexistence of a process that can affect the test, such as the finding of an elevated level of CK (creatine kinase) in a patient who has undergone strenuous exercise and is being evaluated for chest pain.

Because no single value or cutoff point of an individual test can be expected to have both a perfect sensitivity and a perfect specificity, it is often necessary to determine which value or cutoff point is the most appropriate to guide decision making. A graph (Fig. 3-1) of the test's *receiver operating characteristic curve*, which displays the inevitable trade-off between emphasizing a high sensitivity, such as defining an exercise electrocardiogram as abnormal if it shows ≥0.5 mm of ST-segment depression, versus emphasizing a high specificity, such as defining an exercise electrocardiogram as abnormal only if it shows ≥2.0 mm of ST-segment depression, can help the clinician understand the implications of various definitions of a "positive" test result. Such a graph demonstrates that different definitions of normal versus abnormal may be appropriate depending on whether one wishes to rule in the disease via a positive result on a test that has a high specificity or to exclude the disease via a negative result on a test that has a high sensitivity. Different tests may have different sensitivities and specificities, and better tests may have both a higher sensitivity and a higher specificity than poorer tests.

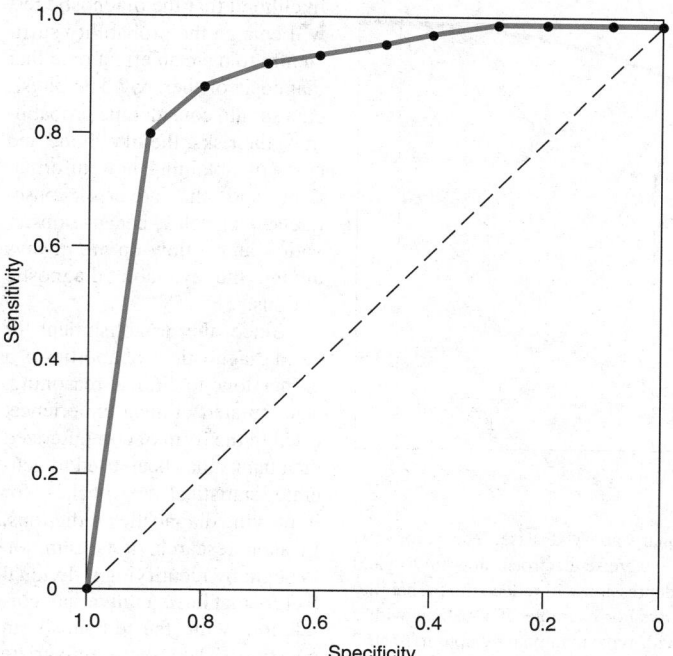

FIGURE 3-1 The inherent trade-off between sensitivity and specificity. For any diagnostic test, an increase in sensitivity will be associated with a decline in specificity. The closer this curve comes to the upper-left-hand corner, the more useful the test; the closer to the broken line, the less useful it is. When deciding on the cutoff between normal versus abnormal, one must determine what sensitivity and specificity are most useful clinically.

One example of a sensitive test is an enzyme-linked immunosorbent assay (ELISA) to test for the presence of antibodies to human immunodeficiency virus type 1 (HIV-1). This relatively inexpensive test has a high sensitivity for detecting HIV-1 antibodies but is not sufficiently specific to be used as the basis for making a firm diagnosis. Thus, if the ELISA assay is positive, it is commonly repeated. Confirmation of the diagnosis of HIV-1 antibody positivity requires a western blot, or an equivalently specific test, to exclude the possibility of a false-positive ELISA assay (see Chap. 308). A common example of a reasonably specific test would be an electrocardiogram to diagnose acute myocardial infarction. While the precise specificity depends on the spectrum of patients being tested, the presence of new ST-segment elevations exceeding 1.0 mm in two or more electrically contiguous leads in patients who present to an emergency department with prolonged acute chest pain consistent with myocardial ischemia is sufficiently specific, i.e., sufficiently unlikely to be a false-positive result, that admission to an intensive care unit and treatment with either intravenous thrombolysis or emergent percutaneous transluminal coronary angioplasty is virtually always recommended. However, this test is not sensitive, and if admission to the hospital were restricted to patients with this electrocardiographic finding, almost half of patients with myocardial infarctions presenting to hospital emergency departments would be missed.

INTEGRATION OF CLINICAL DATA AND TEST RESULTS Although, as we have seen, neither clinical data nor test results may be entirely accurate, the integration of the two can lead to better diagnostic predictions than either alone. By knowing the probability that the patient has a particular condition before a test is performed (the prior, or pretest, probability), and by knowing the sensitivity and the specificity of the test, the posttest probability can be calculated. A common mathematical technique for integrating clinical data and a test result is the odds-likelihood form of Bayesian analysis (Table 3-4). A pretest probability can be expressed as odds (as in a horse race, for example) and multiplied by the likelihood ratio (which is the sensitivity of the test divided by 1 minus the specificity of the test) to yield the posttest odds, which may be transformed back into a posttest probability. This approach can be employed in any situation in which the physician can use clinical findings to estimate a pretest diagnostic probability and integrate this with the result as well as the sensitivity and specificity of the diagnostic test. Many clinical situations may be so complex that it is not practical to estimate the prior probabilities of all likely diagnoses or to know the sensitivities and specificities of each of the tests that might be performed individually or in sequence. Nevertheless, attempts in this direction will stimulate critical thinking, expose uncertainties, and generate ideas for original investigations or a review of past experiences to facilitate the application of Bayesian analysis to the integration of clinical data and laboratory tests.

The results of Bayesian analyses often can be expressed in graphic form, such as the value of exercise electrocardiograms for predicting the presence of coronary artery disease (Fig. 3-2). This series of curves also demonstrates how to consider a test whose result may be in the "gray zone" rather than clearly positive or clearly negative.

One of the key assumptions inherent in most such analyses is that the correlation between the pretest probability and the test result is no greater than expected by chance. If the diagnostic test simply duplicates information that has already been obtained by the clinical examination, it will not have any additional benefit for predicting whether or not the disease is present. For example, in trying to determine whether or not a patient with carcinoma of the colon has hepatic metastases, the finding of jaundice on physical examination should be a strong predictor. The degree of hyperbilirubinemia also can be measured, but the bilirubin level in a patient with clinical jaundice does not add substantial *independent* information to that obtained by a careful physical examination. When integrating a diagnostic test with clinical information, the test is helpful only when it adds incremental

Table 3-4

Example of the Use of Bayesian Analysis to Integrate the Pretest Probability with the Test Result to Calculate a Posttest Probability

Example 1: Prior probability of disease = 25%; a test with a sensitivity (true-positive rate) of 90% and a specificity of 80% (which implies a false-positive rate of 20%) gives a positive result

Example 2: Same pretest probability and test, but now the test gives a negative result. Here the true-negative rate would be 80% and the false-negative rate (which is 1 − sensitivity) would be 10%.

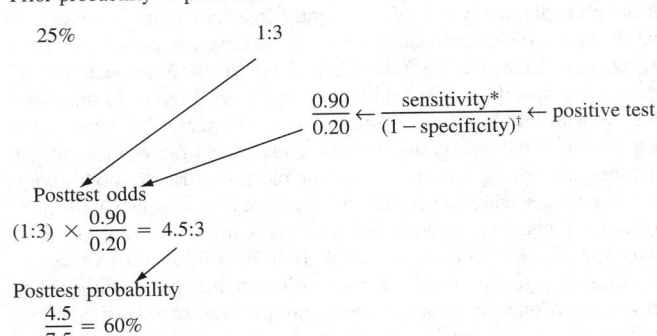

Clinical data

↓

Prior probability → prior odds

25%   1:3

$$\frac{0.90}{0.20} \leftarrow \frac{\text{sensitivity*}}{(1-\text{specificity})^\dagger} \leftarrow \text{positive test}$$

Posttest odds

$(1:3) \times \dfrac{0.90}{0.20} = 4.5:3$

Posttest probability

$\dfrac{4.5}{7.5} = 60\%$

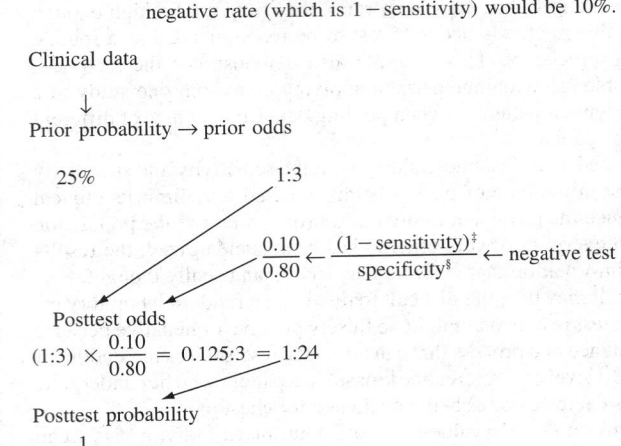

Clinical data

↓

Prior probability → prior odds

25%   1:3

$$\frac{0.10}{0.80} \leftarrow \frac{(1-\text{sensitivity})^\ddagger}{\text{specificity}^\S} \leftarrow \text{negative test}$$

Posttest odds

$(1:3) \times \dfrac{0.10}{0.80} = 0.125:3 = 1:24$

Posttest probability

$\dfrac{1}{25} = 4\%$

---

* Sensitivity = probability of a positive test result in a patient with the disease
† (1 − specificity) = probability of a positive test result in a patient without the disease

‡ (1 − sensitivity) = probability of a negative test result in a patient with the disease.
§ Specificity = probability of a negative test result in a patient without the disease.

---

information to what can be inferred based on the history and physical examination and on prior, less costly or less risky diagnostic tests. If a diagnostic test (such as a retrograde cholangiogram in a patient with hyperbilirubinemia) provides information that cannot be inferred directly, it is less likely that its results are associated with pretest probabilities to an extent greater than would be expected by chance.

A diagnostic test has an impact on the evaluation of a specific patient only if it changes the diagnostic probability to the extent that the new probability dictates a change in the diagnostic strategy or therapeutic plans or if the test serves as part of a sequence of tests that moves the probability across such a threshold. An example is a patient suspected of having a pulmonary embolism, with an estimated probability of 50 percent based on clinical data alone. The finding of a "low probability for pulmonary embolus" pulmonary ventilation-perfusion scan may reduce the probability of pulmonary embolism, but if the goal is to exclude pulmonary embolism with the highest possible degree of certainty, a pulmonary angiogram would be required (Chap. 261).

Because diagnostic tests often do not provide important new information even when their results are accurate, several questions should be considered in deciding when to order diagnostic tests. First, how likely is the disease in question? Second, what would be the clinical consequences if the diagnosis were missed or if the patient were mistakenly treated for a disease that is not present? Third, what is the likelihood that the diagnostic test will change the probability sufficiently to have an effect on either diagnosis or therapy? The physician should consider the probabilities, the risks, the likelihood and costs of obtaining new information, and the adverse consequences of delay, because observation and follow-up are always among the available diagnostic options.

Since the establishment of valid diagnostic probabilities is a cornerstone to clinical reasoning, accumulated clinical experience, often in the form of computerized data banks, has been used to generate statistical approaches for improving diagnostic predictions. In such research, it is common to begin by identifying individual factors that have a univariate correlation with the diagnosis in question. Then these univariate correlates may be included in a multivariate analysis to determine which of them are significant independent predictors of the diagnosis. Some analyses may identify the important predictive

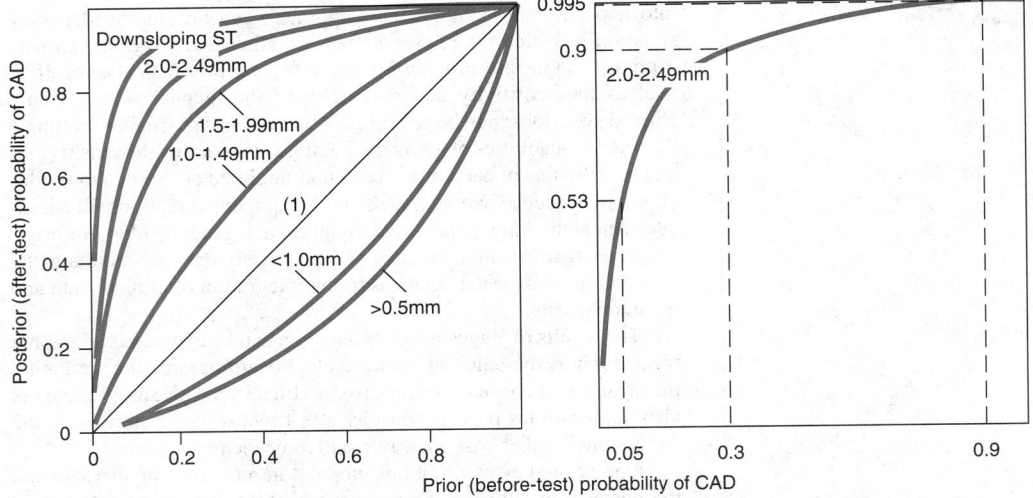

FIGURE 3-2 How the exercise tolerance test affects the probability of coronary artery disease. The before-test probability of coronary artery disease (CAD) will be modified by the result of the exercise electrocardiogram to yield an after-test probability of CAD. Note that the finding of <1 mm of ST-segment depression will reduce the probability of CAD, whereas ≥1 mm of ST-segment depression will increase the probability. For example, if a patient with a before-test probability of CAD of 90 percent (about that of a middle-aged man with typical anginal symptoms) had 2 to 2.49 mm on ST-segment depression on exercise testing, the after-test probability of CAD would be 99.5 percent. In contrast, the same exercise test result in a patient with 30 percent before-test probability of CAD (about that of a patient with atypical anginal symptoms) would yield an after-test probability of about 90 percent. In an asymptomatic patient, with a before-test probability of about 5 percent, the same exercise test result would yield an after-test probability of about 50 percent. Thus the same test yields different after-test probabilities in patients with different before-test probabilities. *(Adapted, with permission of the New England Journal of Medicine, from RD Rifkin, WB Hood, Bayesian analysis of electrocardiographic exercise stress testing. N Engl J Med 297:684, 1977.)*

factors and then assign them "weights," which can be transformed to calculate a probability. Alternatively, the analysis may result in a limited number of categories of patients, each with a discrete probability of the diagnosis.

These quantitative approaches to the estimation of various diagnostic probabilities, which are often termed "prediction rules," are especially helpful if they are in a format that is readily usable by the clinician and if they have been validated prospectively on a sufficient number and spectrum of patients. For example, by carefully defining the key historical questions, findings on physical examination, and electrocardiographic abnormalities that might predict the probability of acute myocardial infarction among emergency department patients with chest pain, accurate guidelines can be developed for the triage of patients to settings ranging from intensive care to discharge home. For such prediction rules to be useful to the clinician, they must be derived from relevant patient populations and use tests that are reproducible and readily available so that the results can be extrapolated to local medical practice.

COMPARING RISKS AND BENEFITS: DECISION ANALYSIS Inherent in the concept that probabilities can guide decision making is the assumption that one can arrive at a reasonable threshold by knowing the relative risks (or costs) and benefits of various options and deciding at what probability this ratio changes to favor an alternative strategy. Decision analysis is an organized process for evaluating such situations and identifies the key issues and problems.

One problem with applying decision-analysis techniques to difficult clinical problems is that the decision analysis is no better than the data on which it is based. In some instances, an attempted decision analysis of a complex clinical problem may yield no more information than that the critical data required for the analysis are missing and that more research in the field needs to be performed. In addition, when clinicians are uncertain about diagnostic or therapeutic strategies, formal analyses may indicate that the differences in outcome among various strategies are very small. In such cases, the formal analysis may have such inherent error that it is not definitive. Even when decision analysis is potentially helpful, it may not be feasible to complete the detailed estimations and calculations within the time constraints of bedside decision making. Nevertheless, the value of the analytic approach to decision making is that it integrates available data, mandates rigorous thinking, and exposes areas of uncertainty or ignorance.

Decision analysis depicts graphically two types of issues in the decision-making process: first, the decisions (or choices) available to the physician and, second, the probabilities of all the events that may result from each decision. To illustrate how this process works, consider a very simplified decision analysis of whether to use an intravenous thrombolytic agent in a patient with a suspected acute myocardial infarction (see Chap. 243). Figure 3-3 depicts the simplified decision tree for this problem. The square box or "node" labeled *A* indicates a decision that the physician must make. The circular nodes, labeled *B* through *O*, indicate where different outcomes, each of which has an estimable probability, could occur. In this analysis, the initial choices were to treat the patient with an intravenous thrombolytic agent or not to treat. The use of such an agent may or may not result in serious complications of therapy, especially bleeding and intracranial hemorrhage.

Each of the possible outcomes for a patient is typically assigned a "utility," which is the relative preference for the outcome, where 1.0 is a perfect outcome and 0 is the worst possible outcome. Each terminal branch of the decision tree is assigned the utility corresponding to its outcome, and the "expected value" of each terminal branch is calculated by multiplying its probability by its utility. To calculate the expected value of each of the two possible courses of action (see Fig. 3-3, node *A*), the expected values of each of the terminal branches that originate from it would be summed. The preferred course of action is the one which, when all possible outcomes are considered, including the risks and benefits of therapy, yields the highest expected value, which is the sum of the product of the probability multiplied by the utility for each of its possible outcomes.

In performing any decision analysis, the relevant probabilities must be known or estimated, a process that sometimes requires guess-

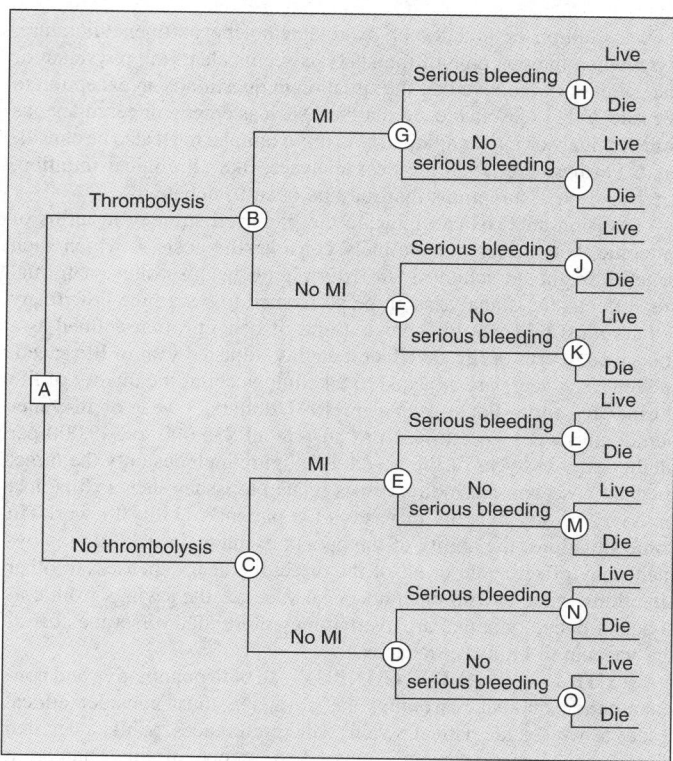

FIGURE 3-3 Simplified decision tree for the decision of whether or not to use an intravenous thrombolytic agent in a patient with a suspected acute myocardial infarction. The square node represents the decision point, and the round nodes denote chance events (see text for details).

work. Next, utilities could be assigned to each of these outcomes. A major practical limitation of decision analysis is the subjective judgment often required to estimate utilities. It is also difficult to adjust future years of life for their quality in any numerical fashion, e.g., in considering how treatment complications, such as an intracranial hemorrhage, or the advantages of treatment, such as congestive heart failure averted because an infarction was smaller, affect the quality of future years of life.

The results and usefulness of a decision analysis depend on the probabilities and utilities that are used in the calculation, and it is imperative for decision analyses to include a *sensitivity analysis*, in which various estimates for each probability are included in the analysis to determine if the conclusions would be changed. For example, in the analysis in Fig. 3-3, some range of probabilities must be assumed for the risk of serious bleeding complications and for the likelihood that any particular patient is having an acute myocardial infarction. If the conclusions of an analysis were altered by relatively minor changes in the assumptions on which it was based, the analysis would not be sufficiently reliable to become the basis for decision making. Because of the impressive benefit of thrombolysis for improving survival in patients with acute myocardial infarctions presenting early after the onset of symptoms, decision analyses have shown treatment to be the preferred option even when an acute myocardial infarction is not certain and even in most elderly patients.

Decision analysis sometimes demonstrates a clear and dramatic advantage with one particular option. In other circumstances, there may be little difference between two options; either option may be reasonable, or secondary issues that cannot be taken into account in the formal analysis, such as the patient's feelings about taking risks or the recent local experience with particular interventions, should be the final determinants in the decision. Physicians who perform a decision analysis therefore must determine the probabilities of each of the possible events by reviewing the pertinent patient experience at their own institution or practice or by reviewing the pertinent literature. Even when the outcome of the analysis seems clear, the physician or the patient may believe that the situation in question is an exception to the rule. Other reasonable alternatives, such as emergent percutaneous transluminal coronary angioplasty in this example, must also be considered. Furthermore, even the best analyses, like all clinical intuition, are based on assumptions that may be open to debate.

Decision analysis can indicate the preferred strategy in terms of outcome, but it does not routinely consider the costs at which such benefits might be achieved. In determining health policy, a formal cost-effectiveness analysis can be performed to determine how many dollars must be spent to achieve a unit of benefit, often defined as a life saved, a year of life saved, or a quality-adjusted year of life saved, in which the years are adjusted to take into account the quality of life during that time. For example, in 1997 dollars, 1 year of in-center hemodialysis can be estimated to cost about $35,000 to $45,000 per quality-adjusted year of life saved; this figure includes only the direct medical costs and not indirect costs related to issues such as time lost or travel or any benefits in terms of a patient's ability to work. In some situations, the ability of the patient to maintain gainful employment may offset some or all of the direct medical expenses. In other situations, such as with pneumococcal vaccine, the savings from episodes of pneumonia that are averted may more than offset the cost of the vaccine in high-risk persons.

ETHICS AND PATIENT INPUT   In both quantitative and non-quantitative clinical reasoning, the physician must consider ethical issues as well as the patient's values and preferences. While a detailed discussion of these issues is beyond the scope of this chapter, it is important to emphasize that patients' preferences for alternative therapies may not agree with the preferences that the physicians propose on the basis of their own clinical judgment or the results of a decision-analysis approach. For example, the preferred treatment for many patients with benign prostatic hypertrophy depends critically on how much the patient is bothered by urinary symptoms. It is imperative that physicians assess those characteristics of life which the patient prizes most (the elusive "quality of life") prior to basing controversial decisions solely on quantitative approaches, the physicians' own subjective impressions of the likely medical benefits, their own personal preferences, or their assumptions about the patient's preferences. While quantitative analyses may apply to groups of patients, judgment must be exercised when adapting them to the individual patient. Therefore, the final plan should reflect an agreement between a well-informed patient and a sympathetic physician who has detailed knowledge of the relevant medical issues and of the impact of the various possible outcomes on the specific patient.

BIBLIOGRAPHY

GASPOZ et al: Cost-effectiveness of a new short-stay unit to "rule out" acute myocardial infarction in low risk patients. J Am Coll Cardiol 24:1249, 1994

HULL RD et al: A non-invasive strategy for the treatment of patients with suspected pulmonary embolism. Arch Intern Med 154:289, 1994

KASSIRER JP: Teaching problem solving—how are we doing? N Engl J Med 332:1507, 1995

SACKETT DL et al: *Clinical Epidemiology: A Basic Science for Clinical Medicine*, 2d ed. Boston, Little, Brown, 1991

SLOAND EM et al: HIV testing: State of the art. JAMA 266:2861, 1991

SOX HC JR (ed): *Common Diagnostic Tests: Use and Interpretation*, 2d ed. Philadelphia, American College of Physicians, 1990

ST CLAIR EW et al: Assessing housestaff diagnostic skills using a cardiology patient simulator. Ann Intern Med 117:751, 1992

TORIBARA NW et al: Screening for colorectal cancer. N Engl J Med 332:861, 1995

VAN DEN HOOGEN HM et al: On the accuracy of the history, physical examination, and erythrocyte sedimentation rate in diagnosing low back pain in general practice. A criteria-based review of the literature. Spine 20:318, 1995

WASSON JH et al: A comparison of transurethral surgery with watchful waiting for moderate symptoms of benign prostatic hypertrophy. N Engl J Med 332:75, 1995

HOST AND DISEASE: INFLUENCE OF DEMOGRAPHIC AND SOCIOECONOMIC FACTORS*

Marked variations in disease occurrence and survival exist among different subgroups of the U.S. population. Some of these are attributable to demographic and social factors such as age, gender, race/ethnicity, sexual orientation, geographic location, and socioeconomic status (SES). Although individual physicians have limited ability to influence these characteristics, it is important to recognize the role of these factors in determining environmental exposures, behavioral risk factors, access to health care, and compliance with recommended preventive and therapeutic regimens, all of which can influence disease etiology and prognosis. Although not reviewed here, other social factors including culture and acculturation, religion, and psychosocial factors (e.g., life events, social mobility, and social networks) also affect the impact of disease.

This chapter describes variations in measures of health across demographic and socioeconomic subgroups. Improvements in mortality and life expectancy have occurred during the twentieth century, but despite overall improvements, differences in morbidity, quality of survival, and mortality continue to exist across racial/ethnic groups. Individuals of lower SES experience greater morbidity and mortality, and differences in SES explain many of the variations in health status across racial/ethnic groups. Differences in behavioral risk factors explain many, but not all, of the differences in disease prevalence across sociodemographic groups. For the already advantaged segments of our population, future improvements in health status will likely result in only minor increases in average life expectancy but may lengthen the period of "healthy life."

DEMOGRAPHIC FACTORS   Age   The specialties of pediatrics, adolescent medicine, and geriatrics developed because the clinical expressions of disease differ across the age spectrum. The biologic, medical, and sociologic characteristics of persons in these age groups are discussed in other chapters. Within the adult range, mortality rates from the leading causes of death vary widely by age group. Additionally, the prevalence of health risk behaviors such as smoking and alcohol use varies by age.

Gender   Although most illnesses affect both men and women, there are notable exceptions. By definition, many disorders of the reproductive tract occur exclusively in one gender. Others, such as carcinoma of the breast, rarely occur in men, whereas recessive disorders linked to the X chromosome, such as hemophilia and Duchenne's muscular dystrophy, are more common in males. Other conditions occur regularly in both sexes but predominate or tend to be more severe in one or the other. Examples include diabetes mellitus, connective tissue diseases, iron deficiency anemia, and osteoporosis in women; coronary atherosclerosis in young and middle-aged men; and gout in men. Other aspects of women's health are discussed in Chap. 6.

Race/Ethnicity   Race and ethnicity also play an important role in the expression of disease. In addition to genetic factors, persons with similar ethnic backgrounds share cultural, nutritional, environmental, economic, and social characteristics that influence disease. There are numerous examples of differences in the risk, incidence, and expression of disease across ethnic groups: sickle cell anemia and other hemoglobinopathies are found almost exclusively in persons of African, Arabic, Indian, Greek, and Italian ancestry; the age-adjusted prevalence of hypertension in African-Americans is two to four times that of whites (with the highest rates in black women); the prevalence of non-insulin diabetes mellitus is approximately twice as high in African-Americans and Native Americans as in whites; the age-adjusted mortality rates for stroke and sudden death are higher in blacks than in whites; the rates for symptomatic coronary artery disease are higher in black than in white women; the prevalence and incidence of tubercu-

*This chapter includes the contributions of Eugene Braunwald and Jean Wilson from prior editions.

losis are approximately twice as high in blacks as in whites; osteoporosis and vertebral fractures occur more frequently in women than in men and in white than in black women; and ankylosing spondylitis and Reiter's syndrome are more common in whites.

Social class, racism, and other sociocultural factors affect health-related behaviors and outcomes across racial/ethnic groups. Even when income, health status, age, sex, and history of chronic disease are taken into account, blacks in the United States have fewer ambulatory visits and are less likely to see a physician, suggesting disadvantages in access to care.

Less is known about the mortality and morbidity data for racial/ethnic groups other than whites and blacks. Moreover, there are serious concerns about the accuracy of such data as do exist, given documented discrepancies in the coding of race/ethnicity among agencies that collect vital statistics. Broad categories such as "Hispanic," "Asian," or "Native American" include diverse populations with diverse disease risks. For example, Mexican-Americans appear to have a low risk of cerebrovascular disease, whereas Puerto Ricans have a high risk of stroke, which would make it difficult to interpret statistics for Hispanics based on the combined experience. More precise ethnic categories, particularly for Asians and Pacific Islanders, often have too few individuals for reliable calculation of cause-specific death rates. Furthermore, the increasing interracial admixture of the population makes traditional racial categories less meaningful over time.

Sexual Orientation   The incidence of some diseases varies greatly in subgroups of the population defined by sexual orientation and practices. For example, the incidence of AIDS, gonorrhea, syphilis, and hepatitis B is higher among homosexual than among heterosexual men. Colitis due to parasites ("gay-bowel syndrome") and anal and oropharyngeal carcinomas also occur more frequently in homosexual men. The increased incidence of these conditions is related to the numbers of sexual partners and sexual practices and not to homosexuality itself. Among lesbians, rates of infection with syphilis, gonorrhea, chlamydia, herpesvirus, and human papillomavirus appear to be lower than among heterosexual women. Many lesbians are nulliparous, and nulliparous women are at increased risk for breast and ovarian cancer.

Geography   Geography can influence disease incidence in several ways. Some diseases occur only in those who have resided for long periods in specific areas. Goiter caused by iodine deficiency occurs mainly in people who live in areas previously covered by glaciers; toxic waste syndromes usually require prolonged residence in an area exposed to toxins; pulmonary hypertension is more common in those living at high altitudes; sarcoidosis is more common in residents of the coniferous belt of the southern United States; multiple sclerosis is more common in temperate climates. Some infectious diseases (e.g., melioidosis, leprosy, leishmaniasis, Chagas' disease, and filariasis) tend to occur in people who live in specific locations for a long time. The advent of widespread airborne travel, refugee resettlement, and immigration requires that clinicians in the United States consider a broad differential diagnosis of disease encompassing conditions related to geographic exposure.

Health indicators and practice patterns differ among diverse geographic regions. In 1990 to 1992, the age-adjusted death rate for residents of large cities in the United States was 19 percent greater than in suburbs around large cities. One study found substantial regional variation in the use of cardiac medications and procedures for the management of acute myocardial infarction in the United States.

THE RELATIONSHIP OF AGE, GENDER, AND RACE/ETHNICITY TO MEASURES OF HEALTH   Life Expectancy
Since 1900, life expectancy in the United States increased by nearly 60 percent for whites and 100 percent for blacks. By 1992, average life expectancy at birth was 73.2 and 79.8 years, respectively, for white males and females and 65.0 and 73.9 years for black males and females (Table 4-1). These gains in life expectancy are the result of declines in age-adjusted mortality rates (Fig. 4-1). Nevertheless, there is a continuing gap in life expectancy between blacks and whites, a slowing of life expectancy gains in blacks beginning in the mid-1980s, and a persistent twofold excess in infant mortality among blacks.

The male-female gap in life expectancy widened and then narrowed during this century, consistent with the pattern of cigarette

Table 4-1

Life Expectancy at Birth for Whites and Blacks, by Gender: United States, 1900–1992

	White		Black	
	Male	Female	Male	Female
1900	46.6	48.7	32.5	33.5
1950	66.5	72.2	58.9	62.7
1960	67.4	74.1	60.7	65.9
1970	68.0	75.6	60.0	68.3
1980	70.7	78.1	63.8	72.5
1990	72.7	79.4	64.5	73.6
1991	72.9	79.6	64.6	73.8
1992	73.2	79.8	65.0	73.9

SOURCE: National Center for Health Statistics.

smoking, first by men and later by women. Life expectancy among whites was on average 2.1 years longer for women than men in 1900, 7.6 years longer in 1970, and 6.6 years longer in 1992.

Mortality Rates   Since the mid-1960s, most of the decline in overall mortality rates in the United States is due to reductions in death from coronary heart disease (CHD) and stroke, affecting primarily the older age groups. Age-adjusted CHD death rates have declined by more than 40 percent since 1970; between 1980 and 1992 alone, age-adjusted heart disease mortality rates in the population aged 55 to 64 years declined 30 percent, from 494.1 to 346.5 per 100,000. For all of the leading causes of death (except diabetes mellitus) in the United States, there is a male excess in age-adjusted death rates; the excess is greater than twofold for deaths due to accidents, suicide, chronic liver disease and cirrhosis, homicide, and human immunodeficiency virus infection (Table 4-2). Data on disease rates among Hispanics,

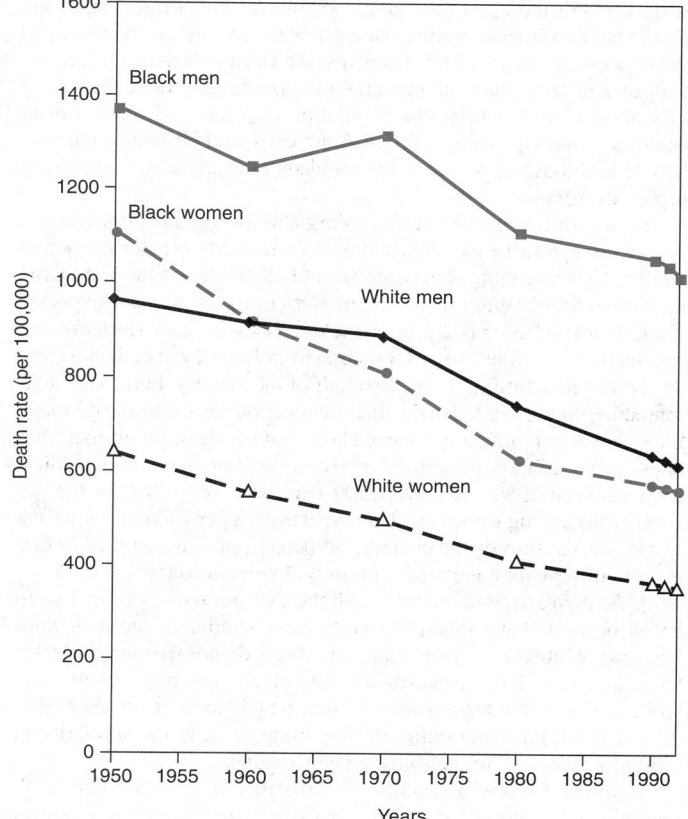

FIGURE 4-1   Age-adjusted death rates per 100,000, 1950–1992, for white and black males and females, age-adjusted to the 1940 U.S. population. (*After National Center for Health Statistics.*)

Table 4-2

Age-Adjusted Death Rates (per 100,000 Population) and Ratios for the Leading Causes of Death by Gender and Race: United States, 1992

Causes	White		Black		Ratio of white male rate to white female rate	Ratio of black male rate to black female rate	Ratio of black male rate to white male rate	Ratio of black female rate to white female rate
	Male	Female	Male	Female				
Heart disease	190.3	98.1	264.1	162.4	1.9	1.6	1.4	1.7
Malignant neoplasms	157.3	110.3	238.1	136.6	1.4	1.7	1.5	1.2
Cerebrovascular diseases	26.3	22.5	52.0	39.9	1.2	1.3	2.0	1.8
Chronic obstructive pulmonary diseases	26.8	16.1	24.8	11.2	1.7	2.2	0.9	0.7
Motor vehicle crashes	22.2	9.6	25.0	8.7	2.3	2.9	1.1	0.9
Pneumonia and influenza	15.8	9.7	25.0	12.2	1.6	2.0	1.6	1.3
Human immunodeficiency virus infection	18.1	1.6	61.8	14.3	11.3	4.3	3.4	8.9
Diabetes mellitus	11.6	9.6	24.2	25.8	1.2	0.9	2.1	2.7
Suicide	19.5	4.6	12.4	2.1	4.2	5.9	0.6	0.5
Homicide and legal intervention	9.3	2.8	68.1	13.0	3.3	5.2	7.3	4.6
Chronic liver disease and cirrhosis	11.1	4.6	17.2	6.9	2.4	2.5	1.5	1.5
Alcohol-induced causes	9.9	2.6	22.3	6.3	3.8	3.5	2.3	2.4
Drug-induced causes	5.5	2.7	10.6	3.6	2.0	2.9	1.9	1.3
All causes	620.9	359.9	1026.9	568.4	1.7	1.8	1.7	1.6

SOURCE: National Center for Health Statistics.

Asians/Pacific Islanders, and Native American/Alaskan Native populations, as well as blacks and whites, assembled by the National Center for Health Statistics, suggest the following: (1) for all age groups, overall death rates are lowest among Asians; (2) blacks have the highest overall death rates for all age groups except ages 15 to 24, when rates are slightly higher for Native American/Alaskan Natives; (3) in all age groups under 65, overall death rates among whites and Hispanics are intermediate between the low rates of Asians and the high rates of blacks; (4) in young people aged 15 to 24, blacks are seven times more likely, and Hispanics and Native Americans are three to four times more likely, to die of homicide than Asians and whites; (5) in the age group under 45, unintentional injury rates are particularly excessive among Native American/Alaskan Natives; (6) in the age groups 25 to 64, heart disease rates in blacks are higher, and rates in Hispanics and especially in Asians are lower, than those of whites; and (7) among the population 65 years and older, cancer death rates among Asians, Native Americans, and Hispanics are only half or less those of whites, whereas black rates are about 20 percent higher than whites.

In the Harlem district of New York City, where the population is 96 percent black, the age-adjusted overall mortality rate for the period 1979 to 1981 was more than twice that of U.S. whites; in the population under age 65, the ratio of deaths in Harlem to the number expected was 2.9 for males and 2.7 for females. Black men in Harlem were less likely to survive to age 65 than men in less-developed countries.

Infant Mortality In the first half of the century, improved environmental conditions led to declines in infectious diseases and dramatic improvements in infant and early childhood survival. Infant mortality rates have continued to decline, largely due to improvements in medical care; between 1950 and 1992, rates decreased from 26.8 to 6.9 per 1000 births among whites and from 43.9 to 16.8 per 1000 births among blacks. At the turn of the century, 30 percent of children died before the age of 5 years compared with only 2 percent today.

U.S.-born Hispanic infants, with the exception of those of Puerto Rican descent, have infant mortality rates similar to those of non-Hispanic whites, i.e., about one-half those of non-Hispanic blacks. Even among college-educated parents, blacks are more likely than whites to have low birth weight babies, which account for the higher overall black infant mortality in this group, despite the similarity in mortality rates for normal birth weight infants.

Leading Causes of Death For the period 1980 to 1986, U.S. mortality rates due to 12 causes considered preventable by medical intervention (tuberculosis, cervical cancer, Hodgkin's disease, rheumatic heart disease, hypertensive heart disease, acute respiratory disease, pneumonia and bronchitis, influenza, asthma, appendicitis, her-

nias, and cholecystitis) were 4.5 times higher in blacks than whites, with highest relative differences for tuberculosis, hypertensive heart disease, and asthma.

Morbidity Morbidity data are consistent with the mortality data. In 1988, 16.3 percent of blacks and 12.8 percent of whites reported limitation of their activity due to chronic conditions. In a study in Manhattan (New York), incidence rates of Parkinson's disease were highest for black men. One population-based study reported hypertensive end-stage renal disease rates in blacks to be 4.5 times higher than in whites, adjusting for age, prevalence of hypertension, diabetes, and education level. On the other hand, malignant melanoma is more common in whites than in blacks.

Access to Care In Massachusetts, black patients with ischemic heart disease undergo coronary angiography and coronary artery bypass grafting less often than whites, even controlling for age, sex, income, source of payment, primary diagnosis, and the number of secondary diagnoses. In Los Angeles County from 1986 through 1988, blacks and Latinos were less likely than whites and Asians to undergo bypass surgery. Among Medicare patients, sex- and age-adjusted rates for coronary artery bypass grafting among blacks were about one-third those among whites in 1986 and were not related to admission rates for acute myocardial infarction. Many of the residual differences may be due to inadequate control for SES, but the disparities exist nonetheless.

SOCIOECONOMIC STATUS Socioeconomic status is measured in various ways, including education, income, occupation, population density, poverty area residence, and combined indices. Different measures of SES are not necessarily interchangeable; it is preferable to have more than one indicator. When a single SES indicator must suffice, education appears to provide the most valid measure. However measured, low SES has adverse health consequences and appears to be largely responsible for the differences in health status between whites and other racial/ethnic groups, especially blacks, in the United States (see below). Increasing attention is being given to understanding mediators of this impressive relationship of SES to disease.

RELATIONSHIP OF SOCIOECONOMIC STATUS TO MEASURES OF HEALTH Mortality Data In a study of 340,000 individuals who died in 1960, clear inverse gradients were found in mortality by education, income, and occupation for white and nonwhite males and females. The mortality of white females with 4 or more years of college education, for example, was only 71 percent of the overall rate for white females, whereas those with fewer than 5 years of education had a mortality ratio of 127 percent. Similarly, life expectancy for white women aged 25 with at least 1 year of college education was almost 10 years greater (56.4 years) than for those with fewer than 5 years of schooling. The decline in heart disease mortality among males between 1960 and 1971 to 1984 was sharpest for those with more years of education.

Mortality differentials by occupational status have been well documented, and social class differences in mortality in Britain may be widening. In the United States, a population-based 18-year follow-up study in Alameda County, California, found that death rates in individuals with inadequate family income were twice as high as in those with adequate income. The Western Collaborative Group Study of 3154 employed, middle-aged men showed an association between SES and mortality, even after adjustment was made for other causes of mortality.

Incidence of Disease When SES is controlled, black/white differences in the incidence of some cancers, including invasive cervical cancer and male lung cancer, are reduced or disappear. In fact, unadjusted for SES, overall cancer rates are higher in blacks compared with whites in the United States, but adjusted rates are higher in whites than in blacks. Differences in heart disease rates across occupational groups in the United States are greater than differences between blacks and whites. Even the onset of the decline in CHD rates among white women in the United States occurred first in geographic areas where average income, education, and occupational levels were highest.

Survival Black women have poorer survival from breast cancer than white women, but race is not significant if SES is controlled. Although infant mortality rates are twice as high among normal birth weight black babies compared with white babies in the general population, no differences are found in comparisons of normal birth weight infants born to black and white college-educated parents. In one study, those with annual household incomes of $40,000 or greater were about half as likely to die within 5 years as patients with lower incomes.

Morbidity Morbidity is also inversely related to income. In the United States in 1993, 26.0 percent of individuals whose family income was less than $14,000 reported limitation of activity due to chronic conditions, compared with only 9.2 percent of those whose income was $50,000 or greater (Table 4-3). Other analyses demonstrate that most preventable morbidity and functional limitation in the U.S. population before age 75 occurs in the lower SES strata. Even among children the average number of disability days in 1980 was 9.1 for those whose families had annual incomes of $5000, compared with 4 days for those from families with incomes of $25,000 or more. The incidence of lower respiratory illness is inversely related to educational level of the head of household, and in one study the lowest income group had a threefold increase in the odds of CHD compared with the highest income group. The pattern was similar in blacks and whites.

There are notable exceptions to the inverse gradient between SES and disease. For example, the incidence of breast cancer is higher in upper SES groups. However, the general validity of the inverse gradient of social class to so many seemingly unrelated causes of disease is impressive.

Differences in health status across SES and racial groups are partially due to differences in the distribution of known disease risk factors. Cigarette smoking, the leading cause of preventable death in the United States, shows a strong inverse relationship to SES. In the population 18 years of age and older, 37.3 percent of males and 27.1 percent of females with less than a high school education were current smokers in 1990, compared with 14.5 percent and 12.3 percent, respectively, of college graduates. The inverse relation of smoking prevalence

Table 4-4

Age-Adjusted Prevalence of Current Cigarette Smoking by Persons 25 Years of Age and Over, by Sex, Race, and Education: United States, 1993

Education, years	Male		Female	
	White	**Black**	**White**	**Black**
<12	39.7	47.2	31.7	29.8
12	29.7	36.4	27.6	23.9
13–15	26.9	30.1	21.9	22.7
>16	14.1	16.0*	12.5	13.3*
Total	26.3	36.0	23.1	22.2

* These age-adjusted percents should be considered unreliable because of small sample size.

SOURCE: National Center for Health Statistics.

and educational status is seen for both white and black, males and females (Table 4-4). It is projected that by the year 2000 smoking prevalence among those with a high school education or less will be about 30 percent, whereas it will be less than 10 percent among college graduates. In California between 1984 and 1989, smoking, nonuse or infrequent use of seat belts, not exercising outside of work, being overweight, and hypertension among women were all more common in those with a high school education or less (Table 4-5). Nationwide data for 1987 to 1989 indicate that self-reports of mammographic screening and of having had a Pap smear within the previous year are positively associated with income level. Finally, the proportion of children in the United States who are vaccinated for measles, rubella, diphtheria/tetanus/pertussis (DTP), polio, and mumps is about 15 to 20 percent higher among white children compared with children of other racial groups (Table 4-6), which may largely reflect SES differences.

For many diseases, however, control for differences in known risk factors diminishes but does not eliminate differences across SES and racial groups. In British civil servants, about 40 percent of the differential in CHD mortality across different employment grades remained after controlling for serum cholesterol, systolic blood pressure, smoking, physical activity, body mass, and other factors. Similarly, adjustment for age and risk factors resulted in only modest reductions in the elevated relative risks of death from heart disease among the least educated men and women aged 45 to 74 in one survey. An examination of follow-up data from the same survey for adults aged 35 to 54 found that the ratio of black to white mortality rates decreased from 2.3 to 1.9 when adjusted for six risk factors (smoking, systolic blood pressure, cholesterol level, body-mass index, alcohol intake, and diabetes) and was further reduced

Table 4-3

Limitation of Activity due to Chronic Conditions by Family Income, United States, 1993

Family Income, $	Percent of Population
<14,000	26.0
14,000–24,999	17.3
25,000–34,999	13.4
35,000–49,999	11.1
50,000 or more	9.2

SOURCE: National Center for Health Statistics.

Table 4-5

Prevalence of Behavioral Risk Factors by Education Level in California, Ages 35–44, 1984–1989

Risk Factor	Males		Females	
	≤ High School, %	> High School, %	≤ High School, %	> High School, %
Current smoking	40.7	25.6	30.1	19.1
Irregular, nonuse of seatbelts	29.6	17.8	20.9	10.9
No exercise outside of work	39.4	14.4	31.9	20.2
Overweight	33.1	19.6	21.6	14.1
Hypertension	13.1	20.0	15.9	10.9
Chronic drinking	13.9	12.8	4.0	2.5
Drinking and driving	6.7	5.2	1.1	1.3

SOURCE: Based on responses to telephone interviews conducted as part of the CDC's ongoing Behavioral Risk Factor Survey. $n = 10,650$ California participants during 1984–1989.

Table 4-6

Vaccination of White and Black Children Aged 19–35 Months for Selected Diseases, by Race, United States, 1993

	White	Black
Measles	84.2	80.8
DTP*	88.3	78.0
Polio	74.7	67.4
Haemophilus b	64.4	46.5

* Diphtheria/tetanus/pertussis.
SOURCE: National Center for Health Statistics.

to 1.4 when adjustment for family income was included; 31 percent of the excess mortality in blacks was, therefore, due to the six risk factors, and 38 percent was due to family income, leaving 31 percent unexplained. On the other hand, lower cardiovascular disease mortality has been reported in Mexican-American compared to white males, despite higher levels of cardiovascular risk factors in the former.

One theme under consideration is the role of relative deprivation, as opposed to absolute levels of income or other measures of SES, in determining health status in developed countries. In Britain, for example, among individuals in nonmanual occupations who are homeowners, mortality is still lower in those with two cars compared to those with only one car. Across the 12 countries of the European Community, a strong correlation between income distribution and life expectancy has been reported.

Nevertheless, avoidable risk factors account for part of the differences in disease status in all SES groups, even among the elderly. Priority areas for health promotion (individual behaviors), health protection (environmental and regulatory measures), and preventive services (counseling, screening, immunization, or chemoprophylactic intervention in clinical settings) are extensively documented. Attempts to promote healthy lifestyles among the socially disadvantaged deserve high priority. In the face of the difficulties of daily life, however, such efforts may not be a high priority for the individuals who are in greatest need, and such education will have little impact unless coupled with adequate income, employment, and housing. It is disturbing that social class disparities, as measured by income, are widening, and it is important that the paucity of national disease data by social class be corrected.

THE FUTURE: IMPROVEMENTS IN YEARS OF HEALTHY LIFE VS. LENGTH OF LIFE It is not clear whether it is biologically possible to extend average life expectancy much beyond that presently attained by the most advantaged members of our society, i.e., around 85 years of age. If it is not possible, our major goal in health promotion should be the "compression of morbidity," i.e., postponement of debilitating illness until as close as possible to the time of death. Stated otherwise, we should focus on the morbidity and quality-of-life outcomes of our prevention efforts: "Add life to your years, not years to your life."

That said, it is important to acknowledge that sizable disadvantaged segments of our population have yet to approximate the purported maximum life span and that attempts to change established behavioral risk factors, while critically important, will not compress morbidity for the population as a whole. Improvements in SES and recognition of the continuing impact of racism on health outcomes are fundamental to achieving that goal.

BIBLIOGRAPHY

ADLER NE et al: Socioeconomic inequalities in health. No easy solution. JAMA 269:3140, 1993

BRAUNWALD E, WILSON JD: Host and disease: Influence of demographic factors, in *Harrison's Principles of Internal Medicine*, 13th ed, KJ Isselbacher et al (eds). New York, McGraw-Hill, 1994, pp 8–10

BUCHER HC et al: Socioeconomic indicators and mortality from coronary heart disease and cancer: A 22-year follow-up of middle-aged men. Am J Public Health 85:1231, 1995

CARLISLE DM et al: Racial and ethnic differences in the use of invasive cardiac procedures among cardiac patients in Los Angeles County, 1986 through 1988. Am J Public Health 85:352, 1995

DENENBERG R: Report on lesbian health. Womens Health Issues 5:81, 1995

DIEZ-ROUX AV et al: Social inequalities and atherosclerosis: The atherosclerosis risk in communities study. Am J Epidemiol 141:960, 1995

DOLL R: Health and the environment in the 1900s. Am J Public Health 82:933, 1992

HAHN RA: The state of federal health statistics on racial and ethnic groups. JAMA 267:268, 1992

KRIEGER N et al: Social class: The missing link in U.S. health data. Int J Health Serv 24:25, 1994

LEE PR et al: Measuring social inequalities in health. Report on the Conference of the National Institutes of Health. Public Health Rep 110:302, 1995

MAYEUX R et al: The frequency of idiopathic Parkinson's disease by age, ethnic group, and sex in northern Manhattan, 1988–1993. Am J Epidemiol 142:820, 1995

NATIONAL CENTER FOR HEALTH STATISTICS: *Health, United States, 1994.* DHHS publication No. (PHS) 95-1232, Hyattsville, MD, 1995

PILOTE L et al: Regional variation across the United States in the management of acute myocardial infarction. N Engl J Med 333:565, 1995

US DEPARTMENT OF HEALTH AND HUMAN SERVICES: *Healthy People 2000.* DHHS publication No. (PHS) 91-50213, Washington, DC, 1990

WHITE et al: Lesbian health care. What a primary care physician needs to know. Western J Med 162:463, 1995

WILKINSON RG: National mortality rates: The impact of inequality? Am J Public Health 82:1082, 1992

---

5 *Howard Hu, Frank E. Speizer*

INFLUENCE OF ENVIRONMENTAL AND OCCUPATIONAL HAZARDS ON DISEASE

Exposures to hazardous materials and processes in the home, the workplace, and the community can cause or exacerbate a multitude of diseases. Physicians commonly treat the sequelae of such diseases in the practice of medicine; however, unless the underlying connection with hazardous exposures is identified and mitigated, treatment of manifestations rather than the cause at best only ameliorates the condition. At worst, the neglect of hazardous exposures may lead to both failure of treatment and failure to recognize a public health problem with wide significance.

No existing surveillance or reporting system can estimate the total contribution of hazardous exposures to morbidity and mortality. However, careful histories have identified occupational factors as etiologic in more than 10 percent of all admissions to general internal medicine wards in hospitals, with even higher percentages when the primary illness is either respiratory or musculoskeletal. Estimates of the number of new cases of disease due to work in the United States range from 125,000 to 350,000 per year; these cases do not include 5.3 million work-related injuries.

Environmental exposures are increasingly associated with decrements in measures of health whose outcomes range from subclinical to clinically catastrophic. For example, exposure to lead at levels that are common in the general population has been associated with increased blood pressure and decreased creatinine clearance. Ambient air pollution with respect to levels of ozone and fine-particulate matter recently has been related to increased rates of hospital admissions for respiratory and cardiovascular diseases and to increased mortality, respectively. Indoor exposures to radon and passive environmental tobacco smoke have been linked with an increased risk of lung cancer. While such data are suggestive but not necessarily conclusive with respect to causation, there is pressure on clinicians to be aware of and act on this type of information.

Patients are becoming increasingly concerned about hazardous exposures. More than 15 percent of patients seen in one study conducted in a primary care clinic expressed the opinion that their health problems were work-related, and 75 percent of this subgroup of patients reported exposure to one or more recognized toxic agents. Patients often want answers to very specific questions, such as: Is the water in our town safe to drink? Could my breathing problem be related to the new roofing sealant used in my building at work? Physicians are consulted because they are the most trusted sources of information on health risks, including chemical risks. Unfortunately, few physicians have more than rudimentary training in environmental and occupational medicine. Therefore, it becomes important for primary care physicians to be able to recognize cases having these elements and either to manage them or to make appropriate referrals.

Many manifestations of exposure-related illnesses are nonspecific (e.g., dizziness, headache) or are commonly encountered in general internal medicine (e.g., myocardial infarction, cancer). The establishment of a connection with a hazard requires a high index of suspicion and the application of fundamental concepts of environmental/occupational medicine. Furthermore, early recognition by physicians of unusual patterns of illness or of evidence of asymptomatic exposure to toxins with low-level effects (e.g., an elevated blood lead level) can alert health officials to the need for control measures. Case reports either sent to local authorities or published in the literature often prompt follow-up studies that can lead to the identification of new hazards. In many states and countries, the reporting by physicians of occupational/environmental diseases is mandatory. For instance, beginning in 1992, physicians in Massachusetts were required to report cases of pneumoconiosis, occupational asthma, carpal tunnel syndrome, and carbon monoxide poisoning, among other conditions. Identification of an environmental/occupational etiology of an illness may have important economic ramifications for the patient (e.g., the awarding of worker's compensation, which covers medical bills as well as lost wages). Finally, physicians are frequently asked to provide expert medical testimony during litigation on the causal relationship between toxic exposures and diseases. In this setting, the more knowledgeable the physician is about potential hazardous exposures, the better prepared he/she is to serve the patient.

THE ILL PATIENT: RECOGNIZING A CHEMICAL OR OTHER ENVIRONMENTAL ETIOLOGY

DEFINITION OF ENVIRONMENTAL/OCCUPATIONAL HAZARDS The term *hazards* encompasses chemical factors as well as other risks posed by the physical environment (changes in temperature and in altitude and/or pressure, exposures to ionizing and nonionizing radiation) and by selected natural phenomena (venoms and stings). A detailed discussion of specific hazards can be found in Part 15. Unless otherwise defined, the terms *toxins* and *toxic exposures* are synonymous with *hazards*. These hazards may exist in the general environment or in the workplace. Strictly speaking, smoking, alcohol ingestion, nutritional factors, and infectious diseases can also be considered chemical or environmental hazards.

THE ENVIRONMENTAL/OCCUPATIONAL HISTORY For a physician, the most critical steps toward recognizing these disorders are remembering to consider them in the differential diagnosis and taking an appropriate environmental/occupational history as part of the medical workup. The level of detail that is called for depends on the clinical situation. *Information should always be obtained on current and major past occupations, and patients should be asked whether they think their health problem is related to their work or to any particular environment or exposure.* In the review of systems, patients should also be asked if they have been exposed to dusts, fumes, chemicals, radiation, or loud noise. When patient and physician are confronted with an illness of uncertain etiology, these factors should be explored in more detail, with the environmental/occupational history as the point of departure. (A brief outline of a sample history is shown in Table 5-1.)

Table 5-1

Initial Clinical Approach to the Recognition of Illness Caused by Environmental or Occupational Hazards

A. Screening questions
  1. Chief symptom and history of present illness
    • What kind of work do you do?
    • Do you think your health problems are related to your work, home, or any other particular environment or exposures?
    • Does the timing of your symptoms have any relation to being at work or at home or to any other particular exposures or activities?
  2. Review of systems
    • Are you now or have you previously been exposed to dusts, fumes, chemicals, radiation, or loud noise?
B. Detailed questioning based on initial suspicion
  • Chronology of jobs: Job title, type of industry, dates of work, description of job, a typical day, potentially hazardous exposures, protective equipment used
  • Chronology of residences: Description of potentially hazardous exposures (e.g., furnaces, pesticide application, home hobbies involving chemicals)
  • Identification of other employees or household members who have similar health problems
  • Exploration in detail of the temporal link between potential exposures and the chief symptom
  • Clinical clues (suspicious scenarios; see text)

SOURCE: Adapted from Newman, 1995.

The identification of specific chemical exposures can be difficult. Household products must list chemical ingredients on their labels, and this information may prove useful. For workplace exposures, the U.S. Occupational Safety and Health Administration (OSHA) requires chemical suppliers to provide material safety data sheets with their products and requires employers to retain these sheets and make them available to employees. The data sheets can be obtained by the physician or employee by a telephoned or written request; failure of an employer to provide them within 30 days of such a request is a violation of OSHA regulations and is punishable by fines. In addition to providing information on chemical ingredients and percent composition, the material safety data sheets provide basic information on toxicity. This information is seldom adequate from a clinical perspective but may indicate the general type of toxicity to be anticipated.

EVALUATION OF POSSIBLE CHEMICAL OR ENVIRONMENTAL HAZARDS Given the wide variety of toxic exposures that may be uncovered during a workup, a clinician should routinely consult additional reference material to evaluate whether particular hazards may be associated with the illness at hand. Many sources of information exist. OSHA and some regional poison-control centers have extensive information on hazards and brief summary documents that can be transmitted by telephone or facsimile. Depending on the area, other resources may include county and state health departments; regional offices of the National Institute for Occupational Safety and Health and the Environmental Protection Agency; the Consumer Products Safety Commission in Washington, D.C.; academic institutions; and individual toxicologists, occupational/environmental medicine specialists, or industrial hygienists. Sophisticated computerized databases are also available, including detailed listings on CD-ROM information systems. MEDLARS, the electronic database maintained by the National Library of Medicine, is accessible by modem and is familiar to many physicians. Files other than MEDLINE, such as the Hazardous Substances Databank, provide specific toxicity information on chemicals and include toxicologic references not covered by MEDLINE. Many of these databases can also be accessed through the Internet.

As with any other illness, laboratory investigation may be crucial. For example, tests of carboxyhemoglobin level to document carbon monoxide exposure or of serum anticholinesterase level to document organophosphate pesticide absorption should be performed within hours of exposure. As in cases of acute drug overdose, it is useful to freeze samples of urine and serum from any patient suspected of having had an acute chemical exposure; such specimens can be analyzed at a later date by sensitive methods of detection. Use of other tests must rely on knowledge of the specific hazard or illness in question.

SUSPICIOUS SCENARIOS   Some medical problems or clinical scenarios demand a particularly high degree of suspicion of occupational or environmental factors as causative or contributing agents.

Respiratory Disease   The contribution of occupational/environmental factors to respiratory disease is generally underrecognized, particularly among patients who smoke and among the elderly (see Chap. 254). For instance, asthma related to chemical exposure may be treated without regard to cause or may be erroneously diagnosed as acute tracheobronchitis. Shortness of breath from asbestosis may be attributed to chronic obstructive pulmonary disease. Chemical pneumonitis may be misdiagnosed as a bacterial infection.

Cancer   Many cancers are thought to be causally related to occupational and environmental factors in addition to tobacco. Some are particularly likely to have a chemical etiology or another environmental cause, including cancers of the skin (solar radiation, arsenic, coal tar, soot); lung (asbestos, arsenic, nickel, radon); pleura (almost exclusively asbestos); nasal cavity and sinuses (chromium, nickel, wood and leather dusts); liver (arsenic, vinyl chloride); bone marrow (benzene, ionizing radiation); and bladder (aromatic amines).

Coronary Disease   Carbon monoxide exposure is common, particularly in homes with malfunctioning furnaces or in workplaces close to motor vehicle exhaust. By reducing oxygen transport by hemoglobin and inhibiting mitochondrial metabolism, carbon monoxide can aggravate coronary disease. Methylene chloride, a solvent used in paint stripping, is converted to carbon monoxide and thus poses the same risk. Exposure to carbon disulfide, a chemical used in the production of rayon, accelerates the rate of atherosclerotic plaque formation.

Hepatitis/Chronic Liver Disease   In the absence of evidence that a virus infection, alcohol ingestion, or drug use is the main cause of hepatitis (see Chaps. 295, 296, and 297), the involvement of a toxin must be considered. Toxin-induced hepatic injury may be cytotoxic, cholestatic, or both. The list of hepatotoxic agents is long, including organic synthetic compounds such as carbon tetrachloride (used in solvents and cleaning fluids) and methylene diamine (a resin hardener); pesticides such as chlordecone (Kepone); metals, particularly arsenic (used in pesticides and paints and found in well water); and natural toxins such as the pyrrolidizine alkaloids.

Kidney Disease   Many chemical and environmental factors can cause renal injury (see Chap. 270). The etiology of much chronic kidney disease, however, remains unknown. An increasing body of evidence now links chronic renal failure with hypertension to lead exposure. Some studies suggest that chronic exposure to hydrocarbons (e.g., gasoline, paints, solvents) may lead to various types of glomerulonephritis, including Goodpasture's syndrome.

Peripheral Neuropathy   Organic solvents such as *n*-hexane, heavy metals such as lead and arsenic, and some organophosphate compounds can damage the axons of peripheral nerves. Dimethylaminopropionitrile, an industrial catalyst, causes bladder neuropathy. Nerve entrapment syndromes of the upper extremity, such as carpal tunnel syndrome, may be caused by jobs that involve repetitive motion, especially those requiring the maintenance of awkward positions.

Neuropsychiatric Symptoms   Fatigue, memory loss, difficulty in concentration, and emotional lability have been linked to chronic exposure to solvents such as toluene and perchloroethylene. Painters, metal degreasers, plastics workers, and cleaners are commonly exposed to solvents and develop these symptoms at a high rate. Characteristic patterns on formal neurobehavioral testing and stabilization of symptoms with gradual improvement after discontinuation of the exposure are among the features that distinguish these patients. Other substances associated with neurobehavioral dysfunction include metals, particularly lead, mercury, arsenic, and manganese; pesticides, such as organophosphates and organochlorines; and gases such as carbon monoxide.

Teratogenesis and Reproductive Problems   Toxins can impair successful reproduction at a variety of levels. Examples include insecticides and herbicides, PCBs (polychlorinated biphenyls) and PBBs (polybrominated biphenyls), ethylene oxide (a sterilizing gas used in hospitals), metals (lead, arsenic, cadmium, mercury), and solvents. Dibromochloropropane, a nematocide, suppresses spermatogenesis. Some toxins, such as PCBs, PBBs, and chlorinated pesticides, are concentrated in milk.

Immunosuppression, Autoimmunity, and Hypersensitivity   Evidence is increasing that exposures to some chemical agents can compromise the immune system, thereby leading to a generalized increased incidence of tumors (e.g., exposure to PBBs) or infections (e.g., respiratory infections after exposure to common air pollutants). Mercury, dieldrin, and methylcholanthrene are known to elicit autoimmune responses. Some chemicals are potent allergic sensitizers that cause dermal and respiratory problems (see Chaps. 254 and 311).

BIOLOGICAL MARKERS   An increasing number of methods are available for measuring and interpreting toxic exposure, including (1) the internal dose of specific toxins and (2) markers of the biological effects of toxins. Internal-dose markers are relevant for toxins that are sequestered in the human body, such as lead (in blood), arsenic (in hair), and other metals (see Chap. 397), and halogenated compounds (such as PCBs). Markers of the biological effects of toxins include depressed levels of acetylcholinesterase in serum after exposure to organophosphate pesticides and sister chromatid exchanges in peripheral lymphocytes after exposure to the carcinogen ethylene oxide.

MANAGING A HAZARD-RELATED ILLNESS

Once a chemical or another environmental hazard has been identified as an important contributor to an illness, the next step is to prevent further exposure. For chronic diseases such as cancer, this step is irrelevant; the illness remains when the exposure has come and gone. For others, the physician *must be willing to become an active advocate for the patient*. This advocacy may involve writing a letter stating that the patient should no longer be exposed to a hazard or should remain out of work. Alternatively, it may involve contacting appropriate officials in government, industry, or labor or other advocates who can deal with a hazardous exposure. Treatment is dependent on the specific hazard.

In few areas of medicine does a physician deal with more scientific uncertainty. Comprehensive information on toxicants is available for only a small percentage of chemicals. In general, the physician should take a conservative approach (i.e., advise the patient to avoid a hazard likely to have contributed to illness) and should use common sense and up-to-date information to evaluate causal relationships.

LOW-LEVEL EXPOSURES AND THEIR EFFECTS

The subclinical effects of toxins that are widespread in our environment and our workplaces are of increasing concern. Given the absence of any demonstrable effect threshold, low-level exposure to carcinogens should be avoided; not only carcinogenic but also noncarcinogenic effects of chronic low-level exposure to these substances are important.

Perhaps lead provides the most important example of low-level noncarcinogenic effects that constitute a major public health problem. Multiple pathways of exposure, including the combustion of leaded gasoline, the use of lead-based paints and solder, and the presence of lead in cans containing food, have contributed to exposure of the entire population. Such low-level exposures can impair neurobehavioral development in infants and children and can raise blood pressure in adults. Furthermore, absorbed lead is stored in the skeleton and may reenter the circulation at times of heightened bone turnover (e.g., pregnancy, lactation, osteoporosis, hyperthyroidism). Subclinical toxic effects can be prevented if chronic low-level exposure is detected early and curtailed. In the case of lead, such exposure is detected by tests of blood lead level, which should be performed regularly in young children living in old neighborhoods and as a precautionary measure in adults with a history of lead exposure.

BIBLIOGRAPHY

BALMES J et al: Hospital records as a data source for occupational disease surveillance: A feasibility study. Am J Ind Med 21:341, 1992

DOCKERY DW et al: An association between air pollution and mortality in six U.S. cities. N Engl J Med 329:1753, 1993

GENNART J-P et al: Importance of accurate employment histories of patients admitted to units of internal medicine. Scand J Work Environ Health 17:386, 1991

HIMMELSTEIN JS, FRUMKIN H: The right to know about toxic exposures: Implications for physicians. N Engl J Med 312:687, 1985

INSTITUTE OF MEDICINE: *Role of the Primary Care Physician in Occupational and Environmental Medicine.* Washington, DC, National Academy Press, 1988

————: *Environmental Medicine—Integrating a Missing Element into Medical Education*, AM Pope, DP Rall (eds). Washington, DC, National Academy Press, 1995

KNEIP TJ, CRABLE JV: *Methods for Biological Monitoring—A Manual for Assessing Human Exposure to Hazardous Substances.* Washington, DC, American Public Health Association, 1988

MORRIS RD et al: Ambient air pollution and hospitalization for congestive heart failure among elderly people in seven large U.S. cities. Am J Public Health 85:1361, 1995

MULLAN RJ, MURTHY LI: Occupational sentinel health events: An up-dated list for physician recognition and public health surveillance. Am J Ind Med 19:775, 1991

NEWMAN LS: Current concepts: Occupational illness. N Engl J Med 333:1128, 1995

PAUL M (ed): *Occupational/Environmental Hazards and Reproductive Health: A Guide for Clinicians.* Baltimore, Williams & Wilkins, 1992

ROSENSTOCK L, CULLEN MR (eds): *Textbook of Clinical Occupational and Environmental Medicine.* Philadelphia, WB Saunders, 1994

SULLIVAN JB JR, KRIEGER GR (eds): *Hazardous Materials Toxicology.* Baltimore, Williams & Wilkins, 1992

| 6 | *Anthony L. Komaroff, Celeste Robb-Nicholson, Beverly Woo* |

WOMEN'S HEALTH

In recent years, the medical problems and health care of women have received increasing attention. There are differences in morbidity and mortality between men and women. Most illnesses that can affect both men and women have not been as well studied in women. Many research studies of disease prevention and pathophysiology have included only male subjects. There are poorly understood differences in the expression of diseases in the two sexes. Finally, it appears that women receive different care than men for certain health problems that are common to both sexes.

MORBIDITY AND MORTALITY IN WOMEN **Morbidity** Over and above obstetric and gynecologic conditions, women experience or report greater morbidity than men. Studies have found that women experience a 25 percent higher rate of restricted activity and a 40 percent higher rate of bed disability, adjusted across all ages. Women also make more visits to physicians, particularly for acute self-limited illnesses. It is unclear whether there are real differences in the prevalence of morbidity or differences in care-seeking behavior following the perception of symptoms.

Mortality In the developed nations, women live longer than men. In 1995, in the United States, the projected average life expectancy from birth is 79.7 years for females and 72.8 years for males. Although more male fetuses are conceived than female fetuses, females have a survival advantage over males in all age groups. The longer life expectancy of women in developed countries, compared to men, is due in large part to the difference in mortality caused by ischemic heart disease (IHD).

As shown in Table 6-1, the leading causes of death among young women in the United States are accidents, homicide, and suicide. During the middle years, breast cancer is a slightly more common cause of death than IHD and lung cancer. In women between ages 65 and 74, IHD, lung cancer, and cerebrovascular disease overtake breast cancer as the leading causes of death. Among women of *all* ages, IHD is the leading cause of death, by a substantial margin, with a mortality rate five to sixfold higher than the rate for either lung or breast cancer. Nevertheless, a recent Gallup poll found that U.S. women believe breast cancer poses the greatest threat to their lives.

Social Factors Influencing Morbidity and Mortality Gender differences in morbidity and mortality may be explained in part by psychosocial factors such as socially defined gender roles, poverty, participation in the work force, health insurance, and life-style factors.

In the past 30 years in the United States, there has been a "feminization of poverty"—i.e., a rapid growth in the relative percentage of people in female-headed households who are living in poverty. One-third of families headed by women currently live in poverty, and the fraction is greater than one-half for African-American and Latina women. Almost a fifth of women over age 65 in the United States live below the poverty level. Women constitute a majority of the poor in all societies. People of lower socioeconomic status experience poorer health and a higher mortality rate than those in higher income groups. Although women of lower socioeconomic status have a smaller risk of breast cancer than women of higher socioeconomic status, they are less likely to be diagnosed at an early stage of the disease. The poor are more likely to smoke and less likely to use recommended preventive measures, including cancer screening. Lack of adequate health insurance is a major problem for many women, especially minority women, poor and low-income women, and women of reproductive age. Women in general are more likely than men to have low-paying, part-time, non-union jobs that do not provide health insurance. Women who are divorced or widowed may also lose health insurance that they had through their husbands.

Biological Factors Influencing Morbidity and Mortality Certain biological differences also contribute to the greater longevity of women. The most obvious is the exposure to estrogen that most women experience for about 40 years of their lives, which may provide some protection from IHD.

PREVENTION (See also Chap. 10) Primary prevention and screening are crucial elements in improving the health of women. Although there are few definitive clinical trials of preventive interventions in women, a growing number of large case-control and prospec-

Table 6-1

Death Rates (per 100,000) for the Leading Causes of Death in U.S. Women, 1990

Ages 24–34 Total: 74.2	Ages 45–54 Total: 342.7	Ages 65–74 Total: 1991.2	All Ages Total: 812.0
1. Motor vehicle accidents (11.5)	1. Breast cancer (45.4)	1. Ischemic heart disease (415.2)	1. Ischemic heart disease (185.6)
2. Homicide (7.2)	2. Ischemic heart disease (33.6)	2. Lung cancer* (181.7)	2. Cerebrovascular disease (68.6)
3. Suicide (5.6)	3. Lung cancer* (35.3)	3. Cerebrovascular disease (126.9)	3. Lung cancer* (40.4)
4. Non-motor vehicle accidents (4.6)	4. Cerebrovascular disease (17.0)	4. Breast cancer (111.7)	4. Breast cancer (34.0)

* Cancer of respiratory and intrathoracic organs, predominantly lung cancer.

SOURCE: Adapted from National Center for Health Statistics: *Vital Statistics of the United States, 1990*, vol II: *Mortality*, Part A. Washington, Public Health Service, 1994. DHHS Publication No. (PHS)95-1101, pp 40–52.

tive cohort observational studies (such as the Nurses' Health Study) have evaluated the prevention of disease in women. Based on available literature and experience, various authoritative organizations (e.g., the U.S. Preventive Services Task Force, Canadian Task Force, American College of Physicians, American Heart Association, American Cancer Society) have published guidelines on preventive practices in women.

While the annual comprehensive physical examination is no longer recommended, most physicians believe that a baseline history and physical examination is useful to set the stage for preventive measures appropriate to each patient. Most authorities recommend that blood pressure be measured every other year throughout life. Counseling on diet, smoking cessation, exercise, and use of seatbelts are of demonstrated value in the primary prevention of diseases and accidents. Counseling about safe sexual practices, alcohol abuse, and violence are recommended.

Screening for glaucoma is recommended for African-American women over age 40 and for Caucasian women over age 50. Yearly examinations to test visual acuity are recommended for women over age 70.

Regular screening for breast, cervical, and colorectal cancer is recommended, but how often tests should be performed and which tools to use are controversial. Most authorities recommend annual clinical breast examination in all women beginning at age 35 to 40. There is strong evidence to support the efficacy of annual mammography in women aged 50 to 59. For women aged 60 and older, the evidence for screening is less strong. Screening for women between the ages of 40 and 49 remains controversial.

Most authorities recommend Pap-smear screening beginning at age 18 or when a woman becomes sexually active. After two or three consecutive normal Pap smears, most groups recommend Pap smear testing every 3 years. If Pap smears have been normal for 10 years, they can be discontinued in women after age 65.

Recommendations for colorectal cancer screening vary, and there are no randomized controlled trials that have demonstrated a benefit. Rectal examination and fecal occult blood testing lack sensitivity and specificity. Randomized trials are underway to evaluate the benefit of flexible sigmoidoscopy.

One major risk factor, cigarette smoking, has been well studied in women. In 1990, 28 percent of men and 23 percent of women were regular smokers. Over the past 60 years there has been a sharp decline in smoking among men, but not among women. "Low-yield" cigarettes are marketed heavily to women; however, users of these cigarettes have the same risk of myocardial infarction as users of higher-yield brands. The Nurses' Health Study showed that one-third of the excess risk of IHD was eliminated two years after smoking cessation, and that all of the excess risk was eliminated by 10 to 14 years after smoking cessation.

Although reduction of serum cholesterol has been associated with a decreased risk of IHD in men, primary prevention studies have included far smaller numbers of women. It is likely that improvement of lipid profiles will decrease the risk of IHD in women, but that has not been proved. The National Cholesterol Education Program recommends that total cholesterol and high-density lipoprotein (HDL) levels be measured once. If both are normal, a repeat test after 5 years is recommended.

Postmenopausal estrogen therapy is associated with a 40 to 50 percent reduction in deaths due to IHD, a finding supported by several case-control studies. Calcium and estrogen replacement therapy have been shown to slow the development of osteoporosis and to reduce the frequency of hip and vertebral fracture in the postmenopausal woman.

Considerable research indicates that a relatively high dietary intake of various antioxidants (including vitamins C and E) is associated with lower rates of vascular disease and malignancies. Randomized trials of supplemental antioxidants are under way. Preliminary research indicates that regular aspirin use is associated with reduced rates of IHD and colorectal carcinoma.

GENDER DIFFERENCES IN DISEASE Obviously, some diseases and conditions occur exclusively (or nearly exclusively) in women—e.g., menopause and various breast and gynecologic disorders. These are discussed elsewhere in this book (Chaps. 48, 91, 337, 338). In this chapter, we seek primarily to highlight some gender differences in diseases that occur in both women and men.

Ischemic Heart Disease (See also Chap. 244)   Many persons think of IHD as primarily a problem of men, perhaps because men have more than twice the total incidence of cardiovascular morbidity and mortality than women between the ages of 35 and 84. However, as stated earlier, in the United States IHD is the leading cause of death among women as well as men (Table 6-1), although the curve for mortality rate from IHD lags behind that for men by about a decade. Nearly 250,000 women die annually from IHD; after age 40, one in three women will die from heart disease. Although IHD mortality has been falling in the United States over the past 30 years, the rate of decline has been lower in women than in men.

Why are rates of IHD lower in women? Women have a more favorable risk profile in some respects: higher HDL cholesterol levels, lower triglyceride levels, and less upper-body obesity than men. But women also have a less favorable risk profile in other respects: more obesity, higher blood pressure, higher plasma cholesterol levels, higher fibrinogen levels, and more diabetes. The simplest explanation for the sex differential in IHD is a "cardioprotective" effect of estrogen, due to improvement of the lipid profile, a direct vasodilatory effect, and perhaps other factors. HDL cholesterol levels appear to be a particularly important risk factor for IHD in women. HDL levels are higher in all age groups in women compared to men, and are higher in premenopausal and estrogen-treated postmenopausal women than in non-estrogen-treated postmenopausal women. Smoking is the most important risk factor for IHD in women.

IHD presents differently in men and women. In the Framingham study, angina was the most frequent initial symptom of IHD in women, occurring in 47 percent of women. Myocardial infarction was the most frequent initial symptom in men, occurring in 46 percent of men. The exercise electrocardiogram appears to have a lower specificity for IHD in women than in men.

Women, particularly African-American women, have higher risks of morbidity and mortality than men following a myocardial infarction. Compared to men, women having coronary artery bypass graft surgery have more advanced disease, a higher perioperative mortality rate, less relief of angina, and less graft patency, but similar 5 and 10 year survival rates. Women undergoing percutaneous transluminal coronary angioplasty have lower rates of clinical and angiographic success than men, but also a lower rate of restenosis and a better long-term outcome. Women may benefit less and have more frequent serious bleeding complications from thrombolytic therapy than do men. Factors such as older age, more comorbid conditions, and more severe IHD in women at the time of events or procedures appear to account for at least part of the gender differences observed. As demonstrated in the CARE trial, women with IHD benefit at least as much as men, and perhaps more, from reductions in cholesterol level.

Hypertension (See also Chap. 246)   Hypertension is more common in U.S. women than men, largely owing to the high prevalence of hypertension in older age groups and the longer survival of women. Renovascular hypertension from fibromuscular dysplasia occurs more often in women. Other causes of secondary hypertension occur with equal frequency in women and men. Both the effectiveness and the adverse effects of various antihypertensive drugs appear to be comparable in women and men. Benefits of treatment for severe hypertension have been dramatic in both women and men. However, in clinical trials of the treatment of mild to moderate hypertension, women have had a smaller decrease in morbidity and mortality than men, perhaps because women have a lower risk of myocardial infarction and stroke than men to begin with. Older women benefit at least as much as men from treatment, as demonstrated by the Systolic Hypertension in the Elderly study. When oral contraceptives were first introduced, many women had a small increase in blood pressure, with 5 percent showing an increase to above 140/90 over a 5-year period. The incidence of hypertension appears to be lower with the current low-dose oral contraceptives. Postmenopausal estrogen therapy is not associated with increases in blood pressure.

Immune-Mediated Diseases Several immune-mediated diseases—e.g., rheumatoid arthritis, systemic lupus erythematosus, multiple sclerosis, Graves' disease, and thyroiditis—occur much more frequently in women than in men. In animal models of rheumatoid arthritis, lupus, and multiple sclerosis, for example, it is females that are predominantly affected. On the other hand, animal studies indicate that females are less susceptible to infection.

In short, women and female animals appear to have more vigorous immune responses, with both beneficial and adverse consequences. Increasing evidence indicates that estrogens up-regulate both cellular and humoral immunity. Some immunocytes contain receptors for estrogen, progestin, and androgens, and the uterus produces a variety of cytokines. The reproductive and immune systems clearly interact in a complex way.

Osteoporosis Estrogen secretion also appears to play an important role in the control of bone density. While it is clear that the risk of osteoporosis in postmenopausal women is much greater than in men of the same age, and while postmenopausal estrogen supplementation is associated with a decreased incidence of osteoporosis, the mechanisms by which estrogen exerts its protective effects are not fully elucidated.

Psychological Disorders Depression, bulimia, and anorexia nervosa occur more often in women, as may anxiety disorders. Epidemiologic studies from both developed and developing nations consistently find major depression to be twice as common in women as in men, with the gender disparity becoming evident in early adolescence. The incidence of major depression in women diminishes after age 45. Interestingly, the incidence of depression does not increase with the onset of menopause, a time of symbolic and actual loss. Depression in women also appears to have a worse prognosis than in men: episodes of depression last longer, and there is a lower rate of spontaneous remission.

Depression occurs in 10 percent of women during pregnancy and in 10 to 15 percent of women during the first several months of the postpartum period. The treatment of depression during pregnancy or in the postpartum nursing mother is problematic: Relatively little is known about the possible teratogenic effects of many antidepressants, and it is uncertain whether the dosing of psychotropic drugs should be different in pregnancy.

Social factors may account for the greater prevalence of some disorders in women; the traditionally subordinate role of women in society may generate helplessness and frustration which, in turn, contribute to psychiatric illness. In addition, it is likely that biological factors, including hormonally influenced neurochemical changes, also play an important role. The limbic system and hypothalamus, areas of the brain thought to subserve appetite, satiety, and emotion, contain estradiol and testosterone receptors.

Alcohol Abuse One-third of Americans who suffer from alcoholism are women. Women alcoholics are less likely to be diagnosed than men. On average, alcoholic women drink less than alcoholic men but exhibit the same degree of impairment. Blood alcohol levels are higher in women than in men after drinking equivalent amounts of alcohol (adjusted for body weight). This greater bioavailability of alcohol in women is probably due to the higher proportion of body fat and to a lower gastric "first-pass metabolism" of alcohol, associated with lower activity of gastric alcohol dehydrogenase. In addition, alcoholic women are more likely than alcoholic men to abuse tranquilizers, sedatives, and amphetamines.

Women alcoholics have a higher mortality rate than both nonalcoholic women and alcoholic men. Compared to men, women also appear to develop alcoholic liver disease and other alcohol-related diseases with shorter drinking histories and lower levels of alcohol consumption. Alcohol abuse also poses special risks to a woman, adversely affecting fertility and the health of the baby (fetal alcohol syndrome).

Human Immunodeficiency Virus Infection (See also Chap. 308) In the United States, more than 20,000 women have developed AIDS, and an estimated 80,000 to 140,000 women have been infected with human immunodeficiency virus (HIV). In 1994, 18 percent of the reported cases of AIDS in persons over age 12 occurred in women, compared to 7 percent of the reported AIDS cases in 1985. The disease continues to affect women in racial/ethnic minorities and lower socioeconomic classes disproportionately. More than half of American women with AIDS are current or past users of intravenous drugs, compared to more than 70 percent of American men with AIDS. Heterosexual contact with an at-risk partner is the fastest-growing transmission category for women and is associated with most of the cases in non-intravenous drug users. About half of women who apparently were infected with HIV by heterosexual transmission did not know that they had been exposed to HIV.

Studies have not consistently demonstrated gender-related differences in the natural history of HIV infection. Compared with men, HIV-infected women more frequently suffer from esophageal candidiasis and less frequently develop Kaposi's sarcoma. Preventive and therapeutic measures appear to be comparably effective for HIV-infected women and men. Some studies have found that women have less access to care than do men.

Violence Against Women There has been a growing awareness of the enormous problem of violence against women, both rape and domestic violence. Rape has been redefined recently in many statutes as "nonconsensual sexual penetration of an adolescent or adult obtained by physical force, by threat of bodily harm, or when the victim is incapable of giving consent by virtue of mental illness, mental retardation, or intoxication." Epidemiologic studies in the United States suggest that at least 20 percent of adult women have experienced sexual assault during their lifetime. Nearly 100,000 cases of rape are reported annually in the United States, and this undoubtedly represents only a fraction of the actual number of cases. Adult women are much more likely to be raped by a spouse, ex-spouse, or acquaintance than by a stranger.

Domestic violence is an enormous problem in the United States. The American Medical Association guidelines define domestic violence as "an ongoing, debilitating experience of physical, psychologic, and/or sexual abuse in the home, associated with increasing isolation from the outside world and limited personal freedom and accessibility to resources." Every year in the United States, more than two million women (likely a low estimate, owing to underreporting) are severely injured and more than 1000 women are killed by their current or former male partner. Domestic violence is the most common cause of physical injury in women, exceeding the combined incidence of all other types of injury (such as from rape, mugging, and auto accidents). Surveys of women seeking medical care for any reason in internal medicine and emergency room practices have reported that the prevalence of domestic violence is an astonishing 15 to 30 percent. Domestic violence is a major health problem in women from all age, ethnic, and socioeconomic groups.

Women who have been raped or injured, as well as women who have been molested during childhood, frequently seek medical care for headaches, sleep and eating disorders, abdominal or pelvic pain, vaginal discharge, or musculoskeletal symptoms. They may also present to physicians with depression, suicidal ideation, and substance abuse. Given this indirect presentation of the consequences of violence, and the high prevalence of violence, clinicians should have a low threshold for pursuing the possibility of violence in female patients, particularly those with vague symptoms and psychological disorders.

The immediate treatment of rape and domestic violence is focused on assessing and treating physical injuries, on providing emotional support, on assessing and dealing with the risks of sexually transmitted infection and pregnancy, on evaluating the safety of the patient and other family members, and on documenting the patient's history and physical examination findings. In addition to dealing with the medical and psychological issues, appropriate care includes providing information about legal services, shelters and safe houses, hotlines, support groups, and counseling services.

RESEARCH IN WOMEN'S HEALTH Although women seek medical attention and use medications more frequently than men, historically relatively few women had been involved in studies of the prevention, pathophysiology, and treatment of diseases that involve both women and men. However, the growing recognition of the importance of women's health has spawned a number of research efforts. The U.S. National Institutes of Health (NIH) has introduced guidelines to mandate the inclusion of women in clinical studies.

Studies of Prevention The Framingham Study, an observational study of men and women under way since 1947, has been increasingly analyzing data specific to women. Since 1976, the Nurses' Health Study has been following more than 120,000 women, prospectively collecting data about their smoking, diet, physical activity, medications, prevention and screening behaviors, and some psychosocial factors. This study already has revealed information about how these factors contribute to the relative risk of developing a number of medical disorders, including breast cancer, ischemic heart disease, stroke, diabetes, and fracture, as well as to causes of mortality.

The Postmenopausal Estrogens/Progestins Intervention (PEPI) Trial was the first major trial testing the effects of postmenopausal hormone replacement therapy. It was a 3-year, multicenter, randomized, double-blind, placebo-control trial of the effects of three estrogen/progestin regimens on risk factors for cardiovascular disease, bone mineral density, and endometrial tissue. Thus far, the study has reported that estrogen alone or in combination with progestin increased serum levels of HDL and decreased low-density lipoprotein (LDL) and fibrinogen levels. While unopposed estrogen (without progestins) resulted in the most beneficial effects on lipids, it also was associated with an increased risk of endometrial hyperplasia.

In 1992, the NIH funded the Women's Health Initiative (WHI)—a study of the health of postmenopausal women. The WHI, the largest research study ever funded by the NIH, will involve 160,000 postmenopausal women at 45 clinical centers across the United States through the year 2002. The WHI includes both a prospective observational study and an interventional randomized trial designed to test strategies to prevent cardiovascular disease, breast cancer, and osteoporotic fractures—among the leading causes of death, disability, and diminished quality of life for older women. The clinical trial component of the WHI will involve 63,000 women in a randomized, controlled trial of the effects of a low-fat diet, hormone replacement therapy, and calcium and vitamin D supplementation on the risks for the illnesses cited above.

There are many other ongoing studies of the pathophysiology and prevention of diseases that affect women, and the next decade should be rich in data from this research.

Pharmacologic Treatment Over $30 billion worth of pharmaceuticals are sold each year in the United States, and the great majority are used by women. Women have been underrepresented in drug trials. In 1992, the U.S. Government Accounting Office reviewed pharmaceutical products that received Food and Drug Administration (FDA) approval between 1988 and 1991. The review concluded that 25 percent of the trials did not actively recruit women, that 30 percent included a smaller number of women than the FDA had recommended, and that in 60 percent of trials women were underrepresented relative to the gender distribution of the disease being treated. Two reasons are commonly given for conducting most clinical pharmacologic studies in men. First, cyclic hormonal changes in females could make experiments more difficult to control and interpret. Second, particularly with new drugs, concern about unsuspected pregnancy and subsequent teratogenic effects have discouraged the recruitment of female subjects.

The underrepresentation of women in drug trials is changing. The FDA now requires information on the safety and effectiveness of experimental drugs in women, on the effects of the menstrual cycle and menopause on a drug's pharmacokinetics, as well as on a drug's influence on the effectiveness of oral contraceptives. The increased emphasis on women in drug trials is likely to yield important information. Those studies that have included women indicate that there are clinically significant differences in the way women respond to a number of frequently prescribed pharmaceuticals, including sedative-hyp-

notics, antidepressants, antipsychotics, anticonvulsants, and beta-adrenoceptor blocking agents. The 1992 FDA Annual Adverse Experience Report found that women have a higher frequency of adverse drug reactions than men. Other studies suggest that the efficacy of many drugs may be different in women. For example, women require lower doses of neuroleptics to control schizophrenia than men do. The reasons for these differences are not clear. Estrogens may affect drug clearance via the cytochrome P450 oxidase system. In some instances, drug pharmacokinetics may change during the menstrual cycle. For example, there is reasonable evidence that some anticonvulsants and lithium may be metabolized more rapidly in the premenstrual period, resulting in an increased frequency of premenstrual ("catamenial") seizures and increased symptoms of bipolar disorder, respectively, in women treated with these drugs.

WOMEN AND HEALTH CARE REFORM The U.S. health care system is in the midst of major changes. Women, as the chief consumers of health care, and supported by an effective lay health movement, are having an increasing voice in this change. A number of women are seeking health care in multidisciplinary women's health units that combine expertise in gynecology, psychiatry, and internal or family medicine. Some internal medicine residency training programs are establishing tracks in women's health. The number of women physicians has grown by 300 percent between 1970 and 1990, and more than 40 percent of all U.S. medical students now are women. This infusion of women into the physician work force is likely to encourage the trend toward a greater recognition of the unique aspects of health and disease of women.

BIBLIOGRAPHY

BLUME SB: Women and alcohol. A review. JAMA 256:1467, 1986

BLUMENTHAL SJ et al: *Towards a Women's Health Research Agenda. Findings of the Scientific Advisory Meeting.* Washington, DC, Bass and Howes, 1991

BRAVEMAN P et al: Women without health insurance: Links between access, poverty, ethnicity, and health. West J Med 149:708, 1988

COLDITZ GA: The Nurses' Health Study: A cohort of U.S. women followed since 1976. JAMWA 50:40, 1995

COUNCIL ON SCIENTIFIC AFFAIRS, AMERICAN MEDICAL ASSOCIATION: Violence against women. Relevance for medical practitioners. JAMA 267:3184, 1992

GIJSBERS VAN WIJK CMT et al: Symptom sensitivity and sex differences in physical morbidity: A review of health surveys in the United States and the Netherlands. Women Health 17:91, 1991

KAPLAN NM: The treatment of hypertension in women. Arch Intern Med 185:563, 1995

MINKOFF HL, DEHOVITZ JA: Care of women infected with the human immunodeficiency virus. JAMA 266:2253, 1991

MURABITO JM: Women and cardiovascular disease: Contributions from the Framingham Heart Study. JAMWA 50:35, 1995

RICH-EDWARDS JW et al: The primary prevention of coronary heart disease in women. N Engl J Med 332:1758, 1995

RODIN J, ICKOVICS JR: Women's health. Review and research agenda as we approach the 21st century. Am Psychol 45:1018, 1990

THE WRITING GROUP FOR THE PEPI TRIAL: Effects of estrogen or estrogen/progestin regimens on heart disease risk factors in postmenopausal women: The Postmenopausal Estrogen/Progestin Interventions Trial. JAMA 273:199, 1995

VERBRUGGE LM, WINGARD DL: Sex differentials in health and mortality. Women Health 12:103, 1987

WEISSMAN MM, OLFSON M: Depression in women: Implications for health care research. Science 269:799, 1995

---

7   *Thomas F. Ferris*

MEDICAL DISORDERS DURING PREGNANCY

Pregnancy may be complicated by chronic disease or a new illness. In the past, many disorders were considered contraindications to pregnancy, but now, with appropriate care, excellent outcomes for both mother and child are the rule.

Systemic vascular resistance is reduced in pregnancy. In spite of a 40 percent increase in cardiac output during the second trimester, blood pressure falls (usually to 100/70 mmHg or lower). Although a modest rise may occur during the last month of normal pregnancy, an increase in systolic pressure of 30 mmHg or in diastolic pressure of 15 mmHg at any time during gestation is abnormal. Perinatal mortality increases with blood pressure levels that would be normal in nonpregnant women. For example, when mean arterial blood pressure (diastolic plus one-third of the pulse pressure) is 90 mmHg or higher during the second trimester, there is a greater risk for stillbirth, fetal growth retardation, and preeclampsia.

Hypertension during pregnancy usually has one of four causes: (1) preeclampsia (toxemia); (2) chronic essential hypertension; (3) gestational hypertension; and (4) renal disease.

PREECLAMPSIA (TOXEMIA) Preeclampsia is a disease of late pregnancy in which hypertension is associated with hepatic, neurologic, hematologic, or renal involvement. Rapid development of edema, particularly of the face and hands, along with a rise in blood pressure, often signals the onset of this condition. Jaundice and abnormal liver function may be present. Hyperreflexia, visual disturbances, and headache indicate neurologic involvement and raise concern for the development of convulsions, termed "eclampsia." Hematologic manifestations of preeclampsia include thrombocytopenia with elevated levels of lactate dehydrogenase (LDH), microangiopathic hemolytic anemia, and thrombocytopenia. This condition is termed HELLP (*h*emolysis, *e*levated *l*iver function tests, *l*ow *p*latelets). In fulminant preeclampsia, disseminated intravascular coagulation may cause a reduction in plasma fibrinogen and elevated circulating fibrin degradation products (Chap. 119).

Proteinuria indicates renal involvement, and is one of the hallmarks of preeclampsia. Since the glomerular filtration rate (GFR) increases by about 50 percent in normal gestation, a reduction in GFR heralds the onset of preeclampsia even with normal levels of blood urea nitrogen (BUN) and serum creatinine. Indeed, a BUN of 6.4 mmol/L (18 mg/dL) or a creatinine level of 90 μmol/L (1 mg/dL) during pregnancy may reflect a 50 percent decline in GFR. In preeclampsia, urate clearance decreases, because of increased proximal tubular reabsorption of urate, which in turn is probably due to the reduction of vascular volume. Hyperuricemia usually precedes the rise in serum creatinine and BUN; in fact, a plasma uric acid level above 270 μmol/L (4.5 mg/dL) in a hypertensive pregnant woman suggests preeclampsia. Volume contraction is similar to that in some other hypertensive states in which venoconstriction causes capillary pressure to rise, with expansion of interstitial volume at the expense of intravascular volume, but a generalized increase in capillary permeability may contribute also.

Fibrin deposits in the glomeruli, with characteristic swelling of the glomerular endothelial cells, are evident in renal biopsies; peripheral necrosis with fibrin deposits in the sinusoids may be present in the liver. Tomographic scanning techniques [computed tomography (CT) or magnetic resonance imaging (MRI)] reveal hypodense areas consistent with small cerebral infarctions in approximately half of the women with eclampsia.

An abnormality in endothelial integrity has been proposed as the cause of the widespread fibrin deposits. Increased synthesis of two vasodilator prostaglandins—prostaglandin (PGE_2) and prostacyclin (PGI_2)—may explain the vasodilation and resistance to angiotensin II in normal pregnancy. In preeclampsia, the synthesis of PGI_2 decreases while sensitivity to angiotensin II increases, and the balance that normally exists between the platelet-aggregative and vasoconstrictor effects of thromboxane A_2 (produced by platelets) and the counteracting antiaggregative and vasodilating effects of PGI_2 (produced by endothelial cells) may be lost, contributing to hypertension and platelet aggregation. The incidence of preeclampsia may be reduced in high-risk women when low-dose aspirin (an inhibitor of thromboxane A_2 synthesis) is administered throughout pregnancy. However, no benefit from low-dose aspirin therapy has been demonstrated in low-risk women.

TREATMENT

Once preeclampsia is diagnosed, hospitalization is indicated, since the disease can progress rapidly to multisystem involvement, including eclampsia, characterized by convulsions. The definitive treatment of preeclampsia and eclampsia is delivery of the conceptus, which should be carried out promptly if fetal size and maturity are adequate. If the fetus is immature, bed rest, restriction of sodium intake to 2 g/d or less, and antihypertensive therapy may be attempted. However, if clinical deterioration occurs in the mother or fetus despite these measures, the fetus should be delivered regardless of gestational age. Beta blockers, calcium antagonists, hydralazine, and central sympathetic antagonists are all useful agents. Angiotensin converting enzyme (ACE) inhibitors are *contraindicated in pregnancy* since they increase the risk for fetal loss.

If an immediate reduction in blood pressure is needed, as in other forms of severe, uncontrolled hypertension (Chap. 246), several agents are useful. These include intravenous hydralazine (10 mg every 15 min until the desired effect is maintained); 500 mg α-methyldopa given over 30 min; and labetalol (1 mg/kg given intravenously, followed by a continuous infusion of 20 mg/h). Intravenous magnesium sulfate is an anticonvulsant and vasodilator that increases the synthesis of PGI_2 by endothelial cells and is used to prevent the development or recurrence of eclampsia. Recently, magnesium sulfate has been shown to be superior to phenytoin or diazepam in this regard.

CHRONIC ESSENTIAL HYPERTENSION (Chap. 246) Like normal women, those with chronic essential hypertension experience a reduction in peripheral resistance during pregnancy. Indeed, a "normal" blood pressure may be obtained for the first time during pregnancy. Women with chronic hypertension are at higher risk for preeclampsia. Careful monitoring for proteinuria and of serum levels of creatinine and uric acid are important in detecting the onset of this complication. There is no evidence that pregnancy has an adverse effect on the course of chronic essential hypertension. Thus, antihypertensive medication (other than ACE inhibitors) should be continued throughout pregnancy in women with essential hypertension. α-Methyldopa has been used extensively in pregnancy, and children born to mothers who have taken this drug throughout pregnancy develop normally.

GESTATIONAL HYPERTENSION Hypertension that develops late in pregnancy (with no end-organ manifestations characteristic of preeclampsia) and disappears after delivery is termed *gestational hypertension*. Usually, women with this condition are overweight; others have a family history of hypertension, develop chronic essential hypertension later in life, and have a high incidence of recurrence during subsequent pregnancies. Attention must be directed toward detecting increases in urinary protein and serum levels of uric acid, creatinine, or BUN, since these remain normal in gestational hypertension and become elevated in preeclampsia. A beta blocker or α-methyldopa are usually effective in lowering blood pressure.

RENAL DISEASE

The increase in GFR during normal pregnancy is due to a rise in renal plasma flow without a concomitant elevation in glomerular pressure. However, in renal disease, any rise in GFR depends on an elevation in glomerular pressure, which can increase proteinuria and worsen the underlying disease. Hypertension becomes more severe during pregnancy in most women with chronic renal disease, and proteinuria increases in approximately 20 percent. Since autoregulation of renal blood flow may be impaired in renal disease, any increase in blood pressure is more apt to raise glomerular pressure. The development or worsening of hypertension during pregnancy in patients with renal disease may be due to preeclampsia superimposed on renal disease.

It is desirable to maintain blood pressure below 120/80 mmHg in pregnant women with chronic renal disease. The 24-h urine protein excretion should be assessed throughout pregnancy, and an increase in proteinuria with no clinical evidence of toxemia usually reflects elevated glomerular pressure. Antihypertensive drugs other than ACE inhibitors should be used.

Many women have had successful pregnancies after renal transplantation. Although these patients receive chronic immunosuppressive therapy throughout gestation, the incidence of congenital malformations does not appear to be increased.

If systemic lupus erythematosus (SLE) (Chap. 312) is quiescent for 12 to 18 months prior to conception, pregnancy does not appear to activate the disease. In nonpregnant women, flare-ups of lupus nephropathy are usually associated with extrarenal manifestations of the disease, i.e., arthritis, rash, and fever, accompanied by a reduction in serum complement and a rise in anti-DNA antibodies. In contrast, pregnant women with SLE may manifest an increase in blood pressure and proteinuria along with a reduction in renal function in the absence of extrarenal manifestations. The renal exacerbations may be due to superimposed preeclampsia or to the effect of hypertension on the nephropathy, since there is no clinical evidence of lupus activity and no increase in anti-DNA antibodies. This is an important distinction, because these women may be treated inappropriately with higher doses of glucocorticoids or immunosuppressive agents (which may exacerbate hypertension) when antihypertensive therapy or delivery (depending on gestational age and maternal condition) is indicated instead. Conversely, women with active SLE who could be treated with glucocorticoids are often delivered inappropriately early for the mistaken diagnosis of preeclampsia.

CARDIAC DISEASE

As noted above, pregnancy is associated with a reduction in systemic vascular resistance. Normally, increases occur in blood volume, stroke volume, heart rate, and cardiac output; these changes often produce systolic (flow) murmurs and third heart sounds. The rise in cardiac output exceeds the increase in oxygen consumption, so the arteriovenous oxygen difference falls. Marked fluctuations in cardiac output occur during normal labor and delivery, and the following four cardiac disorders are adversely affected by pregnancy: (1) valvular heart disease; (2) primary pulmonary hypertension; (3) the Eisenmenger syndrome; and (4) the Marfan syndrome. Delivery or pregnancy termination appear to be the times of greatest risk for these patients.

VALVULAR HEART DISEASE (See Chap. 237) The increased cardiac output associated with pregnancy may cause deterioration in women with *mitral stenosis*. If severe mitral stenosis is identified *prior* to pregnancy, valvulotomy should be carried out before conception, if possible. Asymptomatic pregnant women with mitral stenosis require close observation but not definitive therapy. However, if symptoms of pulmonary congestion develop, diuretics and restriction of activity are indicated. Atrial fibrillation should be treated with oral digoxin and/or a beta blocker to slow the ventricular rate. The latter type of agent may also be useful in patients with sinus rhythm and relatively rapid heart rates (>80 beats per minute). Thromboembolism associated with mitral stenosis necessitates anticoagulation with intravenous heparin; warfarin is *contraindicated* in pregnancy because of its teratogenic effects. A closed mitral valvulotomy (surgical or, preferably, by balloon mitral valvuloplasty) can be carried out during pregnancy when symptoms of mitral stenosis are severe; open-heart surgery is associated with an increase in fetal loss.

Mitral regurgitation is usually well tolerated during pregnancy, presumably because peripheral resistance is lower. Critical *aortic stenosis* is a contraindication for pregnancy until the lesion has been corrected. A maternal mortality rate of 15 percent has been reported in women with critical aortic stenosis.

Balloon flotation (Swan-Ganz) catheters allow precise hemodynamic assessment and control during labor and delivery and in the immediate postpartum period.

Artificial heart valves in pregnant women are associated with many problems. It is mandatory to continue full anticoagulation in patients with mechanical valvular prostheses. Warfarin is contraindicated because of its teratogenic effects; subcutaneous heparin is preferable but may cause bleeding and fetal loss. Tissue valves are less thrombogenic, but their limited durability in young adults is a serious disadvantage. Therefore, in women with serious valvular heart disease, every effort should be made to allow pregnancy to go to completion prior to valve replacement, and subsequent pregnancies should be avoided once a mechanical valve has been implanted.

In women with prosthetic valves, antibiotic prophylaxis with agents effective against genitourinary organisms is mandatory during the peripartum period.

PULMONARY HYPERTENSION AND EISENMENGER SYNDROME (See Chaps. 260 and 235) Pulmonary hypertension of all causes is a strong contraindication for pregnancy. If moderate or severe pulmonary hypertension (systolic pulmonary artery pressure >45 mmHg) is detected during the first trimester, termination of the pregnancy is advisable. In women with congenital heart disease, pulmonary hypertension, and a right-to-left shunt—i.e., the Eisenmenger syndrome, both maternal and fetal mortality are high, the latter increasing with the severity of maternal cyanosis. Bed rest may be required in severe cases. Systemic hypotension increases the right-to-left shunt in such patients and must be avoided.

MARFAN SYNDROME (See Chap. 348) Cardiovascular manifestations of the Marfan syndrome include mitral valve prolapse, mitral and aortic valve abnormalities, and aortic regurgitation due to enlargement of the aortic root. When the aortic root diameter as measured by echocardiography exceeds 40 mm, the risk of aortic dissection and rupture during pregnancy is increased. Women with the Marfan syndrome, especially those with a dilated aortic root, should avoid pregnancy; however, if such women become pregnant and refuse abortion, beta-adrenoceptor blocker therapy should be instituted to reduce the force of myocardial contraction and the resultant shear stress on the aorta.

OTHER FORMS OF CARDIAC DISEASE In the absence of pulmonary hypertension, atrial septal defect (p. 1303) is well tolerated by pregnant women, although the risk of fetal loss is increased. Patients with ventricular septal defect (p. 1304) without pulmonary hypertension also tolerate pregnancy well, but this lesion may be complicated by infective endocarditis, so antibiotic prophylaxis at the time of delivery is mandatory. Mitral valve prolapse (p. 1316), which is common among pregnant women, does not appear to complicate the pregnancy, nor does pregnancy complicate prolapse, although antibiotic prophylaxis is warranted. Women with hypertrophic cardiomyopathy (p. 1330) generally tolerate pregnancy well; indeed, the gestational hypervolemia may be associated with a reduction of the intraventricular pressure gradient and thus ameliorate symptoms. Because of its poor prognosis, chronic dilated cardiomyopathy (p. 1328) accompanied by heart failure is a contraindication to pregnancy.

Peripartum cardiomyopathy, a form of acute dilated cardiomyopathy that may be associated with a myocarditis, appears around the time of delivery (most frequently during the first 6 weeks postpartum), is sometimes associated with preeclampsia, and may actually be caused by pregnancy (p. 1330). Infant mortality is high if congestive heart failure ensues, and maternal mortality may be as high as 30 percent within the first few months. Treatment should include bed rest, digitalis, diuretics, and a vasodilator (other than an ACE inhibitor). About one-third of patients show functional recovery, but one-third have persistent severely impaired left ventricular function. Subsequent pregnancies should be avoided, since peripartum cardiomyopathy may recur.

Premature atrial or ventricular systoles occurring during pregnancy can be treated by the elimination of stimulants, avoidance of excessive fatigue, and reassurance. Drug therapy should be avoided, if possible, but cardioversion has been used safely for tachyarrhythmias during pregnancy.

PULMONARY EMBOLISM (See also Chap. 261)

In pregnancy, the levels of all of the coagulation factors (except factors XI and XIII) are increased, and the level of antithrombin III, a major inhibitor of coagulation, is reduced. Pulmonary embolism occurs about once per 750 pregnancies. Because of the immediate need to prevent embolism and the other long-term complications of deep vein thrombosis (DVT), it is important to recognize the latter condition. DVT may occur during pregnancy owing to compression of the iliac veins by the enlarged uterus as well as to changes in the coagulation and fibrinolytic systems that favor thrombosis. DVT also occurs at an increased incidence in the postpartum period. Impedance plethysmography and Doppler ultrasonography are noninvasive, nonradiologic techniques useful in documenting DVT. When pulmonary embolism is suspected, perfusion lung scanning can be accomplished with smaller quantities of isotope, and pulmonary angiography can be carried out if the abdomen is shielded. Despite the potential small hazard of fetal irradiation posed by the latter procedures, it is extremely important to diagnose pulmonary embolism.

 TREATMENT

Anticoagulant therapy is indicated in pregnant women with DVT, to prevent pulmonary embolism. Heparin, which does not cross the placenta, can be administered at a dose of 1000 U/h by continuous infusion until early during labor. Protamine can then be used to reverse the drug's effects, and heparin can be restarted within 2 h of delivery and continued for 3 to 4 days, after which subcutaneous heparin or oral warfarin therapy may be instituted for 6 months. When venous thrombosis or pulmonary embolism occurs in the early postpartum period, heparin treatment should be instituted for 7 to 10 days, followed by warfarin for about 3 months.

DIABETES MELLITUS (See also Chap. 334)

In pregnancy, there are two major opposing metabolic states: accelerated starvation and insulin resistance. Blood sugar and amino acids are low, while plasma free fatty acids, ketones, and triglycerides are increased. After an overnight fast, plasma glucose is lower by 0.8 to 1.1 mmol/L (15 to 20 mg/dL) than in nonpregnant women; when fasting lasts longer than 12 h, plasma glucose may fall to 2.2 to 2.5 mmol/L (40 to 45 mg/dL), while plasma hydroxybutyrate and acetoacetate rise to levels two to four times higher than in nonpregnant women. As a consequence, ketoacidosis develops in the absence of striking hyperglycemia in pregnant diabetics. Maternal insulin and glucagon do not cross the placenta, but acetoacetate and β-hydroxybutyrate cross readily and are oxidized by the fetal brain and liver.

In spite of the fetal demand for glucose, pregnancy is also a diabetogenic state by virtue of the development of insulin resistance. Elevation of several hormones in pregnancy may be responsible for insulin resistance, including progesterone, estrogen, prolactin, and human placental lactogen.

PREGNANCY IN INSULIN-DEPENDENT AND NON-INSULIN DEPENDENT DIABETES MELLITUS Pregnancy in diabetics is associated with a higher perinatal mortality (3 to 5 percent, vs. 1 to 2 percent in nondiabetic women) and a higher incidence of congenital anomalies (6 to 12 percent, vs. 2 to 3 percent in nondiabetics). Therapeutic control of blood glucose, particularly during organogenesis, reduces the incidence of congenital anomalies. Counseling should emphasize the importance of home monitoring of glucose levels and the need to adjust the insulin dose to maintain fasting blood sugar at a normal level and postprandial glucose no higher than 7.8 mmol/L (140 mg/dL), both prior to conception and throughout pregnancy. Glycosylated hemoglobin should also be monitored during pregnancy. Ultrasound evaluation of the fetus should be carried out during the second trimester, and alpha-fetoprotein levels should be assessed in the 20th week to detect neural tube defects.

Women with diabetic nephropathy have an excellent chance of a normal pregnancy, the rate of perinatal survival being approximately 90 percent. As with other renal diseases, hypertension can worsen late in pregnancy, with an increase in proteinuria and a decrease in creatinine clearance that represent either superimposed preeclampsia or a rise in glomerular pressure. There is no evidence that pregnancy worsens diabetic nephropathy, but care of pregnant women with diabetic nephropathy requires management by obstetricians skilled in high-risk pregnancies and by neonatologists, diabetologists, and nephrologists. Hypertension should be treated as described earlier in this chapter.

GESTATIONAL DIABETES The insulin resistance of normal pregnancy may also contribute to gestational diabetes in women in whom the capacity for insulin secretion is not sufficient to meet the increased insulin demands of pregnancy. The overall prevalence of gestational diabetes is between 1 and 3 percent. An important reason for recognizing the disorder early is that, because glucose crosses the placenta, the condition results in excessive fetal insulin secretion, which in turn can cause fetal macrosomia and increase the risk of birth trauma, need for cesarean section, and neonatal hypoglycemia.

There are no universally accepted criteria for the diagnosis or screening for gestational diabetes if the fasting glucose is normal. Some obstetricians recommend "universal" screening of all pregnant women with normal fasting blood sugar levels between the 24th and 28th weeks of gestation using a 50-g oral glucose load. If the 1-h glucose level exceeds 7.8 mmol/L (140 m/dL), a 100-g oral glucose test is performed after an overnight fast. A diagnosis of gestational diabetes is made if any two of the following values are reached: 1 h, >10.5 mmol/L (>190 ng/dL); 2 h, >9.2 mmol/L (>165 ng/dL); 3 h, >8.0 mmol/L (>145 ng/dL). In contrast, the American College of Obstetricians and Gynecologists recommends screening only for women at high risk, namely women over age 30; women with previous macrosomic, malformed, or stillborn infants; and those with obesity, hypertension, or glycosuria.

 TREATMENT

Gestational diabetes is treated first with dietary measures. If the fasting or postprandial glucose level remains elevated, insulin therapy should be started. Following delivery, carbohydrate tolerance may return to normal, but 30 percent or more of women with gestational diabetes develop diabetes mellitus within 5 years of the pregnancy.

THYROID DISEASE (See also Chap. 331)

The diagnosis of thyroid disease in pregnancy is complicated by the increases in thyroid size, radioactive iodine uptake, basal metabolic rate, and thyroxine-binding globulin level during normal pregnancy. Plasma T_3 and T_4 levels are elevated, but levels of free T_3, T_4, and thyroid-stimulating hormone (TSH) usually remain normal, while the T_3 resin uptake value is in the hypothyroid range. Maternal thyrotoxicosis occurs about once per 500 pregnancies, and the diagnosis may be difficult because the increase in cardiac output, tachycardia, skin warmth, and heat intolerance that are typical of pregnancy can mimic hyperthyroidism. Values of T_4 concentration above 154 mmol/L (12 μg/dL) with a resin T_3 uptake in the euthyroid range (25 to 35 percent) suggests hyperthyroidism in a pregnant woman. Pregnant women can tolerate mild degrees of hyperthyroidism without difficulty, and thyrotoxicosis does not increase fetal loss. Although hyperthyroidism may worsen in the first trimester, it is often more easily controlled in the third trimester. The treatment of gestational thyrotoxicosis involves a choice between antithyroid drugs and ablative surgery. Propylthiouracil is the drug of choice, since methimazole has been associated with aplasia cutis in the fetus. The goal should be to maintain the maternal T_4 concentration in the upper part of the normal range, because at that level fetal thyroid function is normal. The lowest possible dose of propylthiouracil should be used, because the drug crosses the placenta and inhibits fetal synthesis of thyroxine. If the mother is overtreated, fetal goiter occasionally develops owing to stimulation of fetal TSH. When surgery is planned for the treatment of thyrotoxicosis, propylthiouracil should be administered preoperatively to control the hyperthyroid state.

℞ TREATMENT

Hypothyroidism during pregnancy should be treated with hormone replacement, with the knowledge that the dose requirement may increase. The increase in dose requirement has been shown to occur as early as 8 weeks of gestation. The reason for this increased requirement is unclear and may involve the increase in concentration of binding proteins, transplacental transfer of T_4, or placental metabolism of T_4.

DISORDERS OF CALCIUM METABOLISM (See also Chap. 354)

Although the serum calcium level normally falls in pregnancy because of the decrease in serum albumin, the concentration of ionized calcium remains unchanged. Earlier studies of parathyroid hormone (PTH) levels, which used assays that measure PTH fragments, suggested that PTH levels increase during pregnancy with no change in phosphate clearance. However, more recent studies using assays that measure intact PTH have demonstrated a fall in PTH levels in pregnancy. Urinary calcium excretion is approximately 7.5 mmol/d (300 mg/d), compared with 2.5 mmol/d (100 mg/d) in nonpregnant women, and urinary calculi develop in about one of 2000 pregnant women. It may be that the increase in 1,25-dihydroxyvitamin D (which has a placental contribution) is the primary event leading to increased calcium absorption, a fall in PTH, and hypercalciuria. When hyperparathyroidism with hypercalcemia occurs during pregnancy, the neonate may exhibit tetany because of the suppression of fetal PTH secretion.

HEMATOLOGIC DISORDERS

During pregnancy, plasma volume increases more than does red cell mass, so that a fall in hemoglobin concentration of 10 to 20 g/L (1 to 2 g/dL) is usual. Two potential causes of anemia during pregnancy are deficiencies of iron or folate. Since the developing fetus uses these substances in large amounts, these deficiencies may be prevented by providing iron and folate supplements. Pregnancy also results in a leukocytosis that can sometimes reach 18,000 μL.

Sickle cell anemia (Chap. 107) may be complicated by pregnancy, and vasoocclusive crises become more frequent, particularly during labor and the postpartum period. The risks of spontaneous abortion, prematurity, and neonatal death are high.

Thrombocytopenia in pregnancy is most often due to preeclampsia, although sepsis and idiopathic thrombocytopenic purpura may also be responsible. In the last-named condition, antiplatelet antibodies cross the placenta and can cause thrombocytopenia in the fetus as well. Cesarean section is indicated if the fetal platelet count obtained by percutaneous umbilical cord sampling performed at 36 to 37 weeks is less than 50,000/ml.

Stillbirth, often associated with placental venous thrombosis, occurs in women with the so-called lupus anticoagulant (Chap. 312), an immunoglobulin that binds to negatively charged phospholipids and interferes with vitamin K–dependent coagulation factors. The lupus anticoagulant is actually more apt to cause thrombosis than bleeding, and treatment with low-dose aspirin and prednisone throughout pregnancy may reduce the rate of fetal loss.

Disseminated intravascular coagulation may occur as a result of abruptio placentae, a retained dead fetus, amniotic fluid embolism, saline-induced abortion, or fulminant preeclampsia and can be cured by treating the underlying cause.

GASTROINTESTINAL AND LIVER DISEASES

Nausea and vomiting occur in approximately 90 percent of women between the 6th and 16th weeks of pregnancy. When severe, the problem can be treated with oral dimenhydrinate, 50 to 100 mg every 4 h, or D-oxylamine, 12.5 mg every 4 h. In its severe form, *hyperemesis gravidarum* can cause dehydration that requires parenteral feeding. Heartburn, which may be due to relaxation of the lower esophageal sphincter, is usually responsive to treatment with antacids and H_2 receptor blocking agents.

Pregnancy in women with inflammatory bowel disease may be uncomplicated, but it is difficult to anticipate the course in advance. Most patients do well, but in some the pregnancy may exacerbate the disease; rarely the pregnancy may need to be terminated. If the disease is active at the time of conception, the incidence of spontaneous abortion is higher than in normal pregnancy.

Although pregnancy is associated with supersaturation of the bile with cholesterol, the incidence of cholelithiasis in a first pregnancy does not appear to be increased. However, the risk for this complication increases with multiparity. The serum triglyceride and cholesterol levels are elevated during pregnancy; although serum bilirubin remains normal, there is a striking rise in the level of alkaline phosphatase (which originates from the placenta); this level may reach a peak two to four times normal at term.

Although total serum protein concentration declines by approximately 20 percent in midpregnancy because of a decrease in albumin, hepatic synthesis of other plasma proteins increases. In a normal pregnancy, the serum levels of γ-glutamyl transpeptidase and LDH are increased, whereas serum levels of aminotransferases and aspartate aminotransferase are normal.

Intrahepatic cholestasis of pregnancy usually appears in the third trimester and is manifested by pruritus, with bilirubin levels usually less than 100 μmol/L (6 mg/dL). Although bilirubin levels usually remain in the range of 34 to 86 μmol/L (2 to 5 mg/dL), there is a striking increase in the alkaline phosphatase level. The cholestasis and pruritus disappear promptly after delivery, but the syndrome may recur with subsequent pregnancies. Aside from pruritus, the mother does not suffer any adverse effect. However, there appears to be an increase in stillbirths, which is thought to be secondary to the toxicity of bile acids to the fetus. Therefore, fetal surveillance should be carried out once the diagnosis of intrahepatic cholestasis of pregnancy is established. Treatment of pruritus consists of antihistamines and of cholestyramine, 4 g four times a day.

Acute fatty liver of pregnancy, with histologic changes showing hepatocytes with increased microvesicular fat and fibrin deposits in the hepatic sinusoids, may occur late in pregnancy and may be associated with preeclampsia. The serum bilirubin level may exceed 170 μmol/L (10 mg/dL), and the levels of aspartate aminotransferase and alanine aminotransferase are in the range of 5 to 8 μkat/L (300 to 500 U/L). Prothrombin time may be prolonged, and disseminated intravascular coagulation may cause depressed fibrinogen levels, an increase in fibrin degradation products, and thrombocytopenia. Maternal deaths may occur, but this condition usually ameliorates following delivery.

Hepatitis B (Chap. 295) during pregnancy increases the rates of prematurity and fetal death, with a high risk of transmission to the infant, particularly in mothers who are positive for the HBe antigen at the time of delivery. Women who are positive for the HBs antigen and negative for the HBe antigen transmit the disease less frequently. Approximately 5 to 10 percent of infants infected with hepatitis B acquire the disease by the transplacental route. Infants born to mothers with hepatitis B should be treated with both hepatitis B immune globulin and hepatitis B vaccine.

The severity of viral hepatitis A is not altered by pregnancy, and the risk of transmission to the neonate is small.

INFECTIONS

Infectious diseases constitute a serious risk to both the pregnant woman and the fetus.

BACTERIAL INFECTIONS Urinary tract infections (see Chap. 131) are the most common type of bacterial infection in pregnancy. Asymptomatic bacteriuria occurs in up to 7 percent of pregnancies. Physiologic changes in pregnancy, such as hormone-induced dilation of the urinary tract, hydroureter, and vesicoureteral reflux predispose to asymptomatic bacteriuria, and one-third of patients with these conditions develop pyelonephritis, usually during the last trimester. Most cases of pyelonephritis developing late in pregnancy were preceded by asymptomatic bacteriuria early in the pregnancy. Therefore, over 75 percent of cases of pregnancy-associated acute pyelonephritis can be avoided by treating asymptomatic bacteriuria, and screening for bacteriuria at the first prenatal visit is recommended. *Escherichia coli* is the most commonly isolated organism, and treatment of asymptomatic bacteriuria for 3 days with ampicillin, cephalexin, nitrofurantoin, or sulfisoxazole is appropriate, although the latter drug should not be used during the final month of gestation because it may cause jaundice in the infant. In women with asymptomatic bacteriuria, urine cultures should be obtained at monthly intervals for the remainder of the pregnancy. Relapse requires retreatment.

Intrauterine infection occurs in up to 4 percent of pregnancies and is associated with increased rates of morbidity and mortality in the prenatal period. Intraamniotic infection is most common when ascending infection follows rupture of the membranes, but it is also seen with intact membranes, especially in cases of preterm labor. Infection is usually polymicrobial, involving *E. coli* anaerobes, genital mycoplasmas, *Gardnerella vaginalis*, and group B streptococci. Since early clinical signs may be subtle, diagnosis requires a high degree of suspicion. Clinical clues include fever, maternal or fetal tachycardia, uterine tenderness, uncommonly foul-smelling amniotic fluid, and leukocytosis. In addition to the clinical findings, the diagnosis is based on the results of Gram's staining of amniotic fluid and on the glucose concentration and leukocyte esterase activity of amniotic fluid. Delivery of the fetus is indicated. Antibiotic therapy should begin during labor, rather than afterward. Antibiotics with broad coverage, such as ampicillin and gentamicin, are indicated.

Postpartum infections remain the most common cause of maternal mortality in the United States. Most of these deaths are related to postpartum endometrial infections complicated by pelvic abscess, peritonitis, or pelvic thrombophlebitis. Rates of endometritis vary from 1 to 3 percent after vaginal delivery and from 6 to 18 percent after cesarean section. Endometritis should be suspected when a patient has a fever developing 1 to 2 days after delivery. Rupture of the membranes and cesarean delivery following onset of labor are important risk factors for postpartum endometritis. Few patients exhibit all of the classical manifestations, such as fever, abdominal pain, malaise, and purulent or foul-smelling lochia. The workup should include a complete blood count, blood cultures, and a genital tract culture. Postpartum endometritis is usually a polymicrobial infection. The most common bacterial pathogens responsible for the condition are group B streptococci, mixed anaerobic and aerobic organisms, *E. coli*, and enterococci. Group B streptococci are the most frequent blood culture isolates in patients with endometritis. Treatment depends on the organism cultured, but broad-spectrum antibiotics or combinations such as ampicillin, an aminoglycoside, and clindamycin are usually used.

Group B *Streptococcus* (Chap. 143) has become a major cause of postpartum bacteremia, accounting for 10 to 20 percent of blood culture isolates from women admitted to obstetrical services. The source of these infections is group B streptococci colonizing the female genital tract. Although most of these patients have an uncomplicated course following appropriate antibiotic therapy, complications such as pelvic abscesses, septic shock, and septic thrombophlebitis are occasionally seen. Most severe group B *Streptococcus* infections in pregnancy are associated with an identifiable source, such as endometritis or a urinary tract infection. Group B streptococci may be transmitted to the neonate during the perinatal period. The attack rate of serious group B streptococcal infections in newborns is 1.8 per 1000 live births.

Listeria monocytogenes (see Chap. 145) is another bacterial pathogen that can produce specific pregnancy-related morbidity. Infection can occur at any time during pregnancy, but it is most common during the third trimester. Symptoms are frequently suggestive of a urinary tract infection, but urine cultures are sterile. Diagnosis is made by a positive blood culture. The infection can range in clinical severity from a mild febrile illness to severe illness. This infection can precipitate labor and result in premature birth of a dead or infected infant. Treatment should be with ampicillin or penicillin.

Neisseria gonorrhoeae (see Chap. 150) can be transmitted from mother to infant in utero, during delivery, or in the postpartum period. The most common clinical problem caused by this transmission is gonococcal conjunctivitis of the newborn. Conjunctival instillation of a 1% aqueous solution of silver nitrate is effective in preventing blindness caused by this infection. Congenital syphilis (see Chap. 174) occurs by infection of the fetus in utero. Transmission of *Treponema pallidum* to the fetus, which is most common in the early stages of syphilis, can occur at any time during pregnancy. Infection of the fetus before the fourth month is rare. Syphilis can have severe effects on the offspring, including stillbirth, neonatal disease, or latent infection.

VIRAL INFECTIONS These are of major concern during pregnancy because of the consequences to the fetus. Since transplacental transmission may occur, maternal infections with cytomegalovirus (CMV), rubella, varicella zoster, and herpes simplex virus have the greatest teratogenic potential, particularly during the first trimester. Perinatal infection can result from transmission of the virus to the infant during passage through an infected uterine cervix.

CMV (see Chap. 187) is the most common cause of congenital viral infection. The virus is ubiquitous; 35 to 100 percent of the adult population have evidence of prior infection, with the highest prevalence among lower socioeconomic groups. CMV is usually acquired by the oral-respiratory route, through sexual contact, or by blood transfusion. CMV infection establishes a lifelong latent infection in the host, which can be reactivated later by immunosuppression. Rates of cervical infection with CMV increase in later stages of pregnancy. Although during pregnancy CMV can be shed with no evidence of clinical disease in the mother, high numbers of CMV in the cervix suggest that the neonate is at risk during birth. Approximately 1 to 2 percent of all newborn infants in the United States are infected with CMV in utero, but the vast majority of these infants are normal. Clinically apparent congenital infections are most common in the first infant of mothers with primary infection during pregnancy. CMV disease occurs in infants whose mothers are not immune. Cytomegalic inclusion disease is characterized by jaundice, hepatosplenomegaly, a petechial rash, and multiple system and organ involvement. Other manifestations range from subtle neurologic sequelae to severe microcephaly.

Rubella (see Chap. 197) can have severe outcomes in the fetus, including fetal death and premature delivery, if the mother is infected during early pregnancy. A variety of congenital defects are caused by rubella, including cataracts, cardiac abnormalities, deafness, and mental retardation. Fetal abnormalities are greatest when maternal rubella occurs during the first trimester, with 80 percent of children affected; the percentage falls to about 25 percent when infection occurs at the end of the second trimester. Congenital infection can be diagnosed prenatally by detecting rubella IgM antibody in fetal blood obtained under ultrasound guidance. In places where immunization programs have been widely used, the problem has been eliminated. The vaccine can be administered during pregnancy without harm to the fetus. Infection during pregnancy with varicella zoster virus (VZV) represents a health risk to the mother (see Chap. 185). There is nearly a 10 percent risk for severe pneumonia. Antiviral therapy should be instituted early if there is any suspicion of chickenpox-related pneumonia. Although most infants born to VZV-infected mothers are normal, there is a risk to the unborn child of developing congenital teratogenic infection.

Infection of the newborn with herpes simplex virus (HSV) can range from mild localized infection to fatal dissemination (see Chap. 184). Retrograde infection or birth through a maternal genital tract infected with HSV-2 can result in serious disseminated neonatal infection.

OTHER INFECTIONS OF PREGNANCY *Vulvovaginal candidiasis* (see Chap. 207) is more common in pregnant than nonpregnant women. High estrogen levels apparently encourage growth of this organism. Infection rates increase as the gestational period progresses, with up to 55 percent of third-trimester women being colonized and with symptomatic disease developing in most of those colonized.

Toxoplasmosis (see Chap. 219) causes symptoms in only 10 to 20 percent of women infected during pregnancy. Unfortunately, the fetus is at risk whether or not the mother is symptomatic. Transmission to the fetus can occur transplacentally or at birth. One-third of infants born to mothers infected during pregnancy become infected. The risk for congenital infection is greater when maternal infection occurs during the third trimester than the first, although the risk of spontaneous abortion is highest when infection is acquired in the first trimester. Infected infants may have no symptoms at birth but may develop symptoms, particularly chorioretinitis, by adolescence. Less common manifestations include strabismus, epilepsy, and psychomotor retardation. Toxoplasmosis does not cause fetal malformation. Treatment of acutely infected pregnant women decreases the incidence and attenuates the severity of fetal infections.

HUMAN IMMUNODEFICIENCY VIRUS INFECTION

Approximately 80 percent of women with AIDS are of childbearing age. The incidence of infection with human immunodeficiency virus (HIV) will increase in women in the United States during the 1990s (see also Chap. 308). Worldwide, particularly in developing countries, HIV infection is spread mainly heterosexually, with the male-to-female ratio in certain countries approaching 1. Currently, most of the women in the United States who have AIDS are either intravenous drug users (IVDUs) or the heterosexual partners of IVDUs. The geographic distribution of HIV infection among women closely parallels that among IVDUs, with the highest incidence in the Northeast and Southeast seaboard states and Puerto Rico.

EFFECT OF HIV INFECTION ON PREGNANCY Although earlier studies suggested that HIV-positive women were at a higher risk of an unfavorable outcome of pregnancy, at present the accumulating evidence indicates that HIV infection alone does not impose a significant negative effect on pregnancy, particularly when the infection is in the asymptomatic stage. An acceleration of HIV disease during pregnancy is uncommon and may be due to other factors associated with confounding issues present in the women most likely to be infected, such as intravenous drug use and inadequate access to prenatal care.

Primary infection is generally associated with a burst of viremia with or without an acute HIV syndrome, the latter occurring in approximately 50 to 70 percent of individuals following initial infection. It is unclear what effect this burst of viremia has on the pregnancy itself; however, given the strong association between high levels of viremia and transmission of infection to the fetus, it is highly likely that primary infection of the mother during pregnancy increases the chances of transmission of HIV to the fetus.

TRANSMISSION OF HIV TO THE FETUS/INFANT The rate of transmission of HIV from mother to fetus/infant averages approximately 30 percent, ranging from 13 percent in a European collaborative study to 45 percent in Central Africa (see Chap. 308). Higher rates of transmission have been associated with the symptomatic stage in the mother with high levels of plasma viremia in the mother, and with low maternal CD4+ T lymphocyte counts. Although infection of the fetus can occur throughout pregnancy, transmission is thought to occur most often during the perinatal period. Nonetheless, caesarean sections are not currently recommended unless there are other, obstetrical reasons for performing one. Postnatal transmission from mother to infant has been documented, and colostrum and breast milk have been clearly implicated.

In developed countries where other forms of nutrition are available to the infant, breast feeding by an infected mother is absolutely contraindicated.

 TREATMENT

In HIV-infected pregnant women, administration of zidovudine to the mother before and during delivery and to the newborn for 6 weeks reduced the risk of maternal-infant HIV transmission by approximately 66 percent.

NEOPLASTIC DISEASES

Transmission of leukemia or lymphoma to the fetus has not been reported, and there is no clear evidence that pregnancy adversely affects the course of any type of malignancy; however, it is possible that the high estrogen levels of pregnancy accelerate the course of breast cancer.

Deciding whether a pregnancy should be terminated in a woman with a neoplastic disease requires judgment about whether the pregnant state presents a significant obstacle to effective therapy and whether the fetus will be harmed as a result of such therapy. Although most antineoplastic agents are potentially teratogenic or cause fetal wastage, many healthy full-term infants have been born despite active maternal chemotherapy at the time of conception or during the first trimester. Thus, while it would be safer to avoid fetal exposure, the decision to terminate a pregnancy must take into account the parents' desire to have a child. Pregnant women with leukemia who are given the usual chemotherapy for this condition have done surprisingly well; in some studies, the maternal survival rate has been 100 percent, and the incidence of congenital abnormalities in the newborn is less than 10 percent.

BIBLIOGRAPHY

BRIGGS GG et al: *Drugs in Pregnancy and Lactation*, 3d ed. Baltimore, Williams & Wilkins, 1990
BURROW GN, FERRIS TF: *Medical Complications During Pregnancy*, 4th ed. Philadelphia, Saunders, 1994
CLASP (COLLABORATIVE LOW-DOSE ASPIRIN STUDY IN PREGNANCY) COLLABORATIVE GROUP: CLASP: A randomised trial of low-dose aspirin for the prevention and treatment of pre-eclampsia among 9364 pregnant women. Lancet 343:619, 1994
CONNOR EM et al: Reduction of maternal-infant transmission of HIV type 1 with zidovudine treatment. N Engl J Med 331:1173, 1994
LUCAS MJ et al: A comparison of magnesium sulfate with phenytoin for the prevention of eclampsia. N Engl J Med 333:201, 1995
MANDEL SJ et al: Increased need for thyroxine during pregnancy in women with primary hypothyroidism. N Engl J Med 323:91, 1990

| 8 | *Charles E. Irwin, Jr., Mary-Ann Shafer* |

ADOLESCENT HEALTH PROBLEMS

———————— *Approach to the Patient* ————————

Adolescence is the period between childhood and adulthood. This period is usually defined by the rapid onset of biological and psychological growth and development prior to or at the second decade of life and ending before age 20. Major social and environmental factors influence the onset, duration, and completion of adolescence. Over the next decade, the numbers of adolescents will increase, adolescents will include more ethnic and racial minorities than the general population, and the adolescent population will become more impoverished, thereby decreasing their access to health care. Currently, the adolescent population in the United States is the group least likely to have health insurance. Physicians need a careful understanding of the biological and psychosocial changes of adolescence, the associated environmental

Table 8-1

CHAPTER 8
Adolescent Health Problems

31

Sexual Maturity Ratings for Females

A Pubertal development in size of female breasts
Stage 1: Prepubertal. Elevation of the papilla only.
Stage 2: Breast bud stage. A small mound of breast tissue causes elevation of the breast contour and papilla. Areolar diameter enlarges.
Stage 3: Further enlargement of breast and areola with no separation of their contours.
Stage 4: Projection of the areola and papilla to form a secondary mound above the level of the breast.
Stage 5: Adult. The breasts resemble those of a mature female. The areola has recessed to become contiguous with the contour of the breast.

B Pubertal development of female pubic hair
Stage 1: Prepubertal. There is no pubic hair.
Stage 2: Sparse growth of long, slightly pigmented, downy hair, straight or only slightly curled, primarily along the labia majora.
Stage 3: The hair becomes darker, coarser, and more curled and spreads sparsely over the junction of the pubes.
Stage 4: The hair, now adult in type, covers a smaller area than in the adult and does not extend onto the medial surface of the thighs.
Stage 5: Adult. The hair is adult in quantity and type, with extension onto the thighs.

SOURCE: Modified from van Wieringen JC et al: *Growth Diagrams*. Gronigen, Neth., Woplter-Noorhoff Publishing, 1971.

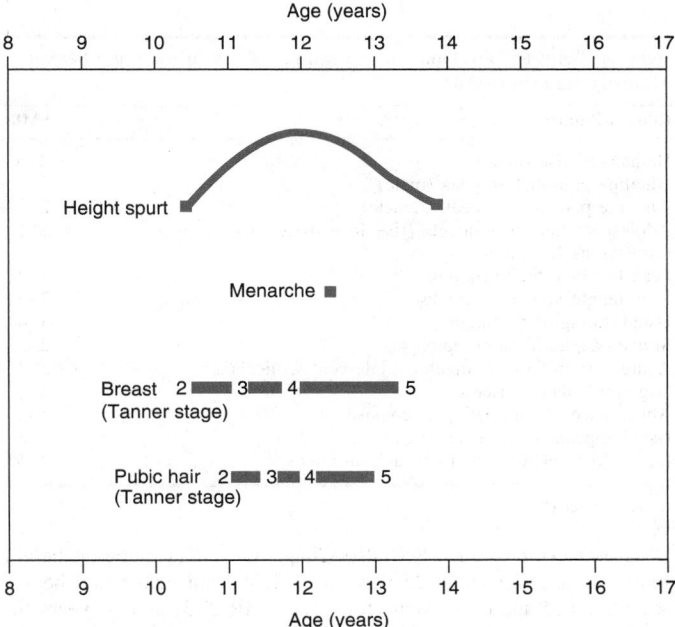

FIGURE 8-1 Pubertal events in females.

changes, and the legal and ethical issues that affect the provision of health care services to adolescents.

__Biological Maturation__ PUBERTY (See also Chaps. 336 and 337) Puberty is defined as the sequential biological processes that ultimately lead to reproductive capacity. The onset and tempo of puberty vary by sex, population group, and individual. During puberty, major alterations in the hormonal regulatory systems in the central nervous system, gonads, and adrenals cause changes in skeletal growth and body composition and the acquisition of secondary sexual characteristics. The mechanisms responsible for the initiation of puberty through activation of the hypothalamic-pituitary-gonadal axis remain undefined.

The sexual maturity ratings (SMRs) of Marshall and Tanner are helpful in monitoring the development of secondary sexual characteristics of pubertal maturation, which are the somatic manifestations of adrenal and gonadal activity. These ratings correlate more closely with bone age than chronologic age. The SMRs for girls are based upon breast and pubic hair development, each in five stages (Table 8-1).

The ratings for boys are based upon genital and pubic hair development (Table 8-2).

The mean age of onset of puberty for girls as defined by breast budding is 11.2 ± 1.6 years, and the mean age of onset for boys as defined by enlargement of testes is 11.6 ± 1.1 years. The mean age of menarche in the United States is 13.3 ± 1.3 years, and the mean age for spermarche is between 13.5 and 14.5 years. The average duration of puberty for girls is 4 years, with a range of 1.5 to 8 years, and for boys is 3 years, with a range of 2 to 5 years. Even though the timing and duration of the events vary, each adolescent follows an orderly sequence in somatic growth and development (Figs. 8-1 and 8-2). Monitoring these events by history and physical examination is helpful in identifying disorders that become manifest during adolescence (Table 8-3).

Table 8-2

Sexual Maturity Ratings for Males

A Pubertal development in size of male genitalia
Stage 1: Prepubertal. Penis, testes, and scrotum are of childhood size.
Stage 2: The scrotum and testes enlarge with testicular measurement greater than 2.5 cm in length (testicular volume, 4–7 mL). Penis usually shows no growth. Scrotal skin reddens or darkens.
Stage 3: Further growth of testes (testicular volume, 8–10 mL) and scrotum with enlargement of penis, mainly in length.
Stage 4: Continued growth of the testes (testicular volume, 10–15 mL) and scrotum with increased size of the penis, especially in breadth.
Stage 5: Adult. The genitalia are adult in size (testicular volume, 20–25 mL) and shape.

B Pubertal development of male pubic hair
Stage 1: Prepubertal. Pubic hair is absent.
Stage 2: Sparse growth of long, slightly pigmented, downy hair, straight or only slightly curled, primarily at the base of the penis.
Stage 3: The hair is considerably darker, coarser, and more curled. The hair spreads sparsely over the junction of the pubes.
Stage 4: The hair, now adult in type, covers a smaller area than in the adult and does not extend onto the medial surface of the thighs.
Stage 5: Adult. The hair is adult in quantity and type, with extension onto the thighs.

SOURCE: Modified from van Wieringen JC et al: *Growth Diagrams*. Gronigen, Neth. Woplter-Noorhoff Publishing, 1971.

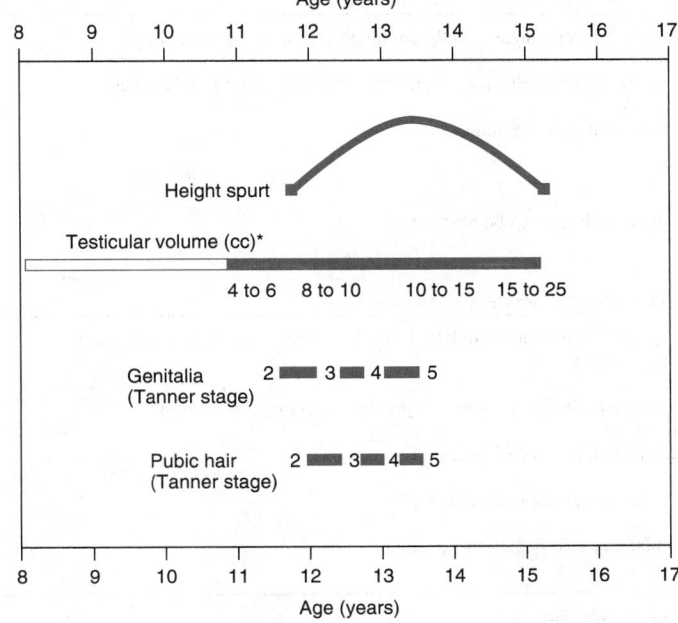

FIGURE 8-2 Pubertal events in males.

Table 8-3

Relation Between Development of Features of Maturation and Sexual Maturity Ratings (SMR)

Clinical Feature	SMR
Hematocrit rise (male)	2–5
Alkaline phosphatase peak (male)	3
Alkaline phosphatase peak (female)	2
Adolescent hormonal levels (rise in estrogen for females, testosterone for males)	2–5
Peak height velocity (male)	3–4
Peak height velocity (female)	2–3
Usual timing of menarche	3–4
Slipped capital femoral epiphysis	2–3
Acute worsening of idiopathic adolescent scoliosis	2–4
Osgood-Schlatter disease	3
Appearance of "normal" gynecomastia	2–3
Usual appearance of acne vulgaris	2–3
Increased levels of serum uric acid in males	2–5

SOURCE: After Daniel.

SKELETAL GROWTH (See also Chap. 329) The pubertal height spurt accounts for about 25 percent of final adult height and begins at an average age of 12 years for girls (SMR 2–3) and 14 years for boys (SMR 3–4). During this spurt, females gain 9.0 ± 1.03 cm/year and reach a final mean adult height of 163 cm at 16 years; males gain 10.3 ± 1.54 cm/year and reach a final mean adult height of 177 cm at 18 years. Assessment of skeletal growth during adolescence should be done through a height velocity curve with consideration of the sexual maturity rating. Bone age can be determined through the utilization of hand roentgenograms.

CHANGES IN BODY COMPOSITION Weight gain during the growth spurt accounts for 40 percent of ideal body weight. Lean body mass increases in boys from 80 to 90 percent and decreases in girls from 80 to 75 percent. In boys mean body fat increases from 4.3 to 11.2 percent by late puberty and is distributed primarily in the truncal area. In girls, mean body fat increases from 15.7 to 26.7 percent and is deposited in the pelvic, breast, upper back, and arm areas. Shortly after the growth spurt is completed, muscle mass peaks and is greater in boys than in girls.

CARDIORESPIRATORY CHANGES At puberty stroke volume, cardiac output, and blood pressure increase, and heart rate decreases. The lungs increase in size. The male larynx, under the influence of androgens, develops an acute 90-degree angle in the anterior thyroid cartilage; male vocal cords are three times the length of those in females. These changes account for the deepening of the voice.

Psychological Development Adolescence is often viewed as a tumultuous period (Table 8-4). However, most adolescents pass through puberty without disruption in their lives. The clinician must assess whether psychosocial development of the adolescent is normal. Adolescence involves a series of changes, which, if mastered, allow normal function as an adult. These changes include separation from the family, maturation of sexual identity, planning for education and career, and development of the capacity for intimacy. Adolescents also undergo cognitive changes with behavioral and social sequelae. The functional and cognitive changes do not necessarily correlate with physical maturation. The early adolescent (ages 10 to 13) tends to focus on the physical changes in his or her body and may have concerns about the maturation process.

Table 8-4

Biopsychosocial Development During Adolescence

Characteristics	Impact
EARLY ADOLESCENCE (Age 10 to 13 Years)	
Onset of puberty, becomes concerned with developing body	Major questions concerning normality of physical maturation; often concerned about the stages of sexual development and how the process relates to peers of same gender. Masturbation begins.
Begins to expand social radius beyond family and concentrate on relationships with peers	Encourage some external responsibilities alone in consultation with parents, i.e., visit with health care provider, contacts with school counselors.
Cognition is usually concrete	Concrete thinking requires dealing with most health situations in a simple, explicit manner using visual and verbal cues.
MIDDLE ADOLESCENCE (Age 14 to 16 Years)	
Pubertal development usually complete and sexual drives emerge	Explores ability to attract opposites. Sexual behavior and experimentation (same and opposite sex) begin. Masturbation increases.
Peer group sets behavioral standards, although some family values persist	Peer group affects compliance, and peers rather than parents offer key support.
Conflicts over independence	Increased assumption of independent action, together with continued need for parental support and guidance; able to discuss and negotiate changes in rules; ambivalence on part of adolescent in discussion and negotiation.
Cognition begins to be abstract	Begins to consider full range of possibilities with poor ability to integrate into real life because of immaturity and incomplete cognitive development.
LATE ADOLESCENCE (Age 17 to 21 Years)	
Physical maturation complete. Body image and gender role definition are secured	Begins to feel comfortable with relationships and decisions regarding sexuality and preference. Individual relationships become more important than peer group.
Narcissism declines; there is a process of giving and sharing	More open to specific questioning regarding behavior.
Idealistic	Idealism may lead to conflicts with family and other authority figures.
Emancipation is nearly secured	With emancipation, more awareness about consequences of personal actions.
Cognitive development is complete	Most are capable of understanding a full range of options for health issues.
Functional role begins to be defined	Often interested in significant discussion of life goals because this is the primary function of this stage.

SOURCE: After Shafer and Irwin.

Middle adolescence (ages 14 to 16 years) is the period of rapid cognitive growth when formal operational thinking emerges. Adolescents begin to understand abstract concepts and may question the judgment of adults. The individual then shifts from the egocentric world of the early adolescent to the sociocentric world of the middle and late adolescent and begins to modulate impulsive behavior.

Late adolescence (ages 17 to 21 years) is the period of establishment of personal identity and intimate relationships and the beginning of the assumption of a role in society. The late adolescent views life in a more sociocentric view, characteristic of adulthood. The late adolescent may be altruistic, and conflicts with the family and society may center on moral issues rather than egocentric considerations.

Families can facilitate adolescence by providing a graduated increase in independence and in responsibilities. Adolescents require both individuality and involvement with family and society to facilitate development of identity and of rational competence. Clinicians should support this process by encouraging adolescents to make their own appointments, assisting the chronically ill adolescent in assuming more responsibility for his or her health care, and encouraging parents to decrease their role in clinical management issues.

Psychological Changes Associated with Pubescence HOR-MONES AND BEHAVIOR Specific behavioral changes are associated with puberty and its timing. Androgens are involved in this process. During peak height velocity (stages 3 to 4), boys tend to have conflicts with their mothers, and as boys complete puberty mothers tend to defer more to their sons. Girls also tend to have more conflict with their mothers and to decrease interactions with their fathers. Other activities associated with changes in androgens include heterosocial and heterosexual behavior. Boys with rising levels of testosterone tend to initiate sexual intercourse and are reported to be more impatient, irritable, and aggressive. Rising levels of adrenal androgens correlate with increased masturbatory activity and heterosocial behavior in girls.

TIMING OF MATURATION Timing of puberty is associated with psychological and behavioral sequelae. Earlier physical maturation in girls is associated with more dissatisfaction with their bodies, lower self-esteem, and general unhappiness. Early-developing girls also receive less support from peer groups and may associate with older adolescents. The early-developing girl initiates sexual behavior before her age peers, experiences an early identity crisis, has greater interest in independence and decision-making, and tends to have more behavioral problems and less interest in academic activities. Early physical maturation in boys is associated with earlier initiation of sexual behavior, and late maturation in boys is more often associated with negative psychological sequelae. The late-maturing boy tends to have a negative self-concept and body image and an increased frequency of identity crises.

Environmental Changes SOCIAL ENVIRONMENT Changes in the social environment during the second decade may affect health status. The family tends to provide less supervision and allow more freedom in choices regarding free time, often providing the adolescent opportunity to engage in risky behaviors. Schools are transformed from supportive elementary schools to the large, impersonal, and less structured environments of middle/junior high schools, high schools, and colleges. Work environments provide even less supervision and on-the-job guidance for the adolescent. With the ongoing restructuring of social programs of the 1990s fewer nurturing programs are available for youth after school. Increased poverty has had a negative effect on the health status of children and adolescents.

LEGAL ENVIRONMENT The law in most states requires consent of a parent for medical care for children below age 18. The involvement of parents is usually not a barrier to the provision of health services, but some sensitive health issues (e.g., sexual behavior and substance use) may interfere with access to health care for adolescents. The Mature Minor Doctrine generally allows adolescents to seek health care independently if they are capable of understanding the risks and benefits of the proposed treatment and therefore capable of informed consent. There is usually little risk of liability in providing health care to the older mature minor (14 years or older) if the care is for the

individual's benefit or is an emergency. In many states adolescents can seek care without parental permission for sensitive issues such as sexually transmitted diseases, contraception, pregnancy, substance use, and some psychiatric problems. Adolescents may also be treated without parental permission if the condition is an emergency and a delay in treatment would be detrimental. Emancipated minors (adolescents who live away from home, are no longer subject to parental control, are economically self-supporting, are married, or are members of the military service) may also consent to their own health care.

MORBIDITY AND MORTALITY

The concept that adolescence is the healthiest period of life is based on measures of mortality and morbidity that do not include functional assessment of health status or the effects of behaviors initiated during adolescence on adult mortality and morbidity.

MORTALITY Mortality rates are low, but since 1985, there has been an increase in mortality for adolescents and young adults. Mortality (per 100,000) increases from 26 in 10 to 14 year olds to 88 in 15 to 19 year olds to 110 in 20 to 24 year olds. Most adolescent mortality is due to violence, particularly motor vehicle accidents, homicide, and suicide. In 1990 injuries accounted for most deaths between the ages of 10 and 24, and mortality rates for males are double those of females. Ethnic and racial groups differ in respect to the cause of death: black males of 15 to 19 years old have a ninefold greater rate of death from homicide than white males and the lowest life expectancy of all adolescents. In contrast, white male adolescents have higher death rates from suicide and motor vehicle accidents. Unintentional injuries account for more than half of deaths in the second decade. Risky driving habits account for half of fatal crashes, and adolescent and young adult (ages 15 to 24) drivers have the highest rates of motor vehicle fatalities. Alcohol is also implicated in fatal bicycle, boating, skateboard, and swimming accidents. Suicide is responsible for 13 percent of deaths between ages 15 and 24. Native American males have high rates, and black adolescents have low rates of suicide. Between ages 15 and 24 homicide accounts for 14 percent of deaths. Homicide is the leading cause of death in black male adolescents and young adults, accounting for 58 percent and 54 percent of the deaths, respectively. Adolescents in impoverished metropolitan areas are more likely to be victims of homicide. Cardiovascular diseases account for 1.4 to 4.1 deaths, and malignancies cause 3.1 to 5.5 deaths per 100,000 persons aged 10 to 24.

MORBIDITY Most morbidity during adolescence originates from substance abuse, sexual activity, and injuries. Additional causes include mental health problems and skeletal and reproductive disorders.

Skeletal System (See also Chap. 329) Rapid growth of the long bones and closure of the epiphyses are associated with several orthopedic problems. Slipped capital femoral epiphyses occur primarily at the time of rapid growth spurt and are more common in the obese. Osgood-Schlatter disease (osteochondrosis of the tibial tuberosity) and idiopathic scoliosis are disorders of adolescence, and neoplasms of osseous origins peak during adolescence. Fractures due to injuries are common throughout adolescence.

Female Reproductive Health Problems Reproductive problems are a common cause of morbidity in young women.

Anovulatory cycles (See also Chap. 337) Dysfunctional uterine bleeding (DUB) is characterized by frequent, irregular, painless menses. Primary DUB results from anovulatory cycles, i.e., oscillations of estrogen levels that lack the characteristic surge in luteinizing hormone and subsequent corpus luteum development, progesterone production, and endometrial maturation of a mature cycle. Without progesterone, the endometrial lining becomes thickened and fragile, resulting in intermittent sloughing and irregular, frequently excessive menstrual bleeding. The differential diagnosis includes pregnancy, stress, rapid weight change, chronic illness, substance abuse, disorders of coagulation, and disorders of the vagina, cervix, uterus, and ovary. Anovulatory cycles may persist for 5 years following menarche.

Dysmenorrhea Dysmenorrhea, both primary and secondary, is a major complaint of menstruating adolescents and a major cause of school absenteeism. Primary dysmenorrhea is due to prostaglandin-stimulated myometrial contractions during ovulatory cycles. Secondary dysmenorrhea is associated with pelvic infections, intrauterine and extrauterine pregnancy, intrauterine devices, and congenital anomalies. Primary dysmenorrhea is treated by suppressing production of the prostaglandins and/or inhibiting ovulation. If the subject fails to respond to oral contraceptives and prostaglandin inhibitors, further evaluation is required.

Sexually transmitted diseases (STD) (See also Chap. 129) Sexually active adolescents have the highest rates of STD of any age group in the United States. Complications include cervical intraepithelial neoplasia, pelvic inflammatory disease, ectopic pregnancy, infertility, genital cancers, neonatal infections, and AIDS. As of June 1995, 2184 cases of AIDS had been diagnosed in 13 to 19 year olds and 17,745 cases in the 20- to 24-year-old cohort. The extent of seroprevalence of human immunodeficiency virus in adolescents is not well defined. When one STD is diagnosed, the clinician must screen for other STDs and counsel the young patient about risks.

Male Reproductive Health Problems (See also Chap. 336) Testicular masses and varicoceles may become evident during puberty and are usually discovered during a routine physical examination. Surgical repair may be indicated to enhance fertility and in the following situations: genital discomfort, testicular volume loss, abnormal semen analysis, or abnormal luteinizing hormone–releasing hormone stimulation test. Testicular cancer is rare in adolescents, but teaching young men to perform self testicular examinations may increase early identification of tumors.

RISK-TAKING BEHAVIORS

SUBSTANCE USE AND ABUSE Since 1991 there has been a reversal in the downward trends of substance use that occurred in the 1980s. This increase in substance abuse has been accompanied by a decrease in the perception of harm by such behavior. In 1994 45.6 percent of high school seniors reported illicit substance use at some time. Rates of lifetime use of LSD and heroin among high school seniors increased to 10.5 and 1.2 percent respectively, and 3 percent of high school seniors reported use of crack cocaine. Lifetime alcohol and tobacco use approximated 87 percent and 62 percent, respectively, among high school seniors in 1994. Binge drinking (the consumption of at least five drinks or more in a row at least once in the previous 2 weeks) was reported by 31 percent of high school seniors and by 40 percent of college students. Initiation of substance abuse during adolescence has major negative health consequences in adulthood, including more common habituation. Girls consistently report greater use of cigarettes, whereas boys use alcohol more commonly. Approximately 19 percent of adolescents leave high school as smokers, and 21 percent of young adults are regular smokers. The lower rates of cigarette smoking in boys may be due to the increase in use of snuff and chewing tobacco.

Surveys may underestimate the true prevalence of substance use, but it is clear that patterns of substance use vary by region, age, gender, and ethnicity. Substance use generally increases with age. Native American adolescents have the highest prevalence rates for cigarettes, alcohol, and most illicit drugs, followed by rates for whites, Hispanics, African-Americans, and Asian-Americans.

UNINTENTIONAL INJURIES Injuries, particularly motor vehicle accidents, account for more than half of deaths in adolescents, and hospitalization for injury accounts for the largest number of hospital days. Alcohol, high speed, and reckless behavior play important roles in these injuries and are also implicated in injuries with bicycles,

skateboards, swimming, and boating. Males outnumber females by greater than 2 to 1 in all injury situations.

SEXUAL BEHAVIOR Adolescents now initiate heterosexual behavior earlier than cohorts of previous generations. By age 15, 26 percent of white females and males, 24 percent of black females, and 69 percent of black males experience coitus. By age 19 these figures increase to 76 percent of white females, 85 percent of white males, 83 percent of black females, and 96 percent of black males. White adolescent females report more frequent sexual intercourse and more partners than their age-related black cohorts. Adolescent females with earlier menarche begin to have intercourse earlier than those with a later menarche. Adolescents who initiate sexual behavior early tend to have more sexual partners and are more likely to acquire a sexually transmitted disease or become pregnant. Fewer than half of sexually active adolescents use condoms. Reported rates of unprotected heterosexual anal intercourse are from 12 percent to 26 percent. Reliable data on same-sex behavior during adolescence are not available, but rates may approximate 5 to 10 percent. Retrospective studies of adult homosexual and bisexual men indicate that half initiated same-sex sexual behavior by age 16.

Overall birth rates have declined over the past decade, but the number of births to unmarried adolescent girls has increased. Furthermore, there were an estimated 412,275 abortions in adolescents in 1992. Pregnancy, birth, and abortion rates vary by race and ethnicity.

COVARIATION OF RISK BEHAVIORS The practice of one risk behavior is associated with a greater likelihood for initiation of another in the near future. The association between alcohol abuse and injury is well established. Other activities that predispose to injury include reckless driving and failure to use seat belts and helmets.

The strongest evidence for covariation is in substance abuse, sexual activity, and delinquent behavior. The major risk for initiation of cigarette, alcohol, and marijuana use is by age 20 and for illicit substance use is by age 21. Young adults who have not used these substances are unlikely to do so thereafter. During early and middle adolescence, less serious substance use predicts subsequent use of more serious substances. Alcohol use precedes marijuana use, and marijuana use precedes other illicit drugs (including psychedelics, cocaine, heroin, and nonprescribed stimulants, sedatives, and tranquilizers). In girls, cigarette use is predictive of subsequent substance use. The influence of alcohol and tobacco use on subsequent marijuana use is independent of age. The earlier adolescents begin using marijuana the more likely the use of other illicit substances. Substance use is also correlated with delinquent behavior, violent behavior, suicide, homicide, early sexual debut, and less effective contraceptive use.

MENTAL HEALTH PROBLEMS

Approximately 10 percent of adolescents have symptoms of psychological distress. Psychiatric conditions that may begin in childhood include anxiety and panic disorders, personality disorders, schizophrenia, suicide, and eating disorders. Three common problems during adolescence are suicide, depression, and eating disorders.

SUICIDE Suicide is the fourth leading cause of death in early adolescence (10 to 14 years old) and the third leading cause in late adolescence and young adulthood. The greatest increase in suicide rates since 1970 is among men aged 15 to 24. Suicide is relatively uncommon before puberty and increases after age 16 with most occurring between ages 18 and 24, particularly in white and Native American late adolescent boys and young men. The relationship between male sex and substance abuse and conduct disorders may be responsible for this predominance. For every completed suicide, there may be 20 to 50 attempted suicides, with a female preponderance. Differences in methods may be responsible for the sex differences between fatal and attempted suicides. Methods for fatal suicide include firearms, hanging, and jumping from heights. Drug ingestion, which rarely causes fatality, is the most common method for suicide attempts in adolescents.

Etiology of Suicide Common factors in suicidal adolescents include a history of suicide in family members, alcohol and substance abuse, attention deficit disorder, conduct disorders, depression, anxiety states, and knowing someone who has committed or attempted suicide. Precipitating factors include acute stress, trouble with the law, trouble at school such as cheating or truancy, substance abuse, pregnancy or fear of pregnancy, hypochondriasis, social isolation, and anxiety. In occasional girls perfectionism and anxiety about academic performance (in the presence of average intelligence) or environmental change appear to be causal. Many suicide victims are intoxicated at the time of death.

Recognition of the At-Risk Suicidal Adolescent   Recognition of the suicidal adolescent may be difficult. The most common underlying psychiatric factor in suicidal adolescents is depression, manifested by feelings of hopelessness, low self-esteem, despair, and somatic complaints. In the younger adolescent, depressive equivalents of school problems and acting-out behavior may include legal problems. The younger adolescent may also have difficulty in describing his or her feelings. In the older adolescent, substance abuse is more common. Injured adolescents should be queried about the cause of the injury to rule out suicidal behavior. Adolescents with a family history of suicide, a history of psychiatric disorders, or a past history of suicidal behavior need to be screened for suicide risk. The depressed adolescent contemplating suicide usually welcomes the opportunity to communicate his or her feelings.

Once a suicidal adolescent is identified, an extensive evaluation is required to assess the problem. Comprehensive workup should include evaluation of the adolescent, the family, and the family together with the adolescent. Confidentiality is immaterial in the face of potential suicide, and parents and/or guardians should be informed immediately about the suicidal behavior. Suicidal intent is as important as the lethality of the method. Many adolescents have little knowledge of lethality. Evaluation should focus on mental health disorders in the family, past history of mental health problems in the adolescent, sexual abuse, and sexual behavior including same-sex behavior, since homosexual adolescents appear to be at greater risk for suicide. All suicidal adolescents need evaluation by a psychiatrist as soon as possible.

In emergencies, the physician must decide if outpatient or inpatient care is appropriate. If immediate treatment is needed, psychiatric consultation is obtained when the patient is stable medically. If the patient is initially medically stable, the physician must decide whether he or she is at continuing risk for suicide. Some programs recommend hospitalization for all suicidal adolescents, and hospitalization is always advisable for the following groups: (1) those still intent on suicide; (2) those with previous suicide attempts; (3) all males; (4) all severely depressed patients; (5) those impaired by substance abuse; (6) those whose attempt was with a lethal method (e.g., firearm, hanging, or jumping from a high place); and (7) those without a supportive environment at home.

When the patient is discharged, the physician needs to monitor compliance with the mental health treatment program and to query the family about the availability of firearms at home. Adolescents who are depressed or suicidal are difficult to engage in treatment programs, and a follow-up appointment with the primary care physician is the best way to monitor compliance. If the adolescent fails to keep the appointment, the physician should telephone and reschedule it.

Depression   (See also Chap. 385)   Depression is the most common feature in patients who attempt suicide. The prevalance of major depressive disorders in adolescence is between 4 and 6 percent with a slight preponderance of females to males. The diagnostic criteria for depression during adolescence are the same as in adulthood (Table 8-5) and include changes in mood and relationships, cognitive functioning, and bodily functioning. Depressive equivalents in the adolescent include hypochondriasis, substance abuse, decrements in school functioning, problems with the law, and major family conflicts.

EATING DISORDERS   (See also Chap. 76)   Eating disorders generally have their onset in postpubertal adolescents, and adolescents may fulfill the DSM-IV criteria for anorexia nervosa or bulimia nervosa prior to the completion of puberty (See Tables 76-1 and 76-2). Adolescents with subclinical eating disorders may need the same treatment

Table 8-5

DSM-III-R Criteria for Diagnosis of Major Depression

Diagnosis requires symptom 1 or 2 and at least four other symptoms for a 2-week period

1. Depressed or irritable mood
2. Diminished interest or pleasure
3. Weight loss or weight gain
4. Insomnia or hypersomnia
5. Psychomotor agitation or retardation
6. Fatigue or loss of energy
7. Feelings of worthlessness or excessive guilt
8. Decreased concentration or indecisiveness
9. Thoughts of death, suicidal ideation, or suicide attempt

SOURCE: After American Psychiatric Association, p 217.

as adolescents with full-fledged disorders. While the eating patterns in many adolescents appear abnormal, and adolescent girls commonly have dissatisfaction with weight and shape and some fear of gaining weight, these feelings and fears are extreme in the adolescent with an eating disorder.

THE CLINICAL VISIT OF THE ADOLESCENT

TRANSITION INTERVIEW   Establishing an effective doctor-patient relationship with the adolescent is a formidable task for the physician whose practice is primarily with adults. A transition interview for the adolescent and family helps to define the relationship between the physician and the emerging adult. Areas to be emphasized include the necessity for the physician to interview and examine the adolescent privately and the need for the patient to generate his or her own questions including initiating appointments. Normal adolescence and the continuing need for some decisions to be made with family guidance and support should be discussed. The payment mechanisms and responsibility for fees should be clarified. During this interview, the physician should inquire about the previous health care and request authorization to contact the former physician.

CONFIDENTIALITY   Confidentiality is fundamental to any doctor-patient relationship. Adolescents need to be able to discuss all matters with the physician openly, honestly, and confidentially, and the physician must provide assurance of the confidential nature of all information. Prior to queries about sexual behavior or substance use, it may be useful to restate the confidential nature of the questioning. With life-threatening behaviors or diseases (e.g., suicidal behavior or management of chronic disease), the physician generally has the right to intervene including identification of a parent, guardian, or supportive adult to assist in the management.

OBTAINING THE HISTORY   History taking should be guided by the developmental stage of the patient (Table 8-4). The adolescent may not disclose his or her primary concern until a secure and confidential relationship has been established. General screening should be undertaken for the major health-damaging behaviors of adolescence, including sexual activity, substance use, depression and its equivalents, and dietary changes suggestive of an eating disorder. Distinguishing between risk-taking behaviors that are temporary, though dangerous, and those that are pathologic is a challenge. This judgment requires assessing the effects of risky behavior on the health status and the motivation for engaging in them and determining whether normal psychosocial development is impaired. Figure 8-3 summarizes the biopsychosocial and environmental factors that increase vulnerability for initiating risky behaviors. Male sex, positive attitudes toward risky behaviors, lack of parental supervision, contact with peers engaging in the behavior, and multiple school transitions are associated with an increased propensity for risky behaviors. The physician should be

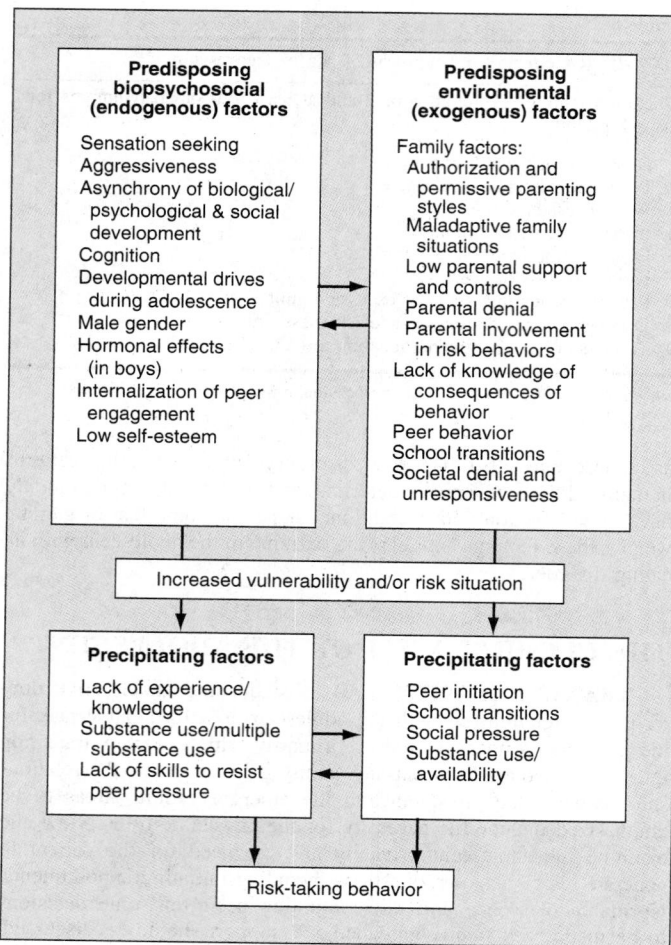

FIGURE 8-3 Principal factors in risk-taking behaviors. (Adapted from Irwin and Millstein.)

specific in questioning about individual risk behaviors, including their frequency and their intensity. One behavior may serve as a warning sign for another risky behavior. For example, early substance abuse correlates with early sexual activity. Guidelines have been developed to assist physicians in screening youth at risk, including *Bright Futures* (Green, 1995) and *Guidelines for Adolescent Preventive Services* (Elster and Kuznets, 1994) (see "Bibliography").

Frequently, adolescents do not want to disclose current behavior, and the physician may query instead about general risk taking and the behavior of peer groups. The physical signs and symptoms associated with risky behaviors are similar to those in adults, but the consequences of such behaviors may have a greater effect on the adolescent, including more family conflicts, impaired academic performance, unwise peer relationships and activities, and changes in extracurricular activities.

Immunization history needs to be reviewed. Previously immunized adolescents who received a complete series of immunizations prior to 5 years of age need to receive a second vaccination for measles alone or for measles, mumps, and rubella. Adolescents who have never been immunized or for whom the immunization history is not available should receive a three-dose primary series of immunizations for tetanus, diphtheria, and poliomyelitis and a two-dose primary series for measles, mumps, rubella, and hepatitis B. Hepatitis A vaccine should be given to sexually active adolescents.

The physical examination and laboratory assessment are guided by the general complaints and the associated physical stigmata of risky behaviors.

BIBLIOGRAPHY

ADAMS LB, SHAFER MA: Early manifestations of eating disorders in adolescents: Defining those at risk. J Nutr Ed 20:307, 1988

AMERICAN PSYCHIATRIC ASSOCIATION: *Diagnostic and Statistical Manual of Mental Disorders*, 4th ed. Washington, DC, The American Psychiatric Association, 1994

BACHMAN JAG et al: Racial/ethnic differences in smoking, drinking and illicit drug use among American high school seniors, 1976–89. Am J Public Health 81:372, 1991

BLUMENTHAL SJ, KUPFER DJ: *Suicide over the Life Cycle.* Washington, DC, American Psychiatric Press, 1990

CENTERS FOR DISEASE CONTROL: *HIV/AIDS Surveillance Report, 1995*, 7(No. 1). Atlanta, Centers for Disease Control and Prevention. 1995

————: Premarital sexual experience among adolescent women—United States, 1970–1988. MMWR 39:929, 1991

COPELAND KC et al: Assessment of pubertal development. Ross Laboratories PREP series. Columbus, Ross Laboratories, 1986

DANIEL WA: Growth at adolescence: Clinical correlates. Semin Adolesc Med 1:15, 1985

ELSTER AB, KUZNETS NJ: AMA Guidelines for Adolescent Preventive Services (GAPS): Recommendations and Rationale. Baltimore, Williams & Wilkins, 1994

ENGLISH A: Treating adolescents: Legal and ethical considerations. Med Clin North Am 74:1097, 1990

FELDMAN SS, ELLIOTT GR: *At the Threshold: The Developing Adolescent.* Cambridge, Harvard University, 1990

FRIEDMAN SB et al (eds): *Comprehensive Adolescent Health Care.* St. Louis, Quality Medical Publishing, 1992

GREEN M: Bright Futures. Arlington, VA, National Center for Education in Maternal and Child Health, 1995

GREULICH WW, PYLE SI: *Radiographic Atlas of Skeletal Development of the Hand and Wrist*, 2d ed. Stanford, Stanford University, 1959

IRWIN CE JR: The theoretical concept of at-risk adolescents. Adolesc Med: State Art Rev 1:1, 1990

————, MILLSTEIN SG: Biopsychosocial correlates of risk taking behavior during adolescence: Can the physician intervene? J Adolesc Health Care 7:82S, 1986

————, SHAFER MA: Adolescent sexuality: Negative outcomes of a normative behavior, in *Adolescents at Risk: Medical and Social Perspectives*, DE Rogers, E Ginzberg (eds). Boulder, Westview Press, 1992, pp 35–79

JOHNSTON LD et al: *National Survey Results on Drug Use from the Monitoring the Future Study, 1975–94.* Vol 1, *Secondary Students.* Rockville, MD, NIH Publication No. 95-4026, 1995

KASS EJ: Adolescent varicocele: Current concepts. Semin Urol 6:140, 1988

MARSHALL W, TANNER JM: Variation in the pattern of pubertal changes in boys. Arch Dis Child 45:13, 1970

————, ————: Variation in the pattern of pubertal changes in girls. Arch Dis Child 44:291, 1969

McANARNEY ER et al: *Textbook of Adolescent Medicine.* Philadelphia, Saunders, 1992

MILLSTEIN SG et al: Health risk behaviors among young adolescents. Pediatrics 89:422, 1992

————: *Promoting the Health of Adolescents.* New York, Oxford University, 1994

NATIONAL CENTER FOR HEALTH STATISTICS: *Vital Statistics of the United States, 1990*, vol 2, *Mortality, part A.* DHHS publication no (PHS) 95-1101, 1994, pp 14–39

NEWACHECK PW et al: Health insurance coverage of adolescents: A current profile and assessment of trends. Pediatrics 90:589, 1992

NOTTELMANN ED et al: Developmental processes in early adolescence: Relations between adolescent adjustment problems and chronologic age, pubertal stage and puberty-related hormones. J Pediatr 110:473, 1987

SHAFER MAB, IRWIN CE JR: The adolescent patient, in *Rudolph's Pediatrics*, 20th ed, A Rudolph (ed). Norwalk, Appleton and Lange, 1995

SHAFFER D et al: Preventing teenage suicide: A critical review. J Am Acad Child Adolesc Psychiatry 27:675, 1988

SINGER MI et al: *Handbook for Screening Adolescents at Psychosocial Risk.* New York, Lexington Books, 1993

STYNE D, GRUMBACH MM: Disorders of puberty in males and females, in *Reproductive Endocrinology*, SS Yen, RB Jaffee (eds). Philadelphia, Saunders, 1991, pp 511–54

SUBSTANCE ABUSE AND MENTAL HEALTH SERVICES ADMINISTRATION, US DHHS: *Preliminary Estimates from the 1993 National Household Survey on Drug Abuse*, 1993

TANNER JM, DAVIES PSW: Clinical longitudinal standards for height and weight velocity for North American Children. J Pediatr 107:317, 1985

UDRY JR: Biological predispositions and social control in adolescent sexual behavior. Am Soc Rev 53:709, 1988

US Dept. of Health and Human Services (PHS), Division of STD Prevention: *Sexually Transmitted Disease Surveillance, 1994*. Atlanta, Centers
for Disease Control and Prevention, 1995

US Office of Technology Assessment: *Adolescent Health*, vol III, *Cross-
cutting Issues in the Delivery of Health and Related Services*, OTA-H-
467, Washington, DC, 1991

US Preventive Services Task Force: *Guide to Clinical Preventive Services:
An Assessment of the Effectiveness of 169 Interventions*. Baltimore, Williams & Wilkins, 1989

9   *Neil M. Resnick*

GERIATRIC MEDICINE

Of all the people who have ever lived to age 65, more than half are now alive. This statistic has important demographic and economic implications, and its impact on medical care is also substantial.

BIOLOGY OF AGING

Numerous molecular concomitants of aging have been described. For instance, there is an increase in chromosome structural abnormalities, DNA cross-linking, and frequency of single-strand breaks, a decline in DNA methylation, and loss of DNA telomeric sequences. The primary structure of proteins is unaltered, but posttranslational changes, such as deamidation, oxidation, cross-linking, and nonenzymatic glycation, increase. Mitochondrial structure also deteriorates, albeit not universally.

However, the biological changes are clearer than the mechanisms that mediate them. In fact, although the senescent phenotype appears to be ubiquitous, biologists disagree about whether senescence even exists beyond zoos and civilized societies and whether it occurs at all in many species. There is little evolutionary rationale for a process that happens after reproduction is complete, particularly one associated with such a long and complex course. In nature, senescence is most notable for its absence; nearly all animals die of predation, disease, or environmental hazards rather than aging. The argument that different species have different maximum lifespans can be explained without invoking a specific aging process: while growth and development are based on a genetic template, aging may reflect merely the accumulation of random damage rather than a specific mechanism.

If aging exists as a distinct process, there is consensus that the mechanisms are likely multifactorial and species-specific, if not organ-and cell-specific, making the paucity of available human data particularly problematic. As a result, there are nearly as many theories of aging as investigators. Most theories overlap or are not mutually exclusive, and none is completely compatible with the dearth of data. As a group, the theories can be divided into two broad categories, based on whether they attribute aging to a genetic program or to progressive and random damage to homeostatic systems. Of the genetic theories, "pleiotropic antagonism" is the only viable one compatible with the limited evolutionary selection pressure present following completion of reproduction. Proposed 35 years ago and still inadequately investigated, it suggests that aging may be caused by the late and deleterious effects of genes that are conserved because of their beneficial effects prior to reproduction. The "random damage" theories are based on the possibility that the balance between ongoing damage and repair is disrupted. The theories differ in the emphasis placed on increased damage (e.g., by free radicals, oxidation, or glycation) versus deficient repair and about the mechanisms that might mediate each. Although such theories are attractive, it remains unclear whether the described abnormalities are the cause or the result of senescence.

Many mechanisms previously postulated to mediate aging have not been borne out, including the somatic mutation theory (in which aging would result from cumulative spontaneous mutations), the error catastrophe theory (in which aging would result from errors in the synthesis of proteins critical to the synthesis of genetic material or protein-synthesizing machinery), and the intrinsic mutagenesis theory (in which aging is the result of ongoing intrinsic DNA rearrangements).

To date, the only intervention known to delay aging is caloric restriction. Its salutary effect has been documented in multiple species, from single-cell organisms to rodents. In rodents, it not only increases average life expectancy and maximum life span but also delays the onset of some typical age-associated diseases as well as deterioration of physiologic systems (e.g., immune responsiveness, glucose metabolism, muscle atrophy). The mechanism is still not determined, but it is specific to caloric restriction rather than to reduction of any dietary component (e.g., fat intake) or supplements with vitamins or antioxidants. Unfortunately, adequate data from primates are not yet available, and the impact of caloric restriction in humans is still unknown. •

PRINCIPLES OF GERIATRIC MEDICINE

Despite the biological controversy, from a physiologic standpoint human aging is characterized by progressive constriction of the homeostatic reserve of every organ system. This decline, often referred to as *homeostenosis*, is evident by the third decade and is gradual and progressive, although the rate and extent of decline vary. The decline of each organ system (Table 9-1) appears to occur independently of changes in other organ systems and is influenced by diet, environment, and personal habits as well as by genetic factors.

Several important principles follow from these facts: (1) Individuals become more dissimilar as they age, belying any stereotype of aging; (2) an *abrupt* decline in any system or function is always due to disease and not to "normal aging"; (3) "normal aging" can be attenuated by modification of risk factors (e.g., increased blood pressure, smoking, sedentary lifestyle); and (4) "healthy old age" is not an oxymoron. In fact, *in the absence of disease, the decline in homeostatic reserve causes no symptoms and imposes few restrictions on activities of daily living regardless of age.*

Appreciation of these facts may make it easier to understand the striking increases that have occurred in life expectancy. Average life expectancy is now 17 years at age 65, 11 years at age 75, 6 years at age 85, 4 years at age 90, and 2 years at age 100. Moreover, the bulk of these years is characterized by a lack of significant impairment (Table 9-2)—only 35 percent of people over age 85 are impaired in any activity required for daily living, and only 20 percent reside in a nursing home. Yet, as individuals age they are more likely to suffer from disease, disability, and the side effects of drugs, all of which, when combined with the decrease in physiologic reserve, make the older person more vulnerable to environmental, pathologic, and pharmacologic challenges.

The following concepts underlie the remainder of the chapter:

1. The onset of a new disease in the elderly (usually defined as over age 75 to 80) generally affects the organ system made most vulnerable by prior physiologic and pathologic changes. Because this organ system often differs from the newly diseased organ system, disease presentation in the elderly is often atypical. For example, fewer than one-fourth of older patients with hyperthyroidism present with goiter, tremor, and exophthalmos; more likely are atrial fibrillation, confusion, depression, syncope, and weakness. Significantly, because the "weakest link" is so often the brain, the lower urinary tract, or the cardiovascular or musculoskeletal system, a limited number of presenting symptoms predominate—acute confusion, depression, incontinence, falling, and syncope—no matter what the underlying disease. Thus for the most common geriatric syndromes, regardless of the presenting symptom, the differential diagnosis is often largely similar. The corollary is equally important: The organ system usually associated with a particular symptom is less likely to be the source of that symptom in older individuals than in younger ones. Compared with middle-aged individuals, for example, acute confusion in older patients is less often due to a new brain lesion, depression to a psychiat-

ric disorder, incontinence to bladder dysfunction, falling to a neuropathy, or syncope to heart disease.

2. Because of decreased physiologic reserve, older patients often develop symptoms at an earlier stage of their disease. For example, heart failure may be precipitated by mild hyperthyroidism, cognitive dysfunction by mild hyperparathyroidism, urinary retention by mild prostatic enlargement, and nonketotic hyperosmolar coma by mild glucose intolerance. Paradoxically, therefore, treatment of the underlying disease may be easier because it is frequently less advanced at the time of presentation. A corollary is that drug side effects can occur with drugs and drug doses unlikely to produce side effects in younger people (Chap. 69). For instance, an antihistamine may cause confusion,

diuretics may precipitate urinary incontinence, digoxin may induce depression even with normal serum levels, and over-the-counter sympathomimetics may precipitate urinary retention in men with mild prostatic obstruction.

Unfortunately, the predisposition to develop symptoms at an earlier stage of disease is often offset by the change in illness behavior that occurs with age. Raised at a time when symptoms and debility were accepted as normal consequences of aging, the elderly are less likely to seek attention until symptoms become disabling. Thus, any symptom, particularly those associated with a change in functional status, must be taken seriously and evaluated promptly.

3. Since many homeostatic mechanisms may be compromised concurrently, there are usually multiple abnormalities amenable to treatment, and small improvements in each may yield dramatic benefits overall. For instance, cognitive impairment in patients with Alz-

Table 9-1

Selected Age-Related Changes and Their Consequences

Organ/System	Age-Related Physiologic Change*	Consequences of Age-Related Physiologic Change	Consequences of Disease, not Age
General	↑Body fat	↑Volume of distribution for fat soluble drugs	Obesity
	↓Total body water	↓Volume of distribution for water soluble drugs	Anorexia
Eyes/ears	Presbyopia	↓Accommodation	
	Lens opacification	↑Susceptibility to glare Need for increased illumination	Blindness
	↓High-frequency acuity	Difficulty discriminating words if background noise is present	Deafness
Endocrine	Impaired glucose homeostasis	↑Glucose level in response to acute illness	Diabetes mellitus
	↓Thyroxine clearance (and production)	↓T_4 dose required in hypothyroidism	Thyroid dysfunction
	↑ADH, ↓renin, and ↓aldosterone		↓Na^+, ↑K^+
	↓Testosterone		Impotence
	↓Vitamin D absorption and activation	Osteopenia	Osteomalacia, fracture
Respiratory	↓Lung elasticity and ↑chest wall stiffness	Ventilation/perfusion mismatch and ↓P_{O_2}	Dyspnea, hypoxia
Cardiovascular	↓Arterial compliance and ↑ systolic BP →LVH	Hypotensive response to ↑HR, volume depletion, or loss of atrial contraction	Syncope
	↓β-adrenergic responsiveness	↓Cardiac output and HR response to stress	Heart failure
	↓Baroreceptor sensitivity and ↓SA node automaticity	Impaired blood pressure response to standing, volume depletion	Heart block
Gastrointestinal	↓Hepatic function	Delayed metabolism of some drugs	Cirrhosis
	↓Gastric acidity	↓Ca^+ absorption on empty stomach	Osteoporosis, B_{12} deficiency
	↓Colonic motility	Constipation	Fecal impaction
	↓Anorectal function		Fecal incontinence
Hematologic/immune system	↓Bone marrow reserve(?)		Anemia
	↓T cell function	False-negative PPD response	
	↑Autoantibodies	False-positive rheumatoid factor, antinuclear antibody	Autoimmune disease
Renal	↓GFR	Impaired excretion of some drugs	↑Serum creatinine
	↓Urine concentration/dilution (see also "Endocrine")	Delayed response to salt or fluid restriction/overload; nocturia	↓↑Na^+
Genitourinary	Vaginal/urethral mucosal atrophy	Dyspareunia, bacteriuria	Symptomatic UTI
	Prostate enlargement	↑Residual urine volume	Urinary incontinence; urinary retention
Musculoskeletal	↓Lean body mass, muscle		Functional impairment
	↓Bone density	Osteopenia	Hip fracture
Nervous system	Brain atrophy	Benign senescent forgetfulness	Dementia, delirium
	↓Brain catechol synthesis		Depression
	↓Brain dopaminergic synthesis	Stiffer gait	Parkinson's disease
	↓Righting reflexes	↑Body sway	Falls
	↓Stage 4 sleep	Early wakening, insomnia	Sleep apnea

* Changes generally observed in healthy elderly subjects free of symptoms and detectable disease in the organ system studied. The changes are usually important only when the system is stressed or other factors are added (e.g., drugs, disease, or environmental challenge); they rarely result in symptoms otherwise. Abbreviations: T_4, thyroxine; BP, blood pressure; HR, heart rate; ADH, antidiuretic hormone; GFR, glomerular filtration rate.

Table 9-2

CHAPTER 9
Geriatric Medicine

39

Life Expectancy and Number of Remaining Years Free of Dependency in Activities of Daily Living

Age	Life Expectancy*, av		Disability-Free Years Remaining	
	Men	Women	Men	Women
65–69	13	20	9	11
70–74	12	16	8	8
75–79	10	13	7	7
80–84	7	10	5	5
≥85	7	8	3	3

* For independent noninstitutionalized elderly men and women in Massachusetts. Longevity and disability-free longevity are surprisingly long and must be incorporated into treatment decisions. Av, average. All figures rounded to nearest year. See text for more recent data on longevity alone.

SOURCE: S Katz et al, N Engl J Med 309:1218, 1983.

heimer's disease may be exacerbated by hearing or visual impairment, depression, heart failure, and electrolyte imbalance. Similarly, urinary incontinence can be worsened by fecal impaction, medications, and excess urinary output. In each case, substantial functional improvement can result from treating the contributing factors even if—as in Alzheimer's disease—the disease itself is untreatable.

4. Many findings that are abnormal in younger patients are relatively common in older people—e.g., bacteriuria, premature ventricular contractions, low bone mineral density, impaired glucose tolerance, and uninhibited bladder contractions. However, they may not be responsible for a particular symptom but only be incidental findings that result in missed diagnoses and misdirected therapy. For instance, the finding of bacteriuria should not end the search for a source of fever in an acutely ill older patient, nor should an elevated random blood sugar—especially in an acutely ill patient—be incriminated as the cause of neuropathy. On the other hand, certain other abnormalities must not be dismissed as due to old age—e.g., there is no anemia, impotence, depression, or confusion of old age.

5. Because symptoms in older people are often due to multiple causes, the diagnostic "law of parsimony" often does not apply. For instance, fever, anemia, retinal embolus, and a heart murmur prompt almost a reflex diagnosis of infective endocarditis in a younger patient but may reflect aspirin-induced blood loss, a cholesterol embolus, insignificant aortic sclerosis, and a viral illness in an older patient.

6. Because the older patient is more likely to suffer the adverse consequences of disease, treatment—and even prevention—may be equally or even more effective. For instance, the benefits of thrombolysis and beta-blocker therapy after a myocardial infarction are as impressive in older patients as in younger ones; and treatment of hypertension and transient ischemic attacks, as well as immunization against influenza and pneumococcal pneumonia are more effective in older patients. In addition, prevention in older patients often must be seen in a broader context. For instance, although interventions to increase bone density may be limited in older patients, fracture still may be prevented by efforts to improve balance, strengthen legs, reduce peripheral edema, treat other contributing medical conditions, replete nutritional deficits, eliminate environmental hazards, and remove adverse medications—not so much those that affect bone metabolism, but rather those that induce orthostasis, confusion, and extrapyramidal stiffness.

HISTORY TAKING IN ELDERLY PATIENTS Most older patients are able to provide a reliable medical history; however, a multitude of complaints may make obtaining a history more difficult and adequate time must be allotted. If the patient is unable to comprehend or communicate, data should be sought from family, friends, and caregivers. The history also should include drug ingestion; a dietary history; and history of falling, of incontinence, and of depression and anxiety.

Advance Directives All older patients should be asked whether they have drafted advance health care directives, and, if they have, a copy should be placed in the record. Such directives may consist of a health care proxy or durable power of attorney for health care, in which patients designate a surrogate decision-maker who makes health care decisions if the patient cannot, and/or a living will or medical directive, in which patients specify their desires for treatment in specific situations if they cannot communicate at the critical time.

Whether or not the patient has formally drafted these directives, it is useful to indicate in the record who should make health care decisions if the patient is no longer able to do so. Patients should then be encouraged to discuss with the physician as well as the designated proxy their feelings about resuscitation, intubation, feeding tubes, hospitalization, etc., in their current state of health and possible future declining states of health. The early elicitation of a patient's preferences and values can often help both physicians and families in subsequent difficult decisions by giving surrogate decision-makers the sense that they are doing as the patient would have wanted.

PHYSICAL EXAMINATION Certain features of the examination should receive special attention, depending in part on clues from the history. Weight and postural blood pressure should be measured at each visit. Vision and hearing should be checked; if hearing is impaired, excess cerumen should be removed from the external auditory canals. Denture fit should be assessed, and the oral cavity should be inspected with the dentures removed. Although thyroid disease becomes more common with age, the sensitivity and specificity of related findings are substantially lower than in younger individuals; consequently, the physical examination can rarely corroborate or exclude thyroid dysfunction in older patients. The breasts should not be overlooked, since older women are more likely to have breast cancer and less likely to do breast self-examination. The systolic murmur of aortic sclerosis is common and may be difficult to differentiate from aortic stenosis, especially since the presence of a fourth heart sound in an elderly person does not imply significant cardiac disease, and the carotid upstroke normally increases owing to age-related arterial stiffening.

In inactive patients and those with fecal or urinary incontinence, one should check for fecal impaction. In patients with urinary incontinence—especially men—a distended bladder must be looked for, since it may be the only finding in urinary retention; perineal sensation and the bulbocavernosus reflex also should be tested. Patients who fall should be observed standing up from a chair, bending down, reaching up, walking 10 feet, turning, returning, and sitting again; abnormalities of gait and balance should be evaluated with the patient's eyes open and closed and in response to a sternal push. It should be appreciated that "frontal release signs" (e.g., "snout," "glabellar," or palmomental reflexes) and absent ankle jerks and vibratory sense in the feet may be normal in the elderly.

MENTAL STATUS EXAMINATION In addition to evaluating mood and affect, some form of cognitive testing is essential in all elderly patients, even if it involves only checking different components of the history for consistency. People with mild degrees of dementia usually retain their social graces and may mask intellectual impairment by a cheerful and cooperative manner. Thus, the examiner should always probe for content. For patients who follow the news, one can ask what stories they are particularly interested in and why; the same applies to reading, social events—even the soap operas on television.

If there is any suspicion of a cognitive deficit after this kind of conversational probing, further questioning is indicated. An examination that tests only orientation as to person, place, and time is insufficient to detect mild or moderate intellectual impairment. As a quick screen, simply assessing orientation and asking the patient to draw a clock with the hands at a set time (e.g., 10 min before 2:00) can be very informative regarding cognitive status, visuospatial deficits, ability to comprehend and execute instructions in logical sequence, and presence or absence of perseveration. For slightly more detailed examinations, many practical mental status tests are available. The most widely used is the Mini-Mental Status Examination of Folstein (Chap. 24), which provides a numerical score that can be obtained in 5 to 10 min. Regardless of the test employed, the total score is less useful diagnostically than is knowledge of the specific domain of the deficit. As a general rule, disproportionate difficulty with immediate recall (e.g., of a list of three items) suggests depression, while predominant difficulty with recalling the items 5 min later suggests dementia. For patients with deficits of attention—recognized by inability to spell simple words backwards, repeat five digits, or recite the months of the year backwards—delirium is probably present, and the accuracy of the remainder of the test is dubious. However, the test can be interpreted accurately only in the context of a comprehensive evaluation.

EVALUATION OF FUNCTIONAL CAPACITY A clear description of the patient's degree of functional incapacity based on both medical and psychosocial problems is essential. The functional assessment includes determination of the patient's ability to perform basic activities of daily life (ADL), which are those needed for personal self-care, as well as the ability to perform more complex tasks required for independent living, the instrumental activities of daily living (IADL). ADLs include bathing, dressing, toileting, feeding, getting in and out of chairs and bed, and walking. IADLs include shopping, cooking, money management, housework, using a telephone, and traveling outside the home. For frail patients, an assessment in the home by a trained observer may be required, but for most patients a questionnaire dealing with these activities can be completed by the family or patient. In either case, the physician must determine the cause of any impairment and whether it can be treated. The assessment should conclude with determination of the socioeconomic circumstances and social support systems.

Since disease can present atypically in the elderly, acute functional decline may represent the first sign of serious acute illness. Thus, *acute functional decline presenting as the onset or worsening of falls, confusion, depression, or incontinence should prompt immediate medical evaluation.*

MANAGEMENT OF COMMON GERIATRIC CONDITIONS

Diseases more common in the elderly are covered elsewhere in the text. The medical problems discussed below do not usually present as clear-cut organ-specific diagnoses and are most common in the frail elderly, especially those over 80 years of age.

INTELLECTUAL IMPAIRMENT The predominant causes of impaired mentation in older patients are delirium, dementia, and depression. Each condition is covered elsewhere in the text in detail (Chaps. 24 and 367), but their management in the elderly is discussed here.

Differentiating the causes of impaired mentation is important, but in older patients they frequently coexist. Thus, the most important first step is to search for and correct all factors that may contribute to cognitive impairment, even in patients with dementia. Evidence of dangerous behavior also should be sought (e.g., leaving the stove on, wandering, and getting lost) and plans should be devised to deal with it. Although there is no specific pharmacologic treatment for Alzheimer's disease and agents such as tacrine are of limited efficacy and tolerability, this does not mean that the physician has no further role in treating the patient and family. In addition to discontinuing all nonessential medications and treating new intercurrent illness, the physician should help the family and patient predict and deal with the disease; indeed, the family often needs the physician's support more than the patient does.

℞ **TREATMENT**
Community services should be suggested as needed, including a visiting nurse, a home health aid to assist with personal hygiene, a homemaker to assist with housework, meal delivery and transportation services, day health centers, and respite care to ease the burden on family members. Support groups such as the Alzheimer's Associ-

ation often are of value to the family and help them to anticipate problems. Signs of patient abuse by an overstressed caregiver should be watched for. Legal counsel should be recommended to help the patient and family devise plans for ongoing management and ultimate disposition of assets.

Finally, abrupt worsening of mentation or the onset of disruptive behavior should always prompt a search for new illness or medication. Exacerbation of cognitive dysfunction may occur with mild infections (e.g., subungual toe abscess, vaginitis, or pressure ulcer); with "therapeutic" levels of many drugs; with use of nonprescribed drugs or alcohol; with modest abnormalities of serum sodium, calcium, glucose, or thyroxine; with mild hypoxia; with borderline nutritional deficiencies; and with the development of fecal impaction, urinary retention, pain, or change in environment, particularly in frail older patients. However, if a cause is not found and behavior does not respond to environmental manipulation, low doses of an antipsychotic medication may be helpful (e.g., haloperidol 0.25 to 2 mg per day orally; see below).

DEPRESSION Depression of significant degree occurs in 5 to 10 percent of community-dwelling elderly but is often overlooked. At highest risk are individuals with recent medical illness (e.g., stroke), bereavement, lack of social supports, recent nursing home admission, or psychiatric history (including alcohol abuse). The diagnosis requires the presence of a depressed mood for at least two consecutive weeks plus at least four of the following eight signs: sleep disturbance, lack of interest, feelings of guilt, decreased energy, decreased concentration, decreased appetite, psychomotor agitation/retardation, and suicidal ideation. Also helpful diagnostically are a personal or family history of depression, anhedonia (loss of pleasure), and past response to an antidepressant. It is essential to bear in mind that depression in older patients is often caused or contributed to by drugs or a systemic illness.

℞ **TREATMENT**
For the hospitalized patient in whom acute depression delays recovery or rehabilitation—when correction of medical and pharmacologic contributing factors is ineffective and there is no prior history of mania or major depression—methylphenidate, 5 to 10 mg at 8 A.M. and noon (to avoid insomnia) is often very effective, with benefits discernible within a few days. For patients with major depression, there is no ideal antidepressant drug. All are about equally effective, but the side effects differ (see below and Chap. 385). Consequently, one should become familiar with one or two agents for patients with psychomotor retardation (e.g., desipramine, sertraline) and for those with agitation (e.g., nortriptyline or trazodone). Because of its potent anticholinergic and orthostatic side effects, amitriptyline should be avoided whenever possible in older patients. Initial low dosages should be increased slowly to avoid serious side effects; low doses of each medication (e.g., nortriptyline, 10 to 50 mg daily; desipramine, 25 to 75 mg daily; or sertraline 50 to 150 mg daily) are often effective in the elderly. Careful follow-up is required to anticipate and minimize anticholinergic side effects, orthostatic hypotension, sedating effects, confusion, bizarre mental symptoms, cardiovascular complications, and drug overdose with suicidal intent. Adverse drug reactions should not be assumed to be due to the aging process.

Cautious use of the monoamine oxidase inhibitors is sometimes of benefit when other antidepressants are ineffective. Monoamine oxidase inhibitors should not be used in combination with the cyclic compounds. Electroconvulsive therapy has been successful and is usually well tolerated by elderly patients who remain severely depressed despite drug treatment, particularly if they also have delusions.

URINARY INCONTINENCE **Transient Incontinence** (Table 9-3) Because urinary continence requires adequate mobility, mentation, motivation, and manual dexterity—in addition to integrated

Table 9-3

CHAPTER 9
Geriatric Medicine

41

Classification of Incontinence

TRANSIENT

Delirium/confusional state
Infection—urinary (symptomatic)
Atrophic urethritis/vaginitis
Pharmaceuticals
Psychological, especially depression
Excessive urine output (e.g., CHF, hyperglycemia)
Restricted mobility
Stool impaction

ESTABLISHED

Detrusor overactivity
Detrusor underactivity
Urethral obstruction
Urethral incompetence

SOURCE: Adapted from NM Resnick, Medical Grand Rounds 3:281, 1984.

control of the lower urinary tract—problems outside the bladder can result in incontinence.

1. *Delirium.* A clouded sensorium impedes recognition of both the need to void and the location of the nearest toilet; once delirium clears, incontinence resolves.

2. *Infection.* Symptomatic urinary tract infection commonly causes or contributes to incontinence; asymptomatic infection does not.

3. *Atrophic urethritis/vaginitis.* Atrophic urethritis/vaginitis, characterized by the presence of vaginal telangiectasia, petechiae, erosions, erythema, or friability, commonly contributes to incontinence in women and responds to a short course of low-dose estrogen or vaginal estrogen creams.

4. *Pharmaceutical.* The drugs most commonly causing transient incontinence are listed in Table 9-4.

5. *Psychologic.* Depression and psychosis are uncommon but treatable causes.

6. *Excess urine output.* Excess urine output may overwhelm the ability to reach a toilet in time. Causes include diuretics, excess fluid intake, and metabolic abnormalities (e.g., hyperglycemia, hypercalcemia, diabetes insipidus); nocturnal incontinence may result from mobilization of peripheral edema.

7. *Restricted mobility.* If mobility cannot be improved, access to a urinal or commode may restore continence. (See "Immobility" below.)

8. *Stool impaction.* This is a common cause of urinary incontinence, especially in hospitalized or immobile patients. Although the mechanism is unknown, a clue to its presence is the coexistence of both urinary and fecal incontinence. Disimpaction restores continence.

Established Incontinence (Table 9-3) The causes of established incontinence include irreversible functional deficits, such as *end-stage* Alzheimer's disease, and intrinsic lower urinary tract dysfunction. Lower urinary tract dysfunction should be sought after transient causes have been excluded.

Detrusor Overactivity This disorder (involuntary bladder contraction) accounts for two-thirds of geriatric incontinence in both sexes, regardless of whether patients are demented. Detrusor overactivity can be diagnosed presumptively in a woman when leakage occurs in the absence of stress maneuvers or urinary retention and is preceded by the abrupt onset of an intense urge to urinate that cannot be forestalled. In men, the symptoms are similar, but since detrusor overactivity often coexists with urethral obstruction, urodynamic testing should be done if prescription of a bladder relaxant is planned. Because detrusor overactivity also may be due to bladder stones or tumor, the abrupt onset of otherwise unexplained urge incontinence—especially if accompanied by perineal/suprapubic discomfort or sterile hematuria—should prompt cystoscopy and cytologic examination.

Table 9-4

Commonly Used Medications That May Affect Continence

Type of Medication	Examples	Potential Effects on Continence
Sedatives/hypnotics	Long-acting benzodiazepines (e.g., diazepam, flurazepam)	Sedation, delirium, immobility
Alcohol		Polyuria, frequency, urgency, sedation, delirium, immobility
Anticholinergics	Dicyclomine, disopyramide, antihistamines	Urinary retention, overflow incontinence, delirium, impaction
Antipsychotics	Thioridazine, haloperidol	Anticholinergic actions, sedation, rigidity, immobility
Antidepressants	Amitriptyline, desipramine	Anticholinergic actions, sedation
Antiparkinsonians	Trihexyphenidyl, benztropine mesylate (not L-dopa/selegiline)	Anticholinergic actions, sedation
Narcotic analgesics	Opiates	Urinary retention, fecal impaction, sedation, delirium
Alpha-adrenergic antagonists	Prazosin, terazosin, doxazosin	Urethral relaxation may precipitate stress incontinence in women
Alpha-adrenergic agonists	Nasal decongestants	Urinary retention in men
Calcium channel blockers	All dihydropyridines*	Urinary retention; nocturnal diuresis due to fluid retention
Potent diuretics	Furosemide, bumetanide	Polyuria, frequency, urgency
Angiotensin-converting enzyme inhibitors	Captopril, enalapril, lisinopril	Drug-induced cough can precipitate stress incontinence in women and in some men with prior prostatectomy
Vincristine		Urinary retention

* Examples include nifedipine, nicardipine, israpidine, felodipine, nimodipine.

SOURCE: Adapted from NM Resnick, in Current Medical Diagnosis and Treatment, LT Tierney et al (eds), Norwalk, Appleton & Lange, 1993.

 TREATMENT

The cornerstone of treatment is behavioral therapy. Patients without dementia are instructed to void every 1 to 2 h (while awake only) and to suppress urgency in between; once daytime continence is restored, the interval between voiding can be progressively increased. Demented patients are "prompted" to void at similar intervals. When drugs are necessary, they should be added to these regimens and monitored to avoid inducing urinary retention. Effective drugs include anticholinergics (e.g., propantheline, 7.5 to 30 mg three to five times daily), oxybutynin (2.5 to 5 mg three or four times daily), dicyclomine (10 to 30 mg three times daily), and imipramine or doxepin (25 to 100 mg at bedtime).

Indwelling catheterization is rarely indicated for detrusor overactivity. If all measures fail, an external collection device or protective pad or undergarment may be required.

Stress incontinence This disorder, the second most common cause of established incontinence in older women (it is rare in men), is characterized by symptoms and evidence of *instantaneous* leakage of urine in response to stress. Leakage is worse or occurs only during the day unless another abnormality (e.g., detrusor overactivity) is also present. On examination, with the bladder full and the perineum relaxed, instantaneous leakage upon coughing strongly suggests stress incontinence, especially if it reproduces symptoms and if urinary retention has been excluded by a postvoiding residual determination; a several-second delay suggests that leakage is instead caused by an involuntary bladder contraction induced by coughing.

 TREATMENT

Surgery is the most effective treatment with a cure rate of 75 to 85 percent. For women who can comply indefinitely, pelvic muscle exercises are an option for mild to moderate stress incontinence; if not contraindicated, an alpha-adrenergic agonist (e.g., phenylpropanolamine) is also helpful in such cases, especially if combined with estrogen. Occasionally, a pessary or even a tampon (for women with vaginal stenosis) provides some relief.

Urethral obstruction Rarely present in women, urethral obstruction (due to prostatic enlargement, urethral stricture, bladder neck contracture, or prostate cancer) is the second most common cause of established incontinence in older men. It can present as dribbling incontinence after voiding, urge incontinence due to detrusor overactivity (which coexists in two-thirds of cases), or overflow incontinence due to urinary retention. Renal ultrasound is recommended to exclude hydronephrosis in men whose postvoiding residual volume exceeds 100 to 200 mL; in older men for whom surgery is planned, urodynamic confirmation of obstruction is strongly advised.

TREATMENT

Surgical decompression is the most effective treatment for obstruction, especially if there is urinary retention. For a nonoperative candidate, intermittent or indwelling catheterization is used; a condom catheter is contraindicated when urinary retention is present. For a man with prostatic obstruction who is not in retention, treatment with an alpha-adrenergic antagonist (e.g., terazosin 5 to 10 mg daily) may lessen symptoms in a few weeks. The 5α-reductase inhibitor finasteride also may ameliorate symptoms in a third or more of patients, but its impact is modest and not apparent for many months. Combined treatment with both agents has proved no better than treatment with an alpha blocker alone.

Detrusor underactivity Whether idiopathic or due to sacral lower motor nerve dysfunction, this is the least common cause of incontinence (<10 percent of cases). When it causes incontinence, detrusor underactivity is associated with urinary frequency, nocturia, and frequent leakage of small amounts. The elevated postvoiding residual volume (generally over 450 mL) distinguishes it from detrusor overactivity and stress incontinence, but only urodynamic testing (rather than cystoscopy or intravenous urography) differentiates it from urethral obstruction in men; such testing usually is not required in women, in whom obstruction is rare.

TREATMENT

For the patient with a poorly contractile bladder, augmented voiding techniques (e.g., double voiding or applying suprapubic pressure) are often effective; pharmacologic agents (e.g., bethanechol) are rarely effective. If further emptying is needed or for the patient with an acontractile bladder, intermittent or indwelling catheterization is the only option. Antibiotics should be used for symptomatic upper tract infection, or as prophylaxis for recurrent symptomatic infections only in a patient using intermittent catheterization; they should not be used as prophylaxis with an indwelling catheter.

FALLS Falls are a major problem for elderly people, especially women. Thirty percent of community-dwelling elderly fall each year, and the proportion increases with age. Nonetheless, falling must *not* be viewed as accidental, inevitable, or untreatable.

Causes of Falls Balance and ambulation require a complex interplay of cognitive, neuromuscular, and cardiovascular function and the ability to adapt rapidly to an environmental challenge. Balance becomes impaired and sway increases with age. The resulting vulnerability predisposes the older person to fall when challenged by an additional insult to *any* of these systems. Thus, a seemingly minor fall may be due to a serious problem, such as pneumonia or a myocardial infarction.

Much more commonly, however, falls are due to the complex interaction between a variably impaired patient and an environmental challenge. While a warped floorboard may pose little problem for a vigorous, unmedicated, alert person, it may be sufficient to precipitate a fall and hip fracture in the patient with impaired vision, strength, balance, or cognition. Thus, falls in older people are rarely due to a single cause, and effective prevention entails a comprehensive assessment of the patient's intrinsic deficits (usually diseases and medications), the routine activities, and the environmental obstacles.

Intrinsic deficits are those that impair sensory input, judgment, blood pressure regulation, reaction time, and balance and gait (Table 9-5). Medications and alcohol use are among the most common, significant, and reversible causes of falling. Other treatable contributors include postprandial hypotension (which peaks 30 to 60 min after a meal), insomnia, urinary urgency, foot problems, and peripheral edema (which can burden impaired leg strength and gait with an additional 5 to 10 pounds).

Environmental obstacles are listed in Table 9-6. Since most falls occur in or around the home, a visit by a visiting nurse, physical therapist, or physician often reaps substantial dividends.

Complications of Falls and Treatment One out of four people who fall suffers serious injury. Five percent of falls result in fractures, and an equal proportion cause serious soft tissue damage. Falls are the sixth leading cause of death for older people and a contributing factor in 40 percent of admissions to nursing homes. Resultant hip problems and fear of falls are major causes of loss of independence.

Subdural hematoma is a treatable but easily overlooked complication of falls that must be considered in any elderly patient presenting with new neurologic signs, including confusion alone, even in the absence of a headache. Dehydration, electrolyte imbalance, pressure sores, and hypothermia also may occur and endanger the patient's life following a fall.

The risk of falling and consequent injury, disability, and potential institutionalization can be reduced by modifying where possible those factors outlined above and in Tables 9-5 and 9-6. Gait training by a physical therapist often alleviates fear of falling. Ensuring the availability of phones at floor level, a portable phone, or a lightweight radio call system is also important.

IMMOBILITY The main causes of immobility are weakness, stiffness, pain, imbalance, and psychological problems. Weakness may result from disuse of muscles, malnutrition, electrolyte disturbances, anemia, neurologic disorders, or myopathies. The most common cause of stiffness in the elderly is osteoarthritis; however, Parkinson's disease, rheumatoid arthritis, gout, pseudogout, and antipsychotic drugs such as haloperidol may also contribute. Pain, whether from bone (e.g., osteoporosis, osteomalacia, Paget's disease, metastatic bone cancer, trauma), joints (e.g., osteoarthritis, rheumatoid arthritis, gout), bursa, muscle (e.g., polymyalgia rheumatica, intermittent claudication, or "pseudoclaudication"), or foot problems may immobilize the patient.

Imbalance and fear of falling are major causes of immobilization. Imbalance may result from general debility, neurologic causes (e.g., stroke; loss of postural reflexes; peripheral neuropathy due to diabetes mellitus, alcohol, or malnutrition; and vestibulocerebellar abnormalities), orthostatic or postprandial hypotension, or drugs (e.g., diuretics, antihypertensives, neuroleptics, and antidepressants) or may occur following prolonged bed rest. Psychological conditions such as severe anxiety or depression also may contribute to immobilization.

Consequences In addition to thrombophlebitis and pulmonary embolus, there are multiple hazards of bed rest in the elderly. Deconditioning of the cardiovascular system occurs within days and involves fluid shifts, fluid loss, decreased cardiac output, decreased peak oxygen uptake, and increased resting heart rate. Striking changes also occur in skeletal muscle. At the cellular level, intracellular ATP and glycogen concentrations decrease, rates of protein degradation increase, and contractile velocity and strength decline, while at the whole-muscle level, atrophy, weakness, and shortening are seen. Pressure sores are another serious complication; mechanical pressure, moisture, friction, and shearing forces all predispose to their development. As a result, within days of being confined to bed, the risk of postural hypotension, falls, and skin breakdown rises. Moreover, these changes usually take weeks to months to reverse.

℞ TREATMENT

The most important step is preventive—to avoid bedrest whenever possible. When it cannot be avoided, several measures can be employed to minimize its consequences. Patients should be positioned as close to the upright position as possible several times daily. Range of motion exercises should begin immediately, and the skin over pressure points should be inspected frequently. Isometric and isotonic exercises should be performed while the patient is in bed, and whenever possible patients should assist their own positioning, transferring, and self-care. As mobility becomes feasible, graduated ambulation should begin. For individuals confined to a wheelchair, ring-shaped devices ("donuts") should not be used to prevent pressure ulcers since they cause venous congestion and edema and actually increase the risk.

If a pressure ulcer develops, therapy depends on its stage. Stage 1 ulcers are characterized by nonblanchable erythema of intact skin; stage 2 lesions involve an ulcer of the epidermis, dermis, or both; stage 3 ulcers extend to the subcutaneous tissue; and stage 4 lesions involve muscle, bone, and/or the supporting tissues. For stage 1 lesions, eliminating excess pressure and ensuring adequate nutrition and hygiene are sufficient. For the remaining types, the caregiver must also ensure that the wound stays clean and moist; thus, if saline dressings are used they should be changed when they are damp rather than dry. Synthetic dressings are more expensive than saline but are more effective because they require fewer changes (with less disruption of reepithelialization) and protect against contamination. Because bacterial colonization of pressure ulcers is universal, swab cultures should not be performed and topical treatment should be considered only for patients whose ulcers have not healed after 2 weeks of therapy. By contrast, associated cellulitis, osteomyelitis, or sepsis requires systemic therapy after cultures of blood and the wound border (by needle aspiration or biopsy) have been obtained. Surgical or enzymatic debridement is required for stage 3 and 4 lesions. In addition to a daily multivitamin, prescribing vitamin C (500 mg twice daily) is also useful. For debilitated patients, special mattresses are beneficial, including those that reduce pressure (e.g., static air mattress or foam) and those that relieve it (e.g., dynamic units that sequentially inflate and deflate).

In addition to treating all identified factors that contribute to immobility, consultation with a physical therapist should be sought. Installing handrails, lowering the bed, and providing chairs of proper height with arms and rubber skid guards may allow the patient to be safely mobile in the home. A properly fitted cane or walker may be helpful.

IATROGENIC DRUG REACTIONS For several reasons, older patients are two or three times more likely to have adverse drug reactions (Chap. 69). Drug clearance is often markedly reduced. This

Table 9-5

Intrinsic Risk Factors for Falling, and Possible Interventions

Risk Factor	Interventions	
	Medical	Rehabilitative or Environmental
Reduced visual acuity, dark adaptation, and perception	Refraction; cataract extraction	Home safety assessment
Reduced hearing	Removal of cerumen; audiologic evaluation	Hearing aid if appropriate (with training); reduction in background noise
Vestibular dysfunction	Avoidance of drugs affecting the vestibular system; neurologic or ear, nose, and throat evaluation, if indicated	Habituation exercises
Proprioceptive dysfunction, cervical degenerative disorders, and peripheral neuropathy	Screening for vitamin B_{12} deficiency and cervical spondylosis	Balance exercises; appropriate walking aid; correctly sized footwear with firm soles; home safety assessment
Dementia	Detection of reversible causes; avoidance of sedative or centrally acting drugs	Supervised exercise and ambulation; home safety assessment
Musculoskeletal disorders	Appropriate diagnostic evaluation	Balance-and-gait training; muscle-strengthening exercises; appropriate walking aid; home safety assessment
Foot disorders (calluses, bunions, deformities, edema)	Shaving of calluses; bunionectomy; treatment of edema	Trimming of nails; appropriate footwear
Postural hypotension	Assessment of medications; rehydration; possible alteration in situational factors (e.g., meals, change of position)	Dorsiflexion exercises; pressure-graded stockings; elevation of head of bed; use of tilt table if condition is severe
Use of medications (sedatives: benzodiazepines, phenothiazines, antidepressants; antihypertensives; others: antiarrhythmics, anticonvulsants, diuretics, alcohol)	Steps to be taken: 1. Attempted reduction in the total number of medications taken 2. Assessment of risks and benefits of each medication 3. Selection of medication, if needed, that is least centrally acting, least associated with postural hypotension, and has shortest action 4. Prescription of lowest effective dose 5. Frequent reassessment of risks and benefits	

SOURCE: After ME Tinetti and M Speechley, N Engl J Med 320:1055, 1989.

Table 9-6

Environmental Factors Affecting the Risk of Falling

Environmental Area or Factor	Objective and Recommendations
All areas	
Lighting	Adequacy of illumination (older people need twice as much as younger people); absence of glare and shadows; accessible switches at room entrances; night light in bedroom, hall, bathroom
Floors	Nonskid backing for throw rugs; carpet edges tacked down; carpets with shallow pile; nonskid wax on floors; cords out of walking path; small objects (e.g., clothes, shoes) off floor
Stairs	Lighting sufficient, with switches at top and bottom of stairs; securely fastened bilateral handrails that stand out from wall; top and bottom steps marked with bright, contrasting tape; stair rises of no more than 6 in; steps in good repair; no objects stored on steps
Kitchen	Items stored so that reaching up and bending over are not necessary; secure step stool available if climbing is necessary; firm, nonmovable table
Bathroom	Grab bars for tub, shower, and toilet; nonskid decals or rubber mat in tub or shower; shower chair with handheld shower; nonskid rugs; raised toilet seat; door locks removed to ensure access in an emergency
Yard and entrances	Repair of cracks in pavement, holes in lawn; removal of rocks, tools, and other tripping hazards; well-lit walkways, free of ice and wet leaves; stairs and steps as above
Institutions	All the above; bed at proper height (not too high or low); spills on floor cleaned up promptly; appropriate use of walking aids and wheelchairs
Footwear	Shoes with firm, nonskid, nonfriction soles; low heels (unless person is accustomed to high heels); avoidance of walking in stocking feet or loose slippers

SOURCE: After ME Tinetti and M Speechley, N Engl J Med 320:1055, 1989.

is due to a decrease in renal plasma flow and glomerular filtration rate and a reduced hepatic clearance. The last is due to a decrease in activity of the drug-metabolizing microsomal enzymes and an overall decline in blood flow to the liver with aging. The volume of distribution of drugs also is affected, since the elderly have a decrease in total body water and a relative increase in body fat. Thus, water-soluble drugs become more concentrated, and fat-soluble drugs have longer half-lives. In addition, serum albumin levels decline, particularly in sick patients, so that there is a decrease in protein binding of some drugs (e.g., warfarin, phenytoin), leaving more free (active) drug available.

In addition to impaired drug clearance, which alters pharmacokinetics, older patients have altered responses to similar serum drug levels, a phenomenon known as altered pharmacodynamics. They are more sensitive to some drugs (e.g., opiates, anticoagulants) and less sensitive to others (e.g., beta-adrenergic agents). Finally, the older patient with multiple chronic conditions is likely to be taking several drugs, including nonprescribed agents. Thus, adverse drug reactions and dosage errors are more likely to occur, especially if the patient has visual, hearing, or memory deficits.

Precautions to Avoid Drug Toxicity   *Drug selection and administration*   Before initiating treatment, the physician should first ensure that the symptom requiring treatment is not itself due to another drug. For example, antipsychotic agents can cause symptoms that mimic depression (flat affect, restlessness, and pacing); such symptoms should prompt lowering of the dose rather than initiation of an antidepressant. In addition, drug therapy should be employed only after nonpharmacologic means have been considered or tried and only when the benefit clearly outweighs the risk.

Once pharmacotherapy has been decided upon, it should begin at less than the usual adult dosage and the dose should be increased slowly. However, given the marked variability in pharmacokinetics and pharmacodynamics in the elderly, dose escalation should continue until either a successful endpoint is reached or an intolerable side effect is encountered. The final dosage schedule should be kept as simple as possible and the number of pills should be kept as low as possible. Serum drug levels are often useful in older patients, especially for monitoring drugs with narrow therapeutic indices such as phenytoin, theophylline, quinidine, aminoglycosides, lithium, and psychotropic agents such as nortriptyline. However, toxicity can occur even with "normal" therapeutic levels of some drugs (e.g., digoxin, phenytoin).

Over-the-counter agents   Nearly three-quarters of the elderly regularly use nonprescribed drugs, many of which cause significant symptoms. Frequent offenders include nonprescribed agents for insomnia (all of which are anticholinergics), and nonsteroidal anti-inflammatory drugs (NSAIDs), which can hamper control of hypertension in addition to causing renal dysfunction, and gastrointestinal bleeding. Because older patients often consider such agents "nostrums" rather than drugs, the physician must ask about them directly.

Sedative-hypnotics   If nonpharmacologic treatment of insomnia is unsuccessful, short-term use of an intermediate-acting agent whose metabolism is not affected by age (e.g., oxazepam, 10 to 30 mg/d) may be useful. Because of the increased risk of confusion and other adverse effects, benzodiazepines with either short (e.g., triazolam) or long duration of action (e.g., flurazepam and diazepam) should be avoided. An antidepressant should not be prescribed for insomnia unless the patient is depressed.

Antibiotics   Serum creatinine is not a good index of renal function in old people; however, when it is elevated special care must be taken with the administration of drugs normally excreted by the kidneys. Concentrations of relevant antibiotics should be measured directly.

Cardiac drugs   In older patients, digitalis, procainamide, and quinidine have prolonged half-lives and narrow therapeutic windows; toxicity is common at the usual dosages. For example, digoxin toxicity—especially anorexia, confusion, or depression—can occur even with therapeutic digoxin levels.

H_2 *receptor antagonists*   Most of these agents interfere with hepatic metabolism of other drugs, and all can produce confusion in the elderly. Because they are renally excreted, lower doses should be used to minimize the risk of toxicity in older individuals.

Antidepressants and antipsychotics   These drugs can produce anticholinergic side effects in old people (e.g., confusion, urinary retention, constipation, dry mouth). This can be minimized by switching to a nonanticholinergic agent (e.g., sertraline or trazodone) or one with less anticholinergic effect (e.g., desipramine). In general, the least potent agents for psychosis (e.g., chlorpromazine) have the most sedating and anticholinergic effects and are the most likely to induce postural hypotension. By contrast, the most potent antipsychotic agents (e.g., haloperidol) have the least sedating, anticholinergic, and hypotensive side effects but cause extrapyramidal side effects, including dystonia, akathisia, rigidity, and tardive dyskinesia. Thus all of these agents are potentially toxic. Moreover, since both depression and agitation often remit spontaneously, cautious discontinuation of these drugs should be considered periodically.

Glaucoma medications   Both topical beta-blockers and carbonic anhydrase inhibitors can cause systemic side effects. The latter can cause malaise and anorexia independent of the induced metabolic acidosis.

Anticoagulants   Elderly patients benefit from anticoagulation as much as do younger individuals but are more vulnerable to serious bleeding. Hence, more careful monitoring and less aggressive anticoagulation are advisable.

Avoid overtreatment   Drugs are not necessarily indicated in some common clinical situations. For instance, antibiotics need not be given for asymptomatic bacteriuria unless obstructive uropathy, other anatomic abnormalities, or stones are also present. Ankle edema is often due to venous insufficiency, drugs such as NSAIDs or some calcium antagonists, or even inactivity or malnutrition in chairbound patients. Diuretics are usually not indicated unless edema is associated with heart failure. Fitted, pressure gradient stockings are often helpful. Regular exercise is much more useful for claudication than is pentoxyfylline. Finally, since older patients generally tolerate aspirin and other NSAIDs less well than do younger patients, localized pain should be treated when possible with local measures such as injection, physical therapy, heat, ultrasound, or transcutaneous electrical stimulation (see Chap. 12).

PREVENTION

Much can be done to prevent the progression and even the onset of disease in older people. Dietary inadequacies in the elderly should be corrected. Daily calcium intake should approximate 1500 mg, and most elderly people should take 400 to 800 IU of vitamin D daily (contained in one to two multivitamin tablets). Tobacco and alcohol use should be minimized, since the benefits of discontinuing these accrue even to individuals over age 65. The importance of reviewing all of a patient's medications and discontinuing them whenever feasible cannot be overemphasized.

The benefits of treating both isolated systolic hypertension and combined systolic and diastolic hypertension in ambulatory elderly have now been documented. Treatment reduces the risk of stroke and the risk of death due to cardiovascular causes in this age group. Conclusive results have been achieved using *low doses* of a thiazide-like diuretic (e.g., chlorthalidone, 12.5 to 25 mg/d) as the first step (alone effective in almost half of patients) and adding low-dose reserpine (0.05 to 0.1 mg/d) or atenolol (25 to 50 mg/d) only as needed. Benefits are dramatic, side effects are minimal, cost is trivial, and concerns about potential toxicity have not been borne out.

Because of the prevalence, functional impact, and ease of treatment, glaucoma should be screened for, and visual and auditory impairment should be corrected. Dentures should be assessed for their fit, and oral lesions beneath them should be detected.

Because thyroid dysfunction is more prevalent in the elderly, difficult to detect clinically, and treatable, serum levels of thyroid-stimulating hormone should be measured at least once in asymptomatic older people. Serum cholesterol is worth measuring in those with established coronary heart disease, but in those without apparent disease, screening for hypercholesterolemia is controversial. It seems reasonable to screen those who would be willing to comply with therapy, whose quality of life is good (from the patient's viewpoint), whose life expectancy exceeds several years (long enough to potentially benefit from therapy), and whose other risk factors—for which benefit of treatment has been definitely established—have already been addressed. A Papanicolaou test should be done in women who have not had one before, since the incidence of both preventable cervical carcinoma and associated death increases with age, especially in this group; it should be repeated triennially in all older women unless two previous tests have been normal. Immunizations for influenza, pneumococcal pneumonia, and tetanus should be current. PPD testing should be done on residents of chronic care facilities and on others at high risk of tuberculosis; those who have recently converted probably should be treated. Since responsiveness wanes with age, the test, if negative, should be repeated in a week to increase the chances of detecting all exposed patients. Because older women with breast cancer are more likely to die *of* it than *with* it, screening mammography is indicated every 1 to 2 years at least until age 75 and thereafter if a positive finding would result in therapeutic intervention. The relative risks and benefits of low-dose aspirin and (for women) estrogen replacement therapy have not yet been elucidated sufficiently in the elderly to warrant routine use, but they should be considered on an individual basis.

Exercise should be encouraged not only because of its beneficial effects on blood pressure, cardiovascular conditioning, glucose homeostasis, bone density, and functional status, but also because it may improve mood and social interaction, reduce insomnia and constipation, and prevent falls. Spinal flexion exercises should be avoided in patients with osteopenia; consultation with a physical therapist may be helpful.

Measures should be taken to prevent falling, as outlined in Tables 9-5 and 9-6. Counseling about driving is important, especially for patients with cognitive impairment. But perhaps the most valuable procedure for prevention of disease in old people is to take a careful history, focusing not only on the "chief complaint" but also on common and often hidden conditions such as falls, confusion, depression, sexual dysfunction, and incontinence. In addition, one should always identify the complications for which the specific patient is at risk and take steps to avert them. For instance, a patient with cognitive impairment who smokes is at risk not only for lung cancer but also for starting a fire, and a patient who requires narcotics is at risk for fecal impaction, delirium, urinary retention, and confusion. Community-dwelling patients who are at highest risk of rapid deterioration and institutionalization and who should be monitored more closely include those over age 80, those who live alone, those who are bereaved or depressed, and those who are intellectually impaired.

BIBLIOGRAPHY

BIOLOGY OF AGING

MASORO EJ (ed): *Handbook of Physiology*. Section 11: *Aging*. New York: Oxford Univ Press (for the American Physiological Society), 1995
RUSTING RL: Why do we age? Sci Am 12:130, 1992
VIJG J, WEI JY: Understanding the biology of aging: The key to prevention and therapy. J Am Geriatr Soc 43:426, 1995
WEINDRUCH R: Caloric restriction and aging. Sci Am 273(1):46, 1996

FUNCTIONAL ASSESSMENT

CORTI M-C et al: Serum albumin and physical disability as predictors of mortality in older persons. JAMA 272:1036, 1994
GURALNIK JM et al: Lower-extremity function in persons over the age of 70 years as a predictor of subsequent disability. N Engl J Med 332:556, 1995
IKEGAMI N: Functional assessment and its place in health care. N Engl J Med 332:598, 1995
LACHS MS et al: A simple procedure for general screening for functional disability in elderly patients. Ann Intern Med 112:699, 1990

DEMENTIA, DELIRIUM, DEPRESSION

CARLSON DL et al: Management of dementia-related behavioral disturbances: A nonpharmacologic approach. Mayo Clin Proc 70:1108, 1995
FLEMING KC, EVANS MD: Pharmacologic therapies in dementia. Mayo Clin Proc 70:1116, 1995
INOUYE SK: The dilemma of delirium: Clinical and research controversies regarding diagnosis and evaluation of delirium in hospitalized elderly medical patients. Am J Med 97:278, 1994
NIH CONSENSUS DEVELOPMENT PANEL: Diagnosis and treatment of depression in late life. JAMA 268:1018, 1992
RUMMANS TA et al: Delirium in elderly patients: Evaluation and management. Mayo Clin Proc 70:989, 1995

URINARY INCONTINENCE

OUSLANDER JG, SCHNELLE JF: Incontinence in the nursing home. Ann Intern Med 122:438, 1995
RESNICK NM: Urinary incontinence. Lancet 346:94, 1995

FALLS/IMMOBILITY/PRESSURE ULCERS

BERGSTROM N et al: *Treatment of Pressure Ulcers*. Clinical Practice Guideline, No. 15. Rockville, MD: US Department of Health and Human Services, Public Health Service, Agency for Health Care Policy and Research (AHCPR) publication NO. 95-0652. December 1994
RUBENSTEIN LZ et al: Falls in the nursing home. Ann Intern Med 121:442, 1994
TINETTI ME et al: A multifactorial intervention to reduce the risk of falling among elderly people living in the community. N Engl J Med 331:821, 1994

GERIATRIC PHARMACOLOGY

AVORN J, GURWITZ JH: Drug use in the nursing home. Ann Intern Med 123:195, 1995
NIH CONSENSUS CONFERENCE: Optimal calcium intake. JAMA 272:1942, 1994
ROCHON PA, GURWITZ JH: Drug therapy. Lancet 346:32, 1995

PREVENTION

DENKE MA, WINKER MA: Cholesterol and coronary heart disease in older adults: No easy answers. JAMA 274:575, 1995

FABACHER D et al: An in-home preventive assessment program for independent older adults: A randomized controlled trial. J Am Geriatr Soc 42:630, 1994

FIATARONE MA et al: Exercise training and nutritional supplementation for physical frailty in very old people. N Engl J Med 330:1769, 1994

FLAHERTY JH: Driving and older persons. Clin Geriat 3(3):44, 1995

KERLIKOWSKE K et al: Efficacy of screening mammography. A meta-analysis. JAMA 273:149, 1995

MARTINEZ R: Older drivers and physicians. JAMA 274:1060, 1995

MULROW CD et al: Hypertension in the elderly. JAMA 272:1932, 1994

US PREVENTIVE SERVICE TASK FORCE: Guide to Clinical Preventive Services, 2d ed. Baltimore, Williams & Wilkins, 1996

MISCELLANEOUS

HARRIS J: The treatment of cancer in an aging population. JAMA 268:96, 1992

JANSEN REMM, LIPSITZ LA: Postprandial hypotension: Epidemiology, pathophysiology, and clinical management. Ann Intern Med 122:286, 1995

LIBOW LS, STARER P: Care of the nursing home patient. N Engl J Med 321:93, 1989

WEBER DC et al: Rehabilitation of geriatric patients. Mayo Clin Proc 70:1198, 1995

10   *Maureen T. Connelly, Thomas S. Inui*

PRINCIPLES OF DISEASE PREVENTION

PERSPECTIVES ON PREVENTION

The primary goals of prevention in medicine are to prolong life, to decrease morbidity, and to improve quality of life—all with the available resources. Working in partnership with patients, physicians play critical roles as educators, managers of access to screening and intervention services, and interpreters of divergent recommendations for promoting health. Despite evidence of the effectiveness of many preventive services in prolonging healthy life and decreasing medical costs, physicians frequently do not integrate appropriate preventive practices into their care. Obstacles to providing optimal preventive care include lack of appropriate training, doubt about the effectiveness of preventive interventions, skepticism about patients' commitment to change, limited reimbursement and time, and conflicting professional recommendations. Success achieved for populations may not be visible to individuals, and physicians may not appreciate the cumulative benefit of their efforts. Despite considerable success in some areas, such as the reduction of smoking by U.S. adults from 40 percent to 25 percent in the last 30 years, effective behavior change in other domains is often elusive, challenging and frustrating physicians and patients alike.

DEFINITIONS This chapter will be devoted to a discussion of *primary* and *secondary* prevention. Primary prevention, including various forms of health promotion and vaccination, is care intended to minimize risk factors and the subsequent incidence of disease. Secondary prevention is screening for detection of early disease, for example the use of mammography to detect preclinical breast cancer. While the term *secondary prevention* is also sometimes used for the prevention of recurrent episodes of an existing illness, most would consider this activity to be *tertiary prevention*, care intended to ameliorate the course of established disease.

Deciding what types of primary and secondary preventive care clinicians should offer to their patients is not a trivial matter. The United States Preventive Services Task Force (USPSTF), The Canadian Task Force on the Periodic Health Examination, and the American College of Physicians, among other organizations, have critically re-viewed the strength of available evidence for preventive practices and have made recommendations. Adopting an evidence-based approach to the development of preventive practices policy is an essential step to assuaging provider concerns about the validity of particular recommendations, to identifying the specific basis of controversies in prevention, and to reassuring patients that certain interventions will do more good than harm.

PRIMARY PREVENTION

RISK MODIFICATION Of the more than 2 million deaths that occur in the United States each year, as many as half may be due to preventable causes (Table 10-1). Life-style and behavior play a central role in the primary causes of morbidity and mortality for adults—coronary heart disease, cancer, and injuries.

Tobacco Perhaps the largest potentially modifiable risk to health is the abuse of tobacco products. Responsible for more than 400,000 deaths each year and an estimated annual cost to society as high as $50 billion, tobacco abuse accounts for a substantial fraction of cardiovascular, cancer, and pulmonary morbidity and mortality. Recent evidence also suggests that passive exposure to tobacco smoke results in chronic pulmonary disease as well as lung cancer for some adults. Because of the addictive properties of nicotine, preventing the initiation of tobacco abuse is the tobacco control intervention of choice. Most adult smokers acquire their habit as teenagers, and primary efforts to discourage initial tobacco use must engage younger audiences.

Counseling regarding the health risks of tobacco and methods for quitting is advised by all prevention advisory panels. Particular attention should be paid to groups at highest risk for tobacco abuse, such as men, blacks, and those with only a high school education or less. Because 70 percent of smokers come into contact with health professionals each year, the medical encounter provides an opportunity to address the health implications of tobacco abuse. Ninety percent of successful quitters will stop smoking without the aid of programmatic interventions. A review of smoking habits, recommendation to stop, and support from a health care provider may generate the impetus for an individual to make an effort to stop smoking. Respect for patients' self-efficacy, reflected in questions such as "What do you understand about the health consequences of smoking?", "Are you ready to quit?", and "What would it take for you to stop smoking?" has been suggested as a means to engage patients in the process. Setting a date to quit, arranging follow-up visits or phone calls during the initial quitting period, providing literature, and considering the use of nicotine replacement systems for those who will completely desist from the use of other tobacco products are all interventions that may improve the quitting success rate.

Table 10-1

Actual Causes of Preventable Deaths in the United States in 1990

	Deaths	
Cause	Estimated No.*	Percentage of Total Deaths
Tobacco	400,000	19
Diet/activity patterns	300,000	14
Alcohol	100,000	5
Microbial agents	90,000	4
Toxic agents	60,000	3
Firearms	35,000	2
Sexual behavior	30,000	1
Motor vehicles	25,000	1
Illicit use of drugs	20,000	<1
TOTAL	1,060,000	50

* Composite approximation drawn from studies that use different approaches to derive estimates, ranging from actual counts (e.g., firearms) to population attributable risk calculations (e.g., tobacco). Numbers over 100,000 are rounded to the nearest 100,000; those over 50,000 are rounded to the nearest 10,000; those below 50,000 are rounded to the nearest 5000.

SOURCE: McGinnis JM, Foege WH: Actual causes of death in the United States. JAMA 270:2207, 1993.

Alcohol and Drugs   The use of alcohol and drugs accounts for more than 100,000 deaths annually. While the ability of health care providers to prevent the initiation of such behaviors has not been proven, screening for exposure and addiction could potentially direct medical effort to the prevention of alcohol and drug-associated problems such as injury, violence, and medical complications of drug abuse. Although instruments such as the CAGE questionnaire have proven to be valuable for detection of alcohol abuse, no comparable brief screening strategy is available for the routine identification of illicit drug abuse. Health care providers screen inadequately for both disorders, despite evidence for effective early treatment of addictions and their complications. Recent data suggesting that moderate alcohol intake may prevent heart disease for some individuals and the lack of a biologic "gold standard" criterion for alcoholism contribute to difficulties in diagnosing alcohol abuse. Legal implications of identifying illicit drug use may hinder detection of this problem. When screening for these disorders is feasible, interventions that have proven effective include brief counseling, referral to ambulatory and in-patient treatment programs, use of 12-step and other community organizations, and appropriate use of medications such as methadone for heroin abuse.

Diet   Mounting evidence suggests that modification of caloric intake, both quantity and quality, can result in decreased morbidity and mortality from cardiovascular disease, cancer, and diabetes. Excess weight is an independent risk factor for coronary disease, in addition to its contribution to the incidence of diabetes, hyperlipidemia, and hypertension. Between 20 and 30 percent of Americans are overweight, defined as 20 percent above the acceptable body-mass index (kg/m^2), and more than 40 percent of certain subpopulations, such as black, Native American, and Mexican-American women, are overweight.

Americans derive excess calories from fats, particularly saturated fats, rather than from more beneficial sources such as complex carbohydrates and fiber. Since intake of saturated fat correlates with cholesterol level, and coronary heart disease is reduced by 2 to 3 percent for every 1 percent reduction in plasma cholesterol level, dietary modification will play a central role in decreasing the primary cause of mortality in America. Excess dietary fat intake has also been associated with breast, colon, prostate, and lung cancer in epidemiologic studies. Reducing calories from all fats to 30 percent and from saturated fat to 10 percent are widely accepted goals. Increasing the intake of dietary fiber, such as from plant, legume, and grain sources, may contribute specifically to a decrease in colon cancer incidence.

Dietary sodium restriction may benefit those who have salt-sensitive hypertension, although the need for such restriction in the general population is unclear. Calcium and vitamin D are protective against osteoporosis, particularly in young women prior to reaching menopause, and evidence suggests that females at all ages have an inadequate intake. Menstruating women are at risk for iron-deficiency anemia. To achieve the recommended daily intake of vitamins and minerals, a varied diet including fish, lean meats, dairy products, whole grains, and five to six servings of fruits and vegetables daily is recommended, rather than the use of vitamin supplements. While evidence supporting the use of antioxidants such as vitamins E and C is still incomplete, the recommended quantities of these micronutrients can be obtained from a balanced diet.

Physicians play a critical role in effecting dietary change in their patients. The value of providing counseling and literature, referring patients to appropriate community groups and nutrition professionals, and helping patients set goals and limits for diet modification cannot be overemphasized. Despite concern about the risk of weight cycling, the health hazards of obesity appear to outweigh the potential harm of repeated weight loss and gain.

Physical Activity   A key counterpart to decreased caloric intake is increased energy expenditure. Not only can increased physical activity decrease obesity, but avoiding a sedentary life-style can also decrease the incidence of cardiac disease, hypertension, diabetes, and osteoporosis. It is estimated that only 22 percent of U.S. adults engage in at least light to moderate physical activity, such as walking for 30 min three to five times per week. A full quarter of the population pursues no vigorous physical activity at all. The magnitude of benefit derived from physical activity may be as great as a 35 percent reduction in coronary heart disease, and even light exercise is preferable to no exercise. While the ultimate goal for optimal cardioprotective physical activity is 20 to 30 min of vigorous activity most days of the week, patients should be encouraged to approach this level gradually. A sudden onset of vigorous activity in the unfit may increase the risk for myocardial infarction and sudden death. Patients should be informed that, despite previous physical inactivity, the incremental adoption of a regular fitness program can decrease their risk of cardiovascular and other diseases to the level of those who have remained fit throughout their lives. Successful exercise programs are integrated into daily routines, self-directed, and injury-free.

Sexual Behavior   Because of the substantial risks of infectious diseases and unwanted pregnancy from unprotected sexual activity, patients should be strongly advised to use barrier methods for all high-risk practices such as oral, anal, and vaginal intercourse as well as additional contraceptive methods when pregnancy would not be welcome.

Environment   Physicians should adopt a broad construction of environmental risks to health, considering the physical, social, and occupational environments of their patients. Taking a complete exposure history, focusing on home, work, neighborhood, hobbies, and dietary habits can help direct interventions and recommendations. While local circumstances will dictate specific risks to which patients should be alerted, such as regional infectious diseases or particular toxic exposures produced by local industry, certain general recommendations should be adopted universally for health promotion.

Since skin cancers, the vast majority of them secondary to sun exposure, constitute the most common form of malignancy, all patients should be counseled to avoid sun overexposure and to use sunscreens. Patients should be encouraged to consider potential toxin exposures, such as those due to air pollution, household smoking, or carbon monoxide and radon gases, and be informed of the medical symptoms and consequences of such exposures. Proper food preparation and storage decrease the incidence of food-borne infectious disease.

Unintended injury constitutes a significant preventable burden of morbidity and mortality and is the leading cause of death for the general population under 40. Automobile accidents are the leading cause of unintentional injuries. The risk of being involved in a disabling traffic accident may be as high as 30 percent in the course of an individual's lifetime, and 50 percent of deaths from automobile accidents could be prevented with regular seatbelt use. Physicians should recommend seatbelt use, as well as helmet use for motorcycle and bicycle riders, since evidence supports a higher likelihood of use among patients who receive such advice. Clinicians should also recommend against operating a motor vehicle after drinking, since alcohol (and illicit drugs) is a clear-cut risk cofactor.

Smoke detectors are underused, being found in only 80 percent of homes. Since most deaths due to fire occur in the residential setting, patients should be encouraged to install at least one on each floor of their home.

Attention to health hazards in the workplace can identify those at risk and prevent long-term consequences of exposure. Evaluation of the work environment should include questions about exposure to metals, dusts, fibers, chemicals, fumes, radiation, loud noises, extreme temperatures, and biologic agents.

Community and family violence, particularly through the misuse of firearms, is the second leading cause of death from unintentional injury. Firearms, especially handguns, are far more likely to injure a family member than an intruder and are associated with increased rates of suicide and harm to children. Patients should be encouraged to remove their weapons from the home and should be informed of the risks associated with improper security and storage of firearms. While community and family violence are epidemic in the United States, interventions to curtail violent behavior are not well established. Screening for exposure to relationship violence, developing plans for safe havens, and referrals to appropriate community and government agencies can prevent continued abuse.

IMMUNIZATION As many as 70,000 deaths due to influenza, pneumococcal infections, and hepatitis B occur in the United States annually. Despite good availability and evidence for the cost-effectiveness of recommended vaccinations for adults, only 40 percent or fewer members of target populations are immunized. Factors explaining poor adherence to adult immunization guidelines include lack of confidence in vaccine efficacy among providers and patients, underestimation of the severity of the target diseases, incomplete reimbursement, lack of systems to identify and vaccinate high-risk populations, and the absence of an adult requirement for vaccination equivalent to our vaccination policies for school-age children. Table 10-2 lists recommended adult immunizations.

CHEMOPROPHYLAXIS There is significant supportive evidence for the use of certain medications in primary prevention. Therapy of this nature in the otherwise healthy person, however, is not risk-free. The use of aspirin for the prevention of cardiovascular disease or colorectal cancer, for example, is supported by evidence from cohort and, in the case of cardiovascular disease, randomized controlled trials. The potential for cerebral bleeds and gastrointestinal intolerance, however, must be balanced against a patient's individual risk for the target diseases. Although no randomized trials have measured the impact on mortality, postmenopausal hormone replacement therapy is another therapy given to healthy women for the prevention of future disease (coronary heart disease and osteoporosis), as well as to control menopausal symptoms. These benefits must be weighed against the risks of possible breast and endometrial cacinoma. Patient involvement in the decision-making process, perhaps even informed consent, is

Table 10-2

Recommendations for Preventive Medical Care

Screening
  Blood pressure
  Height and weight
  Pap smear
  FOBT and/or sigmoidoscopy*
  Mammography ± breast exam†
  Assess for problem drinking
  Total blood cholesterol (men aged 35 to 64, women aged 45 to 64>
  Vision screening‡
  Assess for hearing impairment‡
Counseling
  Tobacco cessation
  Avoidance of alcohol and drugs when driving, swimming, boating
  Limitation of fat, cholesterol
  Maintenance of caloric balance
  Emphasis on grains, fruits, vegetables in diet
  Adequate calcium
  Physical activity
  Lap/shoulder belts
  Motorcycle and bicycle helmets
  Smoke detectors
  Storage or removal of firearms
  STD prevention
  Dental visits, fluoride, flossing
  Contraception
  Fall prevention‡
  CPR training for household‡
  Hot water heater at <120°‡
Immunization
  Tetanus-diphtheria (Td)
  Pneumococcal vaccine‡
  Influenza vaccine‡
Chemoprophylaxis
  Discussion of hormone replacement therapy with perimenopausal women

* After age 49
† After age 49; before age 70
‡ Ages 65 +

SOURCE: Adapted from the U.S. Preventive Services Task Force *Guide to Clinical Preventive Services.* Consult full report for details and recommendations for high-risk individuals.

recommended to ensure compliance, proper use of medication, and sustained monitoring for side effects.

SECONDARY PREVENTION

SCREENING Widespread screening for the presence of existing diseases should meet the following criteria:

1. The targeted disease must be sufficiently burdensome to the population that a screening program is warranted. Minor changes in relative risk should have a substantial impact on the absolute risk within the population.
2. The target disease must have a well-understood natural history with a long preclinical latent period.
3. The screening method must have acceptable technical performance parameters, detecting the disease at an earlier stage than would be possible without screening and minimizing false-positive and false-negative results.
4. Efficacious treatment for the target illness must be available.
5. Early detection must improve disease outcome.
6. Cost, feasibility, and acceptability of screening and early treatment should be established.

While physicians underprovide certain screening services that have met these criteria (for example, regular mammograms for women over age 50 years), it is also the case that some prevalent screening practices today are not solidly rooted in evidence. Screening tests such as measurement of prostate-specific antigen and mammography in women under 50 have been adopted for use by many clinicians despite lack of complete current evidence that these services will decrease the risk of morbidity or mortality or improve the quality of life. See Table 10-2 recommendations of the USPSTF for screening of adults who are at average risk for target conditions. Recommendations for special-risk and vulnerable populations are available in the USPSTF *Guide.*

COMMUNITY HEALTH ADVOCACY

In addition to the direct clinical provision of preventive and health-promoting services, physicians can bring their knowledge, expertise, clinical experience, and influence to bear at the community level to promote health. Whether arguing for the denormalization of tobacco use or providing data about the health risks of local incinerators, physicians are the important sources of information and support for improving health beyond the clinical office. Such activities are consistent with the overall objective of caring for patients and may have a substantial impact on decreasing the prevalence of the root causes of disease.

BIBLIOGRAPHY

AMERICAN COLLEGE OF PHYSICIANS: Preventing firearm violence: A public health imperative. Ann Intern Med 122:311, 1995
FEDSON DS: Adult immunization: Summary of the National Vaccine Advisory Committee Report. JAMA 272:1133, 1994
Healthy People 2000: National Health Promotion and Disease Prevention Objectives. Department of Health and Human Services Publication (PHS) 91-50213, 1991
HELZLSOUER KJ et al: Summary of the round table discussion on strategies for cancer prevention: Diet, food, additives, supplements, and drugs. Cancer Res 54:2044s, 1994
MCCORMICK WC, INUI TS: Geriatric preventive care: Counseling techniques in practice settings. Clin Geriat Med 8:215, 1992
POPE AM, RALL DP (eds): *Environmental Medicine: Integrating a Missing Element into Medical Education.* Washington, DC, National Academy Press, 1995
SCHWARTZ JS et al: Internists' practices in health promotion and disease prevention. Ann Intern Med 114:46, 1991
SOX HC: Preventive health services in adults. N Engl J Med 330:1589, 1994
U.S. PREVENTIVE SERVICES TASK FORCE: *Guide to Clinical Preventive Services,* 2d ed. Baltimore, Williams & Wilkins, 1995
WILLIAMS GC et al: "The facts concerning the recent carnival of smoking in Connecticut" and elsewhere. Ann Intern Med 115:59, 1991

COST AWARENESS IN MEDICINE

COSTS OF HEALTH CARE IN THE UNITED STATES

Through the 1980s and early 1990s, health care expenditures in the United States rose at a rate of more than 10 percent per year, which exceeded the rates of inflation and of growth in the gross national product (GNP). As a consequence, the percentage of the GNP that is spent on health care increased from about 7 percent in 1970 to 9 percent in 1980 and to more than 12 percent by the early 1990s. This escalation exceeded the increases in other western countries, such as the United Kingdom and Canada. Much of the difference between the United States and Canada is explained by higher physician fees rather than by a higher per capita use of services. The United States also spends substantially more on the administrative costs of health care than Canada or Great Britain.

The reasons for the increase in health care costs are multifactorial. The aging of the population and the availability of new diagnostic and therapeutic advances have increased the demand for health care. Furthermore, the supply of specialists has increased dramatically, providing Americans with easier access to advanced medical services but also suggesting than an oversupply of physicians contributed to an excessive escalation in costs. The costs of care are especially influenced by decisions regarding hospital admission and surgery and by decisions affecting the use of intensive care units, life-sustaining treatments, and long-term care facilities. Efforts at cost-containment have attempted to identify unnecessary services, such as routine preoperative electrocardiograms in healthy young patients, or situations in which extraordinary expenses occur, such as in the last 6 months of life. Attempts to reduce "fat" in the health care system may be counterbalanced, at least in part, by growth in the number and age of the population and by continued advances in technology.

Despite these rising costs, an estimated 40 million Americans, or about 15 percent of the population, do not have health care insurance of any kind, even though nearly half are in households in which someone is employed. This lack of insurance coverage and access to health care is often blamed for the fact that the United States, despite its high expenditures on health care, ranks about twentieth in the world in infant mortality and is not in the top ten in life expectancy.

HEALTH INSURANCE   Traditional fee-for-service insurance reimburses the hospital and the physician for services rendered but frequently does not cover preventive care. Even when insurance provides coverage for a service, the patient may be responsible for an initial "deductible" and a copayment, which is usually a fixed percentage of the entire amount charged.

Patients who must pay such out-of-pocket charges for some of their medical care seek less care than those whose care is fully covered by insurance. In the working poor this may result in reduced utilization of services and in an increase in the prevalence of serious disease. When adults of all socioeconomic classes lose health insurance coverage, they may use fewer medical services; as a result, their health status tends to decline.

Most alternatives to traditional fee-for-service medical care require enrolled persons to prepay a fixed premium, which, except when a relatively small copayment is required, usually covers acute, chronic, and preventive medical services and sometimes covers medications and other health care needs. Prepaid plans have varying organizational and financial structures. Early on in their development, staff-model health maintenance organizations (HMOs) were among the most popular formats. In this model, groups of salaried physicians practiced physically together in one or a few central facilities to provide prepaid care. In recent years, independent practice associations (IPAs) have shown the most rapid growth. IPAs provide prepaid care to the patient by contracting with office-based practitioners who agree to see patients on a prenegotiated fee schedule or for a fixed monthly per-patient capitated payment. To balance the normal fee-for-service incentives and control utilization, IPAs employ various forms of administrative controls and review. The number of days of hospitalization have been markedly reduced among enrollees in HMOs, and HMOs have been among the leaders in attempts to reduce hospital costs and lengths of stay.

REIMBURSEMENT OF HOSPITALS AND PHYSICIANS   In 1983, Medicare introduced a system of prospective reimbursement using diagnosis-related groups (DRGs), whereby hospitals were paid a predetermined sum based on the patient's principal diagnosis, procedures, complications, and comorbidities regardless of the costs or charges that were actually generated by the hospital stay. This reimbursement system was designed to reward hospitals for being more efficient, and hospitals could actually be paid more than their costs. While the prospective reimbursement system has undoubtedly stimulated efficiency, it also has raised concerns about the practice of discharging patients prematurely or transferring them to other institutions if the projected cost of caring for them exceeds the expected reimbursement.

Since the introduction of federal prospective reimbursement, the number of inpatient hospital days has decreased. This reduction has been accompanied by a marked increase in ambulatory services, including a shift to the outpatient arena of services that previously were delivered only on an inpatient basis. This shift should lower the cost of delivering an individual unit of service, such as the cost of a breast biopsy, but the overall cost of medical care will rise if, for example, the breast biopsy is performed on an ambulatory basis *and* the inpatient resources that the breast biopsy patient would have used are now consumed by new services such as the treatment of a breast cancer patient with bone marrow transplantation.

Methods of physician payment also have been revised. Physician reimbursement in the United States, whether by Medicare or by private insurers, traditionally was a direct payment based on the doctor's "usual and customary" fee. Medicare changed this approach when it adopted the *relative value scale*, which is based on the concept that payment rates for medical services should, as with other economic "goods," reflect the costs of producing those services. This change suggests that procedural tasks were being reimbursed at rates exceeding those of nonprocedural tasks that require comparable time, skill, and experience. Medicare's relative rates are similar to preexisting fee schedules in Canada.

CONTROL OF HEALTH CARE COSTS   Two different approaches have been suggested to control health care costs: regulation and competition. Regulations, such as per diem rate setting, attempt to control costs by setting and enforcing practice or reimbursement standards. Other regulatory means of attempting to reduce costs include mandatory second opinions prior to elective hospitalization or surgery, but such programs usually do not save more than the costs of administration of the programs themselves.

The competitive approach encourages hospitals and providers to bid in a free-market atmosphere, in which consumers will presumably make rational choices based on the perceived cost and quality of the available alternatives. Insurance plans that utilize deductibles and copayments reflect this approach. It also has been proposed that physicians who practice inexpensively should be rewarded financially, but if physicians are paid to perform fewer services, the quality of care may suffer. In the absence of legislative reform, the U.S. health care system has been changing rapidly in response to competitive forces. In some parts of the country, employers have joined together to demand lower insurance premiums or to contract directly with hospitals and physicians. In other areas, hospitals, doctors, or doctors with their hospitals have contracted with insurance carriers to establish comprehensive systems that can deliver the full range of health services to a large population of individuals. For-profit insurers and hospitals often compete actively with more traditional not-for-profit entities.

Much of the new competition is in "managed care," by which physicians and institutions agree to provide services for a predetermined price. This price may be a discount of historic fee-for-service prices or it may be negotiated for a specific package of services on behalf of multiple providers, such as when physicians and their hospital agree to perform a kidney transplantation, as well as pre- and posttransplant services, for a specific price. In this arrangement, the various providers then divide the total reimbursement according to an internally negotiated formula. Increasingly, however, physicians, often in conjunction with their hospitals, are negotiating full-risk capitation contracts with employers and insurers. Under this arrangement, providers agree to deliver comprehensive medical services, commonly including preventive and long-term care, to a panel of subscribers for a negotiated reimbursement per member per month. The providers who take responsibility for the care of a panel of patients will not be paid more if their expenses exceed their contracted capitation price, but they are able to retain any prenegotiated payments that are in excess of the costs of the services they provide. In many capitated settings, risk-sharing arrangements are used to dissuade individual physicians from utilizing more tests or procedures than desired by the health care system. For example, a portion of the payment earned by a physician, either via a modified fee-for-service arrangement or as part of a monthly capitated fee, may be "withheld" until the overall financial performance of the system is known not to be in deficit. By 1995, about 20 percent of the U.S. population was in managed care plans, and in some parts of the United States the enrollment was above 50 percent. It is projected that 70 percent or more of the population will be in managed care plans by the end of the century.

Reimbursement mechanisms that give physicians incentives to ration services or that directly link the financial stability of the physician's employer to the ability to reduce costs create an inherent conflict of interest. Of course, a different type of conflict of interest exists under traditional fee-for-service reimbursement, by which a physician is paid more to do more.

In managed care systems, the utilization of health services, particularly specialty care, tends to decline. As a result, current forecasts suggest a substantial excess of specialty physicians and hospital beds. Primary care physicians are thought to be inequitably distributed nationwide but only slightly, if at all, insufficient in numbers.

In the presence of competition and an oversupply of hospital beds and specialist physicians, insurers can negotiate lower prices. As a result, insurance premiums are declining in many parts of the United States, even as the insurers keep an increasing percentage of the premium and distribute a smaller percentage to physicians and hospitals. Total reimbursements to all physicians and hospitals are projected to decline by as much as 25 percent in the coming years.

COSTS AND COST-EFFECTIVENESS

The costs of medical care include direct costs, such as the salaries of health personnel, and indirect costs, such as utilities, maintenance, and mortgage payments. Some costs are fixed (i.e., they do not vary with the volume of services provided), and other costs are variable (i.e., they depend on volume). For example, consider a situation in which a new instrument to perform a blood chemistry test costs $1000 and will last for 1 year. Also assume that each individual chemical analysis has an incremental cost of $10 in reagents, personnel time, and other resource inputs. If the laboratory utilizes the instrument to analyze 100 specimens in a year, the average cost per specimen is $20 ($10 each in fixed and variable costs), but if it analyzes 10,000 specimens, the average cost per specimen is $10.10 ($0.10 in fixed costs and $10.00 in variable costs) because the fixed costs are spread over more specimens.

The charges for medical services do not necessarily correspond

to the true costs of providing the services. This occurs in part because the costs are difficult to measure and in part because charges are usually fixed regardless of volume, while costs vary with volume. Many analyses of cost and cost-effectiveness in medicine are based on charges rather than on true costs.

The net costs for a health care program include the costs of providing the program, costs that are generated by adverse side effects of treatment, and costs for treating disease that would not have occurred if the patient had not lived longer as a result of the original treatment. From these costs, the savings in health care, rehabilitation, or custodial costs due to prevention or alleviation of disease are subtracted to determine the net cost. For example, consider a program to perform mammography in women over age 40. The program would have its own direct costs related to advertising, screening, mammography, physician visits, breast biopsy, etc. Some women would have false-positive mammograms and would receive unnecessary breast biopsies. Other women would live longer as a result of early diagnosis and treatment of breast cancer, but they might develop other illnesses, such as coronary disease, in the interim. If they developed conditions such as Alzheimer's disease, the custodial costs might be substantial. However, these costs would be countered by savings from hospitalizations for advanced cancer and by a potential increase in productive wage-earning years.

In all analyses of costs, it is important to consider *when* the costs will be incurred and *when* the effects in health benefits may be realized. Present dollars or health benefits are considered to have greater worth than a promise of future dollars or health benefits for several reasons. Other events may intercede so that a projected future cost or benefit may never occur, and there is always the possibility that money spent now will not achieve the desired effect at some time in the future. Furthermore, another illness may intervene, or there might be better ways to spend the money in the future. The principle by which future dollars and benefits are less highly valued than known immediate costs and benefits is termed *discounting*. It is independent of monetary inflation. By this concept, it is preferable to spend $1000 today to prevent someone from dying today than it is to spend $1000 today in the expectation that someone will not die 10 years from now.

It is unusual for any program simultaneously to achieve the greatest possible benefit and have the lowest possible cost. Instead, one usually either determines the desired benefit and then finds the lowest cost needed to achieve it or determines the resources available and then finds the greatest possible benefit that can be achieved.

Analyses of cost-effectiveness commonly examine the ratio of cost to effectiveness, i.e., the number of dollars required to save a year of life or a quality-adjusted year of life, in which the analysis considers not only the quantity but also the patient-assessed quality of the health benefit. Such analyses are relevant to medicine because interventions only rarely both save lives and reduce costs. Hence it is important to estimate the tradeoff of costs for gains in health. Two strategies with the same ratio may have quite different absolute costs and absolute benefits. For example, a program that saves 100 lives for $100,000 has the same cost-effectiveness ratio as one that saves 1000 lives for $1 million, but the absolute costs and absolute benefits vary tenfold. The choice between these two programs may depend on how much money is available to spend. In assessing any program, it is important to measure incremental costs and effects rather than average costs and effects. For example, consider two programs to reduce death from lung cancer. If, on average, program A costs $100 million to save 100,000 years of life (average of $1000 per year of life) and program B costs $200 million to save 100,100 years of life (about $2000 per year of life), the *incremental* cost of program B versus program A is $1 million per year of life saved.

The cost-effectiveness of an intervention depends on its own cost, the costs it may avert or induce, and the patient's risks. The cost-effectiveness of an intervention will vary dramatically depending on the type of patient to whom it is applied (Table 11-1).

SOCIETAL ISSUES IN COSTS It is rare to find a medical intervention, such as measles vaccination programs, that both saves lives and reduces overall costs because the savings from disease prevention more than outweigh the expenses of the treatment itself. More commonly, medical practices that are truly of benefit also cause an associated increase in medical care costs. Among the more cost-effective examples is coronary artery bypass surgery in patients with left main coronary artery disease, which costs under $10,000 per year of life saved.

The shift of services from the inpatient to the outpatient setting or from the hospital to the home generally reduces the expense of delivery of that aspect of medical care. For example, home dialysis is less expensive than dialysis in an outpatient center, which in turn is less expensive than dialysis in a hospital. Similarly, the administration of parenteral nutrition and intravenous antibiotics at home and the home care for patients with AIDS have greatly reduced the need for hospitalization for conditions in which skilled nursing care is otherwise not required. However, a by-product of this strategy is an increased percentage of severely ill hospital inpatients who require more intensive and expensive care than the less sick patients who otherwise might have occupied hospital beds.

Even now, society has been reluctant to make ethical decisions regarding the amount of cost appropriate for any particular net benefit. Neither medicine nor society is accustomed to placing a dollar value on a life or a year of life. In many analyses, however, the projected annual costs of approximately $35,000 to $45,000 (in 1997 dollars) for renal dialysis for 1 year of useful life have been used as a benchmark of how much the United States is willing to spend to save a year of life, because such a program is supported with tax dollars and presumably is a reasonable reflection of national priorities.

HEALTH SCREENING   *Screening* refers to the performance of a medical evaluation and/or diagnostic tests in asymptomatic persons in the hope that early diagnosis may lead to improved outcome. This important subject is discussed in Chap. 10.

HEALTH PROMOTION AND DISEASE PREVENTION Health promotion and disease prevention require investment of time, energy, and resources in the hope that the yield in terms of improved health warrants this investment. Unfortunately, there is limited information on the effectiveness of health promotion and disease prevention efforts. Interventions that result in a specified *relative* reduction in adverse outcomes have a greater *absolute* effect in higher-risk populations. For example, the same relative reduction in serum cholesterol will be of greater absolute benefit in persons with higher serum cholesterol levels or other unfavorable risk factors. In general, interventions to alter risk factors have a diminishing effect as risk factors decrease in severity.

Both patients and society commonly expect physicians to play a leadership role in health promotion and disease prevention. Patients expect and desire their physicians to make recommendations regarding physical activity, diet, and other lifestyle issues, and physicians often fail in this regard. If physicians do not become involved, patients seek advice elsewhere, risking the possibility that fads or other erroneous sources may influence their choices.

When physicians become actively involved in health promotion, patients respond frequently and make appropriate behavior changes. For example, a physician's encouragement to increase physical activity, especially if combined with explicit suggestions, is likely to lead to changes in behavior so that the time spent by the physician appears to be cost-effective. Advice by a physician that a patient should lose weight or discontinue smoking is successful in only a small minority of cases, but it is an excellent first step toward health promotion and disease prevention (Chap. 389).

Physician-directed dietary interventions commonly lower the serum cholesterol level by as much as 8 percent. Drug treatment may be more effective but is more expensive. For example, treatment with lovastatin in men for the primary prevention of coronary heart disease costs more than $50,000 per year of life saved except in very high risk persons. Treatment strategies for hypertension are more cost-effective; the approximate cost of screening and treating hypertension, given the average medication compliance rates and treatment with a generic beta-adrenergic antagonist, ranges from a projection of about $15,000 per year of life saved for a patient with a diastolic blood pressure of 105 mmHg or higher to about $25,000 to $30,000 for a person with a diastolic blood pressure of 95 to 104 mmHg. Costs would be higher with more expensive medications, although the cost could be warranted if a reduction in side effects led to an improvement in an individual's quality of life.

Immunizations, including pneumococcal and influenza vaccination in elderly and high-risk patients, are effective ways to reduce disease and its associated costs (see Chap. 122).

DIAGNOSTIC TESTING   As detailed in Chap. 3, diagnostic tests are valuable only to the extent that they provide new, *incremental* information that cannot be obtained less expensively from the history, physical examination, or other less expensive tests. Although these tests may often be of psychological benefit in reassuring the patient or the physician, they commonly generate redundant information, often result in a needless expense, and may entail risk. For example, in the evaluation of left ventricular function, the physician must decide whether a two-dimensional echocardiogram is sufficient or the more precise but more expensive measurement by radionuclide ventriculog-

Table 11-1

Example of Costs, Effectiveness, and Cost-Effectiveness for a Hypothetical Intervention in 10,000 Patients for 5 Years* (High-Risk Patients Compared with Low-Risk Patients)

	High Risk		Low Risk	
	Untreated	Treated	Untreated	Treated
Annual death rate	10%	5%	1%	0.5%
Years of life saved[†]	0	5209	0	614
Cost of treatment (in $ millions) at $2000 per year	0	90.5	0	99.0
Annual CABG rate	6%	3%	0.6%	0.3%
Cost per CABG	$20,000	$20,000	$20,000	$20,000
Annual MI rate	4%	2%	0.4%	0.2%
Cost per MI	$10,000	$10,000	$10,000	$10,000
Annual rate of other events	4%	2%	0.4%	0.2%
Cost per other event	$5000	$5000	$5000	$5000
Medical costs (in $ millions)	70.0	39.7	8.8	4.4
Total cost (in $ millions)	70.0	130.2	8.8	103.4
Total cost difference (in $ millions)		60.2		94.8
Approximate cost per year of life saved		$11,500*		$155,000*

* Simplified so that the intervention reduces all risks by 50%, neither costs nor health effects are discounted, all patients are assumed to die at midyear, and the analysis considers only the first 5 years.
† By life-table analysis.
NOTE: CABG, coronary artery bypass grafting; MI, myocardial infarction.
SOURCE: Reprinted from L Goldman et al, J Am Coll Cardiol 27:1020, 1996.

raphy is worthwhile. The physician faces analogous choices when deciding whether to obtain both an abdominal ultrasound examination and an abdominal computed tomography (CT) scan or, in a different case, whether CT and magnetic resonance imaging of the head are both required.

Ideally, each test should be ordered in sequence only to the extent that it is expected to add to the data available. However, this iterative approach can be expensive in hospitalized patients, where the sequencing of tests may lead to delays in scheduling and performing them. In these situations, the expense of the additional days of waiting may more than offset the savings from possibly avoiding a particular test. Usually, careful consideration of the problem by a physician is one of the most cost-effective ways to evaluate the patient. Expert consultation may be more cost-effective and helpful than ordering more diagnostic tests. Although interventions designed to reduce utilization have met with variable success, those that have been successful have generally included educational components, full endorsement by locally respected leaders, frequent reinforcement and attempts to modify the system by which care is delivered.

TREATMENT CHOICES In choosing among various treatments, physicians try to enhance the likelihood of an optimal outcome. It is important to consider whether an equivalent outcome could be achieved at a lower cost. For example, generic medications may be substituted for more expensive brand-name counterparts. Similarly, outcome is not usually compromised by interventions designed to encourage the use of less expensive antibiotic regimens. Endorsement by the medical profession of restricted indications for procedures such as pacemaker implantation and tonsillectomy have led to decreased utilization without any detectable reduction in life expectancy or quality of life. Whenever possible, diagnostic and therapeutic options should be subjected to strict evaluation of both benefit and cost-effectiveness, and physicians have responsibility to assist in such evaluations and to learn from their results.

INDIVIDUALIZATION

The physician has a unique responsibility. On the one hand, the physician must serve as an advocate for the individual patient, within the limits set by society, and recommend the course of action most likely to be beneficial to the patient. The overriding nature of the patient-physician relationship is the cornerstone of humane medical care. On the other hand, physicians must understand the costs as well as the benefits of medical interventions so that they can choose from among the wide range of options. The physician must serve as the advocate for providing the best options to the individual patient and should know which options are of little or no value or are more likely to do harm than good. The physician must, with the assistance and consent of the patient and the family, set priorities for the patient's management within any limits or restrictions imposed by society; such limits may be expressed, for example, in a finite number of dollars available for the treatment of a specific illness.

In addition, physicians have a broad role in determining health costs. Individually and through various professional organizations, physicians have a responsibility to help set national priorities, based on their appreciation of the finite resources available for health care and their knowledge of the relative benefits and costs of various diagnostic and therapeutic options in particular types of patients. The financial incentives of capitation, by which physicians are paid a fixed amount per patient per month regardless of what services are delivered, presents a new series of ethical challenges for physicians to avoid incentives toward underutilization. These challenges are magnified by the pressures of insurers and health care systems to reduce costs. Inappropriate attempts to reduce costs, exemplified by limiting Medicaid payments for effective medications, are counterproductive in that they worsen health and ultimately lead to increased overall costs.

Special consideration revolves around the use of expensive procedures in medical care, such as liver, heart, lung, and bone marrow transplantation. In these situations, the limited availability of donors makes it necessary to choose the best possible recipients from among a wide range of potential candidates and to "ration." Although rationing is not pleasant, physicians have often responded well in situations with limited resources. For example, when faced with a reduction in intensive care unit availability, physicians are usually successful at maintaining normal admission rates for patients who most require intensive care so that little, if any, adverse effects occur in those excluded from intensive care.

There is marked variability in the rates at which various procedures are performed in different geographic areas, even though there are no obvious differences in the types or ages of patients. To date, relatively little difference in health care outcomes can be detected despite wide differences in the rates of various procedures, suggesting that lower utilization rates often do not adversely affect the quality of care. In some circumstances, however, lower rates of expensive and potentially risky procedures have been associated with poorer functional status, indicating that variations may in part be related to patients' preferences and in part to differing beliefs among physicians regarding optimal medical care choices. When the records of patients who have undergone such procedures are reviewed to determine how the indications for their procedure compared with the standards recommended by experts, a substantial proportion of procedures are deemed inappropriate. However, so far there is no close correlation between the percentage of cases deemed inappropriate and the rate at which the procedure is performed in a given location. There is no definitive evidence that high rates of performance can be equated with a high rate of unnecessary use.

The variations in rates of utilization, the proportion of cases in which some procedures seem not to be necessary, and the ability of physicians to respond to situations in which rationing is necessary suggest that in many situations the quality of medical care and the likelihood of a favorable outcome can be maintained while lowering costs. Society, with the input of physicians, must exercise this role without compromising the physician's responsibility to the individual patient and without restricting access on the basis of sex, socioeconomic status, or ethnic background.

BIBLIOGRAPHY

BARR DA: The effects of organizational structure on primary care outcomes under managed care. Ann Intern Med 122:353, 1995

COUNCIL ON ETHICAL AND JUDICIAL AFFAIRS, AMERICAN MEDICAL ASSOCIATION: Ethical issues in managed care. JAMA 273:330, 1995

EPSTEIN AM: US teaching hospitals in the evolving health care system. JAMA 273:1203, 1995

GOLBERG MA et al: The relation between universal health care insurance and cost control. N Engl J Med 332:742, 1995

GOLDMAN L: Cost-effective strategies in cardiology, in *Heart Disease*, 5th ed, E Braunwald (ed). Philadelphia, Saunders, 1997, pp 1741–1756

HYAMS AL et al: Practice guidelines and malpractice litigation: A two-way street. Ann Intern Med 122:450, 1995

IGLEHART JK: Recent changes for academic medical centers. N Engl J Med 332:407, 1995

KUPERSMITH J et al: Cost effectiveness analysis in heart disease. Part III: Ischemia, congestive heart failure, and arrhythmias. Prog Cardiovasc Dis 37:307, 1995

LINDFORS KK et al: The cost-effectiveness of mammographic screening strategies. JAMA 274:881, 1995

LUBITZ J et al: Longevity and medicare expenditures. N Engl J Med 332:999, 1995

McGLYNN EA et al: Comparison of the appropriateness of coronary angiography and coronary artery bypass graft surgery between Canada and New York state. JAMA 272:934, 1994

PILOTE L et al: Regional variation across the United States in the management of acute myocardial infarction. N Engl J Med 333:565, 1995

RASELL ME: Cost-sharing in health insurance—a reexamination. N Engl J Med 332:1164, 1995

SCHROEDER SA: The latest forecast. Managed care collides with physician supply. JAMA 272:239, 1994

SECTION 1
PAIN

12 | *Howard L. Fields, Joseph B. Martin*

PAIN: PATHOPHYSIOLOGY AND MANAGEMENT

The task of medicine is to preserve and restore health and to relieve suffering. Understanding pain is essential to both these goals. Because pain is universally understood as a signal of disease, it is the most common symptom that brings a patient to a physician's attention. The function of the pain sensory system is to detect, localize, and identify tissue-damaging processes. Since different diseases produce characteristic patterns of tissue damage, the quality, time course, and location of a patient's pain complaint and the location of tenderness provide important diagnostic clues and are used to evaluate the response to treatment.

THE PAIN SENSORY SYSTEM

Pain is an unpleasant sensation localized to a part of the body. It is often described in terms of a penetrating or tissue-destructive process (e.g., stabbing, burning, twisting, tearing, squeezing) and/or of a bodily or emotional reaction (e.g., terrifying, nauseating, sickening). Furthermore, any pain of moderate or higher intensity is accompanied by anxiety and the urge to escape or terminate the feeling. These properties illustrate the duality of pain: It is both sensation and emotion. When it is acute, pain is characteristically associated with behavioral arousal and a stress response consisting of increased blood pressure, heart rate, pupil diameter, and plasma cortisol levels. In addition, local muscle contraction (e.g., limb flexion, abdominal wall rigidity) is often seen.

THE PRIMARY AFFERENT NOCICEPTOR A peripheral nerve consists of the axons of three different types of neurons: primary sensory afferents, motor neurons, and sympathetic postganglionic neurons (Fig. 12-1). The cell bodies of primary afferents are located in the dorsal root ganglia in the vertebral foramina. The primary afferent axon bifurcates to send one process into the spinal cord and the other to innervate tissues. Primary afferents are classified by their diameter, degree of myelination, and conduction velocity. The largest-diameter fibers, A-beta, respond maximally to light touch and/or moving stimuli; they are present primarily in nerves that innervate the skin. In normal individuals, the activity of these fibers does not produce pain. There are two other classes of primary afferents: the small-diameter myelinated (A-delta) and the unmyelinated (C fiber) axons (see Fig. 12-1). These fibers are present in the nerves to the skin and to deep somatic and visceral structures. Some tissues, such as the cornea, are innervated only by A-delta and C afferents. Most A-delta and C afferents respond maximally only to intense (painful) stimuli and produce the subjective experience of pain when they are electrically stimulated; this de-

fines them as *primary afferent nociceptors (pain receptors)*. The ability to detect painful stimuli is completely abolished when A-delta and C axons are blocked.

Individual primary afferent nociceptors can respond to several different types of noxious stimuli. For example, most nociceptors respond to heating, intense mechanical stimuli such as a pinch, and application of irritating chemicals.

Sensitization When intense, repeated, or prolonged stimuli are applied in the presence of damaged tissue or inflammation, the threshold for activating primary afferent nociceptors is lowered and the frequency of firing is higher for all stimulus intensities. Inflammatory mediators such as bradykinin, some prostaglandins, and leukotrienes contribute to this process, which is called *sensitization*. In sensitized tissues normally innocuous stimuli can produce pain. Sensitization is a clinically important process that contributes to tenderness, soreness, and hyperalgesia. A striking example of sensitization is sunburned skin, in which severe pain can be produced by a gentle slap on the back or a warm shower.

Compared with superficial structures (e.g., skin, cornea), viscera are relatively insensitive to noxious stimuli under normal conditions. In contrast, when affected by a disease process with an inflammatory component, deep structures such as joints or hollow viscera characteristically become exquisitely sensitive to mechanical stimulation.

A large proportion of A-delta and C afferents innervating viscera are completely insensitive in normal noninjured, noninflamed tissue. That is, they cannot be activated by known mechanical or thermal stimuli and are not spontaneously active. However, in the presence of inflammatory mediators, these afferents become sensitive to mechanical stimuli. Such afferents have been termed *silent nociceptors*, and their characteristic properties may explain how under pathologic conditions the relatively insensitive deep structures can become the source of severe and debilitating pain and tenderness.

Nociceptor-Induced Inflammation One important concept to emerge in recent years is that afferent nociceptors also have a neuroeffector function. Most nociceptors contain polypeptide mediators that are released from their peripheral terminals when they are activated

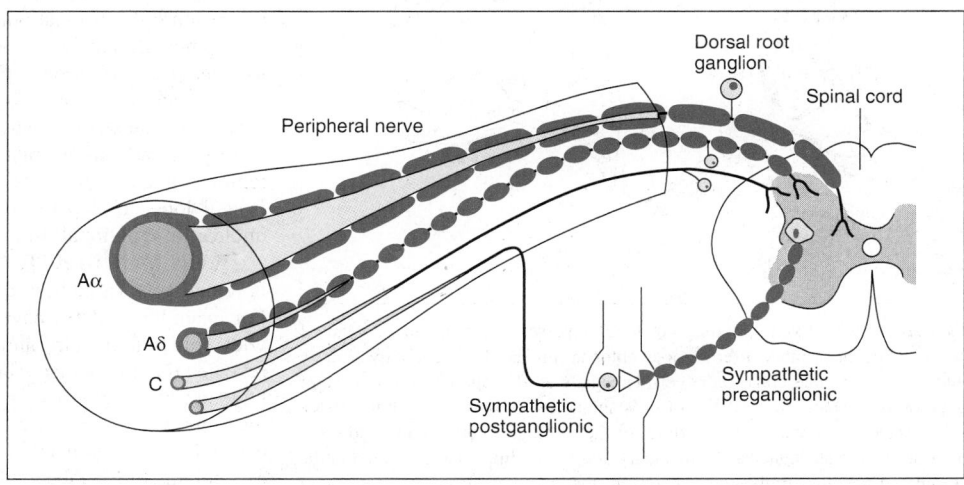

FIGURE 12-1 Components of a typical cutaneous nerve. There are two distinct functional categories of axons: primary afferents with cell bodies in the dorsal root ganglion and sympathetic postganglionic fibers with cell bodies in the sympathetic ganglion. Primary afferents include those with large-diameter myelinated (A-β), small-diameter myelinated (A-δ), and unmyelinated (C) axons. All sympathetic postganglionic fibers are unmyelinated.

(Fig. 12-2). An example is substance P, an 11-amino-acid peptide. Substance P is released from primary afferent nociceptors and has multiple biologic activities. It is a potent vasodilator, degranulates mast cells, is a chemoattractant for leukocytes, and increases the production and release of inflammatory mediators. Interestingly, depletion of substance P from joints reduces the severity of experimental arthritis. Primary afferent nociceptors are not simply passive messengers of threats to tissue injury but also play an active role in tissue protection through these neuroeffector functions.

CENTRAL PATHWAYS FOR PAIN   **The Spinal Cord and Referred Pain**   The axons of primary afferent nociceptors enter the spinal cord via the dorsal root. They terminate in the dorsal horn of the spinal gray matter (Fig. 12-3). The terminals of primary afferent axons contact spinal neurons that transmit the pain signal to brain sites involved in pain perception. The axon of each primary afferent contacts many spinal neurons, and each spinal neuron receives convergent inputs from many primary afferents.

From a clinical standpoint, the convergence of many sensory inputs to a single spinal pain-transmission neuron is of great importance

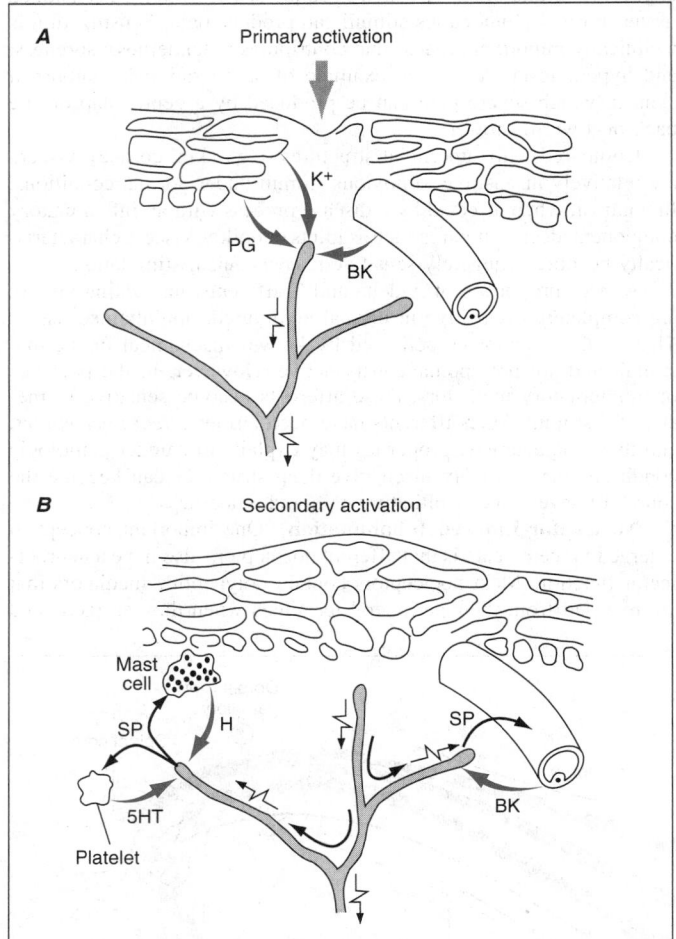

FIGURE 12-2   Events leading to activation, sensitization, and spread of sensitization of primary afferent nociceptor terminals. *A.* Direct activation by intense pressure and consequent cell damage. Cell damage leads to release of potassium (K^+) and to synthesis of prostaglandins (PG) and bradykinin (BK). Prostaglandins increase the sensitivity of the terminal to bradykinin and other pain-producing substances. *B.* Secondary activation. Impulses generated in the stimulated terminal propagate not only to the spinal cord but also into other terminal branches where they induce the release of peptides, including substance P (SP). Substance P causes vasodilation and neurogenic edema with further accumulation of bradykinin. Substance P also causes the release of histamine (H) from mast cells and serotonin (5HT) from platelets.

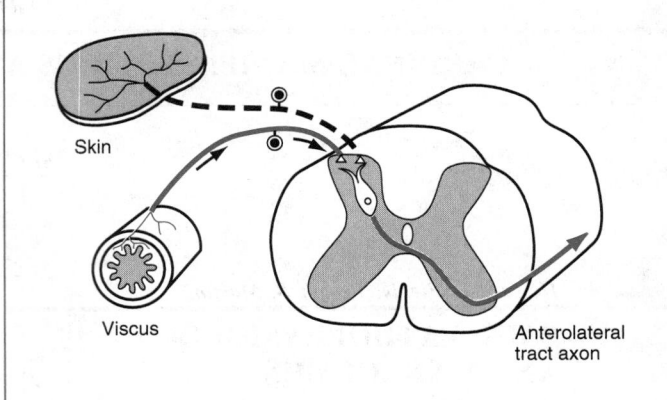

FIGURE 12-3   The convergence-projection hypothesis of referred pain. According to this hypothesis, visceral afferent nociceptors (S) converge on the same pain-projection neurons as the afferents from the somatic structures in which the pain is perceived. The brain has no way of knowing the actual source of input and mistakenly "projects" the sensation to the somatic structure.

because it underlies the phenomenon of referred pain. All spinal neurons that receive input from the viscera and deep musculoskeletal structures also receive input from the skin. The convergence patterns are determined by the spinal segment of the dorsal root ganglion that supplies the afferent innervation of a structure. For example, the afferents that supply the central diaphragm are derived from the third and fourth cervical dorsal root ganglia. Primary afferents with cell bodies in these same ganglia supply the skin of the shoulder and lower neck. Thus sensory inputs from both the shoulder skin and the central diaphragm converge on pain-transmission neurons in the third and fourth cervical spinal segments. *Because of this convergence and the fact that the spinal neurons are most often activated by inputs from the skin, activity evoked in spinal neurons by input from deep structures is mislocalized by the patient to a place that is roughly coextensive with the region of skin innervated by the same spinal segment.* Thus inflammation near the central diaphragm is usually reported as discomfort near the shoulder. This spatial displacement of pain sensation from the site of the injury that produces it is known as *referred pain.*

Ascending Pathways for Pain   A majority of spinal neurons contacted by primary afferent nociceptors send their axons to the contralateral thalamus. These axons form the contralateral spinothalamic tract which lies in the anterolateral white matter of the spinal cord, the lateral edge of the medulla, and the lateral pons and midbrain. The spinothalamic pathway is crucial for pain sensation in humans. Interruption of this pathway produces permanent deficits in pain and temperature discrimination.

Spinothalamic tract axons connect to thalamic neurons that project to somatosensory cortex (Fig. 12-4). This pathway from spinal cord to thalamus to somatosensory cortex appears to be particularly important for the sensory aspects of pain, i.e., its location, intensity, and quality. Spinothalamic tract axons also connect to thalamic and cortical regions linked to emotional responses, such as the cingulate gyrus and frontal lobe. This pathway is thought to subserve the affective or unpleasant emotional dimension of pain.

PAIN MODULATION   The pain produced by similar injuries is remarkably variable in different situations and in different people. For example, athletes have been known to sustain serious fractures with only minor pain, and Beecher's classic World War II survey revealed that many men were unbothered by battle injuries that would have produced agonizing pain in civilian patients. Furthermore, even the suggestion of relief can have a significant analgesic effect (placebo). On the other hand, many patients find even minor injuries (such as venipuncture) unbearable, and the expectation of pain has been demonstrated to induce pain *without a noxious stimulus.*

The powerful effect of expectation and other psychological variables on the perceived intensity of pain implies the existence of brain circuits that can modulate the activity of the pain-transmission path-

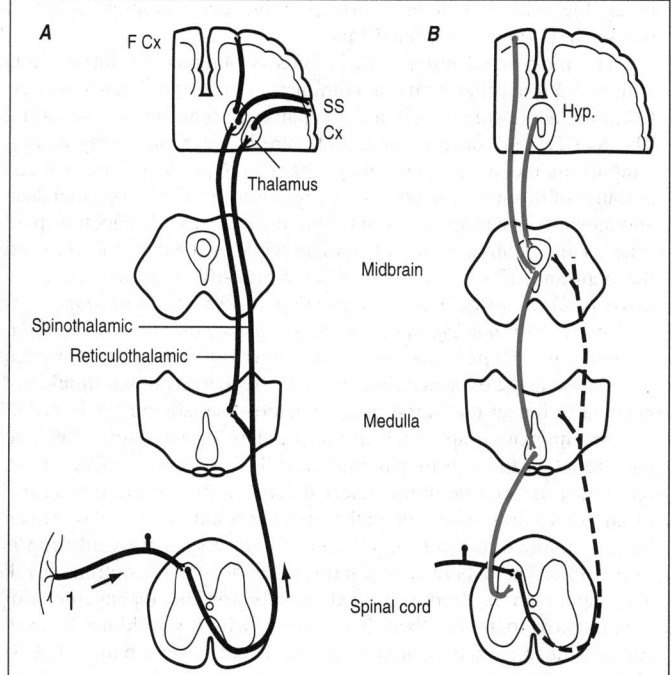

FIGURE 12-4 *A.* Transmission system for nociceptive messages. Noxious stimuli activate the sensitive peripheral ending of the primary afferent nociceptor by the process of transduction (1). The message is then transmitted over the peripheral nerve to the spinal cord, where it synapses with cells of origin of the two major ascending pain pathways, the spinothalamic and spinoreticulothalamic. The message is relayed in the thalamus to both the frontal (F Cx) and the somatosensory cortex (SS Cx). *B.* Pain-modulation network. Inputs from frontal cortex and hypothalamus (Hyp.) activate cells in the midbrain, that control spinal pain-transmission cells via cells in the medulla.

ways. Although there are probably several circuits that can modulate pain, only one has been studied extensively. This circuit has links in the hypothalamus, midbrain, and medulla, and it selectively controls spinal pain-transmission neurons through a descending pathway (see Fig. 12-4).

There is good evidence that this pain-modulating circuit contributes to the pain-relieving effect of narcotic analgesic medications. Each of the component structures of the pathway contains opioid receptors and is sensitive to the direct application of opioid drugs. Furthermore, lesions of the system reduce the analgesic effect of systemically administered opioids such as morphine. Along with the opioid receptor, the component nuclei of this pain-modulating circuit contain endogenous opioid peptides such as the enkephalins and beta-endorphin.

The most reliable way to activate this endogenous opioid-mediated modulating system is by prolonged pain and/or fear. There is evidence that pain-relieving endogenous opioids are released following operative procedures and in patients given a placebo for pain relief.

Pain modulation is bidirectional. Pain-modulating circuits not only produce analgesia but are also capable of increasing pain. Both pain-inhibiting and pain-facilitating neurons in the medulla project to and control spinal pain-transmission neurons. Since pain-transmission neurons can be activated by modulatory neurons, it is theoretically possible to generate a pain signal with no peripheral noxious stimulus. Some such mechanism could account for the finding that pain can be induced by suggestion alone and may provide a framework for understanding how psychological factors can contribute to chronic pain.

NEUROPATHIC PAIN   The normal nervous system transmits coded signals that result in pain. Thus lesions of the peripheral or central nervous system may result in a loss or impairment of pain sensation. Paradoxically, damage or dysfunction of the nervous system can produce pain. For example, damage to peripheral nerves, as occurs

in diabetic neuropathy, or to primary afferents, as in herpes zoster, can result in pain that is referred to the body region innervated by the damaged nerves. Though rare, pain also may be produced by damage to the central nervous system, particularly the spinothalamic pathway or thalamus. Such neuropathic pains are often severe and are notoriously intractable to standard treatments for pain.

Neuropathic pains typically have an unusual burning, tingling, or electric shock–like quality and may be triggered by very light touch. These features are rare in other types of pain. On examination, a sensory deficit is characteristically present in the area of the patient's pain.

A variety of mechanisms contribute to neuropathic pain. As with sensitized primary afferent nociceptors, damaged primary afferents, including nociceptors, become highly sensitive to mechanical stimulation and begin to generate impulses in the absence of stimulation. Damaged primary afferents also may develop sensitivity to norepinephrine. Interestingly, spinal pain-transmission neurons cut off from their normal input may become spontaneously active. Thus both central and peripheral nervous system changes may contribute to neuropathic pain.

Sympathetically Maintained Pain   A certain percentage of patients with peripheral nerve injury develop a severe burning pain (causalgia) in the region innervated by the nerve. The pain typically begins after a delay of hours to days or even weeks. The pain is accompanied by swelling of the extremity, periarticular osteoporosis, and arthritic changes in the distal joints. A similar syndrome called *reflex sympathetic dystrophy* can be produced without obvious nerve damage by a variety of injuries, including fractures of bone, soft tissue trauma, myocardial infarction, and stroke (see Chap. 371). Although the pathophysiology of this condition is poorly understood, the pain can be relieved within minutes by blocking the sympathetic nervous system. This implies that sympathetic activity activates nociceptors even if they are not obviously damaged. These results also suggest that the sympathetic nervous system can, under some circumstances, play an active role in inflammation.

℞ TREATMENT

The ideal treatment for any pain is to remove the cause. Sometimes this is possible, but more often after diagnosis and initiation of appropriate treatments for the cause, there is a lag period before the pain subsides. Furthermore, some conditions are so painful that rapid and effective analgesia is essential (e.g., the postoperative state, burns, trauma, cancer, sickle cell crisis). Analgesic medications are a first line of treatment in these cases, and their use should be familiar to all practitioners.

Aspirin, Acetaminophen, and Nonsteroidal Anti-Inflammatory Agents (NSAIDS)   These drugs are considered together because they are used for similar problems and may have a similar mechanism of action (Table 12-1). All these compounds inhibit cyclooxygenase and, except for acetaminophen, all have anti-inflammatory actions, especially at higher dosages. They are particularly effective for mild to moderate headache and for pain of musculoskeletal origin.

Since they are effective for these common types of pains and are available without prescription, cyclooxygenase inhibitors are by far the most commonly used analgesics. They are absorbed well from the gastrointestinal tract and, with occasional use, side effects are minimal. With chronic use, gastric irritation is a common side effect of aspirin and NSAIDs and the problem that most frequently limits the dose that can be given. Gastric irritation is most severe with aspirin, which may cause erosion of the gastric mucosa, and because aspirin irreversibly acetylates platelets and interferes with coagulation of the blood, gastrointestinal bleeding is a risk. The NSAIDs are less problematic in this regard. Although toxic to the liver when taken in a high dose, acetaminophen rarely produces gastric irritation and does not interfere with platelet function. Table 12-1 lists the dosages and durations of action of the commonly used drugs of this class.

The introduction of a parenteral form of NSAID, ketorolac, extends the usefulness of this class of compounds in the management of acute severe pain. Ketorolac is sufficiently potent and rapid in onset to supplant opioids for many patients with acute severe headache and musculoskeletal pain.

Opioid Analgesics Opioids are the most potent pain-relieving drugs currently available. Furthermore, of all analgesics, they have the broadest range of efficacy, providing the most reliable method for rapidly relieving pain. Although side effects are common, except for respiratory depression, they are usually not serious and can be reversed rapidly with the narcotic antagonist naloxone. The physician should not hesitate to use opioid analgesics in patients with acute severe pain. Table 12-1 lists the most commonly used opioid analgesics.

Opioids produce analgesia by actions in the central nervous system. They activate pain-inhibitory neurons and directly inhibit pain-transmission neurons. Most of the commercially available opioid analgesics act at the same opiate receptor (mu receptor), differing mainly in potency, speed of onset, duration of action, and optimal route of administration. Although the dose-related side effects (sedation, respiratory depression, pruritus, constipation) are similar among the different opioids, some side effects are due to accumulation of nonopioid metabolites that are unique to individual drugs. One striking example of this is normeperidine, a metabolite of meperidine. Normeperidine produces hyperexcitability and seizures that are not reversible with naloxone. Normeperidine accumulation is much greater in patients with renal failure.

The most rapid relief with opioids is obtained by intravenous administration; relief with oral administration is significantly slower. Common acute side effects include nausea, vomiting, and sedation. These effects are dose-related, and there is great variability among patients in the doses that relieve pain and produce side effects. Because of this, initiation of therapy requires titration to optimal dose and interval. The most important principle is to provide adequate pain relief. This requires asking the patient whether the drug has relieved the pain and, if so, when the relief wears off. *The most common error made by physicians in managing severe pain with opioids is to prescribe an inadequate dose. Since many patients are reluctant to complain, this practice leads to needless suffering.* In the absence of sedation at the expected time of peak effect, a physician should not hesitate to repeat the initial dose to achieve satisfactory pain relief.

An innovative approach to the problem of achieving adequate pain relief is the use of patient-controlled analgesia (PCA). PCA requires a device that immediately delivers a pre-programmed dose of an opioid drug when the patient pushes a button. The device can be programmed to limit the total hourly dose so that overdosing is impossible. The patient can then titrate the dose to the optimal level. This approach is used most extensively for the management of postoperative pain, but there is no reason why it should not be used for any hospitalized patient with persistent severe pain. PCA is also used for home care of patients with intractable pain, such as metastatic cancer.

Table 12-1

Drugs for Relief of Pain

NONNARCOTIC ANALGESICS: USUAL DOSES AND INTERVALS

Generic Name	Dose, mg	Interval	Comments
Acetylsalicylic acid	650 PO	q 4 h	Enteric-coated preparations available
Acetaminophen	650 PO	q 4 h	Side effects uncommon
Ibuprofen	400 PO	q 4–6 h	Available without prescription
Naproxen	250–500 PO	q 12 h	Delayed effects may be due to long half-life
Fenoprofen	200 PO	q 4–6 h	pa
Indomethacin	25–50 PO	q 8 h	Gastrointestinal side effects common
Ketorolac	15–60 IM	q 4–6 h	Available for parenteral use (IM)

NARCOTIC ANALGESICS: USUAL DOSES AND INTERVALS

Generic Name	Parenteral Dose, mg	PO Dose, mg	Comments
Codeine	30–60 q 4 h	30–60 q 4 h	Nausea common
Oxycodone	—	5–10 q 4–6 h	Usually available with acetaminophen or aspirin
Morphine	10 q 4 h	60 q 4 h	
Morphine sustained release	pa	60–180 bid to tid	Oral slow-release preparation
Hydromorphone	1–2 q 4 h	2–4 q 4 h	Shorter acting than morphine sulfate
Levorphanol	2 q 6–8 h	4 q 6–8 h	Longer acting than morphine sulfate; absorbed well PO
Methadone	10 q 6–8 h	20 q 6–8 h	Delayed sedation due to long half-life
Meperidine	75–100 q 3–4 h	300 q 4 h	Poorly absorbed PO; normeperidine a toxic metabolite
Butorphanol	—	1–2 q 4 h	Intranasal spray
Fentanyl	—	—	Transdermal patch

ANTICONVULSANTS AND ANTIARRHYTHMICS

Generic Name	PO Dose, mg	Interval
Phenytoin	300	daily/qhs
Carbamazepine	200–300	q 6 h
Clonazepam	1	q 6 h
Mexiletine	150–300	q 6–12 h

TRICYCLIC ANTIDEPRESSANTS

Generic Name	Uptake Blockade		Sedative Potency	Anticholinergic Potency	Orthostatic Hypotension	Cardiac Arrhythmia	Average Dose, mg/day	Range, mg/day
	5HT	NE						
Doxepin	+ +	+	High	Moderate	Moderate	Less	200	75–400
Amitriptyline	+ + + +	+ +	High	Highest	Moderate	Yes	150	25–300
Imipramine	+ + + +	+ +	Moderate	Moderate	High	Yes	200	75–400
Nortriptyline	+ + +	+ +	Moderate	Moderate	Low	Yes	100	40–150
Desipramine	+ + +	+ + + +	Low	Low	Low	Yes	150	50–300

Many physicians, nurses, and patients have a certain trepidation about using opioids that is based on an exaggerated fear of patients becoming addicted. In fact, there is a vanishingly small chance of patients becoming addicted to narcotics as a result of their appropriate medical use.

The availability of new routes of administration has extended the usefulness of opioid analgesics. Most important is the availability of spinal administration. Opioids can be infused through a spinal catheter placed either intrathecally or epidurally. By applying opioids directly to the spinal cord, regional analgesia can be obtained using a relatively low total dose. In this way, such side effects as sedation, nausea, and respiratory depression can be minimized. This approach has been used extensively in obstetrical procedures and for lower-body postoperative pain. Opioids also can be given intranasally (butorphanol), rectally, and transdermally (fentanyl), thus avoiding the discomfort of frequent injections in patients who cannot be given oral medication.

OPIOID AND CYCLOOXYGENASE INHIBITOR COMBINATIONS When used in combination, opioids and cyclooxygenase inhibitors have additive effects. Because a lower dose of each can be used to achieve the same degree of pain relief and their side effects are nonadditive, such combinations can be used to lower the severity of dose-related side effects. Fixed-ratio combinations of an opioid with acetaminophen carry a special risk. Dose escalation as a result of increased severity of pain or decreased opioid effect as a result of tolerance may lead to levels of acetaminophen that are toxic to the liver.

CHRONIC PAIN

PATIENT EVALUATION Managing patients with chronic pain is intellectually and emotionally challenging. The patient's problem is often difficult to diagnose: such patients are demanding of the physician's time and often appear emotionally distraught. The traditional medical approach of seeking an obscure organic pathology is usually unhelpful. On the other hand, psychological evaluation and behaviorally based treatment paradigms are frequently helpful, particularly in the setting of a multidisciplinary pain-management center.

There are several factors that can cause, perpetuate, or exacerbate chronic pain. First, of course, the patient may simply have a disease that is characteristically painful for which there is presently no cure. Arthritis, cancer, migraine headaches, fibromyalgia, and diabetic neuropathy are examples of this. Second, there may be secondary perpetuating factors that are initiated by a bodily disease and persist after that disease has resolved. Examples include damaged sensory nerves, sympathetic efferent activity, and painful reflex muscle contraction. Finally, a variety of psychological conditions can exacerbate or even cause pain.

There are certain areas to which special attention should be paid in the medical history. Because depression is the most common emotional disturbance in patients with chronic pain, they should be questioned about their mood, appetite, sleep patterns, and daily activity. A simple standardized questionnaire, such as the Beck Depression Inventory, can be a useful screening device. It is important to remember that major depression is a common, treatable, and potentially fatal illness.

Other clues that a significant emotional disturbance is contributing to a patient's chronic pain complaint include: pain occurs in multiple unrelated sites; a pattern of recurrent, but separate, pain problems beginning in childhood or adolescence; pain beginning at a time of emotional trauma, such as the loss of a parent or spouse; a history of physical or sexual abuse; and past or present substance abuse.

On examination, special attention should be paid to whether the patient guards the painful area and whether certain movements or postures are avoided because of pain. Discovering a mechanical component to the pain can be useful both diagnostically and therapeutically. Painful areas should be examined for deep tenderness, noting whether this is localized to muscle, ligamentous structures, or joints. Chronic myofascial pain is very common, and in these patients deep palpation may reveal highly localized trigger points that are firm bands or knots in muscle. If injection of local anesthetic into these trigger points

relieves the pain, it supports the diagnosis. A neuropathic component to the pain is indicated by evidence of nerve damage, such as sensory impairment, exquisitely sensitive skin, weakness and muscle atrophy, or loss of deep tendon reflexes. Evidence suggesting sympathetic nervous system involvement includes the presence of diffuse swelling, changes in skin color and temperature, and hypersensitive skin and joint tenderness compared with the normal side. Relief of the pain with a sympathetic block is diagnostic.

A guiding principle in evaluating patients with chronic pain is to assess both emotional and organic factors before initiating therapy. Addressing these issues together, rather than waiting to "rule out" organic causes of the pain, improves compliance in part because it assures patients that a psychological evaluation does not mean that the physician is questioning the validity of their complaint. Even when an organic cause for a patient's pain can be found, it is still wise to look for other factors. For example, cancer patients with painful bony metastases also may have pain due to nerve damage and significant depression. Optimal therapy requires that each of these factors be looked for and treated.

℞ TREATMENT

Once the evaluation process has been completed and the likely causative and exacerbating factors identified, an explicit treatment plan should be developed. An important part of this process is to identify specific and realistic functional goals for therapy, such as getting a good night's sleep, being able to go shopping, or returning to work. A multidisciplinary approach that utilizes medications, counseling, physical therapy, nerve blocks, and even surgery may be required to improve the patient's quality of life. This may require referral to a pain clinic; however, this is not necessary for all chronic pain patients. For some, pharmacologic management alone can provide significant help.

Antidepressant Medications The tricyclic antidepressants (see Table 12-1) are extremely useful for the management of patients with chronic pain. Although developed for the treatment of depression, the tricyclics have a spectrum of dose-related biologic activities that include the production of analgesia in a variety of clinical conditions. Although the mechanism is unknown, the analgesic effect of tricyclics has a more rapid onset of action and occurs at a lower dose than is typically required for the treatment of depression. Furthermore, patients with chronic pain who are not depressed obtain pain relief with antidepressants. There is evidence that tricyclic drugs potentiate opioid analgesia, so they are useful adjuncts for the treatment of severe persistent pain such as occurs with malignant tumors. Table 12-2 lists some of the painful conditions that respond to tricyclics. Tricyclics are of particular value in the management of neuropathic pains such as painful diabetic neuropathy and postherpetic neuralgia, for which there are few other therapeutic options.

The tricyclics that have been shown to relieve pain have significant side effects. Unfortunately, some of the newer antidepressants such as fluoxetine (Prozac) that have fewer and less serious side effects have not been shown to provide pain relief.

Table 12-2

Painful Conditions that Respond to Tricyclic Antidepressants

Postherpetic neuralgia*
Diabetic neuropathy*
Tension headache*
Migraine headache*
Rheumatoid arthritis*†
Chronic low back pain†
Cancer

* Controlled trials demonstrate analgesia.
† Controlled studies indicate benefit but not analgesia.
SOURCE: Fields, 1987, p 291.

Anticonvulsants and Antiarrhythmics (See Table 12-1) These drugs are useful primarily for patients with neuropathic pain. Phenytoin (Dilantin) and carbamazepine (Tegretol) were first shown to relieve the pain of trigeminal neuralgia. This pain has a characteristic brief, shooting, electric shock–like quality. In fact, anticonvulsants seem to be helpful largely for pains that have such a lancinating quality.

Antiarrhythmic drugs such as low-dose lidocaine and mexiletine (Mexitil) are also effective for neuropathic pains. These drugs block the spontaneous activity of primary afferent nociceptors that appears when they are damaged.

Chronic Opioid Medication The long-term use of opioids is accepted for patients with pain due to malignant disease. Although its use for chronic pain of nonmalignant origin is controversial, it is clear that for many such patients opioid analgesics are the only option available for obtaining effective relief. This is understandable since opioids are the most potent and have the broadest range of efficacy of any analgesic medications. Although addiction is rare in patients who first use opioids for pain relief, some degree of tolerance and physical dependence are likely to occur with long-term use. Therefore, before embarking on opioid therapy, other options should be explored, and the limitations and risks of opioids should be explained to the patient. It is also important to point out that some opioid analgesic medications have mixed agonist-antagonist properties (e.g., pentazocine and butorphanol). From a practical standpoint, this means that they may worsen pain by inducing an abstinence syndrome in patients who are physically dependent on other opioid analgesics.

With long-term outpatient use of orally administered opioids it is desirable to use long-acting compounds such as levorphanol, methadone, or sustained-release morphine (see Table 12-1). The pharmacokinetic profile of these drugs enables prolonged pain relief, minimizes side effects such as sedation that are associated with high peak plasma levels, and, perhaps, reduces the likelihood of rebound pain associated with a rapid fall in plasma opioid concentration. Constipation is a virtually universal side effect of opioid use and should be treated expectantly.

It is worth emphasizing, in conclusion, that many patients, especially those with chronic pain, seek medical attention primarily because they are suffering and because only physicians can provide the medications required for their relief. Clearly, it is a primary responsibility of all physicians to attempt to minimize the physical and emotional discomfort of their patients. Familiarity with pain mechanisms and analgesic medications is an important step toward accomplishing this aim.

BIBLIOGRAPHY

BASBAUM AI, FIELDS HL: Endogenous pain control systems: Brainstem spinal pathways and endorphin circuitry. Ann Rev Neurosci 7:309, 1984

FIELDS HL (ed): *Pain Syndromes in Neurology.* London, Butterworth, 1990

————: *Pain.* New York, McGraw-Hill, 1987

————, LIEBESKIND JC (eds): *Pharmacological Approaches to the Treatment of Chronic Pain: New Concepts and Critical Issues.* Seattle, IASP Press, 1994

GALER BS: Neuropathic pain of peripheral origin: Advances in pharmacologic treatment. Neurology 45:517, 1995

MELZACK R, CASEY KL: Sensory, motivational, and central control determinants of pain, in *International Symposium on the Skin Senses*, DR Kenshalo (ed). Springfield, Ill, Charles C Thomas, 1968, p 423

ROWBOTHAM MC: Chronic pain: From theory to practical management. Neurology 45:5, 1995

STEIN C: The control of pain in peripheral tissue by opioids. N Engl J Med 332:1685, 1995

WALL PD, MELZACK R (eds): *Textbook of Pain* 3d ed. New York, Churchill Livingstone, 1994

WILLIS WD (ed): *Hyperalgesia and Allodynia.* New York, Raven Press, 1992

————, COGGESHALL RE: *Sensory Mechanism of the Spinal Cord.* New York, Plenum Press, 1991

13   *Lee Goldman*

CHEST DISCOMFORT AND PALPITATION

CHEST DISCOMFORT

Chest discomfort is one of the most frequent complaints for which patients seek medical attention; the potential benefit (or harm) resulting from the proper (or improper) assessment and management of the patient with this complaint is enormous. Failure to recognize a serious disorder, such as ischemic heart disease, may result in the dangerous delay of much-needed treatment, while an incorrect diagnosis of a potentially hazardous condition such as angina pectoris is likely to have harmful psychological and economic consequences and may lead to unnecessary cardiac catheterization. There is little relation between the severity of chest discomfort and the gravity of its cause. Therefore, a frequent problem in patients who complain of chest discomfort or pain is distinguishing trivial complaints from coronary artery disease and other serious disorders (Table 13-1).

CAUSES OF CHEST DISCOMFORT Discomfort due to **Myocardial Ischemia** Discomfort due to myocardial ischemia occurs when the oxygen supply to the heart is deficient in relation to

Table 13-1

Some Causes of Chest Discomfort and the Types of Discomfort Associated with Them

Cause	New, Acute, Often Ongoing	Recurrent, Episodic	Persistent, Even for Days
CARDIAC			
Coronary artery disease	+	+	—
Aortic stenosis	—	+	—
Hypertropic cardiomyopathy	—	+	—
Pericarditis	+	+	+
VASCULAR			
Aortic dissection	+	—	—
Pulmonary embolism	+	+	—
Pulmonary hypertension	+	+	—
Right ventricular strain	+	+	—
PULMONARY			
Pleuritis or pneumonia	+	+	+
Tracheobronchitis	+	+	+
Pneumothorax	+	—	+
Tumor	—	—	+
Mediastinitis or mediastinal emphysema	+	—	+
GASTROINTESTINAL			
Esophogeal reflux	+	+	+
Esophogeal spasm	+	+	+
Mallory-Weiss tear	+	—	—
Peptic ulcer disease	+	+	—
Biliary disease	+	+	—
Pancreatitis	+	+	+
MUSCULOSKELETAL			
Cervical disk disease	—	+	+
Arthritis of the shoulder or spine	—	+	+
Costochondritis	+	+	+
Intercostal muscle cramps	+	+	+
Interscalene or hyperabduction syndromes	—	+	+
Subacromial bursitis	+	+	+
OTHER			
Disorders of the breast	—	+	+
Chest wall tumors	—	—	+
Herpes zoster	+	—	+
Emotional	+	+	+

the oxygen need. The blood flow through the coronary arteries is directly proportional to the pressure gradient between the aorta and the ventricular myocardium (during systole) or the ventricular cavity (during diastole). However, in the presence of critical stenosis, it is also proportional to the fourth power of the radius of the coronary arteries. A relatively slight alteration in coronary luminal diameter below a critical level can produce a large decrease in coronary flow, provided that other factors remain constant. Coronary blood flow occurs primarily during diastole, when it is unopposed by systolic myocardial compression of the coronary vessels.

When the epicardial coronary arteries are narrowed critically (>70 percent stenosis of the luminal diameter), the intramyocardial coronary arterioles dilate in an effort to maintain total flow at a level that will avert myocardial ischemia at rest. The further dilation that would normally occur during exercise is, therefore, not possible. Hence, any condition in which increased heart rate, arterial pressure, or myocardial contractility occurs in the presence of coronary obstruction tends to precipitate anginal attacks by increasing myocardial oxygen needs in the face of a fixed oxygen supply.

By far the most frequent underlying cause of myocardial ischemia is organic narrowing of the coronary arteries secondary to coronary atherosclerosis (see also Chap. 244). Acute thrombosis superimposed on an atherosclerotic plaque is frequently the cause of unstable angina and acute myocardial infarction (see Chaps. 243 and 244).

Aside from conditions that narrow the lumen of the coronary arteries, the only other frequent causes of myocardial ischemia are disorders such as valvular aortic stenosis (Chap. 237) or hypertrophic cardiomyopathy (Chap. 239), which cause a marked disproportion between the coronary perfusion pressure and the heart's oxygen requirements. Under such conditions, the rise in left ventricular systolic pressure is not, as in hypertensive states, balanced by a corresponding elevation of aortic perfusion pressure. Epidemiologic studies indicate that chest pain is no more common in patients with mitral valve prolapse than in those without it.

The chest discomfort of myocardial ischemia, most commonly from coronary artery disease but also occasionally from the other causes of ischemia noted above, is angina pectoris. Myocardial ischemia secondary to coronary atherosclerosis is more common in adults, especially the elderly who have hypercholesterolemia, diabetes mellitus, hypertension, obesity, or who smoke cigarettes (Chap. 242). Toxins, including cocaine ingestion or withdrawal of chronic exposure to nitroglycerin, can cause sufficient coronary vasoconstriction to result in myocardial ischemia, and cocaine also can cause myocardial infarction.

Angina pectoris (See also Chap. 244) Angina pectoris is usually described as a heaviness, pressure, squeezing, or sensation of strangling or constriction in the chest, but it also may be described as an aching or burning pain, or even as indigestion. Some patients steadfastly deny pain but will admit to a discomfort or unusual feeling or may complain of difficulty in breathing.

Typically, angina pectoris develops gradually during exertion, after heavy meals, and with anger, excitement, frustration, and other emotional states; it is not precipitated by coughing, respiratory movements, or other motion. When angina is induced by walking, it often forces the patient to stop or to reduce speed. Anginal pain typically resolves within 5 to 30 min. More prolonged myocardial ischemia often represents a myocardial infarction, while more prolonged pain without other evidence for myocardial ischemia suggests a noncoronary etiology.

The correct diagnosis of angina pectoris may be aided by noting that the pain disappears more rapidly (usually within 5 min) and more completely when sublingual nitroglycerin is used. The demonstration that the time required for a given exercise to produce pain is consistently and considerably longer when it is undertaken within a few minutes after a sublingual nitroglycerin pill than after a placebo may, in some instances, be powerful clinical evidence for the diagnosis of angina pectoris. Angina is rarely relieved within a few seconds of lying down. It is not precipitated by stooping forward or by chest palpation, deep breathing, or simple changes in position.

Angina occurs most typically in the substernal region, anteriorly across the midthorax; it may radiate to or rarely occur alone in the intercapsular region, arms, shoulders, teeth, or abdomen. It rarely radiates to below the umbilicus, to the back of the neck, or to the occiput. Although the radiation of chest discomfort to the left arm increases the likelihood that myocardial ischemia or infarction is present, impulses from the skin and from visceral structures, such as the esophagus and heart, converge on a common pool of neurons in the posterior horn of the spinal cord, and their origin may be confused by the cerebral cortex.

An increase in heart rate is especially harmful in patients with coronary atherosclerosis or with aortic stenosis, because it both increases myocardial oxygen need and shortens diastole more than systole, thereby decreasing the total available perfusion time per minute. Tachycardia, a decline in arterial pressure, thyrotoxicosis, and diminution in arterial oxygen content (such as occurs in anemia or arterial hypoxia) are precipitating and aggravating factors rather than underlying causes of angina.

Patients with marked *right ventricular hypertension* may have exertional pain that is quite similar to that of angina. This discomfort probably results from relative ischemia of the right ventricle brought about by the increased oxygen needs and by the elevated intramural resistance, with reduction of the normally large systolic pressure gradient that perfuses this chamber.

Myocardial infarction Myocardial infarction is usually associated with a discomfort that is similar in quality and distribution to that of angina but of longer duration (usually 30 min) and usually of greater intensity. In contrast to angina, the pain of myocardial infarction is not rapidly relieved by rest or by coronary dilator drugs and may require large doses of narcotics. It may be accompanied by diaphoresis, nausea, and hypotension (see Chap. 243).

Physical examination The results of physical examination may be normal in patients with myocardial ischemia caused by coronary atherosclerosis. However, myocardial ischemia can cause a third or fourth heart sound because of an impairment of myocardial contraction or relaxation. Ischemic papillary muscle dysfunction can cause transient mitral regurgitation and its associated murmur. Myocardial infarction and, less commonly, severe and generalized ischemia can cause congestive heart failure.

The chest discomfort from myocardial ischemia that is caused by aortic stenosis, hypertrophic cardiomyopathy, and nonatherosclerotic causes of coronary artery disease is generally similar to that of angina pectoris from coronary atherosclerosis. However, in these conditions the physical examination will usually reveal classic findings of an aortic systolic murmur in patients with aortic stenosis (see Chap. 237) and will reveal dynamic outflow obstruction in many patients with hypertrophic cardiomyopathy (see Chap. 239).

Chest Pain due to Pericarditis The visceral surface of the pericardium ordinarily is insensitive to pain, as is the parietal surface, except in its lower portion, which has a relatively small number of pain fibers carried in the phrenic nerves. The pain associated with pericarditis is believed to be due to inflammation of the adjacent parietal pleura. These observations explain why noninfectious pericarditis (e.g., that associated with uremia and with myocardial infarction) and cardiac tamponade with relatively mild inflammation are usually painless or accompanied by only mild pain, whereas infectious pericarditis, being nearly always more intense and spreading to the neighboring pleura, is usually associated with pain (Chap. 240).

Pericarditis can cause pain in several locations (see Chap. 240). Since the central part of the diaphragm receives its sensory supply from the phrenic nerve (which arises from the third to fifth cervical segments of the spinal cord), pain arising from the lower parietal pericardium and central tendon of the diaphragm is felt characteristically at the tip of the shoulder, the adjoining trapezius ridge, and the neck. Involvement of the more lateral part of the diaphragmatic pleura, supplied by branches from the sixth to ninth intercostal nerves, causes pain not only in the anterior part of the chest but also in the upper part of the abdomen or corresponding region of the back, sometimes simulating the pain of acute cholecystitis or pancreatitis.

Pericardial pain commonly has a pleuritic component; i.e., it is related to respiratory movements and aggravated by cough and/or deep inspiration, because of pleural irritation. It is sometimes brought on by swallowing, because the esophagus lies just behind the posterior portion of the heart, and is often altered by a change of body position, becoming sharper and more left-sided in the supine position and milder when the patient sits upright, leaning forward.

In some patients, however, pericardial pain may be described as a steady substernal discomfort that can mimic the pain of acute myocardial infarction. The mechanism of this steady substernal pain is not certain, but it may arise from marked inflammation of the relatively insensitive inner parietal surface of the pericardium or from irritated afferent cardiac nerve fibers lying in the periadventitial layers of the superficial coronary arteries. Occasionally, both pleuritic and steady pain may be present simultaneously.

Vascular Causes of Chest Pain *Aortic dissection* develops as a result of a subintimal hematoma, which may start either because a tear has developed in the intima of the aorta or because of bleeding into the vasa vasorum. Antegrade movement of this hematoma can compromise major branches off the aorta, while retrograde spread can occlude a coronary artery, disrupt the aortic valve annulus, or rupture into the pericardial space.

The pain due to *acute dissection of the aorta* (Chap. 247) or to an expanding aortic aneurysm results from stimulation of nerve endings in the adventitia. The pain usually begins abruptly, reaches an extremely severe peak rapidly, is felt in the center of the chest and/or in the back depending on the site of the dissection, lasts for hours, and requires unusually large amounts of analgesics for relief. Patients commonly describe a true pain rather than the vague discomfort that is sometimes described with myocardial ischemia. The pain is not aggravated by changes in position or respiration.

Chest Pain due to Pulmonary Embolism The acute pain from massive *pulmonary emboli* (Chap. 261) is thought to be related to pulmonary hypertension and to distention of the pulmonary artery. Infarction of a segment of the lung that is adjacent to the pleura commonly irritates the pleural surface and causes chest discomfort hours or even days later. The pain resulting from pulmonary embolism may resemble that of acute myocardial infarction, and in cases of massive embolism it is located substernally. In patients with smaller emboli, the pain is caused by focal pulmonary infarction and is usually located more laterally, is pleuritic in nature, and sometimes is associated with hemoptysis.

Other Pulmonary Causes of Chest Discomfort A variety of diseases of the lung can cause chest discomfort. Pleural pain, which is usually a brief, sharp, knifelike pain that is precipitated by inspiration or coughing, is very common and generally results from stretching of a parietal pleura that is inflamed by fibrinous pleurisy or any pneumonic process (see Chap. 262).

Gastrointestinal Causes of Chest Discomfort *Esophageal pain* commonly presents as a deep thoracic burning discomfort, which is the hallmark of acid-induced pain. Ingestion of aspirin, alcohol, or certain foods typically exacerbates this burning discomfort, and the discomfort may be relieved promptly by antacids or even by one or two swallows of food or water. Patients may have accompanying dysphagia, regurgitation of undigested food, or weight loss. The symptoms of a hiatus hernia tend to be exacerbated by lying down, and all forms of acid-peptic disease may be worse in the early morning, when acidic secretions are not neutralized by food. Esophageal spasm, which may be induced by reflux of gastric acid into an esophagus in which the mucosa has been previously irritated, can cause a squeezing pain that may be indistinguishable from that of myocardial ischemia and that may even have a similar pattern of radiation. Pain resulting from injury of the esophagus, such as in the case of a Mallory-Weiss tear that is caused by severe vomiting, can cause severe acute chest pain (Chap. 283).

Occasionally, other gastrointestinal diseases, including *peptic ulcer disease, biliary disease*, and *pancreatitis*, may present with chest discomfort as well as abdominal discomfort. Pain resulting from gastric or duodenal ulcer (Chap. 284) is epigastric or substernal, usually commences about 1 to 1.5 h after meals, and is usually relieved in several minutes by antacids or milk.

The discomfort caused by acute cholecystitis is more commonly described as an ache, which may be epigastric or substernal. It most commonly occurs an hour or so after meals and not in relation to exertion. The presence of an abdominal disorder, such as a hiatus hernia or a duodenal ulcer, does not constitute proof that the patient's chest pain is related to it. Such disorders are frequently asymptomatic and are not at all uncommon in patients who also have myocardial ischemia.

Neuromusculoskeletal Causes of Chest Discomfort Neuromusculoskeletal chest discomfort can be caused by *cervical disk disease* because of compression of nerve roots, by *arthritis of the shoulder or spine*, or by *costochondritis*, which is an inflammation of the costochondral junctions. Inflammation of the subacromial bursa or, less commonly, the supraspinatus or deltoid tendon may cause pain that radiates to the chest. *Intercostal muscle cramps* may occur throughout the chest. Anterior scalene and hyperabduction syndromes also can cause chest discomfort.

The *costochondral and chondrosternal articulations* are the most common sites of anterior musculoskeletal chest pain. Objective signs in the form of swelling (Tietze's syndrome), redness, and heat are rare, but sharply localized tenderness is common. The pain may be darting and last for only a few seconds or may be a dull ache enduring for hours or days. An associated feeling of tightness due to muscle spasm (see below) is frequent. *Pressure on the chondrosternal and costochondral junctions and on the pectoralis muscles is an essential part of the examination of every patient with chest pain* and will reproduce the pain arising from these tissues.

Emotional Causes of Chest Pain Emotional disorders are commonly associated with chest pain. Usually, the discomfort is experienced as a sense of "tightness," sometimes called "aching," and occasionally it may be designated as a pain of considerable magnitude. Since the discomfort may be described as a tightness or constriction and is often localized at least in part beneath the sternum, it is not surprising that this type of discomfort is frequently confused with that of myocardial ischemia. Ordinarily, it lasts for a half hour or more, is unrelated to exertion, and fluctuates slowly in intensity. The association with fatigue or emotional strain is usually clear, although this may not be volunteered by the patient. Associated hyperventilation can cause innocent changes in the T waves and ST segments, which can be confused with coronary artery disease. Alternatively, chest pain associated with emotional disorders may be sharp and very brief and located near the left nipple.

DIFFERENTIAL DIAGNOSIS OF CHEST DISCOMFORT
The key issue in the evaluation of the patient with chest discomfort is to distinguish potentially life-threatening conditions such as coronary artery disease, aortic dissection, or pulmonary embolism from other causes of chest discomfort. Even patients who have brief episodes of pain and are otherwise in apparently excellent health may have intermittent myocardial ischemia or recurrent pulmonary emboli. One useful approach to the patient with chest pain is to determine whether the syndrome represents new, acute, and often ongoing pain; recurrent, episodic pain; or pain that is persistent, perhaps for days (Fig. 13-1). The various causes of chest pain (Table 13-1) can, in part, be distinguished by their likelihood to present in these three different ways.

New, Acute, often Ongoing Pain In a patient who presents with this syndrome, the physician must immediately distinguish whether the pain represents a condition for which acute circulatory or respiratory insufficiency is a substantial risk (Fig. 13-2). Emergent stabilization and treatment must precede detailed diagnostic evaluation.

In the patient with acute chest discomfort, the diagnostic evaluation begins with a focused history and physical examination that is designed to evaluate the likelihood of conditions, such as acute myocardial

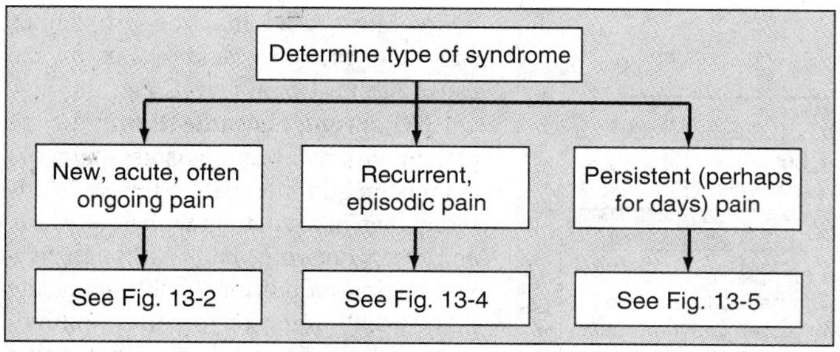

Determine type of syndrome

New, acute, often ongoing pain → See Fig. 13-2

Recurrent, episodic pain → See Fig. 13-4

Persistent (perhaps for days) pain → See Fig. 13-5

FIGURE 13-1   Approach to the patient with chest pain.

infarction, aortic dissection, or pulmonary embolism, that could be life-threatening even in a patient who currently appears to be stable. Accumulated data from large numbers of patients who have presented to emergency departments with acute chest pain can aid in the assessment of the probability that an individual is experiencing an acute myocardial infarction. In this setting, an emergent electrocardiogram is the single best diagnostic test (Fig. 13-3). In patients in whom the electrocardiogram shows Q waves of at least 0.04 s duration or ST-segment elevation that is not known to be old in two more leads, the probability of acute myocardial infarction is 75 percent. In patients in whom the electrocardiogram shows evidence of ST-segment depression of 1 mm or more or T-wave inversion that is not known to be old in two or more leads, the probability of acute myocardial infarction is about 20 percent. On the basis of substantial empirical data, patients with either of these electrocardiographic changes and a clinical syndrome suspicious for acute myocardial ischemia require urgent admission to an intensive care unit, partly for further evaluation but mainly because of the substantial short-term risk of developing life-threatening complications (see Chap. 243). For patients with ST-segment elevation, the likelihood of occlusion of an infarct-related artery mandates urgent reperfusion unless otherwise contraindicated or unless a diagnosis other than acute myocardial infarction is being considered very seriously. For patients with changes suggesting ischemia but without ST elevation, treatment is usually for presumed unstable angina (see Chap. 244).

For patients without electrocardiographic changes of new (or presumably new) ischemia or infarction, further observation with serial electrocardiograms and cardiac enzymes is useful if the clinical presentation nevertheless raises a reasonable likelihood of acute myocardial infarction or acute myocardial ischemia. In this assessment, multiple factors must be taken into account, especially in patients who do not have evident changes on the initial electrocardiogram. For example, a patient is more likely to be having acute myocardial ischemia if the pain is clearly similar to prior known angina pectoris but somehow worse in terms of intensity, duration, or failure to respond to usual measures. In patients wih no prior history of ischemic heart disease, multiple factors, including the patient's age and gender and the location and description of pain, influence whether further observation is required. New approaches to these patients include admission to chest pain observation units in which patients are

watched for up to 6 to 12 h with serial testing. After this observation period, further cardiac testing with a standard exercise electrocardiogram, a myocardial perfusion scintiscan, or a stress echocardiogram may aid in establishing the diagnosis. In patients in whom no myocardial cause is evident, a musculoskeletal and/or gastrointestinal evaluation may be helpful, but such testing can usually be performed on an outpatient basis.

Acute aortic dissection (Chap. 247) may be suggested by the sudden onset of symptoms, the finding of asymmetric pulses, and a history of hypertension or Marfan's syndrome. The routine chest radiograph may show a dilated aortic root to suggest or support this diagnosis, which may then be established by transesophageal echocardiography, computed tomography, or magnetic resonance imaging. Aortography has traditionally been the definitive test, but, because of its invasiveness, it is often now replaced by magnetic resonance imaging in hemodynamically stable patients and preceded by a screening transesophageal echocardiogram in unstable patients.

Acute pulmonary embolism (Chap. 261) may be suggested on the basis of respiratory symptoms, hemoptysis, pleuritic chest discomfort, or a history of deep venous thrombosis or coagulation abnormalities. The evaluation usually requires a lung scan and/or pulmonary arteriogram to evaluate pulmonary perfusion.

Of the various potential gastrointestinal causes of chest discomfort, the most worrisome include a Mallory-Weiss esophageal tear, acute cholecystitis, pancreatitis, and a perforating gastric or duodenal ulcer. For peptic ulcer disease, cholecystitis, and pancreatitis, the abdominal examination usually is critical to the diagnosis. Mallory-Weiss tears

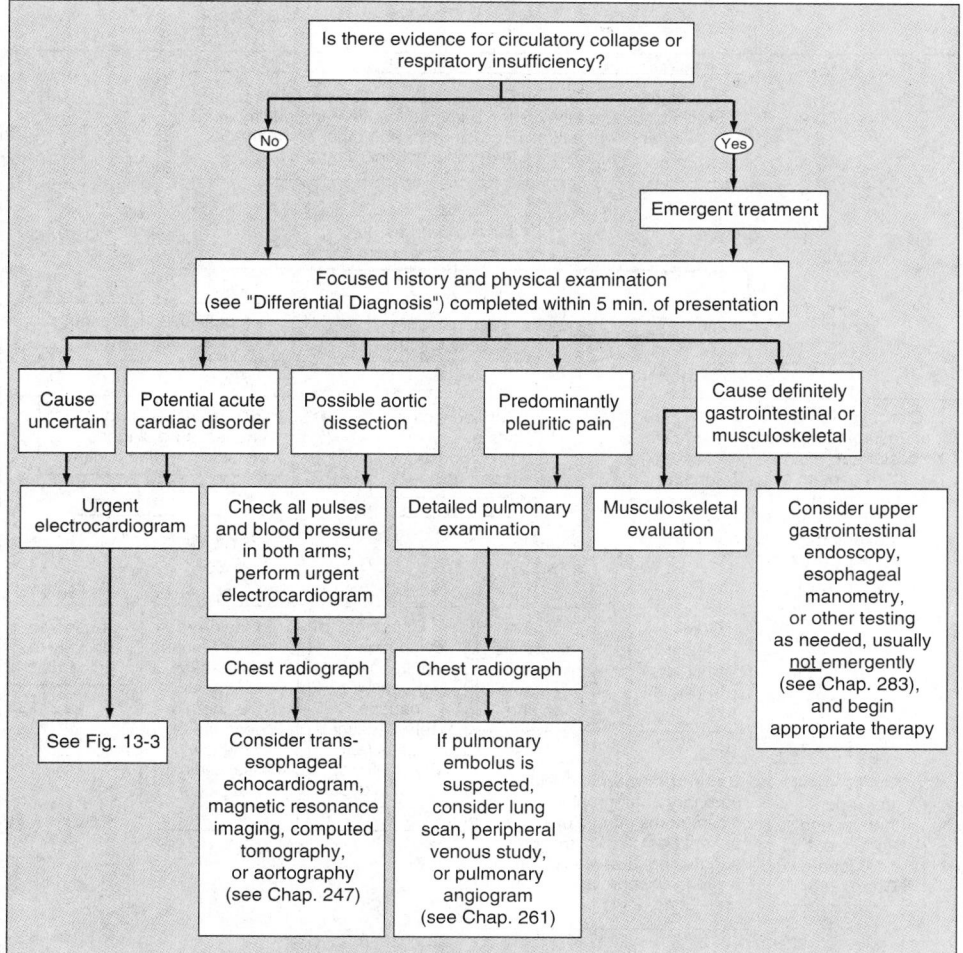

FIGURE 13-2   Approach to the patient with new, acute, often ongoing pain.

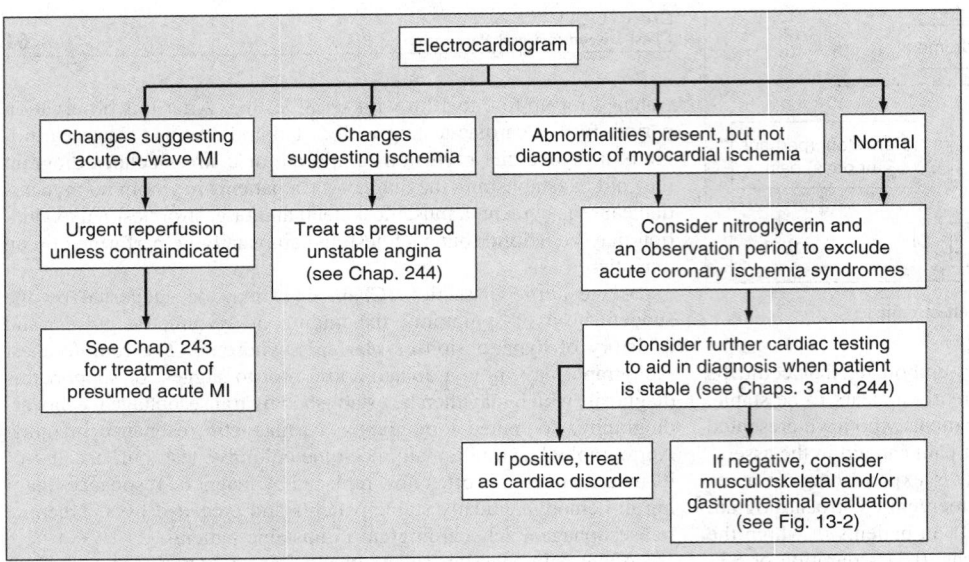

FIGURE 13-3 Approach to the patient with new, acute, often ongoing pain potentially of cardiac etiology or of uncertain cause. (MI, myocardial infarction.)

are commonly associated with hematemesis. In the acute setting, esophageal disease may be a diagnosis of exclusion in patients who have no evidence for cardiac, pulmonary, or vascular causes. Upper gastrointestinal endoscopy or an upper gastrointestinal roentgenogram can diagnose esophageal or peptic ulcer disease. Esophageal manometry and measurement of lower esophageal sphincter pressure are useful in identifying esophageal spasm. The Bernstein acid perfusion test, in which an attempt is made to reproduce the pain by infusion of

hydrochloric acid into the esophagus, can help establish acid reflux as the cause of chest pain (see Chap. 283).

Recurrent Episodic Pain In the patient with recurrent, episodic pain, the diagnostic and therapeutic tempo is different than in the patient with new, acute, and often ongoing pain. Although life-threatening conditions such as acute myocardial infarction, recurrent pulmonary emboli, or even aortic dissection can sometimes present in this way, patients with recurrent, episodic pain are more likely to have a variety of less critical diagnoses (Table 13-1).

In this setting, a detailed and meticulous history of the behavior of the pain is the cornerstone of the evaluation (Fig. 13-4). One useful approach is to divide recurrent, episodic pain into those syndromes that represent a high likelihood for angina, those that are atypical but possibly represent angina, and those that are very unlikely to be caused by angina or myocardial ischemia. The history, physical examination, and subsequent diagnostic testing can be guided by this approach.

The *history* should focus on the behavior of the pain as the cornerstone of the evaluation. The location, radiation, quality, intensity, and duration of the episodes are important. Even more so is the story of the aggravating and alleviating factors. A history of intense aggravation by breathing, coughing, or other respiratory movements will usually point toward the pleura and pericardium or mediastinum as the site, although chest wall pain is likewise affected by respiratory motion. Similarly, a pain that regularly appears on rapid walking, or with other exertion such as sexual activity, and vanishes a few minutes after stopping suggests the diagnosis of angina pectoris, although a similar story will occasionally be obtained from patients with skeletal disorders.

A thorough *physical examination* can provide important clues to the cause of chest discomfort. Blood pressure should be checked in both arms if aortic dissection is being considered. Examination of the skin may reveal cyanosis, which suggests hypoxemia from either diminished cardiac output or impaired respiratory function, or xanthelasma, which would suggest hyperlipidemia and associated coronary disease. The finding of lymphadenopathy suggests a tumor. The examination of the chest wall should include both inspection and palpation to search for costochondritis and other musculoskeletal abnormalities. Lung examination may reveal a pleural rub, signs of pneumonic consolidation, or evidence of congestive heart failure. The physical examination may be totally normal in persons with severe myocardial ischemia, but it also may demonstrate abnormalities of vital signs, a third or fourth heart sound, or mitral regurgitation from papillary muscle dysfunction. Aortic stenosis will be accompanied by its typical murmur (Chap. 237). The cardiac examination also

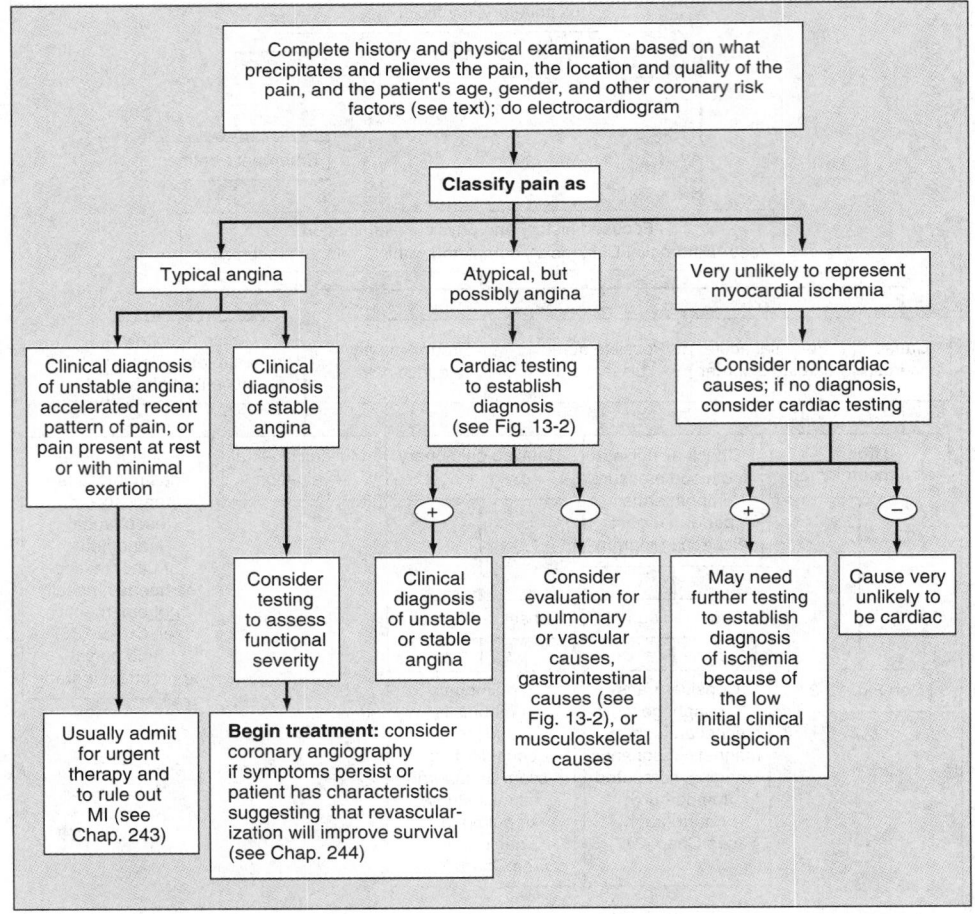

FIGURE 13-4 Approach to the patient with recurrent episodic pain. (MI, myocardial infarction.)

should search for an increased pulmonic second sound that may indicate elevated pulmonary artery pressure, such as is found in pulmonary embolism, and the pericardial friction rub that strongly suggests pericarditis. A careful upper abdominal examination may be the first clue to peptic ulcer disease or cholecystitis.

Critical information can often be obtained by attempts to produce or alleviate the pain, such as with nitroglycerin. Careful palpation of the chest wall, subacromial bursa, deltoid tendon, abdomen, and other structures may be very helpful if it reproduces the chest discomfort. Shoulder and arm motion commonly reproduces pain related to these structures. Evaluation of the patient at the time of a spontaneous episode, such as with an electrocardiogram during pain, is also extremely helpful.

Persistent Chest Discomfort Pain that persists unabated for many hours or days is more likely to represent a noncoronary cause, such as pericarditis, a musculoskeletal condition, a pulmonary abnormality, or one of several gastrointestinal conditions. Once again, a complete history and physical examination is mandatory, and further testing is guided by the findings (Table 13-2). If pericarditis is suspected, an electrocardiogram, chest radiograph, and echocardiogram may establish or exclude the diagnosis. Potential pulmonary conditions are commonly evaluated with a chest radiograph. Suspected musculoskeletal abnormalities may be confirmed, if necessary, by radiographic studies and/or the response to targeted therapies, including a local injection of lidocaine. Potential gastrointestinal causes may be evaluated with a variety of tests as described above. Although acute myocardial infarction, pulmonary embolism, and aortic dissection rarely present as persistent pain, these diagnoses must also be considered in patients in whom the more common causes of persistent pain are not found.

In considering diagnostic tests for all the various causes of chest discomfort, the clinician must remember that a useful test result is commonly one that moves the likelihood of a diagnostic possibility across a threshold, so the test result would lead to a change in management, either by influencing the decision to order additional tests or by causing a change in treatment. In the case of chest discomfort, the decisions cannot be based on a 50 percent threshold: Probabilities of coronary artery disease, pulmonary embolism, or aortic dissection that are well below 50 percent may still demand further evaluation because of the dire consequences of missing one of these important diagnoses. The physician must be prepared to embark on an appropriate evaluation when the history and physical examination do not exclude these diagnoses with a reasonable degree of certainty. The degree of certainty must be determined for the individual condition and patient at hand, typically after an appropriately full and frank discussion between the patient and the physician.

Weighing the Evidence The assessment of the probability of the various causes of chest pain requires the integration of multiple pieces of data, because no single clinical feature can be considered decisive. Each of the conditions that can cause chest discomfort can have varied presentations, and the diagnostic tests upon which physicians often rely can also have false-positive or false-negative results. Thus the principles of clinical reasoning (Chap. 3) should be applied to the evaluation of the patient with chest discomfort.

The information obtained from a careful medical history and physical examination can be used to develop a differential diagnosis of the causes of chest discomfort in an individual patient, to rank these diagnostic possibilities, and often to assign approximate percent probabilities to them. Although the various causes of chest discomfort have typical characteristics, these characteristics must be interpreted in light of the prior probability that a person with a given age and sex and with a particular past medical history would have such a cause of chest discomfort. For example, the possibility of angina pectoris as a cause of precordial or substernal discomfort must be seriously considered in a middle-aged man with coronary risk factors such as hypercholesterolemia and smoking, even if the description of the discomfort is not perfectly typical for angina pectoris. Conversely, when a 20-year-old woman describes the onset of new discomfort in a way that is seemingly classic for angina pectoris, such a diagnosis is relatively

unlikely because the prior probability of ischemic heart disease, given her age and sex, is so low.

Although it is not always possible to assign numerical probabilities to the various causes of chest discomfort in an individual patient, experienced clinicians either implicitly or explicitly assess the relative likelihoods of various potential explanations for any chest discomfort syndrome to help guide their future diagnostic evaluations and therapy. For example, a middle-aged or elderly man with typical characteristics for angina pectoris has about an 85 percent probability of having hemodynamically significant coronary artery disease. By comparison, the same man with a history of chest discomfort that has some characteristics that are typical for angina pectoris but other characteristics that are atypical has a probability of important coronary disease ranging from about 30 to 60 percent. Even persons with chest pain that is decidedly unlikely to represent coronary disease still have some finite possibility of coronary disease, with a likelihood ranging from exceedingly small in a young woman to somewhere in the 10 percent range in a middle-aged man with many coronary risk factors.

Diagnostic tests Although myocardial ischemia commonly is associated with electrocardiographic changes (Chap. 244), many patients have normal tracings between attacks, and in some the electrocardiogram may even be normal during an episode of pain. However, depression of the ST segments, caused by myocardial ischemia, typically occurs during exertion and is accompanied by anginal discomfort; moreover, electrocardiographic evidence of myocardial ischemia may occur at rest and with or without accompanying chest discomfort. The finding of flat or down-sloping ST-segment depressions of 0.1 mV or greater during an attack of pain substantially increases the likelihood that the pain is anginal in origin. Exercise electrocardiography will show ischemic changes in about 50 to 80 percent of persons with symptomatic coronary disease but also in about 10 to 15 percent of patients who do not have coronary disease. The accuracy of ambulatory ischemia monitoring in the general population is less clear.

Although exercise electrocardiography and exercise thallium scintigraphy are of value in distinguishing between cardiac and noncardiac causes of chest discomfort, the results must be interpreted in light of the prior probability of coronary artery disease, which is the probability that the patient has coronary disease based on the presenting clinical characteristics, age, and sex (see Fig. 3-2). Since exercise perfusion scintigraphy appears to provide information that is correlated with the standard exercise electrocardiogram no more than would be expected by chance, it can provide additional independent information (Chap. 3) and further change the probability of coronary artery disease (Fig. 13-1). If absolute diagnostic knowledge is required, cardiac catheterization with coronary angiography serves as the gold standard—i.e., the test that is considered definitive regarding the presence or absence of coronary disease—even though the presence of anatomic disease does not guarantee that the coronary stenoses are causing the chest discomfort.

A sequence of consistently negative cardiologic test results reduces the probability of coronary artery disease to below 10 percent in patients with atypical chest discomfort. However, even after a normal exercise electrocardiogram and exercise perfusion scintigram, the probability of coronary disease will still be about 30 percent in a

Table 13-2

Approach to the Patient with Persistent Pain (Lasting Perhaps for Days)

1. Complete history and physical examination
2. Testing guided by data may include:
   Electrocardiogram
   Chest radiograph
   Computed tomography of chest
   Gastrointestinal evaluation (see Fig. 13-2)
   Spine, shoulder, or rib radiographs
   Echocardiogram

middle-aged or elderly patient with a typical history of angina pectoris (Fig. 13-2). By recognizing the potential change in probabilities that can be obtained with positive and negative results of the diagnostic tests that are planned, the physician can decide whether these potential changes in probability are sufficient to warrant the test. For example, the physician should commonly decide that a patient with typical angina pectoris and a positive exercise electrocardiogram does not require an exercise thallium scintigram to *diagnose* coronary disease, although under some circumstances this examination might aid in the estimation of the patient's subsequent prognosis.

PALPITATIONS

Palpitations are a common, disagreeable symptom that may be defined as an awareness of the beating of the heart, an awareness most commonly brought about by a change in the heart's rhythm or rate or by an augmentation of its contractility. Palpitations are not pathognomonic of any particular group of disorders; indeed, often they signify not a primary physical disorder but rather a psychological disturbance. Even when they occur as a more or less prominent complaint, the diagnosis of the underlying disease is made largely on the basis of other associated symptoms and data. Nevertheless, palpitations are frequently of considerable importance in the minds of patients, who fear they may indicate heart disease. Concern is all the more pronounced in patients who have been told that they *may* have heart disease; to them palpitations may seem to be an omen of impending disaster. Since the resulting anxiety may be associated with increased activity of the autonomic nervous system, with consequent increases in the cardiac rate and rhythm and the vigor of contraction, the patient's awareness of these changes may then lead to a vicious cycle, which may ultimately be responsible for incapacitation.

Palpitations may be described by the patient in various terms, such as "pounding," "fluttering," "flopping," and "skipping," and in most cases it will be obvious that the complaint is of a sensation of disturbed heartbeat. The sensitivity to alterations in cardiac activity among different individuals varies widely. Some patients seem to be unaware of the most serious and chaotic dysrhythmias; others are seriously troubled by an occasional extrasystole. Patients with anxiety states often exhibit a lowered threshold at which disorders of rate and rhythm result in palpitation. The awareness of the heartbeat also tends to be more common at night and during introspective moments than during activity. Patients with organic heart disease and chronic disorders of cardiac rate, rhythm, or stroke volume tend to accommodate to these abnormalities and are often less sensitive than normal persons to such events. Persistent tachycardia and/or atrial fibrillation may not be accompanied by continuous palpitations, in contrast to a sudden, brief alteration in cardiac rate or rhythm, which often causes considerable subjective discomfort. Palpitations are particularly prominent when the precipitating cause for increased heart rate or contractility or arrhythmia is recent, transient, and episodic. Conversely, in emotionally well-adjusted individuals, palpitations commonly become progressively less disconcerting as they become more chronic.

DIFFERENTIAL DIAGNOSIS The patient's description of palpitations represents the most important clue to their etiology (Fig. 13-5). Every effort should be made to ask the patient to check the radial pulse during episodes of palpitation to assist in the diagnosis. If the rhythm is steady and regular and the rate is normal, the patient may be aware of an abnormal stroke volume from a condition such as aortic regurgitation but more likely is reporting a heightened awareness of normal cardiac function, sometimes in response to routine stress. Conversely, if the rhythm is steady and regular but the rate is clearly increased, especially above 120 beats per minute at a time when activity or other stresses should not result in tachycardia, the papitations may well represent a supraventricular or sometimes even a ventricular tachycardia.

An irregular pulse noted during an episode of palpitation virtually

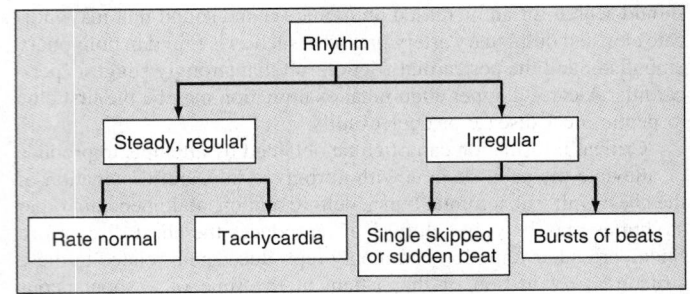

FIGURE 13-5 Flowchart for the description of palpitations.

always represents a true arrhythmia. The arryhthmia may be as simple as an occasional extrasystole. The premature contraction and post-premature beat after an extrasystole are often described as a "flopping," or the patient may say that it feels as if "the heart were turning over." The pause following the premature contraction may be felt as an actual cessation of the heart beat. The first ventricular contraction after the pause may be felt as an unusually vigorous beat and often be described as "pounding" or "thudding." By the patient's account alone, numerous extrasystoles may be difficult to distinguish from atrial fibrillation (Chap. 231). Bursts of beats may represent atrial fibrillation or brief episodes of a supraventricular or ventricular tachycardia.

Ectopic tachycardias commonly begin instantaneously and stop suddenly, sometimes followed by a pause before sinus rhythm resumes. Patients are usually acutely aware of both the onset and ending of the arrhythmia. A variety of vagal maneuvers (Chap. 231) may already have been used by the patient or may be suggested by the physician to aid in cessation of the ectopic arrhythmia.

All of the various arrhythmic causes of palpitations may be more common in the setting of thyrotoxicosis (Chap. 331), hypoglycemia (Chap. 335), pheochromocytoma (Chap. 333), fever (Chap. 17), and certain drugs. These arrhythmias may also be precipitated by tobacco, coffee, tea, alcohol, epinephrine, ephedrine, aminophylline, atropine, or thyroid medication. The physical examination should include a search for evidence of valvular heart disease, hyperthyroidism, and pulmonary disease.

ASSOCIATED SYMPTOMS While palpitations are extremely common in healthy individuals, regardless of whether they are caused by a true arrhythmia or not, the presence of associated signs, symptoms, or other conditions helps to determine the potential seriousness of palpitations. Palpitations associated with symptoms of dizziness, shortness of breath, or chest discomfort, or occurring in a patient with an underlying history of cardiac disease, often require further evaluation. In such individuals, palpitations may be a manifestation of important arrhythmias that influence prognosis and, in some situations, require treatment (Chap. 231).

Approach to the Patient

The most common initial test for a patient with palpitations is a continuous (Holter) monitor, especially if the palpitations occur on a daily basis. For individuals with less frequent symptoms, a variety of loop recorders can be worn for days and activated by the patient at the time that the palpitations are experienced. It should be remembered that many patients have asymptomatic irregularities of the heart rhythm.

In addition to ambulatory electrocardiographic monitoring, exercise testing is sometimes of value in reassuring both the patient and the physician that vigorous exercise does not produce a worrisome arrhythmia. In general, arrhythmias that disappear with exercise are more likely to be more benign than those that are precipitated by it.

The management of palpitations focuses on the treatment of specifically diagnosed arrhythmias, on the elimination of precipitating factors (medications, tobacco, coffee, tea, alcohol), or on the recognition of associated syndromes, including hyperthyroidism, pheochromocytoma, hypoglycemia, menopausal symptoms, or an anxiety state.

As a rule, palpitations themselves often produce anxiety and fear out of proportion to the seriousness to the underlying condition. When the cause has been accurately determined and the significance is explained to the patient, concern is often ameliorated or eliminated. In patients with no important cause, evaluation and appropriate reassurance may be critical to helping the patient regain confidence and return to a normal quality of life.

BIBLIOGRAPHY

ACC/AHA Task Force: Guidelines for clinical use of cardiac radionuclide imaging. J Am Coll Cardiol 25:521, 1995

Barsky AJ et al: The clinical course of palpitations in medical outpatients. Arch Intern Med 155:1782, 1995

Gersh B et al: Chronic ischemic heart disease, in *Heart Disease*, 5th ed, E Braunwald (ed). Philadelphia, Saunders, 1997, pp 1289–1365

Lam HGT et al: Acute noncardiac chest pain in a coronary care unit: Evaluation by a 24-hour pressure and pH recording of the esophagus. Gastroenterology 102:453, 1992

Nienaber CA et al: The diagnosis of thoracic aortic dissection by noninvasive imaging procedures. N Engl J Med 328:1, 1993

Singh S et al: The contribution of gastroesophageal reflux to chest pain in patients with coronary artery disease. Ann Intern Med 117:824, 1992

Wolf MA: Palpitations and disturbances of cardiac rhythm, in *Office Practice of Medicine*, 3d ed, WT Branch Jr (ed). Philadelphia, Saunders, 1994

---

14 *William Silen*

ABDOMINAL PAIN

The correct interpretation of acute abdominal pain is one of the most challenging demands made of any physician. Since proper therapy may require urgent action, the luxury of the leisurely approach suitable for the study of other conditions is sometimes denied. Few other clinical situations demand greater experience and judgment, because the most catastrophic of events may be forecast by the subtlest of symptoms and signs. Nowhere in medicine is a meticulously executed, detailed history and physical examination of greater importance. The etiologic classification in Table 14-1, although not complete, forms a useful frame of reference for the evaluation of patients with abdominal pain.

The diagnosis of "acute or surgical abdomen" so often heard in emergency wards is not an acceptable one because of its often misleading and erroneous connotation. The most obvious of "acute abdomens" may not require operative intervention, and the mildest of abdominal pains may herald the onset of an urgently correctable lesion. Any patient with abdominal pain of recent onset requires early and thorough evaluation with specific attempts at accurate diagnosis.

SOME MECHANISMS OF PAIN ORIGINATING IN THE ABDOMEN   Inflammation of the Parietal Peritoneum   The pain of parietal peritoneal inflammation is steady and aching in character and is located directly over the inflamed area, its exact reference being possible because it is transmitted by somatic nerves supplying the parietal peritoneum. The intensity of the pain is dependent on the type and amount of foreign substance to which the peritoneal surfaces are exposed in a given period of time. For example, the sudden release into the peritoneal cavity of a small quantity of *sterile* acid gastric juice causes much more pain than the same amount of grossly contaminated neutral fecal material. Enzymatically active pancreatic juice incites more pain and inflammation than does the same amount of sterile bile containing no potent enzymes. Blood and urine are often so bland as to go undetected if exposure of the peritoneum has not been sudden and massive. In the case of bacterial contamination, such as in pelvic inflammatory disease, the pain is frequently of low intensity early in the illness until bacterial multiplication has caused the elaboration of irritating substances.

So important is the rate at which the irritating material is applied to the peritoneum that cases of perforated peptic ulcer may be associ-

Table 14-1

Some Important Causes of Abdominal Pain

PAIN ORIGINATING IN THE ABDOMEN

1. Parietal peritoneal inflammation
   a. Bacterial contamination, e.g., perforated appendix, pelvic inflammatory disease
   b. Chemical irritation, e.g., perforated ulcer, pancreatitis, mittelschmerz
2. Mechanical obstruction of hollow viscera
   a. Obstruction of the small or large intestine
   b. Obstruction of the biliary tree
   c. Obstruction of the ureter
3. Vascular disturbances
   a. Embolism or thrombosis
   b. Vascular rupture
   c. Pressure or torsional occlusion
   d. Sickle cell anemia
4. Abdominal wall
   a. Distortion or traction of mesentery
   b. Trauma or infection of muscles
5. Distention of visceral surfaces, e.g., hepatic or renal capsules

PAIN REFERRED FROM EXTRAABDOMINAL SOURCE

1. Thorax, e.g., pneumonia, referred pain from coronary occlusion
2. Spine, e.g., radiculitis from arthritis
3. Genitalia, e.g., torsion of the testicle

METABOLIC CAUSES

1. Exogenous
   a. Black widow spider bite
   b. Lead poisoning and others
2. Endogenous
   a. Uremia
   b. Diabetic ketoacidosis
   c. Porphyria
   d. Allergic factors (C′1 esterase inhibitor deficiency)

NEUROGENIC CAUSES

1. Organic
   a. Tabes dorsalis
   b. Herpes zoster
   c. Causalgia and others
2. Functional

---

ated with entirely different clinical pictures dependent only on the rapidity with which the gastric juice enters the peritoneal cavity.

The pain of peritoneal inflammation is invariably accentuated by pressure or changes in tension of the peritoneum, whether produced by palpation or by movement, as in coughing or sneezing. The patient with peritonitis lies quietly in bed, preferring to avoid motion, in contrast to the patient with colic, who may writhe incessantly.

Another characteristic feature of peritoneal irritation is tonic reflex spasm of the abdominal musculature, localized to the involved body segment. The intensity of the tonic muscle spasm accompanying peritoneal inflammation is dependent on the location of the inflammatory process, the rate at which it develops, and the integrity of the nervous system. Spasm over a perforated retrocecal appendix or perforated ulcer into the lesser peritoneal sac may be minimal or absent because of the protective effect of overlying viscera. A slowly developing process also often greatly attenuates the degree of muscle spasm. Catastrophic abdominal emergencies such as a perforated ulcer have been repeatedly associated with minimal or occasionally no detectable pain or muscle spasm in obtunded, seriously ill, debilitated elderly patients or in psychotic patients.

Obstruction of Hollow Viscera   The pain of obstruction of hollow abdominal viscera is classically described as intermittent, or colicky. Yet the lack of a truly cramping character should not be misleading, because distention of a hollow viscus may produce steady pain with only very occasional exacerbations. Although not nearly as well localized as the pain of parietal peritoneal inflammation, some useful generalities can be made concerning its distribution.

The colicky pain of obstruction of the small intestine is usually periumbilical or supraumbilical and is poorly localized. As the intestine becomes progressively dilated with loss of muscular tone, the colicky nature of the pain may become less apparent. With superimposed strangulating obstruction, pain may spread to the lower lumbar region if there is traction on the root of the mesentery. The colicky pain of colonic obstruction is of lesser intensity than that of the small intestine and is often located in the infraumbilical area. Lumbar radiation of pain is common in colonic obstruction.

Sudden distention of the biliary tree produces a steady rather than colicky type of pain; hence the term *biliary colic* is misleading. Acute distention of the gallbladder usually causes pain in the right upper quadrant with radiation to the right posterior region of the thorax or to the tip of the right scapula, and distention of the common bile duct is often associated with pain in the epigastrium radiating to the upper part of the lumbar region. Considerable variation is common, however, so that differentiation between these may be impossible. The typical subscapular pain or lumbar radiation is frequently absent. Gradual dilatation of the biliary tree, as in carcinoma of the head of the pancreas, may cause no pain or only a mild aching sensation in the epigastrium or right upper quadrant. The pain of distention of the pancreatic ducts is similar to that described for distention of the common bile duct but, in addition, is very frequently accentuated by recumbency and relieved by the upright position.

Obstruction of the urinary bladder results in dull suprapubic pain, usually low in intensity. Restlessness without specific complaint of pain may be the only sign of a distended bladder in an obtunded patient. In contrast, acute obstruction of the intravesicular portion of the ureter is characterized by severe suprapubic and flank pain which radiates to the penis, scrotum, or inner aspect of the upper region of the thigh. Obstruction of the ureteropelvic junction is felt as pain in the costovertebral angle, whereas obstruction of the remainder of the ureter is associated with flank pain that often extends into the corresponding side of the abdomen.

Vascular Disturbances A frequent misconception, despite abundant experience to the contrary, is that pain associated with intraabdominal vascular disturbances is sudden and catastrophic in nature. The pain of embolism or thrombosis of the superior mesenteric artery or that of impending rupture of an abdominal aortic aneurysm certainly may be severe and diffuse. Yet, just as frequently, the patient with occlusion of the superior mesenteric artery has only mild continuous diffuse pain for 2 or 3 days before vascular collapse or findings of peritoneal inflammation appear. The early, seemingly insignificant discomfort is caused by hyperperistalsis rather than peritoneal inflammation. Indeed, absence of tenderness and rigidity in the presence of continuous, diffuse pain in a patient likely to have vascular disease is quite characteristic of occlusion of the superior mesenteric artery. Abdominal pain with radiation to the sacral region, flank, or genitalia should always signal the possible presence of a rupturing abdominal aortic aneurysm. This pain may persist over a period of several days before rupture and collapse occur.

Abdominal Wall Pain arising from the abdominal wall is usually constant and aching. Movement, prolonged standing, and pressure accentuate the discomfort and muscle spasm. In the case of hematoma of the rectus sheath, now most frequently encountered in association with anticoagulant therapy, a mass may be present in the lower quadrants of the abdomen. Simultaneous involvement of muscles in other parts of the body usually serves to differentiate myositis of the abdominal wall from an intraabdominal process that might cause pain in the same region.

REFERRED PAIN IN ABDOMINAL DISEASES Pain referred to the abdomen from the thorax, spine, or genitalia may prove a vexing diagnostic problem, because diseases of the upper part of the abdominal cavity such as acute cholecystitis or perforated ulcer are frequently associated with intrathoracic complications. A most important, yet often forgotten dictum is that the possibility of intrathoracic disease must be considered in every patient with abdominal pain, especially if the pain is in the upper part of the abdomen. Systematic questioning and examination directed toward detecting the presence or absence of myocardial or pulmonary infarction, pneumonia, pericarditis, or esophageal disease (the intrathoracic diseases that most often masquerade as abdominal emergencies) will often provide sufficient clues to establish the proper diagnosis. Diaphragmatic pleuritis resulting from pneumonia or pulmonary infarction may cause pain in the right upper quadrant and pain in the supraclavicular area, the latter radiation to be sharply distinguished from the referred subscapular pain caused by acute distention of the extrahepatic biliary tree. The ultimate decision as to the origin of abdominal pain may require deliberate and planned observation over a period of several hours, during which time repeated questioning and examination will provide the proper explanation.

Referred pain of thoracic origin is often accompanied by splinting of the involved hemithorax with respiratory lag and decrease in excursion more marked than that seen in the presence of intraabdominal disease. In addition, apparent abdominal muscle spasm caused by referred pain will diminish during the inspiratory phase of respiration, whereas it is persistent throughout both respiratory phases if it is of abdominal origin. Palpation over the area of referred pain in the abdomen also does not usually accentuate the pain and in many instances actually seems to relieve it. The frequent coexistence of thoracic and abdominal disease may be misleading and confusing, so differentiation may be difficult or impossible. For example, the patient with known biliary tract disease often has epigastric pain during myocardial infarction, or biliary colic may be referred to the precordium or left shoulder in a patient who has suffered previously from angina pectoris. → *For an explanation of the radiation of pain to a previously diseased area, see Chap. 12.*

Referred pain from the spine, which usually involves compression or irritation of nerve roots, is characteristically intensified by certain motions such as cough, sneeze, or strain and is associated with hyperesthesia over the involved dermatomes. Pain referred to the abdomen from the testicles or seminal vesicles is generally accentuated by the slightest pressure on either of these organs. The abdominal discomfort is of dull aching character and is poorly localized.

METABOLIC ABDOMINAL CRISES Pain of metabolic origin may simulate almost any other type of intraabdominal disease. Here several mechanisms may be at work. In certain instances, such as hyperlipidemia, the metabolic disease itself may be accompanied by an intraabdominal process such as pancreatitis, which can lead to unnecessary laparotomy unless recognized. $C'1$ esterase deficiency associated with angioneurotic edema is also often associated with episodes of severe abdominal pain. Whenever the cause of abdominal pain is obscure, a metabolic origin always must be considered. Abdominal pain is also the hallmark of familial Mediterranean fever (Chap. 288).

The problem of differential diagnosis is often not readily resolved. The pain of porphyria and of lead colic usually is difficult to distinguish from that of intestinal obstruction, because severe hyperperistalsis is a prominent feature of both. The pain of uremia or diabetes is nonspecific, and the pain and tenderness frequently shift in location and intensity. Diabetic acidosis may be precipitated by acute appendicitis or intestinal obstruction, so if prompt resolution of the abdominal pain does not result from correction of the metabolic abnormalities, an underlying organic problem should be strongly suspected. Black widow spider bites produce intense pain and rigidity of the abdominal muscles and of the back, an area infrequently involved in disease of intraabdominal origin.

NEUROGENIC CAUSES Causalgic pain may occur in diseases that injure nerves of sensory type. It has a burning character and is usually limited to the distribution of a given peripheral nerve. Normal stimuli such as touch or change in temperature may be transformed into this type of pain, which is also frequently present in a patient at rest. A helpful finding is the demonstration that cutaneous pain spots are irregularly spaced, and this may be the only indication of an old nerve lesion underlying causalgic pain. Even though the pain may be precipitated by gentle palpation, rigidity of the abdominal muscles is absent, and the respirations are not disturbed. Distention of the abdomen is uncommon, and the pain has no relationship to the intake of food.

Pain arising from spinal nerves or roots comes and goes suddenly and is of a lancinating type (see Chap. 16). It may be caused by herpes zoster, impingement by arthritis, tumors, herniated nucleus pulposus, diabetes, or syphilis. Again, it is not associated with food intake, abdominal distention, or changes in respiration. Severe muscle spasm, as in the gastric crises of tabes dorsalis, is common but is either relieved or is not accentuated by abdominal palpation. The pain is made worse by movement of the spine and is usually confined to a few dermatome segments. Hyperesthesia is very common.

Psychogenic pain conforms to none of the aforementioned patterns of disease. Here the mechanism is hard to define. The most common problem is the hysterical adolescent or young person who develops abdominal pain and who frequently loses an appendix or other organs because of it. Ovulation or some other natural event that causes brief mild abdominal discomfort may sometimes be experienced as an abdominal catastrophe.

Psychogenic pain varies enormously in type and location but usually has no relation to meals. It is often at its onset markedly accentuated during the night. Nausea and vomiting are rarely observed, although occasionally the patient reports these symptoms. Spasm is seldom induced in the abdominal musculature and, if present, does not persist, especially if the attention of the patient can be distracted. Persistent localized tenderness is rare, and if found, the muscle spasm in the area is inconsistent and often absent. Restriction of the depth of respiration is the most common respiratory abnormality, but this is in the nature of a smothering or choking sensation and is part of an anxiety state. It occurs in the absence of thoracic splinting or change in the respiratory rate.

Approach to the Patient

There are few abdominal conditions that require such urgent operative intervention that an orderly approach need be abandoned, no matter how ill the patient. Only those patients with exsanguinating hemorrhage must be rushed to the operating room immediately, but in such instances, only a few minutes are required to assess the critical nature of the problem. Under these circumstances, all obstacles must be swept aside, adequate access for intravenous fluid replacement obtained, and the operation begun. Many patients of this type have died in the radiology department or the emergency room while awaiting such unnecessary examinations as electrocardiograms or films of the abdomen. *There are no contraindications to operation when massive hemorrhage is present.* Although exceedingly important, this situation fortunately is relatively rare.

Nothing will supplant an orderly, painstakingly *detailed history*, which is far more valuable than any laboratory or roentgenologic examination. This kind of history is laborious and time-consuming, making it not especially popular, even though a reasonably accurate diagnosis can be made on the basis of the history alone in the majority of cases. Recent studies of computer-aided diagnosis of abdominal pain indicate that this technique provides no advantage over clinical assessment alone. In cases of *acute* abdominal pain, a diagnosis is readily established in most instances, whereas success is not so frequently achieved in patients with *chronic* pain. Since the irritable bowel syndrome is one of the most common causes of abdominal pain, the possibility of this diagnosis must always be kept in mind (see Chap. 287). The *chronological sequence of events* in the patient's history is often more important than emphasis on the location of pain. If the examiner is sufficiently open-minded and unhurried, asks the proper questions, and listens, the patient will usually provide the diagnosis. Careful attention should be paid to the extraabdominal regions that may be responsible for abdominal pain. An accurate menstrual history in a female patient is essential. Narcotics or analgesics should be withheld until a definitive diagnosis or a definitive plan

has been formulated, because these agents often make it more difficult to secure and to interpret the history and physical findings.

In the examination, simple critical inspection of the patient, e.g., of facies, position in bed, and respiratory activity, may provide valuable clues. The amount of information to be gleaned is directly proportional to the *gentleness* and thoroughness of the examiner. Once a patient with peritoneal inflammation has been examined brusquely, accurate assessment by the next examiner becomes almost impossible. For example, eliciting rebound tenderness by sudden release of a deeply palpating hand in a patient with suspected peritonitis is cruel and unnecessary. The same information can be obtained by gentle percussion of the abdomen (rebound tenderness on a miniature scale), a maneuver that can be far more precise and localizing. Asking the patient to cough will elicit true rebound tenderness without the need for placing a hand on the abdomen. Furthermore, the forceful demonstration of rebound tenderness will startle and induce protective spasm in a nervous or worried patient in whom true rebound tenderness is not present. A palpable gallbladder will be missed if palpation is so brusque that voluntary muscle spasm becomes superimposed on involuntary muscular rigidity.

As in history taking, there is no substitute for sufficient time spent in the examination. It is important to remember that abdominal signs may be minimal but nevertheless, if accompanied by consistent symptoms, may be exceptionally meaningful. Signs may be virtually or actually totally absent in cases of pelvic peritonitis, so careful *pelvic and rectal examinations are mandatory in every patient with abdominal pain.* The presence of tenderness on pelvic or rectal examination in the absence of other abdominal signs must lead the examiner to consider such important operative indications as perforated appendicitis, diverticulitis, twisted ovarian cyst, and many others.

Much attention has been paid to the presence or absence of peristaltic sounds, their quality, and their frequency. Auscultation of the abdomen is probably one of the least rewarding aspects of the physical examination of a patient with abdominal pain. Severe catastrophes, such as strangulating small intestinal obstruction or perforated appendicitis, may occur in the presence of normal peristalsis. Conversely, when the proximal part of the intestine above an obstruction becomes markedly distended and edematous, peristaltic sounds may lose the characteristics of borborygmi and become weak or absent even when peritonitis is not present. It is usually the severe chemical peritonitis of sudden onset that is associated with the truly silent abdomen. Assessment of the patient's state of hydration is important. The hematocrit and urinalysis permit an accurate estimate of the severity of dehydration so that adequate replacement can be carried out.

Laboratory examinations may be of enormous value in assessment of the patient with abdominal pain, yet with but a few exceptions they rarely establish a diagnosis. Leukocytosis should never be the single deciding factor as to whether or not operation is indicated. A white blood cell count greater than $20,000/\mu L$ may be observed with perforation of a viscus, but pancreatitis, acute cholecystitis, pelvic inflammatory disease, and intestinal infarction may be associated with marked leukocytosis. A normal white blood cell count is by no means rare in cases of perforation of abdominal viscera. The diagnosis of anemia may be more helpful than the white blood cell count, especially when combined with the history.

The urinalysis is also of great value in indicating to some degree the state of hydration or to rule out severe renal disease, diabetes, or urinary infection. Determination of the blood urea nitrogen, blood sugar, and serum bilirubin levels also may be helpful. The serum amylase determination is overrated. Since many diseases other than pancreatitis, e.g., perforated ulcer, strangulating intestinal obstruction, and acute cholecystitis, may be associated with very marked increase in the serum amylase, great care must be exercised in denying an operation to a patient solely on the basis of an elevated serum amylase level. The determination of the serum lipase may have a somewhat greater accuracy than the serum amylase.

Plain and upright or lateral decubitus roentgenograms of the abdomen may be of the greatest value. They are usually unnecessary in patients with acute appendicitis or strangulated external hernias. However, in cases of intestinal obstruction, perforated ulcer, and a variety of other conditions, films may be diagnostic. In rare instances, barium or water-soluble medium examination of the upper part of the gastrointestinal tract may demonstrate partial intestinal obstruction that may elude diagnosis by other means. If there is any question of obstruction of the colon, oral administration of barium sulfate should be avoided. On the other hand, barium enema is of inestimable value in cases of colonic obstruction and should be used with greater frequency where the possibility of perforation does not exist.

Peritoneal lavage is a safe and effective diagnostic maneuver in patients with acute abdominal pain. It is of special value in patients with blunt trauma to the abdomen, in whom evaluation of the abdomen may be difficult because of other multiple injuries to the spine, pelvis, or ribs and in whom blood in the peritoneal cavity produces only a very mild peritoneal reaction. In the absence of trauma, peritoneal lavage has been replaced by ultrasound, computed tomography (CT), and laparoscopy. Ultrasonography has proved to be useful in detecting an enlarged gallbladder or pancreas, the presence of gallstones, an enlarged ovary, or a tubal pregnancy. Laparoscopy is especially helpful in diagnosing pelvic conditions, such as ovarian cysts, tubal pregnancies or salpingitis, and acute appendicitis. Radioisotopic scans (HIDA) may help differentiate acute cholecystitis from acute pancreatitis. A CT scan may demonstrate an enlarged pancreas, ruptured spleen, or thickened colonic wall and streaking of the mesocolon characteristic of diverticulitis.

Sometimes, even under the best of circumstances with all available auxiliary aids and with the greatest of clinical skill, a definitive diagnosis cannot be established at the time of the initial examination. Nevertheless, despite lack of a clear anatomic diagnosis, it may be abundantly clear to an experienced and thoughtful physician and surgeon that on clinical grounds alone operation is indicated. Should that decision be questionable, watchful waiting with repeated questioning and examination will often elucidate the true nature of the illness and indicate the proper course of action.

BIBLIOGRAPHY

ATTARD AR et al: Safety of early pain relief for acute abdominal pain. BMJ 305:554, 1992

BUGLIOSI TF et al: Acute abdominal pain in the elderly. Ann Emerg Med 19:1383, 1990

DAVIES AH et al: Ultrasonography in the acute abdomen. Br J Surg 78:1178, 1991

GATZEN C et al: Management of acute abdominal pain: Decision making in the accident and emergency department. J R Coll Surg Edinb 36:121, 1991

LEEK BF: Abdominal and pelvic visceral receptors. Br Med Bull 33:163, 1977

SCOTT HJ, ROSIN RD: The influence of diagnostic and therapeutic laparoscopy on patients presenting with an acute abdomen. J R Soc Med 86:699, 1993

TAOUREL P et al: Acute abdomen of unknown origin: Impact of CT on diagnosis and management. Gastrointest Radiol 17:287, 1992

| 15 | *Neil H. Raskin* |

HEADACHE

Few of us are spared the experience of head pain during our lifetimes; indeed, severe, disabling headache is reported to occur at least annually by 40 percent of individuals worldwide. This incidence occurs whether subjects live in large urban environments or in rural villages. In some individuals, stress and anxiety may trigger "benign" headaches, but emotional factors are not necessary for the symptom to occur. The more severe the headache, the more likely it is to be associated with nausea and to be experienced as a pulsing or pounding discomfort; photophobia and hyperacusis are also more likely to be reported. Moreover, there does not appear to be any utility in having headache; most sufferers report the contrary. A useful classification of the many causes of headache, adapted from recommendations of the International Headache Society, is shown in Table 15-1.

Headache is usually a benign symptom, and only occasionally is it the manifestation of a serious illness such as brain tumor, subarachnoid hemorrhage, meningitis, or giant cell arteritis. Even in emergency settings, only 5 percent of patients who present with headache are found to have a serious underlying neurologic disorder. Nonetheless, it is imperative that these serious conditions be recognized and treated appropriately. Thus, the first issue to resolve in confronting the patient who complains of headache is to make the distinction between benign and more ominous etiologies.

GENERAL CONSIDERATIONS

The quality, location, duration, and time course of the headache and the conditions that produce, exacerbate, or relieve it should be carefully reviewed.

Ascertaining the *quality* of cephalic pain is occasionally helpful. Most headaches are dull, deeply located, and aching. Superimposed on such nondescript pain may be other types of pain that have greater diagnostic value. It is useful to identify *all* types of pain that have been experienced by the patient, regardless of their frequency or intensity. A throbbing quality and tight muscles about the head, neck, and shoulder girdle are common nonspecific accompaniments of headache. It was formerly believed that tight "hat-band" headaches indicated stress, anxiety, or depression, but investigations have not supported this view. Jabbing, brief, sharp cephalic pain, often occurring multifocally (ice pick-like pain), is the signature of a benign disorder.

Pain *intensity* seldom has diagnostic value—in the head or in any other somatic location. From the patient's perspective, it is, of course, the single aspect of pain that is most important. Physicians should be cautious about assessing pain intensity by visually inspecting a patient. People respond to pain in a variety of ways that range from overt histrionic behavior to stoicism. It is of more value to inquire as to how pain disturbs day-to-day function. *Response to placebo medication or procedures produces no useful information*—either diagnostic or therapeutic. It simply identifies a "placebo responder," about 30 percent of the population. There is no evidence that placebo responders have lower pain levels than nonresponders or do not really have pain. Patients entering emergency departments with the most severe headache of their lives usually have migraine. Meningitis, subarachnoid hemorrhage, and cluster headache also produce intense cranial pain. Contrary to common belief, the headache produced by a brain tumor is not usually distinctive or severe.

Data regarding *location* of headache may be informative. If the source is an extracranial structure, as in giant cell arteritis, the correspondence with the site of pain is fairly precise. Inflammation of an extracranial artery causes pain and exquisite tenderness localized to the site of the vessel. Lesions of paranasal sinuses, teeth, eyes, and upper cervical vertebrae induce less sharply localized pain, but pain that is still referred in a regional distribution. Intracranial lesions in the posterior fossa cause pain that is usually occipitonuchal, and supratentorial lesions most often induce frontotemporal pain.

Duration and *time-intensity* curves of headaches are diagnostically useful. A ruptured aneurysm results in head pain that peaks in an instant, thunderclap-like; much less often, unruptured aneurysms may signal their presence in the same way. Cluster headache attacks reach their peak over 3 to 5 min, remain at maximal levels for about 45 min, and then taper off. Migraine attacks build up over hours, are maintained for several hours to days, and are characteristically relieved by sleep. Sleep disruption is characteristic of headaches produced by brain tumors.

Recurrent headache may bear a relationship to certain biologic events or environmental exposures. The following exacerbating phenomena make a benign etiology highly probable: provocation by red wine, sustained exertion, organic odors, hunger, lack of sleep, weather change, and menses. The association of diarrhea with attacks and the amelioration of headache during pregnancy, especially the second and third trimesters, are pathognomonic of migraine. Patients with continuous benign headaches often observe a pain-free interlude of several minutes upon awakening before head pain commences. This phenomenon occurs with other pain syndromes, such as thalamic pain, but does not occur when inflammation (meningitis or giant cell arteritis) is the cause of pain. When attempts are made to elicit this information, patients commonly respond negatively to initial inquiries because the provocative stimuli or quality of the pain may be variable or inconsistent. Induction of pain by red wine and hunger, for example, is *always* inconsistent, for reasons that are unclear. It is important that patients understand that recollection of inciting factors for even some of their headaches may be of diagnostic value and may save unnecessary neuroimaging procedures.

A history of amenorrhea or galactorrhea should lead one to question whether the polycystic ovary syndrome or a prolactin-secreting pituitary adenoma is the source of headache. Headache arising de novo in a patient with known malignancy suggests either cerebral metastases and/or carcinomatous meningitis. When there is striking accentuation of pain with eye movement, a systemic infection and particularly meningitis should be seriously considered. Head pain appearing abruptly after bending, lifting, or coughing can be the clue to a posterior fossa mass or the Arnold-Chiari malformation. Orthostatic headache occurs after lumbar puncture and also with subdural hematoma and benign intracranial hypertension. The eye itself is seldom the cause of acute orbital pain if the sclerae are white and not injected; a "red eye" is the sign of ophthalmic disease. In optic neuritis, pain is typically localized to the eye or supraorbital region and is exacerbated by eye movements. Similarly, acute sinusitis nearly always declares itself through a dark green, purulent nasal exudate.

The analysis of facial pain requires a different approach. Trigeminal and less commonly glossopharyngeal neuralgia are frequent causes of facial pain (see Chap. 372). "Neuralgias" are painful disorders characterized by paroxysmal, fleeting, often electric shock–like episodes that are often caused by demyelinating lesions of nerves (the trigeminal or glossopharyngeal nerves in cranial neuralgias). Certain maneuvers characteristically trigger paroxysms of pain. However, the most common cause of facial pain by far is dental; provocation by hot, cold, or sweet foods is typical. The application of a cold stimulus will repeatedly induce dental pain, whereas in neuralgic disorders a refractory period usually occurs after the initial response so that pain cannot be repeatedly induced. The presence of refractory periods can nearly always be elicited in the history so that patients need not be put through a painful experience.

The effect of eating on facial pain may provide insight into its

Table 15-1

The Classification of Headache

1. **Migraine**	7. **Headache associated with nonvascular intracranial disorder (cont.)**
Migraine without aura	Sarcoidosis and other noninfectious inflammatory diseases
Migraine with aura	Related to intrathecal injections
Ophthalmoplegic migraine	Intracranial neoplasm
Retinal migraine	Associated with other intracranial disorder
Childhood periodic syndromes that may be precursors to or associated with migraine	
Migrainous disorder not fulfilling above criteria	8. **Headache associated with substances or their withdrawal**
	Headache induced by acute substance use or exposure
2. **Tension-type headache**	Headache induced by chronic substance use or exposure
Episodic tension-type headache	Headache from substance withdrawal (acute use)
Chronic tension-type headache	Headache from substance withdrawal (chronic use)
3. **Cluster headache and chronic paroxysmal hemicrania**	9. **Headache associated with noncephalic infection**
Cluster headache	Viral infection
Chronic paroxysmal hemicrania	Bacterial infection
	Other infection
4. **Miscellaneous headaches not associated with structural lesion**	
Idiopathic stabbing headache	10. **Headache associated with metabolic disorder**
External compression headache	Hypoxia
Cold stimulus headache	Hypercapnia
Benign cough headache	Mixed hypoxia and hypercapnia
Benign exertional headache	Hypoglycemia
Headache associated with sexual activity	Dialysis
	Other metabolic abnormality
5. **Headache associated with head trauma**	
Acute posttraumatic headache	11. **Headache or facial pain associated with disorder of facial or cranial structures**
Chronic posttraumatic headache	Cranial bone
	Eyes
6. **Headache associated with vascular disorders**	Ears
Acute ischemic cerebrovascular disorder	Nose and sinuses
Intracranial hematoma	Teeth, jaws, and related structures
Subarachnoid hemorrhage	Temporomandibular joint disease
Unruptured vascular malformation	
Arteritis	12. **Cranial neuralgias, nerve trunk pain, and deafferentation pain**
Carotid or vertebral artery pain	Persistent (in contrast to ticlike) pain of cranial nerve origin
Venous thrombosis	Trigeminal neuralgia
Arterial hypertension	Glossopharyngeal neuralgia
Other vascular disorder	Nervus intermedius neuralgia
	Superior laryngeal neuralgia
7. **Headache associated with nonvascular intracranial disorder**	Occipital neuralgia
High CSF pressure	Central causes of head and facial pain other than tic douloureux
Low CSF pressure	
Intracranial infection	13. **Headache not classifiable**

SOURCE: After Olesen; and Dalessio.

cause. Is it the chewing, swallowing, or taste of the food that elicits pain? Chewing points toward trigeminal neuralgia, temporomandibular joint dysfunction, or giant cell arteritis ("jaw claudication"), whereas swallowing *and* taste provocation points toward glossopharyngeal neuralgia. Pain upon swallowing is common among patients with carotidynia (see Chap. 364) because the inflamed, tender carotid artery abuts the esophagus during deglutition.

Many patients with facial pain do not experience stereotypic neuralgias; the term *atypical facial pain* has been used in this setting. Vague, poorly localized, continuous facial pain is *characteristic* of nasopharyngeal carcinoma; a burning pain often develops as deafferentation occurs and evidence of cranial neuropathy appears. Burning facial pain may also occur with tumors of the fifth cranial nerve (meningioma or schwannoma) or with lesions of the pons that interrupt the dorsal root entry zone of the nerve (multiple sclerosis). In patients with facial pain, the finding of objective sensory loss is an important clue to a serious underlying disorder. Occasionally, the cause of a pain problem cannot be resolved promptly, necessitating periodic follow-up until further signs appear.

PAIN-SENSITIVE STRUCTURES OF THE HEAD

Pain is most commonly due to tissue injury resulting in stimulation of peripheral nociceptors in an intact nervous system, as in the pain of scalded skin or appendicitis. Pain can also result from damage to or anomalous activation of pain-sensitive pathways of the peripheral or central nervous system. Headache may originate from either mechanism. The following cranial structures are sensitive to mechanical stimulation: the scalp and aponeurotica, middle meningeal artery, dural sinuses, falx cerebri, and the proximal segments of the large pial arteries. The ventricular ependyma, choroid plexus, pial veins, and much of the brain parenchyma are pain-insensitive. Electrical stimulation of the midbrain in the region of the dorsal raphe has resulted in migraine-like headaches. Thus whereas most of the brain is insensitive to electrode probing, a site in the midbrain represents a possible source of headache generation.

Sensory stimuli from the head are conveyed to the central nervous system via the trigeminal nerves for structures above the tentorium in the anterior and middle fossae of the skull and via the first three cervical nerves for those in the posterior fossa and the inferior surface of the tentorium. The ninth and tenth cranial nerves supply part of the posterior fossa and refer pain to the ear and throat.

Headache can occur as the result of (1) distention, traction, or dilation of intracranial or extracranial arteries; (2) traction or displacement of large intracranial veins or their dural envelope; (3) compression, traction, or inflammation of cranial and spinal nerves; (4) spasm, inflammation, or trauma to cranial and cervical muscles; (5) meningeal irritation and raised intracranial pressure; and (6) possibly, perturbation of intracerebral serotonergic projections. By and large, intracranial masses cause headache when they deform, displace, or exert traction on vessels, dural structures, or cranial nerves at the base of the brain; this often happens long before intracranial pressure rises. Such mechanical displacement mechanisms do not explain the headaches resulting from cerebral ischemia or from benign intracranial hypertension after the pressure is reduced, nor the headaches that are so common in febrile illnesses and systemic lupus erythematosus. Perturbation of intracerebral serotonergic projections has been suggested as a possible mechanism for these phenomena.

PRINCIPAL CLINICAL VARIETIES OF HEADACHE

Normally there is little difficulty in diagnosing the headache of glaucoma, purulent sinusitis, bacterial meningitis, and brain tumor because of the clues provided by the associated symptoms and signs. The headache symptom alone is often nondescript. It is when headache is chronic, recurrent, and unattended by other important signs of disease that the physician faces a challenging but ultimately gratifying medical problem. The headache syndromes described below should be considered (see also Table 15-2).

MIGRAINE A useful definition of migraine is a benign and recurring syndrome of headache, nausea, vomiting, and/or other symptoms of neurologic dysfunction in varying admixtures. Migraine can often be recognized by its activators (red wine, menses, hunger, lack of sleep, glare, estrogen, worry, perfumes, let-down periods) and its deactivators (sleep, pregnancy, exhilaration, sumatriptan). → *Migraine, by far the most common cause of headache, is considered in detail in Chap. 364.*

CLUSTER HEADACHE The most common form of this syndrome is manifested by one to three short-lived daily attacks of periorbital pain over a 4- to 8-week interval followed by a pain-free interval that averages 1 year. The painful attacks are often associated with a homolateral red, tearing eye, nasal stuffiness, and ptosis. → *This subject is further discussed in Chap. 364.*

TENSION HEADACHE The term *tension headache* is still commonly used to describe a chronic head pain syndrome characterized by tight bandlike discomfort. Patients may report that the head feels as if it is in a vise or that the posterior neck muscles are tight. The pain typically builds slowly, fluctuates in severity, and may persist more or less continuously for many days. In some patients, anxiety or depression coexist with tension headache. Many investigators believe that periodic tension headache is biologically indistinguishable from migraine (Chap. 364).

LUMBAR PUNCTURE HEADACHE Headache following lumbar puncture (Chap. 360) usually begins within 48 h but may be delayed for up to 12 days. Its incidence is between 10 and 30 percent. Head pain is dramatically positional; it begins when the patient sits or stands upright; there is relief upon reclining or with abdominal compression. The longer the patient is upright, the longer the latency before head pain subsides. It is worsened by head shaking and jugular vein compression. The pain is usually a dull ache but may be throbbing; its location is occipitofrontal. Nausea and stiff neck often accompany headache, and occasional patients report blurred vision, photophobia, tinnitus, and vertigo. The symptoms resolve over a few days but may on occasion persist for weeks to months.

Loss of cerebrospinal fluid (CSF) volume decreases the brain's supportive cushion, so that when a patient is upright there is probably dilation and tension placed on the brain's anchoring structures, the pain-sensitive dural sinuses, resulting in pain. Intracranial hypotension often occurs, but severe lumbar puncture headache may be present even in patients who have normal CSF pressure.

Treatment with intravenous caffeine sodium benzoate given over a few minutes as a 500-mg dose will promptly terminate headache in 75 percent of patients; a second dose given in 1 h brings the total success rate to 85 percent. An epidural blood patch accomplished by injection of 15 mL of autologous whole blood rarely fails for those who do not respond to caffeine. The mechanism for these treatment effects is not straightforward. The blood patch has an *immediate* effect, making it unlikely that sealing off a dural hole with blood clot is its mechanism of action.

POSTCONCUSSION HEADACHES Following seemingly trivial head injuries and particularly after rear-end motor vehicle collisions, many patients report varying combinations of headache, dizziness, vertigo, and impaired memory. Anxiety, irritability and difficulty with concentration are other hallmarks of this syndrome. Symptoms may remit after several weeks or persist for months and even years after the injury. Postconcussion headaches may occur whether or not a person was rendered unconscious by head trauma. Typically, the neurologic examination is normal with the exception of the behavioral abnormalities, and computed tomography (CT) or magnetic resonance imaging (MRI) studies are unrevealing. Chronic subdural hematoma may on occasion mimic this disorder. Although the cause of postconcussive headache disorder is not known, it should not in general be viewed as a primary psychological disturbance. It often persists long after the settlement of pending lawsuits. The treatment is symptomatic support. Repeated encouragement that the syndrome eventually remits is important.

TEMPORAL ARTERITIS (See also Chaps. 28 and 319) Temporal (giant cell) arteritis is an inflammatory disorder of arteries that frequently involves the extracranial carotid circulation. This is a common disorder of the elderly; its average annual incidence is 77:100,000 in individuals aged 50 and older. The average age of onset is 70 years, and women account for 65 percent of cases. Fifty percent of patients with untreated temporal arteritis develop blindness due to involvement of the ophthalmic artery and its branches; indeed, the ischemic optic neuropathy induced by giant cell arteritis is the major cause of rapidly developing bilateral blindness in the patient over 60 years of age. Because treatment with glucocorticoids is effective in preventing this complication of temporal arteritis, prompt recognition of this disorder is important.

Typical presenting symptoms include headache, polymyalgia rheumatica (Chap. 319), jaw claudication, fever, and weight loss. Headache is the dominant symptom and often appears in association with malaise and muscle aches. Head pain may be unilateral or bilateral and is located temporally in 50 percent of patients but may involve any and all aspects of the cranium. Pain usually appears gradually over a few hours before peak intensity is reached; occasionally, it is explosive in onset. The quality of pain is only seldom throbbing; it is almost invariably described as dull and boring with superimposed episodic ice pick–like lancinating pains similar to the sharp pains that appear in migraine. Most patients can recognize that the origin of their head pain is superficial, external to the skull, rather than originating deep within the cranium (the pain site for migraineurs). Scalp tenderness is present, often to a marked degree; brushing the hair or resting the head on a pillow may be impossible because of pain. Headache is usually worse at night and is often aggravated by exposure to cold. Reddened, tender nodules or red streaking of the skin overlying the temporal arteries may be found in patients with headache, as is tenderness of the temporal, or less commonly, the occipital arteries.

The erythrocyte sedimentation rate (ESR) is often but not always elevated; a normal ESR does not exclude giant cell arteritis. A temporal artery biopsy and the initiation of prednisone at 80 mg daily for the first 4 to 6 weeks should be instituted when clinical suspicion is high. The prevalence of migraine among the elderly is substantial, considerably higher than that of giant cell arteritis. Migraineurs often report amelioration of their headaches with prednisone, so that one must be cautious about interpreting the therapeutic response.

COUGH HEADACHE A male-dominated (4:1) syndrome, cough headache is characterized by transient, severe head pain upon coughing, bending, lifting, sneezing, or stooping. Head pain persists for seconds to a few minutes. Many patients date the origins of the syndrome to a lower respiratory infection accompanied by severe coughing or to strenuous weight-lifting programs. Headache is usually diffuse but is lateralized in about one-third of patients. The incidence of serious intracranial structural anomalies causing this condition is about 25 percent; the Arnold-Chiari malformation (Chap. 373) is a common cause. Thus, MRI is indicated for most patients with cough headache. The benign disorder may persist for a few years; it responds dramatically to indomethacin at doses ranging from 50 to 200 mg daily. Approximately half of patients will also show a response to therapeutic lumbar puncture with removal of 40 mL of CSF.

Many patients with migraine note that attacks of headache may be provoked by *sustained* physical exertion, such as during the third mile of a 5-mile run. Such headaches build up over hours, in contrast to cough headache. The term *effort migraine* has been used for this syndrome to avoid the ambiguous term *exertional headache*.

Table 15-2

Common Types of Headaches

Type	Usual Site	Age and Sex	Clinical Features	Life Profile
Migraine, with or without aura	Frontotemporal, uni- or bilateral	All ages; highest incidence in children and young adults Female > male in adults Female = male in children	Onset after awakening; quelled by sleep Provoked by menses, odors, foods Stops after 2d trimester of pregnancy Duration: 6 h to 2 days	Cycles of several months to years Less frequent and less severe with aging
Cluster headache	Lateralized, orbital or temporal	All ages above 10; peaks at 30–50 Male preponderance (90%) Provoked by alcohol	Periodic attacks 1–2 attacks per day, commonly awakens from sleep Duration: 45 min Associated with red eye and stuffy nose homolaterally	Daily attacks for 6 weeks with annual recurrence of bout
Tension headache	Generalized	All ages; principally young adults Female preponderance	Nondescript, tight bandlike discomfort continuously Exacerbations provoked by factors similar to migraine	Cycles of several years
Brain tumor	Variable	All ages, both sexes	Interrupts sleep, unrelieved by sleep Exacerbated by orthostatic changes Steadily worsening pain; may be preceded by days to weeks of nausea and vomiting	Monophasic illness lasting weeks to months
Giant cell arteritis	Lateralized, temporal or occipital	Over 55 years, either sex	Marked scalp tenderness with superimposed jabbing and jolting pain Deep, intermittent throbbing Associated with malaise and morning stiffness and pain in shoulders and hips	Monophasic illness lasting weeks to months
Lumbar puncture headache	Bifrontal and/or bioccipital	Over 10 years, either sex	Orthostatic; head pain present with patient sitting or standing and disappears in prone or supine positions	Arises 1–2 days after lumbar puncture and persists for 3–4 days

COITAL HEADACHE This is another male-dominated (4:1) syndrome. Attacks occur periorgasmically, are very abrupt in onset, and subside in a few minutes if coitus is interrupted. These are nearly always benign events and usually occur sporadically; if they persist for hours or are accompanied by vomiting, subarachnoid hemorrhage must be excluded (Chap. 366).

BRAIN TUMOR HEADACHE About 30 percent of patients with brain tumors consider headache to be their chief complaint. The head pain syndrome is usually nondescript—an intermittent deep, dull aching of moderate intensity, which may worsen with exertion or change in position and may be associated with nausea and vomiting. This pattern of symptoms results from migraine far more often than from brain tumor. Headache of brain tumor disturbs sleep in about 10 percent of patients. Vomiting that precedes the appearance of headache by weeks is highly characteristic of posterior fossa brain tumors. → *A detailed discussion of brain tumors can be found in Chap. 375.*

PSEUDOTUMOR CEREBRI Headache, clinically resembling that of brain tumor, is a common presenting symptom of pseudotumor cerebri, an unusual disorder of raised intracranial pressure probably resulting from impaired CSF absorption by the arachnoid villi. Transient visual obscurations, and papilledema with enlarged blind spots and loss of peripheral visual fields, are additional manifestations. Most patients are young, female, and obese. → *Treatment of pseudotumor cerebri is discussed in Chap. 28.*

HEADACHE CAUSED BY SYSTEMIC ILLNESS There is hardly any illness that is never manifested by headache; however, some illnesses are *characteristically* associated with headache. These include infectious mononucleosis, systemic lupus erythematosus, chronic pulmonary failure with hypercapnia (early morning headaches), Hashimoto's thyroiditis, inflammatory bowel disease, many of the illnesses associated with human immunodeficiency virus, and the acute blood pressure elevations that occur in pheochromocytoma and in malignant hypertension. The last two examples are the exceptions to the generalization that hypertension per se is a very uncommon cause of headache; diastolic pressures of at least 120 mmHg are requisite for hypertension to cause headache. Some drugs and drug-withdrawal states, for example oral contraceptives, ovulation-promoting medications, and glucocorticoid withdrawal, are also associated with headache in some individuals.

Approach to the Patient

Entirely different diagnostic possibilities are raised by a patient who presents with the first severe headache ever and a patient who has had recurrent headache over many years. In the first instance, the probability of finding a potentially serious cause is considerably greater than in the second; some of the causes that should be considered include meningitis, subarachnoid hemorrhage, epidural or subdural hematoma, glaucoma, and purulent sinusitis. In general, acute, severe headache with stiff neck and fever suggests meningitis and without fever suggests subarachnoid hemorrhage; in the former case, lumbar puncture is mandatory, whereas in the latter case a neuroimaging procedure (CT) is the study of choice. Acute persistent headache and fever are often the manifestations of an acute systemic viral infection; if the neck is supple in such a patient, lumbar puncture may be deferred. There is always the possibility of a first attack of migraine, but fever would be a rare associated feature. Clinical features that indicate a possible serious underlying etiology to a headache are summarized in Table 15-3.

A complete neurologic examination is an essential first step in the evaluation of chronic headache. In most cases, an abnormal examination should be followed by a CT or MRI study. In patients with recurrent migraine headaches and a normal examination, neuroimaging procedures are not indicated. In other patterns of headache and a normal examination, imaging studies may be indicated, although their

Table 15-3

Headache Symptoms That Suggest a Serious Underlying Disorder

First severe headache ever
Subacute worsening over days or weeks
Disturbs sleep or present immediately upon awakening
Abnormal neurologic examination
Fever or other unexplained systemic signs
Vomiting precedes headache
Induced by bending, lifting, cough
Known systemic illness (e.g., cancer, collagen-vascular disease)
Onset age 55 or older

yield is low. As a screening procedure for intracranial pathology in this setting, CT and MRI methods appear to be equally sensitive.

A general evaluation of recurring headache should consider the investigation of cardiovascular and renal status by blood pressure monitoring and urine examination; eyes by fundoscopy, intraocular pressure measurement, and refraction; cranial arteries by palpation; cervical spine by the effect of passive movement of the head and imaging; and the psychological state of the patient.

The adolescent with chronic daily frontal or holocephalic headache represents a special type of problem. Extensive diagnostic batteries are most often unrevealing, including the psychiatric assessment. Fortunately, the headaches tend to stop after a few years, and symptomatic management with analgesics can enable these teenagers to move through secondary school and enter college. By the time they reach the late teens, the cycle has usually ended.

The relationship of head pain to depression is not straightforward. Many patients in chronic daily pain cycles become depressed, a not unreasonable sequence of events; moreover, there is a greater-than-chance coincidence of migraine with both bipolar (manic depressive) and unipolar major depressive disorders. Yet studies of large populations of depressed patients do not reveal headache prevalence rates that are different from the general population; the high prevalence of headache in the population at large may account for this apparent paradox. The physician should be cautious about assigning depression as the cause of recurring headache; drugs with antidepressant actions are also effective in migraine.

Finally, a note on recurring headache that may be pain-driven. Temporomandibular joint dysfunction is an example; in general, it produces preauricular pain that is associated with chewing food. The pain may radiate to the head but is not easily confused with headache per se. On the other hand, headache-prone patients may observe that headaches are more frequent and severe in the presence of a painful temporomandibular joint problem. Similarly, headache disorders may be activated by pain that follows otologic or endodontic surgical procedures. Treatment of the headache problem is largely ineffective until the cause of the primary pain problem is dealt with. Thus pain about the head as the result of diseased tissue or trauma may reawaken an otherwise quiescent migrainous syndrome.

BIBLIOGRAPHY

Couch JR: Headache to worry about. Med Clin North Am 77:141, 1993
Dalessio DJ: Diagnosing the severe headache. Neurology 44(Suppl 3): 56,1994
Frishberg BM: The utility of neuroimaging in the evaluation of headache in patients with normal examination. Neurology 44:1191, 1994
Johns D: Benign sexual headache within a family. Arch Neurol 43:1158, 1986
Lance JW: *Mechanism and Management of Headache*, 5th ed. London, Butterworth Scientific, 1993
Olesen J: Headache Classification Committee of the International Headache Society. Classification and diagnostic criteria for headache disorders, cranial neuralgia, and facial pain. Cephalalgia 8(Suppl 7): 1, 1988
Pascual J, Iglesias F, Oterino A, Vazquez-Barquero A, Berciano J: Cough, exertional, and sexual headaches: An analysis of 72 benign and symptomatic cases. Neurology 46:1520, 1996
Raskin NH: Lumbar puncture headache: A review. Headache 30:197, 1990
———: The cough headache syndrome: Treatment. Neurology 45:1784, 1995
———: *Headache*, 2d ed. New York, Churchill Livingstone, 1988
Rasmussen BK, Olesen J: Symptomatic and nonsymptomatic headaches in a general population. Neurology 42:1225, 1992

BACK AND NECK PAIN

The importance of back and neck pain in our society is underscored by the following: (1) the annual societal cost of back pain in the United States is estimated to be between $20 and $50 billion, (2) back symptoms are the most common cause of disability in patients under 45 years of age, (3) 50 percent of working adults, in one survey, admitted to having a back injury each year, and (4) approximately 1 percent of the U.S. population is chronically disabled because of back pain.

There is enormous economic pressure to provide rational and efficient care of patients with back pain. As a result, clinical practice guidelines (CPGs) for patients with back pain are evolving rapidly. CPGs are defined as evaluation or treatment algorithms based upon indications for tests or treatment at specific steps in patient care. CPGs for *acute back pain* are based upon incomplete evidence (see algorithms, Fig. 16-7) but reflect common medical practice. Major revisions in these CPGs can be anticipated in the future. Management of patients with *chronic low back pain* (CLBP) is complex and not amenable yet to a simple algorithmic approach.

A clear understanding of spine anatomy, pertinent features of history and examination, relevant laboratory studies, causes of back pain, and management will optimize patient care.

RELEVANT ANATOMY OF THE SPINE

The anterior portion of the spine consists of cylindrical vertebral bodies separated by intervertebral disks and held together by the anterior and posterior longitudinal ligaments. The intervertebral disks are composed of a central gelatinous nucleus pulposus surrounded by a tough cartilagenous ring, the annulus fibrosis; they are responsible for one-fourth of the length of the spinal column (Figs. 16-1 and 16-2). The disks are thickest in the cervical and lumbar regions where movements of the spine are greatest. The disks are elastic in youth and allow the bony vertebrae to move easily upon each other. Elasticity is lost with age. The function of the anterior spine is to absorb the shock of body movements that comprise motor activities of daily living (walking, running).

The posterior portion of the spine consists of the vertebral arches and seven processes. Each arch consists of paired cylindrical pedicles anteriorly and paired laminae posteriorly (Fig. 16-1). The vertebral arch gives rise to two transverse processes laterally, one spinous process posteriorly, and two superior and two inferior articular facets. The functions of the posterior spine are to protect the spinal cord and nerves within the spinal canal and to stabilize the spine by providing sites for the attachment of muscles and ligaments. The contraction of muscles attached to the spinous and transverse processes produces a system of pulleys and levers that results in flexion, extension, and lateral bending movements of the spine. Normal upright posture in humans places the center of gravity anterior to the spine. The graded contraction of well-developed paraspinal muscles attached to the laminae, transverse processes, and spinous processes is necessary to maintain normal upright posture.

Some anatomic features are of considerable clinical importance. The nerve roots exit at a level above their respective vertebral bodies in the cervical region (the C7 nerve root exits at the C6-C7 level) and below their respective vertebral bodies in the thoracic and lumbar regions (the L4 nerve root exits at the L4-L5 level). The spinal cord ends at the L1 or L2 level of the bony spine. As a consequence, the lumbar nerve roots follow a long course within the lumbar spinal canal and can be injured anywhere from the upper lumbar spine to their exit at the intervertebral foramen. For example, it is common for disk herniation at the L4-L5 level to produce compression of the S1 nerve root (Fig. 16-3). In contrast, cervical nerve roots follow a short intraspinal course and exit at the level of their respective spinal cord segments (upper cervical) or one segment below the corresponding levels (lower

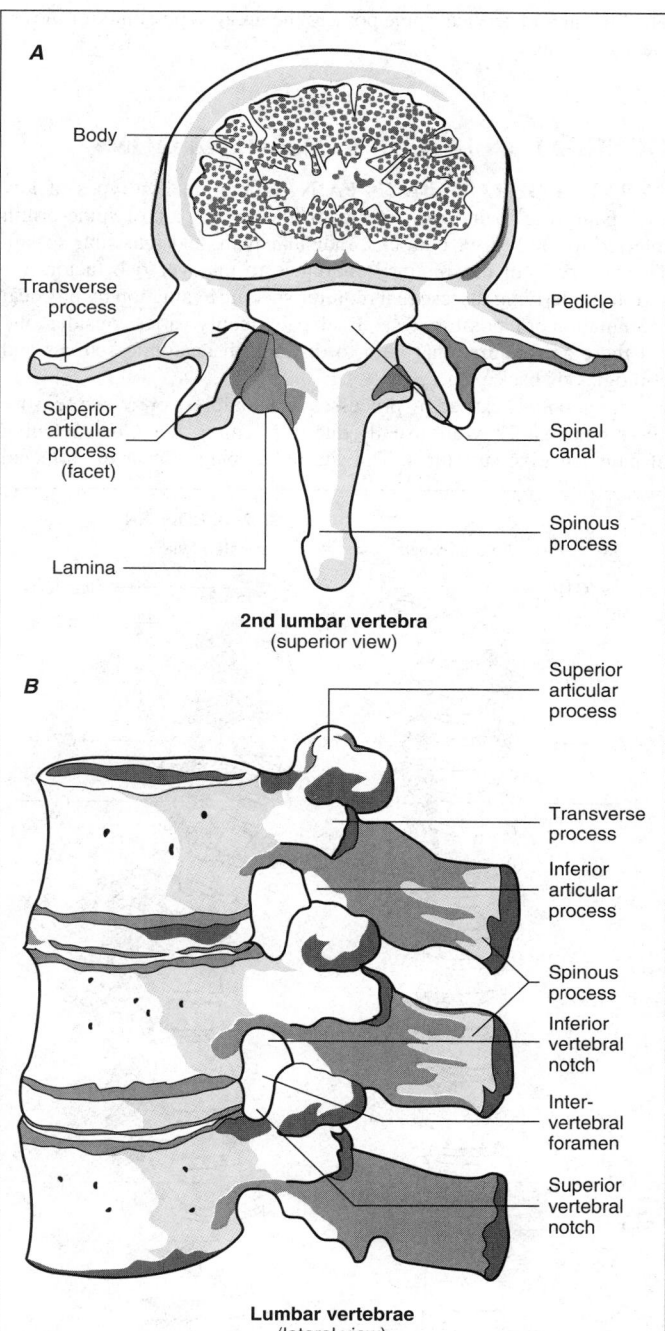

FIGURE 16-1 Vertebral anatomy. (*Copyright 1983. Novartis. Reprinted with permission from The Ciba Collection of Medical Illustrations, Vol. 1, Part I, illustrated by Frank H. Netter, MD. All rights reserved.*)

cervical cord). Cervical spine pathology can result in spinal cord compression, but lumbar spine pathology cannot. Pain-sensitive structures in the spine include the vertebral body periosteum, dura, facets, annulus fibrosus of the intervertebral disk, epidural veins, and the posterior longitudinal ligament. Damage to these nonneural structures may be the source of referred pain. The nucleus pulposus of the intervertebral disk is not pain-sensitive. Pain sensation is provided by the sinuvertebral nerve that arises from the spinal nerve at each spine segment and reenters the spinal canal through the intervertebral foramen at the same level. Disease of these pain-sensitive spine structures may explain many cases of back pain without nerve root compression.

The lumbar and cervical spine possess the greatest potential for movement and injury.

GENERAL CLINICAL CONSIDERATIONS

TYPES OF LOW BACK PAIN There are five types of low back pain: local pain, pain referred to the spine, pain of spine origin referred to the legs or buttocks, radicular pain, and muscular spasm. The history is of paramount importance to uncover risk factors for serious underlying disease that requires specific evaluation by physical examination or laboratory tests. Back pain quality varies considerably, but there are features that help to distinguish anatomic sources and etiologies of back pain.

Local pain is caused by processes that compress or irritate sensory nerve endings. They are usually due to fractures, tears, or stretching of pain-sensitive structures. The site of the pain is near the affected part of the spine. Local pain that does not vary with changes in position suggests spine tumor or infection.

Pain referred to the spine may arise from abdominal or pelvic viscera. The pain is usually described as abdominal or pelvic as well as spinal and is often unaffected by position of the spine. This type of pain may be described occasionally as back pain only.

Pain of spine origin may be referred to the buttocks and legs. Diseases affecting the upper lumbar spine may refer pain to the lumbar region, groin, or anterior thighs. Diseases affecting the lower lumbar spine may result in pain referred to the buttocks, posterior thighs, or rarely the calves or feet. Provocative injections into pain-sensitive structures of the spine (diskography) may produce leg pain that does not follow a dermatomal distribution. The exact pathogenesis of this "sclerotomal" pain is unclear.

Classic *radicular back pain* is usually sharp and radiates from the spine to the leg within the territory of a nerve root (see "Lumbar Disk Disease"). Coughing, sneezing, or voluntary contraction of abdominal muscles (lifting heavy objects or straining at stool) often elicits radiating pain. The patient notices increased pain in postures that stretch the nerves and nerve roots. Sitting stretches the sciatic nerve (L5 and S1 roots) because the nerve passes posterior to the hip. The femoral nerve (L2, L3, and L4 roots) passes anterior to the hip and is not stretched by sitting. The description of the pain alone usually fails to distinguish clearly between pain of bony spine origin and radiculopathy.

The *pain associated with muscle spasm*, although of obscure origin, is commonly associated with many spine disorders. The spasms are accompanied by abnormal posture, taut paraspinal muscles, and dull pain.

Back pain at rest or unassociated with posture should raise the index of suspicion for underlying spine tumor, fracture, infection, or referred pain from visceral structures. Leg pain initiated by ambulation or standing and relieved by the sitting or supine position is suggestive of spinal stenosis. Knowledge of the circumstances associated with back pain onset are important when weighing possible serious underlying causes for the pain. The diagnostic utility of back symptoms and signs suggestive of a serious underlying cause are discussed in the management section. Some patients involved in accidents or work injuries may exaggerate their pain for the purpose of compensation or for psychological reasons.

EXAMINATION OF THE LOW BACK A general physical examination that includes the abdomen and rectum is advisable. Back pain referred from visceral organs may be reproduced during palpation of the abdomen (pancreatitis, abdominal aortic aneurysm) or percussion over the costovertebral angles (pyelonephritis, adrenal disease, L1-L2 transverse process fracture).

Inspection of the normal spine (Fig. 16-2) reveals a normal thoracic kyphosis, lumbar lordosis, and cervical lordosis. Exaggeration of these normal alignments may result in hyperkyphosis (lameback) or hyperlordosis (swayback) of the lumbar spine. Spasm of lumbar

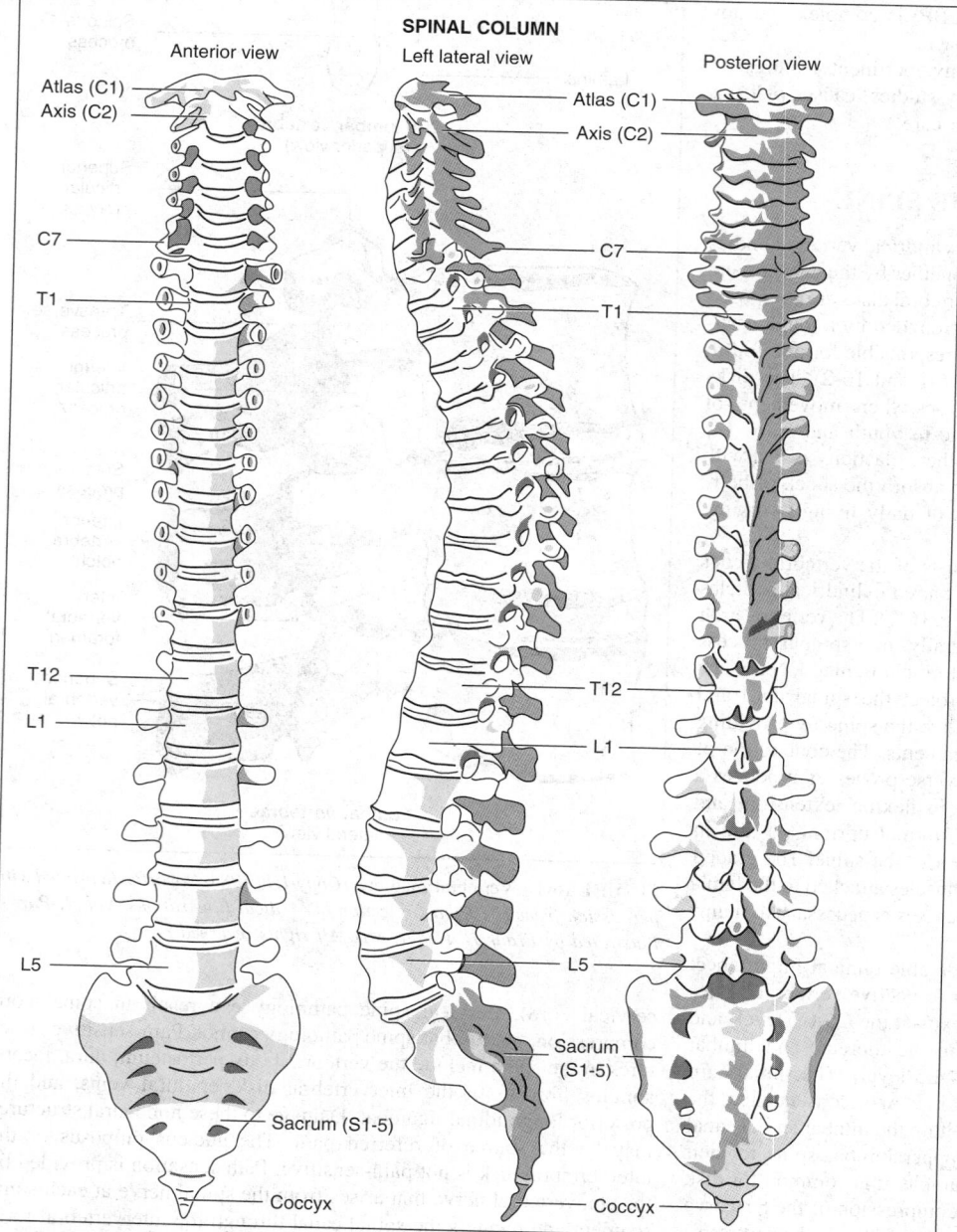

SPINAL COLUMN

Anterior view | Left lateral view | Posterior view

Atlas (C1)
Axis (C2)
C7
T1
T12
L1
L5
Sacrum (S1-5)
Coccyx

Atlas (C1)
Axis (C2)
C7
T1
T12
L1
L5
Sacrum (S1-5)
Coccyx

FIGURE 16-2 Spinal column. (*Copyright 1983. Novartis. Reprinted with permission from The Ciba Collection of Medical Illustrations, Vol. 1, Part I, illustrated by Frank H. Netter, MD. All rights reserved.*)

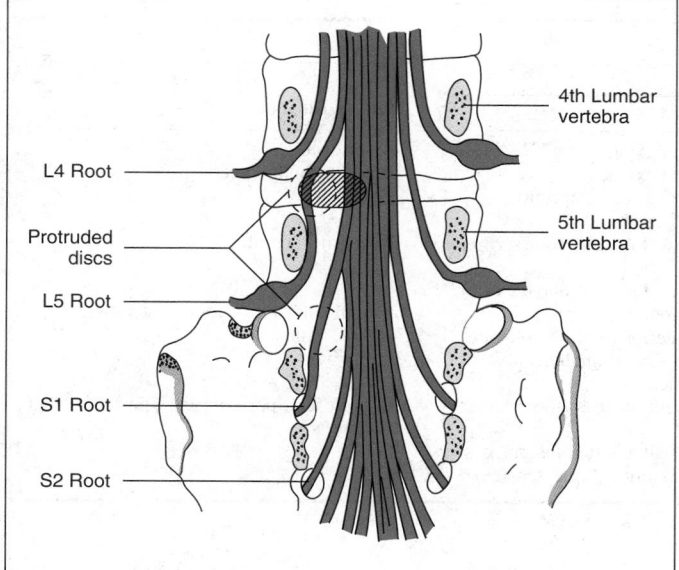

FIGURE 16-3 Locations of compression of lumbar and sacral roots by herniated disks. (*From RD Adams, M Victor, A Ropper, Prinicples of Neurology, 7th ed, New York, McGraw-Hill, 1997, with permission.*)

paraspinal muscles results in flattening of the usual lumbar lordosis. Inspection may reveal lateral curvature of the spine (scoliosis) or an asymmetry in the appearance of the paraspinal muscles, suggesting muscle spasm. Taut paraspinal muscles limit the motion of the lumbar spine in coronal and sagittal planes. Local back pain is often reproduced by palpation or percussion over the spinous process of the affected vertebrae.

Forward bending is frequently limited by paraspinal muscle spasm which accompanies disease of pain-sensitive spine structures. Flexion of the hips is normal in patients with lumbar spine disease (spondylosis), but flexion of the lumbar spine is limited and sometimes painful. Lateral bending to the side opposite the injured spinal element may stretch the damaged tissues, worsen pain, and result in limited motion. Hyperextension of the spine (with the patient prone or standing) is limited when nerve root compression or bony spine disease is present.

Pain from hip disease may mimic the pain of lumbar spine disease. The first movement to be limited is internal rotation of the hip. Manual internal and external rotation at the hip with the knee and hip in flexion may reproduce the pain, as may percussion of the patient's heel with the palm of the examiner's hand.

Passive flexion of the thigh on the abdomen while the knee is extended produces stretching of the L5 and S1 nerve roots and the sciatic nerve. The sciatic nerve passes posterior to the hip. Passive dorsiflexion of the foot during the maneuver adds to the stretch. Flexion to at least 80° is normally possible without causing pain, but tight hamstrings may limit motion. This *straight leg–raising* (SLR) *sign* is positive if the maneuver reproduces the patient's pain. The SLR sign may be elicited in the sitting position to determine if the finding is reproducible. The patient may describe pain in the low back, buttocks, posterior thigh, or lower leg. The *crossed SLR sign* is positive when performance of the maneuver on one leg reproduces the patient's pain symptoms in the opposite leg or buttocks. The nerve or nerve root lesion is always on the side of the pain. The *reverse SLR sign* is elicited by placing the patient in the prone position and passively extending the thigh. This maneuver stretches the L2-L4 nerve roots and the femoral nerve, which pass anterior to the hip. The reverse SLR test is positive if the maneuver reproduces the patient's pain.

The neurologic examination includes a search for weakness, atrophy, asymmetric or age-inappropriate absence of reflexes, diminished sensation in the legs, and signs of spinal cord injury. Examination findings that can be found with specific nerve root lesions are shown in Tables 16-1 and 16-2 and are discussed further in the sections on lumbar and cervical disk disease.

LABORATORY STUDIES "Routine" laboratory studies are rarely needed for the initial evaluation of acute (<3 months), nonspecific, low back pain. If risk factors for underlying serious disease are present (see "Treatment" and algorithms, Fig. 16-7), then laboratory studies (guided by the history and examination) may be helpful. Simple screening tests used in the setting of suspected malignancy or infection include a complete blood count, erythrocyte sedimentation rate, and urinalysis.

Plain films of the lumbar or cervical spine are helpful when risk factors for vertebral fracture (trauma, chronic steroid use) are present. *In the absence of risk factors, routine x-rays of the lumbar spine in the setting of acute, nonspecific, low back pain are expensive and not helpful.* Magnetic resonance imaging (MRI) and CT-myelography

Table 16-1

Cervical Radiculopathy—Neurologic Findings

| Cervical Nerve Roots | Changes | | | Pain Distribution |
	Reflex	Sensory	Motor	
C5	Biceps	Over deltoid +/− Thumb, index finger	Supraspinatus* (initial arm abduction) Infraspinatus* (arm external rotation) Deltoid* (arm abduction) Biceps (arm flexion)	Lateral arm, medial scapula
C6	Biceps	Thumb, index fingers Radial hand/forearm	Biceps (arm flexion) Pronator teres (internal forearm rotation)	Lateral forearm, thumb, index finger
C7	Triceps	Middle fingers Dorsum forearm	Triceps* (arm extension) Wrist extensors* Extensor digitorum* (finger extension) Pronator teres (internal forearm rotation)	Posterior arm, dorsal forearm, lateral hand
C8	Finger flexors	Little finger Medial hand and forearm	Abductor pollicis brevis (abduction D2) First dorsal interosseous (abduction D1) Abductor digit minimi (abduction D5)	4th and 5th fingers, medial forearm
T1	Finger flexors	Axilla and medial arm	Abductor pollicis brevis (abduction D2) First dorsal interosseous (abduction D1) Abductor digit minimi (abduction D5)	Medial arm, axilla, deep shoulder

* These muscles receive the majority of innervation from the root in the same horizontal row.

Table 16-2

Lumbosacral Radiculopathy—Neurologic Findings

Lumbosacral Nerve Roots	Changes			Pain Distribution
	Reflex	Sensory	Motor	
L2†	—	Upper anterior thigh	Psoas (hip flexion)	Anterior thigh
L3†	—	Lower anterior thigh	Psoas (hip flexion)	Anterior thigh, knee
		Anterior knee	Quadriceps (knee extension)	
			Thigh adduction	
L4†	Quadriceps (knee)	Medial calf	Quadriceps (knee extension)*	Knee, medial calf
			Thigh adduction	
			Tibialis anterior (foot dorsiflexion)	
L5‡	—	Dorsal surface—foot	Peroneii (foot eversion)*	Lateral calf, dorsal foot, posterolateral thigh, buttocks
		Lateral calf	Tibialis anterior (foot dorsiflexion)	
			Gluteus medius (hip abduction)	
			Toe dorsiflexors	
S1‡	Gastrocnemius/soleus (ankle)	Plantar surface—foot	Gastrocnemius/soleus (foot plantar flexion)*	Bottom foot, posterior calf, posterior thigh, buttocks
		Lateral aspect—foot	Abductor hallucis (toe flexors)*	
			Gluteus maximus (hip extension)	

* These muscles receive the majority of innervation from the root in the same horizontal row.
† Reverse straight-leg raising sign present—see examination of the spine.
‡ Straight-leg raising sign present—see examination of the spine.

have emerged as the radiologic texts of choice for evaluation of most spinal diseases; specific indications appear below.

CONDITIONS CAUSING DISABLING PAIN IN THE LOW BACK

CONGENITAL ANOMALIES OF THE LUMBAR SPINE
Spondylolysis consists of a bony defect probably caused by a stress fracture to a congenitally abnormal segment in the pars interarticularis (a segment near the junction of the pedicle with the lamina) of the vertebra. The defect (usually bilateral) is best visualized on oblique projections in plain x-rays or by computed tomography (CT) scan and occurs in the setting of a single injury, repeated minor injuries, or growth. The vertebral body, pedicles, and superior articular facets may slip anteriorly and leave the posterior elements behind. This latter abnormality (*spondylolisthesis*) more often results in symptoms. The patient may complain of pain in the low back radiating into the legs, and tenderness may be elicited near the segment that has "slipped" forward (most often L5 on S1 or occasionally L4 on L5). A "step" may be present on deep palpation of the posterior elements of the segment above the spondylolisthetic joint. The trunk may be shortened and the abdomen protuberant as a result of extreme forward displacement of L5 on S1 in severe degrees of spondylolisthesis. In these cases, cauda equina syndrome may occur (Chap. 373).

TRAUMA TO THE LOW BACK AND NECK
Trauma constitutes an important cause of acute low back and neck pain. These patients require careful initial evaluation. A patient complaining of back or neck pain and inability to move the legs may have a spine fracture. In acute injuries that may involve fracture or dislocation of the vertebral segments, the examining physician must be careful to avoid further damage to the spinal cord or nerve roots. The neck or back (depending on the location of the trauma) should be immobilized pending plain x-rays to exclude the presence of a fracture or dislocation.

Sprains and Strains The terms *lumbosacral sprain* and *strain* are used loosely by patients and physicians and do not clearly describe a specific anatomic lesion. The terms *low back strain*, *sprain*, or *mechanically induced muscle spasm* are used for minor, self-limited injuries associated with lifting a heavy object, a fall, or a sudden deceleration as occurs in an automobile accident. Patients with low back pain often assume unusual postures related to paraspinal muscle spasm. The pain is usually confined to the lower back, and there is no radiation to the buttocks or legs.

Vertebral Fractures Most traumatic fractures of the lumbar vertebral bodies result from compression or flexion injuries and consist of anterior wedging or compression. With more severe trauma, the patient may sustain a fracture dislocation or a "burst" fracture involving not only the vertebral body but posterior elements as well. Vertebral fractures are caused by falls from a height (a pars interarticularis fracture of the L5 vertebra is common), sudden deceleration in an automobile accident, or direct injury. Neurologic impairment is commonly associated with these injuries, and early treatment produces a more favorable outcome. When fractures occur with minimal or no trauma, the bone is presumed to be weakened by a pathologic process. The cause is usually postmenopausal (type 1) or senile (type 2) osteoporosis (see Chap. 355), but underlying systemic disorders such as osteomalacia, hyperparathyroidism, hyperthyroidism, multiple myeloma, metastatic carcinoma, or glucocorticoid use may also weaken the vertebral body. The clinical context (trauma, patient age, steroid use), examination findings (neurologic deficit, paraspinal muscle spasm), and x-ray appearance of the spine will establish the diagnosis.

Transverse process fractures are associated with severe injury to the paravertebral muscles—principally the psoas. Associated retroperitoneal hemorrhage may result in a low hematocrit or hypovolemic shock. Such injuries may produce deep tenderness at the injury site and limitation of all lumbar movements. CT or MRI scans establish the diagnosis.

Lumbar Disk Disease This disorder is a common cause of chronic or recurrent low back and leg pain. Disk disease is most likely to occur at the L4-L5 and L5-S1 levels, but upper lumbar levels are involved occasionally. The cause of the disk injury is often unknown. Degeneration of the nucleus pulposus and the annulus fibrosus, which increases with age, may have been asymptomatic or painful. A sneeze, cough, or trivial movement may cause the nucleus pulposus to prolapse, pushing the frayed and weakened annulus posteriorly. In severe disk disease, the nucleus may protrude through the annulus (herniation) or become extruded to lie as a free fragment in the vertebral canal.

The symptoms of a ruptured intervertebral disk consist of pain, abnormal posture, and limitation of spine motion (particularly flexion), or radicular pain. The pattern of radicular pain may suggest involvement of one or several nerve roots. A dermatomal pattern of sensory disturbance (paresthesia, hypersensitivity, or hyposensitivity) or asymmetric reduction or loss of a deep tendon reflex is more suggestive of a specific root lesion than the pain pattern. Motor abnormalities (focal weakness or fasciculations, muscle atrophy) occur less frequently, but a myotomal pattern of involvement can suggest specific nerve root involvement. Lumbar disk disease is usually unilateral (Fig. 16-4), but bilateral involvement can be seen with large

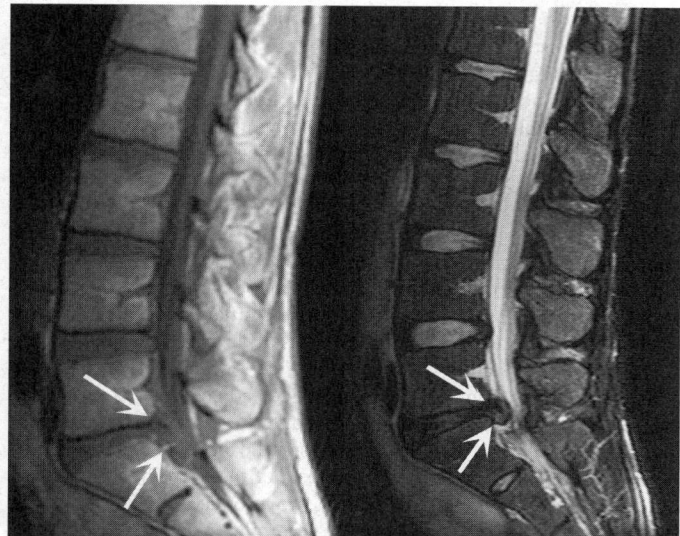

FIGURE 16-4 Lumbar herniated disk; left S1 radiculopathy. Sagittal T1-weighted image on the left with arrows outlining disk margins. Sagittal T2 image on the right reveals a protruding disk at the L5-S1 level (*arrows*) which displaces the central thecal sac.

central disk herniations that compress several nerve roots at the same level. Reflex, sensory, motor, and pain distribution findings pertinent to specific lumbosacral nerve root lesions are summarized in Table 16-2.

The examiner must be cautious to avoid overinterpretation of individual neurologic findings. The suggestion of a nerve root lesion by history and examination does not specify the underlying cause. Epidural abscesses or tumors may produce a syndrome similar to a herniated disk. Fever, constant pain uninfluenced by position, sphincter abnormalities, or signs of spinal cord disease suggest an etiology other than lumbar disk disease. Bilateral absence of ankle reflexes can be a normal finding in old age or a sign of bilateral S1 radiculopathy. An absent deep tendon reflex or focal sensory loss may reflect injury to a nerve root, but other sites of injury along the nerve must also be considered. For example, an absent knee reflex may be due to a femoral neuropathy rather than an L4 nerve root injury. A focal decrease in sensation over the foot and distal lateral calf may result from a peroneal neuropathy rather than an L5 nerve root injury. Paresthesia, when present, may be in the entire cutaneous distribution of the root or in only a portion of the distal nerve root territory. "Weakness" may be due to unsustained effort (breakaway weakness) associated with radicular pain, true weakness, or both. Electromyography (EMG) can often distinguish true weakness from breakaway weakness. Asymmetric muscle atrophy may reflect chronic motor axonal loss associated with nerve root injury, nerve injury, or disuse.

There are five indications for disk surgery: (1) progressive motor weakness from nerve root injury, (2) progressive impairment demonstrated by EMG and nerve conduction studies, (3) abnormal bowel or bladder function or other signs of spinal cord disease, (4) incapacitating nerve root pain despite conservative treatment for at least 4 weeks, and (5) recurrent incapacitating pain despite conservative treatment. The latter two criteria are more subjective and less well established than the first three indications.

Degeneration of the intervertebral disk without frank extrusion of disk tissue may give rise to low back pain with little or no leg pain or, occasionally, leg pain with little or no discomfort in the back. There are no signs of nerve root involvement, but the back pain may be referred to the thigh or leg. Lumbar disk syndromes are usually unilateral, but large central disk herniations (with or without extrusion of a large, free fragment into the spinal canal) can cause bilateral symptoms and signs. Large central disk herniations may result in

cauda equina syndrome with bilateral symptoms and signs from involvement of lumbosacral roots.

Diagnosis is straightforward when all the symptoms and signs indicative of disk disease with radiculopathy are present. When one symptom is present (particularly backache), a specific diagnosis can be difficult. Spine MR scans yield exquisite views of intraspinal and adjacent soft tissue anatomy and are more likely to establish a specific diagnosis or "road map" for surgical therapy than plain films or myelography. Occasional lateral recess or intervertebral foramen bony lesions may be seen with optimal clarity on CT-myelographic studies.

OTHER CAUSES OF LOW BACK PAIN Spinal stenosis, facet hypertrophy, lumbar adhesive arachnoiditis, and failed back syndrome are other sources of back pain.

Spinal stenosis is caused by a narrowed spinal canal. The symptoms include back and leg pain induced by walking or standing (pseudoclaudication) and relieved by the sitting or supine positions. Symptoms in the legs are usually bilateral. Focal weakness, sensory loss, or reflex changes may occur. Unlike vascular claudication, the symptoms are usually provoked by standing without walking. Unlike lumbar disk disease, the symptoms are usually relieved by sitting. Severe neurologic deficits, including paralysis and urinary incontinence, occur in a small minority of patients. Spinal stenosis usually results from acquired (75 percent), congenital, or mixed acquired/congenital factors. Congenital forms (achondroplasia, idiopathic) are characterized by short, thick pedicles that produce both anteroposterior (central) spinal canal stenosis and lateral recess stenosis. Acquired factors that may contribute to spinal stenosis include degenerative diseases (spondylosis, spondylolisthesis, scoliosis), trauma, spine psurgery (postlaminectomy, fusion), metabolic or endocrine disorders (epidural lipomatosis, osteoporosis, acromegaly, renal osteodystrophy, hypoparathyroidism), and Paget's disease. MRI or CT-myelography provide the best definition of the abnormal anatomy (Fig. 16-5).

Conservative treatment includes nonsteroidal anti-inflammatory drugs (NSAIDs), exercise programs, and symptomatic treatment of acute pain exacerbations. Surgical therapy is considered when medical therapy does not relieve pain sufficiently to allow for activities of daily living or when significant focal neurologic signs are present. Between 65 and 80 percent of patients treated surgically experience greater than 75 percent relief of back and leg pain. Up to 25 percent develop recurrent stenosis at the same spinal level or an adjacent level 5 years after the initial surgery; recurrent symptoms usually respond to a second surgical decompression.

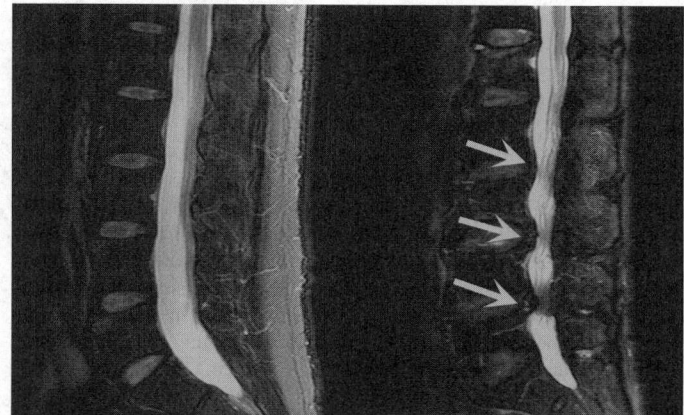

FIGURE 16-5 Spinal stenosis; back pain and leg claudication induced by walking and relieved by sitting. Sagittal T2 fast spin echo MRI of a normal (left) and stenotic (right) lumbar spine, revealing multifocal narrowing of the CSF spaces surrounding the nerve roots within the thecal sac.

Unilateral *facet joint hypertrophy* can produce radicular pain that is exacerbated and relieved by many of the same factors that influence disk-related radiculopathies. Patients often exhibit back pain and a SLR sign. Focal motor weakness, hyporeflexia, and sensory loss may occur. MRI, CT-myelography, and surgical exploration reveal hypertrophic superior or inferior facets. Foraminotomy and facetectomy result in long-term relief of leg and back pain in 80 to 90 percent of patients.

Lumbar adhesive arachnoiditis with radiculopathy is the result of a fibrotic process following an inflammatory response to local tissue injury within the subarachnoid space. The fibrosis results in nerve root adhesions, producing back and leg pain associated with motor, sensory, and reflex deficits. The classic clinical setting is in patients who have had multiple lumbar operations or oil-based myelography (Pantopaque). Myelography-induced arachnoiditis has become rare with the abandonment of oil-based contrast and the maturation of noninvasive imaging techniques (CT and MRI). Other causes of arachnoiditis include chronic spinal infections, spinal cord injury, intrathecal hemorrhage, intrathecal injection of steroids and anesthetics, and foreign bodies. MRI is the method of choice to demonstrate arachnoiditis. The nerve roots may clump together centrally or adhere to the dura peripherally or loculations of cerebrospinal fluid (CSF) may form within the thecal sac that obscure visualization of the roots. Treatment is unsatisfactory. Microsurgical lysis of adhesions, dorsal rhizotomy, and dorsal root ganglionectomy have produced poor results. Dorsal column stimulation for pain relief has produced varying results. Epidural steroid injections have been of limited value.

The cause of the low back pain sometimes remains unclear. Some patients have had multiple operations for disk disease but have persistent pain and disability. The original indications for surgery may have been questionable with back pain only, no definite neurologic signs, and a minor disk bulge noted on CT or MRI. Scoring systems based upon neurologic signs, psychological factors, physiologic studies, and imaging studies have been devised to minimize the likelihood of unsuccessful surgical explorations and to avoid selection of patients with psychological profiles that predict poor functional outcomes.

Surgical treatment should be considered if the pain and/or neurologic findings do not disappear or substantially improve within 3 to 4 weeks and in patients with worsening symptoms. Surgery must be preceded by a lumbar CT or MRI to determine the location and type of pathology (disk herniation or, rarely, intra- or extradural tumor). The usual surgical procedure is a partial hemilaminectomy with excision of the involved prolapsed intervertebral disk. Arthrodesis of the involved segments is rarely indicated and should be considered only in the presence of significant spinal instability such as degenerative spondylolisthesis or isthmic spondylolysis. In the cervical spine, herniated disks are usually managed surgically through the anterior approach. Diskectomy is usually followed by an anterior interbody fusion.

ARTHRITIS Arthritis of the spine is a major cause of back and neck pain.

Spondylosis Osteoarthritic spine disease occurs in later life and primarily involves the cervical and lumbosacral spine. Patients often complain of pain centered in the spine that is increased by motion and associated with stiffness and limitation of motion. The relationship between clinical symptoms and radiologic findings is often not straightforward; pain may be prominent when x-ray findings are minimal and large osteophytes can be seen in asymptomatic patients in middle and later life. Hypertrophied facets and osteophytes may compress nerve roots in the lateral recess or intervertebral foramen. Osteophytes arising from the vertebral body may cause central spinal canal stenosis. Loss of intervertebral disk height reduces the vertical dimensions of the intervertebral foramen, causing the descending pedicle to compress the nerve root exiting at that level. Osteoarthritic changes in the lumbar spine may on occasion compress the cauda equina. Degenerative spondylolisthesis (slipping of a vertebral body over the vertebra below) occurs most often at the L5-S1 level and may further contribute to

root compression. Surgical procedures should be considered only after failure of conservative management.

Ankylosing Spondylitis (See also Chap. 317) This distinctive form of arthritic spine disease typically presents with the insidious onset of low back and buttock pain in a man under the age of 40 years and is associated with morning back stiffness, nocturnal back pain, back pain unrelieved by rest, an elevated sedimentation rate, and the presence of histocompatibility antigen HLA-B27. The differential diagnosis in early stages includes tumor and infection, but the back pain of ankylosing spondylitis characteristically improves with exercise. Loss of the normal lumbar lordosis and exaggeration of thoracic kyphosis are seen as the disease progresses. Inflammation and erosion of the outer fibers of the annulus fibrosus at the point of contact with the vertebral body are followed by ossification and growth of bone. This bony growth (syndesmophyte) bridges adjacent vertebral bodies and results in reduced spine mobility for anterior flexion, lateral flexion, and extension. The radiologic hallmarks of the disease are periarticular destructive changes, subsequent sclerosis of the sacroiliac joints, and bridging of vertebral bodies by bone to produce the characteristic immobile and fused "bamboo spine." Similar patterns of restricted movement may accompany Reiter's syndrome, psoriatic arthritis, and chronic inflammatory bowel disease. Stress fractures through the spontaneously ankylosed posterior bony elements of the rigid, osteoporotic spine may result in focal spine pain and either spinal cord compression or cauda equina syndrome. Occasional atlantoaxial subluxation with spinal cord compression occurs. Bilateral ankylosis of the ribs to the spine and a decrease in the height of axial thoracic structures may cause marked impairment of respiratory function.

OTHER DESTRUCTIVE DISEASES **Neoplasm** (See also Chap. 373) Back pain was the most common neurologic symptom among patients with systemic cancer in one large series. One-third of the patients with undiagnosed back or neck pain and systemic cancer had epidural extension or metastasis, and one-third had pain associated with vertebral metasases alone. Eleven percent had back pain unrelated to metastatic disease. Metastatic carcinoma (breast, lung, prostate, thyroid, kidney, gastrointestinal tract), multiple myeloma, and non-Hodgkin's and Hodgkin's lymphomas are malignant tumors that frequently involve the spine. Back pain may be the presenting symptom because the primary tumor site may be overlooked or asymptomatic. The pain tends to be constant, dull, unrelieved by rest, and worse at night. In contrast, mechanical low back pain is usually improved with rest. Radiographic changes are manifest usually as destructive lesions in one or several vertebral bodies without involvement of the disk space. Disk space involvement increases the likelihood of an infectious process. MRI or CT-myelography are the studies of choice in the setting of suspected spinal metastasis. Debate over which test is preferred continues, but the trend of evidence favors the use of MRI. As a practical matter, the test most rapidly available is the procedure of choice because the patient may worsen during a diagnostic delay.

Infection *Vertebral osteomyelitis* is usually caused by staphylococci, but other bacteria or the tubercle bacillus (Pott's disease) may be the responsible organisms. In 40 percent of patients a primary source of infection can be identified, most often from the urinary tract, skin, or lungs. Intravenous drug use is a well-recognized risk factor. Back pain exacerbated by motion and unrelieved by rest, spine tenderness over the involved spine segment, and an elevated erythrocyte sedimentation rate are the most common findings. Fever is present in only one-fourth, and an elevated white blood cell count in only one-third, of patients. Plain radiographs may show narrowing of a disk space with erosion and destruction of adjacent vertebrae, but these diagnostic changes may take weeks or even months to appear. MRI is highly sensitive and specific for osteomyelitis; definition of soft tissue detail is exquisite. CT scan is also sensitive and specific, and compared to MRI may be more readily available and better tolerated by some patients with severe back pain.

Spinal epidural abscess (discussed in Chap. 373) presents with back pain (aggravated by palpation or movement) and fever. The patient may have radicular complaints, often bilateral, which can progress to spinal cord compression with focal sensory loss, focal weakness, incontinence, and paraplegia. Spine MRI best defines the extent of this lesion, which may extend over multiple spinal levels.

Osteoporosis and Osteosclerosis A considerable loss of bone substance may occur with or without symptoms in many medical disorders, including hyperparathyroidism, chronic steroid use, or immobilization. Compression fractures occur in up to half of patients with severe osteoporosis. The sole manifestation of a compression fracture may be a complaint of focal aching (often after a trivial injury) in the lumbar or thoracic spine, which is exacerbated by movement. Other patients may experience thoracic or upper lumbar radicular pain. Focal spine tenderness is common. When compression fractures are found, treatable risk factors for additional fractures and possible underlying causes should be considered carefully. Compression fractures above the midthoracic region are suggestive of malignancy. Paget's disease of the spine is readily identifiable as osteosclerosis on routine x-ray studies and may result in back pain (related to involvement of pain-sensitive structures or secondary anatomic distortion of these structures) or be painless. Spinal cord or nerve root compression may occur due to bony encroachment on the spinal canal or intervertebral foramina. Single dual-beam photon absorptiometry or quantitative CT can be used to detect small changes in bone mineral density. → *For further discussion of these bone disorders, see Chaps. 354, 355, and 358*.

REFERRED PAIN FROM VISCERAL DISEASE Diseases of the pelvis, abdomen, or thorax may produce local pain or referred pain to the posterior portion of the spinal segment that innervates the diseased organ. Occasionally, back pain may be the first and only sign. In general, pelvic diseases refer pain to the sacral region, lower abdominal diseases to the lumbar region (around the second to fourth lumbar vertebrae), and upper abdominal diseases to the lower thoracic or upper lumbar spine (eighth thoracic to the first and second lumbar vertebrae). Local signs (pain with spine palpation, paraspinal muscle spasm) are absent, and little or no pain accompanies normal movements of the spine.

Low Thoracic and Upper Lumbar Pain in Abdominal Disease Peptic ulcer or tumor of the posterior wall of the stomach or duodenum typically results in epigastric pain (see Chaps. 92 and 284), but spinal pain may be produced if there is retroperitoneal extension. The pain may be midline, paraspinal, or both. Other characteristics of the pain may provide clues to its origin. For example, back pain due to peptic ulcer may be induced after ingestion of an orange, alcohol, or coffee and relieved by food and antacids. Fatty foods are more likely to induce back pain associated with biliary disease. Diseases of the pancreas (pancreatitis, cyst, or tumor) may cause back pain to the right of the spine (if the head of the pancreas is involved) or to the left (if the body or tail are involved). Diseases of retroperitoneal structures (hemorrhage, tumors, pyelonephritis) may produce paraspinal pain with radiation to the lower abdomen, groin, or anterior thighs. A mass in the iliopsoas region often produces unilateral lumbar pain with radiation toward the groin, labia, or testicle. The sudden appearance of lumbar pain in a patient receiving anticoagulants should raise the suspicion of retroperitoneal hemorrhage.

Isolated low back pain occurs in 15 to 20 percent of patients with rupture of an abdominal aortic aneurysm. The classic triad of abdominal pain, shock, and back pain in an elderly man occurs in fewer than 20 percent of patients. Two of the three clinical features are present in two-thirds of patients; hypotension is present in half. This condition has a high mortality rate if untreated, thus it is essential to consider the possibility of a ruptured aneurysm in the appropriate clinical context. The diagnosis is initially missed in one-third of patients, in part because the symptoms and signs can be nonspecific. Common misdiagnoses include nonspecific back pain, diverticulitis, renal colic, sepsis, and myocardial infarction. A careful abdominal examination revealing a pulsatile mass (present in 50 to 75 percent of patients) is the most important physical finding.

Lumbar Pain with Lower Abdominal Diseases Inflammatory bowel disorders (colitis, diverticulitis) or colonic neoplasms may cause lower abdominal pain (between the umbilicus and pubis) and/or pain in the midlumbar spine region. The pain may have a beltlike distribution around the body. A lesion in the transverse colon or first part of the descending colon may cause midline or left-sided pain referred to the L2-L3 level in the back. Sigmoid colon disease may refer pain to the upper sacral region, midline suprapubic region, or left lower quadrant of the abdomen.

Sacral Pain in Gynecologic and Urologic Disease Pelvic organs are rarely the cause of low back pain, although gynecologic disorders that involve the uterosacral ligaments are an important source of chronic back pain. Endometriosis or carcinoma of the uterus (body or cervix) may invade the uterosacral ligaments, while malposition of the uterus may cause uterosacral ligament traction. The pain is referred to the sacral region. In endometriosis, the pain begins during the premenstrual phase and often continues until it merges with menstrual pain. Malposition of the uterus (retroversion, descensus, and prolapse) may lead to sacral pain after standing for several hours.

Menstrual pain may be felt in the sacral region. It is a poorly localized, cramping pain that can radiate down the legs. Other pelvic sources of low back pain include neoplastic invasion of pelvic nerves, radiation necrosis, and pregnancy. Pain due to neoplastic infiltration of nerves is typically continuous, progressive in severity, and unrelieved by rest at night. X-ray therapy of pelvic tumors may produce sacral pain from late radiation necrosis of tissue or nerves. Low back pain with radiation into one or both thighs is common in the last weeks of pregnancy.

Urologic sources of sacral back pain include chronic prostatitis, prostate carcinoma with spinal metastasis, and diseases of the kidney and ureter. Lesions of the bladder and testes do not usually produce back pain. The diagnosis of metastatic prostate carcinoma is established by rectal examination, spine imaging studies (MRI or CT), and measurement of prostate-specific antigen (PSA) (Chap. 97). Infectious, inflammatory, or neoplastic renal diseases may result in ipsilateral lumbar pain, as can renal artery or vein thrombosis. Ureteral obstruction due to renal stones may produce paraspinal lumbar pain.

Postural Back Pain There is a group of patients with chronic, nonspecific low back pain in whom no anatomic or pathologic lesion can be found despite exhaustive investigation. Some of these individuals complain of vague, diffuse back pain with prolonged sitting or standing that is relieved by rest. The physical examination is unrevealing except for "poor posture." Imaging studies and laboratory evaluations are normal. Exercises to strengthen the paraspinal and abdominal muscles are sometimes therapeutic.

Psychiatric Disease CLBP may be encountered in patients with compensation hysteria, malingering, substance abuse, chronic anxiety states, or depression. Many patients with CLBP managed medically or with unsuccessful spine surgery have a history of psychiatric illness (depression, anxiety, substance abuse) or childhood trauma (physical or sexual abuse) that antedates the onset of back pain. Preoperative psychological assessment has been used to exclude patients with marked psychological impairment who are at high risk for a poor surgical outcome. These considerations not withstanding, it is important to be certain that back pain in these patients does not represent serious spine or visceral pathology in addition to the impaired psychological state.

PAIN IN THE NECK AND SHOULDER

Neck pain commonly arises from diseases of the cervical spine and soft tissues of the neck. Neck and low back pain share many clinical features. Neck pain arising from the cervical spine may be precipitated by neck movements and accompanied by focal spine tenderness and limitation of motion. Pain arising from the brachial plexus, shoulder, or peripheral nerves can occasionally be confused with cervical spine disease, but the history and examination usually identify a more distal site of origin for the pain.

CERVICAL SPINE TRAUMA Unlike injury to the low back, trauma to the cervical spine (fractures, subluxation) places the spinal cord at risk for compression. The resulting bladder dysfunction, quadriparesis, and respiratory failure (with upper cervical cord compression; see Chap. 373) can be devastating. Immobilization of the neck is a top priority to minimize further cord injury due to movement of unstable cervical spine segments. The patient may also exhibit combined spinal cord and nerve root findings (myeloradiculopathy).

Whiplash injury is due to trauma (usually in automobile accidents) causing cervical musculoligamental sprain or strain due to hyperflexion or hyperextension. This diagnosis excludes patients with fractures, disk herniation, head injury, or alteration of consciousness. A prospective study of patients with whiplash injury found that 18 percent had persistent injury-related symptoms 2 years after the car accident. Such patients were older, had a higher incidence of inclined or rotated head position at impact, greater intensity of initial neck and head pain, greater number of initial symptoms, and more osteoarthritic changes on cervical spine x-rays at baseline compared to patients in remission. Objective data on the pathology of the soft tissue injuries is lacking. In general, patients with severe initial injury are at increased risk for poor long-term outcome.

CERVICAL DISK DISEASE   Acute or subacute lower cervical disk herniation is a common cause of neck, shoulder, arm, and hand pain. Neck pain (worse with neck movement), stiffness, and limited range of motion are the rule. Nerve root compression may cause radiation of pain into the shoulder or arm. Extension and lateral rotation of the neck (Spurling's sign) may narrow the neural foramen and reproduce the radicular symptoms. Acute cervical nerve root compression from a ruptured disk is often due to trauma in young individuals and is less common than acute lumbar nerve root compression. Subacute radiculopathy is less likely to be related to a specific traumatic incident and may involve both disk disease and spondylosis. Cervical disk herniations are usually posterolateral near the lateral recess and intervertebral foramen. The usual patterns of reflex, sensory, and motor changes and pain distribution with common cervical nerve root lesions are listed in Table 16-2. Nerve root function normally varies somewhat from patient to patient, and overlap in function between nerve roots is common. The anatomic pattern of pain is the most variable of the clinical features. The distribution of symptoms and signs often occupies only part of the associated nerve root territory.

CERVICAL SPONDYLOSIS   Osteoarthritis of the cervical spine may cause neck pain that radiates into the back of the head, shoulders, or arms. Arthritic or other pathologic conditions of the upper cervical spine may be the source of headaches in the posterior occipital region (supplied by the C2-C4 nerve roots). Cervical spondylosis with osteophyte formation in the lateral recess or hypertrophic facet joints may result in a monoradiculopathy (Fig. 16-6). Narrowing of the spinal canal by osteophyte formation, ossification of the posterior longitudinal ligament, or herniation of a large central disk may result in spinal cord compression with bladder symptoms and motor, sensory, and reflex changes. An electrical sensation elicited by neck flexion and radiating down the spine (Lhermitte's symptom) indicates spinal cord involvement. When little or no neck pain accompanies the cord compression, the diagnosis may be confused with amyotrophic lateral sclerosis (Chap. 370), multiple sclerosis (Chap. 376), spinal cord tumors (Chap. 373), or syringomyelia (Chap. 373). The possibility of treatable cervical spinal cord disease must be considered even when the patient presents with complaints in the legs only. In some patients, a combination of spondylitic changes results in cervical spinal stenosis with myeloradiculopathy. Lumbar spinal stenosis may mask associated findings of coexistent cervical myelopathy. MRI or CT-myelography will reveal the full extent of the anatomic abnormalities in cervical spondylosis and cervical disk disease. EMG and nerve conduction studies are useful to quantify the severity and localize the levels of nerve root injury.

OTHER CAUSES OF NECK PAIN   Rheumatoid arthritis (RA) (see Chap. 313) of the cervical apophyseal joints results in neck pain, stiffness, and limitation of motion. The diagnosis of RA is straightforward in typical cases with symmetric inflammatory polyarthritis. In advanced RA, synovitis of the atlantoaxial joint (C1-C2; see Fig. 16-2) may damage the transverse ligament of the atlas, producing forward displacement of the atlas on the axis (atlantoaxial subluxation). Atlantoaxial subluxation occurs radiographically in 30 percent of patients with RA, and the degree of subluxation correlates with the severity of erosive disease. When subluxation is present, neurologic examination and MR or CT scans are useful to assess the presence and clinical importance of any associated spinal cord compression. Occasional patients develop high spinal cord compression, leading to quadriparesis, respiratory insufficiency, and death. Although low back pain is common in RA patients, the frequency of facet disease, fracture, and spondylolisthesis is no greater than among age- and sex-matched controls with mechanical low back pain.

Ankylosing spondylitis can cause neck pain and occasional atlantoaxial subluxation with spinal cord compression. Herpes zoster may cause neck and posterior occipital pain in a C2-C3 distribution prior to the outbreak of vesicles. Neoplasms metastatic to the cervical spine, infections (osteomyelitis and epidural abscess), and metabolic bone

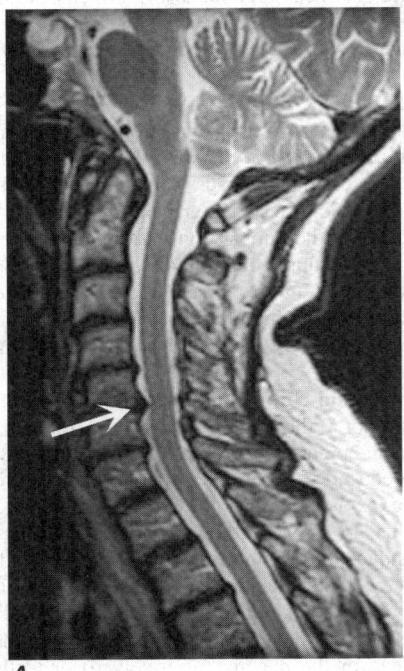

A

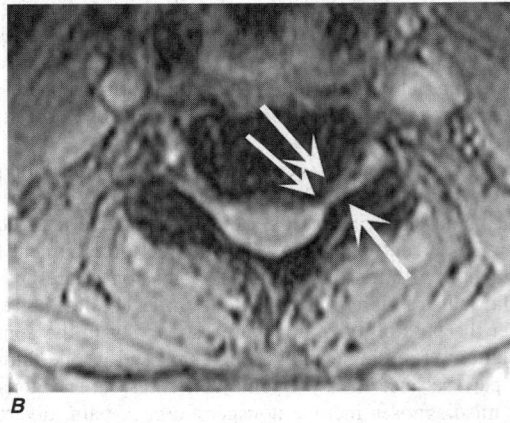

B

FIGURE 16-6   Cervical spondylosis; left C6 radiculopathy. *A.* Sagittal T2 fast spin echo MRI reveals a hypointense osteophyte which protrudes from the C5-C6 level into the thecal sac, displacing the spinal cord posteriorly (*white arrow*). *B.* Axial 2-mm section from a 3-D volume gradient echo sequence of the cervical spine. The high signal of the right C5-C6 intervertebral foramen contrasts with the narrow high signal of the left C5-C6 intervertebral foramen produced by osteophytic spurring (*arrows*).

diseases may also cause neck pain. Diagnostic considerations are similar to those described above for low back pain. Neck pain may be referred from the heart in coronary artery ischemia (cervical angina syndrome).

THORACIC OUTLET The thoracic outlet is an anatomic region containing the first rib, the subclavian artery and vein, the brachial plexus, the clavicle, and the lung apex. Injury to these structures may produce thoracic outlet syndrome (TOS), characterized by pain around the shoulder and supraclavicular region induced by certain tasks and positions. There are at least three subtypes of TOS. *True neurogenic thoracic outlet syndrome* results from compression of the lower trunk of the plexus by an anomalous band of tissue connecting an elongate transverse process at C7 with the first rib. Neurologic deficits include weakness of intrinsic muscles of the hand and diminished sensation on the palmar aspect of the 4th and 5th digits. EMG and nerve conduction studies confirm the diagnosis. The *arterial thoracic outlet syndrome* results from compression of the subclavian artery by a cervical rib; the compression results in poststenotic dilatation of the artery and thrombus formation. A reduced blood pressure in the affected limb may be accompanied by signs of emboli in the hand. Neurologic signs are absent. Noninvasive Doppler techniques confirm the diagnosis. The *disputed thoracic outlet syndrome* includes a large number of patients with chronic arm and shoulder pain of unclear cause. The lack of sensitive and specific changes on physical examination or laboratory markers for this condition frequently results in diagnostic uncertainty, and treatment of this form of TOS is often unsuccessful.

BRACHIAL PLEXUS AND NERVES Pain from injury to the brachial plexus or peripheral nerves can on occasion be confused with pain of neck origin. Infiltration of peripheral nerves by neoplasm may occur in the lower trunk of the brachial plexus and produce shoulder pain radiating down the arm, numbness of the fourth and fifth fingers, and weakness of intrinsic hand muscles innervated by the ulnar and median nerves. Postradiation fibrosis (breast carcinoma is the most common setting) or a Pancoast tumor of the lung (Chap. 90) may produce similar findings. A Horner's syndrome is present in two-thirds of patients with Pancoast tumor. Suprascapular neuropathy may produce severe shoulder pain, weakness, and wasting of the supraspinatous and infraspinatous muscles. Acute brachial neuritis is often confused with radiculopathy. The acute onset of severe shoulder or scapular pain is followed over days to weeks by weakness of the proximal arm and shoulder girdle corresponding to muscles innervated by the upper trunk of the plexus. Antecedent infection and immunization have been associated with acute brachial neuritis, but a causal link is circumstantial. Identification of this syndrome is important because slow, complete recovery occurs in 75 percent of patients after 2 years and in 89 percent after 3 years. Occasional cases of carpal tunnel syndrome produce pain and paresthesia extending into the forearm, arm, and shoulder resembling a C5 or C6 root lesion. Lesions of the radial or ulnar nerve can mimic a radiculopathy at C7 or C8, respectively. EMG and nerve conduction studies can accurately localize lesions to the nerve roots, brachial plexus, or nerves. Peripheral nerve disorders are discussed more fully in Chap. 381.

SHOULDER Pain in the shoulder region can be difficult to separate clearly from neck pain. If the symptoms and signs of radiculopathy are absent, then the differential diagnosis includes mechanical shoulder pain (tendonitis, bursitis, rotator cuff tear, partial cuff tear, adhesive capsulitis, and cuff impingement under the acromion) and referred pain (subdiaphragmatic irritation, angina, Pancoast tumor). Mechanical pain is often worse at night, associated with local shoulder tenderness, and aggravated by abduction, internal rotation, or extension of the arm. The pain of shoulder disease may at times radiate into the arm or hand, but the sensory, motor, and reflex changes that indicate disease of the nerve roots, plexus, or peripheral nerves are absent.

℞ TREATMENT

Acute Low Back Pain A practical approach to the management of low back pain is to consider acute and chronic presentations separately. Acute low back pain is defined as pain of less than 3 months' duration. Full recovery can be expected in 85 percent of patients with acute low back pain unaccompanied by leg pain. Most of these patients exhibit "mechanical" symptoms—pain that is aggravated by motion and relieved by rest. Despite the staggering annual costs of back pain to society, there is a paucity of well-controlled clinical trials in this area.

Recent observational, population-based studies (North Carolina Back Pain Project) have been used to justify a minimalist approach to individual patient care. These studies share a number of limitations: (1) comparison of treatment groups often lacks a true placebo control group, (2) it is assumed that patients who consult different provider groups (generalists, orthopedists, neurologists) have similar etiologies for their back pain, (3) no information is provided about the details of treatment within each provider group or between provider groups, and (4) there is no attempt to tabulate serious causes of low back pain. The appropriateness of specific diagnostic procedures or therapeutic interventions for low back pain cannot be assessed from these studies.

Competitive pressures in the health care marketplace have encouraged the rapid development of CPGs for the treatment of back pain. In December 1994, the Agency for Health Care Policy and Research (AHCPR) published a summary guideline entitled "Acute Low Back Problems in Adults." The following characteristics of evidence were considered in developing the guidelines: the quality and amount of evidence for efficacy, the strength of an effect for the diagnostic/therapeutic method, the consistency of findings between studies when multiple studies were available, the clinical applicability of the evidence to adult patients, and evidence on complications or cost.

Entry into the AHCPR guideline begins with adults (patients > 18 years of age) who have less than 3 months of activity intolerance due to low back pain and/or back-related leg symptoms. The term *back problems* was defined as pain of sufficient magnitude to limit a return to functional activities. The next guideline phase focused on the use of the medical history and physical examination to divide patients into management subcategories. "Red flags" were used to identify features that raised the likelihood that a serious underlying disease requiring rapid evaluation and treatment was present. Findings on neurologic examination were heavily weighted in the initial screen. If the history, physical examination, and neurologic screening examination did not yield red flags, then patients were treated symptomatically. No diagnostic tests were deemed necessary. The common serious etiologies considered as red flags were cancer metastatic to spine, spine fracture, and spine infection.

The guidelines attempted to use available medical literature to create management recommendations and often quoted specific values for the sensitivity and specificity (SAS) of certain tests. However, the applicability of these values to common outpatient clinical settings is limited for numerous reasons: (1) many of the studies used to calculate SAS were retrospective series comprising patients who ultimately had surgery, and they excluded nonsurgical patients with abnormal findings on examination (e.g., SLR) who never underwent surgery; (2) patients were preselected by virtue of referral to orthopedic surgeons and thus may not have reflected a general medical population; (3) different entry criteria and protocols for evaluation were employed in different studies; (4) many studies were performed prior to the era of modern neuroimaging; (5) surgical outcome was assessed by anatomic endpoints (compression of nerve roots) and not by functional status; and (6) none of the studies documented the natural history of disk lesions associated with a focal neurologic deficit. These limitations emphasize the point that the use of current CPGs for the treatment of low back pain should not substitute for sound clinical judgment in specific circumstances.

The proposed algorithms (Fig. 16-7) for management of acute back pain draw considerably from published guidelines. The initial assessment must exclude serious causes of spine pathology that require urgent intervention, including infection, cancer, and trauma. Risks factors for a possible serious underlying cause of back pain include: age > 50 years, prior diagnosis of cancer or other serious medical illness, bed rest without relief, duration of pain > 1 month, urinary incontinence or recent nocturia, focal leg weakness or numbness, pain radiating into the leg(s) from the back, intravenous drug use, chronic infection (pulmonary or urinary), pain increasing with standing and relieved by sitting, history of spine trauma, and glucocorticoid use. Clinical signs associated with a possible serious etiology include unexplained fever, well-documented and unexplained weight loss, positive SLR sign, reverse SLR sign, crossed SLR sign, percussion tenderness over the spine or costovertebral angle, an abdominal mass (pulsatile or non-pulsatile), a rectal mass, focal sensory loss (saddle anesthesia or focal limb sensory loss), or leg weakness, spasticity, and asymmetric leg reflexes. Laboratory studies are unnecessary at this time unless a serious underlying cause is suspected based upon the symptoms and signs (Fig. 16-7, Algorithms

1 and 2). Plain spine films are rarely indicated in the first month of symptoms unless a spine fracture is suspected.

The roles of bed rest, early exercise, and traction in the treatment of acute low back pain among patients lacking clinical features to suggest a serious underlying cause have been the subject of recent studies. Clinical trials fail to demonstrate any benefit of prolonged (>2 days) bed rest. Theoretical advantages of early activity following the onset of acute low back pain include maintenance of cardiovascular conditioning, improved disk and cartilage nutrition, improved bone and muscle strength, and increased endorphin levels. A recent trial did not show benefit from an early *vigorous* exercise program, but the benefits of less vigorous exercise or other exercise programs remain unknown. The effect of bed rest on patients with sciatica or acute back pain and focal neurologic findings is also unknown. Early resumption of usual physical activity (without heavy manual labor) is beneficial. Well-designed clinical studies of traction, which include a sham traction group, fail to show a benefit of this treatment for acute low back pain. Despite this knowledge, a recent study of physician perceptions of treatment effectiveness identified strict bed rest for more than 3 days, trigger point injections (see below), and physical therapy as beneficial in over 50 percent of patients with acute low back pain. A highly variable perception of treatment effectiveness was present between physicians within a given specialty. In many instances, the behavior of treating physicians does not reflect the current medical literature.

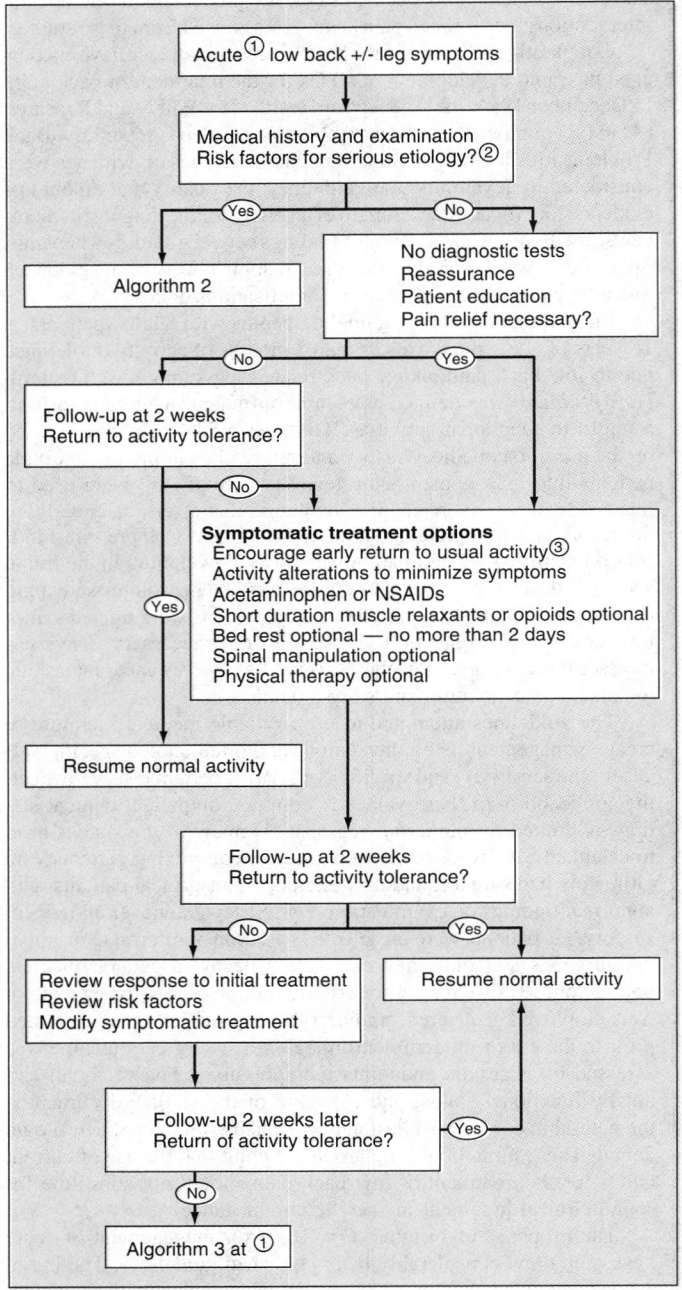

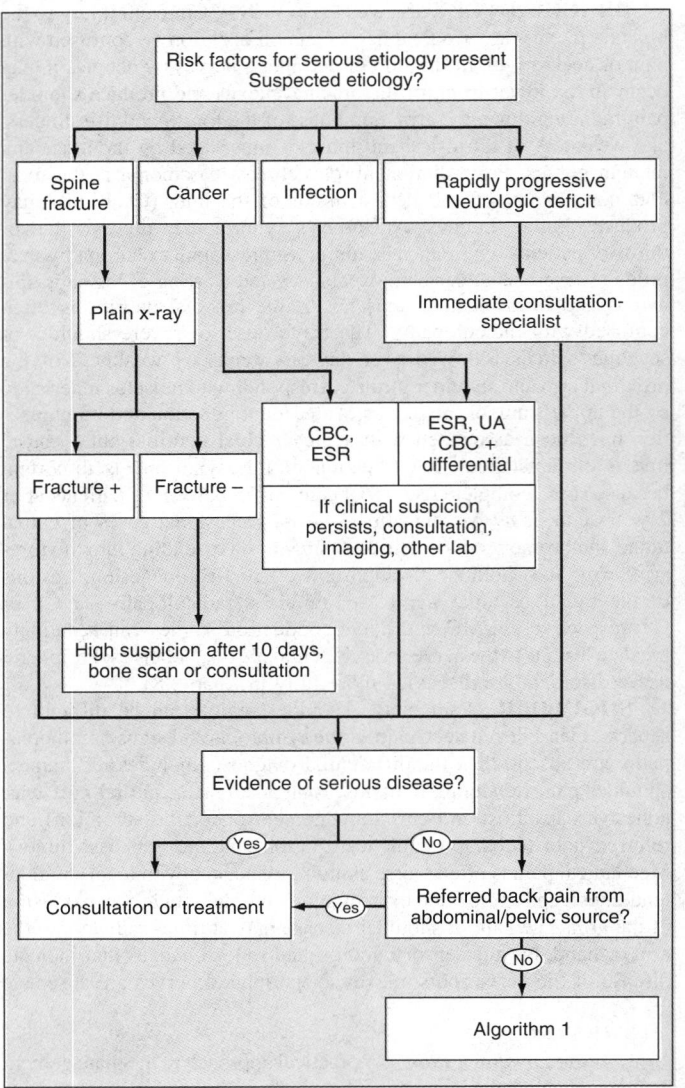

FIGURE 16-7　Algorithms for management of acute low back pain. Algorithm 1: First 4 weeks; ①, adults ≥18 years of age, symptoms <3 months; ②, see Algorithm 2; ③, excluding heavy manual labor.

FIGURE 16-7 *(continued)*　Algorithm 2: Low back pain of possible serious etiology.

Proof is lacking to support the treatment of acute back and neck pain with acupuncture, transcutaneous electrical nerve stimulation, massage, ultrasound, diathermy, or electrical stimulation. Cervical collars can limit spontaneous and reflex neck movements that exacerbate pain. Evidence regarding the efficacy of self-application of ice and heat or use of shoe insoles is lacking. These interventions remain a therapeutic option given the lack of negative evidence, low cost, and low risk. Biofeedback has not been studied rigorously. Facet joint, trigger point, and ligament injections are not recommended in the treatment of acute low back pain.

A beneficial role of specific exercises or modification of posture has not been validated by rigorous clinical studies. As a practical matter, temporary suspension of activity known to increase mechanical stress on the spine such as heavy lifting, prolonged sitting, bending or twisting, or straining at stool may be helpful.

Patient education is an important part of treatment. Clinical studies reveal that patient satisfaction and the likelihood of follow-up increases when patients are educated about prognosis, treatment methods, activity modifications, and strategies to prevent future exacerbations. In one study, patients who felt they did not receive an adequate explanation for their symptoms wanted more diagnostic tests. The evidence for the efficacy of structured education programs about low back pain ("back school") is inconclusive; in one controlled study, patients attending back school had a shorter duration of sick leave during the initial episode but not during subsequent episodes.

Medications used in the treatment of acute low back pain include NSAIDs, acetaminophen, muscle relaxants, and opioids. NSAIDs are superior to placebo for back pain relief. Acetaminophen is superior to placebo in the treatment of other types of pain but has not been compared against placebo for low back pain. Muscle relaxants provide short-term (4 to 7 days) benefit compared with placebo, but drowsiness often limits their use. The efficacy of muscle relaxants compared to NSAIDs or in combination with NSAIDs is unclear. Opioid analgesics have not been shown to be more effective than NSAIDs or acetaminophen for relief of acute low back pain or likelihood of return to work. Short-term use of opioids in selected patients unresponsive to or unable to take acetaminophen or NSAIDs may be helpful. There is no evidence to support the use of oral glucocorticoids or tricyclic antidepressants in treatment of acute low back pain. Equivocal data suggests that epidural steroids may occasionally produce short-term pain relief in patients with acute low back pain and radiculopathy, but proof is lacking for pain relief beyond 1 month. Epidural anesthetics, steroids, or opioids are not indicated as initial treatment for patients with acute low back pain unaccompanied by radiculopathy.

A short course of spinal manipulation for symptomatic relief of uncomplicated, acute low back pain is an option. A mild benefit of manipulation is seen only during the first 2 weeks after onset of treatment but may lessen pain and improve daily function in this situation. Treatment longer than 1 month or treatment of patients with radiculopathy is of unknown value and carries potential risk. The appropriate frequency or duration of spinal manipulation has not been adequately addressed.

CHRONIC LOW BACK PAIN CLBP is defined as pain lasting longer than 12 weeks. Patients with CLBP comprise 5 percent of all back pain patients but consume 50 percent of back pain costs. The initial approach to these patients is similar to that for acute low back pain. The differential diagnosis of CLBP includes most of the conditions described in this chapter. Treatment of this heterogeneous group of patients is based upon identification of the underlying cause.

Many diseases that result in CLBP can be defined by the combination of neuroimaging and electrophysiologic studies. MRI, CT, or CT-myelography are not indicated within the first month of back pain symptoms in the absence of risk factors for a serious underlying cause. Spine MRI or CT-myelography is the technique of choice; their sensitivity and specificity in the diagnosis of lumbar disk disease and lumbar spinal stenosis are equivalent, but MRI does not expose the patient to ionizing radiation and the definition of soft tissue structures by MRI is superior. Both techniques are noninvasive. CT-myelography provides optimal imaging of bony lesions in the region of the lateral recess and intervertebral foramen and is tolerated by claustrophobic patients. With rare exceptions, conventional myelography and bone scan are inferior to MRI and CT-myelography. The selection of diagnostic procedures for individual patients is often aided by appropriate neurologic, surgical, or medical consultation. Imaging studies should be performed only in circumstances where the results are likely to influence surgical or medical treatment.

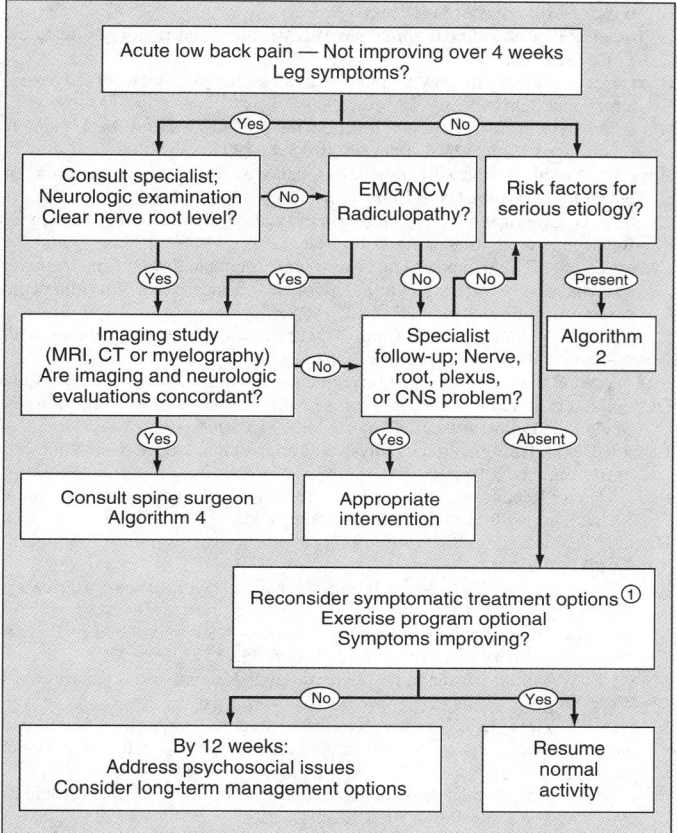

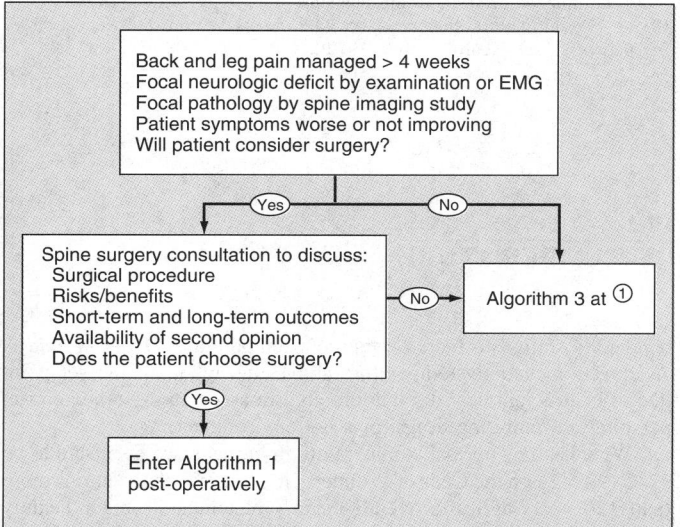

FIGURE 16-7 *(continued)* *Top.* Algorithm 3: Management for weeks 4 to 12; ①, entry point from Algorithm 4 postoperatively or if patient declines surgery. *Bottom.* Algorithm 4: Surgical options.

Diskography is of questionable value in the evaluation of back pain. No additional anatomic information is provided beyond what is available by MRI scan. Reproduction of the patient's typical pain with the injection provides evidence for a specific disk as a pain generator, but controversy exists regarding how to use this information to decide whether or not to operate. There is no proven role for thermography in the management of radiculopathy.

Sensory nerve conduction studies, motor nerve conduction studies, and needle EMG (Chap. 361) are used to assess the functional integrity of the peripheral nervous system in the setting of back pain. Sensory nerve conduction studies are normal when a circumscribed sensory loss is due to nerve root damage proximal to the dorsal root ganglion (DRG). The amplitude of motor nerve compound muscle action potentials (CMAP) may be reduced when there is significant loss of motor axons in a damaged nerve root. The diagnostic yield of needle EMG is higher than that of nerve conduction studies for radiculopathy. Denervation changes in a myotomal (segmental) distribution are detected by sampling multiple muscles supplied by different nerve roots and nerves; the pattern of muscle involvement indicates the nerve root(s) responsible for the injury. Needle EMG can also provide objective information about motor nerve fiber injury when the clinical evaluation of weakness is limited by pain or lack of patient effort. EMG and nerve conduction studies will be normal when only limb pain or sensory nerve root injury or irritation is present. Mixed nerve somatosensory evoked potentials and F-wave studies are of uncertain value in the evaluation of nerve root lesions.

The diagnosis of nerve root injury is most secure when the history and examination and results of imaging studies and EMG are concordant. The correlation between CT and EMG for localization of nerve root injury is between 65 and 73 percent. Up to 25 percent of asymptomatic individuals have a herniated disk detected by CT or MRI scans. Thus, surgical intervention based solely upon radiologic findings and pain increases the likelihood of an unsuccessful outcome.

CLBP can be treated with a variety of conservative measures. Acute and subacute exacerbations are managed with NSAIDs and comfort measures. Bed rest should not exceed 2 days. Activity tolerance is the primary goal, while pain relief is secondary. Exercise programs can reverse type II muscle fiber atrophy in paraspinal muscles and result in improved trunk extension strength. Supervised, intensive physical exercise or "work hardening" regimens (under the guidance of a physical therapist) have been effective in returning patients to work, improving walking distances, and diminishing pain. The benefit can be sustained among patients who follow home exercise regimens. Compliance with the exercise regimen strongly influences outcome. A reduction in sick leave days, long-term health care utilization, and pension expenditures may offset the initial expense of multidisciplinary treatment programs. Hydrotherapy resulted in diminished duration and intensity of back pain, reduced analgesic drug consumption, improved spine mobility, and improved functional score in one study comparing 3 weeks of hydrotherapy versus routine ambulatory care. Functional score returned to baseline at the 9-month follow-up, but all other beneficial effects were sustained.

BIBLIOGRAPHY

AGENCY FOR HEALTH CARE POLICY AND RESEARCH (AHCPR): *Acute Low Back Problems in Adults*. U.S. Department of Health and Human Services. Public Health Service. ACHPR Publication No. 95-0642. Rockville, MD

AMINOFF MJ et al: Electrophysiologic evaluation of lumbosacral radiculopathies: Electromyography, late responses, and somatosensory evoked potentials. Neurology 35:1514, 1985

AMUNDSEN T et al: Lumbar spinal stenosis. Clinical and radiologic features. Spine 20:1178, 1995

BATEMAN JL, PEVZNER MM: Spinal osteomyelitis: A review of 10 years' experience. Orthopedics 18:561, 1995

BEURSKENS AJ et al: Efficacy of traction for non-specific low back pain: A randomised clinical trial. Lancet 346:1596, 1995

BODEN SD et al: Abnormal magnetic-resonance scans of the lumbar spine in asymptomatic subjects. J Bone Joint Surg 72A:403, 1990

CAPUTY AJ, LUESSENHOP AJ: Long-term evaluation of decompressive surgery for degenerative lumbar stenosis. J Neurosurg 77:669, 1992

CAREY TS et al: The outcomes and costs of care for acute low back pain among patients seen by primary care practitioners, chiropractors, and orthopedic surgeons. N Engl J Med 333:913, 1995

CLOUSTON PD et al: The spectrum of neurological disease in patients with systemic cancer. Ann Neurol 31:268, 1992

DAROUICHE RO et al: Bacterial spinal epidural abscess. Medicine 71:369, 1992

DEYO RA et al: How many days of bed rest for acute low back pain? A randomized clinical trial. N Engl J Med 315:1064, 1986

ELAM KC et al: How emergency physicians approach low back pain: Choosing costly options. J Emerg Med 13:143, 1995

FROST H et al: Randomised controlled trial for evaluation of fitness programme for patients with chronic low back pain. BMJ 310:151, 1995

HELLER JG: The syndromes of degenerative cervical disease. Orthop Clin North Am 23:381, 1992

KORI SH et al: Brachial plexus lesions in patients with cancer: 100 cases. Neurology 31:45, 1981

MALMIVAARA A et al: The treatment of acute low back pain—bed rest, exercises, or ordinary activity? N Engl J Med 332:351, 1995

MARSTON WA et al: Misdiagnosis of ruptured abdominal aortic aneurysms. J Vasc Surg 16:17, 1992

MARTIN RJ, YUAN HA: Neurosurgical care of spinal epidural, subdural, and intramedullary abscesses and arachnoiditis. Orthop Clin North Am 27:125, 1996

PEARSON SD et al: Critical pathways as a strategy for improving care: Problems and potential. Ann Intern Med 123:941, 1995

STURZENEGGER M et al: Presenting symptoms and signs after whiplash injury: The influence of accident mechanisms. Neurology 44:688, 1994

TSAIRIS P et al: Natural history of brachial plexus neuropathy: Report on 99 patients. Arch Neurol 27:109, 1972

SECTION 2
ALTERATIONS IN BODY TEMPERATURE

17

Jeffrey A. Gelfand, Charles A. Dinarello

FEVER AND HYPERTHERMIA

Fever is an elevation of body temperature above the normal circadian range as the result of a change in the thermoregulatory center located in the anterior hypothalamus. A normal body temperature is ordinarily maintained, despite environmental variations, through the ability of the thermoregulatory center to balance heat production by the tissues (notably, muscles and the liver) with heat dissipation. With fever, the balance is shifted to increase the core temperature. *Hyperthermia* is an elevation of body temperature above the hypothalamic set point due to insufficient heat dissipation (e.g., in association with exercise, perspiration-inhibiting drugs, or a hot environment).

Whereas the "normal" temperature in humans has been said to be 37°C (98.6°F) on the basis of Wunderlich's original observations more than 120 years ago, the overall mean oral temperature for healthy individuals aged 18 to 40 years is actually 36.8 ± 0.4°C (98.2 ± 0.7°F), with a nadir at 6 A.M. and a zenith at 4 to 6 P.M. The maximum normal oral temperature at 6 A.M. is 37.2°C (98.9°F), and the maximum normal oral temperature at 4 P.M. is 37.7°C (99.9°F)—both values defining the 99th percentile for healthy individuals. Given these criteria, *an A.M. temperature of greater than 37.2°C (98.9°F) or a P.M. temperature of greater than 37.7°C (99.9°F) would define a fever.* Rectal temperatures are generally 0.6°C (1°F) higher. Lower esophageal temperatures closely reflect core temperature. The temperature of a freshly passed urine specimen is close to rectal values. The normal 24-h circadian temperature rhythm is associated with temperatures varying typically by 0.5°C (0.9°F) but occasionally by as much as 1°C between the A.M. nadir and the P.M. peak. This morning-low and evening-high pattern is usually preserved in febrile diseases but not in hyperthermia. In menstruating women, the A.M. temperature is generally lower in the 2 weeks prior to ovulation, rising by about 0.6°C (1°F) with ovulation and remaining at that level until menses occur. In addition, there may be a seasonal variation in body temperature. Finally, such physiologic factors as postprandial state, pregnancy, endocrine alterations, and age may affect baseline temperatures.

PYROGENS Substances that cause fever are called *pyrogens* and may be either exogenous or endogenous. *Exogenous pyrogens* come from outside the host, whereas endogenous pyrogens are produced by the host, generally in response to initiating stimuli that are usually triggered by infection or inflammation. The majority of exogenous pyrogens are microorganisms, their products, or toxins. The best-characterized type of exogenous pyrogen consists of a heterogeneous group of molecules that is common to all gram-negative bacteria and is referred to as *endotoxin* (lipopolysaccharide, LPS). LPS, which is found in the outer membrane of all gram-negative bacteria, comprises lipid A and a polysaccharide core linked to an O-polysaccharide side chain composed of repeating units of sugars that vary with the gram-negative organism. Gram-positive organisms also are sources of potent pyrogens. These include cell wall–derived lipoteichoic acid and peptidoglycans. Several exotoxins and enterotoxins produced by pathologic strains of streptococci and staphylococci act as bacterial superantigens—polyclonal T-lymphocyte activators that bind to the variable region of the T-cell receptor rather than in the antigen-binding pocket of the receptor. This binding leads to the activation of cells of many specificities, with resultant mediator release and tissue damage. These toxins are thought to contribute to both staphylococcal and streptococcal toxic shock. In vivo, as little as 1 ng of LPS/kg is capable of producing fever in humans; although there are no in vivo data for humans, gram-positive cell-wall constituents generally require a 2- to 3-log larger amount of material by weight to induce the production of endogenous pyrogens in vitro.

In general, exogenous pyrogens act primarily by inducing the formation of endogenous pyrogens through stimulation of the host's cells—usually monocytes and macrophages. However, the distinction between exogenous and endogenous pyrogens is sometimes blurred. For example, LPS may act directly on endothelial cells in the brain to generate fever, whereas many exogenous products result in the release of endogenous pyrogens, thereby causing fever. Such endogenous substances include antigen-antibody complexes with complement, complement cleavage products, steroid hormone metabolites, bile acids, and some cytokines.

Endogenous pyrogens are polypeptides produced by a variety of host cells, particularly monocytes/macrophages. Endogenous pyrogens, produced either systemically or locally, gain entrance to the circulation and produce fever at the level of the thermoregulatory center of the hypothalamus.

It was originally thought that there was a single endogenous pyrogen. The standard experimental model utilized injection of leukocyte supernatants or sera from febrile rabbits into normal rabbits. It was then realized that there are two leukocyte endogenous pyrogens: interleukin (IL) 1α and IL-1β. These two interleukins have a common molecular weight of approximately 17.5 kDa, have only 26 percent amino acid sequence homology, and bind to the same receptors. Originally thought to be produced only by phagocytic cells, IL-1α or IL-1β is also produced by endothelial cells, B lymphocytes, natural killer cells, fibroblasts, smooth-muscle cells, keratinocytes, and glial cells. Because of the ubiquitous production of these and other interleukins, cell-derived inflammatory polypeptides, and growth-promoting

peptides, the more general term *cytokine* has been adopted to refer to these substances. Cytokines are regulatory polypeptides produced by a large variety of nucleated cells. Specifically, cytokines are produced by monocytes/macrophages, lymphocytes, endothelial cells, hepatocytes, epithelial cells, keratinocytes, and fibroblasts as well as other cells. Cytokines typically act locally, initiating autocrine (self-stimulating) or paracrine (nearby-stimulating) effects. When found in the circulation, cytokines are usually present in picogram-per-milliliter concentrations.

The major fever-inducing cytokines appear to be IL-1α, IL-1β, tumor necrosis factor α (TNFα), interferon (IFN) α, and IL-6. When any of these cytokines is administered intravenously to humans, chills and fever develop within 1 h. IL-1α and -1β are the most pyrogenic, with temperatures of 39°C developing in response to doses of 1 to 10 ng/kg of body weight. Doses of 100 ng/kg have caused higher fevers and rigors. TNFα produces chills and a temperature of 39°C at somewhat higher doses (50 to 100 ng/kg). IL-6 is the least pyrogenic of these cytokines, producing a temperature of 39°C at 10 μg/kg. IFNα and IFNγ have been administered primarily by the subcutaneous route; therefore, chills and fever develop after 3 to 4 h. On a weight basis, the interferons are less potent than IL-1 or TNFα and similar to IL-6. Moreover, the degree of fever elicited decreases with repeated injections of interferon. Studies with genetically altered mice have revealed that IL-1 and TNFα cause fever by inducing IL-6 in the brain.

HYPOTHALAMIC CONTROL OF TEMPERATURE Body temperature is controlled by the hypothalamus. Neurons in both the preoptic anterior hypothalamus and the posterior hypothalamus receive two kinds of signals—one from peripheral nerves that reflect receptors for warmth and cold and the other from the temperature of the blood bathing the region. These two signals are integrated by the thermoregulatory center of the hypothalamus to maintain normal temperature. In a neutral environment, the metabolic rate of humans consistently produces more heat than is necessary to maintain the core body temperature at 37°C. Therefore, the hypothalamus controls temperature by mechanisms of heat loss.

Clusters of neurons in the preoptic/anterior hypothalamus are supplied by a rich and permeable vascular network with limited blood-brain barrier function. The specialized vascular network is called the *organum vasculosum laminae terminalis*. It is likely that the endothelial cells of this network release arachidonic acid metabolites when exposed to endogenous pyrogenic cytokines from the circulation. The arachidonic acid metabolites—mainly prostaglandin E$_2$ (PGE$_2$)—then presumably diffuse into the preoptic/anterior hypothalamic region and initiate fever. It is also possible that PGE$_2$ or other arachidonic acid products induce a second messenger such as cyclic AMP, which in turn raises the thermoregulatory set point. PGE$_2$ is the most potent of the fever-producing arachidonic acid derivatives when injected directly into the hypothalamus and is believed to mediate the rise in the thermoregulatory set point. With the new, higher "thermostatic setting," signals go to various efferent nerves, particularly those sympathetic fibers innervating the peripheral blood vessels, which in turn initiate vasoconstriction and promote heat conservation. The thermoregulatory center also sends signals to the cerebral cortex, initiating behavioral changes such as seeking a warm environment, putting on more clothes, and special posturing. With the shunting of blood from the periphery and these behavioral changes, the body temperature usually rises by 2 to 3°C; if the hypothalamus calls for more heat, shivering (involuntary muscle contraction) is triggered to increase heat production. The combination of heat conservation and increased heat production continues until the temperature of the blood bathing the anterior hypothalamic neurons matches the new "setting." At that point, the hypothalamus maintains the new febrile temperature (Fig. 17-1).

The hypothalamic set point is reset downward by the disappearance of stimulating pyrogenic cytokines or by the inhibition of local prostaglandin synthesis by cyclooxygenase inhibitors such as aspirin and ibuprofen. The reduction of fever by acetaminophen involves the metabolism of the drug by brain cytochromes and the subsequent inhibition of brain cyclooxygenase by the metabolites. Vasodilation and sweating dissipate heat through radiation and conduction from the skin. Behavioral changes, such as the removal of insulating clothing or bedding, may be triggered. There are also endogenous antipyretic substances. These include arginine vasopressin, adrenocorticotropin, α-melanocyte-stimulating hormone, and corticotropin-releasing hormone, each of which appears to alter the ability of endogenous pyrogens to stimulate prostaglandin production.

Specific cytokine antagonists and inhibitory cytokines may play a role in modulating fever. The IL-1 receptor antagonist (IL-1Ra) is a 23- to 25-kDa protein that blocks the binding of IL-1 to its receptors. Whereas IL-1Ra blocks the hypotensive effects of IL-1 and gram-negative and gram-positive bacteremia in experimental animals, in volunteers it has failed to prevent fever in response to small doses of intravenous LPS. Peak molar concentrations of IL-1Ra may exceed those of IL-1β by 100-fold, but these levels tend to be reached 1 h after the IL-1β peak and may be part of the recovery process.

Endogenous binding proteins for TNFα are produced by cleavage of the extracellular domains of the two TNFα receptors. Circulating levels of these two soluble TNFα receptor fragments (type I and type II) are higher than circulating levels of TNFα. In addition, cytokines that inhibit the production of the major pyrogens IL-1 and TNFα include transforming growth factor β, IL-4, and IL-10. There is little information on the role of these cytokines in modulating the febrile response.

BIOLOGIC ACTIVITIES OF IL-1, TNFα, AND IL-6 It is important to distinguish between the critical physiologic roles of local IL-1 and TNFα and the high systemic blood levels of these cytokines that are often seen with severe and life-threatening diseases. IL-1 and TNFα mediate local phagocytic-cell emigration and activation as well as the release of lipid-derived mediators such as PGE₂, thromboxane,

and platelet-activating factor. IL-1 induces the synthesis of IL-8, which in turn is a potent neutrophil and monocyte chemotactic factor. IL-8 stimulates the release of enzymes from neutrophils, further enhancing the host's attack on invading microbes. Vasodilation, the induction of adhesive glycoproteins, the activation of T and B lymphocytes, and the enhancement of killing by phagocytic cells are directly or indirectly mediated by these pyrogenic cytokines. The acute-phase response is stimulated, resulting in changes in protein synthesis in the liver. Serum albumin levels decrease, and the production of acute-phase proteins, including antiproteases, complement components, fibrinogen, ceruloplasmin, ferritin, and haptoglobin, is increased. Levels of C-reactive protein, which binds to damaged and necrotic cells and to some microorganisms, may increase by 1000-fold. Concentrations of serum amyloid A protein also may increase markedly, with the protein deposited in various organs to cause secondary amyloidosis. Decreases in serum iron and zinc levels deprive invading microbes of these critical growth factors. Although IL-1 and TNFα can induce these hepatic changes, IL-6 is thought to be the prime mediator of the acute-phase response.

IL-1 and TNFα act synergistically to mediate local and systemic inflammatory effects. Amounts of each cytokine that cause little inflammation individually produce refractory hypotension and the failure of mutiple organ systems in combination. Suppression of either of these two cytokines may have a significant therapeutic effect by blocking this synergistic toxicity. Furthermore, IL-1–induced activation of T and B cells is greater at 39°C than at 37°C. Both IL-1 and TNFα increase the loss of mean body mass and cause anorexia, contributing to the cachexia of chronic febrile states. IL-1 and TNFα are found in the circulation only briefly but nevertheless induce IL-6. Levels of IL-6 correlate better with the degree of fever and other pathologic findings in a variety of infectious diseases than do levels of IL-1 or TNFα because of the persistence of IL-6 in the circulation. However, there is little or no evidence that IL-6 is—like IL-1 and TNFα—a lethal cytokine.

WHY FEVER? From an evolutionary perspective, the phenomenon of fever has been operative for hundreds of millions of years. Fish, amphibians, and reptiles develop fever. When fish are injected with bacterial endotoxin or gram-negative bacteria, they raise their body temperature by swimming to warmer water. When lizards are injected with bacteria or pyrogens, they generate fever by basking in the sun to raise their core temperature to "febrile" levels. In many situations, the elevation of body temperature increases chances for survival. The growth and virulence of several bacterial species are impaired at high temperatures; thus, for example, fever therapy was used in neurosyphilis before antibiotics became available. Type III pneumococci are particularly sensitive to high temperature and at 41°C grow poorly and may autolyze. Inhibition of fever in rabbits infected with type III pneumococci increases the mortality rate. Temperatures in the febrile range appear to increase the phagocytic and bactericidal activity of neutrophils and the cytotoxic effects of lymphocytes. Thus fever probably enhances the ability to survive infection. Redundancies among the pyrogens (IL-1β, IL-1α, TNFα, IL-6, interferons) suggest that it is beneficial to preserve a number of pathways for eliciting this response.

However, fever involves considerable "costs" to the host in addition to discomfort. For each elevation of body temperature by 1°C, there is an increase in O₂ consumption of 13 percent and an increase in caloric and fluid requirements. The increased metabolic demand may stress fetuses as well as patients with marginal cardiac or cerebral vascular supply. IL-1 and TNFα accelerate muscle catabolism, an effect leading to a loss of body weight and a negative nitrogen balance. Essentially, skeletal muscle is utilized as an energy source, with liberation of amino acids for gluconeogenesis and for the synthesis of acute-phase proteins and formation of clones of immune cells. Fever reduces mental acuity and can produce delirium and stupor. Children are prone to develop seizures with fevers, particularly if they have a history of seizures. A single episode of a temperature of ≥37.8°C (100°F) in the first trimester of pregnancy doubles the risk of neural tube defects in the fetus.

ACCOMPANIMENTS OF FEVER Not surprisingly, many features associated with fever, including back pain, generalized myal-

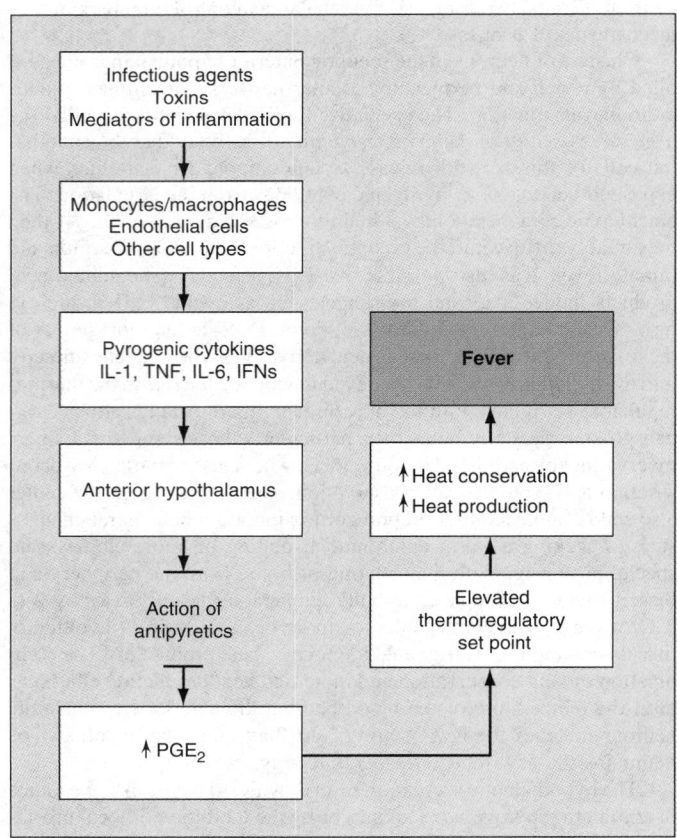

FIGURE 17-1 Chronology of events required for the induction of fever.

gias, arthralgias, anorexia, and somnolence, can be reproduced by infusions of purified cytokines. These symptoms may be reduced by cyclooxygenase inhibitors. *Chills*, a sensation of cold occurring in most fevers, are part of the central nervous system (CNS) response to the thermoregulatory set point's call for more heat. A *rigor*, a profound chill with piloerection ("goose flesh") accompanied by chattering of the teeth and severe shivering, is common in bacterial, rickettsial, and protozoal diseases and in influenza (but not in other viral diseases). Rigors can be produced by sepsis; by systemic infections such as leptospirosis, brucellosis, rat-bite fever, and endocarditis; by malaria; by the intermittent sepsis seen with abscesses; and by lymphoma, leukemia, renal cell carcinoma, and hepatoma. Rigors are also common with drug-induced fevers. *Sweats* occur with the activation of heat-loss mechanisms by antipyretic treatment, by attainment of a new "thermal ceiling," or by elimination of the febrile stimulus. The intermittent administration of antipyretics may exaggerate swings of temperature, thereby causing chilliness, discomfort, and exhaustion. Hypothalamic reflexes trigger sweating, which allows rapid dissipation of heat by evaporative loss.

Alterations of mental status and convulsions are common among the very young and the very old and among patients with dementia, hepatic failure, or chronic renal failure. A progression from irritability to delirium to frank obtundation usually clears with the abating of fever.

Convulsions typically develop in febrile infants and in febrile children less than 5 years old, being particularly common at the onset of febrile disease and at higher temperatures (>40°C). Febrile convulsions in children are not necessarily a sign of significant cerebral disease, but a CNS disorder must be excluded in these cases. Fever may precipitate seizures in epileptic adults as well.

Approach to the Patient

History   It is in the diagnosis of a febrile illness that the science and art of medicine come together. In no other clinical situation is a meticulous history more important. Painstaking attention must be paid to the chronology of symptoms in relation to the use of drugs (including those taken without a physician's supervision) or treatments such as surgical or dental procedures. The exact nature of any prosthetic materials and/or implanted devices should be ascertained. A careful occupational history should include exposures to animals; toxic fumes; potential infectious agents; possible antigens; or other febrile or infected individuals in the home, workplace, or school. A history of the geographic areas in which the patient has lived and a travel history should include locations during military service. Information on unusual hobbies, dietary proclivities (such as raw or poorly cooked meat, raw fish, and unpasteurized milk or cheeses), and household pets should be elicited, as should that on sexual orientation and practices, including precautions taken or omitted. Attention should be directed to the use of tobacco, marijuana, intravenous drugs, or alcohol; trauma; animal bites; tick or other insect bites; and prior transfusions, immunizations, drug allergies, or hypersensitivities. A careful family history should include information on family members with tuberculosis, other febrile or infectious diseases, arthritis or collagen vascular disease, or unusual familial symptomatology such as deafness, urticaria, fevers and polyserositis, bone pain, or anemia. Ethnic origin may be critical. For example, blacks are more likely than persons in other groups to have hemoglobinopathies. Turks, Arabs, Armenians, and Sephardic Jews are especially likely to have familial Mediterranean fever.

Patterns of Fever   The widespread use of antipyretics, glucocorticoids, and antibiotics can alter the course of fever so that "classic" fever patterns are not seen. Some patterns are clinically informative, however. Whereas the circadian temperature pattern is preserved and in fact exaggerated in most fevers, it may be reversed in typhoid fever and disseminated tuberculosis. Temperature-pulse dissociation (relative bradycardia) is seen in typhoid fever as well as in brucellosis, leptospirosis, some drug-associated fevers, and many factitious fevers. Bradycardia in the presence of fever also may signify cardiac conduction abnormalities, as it does in acute rheumatic fever, Lyme disease, viral myocarditis, or valve-ring abscess complicating bacterial endocarditis.

Fever may be sustained, intermittent, remittent, or relapsing. A *sustained* fever is one in which temperature elevation is persistent, with minimal variation. With *intermittent* fever, there is an exaggeration of the normal circadian rhythm; when this variation is extremely large, the fever is termed *hectic* or *septic*. Intermittent, hectic, and septic patterns are common in deep-seated or systemic infections, malignancy, and drug fevers. When hectic fevers occur daily, they are sometimes termed *quotidian*.

Remittent fever, in which the temperature falls each day but not to normal, is typical for tuberculosis, viral diseases, many bacterial infections, and noninfectious conditions. It should be emphasized that newborns, the elderly, patients with chronic renal or hepatic failure, patients taking glucocorticoids, or patients with bacteremic shock may fail to generate fever altogether; in these individuals, *hypothermia* may be a sign of severe infection.

With *relapsing* fevers, febrile episodes are separated by intervals of normal temperature; when paroxysms occur on the first and third days, the fever is called *tertian*. *Plasmodium vivax* causes tertian fevers. *Quartan* fevers are associated with paroxysms on the first and fourth days and are seen with *Plasmodium malariae*. Other relapsing fevers are related to *Borrelia* infections and rat-bite fever, which are both associated with days of fever followed by a several-day afebrile period and then a relapse of days of fever. Pel-Ebstein fever, with fevers lasting 3 to 10 days followed by afebrile periods of 3 to 10 days, is classic for Hodgkin's disease and other lymphomas. Another characteristic fever is that of cyclic neutropenia, in which fevers occur every 21 days and accompany the neutropenia.

Physical Examination   A meticulous physical examination should be repeated on a regular basis. All the vital signs are relevant. The temperature may be taken orally or rectally, but the site used should be consistent. Axillary temperatures are notoriously unreliable, as are oral temperatures taken after recent consumption of hot or cold drinks, smoking, or hyperventilation.

In some cases, patients are thoroughly examined at the time of initial evaluation, but the diagnostic emphasis then shifts to laboratory data and other diagnostic procedures. Particular attention should be paid to daily (or sometimes more frequent) physical examination, which should continue until the diagnosis is certain and the anticipated response has been achieved. Special attention should be paid to the skin, lymph nodes, eyes, nail beds, cardiovascular system, chest, abdomen, musculoskeletal system, and nervous system. Rectal examination is imperative. The penis, prostate, scrotum, and testes should be examined carefully, and the foreskin, if present, retracted. Pelvic examination must be part of every complete physical examination of a woman.

Laboratory Tests   Few signs and symptoms in medicine have as many diagnostic possibilities as fever. If the history, epidemiologic situation, or physical examination suggests more than a simple viral illness or streptococcal pharyngitis, then laboratory testing is indicated. The tempo and complexity of the workup will depend on the pace of the illness, diagnostic considerations, and the immune status of the host. If findings are focal or if the history, epidemiologic setting, or physical examination suggests certain diagnoses, the laboratory examination can be focused. If fever is undifferentiated, the "diagnostic nets" must be cast farther, and certain guidelines are indicated, as follows.

CLINICAL PATHOLOGY   The workup should include a complete blood count; a differential count should be performed manually or with an instrument sensitive to the identification of eosinophils, juvenile or band forms, toxic granulations, and Döhle bodies, the last three of which are suggestive of bacterial infection. Neutropenia may be seen with some viral infections, particularly parvovirus B19 infection; drug reactions; systemic lupus erythematosus; typhoid; brucellosis; and infiltrative diseases of the bone marrow, including lymphoma, leukemia, tuberculosis, and histoplasmosis. Lymphocytosis may be seen with typhoid, brucellosis, tuberculosis, and viral disease. Atypical lymphocytes are documented in many viral diseases, including infection with

Epstein-Barr virus, cytomegalovirus, or human immunodeficiency virus; dengue; rubella; varicella; measles; and viral hepatitis. This abnormality also occurs in serum sickness and toxoplasmosis. Monocytosis is a feature of typhoid, tuberculosis, brucellosis, and lymphoma. Eosinophilia may be associated with hypersensitivity drug reactions, Hodgkin's disease, adrenal insufficiency, and certain metazoan infections. If the febrile illness appears to be severe or is prolonged, the smear should be examined carefully and the erythrocyte sedimentation rate should be determined. Urinalysis, with examination of urinary sediment, is indicated. It is axiomatic that any abnormal fluid accumulation (pleural, peritoneal, joint), even if previously sampled, merits reexamination in the presence of undiagnosed fever. Joint fluids should be examined for crystals. Bone marrow biopsy (not simple aspiration) for histopathologic studies (as well as culture) is indicated when marrow infiltration by pathogens or tumor cells is possible. Stool should be inspected for occult blood; an inspection for fecal leukocytes, ova, or parasites also may be indicated.

CHEMISTRY Electrolyte, glucose, blood urea nitrogen, and creatinine levels should be measured. Liver function tests are usually indicated if efforts to identify the cause of fever do not point to the involvement of another organ. Additional assessments (e.g., measurement of creatine phosphokinase) can be added as the workup progresses.

MICROBIOLOGY Smears and cultures of specimens from the throat, urethra, anus, cervix, and vagina should be assessed in appropriate situations. Sputum evaluation (Gram's staining, staining for acid-fast bacilli, culture) is indicated for any patient with fever and cough. Cultures of blood, abnormal fluid collections, and urine are indicated when fever is thought to indicate more than uncomplicated viral illness. Cerebrospinal fluid should be examined and cultured if meningismus, severe headache, or a change in mental status is noted.

RADIOLOGY A chest x-ray is usually part of the evaluation for any significant febrile illness.

Outcome of Diagnostic Efforts In most cases of fever, either the patient recovers spontaneously or the history, physical examination, and initial screening laboratory studies lead to a diagnosis. In the former case, a viral illness is usually considered to have been the source of the fever. When fever continues for 2 to 3 weeks, during which time repeat physical examinations and laboratory tests are unrevealing, the patient is provisionally diagnosed as having fever of unknown origin (see Chap. 125).

℞ TREATMENT

When to Treat Fever It is distressingly common in hospitals to find "routine," "standing," or "prn" orders for the use of antipyretics (such as acetaminophen) for a temperature above an arbitrary level; it is also common to find patients awake and alert but most uncomfortable, shivering on a cooling blanket. Such therapies have their appropriate application but are frequently used without therapeutic rationale. The first decision to make is whether an elevated temperature in fact reflects *fever* or *hyperthermia*.

Hyperthermia is an elevation of core temperature *without elevation of the hypothalamic set point*. Hyperthermia is most commonly due to inadequate heat dissipation, though more rarely the primary cause is excessive heat production with heat dissipation inadequate to compensate. The various syndromes of hyperthermia, as distinguished from true elevation of the hypothalamic set point, or fever, are listed in Table 17-1.

Heat stroke, caused by thermoregulatory failure in association with a warm environment, may be categorized as exertional or nonexertional. *Exertional heat stroke* typically occurs in younger individuals exercising at ambient temperatures and/or humidities that are higher than normal. Even in normal individuals, dehydration or the use of common medications (e.g., over-the-counter antihista-

mines with anticholinergic side effects) may help to precipitate exertional heat stroke.

Nonexertional or *classic heat stroke* typically occurs in elderly individuals, particularly during heat waves. For example, in Chicago in July 1995, a total of 465 deaths were certified as heat related. The elderly, the bedridden, persons taking anticholinergic or antiparkinsonian drugs or diuretics, and individuals confined to poorly ventilated and un-air-conditioned environments are most susceptible.

Drug-induced hyperthermia has become increasingly common as a result of the increased use of prescription psychotropic drugs and illicit drugs. Drug-induced hyperthermia may be caused by monoamine oxidase inhibitors, tricyclic antidepressants, and amphetamines and by the illicit use of phencyclidine, lysergic acid diethylamide (LSD), or cocaine.

Malignant hyperthermia is an inherited abnormality of skeletal-muscle sarcoplasmic reticulum that causes a rapid increase in intracellular calcium levels in response to halothane and other inhalational anesthetics or to succinylcholine. Elevated temperature, increased muscle metabolism, rigidity, rhabdomyolysis, acidosis, and cardiovascular instability develop rapidly. Cessation of anesthesia and administration of dantrolene sodium are the immediately indicated therapies. The *neuroleptic malignant syndrome* can occur with phenothiazines and other drugs such as haloperidol and is characterized by muscle rigidity, autonomic dysregulation, and hyperthermia. This disorder appears to be caused by the inhibition of central dopamine receptors in the hypothalamus, which results in increased heat generation and decreased heat dissipation. Thyrotoxicosis and pheochromocytoma can also cause increased thermogenesis.

A high core temperature in a patient likely to have hyperthermia (due to environmental exposure or treatment with anticholinergic or neuroleptic drugs, tricyclic antidepressants, succinylcholine, or halothane) along with appropriate clinical findings (dry skin, hallucinations, delirium, pupil dilation, muscle rigidity, and/or elevated levels of creatine phosphokinase) is characteristic of hyperthermia. The attempt to lower the already-normal hypothalamic set point is of little use. Physical cooling with sponging, fans, cooling blankets, and even ice baths should be initiated immediately in conjunction with the administration of intravenous fluids and appropriate pharmacologic agents (such as dantrolene for malignant hyperthermia and the neuroleptic malignant syndrome or physostigmine for tricyclic antidepressant overdose). If insufficient cooling is achieved by external means, internal cooling can be achieved by gastric or peritoneal lavage with iced saline. In extreme circumstances, hemodialysis or even cardiopulmonary bypass with cooling of blood may be performed.

Malignant hyperthermia should be treated immediately with intravenous dantrolene. The recommended dose of dantrolene is 1 to

---

Table 17-1

Causes of Hyperthermia Syndromes

Heat stroke
    Exertional: Exercise in higher-than-normal heat and/or humidity
    Nonexertional: Anticholinergics, including antihistamines; antiparkinsonian drugs; diuretics; phenothiazines

Drug-induced hyperthermia
    Amphetamines; monoamine oxidase inhibitors; cocaine; phencyclidine; tricyclic antidepressants; LSD

Neuroleptic malignant syndrome
    Phenothiazines; butyrophenones, including haloperidol and bromperidol; fluoxetine; loxapine; tricyclic dibenzodiazepines; metoclopramide; domperidone; thiothixene; molindone

Malignant hyperthermia
    Inhalational anesthetics; succinylcholine

Endocrinopathy
    Thyrotoxicosis
    Pheochromocytoma

SOURCE: After FJ Curley, RS Irwin.

2.5 mg/kg of body weight given intravenously every 6 h for at least 24 to 48 h—until oral dantrolene can be administered, if needed. Procainamide should also be administered to patients with malignant hyperthermia because of the likelihood of ventricular fibrillation in this syndrome. Dantrolene at similar doses is indicated in the neuroleptic malignant syndrome and drug-induced hyperthermia and may even be useful in the hyperthermia of thyrotoxicosis. The neuroleptic malignant syndrome may also be treated with bromocriptine, levodopa, amantadine, or nifedipine or by induction of muscle paralysis with curare and pancuronium.

With *hyperpyrexia* (temperature $\geq 41°C$), treatment with antipyretics is clearly indicated, and physical cooling while "resetting" the hypothalamic set point with antipyretics will speed the process. Antipyretics also suppress the constitutional symptoms that accompany fever (myalgias, chills, headache.). However, there is little evidence that low-grade or moderate fever is harmful or that antipyretic therapy for such fever is beneficial, with the aforementioned exceptions—children with febrile seizures, pregnant women, and patients with impaired cardiac, pulmonary, or cerebral function. Temperature is often suppressed needlessly, and "routine" antipyretic orders may obscure the important clinical information to be gained by following the upward or downward course of a patient's temperature. Nonsteroidal anti-inflammatory drugs (NSAIDs) and glucocorticoids may mask the inflammatory features of a localized infection, thus preventing its detection and even encouraging its spread. In addition, the drugs themselves may cause adverse effects. The administration of aspirin to children with viral diseases is to be avoided because of the possibility of Reye's syndrome, which occurs in association with influenza and varicella and occasionally with enterovirus infection. The antiplatelet and even antiphagocytic effects of aspirin have led to the general use of acetaminophen. Acetaminophen is a poor cyclooxygenase inhibitor in peripheral tissue and thus lacks anti-inflammatory activity; in the CNS, the oxidation of acetaminophen converts it to an active cyclooxygenase inhibitor—an event explaining its antipyretic effect. Ibuprofen may be safe for children, with possibly more pronounced and more prolonged temperature reduction at doses similar to those of acetaminophen. Ibuprofen does not appear to pose a risk of Reye's syndrome, but the caveat about bacterial infections remains. Other NSAIDs, particularly indomethacin and naproxen, are also useful as antipyretics.

Glucocorticoids are potent antipyretics. They inhibit PGE_2 synthesis by inhibiting phospholipase A_2, and they block both mRNA transcription for IL-1 and $TNF\alpha$ and translation of these cytokines. The potent immunosuppressive and antiphagocytic effects of glucocorticoids limit their use as antipyretics to febrile states in which inflammation is a major pathogenic factor—such as bacterial meningitis, tuberculous pericarditis, and vasculitis. The severe rigors that accompany some fevers can be reduced with meperidine, morphine sulfate, prochlorperazine, or chlorpromazine. These two classes of agents combined have an additive suppressive effect on rigors; however, care must be taken to avoid hypotension when these agents are administered either singly or together.

Specific Therapy The advantages and disadvantages of antipyretic therapy have just been discussed. More specific therapy is based on the differential diagnosis for a given patient, including the relative probabilities of syndromes that are imminently life-threatening, the risks of not treating, and the risks of treatment itself. Sepsis of various etiologies is a leading consideration in determining the need for therapy.

Sepsis is defined as evidence of infection with a systemic response. *Sepsis syndrome* refers to a systemic response sufficient to produce organ dysfunction, and *septic shock* is the sepsis syndrome with documented hypotension. In a nonimmunocompromised adult with sepsis, gram-positive infection, gram-negative rod infection, and meningococcal infection can be "covered" by a variety of antibiotic combinations, including imipenem, ticarcillin/clavulanate, or a third-generation cephalosporin. The suspected involvement of a methicillin-resistant strain of *Staphylococcus aureus* dictates the addition of vancomycin to the regimen. If the patient has had a

splenectomy, therapy with ampicillin/sulbactam, ceftriaxone, cefotaxime, or cefuroxime is indicated. Suspicion of *Legionella* dictates the addition of erythromycin (possibly with rifampin) or, alternatively, of clarithromycin or azithromycin. In appropriate settings, the involvement of rickettsiae should be suspected, and the administration of either doxycycline or chloramphenicol is indicated. If a case of septic shock has no evident source, the differential diagnosis should include meningococcemia, staphylococcal and streptococcal toxic shock syndromes, and (rarely) gram-negative bacteremia. A combination of high-dose penicillin and penicillinase-resistant synthetic penicillins (nafcillin, oxacillin) will cover these cocci. Clindamycin and early fasciotomy of any putative soft-tissue lesion should be considered in cases of streptococcal toxic shock; tampons or wounds should be sought in staphylococcal toxic shock. A third-generation cephalosporin suffices to treat gram-negative bacteremia. Ticarcillin/clavulanate or piperacillin/tazobactam is an alternative. If a typhoidal syndrome is suspected, therapy with a fluoroquinolone such as ciprofloxacin or ofloxacin is indicated. Intravenous penicillin should be used if leptospirosis is suspected. In appropriate geographic areas, plague is a consideration; treatment with an aminoglycoside or chloramphenicol is indicated in this situation. Suspected endocarditis should be treated with a combination of penicillin, oxacillin/nafcillin, or vancomycin and gentamicin, depending on the type of patient and the suspected origin of infection. In intravenous drug users, the involvement of methicillin-sensitive or -resistant *S. aureus* and gram-negative bacilli should also be considered.

A febrile patient with headache, myalgia, cough, abdominal pain, nausea, or vomiting who develops interstitial infiltrates and/or respiratory distress may be infected with hantavirus. A controlled trial of intravenous ribavirin, performed in China with the Korean form of the disease, suggested benefit from therapy.

Consideration must also be given to acute febrile conditions in which the prevention of tissue damage requires immediate therapeutic intervention with agents other than anti-infectives. Examples include aspirin for acute rheumatic fever, intravenous gamma globulin for the Kawasaki syndrome, and glucocorticoids and/or cyclophosphamide for various forms of acute vasculitis.

Ultimately, the physician's task in dealing with these diverse diagnostic and therapeutic possibilities is to thoughtfully distill the data acquired by meticulous history-taking, physical examination, and laboratory studies; to narrow the possibilities; and to make a risk-benefit assessment regarding empirical therapy. In the "art" of medicine, this skill is known as "judgment." There is no formula for this type of judgment in any textbook.

BIBLIOGRAPHY

ATKINS E: Fever: Historical aspects, in *Interleukin-1, Inflammation, and Disease,* R Bomford, B Henderson (eds). New York, Elsevier Science Publishers, 1989, pp 3–15

CANNON JG et al: Circulating interleukin-1 and tumor necrosis factor in septic shock and experimental endotoxin fever. J Infect Dis 161:79, 1990

CENTERS FOR DISEASE CONTROL AND PREVENTION: Heat-related mortality—Chicago. MMWR 44:577, 1995

CURLEY FJ, IRWIN RS: Disorders of temperature control. Hyperthermia, in *Intensive Care Medicine,* 3d ed, JM Rippe et al (eds). Boston, Little, Brown, 1996, pp 859–873

DINARELLO CA: Interleukin-1 and interleukin-1 antagonism. Blood 77: 1627, 1991

——, WOLFF SM: Pathogenesis of fever, in *Principles and Practice of Infectious Diseases,* 3d ed, GL Mandell et al (eds). New York, Wiley, 1990, pp 462–467

—— et al: New concepts on the pathogenesis of fever. Rev Infect Dis 10:168, 1988

HECKER RB et al: Bayesian analysis of noninvasive versus oral temperature measurements to determine hypothermia in postoperative patients. South Med J 89:71, 1996

MACKOWIAK PA et al: A critical appraisal of 98.6°F, the upper limit of the normal body temperature, and other legacies of Carl Reinhold August Wunderlich. JAMA 268:1578, 1992

————: Carl Reinhold August Wunderlich and the evolution of clinical thermometry. Clin Infect Dis 18:458, 1994

MILENO MD et al: Coagulation of whole blood stimulates interleukin-1β gene expression. J Infect Dis 172:308, 1995

MILUNSKY A et al: Maternal heat exposure and neural tube defects. JAMA 268:882, 1992

STEINMETZ HT et al: Increase in interleukin-6 serum level preceding fever in granulocytopenia and correlation with death from sepsis. J Infect Dis 171:225, 1995

18 Elaine T. Kaye, Kenneth M. Kaye

FEVER AND RASH

The acutely ill patient with fever and rash often presents a diagnostic challenge for physicians. The distinctive appearance of an eruption in concert with a clinical syndrome may facilitate a prompt diagnosis and the institution of life-saving therapy or critical infection-control interventions.

Approach to the Patient

A thorough history of patients with fever and rash includes the following relevant information: immune status, medications taken within the previous month, specific travel history, immunization status, exposure to domestic pets and other animals, history of animal or arthropod bites, existence of cardiac abnormalities, presence of prosthetic material, recent exposure to ill individuals, and exposure to sexually transmitted diseases. The history should also include the site of onset of the rash and its direction and rate of spread.

A thorough physical examination entails close attention to the rash, with an assessment and precise definition of its salient features. First, it is critical to determine the *type* of lesions that make up the eruption. *Macules* are flat lesions defined by an area of changed color (i.e., a blanchable erythema). *Papules* are raised, solid lesions <5 mm in diameter; *plaques* are lesions >5 mm in diameter with a flat, plateau-like surface; and *nodules* are lesions >5 mm in diameter with a more rounded configuration. *Wheals* (urticaria, hives) are papules or plaques that are pale pink and may appear annular (ringlike) as they enlarge; classic (nonvasculitic) wheals are transient, lasting only 24 to 48 h in any defined area. *Vesicles* (<5 mm) and *bullae* (>5 mm) are circumscribed, elevated lesions containing fluid. *Pustules* are raised lesions containing purulent exudate; vesicular processes such as varicella or herpes simplex may evolve to pustules. *Nonpalpable purpura* is a flat lesion that is due to bleeding into the skin; if <3 mm in diameter, the purpuric lesions are termed *petechiae*; if >3 mm, they are termed *ecchymoses*. *Palpable purpura* is a raised lesion that is due to inflammation of the vessel wall (vasculitis) with subsequent hemorrhage.

Other pertinent features of rashes include their *configuration* (i.e., annular or target), the *arrangement* of their lesions, and their *distribution* (i.e., central or peripheral). → *For further discussion, see Chaps. 54 and 57.*

CLASSIFICATION OF RASH This chapter reviews rashes that reflect systemic disease but does not include localized skin eruptions (i.e., cellulitis, impetigo) that may also be associated with fever (see Chap. 133). Rashes are classified herein on the basis of the morphology and distribution of lesions. For practical purposes, this classification system is based on the most typical disease presentations. However, morphology may vary as rashes evolve, and the presentation of diseases with rashes is subject to many variations (see Chap. 57). For instance, the classic petechial rash of Rocky Mountain spotted fever (RMSF) may initially consist of blanchable erythematous macules on the hands and feet; at times, the rash associated with RMSF may not be predominantly acral, or a rash may not develop at all.

Diseases with fever and rash may be classified by type of eruption: centrally distributed maculopapular, peripheral, confluent desquamative erythematous, vesiculobullous, urticarial, nodular, and purpuric (Table 18-1). For a more detailed discussion of each disease associated with a rash, the reader is referred to the chapter dealing with that specific disease. (Reference chapters are cited in the text and listed in Table 18-1.)

Centrally Distributed Maculopapular Eruptions Centrally distributed rashes, in which lesions are primarily truncal, are the most common type of eruption. The rash of *measles* (rubeola) starts at the hairline 2 to 3 days into the illness and moves down the body, sparing the palms and soles (see Chap. 196). It begins as discrete erythematous lesions, which become confluent as the rash spreads. Koplik's spots (1- to 2-mm white or bluish lesions with an erythematous halo on the buccal mucosa) are pathognomonic for measles and are generally seen during the first 2 days of symptoms. They should not be confused with Fordyce's spots (ectopic sebaceous glands), which have no erythematous halos and are found in the mouth of healthy individuals. Koplik's spots may briefly overlap with the measles exanthem.

German measles (rubella) also spreads from the hairline downward; unlike that of measles, however, the rash of rubella tends to clear from originally affected areas as it migrates and may be pruritic (see Chap. 197). Forchheimer spots (palatal petechiae) may develop but are nonspecific since they also develop in mononucleosis (Chap. 186) and scarlet fever (Chap. 143). Postauricular and suboccipital adenopathy and arthritis are common among adults with German measles. Exposure of pregnant women to ill individuals should be avoided, as rubella causes severe congenital abnormalities. Numerous strains of enteroviruses (Chap. 195), primarily echoviruses and coxsackieviruses, cause nonspecific syndromes of fever and eruptions that may mimic rubella or measles. Both infectious mononucleosis caused by Epstein-Barr virus and primary infection with human immunodeficiency virus (HIV; Chap. 308) may also include pharyngitis, lymphadenopathy, and a nonspecific maculopapular exanthem.

The rash of *erythema infectiosum* (fifth disease), which is caused by human parvovirus B19, primarily affects children 3 to 12 years old; it develops after fever has resolved as a bright blanchable erythema on the cheeks ("slapped cheeks") with perioral pallor (Chap. 189). A more diffuse rash (often pruritic) appears the next day on the trunk and extremities and then rapidly develops into a lacy reticular eruption that may wax and wane (especially with temperature change) over 3 weeks. Adults with fifth disease often have arthritis, and fetal hydrops can develop in association with this condition in pregnant women.

Exanthem subitum (roseola) is most common among children under 3 years of age (Chap. 187). As in erythema infectiosum, the rash usually appears after fever has subsided. It consists of 2- to 3-mm rose-pink macules and papules that rarely coalesce, occur initially on the trunk and sometimes on the extremities (sparing the face), and fade within 2 days.

Though drug reactions have many manifestations, including urticaria, exanthematous *drug-induced eruptions* (Chap. 56) are most common and are often difficult to distinguish from viral exanthems. Eruptions elicited by drugs are usually more intensely erythematous and pruritic than viral exanthems, but this distinction is not reliable. A history of new medications and an absence of prostration may help to distinguish a drug-related rash from an eruption of another etiology. Rashes may persist for up to 2 weeks after administration of the offending agent is discontinued. Certain populations are more prone than others to drug rashes. Of HIV-infected patients, 50 to 60 percent develop a rash in response to sulfa drugs; 50 to 100 percent of patients with mononucleosis due to Epstein-Barr virus develop a rash when given ampicillin.

Rickettsial illnesses (Chap. 179) should be considered in the evaluation of individuals with centrally distributed maculopapular eruptions. The usual setting for *epidemic typhus* is a site of war or natural disaster in which people are exposed to body lice. A diagnosis of recrudescent typhus should be considered in European immigrants to the United States. However, an indigenous form of typhus, presumably transmitted by flying squirrels, has been reported in the southeastern United

Table 18-1

Diseases Associated with Fever and Rash

Disease	Etiology	Description	Group Affected/ Epidemiological Factors	Clinical Syndrome	Chapter Reference
CENTRALLY DISTRIBUTED MACULOPAPULAR ERUPTIONS					
Measles (rubeola, first disease)	Paramyxovirus	Discrete lesions that become confluent as rash spreads from hairline downward, sparing palms and soles; lasts ≥3 d; Koplik's spots	Nonimmune individuals	Cough, conjunctivitis, coryza, severe prostration	196
German measles (rubella, third disease)	Togavirus	Spreads from hairline downward, clearing as it spreads; Forchheimer spots	Nonimmune individuals	Adenopathy, arthritis	197
Erythema infectiosum (fifth disease)	Human parvovirus B19	Bright-red "slapped-cheek" appearance followed by diffuse lacy reticular rash that waxes and wanes over 3 weeks	Most common in children aged 3–12 years; occurs in winter and spring	Mild fever; arthritis in adults	189
Exanthem subitum (roseola, sixth disease)	Human herpesvirus 6	Diffuse maculopapular eruption (sparing face); resolves within 2 d	Usually affects children <3 years old	Rash following resolution of fever; similar to Boston exanthem (echovirus 16)	187
Primary HIV infection	HIV	Nonspecific diffuse macules and papules; may be urticarial; palatal ulcers in some cases	Individuals recently infected with HIV	Pharyngitis, adenopathy, arthralgias	308
Infectious mononucleosis	Epstein-Barr virus	Diffuse maculopapular eruption (10–15% of cases; 90% if ampicillin is given); urticaria in some cases; periorbital edema (50%); palatal petechiae (25%)	Adolescents, young adults	Hepatosplenomegaly, pharyngitis, cervical lymphadenopathy, atypical lymphocytosis, heterophile antibody	186
Other viral exanthems	Echoviruses 2, 4, 9, 11, 16, 19, and 25; coxsackieviruses A9, B1, and B5	Skin findings mimicking rubella or measles	Affect children more commonly than adults	Nonspecific viral syndromes	195
Exanthematous drug-induced eruption	Drugs (antibiotics, anticonvulsants, diuretics, etc.)	Intensely pruritic, bright-red macules and papules, symmetric on trunk and extremities; may become confluent	Occurs 2–3 d after exposure in those previously sensitized; otherwise, after 2–3 weeks (but can occur anytime, even after drug is discontinued)	Variable findings: fever and eosinophilia	56
Epidemic typhus	Rickettsia prowazekii	Maculopapular eruption, usually sparing face, palms, soles; evolves from blanchable macules to confluent eruption with petechiae; rash evanescent in recrudescent typhus (Brill-Zinsser disease)	Exposure to body lice; occurrence of recrudescent typhus as relapse after 30–50 years	Headache, myalgias; 10–40% mortality if untreated; milder clinical presentation in recrudescent form	179
Endemic (murine) typhus	Rickettsia typhi	Maculopapular eruption, usually sparing palms, soles	Exposure to rat or cat fleas	Headache, myalgias	179
Scrub typhus	Rickettsia tsutsugamushi	Diffuse macular rash starting on trunk; eschar at site of mite bite	Endemic in South Pacific, Australia, Asia; transmitted by mites	Headache, myalgias, regional adenopathy, mortality up to 30% if untreated	179
Rickettsial spotted fevers	Rickettsia conorii (boutonneuse fever), Rickettsia australis (North Queensland tick typhus), Rickettsia sibirica (Siberian tick typhus)	Eschar at site of bite; maculopapular (rarely, vesicular and petechial) eruption on proximal extremities, spreading to trunk and face	Exposure to ticks; R. conorii in Mediterranean region, India, Africa; R. australis in Australia; R. sibirica in Siberia, Mongolia	Headache, myalgias, regional adenopathy	179
Ehrlichiosis	Ehrlichia species	Maculopapular eruption (40% of cases), sparing extremities, palms, soles; feature distinguishing from RMSF is central distribution with peripheral sparing	Tick-borne; most common in U.S. Southeast and southern Midwest	Headache, myalgias, leukopenia	179

(continued)

Table 18-1—*(Continued)*

Diseases Associated with Fever and Rash

Disease	Etiology	Description	Group Affected/ Epidemiological Factors	Clinical Syndrome	Chapter Reference
Leptospirosis	*Leptospira interrogans*	Maculopapular eruption; conjunctivitis; scleral hemorrhage in some cases	Exposure to water contaminated with animal urine	Myalgias; aseptic meningitis; *fulminant form*: icterohemorrhagic fever (Weil's disease)	176
Lyme disease	*Borrelia burgdorferi*	Papule expanding to erythematous annular lesion with central clearing (ECM; average diameter, 15 cm), sometimes with concentric rings, sometimes with indurated or vesicular center; multiple secondary ECM lesions in some cases	Bite of tick vector	Headache, myalgias, chills, photophobia occurring acutely; CNS disease, myocardial disease, arthritis weeks to months later in some cases	178
Typhoid fever	*Salmonella typhi*	Blanchable erythematous macules and papules, 2–4 mm, usually on trunk (rose spots)	Ingestion of contaminated food or water (rare in U.S.)	Variable abdominal pain and diarrhea; headache, myalgias, hepatosplenomegaly	158
Rat-bite fever (sodoku)	*Spirillum minus*	Eschar at site of bite; then blotchy violaceous or red-brown central rash	Rate bite; primarily found in Asia; rare in U.S.	Regional adenopathy, recurrent fevers if untreated	135
Relapsing fever	*Borrelia* species	Central rash at end of febrile episode; petechiae in some cases	Exposure to ticks or body lice	Recurrent fever, headache, myalgias, hepatosplenomegaly	177
Erythema marginatum (rheumatic fever)	Group A *Streptococcus*	Erythematous annular papules and plaques occurring as polycyclic lesions in waves over trunk, proximal extremities; evolving and resolving within hours	Patients with rheumatic fever	Pharyngitis preceding polyarthritis, carditis, subcutaneous nodules, chorea	236
Systemic lupus erythematosus	Autoimmune disease	Macular and papular erythema, often in sun-exposed areas; discoid lupus lesions (local atrophy, scale, pigmentary changes); periungual telangiectasis; malar rash; vasculitis sometimes causing urticaria, palpable purpura; oral erosions in some cases	Most common in young to middle-aged women; flares precipitated by sun exposure	Arthritis; cardiac, pulmonary, renal, hematologic, and vasculitic disease	312
Adult-onset Still's disease	Autoimmune disease	Transient 2- to 5-mm erythematous papules appearing at height of fever on trunk, proximal extremities; lesions evanescent	Young adults; more common in females	High spiking fever, polyarthritis, splenomegaly; erythrocyte sedimentation rate, >100 mm/h	326

PERIPHERAL ERUPTIONS

Disease	Etiology	Description	Group Affected/ Epidemiological Factors	Clinical Syndrome	Chapter Reference
Chronic meningococcemia, disseminated gonococcal infection*	—	—	—	—	149, 150
RMSF	*Rickettsia rickettsii*	Rash beginning on wrists and ankles and spreading centripetally; appears on palms and soles late in disease; lesion evolution from blanchable macules to petechiae	Tick vector; widespread but more common in southeastern and southwest-central U.S.	Headache, myalgias, abdominal pain; mortality up to 40% if untreated	179
Secondary syphilis	*Treponema pallidum*	Coincident primary chancre in 10% of cases; copper-colored, scaly papular eruption, diffuse but prominent on palms and soles; rash never vesicular in adults; condyloma latum, mucous patches, and alopecia in some cases	Sexually transmitted	Fever, constitutional symptoms	174

(continued)

Disease	Etiology	Description	Group Affected/ Epidemiological Factors	Clinical Syndrome	Chapter Reference
Atypical measles	Paramyxovirus	Maculopapular eruption beginning on distal extremities and spreading centripetally; may evolve into vesicles or petechiae; edema of extremities; Koplik's spots absent	Individuals contracting measles who received killed measles vaccine between 1963 and 1967 in U.S.	Headache, nodular pneumonia	196
Hand-foot-and-mouth disease	Coxsackievirus A16	Tender vesicles, erosions in mouth; 0.25-cm papules on hands and feet with rim of erythema evolving into tender vesicles	Summer and fall; primarily children under 10 years; multiple family members	Transient fever	195
Erythema multiforme	Drugs, infection, idiopathic causes	Target lesions (central erythema surrounded by area of clearing and another rim of erythema) up to 2 cm; symmetric on knees, elbows, palms, soles; may become diffuse; may involve mucosal surfaces	Drug intake (i.e., sulfa, phenytoin, penicillin); herpes simplex or *Mycoplasma pneumoniae* infection	Varies with predisposing factor	—†
Rat-bite fever (Haverhill fever)	*Streptobacillus moniliformis*	Maculopapular rash over palms, soles, extremities; may be purpuric; may desquamate	Rat bite	Myalgias; arthritis (50%); fever recurrence in some cases	135
Bacterial endocarditis	*Streptococcus*, *Staphylococcus*, etc.	*Subacute course*: Osler's nodes (tender pink nodules on finger or toe pads); petechiae on skin and mucosa; splinter hemorrhages. *Acute course* (*S. aureus*): Janeway lesions (painless erythematous or hemorrhagic macules on palms and soles)	Abnormal heart valve, intravenous drug use	New heart murmur	126

CONFLUENT DESQUAMATIVE ERYTHEMAS

Disease	Etiology	Description	Group Affected/ Epidemiological Factors	Clinical Syndrome	Chapter Reference
Scarlet fever (second disease)	Group A *Streptococcus* (pyrogenic exotoxins A, B, C)	Diffuse blanchable erythema beginning on face and spreading to trunk and extremities; circumoral pallor; "sandpaper" texture to skin; accentuation of linear erythema in skin folds (Pastia's lines); enanthem of white evolving into red "strawberry" tongue; desquamation in second week	Most common in children aged 2–10 years; usually follows group A streptococcal pharyngitis	Fever, pharyngitis, headache	143
Kawasaki disease	Idiopathic causes	Rash similar to scarlet fever (scarlatiniform) or erythema multiforme; fissuring of lips, strawberry tongue; conjunctivitis; edema of hands, feet; desquamation later in disease	Children under 8 years	Cervical adenopathy, pharyngitis, coronary artery vasculitis	57, 319
Streptococcal toxic shock syndrome	Group A *Streptococcus* (associated with pyrogenic exotoxin A or certain M types)	When present, rash often scarlatiniform	May occur in setting of severe group A streptococcal infections, such as necrotizing fasciitis, bacteremia, pneumonia	Multiorgan failure, hypotension; 30% mortality rate	143
Staphylococcal toxic shock syndrome	*S. aureus* (toxic shock syndrome toxin 1, enterotoxin B or C)	Diffuse erythema involving palms; pronounced erythema of mucosal surfaces, conjunctivitis; desquamation 7–10 d into illness	Colonization with toxin-producing *S. aureus*	Fever >39°C (102°F), hypotension, multiorgan dysfunction	142

(continued)

Table 18-1—*(Continued)*

Diseases Associated with Fever and Rash

Disease	Etiology	Description	Group Affected/ Epidemiological Factors	Clinical Syndrome	Chapter Reference
Staphylococcal scalded-skin syndrome	*S. aureus*, phage group II	Diffuse tender erythema, often with bullae and desquamation; Nikolsky's sign	Colonization with toxin-producing *S. aureus*; occurs in children under 10 (termed "Ritter's disease" in neonates) or adults with renal dysfunction	Irritability; nasal or conjunctival secretions	142
Exfoliative erythroderma syndrome	Underlying psoriasis, eczema, drug eruption, mycosis fungoides	Diffuse erythema (often scaling) interspersed with lesions of underlying condition	Usually occurs in adults over age 50; more common in men	Fever, chills (i.e., difficulty with thermoregulation); lymphadenopathy	55, 56
Toxic epidermal necrolysis	Drugs, other causes (infection, neoplasm, graft-vs.-host disease)	Diffuse erythema or target-like lesions progressing to bullae, with sloughing and necrosis of the entire epidermis; Nikolsky's sign	Uncommon in children; more common in patients with HIV infection or graft-vs.-host disease	Dehydration, sepsis sometimes resulting from lack of normal skin integrity; 25% mortality	56, 308

VESICULOBULLOUS ERUPTIONS

Disease	Etiology	Description	Group Affected/ Epidemiological Factors	Clinical Syndrome	Chapter Reference
Hand-foot-and-mouth syndrome‡; staphylococcal scalded-skin syndrome, toxic epidermal necrolysis§	—	—	—	—	—†
Varicella (chickenpox)	Varicella-zoster virus	Macules (2–3 mm) evolving into papules, then vesicles (sometimes umbilicated), on an erythematous base ("dewdrops on a rose petal"); pustules then forming and crusting; lesions appearing in crops; may involve scalp, mouth; intensely pruritic	Usually affects children; 10% of adults susceptible; most common in late winter and spring	Malaise; mild disease in healthy children; more severe disease with complications in adults and immunocompromised children	185
Rickettsialpox	*Rickettsia akari*	Eschar found at site of mite bite; diffuse rash involving face, trunk, extremities; 2- to 10-mm papules and plaques evolving into vesicles and then crusting	Seen in urban settings; transmitted by mouse mites	Headache, myalgias, regional adenopathy; mild disease	179
Disseminated *Vibrio vulnificus* infection	*V. vulnificus*	Erythematous lesions evolving into hemorrhagic bullae and then into necrotic ulcers	Patients with cirrhosis; exposure by ingestion of contaminated saltwater seafood	Hypotension; 50% mortality	161
Ecthyma gangrenosum	*Pseudomonas aeruginosa*, other gram-negative rods, fungi	Indurated plaque evolving into hemorrhagic bulla or pustule that sloughs, resulting in eschar formation; erythematous halo; most common in axillary, groin, perianal regions	Usually affects neutropenic patients; occurs in up to 28% of individuals with *Pseudomonas* bacteremia	Clinical signs of sepsis	157

URTICARIAL ERUPTIONS

Disease	Etiology	Description	Group Affected/ Epidemiological Factors	Clinical Syndrome	Chapter Reference
Urticarial vasculitis	Serum sickness, connective-tissue disease, infection, idiopathic causes	Erythematous, circumscribed areas of edema; occasionally indurated; pruritic or burning; lesions sometimes purpuric; individual lesions lasting up to 5 d	In serum sickness, occurs 8–14 d after antigen exposure in nonsensitized individuals; may occur within 36 h in sensitized individuals	Malaise, lymphadenopathy, myalgias, arthralgias	319†

(continued)

Disease	Etiology	Description	Group Affected/ Epidemiological Factors	Clinical Syndrome	Chapter Reference
NODULAR ERUPTIONS					
Disseminated infection	Fungi (e.g., candidiasis, histoplasmosis, cryptococcosis, sporotrichosis, coccidioidomycosis); mycobacteria	Subcutaneous nodules (up to 3 cm); fluctuance, draining common with mycobacteria; necrotic nodules (extremities, periorbital or nasal regions) common with *Aspergillus, Mucor*	Immunocompromised hosts (i.e., bone marrow transplant recipients, patients undergoing chemotherapy, HIV-infected patients, alcoholics)	Features vary with organism	—†
Erythema nodosum (septal panniculitis)	Infections (e.g., streptococcal, fungal, mycobacterial, yersinial); drugs (e.g., sulfas, penicillins, oral contraceptives); sarcoidosis; idiopathic causes	Large, violaceous, nonulcerative, subcutaneous nodules; exquisitely tender; usually on lower legs but also on upper extremities	More common in females aged 15–30	Arthralgias (50%); features vary with associated condition	—†
Sweet's syndrome (acute febrile neutrophilic dermatosis)	Yersinial infection; lymphoproliferative disorders; idiopathic causes	Tender edematous nodules giving impression of vesiculation; usually on face, neck, upper extremities; when on lower extremities, may mimic erythema nodosum	More common in women and in persons aged 30–60	Headache, arthralgias, leukocytosis	57
PURPURIC ERUPTIONS					
RMSF, rat-bite fever, endocarditis‡; epidemic typhus¶	—	—	—	—	—†
Acute meningococcemia	*Neisseria meningitidis*	Petechiae rapidly becoming numerous, sometimes enlarging and becoming vesicular; trunk, extremities most commonly involved; may appear on face, hands, feet; may include purpura fulminans reflecting DIC (see below)	Most common in children, individuals with asplenia or terminal complement component deficiency (C5-C8)	Hypotension, meningitis (sometimes preceded by upper respiratory infection)	149
Purpura fulminans	Severe DIC	Large ecchymoses with sharply irregular shapes evolving into hemorrhagic bullae and then into black necrotic lesions	Individuals with sepsis (e.g., involving *N. meningitidis*), malignancy, or massive trauma; asplenic patients at high risk for sepsis	Hypotension	124, 149
Chronic meningococcemia	*N. meningitidis*	Variety of recurrent eruptions, including pink maculopapular; nodular (usually on lower extremities); petechial (sometimes developing vesicular centers); purpuric areas with pale blue-gray centers	Individuals with complement deficiencies	Fevers, sometimes intermittent; arthritis, myalgias, headache	149
Disseminated gonococcal infection	*Neisseria gonorrhoeae*	Papules (1–5 mm) evolving over 1–2 d into hemorrhagic pustules with gray necrotic centers; hemorrhagic bullae occurring rarely; lesions (usually fewer than 40) distributed peripherally near joints (more commonly on upper extremities)	Sexually active individuals (more often females), some with complement deficiency	Low-grade fever, tenosynovitis, arthritis	150
Enteroviral petechial rash	Usually echovirus 9 or coxsackievirus A9	Disseminated petechial lesions (may also be maculopapular, vesicular, or urticarial)	Often occurs in outbreaks	Pharyngitis, headache; aseptic meningitis with echovirus 9	195

(continued)

Table 18-1—(*Continued*)

Diseases Associated with Fever and Rash

Disease	Etiology	Description	Group Affected/ Epidemiological Factors	Clinical Syndrome	Chapter Reference
Viral hemorrhagic fever	Arboviruses and arenaviruses	Petechial rash	Residence in or travel to endemic areas	Triad of fever, shock, hemorrhage from mucosa or gastrointestinal tract	200, 201
Thrombotic thrombocytopenic purpura	Idiopathic causes	Petechiae	Usually affects young adults; more common in women; hemolytic-uremic syndrome seen in children after gastroenteritis caused by *Escherichia coli* O157:H7	Fever, hemolytic anemia, thrombocytopenia, neurologic and renal dysfunction; coagulation studies normal	57, 109, 117

* See "Purpuric eruptions."
† See etiology-specific chapters.
‡ See "Peripheral eruptions."
§ See "Confluent desquamative erythemas."
¶ See "Centrally distributed maculopapular eruptions."
NOTE: DIC, disseminated intravascular coagulation; ECM, erythema chronicum migrans; HIV, human immunodeficiency virus; RMSF, Rocky Mountain spotted fever.

States. *Endemic typhus* or *leptospirosis* (caused by a spirochete; see Chap. 176) may be seen in urban environments where rodents proliferate. Outside the United States, other rickettsial diseases cause a spotted-fever syndrome and should be considered in residents of or travelers to endemic areas. Similarly, *typhoid fever*, a nonrickettsial disease caused by *Salmonella typhi* (Chap. 158), is usually acquired during travel outside the United States.

Some centrally distributed maculopapular eruptions have distinctive features. Erythema chronicum migrans (ECM), the rash of Lyme disease (Chap. 178), typically manifests as singular or multiple annular plaques. Untreated ECM lesions usually fade within a month but may persist for more than a year. *Erythema marginatum*, the rash of acute rheumatic fever (Chap. 236), has a distinctive pattern of enlarging and shifting transient annular lesions.

Collagen vascular diseases may cause fever and rash. Patients with *systemic lupus erythematosus* (Chap. 312) typically develop a sharply defined, erythematous eruption in a butterfly distribution on the cheeks (malar rash) as well as many other skin manifestations. *Still's disease* (Chap. 326) manifests as an evanescent salmon-colored rash on the trunk that coincides with fever spikes.

Peripheral Eruptions These rashes are alike in that they are most prominent peripherally or begin in peripheral (acral) areas before spreading centripetally. Early diagnosis and therapy are critical in RMSF (Chap. 179) because of its grave prognosis if untreated. Lesions evolve from macular to petechial, start on the wrists and ankles, spread centripetally, and appear on the palms and soles only later in the disease. The rash of *secondary syphilis* (Chap. 174), which may be diffuse but is prominent on the palms and soles, should be considered in the differential diagnosis of pityriasis rosea, especially in sexually active patients. *Atypical measles* (Chap. 196) is seen in individuals contracting measles who received the killed measles vaccine between 1963 and 1967 in the United States and who were not subsequently protected with the live vaccine. *Hand-foot-and-mouth disease* (Chap. 195) is distinguished by tender vesicles distributed peripherally and in the mouth; outbreaks commonly occur within families. The classic target lesions of *erythema multiforme* appear symmetrically on the elbows, knees, palms, and soles. In relatively severe cases, these lesions may spread diffusely and involve mucosal surfaces. Lesions may develop on the hands and feet in *endocarditis* (Chap. 126).

Confluent Desquamative Erythemas These eruptions consist of diffuse erythema, often followed by desquamation. The eruptions caused by group A *Streptococcus* or *Staphylococcus aureus* are toxin mediated. Certain disease features may provide diagnostic clues. *Scarlet fever* (Chap. 143) usually follows pharyngitis; patients have a facial flush, a "strawberry" tongue, and accentuated petechiae in body folds (Pastia's lines). *Kawasaki disease* (Chaps. 57 and 319) presents in the pediatric population as fissuring of the lips, a strawberry tongue, conjunctivitis, adenopathy, and sometimes cardiac abnormalities. *Streptococcal toxic shock syndrome* (Chap. 143) manifests with hypotension, multiorgan failure, and often a severe group A streptococcal infection (e.g., necrotizing fasciitis). *Staphylococcal toxic shock syndrome* (Chap. 142) also presents with hypotension and multiorgan failure, but usually only *S. aureus* colonization—not a severe *S. aureus* infection—is documented. *Staphylococcal scalded-skin syndrome* (Chap. 142) is seen primarily in children and in immunocompromised adults. Generalized erythema is often evident during the prodrome of fever and malaise; profound tenderness of the skin is distinctive. In the exfoliative stage, the skin can be induced to form bullae with light lateral pressure (Nikolsky's sign). In a mild form, a scarlatiniform eruption mimics scarlet fever, but the patient does not exhibit a strawberry tongue or circumoral pallor. In contrast to the staphylococcal scalded-skin syndrome, in which the cleavage plane is superficial in the epidermis, *toxic epidermal necrolysis* (Chap. 56) involves sloughing of the entire epidermis, resulting in severe disease. This condition is uncommon among children and relatively common among HIV-infected patients (Chap. 308). *Exfoliative erythroderma syndrome* (Chaps. 55 and 56) is a serious reaction associated with systemic toxicity that is often due to eczema, psoriasis, mycosis fungoides, or a severe drug reaction.

Vesiculobullous Eruptions *Varicella* (Chap. 185) is highly contagious, often occurring in winter or spring. At a given time within a given region of the body, varicella lesions are in different stages of development. In immunocompromised hosts, varicella vesicles may lack the characteristic erythematous base or may appear hemorrhagic. *Rickettsialpox* (Chap. 179) is often documented in urban settings and is characterized by vesicles and pustules. It can be distinguished from varicella by an eschar at the side of the mouse-mite bite. *Disseminated Vibrio vulnificus infection* (Chap. 161) or *ecthyma gangrenosum* due to *Pseudomonas aeruginosa* (Chap. 157) should be considered in immunosuppressed individuals with sepsis and hemorrhagic bullae.

Urticarial Eruptions Individuals with classic urticaria ("hives") usually have a hypersensitivity reaction without associated fever. In the presence of fever, urticarial eruptions are usually due to *urticarial vasculitis* (Chap. 319). Unlike individual lesions of classic urticaria, which last up to 48 h, these lesions may last up to 5 days. Etiologies include serum sickness (often induced by drugs such as penicillins, sulfas, salicylates, or barbiturates), connective-tissue disease (e.g., systemic lupus erythematosus or Sjögren's syndrome), and infection (e.g., with hepatitis B virus, coxsackievirus A9, or parasites). Malignancy may be associated with fever and chronic urticaria (Chap. 57).

Nodular Eruptions In immunocompromised hosts, nodular lesions often represent disseminated infection. Patients with disseminated *candidiasis* (often due to *Candida tropicalis*) may have a triad of fever, myalgias, and eruptive nodules (Chap. 207). Disseminated *cryptococcosis* lesions (Chap. 206) may resemble molluscum contagiosum. Necrosis of nodules should raise the suspicion of *aspergillosis* (Chap. 208) or *mucormycosis* (Chap. 209). *Erythema nodosum* presents with exquisitely tender nodules on the lower extremities. *Sweet's syndrome* (Chap. 57) should be considered in individuals with multiple nodules and plaques, often so edematous that they give the appearance of vesicles or bullae. Sweet's syndrome may affect either healthy individuals or persons with lymphoproliferative disease.

Purpuric Eruptions *Acute meningococcemia* (Chap. 149) classically presents in children as a petechial eruption, but initial lesions may appear as blanchable macules or urticaria. RMSF should be considered in the differential diagnosis of acute meningococcemia. *Echovirus 9 infection* (Chap. 195) may mimic acute meningococcemia; patients should be treated as if they have bacterial sepsis since prompt differentiation of these conditions may be impossible. Large ecchymotic areas of *purpura fulminans* reflect severe underlying disseminated intravascular coagulation, which may be due to infectious or noninfectious causes. The lesions of *chronic meningococcemia* (Chap. 149) may have a variety of morphologies, including petechial. Purpuric nodules may develop on the legs and resemble erythema nodosum but lack its exquisite tenderness. Lesions of *disseminated gonococcemia* (Chap. 150) are distinctive, sparse, countable hemorrhagic pustules, usually located near joints. The lesions of chronic meningococcemia and those of gonococcemia may be indistinguishable in terms of appearance and distribution. *Viral hemorrhagic fever* (Chaps. 200 and 201) should be considered in patients with an appropriate travel history and a petechial rash. *Thrombotic thrombocytopenic purpura* (Chaps. 57, 109, and 117) is a noninfectious cause of fever and petechiae.

BIBLIOGRAPHY

CHERRY JD: Contemporary infectious exanthems. Clin Infect Dis 16:199, 1993
———: Cutaneous manifestations of systemic infections, in *Textbook of Pediatric Infectious Diseases*, vol. 1, 3d ed, RD Feigin and JD Cherry (eds). Philadelphia, Saunders, 1992, pp 755–782
FITZPATRICK TB et al (eds): *Dermatology in General Medicine*, 4th ed. New York, McGraw-Hill, 1993
HURWITZ S (ed): *Clinical Pediatric Dermatology*. Philadelphia, Saunders, 1981
LEVIN S, GOODMAN LJ: An approach to acute fever and rash (AFR) in the adult. Curr Clin Top Infect Dis 15:19, 1995
WEBER DJ, COHEN MS: The acutely ill patient with fever and rash, in *Principles and Practice of Infectious Diseases*, vol 1, 4th ed, GL Mandell et al (eds). New York, Churchill Livingstone 1995, pp 549–561
WENNER HA: Virus diseases associated with cutaneous eruptions. Prog Med Virol 16:269, 1973

19 *Kevin J. Petty*

HYPOTHERMIA

Hypothermia is defined arbitrarily as a core body temperature of 35°C or below and is classified as mild (35 to 32°C), moderate (< 32 to 28°C), or severe (< 28°C). Hypothermia can have several causes and is usually multifactorial in origin. Precise estimates of the incidence are difficult to obtain because nonfatal hypothermia is often not detected or reported and fatal hypothermia is probably underreported. Between 1979 and 1991 approximately 770 deaths per year occurred in the United States due to environmental hypothermia. Among those deaths,

67 percent were men, 61 percent were white, and more than half were above 65 years of age. Most cases occur in the winter months in areas with cold climates, but hypothermia can occur in mild climates at any season. Risk factors include extremes of age (especially the elderly), homelessness, ethanol use, malnutrition, poverty, mental illness, use of neuroleptic medications, and hypothyroidism. A common setting is chronic indoor cold exposure in an impoverished elderly person with underlying illnesses and immobility. Homeless male alcoholics are at great risk.

THERMOREGULATION Heat is generated in most tissues of the body and is lost by radiation (55 percent), evaporation (5 percent from airways, 25 percent from skin), conduction (15 percent), and convection (5 percent). Immersion in water results in hypothermia more rapidly because the thermal conductivity of water is 20 to 30 times greater than that of air. The balance between heat production and heat loss in the body is regulated by the hypothalamus (preoptic and posterior regions). Exposure to cold activates cutaneous cold receptors that transmit the signal via the lateral spinothalamic tracts to the preoptic nuclei of the hypothalamus. The posterior hypothalamus activates the sympathetic nervous system to increase muscle tone and cause shivering, which in turn increases the metabolic rate from a normal level of 40 to 60 kcal/h to as high as 300 kcal/h. Even at maximum metabolic rates, heat loss from the body can exceed heat production. As the body temperature drops below 30°C, metabolic processes slow and shivering stops, thereby accelerating the development of hypothermia.

CAUSES Extreme environmental conditions can cause hypothermia in healthy individuals, but it rarely requires medical attention. Most severe hypothermia occurs in persons with underlying medical conditions that lead to excessive heat loss (usually involving environmental exposure) or inadequate heat production, and both processes are usually involved (Table 19-1). It is worthwhile keeping in mind that body temperature never falls below the environmental temperature.

Most environmental exposures are accidental. Iatrogenic hypothermia can occur when obtunded patients are left uncovered in hospital rooms or during surgical procedures when large body surface areas are exposed for long periods in the operating room. The shivering response is inhibited by anesthesia, enhancing the likelihood of hypothermia. Its only manifestation in this setting may be difficult in achieving hemostasis due to inactivation of clotting factors at low temperatures. Enhanced blood flow to the skin (burns, psoriasis) can also produce hypothermia in the presence of slight environmental challenge because heat conservation via peripheral vasoconstriction is impaired.

Decreased heat production can contribute to the development of hypothermia. Malnutrition and/or starvation deplete the stores of glycogen and fat necessary for effective heat production. Hypothermia occurs in more than 10 percent of patients with sepsis (usually bacterial) and is often associated with a poor prognosis. Approximately 40 percent of resting oxygen consumption is regulated by thyroid hormone, and hypothermia is common in severe hypothyroidism where the metabolic rate can be reduced to as much as 40 percent below normal. Hypothermia in hepatic failure is often due to a combination of hypoglycemia from inadequate hepatic gluconeogenesis and altered hypothalamic function (decreased shivering). Hypoglycemia from any cause (glucocorticoid deficiency, ethanol use, hyperinsulinism), uremia, and diabetic ketoacidosis also predispose to hypothermia.

Hypothalamic lesions (tumor, inflammation) can cause thermoregulatory instability and hypothermia. Spinal cord lesions at the first thoracic nerve root or above can lead to hypothermia by blocking shivering and interrupting cold-induced compensatory reflexes mediated by the lateral spinothalamic tracts. Episodic spontaneous hypothermia with hyperhidrosis is a rare disorder associated with excessive sweating in the absence of shivering; nearly half of these patients have agenesis of the corpus callosum (Shapiro's syndrome), suggesting a central nervous system (CNS) etiology.

Table 19-1

Causes of Hypothermia

I. Excessive heat loss
  A. Environmental exposure
    1. Accidental
    2. Iatrogenic
  B. Increased cutaneous blood flow—burns, psoriasis, toxic epidermal necrolysis
II. Inadequate heat production
  A. Decreased metabolism
    1. Malnutrition
    2. Hypothyroidism
    3. Adrenal insufficiency
    4. Hepatic failure
    5. Hypoglycemia
    6. Diabetic ketoacidosis
  B. Altered thermoregulation
    1. Sepsis
    2. Uremia
    3. Hypothalamic dysfunction
    4. Spinal cord injury—T1 or above
    5. Episodic spontaneous hypothermia with hyperhidrosis
  C. Drug-induced
    1. Phenothiazines
    2. Barbiturates
    3. Ethanol
    4. Opiates
    5. Clonidine
    6. Lithium
    7. Benzodiazepines

Several drugs can contribute to hypothermia. Phenothiazines, barbiturates, opiates, benzodiazepines, and ethanol inhibit shivering through their CNS effects. Ethanol inhibits shivering, impairs hepatic gluconeogenesis, and enhances heat loss by inducing peripheral vasodilatation. Clonidine inhibits central sympathetic outflow.

EFFECTS ON ORGAN SYSTEMS Acute cold exposure causes tachycardia, increased cardiac output, peripheral vasoconstriction, and increased peripheral vascular resistance secondary to sympathetic stimulation. As body temperature drops below 32°C, cardiac conduction becomes impaired, and heart rate and cardiac output decrease. Atrial fibrillation with slow ventricular response is common below 32°C, and ventricular fibrillation may occur below 28°C. Electrocardiographic changes include the characteristic Osborn (J) wave (a positive deflection occurring at the junction of the QRS complex and the ST segment).

Peripheral vasoconstriction shunts blood to the central circulation and increases central blood volume; a diuresis (cold diuresis) ensues, tending to lower intravascular volume in a compensatory fashion. With prolonged cold exposure the combination of cold diuresis, additional volume losses due to impaired sodium and water reabsorption by the kidneys (due to impaired function of epithelial transport mechanisms), and intravascular fluid shifts with intracellular and peripheral edema can cause severe volume depletion and hypotension. Volume depletion in turn leads to hemoconcentration and increased blood viscosity that predispose to thrombosis. Conversely, bleeding due to inefficient clotting at lower temperatures, thrombocytopenia, and disseminated intravascular coagulation can cause even minor trauma to result in significant blood loss.

The acid-base and electrolyte derangements depend on the duration of cold exposure. Lactic acidosis due to decreased peripheral tissue perfusion can lead to a compensatory respiratory alkalosis. In severe hypothermia depression of respiration can cause respiratory acidosis. Levels of serum electrolytes are usually normal, but movement of potassium into cells can cause hypokalemia in the absence of trauma or rhabdomyolysis.

Cold exposure can induce bronchorrhea and bronchospasm. Early tachypnea is followed by hypoventilation as hypothermia becomes more severe. Decreased mental status predisposes to aspiration because of loss of coughing and gag reflex, and pulmonary edema can occur. Shift of the oxygen dissociation curve of hemoglobin to the left at lower temperatures impairs oxygen delivery to hypothermic tissues, an impairment mitigated by decreased tissue oxygen requirements due to decreased metabolism.

The nervous system manifestations are diverse. Cerebral blood flow decreases, and nerve conduction velocity slows as neuronal metabolism declines. Manifestations include dysarthria, ataxia, amnesia, hallucinations, confusion, slow pupillary reflexes, and delayed deep tendon reflexes; the latter phenomenon may make it hard to recognize hypothyroidism in the presence of hypothermia. Chronic hypothermia can be a primary or contributing cause of altered mental status in the elderly. Hypothermic individuals may remove their clothing because of feeling warm ("paradoxical undressing"). In severe hypothermia coma can be associated with an isoelectric electroencephalogram (EEG); in this setting an isoelectric EEG is not indicative of brain death and may be reversible.

Enhanced secretion of hypothalamic-releasing hormones by acute cold exposure results in increased secretion of ACTH and thyroid-stimulating hormone (TSH). Levels of serum cortisol and catecholamines increase as with other acute stresses. The acute release of vasopressin by expansion of the central blood volume contributes to cold diuresis. Levels of serum thyroid hormones increase only slightly, and serum free thyroxine levels remain normal in euthyroid individuals. Moderate to severe hypothermia inhibits insulin action and leads to decreased glucose utilization and hyperglycemia except when hypoglycemia is a cause of the hypothermia. Severe hypothermia eventually inhibits the release and action of ACTH and steroid hormones.

Intestinal hypomotility is common in moderate hypothermia. Decreased hepatic metabolism can prolong the serum half-life of compounds normally cleared by the liver. Pancreatitis and hyperamylasemia occur in as many as half of patients after rewarming. It is unclear whether hypothermia per se causes pancreatitis because ethanol abuse, a common factor in hypothermia, is an independent cause of pancreatitis.

DIAGNOSIS Oral thermometers are often calibrated only down to 34.4°C. Accurate temperature measurement in the low range requires the use of a thermometer capable of reading down to 15°C or preferably a rectal thermocouple probe inserted at least 15 cm. The reliability of infrared tympanic thermography in this setting has not been established. Therefore, when an initial body temperature of 35°C or less is obtained, it is important to remeasure core temperature accurately.

Historical data, when available, are often helpful in determining the cause and duration of the hypothermia. Preexisting medical conditions, medications, home environment, and the length and severity of exposure should be ascertained. Due to vasoconstriction blood pressure may be difficult to obtain without the use of Doppler ultrasound. Pulse oximetry is of little value for the same reason. Evidence of trauma and of coexisting medical conditions should be carefully sought. The ingestion of alcohol (which may be detected on the breath) is a common contributing factor. Neurologic function can range from alertness to obtundation and correlates with the severity of hypothermia. Focal findings on neurologic examination should prompt a search for specific intracranial lesions.

Initial laboratory evaluation should include a complete biochemical profile [electrolytes, blood urea nitrogen (BUN), creatinine, calcium, phosphorous, magnesium, glucose, liver function], measurement of amylase levels, complete blood count, prothrombin/partial thromboplastin times (PT/PTT), electrocardiogram, chest x-ray, urinalysis, arterial blood gas analysis, and toxicologic screen. Blood and urine cultures should be obtained because of the relatively high prevalence of bacteremia and sepsis in hypothermic patients (nearly 40 percent in one urban hospital). Serum TSH should be measured in most, if not all, hypothermic patients to assess for hypothyroidism. Appropriate imaging studies (computed tomography, magnetic resonance imaging) should be obtained when trauma or head injury is suspected. Arterial blood gas is usually analyzed at 37°C and should not be corrected for the body temperature.

Rewarming techniques can be active or passive, internal or external. Passive external rewarming involves covering the patient with blankets and clothing in a warm environment to allow endogenous heat production to correct the hypothermia; it is important to keep the head covered because up to 30 percent of body heat can be lost from the head. This is the easiest and safest method and should be used first in most patients with mild hypothermia. Body temperature increases of 0.5 to 2.0°C/h can be expected.

Active external rewarming involves direct application of heat sources (heating blankets, heat lamps, warm water immersion) to external body surfaces. This procedure can worsen the condition in two ways if not performed properly. First, the direct application of heat to the skin can produce shock by relieving cold-induced vasoconstriction, thereby removing an important support for maintenance of blood pressure in the volume-depleted patient. Second, the relief of peripheral vasoconstriction allows cooler peripheral blood to enter the central circulation and can cause core temperature to drop even further (a phenomenon referred to as "afterdrop"). There is a risk of burn injury when heat sources are applied directly to the skin. Direct heat should be applied only to the thorax if active external rewarming is used.

Active internal rewarming can be achieved by several techniques. The simplest method is airway rewarming in which the patient inspires humidified oxygen heated to 42°C via face mask or endotracheal tube. Rewarming rates of 1 to 2°C/h can be achieved with airway rewarming. Intravenous fluids should be heated to 40°C, but their use has minimal effects on core rewarming. Lavage of the stomach, bladder, or colon with warmed fluids produces limited warming and generally is not used if rapid rewarming is needed. Peritoneal and pleural lavage induce warming rates of 2 to 4°C/h but should be used only in moderate to severe hypothermia where there is cardiovascular instability or when external rewarming is ineffective.

The most efficient rewarming technique is extracorporeal blood warming by hemodialysis or cardiopulmonary bypass. Both methods involve continuous removal of blood that is circulated and warmed externally before being reinfused. Cardiopulmonary bypass is the most efficient technique and can increase core temperature 1 to 2°C every 3 to 5 min. These procedures are reserved for the most severe cases of hypothermia (e.g., cardiac arrest) and when peritoneal and/or pleural lavage are ineffective.

The volume depletion should be corrected with isotonic fluids. Warmed normal saline (or 5% dextrose/normal saline) should be given intravenously. Lactated Ringer's solution should be avoided because lactate metabolism is impaired by hypothermia. Physical manipulation of the patient should be minimized, and central vein lines, nasogastric tubes, and endotracheal tubes should be inserted carefully because of the possibility of cardiac arrhythmia. Treatment of acidosis is usually not necessary since rewarming corrects most abnormalities, and drugs should be administered with caution because their effectiveness may be impaired at lower body temperatures and because their metabolic clearance is prolonged. If sepsis is a possibility, it is appropriate to administer empiric broad-spectrum antibiotics until the results of blood cultures are available (see Chap. 124).

Rewarming often corrects hyperglycemia. Insulin is inactive at body temperatures below 32°C, and excess insulin can produce late hypoglycemia when body temperature is raised. Furthermore, prolonged shivering can cause depletion of muscle glycogen and predispose to hypoglycemia. Therefore, insulin should not be administered until it is clear that hyperglycemia persists after rewarming. Hypokalemia may correct with rewarming alone as potassium shifts to the extracellular space, but serum potassium levels should be monitored during rewarming. Development of hyperkalemia during hypothermia suggests significant tissue necrosis (rhabdomyolysis) with or without renal failure.

Continuous cardiac monitoring is essential. Atrial arrhythmias are common and are usually reversible with rewarming alone. Antiarrhythmic or vasopressor drugs should not be administered until body temperature is normal. Ventricular arrhythmias in the hypothermic patient tend to be refractory to drugs and to defibrillation. Bretylium tosylate is the drug of choice for ventricular fibrillation. Only one attempt at electrical defibrillation should be made when the core temperature is <30°C. When cardiac arrest is present, active internal rewarming and cardiopulmonary resuscitation should be initiated simultaneously.

It is occasionally difficult to distinguish reversible from irreversible hypothermia. Apnea, asystole, and absence of brain activity are usually signs of death but can also be present in severe, reversible hypothermia, particularly in victims of immersion hypothermia and near-drowning. The lowest recorded body temperature in a patient who was resuscitated successfully was 15.2°C in a 23-day-old infant. Generally, cardiopulmonary resuscitation of hypothermic patients should continue until core body temperature has been raised at least to 32°C or until cardiovascular status has stabilized.

Once body temperature is corrected and the patient is stabilized, a search should be made for precipitating causes. Empiric broad-spectrum antibiotic therapy may be given because the usual manifestations of infection are masked. A careful neurologic examination should be performed. Coexisting medical conditions (myocardial infarction, diabetic ketoacidosis, renal failure, hepatic failure, gastrointestinal bleeding, pancreatitis, rhabdomyolysis, hypothyroidism) should be treated aggressively if present.

Preventive measures in high-risk individuals such as the elderly include use of layered clothing and headgear, adequate shelter, increased caloric intake, and avoidance of ethanol.

BIBLIOGRAPHY

DANZL DF, POZOS RS: Accidental hypothermia. N Engl J Med 331:1756, 1994
HARCHELROAD F: Acute thermoregulatory disorders. Clin Geriatr Med 9:621, 1993
JOLLY B, GHATS K: Accidental hypothermia. Emerg Med Clin North Am 10:311, 1992
KOLODZIK PW: Hypothermia, in *Presenting Signs and Symptoms in the Emergency Department*, GC Hamilton (ed). Baltimore, Williams & Wilkins, 1993, p 248

20   *Robert B. Daroff, Joseph B. Martin*

FAINTNESS, SYNCOPE, DIZZINESS, AND VERTIGO

Syncope is defined as transient loss of consciousness with postural collapse caused by an acute decrease in cerebral blood flow. Although often preceded by faintness or light-headedness (presyncope), it may not be when caused by cardiac asystole or ventricular tachycardia. Presyncope symptoms may be manifest as "dizziness," always without true vertigo, or may be mimicked by a warning (aura) prior to a seizure. The sequence of symptoms is reasonably stereotyped and includes increasing lightheadedness, visual blurring proceeding to blindness, diaphoresis, and heaviness in the lower limbs progressing to postural sway. These symptoms increase in severity until consciousness is lost or the ischemia is corrected, often by assuming the recumbent position. The differentiation of syncope from seizure is an important, sometimes difficult, diagnostic problem.

In this chapter syncope and dizziness are considered with particular reference to clinical manifestations, differential diagnosis, and treatment.

SYNCOPE

At the beginning of a syncopal attack, the patient is nearly always in the upright position, either sitting or standing. A cardiac etiology, such as a Stokes-Adams attack, is exceptional in this respect (see Chap. 230). The patient is warned of the impending faint by a sense of "feeling bad," of giddiness, and of movement or swaying of the floor or surrounding objects. The patient becomes confused and may yawn, visual spots and dimming may occur, and the ears may ring. Nausea and sometimes vomiting accompany these symptoms. There is a striking pallor or ashen gray color of the face, and generalized perspiration ensues. In some patients, a deliberate onset with presyncopal symptoms may allow time for protection against injury; in others, the syncope is sudden and without warning. The onset varies from instantaneous to 10 to 30 s, rarely longer.

The depth and duration of unconsciousness vary. Sometimes the patient remains partly aware of the surroundings, or there may be profound coma. The patient may remain in this state for seconds to minutes or even as long as half an hour. Usually the patient lies motionless with skeletal muscles relaxed, but a few clonic jerks of the limbs and face may occur shortly after the beginning of the unconsciousness. In some situations there may be a brief tonic-clonic seizure. Sphincter control is usually maintained. The pulse is feeble or apparently absent, the blood pressure may be low to undetectable, and breathing may be almost imperceptible. Once the patient is in a horizontal position, gravity no longer hinders the flow of blood to the brain. The strength of the pulse may then improve, color begins to return to the face, breathing becomes quicker and deeper, and consciousness is regained. There is usually an immediate recovery of consciousness. Some patients may, however, be keenly aware of physical weakness, and rising too soon may precipitate another faint. In other patients, particularly those with transient tachyarrhythmias, there may be no residual symptoms following the initial syncope. Headache and drowsiness, which, with mental confusion, are the usual sequelae of a convulsion, do not follow a syncopal attack.

ETIOLOGY   The list of causes in Table 20-1 is based on established or assumed physiologic mechanisms. The more common types of faint are reducible to a few simple mechanisms. Syncope results from a sudden impairment of brain metabolism usually brought about by hypotension with reduction of cerebral blood flow.

Several mechanisms subserve circulatory adjustments to the upright posture. Approximately three-fourths of the systemic blood volume is contained in the venous bed, and any interference with venous return may lead to a reduction in cardiac output. Cerebral blood flow may still be maintained, as long as systemic arterial vasoconstriction occurs, but when this adjustment fails, serious hypotension with resultant cerebral underperfusion to less than half normal results in syncope. Normally, the pooling of blood in the lower parts of the body is prevented by (1) pressor reflexes that induce constriction of peripheral arterioles and venules, (2) reflex acceleration of the heart by means of aortic and carotid reflexes, and (3) improvement of venous return to the heart by activity of the muscles of the limbs. Placing a normal person on a tilt table to relax the muscles and tilting upright slightly diminishes cardiac output and allows the blood to accumulate in the legs to a slight degree; this may then be followed by a slight transitory

Table 20-1

Causes of Faintness and Disturbances of Consciousness

I. Circulatory (reduced cerebral blood flow)
  A. Inadequate vasoconstrictor mechanisms
    1. Vasovagal (vasodepressor)
    2. Postural hypotension
    3. Primary autonomic insufficiency
    4. Sympathectomy (pharmacologic, due to antihypertensive medications such as methyldopa and hydralazine, or surgical)
    5. Diseases of central and peripheral nervous systems, including autonomic nerves (Chaps. 371 and 381)
    6. Carotid sinus syncope (see also "Bradyarrhythmias," below)
    7. Hyperbradykininemia
  B. Hypovolemia
    1. Blood loss—gastrointestinal hemorrhage
    2. Addison's disease
  C. Mechanical reduction of venous return
    1. Valsalva maneuver
    2. Cough
    3. Micturition
    4. Atrial myxoma, ball valve thrombus
  D. Reduced cardiac output
    1. Obstruction to left ventricular outflow: aortic stenosis, hypertrophic subaortic stenosis
    2. Obstruction to pulmonary flow: pulmonic stenosis, primary pulmonary hypertension, pulmonary embolism
    3. Myocardial: massive myocardial infarction with pump failure
    4. Pericardial: cardiac tamponade
  E. Arrhythmias (Chaps. 230 and 231)
    1. Bradyarrhythmias
      a. Atrioventricular (AV) block (second- and third-degree), with Stokes-Adams attacks
      b. Ventricular asystole
      c. Sinus bradycardia, sinoatrial block, sinus arrest, sick-sinus syndrome
      d. Carotid sinus syncope (see also inadequate vasoconstrictor mechanisms, above)
      e. Glossopharyngeal neuralgia (and other painful states)
    2. Tachyarrhythmias
      a. Episodic ventricular tachycardia with or without associated bradyarrhythmias
      b. Supraventricular tachycardia without AV block
II. Other causes of disturbances of consciousness
  A. Altered state of blood to the brain
    1. Hypoxia
    2. Anemia
    3. Diminished carbon dioxide due to hyperventilation (faintness common, syncope seldom occurs)
    4. Hypoglycemia (episodic weakness common, faintness occasional, syncope rare)
  B. Cerebral
    1. Cerebrovascular disturbances (cerebral ischemic attacks, see Chap. 366)
      a. Extracranial vascular insufficiency (vertebral-basilar, carotid)
      b. Diffuse spasm of cerebral arterioles (hypertensive encephalopathy)
    2. Emotional disturbances, anxiety attacks, and hysterical seizures

fall in systolic arterial pressure and, in patients with defective vasomotor reflexes, may produce faints.

TYPES OF SYNCOPE **Vasodepressor (Vasovagal) or Neurocardiogenic Syncope** This form of syncope is the common faint that may be experienced by normal persons and accounts for about 50 percent of all instances of syncope. It is frequently recurrent and commonly precipitated by emotional stress (especially in a warm, crowded room), fear (e.g., in a dentist's chair), extreme fatigue, injury, or pain. Many episodes, however, occur without obvious antecedent cause. In its classic form, vasodepressor syncope comprises a constellation of symptoms including hypotension, bradycardia, nausea, pallor, and diaphoresis. Syncope typically occurs in the setting of diminished venous return that leads to reduced stroke volume and a reflex increase in sympathetic activity. In susceptible individuals, this increase in sympathetic activity causes cardiac hypercontractility and excessive stimulation of ventricular mechanoreceptors (afferent vagal C fibers), which, in turn, leads to sympathetic withdrawal and activation of the parasympathetic nervous system via a centrally mediated vasomotor reflex. The net result is a vicious cycle of *inappropriate peripheral vasodilatation* and *relative bradycardia* leading to progressive hypotension and syncope that can be reversed by assumption of supine posture and elevation of the legs. Orthostatic stress induced by prolonged upright tilt testing at 60 to 80 degrees is a sensitive technique for reproducing syncope in many patients with this syndrome. The use of low-dose isoproterenol infusion enhances the sensitivity of upright tilt testing but leads to false-positive tests when used in high doses. Vasodepressor syncope may occur with sudden severe pain, particularly if it originates in the viscera, and may also rarely accompany a severe migraine headache.

Postural (Orthostatic) Hypotension with Syncope This type of syncope affects persons who have a chronic defect in, or variable instability of, vasomotor reflexes. The fall in blood pressure on assumption of upright posture is due to a loss of vasoconstriction reflexes in resistance and capacitance vessels of the lower extremities. Although the syncopal attack differs little from vasodepressor syncope, the effect of posture is critical. Sudden arising from a recumbent position or standing quietly are precipitating circumstances.

Postural syncope may occur in the following conditions:

1. In otherwise normal persons who have defective postural reflexes. In such individuals, fainting may occur when they are tilted on a table. Under such circumstances the blood pressure at first diminishes slightly and then stabilizes at a lower level. Shortly thereafter, the compensatory reflexes suddenly fail and the arterial pressure falls precipitously. The condition is often familial.
2. In *primary autonomic insufficiency* and in the *dysautonomias*. Three syndromes have been delineated:

Acute or subacute dysautonomia In this rare condition, an otherwise healthy adult or child develops, over a period of a few days or weeks, a partial or complete paralysis of the parasympathetic and sympathetic nervous systems. Pupillary reflexes are lost, and lacrimation, salivation, and sweating are absent or diminished. Impotence, paresis of bladder and bowel musculature, and orthostatic hypotension are present. The cerebrospinal fluid (CSF) protein is often increased. Sensory and motor nerves are intact, but unmyelinated autonomic nerves degenerate. The disease appears to represent a variant of Guillain-Barré syndrome, and recovery usually occurs within a few months.

Chronic postganglionic autonomic insufficiency This is a disease of the middle-aged and elderly who gradually develop chronic orthostatic hypotension, sometimes in conjunction with impotence and sphincter disturbances. Typically, after standing for 5 to 10 min, the blood pressure falls by at least 35 mmHg, the pulse pressure narrows, and there is no compensatory tachycardia, pallor, or nausea. Men are more often affected than women.

Chronic preganglionic autonomic insufficiency In this condition, orthostatic hypotension with anhidrosis, impotence, and sphincter disturbances is combined with a disorder of the central nervous system (CNS). These disorders, designated *multisystem atrophies*, include

syndromes characterized by (1) tremor, extrapyramidal rigidity, and akinesia (Shy-Drager syndrome); (2) progressive cerebellar degeneration, some instances of which are familial; and (3) a more variable extrapyramidal and cerebellar disorder (striatonigral degeneration). These syndromes lead to severe disability and often death within a few years (see Chaps. 368 and 371).

The differentiation of chronic peripheral postganglionic and central preganglionic insufficiency is based on pathologic and pharmacologic evidence. In the postganglionic type, neurons of the sympathetic ganglia degenerate, whereas in the central type, intermediolateral horn preganglionic cells of the thoracic spinal cord degenerate. In the postganglionic peripheral type, resting levels of norepinephrine are subnormal because of failure to release norepinephrine from postganglionic endings, and there is hypersensitivity to injected norepinephrine. In the central type, resting levels of norepinephrine are normal. On standing, unlike the reaction in the normal individual, there is little, if any, rise in norepinephrine levels in either type. And in both types, the levels of plasma dopamine β-hydroxylase (the enzyme that converts dopamine to norepinephrine) are subnormal.

Other causes of postural syncope (1) After physical deconditioning, e.g., after prolonged illness with recumbency, especially in elderly individuals with reduced muscle tone, or after prolonged weightlessness, as in space flight. (2) After a sympathectomy that has abolished vasopressor reflexes. (3) In diabetic, alcoholic, and other neuropathies. The most common neurogenic orthostatic hypotension accompanies diseases of the peripheral nervous system. Diabetic polyneuropathy, beriberi, amyloid polyneuropathy, and the Adie syndrome are examples. Usually the orthostatic hypotension is associated with disturbances in sweating, impotence, and sphincter difficulties. Presumably the lesion involves postganglionic, unmyelinated fibers in peripheral nerves. (4) In patients receiving antihypertensive and vasodilator drugs as well as those who may be hypovolemic because of diuretics, excessive sweating, or adrenal insufficiency.

Micturition syncope, a condition usually seen in elderly men during or after urination, particularly after arising from sleep, is probably a special type of vasodepressor syncope. Release of intravesicular pressure may trigger vasodilatation and vagally mediated bradycardia.

Cardiac Syncope Cardiac syncope results from a sudden reduction in cardiac output, caused most commonly by a cardiac arrhythmia. In normal individuals, slow ventricular rates, but above 35 to 40 beats per minute, and fast rates not exceeding 180 beats per minute do not reduce cerebral blood flow, especially if the person is in the supine position. However, changes in pulse rate outside these limits may impair cerebral circulation and function. Upright posture, cerebrovascular disease, anemia, and coronary, myocardial, or valvular disease all reduce the tolerance to alterations in rate.

Atrioventricular block High-degree atrioventricular block is commonly associated with fainting (*Stokes-Adams-Morgagni syndrome*; see Chap. 230). In patients with these attacks, the block may be persistent or intermittent. When the block is high-grade or complete and the pacemaker below the block fails to function, or functions at too slow a rate, syncope occurs. Stokes-Adams attacks occur precipitously, usually without warning symptoms. Should cardiac asystole persist more than 8 to 10 s, the patient turns pale, falls unconscious, and may exhibit a few clonic jerks. With longer periods of asystole, cyanosis ensues, breathing is irregular, and fixed pupils, incontinence, and bilateral Babinski signs may be present. While recovery following a Stokes-Adams attack is usually prompt and complete, prolonged confusion and neurologic signs due to cerebral ischemia may occur in some patients, and permanent impairment of mental function may occasionally result, although focal neurologic signs are rare. The patient usually does not recall presyncopal symptoms. Cardiac faints of this type may recur several times a day. Commonly the heart block is transitory, and the electrocardiogram (ECG) taken later may not show any arrhythmia. Ventricular tachycardia or fibrillation may follow a period of asystole, resulting in prolonged coma or sudden death.

Sinus node disorders Disorders of sinus node automaticity or sinoatrial conduction may result in asystole or bradycardia of sufficient severity to cause presyncope or syncope. This disorder is most frequently detected with ambulatory ECG monitoring. Findings consistent with a diagnosis of sinus node dysfunction include symptomatic sinus pauses (>3 s) resulting from sinus arrest or sinoatrial block and severe unexplained sinus bradycardia (<40 beats per minute). The *bradycardia-tachycardia syndrome* is a common form of sinus node dysfunction in which syncope generally occurs as a result of marked sinus pauses following termination of paroxysmal supraventricular tachycardia. Electrophysiologic testing is sometimes helpful in unmasking diagnostic abnormalities in patients with syncope and suspected sinus node dysfunction in whom the diagnosis is not established by ambulatory ECG recording.

Tachyarrythmias Recurrent paroxysmal tachyarrhythmias also may cause presyncope and syncope as a result of a sudden reduction in cardiac output. The magnitude of tachycardia-induced hypotension is dependent on the interaction of several variables, including the rate and mechanism of the tachycardia, the type and severity of underlying cardiac disease, the patient's posture and activity level at the onset of the tachycardia, the sensitivity of the tachycardia to endogenous catecholamines, and the integrity of compensatory autonomic reflexes. *Supraventricular tachyarrhythmias* are not commonly associated with syncope. However, even in the absence of structural heart disease, the extremely high heart rates may impair cardiac filling and output sufficiently to cause loss of consciousness. These tachycardias result most commonly from the occurrence of paroxysmal atrial flutter, atrial fibrillation, or reentry involving the atrioventricular (AV) node or accessory pathways that bypass part or all of the AV conduction system (see Chap. 230). Patients with the Wolff-Parkinson-White syndrome are susceptible to several forms of supraventricular tachycardia, the most dangerous of which is atrial fibrillation with rapid antegrade conduction to the ventricles over an accessory AV connection that may result in syncope and, in rare instances, sudden death. When abnormal conduction over an accessory AV connection or an AV nodal reentry rhythm is suspected as a cause of syncope, electrophysiologic testing is indicated to define the mechanism and pathway of the tachycardia and to facilitate the selection of an effective therapeutic intervention (see also Chap. 230).

Paroxysmal ventricular tachycardia is a relatively common cause of syncope, particularly in patients with structural heart disease. Typically, the tachycardias are rapid and associated with abrupt loss of consciousness without premonitory symptoms. Usually the patient is unaware of palpitations, and recovery following an episode is prompt and complete without residual neurologic or cardiac sequelae. Unexplained syncope in a patient with structural heart disease is a potentially ominous finding and merits careful evaluation. The presence of pathologic Q waves on the ECG, indicative of a prior transmural myocardial infarction, is strongly associated with ventricular tachycardia as a cause of syncope in patients with ischemic heart disease. Other forms of heart disease such as hypertrophic and dilated cardiomyopathy, right ventricular dysplasia, and the long-QT-interval syndromes are also frequently associated with paroxysmal ventricular tachycardia and syncope (see Chap. 231).

Reflexive heart block In another form of cardiac syncope, the heart block is reflexive and is due to irritation of the vagus nerves. Examples of this phenomenon have been observed in patients with esophageal diverticula, mediastinal tumors, gallbladder disease, carotid sinus disease, glossopharyngeal neuralgia, and pleural and pulmonary irritation. In these conditions, reflex bradycardia is more commonly of the sinoatrial than the atrioventricular type.

Other causes Cardiac syncope also may result from *acute massive myocardial infarction*, particularly when associated with cardiogenic shock. *Aortic stenosis* often sets the stage for exertional syncope, most commonly by limiting cardiac output in the face of peripheral vasodilatation, with resultant myocardial and cerebral ischemia and occasionally arrhythmias. *Idiopathic hypertrophic subaortic stenosis* also may lead to exertional syncope because of intensified obstruction, ventricular arrhythmias, or both (Chap. 239). In *primary pulmonary hypertension*, a relatively fixed cardiac output and bouts of acute right ventricular failure may be associated with syncope (Chap. 238). However, vagal reflexes may be involved in this condition as well as in the syncope that occurs with *pulmonary embolism*. Ball-valve thrombus in the left atrium, left atrial myxoma, or thrombosis or malfunction of a prosthetic valve may produce sudden mechanical obstruction of the circulation and syncope. *Tetralogy of Fallot* is the congenital cardiac malformation most commonly responsible for syncope. In this condition, systemic vasodilatation, perhaps associated with infundibular spasm, greatly increases the right-to-left shunt and produces arterial hypoxia, which leads to syncope (Chap. 235).

Carotid Sinus Syncope The carotid sinus is normally sensitive to stretch and gives rise to sensory impulses carried via the nerve of Hering, a branch of the glossopharyngeal nerve, to the medulla oblongata. Massage of one or both of the carotid sinuses, particularly in elderly persons, causes (1) a reflex cardiac slowing (sinus bradycardia, sinus arrest, or even AV block), the so-called vagal type of response, and (2) a fall of arterial pressure without cardiac slowing, the so-called depressor type of response. Both types of carotid sinus response may coexist.

Syncope due to carotid sinus sensitivity is extremely uncommon and said to be initiated by turning of the head to one side, by a tight collar, or by shaving over the region of the sinus. In a patient displaying faintness on compression of one carotid sinus, it is important to distinguish between the benign disorder (carotid sinus hypersensitivity) and a much more serious condition such as carotid artery stenosis on the opposite side (see Chap. 366). Thus, carotid compression is a risky maneuver that may lead to cerebral ischemia.

Glossopharyngeal Neuralgia This painful disorder may induce reflex fainting. The sequence is always pain, followed by syncope. The pain is localized to the jaw, base of the tongue, pharynx or larynx, tonsillar area, and ear. The cardiovascular effects are attributable to excitation of the dorsal motor nucleus of the vagus via collateral fibers from the nucleus of the tractus solitarius. Treatment of the neuralgia with carbamazepine is often effective for the syncope, as well as for the pain.

Cough Syncope This is a rare condition that follows paroxysm of coughing, usually in chronic bronchitis. After forceful coughing, the patient suddenly becomes weak and loses consciousness momentarily. The coughing increases intrathoracic pressure and the elevated pressure is transmitted via the great veins to the intracranial compartment, causing increased intracranial pressure and secondarily decreased cerebral blood flow. At a critically low blood flow, syncope ensues.

Stretch Syncope This is a rare condition that occurs in otherwise normal adolescents. The provoking maneuver is simultaneous neck extension and upper limb stretching. The mechanism seems to be compression of the vertebral arteries in the neck.

DIFFERENTIAL DIAGNOSIS Anxiety Attacks and the Hyperventilation Syndrome Anxiety, such as occurs in panic attacks, is frequently interpreted as a feeling of faintness or dizziness without loss of consciousness. The symptoms are not accompanied by facial pallor and are not relieved by recumbency. The diagnosis is made on the basis of the associated symptoms, and the attack can be reproduced by hyperventilation. Hyperventilation results in hypocapnia, alkalosis, increased cerebrovascular resistance, and decreased cerebral blood flow. The release of epinephrine in anxiety states also contributes to the symptoms.

Hypoglycemia Severe hypoglycemia is usually traceable to a serious disease such as a tumor of the islets of Langerhans; advanced adrenal, pituitary, or hepatic disease; or to excessive administration of insulin; it leads to confusion or loss of consciousness. Mild hypoglycemia, often reactive type and occurring 2 to 5 h after eating, is not usually associated with a disturbance of consciousness.

Acute Hemorrhage Acute hemorrhage, usually within the gastrointestinal tract, is an occasional cause of syncope. In the absence of pain and hematemesis, the cause of the weakness, faintness, or even unconsciousness may remain obscure until the passage of a black stool.

Cerebral Transient Ischemic Attacks (TIAs) TIAs occur in patients with atherosclerotic narrowing, occlusion, or emboli to the major arteries of the brain. The symptoms are manifold (see Chap. 366). Sudden drop attacks may mimic syncope. Isolated loss of consciousness is rare.

Hysterical Fainting The attack is usually unattended by an outward display of anxiety. Lack of change in pulse and blood pressure or color of the skin and mucous membranes distinguishes it from the vasodepressor faint.

Approach to the Patient

Type of Onset (see Fig. 20-1) The timing and type of onset may assist in determining the cause. Syncope that begins over a period of a few seconds is most likely due to postural hypotension, sudden AV block, asystole, or ventricular tachycardia. When symptoms develop gradually during a period of several minutes, hyperventilation or hypoglycemia should be considered. Onset of syncope during or immediately after exertion suggests aortic stenosis, idiopathic hypertrophic subaortic stenosis or excessive bradycardia, and, in elderly subjects, postural hypotension. Exertional syncope is seen occasionally in persons with aortic insufficiency. In patients with ventricular standstill or ventricular fibrillation, loss of consciousness occurs 8 to 10 s later and then often by brief clonic muscle contractions.

Position at Onset of Attack Epilepsy and syncopal attacks due to hypoglycemia, hyperventilation, or heart block are likely to be independent of posture. Faintness associated with a drop in blood pressure and with ectopic tachycardia usually occurs only in the sitting or standing position, whereas faintness resulting from orthostatic hypotension is apt to begin shortly after change from the recumbent to the standing position.

Associated Symptoms Symptoms such as palpitation may be present when the attack is due to anxiety or hyperventilation, ectopic tachycardia, or hypoglycemia. Numbness and tingling in the hands and face are frequent accompaniments of hyperventilation. Genuine convulsions during the attack may occasionally occur with heart block, asystole, or ventricular tachycardia.

In patients with recurrent syncope an attempt to reproduce an attack may assist in diagnosis.

Symptoms induced by hyperventilation can be reproduced readily by having the subject breathe rapidly and deeply for 2 to 3 min. Anxiety attacks induced by hyperventilation tend to be lessened when the patient learns that the symptoms can be produced and alleviated at will simply by controlling breathing.

Other conditions in which the diagnosis is commonly clarified by reproducing the attacks are orthostatic hypotension and orthostatic tachycardia (observations of pulse rate, blood pressure, and symptoms in the recumbent and standing positions), and cough syncope (by inducing the Valsalva maneuver). In each instance, the crucial point is not whether symptoms are produced (the procedures mentioned frequently induce symptoms in healthy persons) but whether the exact pattern of symptoms that occurs in the spontaneous attacks is reproduced in the artificial ones. Continuous ambulatory ECG monitoring is essential to identify arrhythmias responsible for syncope, particularly in patients with frequently recurring symptoms. Monitoring is diagnostic if it shows episodes of asystole, extreme bradycardia, or tachyarrhythmia.

In cases of recurrent syncope of unknown cause in which ambulatory ECG monitoring is unrevealing and there is underlying heart disease, particularly ischemic and prior myocardial infarction, the use of intracardiac electrophysiologic techniques with programmed stimulation can be helpful in detecting cardiac rhythm abnormalities and in establishing effective treatment. During stimulation, up to two-thirds of such patients can be shown to have rapid ventricular tachycardia. Occasionally, intracardiac electrophysiologic studies are helpful in identifying significant His bundle conduction delays or sick-sinus syndrome. The diagnostic yield of intracardiac electrophysiologic test-

ing is lower in patients with nonischemic heart disease and in patients with structurally normal hearts than in patients with ischemic heart disease. Recently, the signal-averaged ECG has proved to be useful in identifying patients with unexplained syncope who are likely to have ventricular tachycardia induced by electrophysiologic study.

Head-up tilt testing is a useful provocative technique for the diagnosis of vasodepressor syncope. Upright tilt to a maximum of 60 to 70 degrees usually precipitates symptomatic hypotension or syncope within 10 to 30 min in patients with this syndrome. In normal subjects, passive tilting to 60 degrees causes a small decrease in systolic blood pressure and an increase in diastolic blood pressure and heart rate. Recently, tilt testing has been used in conjunction with electrophysiologic testing to assess the efficacy of prophylactic pacing in selected patients with vasodepressor syncope and to evaluate the impact of posture on the hemodynamic consequences of some tachyarrhythmias. Sublingual nitroglycerine administered during head-up tilt testing may unmask certain vasovagal-induced causes of syncope.

Syncope should be distinguished from disturbances of cerebral function caused by a seizure. A seizure may occur day or night, regardless of the position of the patient; syncope rarely appears when the patient is recumbent, the only common exception being the Stokes-Adams attack. The patient's color may not change in seizures, though there may be cyanosis; pallor is an early and invariable finding in all types of syncope, except chronic orthostatic hypotension and hysteria, and it precedes unconsciousness. Seizures are often heralded by an aura, which is caused by a focal seizure discharge and hence has brain-localizing significance. The aura is usually followed by rapid return to normal or by loss of consciousness. The onset of syncope is usually more deliberate and without aura. Injury from falling is frequent in a

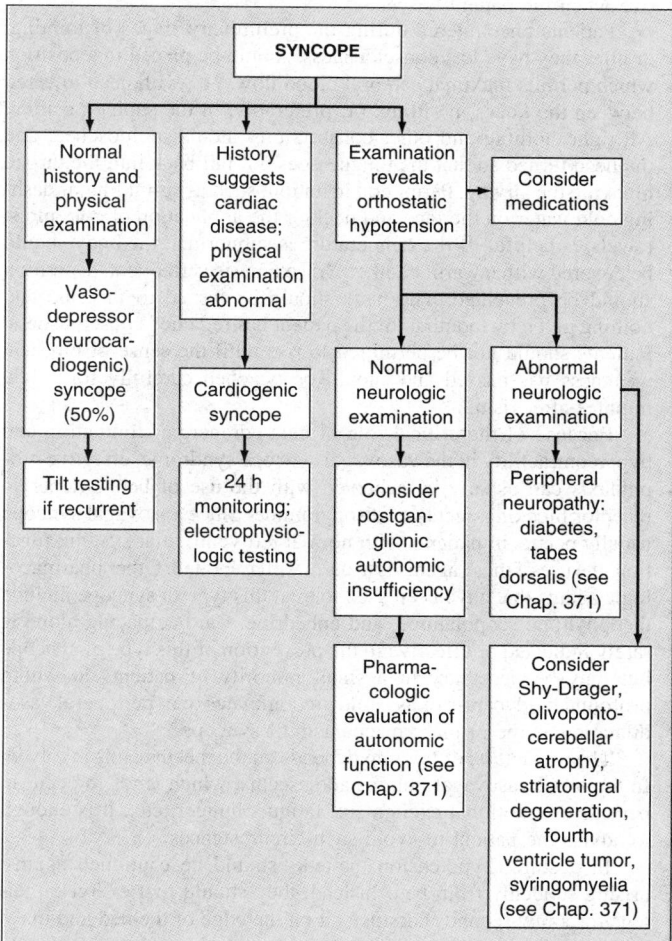

FIGURE 20-1 Approach to the patient with syncope.

seizure and rare in syncope for the reason that only in seizures are protective reflexes abolished instantaneously. Tonic-convulsive movements are a feature of seizures and usually do not occur with syncope, although, as stated above, brief tonic clonic seizurelike activity can accompany fainting episodes. Upward deviation of the eyes occurs with both conditions. The period of unconsciousness tends to be longer in seizures than in syncope. Urinary incontinence is frequent in seizures and rare in syncope. The return of consciousness is prompt in syncope, slow after a seizure. Mental confusion, headache, and drowsiness are common sequelae of seizures; physical weakness with a clear sensorium characterizes the postsyncopal state. Repeated spells of unconsciousness in a young person at a rate of several per day or month are more suggestive of epilepsy than of syncope.

The electroencephalogram (EEG) may be helpful in differentiating syncope from seizures. In the interval between epileptic seizures, it may show some degree of abnormality in up to 80 percent of patients. In the interval between syncopal attacks, the EEG should be normal.

℞ TREATMENT

The treatment of cardiac arrythmias is given in Chap. 230. In most instances, fainting is relatively benign. In dealing with patients who have fainted, the physician should think first of those causes of fainting that constitute a therapeutic emergency. Among them are massive internal hemorrhage and myocardial infarction, which may be painless, and cardiac arrhythmias. In elderly persons, a sudden faint, without obvious cause, should arouse the suspicion of complete heart block or a tachyarrhythmia, even though all findings are negative when the patient is seen.

Patients encountered during the preliminary stages of fainting, or after they have lost consciousness, should be placed in a position which permits maximal cerebral blood flow, i.e., with head lowered between the knees, if sitting, or, preferably, in the supine position. All tight clothing and other constrictions should be loosened, and the head turned so that the tongue does not fall back into the throat, blocking the airway. Peripheral irritation, such as sprinkling or dashing cold water on the face and neck or the application of cold moist towels, is helpful. If the temperature is subnormal, the body should be covered with a warm blanket. Since emesis is frequent, aspiration should be prevented. The head should be turned to the side and nothing given by mouth until the patient has regained consciousness. Patients should not be permitted to rise until the sense of physical weakness has passed and should be watched carefully for a few minutes after rising.

Because of the critical role of beta-adrenergic stimulation and hypercontractility in the vasovagal syncope syndrome, effective prophylaxis can usually be achieved with the use of beta-adrenergic receptor blocking agents or disopyramide. Since vasovagal syncope usually occurs in patients with normal left ventricular systolic function, the use of these agents is usually well tolerated. Other pharmacologic agents that have been used to treat this type of syncope include theophylline, scopolamine, and ephedrine. Cardiac pacing alone is rarely indicated or effective in the prevention of this type of syncope but may be necessary in a small minority of patients in whom profound bradycardia or asystole predominates over peripheral vasodilatation as the primary mechanism of syncope.

The *prevention* of fainting depends on the mechanisms involved. In the usual vasovagal faint of adolescents, which tends to occur in periods of emotional excitement, fatigue, hunger, etc., it is enough to advise the patient to avoid such circumstances.

In postural hypotension, patients should be cautioned against arising suddenly from bed. Instead, they should first exercise their legs for a few seconds and then sit on the edge of the bed and make certain they are not lightheaded or dizzy before starting to walk. Sleeping with the headposts of the bed elevated on wooden blocks 8 to 12 in. high and wearing a snug elastic abdominal binder and elastic stockings are often helpful. The distinction made between the various types of orthostatic hypotension has therapeutic significance. In the peripheral postganglionic type, the most effective treatment is 9α-fluorohydrocortisone (oral dose 0.1 to 0.2 mg/d) and salt loading to increase blood volume, supplemented by mechanical devices to prevent pooling of blood in the legs and lower trunk (g suit). However, salt together with mineralocorticoids may induce serious supine hypertension, and the dose of the drug must be adjusted for this. For the central preganglionic type, there has been greater success with use of a sympathomimetic amine such as tyramine (which releases norepinephrine from intact postganglionic endings) supplemented by a monoamine oxidase inhibitor (to prevent destruction of the amine) and possibly propranolol. Levodopa has been effective in some cases. In the postganglionic type, judicious use of phenylephrine or ephedrine may be beneficial if they do not cause insomnia. If there are no contraindications, a high intake of sodium chloride, which expands the extracellular fluid volume, may be tried.

The treatment of carotid sinus syncope involves first of all instructing the patient in measures that minimize the hazards of a fall (see below). Loose collars should be worn, and the patient should learn to turn the whole body, rather than the head alone, when looking to one side. Atropine or the ephedrine group of drugs should be used, respectively, in patients with pronounced bradycardia or hypotension during attacks. The treatment of the various cardiac arrhythmias that may induce syncope is discussed in Chap. 230. The treatment of hypoglycemia is found in Chap. 335.

The chief hazard of a faint in most elderly persons is not the underlying disease but fracture or other trauma due to the fall. Therefore, patients subject to recurrent syncope should cover the bathroom floor and bathtub with rubber mats and should have as much of their home carpeted as is feasible. Especially important is the floor space between the bed and the bathroom, because faints are common in elderly persons when walking from bed to toilet. Outdoor walking should be on soft ground rather than hard surfaces, and the patient should avoid standing still, which is more likely than walking to induce an attack.

DIZZINESS AND VERTIGO

Dizziness is a common and often vexing symptom. Patients use the term to encompass a variety of sensations, including those that seem semantically appropriate (e.g., lightheadedness, faintness, spinning, giddiness, etc.) and those that are misleadingly inappropriate, such as mental confusion, blurred vision, headache, tingling, or "walking on cotton." Moreover, some patients with gait disturbances and no abnormal cephalic sensations will describe their problem as "dizziness." A careful history is necessary to determine exactly what a patient who states, "Doctor, I'm dizzy," is experiencing.

After eliminating the misleading symptoms such as confusion, "dizziness" usually means either *faintness* (analogous to the feelings that precede syncope) or *vertigo* (an illusory or hallucinatory sense of environmental or self-movement). In other instances, neither of these terms accurately describes a patient's symptoms, and the explanation may only become apparent when the neurologic examination reveals spasticity, parkinsonism, or other ambulation disturbances as the cause of the complaint. Operationally, dizziness is classified into four categories: (1) faintness, (2) vertigo, (3) miscellaneous head sensations, and (4) gait disturbances.

FAINTNESS Fainting (syncope) is a loss of consciousness secondary to cerebral ischemia, more specifically ischemia to the brainstem. Prior to the actual faint, there are often prodromal symptoms (faintness) reflecting ischemia to a degree insufficient to impair consciousness (see above).

VERTIGO Vertigo is a hallucination of self- or environmental movement, most commonly a feeling of spinning, usually due to a disturbance in the vestibular system. The end organs of this system, situated in the bony labyrinths of the inner ears, consist of the three semicircular canals and the otolithic apparatus (utricle and saccule) on each side. The canals transduce angular acceleration, while the otoliths transduce linear acceleration and static gravitational forces, the latter providing a sense of head position in space. The neural output of the end organs is conveyed to the vestibular nuclei in the brainstem via the eighth cranial nerve. The principal projections from the vestibular nuclei are to the nuclei of cranial nerves III, IV, and VI, the spinal cord, the cerebral cortex, and the cerebellum. The vestibuloocular reflex (VOR) serves to maintain visual stability during head movement and depends on direct projections from the vestibular nuclei to the sixth cranial nerve (abducens) nuclei in the pons and, via the medial longitudinal fasciculus, to the third (oculomotor) and fourth (trochlear) cranial nerve nuclei in the midbrain. These connections account for the nystagmus (to-and-fro oscillation of the eyes) that is an almost invariable accompaniment of vestibular dysfunction. The vestibulospinal pathways assist in the maintenance of postural stability. Projections to the cerebral cortex, via the thalamus, provide conscious awareness of head position and movement. The vestibular nerves and nuclei project to areas of the cerebellum (primarily the flocculus and nodulus) that modulate the VOR.

The vestibular system is one of three sensory systems subserving spatial orientation and posture; the other two are the visual system (retina to occipital cortex) and the somatosensory system that conveys peripheral information from skin, joint, and muscle receptors. The three stabilizing systems overlap sufficiently to compensate (partially or completely) for each other's deficiencies. Vertigo may represent either physiologic stimulation or pathologic dysfunction in any of the three systems.

Physiologic Vertigo   This occurs when (1) the brain is confronted with a mismatch among the three stabilizing sensory systems; (2) the vestibular system is subjected to unfamiliar head movements to which it has never adapted, such as in seasickness; or (3) unusual head/neck positions, such as the extreme extension when painting a ceiling. Intersensory mismatch explains carsickness, height vertigo, and the visual vertigo most commonly experienced during motion picture chase scenes; in the latter, the visual sensation of environmental movement is unaccompanied by concomitant vestibular and somatosensory movement cues. *Space sickness*, a frequent transient effect of active head movement in the weightless zero-gravity environment, is another example of physiologic vertigo.

Pathologic Vertigo   This results from lesions of the visual, somatosensory, or vestibular systems. Visual vertigo is caused by new or incorrect spectacles or by the sudden onset of an extraocular muscle paresis with diplopia; in either instance, CNS compensation rapidly counteracts the vertigo. Somatosensory vertigo, rare in isolation, is usually due to a peripheral neuropathy that reduces the sensory input necessary for central compensation when there is dysfunction of the vestibular or visual systems.

The most common cause of pathologic vertigo is vestibular dysfunction. The vertigo is frequently accompanied by nausea, jerk nystagmus, postural unsteadiness, and gait ataxia. Since vertigo increases with rapid head movements, patients tend to hold their heads still.

Labyrinthine dysfunction   This causes severe rotational or linear vertigo. When rotational, the hallucination of movement, whether of environment or self, is directed away from the side of the lesion. The fast phases of nystagmus beat away from the lesion side, and the tendency to fall is toward the side of the lesion.

When the head is straight and immobile, the vestibular end organs generate a tonic resting firing frequency that is equal from the two sides. With any rotational acceleration, the anatomic positions of the semicircular canals on each side necessitate an increased firing rate from one and a commensurate decrease from the other. This change in neural activity is ultimately projected to the cerebral cortex, where it is summed with inputs from the visual and somatosensory systems to produce the appropriate conscious sense of rotational movement. After cessation of movement, the firing frequencies of the two end organs reverse; the side with the initially increased rate decreases, and the other side increases. A sense of rotation in the opposite direction is experienced; since there is no actual head movement, this hallucinatory sensation is *vertigo*. Any disease state that changes the firing frequency of an end organ, producing unequal neural input to the brainstem and ultimately the cerebral cortex, causes vertigo. The symptom can be conceptualized as the cortex inappropriately interpreting the abnormal neural input from the brainstem as indicating actual head rotation. Transient abnormalities produce short-lived symptoms. With a fixed unilateral deficit, central conpensatory mechanisms ultimately diminish the vertigo. Since compensation depends on the plasticity of connections between the vestibular nuclei and the cerebellum, patients with brainstem or cerebellar disease have diminished adaptive capacity, and symptoms may persist indefinitely. Compensation is always inadequate for severe fixed bilateral lesions despite normal cerebellar connections: these patients are permanently symptomatic.

Acute unilateral labyrinthine dysfunction is caused by infection, trauma, and ischemia. Often, no specific etiology is uncovered, and the nonspecific terms *acute labyrinthitis*, *acute peripheral vestibulopathy*, or *vestibular neuritis* are used to describe the event. It is impossible to predict whether a patient recovering from the first bout of vertigo will have recurrent episodes.

Acute bilateral labyrinthine dysfunction is usually the result of toxins such as drugs or alcohol. The most common offending drugs are the aminoglycoside antibiotics.

Schwannomas involving the eighth cranial nerve (*acoustic neuroma*) grow slowly and produce such a gradual reduction of labyrinthine output that central compensatory mechanisms can prevent or minimize the vertigo; auditory symptoms of hearing loss and tinnitus are the most common manifestations. While lesions of the brainstem or cerebellum can cause acute vertigo, associated signs and symptoms usually permit distinction from a labyrinthine etiology (Table 20-2). However, labyrinthine ischemia may be the sole manifestation of vertebrobasilar insufficiency. Occasionally, an acute lesion of the vestibulocerebellum may present with monosymptomatic vertigo indistinguishable from a labyrinthopathy.

Table 20-2

Differentiation of Peripheral and Central Vertigo

Sign or Symptom	Peripheral (Labyrinth)	Central (Brainstem or Cerebellum)
Direction of associated nystagmus	Unidirectional; fast phase opposite lesion*	Bidirectional or unidirectional
Purely horizontal nystagmus without torsional component	Uncommon	Common
Vertical or purely torsional nysagmus	Never present	May be present
Visual fixation	Inhibits nystagmus and vertigo	No inhibition
Severity of vertigo	Marked	Often mild
Direction of spin	Toward fast phase	Variable
Direction of fall	Toward slow phase	Variable
Duration of symptoms	Finite (minutes, days, weeks) but recurrent	May be chronic
Tinnitus and/or deafness	Often present	Usually absent
Associated central abnormalities	None	Extremely common
Common causes	Infection (labyrinthitis), Ménière's, neuronitis, ischemia, trauma, toxin	Vascular, demyelinating, neoplasm

* In Ménière's disease, the direction of the fast phase is variable.

Recurrent unilateral labyrinthine dysfunction, in association with signs and symptoms of cochlear disease (progressive hearing loss and tinnitus), is usually due to Ménière's disease. When auditory manifestations are absent, the term *vestibular neuronitis* denotes recurrent monosymptomatic vertigo. TIAs of the posterior cerebral circulation (vertebrobasilar insufficiency) very infrequently cause recurrent vertigo without concomitant motor, sensory, visual, cranial nerve, or cerebellar signs.

Positional vertigo is precipitated by a recumbent head position, either to the right or to the left. Benign paroxysmal positional (or positioning) vertigo (BPPV) is particularly common. Although the condition may be due to head trauma, usually no precipitating factors are identified. It generally abates spontaneously after weeks or months. The vertigo and accompanying nystagmus have a distinct pattern of latency, fatigability, and habituation that differs from the less common central positional vertigo (Table 20-3) due to lesions in and around the fourth ventricle. Moreover, the pattern of nystagmus in BPPV is distinctive. The lower eye displays a large-amplitude torsional nystagmus, and the upper eye has a lesser degree of torsion combined with upbeating nystagmus. If the eyes are directed to the upper ear, the vertical nystagmus in the upper eye increases in amplitude.

Vestibular epilepsy, vertigo secondary to temporal lobe epileptic activity, is rare and almost always intermixed with other epileptic manifestations.

Psychogenic vertigo, usually a concomitant of agoraphobia (fear of large open spaces, crowds, or leaving the safety of home), should be suspected in patients so "incapacitated" by their symptoms that they adopt a prolonged housebound status. Despite their discomfort, most patients with organic vertigo attempt to function. Organic vertigo is accompanied by nystagmus; a psychogenic etiology is almost certain when nystagmus is absent during a vertiginous episode.

Evaluation of patients with pathologic vestibular vertigo The evaluation depends on whether a central etiology is suspected (see Table 20-2). If so, magnetic resonance imaging of the head is mandatory. Such an examination is rarely helpful in cases of recurrent monosymptomatic vertigo with a normal neurologic examination. Typical BPPV requires no investigation after the diagnosis is made (see Table 20-3).

Vestibular function tests serve to (1) demonstrate an abnormality when the distinction between organic and psychogenic is uncertain, (2) establish the side of the abnormality, and (3) distinguish between peripheral and central etiologies. The standard test is electronystagmography, where warm and cold water (or air) are applied, in a prescribed fashion, to the tympanic membranes, and the slow-phase velocities of the resultant nystagmus from the right and left ears are compared. A velocity decrease from one side indicates hypofunction ("canal paresis"). An inability to induce nystagmus with ice water denotes a "dead labyrinth." Some institutions have the capability of quantitatively determining various aspects of the vestibuloocular reflex using computer-driven rotational chairs and precise oculographic recording of the eye movements.

℞ **TREATMENT**

Treatment of acute vertigo consists of bed rest and vestibular suppressant drugs such as antihistaminics (meclizine, dimenhydrinate, promethazine), centrally acting anticholinergics (scopolamine), or a tranquilizer with GABA-ergic effects (diazepam). If the vertigo persists beyond a few days, most authorities advise ambulation in an attempt to induce central compensatory mechanisms, despite the short-term discomfiture to the patient. Chronic vertigo of labyrinthine origin may be treated with a systematized exercise program to facilitate compensation.

Prophylactic measures to prevent recurrent vertigo are variably effective. Antihistamines are commonly utilized. Ménière's disease may respond to a very low salt diet (1 g/day). Persisting (beyond 4 to 6 weeks) BPPV responds dramatically to specific exercise programs.

There are a variety of inner ear surgical procedures for all forms of refractory chronic or recurrent vertigo, but these are only rarely necessary.

Miscellaneous Head Sensations This designation is used, primarily for purposes of initial classification, to describe dizziness that is neither faintness nor vertigo. Cephalic ischemia or vestibular dysfunction may be of such low intensity that the usual symptomatology is not clearly identified. For example, a small decrease in blood pressure or a slight vestibular imbalance may cause sensations different from distinct faintness or vertigo but that may be identified properly during provocative testing techniques. Other causes of dizziness in this category are hyperventilation syndrome, hypoglycemia, and the somatic symptoms of a clinical depression; these patients should have normal neurologic examinations and vestibular function tests.

Gait Disturbances Some individuals with gait disorders complain of dizziness despite the absence of vertigo or other abnormal cephalic sensations. The causes include peripheral neuropathy, myelopathy, spasticity, parkinsonian rigidity, and cerebellar ataxia. In this context, the term *dizziness* is being used to describe disturbed mobility. There may be mild associated lightheadedness, particularly with impaired sensation from the feet or poor vision; this is known as *multiple-sensory-defect dizziness* and occurs in elderly individuals who complain of dizziness only during ambulation. Decreased position sense (secondary to neuropathy or myelopathy) and poor vision (from cataracts or retinal degeneration) create an overreliance on the aging vestibular apparatus. A less precise, but sometimes comforting, designation is *benign dysequilibrium of aging*.

Approach to the Patient

The most important diagnostic tool is a careful history focused on the meaning of "dizziness" to the patient. Is it faintness? Is there a sensation of spinning? If either of these is affirmed and the neurologic examination is normal, appropriate investigations for the multiple etiologies of cephalic ischemia or vestibular dysfunction are undertaken.

When the meaning of "dizziness" is uncertain, provocative tests may be helpful. These office procedures simulate either cephalic ischemia or vestibular dysfunction. Cephalic ischemia is obvious if the dizziness is duplicated during orthostatic hypotension. Further provocation involves the Valsalva maneuver, which decreases cerebral blood flow and should reproduce ischemic symptoms.

The simplest provocative test for vestibular dysfunction is rapid rotation and abrupt cessation of movement in a swivel chair. This always induces vertigo that the patients can compare with their symptomatic dizziness. The intense induced vertigo may be unlike the spontaneous symptoms, but shortly thereafter, when the vertigo has all but subsided, a lightheadedness supervenes that may be identified as "my dizziness." When this occurs, the dizzy patient, originally classified as suffering from "miscellaneous head sensations," is now properly diagnosed as having mild vertigo secondary to a vestibulopathy.

Table 20-3

Benign Paroxysmal Positional Vertigo (BPPV) and Central Positional Vertigo

Features	BPPV	Central
Latency*	3–40 s	None: immediate vertigo and nystagmus
Fatigability†	Yes	No
Habituation‡	Yes	No
Intensity of vertigo	Severe	Mild
Reproducibility§	Variable	Good

* Time between attaining head position and onset of symptoms.
† Disappearance of symptoms with maintenance of offending position.
‡ Lessening of symptoms with repeated trials.
§ Likelihood of symptom production during any examination session.

Patients with symptoms of positional vertigo should be appropriately tested (see Table 20-3); positional testing is more sensitive with special spectacles that preclude visual fixation (Frenzel lenses).

A final provocative test, requiring the use of Frenzel lenses, is vigorous head shaking in the horizontal plane for about 10 s. If nystagmus develops after the shaking stops, even in the absence of vertigo, vestibular dysfunction is demonstrated. The maneuver can then be repeated in the vertical plane. If the provocative tests establish the dizziness as a vestibular symptom, the previously described evaluation of vestibular vertigo is undertaken.

Hyperventilation is the cause of dizziness in many anxious individuals; tingling of the hands and face may be absent. Forced hyperventilation for 1 min is indicated for patients with enigmatic dizziness and normal neurologic examinations. Similarly, depressive symptoms (which patients usually insist are "secondary" to the dizziness) must alert the examiner to a clinical depression as the *cause*, rather than the effect, of the dizziness.

CNS disease can produce dizzy sensations of all types. Consequently, a neurologic examination is always required even if the history or provocative tests suggest a cardiac, peripheral vestibular, or psychogenic etiology. Any abnormality on the neurologic examination should prompt appropriate neurodiagnostic studies.

BIBLIOGRAPHY

BALOH RW: Approach to the evaluation of the dizzy patient. Otolaryngol Head Neck Surg 112:3, 1995

BRANDT T et al: Therapy for benign paroxysmal positioning vertigo, revisited. Neurology 44:796, 1994

BRIGNOLE M et al: Mechanisms of syncope caused by transient bradycardia and the diagnostic value of electrophysiologic testing and cardiovascular reflexivity maneuvers. Am J Cardiol 76:273, 1995

BRUNI J: Episodic impairment of consciousness, in *Neurology in Clinical Practice*, WG Bradley et al (eds). Boston, Butterworth-Heinemann, 1996, chap 2

CALKINS H et al: Clinical presentation and long-term follow-up of athletes with exercise-induced vasodepressor syncope. Am Heart J 129:1159, 1995

———— et al: The value of the clinical history in the differentiation of syncope due to ventricular tachycardia, atrioventricular block, and neurocardiogenic syncope. Am J Med 98:365, 1995

EVANS RW: Neurologic aspects of hyperventilation syndrome. Semin Neurol 15:115, 1995

FERRANTE L et al: Glossopharyngeal neuralgia with cardiac syncope. Neurosurgery 36:58, 1995

GOMEZ CR et al: Isolated vertigo as a manifestation of vertebrobasilar ischemia. Neurology 47:94, 1996

KLEIN GJ et al: Electrophysiological testing: The final court of appeal for diagnosis of syncope? Circulation 92:1332, 1995

KUSUMOTO FM, GOLDSCHLAGER N: Cardiac pacing. N Engl J Med 334:89, 1996

LANDAU WM: Neuroskepticism: Sovereign remedy for the carotid sinus syndrome. Neurology 44:1570, 1994

————, NELSON DA: Feinting science: Neurocardiogenic syncope and collateral vasovagal confusion. Neurology 46:609, 1996

———— et al: Benign positional vertigo: Recognition and treatment. BMJ 311:489 and 799, 1995

LEMPERT T et al: Syncope: A videometric analysis of 56 episodes of transient cerebral hypoxia. Ann Neurol 36:233, 1994

———— LEMPERT T et al: The eye movements of syncope. Neurology 46:1086, 1996

LIPPMAN N et al: Failure to decrease parasympathetic tone during upright tilt predicts a positive tilt-table test. Am J Cardiol 75:591, 1995

LOW PA: Update on the evaluation, pathogenesis, and management of neurogenic orthostatic hypotension. Neurology 45:suppl 5, 54–532, 1995

MATHIAS CJ: Disorders of the autonomic nervous system, in *Neurology in Clinical Practice*, WG Bradley et al (eds). Boston, Butterworth-Heinemann, 1996, chap 82

MATTLE HP et al: Transient cerebral circulatory arrest coincides with fainting in cough syncope. Neurology 45:498, 1995

NADOL JB: Vestibular neuritis. Otolaryngol Head Neck Surg 112:162, 1995

SHARPE JA: Neuro-ophthalmic implications of vestibular disorders, in *Neuro-Ophthalmological Disorders*, RJ Tusa, SA Newman (eds). New York, Dekker, 1995, chap 18

STURZENEGGER M et al: Transcranial Doppler and angiographic findings in adolescent stretch syncope. J Neurol Neurosurg Psychiatry 58:367, 1995

TROOST BT: Dizziness and vertigo, in *Neurology in Clinical Practice*, WG Bradley et al (eds). Boston, Butterworth-Heinemann, 1996, chap 18

21   *Richard K. Olney, Michael J. Aminoff*

WEAKNESS, ABNORMAL MOVEMENTS, AND IMBALANCE

Motor dysfunction may result from weakness, movement disorders, ataxia, imbalance, and other disturbances in the initiation or coordination of movement. In this chapter, we describe the normal anatomy and physiology of the neural structures that subserve these functions, review the manner in which this physiology is altered to produce symptoms, and present a clinical approach toward the diagnosis of these various types of motor dysfunction.

WEAKNESS

Weakness is a reduction in normal power of one or more muscles. Patients may use the term differently; thus one or more specific examples of weakness should be elicited during the history. Increased fatigability or limitation in function due to pain is often confused with weakness by patients. Increased fatigability is the inability to sustain the performance of an activity that should be normal for a person of the same age, gender, and size.

Weakness is commonly described by severity and distribution. Paralysis and the suffix "-plegia" indicate weakness that is so severe that it is complete or nearly complete. "Paresis" refers to weakness that is mild. The prefix "hemi-" refers to one half of the body, "para-" to both legs, and "quadri-" to all four limbs.

Recognition of altered tone is important in localizing the cause of weakness. *Tone* is the resistance of a muscle to passive stretch. Central nervous system abnormalities that cause weakness generally produce *spasticity*, an increase in tone due to upper motor neuron disease. Spasticity is velocity dependent, has a sudden release after reaching a maximum (the "clasp-knife" phenomenon), and predominantly affects antigravity muscles (i.e., upper limb flexors more than extensors and lower limb extensors more than flexors). Spasticity is distinct from rigidity and paratonia, two other types of increased tone. *Rigidity* is increased tone that is present throughout the range of motion (a "lead pipe" or "plastic" stiffness) and affects flexors and extensors equally. In some patients, rigidity has a cogwheel quality that is enhanced by voluntary movement of the contralateral limb (reinforcement). Rigidity occurs with certain extrapyramidal disorders. *Paratonia*, also referred to as *gegenhalten*, is increased tone that varies irregularly in a manner that may seem related to the degree of relaxation, is present throughout the range of motion, and affects flexors and extensors equally. Paratonia usually results from disease of the frontal lobes. Weakness with decreased tone (flaccidity) or normal tone occurs with disorders of the *motor unit*, that is, a single lower motor neuron and all of the muscle fibers it innervates.

Three basic patterns of weakness can usually be recognized based on the signs summarized in Table 21-1. One results from upper motor neuron pathology, and the other two from disorders of the motor unit (lower motor neuron and myopathic weakness). Fasciculations and the early presence of atrophy help to distinguish lower motor neuron (neurogenic) weakness from myopathic weakness. A *fasciculation* is a visible or palpable twitch within a single muscle due to the spontaneous discharge of one motor unit. Neurogenic weakness also produces more prominent hypotonia and greater depression of tendon reflexes than myopathic weakness.

PATHOGENESIS OF WEAKNESS   **Upper Motor Neuron Weakness**   This pattern of weakness results from disorders that affect the upper motor neurons or their axons in the cerebral cortex, subcortical white matter, internal capsule, brainstem, or spinal cord.

Upper motor neurons have their cell bodies in layer V of the cerebral cortex. Most are contained in the primary motor cortex (the precentral gyrus, or Brodmann's area 4) and in the premotor and

Table 21-1

Signs that Distinguish Patterns of Weakness

Sign	Upper Motor Neuron	Lower Motor Neuron	Myopathic
Atrophy	None	Severe	Mild
Fasciculations	None	Common	None
Tone	Spastic	Decreased	Normal/decreased
Distribution of weakness	Pyramidal/regional	Distal/segmental	Proximal
Tendon reflexes	Hyperactive	Hypoactive/absent	Normal/hypoactive
Babinski's sign	Present	Absent	Absent

supplemental motor cortex (area 6). A significant minority are in the primary sensory cortex (areas 3, 1, and 2) and the superior parietal lobule (areas 5 and 7). The upper motor neurons in the primary motor cortex are somatotopically organized. Those that activate facial muscles are at the lower end of the precentral gyrus, those that activate arm and hand muscles are higher in this gyrus, and those that activate the leg muscles are in the paracentral lobule over the medial surface of the cerebral hemisphere. Somatotopic organization of the upper motor neurons is also preserved in other cortical motor areas (e.g., premotor and supplemental motor cortices).

Axons of the upper motor neurons descend through the subcortical white matter and the posterior limb of the internal capsule. Those axons that comprise the *pyramidal* or *corticospinal system* descend through the brainstem in the cerebral peduncles of the midbrain, the basis pontis, and the medullary pyramids (Fig. 21-1). At the cervicomedullary junction, most pyramidal axons decussate into the contralateral corticospinal tract of the lateral spinal cord, but 10 to 30 percent remain ipsilateral in the anterior spinal cord. Pyramidal neurons include both the large corticomotoneurons and the smaller corticospinal neurons. The corticomotoneurons are glutamatergic and make direct monosynaptic connections with lower motor neurons. They innervate most densely the lower motor neurons of hand muscles and are involved in the execution of learned, fine movements. The corticospinal neurons are also glutamatergic, but they synapse on neurons in the dorsal horn and interneurons in the intermediate zone of the spinal cord to facilitate cortically initiated movements. Corticobulbar neurons are upper motor neurons that are similar to corticospinal neurons but innervate brainstem motor nuclei. Although analogous in function and often referred to as pyramidal in general contexts, corticobulbar neurons are not strictly part of the pyramidal system, as their axons never traverse the medullary pyramids.

Bulbospinal upper motor neurons influence strength and tone but are not part of the pyramidal system (Fig. 21-1). Corticorubral, corticoreticular, corticopontine, and other cortical-brainstem pathways contribute to lower motor neuron activity indirectly through these pathways. The cortical neurons influence the red nucleus and superior colliculus of the midbrain and the vestibular nuclei, the inferior olivary nucleus, and reticular formation of the pons and medulla. The descending *ventromedial bulbospinal pathways* originate in the tectum of the midbrain (tectospinal pathway), the lateral and medial vestibular nuclei (vestibulospinal pathway), and the reticular formation (reticulospinal pathway). These pathways influence axial and proximal muscles and are involved in the maintenance of posture and integrated movements of the limbs and trunk. The

descending *ventrolateral bulbospinal pathways*, which originate predominantly in the magnocellular portion of the red nucleus (rubrospinal pathway), facilitate distal limb muscles. The bulbospinal system is sometimes referred to as the *extrapyramidal upper motor neuron system*.

The pyramidal and bulbospinal pathways contribute to normal strength, tone, coordination, and gait. Clinical lesions generally affect both pyramidal and bulbospinal pathways and are rarely purely pyramidal. Purely pyramidal lesions in animals produce an acute flaccid contralateral hemiplegia that spares the face and is associated with an extensor plantar (Babinski) response; strength recovers over weeks to months, and spasticity and hyperreflexia do not develop. In upper motor neuron weakness in humans, the development of spasticity and hyperreflexia has been reported with the rare cases of pure bilateral pyramidal infarction.

Upper motor neuron lesions produce weakness through decreased activation of the lower motor neurons that innervate muscles in one or more regions of the body. Upper motor neuron weakness always affects more than one muscle group and uncommonly affects all muscles within a limb. In general, distal muscle groups are affected more severely than proximal ones, and axial movements are spared unless the lesion is severe and bilateral. With corticobulbar involvement, weakness is usually observed only in the lower face and tongue; extraocular, upper facial, pharyngeal, and jaw muscles are almost always spared. With bilateral corticobulbar lesions, *pseudobulbar palsy* often develops, in which dysarthria, dysphagia, dysphonia, and emotional lability accompany bilateral facial weakness. Spastic tone accompanies upper motor neuron weakness, unless it is acute. Acute

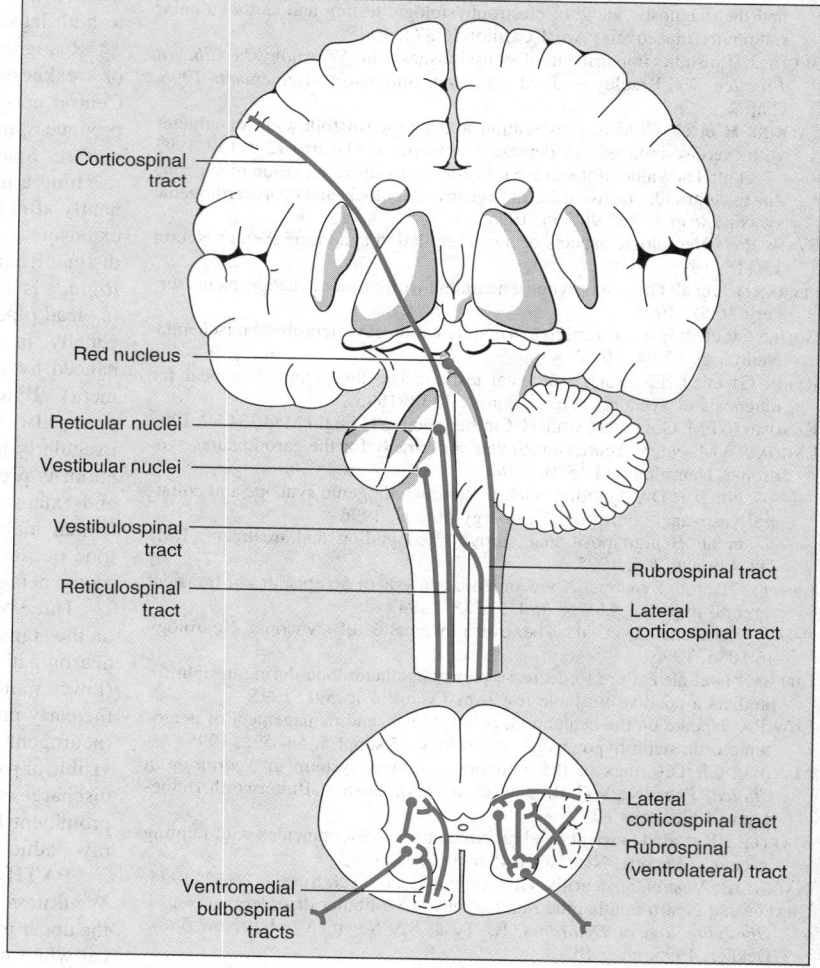

Corticospinal tract

Red nucleus

Reticular nuclei

Vestibular nuclei

Vestibulospinal tract

Reticulospinal tract

Rubrospinal tract

Lateral corticospinal tract

Lateral corticospinal tract

Rubrospinal (ventrolateral) tract

Ventromedial bulbospinal tracts

FIGURE 21-1   The corticospinal and bulbospinal upper motor neuron pathways. The axons of the bulbospinal neurons are contained in both ventromedial and ventrolateral tracts. In all figures, nerve cell bodies and axon terminals are shown, respectively, as closed circles and forks.

lesions below the foramen magnum usually produce *spinal shock* if weakness is severe. During spinal shock, tendon reflexes are absent and tone is flaccid. Spasticity subsequently develops over days to weeks.

Upper motor neuron lesions also cause incoordination that is manifest as slow, coarse movements for which normal rhythmicity is maintained. Finger-nose-finger and heel-knee-shin are performed slowly but adequately. The incoordination is more obvious with rapidly repeated movements, such as tapping the index finger on the thumb.

Lower Motor Neuron Weakness   This pattern results from disorders of cell bodies of lower motor neurons in the brainstem motor nuclei and the anterior horn of the spinal cord, or from dysfunction of the axons of these neurons as they pass to skeletal muscle.

Lower motor neurons are divided into alpha and gamma types (Fig. 21-2). Gamma motor neurons are smaller than alpha motor neurons and innervate the intrafusal muscle fibers of the muscle spindle. Activation of the gamma motor neuron increases the tension on muscle spindles and facilitates stretch reflexes and other local reflex mechanisms that activate a muscle through the alpha motor neurons. Each muscle is innervated by many (usually several hundred) alpha motor neurons. Each alpha motor neuron activates many extrafusal muscle fibers, several hundred for limb and axial muscles or fewer than twenty for extraocular muscles, through release of acetylcholine.

Lower motor neuron axons exit the brainstem in certain cranial nerves and the spinal cord in the ventral roots. The ventral roots fuse with the dorsal roots at the intervertebral foramen to form spinal nerves. For innervation of limb muscles, several adjacent spinal nerves fuse to form plexuses before dividing into peripheral nerves. Most peripheral nerves branch one or more times as they innervate different muscles. Each alpha motor axon extensively arborizes just before reaching the many muscle fibers that it innervates.

The alpha motor neuron receives direct excitatory, glutamatergic input from corticomotoneurons and primary muscle spindle afferents. The alpha and gamma motor neurons also receive direct or indirect excitatory input from other descending upper motor neuron pathways, segmental sensory inputs, and interneurons. The alpha motor neurons in the spinal cord receive direct postsynaptic inhibition from Renshaw cell interneurons, which release glycine. Other interneurons produce presynaptic inhibition on dorsal horn neurons through release of gamma-aminobutyric acid (GABA); this indirectly inhibits the alpha and gamma motor neurons. Other descending upper motor neuron pathways and segmental sensory inputs also produce direct or indirect inhibition of the alpha and gamma motor neurons.

When the balance of descending upper motor neuron and segmental inputs is excitatory, the pool of lower motor neurons that innervates a muscle is activated in an orderly manner. The lower motor neurons with the smallest cell bodies are activated first. With increasing effort,

these motor units discharge more rapidly, and larger motor units are then gradually recruited. With maximum effort, the entire lower motor neuron pool is activated to produce maximum power.

Lower motor weakness is produced by a decrease in the number of motor units that can be activated, due to a loss of the alpha motor neurons or disruption of their connections to muscle. With a decreased number of motor units, fewer muscle fibers are activated with full effort and maximum power is reduced. Loss of gamma motor neurons does not cause weakness but decreases tension on the muscle spindles. Muscle tone and tendon reflexes depend on gamma motor neurons, muscle spindles, their afferent fibers, and the alpha motor neurons. A tap on a tendon stretches muscle spindles and activates the primary spindle afferent fibers. These monosynaptically stimulate the alpha motor neurons in the spinal cord through release of glutamate. The activated alpha motor neurons produce a brief muscle contraction, which is the familiar tendon reflex. Loss of the gamma motor neuron input to the intrafusal muscle fibers decreases both continuous discharge of spindle afferents (which increase muscle tone) and phasic discharge of spindle afferents in response to stretch (which produces the tendon reflex).

When a motor unit becomes diseased, especially in anterior horn cell diseases, it may spontaneously discharge, producing a fasciculation, without being recruited in the normal manner. These isolated small twitches may be seen or felt clinically or recorded by electromyography (EMG) (See Chap. 361). When alpha motor neurons or their axons degenerate, the denervated muscle fibers spontaneously discharge in a manner that cannot be seen or felt but can be recorded with EMG. These small single muscle fiber discharges are called *fibrillation potentials*. The recruitment of surviving motor units can be assessed with EMG. If significant lower motor neuron weakness is present, recruitment of motor units is delayed or reduced, meaning that fewer than normal are activated at a given discharge frequency. This contrasts with upper motor neuron weakness, in which a normal number of motor units are activated at a given frequency but in which the maximum discharge frequency is decreased.

Myopathic Weakness   This pattern of weakness is produced by disorders within the motor unit that affect the muscle fibers or the neuromuscular junctions.

Two types of muscle fibers exist. Type I muscle fibers are rich in mitochondria and oxidative enzymes, produce relatively low force, but have low energy demands that can be supplied by ongoing aerobic metabolism. They produce sustained postural and nonforceful movements. Type II muscle fibers are rich in glycolytic enzymes, can produce relatively high force, but have high energy demands that cannot be supplied for long by ongoing aerobic metabolism. Thus, these units can be activated maximally for only brief periods of time to produce high-force movements.

For graded voluntary movements, type I muscle fibers are activated earliest in recruitment. For each muscle fiber, if the nerve terminal releases a normal number of acetylcholine molecules presynaptically and a sufficient number of postsynaptic acetylcholine receptors are opened, the end plate reaches threshold and thereby generates an action potential that spreads across the muscle fiber membrane and into the transverse tubular system. This electrical excitation activates intracellular events that produce an energy-dependent contraction of the muscle fiber (excitation–contraction coupling).

Myopathic weakness is produced by a decrease in the number or contractile force of muscle fibers activated within the motor unit. With muscular dystrophies, inflammatory myopathies, or myopathies with muscle fiber necrosis, decreased numbers of muscle fibers survive within many motor units. As demonstrated with EMG, the size of each motor unit action potential is decreased so that motor units must be recruited more rapidly than normal to produce the power necessary for a certain movement. Neuromuscular junction diseases produce weakness in a similar manner, although the loss of muscle fibers within the motor unit is functional rather than actual. Furthermore, the number

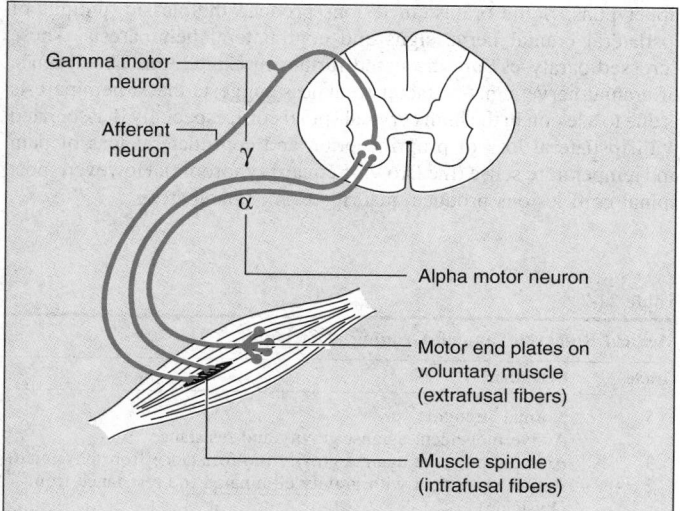

FIGURE 21-2   Alpha and gamma motor neurons and the primary spindle afferent neuron.

of muscle fibers activated can vary over time, depending on the state of rest of the neuromuscular junctions. Some myopathies produce weakness through loss of contractile force of muscle fibers. These may not affect the size of the motor unit action potentials and are detected by a discrepancy between the electrical activity and force of a muscle.

Nonparalytic Disorders of Movement Other disorders of movement occur that do not cause weakness. Those that are classified as movement disorders or as imbalance and ataxia will be discussed later in this chapter. Others are caused by disorders in initiation or integration of movement. Such disorders are produced by diseases that affect the cerebral hemispheres without causing obvious upper motor neuron weakness.

Most functional movements require the integrated coordination of many muscle groups. For example, consider a simple movement, such as grasping a ball. The primary movement is a flexion of the thumb and fingers of one hand, with opposition of the thumb and little finger. This requires the contraction of several muscles, including flexor digitorum superficialis, flexor digitorum profundus, flexor pollicis longus, flexor pollicis brevis, opponens pollicis, and opponens digiti minimi. These prime movers for this action are called *agonists*. In order for the grasping to be smooth and forceful, the thumb and finger extensors need to relax at the same rate as the flexors contract. The muscles that act in a directly opposing manner to the agonists are *antagonists*. A secondary action of the thumb and finger flexors is to flex the wrist; because wrist flexion tends to weaken finger flexion if both occur, activation of wrist extensors assists the grasping movement. Muscles that produce such complementary movements are *synergists*. Finally, the arm needs to be held in a stable position as the grasp occurs, so that the ball is not knocked away before it is secured. Muscles that stabilize the arm position are *fixators*.

The coordination of activity by agonists, antagonists, synergists, and fixators is regulated by a three-level hierarchy of motor control. The lowest level of control is mediated through segmental reflexes in the spinal cord. These reflexes facilitate agonists and reciprocally inhibit the antagonists. Spinal segments also control rhythmic patterns of movement that involve more than a single pair of agonists and antagonists. For example, the lumbosacral spinal cord contains the basic programming for cyclical stepping movements that involve the synergistic activation of different muscle groups over time. The intermediate level of control is mediated through the descending bulbospinal pathways, which integrate visual, proprioceptive, and vestibular feedback into the execution of an action (discussed later). For example, the locomotor center in the mesencephalon is required to modify the cyclical stepping movements in order that balance be maintained and forward movement occur. The highest level of control is mediated by the cerebral cortex. Superimposition of this highest level of control is necessary for activities, such as walking, to be goal-directed. Precise movements that are learned and improved through practice are also initiated and controlled by the motor cortex. Although only the agonists are directly activated, during the course of a complex sequence of actions, such as playing the piano, the sequential activation of different groups of agonists for each note or chord is a part of the learned motor program. Further, the execution of these actions also involves input from the basal ganglia and cerebellar hemispheres to facilitate agonists, synergists, and fixators and to inhibit undesired antagonists.

Apraxia is a disorder of initiating and planning movement (see also Chap. 25). Unilateral apraxia of the right hand may be due to a lesion of the left frontal lobe (especially anterior or inferior), the left temporoparietal region (especially the supramarginal gyrus), or their connections. Left body apraxia is produced by lesions of these regions in the right hemisphere or by lesions in the corpus callosum that disconnect the right temporoparietal or frontal regions from those on the left. Bilateral apraxia is often due to bilateral frontal lobe lesions or diffuse bilateral hemispheric disease.

DIAGNOSTIC APPROACH AND DIFFERENTIAL DIAGNOSIS FOR COMMON CLINICAL PRESENTATIONS OF WEAKNESS Clinical Assessment of Weakness When there is a discrepancy between the history and physical findings, it is usually because the patient complains of weakness, whereas symptoms are actually due to other causes, such as incoordination. The proper approach to weakness requires that its mode of onset, distribution, and associated features be carefully defined in order to identify the responsible anatomic lesion and the likely etiology.

Power may be examined in a variety of ways. Direct testing is most often used to determine whether weakness is present and to assess its distribution. The patient is asked to push or pull in a specified direction against the resistance of the physician, and the strength in each muscle group is graded from 0 to 5 by the scale developed by the Medical Research Council (Table 21-2). A second method is indirect testing through observation of task performance such as holding the arms outstretched. This is especially useful in detecting mild, asymmetric upper motor neuron weakness through the observation of a downward drift with pronation of the forearm on one side. A third method is functional testing, which involves quantitation of activities. Common tests include counting the number of times a person can perform a deep-knee bend or step on a stool or chair, or timing the length of time the arms can be held abducted to 90 degrees. Functional testing for weakness is time-consuming and any weakness is difficult to localize to a specific muscle or group of muscles; however, it provides reproducible data for assessment of changes in the patient's status over time.

Other essential parts of the motor examination include appraisal of muscular bulk, inspection for fasciculations, and assessment of tone in all four limbs. The presence of fasciculations is most easily determined by observing relaxed limbs that are illuminated from behind. Fasciculations can also be palpated as irregular low-amplitude twitches within the muscle. Tone is assessed by passive movement of each limb at its various joints and at several different speeds. In the clinical context of weakness, tone may be spastic or decreased. The presence of cogwheel rigidity, lead-pipe rigidity, or paratonia suggests a nonparalytic disorder of movement.

Hemiparesis Hemiparesis results from an upper motor neuron lesion above the midcervical spinal cord; most lesions that produce hemiparesis are located above the foramen magnum. More precise localization of the lesion is aided by recognition of associated signs. Language disorders, cortical sensory disturbances, cognitive disorders, disorders of visual-spatial integration, apraxia, and seizures identify a cortical lesion. Homonymous visual field defects reflect either a cortical or a subcortical hemispheric lesion. A hemiparesis of the face, arm, and leg without associated signs indicates a small, discrete lesion in the posterior limb of the internal capsule, cerebral peduncle, or upper pons. Some brainstem lesions produce the classic findings of ipsilateral cranial nerve signs and contralateral hemiparesis. These "crossed paralyses" are discussed further in Chap. 366. The absence of cranial nerve signs or facial weakness suggests that a hemiparesis is due to a lesion in the high cervical spinal cord, especially if associated with ipsilateral loss of proprioception and contralateral loss of pain and temperature sense (the Brown-Séquard syndrome). However, most spinal cord lesions produce quadriparesis or paraparesis.

Table 21-2

Medical Research Council Grading of Strength

Grade	Definition
5	Normal strength
4	Active movement against gravity and resistance
3	Active movement against gravity (no resistance from physician)
2	Active movement with gravity eliminated (no resistance from physician)
1	Flicker or trace contraction
0	No visible or palpable contraction

Acute hemiparesis usually has a vascular pathogenesis (Chap. 366). Less commonly, hemorrhage may occur into primary or metastatic brain tumors (Chap. 375) or from rupture of normal vessels due to trauma (Chap. 374); the trauma may be trivial in patients who are anticoagulated or elderly. Less likely possibilities include a focal inflammatory lesion from multiple sclerosis or sarcoidosis (Chap. 376), or an acute bacterial abscess (Chap. 377). The diagnostic approach begins immediately with a computed tomography (CT) scan of the brain, and subsequent decisions are based upon the result (Fig. 21-3). If CT of the brain is normal and an ischemic stroke is unlikely, magnetic resonance imaging (MRI) of the brain or cervical spine may be required.

Subacute hemiparesis has a long differential diagnosis. Subacute subdural hematoma is a common cause of hemiparesis that develops over days to a few weeks; this readily treatable condition must always be considered, especially in elderly patients or those who are anticoagulated, even in the absence of a history of trauma (Chap. 374). Infectious possibilities include cerebral bacterial abscess (Chap. 377), fungal granuloma or meningitis (Chap. 378), and parasitic infection. Weakness from malignant primary and metastatic neoplasms may evolve over days to weeks (Chap. 375). AIDS (Chap. 308) may present with subacute hemiparesis due to toxoplasmosis or primary central nervous system lymphoma. Noninfectious inflammatory processes, such as multiple sclerosis (Chap. 376) or, less commonly, sarcoidosis, are further considerations. The diagnostic approach is summarized in Fig. 21-3; if the brain MRI is normal, MRI of the cervical spine may be required.

Chronic hemiparesis that develops over months (as opposed to one that develops acutely and then persists for months) is usually due to a histologically benign neoplasm (Chap. 375), an unruptured arteriovenous malformation (Chap. 366), a chronic subdural hematoma (Chap. 374), or a degenerative disease (Chaps. 368 to 371). The initial diagnostic test is often an MRI of the brain, especially if the clinical findings suggest brainstem pathology. If MRI of the brain is normal, less likely possibilities of a foramen magnum or high cervical spinal cord lesion should be considered (Fig. 21-3).

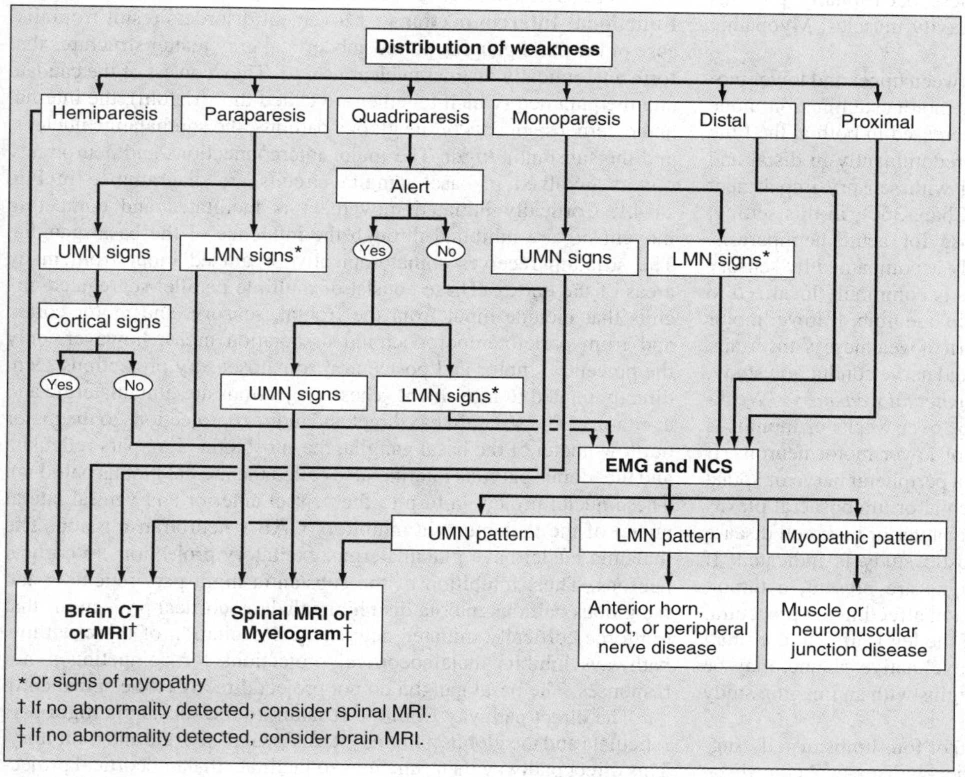

Paraparesis Paraparesis most commonly results from an intraspinal lesion at or below the upper thoracic spinal cord level. A sensory level over the trunk identifies the approximate level of the cord lesion. Other causes for paraparesis include other upper motor neuron lesions (parasagittal lesions and hydrocephalus) and lower motor neuron lesions (anterior horn cell disorders, cauda equina syndromes, and atypical peripheral neuropathies).

Acute paraparesis due to spinal cord disease may be difficult to distinguish from disorders affecting lower motor neurons or cerebral hemispheres. With paraparesis or paraplegia from acute spinal cord disease, the upper motor neuron deficit is usually associated with urinary and fecal incontinence and often lower limb numbness that extends rostrally to a level on the trunk; tone is typically flaccid, and tendon reflexes absent. With a sensory level and sphincter involvement, the diagnostic approach starts with an imaging study of the spinal cord (Fig. 21-3). The diagnostic possibilities include epidural metastasis, epidural hematoma, and spinal cord ischemia from a dural arteriovenous fistula or other vascular anomaly, each of which requires acute intervention. These need to be distinguished from transverse myelitis and lesions outside the spinal cord (Chap. 373). Diseases of the cerebral hemispheres that result in acute paraparesis include anterior cerebral artery ischemia, superior sagittal sinus thrombosis, cortical venous thrombosis, or acute hydrocephalus. If upper motor neuron signs are associated with drowsiness, confusion, seizures, or other cortical signs but not a sensory level over the trunk, the diagnostic approach starts with an MRI of the brain. Paraparesis is part of the cauda equina syndrome, which may result from trauma to the low back, a midline disk herniation, or lumbar intraspinal metastasis; although sphincters are affected, hip flexion is often spared as is sensation over the anterolateral thighs. Paraparesis is rarely caused by acute demyelinating polyneuropathy (the most common form of Guillain-Barré syndrome) or, rarely, a myopathy. In such cases, electrophysiologic studies are diagnostically helpful and refocus the subsequent evaluation (Chaps. 381 and 383).

Subacute or *chronic paraparesis* with spasticity is caused by upper motor neuron disease. When paraparesis develops over weeks or months with lower limb sensory loss and sphincter involvement, possible spinal cord disorders include multiple sclerosis, intraparenchymal tumor, chronic spinal cord compression from degenerative disease of the spine, subacute combined degeneration due to vitamin B_{12} deficiency, and hereditary diseases. Chronic progressive multiple sclerosis usually presents in the fourth or fifth decade with progressive paraparesis (Chap. 376). Primary spinal cord gliomas typically produce a progressive myelopathy that is painful (Chap. 375). The clinical approach begins with MRI or myelography to image the spinal cord. If the imaging study is normal and spasticity is present, MRI of the brain may also be indicated. If cortical signs are present, parasagittal meningioma or chronic hydrocephalus is likely and MRI of the brain is the initial test. Progression over months to years may also be due to degenerative disorders, such as primary lateral sclerosis (Chap. 370) or hereditary disorders, such as familial spastic paraparesis and adrenomyeloneuropathy (Chap. 373). In

FIGURE 21-3 An algorithm for the initial work-up of a patient with weakness. CT, computed tomography; EMG, electromyography; LMN, lower motor neuron; MRI, magnetic resonance imaging; NCS, nerve conduction studies; UMN, upper motor neuron.

the rare situations in which a chronic paraparesis is due to lower motor neuron or myopathic weakness, the localization is usually suspected on clinical grounds and confirmed by EMG and nerve conduction tests.

Quadriparesis   Quadriparesis can result from upper motor neuron disease (localized to the upper cervical spinal cord or above), diffuse lower motor neuron disease, or a myopathy.

Acute quadriparesis   The differential diagnosis for acute quadriparesis with onset over minutes includes many diseases of upper motor neurons (e.g., anoxia, hypotension, brainstem or cervical cord ischemia, trauma, and systemic metabolic abnormalities) and also rare forms of myopathic weakness (systemic toxins or periodic paralyses). Onset over hours to a few days may be due to upper motor neuron, lower motor neuron, or myopathic disorders. All three patterns of weakness are usually associated initially with hypotonia. If the acute quadriparesis is associated with stupor or coma, the evaluation begins with a CT scan of the brain. If upper motor neuron signs are present but the patient is alert, the initial test is usually an MRI of the cervical cord. If weakness is lower motor neuron, myopathic, or uncertain in origin, the clinical approach starts with an electrodiagnostic study. Acute demyelinating polyneuropathy (Chap. 381) is an important diagnostic possibility in this setting.

Subacute or chronic quadriparesis   When quadriparesis due to upper motor neuron disease develops over weeks, months, or years, the distinction between disorders of the cerebral hemispheres, brainstem, and cervical spinal cord is usually possible by clinical criteria alone. The diagnostic approach begins with an MRI of the clinically suspected site of pathology. Lower motor neuron disease presents with weakness that is most profound distally, whereas myopathic weakness is typically proximal (Chaps. 381 and 383). The evaluation then begins with EMG and nerve conduction studies.

Monoparesis or Weakness within One Limb   This is usually due to lower motor neuron disease, with or without associated sensory involvement. Upper motor neuron weakness occasionally presents with a monoparesis of distal and nonantigravity muscles. Myopathic weakness is rarely limited to one limb.

Acute monoparesis   Distinguishing between upper and lower motor neuron disorders may be difficult with motor examination alone because tone and reflexes are frequently decreased in both at the time of acute presentation. If the weakness is predominantly in distal and nonantigravity muscles and not associated with sensory impairment or pain, focal cortical ischemia is likely (Chap. 366); in this setting, diagnostic possibilities are similar to those for acute hemiparesis. Acute lower motor neuron disease is usually accompanied by sensory loss and pain. The distribution of weakness is commonly localized to a single nerve root or peripheral nerve within one limb. If lower motor neuron weakness is suspected, or if the pattern of weakness is uncertain, the clinical approach begins with an EMG and nerve conduction study.

Subacute or chronic monoparesis or segmental weakness   Weakness with atrophy of one limb that develops over weeks or months is almost always due to a localized disorder of lower motor neurons. If the weakness is associated with numbness, a peripheral nerve or spinal root origin is likely; uncommonly, the brachial or lumbosacral plexus is affected. If numbness is absent, segmental anterior horn cell disease is likely. In either case, an electrodiagnostic study is indicated. If upper rather than lower motor neuron signs are present, a tumor, vascular malformation, or other cortical lesion affecting the precentral gyrus may be responsible. Alternatively, if the leg is affected, a small thoracic cord lesion, often a tumor or demyelinative plaque, may be present. In these situations, the approach begins with an imaging study of the suspicious area.

Distal Weakness   Involvement of two or four limbs distally suggests lower motor neuron or peripheral nerve disease. Acute distal lower limb weakness occurs occasionally from an acute toxic polyneuropathy or cauda equina syndrome. Distal symmetric weakness usually develops over weeks, months, or years and is due to metabolic, toxic,

hereditary, degenerative, or inflammatory diseases of peripheral nerves (Chap. 381). With peripheral nerve disease, weakness is usually less severe than numbness. Anterior horn cell disease may begin distally but is typically asymmetric and is not associated with numbness (Chap. 370). Rarely, myopathies also present with distal weakness without associated numbness (Chap. 383). The first step in evaluation is to obtain an electrodiagnostic study (Fig. 21-3).

Proximal Weakness   Proximal weakness of two or four limbs suggests a disorder of muscle or, less commonly, neuromuscular junction or anterior horn cell. Proximal weakness that develops over weeks, months, or years is usually due to hereditary, inflammatory, metabolic, or endocrine disease. Myopathy often produces symmetric weakness of the pelvic or shoulder girdle muscles (Chap. 383). Diseases of the neuromuscular junction (such as myasthenia gravis) may present with symmetric proximal weakness (Chap. 382), often associated with ptosis, diplopia, or bulbar weakness and fluctuating in severity during the day. The proximal weakness of anterior horn cell disease is most often asymmetric, but may be symmetric if familial (Chap. 370). Numbness does not occur with any of these diseases. The evaluation usually begins with determination of the serum creatine kinase level and electrophysiologic studies.

MOVEMENT DISORDERS

Movement disorders are neurologic syndromes in which abnormal movements (or *dyskinesias*) occur due to a disturbance of fluency and speed of voluntary movement or the presence of unintended extra movements. Because they are so distinct from the pyramidal disorders that cause upper motor neuron weakness, movement disorders are often referred to as *extrapyramidal diseases*. Movement disorders are divided into hypokinetic and hyperkinetic types. *Hypokinetic movement disorders* are characterized by *akinesia* or *bradykinesia*, in which purposeful motor activity is absent or reduced. This is often described as "poverty of movement." *Hyperkinetic movement disorders* are those in which an excessive amount of spontaneous motor activity is seen or in which abnormal involuntary movements occur.

PATHOGENESIS OF MOVEMENT DISORDERS   Normal Functional Interconnections   Movement disorders result from disease of the basal ganglia, paired subcortical gray matter structures that form anatomically distinct nuclear groups. They consist of the caudate and the putamen (which together are called the striatum), the internal and external segments of the globus pallidus, the subthalamic nucleus, and the substantia nigra. The major interconnections and neurotransmitters involved in basal ganglia circuits are diagrammed in Fig. 21-4A. Cortically initiated movement is facilitated and competing movements are inhibited through the influence of the basal ganglia. The striatum receives somatotopically organized input from many areas of the cortex. These consist of multiple parallel segregated circuits that include input from the frontal, sensory, and motor cortex and from parietotemporooccipital association areas; however, only the precentral motor and postcentral somatosensory projections seem directly related to movement. These projections are glutamatergic and excitatory. The striatum has direct and indirect projections to the major outflow nuclei of the basal ganglia, the substantia nigra pars reticulata and the globus pallidus interna (also called the medial globus pallidus). These nuclei project in turn to the ventral anterior and ventral lateral nuclei of the thalamus via inhibitory GABA neurotransmission. The thalamic nuclei have glutamatergic, excitatory projections to cortical neurons. Thus, inhibition of the substantia nigra pars reticulata and the globus pallidus interna disinhibits thalamocortical projections that reinforce cortically initiated activity, and excitation of these outflow pathways inhibits thalamocortical projections for competing motor responses. The basal ganglia do not project directly to the spinal cord.

The direct pathway from the striatum to the substantia nigra pars reticulata and the globus pallidus interna is GABA-ergic and inhibitory. This direct pathway then functions to facilitate thalamocortical projections that reinforce cortically initiated movement. The indirect pathway is more complex and functions to inhibit thalamocortical projections to other areas of the motor cortex. The first connection of the indirect pathway is GABA-ergic; it inhibits activity in the globus pallidus externa (also called the lateral globus pallidus). The globus pallidus externa has GABA-ergic, inhibitory input on the subthalamic nucleus. The subthalamic nucleus has excitatory, glutamatergic feedback on the globus pallidus externa and excitatory, glutamatergic input on the substantia nigra pars reticulata and the globus pallidus interna. Thus, activation of the indirect pathway increases outflow from the substantia nigra pars reticulata and the globus pallidus interna, in contrast to the decreased outflow that is produced by activation of the direct pathway.

The direct and indirect pathways are influenced also by input from the substantia nigra pars compacta. This dopaminergic input on the striatum activates direct pathway neurons that predominantly express D_1 dopamine receptors and inhibits indirect pathway neurons that predominantly express D_2 dopamine receptors. The striatum also has GABA-ergic, inhibitory feedback connections with the pars compacta. Striatal activity is further modulated by cholinergic interneurons within the striatum, which are functionally antagonistic to the dopaminergic projections.

Hypokinetic Movement Disorders This model explains well the *hypokinetic movement disorders*. As diagrammed in Fig. 21-4*B*, the fundamental abnormality of Parkinson's disease consists of a loss of dopaminergic neurons in the substantia nigra pars compacta. This causes a loss of excitation of the D_1 striatal neurons in the direct pathway and a loss of inhibition of the D_2 striatal neurons in the indirect pathway. This combination of changes increases outflow from the substantia nigra pars reticulata and the globus pallidus interna, which increases inhibition of thalamocortical projections and results in loss of facilitation of cortically initiated movement. The resting tremor of Parkinson's disease is less readily explained by this model but may result from effects on cholinergic interneurons in the striatum.

Hyperkinetic Movement Disorders As diagrammed in Fig. 21-4*C*, the pathogenesis of chorea in Huntington's disease is an initial loss of the striatal neurons that express D_2 receptors and normally project GABA-ergic inhibition through the indirect pathway. This disinhibits the globus pallidus externa, which in turn increases inhibition of the subthalamic nucleus. Because the glutamatergic input from the subthalamic nucleus is the primary source of excitation on the

substantia nigra pars reticulata and the globus pallidus interna, loss of this excitation reduces inhibition of the thalamus and cortically initiated movements are facilitated without normal feedback control. The pathogenesis of hemiballismus is similar but less complicated— a direct lesion of the glutamatergic neurons in the subthalamic nucleus leads to disinhibition of thalamocortical projections.

Some movement disorders, for example parkinsonism and chorea, may result from changes in discrete populations of neurons that use a specific neurotransmitter. Such selective vulnerability is commonly present in degenerative neurologic diseases, both hereditary and sporadic, and in toxic, nutritional, and inflammatory conditions. Structural disease that affects more than one cell type is common only in hemiballismus, in which a lesion of the subthalamic nucleus, usually a stroke, is almost always found.

DIAGNOSTIC APPROACH AND DIFFERENTIAL DIAGNOSIS FOR COMMON CLINICAL PRESENTATIONS OF MOVEMENT DISORDERS An algorithm for the interpretation of abnormal movements is illustrated in Fig. 21-5. The initial step is to determine if the movement disorder is due to an excess or a poverty of movement (e.g., a hyperkinetic or a hypokinetic movement disorder).

Hyperkinetic Movement Disorders Abnormal involuntary movements are divided into those that are rhythmical and those that are irregular. Those that are rhythmical are termed *tremors*. Tremors are divided into three types: rest tremor, postural tremor, and intention tremor. A *rest tremor* is maximal at rest and becomes less prominent with activity. It is characteristic of parkinsonism, a hypokinetic movement disorder, and is therefore commonly associated with bradykinesia and cogwheel rigidity. A rest tremor that develops acutely is usually due to toxins [such as exposure to 1-methyl-4-phenyl-1,2,3,6-tetrahydropyridine (MPTP)] or dopamine blocking drugs (such as phenothiazines). If insidious in onset, the diagnostic approach is the same as for Parkinson's disease (Chap. 368). A *postural tremor* is maximal while limb posture is actively maintained against gravity; it is lessened

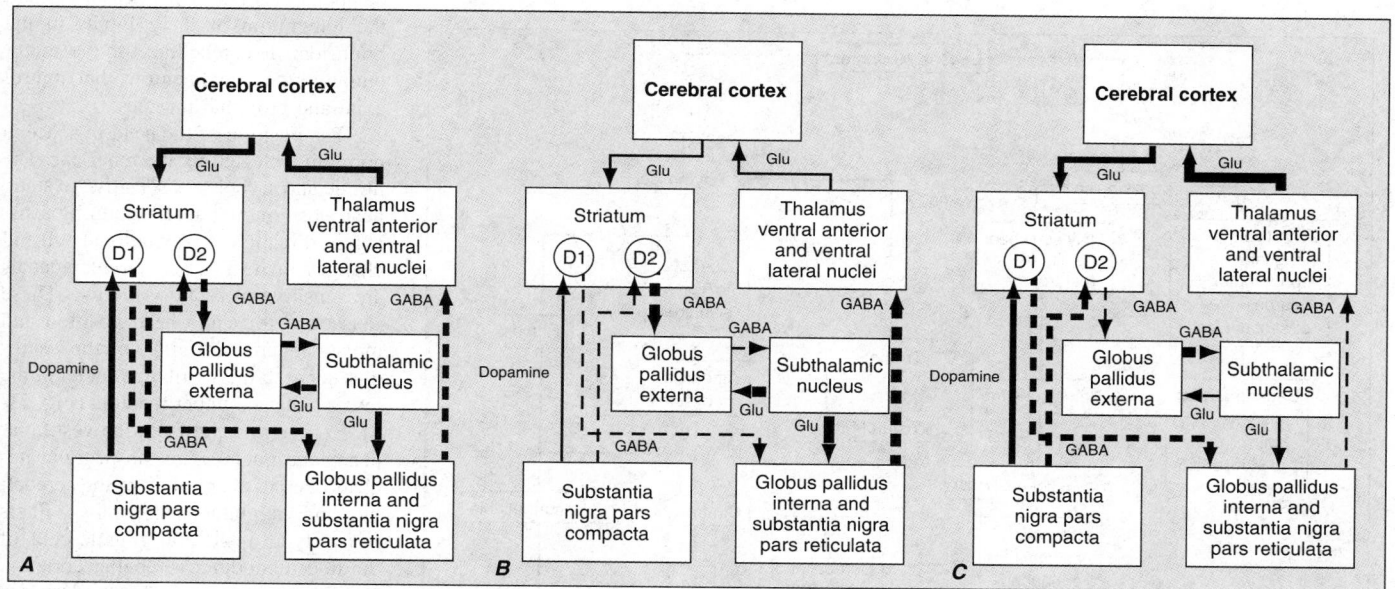

FIGURE 21-4*A, B, C* Diagram of the normal major functional connections and neurotransmitters involved in the basal ganglia circuits. *A.* The striatum receives glutamatergic afferents from the sensorimotor cortex and dopaminergic afferents from the substantia nigra pars compacta. The major output of the basal ganglia is GABA-ergic inhibition from the globus pallidus interna and the substantia nigra pars reticulata to the ventral anterior and ventral lateral nuclei of the thalamus. The striatum projects to the output nuclei by a direct and an indirect pathway. *B.* Parkinson's disease results from a loss of dopaminergic projections from the substantia nigra pars compacta to the striatum. Loss of D_1 receptor stimulation results in disinhibition of the output nuclei by the direct pathway. Loss of D_2 receptor inhibition results in excitation of the output nuclei by the indirect pathway. Thus, inhibition of the thalamus is abnormally increased and cortically initiated movements are not facilitated. *C.* Huntington's chorea results from early loss of striatal neurons that express D_2 receptors and normally project GABA-ergic inhibition to the globus pallidus externa. This causes disinhibition of the thalamus and excess thalamocortical excitation of movements. GABA, gamma-aminobutyric acid; Glu, glutamate; ⟶, excitatory; ⇢, inhibitory.

by rest and is not markedly enhanced during voluntary movement toward a target. A postural tremor that develops acutely is usually due to toxic or metabolic factors (for example, hyperthyroidism) or stress. The insidious onset of a postural tremor suggests a benign or familial essential tremor (Chap. 368). An *intention tremor* is most prominent during voluntary movement toward a target and is not present during postural maintenance or at rest. It is a sign of cerebellar disease (Chap. 369). *Asterixis*, which may superficially resemble a tremor, is an intermittent inhibition of muscle contraction that occurs with metabolic encephalopathy. This leads, for example, to a momentary and repetitive partial flexion of the wrists during attempted sustained wrist extension (Chap. 380).

Abnormal involuntary movements that are irregular are characterized further by their speed and site of occurrence and by whether they can be suppressed voluntarily. The slowest are athetosis and dystonia. *Athetosis* is a slow writhing, sinuous movement that occurs nearly continuously in distal muscles. *Dystonia* is a slowly varying but nearly continuous deviation of posture about one or more joints; it may occur in a proximal or distal limb or in axial structures. Dystonia is a more sustained deviation of posture than athetosis, although these two phenomena overlap considerably. The further evaluation of athetosis and dystonia are discussed in Chap. 368.

Among the rapid irregular movements, *tics* are controlled with voluntary effort, while the others are not. Tics often occur repetitively in a single location but are sometimes multifocal (Chap. 368).

Chorea, hemiballismus, and myoclonus are rapid, irregular jerks that cannot be consciously suppressed. *Hemiballismus* is the most distinctive among them. It is manifest as a sudden and often violent flinging movement of a proximal limb, usually an arm (Chap. 368). Hemiballismus usually develops acutely due to infarction of the contralateral subthalamic nucleus but occasionally develops subacutely or chronically due to other lesions of this nucleus.

Chorea is a rapid, jerky, irregular movement that tends to occur in the distal limbs or face but may also occur in proximal limb and axial structures. Acute onset is usually toxic due to excess levodopa or dopamine-agonist therapy. In children, it may be associated with rheumatic fever and, in such cases, is referred to as *Sydenham's chorea*. The gradual onset of chorea is typical of degenerative neurologic diseases, such as Huntington's chorea (Chap. 367).

Myoclonus is a rapid, brief, irregular movement that is usually multifocal. Myoclonus can occur spontaneously at rest, in response to sensory stimuli, or with voluntary movements. It is a symptom that occurs in a wide variety of metabolic and neurologic disorders. Posthypoxic intention myoclonus is a special myoclonic syndrome that occurs as a sequel to transient cerebral anoxia. Myoclonus may result from lipid storage disease, encephalitis, Creutzfeldt-Jakob disease, or metabolic encephalopathies due to respiratory failure, chronic renal failure, hepatic failure, or electrolyte imbalance. Myoclonus is also a feature of certain types of epilepsy, as discussed in Chap. 365.

Hypokinetic Movement Disorders These syndromes are manifest as bradykinesia, with a masked expressionless facial appearance, loss of associated limb movements during walking, and rigid en bloc turning. If bradykinesia is associated only with a rest tremor, cogwheel rigidity, or impairment of postural reflexes (especially with a tendency to fall backwards), Parkinson's disease is likely (Chap. 368). If cognitive, language, upper motor neuron, sensory, or autonomic signs are also present, a multisystem *degenerative neurologic disease* is present. → *These disorders are discussed in Chaps. 368, 369, and 371.*

IMBALANCE AND DISORDERS OF GAIT

Imbalance is the impaired ability to maintain the intended orientation of the body in space. It is generally manifest as difficulty in maintaining an upright posture while standing or walking; a severe imbalance may also affect the ability to maintain posture while seated. Patients with imbalance commonly complain of a feeling of unsteadiness or dysequilibrium. Whereas imbalance and unsteadiness are synonymous, *dysequilibrium* implies the additional component of impaired spatial orientation even while lying down. Patients with dysequilibrium commonly also experience *vertigo*, defined as an hallucination of rotatory movement.

PATHOGENESIS OF IMBALANCE AND DISORDERS OF GAIT Imbalance Imbalance results from disorders of the spinocerebellar or vestibular sensory input, the integration of these inputs in the brainstem or cerebellum, or the motor output to the spinal neurons that control axial and proximal muscles.

The position of the head in space is normally detected by the inner ear. The utricle and saccule are sensitive to static head position and acceleration by sensing the direction of gravitational pull and changes in it. The semicircular canals are sensitive to rotatory motion. These sensations for static head position and movement are transmitted by the vestibular nerve to the vestibular nuclei in the lower pons and upper medulla (Fig. 21-6). Excitatory input from the vestibular nerve and nuclei is to the fastigial nucleus deep in the midline of the cerebellum and via glutamatergic mossy fibers to overlying ipsilateral granule cells of the flocculonodular cerebellar cortex.

The position of the head relative to the limbs and trunk is detected by receptors that respond to joint position, joint movement, and shortening or lengthening of muscle spindles in axial and proximal limb muscles. This sensory input is transmitted both along the posterior column and medial lemniscal pathways to the cerebrum and the spinocerebellar

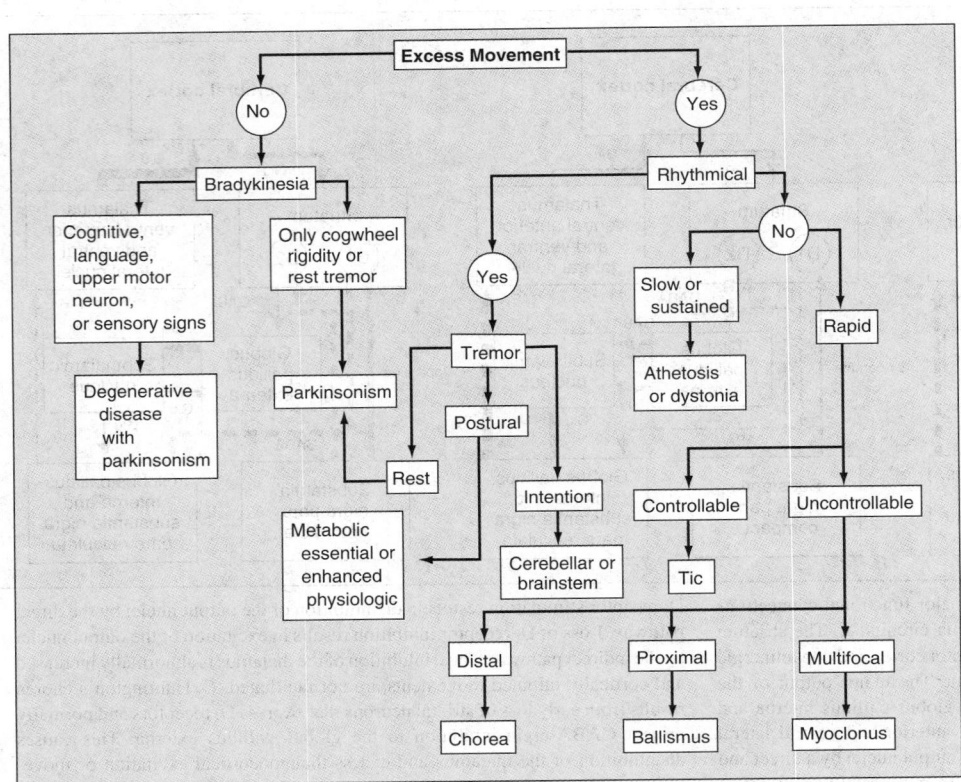

FIGURE 21-5 An algorithm for interpretation of abnormal movements.

proprioceptive sensory input ascends up the spinal cord in the ventral
and dorsal spinocerebellar tracts and, for the head position, the cuneo-
cerebellar tracts (Fig. 21-6). These enter the cerebellum as excitatory,
glutamatergic mossy fiber inputs to the granule cells in the ipsilateral
midline vermal cerebellar cortex and the ipsilateral fastigial nucleus.
Visual input, by way of the tectum of the midbrain, is transmitted to
the cerebellum through similar, excitatory mossy fibers.

The midline cerebellar cortex and nuclei are of paramount importance in the integration of these inputs and in control of appropriate
motor responses required to maintain normal balance. In both midline
and lateral cerebellar cortices, several neuronal cell types mediate
these complex interactions. The Purkinje cells of the middle cortical
layer are the principal outflow neurons of cerebellar cortical activity.
They have inhibitory GABA-ergic projections to the deep cerebellar
nuclei. The granule cells of the inner cellular layer project an extensive
network of axons to the outer molecular layer as parallel fibers, which
run parallel to the long axis of the folia. The parallel fibers produce
a weak excitatory, glutamatergic influence on the dendrites of many
Purkinje cells in the molecular layer and on the basket and stellate
cells, which are the interneurons of the molecular layer. Both basket
and stellate cells have inhibitory projections onto the Purkinje cells.
Basket cell axons run perpendicular to the parallel fibers and produce
GABA-ergic inhibition on Purkinje cell bodies just outside the band
of parallel fiber excitation. Thus, basket cells provide center-surround
antagonism in the cerebellar cortex. A third inhibitory neuron that
acts in the cerebellar cortex is the Golgi cell, which is found at the
outer border of the granular layer. Golgi dendrites project to the

molecular layer, where they receive excitatory parallel fiber input. The
Golgi cells exert GABA-ergic feedback inhibition to the granule cells.
The major output of the cerebellar cortex is inhibition of the deep
cerebellar nuclei by the Purkinje cells. The deep cerebellar nuclei
receive excitatory input from mossy fibers.

The major cerebellar output for balance is from the fastigial nuclei
to the vestibular nuclei and reticular formation and, to a lesser extent,
directly from the midline Purkinje cells to the vestibular nuclei. Vestibular nuclei and reticular formation project descending vestibulospinal
and reticulospinal output via the ventromedial pathways to control the
axial and proximal muscles of the limbs and trunk (Fig. 21-1).

The speed, fluency, and integration of limb movements are also
controlled by the cerebellum. Spinocerebellar proprioceptive feedback
from the limbs projects onto the granule cells in the ipsilateral intermediate cerebellar cortex and the ipsilateral interposed (globose and
emboliform) nuclei as excitatory, glutamatergic mossy fiber inputs
(Fig. 21-7). The major output system from the interposed nuclei is to
the magnocellular portion of the contralateral red nucleus and then to
the descending rubrospinal pathway, which is the major ventrolateral
bulbospinal pathway that facilitates limb movements, in part through
activation of gamma motor neurons.

The lateral cerebellar hemispheres coordinate a complex feedback
circuit that modulates cortically initiated limb movement. Cortical
motor commands influence the cerebellar hemispheres indirectly
through pontocerebellar mossy fibers and olivocerebellar climbing
fibers (Fig. 21-8). Descending corticopontine fibers excite the ipsilateral pontine nuclei. The pontocerebellar fibers decussate in the pons, project
to the cerebellum through the middle cerebellar
peduncle, and excite the granule cells and the dentate nucleus of the contralateral cerebellar hemisphere. The inferior olivary nucleus of the medulla
receives input from the cortex as collaterals from
corticospinal axons and from the basal ganglia,
red nucleus, and reticular formation. Excitatory,
climbing fibers from the inferior olivary nuclei
decussate, pass through the inferior cerebellar peduncle, and stimulate the Purkinje cells of the
lateral cerebellar hemispheres and dentate nuclei.
The excitatory climbing fibers use aspartate as a
neurotransmitter. The output from the cerebellar
hemispheres is predominantly via the dentate nuclei to the parvocellular component of the contralateral red nucleus, to the ventrolateral nucleus of
the thalamus, and then to the motor and premotor
cerebral cortex. Lesions along this circuit result
in cerebellar limb ataxia.

Sensory ataxia is caused by lesions that affect
the peripheral sensory fibers, dorsal root ganglia
cells, posterior columns of the spinal cord, lemniscal system in the brainstem, thalamus, or parietal
cortex; relevant anatomy is discussed in Chap. 23.
Impairment of the proprioceptive sensory feedback to the cerebellum, basal ganglia, and cortex
produces sensory ataxia. Sensory ataxia results in
imbalance and disturbs the fluency and integration
of movements that can be partially alleviated by
visual feedback.

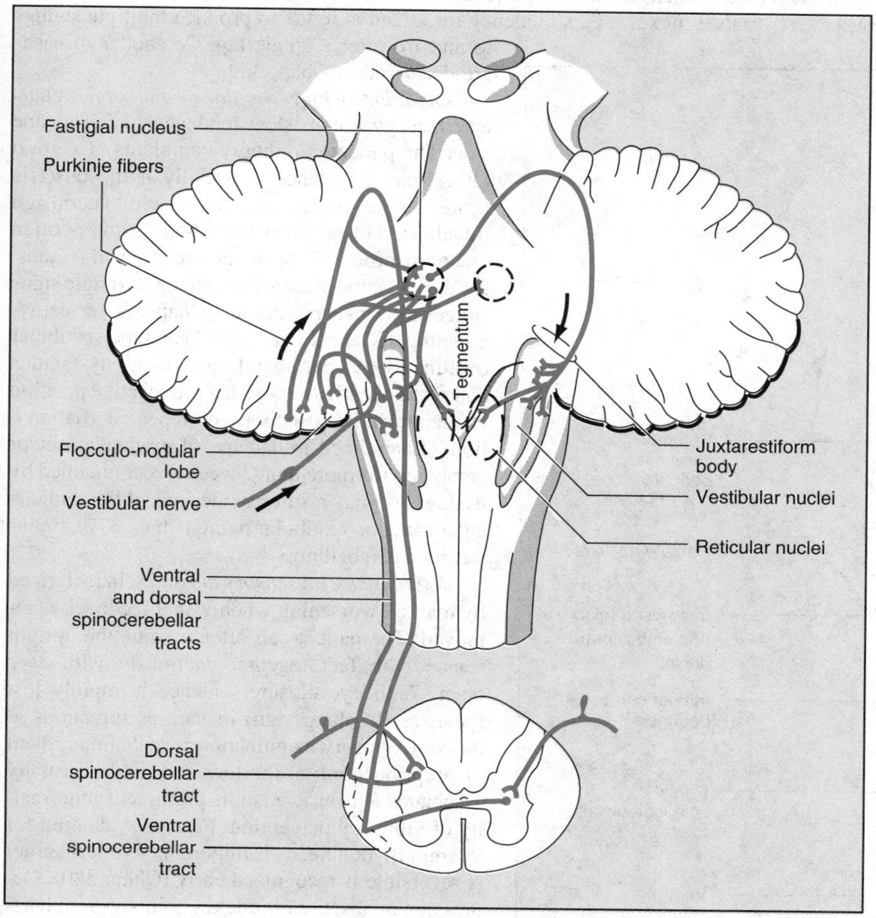

Disorders of Gait Walking is one of the most
complicated and common motor activities of daily
life. Essentially all structures discussed in this chapter participate in normal walking. Cyclical stepping
movements produced by the lumbosacral spinal
cord centers are modified by cortical, basal ganglionic, brainstem, and cerebellar influences based on
proprioceptive, vestibular, and visual feedback.

FIGURE 21-6 Cerebellar control of balance. The vestibular and spinocerebellar mossy fiber afferents excite the granule cells in the flocculonodular and vermal cortex and the fastigial nuclei. The
Purkinje cells of the cerebellar cortex inhibit the fastigial nuclei. The major efferent projections are
from the fastigial nucleus to the vestibular nuclei and the reticular formation. The vermis is a central
portion of the cerebellum that is not illustrated in the figure because it overlies the brainstem and
fastigial nuclei.

DIAGNOSTIC APPROACH AND DIFFERENTIAL DIAGNOSIS FOR COMMON CLINICAL PRESENTATIONS OF IMBALANCE AND ABNORMAL GAIT   Examination for Imbalance, Incoordination, and Abnormal Gait   Neurologic examination of coordination, balance, and gait is typically performed together. The patient performs several maneuvers with each limb while coordination is assessed. The finger-nose-finger and the heel-knee-shin maneuvers are observed for signs of incoordination in general and dysmetria in particular. *Dysmetria* consists of irregular errors in the distance and force of limb movements. This is accentuated near the target or point of intention and hence termed *intention tremor*. The patient is also asked to maintain the arms outstretched against a resistance that is suddenly removed; excessive rebound indicates cerebellar dysfunction. The ability of the patient to rapidly and repetitively tap the hands and feet is assessed for speed and rhythmicity. Slow, coarse, but rhythmical movements indicate upper motor neuron incoordination. Errors in rhythm and irregular rate indicate cerebellar disease; this is most readily demonstrated by asking the patient to perform rapidly alternating movements. During attempts to tap alternately the dorsal and palmar surfaces of the hand as rapidly as possible, the rate, rhythm, and regularity of force cannot be sustained, a sign called *dysdiadochokinesia*. The patient is asked to demonstrate how to comb the hair or brush the teeth to assess the ability to initiate and execute a simple sequence of activity. Balance is examined by having the patient stand stationary with the feet together. If this position can be maintained, the eyes are closed for 5 to 10 s. Accentuation of sway or actual loss of balance is assessed. If balance is momentarily lost, several trials

may be necessary to determine if the loss is consistently in the same direction. Walking along an uncrowded space, such as a hallway, is observed for 20 m or more. Symmetry of arm swing and various phases of the gait cycle are observed. Walking is then performed for several steps on the heels, on the toes, and in tandem.

Imbalance   An algorithm for the interpretation of imbalance is presented in Fig. 21-9.

Cerebellar ataxia results from disorders of the cerebellum or of its afferent inputs or efferent projections. The examination frequently assists in localizing the anatomic site responsible for the ataxia. Abnormalities of the midline cerebellar vermis or the flocculonodular lobe are usually revealed during the process of rising from a chair, assuming the upright stance with the feet together, or performing some other activity while standing. Once a desired position is reached, imbalance may be surprisingly mild. As walking begins, the imbalance recurs. Patients usually learn to lessen the imbalance by walking with the legs widely separated. The imbalance is usually not lateralized and may be accompanied by symmetric nystagmus if the flocculonodular lobe or its connections are affected. These abnormalities of the midline vermis characteristically produce truncal ataxia; dysmetria of the lower limbs with intention tremor may also be present.

Abnormalities of the intermediate and lateral portions of the cerebellum typically produce impaired limb movements rather than truncal ataxia. If involvement is asymmetric, lateralized imbalance is common and usually associated with asymmetric nystagmus. Clinical signs of cerebellar limb ataxia include dysmetria, intention tremor, dysdiadochokinesia, and abnormal rebound. Muscle tone is often modestly reduced; this contributes to the abnormal rebound due to decreased activation of segmental spinal cord reflexes and also to pendular reflexes, i.e., a tendency for a tendon reflex to produce multiple swings to and fro after a single tap. Cerebellar diseases are discussed in Chap. 369.

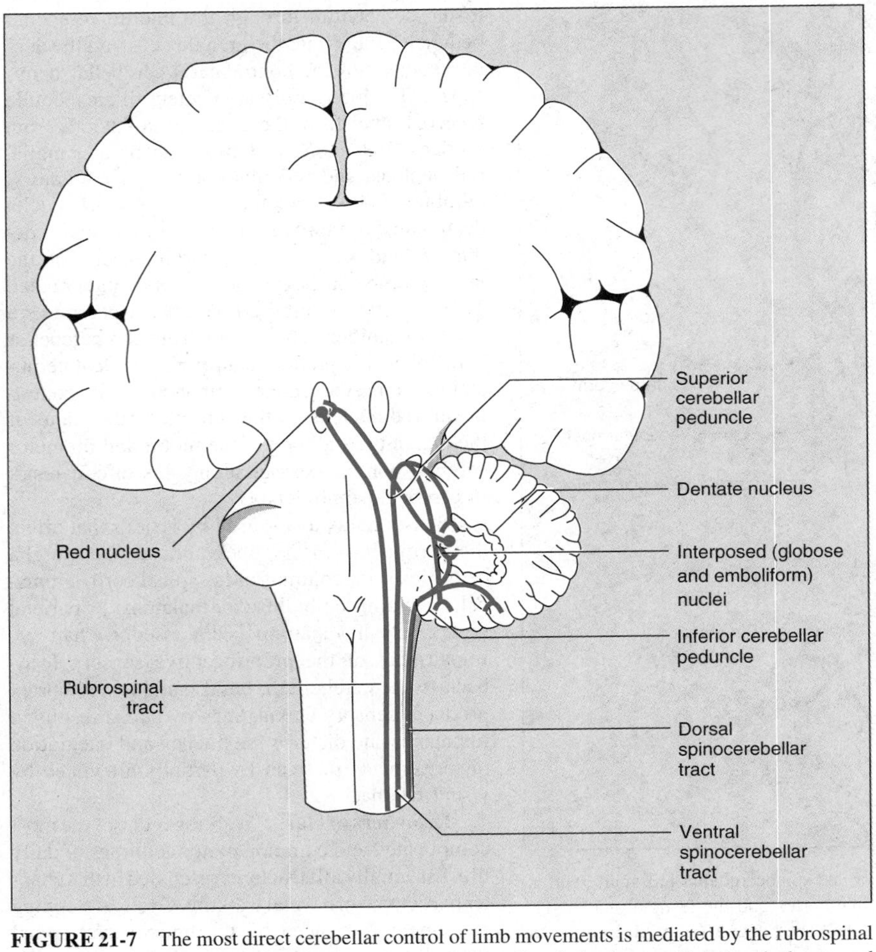

Imbalance with vestibular dysfunction is characterized by a consistent tendency to fall to one side. The patient commonly complains of vertigo rather than imbalance, especially if the onset is acute. Acute vertigo associated with lateralized imbalance but no other neurologic signs is often due to disorders of the semicircular canal (Chaps. 20 and 372); the presence of other neurologic signs suggests brainstem ischemia (Chap. 366) or demyelinating disease (Chap. 376). When the vestibular dysfunction is peripheral, positional nystagmus and vertigo tend to resolve if a provocative position is maintained (extinction) or repeated (habituation). Lateralized imbalance of gradual onset or persisting for more than 2 weeks, accompanied by nystagmus, may result from lesions of the semicircular canal or vestibular nerve (Chap. 372), brainstem, or cerebellum.

Imbalance with sensory ataxia is characterized by marked worsening when visual feedback is removed. The patient can often assume the upright stance with feet together cautiously with eyes open. With eye closure, balance is rapidly lost (positive Romberg sign) in various directions at random. Sensory examination reveals impairment of proprioception at the toes and ankles, usually associated with an even more prominent abnormality of vibratory perception. Prompt evaluation for vitamin B_{12} deficiency is important, as this disorder is reversible if recognized early (Chap. 380). Depression or absence of reflexes points to peripheral nerve disorders (Chap. 381). Spasticity with extensor plantar responses suggest posterior column and spinal cord disorders (Chap. 373). Rarely, sensory ataxia produces lateralized imbalance. In these cases, the disorder is usually in the parietal lobe or thalamus (Chap. 23), but may also be due to

Superior cerebellar peduncle

Dentate nucleus

Interposed (globose and emboliform) nuclei

Inferior cerebellar peduncle

Red nucleus

Rubrospinal tract

Dorsal spinocerebellar tract

Ventral spinocerebellar tract

FIGURE 21-7   The most direct cerebellar control of limb movements is mediated by the rubrospinal pathway. Spinocerebellar afferents excite the granule cells of the intermediate hemispheres and the interposed nuclei. The interposed nuclei excite the magnocellular portion of the contralateral red nucleus.

an asymmetric sensory neuropathy (Chap. 381) or posterior column disease (Chap. 373).

Sensory limb ataxia is similar to cerebellar limb ataxia but is markedly worse when the eyes are closed. Examination also reveals abnormal proprioception and vibratory perception. The approach focuses on localizing the proprioceptive impairment to the peripheral nerves (Chap. 381), the posterior columns of the spinal cord (Chap. 373), or rarely the parietal lobe.

Other forms of imbalance occur, but the fundamental problem is usually a primary disorder of strength, extrapyramidal function, or cortical initiation of movement.

Abnormal Gait Each of the disorders discussed in this chapter produces a characteristic gait disturbance. If the neurologic examination is normal, except for an abnormal gait, diagnosis may be difficult, even for the experienced clinician.

Hemiparetic gait characterizes spastic hemiparesis. In its most severe form, an abnormal posture of the limbs is produced by spasticity. The shoulder is adducted and internally rotated, with flexion of the elbow, wrist, and fingers and with extension of the hip, knee, and ankle. Forward swing of the spastic leg during walking requires abduction and circumduction at the hip, often with contralateral tilt of the trunk. In its mildest form, the affected arm is held in a normal position, but swings less than the normal arm. The affected leg is flexed less than the normal leg during its forward swing and is more externally rotated. A hemiparetic gait is a common residual sign of a stroke (Chap. 366).

Paraparetic gait is a walking pattern in which both legs are moved in a slow, stiff manner with circumduction, similar to the leg movement in an hemiparetic gait. In many patients, the legs tend to cross with each forward swing ("scissoring"). A paraparetic gait is a common sign of spinal cord disease (Chap. 373) and also occurs in cerebral palsy.

Steppage gait is produced by weakness of ankle dorsiflexion. Because of the partial or complete foot drop, the leg must be lifted higher than usual to avoid catching the toe on the floor during the forward swing of the leg. If unilateral, steppage gait is usually due to L5 radiculopathy, sciatic neuropathy, or peroneal neuropathy (Chap. 381). If bilateral, it is the common result of a distal polyneuropathy or lumbosacral polyradiculopathy (Chap. 381).

Waddling gait results from proximal lower limb weakness, most often from myopathy (Chap. 383) but occasionally from neuromuscular junction disease (Chap. 382) or a proximal symmetric spinal muscular atrophy (Chap. 370). With weakness of hip flexion, the trunk is tilted away from the leg that is being moved to lift the hip and provide extra distance between the foot and the floor, and the pelvis is rotated forward to assist with forward motion of the leg. Because pelvic girdle weakness is customarily bilateral, the pelvic lift and rotation alternates from side to side, giving the waddling appearance to the gait.

Parkinsonian gait is characterized by a forward stoop, with modest flexion at the hips and knees. The arms are flexed at the elbows and adducted at the shoulders, often with a 4- to 6-Hz resting pronation-supination tremor but little other movement, even during walking. Walking is initiated slowly by leaning forward and maintained with short rapid steps, during which the feet shuffle along the floor. The pace tends to accelerate (festinate) as the upper body gradually leans further ahead of the feet, whether movement is forwards (propulsion) or backwards (retropulsion). The postural instability leads to falls (Chap. 368).

Apraxic gait results from bilateral frontal lobe disease with impaired ability to plan and execute sequential movements. This gait superficially resembles that of parkinsonism, in that the posture is stooped and any steps taken are short and shuffling. However, initiation and maintenance of walking are impaired in a different manner. Each movement that is required for walking can usually be performed, if tested in isolation while sitting or lying. However, when asked to step forward while standing, a long pause often occurs before any attempt is made to flex at the hip and advance. Furthermore, once walking is initiated, it is not maintained, even in an abnormal festinating manner. Rather, after one or several steps are taken, walking is stopped for several seconds or longer. The process is then repeated. This gait is usually accompanied by dementia (Chap. 367).

Choreoathetotic gait is characterized by an intermittent, irregular movement that disrupts the smooth flow of a normal gait. Flexion or extension movements at the hip are common and unpredictable but readily observed as a pelvic lurch (Chap. 368).

Cerebellar ataxic gait is a broad-based gait disorder in which the speed and length of stride varies irregularly from step to step. With midline cerebellar disease, as in alcoholics (Chap. 380), posture is erect but the feet are separated; lower limb ataxia is commonly present as well. Assumption of a particular stance or a change in position may cause instability, yet balance can usually be maintained well with the eyes open or closed. Walking may be rapid but cadence is irregular. Although patients commonly lack confidence in the stability of their walking, minimal support is often required for reassurance. With disease of the cerebellar hemispheres, limb ataxia and nystagmus are commonly present as well (Chap. 369).

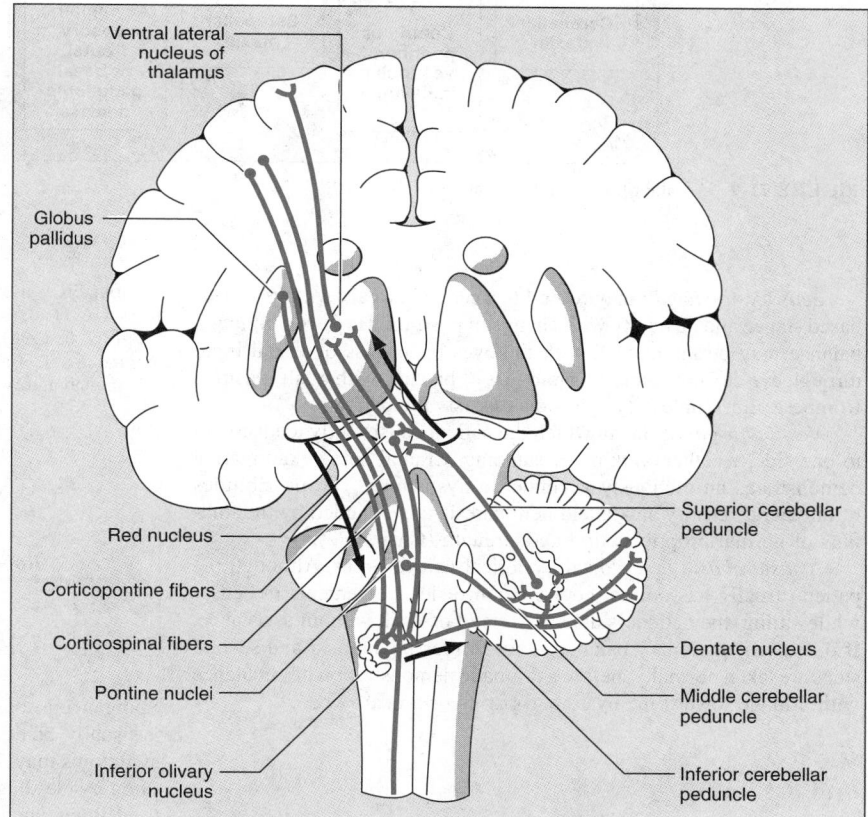

FIGURE 21-8 Cerebellar modulation of cortically initiated movement is mediated by a complex feedback circuit that involves the lateral cerebellar hemispheres. In response to stimulation by corticopontine fibers, pontocerebellar fibers decussate in the pons, project to the cerebellum through the middle cerebellar peduncle, and excite the granule cells and the dentate nucleus of the contralateral cerebellar hemisphere. The inferior olivary nucleus of the medulla projects excitatory, climbing fibers to the Purkinje cells of the contralateral lateral cerebellar hemispheres and dentate nuclei. The cerebellar output is predominantly to the contralateral red nucleus, to the ventrolateral nucleus of the thalamus, and from there to the motor and premotor cerebral cortex.

Labels in figure: Ventral lateral nucleus of thalamus; Globus pallidus; Red nucleus; Corticopontine fibers; Corticospinal fibers; Pontine nuclei; Inferior olivary nucleus; Superior cerebellar peduncle; Dentate nucleus; Middle cerebellar peduncle; Inferior cerebellar peduncle

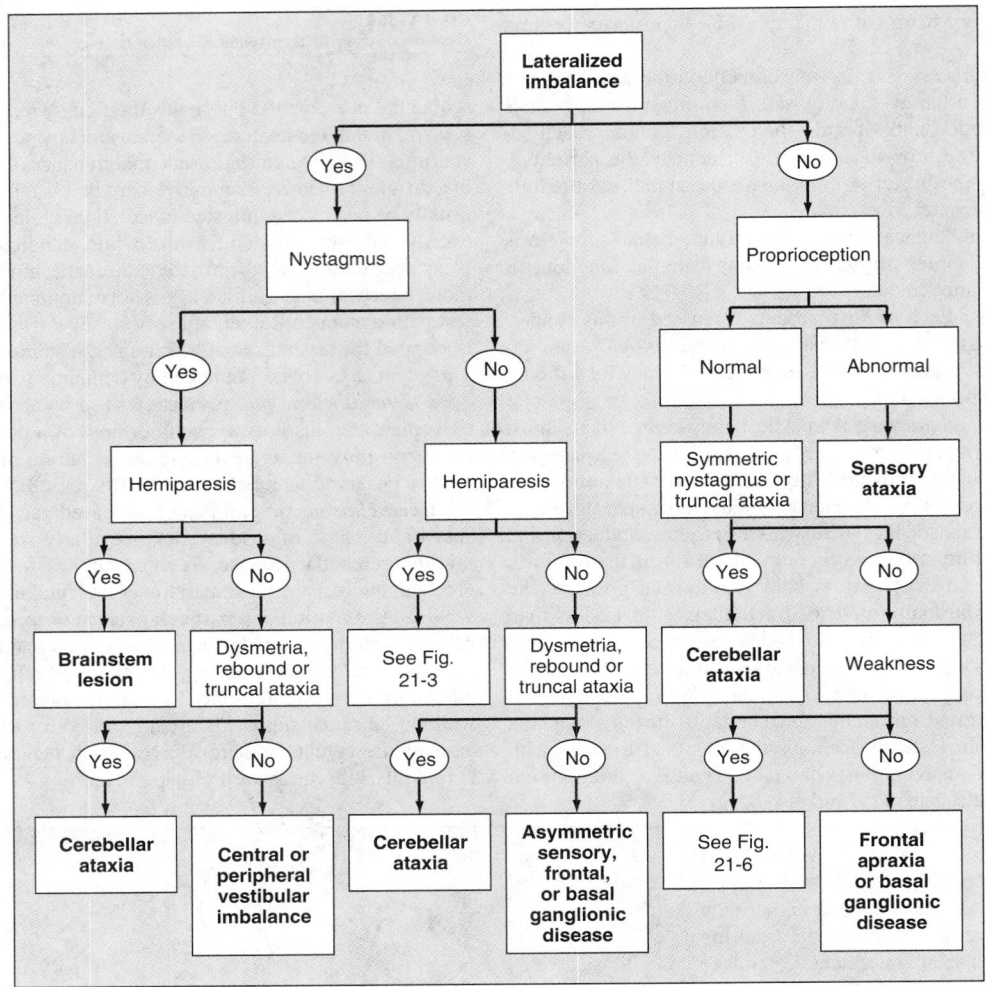

FIGURE 21-9 An algorithm for interpretation of imbalance.

Sensory ataxic gait may resemble a cerebellar gait, with its broad-based stance and difficulty with change in position. However, although balance may be maintained with the eyes open, loss of visual input through eye closure results in rapid loss of balance with a fall (positive Romberg sign), unless the physician assists the patient.

Vestibular gait is one in which the patient consistently tends to fall to one side, whether walking or standing. Cranial nerve examination demonstrates an obviously asymmetric nystagmus. The possibilities of unilateral sensory ataxia and hemiparesis are excluded by the findings of normal proprioception and strength (Chap. 372).

Astasia-abasia is a typical hysterical gait disorder. Although the patient usually has normal coordination of leg movements in bed or while sitting, the patient is unable to stand or walk without assistance. If distracted, stationary balance is sometimes maintained and several steps are taken normally, before a dramatic demonstration of imbalance with a lunge toward the examiner's arms or a nearby bed.

BIBLIOGRAPHY

ALBIN RL et al: The functional anatomy of disorders of the basal ganglia. Trends Neurosci 18:63, 1995

BRODAL A: *Neurological Anatomy in Relation to Clinical Medicine*, 3d ed. Oxford, Oxford University Press, 1981

COLES SK et al: The mesencephalic centre controlling locomotion in the rat. Neuroscience 28:149, 1989

HORE J et al: Cerebellar dysmetria at the elbow, wrist, and fingers. J Neurophysiol 65:563, 1991

JAGIELLA WM, SUNG JH: Bilateral infarction of the medullary pyramids in humans. Neurology 39:21, 1989

KANDEL ER et al: *Principles of Neural Science*, 3d ed. New York, Elsevier, 1991

ROSS CA et al: Messenger molecules in the cerebellum. Trends Neurosci 13:216, 1990

WICHMANN T et al: Parkinson's disease and the basal ganglia: Lessons from the laboratory and from neurosurgery. Neuroscientist 1:236, 1995

22 *Robert C. Griggs*

EPISODIC MUSCLE SPASMS, CRAMPS, AND WEAKNESS

Spontaneous or exercise-related discomfort from muscles or joints is usually benign and does not signal neuromuscular disease. Such symptoms may, however, provide clues to disabling disorders that too often evade diagnosis. The terms *pain*, *spasm*, and *cramp* are often used interchangeably by patients to describe symptoms referable to muscles. Other terms including *aching*, *heaviness*, and *stiffness* are also used and usually connote less certainty about the localization of the discomfort. In clinical terminology, *spasm* refers to a brief, unsustained contraction of a single or multiple muscles. *Cramp* is a paroxysmal, spontaneous, prolonged, and painful contraction of one or more muscles. Muscle pain may be associated with fatigue (asthenia) or weakness. This chapter discusses both fatigue and episodic weakness. The usual causes of weakness are considered in Chap. 21.

SPASMS Abnormal movements of muscle may arise from abnormal electrical activity of the central nervous system (CNS) mediated via the motor neuron or occur within the motor neuron or muscle fiber itself. It may be difficult on clinical grounds alone to determine the precise site of origin of the abnormal motor activity. In general, movements originating in the CNS affect the entire side of the body, an entire limb, or a group of muscles. Central disorders may be rhythmic or intermittent; those arising in the periphery are usually random. The electroencephalogram (EEG) may provide evidence for altered cortical activity in some conditions with a CNS etiology. The electromyogram (EMG) is less helpful because it reflects motor activity from any cause. EMG evidence of an underlying nerve or muscle disease may, however, be helpful in diagnosis (see Chap. 361).

Intermittent, nonrhythmic movements of an entire limb, of the trunk, or of a portion of the face may result from cerebral seizure activity (Chap. 361) or from myoclonus (Chap. 21). Flexor and extensor spasms of an entire side or of the lower limbs result from a loss of motor inhibition within the CNS (Chap. 21). *Segmental myoclonus* results from focal disease within the brainstem or spinal cord that causes an abnormal discharge of groups of motor neurons. Localized vascular disease, tumor, or another lesion may be implicated.

Abnormal Facial Movements *Hemifacial spasm* results from paroxysmal facial nerve activity, sometimes triggered by pressure from a tortuous blood vessel adjacent to the facial nerve as it leaves the brainstem. Hemifacial spasm commonly occurs in muscles about the eye but also may involve or spread to the entire side of the face. Symptoms are often intermittent and intensified when patients are using facial muscles in activities such as speaking. Hemifacial spasm is painless but embarrassing, especially to individuals dealing with the public. Since it is often intensified and more severe when the patient is in stressful situations, an erroneous diagnosis of tic is often made. Cerebellopontine angle lesions can occasionally produce a similar disorder. Neuroradiologic investigation is indicated in patients with hemifacial spasm. Injection of botulinum toxin into involved muscles alleviates spasm for up to 3 months; surgical exploration and shielding of the facial nerve from the adjacent vessel is often curative (Chap. 372).

Facial *tics* are stereotyped movements of the face such as eye blinking, head turning, or grimacing that are under voluntary control but may be suppressed only by effort and anxiety on the part of the subject (see Chap. 21). Some tics are so frequently encountered as to be considered mannerisms, analogous to excessive clearing of the throat. The repetitive elevation of the eyebrows by frontalis muscle contraction is an example. Certain hereditary movement disorders such as Gilles de la Tourette syndrome are characterized by multiple tics. Tics can often be controlled by neuroleptic agents (Chap. 21).

Synkinesias of the face result from aberrant regeneration of the facial nerve following facial paralysis from Bell's palsy or other facial nerve lesions. Nearly 50 percent of patients who recover from Bell's palsy display such movements; an example is *jaw winking*, where voluntary movements of the lower face elicit contraction of the orbicularis oculi muscle with unilateral eye closure (see Chap. 372).

Trigeminal neuralgia (tic douloureux) is characterized by brief, paroxysmal, lancinating pain in one side of the face (see Chap. 372). Although the portion of the nerve involved is almost exclusively sensory, the severity of the pain causes involuntary contraction of facial muscles, hence the name *tic*. Abnormal movements do not occur in the absence of pain.

Facial myokymia refers to a nearly continuous twitching of facial muscles. Although often benign, it may result from lesions of the pons such as a neoplasm or multiple sclerosis. Facial and limb myokymia occur in association with episodic ataxia in hereditary defects of nerve potassium ion channels. Similar movements occur in motor neuron diseases such as amyotrophic lateral sclerosis (see Chaps. 363 and 383).

Abnormal Limb Movements No movement should be visible in totally relaxed muscles. Diseases of motor neurons or their proximal axons are often associated with *fasciculations*, the spontaneous firing of an entire motor unit. Fasciculations are visible on inspection of muscle or perceived by the patient as a pulsation or quivering within

muscle. Fasciculations occur at times in most normal individuals, and unless weakness is present, they are seldom of any significance. Fasciculations are normal if observed in incompletely relaxed muscles and are frequently observed at rest in the calves of normal individuals. *Myokymia*, consisting of numerous, repetitive fasciculations, also may occur in limb muscles, giving a writhing appearance. Myokymia disappears with neuromuscular blockade, proving that the activity originates in anterior horn cells or in peripheral nerve. In patients with longstanding muscle denervation and reinnervation, motor unit size enlarges and fasciculations may be so large as to produce movement of the limbs, particularly of the fingers, a condition termed *minipolymyoclonus*.

Certain conditions are characterized by a compulsion to move the extremities. *Akathisia*, or motor restlessness, occurs in Parkinson's disease and other disorders of the basal ganglia, including drug-induced movement disorders. The *restless legs syndrome* describes an uncomfortable sensation in muscles, usually in the legs and thighs, that occurs most commonly in middle-aged women. Patients feel they need to move their legs to relieve the abnormal sensation. The restless legs syndrome is frequent in uremia and may occur in other neuropathies, suggesting that the sensation is caused by an underlying neuropathy. It also may be familial, and detailed study of such patients has failed to demonstrate any evidence of neuropathy. The restless sensation may be accompanied by myoclonic jerks of muscle. These myoclonic jerks are similar to the myoclonus observed in normal individuals entering REM sleep (see Chap. 27).

These forms of muscle spasm and myoclonus are somewhat similar to a group of unusual *startle* syndromes or *hyperexplexias* characterized by sudden jerking of limbs or occasionally of trunk muscles. Sudden noise or touch may cause a patient to jump or to fling an extremity. Hyperexplexias result from mutations in the glycine receptor (see Chap. 363).

SUSTAINED MUSCLE CONTRACTIONS Distinguishing central from peripheral causes of sustained muscle contraction is often difficult. Abnormal muscle contractions with increased muscle tone usually result from CNS disease. Thus loss or disturbance of CNS inhibition may lead to abnormal muscle contraction characteristic of spasticity, rigidity, or "paratonic" rigidity. In most instances there is other evidence of CNS disorder (Chap. 21). Diseases of the basal ganglia, many of them hereditary, may lead to dystonia (see Chaps. 21 and 363).

Abnormal muscle contractions also may arise from repetitive depolarization of the component portions of the motor unit: the motor neuron, the peripheral axon of the neuron, the neuromuscular junction, or muscle fibers. Electrically inactive contractions may arise from disorders of the muscle contractile system.

Motor Neuron Disorders *Cramp* is a term often used by patients to refer to a painful, involuntary contraction of a single muscle or a muscle group. Muscle cramps can arise from spontaneous firing of groups of anterior horn cells followed by contraction of many motor units. EMG recordings indicate that motor units fire at a rate of up to 300 per second, much higher than occurs with voluntary contraction. Cramps occur frequently in the legs in elderly patients and, when severe, are followed by residual tenderness and evidence of muscle fiber necrosis, including elevation of serum creatine kinase. Cramps in the calf muscles are so common as to be considered normal, but more generalized cramps may be a sign of chronic disease of the motor neuron, such as amyotrophic lateral sclerosis. They may be particularly troublesome during pregnancy, in patients with electrolyte disturbances (hyponatremia), and in patients on hemodialysis. When recurrent and localized to one muscle group, they suggest nerve root disease. In many instances, however, it is impossible to determine the cause of cramps. Benign cramps, occurring commonly at night, may be relieved by quinine sulfate. Other causes of contractions arising from the motor neuron include *tetanus* (Chap. 146) and the *stiff-man syndrome*. In both disorders, a loss of inhibitory neuronal input to anterior horn cells may result in repeated firing of motor neurons, producing severe, painful muscle contraction. Antibodies to glutamic acid decarboxylase are often present in the stiff-man syndrome, and the disorder may respond to plasma exchange. A similar clinical picture may occur acutely with *strychnine poisoning*. Diazepam improves these spasms but may cause respiratory depression in doses sufficient to alleviate muscle contraction.

Peripheral Nerve Disorders *Tetany* is characterized by contractions of predominantly distal muscles, particularly in the hand (carpal spasm) and feet (pedal spasm). Laryngospasm also may occur. Tetany results from increased excitability of peripheral nerves. The muscle contractions are initially painless, but if sustained, they may cause muscle damage with pain. Severe tetany may involve spine musculature to produce opisthotonus. Tetany is usually caused by hypocalcemia, but it may occur with hypomagnesemia or severe respiratory alkalosis (see Chap. 354). Idiopathic normocalcemic tetany, *spasmophilia*, occurs in both hereditary and acquired forms. The acquired disorder is similar to Isaac's syndrome (neuromyotonia), in which hyperexcitability of peripheral nerve leads to muscle cramps and twitching. Such patients have responded to plasma exchange and it may be mediated by IgG autoantibodies to nerve membrane potassium channels.

Muscle Disorders *Myotonia* Repetitive depolarization of muscle cells can cause muscle contraction resulting in muscle stiffness and impaired relaxation. Myotonia is usually painless, but it may disable patients by interfering with fine hand movements or by slowing ambulation. Myotonic dystrophy is the most common disorder associated with myotonia, although other manifestations of the disease such as cataracts and muscle weakness are usually more symptomatic. A similar disorder, proximal myotonic myopathy (PROMM), is associated with muscle pain (see Chap. 383). Myotonia congenita and paramyotonia congenita are less common but more troublesome in terms of severity of myotonia. Myotonia is often worsened by cold and characteristically is attenuated by repeated muscle activity. *Myotonia congenita* has both autosomal dominant and recessive variants. Myotonia results from defects in chloride channel function and can also result from defects of sodium channel function. One such disorder is paramyotonia congenita, which is characterized by *paradoxical myotonia*: myotonia that worsens with repeated activity. These patients also suffer from episodic and cold-induced weakness (see Chap. 383). Myotonia can often be alleviated by quinine, phenytoin, or mexiletine.

Contracture Muscle contracture is a painful shortening of a muscle unassociated with muscle membrane depolarization. It occurs in disorders where a metabolic defect such as myophosphorylase deficiency limits the production of high-energy phosphates. Contractures are precipitated by exercise, are usually intensely painful, and result in muscle damage; widespread muscle contractures may cause sufficient myoglobinuria to precipitate renal failure. This use of the term *contracture* is confusing because the same word is used to describe the unrelated limitation of joint movement by shortening of muscle tendons seen in rheumatologic disorders, cerebral palsy, or chronic myopathies. Muscle rigidity from metabolic contracture can occur in the malignant hyperthermia syndrome, usually associated with general anesthesia. In the neuroleptic malignant syndrome, muscle rigidity arises from CNS overactivity, and intense electrical activity is present in muscle.

MUSCLE PAIN, ACHING, AND TENDERNESS Painful muscles do not always imply muscle disease. Joint and bone disease frequently produces complaints of muscle pain and may further confuse the anatomic localization of symptoms by resulting in disuse atrophy and moderate muscle weakness. Pain from disease of overlying subcutaneous tissue or fascia and of tendons also may be referred to muscle. Additionally, disease of major peripheral nerves or of their small intramuscular branches may produce both muscle pain and weakness. Muscle pain may be a major symptom in inflammatory, metabolic, endocrine, and toxic myopathies (see Chaps. 315 and 383).

Muscle Trauma Vigorous activity, even in conditioned athletes, may be associated with muscle and tendon tears, which lead to temporary acute muscle pain, swelling, and tenderness. Rupture of muscle tendons such as the biceps or gastrocnemius muscle may produce visible muscle shortening. Many such tears resolve without surgery but leave an abnormal appearance to the muscle belly.

The almost-pleasurable ache and fatigue of muscles after strenuous activity is separable only by degree from more severe, but still normal pain following severe, unaccustomed activity. Such symptoms are often associated with laboratory evidence of profound muscle damage, including a rise in serum enzymes (creatine kinase), focal edema on magnetic resonance imaging (MRI), and widespread muscle necrosis on biopsy. Myoglobinuria may occur. Particularly likely to produce muscle pain and necrosis are certain types of exercise: brief periods of contracting a muscle while it is lengthening (eccentric contractions) and prolonged exercise such as marathon running. The point at which such symptoms become abnormal is not clear. Many patients have pain with moderate activity. Such exertional muscle pain is also characteristic of metabolic disorders of muscle such as carnitine palmitoyl transferase deficiency; patients with partial defects in *dystrophin* may have recurrent exercise-induced myalgias. Complete deficiency of this protein causes Duchenne muscular dystrophy (see Chap. 383). Deficiencies of enzymes of glycolysis are more commonly associated with contractures (see Chap. 383). The majority of patients with exertional and postexertional muscle pain do not have a definable abnormality.

Diffuse Myalgias Muscle pain in the absence of muscle weakness can occur in acute infections caused by influenza virus and coxsackievirus. Fibrositis, fibromyalgia, and fibromyositis are synonyms for a disorder associated with pain and tenderness of muscle and adjacent connective tissue. Focal "trigger points" of tenderness can be identified, and systemic symptoms such as fatigue, insomnia, and depression are frequently present (see Chap. 315). Although patients often identify painful swellings, histologic evaluation discloses no abnormality of muscle or connective tissue. Symptoms may respond partially to amitriptyline or nonsteroidal anti-inflammatory agents, but the disorder tends to be chronic and unrelenting. A supportive program of physical reconditioning is sometimes helpful. Patients whose symptoms persist for months or years are often considered to be depressed; whether depression causes or results from symptoms is unclear.

Polymyalgia rheumatica occurs in patients over age 50 and is characterized by stiffness and pain in shoulder and hip musculature. Despite symptoms of pain localized to muscles, there is convincing evidence that the disease includes a proximal, inflammatory arthritis; joint effusions are often present in knees and other peripheral joints as well. Patients often develop profound disuse atrophy of muscles and complain of weakness, giving rise to a suspicion of polymyositis. However, creatine kinase levels are usually normal, and muscle biopsy shows atrophy without evidence of muscle necrosis or inflammation. The erythrocyte sedimentation rate is elevated in most patients, and temporal arteritis may be present (see Chap. 319). Treatment with nonsteroidal anti-inflammatory agents is advocated except in patients with temporal arteritis, for whom prednisone (40 to 60 mg/d) is recommended. Patients with polymyalgia rheumatica who fail to respond to nonsteroidal anti-inflammatory agents may require low-dose prednisone (10 to 20 mg/d). Myalgias are also frequent in other rheumatologic disorders, including rheumatoid arthritis, systemic lupus erythematosus, polyarteritis nodosa, scleroderma, and the mixed connective tissue syndrome. Patients with polymyositis and dermatomyositis may have myalgias, although in the majority muscles are not painful (see Chap. 315).

Diagnostic Algorithm Complaints of muscle pain and fatigue are among the most frequent symptoms offered by patients. The decision as to which patients require extensive diagnostic tests can usually be made by history, examination, and routine blood studies (Fig. 22-1).

EPISODIC WEAKNESS The term *weakness* is often used by a patient to describe a loss of stamina or decreased "energy." Even careful efforts at eliciting a history of true as opposed to subjective weakness may fail to distinguish the two conditions. The most helpful strategy is to ask the patient to identify whether a discrete loss of

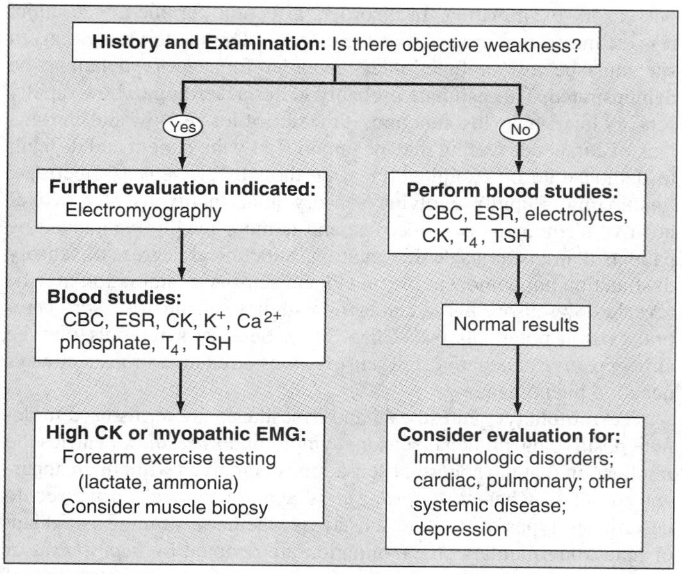

```
┌─────────────────────────────────────────────────────┐
│   History and Examination: Is there objective weakness? │
│                                                         │
│              ┌────┐              ┌────┐                 │
│              │Yes │              │ No │                 │
│              └────┘              └────┘                 │
│                                                         │
│  ┌─────────────────────┐   ┌─────────────────────┐    │
│  │ Further evaluation   │   │ Perform blood studies:│   │
│  │ indicated:           │   │ CBC, ESR, electrolytes,│  │
│  │ Electromyography     │   │ CK, T₄, TSH           │   │
│  └─────────────────────┘   └─────────────────────┘    │
│                                                         │
│  ┌─────────────────────┐   ┌─────────────────────┐    │
│  │ Blood studies:       │   │  Normal results      │    │
│  │ CBC, ESR, CK, K⁺, Ca²⁺│  └─────────────────────┘    │
│  │ phosphate, T₄, TSH   │                              │
│  └─────────────────────┘                              │
│                                                         │
│  ┌─────────────────────┐   ┌─────────────────────┐    │
│  │ High CK or myopathic │   │ Consider evaluation for:│ │
│  │ EMG:                 │   │ Immunologic disorders;  │ │
│  │ Forearm exercise      │   │ cardiac, pulmonary; other│ │
│  │ testing               │   │ systemic disease;       │ │
│  │ (lactate, ammonia)    │   │ depression              │ │
│  │ Consider muscle biopsy│   └─────────────────────┘    │
│  └─────────────────────┘                              │
└─────────────────────────────────────────────────────┘
```

FIGURE 22-1 Evaluation of muscle pain and fatigue. CBC, complete blood count; ESR, erythrocyte sedimentation rate; T_4, thyroxine; TSH, thyroid-stimulating hormone.

function has occurred and to elicit the circumstances in which symptoms are noted.

Weakness, whether true or perceived, may be due to disorders of the central or peripheral nervous system. Weakness from CNS disorders such as transient cerebral ischemia is usually associated with a change in level of consciousness or cognition, with increased muscle tone and muscle stretch reflexes, and often with alterations of sensation. Most neuromuscular causes of intermittent weakness are associated with normal mental function, diminished muscle tone, and muscle stretch reflexes. The major causes of intermittent weakness are listed in Table 22-1. Central causes are considered in Chaps. 21 and 366.

Episodic Asthenia Patients who describe intermittent "weakness" but actually have *fatigue*, suffer from asthenia, which can be separated from true weakness by the fact that patients do not lack the ability to do a task but rather the ability to perform it repetitively. Asthenia is a major problem in many patients with serious renal, hepatic, cardiac, or pulmonary disease. Examination of such patients usually confirms their ability to do all functional activities at least once, such as rising from a knee bend, climbing stairs, or rising from a chair. Fatigue is also characteristic of relatively selective damage to CNS descending motor tracts, in which signs of neurologic abnormality may be minimal. Fatigue that is worsened by activity is characteristic of *chronic fatigue syndrome* (see Chap. 384).

Intermittent weakness due to peripheral neuromuscular disease may result from abrupt changes in peripheral nerve function, intermittent destruction of muscle, alterations of electrophysiologic properties of muscle from abnormalities of blood electrolytes, genetic diseases of muscle ion channels, and intermittent failure of neuromuscular transmission.

Failure of Peripheral Nerve Conduction A number of uncommon peripheral neuropathies are associated with recurrent weakness. *Hereditary liability to pressure palsies*, often termed *tomaculous neuropathy* because of the sausage-like appearance of myelin on nerve biopsy, is characterized by abrupt paralysis following compression of a peripheral nerve. The disease is autosomal dominant and results in many families from an abnormality in peripheral myelin protein (PMP–22) (see Chap. 363). The paralysis is usually self-limited, lasting days to weeks. Other types of peripheral neuropathy also may predispose to the development of reversible, compressive neuropathies (see Chap. 381).

Disordered Neuromuscular Junction Transmission *Myasthenia gravis*, particularly in its initial manifestations, is characterized by transient weakness. Cranial muscles are usually affected first, caus-

ing double vision, ptosis, dysphagia, and dysarthria. Rarely, limb weakness may herald the onset of myasthenia gravis and in the absence of cranial muscle dysfunction may escape diagnosis for months. Diurnal variation in strength is typical, with weakness worsening as the day wears on. Other, less-common defects of the neuromuscular junction such as the Lambert-Eaton syndrome also may present with intermittent weakness (see Chap. 382).

Intermittent Alterations in Electrolytes Transient shifts in serum potassium are associated with profound alterations in muscle strength. Although the primary periodic paralyses (hypo- and hyperkalemic periodic paralysis) spring to mind in a patient with weakness and an abnormality in serum potassium, other causes of abnormal serum potassium are more frequently behind episodic weakness (see Chap. 383). Familial periodic paralysis seldom presents after age 30; other causes are usually present in older patients. Hypokalemic periodic paralysis may occur in patients with hyperthyroidism. Episodic weakness due to hypokalemia may occur with renal or gastrointestinal potassium loss (see Table 22-1).

Hyperkalemic weakness usually occurs in the setting of chronic renal or adrenal disease. Other electrolyte disturbances may produce intermittent weakness as the initial clinical manifestation of a severe metabolic abnormality (see Table 22-1). Correction of the metabolic derangement improves the weakness.

Metabolic Muscle Disease A number of uncommon defects in glycogen and lipid utilization are associated with impaired energy production by muscle and cause intermittent weakness, usually accompanied by muscle pain and evidence of muscle damage. Carnitine palmitoyl transferase deficiency is one such condition. Mitochondrial disorders such as cytochrome oxidase deficiency may produce severe exercise intolerance with fatigue and weakness associated with lactic acidosis. Muscle pain and destruction seldom occur. (See also Chap. 383.)

Other Disorders Recurrent attacks of a feeling of "weakness" often occur in patients with the *hyperventilation syndrome*; such patients are, however, of normal strength when tested. Similarly, *recurrent hypoglycemic episodes* are associated with subjective weakness, although hypoglycemia is uncommon as the cause of this symptom.

Table 22-1

Causes of Episodic Generalized Weakness

1. Electrolyte disturbances
   a. Hypokalemia: Primary aldosteronism (Conn's syndrome); barium poisoning; renal tubular acidosis; juxtaglomerular apparatus hyperplasia (Bartter's syndrome); villous adenoma of colon; alcoholism; diuretics; licorice; para-aminosalicylic acid; glucocorticoids
   b. Hyperkalemia: Addison's disease; chronic renal failure; hyporeninemic hypoaldosteronism
   c. Hypercalcemia
   d. Hypocalcemic tetany
   e. Hyponatremia
   f. Hypophosphatemia
   g. Hypermagnesemia
2. Neuromuscular junction disorders
   a. Myasthenia gravis
   b. Lambert-Eaton syndrome
3. Muscle disorders
   a. Sodium and chloride channelopathies: Periodic paralyses and myotonias
   b. Metabolic defects of muscle (impaired carbohydrate or fatty acid utilization)
4. Central nervous system causes
   a. Cataplexy and sleep paralysis associated with narcolepsy
   b. Multiple sclerosis
   c. Transient ischemic attacks
5. Disorders with only subjective weakness: Hyperventilation, hypoglycemia

Central nervous system disorders may cause generalized weakness without an associated alteration of consciousness. *Drop attacks* resulting from impaired blood supply to the motor pathways of the brainstem cause sudden paraparesis or quadriparesis, usually lasting only a few seconds. Patients with narcolepsy may have sudden loss of muscle strength and tone during episodes of *cataplexy*. A disorder of the reticular activating system is responsible for these episodes as well as for *sleep paralysis* that occurs as narcoleptic patients are falling asleep or awakening (see Chap. 27).

BIBLIOGRAPHY

ARGOV Z: Phosphorus magnetic resonance spectroscopy (^{31}P MRS) in neuromuscular disorders. Ann Neurol 30:90, 1991

BERTOLASI L et al: The influence of muscular lengthening on cramps. Ann Neurol 33:176, 1993

DEMIRKIRAN M, JANKOVIC J: Paroxysmal dyskinesias: Clinical features and classification. Ann Neurol 38:571, 1995

EDWARDS RHT et al: Muscle biochemistry and pathophysiology in postviral fatigue syndrome. Br Med Bull 47:826, 1991

GRIGGS RC et al: *Evaluation and Treatment of Myopathies*. Philadelphia, F.A. Davis, 1995

LAYZER RB: Muscle pain, cramps, and fatigue, in *Myology*, AG Engel, C Franzini-Armstrong (eds). New York, McGraw-Hill, 1994, pp 1754–1768

O'KEEFFE ST: Restless legs syndrome. Arch Intern Med 156:243, 1996

PTACEK LJ et al: Genetics and physiology of the myotonic muscle disorders. N Engl J Med 328:482, 1993

| **23** | *Arthur K. Asbury* |

NUMBNESS, TINGLING, AND SENSORY LOSS

Normal somatic sensation is a continuous process that commands considerable moment-to-moment nervous system activity. Little of the activity intrudes on consciousness or exacts notice. In contrast, disordered sensation, particularly pains and paresthesias, may be highly intrusive, alarming, tenacious, and may dominate attention. Abnormalities of sensation tend to make patients seek prompt medical attention. When abnormal sensations are perceived as painful, medical advice is sought even more quickly. For a consideration of pain, see Chap. 12. The physician must be able to assess abnormal sensations, estimate their likely site of origin, and recognize their implications.

POSITIVE AND NEGATIVE PHENOMENA All abnormal sensory phenomena may be divided into two categories, positive and negative. Positive phenomena include tingling, pins-and-needles, pricking, bandlike sensations, lightning-like shooting feelings (lancinations), aching, and knifelike, twisting, drawing, pulling, tightening, burning, searing, electrical, and raw sensations. These descriptors are frequently the actual words used by patients. Such sensations may or may not be experienced as painful. The basis for positive phenomena is thought to be ectopic generation of volleys of impulses at a site of lowered neural threshold along the sensory pathways, either in peripheral or central sensory fibers. Such trains of ectopically generated afferent impulses determine the nature of the abnormal sensation experienced, depending on the number, rate, and distribution of impulses and the type and function of nerve fibers in which they arise.

Positive phenomena represent heightened activity in sensory pathways; therefore, they are not necessarily associated with any sensory deficit upon examination.

Negative phenomena result from loss of sensory function and are characterized by diminution or absence of feeling, often experienced as numbness, in a particular distribution. Negative phenomena, in contrast to positive phenomena, are accompanied by abnormal findings on sensory examination. In disorders affecting peripheral sensation, it is estimated that at least half the afferent fibers innervating a given site must be lost or functionless in order for sensory deficit to be demonstrated. This estimate probably varies according to how rapidly sensory fibers have lost function. If the rate of loss is slow and chronic, lack of cutaneous feeling may be unnoticed by the patient and difficult to demonstrate on examination, even though few sensory fibers are functioning. Rapidly evolving sensory abnormality usually evokes positive phenomena of some type and is more readily recognized by patients than insidious deafferentation. Subclinical degrees of sensory dysfunction not demonstrable on clinical sensory examination may be revealed by sensory nerve conduction studies or somatosensory cerebral evoked potentials (see Chap. 361). Sensory symptoms may be either positive or negative, but sensory signs on examination are always negative phenomena.

Terminology Paresthesia and dysesthesia are terms used to denote positive phenomena (sensory symptoms). *Paresthesia* carries the implication that the abnormal sensation is perceived without an apparent stimulus, whereas *dysesthesia* is a more general term used to describe all types of positive sensations whether a stimulus is evident or not. Abnormalities on examination are denoted by *hypesthesia* or *hypoesthesia* (reduction of cutaneous sensation to a specific type of testing such as pressure, light touch, and warm or cold stimuli); *anesthesia* (complete absence of skin sensation to the same stimuli plus pinprick); and *hypalgesia* (referring to loss of pain perception, i.e., nociception, such as the pricking quality elicited by a pin). *Hyperesthesia* means exaggerated perception of sensations in response to mild stimuli (light touch or stroking of the skin). Similarly, *allodynia* describes the situation in which an ordinarily nonpainful stimulus, once perceived, is experienced as painful, even excruciating. An example is elicitation of a painful sensation by application of a vibrating tuning fork. *Hyperalgesia* denotes an exaggerated response to a noxious stimulus, and *hyperpathia*, a broad term, encompasses all the phenomena described by hyperesthesia, allodynia, and hyperalgesia.

Disorders of deep sensation, arising from muscle spindles, tendons, and joints, affect proprioception (position sense). Manifestations include imbalance, particularly with eyes closed or in the dark, clumsiness of precision movements, and unsteadiness of gait, which are referred to collectively as *sensory ataxia* (see Chap. 21). Other findings on examination include reduced or absent joint position and vibratory sensibility and absent deep tendon reflexes in the affected limbs. Romberg's sign is positive, which means that the patient sways or topples when asked to stand with feet close together and eyes closed.

In severe states of deafferentation involving deep sensation, the patient cannot walk or stand unaided or even sit unsupported. Continuous, sometimes wormlike involuntary movements, called *pseudoathetosis*, of the hands and arms occur, particularly with eyes closed. Such patients are severely disabled.

Normal Sensation Cutaneous afferent innervation is subserved by a rich variety of receptors, both naked endings (nociceptors and thermoreceptors) and encapsulated terminals (mechanoreceptors). Each has its own set of sensitivities to specific stimuli, size and distinctness of receptive fields, and adaptational qualities. Much of the knowledge about these receptors has come from the development of techniques to study single intact nerve fibers intraneurally in awake unanesthetized human subjects. It is possible not only to record from single nerve fibers, large or small, but also to stimulate single fibers in isolation. A single impulse, whether elicited by a natural stimulus or evoked by electrical microstimulation, in a large myelinated afferent fiber may be both perceived and localized.

Afferent fibers in peripheral nerve trunks traverse the dorsal roots and enter the dorsal horn of the spinal cord. From there the polysynaptic projections of the smaller fibers (unmyelinated and small myelinated), which in general subserve nociception and temperature sensibility, cross and ascend in the contralateral spinothalamic tract through spinal cord, through brainstem, to the ventral posterolateral nucleus (VPL) of the thalamus, and ultimately project to the postcentral gyrus of the parietal cortex (see Chap. 12). This is the *spinothalamic* pathway. The larger fibers that subserve tactile and position sense and kinesthesia project rostrally in the ipsilateral posterior column of the spinal cord and finally make their first synapse in the gracile or cuneate nuclei of the lower medulla (see Fig. 23-1). The second-order neuron decussates and ascends in the medial lemniscus located medially in the medulla and in the tegmentum of the pons and midbrain and synapses in the VPL. The third-order neuron projects to parietal cortex; this entire system is referred to as *lemniscal*.

Although the fiber types and functions that make up the spinothalamic and lemniscal systems are relatively well known, it has been found that many other fibers, particularly those associated with touch, pressure, and position sense, ascend in a diffusely distributed pattern both ipsilaterally and contralaterally in the anterolateral quadrants of the spinal cord. These anatomic facts explain why an individual with a known complete lesion of the posterior columns of the spinal cord may have little sensory deficit on examination.

EXAMINATION OF SENSATION   The initial step in examination of the somatosensory system is to conduct the tests of primary sensation, which by convention include the sense of pain, touch, vibration, joint position, and thermal sensation, both hot and cold (see Table 23-1).

Some general principles pertain. First, the examiner must depend on subjective patient response, which in turn depends on the level of alertness, motivation, and intelligence of the patient and also on the skill with which the examiner has made the task clear. In a stupefied or obtunded patient, sensory examination is reduced to observing the briskness of withdrawal and the complexity of defensive movements of the patient in response to a pinch or other noxious stimulus. In the alert but uncooperative patient, it is often possible to get some idea of proprioceptive function by noting covertly the patient's best performance of movements requiring balance and precision. Cutaneous sensation may be unexaminable.

Second, sensory examination should not be pressed if the patient is fatigued. An abbreviated survey will suffice until a more extensive examination can be carried out when the patient has rested. Third, sensory examination in a patient who has no neurologic complaints should be quite abbreviated and may consist of pin, touch, and vibration testing in the hands and feet plus evaluation of station and gait, including Romberg's maneuver, which also tests the integrity of motor and cerebellar systems. Fourth, patients should be tested with their eyes closed or covered during both primary sensation and cortical sensory function examination.

Primary Sensation   (See Table 23-1)   The sense of pain is usually tested with a pin, asking the patient to focus on the pricking or unpleasant quality of the stimulus and not just the pressure or touch sensation elicited. Areas of hypalgesia should be mapped by proceeding from the most hypalgesic zones to less affected ones (see Figs. 23-2 and 23-3).

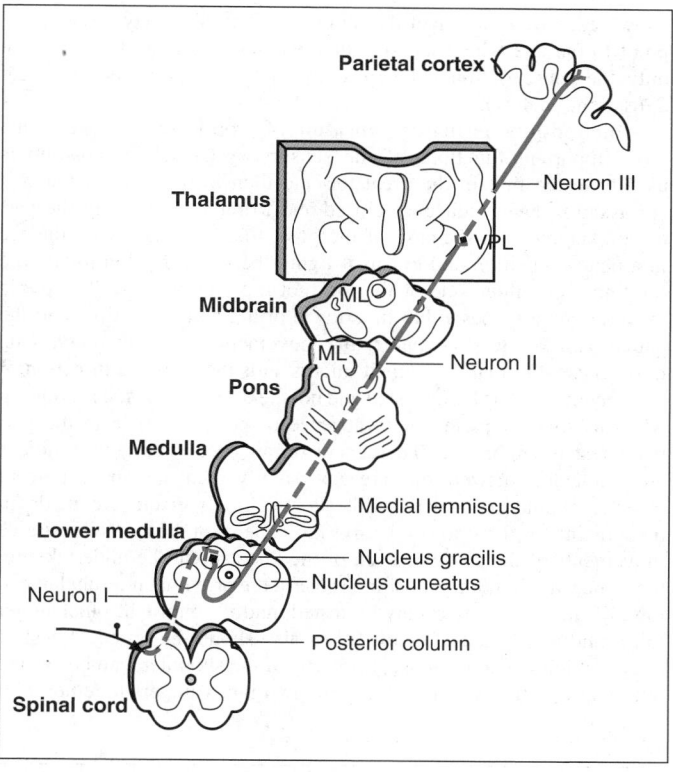

Figure 23-1   Schematic diagram of lemniscal system, which subserves proprioception and discriminative touch.

Temperature sensation, both to hot and to cold, is probably best tested by touching the skin for a couple of seconds with a water flask filled with water of the desired temperature, using a thermometer to verify the temperature. For most purposes, it is satisfactory if a patient can identify as warm the flask that is 35 or 36°C and as cool the one that is 28 to 32°C. Between 28 and 32°C, most individuals can distinguish temperature differences in 1°C steps. Both cold and warm should be tested because different receptors respond to each.

Touch is usually tested with a wisp of cotton or a fine camel's hair brush. In general, it is better to avoid testing touch on hairy skin because of the profusion of sensory endings that surround each hair follicle. The patients, whose eyes are covered, should be asked to say

Table 23-1

Testing Primary Sensation

Sense	Test Device	Endings Activated	Fiber Size Mediating	Central Pathway*
Pain	Pinprick	Cutaneous nociceptors	Small	SpTh, also D
Temperature, heat	Flask with warm water	Cutaneous thermoreceptors for hot	Small	SpTh
Temperature, cold	Flask with cold water	Cutaneous thermoreceptors for cold	Small	SpTh
Touch	Cotton wisp, fine brush	Cutaneous mechanoreceptors, also naked endings	Large and small	Lem, also D and SpTh
Vibration	Tuning fork, 128 Hz	Mechanoreceptors, especially pacinian corpuscles	Large	Lem, also D
Joint position	Passive movement of specific joints	Joint capsule and tendon endings, muscle spindles	Large	Lem, also D

* D, diffuse ascending projections in ipsilateral and contralateral anterolateral columns; SpTh, spinothalamic projection, contralateral; Lem, posterior column and lemniscal projection, ipsilateral.

"now" each time they feel the stimulus. They also may be asked to point to the site where the stimulus was felt, although this tests not only the sense of touch but also touch localization (see "Cortical Sensation," below).

Joint position testing is a measure of proprioception, one of the most important functions of the sensory system. Joint position is usually tested first in the great toe and then in the fingers. Patients are asked to keep their eyes closed and to relax completely the part to be examined. In the case of the great toe, one starts with the toe in a neutral position and grasps it lightly between the thumb and the forefinger on either side of the toe (not top and bottom). The toe is moved a few degrees either in a dorsal or a plantar direction, and the patient is asked to say whether the movement was up or down. One must make sure that the patient understands that it is the direction of movement which is being tested and not the direction the toe is pointing when it stops. A patient with absence of position sense in the part being tested will have a 50 percent error rate because only two choices are available. Answers that are consistently greater than 50 percent in error should be viewed with skepticism. If errors are made in recognizing the direction of passive movements of the toe, then passive movements of the ankle or even of the knee should be undertaken in the same way. Similarly, position sense at the proximal interphalangeal joint of the index finger may be tested, and if abnormal, other finger joints and the wrist and elbow joints also should be tested. A test of proximal joint position sense, primarily at the shoulder, can be carried out by asking the patient to bring the two index fingers together with

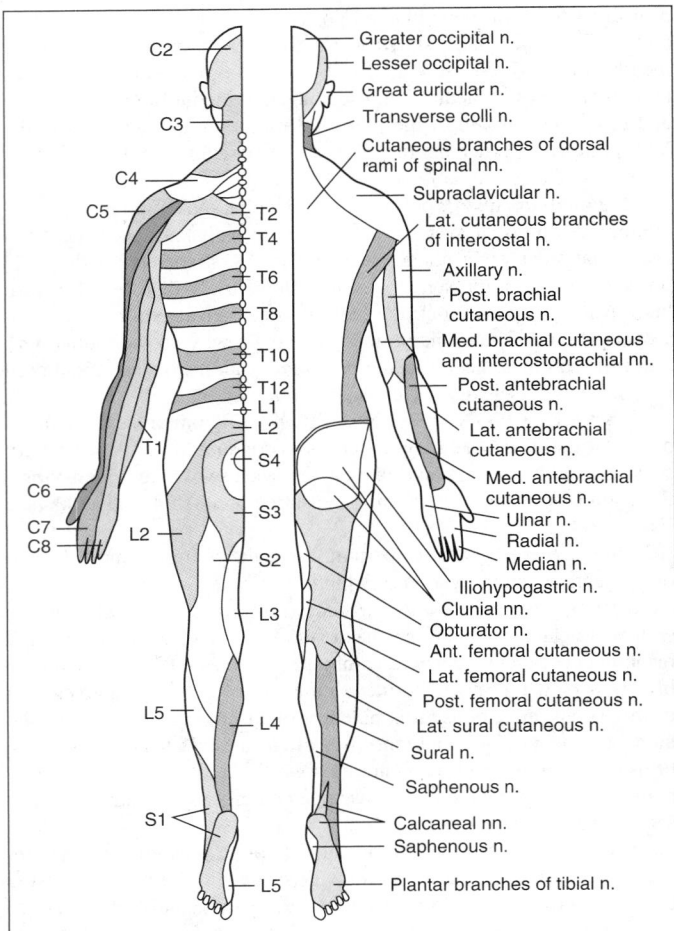

Figure 23-3 Posterior view of dermatomes *(left)* and cutaneous areas supplied by individual peripheral nerves *(right)*. *(Modified from MB Carpenter and J Sutin, in Human Neuroanatomy, 8th ed, Baltimore, Williams & Wilkins, 1983.)*

the arms extended and the eyes closed. Normal individuals should be able to do this quite accurately with errors of a centimeter or less.

The sense of vibration is tested with a tuning fork, preferably a large one that vibrates at 128 Hz. The decay of vibration using this fork is slow enough to be of quantitative use because it takes 15 to 20 s to decay below threshold. Vibration is usually tested at bony prominences, specifically the malleoli at the ankles, the patella, the anterior iliac spine, the spinous processes of the vertebral bodies, the metacarpal-phalangeal joints (knuckles), the styloid process of the ulna, the elbow, and the acromion of the shoulder. Control sites at which to test vibration are the sternum and the forehead. The examiner can compare the threshold at a given site in both patient and self. A crude approximation of degree of vibratory sense loss can be made by counting the seconds that the examiner can feel the sense of vibration longer than the patient. It must be clear to the patient that it is the sense of vibration and not just the pressure of the end of the tuning fork to which attention is directed.

Cortical Sensation Cortical sensory testing includes two-point discrimination, touch localization, stereognosis, graphesthesia, and bilateral simultaneous stimulation, to name the most commonly used methods. Abnormalities of these sensory tests, in the presence of normal primary sensation in an alert cooperative patient, signify a lesion of the parietal cortex or thalamocortical projections to the parietal lobe. If primary sensation is altered, it is not possible to test for these cortical discriminative functions.

Two-point discrimination is tested by special calipers whose points may be set from 2 mm to several centimeters apart and then applied simultaneously to the site to be tested. The pulp of the fingertips is a common site to test; a normal individual can distinguish about 3-mm

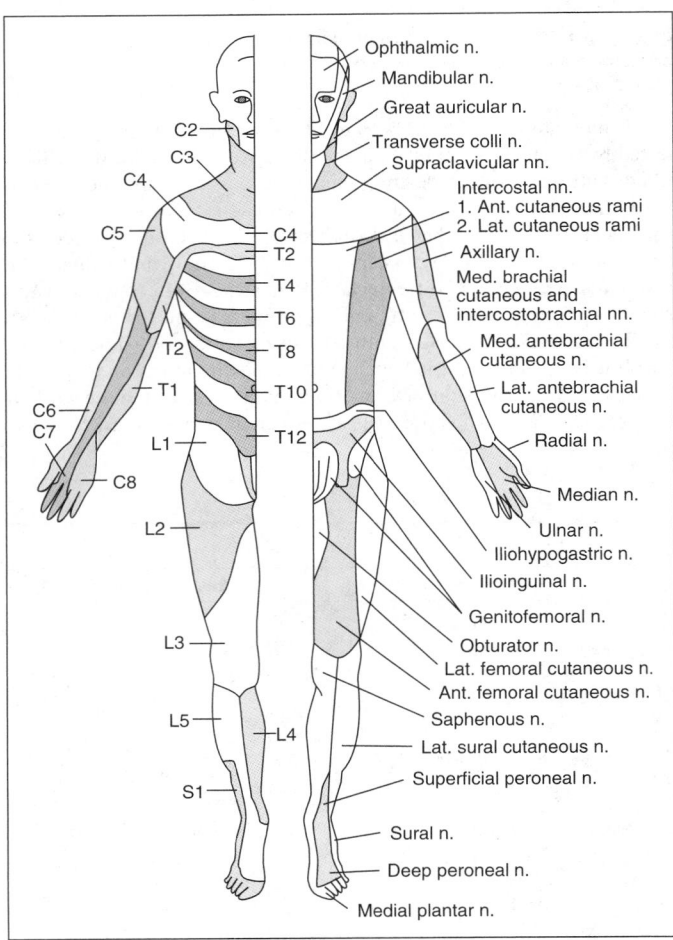

Figure 23-2 Anterior view of dermatomes *(left)* and cutaneous areas supplied by individual peripheral nerves *(right)*. *(Modified from MB Carpenter and J Sutin, in Human Neuroanatomy, 8th ed, Baltimore, Williams & Wilkins, 1983.)*

separation of points there. One can distinguish more closely set points on the tongue and lips, but the threshold for discriminating two points may be centimeters at other sites on the body. Comparisons should always be made between analogous sites on the two sides of the body, since the deficit, with a specific parietal lesion, is likely to be hemilateral. This point holds true for all cortical sensory testing.

Touch localization is usually carried out by light pressure with the examiner's fingertip, asking the patient, whose eyes are closed, to identify the site of touch. It is usual to ask the patient to touch the same site with a fingertip. Bilateral simultaneous stimulation at analogous sites (e.g., the dorsa of both hands) can be carried out to determine whether the perception of touch is extinguished consistently on one side or the other. The phenomenon is referred to as *extinction* on bilateral simultaneous stimulation.

Graphesthesia means the capacity to recognize with eyes closed letters or numbers drawn by the examiner's fingertip on various parts of the body. The usual comparison is the palm of one hand versus the palm of the other. Numbers should be drawn large enough to occupy most of the palm. Once again, the comparison of one side with the other is of prime importance. Failure to recognize numbers or letters is termed *agraphesthesia*.

Stereognosis refers to the ability to identify common objects by palpation, recognizing their shape, texture, and size. Common standard objects are the best test objects, such as a marble, a paper clip, a small rubber ball, or coins. Patients with normal stereognosis should be able to distinguish a dime from a penny and certainly a nickel from a quarter. Patients should only be allowed to feel the object with one hand at a time. If they are unable to identify it in one hand, it should be placed in the other for comparison. Individuals unable to identify common objects and coins in one hand who can do so in the other are said to have *astereognosis* of the abnormal hand. Note that the major comparison is one side of the body with the other.

Localization of Sensory Abnormalities Peripheral neuropathies are generally graded, distal, and symmetric in distribution of deficit. Although most peripheral neuropathies are pansensory and affect all modalities of sensation, selective sensory dysfunction according to nerve fiber size may occur. In small fiber neuropathies, the hallmark is burning, painful dysesthesias with reduced pinprick and thermal sensation but with sparing of proprioception, motor function, and even deep tendon jerks. Touch is variably involved, but when spared, the sensory pattern is referred to as *sensory dissociation* (see below). In contrast to small fiber neuropathies, large fiber neuropathies are characterized by position sense deficit, imbalance, absent tendon jerks, and variable motor dysfunction but preservation of most cutaneous sensation and few or no dysesthesias.

Paresthesias and dysesthesias may be of either peripheral nerve or spinal cord origin and probably can arise in the brainstem, but in every instance they are thought to represent abnormal showers of impulses generated from an ectopic focus or foci. By themselves, paresthesias may not be localizable, but when accompanied by other signs of neuropathy or of myelopathy, the correct site of origin may be deduced.

Dissociated sensory deficit patterns, in which pinprick and thermal sensation are lost but touch is spared, are usually a sign of spinothalamic tract involvement in the spinal cord, especially if the deficit is unilateral and has an upper level on the torso. Bilateral spinothalamic tract involvement occurs with lesions affecting the center of the spinal cord, such as happens with expansion of the central canal in syringomyelia. Sensory dissociation also may occur in peripheral neuropathies in which afferent cutaneous nerve fibers of small diameter are preferentially affected. Neuropathies in which sensory dissociation may occur include leprous neuritis, hereditary sensory neuropathy, and certain cases of amyloid and diabetic polyneuropathy (see Chap. 381).

Hemisensory disturbance with tingling numbness from head to foot is often thalamic in origin but can also be anterior parietal. If abrupt in onset, the lesion is likely to be due to a small stroke (lacunar infarction), particularly if localized to the thalamus. Occasionally, with lesions affecting the posterolateral thalamus (VPL) or adjacent white matter, a syndrome of thalamic pain, also called *Déjerine-Roussy*

syndrome, may ensue. This is a persistent unrelenting hemipainful state often described in dramatic terms such as "like the flesh is being torn from my limbs" or "as though that side is bathed in acid" (see Chap. 12). Harlequin patterns of sensory disturbance, in which one side of the face and the opposite side of the body are affected, localize to the lateral medulla, where a small lesion may damage both the ipsilateral descending trigeminal tract and ascending spinothalamic fibers (lateral lemniscus) subserving the opposite arm, leg, and hemitorso (see "Lateral Medullary Syndrome" in Fig. 366-7).

With lesions of the parietal lobe, either of the cortex or of subjacent white matter, the most prominent symptoms are contralateral hemineglect, hemi-inattention, and a tendency not to use the contralateral hand and arm. Tests of primary sensation may be normal or altered. Anterior parietal infarction may present as a pseudothalamic syndrome with hemilateral loss of primary sensation. Dysesthesias, or even a sense of numbness, also occur except in the special circumstance of focal sensory seizures. These are generally due to lesions in or near the postcentral gyrus. Symptoms of focal somatosensory seizures are usually combinations of numbness and tingling but frequently, additional, more complex sensations are present, such as a rushing feeling, a sense of warmth, a sense of movement without visible motion, or an unpleasantly dysesthetic quality. Duration of seizures is variable; they may be transient, lasting only seconds, or they may persist for hours. Focal motor features (clonic jerking) may supervene, and seizures can become generalized with loss of consciousness. Likely sites of symptoms are unilaterally in the lips, face, digits, or foot, and symptoms may spread as in a Jacksonian march. On occasion, symptoms may occur in a symmetric bilateral fashion, for instance, in both hands; this results from involvement of the second sensory area (unilaterally) located in the rolandic area at and just above the Sylvian fissure.

BIBLIOGRAPHY

BASSETTI C et al: Sensory syndromes in parietal stroke. Neurology 43:1942, 1993

LIGHT AR, PERL ER: Peripheral sensory systems, in *Peripheral Neuropathy*, PJ Dyck et al (eds). Philadelphia, Saunders, 1993, pp 149–165

OCHOA JL: Positive sensory symptoms in neuropathy: Mechanisms and aspects of treatment, in *Peripheral Nerve Disorders*, AK Asbury and PK Thomas (eds). Oxford, Butterworth-Heinemann, 1995, pp 44–58

24	*Allan H. Ropper, Joseph B. Martin*

ACUTE CONFUSIONAL STATES AND COMA

Confusional states and coma are among the most common problems in general medicine. It is estimated that over 5 percent of admissions to the emergency ward of large municipal hospitals are due to diseases that cause a disorder of consciousness. Because a clouding of consciousness (confusion) cannot easily be separated from a diminished level of consciousness (drowsiness, stupor, and coma) and the two are produced by many of the same medical disorders, these conditions are presented here.

Although the interpretation of consciousness is a psychological and philosophical matter, the distinction between *level* of consciousness, or wakefulness, and *content* of consciousness, or awareness, has neurologic significance. Wakefulness-alertness is maintained by a system of upper brainstem and thalamic neurons, the reticular activating system (RAS), and its broad connections to the cerebral hemispheres. Therefore, reduced wakefulness results from depression of the neuronal activity in either the cerebral hemispheres or in the RAS. *Awareness* and *thinking* are dependent on integrated and organized thoughts, subjective experiences, emotions, and mental processes, each of which resides to some extent in anatomically defined regions of the brain. Self-awareness requires that the organism senses this personal stream of thoughts and emotional experiences. The inability to maintain a coherent sequence of thoughts, accompanied usually by inattention and disorientation, is the best definition of *confusion* and is a disorder of the content of consciousness.

STATES OF REDUCED ALERTNESS The unnatural condition of reduced alertness and lessened responsiveness is a continuum that in extreme form characterizes the deep sleeplike state from which the patient cannot be aroused, called *coma*. *Drowsiness* is a disorder that simulates light sleep from which the patient can be easily aroused by touch or noise and can maintain alertness for some time. *Stupor* defines a state in which the patient can be awakened only by vigorous stimuli, and an effort to avoid uncomfortable or aggravating stimulation is displayed. As already indicated, both drowsiness and stupor are usually attended by some degree of mental confusion. Verbal responses in these states are therefore incorrect, slow, or absent during periods of arousal. *Coma* indicates a state from which the patient cannot be aroused by stimulation, and no purposeful attempt is made to avoid painful stimuli.

In clinical practice these terms must be supplemented by a narrative description of the behavioral state of the patient and of responses evoked by various stimuli precisely as they are observed at the bedside. Such descriptions are preferable to ambiguous summary terms such as semicoma or obtundation, the definitions of which differ between observers.

THE CONFUSIONAL STATE Confusion is a behavioral state of reduced mental clarity, coherence, comprehension, and reasoning. *Inattention and disorientation are the main early signs*; however, as an acute confusional state worsens there is deterioration in memory, perception, comprehension, problem solving, language, praxis, visuospatial function, and various aspects of emotional behavior that are each identified with particular regions of the brain. Early in the process it is difficult to know if these complex mental functions are reduced solely as a result of the pervasive defect in attention, but global cortical dysfunction is expected from the metabolic diseases and pharmacologic agents that are the most common sources of the acute confusional state. When there is in addition to confusion an element of drowsiness, the patient is said to have an *encephalopathy*.

Confusion may be a feature of a dementing illness, in which case the chronicity of the process and often a disproportionate effect on memory distinguish it from acute confusion. The confusional state may also derive from a single cortical deficit in higher mental function such as impaired language comprehension, loss of memory, or lack of appreciation of space, in which case each state is defined by the dominant behavioral change (namely, aphasia, dementia, agnosia) rather than characterizing the state as confusion (see Chap. 25).

The drowsiness caused by systemic metabolic changes or by brain lesions is typically accompanied by confusion (encephalopathy). In these instances the primary problem that is causing a diminished level of consciousness should be addressed. A difficult circumstance arises when a process that ultimately leads to drowsiness or stupor begins with confusion or delirium in a fully awake patient.

The confused patient is usually subdued, not inclined to speak, and is inactive physically. In certain cases confusion is accompanied by illusions (misperceptions of environmental sight, sound, or touch) or hallucinations (spontaneous endogenous perceptions). While psychiatrists use the term *delirium* interchangeably with confusion, neurologists prefer to reserve it as a description for an agitated, hypersympathotonic, hallucinatory state most often due to alcohol or drug withdrawal or to hallucinogenic drugs.

COMALIKE SYNDROMES AND RELATED STATES Coma is characterized by complete unarousability. Several other syndromes render patients apparently unresponsive or insensate but are considered separately because of their special significance. The *vege-*

tative state, an unfortunate term, describes patients who were earlier comatose but whose eyelids have after a time opened, giving the appearance of wakefulness. There may be yawning, grunting, and random limb and head movements, but there is an absolute absence of response to commands and an inability to communicate—in essence, an "awake coma." There are accompanying signs of extensive damage to both cerebral hemispheres, i.e., Babinski signs, decerebrate or decorticate limb posturing, and absent response to visual stimuli. Autonomic nervous system functions such as cardiovascular, thermoregulatory, and neuroendocrine control are preserved and may be subject to periods of overactivity. The vegetative state results from global damage to the cerebral cortex, most often from cardiac arrest or head injury as discussed further in Chaps. 366 and 374. *Akinetic mutism* refers to a partially or fully awake patient who when unstimulated remains immobile and silent. The state may result from hydrocephalus, from masses in the region of the third ventricle, or from large bilateral lesions in the cingulate gyrus or other portions of both frontal lobes. Lesions in the periaqueductal or low diencephalic regions may cause a similar state. *Abulia* can be viewed as a mild form of akinetic mutism with the same anatomic origins. The abulic patient is hypokinetic and slow to respond but generally gives correct answers. It is typical to halt while reciting numbers or sequential calculations and, with a delay, to resume correctly. The *locked-in state* describes a pseudocoma in which patients are awake but deefferented, i.e., have no means of producing speech or limb, face, or pharyngeal movements. Infarction or hemorrhage of the ventral pons, which transects all descending corticospinal and corticobulbar pathways are the usual causes. The RAS arousal system, vertical eye movements, and lid elevation remain unimpaired. Such eye movements can be used by the patient to signal to the examiner. A similar awake state simulating unresponsiveness may occur as a result of total paralysis of limb, ocular, and oropharyngeal musculature in severe cases of acute Guillain-Barré syndrome (a peripheral nerve disease) (see Chap. 381). Unlike brainstem stroke, vertical eye movements are not selectively spared.

Certain psychiatric states can mimic coma by producing an apparent unresponsiveness. *Catatonia* is a peculiar hypomobile syndrome associated with major psychosis. In the typical form patients appear awake with eyes open but make no voluntary or responsive movements, although they blink spontaneously and may not appear distressed. It is characteristic but not invariable to have a "waxy flexibility," in which limbs maintain their posture when lifted by the examiner. Upon recovery, such patients have some memory of events that occurred during their catatonic stupor. Patients with *hysterical* or *conversion pseudocoma* show signs that indicate voluntary attempts to appear comatose, though it may take some ingenuity on the part of the examiner to demonstrate these. Eyelid elevation is actively resisted, blinking occurs to a visual threat when the lids are held open, and the eyes move concomitantly with head rotation, all signs belying brain damage.

ANATOMIC CORRELATES OF CONSCIOUSNESS A normal level of consciousness (wakefulness) depends upon activation of the cerebral hemispheres by neurons located in the brainstem RAS. Both of these components and the connections between them must be preserved for normal consciousness to be maintained. The principal causes of coma are therefore: (1) widespread damage in both hemispheres from ischemia, trauma, or other less common brain diseases; (2) suppression of cerebral function by extrinsic drugs, toxins, or hypoxia or by internal metabolic derangements such as hypoglycemia, azotemia, hepatic failure, or hypercalcemia; and (3) brainstem lesions that cause proximate damage to the RAS.

The RAS is a physiologic system contained within the rostral portion of the reticular formation; it consists of neurons located bilaterally in the medial tegmental gray matter of the brainstem that extends from the medulla to the diencephalon. Animal experiments and human clinicopathologic observations have established that the region of the reticular formation that is of critical importance for maintaining wakefulness extends from the rostral pons to the caudal diencephalon. A practical consideration follows: *Destructive lesions that produce coma also affect adjacent brainstem structures of the upper pons, midbrain, and diencephalon that are concerned with pupillary function and eye movements.* Abnormalities in these systems provide convenient, albeit indirect, evidence of direct brainstem damage as the source of coma. Lesions confined to the cerebral hemispheres do not immediately affect the brainstem RAS, although secondary dysfunction of the upper brainstem often results from compression by a mass in a cerebral hemisphere (see transtentorial herniation below).

Brainstem RAS neurons project rostrally to the cortex, primarily via thalamic relay nuclei that exert a tonic influence on the activity of the cerebral cortex. Experimental work in primates suggests that the brainstem RAS affects the level of consciousness by suppressing the activity of the nonspecific nuclei that, in turn, have a predominantly inhibitory effect on the cortex, but this is an oversimplification. It is believed that high-frequency (30 to 40 Hz) rhythms synchronize cortical and thalamic neurons during wakefulness. The basis of behavioral arousal by environmental stimuli (somesthetic, auditory, and visual) is related to the rich innervation that the RAS receives from these sensory systems.

The relays between the RAS and the thalamic and cortical areas are accomplished by neurotransmitters. Of these, the influences on arousal of acetylcholine and biogenic amines have been studied most extensively. Cholinergic fibers connect the midbrain to other areas of the upper brainstem, thalamus, and cortex. Serotonin and norepinephrine also subserve important functions in the regulation of the sleep-wake cycle (see Chap. 27). Their roles in arousal and coma have not been clearly established, although the alerting effects of amphetamines are likely to be mediated by catecholamine release.

A reduction in alertness is related in a semiquantitative way to the total mass of damaged cortex or RAS and is not focally represented in any region of the hemispheres, with the exception that large, acute, and purely unilateral hemispheral lesions, particularly on the left, may cause transient drowsiness even in the absence of damage to the opposite hemisphere or RAS. *Hemispheral lesions in most instances cause coma indirectly when a large mass in one or both hemispheres secondarily compresses the upper brainstem and diencephalic RAS.* This is most typical of cerebral hemorrhages and rapidly expanding tumors. The magnitude of decrease in alertness is also related to the rapidity of onset of the cortical dysfunction or RAS compression.

This secondary compressive effect has led to a concept of *transtentorial herniation* with progressive brainstem dysfunction to explain the neurologic signs that accompany coma from supratentorial mass lesions. Herniation refers to displacement of brain tissue away from a mass, past a less mobile structure such as the dura, and into a space that it normally does not occupy. The common herniations seen at postmortem examinations are transfalcial (displacement of the cingulate gyrus under the falx in the anterior midline), transtentorial (medial temporal lobe displacement into the tentorial opening), and foraminal (the cerebellar tonsils forced into the foramen magnum). Uncal transtentorial herniation, or impaction of the anterior medial temporal gyrus into the anterior portion of the tentorial opening, causes compression of the third nerve with pupillary dilation. Subsequent coma may be due to midbrain compression by the parahippocampal gyrus. Central transtentorial herniation denotes symmetric downward movement of the upper diencephalon (thalamic region) through the tentorial opening in the midline and is heralded by miotic pupils and drowsiness. These shifts in brain are thought to cause a progression of rostral to caudal brainstem compression of first the midbrain, then the pons, and finally the medulla, leading to the sequential appearance of neurologic signs corresponding to the level damaged and to progressively diminished alertness. However, many patients with supratentorial masses do not follow these stereotypic patterns; for example, an orderly progression of signs from midbrain to medulla is often bypassed in catastrophic lesions where all brainstem functions are lost almost simultaneously. Furthermore, drowsiness and stupor typically occur with moderate lateral shifts at the level of the diencephalon when there is only minimal vertical displacement of structures near the tentorial opening and well before downward herniation is evident on computed tomgaphy (CT) scan or magnetic resonance imaging (MRI).

PATHOPHYSIOLOGY OF COMA AND CONFUSION

Coma of metabolic origin is produced by interruption of energy substrate delivery (hypoxia, ischemia, hypoglycemia) or by alteration of the neurophysiologic responses of neuronal membranes (drug or alcohol intoxication, toxic endogenous metabolites, anesthesia, or epilepsy). These same metabolic abnormalites can cause widespread neuronal dysfunction in the cortex that reduces all aspects of mentation and results in an acute confusional state. In this way, acute confusion and coma can be viewed as a continuum in metabolic encephalopathy.

The neurons of the brain are dependent on cerebral blood flow (CBF), oxygen, and glucose. CBF is approximately 75 mL per 100 g/min in gray matter and 30 mL per 100 g/min in white matter (mean = 55 mL per 100 g/min). Oxygen consumption is 3.5 mL per 100 g/min, and glucose consumption is 5 mg per 100 g/min. Brain stores of glucose provide energy for approximately 2 min after blood flow is interrupted, and consciousness is lost within 8 to 10 s. Hypoxia and ischemia simultaneously exhaust glucose more rapidly. The EEG becomes diffusely slowed (typical of metabolic encephalopathies) when mean CBF is below 25 mL per 100 g/min; at 15 mL per 100 g/min, all recordable brain electrical activity ceases. If all other conditions such as temperature and arterial oxygenation remain normal, CBF less than 10 mL per 100 g/min causes irreversible brain damage. The rapidity of the development of ischemia and its duration are also important determinants of irreversible damage.

Confusion and coma due to hyponatremia, hyperosmolarity, hypercapnia, hypercalcemia, and the encephalopathies of hepatic and renal failure are associated with a variety of metabolic derangements of neurons and astrocytes. The reversible toxic effects of these conditions on the brain are not understood but may, in different cases, impair energy supplies, change ion fluxes across neuronal membranes, and cause neurotransmitter abnormalities. In some instances there are specific morphologic changes of nerve cells (see Chap. 380). For example, the high brain ammonia concentration associated with *hepatic coma* interferes with cerebral energy metabolism and the Na^+, K^+-ATPase pump, increases the number and size of astrocytes, causes increased concentrations of potentially toxic products of ammonia metabolism, and results in abnormalities of neurotransmitters, including possible "false" neurotransmitters, which may act competitively at receptor sites. Ammonia or other metabolites also may bind to benzodiazepine–gamma-aminobutyric acid receptors to cause central nervous system (CNS) depression by an endogenous mechanism. Furthermore, these changes are not mutually exclusive.

The mechanism of the encephalopathy of *renal failure* is also poorly understood. Unlike ammonia, urea itself does not produce CNS toxicity. A multifactorial cause has been proposed including an increased permeability of the blood-brain barrier to toxic substances such as organic acids and an increase in brain calcium or cerebrospinal fluid (CSF) phosphate content.

Abnormalities of *osmolarity* are involved in the coma and seizures caused by several systemic medical disorders, including diabetic ketoacidosis, the nonketotic hyperosmolar state, and hyponatremia. Brain water volume correlates best with level of consciousness in hyponatremic–hypoosmolar states, but other factors probably also play a role. Sodium levels below 125 mmol/L cause acute or subacute confusion and below 115 mmol/L are associated with coma and convulsions, depending on the rapidity with which the hyponatremia develops. Serum osmolarity is generally above 350 mosmol/L in hyperosmolar coma.

Hypercapnia produces a diminished level of consciousness proportional to the P_{CO_2} tension in the blood and to the rapidity of onset. A relationship between CSF acidosis and the severity of symptoms has been established. The pathophysiology of other metabolic encephalopathies such as hypercalcemia, hypothyroidism, vitamin B_{12} deficiency, and hypothermia are incompletely understood but must also reflect derangements of CNS biochemistry and membrane functioning.

The large group of *drugs* that depress the CNS, anesthetics, and some endogenous toxins appear to produce coma by suppression of both the RAS and the cerebral cortex. For this reason, combinations of cortical and brainstem signs occur in drug overdose and some other metabolic comas, which may lead to a specious diagnosis of structural brainstem damage.

Although all metabolic derangements alter neuronal electrophysiology, the only primary disturbance of brain electrical activity encountered in clinical practice is *epilepsy*. Continuous, generalized electrical discharges of the cortex (seizures) are associated with coma even in the absence of epileptic motor activity (convulsions). Coma following seizures, termed the *postictal state*, may be due to exhaustion of energy metabolites or be secondary to locally toxic molecules produced during the seizures. Recovery from postictal unresponsiveness occurs when neuronal metabolic balance is restored. The postictal state produces a pattern of continuous, generalized slowing of the background EEG activity similar to that of metabolic encephalopathy.

Approach to the Patient

In Coma   The diagnosis and acute management of coma depend on knowledge of its main causes in clinical practice, an interpretation of certain clinical signs, notably the brainstem reflexes, and the efficient use of diagnostic tests. It is common knowledge that acute respiratory and cardiovascular problems should be attended to prior to neurologic diagnosis. A complete medical evaluation, except for the vital signs, funduscopy, and examination for nuchal rigidity, may be deferred until the neurologic evaluation has established the severity and nature of coma.

HISTORY   In many cases, the cause of coma is immediately evident (e.g., trauma, cardiac arrest, or known drug ingestion). In the remainder, historical information about the onset of coma is often sparse. The most useful historical points are (1) the circumstances and temporal profile of the onset of neurologic symptoms; (2) the precise details of preceding neurologic symptoms (confusion, weakness, headache, seizures, dizziness, diplopia, or vomiting); (3) the use of medications, illicit drugs, or alcohol; and (4) a history of liver, kidney, lung, heart, or other medical disease. Telephone calls to family and observers on the scene are an important part of the initial evaluation. Ambulance attendants often provide the best information in an enigmatic case.

PHYSICAL EXAMINATION AND GENERAL OBSERVATIONS   The temperature, pulse, respiratory rate and pattern, and blood pressure should be measured. Fever suggests systemic infection, bacterial meningitis, encephalitis, or a brain lesion that has disturbed the temperature-regulating centers. High body temperature, 42° to 44°C, associated with dry skin should arouse the suspicion of heat stroke or anticholinergic drug intoxication. Hypothermia is observed with bodily exposure to lowered environmental temperature; alcoholic, barbiturate, sedative, or phenothiazine intoxication; hypoglycemia; peripheral circulatory failure; or hypothyroidism. Hypothermia itself causes coma only when the temperature is below 31°C. Aberrant respiratory patterns that may reflect brainstem disorders are discussed below. A change of pulse rate combined with hyperventilation and hypertension may signal an increase in intracranial pressure. Marked hypertension is a very helpful signature of hypertensive encephalopathy, cerebral hemorrhage, or hydrocephalus and occurs acutely, but to lesser degree, after head trauma. Hypotension is characteristic of coma from alcohol or barbiturate intoxication, internal hemorrhage, myocardial infarction, septicemia, and Addisonian crisis. The funduscopic examination is used to detect subarachnoid hemorrhage (subhyaloid hemorrhages), hypertensive encephalopathy (exudates, hemorrhages, vessel-crossing changes), and increased intracranial pressure (papilledema). Generalized cutaneous petechiae suggest thrombotic thrombocytopenic purpura or a bleeding diathesis associated with intracerebral hemorrhage.

GENERAL NEUROLOGIC ASSESSMENT   An exact description of spontaneous and elicited movements is of great value in establishing the level of neurologic dysfunction. The patient's state should be observed first without examiner intervention. The nature of respirations and spontaneous movements are noted. Patients who toss about, reach up toward the face, cross their legs, yawn, swallow, cough, or moan are closest to being awake. The only sign of seizures may be small excursion twitching of a foot, finger, or facial muscle. An outturned leg at rest or lack of restless movements on one side suggests a hemiparesis.

The terms *decorticate* and *decerebrate rigidity*, or "posturing," describe stereotyped arm and leg movements occurring spontaneously or elicited by sensory stimulation. Flexion of the elbows and wrists and arm supination (decortication) suggest severe bilateral damage in the hemispheres above the midbrain, whereas extension of the elbows and wrists with pronation (decerebration) suggests damage to the corticospinal tracts in the midbrain or caudal diencephalon. Arm extension with minimal leg flexion or flaccid legs has been associated with lesions in the low pons. These terms, however, have been adapted from animal work and cannot be applied with the same precision to coma in humans. Acute lesions of any type frequently cause limb extension regardless of location, and almost all extensor posturing becomes flexion as time passes, so posturing alone cannot be utilized to make an anatomic localization. Metabolic coma, especially after acute hypoxia, also may produce vigorous spontaneous extensor (decerebrate) rigidity. Posturing may coexist with purposeful limb movements, usually reflecting subtotal damage to the motor system. Multifocal myoclonus is almost always an indication of a metabolic disorder, particularly azotemia, anoxia, or drug ingestion. In a drowsy and confused patient bilateral asterixis is a certain sign of metabolic encephalopathy or drug ingestion (see below).

ELICITED MOVEMENTS AND LEVEL OF AROUSAL   If the patient is not aroused by conversational voice, a sequence of increasingly intense stimuli is used to determine the patient's best level of arousal and the optimal motor response of each limb. It should be recognized that the results of this testing may vary from minute to minute and that serial examinations are most useful. Nasal tickle with a cotton wisp is a strong arousal stimulus. Pressure on the knuckles or bony prominences is the preferred and humane form of noxious stimulus. Pinching the skin over the face, chest, or limbs causes unsightly ecchymoses and is not necessary.

Responses to noxious stimuli should be appraised critically. Abduction avoidance movement of a limb is usually purposeful and denotes an intact corticospinal system to that limb. Stereotyped posturing following stimulation of a limb indicates severe dysfunction of the corticospinal system. Adduction and flexion of the stimulated limbs may be reflex movements and imply corticospinal system damage. Brief clonic or twitching limb movements occur at the end of extensor posturing excursions and should not be mistaken for convulsions.

BRAINSTEM REFLEXES   Brainstem signs are a key to localization of the lesion in coma (Fig. 24-1). As a rule, coma associated with normal brainstem function indicates widespread and bilateral hemispheral disease or dysfunction. The brainstem reflexes that allow convenient examination are pupillary light responses, eye movements, both spontaneous and elicited, and respiratory pattern.

Pupillary reaction is examined with a bright, diffuse light and, if the response is absent, confirmed with a magnifying lens. Light reaction in pupils smaller than 2 mm is often difficult to appreciate, and excessive room lighting mutes pupillary reactivity. Symmetrically reactive round pupils (2.5 to 5 mm in diameter) usually exclude midbrain damage as the cause of coma. One enlarged (greater than 5 mm) and unreactive or poorly reactive pupil results either from an intrinsic midbrain lesion (on the same side) or, far more commonly, is secondary to compression or stretching of the third nerve by the secondary effects of a mass. Unilateral pupillary enlargement usually denotes an ipsilateral mass, but this sign occasionally occurs contralaterally, possibly by compression of the midbrain or third nerve against the opposite tentorial margin. Oval and slightly eccentric pupils accompany early midbrain–third nerve compression. Bilaterally dilated and unreactive pupils indicate severe midbrain damage, usually from secondary compression by transtentorial herniation or from ingestion of drugs with anticholinergic activity. The use of mydriatic eye drops by a previous examiner, self-administration by the patient, or direct ocular trauma may cause misleading pupillary enlargement. Reactive and bilaterally small but not pinpoint pupils (1 to 2.5 mm) are most commonly seen in metabolic encephalopathy or after deep bilateral hemispheral lesions such as hydrocephalus or thalamic hemorrhage. This has been attributed to dysfunction of sympathetic nervous system efferents emerging from the posterior hypothalamus. Very small but reactive pupils (less than 1 mm) characterize narcotic or barbiturate overdose but also occur with acute, extensive bilateral pontine damage, usually from hemorrhage. The response to naloxone and the presence of reflex eye movements distinguish these. The unilaterally small pupil of a Horner's syndrome is detected by failure of the pupil to enlarge in the dark. It is rare in coma but may occur ipsilateral to a large cerebral hemorrhage that affects the thalamus. Lid tone, tested by lifting the eyelids, palpating resistance to opening, and speed of closure, is reduced progressively as coma deepens.

Eye movements are the second foundation of physical diagnosis in coma because their examination permits an analysis of a large portion of the brainstem. The eyes are first observed by elevating the lids and noting the resting position and spontaneous movements of the globes. Horizontal divergence of the eyes at rest is normally observed in drowsiness. As patients either awaken or coma deepens, the ocular axes become parallel again. An adducted eye at rest indicates lateral rectus paresis (weakness) due to a sixth nerve lesion, and when bilateral, it is often a sign of increased intracranial pressure. An abducted eye at rest, often accompanied by ipsilateral pupillary enlargement, indicates medial rectus paresis due to third nerve dysfunction. With few exceptions, vertical separation of the ocular axes, or *skew deviation*, results from pontine or cerebellar lesions.

Spontaneous eye movements in coma generally take the form of conjugate horizontal roving. This motion exonerates the midbrain and pons and has the same meaning as normal reflex eye movements (see below). Cyclic vertical downward movements are seen in specific

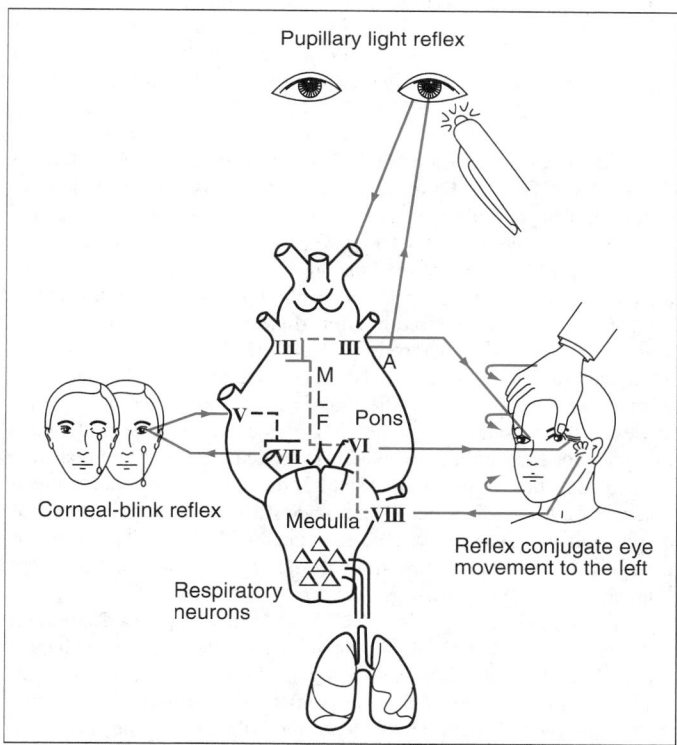

FIGURE 24-1 Brainstem reflexes in the coma examination. Midbrain and third nerve function are tested by pupillary reaction to light, pontine function by spontaneous and reflex eye movements and corneal responses, and medullary function by respiratory and pharyngeal responses.

Reflex conjugate, horizontal eye movements are dependent on the medial longitudinal fasciculus (MLF) interconnecting the sixth and contralateral third nerve nuclei. Eye movements are elicited by head rotation (oculocephalic reflex) or caloric stimulation of the labyrinths (oculovestibular reflex). These reflex movements are suppressed in the awake patient by the cerebral hemispheres via their connections to the brainstem.

circumstances. "Ocular bobbing" describes a brisk downward and slow upward movement of the globes associated with loss of horizontal eye movements and is diagnostic of bilateral pontine damage. "Ocular dipping" is a slower, arrhythmic downward movement followed by a faster upward movement in patients with normal reflex horizontal gaze and denotes diffuse anoxic damage to the cerebral cortex. The eyes may turn down and inward in thalamic and upper midbrain lesions.

"Doll's-eye," or *oculocephalic*, responses are reflex movements tested by moving the head from side to side or vertically, first slowly then briskly; eye movements are evoked in the opposite direction to head movement (see Fig. 24-1). These responses are generated by brainstem mechanisms originating in the labyrinths and cervical proprioceptors. They are normally suppressed by visual fixation mediated by the cerebral hemispheres in awake patients but appear as the hemispheres become suppressed or inactive. The neuronal pathways for reflex horizontal eye movements require integrity of the region surrounding the sixth nerve nucleus and are yoked to the contralateral third nerve via the medial longitudinal fasciculus (MLF) (see Fig. 24-1). Two disparate pieces of information are obtained from the reflex eye movements. First, in coma resulting from bihemispheral disease or metabolic or drug depression, the eyes move easily or "loosely" from side to side in a direction opposite to the direction of head turning. The ease with which the globes move toward the opposite side is a reflection of disinhibition of brainstem reflexes by damaged cerebral hemispheres. Second, conjugate oculocephalic movements demonstrate the integrity of brainstem pathways extending from the high cervical spinal cord and medulla, where vestibular and proprioceptive input from head turning originates, to the midbrain, at the level of the third nerve. Thus full and conjugate eye movements that are induced by the oculocephalic maneuver demonstrate the intactness of a large segment of brainstem and virtually exclude a primary lesion of the brainstem as the cause of coma.

Incomplete ocular adduction indicates an ipsilateral midbrain (third nerve) lesion or damage to the pathways mediating reflex eye movements in the MLF (i.e., internuclear ophthalmoplegia). Third nerve damage is usually associated with an enlarged pupil and horizontal ocular divergence at rest, whereas MLF lesions are unrelated to pupillary function and leave the globe in the primary position. Adduction of the globes is by nature more difficult to obtain than abduction, and subtle abnormalities in the doll's-eye maneuver should be interpreted with caution.

Caloric stimulation of the vestibular apparatus (*oculovestibular* response) is an adjunct to the oculocephalic test, acting as a stronger stimulus to reflex eye movements but giving fundamentally the same information. Irrigation of the external auditory canal with cool water causes convection currents in the endolymph of the labyrinths of the inner ear. An intact brainstem pathway from the labyrinths to the oculomotor nuclei of the midbrain is indicated, with brief latency, by tonic deviation of both eyes (lasting 30 to 120 s) to the side of cool-water irrigation. Bilateral conjugate eye movements therefore have similar significance as full oculocephalic responses. If the cerebral hemispheres are functioning properly, as in hysterical coma, an obligate rapid corrective movement is generated away from the side of tonic deviation. The absence of this nystagmus-like quick phase signifies that the cerebral hemispheres are damaged or suppressed.

Conjugate horizontal ocular deviation at rest or incomplete conjugate eye movements with head turning indicate damage in the pons on the side of the gaze paresis or frontal lobe damage on the opposite side. This phenomenon may be summarized by the following aphorism: *The eyes look toward a hemispheral lesion and away from a brainstem lesion.* It is usually possible to overcome the ocular deviation associated with frontal lobe damage by oculocephalic testing. Seizures also may cause aversive (opposite) eye deviation with rhythmic, jerky movements to the side of gaze. On rare occasions, the eyes may turn paradoxically away from the side of a deep hemispheral lesion ("wrong-way eyes"). In hydrocephalus with dilatation of the third ventricle, the globes frequently rest below the horizontal meridian. Two types of rapid rhythmic eye movements may occur in stupor or coma. *Ocular myoclonus* is a rapid horizontal oscillatory nystagmus usually associated with a similar movement of the palate and due to damage to the central tegmental fasciculus, a longitudinal tract in the brainstem. *Opsoclonus* is an irregular, jerky, saccadic movement varying in direction that results from cerebellar lesions.

A major pitfall in coma diagnosis may occur when reflex eye movements are suppressed by drugs. The eyes then move with the head as it is turned as if the globes locked in place, thus spuriously suggesting brainstem damage. Overdoses of phenytoin, tricyclic antidepressants, and barbiturates are commonly implicated as well as, on occasion, alcohol, phenothiazines, diazepam, and neuromuscular blockers such as pancuronium. The presence of normal pupillary size and light reaction will distinguish most drug-induced comas from brainstem damage. Small to midposition, 1- to 3-mm nonreactive pupils may occur with very high serum levels of barbiturates or secondary to hydrocephalus (see below).

Although the *corneal reflexes* are rarely useful alone, they may corroborate eye movement abnormalities because they also depend on the integrity of pontine pathways. By touching the cornea with a wisp of cotton, a response consisting of brief bilateral lid closure may be observed. The corneal response may be lost if the reflex connections between the fifth and seventh cranial nerves within the pons are damaged. The normal efferent response is bilateral, with closure of both eyelids. CNS depressant drugs diminish or eliminate the corneal responses soon after the reflex eye movements become paralyzed but before the pupils become unreactive to light.

RESPIRATION Respiratory patterns have received much attention in coma diagnosis but are of inconsistent localizing value. Shallow, slow, but well-timed regular breathing suggests metabolic or drug depression. Rapid, deep (Kussmaul) breathing usually implies metabolic acidosis but also may occur with pontomesencephalic lesions. Cheyne-Stokes respiration in its classic cyclic form, ending with a brief apneic period, signifies mild bihemispheral damage or metabolic suppression and commonly accompanies light coma. Agonal gasps reflect bilateral lower brainstem damage and are well known as the terminal respiratory pattern of severe brain damage. In brain-dead patients, shallow respiratory-like movements with irregular, nonrepetitive back arching may be produced by hypoxia and are probably generated by the surviving cervical spinal cord and lower medulla. Other cyclic breathing variations are not usually diagnostic of specific local lesions.

Approach to the Patient

With Acute Confusion Acute confusion is characterized by difficulty in maintaining a coherent stream of thinking and mental performance. This is manifested most obviously by inattention and disorientation, which in turn may generate difficulty with memory and all mental activities. Attention may be gauged by the clarity of and speed of response while the history is being taken but should also be examined by having the patient repeat strings of numbers (most adults easily retain seven digits forward and four backward) or perform serial calculations that require holding the result of one calculation in a working memory in order to pursue the next step—the serial 3-from-30 subtraction test is the usual paradigm. Orientation and memory are tested by asking the patient in a forthright manner the date, inclusive of month, day, year, and day of week; the precise place; and some items of generally acknowledged and universally known information (the name of the President, a recent national catastrophe, the state capital). Further probing may be necessary to reveal a defect—why is the patient in the hospital; what is his or her address, zip code, telephone number, social security number? Problems of increasing complexity may be

pursued but they give little more practical information once a confusional state has been established.

Evidence of drug ingestion should be sought on general physical examination. Other salient neurologic findings are the level of alertness, which typically fluctuates in acute cases; indications of focal damage of the cerebrum such as hemiparesis, hemianopia, and particularly aphasia; adventitious movements of myoclonus; or convulsions. The most pertinent sign of a metabolic encephalopathy is *asterixis*, which is an arrhythmic flapping tremor that is typically elicited by asking the patient to hold the arm out straight with the wrist fully extended. After a few seconds, a large jerking lapse in the posture of the hand occurs and then a rapid return to the original position. The same can be appreciated in any tonically held posture, even of the tongue, and in extreme form the movements may intrude on voluntary limb motion. Bilateral asterixis always signifies a metabolic encephalopathy, for example, from hepatic failure or from drug ingestion, especially with anticonvulsants. Myoclonic jerking and tremor in an awake patient are typical of uremic encephalopathy or antipsychotic (butyrophone) drug ingestion.

The language of the confused patient may be disorganized and rambling, even to the extent of incorporating paraphasic words. These features, along with impaired comprehension that is due to inattention, may be mistaken for aphasia.

Distinguishing dementia from confusion is a great problem. The memory loss of dementia necessarily engenders a confusional state that varies in severity from hour to hour and day to day. Poor mental performance is derived mainly from incomplete recollection, inadequate access to names and ideas, and on the inability to retain new information, thus affecting orientation and factual knowledge; attention is preserved in the early stages of the process. Depending upon the nature of the dementing disease, there may be added specific deficits of language, praxis, visual-spatial performance, or a slowed frontal lobe state. Eventually dementia produces a chronic confusion with breakdown of all types of mental performance, and the distinction from confusion depends simply on the chronic nature of the condition.

LABORATORY EXAMINATION FOR ACUTE CONFUSION AND COMA Four laboratory tests are used most frequently in the diagnosis of confusion and coma: chemical-toxicologic analysis of blood and urine, CT or MRI, EEG, and CSF examination.

Chemical blood determinations are made routinely to investigate metabolic, toxic, or drug-induced encephalopathies. The major metabolic aberrations encountered in clinical practice are those of electrolytes, calcium, blood urea nitrogen (BUN), glucose, plasma osmolarity, and hepatic dysfunction (NH_3). Toxicologic analysis is of great value in any case of coma where the diagnosis is not immediately clear. However, the presence of exogenous drugs or toxins, especially alcohol, does not ensure that other factors, particularly head trauma, may not also contribute to the clinical state. Ethanol levels in nonhabituated patients of 200 mg/dL generally cause confusion and impaired mental activity and above 300 mg/dL are associated with stupor. The development of tolerance may allow the chronic alcoholic to remain awake at levels over 400 mg/dL.

The increased availability of CT and MRI has focused attention on causes of coma that are radiologically detectable (e.g., hemorrhages, tumors, or hydrocephalus). This approach, although at times expedient, is imprudent because most cases of confusion and coma are metabolic or toxic in origin. The notion that a normal CT scan excludes anatomic lesions as the cause of coma is also erroneous. Early bilateral hemisphere infarction, small brainstem lesions, encephalitis, meningitis, mechanical shearing of axons as a result of closed head trauma, absent cerebral perfusion associated with brain death, sagittal sinus thrombosis, and subdural hematomas that are isodense to adjacent brain are some of the lesions that may be overlooked by CT. Even MRI may fail to demonstrate these processes early in their evolution. Nevertheless, in coma of unknown etiology, a CT or MRI scan should be obtained. In those cases in which the etiology is clinically apparent, these provide verification and define the extent of the lesion (Fig. 24-2).

With acute mass lesions, 3 to 5 mm of horizontal displacement of the pineal body from the midline generally corresponds to drowsiness, 5 to 8 mm corresponds to stupor, and greater than 8 mm corresponds to coma. As a supratentorial mass enlarges, the opposite perimesencephalic cistern is first compressed from lateral movement of the brainstem, the ipsilateral cistern is widened, and finally, both are compressed from the lateral mass effect. The lateralventricle opposite the mass becomes enlarged as the third ventricle is compressed. These radiologic features of tissue shifts near the tentorial opening are helpful in correlating the clinical state with the progress of a mass lesion on scans (Fig. 24-3). For technical reasons, MRI is difficult to perform in comatose patients, and it also does not demonstrate hemorrhages as well as CT (see Chap. 362).

The EEG is useful in metabolic or drug-induced confusional states but is rarely diagnostic in coma, with the exception of comas due to clinically unrecognized seizures, herpes virus encephalitis, and Creutzfeldt-Jakob disease. The amount of background slowing of the EEG is a useful gauge of the severity of any diffuse encephalopathy. Predominant high-voltage slowing (delta waves) in the frontal regions is typical of metabolic coma, as from hepatic failure and widespread fast (beta) activity implicates the effects of sedative drugs. A pattern of "alpha coma" is defined by widespread, invariant 8- to 12-Hz activity superficially resembling the normal alpha rhythm of waking but unresponsive to environmental stimuli. Alpha coma results from either high pontine or diffuse cortical damage and is associated with a poor prognosis. Coma due to persistent epileptic discharges that are not clinically manifested may be revealed by EEG recordings. Normal alpha activity on the EEG also may alert the clinician to the locked-in syndrome or a hysterical case. Computed on-line EEG analysis and evoked potential recordings (auditory and somatosensory) are useful additional methods for coma diagnosis and monitoring.

Lumbar puncture is now used more judiciously in cases of coma or confusion because the CT scan excludes intracerebral hemorrhages and most subarachnoid hemorrhages. The use of lumbar puncture in coma is limited to diagnosis of meningitis or encephalitis and instances of suspected subarachnoid hemorrhage in which the CT is normal. Lumbar puncture should not be deferred if meningitis is a strong clinical possibility. Xanthochromia is documented by spinning the CSF in a large tube and comparing the supernatant to water. This yellow coloration indicates preexisting blood in the CSF (or very high protein levels) and permits exclusion of a traumatic puncture. In addition, initial and final tubes should be inspected for a decrement in the number of erythrocytes, indicating traumatic puncture. Knowing the pressure within the subarachnoid space is of further help in interpreting abnormalities of the cell count and protein content of the CSF.

DIFFERENTIAL DIAGNOSIS OF CONFUSION AND COMA In most instances, confusion and coma are part of an obvious medical problem such as known drug ingestion, hypoxia, stroke, trauma, or liver or kidney failure. Attention is then appropriately focused on the primary illness. A complete listing of all diseases that cause confusion and coma would serve little purpose, since it would not aid diagnosis. Some general rules, however, are helpful. Illnesses that cause sudden or acute coma are due to drug ingestion or to one of the catastrophic brain lesions—hemorrhage, trauma, hypoxia, or, rarely, acute basilar artery occlusion. Coma that appears subacutely is usually related to preceding medical or neurologic problems, including the secondary brain swelling that surrounds a preexisting lesion. Coma diagnosis, therefore, requires familiarity with the common intracerebral catastrophes. These are described in more detail in Chap. 366 but may be summarized as follows: (1) basal ganglia and thalamic hemorrhage (acute but not instantaneous onset, vomiting, headache, hemiplegia, and characteristic eye signs); (2) subarachnoid hemorrhage (instantaneous onset, severe headache, neck stiffness, vomiting, third or sixth nerve lesions, transient loss of consciousness, or sudden coma with vigorous extensor posturing); (3) pontine hemorrhage (sudden onset, pinpoint pupils, loss of reflex eye movements and corneal responses, ocular bobbing, posturing, hyperventilation, and sweating); (4) cerebellar hemorrhage (occipital headache, vomiting, gaze paresis, and inability to stand); and (5) basilar artery thrombosis (neurologic prodrome or warning spells, diplopia, dysarthria, vomiting, eye movement and corneal response abnormalities, and asymmetric limb paresis). The most common stroke, namely, infarction in the territory of the middle cerebral artery, does not cause coma acutely. The syndrome of acute hydrocephalus causing coma may accompany many intracranial catastrophes, particularly subarachnoid hemorrhage. Acute symmetric enlargement of both lateral ventricles causes headache and sometimes vomiting followed by drowsiness that may progress quickly to coma, with extensor posturing of the limbs, bilateral Babinski signs, small nonreactive pupils, and impaired vertical oculocephalic movements.

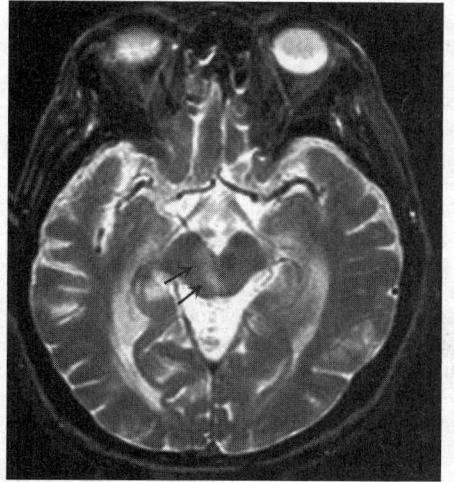 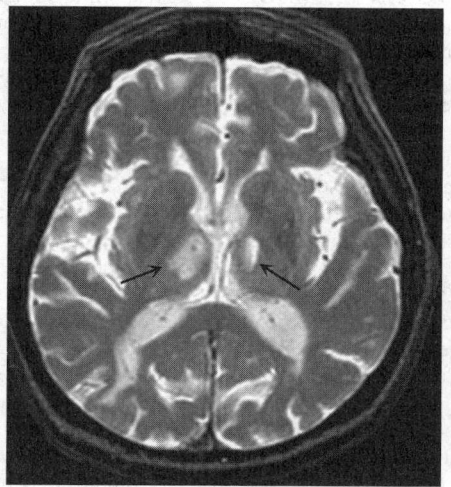 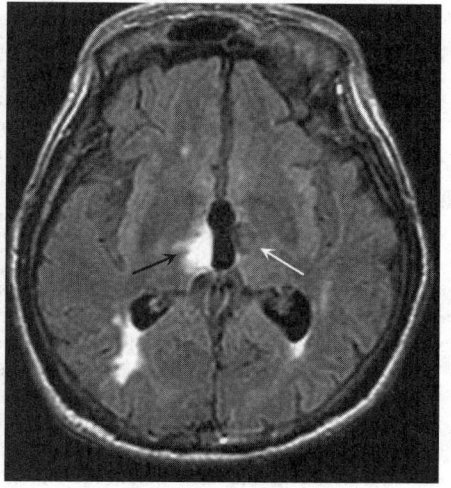

A   *B*   *C*

FIGURE 24-2 Coma with right 3d nerve palsy due to stroke. *A.* T2-weighted fast spin echo MR image demonstrates a wedge-shaped area of abnormal signal intensity consistent with infarction within the midbrain extending from the aqueduct ventrally along the course of the 3d cranial nerve (arrows). *B.* T2-weighted image demonstrates bilateral thalamic infarctions (arrows). This area is perfused by the perforating arteries arising from the tip of the basilar artery. *C.* T2-weighted image with fluid attentuation (FLAIR). Note that the right thalamic infarction (*black arrow*) has abnormal high signal intensity while the left thalamic infarction (*white arrow*) has low signal intensity indicating a more chronic cavitated process. Also note the abnormal signal intensities along both trigones of the lateral ventricles consistent with small vessel ischemic disease. This patient suffered brainstem and bithalamic infarctions secondary to occlusion of the top of the basilar artery. (Prepared by William Dillon, M.D.)

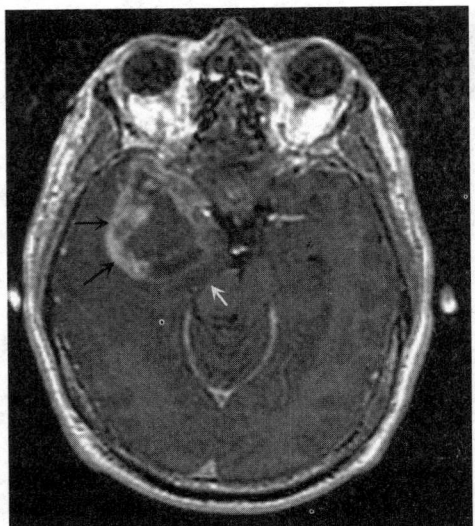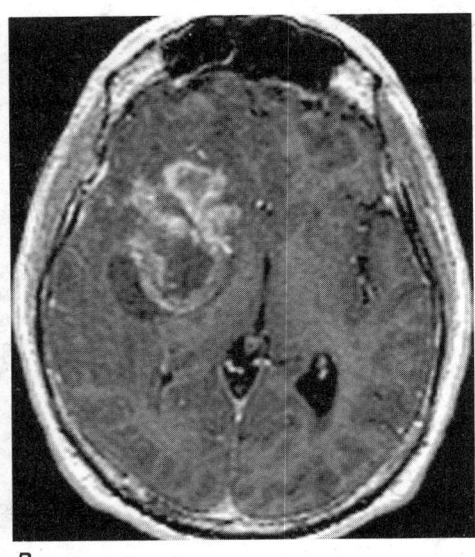

FIGURE 24-3 Unilateral intracranial mass lesion: coma, seizures, and right third nerve palsy. Axial post-contrast T$_1$-weighted MRI images through the suprasellar cistern (*A*) and third ventricle (*B.*) A heterogeneously enhancing mass in the right temporal lobe (*arrows*) compresses the right cerebral peduncle and midbrain (*white arrow*). This glioblastoma multiforme was resected and treated with a combination of radiation and chemotherapy. (Prepared by William Dillon, M.D.)

If the history and examination are not typical for any neurologic diagnosis and metabolic or drug causes are excluded, then information obtained from CT or MRI may be used as outlined in Table 24-1. The CT scan is useful to focus the differential diagnosis, and because of its accuracy and general availability, the diagnoses that it facilitates are listed in the table. As mentioned earlier, the majority of medical causes of coma are established without a CT or with the study being normal.

COMA AFTER HEAD TRAUMA Concussion is a common form of transient coma that results from torsion of the hemispheres about the midbrain-diencephalic junction with brief interruption of RAS function. Persistent coma after head trauma presents a more complex and serious problem (Chap. 374). The main causes are subdural or epidural hemorrhage, deep cerebral hemorrhage, bilateral frontotemporal contusions, and extensive white matter damage.

COMA WITH ISCHEMIC-ANOXIC BRAIN DAMAGE There are widespread and complex changes in the CNS following cardiac arrest, profound hypotension, or anoxia. Some of these are physiologic and mediated by alterations in electrical and neurotransmitter function, and others may result from endogenously released neurotoxins that ultimately lead to neuronal death. Several clinically recognizable patterns emerge that occur usually in pure form but that may coexist: (1) a deep coma with preserved brainstem function that evolves to the vegetative state or to a dementia, reflecting damage to neurons throughout the cortex—brainstem function may be suppressed in the first hours, thus emulating brain death, and the limbs may be either flaccid or show vigorous extensor posturing or myoclonic jerks; (2) syndromes of proximal bibrachial and paraparetic weakness or of cortical blindness that are due to bilateral infarctions of the watershed regions between major cortical vessel territories from diminished blood flow; (3) a Korsakoff-amnestic state that indicates the selective vulnerability of neurons in the hippocampal cortex; and infrequently (4) a cerebellar syndrome.

Brain Death Brain death is a state of total cessation of cerebral blood flow and global infarction of the brain at a time when respiration is preserved by artificial support and the heart continues to function. It is the only type of irrevocable loss of brain function currently recognized as equivalent to death. Many sets of roughly equivalent criteria have been advanced for the diagnosis of brain death, and it is essential to adhere to those endorsed as standard practice by the local medical community. Ideal criteria are simple, conducted at the bedside, and allow no chance of diagnostic error. There are three essential elements: (1) widespread cortical destruction shown by deep coma; (2) global brainstem damage demonstrated by absent pupillary light reaction, and absent oculovestibular and corneal reflexes; and (3) medullary destruction indicated by complete apnea. The pulse rate is also invariant and unresponsive to atropine. Most patients have diabetes insipidus, but in some it develops after the clinical signs of brain death. The pupils need not be enlarged but should not be constricted. The absence of deep tendon reflexes is not required because the spinal cord may remain functional.

The possibility of profound drug-induced or hypothermic CNS depression should always be excluded. Some period of observation, usually 6 to 24 h, is desirable during which this state is shown to be sustained. It is often advisable to delay clinical testing for up to 24 h if a cardiac arrest has caused brain death or if the inciting disease is not known.

Demonstration of apnea generally requires that the P$_{CO_2}$ be high enough to stimulate respiration. This can be accomplished safely in most patients by removal of the respirator and use of diffusion oxygenation sustained by a tracheal cannula connected to an oxygen supply. In brain-dead patients, CO$_2$ tension increases approximately 0.3 to 0.4 kPa/min (2 to 3 mmHg/min) during apnea. At the end of an appropriate interval, arterial P$_{CO_2}$ should be at least above 6.6 to 8.0 kPa (50 to 60 mmHg) for the test to be valid. Large posterior fossa lesions that compress the brainstem, CNS-depressant drugs, and profound hypothermia can simulate brain death, but adherence to recognized protocols for diagnosis will prevent these errors.

An isoelectric EEG is often used as a confirmatory test for total cortical damage, but it is not absolutely necessary. Radionuclide brain scanning, cerebral angiography, or transcranial Doppler measurements may also be used to demonstrate the absence of cerebral blood flow, but with the exception of the latter, they are cumbersome and have not been correlated extensively with pathologic material.

There is no explicit reason to make the diagnosis of brain death except when organ transplantation or difficult resource-allocation (intensive care) issues are involved. Although it is commonly accepted that the respirator can be disconnected from a brain-dead patient, most problems arise because of inadequate explanation and preparation of the family by the physician.

℞ TREATMENT

The immediate goal in acute coma is the prevention of further nervous system damage. Hypotension, hypoglycemia, hypercalcemia, hypoxia, hypercapnia, and hyperthermia should be corrected rapidly and assiduously. An oropharyngeal airway is adequate to keep the pharynx open in drowsy patients who are breathing normally. Tracheal intubation is indicated if there is apnea, upper airway obstruction, hypoventilation, or emesis, or if the patient is liable to aspirate. Mechanical ventilation is required if there is hypoventilation or if there is an intracranial mass and induced hypocapnia is necessary. Intravenous access is established, and naloxone and dextrose are administered if narcotic overdose or hypoglycemia are even remote possibilities. Thiamine is administered with glucose in order to avoid eliciting Wernicke's encephalopathy in malnourished patients. The veins of intravenous drug abusers may be difficult to cannulate; in such cases, naloxone can be injected sublingually through a small-guage needle. In cases of suspected basilar thrombosis with brainstem ischemia, intravenous heparin or a thrombolytic agent is administered after obtaining a CT scan, keeping in mind that cerebellar and pontine hemorrhages resemble the syndrome of basilar artery occlusion. Physostigmine, when used by experienced physicians with careful monitoring, may awaken patients with anticholinergic-type drug overdose, but many physicians believe that this is justified only to treat cardiac arrhythmias resulting from these overdoses. The use of benzodiazepine antagonists is promising for treatment of overdoses and has transient benefit in hepatic encephalopathy. Intravenous administration of water should be monitored carefully in any serious acute CNS illness because of the potential for exacerbating brain swelling. Neck injuries must not be overlooked, particularly prior to attempting intubation or eliciting oculocephalic responses. Headache accompanied by fever and meningismus indicates an urgent need for examination of the CSF to diagnose meningitis, and *lumbar puncture should not be delayed while awaiting a CT scan.*

Table 24-1

Approach to the Differential Diagnosis of Coma

NORMAL BRAINSTEM REFLEXES, NO LATERALIZING SIGNS

A. Bilateral hemispheral dysfunction without mass lesion (CT or MRI normal; primary test used for diagnosis is indicated in parentheses)
   1. Drug-toxin ingestion (toxicologic analysis)
   2. Endogenous metabolic encephalopathy (glucose, ammonia, calcium, osmolarity, P_{O_2}, P_{CO_2}, urea, sodium)
   3. Shock, hypertensive encephalopathy
   4. Meningitis (CSF analysis)
   5. Nonherpetic viral encephalitis (CSF analysis)
   6. Epilepsy (EEG)
   7. Reye's syndrome (ammonia, increased intracranial pressure)
   8. Fat embolism
   9. Subarachnoid hemorrhage with normal CT (CSF analysis)
   10. Creutzfeldt-Jakob disease (EEG)
   11. Hysterical coma or catatonia
B. Anatomic lesions of hemisphere found by CT or MRI
   1. Hydrocephalus
   2. Bilateral subdural hematomas
   3. Bilateral contusions, edema, or axonal shearing of hemispheres due to closed head trauma
   4. Subarachnoid hemorrhage
   5. Acute disseminated encephalomyelitis (CSF analysis)

NORMAL BRAINSTEM REFLEXES (WITH/WITHOUT UNILATERAL THIRD NERVE PALSY), LATERALIZING MOTOR SIGNS (CT OR MRI ABNORMAL)

A. Unilateral mass lesion
   1. Cerebral hemorrhage (basal ganglia, thalamus)
   2. Large infarction with surrounding brain edema
   3. Herpes virus encephalitis (temporal lobe lesion)
   4. Subdural or epidural hematoma
   5. Tumor with edema
   6. Brain abscess with edema
   7. Vasculitis with multiple infarctions
   8. Metabolic encephalopathy superimposed on preexisting focal lesions (i.e., stroke with hyperglycemia, hyponatremia, etc.)
   9. Pituitary apoplexy
B. Asymmetric signs accompanied by diffuse hemispheral dysfunction
   1. Metabolic encephalopathies with asymmetric signs (blood chemical determinations)
   2. Isodense subdural hematoma (MRI, CT with contrast)
   3. Thrombotic thrombocytopenic purpura (blood smear, platelet count)
   4. Epilepsy with focal seizures or postictal state (EEG)

MULTIPLE BRAINSTEM REFLEX ABNORMALITIES

A. Anatomic lesions in brainstem
   1. Pontine, midbrain hemorrhage
   2. Cerebellar hemorrhage, tumor, abscess
   3. Cerebellar infarction with brainstem compression
   4. Mass in hemisphere causing advanced upper brainstem compression
   5. Primary brainstem tumor, demyelination, or abscess
   6. Traumatic brainstem contusion-hemorrhage
B. Brainstem dysfunction without mass lesion
   1. Basilar artery thrombosis causing brainstem infarction (clinical signs, angiogram)
   2. Severe drug overdose (toxicologic analysis)
   3. Brainstem encephalitis
   4. Basilar artery migraine

Enlargement of one pupil usually indicates secondary midbrain compression by a hemispherical mass and demands immediate reduction of intracranial pressure (ICP) as discussed further in Chap. 374. Surgical evacuation of the mass may be appropriate. Medical management to reduce intracranial pressure consists of intravenous fluid normal saline (the safest fluid because it is slightly hyperosmolar in most patients). Therapeutic hyperventilation may be used to achieve an arterial P_{CO_2} of 3.7 to 4.2 kPa (28 to 32 mmHg), but its effects are brief. Hyperosmolar therapy with mannitol or an equivalent is the mainstay of ICP reduction. It may be used simultaneously with hyperventilation in critical cases. A ventricular puncture is necessary to decompress hydrocephalus if medical measures fail to improve alertness. The use of high-dose barbiturates and other neuronal sparing agents soon after cardiac arrest has not been shown in clinical studies to be beneficial and corticosteroids have no proven value except in cases of brain tumor.

PROGNOSIS OF COMA AND THE VEGETATIVE STATE Interest in predicting the outcome of coma is oriented toward allocating medical resources and limiting the support of hopeless cases. To date, no collection of clinical signs except those of brain death assuredly predicts outcome of coma, but certain constellations have prognostic value. Children and young adults may have ominous early clinical findings such as abnormal brainstem reflexes and yet recover. All schemes for prognosis should be taken as only approximate indicators, and medical judgments must be tempered by other factors such as age, underlying disease, and general medical condition. In an attempt to collect prognostic information from large numbers of patients with head injury, the Glasgow Coma Scale was devised; empirically it has predictive value in cases of brain trauma (see Chap. 374). Major points include a 95 percent death rate in patients whose pupillary reaction or reflex eye movements are absent 6 h after onset of coma, and a 91 percent death rate if the pupils are unreactive at 24 h (although roughly 5 percent make a good recovery).

Prognostication of nontraumatic coma is difficult because of the heterogeneity of contributing diseases. Metabolic coma generally has a more favorable prognosis than anoxic or traumatic coma. Unfavorable signs in the first hours after admission are the absence of any two of pupillary reaction, corneal reflex, or the oculovestibular response. One day after the onset of coma, the preceding signs, in addition to absence of eye opening and muscle tone, predict death or severe disability, and the same signs at 3 days strengthen the prediction of a poor outcome. In many patients, precise combinations of predictive signs do not occur, and coma scales lose their value. The use of evoked potentials aids prognostication in head-injured and post–cardiac arrest patients. Bilateral absence of cortical somatosensory evoked potentials is associated with death or a vegetative state in most cases. Medical practitioners are becoming less reluctant to withdraw support from non–brain-dead but severely neurologically injured patients as predictions become more reliable and resources more limited.

The prognosis for regaining full mental faculties once the vegetative state has supervened is almost nil. Most instances of dramatic recovery, when investigated carefully, yield to the usual rules for prognosis, but it must be acknowledged that rare instances of awakening to a condition of dementia or paralysis after months or years in this state have been documented.

BIBLIOGRAPHY

CELESIA GG et al: Persistent vegetative state—Report of the American Neurological Association Committee on Ethical Affairs. Ann Neurol 33:386, 1993
IVAN L, BRUCE D: *Coma.* Springfield, IL, Charles C Thomas, 1982
JENNET B et al: Prognosis of patients with severe head injury. Neurosurgery 4:283, 1979
LEVY D et al: Prognosis in non-traumatic coma. Ann Intern Med 94:229, 1981

PLUM F, POSNER J: *The Diagnosis of Stupor and Coma*, 3d ed. Philadelphia, Davis, 1980

ROPPER AH: Lateral displacement of the brain and level of consciousness in patients with an acute hemispheral mass. N Engl J Med 314:953, 1986

————: Coma and acutely raised intracranial pressure, in *Diseases of the Nervous System*, 2d ed, A Asbury et al (eds). Philadelphia, Saunders, 1992

————: *Neurological and Neurosurgical Intensive Care*, 3d ed. New York, Raven, 1992

YOUNG BY et al: *Coma and Impaired Consciousness*. New York, McGraw-Hill, 1997

25 M.-Marsel Mesulam

APHASIAS AND OTHER FOCAL CEREBRAL DISORDERS

The cerebral cortex is subdivided into five functional zones designated as (1) primary sensorimotor, (2) unimodal association, (3) heteromodal association, (4) paralimbic, and (5) limbic (Table 25-1, Fig. 25-1). The *primary sensorimotor zone*, devoted to elementary sensory and motor functions, takes up less than 10 percent of the cerebral cortex. The remaining four zones, collectively known as the *association cortex*, account for the vast majority of the cerebral cortex and sustain complex cognitive and behavioral functions. The conventional neurologic examination places a greater emphasis on testing of sensorimotor than cognitive function. Hence, detection of disease in the sensorimotor cortex and related pathways is more precise than detection of disease confined to the association cortex. A "normal" neurologic examination in a patient with a large frontal, parietal, or temporal lobe lesion is not uncommon in clinical experience. A systematic testing of cognitive function is necessary if the clinical assessment of the association cortex

Table 25-1

Types of Cortical Areas and Their Corresponding Brodmann Numbers

PRIMARY SENSORY AND MOTOR CORTEX

Primary visual (area 17, striate cortex)
Primary auditory (areas 41, 42)
Primary somatosensory (areas 3, 1, 2 but mostly area 3b)
Primary motor (area 4)

UNIMODAL ASSOCIATION CORTEX

Unimodal visual [areas 18–19 (peristriate cortex, upstream visual association); 20–21, ?37 (downstream visual association)]
Unimodal auditory (area 22)
Unimodal somatosensory (area 5, rostral area 7)
Unimodal motor (areas 6, ?caudal 8, ?44, premotor cortex)

HETEROMODAL ASSOCIATION CORTEX

Heteromodal prefrontal (areas 9, 10, 45, 46, 47, rostral parts of areas 11, 12, 32)
Heteromodal parietotemporal (areas 39, 40, caudal parts of area 7, banks of superior temporal sulcus, ?area 36)

PARALIMBIC CORTEX

Insula (areas 14, 15), temporopolar cortex (area 38), caudal orbitofrontal cortex (caudal areas 11, 12), cingulate complex (areas 23, 24, ?31, 33, 25, 26, 29, caudal parts of area 32), parahippocampal cortex (areas 28, 34, 35, 30)

CORE LIMBIC AREAS

Corticoid formations (amygdala, substantia innominata, septal nuclei)
Allocortex (hippocampus, pyriform olfactory cortex)

is to be guided by the same rational approach that guides the assessment of other components of the nervous system.

The interpretation of the traditional neurologic examination tends to be based on relatively invariant relationships between anatomy and function. Damage to the optic tract or striate cortex, for example, always leads to contralateral homonymous hemianopic visual field defects. The destruction of the sciatic nerve always leads to loss of the ankle jerk. The approach to higher cortical function was initially based on the expectation that analogous relationships would be uncovered in the association cortex; that it would be possible to identify centers for "hearing words," "perceiving space," or "storing memories"; and that it would consequently be possible to devise specific bedside tests for the precise localization of association cortex lesions. These expectations now need to be modified to incorporate more modern models of localization based on an understanding of *large-scale neural networks* and *selectively distributed processing*.

According to current thinking, cognitive and behavioral functions (domains) are coordinated by intersecting neural networks that contain interconnected cortical and subcortical components. The network approach to higher cortical function has at least four implications of clinical relevance: (1) a single domain such as language or memory can be disrupted by damage to any one of several areas, as long as

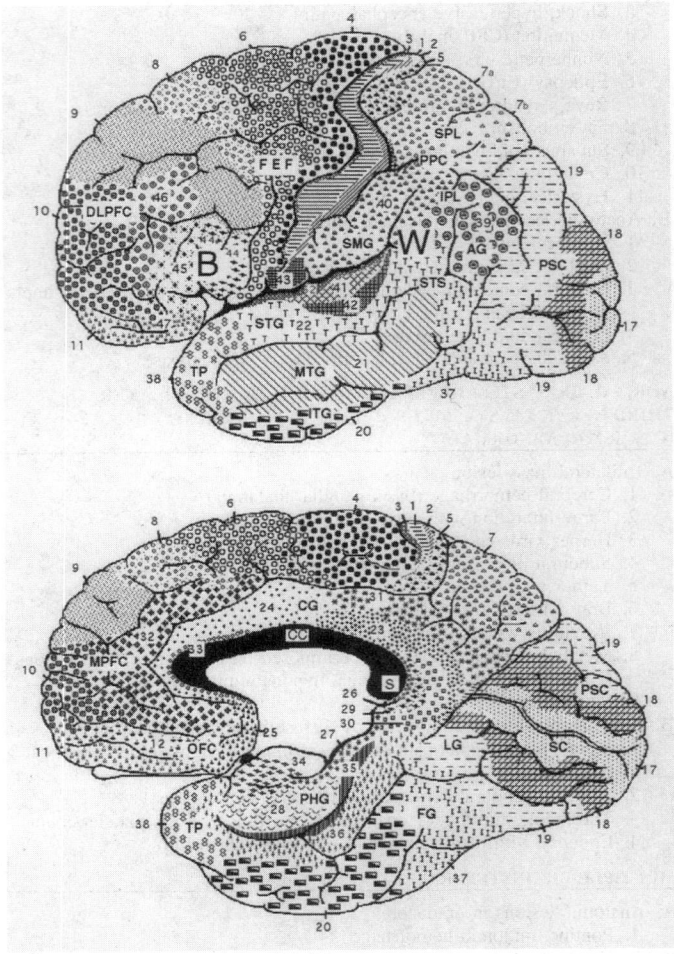

FIGURE 25-1 Lateral (*top*) and medial (*bottom*) views of the cerebral hemispheres. The numbers refer to the Brodmann cytoarchitectonic designations. AG, angular gyrus; B, Broca's area; CC, corpus callosum; CG, cingulate cortex; DLPFC, dorsolateral prefrontal cortex; FEF, frontal eye fields (premotor cortex); FG, fusiform gyrus; IPL, inferior parietal lobule; ITG, inferior temporal gyrus; LG, lingual gyrus; MPFC, medial prefrontal cortex; MTG, middle temporal gyrus; OFC, orbitofrontal gyrus; PHG, parahippocampal gyrus; PPC, posterior parietal cortex; PSC, peristriate cortex; SC, striate cortex; SMG, supramarginal gyrus; SPL, superior parietal lobule; STG, superior temporal gyrus; STS, superior temporal sulcus; TP, temporopolar cortex; W, Wernicke's area.

these areas belong to the same network; (2) damage confined to a single area can give rise to multiple deficits, involving the functions of all networks that intersect in that region; (3) damage to a network component may give rise to minimal or transient deficits in the relevant domain if other parts of the network undergo compensatory reorganization; and (4) individual anatomic sites within a network display a relative (but not absolute) specialization for different behavioral aspects of the relevant function. Thus, damage to each anatomic component of a network may lead to impairments of the same domain but with different clinical patterns. Five anatomically defined large-scale networks are most relevant to clinical practice: a perisylvian network for language; a parietofrontal network for spatial orientation; an occipitotemporal network for object recognition; a limbic network for retentive memory; and a prefrontal network for attention and comportment (see Fig. 25-1).

THE LEFT PERISYLVIAN NETWORK FOR LANGUAGE: APHASIAS AND RELATED CONDITIONS   **Definitions**   Language allows the communication and reshaping of thoughts and experiences by linking them to arbitrary symbols known as words. The neural substrate of language is composed of a distributed network centered in the perisylvian region of the *left* hemisphere. The posterior pole of this network is known as *Wernicke's area* and includes the posterior third of the superior temporal gyrus and a surrounding rim of the inferior parietal lobule. An essential function of Wernicke's area is to transform sensory inputs into their neural word representations so that these can enter the distributed associations that lead to meaning. The anterior pole of the language network, known as *Broca's area*, includes the posterior part of the inferior frontal gyrus and a surrounding rim of prefrontal heteromodal cortex. An essential function of this area is to transform neural word representations into their articulatory sequences so that the words can be uttered in the form of spoken language. The sequencing function of Broca's area also appears to involve the ordering of words into sentences so that the resulting statement has a meaning-appropriate *syntax* (grammar). Wernicke's and Broca's areas are interconnected with each other and with additional perisylvian, temporal, prefrontal, and posterior parietal regions, making up a neural network subserving the various aspects of language function. Damage to any one of these components or to their interconnections can give rise to language disturbances (*aphasia*). Aphasia should be diagnosed only when there are deficits in the formal aspects of language such as naming, word choice, comprehension, spelling, and syntax. Dysarthria and mutism do not, by themselves, lead to a diagnosis of aphasia. The language network shows a left hemisphere dominance pattern in the vast majority of the population. In approximately 90 percent of right handers and 60 percent of left handers, aphasia occurs only after lesions of the left hemisphere. In some individuals no hemispheric dominance for language can be discerned, and in some others (including a small minority of right handers) there is a right hemisphere dominance for language. A language disturbance occurring after a right hemisphere lesion in a right hander is called *crossed aphasia*.

Clinical Examination   The clinical examination of language should include the assessment of naming, spontaneous speech, comprehension, repetition, reading, and writing. A deficit of naming (*anomia*) is the single most common finding in aphasic patients. When asked to name common objects (pencil or wristwatch) or their parts (eraser, lead, stem, band), the patient may fail to come up with the appropriate word, may provide a circumlocutious description of the object ("the thing for writing"), or may come up with the wrong word (*paraphasia*). If the patient offers an incorrect but legitimate word ("pen" for "pencil"), the naming error is known as a *semantic paraphasia*; if the word approximates the correct answer but is phonetically inaccurate ("plentil" for "pencil") it is known as a *phonemic paraphasia*. Asking the patient to name body parts, geometric shapes, and component parts of objects (lapel of coat, cap of pen) can elicit mild forms of anomia in patients who can otherwise name common objects. In most anomias, the patient cannot retrieve the appropriate name when shown an object but can point to the appropriate object when the name is provided by the examiner. This is known as a one-way naming deficit. A two-way

naming deficit exists if the patient can neither provide nor recognize the correct name, a condition always associated with impairments of language comprehension. *Spontaneous speech* is described as "fluent" if it maintains appropriate phrase length and melody or as "nonfluent" if it is halting, dysarthric, and average phrase length is below four words. The examiner should also note if the speech is paraphasic or circumlocutious; if it shows a relative paucity of substantive nouns and action verbs versus function words (prepositions, conjunctions); and if word order, tenses, suffixes, prefixes, plurals, and possessives are appropriate. *Comprehension* can be tested by assessing the patient's ability to follow conversation, by asking yes-no questions ("Can a dog fly?", "Does it snow in summer?") or asking the patient to point to appropriate objects ("Where is the source of illumination in this room?"). Statements with embedded clauses or passive voice construction ("If a tiger is eaten by a lion, which animal stays alive?") help to assess the ability to comprehend complex syntactic structure. Commands to close or open the eyes, stand up, sit down, or roll over should not be used to assess overall comprehension since appropriate responses aimed at such axial movements are subserved by neural systems outside of the language network and can be preserved in patients who otherwise have profound comprehension deficits.

Repetition is assessed by asking the patient to repeat single words, short sentences, or strings of words such as "No ifs, ands, or buts". The testing of repetition with tongue-twisters such as "hippopotamus" or "Irish constabulary" provides a better assessment of dysarthria than aphasia. Aphasic patients may have little difficulty with tongue-twisters but have a particularly hard time repeating a string of function words. It is important to make sure that the number of words does not exceed the patient's attention span. Otherwise, the failure of repetition becomes a reflection of the narrowed attention span rather than an indication of an aphasic deficit. *Reading* should be assessed for deficits in reading aloud as well as comprehension. *Writing* is assessed for spelling errors, word order, and grammar. *Alexia* describes an inability to either read aloud or comprehend single words and simple sentences; *agraphia* (or dysgraphia) is used to describe an acquired deficit in the spelling or grammar of written language.

Each sector of the language network participates in several language functions but also displays local specializations. For example, Wernicke's area occupies the lexical-semantic pole of the language network, whereas Broca's area occupies its syntactic pole. This organization allows the classification of aphasic patients into specific clinical syndromes and helps to determine the most likely anatomic distribution of the underlying neurologic disease. It also has implications for etiology and prognosis (Table 25-2). The syndromes outlined below are idealizations; pure syndromes occur rarely. The correspondence between individual deficits of language function and lesion location does not display a rigid one-to-one relationship and should be conceptualized within the context of the distributed network model. With these considerations in mind, the aphasic syndromes can be divided into "central" syndromes, which result from damage to the two centers of the language network (Broca's and Wernicke's areas), and "disconnection" syndromes, which arise from lesions that interrupt the connections of these centers with each other and with the other components of the language network.

Wernicke's aphasia   Comprehension is impaired for spoken and written language. Language output is fluent and maintains appropriate melody but is highly paraphasic and circumlocutious. The tendency for paraphasic errors may be so pronounced that it leads to strings of neologisms, which form the basis of what is known as "jargon aphasia." Speech contains large numbers of function words (e.g., prepositions, conjunctions) but few substantive nouns or verbs that refer to specific actions. The output is therefore voluminous but uninformative. For example, a 76-year-old man was brought to the emergency room because he started to talk "funny" while playing cards. In the following passage he is trying to describe how his wife accidentally threw away something important, perhaps his dentures: "We don't need it anymore, she says. And with it when that was downstairs was my teethtick . . . a . . . den . . . dentith . . . my dentist. And they happened to be in that bag . . . see? How could this have happened? How could a thing like this happen . . . So she says we won't need it anymore . . . I didn't think we'd use it. And now if I have any problems anybody coming a month from now, four months from now, or six months from now, I have a new dentist. Where my two . . . two little pieces of dentist that I use . . . that I . . . all gone. If she throws the whole thing away . . . visit some friends of hers and she can't throw them away."

Gestures and pantomime do not improve communication. The patient does not seem to realize that his or her language is incomprehensible and may appear angry and impatient when the examiner fails to decipher the meaning of a severely paraphasic statement. In some patients this type of aphasia can be associated with severe agitation and paranoid behaviors. One area of comprehension that may be preserved is the ability to follow commands aimed at axial musculature. The dissociation between the failure to understand simple questions ("What is your name") in a patient who rapidly closes his or her eyes, sits up, or rolls over when asked to do so is characteristic of Wernicke's aphasia and helps to differentiate it from deafness, psychiatric disease, or malingering. Patients with Wernicke's aphasia cannot express their thoughts in meaning-appropriate words and cannot decode the meaning of words in any modality of input. This aphasia therefore has expressive as well as receptive components and should not be designated as a "sensory aphasia" or "receptive aphasia," two terms often used as synonyms for Wernicke's aphasia. In addition to the paraphasic speech and poor comprehension of spoken language, patients with Wernicke's aphasia also have impaired repetition, naming, reading, and writing.

The lesion site most commonly associated with Wernicke's aphasia is the posterior portion of the language network and tends to involve at least parts of Wernicke's area. An embolus to the inferior division of the middle cerebral artery, and to the posterior temporal or angular branches in particular, is the most common etiology (Chap. 366). Intracerebral hemorrhage, venous infarction, severe head trauma, or neoplasm are other causes. A coexisting right hemi- or superior quadrantanopia is common in patients with Wernicke's aphasia, and mild right nasolabial flattening may be found, but otherwise the examination is often unrevealing. The paraphasic, neologistic speech in an agitated patient with an otherwise uneventful neurologic examination may lead to the suspicion of a primary psychiatric disorder such as schizophrenia or mania, but the other components characteristic of acquired aphasia and the absence of prior psychiatric disease usually settle the issue. The prognosis for recovery is guarded in most cases; some patients with Wernicke's aphasia due to intracerebral hemorrhage or head trauma may improve as the hemorrhage or the injury heals.

Broca's aphasia Speech is nonfluent, labored, dysarthric, and interrupted by many word-finding pauses. It is impoverished in function words but enriched in meaning-appropriate nouns and verbs. Abnormal word order and the inappropriate deployment of *bound morphemes* (word endings used to denote tenses, possessives, or plurals) lead to a characteristic agrammatism. Speech is telegraphic and pithy but quite informative. In the following passage, a 45-year-old man with Broca's aphasia describes his medical history: "I see . . . the dotor, dotor sent me . . . Bosson. Go to hospital. Dotor . . . kept me beside. Two, tee days, doctor send me home."

Output may be reduced to a grunt or single word ("yes" or "no") which is emitted with different intonations in an attempt to express approval or disapproval. In addition to fluency, naming and repetition are also impaired. Comprehension of spoken language is intact, except for syntactically difficult sentences with passive voice structure or embedded clauses. Reading comprehension is also preserved, with the occasional exception of a specific inability to read small grammatical words such as conjunctions and pronouns. The last two features indicate that Broca's aphasia is not just an "expressive" or "motor" disorder and that it may also involve a comprehension deficit for function words and syntax. Patients with Broca's aphasia can be tearful, easily frustrated, and profoundly depressed. Insight into their condition is preserved, in contrast to Wernicke's aphasia. Even when spontaneous speech is severely dysarthric, the patient may be able to display a relatively normal articulation of words when singing. This dissociation has been used to develop specific therapeutic approaches (melodic intonation therapy) for treating patients with Broca's aphasia. Additional neurologic deficits that are usually encountered in these patients include right facial weakness, hemiparesis or hemiplegia, and a buccofacial apraxia characterized by an inability to carry out motor commands involving oropharyngeal and facial musculature (for example, show me how you would blow out a match, suck through a straw). Visual fields are intact. The cause is most often infarction of Broca's area (the inferior frontal convolution; see Fig. 25-1) and surrounding anterior perisylvian and insular cortex, due to occlusion of the superior division of the middle cerebral artery (Chap. 366). Mass lesions including tumor (either primary or metastatic), intracerebral or subdural hemorrhage, or abscess can also present as Broca's aphasia. Small lesions confined to the posterior part of Broca's area may lead to a nonaphasic and often reversible deficit of speech articulation. In these cases, the remaining parts of the language network appear sufficient for sustaining essential language functions. Patients frequently have limited motor deficits at presentation, for example, isolated facial weakness. By contrast, patients with dense hemiparesis or hemiplegia have larger lesions and less favorable prospects for recovery. When the cause is stroke, recovery of language function generally peaks within several months, after which time no further progress is made.

Global aphasia Speech output is nonfluent, and comprehension of spoken language is severely impaired. Naming, repetition, reading, and writing are also impaired. This syndrome represents the combined involvement of Broca's and Wernicke's areas and usually results from strokes that involve the entire middle cerebral artery distribution in the left hemisphere. Most patients are initially mute or say a few words, such as "hi" or "yes." Related signs include right hemiplegia, hemisensory loss, and homonomous hemianopia. Occasionally, a patient with a lesion in Wernicke's area will present with a global aphasia that soon resolves into Wernicke's aphasia. In this circumstance, the impaired fluency (which gives the initial impression of global aphasia) arises from a mechanism analogous to spinal shock or dias-

Table 25-2

Clinical Features of Aphasias and Related Conditions

	Comprehension	Repetition of Spoken Language	Naming	Fluency
Wernicke's	Impaired	Impaired	Impaired	Preserved or increased
Broca's	Preserved (except grammar)	Impaired	Impaired	Decreased
Global	Impaired	Impaired	Impaired	Decreased
Conduction	Preserved	Impaired	Impaired	Preserved
Nonfluent (motor) transcortical	Preserved	Preserved	Impaired	Impaired
Fluent (sensory) transcortical	Impaired	Preserved	Impaired	Preserved
Isolation	Impaired	Echolalia	Impaired	No purposeful speech
Anomic	Preserved	Preserved	Impaired	Preserved except for word-finding pauses
Pure word deafness	Impaired only for spoken language	Impaired	Preserved	Preserved
Pure alexia	Impaired only for reading	Preserved	Preserved	Preserved

chisis, where acute dysfunction in a network component leads to a remote and reversible dysfunction in other network components.

CHAPTER 25
Aphasias and Other Focal Cerebral Disorders 137

Conduction aphasia Speech output is fluent but paraphasic; comprehension of spoken language is intact; repetition is severely impaired. Naming and writing are also impaired. Reading aloud is impaired, but reading comprehension is preserved. This type of aphasia represents a disconnection between the anterior and posterior poles of the language network. As a consequence of this disconnection, neural word representations formed in Wernicke's area and adjacent regions cannot be conveyed to Broca's area for assembly into corresponding articulatory patterns. The lesion sites spare Broca's and Wernicke's areas but involve projection paths that link the two or adjacent perisylvian regions such as the insula or supramarginal gyrus. Occasionally, a Wernicke's area lesion gives rise to a transient Wernicke's aphasia that rapidly resolves into a conduction aphasia. The paraphasic output in conduction aphasia interferes with the ability to express meaning, but this deficit is not nearly as severe as the one displayed by patients with Wernicke's aphasia. Associated neurologic signs in conduction aphasia vary according to the primary lesion site.

Nonfluent transcortical aphasia (transcortical motor aphasia) The clinical features are somewhat similar to those of Broca's aphasia, but repetition is intact and the agrammatism may be less pronounced. The rest of the neurologic examination may be intact, but a right hemiparesis can also exist. The lesion site is one that leaves the core of the language network intact but that disconnects it from prefrontal areas of the brain. Characteristic lesion sites include the anterior half of the vascular watershed zone between anterior and middle cerebral artery territories or the supplementary motor cortex in the territory of the anterior cerebral artery.

Fluent transcortical aphasia (transcortical sensory aphasia) Clinical features are similar to those of Wernicke's aphasia, but repetition is intact. The lesion site disconnects the intact core of the language network from other temporoparietal association areas. Associated neurologic findings may include hemianopia. Fluent transcortical aphasia can be associated with cerebrovascular lesions (e.g., infarctions in the posterior part of the watershed zone) or neoplasms that involve the temporoparietal cortex posterior to Wernicke's area.

Isolation aphasia This rare syndrome represents a combination of the two transcortical aphasias. Comprehension is severely impaired, and there is no purposeful speech output. The patient may parrot fragments of heard conversations (*echolalia*), indicating that the neural mechanisms for repetition are relatively spared. This condition represents the pathologic function of the language network when it is isolated from other regions of the brain. Lesions are patchy and can be associated with anoxia, carbon monoxide poisoning, or complete watershed zone infarctions. Broca's and Wernicke's areas tend to be spared, but there is damage in surrounding frontal, parietal, and temporal cortex.

Anomic aphasia This type of aphasia could be considered as the "minimal dysfunction" syndrome of the language network. Articulation, comprehension, and repetition are intact but confrontation naming, word finding, and spelling are impaired. Speech is enriched in function words but impoverished in substantive nouns and verbs denoting specific actions. Language output is fluent but paraphasic, circumlocutious, and uninformative. The lesion sites can be anywhere within the left hemisphere language network, including the middle and inferior temporal gyri. *Anomic aphasia is the single most common language disturbance seen in head trauma and metabolic encephalopathy.* This is also the most common aphasia seen in Alzheimer's disease. The language impairment of Alzheimer's disease almost always leads to fluent aphasias (e.g., anomic, Wernicke's, conduction, or fluent transcortical aphasia). The insidious onset and relentless progression of nonfluent language disturbances (Broca's or nonfluent transcortical aphasia) can be seen in patients with the syndrome of *primary progressive aphasia*, a degenerative disease that is most commonly associated with focal nonspecific neuronal loss or Pick's disease.

Pure word deafness This is not a true aphasic syndrome because the language deficit is modality-specific. The most common lesions are either bilateral or left-sided in the superior temporal gyrus. The net effect of the underlying lesion is to interrupt the flow of information from the unimodal auditory association cortex to Wernicke's area. Patients with this syndrome have no difficulty understanding written language and can express themselves very well in spoken or written language. These patients are not deaf in the traditional sense and have no difficulty interpreting and reacting to environmental sounds since primary auditory cortex and subcortical auditory relays are intact. Since auditory information cannot be conveyed to the language network, however, it cannot be decoded into neural word representations and the patient reacts to speech as if it were in an alien tongue that cannot be deciphered. Patients with this syndrome cannot repeat spoken language but have no difficulty naming objects. In time, patients with pure word deafness teach themselves lip reading and may appear to have improved upon superficial bedside examination. There may be no additional neurologic findings, but agitated paranoid reactions are frequent. Cerebrovascular lesions are the most frequent causes of this syndrome.

Pure alexia without agraphia This is the visual equivalent of pure word deafness. The lesions (usually a combination of damage to the left occipital cortex and to a posterior sector of the corpus callosum—the splenium) interrupt the flow of visual input into the language network. There is usually a right hemianopia, but the core language network remains unaffected. The patient can understand and produce spoken language, name objects in the left visual hemifield, repeat, and write. However, the patient acts as if he or she is completely illiterate when asked to read even the simplest sentence because the visual information from the written words (presented to the intact left visual hemifield) cannot reach the language network. According to Geschwind, objects in the left hemifield can be named accurately because they activate nonvisual associations in the right hemisphere, which, in turn, can access the language network through transcallosal pathways anterior to the splenium. Patients with this syndrome may also lose the ability to name colors, although they can match colors. This is known as a *color anomia*. The most common etiology of pure alexia is a cerebrovascular lesion in the distribution of the posterior cerebral artery or an infiltrating neoplasm in the left occipital cortex that involves the optic radiations as well as the crossing fibers of the splenium. Since the posterior cerebral artery also supplies medial temporal components of the limbic system, the patient with pure alexia may also experience an amnesia, but this is usually transient.

Aphemia There is an acute onset of severely impaired fluency (often mutism) that resolves, in time, into a hoarse whisper. Writing, reading, and comprehension are intact, so this is not a true aphasic syndrome. Partial lesions of Broca's area or subcortical lesions that undercut its connections with other parts of the brain may be present. Occasionally, the lesion site is on the medial aspects of the frontal lobes and may involve the supplementary motor cortex of the left hemisphere.

Apraxia Apraxia is a generic term that designates a complex motor deficit that cannot be attributed to pyramidal, extrapyramidal, cerebellar, or sensory dysfunction and that does not arise from the patient's failure to understand the nature of the task. The one form that is most frequently encountered in clinical practice is known as *ideomotor apraxia*. Commands to perform a specific motor act ("cough," "blow out a match") or to pantomime the use of a common tool (a comb, hammer, straw, or toothbrush) in the absence of the real object cannot be followed. The patient's ability to comprehend the command is ascertained by demonstrating multiple movements and establishing that the correct one can be recognized. Some patients with this type of apraxia can imitate the appropriate movement (when it is demonstrated by the examiner) and show no impairment when handed the real object, indicating that the sensorimotor mechanisms necessary for the movement are intact. Ideomotor apraxia represents a disconnection of the language network from pyramidal motor systems: commands to execute complex movements are understood but cannot be conveyed to the appropriate motor areas, even though the relevant motor mechanisms are intact. *Buccofacial apraxia* involves apraxic deficits in movements of the face and mouth. *Limb apraxia* encompasses apraxic deficits in movements of the arms and legs. Ideomotor apraxia is commonly associated with aphasic syndromes, especially Broca's aphasia and conduction aphasia. Its presence cannot be ascertained in patients with language comprehension deficits. As indicated above, the ability to follow commands aimed at axial musculature ("close the eyes," "stand up") is subserved by different pathways and may be intact in otherwise severely aphasic and apraxic patients. Patients with lesions of the anterior corpus callosum can display a special type of ideomotor apraxia confined to the left side of the body. Since the handling of real objects is not impaired, ideomotor apraxia, by itself, causes no limitation of daily living activities.

Two other types of apraxia are ideational apraxia and limb-kinetic apraxia. *Ideational apraxia* refers to a deficit in the execution of a goal-directed sequence of movements in patients who have no difficulty executing the individual components of the sequence. For example, when asked to pick up a pen and write, the sequence of uncapping the pen, placing the cap at the opposite end, turning the point towards the writing surface, and writing may be disrupted and the patient may be seen trying to write with the wrong end of the pen or even with the removed cap. These motor sequencing problems are usually seen in the context of confusional states and dementias rather than focal lesions associated with aphasic conditions. *Limb-kinetic apraxia* involves a clumsiness in the actual use of tools that cannot be attributed to sensory, pyramidal, extrapyramidal, or cerebellar dysfunction. This condition can emerge in the context of focal premotor cortex lesions or *corticobasal ganglionic degeneration*.

Gerstmann's syndrome The combination of *acalculia* (impairment of simple arithmetic), *dysgraphia* (impaired writing), *finger anomia* (an inability to name individual fingers such as the index or thumb), and *right-left confusion* (an inability to tell whether a hand, foot, or arm of the patient or examiner is on the right or left side of the body) is known as Gerstmann's syndrome. In making this diagnosis it is important to establish that the finger and left-right naming deficits are not part of a more generalized anomia and that the patient is not otherwise aphasic. When Gerstmann's syndrome is seen in isolation, it is commonly associated with damage to the inferior parietal lobule (especially the angular gyrus) in the left hemisphere.

Aprosodia Variations of melodic stress and intonation influence the meaning and impact of spoken language. For example, the two statements "He is clever." and "He is clever?" contain an identical word choice and syntax but convey vastly different messages because of differences in the intonation and stress with which the statements are uttered. This aspect of language is known as *prosody*. Damage to perisylvian areas in the right hemisphere can interfere with speech prosody and can lead to syndromes of aprosodia. Ross has pointed out that damage to right hemisphere regions corresponding to Wernicke's area yields a greater impairment in the decoding of speech prosody, whereas damage to right hemisphere regions corresponding to Broca's area yields a greater impairment in the ability to introduce meaning-appropriate prosody into spoken language. The latter deficit is the most common type of aprosodia identified in clinical practice—the patient produces grammatically correct language with accurate word choice but the statements are uttered in a monotone that interferes with the ability to convey the intended stress and affect. Patients with this type of aprosodia give the mistaken impression of being depressed or indifferent.

Subcortical aphasias The major aphasic syndromes in Table 25-2 are classified according to cortical lesion sites. However, damage to subcortical components of the language network (e.g., the head of the caudate and thalamus of the left hemisphere) can also lead to aphasia. The resulting syndromes contain combinations of deficits in the various aspects of language but rarely fit the specific patterns described in Table 25-2. An anomic aphasia accompanied by dysarthria

or a fluent aphasia with hemiparesis represents deviation from the major syndromes listed in Table 25-2 and should raise the suspicion of a subcortical lesion site.

THE PARIETOFRONTAL NETWORK FOR SPATIAL ORIENTATION: NEGLECT AND RELATED CONDITIONS

A number of clinical syndromes are recognizable with deficits in this network. They include hemispatial neglect, Balint's syndrome, simultanagnosia, dressing apraxia, and construction apraxia.

Hemispatial Neglect Adaptive orientation to significant events within the extrapersonal space is subserved by a large-scale network containing three major cortical components. The *cingulate cortex* provides access to a limbic-motivational mapping of the extrapersonal space, the *posterior parietal cortex* to a sensory-representational mapping, and the *frontal eye fields* in the frontal lobe to a motor-exploratory mapping. Subcortical components of this network include the striatum and the pulvinar nucleus of the thalamus. Contralesional hemispatial neglect represents one outcome of damage to any of the cortical or subcortical components of this network. *The traditional view that hemispatial neglect always denotes a parietal lobe lesion is inaccurate.* In keeping with this anatomic organization, the clinical manifestations of neglect display three behavioral components: sensory events (or their mental representations) within the neglected hemispace have a lesser impact on overall awareness; there is a paucity of exploratory and orienting acts directed toward the neglected hemispace; and the patient behaves as if the neglected hemispace was motivationally devalued.

The neural organization of spatial orientation displays a right hemisphere dominance pattern. The right hemisphere directs attention to the *entire* extrapersonal space, whereas the left hemisphere directs attention only to the contralateral right hemispace. Unilateral left hemisphere lesions do not give rise to contralesional neglect since the ipsiversive attentional mechanisms of the right hemisphere can compensate for the loss of the *contralaterally* directed attentional functions of the left hemisphere. Unilateral right hemisphere lesions, however, give rise to severe contralesional left hemispatial neglect because the unaffected left hemisphere does not contain ipsiversive attentional mechanisms. Contralesional neglect is consequently more common, severe, and lasting after damage to the right hemisphere than after damage to the left hemisphere. Severe neglect for the right hemispace is rare, even in left handers with left hemisphere lesions.

Patients with severe neglect may fail to dress, shave, or groom the left side of the body; may fail to eat food placed on the left side of the tray; and may fail to read the left half of sentences. When the examiner draws a large circle [12 to 16 cm (5 to 6 in.) in diameter] and asks the patient to place the numbers 1 to 12 as if the circle represented the face of a clock, there is a tendency to crowd the numbers on the right side and leave the left side empty. When asked to copy a simple line drawing, the patient fails to copy detail on the left; and when asked to write, there is a tendency to leave an unusually wide margin on the left.

Two bedside tests that are useful in assessing neglect are *simultaneous bilateral stimulation* and *visual target cancellation*. In the former, the examiner provides either unilateral or simultaneous bilateral stimulation in the visual, auditory, and tactile modalities. Following right hemisphere injury, patients who have no difficulty detecting unilateral stimuli on either side experience the bilaterally presented stimulus as coming only from the right. This phenomenon is known as *extinction* and is a manifestation of the sensory-representational aspect of hemispatial neglect. In the target detection task, targets (e.g., A's) are interspersed with foils (e.g., other letters of the alphabet) on a 21.5 × 28.0 cm (8.5 × 11 in.) sheet of paper and the patient is asked to circle all the targets. A failure to detect targets on the left is a manifestation of the exploratory deficit in hemispatial neglect. Hemianopia, by itself, does not interfere with performance in this task since the patient is free to turn the head and eyes to the left. The normal tendency in target detection tasks is to start from the left upper quadrant and move systematically in horizontal or vertical sweeps. Some patients show a tendency to start the process from the right and proceed in a haphazard fashion. This represents a subtle manifestation of left neglect, even if the patient eventually manages to detect all the appropriate targets. Some patients with neglect may also deny the existence of hemiparesis or hemihypesthesia and may even deny ownership of the paralyzed limb, a condition known as *anosognosia*.

The clinical manifestations of neglect are not identical in all patients. In general, lesions that are centered around the frontal component of the network for spatial orientation are likely to result in neglect syndromes with relatively more salient motor-exploratory deficits, whereas lesions centered around the parietal component are likely to result in neglect syndromes with more salient sensory-representational deficits. Cerebrovascular lesions and neoplasms in the right hemisphere are the most common causes of hemispatial neglect. Depending on the site of the lesion, the patient with neglect may also have hemiparesis, hemihypesthesia, and hemianopia on the left, but these are not invariant findings.

Balint's Syndrome, Simultanagnosia, Dressing Apraxia, and Construction Apraxia   Bilateral involvement of the network for spatial orientation, especially its parietal components, leads to a state of severe spatial disorientation known as *Balint's syndrome*. Balint's syndrome involves deficits in the orderly visuomotor scanning of the environment (*oculomotor apraxia*) and in accurate manual reaching toward visual targets (*optic ataxia*). The third and most dramatic component of Balint's syndrome is known as *simultanagnosia* and reflects an inability to integrate visual information in the center of gaze with more peripheral information. The patient gets stuck on the detail that falls in the center of gaze without attempting to scan the visual environment for additional information. The patient with simultanagnosia "misses the forest for the trees." Complex visual scenes cannot be grasped in their entirety, leading to severe limitations in the visual identification of objects and scenes. For example, a patient who is shown a table lamp and asked to name the object may look at its circular base and call it an ash tray. Some patients with simultanagnosia report that objects they look at may suddenly vanish, probably indicating an inability to look back at the original point of gaze after brief saccadic displacements. Movement and distracting stimuli greatly exacerbate the difficulties of visual perception. Simultanagnosia can sometimes occur without the other two components of Balint's syndrome.

A modification of the letter cancellation task described above can be used for the bedside diagnosis of simultanagnosia. In this modification, some of the targets (e.g., A's) are made to be much larger than the others [7.5 to 10 cm vs. 2.5 cm (3 to 4 in. vs. 1 in.) in height], and all targets are embedded among foils. Patients with simultanagnosia display a counterintuitive but characteristic tendency to miss the larger targets (Fig. 25-2). This occurs because the information needed for the identification of the larger targets cannot be confined to the immediate line of gaze and requires the integration of visual information across a more extensive field of view. The greater difficulty in the detection of the larger targets also indicates that poor acuity is not responsible for the impairment of visual function and that the problem is central rather than peripheral. Balint's syndrome results from bilateral dorsal parietal lesions; common settings include watershed infarction between the middle and posterior cerebral artery territories, hypoglycemia, sagittal sinus thrombosis, or degenerative diseases such as Alzheimer's disease. In patients with Balint's syndrome due to stroke, bilateral visual field defects (usually inferior quadrantanopsias) are common.

Another manifestation of bilateral (or right sided) dorsal parietal lobe lesions is *dressing apraxia*. The patient with this condition is unable to align the body axis with the axis of the garment and can be seen struggling as he or she holds a coat from its bottom or extends his or her arm into a fold of the garment rather than into its sleeve. Lesions that involve the posterior parietal cortex in the right hemisphere also lead to severe difficulties in copying simple line drawings. This is known as a *construction apraxia*. In some patients, the drawing difficulties are confined to the left side of the figure and represent a manifestation of hemispatial neglect; in others, there is a more universal deficit in reproducing contours and three-dimensional perspective. Dressing apraxia and construction apraxia represent special instances of a more general disturbance in spatial orientation.

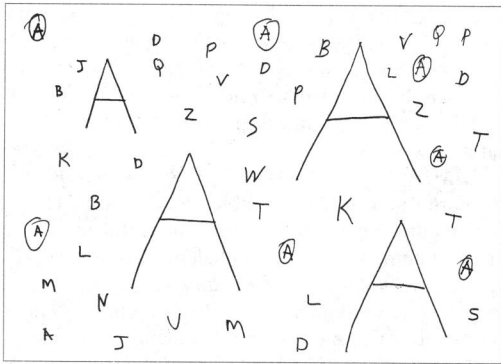

FIGURE 25-2   This 70-year-old woman with a 2-year history of degenerative dementia was asked to circle all the A's. She detects most of the small targets but ignores the larger ones. This is a manifestation of simultanagnosia.

THE OCCIPITOTEMPORAL NETWORK FOR OBJECT RECOGNITION: PROSOPAGNOSIA AND OBJECT AGNOSIA   Perceptual information about faces and objects is initially encoded in primary (striate) visual cortex and adjacent (upstream) peristriate visual association areas. This information is subsequently relayed first to the downstream visual association areas of occipitotemporal cortex and then to other heteromodal and paralimbic areas of the cerebral cortex. Bilateral lesions in the fusiform and lingual gyri of occipitotemporal cortex disrupt this process and interfere with the ability of otherwise-intact perceptual information to activate the distributed multimodal associations that lead to the recognition of faces and objects. The resultant face and object recognition deficits are known as *prosopagnosia* and *visual object agnosia*.

The patient with prosopagnosia cannot recognize familiar faces, including, sometimes, the reflection of his or her own face in the mirror. This is not a perceptual deficit since prosopagnosic patients can easily tell if two faces are identical or not. Furthermore, a prosopagnosic patient who cannot recognize a familiar face by visual inspection alone can use auditory cues to reach appropriate recognition if allowed to listen to the person's voice. The deficit in prosopagnosia is therefore modality-specific and reflects the existence of a lesion that prevents the activation of otherwise intact multimodal templates by relevant visual input. Damasio has pointed out that the deficit in prosopagnosia is not limited to the recognition of faces but that it can also extend to the recognition of individual members of larger generic object groups. For example, prosopagnosic patients characteristically have no difficulty with the generic identification of a face as a face or of a car as a car, but they cannot recognize the identity of an individual face or the make of an individual car. This reflects a visual recognition deficit for proprietary features that characterize individual members of an object class. When recognition problems become more generalized and extend to the generic identification of common objects, the condition is known as visual object agnosia. In contrast to prosopagnosic patients, those with object agnosia cannot recognize a face as a face or a car as a car. It is important to distinguish visual object agnosia from anomia. The patient with anomia cannot name the object but can describe its use. In contrast, the patient with visual agnosia is unable either to name a visually presented object or to describe its use. The characteristic lesions in prosopagnosia and visual object agnosia consist of bilateral infarctions in the territory of the posterior cerebral arteries and involve the lingual and fusiform gyri. Associated deficits can include visual field defects (especially superior quadrantanopias) or a centrally based color blindness known as achromatopsia. Rarely, the responsible lesion is unilateral. In such cases, prosopagnosia is associated with lesions in the right hemisphere and object agnosia with lesions in the left.

As noted above, patients with Balint's syndrome also experience severe visual recognition difficulties based on abnormalities in the integration of visual percepts. The resulting face and object recognition deficits of Balint's syndrome are known as *apperceptive visual agnosias*, whereas the prosopagnosia and visual object agnosias described in this section are known as *associative agnosias* because they result from the failure of an intact percept to evoke the relevant multimodal associations.

THE LIMBIC NETWORK FOR MEMORY: AMNESIAS The core limbic and paralimbic areas listed in Table 25-1, the anterior and medial nuclei of the thalamus, the medial and basal parts of the striatum, and the hypothalamus collectively constitute a distributed network known as the *limbic system*. The behavioral affiliations of this network include the coordination of emotion, motivation, autonomic tone, and endocrine function. An additional area of specialization for the limbic network, and the one which is of most relevance to clinical practice, is that of declarative (conscious) memory for events and experiences. Damage to components of the limbic network can give rise to severe and global disturbances of retentive memory. This type of memory disturbance is known as an amnestic state. In the absence of deficits in motivation, attention, language, or visuospatial function, the clinical diagnosis of a persistent global amnestic state implies a primary disturbance in the core process of retentive memory and is always associated with bilateral lesions within the limbic network.

The memory disturbance in the amnestic state is multimodal and includes retrograde and anterograde components. The *retrograde amnesia* involves an inability to recall experiences that occurred before the onset of the amnestic state. Relatively recent events are more vulnerable to retrograde amnesia than more remote events. This is known as Ribot's gradient and explains why patients with even very severe retrograde amnesia rarely forget events of early childhood. A patient who comes to the emergency room complaining that he cannot remember his identity but who can remember the events of that day is almost certainly not suffering from a neurologic cause of memory disturbance. The second and most important component of the amnestic state is the *anterograde amnesia*, which indicates an inability to store, retain, and recall new knowledge. Patients with amnestic states are perfectly alert and motivated but cannot remember what they ate a few minutes ago or the details of an important event they may have experienced a few hours ago. In the acute stages, there may also be a tendency to fill in memory gaps with inaccurate, fabricated, and often implausible information. This is known as *confabulation*. Patients with the amnestic syndrome forget that they forget and tend to deny the existence of a memory problem when questioned.

The patient with an amnestic state is almost always disoriented, especially to time. Accurate temporal orientation and accurate knowledge of current news rule out a major amnestic state. Memory can be tested with a list of four to five words read aloud by the examiner up to five times or until the patient can immediately repeat the entire list without intervening delay. In the next phase of testing, no distraction is provided and the patient is allowed to concentrate on the words and to rehearse them internally for 1 min before being asked to recall them. Accurate performance in this phase indicates that the patient is motivated and sufficiently attentive to hold the words in consciousness for at least 1 min. The final phase of the testing involves a retention period of 5 to 10 min during which the patient is engaged in other tasks. Adequate recall at the end of this interval requires encoding, retention, and retrieval. Amnestic patients fail this phase of the task and may even forget that they were given a list of words to remember. Accurate recognition of the words by multiple choice in a patient who cannot recall them indicates a less severe memory disturbance that affects mostly the retrieval stage of memory.

Many neurologic diseases can give rise to an amnestic state. These include tumors (of the sphenoid wing, posterior corpus callosum, thalamus, or medial temporal lobe), infarctions (in the territories of the anterior or posterior cerebral arteries), head trauma, herpes simplex encephalitis, Wernicke-Korsakoff encephalopathy, paraneoplastic lim-

bic encephalitis, and degenerative dementias such as Alzheimer's or Pick's disease. The one common denominator of all these diseases is that they lead to the bilateral involvement of one or more components in the limbic network. Occasionally, unilateral left sided lesions can give rise to an amnestic state, but the memory disorder tends to be transient. Depending on the nature and distribution of the underlying neurologic disease, the patient may also have visual field deficits, eye movement limitations, or cerebellar findings. In many patients there are no associated neurologic findings, and the differential diagnosis of psychiatric disease may occasionally be entertained. In this setting, the amnesia may remain undetected and lead to the inappropriate management of patients with head trauma or herpes simplex encephalitis.

Transient global amnesia is a distinctive syndrome usually seen in late middle age. Patients become acutely disoriented and repeatedly ask who they are, where they are, what they are doing. The spell is characterized by anterograde amnesia (inability to retain new information) and a retrograde amnesia for relatively recent events that occurred before the onset. The syndrome usually resolves within 24 to 48 h and is followed by the filling-in of the period affected by the retrograde amnesia, although there is persistent loss of memory for the events that occurred during the ictus. Recurrences are noted in approximately 20 percent of patients. Migraine, temporal lobe seizures, and transient ischemic events in the posterior cerebral territory (artery of Percheron; see Chap. 366) have been postulated as causes of transient global amnesia.

Although the limbic network is the site of damage for amnestic states, it is almost certainly not the storage site for memories. Memories are stored in widely distributed form throughout association cortex. The role attributed to the limbic network is to bind these distributed fragments into coherent events and experiences that can sustain conscious recall. Damage to the limbic network does not necessarily destroy memories but interferes with their conscious (declarative) recall in coherent form. The individual fragments of information remain preserved despite the limbic lesions and can sustain what is known as *implicit memory*. For example, patients with amnestic states can acquire new motor or perceptual skills, even though they may have no conscious knowledge of the experiences that led to the acquisition of these skills.

THE PREFRONTAL NETWORK FOR ATTENTION AND COMPORTMENT Approximately one-third of all the cerebral cortex in the human brain is located in the frontal lobes. The frontal lobes can be subdivided into motor-premotor, dorsolateral prefrontal, medial prefrontal, and orbitofrontal components. The terms *frontal lobe syndrome* and *prefrontal cortex* refer only to the last three of these four components. These are the parts of the cerebral cortex that show the greatest phylogenetic expansion in primates and especially in humans. The dorsolateral prefrontal, medial prefrontal, and orbitofrontal areas, and the subcortical structures with which they are interconnected (i.e., the head of the caudate and the dorsomedial nucleus of the thalamus), collectively make up a large-scale prefrontal network that coordinates exceedingly complex aspects of human cognition and comportment.

The orbitofrontal cortex provides a convergence site for neural inputs from association, paralimbic, and limbic cortices and constitutes a zone of intersection for the prefrontal and limbic networks. In keeping with this organization, the prefrontal network plays an important role in behaviors that require an integration of thought with emotion and motivation. There is no simple formula for summarizing the diverse functional affiliations of the prefrontal network. Its integrity appears important for the simultaneous (on-line) awareness of context, options, consequences, relevance, and perspectives so as to allow the formulation of adaptive inferences, decisions, and actions. Damage to this part of the brain impairs mental flexibility, foresight, judgment, and the ability to inhibit inappropriate responses. Behaviors impaired by prefrontal cortex lesions are often referred to as "executive functions."

Even very large bilateral prefrontal lesions may leave all sensory, motor, and basic cognitive functions intact while leading to isolated but dramatic alterations of personality and comportment. The associated impairments may emerge only in real-life situations when behavior is under minimal external control and may not be apparent within the structured environment of the medical office. The physician must therefore be prepared to make a diagnosis of frontal lobe disease on the basis of historical information alone even when the office examination of mental state may be quite intact. The most common clinical manifestations of damage to the prefrontal network take the form of two relatively distinct syndromes. In the *frontal abulic syndrome*, the patient shows a loss of initiative, creativity, and curiosity and displays a pervasive emotional blandness and apathy. In the *frontal disinhibition syndrome*, the patient becomes socially disinhibited and shows severe impairments of judgment, insight, and foresight. The dissociation between intact intellectual function and a total lack of even rudimentary common sense is striking. Despite the preservation of all essential memory functions, the patient cannot learn from experience and continues to display inappropriate behaviors without appearing to experience emotional pain, guilt, or regret when such behaviors repeatedly lead to disastrous consequences. Testing judgment by asking patients what they would do if they detected a fire in a theater or found a stamped and addressed envelope on the road is not very informative since patients who answer these questions wisely in the office may still do the wrong thing in the more complex real-life setting.

The abulic syndrome tends to be associated with damage to the dorsolateral prefrontal cortex, and the disinhibition syndrome with the medial prefrontal or orbitofrontal cortex. These syndromes tend to arise almost exclusively after bilateral lesions, most frequently in the setting of head trauma, stroke, ruptured aneurysms, hydrocephalus, or tumors (including metastases, glioblastoma, and falx or olfactory groove meningiomas). Unilateral lesions confined to the prefrontal cortex may remain silent until the pathology spreads to the other side. The emergence of developmentally primitive reflexes such as grasping, rooting, and sucking are also signs of frontal lobe disease. However, these reflexes are seen primarily in patients with large structural lesions that extend into the premotor components of the frontal lobes or in the context of metabolic encephalopathies. The vast majority of patients with prefrontal lesions and frontal lobe behavioral syndromes do not display these reflexes. Absent suck, root, and grasp reflexes therefore do not exclude a frontal lobe lesion.

Involvement of the prefrontal network impairs reasoning, abstract thinking, and hypothesis formation and leads to a stimulus-bound, concrete, and impulsive mode of mental functioning. Damage to this part of the brain also disrupts a variety of attention-related functions including concentration span, verbal fluency, the inhibition of immediate but inappropriate responses, and mental flexibility. Digit span (which should be seven forward and five reverse) is decreased; the recitation of the months of the year in reverse order (which should take less than 15 s) is slowed; and the number of words starting with a, f, or s that can be generated in 1 min (normally 12 or more per letter) is diminished even in nonaphasic patients. Characteristically, there is a progressive slowing of performance as the task proceeds; e.g., the patient asked to count backwards from 20 responds "20, 19, 18 . . . 17, ... 16," etc., and may not complete the task. In go–no go tasks (where the instruction is to raise the finger upon hearing one tap but to keep it still upon hearing two taps), the patient shows a characteristic inability to keep still in response to the "no go" stimulus; mental flexibility (tested by the ability to shift from one criterion to another in sorting or matching tasks) is impoverished; distractibility by irrelevant stimuli is increased; and there is a pronounced tendency for impersistence and perseveration. The effective scanning of internal information stores, the capacity for focusing on a trend of thought, and the ability to shift the focus of attention flexibly from one thought or stimulus to another are also impaired.

These attentional deficits contribute to the emergence of "working memory" impairments. The capacity for working memory refers to the amount of information that can be kept *on-line* at any given time. Working memory impairments interfere with the ability to maintain a coherent trend of thought and lead to confusion, especially in complex situations that require the simultaneous consideration of several variables. The attentional deficits disrupt the registration and retrieval of new information and lead to secondary memory deficits. These mem-

ory difficulties can be differentiated from those of the amnestic state by showing that they improve when the attentional load of the task is decreased. Working memory (also known as immediate memory) is an attentional function based on the temporary on-line holding of information. It is closely associated with the integrity of the prefrontal network and the ascending reticular activating system. Retentive memory, on the other hand, depends on the stable (off-line) storage of information and is associated with the integrity of the limbic network. The distinction of the underlying neural mechanisms is illustrated by the observation that severely amnestic patients who cannot remember events that occurred a few minutes ago may have intact if not superior working memory capacity as shown in tests of digit span. Working memory is closely related to the integrity of the dorsolateral prefrontal cortex, whereas other attentional functions such as the ability to inhibit inappropriate responses (as assessed by the go–no go task) depend primarily on the integrity of the medial prefrontal or orbitofrontal cortex.

The network approach postulates that the same cognitive domain can be impaired after damage to different parts of the brain as long as these parts belong to the same large-scale neural network. Accordingly, lesions in the caudate nucleus or in the dorsomedial nucleus of the thalamus (structures that can be considered as subcortical components of the prefrontal network) can also give rise to the clinical picture of a frontal lobe syndrome. This is one reason why the mental state changes associated with degenerative basal ganglia diseases, such as Parkinson's or Huntington's disease, may take the form of a frontal lobe syndrome. Because of its widespread connections with other regions of association cortex, one essential computational role of the prefrontal network is to function as an integrator or orchestrator for other networks. Bilateral multifocal lesions of the cerebral hemispheres, none of which are individually large enough to cause specific cognitive deficits such as aphasia or neglect, can collectively interfere with the connectivity and integrating function of prefrontal cortex. This is one reason why a frontal lobe syndrome is the single most common behavioral profile associated with a variety of bilateral multifocal brain diseases including metabolic encephalopathy, multiple sclerosis, Vitamin B_{12} deficiency, and others. In fact, the vast majority of patients with the clinical diagnosis of a frontal lobe syndrome tend to have lesions that do not involve prefrontal cortex but that involve either the subcortical components of the prefrontal network or its connections with other parts of the brain. In order to avoid the paradox of making a diagnosis of "frontal lobe syndrome" in a patient with no evidence of frontal cortex disease, it is advisable to use the diagnostic term *prefrontal network syndrome*, with the understanding that the responsible lesions can lie anywhere within this distributed network.

The patient with frontal lobe disease raises potential dilemmas in differential diagnosis: the abulia and blandness may be misinterpreted as depression, and the disinhibition as mania or acting-out. Appropriate intervention may be delayed while a treatable tumor keeps expanding. An informed approach to frontal lobe disease and its comportmental manifestations may help to avoid such errors.

CARING FOR THE PATIENT WITH DEFICITS OF HIGHER CORTICAL FUNCTION Some of the deficits described in this chapter are so complex that they may bewilder not only the patient and family but also the physician. It is imperative to carry out a systematic clinical evaluation in order to characterize the nature of the deficits and explain them in lay terms to the patient and family. Such an explanation can allay at least some of the anxieties, address the mistaken impression that the deficit (e.g., social disinhibition or inability to recognize family members) is psychologically motivated, and lead to practical suggestions for daily living activities. Patients with simultanagnosia, for example, should be given the counterintuitive instruction to stand back when they cannot find an item so that a greater search area falls within the immediate field of gaze. Physicians tend to place a great emphasis on signs that are elicited during the clinical examination. In some patients, however, the history may be more important and may conflict with the bedside examination. For example, patients with frontal lobe disease can be extremely irritable and abusive to spouses and yet display all the appropriate social graces during the visit to the medical office.

Reactive depression is common in patients with higher cortical dysfunction and should be treated. These patients may be sensitive to the usual doses of antidepressants or anxiolytics and deserve a careful titration of dosage. Brain damage may cause a dissociation between feeling states and their expression so that a patient who may superficially appear jocular could still be suffering from an underlying depression that deserves to be treated. In many cases, agitation may be controlled with reassurance. In other cases, treatment with benzodiazepines or sedating antidepressants may become necessary. The use of neuroleptics for the control of agitation should be reserved only for refractory cases since extrapyramidal side effects are frequent in patients with coexisting brain damage.

The assessment of higher cortical function can be as systematic as the rest of the neurologic examination but requires time and familiarity with specialized tests. The consultation of a skilled neuropsychologist may aid in the formulation of diagnosis and management. The availability of computed tomography, magnetic resonance imaging, positron emission tomography, and single-photon emission computed tomography does not obviate the need for careful clinical assessment since the complex results and implications of these diagnostic procedures can be interpreted fully only in the light of a thorough clinical evaluation.

Spontaneous improvement of cognitive deficits due to acute neurologic lesions is common. It is most rapid in the first few weeks but may continue for up to 2 years, especially in young individuals with single brain lesions. The mechanisms for this recovery are incompletely understood. Some of the initial deficits appear to arise from remote dysfunction (diaschisis) in parts of the brain that are interconnected with the site of initial injury. Improvement in these patients may reflect, at least in part, a normalization of the remote dysfunction. Other mechanisms may involve functional reorganization in surviving neurons adjacent to the injury or the compensatory use of homologous structures, for example, the right superior temporal gyrus with recovery from Wernicke's aphasia. Cognitive rehabilitation procedures have been used in the treatment of higher cortical deficits. There are few controlled studies, but some do show a benefit of rehabilitation in the recovery from hemispatial neglect and aphasia. In some of these patients, the recovery of cognitive deficits reflects the development of compensatory strategies. In other patients, recovery may involve a reorganization of the relevant neural networks. Some types of deficits may be more prone to recovery than others. For example, patients with nonfluent aphasias are more likely to benefit from speech therapy than patients with fluent aphasias and comprehension deficits. In general, lesions that lead to a denial of illness (e.g., anosognosia) are associated with cognitive deficits that are more resistant to rehabilitation. The recovery of higher cortical dysfunction is rarely complete. Periodic neuropsychological assessment is necessary for quantifying the pace of the improvement and for generating specific recommendations for cognitive rehabilitation, modifications in the home environment, and the time-table for returning to school or work.

BIBLIOGRAPHY

BENSON F: Aphasia and related disorders: A clinical approach, in *Principles of Behavioral Neurology*, M-M Mesulam (ed). Philadelphia, Davis, 1985, pp 193–238

DAFFNER KR et al: Dissociated neglect behavior following sequential strokes in the right hemisphere. Ann Neurol 28:97, 1990

DAMASIO AR: Disorders of complex visual processing: Agnosias, achromatopsia, Balint's syndrome, and related difficulties of orientation and construction, in *Principles of Behavioral Neurology*, M-M Mesulam (ed). Philadelphia, Davis, 1985, pp 259–288.

———: Aphasia. N Engl J Med 326:531, 1992

DEUEL RK, COLLINS RC: Recovery from unilateral neglect. Exp Neurol 81:733, 1983

GESCHWIND N: Disconnection syndromes in animals and man. Brain 88:237, 1965

GITELMAN DR et al: Functional imaging of human right hemispheric activation for exploratory movements. Ann Neurol 39:174, 1996

GRENSHAM GE et al: *Post-Stroke Rehabilitation*. In: U. S. Department of Health and Human Services Agency for Health Care Policy and Research, Publication No. 95-0662. Rockville, Maryland 1995

HEILMAN KM et al: Neglect and related disorders, in *Clinical Neuropsychology*, KM Heilman, E Valenstein (eds). New York, Oxford University Press, 1985, pp 279–336

MESULAM M-M: Patterns in behavioral neuroanatomy: Association areas, the limbic system, and hemispheric specialization, in *Principles of Behavioral Neurology*, M-M Mesulam (ed). Philadelphia, Davis, 1985, pp 1–70

———: Frontal cortex and behavior. Ann Neurol 19:320, 1986

———: Primary progressive aphasia—differentiation from Alzheimer's disease [editorial]. Ann Neurol 22:533, 1987

———: Large-scale neurocognitive networks and distributed processing for attention, language, and memory. Ann Neurol 28:597, 1990

———: Higher visual functions of the cerebral cortex and their disruption in clinical practice, in *Principles and Practice of Ophthalmology*, DM Albert, FA Jakobiec (eds). Philadelphia, Saunders, 1994, pp 2640–2653

MOHR JR et al: Broca's aphasia: Pathologic and clinical. Neurology 28:311, 1978

NAESER MA, HELM-ESTABROOKS N: CT scan lesion localization and response to melodic intonation therapy with nonfluent aphasia cases. Cortex 21:203, 1985

PRICE BH et al: Neuropsychological patterns and language deficits in 20 consecutive cases of autopsy-confirmed Alzheimer's disease. Arch Neurol 50:931, 1993

ROSS ED: Nonverbal aspects of language. Neurol Clin 11:9, 1993

SEECK M et al: Selectively distributed processing of visual object recognition in the temporal and frontal lobes of the human brain. Ann Neurol 37:538, 1995

SIGNORET J-L: Memory and amnesias, in *Principles of Behavioral Neurology*, M-M Mesulam (ed). Philadelphia, Davis, 1985, pp 169–192

TURNER RS et al: Clinical, neuroimaging, and pathologic features of progressive nonfluent aphasia. Ann Neurol 39:166, 1996

WEILLER C et al: Recovery from Wernicke's aphasia: A positron emission tomographic study. *Ann Neurol* 37:723, 1995

WEINTRAUB S, MESULAM M-M: The examination of mental state, in *Principles of Behavioral Neurology*, M-M Mesulam (ed). Philadelphia, Davis, 1985, pp 71–123

26   *Thomas D. Bird*

MEMORY LOSS AND DEMENTIA

DEFINITION Dementia is a serious and common problem that affects more than 4 million Americans and costs society more than $50 billion annually. Ten percent of persons over age 70 and 20 to 40 percent of individuals over age 85 have clinically identifiable memory loss. Dementia is a syndrome with many causes. A simple definition of dementia is a deterioration in cognitive abilities that impairs the previously successful performance of activities of daily living. Memory is the most common and most important cognitive ability that is lost. Other mental faculties may also be affected such as attention, judgment, comprehension, orientation, learning, calculation, problem solving, mood, and behavior. Agitation or withdrawal, hallucinations, delusions, insomnia, and loss of inhibitions are also common. Individuals with mental retardation and psychosis may become demented if a decline in intellectual function occurs. Many common forms of dementia are progressive, but some dementing illnesses are static and unchanging. Dementia is a chronic condition, whereas delirium is an acute confusional state associated with a change in level of consciousness (ranging from lethargy to agitation).

Memory is a complex function of the brain that has fascinated philosophers and scientists for centuries. Memory is currently viewed as a mental process using several storage buffers of differing capacity and duration (Table 26-1). Sensory memory lasts for about 250 ms in the visual mode (iconic memory) and 1 to 2 s in the auditory mode (echoic memory). Immediate (short-term or primary) memory has a duration of about half a minute and a limited capacity of approximately 5 to 10 items. Immediate memory is highly vulnerable to distraction, requiring attention and vigilance to maintain the content. It is often tested at the bedside by asking the patient to recall several digits forward and backward. Recent, or secondary, memory has been called both "short-term" and "long-term." It has a duration of minutes to weeks and exhibits a larger storage capacity than immediate memory. On entering this buffer, information undergoes a process of consolidation of variable duration. Recent memory is commonly tested in the clinical setting by asking a patient to recall three words after 3 to 5 min. Remote, or long-term, memory stores information lasting weeks to a lifetime and contains most of our personal experiences and knowledge. Some information appears to be stored accurately for an indefinite time, whereas other items fade or become distorted. Memory function includes registration (encoding or acquisition), retention (storage or consolidation), stabilization, and retrieval (decoding or recall). Registration and retrieval are conscious processes. Animal experiments have shown that long-term memory requires new protein synthesis, and the stabilization process probably involves physical changes at neuronal synapses.

Several additional classifications of memory are sometimes used by psychologists, particularly in reference to the content or use of the memory stores. Reference memory refers to a filing system that contains recent and remote information gained from previous experience. Working memory refers to an active process that is being updated continually by current experience. Episodic memory contains information about events occurring in a specific place and time. Semantic memory contains unchanging facts, principles, associations, and rules (for example, state capitals and the number of days in a week). Declarative (explicit) memory refers to facts about the world and past personal events that must be consciously retrieved to be remembered. Procedural (implicit) memory, in contrast, is involved in learning and retaining a skill or procedure such as how to ride a bicycle, get dressed, or drive a car. Abilities stored in procedural memory become automatic and do not require conscious implementation.

Finally, the term *executive function* refers to mental activity involved in planning, initiating, and regulating behavior. It is considered the central organizing function of the brain that results in systematic, goal-directed activity. Executive functions are active in nonroutine situations where reflex or automatic behavior is not adequate. The anatomic and physiologic substrates of executive function are presumed to involve the frontal lobes (see Chap. 25). Deficits in executive function occur frequently in patients with dementia.

FUNCTIONAL ANATOMY AND PATHOGENESIS Dementia results from disorders of cerebral neuronal circuits and is a result of the total quantity of neuronal loss combined with the specific location of such loss (Chap. 25). The anatomic basis of memory was initially clarified from study of the alcohol/thiamine deficiency syndrome of Korsakoff and the consequences of temporal lobe surgery performed for the treatment of epilepsy. In Korsakoff's syndrome lesions in the hypothalamus, mammillary bodies, and dorsomedial nuclei of the thalamus showed that these areas were important for learning, recall, and recognition. Unilateral temporal lobe surgery for epilepsy produced mild to moderate amnesia for either verbal or nonverbal material. Bilateral medial temporal lobe excision involving the hippocampal formation, the parahippocampal gyrus, and part of the amygdala produced a severe anterograde learning disorder, i.e., an inability to store new memories, often with retained ability to recall old ones. The components of the medial temporal lobe memory system include the hippocampus and adjacent cortex, including the entorhinal, perirhinal, and parahippocampal regions (Fig. 26-1). This includes a circular pathway of neurons from entorhinal cortex to dentate gyrus, CA3 and CA1 neurons of hippocampus to subiculum, and back to entorhinal cortex; this pathway is heavily damaged in Alzheimer's disease (AD). This system is fast, has limited capacity, and performs a crucial function at the time of learning and establishing declarative memory. Its role continues after learning during a lengthy period of reorganization and consolidation whereby memory stored in neocortex eventually becomes independent of the medial temporal lobe memory system. This process, by which the burden of long-term (permanent) memory storage is gradually assumed by neocortex, assures that the medial temporal lobe system is always available for the acquisition of new information. Recent functional brain imaging studies indicate that learning and memory involve many of the same regions of the cortex that process sensory information and control motor output. The forms of perceptual and motor learning that can occur without conscious recollections are mediated in part by contractions and expansions of representations in the sensory and motor cortex. One study, for example, has shown that the cortical representation of the fingers of the left hand of musical string players is larger than that in controls, suggesting that the representation of different parts of the body in the primary somatosensory cortex of humans depends on use and changes to conform to the current needs and experiences of the individual. Discrete cortical regions exist in which object knowledge (such as words related to color, animals, tools, or action) is organized as a distributed system in which the attributes of an object are stored close to the regions of the cortex that mediate perception of those attributes (Chap. 25). That is, brain regions active during object identification are partly dependent on the intrinsic properties of the object. Procedural (implicit) memory appears to involve centers outside the hippocampus such as amygdala, cerebellum, and sensory cortex.

Biochemically, the cholinergic system plays an important role in memory. Anticholinergic agents such as atropine and scopolamine interfere with memory. Choline acetyl transferase (the enzyme catalyzing the formation of acetylcholine) and nicotinic cholinergic receptors

Table 26-1

Classification of Memory

Type	Time Interval	Test/Example	Probable Cerebral Location
Sensory			
Iconic (visual)	<1 s	After image	Visual cortex
Echoic (auditory)	1–2 s	Cough/dog bark	Auditory cortex
Immediate (primary/working)	30 s	Digit span	Perisylvian cortex, frontal lobe
Recent (secondary/reference)	Minutes–weeks/months	Recall 3 words after 3–5 min	Hippocampus, mamillothalamic tract, dorsomedial thalamus
Declarative (explicit)			
Episodic		Recall trip last week	
Semantic		Recall names of months	
Procedural (implicit)		Ride a bike	Amygdala, cerebellum, association cortex,
		Get dressed	frontal lobe, ? other
Remote (reference)	Months–years	Recall high school graduation	Association cortex, ? other

SOURCE: Modified from Erickson.

are known to be deficient in the cortex of patients with AD. The brains of AD patients show severe neuronal loss in the nucleus basalis of Meynert, a major source of cholinergic input to the cerebral cortex. These findings form the basis for the use of tacrine (a cholinesterase inhibitor) in the treatment of AD, its modest benefit presumably arising from increased available levels of acetylcholine. Behavior and mood are modulated by noradrenergic, serotonergic, and dopaminergic pathways, and norepinephrine has been shown to be reduced in the brainstem locus coeruleus in AD. Neurotrophins are also postulated to play a role in memory in part by preserving cholinergic neurons.

Long-term potentiation (LTP), which refers to a long-lasting enhancement of synaptic transmission resulting from repetitive stimulation of excitatory synapses, is presumed to be involved in memory acquisition and storage. LTP occurs in hippocampus and is mediated by N-methyl-D-aspartate (NMDA) receptors. Gene knockout mouse models have been useful in the definition of secondary messenger systems that play a role in hippocampal LTP. For example, disruption of either calcium/calmodulin-dependent protein kinase or cytoplasmic tyrosine kinase (fyn) results in deficient hippocampal LTP and impaired spatial learning. On the other hand, mice in which a neuronal glycoprotein thy-1 has been inactivated show regionally selective impairment of LTP but intact spatial learning, suggesting that LTP in the entorhinal projection to the dentate gyrus of the hippocampus (Fig. 26-1) may not be necessary for some forms of spatial learning.

Most diseases causing dementia do not have highly restricted regions of pathology. Disorders such as AD appear to represent relatively diffuse neuronal deterioration throughout the cerebral cortex, whereas multi-infarct dementia associated with recurrent strokes causes more focal damage in a random patchwork of cortical regions. Diffuse white matter damage may disrupt intracerebral connections and cause dementia syndromes such as those associated with leukodystrophies, multiple sclerosis, and Binswanger's disease. Subcortical

structures such as the caudate, putamen, thalamus, and substantia nigra also modulate cognition and behavior in ways that are not yet well understood. Some investigators distinguish between cortical and subcortical types of dementia. Cortical dementia such as AD and Pick's disease primarily present as memory loss and are often associated with aphasia or other disturbance of language. Patients with subcortical dementia such as Huntington's disease (HD) are less likely to have memory and language problems and more likely to have difficulties with attention, judgment, and behavior. Both the clinical and anatomic characteristics of the cortical and subcortical dementias show considerable overlap, and the conditions are often not distinct.

Lesions of some relatively specific cortical-subcortical pathways may have significant effects on behavior (Chap. 25). The dorsolateral prefrontal cortex has connections with dorsolateral caudate, globus pallidus, and thalamus. Lesions of these pathways result in poor organization and planning, perseveration, and decreased cognitive flexibility with impaired judgment. The lateral orbital frontal cortex connects with the ventromedial caudate, globus pallidus, and thalamus. Lesions of these connections cause irritability, impulsiveness, and distractibility. The anterior cingulate cortex connects with the nucleus accumbens, globus pallidus, and thalamus. Interruption of these connections produces apathy and poverty of speech or even akinetic mutism.

The single strongest risk factor for dementia is increasing age. The prevalence of disabling memory loss increases with each decade over age 50 and is associated most often with the microscopic changes of AD at autopsy. Slow accumulation of mutations in neuronal mitochondria is hypothesized to contribute to the increasing prevalence of dementia with age. Yet many centenarians have intact memory function and no evidence of clinically significant dementia. Whether dementia is an inevitable consequence of normal human aging remains controversial.

DIFFERENTIAL DIAGNOSIS The many causes of dementia are listed in Table 26-2. The frequency of each condition depends on the age group under study, the country of origin, and perhaps racial or ethnic variations. AD is the most common cause of dementia in

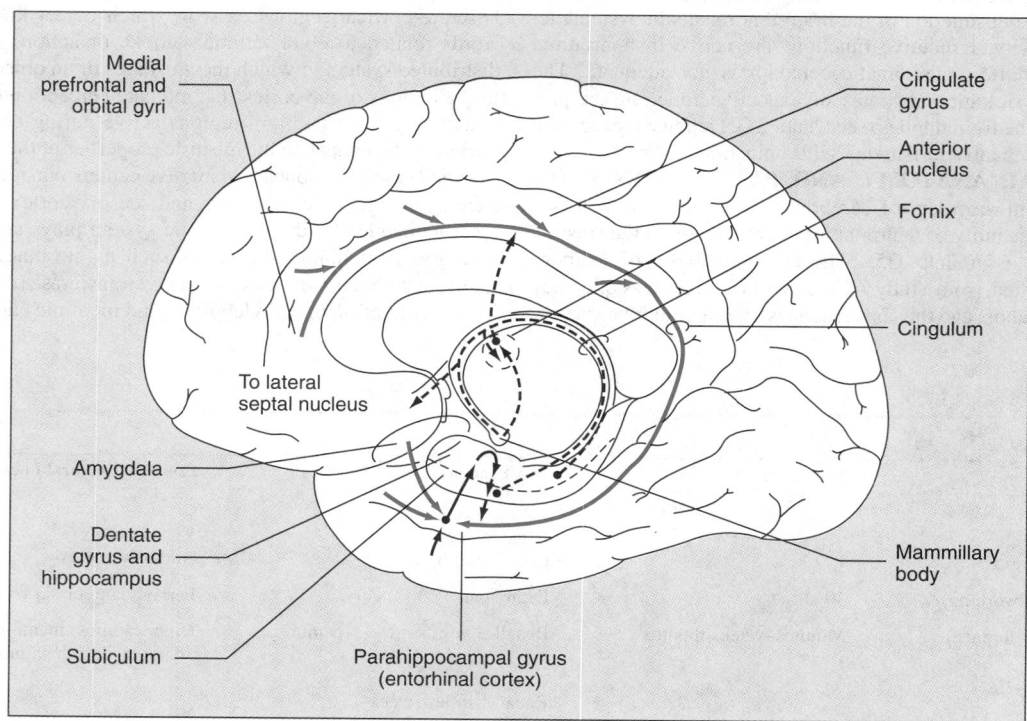

FIGURE 26-1 The principal connections of the hippocampus. Afferent connections (*blue arrows*) from the cingulate gyrus (cortical association fibers) and amygdala converge on the entorhinal cortex (part of the parahippocampal gyrus) and connect with the hippocampus via a polysynaptic circuit (*black arrows*) from dentate to CA3, CA1, and subiculum neurons with output back to the entorhinal cortex. Efferent connections (*broken arrows*) are principally via the fornix to the anterior nucleus of the thalamus, septal nuclei, and mamillary body.

Vascular disease is the second most common cause of dementia in the United States, representing 20 to 25 percent, but is more common than AD in some Asian countries. Dementia associated with chronic alcoholism and Parkinson's disease (PD) represent the next two most common categories. Chronic intoxications including those resulting from prescription drugs are an important, potentially treatable cause of dementia. Other disorders listed in the table are uncommon but important because many are reversible. The classification of dementing illnesses into two broad groups of treatable and untreatable disorders is a useful approach to the differential diagnosis of dementia.

Subtle cumulative memory loss is a natural part of aging. This frustrating experience, often the source of jokes and humor, is referred to as *benign forgetfulness of the elderly*. Benign means that it is not so progressive or serious that it impairs reasonably successful and productive daily functioning, although the distinction between benign and more significant memory loss can be difficult to make. A proportion of persons with benign memory loss progress to frank dementia, usually caused by AD. It remains unclear why some individuals show progression and others do not. It was once assumed that a cumulative loss of hippocampal neurons with normal aging might underlie this forgetfulness, but recent quantitative neuronal counts indicate that this "natural" neuronal loss may not occur.

Alzheimer's disease is a slowly progressive dementing illness associated with diffuse cortical atrophy and specific neuropathologic hallmarks of amyloid plaques and neurofibrillary tangles. Although quite common in the elderly, it remains a diagnosis of exclusion to be confirmed definitively only at autopsy. The clinical diagnosis of AD established by experienced neurologists proves to be correct at autopsy approximately 85 to 90 percent of the time. → *This condition is described in greater detail in Chap. 367.*

Two major types of vascular dementia can be identified (Chap. 367). The first, often called multi-infarct dementia, results from an accumulation of discrete cerebral strokes that produce disabling deficits of memory, behavior, and other cognitive abilities. Such patients usually give a history of sudden, separate stroke episodes with stepwise deterioration. On examination, focal neurologic deficits such as hemiparesis, unilateral Babinski reflex, aphasia, or visual field defect are common. Brain imaging shows multiple areas of stroke, which may have been ischemic or hemorrhagic. A second, more subtle and insidious type of vascular dementia, Binswanger's disease, is a dementing illness associated with diffuse, subcortical white matter damage often occurring in patients with chronic hypertension and/or severe atherosclerosis. The white matter changes are dramatically visualized by magnetic resonance imaging (MRI). The pathogenesis of Binswanger's disease is unknown. Because AD and vascular dementia are common, occasional patients may have both conditions.

Dementia commonly accompanies *chronic alcoholism* (Chap. 380). This may be a result of associated malnutrition, especially of B vitamins and particularly thiamine. However, other as yet poorly defined aspects of chronic alcohol ingestion may also produce cerebral damage and atrophy. A rare idiopathic syndrome of dementia and seizures with degeneration of the corpus callosum has been reported primarily in male Italian drinkers of red wine (MarchiafavaBignami disease).

Thiamine (vitamin B_1) deficiency causes Wernicke's encephalopathy (Chap. 380). The clinical presentation is a malnourished individual (frequently but not necessarily alcoholic) with confusion, ataxia, and diplopia from ophthalmoplegia (Charcot's triad). Thiamine deficiency damages the thalamus, mammillary bodies, midline cerebellum, periaquaductal gray matter of the midbrain, and peripheral nerves. Damage to medial thalamic regions correlates most closely with memory loss. Prompt administration of parenteral thiamine (100 mg intravenously for 3 days followed by daily oral dosage) may reverse the disease if given in the first few days of symptom onset. However, prolonged untreated thiamine deficiency can result in an irreversible dementia/amnestic syndrome (Korsakoff's psychosis) or even death.

In *Korsakoff's syndrome*, the patient is unable to recall new information despite normal immediate memory, attention span, and level of consciousness. Memory for new events is seriously impaired, whereas memory of knowledge prior to the illness is relatively intact. Patients are easily confused, disoriented, and incapable of recalling new infor-

Table 26-2

Differential Diagnosis of Dementia

MOST COMMON CAUSES OF DEMENTIA

Alzheimer's disease	Alcoholism*
Vascular dementia	Parkinson's disease
Multi-infarct	Drug/medication intoxication*
Diffuse white matter disease (Binswanger's)	

LESS COMMON CAUSES OF DEMENTIA

Vitamin deficiencies	Toxic disorders
Thiamine (B_1): Wernicke's encephalopathy*	Drug, medication, and narcotic poisoning*
B_{12} (Pernicious anemia)*	Heavy metal intoxication*
Nicotinic acid (pellagra)*	Dialysis dementia (aluminum)
Endocrine and other organ failure	Organic toxins
Hypothyroidism*	Psychiatric
Adrenal insufficiency and Cushing's syndrome*	Depression (pseudodementia)*
Hypo- and hyperparathyroidism*	Schizophrenia*
Renal failure*	Conversion reaction*
Liver failure*	Degenerative disorders
Pulmonary failure*	Huntington's disease
Chronic infections	Pick's disease
HIV	Diffuse Lewy body disease
Neurosyphilis*	Progressive supranuclear palsy (Steel-Richardson syndrome)
Papovavirus (progressive multifocal leukoencephalopathy)	Multisystem degeneration (Shy-Drager syndrome)
Prion (Creutzfeldt-Jakob and Gerstmann-Sträussler-Scheinker diseases)	Hereditary ataxias (some forms)
Tuberculosis, fungal, and protozoal*	Motor neuron disease [amyotrophic lateral sclerosis (ALS); some forms]
Sarcoidosis*	Frontal lobe dementia
Whipple's disease*	Cortical basal degeneration
Head trauma and diffuse brain damage	Multiple sclerosis
Dementia pugilistica	Adult Down's syndrome with Alzheimer's
Chronic subdural hematoma*	ALS–Parkinson's–Dementia complex of Guam
Postanoxia	Miscellaneous
Postencephalitis	Vasculitis*
Normal-pressure hydrocephalus*	Acute intermittent porphyria*
Neoplastic	Recurrent nonconvulsive seizures*
Primary brain tumor*	Additional conditions in children or adolescents
Metastatic brain tumor*	Hallervorden-Spatz disease
Paraneoplastic limbic encephalitis	Subacute sclerosing panencephalitis
	Metabolic disorders (e.g., Wilson's and Leigh's diseases, leukodystrophies, lipid storage diseases, mitochondrial mutations)

* Potentially treatable dementia.

mation for more than a brief interval. Superficially, they may be conversant, entertaining, able to perform simple tasks, and follow immediate commands. Confabulation is common, although not always present, and may result in obviously erroneous statements and elaborations. There is no specific treatment because the previous thiamine deficiency has produced irreversible damage to the medial thalamic nuclei and mammillary bodies. Mammillary body atrophy may be visible on high-resolution MRI.

Vitamin B$_{12}$ deficiency, as can occur in pernicious anemia, causes a macrocytic anemia and may also damage the nervous system (Chaps. 373 and 380). Neurologically it most commonly produces a spinal cord syndrome (myelopathy) affecting the posterior columns (loss of position and vibratory sense) and the lateral corticospinal tracts (hyperactive tendon reflexes and Babinski responses); it also damages peripheral nerves, resulting in sensory loss with depressed tendon reflexes. Damage to cerebral myelinated fibers may also cause dementia. The mechanism of neurologic damage is unclear but may be related to a deficiency of *S*-adenosylmethionine (required for methylation of myelin phospholipids) due to reduced methionine synthase activity or accumulation of methylmalonate and propionate, providing abnormal substrates for fatty acid synthesis in myelin. The neurologic signs of vitamin B$_{12}$ deficiency are usually associated with macrocytic anemia, but on occasion may occur in its absence. Treatment with parenteral vitamin B$_{12}$ (1000 μg intramuscularly daily for a week, weekly for a month, and monthly for life for pernicious anemia) stops progression of the disease if instituted promptly, but reversal of advanced nervous system damage will not occur.

Deficiency of nicotinic acid (pellagra) is associated with sun-exposed skin rash, glossitis, and angular stomatitis (Chaps. 79 and 380). Severe dietary deficiency of nicotinic acid along with other B vitamins such as pyridoxine may result in spastic paraparesis, peripheral neuropathy, fatigue, irritability, and dementia. This syndrome has been seen in prisoner-of-war and concentration camps. Low serum folate levels appear to be a rough index of malnutrition, but isolated folate deficiency has not been proven to be a specific cause of dementia.

Approximately 20 percent of patients with PD (Chap. 368) eventually develop dementia. Treatment with L-dopa neither accelerates nor prevents this process. Some PD patients with dementia have cytoplasmic neuronal inclusions (Lewy bodies) or AD changes in cerebral cortex, but others have no specific identifiable cortical pathology.

Infections of the central nervous system (CNS) usually cause delirium and other acute neurologic syndromes. However, some chronic CNS infections such as tuberculosis or cryptococcosis may produce a dementing illness (Chap. 378). Between 20 and 30 percent of patients in the advanced stages of infection with human immunodeficiency virus (HIV) become demented (Chap. 308). Cardinal features include psychomotor retardation, apathy, and impaired memory. This may result from secondary opportunistic infections but can also be caused by direct involvement of CNS neurons with HIV, where there is a multinucleated giant cell encephalitis and diffuse pallor of white matter. The neuronal toxicity may be mediated by cytokines or the direct neurotoxic effect of the gp 120 envelope glycoprotein. In the absence of CNS opportunistic infection, elevated β2 microglobulin in CSF is a useful marker for HIV dementia. Herpes simplex encephalitis (Chap. 379) has a predilection for the inferior temporal lobes and may present as subacute confusion and disorientation but more often as an acute syndrome rather than a chronic dementia. Computed tomography (CT), MRI, and electroencephalogram (EEG) may all demonstrate the temporal lobe location of the lesions. Cerebrospinal fluid (CSF) usually shows increased protein and a lymphocytic pleocytosis. CNS syphilis (Chap. 174) was a common cause of dementia in the preantibiotic era; it is uncommon nowadays but can still be encountered in the population with multiple sex partners. Characteristic CSF changes consist of pleocytosis, increased protein, and positive VDRL test.

Prion disorders such as Creutzfeldt-Jakob disease (CJD) (Chap. 379) are very rare conditions (approximately 1 per million population) that commonly produce dementia. CJD is usually a rapidly progressive disease associated with dementia, rigidity, and myoclonus, causing death in less than 1 to 2 years. These clinical characteristics may also rarely be seen in AD, and the differential diagnosis usually depends on the slower progression of AD and the markedly abnormal periodic EEG discharges seen in CJD. Ataxia or cortical blindness may also accompany CJD. The transmissible agent, or prion, consists principally of an abnormal isoform of a host-encoded protein, the prion protein (PrP), which accumulates in affected brains. The abnormal disease-causing prion protein (PrP^{SC}) is derived from the normal prion protein (PrP^C) by a posttranslation mechanism that may represent a physical conformational change. PrP^{SC} apparently acts as a template that promotes the conversion of PrP^C to PrP^{SC}, and this cascading conformational change somehow produces neuronal damage and death. The disease is transmissible by tissue transplantation to animals or other humans and is occasionally inherited (familial CJD, or Gerstmann-Sträussler-Scheinker disease). The inherited variety has the unique characteristic of being both a genetic and a transmissible disorder. Sporadic cases are not inherited. CJD is not contagious by touch or airborne spread. Bovine spongiform encephalopathy in the United Kingdom is thought to have resulted from cattle feed containing sheep tissues contaminated with infectious prions (PrP scrapie). Possible transmission to the human population is under investigation. Immunoassay for a 14-3-3 brain protein in CSF may be a useful marker for transmissible spongiform encephalopathies in patients with dementia.

Primary and metastatic *neoplasms of the* CNS (Chap. 375) usually produce focal neurologic findings and seizures rather than dementia. However, if tumor growth begins in the frontal or temporal lobes, the initial manifestations may be memory loss or behavioral changes. A rare paraneoplastic syndrome of dementia associated with occult carcinoma (usually small cell lung cancer) has been termed *limbic encephalitis* (Chap. 103). In this syndrome, confusion, agitation, seizures, poor memory, and frank dementia may occur in association with sensory neuropathy. The CSF often shows an increase in cells and protein. There is neuronal loss and perivascular lymphocytic infiltration in the hippocampus, amygdala, and cingulate and frontal cortex. Circulating antineuronal nuclear antibodies may be present. There is no specific treatment.

The syndrome of *normal-pressure hydrocephalus* (Chap. 367) is frequently discussed but difficult to diagnose. Clinically, a triad of memory loss, gait disturbance, and bladder incontinence is typical. The gait abnormality is often the initial symptom, and the dementia is usually mild. On imaging studies, the lateral ventricles are enlarged but there is minimal or no cortical atrophy. Lumbar puncture shows a normal or slightly elevated opening pressure with normal CSF. The condition may be idiopathic or the result of previous meningitis or subarachnoid blood from a ruptured aneurysm or head trauma. The pathogenetic mechanism is presumably a block of normal CSF flow over the convexity and delayed absorption into the venous system, with resulting stretch and distortion of white matter tracts within the corona radiata. Some individuals improve with ventricular shunting but many do not. The condition is difficult to distinguish from AD (see Chap. 367).

A nonconvulsive *seizure disorder* may underlie a syndrome of confusion, clouding of consciousness, and garbled speech. Psychiatric disease is often suspected, but an EEG demonstrates the seizure discharges. If recurrent or persistent, the condition may be termed *complex partial status epilepticus*. The cognitive disturbance often responds to anticonvulsant therapy. The etiology may be previous small strokes or head trauma; some cases are idiopathic.

It is important to recognize systemic diseases that indirectly affect the brain and produce chronic confusion or dementia. Such conditions include dysthyroid states (especially hypothyroidism), vasculitis, and hepatic, renal, or pulmonary disease. Hepatic encephalopathy may begin with irritability and confusion and slowly progress to agitation, lethargy, and coma (Chap. 380).

Isolated angiitis of the CNS (CNS granulomatous angiitis) (Chaps. 319 and 366) occasionally causes a chronic encephalopathy associated with confusion, disorientation, and clouding of consciousness. Headache is common, and strokes and cranial neuropathies may occur. Brain imaging studies may be normal or nonspecifically abnormal. CSF studies reveal a mild pleocytosis or elevation in the protein level in half of the cases. Cerebral angiography often shows multifocal stenosis and narrowing of vessels. A few patients have only small-vessel disease that is not revealed on angiography. The angiographic appearance is not specific and may be mimicked by atherosclerosis, infection, or other causes of vascular disease. Brain or meningeal biopsy demonstrates abnormal arteries with endothelial cell proliferation and infiltrates of mononuclear cells. Autoantibodies and immune complexes are not present, and a cell-mediated process appears most likely. The prognosis is poor, but some patients respond to glucocorticoids or chemotherapy.

Chronic metal intoxications may also produce a dementing syndrome. The key to diagnosis is to elicit a history of exposure at work, home, or even as a consequence of a medical procedure such as dialysis. Lead poisoning has highly variable neurologic manifestations. Fatigue, depression, and confusion may be associated with episodic abdominal pain and peripheral neuropathy. Gray lead lines may appear in the gums. There is usually an associated anemia with basophilic stippling of red cells. The clinical presentation can resemble that of acute intermittent porphyria, including elevated levels of urine porphyrins as a result of the inhibition of δ-aminolevulinic acid dehydratase. Chronic lead poisoning from inadequately fired glazed pottery has been reported. The treatment is chelation therapy with agents such as EDTA. Chronic mercury poisoning may produce dementia, peripheral neuropathy, and a fine tremulousness that may progress to a cerebellar intention tremor or choreoathetosis. The confusion and memory loss of chronic arsenic intoxication is also associated with nausea, weight loss, peripheral neuropathy, pigmentation and scaling of the skin, and transverse white lines of the fingernails (Mee's lines). Treatment is chelation therapy with dimercaprol (BAL). Aluminum poisoning has been best documented with the dialysis dementia syndrome in which water used during renal dialysis was contaminated with excessive amounts of aluminum. This resulted in a progressive encephalopathy associated with confusion, memory loss, agitation, and, later, lethargy and stupor. Speech arrest and myoclonic jerking was common and associated with severe and generalized EEG changes. The condition was often fatal. There were no specific pathologic findings, but elevated brain aluminum content was documented. The condition has been eliminated by use of deionized water for dialysis. Although aluminum injected into experimental animals may produce neurofibrillary tangles, dialysis dementia patients had neither tangles nor amyloid plaques, and there has been no direct association of aluminum poisoning with AD.

Recurrent head trauma in professional boxers may lead to dementia, sometimes called the "punch drunk" syndrome or *dementia pugilistica.* The symptoms can be progressive and may begin late in a boxer's career or even long after retirement. The severity of the syndrome correlates with the length of the boxing career and the total number of bouts. Early in the condition there occurs a personality change associated with social instability and sometimes paranoia and delusions. Later, memory loss progresses to full dementia, often associated with parkinsonian signs and ataxia or intention tremor. At autopsy, the cerebral cortex may show changes similar to AD, although neurofibrillary tangles are usually more predominant than amyloid plaques (which are usually diffuse rather than neuritic). There may also be loss of neurons in the substantia nigra. Chronic subdural hematoma is also occasionally associated with dementia, often in the context of underlying cortical atrophy from conditions such as AD or HD. In these latter cases, evacuation of the subdural hematoma will not alter the underlying degenerative process.

Head injury (Chap. 374) may also be associated with temporary amnesia. The memory disturbance may include events that occurred both prior to the injury (retrograde amnesia) and during the postinjury period (posttraumatic or anterograde amnesia). Retrograde amnesia following severe head injury may extend back for hours or weeks prior to the injury; remote memory is usually intact. As patients recover, the extent of retrograde amnesia shrinks and may disappear. Often, retrograde amnesia causes permanent inability to recall the few minutes prior to the head injury, implying disruption of the immediate memory system and failure to register long-term memory. The length of posttraumatic amnesia generally corresponds to the length of the postconcussive confusional state but posttraumatic amnesia may persist even in the presence of normal immediate memory and digit span. The duration of posttraumatic amnesia indicates the severity of head injury; the ability to learn new material is often the last cognitive deficit to recover. There are reports of recovery from retrograde amnesia occurring months or years after the initial brain insult, the recovery sometimes stimulated by hypnosis, amobarbital interview, or electrical stimulation. One theory of such recovery envisions a resetting of distorted patterns of neuronal matrices subserving memory.

Transient global amnesia (TGA) is characterized by sudden onset of complete anterograde loss of memory and learning abilities, usually occurring in persons over age 50. Onset of memory loss may occur in the context of an emotional stimulus or physical exertion. During the attack the individual is alert and communicative, general cognition seems intact, and there are no other neurologic signs or symptoms. The patient may seem confused and repeatedly ask about present events. Ability to form new memories returns after a period of hours, and the individual returns to normal but has no recall for the period of the attack. Frequently no cause can be determined, but cerebrovascular disease, epilepsy (7 percent in one study), migraine, or cardiac arrhythmia are sometimes implicated. A Mayo Clinic review of 277 patients with TGA found a past history of migraine in 14 percent and cerebrovascular disease in 11 percent, but these conditions were not temporally related to the TGA episodes. About one-fourth of the patients had recurrent attacks, but they were not at increased risk for subsequent stroke. Rare instances of permanent memory loss after sudden onset have been reported.

Psychogenic amnesia for personally important memories is common, although whether this results from deliberate avoidance of unpleasant memories or from unconscious repression may be impossible to establish. The event-specific amnesia is particularly common after violent crimes such as homicide of a close relative or friend or sexual abuse. It also may occur with severe drug or alcohol intoxication and sometimes with schizophrenia. More prolonged psychogenic amnesia occurs in fugue states that also commonly follow severe emotional stress. The patient with a fugue state suffers from a sudden loss of personal identity and may be found wandering far from home. In contrast to organic amnesia, fugue states are associated with amnesia for personal identity and events closely associated with the personal past. At the same time, memory for other recent events and the ability to learn and use new information are preserved. The episodes usually last hours or days and occasionally weeks or months while the patient takes on a new identity. On recovery, there is a residual amnesic gap for the period of the fugue.

Psychiatric diseases may mimic dementia. Severely depressed individuals may appear demented, a phenomenon called *pseudodementia.* Unlike cortical dementias, memory and language are usually intact when carefully tested in depressed persons. The patients may feel confused and are unable to accomplish routine tasks. Vegetative symptoms are common, such as insomnia, lack of energy, poor appetite, and concern with bowel function. The psychosocial milieu may suggest prominent reasons for depression. The patients respond to antidepressant treatment. Schizophrenia is usually not difficult to distinguish from dementia but occasionally the distinction can be problematic. (Kraepelin's original term for schizophrenia was *dementia praecox.*) Schizophrenia usually has a much earlier age of onset (second and third decades) than most dementing illnesses, is associated with intact memory, and the delusions and hallucinations of schizophrenia are usually more complex and bizarre than those of dementia. Some chronic schizophrenics develop an unexplained progressive dementia late in life that is not related to AD. Memory loss may also be part of a conversion reaction. In this situation, patients commonly complain bitterly of memory loss but careful cognitive testing either does not confirm the deficits or demonstrates inconsistent or unusual patterns of cognitive problems. The patients' behavior and "wrong" answers to questions often indicate that they both understand the question and know the answer.

Clouding of cognition by chronic drug or medication use, often prescribed by physicians, is an important cause of dementia. Sedatives, tranquilizers, and analgesics used to treat insomnia, pain, anxiety, or agitation may cause confusion, memory loss, and lethargy, especially in the elderly. Discontinuation of such medication often improves mentation.

Approach to the Patient

The approach to the patient with dementia should always keep two major issues in the forefront: What is the most accurate diagnosis and is there a treatable condition? A broad overview of this approach is shown in Table 26-3.

History The history should concentrate on the onset, duration, and tempo of the memory loss. Acute or subacute confusion may represent delirium and suggests intoxication, infection, or metabolic derangement. An elderly person with slowly progressive memory loss over several years is likely to have AD. Initial symptoms often are difficulty with managing money, driving, shopping, following instructions, or finding one's way around town. A change in personality is also common. A history of sudden stroke with an irregular stepwise progression suggests multi-infarct dementia. Stroke is also commonly associated with a history of hypertension, atrial fibrillation, peripheral vascular disease, and diabetes. Rapid progression with rigidity and myoclonus suggests CJD. Seizures may indicate strokes or neoplasm. Trouble in walking may suggest PD or normal-pressure hydrocephalus, especially the latter when associated with bladder incontinence. Multiple sex partners or intravenous drug use may indicate CNS infection, especially with HIV. A history of recurrent head trauma could indicate chronic subdural hematoma, dementia pugilistica, or normal-pressure hydrocephalus. Alcoholism may suggest malnutrition and thiamine deficiency. A remote history of gastric surgery resulting in loss of intrinsic factor might indicate vitamin B$_{12}$ deficiency. Certain occupations such as working in a battery or chemical factory might indicate heavy metal intoxication. Careful review of medication intake, especially of sedatives and tranquilizers, may raise the issue of chronic drug intoxication. A positive family history of dementia would be elicited in HD or familial AD. Recent death of a loved one, insomnia, or poor appetite suggest depression.

Physical Examination A careful examination is essential to document the dementia, look for other signs of nervous system involvement, and search for clues suggesting other systemic disease. Cognitive function should be assessed in terms of orientation, recent and remote memory, and calculation. Many of the simple, commonly used bedside tests of cognitive function (such as serial 7s, digits forward and backward) are most useful when they are performed normally; this makes the diagnosis of dementia more difficult to interpret and are of less diagnostic importance. Drawing a clock and the trail-making test are frequently used tests of immediate memory and visual-spatial abilities. The mini-mental status exam (MMSE) is an easily administered 30-points test of cognitive function (Table 26-4). It is used to indicate a dementing process quickly, provide a rough assessment of its severity, and follow progression of the illness. The MMSE is influenced by culture and education and is less useful in the early and late stages of dementia. Language function should be tested by ability to read, write, comprehend, and name objects. Resting tremor, cogwheel rigidity, bradykinesia, and festinating gait indicates a parkinsonian syndrome. Gait ataxia or apraxia (inability to initiate and coordinate steps in a sequential fashion) suggests normal-pressure hydrocephalus. Confusion, sixth cranial nerve paresis, and ataxia suggests thiamine deficiency. Myoclonic jerks are present in CJD but also occur in AD. Hemiparesis or other focal neurologic deficits may occur in multi-infarct dementia or brain tumor. Bilateral hyperactive tendon reflexes, Babinski responses, and loss of vibration and position sensation suggest a myelopathy, such as occurs in vitamin B$_{12}$ deficiency. Stocking-glove sensory loss and diminished tendon reflexes suggest a peripheral neuropathy, which could indicate underlying diabetes, vitamin deficiency, or heavy metal intoxication. Dry cool skin, hair loss, and bradycardia suggest hypothyroidism. Confusion associated with repetitive stereotyped movements may indicate ongoing seizure activity. Hearing impairment or visual loss may produce confusion and disorientation misinterpreted as dementia. Such sensory deficits are common in the elderly.

Laboratory Tests The use of multiple laboratory tests in the evaluation

---

Table 26-3

Evaluation of the Demented Patient

Routine Evaluation	Optional Focused Tests	Occasionally Helpful Tests
History	HIV	EEG
Physical examination	Chest x-ray	Parathyroid function
Laboratory tests	Lumbar puncture	Adrenal function
Thyroid function (TSH)	Liver function	Urine heavy metals
Vitamin B$_{12}$	Renal function	RBC sedimentation rate
Complete blood count	Urine toxin screen	Angiogram
Electrolytes	Psychometric testing	Brain biopsy
VDRL	Apolipoprotein E	
CT/MRI		

DIAGNOSTIC CATEGORIES

Treatable Causes	Untreatable/Degenerative Dementias	Psychiatric Disorders
Examples	Examples	Depression
Hypothyroidism	Alzheimer's	Schizophrenia
Thiamine deficiency	Pick's	Conversion reaction
Vitamin B$_{12}$ deficiency	Huntington's	
Normal-pressure	Diffuse Lewy body disease	
hydrocephalus	Multi-infarct	
Chronic infection	Leukoencephalopathies	
Brain tumor	Parkinson's	
Drug intoxication		
	Associated Treatable Conditions	
	Depression	
	Seizures	
	Insomnia	
	Agitation	
	Caregiver "burnout"	
	Drug side effects	

of dementia is controversial. The physician does not want to miss a treatable cause, yet no single treatable cause stands out as common; thus a screen must employ multiple different tests, each of which has a low yield. Therefore, cost/benefit ratios are difficult to assess, and many laboratory screening algorithms for dementia discourage multiple tests. Nevertheless, even a test with only a 1 to 2 percent positive rate is probably worth undertaking if the alternative is missing a treatable cause of dementia. The algorithm in Table 26-3 lists most screening tests for dementia. Neuroimaging studies (CT and MRI) are especially controversial because of their costs. However, they are clearly of value to identify primary and secondary neoplasms, locate areas of infarction, or suggest normal-pressure hydrocephalus or diffuse white matter disease. They also lend support to the diagnosis of AD, especially if there is hippocampal atrophy in addition to diffuse cortical atrophy. On the other hand, attempts to relate cognition to neuroimaging measures of atrophy and white matter changes have only shown modest correlations. A diagnosis of AD is reached primarily by exclusion of other causes of dementia. (The indications for apolipoprotein E testing for AD are discussed in Chap. 367.) Serum levels of vitamin B_{12} and thyroid-stimulating hormone, complete blood count, electrolyte measurements, and VDRL are reasonable routine screening tests because they detect treatable conditions. Lumbar puncture need not be done routinely in the evaluation of dementia, but is indicated if CNS infection is a serious consideration, for example, in patients with delirium, fever, or nuchal rigidity. CSF levels of tau protein are increased, and $A\beta$ amyloid decreased, in some AD patients; however, the clinical utility of these changes is not yet clear. Formal psychometric testing is not necessary in every patient with dementia, but can be used to document the severity of dementia, suggest psychogenic causes, and provide a semiquantitative method for following the disease course. EEG is rarely helpful except to suggest CJD (repetitive bursts of diffuse high voltage sharp waves) or an underlying nonconvulsive seizure disorder (epileptiform discharges). Brain biopsy (including meninges) is not commonly advised except to diagnose vasculitis, potentially treatable neoplasms, unusual infections (such as sarcoid), or in young persons where the diagnosis is in doubt. Angiography is not likely to be of use except when multiple strokes or cerebral vasculitis is a possible cause of the dementia.

Table 26-4

The Mini-Mental Status Examination

	Points
Orientation	
Name: season/date/day/month/year	5 (1 for each name)
Name: hospital/floor/town/state/country	5 (1 for each name)
Registration	
Identify three objects by name and ask patient to repeat	3 (1 for each object)
Attention and calculation	
Serial 7s; subtract from 100 (e.g., 93–86–79–72–65)	5 (1 for each subtraction)
Recall	
Recall the three objects presented earlier	3 (1 for each object)
Language	
Name pencil and watch	2 (1 for each object)
Repeat "No ifs, ands, or buts"	1
Follow a 3-step command (e.g., "Take this paper, fold it in half, and place it on the table")	3 (1 for each command)
Write "close your eyes" and ask patient to obey written command	1
Ask patient to write a sentence	1
Ask patient to copy a design (e.g., intersecting pentagons)	1
TOTAL	30

℞ TREATMENT

The two major goals of management are, first, to treat any correctable cause of the dementia and, second, to provide comfort and support to the patient and caregivers. Treatment of underlying causes might include thyroid replacement for hypothyroidism, vitamin therapy for thiamine and B_{12} deficiency, antibiotics for opportunistic infections, ventricular shunting for normal-pressure hydrocephalus, and appropriate surgical, radiation, and/or chemotherapy for CNS neoplasms. Removal of sedating or cognition-impairing drugs and medications is often beneficial. If the patient is depressed rather than demented (pseudodementia), the depression should be vigorously treated. Patients with degenerative diseases such as AD and HD may also be depressed, and that portion of their condition may respond to antidepressant therapy. Antidepressants should be used with caution in demented patients because they may produce delirium. Antidepressants that are low in cognitive side effects, such as selective serotonin reuptake inhibitors, and tricyclic antidepressants with low anticholinergic activity, such as desipramine and nortriptyline, are advisable. Anticonvulsants are used to control seizures. Agitation, hallucinations, delusions, and confusion are difficult to treat. These behavioral problems represent major causes for nursing home placement and institutionalization. Drugs such as phenothiazines, haloperidol, and benzodiazepines may ameliorate the behavior problems but have untoward side effects such as sedation, rigidity, and dyskinesias. Medications that may calm agitation and insomnia without worsening dementia include low-dose haloperidol (0.5 to 2 mg), trazodone, buspirone, and propranolol. When patients do not respond it is usually a mistake to advance to higher doses or to use anticholinergics or sedatives (such as barbiturates or benzodiazepines).

Nondrug behavior therapy has an important place in the management of dementia. The primary goal is to make the demented patient's life comfortable, uncomplicated, and safe. Preparing lists, schedules, calendars, and labels can be helpful. It is also useful to stress familiar routines, short-term tasks, brief walks, and simple physical exercises. For many demented patients, the memory for facts is worse than that for routine activities, and they still may be able to take part in remembered physical activities such as walking, bowling, dancing, and golf. Demented patients usually object to losing control over familiar tasks such as driving, cooking, and handling finances. Attempts to help or take over may be greeted with complaints, depression, or anger. Hostile responses on the part of the caretaker are useless and sometimes harmful. Explanation, reassurance, distraction, and calm statements are more productive responses in this setting. Eventually, tasks such as finances and driving must be assumed by others, and the patient will conform and adjust. Safety is an important issue that includes not only driving but the environment of the kitchen, bathroom, and sleeping area. These areas need to be monitored, supervised, and made as safe as possible. A move to a retirement home, assisted-living center, or nursing home can initially increase confusion and agitation. Repeated reassurance, reorientation, and careful introduction to the new personnel will help to smooth the process. Provision of activities that are known to be enjoyable to the patient can be of considerable benefit. Attention should also be paid to frustration and depression in family members and caregivers. Caregiver guilt and burn-out are common. Family members often feel overwhelmed and helpless and may vent their frustrations on the patient, each other, and healthcare providers. Caregivers should be encouraged to take advantage of day-care facilities and respite breaks. Education and counseling about dementia are important. Local and national support groups can be of considerable help, such as the Alzheimer's Disease and Related Disorders Association.

BIBLIOGRAPHY

COREY-BLOOD J et al: Diagnosis and evaluation of dementia. Neurology 45:211, 1995

CUMMINGS JK: *Dementia: A Clinical Approach*, 2d ed. Boston, Butterworth-Heinemann, 1992

EBLY EM et al: Prevalence and types of dementia in the very old: Results from the Canadian Study of Health and Aging. Neurology 44:1593, 1994

ERICKSON K: Amnestic disorders. Pathophysiology and patterns of memory dysfunction. West J Med 152:159, 1990

FLEMING KC, EVANS JM: Pharmacologic therapies in dementia. Mayo Clin Proc 70:1116, 1995

HODGES JR, WARLOW CP: Syndromes of transient amnesia: Towards a classification. A study of 153 cases. J Neurol Neurosurg Psychiatry 53:834, 1990

MARTIN LM, FLEMING KC et al: Recognition and management of anxiety and depression in elderly patients. Mayo Clin Proc 70:999, 1995

SIU AL: Screening for dementia and investigating its causes. Ann Intern Med 115:122, 1991

WILLMER J et al: The usefulness of CT scanning in diagnosing dementia of the Alzheimer type. Can J Neurol Sci 20:210, 1993

27	*Charles A. Czeisler, Gary S. Richardson*

DISORDERS OF SLEEP AND CIRCADIAN RHYTHMS

Disturbed sleep is among the most frequent health complaints physicians encounter. One-third of adults in the United States experience occasional or persistent sleep disturbances. Sleep deprivation or disruption of the circadian timing system can lead to serious impairment of daytime functioning. Sleep disorders may either contribute to or result from related medical or psychiatric conditions. Twenty-five years ago, many such complaints were treated with hypnotic medications without further diagnostic evaluation. Since then, a distinct class of sleep and arousal disorders has been identified, and the field of sleep disorders is now an established clinical discipline. Two principal neurobiologic systems govern the sleep-wake cycle: one that actively generates sleep and sleep-related processes and another that times sleep within the 24-h day. Either intrinsic abnormalities in these systems or extrinsic disturbances (environmental, drug- or illness-related) can lead to sleep or circadian rhythm disorders.

PHYSIOLOGY OF SLEEP AND WAKEFULNESS

Most adults sleep 7 to 8 h per night, although the timing, duration, and internal structure of sleep vary among apparently healthy individuals and as a function of age. At the extremes, infants and the elderly have frequent interruptions of sleep. In the United States, adults of intermediate age tend to have one consolidated sleep episode per day, although in some cultures sleep may be divided into a midafternoon nap and a shortened night sleep. While there is a wide range of normal sleep lengths, epidemiologic studies suggest that adults with habitual sleep durations of fewer than 4 h or greater than 9 have increased mortality rates as compared to those who sleep 7 to 8 h per night.

STATES AND STAGES OF SLEEP States and stages of human sleep are defined on the basis of characteristic patterns in the electroencephalogram (EEG), the electrooculogram (EOG—a measure of eye-movement activity), and the surface electromyogram (EMG).

The continuous recording of this array of electrophysiologic parameters to define sleep and wakefulness is termed *polysomnography*.

Polysomnographic profiles define two states of sleep: (1) rapid-eye-movement (REM) sleep, and (2) non-rapid-eye-movement (NREM) sleep. NREM sleep is in turn subdivided into four stages, characterized by increasing arousal threshold and slowing of the cortical EEG (Fig. 27-1). REM sleep is characterized by a low-amplitude, mixed-frequency EEG similar to that of NREM stage 1 (Fig. 27-1). The EOG shows bursts of REM similar to those seen during eyes-open wakefulness. EMG activity is absent, reflecting the complete brainstem-mediated muscle atonia that is characteristic of that state.

ORGANIZATION OF HUMAN SLEEP Normal nocturnal sleep in adults displays a consistent organization from night to night (Fig. 27-2). After sleep onset, sleep usually progresses through NREM stages 1 to 4 within 45 to 60 min. Slow-wave sleep predominates in the first third of the night and comprises 15 to 25 percent of total nocturnal sleep time in young adults. The percentage of slow-wave sleep is influenced by several factors, most notably age (see below). Prior sleep deprivation increases the rapidity of sleep onset and both the intensity and amount of slow-wave sleep.

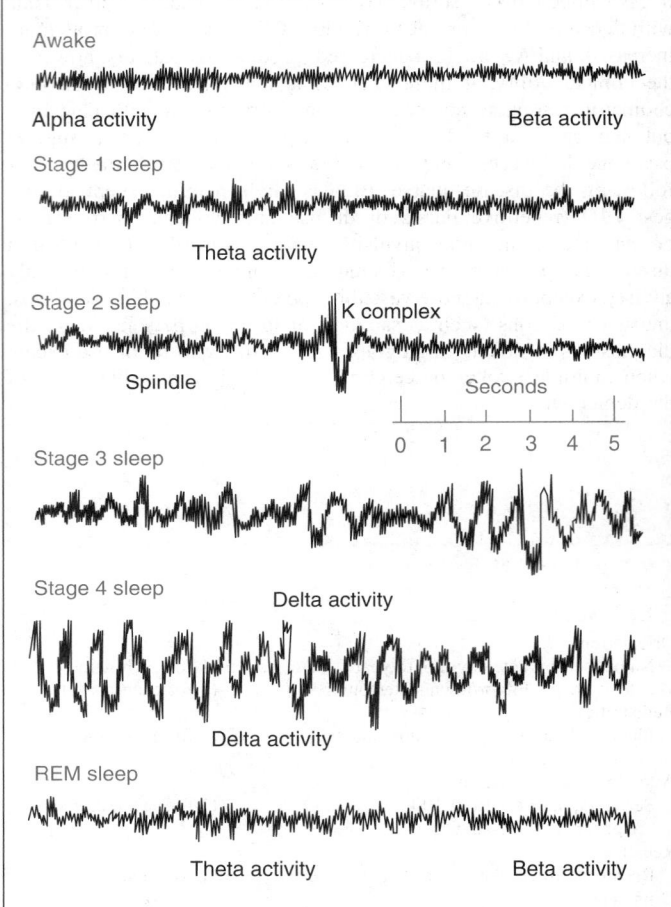

FIGURE 27-1 Electroencephalogram of human sleep stages. The first trace illustrates alpha activity seen in quiet wakefulness (eyes closed) and the beta activity of an alert subject. Stage 1 theta activity is seen in the second trace; stage 2 sleep (with associated sleep spindle and K complex) in the third. The fourth and fifth traces show slow-wave (stages 3 and 4) sleep, with prominent delta activity. This synchronous activity is absent in REM sleep (sixth trace), which resembles stage 1 EEG. However, REM sleep is accompanied by rapid eye movements and muscle paralysis. (*Reproduced from J Horne, Why We Sleep: The Functions of Sleep in Humans and Other Mammals. Oxford, Oxford University Press, 1988.*)

The first REM sleep episode usually occurs in the second hour of sleep. More rapid onset of REM sleep in a young adult may (particularly if less than 30 min) suggest pathology such as endogenous depression, narcolepsy, circadian rhythm disorders, or drug withdrawal. NREM and REM alternate through the night with an average period of 90 to 110 min (the "ultradian" cycle). Overall, REM sleep constitutes 20 to 25 percent of total sleep, and NREM stages (1 and 2) are 50 to 60 percent (increasing in elderly subjects).

Age has a large impact on sleep state organization (Fig. 27-2). Slow-wave sleep is most prominent during childhood, decreasing sharply at puberty and across the second and third decades of life. After age 30, there is a progressive, almost linear decline in the amount of slow-wave sleep, and the amplitude of delta EEG activity comprising slow-wave sleep is reduced. In the otherwise healthy elderly person, slow-wave sleep may be completely absent, particularly in males.

A different age profile exists for REM sleep. In infancy, REM sleep may comprise 50 percent of total sleep time, and the percentage is inversely proportional to developmental age. The amount of REM sleep falls off sharply over the first postnatal year as a mature REM-NREM cycle develops. During the rest of life into extreme old age, REM sleep occupies a more constant percentage of total sleep time than does slow-wave sleep.

BEHAVIORAL CORRELATES OF SLEEP STATES AND STAGES Polysomnographic staging of sleep correlates with behavioral changes during specific states and stages. Awakenings from REM sleep are associated with recall of vivid dream imagery more than 80 percent of the time. The reliability of dream recall increases with REM sleep episodes occurring later in the night. Imagery may also be reported after NREM sleep interruptions, though these typically lack the detail and vividness of REM sleep dreams. The incidence of NREM sleep dream recall can be increased by selective REM sleep deprivation, suggesting that REM sleep and dreaming per se are not inexorably linked. Sleep onset is associated with marked decrements in perception of both auditory and visual stimuli and lapses of consciousness. During stage 1 sleep, subjects may respond to faint auditory or visual signals without "awakening." Furthermore, memory incorporation is inhibited at the onset of NREM stage 1, and subjects aroused from that stage frequently deny having been asleep. At the same time, it is possible to continue performing routine and familiar motor tasks, such as driving an automobile, during the transitional state between wakefulness and sleep (stage 1 sleep) that often intrudes upon behavioral wakefulness in the sleepy individual. During such intrusions, typically lasting only seconds but known on occasion to persist for longer durations, visual and auditory perception are attenuated and reaction time is prolonged. Subsequently, the sleepy individual may be unaware that such an event has occurred. The dramatic perceptual and cognitive deficits associated with frequent brief intrusions of stage 1 sleep into behavioral wakefulness are a major component of the impaired psychomotor performance seen with sleepiness.

PHYSIOLOGIC CORRELATES OF SLEEP STATES AND STAGES All major physiologic systems are influenced by sleep. In some cases, concomitant behavior changes such as supine posture or inactivity are the proximal causes of altered physiologic function, but in most cases the sleep state itself appears to be responsible. Changes in cardiovascular function include a decrease in blood pressure and heart rate during NREM, and particularly during slow-wave, sleep. During REM sleep, phasic activity (bursts of eye movements) is associated with variability in both blood pressure and heart rate mediated principally by the vagus. Cardiac dysrhythmias may occur selectively during REM sleep. Respiratory function also changes (see Chap. 263). In comparison to relaxed wakefulness, respiratory rate becomes more regular during NREM sleep (especially slow-wave sleep) and tonic REM sleep and becomes very irregular during phasic REM sleep. Minute ventilation decreases in NREM sleep out of proportion to the decrease in metabolic rate at sleep onset, resulting in a higher P_{CO_2}. Multiple factors contribute to these sleep-related changes in breathing: (1) decreased upper airway patency and consequent increased upper airway resistance, likely the result of sleep-related relaxation of a subset of tonically active upper airway muscles that lack a clear pattern of respiratory activation; (2) change in responsiveness of the respiratory system to chemical stimuli, namely P_{CO_2} and P_{O_2}; (3) loss of respiratory responses to wakeful stimuli; and (4) decreased metabolic rate. In addition, the cough reflex is attenuated or absent during sleep. These changes in respiratory function may be relevant to the pathogenesis of obstructive sleep apnea and sudden infant death syndrome (see Chap. 263).

Endocrine function also varies with sleep. The most prominent changes are apparent in neuroendocrine parameters. Slow-wave sleep is associated with secretion of growth hormone, while sleep in general is associated with augmented secretion of prolactin. Sleep has a complex effect on the secretion of luteinizing hormone (LH); during puberty, sleep is associated with increased LH secretion, whereas sleep in the mature woman inhibits LH secretion in the early follicular phase of the menstrual cycle. Sleep onset (and probably slow-wave sleep)

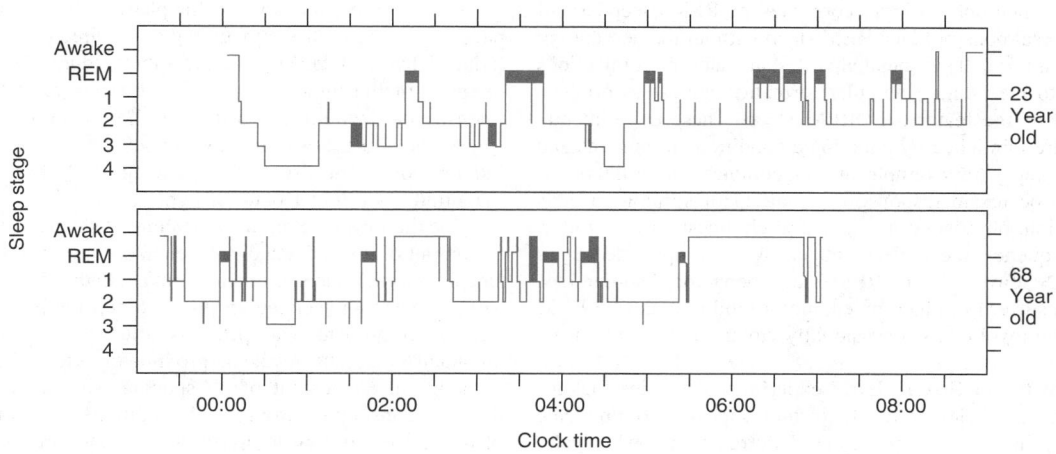

FIGURE 27-2 Plots of the stages of REM sleep (solid bars), the four stages of NREM sleep and wakefulness over the course of the entire night for representative young (upper panel, age 23) and elderly (lower panel, age 68) adult men. The recording in the elderly subject illustrates the reduction of slow-wave sleep, frequent spontaneous awakenings, early sleep onset, and early morning awakening that are characteristic features of sleep in the aged, even in the absence of specific medical or psychiatric pathology. *(From the Circadian, Neuroendocrine, and Sleep Disorders Section, Endocrine Division, Brigham and Womens' Hospital.)*

is associated with inhibition of thyroid-stimulating hormone and of the adrenocorticotropic hormone–cortisol axis, an effect that is superimposed on the circadian rhythms in the two systems. The pineal hormone melatonin is secreted predominantly at night, in both day- and night-active species, reflecting the direct modulation of pineal activity by the circadian pacemaker in the anterior hypothalamus (see below). Melatonin secretion is not dependent upon the occurrence of sleep, persisting in individuals kept awake at night. In addition, some recent data suggest that exogenous melatonin may increase sleepiness and potentiate sleep, particularly when administered during daylight hours when endogenous melatonin levels are low. However, further studies are required to verify and quantify putative sleep-promoting properties of melatonin.

Sleep is also associated with alterations of thermoregulatory function. NREM sleep is associated with an attenuation of thermoregulatory responses to either heat or cold stress, and animal studies of thermosensitive neurons in the hypothalamus document a NREM-sleep-dependent reduction of the thermoregulatory set-point. REM sleep is associated with complete absence of thermoregulatory responsiveness, effectively resulting in functional poikilothermy. However, the potential adverse impact of this failure of thermoregulation is blunted by inhibition of REM sleep by extreme ambient temperatures.

Neuroanatomy of Sleep   Lesion studies in animals and neurologic diseases in humans have suggested distinct neuroanatomic sites in the generation of normal sleep and wakefulness. The studies of von Economo of patients with encephalitis lethargica suggested that the anterior hypothalamus contained a "sleep center" while the posterior hypothalamus contained a "wake center." Experimental studies in animals have variously implicated the medullary reticular formation, the thalamus, and the basal forebrain in the generation of sleep, while the brainstem reticular formation, the midbrain, the subthalamus, the thalamus, and the basal forebrain have all been suggested to play a role in the generation of wakefulness or EEG arousal (see also Chap. 24).

Despite many studies, there is little evidence for either a single, discrete "sleep center" or a single, discrete "wake center." Current hypotheses suggest that the capacity for sleep and wakefulness generation is distributed along an axial "core" of neurons extending from the brainstem rostrally to the basal forebrain. Complex commingling of neuronal groups occurs at many points along this brainstem-forebrain axis.

Nonetheless, the neuroanatomic correlates of REM sleep appear to be discretely localized. Specific regions in the pons are associated with each of the neurophysiologic correlates of REM sleep. Small lesions in the dorsal pons produce REM sleep without the descending muscle inhibition normally associated with that state; microinjections of carbachol into the pontine reticular formation appear to produce a state with all of the features of REM sleep. These experimental manipulations are mimicked by pathologic conditions in humans and animals. In narcolepsy, for example, abrupt, complete, or partial paralysis (cataplexy) occurs in response to a variety of stimuli. In dogs with this condition, physostigmine, a central cholinesterase inhibitor, increases the frequency of cataplectic attacks while atropine decreases their frequency. Conversely, in REM sleep behavior disorder (see below), patients suffer from incomplete motor inhibition during REM sleep, resulting in involuntary, occasionally violent movement during REM sleep.

Neurochemistry of Sleep   Early experimental studies that focused on the raphe nuclei of the brainstem appeared to implicate serotonin as the primary sleep-promoting neurotransmitter, while catecholamines were considered to be responsible for wakefulness. Subsequent work has demonstrated that the raphe-serotonin system may facilitate sleep but is not necessary to its expression. The extensive pharmacology of sleep and wakefulness suggests roles for other neurotransmitters as well. Cholinergic neurotransmission is known to play a role in REM sleep generation. The alerting influence of caffeine

implicates adenosine, whereas the hypnotic effect of benzodiazepines and barbiturates suggests a role for endogenous ligands of the GABA-A receptor complex.

A variety of sleep-promoting substances have been identified. These include prostaglandin D_2, delta sleep–inducing peptide, muramyl dipeptide, interleukin 1, fatty acid primary amides, and melatonin (see above), and the hypnotic effect is commonly limited to NREM or slow-wave sleep, although peptides that increase REM sleep have also been reported. Many putative "sleep factors," including interleukin 1 and prostaglandin D_2, are immunologically active as well, suggesting a link between immune function and sleep-wake states.

PHYSIOLOGY OF CIRCADIAN RHYTHMICITY   The sleep-wake cycle is the most evident of the many 24-h rhythms in humans. Prominent daily variations also occur in endocrine, thermoregulatory, cardiac, pulmonary, renal, gastrointestinal, and cognitive functions. However, in evaluating a daily variation, it is important to distinguish between those rhythmic components passively evoked by periodic environmental or behavioral changes (e.g., the increase in blood pressure and heart rate upon assumption of the upright posture), and those actively driven by an endogenous oscillatory process (e.g., the circadian variation in plasma cortisol that persists under a variety of environmental and behavioral conditions).

The suprachiasmatic nuclei (SCN) of the hypothalamus act as the central neural pacemakers driving endogenous circadian rhythms in mammals. Bilateral destruction of these nuclei results in a loss of endogenous circadian rhythmicity that can only be restored by transplantation of the same structure(s) from a donor animal. The period and phase of the endogenous neural oscillator are normally synchronized to the 24-h period of the environmental light-dark cycle. Entrainment of mammalian circadian rhythms by the light-dark cycle is mediated via the retinohypothalamic tract, a monosynaptic pathway that links the retina to the SCN.

The principal properties characterizing an endogenous circadian pacemaker are its *intrinsic period*, *entrained phase*, *amplitude*, and *resetting capacity*. In human subjects living in controlled laboratory environments free of time cues (*free-running*), the duration of the behavioral rest-activity cycle averages 25 h. However, the timing of the light-dark cycle has generally been uncontrolled in such free-running studies, with the subjects choosing to be exposed to light during their "subjective days" and to darkness during their "subjective nights." Recent work suggests that when the light-dark cycle is controlled, the observed period of the human circadian pacemaker is much closer to 24 h. Nonetheless, synchronization of the endogenous circadian pacemaker to the 24-h day requires that the pacemaker be reset each day, which is normally achieved by exposure to the environmental light-dark cycle.

Exposure to light can shift the phase of the endogenous circadian pacemaker, but both the magnitude and the direction of the phase shifts induced by light depend on the timing, duration, wavelength, and intensity of the light. Properly timed exposure to light of sufficient intensity can, within 2 to 3 d, reset the human circadian pacemaker (presumably the SCN) to any desired hour. Exposure to ordinary indoor room light also shifts circadian phase but not by as great a magnitude as brighter outdoor light.

The timing and internal architecture of sleep are directly coupled to the output of the endogenous pacemaker. Spontaneous sleep duration, sleepiness, REM sleep propensity, and both the ability and the tendency to sleep vary with circadian phase. Sleep tendency, sleepiness, and REM sleep propensity all peak just after the nadir of the endogenous circadian temperature cycle (approximately 1 to 3 h before awakening). In addition, 85 percent of all spontaneous awakenings of subjects living in constant environmental conditions occur on the rising slope of the temperature cycle. Furthermore, there are certain times (wake maintenance zones) when it is very difficult to fall asleep, even for subjects who are sleep-deprived. Misalignment of the output of the endogenous circadian pacemaker with the desired sleep-wake cycle is thought to be responsible for certain types of insomnia, as well as for the decrements of alertness and performance in night-shift workers and after jet lag.

DISORDERS OF SLEEP AND WAKEFULNESS

An international classification of sleep disorders (Table 27-1) divides these conditions into three major groups: dyssomnias, parasomnias, and medical psychiatric sleep disorders. A detailed description of each of these disorders may be found in the publication of the American Sleep Disorders Association.

Approach to the Patient

With a Sleep Complaint Patients may seek help from a physician because of: (1) an acute or chronic inability to sleep adequately at night; (2) chronic fatigue, sleepiness, or tiredness during the day; or (3) a behavioral manifestation associated with sleep itself. Disruption or disturbance of nocturnal sleep is directly related to decreased alertness and impairment of daytime cognitive and psychomotor performance, which is often of serious concern to the patient. Table 27-2 outlines the most common pathways encountered in the evaluation of the patient with a complaint of excessive daytime sleepiness.

Taking a careful history is critical in the evaluation of the patient with a sleep complaint. In particular, the duration, severity, and consistency of the complaint are important, along with the patient's esti-

mate—in the case of an insomnia complaint—of the consequences of reported sleep loss on subsequent waking function. Information from a friend or family member can be an invaluable aid in assessing the severity of the complaint on daytime functioning, as some patients will underreport such potentially embarrassing symptoms as heavy snoring or falling asleep while driving.

Retrospective completion by the physician and patient of a day-by-day sleep-work-drug log in reverse chronologic order can help the physician better understand the nature of the complaint. Work times should be specified each day. Drug and alcohol use, including caffeine and hypnotics, should be noted each day. This log should be compared with a prospective sleep-work-drug log (including daytime naps and nocturnal awakenings) as recorded by the patient for at least 2 weeks. The sleep times should be plotted to facilitate recognition of circadian rhythm sleep disorders such as delayed sleep phase syndrome (see below).

Laboratory evaluation of objective sleep measures is necessary in the diagnosis of specific disorders such as narcolepsy and sleep apnea and may be of utility in other settings as well. In addition to the three electrophysiologic variables used to define sleep states and stages, the standard clinical polysomnogram includes measures of respiration (respiratory effort, air flow, and oxygen saturation), anterior tibialis EMG, and ECG. Evaluation of penile tumescence during nocturnal sleep also can be used to help determine whether the cause of erectile dysfunction in a patient is psychogenic or organic (see Chap. 51).

Table 27-1

International Classification of Sleep Disorders

DYSSOMNIAS

Intrinsic sleep disorders	Extrinsic sleep disorders
Psychophysiologic insomnia	Inadequate sleep hygiene
Idiopathic insomnia	Environmental sleep disorder
Narcolepsy	Altitude insomnia
Recurrent or idiopathic hypersomnia	Adjustment sleep disorder
Posttraumatic hypersomnia	Sleep-onset association disorder
Sleep apnea syndromes	Food allergy insomnia
Periodic limb movement disorder	Nocturnal eating (drinking) syndrome
Restless legs syndrome	Drug- or alcohol-dependent sleep disorders
Circadian rhythm sleep disorders	
Time-zone change (jet lag) syndrome	
Shift-work sleep disorder	
Delayed sleep phase syndrome	
Advanced sleep phase syndrome	
Non-24-h sleep-wake disorder	

PARASOMNIAS

Arousal disorders	Parasomnias usually associated with REM sleep
Confusional arousals	Nightmares
Sleepwalking	Sleep paralysis
Sleep terrors	Impaired sleep-related penile erections
Sleep-wake transition disorders	Sleep-related painful erections
Rhythmic movement disorder	REM sleep-related cardiac arrhythmias
Sleep talking	REM sleep behavior disorder
Nocturnal leg cramps	Other parasomnias
	Sleep bruxism
	Sleep enuresis
	Nocturnal paroxysmal dystonia

SLEEP DISORDERS ASSOCIATED WITH MEDICAL/PSYCHIATRIC DISORDERS

Associated with mental disorders	Associated with other medical disorders
Associated with neurologic disorders	Sleeping sickness
Cerebral degenerative disorders	Nocturnal cardiac ischemia
Parkinsonism	Chronic obstructive pulmonary disease
Fatal familial insomnia	Sleep-related asthma
Sleep-related epilepsy	Sleep-related gastroesophageal reflux
Sleep-related headaches	Peptic ulcer disease
	Fibrositis syndrome

SOURCE: Modified from the Diagnostic Classification Steering Committee.

DAYTIME CONSEQUENCES OF SLEEP DISORDERS

While the experience of disrupted nocturnal sleep may be the most prominent symptom for patients with sleep disorders, particularly those with insomnia, the impact of this sleep disruption on daytime function is arguably the more important aspect from both clinical and public health perspectives. Sleepiness-related automobile accidents, for example, constitute an important health risk for the patient with disrupted sleep.

Daytime impairment due to sleep loss may be difficult to quantify in the clinical setting for several reasons. First, sleepiness is not necessarily proportional to subjectively assessed sleep deprivation. In obstructive sleep apnea, for example, the repeated brief interruptions of sleep associated with resumption of respiration at the end of apneic episodes result in significant waking impairment, despite the fact that the patient may be unaware of the sleep fragmentation. Second, subjective descriptions of waking impairment vary from patient to patient. Patients may describe themselves as "sleepy," "fatigued," or "tired" and may have a clear sense of the meaning of those terms, while others may use the same terms to describe a completely different condition. Third, sleepiness, particularly when profound, may affect judgment in a manner analogous to ethanol, such that subjective awareness of the condition and the consequent cognitive and motor impairments is reduced. Finally, patients may be reluctant to admit that sleepiness is a problem, both because they are generally unaware of what constitutes normal alertness and because sleepiness is generally viewed pejoratively, ascribed more often to a deficit in motivation than to an inadequately addressed physiologic need.

In assessing sleepiness in the clinical setting, specific questioning about the occurrence of sleep episodes during normal waking hours, both intentional and unintentional, can overcome the inconsistencies among subjective characterizations and will simultaneously provide an index of the adverse impact of sleepiness on daytime function. Specific areas to be addressed include the occurrence of inadvertent sleep episodes while driving or in other safety-related settings, sleepiness while at work or school (and the relationship of sleepiness to work and school performance), and the effect of sleepiness on social and family life. Evidence for significant daytime impairment (typically in association with the diagnosis of a primary sleep disorder such as narcolepsy or sleep apnea) raises the question of the physician's responsibility to notify licensing authorities of the increased risk of sleepiness-related vehicle accidents. As with epilepsy, legal requirements vary from state to state, and existing legal precedents typically do not provide a consistent interpretation of the balance between the physician's responsibility and the patient's right to privacy. At a minimum, physicians should document discussions with the patient regarding the increased risk of operating a vehicle, as well as a recommendation that driving be suspended until successful treatment can be instituted.

Differentiation of sleepiness from fatigue can be difficult, particularly given the imprecise use of these terms by patients in describing subjective symptoms. The distinction can be useful in the differentiation of patients with complaints of fatigue or tiredness in the setting of disorders such as fibromyalgia, chronic fatigue syndrome (see Chap. 384), or endocrine deficiencies such as hypothyroidism or Addison's disease. While patients with these disorders can typically distinguish their daytime symptoms from the sleepiness that occurs with sleep deprivation, substantial overlap can occur. This is particularly true when the primary disorder also results in chronic sleep disruption (e.g., sleep apnea in hypothyroidism) or in abnormal sleep (e.g., fibromyalgia).

While clinical evaluation of the complaint of excessive sleepiness is usually adequate, objective quantification is sometimes necessary for diagnostic purposes or for the evaluation of treatment response. Assessment of daytime functioning as an index of the adequacy of sleep can be made with the multiple sleep latency test (MSLT), which involves repeated measurement of sleep latency (time to onset of sleep) under standardized conditions during a day following quantified nocturnal sleep. The average latency across four to six tests (administered every 2 h across the waking day) is taken as an objective measure of daytime sleep tendency. Disorders of sleep that result in pathologic daytime somnolence can be reliably distinguished with the MSLT. In addition, the multiple measurements of sleep onset may identify direct transitions from wakefulness to REM sleep that are suggestive of specific pathologic conditions (e.g., narcolepsy).

INSOMNIA Insomnia is the complaint of inadequate sleep; it can be classified according to the nature of sleep disruption and the duration of the complaint. The nature of the sleep disruption provides important information about the possible etiology of the insomnia and is also central to the selection of specific and appropriate treatment. Insomnia is subdivided into difficulty falling asleep (*sleep onset insomnia*), frequent or sustained awakenings (*sleep maintenance insomnia*), early morning awakenings (*sleep offset insomnia*), or persistent sleepiness despite sleep of adequate duration (*nonrestorative sleep*). Simi-

larly, the duration of the symptom is an important determinant of the nature of appropriate treatment. An insomnia complaint lasting one to several nights (within a single episode) is termed *transient insomnia*. Transient insomnia is typically the result of situational stress or a change in sleep schedule or environment (e.g., jet lag). *Short-term insomnia* lasts from a few days to 3 weeks. Disruption of this duration is usually associated with more protracted stress, such as recovery from surgery or short-term illness. *Long-term* or *chronic insomnia* lasts for months or years and commonly reflects perpetuating factors associated with a primary sleep disorder (see below). Chronic insomnia may present as recurrent episodes of insomnia, not necessarily associated with parallel variation in the underlying cause. Although some clinicians refer to this as recurrent insomnia, others suggest that this may be the typical pattern of all chronic insomniacs.

While an occasional night of poor sleep, typically in the setting of stress or excitement about external events, is both common and without lasting consequences, persistent insomnia can have important adverse consequences in the form of impaired daytime function, mood disturbances, and increased risk of injury due to accidents.

Psychophysiologic Insomnia Persistent psychophysiologic insomnia is a behavioral disorder in which patients are preoccupied with a perceived inability to sleep adequately at night. The sleep disturbance is often triggered by an emotionally stressful event; however, the poor sleep habits acquired during the stressful period persist long after the initial incident. Such patients become hyperaroused by their own persistent efforts to sleep and/or the sleep environment, and the insomnia is a conditioned or learned response. Patients with psychophysiologic insomnia fall asleep more easily at unscheduled times (when not trying) or outside the home environment. In these cases, polysomnographic recording reveals an objective sleep disturbance, often with an abnormally long sleep latency, frequent nocturnal awakenings, and an increased amount of stage 1 transitional sleep. Extrinsic factors may contribute to this condition (see below). Rigorous attention should be paid to sleep hygiene (see below) and correction of counterproductive, arousing behaviors before bedtime. Behavioral therapy (i.e., sleep hygiene, relaxation training, stimulus control therapy, sleep restriction therapy) is the treatment modality of choice for psychophysiologic insomnia, and such therapy appears best instituted without medication.

Extrinsic Insomnia A number of sleep disorders are the result of extrinsic factors that interfere with sleep. *Adjustment sleep disorder*, also called *transient situational insomnia*, can occur after a change in the sleeping environment (e.g., in an unfamiliar hotel or hospital bed) or before or after a significant life event, such as a change of occupation, loss of a loved one, illness, or anxiety over a deadline or examination. Increased sleep latency, frequent awakenings from sleep, and early morning awakening can all occur. Recovery generally occurs rapidly, certainly within 2 to 3 weeks. *Inadequate sleep hygiene* is characterized

Table 27-2

Evaluation of the Patient with the Complaint of Excessive Daytime Somnolence

Findings on History and Physical Examination	Diagnostic Evaluation	Diagnosis	Therapy
Obesity, snoring, hypertension	Polysomnography with respiratory monitoring	Obstructive sleep apnea	Continuous positive airway pressure; ENT surgery (e.g., uvulopalatopharyngoplasty); dental appliance; pharmacologic therapy (e.g., protriptyline); weight loss; (see Chap. 264)
Cataplexy, hypnogogic hallucinations, sleep paralysis, family history	Polysomnography with multiple sleep latency test	Narcolepsy-cataplexy syndrome	Stimulants (e.g., methylphenidate, pemoline); REM-suppressant antidepressants (e.g., protriptyline); genetic counseling
Restless legs syndrome, disturbed sleep, predisposing medical condition (e.g., anemia or renal failure)	Polysomnography with bilateral anterior tibialis EMG	Periodic limb movements of sleep	Treatment of predisposing condition, if possible; dopamine agonists (e.g., levodopa-carbidopa); benzodiazepines (e.g., clonazepam)
Disturbed sleep, predisposing medical conditions (e.g., asthma) and/or predisposing medical therapies (e.g., theophylline)	Sleep-wake diary	Insomnias (see text)	Treatment of predisposing condition and/or change in therapy, if possible; behavioral therapy; short-acting benzodiazepine receptor agonist (e.g., zolpidem)

NOTE: ENT, ears, nose, throat; REM, rapid eye movement; EMG, electromyogram.

by a behavior pattern prior to sleep and/or a bedroom environment that is not conducive to sleep. Noise and/or light in the bedroom can interfere with sleep, as can a bed partner with periodic limb movements during sleep or one who snores loudly. Luminous clocks can arouse the patient, heightening anxiety about the time it has taken to fall asleep. Drugs that act on the central nervous system, large meals, vigorous exercise, or hot showers just before sleep may interfere with sleep onset. In preference to hypnotic medications, patients should be counseled to develop a soporific bedtime ritual and to prepare and reserve the bedroom environment for sleeping. Consistent, regular rising times should be charted daily; total time in bed should be restricted to actual sleep time.

Altitude Insomnia Sleep disturbance is a common consequence of exposure to high altitude. Periodic breathing of the Cheyne-Stokes type occurs during NREM sleep about half the time at altitude, with restoration of a regular breathing pattern during REM sleep. Central rather than obstructive sleep apnea appears to be responsible, characterized by regular respiratory pauses. Both hypoxia and hypocapnia are thought to be involved in the development of periodic breathing. Frequent awakenings and poor quality sleep characterize altitude insomnia, which is generally worst on the first few nights at high altitude but may persist. The duration of sleep is unchanged, but there are more arousals after sleep onset and less time in slow-wave (stages 3 and 4) sleep. Treatment with acetazolamide can decrease time spent in periodic breathing and substantially reduce hypoxia during sleep. Medroxyprogesterone acetate also reduces hypoxia but does not significantly reduce periodic breathing during sleep at altitude.

Drug- or Alcohol-Dependent Sleep Disorders Disturbed sleep can result from ingestion of a wide variety of agents. Caffeine is perhaps the most common pharmacologic cause of insomnia in sensitive patients. It produces increased latency to sleep onset, more frequent arousals during sleep, and a reduction in total sleep time for up to 8 to 14 h after ingestion. Occasional patients are surprised to learn that their insomnia may be related to coffee consumption; a careful history will reveal that such patients may drink 15 to 20 cups per day. As few as 3 to 5 cups of coffee can significantly disturb sleep in some patients; therefore, a 1- to 2-month caffeine withdrawal period should be attempted in patients with these symptoms. Similarly, alcohol and nicotine can interfere with sleep, although many patients use them to relax and promote sleep. Although alcohol can increase drowsiness and shorten sleep latency, even moderate amounts of alcohol increase awakenings after sleep onset by interfering with the ability of the brain to maintain sleep. In addition, alcohol ingestion prior to sleep is contraindicated in patients with sleep apnea because of the inhibitory effects of alcohol on upper airway muscle tone. Acutely, amphetamines and cocaine suppress both REM sleep and total sleep time, which return to normal with chronic use. Withdrawal leads to a REM sleep rebound. Finally, rebound insomnia associated with the acute withdrawal of hypnotics can be severe, especially following the use of high doses of benzodiazepines with a short half-life. For this reason, hypnotics should rarely be prescribed for habitual use; doses should be low to moderate, the total duration of hypnotic therapy should be limited to 2 to 3 weeks, and drug dosage should be reduced prior to withdrawal.

NARCOLEPSY Excessive daytime sleepiness with involuntary daytime sleep episodes, disturbed nocturnal sleep, and cataplexy (sudden weakness or loss of muscle tone without loss of consciousness that is elicited by emotion) are the most common symptoms of narcolepsy (see Table 27-3). Some patients also experience muscular paralysis and/or hallucinations at sleep onset or upon awakening. The severity varies. Patients may have two to three cataplectic attacks per day or per decade, and the extent and duration of an attack may vary from a transient sagging of the jaw lasting a few seconds to flaccid paralysis of the entire voluntary musculature for up to 20 to 30 min, in rare cases.

Narcolepsy affects about 1 in 4000 people in the United States and appears to have a genetic basis. Experiments in some canine models of narcolepsy suggest an autosomal recessive pattern of inheritance. First-degree relatives of narcoleptic patients have about a 1 percent incidence of narcolepsy, much higher than the general popula-

tion. In addition, nearly all narcoleptics are positive for the human leukocyte antigen DR15 (ordinarily found in 20 to 30 percent of the general population) (see Chap. 306). A high rate of discordance in identical twins indicates that one or more nonheritable factors contributes to its development.

Symptoms typically begin in the second decade, although the onset ranges from ages 5 to 50. Once established, the disease is chronic without remissions.

Diagnosis Classically, the diagnosis of narcolepsy required the presence of the "narcolepsy tetrad," consisting of (1) excessive daytime somnolence, (2) cataplexy, (3) hypnogogic hallucinations (the occurrence of vivid hallucinatory dream imagery at sleep onset), and (4) sleep paralysis (an awareness that voluntary musculature is paralyzed coincident with the onset of sleep). The last three symptoms of the tetrad are all manifestations of the abnormal REM sleep regulation inherent in the syndrome. All patients with narcolepsy have objectively verifiable daytime somnolence, but the other three symptoms are variably present, and only cataplexy is unique to narcolepsy. At least half have cataplexy of some degree, and similar percentages report hypnogogic hallucinations and/or sleep paralysis. Other associated symptoms are useful but not specific. A history of "automatic behavior" during wakefulness (a trancelike state during which simple motor behaviors persist) serves principally to corroborate the presence of daytime somnolence but is not specific for mechanism. Patients with narcolepsy also commonly report severe disruption of nocturnal sleep.

A family history is important in the evaluation of the patient with excessive daytime somnolence. Careful observation of the children and siblings of known narcoleptics, particularly at the typical age of onset (second decade), can lead to early diagnosis. The diagnosis of narcolepsy in a patient with a suggestive history depends upon (1) objective verification of excessive daytime somnolence, typically using the MSLT after nocturnal sleep recording; (2) a history of unambiguous cataplexy; (3) documentation of abnormal REM sleep regulation as evidenced by REM sleep onset within 10 min of sleep onset, either during the nocturnal recording or on one or more of the MSLT determinations; and (4) exclusion of other disorders, such as sleep apnea, that cause excessive sleepiness.

℞ TREATMENT

The treatment of narcolepsy is symptomatic. Somnolence is treated with stimulants. Methylphenidate is considered the drug of choice by most. Pemoline, a common second choice, has a longer half-life and is associated with fewer side effects but may not be as effective. Dextroamphetamine and methamphetamine are also frequently used, particularly when methylphenidate and pemoline are inadequate.

Treatment of cataplexy, hypnogogic hallucinations, and sleep paralysis requires antidepressants, which are effective, in part, because of potent REM-suppressive effects. Protriptyline, imipramine, and clomipramine are commonly used in the United States. Efficacy is limited largely by anticholinergic side effects. Fluoxetine and other serotonin reuptake inhibitors are often effective for this condition.

Table 27-3

Prevalence of Symptoms in Narcolepsy

Symptom	Prevalence, %
Excessive daytime somnolence	100
Disturbed sleep	87
Cataplexy	76
Hypnogogic hallucinations	68
Sleep paralysis	64
Memory problems	50

SOURCE: Modified from TA Roth, L Merlotti in SA Burton et al (eds), *Narcolepsy 3rd International Symposium: Selected Symposium Proceedings*, Chicago, Matrix Communications, 1989.

SLEEP APNEA SYNDROMES Respiratory dysfunction during sleep is a common, serious cause of excessive daytime somnolence as well as of disturbed nocturnal sleep. An estimated 2 to 5 million people in the United States stop breathing for 10 to 150 s, from thirty to several hundred times every night during sleep. These cessations of breathing may be due to either an occlusion of the airway (*obstructive sleep apnea*), absence of respiratory effort (*central sleep apnea*), or a combination of these factors (*mixed sleep apnea*). Failure to recognize and appropriately treat these conditions may lead to serious cardiovascular complications and increased mortality. This problem is particularly prevalent in overweight men and in the elderly and is often associated with hypertension. Occult sleep-related breathing disorders may result in significant impairment of daytime alertness and functioning in otherwise healthy elderly persons. → *Readers are referred to Chap. 263 for a comprehensive review of the diagnosis and treatment of patients with these conditions.*

DYSSOMNIA ASSOCIATED WITH LIMB MOVEMENTS
Restless Legs Syndrome Patients with dyssomnia associated with the restless legs syndrome (RLS) report an irresistible urge to move their legs when awake and inactive, especially when lying in bed just prior to sleep. This interferes with the ability to fall asleep. They report a creeping or crawling sensation deep within the calves or thighs, or sometimes even in the upper limbs, that is only relieved briefly by movement, particularly walking. In contrast, paresthesia secondary to peripheral neuropathy persists with activity. The severity of this chronic, idiopathic disorder may wax and wane with time and can be exacerbated by caffeine and pregnancy. Iron- or folic acid-deficiency anemia and renal failure may actually cause RLS, which is then considered secondary RLS. Nearly all patients with restless legs also experience periodic limb movement disorder during sleep, although the reverse is not the case.

Periodic Limb Movement Disorder Periodic limb movement disorder, also known as *nocturnal myoclonus*, is the principal objective polysomnographic finding in 17 percent of patients with insomnia and 11 percent of those with excessive daytime somnolence. This condition can be documented in one-sixth of patients with insomnia seen at sleep disorders centers, although it is often thought to be an incidental finding rather than the cause of disturbed sleep. Stereotyped, rhythmic, 0.5- to 5.0-s extensions of the great toe and dorsiflexion of the foot recur every 20 to 40 s during NREM stages 1 and 2 sleep, in episodes lasting from minutes to hours. Most such episodes occur during the first half of the night. The disorder occurs in a wide variety of sleep disorders (including narcolepsy, sleep apnea, REM sleep behavior disorder, and various forms of insomnia) and is associated with frequent arousals and an increased number of sleep-stage transitions. However, it has not been demonstrated that these sleep disturbances always lead to insomnia. In fact, periodic limb movement may be secondary to chronic sleep-wake disturbance rather than the cause of it. The incidence increases with age; 44 percent of healthy subjects over age 65 without a sleep complaint and almost all patients with RLS have periodic limb movements. The pathophysiology is not well understood. Polysomnography with bilateral surface EMG recording of the anterior tibialis, extensor carpi radialis, triceps and/or biceps is used to establish the diagnosis. Treatment options are limited; some patients may respond to a combination of carbidopa and levodopa, clonazepam, or levodopa alone.

PARASOMNIAS The term *parasomnia* refers to behavioral disorders during sleep that are associated with brief or partial arousals but not with marked sleep disruption or impaired daytime alertness. The presenting complaint is usually related to the behavior itself. Most are more common in children but may persist into adulthood when their occurrence may have more pathologic significance.

Sleepwalking (Somnambulism) Patients affected by this disorder carry out automatic motor activities that range from minor to complex. Individuals may leave the bed, walk, urinate inappropriately, or exit from the house while remaining unconscious or uncommunica-

tive. Arousal is difficult, and untoward or even fatal activities can occur. Sleepwalking occurs in stage 3 or 4 NREM sleep. It is most common in children and adolescents. Episodes are usually isolated but may be recurrent in 1 to 6 percent of patients. The cause is unknown.

Sleep Terrors This disorder, also called *pavor nocturnus*, occurs primarily in young children during the first several hours after sleep onset, in stages 3 and 4 of NREM sleep. The child suddenly screams, exhibiting autonomic arousal with sweating, tachycardia, and hyperventilation. The individual may be difficult to arouse and rarely recalls the episode on awakening in the morning. Recurrent attacks are rare, and treatment is usually by way of reassurance of parents. Both sleep terrors and sleepwalking represent abnormalities of arousal. In contrast, *nightmares* (dream anxiety attacks) occur during REM sleep and cause full arousal, with memory for the dream-associated unpleasant episode.

REM Sleep Behavior Disorder This is a rare parasomnia arising from REM sleep instead of slow-wave sleep, as is characteristic of the other, more common parasomnias. It primarily afflicts men of middle age or older, many of whom have a history of prior neurologic disease (e.g., degenerative diseases, Guillain-Barré syndrome, dementia, subarachnoid hemorrhage, stroke). Presenting symptoms are of violent behavior during sleep, reported by a bed partner. In contrast to typical somnambulism, injury to patient or bystander is common, and, upon awakening, the patient reports vivid, often unpleasant dream imagery. The principal differential diagnosis is that of nocturnal seizures, which can be excluded with polysomnography. In REM sleep behavior disorder, seizure activity is absent, and the EEG/EOG REM sleep pattern exhibits a high-amplitude EMG. Complex, purposeful motor behavior occurs during REM sleep episodes. The pathogenesis is unclear, but the preexisting neurologic disease may have involved brainstem areas responsible for descending motor inhibition during REM sleep. In support of this hypothesis are the remarkable similarities between the REM sleep behavior disorder and the sleep of animals with bilateral lesions of the pontine tegmentum in areas controlling REM sleep motor inhibition. Treatment with clonazepam provides sustained improvement in almost all reported cases.

Sleep Bruxism Bruxism is an involuntary, forceful grinding of teeth during sleep that affects 10 to 20 percent of the population. The patient is usually unaware of the problem, and data on this parasomnia come from roommates and bed partners, alarmed by the loud grinding noise, and from dentists who see evidence of destruction of tooth enamel and dentum. The typical age of onset is 17 to 20 years, and spontaneous remission usually occurs by age 40. Sex distribution appears to be equal.

Hypotheses about the pathophysiology suggest contributory roles for dental abnormalities, e.g., malocclusion, and for central neural mechanisms. Psychological factors may also play a role in that stress exacerbates the disorder. Treatment is dictated by the risk of dental injury. In many cases, the diagnosis is made during dental examination, damage is minor, and no treatment is indicated. In more severe cases, treatment with a rubber tooth guard is necessary to prevent permanent and disfiguring tooth injury. Stress management or, in some cases, biofeedback can be useful when bruxism is a manifestation of severe stress. Useful pharmacologic therapy has not been described.

Sleep Enuresis Bedwetting, like sleepwalking and night terrors, is another parasomnia occurring during slow-wave sleep in the young. Before age 5 or 6, nocturnal enuresis should probably be considered a normal feature of development. The condition usually spontaneously improves at puberty, has a prevalence in late adolescence of 1 to 3 percent, and is rare in adulthood. The age threshold for initiation of treatment depends on parental and patient concern about the problem. Persistence of enuresis into adolescence or adulthood may reflect a variety of underlying conditions. In older patients with enuresis a distinction must be made between primary and secondary enuresis, the latter being defined as bedwetting in patients who have been fully continent for 6 to 12 months. Treatment of primary enuresis is reserved for patients of appropriate age (older than 5 or 6 years) and consists of bladder training exercises and behavioral therapy. Urologic abnormalities are more common in primary enuresis and must be assessed by urologic examination. Important causes of secondary enuresis include emotional disturbances, urinary tract infections, cauda equina lesions, epilepsy, sleep apnea, and urinary tract malformations. In the patient for whom enuresis may be a source of significant stress, symptomatic pharmacotherapy may be appropriate while attention is also paid to underlying causes. This is usually accomplished with oxybutynin chloride or imipramine. Intranasal desmopressin has been used in some patients.

Miscellaneous Parasomnias Other clinical entities fulfill the definition of a parasomnia in that they occur selectively during sleep and are associated with some degree of sleep disruption. Examples include *jactatio capitis nocturna* (nocturnal headbanging), sleep talking, and nocturnal leg cramps.

SLEEP DISORDERS ASSOCIATED WITH MEDICAL/ PSYCHIATRIC DISORDERS **Sleep Disorders Associated with Mental Disorders** Sleep architecture and physiology are disturbed in *schizophrenia* (with a decreased amount of stage 4 sleep and a lack of augmentation of REM sleep following REM sleep deprivation); chronic schizophrenics usually show day-night reversal, sleep fragmentation, and insomnia. Patients with other psychiatric disorders (anxiety disorders, affective illness, obsessive-compulsive disorders, and chronic alcoholism) also often sleep poorly. There is considerable heterogeneity, however, in the nature of the sleep disturbance both between conditions and among patients with the same condition.

Depression can be associated with sleep onset insomnia, sleep maintenance insomnia, and/or early morning wakefulness. However, hypersomnia occurs in some depressed patients, especially adolescents and those with either bipolar or seasonal (fall/winter) depression (see also Chap. 385). Indeed, sleep disturbance is an important vegetative sign of depression and may commence before any mood changes are perceived by the patient. Consistent polysomnographic findings in depression include decreased REM sleep latency, lengthened first REM sleep episode, and shortened first NREM sleep episode; however, these findings are not specific for depression, and the extent of these changes varies with age and symptomatology. Depressed patients also show decreased slow-wave sleep and reduced sleep continuity.

In *mania* and *hypomania*, sleep latency is increased and total sleep time can be reduced. Patients with *anxiety disorders* tend not to show the changes in REM sleep and slow-wave sleep seen in endogenously depressed patients. Finally, *chronic alcoholics* lack slow-wave sleep, have decreased amounts of REM sleep (as an acute response to alcohol), and have frequent arousals throughout the night. This is associated with impaired daytime alertness. The sleep of chronic alcoholics remains disturbed for years after discontinuance of alcohol usage.

Sleep Disorders Associated with Neurologic Disorders A variety of neurologic diseases result in sleep disruption through both indirect, nonspecific mechanisms (e.g., pain in cervical spondylosis or low back pain) or by impairment of central neural structures involved in the generation and control of sleep itself.

For example, the dementias have long been associated with disturbances in the timing of the sleep-wake cycle, often characterized by nocturnal wandering and an exacerbation of symptomatology at night (so-called sundowning). Such clinical observations are consistent with the neuropathologic report that 80 percent of the cells in the hypothalamic circadian pacemaker (the SCN) are lost in patients with senile dementia (Alzheimer's disease), though the report has not been replicated and a causal association remains unproven.

Epilepsy may rarely present as a sleep complaint (see also Chap. 365). Often the history is of abnormal behavior, at times with convulsive movements, during sleep, and the differential diagnosis includes REM sleep behavior disorder, sleep apnea syndrome, and periodic movements of sleep (see above). Diagnosis requires nocturnal EEG recording. Other neurologic diseases associated with abnormal movements, such as *Parkinson's disease, hemiballismus, Huntington's chorea,* and *Gilles de la Tourette syndrome*, are also associated with disrupted sleep, presumably through secondary mechanisms. Headache syndromes may show sleep-associated exacerbations (*migraine* or *cluster headache*) (see also Chaps. 15 and 364). The mechanism of association between sleep and headache is unknown.

Fatal familial insomnia is a rare hereditary disorder caused by bilateral degeneration of anterior and dorsomedial nuclei of the thalamus. Insomnia is a prominent early symptom. Progressively, the syndrome produces autonomic dysfunction, dysarthria, myoclonus, coma, and death. The pathogenesis of the thalamic destruction is unknown.

Sleep Disorders Associated with Other Medical Disorders A number of medical conditions are associated with disruptions of sleep. The association may be nonspecific, for example, that between sleep disruption and chronic pain from rheumatologic disorders. Attention to this association is important in that sleep-associated symptoms are the presenting complaint of many such patients. In addition, sleep disruption may stem from the appropriate use of drugs such as steroids or from the symptoms of another illness.

Among the most prominent associations is that between sleep disruption and *asthma*. In many asthmatics there is a prominent daily variation in airway resistance that results in marked increases in asthmatic symptoms at night, especially during sleep. In addition, treatment of asthma with theophylline-based compounds, adrenergic agonists, or glucocorticoids can independently disrupt sleep. When sleep disruption is a prominent side effect of asthma treatment, inhaled steroids (e.g., beclomethasone) that do not disrupt sleep may provide a useful alternative.

Cardiac ischemia may also be associated with sleep disruption. Variability in autonomic nervous system function during REM sleep may account for the association of sleep and angina, although this remains unproven. Patients may present with complaints of nightmares or vivid, disturbing dreams, with or without awareness of the more classical symptoms of angina. Recent work suggests that patients with nocturnal angina are likely to have obstructive sleep apnea, treatment of which may substantially improve the nocturnal angina symptoms. *Paroxysmal nocturnal dyspnea* can also occur as a consequence of sleep-associated cardiac ischemia that causes pulmonary congestion exacerbated by recumbent posture.

Chronic obstructive pulmonary disease is also associated with sleep disruption. Other conditions associated with sleep disruption include *cystic fibrosis, menopause, hyperthyroidism, gastroesophageal reflux, chronic renal failure,* and *liver failure.*

CIRCADIAN RHYTHM SLEEP DISORDERS

A subset of patients presenting with either insomnia or hypersomnia may have a disorder of sleep *timing* rather than sleep *generation.* Disorders of sleep timing can either be organic (i.e., due to an intrinsic defect in the circadian pacemaker or its input from entraining stimuli) or environmental (i.e., due to a disruption of exposure to entraining stimuli from the environment). Regardless of etiology, the symptoms reflect the influence of the underlying circadian pacemaker on sleep-wake function. Thus, effective therapeutic approaches should aim to entrain the oscillator at an appropriate phase.

RAPID TIME-ZONE CHANGE (JET LAG) SYNDROME More than 60 million people experience transmeridian air travel annually, which is often associated with excessive daytime sleepiness, sleep onset insomnia, and frequent arousals from sleep, particularly in the latter half of the night. Gastrointestinal discomfort is common. The syndrome is transient, typically lasting 2 to 14 d depending on the number of time zones crossed, the direction of travel, and the traveler's age and phase-shifting capacity. Travelers who spend more time outdoors reportedly adapt more quickly than those who remain in hotel rooms, presumably due to bright (outdoor) light exposure.

SHIFT-WORK SLEEP DISORDER About 7 million workers in the United States regularly work at night, either on a permanent or rotating schedule. In addition, each week millions of Americans elect to remain awake at night to meet deadlines, drive long distances, or participate in recreational activities, leading to an inversion of their sleep-wake cycle. Studies of regular night-shift workers indicate that the circadian timing system typically fails to adapt successfully to such inverted schedules. This leads to a misalignment between the desired work-rest schedule and the output of the pacemaker and in disturbed daytime sleep. Consequent sleep deprivation, increased length of time awake prior to work, and misalignment of circadian phase produce decreased alertness and performance and cause increased safety hazards among night workers. Routine tasks such as highway driving are particularly vulnerable to sleep-related accidents. There is a marked increase in the risk of fatal-to-the-driver road accidents between midnight and 6 A.M., even when alcohol is eliminated as a causal factor. In addition, chronic shift workers have higher rates of cardiac, gastrointestinal, and reproductive disorders.

Interventions should promote increased awareness of the hazards associated with night work and should be aimed at minimizing both circadian disruption and sleep deprivation. The work schedule should minimize: (1) exposure to night work; (2) the frequency of shift rotation so that shifts do not rotate more than once every 2 to 3 weeks; (3) the number of consecutive night shifts worked from seven (which is typical) to four or five; and (4) the duration of night shifts. In addition, strategic use of bright-light exposure can facilitate rapid adaptation to night-shift work, where feasible. These steps can lead to marked improvements in employee health and performance and to reduced accident rates among shift workers.

DELAYED SLEEP PHASE SYNDROME Delayed sleep phase syndrome is characterized by: (1) reported sleep onset and wake times intractably later than desired; (2) actual sleep times at nearly the same clock hours daily; and (3) essentially normal all-night polysomnography except for delayed sleep onset. Patients exhibit an abnormally delayed endogenous circadian phase, with the temperature minimum during the constant routine occurring later than normal. This delayed phase could be due to: (1) an abnormally long intrinsic period of the endogenous circadian pacemaker; (2) an abnormally reduced phase-advancing capacity of the pacemaker; or (3) an irregular prior sleep-wake schedule, characterized by frequent nights when the patient chooses to remain awake well past midnight (for social, school, or work reasons). In most cases, it is difficult to distinguish among these factors, since patients with an abnormally long intrinsic period are more likely to "choose" such late-night activities because they are unable to sleep at that time. Patients tend to be young adults. This self-perpetuating condition can persist for years and does not usually respond to attempts to reestablish normal bedtime hours.

Patients respond to a rescheduling regimen in which bedtimes are successively delayed by about 3 h/d until the desired (and earlier) bedtime is achieved. Treatment methods involving bright-light phototherapy during the morning hours also show promise in these patients.

ADVANCED SLEEP PHASE SYNDROME Advanced sleep phase syndrome is the converse of the delayed sleep phase syndrome and tends to occur in the elderly. Patients with this condition report excessive daytime sleepiness during the evening hours, when they have great difficulty remaining awake, even in social settings. The patients awaken from 3 to 5 A.M. each day, often several hours before their desired wake times. Although such patients have not been studied extensively, some of these patients may benefit from bright-light phototherapy during the evening hours, designed to reset the circadian pacemaker to a later hour.

NON-24-H SLEEP-WAKE DISORDER This condition can occur when the maximal phase-advancing capacity of the circadian pacemaker is not adequate to accommodate the difference between the 24-h geophysical day and the intrinsic period of the pacemaker in the patient. Alternatively, patients' self-selected exposure to artificial light may drive the circadian pacemaker to a longer than 24-h schedule. Patients affected are not able to maintain a stable phase relationship between the output of the pacemaker and the 24-h day. Such patients typically present with an incremental pattern of successive delays in sleep onsets and wake times, progressing in and out of phase with local time. When the patient's endogenous rhythms are out of phase with the local environment, insomnia coexists with excessive daytime sleepiness. Conversely, when the endogenous rhythms are in phase with the local environment, symptoms remit. The intervals of alternation between symptomatic vs. asymptomatic intervals may last several weeks to several months. Blind individuals unable to perceive light are particularly susceptible to this disorder.

MEDICAL IMPLICATIONS OF CIRCADIAN RHYTHMIC-ITY Understanding the role of circadian rhythmicity in the pathophysiology of illness may lead to improvements in diagnosis and treatment. For example, prominent circadian variations have been reported in the incidence of *acute myocardial infarction*, *sudden cardiac death*, and *stroke*, the leading causes of death in the United States. Platelet aggregability is increased after arising in the early morning hours, coincident with the peak incidence of these cardiovascular events. A better understanding of the possible role of circadian rhythmicity in the acute destabilization of a chronic condition such as atherosclerotic disease could improve the understanding of the pathophysiology.

Diagnostic and therapeutic procedures may also be affected by the time of day at which data are collected. Examples include blood pressure, body temperature, the dexamethasone suppression test, and plasma cortisol levels. The timing of chemotherapy administration has been reported to have an effect on the outcome of treatment. Few physicians realize the extent to which routine measures are affected by the time (or sleep/wake state) when the measurement is made.

In addition, both the toxicity and effectiveness of drugs can vary during the day. For example, more than a fivefold difference has been observed in mortality rates following administration of toxic agents to experimental animals at different times of day. Anesthetic agents are particularly sensitive to time-of-day effects.

Finally, it should be noted that the risk of errors and accidents due to inattention and/or sleepiness varies markedly with the time of day. Single-vehicle truck accidents, industrial errors and accidents, and lapses of attention all peak during a critical zone of vulnerability that typically occurs during the latter half of the night, coincident with maximal sleep drive within the brain. The physician must be increasingly aware of the public health risks associated with the ever-increasing demands made by the duty-rest-recreation schedules in our round-the-clock society.

BIBLIOGRAPHY

ALDRICH MS: Narcolepsy. Neurology 42 (Suppl 6):34, 1992

BECKER PM et al: Dopaminergic agents in restless legs syndrome and periodic limb movements of sleep: Response and complications of extended treatment in 49 cases. Sleep 16:713, 1993

BENCA RM et al: Sleep and psychiatric disorders. A meta-analysis. Arch Gen Psychiatry 49:651, 1992

BLIWISE DL: Sleep in normal aging and dementia. Sleep 16:40, 1993

CZEISLER CA et al: Exposure to bright light and darkness to treat physiologic maladaptation to night work. N Engl J Med 322:1253, 1990

———— et al: Association of sleep-wake habits in older people with changes in output of circadian pacemaker. Lancet 340:933, 1992

———— et al: Suppression of melatonin secretion in some blind patients by exposure to bright light. N Engl J Med 332:6, 1995

DIAGNOSTIC CLASSIFICATION STEERING COMMITTEE, THORPY MJ(chairman): *International Classification of Sleep Disorders: Diagnostic and Coding Manual*. Rochester, MN, American Sleep Disorders Association, 1990

DIJK D-J, CZEISLER CA: Contribution of the circadian pacemaker and the sleep homeostat to sleep propensity, sleep structure, electroencephalographic slow waves, and sleep spindle activity in humans. J Neurosci 15:3526, 1995

FARNEY RJ, WALKER JM: Office management of common sleep-wake disorders. Med Clin North Am 79:391, 1995

FINDLEY LJ et al: Drivers with untreated sleep apnea. A cause of death and serious injury. Arch Intern Med 151:1451, 1991

FRANKLIN KA et al: Sleep apnea and nocturnal angina. Lancet 345:1085, 1995

GUILLEMINAULT C et al: Nondrug treatment trials in psychophysiologic insomnia. Arch Intern Med 155:838, 1995

KRYGER MH et al (eds): *Principles and Practice of Sleep Medicine*, 2d ed. Philadelphia, Saunders, 1994

LYDIC R et al: Cholinergic reticular mechanisms influence state-dependent ventilatory response to hypercapnia. Am J Physiol 261:R738, 1991

Polo O et al: Management of obstructive sleep apnoea/hypopnoea syndrome. Lancet 344:656, 1994

Radecki SF, Brunton SA: Management of insomnia in office-based practice: National prevalence and therapeutic patterns. Arch Fam Med 2:1129, 1993

Schwartz WJ: A clinician's primer on the circadian clock: Its localization, function, and resetting. Adv Intern Med 38:81m, 1993

Sherin JE et al: Activation of ventrolateral preoptic neurons during sleep. Science 271:216, 1996

Tateishi J et al: First experimental transmission of fatal familial insomnia. Nature 376:434, 1995

U.S. Congress, Office of Technology Assessment: *Biological Rhythms: Implications for the Worker*, OTA-BA-463. Washington, DC, U.S. Government Printing Office, September, 1991

SECTION 4

DISORDERS OF EYES, EARS, NOSE, AND THROAT

---

28 *Jonathan C. Horton*

DISORDERS OF THE EYE

THE HUMAN VISUAL SYSTEM

The visual system provides a supremely efficient means for the rapid assimilation of information from the environment to aid in the guidance of behavior. The act of seeing begins with the capture of images focused by the cornea and lens upon a light-sensitive membrane in the back of the eye, called the *retina*. The retina is actually part of the brain, banished to the periphery to serve as a transducer for the conversion of patterns of light energy into neuronal signals. Light is absorbed by photopigment in two classes of receptors: rods and cones. There are approximately 100 million rods and 5 million cones in the human retina. The rods are operative under scotopic, or dim, illumination. The cones, active under photopic, or daylight, conditions, are specialized for color perception and high spatial resolution. The majority of cones are located within the macula, the portion of the retina serving the central 10° of vision. In the middle of the macula a small pit termed the *fovea*, packed exclusively with cones, provides best visual acuity.

Photoreceptors hyperpolarize to light, activating bipolar, amacrine, and horizontal cells in the inner nuclear layer. After processing of the photoreceptor response by this complex retinal circuit, the flow of sensory information ultimately converges upon a final common pathway: the ganglion cells. These cells translate the visual image impinging upon the retina into a continuously varying barrage of action potentials that propagates along the primary optic pathway to visual centers within the brain. There are a million ganglion cells in each retina, and hence a million fibers in each optic nerve.

Ganglion cell axons sweep along the inner surface of the retina in the nerve fiber layer, exit the eye at the optic disc, and travel through the optic nerve, optic chiasm, and optic tract to reach targets in the brain. The majority of fibers synapse upon cells in the lateral geniculate body, a thalamic relay station. Cells in the lateral geniculate body project in turn to the primary visual cortex. This massive afferent retinogeniculocortical sensory pathway provides the neural substrate for visual perception. Although the lateral geniculate body is the main target of the retina, separate classes of ganglion cells project to other subcortical visual nuclei involved in different functions. The pupillary reflex is mediated by input to the pretectal olivary nuclei in the midbrain. These pretectal nuclei send their output to the ipsilateral and contralateral Edinger-Westphal nuclei of the oculomotor nuclear complex. Cells in the Edinger-Westphal nuclei provide parasympathetic innervation to the iris sphincter via an interneuron in the ciliary ganglion. Circadian rhythms are timed by a retinal projection to the suprachiasmatic nucleus. Visual orientation and eye movements are served by retinal input to the superior colliculus. Gaze stabilization and optokinetic reflexes are governed by a group of small retinal targets known collectively as the *brainstem accessory optic system.*

Finally, there is a sizeable retinal projection to the pulvinar, a large thalamic visual nucleus of obscure function.

The eyes must be rotated constantly within their orbits to place and maintain targets of visual interest upon the fovea. This activity, called *foveation*, or *looking*, is governed by an elaborate efferent motor system. Each eye is moved by six extraocular muscles, supplied by cranial nerves from the oculomotor (III), trochlear (IV), and abducens (VI) nuclei. Activity in these ocular motor nuclei is coordinated by pontine and midbrain mechanisms for smooth pursuit, saccades, and gaze stabilization during head and body movements. Large regions of the frontal and parietooccipital cortex control these brainstem eye movement centers by providing descending supranuclear input.

Visual function can be disturbed in myriad ways. The eyes are mounted in a prominent position on the head, where they are vulnerable to trauma, exposure, and infection. Vision can be damaged by diseases intrinsic to the eye, such as glaucoma, cataract, or retinal detachment. Many neurologic diseases produce ocular symptoms, because extensive areas of the cortex, thalamus, and brainstem are devoted to visual perception or to the execution of eye movements. In genetic disorders, eye manifestations are common and often help the clinician to recognize a rare syndrome. Finally, the eyes are affected frequently by acquired systemic diseases.

The eye is a specialized organ, requiring unique optical instruments for proper examination. The slit lamp and ophthalmoscope proffer a beautiful, magnified view of the transparent anatomy of the eye and afford the only opportunity for direct inspection of blood vessels in a living subject. Some physicians do not acquire sufficient facility with these instruments and consequently feel unable to care for patients with eye problems. Although it may be determined that a patient requires specialized eye care, the initial evaluation of ocular symptoms lies within the purview of all physicians, and the assessment of visual acuity, pupils, eye movements, visual fields, and the fundi remain part of any complete physical examination.

CLINICAL ASSESSMENT OF VISUAL FUNCTION

REFRACTIVE STATE In approaching the patient with reduced vision, the first step is to decide whether refractive error is responsible. In *emmetropia*, parallel rays from infinity are focused perfectly upon the retina. Sadly, this condition is enjoyed by only a minority of the population. In *myopia*, the globe is too long, and light rays come to a focal point in front of the retina. Near objects can be seen clearly, but distant objects require a diverging lens in front of the eye. In *hyperopia*, the globe is too short, and hence a converging lens is used to supplement the refractive power of the eye. In *astigmatism*, the corneal surface is not perfectly spherical, necessitating a cylindrical corrective lens. With the onset of middle age, *presbyopia* develops as the lens within the eye becomes unable to increase its refractive power to accommodate upon near objects. To compensate for presbyopia, the emmetropic patient must use reading glasses. The patient already wearing glasses for distance correction usually switches to bifocals. The only exception is the myope, who may achieve clear vision at near simply by removing glasses containing the distance prescription.

Refractive errors usually develop slowly and remain stable after adolescence, except in unusual circumstances. For example, the acute onset of diabetes mellitus can produce sudden myopia because of fluid imbibition and swelling of the lens induced by hyperglycemia. Testing vision through a pinhole aperture is a useful way to screen quickly for refractive error. If the visual acuity is better through a pinhole than with the unaided eye, the patient needs a formal refraction screening.

VISUAL ACUITY The Snellen chart is used to test acuity at a distance of 6 m (20 ft). For convenience, a scale version of the Snellen chart, called the Rosenbaum card, is held at 36 cm (14 in) from the patient (Fig. 28-1). All subjects should be able to read the 6/6 m (20/20 ft) line with each eye using the proper refractive correction. Patients who need reading glasses must wear them for accurate testing. If 6/6 (20/20) acuity is not present in each eye, the deficiency in vision must be explained. For acuity worse than 6/240 (20/800), the ability to count fingers, see hand motions, or perceive a bright light should be recorded. Legal blindness is defined by the Internal Revenue Service as a best corrected acuity of 6/60 (20/200) or less in the better eye, or a binocular visual field subtending 20° or less. For driving the laws vary by state, but most require a corrected acuity of 6/12 (20/40) in at least one eye. Patients with a homonymous hemianopia cannot drive.

PUPILS The pupils should be tested individually in dim light with the patient fixating upon a distant target. If they respond briskly to light, there is no need to check the near response, because isolated loss of constriction (miosis) to accommodation does not occur. For this reason, the ubiquitous abbreviation PERRLA (pupils equal, round, and reactive to light and accommodation) implies a wasted effort with the last step. However, it is important to test the near response if the light response is poor or absent. Light-near dissociation occurs with neurosyphilis (Argyll Robertson pupil), lesions of the dorsal midbrain (obstructive hydrocephalus, pineal region tumors), and after aberrant regeneration (oculomotor nerve palsy, Adie's tonic pupil).

An eye with no light perception has no pupillary response to direct light stimulation. If the retina or optic nerve is only partially injured, the direct pupillary response will be less than the consensual pupillary response evoked by shining a light into the other eye. This *relative afferent pupillary defect* (Marcus Gunn pupil) can be elicited with the swinging flashlight test (Fig. 28-2). It is an extremely useful sign in retrobulbar optic neuritis and other optic nerve diseases, where it may be the sole objective evidence for disease.

Subtle inequality in pupil size, up to 0.5 mm, is a fairly common finding in normal subjects. The diagnosis of essential or physiologic anisocoria is secure as long as the relative pupil asymmetry remains constant as ambient lighting varies. Anisocoria that increases in dim light indicates a sympathetic paresis of the iris dilator muscle. The triad of miosis with ipsilateral ptosis and anhidrosis constitutes Horner's syndrome, although anhidrosis is often absent. Brainstem stroke, carotid dissection, or neoplasm impinging upon the sympathetic chain are occasionally identified as the cause of Horner's syndrome, but the majority of cases are idiopathic.

Anisocoria that increases in bright light suggests a parasympathetic palsy. The first concern is an oculomotor nerve paresis. This possibility is excluded if the eye movements are full and the patient has no ptosis or diplopia. Acute pupillary dilation (mydriasis) can occur from damage to the ciliary ganglion in the orbit. Common mechanisms are infection (herpes zoster, influenza), trauma (blunt, penetrating, surgical), or ischemia (diabetes, temporal arteritis). After denervation of the iris sphincter the pupil does not respond well to light, but the response to near is often relatively intact. When the near stimulus is removed, the pupil redilates very slowly compared with the normal

pupil, hence the term *tonic pupil*. In Adie's syndrome, a tonic pupil occurs in conjunction with weak or absent tendon reflexes in the lower extremities. This benign disorder, which occurs predominantly in healthy young women, is assumed to represent a mild dysautonomia. Tonic pupils are also associated with Shy-Drager syndrome, segmental hypohidrosis, diabetes, and amyloidosis. Occasionally, a tonic pupil is discovered incidentally in an otherwise completely normal, asymptomatic individual. The diagnosis is confirmed by placing a drop of dilute (0.125%) pilocarpine into each eye. Denervation hypersensitivity produces pupillary constriction in a tonic pupil, whereas the normal pupil shows no response. Pharmacologic dilation from accidental or deliberate instillation of anticholinergic agents (atropine, scopolamine drops) into the eye can also produce pupillary mydriasis. In this situation, normal strength (1%) pilocarpine causes no constriction.

Both pupils are affected equally by systemic medications. They are small with narcotic use (morphine, heroin) and large with anticholinergics (scopolamine). Parasympathetic agents (pilocarpine, demecarium bromide) used to treat glaucoma produce miosis. In any patient with an unexplained pupillary abnormality, a slit-lamp examination

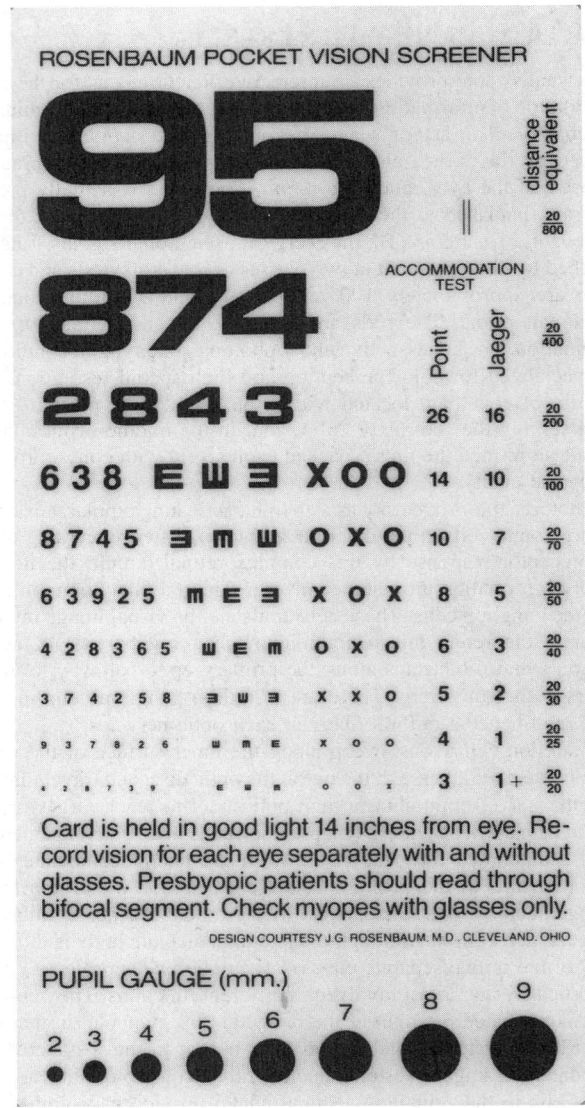

FIGURE 28-1 The Rosenbaum card is a miniature, scale version of the Snellen chart for testing visual acuity at near. When the visual acuity is recorded, the Snellen distance equivalent should bear a notation indicating that vision was tested at near, not at 6 m (20 ft), or else the Jaeger number system should be used to report the acuity.

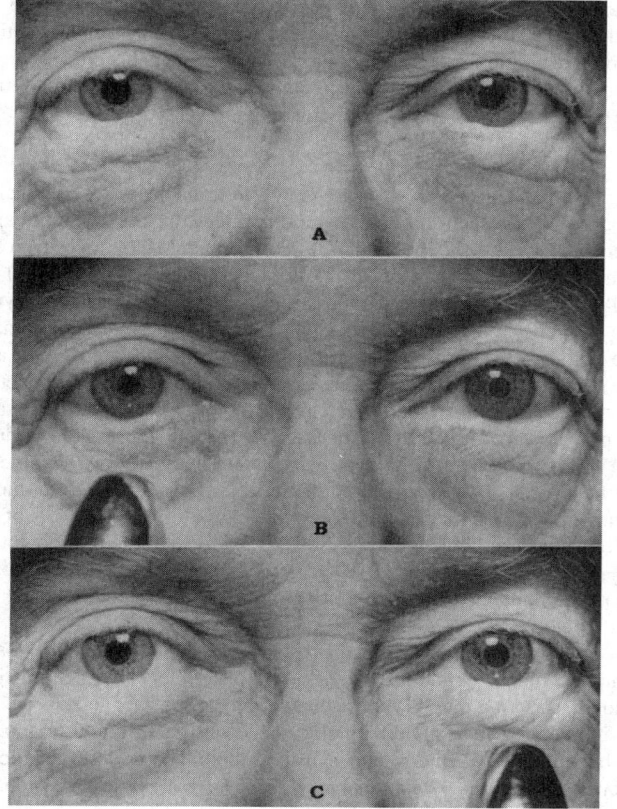

FIGURE 28-2 Demonstration of a relative afferent pupil defect (Marcus Gunn pupil) in the left eye, done with the patient fixating upon a distant target. *A.* With dim background lighting, the pupils are equal and relatively large. *B.* Shining a flashlight into the right eye evokes equal, strong constriction of both pupils. *C.* Swinging the flashlight over to the damaged left eye causes dilation of both pupils, although they remain smaller than in *A.* Swinging the flashlight back over to the healthy right eye would result in symmetric constriction back to the appearance shown in *B.* Note that the pupils always remain equal; the damage to the left retina/optic nerve is revealed by weaker bilateral pupil constriction to a flashlight in the left eye compared with the right eye. (*From P Levatin, Arch Ophthalmol 62:768, 1959.*)

is helpful to exclude surgical trauma to the iris, an occult foreign body, perforating injury, intraocular inflammation, adhesions (synechia), angle-closure glaucoma, and iris sphincter rupture from blunt trauma.

EYE MOVEMENTS AND ALIGNMENT Eye movements are tested by asking the patient with both eyes open to pursue a small target such as a penlight into the cardinal fields of gaze. Normal ocular versions are smooth, symmetric, full, and maintained in all directions without nystagmus. Saccades, or quick refixation eye movements, are assessed by having the patient look back and forth between two stationary targets. The eyes should move rapidly and accurately in a single jump to their target. Ocular alignment can be judged by holding a penlight directly in front of the patient at about 1 m. If the eyes are straight, the corneal light reflex will be centered in the middle of each pupil. To test eye alignment more precisely, the cover test is useful. The patient is instructed to gaze upon a small fixation target in the distance. One eye is covered suddenly while observing the second eye. If the second eye shifts to fixate upon the target, it was misaligned. If it does not move, the first eye is uncovered and the test is repeated on the second eye. If neither eye moves, the eyes are aligned orthotropically. If the eyes are orthotropic in primary gaze but the patient complains of diplopia, the cover test should be performed with the head tilted or turned in whatever direction elicits the patient's diplopia. With practice the examiner can detect an ocular deviation (hetero-

tropia) as small as 1 to 2° with the cover test. Deviations can be measured by placing prisms in front of the misaligned eye to determine the power required to neutralize the fixation shift evoked by covering the other eye.

STEREOPSIS Stereoacuity is determined by presenting targets with retinal disparity separately to each eye using polarized images. The most popular office tests measure a range of thresholds from 800 to 40 seconds of arc. Normal stereoacuity is 40 seconds of arc. If a patient achieves this level of stereoacuity, one is assured that the eyes are aligned orthotropically and that vision is intact in each eye. Random dot stereograms have no monocular depth cues and provide an excellent screening test for strabismus and amblyopia in children.

COLOR VISION The retina contains three classes of cones, with visual pigments of differing peak spectral sensitivity: red (560 nm), green (530 nm), and blue (430 nm). The red and green cone pigments are encoded on the X chromosome; the blue cone pigment on chromosome 7. Mutations of the blue cone pigment are exceedingly rare. Mutations of the red and green pigments cause congenital X-linked color blindness in 8 percent of males. Affected individuals are not truly color blind, rather, they differ from normal subjects in how they perceive color and how they combine primary monochromatic lights to match a given color. Anomalous trichromats have three cone types, but a mutation in one cone pigment (usually red or green) causes a shift in peak spectral sensitivity, altering the proportion of primary colors required to achieve a color match. Dichromats have only two cone types and will therefore accept a color match based upon only two primary colors. Anomalous trichromats and dichromats have 6/6 (20/20) visual acuity, but their hue discrimination is impaired. Ishihara color plates can be used to detect red-green color blindness. The test plates contain a hidden number, visible only to subjects with color confusion from red-green color blindness. Because color blindness is almost exclusively X-linked, it is worth screening only male children.

The Ishihara plates are often used to test patients with acquired defects of color vision. Although they are not intended for this purpose, no other simple, convenient method for quantitative color vision testing is available for regular office use. Acquired defects in color vision frequently result from disease of the macula or optic nerve. For example, patients with a history of optic neuritis often complain of color desaturation long after their visual acuity has returned to normal. Color blindness can also occur from bilateral strokes involving the ventral portion of the occipital lobe (cerebral achromatopsia). Such patients can perceive only shades of gray and may also have difficulty recognizing faces (prosopagnosia). Infarcts of the dominant occipital lobe sometimes give rise to color anomia. Affected patients can discriminate colors, but they cannot name them.

VISUAL FIELDS Vision can be impaired by damage to the visual system anywhere from the eyes to the occipital lobes. One can localize the site of the lesion with considerable accuracy by mapping the visual field deficit by finger confrontation and then correlating it with the topographic anatomy of the visual pathway (Fig. 28-3). More quantitative data can be obtained by formal perimetric examination of the visual fields. In kinetic perimetry, the patient faces a tangent screen or a hemispheric bowl (Goldmann perimeter) while the examiner moves a small light target from the periphery towards the center. Such manual techniques largely have been supplanted by computer-driven perimeters (Humphrey, Octopus) that present a target of variable intensity at fixed positions in the visual field (Fig. 28-3*A*). By generating an automated printout of light thresholds, these static perimeters provide a sensitive means of detecting scotomas in the visual field. They are also useful for serial assessment of visual function in chronic diseases like glaucoma or pseudotumor cerebri.

The crux of visual field analysis is to decide whether a lesion is before, at, or behind the optic chiasm. If a scotoma is confined to one eye, it must be due to a lesion anterior to the chiasm, involving either the optic nerve or retina. Retinal lesions produce scotomas that correspond optically to their location in the fundus. For example, a superior-nasal retinal detachment results in an inferior-temporal field cut. Damage to the macula causes a central scotoma (Fig. 28-3*B*).

Optic nerve disease produces characteristic patterns of visual field loss. Glaucoma selectively destroys axons that enter the superotemporal or inferotemporal poles of the optic disc, resulting in arcuate scotomas shaped like a Turkish scimitar, which emanate from the blind spot and curve around fixation to end flat against the horizontal meridian (Fig. 28-3*C*). This type of field defect mirrors the arrangement of the nerve fiber layer in the temporal retina. The superb acuity of humans is achieved by thrusting aside all retinal elements at the fovea except photoreceptors, to minimize absorption and scattering of light. To avoid passing over the fovea, axons from cells in the temporal retina must follow an indirect course arching around the fovea to reach the optic disc. Arcuate or nerve fiber layer scotomas also occur from optic neuritis, ischemic optic neuropathy, optic disc drusen, and branch retinal artery occlusion.

Damage to the entire upper or lower pole of the optic disc causes an altitudinal field cut that follows the horizontal meridian (Fig. 28-3*D*). This pattern of visual field loss is typical of ischemic optic neuropathy but also occurs from retinal vascular occlusion, advanced glaucoma, and optic neuritis.

About half the fibers in the optic nerve originate from ganglion cells serving the macula. Damage to papillomacular fibers causes a cecocentral scotoma encompassing the blind spot and macula (Fig. 28-3*E*). If the damage is irreversible, pallor eventually appears in the temporal portion of the optic disc. Temporal pallor from a cecocentral scotoma may develop in optic neuritis, nutritional optic neuropathy, toxic optic neuropathy, Leber's hereditary optic neuropathy, and compressive optic neuropathy. It is worth mentioning that the temporal side of the optic disc is slightly more pale than the nasal side in most normal subjects. Therefore, it can sometimes be difficult to decide whether the temporal pallor visible on fundus examination represents a pathologic change. Pallor of the nasal rim of the optic disc is a less equivocal sign of optic atrophy.

At the optic chiasm, fibers from nasal ganglion cells decussate into the contralateral optic tract. For unknown reasons, crossed fibers are damaged more by compression than uncrossed fibers. As a result, mass lesions of the sellar region cause a temporal hemianopia in each eye. Tumors anterior to the optic chiasm, such as meningiomas of the tuberculum sella, produce a junctional scotoma characterized by an optic neuropathy in one eye and a superior temporal field cut in the other eye (Fig. 28-3*G*). More symmetric compression of the optic chiasm by a pituitary adenoma (Fig. 28-4), meningioma, craniopharyngioma, glioma, or aneurysm results in a bitemporal hemianopia (Fig. 28-3*H*). The insidious development of a bitemporal hemianopia often goes unnoticed by the patient and will escape detection by the physician unless each eye is tested separately.

It is difficult to localize a postchiasmal lesion accurately, because injury anywhere in the optic tract, lateral geniculate body, optic radiations, or visual cortex can produce a homonymous hemianopia, i.e., a temporal hemifield defect in the contralateral eye and a matching nasal hemifield defect in the ipsilateral eye (Fig. 28-3*I*). A unilateral postchiasmal lesion leaves the visual acuity in each eye unaffected, although the patient may read the letters on only the left or right half of the eye chart. Lesions of the optic radiations tend to cause poorly matched or incongruous field defects in each eye. Damage to the optic radiations in the temporal lobe (Meyer's loop) produces a superior quandrantic homonymous hemianopia (Fig. 28-3*J*), whereas injury to the optic radiations in the parietal lobe results in an inferior quandrantic homonymous hemianopia (Fig. 28-3*K*). Lesions of the primary visual cortex give rise to dense, congruous hemianopic field defects. Occlusion of the posterior cerebral artery supplying the occipital lobe is a frequent cause of total homonymous hemianopia. Some patients with hemianopia after occipital stroke have macular sparing, because the macular representation at the tip of the occipital lobe is supplied by collaterals from the middle cerebral artery (Fig. 28-3*L*). Destruction of both occipital lobes produces cortical blindness. This condition can be distinguished from bilateral prechiasmal visual loss by noting that the pupil responses and optic fundi remain normal.

Approach to the Patient

Red or Painful Eye *Corneal abrasions* are seen best by placing a drop of fluorescein in the eye and looking with the slit lamp using a cobalt-blue light. A penlight with a blue filter will suffice if no slit lamp is available. Damage to the corneal epithelium is revealed by yellow fluorescence of the exposed basement membrane underlying the epithelium. It is important to check for foreign bodies. To search the conjunctival fornices, the lower lid should be pulled down and the upper lid everted. A foreign body can be removed with a moistened cotton-tipped applicator after placing a drop of topical anesthetic, such as proparacaine, in the eye. Alternatively, it may be possible to flush the foreign body from the eye by irrigating copiously with saline or artificial tears. If the corneal epithelium has been abraded, antibiotic ointment and a patch should be applied to the eye. A drop of an intermediate-acting cycloplegic such as cyclopentolate hydrochloride 1%, helps to reduce pain by relaxing the ciliary body. The eye should be reexamined the next day. Minor abrasions may not require patching and cycloplegia.

Subconjunctival hemorrhage results from rupture of small vessels bridging the potential space between the episclera and conjunctiva. Blood dissecting into this space can produce a spectacular red eye, but vision is not affected and the hemorrhage resolves without treatment. Subconjunctival hemorrhage is usually spontaneous but can occur from blunt trauma, eye rubbing, or vigorous coughing. Occasionally it is a clue to an underlying bleeding disorder.

A *pinguecula* is a small, raised conjunctival nodule at the temporal or nasal limbus. In adults such lesions are extremely common and have little significance, unless they become inflamed (pingueculitis). A *pterygium* resembles a pinguecula but has crossed the limbus to encroach upon the corneal surface. Removal is justified when symptoms of irritation or blurring develop, but recurrence is a common problem.

Blepharitis refers to inflammation of the eyelids. The most common form occurs in association with acne rosacea or seborrheic dermatitis. The eyelid margins are usually colonized heavily by staphylococcus. Upon close inspection, they appear greasy, ulcerated, and crusted with scaling debris that clings to the lashes. Treatment consists of warm compresses, strict eyelid hygiene, and topical antibiotics such as erythromycin. An external *hordeolum* (sty) is caused by staphylococcal infection of the superficial accessory glands of Zeis or Moll located in the eyelid margins. An internal hordeolum occurs after suppurative infection of the oil-secreting meibomian glands within the tarsal plate of the eyelid. Systemic antibiotics, usually tetracyclines, are sometimes necessary for treatment of meibomian gland inflammation (meibomitis) or chronic, severe blepharitis. A *chalazion* is a painless, granulomatous inflammation of a meibomian gland that produces a pealike nodule within the eyelid. It can be incised and drained, or injected with glucocorticoids. Basal cell, squamous cell, or meibomian gland carcinoma should be suspected for any nonhealing, ulcerative lesion of the eyelids.

Dacrocystitis, or inflammation of the lacrimal drainage system, can produce epiphora (tearing) and ocular injection. Gentle pressure over the lacrimal sac evokes pain and reflux of mucus or pus from the tear puncta. Dacrocystitis usually occurs after obstruction of the lacrimal system. It is treated with topical and systemic antibiotics, followed by probing or surgery to reestablish patency. *Entropion* (inversion of the eyelid) or *ectropion* (sagging or eversion of the eyelid) can also lead to epiphora and ocular irritation.

Conjunctivitis is the most common cause of a red, painful eye. Pain is minimal, and the visual acuity is reduced only slightly. The most common viral etiology is adenovirus infection. It causes a watery discharge, mild foreign-body sensation, and photophobia. Bacterial infection tends to produce a more mucopurulent exudate. Mild cases

Monocular Pre-chiasmal Field Defects:

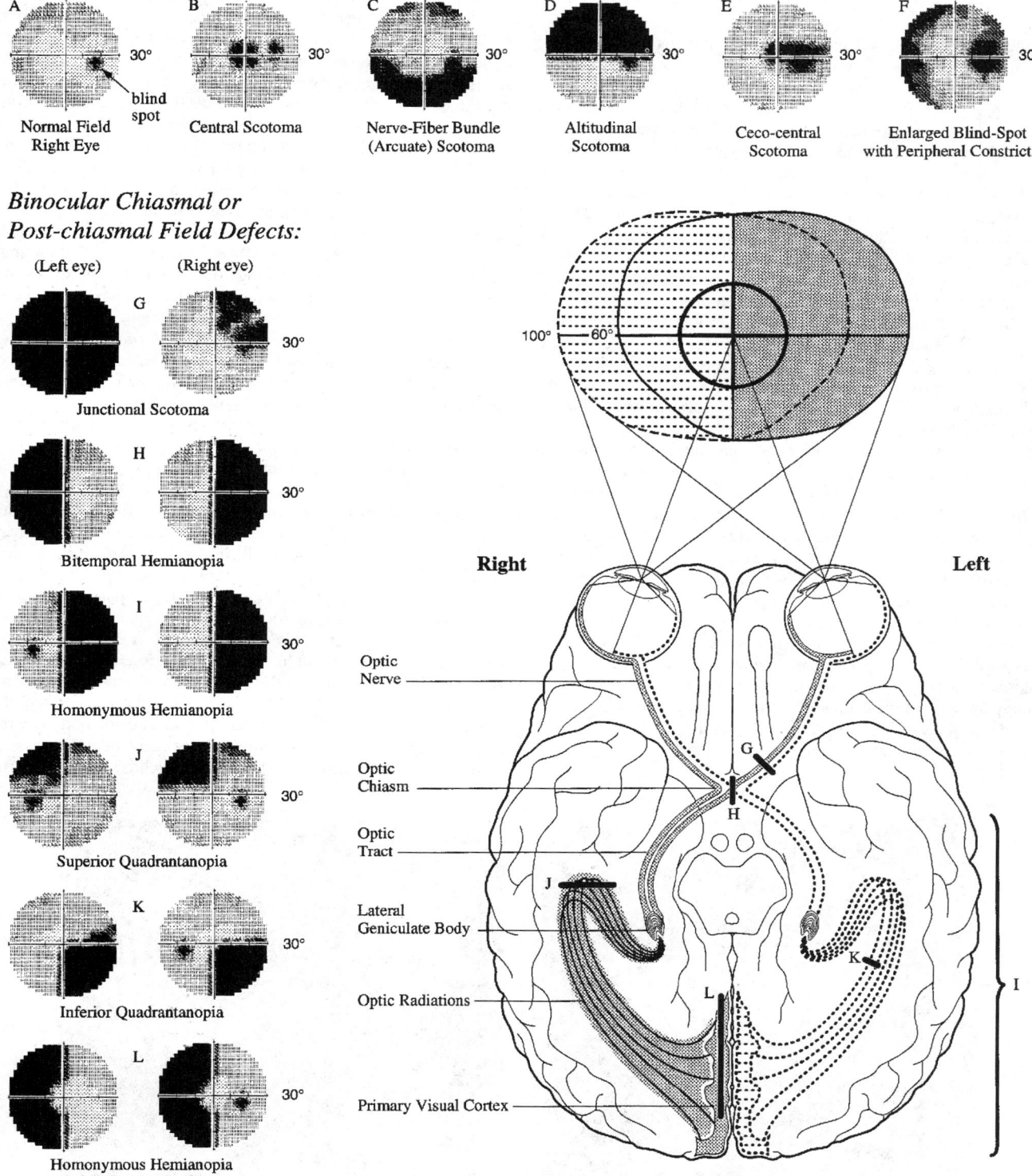

A — Normal Field Right Eye (blind spot) — 30°

B — Central Scotoma — 30°

C — Nerve-Fiber Bundle (Arcuate) Scotoma — 30°

D — Altitudinal Scotoma — 30°

E — Ceco-central Scotoma — 30°

F — Enlarged Blind-Spot with Peripheral Constriction — 30°

Binocular Chiasmal or Post-chiasmal Field Defects:

(Left eye)   (Right eye)

G — Junctional Scotoma — 30°

H — Bitemporal Hemianopia — 30°

I — Homonymous Hemianopia — 30°

J — Superior Quadrantanopia — 30°

K — Inferior Quadrantanopia — 30°

L — Homonymous Hemianopia with Macular Sparing — 30°

Right   Left

Optic Nerve
Optic Chiasm — G, H
Optic Tract — J
Lateral Geniculate Body — K
Optic Radiations — L
Primary Visual Cortex

I

FIGURE 28-3 Ventral view of the brain, correlating patterns of visual field loss with the sites of lesions in the visual pathway. The visual fields overlap partially, creating 120° of central binocular field flanked by a 40° monocular crescent on either side. The visual field maps in this figure were done with a computer-driven perimeter (Humphrey Instruments, Carl Zeiss, Inc.). It plots the retinal sensitivity to light in the central 30° using a gray scale format. Areas of visual field loss are shown in black. The examples of common monocular, prechiasmal field defects are all shown for the right eye. By convention, the visual fields are always recorded with the left eye's field on the left, and the right eye's field on the right, just as the patient sees the world.

of infectious conjunctivitis usually are treated empirically with broad-spectrum topical ocular antibiotics, such as sulfacetamide 10%, poly-mixin-bacitracin-neomycin, or trimethoprim-polymixin combination. Smears and cultures are usually reserved for severe, resistant, or recurrent cases of conjunctivitis. To prevent contagion, patients should be admonished to wash their hands frequently, not to touch their eyes, and to avoid direct contact with others.

Allergic conjunctivitis is extremely common and often mistaken for infectious conjunctivitis. Three forms are recognized, with closely overlapping manifestations. *Hay fever conjunctivitis* has a seasonal incidence, related to the release of airborne antigens into the air by plants. IgE-mediated activation of mast cells in the conjunctiva causes itching, redness, and edema. *Vernal conjunctivitis* is also seasonal, becoming worse during warm months. It affects exclusively children or adolescents and is more common in boys. The cause is unknown, but airborne antigens are thought to trigger symptoms. Itching, photophobia, epiphora, and mucous discharge are typical. The palpebral conjunctiva may become hypertropic with giant excrescences called cobblestone papillae. Irritation from contact lenses or any chronic foreign body can also induce formation of cobblestone papillae. *Atopic conjunctivitis* occurs in subjects with atopic dermatitis or asthma. Symptoms caused by allergic conjunctivitis can be alleviated with cold compresses, topical vasoconstrictors, antihistamines, and mast-cell stablizers such as cromolyn sodium. Topical glucocorticoid solutions provide dramatic relief of immune-mediated forms of conjunctivitis, but their long-term use is ill-advised because of the complications of glaucoma, cataract, and secondary infection. Topical nonsteroidal anti-inflammatory agents (NSAIDs) like ketorolac tromethamine are a better alternative.

Keratoconjunctivitis sicca, or dry eye, produces burning, foreign-body sensation, injection, and photophobia. In mild cases the eye appears surprisingly normal, but tear production measured by wetting of a filter paper (Schirmer strip) is deficient. A variety of systemic drugs, including antihistaminic, anticholinergic, and psychotropic medications, result in dry eye by reducing lacrimal secretion. Disorders that involve the lacrimal gland directly, such as sarcoidosis or Sjögren's syndrome, also cause dry eye. Patients may develop dry eye after radiation therapy if the treatment field includes the orbits. Problems with ocular drying are also common after lesions affecting cranial nerves V or VII. Corneal anesthesia is particularly dangerous, because the absence of a normal blink reflex exposes the cornea to injury without pain to warn the patient. Dry eye is managed by frequent and liberal application of artificial tears and ocular lubricants. In severe cases the tear puncta can be plugged or cauterized to reduce lacrimal outflow.

Keratitis is a threat to vision because of the risk of corneal clouding, scarring, and perforation. Worldwide, the two leading causes of blindness from keratitis are trachoma from chlamydial infection and vitamin A deficiency related to malnutrition. In the United States, contact lenses play a major role in corneal infection and ulceration. They should not be worn by anyone with an active eye infection. In evaluating the cornea, it is important to differentiate between a superficial infection (*keratoconjunctivitis*) and a deeper, more serious ulcerative process. The latter is accompanied by greater visual loss, pain, photophobia, redness, and discharge. Slit-lamp examination shows disruption of the corneal epithelium, a cloudy infiltrate or abscess in the stroma, and an inflammatory cellular reaction in the anterior chamber. In severe cases, pus settles at the bottom of the anterior chamber, giving rise to a hypopyon. Immediate empiric antibiotic therapy should be initiated after corneal scrapings are obtained for Gram's stain, Giemsa stain, and cultures. Fortified topical antibiotics are most effective, supplemented with subconjunctival antibiotics as required. The most frequent bacterial pathogens are *Staphylococcus*, *Streptococcus* (particularly *S. pneumoniae*), *Pseudomonas*, Enterobacteriaceae, *Haemophilus*, and *Neisseria*. For *Neisseria*, systemic antibiotics should be given in addition to topical antibiotics to eliminate systemic infection. A fungal etiology should always be considered in the patient with keratitis. Fungal infection is common in warm humid climates, especially after penetration of the cornea by plant or vegetable material.

The *herpes viruses* are a major cause of blindness from keratitis. Most adults in the United States have serum antibodies to herpes simplex, indicating prior viral infection (Chap. 184). Primary ocular infection generally is caused by herpes simplex type 1, rather than type 2. It manifests as a unilateral follicular blepharoconjunctivitis, easily confused with adenoviral conjunctivitis, unless telltale vesicles appear on the periocular skin or conjunctiva. A dendritic pattern of corneal epithelial ulceration revealed by fluorescein staining is pathognomonic for herpes infection but is seen in only a minority of primary infections. Recurrent ocular infection arises from reactivation of the latent herpes virus. Viral eruption in the corneal epithelium may result in the characteristic herpes dendrite. Involvement of the corneal stroma produces edema, vascularization, and iridocyclitis. Herpes keratitis is

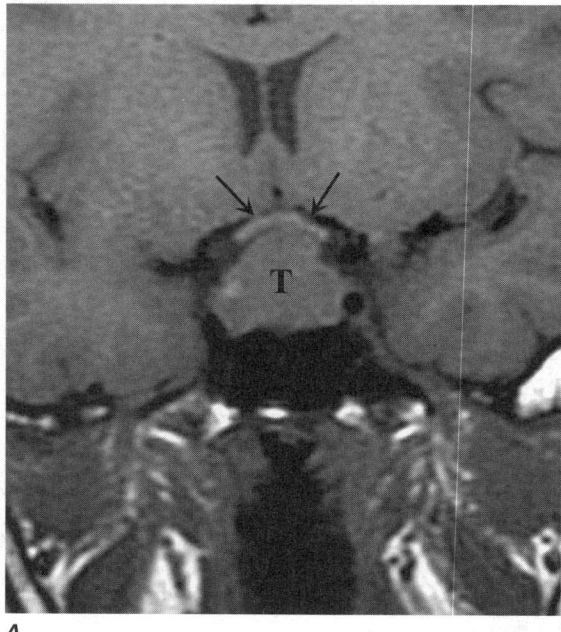

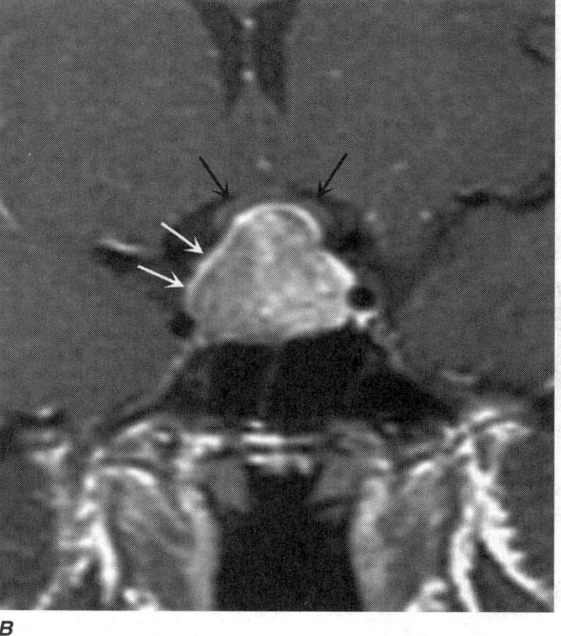

A

B

FIGURE 28-4 Pituitary adenoma: Coronal precontrast (*A*) and postcontrast (*B*) T1-weighted MRI through the sella turcica shows a large tumor (T) arising from the pituitary fossa. The optic chiasm (*black arrows*) is elevated and compressed, producing a visual field defect resembling that shown in Fig.

28-3H. There is peripheral enhancement around the mass due to displaced normal pituitary tissue (*white arrows*) and heterogeneous enhancement of the mass itself. The patient presented with decreased vision in both eyes of several years duration and optic pallor.

treated with topical antiviral agents, cycloplegics, and oral acyclovir. Topical glucocorticoids are effective in mitigating corneal scarring but must be used with extreme caution because of the danger of corneal melting and perforation. Topical steroids also carry the risk of prolonging infection and inducing glaucoma.

Herpes zoster from reactivation of latent varicella (chickenpox) virus causes a dermatomal pattern of painful vesicular dermatitis. Ocular symptoms can occur after zoster eruption in any branch of the trigeminal nerve but are particularly common when vesicles form on the nose, reflecting nasociliary (V1) nerve involvement (Hutchinson's sign). Herpes zoster ophthalmicus produces corneal dendrites, which can be difficult to distinguish from those seen in herpes simplex. Stromal keratitis, anterior uveitis, raised intraocular pressure, ocular motor nerve palsies, acute retinal necrosis, and postherpetic scarring and neuralgia are other common sequelae. Herpes zoster ophthalmicus is treated with antiviral agents and cycloplegics. In severe cases, steroids may be added to prevent permanent visual loss from corneal scarring.

Episcleritis is an inflammation of the episclera, a thin layer of connective tissue between the conjunctiva and sclera. Episcleritis resembles conjunctivitis but is a more localized process and discharge is absent. Most cases of episcleritis are idiopathic, but some occur in the setting of an autoimmune disease. *Scleritis* refers to a deeper, more severe inflammatory process, frequently associated with a connective tissue disease such as rheumatoid arthritis, lupus erythematosus, polyarteritis nodosa, Wegener's granulomatosis, or relapsing polychondritis. The inflammation and thickening of the sclera can be diffuse or nodular. In anterior forms of scleritis, the globe assumes a violet hue and the patient complains of severe ocular tenderness and pain. With posterior scleritis the pain and redness may be less marked, but there is often proptosis, choroidal effusion, reduced motility, and visual loss. Episcleritis and scleritis should be treated with NSAIDs. If these agents fail, topical or even systemic glucocorticoid therapy may be necessary, especially if an underlying autoimmune process is active.

Uveitis involving the anterior structures of the eye is called *iritis* or *iridocyclitis*. The diagnosis requires slit-lamp examination to identify inflammatory cells floating in the aqueous humor or deposited upon the corneal endothelium (keratic precipitates). Anterior uveitis develops in sarcoidosis, ankylosing spondylitis, juvenile rheumatoid arthritis, inflammatory bowel disease, psoriasis, Reiter's syndrome, and Behçet's disease. It is also associated with herpes infections, syphilis, Lyme disease, onchocerciasis, tuberculosis, and leprosy. Although anterior uveitis can occur in conjunction with many diseases, no cause is found to explain the majority of cases. For this reason, laboratory evaluation usually is reserved for patients with recurrent or severe anterior uveitis. Treatment is aimed at reducing inflammation and scarring by judicious use of topical steroids. Dilation of the pupil reduces pain and prevents the formation of synechiae.

Posterior uveitis is diagnosed by observing inflammation of the vitreous, retina, or choroid on fundus examination. It is more likely than anterior uveitis to be associated with an identifiable systemic disease. Some patients have panuveitis, or inflammation of both the anterior and posterior segments of the eye. Posterior uveitis is a manifestation of autoimmune diseases such as sarcoidosis, Behçet's disease, Vogt-Koyanagi-Harada syndrome, and inflammatory bowel disease. It also accompanies diseases such as toxoplasmosis, onchocerciasis, cysticercosis, coccidioidomycosis, toxocariasis, and histoplasmosis; infections caused by organisms such as *Candida*, *Pneumocystis carinii*, *Cryptococcus*, *Aspergillus*, herpes, and cytomegalovirus **(Plate III-1)**; and other diseases such as syphilis, Lyme disease, tuberculosis, cat-scratch disease, Whipple's disease, and brucellosis. In multiple sclerosis, chronic inflammatory changes can develop in the extreme periphery of the retina (pars planitis or intermediate uveitis).

Acute angle-closure glaucoma is a rare and frequently misdiagnosed cause of a red, painful eye. Susceptible eyes have a shallow anterior chamber, either because the eye has a short axial length (hyperopia) or a lens enlarged by the gradual development of cataract.

When the pupil becomes mid-dilated, the peripheral iris blocks aqueous outflow via the anterior chamber angle and the intraocular pressure rises abruptly, producing pain, injection, corneal edema, obscurations, and blurred vision. In some patients, ocular symptoms are overshadowed by nausea, vomiting or headache, prompting a fruitless workup for abdominal or neurologic disease. The diagnosis is made by measuring the intraocular pressure during an acute attack or by performing gonioscopy to reveal the narrowed chamber angle by means of a specially mirrored contact lens. Acute angle closure is treated with oral or intravenous acetazolamide, topical beta blockers, and pilocarpine to induce miosis. If these measures fail, a laser can be used to create a hole in the peripheral iris to relieve pupillary block. Many physicians are reluctant to dilate patients routinely for fundus examination because they fear precipitating an angle-closure glaucoma. The risk is actually remote and more than outweighed by the potential benefit to patients of discovering a hidden fundus lesion visible only through a fully dilated pupil. Moreover, a single attack of angle closure after pharmacologic dilation rarely causes any permanent damage to the eye and serves as an inadvertent provocative test to identify patients with narrow angles who would benefit from prophylactic laser iridectomy.

Endophthalmitis occurs from bacterial, viral, fungal, or parasitic infection of the internal structures of the eye. It is usually acquired by hematogenous seeding from a remote site. Chronically ill, diabetic, or immunosuppressed patients, especially those with a history of indwelling intravenous catheters or positive blood cultures, are at greatest risk for endogenous endophthalmitis. Although most patients have ocular pain and injection, visual loss is sometimes the only symptom. Septic emboli, from a diseased heart valve or a dental abscess, that lodge in the retinal circulation can give rise to endophthalmitis. White-centered retinal hemorrhages (Roth's spots) are considered pathognomonic for subacute bacterial endocardititis, but they also appear in leukemia, diabetes, and many other conditions. Endophthalmitis also occurs as a complication of ocular surgery, occasionally months or even years after the operation. An occult penetrating foreign body or unrecognized trauma to the globe should be considered in any patient with unexplained intraocular infection or inflammation.

Transient or Sudden Visual Loss Transient ischemic attack of the retina is called *amaurosis fugax*. Because neural tissue has a high rate of metabolism, interruption of blood flow to the retina for more than a few seconds results in *transient monocular blindness*, a term used interchangeably with amaurosis fugax. Patients describe a rapid fading of vision like a curtain descending, sometimes affecting only a portion of the visual field. Amaurosis fugax usually occurs from an embolus that becomes stuck within a retinal arteriole **(Plate III-2)**. If the embolus breaks up or passes, flow is restored and vision returns quickly to normal without permanent damage. With prolonged interruption of blood flow, the inner retina suffers infarction. Ophthalmoscopy reveals zones of whitened, edematous retina following the distribution of branch retinal arterioles. Complete occlusion of the central retinal artery produces arrest of blood flow and a milky retina with a cherry-red fovea. Emboli are composed of either cholesterol (Hollenhorst plaque), calcium, or platelet-fibrin debris. The most common source is an atherosclerotic plaque in the carotid artery or aorta, although emboli can also arise from the heart, especially in patients with diseased valves, atrial fibrillation, or wall motion abnormalities.

In rare instances, amaurosis fugax occurs from low central retinal artery perfusion pressure in a patient with a critical stenosis of the ipsilateral carotid artery and poor collateral flow via the circle of Willis. In this situation, amaurosis fugax develops when there is a dip in systemic blood pressure or a slight worsening of the carotid stenosis. Sometimes there is contralateral motor or sensory loss, indicating concomitant hemispheric cerebral ischemia.

Amaurosis fugax warns of a patient at high risk for stroke. The carotid arteries should be studied by ultrasound. Endarterectomy for a stenosis of 60 percent or more, even in asymptomatic patients, has been shown to reduce the subsequent rate of ipsilateral stroke (Chap. 366). Therapy with aspirin, warfarin, or other anticoagulants is appropriate in selected patients. If no carotid lesion is found, cardiac ultrasound and ambulatory ECG monitoring should be undertaken.

Marked *systemic hypertension* causes sclerosis of retinal arterioles, splinter hemorrhages, focal infarcts of the nerve fiber layer (cotton-wool spots), and leakage of lipid and fluid (hard exudate) into the macula **(Plate III-3).** In hypertensive crisis, sudden visual loss can result from vasospasm of retinal arterioles and consequent retinal ischemia. In addition, acute hypertension may produce visual loss from ischemic swelling of the optic disc. Patients with acute hypertensive retinopathy should be treated by lowering the blood pressure. However, the blood pressure should not be reduced precipitously, because there is a danger of optic disc infarction from sudden hypoperfusion.

Impending *branch* or *central retinal vein occlusion* can produce prolonged visual obscurations that resemble those described by patients with amaurosis fugax. The veins appear engorged and phlebitic, with numerous retinal hemorrhages **(Plate III-4).** In some patients, venous blood flow recovers spontaneously, while others evolve a frank obstruction with extensive retinal bleeding ("blood and thunder" appearance), infarction, and visual loss. Venous occlusion of the retina is often idiopathic, but hypertension, diabetes, and glaucoma are prominent risk factors. The benefit of treatment with anticoagulants is unproven and carries the risk of hemorrhage into the vitreous. Polycythemia, thrombocythemia, or other factors leading to an underlying hypercoagulable state should be corrected.

Anterior ischemic optic neuropathy (AION) is caused by insufficient blood flow through the posterior ciliary arteries supplying the optic disc. It produces sudden, painless, monocular visual loss, although patients occasionally report premonitory obscurations. The optic disc appears swollen and surrounded by nerve fiber layer splinter hemorrhages **(Plate III-5).** AION is divided into two forms: arteritic and nonarteritic. The nonarteritic form of AION is most common. No specific cause can be identified, although diabetes and hypertension are frequent risk factors. No treatment is available. About 5 percent of patients, especially those over age 65, develop the arteritic form of AION in conjunction with giant cell (temporal) arteritis (Chap. 319). It is urgent to identify patients with arteritic AION so that glucocorticoid therapy can be instituted immediately to prevent blindness in the second eye. Symptoms of polymyalgia rheumatica may be present, and the sedimentation rate is usually elevated. In a patient with visual loss from suspected arteritic AION, temporal artery biopsy is helpful to confirm the diagnosis, but steroid treatment should be started without waiting for the biopsy to be completed. The diagnosis of arteritic AION is difficult to sustain in the face of a normal sedimentation rate and a negative temporal artery biopsy, but such cases do occur rarely.

Posterior ischemic optic neuropathy is an infrequent cause of acute visual loss. It is induced by the combination of severe anemia and hypotension, causing infarction of the retrobulbar optic nerve. Cases have been reported after major blood loss during surgery, exsanguinating trauma, gastrointestinal bleeding, and renal dialysis. The fundus usually appears normal, although optic disc swelling develops if the process extends far enough anteriorly. Vision can be salvaged in some patients by prompt blood transfusion and reversal of hypotension.

Optic neuritis is a common inflammatory disease of the optic nerve. In the recent Optic Neuritis Treatment Trial, the mean age of patients was 32 years, 77 percent were female, 92 percent had ocular pain (especially with eye movements), and 35 percent had optic disc swelling. In the majority of patients, the demyelinating event was retrobulbar and the ocular fundus appeared normal on initial examination **(Plate III-6),** although optic disc pallor slowly developed over subsequent months. Many patients with optic neuritis eventually develop multiple sclerosis, but for some patients optic neuritis remains an isolated event. Virtually all patients experience a gradual recovery of vision after a single episode of optic neuritis, even without treatment. This rule is so reliable that failure of vision to improve substantially after a first attack of optic neuritis casts doubt upon the original diagnosis.

Treatment of optic neuritis with glucocorticoids is controversial. The Optic Neuritis Treatment Trial showed that patients treated with a conventional dose of oral steroids (prednisone, 1 mg/kg per day for 14 days) did no better than patients treated with a placebo. Surprisingly, patients who received oral prednisone appeared to have an increased recurrence rate of optic neuritis. From these results, it is apparent that treatment of optic neuritis with oral glucocorticoids is of no help and may even heighten the risk of further attacks. High-dose intravenous methylprednisolone (250 mg every 6 h for 3 days) followed by oral prednisone (1 mg/kg per day for 11 days) led to a slightly faster recovery of visual function, but final acuity 6 months later was not significantly different in patients treated with a placebo. Remarkably, intravenous glucocorticoids were associated with a reduced rate of development of multiple sclerosis over a 2-year follow-up period, especially in the subgroup of patients with multiple foci of demyelination on their magnetic resonance (MR) scan. However, by the end of a 3-year follow-up period, patients treated with intravenous glucocorticoids versus placebo showed no difference in the rate of multiple sclerosis. Moreover, intravenous steroids did not reduce the likelihood of subsequent attacks of optic neuritis. To summarize: the study authors recommend an MR scan in patients with optic neuritis. If two or more foci of demyelination are found or visual loss is severe, they suggest treatment with intravenous steroids. The potential benefits of intravenous steroids are: (1) a slightly faster recovery of visual function, and (2) a potential reduction in the risk of subsequent neurologic events that would signify multiple sclerosis. Critics of the Optic Neuritis Treatment Trial have questioned these recommendations, pointing out that: (1) visual outcome is the same in the long run, (2) evidence indicating a reduced risk of eventual multiple sclerosis with intravenous steroid treatment is based upon follow-up data in a rather small number of patients, and (3) the protection against multiple sclerosis is transient, and no longer apparent 3 years later. In cases of unilateral optic neuritis, the decision whether to obtain an MR scan or to treat with intravenous steroids should be based upon clinical judgment and careful discussion with the patient. In cases of bilateral, simultaneous optic neuritis, the rationale for intravenous steroids is stronger.

Leber's hereditary optic neuropathy (Chap. 380) is a disease of young men, characterized by onset over a few weeks of painless, severe, central visual loss in one eye, followed weeks or months later by the same process in the other eye. Acutely, the optic disc appears mildly plethoric with surface capillary telangiectases, but no vascular leakage on fluorescein angiography. Eventually optic atrophy ensues. There is no treatment. Recently, Wallace discovered that Leber's optic neuropathy is caused by a point mutation at codon 11778 in the mitochondrial gene encoding nicotinamide adenine dinucleotide dehydrogenase (NADH) subunit 4. Subsequently, additional mutations responsible for the disease have been identified, most in mitochondrial genes encoding proteins involved in electron transport. Mitochrondrial mutations causing Leber's neuropathy are inherited from the mother by all her children, but usually only sons develop symptoms. This curious male predilection is a mystery.

Toxic optic neuropathy can result in acute visual loss with bilateral optic disc swelling and central or cecocentral scotomas. Such cases have been reported from ethambutol, methyl alcohol (moonshine), ethylene glycol (antifreeze), and carbon monoxide. In toxic optic neuropathy, visual loss can also develop gradually and produce optic atrophy without a phase of acute optic disc edema **(Plate III-7).** Many agents have been implicated as a cause of toxic optic neuropathy, but the evidence supporting the association for many is weak. The following is a partial list of potential offending drugs or toxins: disulfiram, ethchlorvynol, chloramphenicol, amiodarone, monoclonal anti-CD3 antibody, ciprofloxacin, digitalis, streptomycin, lead, arsenic, thallium, D-penicillamine, isoniazid, emetine, and sulfonamides. Deficiency states, induced either by starvation, malabsorption, or alcoholism, can lead to insidious visual loss. Thiamine, vitamin B_{12}, and folate levels should be checked in any patient with unexplained, bilateral central scotomas and optic pallor.

Papilledema connotes bilateral optic disc swelling from raised intracranial pressure **(Plate III-8)**. Headache is a frequent, but not invariable, accompaniment. All other forms of optic disc swelling, e.g., from optic neuritis or ischemic optic neuropathy, should be called "optic disc edema." This convention is arbitrary but serves to avoid confusion. Often it is difficult to differentiate papilledema from other forms of optic disc edema by fundus examination alone. Transient visual obscurations are a classic symptom of papilledema. They can occur in only one eye or simultaneously in both eyes. They usually last seconds but can persist for minutes if the papilledema is fulminant. Obscurations follow abrupt shifts in posture or happen spontaneously. When obscurations are prolonged or spontaneous, the papilledema is more threatening. Visual acuity is not affected by papilledema, unless the papilledema is severe, long-standing, or accompanied by macular edema and hemorrhage. Visual field testing shows enlarged blind spots and peripheral constriction (Fig. 28-3*F*). With unremitting papilledema, peripheral visual field loss progresses in an insidious fashion while the optic nerve develops atrophy. In this setting, reduction of optic disc swelling is an ominous sign of a dying nerve rather than an encouraging indication of resolving papilledema.

Evaluation of papilledema requires computed tomography (CT) or MR imaging to exclude a brain tumor. If none is found, MR angiography is appropriate in selected cases to investigate the possibility of a dural venous sinus occlusion or an arteriovenous shunt. If neuroradiologic studies are normal, the subarachnoid opening pressure should be measured by lumbar puncture to confirm that it is elevated. If it is elevated, without explanation, the diagnosis of *pseudotumor cerebri* (idiopathic intracranial hypertension) is made by exclusion. The majority of patients are young, female, and obese. Treatment with a carbonic anhydrase inhibitor such as acetazolamide lowers intracranial pressure by reducing the production of cerebrospinal fluid. Weight reduction is exceedingly important but often unsuccessful. If acetazolamide and weight loss fail, and visual field loss is progressive, lumboperitoneal shunting or optic nerve sheath fenestration should be undertaken without delay, when required, to prevent blindness.

Optic disc drusen are refractile deposits within the substance of the optic nerve head **(Plate III-9)**. They are unrelated to drusen of the retina, which occur in age-related macular degeneration. Optic disc drusen are most common in people of northern European descent, with an incidence of 3 to 4 per thousand. Their diagnosis is obvious when they are visible as glittering particles upon the surface of the optic disc. However, in many patients they are hidden beneath the surface, producing an elevated optic disc with blurred margins that is easily mistaken for papilledema. It is important to recognize pseudopapilledema due to optic disc drusen to avoid an unneccessary evaluation for papilledema. Ultrasound or CT scanning are sensitive for detection of buried optic disc drusen because they contain calcium. In most patients, optic disc drusen are an incidental, innocuous finding, but they can produce visual obscurations. On perimetry they give rise to enlarged blind spots and arcuate scotomas from damage to the optic disc. With increasing age, drusen tend to become more exposed on the disc surface as optic atrophy develops. Hemorrhage, choroidal neovascular membrane, and anterior ischemic optic neuropathy are more likely to occur in patients with optic disc drusen. No treatment for drusen is available.

Vitreous degeneration occurs in all individuals with advancing age, leading to chronic and acute visual symptoms. Opacities develop in the vitreous, casting annoying shadows upon the retina. As the eye moves, these distracting "floaters" move synchronously, with a slight lag caused by inertia of the vitreous gel. Vitreous traction upon the retina causes mechanical stimulation, resulting in perception of flashing lights. This photopsia is brief and confined to one eye, in contrast to the bilateral, prolonged scintillations of cortical migraine. Contraction of the vitreous can result in sudden separation from the retina, heralded by an alarming shower of floaters and photopsia. This process, known as *vitreous detachment*, is a frequent involutional event in the elderly. It is not harmful unless it damages the retina. A careful examination of the dilated fundus is mandatory in any patient complaining of floaters or photopsia to search for peripheral tears or holes. If such a lesion is found, laser application or cryotherapy can forestall a retinal detachment. Occasionally a tear ruptures a retinal blood vessel, causing vitreous hemorrhage and sudden loss of vision. On attempted ophthalmoscopy the fundus is hidden by a dark red haze of blood. Ultrasound is required to examine the interior of the eye for a retinal tear or detachment. If the hemorrhage does not resolve spontaneously, the vitreous can be removed surgically. Vitreous hemorrhage also occurs from the fragile neovascular vessels that proliferate on the surface of the retina in diabetes, sickle cell anemia, and other ischemic ocular diseases.

Retinal detachment produces symptoms of floaters, flashing lights, and a scotoma in the peripheral visual field corresponding to the detachment **(Plate III-10)**. If the detachment includes the fovea, there is an afferent pupil defect and the visual acuity is reduced. In most eyes, retinal detachment starts with a hole, flap, or tear in the peripheral retina (rhegmatogenous retinal detachment). Patients with peripheral retinal thinning (lattice degeneration) are particularly vulnerable to this process. Once a break has developed in the retina, liquified vitreous is free to enter the subretinal space, separating the retina from the pigment epithelium. The combination of vitreous traction upon the retinal surface and passage of fluid behind the retina leads inexorably to detachment. Patients with a history of myopia, trauma, or prior cataract extraction are at greatest risk for retinal detachment. The diagnosis is confirmed by ophthalmoscopic examination of the dilated eye.

Classic migraine (Chap. 364) usually occurs with a visual aura lasting about 20 min. In a typical attack, a small central disturbance in the field of vision marches toward the periphery, leaving a transient scotoma in its wake. The expanding border of migraine scotoma has a scintillating, dancing, or zig-zag edge, resembling the bastions of a fortified city, hence the term "fortification spectra." Patients' descriptions of fortification spectra vary widely and can be confused with amaurosis fugax. Migraine patterns usually last longer and are perceived in both eyes, whereas amaurosis fugax is briefer and occurs in only one eye. Migraine phenomena also remain visible in the dark or with the eyes closed. Generally they are confined to either the right or left visual hemifield, but sometimes both fields are involved simultaneously. Patients often have a long history of stereotypic attacks. After the visual symptoms recede, headache develops in most patients.

Transient ischemic attacks from *vertebrobasilar insufficiency* result in acute homonymous visual symptoms. Many patients mistakenly describe symptoms in their left or right eye, when in fact they are occurring in the left or right hemifield of both eyes. Interruption of blood supply to the visual cortex causes a sudden fogging or graying of vision, occasionally with flashing lights or other positive phenomena that mimic migraine. Cortical ischemic attacks are briefer in duration than migraine, occur in older patients, and are not followed by headache. There may be associated signs of brainstem ischemia, such as diplopia, vertigo, numbness, weakness, or dysarthria.

Stroke occurs when interruption of blood supply from the posterior cerebral artery to the visual cortex is prolonged. The only finding on examination is a homonymous visual field defect that stops abruptly at the vertical meridian. Occipital lobe stroke is usually due to thrombotic occlusion of the vertebrobasilar system, embolus, or dissection. Lobar hemorrhage, tumor, abscess, and arteriovenous malformation are other common causes of hemianopic cortical visual loss.

Factitious (functional, nonorganic) *visual loss* is claimed by hysterics or malingerers. The latter comprise the vast majority, seeking sympathy, special treatment, or financial gain by feigning loss of sight. The diagnosis is suspected when the history is atypical, physical findings are lacking or contradictory, inconsistencies emerge on testing, and a secondary motive can be identified. In our litigious society, the fraudulent pursuit of recompense has spawned an epidemic of factitious visual loss.

Chronic Visual Loss *Cataract* is a clouding of the lens sufficient to reduce vision. Most cataracts develop slowly as a result of aging, leading to gradual impairment of vision. The formation of cataract occurs more rapidly in patients with a history of ocular trauma, uveitis, or diabetes mellitus. Cataracts are acquired in a variety of genetic diseases, such as myotonic dystrophy, neurofibromatosis type 2, and galactosemia. Radiation therapy and glucocorticoid treatment can induce cataract as a side effect. The cataracts associated with radiation or steroids have a typical posterior subcapsular location. Cataract can be detected by noting an impaired red reflex when viewing light reflected from the fundus with an ophthalmoscope or by examining the dilated eye at the slit lamp.

The only treatment for cataract is surgical extraction of the opacified lens. Over a million cataract operations are performed each year in the United States. The operation is generally done under local retrobulbar anesthesia on an outpatient basis. Remarkable technical innovations have made it possible to aspirate the cataract while leaving the lens capsule intact (extracapsular cataract extraction), rather than removing the entire lens with its capsule (intracapsular cataract extraction). A plastic or silicone intraocular lens is then placed within the empty lens capsule in the posterior chamber, substituting for the natural lens, and leading to rapid recovery of sight. More than 95 percent of patients who undergo cataract extraction can expect an improvement in vision. In many patients, the lens capsule remaining in the eye after cataract extraction eventually turns cloudy, causing a secondary loss of vision. A small opening is made in the lens capsule with a laser to restore clarity.

Glaucoma is a slowly progressive, insidious optic neuropathy, usually associated with chronic elevation of intraocular pressure. In Americans of African descent it is the leading cause of blindness. The mechanism whereby raised intraocular pressure injures the optic nerve is not understood. Axons entering the inferotemporal and superotemporal aspects of the optic disc are damaged first, producing typical nerve fiber bundle or arcuate scotomas on perimetric testing. As fibers are destroyed, the neural rim of the optic disc shrinks and the physiologic cup within the optic disc enlarges (**Plate III-11**). This process is referred to colloquially as pathologic "cupping." The cup-to-disc diameter is expressed as a ratio, e.g., 0.2/1. The cup-to-disc ratio ranges widely in normal subjects, making it difficult to diagnose glaucoma reliably simply by observing an unusually large or deep optic cup. Careful documentation of serial prospective examinations is helpful. In the patient with physiologic cupping, the large cup remains stable, whereas in the patient with glaucoma it expands relentlessly over the years. Detection of visual field loss on formal perimetry also contributes to the diagnosis of glaucoma. Finally, most patients with glaucoma have raised intraocular pressure. However, a surprising number of patients with typical glaucomatous cupping and visual field loss have an intraocular pressure that apparently never exceeds the normal limit of 20 mmHg (so-called low-tension glaucoma).

In acute angle-closure glaucoma, the eye is red and painful due to abrupt, severe elevation of intraocular pressure. Such cases account for only a handful of patients with glaucoma. Most patients with glaucoma have open, nonoccludable anterior chamber angles. In open-angle glaucoma the cause of the raised intraocular pressure is unknown. Because the elevation of intraocular pressure develops gradually and is less marked than in angle-closure glaucoma, there is no pain or ocular injection. The central visual field and foveal acuity are spared until end-stage disease is reached. For these reasons, severe and irreversible damage can occur before either the patient or physician recognizes the diagnosis. Screening of patients for glaucoma by noting the cup-to-disc ratio on ophthalmoscopy and by measuring intraocular pressure (using a Schiotz, Tonopen, or Goldmann tonometer) is vital. Glaucoma is treated with topical adrenergic agonists (epinephrine, dipivefrin, apraclonidine), cholinergic agonists (pilocarpine), and beta blockers (betaxolol, carteolol, levobunolol, metipranolol, and timolol). Occasionally, systemic absorption of beta blocker from an eye drop can be sufficient to cause side effects of bradycardia, hypotension, heart block, bronchospasm, impotence, or depression. Topical or oral carbonic anhydrase inhibitors are used to lower intraocular pressure by reducing aqueous production. Laser treatment of the trabecular meshwork in the anterior chamber angle improves aqueous outflow from the eye. If medical or laser treatments fail to halt optic nerve damage from glaucoma, a filter must be constructed surgically (trabeculectomy) to release aqueous from the eye in a controlled fashion.

Macular degeneration is a major cause of gradual, painless, bilateral central visual loss in the elderly. The old term, "senile macular degeneration," misinterpreted by many patients as an unflattering reference, has been replaced with "age-related macular degeneration." It occurs in a nonexudative (dry) form and an exudative (wet) form. The nonexudative process begins with the accumulation of extracellular deposits, called drusen, underneath the retinal pigment epithelium. On ophthalmoscopy they are pleomorphic but generally appear as small discrete yellow lesions clustered in the macula (**Plate III-12**). With time they become larger, more numerous, and confluent. The retinal pigment epithelium becomes focally detached and atrophic, causing visual loss by interfering with photoreceptor function. There is currently no way to prevent the development of age-related macular degeneration. Concoctions of various vitamins (A, C, and E) and minerals (zinc, copper, and selenium) have been marketed, without good evidence that they retard the process of macular degeneration.

Exudative macular degeneration, which develops in only a minority of patients, occurs when neovascular vessels from the choroid grow through defects in Bruch's membrane into the potential space beneath the retinal pigment epithelium. Leakage from these vessels produces elevation of the retina and pigment epithelium, with distortion (metamorphopsia) and blurring of vision. Although onset of these symptoms is usually gradual, bleeding from subretinal choroidal neovascular membranes sometimes causes acute visual loss. The neovascular membranes can be difficult to see on fundus examination because they are beneath the retina. Fluorescein angiography is extremely useful for their detection. In some patients, prompt laser ablation of choroidal neovascular membranes seen on fluorescein angiography can halt the exudative process. However, the neovascular membranes frequently recur, requiring constant vigilance and repeated photocoagulation.

Major or repeated hemorrhage under the retina from neovascular membranes results in fibrosis, development of a round (disciform) macular scar, and permanent loss of central vision. Surgical attempts to remove subretinal membranes in age-related macular degeneration have not improved vision in most patients. However, outcomes have been more encouraging for patients with choroidal neovascular membranes from ocular histoplasmosis syndrome.

Central serous chorioretinopathy primarily affects males between the ages of 20 and 50. Leakage of serous fluid from the choroid causes small, localized detachment of the retinal pigment epithelium and the neurosensory retina. These detachments produce acute or chronic symptoms of metamorphopsia and blurred vision when the macula is involved. They are difficult to visualize with a direct ophthalmoscope because the detached retina is transparent and only slightly elevated. Diagnosis of central serous chorioretinopathy is made easily by fluorescein angiography, which shows dye streaming into the subretinal space. The cause of central serous chorioretinopathy is unknown. Symptoms may resolve spontaneously if the retina reattaches, but recurrent detachment is common. Laser photocoagulation has benefited some patients with this condition.

Diabetic retinopathy was a rare disease until 1921, when the discovery of insulin resulted in a dramatic improvement in life expectancy for patients with diabetes mellitus. It is now a leading cause of blindness in the United States. The retinopathy of diabetes takes years to develop but eventually appears in nearly all cases. Regular surveillance of the dilated fundus is crucial for any patient with diabetes. In advanced diabetic retinopathy, the proliferation of neovascular vessels leads to blindness from vitreous hemorrhage, retinal detachment, and glaucoma (**Plate III-13**). These complications can be avoided in most patients by administration of panretinal laser photocoagulation at the appropriate point in the evolution of the disease. → *The manifestations* and management of diabetic retinopathy are discussed further in Chap. 334.

CHAPTER 28
Disorders of the Eye **169**

Retinitis pigmentosa is a general term for a disparate group of rod and cone dystrophies characterized by progressive night blindness (nyctalopia), visual field constriction with a ring scotoma, loss of acuity, and an abnormal electroretinogram (ERG). It occurs sporadically or in an autosomal recessive, dominant, or X-linked pattern. Irregular black deposits of clumped pigment in the peripheral retina, called bone spicules because of their vague resemblance to the spicules of cancellous bone, give the disease its name (**Plate III-14**). The name is actually a misnomer because retinitis pigmentosa is not an inflammatory process. Most cases are due to a mutation in the gene for rhodopsin, the rod photopigment, or in the gene for peripherin, a glycoprotein located in photoreceptor outer segments. There is no effective treatment for retinitis pigmentosa. Vitamin A (15,000 IU/day) slightly retards the deterioration of the ERG but has no beneficial effect upon visual acuity or visual fields. Some forms of retinitis pigmentosa occur in association with rare, hereditary systemic diseases (olivopontocerebellar degeneration, Bassen-Kornzweig disease, Kearns-Sayre syndrome, Refsum's disease). Chronic treatment with chloroquine, hydroxychloroquine, and phenothiazines (especially thioridazine) can produce visual loss from a toxic retinopathy that resembles retinitis pigmentosa.

Epiretinal membrane refers to a fibrocellular tissue that grows across the inner surface of the retina, causing metamorphopsia and reduced visual acuity from distortion of the macula. With the ophthalmoscope one can see a crinkled, cellophane-like membrane on the retina. Epiretinal membrane is most common in patients over 50 years of age and is usually unilateral. Most cases are idiopathic, but some occur as a result of hypertensive retinopathy, diabetes, retinal detachment, or trauma. When visual acuity is reduced to the level of about 6/24 (20/80), vitrectomy and surgical peeling of the membrane to relieve macular puckering are recommended. Contraction of an epiretinal membrane sometimes gives rise to a *macular hole*. Most macular holes, however, are caused by local vitreous traction within the fovea. Vision is usually depressed to the level of 6/30 (20/100) or worse. Vitrectomy may improve visual acuity in some patients with macular hole. Fortunately, fewer than 10 percent of patients with macular hole develop a hole in their other eye.

Melanoma of the choroid is the most common primary tumor of the eye (**Plate III-15**). It causes photopsia, an enlarging scotoma, and loss of vision. A small melanoma is often difficult to differentiate from a benign choroidal nevus. Careful serial examinations are required to document a malignant pattern of growth. Treatment of melanoma is controversial. Options include enucleation, local resection, and irradiation. *Metastatic tumors* to the eye outnumber primary tumors of uveal origin. Breast and lung carcinoma have a special propensity to spread to the choroid or iris. Leukemia and lymphoma also commonly invade ocular tissues. Sometimes their only sign on eye examination is a cellular debris in the vitreous, which can masquerade as a chronic posterior uveitis. *Retrobulbar tumor* of the optic nerve (meningioma, glioma) or *chiasmal tumor* (pituitary adenoma, meningioma) produces gradual visual loss with few objective findings, except for optic disc pallor. Rarely, sudden expansion of a pituitary adenoma from infarction and bleeding (*pituitary apoplexy*) causes acute retrobulbar visual loss, with headache, nausea, and ocular motor nerve palsies. In any patient with visual field loss or optic atrophy, CT or MR scanning should be considered if the cause remains unknown after careful review of the history and thorough examination of the eye (Fig. 28-4).

Proptosis Proptosis is an abnormal forward protrusion of one or both eyes. It is measured using a Hertel exophthalmometer, a handheld instrument that records the position of the anterior corneal surface relative to the lateral orbital rim. If this instrument is not available, relative eye position can be judged by bending the patient's head forward and looking down upon the orbits. A proptosis of only 2 mm in one eye is detectable from this perspective. The development of proptosis implies a space-occupying lesion in the orbit. A CT or MR scan should be obtained in any patient with proptosis, unless the diagnosis of Graves' ophthalmopathy is certain.

Graves' ophthalmopathy is the leading cause of proptosis in adults (Chap. 331). Orbital inflammation and engorgement of the extraocular muscles, particularly the medial rectus and the inferior rectus, account for the protrusion of the globe. Corneal exposure, lid retraction, conjunctival injection, restriction of gaze, diplopia, and visual loss from optic nerve compression are cardinal symptoms. Optic nerve compression should be relieved promptly with radiation therapy or orbital decompression to prevent permanent visual loss.

Orbital pseudotumor is an idiopathic, inflammatory orbital syndrome, frequently confused with Graves' ophthalmopathy. Symptoms are pain, limited eye movements, proptosis, and congestion. Evaluation for sarcoidosis, Wegener's granulomatosis, and other types of orbital vasculitis or collagen-vascular disease is negative. Imaging often shows swollen eye muscles (orbital myositis) with enlarged tendons. By contrast, in Graves' ophthalmopathy the tendons of the eye muscles usually are spared. The Tolosa-Hunt syndrome may be regarded as an extension of orbital pseudotumor through the superior orbital fissure into the cavernous sinus. The diagnosis of orbital pseudotumor is difficult. Biopsy of the orbit frequently yields nonspecific evidence of fat infiltration by lymphocytes, plasma cells, and eosinophils. A dramatic response to a therapeutic trial of systemic glucocorticoids indirectly provides the best confirmation of the diagnosis.

Orbital cellulitis causes pain, lid erythema, proptosis, conjunctival chemosis, restricted motility, decreased acuity, afferent pupillary defect, fever, and leukocytosis. It often arises from a paranasal sinus, especially by contiguous spread of infection from the ethmoid sinus through the thin lamina papyracea of the medial orbit. A history of recent upper respiratory tract infection, chronic sinusitis, thick mucous secretions, or dental disease is significant in any patient with suspected orbital cellulitis. Blood cultures should be obtained, but they are usually negative. Most patients respond to empiric therapy with broad-spectrum intravenous antibiotics. Occasionally, orbital cellulitis follows an overwhelming course, with massive proptosis, blindness, septic cavernous sinus thrombosis, and meningitis. To avert this disaster, orbital cellulitis should be managed aggressively in the early stages, with immediate antibiotic therapy and imaging of the orbits. Prompt surgical drainage of an orbital abscess or paranasal sinusitis is indicated if optic nerve function deteriorates despite antibiotics.

Tumors of the orbit cause painless, progressive proptosis. The most common primary tumors are hemangioma, lymphangioma, neurofibroma, dermoid cyst, optic nerve glioma, optic nerve meningioma, and benign mixed tumor of the lacrimal gland. Metastatic tumor to the orbit occurs frequently in breast carcinoma, lung carcinoma, and lymphoma. Diagnosis by fine-needle aspiration followed by urgent radiation therapy can sometimes preserve vision.

Carotid cavernous fistulas with anterior drainage through the orbit produce proptosis, diplopia, glaucoma, and tortuous, red conjunctival vessels. Direct fistulas usually result from trauma. They are easily diagnosed because of the dramatic signs produced by high-flow, high-pressure shunting. Indirect fistulas, or dural arteriovenous malformations, are more likely to occur spontaneously, especially in older women. The signs are more subtle and the diagnosis is frequently missed. The combination of slight proptosis, diplopia, enlarged muscles, and an injected eye is often mistaken for thyroid ophthalmopathy. A bruit heard upon auscultation of the head, or reported by the patient, is a valuable diagnostic clue. Imaging shows an enlarged superior ophthalmic vein in the orbits. Carotid cavernous shunts can be eliminated by intravascular embolization.

Ptosis *Blepharoptosis* is an abnormal drooping of the eyelid. Unilateral or bilateral ptosis can be congenital, from dysgenesis of the levator palpebrae superioris, or from abnormal insertion of its aponeurosis into the eyelid. Acquired ptosis can develop so gradually that the patient is unaware of the problem. Inspection of old photographs is helpful in dating the onset. A history of prior trauma, eye surgery, contact lens use, diplopia, systemic symptoms (e.g., dysphagia or peripheral muscle weakness), or a family history of ptosis should be sought. Fluctuating ptosis that worsens late in the day is typical of myasthenia gravis. Examination should focus upon evidence for proptosis, eyelid masses or deformities, inflammation, pupil inequality, or limitation of motility. The width of the palpebral fissures is measured in primary gaze to quantitate the degree of ptosis. The ptosis will be underestimated if the patient is compensating by lifting the brow with the frontalis muscle.

Mechanical ptosis occurs in many elderly patients from stretching and redundancy of eyelid skin and subcutaneous fat (dermatochalasis). The extra weight of these sagging tissues causes the lid to droop. Enlargment or deformation of the eyelid from infection, tumor, trauma, or inflammation also results in ptosis on a purely mechanical basis.

Aponeurotic ptosis is an acquired dehiscence or stretching of the aponeurotic tendon, which connects the levator muscle to the tarsal plate of the eyelid. It occurs commonly in older patients, presumably from loss of connective tissue elasticity. Aponeurotic ptosis is also a frequent sequela of eyelid swelling from infection or blunt trauma to the orbit, cataract surgery, or hard contact lens usuage.

Myogenic ptosis includes myasthenia gravis (see Chap. 382) and a number of rare myopathies that manifest with ptosis. The term *chronic progressive external ophthalmoplegia* refers to a spectrum of systemic diseases caused by mutations of mitochrondrial DNA. As the name implies, the most prominent findings are symmetric, slowly progressive ptosis and limitation of eye movements. In general, diplopia is a late symptom because all eye movements are reduced equally. In the *Kearns-Sayre* variant, retinal pigmentary changes and abnormalities of cardiac conduction develop. Peripheral muscle biopsy shows characteristic "ragged-red fibers." *Oculopharyngeal dystrophy* is a distinct autosomal dominant disease with onset in middle age, characterized by ptosis, limited eye movements, and trouble swallowing. *Myotonic dystrophy*, another autosomal dominant disorder, causes ptosis, ophthalmoparesis, cataract, and pigmentary retinopathy. Patients have muscle wasting, myotonia, frontal balding, and cardiac abnormalities.

Neurogenic ptosis results from a lesion affecting the innervation to either of the two muscles that open the eyelid: Muller's muscle or the levator palpebrae superioris. Examination of the pupil helps to decide between these two possibilities. In Horner's syndrome, the eye with ptosis has a smaller pupil and the eye movements are full. In an oculomotor nerve palsy, the eye with the ptosis has a larger, or a normal, pupil. If the pupil is normal but there is limitation of adduction, elevation, and depression, a pupil-sparing oculomotor nerve palsy is likely (see next section). Rarely, a lesion affecting the small, central subnucleus of the oculomotor complex will cause bilateral ptosis with normal eye movements and pupils.

Double Vision   The first point to clarify is whether diplopia persists in either eye after covering the fellow eye. If it does, the diagnosis is monocular diplopia. The cause is usually intrinsic to the eye and therefore has no dire implications for the patient. Corneal aberrations (e.g., keratoconus, pterygium), uncorrected refractive error, cataract, or foveal traction may give rise to monocular diplopia. Occasionally it is a symptom of malingering or psychiatric disease. Diplopia alleviated by covering one eye is binocular diplopia and is caused by disruption of ocular alignment. Inquiry should be made into the nature of the double vision (purely side-by-side versus partial vertical displacement of images), mode of onset, duration, intermittency, diurnal variation, and associated neurologic or systemic symptoms. If the patient has diplopia while being examined, motility testing should reveal a deficiency corresponding to the patient's symptoms. However, subtle limitation of ocular excursions is often difficult to detect. For example, a patient with a slight left abducens nerve paresis may appear to have full eye movements, despite a complaint of horizontal diplopia upon looking to the left. In this situation, the cover test provides a more sensitive method for demonstrating the ocular malalignment. It should be conducted in primary gaze, and then with the head turned and tilted in each direction. In the above example, a cover test with the head turned to the right will maximize the fixation shift evoked by the cover test.

Occasionally, a cover test performed in an asymptomatic patient during a routine examination will reveal an ocular deviation. If the eye movements are full and the ocular misalignment is equal in all directions of gaze (concomitant deviation) the diagnosis is strabismus. In this condition, which affects about 1 percent of the population, fusion is disrupted in infancy or early childhood. To avoid diplopia, vision is suppressed from the nonfixating eye. In some children, this leads to impaired vision (amblyopia, or "lazy" eye) in the deviated eye.

Binocular diplopia occurs from a wide range of processes: infectious, neoplastic, metabolic, degenerative, inflammatory, and vascular. One must decide if the diplopia is neurogenic in origin or due to restriction of globe rotation by local disease in the orbit. Orbital pseudotumor, myositis, infection, tumor, thyroid disease, and muscle entrapment (e.g., from a blowout fracture) cause restrictive diplopia. The diagnosis is confirmed by performing a forced duction test in the office. After applying topical anesthesia, the physician grasps the eye with forceps and pulls it toward the direction of deficient motion. If rotation of the globe is prevented by tethering, a restrictive process is at work. The utility of this test is limited by its unpopularity with patients; in practice, the diagnosis of restriction is made by recognizing other associated signs and symptoms of local orbital disease.

Myasthenia gravis (Chap. 382) is a major cause of diplopia. The diplopia is often intermittent, variable, and not confined to any single ocular motor nerve distribution. The pupils are always normal. Fluctuating ptosis may be present. Many patients have a purely ocular form of the disease, with no evidence of systemic muscular weakness. The diagnosis can be confirmed by an intravenous edrophonium injection or by an assay for antiacetylcholine receptor antibodies. Negative results from these tests do not exclude the diagnosis. *Botulism* from food or wound poisoning can mimic ocular myasthenia.

After restrictive orbital disease and myasthenia gravis are excluded, a lesion of a cranial nerve supplying innervation to the extraocular muscles is the most likely cause of binocular diplopia.

The *oculomotor nerve* (third cranial nerve) innervates the medial, inferior, and superior recti; inferior oblique; levator palpebrae superioris; and the iris sphincter. Total palsy of the oculomotor nerve lesion causes ptosis, a dilated pupil, and leaves the eye "down and out" because of the unopposed action of the lateral rectus and superior oblique. This combination of findings is obvious. More challenging is the diagnosis of an early or partial oculomotor nerve palsy. In this setting, any combination of ptosis, pupil dilation, and weakness of the eye muscles supplied by the oculomotor nerve may be encountered. Frequent serial examinations during the evolving phase of the palsy and a high index of suspicion help ensure that the diagnosis is not missed. The advent of an oculomotor nerve palsy with any degree of pupil involvement in an otherwise healthy patient, especially when accompanied by pain, raises the specter of a circle of Willis aneurysm. If an MR scan shows no compressive lesion, an arteriogram must be performed to rule out an aneurysm of either the posterior communicating artery or the basilar artery. If the pupil is entirely normal, with all other components of an oculomotor palsy present, aneurysm is so rare that an angiogram is seldom indicated.

A lesion of the oculomotor nucleus in the rostral midbrain produces signs that differ from those caused by a lesion of the nerve itself. There is bilateral ptosis because the levator muscle is innervated by a single central subnucleus. There is also weakness of the contralateral superior rectus, because it is supplied by the oculomotor nucleus on the other side. Occasionally both superior recti are weak. Isolated nuclear oculomotor palsy is quite rare. Usually neurologic examination reveals additional signs to suggest brainstem damage from infarction, hemorrhage, tumor, or infection.

Injury to structures surrounding fascicles of the oculomotor nerve descending through the midbrain has given rise to a number of classic eponymic designations. In *Nothnagel's syndrome*, injury to the superior cerebellar peduncle causes ipsilateral oculomotor palsy and contralateral cerebellar ataxia. In *Benedikt's syndrome*, injury to the red nucleus results in ipsilateral oculomotor palsy and contralateral tremor, chorea, and athetosis. *Claude's syndrome* incorporates features of both the aforementioned syndromes, by injury to both the red nucleus and the superior cerebellar peduncle. Finally, in *Weber's syndrome*, injury to the cerebral peduncle causes ipsilateral oculomotor palsy with contralateral hemiparesis.

In the subarachnoid space the oculomotor nerve is vulnerable to aneurysm, meningitis, tumor, infarction, and compression. In cerebral herniation the nerve becomes trapped between the edge of the tentorium and the uncus of the temporal lobe. Oculomotor palsy can also occur from midbrain torsion and hemorrhages during herniation. In the cavernous sinus, oculomotor palsy arises from carotid aneurysm, carotid cavernous fistula, cavernous sinus thrombosis, tumor (pituitary adenoma, meningioma, metastasis), herpes zoster infection, and the Tolosa-Hunt syndrome.

The etiology of an isolated, pupil-sparing oculomotor palsy often remains obscure, even after neuroimaging and extensive laboratory testing. Most cases are thought to result from microvascular infarction of the nerve, somewhere along its course from the brainstem to the orbit. Usually the patient complains of pain. Diabetes, hypertension, and vascular disease are major risk factors. Spontaneous recovery over a period of months is the rule. If this fails to occur, or if new findings develop, the diagnosis of microvascular oculomotor nerve palsy should be reconsidered. Aberrant regeneration is common when the oculomotor nerve is injured by trauma or compression (tumor, aneurysm). Miswiring of sprouting fibers to the levator muscle and the rectus muscles results in elevation of the eyelid upon downgaze or adduction. The pupil also constricts upon attempted adduction, elevation, or depression of the globe. Aberrant regeneration is not seen after oculomotor palsy from microvascular infarct and hence vitiates that diagnosis.

The *trochlear nucleus* (fourth cranial nerve) is located in the midbrain, just caudal to the oculomotor nerve complex. Its fibers exit the brainstem dorsally and cross to innervate the contralateral superior oblique. The principal actions of this muscle are to depress and to intort the globe. A palsy therefore results in hypertropia and excyclotorsion. The cyclotorsion is seldom noticed by patients. Instead, they complain of vertical diplopia, especially upon reading or looking down. The vertical diplopia also is exacerbated by tilting the head toward the side with the palsy, and alleviated by tilting it away. This "head tilt test" is a cardinal diagnostic feature.

Isolated trochlear nerve palsy occurs from all the causes listed above for the oculomotor nerve, except aneurysm. The trochlear nerve is particularly apt to suffer injury after closed head trauma. The mechanism is unknown, but the free edge of the tentorium may impinge upon the nerve during a concussive blow. Most isolated trochlear nerve palsies are idiopathic and hence diagnosed by exclusion as "microvascular." Spontaneous improvement occurs over a period of months in most patients. A base-down prism (conveniently applied to the patient's glasses as a stick-on Fresnel lens) may serve as a temporary measure to alleviate diplopia. If the palsy does not resolve, the eyes can be realigned by surgically adjusting other eye muscles.

The *abducens nerve* (sixth cranial nerve) innervates the lateral rectus muscle. A palsy produces horizontal diplopia, worse on gaze to the side of the lesion. A nuclear lesion has different consequences, because the abducens nucleus contains interneurons that project via the medial longitudinal fasciculus to the medial rectus subnucleus of the contralateral oculomotor complex. Therefore, an abducens nuclear lesion produces a complete lateral gaze palsy, from weakness of both the ipsilateral lateral rectus and the contralateral medial rectus. *Foville's syndrome* following dorsal pontine injury includes lateral gaze palsy, ipsilateral facial palsy, and contralateral hemiparesis incurred by damage to descending corticospinal fibers. *Millard-Gubler syndrome* from ventral pontine injury is similar, except for the eye findings. There is lateral rectus weakness only, instead of gaze palsy, because the abducens fascicle is injured rather than the nucleus. Infarct, tumor, hemorrhage, vascular malformation, and multiple sclerosis are the most common etiologies of brainstem abducens palsy.

After leaving the ventral pons, the abducens nerve runs forward along the clivus to pierce the dura at the petrous apex where it enters the cavernous sinus. Along its subarachnoid course it is susceptible to meningitis, tumor (meningioma, chordoma, carcinomatous meningitis), subarachnoid hemorrhage, trauma, and compression by aneurysm or dolichoectatic vessels. At the petrous apex, mastoiditis can produce deafness, pain, and ipsilateral abducens palsy (*Gradenigo's syndrome*). In the cavernous sinus, the nerve can be affected by carotid aneurysm, carotid cavernous fistula, tumor (pituitary adenoma, meningioma, nasopharyngeal carcinoma), herpes infection, and Tolosa-Hunt syndrome.

Unilateral or bilateral abducens palsy is a classic sign of raised intracranial pressure. The diagnosis can be confirmed if papilledema is observed on fundus examination. The mechanism is still debated but is probably related to rostral-caudal displacement of the brainstem. The same phenomenon accounts for abducens palsy from low intracranial pressure (e.g., after lumbar puncture, spinal anesthesia, or spontaneous dural cerebrospinal fluid leak).

Treatment of abducens palsy is aimed at prompt correction of the underlying cause. However, the cause remains obscure in many instances, despite diligent evaluation. As mentioned above for isolated trochlear or oculomotor palsy, most cases are assumed to represent microvascular infarcts because they often occur in the setting of diabetes or other vascular risk factors. Some cases may develop as a postinfectious mononeuritis (e.g., following a viral flu). Patching one eye or applying a temporary prism will provide relief of diplopia until the palsy resolves. If recovery is incomplete, eye muscle surgery can nearly always realign the eyes, at least in primary position. A patient with an abducens palsy that fails to improve should be reevaluated for an occult etiology (e.g., chordoma, carcinomatous meningitis, carotid cavernous fistula, myasthenia gravis).

Multiple ocular motor nerve palsies should not be attributed to spontaneous microvascular events affecting more than one cranial nerve at a time. This remarkable coincidence does occur, especially in diabetic patients, but the diagnosis is made only in retrospect after exhausting all other diagnostic alternatives. Neuroimaging should focus on the cavernous sinus, superior orbital fissure, and orbital apex, where all three ocular motor nerves are in close proximity. In the diabetic or compromised host, fungal infection (*Aspergillus*, Mucorales, *Cryptococcus*) is a frequent cause of multiple nerve palsies. In the patient with systemic malignancy, carcinomatous meningitis is a likely diagnosis. Cytologic examination may be negative despite repeated sampling of the cerebrospinal fluid. The cancer-associated Eaton-Lambert myasthenic syndrome can also produce ophthalmoplegia. Giant cell (temporal) arteritis occasionally manifests as diplopia from ischemic palsies of extraocular muscles. Fisher's syndrome, an ocular variant of Guillain-Barré, can produce ophthalmoplegia with areflexia and ataxia. Often the ataxia is mild, and the areflexia is overlooked because the physician's attention is focused upon the eyes.

Supranuclear disorders of gaze are often mistaken for multiple ocular motor nerve palsies. For example, Wernicke's encephalopathy can produce nystagmus and a partial deficit of horizontal and vertical gaze that mimics a combined abducens and oculomotor nerve palsy. The disorder occurs in malnourished or alcoholic patients and can be reversed by giving thiamine. Infarct, hemorrhage, tumor, multiple sclerosis, encephalitis, vasculitis, and Whipple's disease are other important causes of supranuclear gaze palsy.

The *frontal eye field* of the cerebral cortex is involved in generation of saccades to the contralateral side. After hemispheric stroke, the eyes usually deviate towards the lesioned side because of the unopposed action of the frontal eye field in the normal hemisphere. With time, this deficit resolves. Seizures generally have the opposite effect: the eyes deviate conjugately away from the irritative focus. *Parietal lesions* disrupt smooth pursuit of targets moving toward the side of the lesion. Bilateral parietal lesions produce Balint's syndrome, characterized by impaired eye-hand coordination (optic ataxia), difficulty initiating voluntary eye movements (ocular apraxia), and visuospatial disorientation (simultanagnosia).

Descending cortical inputs mediating *horizontal gaze* ultimately converge at the level of the pons. Neurons in the paramedian pontine reticular formation are responsible for controlling conjugate gaze toward the same side. They project directly to the ipsilateral abducens nucleus. A lesion of either the paramedian pontine reticular formation or the abducens nucleus causes an ipsilateral conjugate gaze palsy. Lesions at either locus produce nearly identical clinical syndromes, with the following exception: vestibular stimulation (oculocephalic maneuver or caloric) will succeed in driving the eyes conjugately to the side in a patient with a lesion of the paramedian pontine reticular formation, but not in a patient with a lesion of the abducens nucleus.

Internuclear ophthalmoplegia results from damage to the medial longitudinal fasciculus ascending from the abducens nucleus in the pons to the oculomotor nucleus in the midbrain (hence, "internuclear"). Damage to fibers carrying the conjugate signal from abducens interneurons to the contralateral medial rectus motoneurons results in a failure of adduction on attempted lateral gaze. For example, a patient with a left internuclear ophthalmoplegia will have slowed or absent adducting movements of the left eye. A patient with bilateral injury to the medial longitudinal fasciculus will have bilateral internuclear ophthalmoplegia. Multiple sclerosis is the most common cause, although tumor, stroke, trauma, or any brainstem process may be responsible. One-and-a half syndrome is due to a combined lesion of the medial longitudinal fasciculus and the abducens nucleus on the same side. The patient's only horizontal eye movement is abduction of the eye on the other side.

Vertical gaze is controlled at the level of the midbrain. The neuronal circuits affected in disorders of vertical gaze are not well elucidated, but lesions of the rostral interstitial nucleus of the medial longitudinal fasciculus and the interstitial nucleus of Cajal cause supranuclear paresis of upgaze, downgaze, or all vertical eye movements. Distal basilar artery ischemia is the most common etiology. *Skew deviation* refers to a vertical misalignment of the eyes, usually constant in all positions of gaze. The finding has poor localizing value because skew deviation has been reported after lesions in widespread regions of the brainstem and cerebellum.

Parinaud's syndrome (dorsal midbrain syndrome) is a distinct supranuclear vertical gaze disorder from damage to the posterior commissure. It is a classic sign of hydrocephalus from aqueductal stenosis. Pineal region tumors (germinoma, pineoblastoma), cysticercosis, and stroke also cause Parinaud's syndrome. Features include loss of upgaze (and sometimes downgaze), convergence-retraction nystagmus on attempted upgaze, downwards ocular deviation (setting sun sign), lid retraction (Collier's sign), skew deviation, pseudoabducens palsy, and light-near dissociation of the pupils. Disorders of vertical gaze, especially downwards saccades, are an early feature of progressive supranuclear palsy. Smooth pursuit is affected later in the course of the disease. Parkinson's disease, Huntington's chorea, and olivopontocerebellar degeneration can also affect vertical gaze.

Nystagmus is a rhythmical oscillation of the eyes, occurring normally from vestibular and optokinetic stimulation or abnormally in a wide variety of diseases. Blindness from anterior visual pathway disease in early life causes a complex, searching nystagmus with irregular pendular (sinusoidal) and jerk features. This nystagmus is commonly referred to as *congenital nystagmus*, a poor term, given that it is acquired often in early childhood. Sometimes it develops in a perfectly normal child.

Jerk nystagmus is characterized by a slow drift off the target, followed by a fast corrective saccade. By convention, the nystagmus is named after the quick phase. Jerk nystagmus can be downbeat,

upbeat, horizontal (left or right), and torsional. The pattern of nystagmus may vary with gaze position. Some patients will be oblivious to their nystagmus. Others will complain of a subjective, to-and-fro movement of the environment (oscillopsia), corresponding to their nystagmus. Fine nystagmus may be difficult to see upon gross examination of the eyes. Observation of nystagmoid movements of the optic disc on ophthalmoscopy is a sensitive way to detect subtle degrees of nystagmus. The slit lamp is also useful.

Gaze-evoked nystagmus is the most common form of jerk nystagmus. When the eyes are held eccentrically in the orbits, they have a natural tendency to drift back to primary position. The subject compensates by making a corrective saccade to maintain the deviated eye position. Many normal patients have mild gaze-evoked nystagmus. Exaggerated gaze-evoked nystagmus can be induced by drugs (sedatives, anticonvulsants, alcohol), muscle paresis, myasthenia, demyelinating disease and, cerebellopontine angle, brainstem, and cerebellar lesions.

Vestibular nystagmus results from dysfunction of the labyrinth (Ménière's disease), vestibular nerve, or vestibular nucleus in the brainstem. Peripheral vestibular nystagmus often occurs in discrete attacks, with symptoms of nausea and vertigo. There may be associated tinnitus and hearing loss. Sudden shifts in head position may provoke or exacerbate symptoms.

Downbeat nystagmus occurs from lesions near the craniocervical junction (Chiari malformation, basilar invagination). It has also been reported in brainstem or cerebellar stroke, lithium or anticonvulsant intoxication, and multiple sclerosis. *Upbeat nystagmus* is associated with damage to the pontine tegmentum, from stroke, demyelination, or tumor.

Opsoclonus is a rare, dramatic disorder of eye movements consisting of bursts of consecutive saccades (saccadomania). When the saccades are confined to the horizontal plane, the term *ocular flutter* is preferred. It is a sign of neuroblastoma, encephalitis, trauma, or paraneoplastic syndrome. It has been reported as a benign, transient phenomenon in otherwise healthy patients, probably as a consequence of a mild, occult viral encephalitis.

BIBLIOGRAPHY

ALBERT DM, JAKOBIEC FA (eds): *Principles and Practice of Ophthalmology.* Philadelphia, Saunders, 1994

BECK RW et al: A randomized controlled trial of corticosteroids in the treatment of acute optic neuritis. N Engl J Med 326:581, 1992

———— et al: The effect of corticosteroids for acute optic neuritis on the subsequent development of multiple sclerosis. N Engl J Med 329:1764, 1993

BURDE RM et al: *Clinical Decisions in Neuro-ophthalmology*, 2d ed. St. Louis, Mosby, 1992

DUANE T (ed): *Clinical Ophthalmology.* Philadelphia, Lippincott, 1994

EXECUTIVE COMMITTEE FOR THE ASYMPTOMATIC CAROTID ATHEROSCLEROSIS STUDY: Endarterectomy for asymptomatic carotid artery stenosis. JAMA 273:1421, 1995

GASS JD: *Stereoscopic Atlas of Macular Diseases*, 4th ed. St. Louis, Mosby, 1996

GOLD DH, WEINGEIST TA (eds): *The Eye in Systemic Disease.* Philadelphia, Lippincott, 1990

LEIGH RJ, ZEE DS: *The Neurology of Eye Movements*, 2d ed. Philadelphia, Davis, 1991

MILLER NR: *Walsh and Hoyt's Clinical Neuroophthalmology*, 4th ed. Baltimore, Williams & Wilkins, 1995

NATHAN J et al: Molecular genetics of inherited variation in human color vision. Science 232:203, 1986

SINGH G: A mitochondrial DNA mutation as a cause of Leber's hereditary optic neuropathy. N Engl J Med 320:1300, 1989

SMOLIN G, THOFT RA (eds): *The Cornea*, 3d ed. Boston, Little, Brown, 1994

VAUGHN D et al: *General Ophthalmology*, 14th ed. Norwalk, Appleton & Lange, 1995

DISORDERS OF SMELL, TASTE, AND HEARING

SMELL

The sense of smell determines the flavor and palatability of food and drink. It serves along with the trigeminal system as a monitor of inhaled chemicals, including dangerous substances such as natural gas, smoke, and air pollutants. Although qualitative sensations of smell are subserved by the olfactory neuroepithelium, many substances are capable of producing somatic sensations of coolness, warmth, and irritation through the trigeminal, glossopharyngeal, and vagal afferents in the nose, oral cavity, tongue, pharynx, and larynx. The sense of smell should be considered as one of several chemosensory systems, since most chemical substances initiate olfactory, trigeminal, and taste perceptions.

The *olfactory neuroepithelium* is located in the superior part of the nasal cavities. It contains an orderly arrangement of bipolar olfactory receptor cells, microvillar cells, sustentacular cells, and basal cells. The dendritic process of the bipolar cell has a bulb-shaped knob or vesicle that projects into the mucous layer and bears six to eight cilia. The receptor sites for odorant molecules are located on the cilia. The microvillar cells are located adjacent to the receptor cells on the surface of the neuroepithelium. The sustentacular cells, unlike their counterparts in the respiratory epithelium, are not specialized to secrete mucus. Their function is unknown. The basal cells are progenitors of other cell types in the olfactory neuroepithelium, including the bipolar receptor cells. There is a regular turnover of the bipolar receptor cells, which function as the primary sensory neurons. In addition, with injury to the cell body or its axon, the receptor cell is replaced by a differentiated basal cell which reestablishes a central neural connection. *Hence these primary sensory neurons are unique among sensory systems in that they are regularly replaced and regenerate after injury.*

The unmyelinated axons of the receptor cells form the fila of the olfactory nerve, pass through the cribriform plate, and terminate within spherical masses of neuropil, termed *glomeruli*, in the olfactory bulb. The glomeruli are the focus of a high degree of convergence of information, since many more fibers enter than leave them. The main second-order neurons are the mitral cells. The primary dendrite of each mitral cell extends into a single glomerulus. Axons of the mitral cells project along with the axons of adjacent tufted cells to the limbic system, including the anterior olfactory nucleus, the prepiriform cortex, the periamygdaloid cortex, the olfactory tubercle, the nucleus of the lateral olfactory tract, and the corticomedial nucleus of the amygdala. Cognitive awareness of smell requires stimulation of the prepiriform cortex or the amygdaloid nuclei.

Odorants are absorbed into the mucus overlying the olfactory neuroepithelium, diffuse to the cilia, and reversibly bind to membrane receptor sites. The process causes conformational changes in the receptor proteins which induce a chain of biochemical events that results in generation of action potentials in the primary neurons. Transduction depends on the activation of G protein–coupled second messengers. Intensity appears to be coded by the amount of firing in the afferent neurons. Indeed, a clear relationship exists in humans between psychophysical measures of intensity and the magnitude of the evoked potential from the olfactory neuroepithelium. The discovery of a large family of receptor genes suggests that there may be specific receptors for each odorant. A single receptor neuron expresses only one receptor subtype of the multigene family. All receptor neurons expressing a given receptor subtype project their axons to one or two glomeruli in the olfactory bulb.

DISORDERS OF THE SENSE OF SMELL
Disorders of the sense of smell are caused by conditions that interfere with the access of the odorant to the olfactory neuroepithelium (transport loss), injure the receptor region (sensory loss), or damage central olfactory pathways (neural loss).

Transport olfactory loss can result from swollen nasal mucous membrane in acute viral upper respiratory infections, bacterial rhinitis and sinusitis, allergic rhinitis, and structural changes in the nasal cavity such as deviations of the nasal septum, polyps, and neoplasms. It is also likely that abnormalities of mucus secretion in which the olfactory cilia are immersed could result in a loss of olfactory sensitivity.

Sensory olfactory losses are caused by destruction of the olfactory neuroepithelium by viral infections, neoplasms, the inhalation of toxic chemicals, drugs that affect cell turnover, and radiation therapy to the head. *Neural olfactory losses* occur in head trauma, with or without fracture of the base of the anterior cranial fossa or cribriform plate area; Parkinson's disease, Alzheimer's disease, Korsakoff's psychosis, and vitamin B$_{12}$ deficiency; neoplasms of the anterior cranial fossa; neurosurgical procedures; administration of neurotoxic agents (e.g., ethanol, amphetamines, topical cocaine, aminoglycosides, tetracycline, cigarette smoke); and in some congenital disorders such as Kallmann's syndrome. Other endocrine disorders, including Cushing's syndrome, hypothyroidism, and diabetes mellitus, can affect smell perception.

From the psychophysical point of view, disorders of the sense of smell may be categorized by either the patient's complaint or the objective sensory measurements as *total anosmia* (general anosmia)—inability to detect any qualitative olfactory sensations; *partial anosmia*—ability to detect some, but not all, qualitative olfactory sensations; *specific anosmia*—loss of ability to appreciate only one or a very limited number of odorants; *total hyposmia* (general hyposmia)—decreased sensitivity to all odorants; *partial hyposmia*—decreased sensitivity to some odorants; *dysosmia* (cacosmia or paraosmia)—distortion in the perception of an odor, i.e., the perception of an unpleasant odor when a pleasant odorant is being presented or the perception of an odor when there is no odorant in the environment; *total hyperosmia* (general hyperosmia)—increased sensitivity to all odorants; *partial hyperosmia*—increased sensitivity to some odorants; and *agnosia*—inability to classify, contrast, or identify odor sensations verbally, even though the ability to distinguish between odorants or to recognize them may be normal.

Clinical Evaluation The history of the onset and development of the disorder of the sense of smell may be of paramount importance in making an etiologic diagnosis. Unilateral anosmia is rarely a complaint. Only by separate testing of smell in each nasal cavity can it be recognized. Bilateral anosmia, on the other hand, does bring patients to medical attention. Anosmic patients usually complain of a loss of the sense of taste even though their taste thresholds may be within normal limits. In actuality, they are complaining of a loss of flavor detection, which is mainly an olfactory function. Flavor appreciation depends on the olfactory detection of volatile substances in food and beverages as well as the sense of taste. The physical examination should include a complete examination of the ears, upper respiratory tract, and head and neck. A neurologic examination emphasizing the cranial nerves is essential. Computed tomography (CT) scans of the head with enhancement are required to rule out neoplasms of the anterior cranial fossa, unsuspected fractures of the anterior cranial fossa, paranasal sinusitis, and neoplasms of the nasal cavity and paranasal sinuses.

The sensory evaluation of olfactory function is necessary for corroboration of the patient's complaint, evaluation of the efficacy of treatment, and determination of the degree of permanent impairment. The first step in the sensory evaluation is to determine the degree to which qualitative sensations are present. For this assessment, a smell identification test is used that consists of a 40-item, forced choice, microencapsulated odor, scratch-and-sniff paradigm. For example, one of the items reads, "This odor smells most like (a) chocolate, (b) banana, (c) onion, or (d) fruit punch," and the patient is instructed to answer one of the alternatives. The test is highly reliable (short-term test-retest reliability $r = 0.95$) and is sensitive to age and sex differences (Fig. 29-1). It is an accurate quantitative determination of the relative degree of olfactory deficit. Persons with a total loss of smell function score in the range of 7 to 19 out of 40. The average score for total anosmics is slightly higher than that expected on the basis of chance because of the inclusion of some odorants that act by trigeminal stimulation.

The second step is to establish a detection threshold for the odorant phenyl ethyl alcohol, using a graduated stimulus. Sensitivity for each side of the nose is determined with a detection threshold for phenyl ethyl methyl ethyl carbinol. Nasal resistance is measured with anterior rhinomanometry for each side of the nose.

Techniques have been developed to biopsy the olfactory neuroepithelium, but in view of the widespread degeneration of the olfactory neuroepithelium and intercalation of respiratory epithelium in the olfactory area of adults with no apparent olfactory dysfunction, biopsy material must be interpreted cautiously.

Differential Diagnosis At the present time, there are no psychophysical methods to differentiate sensory from neural olfactory losses. Fortunately, the history of the disease provides important clues to the cause. The leading causes of olfactory disorders are head trauma and viral infections. Head trauma is a more frequent cause of anosmia in children and young adults, and viral infections are more important causes of anosmia in older adults.

Cranial trauma is followed by uni- or bilateral impairment of smell in 5 to 10 percent of cases. Frontal injuries and fractures disrupt the cribriform plate and olfactory axons that perforate it. Sometimes there is an associated cerebrospinal fluid (CSF) rhinorrhea resulting from a tearing of the dura overlying the cribriform plate and paranasal sinuses. Anosmia also may follow blows to the occiput. Once traumatic anosmia develops, it is usually permanent; only about 10 percent of patients ever improve or recover. Perversion of the sense of smell may occur as a phase in the recovery process.

Viral infections destroy the olfactory neuroepithelium, and it is replaced by respiratory epithelium. Congenital anosmias are rare but important. Kallmann's syndrome is a neuronal migration defect for which the X-linked gene (KAL) has been cloned. It is characterized by congenital anosmia and hypogonadotropic hypogonadism (see Chap. 328). The hypothalamic and olfactory bulb defects result from failure of migration from the olfactory placode of olfactory receptor neurons and neurons synthesizing gonadotropin-releasing hormone. Anosmia also can occur in albinos. The receptor cells are present but are hypoplastic, lack cilia, and do not project above the surrounding supporting cells.

Meningioma of the inferior frontal region is the most frequent neoplastic cause of anosmia; rarely, anosmia can occur with glioma of the frontal lobe. Occasionally, pituitary adenomas, craniopharyngiomas, suprasellar meningiomas, and aneurysms of the anterior part of the circle of Willis extend forward and damage olfactory structures. These tumors and hamartomas also may induce seizures with olfactory hallucinations, indicating involvement of the uncus of the temporal lobe.

Dysosmia, subjective distortions of olfactory perception, may occur with intranasal disease that partially impairs smell or may represent a phase in the recovery from a neurogenic anosmia. Most dysosmic disorders consist of disagreeable or foul odors, and they may be accompanied by distortions of taste. Dysosmia is associated with depression.

℞ TREATMENT

Therapy for patients with transport olfactory losses due to allergic rhinitis, bacterial rhinitis and sinusitis, polyps, neoplasms, and structural abnormalities of the nasal cavities can be undertaken rationally and with a high chance of improvement. Allergy management, antibiotic therapy, topical and systemic glucocorticoid therapy, and operations for nasal polyps, deviation of the nasal septum, and chronic hyperplastic sinusitis are frequently effective in restoring the sense of smell.

There is no treatment with demonstrated efficacy for sensorineural olfactory losses. Fortunately, spontaneous recovery often occurs. Zinc and vitamin therapy are advocated by some. Profound zinc deficiency can undoubtedly result in losses and distortion of the sense of smell, but it is not a clinical problem except in very limited geographic areas. Vitamin therapy has mainly been in the form of vitamin A. The epithelial degeneration associated with vitamin A deficiency can cause anosmia, but vitamin A deficiency is not a common clinical problem in the United States.

TASTE

Many patients with a loss of olfactory sensitivity also complain of a loss of the sense of taste. On psychophysical testing, most of these patients have normal detection thresholds for taste. Disturbances of the sense of taste are far less frequent than disturbances of the sense of smell.

The taste receptor cells are located in the taste buds, spherical groups of cells arranged like the segments of a citrus fruit. At the surface, the taste bud has a pore into which microvilli of the receptor cells project. Taste buds have a similar appearance wherever they are located. Unlike the olfactory system, the receptor cell is not the primary neuron. Instead, gustatory afferent nerve fibers contact individual taste receptor cells. Transduction depends on activation of G protein–coupled second messengers but differs in details for each taste quality.

The sense of taste is mediated through the facial, glossopharyngeal, and vagal nerves. The gustatory system consists of at least five receptor populations. Taste buds are located in the foliate papillae along the lateral margin of the tongue, in the fungiform papillae throughout the dorsum of the tongue, in the circumvallate papillae at the junction of the dorsum and the base of the tongue, and in the palate, epiglottis, larynx, and esophagus. The chorda tympani branch of the facial nerve subserves taste from the anterior two-thirds of the tongue. The posterior third of the tongue is supplied by the lingual branch of the glossopharyngeal nerve. Afferents from the palate travel with the greater superficial petrosal nerve to the geniculate ganglion and thence via the facial nerve to the brainstem. The internal branch of the superior laryngeal nerve of the vagus nerve contains the taste afferents from the larynx including the epiglottis and esophagus.

The central connections of the nerves terminate in the brainstem in the nucleus of the tractus solitarius. The fibers of the chorda tympani and greater superficial petrosal nerves go to the cephalic portion of the nucleus. The glossopharyngeal gustatory fibers go to the middle, and the superior laryngeal nerve fibers go to the caudal portion of the nucleus. The central pathway from the nucleus of the tractus solitarius projects to the ipsilateral parabrachial nuclei of the pons. Two divergent pathways project from the parabrachial nuclei. One ascends to the gustatory relay in the dorsal thalamus, synapses, and continues to the

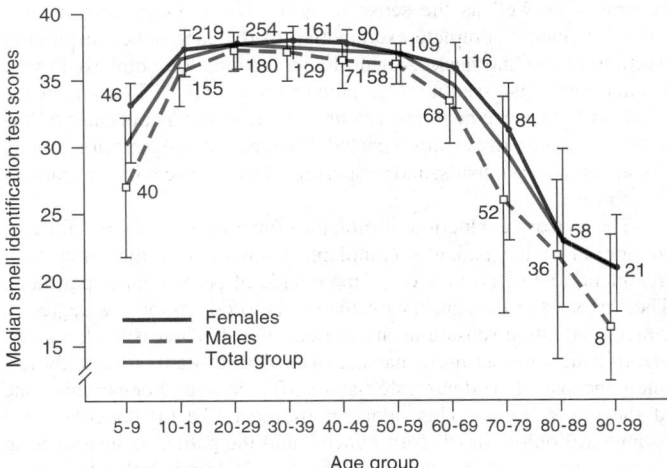

FIGURE 29-1 Smell identification test. Scores for a group of male and female subjects 5 to 99 years in age are shown. (*Reprinted with permission from RL Doty et al. Copyright 1984 by the AAAS.*)

cortex of the insula. There is also evidence for a direct pathway from

CHAPTER 29
Disorders of Smell, Taste, and Hearing

175

the parabrachial nuclei to the cortex. (Olfaction and gustation appear to be unique among sensory systems in that at least some fibers bypass the thalamus.) The other pathway from the parabrachial nuclei goes to the ventral forebrain, including the lateral hypothalamus, substantia innominata, central nucleus of the amygdala, and the stria terminalis.

Tastants gain access to the receptor cells through the taste pore. Four classes of taste are recognized: sweet, salt, sour, and bitter. Individual gustatory afferent fibers almost always respond to a number of different chemicals. Response patterns of gustatory afferent axons can be grouped into classes based on the stimulus chemical that produces the largest response. For example, for sucrose–best response neurons, the second-best stimulus is almost always sodium chloride. The fact that individual gustatory afferent fibers respond to a large number of different chemicals led to the *across-fiber-pattern* theory of gustatory coding, while the best-stimulus analysis led to the concept of *labeled* afferents. It appears that labeled fibers are important for establishing gross quality, but the across-fiber pattern within a best-stimulus category, and perhaps among categories, is needed for discriminating chemicals within qualities. For example, sweetness may be carried by sucrose-best neurons, but the differentiation of sucrose and fructose may require a comparison of the relative activity among sucrose-best, salt-best, and quinine-best neurons. As with olfaction and other sensory systems, intensity appears to be encoded by the quantity of neural activity.

DISORDERS OF THE SENSE OF TASTE Disorders of the sense of taste are caused by conditions that interfere with the access of the tastant to the receptor cells in the taste bud (transport loss), injure receptor cells (sensory loss), or damage gustatory afferent nerves and central gustatory pathways (neural loss).

Transport gustatory losses result from xerostomia due to many causes, including Sjögren's syndrome, heavy-metal intoxication, and bacterial colonization of the taste pore. The salivary milieu of the receptors may prove to be important to diverse causes of gustatory loss.

Sensory gustatory losses are caused by inflammatory and degenerative diseases in the oral cavity; a vast number of drugs, particularly those that interfere with cell turnover such as antithyroid and antineoplastic agents; radiation therapy to the oral cavity and pharynx; viral infections; endocrine disorders; neoplasms; and aging.

Neural gustatory losses occur with neoplasms, trauma, and operations in which the gustatory afferents are injured. Taste buds degenerate when their gustatory afferents are transected but remain when their somatosensory afferents are severed.

Clinical Manifestations From the psychophysical point of view, disturbances of the sense of taste may be categorized by either the patient's complaint or the objective sensory measurements as *total ageusia*—inability to detect the qualities of sweet, salt, bitter, or sour; *partial ageusia*—ability to detect some of but not all the qualitative gustatory sensations; *specific ageusia*—inability to detect the taste quality of certain substances; *total hypogeusia*—decreased sensitivity to all tastants; *partial hypogeusia*—decreased sensitivity to some tastants; and *dysgeusia*—distortion in the perception of a tastant, i.e., the perception of the wrong quality when a tastant is presented or the perception of a taste when there has been no tastant ingested. Confusions of sour and bitter are common and, at times, may be semantic misunderstandings. Frequently, however, they have physiologic or pathophysiologic bases.

It may be possible to differentiate between the loss of flavor recognition in patients with olfactory losses who complain of a loss of taste as well as smell by asking if they are able to taste sweetness in sodas, saltiness in potato chips, etc.

Patients who complain of loss of taste should be evaluated psychophysically for gustatory function in addition to being evaluated for olfactory function. The first step is to perform suprathreshold whole-mouth taste testing for quality, intensity, and pleasantness perception with sucrose, citric acid, caffeine, and sodium chloride. In the quantification of the sense of taste, detection thresholds are obtained by applying graduated dilutions to the tongue quadrants or by whole-mouth sips. Finally, suprathreshold magnitude estimation may be used

to shed further light on the patient's complaint. Electric taste testing (*electrogustometry*) is used clinically to identify taste deficits in specific quadrants of the tongue.

Biopsy of the foliate or fungiform papillae for histopathologic study of taste buds remains experimental but holds promise of shedding light on the categorization of taste disorders.

Differential Diagnosis As with olfaction, psychophysical methods for differentiating transport, sensory, and neural gustatory losses are not available. Once there is objective evidence of a disorder of taste, it is important to establish, as is done in other neurologic deficits, an anatomic diagnosis before proceeding to an etiologic diagnosis. The history of the disease often provides important clues to the cause. For example, absence of taste on the anterior two-thirds of the tongue associated with a facial paralysis indicates that the lesion is proximal to the point of junction of the chorda tympani branch with the facial nerve in the mastoid.

℞ TREATMENT

Therapy for gustatory losses remains limited. Artificial saliva benefits some patients with a disturbed salivary milieu. Treatment for bacterial and fungal infections of the oral cavity is appropriate and may be helpful. Withdrawal of drugs affecting cell turnover is usually helpful if the patient's general condition permits. Zinc and vitamin therapy for gustatory losses is advocated by some but lacks demonstrated efficacy. No therapeutic strategies exist for the sensorineural disorders of taste.

HEARING

Hearing occurs by air conduction and bone conduction. In air conduction, sound waves reach the ear by propagation in air, enter the external auditory canal, and set the tympanic membrane in motion, which in turn moves the malleus, incus, and stapes. Movement of the footplate of the stapes causes pressure changes in the fluid-filled inner ear eliciting a traveling wave in the basilar membrane of the cochlea. Hearing by bone conduction occurs when the sounding source, in contact with the head, results in vibration of the bones of the skull, including the temporal bone, producing a traveling wave in the basilar membrane. In either case, the traveling wave moves from the base to the apex of the cochlea. Hairs (stereocilia) of the hair cells of the organ of Corti, which rests on the basilar membrane, are in contact with the tectorial membrane and are deformed by the traveling wave. A point of maximal displacement of the basilar membrane determined by the frequency of the stimulating tone occurs with each traveling wave. High-frequency tones cause maximal displacement of the basilar membrane near the base of the cochlea. As the frequency of the stimulating tone decreases, the point of maximal displacement moves toward the apex of the cochlea.

The inner and outer hair cells of the organ of Corti have different innervation patterns, but both are mechanoreceptors. The afferent innervation relates principally to the inner hair cells, and the efferent innervation relates principally to outer hair cells. The outer hair cells have an internal organization that is in certain respects similar to muscle cells. Not only does the organ of Corti respond to acoustic stimulation, it also produces acoustic energy that can be detected in the external auditory canal with sensitive microphones. These otoacoustic emissions (OAE) occur spontaneously and can be evoked by acoustic stimulation. The sources of this acoustic energy are the outer hair cells.

Motility of outer hair cells occurs with mechanical (acoustical) and electrical stimulation, iontophoretically applied acetylcholine, and changes in their internal and external ionic milieu and is modulated by stimulation of the efferent olivocochlear bundle.

The outer hair cells are capable of slow and fast motility. Slow elongation and contraction occur with increased intracellular calcium in the presence of ATP, the application of acetylcholine, and changes in the ionic environment (increased potassium, which depolarizes the cell), while rapid motility occurs with mechanical (acoustic) and direct-current electrical stimulation. The electrokinetic membrane is located in the outer or lateral wall of the outer hair cell. Fast contractile activity occurs with changes in the membrane potential. The electromotility is driven by a novel and perhaps unique membrane-based force generator that can achieve audible frequencies.

The motility of the outer hair cells alters the micromechanics of the inner hair cells and thereby satisfies the long-sought cochlear amplifier required to explain the exquisite sensitivity and frequency selectivity of the cochlea.

A resting direct-current potential, the *endocochlear potential*, exists in the scala media and at the stereocilia end of the hair cells. It is generated by the stria vascularis. It is present whether there is acoustic stimulation or not. It has a magnitude of 80 mV, not unlike the intracellular potential, but its polarity is positive within the endolymph relative to the perilymph. It increases the potential differential at the stereocilia end of the hair cell, which undoubtedly is of importance in transduction.

As the traveling wave moves along the basilar membrane, the stereocilia are deformed and several receptor potentials are produced: the cochlear microphonic and the positive and negative summating potentials. It is thought that these receptor potentials arise at the apical end of the stereocilia. It may be that the summating potentials are generated largely by the inner hair cells and the cochlear microphonic potential is generated by the outer hair cells. The summating potential represents a direct-current shift that approximates the "envelope" of the acoustical stimulus. The cochlear microphonic potential is an alternating-current response that faithfully represents the frequency and intensity of the stimulating tone.

The current concept of cochlear transduction is that displacement of the tips of the stereocilia cause tip links between stereocilia to allow potassium to flow into the cell, resulting in its depolarization. The potassium causes calcium channels near the base to open and allow calcium to enter the cell. The calcium ions stimulate transmitter release. The action potential in the eighth nerve occurs 0.5 ms after the onset of the cochlear microphonic potential. The neurotransmitter at the hair cell and cochlear nerve dendrite interface is thought to be glutamate. Each of the cochlear nerve neurons can be activated at a frequency and intensity specific for that cell. This phenomenon of the characteristic or best frequency occurs at each point of the central auditory pathway: dorsal and ventral cochlear nuclei, trapezoid body, superior olivary complex, lateral lemniscus, inferior colliculus, medial geniculate body, and auditory cortex. At low frequencies, individual auditory nerve fibers can respond more or less synchronously with the stimulating tone. At higher frequencies, phase-locking occurs so that neurons take turns in responding to particular phases of the cycle of the sound wave. Intensity is encoded by the amount of neural activity in individual neurons, the number of neurons that are active, and the specific neurons that are activated.

DISORDERS OF THE SENSE OF HEARING A loss of hearing can result from lesions in the external auditory canal, middle ear, inner ear, or central auditory pathways. Lesions in the external auditory canal or middle ear cause conductive hearing losses, while lesions in the inner ear or eighth nerve cause sensorineural hearing losses.

Conductive hearing losses result from obstruction of the external auditory canal by cerumen, debris, and foreign bodies; swelling of the lining of the canal; stenosis and neoplasms of the canal; perforations of the tympanic membrane, as in chronic otitis media; disruption of the ossicular chain, as occurs with necrosis of the long process of the incus in trauma or infection; fixation of the ossicles, as in otosclerosis; and fluid, scarring, or neoplasms in the middle ear. *Sensory hearing losses* are due principally to damage to the hair cells of the organ of Corti caused by intense noise, viral infections, ototoxic drugs, fractures of the temporal bone, meningitis, cochlear otosclerosis, Ménière's disease, and aging. Neural hearing losses are due mainly to cerebellar

angle tumors such as vestibular schwannomas (acoustic neuromas) but also may result from any neoplastic, vascular, demyelinating, infectious, or degenerative disease or trauma affecting the central auditory pathways.

Clinical Evaluation of Hearing The physical examination should evaluate the external ear canal and tympanic membrane. Careful inspection of the nose, nasopharynx, and upper respiratory tract is indicated. The other cranial nerves should be carefully evaluated. Conductive and sensorineural hearing losses can be differentiated by comparing the threshold of hearing by air conduction with that elicited by bone conduction. Testing the hearing by air conduction is accomplished by presenting the stimulus in air. Hearing by air conduction is affected by the patency of the external auditory canal, the efficiency of the middle ear, and the integrity of the inner ear, eighth nerve, and central auditory pathways. Testing the hearing by bone conduction is accomplished by placing the stem of a vibrating tuning fork or an oscillator of an audiometer in contact with the head. Hearing by bone conduction bypasses the external auditory canal and middle ear and tests the integrity of the inner ear, eighth nerve, and central auditory pathways. If air-conduction thresholds are elevated and bone-conduction thresholds are in the normal range, the lesion causing hearing loss is in the external auditory canal or middle ear. If both air-conduction and bone-conduction thresholds are elevated, the lesion is in the inner ear, eighth nerve, or central auditory pathways. Of course, conductive and sensorineural hearing losses can coexist, in which case both the air-conduction and bone-conduction thresholds are elevated, but in this case, air-conduction thresholds are elevated more than bone-conduction thresholds.

The Weber and Rinne tuning fork tests are used to differentiate conductive from sensorineural hearing losses. The Weber tuning fork test may be performed with a 256- or 512-Hz fork. The Rinne tuning fork test is most sensitive in detecting mild conductive hearing losses if a 256-Hz fork is used. Weber's test is performed by placing the stem of a vibrating tuning fork on the head in the midline and asking the patient whether the tone is heard in both ears or better in one ear than in the other. With a unilateral conductive hearing loss, the tone is perceived in the affected ear. With a unilateral sensorineural hearing loss, the tone is perceived in the unaffected ear. Rinne's test compares the ability to hear by air conduction with the ability to hear by bone conduction. The tines of a vibrating tuning fork are held near the opening of the external auditory canal, and then the stem is placed on the mastoid process. The patient is asked to indicate whether the tone is louder by air conduction or bone conduction. Normally, a tone is heard louder by air conduction than by bone conduction. With a conductive hearing loss, the bone-conduction stimulus is perceived as louder than the air-conduction stimulus. With sensorineural hearing losses, both air-conduction and bone-conduction perceptions are reduced, but the air-conduction stimulus is perceived as louder, as it is in normal hearing. The combined information from the Weber and Rinne tests permits a tentative conclusion as to whether a conductive or sensorineural hearing loss is present.

Laboratory Assessment of Hearing Quantification of hearing loss is obtained with an audiometer, an electronic device that allows the presentation of specific frequencies at specific intensities to each ear by either air or bone conduction. The testing is done in a sound-attenuated chamber, and masking, usually with broad-spectrum noise, is presented to the nontest ear so that responses are based on perception from the ear under test. Frequencies from 250 to 8000 Hz are used in clinical testing. The responses are measured in decibels. A decibel (dB) is equal to 10 times the logarithm of the ratio of the acoustic power required to achieve threshold in the patient to the acoustic power required to achieve threshold in a normal hearing person. An *audiogram* is a plot of intensity in decibels required to achieve threshold versus frequency.

The audiometric pattern of hearing loss is often of diagnostic value. Conductive hearing losses usually have a fairly equal threshold elevation for each frequency. Conductive hearing losses with a large mass component, as is often seen in middle-ear effusions, have a greater elevation of thresholds in the higher frequencies. Conductive hearing losses with a large stiffness component, as in fixation of the footplate of the stapes in early otosclerosis, have a greater elevation of thresholds in the lower frequencies. In general, sensorineural hearing losses tend to have a greater threshold elevation at each higher frequency. Interesting exceptions to this generalization are noise-induced hearing loss, in which the loss at 4000 Hz is greater than it is at higher frequencies, and in Ménière's disease, particularly in the early stages of the disease, where thresholds are elevated more in lower than in higher frequencies.

Speech audiometry provides essential additional information. The *spondee threshold* is defined as the intensity at which speech is recognized as a meaningful symbol and is obtained by presenting through an audiometer two-syllable words with an equal accent on each syllable. The intensity at which the patient can repeat 50 percent of the words correctly is the spondee threshold and usually approximates the average threshold at the speech frequencies (500, 1000, and 2000 Hz). Once the spondee threshold is determined, the discrimination, or word-recognition ability, is tested by presenting one-syllable words at 25 to 40 dB above the spondee threshold. The words are phonetically balanced (PB) in that the phonemes (speech sounds) occur in the list of words at the same frequency that they occur in ordinary conversational English. An individual with normal hearing can repeat 90 to 100 percent of the PB words correctly. Likewise, individuals with a conductive hearing loss do well in discrimination testing. On the other hand, patients with a sensorineural hearing loss have a loss of discrimination attributable to the loss of peripheral analysis of sound in the inner ear or eighth nerve. With a lesion in the inner ear, the discrimination is moderately affected, usually in the 50 to 80 percent range, while with neural lesions, the discrimination is severely affected, often in the 0 to 50 percent range.

The discrimination testing may then be done at higher intensities than 25 to 40 dB above the spondee threshold to determine the performance-intensity function. A deterioration in discrimination ability at higher intensities suggests a lesion in the eighth nerve or central auditory pathways.

Tympanometry measures the impedance of the middle ear to sound. A sounding source and microphone are introduced into the ear canal with an airtight seal. The amount of sound that is absorbed through the middle ear or reflected from the middle ear is measured at the microphone. In conductive hearing losses, more sound is reflected than in the normal middle ear. The pressure in the ear canal can be increased or decreased from atmospheric pressure. Normally, the middle ear is most compliant at atmospheric pressure. With a negative pressure in the middle ear, as with eustachian tube obstruction, the point of maximal compliance occurs with negative pressure in the ear canal. With discontinuity of the ossicular chain, no point of maximal compliance can be obtained. Tympanometry is particularly useful in the identification and diagnosis of middle-ear effusions in children.

During tympanometry, an intense tone (80 dB above the hearing threshold) elicits contraction of the stapedius muscle. The change in compliance of the middle ear with contraction of the stapedius muscle can be detected. The presence or absence of this *acoustic reflex* is important in the anatomic localization of facial nerve paralysis. The presence or absence of *acoustic reflex decay* helps differentiate sensory from neural hearing losses. In neural hearing loss, the reflex adapts or decays with time.

In order to evaluate a patient with a loss of hearing, the minimum audiologic assessment should include the measurement of pure tone air-conduction and bone-conduction thresholds, spondee threshold, discrimination score, performance-intensity function, OAE, tympanometry, acoustic reflexes, and acoustic-reflex decay. This information provides a comprehensive screening evaluation of the whole auditory system and allows one to determine whether further differentiation of a sensory (cochlear) from a neural (retrocochlear) hearing loss is indicated.

In addition to these tests, testing for recruitment, the short increment sensitivity index, tone decay, Békésy audiometry, and auditory brainstem evoked responses (ABR) help differentiate sensory from neural hearing losses. Of these, ABR is the most powerful means of differentiating the site of sensorineural hearing loss (see Chap. 361). In response to sound, five distinct waves can be recorded with computer averaging from scalp surface electrodes. Poor or absent waveforms, abnormal latency of waves, and abnormal interwave latency are evidence of lesions in the eighth nerve and brainstem. In addition, ABR is valuable in situations in which patients cannot or will not give reliable voluntary thresholds. It is also used to measure auditory function in neonates and young children and to monitor the integrity of the auditory nerve and brainstem in various clinical situations, including intraoperatively and in determination of brain death.

Otoacoustic emissions can be measured with sensitive microphones inserted into the external auditory canal in infants, children, and adults. The emissions may be spontaneous or evoked with sound stimulation. The presence of OAE indicates that the outer hair cells are intact and can be used as important evidence in distinguishing sensory from neural hearing losses. Otoacoustic emissions are particularly robust in infants.

The measurement of OAE can be done rapidly and with limited technical expertise in newborns. It is uncertain whether this technique or automated ABR will become the preferred method of screening neonates for hearing impairment. One strategy is to screen all neonates with OAE and to confirm hearing impairment with ABR. High-risk factors include a family history of hearing impairment, prenatal infection, prematurity, low birth weight, neonatal anoxia, a low Apgar score, neonatal jaundice, and neonatal infection. Unfortunately, ABR fails to identify 50 percent of infants with profound hearing impairment among high-risk infants. In the United States, the average age of identification of profound hearing impairment is 2½ years.

The natural acquisition and development of oral speech and language depend on hearing language. The critical period for language acquisition is the first 2 years of life. Therefore, the early identification of hearing impairment in infants is of the greatest importance so that amplification with a hearing aid and special education can commence within the first several months of life.

In addition to the universal screening of infants for hearing impairment, hearing should be assessed in all children before the first formal educational experience (preschool or kindergarten). Hearing also should be measured in the late teenage period when otosclerosis and noise-induced hearing loss begin to appear and in the sixth decade of life when presbycusis makes its appearance. Known causes of hearing impairment in addition to the risk factors already mentioned are meningitis, cytomegalovirus infections, head trauma, middle-ear infections and effusions, administration of ototoxic drugs (e.g., salicylates, quinine and its synthetic analogues, aminoglycoside antibiotics, loop diuretics such as furosemide and ethacrynic acid, and cancer chemotherapeutic agents such as *cis*-platinum), and noise exposure. At any time in life when one of these hearing risks is encountered, an audiologic assessment should be carried out.

Ten million Americans have noise-induced hearing loss, and 20 million are exposed to hazardous noise in their employment. Noise-induced hearing loss results from recreational as well as occupational activities and begins in adolescence, particularly among boys as they begin to engage in high-risk activities, such as wood and metal working with electrical equipment and target practice and hunting with small firearms. All internal-combustion and electric engines, including snow and leaf blowers, snowmobiles, outboard motors, and chain saws, require protection of the user with hearing protectors such as ear plugs or fluid-filled ear muffs. Virtually all noise-induced hearing loss is preventable through education, which should begin before the teenage years.

Programs of industrial conservation of hearing are required when the exposure over an 8-h period averages 85 dB on the A scale. Workers in such noisy environments can be protected with preemployment audiologic assessment, the mandatory use of hearing protectors, and annual audiologic assessments.

--- *Approach to the Patient* ---

Clinical Assessment of a Complaint of Hearing Loss In evaluating patients who complain of loss of hearing, associated symptoms of tinnitus, vertigo, difficulty with balance, earache, otorrhea, and aural fullness should be sought along with a careful reconstruction of the history of evolution of the hearing deficit. A sudden onset of unilateral hearing loss, with or without tinnitus, may represent a viral infection in the inner ear. Gradual progression in a hearing deficit is common with otosclerosis, noise-induced hearing loss, vestibular schwannoma, or Ménière's disease. In the latter case, intermittent tinnitus and vertigo are usual. Hearing loss can occur with demyelinative lesions in the brainstem.

The genetic basis of hearing impairment is apparent in families in which hearing impairment occurs in multiple generations. Hearing impairment is also genetically predetermined in instances in which there are obvious environmental factors. For example, in certain Asian families the susceptibility to aminoglycoside ototoxicity is transmuted through a mitochondrial mutation. The variation in individual and familial susceptibility to noise-induced hearing loss and presbycusis is also probably genetically determined.

One in 1000 infants is born with profound hearing impairment. At least 50 percent of congenital deafness has a genetic basis. A larger number of individuals develop hereditary hearing impairment in childhood and later in life. Between 70 and 80 percent of hereditary hearing impairment is autosomal recessive, and between 15 and 20 percent is autosomal dominant. Less than 5 percent is X-linked. Hereditary hearing impairment also occurs in syndromes in which other organ systems are affected. Greater progress has been made in finding the genes for syndromes of hereditary deafness because of the ease of making the determination of the hereditary basis of the hearing impairment. The genes for Waardenburg's syndrome (failure of melanocytes to migrate from the neural crest, resulting in deafness and pigmentary and integumentary changes) have been mapped to chromosome 2 (type 1) and chromosome 3 (type 2), and the genes for Usher's syndrome (deafness, vestibular loss, and blindness due to retinitis pigmentosa) have been mapped to chromosome 1 (type 2) and chromosome 2 (type 1). The genes for one form of Alport's syndrome (deafness and glomerulonephritis leading to renal failure), albinism, and neurofibromatosis type 2 (bilateral acoustic neurinomas) have been found. The first nonsyndromic deafness gene was found in a Costa Rican kindred with an autosomal dominant hearing impairment on the long arm of chromosome 5. Several genes responsible for recessive nonsyndromic hereditary hearing impairment in isolated, consanguineous families have been located.

Between 30 and 35 percent of individuals over 65 years of age have a hearing loss that is sufficiently great to require a hearing aid. Presbycusis is characterized by a loss of discrimination for phonemes, recruitment (abnormal growth of loudness), and particular difficulty in understanding speech in noisy environments.

Tinnitus is defined as the perception of a sound when there is no sound in the environment. It may have a buzzing, roaring, or ringing quality and may be pulsatile (synchronous with the heartbeat). Tinnitus is usually associated with a conductive or sensorineural loss of hearing. The pathophysiology of tinnitus is not well understood. The cause of the tinnitus can usually be determined by finding the cause of the associated hearing loss. Tinnitus may be the first symptom of a serious condition such as a vestibular schwannoma. Pulsatile tinnitus requires evaluation of the vascular system of the head to exclude vascular tumors such as glomus jugulare tumors, aneurysms, and stenotic lesions.

Differential Diagnosis Many patients with sensorineural hearing losses should have the vestibular system evaluated with electronystagmography and caloric testing (see Chap. 20). Most patients with conductive hearing losses should have CT of the temporal bones. Patients with unilateral or asymmetric sensorineural hearing losses should have

magnetic resonance imaging of the head with gadolinium enhancement.

Prevention Conductive hearing losses may be prevented by prompt and appropriate antibiotic therapy of adequate duration for acute otitis media and by reventilation of the middle ear with tympanostomy tubes in middle-ear effusions lasting 6 weeks or longer. Loss of vestibular function and deafness due to aminoglycoside antibiotics can largely be prevented by careful monitoring of serum peak and trough levels. Noise-induced hearing loss can be prevented by avoidance of exposure to loud noise or by regular use of ear plugs or fluid-filled muffs to attenuate intense sound. Vaccination of infants against type B *Haemophilus influenzae* meningitis will prevent a major cause of acquired deafness, as has immunization for measles, mumps, and rubella.

℞ **TREATMENT**

Most patients with conductive hearing losses can have the middle ear reconstructed using procedures such as tympanoplasty after chronic otitis media and trauma and stapedectomy for otosclerosis. Tympanostomy tubes allow the prompt return of hearing to normal in children and adults with middle-ear effusions. Hearing aids are effective and well-tolerated for patients with conductive hearing losses. Patients with mild, moderate, and severe sensorineural hearing losses are regularly rehabilitated with hearing aids of varying configuration and strength. However, the problem of understanding conversation with a hearing aid in noise remains. Hearing aids have been improved to provide greater fidelity and have been miniaturized. High-frequency emphasis, needed for many sensorineural hearing losses, has been achieved principally by venting the ear mold and with filters. The augmentation of soft sounds and the nonamplification of intense sounds has been achieved. Digital hearing aids lend themselves to programming for the individual, and multiple and directional microphones at the ear level help some with difficulty of hearing with a hearing aid in noisy surroundings. Since all hearing aids amplify noise as well as speech, the only absolute solution to the problem found so far is to place the microphone closer to the speaker than the noise source. This arrangement is not possible with a self-contained, cosmetically acceptable device. It is cumbersome and requires a user-friendly environment.

In many situations, including lectures and the theater, hearing-impaired persons benefit from assistive devices that are based on the principle of having the speaker closer to the microphone than any source of noise. Assistive devices include infrared and FM transmission as well as an electromagnetic loop around the room for transmission to the individual's hearing aid. Hearing aids with telecoils also can be used with properly equipped telephones in the same way.

Cochlear implants are neural prostheses that convert sound energy to electrical energy and can be used to stimulate the auditory division of the eighth nerve directly. Cochlear implants consist of electrodes that are inserted into the cochlea, speech processors that extract acoustical elements of speech for conversion to electric currents, and a means of transmitting the electrical energy through the skin. Most commonly for this purpose an induction coil is held over an implanted induction coil with magnets in each coil. In most causes of profound hearing impairment, the auditory hair cells are lost, but the ganglionic cells of the auditory division of the eighth nerve are preserved. Cochlear implants are appropriate for children with congenital and acquired profound hearing impairment and adults with hearing impairment that is so severe that less than 30 percent of speech can be understood with a hearing aid in ideal listening circumstances. Worldwide, more than 14,000 deaf individuals, 2000 of whom are children, have had cochlear implants. They experience sound that helps with speech reading and allows some open-set word recognition. It is anticipated that improvements in the electrode design and speech processors will permit further improvement in understanding speech. The implant also allows the recipient to hear and identify environmental sounds and distinguish between men's and women's voices. It is also a help in modulating the person's own voice.

For individuals who have had both eighth nerves destroyed by trauma or bilateral vestibular schwannomas, a brainstem auditory implant has been placed near the cochlear nucleus on a limited, experimental basis. Recipients of the brainstem implant derive benefit similar to those with the cochlear implant.

The treatment of tinnitus is particularly problematic. The frequency range and intensity of tinnitus can often be matched with the use of an audiometer. Relief of the tinnitus may be obtained by masking it with background music. Hearing aids also are helpful in tinnitus suppression, as are tinnitus maskers, devices that present a sound to the affected ear that is more pleasant to listen to than the tinnitus. The use of a tinnitus masker is often followed by several hours of inhibition of the tinnitus.

Communicating with Hard-of-Hearing Individuals First of all, unnecessary noise should be eliminated or reduced. The radio and television should be turned off. Persons with hearing impairment depend on speech reading. They should be allowed to see the face of the speaker at all times. Speaking directly into the ear is occasionally helpful, but usually more is lost in communication than gained when the speaker's face cannot be seen. The lighting of the face of the speaker should be considered. The hard-of-hearing person should sit with his or her back to the window so that the light will be on the speaker's face. Speech should be slow enough to make each word distinct, but overly slow speech is distracting and loses contextual and speech-reading benefits. Although speech should be in a loud, clear voice, one should be aware that in sensorineural hearing losses in general and in elderly hard-of-hearing persons in particular, recruitment (the ability to hear loud sounds normally loud) may be troublesome. Above all, optimal communication cannot take place without both parties giving it their full and undivided attention.

BIBLIOGRAPHY

BALLENGER JJ, SNOW JB (eds): *Otorhinolaryngology Head and Neck Surgery*, 15th ed. Baltimore, Williams & Wilkins, 1995

DOTY RL et al: Smell identification ability: Changes with age. Science 226:1441, 1984

FIRESTEIN S, SHEPHERD GM: Interaction of anionic and cationic currents leads to a voltage dependence in the odor response of olfactory receptor neurons. J Neurophys 73:562, 1995

FRANCO B et al: A gene deleted in Kallmann's syndrome shares homology with neural cell adhesion and axonal path-finding molecules. Nature 353:529, 1991

GETCHELL TV et al: *Smell and Taste in Health and Disease*. New York, Raven Press, 1991

KALINEC F et al: A membrane-based force generation mechanism in auditory sensory cells. Proc Natl Acad Sci USA 89:8671, 1992

PREZANT TR: Mitochondrial ribosomal RNA mutation associated with antibiotic-induced and nonsyndromic deafness. Nat Genet 4:288, 1993

RUSSLER KJ et al: A zonal organization of odorant receptor gene expression in the olfactory epithelium. Cell 73:597, 1993

WARCHOL ME et al: Regenerative proliferation in inner ear sensory epithelia from adult guinea pigs and humans. Science 259:1619, 1993

30	*Marlene Durand, Michael Joseph, Ann Sullivan Baker**

INFECTIONS OF THE UPPER RESPIRATORY TRACT

Infections of the upper respiratory tract include some of the most common infectious diseases encountered by internists and other primary-care physicians. Pharyngitis, laryngitis, rhinitis, sinusitis, otitis externa, and otitis media account for millions of visits to physicians annually. Although these infections are usually mild enough to be

*Deceased.

treated on an outpatient basis, the primary-care physician must be able to recognize their serious complications, such as peritonsillar abscess from pharyngitis, subperiosteal abscess from frontal sinusitis, and temporal-bone osteomyelitis from invasive otitis externa. The physician must also identify potentially life-threatening infections of the head and neck, such as epiglottitis, Ludwig's angina, and rhinocerebral mucormycosis.

INFECTIONS OF THE NOSE AND FACE

Skin infections that commonly affect the nose and face include folliculitis, furunculosis, impetigo, and erysipelas. These are discussed in detail elsewhere (see Chap. 133, in particular Table 133-1).

Infection of the mucosal surface of the nose is most commonly due to respiratory viruses (e.g., rhinovirus) and presents as acute rhinitis. There are several rare, chronic intranasal infections. *Ozena*, or atrophic rhinitis, is characterized by atrophied mucosa overlaid by foul-smelling dry crusts (Greek *ozein*, "stench"). *Klebsiella ozaenae* is often isolated from nasal cultures, but whether it is a cause of illness or merely a colonizer is unclear. Intranasal irrigation with aminoglycosides (e.g., tobramycin ophthalmic solution) or oral administration of ciprofloxacin has resulted in clinical improvement in some cases. *Klebsiella rhinoscleromatis* causes *rhinoscleroma*, a chronic granulomatous disease of the upper respiratory tract mucosa that is seen in inhabitants of parts of Africa, Asia, and Latin America and was recently described in two patients positive for human immunodeficiency virus (HIV). Mikulicz cells (foamy histiocytes) are seen in the submucosa of biopsy specimens. Rhinoscleroma can be treated with streptomycin, trimethoprim-sulfamethoxazole, a quinolone, or tetracycline for 2 months. *Pseudomonas mallei* causes *glanders*, a respiratory disease of horses. Infection is rare in humans; nasal inoculation may produce a purulent nasal discharge followed by granulomatous intranasal lesions that ulcerate. Treatment with sulfadiazine is administered.

Neonatal congenital syphilis may present as rhinitis (snuffles), and the generalized osteochondritis that follows may result in a "saddle-nose" deformity. In *leprosy*, *Mycobacterium leprae* infiltrates the nasal mucosa and may cause chronic nasal congestion and nosebleeds. Involvement of the nasal cartilage may also result in a saddle nose.

Rhinosporidium seeberi is a fungus-like organism, not yet cultured, that causes *rhinosporidiosis*. Pedunculated nasal masses that grow over months or years cause obstruction and a foul odor and must be surgically excised. *Blastomyces dermatitidis*, a fungus prevalent in the Mississippi and Ohio River valleys, usually causes pulmonary disease but may cause chronic ulcerative lesions of the skin and nasal mucosa. *Mucormycosis*, a life-threatening fungal illness that occurs primarily in diabetic patients, may present as black eschars in the nasal cavity (see "Fungal Sinusitis").

SINUSITIS

The paranasal sinuses are aerated cavities in the bones of the face that develop as outpouches of the nasal cavity and communicate with this cavity throughout life. The maxillary and ethmoid sinuses are present at birth; the frontal and sphenoid sinuses develop after ages 2 and 7, respectively. Like the nose, the sinuses are lined with respiratory epithelium that includes mucus-producing goblet cells and ciliated cells. The mucous blanket is carried toward the sinus openings (ostia) at a speed of up to 1 cm/min by the beating of the cilia. The ostia are small; the ethmoid sinus ostia, for example, are only 1 to 2 mm in diameter. Delay in the mucociliary transport time or—more important—obstruction of the ostia may lead to retained secretions and sinusitis.

Sinusitis is a common problem. In the United States, this infection accounts for millions of office visits annually. The most common type, maxillary sinusitis, is followed in frequency by ethmoid, frontal, and sphenoid sinusitis. A viral infection of the upper respiratory tract is the most common precursor of sinusitis, although only about 0.5 percent of such infections are complicated by clinically evident acute bacterial sinusitis. Sinusitis develops primarily through ostial obstruction due to mucosal edema. Viral upper respiratory infections also increase the amount of mucus produced and may damage ciliated cells, thereby delaying mucus transport time. Allergic rhinitis is another common cause of ostial obstruction, either by mucosal edema or by polyps. Nasotracheal or nasogastric intubation can result in obstruction of the ostia and is a major risk factor for nosocomial sinusitis in intensive care units. Dental infections may cause 5 to 10 percent of all cases of maxillary sinusitis; the roots of the upper back teeth (second bicuspid, first and second molars) abut the floor of the maxillary sinus. Other causes of sinusitis include barotrauma from deep-sea diving or airplane travel, mucus abnormalities (e.g., cystic fibrosis), and chemical irritants. Foreign bodies, tumors (e.g., midline granuloma, intranasal lymphoma, or squamous cell carcinoma), and granulomatous diseases (e.g., Wegener's granulomatosis or rhinoscleroma) may all cause sinusitis secondary to obstruction.

ACUTE BACTERIAL SINUSITIS **Manifestations** Symptoms of acute sinusitis include purulent nasal or postnasal drainage, nasal congestion, and sinus pain or pressure whose location depends on the sinus involved. Maxillary sinus pain is often perceived as being located in the cheek or upper teeth; ethmoid sinus pain, between the eyes or retroorbital; frontal sinus pain, above the eyebrow; and sphenoid sinus pain, in the upper half of the face or retroorbital with radiation to the occiput. Sinus pain is frequently worse when the patient bends over or is supine. Fever develops in about half of patients with acute maxillary sinusitis.

Diagnosis The diagnosis of bacterial sinusitis may be difficult, as symptoms may resemble those of the inciting upper respiratory infection. The persistence of cold symptoms for 7 to 10 days (or longer than usual for a particular patient) is the most consistent clinical feature of bacterial sinusitis, according to some authors. Complete opacification of sinus, shown by transillumination of maxillary and frontal sinuses with a strong flashlight in a dark room, constitutes good evidence of sinusitis; normal light transmission correlates well with an absence of infection. Partial transmission (dullness) is not diagnostically helpful, as it indicates infection in only one-quarter of cases. Transillumination is not of diagnostic value in patients with increased sinus-bone thickness, including children under age 10 and patients with chronic sinusitis. Four-view sinus x-rays are helpful in the diagnosis of acute sinusitis: radiologic opacity, an air-fluid level, or 4 mm or more of sinus mucosal thickening correlates well with active bacterial infection. Computed tomography (CT) of the sinus is much more sensitive than routine radiography, particularly for ethmoid and sphenoid disease. Its use should be reserved for complicated cases and for cases in hospitalized patients, however. In light of the recent finding that sinus CT often shows reversible acute changes in patients with common colds, it is apparent that routine early use of CT would lead to overdiagnosis of bacterial sinusitis.

Etiology The bacteriology of acute community-acquired maxillary sinusitis has been well defined by studies using direct sinus puncture and aspiration. In children and adults, *Streptococcus pneumoniae* and *Haemophilus influenzae* (not type b), the most common pathogens, cause about one-third and one-fourth of cases, respectively. In children, *Moraxella catarrhalis* is also important, accounting for 20 percent of cases. In adults, gram-negative bacilli play a role (9 percent of cases), and anaerobes (6 percent) are especially important in cases associated with dental infections. How often *Chlamydia pneumoniae* causes sinusitis is not known. Rhinoviruses as well as influenza and parainfluenza viruses are found alone or with bacteria in one-fifth of adult cases.

℞ **TREATMENT**
Empiric therapy for acute bacterial sinusitis should be directed against the common bacterial pathogens; sinus puncture is not indicated in routine cases, and cultures of nasal drainage are not very reliable. Amoxicillin or trimethoprim-sulfamethoxazole may be effective in the treatment of first-time cases. Other effective but more expensive antibiotics include amoxicillin/clavulanate, cefuroxime axetil, and loracarbef. Treatment should be given for 1 to 2 weeks. Intravenous administration of antibiotics may be necessary for the treatment of patients with severe disease who appear toxic. In nosocomial sinusitis, *Staphylococcus aureus* and gram-negative bacilli are most common, and sinus cultures are indicated as an aid in tailoring therapy. Initial broad-spectrum intravenous therapy (e.g., with nafcillin and ceftriaxone) should be adjusted on the basis of culture results. Surgery to widen the ostia and drain thick secretions may be essential in severe acute sinusitis, particularly when ethmoid, frontal, or sphenoid disease fails to respond to initial intravenous therapy.

CHRONIC BACTERIAL SINUSITIS **Manifestations** Chronic sinusitis is characterized by symptoms of sinus inflammation lasting 3 months or more. Most experts believe that this condition is caused by dysfunction of the mucociliary blanket, usually as a result of repeated past infections, rather than by the persistence of bacterial infection. Patients complain of constant sinus pressure, nasal congestion, and postnasal drainage, especially in the morning. A temperature of $\geq 38°C$ (100.5°F) is rare and may signify a superimposed acute bacterial infection. Many patients also note a change in nasal discharge (to thick and green) with acute exacerbations.

Diagnosis Sinus CT should be used in all cases of chronic sinusitis to define the extent of disease and to help exclude other diagnoses, such as an obstructing tumor or a granulomatous process. Patients should also be evaluated for allergies and immunodeficiencies (e.g., hypogammaglobulinemia). Evaluation by an otolaryngologist is essential, as this specialist will be able to obtain additional information by an office nasal endoscopic examination. Surgery, now usually done endoscopically, may be necessary to correct blockage of the sinus ostia. This blockage occurs most often in the osteomeatal complex that drains the maxillary, frontal, and anterior ethmoid sinuses. Samples of sinus secretions obtained intraoperatively should be cultured for anaerobes, aerobes, and fungi. Fungal sinusitis may mimic chronic bacterial infection (see "Fungal Sinusitis").

Etiology The bacteriology of chronic sinusitis is not well defined. Nearly all patients with chronic disease, especially those who have had prior sinus surgery, have sinus cultures positive for bacteria, which often represent colonization rather than infection. Patients who have received multiple courses of antibiotics may be colonized by *S. aureus* or by resistant species of gram-negative bacilli.

℞ **TREATMENT**
The need for antibiotic therapy must be assessed on an individual basis, with antibiotics chosen in light of recent culture results.

COMPLICATIONS OF BACTERIAL SINUSITIS The most common complication of sinusitis is orbital cellulitis. This condition is usually secondary to ethmoid sinusitis, since the ethmoid is separated from the orbit by only a very thin bone (the lamina papyracea). Patients present with fever, periorbital edema and erythema, conjunctival injection and chemosis, and proptosis. CT or magnetic resonance imaging (MRI) should be used to rule out a drainable orbital abscess, especially in patients with decreased eye movement. Treatment with broad-spectrum antibiotics (e.g., nafcillin and ceftriaxone) should be started immediately. If there is no improvement within 24 h, the ethmoid sinus should be drained.

Another extracranial complication of sinusitis is frontal subperiosteal abscess (Pott's puffy tumor) from frontal sinusitis. Patients present with a tender doughy swelling over the forehead. Treatment consists of surgical drainage of the abscess and the frontal sinus and 6 weeks of intravenous antibiotic therapy.

Intracranial complications such as epidural abscess, subdural empyema, meningitis, cerebral abscess, and dural-vein thrombophlebitis may result from sinusitis, particularly from frontal or sphenoid infections. Because the sphenoid sinus sits between the two cavernous sinuses, sphenoid sinusitis is a major cause of cavernous sinus thrombophlebitis.

FUNGAL SINUSITIS Fungal sinusitis is categorized as noninvasive or invasive. *Noninvasive* disease is chronic and occurs in immunocompetent hosts. It has two forms that are analogous to the noninvasive pulmonary diseases of aspergilloma and allergic bronchopulmonary aspergillosis. A fungus ball (aspergilloma) inside a sinus may cause symptoms of obstruction without invading the mucosa. Typically, only one sinus (often maxillary) is affected, and patients have unilateral symptoms and opacification of only that sinus on CT. Treatment is surgical only, unless special fungal stains show tissue invasion on histopathology. Allergic fungal sinusitis was first described in 1983 and is seen mainly in patients with a history of nasal polyposis and asthma. It is characterized by extremely thick sinus mucus ("allergic mucin") that, on histopathologic examination, is found to contain numerous Charcot-Leyden crystals, eosinophils, and rare fungal hyphae. There is no evidence of tissue invasion. Surgical removal of the inspissated mucus may be curative, although some experts recommend the use of intranasal or systemic glucocorticoids to prevent recurrences.

Invasive fungal sinusitis presents differently in immunocompetent and immunocompromised hosts. In immunocompromised individuals, fungal disease has an acute presentation. Rhinocerebral mucormycosis is a life-threatening infection due to fungi of the order Mucorales (*Rhizopus, Mucor, Absidia*) that usually involves diabetic patients with ketoacidosis but may also involve leukemic patients with prolonged neutropenia as well as transplant recipients. The affected patients have facial pain, headache, and fever; there may be early signs of orbital cellulitis and altered mental status. Black eschars overlying necrotic tissue may be seen in the nasal passages and should be biopsied emergently. The finding of tissue invasion by broad-based, nonseptate hyphae necessitates extensive surgical debridement and intravenous therapy with amphotericin B. *Aspergillus* and other fungi may also cause invasive sinus disease.

Immunocompetent hosts with invasive fungal sinusitis, in contrast, have slowly progressive disease. Fungi in ethmoid and sphenoid sinuses may invade the orbital apex, causing proptosis, ptosis, limitation of eye movement, and decreased vision. Patients may mistakenly be treated with glucocorticoids for presumed optic neuritis or orbital pseudotumor until sinus disease is recognized and biopsies are undertaken. Treatment consists of surgical debridement of the sinuses involved and prolonged intravenous therapy with amphotericin B. In all cases of invasive fungal sinusitis, follow-up CT and MRI should be conducted frequently to evaluate the progression of disease.

Mortality from fungal sinusitis is high, even among immunocompetent hosts.

EAR AND MASTOID INFECTIONS

AURICULAR CELLULITIS AND PERICHONDRITIS *Auricular cellulitis* usually presents as a swollen, erythematous, hot, mildly tender ear. The lobule is especially swollen and red. There may be a history of minor trauma to the ear (e.g., involving earrings, cotton swabs, or scratching). Treatment consists of warm compresses and intravenous administration of antibiotics active against *S. aureus* and streptococci.

Perichondritis, an infection of the perichondrium of the ear, is often accompanied by infection of the underlying cartilage of the pinna (chondritis). Associated interruption of the blood supply to the cartilage may lead to ear deformity. Patients present with a swollen, hot, red, and exquisitely tender pinna, usually with sparing of the lobule. The most common antecedents of the infection are burns or significant trauma to the ear (e.g., as a result of boxing). *Pseudomonas aeruginosa* and *S. aureus* are the most common pathogens. Perichondritis should be treated with antibiotics, such as intravenous ticarcillin/clavulanic acid or intravenous nafcillin plus oral ciprofloxacin, for at least 4 weeks. Incision and drainage may be helpful for culture and for resolu-

tion of infection, which is often slow. This infection must be distinguished from relapsing polychondritis, a rheumatologic condition (see Chap. 326).

OTITIS EXTERNA The external auditory canal is about 2.5 cm long and is lined by skin. Beneath this skin is cartilage in the lateral half of the canal, temporal bone in the medial half. The skin in the bony portion lacks a subcutaneous layer and is attached directly to the periosteum, an important feature in the pathogenesis of invasive otitis externa (see below). Cerumen, secreted by glands, acidifies the canal and suppresses bacterial growth. However, desquamated skin and retained moisture make the canal especially susceptible to the hydrophilic organism *P. aeruginosa*.

Acute otitis externa, or swimmer's ear, occurs mostly in the summer and may be due to a decrease in canal acidity and resulting bacterial overgrowth. The ear is pruritic and painful, and the canal appears swollen and red. The most common pathogens are *P. aeruginosa*, *S. aureus*, and streptococci. Treatment consists of cleansing of the ear with alcohol–acetic acid mixtures and the administration of topical antibiotic ear drops, such as polymyxin-neomycin (4 drops four times daily for 5 days). Herpes zoster in the external canal causes severe otalgia and is often accompanied by ipsilateral facial paralysis due to the involvement of the geniculate ganglion of cranial nerve VII (Ramsay Hunt syndrome). Recent reports suggest that treatment with intravenous acyclovir decreases the incidence of permanent facial-nerve palsy, but the results of relevant controlled trials have not yet been published.

Chronic otitis externa causes pruritus rather than ear pain and is often due to irritation from either repeated minor trauma to the canal (e.g., scratching or use of cotton swabs) or drainage of a chronic middle-ear infection. In the latter situation, treatment of chronic otitis media with oral antibiotics will also cover this condition.

Invasive ("malignant") otitis externa is a potentially life-threatening infection, usually due to *P. aeruginosa*, that slowly invades from the external canal into adjacent soft tissues, mastoid, and temporal bone and eventually spreads across the base of the skull. It occurs primarily in diabetic patients whose diabetes, unlike that of patients with mucormycosis, is usually under control. There is often a history of ear pain and drainage of several months' duration. Examination reveals an edematous canal, with granulation tissue in the posterior wall about halfway down the canal (the region of the cartilage-bone junction). Trismus or partial facial paralysis (cranial nerve VII) is evident in some instances. Cranial nerves IX, X, and XI are occasionally affected as well. Signs of intradural involvement, such as meningitis, temporal-lobe cerebritis, or brain abscess, are rare. Fever is rare in invasive otitis externa and when it does develop is usually low-grade.

Laboratory studies usually reveal a normal white blood cell count but a high sedimentation rate. CT and MRI studies are essential for defining the extent of bone and soft-tissue involvement and for helping the ear, nose, and throat surgeon decide on the optimal location for biopsy. Cultures of discharge from the external canal may be unreliable, and in nearly all cases antibiotics should be withheld until a deep-tissue specimen is obtained for culture and pathologic examination. Once this specimen has been collected, empiric therapy with intravenous antibiotics active against *Pseudomonas* (e.g., ticarcillin, pipericillin, or ceftazidime, plus an aminoglycoside) may be started intraoperatively. In more than 95 percent of cases, *P. aeruginosa* is the pathogen involved; in the remaining cases, the pathogens include *Staphylococcus epidermidis*, *Aspergillus*, *Fusobacterium*, and *Actinomyces*. Intravenous antibiotic treatment should be continued for 6 to 8 weeks in advanced cases; in early cases, oral ciprofloxacin alone (750 mg twice daily for 6 weeks) may follow the initial 2 weeks of combination intravenous therapy if intraoperative cultures reveal a *Pseudomonas* strain sensitive to this drug.

ACUTE OTITIS MEDIA The middle ear is connected to the nasopharynx via the eustachian tube. When this tube is blocked, fluid collects in the middle-ear and mastoid cavities, providing a culture medium for any bacteria present. Acute otitis media (AOM), or middle-ear infection, may result. Viral upper respiratory infections, which can cause edema of the eustachian tube mucosa, often precede or accompany episodes of AOM. Otitis media, like upper respiratory tract infections, is most common in fall, winter, and spring. The incidence of AOM declines with age. More than two-thirds of children under age 3 have had at least one episode of AOM; the prevalence among adults is only 0.25 percent.

Symptoms include ear pain, fever, and decreased hearing acuity. On examination, the tympanic membrane moves poorly with insufflation and is usually red, opaque, bulging, or retracted. Spontaneous perforations of the tympanic membrane and otorrhea are occasionally documented.

The bacteriology of AOM has been delineated for pediatric disease: *S. pneumoniae* (35 percent), *H. influenzae* (25 percent), and *M. catarrhalis* (15 percent) are the most common organisms in nonneonates; group B streptococci and gram-negative bacilli are important in neonates. Viruses, either alone or with bacteria, are found in one-quarter of pediatric cases. Small studies of AOM in adults have also found *S. pneumoniae* (21 percent) and *H. influenzae* (26 percent) to be the most common pathogens. About 90 percent of the *H. influenzae* infections are due to nontypable strains: those due to type b may be accompanied by bacteremia or meningitis.

℞ TREATMENT

Treatment of otitis media is empiric, as diagnostic tympanocentesis is indicated only for patients who appear toxic, who are immunocompromised, or whose infection is refractory to initial therapy. Although about one-third of *H. influenzae* strains and at least three-quarters of *M. catarrhalis* strains are β-lactamase producers, most authorities still find amoxicillin therapy to be successful in routine cases. Other drugs effective against most β-lactamase-positive strains include amoxicillin/clavulanate, trimethoprim-sulfamethoxazole, erythromycin-sulfisoxazole, clarithromycin, and second-generation oral cephalosporins (e.g., loracarbef, cefpodoxime proxetil, and cefuroxime axetil). Penicillin resistance in pneumococci, an increasing problem, is not mediated by β-lactamase. Resistant strains may respond to therapy with erythromycin or sulfa drugs; serious infections require treatment with intravenous vancomycin or a third-generation cephalosporin (e.g., ceftriaxone). Adjunctive treatment of AOM with antihistamines is of no proven benefit.

Recurrent episodes of AOM in children are due to the same pathogens that cause primary AOM (*S. pneumoniae*, *H. influenzae*, and *M. catarrhalis*). Most early recurrences (75 percent), however, are not relapses but are due to different organisms or to different strains of the organism that caused the initial episode. The pattern of recurrent AOM in adults is presumably similar but has not been well studied. Treatment for recurrent AOM should include drugs with activity against β-lactamase-positive strains. Patients with frequent recurrences (e.g., three episodes within 6 months) may benefit from antibiotic prophylaxis with once-daily amoxicillin or sulfisoxazole during the winter months, although this benefit must be weighed against the risk of selecting more antibiotic-resistant strains of bacteria.

SEROUS OTITIS MEDIA Otitis media with effusion, or serous otitis media, is characterized by the persistence of middle-ear fluid for several months without other signs of infection. This condition is associated with a 25-dB hearing loss in the affected ear. Cultures of middle-ear fluid are frequently negative, although effusions have resolved more quickly in antibiotic-treated children than in controls in several clinical trials. Adenoidectomy, myringotomy, or tympanostomy tubes have been shown to decrease the duration of effusion in some children.

CHRONIC SUPPURATIVE OTITIS MEDIA In chronic suppurative otitis media, patients discharge chronic purulent drainage from their ears through perforated tympanic membranes. Patients with chronic suppurative otitis media are divided into two groups: those with and those without cholesteatoma. Aerobic culture of draining fluid from both children and adults reveals a high percentage of *S. aureus*, *P. aeruginosa*, and enteric gram-negative bacilli (*Klebsiella, Escherichia coli, Proteus*). Anaerobes, including *Prevotella, Fusobacterium, Porphyromonas,* and some *Bacteroides* species, are found in 50 percent of cases, usually in mixed culture with aerobes. CT should be used to rule out a surgically treatable nidus of infection, such as an infected cholesteatoma or mastoid sequestrum. Surgical drainage of infected areas of the middle ear, followed by a prolonged course of topical antibiotic drops, has been the mainstay of therapy for chronic suppurative otitis media. Recent reports of nonsurgical cure of chronic suppurative otitis media in children without cholesteatoma by intravenous antibiotic therapy based on culture results are encouraging, however.

Tuberculous otitis media, a rare but frequently misdiagnosed cause of chronic suppurative otitis media, is characterized by a tympanic membrane with multiple perforations, extensive granulation tissue, and severe hearing loss. Antituberculous therapy should be administered.

MASTOIDITIS The mastoid is the portion of the temporal bone posterior to the ear that contains a honeycomb of air cells lined with respiratory epithelium. These air cells connect with the middle ear. Fluid in the middle ear, a prelude to otitis media, is almost always accompanied by fluid in the mastoid. True mastoiditis, however, has become rare in the antibiotic era, probably because of prompt treatment of otitis media.

Mastoiditis is characterized by erosion of the bony partitions between the mastoid air cells. Patients with acute mastoiditis present with pain, tenderness, and swelling over the mastoid. When there is an overlying subperiosteal abscess or cellulitis, the pinna is pushed out and forward. CT may show bony destruction or a drainable mastoid abscess.

The reported bacteriology of mastoiditis has varied. Some cases involve organisms similar to those implicated in AOM (*S. pneumoniae, H. influenzae*); others are attributable to *S. aureus* and gram-negative bacilli, including *Pseudomonas*. Ideally, therapy should be guided by the results of cultures of middle-ear fluid obtained by tympanocentesis. Initial broad-spectrum therapy, such as that with intravenous ticarcillin/clavulanate plus gentamicin, can later be narrowed.

COMPLICATIONS OF OTITIS MEDIA AND MASTOIDITIS Extracranial complications include hearing loss, labyrinthitis and resulting vertigo, and facial-nerve palsy. Additional complications from mastoiditis develop when infection tracks under the periosteum of the temporal bone to cause a subperiosteal abscess or breaks through the mastoid tip to cause a neck abscess deep to the sternocleidomastoid muscle (Bezold's abscess). Intracranial complications include epidural abscess, dural venous thrombophlebitis (usually sigmoid sinus), meningitis, and brain abscess.

INFECTIONS OF THE ORAL CAVITY AND PHARYNX

ORAL CAVITY INFECTIONS The oral cavity extends from the lips to the circumvallate papillae of the tongue and is heavily colonized with viridans streptococci and anaerobes. These organisms can cause several infections in this area. *Gingivitis* is an infection of the gums, the earliest form of periodontal disease. Anaerobes residing in the mouth, especially anaerobic gram-negative rods such as *Prevotella intermedia,* are the most common pathogens. Patients with *Vincent's angina,* also called *acute necrotizing ulcerative gingivitis* or *trench mouth,* have halitosis and ulcerations of the interdental papillae. Oral anaerobes are the cause, and therapy with oral penicillin plus metronidazole or with clindamycin alone is effective in both this condition and gingivitis.

Ludwig's angina is a rapidly spreading, life-threatening cellulitis of the sublingual and submandibular spaces that usually starts in an infected lower molar. Patients are febrile and may drool the secretions they cannot swallow. A brawny, boardlike edema in the sublingual area pushes the tongue up and back, sometimes causing airway obstruction. Treatment with intravenous antibiotics active against streptococci and oral anaerobes (e.g., ampicillin/sulbactam or high-dose penicillin plus metronidazole) and airway monitoring are essential. Intubation or tracheostomy may be necessary. Surgical opening of the infected tissue compartments is usually necessary.

Noma, or *cancrum oris*, is a fulminant gangrenous infection of the oral and facial tissues that occurs in severely malnourished and debilitated patients and is especially common among children. Beginning as a necrotic ulcer in the gingiva of the mandible, noma is caused by oral anaerobes, especially fusospirochetal organisms (e.g., *Fusobacterium nucleatum*). It is treated with high-dose penicillin, debridement, and correction of the underlying malnutrition.

Herpes simplex commonly causes cold sores of the lips but may also cause painful vesicles on the tongue and buccal mucosa. Primary infection may require intravenous hydration and should be treated with acyclovir. *Thrush*, a condition caused by an overgrowth of yeast (usually *Candida* species) that occurs in immunocompromised patients, is treated with topical antifungal solutions (e.g., nystatin) or with oral fluconazole.

PHARYNGITIS   Most cases of pharyngitis are thought to be viral. Many occur as part of common colds caused by rhinovirus, coronavirus, or parainfluenza virus. Patients have a scratchy or sore throat as well as coryza and cough. The pharynx is inflamed and edematous, but no exudate is evident. Influenza virus and adenovirus may cause a particularly severe sore throat, along with fever and myalgias. In infection with either of the latter viruses, there is pharyngeal erythema and edema; however, adenovirus infection also commonly causes an exudate, thus mimicking streptococcal pharyngitis. *Infectious mononucleosis* due to Epstein-Barr virus often causes a severe sore throat. Exudative pharyngitis or tonsillitis is documented in half of mononucleosis cases and may also mimic streptococcal infection. *Herpangina*, caused by coxsackievirus, is characterized by fever, sore throat, myalgias, and a vesicular enanthem on the soft palate between the uvula and the tonsils. There are usually only two to six lesions, which begin as small papules that vesiculate and then ulcerate. Fever and nonexudative pharyngitis are common symptoms of the acute retroviral syndrome that develops several weeks after infection with HIV.

The most important bacterial cause of pharyngitis is group A *Streptococcus* (*Streptococcus pyogenes*). This organism is responsible for about 15 percent of all cases of pharyngitis and can cause important complications, both suppurative (peritonsillar and retropharyngeal abscess) and nonsuppurative (scarlet fever, streptococcal toxic shock syndrome, rheumatic fever, acute poststreptococcal glomerulonephritis). Fever, severe sore throat, cervical adenopathy, and inflammation of the tonsils and pharynx (which are covered with exudate) are classic findings. However, many cases of streptococcal pharyngitis are mild, with minimal erythema and no exudate, and mimic the pharyngitis of the common cold. Although some patients may in fact have viral pharyngitis and may simply be colonized with group A streptococci, these individuals must nevertheless be treated for presumed streptococcal pharyngitis. Diagnosis is made by culture. Recently, rapid antigen tests have become available. These tests are specific but not very sensitive: a positive test may be considered equivalent to a positive culture, but a negative test requires culture confirmation. Ten days of treatment with oral penicillin (or with erythromycin in penicillin-allergic patients) are required; shorter courses do not eradicate the organism. A single dose of intramuscular benzathine penicillin is an alternative of equal efficacy. Other antibiotics active against streptococci may be used (e.g., cephalexin, amoxicillin, cefuroxime, or cefprozil), although studies of the prevention of rheumatic fever are available only for penicillin (see Chap. 236).

Other bacterial causes of pharyngitis include groups C and G *Streptococcus*, *Neisseria gonorrhoeae* (see Chap. 150), *Arcanobacterium haemolyticum*, *Yersinia enterocolitica*, and—very rarely—*Corynebacterium diphtheriae* (see Chap. 144). In addition, *Mycoplasma pneumoniae* (Chap. 180) and *C. pneumoniae* (Chap. 181) can cause pharyngitis.

A peritonsillar abscess (*quinsy*) may follow untreated streptococcal pharyngitis. Oral anaerobes also play a role in quinsy. Patients have a severe sore throat and speak with a "hot-potato" voice. Examination reveals pronounced unilateral peritonsillar swelling and erythema causing deviation of the uvula. Immediate aspiration by an otolaryngologist is required in conjunction with antibiotic therapy with penicillin plus metronidazole, clindamycin, or ampicillin/sulbactam.

LARYNGITIS, CROUP, AND EPIGLOTTITIS

LARYNGITIS   Laryngitis is characterized by hoarseness. Most cases of acute laryngitis are caused by viruses (rhinovirus, influenza virus, parainfluenza virus, coxsackievirus, adenovirus, or respiratory syncytial virus). Acute laryngitis may also be associated with group A *Streptococcus* and *M. catarrhalis*. Laryngitis must be differentiated from epiglottitis (see below). The goal of treatment is merely the relief of symptoms except when throat cultures are positive for group A *Streptococcus* (in which case penicillin should be used) or possibly for *M. catarrhalis* (in which case erythromycin should be used).

Chronic laryngitis due to infection is rare and must be distinguished from hoarseness of neoplastic etiology. *Tuberculous laryngitis* may be mistaken for laryngeal cancer when assessed by direct laryngoscopy. Laryngeal and supraglottic lesions include mucosal hyperemia and thickening, nodules, and ulcerations. In a recent study, a history of fever and night sweats was rare, and the most common chest radiographic finding was apical thickening and fibrosis. Biopsy reveals granulomas with acid-fast bacilli. Cultures should be performed to confirm the diagnosis and evaluate the sensitivities of the pathogen. Laryngeal tuberculosis is highly contagious and should be managed with the same precautions and therapy used for active pulmonary disease (see Chap. 171). Fungal infections causing laryngitis include histoplasmosis (Chap. 203), blastomycosis (Chap. 205), and candidiasis (Chap. 207). *Histoplasma* and *Blastomyces* may cause nodules on the larynx, with or without ulcerations. *Candida* may cause laryngitis, along with thrush, in immunosuppressed patients or in patients with chronic mucocutaneous candidiasis.

CROUP   Croup, or acute laryngotracheobronchitis, is an infection of the upper and lower respiratory tract that causes marked subglottic edema. It mainly affects 2- and 3-year-old children and usually follows the onset of upper respiratory tract infection by 1 to 2 days. Symptoms include fever, hoarseness, a "seal's bark" cough, and inspiratory stridor. The most common etiology is parainfluenza virus, although croup may also be caused by other respiratory viruses (e.g., influenza or respiratory syncytial virus) and by *M. pneumoniae*.

Croup must be differentiated from epiglottitis (see below). Epiglottitis usually progresses more rapidly and produces a more toxic appearance. Neck x-rays may be helpful but do not reliably exclude epiglottitis. In croup, the anterior-posterior neck x-ray shows subglottic edema (the "hourglass sign"); in epiglottitis, the lateral neck view shows a thick epiglottis.

Patients with severe croup should be hospitalized, monitored for hypoxemia through pulse oximetry, and watched for airway obstruction requiring intubation. Humidification is commonly prescribed, but few controlled trials have assessed its benefit. Nebulized epinephrine provides temporary (2-h) improvement in patients with marked stridor, but such patients must be observed for rebound edema. Glucocorticoid therapy is controversial.

EPIGLOTTITIS   Acute epiglottitis (supraglottitis) is a life-threatening, rapidly progressive cellulitis of the epiglottis that may cause complete airway obstruction. It begins as a cellulitis between the tongue base and the epiglottis that pushes the epiglottis posteriorly. The epiglottis itself then becomes swollen, threatening the airway. Epiglottitis is most common among children 2 to 4 years old but may also affect older children and adults. Since the advent of vaccination against *H. influenzae* type b in 1985, the overall incidence of epiglottitis among children has decreased.

The typical young child with epiglottitis has a several-hour history of fever, irritability, dysphonia, and dysphagia and presents sitting forward and drooling. Some adolescents and adults may have a less fulminant presentation, with symptoms (especially sore throat) of 1 or 2 days' duration. Adults may present with dyspnea (25 percent), drooling (15 percent), and stridor (10 percent). Epiglottitis constitutes a medical emergency, as airway occlusion may occur suddenly. Lateral neck films showing an enlarged epiglottis (the "thumb sign") are helpful if positive but may be falsely negative. The value of obtaining these films has also been questioned because doing so may cause a critical delay in securing the airway. Direct viewing of the pharynx by use of a tongue blade should not be attempted, as immediate laryngospasm and airway obstruction may result. Instead, a child with suspected epiglottitis should be transported—while sitting up—to the operating room for visualization of the epiglottis with a fiberoptic laryngoscope, with preparations made for immediate airway control. If the epiglottis is cherry-red, an uncuffed endotracheal tube should be placed. Diagnosis in adults is also made by direct viewing of the epiglottis with a flexible fiberoptic laryngoscope, again only after preparations are made to secure the airway.

All patients must be closely monitored in an intensive care unit and should be given antibiotics active against *H. influenzae*. This organism is responsible for nearly all pediatric cases and is isolated from the blood in almost 100 percent. In adults, blood cultures are positive in about 25 percent of cases, all of which are due to *H. influenzae*. Other pathogens isolated from the pharynx of adults with epiglottitis include *Haemophilus parainfluenzae*, *S. pneumoniae*, group A *Streptococcus*, and (rarely) *S. aureus*; the correlation between throat and epiglottis cultures is unclear, however. Children may be treated with intravenous cefuroxime, ceftriaxone, ampicillin/sulbactam, or trimethoprim-sulfamethoxazole. Adults may be treated with cefuroxime, ampicillin/sulbactam, or nafcillin plus ceftriaxone; those highly allergic to penicillin may be given clindamycin plus trimethoprim-sulfamethoxazole. If the patient with *H. influenzae* epiglottitis has household contacts that include an unvaccinated child under age 4, all members of the household and the patient should receive prophylactic rifampin to eradicate the carriage of *H. influenzae*.

DEEP NECK INFECTIONS

Deep neck infections may be life-threatening because of airway compromise, involvement of the carotid sheath, or spread into the mediastinum.

SUBMANDIBULAR SPACE INFECTIONS See *Ludwig's angina* above (under "Oral Cavity Infections").

LATERAL PHARYNGEAL SPACE INFECTIONS The lateral pharyngeal space, also called the parapharyngeal or pharyngomaxillary space, is in the superior lateral portion of the neck and extends from the hyoid bone to the base of the skull. It lies deep to the lateral wall of the pharynx and is lateral to the tonsil and carotid sheath and medial to the parotid gland. Infection in this space may follow tonsillitis, pharyngitis with adenoid involvement, parotitis, mastoiditis, or periodontal infection.

On presentation, most patients appear toxic and have fever, sore throat, pain on swallowing, and leukocytosis. Infection confined to the posterior (retrostyloid) portion of the lateral pharyngeal space causes swelling of the lateral pharyngeal wall, which may be missed because it is behind the palatopharyngeal arch. Involvement of the anterior portion of this space causes medial displacement of the tonsil, swelling over the parotid gland, and trismus. Rigidity of the neck or torticollis toward the opposite side may develop. Diagnosis is confirmed by CT with contrast.

Treatment includes securing of the airway, surgical drainage in the operating room, and administration of intravenous antibiotics active against streptococci and oral anaerobes (e.g., ampicillin/sulbactam). Major complications result from involvement of the carotid sheath and the vessels it contains. These complications are frequently fatal and include jugular vein thrombophlebitis, erosion into the carotid artery, and mediastinitis. Jugular vein thrombophlebitis is characterized by high fevers, chills, and neck tenderness at the angle of the mandible. Erosion into the carotid artery is usually heralded by repeated small bleeds into the mouth. The involvement of adjacent cranial nerves may result in ipsilateral Horner's syndrome, hoarseness, or unilateral tongue paresis. Extension of infection along the carotid sheath into the posterior mediastinum results in mediastinitis and a mortality of 50 percent. MRI is useful in delineating carotid and jugular involvement.

RETROPHARYNGEAL SPACE INFECTION The retropharyngeal space lies between the pharynx and the prevertebral fascia and extends from the base of the skull into the mediastinum. Infection in this space may result from the spread of lateral pharyngeal space infection or from the lymphatic spread of infection in more cephalad sites (posterior sinuses, adenoids, nasopharynx) to the retropharyngeal lymph nodes. Retropharyngeal abscess is most common among infants and young children, probably because the retropharyngeal nodes later involute. Retropharyngeal abscess may also follow trauma to the posterior pharynx (e.g., endoscopy in adults, lollipop-stick perforation in children) or may result from anterior extension of infection from cervical osteomyelitis.

Symptoms include fever, marked difficulty and pain with swallowing, and a "hot-potato" voice. Physical examination may document drooling, nuchal rigidity, and bulging of the posterior pharyngeal wall. Advanced cases include dyspnea and stridor. Diagnosis may be confirmed by a lateral neck soft-tissue x-ray or CT scan. Treatment requires securing of the airway and emergency surgical drainage. Intravenous antibiotics should be given; the agents chosen should be active against streptococci, oral anaerobes, *S. aureus*, and *H. influenzae* (e.g., ampicillin/sulbactam alone or clindamycin plus ceftriaxone). Potential complications include airway obstruction, intraoral rupture of the abscess causing aspiration pneumonia, and mediastinitis.

BIBLIOGRAPHY

BAKER AS, MONTGOMERY WW: Oropharyngeal space infections. Curr Clin Top Infect Dis 8:227, 1987

CHOW AW: Life-threatening infections of the head and neck. Clin Infect Dis 14:991, 1992

CODY DT II et al: Allergic fungal sinusitis: The Mayo Clinic experience. Laryngoscope 104:1074, 1994

DEL BECCARO MA et al: Bacteriology of acute otitis media: A new perspective. J Pediatr 120:81, 1992

DONALD PJ et al (eds): *The Sinuses.* New York, Raven Press, 1995

EVANS FO et al: Sinusitis of the maxillary antrum. N Engl J Med 293:735, 1974

GWALTNEY JM JR et al: Computed tomographic study of the common cold. N Engl J Med 330:25, 1994

HARRIS JP, DARROW DH: Complications of chronic otitis media, in *Surgery of the Ear and Temporal Bone*, JB Nadol Jr, HF Schuknecht (eds). New York, Raven Press, 1993, p 171

KLEIN JO: Otitis externa, otitis media, mastoiditis, in *Principles and Practice of Infectious Diseases*, 4th ed, GL Mandell et al (eds). New York, Churchill Livingstone, 1995, p 579

LIM DJ, BLUESTONE CD (eds): Recent advances in otitis media: Report of the Fifth Research Conference. Ann Otol Rhinol Laryngol 103(Suppl 164), 1994

PARADISE JL: Etiology and management of pharyngitis and pharyngotonsillitis in children: A current review. Ann Otol Rhinol Laryngol 155:51, 1992

SCHWARTZ LE, BROWN RB: Purulent otitis media in adults. Arch Intern Med 152:2301, 1992

SINAVE CP et al: The Lemierre syndrome: Suppurative thrombophlebitis of the internal jugular vein secondary to oropharyngeal infection. Medicine 68:85, 1989

WASHBURN RG et al: Chronic fungal sinusitis in apparently normal hosts. Medicine 67:231, 1988

ORAL MANIFESTATIONS OF DISEASE

A thorough oral examination, to include the oral and pharyngeal soft tissues as well as the teeth, is an important part of the physical examination. The common oral diseases are due to infection by bacteria, fungi, or viruses. The complex development of the orofacial structures leads to close interposition of a wide range of tissues, most of which are prone to developmental anomalies, growth disturbances, and neoplasia.

DISEASES OF THE TEETH

DENTAL CARIES, PULPAL AND PERIAPICAL DISEASE, AND COMPLICATIONS Dental caries is a destructive disease of the hard tissues of the teeth due to infection with *Streptococcus mutans* and other bacteria. Formerly one of the most common human diseases, caries has shown marked changes in recent years. In the United States, fewer than half of those 17 years and younger now have carious lesions, although in many segments of the population and in developing countries this decrease has not occurred. Much of the decline is due to artificial fluoridation of drinking water to a level of 1 part per million, with additional effects due to fluoride-containing toothpastes and topical fluoride administration. Conversely, retention of teeth and the aging of the population have led to an increase in root caries. Increasing numbers of patients surviving with the consequences of cancer therapy and other special populations (diabetics and those with xerostomia due to Sjögren's syndrome or to medications) may experience severe caries unless appropriate topical fluoride prophylaxis is used. Treatment of caries involves removal of the softened and infected hard tissues, sealing of the exposed dentine, and restoration of the lost tooth structure with silver amalgam, composite plastic, gold, or porcelain.

If the carious lesion progresses, infection of the dental pulp may occur, causing *acute pulpitis*. The tooth may become sensitive to hot or cold, and then severe continuous throbbing pain ensues. At this stage, pulp damage is irreversible, and root canal therapy becomes necessary. The contents of the pulp chamber and root canals are removed, followed by thorough cleaning, antisepsis, and filling with an inert material. Alternatively, extraction of the tooth may be indicated.

If the pulpitis is not treated successfully, infection may spread beyond the tooth apex into the periodontal ligament. If the infection causes acute inflammation, pain on chewing or on percussion is present, and a *periapical abscess* may form, while chronic inflammation can produce a *periapical granuloma* within the alveolar bone. This may cause slight pain and tenderness or may be asymptomatic. Proliferation of epithelial cell rests may convert the granuloma into a *periapical cyst*. Both the granuloma and the cyst produce periapical radiolucencies, whereas the periapical abscess does not do so unless it forms as a complication of one of the other two lesions. The pus in the periapical abscess may track through the alveolar bone into soft tissues, causing cellulitis and bacteremia, or may discharge into the oral cavity (*parulis* or *gumboil*), into the maxillary sinus, or through the skin of the face or submandibular area. A severe form of cellulitis, *Ludwig's angina*, originates from an infected mandibular molar, involves the submandibular space, and extends throughout the floor of the mouth, with elevation of the tongue, dysphagia, and difficulty in breathing. Glottal edema may occur, necessitating emergency tracheotomy.

EFFECT OF SYSTEMIC FACTORS ON TEETH Systemic factors, occurring in utero or in infancy during the stages of crown formation, may influence the development and structure of the teeth. Enamel hypoplasia of the primary and/or permanent teeth, manifested by alterations ranging from white spots to gross defects in the surface structure of the crowns, may be caused by disturbances of calcium and phosphate metabolism such as are found in vitamin D–resistant rickets, hypoparathyroidism, gastroenteritis, and celiac disease. Prema-

ture birth or high fevers also may give rise to enamel hypoplasia. Tetracycline, when given during the second half of pregnancy, in infancy, and in childhood up to 8 years of age, causes both a permanent discoloration of the teeth and enamel hypoplasia. Daily ingestion of more than 1.5 mg fluoride can result in enamel discoloration (*mottling*). Prenatal factors appear to influence crown size. Larger teeth are associated with maternal diabetes, maternal hypothyroidism, and large birth size. Tooth size is reduced in Down's syndrome. Premature loss of the deciduous dentition is frequently the first symptom in juvenile hypophosphatasia. Systemic disease may give rise to pain that simulates pulpal disease. Maxillary sinusitis is frequently manifested as pain in the maxillary teeth, including sensitivity to thermal changes and percussion. Cardiac disease with angina pectoris may result in pain referred to the lower jaw, probably through the vagus nerve.

PERIODONTAL DISEASES

In adults, chronic destructive periodontal disease becomes responsible for more loss of teeth than caries, particularly in the aged. However, the prevalence and incidence of periodontal disease also appears to be declining in the United States. The most common form of periodontal disease starts as inflammation of the marginal gingiva (*gingivitis*) which is painless, although the gingiva may bleed on brushing. The disease spreads to involve the periodontal ligament and alveolar bone. As the latter is slowly resorbed, there is loss of periodontal ligament attachment between tooth and bone. The soft tissue separates from the tooth surface, causing "pocket" formation with bleeding on probing and during chewing. Acute inflammation may become superimposed on this chronic process, with the production of pus and the formation of a *periodontal abscess*. Ultimately, extreme bone loss, tooth mobility, and recurrent abscess formation lead to tooth exfoliation or may mandate tooth extraction.

Gingivitis and periodontitis are infections associated with the accumulation of *bacterial plaque*, which may become mineralized (*calculus*) and which can be prevented by appropriate *oral hygiene* measures, including tooth brushing, flossing, antibacterial mouth rinses, and the removal of impacted food debris. Poorly fabricated or deteriorated restorations may contribute through overextended or inadequate margins, while the role of occlusal trauma is unclear. Therapy is directed at the causative microflora and consists of removal of plaque and calculus, debridement of the pocket lining and superficial infected cementum, and elimination of other contributing factors.

Periodontal disease appears to be a group of conditions, including *adult periodontitis*, associated with *Porphyromonas gingivalis*, *Prevotella intermedia*, and other gram-negative organisms. *Localized juvenile periodontitis* (LJP) causes rapid, severe pocketing and bone loss and is associated with *Actinobacillus actinomycetemcomitans*, *Capnocytophaga*, *Eikenella corrodens*, and other anaerobes. *Acute necrotizing ulcerative gingivitis* (ANUG) involves sudden inflammation of the gingivae with necrosis, tissue loss, pain, bleeding, and halitosis and is associated with *P. intermedia* and spirochetes. ANUG and an aggressive and rapid form of periodontitis (*necrotizing ulcerative periodontitis*) are seen in association with human immunodeficiency virus (HIV) infection. Some of these cases progress to a destructive gangrene-like lesion of oral soft tissues and bone (*necrotizing stomatitis*) resembling the *noma* formerly seen in severely malnourished populations. Therapy involves local antibacterial measures, debridement, and, in severe cases, systemic antibiotics effective against gram-negative anaerobes.

Host factors may be involved in the pathogenesis of periodontal disease in other populations as well. Thus familial defects in neutrophil chemotaxis are found in LJP, and these may predispose to tissue destruction caused by the toxins of *A. actinomycetemcomitans*, including leucotoxin, collagenase, endotoxin, and a factor further inhibiting neutrophil chemotaxis. Patients with IgA deficiency and agammaglobulinemia probably have less periodontal disease than matched healthy individuals, whereas in *Down's syndrome* and *diabetes mellitus* severe periodontal disease may occur. During pregnancy there may be severe gingivitis and the formation of localized *pyogenic granulomas*. Certain drugs, notably the anticonvulsant *phenytoin* and the antiangina calcium channel blocker *nifedipine*, cause *fibrous hyperplasia* of the gingiva, which may cover the teeth, interfere with eating, and be unsightly. Similar clinical appearances can be due to *idiopathic familial gingival fibromatosis*. Surgical management is used for both conditions, although a change in medication may be appropriate for the drug-induced form.

Periapical and periodontal bacterial infections can cause transient bacteremia after tooth extraction and even routine dental prophylaxis. These can lead to bacterial endocarditis in patients with a history of rheumatic fever, other valvular disease, valvular graft, or heart or joint prostheses. Antibiotic coverage is appropriate in such cases.

DISEASES OF THE ORAL MUCOSA

INFECTIONS Most oral mucosal diseases involve microorganisms (see Table 31-1).
PIGMENTED LESIONS See Table 31-2
DERMATOLOGIC DISEASES See Tables 31-1, -2, and -3 and Chaps. 54 to 58
DISEASES OF THE TONGUE See Table 31-4
HALITOSIS See Table 31-5
HIV DISEASE AND AIDS (See Table 31-6 and Chaps. 192 and 308) Immunosuppression induced by HIV infection predisposes to numerous oral infections, neoplasms, and autoimmune and idiopathic lesions. Some of these, such as *oral candidiasis* (**Plate ID-42**) and *hairy leukoplakia* (**Plate ID-41**) [a benign epithelial hyperplasia associated with Epstein-Barr virus (EBV)], are common features of HIV disease and often precede or accompany full-blown AIDS. Some, such as oral Kaposi's sarcoma and lymphoma, are diagnostic of AIDS. Oral candidiasis is easily treated with topical or systemic antifungals. These include nystatin oral pastilles, clotrimazole oral troches, nystatin vaginal tablets used orally, fluconazole, and ketoconazole. While most oral lesions of HIV disease are also found in the general population, both hairy leukoplakia and necrotizing ulcerative periodontal disease are strongly associated with HIV infection and are seen only very rarely in other circumstances. Only small and variable amounts of HIV can be found in saliva, but blood, tissue fluid, and gingival crevicular exudate, found in the mouth as a result of lesions or of clinical manipulation, are certainly sources of other viruses, such as herpes simplex virus (HSV) and EBV, and the same may be true for HIV.

HEMATOLOGIC AND NUTRITIONAL DISEASE Gingival bleeding, necrotic ulcers, and enlargement due to malignant infiltrates are seen in all forms of leukemia, particularly *monocytic leukemia*. In *agranulocytosis* severe oral mucosal ulcers are seen, while in *thrombocytopenia* oral petechiae, ecchymoses, and gingival bleeding occur. In *Plummer-Vinson syndrome* (see Chap. 106), atrophy of oral mucosa, particularly the tongue papillae, causes redness and soreness as well as dysphagia. This is associated with increased susceptibility to oral cancer. A smooth tongue also can be seen in *pernicious anemia* (Chap. 108). Severe oral mucositis with ulcers, candidiasis, bacterial infections, and xerostomia complicate local radiotherapy for head and neck malignancies as well as chemotherapy for both local and other malignancies. Although now rarely seen in the United States, oral features of vitamin deficiency include oral mucositis and ulcers, glossitis, and burning sensations in the tongue (*B group vitamin deficiency*) and petechiae, gingival swelling, bleeding, and ulceration as well as loosening of teeth (*scurvy* of vitamin C deficiency).

DISEASES OF THE SALIVARY GLANDS

The major and minor salivary glands can be involved in mumps, sarcoidosis, tuberculosis, lymphoma, and Sjögren's syndrome (Chap.

316). The latter may cause dry eyes and dry mouth (*xerostomia*) and be associated with features of connective tissue diseases, including rheumatoid arthritis or systemic lupus erythematosus. Xerostomia also may be due to medications such as diuretics, antihistamines, or tricylic antidepressants as well as therapeutic irradiation for head and neck cancer. It may cause *cervical or incisal caries* and oral candidiasis. Management includes fluoride mouth rinses and topical applications, saliva substitutes, salivary stimulation with sugarless candies, and the avoidance of sugar-containing drinks or food. Candidiasis is treated with nystatin or other antifungals. Salivary stones (*sialolithiasis*), usually in the duct of a major salivary gland, cause *sialoadenitis* with pain and swelling, often on eating. Recurrent *parotitis* without apparent cause is seen in children.

The most common neoplasm of the salivary glands is the *pleomorphic adenoma*, which is benign but will recur unless fully enucleated; malignant tumors include *mucoepidermoid carcinoma*, *adenoid cystic carcinoma*, and *adenocarcinoma*. The pleomorphic adenoma causes a firm, slowly growing mass in the parotid, palate, or cheek, whereas malignant tumors grow faster and can cause ulceration and invade nerves, producing numbness or facial paralysis.

NEUROLOGIC DISTURBANCES AND OROFACIAL PAIN

The mouth and face may be the site of pain from a number of vascular, neurologic, muscle/connective tissue, or joint conditions. Interdisciplinary diagnosis and management programs involving neurologists, restorative dentists, oral surgeons, otorhinolaryngologists, and other specialists, together with new imaging techniques to diagnose or exclude organic lesions, have begun to clarify this complex field. *Temporal arteritis* causes pain in the face, jaws, and tongue and may mimic temporomandibular joint disease. Glucocorticoids may provide relief. *Myofascial pain* is a dull, constant ache with local tenderness in the muscles of the jaws and difficulty in opening the mouth. This may be related to clenching and grinding habits (*bruxism*). *Arthralgia* of the temporomandibular joint causes local pain, which may extend to the face and head. Both myofascial pain and arthralgia can be relieved with heat, rest, and anti-inflammatory agents. Displacement of the meniscus or condyle may cause pain, clenching, or locking of the mandible in the open position. The joint may become involved in *osteoarthritis* with minimal symptoms, whereas *rheumatoid arthritis* causes pain and swelling in the joint, limitation of movement, and, in the *juvenile* form, severe malocclusion in children. *Ankylosis* may occur, necessitating condylectomy (see Chap. 313).

Trigeminal neuralgia (tic douloureux) causes sudden, severe, unilateral lancinating pain initiated by touching a "trigger zone" or occurring spontaneously. Confusion with pulpal or periapical pain is common, leading to inappropriate endodontic or surgical therapy. Many cases respond to carbamazepine and phenytoin, but for a few, surgical intervention to decompress the trigeminal nerve is indicated. Similar symptoms in the distribution of the ninth cranial nerve (tongue, pharynx, soft palate) are due to *glossopharyngeal neuralgia*, which may be triggered by swallowing and may produce referred pain in the temporomandibular joint. *Postherpetic neuralgia* may follow trigeminal herpes zoster (see Chap. 372) and cause burning, aching, and long-lasting pain. *Facial palsy* is usually unilateral and may be due to trauma, surgical intervention, tumor, or infection of the seventh cranial nerve. *Bell's palsy* is a form with acute onset and unknown cause, possibly viral infection such as herpes zoster. The corner of the mouth droops, and there may be difficulty in speech, eating, and in closing the eye. The symptoms usually disappear spontaneously, but residual facial immobility and lip drooping may persist. Abnormal or reduced *taste sensation* may be due to xerostomia, disturbances of the facial and glossopharyngeal nerves or their central connections, aging, or the wearing of dentures. Disease involving the hypoglossal nerve may cause atrophy of the tongue muscles with protrusion, if bilateral, or deviation toward the affected side, if unilateral.

Table 31-1

Vesicular, Bullous, or Ulcerative Lesions of the Oral Mucosa

Condition	Usual Location	Clinical Features	Course
VIRAL DISEASES			
Primary acute herpetic gingivo-stomatitis (herpes simplex virus type 1, rarely type 2)	Lip and oral mucosa	Labial vesicles that rupture and crust, and intraoral vesicles that quickly ulcerate; extremely painful; acute gingivitis, fever, malaise, foul odor, and cervical lymphadenopathy; occurs primarily in infants, children, and young adults	Heals spontaneously in 10–14 days unless secondarily infected
Recurrent herpes labialis	Mucocutaneous junction of lip, perioral skin	Eruption of groups of vesicles that may coalesce then rupture and crust; painful to pressure or spicy foods	Lasts about 1 week, but condition may be prolonged if secondary infection occurs
Recurrent intraoral herpes simplex	Palate and gingiva	Small vesicles that rupture and coalesce; painful	Heal spontaneously in about 1 week
Chickenpox (varicella-zoster virus)	Gingiva and oral mucosa	Skin lesions may be accompanied by small vesicles on oral mucosa that rupture to form shallow ulcers; may coalesce to form large bullous lesions that ulcerate; mucosa may have generalized erythema	Lesions heal spontaneously within 2 weeks
Herpes zoster (reactivation of varicella-zoster virus)	Cheek, tongue, gingiva, or palate	Unilateral vesicular eruption and ulceration in linear pattern following sensory distribution of trigeminal nerve or one of its branches	Gradual healing without scarring; postherpetic neuralgia is common
Infectious mononucleosis (Epstein-Barr virus)	Oral mucosa	Fatigue, sore throat, malaise, low-grade fever, and enlarged cervical lymph nodes; numerous small ulcers usually appear several days before lymphadenopathy; gingival bleeding and multiple petechiae at junction of hard and soft palates	Oral lesions disappear during convalescence
Warts (papillomavirus)	Anywhere on skin and oral mucosa	Single or multiple papillary lesions, with thick, white keratinized surfaces containing many pointed projections; cauliflower lesions covered with normal-colored mucosa or multiple pink or pale bumps (focal epithelial hyperplasia)	Lesions grow rapidly and spread
Herpangina (coxsackievirus A; also possibly coxsackievirus B and echovirus)	Oral mucosa, pharynx, tongue	Sudden onset of fever, sore throat, and oropharyngeal vesicles, usually in children under 4 years, during summer months; diffuse pharyngeal congestion and vesicles (1–2 mm), grayish-white surrounded by red areola; vesicles enlarge and ulcerate	Incubation period 2–9 days; fever for 1–4 days; recovery uneventful
Hand, foot, and mouth disease (type A coxsackieviruses)	Oral mucosa, pharynx, palms, and soles	Fever, malaise, headache with oropharyngeal vesicles that become painful, shallow ulcers	Incubation period 2–18 days; lesions heal spontaneously in 2–4 weeks
Primary HIV infection	Gingiva, palate, and pharynx	Acute gingivitis and oropharyngeal ulceration, associated with febrile illness resembling mononucleosis and including lymphadenopathy	Followed by HIV seroconversion, asymptomatic HIV infection, and usually ultimately by HIV disease
BACTERIAL OR FUNGAL DISEASES			
Acute necrotizing ulcerative gingivitis ("trench mouth," Vincent's infection)	Gingiva	Painful, bleeding gingiva characterized by necrosis and ulceration of gingival papillae and margins plus lymphadenopathy and foul odor	Continued destruction of tissue followed by remission, but may recur
Prenatal (congenital) syphilis	Palate, jaws, tongue, and teeth	Gummatous involvement of palate, jaws, and facial bones; Hutchinson's incisors, mulberry molars, glossitis, mucous patches, and fissures of corners of mouth	Tooth deformities in permanent dentition irreversible
Primary syphilis (chancre)	Lesion appears where organism enters body; may occur on lips, tongue, or tonsillar area	Small papule developing rapidly into a large, painless ulcer with indurated border; unilateral lymphadenopathy; chancre and lymph nodes containing spirochetes; serologic tests positive by third to fourth weeks	Healing of chancre in 1–2 months, followed by secondary syphilis in 6–8 weeks
Secondary syphilis	Oral mucosa frequently involved with mucous patches, primarily on palate, also at commissures of mouth	Maculopapular lesions of oral mucosa, 5–10 mm in diameter with central ulceration covered by grayish membrane; eruptions occurring on various mucosal surfaces and skin accompanied by fever, malaise, and sore throat	Lesions may persist from several weeks to a year
Tertiary syphilis	Palate and tongue	Gummatous infiltration of palate or tongue followed by ulceration and fibrosis; atrophy of tongue papillae produces characteristic bald tongue and glossitis	Gumma may destroy palate, causing complete perforation

(continued)

Table 31-1—*(continued)*

Vesicular, Bullous, or Ulcerative Lesions of the Oral Mucosa

Condition	Usual Location	Clinical Features	Course
Gonorrhea	Lesions may occur in mouth at site of inoculation or secondarily by hematogenous spread from a primary focus elsewhere	Earliest symptoms are burning or itching sensation, dryness, or heat in mouth followed by acute pain on eating or speaking; tonsils and oropharynx most frequently involved; oral tissues may be diffusely inflamed or ulcerated; saliva develops increased viscosity and fetid odor; submaxillary lymphadenopathy with fever in severe cases	Lesions may resolve with appropriate antibiotic therapy
Tuberculosis	Tongue, tonsillar area, soft palate	A solitary, irregular ulcer covered by a persistent exudate; ulcer has an undermined, firm border	Lesions may persist
Cervicofacial actinomycosis	Swellings in region of face, neck, and floor of mouth	Infection may be associated with an extraction, jaw fracture, or eruption of molar tooth; in acute form resembles an acute pyogenic abscess, but contains yellow "sulfur granules" (gram-positive mycelia and their hyphae)	Acute form may last a few weeks; chronic form lasts months or years; prognosis excellent; actinomycetes respond to antibiotics (tetracyclines or penicillin) but not to antifungal drugs
Histoplasmosis	Any area in mouth, particularly tongue, gingiva, or palate	Numerous small nodules that may ulcerate; hoarseness and dysphagia may occur because of lesions in larynx, usually associated with fever and malaise	May be fatal
Candidiasis	Any area of oral mucosa	Pseudomembranous form has white patches that are easily wiped off leaving red, bleeding, sore surface; erythematous form is flat and red; rarely, candidal leukoplakia appears as white patch in tongue that does not rub off; angular cheilitis due to *Candida* involves sore cracks and redness at angle of mouth; *Candida* seen on KOH preparation in all forms	Responds to antifungals

DERMATOLOGIC DISEASES

Condition	Usual Location	Clinical Features	Course
Mucous membrane pemphigoid	Primarily mucous membranes of the oral cavity, but may also involve the eyes, urethra, vagina, and rectum	Painful, grayish-white collapsed vesicles or bullae with peripheral erythematous zone; gingival lesions desquamate, leaving ulcerated area	Protracted course with remissions and exacerbations; involvement of different sites occurs slowly; glucocorticoids may temporarily reduce symptoms but do not control the disease
Erythema multiforme (Stevens-Johnson syndrome)	Primarily the oral mucosa and skin of hands and feet	Intraoral ruptured bullae surrounded by an inflammatory area; lips may show hemorrhagic crusts; the "iris," or "target" lesion, on the skin is pathognomonic; patient may have severe signs of toxicity	Onset very rapid; condition may last 1–2 weeks; may be fatal; acute episodes respond to steroids
Pemphigus vulgaris	Oral mucosa and skin	Ruptured bullae and ulcerated oral areas; mostly in older adults	With repeated recurrence of bullae, toxicity may lead to cachexia, infection, and death within 2 years; often controllable with steroids
Lichen planus	Oral mucosa and skin	White striae in mouth; purplish nodules on skin at sites of friction; occasionally causes oral mucosal ulcers and erosive gingivitis	Protracted course, may respond to topical steroids

OTHER CONDITIONS

Condition	Usual Location	Clinical Features	Course
Recurrent aphthous ulcers	Anywhere on nonkeratinized oral mucosa (lips, tongue, buccal mucosa, floor of mouth, soft palate, oropharynx)	Single or clusters of painful ulcers with surrounding erythematous border; lesions may be 1–2 mm in diameter in crops (herpetiform), 1–5 mm (minor), or 5–15 mm (major)	Lesions heal in 1–2 weeks but may recur monthly or several times a year; topical steroids give symptomatic relief; systemic glucocorticoids may be needed in severe cases; a tetracycline oral suspension may decrease severity of herpetiform ulcers
Behçet's syndrome	Oral mucosa, eyes, genitalia, gut, and CNS	Multiple aphthous ulcers in mouth; inflammatory ocular changes, ulcerative lesions on genitalia; inflammatory bowel disease and CNS disease	Ulcers may persist for several weeks and heal without scarring
Traumatic ulcers	Anywhere on oral mucosa; dentures frequently responsible for ulcers in vestibule	Localized, discrete ulcerated lesion with red border; produced by accidental biting of mucosa, penetration by a foreign object, or chronic irritation by a denture	Lesions usually heal in 7–10 days when irritant is removed, unless secondarily infected

Table 31-2

Pigmented Lesions of the Oral Mucosa

Condition	Usual Location	Clinical Features	Course
Oral melanotic macule	Any area of the mouth	Discrete or diffuse localized, brown to black macule	Remains indefinitely
Diffuse melanin pigmentation	Any area of the mouth	Diffuse pale to dark-brown pigmentation; may be physiologic ("racial") or due to smoking	Remains indefinitely
Nevi	Any area of the mouth	Discrete, localized, brown to black pigmentation	Remains indefinitely
Malignant melanoma	Any area of the mouth	Can be flat and diffuse, painless, brown to black, or can be raised and nodular	Expands and invades early; metastasis leads to death
Addison's disease	Any area in mouth but mostly on buccal mucosa	Blotches or spots of bluish-black to dark-brown pigmentation occurring early in the disease, accompanied by diffuse pigmentation of skin; other symptoms of adrenal insufficiency	Condition controlled by steroid therapy
Peutz-Jeghers syndrome	Any area in mouth	Dark-brown spots on lips, buccal mucosa, with characteristic distribution of pigment around lips, nose, eyes, and on hands; concomitant intestinal polyposis	Pigmented lesions remain indefinitely; polyps may become malignant
Drug ingestion (tranquilizers, oral contraceptives, antimalarials)	Any area in mouth	Brown, black, or gray areas of pigmentation	Disappears following cessation of drug
Amalgam tattoo	Gingiva and mucobuccal fold	Small blue-black pigmented areas associated with embedded amalgam particles in soft tissues; these may show up on radiographs as radiopaque particles in some cases	Remains indefinitely
Heavy metal pigmentation (bismuth, mercury, lead)	Gingival margin	Thin blue-black pigmented line along gingival margin; due to prior treatment for syphilis with bismuth or mercury or to accidental absorption of lead	Long-lasting
Black hairy tongue	Dorsum of tongue	Elongation of filiform papillae of tongue, which take on a brown to black coloration	Long-lasting but may disappear spontaneously
Fordyce's "disease"	Buccal and labial mucosa	Aggregation of numerous small yellowish spots just beneath mucosal surface; no symptoms; due to hyperplasia of sebaceous glands	Remains without apparent change indefinitely

Table 31-3

White Lesions of Oral Mucosa

Condition	Usual Location	Clinical Features	Course
Lichen planus	Buccal mucosa, tongue, gingiva, and lips; skin	Striae, white plaques, red areas, ulcers in mouth; purplish papules on skin; may be asymptomatic, sore, or painful; lichenoid drug reactions may look similar	Protracted; responds to topical steroids
White sponge nevus	Oral mucosa, vagina, anal mucosa	Painless white thickening of epithelium; adolescent/early adult onset; familial	Benign and permanent
Smoker's leukoplakia and smokeless tobacco lesions	Any area of oral mucosa, sometimes related to location of habit	White patch that may become firm, rough, or red-fissured and ulcerated; may become sore and painful but usually painless	Occasionally premalignant; may or may not resolve on cessation of habit
Nicotinic stomatitis	Palate in pipe smokers	White nodular elevations on hard palate with central red areas	Benign; usually resolves on cessation of pipe smoking
Frictional keratosis	Any area in mouth	Elevated white lesion due to hyperkeratosis and thickening of the oral epithelium secondary to chronic irritation	Removal of irritant leads to healing in 2–3 weeks
Candidiasis ("candidosis," "moniliasis")	Any area in mouth	*Pseudomembranous type* ("thrush"): creamy white curdlike patches that reveal a raw, bleeding surface when scraped; found in sick infants, debilitated elderly patients receiving high doses of glucocorticoids or broad-spectrum antibiotics, or in patients with AIDS	Responds favorably to antifungal therapy and correction of predisposing causes where possible
		Erythematous type: flat, red, sometimes sore areas, same groups of patients	Course same as for pseudomembranous type
		Candidal leukoplakia: nonremovable white thickening of epithelium due to *Candida*	Responds to prolonged antifungals
		Angular cheilitis: sore fissures at corner of mouth	Responds to topical antifungals
Hairy leukoplakia	Usually lateral tongue, rarely elsewhere on oral mucosa	White areas ranging from small and flat to extensive and "hairy"; found in HIV carriers in all risk groups for AIDS; rarely causes discomfort	Due to EBV; many patients develop AIDS; responds to high dose acyclovir but recurs
Chemical burns	Any area in mouth	White slough due to necrosis of epithelium and underlying connective tissue caused by contact with agents (e.g., aspirin) applied locally or the use of undiluted sodium perborate or hydrogen peroxide as a mouthwash; removal of slough leaves a raw, painful surface	Lesion heals in several weeks if not secondarily infected

Table 31-4

Alterations of the Tongue

Type of Change	Clinical Features
SIZE OR MORPHOLOGY CHANGES	
Macroglossia	Enlarged tongue that may be part of a syndrome found in developmental conditions such as Down's syndrome; may be due to tumor (hemangioma or lymphangioma), metabolic disease (such as primary amyloidosis), or endocrine disturbance (such as acromegaly or cretinism)
Fissured ("scrotal") tongue	Dorsal surface and sides of tongue covered by painless shallow or deep fissures that may collect debris and become irritated
Median rhomboid glossitis	Congenital abnormality of tongue with ovoid, denuded area in median posterior portion of the tongue; may be associated with candidiasis and may respond to antifungals
COLOR CHANGES	
"Geographic" tongue (benign migratory glossitis)	Asymptomatic inflammatory condition of the tongue, with rapid loss and regrowth of filiform papillae, leading to appearance of denuded red patches "wandering" across the surface of the tongue
Hairy tongue	Elongation of filiform papillae of the medial dorsal surface area due to failure of keratin layer of the papillae to desquamate normally; brownish-black coloration may be due to staining by tobacco, food, or chromogenic organisms
"Strawberry" and "raspberry" tongue	Appearance of tongue during scarlet fever due to the hypertrophy of fungiform papillae plus changes in the filiform papillae
"Bald" tongue	Atrophy may be associated with xerostomia, pernicious anemia, iron-deficiency anemia, pellagra, or syphilis; may be accompanied by painful burning sensation; may be an expression of erythematous candidiasis and respond to antifungals

Table 31-5

Causes of Halitosis

1. Upper respiratory infection
   a. Bronchiectasis
   b. Lung abscess
2. Oral infection
   a. Acute primary herpetic gingivostomatitis
   b. Acute necrotizing ulcerative gingivitis
   c. Periodontal disease
   d. Caries
3. Smoking
4. Hepatic failure (fishy odor)
5. Azotemia (ammoniacal or urinary odor)
6. Diabetic ketoacidosis (sweet, fruity odor)

Table 31-6

Oral Lesions of HIV Disease and AIDS

I. Fungal
   A. Candidiasis
      1. Pseudomembranous
      2. Erythematous
      3. Angular cheilitis
   B. Histoplasmosis
   C. Cryptococcosis
II. Bacterial
   A. Acute necrotizing ulcerative gingivitis
   B. Necrotizing ulcerative periodontitis
   C. Necrotizing stomatitis
   D. *M. avium* complex and tuberculosis
   E. Stomatitis due to enteric organisms
III. Viral
   A. Herpes simplex
   B. Herpes zoster
   C. Hairy leukoplakia
   D. Warts
IV. Neoplastic
   A. Kaposi's sarcoma
   B. Lymphoma
V. Other
   A. Recurrent aphthous ulcers
   B. Immune thrombocytopenic purpura
   C. Xerostomia
   D. Salivary gland enlargement

BIBLIOGRAPHY

BARKER FG et al: The long-term outcome of microvascular decompression for trigeminal neuralgia. N Engl J Med 334:1077, 1996

GENCO R et al: *Contemporary Periodontics*. St. Louis, Mosby, 1990

GREENSPAN D et al: *AIDS and the Mouth*. Chicago, Year Book, 1990

LYNCH MA et al: *Burket's Oral Medicine, Diagnosis and Treatment*, 8th ed. Philadelphia, Lippincott, 1994

NEWBRUN E: *Cariology*, 3d ed. Chicago, Quintessence, 1989

SECTION 5

ALTERATIONS IN CIRCULATORY AND RESPIRATORY FUNCTIONS

32

Roland H. Ingram, Jr., Eugene Braunwald

DYSPNEA AND PULMONARY EDEMA

DYSPNEA

The breathing pattern is controlled by a series of central and peripheral mechanisms that can adjust ventilation appropriate to increased metabolic demands during physical activity. It can also increase ventilation in excess of metabolic demands in conditions such as anxiety and fear. A normal resting person is unaware of the act of breathing, and while he or she may become conscious of breathing during mild to moderate exertion, no discomfort is experienced. However, during and following exhausting exertion, an individual may become unpleasantly aware of breathing yet feel reasonably assured that the sensation will be transitory and is appropriate to the level of exercise. Therefore, as a cardinal symptom of diseases affecting the cardiorespiratory system, *dyspnea* is defined as an *abnormally uncomfortable awareness of breathing*.

Although dyspnea is not painful in the usual sense of the word, it is, like pain, involved with both the perception of a sensation and the reaction to that perception. Patients experience a number of uncomfortable sensations related to breathing and use an even larger number of verbal expressions to describe these sensations, such as "cannot get enough air," "air does not go all the way down," "smothering feeling or tightness or tiredness in the chest," and a "choking sensation." It may be necessary, therefore, to review meticulously the patient's history in order to ascertain whether the more abstruse descriptions do, in fact, represent dyspnea. Once it is established that a patient does have dyspnea, it is of paramount importance to define the circumstances in which it occurs and to assess associated symptoms. There are situations in which breathing appears labored but in which dyspnea does not occur. For example, the hyperventilation associated with metabolic acidemia is rarely accompanied by dyspnea. On the other hand, patients with apparently normal breathing patterns may complain of shortness of breath.

QUANTITATION OF DYSPNEA The gradation of dyspnea may usefully be based on the amount of physical exertion required to produce the sensation. In assessing the severity of dyspnea, it is important to obtain a clear understanding of the patient's general physical condition, work history, and recreational habits. For example, the development of dyspnea in a trained runner upon running 2 mi may signify a much more serious disturbance than a similar degree of breathlessness in a sedentary person upon running a fraction of this distance. Interindividual variation in perception must also be considered. Some patients with severe disease may complain of only mild dyspnea; others with mild disease may experience more severe shortness of breath. Some patients with lung or heart disease may have such reduced capabilities due to other disease (e.g., peripheral vascular insufficiency or severe osteoarthritis of the hips or knees) that exertional dyspnea is precluded despite serious impairment of pulmonary or cardiac function.

Some patterns of dyspnea are not directly related to physical exertion. Sudden and unexpected dyspneic episodes at rest can be associated with pulmonary emboli, spontaneous pneumothorax, hypercapnea secondary to breath holding, or anxiety. Nocturnal episodes of severe paroxysmal dyspnea are characteristic of left ventricular failure. Dyspnea upon assuming the supine posture, *orthopnea* (see below), thought to be mainly characteristic of congestive heart failure, also may occur in some patients with asthma and chronic obstruction of the airways and is a regular finding in the rare occurrence of bilateral diaphragmatic paralysis. *Trepopnea* is used to describe the unusual circumstance in which dyspnea occurs only in a lateral decubitus position, most often in patients with heart disease, while *platypnea* is dyspnea that occurs only in the upright position. Positional alterations in ventilation-perfusion relationships (see Chap. 250) have been invoked to explain these patterns. Platypnea can also be seen with deficient abdominal musculature, a deficiency that results in loss of diaphragmatic support due to anterior protrusion of abdominal viscera in the upright posture. Upon lying down, the viscera resume support of the diaphragm, stretching it to its optimal operational length. This form of platypnea is alleviated by use of an abdominal binder.

MECHANISMS OF DYSPNEA (See Fig. 32-1) Physicians usually relate the symptom of dyspnea to a process such as obstruction of the airways or congestive heart failure and generally proceed with further diagnostic and/or therapeutic attempts, having satisfied themselves that they understand the mechanism of the dyspnea. In fact, elucidation of the *actual* mechanism(s) of dyspnea has eluded clinical investigators.

Dyspnea occurs whenever the work of breathing is excessive. Increased force generation is required of the respiratory muscles to produce a given volume change if the chest wall or lungs are less compliant or if resistance to airflow is increased. Increased work of breathing also occurs when the ventilation is excessive for the level of activity. Although an individual is more apt to become dyspneic when the work of breathing is increased, the work theory does not account for the perceptual difference between a deep breath with a normal mechanical load and a normal-sized breath with an increased mechanical load. The work might be the same with both breaths, but the normal one with the increased load will be associated with discomfort. In fact, with respiratory loading, such as adding a resistance at the mouth, there is an increase in respiratory center output that is disproportionate to the increase in the work of breathing. It has been postulated that whenever the force that muscles actually generate during breathing approaches some fraction of their maximal force-generating ability, which may vary among individuals, dyspnea ensues due to transduction of mechanical to neural stimuli. Such a theory would still not explain why patients who are completely paralyzed, either by cord transections or neuromuscular blockade, experience dyspnea although aided by a mechanical ventilator. It is probable, in these circumstances, that signals from the lungs and/or airways travel via the vagus nerve to the central nervous system to account for the sensation.

In all likelihood, several different mechanisms operate to different degrees in the various clinical situations in which dyspnea occurs. In some circumstances, dyspnea is evoked by stimulation of receptors in the upper respiratory tract; in others it may originate from receptors in the lungs, airways, respiratory muscles, chest wall, or some combination of these structures. In any event, dyspnea is characterized by an excessive or abnormal activation of the respiratory centers in the brainstem. This activation comes about from stimuli transmitted from

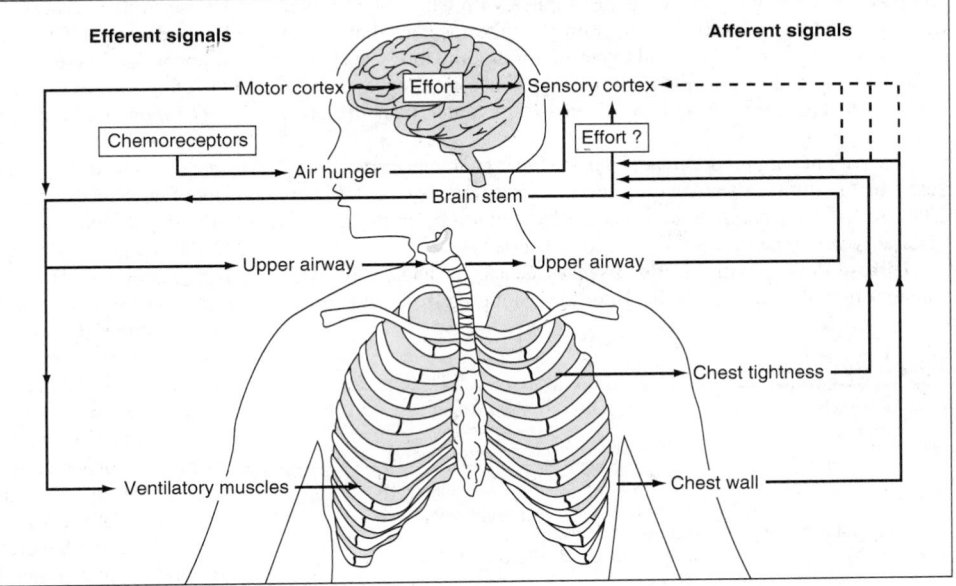

FIGURE 32-1 Efferent and afferent signals that contribute to the sensation of dyspnea. There is evidence that the sense of respiratory effort arises from a signal transmitted from the motor cortex to the sensory cortex simultaneously with the outgoing motor command to the ventilatory muscles. The motor output of the brainstem may also contribute to the sense of effort, as shown in the arrow from the brainstem to the sensory cortex. The sense of air hunger arises, in part, from increased respiratory activity within the brainstem, and the sensation of chest tightness probably results from stimulation of vagal-irritant receptors. While afferent information from airway, lung, and chest-wall receptors probably passes through the brainstem before reaching the sensory cortex, the dashed lines indicate uncertainty about whether some afferents bypass the brainstem and project directly to the sensory cortex. (*From Manning and Schwartzstein, with permission.*)

or through a variety of structures and pathways, including (1) intrathoracic receptors via the vagi; (2) afferent somatic nerves, particularly from the respiratory muscles and chest wall, but also from other skeletal muscles and joints; (3) chemoreceptors in the brain, aortic and carotid bodies, and elsewhere in the circulation; (4) higher (cortical) centers; and perhaps (5) afferent fibers in the phrenic nerves. In general, despite the interindividual variations described above, there is a reasonable correlation between the severity of dyspnea and the magnitude of disturbances of pulmonary or cardiac function that are responsible.

The mechanisms responsible for dyspnea may vary in different conditions (Table 32-1).

DIFFERENTIAL DIAGNOSIS   Obstructive Disease of Airways (See also Chaps. 252 and 258)   Obstruction to airflow can be present anywhere from the extrathoracic airways out to the small airways in the periphery of the lung. Large extrathoracic airway obstruction can occur acutely, as with aspiration of food or a foreign body or with angioedema of the glottis. Circumstantial evidence or testimony from witnesses should cause the physician to suspect aspiration, and an allergic history together with a few scattered hives should raise the possibility of glottic edema. The acute form of upper airway obstruction is a medical emergency. More chronic forms can occur with tumors or with fibrotic stenosis following tracheostomy or prolonged endotracheal intubation. Whether acute or chronic, the cardinal symptom is dyspnea, and the characteristic signs are stridor and retraction of the supraclavicular fossae with *inspiration*.

Obstruction of intrathoracic airways can occur acutely and intermittently or can be present chronically with worsening during respiratory infections. Acute intermittent obstruction with wheezing is typical of *asthma* (Chap. 252). Chronic cough with expectoration is typical of *chronic bronchitis* (Chap. 258) and *bronchiectasis* (Chap. 256). Most often there is a prolongation of expiration and coarse rhonchi, which are generalized in chronic bronchitis and may be localized in the case of bronchiectasis. Intercurrent infection results in worsening of the cough, increased expectoration of purulent sputum, and more severe dyspnea. During such episodes, the patient may complain of nocturnal paroxysms of dyspnea with wheezing relieved by cough and expectoration of sputum. Despite the fact that severe limitation of expiratory flow and hyperinflation of the lung are characteristic of these diseases, the sensory experience is often that of an inability to take in a sufficiently deep breath rather than difficulty in exhaling.

The patient with predominant *emphysema* is characterized by many years of exertional dyspnea progressing to dyspnea at rest (Chap. 258). Although a parenchymal disease by definition, emphysema is invariably accompanied by obstruction of airways.

Diffuse Parenchymal Lung Diseases (See also Chap. 259)   This category includes a large number of diseases ranging from acute pneumonia to chronic disorders such as sarcoidosis and the various forms of *pneumoconiosis* (Chap. 254). History, physical findings, and radiographic abnormalities often provide clues to the diagnosis. The patients are often tachypneic with arterial P_{CO_2} and P_{O_2} values below normal. Exertion often further reduces the arterial P_{O_2}. Lung volumes are decreased, and the lungs are stiffer, i.e., less compliant than normal.

Pulmonary Vascular Occlusive Diseases (See also Chap. 261) Repeated episodes of dyspnea at rest often occur with recurrent pulmonary emboli. Evidence of a source for emboli, such as phlebitis of a lower extremity or the pelvis, is quite helpful in leading the physician to suspect the diagnosis. Arterial blood gases are most often abnormal, but lung volumes are frequently normal or only minimally abnormal.

Diseases of the Chest Wall or Respiratory Muscles (See also Chap. 263)   The physical examination establishes the presence of a chest wall disease such as severe kyphoscoliosis, pectus excavatum, or ankylosing spondylitis. Although all three of these deformities may be associated with dyspnea, only severe kyphoscoliosis regularly interferes with ventilation sufficiently to produce chronic cor pulmonale and respiratory failure.

Both weakness and paralysis of respiratory muscles can lead to respiratory failure and dyspnea (Chap. 263), but most often the signs and symptoms of the neurologic or muscular disorder are more prominently manifested in other systems.

Heart Disease   In patients with cardiac disease, exertional dyspnea occurs most commonly as a consequence of an elevated pulmonary capillary pressure, which in turn may be due to left ventricular dysfunction (Chaps. 232 and 233), reduced left ventricular compliance, and mitral stenosis. The elevation of hydrostatic pressure in the pulmonary vascular bed tends to upset the Starling equilibrium (see "Pulmonary Edema," below) with resulting transudation of liquid into the interstitial space, reducing the compliance of the lungs and stimulating J (juxtacapillary) receptors in the alveolar interstitial space. When it is prolonged, pulmonary venous hypertension results in thickening of the walls of small pulmonary vessels and an increase in perivascular cells and fibrous tissue, causing a further reduction in compliance. The competition for space among vessels, airways, and increased liquid within the interstitial space compromises the lumina of small airways, increasing the airways' resistance. Diminution in compliance and an increase in the airways' resistance increase the work of breathing. In advanced congestive heart failure, usually involving elevation of both pulmonary and systemic venous pressures, hydrothorax may develop, interfering further with pulmonary function and intensifying dyspnea.

Orthopnea, i.e., dyspnea in the recumbent position, and *paroxysmal nocturnal dyspnea*, i.e., attacks of shortness of breath that usually occur at night and awaken the patient from sleep, are characteristic of more advanced forms of heart failure associated with elevations of pulmonary venous and capillary pressures and are discussed in Chap. 233. Orthopnea is the result of the alteration of gravitational forces when the recumbent position is assumed, which elevates pulmonary venous and capillary pressures. These, in turn, increase the pulmonary closing volume (Chap. 250) and reduce the vital capacity.

Paroxysmal (nocturnal) dyspnea   Also known as *cardiac asthma*, this condition is characterized by attacks of severe shortness of breath that generally occur at night and usually awaken the patient from sleep. The attack is precipitated by stimuli that aggravate the previously existing pulmonary congestion; frequently, the total blood volume is augmented at night because of the reabsorption of edema from dependent portions of the body during recumbency. A sleeping patient can tolerate relatively severe pulmonary engorgement and may awaken only when actual pulmonary edema and bronchospasm have developed, with the feeling of suffocation and with wheezing respirations. Two other forms of nocturnal dyspnea must be distinguished from that due to heart failure. Chronic bronchitis is characterized by mucus hypersecretion and, after a few hours sleep, secretions can accumulate and produce dyspnea and wheezing, both of which are relieved by cough and expectoration of sputum. Asthma patients have circadian variations in their degree of airway obstruction. The obstruction becomes most severe between 1 A.M. and 2 A.M. and can be sufficiently severe that the patient awakens with a sense of suffocation, extreme

Table 32-1

Possible Mechanisms of Dyspnea in Selected Conditions

Condition	Mechanism
Asthma	Increased sense of effort
	Stimulation of irritant receptors in airways
Neuromuscular disease	Increased sense of effort
COPD	Increased sense of effort
	Hypoxia
	Hypercapnia
	Dynamic airway compression
Mechanical ventilation	Afferent mismatch
	Factors associated with the underlying condition
Pulmonary embolism	Stimulation of pressure receptors in pulmonary vasculature or right atrium (?)

NOTE: COPD, chronic obstructive pulmonary disease.

SOURCE: From Manning and Schwartzstein, with permission.

dyspnea, and wheezing. Although there is a prominent inflammatory component to nocturnal asthma, inhaled bronchodilators usually improve symptoms quickly.

Cheyne-Stokes respiration → *See Chap. 233.*

Diagnosis The diagnosis of cardiac dyspnea depends on the recognition of heart disease on the basis of the clinical examination supplemented by noninvasive testing. There may be a history of antecedent myocardial infarction, third and fourth heart sounds may be audible, and/or there may be evidence of left ventricular enlargement, jugular neck vein distention, and/or peripheral edema. Often there are radiographic signs of heart failure, with evidence of interstitial edema, pulmonary vascular redistribution, and accumulation of liquid in the septal planes and pleural cavity. Transthoracic echocardiography is particularly useful in establishing the diagnosis of structural heart disease, which can be responsible for dyspnea. Specifically, left atrial and/or left ventricular dilatation, left ventricular hypertrophy, a reduced left ventricular ejection fraction, and disorders of left ventricular wall motion may be clues to the presence of a cardiac etiology of otherwise unexplained dyspnea.

Differentiation between Cardiac and Pulmonary Dyspnea In most patients with dyspnea there is obvious clinical evidence of disease of the heart and/or lungs. Like patients with cardiac dyspnea, patients with chronic obstructive lung disease also may waken at night with dyspnea, but, as pointed out above, this is usually associated with sputum production; the dyspnea is relieved after these patients rid themselves of secretions. The difficulty in the distinction between cardiac and pulmonary dyspnea may be compounded by the coexistence of diseases involving both organ systems.

In patients in whom the etiology of dyspnea is not clear, it is desirable to carry out pulmonary function testing, for these tests may be helpful in determining whether dyspnea is produced by heart disease, lung disease, abnormalities of the chest wall, or anxiety (Chap. 250). In addition to the usual means of assessing patients for heart disease, determination of the ejection fraction at rest and during exercise by echocardiography or radionuclide ventriculography is helpful in the differential diagnosis of dyspnea. The left ventricular ejection fraction is depressed in left ventricular failure, while the right ventricular ejection fraction may be low at rest or may decline during exercise in patients with severe lung disease. Both left and right ventricular ejection fractions are normal at rest and during exercise in dyspnea due to anxiety or malingering. Careful observation during the performance of an exercise treadmill test will often help in the identification of the patient who is malingering or whose dyspnea is secondary to anxiety. Under these circumstances, the patient usually complains of severe shortness of breath but appears to be breathing either effortlessly or totally irregularly.

Anxiety Neurosis Dyspnea experienced by a patient with an anxiety neurosis is difficult to evaluate. The signs and symptoms of acute and chronic hyperventilation do not serve to distinguish between anxiety neurosis and other processes, such as recurrent pulmonary emboli. Another potentially confusing situation is seen when chest pain and electrocardiographic changes accompany the hyperventilation syndrome. When present and attributable to this condition, often referred to as *neurocirculatory asthenia* (Chap. 13), the chest pain is often sharp, fleeting, and in various loci, and the electrocardiographic changes are most often seen during repolarization. Frequent sighing respirations and an irregular breathing pattern point to a psychogenic origin of the dyspnea.

PULMONARY EDEMA See Table 32-2

CARDIOGENIC PULMONARY EDEMA (See Table 32-2, IA) An increase in pulmonary venous pressure, which results initially in engorgement of the pulmonary vasculature, is common in most instances of dyspnea in association with congestive heart failure. The lungs become less compliant, the resistance of small airways increases, and there is an increase in lymphatic flow that apparently serves to maintain a constant pulmonary extravascular liquid volume. Mild

tachypnea is present. If it is sufficient both in magnitude and duration, the increase in intravascular pressure results in a net gain of liquid in the extravascular space, i.e., *interstitial* edema develops. At this point symptoms worsen, tachypnea increases, gas exchange deteriorates further, and radiographic changes, such as Kerley B lines and loss of distinct vascular margins, are seen. At this stage, the capillary endothelial intercellular junctions have widened and allow passage of macromolecules into the interstices.

Further elevations in intravascular pressure result in disruption of the tight junctions between alveolar lining cells, and alveolar edema ensues with outpouring of liquid that contains both red blood cells and macromolecules. At this point *alveolar* edema is present. With yet more severe disruption of the alveolar-capillary membrane, edematous liquid floods the alveoli and airways. At this point, full-blown clinical pulmonary edema with bilateral wet rales and rhonchi occurs, and the chest radiograph may show diffuse haziness of the lung fields with greater density in the more proximal hilar regions. Typically, the patient is anxious and perspires freely, and the sputum is frothy and blood-tinged. Gas exchange is more severely compromised with worsening hypoxia. Without effective treatment (Chap. 233), progressive acidemia, hypercapnia, and respiratory arrest ensue.

Table 32-2

Classification of Pulmonary Edema Based on Initiating Mechanism

I. Imbalance of Starling forces
   A. Increased pulmonary capillary pressure
      1. Increased pulmonary venous pressure without left ventricular failure (e.g., mitral stenosis)
      2. Increased pulmonary venous pressure secondary to left ventricular failure
      3. Increased pulmonary capillary pressure secondary to increased pulmonary arterial pressure (so-called overperfusion pulmonary edema)
   B. Decreased plasma oncotic pressure
      1. Hypoalbuminemia
   C. Increased negativity of interstitial pressure
      1. Rapid removal of pneumothorax with large applied negative pressures (unilateral)
      2. Large negative pleural pressures due to acute airway obstruction alone with increased end-expiratory volumes (asthma)
II. Altered alveolar-capillary membrane permeability (acute respiratory distress syndrome)
   A. Infectious pneumonia—bacterial, viral, parasitic
   B. Inhaled toxins (e.g., phosgene, ozone, chlorine, Teflon fumes, nitrogen dioxide, smoke)
   C. Circulating foreign substances (e.g., snake venom, bacterial endotoxins)
   D. Aspiration of acidic gastric contents
   E. Acute radiation pneumonitis
   F. Endogenous vasoactive substances (e.g., histamine, kinins)
   G. Disseminated intravascular coagulation
   H. Immunologic—hypersensitivity pneumonitis, drugs (nitrofurantoin), leukoagglutinins
   I. Shock lung in association with nonthoracic trauma
   J. Acute hemorrhagic pancreatitis
III. Lymphatic insufficiency
   A. After lung transplant
   B. Lymphangitic carcinomatosis
   C. Fibrosing lymphangitis (e.g., silicosis)
IV. Unknown or incompletely understood
   A. High-altitude pulmonary edema
   B. Neurogenic pulmonary edema
   C. Narcotic overdose
   D. Pulmonary embolism
   E. Eclampsia
   F. After cardioversion
   G. After anesthesia
   H. After cardiopulmonary bypass

SOURCE: From Braunwald et al., with permission.

The earlier sequence of liquid accumulation described above follows the Starling law of capillary–interstitial liquid exchange:

$$\text{Liquid accumulation} = K[(P_c - P_{IF}) - \sigma(\pi_{pl} - \pi_{IF})] - Q_{lymph}$$

where K = hydraulic conductance (directly proportional to membrane surface area and inversely proportional to membrane thickness)

P_c = mean intracapillary pressure
π_{IF} = oncotic pressure of interstitial liquid
σ = reflection coefficient of macromolecules
P_{IF} = mean interstitial liquid pressure
π_{pl} = oncotic pressure of the plasma
Q_{lymph} = lymphatic flow

The pressures tending to move liquid out of the vessel are P_c and π_{IF}, which are normally more than offset by pressures tending to move liquid back into the vasculature, i.e., the algebraic sum of P_{IF} and π_{pl}. Implicit in the preceding equation is that lymphatic flow can increase in the case of imbalance of forces and result in no net accumulation of interstitial liquid. Further elevations in P_c not only increase the outward movement of liquid in each capillary region but also recruit more of the capillary bed, which increases K. These two effects lead to liquid filtration that exceeds clearance capability by the lymphatics, and liquid accumulates in the loose interstitial spaces of the lung. Even greater increases in P_c open first the loose endothelial intercellular junctions and later the tight alveolar intercellular junctions with an increase in permeability to macromolecules. This secondary disruption of both the function and structure of the alveolar-capillary membrane leads to alveolar flooding.

NONCARDIOGENIC PULMONARY EDEMA (See Table 32-2, IB, IC, II, III, and IV)   Several clinical conditions are associated with pulmonary edema based on an imbalance of Starling forces other than through primary elevations of pulmonary capillary pressure. Although diminished plasma oncotic pressure in hypoalbuminemic states (e.g., severe liver disease, nephrotic syndrome, protein-losing enteropathy) might be expected to lead to pulmonary edema, the balance of forces normally so strongly favors resorption that even in these conditions some elevation of capillary pressure is usually necessary before interstitial edema develops. Increased negativity of interstitial pressure has been implicated in the genesis of unilateral pulmonary edema following rapid evacuation of a large pneumothorax. In this situation, the findings may be apparent only by radiography, but occasionally the patient experiences dyspnea with physical findings localized to the edematous lung. It has been proposed that large negative intrapleural pressures during acute severe asthma may be associated with the development of interstitial edema. Lymphatic blockade secondary to fibrotic and inflammatory diseases or lymphangitic carcinomatosis may lead to interstitial edema. In such instances, both clinical and radiographic manifestations are dominated by the underlying disease process.

Other conditions characterized by increases in the interstitial liquid content of the lungs appear to be associated primarily with disruption of the alveolar-capillary membranes. Any number of spontaneously occurring or environmental toxic insults, including diffuse pulmonary infections, aspiration, and shock (particularly due to sepsis and hemorrhagic pancreatitis and following cardiopulmonary bypass), are associated with diffuse pulmonary edema that clearly does not have a hemodynamic origin. → *These conditions, which may lead to the acute respiratory distress syndrome, are discussed in Chap. 265.*

Other Forms of Pulmonary Edema   There are three forms of pulmonary edema that have not been clearly related to increased permeability, inadequate lymphatic flow, or an imbalance of Starling forces; hence their precise mechanism remains unexplained. *Narcotic overdose* is a well-recognized antecedent to pulmonary edema. Although illicit use of parenteral heroin is the most frequent cause, parenteral and oral overdoses of legitimate preparations of morphine, methadone,

and dextropropoxyphene also have been associated with pulmonary edema. The earlier idea that injected impurities lead to the disorder is untenable. Available evidence suggests that there are alterations in the permeability of alveolar and capillary membranes rather than an elevation of pulmonary capillary pressure.

Exposure to high altitude in association with severe physical exertion is a well-recognized setting for pulmonary edema in unacclimatized yet otherwise healthy persons. Recent data show that acclimatized high-altitude natives also develop this syndrome upon return to high altitude after a relatively brief sojourn at low altitudes. The syndrome is far more common in persons under the age of 25 years. The mechanism for high-altitude pulmonary edema remains obscure, and studies have been conflicting, some suggesting pulmonary venous constriction and others indicating pulmonary arteriolar constriction as the prime mechanisms. A role for hypoxia at high altitude is suggested by the fact that patients respond to the administration of oxygen and/or return to lower altitudes. Hypoxia per se does not alter permeability of the alveolar-capillary membrane. Hence increased cardiac output and pulmonary arterial pressures with exercise combined with hypoxic pulmonary arteriolar constriction, which is more prominent in young persons, may combine to make this an example of prearteriolar, high-pressure pulmonary edema.

Neurogenic pulmonary edema has been described in patients with central nervous system disorders and without apparent preexisting left ventricular dysfunction. Although most experimental equivalents have implicated sympathetic nervous system activity, the mechanism whereby sympathetic efferent activity leads to pulmonary edema is a matter of speculation. It is known that a massive adrenergic nervous discharge leads to peripheral vasoconstriction with elevation of blood pressure and shifts of blood to the central circulation. In addition, it is probable that a reduction in left ventricular compliance also occurs, and both factors serve to increase left atrial pressures sufficiently to induce pulmonary edema on a hemodynamic basis. Some experimental evidence suggests that stimulation of adrenergic receptors increases capillary permeability directly, but this effect is relatively minor as compared with the imbalance of Starling forces.

TREATMENT OF PULMONARY EDEMA   → *See Chap. 233.*

BIBLIOGRAPHY

BRAUNWALD E et al: Clinical aspects of heart failure; High-output heart failure; Pulmonary edema, in *Heart Disease*, 5th ed, E Braunwald (ed). Philadelphia, Saunders, 1997, p 445
COLICE GL: Detecting the presence and cause of pulmonary edema. Postgrad Med 93:161, 169, 1993
ELLIOTT MW et al: The language of breathlessness: Use of verbal descriptors by patients with cardiopulmonary diseases. Am Rev Respir Dis 144:826, 1991
GILLESPIE DJ, STAATS BA: Unexplained dyspnea. Mayo Clin Proc 69:657, 1994
GROPPER MA et al: Acute cardiogenic pulmonary edema. Clin Chest Med 15:501, 1994
KILLIAN KJ, JONES NL: Mechanisms of exertional dyspnea. Clin Chest Med 15:247, 1994
MANNING HL, SCHWARTZSTEIN RM: Pathophysiology of dyspnea. N Engl J Med 333:1547, 1995

33   *Steven E. Weinberger, Eugene Braunwald*

COUGH AND HEMOPTYSIS

COUGH

Cough is an explosive expiration that provides a protective mechanism for clearing the tracheobronchial tree of secretions and foreign material. However, when excessive or bothersome, it is also one of the most common symptoms for which medical attention is sought. Reasons for the latter include discomfort from the cough itself, interference with normal lifestyle, and concern for the cause of the cough, especially fear of cancer or AIDS.

MECHANISM Coughing may be initiated either voluntarily or reflexively. As a defensive reflex it has both afferent and efferent pathways. The *afferent limb* includes receptors within the sensory distribution of the trigeminal, glossopharyngeal, superior laryngeal, and vagus nerves. The *efferent limb* includes the recurrent laryngeal nerve and the spinal nerves. The *sequence* of a cough starts with a deep inspiration and is followed by glottic closure, relaxation of the diaphragm, and muscle contraction against a closed glottis. The resulting markedly positive intrathoracic pressure causes narrowing of the trachea. Once the glottis opens, the large pressure differential between the airways and the atmosphere coupled with tracheal narrowing produces rapid flow rates through the trachea. The shearing forces that develop aid in the elimination of mucus and foreign materials.

ETIOLOGY As a protective mechanism against foreign or noxious material, cough can be initiated by a variety of airway irritants, which enter the tracheobronchial tree by inhalation (smoke, dust, fumes) or by aspiration (upper airway secretions, gastric contents, foreign bodies). When cough is due to irritation by upper airway secretions (as with postnasal drip) or gastric contents (as with gastroesophageal reflux), the initiating factor may go unrecognized and the cough can be persistent. Additionally, prolonged exposure to such irritants may initiate airway inflammation, which can itself trigger cough and sensitize the airway to other irritants.

Any disorder resulting in inflammation, constriction, infiltration, or compression of airways can be associated with cough. Inflammation commonly results from airway infections, ranging from viral or bacterial bronchitis to bronchiectasis. In viral bronchitis, airway inflammation sometimes persists long after resolution of the typical acute symptoms, thereby producing a prolonged cough, lasting for weeks. Pertussis infection is also a possible cause of persistent cough in adults; however, diagnosis is generally made on clinical grounds (see Chap. 154), and confirmation requires serologic testing for antibodies using an assay which is not readily available. Asthma, which is associated with airway inflammation as well as potentially reversible bronchoconstriction, is a common cause of cough. Although the clinical setting commonly suggests when a cough is secondary to asthma, some patients present with cough in the absence of wheezing or dyspnea, thus making the diagnosis more subtle ("cough variant asthma"). A neoplasm infiltrating the airway wall, such as bronchogenic carcinoma or a carcinoid tumor, is commonly associated with cough. Airway infiltration with granulomas may also trigger a cough, as seen with endobronchial sarcoidosis or tuberculosis. Compression of airways results from extrinsic masses, including lymph nodes, mediastinal tumors, and aortic aneurysms.

Examples of parenchymal lung disease potentially producing cough include interstitial lung disease, pneumonia, and lung abscess. Congestive heart failure may be associated with cough, probably as a consequence of interstitial as well as peribronchial edema. A nonproductive cough complicates the use of angiotensin-converting enzyme (ACE) inhibitors in 5 to 20 percent of patients taking these agents. Onset is usually within 1 week of starting the drug but can be delayed up to 6 months. Although the mechanism is not known with certainty, it may relate to accumulation of bradykinin or substance P, both of which are degraded by ACE.

Approach to the Patient

A detailed history frequently provides the most valuable clues for etiology of the cough. Particularly important questions include:

1. Is the cough acute or chronic?
2. At its onset, were there associated symptoms suggestive of a respiratory infection?
3. Is it seasonal or associated with wheezing?
4. Is it associated with symptoms suggestive of postnasal drip (nasal discharge, frequent throat clearing) or gastroesophageal reflux (heartburn or sensation of regurgitation)?
5. Is it associated with fever or sputum? If sputum is present, what is its character?
6. Does the patient have any associated diseases or risk factors for disease (e.g., cigarette smoking, risk factors for infection with human immunodeficiency virus, environmental exposures)?
7. Is the patient taking an ACE inhibitor?

The general *physical examination* may point to a nonpulmonary cause of cough, such as heart failure, primary nonpulmonary neoplasm, or AIDS. Examination of the oropharynx may provide suggestive evidence for postnasal drip, including oropharyngeal mucus or erythema, or a "cobblestone" appearance to the mucosa. Auscultation of the chest may demonstrate inspiratory stridor (indicative of upper airway disease), rhonchi or expiratory wheezing (indicative of lower airway disease), or inspiratory crackles (suggestive of a process involving the pulmonary parenchyma, such as interstitial lung disease, pneumonia, or pulmonary edema).

Chest radiography may be particularly helpful in suggesting or confirming the cause of the cough. Important potential findings include the presence of an intrathoracic mass lesion, a localized pulmonary parenchymal infiltrate, or diffuse interstitial or alveolar disease. An area of honeycombing or cyst formation may suggest bronchiectasis, while symmetric bilateral hilar adenopathy may suggest sarcoidosis.

Pulmonary function testing (see Chap. 250) is useful for assessing the functional abnormalities that accompany certain disorders producing cough. Measurement of forced expiratory flow rates can demonstrate reversible airflow obstruction characteristic of asthma. When asthma is considered but flow rates are normal, bronchoprovocation testing with methacholine or cold-air inhalation can demonstrate hyperreactivity of the airways to a bronchoconstrictive stimulus. Measurement of lung volumes and diffusing capacity is useful primarily for demonstration of a restrictive pattern, often seen with any of the diffuse interstitial lung diseases.

If *sputum* is produced, gross and microscopic examination may provide useful information. Purulent sputum suggests chronic bronchitis, bronchiectasis, pneumonia, or lung abscess. Blood in the sputum may be seen in the same disorders, but its presence also raises the question of an endobronchial tumor. Gram and acid-fast stains and cultures may demonstrate a particular infectious pathogen, while sputum cytology may provide a diagnosis of a pulmonary malignancy.

More specialized studies are helpful in specific circumstances. *Fiberoptic bronchoscopy* is the procedure of choice for visualizing an endobronchial tumor and collecting cytologic and histologic specimens. Inspection of the tracheobronchial mucosa can demonstrate endobronchial granulomas often seen in sarcoidosis, and endobronchial biopsy of such lesions or transbronchial biopsy of the lung interstitium can confirm the diagnosis. Inspection of the airway mucosa by bronchoscopy can also demonstrate the characteristic appearance of endobronchial Kaposi's sarcoma in patients with AIDS. *High-resolution computed tomography* (HRCT) can confirm the presence of interstitial disease and can sometimes suggest a diagnosis based on the pattern of disease. It is the procedure of choice for demonstrating dilated airways and confirming the diagnosis of bronchiectasis.

A diagnostic algorithm for evaluation of chronic cough is presented in Fig. 33-1.

COMPLICATIONS Paroxysms of coughing may precipitate syncope (cough syncope; see Chap. 20), consequent to markedly positive intrathoracic and alveolar pressures, which diminish venous return, producing a decrease in cardiac output. Although cough fractures of the ribs may occur in otherwise normal patients, their occurrence should at least raise the possibility of pathologic fractures, which are seen with multiple myeloma, osteoporosis, and osteolytic metastases.

℞ TREATMENT

Definitive treatment of cough depends on determining the underlying cause and then initiating specific therapy. Elimination of an exogenous inciting agent (cigarette smoke, ACE inhibitors) or an endogenous trigger (postnasal drip, gastroesophageal reflux) is usually effective when such a precipitant can be identified. Other important management considerations are treatment of specific respiratory tract infections, bronchodilators for potentially reversible airflow obstruction, chest physiotherapy to enhance clearance of secretions in patients with bronchiectasis, and treatment of endobronchial tumors or interstitial lung disease when such therapy is available and appropriate.

Symptomatic or nonspecific therapy of cough should be considered when: (1) the cause of the cough is not known or specific treatment is not possible, and (2) the cough performs no useful function or causes marked discomfort. An irritative, nonproductive cough may be suppressed by an antitussive agent, which increases the latency or threshold of the cough center. Such agents include codeine (15 mg qid) or nonnarcotics such as dextromethorphan (15 mg qid). These drugs provide symptomatic relief by interrupting prolonged, self-perpetuating paroxysms. However, a cough productive of significant quantities of sputum should usually not be suppressed, since retention of sputum in the tracheobronchial tree may interfere with the distribution of ventilation, alveolar aeration, and the ability of the lung to resist infection.

Other agents working by a variety of mechanisms have also been used to control cough, but objective information assessing their benefit is meager. The inhaled anticholinergic agent, ipratropium bromide (2 to 4 puffs qid), has been used with the rationale of inhibiting the efferent limb of the cough reflex. Inhaled glucocorticoids (e.g., beclomethasone or triamcinolone, 8 to 16 puffs per day divided over two to four doses) have been used for patients in whom airway inflammation is thought to be playing a role in the cough.

HEMOPTYSIS

Hemoptysis is defined as the expectoration of blood from the respiratory tract, a spectrum that varies from blood streaking of sputum to coughing up massive amounts of blood (i.e., >100 mL/24 h). Massive hemoptysis can represent an acutely life-threatening problem. Large amounts of blood can fill the airways and the alveolar spaces, not only seriously disturbing gas exchange but potentially causing the patient to suffocate. Expectoration of even relatively small amounts of blood is a frightening symptom, and quantitation by the patient may therefore be unreliable. It can be a marker for potentially serious disease, such as bronchogenic carcinoma.

ETIOLOGY Because blood originating from the nasopharynx or the gastrointestinal tract can mimic blood coming from the lower respiratory tract, it is important to determine initially that the blood is not coming from one of these alternative sites. Clues that the blood is originating from the gastrointestinal tract include a dark red appearance and an acidic pH, in contrast to the typical bright red appearance and alkaline pH of true hemoptysis.

The bronchial arteries, which are part of the high-pressure systemic circulation, originate either from the aorta or from intercostal arteries and are the source of bleeding in bronchitis or bronchiectasis or with endobronchial tumors.

An etiologic classification of hemoptysis can be based on the site of origin within the lungs (see Table 33-1). The most common site of bleeding is the airways, i.e., the tracheobronchial tree, which can be affected by inflammation (acute or chronic bronchitis, bronchiectasis) or by neoplasm (bronchogenic carcinoma, endobronchial metastatic carcinoma, or bronchial carcinoid tumor). Blood originating from the pulmonary parenchyma can be either from a localized source, such as an infection (pneumonia, lung abscess, tuberculosis), or from a process diffusely affecting the parenchyma (as with a coagulopathy or with an autoimmune process such as Goodpasture's syndrome). Disorders primarily affecting the pulmonary vasculature include pulmonary embolic disease and those conditions associated with elevated pulmonary venous and capillary pressures, such as mitral stenosis or left ventricular failure.

Although the relative frequency of the different etiologies of hemoptysis varies from series to series, most recent studies indicate

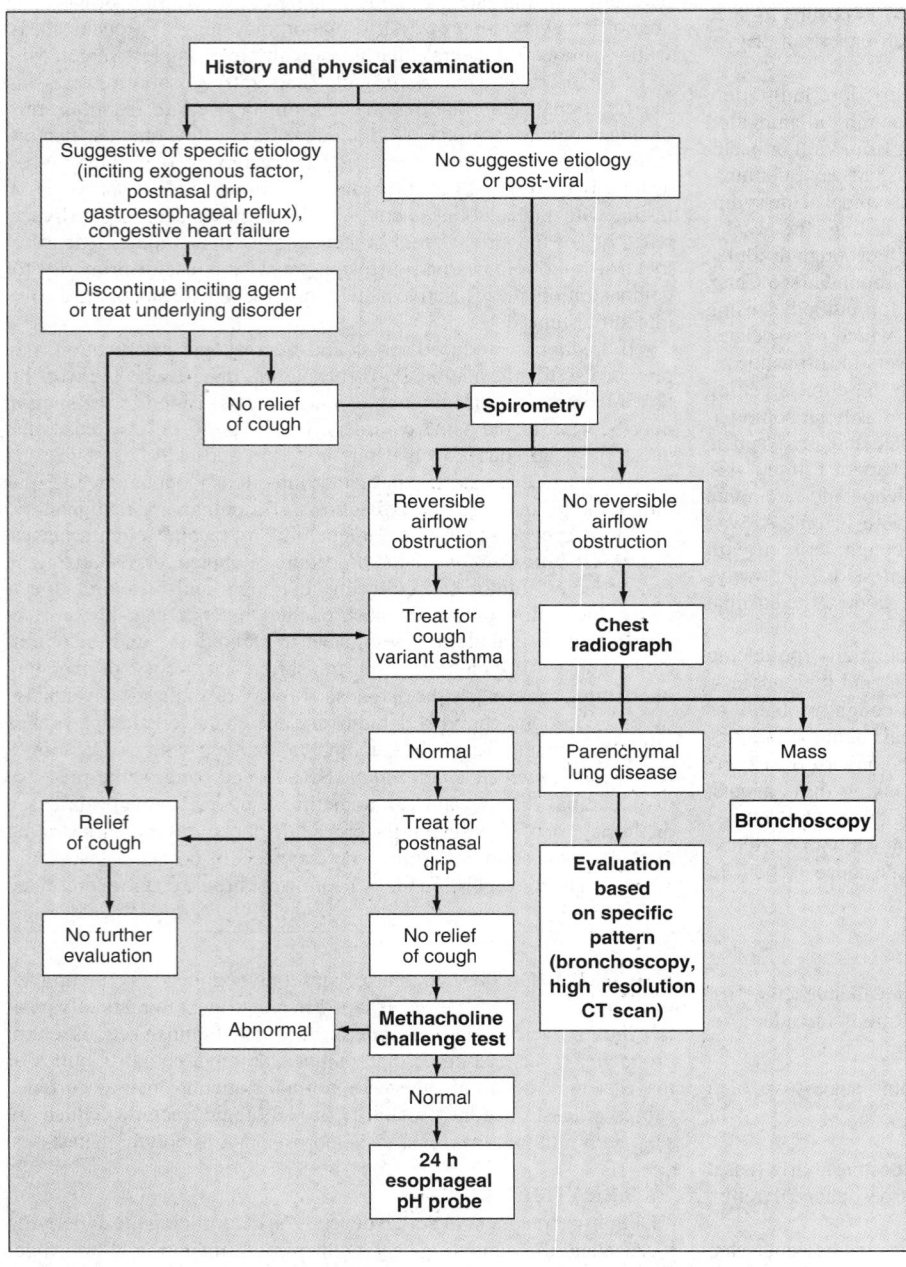

FIGURE 33-1 An algorithm for the evaluation of chronic cough.

that bronchitis and bronchogenic carcinoma are the two most common causes. Despite the lower frequency of tuberculosis and bronchiectasis seen in recent compared to older series, these two disorders still represent the most common causes of massive hemoptysis in several series. Even after extensive evaluation, a sizable proportion of patients (up to 30 percent in some series) have no identifiable etiology for their hemoptysis. These patients are classified as having idiopathic or cryptogenic hemoptysis, and subtle airway or parenchymal disease is presumably responsible for the bleeding.

Approach to the Patient

The history is extremely valuable. Hemoptysis that is described as blood-streaking of mucopurulent or purulent sputum often suggests bronchitis. Chronic production of sputum with a recent change in quantity or appearance favors an acute exacerbation of chronic bronchitis. Fever or chills accompanying blood-streaked purulent sputum suggests pneumonia, whereas a putrid smell to the sputum raises the possibility of lung abscess. When sputum production has been chronic and copious, the diagnosis of bronchiectasis should be considered, although the absence of chronic sputum production does not necessarily exclude a diagnosis of bronchiectasis (so-called dry bronchiectasis). Hemoptysis following the acute onset of pleuritic chest pain and dyspnea is suggestive of pulmonary embolism.

A history of previous or coexisting disorders should be sought, such as renal disease (seen with Goodpasture's syndrome or Wegener's granulomatosis), lupus erythematosus (with associated pulmonary hemorrhage from lupus pneumonitis), or a previous malignancy (either recurrent lung cancer or endobronchial metastasis from a nonpulmonary primary tumor). In a patient with AIDS, endobronchial or pulmonary parenchymal Kaposi's sarcoma should be considered. Risk factors for bronchogenic carcinoma, particularly smoking and asbestos exposure, should be sought. Patients should be questioned about previous bleeding disorders, treatment with anticoagulants, or use of drugs that can be associated with thrombocytopenia.

The *physical examination* may also provide helpful clues to the diagnosis. For example, examination of the lungs may demonstrate a pleural friction rub (pulmonary embolism), localized or diffuse crackles (parenchymal bleeding or an underlying parenchymal process associated with bleeding), evidence of airflow obstruction (chronic bronchitis), or prominent rhonchi, with or without wheezing or crackles (bronchiectasis). Cardiac examination may demonstrate findings of pulmonary arterial hypertension, mitral stenosis, or heart failure. Skin examination may reveal Kaposi's sarcoma, arteriovenous malformations of Osler-Rendu-Weber disease, or lesions suggestive of systemic lupus erythematosus.

Diagnostic evaluation of hemoptysis starts with a chest radiograph to look for a mass lesion, findings suggestive of bronchiectasis (see Chap. 256), or focal or diffuse parenchymal disease (representing either focal or diffuse bleeding or a focal area of pneumonitis). Additional initial screening evaluation often includes a complete blood count, a coagulation profile, and assessment for renal disease with a urinalysis and measurement of blood urea nitrogen and creatinine levels. When sputum is present, examination by Gram and acid-fast stains (along with the corresponding cultures) is indicated.

Fiberoptic bronchoscopy is particularly useful for localizing the site of bleeding and for visualization of endobronchial lesions. When bleeding is massive, rigid bronchoscopy is often preferable to fiberoptic bronchoscopy because of better airway control and greater suction capability. In patients with suspected bronchiectasis, HRCT is now the diagnostic procedure of choice, having replaced bronchography.

A diagnostic algorithm for evaluation of nonmassive hemoptysis is presented in Fig. 33-2.

Table 33-1

Differential Diagnosis of Hemoptysis

Source other than the lower respiratory tract
    Upper airway (nasopharyngeal) bleeding
    Gastrointestinal bleeding

Tracheobronchial source
    Neoplasm (bronchogenic carcinoma, endobronchial metastatic tumor,
      bronchial carcinoid)
    Bronchitis (acute or chronic)
    Bronchiectasis
    Broncholithiasis
    Airway trauma
    Foreign body

Pulmonary parenchymal source
    Lung abscess
    Pneumonia
    Tuberculosis
    Mycetoma ("fungus ball")
    Goodpasture's syndrome
    Idiopathic pulmonary hemosiderosis
    Wegener's granulomatosis
    Lupus pneumonitis
    Lung contusion

Primary vascular disease
    Arteriovenous malformation
    Pulmonary embolism
    Elevated pulmonary venous pressure (esp. mitral stenosis)

Miscellaneous/rare causes
    Pulmonary endometriosis
    Systemic coagulopathy or use of anticoagulants

SOURCE: Adapted from SE Weinberger, Principles of Pulmonary Medicine, 2d ed, Philadelphia, Saunders, 1992

℞ TREATMENT

The rapidity of bleeding and its effect on gas exchange determine the urgency of management. When the bleeding is confined to either blood-streaking of sputum or production of small amounts of pure blood, gas exchange is usually preserved; establishing a diagnosis is the first priority. When hemoptysis is massive, maintaining adequate gas exchange, preventing blood from spilling into unaffected areas of lung, and avoiding asphyxiation are the highest priorities. Keeping the patient at rest and partially suppressing cough may help the bleeding to subside. If the origin of the blood is known and is limited to one lung, the bleeding lung should be placed in the dependent position, so that blood is not aspirated into the unaffected lung.

With massive bleeding, the need to control the airway and maintain adequate gas exchange may necessitate endotracheal intubation and mechanical ventilation. In patients in danger of flooding the lung contralateral to the side of hemorrhage despite proper positioning, isolation of the right and left mainstem bronchi from each other can be achieved with specially designed double-lumen endotracheal tubes. Another option involves inserting a balloon catheter through a bronchoscope by direct visualization and inflating the balloon to occlude the bronchus leading to the bleeding site. This technique not only prevents aspiration of blood into unaffected areas but also may promote tamponade of the bleeding site and cessation of bleeding.

Other available techniques for control of significant bleeding include laser phototherapy, embolotherapy, and surgical resection of the involved area of lung. With bleeding from an endobronchial tumor, the neodymium:yttrium-aluminum-garnet (Nd:YAG) laser can often achieve at least temporary hemostasis by coagulating the bleeding site. Embolotherapy involves an arteriographic procedure in which a vessel proximal to the bleeding site is cannulated, and a material such as Gelfoam is injected to occlude the bleeding vessel. Surgical resection is a therapeutic option either for the emergent therapy of life-threatening hemoptysis that fails to respond to other measures or for the elective but definitive management of localized disease subject to recurrent bleeding.

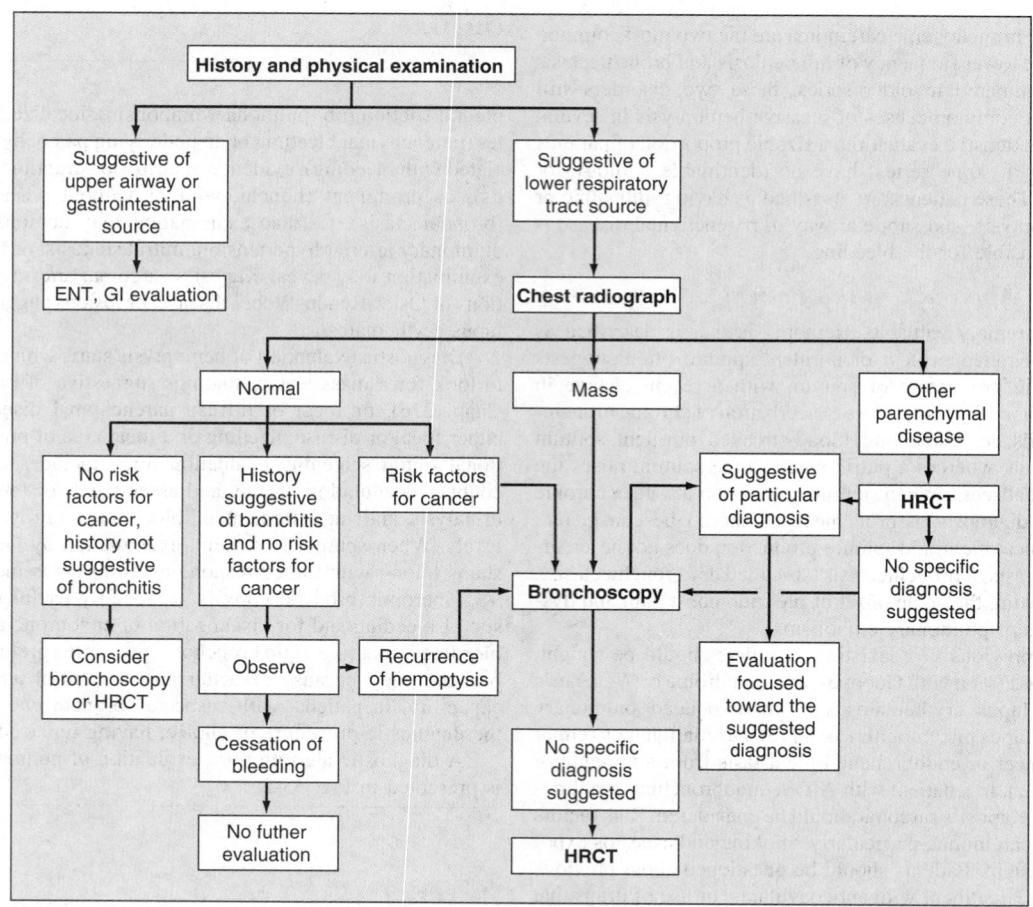

FIGURE 33-2 An algorithm for the evaluation of non-massive hemoptysis. HRCT, High resolution computer tomography.

BIBLIOGRAPHY

COUGH

ING AJ et al: Pathogenesis of chronic persistent cough associated with gastro-esophageal reflux. Am J Respir Crit Care Med 149:160, 1994

IRWIN RS et al: Appropriate use of antitussives and protussives. A practical review. Drugs 46:80, 1993

ISRAILI ZH, HALL WD: Cough and angioneurotic edema associated with angiotensin-converting enzyme inhibitor therapy. Ann Intern Med 117:234, 1992

PATRICK H, PATRICK F: Chronic cough. Med Clin North Am 79:361, 1995

PRATTER MR et al: An algorithmic approach to chronic cough. Ann Intern Med 119:977, 1993

WRIGHT SW et al: Pertussis infection in adults with persistent cough. JAMA 273:1044, 1995

HEMOPTYSIS

CAHILL BC, INGBAR DH: Massive hemoptysis: Assessment and management. Clin Chest Med 15:147, 1994

PRIMACK SL et al: Diffuse pulmonary hemorrhage: Clinical, pathologic, and imaging features. AJR 164:295, 1995

SANTIAGO S et al: A reappraisal of the causes of hemoptysis. Arch Intern Med 151:2449, 1991

THOMPSON AB et al: Pathogenesis evaluation, and therapy for massive hemoptysis. Clin Chest Med 13:69, 1992

| **34** | *Patrick T. O'Gara, Eugene Braunwald* |

APPROACH TO THE PATIENT WITH A HEART MURMUR

Auscultation of the heart constitutes the final step in the cardiovascular examination and for many patients with established or suspected cardiac disease represents the defining moment in the doctor-patient relationship. The examiner must bring to this exercise an integrated approach that incorporates pertinent information simultaneously from several sources. The auscultatory findings must be interpreted in the context of the history and general physical examination and must be consonant with the observations made regarding the venous wave forms and major arterial pulses. In this way, abnormalities of the heart sounds, adventitious sounds, and murmurs can be placed in their proper perspective.

In many patients, a heart murmur is the only or the most conspicuous finding on physical examination. The recognition of a heart murmur commonly leads to additional testing, such as electrocardiography, chest radiography, and echocardiography, and may result in referral to a cardiologist. The differential diagnosis of a heart murmur should more properly begin with an unbiased and systemic evaluation of its major attributes: timing, duration, intensity, quality, frequency, configuration, location, radiation, and response to maneuvers (Table 227-1). Laboratory testing can be pursued thereafter to clarify any remaining ambiguity and to provide additional anatomic and physiologic information that will impact on patient management.

Heart murmurs are defined in terms of their timing within the cardiac cycle. *Systolic murmurs* begin with or after the first heart sound (S_1) and terminate at or before the component (A_2 or P_2) of the second heart sound (S_2) that corresponds to their side of origin (left or right). *Diastolic murmurs* begin with or after the associated component of S_2 and end at or before the subsequent S_1. *Continuous murmurs* are not confined to either phase of the cardiac cycle but rather begin in systole and proceed through S_2 into all or part of diastole.

The appropriate timing of heart murmurs is the first critical step in their identification. The distinction between S_1 and S_2, and, therefore, systole and diastole, is usually a straightforward process but can be difficult in the setting of a tachyarrhythmia, in which case the heart sounds can be distinguished by simultaneous palpation of the carotid arterial pulse. The upstroke should closely follow S_1. The principal causes of heart murmurs are shown in Table 34-1, and the critical importance of the timing of heart murmurs in the differential diagnosis is shown in Fig. 34-1.

SYSTOLIC HEART MURMURS

Systolic heart murmurs derive from the increased turbulence associated with (1) enhanced or accelerated flow across a normal semilunar valve

or into a dilated great vessel, (2) flow across a structurally abnormal semilunar valve or through a narrowed ventricular outflow tract, (3) flow across an incompetent atrioventricular valve, and (4) flow across the interventricular septum. One approach to their differential diagnosis further subdivides these murmurs according to their time of onset and duration within the systolic phase of the cardiac cycle.

EARLY SYSTOLIC MURMURS   Early systolic murmurs begin with S_1 and extend for a variable period of time, ending well before S_2. Their causes are relatively few in number. *Acute severe mitral regurgitation* into a normal-sized, relatively noncompliant left atrium results in an early and attenuated systolic murmur that is decrescendo in configuration and usually best heard at or just medial to the apical impulse (Chap. 237). These characteristics reflect the rapid rise in left atrial pressure caused by the sudden volume load into a nondilated chamber and contrast sharply with the auscultatory features of chronic mitral regurgitation. Clinical settings in which this occurs include: (1) papillary muscle rupture complicating acute myocardial infarction, (2) infective endocarditis, (3) rupture of chordae tendineae, and (4) blunt chest wall trauma.

Table 34-1

Principal Causes of Heart Murmurs

ORGANIC SYSTOLIC MURMURS

Midsystolic (ejection)
  Aortic
    Obstructive
      Supravalvular—supraaortic stenosis, coarctation of the aorta
      Valvular—AS and sclerosis
      Subvalvular—discrete or HOCM
    Increased flow, hyperkinetic states, AR, complete heart block
    Dilatation of ascending aorta, atheroma, aortitis, aneurysm of aorta
  Pulmonary
    Obstructive
      Supravalvular—pulmonary arterial stenosis
      Valvular—pulmonic valve stenosis
      Subvalvular—infundibular stenosis
    Increased flow, hyperkinetic states, left-to-right shunt (e.g., ASD, VSD)
    Dilatation of pulmonary artery
Holosystolic (regurgitant)
  Atrioventricular valve regurgitation (MR, TR)
  Left-to-right shunt at ventricular level

EARLY DIASTOLIC MURMURS

Aortic regurgitation
  Valvular; rheumatic deformity; perforation, postendocarditis, posttraumatic, postvalvulotomy
  Dilatation of valve ring: aorta dissection, annuloectasia, cystic medial necrosis, hypertension
  Widening of commissures: syphilis
  Congenital: bicuspid valve, with VSD
Pulmonic regurgitation
  Valvular: postvalvulotomy, endocarditis, rheumatic fever, carcinoid
  Dilatation of valve ring: pulmonary hypertension; Marfan syndrome
  Congenital: isolated or associated with tetralogy of Fallot, VSD, pulmonic stenosis

MIDDIASTOLIC MURMURS

Mitral stenosis
Carey-Coombs murmur (middiastolic apical murmur in acute rheumatic fever)
Increased flow across nonstenotic mitral valve (e.g., MR, VSD, PDA, high-output states, and complete heart block)
Tricuspid stenosis
Increased flow across nonstenotic tricuspid valve (e.g., TR, ASD, and anomalous pulmonary venous return)
Left and right atrial tumors

CONTINUOUS MURMURS

Patent ductus arteriosus
Coronary AV fistula
Ruptured aneurysm of sinus of Valsalva
Aortic septal defect
Cervical venous hum
Anomalous left coronary artery
Proximal coronary artery stenosis
Mammary souffle
Pulmonary artery branch stenosis
Bronchial collateral circulation
Small (restrictive) ASD with MS
Intercostal AV fistula

NOTE: AR, aortic regurgitation; AS, aortic stenosis; ASD, atrial septal defect; AV, arteriovenous; HOCM, hypertrophic obstructive cardiomyopathy; MR, mitral regurgitation; MS, mitral stenosis; PDA, patent ductus arteriosus; TR, tricuspid regurgitation; VSD, ventricular septal defect.

SOURCE: E Braunwald, in Heart Disease, 4th ed, E. Braunwald (ed), Philadelphia, Saunders, 1992

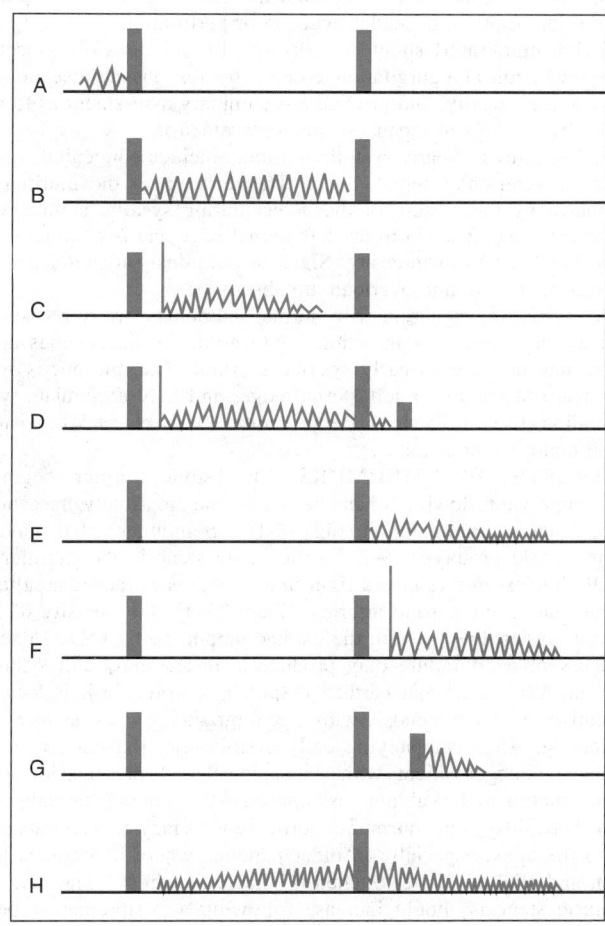

FIGURE 34-1 Diagram depicting principal heart murmurs. *A.* Presystolic murmur of mitral or tricuspid stenosis. *B.* Pansystolic murmur of mitral or tricuspid incompetence or of ventricular septal defect. *C.* Aortic ejection murmur beginning with an ejection click and fading before the second heart sound. *D.* Systolic murmur in pulmonic stenosis spilling through the aortic second sound, pulmonic valve closure being delayed. *E.* Aortic or pulmonary diastolic murmur. *F.* Long diastolic murmur of mitral stenosis following the opening snap. *G.* Short middiastolic inflow murmur following a third heart sound. *H.* Continuous murmur of patent ductus arteriosus. *(Adapted from P Wood, Diseases of the Heart and Circulation, Philadelphia, Lippincott, 1968, with permission.)*

Acute mitral regurgitation from papillary muscle rupture usually accompanies an inferior, posterior, or lateral infarction. The murmur is associated with a precordial thrill in approximately one-half of cases and is to be distinguished from that associated with postinfarction ventricular septal rupture. The latter is more commonly (90 percent) accompanied by a thrill at the left sternal edge, is holosystolic, and complicates anterior infarctions as often as inferior-posterior events. The recognition of either of these mechanical defects mandates aggressive medical stabilization and emergent surgical intervention (Chap. 243).

The other potential causes of acute severe mitral regurgitation may be distinguished on the basis of associated findings. Spontaneous chordal rupture usually occurs on a substrate of myxomatous degeneration, such as that underlying most forms of mitral valve prolapse (Chap. 237). This lesion may be part of a more generalized process, as can occur with the Marfan or Ehlers-Danlos syndromes, or it may be an isolated phenomenon. Infectious endocarditis is associated with fever, peripheral embolic lesions, and positive blood cultures and most commonly occurs on a previously abnormal valvular apparatus (Chap. 126). Trauma is usually self-evident but may be disarmingly trivial (Chap. 241). It can result in papillary muscle contusion and rupture, chordal interruption, or leaflet avulsion or perforation.

Echocardiography should be performed in all cases of suspected acute severe mitral regurgitation to define the responsible mechanism, estimate the severity, and provide a preliminary assessment as to the feasibility of surgical repair (versus replacement).

Other causes of early systolic murmurs include congenital, small muscular ventricular septal defect. The duration of the murmur is attenuated by the closure of the defect during systolic contraction. The murmur is localized to the left sternal edge and is commonly of grade IV/VI or V/VI intensity. Signs of pulmonary hypertension or left ventricular volume overload are absent.

Tricuspid regurgitation with normal pulmonary artery pressures, such as that caused by infectious endocarditis in intravenous drug users, may produce an early systolic murmur. The murmur is soft, best heard at the lower left sternal edge, and may accentuate with inspiration (Carvallo's sign). Regurgitant $c - v$ waves may be visible in the jugular venous pulse.

MIDSYSTOLIC MURMURS Midsystolic murmurs begin at a short interval following S_1, end before S_2, and are usually crescendo-decrescendo in configuration (Fig. 34-1C). Semilunar valve stenosis is the classic prototype. With aortic valve stenosis the murmur is usually loudest in the second right intercostal space (aortic area) and radiates along the carotid arteries (Chap. 237). The intensity of the murmur varies directly with the cardiac output; aortic valve stenosis with severe heart failure may produce a misleadingly soft systolic murmur. With a normal cardiac output, a systolic thrill is usually indicative of severe stenosis with a peak gradient in excess of 50 to 60 mmHg. An accompanying early systolic ejection click may be audible in younger patients with a bicuspid valve; its presence localizes the obstruction to the valvular (as opposed to the sub- or supravalvular) level. The midsystolic murmur of aortic stenosis may be well transmitted to the apex, especially in older patients, where it becomes less harsh and slightly higher pitched (Gallavardin effect). The murmur of aortic stenosis should increase following a postpremature beat, whereas a mitral regurgitant murmur would not be expected to change in intensity.

Sclerosis of the aortic valve produces a murmur of similar location, radiation, and configuration, albeit without the usual signs of hemodynamic significance. The carotid upstroke is well preserved, the murmur peaks in midsystole and is not accompanied by a thrill, and only a modest gradient is estimated by Doppler echocardiography. Noncritical sclerodegenerative thickening of the aortic valve leaflets is perhaps the most common cause of a midsystolic murmur in an older adult. The similar midsystolic murmur of pulmonic valve stenosis, usually introduced by an ejection click, is best appreciated in the second and

third left intercostal spaces (pulmonic area). The murmur lengthens and the intensity of P_2 diminishes with increasing degrees of stenosis. A midsystolic murmur in the aortic position of no functional significance can also be detected in hyperdynamic states (fever, thyrotoxicosis, pregnancy, anemia) and in the presence of isolated aortic regurgitation with the augmented flow into a dilated proximal aorta.

Crescendo-decrescendo midsystolic murmurs of grade II/VI or III/VI intensity heard in the pulmonic area may be innocent (Still's murmur), if unaccompanied by any other signs of cardiac disease in children or young adults, or they may reflect enhanced flow into a normal pulmonary artery in hyperkinetic states or augmented flow into a dilated pulmonary artery. The latter may occur with an atrial septal defect, in which case splitting of S_2 should be abnormal (fixed).

The midsystolic murmur of hypertrophic cardiomyopathy (Chap. 239) is usually loudest between the left sternal edge and apex, of grade II/VI to III/VI intensity, and crescendo-decrescendo in configuration. In contrast to aortic valve stenosis, the murmur does *not* radiate into the neck and the carotid upstrokes are brisk and full and may even be bifid. The intensity of the murmur associated with hypertrophic cardiomyopathy increases following maneuvers that decrease left ventricular volume (strain phase of the Valsalva maneuver, standing, amyl nitrite) or increase myocardial contractility (inotropic therapy). Conversely, the intensity of the systolic murmur decreases with maneuvers that increase ventricular volume (squatting, passive leg raising), impair contractility (beta-adrenoreceptor blockade), or raise preload and systemic afterload (squatting). Among these several maneuvers, auscultation in the standing and squatting positions, if possible, is perhaps the most sensitive technique to elicit a dynamic change in the intensity of the murmur associated with hypertrophic obstructive cardiomyopathy.

LATE SYSTOLIC MURMURS A late systolic murmur begins well after the onset of ejection and is usually best heard at the left ventricular apex or between the apex and the left sternal edge. When introduced by a nonejection click, it is usually indicative of systolic prolapse of the mitral valve leaflet(s) into the left atrium. The click and murmur move closer to S_1 following maneuvers that decrease left ventricular volume (standing, Valsalva) and move oppositely upon increases in volume (leg raising, squatting). The intensity of the murmur augments with increases in systemic afterload (squatting, pressor agents) and decrease with vasodilation (amyl nitrite). Isometric exercise, which also delays the onset of the murmur, accentuates the intensity.

HOLOSYSTOLIC MURMURS These murmurs, also termed *pansystolic murmurs*, begin with S_1 and continue through systole to S_2 (Fig. 34-1C). They are, with rare exception, indicative of atrioventricular valve regurgitation or of a ventricular septal defect; the differential diagnosis is shown in Fig. 34-2. The murmur of mitral regurgitation is loudest at the left ventricular apex. Its radiation reflects the direction of the regurgitant jet. With a flail posterior mitral leaflet due to ruptured chordae tendineae, for example, the jet is directed anterosuperiorly, and the murmur radiates prominently to the base of the heart where it might be confused with aortic valve stenosis unless the carotid upstrokes are carefully examined. Conversely, a flail anterior leaflet is associated with a posteriorly directed jet, which radiates into the axilla and the back. It may even strike the spine and be transmitted to the base of the neck. Severe mitral regurgitation is usually associated with a systolic thrill, a soft S_3, and a short diastolic rumbling murmur best appreciated in the left lateral decubitus position.

The holosystolic murmur of tricuspid regurgitation is generally softer (grades I to III/VI) than that of mitral regurgitation, is loudest at the left lower sternal edge, and increases in intensity upon inspiration. Associated signs include prominent "$c - v$" waves in the jugular venous pulse, systolic hepatic pulsations, and peripheral edema. Among the several causes of tricuspid regurgitation, annular dilatation from right ventricular enlargement in the setting of pulmonary artery hypertension is the most common.

Ventricular septal defect (Chap. 235) also produces a holosystolic murmur, the intensity of which varies inversely with the anatomic size of the defect. It is usually accompanied by a palpable thrill along the mid-left sternal border. The murmur of a ventricular septal defect is louder than that due to tricuspid regurgitation and does not share the latter's inspiratory increase in intensity or associated peripheral signs.

DIASTOLIC HEART MURMURS

Like systolic murmurs, diastolic murmurs also can be subcategorized according to their time of onset.

EARLY DIASTOLIC MURMURS (Fig. 34-1E) Early diastolic murmurs result from semilunar valve incompetence and begin at the valve closure sound (A_2 or P_2), which reflects their side of origin. They are generally high pitched and decrescendo in configuration, especially in states of chronic regurgitation, wherein their duration is a crude index of the severity of the lesion. The murmur of aortic regurgitation is generally, but not always, best heard in the second intercostal space at the left sternal edge. There is a tendency for the murmur associated with primary valvular pathology (e.g., rheumatic deformity, congenital bicuspid valve, endocarditis) to radiate more prominently along the *left* sternal border and to be well transmitted to the apex, while the murmur associated with primary aortic root pathology (e.g., annuloaortic ectasia, aortic dissection) radiates more often along the right sternal edge. It is occasionally necessary to examine the patient sitting forward in full expiration to appreciate the murmur, a maneuver that brings the aortic root closer to the anterior chest wall. Severe aortic regurgitation may be accompanied by a lower-pitched mid- to late-diastolic murmur at the apex (Austin Flint murmur), which is generally thought to reflect turbulence at the mitral inflow area from the mixing of the regurgitant (aortic) and forward (mitral) streams, and should be distinguished from mitral stenosis (see above). In the absence of significant heart failure, chronic severe aortic regurgitation is accompanied by several peripheral signs of significant diastolic runoff, including a wide systemic pulse pressure and water-hammer carotid upstrokes (Corrigan's pulse).

The murmur associated with *acute* aortic regurgitation is notably shorter in duration, lower pitched, and can be difficult to appreciate in the presence of tachycardia. Peripheral signs of significant diastolic runoff may be absent. These attributes reflect the abrupt rise in diastolic pressure within the noncompliant left ventricle, with a correspondingly rapid decline in the aortic diastolic–left ventricular pressure gradient.

The murmur of pulmonic valve regurgitation (Graham Steell murmur) begins with a loud (palpable) pulmonic closure sound (P_2) and is best heard in the pulmonic area with radiation along the left sternal border. Typically, it is high pitched, with a decrescendo quality, and is indicative of significant pulmonary artery hypertension with a diastolic pulmonary artery–right ventricular pressure gradient. Its increase in intensity upon inspiration is one means by which to distinguish it from aortic regurgitation. Signs of right ventricular pressure and volume overload are also usually present. With significant mitral stenosis, an early decrescendo diastolic murmur along the left sternal border is not uncommon and is almost always due to

aortic rather than pulmonic regurgitation, despite the coexistence of pulmonary artery hypertension.

Pulmonic valve regurgitation in the absence of pulmonary artery hypertension can occur on a congenital basis and rarely with infectious endocarditis. In these instances, the early diastolic murmur is softer and lower pitched than the classic Graham Steell murmur. It begins at or even after P_2, which should be easily separable from A_2 and thus produce appreciation of an early diastolic pause.

MIDDIASTOLIC MURMURS Middiastolic murmurs usually result from obstruction and/or augmented flow across the atrioventricular valves. The classic example is that of mitral stenosis due to rheumatic deformity (Fig. 34-1F). In the absence of extensive calcification, the first heart sound (S_1) is loud and the murmur begins after the opening snap; the time interval between S_2 and the opening snap is inversely related to the left atrial–left ventricular pressure gradient. The murmur is low pitched and best heard with the bell of the stethoscope over the apex, particularly in the left lateral decubitus position. While its intensity does not reflect the severity of the obstruction accurately, the duration of the murmur does provide some indication as to the magnitude of the obstruction. A longer murmur denotes persistence of a left atrioventricular pressure gradient over a greater proportion of the diastolic time interval. Presystolic accentuation of the murmur (Fig. 34-1A) is frequently appreciated in the presence of sinus rhythm and reflects a further increase in transmitral flow consequent to mechanical atrial systole.

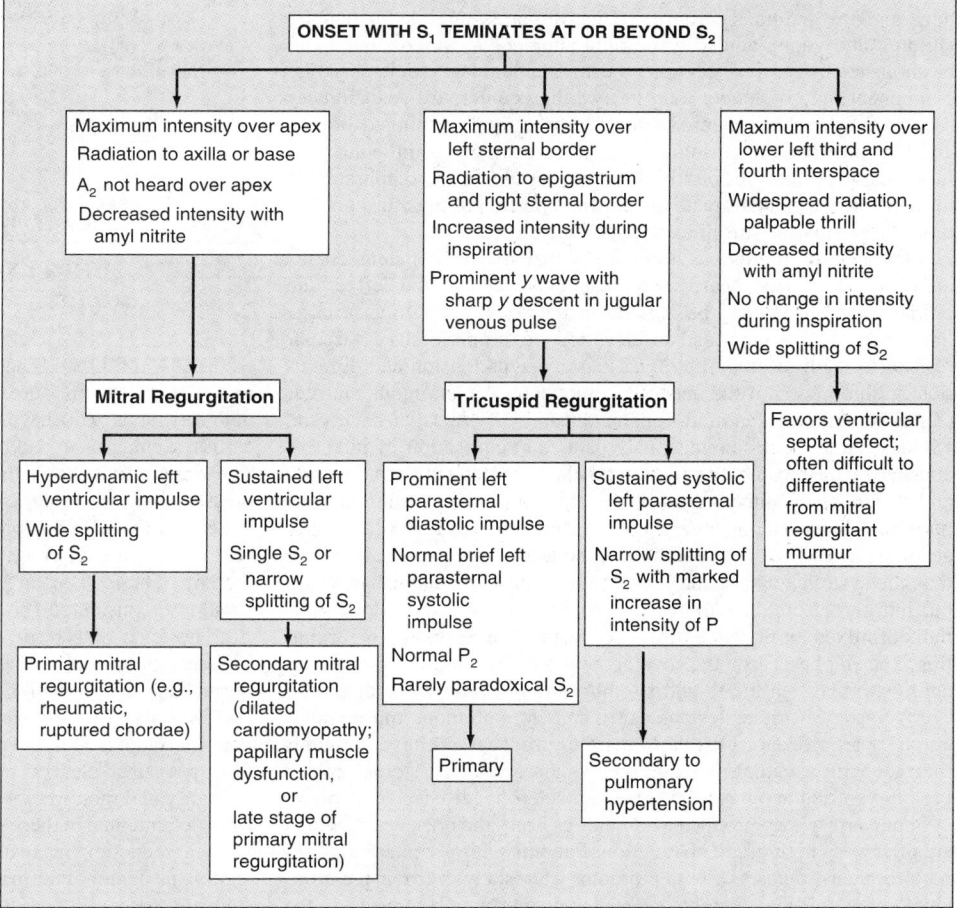

FIGURE 34-2 Differential diagnosis of pansystolic murmur (regurgitant). S_1, first heart sound; S_2, second heart sound; A_2, aortic component of the second heart sound; P_2, pulmonary component of the second heart sound (echo-Doppler evaluation should be considered for differential diagnosis). [*From C Chatterjee, in K Chatterjee et al (eds), Cardiology: An Illustrated Text/Reference, Philadelphia, Lippincott, 1991, with permission.*]

The murmur associated with tricuspid stenosis shares many of these features, but it is best heard at the lower left sternal border and, like most right-sided events, increases in intensity upon inspiration. The observant examiner may discern a prolonged y descent in the jugular venous pulse. Signs of right heart failure may predominate.

There are several other causes of mid-diastolic murmurs that are important to distinguish from mitral stenosis. *Left atrial myxomas* (Chap. 241) may masquerade as mitral stenosis, but the diastolic murmur is not accompanied by an opening snap or pre-systolic accentuation. Augmented flow across the mitral valve in diastole, such as occurs with severe mitral regurgitation or with large left to right intracardiac or great vessel shunts may produce a short, low pitched mid-diastolic apical murmur. The murmur usually follows a soft S_3 that is lower pitched and later in timing than the opening snap (Fig. 34-1*G*). Severe tricuspid regurgitation can also result in enhanced diastolic tricuspid flow and produce a right-sided filling complex similar to that which accompanies severe mitral regurgitation. The Austin Flint murmur of severe aortic regurgitation has been previously described and occurs in the presence of severe aortic regurgitation.

CONTINUOUS MURMURS

Continuous murmurs begin in systole, peak near S_2, and continue into all or part of diastole (Fig. 34-1*H*). Accordingly, they reflect the persistence of flow between two chambers during both phases of the cardiac cycle. The differential diagnosis of continuous murmurs is shown in Table 34-1. Two innocent variants are the cervical venous hum and the mammary souffle. The former is audible in healthy children and young adults in the right supraclavicular fossa and can be abolished by compression over the internal jugular vein. Its diastolic component may be louder than its systolic counterpart. A mammary souffle represents augmented arterial flow through engorged breasts and becomes audible during the late third trimester of pregnancy or in the early postpartum period. Firm pressure with the diaphragm of the stethoscope can eliminate the diastolic portion of the murmur. The murmur dissipates with time after delivery.

The classic continuous murmur is that due to a patent ductus arteriosus. It is best heard at or just above and to the left of the pulmonic area and may be audible in the back. Over time, a large uncorrected shunt may lead to elevation of the pulmonary vascular resistance, with resultant pulmonary artery hypertension and diminution or elimination of the diastolic component. A continuous murmur can also signify a ruptured congenital sinus of Valsalva aneurysm, which occurs either spontaneously or as a complication of infective endocarditis. Here, a high-pressure fistula is created between the aorta and a cardiac chamber, usually the right atrium or ventricle. The murmur is loudest along the right or left sternal border and is frequently accompanied by a thrill. Notably, the diastolic component is louder than the systolic component. It can be difficult to distinguish continuous murmurs from the temporally separate systolic and diastolic murmurs of mixed aortic valve disease or isolated severe aortic regurgitation. The emphasis is on the envelopment of S_2 by continuous murmurs and a gap between the to-and-fro murmurs of aortic valve disease.

A variety of other lesions can result in continuous murmurs. A coronary arteriovenous fistula sometimes produces a faint, continuous murmur with a louder diastolic component at the left sternal border or left ventricular apex. Severe atherosclerotic disease of a major systemic artery may produce a continuous bruit, the presence of which signifies very high grade obstruction. Patients with peripheral pulmonary (branch) stenosis or with pulmonary atresia with extensive bronchial collaterals may also have continuous murmurs best heard in the back or along the lateral thoracic cage. Similar findings are present in patients with severe aortic coarctation, a lesion that should be identifiable on the basis of weak and delayed lower extremity pulses and upper extremity hypertension. The continuous murmurs emanate from the enlarged collateral (intercostal) arteries.

In many patients the cause of a heart murmur can be readily elucidated from careful assessment of the murmur itself, as described in this chapter, when considered in the light of the history, general physical examination, and other features of the cardiac examination, as described in Chap. 227. When the diagnosis is in doubt, or when additional pathoanatomic and physiologic data are necessary in assessing the patient and planning treatment, a transthoracic echocardiogram with Droppler interrogation is of great value in identifying not only the etiology of the murmur but also the severity of the responsible lesion.

The majority of heart murmurs are midsystolic and soft (Grades I to II/VI). When such a murmur occurs in a child or young adult *without* other evidence of heart disease on clinical examination, it is usually benign and echocardiography is not generally required. On the other hand, echocardiographic examination is indicated in patients with loud systolic murmurs ($\geq$III/VI), especially those that are holosystolic, as well as in most patients with diastolic or continuous murmurs.

BIBLIOGRAPHY

GREWE K et al: Differentiation of cardiac murmurs by auscultation. Curr Prob Cardiol 13(10):669, 1988

LEMBO NJ et al: Bedside diagnosis of systolic murmurs. N Engl J Med 318(24):1572, 1988

PERLOFF JK: *The Clinical Recognition of Congenital Heart Disease,* 3d ed. Philadelphia, Saunders, 1987

————, BRAUNWALD E: Physical examination of the heart and circulation, in *Heart Disease,* 5th ed, E Braunwald (ed). Philadelphia, Saunders, 1997, pp 15–52

SAPIRA JD: *The Art and Science of Bedside Diagnosis.* Baltimore, Urban and Schwartzenberg, 1990

WEYMAN AE (ed): *Principles and Practice of Echocardiography,* 2d ed. Philadelphia, Lea & Febiger, 1994

| 35 | *Gordon H. Williams* |

APPROACH TO THE PATIENT WITH HYPERTENSION

DEFINITION Since there is no dividing line between normal and high blood pressure, arbitrary levels have been established to define persons who have an increased risk of developing a morbid cardiovascular event and/or will clearly benefit from medical therapy. These definitions should take into account not only the level of diastolic pressure but also systolic pressure, age, sex, and race. For example, patients with a diastolic pressure greater than 90 mmHg have a significant reduction in morbidity and mortality rate if they receive adequate therapy. These, then, are patients who have hypertension and who should be considered for treatment.

The level of *systolic* pressure is also important in assessing the influence of arterial pressure on cardiovascular morbidity. Males with normal diastolic pressures (<82 mmHg) but elevated systolic pressures (>158 mmHg) have a cardiovascular mortality rate 2.5 times higher than individuals who have similar diastolic pressures but whose systolic pressures clearly are normal (<130 mmHg). A reduction in mortality and morbidity with treatment, specifically in the elderly, has been documented in these patients. This beneficial effect results mainly from a reduction in strokes and occurs in women as well. Other significant factors that modify the influence of blood pressure on the frequency of morbid cardiovascular events are age, race, and sex, with young black males being most adversely affected by hypertension.

When hypertension is suspected, blood pressure should be measured at least twice during two separate examinations after the initial screening. In adults, a *diastolic* pressure below 85 mmHg is considered to be normal; one between 85 and 89 mmHg is high normal; one of

90 to 104 mmHg represents mild hypertension; one of 105 to 114 mmHg represents moderate hypertension; and one of 115 mmHg or greater represents severe hypertension. When the diastolic pressure is below 90 mmHg, a *systolic* pressure below 140 mmHg indicates normal blood pressure; one between 140 and 159 mmHg indicates borderline isolated systolic hypertension; and one of 160 mmHg or higher indicates isolated systolic hypertension. Increasing use of 12- or 24-h blood pressure monitoring may provide additional useful information in patients who are difficult to classify. However, normal values for this procedure and its usefulness in relation to therapeutic outcomes are not currently known. A useful classification of hypertension derived from the Joint Committee on Detection, Evaluation, and Treatment of High Blood Pressure is shown in Table 35-1.

Arterial pressure fluctuates in most persons, whether they are normotensive or hypertensive. Patients who are classified as having *labile hypertension* are those who sometimes, but not always, have arterial pressures in the hypertensive range. These patients are often considered to have borderline hypertension.

Sustained hypertension can become accelerated or enter a malignant phase, although that is unusual in treated patients. Though a patient with *malignant hypertension* often has a blood pressure above 200/140, the condition is defined by the presence of papilledema, usually accompanied by retinal hemorrhages and exudates, rather than by the absolute pressure level. *Accelerated hypertension* is defined as a significant recent increase over previous hypertensive levels associated with evidence of vascular damage on funduscopic examination but without papilledema.

PATIENT EVALUATION   In evaluating patients with hypertension, the initial history, physical examination, and laboratory tests should be directed at (1) uncovering correctable secondary forms of hypertension (see Chap. 246), (2) establishing a pretreatment baseline, (3) assessing factors that may influence the type of therapy or be changed adversely by therapy, (4) determining if target organ damage is present, and (5) determining whether other risk factors for the development of arteriosclerotic cardiovascular disease are present (see Chap. 242). Ideally, this evaluation also would determine the underlying mechanism(s) in essential hypertension, particularly if such information leads to a more specific therapeutic program. Unfortunately, at present this aspect of the evaluation is limited by lack of knowledge of some of the underlying mechanisms, by uncertainty as to the correct treatment for a distinct subset even if the underlying mechanisms are known, or by the prohibitive cost of defining a subset of hypertensive patients even if specific therapy were available. However, with the accumulation of additional information, this sixth component of the evaluation of patients with hypertension may become increasingly important.

Table 35-1

Classification of Blood Pressure for Adults Aged 18 Years and Older

Category	Systolic Pressure, mmHg	Diastolic Pressure, mmHg
Normal*	<130	<85
High normal	130–139	85–89
Hypertension†		
Stage 1 (mild)	140–159	90–99
Stage 2 (moderate)	160–179	100–109
Stage 3 (severe)	180–209	110–119
Stage 4 (very severe)	≥210	≥120

* Optimal blood pressure with respect to cardiovascular risk is <120/80 mmHg. However, unusually low readings should be evaluated for clinical significance.

† Based on the average of ≥2 readings taken at each of two or more visits after an initial screening.

NOTE: Classification of blood pressure for adults aged 18 years and older not taking antihypertensive drugs and not acutely ill. When systolic and diastolic pressures fall into different categories, the higher category should be selected to classify the individual's blood pressure status.

SOURCE: From NK Hollenberg. Summary of the Joint National Committee (JNC)-V and WHO/International Society of Hypertension (ISH) Special Reports, in NK Hollenberg (ed): Hypertension: Mechanisms and therapy, in *Atlas of Heart Diseases*, vol. 1, E Braunwald (series ed). Philadelphia, Current Medicine, 1995, pp 13.1–13.16

Symptoms and Signs   Most patients with hypertension have no specific symptoms referable to their blood pressure elevation and are identified only in the course of a physical examination. When symptoms do bring the patient to the physician, they fall into three categories. They are related to (1) the elevated pressure itself, (2) the hypertensive vascular disease, and (3) the underlying disease, in the case of secondary hypertension. Though popularly considered a symptom of elevated arterial pressure, headache is characteristic only of severe hypertension; most commonly such headaches are localized to the occipital region and are present when the patient awakens in the morning but subside spontaneously after several hours. Other complaints that may be related to elevated blood pressure include dizziness, palpitations, easy fatigability, and impotence. Complaints referable to vascular disease include epistaxis, hematuria, blurring of vision owing to retinal changes, episodes of weakness or dizziness due to transient cerebral ischemia, angina pectoris, and dyspnea due to cardiac failure. Pain due to dissection of the aorta or to a leaking aneurysm is an occasional presenting symptom.

Examples of symptoms related to the underlying disease in secondary hypertension are polyuria, polydipsia, and muscle weakness secondary to hypokalemia in patients with primary aldosteronism or weight gain, and emotional lability in patients with Cushing's syndrome. The patient with a pheochromocytoma may present with episodic headaches, palpitations, diaphoresis, and postural dizziness.

History   A strong family history of hypertension, along with the reported finding of intermittent pressure elevation in the past, favors the diagnosis of essential hypertension. Secondary hypertension often develops before the age of 35 or after 55. A history of use of adrenal steroids or estrogens is of obvious significance. A history of repeated urinary tract infections suggests chronic pyelonephritis, although this condition may occur in the absence of symptoms; nocturia and polydipsia suggest renal or endocrine disease, while trauma to either flank or an episode of acute flank pain may be a clue to the presence of renal injury. A history of weight gain is compatible with Cushing's syndrome, and one of weight loss is compatible with pheochromocytoma. A number of aspects of the history aid in determining whether vascular disease has progressed to a dangerous stage. These include angina pectoris and symptoms of cerebrovascular insufficiency, congestive heart failure, and/or peripheral vascular insufficiency. Other risk factors that should be asked about include cigarette smoking, diabetes mellitus, lipid disorders, and a family history of early deaths due to cardiovascular disease. Finally, aspects of the patient's lifestyle that could contribute to the hypertension or affect its treatment should be assessed, including diet, physical activity, family status, work, and educational level.

Physical Examination   The physical examination starts with the patient's general appearance. For instance, are the round face and truncal obesity of Cushing's syndrome present? Is muscular development in the upper extremities out of proportion to that in the lower extremities, suggesting coarctation of the aorta? The next step is to compare the blood pressures and pulses in the two upper extremities and in the supine and standing positions (for at least 2 min). A rise in diastolic pressure when the patient goes from the supine to the standing position is most compatible with essential hypertension; a fall, in the absence of antihypertensive medications, suggests secondary forms of hypertension. The patient's height and weight should be recorded. Detailed examination of the ocular fundi is mandatory, as funduscopic findings provide one of the best indications of the duration of hypertension and of prognosis. A useful guide is the Keith-Wagener-Barker classification of funduscopic changes (Table 35-2); the specific changes in each fundus should be recorded and a grade assigned. Palpation and auscultation of the carotid arteries for evidence of stenosis or occlusion are important; narrowing of a carotid artery may be a manifestation of hypertensive vascular disease, and it also may be a clue to the presence of a renal arterial lesion, since these two lesions may occur together. In examination of the heart and lungs, evidence of left ventricular hypertrophy and cardiac decompensation should be sought. Is there a left ventricular lift? Are third and fourth heart sounds present? Are there pulmonary rales? A third heart sound and pulmonary rales are unusual in uncomplicated hypertension. Their presence suggests ventricular dysfunction. Chest examination also includes a search for extracardiac murmurs and palpable collateral vessels that may result from coarctation of the aorta.

The most important part of the abdominal examination is auscultation for bruits originating in stenotic renal arteries. Bruits due to renal arterial narrowing nearly always have a diastolic component or may be continuous and are best heard just to the right or left of the midline above the umbilicus or in the flanks; they are present in many patients with renal artery stenosis due to fibrous dysplasia and in 40 to 50 percent of those with functionally significant stenosis due to arteriosclerosis. The abdomen also should be palpated for an abdominal aneurysm and for the enlarged kidneys of polycystic renal disease. The femoral pulses must be carefully felt, and, if they are decreased and/or delayed in comparison with the radial pulse, the blood pressure in the lower extremities must be measured. Even if the femoral pulse is normal to palpation, arterial pressure in the lower extremities should be recorded at least once in patients in whom hypertension is discovered before the age of 30 years. Finally, examination of the extremities for edema and a search for evidence of a previous cerebrovascular accident and/or other intracranial pathology should be performed.

Laboratory Investigation   There is controversy as to what laboratory studies should be performed in patients presenting with hypertension. In general, the disagreement centers on how extensively the patient should be evaluated for secondary forms of hypertension or subsets of essential hypertension. The *basic* laboratory studies that should be performed in all patients with sustained hypertension are described below (Table 35-3). The *secondary studies* that should be added if (1) the initial evaluation indicates a form of secondary hypertension and/or (2) arterial pressure is not controlled after initial therapy as discussed in Chap. 246.

Renal status is evaluated by assessing the presence of protein, blood, and glucose in the urine and measuring serum creatinine and/or blood urea nitrogen. Microscopic examination of the urine is also helpful. The serum potassium level should be measured both as a screen for mineralocorticoid-induced hypertension and to provide a baseline before diuretic therapy is begun.

Other blood chemistry measurements also may be useful, particularly as they often can be ordered as a battery of automated tests at minimal cost to the patient. For example, a blood glucose determination is helpful both because diabetes mellitus may be associated with accelerated arteriosclerosis, renal vascular disease, and diabetic nephropathy in patients with hypertension and because primary aldosteronism, Cushing's syndrome, and pheochromocytoma all may be associated with hyperglycemia. Furthermore, since antihypertensive therapy with diuretics, for example, can raise the blood glucose level, it is important to establish a baseline. The possibility of hypercalcemia also may be investigated. Serum uric acid determination is useful because of the increased incidence of hyperuricemia in patients with renal and essential hypertension and because, as with blood glucose, the level may be raised subsequently by treatment with diuretics. Serum cholesterol, high density lipoprotein cholesterol, and triglycerides may be measured to identify other factors that predispose to the development of arteriosclerosis.

An electrocardiogram should be obtained in all cases to permit assessment of cardiac status, particularly if left ventricular hypertrophy

Table 35-3

Laboratory Tests for Evaluation of Hypertension

BASIC TESTS FOR INITIAL EVALUATION

A. Always included:
1. Urine for protein, blood, and glucose
2. Hematocrit
3. Serum potassium
4. Serum creatinine and/or blood urea nitrogen
5. Electrocardiogram
B. Usually included, depending on cost and other factors:
1. Microscopic urinalysis
2. White blood cell count
3. Plasma/blood glucose, cholesterol, HDL cholesterol, and triglycerides
4. Serum calcium, phosphate, and uric acid
5. Chest x-ray; echocardiogram

SPECIAL STUDIES TO SCREEN FOR SECONDARY HYPERTENSION

A. Renovascular disease: angiotensin converting enzyme inhibitor renogram, renal duplex ultrasound
B. Pheochromocytoma: 24-h urine assay for creatinine, metanephrines, and catecholamines or plasma catecholamines
C. Cushing's syndrome: overnight dexamethasone suppression test or 24-h urine cortisol

Table 35-2

Classification of Hypertensive and Arteriolosclerotic Retinopathy

| | Hypertension | | | | | | Arteriosclerosis | |
| | Arterioles | | | | | | | |
Degree	General Narrowing, AV ratio*	Focal Spasm†	Hemorrhages	Exudates	Papilledema		Arteriolar Light Reflex	AV Crossing Defects‡
Normal	3:4	1:1	0	0	0		Fine yellow line, red blood column	none
Grade I	1:2	1:1	0	0	0		Broadened yellow line, red blood column	Mild depression of vein
Grade II	1:3	2:3	0	0	0		Broad yellow line, "copper wire," blood column not visible	Depression or humping of vein
Grade III	1:4	1:3	+	+	0		Broad white line, "silver wire," blood column not visible	Right-angle deviation, tapering, and disappearance of vein under arteriole; distal dilation of vein
Grade IV	Fine, fibrous cords	Obliteration of distal flow	+	+	+		Fibrous cords, blood column not visible	Same as grade III

* Ratio of arteriolar to venous diameters.
† Ratio of diameters of region of spasm to proximal arteriole.
‡ Arteriolar length and tortuosity increase with severity.

is present, and to provide a baseline. The echocardiogram is more sensitive than either the electrocardiogram or physical examination in determining whether cardiac hypertrophy is present. Thus, in some circumstances, this modality may be a useful addition to the *baseline* evaluation of a hypertensive patient, particularly as left ventricular hypertrophy is an independent cardiovascular risk factor and its presence suggests the need for vigorous antihypertensive therapy. Furthermore, while a substantial increase in arterial pressure usually correlates with the presence of left ventricular hypertrophy, a mild increase may not. Thus, one cannot use the blood pressure as a surrogate marker for the presence or absence of left ventricular hypertrophy. On the other hand, because of the cost of an echocardiogram and the uncertainty as to whether the resultant information would modify therapy, it is unclear that routine *follow-up* echocardiograms during therapy are justified. The chest roentgenogram also may be helpful by providing the opportunity to identify aortic dilation or elongation and the rib notching that occurs in coarctation of the aorta.

Certain clues from the history, physical examination, and basic laboratory studies may suggest an unusual cause for the hypertension and dictate the need for special studies, which are outlined in Chap. 246.

℞ TREATMENT
See Chap. 246.

BIBLIOGRAPHY

GIFFORD RW et al: Office evaluation of hypertension: A statement for health professionals by a writing group of the Council for High Blood Pressure Research, American Heart Association. Circulation 79:721, 1989

GLYNN RJ et al: Evidence for a positive linear relation between blood pressure and mortality in elderly people. Lancet 345:825, 1995

JOINT NATIONAL COMMITTEE ON DETECTION, EVALUATION AND TREATMENT OF HIGH BLOOD PRESSURE: The fifth report. Arch Intern Med 153:154, 1993

KURTZ TW, SPENCE MA: Genetics of essential hypertension. Am J Med 94:77, 1993

LITTENBERG B et al: Screening for hypertension. Ann Intern Med 112:192, 1990

NATIONAL HIGH BLOOD PRESSURE EDUCATION PROGRAM WORKING GROUP: National High Blood Pressure Education Program Working Group report on hypertension in the elderly. Hypertension 23:145, 1994

SAGIE A et al: The natural history of borderline isolated systolic hypertension. N Engl J Med 329:1912, 1993

STAMLER J et al: Blood pressure, systolic and diastolic, and cardiovascular risks. US population data. Arch Intern Med 153:598, 1993

WEBER MA et al: Diagnosis of mild hypertension by ambulatory blood pressure monitoring. Circulation 90:2291, 1994

36 *Eugene Braunwald*

HYPOXIA, POLYCYTHEMIA, AND CYANOSIS

HYPOXIA

The fundamental purpose of the cardiorespiratory system is to deliver oxygen (and substrates) to the cells and to remove carbon dioxide (and other metabolic products) from them. Proper maintenance of this function depends on intact cardiovascular and respiratory systems and a supply of inspired gas containing adequate oxygen. Changes in oxygen and in carbon dioxide tension as well as changes in the intraerythrocytic concentration of certain *organic phosphate compounds*, especially 2,3-bisphosphoglyceric acid (2,3-BPG), cause shifts in the oxygen dissociation curve (see Fig. 107-1). When hypoxia occurs consequent to respiratory failure, Pa_{CO_2} usually rises (Chap. 250), and the oxygen dissociation curve is displaced to the right. Under these conditions or when the concentration of 2,3-BPG rises, the percentage saturation of the hemoglobin in the arterial blood at a given level of alveolar oxygen tension (Pa_{O_2}) declines. Thus arterial hypoxia and cyanosis are likely to be more marked in proportion to the degree of depression of Pa_{O_2} when such depression results from pulmonary disease than when the depression occurs as the result of a decline in the partial pressure of oxygen in the inspired air, in which case Pa_{CO_2} falls secondary to anoxia-induced hyperventilation and the oxygen dissociation curve is displaced to the left, limiting the decline in O_2 saturation of hemoglobin.

DIFFERENTIAL DIAGNOSIS **Anemic Hypoxia** Any decrease in hemoglobin concentration is attended by a corresponding decline in the oxygen-carrying capacity of the blood. The Pa_{O_2} remains normal, but the absolute amount of oxygen transported per unit volume of blood is diminished. As the anemic blood passes through the capillaries and the usual amount of oxygen is removed from it, the P_{O_2} in the venous blood declines to a greater degree than would normally be the case.

Carbon Monoxide Intoxication (Chap. 391) The hemoglobin that is combined with carbon monoxide (carboxyhemoglobin) is unavailable for oxygen transport. In addition, the presence of carboxyhemoglobin shifts the hemoglobin dissociation curve to the left so that the oxygen can be unloaded only at lower tensions. By such formation of carboxyhemoglobin, a given degree of reduction in oxygen-carrying power produces a far greater degree of tissue hypoxia than the equivalent reduction in hemoglobin due to simple anemia.

Respiratory Hypoxia Arterial unsaturation is a common finding in advanced pulmonary disease. The most common cause of respiratory hypoxia is ventilation-perfusion mismatch, which results from perfusion of poorly ventilated alveoli. As discussed in Chap. 250, it may also be caused by hypoventilation, and it is then associated with an elevation of Pa_{CO_2}. These two forms of respiratory hypoxia are usually readily correctable by inspiring 100% O_2. A third cause is shunting of blood from right to left by perfusion of nonventilated portions of the lung, as in pulmonary atelectasis or through vascular abnormalities of the lung with arteriovenous connections. The low Pa_{O_2} in this situation is *not* correctable by inspiring 100% O_2.

Hypoxia Secondary to Right-to-Left Extrapulmonary Shunting From a physiologic viewpoint, this cause of hypoxia resembles intrapulmonary right-to-left shunting but is caused by congenital cardiac malformations such as tetralogy of Fallot, transposition of the great arteries, and Eisenmenger's complex (Chap. 235). As in pulmonary right-to-left shunting, the Pa_{O_2} cannot be brought to normal with inspiration of 100% O_2.

Circulatory Hypoxia As in anemic hypoxia, Pa_{O_2} is normal, but venous and tissue P_{O_2} values are reduced as a consequence of reduced tissue perfusion in the face of normal tissue oxygen consumption. Generalized circulatory hypoxia occurs in heart failure (Chap. 233) and in most forms of shock (Chap. 38).

Specific Organ Hypoxia Decreased circulation to a specific organ resulting in localized circulatory hypoxia may be due to organic arterial obstruction or may occur as a consequence of vasoconstriction (Chap. 248). The latter is seen in the upper extremities in Raynaud's phenomenon. In an attempt to maintain adequate perfusion to more vital organs, reduced circulation may occur in all limbs in patients with heart failure or hypovolemic shock. Ischemic hypoxia with accompanying pallor occurs in organic arterial obliterative disease. Localized hypoxia also may result from venous obstruction and the resultant congestion and reduced arterial inflow. Edema, which increases the distance through which oxygen diffuses before it reaches the cells, also can cause localized hypoxia.

Increased Oxygen Requirements If the oxygen consumption of the tissues is elevated without a corresponding increase in volume flow per unit of time, the P_{O_2} in venous blood (and hence capillary and tissue P_{O_2}) may be reduced. This will occur even if oxygen diffusion into blood perfusing the pulmonary capillary bed is normal and the hemoglobin is qualitatively and quantitatively normal. Such a situation may be encountered when fever or thyrotoxicosis occurs in patients in whom the cardiac output is fixed and cannot rise normally. Under these conditions, the circulation may be considered deficient relative to the metabolic requirements.

Ordinarily, the clinical picture of patients with hypoxia due to an elevated metabolic rate is quite different from that in other types of hypoxia; the skin is warm and flushed, owing to increased cutaneous blood flow which dissipates the excessive heat produced, and cyanosis is usually absent.

Exercise is a classic example of increased tissue oxygen requirements. These increased demands are normally met by several mechanisms operating simultaneously: (1) increasing the cardiac output and ventilation and thus oxygen delivery to the tissues; (2) preferentially directing the blood to the exercising muscles and away from resting muscles, skin, and viscera (by changing vascular resistances in various circulatory beds, directly and/or reflexly); (3) increasing oxygen extraction from the delivered blood and widening the arteriovenous oxygen differences; and (4) reducing the pH of the tissues and capillary blood, thereby unloading more oxygen from hemoglobin. If the capacity of these mechanisms is exceeded, then hypoxia, especially of the exercising muscles, will result.

Improper Oxygen Utilization Cyanide (Chap. 391) and several other similarly acting poisons cause a paradoxic state in which the tissues are unable to utilize oxygen, and as a consequence, the venous blood tends to have a high oxygen tension. This condition has been termed *histotoxic hypoxia*. Cyanide produces cellular hypoxia by paralyzing the electron-transfer function of cytochrome oxidase so that it cannot pass electrons to oxygen, whereas diphtheria toxin is believed to inhibit the synthesis of one of the cytochromes and thus interfere with oxygen consumption and energy production by the cells involved.

EFFECTS OF HYPOXIA Changes in the central nervous system, particularly the higher centers, are especially important. Acute hypoxia produces impaired judgment, motor incoordination, and a clinical picture closely resembling that of acute alcoholism. When hypoxia is long-standing, fatigue, drowsiness, apathy, inattentiveness, delayed reaction time, and reduced work capacity occur. As hypoxia becomes more severe, the centers of the brainstem are affected, and death usually results from respiratory failure. With reduction of Pa_{O_2}, cerebrovascular resistance decreases and cerebral blood flow increases, which tends to reduce the cerebral hypoxia. On the other hand, when the reduction of Pa_{O_2} is accompanied by hyperventilation and diminution of Pa_{CO_2}, cerebrovascular resistance rises, blood flow falls, and hypoxia is enhanced. Compared with the brain, the phylogenetically older spinal cord and peripheral nerves are relatively insensitive to hypoxia. Hypoxia also causes pulmonary arterial constriction, which serves the useful function of shunting blood away from poorly ventilated areas toward better-ventilated portions of the lung. However, it has the disadvantage of causing increased pulmonary vascular resistance and increased right ventricular afterload.

A complex disturbance of cellular functions results from the metabolic effects of severe acute hypoxia. In liver and muscles, the metabolism of the primary foodstuff, carbohydrate, normally proceeds anaerobically (i.e., without oxidation) to the stage of formation of pyruvic acid. The breakdown of pyruvate requires oxygen, and when this is deficient, increasing proportions of pyruvate are reduced to lactic acid, which cannot be broken down further. Hence there is an increase in the blood lactate, with decrease in bicarbonate and a corresponding metabolic acidosis. Under these circumstances, the total energy obtained from foodstuff breakdown is greatly reduced, and the amount of energy available for continuing resynthesis of energy-rich phosphate compounds becomes inadequate, leading to a complex disturbance of cellular function.

Most of the useful respiratory response to hypoxia originates in special chemosensitive cells in the carotid and aortic bodies, although the respiratory center in the brainstem is also stimulated directly by oxygen lack. The resultant increase in ventilation, with loss of carbon dioxide, leads to respiratory alkalosis. On the other hand, the diffusion of additional quantities of lactic acid from the tissues into the blood tends to produce metabolic acidosis. In either case, the total amount

of bicarbonate, and hence the carbon dioxide–combining power, tends to be diminished (Chap. 50).

Diminished oxygen tension in any tissue results in local vasodilatation, and the diffuse vasodilatation that occurs in generalized hypoxia causes an elevation of total cardiac output. In patients with preexisting heart disease, the development of hypoxia and the requirements of the peripheral tissues for an increase of cardiac output may precipitate congestive heart failure. In patients with ischemic heart disease, a reduced Pa_{O_2} may intensify ischemia and further impair left ventricular function. Prolonged or severe hypoxia also may impair hepatic and renal function.

One of the important mechanisms of compensation for prolonged hypoxia is an increase in the hemoglobin concentration. This is due not to direct stimulation of the bone marrow but to the effect of erythropoietin. Assayable levels of erythropoietin are increased by hypoxia, and its production has been found to be regulated by the balance between tissue oxygen supply and demand.

POLYCYTHEMIA (See also Chap. 111)

The term *polycythemia* signifies an increase above normal in the number of red blood cells in the circulating blood. This elevation is usually, although not always, accompanied by a corresponding increase in the quantity of hemoglobin and in the hematocrit. The increase may or may not be associated with an elevation in the total quantity of red blood cells in the body. It is important to distinguish between *absolute* polycythemia (an increase in the total red cell mass) and *relative* (sometimes termed *spurious*), polycythemia, which occurs when, through loss of blood plasma, the *concentration* of the red cells in the circulating blood becomes greater than normal. This may be the consequence of abnormally lowered fluid intake, of the loss of plasma into the interstitial fluid, or of the marked loss of body fluids, such as occurs in persistent vomiting, severe diarrhea, copious sweating, or acidosis.

Because the term *polycythemia* is used loosely to refer to all varieties of increase in the number of red cells, the terms *erythrocytosis* and *erythremia* are preferred in referring to two forms of absolute polycythemia. Erythrocytosis denotes absolute polycythemia that occurs in response to some known stimulus, most commonly hypoxemia (secondary polycythemia); erythremia refers to the disease of unknown etiology—polycythemia vera. In secondary polycythemia, but not in polycythemia vera, the absolute increase in red cell mass is due to an increased production of erythropoietin. Erythrocytosis develops as a consequence of a variety of factors and represents a physiologic response to hypoxia. An approach to the differential diagnosis of erythrocytosis should begin with a consideration of its mechanisms (see Chap. 111).

Stress Erythrocytosis (Gaisböck's Syndrome) These terms have been applied to the polycythemia seen occasionally in active, hard-working, middle-aged white males who are typically hypertensive, overweight, and in a state of anxiety and who appear florid but have none of the other characteristic signs of polycythemia vera, i.e., no splenomegaly or leukocytosis with immature white blood cells. In such persons, the total red blood cell mass is normal, and the plasma volume is below normal. Thus they have a moderately elevated hematocrit, usually 50 to 60 percent, and *relative* polycythemia. *Smokers' polycythemia* is a closely related condition, but the high carboxyhemoglobin concentration may cause a small absolute increase in red cell mass which is often associated with a reduced plasma volume. Smoking should be discontinued.

SECONDARY POLYCYTHEMIA Sojourn at high altitudes leads to defective saturation of arterial blood with oxygen and stimulates the production of more red cells. The oxygen saturation, rather than oxygen tension, appears to be the more important determinant of the erythropoietic response to chronic hypoxia. A condition known as *chronic mountain sickness* or *soroche* (Monge's disease) may set in insidiously after several years of continued residence at high altitude. This condition appears to be caused by the development of alveolar hypoventilation superimposed on a lowered inspired O_2 concentration.

Prominent manifestations are a florid color that turns to cyanosis on mild exertion, impaired mental acuity, fatigue, and headache. Those affected are usually in the fourth to sixth decades. Return to sea level promptly relieves the symptoms. Living at high altitudes also evokes a number of compensatory reactions which act to increase oxygen delivery to the tissues. These include hyperventilation (which reduces the oxygen gradient between inspired and alveolar air), erythrocytosis, an augmentation of pulmonary capillary blood volume, an increase of pulmonary diffusing capacity, and an increase in cardiac output.

Any pulmonary disease that produces chronic hypoxia may lead to erythrocytosis. The increased blood viscosity secondary to the polycythemia elevates pulmonary arterial pressure and, combined with the elevation of pulmonary vascular resistance resulting from hypoxia, further elevates right ventricular pressure, contributing to the development or intensification of cor pulmonale (Chap. 238). The *abnormal ventilatory conditions* present in very obese individuals may cause alveolar hypoventilation and result in arterial unsaturation, erythrocytosis, hypercapnia, and somnolence (the Pickwickian syndrome; Chap. 263). This syndrome is also observed in nonobese persons (sleep-apnea syndrome) in whom decreased sensitivity of the respiratory center to CO_2 may play a role (Chap. 263).

The partial shunting of blood from the pulmonary circuit (right-to-left shunts), such as occurs in *congenital heart disease*, causes the most striking erythrocytosis resulting from abnormalities in the heart or lungs (Chap. 235). Erythrocyte counts as high as $12 \times 10^6/\mu L$, which are possible only when the red corpuscles are smaller than normal, have been observed in such patients, with a hematocrit as high as 86 percent. As the polycythemia develops, there is a progressive elevation of blood viscosity, which rises logarithmically when the volume of packed red blood cells exceeds 55 percent. The most common defects producing such polycythemia in the adult are tetralogy of Fallot and Eisenmenger syndrome. Other congenital cardiac malformations commonly responsible for polycythemia, but occurring more commonly in neonates, include transposition of the great arteries, tricuspid atresia, and persistent truncus arteriosus.

Rarely, patients with hepatic cirrhosis are hypoxemic secondary to intrapulmonary shunts or to right-to-left shunts from the portal to the pulmonary veins. The polycythemia of cyanotic congenital heart disease may lead to spontaneous thrombosis at any site, including the central nervous system.

The increase in hematocrit and the sharp increase in viscosity that occur when patients with congenital heart disease, large right-to-left shunts, and secondary polycythemia become dehydrated are particularly hazardous. Symptoms due to increased blood viscosity include reduced mentation, headache, fatigue, visual disturbance, and dizziness. This condition also may be accompanied by a variety of blood coagulation defects, including reduced fibrinogen and prothrombin concentrations, as well as thrombocytopenia. Reduction in red blood cell volume (phlebotomy with reinfusion of the plasma) is sometimes performed in severely symptomatic patients with extremely high hematocrit levels, usually exceeding 65 percent. It must be carried out slowly, with caution, and with the realization that the polycythemia is, in fact, an important compensatory mechanism. However, reduction of red blood cell volume may result in a reduction of the elevated blood viscosity which improves blood flow.

The excessive use of coal-tar derivatives and other forms of chronic poisoning, by producing abnormal hemoglobin pigments such as *methemoglobin* and *sulfhemoglobin* (Chap. 107), also may cause erythrocytosis. The production of erythropoietin and a secondary erythrocytosis *unassociated* with leukocytosis or thrombocytosis is stimulated in patients with abnormal hemoglobins that displace the oxygen dissociation curve to the left and interfere with oxygen unloading in the tissues (Chap. 107). Reductions in the synthesis of 2,3-bisphosphoglycerate also causes a shift to the left of the oxygen-hemoglobin dissociation curve.

Mild erythrocytosis is sometimes found in *Cushing's syndrome* and can be produced by the administration of large amounts of adrenocortical steroids and androgens. Especially intriguing are the instances of erythrocytosis observed in association with various *tumors* that produce erythropoietin or an erythropoietin-like substance. These include vascular tumors (hemangioblastomas) in the posterior fossa, renal tumors (renal cell carcinoma, adenoma, and sarcoma), uterine myoma, hepatic carcinoma, and pheochromocytoma. Erythrocytosis also occurs occasionally in patients with solitary and polycystic disease of the kidneys, hydronephrosis, and renal artery stenosis. Plasma erythropoietin levels have been found to be elevated in a number of these patients with tumors and indeed all forms of secondary polycythemia. Erythropoietin-like activity has been demonstrated in tumor extracts and in renal cyst fluid, and erythrocytosis has disappeared after the associated tumor was removed.

CLINICAL FEATURES AND DIFFERENTIAL DIAGNOSIS Patients with polycythemia present with (in addition to the symptoms of the underlying condition) a characteristic "ruddy" cyanosis, dizziness, headache, epistaxes, and an increased incidence of thrombotic complications.

The *differential diagnosis* of absolute polycythemia is shown in Fig. 36-1 and is discussed further in Chap. 111. In polycythemia vera, erythropoietin levels are usually absent or below normal; leukocyte alkaline phosphatase, vitamin B_{12} binding capacity, vitamin B_{12} levels, and platelet and total white blood cell counts are usually elevated; and splenomegaly is common. Serum uric acid and lactate dehydrogenase (LDH) levels may be increased. The bone marrow shows hyperplasia of all elements. In secondary polycythemia with hypoxia, erythropoietin levels are elevated, while levels of leukocyte alkaline phosphatase and serum vitamin B_{12} and the platelet, total white blood cell, and differential counts are all normal. The liver and spleen are not enlarged, and the bone marrow shows only erythroid hyperplasia. In the absence of features of either polycythemia vera or polycythemia secondary to hypoxia or to a tumor, a hemoglobin with a high affinity for oxygen should be sought.

Workup of patients with polycythemia should include a chest roentgenogram, electrocardiogram, and arterial oxygen saturation determination to search for disease of the heart and lungs. In addition, imaging of the spleen should be carried out to assess its size and of the kidney to look for an erythropoietin-producing lesion (such as a renal cell carcinoma, hydronephrosis, or cyst). In patients who do not appear to have polycythemia vera or hypoxemia, the oxygen affinity of the patient's hemoglobin, i.e., the P_{O_2} at which 50 percent of the hemoglobin is deoxygenated (P_{50}) should be measured to detect hemoglobins which fail to release oxygen normally.

CYANOSIS

Cyanosis refers to a bluish color of the skin and mucous membranes resulting from an increased amount of reduced hemoglobin, or of hemoglobin derivatives, in the small blood vessels of those areas. It is usually most marked in the lips, nail beds, ears, and malar eminences. The florid skin characteristic of polycythemia vera (Chap. 111) must be distinguished from the true cyanosis discussed here. A cherry-colored flush, rather than cyanosis, is caused by carboxyhemoglobin (Chap. 391). The degree of cyanosis is modified by the quality of cutaneous pigment and the thickness of the skin, as well as by the state of the cutaneous capillaries. The accurate clinical detection of the presence and degree of cyanosis is difficult, as proved by oximetric studies. In some instances, central cyanosis can be detected reliably when the arterial saturation has fallen to 85 percent; in others, particularly in dark-skinned persons, it may not be detected until the saturation has declined to 75 percent.

The increase in the quantity of reduced hemoglobin in the cutaneous vessels that produces cyanosis may be brought about either by an increase in the quantity of venous blood in the skin as the result of dilatation of the venules and venous ends of the capillaries or by a reduction in the oxygen saturation in the capillary blood. In general, cyanosis becomes apparent when the mean capillary concentration of reduced hemoglobin exceeds 50 g/L (5 g/dL). It is the *absolute* rather than the *relative* quantity of reduced hemoglobin that is important in producing cyanosis. Thus, in a patient with severe anemia, the relative amount of reduced hemoglobin in the venous blood may be very large when considered in relation to the total amount of hemoglobin. However, since the concentration of the latter is markedly reduced, the *absolute* quantity of reduced hemoglobin may still be small, and therefore patients with severe anemia and even *marked* arterial desaturation do not display cyanosis. Conversely, the higher the total hemoglobin content, the greater is the tendency toward cyanosis; thus patients with marked polycythemia tend to be cyanotic at higher levels of arterial oxygen saturation than patients with normal hematocrit values. Likewise, local passive congestion, which causes an increase in the total amount of reduced hemoglobin in the vessels in a given area, may cause cyanosis. Cyanosis also is observed when nonfunctional hemoglobin such as methemoglobin or sulfhemoglobin (Chap. 107) is present in blood.

Cyanosis may be subdivided into central and peripheral types. In the *central* type, there is arterial blood unsaturation or an abnormal hemoglobin derivative, and the mucous membranes and skin are both affected. *Peripheral* cyanosis is due to a slowing of blood flow and abnormally great extraction of oxygen from normally saturated arterial blood. It results from vasoconstriction and diminished peripheral blood flow, such as occurs in cold exposure, shock, congestive failure, and peripheral vascular disease. Often in these conditions the mucous membranes of the oral cavity or those beneath the tongue may be spared. Clinical differentiation between central and peripheral cyanosis may not always be simple, and in conditions such as cardiogenic shock with pulmonary edema there may be a mixture of both types.

DIFFERENTIAL DIAGNOSIS **Central Cyanosis** (See Table 36-1) Decreased arterial oxygen saturation results from a marked reduction in the oxygen tension in the arterial blood. This may be brought about by a decline in the tension of oxygen in the inspired air without sufficient compensatory alveolar hyperventilation to maintain alveolar oxygen tension. Cyanosis does not occur to a significant degree in an ascent to an altitude of 2500 m (8000 ft) but is marked in a further ascent to 5000 m (16,000 ft). The reason for this becomes clear on studying the *S* shape of the oxygen dissociation curve (Fig. 107-1). At 2500 m (8000 ft) the tension of oxygen in the inspired air is about 120 mmHg, the alveolar tension is approximately 80 mmHg, and the hemoglobin is nearly completely saturated. However, at 5000 m (16,000 ft) the oxygen tensions in atmospheric air and alveolar air are about 85 and 50 mmHg, respectively, and the oxygen dissociation curve shows that the arterial blood is only about 75 percent saturated. This leaves 25 percent of the hemoglobin in the reduced form, an amount likely to be associated with cyanosis in the absence of anemia. Similarly, a mutant hemoglobin with a low affinity for oxygen (e.g., Hb Kansas) causes lowered arterial oxygen saturation and resultant central cyanosis (Chap. 107).

Seriously *impaired pulmonary function*, through alveolar hypoventilation or perfusion of unventilated or poorly ventilated areas of the lung, is a common cause of central cyanosis (Chap. 250). This may occur acutely, as in extensive pneumonia or pulmonary edema, or with chronic pulmonary diseases (e.g., emphysema). In the last situation polycythemia is generally present, and clubbing of the fingers may occur. However, in many types of chronic pulmonary disease with fibrosis and obliteration of the capillary vascular bed, cyanosis does not occur because there is relatively little perfusion of underventilated areas.

Another cause of decreased arterial oxygen saturation is *shunting of systemic venous blood into the arterial circuit*. Certain forms of congenital heart disease are associated with cyanosis (Chap. 235). Since blood flows from a higher-pressure to a lower-pressure region, in order for a cardiac defect to result in a right-to-left shunt, it must ordinarily be combined with an obstructive lesion distal to the defect or with elevated pulmonary vascular resistance. The most common congenital cardiac lesion associated with cyanosis in the adult is the combination of ventricular septal defect and pulmonary outflow tract obstruction (tetralogy of Fallot). The more severe the obstruction, the greater the degree of right-to-left shunting and resultant cyanosis. The mechanisms for the elevated pulmonary vascular resistance which may produce cyanosis in the presence of intra- and extracardiac communications without pulmonic stenosis (Eisenmenger syndrome) are discussed in Chap. 235. In patients with patent ductus arteriosus, pulmonary hypertension, and right-to-left shunt, *differential cyanosis* results; i.e., cyanosis occurs in the lower but not in the upper extremities.

Pulmonary arteriovenous fistulas may be congenital or acquired, solitary or multiple, microscopic or massive. The degree of cyanosis produced by these fistulas depends on their size and number. They occur with some frequency in hereditary hemorrhagic telangiectasia. Arterial oxygen unsaturation also occurs in some patients with cirrhosis, presum-

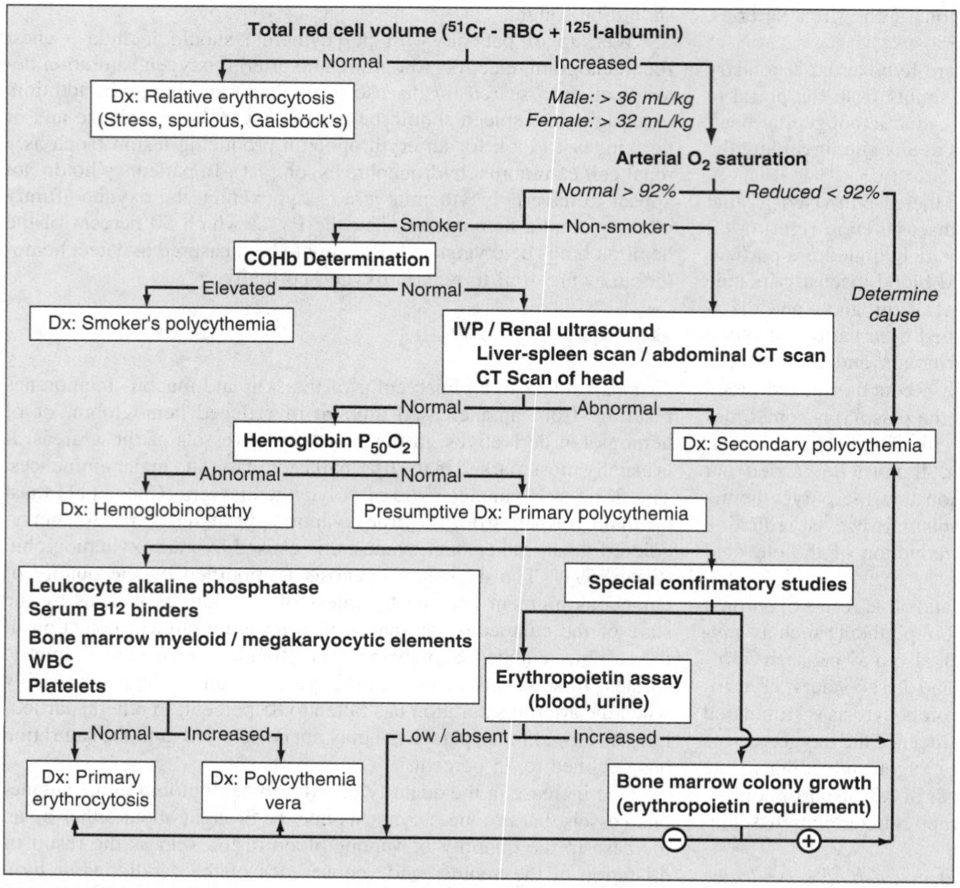

FIGURE 36-1 Algorithm for evaluation of an elevated hematocrit. COHb, carboxyhemoglobin; CT, computed tomography; IVP, intravenous pyelogram; $P_{50}O_2$, the P_{O_2} at which 50% of the hemoglobin is deoxygenated; RBC, red blood cells; WBC, white blood cells. *(From Fruchtman and Berk, with permission.)*

In patients with cardiac or pulmonary right-to-left shunts, the presence and severity of cyanosis depend on the size of the shunt relative to the systemic flow as well as on the oxyhemoglobin saturation of the venous blood. In patients with central cyanosis due to arterial oxygen unsaturation, the severity of cyanosis increases with exercise. With increased extraction of oxygen from the blood by the exercising muscles, the venous blood returning to the right side of the heart is more unsaturated than at rest, and shunting of this blood or its passage through lungs incapable of normal oxygenation intensifies the cyanosis. Also, since the systemic vascular resistance normally decreases with exercise, the right-to-left shunt is augmented by exercise in patients with congenital heart disease and communications between the two sides of the heart. Secondary polycythemia occurs frequently in patients with arterial unsaturation and contributes to the cyanosis.

Cyanosis can be caused by small amounts of circulating methemoglobin and by even smaller amounts of sulfhemoglobin (Chap. 107). Although they are uncommon causes of cyanosis, these abnormal hemoglobin pigments should be sought by spectroscopy when cyanosis is not readily explained by malfunction of the circulatory or respiratory systems. Generally, clubbing does not occur with them. The diagnosis of methemoglobinemia can be suspected, if, on mixing the patient's blood in a test tube and exposing it to air, it remains brown.

Peripheral Cyanosis Probably the most common cause of peripheral cyanosis is generalized vasoconstriction resulting from exposure to cold air or water. This is a normal response. When cardiac output is low, as in severe congestive heart failure or shock, cutaneous vasoconstriction occurs as a compensatory mechanism, so blood is diverted from the skin to more vital areas such as the central nervous system and heart (Chap. 233), and intense cyanosis associated with cool extremities may result. Even though the arterial blood is normally saturated, the reduced volume flow through the skin and the reduced oxygen tension at the venous end of the capillary result in cyanosis.

Arterial obstruction to an extremity, as with an embolus, or arteriolar constriction, as in cold-induced vasospasm (Raynaud's phenomenon; Chap. 248), generally results in pallor and coldness, but there may be associated cyanosis. If there is venous obstruction and the extremity is congested, as with stagnation of blood flow, cyanosis is also present. Venous hypertension, which may be local (as in thrombophlebitis) or generalized (as in tricuspid valve disease or constrictive

Table 36-1

Causes of Cyanosis

CENTRAL CYANOSIS

Decreased arterial oxygen saturation
   Decreased atmospheric pressure—high altitude
   Impaired pulmonary function
      Alveolar hypoventilation
      Uneven relationships between pulmonary ventilation and perfusion
         (perfusion of hypoventilated alveoli)
      Impaired oxygen diffusion
   Anatomic shunts
      Certain types of congenital heart disease
      Pulmonary arteriovenous fistulas
      Multiple small intrapulmonary shunts
   Hemoglobin with low affinity for oxygen
Hemoglobin abnormalities
   Methemoglobinemia—hereditary, acquired
   Sulfhemoglobinema—acquired
   Carboxyhemoglobinemia (not true cyanosis)

PERIPHERAL CYANOSIS

Reduced cardiac output
Cold exposure
Redistribution of blood flow from extremities
Arterial obstruction
Venous obstruction

pericarditis), dilates the subpapillary venous plexuses and thereby intensifies cyanosis.

Approach to the Patient

Certain features are important in arriving at the proper cause of cyanosis:

1. The history, particularly the duration (cyanosis present since birth is usually due to congenital heart disease), and possible exposure to drugs or chemicals that may produce abnormal types of hemoglobin.
2. Clinical differentiation of central as opposed to peripheral cyanosis. Objective evidence by physical or radiographic examination of disorders of the respiratory or cardiovascular systems. Massage or gentle warming of a cyanotic extremity will increase peripheral blood flow and abolish peripheral but not central cyanosis.
3. The presence or absence of clubbing of the fingers (see below). Clubbing without cyanosis is frequent in patients with infective endocarditis and in association with ulcerative colitis; it may occasionally occur in healthy persons, and in some instances it may be occupational, e.g., in jackhammer operators. Slight cyanosis of the lips and cheeks, without clubbing of the fingers, is common in patients with mitral stenosis and is probably due to minimal arterial hypoxia resulting from fibrotic changes in the lungs secondary to long-standing congestion combined with reduction of cardiac output (Chap. 237). The combination of cyanosis and clubbing is frequent in patients with certain types of congenital cardiac disease and is seen occasionally in persons with pulmonary disease such as lung abscess or pulmonary arteriovenous shunts. On the other hand, peripheral cyanosis or acutely developing central cyanosis is not associated with clubbed fingers.
4. Determination of arterial blood oxygen tension or oxygen saturation, spectroscopic and other examinations of the blood for abnormal types of hemoglobin.

CLUBBING

The selective bullous enlargement of the distal segments of the fingers and toes due to proliferation of connective tissue, particularly on the dorsal surface, is termed *clubbing*; an increase occurs in the sponginess of the soft tissue at the base of the nail. Clubbing may be hereditary, idiopathic, or acquired and associated with a variety of disorders, including cyanotic congenital heart disease, infective endocarditis, and a variety of pulmonary conditions (among them primary and metastatic lung cancer, bronchiectasis, lung abscess, cystic fibrosis, and mesothelioma), as well as with some gastrointestinal diseases (including regional enteritis, chronic ulcerative colitis, and hepatic cirrhosis). Clubbing in patients with primary and metastatic lung cancer, mesothelioma, bronchiectasis, and hepatic cirrhosis may be associated with *hypertrophic osteoarthropathy*. In this condition, the subperiosteal formation of new bone in the distal diaphyses of the long bones of the extremities causes pain and symmetric arthritis-like changes in the shoulders, knees, ankles, wrists, and elbows. The diagnosis of hypertrophic osteoarthropathy may be confirmed by bone radiographs and scans. Although the mechanism of clubbing is unclear, it appears to be secondary to a (presumably humoral) substance which causes dilation of the vessels of the fingertip.

BIBLIOGRAPHY

DOLL DC, GREENBERG BR: Cerebral thrombosis in smokers' polycythemia. Ann Intern Med 102:786, 1985
FRUCHTMAN SM, BERK PD: Polycythemia vera and agnogenic myeloid multiplasia, in *Blood: Principles and Practice of Hematology,* RI Handin et al (eds). Philadelphia, Lippincott, 1995, pp 415–438
HANSEN-FLASCHEN J, NORDBERG J: Clubbing and hypertrophic osteoarthropathy. Clin Chest Med 8:287, 1987

HURTADO A: Some clinical aspects of life at high altitudes. Ann Intern Med 53:247, 1960

JANDL JH: Polycythemia: Erythrocytosis, in *Blood: Textbook of Hematology*, JH Jandl (ed). Boston, Little, Brown, 1996, pp 605–614

SCHWARCZ TH et al: Thromboembolic complications of polycythemia: Polycythemia vera vs. smokers' polycythemia. J Vasc Surg 17:518, 1993

SMITH JR, LANDAW SA: Smokers' polycythemia. N Engl J Med 298:6, 1978

SZIDON JP, FISHMAN AP: Cyanosis and clubbing, in *Pulmonary Diseases and Disorders*, 2d ed, A Fishman (ed). Philadelphia, Saunders, 1988, p 351

TERRITO MC, ROSOVE MH: Cyanotic congenital heart disease: Hematologic management. J Am Coll Cardiol 18:320, 1991

37   *Eugene Braunwald*

EDEMA

Edema is defined as a clinically apparent increase in the interstitial fluid volume, which may expand by several liters before the abnormality is evident. Therefore, a weight gain of several kilograms usually precedes overt manifestations of edema, and a similar weight loss from diuresis can be induced in a slightly edematous patient before "dry weight" is achieved. *Ascites* (Chap. 46) and *hydrothorax* refer to accumulation of excess fluid in the peritoneal and pleural cavities, respectively, and are considered to be special forms of edema. *Anasarca* refers to gross, generalized edema.

Depending on its cause and mechanism, edema may be localized or have a generalized distribution; it is recognized in its generalized form by puffiness of the face, which is most readily apparent in the periorbital areas, and by the persistence of an indentation of the skin following pressure; this is known as "pitting" edema. In its more subtle form, it may be detected by noting that after the stethoscope is removed from the chest wall, the rim of the bell leaves an indentation on chest skin for a few minutes. When the ring on a finger fits more snugly than in the past or when a patient complains of difficulty in putting on shoes, particularly in the evening, edema may be present.

PATHOGENESIS   About one-third of the total-body water is confined to the extracellular space. Approximately 25 percent of the latter, in turn, is composed of the plasma volume, and the remainder is interstitial fluid.

Starling Forces   The forces that regulate the disposition of fluid between these two components of the extracellular compartment are frequently referred to as the *Starling forces* (see p. 194). The hydrostatic pressure within the vascular system and the colloid oncotic pressure in the interstitial fluid tend to promote movement of fluid from the vascular to the extravascular space. In contrast, the colloid oncotic pressure contributed by the plasma proteins and the hydrostatic pressure within the interstitial fluid, referred to as the *tissue tension*, promote the movement of fluid into the vascular compartment. Consequently there is a movement of water and diffusible solutes from the vascular space at the arteriolar end of the capillaries. Fluid is returned from the interstitial space into the vascular system at the venous end of the capillary and by way of the lymphatics, and unless these channels are obstructed, lymph flow tends to increase if there is net movement of fluid from the vascular compartment to the interstitium. These forces are usually balanced so that a steady state exists in the sizes of the intravascular and interstitial compartments, and yet a large exchange between them is permitted. However, should any one of the hydrostatic or oncotic forces be altered significantly, a net movement of fluid between the two components of the extracellular space will occur. The development of edema then depends on one or more alterations in the Starling forces so that there is a net movement of fluid from the vascular system into the interstitium or into a body cavity.

An increase in capillary pressure as a cause of edema may result from an elevation of venous pressure due to local obstruction in venous drainage. This increase in capillary pressure may be generalized, as occurs in congestive heart failure. The colloid oncotic pressure of the plasma may be reduced, owing to any factor that may induce severe hypoalbuminemia, such as malnutrition, liver disease, loss of protein into the urine or into the gastrointestinal tract, or a severe catabolic state.

Capillary Damage   Edema may also result from damage to the capillary endothelium, which increases its permeability and permits the transfer of protein into the interstitial compartment. Injury to the capillary wall can result from chemical or bacterial agents as well as from thermal or mechanical trauma. Increased capillary permeability may also be a consequence of a hypersensitivity reaction and is characteristic of immune injury. Damage to the capillary endothelium is presumably responsible for inflammatory edema, which is usually nonpitting, localized, and accompanied by other signs of inflammation—redness, heat, and tenderness.

To formulate a hypothesis about the pathophysiology of an edematous state, it is important to discriminate between the *primary* events, such as venous or lymphatic obstruction, reduction of cardiac output, hypoalbuminemia, trapping of fluid in spaces such as the peritoneal cavity, or an increase in capillary permeability, and the predictable *secondary* consequences, which include the renal retention of salt and water in an attempt to restore the plasma volume. Both the primary event and the secondary consequences may contribute to the formation of edema.

Reduction of Effective Arterial Volume   In many forms of edema the *effective arterial blood volume*, an as yet poorly defined parameter of the filling of the arterial tree, is reduced, and as a consequence a series of physiologic responses designed to restore it to normal are set into motion. A key element of these responses is the retention of an increment of salt and therefore of water, principally by the proximal tubule (Fig. 37-1), and in many instances this repairs the deficit of the effective arterial blood volume; often this occurs without the development of overt edema. If, however, the retention of salt and water is insufficient to restore and maintain the effective arterial blood volume, the stimuli are not dissipated, the retention of salt and water continues, and edema ultimately develops. This sequence of events is operative in dehydration and hemorrhage. Although in these conditions there is a reduction of effective arterial blood volume and activation of the entire sequence shown in the center of Fig. 37-2, including the diminished excretion of salt and water, edema does *not* occur because the net sodium and water balance is negative rather than positive. In most conditions that lead to edema the mechanisms responsible for maintaining a normal effective osmolality in the body fluids operate efficiently so that sodium retention promotes thirst and secretion of the antidiuretic hormone, which, in turn, lead to the ingestion and retention of approximately 1 L of water for each 140 mmol sodium retained. In edematous states, isotonic expansion of the extracellular fluid space may be massive, while the intracellular fluid volume is changed little or not at all.

Reduced Cardiac Output   A reduction of cardiac output, whatever the cause, is associated with a reduction of the effective arterial blood volume as well as of renal blood flow, constriction of the efferent renal arterioles, and an elevation of the filtration fraction, i.e., the ratio of glomerular filtration rate to renal plasma flow. In severe heart failure there is a reduction in the glomerular filtration rate. Activation of the sympathetic nervous system and of the renin-angiotensin systems are responsible for renal vasoconstriction. The finding that alpha-adrenergic blocking agents and/or angiotensin-converting enzyme (ACE) inhibitors augment renal blood flow and induce diuresis supports the role of these two systems in elevating renal vascular resistance and salt and water retention.

Renal Factors   Reduced cardiac output lowers effective arterial blood volume. There is increased reabsorption of glomerular filtrate in both the proximal (Fig. 37-1) and distal increases in sodium reabsorption in heart failure. Alterations in intrarenal hemodynamics appear to play a significant role. Heart failure, and other conditions such as nephrotic syndrome and cirrhosis that reduce effective arterial blood volume, cause renal efferent arteriolar constriction. This, in turn, reduces the hydrostatic pressure and raises the colloid osmotic pressure in the peritubular capillaries, thus enhancing salt and water reabsorption in the proximal tubule as well as in the ascending limb of the loop of Henle.

In addition, the diminished renal blood flow characteristic of states in which the effective arterial blood volume is reduced is translated by the renal juxtaglomerular cells into a signal for increased renin release (Chap. 332). The mechanisms responsible for this release include a baroreceptor response: reduced renal perfusion results in incomplete filling of the renal arterioles and diminished stretch of the juxtaglomerular cells, a signal that provides for the elaboration or release, or both, of renin. A second mechanism for renin release involves the macula densa; as a result of reduced glomerular filtration the sodium chloride load reaching the distal renal tubules is reduced. This is sensed by the macula densa, which signals the neighboring juxtaglomerular cells to secrete renin. A third mechanism involves the sympathetic nervous system and circulating catecholamines. Activation of the beta-adrenergic receptors in the juxtaglomerular cells stimulates renin release. These three mechanisms generally act in concert.

The Renin-Angiotensin-Aldosterone (RAA) System (See Chap. 332) Renin, an enzyme with a molecular weight of about 40,000, acts on its substrate, angiotensinogen, an $alpha_2$ globulin synthesized by the liver, to release angiotensin I, a decapeptide, which is broken down to angiotensin II (AII), an octapeptide. This has generalized vasoconstrictor properties; it is especially active on the efferent arterioles, and independently increases Na^+ reabsorption in the proximal tubule. The RAA system has long been recognized as a hormone system. However, it also operates locally. Both circulating and intrarenally produced AII contribute to renal vasoconstriction and to salt and

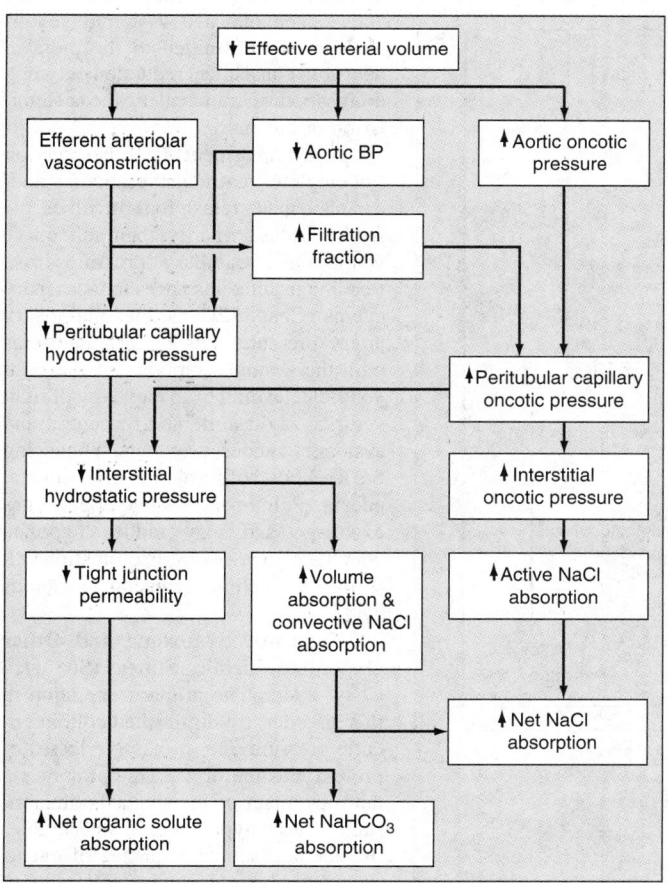

FIGURE 37-1 Effect of hemodynamic changes on proximal tubule solute transport: a summary. Hemodynamic mechanisms by which a reduction of effective arterial volume causes salt and water retention and thereby contributes to the formation of edema. *(From Seldin DW et al, Semin Nephrol 11:212, 1991, with permission.)*

water retention. These renal effects of AII are mediated by activation of AII type 1 receptors, which can be blocked by specific antagonists such as losartan. AII also enters the circulation and stimulates the production of aldosterone by the zona glomerulosa of the adrenal cortex. In patients with heart failure, not only is aldosterone secretion elevated but the biologic half-life of aldosterone is prolonged, which further increases the plasma level of the hormone. A depression of hepatic blood flow, particularly during exercise, secondary to a reduction in cardiac output, is responsible for the reduced hepatic catabolism of aldosterone. Aldosterone, in turn, enhances Na^+ reabsorption (and K^+ excretion) by the collecting tubule. The activation of the RAA system is most striking in the early phase of acute, severe heart failure and is less intense in patients with chronic, stable, compensated heart failure.

Although increased quantities of aldosterone are secreted in heart failure and in other edematous states and although blockade of the action of aldosterone by spironolactone (an aldosterone antagonist) or amiloride (a blocker of epithelial Na^+ channels) often induces a moderate diuresis in edematous states, persistent augmented levels of aldosterone (or other mineralocorticoids) alone do not always promote accumulation of edema, as witnessed by the lack of striking fluid retention in most instances of primary aldosteronism (Chap. 332). Furthermore, although normal individuals retain some salt and water under the influence of a potent mineralocorticoid, such as deoxycorticosterone acetate or fludrocortisone, this accumulation is self-limiting, despite continued exposure to the steroid, a phenomenon known as *mineralocorticoid escape*. The failure of normal individuals receiving large doses of mineralocorticoids to accumulate large quantities of extracellular fluid and to develop edema is probably a consequence of an increase in glomerular filtration rate (pressure natriuresis) and through the action of natriuretic substance(s) (see below). The continued secretion of aldosterone may be more important in the accumulation of fluid in edematous states because patients with edema are generally unable to repair the deficit in effective arterial blood volume. As a consequence they do not develop pressure natriuresis nor do they elaborate normal quantities of atrial natriuretic peptide.

Blockade of the RAA system, by blocking AII receptors or inhibiting the ACE reduces efferent arterial resistance and increases renal blood flow. This action (combined in patients with heart failure with a rise in cardiac output secondary to afterload reduction) as well as reduction in the secretion of aldosterone cause diuresis. However, in patients with moderate or severe impairment of renal function interference with the RAA system can cause paradoxical sodium retention due to intensification of renal failure.

Arginine Vasopressin (AVP) and Endothelin (See also Chap. 330) The secretion of AVP occurs in response to increased intracellular osmolar concentration and by stimulating V_2 receptors increases the reabsorption of free water in the distal tubule, thereby increasing total-body water. Circulating AVP is elevated in many patients with heart failure secondary to an as yet unidentified nonosmotic stimulus, who fail to show the normal reduction of AVP with a reduction of osmolality, contributing to fluid retention and edema formation.

Endothelin This is a potent peptide vasoconstrictor released by endothelial cells; its concentration is elevated in heart failure and contributes to renal vasoconstriction, Na^+ retention, and edema in heart failure.

Natriuretic Peptides Atrial distention and/or a sodium load cause release into the circulation of atrial natriuretic peptide (ANP), a polypeptide; a high-molecular-weight precursor of ANP is stored in secretory granules within atrial myocytes. Release of ANP causes (1) excretion of sodium and water by augmenting glomerular filtration rate, inhibiting sodium reabsorption in the proximal tubule, and inhibiting release of renin and aldosterone; and (2) arteriolar and venous dilatation by antagonizing the vasoconstrictor actions of AII, AVP, and sympathetic stimulation. Thus, ANP has the capacity to oppose sodium retention and arterial pressure elevation in hypervolemic states.

The closely related brain natriuretic peptide (BNP) is stored primarily in cardiac ventricular myocardium and is released when ventricular diastolic pressure rises. Its actions are similar to ANP. Circulating levels of ANP and BNP are elevated in congestive heart failure but obviously not sufficient to prevent edema formation. In addition, in edematous states (particularly heart failure), there is abnormal resistance to the actions of natriuretic peptides.

CLINICAL CAUSES OF EDEMA   Obstruction of Venous (and Lymphatic) Drainage of a Limb   In this condition the hydrostatic pressure in the capillary bed upstream to the obstruction increases so that more fluid than normal is transferred from the vascular to the interstitial space. Since the alternative route (i.e., the lymphatic channels) may also be obstructed, this event causes an increased volume of interstitial fluid in the limb, i.e., a trapping of fluid in the extremity, at the expense of the blood volume in the remainder of the body, thereby reducing effective arterial blood volume and leading to the consequences shown in Fig. 37-2.

When venous and lymphatic drainage are obstructed in a limb, fluid accumulates in the interstitium at the expense of plasma volume. The latter stimulates the retention of salt and water until the deficit in plasma volume has been corrected. Tissue tension rises in the affected limb until it counterbalances the primary alterations in the Starling forces, at which time no further fluid accumulates. The net effect is a local increase in the volume of interstitial fluid. This same

sequence occurs in ascites and hydrothorax, in which fluid is trapped or accumulates in the cavitary space, depleting the intravascular volume and leading to secondary salt and fluid retention, as already described.

Congestive Heart Failure (See also Chap. 233)   In this disorder the defective systolic emptying of the chambers of the heart and/or the impairment of ventricular relaxation promotes an accumulation of blood in the heart and venous circulation at the expense of the arterial volume, and the aforementioned sequence of events (Fig. 37-2) is initiated. In mild heart failure, a small increment of total blood volume may repair the deficit of arterial volume and establish a new steady state because, through the operation of Starling's law of the heart, an increase in the volume of blood within the chambers of the heart promotes a more forceful contraction and may thereby increase the cardiac output (Fig. 233-1). However, if the cardiac disorder is more severe, retention of fluid cannot repair the deficit in effective arterial blood volume. The increment accumulates in the venous circulation, and the increase in capillary and lymphatic hydrostatic pressures promotes the formation of edema. In heart failure, a reduction occurs in baroreflex-mediated inhibition of the vasomotor center, which causes activation of renal vasoconstrictor nerves and the RAA system, causing sodium and water retention.

Incomplete ventricular emptying (systolic heart failure) and/or inadequate ventricular relaxation (diastolic heart failure) both lead to an elevation of ventricular diastolic pressure. If the impairment of cardiac function involves the right ventricle, pressures in the systemic veins and capillaries may rise, thereby augmenting the transudation of fluid into the interstitial space and enhancing the likelihood of peripheral edema in the presence of the accumulation of sodium and water, as described above. The elevated systemic venous pressure is transmitted to the thoracic duct with consequent reduction of lymph drainage, further increasing the accumulation of edema.

If the impairment of cardiac function (incomplete ventricular emptying and/or inadequate relaxation) involves the left ventricle primarily, then pulmonary venous and capillary pressures rise [leading in some instances to pulmonary edema (Chap. 32)], as does pulmonary artery pressure; this in turn interferes with the systolic emptying of the right ventricle, leading to an elevation of right ventricular diastolic and of central and systemic venous pressures, enhancing the likelihood of formation of peripheral edema. Pulmonary edema impairs gas exchange and may induce hypoxia, which embarrasses cardiac function still further, sometimes causing a vicious cycle.

Nephrotic Syndrome and Other Hypoalbuminemic States (See also Chap. 274)   The primary alteration in this disorder is a diminished colloid oncotic pressure due to massive losses of protein into the urine. This promotes a net movement of fluid into the interstitium, causes hypovolemia, and initiates the edema-forming sequence of events described above, including activation of the RAA system. With severe hypoalbuminemia, the salt and water that are retained cannot be restrained within the vascular compartment, total and effective arterial blood volumes decline, and

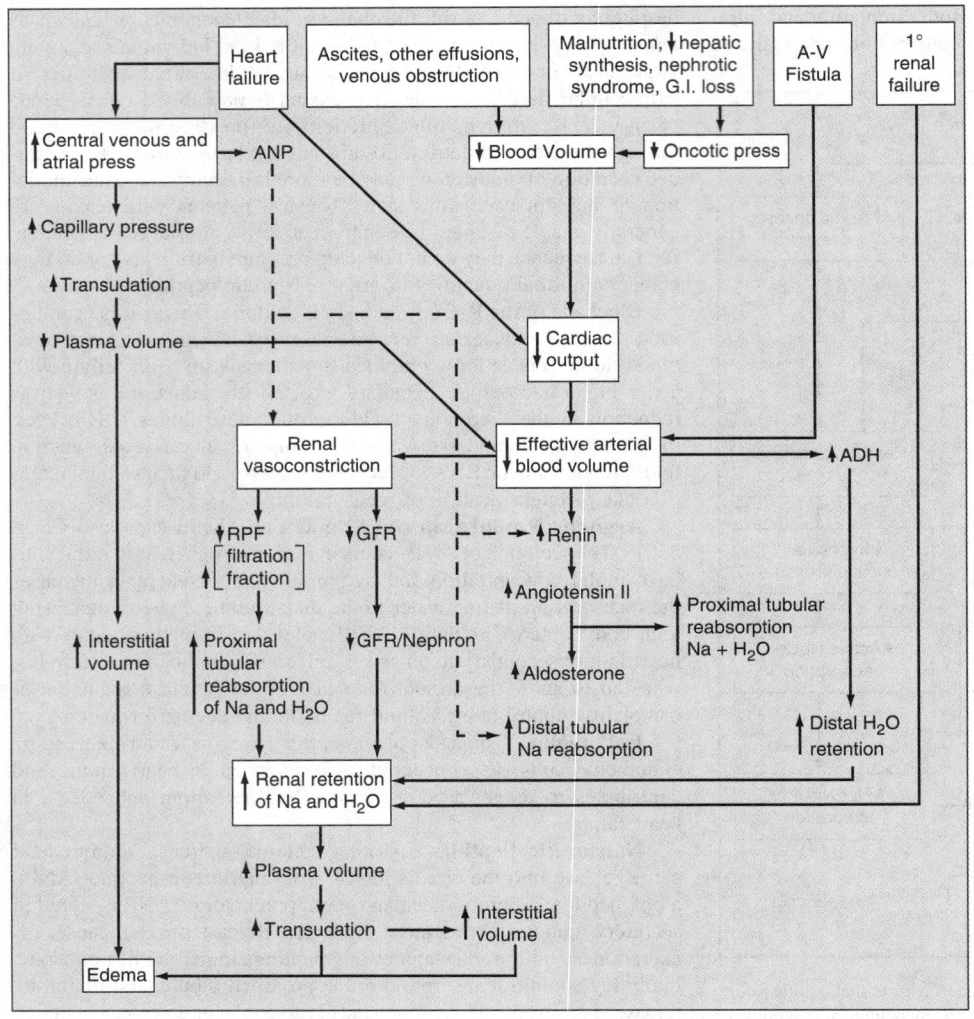

FIGURE 37-2   Sequence of events leading to the formation and retention of salt and water and the development of edema. ANP, atrial natriuretic peptide; RPF, renal plasma flow; GFR, glomerular filtration rate. Inhibitory influences are shown by broken lines. ADH, antidiuretic hormone

hence the stimuli to retain salt and water are not abated. A similar sequence of events occurs in other conditions that lead to *severe* hypoalbuminemia, including severe nutritional deficiency states, protein-losing enteropathy, congenital hypoalbuminemia, and severe, chronic liver disease. However, in the nephrotic syndrome, the impairment of renal function contributes to the retention of sodium.

Cirrhosis (See also Chaps. 46 and 298) This condition is characterized by hepatic venous outflow blockade, which in turn causes expansion of the splanchnic blood volume and increased hepatic lymph formation. Intrahepatic hypertension acts as a potent stimulus for renal Na^+ retention and perhaps systemic vasodilation and a reduction of effective arterial blood volume as well. These alterations are frequently complicated by hypoalbuminemia secondary to reduced hepatic synthesis and reduce the effective arterial blood volume even further, leading to activation of the RAA system, of renal sympathetic nerves and other salt- and water-retaining mechanisms. The concentration of circulating aldosterone is elevated by the liver's failure to metabolize this hormone. Initially, the excess interstitial fluid is localized preferentially upstream to the congested portal venous system and obstructed hepatic lymphatics, i.e., in the peritoneal cavity. In later stages, particularly when there is severe hypoalbuminemia, peripheral edema may develop. The excess production of prostaglandins (PGE_2 and PGI_2) in cirrhosis attenuates renal Na^+ retention. When the synthesis of these substances is inhibited by nonsteroidal antiinflammatory agents, renal function deteriorates and Na^+ retention increases.

Idiopathic Edema This syndrome, which occurs almost exclusively in women, is characterized by periodic episodes of edema (unrelated to the menstrual cycle), frequently accompanied by abdominal distention. Diurnal alterations in weight occur with orthostatic retention of sodium and water, so that the patient may weigh several pounds more after having been in the upright posture for several hours. Such large diurnal weight changes suggest an increase in capillary permeability which appears to fluctuate in severity and to be aggravated by hot weather. There is some evidence that a reduction in plasma volume occurs in this condition with secondary activation of the RAA system and impaired suppression of AVP release. Idiopathic edema should be distinguished from cyclical or premenstrual edema in which the sodium and water retention may be secondary to excessive estrogen stimulation. There are also some cases in which the edema appears to be "diuretic-induced." It has been postulated that in these patients, chronic diuretic administration leads to mild blood volume depletion, which causes chronic hyperreninemia and juxtaglomerular hyperplasia. Salt-retaining mechanisms appear to overcompensate for the direct effects of the diuretics. *Acute* withdrawal of diuretics can then leave the sodium-retaining forces unopposed, leading to fluid retention and edema. Decreased dopaminergic activity and reduced urinary kallikrein and kinin excretion have been reported in this condition and may also be of pathogenetic importance.

℞ **TREATMENT**

The treatment of idiopathic cyclic edema includes a reduction in salt intake, rest in the supine position for several hours each day, the wearing of elastic stockings (which are put on before arising in the morning), and an attempt to understand any underlying emotional problems. A variety of pharmacologic agents including ACE inhibitors, progesterone, the dopamine receptor agonist bromocriptine, and the sympathomimetic amine dextroamphetamine have all been reported to be useful when administered to patients who do not respond to simpler measures. Diuretics may be initially helpful but may lose their effectiveness with continuous administration; accordingly, they should be employed sparingly, if at all. Discontinuation of diuretics paradoxically leads to diuresis in "diuretic-induced" edema, described above.

DIFFERENTIAL DIAGNOSIS

Localized edema can usually be readily differentiated from generalized edema. The great majority of patients with generalized edema suffer from advanced cardiac, renal, hepatic, or nutritional disorders. Conse-

quently, the differential diagnosis of generalized edema should be directed toward identifying or excluding these several conditions.

LOCALIZED EDEMA (See also Chap. 248) Edema originating from inflammation or hypersensitivity is usually readily identified. Localized edema due to venous or lymphatic obstruction may be caused by thrombophlebitis, chronic lymphangitis, resection of regional lymph nodes, filariasis, etc. Lymphedema is particularly intractable because restriction of lymphatic flow results in increased protein concentration in the interstitial fluid, a circumstance that aggravates retention of fluid.

EDEMA OF HEART FAILURE (See also Chap. 233) The presence of heart disease, as manifested by cardiac enlargement and gallop rhythm, together with evidence of cardiac failure, such as dyspnea, basilar rales, venous distention, and hepatomegaly, usually provides an indication on clinical examination that edema results from heart failure. Noninvasive tests such as echocardiography and radionuclide angiography may be helpful in establishing the diagnosis of heart failure.

EDEMA OF THE NEPHROTIC SYNDROME (See also Chap. 274) Marked proteinuria (>3.5 g/d), severe hypoalbuminemia (<2 g/dL), and in some instances hypercholesterolemia are present. This syndrome may occur during the course of a variety of kidney diseases, which include glomerulonephritis, diabetic glomerulosclerosis, and hypersensitivity reactions. A history of previous renal disease may or may not be elicited.

EDEMA OF ACUTE GLOMERULONEPHRITIS AND OTHER FORMS OF RENAL FAILURE The edema occurring during the acute phases of glomerulonephritis is characteristically associated with hematuria, proteinuria, and hypertension. Although some evidence supports the view that the fluid retention is due to increased capillary permeability, in most instances the edema in this disease results from primary retention of sodium and water by the kidneys owing to renal insufficiency. This state differs from congestive heart failure in that it is characterized by a normal (or sometimes even increased) cardiac output and a normal arterial–mixed venous oxygen difference. Patients with edema due to renal failure commonly have evidence of pulmonary congestion on chest roentgenograms before cardiac enlargement is significant, but they usually do not develop orthopnea. Patients with chronic impairment of renal function may also develop edema due to primary renal retention of sodium and water.

EDEMA OF CIRRHOSIS (See also Chap. 298) Ascites and biochemical and clinical evidence of hepatic disease (collateral venous channels, jaundice, and spider angiomas) characterize edema of hepatic origin. The ascites is frequently refractory to treatment because it collects as a result of a combination of obstruction of hepatic lymphatic drainage, portal hypertension, and hypoalbuminemia. Edema may also occur in other parts of the body in these patients as a result of hypoalbuminemia. Furthermore, the sizable accumulation of ascitic fluid may increase intraabdominal pressure and impede venous return from the lower extremities; hence, it tends to promote accumulation of edema in this region as well.

EDEMA OF NUTRITIONAL ORIGIN A diet grossly deficient in protein over a prolonged period may produce hypoproteinemia and edema. The latter may be intensified by the development of beriberi heart disease, also of nutritional origin, in which multiple peripheral arteriovenous fistulas result in reduced effective systemic perfusion and effective arterial blood volume, thereby enhancing edema formation. Edema may actually become intensified when these famished subjects are first provided with an adequate diet. The ingestion of more food may increase the quantity of salt ingested, which is then retained along with water. So-called "refeeding edema" may also be linked to increased release of insulin, which directly increases tubular sodium reabsorption. In addition to hypoalbuminemia, hypokalemia and caloric deficits may be involved in the edema of starvation.

OTHER CAUSES OF EDEMA These include hypothyroidism, in which the edema (myxedema) may be located typically in the pretibial region and which may also be associated with periorbital puffiness. Exogenous hyperadrenocortism, pregnancy, and administration of estrogens and vasodilators, particularly the calcium antagonist nifedipine, may also all cause edema.

DISTRIBUTION OF EDEMA The distribution of edema is an important guide to the cause. Thus, edema limited to one leg or to one or both arms is usually the result of venous and/or lymphatic obstruction. Edema resulting from hypoproteinemia characteristically is generalized, but it is especially evident in the very soft tissues of the eyelids and face and tends to be most pronounced in the morning because of the recumbent posture assumed during the night. Less common causes of facial edema include trichinosis, allergic reactions, and myxedema. Edema associated with heart failure, on the other hand, tends to be more extensive in the legs and to be accentuated in the evening, a feature also determined largely by posture. When patients with heart failure have been confined to bed, edema may be most prominent in the presacral region. Unilateral edema occasionally results from lesions in the central nervous system affecting the vasomotor fibers on one side of the body; paralysis also reduces lymphatic and venous drainage on the affected side.

ADDITIONAL FACTORS IN DIAGNOSIS The color, thickness, and sensitivity of the skin are significant. Local tenderness and increase in temperature suggest inflammation. Local cyanosis may signify a venous obstruction. In individuals who have had repeated episodes of prolonged edema, the skin over the involved areas may be thickened, indurated, and often red.

Measurement or estimation of the venous pressure is of importance in evaluating edema. Elevation in an isolated part of the body usually reflects localized venous obstruction. Generalized elevation of systemic venous pressure usually indicates the presence of congestive heart failure. Ordinarily, significant increase in venous pressure can be recognized by the level at which cervical veins collapse (Chap. 227). In patients with obstruction of the superior vena cava, edema is confined to the face, neck, and upper extremities, where the venous pressure is elevated compared with that in the lower extremities. Measurement of venous pressure in the upper extremities is also useful in patients with massive edema of the lower extremities and ascites; it is elevated when the edema is on a cardiac basis (e.g., constrictive pericarditis or tricuspid stenosis) but is normal when it is secondary to cirrhosis. Severe heart failure may cause ascites that may be distinguished from the ascites caused by hepatic cirrhosis by the jugular venous pressure, which usually is elevated in heart failure and normal in cirrhosis.

Determination of the concentration of serum albumin aids importantly in identifying those patients in whom edema is due, at least in part, to diminished intravascular colloid oncotic pressure. The presence of proteinuria also affords useful clues. The absence of protein in the urine is evidence against renal disease as a cause of edema. Slight to moderate proteinuria is the rule in patients with heart failure, whereas persistent massive proteinuria is characteristic of the nephrotic syndrome.

_____ *Approach to the Patient* _____

An important first question is whether the edema is localized or generalized. If it is localized, those phenomena that may be responsible should be concentrated upon. Hydrothorax and ascites are forms of localized edema. Either may be a consequence of local venous or lymphatic obstruction, as in inflammatory or neoplastic disease

If the edema is generalized, it should be determined, first, if there is serious hypoalbuminemia, e.g., serum albumin <2.5 g/dL. If so, the history, physical examination, urinalysis, and other laboratory data will help evaluate the question of cirrhosis, severe malnutrition, protein-losing gastroenteropathy, or the nephrotic syndrome as the underlying disorder. If hypoalbuminemia is not present, it should be determined if there is evidence of congestive heart failure of a severity to promote generalized edema. Finally, it should be determined whether the patient has an adequate urine output, or if there is significant oliguria or even anuria. These abnormalities are discussed in Chaps. 47, 270, and 271.

BIBLIOGRAPHY

ANAND IS et al: Studies of body water and sodium, renal function, hemodynamic indexes, and plasma hormones in untreated congestive heart failure. Circulation 80:299, 1989
ELLISON DH: Diuretic drugs and the treatment of edema: From clinic to bench and back again. Am J Kidney Dis 23:623, 1994
GOLDEN MHN: Protein deficiency, energy deficiency, and the oedema of malnutrition. Lancet 1:1261, 1982
GOLDSMITH SR: Control of arginine vasopressin and congestive heart failure. Am J Cardiol 71:629, 1993
LEIER C, BOUDOULAS H: Renal disorders and heart disease, in *Heart Disease*, 5th ed, E Braunwald (ed). Philadelphia, Saunders, 1997, pp 1914–1938
MARTIN PY, SCHRIER RW: Renal sodium excretion and edematous disorders. Endocrinol Metab Clin North Am 24:459, 1995
MILLER JA et al: Control of extracellular fluid volume and the pathophysiology of edema formation, in *The Kidney*, 5th ed, BM Brenner (ed). Philadelphia, Saunders, 1996, pp 817–872
PELOSI AJ et al: The role of diuretics in the aetiology of idiopathic oedema. Q J Med 88:49, 1995
STREETEN DH: Idiopathic edema. Pathogenesis, clinical features, and treatment. Endocrinol Metab Clin North Am 24:531, 1995
STRUTHERS AD: Ten years of natriuretic peptide research: A new dawn for their diagnostic and therapeutic use? BMJ 308:1615, 1994

| 38 | *Steven M. Hollenberg, Joseph E. Parrillo* |

SHOCK

Shock is the state in which failure of the circulatory system to maintain adequate cellular perfusion results in widespread reduction in delivery of oxygen and other nutrients to tissues. Circulatory insufficiency causes cellular and then organ dysfunction, which may become irreversible unless corrected promptly. Shock is a syndrome defined by a constellation of clinical signs that may arise from any of several causes. At the onset, the physiologic alterations accompanying shock reflect the nature of the initiating event. As the syndrome progresses, however, a common pattern emerges resulting from the consequences of inadequate tissue perfusion.

CONTROL OF ARTERIAL BLOOD PRESSURE

Maintenance of adequate perfusion of vital organs is critical for survival. Organ perfusion is dependent on arterial pressure, which is determined by two factors: cardiac output and vascular resistance. Hence, organ perfusion can be compromised by a decrease in cardiac output or by maldistribution of cardiac output. Within an organ, distribution of blood flow depends on perfusion pressure, vascular resistance, and patency of nutritional microvessels. Maldistribution of flow can aggravate organ dysfunction. Because the initiating factor in shock is inadequate tissue perfusion, it is important to understand the critical determinants of tissue perfusion. These determinants can be divided into cardiac, vascular, humoral, and microcirculatory factors.

CARDIAC FACTORS Cardiac output is the product of stroke volume and heart rate. Stroke volume, in turn, is determined by three factors: preload, afterload, and myocardial contractility (Chap. 232).

VASCULAR FACTORS Resistance to the flow of blood in a vessel is proportional to vessel length and viscosity of blood and inversely proportional to the fourth power of the vessel radius. Therefore, the cross-sectional area of a vessel is by far the most important determinant of the resistance to flow. Since the major site of resistance in the systemic vasculature is at the arteriolar level, and vascular smooth-muscle tone regulates the radius of the resistance arterioles, arteriolar smooth-muscle tone is the most important determinant of vascular resistance.

Arteriolar tone is regulated by extrinsic factors, which include neural and hormonal regulation, and intrinsic or local factors, which include the myogenic response, metabolic autoregulation, and endothelial-mediated regulation. Resistance arterioles receive a tonic vasoconstrictor stimulus from sympathetic nerves innervating the vascular smooth muscle; sympathetic tone is largely regulated by arterial and cardiopulmonary baroreceptors. Adrenal stimulation results in release of epinephrine and norepinephrine into the systemic circulation. Blood vessels can contract or relax in response to changes in transmural pressure so as to maintain a constant blood flow with changes in perfusion pressure; this *myogenic response* serves to maintain a constant arterial wall tension, ensuring local autoregulation of flow. Metabolic regulation results from release of vasodilators that increase tissue blood flow in response to increased metabolic activity; the most important of these are adenosine and vasodilator prostaglandins. Microvascular vesels also relax in the presence of low oxygen tensions, also due to release of prostaglandins. Vascular endothelial cells secrete a number of substances with local actions, including endothelium-derived relaxing factor (nitric oxide) (Chap. 71); the molecules derived from arachidonic acid, collectively termed *eicosanoids*; the vasoconstrictor peptides endothelin-1 and angiotensin II; and oxygen free radicals. The actions of and interactions among these mediators are important components of regulation of the local environment by endothelial cells.

HUMORAL FACTORS   Circulating humoral substances play important roles in cardiovascular homeostasis. In shock, release of circulating mediators such as renin, vasopressin, prostaglandins, kinins, atrial natriuretic factor, and catecholamines is mediated both by central nervous system activation and by cellular effects of ischemia, toxins, and immunologic mechanisms.

MICROCIRCULATORY FACTORS   Because shock results from microcirculatory failure, the most critical aspects of the pathogenesis of shock take place in the microcirculation. Normal blood delivery to an organ as a whole does not necessarily indicate that perfusion of all segments of that organ is commensurate with regional metabolic demand. Adhesion of leukocytes and platelets to activated or damaged vascular endothelial cells can cause sludging and occlusion of microvessels; activation of the coagulation system with fibrin deposition and accumulation of microthrombi can contribute to microvascular occlusion. Shunting can occur as a result of perfusion of vessels with inadequate capillary exchange. Decreased deformability of erythrocytes can also contribute to decreased microcirculatory flow and capillary exchange.

Microvascular flow is influenced by the balance between colloid osmotic pressure and capillary hydrostatic pressure, which, in turn, determines the balance between intravascular and extravascular fluid. Sympathetic stimulation constricts precapillary resistance vessels, decreasing capillary hydrostatic pressures and facilitating movement of fluid from the extravascular to the intravascular space, but it also constricts postcapillary venules. As severe tissue hypoxia and acidosis supervene, sympathetically mediated arteriolar vasoconstrictive responses can be outweighed by metabolic vasodilation; along with venoconstriction, this can cause extravasation of fluid into the interstitial space. In addition, circulating toxins and adhesion of activated leukocytes can increase capillary permeability, further increasing tissue edema. This process can be exacerbated by loss of plasma proteins into the interstitium, further reducing colloid osmotic pressure, intravascular volume, and tissue perfusion.

CLASSIFICATION OF SHOCK

A classification of shock based on the underlying causes of abnormal tissue perfusion is shown in Table 38-1.

HYPOVOLEMIC SHOCK   Hypovolemic shock is due to a reduction in circulating blood volume, which decreases preload and leads to inadequate ventricular filling, reflected in decreased left and right ventricular end-diastolic volumes and pressures. The result is decreased stroke volume and inadequate cardiac output. Hypovolemic shock may result from hemorrhage or from fluid depletion due to

vomiting, diarrhea, burns, or dehydration. Hypovolemic shock is the most common type of shock seen clinically; it has been well studied, because all gradations of hypovolemia can be reproducibly induced in animal models.

CARDIOGENIC SHOCK   Cardiogenic shock (see also Chap. 243) results from severe depression of cardiac performance. Hemodynamically, it is characterized by a systolic blood pressure <80 mmHg, cardiac index <1.8(L/min)/m², and left ventricular filling pressure >18 mmHg; pulmonary edema is usually present. The most frequent cause is myocardial infarction with loss of substantial muscle mass (usually 40 percent or more of the left ventricular myocardium). Extensive right ventricular infarction can also precipitate cardiogenic shock. Pump failure can also result from acute myocarditis or from depression of myocardial contractility following cardiac arrest or prolonged cardiopulmonary bypass.

Cardiogenic shock can be caused by mechanical abnormalities. Severe valvular stenosis can decrease stroke volume and cardiac output. Acute, massive mitral or aortic regurgitation leads to a reduction in forward cardiac output that may result in pulmonary edema and cardiogenic shock. Acutely acquired ventricular septal defects, which usually occur in the setting of acute myocardial infarction, can also cause cardiogenic shock by reducing forward flow.

EXTRACARDIAC OBSTRUCTIVE SHOCK   This form of shock is best exemplified by pericardial tamponade (Chap. 240). Increased pericardial pressure impairs ventricular diastolic filling, decreasing preload, stroke volume, and cardiac output. Tension pneumothorax can also impair cardiac filling by decreasing venous return to the heart. Massive pulmonary embolism is another form of extracardiac obstructive shock, although the mechanism is different (Chap. 261). When more than 50 to 60 percent of the pulmonary vascular bed is obstructed by thrombus, acute right ventricular failure can occur, and left ventricular filling is impaired.

Table 38-1

Classification of Forms of Shock

CARDIOGENIC SHOCK

Myopathic
  Acute myocardial infarction
  Dilated cardiomyopathy
  Myocardial depression in septic shock
Mechanical
  Mitral regurgitation
  Ventricular septal defect
  Ventricular aneurysm
  Left ventricular outflow track obstruction (aortic stenosis, hypertrophic cardiomyopathy)
Arrhythmic

EXTRACARDIAC OBSTRUCTIVE SHOCK

Pericardial tamponade
Pulmonary embolism (massive)
Severe pulmonary hypertension (primary or Eisenmenger)

HYPOVOLEMIC SHOCK

Hemorrhage
Fluid depletion

DISTRIBUTIVE SHOCK

Septic shock
Toxic products (drug overdose)
Anaphylaxis
Neurogenic shock
Endocrinologic shock

SOURCE: Modified from SM Hollenberg and JE Parrillo, in Surgical Intensive Care, GT Shires, PL Barie (eds), New York, Little, Brown, 1993.

DISTRIBUTIVE SHOCK   Distributive shock is caused by profound peripheral vasodilation; although cardiac output may be normal or high, organ and tissue perfusion pressures are inadequate. The prototype of distributive shock is septic shock, which is the most common cause of death in intensive care units in the United States; the pathogenesis of septic shock is considered in detail below. Other types of distributive shock include anaphylaxis, neurogenic shock, and adrenal insufficiency.

In the clinical setting, patients may demonstrate elements of more than one type of shock simultaneously. For example, during septic shock, elements of distributive and hypovolemic shock can be complicated by myocardial impairment. Traumatic shock can also be complicated by elements of both hypovolemic and distributive shock. In a given patient, the nature of the circulatory disturbance may change with time and with therapy.

PATHOGENESIS

Cellular dysunction in shock is the final outcome of a process with multiple stimuli. In early shock, compensatory mechanisms are activated in an attempt to restore pressure and flow to vital organs. When these compensatory mechanisms begin to fail, impairment of tissue perfusion is manifested as organ dysfunction. Excessive and prolonged reduction of tissue perfusion leads to damage to cellular membranes, leakage of lysosomal enzymes, and reduction in cellular energy stores and may result in cell death. Once a sufficiently large number of cells from vital organs have reached this stage, shock can become irreversible, and death can occur despite correction of the underlying cause. This concept of irreversibility is useful because it emphasizes the need to prevent the progression of shock.

Cellular dysfunction in shock occurs through three main mechanisms: cellular ischemia, inflammatory mediators and free radical injury. With cellular hypoperfusion, oxygen depletion leads to anaerobic glycolysis, which produces only 2 ATP molecules during the breakdown of 1 glucose molecule as opposed to the 36 ATP molecules produced by aerobic glycolysis. This results in depletion of ATP and intracellular energy reserves. Anaerobic glycolysis also causes accumulation of lactic acid, with resultant intracellular acidosis. Failure of energy-dependent ion transport pumps decreases transmembrane potential, causing accumulation of intracellular sodium and water. Normal gradients of potassium, chloride, and calcium cannot be maintained. Intracellular accumulation of calcium further exacerbates mitochondrial dysfunction. Cellular membrane dysfunction is manifested by changes in cellular structure. Initial pathologic changes include enlargement of the endoplasmic reticulum and formation of blebs at the cellular surface; progression leads to mitochondrial condensation. Swelling of the mitochondria heralds irreversible cell injury. Terminal events include accumulation of denatured proteins and chromatin in the cytoplasm, lysosomal breakdown, and fracture of the mitochondria, nuclear envelope, and plasma membrane.

SEPTIC SHOCK   Disruption of cellular metabolism by the effects of inflammatory mediators plays a dominant role in the pathogenesis of septic shock and may be important in other forms of shock as well. Prominent among these mediators are cytokines such as tumor necrosis factor (TNF), interleukin (IL) 1, IL-2, interferon γ, eicosanoids, and platelet activating factor (PAF). TNF activates inflammatory cells, stimulates release of other inflammatory cytokines, promotes the expression of adhesion molecules on both endothelial cells and neutrophils, activates coagulation pathways, decreases transmembrane potential, causes arteriolar vasodilation, increases microvascular permeability, and can directly block intracellular pathways, leading to cellular dysfunction. IL-1 has similar effects and can potentiate the effects of TNF. Interferon γ promotes release of TNF and IL-1 and may act synergistically with these cytokines to produce cytotoxic activity. PAF also promotes release of TNF and eicosanoids and markedly increases microvascular permeability.

Free radicals are reactive oxygen intermediates that react with a variety of other molecules—inactivating proteins, damaging DNA, and, most importantly, inducing lipid peroxidation in the membrane. Massive production of free radicals can occur after ischemia and subsequent reperfusion. In shock, cellular ischemia and intracellular calcium accumulation can activate intracellular proteases and convert the enzyme xanthine dehydrogenase, which recycles ATP, to xanthine oxidase, which oxidizes purines with the formation of the highly toxic superoxide radical. When oxygen is reintroduced suddenly, large amounts of superoxide can be produced, and the cell's endogenous antioxidant defense systems can be overwhelmed. Lipid peroxidation is a self-sustaining process that severely impairs membrane integrity.

GENE EXPRESSION IN SHOCK   Recent studies have suggested two common programs of gene expression in response to stress: the acute-phase response and the heat-shock response. The acute-phase response to adverse stimuli is involved in maintaining *systemic* homeostasis; specific cell types express different genes. This response is identifiable clinically by accumulation in the plasma of proteins collectively known as *acute-phase reactants*, which are synthesized and secreted by the liver. The heat-shock response is a generic cellular response involved in maintaining *intracellular* homeostasis; the proteins synthesized act within cells and cannot be measured in blood. Some heat-shock proteins function as "molecular chaperones," which play a role in folding, stabilizing, and translocating newly synthesized proteins. Other heat-shock proteins appear to be involved in the genetic program of cell death known as *apoptosis*, a physiologic mechanism that normally functions to remove senescent cells. Although induction of heat-shock proteins has been shown to make cells more resistant to subsequent stress, evidence is accumulating to suggest that overexpression of these proteins may be deleterious in shock. Induction of the heat-shock response can preempt expression of both acute-phase and other genes important in synthetic function. This execution of a genetic program of cellular defense by individual cells may not be beneficial for the organism as a whole. In addition to preempting vital programs of gene expression, heat-shock protein induction may also initiate programmed cell death.

TRANSITION TO IRREVERSIBLE DAMAGE   Understanding the transition from reversible cellular dysfunction to irreversible cellular damage is important to an understanding of the pathogenesis of shock. This is thought to occur due to a self-amplifying and self-sustaining inflammatory process. Ordinarily, activation of the inflammatory system engenders counterregulatory anti-inflammatory mechanisms. If the inflammatory stimulus is sufficiently severe or prolonged, however, cellular autocrine and paracrine responses can lead to the development of positive feedback loops. Activation of endothelial cells ordinarily leads to expression of adhesion molecules and release of chemotactic factors and proinflammatory cytokines. In shock, these processes are excessive and unregulated. Adherent neutrophils and macrophages, in turn, become overactivated and release large quantities of inflammatory mediators. Similar self-sustaining mechanisms can be seen after free radical injury, in which lipid peroxidation leads to initiation of a cycle of autooxidation. Finally, accumulated injuries within a cell can reach a threshold at which self-destruction occurs.

ORGAN DYSFUNCTION

The clinical presentation of shock varies because each organ system is affected differently, depending on the severity of the perfusion deficit, the underlying cause of shock, and prior organ dysfunction. If circulatory failure persists and sufficient cellular dysfunction occurs, dysfunction of multiple organ systems results. Multiple organ failure may be fatal, even without massive cell death, if cellular dysfunction is severe enough to interfere with organ function in a manner incompatible with life.

HEART   Cardiac dysfunction is frequent during circulatory shock. In cardiogenic shock, this dysfunction usually results from myocardial infarction or ischemia. Myocardial dysfunction, in turn, can exacerbate myocardial ischemia, setting up a vicious cycle. The increased ventricular diastolic pressures that result from heart failure reduce the pressure gradient for coronary perfusion, and the additional wall stress elevates myocardial oxygen requirements. Tachycardia reduces the time available for diastolic filling, further compromising coronary blood flow. Ischemia also decreases diastolic compliance, further increasing ventricular diastolic pressures.

In other forms of shock, most notably sepsis, ischemia is less important; myocardial dysfunction is associated with release of circulating myocardial depressant substances. Pulmonary hypertension and increased right ventricular afterload can cause right sided heart failure after pulmonary embolism and may contribute to limitation of cardiac output in sepsis. Decreased myocardial responsiveness to catecholamines and diastolic dysfunction may also contribute to myocardial dysfunction in sepsis.

BRAIN Most patients with circulatory failure have abnormalities of mental status, usually manifested as confusion. The etiology is multifactorial; hypoperfusion, hypoxemia, acid-base abnormalities, and electrolyte disturbances all contribute. Cerebral autoregulation compensates to an extent for hypoperfusion, but when mean arterial pressure is <60 mmHg, compensation begins to fail, and critical cerebral hypoperfusion can lead to ischemic injury.

LUNGS Pulmonary dysfunction occurs early in shock. Acute lung injury causes decreased compliance, impaired gas exchange, and shunting of blood through unventilated areas. The clinical consequence of this injury, severe hypoxemia with bilateral pulmonary infiltrates in the setting of normal filling pressures, constitutes the acute respiratory distress syndrome (ARDS) (see Chap. 265). Work of breathing increases, with increased respiratory muscle oxygen requirements in the setting of tissue hypoperfusion. Respiratory muscle fatigue and ventilatory failure can ensue, requiring mechanical ventilation. The pathologic hallmarks of early ARDS are neutrophil-fibrin aggregates within the pulmonary microvasculature. With progression, there is extension of inflammation into the interstitium and alveoli and exudation of proteinaceous fluid into the alveolar space. Consolidation and fibrosis are seen in the end stages.

KIDNEYS Renal perfusion is compromised by circulatory failure, in part because blood flow is directed preferentially toward the heart and brain and away from the kidney. Increased afferent arteriolar tone initially compensates for decreased renal blood flow and maintains glomerular perfusion. When this compensatory mechanism fails, reduction in renal cortical blood flow can lead to acute tubular necrosis and renal failure. Associated insults such as nephrotoxic drugs, intravenous contrast medium, or rhabdomyolysis can exacerbate renal injury in shock.

LIVER AND GASTROINTESTINAL TRACT Hepatic injury results from hypoperfusion, often complicated in septic and traumatic shock by activation of Kuppfer cells and release of cytokines. Derangements of metabolic function of the liver include impairment of both synthesis and detoxification. Phagocytic clearance within the hepatic reticuloendothelial system is also impaired. Increased serum levels of transaminases, lactic dehydrogenase, and bilirubin reflect hepatic parenchymal injury. Decreased levels of albumin and clotting factors indicate decreased synthetic capability. Dramatic increases in transaminases can be seen with profound hypoxemia or hypotension ("shock liver"); these are transient and resolve rapidly with reperfusion. Ischemic liver injury affects the center of the hepatic lobule (venous end) most prominently, with relative sparing of the portal (arterial) end; this is seen pathologically as central congestion and centrilobular necrosis. In septic shock, intrahepatic cholestasis can be present, with marked increases in bilirubin and only modest increases in transaminases; these changes may reflect dysfunction of bile canaliculi due to bacterial toxins.

Splanchnic blood flow is compromised in circulatory shock as blood flow is diverted elsewhere. Intestinal ischemia may occur, and injury may be further exacerbated by subsequent release of oxygen radicals during reperfusion following resuscitation. It has been hypothesized that ischemia/reperfusion injury may compromise the integrity of the intestinal mucosal barrier, leading to translocation of bacterial toxins, although this has not been demonstrated conclusively in patients. Splanchnic hypoperfusion can also lead to stress ulceration,

ileus, and malabsorption, and occasionally acalculous cholecystitis or pancreatitis may occur.

HEMATOLOGIC SYSTEM Abnormalities of coagulation are frequent in both septic and traumatic shock. Thrombocytopenia can result from hemodilution associated with volume repletion. Thrombocytopenia in sepsis is common, usually immunologically mediated, and often complicated by underlying illness and medications. Activation of the coagulation cascade within the microvasculature can lead to disseminated intravascular coagulation (Chap. 118), which leads to thrombocytopenia, microangiopathic hemolytic anemia, decreased fibrinogen, and circulating fibrin split products. Microvascular consumption of clotting factors can lead to their depletion, with subsequent hemorrhage.

PATHOGENESIS OF SPECIFIC FORMS OF SHOCK

The pathogenesis of different forms of shock is shown in Fig. 38-1. In hypovolemic, cardiogenic, and extracardiac obstructive shock, decreased tissue perfusion results from inadequate cardiac output. In distributive shock, decreased arterial pressure results from decreased systemic vascular resistance, and maldistribution of blood flow in the microcirculation is a major contributing factor to multiple organ system failure.

HYPOVOLEMIC SHOCK Hypovolemic shock has been studied extensively and its stages can be easily quantitated in experimental animals by the stepwise removal of blood from the intravascular space. Many of the lessons learned from these studies are applicable to other forms of shock with reduced cardiac output. With the loss of 10 percent of total blood volume, compensatory mechanisms are activated that maintain cardiac output despite decreased filling pressure and stroke volume. Increased adrenergic activity, resulting from both increased sympathetic discharge and adrenal release of catecholamines, leads to arterial vasoconstriction, venoconstriction with augmented venous return, and tachycardia. Reduction in hydrostatic pressure in the capillaries, along with precapillary arteriolar vasoconstriction, favors transudation of fluid from the extracellular space into the vessels. Intravas-

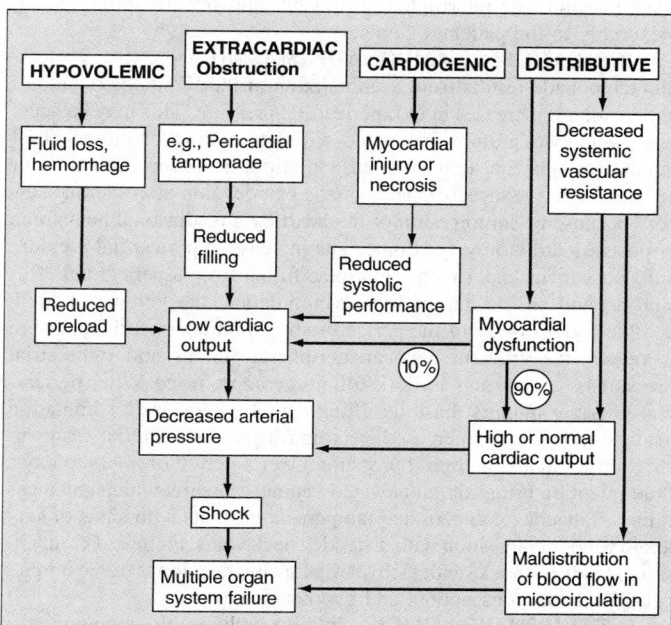

FIGURE 38-1 Pathogenesis of shock in humans. This schematic diagram depicts the present understanding of the pathogenetic relationships among the different types of shock and the cardiovascular abnormalities they usually produce.

cular volume contraction leads to activation of the renin-angiotensin system, increased release of antidiuretic hormone, and elevated levels of ACTH and aldosterone; renal sodium and water retention ensue. These adaptations may be sufficient to maintain arterial pressure, and orthostatic hypotension may be the only sign of early hypovolemia. However, if 20 to 25 percent of the blood volume is lost rapidly, the compensatory mechanisms begin to fail and the clinical shock syndrome ensues. Cardiac output declines, and there is hypotension despite generalized vasoconstriction. Reduced tissue perfusion leads to anaerobic metabolism, manifested by elevated lactate levels and metabolic acidosis. Reflex adrenergic discharge is intensified, and flow is redistributed to maintain perfusion to the brain and heart. This redistribution reflects the predominance of autoregulation of blood flow in the cerebral and coronary systems in contrast to the dependence of flow in other organs on sympathetic tone. Excessive vasoconstriction can reduce flow to the point that cellular damage occurs. Damage to the capillary endothelium leads to loss of fluid and proteins from the circulation, further exacerbating the hypovolemia. Ultimately end-organ damage and multiple organ system failure ensue.

CARDIOGENIC SHOCK (See also Chap. 243) When myocardial function is depressed, several compensatory mechanisms are activated. Sympathetic stimulation increases heart rate and contractility, and renal fluid retention increases preload. If cardiac output cannot be maintained by these mechanisms, blood flow is redistributed to maintain cerebral and cardiac perfusion. In a failing heart, the compensatory mechanisms may ultimately become dysfunctional. Increased heart rate and contractility can raise myocardial oxygen demand and exacerbate ischemia. In addition, tachycardia decreases diastolic filling time, further compromising myocardial perfusion. Fluid retention may increase intravascular volume to the point where pulmonary congestion and hypoxemia occur. Ischemia also decreases ventricular diastolic compliance, further elevating left atrial pressures and worsening pulmonary congestion. Vasoconstriction to maintain blood pressure can compromise renal, splanchnic, and cutaneous perfusion. The increased systemic vascular resistance caused by this vasoconstriction increases myocardial afterload, further impairing cardiac performance and increasing myocardial oxygen demand. This increased demand, in the face of inadequate perfusion, leads to worsening ischemia and a vicious cycle that must be interrupted to prevent a downward spiral leading inexorably to the patient's demise.

PERICARDIAL TAMPONADE (See also Chap. 240) Pericardial tamponade results from accumulation of fluid in the pericardium with resultant increases in intrapericardial pressure. This may be acute (e.g., hemopericardium associated with penetrating or closed chest trauma) or subacute (e.g., uremia, radiation, neoplasm, infection, or connective tissue disease). Tamponade can develop after cardiac surgery because of compression of the heart by a mediastinal hematoma or postpericardiotomy syndrome. The increase in pericardial pressure and consequent impairment of cardiac filling from a pericardial effusion depend on the rate of fluid accumulation, the volume of fluid, and the distensibility of the pericardium. As intrapericardial pressure increases, the gradient between peripheral venous and right atrial pressure is reduced and diastolic filling is compromised. When pericardial pressure impairs diastolic filling acutely, adrenergic stimulation leads to tachycardia, increased ejection fraction, and arterial vasoconstriction to maintain arterial pressure. Over a period of hours to days, fluid retention brings about elevated venous pressure, which enhances filling. Subacute, compensated tamponade presents with signs of systemic venous congestion with distended neck veins. Failure of compensation leads to shock, with tachycardia, tachypnea, low cardiac output, peripheral vasoconstriction, and hypotension.

DISTRIBUTIVE SHOCK In this condition, tissue hypoperfusion results from abnormal shunting of a normal or increased cardiac output. Although the differential diagnosis includes anaphylaxis, drug overdose, neurogenic shock, and Addisonian crisis, the most important and prevalent etiology is septic shock (Chap. 124). In some forms of

distributive shock, organ blood flow appears adequate, but a mediator-induced "metabolic block" exists at the tissue level, preventing adequate utilization of oxygen and other nutrients. Lactate accumulates because cells are unable to use oxidative metabolic pathways normally. Thus, in some patients, blood flow through large vessels to tissues is adequate, but abnormalities of microvascular flow or an inability of cells to utilize nutrients leads to widespread cellular dysfunction and progressive shock.

Septic shock results when infectious agents or infection-induced mediators in the bloodstream induce cardiovascular decompensation. Septic shock is characterized at the onset by a high cardiac output and a low systemic vascular resistance. As shown in Fig. 38-2, septic shock usually begins with a nidus of infection that releases microorganisms into the bloodstream. Toxic effects can result from the organisms

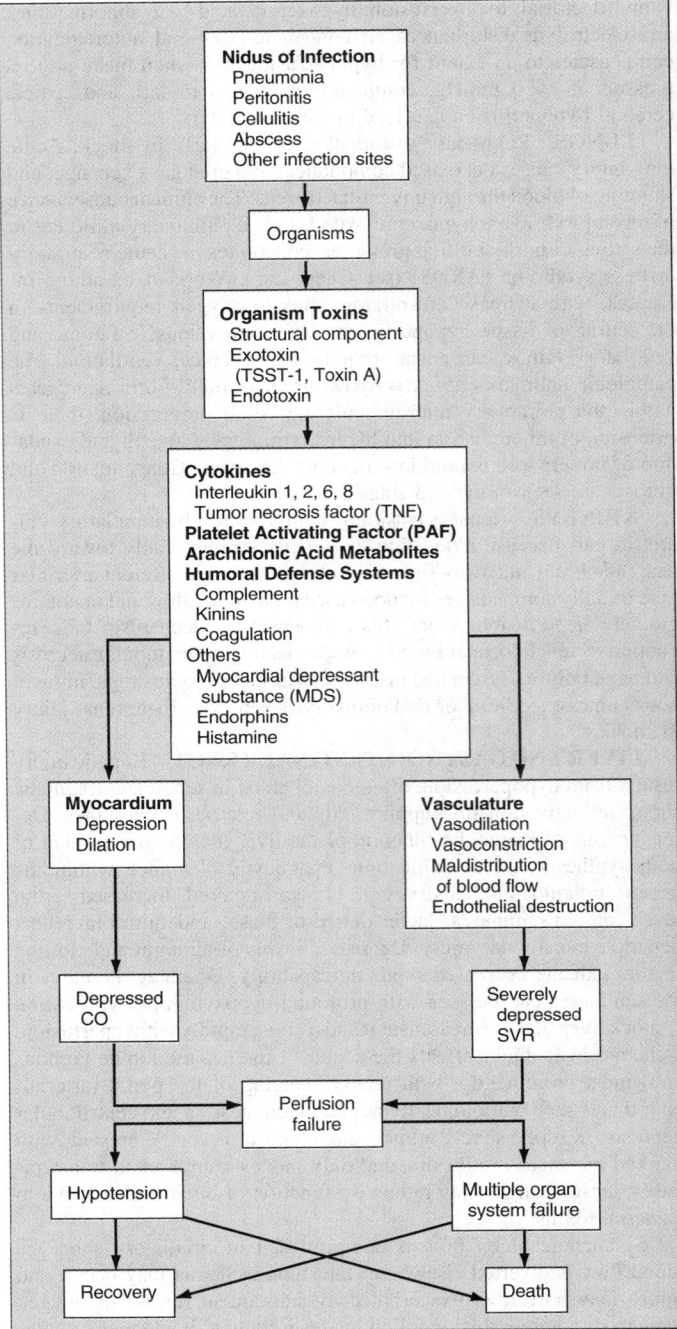

FIGURE 38-2 Pathogenesis of human septic shock. This schematic diagram represents the present understanding of the interrelationships in the pathogenesis of septic shock in humans. CO, cardiac output; SVR, systemic vascular resistance. (*Modified from Parrillo et al, 1990.*)

themselves; from components such as endotoxin, the lipopolysaccharide associated with the outer membrane of gram-negative bacteria; or from elaboration of exotoxins. The most important pathologic effects of these organisms and toxins may result from stimulation of the release of massive quantities of endogenous inflammatory mediators. Endotoxin is a potent trigger for release of cytokines, most notably the interleukins and TNF, which amplify the systemic response to endotoxin by stimulating neutrophils, endothelial cells, and platelets and by causing the release of other mediators, such as PAF, arachidonic acid metabolites, complement, kinins, histamine, and endorphins.

The effects of these mediators can be divided into two broad categories: effects on the peripheral vasculature and effects on the heart. Both exogenous and endogenous mediators have been shown to mediate peripheral vasodilation in sepsis. Administration of small doses of endotoxin to normal volunteers causes a decrease in arterial pressure, an increase in cardiac output, and a decrease in systemic vascular resistance similar to those seen in sepsis. Similar vasodilation with increased cardiac output occurs after administration of TNF, IL-1, or IL-2. A pivotal mediator of vasodilation in response to cytokines is nitric oxide, which is formed from arginine by the enzyme nitric oxide synthase (Chap. 71). Endotoxin, TNF, and interleukins can stimulate inducible nitric oxide synthase in macrophages and vascular smooth muscle cells, with release of large amounts of this vasodilatory molecule.

Endotoxin can also activate the intrinsic coagulation cascade along with the fibrinolytic system; this can lead to deposition of fibrin microaggregates in the microvasculature, obstructing flow and exacerbating tissue hypoxia. TNF and the interleukins activate both endothelial cells and neutrophils, leading to neutrophil aggregation and further microcirculatory insufficiency.

Although patients with septic shock have high cardiac outputs, left and right ventricular ejection fractions are reduced. Dilation of the ventricles allows normal stroke volumes to be maintained despite the depression of myocardial contractility, and tachycardia results in an elevated cardiac output. Septic patients also manifest a decreased ventricular stroke work response to volume infusion, further indicating depressed myocardial performance. The mechanisms responsible have not been completely clarified; it appears that cytokines, particularly TNF and IL-1, play an important role, possibly through generation of nitric oxide.

If septic shock persists, the combination of peripheral vascular abnormalities and myocardial depression results in a mortality of approximately 50 percent (Fig. 38-2). Death results from unrelenting hypotension and/or multiple organ system failure. The hypotension is associated with a severe and irreversible reduction in systemic vascular resistance. Occasionally (in about 10 percent of nonsurvivors) myocardial depression is so severe that cardiac output becomes low, exacerbating the hypotension.

CLINICAL MANIFESTATIONS

Some symptoms and signs are similar for all types of shock. The condition is almost always characterized by hypotension, which in adults generally refers to a mean arterial pressure below 60 mmHg. In interpreting any given level of arterial pressure, however, the chronic level of pressure must be considered; patients with severe chronic hypertension may be relatively hypotensive when their mean arterial pressure declines by 40 mmHg, even if it still exceeds 60 mmHg. Conversely, patients with chronically low arterial pressures may not exhibit clinical abnormalities until mean pressure falls below 50 mmHg. Common manifestations of shock include tachycardia, oliguria, a clouded sensorium, and cool, mottled extremities indicative of reduced blood flow to the skin. Metabolic acidosis, often due to elevated blood lactate levels, reflects prolonged inadequate blood flow to tissues.

Other clinical manifestations are specific to the type of shock. Patients with hypovolemic shock frequently have a history of gastrointestinal bleeding, hemorrhage from another site, or clear evidence of large volume losses via diarrhea and/or vomiting. Patients with

cardiogenic shock usually have symptoms and signs of heart disease, including elevated filling pressures, gallop rhythms, and other evidence of heart failure. Mechanical causes of cardiogenic shock frequently cause heart murmurs, such as those of mitral regurgitation, aortic stenosis, or ventricular septal defect. Patients with pericardial tamponade may demonstrate pulsus paradoxus and distant heart sounds. In patients with distributive shock due to sepsis, there may be evidence of localized infection as well as fever and chills. Patients with sepsis and neutropenia are less likely to have a clinically evident nidus of infection and may be septic from their own skin or bowel flora.

Approach to the Patient

Shock is an emergency. Optimal management entails balancing the need to initiate therapy before shock causes irreversible damage to vital organs against the need to perform the clinical assessment required to understand the cause of shock and target therapy to that cause. A practical approach is to make a rapid evaluation initially, based on a limited history and physical examination, and initiate specific diagnostic procedures directed toward determining the cause and severity of shock. Initial tests ordinarily include a chest x-ray, electrocardiogram, measurement of arterial blood gas and electrolyte levels, a complete blood count, and other tests directed as specific questions raised by the initial examination. Right heart catheterization with a balloon-tipped, flow-directed (Swan-Ganz) catheter is frequently useful. As this initial evaluation is in progress, therapy should be initiated. After stabilization, a more comprehensive diagnostic evaluation should be undertaken, and the response to the initial therapeutic interventions should be assessed.

USE OF RIGHT HEART CATHETERIZATION TO EVALUATE SHOCK The different categories of shock (see Table 38-1) have different hemodynamic profiles (Table 38-2). Patients with mild hypovolemic shock may be treated successfully with simple fluid replacement. In patients with moderate or severe shock, however, right heart catheterization is often useful, not only for providing a diagnostic hemodynamic assessment but also for monitoring the response to therapy, because noninvasive evaluation is frequently incorrect in estimating filling pressures and cardiac output.

Table 38-2 summarizes the usual findings at right heart catheterization in patients with different forms of shock. Individual patients may present with hemodynamic features of more than one type of shock, but when these profiles are combined with clinical findings and the calculation of systemic vascular resistance, the etiology of most cases of shock can be categorized.

℞ TREATMENT

General Principles Whenever possible, patients should be treated in an intensive care unit. Continuous electrocardiographic monitoring should be performed for detection of rhythm disturbances, and an arterial line should be in place for beat-to-beat measurement of arterial pressures. Pulse oximetry is often useful to detect fluctuations in arterial oxygenation. In most case of shock that cannot be reversed rapidly, serial measurements of left and right ventricular filling pressures and cardiac output should be performed. Frequent measurements of arterial blood gases, serum electrolytes, complete blood counts, and coagulation parameters should be done to follow the patient's progress and to monitor the effects of therapy. Serum calcium, phosphorus and magnesium levels should be checked as well, because substantial reductions in these ions can be associated with depression of myocardial and respiratory muscle function. The frequency of measurements should be based on the clinical course and the perceived need to assess responses to therapy.

Guidelines for managing shock are listed in Table 38-3. In general, the goals of treating shock are to maintain mean arterial pressure and to ensure adequate perfusion and delivery of oxygen and other nutrients to the vital organs. Tissue hypoperfusion and

Table 38-2

Use of Right Heart Catheterization to Diagnose the Etiology of Shock

Diagnosis	Pulmonary Capillary Wedge Pressure	Cardiac output (CO)	Miscellaneous Comments
Cardiogenic shock			
Cardiogenic shock due to myocardial dysfunction	↑↑	↓↓	Usually occurs with evidence of extensive myocardial infarction (>40% of LV infarcted), severe cardiomyopathy, or myocarditis
Cardiogenic shock due to a mechanical defect			
Acute ventricular septal defect	↑	LVCO ↓↓ and RVCO > LVCO	Predominant shunt is left to right, pulmonary blood flow is greater than systemic blood flow: oxygen "step-up" occurs at RV level
Acute mitral regurgitation	↑↑	Forward CO ↓↓	V waves in pulmonary capillary wedge pressure tracing
Right ventricular infarction	Normal or ↓	↓↓	Elevated RA and RV filling pressures with low or normal pulmonary capillary wedge pressures
Extracardiac obstructive forms of shock			
Pericardial tamponade	↑	↓ or ↓↓	RA mean, RV end-diastolic pulmonary capillary wedge mean pressures are elevated and within 5 mmHg of one another
Massive pulmonary embolism	Normal or ↓	↓↓	Usual finding is elevated right-sided pressures
Hypovolemic shock	↓↓	↓↓	
Distributive forms of shock			
Septic shock	↓ or normal	↑ or normal, rarely ↓	
Anaphylactic shock	↓ or normal	↑ or normal	

↑↑ or ↓↓ designates a moderate to severe increase or decrease: ↑ or ↓ designates a mild to moderate increase or decrease; CO, cardiac output; RA, right atrium; RV, right ventricle; LV, left vetricle.

NOTE: Systemic vascular resistance is increased, initially, in all forms of shock except distributive shock, in which it is usually reduced.

SOURCE: Modified from SM Hollenberg and JE Parrillo, in Surgical Intensive Care, GT Shires, PL Barie (eds), New York, Little, Brown, 1993.

anaerobic metabolism can lead to formation and release of lactic acid into the bloodstream. A reduction of elevated serum lactate levels is one good indicator of successful resuscitation and is often used as a therapeutic goal. In addition to these general goals, specific forms of shock require therapy directed at the underlying processes.

Hypovolemic Shock Infusion of fluid is the fundamental treatment of acute hypovolemia. The challenge is to restore cardiac filling pressures to optimum levels promptly and adequately without inducing pulmonary edema and compromising oxygenation. A major increase in pulmonary microvascular pressure is the most important determinant of transudation of fluid into the pulmonary interstitium. The clinical implication of this observation is that monitoring of pulmonary hydrostatic pressure, by physical examination or measured hemodynamics, is critical during resuscitation. Regardless of the type and amount of fluid used for resuscitation, it is imperative to use physiologic endpoints to gauge the initial response to treatment and to adjust the therapy to meet the needs of the individual patient.

Crystalloids, either normal saline or Ringer's lactate, are usually used for initial resuscitation for most forms of hypovolemic shock. After the initial resuscitation, with up to several liters of crystalloid

Table 38-3

Guidelines for Managing Shock

Abnormality	Intervention*	Therapeutic Goal
Hypotension	ICU monitoring, volume expansion, vasopressor agents	Mean arterial pressure of at least 60 mmHg Pulmonary capillary wedge pressure between 14 and 18 mmHg
Tissue hypoperfusion	ICU monitoring, volume expansion, vasopressor agents, inotropic agents	Hemoglobin above 10 g/dL Oxygen saturation above 92% Cardiac index above 2.2(L/min)/m² Normal blood lactate concentration
Organ system dysfunction	ICU monitoring, volume expansion, vasopressors, inotropic agents	Normalize values or otherwise reverse evidence of dysfunction in the following systems: Renal—blood urea nitrogen and creatinine levels, urine output Hepatic—bilirubin level Pulmonary—arterial P_{O_2} and alveolar-arterial gradient Central nervous system—mental status
Infection	Appropriate antibiotics and surgical drainage, if necessary	Eradication of infection
Mediators producing toxic effects	Mediator inhibition†	Reversal of toxic effect

* ICU denotes intensive care unit.
† This therapy is still in the experimental phase.

SOURCE: Adapted from Parrillo, 1993

fluid, use of colloids, such as albumin or starch solutions, has been advocated as a more efficient and rapid method of fluid repletion that can help maintain colloid osmotic pressure. However, colloids are expensive, and despite numerous studies, a convincing benefit has not been demonstrated from administration of colloids rather than crystalloids for fluid repletion. Preliminary studies with hypertonic saline solutions suggest that effective resuscitation can be achieved using relatively small volumes of fluid; in some settings, such as burn resuscitation, such limitation of the volume of fluid administered may be important. In hemorrhagic shock, restoration of oxygen-carrying capacity is achieved through transfusion of packed red blood cells; the goal is to maintain a hemoglobin concentration of 10 g/dL.

Cardiogenic Shock In cardiogenic shock due to myocardial infarction (see also Chap. 243), therapy should be directed toward reducing myocardial ischemia and salvaging ischemic but reversibly damaged myocardium at the infarct border. Initial measures include supplemental oxygen and, when systolic blood pressure permits, administration of intravenous nitroglycerin. Insertion of an intraaortic balloon pump decreases ventricular afterload, improving myocardial performance and decreasing myocardial oxygen demand and improving coronary perfusion pressure by increasing aortic diastolic pressure. The possibility of acute mechanical abnormalities such as mitral regurgitation or ventricular septal defect should be excluded, with either echocardiography or right heart catheterization. Where possible, it is probably best to perform emergent coronary angiography to define the coronary anatomy and to attempt revascularization. Trials of revascularization with either angioplasty or bypass surgery for patients with cardiogenic shock have suggested improved survival compared to historical controls. Administration of thrombolytic agents is another alternative, although a mortality benefit for patients who present with myocardial infarction and cardiogenic shock has not been demonstrated in clinical trials.

Cardiogenic shock can also occur after prolonged cardiopulmonary bypass; the stunned myocardium may require hours or days to recover sufficiently to support the circulation. Treatment consists of cardiovascular support with the combination of inotropic agents such as dopamine, dobutamine, or amrinone and intraaortic balloon counterpulsation. Dopamine, which acts directly on myocardial $beta_1$-adrenergic receptors and indirectly by releasing norepinephrine, has both inotropic and vasopressor effects. Tachycardia and increased peripheral resistance with dopamine administration can potentially exacerbate myocardial ischemia. Dobutamine, a selective $beta_1$-adrenergic receptor agonist, can improve myocardial contractility and increase cardiac output without inducing marked changes in heart rate or systemic vascular resistance. Amrinone and milrinone are phosphodiesterase inhibitors with both positive inotropic and vasodilator actions. Amrinone and milrinone have longer half-lives than dobutamine and can cause hypotension, so they are often reserved for use when other agents have proven ineffective. Because they do not act directly through adrenergic receptors, they may be effective in situations in which beta-adrenergic receptors are diminished. The addition of amrinone or milrinone to dopamine or

dobutamine may be considered in patients who fail to respond to one class of agents alone.

Extracardiac Obstructive Shock Pericardial tamponade (Chap. 240) is the prototype of extracardiac obstructive shock and may be recognized by clinical manifestations (hypotension, jugular venous distention, pulsus paradoxus) and characteristic findings on echocardiography. Although intravascular volume expansion and sometimes vasopressor agents are useful temporizing measures, the only effective therapy is pericardial drainage via needle pericardiocentesis or surgery.

Pulmonary embolism (Chap. 261) is usually treated with systemic anticoagulation, but when massive pulmonary embolism causes right ventricular failure and shock, thrombolytic therapy should be strongly considered. In patients with contraindications to thrombolytic therapy, emergency surgical pulmonary embolectomy is an alternative, if there is sufficient time to make the diagnosis, mobilize the surgical team, and institute cardiopulmonary bypass.

Septic Shock (See also Chap. 124) Therapy of septic shock has three main components. First, the nidus of infection must be identified and eliminated, using surgical drainage, antibiotic therapy, or both. Rapid institution of appropriate antibiotic therapy leads to improved survival, but the specific organisms causing sepsis are usually not known when the patient presents. Accordingly, a broad-spectrum antibiotic regimen should be chosen initially that will be effective against all the likely causative microorganisms, given the patient's clinical presentation and the hospital's organism resistance patterns.

Second, while the source of sepsis is being eradicated, adequate organ system perfusion and function must be maintained, guided by cardiovascular monitoring. Since antibiotics usually require 48 h or more to sterilize a septic focus, maintenance of tissue oxygen delivery is crucial to a favorable outcome (Table 38-3). Since oxygen delivery is the product of blood hemoglobin concentration, oxygen saturation, and cardiac output, maintenance of a blood hemoglobin level greater than 10 g/dL, oxygen saturation higher than 92%, and adequate cardiac output are important therapeutic guidelines. Initial cardiovascular therapy should optimize preload by administering volume to attain a pulmonary artery wedge pressure of 14 to 18 mmHg. If the serum albumin level is low (<2 g/dL), concentrated albumin infusions may be used to increase intravascular oncotic pressure. Since tissue hypoperfusion in sepsis results in part from abnormal shunting of cardiac output, some clinicians advocate increasing cardiac output to very high, supranormal levels. However, use of inotropic agents to achieve such supranormal cardiac outputs has not been shown to be beneficial in controlled trials.

If fluid therapy alone fails to restore adequate arterial pressure and organ perfusion, therapy with vasopressor agents should be initiated (Table 38-4). For the persistently hypotensive patient, dopamine (Chap. 70) frequently raises arterial pressure and maintains or enhances blood flow to the renal and splanchnic circulations. Patients

Table 38-4

Commonly Used Vasopressor Agents (Relative Potency*)

Agent	Dose	Cardiac		Peripheral Vascular		
		Heart Rate	Contractility	Vasoconstriction	Vasodilation	Dopaminergic
Dopamine	1–4 (μ/kg)/min	1+	1+	0	1+	4+
	4–20 (μg/kg)/min	2+	2–3+	2–3+	0	2+
Norepinephrine	2–20 μg/min	1+	2+	4+	0	0
Dobutamine	2.5–15 (μg/kg)/min	1–2+	3–4+	0	2+	0
Isoproterenol	1–5 μg/min	4+	4+	0	4+	0
Epinephrine	1–20 μg/min	4+	4+	4+	3+	0
Phenylephrine	20–200 μg/min	0	0	3+	0	0

* The 1 to 4+ scoring system is an arbitrary system to allow a judgment of comparative potency among these vasopressor agents.
SOURCE: Adapted from JE Parrillo, Major Issues in Critical Care Medicine, JE Parrillo, SM Ayres (eds), Baltimore, Williams & Wilkins, 1984.

who remain hypotensive despite dopamine require norepinephrine, a more potent vasopressor. Once hypotension has been corrected, to optimize oxygen delivery to tissues, raising a low cardiac index with dobutamine can be useful.

The third therapeutic goal is to interrupt the pathogenic sequence leading to septic shock. Several multicenter trials have documented that early glucocorticoid therapy fails to improve either morbidity or mortality in septic shock. Newer therapies have focused on inhibiting potentially toxic mediators such as endotoxin, TNF, and IL-1. Trials of inhibitors of the mediators of sepsis, which include anti-endotoxin antibodies, anti-TNF antibodies, IL-1 receptor antagonists, and soluble TNF receptors, have not shown a significant reduction in mortality in septic patients to date. → *For further discussion, see also Chap. 124.*

BIBLIOGRAPHY

BUCHMAN TG et al: Molecular biology of circulatory shock. Part II. Expression of four groups of hepatic genes is enhanced after resuscitation from cardiogenic shock. Surgery 108:559, 1990

CIPOLLE MD et al: Secondary organ dysfunction. From clinical perspectives to molecular markers. Crit Care Clin 9:261, 1993

GATTINONI L et al: A trial of goal-oriented hemodynamic therapy in critically ill patients. N Engl J Med 333:1025, 1995

GOULD SA et al: Hypovolemic shock. Crit Care Clin 9:239, 1993

GUYTON AC: Cardiac output and circulatory shock, in *Human Physiology and Mechanisms of Disease*, 5th ed. Philadelphia, Saunders, 1991, pp 187–200

HOLLENBERG SM, CUNNIN RE: Endothelial and vascular smooth muscle function in sepsis. J Crit Care 9:262, 1994

MARTIN C et al: Norepinephrine or dopamine for the treatment of hyperdynamic septic shock. Chest 103:1826, 1993

MIMOZ O et al: Pulmonary artery catheterization in critically ill patients: A prospective analysis of outcome changes associated with catheter-prompted changes in therapy. Crit Care Med 22:573, 1994

PARRILLO JE: Pathogenetic mechanisms of septic shock. N Engl J Med 328:1471, 1993

——— et al: Septic shock in humans: Advances in the understanding of pathogenesis, cardiovascular dysfunction, and therapy. Ann Intern Med 113:227, 1990

SUFFREDINI AF: Current prospects for the treatment of clinical sepsis. Crit Care Med 22:S12, 1994

39 *Robert J. Myerburg, Agustin Castellanos*

CARDIOVASCULAR COLLAPSE, CARDIAC ARREST, AND SUDDEN CARDIAC DEATH

OVERVIEW AND DEFINITIONS

The vast majority of naturally occurring sudden deaths are caused by cardiac disorders. The magnitude of the problem of *cardiac* causes is highlighted by estimates that more than 300,000 sudden cardiac deaths (SCD) occur each year in the United States, as many as 50 percent of all cardiac deaths. SCD is a direct consequence of cardiac arrest, which is often reversible if responded to promptly. Since resuscitation techniques and emergency rescue systems are available to save patients who have out-of-hospital cardiac arrest, which was uniformly fatal in the past, understanding the SCD problem has practical importance.

SCD must be defined carefully. In the context of time, "sudden" is defined, for most clinical and epidemiologic purposes, as 1 h or less between the onset of the terminal clinical event and death. An exception is unwitnessed deaths in which pathologists may expand the definition of time to 24 h after the victim was last seen to be alive and stable.

Because of community-based interventions, victims may remain biologically alive for days or weeks after a cardiac arrest that has resulted in irreversible central nervous system damage. Confusion in terms can be avoided by adhering strictly to definitions of death, cardiac arrest, and cardiovascular collapse, as outlined in Table 39-1. Death is biologically, legally, and literally an absolute and irreversible event. Death may be delayed in a survivor of cardiac arrest, but "survival after sudden death" is contradictory. Currently, the accepted definition of SCD is *natural death due to cardiac causes,* heralded by abrupt loss of consciousness within *1 h* of the onset of acute symptoms, in an individual who may have known *preexisting* heart disease but in whom the *time* and *mode* of death are *unexpected.* When biologic death of the cardiac arrest victim is delayed because of interventions, the relevant pathophysiologic event remains the sudden and unexpected cardiac arrest that leads ultimately to death, even though delayed by artificial methods. The language used should reflect the fact that the index event was a cardiac arrest and that death was due to its delayed consequences.

ETIOLOGY, INITIATING EVENTS, AND CLINICAL EPIDEMIOLOGY

Extensive epidemiologic studies have identified populations at high risk for SCD. In addition, a large body of pathologic data provides information on the underlying *structural abnormalities* in victims of SCD, and clinical/physiologic studies have begun to identify a group of *transient functional factors* that may convert a long-standing underlying structural abnormality from a stable to an unstable state (Table 39-2). This information is developing into an understanding of the causes and mechanisms of SCD.

Cardiac disorders constitute the most common causes of sudden *natural* death. After an initial peak incidence of sudden death between birth and 6 months of age (the sudden infant death syndrome), the incidence of sudden death declines sharply and remains low through childhood and adolescence. The incidence begins to increase in young adults, reaching a second peak in the age range of 45 to 75 years. Increasing age in this range is a powerful risk factor for sudden *cardiac* death, and the proportion of cardiac causes among all sudden natural deaths increases dramatically with advancing years. From 1 to 13 years of age, only one of five sudden *natural* deaths is due to cardiac causes. Between 14 and 21 years of age, the proportion increases to 30 percent, and then to 88 percent in the middle-aged and elderly.

Young and middle-aged men and women have very different susceptibilities to SCD, but the gender differences decrease with advanc-

Table 39-1

Distinction Between Death, Cardiac Arrest, and Cardiovascular Collapse

Term	Definition	Qualifiers or Exceptions
Death	Irreversible cessation of all biologic functions	None
Cardiac arrest	Abrupt cessation of cardiac pump function which may be reversible by a prompt intervention but will lead to death in its absence	Rare spontaneous reversions; likelihood of successful interventions relates to mechanism of arrest and clinical setting
Cardiovascular collapse	A sudden loss of effective blood flow due to cardiac and/or peripheral vascular factors which may reverse spontaneously (e.g., neurocardiogenic syncope; vasovagal syncope) or only with interventions (e.g., cardiac arrest)	Nonspecific term which includes cardiac arrest and its consequences and also events which characteristically revert spontaneously

ing age. The overall male/female ratio is approximately 4:1, but in the 45- to 64-year-old age group, the male SCD excess is nearly 7:1. It falls to approximately 2:1 in the 65- to 74-year-old age group. The difference in risk for SCD parallels the risks for other manifestations of coronary heart disease in men and women. As the gap for other manifestations of coronary heart disease closes in the seventh and eighth decades of life, the excess risk of SCD also narrows. Despite the lower incidence in women, the classic coronary risk factors still operate in women—cigarette smoking, diabetes, hyperlipidemia, hypertension—and SCD remains an important clinical and epidemiologic problem.

Hereditary factors contribute to the risk of SCD, but largely in a nonspecific manner: They represent expressions of the hereditary predisposition to coronary heart disease. Except for a few specific syndromes, such as the genetic hyperlipoproteinemias (Chap. 341), congenital long QT interval syndromes (Chap. 231), and a number of myopathic and dysplastic syndromes there are no *specific* hereditary risk factors for SCD.

The major categories of structural causes of, and functional factors contributing to, the SCD syndrome are listed in Table 39-2. Worldwide, and especially in western cultures, coronary atherosclerotic heart disease is the most common structural abnormality associated with SCD. Up to 80 percent of all SCDs in the United States are due to the consequences of coronary atherosclerosis. The cardiomyopathies (di-

TABLE 39-2

Cardiac Arrest and Sudden Cardiac Death

STRUCTURAL CAUSES

I. Coronary heart disease
  A. Coronary artery abnormalities
    1. Chronic atherosclerotic lesions
    2. Acute (active) lesions
      (plaque fissuring, platelet aggregation, acute thrombosis)
    3. Anomalous coronary artery anatomy
  B. Myocardial infarction
    1. Healed
    2. Acute
II. Myocardial hypertrophy
  A. Secondary
  B. Hypertrophic cardiomyopathy
    1. Obstructive
    2. Nonobstructive
III. Dilated cardiomyopathy—primary muscle disease
IV. Inflammatory and infiltrative disorders
  A. Myocarditis
  B. Noninfectious inflammatory diseases
  C. Infiltrative diseases
V. Valvular heart disease
VI. Electrophysiologic abnormalities, structural
  A. Anomalous pathways in Wolff-Parkinson-White syndrome
  B. Conducting system disease
  C. Membrane channel structure (e.g., congenital long QT syndrome)

FUNCTIONAL CONTRIBUTING FACTORS

I. Alterations of coronary blood flow
  A. Transient ischemia
  B. Reperfusion after ischemia
II. Low cardiac output states
  A. Heart failure
    1. Chronic
    2. Acute decompensation
  B. Shock
III. Systemic metabolic abnormalities
  A. Electrolyte imbalance (e.g., hypokalemia)
  B. Hypoxemia, acidosis
IV. Neurophysiologic disturbances
  A. Autonomic fluctuations: central, neural, humoral
  B. Receptor function
V. Toxic responses
  A. Proarrhythmic drug effects
  B. Cardiac toxins (e.g., cocaine, digitalis intoxication)
  C. Drug interactions

lated and hypertrophic, collectively, Chap. 239) account for another 10 to 15 percent of SCDs, and all the remaining diverse etiologies cause only 5 to 10 percent of these events. Transient ischemia in the previously scarred or hypertrophied heart, hemodynamic and fluid and electrolyte disturbances, fluctuations in autonomic nervous system activity, and transient electrophysiologic changes caused by drugs or other chemicals (e.g., proarrhythmia) have all been implicated as mechanisms responsible for transition from electrophysiologic stability to instability. In addition, spontaneous reperfusion of ischemic myocardium, caused by vasomotor changes in the coronary vasculature and/or spontaneous thrombolysis, may cause transient electrophysiologic instability and arrhythmias.

PATHOLOGY Data from postmortem examinations of SCD victims parallel the clinical observations on the prevalence of coronary heart disease as the major structural etiologic factor. More than 80 percent of SCD victims have pathologic findings of coronary heart disease. The pathologic description often includes a combination of long-standing, extensive atherosclerosis of the epicardial coronary arteries and acute active coronary lesions, which include a combination of fissured or ruptured plaques, platelet aggregates, hemorrhage, and thombosis. In one study, chronic coronary atherosclerosis involving two or more major vessels with $\geq$75 percent stenosis was observed in 75 percent of the victims. In another study, atherosclerotic plaque fissuring, platelet aggregates, and/or acute thrombosis were observed in 95 of 100 individuals who had pathologic studies after SCD. Most of these acute changes were superimposed on preexisting chronic lesions.

As many as 70 to 75 percent of males who die suddenly have prior myocardial infarctions (MIs), but only 20 to 30 percent have recent acute MIs. A high incidence of left ventricular (LV) hypertrophy coexists with prior MIs.

CLINICAL DEFINITION OF FORMS OF CARDIOVASCULAR COLLAPSE (Table 39-1) *Cardiovascular collapse* is a general term connoting loss of effective blood flow due to acute dysfunction of the heart and/or peripheral vasculature. Cardiovascular collapse may be caused by vasodepressor syncope (vasovagal syncope, postural hypotension with syncope, neurocardiogenic syncope—see Chap. 20), a transient severe bradycardia, or cardiac arrest. The latter is distinguished from the transient forms of cardiovascular collapse in that it usually requires an intervention to achieve resuscitation. In contrast, vasodepressor syncope and many primary bradyarrhythmic syncopal events are transient and non-life-threatening, and the patient will regain consciousness spontaneously.

The most common electrical mechanism for true cardiac arrest is ventricular fibrillation (VF), which is responsible for 65 to 80 percent of cardiac arrests. Severe persistent bradyarrhythmias, asystole, and pulseless electrical activity (an organized electrical activity without mechanical response—formerly called electomechanical dissociation) cause another 20 to 30 percent. Sustained ventricular tachycardia (VT) with hypotension is a less common cause. Acute low cardiac output states, having precipitous onset, also may present clinically as a cardiac arrest. The causes include massive acute pulmonary emboli, internal blood loss from ruptured aortic aneurysm, intense anaphylaxis, cardiac rupture after myocardial infarction, and unexpected fatal arrhythmia due to electrolyte disturbances.

CLINICAL CHARACTERISTICS OF CARDIAC ARREST

PRODROME, ONSET, ARREST, DEATH SCD may be presaged by days, weeks, or months of increasing angina, dyspnea, palpitations, easy fatigability, and other nonspecific complaints. However, these *prodromal complaints* are generally predictive of any major cardiac event; they are not specific for predicting SCD.

The *onset of the terminal event*, leading to cardiac arrest, is defined as an acute change in cardiovascular status preceding cardiac arrest by up to 1 h. When the onset is instantaneous or abrupt, the probability that the arrest is cardiac in origin is >95 percent. Continuous ECG recordings, fortuitously obtained at the onset of a cardiac arrest, commonly demonstrate changes in cardiac electrical activity in the minutes or hours before the event. There is a tendency for the heart rate to increase and for advanced grades of premature ventricular contractions (PVCs) to evolve. Most cardiac arrests that occur by the mechanism of VF begin with a run of sustained or nonsustained VT, which then degenerates into VF.

Sudden unexpected loss of effective circulation may be separated into "arrythmic events" and "circulatory failure." Arrythmic events are characterized by a high likelihood of patients being awake and active immediately prior to the event, are dominated by VF as the electrical mechanism, and have a short duration of terminal illness (<1 h). In contrast, circulatory failure deaths occur in patients who are inactive or comatose, have a higher incidence of asystole than VF, have a tendency to a longer duration of terminal illness, and are dominated by noncardiac events preceding the terminal illness.

The onset of cardiac arrest may be characterized by typical symptoms of an acute cardiac event, such as prolonged angina or the pain of onset of MI, acute dyspnea or orthopnea, or the sudden onset of palpitations, sustained tachycardia, or light-headedness. However, in many patients, the onset is precipitous, without forewarning.

Cardiac arrest is, by definition, abrupt. Mentation may be impaired in patients with sustained VT during the onset of the terminal event. However, complete loss of consciousness is a *sine qua non* in cardiac arrest. Although rare spontaneous reversions occur, it is usual that cardiac arrest progresses to death within minutes (i.e., SCD has occurred) if active interventions are not undertaken promptly.

The ability to resuscitate the victim of cardiac arrest is related to the time from onset to institution of resuscitative efforts, the setting in which the event occurs, the mechanism (VF, VT, pulseless electrical activity, asystole), and the clinical status of the patient prior to the cardiac arrest. Those settings in which it is possible to institute prompt cardiopulmonary resuscitation (CPR) provide a better chance of a successful outcome. However, the outcome in intensive care units and other in-hospital environments is heavily influenced by the patient's preceding clinical status. The immediate outcome is good for cardiac arrest occurring in the intensive care unit in the presence of an acute cardiac event or transient metabolic disturbance, but the outcome for patients with far-advanced chronic cardiac disease or advanced noncardiac diseases (e.g., renal failure, pneumonia, sepsis, diabetes, cancer) is no more successful in hospital than in the out-of-hospital setting.

The success rate for initial resuscitation and ultimate survival from an out-of-hospital cardiac arrest depends in part on the mechanism of the event. When the mechanism is VT, the outcome is best (67 percent); VF is the next most successful (25 percent), and asystole and pulseless electrical activity generate dismal outcome statistics (Fig. 39-1). Advanced age also influences adversely the chances of successful resuscitation.

Progression to biologic death is a function of the mechanism of cardiac arrest and the length of the delay before interventions. VF or asystole, without CPR within the first 4 to 6 min, has a poor outcome, and there are few survivors among patients who had no life-support activities for the first 8 min after onset. Outcome statistics are improved considerably by lay bystander intervention (basic life support—see below) prior to definitive interventions (advanced life support—defibrillation) and by early defibrillation. Death during the hospitalization after a successfully resuscitated cardiac arrest relates closely to the severity of central nervous system injury. Anoxic encephalopathy and infections subsequent to prolonged respirator dependence account for 60 percent of the deaths. Another 30 percent occur as a consequence of low cardiac output states that fail to respond to interventions. Paradoxically, recurrent arrhythmias are the least common cause of death, accounting for only 10 percent of in-hospital deaths.

Among patients who have cardiac arrest in the setting of acute

MI, it is important to distinguish between primary and secondary cardiac arrests. *Primary* cardiac arrests refer to those that occur in the absence of hemodynamic instability, and *secondary* cardiac arrests are those that occur in patients in whom abnormal hemodynamics dominate the clinical picture before cardiac arrest. The success rate for immediate resuscitation in primary cardiac arrest during acute MI in a monitored setting should approach 100 percent. In contrast, as many as 70 percent of patients with secondary cardiac arrest succumb immediately or during the same hospitalization.

IDENTIFICATION OF PATIENTS AT RISK FOR SUDDEN CARDIAC DEATH Primary prevention of cardiac arrest depends on the ability to identify individual patients at high risk. One must view the problem in the context of the total number of events and the population pools from which they are derived. In Fig. 39-2A, the inverted triangle demonstrates that the annual incidence of SCD among an unselected adult population is 1 to 2 per 1000 population, largely reflecting the prevalence of those coronary heart disease patients among whom SCD is the first clinically recognized manifestation (20 to 25 percent of first coronary events are SCD). The incidence (percent per year) increases progressively with addition of identified coronary risk factors to populations free of prior coronary events. The most powerful factors are age, elevated blood pressure, LV hypertrophy, cigarette smoking, elevated serum cholesterol level, obesity, and nonspecific electrocardiographic abnormalities. These coronary risk factors are not specific for SCD but rather represent increasing risk for all coronary deaths. The proportion of coronary deaths that are sudden remains at approximately 50 percent in all risk categories. Despite the marked *relative* increased risk of SCD with addition of multiple risk factors (from 1 to 2 per 1000 population per year in an unselected population to as much as 50 to 60 per 1000 in subgroups having multiple risk factors for coronary artery disease), the *absolute* incidence remains relatively low when viewed as the relationship between the number of individuals who have a preventive intervention and the number of events that can be prevented. Specifically, a 50 percent reduction in annual SCD risk would be a huge *relative* decrease but would require an intervention in up to 200 unselected individuals to prevent one sudden death. These figures highlight the importance of primary prevention of coronary heart disease. Control of coronary risk factors may be the only practical method to prevent SCD in major segments of the population, because of the paradox that the majority of events occur in the large unselected subgroups rather than in the specific high-risk subgroups (compare "Events/Year" with "Percent/Year" in Fig. 39-2A). Under most conditions of higher level of risk,

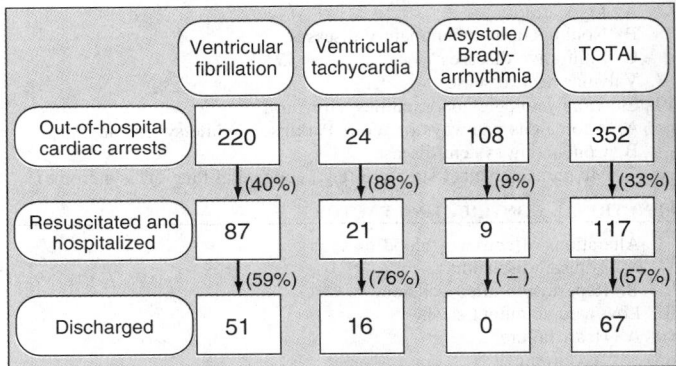

FIGURE 39-1 Initial electrophysiologic mechanisms recorded during out-of-hospital cardiac arrest. The figures highlighted by the boxes indicate the number of patients in each of three mechanism categories (ventricular fibrillation, ventricular tachycardia, and bradyarrhythmia/asystole). In each category, the data indicate the number of prehospital cardiac arrests (*top*), the number of patients successfully resuscitated in the field and transferred to the hospital alive (*middle*), and the number of patients who survived to be discharged from hospital (*bottom*). The percentages in parentheses indicate survivals between each level of care for each category. (*Modified from RJ Myerburg et al: Clinical, electrophysiologic, and hemodynamic profile of patients resuscitated from prehospital cardiac arrest. Am J Med 68:568, 1980, with permission*).

particularly those indexed to a recent major cardiovascular event (e.g., MI, recent onset of heart failure, survival after out-of-hospital cardiac arrest), the highest risk of sudden death occurs within the initial 6 to 18 months and then decreases toward baseline risk of the underlying disease (Fig. 39-2B). Accordingly, preventive interventions are most likely to be effective when initiated early.

For patients with acute or prior clinical manifestations of coronary heart disease, high-risk subgroups having a much higher ratio of SCD risk to population base can be identified. The acute, convalescent, and chronic phases of MI provide large population subsets with more

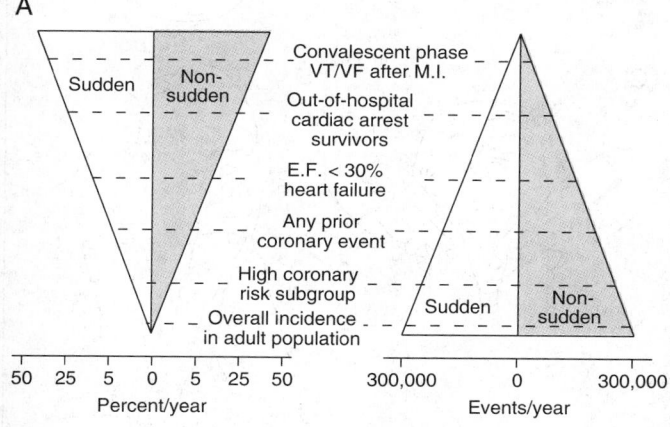

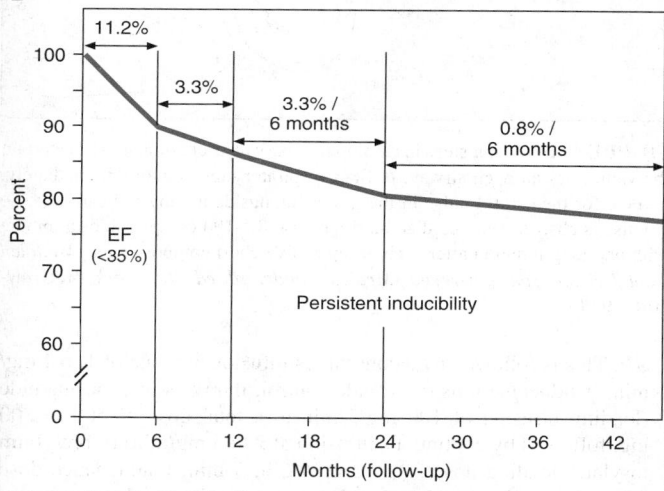

FIGURE 39-2 *A*. Incidence of sudden and nonsudden cardiac deaths in population subgroups, and the relation of total number of events per year to incidence figures. Approximations of subgroup incidence figures, and the related population pool from which they are derived, are presented. Approximately 50 percent of all cardiac deaths are sudden and unexpected. The incidence triangle on the left ("Percent/Year") indicates the approximate percentage of sudden and nonsudden deaths in each of the population subgroups indicated, ranging from the lowest percentage in unselected adult populations (0.1 to 2 percent per year) to the highest percentage in patients with VT or VF during convalescence after an MI (approximately 50 percent per year). The triangle on the right indicates the total number of events per year in each of these groups, to reflect incidence in context with the size of the population subgroups. The highest risk categories identify the smallest number of total annual events, and the lowest incidence category accounts for the largest number of events per year. (EF, ejection fraction; VT, ventricular tachycardia; VF, ventricular fibrillation; MI, myocardial infarction.) *B*. Time dependence of risk among survivors of out-of-hospital cardiac arrest. Recurrence risk is highest in the first 6 months of the index event. Survival is expressed as a percentage. High risk is best predicted initially by an ejection fraction ≤ 35 percent during the first 6 months, and subsequently persistent inducibility of VT during electrophysiologic testing becomes an added major risk. *n* = 101 at *t* = 0. [*After T Furukawa et al, in RJ Myerberg et al, Circulation 85(Suppl 1):2, 1992. Reproduced with permission of the American Heart Association.*]

highly focused risk (Chap. 243). The potential risk of cardiac arrest from the onset through the first 72 h after acute MI (the acute phase) may be as high as 15 to 20 percent. The highest risk of SCD in relation to MI is found in the subgroup that has experienced sustained VT or VF during the convalescent phase (3 days to 8 weeks) after MI. A greater than 50 percent mortality in 6 to 12 months has been observed among these patients, when managed with conservative medical therapy, and at least 50 percent of the deaths are sudden. Since the development of aggressive intervention techniques, the incidence appears to have fallen dramatically.

After the acute phase of MI, long-term risk for total mortality and SCD are predicted by a number of factors. The most important for both SCD and non-SCD is the extent of myocardial damage sustained during the acute event. This is measured by the degree of reduction in the ejection fraction (EF), functional capacity, and/or the occurrence of heart failure. Increasing *frequency* of postinfarction PVCs, with a plateau above the range of 10 to 30 PVCs per hour on 24-h ambulatory monitor recordings, also indicates increased risk, but advanced *forms* (salvos, nonsustained VT) are probably the more powerful predictor. PVCs interact strongly with decreased left ventricular EF. The combination of frequent PVCs, salvos or nonsustained VT, and an EF ≤ 30 percent identifies patients who have an annual risk of 20 percent. The risk falls off sharply with decreasing PVC frequency and the absence of advanced forms, as well as with higher EF. Despite the risk implications of postinfarction PVCs, improved outcome as a result of PVC suppression has not been demonstrated (Chap. 231).

The extent of underlying disease due to any cause and/or prior clinical expression of risk of SCD (i.e., survival after out-of-hospital cardiac arrest not associated with acute MI) identify patients at very high risk for subsequent (recurrent) cardiac arrest. Survival after out-of-hospital cardiac arrest predicts up to a 30 percent 1-year recurrent cardiac arrest rate in the absence of specific interventions (see below).

A general rule is that the risk of SCD is approximately one-half the total cardiovascular mortality rate. Thus, the SCD risk is approximately 20 percent per year for patients with advanced coronary heart disease or dilated cardiomyopathy severe enough to result in a 40 percent 1-year total mortality rate. As shown in Fig. 39-2A, the very high risk subgroups provide more focused population fractions ("Percent/Year") for predicting cardiac arrest or SCD; but the impact on the overall population, indicated by the absolute number of preventable events ("Events/Year"), is considerably smaller. The requirements for achieving a major population impact are effective prevention of the underlying diseases and/or new epidemiologic probes that will allow better resolution of subgroups within large general populations.

℞ TREATMENT

The individual who collapses suddenly is managed in four stages: (1) the initial response and basic life support, (2) advanced life support, (3) postresuscitation care, and (4) long-term management. The initial response and basic life support can be carried out by physicians, nurses, paramedical personnel, and trained lay persons. There is a requirement for increasing skills as the patient moves through the stages of advanced life support, postresuscitation care, and long-term management.

Initial Response and Basic Life Support The initial response will confirm whether a sudden collapse is indeed due to a cardiac arrest. Observations for respiratory movements, skin color, and the presence or absence of pulses in the carotid or femoral arteries will promptly determine whether a life-threatening cardiac arrest has occurred. As soon as a cardiac arrest is suspected or confirmed, contacting an emergency rescue system (e.g., 911) should be the immediate priority.

Agonal respiratory movements may persist for a short time after the onset of cardiac arrest, but it is important to observe for severe stridor with a persistent pulse as a clue to aspiration of a foreign body or food. If this is suspected, a prompt Heimlich maneuver (see below) may dislodge the obstructing body. A precordial blow, or "thump," delivered firmly by the clenched fist to the junction of the middle and lower third of the sternum may occasionally revert VT or VF, but there is concern about converting VT *to* VF. Therefore, it has been recommended to use precordial thumps as an advanced life support technique when monitoring and defibrillation are available. This conservative application of the technique remains controversial.

The third action during the initial response is to clear the airway. The head is tilted back and chin lifted so that the oropharynx can be explored to clear the airway. Dentures or foreign bodies are removed, and the Heimlich maneuver is performed if there is reason to suspect that a foreign body is lodged in the oropharynx. If respiratory arrest precipitating cardiac arrest is suspected, a second precordial thump is delivered after the airway is cleared.

Basic life support, more popularly known as CPR, is intended to maintain organ perfusion until definitive interventions can be instituted. The elements of CPR are the establishment and maintenance of ventilation of the lungs and compression of the chest. Mouth-to-mouth respiration may be used if no specific rescue equipment is immediately available (e.g., plastic oropharyngeal airways, esophageal obturators, masked Ambu bag). Conventional ventilation techniques during CPR require the lungs to be inflated 10 to 12 times per minute, i.e., once every fifth chest compression when two persons are performing the resuscitation and twice in succession every 15 chest compressions when one person is carrying out both ventilation and chest wall compression.

Chest compression is based on the assumption that cardiac compression allows the heart to maintain a pump function by sequential filling and emptying of its chambers, with competent valves maintaining forward direction of flow. The technique is illustrated in Fig. 39-3. The palm of one hand is placed over the lower sternum, with the heel of the other resting on the dorsum of the lower hand. The sternum is depressed, with the arms remaining straight, at a rate of approximately 80 to 100 per minute. Sufficient force is applied to depress the sternum 3 to 5 cm, and relaxation is abrupt.

Advanced Life Support   Advanced life support is intended to achieve adequate ventilation, control cardiac arrhythmias, stabilize the hemodynamic status (blood pressure and cardiac output), and restore organ perfusion. The activities carried out to achieve these goals include (1) intubation with an endotracheal tube, (2) defibrillation/cardioversion and/or pacing, and (3) insertion of an intravenous line. Ventilation with O_2 (room air if O_2 is not immediately available) may promptly reverse hypoxemia and acidosis. The speed with which defibrillation/cardioversion is carried out is an important element for successful resuscitation. When possible, immediate defibrillation should precede intubation and insertion of an intravenous line; CPR should be carried out while the defibrillator is being charged. As soon as a diagnosis of VT or VF is obtained, a 200-J shock should be delivered. Additional shocks at higher energies, up to a maximum of 360 J, are tried if the initial shock does not successfully abolish VT or VF. Epinephrine, 1 mg intravenously, is given after failed defibrillation, and attempts to defibrillate are repeated. The dose of epinephrine may be repeated after intervals of 3 to 5 min.

If the patient is less than fully conscious upon reversion, or if two or three attempts fail, prompt intubation, ventilation, and arterial blood gas analysis should be carried out. Intravenous $NaHCO_3$, which was formerly used in large quantities, is no longer considered routinely necessary and may be dangerous in larger quantities. However, the patient who is persistently acidotic after successful defibrillation and intubation should be given 1 meq/kg $NaHCO_3$ initially and an additional 50 percent of the dose repeated every 10 to 15 min.

After initial unsuccessful defibrillation attempts, or with persistent electrical instability, a bolus of 1 mg/kg lidocaine is given intravenously (Chap. 243), and the dose is repeated in 2 min in those patients who have persistent ventricular arrhythmias or remain in

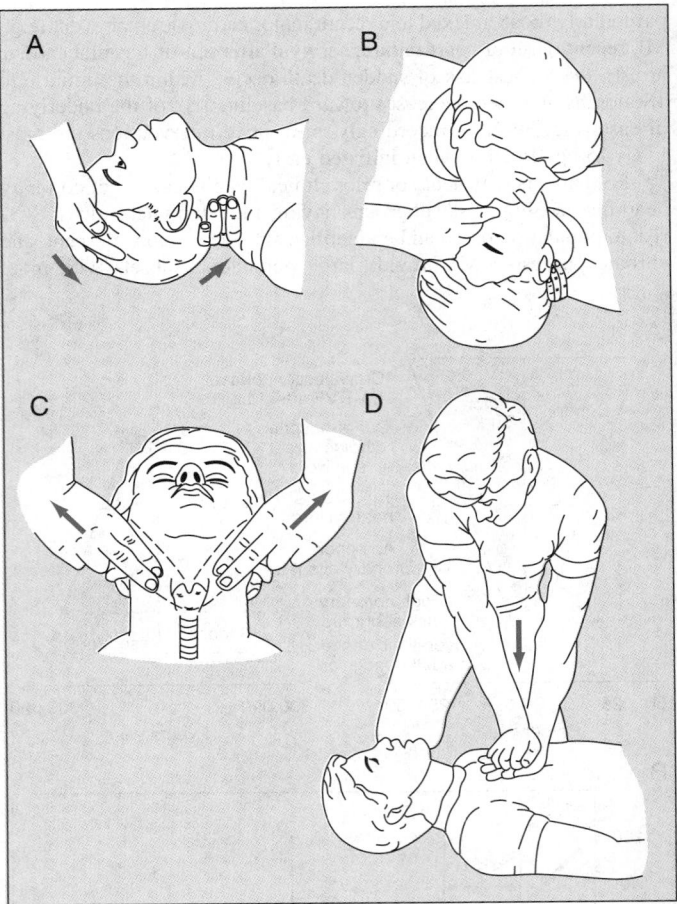

FIGURE 39-3   Major steps in cardiopulmonary resuscitation. *A*. Make certain the victim has an open airway. *B*. Start respiratory resuscitation immediately. *C*. Feel for the carotid pulse in the groove alongside the thyroid cartilage. *D*. If pulse is absent, begin cardiac massage. Use 80–100 compressions a minute with one lung inflation after each group of five chest compressions. *(Modified from J Henderson, Emergency Medical Guide, 4th ed, New York, McGraw-Hill, 1978.)*

VF. This is followed by a continuous infusion at a rate of 1 to 4 mg/min. If lidocaine fails to provide control, intravenous procainamide (loading infusion of 100 mg/5 min to a total dose of 500 to 800 mg, followed by continuous infusion at 2 to 5 mg/min) or bretylium tosylate (loading dose 5 to 10 mg/kg in 5 min; maintenance dose 0.5 to 2 mg/min) may be tried. Intravenous calcium gluconate is no longer considered safe or necessary for routine administration. It is used only in patients in whom acute hyperkalemia is known to be the triggering event for resistant VF, in the presence of known hypocalcemia, or in patients who have received toxic doses of calcium channel antagonists.

Cardiac arrest secondary to bradyarrhythmias or asystole is managed differently. Once it is known that this type of rhythm is present, there is no role for external shock. The patient is promptly intubated, CPR is continued, and an attempt is made to control hypoxemia and acidosis. Epinephrine and/or atropine are given intravenously or by an intracardiac route. External pacing devices are now available to attempt to establish a regular rhythm, but the prognosis is generally very poor in this form of cardiac arrest. The one exception is bradyarrhythmic/asystolic cardiac arrest secondary to airway obstruction. This form of cardiac arrest may respond promptly to removal of foreign bodies by the Heimlich maneuver or, in hospitalized patients, by intubation and suctioning of obstructing secretions in the airway.

Postresuscitation Care   This phase of management is determined by the clinical setting of the cardiac arrest. *Primary VF in acute MI* (Chap. 243) is generally very responsive to life-support techniques and easily controlled after the initial event. Patients are maintained on a lidocaine infusion at the rate of 2 to 4 mg/min for 24 to 72 h after the event. In the in-hospital setting, respirator support is usually not necessary or is needed for only a short time, and hemodynamics stabilize promptly after defibrillation or cardioversion. In *secondary VF in acute MI* (those events in which hemodynamic abnormalities predispose to the potentially fatal arrhythmia), resuscitative efforts are less often successful, and in those patients who are successfully resuscitated, the recurrence rate is high. The clinical picture is dominated by hemodynamic instability. In fact, the outcome is determined more by the ability to control hemodynamic dysfunction than by electrophysiologic abnormalities. Bradyarrhythmias, asystole, and pulseless electrical activity are commonly secondary events in hemodynamically unstable patients and are less responsive to interventions.

The outcome after in-hospital cardiac arrest associated with *noncardiac* diseases is poor, and in the few successfully resuscitated patients, the postresuscitation course is dominated by the nature of the underlying disease. Patients with cancer, renal failure, acute central nervous system disease, and uncontrolled infections, as a group, have a survival rate of less than 10 percent after in-hospital cardiac arrest. Some major exceptions are patients with transient airway obstruction, electrolyte disturbances, proarrhythmic effects of drugs, and severe metabolic abnormalities, most of whom may have an excellent chance of survival if they can be resuscitated promptly and maintained while the transient abnormalities are being corrected.

Long-Term Management After Survival of Out-of-Hospital Cardiac Arrest Patients who do not suffer irreversible injury of the central nervous system and who achieve hemodynamic stability should have extensive diagnostic and therapeutic testing to guide long-term management. This aggressive approach is driven by the fact that statistics from the 1970s indicated survival after out-of-hospital cardiac arrest was followed by a 30 percent recurrent cardiac arrest rate at 1 year, 45 percent at 2 years, and a total mortality rate of almost 60 percent at 2 years. Historical comparisons suggest that these dismal statistics may be significantly improved by newer interventions, but the magnitude of the improvement is unknown because of the lack of concurrently controlled intervention studies.

Among those patients in whom an acute transmural MI is the cause of out-of-hospital cardiac arrest, the management is the same as in any other patient who suffers cardiac arrest during the acute phase of a documented MI (see Chap. 243). For almost all other categories of patients, however, extensive diagnostic studies are carried out to determine etiology, functional impairment, and electrophysiologic instability as guides to future management. In general, patients who have out-of-hospital cardiac arrest due to chronic ischemic heart disease, without an acute MI, are evaluated to determine whether transient ischemia or chronic electrophysiologic instability was the more likely cause of the event. If there is reason to suspect an ischemic mechanism, coronary revascularization or drugs, most commonly beta blockers, are used to reduce ischemia. Electrophysiologic instability is best identified by the use of programmed electrical stimulation to determine whether sustained VT or VF can be induced (Chap. 231). If so, this information can be used as a baseline against which to evaluate drug efficacy for prevention of inducibility or to determine suitability for map-guided antiarrhythmic surgery, or whether an implantable cardioverter/defibrillator (ICD) might be the best strategy. Using this technique in patients with EF of 30 percent or more, the recurrent cardiac arrest rate is less than 10 percent during the first year of follow-up when inducibility is suppressed

by a drug. The outcome is not as good for patients with EF under 30 percent but may be still better than the apparent natural history of survival after cardiac arrest. For patients for whom successful drug therapy cannot be identified by this technique, insertion of an ICD, antiarrhythmic surgery (e.g., coronary bypass surgery, aneurysmectomy, cryoablation), or empiric amiodarone therapy can be considered options (Chap. 231). Primary surgical success, defined as surviving the procedure and reverting to a noninducible status without drug therapy, is better than 90 percent when patients are selecte for ability to be mapped in the operating room. However, only a small fraction of patients meet the criteria. In addition, VT/VF *cannot* be induced in a number of survivors of cardiac arrest (30 to 50 percent), and inducible arrhythmias can be suppressed by drugs in no more than 20 to 30 percent of those whose arrhythmias can be induced. Because of these limitations of drug therapy and surgical approaches, ICD therapy has evolved into the most commonly used strategy for cardiac arrest survivors. ICDs have very good success rates for sensing and reverting life-threatening arrhythmias, but improvement in long-term total survival outcomes remains ill defined.

The ESVEM study has suggested that ambulatory monitor-based suppression of ambient arrhythmias is equivalent to electrophysiologically guided testing in predicting long-term outcome. This conclusion has generated a debate which remains to be resolved.

BIBLIOGRAPHY

AKHTAR M et al: Implantable cardioverter-defibrillator therapy for prevention of sudden cardiac death. Cardiol Clin 11:97, 1993

CRANDALL BG et al: Implantable cardioverter-defibrillator therapy in survivors of out-of-hospital sudden cardiac death without inducible arrhythmias. J Am Coll Cardiol 21:1186, 1993

CUMMINS RO et al: Improving survival from sudden cardiac arrest: The "chain of survival" concept. Circulation 83:1832, 1991

ECHT DS et al: Mortality and morbidity in patients receiving encainide, flecainide, or placebo: The Cardiac Arrhythmia Suppression Trial. N Engl J Med 324:781, 1991

EMERGENCY CARDIAC CARE COMMITTEE AND SUBCOMMITTEES, AMERICAN HEART ASSOCIATION: Guidelines for cardiopulmonary resuscitation and emergency cardiac care. JAMA 268:2172, 1992

HEIMLICH HJ: A life-saving maneuver to prevent food choking. JAMA 234:398, 1975

JASTREMSKI MS: In-hospital cardiac arrest. Ann Emerg Med 22:113, 1993

JOSLYN et al: Survival from out-of-hospital cardiac arrest: Effects of patient age and presence of 911 Emergency Medical Services phone access. Am J Emerg Med 11:200, 1993

KANNEL WB, SCHATZKIN A: Sudden death: Lessons from subsets in population studies. J Am Coll Cardiol 5(suppl 6):141B, 1985

MASON JW, for the Electrophysiologic Study versus Electrocardiographic Monitoring Investigators: A comparison of electrophysiologic testing with Holter monitoring to predict antiarrhythmic drug efficacy for ventricular tachyarrhythmias. N Engl J Med 329:445, 1993

MYERBURG RJ, CASTELLANOS A: Cardiac arrest and sudden cardiac death, in *Heart Disease*, 5th ed, E Braunwald (ed). Philadelphia, Saunders, 1997, pp 742–779

——— et al: Epidemiology, transient risk, and intervention assessment. Ann Intern Med 119:1187, 1993

ORNATO JP: Use of adrenergic agonists during CPR in adults. Ann Emerg Med 22:411, 1993

WILBER DJ et al: Out-of-hospital cardiac arrest: Use of electrophysiologic testing in the prediction of long-term outcome. N Engl J Med 318:19, 1988

WILLICH SN et al: Sudden cardiac death. Support for a role of triggering in causation. Circulation 87:1442, 1993

40 Raj K. Goyal

DYSPHAGIA

Dysphagia is defined as a sensation of "sticking" or obstruction of the passage of food through the mouth, pharynx, or esophagus. It should be distinguished from other symptoms related to swallowing. *Aphagia* signifies complete esophageal obstruction, which is usually due to bolus impaction and represents a medical emergency. *Difficulty in initiating a swallow* occurs in disorders of the voluntary phase of swallowing. However, once initiated, swallowing is completed normally. *Odynophagia* means painful swallowing. Frequently, odynophagia and dysphagia occur together. *Globus pharyngeous* is the sensation of a lump lodged in the throat. However, no difficulty is encountered when swallowing is performed. *Misdirection of food*, resulting in nasal regurgitation and laryngeal and pulmonary aspiration of food during swallowing, is characteristic of oropharyngeal dysphagia. *Phagophobia*, meaning fear of swallowing, and *refusal to swallow* may occur in hysteria, rabies, tetanus, and pharyngeal paralysis due to fear of aspiration. Painful inflammatory lesions that cause odynophagia also may cause refusal to swallow. Some patients may feel the food as it goes down the esophagus. This esophageal sensitivity is not associated with the food sticking or obstruction, however. Similarly, the *feeling of fullness in the epigastrium* that occurs after a meal or after swallowing air should not be confused with dysphagia.

PHYSIOLOGY OF SWALLOWING The process of swallowing begins with a voluntary (oral) phase during which a bolus of food is pushed into the pharynx by the contraction of the tongue. The bolus then activates oropharyngeal sensory receptors that initiate the involuntary (pharyngeal and esophageal) phase, or deglutition reflex. The deglutition reflex is a complex series of events that serves both to propel food through the pharynx and the esophagus and to prevent its entry into the airway. When the bolus is propelled backward by the tongue, the larynx moves forward and the upper esophageal sphincter opens. As the bolus moves into the pharynx, contraction of the superior pharyngeal constrictor against the contracted soft palate initiates a peristaltic contraction that proceeds rapidly downward to move the bolus through the pharynx and the esophagus. The lower esophageal sphincter opens as the food enters the esophagus and remains open until the peristaltic contraction has swept the bolus into the stomach. Peristaltic contraction in response to a swallow involves inhibition followed by sequential contraction of muscles along the entire swallowing passage; this is called *primary peristalsis*. The inhibition that precedes the peristaltic contraction is called *deglutitive inhibition*. Local distention of the esophagus from food activates intramural reflexes in the smooth muscle and results in *secondary peristalsis*, limited to the thoracic esophagus. *Tertiary contractions* are nonperistaltic because they occur simultaneously over a long segment of the esophagus. Tertiary contractions may occur in response to a swallow or esophageal distention, or they may occur spontaneously.

PATHOPHYSIOLOGY OF DYSPHAGIA The normal transport of an ingested bolus through the swallowing passage depends on the size of the ingested bolus; the luminal diameter of the swallowing passage; the peristaltic contraction; and deglutitive inhibition, including normal relaxation of upper and lower esophageal sphincters during swallowing. Dysphagia caused by a large bolus or luminal narrowing is called *mechanical dysphagia*, whereas dysphagia due to incoordination or weakness of peristaltic contractions or to impaired deglutitive inhibition is called *motor dysphagia*.

Mechanical Dysphagia Mechanical dysphagia could be caused by a very large food bolus, intrinsic narrowing, or extrinsic compression of the lumen. In an adult, the esophageal lumen can distend up to a diameter of 4 cm because of the elasticity of the esophageal wall. When the esophagus cannot dilate beyond 2.5 cm in diameter, dysphagia to normal solid food can occur, but it is always present when it cannot distend beyond 1.3 cm. Circumferential lesions produce dysphagia more consistently than do lesions that involve only a portion of circumferences of the esophageal wall, as uninvolved segments retain their distensibility. The causes of mechanical dysphagia are listed in Table 40-1. Common causes include carcinoma, peptic and other benign strictures, and lower esophageal ring.

Motor Dysphagia Motor dysphagia may result from difficulty in initiating a swallow or from abnormalities in peristalsis and deglutitive inhibition due to diseases of the esophageal striated or smooth muscle.

Diseases of the striated muscle involve the pharynx, upper esophageal sphincter, and cervical esophagus. The striated muscle is innervated by a somatic component of the vagus with cell bodies of the lower motor neurons located in the nucleus ambiguus. These neurons are cholinergic and excitatory and are the sole determinant of the muscle activity. Peristalsis in the striated muscle segment is due to sequential central activation of neurons innervating muscles at different levels along the esophagus. Motor dysphagia of the pharynx results from neuromuscular disorders causing muscle paralysis, simultaneous nonperistaltic contraction, or loss of opening of the upper esophageal sphincter. Loss of opening of the upper sphincter is caused by paralysis of geniohyoid and other suprahyoid muscles or loss of deglutitive inhibition of the cricopharyngeus muscle. Because each side of the pharynx is innervated by ipsilateral nerves, a lesion of motor neurons occurring only on one side leads to unilateral pharyngeal paralysis. Although lesions of striated muscle also involve the cervical part of the esophagus, the clinical manifestations of pharyngeal dysfunction usually overshadow the manifestations due to esophageal involvement.

Diseases of the smooth muscle segment involve the thoracic part of the esophagus and the lower esophageal sphincter. The smooth muscle is innervated by the parasympathetic component of the vagal preganglionic fibers and postganglionic neurons in the myenteric ganglia. The vagal pathway consists of parallel excitatory and inhibitory pathways that use acetycholine and nitric oxide as neurotransmitters, respectively. The activation of inhibitory nerves causes inhibition that is followed by rebound contraction. These pathways are involved in the resting tone of the lower esophageal sphincter as well as swallow-induced lower esophageal sphincter opening and inhibition followed by peristaltic contractions in the esophageal body. Dysphagia results when the peristaltic contractions are weak or nonperistaltic or when the lower sphincter fails to open normally. Loss of contractile power occurs due to muscle weakness, as in scleroderma. The nonperistaltic contractions and impaired relaxation of the lower esophageal sphincter result from a defect in inhibitory vagal innervation and account for dysphagia in achalasia.

The causes of motor dysphagia are also listed in Table 40-1. The important causes are pharyngeal paralysis, cricopharyngeal achalasia, scleroderma of the esophagus, achalasia, and diffuse esophageal spasm and related motor disorders.

Approach to the Patient

History The history can provide a correct presumptive diagnosis in over 80 percent of patients. The type of food causing dysphagia provides useful information. Difficulty only with solids implies mechanical dysphagia with a lumen that is not severely narrowed. In advanced obstruction, dysphagia occurs with liquids as well as solids. In contrast, motor dysphagia due to achalasia and diffuse esophageal spasm is equally affected by solids and liquids from the very onset. Patients with scleroderma have dysphagia to solids that is unrelated to posture and to liquids in the recumbent but not in the upright posture. When peptic stricture develops in patients with scleroderma, dysphagia becomes more persistent.

The duration and course of dysphagia are helpful in diagnosis. Transient dysphagia of short duration may be due to an inflammatory process. Progressive dysphagia lasting a few weeks to a few months

Table 40-1

Causes of Dysphagia

MECHANICAL DYSPHAGIA	MOTOR (NEUROMUSCULAR) DYSPHAGIA

MECHANICAL DYSPHAGIA

I. Luminal
   A. Large bolus
   B. Foreign body
II. Intrinsic narrowing
   A. Inflammatory condition causing edema and swelling
      1. Stomatitis
      2. Pharyngitis, epiglottitis
      3. Esophagitis
         a. Viral (herpes simplex, varicella-zoster, cytomegalovirus)
         b. Bacterial
         c. Fungal (candidal)
         d. Mucocutaneous bullous diseases
         e. Caustic, chemical, thermal injury
   B. Webs and rings
      1. Pharyngeal (Plummer-Vinson syndrome)
      2. Esophageal (congenital, inflammatory)
      3. Lower esophageal mucosal ring (Schatzki ring)
   C. Benign strictures
      1. Peptic
      2. Caustic and pill-induced
      3. Inflammatory (Crohn's disease, candidal, mucocutaneous lesions)
      4. Ischemic
      5. Postoperative, postirradiation
      6. Congenital
   D. Malignant tumors
      1. Primary carcinoma
         a. Squamous cell carcinoma
         b. Adenocarcinoma
         c. Carcinosarcoma
         d. Pseudosarcoma
         e. Lymphoma
         f. Melanoma
         g. Kaposi's sarcoma
      2. Metastatic carcinoma
   E. Benign tumors
      1. Leiomyoma
      2. Lipoma
      3. Angioma
      4. Inflammatory fibroid polyp
      5. Epithelial papilloma
III. Extrinsic compression
   A. Cervical spondylitis
   B. Vertebral osteophytes
   C. Retropharyngeal abscess and masses
   D. Enlarged thyroid gland
   E. Zenker's diverticulum
   F. Vascular compression
      1. Aberrant right subclavian artery
      2. Right-sided aorta
      3. Left atrial enlargement
      4. Aortic aneurysm
   G. Posterior mediastinal masses
   H. Pancreatic tumor, pancreatitis
   I. Postvagotomy hematoma and fibrosis

MOTOR (NEUROMUSCULAR) DYSPHAGIA

I. Difficulty in initiating swallowing reflex
   A. Paralysis of the tongue
   B. Oropharyngeal anesthesia
   C. Lack of saliva (e.g., Sjögren's syndrome)
   D. Lesions of sensory components of vagus and glossopharyngeal nerves
   E. Lesions of swallowing center
II. Disorders of pharyngeal and esophageal striated muscle
   A. Muscle weakness
      1. Lower motor neuron lesion (bulbar paralysis)
         a. Cerebrovascular accident
         b. Motor neuron disease
         c. Poliomyelitis, postpolio syndrome
         d. Polyneuritis
         e. Amyotrophic lateral sclerosis
         f. Familial dysautonomia
      2. Neuromuscular
         a. Myasthenia gravis
      3. Muscle disorders
         a. Polymyositis
         b. Dermatomyositis
         c. Myopathies (myotonic dystrophy, oculopharyngeal myopathy)
   B. Nonperistaltic contractions or impaired deglutitive inhibition
      1. Pharynx and upper esophagus
         a. Rabies
         b. Tetanus
         c. Extrapyramidal tract disease
         d. Upper motor neuron lesions (pseudobulbar paralysis)
      2. Upper esophageal sphincter (UES)
         a. Paralysis of suprahyoid muscles (causes same as paralysis of pharyngeal musculature)
         b. Cricopharyngeal achalasia
III. Disorders of esophageal smooth muscle
   A. Paralysis of esophageal body causing weak contractions
      1. Scleroderma and related collagen-vascular diseases
      2. Hollow visceral myopathy
      3. Myotonic dystrophy
      4. Metabolic neuromyopathy (amyloid, alcohol?, diabetes?)
      5. Achalasia (classical)
   B. Nonperistaltic contractions or impaired deglutitive inhibition
      1. Esophageal body
         a. Diffuse esophageal spasm
         b. Achalasia (vigorous)
         c. Variants of diffuse esophageal spasm
      2. Lower esophageal sphincter
         a. Achalasia
            (1) Primary
            (2) Secondary
               (a) Chagas' disease
               (b) Carcinoma
               (c) Lymphoma
               (d) Neuropathic intestinal pseudoobstruction syndrome
               (e) Toxins and drugs
         b. Lower esophageal muscular (contractile) ring

is suggestive of carcinoma of the esophagus. Episodic dysphagia to solids lasting several years indicates a benign disease characteristic of a lower esophageal ring.

The localization of the site of dysphagia by the patient is helpful in determining the site of esophageal obstruction; the lesion is at or below the perceived location of dysphagia.

Associated symptoms provide important diagnostic clues. Nasal regurgitation and tracheobronchial aspiration with swallowing are hallmarks of pharyngeal paralysis or a tracheoesophageal fistula. Tracheobronchial aspiration unrelated to swallowing may be secondary to achalasia, a Zenker's diverticulum, or gastroesophageal reflux.

Severe weight loss that is out of proportion to the degree of dysphagia is highly suggestive of carcinoma. When hoarseness precedes dysphagia, the primary lesion is usually in the larynx. Hoarseness following dysphagia may suggest involvement of the recurrent laryngeal nerve by extension of esophageal carcinoma beyond the walls of

the esophagus. Sometimes hoarseness may be due to laryngitis secondary to gastroesophageal reflux. Association of laryngeal symptoms and dysphagia also occurs in various neuromuscular disorders. Hiccups suggest a lesion in the distal portion of the esophagus. Unilateral wheezing with dysphagia indicates a mediastinal mass involving the esophagus and a large bronchus.

Chest pain with dysphagia occurs in diffuse esophageal spasm and in related motor disorders. Chest pain resembling diffuse esophageal spasms also may occur in esophageal obstruction due to a large bolus. A prolonged history of heartburn and reflux preceding dysphagia indicates peptic stricture. Similarly, a history of prolonged nasogastric intubation, ingestion of caustic agents, ingestion of pills without water, previous radiation therapy, or associated mucocutaneous diseases may provide the cause of esophageal stricture. If odynophagia is present, candidal or herpes esophagitis or pill-induced esophagitis should be suspected.

In patients with AIDS or other immunodeficiency states, esophagitis due to opportunistic infections such as *Candida*, herpes simplex virus, or cytomegalovirus and tumors such as Kaposi's sarcoma and lymphoma should be suspected.

PHYSICAL EXAMINATION Physical examination is important in motor dysphagia due to skeletal muscle, neurologic, and oropharyngeal diseases. Signs of bulbar or pseudobulbar palsy, including dysarthria, dysphonia, ptosis, tongue atrophy, and hyperactive jaw jerk, in addition to evidence of generalized neuromuscular disease, should be carefully searched for. The neck should be examined for thyromegaly or a spinal abnormality. A careful inspection of the mouth and pharynx should disclose lesions that may cause interference with passage of food from the mouth or esophagus because of pain or obstruction. Changes in the skin and extremities may suggest a diagnosis of scleroderma and other collagen-vascular diseases or mucocutaneous diseases such as pemphigoid or epidermolysis bullosa, which may involve the esophagus. Metastatic diseases to lymph nodes and liver may be evident. Pulmonary complications of acute aspiration pneumonia or chronic aspiration may be present.

DIAGNOSTIC PROCEDURES All patients with dysphagia must be thoroughly investigated because the treatment depends on the underlying cause. If oropharyngeal dysphagia is suspected, videofluoroscopy of oropharyngeal swallowing should be obtained. If mechanical dysphagia is suspected on clinical history, barium swallow, esophagogastroscopy and endoscopic biopsies are the diagnostic procedures of choice. Barium swallow and esophageal motility studies are diagnostic tests for motor dysphagia. Esophagogastroscopy may be needed in patients with motor dysphagia to exclude an associated structural abnormality (see Chap. 283).

BIBLIOGRAPHY

CASTELL DO (ed): *The Esophagus*. Boston, Little, Brown, 2d ed, 1995

ENTERLINE H, THOMPSON J: *Pathology of the Esophagus*. New York, Springer-Verlag, 1984

GOYAL RK, PATERSON WG: Esophageal motility, in *Handbook of Physiology: Gastrointestinal System I*. Bethesda, MD, American Physiological Society, 1989, pp 865–908

GOYAL RK, HIRANO I: Mechanisms of disease: The enteric nervous system. N Engl J Med 334:110, 1996

HENDRIX TR: Art and science of history taking in patient with difficulty swallowing. Dysphagia 8:69, 1993

KOCH WM: Swallowing disorders. Diagnosis and therapy. Med Clin North Am 77:571, 1993

MORTON RE et al: Videofluoroscopy in the assessment of feeding disorders of children with neurological problems. J Dev Med Child Neurol 35:388, 1993

SHAKER R et al: Coordination of deglutition and phases of inspiration: Effect of aging, tachypnea, bolus volume, and chronic obstructive pulmonary disease. Am J Physiol 263:G750, 1992

YAMATO S et al: Role of nitric oxide in lower esophageal sphincter relaxation to swallowing. Life Sci 50:1263, 1992

41

Lawrence S. Friedman, Kurt J. Isselbacher

NAUSEA, VOMITING, AND INDIGESTION

NAUSEA AND VOMITING

Nausea and vomiting may occur independently of each other but generally are closely allied and are presumed to be mediated by the same neural pathways, so they may be considered together. *Nausea* denotes the feeling of an imminent desire to vomit, usually referred to the throat or epigastrium. *Vomiting* (or *emesis*) refers to the forceful oral expulsion of gastric contents. *Retching* denotes the labored rhythmic contraction of respiratory and abdominal musculature that frequently precedes or accompanies vomiting.

Nausea often precedes or accompanies vomiting. It is usually associated with diminished functional activity of the stomach (e.g., hypotonicity, hypoperistalsis, and hyposecretion) and altered small-intestinal motility (e.g., hypertonicity and reversed peristalsis of the duodenum). Often accompanying severe nausea is evidence of altered autonomic (especially parasympathetic) activity, such as skin pallor, increased perspiration, hypersalivation, defecation, and, occasionally, hypotension and bradycardia (vasovagal syndrome); anorexia is also usually present.

Nausea, retching, and hypersalivation frequently precede the act of vomiting, which is a highly integrated sequence of involuntary visceral and somatic motor events. The stomach plays a relatively passive role in the vomiting process, the major ejection force being provided by the abdominal musculature. With relaxation of the gastric fundus and gastroesophageal sphincter, a sharp increase in intraabdominal pressure is brought about by forceful contraction of the diaphragm and abdominal wall muscles. This, together with concomitant annular contraction of the gastric pylorus, results in the expulsion of gastric contents into the esophagus. Increased intrathoracic pressure results in the further movement of esophageal contents into the mouth. Reversal of the normal direction of esophageal peristalsis may play a role in this process. Reflex elevation of the soft palate during the vomiting act prevents the entry of the expelled material into the nasopharynx, whereas reflex closure of the glottis and inhibition of respiration help to prevent pulmonary aspiration.

Repeated emesis may have deleterious effects in a number of ways. The process of vomiting, if forceful, may lead to pressure rupture of the esophagus (Boerhaave's syndrome) or to linear mucosal (Mallory-Weiss) tears in the region of the cardioesophageal junction with resulting hematemesis. Prolonged vomiting may lead to dehydration, the loss of gastric secretions (especially hydrochloric acid) resulting in metabolic alkalosis with hypokalemia, malnutrition with various deficiency states, and dental caries. In states of central nervous system depression (e.g., coma), gastric contents may be aspirated into the lungs, with a resulting aspiration pneumonitis.

VOMITING MECHANISM The act of vomiting is under the control of two functionally distinct medullary centers: the *vomiting center* in the dorsal portion of the lateral reticular formation and the *chemoreceptor trigger zone* in the area postrema of the floor of the fourth ventricle. The vomiting center controls and integrates the actual act of emesis. It receives afferent stimuli from the gastrointestinal tract and other parts of the body, from higher brainstem and cortical centers, especially the labyrinthine apparatus, and from the chemoreceptor trigger zone. Persons vary considerably in the threshold of their vomiting centers to different stimuli. The important efferent pathways in vomiting are the phrenic nerves (to the diaphragm), the spinal nerves (to the intercostal and abdominal musculature), and visceral efferent fibers in the vagus nerve (to the larynx, pharynx, esophagus, and stomach). The vomiting center is located near other medullary centers regulating respiratory, vasomotor, and autonomic functions that may be involved in the act of vomiting.

The chemoreceptor trigger zone by itself is incapable of mediating the act of vomiting; rather activation of this zone results in efferent impulses to the medullary vomiting center, which in turn initiates emesis. The chemoreceptor trigger zone is an emetic chemoreceptor that can be activated by a variety of stimuli or drugs, including apomorphine and other opiates, levodopa (after decarboxylation to dopamine), digitalis, bacterial toxins, radiation, and metabolic abnormalities as occur with uremia and hypoxia.

CLINICAL CLASSIFICATION Nausea and vomiting are common manifestations of many organic and functional disorders. The precise mechanisms triggering vomiting in various clinical conditions are not well understood, making classification of mechanisms difficult.

Many *acute abdominal emergencies* that lead to the "surgical abdomen" are associated with nausea and vomiting. Vomiting may be seen with inflammation of a viscus, as in acute appendicitis or acute cholecystitis, intestinal obstruction, or acute peritonitis (see Chap. 288).

Other *disorders of the alimentary tract*, including those associated with chronic indigestion (see below), are frequently accompanied by nausea and vomiting. In peptic ulcer, emesis may be either spontaneous or self-induced and may lead to relief of symptoms, particularly if antral or pyloric edema has resulted in gastric outlet obstruction. Nausea and vomiting are also prominent in patients with disordered gastrointestinal motility, including postvagotomy, diabetic, or idiopathic gastroparesis (gastric atony); other gastric "dysrhythmias" resulting from abnormal myoelectric activity; and intestinal pseudoobstruction due to abnormal intestinal myogenic or neurogenic function. Gastroparesis may be demonstrated by gastric scanning after a radiolabeled meal or by radiography after ingestion of indigestible radiopaque solid markers. Experimentally, some patients with otherwise unexplained nausea and vomiting have been demonstrated to have accelerated ("tachygastria") or irregular ("gastric tachyarrhythmia") gastric electrical activity as measured by electrodes implanted surgically on the serosa of the stomach or placed on the abdominal surface ("electrogastrogram"). Typically, intestinal obstruction of any cause (e.g., adhesions, malignancy, hernia, volvulus) leads to vomiting, as do other disorders of the liver, pancreas, and biliary tract. Nausea and vomiting may accompany the distention and pain seen in the aerophagic syndromes (see below).

Viral, bacterial, and parasitic *infections of the intestinal tract* are typically associated with severe nausea and vomiting, often with diarrhea. *Acute systemic infections* with fever, especially in young children, are also frequently accompanied by vomiting and often by severe diarrhea. The mechanism whereby infections remote from the gastrointestinal tract produce these manifestations may relate to stimulation of the medullary chemoreceptor trigger zone by toxins or abnormal metabolites.

Central nervous system disorders that lead to increased intracranial pressure (e.g., neoplasms, encephalitis, hydrocephalus) may be accompanied by vomiting, which is often *projectile* (intensely forceful). Vertigo due to disorders of the labyrinthine apparatus, such as acute labyrinthitis and Ménière's disease, may be accompanied by vomiting with nausea and retching. Similarly, motion sickness is typically associated with anorexia, nausea, and vomiting as well as apathy, increased salivation, cold sweating, and headache. Additionally, migraine headaches, tabetic crises, acute meningitis, and the reactive phase of hypotension with syncope may be associated with nausea and vomiting.

Nausea and vomiting may be present in *acute myocardial infarction*, especially when posterior in location or transmural in extent, and in *congestive heart failure*, perhaps in relation to congestion of the liver. The possibility that these symptoms also may be due to drugs (e.g., opiates or digitalis) should always be borne in mind in patients with cardiac disease. Nausea and vomiting are common in cancer patients, especially those who are terminally ill.

Nausea and vomiting commonly accompany several *metabolic and endocrinologic disorders*, including uremia, diabetic ketoacidosis, hypo- and hyperparathyroidism, hyperthyroid crisis, and adrenal insufficiency, especially adrenal crisis. The morning sickness of early pregnancy is another instance of nausea and vomiting possibly related to hormonal changes; the term *hyperemesis gravidarum* is applied when fluid and electrolyte disturbances or nutritional deficiencies result.

The *side effects of many drugs and chemicals* include nausea and vomiting. In some cases, drugs have central emetic effects, as with digitalis, morphine, histamine, phenytoin, and some chemotherapeutic agents. In other cases, drug-induced gastric irritation leads to stimulation of the medullary vomiting center, as with salicylates, aminophylline, some antibiotics, and ipecac. The ingestion of a toxin (e.g., food poisoning) also may cause acute vomiting.

Psychogenic vomiting refers to chronic or recurrent vomiting that may result from an emotional or psychological disturbance. Often patients with emotional disorders and chronic vomiting maintain a relatively normal state of nutrition because only a relatively small amount of the ingested food is vomited. In some cases regurgitation rather than vomiting may predominate, and the degree of weight loss

may be out of proportion to the patient's description of the frequency and severity of vomiting. As discussed in Chap. 76, anorexia nervosa and bulimia are emotional disturbances that may be associated with vomiting and weight loss.

DIFFERENTIAL DIAGNOSIS Vomiting should be distinguished from *regurgitation*, which refers to the expulsion of food in the absence of nausea and without the abdominal diaphragmatic muscular contraction associated with vomiting. Regurgitation of esophageal contents may occur with esophageal strictures or diverticula. Regurgitation of gastric contents is generally seen in gastroesophageal reflux disease due to lower esophageal sphincter incompetence, in pyloric spasm or obstruction due to peptic ulcer, or in gastroparesis. *Hiccups* are a distinctive sound caused by contractions of the inspiratory muscles terminated abruptly by closure of the glottis. Brief episodes of hiccups may be caused by gastric distention, a sudden change in temperature, ingestion of alcohol, excess smoking, or excitement, whereas persistent hiccups may signify a serious underlying disease, such as a structural lesion or infection of the central nervous system, diaphragmatic irritation by a tumor or inflammatory process, metabolic derangement, vascular lesion, intraabdominal process, or systemic infection. In addition, a variety of drugs, including barbiturates and sedatives, general anesthesia, and psychogenic factors may lead to hiccups. *Rumination* is the effortless regurgitation of undigested food starting within minutes of a meal, presumably due to intraabdominal muscular contraction and simultaneous voluntary lower esophageal relaxation. It is rare in adults but more common in patients with bulimia nervosa and in infants, children, and mentally deficient persons.

The temporal relationship of vomiting to eating may be of help diagnostically. Vomiting that occurs predominantly in the morning is often seen early in pregnancy and in uremia. Alcoholic gastritis is also commonly accompanied by early-morning retching and emesis, the so-called dry heaves. Vomiting that occurs during or shortly after eating may suggest psychogenic vomiting or peptic ulcer with pylorospasm. Vomiting that occurs 4 to 6 h or longer after eating and involves the elimination of large quantities of undigested food often indicates gastric retention (e.g., pyloric obstruction, gastroparesis) or certain esophageal disorders (achalasia, Zenker's diverticulum). Vomiting that is projectile or without antecedent nausea suggests the possibility of a central nervous system lesion.

Associated symptoms also may provide diagnostic clues. For example, vertigo and tinnitus indicate the possibility of Ménière's disease. A long history of vomiting with little or no weight loss suggests psychogenic vomiting. Relief of abdominal pain with vomiting is typical of peptic ulcer. Early satiety is typical of gastroparesis.

The character of the vomitus also offers clues to the diagnosis. If the vomitus contains large amounts of free hydrochloric acid, gastric outlet obstruction due to an ulcer or a hypersecretory state such as Zollinger-Ellison syndrome should be considered. Absence of free hydrochloric acid is more compatible with gastric malignancy. A feculent or putrid odor reflects the results of bacterial action on the intestinal contents and may occur with distal intestinal obstruction, peritonitis, or gastrocolic fistula. Bile is commonly present in gastric contents whenever vomiting is prolonged; it has no significance unless constantly present in large quantities, when it may signify an obstructing lesion below the ampulla of Vater. The presence of blood in the gastric contents usually denotes bleeding from the esophagus, stomach, or duodenum.

_____ *Approach to the Patient* _____

Every effort should be made to identify the underlying cause of nausea and vomiting. Evaluation should begin with a careful history taking, including a careful drug history; physical examination; and, if necessary, routine laboratory tests such as a complete blood count, erythrocyte sedimentation rate, electrolyte levels including blood urea nitrogen and creatinine, glucose levels, and liver function tests. Additional testing should be dictated by the age of the patient and clinical presentation, particularly when nausea and vomiting are chronic. In women of child-bearing age, a pregnancy test should be obtained. In selected cases urinalysis, cultures, a toxic screen, and tests of endocrine function (thyroid function tests, fasting morning cortisol level) may be indicated. The possibility of an underlying gastrointestinal or hepatobiliary disorder may be evaluated with plain and barium radiography, ultrasound, computed tomography (CT), and endoscopy. If neurologic disease is suspected, a CT scan of the head is indicated.

In over 50 percent of patients with chronic nausea and vomiting, the basic evaluation outlined above will be unrevealing, and in selected cases further specialized testing may be helpful, particularly if a gastrointestinal motility disorder is suspected. An array of tests may be considered, including esophageal motility and 24-h esophageal pH testing, gastric emptying and motility studies, and, if available, electrogastrography and small-intestinal motility testing. In occasional patients, a formal psychiatric consultation may prove to be revealing.

℞ TREATMENT

Effective therapy of nausea and vomiting usually depends on correction of the underlying cause. *Antiemetic agents* vary in their usefulness depending on the cause of the symptoms, responsiveness of the patient, and occurrence of side effects. *Antihistamines* such as dimenhydrinate, meclizine, and promethazine hydrochloride are effective for the control of nausea and vomiting due to motion sickness and other inner-ear disturbances and may be effective in pregnancy, uremia, and postoperative vomiting; they do not act on the chemoreceptor trigger zone and are of little value in other causes of vomiting. *Anticholinergics* such as scopolamine block central muscarinic receptors in afferent pathways of the vomiting reflex and are also effective in motion sickness. *Phenothiazine* derivatives such as prochlorperazine and the structurally related butyrophenone haloperidol inhibit cerebral dopamine receptors and act principally at the chemoreceptor trigger zone. They are often ineffective for severe nausea and vomiting and have the potential for causing sedation, hypotension, and Parkinson-like effects. *Metoclopramide* is the prototype of selective dopamine antagonists called *substituted benzamides*. Metoclopramide is useful in all types of vomiting except motion sickness and inner-ear dysfunction. In contrast to the phenothiazines, which have anticholinergic effects, metoclopramide has powerful peripheral cholinergic effects that enhance gastric emptying. Metoclopramide may be superior to phenothiazines in the treatment of severe nausea and vomiting and is particularly useful in the treatment of gastroparesis. The usual oral dosage is 5 to 20 mg four times daily, but intravenous doses up to 1 to 3 mg/kg, which also inhibit 5-hydroxytryptamine$_3$ receptors, may be effective as prophylaxis prior to potent chemotherapeutic agents (e.g., cisplatin). Unfortunately, neurologic side effects are frequent, including drowsiness, dystonic reactions, anxiety, insomnia, depression, parkinsonism, confusion, and a rise in prolactin level. Alternative newer agents such as *cisapride* and *domperidone* (the latter not yet licensed for use in the United States) exert peripheral antiemetic effects without the central nervous system side effects of metoclopramide. Cisapride has cholinomimetic effects but minimal antidopaminergic activity. The standard dose is 10 to 20 mg four times daily, generally before meals and at bedtime. *Glucocorticoids* are often combined with metoclopramide to control nausea and vomiting due to cancer chemotherapy; the mechanism of action may involve inhibition of prostaglandin formation. The sedative *lorazepam* may be added to this regimen. *Tetrahydrocannabinol*, the active ingredient of marijuana, is marketed as dronabinol for the prevention of nausea and vomiting after cancer chemotherapy; the mechanism of action is unknown. *Ondansetron* and *granisetron*, serotonin antagonists that bind to 5-hydroxytryptamine$_3$ receptors in the chemoreceptor trigger zone and

gut, are particularly effective in preventing chemotherapy-induced nausea and vomiting, especially when combined with intravenous dexamethasone. The recommended dose of ondansetron is 0.15 mg/kg infused intravenously over 15 min and given three times 4 h apart, beginning 30 min before the start of chemotherapy, although lower doses may be effective in some patients. The recommended dose of granisetron is 10 μg/kg intravenously infused over 5 min, beginning 30 min before the start of chemotherapy. The antibiotic *erythromycin*, which binds to motilin receptors in the gut, has been shown in doses as low as 125 mg four times daily to enhance gastric emptying in patients with gastroparesis; however, stimulation of antral contractility by erythromycin leads to abdominal cramps, nausea, and bloating and may limit its usefulness.

INDIGESTION

Indigestion is a term frequently used by patients to describe a variety of symptoms generally appreciated as upper abdominal distress and often associated with the intake of food. The term is nonspecific and may not have the same meaning for the patient and physician. Thus, in approaching the patient with indigestion, it is important for the physician first to elicit a precise description of this complaint. To some patients, indigestion refers to actual abdominal pain or pressure, which may be associated with postprandial fullness, early satiety, nausea, or bloating, and which is generally designated as *dyspepsia*. Others may use the term indigestion to describe either a vague feeling that digestion has not proceeded naturally or that intolerances to specific foods exist. Still others may use it to describe belching, a feeling of excessive gas, or flatulence. When heartburn is the predominant symptom, the patient can be presumed to have *gastroesophageal reflux disease* (see Chap. 283).

After having ascertained the patient's definition of indigestion, it is important to determine (1) the location and duration of the discomfort, (2) the temporal relation of the symptoms to the ingestion of food, and (3) the possible relation of the symptoms to the ingestion of specific types of food (e.g., milk, fatty foods) or drugs.

Indigestion may occur in association with diseases of the gastrointestinal tract or pathologic states in other organ systems. As a result of a systematic clinical and laboratory investigation, a definable pathophysiologic process sometimes can be shown to be responsible for the symptoms in a given case of indigestion. Frequently, however, a clear etiologic explanation for the patient's complaint of indigestion cannot be established, and descriptive designations are applied. For example, the term *nonulcer dyspepsia* is often used to describe ulcerlike symptoms when no ulcer is found. The term *flatulent dyspepsia* is used when belching, abdominal distention, and early satiety are prominent symptoms; the term *dysmotility-like dyspepsia* has been applied to the same constellation of symptoms. Unfortunately, these terms do not imply that the symptoms described are attributable to a particular pathogenic process. The term *functional dyspepsia* is used interchangeably with nonulcer dyspepsia when clinical evaluation fails to reveal an explanation for indigestion. In some cases of functional dyspepsia, sophisticated testing of gastrointestinal electrical activity and manometric studies may reveal disturbances of gastrointestinal motility, although the cause-and-effect relationship between such findings and the patient's symptoms may be difficult to prove. Indeed, some patients with functional dyspepsia also have features of the irritable bowel syndrome, suggesting a diffuse intestinal motility disturbance (see Chap. 287).

SYNDROMES COMMONLY DESCRIBED AS INDIGESTION Pain A careful elucidation of the pattern of pain may provide important diagnostic information. Visceral abdominal pain is mediated by visceral afferent nerves that accompany the abdominal sympathetic pathways (see Chap. 14). Visceral pain is described as dull and aching in nature, with a diffuse midline localization, or as fullness or pressure. The location of the discomfort generally corresponds to the segmental level of neural innervation of the affected organ. Abdominal visceral pain, which can be produced experimentally by artificially increasing pressure in a hollow viscus, results from distention or exaggerated muscular contraction of the viscus. Inflammation generally lowers the threshold for pain from such stimuli.

The visceral pain of indigestion should be distinguished from the sharp, localized pain patterns of many acute abdominal processes involving the peritoneum. In contrast to visceral pain, this somatic pain is mediated by cerebrospinal afferent nerves.

In view of the diffuse nature of visceral abdominal pain, the main clue to the cause comes from the *location* of the pain and the corresponding segmental level of neural innervation; however, in any given segmental region there is no way of determining which of several viscera is the source of the pain (Table 41-1). The following rules, already described in Chap. 14, are useful: *Substernal pain* of gastrointestinal origin usually arises from disorders of the esophagus or cardia of the stomach. Because pain in this area can emanate from the heart, cardiac disease must be carefully considered and excluded. *Epigastric pain* is generally of gastric, duodenal, biliary, or pancreatic origin. (The epigastrium is also a frequent location for "functional" pain.) As pathologic processes in the biliary tract or pancreas become more intense, pain may lateralize and localize, e.g., biliary pain to the right upper quadrant and tip of the scapula and pancreatic pain to the left upper quadrant and back. *Periumbilical pain* is generally associated with disease involving the small intestine. *Pain below the umbilicus* is often of appendiceal, colonic, or pelvic origin.

The unraveling of the *temporal relationships* of the patient's symptoms often provides additional diagnostic clues. It is important to ascertain whether the symptoms are *constant* (continually present over extended periods of time), as may occur with an infiltrating gastric carcinoma, or *intermittent*, as in acute gastritis or biliary colic. The symptoms may have a *diurnal* pattern, as in reflux esophagitis in which pain often occurs nocturnally and with recumbency. Pain that awakens the patient from a sound sleep may occur with duodenal ulcer. Occasionally symptoms are *seasonal*, as in peptic ulcer disease, in which some patients experience more discomfort in the spring and autumn than at other times.

Another helpful diagnostic feature is the relation of pain to *food ingestion*. Early postprandial symptoms may reflect esophageal disease, acute gastritis, or gastric carcinoma. Late postprandial indiges-

tion, i.e., occurring several hours after eating, may reflect failure of the stomach to empty adequately, as in gastric outlet obstruction, gastroparesis and other disorders of gastric motility, or duodenal ulcer, in which case pain results from exposure of ulcerated mucosa to acid secreted by the stomach and unbuffered by food. Conversely, the relief of pain following ingestion of food or antacids is characteristic of duodenal ulcer and is presumably due to the neutralization of acid. Late postprandial indigestion also may result from impaired digestive and absorptive processes, as in pancreatic insufficiency.

It is important to recognize that the pain patterns and relationships to the intake of food described above are generalizations, and many cases do not conform to classic "textbook" descriptions. For example, although pain limited to the right upper quadrant is often caused by gallbladder disease, about half of patients with this condition experience only epigastric pain. Similarly, there are some patients with duodenal ulcer whose pain is not relieved by food or antacids, while there are other patients with functional indigestion and even gastric carcinoma whose pain improves with food or antacids.

Nonulcer Dyspepsia Nonulcer dyspepsia refers to symptoms that suggest a diagnosis of peptic ulcer despite the documented absence of an ulcer by endoscopy or barium x-ray studies and the absence of any other demonstrable organic disorder (e.g., biliary tract disease) or evidence of the irritable bowel syndrome to account for the symptoms. Nonulcer dyspepsia is at least twice as common as peptic ulcer and may affect 20 to 30 percent of the population. Only 20 to 30 percent of patients with dyspepsia seek medical care. The pathogenesis of nonulcer dyspepsia is poorly understood; most patients have normal gastric acid secretion, and a relation between nonulcer dyspepsia and duodenitis or duodenal ulcer has not been demonstrated. Similarly, a role for *Helicobacter pylori* and associated chronic gastritis in causing dyspeptic symptoms in persons without peptic ulcer is unproven (see Chap. 284). Disordered gastroduodenal and small-intestinal motility appears to account for some cases of nonulcer dyspepsia. Between 25 and 50 percent of patients with nonulcer dyspepsia have postprandial antral hypomotility and delayed gastric emptying. Moreover, 50 percent experience abdominal discomfort in response to balloon distention at volumes lower than those that provoke pain in healthy controls, suggesting visceral hypersensitivity.

Heartburn Heartburn, or pyrosis, is a sensation of warmth or burning located substernally or high in the epigastrium with radiation into the neck and occasionally to the arms. Occasional heartburn is common in normal persons, but frequent and severe heartburn is generally a manifestation of esophageal dysfunction. Heartburn may result from abnormal motor activity or distention of the esophagus, sensitivity of the esophageal mucosa to refluxed acid or bile, or esophageal mucosal inflammation (esophagitis).

Heartburn is most often associated with gastroesophageal reflux (see Chap. 283). In this setting, heartburn typically occurs after a large meal, with stooping or bending, or when the patient is supine. It may be accompanied by the spontaneous appearance in the mouth of fluid which may be salty ("water brash"), sour (gastric contents), or bitter and green or yellow (bile). Heartburn may arise following the ingestion of certain foods (e.g., citrus fruit juices) or drugs (e.g., alcohol and aspirin). Characteristically, heartburn is alleviated promptly, even if only temporarily, by antacids.

Food Intolerance In some persons, specific foods or types of foods appear to be related to indigestion. Careful documentation of this relationship is sometimes of great help in arriving at an etiologic diagnosis.

Some foods may be poorly tolerated because of their consistency. Patients with esophageal stricture or carcinoma may tolerate liquids well but may experience discomfort, especially substernal distress, after ingesting solids (see Chaps. 40 and 283). Citrus fruits, perhaps because of their relatively low pH, and spicy foods often provoke symptoms in patients with peptic ulcer disease or peptic esophagitis. Certain foods may be tolerated poorly because of impaired intestinal

Table 41-1

Distribution of Visceral Pain and Examples of Disorders Frequently Involving the Specific Organ

Organ	Common Location of Pain	Examples of Disorders
Esophagus	Substernum, epigastrium	Peptic esophagitis, stricture, esophageal motility disorder, carcinoma
Stomach	Epigastrium	Gastric ulcer, gastritis, carcinoma
Duodenum (first and second portions)	Epigastrium	Duodenal ulcer
Small intestine (excluding first and second portions of duodenum)	Periumbilical region	Infectious gastroenteritis, Crohn's disease, lymphoma, intestinal obstruction
Gallbladder	Epigastrium, right upper quadrant, right upper back	Cholelithiasis, cholecystitis
Pancreas	Epigastrium, left upper quadrant, left side of back	Pancreatitis, pancreatic carcinoma
Liver	Right upper quadrant	Hepatitis, cirrhosis, passive congestion
Colon	Below umbilicus	Infectious colitis, ulcerative or Crohn's colitis, carcinoma, partial obstruction

digestion or absorption, as with the ingestion of fatty foods in patients with pancreatic or biliary tract disease.

Patients may have a congenital or acquired *deficiency of a specific enzyme* required for intestinal absorption of a certain nutrient. One example is the deficiency of lactase, the intestinal mucosal enzyme that catalyzes the hydrolysis of lactose. In persons who are lactase-deficient, the ingestion of milk (which contains lactose) results in abdominal cramps, distention, diarrhea, and flatulence (Chap. 285). Sucrose may lead to similar symptoms in persons with hereditary sucrase-isomaltase deficiency. Certain nutrients may lead to profound systemic effects because of *biochemical defects* in the patient that render the substances particularly hazardous, as in galactose intolerance in persons with galactosemia (see Chap. 351).

Some foods or food additives may initiate *allergic reactions*, which should be suspected when symptoms occur after ingestion of a specific food, recur on challenge testing, and are associated with other features of an allergic reaction, such as lip swelling, urticaria, angioedema, asthma, or, rarely, anaphylactic shock. Acute IgE-mediated reactions are most commonly associated with cow's milk (in infants), shellfish, wheat, eggs, nuts, and chocolate and may be confirmed by the radioallergosorbent test in some cases. Delayed hypersensitivity reactions also may occur; may be associated with less severe symptoms, including joint and muscle pain, fatigue, serous otitis, and altered spacial perception; and are more difficult to relate to specific foods. Some foods may exert *toxic effects* on the intestine in susceptible persons (e.g., gluten in patients with celiac sprue).

In many instances we do not understand the mechanism by which indigestion is associated with the ingestion of specific foods. Thus a history of fatty food intolerance or distress after eating spicy foods is commonly obtained from patients with indigestion; however, the mechanisms leading to these symptoms in these circumstances are often unclear.

Aerophagia In patients with a complaint of *chronic, repetitive eructation* (belching), each belch can often be observed to be preceded by a swallow of air, most of which passes only partway down the esophagus and is then regurgitated. Thus excessive eructation usually results from *aerophagia*, or air swallowing, not from excessive gas production in the stomach or the intestine. A degree of aerophagia occurs in normal persons, but some individuals gulp air excessively because of chronic anxiety, rapid eating, drinking carbonated beverages or any beverage through a straw, gum chewing, sucking on hard candy, smoking cigarettes, postnasal drip, poorly fitting dentures, or esophageal speech. Because eructation that follows aerophagia may provide temporary relief to the patient, a vicious cycle of aerophagia and eructation may ensue.

About 20 to 60 percent of intestinal gas represents swallowed air. Because nitrogen and oxygen are the only gases present in the atmosphere in appreciable concentrations, and because they are not produced in the gastrointestinal tract, their detection on chromatographic analysis of intestinal gas indicates that swallowed air is the source. Swallowed air that is not eructated passes into the stomach and intestine. Accumulation of swallowed air in the stomach may lead to postprandial fullness and pressure and the finding by x-ray of a large amount of air in the gastric fundus. This symptom complex, referred to as the *magenblase* (i.e., gastric bubble) *syndrome*, may occur when a patient lies supine after a large meal, thereby permitting gastric air to be "trapped" below the gastroesophageal junction by overlying fluid and unable to be eructated. Inability to eructate is also thought to underlie the "gas-bloat" syndrome observed after surgical repair of a hiatal hernia. Acute gastric distention by swallowed air can sometimes produce sharp pain, which may mimic angina pectoris. Swallowed air that successfully passes the stomach may either produce diffuse abdominal distention or become trapped in the splenic flexure of the colon. The latter condition, or *splenic flexure syndrome*, is characterized by a sensation of left upper quadrant fullness and pressure with radiation to the left side of the chest. Relief of pain often follows defecation or the expulsion of flatus. The diagnosis is suggested by the finding of increased tympany in the extreme left lateral portion of the upper abdomen on physical examination or of large amounts of air in the splenic flexure of the colon on a plain abdominal radiograph.

Gaseousness, Bloating, and Flatulence Despite the widely held belief that feelings of *diffuse abdominal pain and bloating* are often caused by excessive quantities of intestinal gas, studies employing an intestinal gas wash-out technique suggest that patients complaining of excessive gas actually have normal volumes of intestinal gas. In some cases, the primary abnormality causing functional bloating and pain appears to be a motility disturbance that causes the patient to perceive pain with an intestinal gas volume that is well tolerated by normal subjects. Alternatively, intestinal motility may be normal in such persons, but they may be excessively sensitive to normal impulses arising from the intestinal tract (visceral hypersensitivity).

A major source of intestinal gas is the fermentative action of intestinal bacteria on carbohydrates and proteins within the lumen. Normally such bacteria are limited to the colon, and the principal gases produced are carbon dioxide and hydrogen (in addition to minute quantities of odoriferous gases—indoles, skatols, and sulfur-containing compounds—which give flatus its characteristic odor). In the upper small bowel carbon dioxide is also produced when hydrochloric acid from the stomach or ingested fatty acids are neutralized by bicarbonate. (This may explain, in part, indigestion associated with fatty foods.) About one-third of adults produce appreciable quantities of methane in the colon; this appears to be a familial trait and unrelated to ingestion of specific foods.

An increase in intraluminal gas production resulting in *abdominal distention, bloating, and flatulence* occurs following the ingestion of certain foods, such as legumes and some grains, that contain significant quantities of nonabsorbable complex carbohydrates that pass into the colon, where they supply gas-forming substrates for colonic bacteria. The best-studied example of this is beans, which contain oligosaccharides (stachyose and raffinose) that cannot be split by intestinal mucosal enzymes but are metabolized by colonic bacteria. Less well appreciated is that fructose, a natural or added sweetener in fruit (particularly figs, dates, prunes, and grapes), fruit juices and soft drinks, and present in oligosaccharides in onions, asparagus, and wheat, may be incompletely absorbed in the small intestine and thereby contribute to abdominal distention, bloating, and flatulence. [In contrast, intestinal absorption of fructose is more likely to be complete when fructose is mixed with glucose or ingested as sucrose (glucose-fructose).] Intestinal malabsorption of sorbitol may underlie symptoms of abdominal distention, gaseousness, and diarrhea associated with certain fruits or when sorbitol is used as a sweetener in "sugar-free" gums and candies or as an "inert" ingredient in some medications. Increased intraluminal gas production also may result from abnormal bacterial colonization of the small intestine (bacterial overgrowth syndrome) or infection with *Giardia lamblia*.

Indigestion due to Extraintestinal Disease A number of extraintestinal diseases may lead to indigestion. Thus indigestion may be prominent in congestive heart failure, pulmonary tuberculosis, neoplastic disease, and uremia. Also, a variety of drugs such as aspirin, nonsteroidal anti-inflammatory agents, and glucocorticoids may cause indigestion because of their ulcerogenic properties.

Approach to the Patient

Indigestion represents a challenging and difficult diagnostic problem because of its nonspecific nature. It is essential to obtain a clear and detailed description of the specific symptoms, particularly the patient's definition of the term *indigestion*. The nature of the distress, its frequency and time of occurrence, its relationship to meals, and the special circumstances that lead to its exacerbation or relief should be elicited. Associated intestinal symptoms such as nausea and vomiting, abnormal bowel habits, diarrhea, steatorrhea, and melena should be sought, and an assessment of nutritional status, appetite, and changes in weight should be made. A careful history also should include an assessment of the patient's general health, including the possible presence of extraintestinal disorders that may produce indigestion. A careful dietary history is essential, and asking the patient to keep a diary of foods eaten may prove revealing. Similarly, the patient's medications should be reviewed, particularly for agents that may slow gut transit such as narcotics, anticholinergics, and calcium antagonists. Psychological factors may play an etiologic or contributory role, and the presence of anxiety, depressive symptoms, or hysteria should be noted.

Physical examination rarely establishes the specific diagnosis but may be useful in detecting diseases in other organ systems that can affect intestinal function (e.g., congestive heart failure). Stools should be examined for appearance and occult blood.

Whether further diagnostic studies are indicated depends on the specific nature of the patient's complaints and the patient's age (concern about the possibility of gastrointestinal malignancy being greater in older patients). Abdominal pain may be evaluated with radiologic and imaging studies of the esophagus, stomach, small intestine, colon, pancreas, and biliary tract. Esophagogastroscopy, endoscopic cholangiopancreatography, sigmoidoscopy, or colonoscopy may be considered depending on the specific symptoms. On the other hand, in patients under age 40 with epigastric pain typical of peptic ulcer, routine diagnostic studies are unlikely to disclose serious diseases (such as gastric carcinoma) and are often in fact negative; additional options in such patients include serologic testing for *H. pylori* and empiric treatment with "triple therapy" (a bismuth compound and two antibiotics) in persons who are seropositive or an empiric trial of antacids, H_2-receptor–blocking drugs, or sucralfate (see Chap. 284). In contrast to peptic ulcer, nonulcer dyspepsia improves inconsistently following antacids and other standard ulcer therapy. Esophagogastroscopy may be reserved for patients with symptoms that persist despite therapy or that recur soon after therapy is discontinued. However, in patients with *H. pylori* on endoscopic antral biopsy and no other explanation for indigestion (e.g., no ulcer), eradication of *H. pylori* has not been demonstrated in controlled trials to be of benefit. In fact, the cost-effective approach to the evaluation of dyspepsia, including the relative merits of initial endoscopy versus empiric therapy and the choice of empiric therapy, is still debated. In general, most authorities do not recommend treatment to eradicate *H. pylori* unless a peptic ulcer is confirmed (see Chap. 284). A suggested algorithm for the management of the patient with dyspepsia is shown in Fig. 41-1.

In individuals complaining of excessive eructation, the simple demonstration that aerophagia reproduces the symptoms may suffice to confirm the diagnosis and hopefully break the habit. Patients complaining of excessive gas, bloating, distention, and flatulence must be questioned carefully about dietary preferences and the relation of symptoms to ingestion of specific foods. In some cases, elimination of certain foods (e.g., milk, legumes) from the diet followed by rechallenge may be confirmatory. In other cases, a more detailed assessment, including stool examination for fat and muscle fibers and for parasites such as *G. lamblia*, breath tests to detect carbohydrate malabsorption or bacterial overgrowth, esophageal manometry and ambulatory pH monitoring, measurement of the rate of gastric emptying of a solid meal, and gastrointestinal motility studies, may be desirable. When no precise explanation for gaseousness can be identified, trials of activated charcoal to reduce gaseousness associated with carbohydrate malabsorption or simethicone to alter the elasticity of gas bubbles may be considered, although their value is uncertain.

In many cases of indigestion no clear explanation is obtained, even after careful diagnostic studies and therapeutic trials. Some cases represent gastrointestinal motility disturbances, perhaps due to subtle physiologic derangements not detectable by currently available methods. In some such instances, it may be beneficial to implement an empiric trial of a gastric prokinetic agent (e.g., cisapride, metoclopramide), which augments gastrointestinal motility. Other cases represent early stages of disease processes that may only be diagnosed by conventional methods at a later date. Still others are psychogenic and may respond to appropriate psychiatric measures. The ultimate evaluation of indigestion requires, therefore, the utmost in sensitivity, diligence, and concern on the part of the examining physician.

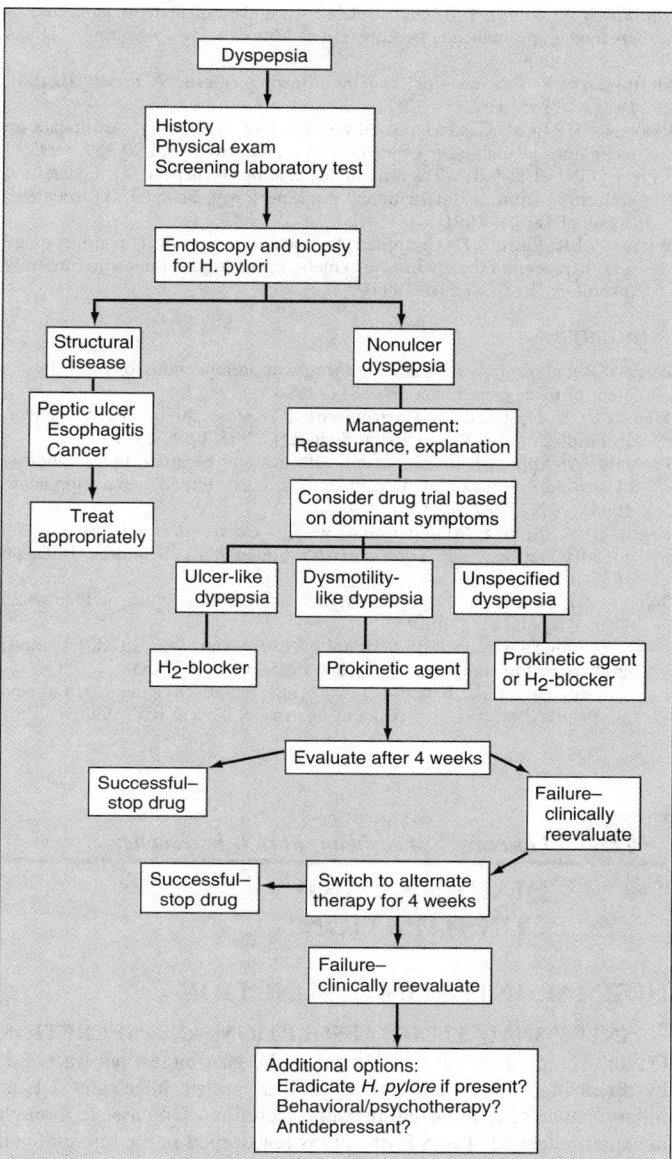

FIGURE 41-1 A suggested approach to the patent with dyspepsia. [Adapted from Talley NJ. Nonulcer dyspepsia, in *Textbook of Gastroenterology*, 2d ed, Yamada T et al (eds). Philadelphia, Lippincott, 1995, p. 1453.]

For further information, see Chap. 38 Agents affecting gastrointestinal water flux and motility, in Goodman and Gilman's The Pharmacological Basis of Therapeutics, *9th ed, New York, McGraw Hill, 1996.*

BIBLIOGRAPHY

NAUSEA AND VOMITING

GRUNBERG SM, HESKETH PJ: Control of chemotherapy-induced emesis. N Engl J Med 329:1790, 1993

KOCH KL: Approach to the patient with nausea and vomiting, in *Textbook of Gastroenterology*, 2d ed, T Yamada et al (eds). Philadelphia, Lippincott, 1995, pp 731–782

LEE M, FELDMAN M: Nausea and vomiting, in *Gastrointestinal Disease*, 5th ed, MH Sleisenger, JS Fordtran (eds). Philadelphia, Saunders, 1993, pp 509–523

MARKHAM A, SORKIN EM: Ondansetron: An update of its therapeutic use in chemotherapy-induced postoperative nausea and vomiting. Drugs 45:931, 1993

MITCHELSON F: Pharmacologic agents affecting emesis: A review (part I). Drugs 43:295, 1992

PARKMAN HP et al: Gastroduodenal motility and dysmotility: An update on techniques available for evaluation. Am J Gastroenterol 90:869, 1995

TYTGAT GNJ et al (eds): Towards understanding dyspepsia: An update and concensus from an International Working Party. Scand J Gastroenterol 26(suppl 182):1, 1991

WISEMAN LR, FAULDS D: Cisapride: An updated review of its pharmacology and therapeutic efficacy as a prokinetic agent in gastrointestinal motility disorders. Drugs 47:116, 1994

INDIGESTION

BYTZER P et al: Empirical H₂ blocker therapy or prompt endoscopy in management of dyspepsia. Lancet 343:811, 1994

MISIEWICZ JJ: Dyspepsia, in *Gastrointestinal Disease*, 5th ed, MH Sleisinger, JS Fordtran (eds). Philadelphia, Saunders, 1993, pp 572–579

PERMAN JA: Approach to the patient with gas and bloating, in *Textbook of Gastroenterology*, 2d ed, T Yamada et al (eds). Philadelphia, Lippincott, 1995, pp 772–782

STROCCHI A, LEVITT MD: Intestinal gas, in *Gastrointestinal Disease*, 5th ed, MH Sleisinger, JS Fordtran (eds). Philadelphia, Saunders, 1993, pp 1035–1042

TALLEY NJ: Non-ulcer dyspepsia: Myths and realities. Aliment Pharmacol Ther 5(suppl 1):145, 1991

———: Nonulcer dyspepsia, in *Textbook of Gastroenterology*, 2d ed, T Yamada et al (eds). Philadelphia, Lippincott, 1995, pp 1446–1455

———: Review article: Functional dyspepsia—should treatment be targeted on disturbed physiology? Aliment Pharmacol Ther 9:107, 1995

42   *Lawrence S. Friedman, Kurt J. Isselbacher*

DIARRHEA AND CONSTIPATION

NORMAL INTESTINAL FUNCTION

INTESTINAL FLUID ABSORPTION AND SECRETION

On an average day, 9 L of fluid enters the gastrointestinal tract: 2 L by direct ingestion, 1 L as saliva, 2 L as gastric juice, and 4 L as biliary, pancreatic, and small intestine secretions. On passage through the small intestine, 4 to 5 L of fluid is reabsorbed in the jejunum and 3 to 4 L in the ileum. Therefore, approximately 1 L of residual fluid enters the colon, where an additional 800 mL is reabsorbed before passage to the rectum and evacuation. Overall, the usual amount of fluid excreted in feces is approximately 200 mL/d.

In the intestine, water absorption follows active and passive sodium (Na^+) and nutrient absorption (Fig. 42-1). In the small intestine, Na^+ is cotransported with chloride (Cl^-) and nutrients such as glucose; in the terminal ileum, Na^+ is cotransported with bile salts; and in the colon, Na^+ is absorbed via Na^+ channels and by the electroneutral NaCl absorptive mechanism used in the small intestine. The cotransport mechanisms for Na^+ and nutrient absorption depend in part on Na^+ gradients across the apical membrane of intestinal epithelial cells created by the Na^+, K^+-ATPase pump of the basolateral membrane. The most important of these clinically is a Na^+-glucose cotransport carrier in the small intestine. Absorption of glucose by this mechanism results in accumulation of glucose in the epithelial cell, followed by its movement across the basolateral membrane by a facilitated transport mechanism, while Na^+ is actively pumped across the basolateral membrane by Na^+, K^+-ATPase. The absorption of Na^+ also promotes absorption of Cl^- through a paracellular pathway. Water absorption follows passively to maintain isoosmolality in the intercellular space. Because the Na^+-glucose cotransport mechanism remains unaffected by most diarrheal diseases, administration of a glucose-salt solution is useful clinically for the management of diarrhea and dehydration regardless of the cause.

Other cotransport mechanisms exist. A Na^+-Cl^- cotransport mechanism is thought actually to be composed of an Na^+-H^+ exchange carrier and a Cl^--HCO_3^- exchange carrier. This mechanism permits entry of both Na^+ and Cl^- into a cell in exchange for H^+ and HCO_3^-. Additional transport mechanisms have been identified for potassium (K^+), which may be absorbed in exchange for H^+, and for calcium (Ca^{2+}), the absorption of which is regulated by vitamin D and 1,25-dihydroxyvitamin D_3, parathyroid hormone, calcitonin, and a number of calcium-binding proteins.

In addition to its absorptive function, the intestine has a secretory function. Cl^- can be secreted by intestinal crypt cells via an electrogenic mechanism, with Na^+, K^+, and water following passively through tight junctions. HCO_3^- is secreted in the duodenum, other parts of the small intestine, and into the bile and pancreatic ducts. Because of the large acid load from the stomach, secreted HCO_3^- is diluted and present in relatively low concentrations. However, in the distal gut, HCO_3^- gradually becomes the predominant anion, permitting conservation of Cl^-, presumably via a Cl^--HCO_3^- exchange mechanism at the apical membrane of the epithelial cells. Intracellular cyclic nucleotides and ionized calcium (Ca^{2+}) initiate and regulate active Cl^- secretion.

COLONIC FUNCTION   As in the small intestine, an Na^+ absorptive mechanism exists in the colon. Na^+ absorption is predominantly electrogenic in that the absorbed Na^+ ion is unaccompanied by cation exchange or anion cotransport. Na^+ enters colonic epithelial cells through channels in the apical membrane and is pumped out across the basolateral membrane by Na^+, K^+-ATPase.

A variety of neural and nonneural mediators regulate colonic ion transport and motility, but the precise mechanisms are not well understood. The colon and rectum are innervated by nerve fibers that release norepinephrine, acetylcholine, and other neurotransmitters. Parasympathetic nerves stimulate peristaltic contraction and electrolyte secretion, whereas adrenergic tone inhibits cholinergic stimulation and increases electrolyte absorption. Additional regulation is provided by local reflex arcs within the autonomous enteric nervous system and intrinsic contractile responses of the colonic smooth muscle.

DEFECATION   The defecatory reflex is initiated by acute distention of the rectum, which results in partial and transient relaxation of the internal anal sphincter via parasympathetic innervation. As sigmoid and rectal contractions increase the pressure within the rectum, the rectosigmoid angle created by tonic contraction of the puborectalis muscle, which forms a sling around the anorectal junction, is obliterated. Contraction of the external anal sphincter, which consists of at least three bundles of striated muscle surrounding the anal canal and innervated by the pudendal nerve, can delay defecation until a socially acceptable time. Concomitant relaxation of the internal and external anal sphincters then permits the evacuation of feces, which can be

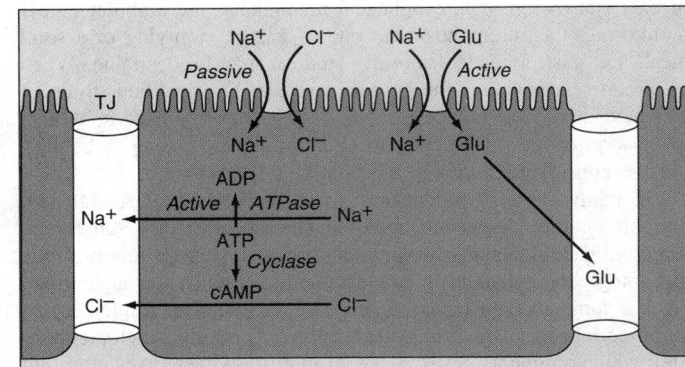

FIGURE 42-1   Sodium, chloride, and glucose transport by intestinal epithelial cells. Passive and active transport mechanisms for sodium (Na^+), chloride (Cl^-), and sodium-glucose coupled uptake are shown. Na^+ is pumped out at basolateral border by the active ATPase pump; Cl^- in part accompanies Na^+ but also is actively extruded by cyclic AMP. TJ, tight junction.

augmented by an increase in intraabdominal pressure created by the Valsalva maneuver.

DIARRHEA

DEFINITION In developed countries, normal stool weight of an adult human is less than 200 g/d; stool water accounts for 60 to 85 percent of the weight. Normal bowel frequency ranges from three times a week to three times a day. Factors that influence stool weight, consistency, and frequency include the fiber content of the diet, gender (the average daily weight of stool in women is less than that of men), ingested medications, and possibly exercise and stress. *Diarrhea* is formally defined as an increase in daily stool weight above 200 g. Typically, the patient also may describe an abnormal increase in stool liquidity and frequency.

Diarrhea must be distinguished from *pseudodiarrhea* or *hyperdefecation*, which is an increased frequency of defecation without an increase in stool weight above normal, as occurs in patients with irritable bowel syndrome, proctitis, or hyperthyroidism. Diarrhea also must be distinguished from fecal *incontinence*, which is the involuntary release of rectal contents. Incontinence is more common when stool is liquid than solid and reflects abnormal function of the anorectum or pelvic muscles. Diarrhea is considered *acute* when lasting less than 7 to 14 days and *chronic* when lasting more than 2 to 3 weeks.

ACUTE DIARRHEA The most common causes of acute diarrhea are infectious agents (Table 42-1). Acute diarrhea also may be caused by ingested drugs or toxins, the administration of chemotherapy, resumption of enteral feeding following a prolonged fast, fecal impaction (overflow diarrhea), or particular situations, such as marathon running. Additionally, acute diarrhea may represent the onset of a chronic diarrheal illness.

Table 42-1

Infectious Diarrhea: Pathophysiologic Mechanisms and Causes

Pathophysiologic Mechanism	Examples
Toxin production	
Preformed toxin	*Bacillus cereus*
	Clostridium perfringens
	Staphylococcus aureus
Enterotoxin	*Aeromonas* sp.
	Enterotoxigenic *E. coli*
	Vibrio cholerae
Cytotoxin	*Clostridium difficile*
	E. coli O157:H7
Enteroadherence	Cryptosporidiosis
	Cyclospora sp. (?)
	Enteroadherent and enteropathogenic *E. coli*
	Helminths
	Giardia
Mucosal invasion	
Minimal	Norwalk virus
	Rotavirus
	Other viruses (e.g., adenovirus, astrovirus, calicivirus, coronavirus, cytomegalovirus, herpes simplex virus)
Variable	*Aeromonas* sp.
	Campylobacter sp.
	Salmonella sp.
	Vibrio parahemolyticus
Severe	*Entamoeba histolytica*
	Enteroinvasive *E. coli*
	Shigella sp.
Systemic infection	Legionellosis
	Listeriosis
	Measles
	Psittacosis
	Rocky Mountain spotted fever
	Toxic shock syndrome
	Viral hepatitis

Infectious Diarrhea (see Chaps. 128, 142, 155, and 158 to 161) Worldwide, acute infectious diarrhea accounts for more than 5 to 8 million deaths each year in children less than age 5, especially in developing nations, where acute infectious diarrhea is a major cause of protein-calorie malnutrition and dehydration. Contributing factors include inadequate sewage disposal and water supplies, lack of refrigeration, overcrowding and lack of personal hygiene, poverty, lack of access to health care, and lack of education. Even in the United States, significant economic loss results from acute infectious diarrhea, which accounts for 250,000 hospital admissions and nearly 8 million office visits to physicians each year.

Most infectious diarrheas are acquired by fecal-oral transmission by way of water or food contaminated by human waste as a result of poor sewage systems or by wild or domestic animal feces in inadequately purified water. Beef, pork, or poultry may be the source of infection (especially with *Escherichia coli* O157:H7) when improperly cooked. Food-preparing surfaces may be contaminated by organisms that are spread to uncooked food. Person-to-person transmission also may occur through aerosolization (Norwalk agent, rotavirus), contamination of hands (*Clostridium difficile*) or surfaces, or sexual activity.

In the United States, groups at particularly high risk of acute infectious diarrhea include travelers to or recently from developing nations, persons who ingest shellfish, male homosexuals (gay bowel syndrome), prostitutes, and intravenous drug users. Persons with AIDS in particular are at risk for a remarkable array of serious enteric infections (Table 42-2). Among children attending day-care centers, acute infectious diarrhea commonly results from person-to-person transmission. The most common organisms involved in day-care outbreaks of diarrhea are *Shigella*, *Giardia lamblia*, and *Cryptosporidium*. Secondary attack rates ranging between 10 and 20 percent represent an important source of infection for parents and siblings. Additional high-risk institutions for outbreaks of acute infectious diarrhea include residential homes for the mentally and developmentally handicapped, nursing homes, and hospitals.

Clinical Features Patients with acute infectious diarrhea typically present with nausea, vomiting, abdominal pain, fever, and diarrhea, which may be watery, malabsorptive, or bloody, depending on the specific pathogen (see Table 42-1). Patients ingesting *toxins* or those with *toxigenic infection* typically have nausea and vomiting as prominent symptoms but rarely a high fever. Abdominal pain is mild, diffuse, and crampy and results from the high volumes of secreted fluid that stimulate peristalsis and cause watery diarrhea. Vomiting

Table 42-2

Possible Causes of Diarrhea in Patients with AIDS

Nonopportunistic pathogens
Shigella
Salmonella
Campylobacter
Entamoeba histolytica
Chlamydia
Neisseria gonorrhoeae
Treponema pallidum and other spirochetes
Giardia lamblia
Opportunistic infections
Protozoa
Cryptosporidium
Isospora belli
Microsporidia
Blastocystis hominis
Viruses
Cytomegalovirus
Herpes simplex
Adenovirus
Human immunodeficiency virus
Bacteria
Mycobacterium avium complex

that begins within several hours of ingesting a food should suggest food poisoning due to a preformed toxin. Parasites that do not invade the intestinal mucosa such as *Giardia lamblia* and *Cryptosporidium* usually cause only mild abdominal discomfort. *Giardia* also may be associated with mild steatorrhea, gaseousness, and bloating. *Invasive bacteria* such as *Campylobacter*, *Salmonella*, and *Shigella* and organisms that produce cytotoxins such as *C. difficile* and enterohemorrhagic *E. coli* (serotype O157:H7) cause severe intestinal inflammation, abdominal pain, and often a high fever; occasionally, peritoneal signs may suggest a surgical abdomen. *Yersinia* often infects the terminal ileum and cecum and presents with right lower quadrant pain and tenderness suggestive of acute appendicitis. Watery diarrhea is typical of organisms that invade the intestinal epithelium with *minimal inflammation*, such as enteric viruses, or organisms that *adhere* to but do not destroy the epithelium, such as enteropathogenic or enteroadherent *E. coli*, protozoa, and helminths. Some organisms such as *Campylobacter*, *Aeromonas*, *Shigella*, and *Vibrio* species (e.g., *Vibrio parahemolyticus* and *V. fulnifice*) both produce enterotoxins and invade the intestinal mucosa; patients therefore often present with watery diarrhea followed within hours or days by bloody diarrhea.

The presence of systemic symptoms may provide additional clues to the underlying cause of diarrhea. Both shigellosis and infection with enterohemorrhagic *E. coli* may be accompanied by the hemolytic-uremic syndrome, particularly in persons who are very young or very old. *Yersinia* infection and occasionally other enteric bacterial infections may be accompanied by Reiter's syndrome (arthritis, urethritis, and conjunctivitis), thyroiditis, pericarditis, or glomerulonephritis.

Differential Diagnosis Virtually any *medication* can cause diarrhea, and a careful drug history should be obtained in any patient with acute diarrhea (Table 42-3). Other ingested toxins also must be considered, including organophosphate insecticides, mushrooms, arsenic, and even caffeine. *Acute diverticulitis* occasionally may present with diarrhea accompanied by fever and abdominal pain (see Chap. 288). In patients with acute bloody diarrhea, diagnostic considerations may include *superior mesenteric arterial* or *venous thrombosis*, *ischemic* or *drug-induced colitis*, or *idiopathic inflammatory bowel disease* (ulcerative colitis or Crohn's disease) (see Chap. 286). In the elderly patient with acute colitis, differentiating an ischemic cause from enterohemorrhagic *E. coli* O157:H7 may be difficult because both diseases may be associated with submucosal hemorrhage that presents as "thumbprinting" on a plain abdominal radiograph. While colonoscopic and radiographic findings may be indistinguishable in infectious colitis and inflammatory bowel disease, histologic findings may be helpful

Table 42-3

Drugs That Commonly Cause Diarrhea

Gastrointestinal drugs	Hypolipidemic agents
Magnesium-containing antacids	Clofibrate
Laxatives	Gemfibrozil
Misoprostol	Lovastatin
Olsalazine	Probucol
Cardiac drugs	Neuropsychiatric drugs
Digitalis	Lithium
Quinidine	Fluoxetine (Prozac)
Procainamide	Alprazolam (Xanax)
Hydralazine	Valproic acid
Beta blockers	Ethosuximide
Angiotensin-converting enzyme	L-Dopa
inhibitors	Others
Diuretics	Theophylline
Antibiotics	Thyroid hormones
Clindamycin	Colchicine
Ampicillin	Nonsteroidal anti-
Cephalosporins	inflammatory drugs
Erythromycin	
Chemotherapeutic agents	

in suggesting one diagnosis or the other, since the inflammatory infiltrate in acute infectious diarrhea consists mainly of polymorphonuclear leukocytes rather than the chronic inflammatory infiltrate with crypt distortion typical of inflammatory bowel disease. The finding of pseudomembranes on colonoscopy points to *C. difficile* as the cause.

Laboratory Diagnosis Acute infectious diarrhea is usually self-limited, often resolving by the time the patient seeks medical attention. Because of the expense of stool cultures and other diagnostic tests, considerable judgment is required in deciding which patients with acute diarrhea should be evaluated and treated with antibiotics. For the patient presenting without high fever, bloody diarrhea, or dehydration, symptomatic therapy with oral fluids in the absence of specific diagnostic testing may suffice. On the other hand, a high fever, systemic toxicity, bloody diarrhea, and dehydration favor diagnostic testing, as do a known outbreak of food poisoning, recent overseas travel, immunocompromise, male homosexuality, or recent antibiotic use. In these situations, freshly collected stool should be examined for *occult blood* and *white blood cells*. The finding of primarily polymorphonuclear leukocytes on a Wright's or methylene blue stain suggests *Salmonella*, *Shigella*, invasive *E. coli*, *Yersinia*, or *Entamoeba histolytica*. Although it is common practice to obtain a qualitative fecal fat determination in patients with acute diarrhea, the presence of a small amount of fat in the stool is not uncommon in patients with acute diarrhea of any cause and provides no particular diagnostic information. The cornerstone of diagnosis in patients with severe and especially bloody diarrhea or a suggestive epidemiologic history is *bacterial culture* and *microscopic examination* of the stool for ova and parasites. Most laboratories routinely examine stool specimens sent for culture for *Salmonella*, *Shigella*, *Yersinia*, and *Campylobacter*, but special requests must be made to identify other organisms, including *C. difficile* (culture and toxin) and enterohemorrhagic *E. coli*. Special cultivation or staining techniques also may be required to identify organisms that cause watery diarrhea, including *Aeromonas*, *Cryptosporidium*, and *Vibrio* species. Certain organisms such as *Giardia* and *Strongyloides* as well as *Cryptosporidium* and *Isospora belli* may be difficult to detect in stool and are better diagnosed by *duodenal aspiration* or intestinal biopsy. Alternatively, a sensitive and specific enzyme-linked immunosorbent assay for *Giardia* antigen in stool may be used to confirm giardiasis. In patients with AIDS, electron microscopic examination of small intestinal biopsy specimens may facilitate detection of *Microsporidia*. *Sigmoidoscopy* and occasionally *colonoscopy* are generally reserved for patients with bloody diarrhea that does not improve within 10 days. As discussed above, mucosal changes may be nonspecific, although in some cases characteristic findings may be observed, such as pseudomembranes in *C. difficile*–induced colitis. *Barium radiographs* are also best deferred until the initial course of illness has been observed and appropriate stool specimens obtained. Even with the application of all available laboratory studies, between 20 and 40 percent of all acute infectious diarrheas remain undiagnosed.

Rx **TREATMENT**

General and nonspecific treatment of acute infectious diarrhea includes rest and fluid replacement. Because death in most instances of acute diarrhea results from dehydration, careful attention must be paid to correction of fluid and electrolyte deficits. Intravenous fluid therapy may be necessary in severely dehydrated individuals, especially infants and the elderly. Oral sugar-electrolyte solutions used in the treatment of patients with cholera can also be considered in patients with acute diarrhea due to other enterotoxin-producing bacteria. Antibiotic therapy in bacterial diarrheas is controversial and generally not necessary in patients with mild or resolving disease but should be considered in patients with shigellosis, traveler's diarrhea, pseudomembranous enterocolitis, cholera, and parasitic diseases. Regardless of the cause of infectious diarrhea, patients should be treated if they are immunocompromised, have a malignancy, have an abnormal heart valve or vascular or orthopedic prosthesis, have hemolytic anemia, or are extremely young or old. Anticholinergic drugs and opiates to control diarrhea should generally be avoided when an enteroinvasive organism is suspected because of the risk of prolonging colonization or causing ileus. However, loperamide and bismuth subsalicylate have been shown to be safe in patients with traveler's diarrhea who have neither a high fever nor blood or pus in the stool.

CHRONIC DIARRHEA Diarrhea that persists for weeks or months, whether constant or intermittent, requires evaluation. Although in the majority of cases the cause will prove to be irritable bowel syndrome, diarrhea may represent a manifestation of an underlying serious illness, and a careful search for disease should be undertaken. Chronic diarrhea can be categorized pathophysiologically as inflammatory, osmotic (malabsorption), secretory, due to intestinal dysmotility, or factitious (Table 42-4).

Inflammatory Diarrhea Inflammatory diarrheas are characterized generally by the presence of fever, abdominal tenderness, and blood or leukocytes in the stool, with inflammatory lesions on intestinal mucosal biopsy. In some cases, hypoalbuminemia, hypoglobulinemia, and protein-losing enteropathy may be present. In addition to inflammation, the mechanism of diarrhea may also be malabsorption or increased intestinal secretion.

In a patient who is not systemically ill, a liquid stool containing overt or occult blood raises the possibility of a *colonic neoplasm*. Patients with *ulcerative proctitis* also may present in this manner. In

a patient who is systemically ill with chronic bloody diarrhea, the diagnosis of *inflammatory bowel disease* (either *ulcerative colitis* or *Crohn's disease*) is suggested. These disorders also should be suspected when chronic diarrhea is associated with prominent extraintestinal manifestations, including arthritis, skin lesions (such as erythema nodosum or pyoderma gangrenosum), uveitis, or vasculitis. Diarrhea in inflammatory bowel disease may result from damage to absorptive surface epithelium as well as the release into the circulation of secretagogues such as leukotrienes, prostaglandins, histamine, and other cytokines that stimulate intestinal secretion or the enteric nervous system.

Inflammatory diarrhea is seen in patients with *chronic radiation enterocolitis* as a result of pelvic irradiation for malignancies of the female urogenital tract or the male prostate. The segments usually involved are the terminal ileum, cecum, and rectosigmoid because they are fixed in the pelvis. The risk of radiation enterocolitis correlates with the radiation dose; the frequency is 1 to 5 percent with doses of 45 to 50 Gy (4500 to 5500 rad) and 35 percent with higher doses. Chronic radiation injury is characterized by progressive swelling of the endothelial cells in small arterioles of the submucosa leading to obliterative endarteritis and vascular thrombosis and resulting in ischemia with fibrosis, bowel wall thickening, ulceration, and fissuring of the mucosa. Colonoscopy may show luminal narrowing, ulceration, diffuse inflammatory changes, and characteristic mucosal telangiectases which may bleed severely. Diarrhea also may result from bile acid malabsorption because of ileal inflammation or bacterial overgrowth resulting from intestinal strictures or stasis.

Eosinophilic gastroenteritis is characterized by infiltration of any portion of the gastrointestinal tract with eosinophils. In addition to diarrhea, patients present with abdominal pain, nausea, vomiting, weight loss, and, in 75 percent of cases, peripheral eosinophilia; some patients may develop steatorrhea and protein-losing enteropathy. Severe *protein-losing enteropathy* is manifested by peripheral edema, ascites, and occasionally anasarca. It may occur in a variety of disease states, including infections (viral gastroenteritis, bacterial overgrowth, parasitic infestation, *C. difficile* enterocolitis, or Whipple's disease), inflammatory bowel disease, splanchnic congestion due to congestive heart failure, lymphoma, or other conditions associated with lymphatic obstruction, such as congenital intestinal lymphangiectasia, Ménétrier's disease, systemic lupus erythematosus, or milk allergy. Recently, an increasing number of infectious causes of chronic diarrhea have been associated with infection caused by the human immunodeficiency virus (HIV) or with AIDS (see Table 39-2 and Chap. 308). In many patients with AIDS and diarrhea, multiple potential pathogens may be present in the stool, although the exact cause of diarrhea may be uncertain because such pathogens may also be found in the stool of AIDS patients without diarrhea. HIV itself is also thought to cause diarrhea in some cases (AIDS enteropathy), but the mechanism is not understood.

Other miscellaneous diseases associated with inflammatory diarrhea include *Behçet's syndrome* and *graft-versus-host disease* following allogeneic bone marrow transplantation.

Osmotic Diarrhea (See Chap. 285) Osmotic diarrhea occurs when an orally ingested solute is not fully absorbed in the small intestine and thereby exerts an osmotic force that draws fluid into the intestinal lumen. The increased luminal fluid volume overwhelms the capacity of the colon for reabsorption. The nonabsorbed solute can be a maldigested or malabsorbed nutrient or drug. Clinical symptoms are usually recognized because of the malabsorption of *fat* (*steatorrhea*) or *carbohydrates*. *Protein* or *amino acid* malabsorption (*azotorrhea*) is generally not recognized clinically unless it is severe enough to cause malnutrition or the consequences of a specific deficiency in an amino acid. The various disorders associated with malabsorption and maldigestion are discussed in more detail in other chapters, specifically, mucosal malabsorptive disorders in Chap. 285 and pancreatic exocrine deficiency and related disorders in Chap. 304.

Table 42-4

Classification of Chronic Diarrhea

Mechanism	Clinical Features	Examples
INFLAMMATORY		
Mucosal and submucosal inflammation Damaged epithelium In some cases impaired intestinal absorption and excessive secretion	Fever, abdominal pain, blood and/or leukocytes in stool	Ulcerative colitis Crohn's disease Radiation enterocolitis Eosinophilic gastroenteritis Infections associated with AIDS
OSMOTIC		
Nonabsorbed or nondigested intraluminal solute	Improvement of diarrhea with fasting Bulky, greasy, foul-smelling stools; weight loss Nutrient deficiencies Osmotic gap in fecal water	Pancreatic insufficiency Bacterial overgrowth Celiac sprue Lactase deficiency Whipple's disease Abetalipoproteinemia Short bowel syndrome
SECRETORY		
Excessive secretion of electrolytes	Watery diarrhea, persists with fasting Dehydration Other systemic effects of hormones Absence of osmotic gap in fecal water	Carcinoid syndrome Zollinger-Ellison syndrome Vasoactive intestinal peptide-secreting pancreatic adenomas Medullary carcinoma of thyroid Villous adenoma of rectum Microscopic colitis Cholerrheic diarrhea
ALTERED INTESTINAL MOTILITY		
Rapid transit In some cases associated bacterial overgrowth	Alternating diarrhea and constipation Neurologic symptoms; bladder involvement	Irritable bowel syndrome Fecal impaction Neurologic diseases
FACTITIOUS		
Self-induced	Usually women Watery diarrhea with hypokalemia, weakness, edema	Laxative abuse

Intraluminal maldigestion may result from *pancreatic exocrine insufficiency*, which occurs when at least 90 percent of the secretory capacity of the pancreas is lost in patients with *chronic pancreatitis* or occasionally *pancreatic ductal obstruction*. Maldigestion and weight loss occur despite preserved appetite. In children, *cystic fibrosis* or *Shwachman's syndrome* may cause chronic pancreatic insufficiency. *Somatostatinoma* is a rare pancreatic islet tumor that leads to gallstones, diabetes, and steatorrhea thought to be caused by inhibition of pancreatic secretion. Intraluminal maldigestion also may result from *bile duct obstruction* as a result of cancer of the head of the pancreas or from severe liver disease with *cholestasis*. Deficiency of intraluminal bile salts usually results in only mild fat malabsorption. *Bacterial overgrowth* in a blind loop of intestine or a segment of stasis (e.g., due to enterocolonic fistula, jejunal diverticulosis, intestinal dysmotility due to scleroderma, diabetes, or chronic intestinal pseudo-obstruction) may result in steatorrhea due to deconjugation of the bile salts and impaired micelle formation; additional factors leading to diarrhea include brush border enzyme injury, mucosal inflammation, and hydroxylation of fat causing fatty acid diarrhea.

Osmotic diarrhea may result from the chronic ingestion of certain fruits or candy, gum, dietetic foods, and medications sweetened with unabsorbed carbohydrates such as sorbitol or fructose. Congenital absence of specific brush border carbohydrate hydrolases and transport proteins also may lead to chronic diarrhea; the most common of these is lactase deficiency resulting in lactose intolerance.

The classic example of *mucosal malabsorption* is *celiac sprue*, or gluten-sensitive enteropathy (see Chap. 285). In addition to presenting with typical symptoms and signs of malabsorption, patients with celiac sprue may have atypical presentations, including failure to thrive, muscle wasting, abdominal distention, and irritability in young children, and iron-deficiency anemia, growth retardation, and anorexia in adolescents or young adults. Later in life, patients may present with insidious nutritional deficiencies, infertility, and neuromuscular disease. Like celiac sprue, *tropical sprue* is characterized by malabsorption and histologic changes in the small bowel of villus atrophy, crypt hyperplasia, damaged surface epithelium, and a mononuclear infiltrate in the lamina propria. A disease affecting residents in certain tropical parts of the world, tropical sprue can occur even in visitors residing for as little as 1 to 3 months in an endemic area. The onset may be acute, suggesting an infectious etiology.

Intestinal malabsorption is typical of *Whipple's disease* due to *Tropheryma whippelii*, which usually affects middle-aged men but may present at any age and in patients of either sex. Additional manifestations include arthralgias, fever and chills, hypotension, lymphadenopathy, and involvement of the central nervous system (see Chap. 285). *Abetalipoproteinemia* is caused by the absence of Apo B resulting in defective chylomicron formation. Children with this disorder present with steatorrhea, acanthocytic red blood cells, ataxia, and retinitis pigmentosa (see Chap. 285). Steatorrhea also may result from infections with *Giardia, Isospora, Strongyloides*, and *Mycobacterium avium* complex. Ingestion of certain *drugs* may result in steatorrhea because of damage to enterocytes; examples include colchicine, neomycin, and *para*-aminosalicylic acid.

Intestinal lymphangiectasia (Chap. 285) causes protein-losing enteropathy with steatorrhea but preserved absorption of carbohydrates and is thus an example of *postmucosal obstruction of lymphatic channels*. The disease may be congenital or acquired as a result of trauma, lymphoma, carcinoma, or Whipple's disease.

Finally, extensive intestinal resection may result in the *short bowel syndrome*, in which steatorrhea results from an inadequate absorptive surface, decreased transit time, and a decreased bile salt pool. Other factors that may contribute to diarrhea in short bowel syndrome include the osmotic effect of nonabsorbed solutes, gastric hypersecretion, and in some cases bacterial overgrowth.

Secretory Diarrhea Secretory diarrhea is characterized by a large volume of fecal output caused by abnormal fluid and electrolyte transport not necessarily related to the ingestion of food. Therefore, diarrhea usually persists with fasting. The term *watery diarrhea* is often used synonymously with secretory diarrhea. Because there is no malabsorbed solute, fecal osmolality in secretory diarrheas can be accounted for by normal ionic constituents with no fecal osmotic gap (see below).

The classic examples of secretory diarrhea are those mediated by hormones (see Chaps. 95 and 284). Patients with metastatic *carcinoid tumors* of the gastrointestinal tract may have watery diarrhea as part of the carcinoid syndrome that includes episodic flushing, telangiectatic skin lesions, cyanosis, pellagra-like skin lesions, bronchospasm, and cardiac murmurs due to right-sided valvular lesions. The carcinoid syndrome results from secretion of a variety of vasoactive substances that are potent intestinal secretagogues, including serotonin, histamine, catecholamines, prostaglandin, and kinins. The *Zollinger-Ellison syndrome* is characterized by recurrent, refractory, and unusually located peptic ulcers due to a gastrinoma; diarrhea occurs in up to one-third of patients and may be the presenting symptom in 10 percent of cases. The diarrhea is due only in part to the high volumes of secreted hydrochloric acid but is also due to maldigestion of fat caused by inactivation of pancreatic lipase and precipitation of bile acids at low pH. *Non-beta cell pancreatic adenomas* may secrete a variety of peptides, including vasoactive intestinal polypeptide (VIP), pancreatic polypeptide, secretin, neurotensin, calcitonin, prostaglandins, and others. Those that secrete VIP may be associated with the *watery diarrhea/hypokalemia achlorhydria* (WDHA) *syndrome*, characterized by often massive secretory diarrhea, achlorhydria, hypokalemia, hypomagnesemia, hypercalcemia without hyperparathyroidism, and, in some cases flushing, myopathy, or nephropathy. Not all patients with WDHA syndrome have a *vipoma*, and in such cases, alternative mediators of intestinal secretion have been postulated. *Medullary carcinoma of the thyroid* (Chap. 331) may be sporadic or a feature of multiple endocrine neoplasia syndrome type IIa with pheochromocytomas and hyperparathyroidism. Watery diarrhea is thought to be mediated by calcitonin produced by the tumor, although in some cases other mediators may be found. The occurrence of diarrhea in medullary carcinoma of the thyroid is usually associated with metastases and a poor prognosis. *Systemic mastocytosis* (Chap. 285), which may be associated with the skin lesion urticaria pigmentosa, also may be associated with diarrhea that is secretory and mediated by histamine or malabsorptive and due to intestinal mucosal infiltration by mast cells.

Diarrhea associated with a *villous adenoma* (Chap. 92) of the rectum or rectosigmoid usually occurs with large tumors, often more than 3 to 4 cm in diameter. Hypokalemia due to potassium loss is common.

Microscopic or *lymphocytic colitis* and *collagenous colitis* (Chap. 286) may represent variants of the same disease. Their hallmarks are a characteristic histologic lesion, despite a normal mucosal appearance on colonoscopy, and diarrhea that is often secretory. In both disorders, histologic findings include infiltration of the lamina propria with inflammatory cells as well as intraepithelial lymphocytes, but only in collagenous colitis is there also a characteristic subepithelial collagen band.

Secretory diarrhea may result from *severe disease, resection*, or *bypass of the distal ileum* when less than 100 cm of the ileum is affected (Chap. 285). Presumably, diarrhea results from stimulation of colonic secretion by dihydroxy bile salts that escape absorption in the terminal ileum (cholerrheic diarrhea). By preventing gallbladder contraction and the delivery of large amounts of bile into the intestine, fasting eliminates this type of secretory diarrhea. When greater than 100 cm of terminal ileum is diseased or resected, hepatic synthesis cannot maintain an adequate intraluminal bile salt pool, and steatorrhea also ensues. Bile acid–induced diarrhea may occur following cholecystectomy because of the loss of the storage capacity of the gallbladder. Rarely, *primary (idiopathic) bile acid malabsorption* by the terminal ileum may account for otherwise unexplained secretory diarrhea. Rapid small intestinal transit resulting in increased delivery of bile acids to the colon also may account for *postvagotomy diarrhea*, which occurs in up to 30 percent of patients undergoing truncal vagotomy with a drainage procedure for peptic ulcer disease; diarrhea is much less common following proximal gastric vagotomy.

Altered Intestinal Motility Diarrhea may be associated with disorders that affect intestinal motility. The most common of these is *irritable bowel syndrome* (Chap. 287), in which diarrhea typically alternates with constipation and is associated with abdominal pain, the passage of mucus, and a sense of incomplete evacuation. However, in some patients, constipation alone with lower abdominal cramps is the predominant clinical manifestation, while others present only with painless diarrhea presumably due to disordered intestinal motility. Diarrhea may occasionally occur paradoxically as a result of *fecal impaction* or an obstructing tumor with the overflow of liquid colonic contents around the impacted stool or obstruction. A variety of *neurologic diseases* also may be associated with diarrhea because of altered autonomic control of bowel function. Profuse watery diarrhea, often with incontinence, may be seen in patients with *type 1 diabetes* and is often associated with severe neuropathy, nephropathy, and retinopathy. Additional contributing factors may include bacterial overgrowth secondary to intestinal dysmotility, pancreatic exocrine insufficiency, or, rarely, celiac sprue. Diarrhea also may occur in patients with *traumatic neuropathy*, the *Shy-Drager syndrome*, or *lesions of the cauda equina*.

Factitious Diarrhea Factitious diarrhea is self-induced by the patient and may result from intestinal infection, the addition of water or urine to the stool, or self-medication with laxatives. Patients are predominantly women with severe chronic watery diarrhea, abdominal pain, nausea and vomiting, weight loss, peripheral edema, and weakness resulting from hypokalemia. The diagnosis of factitious diarrhea should be suspected in a patient with a history of psychiatric disease or multiple previous negative evaluations for diarrhea. Additional diagnoses to consider in patients with chronic diarrhea of obscure origin are listed in Table 42-5.

Approach to the Patient

With Diarrhea A thorough history and physical examination are crucial initial steps in the evaluation of the patient with chronic diarrhea. The history in particular may direct the evaluation toward a general pathophysiologic mechanism or even a specific diagnosis and serves as a useful guide to the selection of a limited number of appropriate diagnostic studies.

Inflammatory diarrheas may be suggested by the presence of fever with abdominal pain, often localized to one of the lower quadrants. Extraintestinal manifestations such as arthritis, skin lesions, or ocular symptoms suggest idiopathic inflammatory bowel disease. The presence of peripheral edema, ascites, or anasarca is compatible with protein-losing enteropathy. Intestinal malabsorption is suggested by (1) bulky or greasy foul-smelling stools that are difficult to flush and leave oil in the bowl, (2) flatulence, and (3) weight loss. Malabsorption of specific essential nutrients may present as anemia, a bleeding tendency, osteopenia, amenorrhea, or infertility. Steatorrhea is typically more severe in pancreatic insufficiency than in intestinal mucosal disease, whereas flatulence and bloating are more typical of intestinal mucosal disease than pancreatic insufficiency because of associated carbohydrate malabsorption. Osmotic diarrhea of any cause often improves or resolves with fasting. In watery diarrheas, weight loss is

Table 42-5

Causes of Chronic Diarrhea of Obscure Origin

Drugs (see Table 42-3)
Laxative abuse
Microscopic or collagenous colitis
Bacterial overgrowth
Carbohydrate malabsorption
Bile acid malabsorption (including after cholecystectomy and ileal resection)
Diabetic diarrhea
Epidemic chronic diarrhea (? contaminated milk or water)
Chronic idiopathic secretory diarrhea
Fecal incontinence

unusual except in patients with advanced neuroendocrine tumors, which also may be suggested by characteristic systemic manifestations such as flushing. Symptoms of autonomic dysfunction such as postural hypotension, impotence, or disordered sweating are often found in patients with diabetic diarrhea. Diarrhea alternating with constipation is typical of the irritable bowel syndrome.

In addition to providing clues to the underlying cause of diarrhea, the physical examination is important in assessing the presence of volume depletion, as manifested by postural hypotension, tachycardia, absence of axillary sweat, decreased skin turgor, mental lethargy, and generalized weakness.

Laboratory studies may be employed in the evaluation of chronic diarrhea, but a "shotgun" approach should be avoided. In many patients it is helpful to start with routine blood studies such as a complete blood count and peripheral smear and serum electrolyte, calcium, phosphate, albumin, and quantitative immunoglobulin determinations.

Inflammatory diarrheas may be associated with leukocytosis, an elevated erythrocyte sedimentation rate, or hypoalbuminemia. The hallmark of inflammatory diarrheas is the presence of either *gross or occult blood and leukocytes* in the stool; leukocytes can be detected by a Wright's or methylene blue stain. Further evaluation usually involves *upper gastrointestinal endoscopy or colonoscopy* with diagnostic biopsies. An *upper gastrointestinal radiograph with a small bowel follow-through* also may be indicated to evaluate the small intestine. In rare instances, [111]*In-labeled white blood cell scans* may be used to detect bowel inflammation not apparent on endoscopy or conventional barium radiography. In patients with AIDS and chronic diarrhea, multiple stool specimens for culture and examination for ova and parasites should be obtained prior to more invasive diagnostic testing.

A wide array of tests may be helpful in evaluating the patient with an osmotic diarrhea. Decreased levels of iron, folate, vitamin B_{12}, and vitamin D may suggest malabsorption. The prothrombin time may be prolonged due to vitamin K deficiency, and serum carotene, cholesterol, and albumin levels may be decreased. A stool pH of less than 5.3 suggests carbohydrate malabsorption. The cornerstone of testing for intestinal malabsorption is the measurement of *fecal fat*, which is described in detail in Chap. 285.

The capacity of the small intestine to absorb simple sugars can be assessed by the D-*xylose absorption test*, in which 25 g of this five-carbon sugar is administered orally and urine is collected for the subsequent 5 h; normally, at least 25 percent of the administered dose is excreted in the urine. The sensitivity of this test may be increased by obtaining a blood sample following the oral dose; a blood level of greater than 30 mg/dL at 2 h is normal (see Chap. 285).

The definitive test for malabsorption due to intestinal mucosal disease is the *small-intestinal biopsy*, which may be performed via upper endoscopy with forceps biopsy of the distal duodenum or with a specialized small bowel biopsy instrument that reaches the jejunum. Small-intestinal biopsy is generally diagnostic in diseases characterized by diffuse involvement of the small intestine such as Whipple's disease, *M. avium complex* infection, or abetalipoproteinemia but may be falsely negative in diseases with a patchy distribution such as lymphoma, eosinophilic gastroenteritis, or amyloidosis. In celiac sprue, histologic findings may be suggestive, but the diagnosis can be confirmed only by demonstrating that the histologic lesion reverses following withdrawal of gluten from the diet. The diagnosis of celiac sprue is also suggested by detection of anti-endomysial and anti-gliadin antibodies in serum.

Protein-losing enteropathy is best confirmed by assaying for α_1-antitrypsin, an endogenous protein, on an aliquot of lyophilized stool (Chap. 285). One screening test of *pancreatic function* available in some countries is the *bentiromide test*, which depends on the ability of pancreatic chymotrypsin to cleave *para*-aminobenzoic acid (PABA) from the synthetic peptide *N*-benzoyl-L-tyrosyl *para*-aminobenzoic acid (bentiromide); the cleaved PABA is absorbed by the intestine, conjugated in the liver, and excreted in the urine. This and other tests of pancreatic function are discussed in Chap. 304.

The *Schilling test*, used in the evaluation of patients with suspected pernicious anemia, also can be used as a diagnostic test for pancreatic insufficiency, in which vitamin B_{12} absorption is impaired because gastric R-proteins are not cleaved from intrinsic factor as a result of diminished pancreatic proteolytic activity in the upper small intestine; vitamin B_{12} absorption improves when the test is repeated following oral administration of pancreatic enzymes.

Bacterial overgrowth may be detected by aspirating fluid from the upper small intestine through an endoscope or a small-intestinal tube placed under fluoroscopic guidance and finding a *bacterial colony count* of greater than 10^5 per mL. Alternatively, the diagnosis of bacterial overgrowth is suggested by an increase in exhaled $^{14}CO_2$ within 60 min of the ingestion of 1 g ^{14}C-D-xylose (*^{14}C-xylose breath test*) or after the ingestion of ^{14}[C]cholylglycine (*bile acid breath test*) or the detection of increased breath H_2 within the first 2 h after ingestion of either glucose or rice flour (*breath hydrogen test*) (see Chap. 285).

Radiologic tests may play a diagnostic role in patients with suspected malabsorption. An abdominal radiograph may demonstrate pancreatic calcification in patients with chronic pancreatitis. *Abdominal ultrasonography*, *computed tomography*, or *endoscopic retrograde cholangiopancreatography* also may be useful in the evaluation of suspected pancreatic disease. Standard *barium radiographs* of the gastrointestinal tract may suggest thickening of the valvulae conniventes due to infiltrative disease such as Whipple's disease, lymphoma, or amyloidosis or dilatation of the small bowel with flocculation of the barium in celiac sprue. Additional relevant findings may include a gastrocolic fistula, blind loop, stricture, or multiple diverticula.

Fecal osmolality measurements may be helpful in distinguishing osmotic from secretory diarrhea when the diarrhea is watery. Measured osmolality can be compared with the calculated fecal osmolality, which is the sum of the measured Na^+ and K^+ concentrations multiplied by 2 (to account for anions). The osmotic gap is the measured fecal osmolality minus the calculated fecal osmolality and corresponds approximately to the concentration of poorly absorbed solutes in fecal water. Measured fecal osmolality should approximate plasma osmolality, which, in general, is 290 mosmol/kg H_2O. (In fact, a measured fecal osmolality greater than 300 mosmol/kg H_2O indicates bacterial degradation of nonabsorbed carbohydrate in the collection jar or the addition of urine to the jar.) A fecal osmotic gap greater than 50 mosmol/kg H_2O is significant and suggests osmotic diarrhea due to a poorly absorbed carbohydrate or excessive ingestion of magnesium-containing laxatives. If the fecal osmolality is much lower than that of the plasma (290 mosmol/kg H_2O), fluid has been added to the stool.

In patients with watery diarrhea, blood levels of *serotonin, gastrin, VIP, calcitonin,* and other potential secretagogues should be obtained, in addition to a *urinary 5-hydroxyindole acetic acid* level. *Flexible sigmoidoscopy* or *colonoscopy* should be considered to exclude villous adenoma of the rectum or sigmoid as well as microscopic or collagenous colitis. Colonoscopy also may reveal melanosis coli due to abuse of anthraquinone laxatives. Ingestion of phenolphthalein laxatives may be detected by *alkalinizing the stool* with either NaOH or KOH, which results in a pink or purple color. When the index of suspicion for laxative abuse is high, a cautious room search may be diagnostic. In addition, spectrophotometry or thin-layer chromatography to detect bisacodyl, phenolphthalein, and anthraquinones can be performed on urine or stool water.

In cases of suspected ileal bile salt malabsorption, a *^{75}selenahomotaurocholic acid* (*^{75}SeHCAT*) *test* may be available in some centers. *^{75}SeHCAT* acid is an analogue of taurocholic acid and is thus absorbed in the terminal ileum; scanning with a gamma camera can be used to quantitate ileal absorption and increased bile acid loss. Alternatively, a therapeutic trial of the bile salt–binding resin *cholestyramine* may be administered.

℞ **TREATMENT**

While every effort should be made to identify and correct the specific cause of diarrhea, in many cases a cause that is specifically treatable may not be identifiable, and symptomatic therapy alone may be indicated. Psyllium and other hydrophilic agents absorb water and thereby enhance stool consistency. Most other available antidiarrheal agents act by altering intestinal motility; some also may have mild proabsorptive or antisecretory activity. *Opiate antidiarrheal agents* such as diphenoxylate and loperamide may be helpful in secretory diarrhea of mild to moderate severity. However, such antimotility agents may be contraindicated in diarrhea due to infectious agents because stasis may enhance tissue invasion by the organisms or delay their clearance from the bowel. In patients with severe inflammatory bowel disease, such drugs may contribute to the development of toxic megacolon and are contraindicated. *Octreotide*, a long-acting synthetic analogue of somatostatin, has a significant antisecretory effect in the carcinoid syndrome and other neuroendocrine tumors because of its specific inhibition of hormone secretion; it also may have some benefit in the short bowel syndrome. *Clonidine*, an alpha₂-adrenergic agonist, may be useful in the diarrhea of opiate withdrawal and diabetic diarrhea. *H^+, K^+-ATPase inhibitors*, such as omeprazole and lansoprazole, and *H_2-receptor antagonists* are useful in the diarrhea that results from gastric hypersecretion in the Zollinger-Ellison syndrome. Other drugs that may have some benefit in the treatment of neuroendocrine tumors or unexplained secretory diarrheas include *phenothiazines* and *calcium channel blockers*. *Indomethacin*, an inhibitor of prostaglandin synthesis and secretion, may have benefit in the diarrhea of medullary carcinoma of the thyroid and villous adenomas. A combination of H_1- and H_2-receptor antagonists may be helpful in treating the diarrhea of systemic mastocytosis. *Cholestyramine* is the drug of choice in diarrhea caused by ileal bile salt malabsorption.

CONSTIPATION

DEFINITION Constipation is a common complaint in clinical practice. Because of the wide range of normal bowel habits, constipation is difficult to define precisely. Most persons have at least three bowel movements per week, and *constipation* has been defined as a frequency of defecation of less than three times per week. However, stool frequency alone is not a sufficient criterion to use, because many constipated patients describe a normal frequency of defecation but subjective complaints of excessive straining, hard stools, lower abdominal fullness, and a sense of incomplete evacuation. Thus a combination of objective and subjective criteria must be used to define constipation.

CAUSES Pathophysiologically, constipation generally results from *disordered colonic transit or anorectal function* as a result of a primary motility disturbance, certain drugs, or in association with a large number of systemic diseases that affect the gastrointestinal tract. Constipation of any cause may be exacerbated by chronic illnesses that lead to physical or mental impairment and result in inactivity or physical immobility. Additional contributing factors may include a lack of fiber in the diet, generalized muscle weakness, and possibly stress and anxiety.

In the patient presenting with the recent onset of constipation, an *obstructing lesion* of the colon should be sought. In addition to a *colonic neoplasm*, other causes of colonic obstruction include *strictures* due to colonic ischemia, diverticular disease, or inflammatory bowel disease; *foreign bodies*; or *anal strictures*. Anal sphincter spasm due to painful *hemorrhoids* or *fissures* also may inhibit the desire to evacuate.

In the absence of an obstructing lesion of the colon, *disturbed colonic motility* may mimic colonic obstruction. Disruption of parasympathetic innervation to the colon as a result of injury or lesions of the lumbosacral spine or sacral nerves may produce constipation with hypomotility, colonic dilatation, decreased rectal tone and sensation, and impaired defecation. In patients with *multiple sclerosis*, constipation may be associated with neurogenic dysfunction of other organs. Similarly, constipation may be associated with *lesions of the central nervous system* caused by parkinsonism or a cerebrovascular accident. In South America, the parasitic infection *Chagas' disease* may result in constipation because of damage to myenteric plexus ganglion cells. *Hirschsprung's disease*, or aganglionosis, is characterized by absence of myenteric neurons in a segment of distal colon just proximal to the anal sphincter. This results in a segment of contracted bowel which produces obstruction and proximal dilatation. In addition, an absent rectosphincteric inhibitory reflex results in the failure of the internal anal sphincter to relax following rectal distention. Most patients with Hirschsprung's disease are diagnosed by 6 months of age, but in occasional cases symptoms are mild enough that the diagnosis may be delayed into adulthood (see Chap. 288).

Drugs that may lead to constipation include those with anticholinergic properties, such as antidepressants and antipsychotics, codeine and other narcotic analgesics, aluminum- or calcium-containing antacids, sucralfate, iron supplements, and calcium channel blockers. In patients with certain endocrinopathies such as *hypothyroidism* and *diabetes mellitus*, constipation is generally mild and responsive to therapy. Rarely, life-threatening megacolon occurs in patients with myxedema. Constipation is common during *pregnancy*, presumably as a result of altered progesterone and estrogen levels which decrease intestinal transit. *Collagen vascular diseases* may be associated with constipation, which may be a particularly prominent feature of *progressive systemic sclerosis*, in which delayed intestinal transit results from atrophy and fibrosis of colonic smooth muscle.

In the large majority of patients with severe constipation, no obvious cause can be identified. In *idiopathic childhood constipation*, both psychological and physiologic factors are thought to play a role. Affected children often have slow colonic transit localized to the distal colon and rectum, and voluntary withholding behavior or abnormal anorectal function has been suggested to play a role in this disorder. Young to middle-aged women may present with severe constipation characterized by infrequent defecation, excessive straining when defecating, and unresponsiveness to fiber supplements or mild laxatives. In 70 percent of such cases, slow colonic transit (colonic inertia) may be demonstrated by the delayed passage of radiopaque markers through the proximal colon. In 30 percent of cases colonic transit is normal, and abnormalities of anorectal sensory and motor function may be demonstrated. The terms *outlet obstruction* and *anismus* have been used to describe this form of constipation, which appears to result from failed relaxation or inappropriate contraction of the puborectalis and external anal sphincter muscles. Because relaxation of these muscles involves cortical inhibition of the spinal reflex during defecation and may be modified by biofeedback, it is speculated that such rectosphincteric dysfunction is an acquired or learned rather than an organic or neurogenic disease. Chronic straining at defecation itself may lead to descent of the perineal floor and stretching of the pudendal nerve, thus leading to an incompetent anal sphincter and fecal incontinence. *Rectal prolapse* may impair defecation as a result of rectal intussusception or chronic pudendal nerve injury. A *rectocele* is an anterior rectal herniation that may interfere with defecation by filling with feces preferentially during attempts at defecation.

Chronic idiopathic intestinal pseudoobstruction is a rare disorder in which episodes of intestinal obstruction are unaccompanied by evidence of mechanical blockage (see Chap. 288). This disorder may be familial as a result of a neuropathy or myopathy involving the bowel and in some cases the bladder. *Idiopathic megacolon* or *megarectum* is characterized by a dilated colon or rectum, respectively, with constipation and defecatory difficulties attributed to neurogenic dysfunction.

In young to middle-aged adults, constipation is most commonly attributable to the *irritable bowel syndrome*. Unlike some of the idiopathic constipation syndromes described above, irritable bowel syndrome is typically accompanied by abdominal pain, especially in the lower abdomen, as well as by the passage of small, hard stools with a sense of incomplete evacuation and excessive straining. Patients also may complain of flatulence, abdominal bloating, heartburn, nausea, dysphagia, back pain, and genitourinary symptoms. Colonic transit is usually normal in such patients, and the precise pathophysiologic basis for the symptoms is uncertain (see Chap. 287).

Approach to the Patient

With Constipation   A precise description of symptoms and their duration should be obtained. A recent change in bowel habits always demands an evaluation for an obstructing neoplasm. A description of the frequency and nature of defecation should be obtained, including the presence of excessive straining, hard scybalous stools, or a sense of incomplete evacuation. The patient should be questioned about associated abdominal pain and bloating and upper gastrointestinal or genitourinary symptoms. It is especially important to obtain a history of prior laxative use and its duration. A gentle but careful assessment should be made for evidence of anxiety, emotional distress, or affective disorders and the use of mood-altering drugs.

Physical examination should be directed toward the detection of nongastrointestinal diseases that may contribute to constipation. Particular attention should be paid to the neurologic examination, including an assessment of autonomic function. The abdomen should be examined for evidence of prior surgery, bowel distention, or retained stool. A careful perineal and anorectal examination should be conducted for evidence of deformity, gluteal muscle atrophy, rectal prolapse, anal stenosis, anal fissure, rectal mass, or fecal impaction. The patient may need to strain to demonstrate evidence of a rectocele or rectal prolapse. A normal "anal wink" may be elicited by demonstrating reflex contraction of the anal canal following pinprick of the perineum. A variety of complications of constipation or its treatment also may be detected and may be the reason the patient seeks medical attention (Table 42-6).

Flexible sigmoidoscopy or *colonoscopy* may demonstrate melanosis coli as a brown-black discoloration of the bowel mucosa resulting from chronic use of anthraquinone laxatives. The absence of haustrations on endoscopy or barium enema suggests a "cathartic colon" due to laxative abuse. *Barium enema* also may demonstrate obstructing lesions of the colon, megacolon, or megarectum and in Hirschsprung's disease will show the characteristic denervated bowel segment with proximal dilatation of the colon. In such cases, rectal biopsies may be obtained to demonstrate the absence of neurons.

Studies of colonic and anorectal function should be reserved for patients with severe idiopathic constipation who fail to respond to simple therapeutic measures (see below). In patients with a complaint of infrequent defecation, *colonic transit studies* may demonstrate colonic inertia. Radiopaque markers are ingested and their transit is monitored by serial abdominal radiographs until at least 80 percent have passed or a defined period of time has elapsed. The upper limit of normal for most adults is approximately 70 h. In patients with suspected outlet obstruction, *anorectal motility studies* provide information about rectal sensation, viscoelasticity, relaxation of the internal anal sphincter, and defecation of air-filled balloons of various sizes inserted into the rectum. Whereas patients with constipation due to irritable bowel syndrome often have a low rectal compliance and tolerate rectal distention poorly, those with megarectum have a very high rectal compliance. The absence of internal anal sphincter relaxation suggests Hirschsprung's disease. In some centers, anorectal manometry is supplemented by *electromyogram studies* to record external anal sphincter function and *defecography*, in which thickened barium approximating the consistency of stool is introduced into the rectum

Table 42-6

Complications of Constipation or Its Treatment

Hemorrhoids	Ischemic colitis
Anal fissure	Colonic volvulus
Rectal prolapse	Colonic perforation
Stercoral ulcer	Fecal incontinence
Melanosis coli	Urinary retention
Cathartic colon	Cardiac and cerebrovascular dysfunction
Fecal impaction	(e.g., syncope, arrhythmias, angina)

and its evacuation monitored by fluoroscopy while the patient sits on a commode.

 TREATMENT

Treatment of constipation must be individualized, taking into account the duration and severity of constipation, potential contributing factors, the age of the patient, and the patient's expectations. Symptomatic therapy is quite empiric in that there is often little objective evidence to support a particular strategy. Initial therapy is usually dietary, with an emphasis on increasing dietary fiber intake. Although there is little evidence that constipated persons consume less dietary fiber than nonconstipated persons, many constipated persons respond to increases in dietary fiber to between 20 and 30 g/d. Fiber supplementation may increase stool weight and the frequency of defecation and decrease gastrointestinal transit time. Fiber supplementation is not appropriate for patients with obstructing lesions of the gastrointestinal tract or those with megacolon or megarectum.

Except for bulk laxatives, routine use of laxatives over long periods of time should be discouraged because of the risk of side effects such as lipid pneumonia due to mineral oil or damage to myenteric plexuses resulting in "cathartic colon" due to stimulant anthraquinone laxatives such as senna. *Bulk-forming laxatives* consist of natural (psyllium) or synthetic polysaccharides or cellulose derivatives that act in a manner similar to fiber. Fluid intake should be increased with the use of these preparations. *Emollient laxatives* include mineral oil, which when given orally or by enema penetrates and softens the stool, and docusate salts, which are anionic surfactants that lower the surface tension of stool to allow mixing of aqueous and fatty substances and thereby soften the stool. *Hyperosmolar agents* include mixed electrolyte solutions containing polyethylene glycol and nonabsorbable sugars such as lactulose and sorbitol, which act as osmotic agents and are used in bowel cleansing prior to colonoscopy. Lactulose may occasionally be prescribed for long-term use. *Saline laxatives* contain cations and anions that exert an osmotic effect to increase intraluminal water content; in elderly patients they may cause fluid retention. *Stimulant laxatives* include castor oil, anthraquinones such as senna, and diphenylmethanes such as phenolphthalein and bisacodyl. Castor oil is converted to ricinoleic acid, which stimulates intestinal secretion and increases intestinal motility. The anthraquinones increase fluid and electrolyte accumulation in the distal ileum and colon. Phenolphthalein and bisacodyl stimulate colonic motor activity and inhibit glucose and sodium absorption. Recently, the prokinetic agent cisapride has been shown to enhance intestinal transit through the proximal colon, but its role in the management of constipation is uncertain. A role for excessive endogenous opioids in constipation related to motility disorders has been hypothesized, and the benefit of opioid receptor antagonists in the treatment of constipation has been reported but requires further study. *Biofeedback* techniques have shown promise in the treatment of constipation resulting from inappropriate contraction of the pelvic floor muscles and external anal sphincter.

Surgical treatment for severe chronic constipation is generally controversial, except in Hirschsprung's disease, in which surgical resection of the aganglionic segment is the treatment of choice. In colonic inertia, subtotal colectomy with ileorectal anastomosis may be indicated in carefully selected patients in whom upper gastrointestinal motility is normal and anorectal dysmotility has been excluded. Surgery to reduce or resect a rectocele, intussusception, or prolapse should be undertaken with caution, because symptoms often are not alleviated.

BIBLIOGRAPHY

BOYCE TG et al: *Escherichia coli* O157:H7 and the hemolytic–uremic syndrome. N. Engl J Med 333:364, 1995

CAMILLERI M et al: Clinical management of intractable constipation. Ann Intern Med 121:520, 1994

DONOWITZ M et al: Evaluation of patients with chronic diarrhea. N Engl J Med 332:725, 1995

EHERER AJ, FORDTRAN JS: Fecal osmotic gap and pH in experimental diarrhea of various causes. Gastroenterology 103:545, 1992

FIELD M (ed): *Diarrheal Diseases.* New York, Elsevier, 1991

———— et al: Intestinal electrolyte transport and diarrheal disease. N Engl J Med 321:800, 1989

FINE KD, FORDTRAN JS: The effect of diarrhea on fecal fat excretion. Gastroenterology 102:1936, 1992

———— et al: Diarrhea, in *Gastrointestinal Disease: Pathophysiology, Diagnosis, Management,* 5th ed, MH Sleisenger, JS Fordtran (eds). Philadelphia, Saunders, 1993, pp 1043-1071

HEATON KW et al: Defecation frequency and timing, and stool form in the general population: A prospective study. Gut 33:818, 1992

PEMBERTON JH et al: Evaluation and surgical treatment of severe chronic constipation. Ann Surg 214:403, 1991

PHILLIPS S et al: Stool composition in factitial diarrhea: A 6-year experience with stool analysis. Ann Intern Med 123:97, 1995

POWELL DW: Approach to the patient with diarrhea, in *Textbook of Gastroenterology,* 2nd ed. T Yamada et al (eds). Philadelphia, Lippincott, 1995, pp 813-863

READ NW et al: Constipation and incontinence in the elderly. J Clin Gastroenterol 20:61, 1995

SCHILLER LR: Review article: Anti-diarrhoeal pharmacology and therapeutics. Aliment Pharmacol Ther 9:87, 1995

WALD A: Approach to the patient with constipation, in *Textbook of Gastroenterology,* 2nd ed, T Yamada et al (eds). Philadelphia, Lippincott, 1995, pp 864-880

WALD A: Colonic and anorectal motility testing in clinical practice. Am J Gastroenterol 89:2109, 1994

WENZL HH et al: Determinants of decreased fecal consistency in patients with diarrhea. Gastroenterology 108:1729, 1995

WISTROM J et al: Empiric treatment of acute diarrheal disease with norfloxacin. Ann Intern Med 117:202, 1992

43   *Daniel W. Foster*

GAIN AND LOSS IN WEIGHT

In normal persons weight is stable over long periods because food intake is matched to energy expenditure by neural activity in the hypothalamus that provides signals to eat or to stop eating. Because the system is usually effective, either weight gain or weight loss may bring a patient to the physician. No history is complete without ascertaining whether weight has been gained or lost and, if so, how much. In general, a change of 5 percent of body weight or 5 kg is considered significant. However, a 5-kg weight loss may not be of importance in a 130-kg man who is trying to lose weight, while a 2-kg weight loss may well be worrisome in a person weighing 40 kg.

WEIGHT GAIN

Weight gain is less likely to have a pathologic cause than weight loss. In most cases it is a consequence of overeating and inadequate exercise, and the diagnosis is usually simple obesity. Occasionally obesity may be the consequence of hypothyroidism, Cushing's syndrome, or hypothalamic disease such as craniopharyngioma (see Chap. 75). Workup for pathologic causes of weight gain is rarely indicated unless accompanying signs suggest an underlying cause. Sometimes weight gain is not fat but fluid, in which case the primary problems to be considered are congestive heart failure, renal failure, or cirrhosis with ascites.

There is an epidemic of obesity in the United States and some European countries such as Italy. The epidemic is almost certainly due to the availability of attractive, tasty food at low cost. Despite multiple studies suggesting altered metabolism or disturbed satiety signals as predisposing factors, one does not become fat without overeating. All obese patients have elevated, not depressed, absolute resting metabolic rates.

This is not to say that pathologic mechanisms may not play a role. Particular interest has focused on the presumed satiety signal, leptin, synthesized in and released from adipose tissue as the product of the *ob* gene. Leptin is believed to act in the hypothalamus to block the synthesis or release of neuropeptide Y, which appears to be a potent feeding signal. Although leptin deficiency is the cause of obesity in some strains of mice, mutations or deletions in the *ob* gene have not proven to be operative in humans. Resistance to leptin may be important in human obesity. However, at the time of this writing it is not documented that defects in leptin synthesis/action play any significant role in the obese state in humans.

Although rarely caused by disease, obesity predisposes to disease, especially diabetes mellitus but also to gall stones, degenerative joint disease, hyperlipidemia, atherosclerosis, hypertension, sleep apnea, and perhaps cancer.

WEIGHT LOSS

In all studies there are patients who lose weight without discernible cause, but significant involuntary weight loss is usually a marker of serious disease. *Even if no disease is found on initial evaluation, it should not be assumed that weight loss is idiopathic.* The patient should be followed at regular intervals with careful repeat examination since occult illness causing weight loss may not become manifest for long periods.

There are three general mechanisms of weight loss, but more than one may be operative in the same patient: increased energy expenditure, increased loss of energy in stool or urine, and decreased food intake. Decreased intake is by far the most common mechanism; it is usually due to loss of appetite but may result from obstruction in the esophagus or stomach secondary to stricture, compressive mass, or infiltrating malignancy. The only common causes of increased metabolism are hyperthyroidism, pheochromocytoma, and major exercise programs. Loss of ingested energy generally is due to either diabetes mellitus with glycosuria or intestinal malabsorption with steatorrhea. Chronic pancreatitis in alcoholics is the most common cause of steatorrhea, but malabsorption can occur with intestinal lymphoma, celiac sprue, islet cell tumors (such as somatostatinomas or gastrinomas), radiation injury, biliary tract obstruction, inflammatory bowel disease, and a variety of other disorders. If weight loss occurs with a history of increased food intake, the diagnosis is usually diabetes mellitus, hyperthyroidism, or malabsorption syndrome. Occasionally leukemias and lymphomas may present with weight loss in the absence of anorexia or even with increased food intake.

Large prospective studies of the causes of weight loss are not available, and the five retrospective studies published since 1981 involve relatively small numbers of patients, rendering all conclusions suspect. In young persons, the most likely diagnoses are diabetes mellitus, hyperthyroidism, anorexia nervosa, or infection, especially human immunodeficiency virus (HIV). In older persons, cancer is the most likely cause of significant weight loss, with psychiatric illness such as Alzheimer's disease and depression being a distant second.

Under most circumstances the diagnosis of the cause of weight loss is not difficult and is revealed by history, physical examination, and routine laboratory screening. The most common occult condition is cancer. Gastrointestinal, pancreatic, and hepatic malignancies are particularly prone to cause early weight loss. Infectious disease may occasionally be symptomatically silent. Weight loss may occur in HIV infection prior to AIDS-defining illness, and tuberculosis, fungal disease, bacterial endocarditis, or hepatitis may present as weight loss in the absence of defining symptoms. Eating disorders, early Alzheimer's disease, and depression may cause unexplained anorexia and weight loss. Uremia and hypercalcemia may be asymptomatic but are easily recognized through screening laboratory examination. Elevated calcium levels not only produce anorexia but sometimes induce nephrogenic diabetes insipidus, compounding the weight loss by volume depletion. Weight loss may or may not be a prominent feature of pheochromocytoma. Pernicious anemia may cause anorexia before hematologic changes occur, and early adrenal insufficiency

can cause weight loss in the absence of electrolyte changes, nausea, vomiting, or hypotension. Other causes of anorexic weight loss are chronic obstructive pulmonary disease/emphysema, congestive heart failure, chronic liver disease, and neurologic diseases such as Parkinsonism. For those returning from foreign countries, parasitic disease must always be considered.

A list of common causes of weight loss is given in Table 43-1.

DIAGNOSIS

Weight gain does not require much diagnostic expenditure since the vast majority of cases are simple obesity, as mentioned above. Three scenarios warrant laboratory testing: symptoms suggesting hypothyroidism [thyroid-stimulating hormone (TSH)]; central obesity, diabetes, and hypertension accompanied by quadriceps weakness and spontaneous bruising raising the possibility of Cushing syndrome (overnight dexamethasone suppression test, 24-h urinary free cortisol); and obesity accompanied by headache and endocrine dysfunction suggesting craniopharyngioma or pituitary tumor compressing or invading the hypothalamus [computed tomography (CT) or magnetic resonance imaging (MRI) of the head].

When weight loss is the chief complaint or cachexia is a major finding on physical examination, the diagnosis is often readily apparent on first evaluation. It is usually helpful to do a two-stage workup (Table 43-2). First-phase tests are done in every patient. The multiple chemistry panel will reveal diabetes mellitus, hypercalcemia, renal failure, liver disease, and electrolyte abnormalities that may suggest adrenal insufficiency or gastrointestinal illness. TSH should be assayed to rule out hyperthyroidism. HIV testing is indicated if risk factors are present. A chest x-ray must always be obtained. The stool should be checked for occult blood.

Second-phase testing is initiated if the cause of weight loss is still not apparent and in most instances begins with an abdominal CT scan. If hypercalcemia is present, measurements should be made of serum parathyroid hormone (PTH), human PTH-related peptide (a cancer marker), and 1,25-dihydroxyvitamin D and angiotensin-converting enzyme (markers for sarcoidosis). Mammography is indicated in women. Weakness, pigmentation, and hypoglycemia, with or without hyponatremia/hyperkalemia, require a short ACTH test to rule out adrenal insufficiency. Febrile weight loss makes it necessary to obtain blood cultures and, at times, bone marrow biopsy and culture. Iron deficiency anemia is an indication for colonoscopy and occasionally upper endoscopy. Weight loss with diarrhea may, in addition, require measure-

Table 43-1

Common Causes of Weight Loss

1. Increased energy expenditure
   a. Hyperthyroidism
   b. Pheochromocytoma
   c. Extensive exercise
2. Increased energy loss
   a. Diabetes mellitus
   b. Malabsorption syndromes
3. Diminished food intake*
   a. Cancer
   b. Infection (HIV, tuberculosis, endocarditis)
   c. Hypercalcemia (malignancy, hyperparathyroidism, sarcoidosis)
   d. Uremia
   e. Obstructive gastrointestinal disease
   f. Anorexia nervosa
   g. Adrenal insufficiency (primary or secondary)
   h. Pernicious anemia
   i. Alzheimer's disease
   j. Depression

---

* Many other diseases can be associated with anorexia, e.g., congestive heart failure, chronic obstructive pulmonary disease, chronic liver disease, neurologic disease, and inflammatory/autoimmune disease. The conditions listed above are emphasized because they have the capacity to be occult.

GASTROINTESTINAL BLEEDING

Table 43-2

Screening Tests for Involuntary Weight Loss

1. First-phase screen*
   a. CBC, erythrocyte sedimentation rate
   b. Urinalysis
   c. Multiphase chemical screen (SMA 20)
   d. TSH
   e. HIV test for persons at risk
   f. Chest x-ray
   g. Stool for occult blood
2. Second-phase screen
   a. Abdominal CT scan
   b. Mammography, serum protein electrophoresis, parathyroid hormone, human PTH-related peptide, angiotensin-converting enzyme, and 1, 25-dihydroxyvitamin D if hypercalcemia is present
   c. Colonoscopy if iron deficiency anemia or melena is found or inflammatory bowel disease is suspected
   d. Upper endoscopy for upper GI bleeding or dysphagia
   e. Short ACTH test for weakness, pigmentation, or hyponatremia/hyperkalemia
   f. Blood cultures for fever of unknown origin with weight loss
   g. Bone marrow biopsy with culture for febrile weight loss with negative blood cultures
   h. 72-h stool fat for weight loss with chronic diarrhea
   i. Head CT or MRI for weight loss with headache, neurologic symptoms, or endocrine deficiency
   j. Spinal MRI if examination suggests paraspinal disease.
   k. Vitamin B_{12}

* First-phase and second-phase screens are arbitrary definitions. The history and physical examination together with initial laboratory tests may move a second-phase test to an early time point. The suggested order is for true occult disease

ment of 72-h stool fat content or hormones such as gastrin, somatostatin, or glucagon. Even in the absence of anemia or macrocytosis, a vitamin B_{12} level should be measured in unexplained weight loss. New or severe headaches with or without neurologic symptoms are indications for CT examination, while back pain with fever and neurologic loss suggest the possibility of paraspinal or epidural abscess due to tuberculosis or staphylococci, especially in intravenous drug users.

SUMMARY

Weight loss is more often a diagnostic problem than a weight gain and is often a sign of serious organic illness. Diagnosis is usually quite straightforward. In cases where no ready explanation is available, persistence is essential. Initially the patient should be reexamined at monthly intervals with complete physical and laboratory examinations. If no cause is found by 6 months, the return intervals can be stretched.

BIBLIOGRAPHY

EZZELL C: Research in focus. Fat times for obesity research: Tons of new information, but how does it all fit together? J NIH Res 7:39, 1995

LEIBEL R et al: Changes in energy expenditure resulting from altered body weight. N Engl J Med 332:621, 1995

MACALLAN DC et al: Energy expenditure and wasting in human immunodeficiency virus and infection. N Engl J Med 333:83, 1995

OLEFSKY JM: Weighing in on the lean genes. J Clin Invest 95:2427, 1995

RABINOVITZ M et al: Unintentional weight loss: A retrospective analysis of 154 cases. Arch Intern Med 146:186, 1986

THOMPSON MP, MORRIS LK: Unexplained weight loss in the ambulatory elderly. J Am Geriatr Soc 39:497, 1991

WOLF-KLINE GP, SILVERSTONE FA: Weight loss and Alzheimer's disease: An international review of the literature. Int Psychogeriatr 6:135, 1994

Hematemesis is defined as the vomiting of blood, and *melena* as the passage of stools rendered black and tarry by the presence of blood. These clinical manifestations of gastrointestinal (GI) hemorrhage suggest a proximal source of bleeding. The color of vomited blood depends on the concentration of hydrochloric acid in the stomach and the duration of its contact with the blood. Thus, if vomiting occurs shortly after the onset of bleeding, the vomitus appears red, and later the appearance will be dark red, brown, or black. Precipitated blood clots and acid-degraded blood in the vomitus will produce a characteristic "coffee grounds" appearance when vomited. Hematemesis usually indicates bleeding proximal to the ligament of Treitz, because blood entering the GI tract below the duodenum rarely enters the stomach.

While bleeding sufficient to produce hematemesis usually results in melena, less than half of patients with melena have hematemesis. Melena usually denotes bleeding from the esophagus, stomach, or duodenum, but lesions in the jejunum, ileum, and even ascending colon may occasionally cause melena provided the gastrointestinal transit time is sufficiently prolonged. Approximately 60 mL of blood is required to produce a single black stool; acute blood loss greater than this may produce melena for as long as 7 days. After the stool color returns to normal, tests for occult blood may remain positive for over a week. The black color of melena results from contact of the blood with hydrochloric acid to produce hematin. Such stools are tarry ("sticky") and have a characteristic odor. This tarry consistency is in contrast to black or dark gray stools occurring after the ingestion of iron, bismuth, or licorice. GI bleeding, even if detected only by positive tests for occult blood, indicates potentially serious disease and must be further investigated.

Hematochezia, the passage of red blood per rectum, generally signifies bleeding from a source distal to the ligament of Treitz. However, brisk proximal bleeding can cause hematochezia due to rapid transit.

The clinical manifestations of GI bleeding depend on the extent and rate of hemorrhage and the presence of coincidental diseases. Blood loss of less than 500 mL is rarely associated with systemic signs; exceptions include bleeding in the elderly or in the anemic patient in whom smaller amounts of blood loss may produce hemodynamic alterations. Rapid hemorrhage of greater volume results in decreased venous return to the heart, decreased cardiac output, and increased peripheral resistance due to reflex vasoconstriction (see Chap. 38). Orthostatic hypotension greater than a change of 10 mmHg usually indicates a 20 percent or greater reduction in blood volume. Concomitant symptoms may include lightheadedness, syncope, nausea, sweating, and thirst. When blood loss is 25 to 40 percent of blood volume, shock frequently ensues with pronounced tachycardia and hypotension. Pallor is prominent, and the skin is cool. However, in the presence of beta-adrenergic and calcium channel blockers, these clinical signs may be blunted.

In the setting of rapid hemorrhage, the initial hematocrit may not accurately reflect the magnitude of blood loss, since equilibration with extravascular fluid and hemodilution often require over 8 h. Common laboratory findings include mild leukocytosis and thrombocytosis which develop within 6 h after the onset of bleeding. The blood urea nitrogen (BUN) may be elevated out of proportion to the creatinine, particularly in upper GI bleeding, due to breakdown of blood proteins to urea by intestinal bacteria as well as mild reduction in the glomerular filtration rate.

Occult bleeding, detected by card test for hemoglobin peroxidase (e.g., Hemocult), is an important means of finding colorectal neoplasia at earlier, potentially curable stages. Testing is advocated for patients over age 50 as a part of the yearly checkup. Multiple stools should be tested (usually two samples from three stools), and if any sample is positive, additional studies should be performed. A positive result can be due to physiologic blood loss, dietary peroxidases, undercooked meat, or any cause of upper or lower GI bleeding. The daily ingestion of over 500 mg of vitamin C may result in a false-negative test. To limit the confounding variables, patients should be tested on a high-fiber and low-meat diet with no ingestion of nonsteroidal anti-inflammatory agents (NSAIDs) or vitamin C, although the daily low dose of aspirin (80 to 325 mg) taken to prevent cardiovascular disease generally does not lead to false-positive results.

ETIOLOGY OF UPPER GI BLEEDING (See Table 44-1)   A careful history and physical examination of the oropharynx and nasal cavity should serve to exclude epistaxis or swallowed blood as a source of hematemesis or melena.

The most common causes of upper gastrointestinal hemorrhage are (1) erosive or hemorrhagic gastropathy, (2) duodenal ulcer, (3) gastric ulcer, (4) Mallory-Weiss tear, (5) varices or portal hypertensive gastropathy, and (6) arteriovenous malformations (AVMs). These entities account for over 90 percent of all cases of upper GI hemorrhage in which a specific source can be found.

Gastric erosions or *erosive, hemorrhagic gastropathy* are often associated with the ingestion of aspirin or other NSAIDs.

Peptic ulcers (either duodenal or gastric) caused by *Helicobacter pylori* are common causes of upper GI bleeding. Because hemorrhage may be the initial clinical manifestation of a peptic ulcer, the diagnosis should be considered even if a history characteristic of ulcer disease is not obtained. Concomitant use of NSAIDs increases the risk of peptic ulcer bleeding and the mortality associated with it.

Bleeding from *varices* or from *portal hypertensive gastropathy* is characteristically abrupt and massive. Bleeding from esophageal or gastric varices is usually the result of portal hypertension secondary to cirrhosis. Although alcoholic cirrhosis is the most prevalent cause in the United States, any condition producing portal hypertension may result in variceal bleeding. Further, while the presence of varices usually connotes long-standing portal hypertension, acute hepatitis or severe fatty infiltration of the liver may rarely produce varices that disappear once the hepatic abnormality resolves. Although upper GI bleeding in a patient with cirrhosis suggests a variceal source, up to one-quarter of those patients will be bleeding from another lesion, such as erosive gastropathy, peptic ulcer, gastritis, or Mallory-Weiss tear. Consequently, it is essential to determine the cause of bleeding promptly so that the appropriate treatment can be instituted.

Mallory-Weiss tears (esophagogastric mucosal tears) occur in the region of the esophagogastric junction and are often characterized historically by retching or nonbloody vomiting followed by hematemesis. However, a history of retching may be lacking in up to half of cases.

Esophagitis mostly due to gastroesophageal reflux may cause bleeding. Esophagitis associated with cancer or due to infections such as cytomegalovirus, herpes virus, or *Candida* rarely causes acute bleeding; however, it may cause chronic blood loss. Chronic blood loss may also result from linear mucosal tears in large sliding hiatal hernias as a result of the shearing effect caused by differences in intrathoracic and intragastric pressure.

Gastric carcinoma, lymphoma, polyps, and other tumors of the stomach and small bowel are uncommon causes of GI hemorrhage. Leiomyoma and leiomyosarcoma are uncommon, but they can lead to massive hemorrhage. Bleeding from duodenal or jejunal diverticula is an unusual cause of GI bleeding.

Rupture of arteriosclerotic aortic aneurysms into the small intestine is almost always fatal. Rupture usually occurs following arterial reconstructive surgery with fistula formation between the synthetic graft and bowel lumen. A small or "herald bleed" may precede a sudden massive hemorrhage from an aortoenteric fistula. Sudden bleeding also may occur from hemobilia following hepatic surgery or trauma.

Primary blood dyscrasias, vasculitis, hereditary hemorrhagic telangiectasia, and connective tissue disorders may result in significant GI bleeding. Uremia may produce gastrointestinal blood loss due to telangiectases throughout the GI tract. Pancreatic cancer may occasionally erode into the duodenum and produce upper GI bleeding.

ETIOLOGY OF LOWER GI BLEEDING (See Table 44-2)

Anal and Rectal Lesions   Small amounts of bright red blood on the surface of the stool and toilet tissue are often caused by hemorrhoids or anal fissures; such bleeding is generally precipitated by the strained passage of a hard stool. Proctitis is another source of rectal bleeding.

Colonic Lesions   Carcinoma of the colon as well as colonic polyps usually produce chronic occult blood loss but occasionally may produce brisk bleeding. Angiodysplasia, a mucosal vascular tuft, is a major source of acute or chronic bleeding in older patients. Bloody diarrhea may be the presenting symptom in patients with ulcerative colitis. Bleeding also may accompany diarrhea due to infections with *Shigella*, *Salmonella*, *Campylobacter jejuni*, *Clostridium difficile*, enterohemorrhagic toxigenic *Escherichia coli* O157:H7, ameba, and other parasites. In the elderly, diabetic patients, and patients with vascular disease, mesenteric ischemia may be a cause of bloody diarrhea.

Diverticula   Bleeding from colonic diverticula is a common cause of lower GI hemorrhage in persons over age 40. The usual presentation of a diverticular hemorrhage is that of the brisk painless passage of a maroon-colored stool. Meckel's diverticulum, a congenital anomaly most often in the distal ileum, is present in about 2 percent of the population and is an important cause of acute hemorrhage in children and young adults.

Approach to the Patient

With Acute Upper GI Bleeding   The approach to the bleeding patient depends on the site, extent, and rate of bleeding. The primary consideration in the care of the bleeding patient is maintaining adequate intravascular volume and hemodynamic stability. When first seen, the patient may be in shock. Prior to taking a history and performing a thorough physical examination, vital signs should be noted, blood sent for typing and cross-matching, and large-bore intravenous lines placed for infusion of saline or packed red blood cells.

HISTORY   A history or symptoms suggestive of peptic ulcer disease may provide a useful clue. Similarly, recent use of NSAIDs should make one suspect erosive gastropathy. If alcohol use has been long-standing and there are stigmata of chronic liver disease, esophageal varices may be a source of hemorrhage. Prior history of GI bleeding or a family history of intestinal disease or hemorrhagic diathesis may provide diagnostic clues. Recent retching followed by hematemesis should suggest the diagnosis of Mallory-Weiss tear.

PHYSICAL EXAMINATION   Following evaluation for orthostatic changes in pulse and blood pressure, clinical assessment of central

---

Table 44-1

Common Causes of Acute Upper GI Bleeding

1. Erosive, hemorrhagic gastropathy (aspirin, other NSAIDs)
2. Duodenal ulcer
3. Gastric ulcer
4. Mallory-Weiss tear
5. Varices / portal hypertensive gastropathy
6. Arteriovenous malformations

Table 44-2

Common Causes of Acute Lower GI Bleeding (in Order of Frequency)

Under Age 55	Over Age 55
1. Anorectal disease (hemorrhoids, fissures)	1. Anorectal disease (hemorrhoids, fissures)
2. Colitis (IBD,* infectious)	2. Diverticulosis
3. Diverticulosis	3. Angiodysplasia
4. Polyps, cancer (hyperplastic, hamartomas)	4. Polyps, cancer
5. Angiodysplasia	5. Enterocolitic (ischemic, infectious, IBD, radiation)

* IBD, inflammatory bowel disease.

venous pressure, and institution of volume repletion, the patient should be examined for clues to the underlying illness. A nonintestinal bleeding source should be excluded by careful examination of the oral cavity and nasopharynx. Dermatologic examination may disclose the characteristic telangiectatic lesions of Osler-Rendu-Weber disease (although these will not be visible if severe anemia is present). Stigmata of chronic liver disease such as spider angiomata, gynecomastia, testicular atrophy, jaundice, ascites, and hepatosplenomegaly suggest portal hypertension with bleeding from esophageal or gastric varices as an important potential source.

LABORATORY STUDIES Initial studies should include the hematocrit, hemoglobin, careful assessment of red blood cell morphologic features (hypochromic, microcytic red blood cells suggest that blood loss is chronic), white blood cell count, differential, and platelet count. Prothrombin time and partial thromboplastin time studies are needed to exclude primary or secondary clotting defects. An increase in BUN and the BUN to creatinine ratio may aid in suggesting upper GI bleeding. Abdominal films are rarely helpful in establishing a diagnosis unless a perforated or ischemic viscus is suspected or if intestinal obstruction is present. Although the initial studies are valuable and essential, repeated evaluation of the laboratory data is important as one follows the clinical course of the bleeding; a flow chart of data is desirable and should include the times that blood products and intravenous fluids were administered and their amounts.

DIAGNOSTIC AND THERAPEUTIC APPROACH (See Fig. 44-1) The diagnostic approach to the patient with GI hemorrhage must be individualized. When there is a history of melena or hematemesis or the suspicion of bleeding from the upper part of the GI tract, a nasogastric tube should be passed to empty the stomach and to determine whether the bleeding is proximal to the ligament of Treitz. If the initial nasogastric aspirate is clear or bilious, current active bleeding is unlikely and the tube may be removed.

If blood or "coffee grounds" material is aspirated from the nasogastric tube, water or saline lavage (at room temperature) should be initiated. Irrigation of the stomach serves two purposes: (1) it provides the clinician with an assessment of the rapidity of the bleeding, and (2) it clears the stomach of blood and blood clots prior to diagnostic endoscopy (EGD), which will improve the ability to view all mucosal surfaces. The pace of subsequent diagnostic evaluation will depend on the character of the nasogastric aspirate as well as on vital signs, transfusion requirements, and the number and color of stools.

Once the patient is hemodynamically stable, EGD should be performed to identify the source of bleeding (see Fig. 44-1). Early EGD also may provide prognostic information as to whether the patient is likely to rebleed and to permit endoscopic therapy. When there is evidence of persistent upper GI bleeding, based on continuing blood in the nasogastric tube drainage or failure of the patient to stabilize hemodynamically, the situation must be viewed as urgent, and EGD should commence as soon as possible. If the source of bleeding is found, the endoscopist needs to determine whether therapy via the endoscope may stop the bleeding. Bleeding from an ulcer may be controlled with injection of a vasoconstricting agent such as epinephrine or a sclerosing agent or by the use of electrocautery, most commonly performed with a bipolar or multipolar probe or a heater probe. Such therapy should be attempted when there is arterial spurting, which is unlikely to subside spontaneously, or when there is a "visible vessel," an exposed arteriole in the ulcer base that connotes a 50 percent bleeding risk. Erosive or hemorrhagic gastropathy (due to aspirin or other NSAIDs) is usually not amenable to endoscopic therapy. Fortunately, this condition often improves with cessation of the offending agent and the administration of H_2-receptor antagonists or proton pump inhibitors. AVMs, when bleeding, are frequently treated with bipolar electrocautery, but when detected they are usually not actively bleeding. Mallory-Weiss tears usually cease bleeding spontaneously but may require cautery or injection therapy if bleeding persists.

Esophageal variceal bleeding usually requires endoscopic intervention. The varices may be actively spurting or oozing blood or may show evidence of recent bleeding by "red wale" marks or cherry red spots. Until now, the most common approach to stop the bleeding has been sclerotherapy. This involves the injection of varices with sclerosing agents such as ethanolamine, sodium tetradecylsulfate, sodium morrhuate, or absolute ethanol. Esophageal variceal banding ligation (similar to rubber band ligation of hemorrhoids) is an increasingly used technique and is associated with a lower risk of esophageal stricture formation and systemic toxicity than sclerotherapy. Systemic infusion of vasopressin together with intravenous nitroglycerin lowers portal venous pressure and may be used adjunctively to control variceal bleeding. Similarly, systemic somatostatin or its analogues (e.g., octreotide) can lower portal pressure and help to control variceal bleeding without the peripheral vasoconstrictive side effects of vasopressin.

If endoscopic or pharmacologic measures fail to stop variceal bleeding, balloon tamponade with the Blakemore or Linton tube may be used to compress the varices directly and thereby stop bleeding temporarily until definitive therapy can be attempted. Another approach is the placement of a transjugular intrahepatic portosystemic

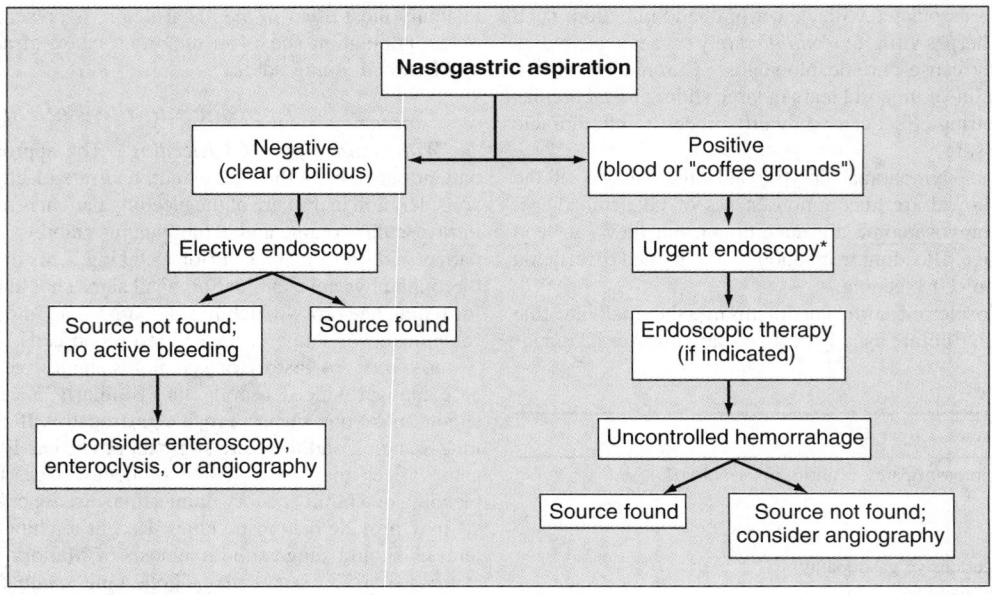

FIGURE 44-1 Approach to the patient with acute upper GI bleeding. (*Request surgical consultation early, in event operative intervention is required.)

shunt. This procedure involves placing an expandable metal stent through the liver to connect the portal and hepatic vein. Occasionally, upper GI bleeding is too brisk to visualize the bleeding site endoscopically; in such cases, angiography, such as selective mesenteric arteriography, may be appropriate. Bleeding of this magnitude usually requires surgical intervention once the bleeding site is localized, but on occasion intraarterial infusion of vasopressin or angiographic injection of Gelfoam or metallic coils may arrest the bleeding.

_____ Approach to the Patient _____

With Acute Lower GI Bleeding The common causes of acute lower GI bleeding vary with age (see Table 44-2 and Fig. 44-2). In all instances, upper GI bleeding should be excluded, if necessary by nasogastric aspirate or even EGD, and there should be careful digital rectal examination and anoscopy to rule out anorectal pathology such as fissures and bleeding from internal hemorrhoids. A flexible sigmoidoscopic examination (after a gentle saline enema) should be performed to exclude rectosigmoid disease.

In the hemodynamically stable patient, elective colonoscopy should be performed after lavage with an oral polyethyleneglycol/electrolyte or phosphosoda solution. The therapeutic endoscopist may remove polyps, cauterize angiodysplastic lesions, and on occasion inject a bleeding diverticulum with epinephrine. If colonoscopy is negative but there is recurrent or intermittent lower GI bleeding, a tagged red blood scan may be considered. Images may be obtained for up to 48 h. If the scan shows a suspicious lesion, elective angiography helps to localize the site of bleeding more accurately. The patient with a torrential lower GI bleed usually cannot be prepped for colonoscopy nor wait for tagged red blood cell images; such a patient should promptly undergo mesenteric angiography after a nasogastric aspirate has ruled out brisk upper GI bleeding. Once the site of bleeding is localized by angiography, surgery is often required.

Acute upper and lower GI bleeding present a challenge both diagnostically and therapeutically. It requires optimal teamwork of emergency and intensive care room staff, internists, gastroenterologists, invasive radiologists and surgeons.

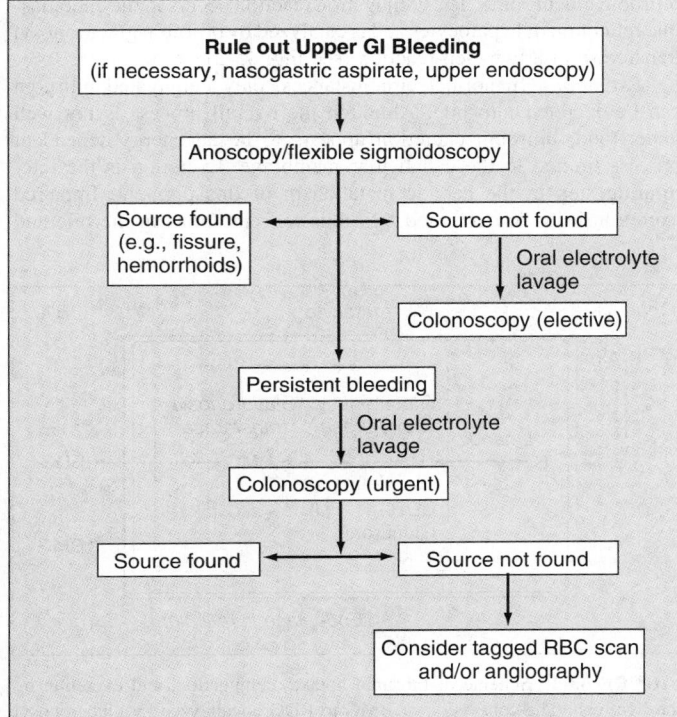

FIGURE 44-2 Approach to the patient with acute lower GI bleeding.

BIBLIOGRAPHY

CELLO JP et al: Endoscopic sclerotherapy versus portacaval shunt in patients with severe cirrhosis and acute variceal hemorrhage: Long-term follow-up. N Engl J Med 316:11, 1987

CHOJKIER M et al: A controlled comparison of continuous intraarterial and intravenous infusions of vasopressin in hemorrhage from esophageal varices. Gastroenterology 77:540, 1979

JENSEN DM, MACHICADO CA: Diagnosis and treatment of severe hemotochezia: The role of urgent colonoscopy after purge. Gastroenterology 95:1569, 1988

KANKARIA RG, FLEISHER DE: Critical management of nonvariceal upper gastrointestinal bleeding. Crit Care Clin 11:347, 1985

LAINE L: Multipolar electrocoagulation in the treatment of active upper gastrointestinal tract hemorrhage. N Engl J Med 316:1613, 1987

PETERSON WL et al: Routine early endoscopy in upper gastrointestinal tract bleeding: A randomized, controlled trial. N Engl J Med 304:925, 1981

REINUS JF, BRANDT LJ: Vascular ectasias and diverticulosis. Common causes of lower intestinal bleeding. Gastroenterol Clin North Am 23:1, 1988

RICHTER JM et al: Angiodysplasia: Clinical presentation and colonoscopic diagnosis. Dig Dis Sci 29:481, 1984

ROSEN RJ, SANCHEZ G: Angiographic diagnosis and management of gastrointestinal hemorrhage. Radiol Clin North Am 32:951, 1994

SUNG JJY et al: Prospective randomized study of the effects of octreotide on rebleeding from esophageal varices after endoscopic ligation. Lancet 346:1666, 1995

45   _Lee M. Kaplan, Kurt J. Isselbacher_

JAUNDICE

Accumulation of bilirubin in the bloodstream causes yellow pigmentation of the plasma, leading to discoloration of heavily perfused tissues. Serum bilirubin levels accumulate when its production from heme exceeds its metabolism and excretion. Imbalance between production and clearance may result either from excess release of bilirubin precursors into the bloodstream or from physiologic processes that impair the hepatic uptake, metabolism, or excretion of this metabolite (see Table 45-1). Clinically, hyperbilirubinemia appears as _jaundice_ or _icterus_, yellow pigmentation of the skin and sclerae. Jaundice can usually be detected when the serum bilirubin level exceeds 34 to 43 μmol/L (2.0 to 2.5 mg/dL), or about twice the upper limit of the normal range, but may be detectable at lower bilirubin levels in patients with fair skin and profound anemia. Conversely, jaundice is frequently obscured in individuals with dark skin or edema. Scleral tissue is rich in elastin, which has a high affinity for bilirubin, so that scleral icterus is usually a more sensitive sign of hyperbilirubinemia than generalized jaundice. A similarly early sign of hyperbilirubinemia is darkening of the urine, which results from renal excretion of bilirubin in the form of bilirubin glucuronide. With pronounced jaundice, the skin may take

Table 45-1

Comparative Properties of Conjugated and Unconjugated Bilirubin

Properties and Reactions	Unconjugated	Conjugated
Water solubility	0	+
Affinity for lipids	+ +	±
Renal excretion	0	+
van den Bergh reaction	Indirect (total minus direct)	Direct
Binding to serum albumin (reversible)	+ + +	+
Formation of bilirubin-albumin complex (irreversible; delta bilirubin)	0	+ *

* Detectable in plasma under conditions of prolonged conjugated hyperbilirubinemia (see text).

on a greenish hue because of oxidation of some of the circulating bilirubin to biliverdin. This effect is seen more commonly with profound or long-standing *conjugated* hyperbilirubinemia such as in cirrhosis (see below). Other causes of yellowed skin include *carotenemia*, usually developing as a result of ingestion and absorption of large amounts of β-carotene and related pigmented compounds. Unlike hyperbilirubinemia, however, carotenemia does not cause scleral icterus.

PRODUCTION AND METABOLISM OF BILIRUBIN
Sources and Chemical Characterization of Serum Bilirubin

Normal serum bilirubin concentrations range from 5 to 17 μmol/L (0.3 to 1.0 mg/dL). More than 90 percent of serum bilirubin in normal individuals is in the unconjugated form, a nonpolar molecule circulating as an albumin-bound complex. The remainder is conjugated to a polar group (primarily glucuronide), rendering it water-soluble and thus able to be filtered and excreted by the kidney. When measured by routine clinical assays, the conjugated, or direct, fraction is frequently overestimated, leading to reported normal values of 1.7 to 8.5 μmol/L (0.1 to 0.5 mg/dL).

Approximately 80 percent of circulating bilirubin is derived from senescent red blood cells. When circulating erythrocytes reach the end of their normal life span of approximately 120 days, they are destroyed by reticuloendothelial cells (Fig. 45-1). Oxidation of the heme moiety dissociated from the hemoglobin within these cells generates biliverdin, which is then metabolized to bilirubin. Approximately 15 to 20 percent of circulating bilirubin is derived from other sources, including (1) ineffective erythropoiesis resulting from destruction of maturing erythroid cells in the bone marrow; and (2) the metabolism of other heme-containing proteins, most notably hepatic cytochromes, muscle myoglobin, and widely distributed heme-containing enzymes.

Unconjugated bilirubin liberated into the plasma is bound tightly, but noncovalently, to albumin. Certain organic anions, such as sulfonamides and salicylates, compete with bilirubin for binding sites on albumin, permitting the released pigment to enter tissues. Neonatal brain cells, especially those of the basal ganglia, have an affinity for unconjugated bilirubin facilitating its retention in the brain. This phenomenon may explain the neurotoxic effects of neonatal hyperbilirubinemia. Conjugated bilirubin is bound to albumin in two forms, reversible and irreversible. Reversible, noncovalent binding is similar to that of unconjugated bilirubin, although the complex is less stable. When present in serum for extended periods of time (e.g., with cholestasis, long-standing biliary obstruction, or chronic active hepatitis), conjugated bilirubin can form an irreversible, covalent complex with albumin referred to as *delta bilirubin* or *biliprotein*. Because of the irreversibility of binding, this complex is not excreted by the kidney. This delta bilirubin has a serum half-life similar to that of albumin (15 to 20 days) and thus remains detectable in serum for up to several weeks after relief of biliary obstruction or during recovery from hepatocellular disease.

Bilirubin is present in body fluids (joint effusions, ascites, pleural effusions, cysts, cerebrospinal fluid, etc.) in proportion to their albumin content and is absent from true secretions such as tears, saliva, and pancreatic juice. The appearance of jaundice is also influenced by blood flow and edema, with paralyzed extremities and edematous areas tending to remain uncolored.

Hepatic Metabolism of Bilirubin

The liver has a central role in the metabolism of the bile pigments. This process can be divided into three distinct phases: (1) hepatic uptake, (2) conjugation, and (3) excretion into bile. Of these three phases, excretion appears to be the rate-limiting step and the one most susceptible to impairment when the liver cell is damaged.

Uptake Unconjugated bilirubin bound to albumin is presented to the liver cell, where the complex dissociates and the nonpolar bilirubin enters the hepatocyte by diffusion or transport across the plasma membrane. The uptake and subsequent hepatocyte storage of bilirubin involve binding of bilirubin to cytoplasmic anion-binding proteins, especially ligandin (glutathione-*S*-transferase B), that prevent efflux of bilirubin back into the plasma.

Conjugation Unconjugated bilirubin is water-insoluble unless complexed to an amphipathic molecule such as albumin. Since albumin is absent from bile, bilirubin must be converted to a water-soluble derivative before biliary excretion. This process is accomplished predominantly by conjugation of bilirubin to glucuronic acid, generating bilirubin glucuronide. The conjugation reaction occurs in the endoplasmic reticulum of hepatocytes and is catalyzed by bilirubin glucuronosyl transferase in a two-step reaction (see Fig. 45-2).

Excretion In normal circumstances, only conjugated bilirubin can be excreted into bile. Although the overall process is not well understood, bilirubin excretion appears to be an energy-dependent process limited to the canalicular membrane. Excretion is the rate-limiting step in the hepatic metabolism of this pigment. Impaired excretion leads to decreased bilirubin concentrations in the bile and

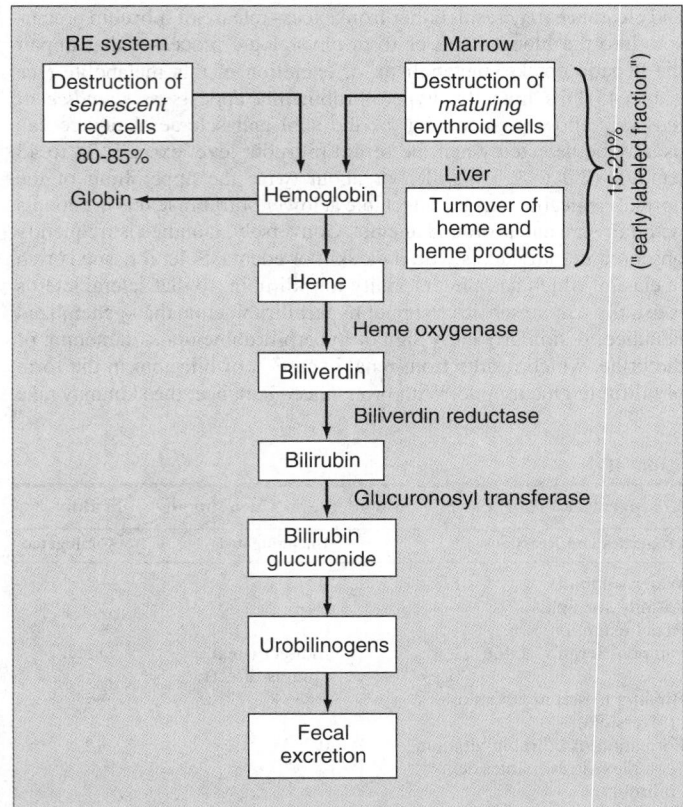

FIGURE 45-1 The sources and precursors of bilirubin and steps in its subsequent metabolism and excretion. RE, reticuloendothelial.

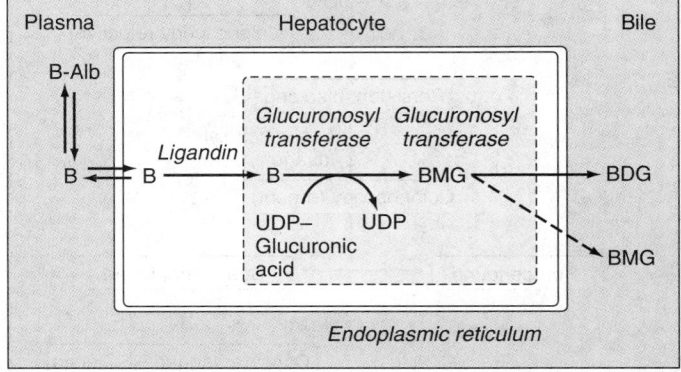

FIGURE 45-2 Scheme of bilirubin uptake, conjugation, and excretion by the liver cell. The conversion of BMG to BDG is catalyzed by glucuronosyl transferase of the endoplasmic reticulum. B, bilirubin; BMG, bilirubin monoglucuronide; BDG, bilirubin diglucuronide; UDP, uridine diphosphate.

concomitant efflux of *conjugated* bilirubin through the sinusoidal membrane of the hepatocyte into the bloodstream. The role of intracellular protein trafficking and membrane transport processes in normal and disordered bilirubin excretion are still incompletely understood.

Intestinal Phase of Bilirubin Metabolism   After secretion into the bile, conjugated bilirubin is transported through the biliary ducts into the duodenum. Conjugated bilirubin is not reabsorbed by the intestinal mucosa. It is either excreted unchanged in the stool or metabolized by ileal and colonic bacteria to *urobilinogen* and related products. Urobilinogen can be reabsorbed from the small intestine and colon and enters the portal circulation. Some of the portal urobilinogen is taken up by the liver and reexcreted into the bile, and the remainder bypasses the liver and is excreted by the kidney. Under normal conditions, the daily urinary excretion of urobilinogen does not exceed 4 mg. When the hepatic uptake and excretion of urobilinogen is impaired (e.g., in hepatocellular disease) or the production of bilirubin is greatly increased (e.g., with hemolysis), daily urinary urobilinogen excretion may increase significantly. In contrast, cholestasis or extrahepatic biliary obstruction interferes with the intestinal phase of bilirubin metabolism and leads to markedly decreased production and urinary excretion of urobilinogen. Measurement of urinary urobilinogen can thus be a useful tool in distinguishing possible causes of hyperbilirubinemia.

Renal Excretion of Bilirubin   The urine normally contains no detectable bilirubin by usual clinical assays, although traces may be detected by sensitive spectrophotometric procedures. Unconjugated bilirubin, being tightly bound into albumin, is not filtered by the renal glomeruli. Because there is no tubular secretory process for bilirubin, unconjugated bilirubin is not excreted in urine. In contrast, conjugated bilirubin is a polar molecule less tightly bound to albumin. A significant fraction circulates unbound, is filtered by the renal glomeruli, and appears in the urine. *The presence of bilirubin in the urine is evidence of conjugated hyperbilirubinemia* and can be a useful differentiating point early in the evaluation of jaundice. Bile salts enhance the glomerular filtration of conjugated bilirubin, and in conditions associated with increased circulating bile salts (e.g., cholestasis, extrahepatic biliary obstruction) renal bilirubin excretion is significantly enhanced. This increased renal excretion may explain the observation that serum conjugated bilirubin tends to plateau at levels below 510 to 680 μmol/L (30 to 40 mg/dL) in patients with *biliary tract obstruction*, while higher levels may occur in patients with severe hepatocellular injury. For additional information about the production, metabolism, and excretion of bilirubin, please refer to Chap. 294.

PATHOPHYSIOLOGIC CONSEQUENCES OF HYPER-BILIRUBINEMIA   In most cases, hyperbilirubinemia itself has little pathophysiologic effect. Unlike circulating bile salts, whose levels are also elevated in cholestasis and biliary obstruction, bilirubin does not become deposited in cutaneous tissues and does not produce pruritus. However, unconjugated plasma bilirubin that is not bound to albumin can cross the blood-brain barrier. In conditions such as neonatal jaundice or type I or II Crigler-Najjar syndrome (see below), extremely high concentrations (>340 μmol/L or >20 mg/dL) of unconjugated bilirubin can accumulate, and the resulting diffusion of bilirubin into the central nervous system can cause encephalopathy (kernicterus) and permanent impairment of nervous function. The risk of kernicterus is increased by conditions that favor elevated circulating levels of *unbound*, unconjugated bilirubin, such as hemolysis, hypoalbuminemia, acidosis, and increased levels of compounds that compete for albumin binding such as free fatty acids and drugs. Circulating concentrations of unconjugated bilirubin can be decreased by removing these contributory factors and by facilitating the biliary excretion of unconjugated bilirubin. Exposure to blue light causes conformational changes in unconjugated bilirubin, rendering it more polar and water-soluble. These *photoisomers* are taken up and excreted by the liver and kidney, without need for conjugation. Intense treatment with blue light can provide sufficient isomerization of unconjugated bilirubin circulating through the skin to prevent kernicterus in patients with neonatal jaundice.

CHEMICAL TESTS FOR BILE PIGMENTS   The most widely employed chemical test for bile pigments in serum is the van

den Bergh reaction. The bilirubin pigments are exposed to sulfanilic acid to generate diazo conjugates, and the chromogenic products are measured colorimetrically. The van den Bergh reaction can be used to distinguish between unconjugated and conjugated bilirubin because of the different solubility properties of the pigments. When the reaction is performed in an aqueous medium, the water-soluble conjugated bilirubin reacts directly with sulfanilic acid, giving a positive *direct* van den Bergh reaction. When the reaction is performed in methanol, the intramolecular hydrogen bonds of unconjugated bilirubin are broken; thus, both conjugated and unconjugated pigments react, giving a measure of the *total* bilirubin level. The *indirect* value, representative of the unconjugated bilirubin fraction, is estimated by subtracting the direct-reacting fraction from the total measured bilirubin. The ability of the direct van den Bergh reaction to distinguish between conjugated and unconjugated bilirubin is dependent on the duration of the reaction. If the reaction is allowed to proceed longer than 1 min, a small amount of unconjugated pigment will react in the aqueous medium, giving a falsely high estimate of the direct-reacting (conjugated) fraction. This observation underscores the importance of considering these reactions as *approximations* rather than actual measurements of the conjugated and unconjugated fractions. More accurate measures of bilirubin fractions in biologic fluids reveal that normal serum contains predominantly (>96 percent) unconjugated bilirubin. This observation confirms the long-held suspicion that the small amount of direct-reacting bilirubin measured in normal serum by the van den Bergh method (2 to 5 μmol/L or 0.1 to 0.3 mg/dL) is an overestimate of the amount actually present. A summary of the key differences in the properties and reactions of the bilirubin pigments is shown in Table 45-1.

Qualitative determination of bilirubin in the urine may be accomplished by specific reaction with Ictotest tablets or dipstick. The foam test also is a simple qualitative test. When normal urine is shaken vigorously in a test tube, the foam is absolutely white. In urine containing bilirubin, the foam will be yellow. This difference may be subtle, becoming evident only after comparison with a similarly shaken specimen from a normal individual. Except for concentrated urine, the most common cause of a deep yellow-brown or dark urine is bilirubinuria. However, other causes of darkened urine need to be considered, including yellow or orange urine due to drugs (e.g., sulfasalazine, rifampin, thiamine), red urine due to porphyria, hemoglobinuria, myoglobinuria, or drugs (e.g., pyridium), and dark brown or black urine due to homogentisic acid (in ochronosis) or melanin (with melanoma).

ETIOLOGIC CONSIDERATIONS IN JAUNDICE   Once jaundice is recognized clinically or chemically, it is important to determine whether it is predominantly due to unconjugated or conjugated hyperbilirubinemia (see Fig. 45-3). In the absence of available chemical determinations, a simple approach is to determine whether bilirubin is present in the urine. Its absence in the urine suggests unconjugated hyperbilirubinemia, since this pigment is not filtered by the renal glomeruli; its presence indicates conjugated hyperbilirubinemia. When chemical analysis (van den Bergh reaction) reveals 80 to 85 percent of the total serum bilirubin to be unconjugated, a patient is considered to have primarily *unconjugated hyperbilirubinemia*. A patient with more than 50 percent direct-reacting (conjugated) serum bilirubin is considered to have predominantly *conjugated hyperbilirubinemia*.

An approach to the classification of jaundice based on this important distinction is presented in Table 45-2. Derangements of bilirubin metabolism may occur through any of four mechanisms: (1) overproduction, (2) decreased hepatic uptake, (3) decreased hepatic conjugation, and (4) decreased excretion of bilirubin into bile (due either to intrahepatic dysfunction or extrahepatic mechanical obstruction). Jaundice may also be described on the basis of the pathogenic mechanisms or disease processes leading to increased bilirubin levels. Thus, the terms *hemolytic jaundice*, *hepatocellular jaundice*, and *obstructive* or *cholestatic jaundice* are often used. Though these classifications are helpful, in any one patient more than a single derangement in bilirubin metabolism may be operative, and more than a single "type" of jaundice may be present. For example, a patient with cirrhosis may have not only impaired hepatocyte function (and hence hepatocellular jaundice) but also hemolysis. Furthermore, as indicated above, obstructive jaundice or cholestasis may be due either to *mechanical* obstruction of the biliary radicles or to impaired *functional* hepatic excretion of bilirubin. This chapter presents a brief description of the major causes of jaundice. A more detailed discussion of individual diseases is found in Chap. 294.

Jaundice with Predominantly Unconjugated Bilirubinemia
Overproduction of bilirubin　An increased amount of hemoglobin released from senescent or hemolyzed red blood cells leads to increased bilirubin production. Erythrocyte destruction leading to hyperbilirubinemia most commonly results from intravascular hemolysis (e.g., autoimmune, microangiopathic, or hemoglobinopathy-associated) or resorption of a large hematoma. Excess bilirubin production is reflected in increased serum bilirubin levels of up to 51 to 68 μmol/L (3 to 4 mg/dL), with a predominance of unconjugated bilirubin. For further discussion of the causes of increased bilirubin production, refer to Chap. 294.

Impaired hepatic uptake of bilirubin　As indicated above, the uptake of bilirubin by hepatocytes requires dissociation of the nonpolar pigment molecule from albumin, transport across the cell membrane,

and binding to ligandin. In rare cases of drug-induced jaundice (e.g., from flavaspidic acid) and possibly in some patients with Gilbert's syndrome, there may be a disruption of this phase of bilirubin handling.

Impaired glucuronide conjugation　Deficiency in glucuronosyl transferase activity can occur as a result of both acquired and genetic defects. In the fetus and neonate, glucuronosyl transferase activity is normally low and the immature hepatocyte has an increased capacity for secretion of unconjugated bilirubin. Although transient, these alterations, together with increased neonatal intestinal absorption of unconjugated bilirubin, contribute to the development of *neonatal jaundice* that occurs between the second and fifth days of life. The significance of inherited deficiencies of glucuronosyl transferase depends on the level of residual enzyme activity. Gilbert's syndrome, associated with a *mild decrease* in activity, produces mild, asymptomatic, unconjugated hyperbilirubinemia. *Moderately decreased* activity occurs in Crigler-Najjar syndrome type II; this enzyme is *totally absent* in Crigler-Najjar syndrome type I, an autosomal recessive disorder associated with kernicterus and childhood mortality from central nervous system dysfunction. Acquired defects in glucuronosyl transferase activity may be induced by drugs (i.e., direct enzyme inhibition) or be associated with liver disease generally. However, in most hepatocellular disorders, bilirubin excretion is impaired to a greater extent than bilirubin conjugation, leading to primarily *conjugated* hyperbilirubinemia.

Jaundice with Predominantly Conjugated Bilirubinemia　*Impaired bilirubin excretion by hepatocytes*　Interference with the biliary excretion of conjugated bilirubin by hepatocytes leads to efflux

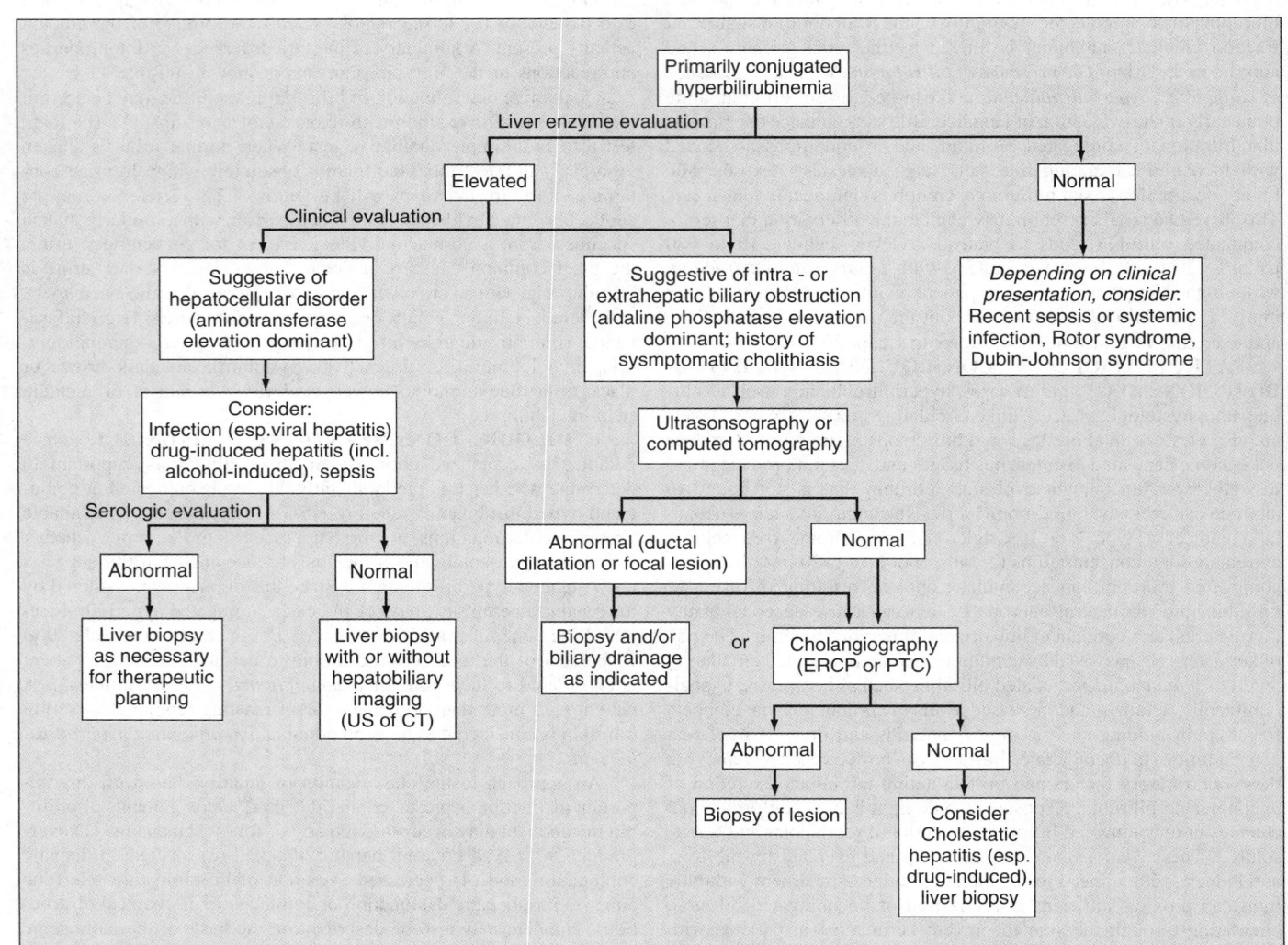

FIGURE 45-3　Algorithm for evaluation of conjugated hyperbilirubinemia. Abbreviations: CT, computed tomography, ERCP, endoscopic retrograde cholangiopancreatography; PTC, percutaneous transhepatic cholangiography; US, ultrasonography.

of this pigment into the systemic circulation, resulting in predominantly conjugated hyperbilirubinemia and consequent bilirubinuria. The mechanism for this efflux is unknown, although it is likely that impaired canalicular excretion leads to increased intracellular levels of conjugated bilirubin, which diffuses or is transported through the sinusoidal membrane into the blood. In addition, hepatocellular necrosis can promote rupture of the bile canaliculi, leading to direct reflux of bile into the hepatic sinusoids. Several mechanisms have been postulated to account for the decreased excretion of conjugated bilirubin in hepatocellular and cholestatic liver disease: (1) occlusion of the canaliculi by inspissated bile, (2) canalicular occlusion by swollen hepatocytes, (3) obstruction of the terminal intrahepatic bile ducts (cholangioles) by inflammatory cells, (4) altered hepatocyte permeability, allowing reuptake of excreted pigment, and (5) specific inhibition of membrane transport proteins.

Table 45-2

Classification of Jaundice Based on Underlying Derangement of Bilirubin Metabolism

PREDOMINANTLY *UNCONJUGATED* HYPERBILIRUBINEMIA

I. Overproduction
    A. Hemolysis (intra- and extravascular)
    B. Ineffective erythropoiesis
II. Decreased hepatic uptake
    A. Prolonged fasting
    B. Sepsis
III. Decreased bilrubin conjugation (decreased hepatic glucuronosyl transferase activity)
    A. Hereditary transferase deficiency
        1. Gilbert's syndrome (*mild* transferase deficiency)
        2. Crigler-Najjar type II (*moderate* transferase deficiency)
        3. Crigler-Najjar type I (*absence* of transferase)
    B. Neonatal jaundice (*transient* transferase deficiency; increased intestinal absorption of unconjugated bilirubin)
    C. Acquired transferase deficiency
        1. Drug inhibition (e.g., chloramphenicol, pregnanediol)
        2. Breast milk jaundice (transferase inhibition by pregnanediol and fatty acids in breast milk)
        3. Hepatocellular disease (hepatitis, cirrhosis)*
    D. Sepsis

PREDOMINANTLY *CONJUGATED* HYPERBILIRUBINEMIA

I. Impaired hepatic excretion (intrahepatic defects)
    A. Familial or hereditary disorders
        1. Dubin-Johnson syndrome
        2. Rotor syndrome
        3. Recurrent (benign) intrahepatic cholestasis
        4. Cholestatic jaundice of pregnancy
    B. Acquired disorders
        1. Hepatocellular disease (e.g., viral or drug-induced hepatitis, cirrhosis)*
        2. Drug-induced cholestasis (e.g., oral contraceptives, androgens, chlorpromazine)
        3. Alcoholic liver disease
        4. Sepsis
        5. Postoperative state
        6. Parenteral nutrition
        7. Biliary cirrhosis (primary or secondary)
II. Extrahepatic biliary obstruction
    A. Intraductal obstruction
        1. Gallstones
        2. Biliary malformation (e.g., stricture, atresia, choledochol cyst)
        3. Infection (e.g., *Clonorchis, Ascaris,* oriental cholangiohepatitis)
        4. Malignancy (cholangiocarcinoma, ampullary carcinoma)
        5. Hemobilia (trauma, tumor)
        6. Sclerosing cholangitis
    B. Compression of biliary ducts
        1. Malignancy (e.g., pancreatic carcinoma, lymphoma, metastases to portal lymph nodes)
        2. Inflammation (e.g., pancreatitis)

---

* In hepatocellular disease (hepatitis and cirrhosis) there is usually interference in the three major steps of bilirubin metabolism—uptake, conjugation, and excretion. However, excretion is the rate-limiting step and is usually impaired to the greatest extent. As a result, conjugated bilirubin predominates in serum.

Hepatocellular disorders in which jaundice may be associated with an obstructive, or cholestatic, phase include (1) drug reactions, especially those due to chlorpromazine or anabolic steroids, (2) alcoholic hepatitis and alcohol-induced fatty liver, (3) jaundice in the last trimester of pregnancy, (4) certain types of postoperative jaundice, (5) benign recurrent intrahepatic cholestasis, (6) Dubin-Johnson and Rotor syndromes, and (7) occasional cases of viral or autoimmune hepatitis. Impairment of bilirubin excretion is common in late-stage cirrhosis from any cause. It occurs much earlier in the course of primary biliary cirrhosis and in the rare cases of biliary cirrhosis occurring secondary to chronic, recurring choledocholithiasis or cholangitis.

Extrahepatic biliary obstruction Complete obstruction of the extrahepatic bile ducts leads to jaundice and predominantly conjugated hyperbilirubinemia associated with marked bilirubinuria and acholic stools. As noted above, the concentration of bilirubin rises progressively and plateaus at a level of 510 to 680 μmol/L (30 to 40 mg/dL). *Partial obstruction* of extrahepatic bile ducts also can lead to jaundice if the clearance of bilirubin into the duodenum is unable to match the level of pigment production. In such cases, intrabiliary pressure is usually increased (to levels approaching 250 mmHg). This increased pressure interferes with hepatocyte bilirubin secretion, further exaggerating the imbalance between bilirubin production and clearance. In partial biliary obstruction, the degree of jaundice and bilirubinuria depends on many factors, including the presence of concurrent hepatocellular disease or cholangitis, which can exacerbate the impairment of hepatocyte bilirubin excretion. The functional reserve of the liver is so great that occlusion of the intrahepatic bile ducts does not give rise to jaundice unless the drainage of bile from a large segment (>75 percent) of the parenchyma is interrupted. In most patients, either of the two major hepatic ducts or a large number of secondary radicles may be occluded without production of jaundice. In contrast, diffuse narrowing of the intrahepatic biliary ducts, even without complete obstruction, may produce jaundice in a manner analogous to partial obstruction of the extrahepatic ducts.

EVALUATION OF JAUNDICE The first task in the evaluation of jaundice is to consider whether the hyperbilirubinemia is due to hemolysis or hepatobiliary disease. This differentiation is most easily accomplished by measuring the direct and indirect bilirubin fractions. Predominantly unconjugated hyperbilirubinemia indicates a hemolytic disorder due to accelerated intravascular red blood cell destruction or resorption of a large hematoma. Exceptions to this rule are Gilbert's syndrome, the other, rare, hereditary disorders of glucuronosyl transferase, and end-stage hepatic failure. Further evaluation of the cause of hemolysis can then proceed as described in Chap. 108, "Megaloblastic Anemia," Chap. 107, "Hemoglobinopathies," and Chap. 109, "Anemias Due to Hemolysis and Acute Bood Loss."

Jaundice associated with predominantly (>50 percent) conjugated hyperbilirubinemia usually results from one of three groups of disorders: hepatocellular disease, intrahepatic biliary obstruction ("cholestasis"), and extrahepatic biliary obstruction. An early goal is the determination of which category of disease explains the patient's jaundice. Central to this determination is a careful *clinical* evaluation, including history, physical examination, basic tests of liver function, and a complete blood count. Using these simple tools, experienced clinicians can determine the overall nature of the jaundice in the majority of cases. Most importantly, however, the results of the clinical evaluation direct the physician to a logical progression of imaging studies, serologic tests, and pathologic evaluation. The initial clinical evaluation should focus on features of the patient's illness that distinguish between hepatocellular disease, intrahepatic cholestasis, and extrahepatic biliary obstruction. A general algorithm for the evaluation of jaundice due to conjugated hyperbilirubinemia is shown in Fig. 45-3.

History Historic evaluation should include determination of the length of symptoms, presence and character of abdominal pain, fever or other symptoms of active inflammation, and changes in appetite, weight, and bowel habits. Specific attention should be directed to a history of blood product transfusions, intravenous drug use, promiscuous sexual activity, and ethanol use. A history of medication use should be sought, particularly drugs known to cause either cholestasis, such as anabolic steroids and chlorpromazine, or hepatocellular necrosis, such as acetaminophen or isoniazid. A history of arthralgias may suggest acute viral hepatitis. Viral disease should also be considered in patients with a history of travel to developing countries endemic for enterally transmitted hepatitis E or East Asian countries, where the parenterally transmitted hepatitis B and C viruses are widespread. Pruritus is most commonly associated with chronic cholestasis, developing from either extrahepatic obstruction or cholestatic liver disease such as sclerosing cholangitis or primary biliary cirrhosis. In contrast, acholic stools develop more commonly in patients with extrahepatic biliary obstruction from tumor, choledocholithiasis, or secondary to a congenital biliary abnormality such as an inflamed choledochal cyst. The presence of acholic and heme-positive stool ("silver stools") should suggest a tumor of the distal biliary tract such as ampullary, periampullary, or cholangiocarcinoma. This combination may also be seen in patients with pancreatic carcinoma eroding into the biliary tract or duodenum. Jaundice, in the setting of previous biliary surgery, may suggest retained or recurrent stones, a biliary stricture, or recurrent obstruction from an enlarging tumor. Finally, a preexisting or underlying condition predisposing to hepatobiliary disease should be solicited. For example, inflammatory bowel disease, particularly ulcerative colitis, may be associated with sclerosing cholangitis. Pregnancy predisposes to cholestasis, steatosis, and acute liver failure. Right heart failure may result in hepatic congestion and cholestasis, and sepsis can cause selective disruption of bilirubin transport or generalized intrahepatic cholestasis.

Physical Examination The examination is also important for directing the subsequent evaluation. Excoriations suggest prolonged cholestasis or high grade biliary obstruction, and a greenish hue to the jaundice is associated with particularly severe or long-standing liver disease, such as biliary cirrhosis, sclerosing cholangitis, severe, chronic hepatitis, or long-standing malignant obstruction. Fever and epigastric or right upper quadrant tenderness are frequently associated with choledocholithiasis and cholangitis or cholecystitis. In contrast, malignant biliary obstruction commonly presents as painless jaundice. An enlarged, tender liver suggests acute hepatic inflammation or a rapidly enlarging hepatic tumor, while a palpable gallbladder suggests distal biliary obstruction from a malignant tumor. The presence of splenomegaly may provide a clue to the presence of portal hypertension, from chronic active hepatitis, severe alcoholic or acute viral hepatitis, or cirrhosis. Cirrhosis is also associated with a hyperestrogenic state that may be reflected in gynecomastia, testicular atrophy, or spider angiomata. Testicular atrophy may be particularly prominent in cirrhosis due to alcoholic liver disease or hemochromatosis. Palmar erythema, facial telangiectasia, and Dupuytren's contractures are also associated with cirrhosis, particularly as a result of chronic ethanol ingestion. Wasting or lymphadenopathy suggests malignancy, and in the presence of splenomegaly, these signs may direct consideration of a pancreatic tumor obstructing the splenic vein or a widely metastatic lymphoma. In patients whose history or examination suggests malignancy, particular attention should be directed toward physical findings suggestive of a primary tumor, including heme-positive stools, abdominal or breast masses, thyroid nodules, and supraclavicular lymphadenopathy. Physical findings associated with specific liver diseases include distended neck veins and hepatojugular reflux (right heart failure), xanthomata (primary biliary cirrhosis), and Kayser-Fleischer rings (Wilson's disease).

Laboratory Tests Initial laboratory evaluation should focus on serum bilirubin fractionation. Predominantly *unconjugated* (indirect) hyperbilirubinemia should prompt consideration of a hemolytic disorder, such as an autoimmune or microangiopathic hemolytic anemia, ineffective erythropoiesis, or resorption of a large hematoma. The most common cause of mild elevations in the unconjugated fraction, however, is Gilbert's syndrome, an inherited condition resulting from a mild deficiency in hepatic glucuronosyl transferase. Individuals with Gilbert's syndrome experience variable elevations in circulating unconjugated bilirubin, especially in association with physical stress, fever, intercurrent infection or surgery, fasting, or heavy ethanol ingestion. This mild metabolic abnormality produces no symptoms other than jaundice, and is *not* associated with liver enzyme abnormalities or adverse long-term effects.

Conjugated (direct) hyperbilirubinemia usually results from hepatocellular or cholestatic liver disease or from extrahepatic biliary obstruction. Because hepatic glucuronosyl transferase activity is normally present in great abundance, adequate bilirubin glucuronide formation can occur even with severe liver disease. In patients with primarily conjugated hyperbilirubinemia, the presence and nature of liver enzyme abnormalities usually provide important clues about the nature of the underlying process. Conjugated hyperbilirubinemia without liver enzyme abnormalities is relatively uncommon but can be seen in pregnancy, sepsis, or after recent surgery. Isolated conjugated hyperbilirubinemia is the primary manifestation of two heritable disorders, Rotor and Dubin-Johnson syndromes, and can also be seen in some patients with the syndrome of recurrent benign intrahepatic cholestasis. As described more fully in Chap. 292, elevation of the aminotransferases out of proportion to other liver enzymes suggests hepatocellular damage, most commonly seen in toxic, viral, or ischemic hepatitis, while prominent elevations of the alkaline phosphatase, 5'-nucleotidase and/or gamma-glutamyl transpeptidase are more suggestive of intrahepatic cholestasis or extrahepatic obstruction. Although these patterns are not invariably diagnostic, they are helpful in directing the ensuing evaluation.

Patients with a clinical evaluation and laboratory findings suggestive of hepatocellular disease should be evaluated for evidence of viral hepatitis, drug toxicity, hepatic congestion, such as that produced by right ventricular failure or acute obstruction of the hepatic veins, or ischemic hepatitis. In the appropriate clinical setting, serologic studies are extremely helpful for establishing or excluding the diagnosis of hepatitis A; acute and chronic hepatitis B; hepatitis C, D, and E; and hepatitis from cytomegalovirus (CMV) or Epstein-Barr virus. Common causes of toxic hepatitis include acetaminophen, isoniazid, and halogenated anesthetic agents. Patients with alcoholic liver disease are particularly susceptible to acetaminophen toxicity, which may occur after therapeutic doses in these individuals. For patients with probable hepatocellular disease, liver biopsy can provide important diagnostic and prognostic information. The results of percutaneous, transjugular, or laparoscopic biopsy may also provide important information for optimal therapy. The role of hepatobiliary imaging in these patients is less clearly defined. In some cases, identification of focal lesions by computed tomography (CT), transabdominal ultrasonography (US), or magnetic resonance imaging (MRI) can increase the diagnostic accuracy of liver biopsy. These imaging techniques can also aid in diagnosis by suggesting the presence of hepatic fat deposition, cirrhosis, or the excessive hepatic iron deposition of hemochromatosis. Ultrasound is an exquisitely sensitive means of detecting ascites. Combined with Doppler flow analysis, it can also determine the patency and direction of flow in the portal and hepatic veins, frequently enabling noninvasive diagnosis of portal vein thrombosis and Budd-Chiari syndrome.

Hepatobiliary Imaging For patients whose clinical evaluation and liver chemistries suggest cholestasis or extrahepatic biliary obstruction, biliary imaging is an important early diagnostic tool to differentiate intrahepatic causes from extrahepatic obstruction. Both US and CT detect dilated extrahepatic biliary ducts with great sensitivity. In the absence of previous hepatobiliary surgery, the specificity of these tests for identifying dilated extrahepatic ducts is well above 90 percent. Both techniques are sensitive indicators of intrahepatic, portal, and pancreatic masses, and either can be effective in diagnosing biliary obstruction from tumors or impacted stones. In addition, US is an extremely effective means of detecting stones within the gallbladder and is somewhat more sensitive than CT. These imaging techniques are considerably less sensitive for detecting choledocholithiasis. Both fail to detect approximately 40 percent of intraductal stones, although selected studies suggest that CT is somewhat better at detecting stones within nondilated ducts.

In patients with clinical and radiographic evidence of extrahepatic biliary obstruction, further evaluation should be directed at determining the cause of the obstruction and providing rapid relief. Masses identified by transabdominal or endoscopic US, CT, or MRI are usually accessible to radiographically directed percutaneous or endoscopic biopsy. Further definition and relief of extrahepatic biliary obstruction can frequently be accomplished by *percutaneous* or *endoscopic cholangiography*. In the hands of experienced practitioners, dilated biliary ducts can be accessed percutaneously in more than 90 percent of patients, nondilated ducts in up to 70 percent. Percutaneous transhepatic cholangiography (PTC) may be particularly useful for imaging and drainage of patients with biliary obstruction well above the bifurcation of the common bile duct and in patients whose obstruction cannot be relieved during endoscopic cholangiography. Collection of bile for cytologic analysis may also allow identification of the obstructing lesion. Endoscopic retrograde cholangiopancreatography (ERCP) is frequently the preferred technique for diagnosing and treating distal biliary obstructions. In addition to cholangiography, ERCP provides the opportunity for inspection and biopsy of the ampulla of Vater and surrounding duodenum (common sites of tumors obstructing the bile ducts), visualization of the pancreatic ducts to detect evidence of pancreatic ductal stones or small pancreatic tumors, and direct biopsy of the bile duct epithelium and pancreatic head. Both PTC and ERCP can afford relief of malignant obstruction and dissolution or fragmenting of ductal stones. ERCP also provides the opportunity for long-term relief of stone disease via endoscopic papillotomy and is the preferred approach to intraductal stones remaining after surgical or laparoscopic cholecystectomy.

For patients with a clinical presentation of cholestasis who have ducts of *normal* caliber, attention should focus on intrahepatic cholestasis caused by primary biliary cirrhosis, drugs or toxins (including ethanol), and extrahepatic obstruction *without* ductal dilation, which can be caused by primary sclerosing cholangitis, primary biliary cirrhosis, or intrahepatic arterial chemotherapy and is occasionally seen in patients with cholangiocarcinoma. A related cholestatic process, termed *vanishing bile duct syndrome* (VBDS), can occur as a result of liver transplant rejection, AIDS, CMV infection, and radiation injury. VBDS is rarely associated with Hodgkin's disease and sarcoidosis and may develop after treatment with flucloxacillin, anticonvulsants, and other medications. If the clinical picture is more suggestive of cholestasis or biliary cirrhosis, liver biopsy may provide the most direct route to diagnosis. In contrast, cholangiography with cytologic analysis of the bile and/or biopsy of the ductal epithelium is indicated in patients whose presentation suggests extrahepatic obstruction, such as patients with jaundice and nondilated ducts in the setting of weight loss, lymphadenopathy, or inflammatory bowel disease.

BIBLIOGRAPHY

AONO S et al: Analysis of genes for UDP-glucuronosyl transferase in Gilbert's syndrome. Lancet 345:958, 1995

CHOWDHURY JR et al: Hereditary jaundice and disorders of bilirubin metabolism, in *The Metabolic Basis of Inherited Disease*, 7th ed. CR Scriver et al (eds). New York, McGraw-Hill, 1995, pp 2161–2208

FRANK BB et al: Clinical evaluation of jaundice: A guideline of the patient care committee of the American Gastroenterological Association. JAMA 262:3031, 1989

LAMONT JT, ISSELBACHER KJ: Postoperative jaundice, in *Wright's Liver and Biliary Disease*, 3d ed. GH Millward-Sadler et al (eds). Philadelphia, Saunders, 1992, pp 1372–1380

LESTER R (ed): The pathogenesis of cholestasis: Past and future trends. Semin Liver Dis 13:219, 1993

ROY-CHOWDHURY J et al: Bilirubin metabolism and its disorders, in *Hepatology,* 3d ed, D Zakim, T Boyer (eds). Philadelphia, Saunders, 1996, p 323

SHERLOCK S, DOOLEY J (eds): *Diseases of the Liver and Biliary System*, 9th ed. Oxford, Blackwell, 1993, pp 199–213

WEISS JS et al: The clinical importance of a protein-bound fraction of serum bilirubin in patients with hyperbilirubinemia. N Engl J Med 309:147, 1983

46

Robert M. Glickman, Kurt J. Isselbacher

ABDOMINAL SWELLING AND ASCITES

ABDOMINAL SWELLING   Abdominal swelling or distention is a common problem in clinical medicine and may be the initial manifestation of a systemic disease or of otherwise unsuspected abdominal disease. *Subjective* abdominal enlargement, often described as a sensation of fullness or bloating, is usually transient and is often related to a functional gastrointestinal disorder when it is not accompanied by objective physical findings of increased abdominal girth or local swelling. *Obesity* and lumbar lordosis, which may be associated with prominence of the abdomen, may usually be distinguished from true increases in the volume of the peritoneal cavity by history and careful physical examination.

Clinical History   Abdominal swelling may first be noticed by the patient because of a progressive increase in belt or clothing size, the appearance of abdominal or inguinal hernias, or the development of a localized swelling. Often, considerable abdominal enlargement has gone unnoticed for weeks or months, either because of coexistent obesity or because the ascites formation has been insidious, without pain or localizing symptoms. Progressive abdominal distention may be associated with a sensation of "pulling" or "stretching" of the flanks or groins and vague low back pain. Localized *pain* usually results from involvement of an abdominal organ (e.g., a passively congested liver, large spleen, or colonic tumor). Pain is uncommon in cirrhosis with ascites, and when it is present, pancreatitis, hepatocellular carcinoma, or peritonitis should be considered. Tense ascites or abdominal tumors may produce increased intraabdominal pressure, resulting in *indigestion* and *heartburn* due to gastroesophageal reflux or *dyspnea*, *orthopnea*, and *tachypnea* from elevation of the diaphragm. A coexistent pleural effusion, more commonly on the right, presumably due to leakage of ascitic fluid through lymphatic channels in the diaphragm, also may contribute to respiratory embarrassment. The patient with diffuse abdominal swelling should be questioned about increased alcohol intake, a prior episode of jaundice or hematuria, or a change in bowel habits. Such historical information may provide the clues that will lead one to suspect an occult cirrhosis, a colonic tumor with peritoneal seeding, congestive heart failure, or nephrosis.

Physical Examination   A carefully executed general physical examination can yield valuable clues concerning the etiology of abdominal swelling. Thus palmar erythema and spider angiomas suggest an underlying cirrhosis, while supraclavicular adenopathy (Virchow's node) should raise the question of an underlying gastrointestinal malignancy.

Inspection of the abdomen is important. By noting the abdominal contour, one may be able to distinguish localized from generalized swelling. The tensely distended abdomen with tightly stretched skin, bulging flanks, and everted umbilicus is characteristic of ascites. A prominent abdominal venous pattern with the direction of flow away from the umbilicus often is a reflection of portal hypertension; venous collaterals with flow from the lower part of the abdomen toward the umbilicus suggest obstruction of the inferior vena cava; flow downward toward the umbilicus suggests superior vena cava obstruction. "Doming" of the abdomen with visible ridges from underlying intestinal loops is usually due to intestinal obstruction or distention. An epigastric mass, with evident peristalsis proceeding from left to right, usually indicates underlying pyloric obstruction. A liver with metastatic deposits may be visible as a nodular right upper quadrant mass moving with respiration.

Auscultation may reveal the high-pitched, rushing sounds of early intestinal obstruction or a succussion sound due to increased fluid and gas in a dilated hollow viscus. Careful auscultation over an enlarged liver occasionally reveals the harsh bruit of a vascular tumor, especially a hepatocellular carcinoma, or the leathery friction rub of a surface nodule. A venous hum at the umbilicus may signify portal hypertension and an increased collateral blood flow around the liver. A fluid wave and flank dullness that shifts with change in position of the patient are important signs that indicate the presence of peritoneal fluid. In obese patients, small amounts of fluid may be difficult to demonstrate; on occasion, the fluid may be detected by abdominal percussion with patients on their hands and knees. Small amounts of ascites often can only be detected by ultrasound examination of the abdomen. Careful percussion should serve to distinguish generalized abdominal enlargement from localized swelling due to an enlarged uterus, ovarian cyst, or distended bladder. Percussion also can outline an abnormally small or large liver. Loss of normal liver dullness may result from massive hepatic necrosis; it also may be a clue to free gas in the peritoneal cavity, as from perforation of a hollow viscus.

Palpation is often difficult with massive ascites, and ballottement of overlying fluid may be the only method of palpating the liver or spleen. A slightly enlarged spleen in association with ascites may be the only evidence of an occult cirrhosis. When there is evidence of portal hypertension, a soft liver suggests that obstruction to portal flow is extrahepatic; a firm liver suggests cirrhosis as the likely cause of the portal hypertension. A very hard or nodular liver is a clue that the liver is infiltrated with tumor, and when accompanied by ascites, it suggests that the latter is due to peritoneal seeding. The presence of a hard periumbilical nodule (Sister Mary Joseph's nodule) suggests metastatic disease from a pelvic or gastrointestinal primary tumor. A pulsatile liver and ascites may be found in tricuspid insufficiency.

An attempt should be made to determine whether a mass is solid or cystic, smooth or irregular, and whether it moves with respiration. The liver, spleen, and gallbladder should descend with respiration unless they are fixed by adhesions or extension of tumor beyond the organ. A fixed mass not descending with respiration may indicate that it is retroperitoneal. Tenderness, especially if localized, may indicate an inflammatory process such as an abscess; it also may be due to stretching of the visceral peritoneum or tumor necrosis. Rectal and pelvic examinations are mandatory; they may reveal otherwise undetected masses due to tumor or infection.

Radiographic and laboratory examinations are essential for confirming or extending the impressions gained on physical examination.

Upright and recumbent films of the abdomen may demonstrate the dilated loops of intestine with fluid levels characteristic of intestinal obstruction or the diffuse abdominal haziness and loss of psoas margins suggestive of ascites. Ultrasonography is often of value in detecting ascites, determining the presence of a mass, or evaluating the size of the liver and spleen. Computed tomography (CT) scanning provides similar information. CT scanning is often necessary to visualize the retroperitoneum, pancreas, and lymph nodes. A plain film of the abdomen may reveal the distended colon of otherwise unsuspected ulcerative colitis and give valuable information as to the size of the liver and spleen. An irregular and elevated right side of the diaphragm may be a clue to a liver abscess or hepatocellular carcinoma. Studies of the gastrointestinal tract with barium or other contrast media are usually necessary in the search for a primary tumor.

ASCITES The evaluation of a patient with ascites requires that the *cause* of the ascites be established. In most cases ascites will appear as a part of a well-recognized illness, i.e., cirrhosis, congestive heart failure, nephrosis, or disseminated carcinomatosis. In these situations, the physician should determine that the development of ascites is indeed a consequence of the basic underlying disease and not due to the presence of a separate or related disease process. This distinction is necessary even when the cause of ascites seems obvious. For example, when the patient with compensated cirrhosis and minimal ascites develops progressive ascites that is increasingly difficult to control with sodium restriction or diuretics, the obvious temptation is to attribute the worsening of the clinical picture to progressive liver disease. However, an occult hepatocellular carcinoma, portal vein thrombosis, spontaneous bacterial peritonitis, or even tuberculosis may be responsible for the decompensation. The disappointingly low success in diagnosing tuberculous peritonitis or hepatocullar carcinoma in the patient with cirrhosis and ascites reflects the too-low index of suspicion for the development of such superimposed conditions. Similarly, the patient with congestive heart failure may develop ascites from a disseminated carcinoma with peritoneal seeding.

Diagnostic paracentesis (50 to 100 mL) should be part of the routine evaluation of the patient with ascites. The fluid should be examined for its gross appearance; protein content, cell count, and differential cell count should be determined, and Gram's and acid-fast stains and culture performed. Cytologic and cell-block examination may disclose an otherwise unsuspected carcinoma. Table 46-1

Table 46-1

Ascitic Fluid Characteristics in Various Disease States

Condition	Gross Appearance	Protein, g/L	Serum-Ascites Albumin Gradient, g/dL	Cell Count Red Blood Cells, >10,000/μL	White Blood Cells, per μL	Other Tests
Cirrhosis	Straw-colored or bile-stained	<25 (95%)	>1.1	1%	<250 (90%);* predominantly mesothelial	
Neoplasm	Straw-colored, hemorrhagic, mucinous, or chylous	>25 (75%)	<1.1	20%	>1000 (50%); variable cell types	Cytology, cell block, peritoneal biopsy
Tuberculous peritonitis	Clear, turbid, hemorrhagic, chylous	>25 (50%)	<1.1	7%	>1000 (70%); usually >70% lymphocytes	Peritoneal biopsy, stain and culture for acid-fast bacilli
Pyogenic peritonitis	Turbid or purulent	If purulent, >25	<1.1	Unusual	Predominantly polymorphonuclear leukocytes	+ Gram's stain, culture
Congestive heart failure	Straw-colored	Variable, 15–53	>1.1	10%	<1000 (90%); usually mesothelial, mononuclear	
Nephrosis	Straw-colored or chylous	<25 (100%)	<1.1	Unusual	<250; mesothelial, mononuclear	If chylous, ether extraction, Sudan staining
Pancreatic ascites (pancreatitis, pseudocyst)	Turbid, hemorrhagic, or chylous	Variable, often >25	<1.1	Variable, may be blood-stained	Variable	Increased amylase in ascitic fluid and serum

* Since the conditions of examining fluid and selecting patients were not identical in each series, the percentage figures (in parentheses) should be taken as an indication of the order of magnitude rather than as the precise incidence of any abnormal finding.

presents some of the features of ascitic fluid typically found in various disease states. In some disorders, such as cirrhosis, the fluid has the characteristics of a transudate (<25 g protein per liter and a specific gravity of <1.016); in others, such as peritonitis, the features are those of an exudate. Rather than the total protein content of ascites, some authors prefer the use of a *serum-ascites albumin gradient* (SAG) to characterize ascites. The gradient correlates directly with portal pressure. A gradient >1.1 g/dL is characteristic of uncomplicated cirrhotic ascites; a gradient <1.1 g/dL is seen in conditions characterized by exudative ascites. Although there is variability of the ascitic fluid in any given disease state, some features are sufficiently characteristic to suggest certain diagnostic possibilities. For example, blood-stained fluid with >25 g protein per liter is unusual in uncomplicated cirrhosis but is consistent with tuberculous peritonitis or neoplasm. Cloudy fluid with a predominance of polymorphonuclear cells and a positive Gram's stain are characteristic of bacterial peritonitis; if most cells are lymphocytes, tuberculosis should be suspected. The complete examination of each fluid is most important, for occasionally only *one* finding may be abnormal. For example, if the fluid is a typical transudate but contains more than 250 white blood cells per microliter, the finding should be recognized as atypical for cirrhosis and should warrant a search for tumor or infection. This is especially true in the evaluation of cirrhotic ascites where occult peritoneal infection may be present with only minor elevations in the white blood cell count of the peritoneal fluid (300 to 500 cells per microliter). Since Gram's stain of the fluid may be negative in a high proportion of such cases, careful culture of the peritoneal fluid is mandatory. Bedside inoculation of blood culture flasks with ascitic fluid results in a dramatically increased incidence of positive cultures when bacterial infection is present (90 versus 40 percent positivity with conventional cultures done by the laboratory). Direct visualization of the peritoneum (laparoscopy) may disclose peritoneal deposits of tumor, tuberculosis, or metastatic disease of the liver. Biopsies are taken under direct vision, often adding to the diagnostic accuracy of the procedure.

Chylous ascites refers to a turbid, milky, or creamy peritoneal fluid due to the presence of thoracic or intestinal lymph. Such a fluid shows Sudan-staining fat globules microscopically and an increased triglyceride content by chemical examination. Opaque milky fluid usually has a triglyceride concentration of >1000 mg/dL. A turbid fluid due to leukocytes or tumor cells may be confused with chylous fluid (pseudochylous), and it is often helpful to carry out alkalinization and ether extraction of the specimen. Alkali will tend to dissolve cellular proteins and thereby reduce turbidity; ether extraction will lead to clearing if the turbidity of the fluid is due to lipid. Chylous ascites is most often the result of lymphatic obstruction from trauma, tumor, tuberculosis, filariasis (see Chap. 223), or congenital abnormalities. It also may be seen in the nephrotic syndrome.

Rarely, ascitic fluid may be *mucinous* in character, suggesting either pseudomyxoma peritonei (Chap. 288) or rarely a colloid carcinoma of the stomach or colon with peritoneal implants.

On occasion, ascites may develop as a seemingly isolated finding in the absence of a clinically evident underlying disease. It is then that a careful analysis of ascitic fluid may indicate the direction the evaluation should take. A useful framework for the workup starts with an analysis of whether the fluid is an exudate or transudate. *Transudative ascites* of unclear etiology is most often due to occult cirrhosis, right-sided venous hypertension raising hepatic sinusoidal pressure, or hypoalbuminemic states such as nephrosis or protein-losing enteropathy. Cirrhosis with well-preserved liver function (normal albumin) resulting in ascites invariably is associated with signifi-

cant portal hypertension (see Chap. 298). Evaluation should include liver function tests, liver-spleen scan, or other hepatic imaging procedure (i.e., CT or ultrasound) to detect nodular changes in the liver or a colloid shift of isotope to suggest portal hypertension. On occasion, a wedged hepatic venous pressure can be useful to document portal hypertension. Finally, if clinically indicated, a liver biopsy will confirm the diagnosis of cirrhosis and perhaps suggest its etiology. Other etiologies may result in hepatic venous congestion and resultant ascites. Right-sided cardiac valvular disease and particularly constrictive pericarditis should raise a high index of suspicion and may require cardiac imaging and cardiac catheterization for definitive diagnosis. Hepatic vein thrombosis is evaluated by visualizing the hepatic veins using imaging techniques (Doppler ultrasound, angiography, CT scans, magnetic resonance imaging) to demonstrate obliteration, thrombosis, or obstruction by tumor. Uncommonly, transudative ascites may be associated with benign tumors of the ovary, particularly fibroma (Meigs' syndrome) with ascites and hydrothorax.

Exudative ascites should initiate an evaluation for primary peritoneal processes, most importantly infection and tumor. Routine bacteriologic culture of ascitic fluid often will yield a specific organism causing infectious peritonitis. Tuberculous peritonitis (see Table 46-1) is best diagnosed by peritoneal biopsy, either percutaneously or via laparoscopy. Histologic examination invariably shows granulomata that may contain acid-fast bacilli. Since cultures of peritoneal fluid and biopsies for tuberculosis may require 6 weeks, characteristic histology with appropriate stains allows antituberculosis therapy to be started promptly. Similarly, the diagnosis of peritoneal seeding by tumor can usually be made by cytologic analysis of peritoneal fluid or by peritoneal biopsy if cytology is negative. Appropriate diagnostic studies can then be undertaken to determine the nature and site of the primary tumor. Pancreatic ascites (see Table 46-1) is invariably associated with an extravasation of pancreatic fluid from the pancreatic ductal system, most commonly from a leaking pseudocyst. Ultrasound or CT examination of the pancreas followed by visualization of the pancreatic duct by direct cannulation (viz., endoscopic retrograde cholangiopancreatography, ERCP) will usually disclose the site of leakage and permit resective surgery to be carried out.

An analysis of the physiologic and metabolic factors involved in the production of ascites (see Chap. 298 for details), coupled with a complete evaluation of the nature of the ascitic fluid, will invariably disclose the etiology of the ascites and permit appropriate therapy to be instituted.

BIBLIOGRAPHY

EPSTEIN M: Treatment of refractory ascites. N Engl J Med 321:1675, 1989

HOEFS JC: Globulin correction of the albumin gradient: Correlation with measured ascites colloid osmotic pressure gradients. Hepatology 16:396, 1992

LIPSKY MS, STERNBACH MR: Evaluation and initial management of patients with ascites. Am Fam Physician 54:1327, 1996

PINTO PC et al: Large volume paracentesis in nonedematous patients with tense ascites: Its effect on intravascular volume. Hepatology 8:207, 1988

RECTOR WG JR, REYNOLDS TB: Superiority of the serum: ascites albumin difference over the ascites total protein concentration in separation of "transudative" and "exudative" ascites. Am J Med 77:83, 1988

RUNYON BA: Care of patients with ascites. N Engl J Med 330:337, 1994

——— et al: The serum-ascites albumin gradient in the differential diagnosis of ascites. Ann Intern Med 117:215, 1992

47

Bradley M. Denker, Barry M. Brenner

CARDINAL MANIFESTATIONS OF RENAL DISEASE

Renal diseases may present to the physician in several different ways depending upon the nature of the illness and the timing of presentation. Some patients with advanced renal disease have signs and symptoms of uremia with unremarkable urinalysis, while others have abnormalities of the urine but few, if any, disturbances in renal function. After a complete history and physical examination, the urinalysis and serum chemistries are essential aids in helping to distinguish among the various etiologies of renal disease. Urine characteristics including volume, specific gravity, electrolyte composition, and sediment (cells, casts, and crystals) can help define the specific process affecting the kidneys. This chapter focuses on the evaluation of patients with reduced glomerular filtration rate (GFR) and/or abnormalities of the urine.

AZOTEMIA

ASSESSMENT OF GLOMERULAR FILTRATION RATE
A reduced GFR leads to retention of nitrogenous waste products (azotemia) such as blood urea nitrogen (BUN) and creatinine. Azotemia may result from reduced renal perfusion, intrinsic renal disease, or postrenal processes (ureteral obstruction). Precise determination of GFR is problematic as commonly used markers (urea and creatinine) are partially handled by tubule transport. An ideal endogenous marker for GFR would be produced at a constant rate, freely filtered at the glomerulus, not protein-bound, and excreted without tubular modification (no reabsorption, secretion, or catabolism). BUN varies directly with protein intake, and urea is readily reabsorbed by the medullary collecting duct. The permeability of the tubule to urea is linked to water reabsorption; it is low in states of diuresis and low levels of arginine vasopressin (AVP) but is enhanced in states of decreased intravascular volume, low tubule fluid flow rate, and increased levels of AVP. Gastrointestinal bleeding, glucocorticoids, and tetracycline can also increase BUN, while reduced levels can be seen in patients with malnutrition and muscle wasting as seen in starvation or chronic liver disease. Urea clearance is generally an underestimate of GFR because of tubule urea reabsorption and may be as low as one-half of GFR measured by other techniques.

Creatinine is a small, freely filtered solute whose production varies little from day to day (since it is derived from metabolism of muscle creatine). However, serum creatinine can increase acutely from dietary ingestion of cooked meat. Creatinine can be secreted by the proximal tubule through an organic cation pathway that is saturable and can be blocked by some commonly used medications including cimetidine, trimethoprim, pyrimethamine, and dapsone. The secreted creatinine component confounds GFR measurements because it can vary within individuals over time; moreover, the proportion of secreted creatinine increases as GFR decreases. Extrarenal clearance of creatinine through gastrointestinal metabolism by bacterial flora can also affect GFR measurements when GFR is reduced. Most autoanalyzers of serum creatinine avoid contributions of noncreatinine chromogens, but high bilirubin levels can cause falsely low creatinine levels. Despite these shortcomings, creatinine clearance remains the most common clinical measure of GFR. The gradual loss of muscle from chronic illness, glucocorticoids, and malnutrition can mask significant changes in GFR through small or imperceptible changes in serum creatinine. More accurate determinations of GFR are available using inulin clearance or radionuclide-labeled markers such as ^{125}I-iothalamate or ^{51}Cr-ethylenediaminetetraacetic acid (EDTA).

Approach to the Patient

With Azotemia Once it has been established that GFR is reduced, the physician must decide if this represents acute or chronic renal failure. The clinical situation, history, and laboratory data often make this an easy distinction. Laboratory abnormalities characteristic of chronic renal failure include anemia, hypocalcemia, hyperphosphatemia, and radiographic evidence of renal osteodystrophy (Chap. 271). The urinalysis and renal ultrasound can also facilitate the distinction between acute and chronic renal failure. An approach to the evaluation of azotemic patients is shown in Fig. 47-1. Patients with advanced chronic renal failure often have some proteinuria, nonconcentrated urine (isosthenuria), and small kidneys on ultrasound, which is characterized by increased echogenicity and cortical thinning. Treatment should be directed toward slowing the progression of renal disease and providing symptomatic relief for edema, acidosis, anemia, and hyperphosphatemia, as discussed in Chap. 271. Acute renal failure can result from processes affecting renal blood flow (prerenal azotemia), intrinsic renal diseases (affecting vessels, glomeruli, or tubules), or postrenal processes (obstruction to urine flow in ureters, bladder, or urethra) (see Chap. 270).

PRERENAL FAILURE Decreased renal perfusion accounts for 40 to 80 percent of acute renal failure and, if appropriately treated, is readily reversible. The etiologies of prerenal azotemia include any cause of decreased circulating blood volume including volume loss (gastrointestinal hemorrhage, burns, diarrhea, diuretics), volume sequestration (pancreatitis, peritonitis, rhabdomyolysis), or decreased effective circulating volume (cardiogenic shock, sepsis). Renal perfusion can also be affected adversely by reductions in cardiac output from peripheral vasodilatation (sepsis, drugs) or profound renal vasoconstriction [severe heart failure, hepatorenal syndrome, drugs (e.g., nonsteroidal anti-inflammatory drugs, or NSAIDs)]. True, or "effective," hypovolemia leads to a fall in mean arterial pressure, which in turn triggers a series of neural and humoral responses that include activation of the sympathetic nervous system and renin-angiotensin-aldosterone system and AVP release. GFR is maintained by prostaglandin-mediated relaxation of afferent arterioles and angiotensin II–mediated constriction of efferent arterioles. Once the mean arterial pressure falls below 80 mmHg, there is a steep decline in GFR. Blockade of prostaglandin production by NSAIDs can result in severe vasoconstriction and acute renal failure in the presence of hypotension. Angiotensin-converting enzyme (ACE) inhibitors decrease efferent arteriolar tone and can thereby reduce glomerular capillary perfusion pressure. Patients on NSAIDs and/or ACE inhibitors are most susceptible to hemodynamically mediated acute renal failure when blood volume is reduced. Patients with renal artery stenosis are dependent upon efferent arteriolar vasoconstriction for maintenance of glomerular filtration pressure and are particularly susceptible to precipitous declines in GFR when given ACE inhibitors.

Prolonged renal hypoperfusion can lead to acute tubular necrosis (ATN), an intrinsic renal disease discussed below. The urinalysis and urinary electrolytes can be useful in distinguishing prerenal azotemia from ATN (Table 47-1). In prerenal failure the tubules are intact, leading to a concentrated urine (>500 mosmol/L), avid Na retention (urine Na concentration < 20 mmol/L; fractional excretion of Na < 1%), and urine/plasma creatinine ratio > 40 (Table 47-1). Urine sediment in prerenal failure is usually normal or has occasional hyaline and granular casts, while the sediment in ATN is usually filled with cellular debris and muddy brown granular casts.

INTRINSIC RENAL DISEASE When prerenal and postrenal azotemia have been excluded as etiologies of renal failure, an intrinsic parenchymal renal disease is present. Intrinsic renal disease can arise from processes involving large renal vessels, microvasculature and glomeruli, or tubular interstitium. Ischemic and toxic ATN account for about 90 percent of acute intrinsic renal failure. As outlined in Fig. 47-1, the clinical setting and urinalysis are helpful in separating the possible etiologies of acute intrinsic renal failure. Prerenal azotemia and ATN are part of a spectrum of renal hypoperfusion: evidence of structural tubule injury is present in ATN, whereas prompt reversibility occurs with prerenal azotemia upon restoration of adequate renal perfusion. Thus, ATN can often be distinguished from prerenal azotemia by urinalysis and urine electrolyte composition (Table 47-1 and Fig. 47-1). Ischemic ATN is observed most frequently in patients who have undergone major surgery, trauma, severe hypovolemia, overwhelming sepsis, or extensive burns. Nephrotoxic ATN complicates the administration of many common medications usually by inducing a combination of intrarenal vasoconstriction, direct tubule toxicity, and/or tubular obstruction. The kidney is vulnerable to toxic injury by virtue of its rich blood supply (25 percent of cardiac output) and its ability to concentrate and metabolize toxins. A diligent search for hypotension and nephrotoxins will usually uncover the specific etiology of ATN. → *An extensive list of potential drugs and toxins implicated in ATN can be found in Chap. 270.*

Processes that involve the tubules and interstitium can lead to acute renal failure. These include drug-induced interstitial nephritis (especially antibiotics, NSAIDs, and diuretics), severe infections (both bacterial and viral), systemic diseases (such as systemic lupus erythematosus), or infiltrative disorders (such as sarcoid, lymphoma, or leukemia) (see Chap. 276). The urinalysis usually shows mild to moderate proteinuria, hematuria, and pyuria and occasionally white blood cell casts. The finding of red blood cell casts in interstitial nephritis has been reported but should prompt a search for glomerular diseases. The finding of eosinophils in the urine is suggestive of allergic interstitial nephritis or atheroemboli.

Occlusion of large renal arteries and veins is an uncommon cause of acute renal failure. A significant reduction in GFR by this mechanism suggests bilateral processes or a unilateral process in a patient with a single functioning kidney. Renal arteries can be occluded with atheroemboli, thromboemboli, in situ thrombosis, aortic dissection, or vasculitis. Atheroembolic renal failure can occur spontaneously but is most often associated with recent aortic instrumentation. The emboli are cholesterol-rich and lodge in medium and small renal arteries, leading to an eosinophil-rich inflammatory reaction. The urinalysis in atheroembolic acute renal failure is usually normal but may contain eosinophils and casts. The diagnosis can be confirmed by renal biopsy, but this is often unnecessary when other stigmata of atheroemboli are present (livido reticularis, distal peripheral infarcts, eosinophilia). Renal artery thrombosis may lead to mild proteinuria and hematuria, whereas renal vein thrombosis usually induces heavy proteinuria and hematuria. → *These vascular catastrophes often require angiography for confirmation (Fig. 47-1) and are discussed in Chap. 277.*

Diseases of glomeruli (glomerulonephritis or vasculitis) and the renal microvasculature (hemolytic uremic syndromes, thrombotic thrombocytopenic purpura, or malignant hypertension) usually present with various manifestations of glomerular injury: proteinuria, hematuria, reduced GFR, and alterations of sodium excretion leading to hyperten-

sion, edema, and circulatory congestion (acute nephritic syndrome). These findings may occur as primary renal diseases or as renal manifestations of systemic diseases. The finding of red blood cell casts in the urine is an indication for early renal biopsy (Fig. 47-1) since the pathologic pattern has important implications for diagnosis, prognosis, and treatment. Hematuria without red blood cell casts can also be an indication of glomerular disease (Figs. 47-1 and 47-2). → *A detailed discussion of glomerulonephritis and diseases of the microvasculature is presented in Chap. 274.*

Table 47-1

Laboratory Findings in Acute Renal Failure

Index	Prerenal Azotemia	Oliguric Acute Renal Failure
BUN/P_{Cr} Ratio	>20:1	10–15:1
Urine sodium (U_{Na}), mEq/L	<20	>40
Urine osmolality, mOsm/L H_2O	>500	<350
Fractional excretion of sodium $$FE_{Na} = \frac{U_{Na} \times P_{Cr} \times 100}{P_{Na} \times U_{Cr}}$$	<1%	>2%
Urine/Plasma Creatinine (U_{Cr}/P_{Cr})	>40	<20

NOTE: BUN, Blood urea nitrogen; P_{Cr}, plasma creatinine; U_{Na}, urine sodium concentration; P_{Na}, plasma sodium concentration; U_{Cr}, urine creatinine concentration.

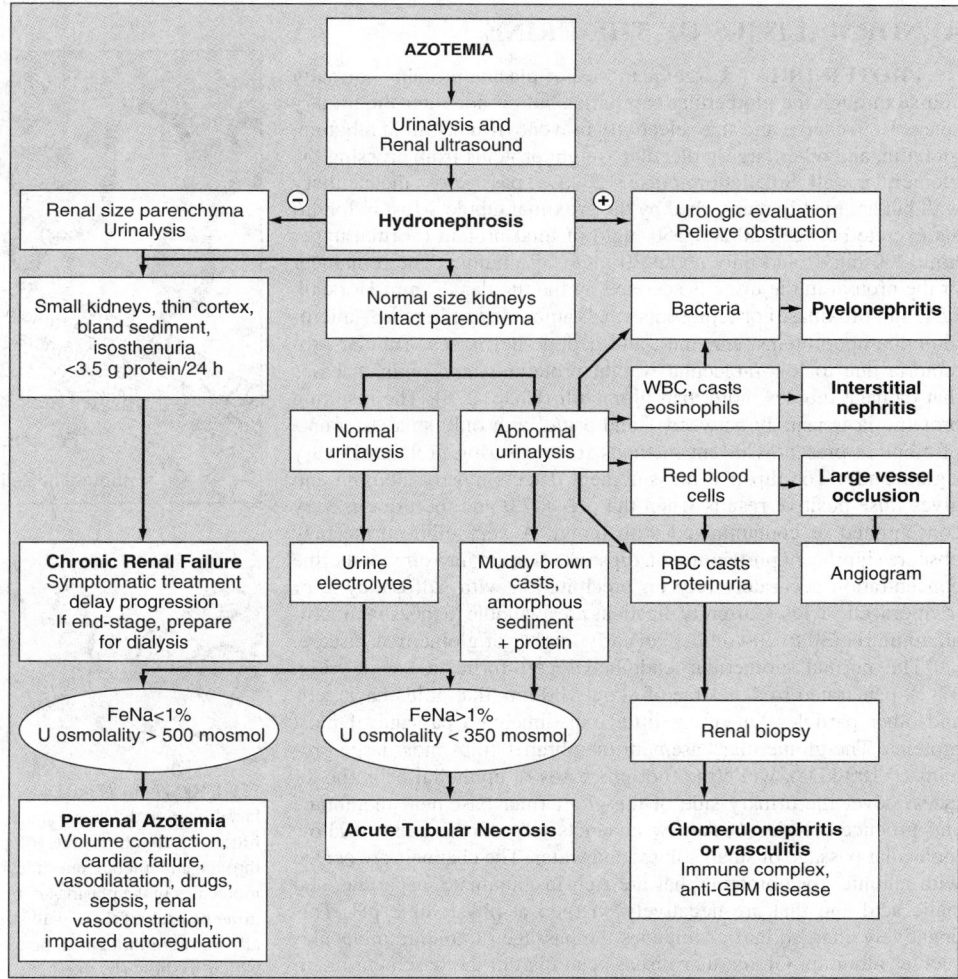

FIGURE 47-1 Approach to the patient with azotemia. (WBC, white blood cell; RBC, red blood cell; GBM, glomerular basement membrane.)

Postrenal azotemia Urinary tract obstruction accounts for fewer than 5 percent of cases of acute renal failure but is usually reversible and must be ruled out early in the evaluation (Fig. 47-1). Since a single kidney is capable of adequate clearance, acute renal failure from obstruction requires either obstruction at the urethra or bladder outlet, bilateral ureteral obstruction, or unilateral obstruction in a patient with a single functioning kidney. Obstruction is usually diagnosed by the presence of ureteral dilatation on renal ultrasound. However, early in the course of obstruction or if the ureters are unable to dilate (such as encasement by pelvic tumors), the ultrasound examination may be negative. → *The specific urologic conditions that cause obstruction are discussed in Chap. 280.*

Oliguria and anuria Oliguria refers to a 24-h urine output of <500 mL, and anuria is the complete absence of urine formation. Anuria can be caused by total urinary tract obstruction, total renal artery or vein occlusion, and shock (manifested by severe hypotension and intense renal vasoconstriction). Cortical necrosis, ATN, and rapidly progressive glomerulonephritis can occasionally cause anuria. Oliguria can accompany any cause of acute renal failure and carries a more serious prognosis for renal recovery in all conditions except prerenal azotemia. Nonoliguria refers to urine output >500 mL/d in patients with acute or chronic azotemia. With nonoliguric ATN, disturbances of potassium and hydrogen balance are less severe than in oliguric patients and recovery to normal renal function is usually more rapid.

ABNORMALITIES OF THE URINE

PROTEINURIA Large quantities of plasma proteins normally course through the glomerular capillaries but do not enter the urinary space. Both charge and size selectivity prevent virtually all of albumin, globulin, and other large-molecular-weight proteins from crossing the glomerular wall. Smaller proteins (<20 kDa) pass across the capillary wall but are readily reabsorbed by the proximal tubule. Most individuals excrete between 30 and 150 mg/d of total protein (normal upper limit 200 mg/d) and only about 30 mg/d of albumin. The remainder of the protein in the urine is secreted by the tubules (Tamm-Horsfall, IgA, and urokinase) or represents small amounts of filtered β_2-microglobulin, apoproteins, enzymes, and peptide hormones. Tubular proteinuria due to low-molecular-weight proteins occurs with diseases that damage tubules more than glomeruli (Chap. 276). The resulting proteinuria is usually between 1 and 3 g/d with only small amounts of albumin present. Current methods for measuring proteinuria vary significantly. The dipstick measurement detects mostly albumin and gives false-positive results when the pH > 7.0 and the urine is very concentrated or contaminated with blood. A very dilute urine may obscure significant proteinuria on dipstick. Tests to measure total urine concentration accurately rely on precipitation with sulfosalicylic or trichloracetic acids. Currently dipsticks are available to measure microalbuminuria (30 to 200 mg/L), an early marker of glomerular disease.

The normal glomerular endothelial cell forms a barrier (Fig. 47-2), penetrated by fenestrae of about 100 nm, that holds back cells and other particles but offers little impediment to passage of most proteins. The glomerular basement membranes traps most large proteins (>100 kDa), while the foot processes of epithelial cells (podocytes) cover the urinary side of the glomerular basement membrane and produce a series of narrow channels (slit diaphragms) to allow molecular passage of small solutes and water. The channels are coated with anionic glycoproteins that are rich in glutamate, aspartate, and sialic acid and that are negatively charged at physiologic pH. This negatively charged barrier impedes the passage of anionic molecules such as albumin. Glomerular disease can disrupt the basement membrane by immune complex deposition, allowing large-protein leakage. Several glomerular diseases affect primarily the epithelial cells and result in loss of foot processes with resulting albuminuria. When the

total daily excretion of protein (mostly albumin) exceeds 3.5 g, there is often associated hypoalbuminemia, hyperlipidemia, and edema (nephrotic syndrome). However, total urinary protein excretion greater than 3.5 g/d does occur without the other features of the nephrotic syndrome in some plasma cell dyscrasias (such as multiple myeloma). These diseases can be associated with large amounts of excreted light chains in the urine which may not be detected by dipstick, which detects mostly albumin. The light chains produced from these disorders are filtered by the glomerulus and overwhelm the reabsorptive capacity of the proximal tubule. A sulfosalicylic acid precipitate that is out of proportion to the dipstick estimate is suggestive of light chains (Bence Jones protein), and light chains typically redissolve upon warming of the precipitate. Renal failure from these disorders occurs through a variety of mechanisms including tubule obstruction (cast nephropathy) and light chain deposition (see Chap. 275).

Hypoalbuminemia in nephrotic syndrome occurs through excessive urinary losses, increased renal catabolism, and inadequate hepatic synthesis. The resulting decrease in plasma oncotic pressure contributes to edema formation by altering the Starling forces and favoring fluid movement from capillaries to interstitium. The resulting homeostatic mechanisms designed to correct the decrease in effective intravascular volume contribute to edema formation. These mechanisms include activation of the renin-angiotensin system, AVP, and the sympathetic nervous system, which contribute to excessive renal salt and water reabsorption and can contribute to unrelenting edema. The severity of edema correlates with the degree of hypoalbuminemia and is modified by other factors such as heart disease or peripheral vascular disease. The diminished plasma oncotic pressure and urinary losses of regulatory proteins appear to stimulate hepatic lipoprotein synthesis. The resulting hyperlipidemia results in lipid bodies (fatty casts, oval

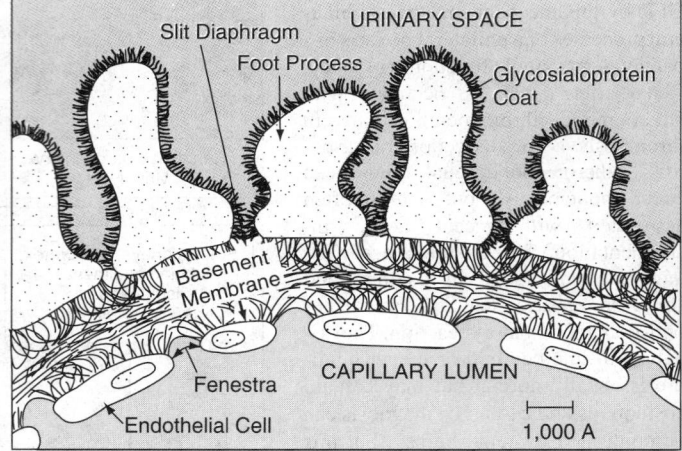

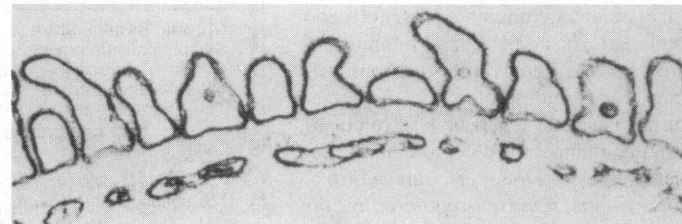

FIGURE 47-2 *(Top)* Diagram showing normal structures separating the capillary lumen and urinary space in the glomerulus. In the process of glomerular filtration, an ultrafiltrate of plasma traverses the glomerular capillary wall through endothelial fenestrae, basement membrane, and slit diaphragms. Macromolecules in the plasma are believed to be restricted from entry into glomerular urine by each of these wall structures. In addition, circulating polyanions (e.g., albumin) are thought to be retarded by negatively charged glycosialoproteins, which, as shown by the shaded area in the upper panel, are distributed throughout the glomerular wall. *(Bottom)* A corresponding electron micrograph of the same structures. *(Drawing by NL Gahan from BM Brenner, R. Beeuwkes, Hosp. Pract., vol. 13, no. 7, 1978. Reproduced with permission.)*

fat bodies) in the urine. Other proteins are lost in the urine, leading to a variety of metabolic disturbances; these proteins include thyroxine-binding globulin, cholecalciferol-binding protein, transferrin, and metal-binding proteins. A hypercoagulable state frequently accompanies severe nephrotic syndrome due to urinary losses of antithrombin III, reduced serum levels of proteins S and C, hyperfibrinogenemia, and enhanced platelet aggregation. Some patients develop severe IgG deficiency with resulting defects in immunity.

HEMATURIA, PYURIA, AND CASTS Isolated hematuria without proteinuria, other cells, or casts is often indicative of bleeding from the urinary tract. Hematuria is defined as two to five red blood cells per high-power field and can be detected by dipstick. Common causes of isolated hematuria include stones, neoplasms, tuberculosis, trauma, and prostatitis. Gross hematuria with blood clots is almost never indicative of glomerular bleeding but rather suggests a postrenal source in the urinary collecting system. Evaluation of patients presenting with microscopic hematuria is outlined in Fig. 47-3. A single urinalysis with hematuria is common and can result from menstruation, viral illness, allergy, exercise, or mild trauma. However, persistent or significant hematuria (> three red blood cells per high-power field on three urinalyses, or single urinalysis with >100 red blood cells, or gross hematuria) identifies significant renal or urologic lesions. Even patients who are chronically anticoagulated should be investigated as outlined in Fig. 47-3.

Hematuria with pyuria and bacteriuria is typical of infection and should be treated with antibiotics after appropriate cultures. Acute cystitis or urethritis in women can cause gross hematuria. Hypercalciuria and hyperuricosuria are also risk factors for unexplained isolated hematuria in both children and adults. In some of these patients (50 to 60 percent), reducing calcium and uric acid excretion through

dietary interventions can eliminate the microscopic hematuria. → *Urologic etiologies of hematuria are discussed in more detail in Chap. 280.*

Isolated microscopic hematuria can be a manifestation of glomerular diseases. The red blood cells of glomerular origin are often dysmorphic when examined by phase-contrast microscopy. Irregular shapes of red blood cells may also occur due to pH and osmolarity changes in the distal tubule. There is, however, significant interobserver variability in detecting dysmorphic red blood cells, especially if a phase-contrast microscope is not available. The most common etiologies of isolated glomerular hematuria are IgA nephropathy (Chap. 275), hereditary nephritis, and thin basement membrane disease. IgA nephropathy and hereditary nephritis can have episodic gross hematuria. A family history of renal failure is often present in patients with hereditary nephritis, and patients with thin basement membrane disease often have other family members with microscopic hematuria. A renal biopsy is needed for the definitive diagnosis of these disorders, which are discussed in more detail in Chap. 275. Hematuria with dysmorphic red blood cells, red blood cell casts, and protein excretion >500 mg/d is virtually diagnostic of glomerulonephritis. Red blood cell casts form as red blood cells, enter the tubular fluid, and become trapped in a cylindrical mold of gelled Tamm-Horsfall protein. Even in the absence of azotemia, these patients should undergo serologic evaluation and renal biopsy as outlined in Fig. 47-3.

Isolated pyuria is unusual since inflammatory reactions in the kidney or collecting system are also associated with hematuria. The presence of bacteria suggests infection, and white blood cell casts with bacteria are indicative of pyelonephritis. White blood cells and/or white blood cell casts may also be seen in tubulointerstitial processes such as interstitial nephritis, systemic lupus erythematosus, and transplant rejection. In chronic renal diseases, degenerated cellular casts called *waxy casts* can be seen in the urine. Broad casts are thought to arise in the dilated tubules of enlarged nephrons that have undergone compensatory hypertrophy in response to reduced renal mass (i.e., chronic renal failure). A mixture of broad casts together with cellular casts and red blood cells may be seen in smoldering processes such as chronic glomerulonephritis with persistent active glomerulitis.

ABNORMALITIES OF URINE VOLUME

The volume of urine produced varies depending upon the fluid intake, renal function, and physiologic demands of the individual. The causes of decreased (oliguria) or absent urine production (anuria) were discussed earlier in this chapter. → *The physiology of free water formation and renal water conservation are discussed in Chap. 269.*

POLYURIA From the history alone, it is often difficult to distinguish urinary frequency (often of small volumes) from polyuria; a 24-h urine collection is needed for evaluation (Fig. 47-4). It is necessary to determine if the polyuria represents a solute or water diuresis and if the diuresis is appropriate for the clinical circumstances. The average person excretes between 600 and 800 mosmol of solutes per day, primarily as urea and electrolytes. The urine osmolality can help distinguish a solute from a water diuresis. If the urine output is >3 L/d (arbitrarily defined as polyuria) and the urine is dilute (<250 mosmol/L), then total mosmol excretion is normal and a water diuresis is present. This circumstance could arise from polydipsia, inadequate secretion of AVP (central diabetes insipidus), or failure of renal tubules to respond to AVP (nephrogenic diabetes insipidus). If the urine volume is >3 L/d and urine osmolality is >300 mosmol/L, then a solute diuresis is clearly present and a search for the responsible solute(s) is mandatory.

Excessive filtration of a poorly reabsorbed solute such as glucose, mannitol, or urea can depress reabsorption of NaCl and water in the proximal tubule and lead to enhanced excretion in the urine. Poorly controlled diabetes mellitus is the most common cause of a solute diuresis, leading to volume depletion and serum hypertonicity. Since

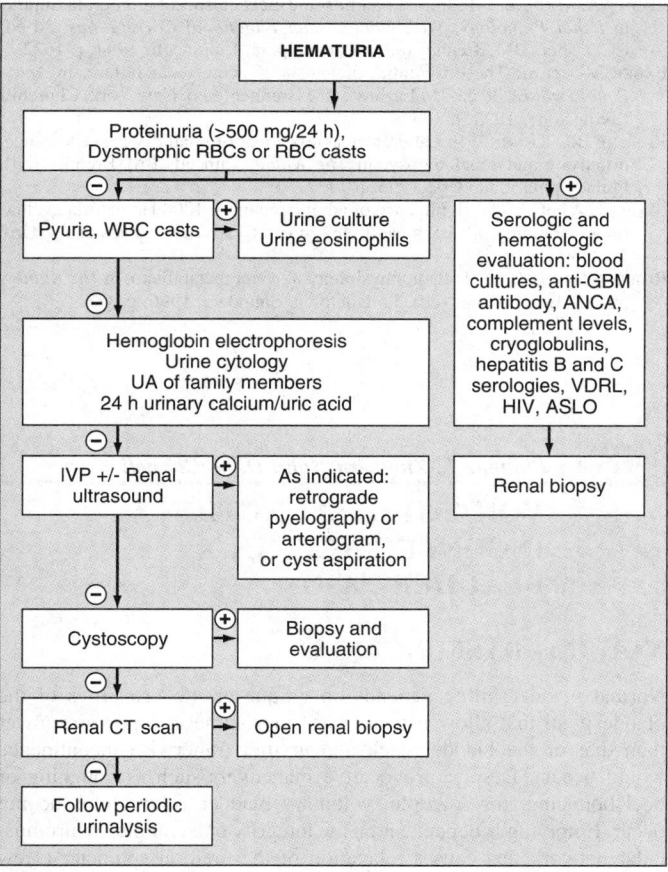

FIGURE 47-3 Approach to the patient with hematuria. (RBC, red blood cell; WBC, white blood cell; GBM, glomerular basement membrane; ANCA, antineutrophil cytoplasmic antibody; VDRL, venereal disease research laboratory; HIV, human immunodeficiency virus; ASLO, antistreptolysin O; UA, urinalysis; IVP, intravenous pyelography; CT, computed tomography.)

the urine Na concentration is less than that of blood, more water than Na is lost, causing hypernatremia and hypertonicity. Common iatrogenic solute diuresis occurs from mannitol administration, radiocontrast media, and high-protein feedings (enterally or parenterally), leading to increased urea production and excretion. Less commonly, excessive Na loss may occur from cystic renal diseases and Bartter's syndrome or during the course of a tubulointerstitial process (such as resolving acute tubular necrosis). In these so-called salt-wasting disorders, the tubule damage results in direct impairment of Na reabsorption and indirectly reduces the responsiveness of the tubule to aldosterone. Usually, the Na losses are mild, and the obligatory urine output is less than 2 L/d. (Resolving acute tubular necrosis and postobstructive diuresis are exceptions and may be associated with significant natriuresis and polyuria.)

Formation of large volumes of dilute urine represent polydipsic states or diabetes insipidus (Chaps. 276 and 330). Primary polydipsia can result from habit, psychiatric disorders, neurologic lesions, or medications. During deliberate polydipsia, extracellular fluid volume is normal or expanded and AVP levels are reduced because serum osmolality tends to be near the lower limits of normal. Reabsorption of water from the distal convoluted tubule and collecting duct is minimal with low AVP levels. The drive for water reabsorption is also reduced from washout of medullary hypertonicity gradients. The serum Na concentration may help to distinguish patients with primary polydipsia from those with diabetes insipidus; patients with polydipsia tend to have low-normal serum sodium concentrations, while patients with diabetes insipidus usually have normal to high-normal concentrations. A water deprivation test (see Chap. 330) may be needed to ascertain the exact diagnosis.

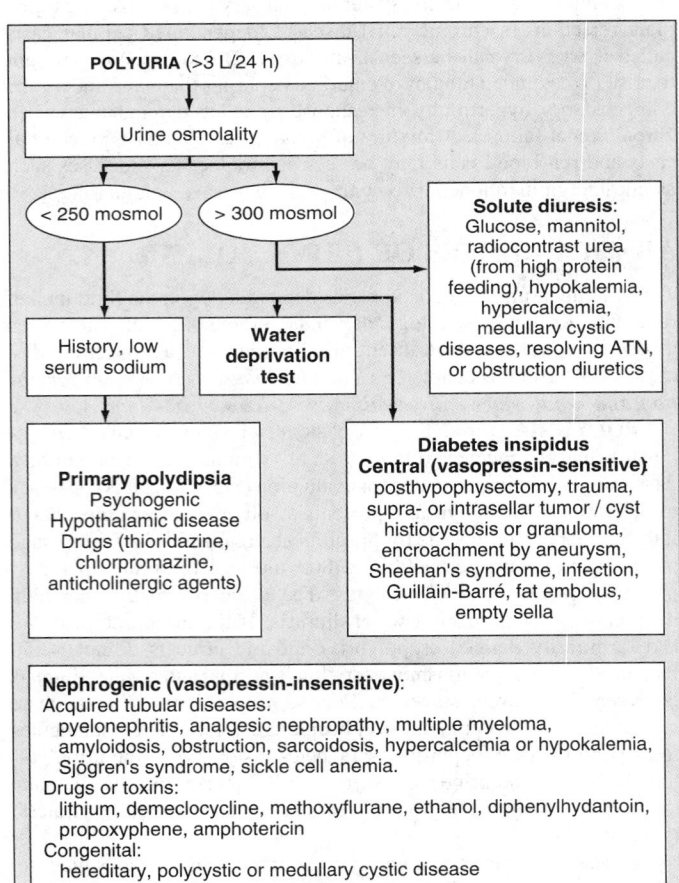

FIGURE 47-4 Approach to the patient with polyuria. (Osm, osmolality; ATN, acute tubular necrosis.)

Central diabetes insipidus may be idiopathic in origin or secondary to a variety of hypothalamic conditions including posthypophysectomy, trauma and neoplastic, inflammatory, vascular, or infectious hypothalamic diseases. Idiopathic central diabetes insipidus is associated with selective destruction of the vasopressin-secreting neurons in the supraoptic and paraventricular nuclei and can be inherited as an autosomal dominant trait or occur spontaneously (Fig. 47-4), (see Chap. 330). Nephrogenic diabetes insipidus can occur in a variety of clinical situations as summarized in Fig. 47-4. Hypercalcemia and hypokalemia are reversible causes of nephrogenic diabetes insipidus, and familial conditions also exist. Usually nephrogenic diabetes insipidus is acquired from renal diseases or medications (Fig. 47-4). In both central and nephrogenic diabetes insipidus, water reabsorption is reduced along the distal nephron. Similar to the washout of medullary gradients seen with polydipsia, diabetes insipidus is also associated with dilution of the medullary solutes. Administering AVP can lead to formation of a more concentrated urine, but the maximal urine osmolality attained is often below normal (see Chap. 330).

Determination of the plasma AVP level is recommended as the best method for distinguishing between central and nephrogenic diabetes insipidus. Alternatively, a water deprivation test (Chap. 330) plus exogenous AVP may also distinguish primary polydipsia from central and nephrogenic diabetes insipidus.

BIBLIOGRAPHY

ANDERSON S et al: Renal and systemic manifestations of glomerular disease, in *The Kidney*, 5th ed, BM Brenner (ed). Philadelphia, Saunders, 1996, p 1981

ANDRES A et al: Isolated hematuria: Hypercalciuria and hyperuricosuria as risk factors. Kidney Int 36:96, 1989

BRADY HR et al: Acute renal failure, in *The Kidney*, 5th ed, BM Brenner (ed). Philadelphia, Saunders, 1996, p 1200

EDDY AA, MICHAEL AF: Immunopathogenic mechanisms of glomerular injury, in *Renal Pathology: With Clinical and Functional Correlations*, 2d ed, CC Tisher, BM Brenner (eds). Philadelphia, Lippincott, 1994, p 1622

FABER MD et al: The differential diagnosis of acute renal failure, in *Acute Renal Failure*, 3d ed, JM Lazarus, BM Brenner (eds). New York, Churchill Livingstone, 1993, p 133

KASISKE BL, KEANE WF: Laboratory assesssment of renal disease: Clearance, urinalysis and renal biopsy, in *The Kidney*, 5th ed, BM Brenner (ed). Philadelphia, Saunders, 1996, p 1137

MARIANI AJ et al: The signiicance of adult hematuria: 1000 Hematuria evaluations including a risk-benefit and cost-effectiveness analysis. J Urol 141:350, 1989

ROBERTSON GL, BERL T: Pathophysiology of water metabolism, in *The Kidney*, 5th ed, BM Brenner (ed). Philadelphia, Saunders, 1996, p 873

48   *Philippe E. Zimmern, John D. McConnell*

VOIDING DYSFUNCTION, INCONTINENCE, AND BLADDER PAIN

VOIDING DYSFUNCTION

Normal bladder filling depends on unique elastic properties of the bladder wall that allow it to increase in volume at a pressure lower than that of the bladder neck and urethra (otherwise incontinence would occur). Despite provocative maneuvers such as coughing or heel bouncing, for example, voluntary bladder contractions do not occur. Emptying is dependent on the integrity of a complex neuromuscular network that causes relaxation of the urethral sphincter a few milliseconds before the onset of the detrusor (bladder muscle) contraction. With normal, sustained detrusor contraction, the bladder empties completely. A bladder that can fill and empty in this manner has a normal detrusor muscle and is described as *stable* according to conventional terminology.

Since the voluntary control of micturition depends on the neural connections between the cerebral cortex and the brainstem, disruption of these pathways (brain tumor, stroke, head trauma, Parkinson's disease) impairs the ability to suppress and control bladder contractions. A bladder contraction "without the owner's permission" (McGuire) characterizes an unstable bladder. Bladder or detrusor instability of neurologic origin is termed *detrusor hyperreflexia*. Conversely, the detrusor muscle that cannot contract during voiding is called *noncontractile* or *underactive*, and underactivity of the detrusor due to a lesion of the sacral cord or pelvic nerves is termed *detrusor areflexia*. These terms that characterize the function of the detrusor muscle and urethra have replaced terms such as atonic, hypotonic, autonomic, or flaccid, which refer to etiologies of dysfunction sometimes difficult to ascertain with certainty.

Contrary to common belief, the center that controls normal micturition is not in the spinal cord but in the brainstem. Proper coordination (synergia) between the detrusor and urethral sphincters requires an intact neural (autonomic and somatic nervous systems) communication between bladder and urethra. Injury to the upper spinal cord, for example, can cause dyssynergia between bladder and urethra that results in urge incontinence, residual urine retention, bladder wall changes (trabeculation and fibrosis), and possibly renal insufficiency.

A simple way to classify voiding dysfunction is to determine whether it is primarily a *storage failure* or an *emptying failure* by asking two questions:

Is the voiding dysfunction due to the bladder or outlet (bladder neck or urethra) (failure to store)?
Is the patient neurologically intact (failure to empty)?

Bladder storage and emptying problems may coexist in the same individual and can cause similar lower urinary tract symptoms (LUTS).

LOWER URINARY TRACT SYMPTOMS IN MEN The most common cause of LUTS in men of middle age and older is prostatic hyperplasia, which causes obstruction to urine flow by encroachment on the urethral lumen (see Chap. 97). Histologically, 50 to 80 percent of the prostatic volume is composed of stromal tissue (smooth muscle), while the remainder is glandular. The transitional zone, which is responsible for benign prostatic growth, comprises 10 to 15 percent of the prostate at the end of puberty but increases in volume after age 40. However, prostatic enlargement is not always accompanied by symptoms because the direction of growth can be outward, so that little change may occur in urine flow (at least up to a certain prostatic volume). Alternatively, men with early histologic evidence of prostatic hyperplasia can experience significant voiding symptoms. The reason for the latter phenomenon is believed to be an increased tone of the prostatic smooth muscle, possibly due to an increase in alpha-adrenergic receptors; in this circumstance enhanced prostatic tension within a nondistensible prostatic capsule can cause obstruction.

In response to obstruction, the bladder smooth muscle cells hypertrophy to generate the higher pressures necessary for voiding, and the increase in bladder muscle mass leads to reduced elasticity, or compliance, and decreased bladder capacity. Detrusor dysfunction from bladder outlet obstruction can cause any combination of the LUTS described above. When the obstruction progresses, infiltration of extracellular matrix between the smooth muscle bundles of the bladder wall can result in a hypocontractile or acontractile bladder (bladder failure).

Other complications such as urinary tract infections or bladder stones secondary to the large postvoid residuals (stasis) and upper tract damage (hydronephrosis, reflux) can develop during the course of the obstructive process. Although prostatic hyperplasia is the most common cause of bladder outlet obstruction in men, other sources of obstruction include prostate cancer, urethral stricture, and lack of proper sphincteric relaxation (neurologic cause). Nonobstructive causes of LUTS include diabetic neuropathy, which can affect the parasympathetic nerves of the bladder. Decreased sensation of bladder fullness leads to incomplete emptying and overdistention of the bladder and in turn to increased frequency and nocturia due to bladder overflow;

these symptoms are frequently made worse by the polydipsia/polyuria of diabetes mellitus. At times, storage symptoms can be caused by other neurologic causes such as stroke, multiple sclerosis, or Parkinson's disease.

The International Prostate Symptom Score (IPSS) is routinely employed to assess the severity of LUTS:

Decreased force of stream—over the past month how often have you had a weak urinary stream?
Intermittency—over the past month how often have you found you stopped and started again several times when urinating?
Incomplete emptying—over the past month how often have you had a sensation of not emptying your bladder completely after finishing urination?
Straining—over the past month how often have you had to push or strain to begin urination?

The IPSS also assesses the impact of storage symptoms:

Frequency—over the past month how often have you had to urinate again within 2 h after urinating?
Urgency—over the past month how often have you found it difficult to postpone urination?
Nocturia—over the past month how many times did you typically get up to urinate between going to bed and getting up in the morning? (Range: none to five or more times.)

Except for nocturia, the answers range from 0 (not at all) to 5 (almost always). A total score less than 8 indicates minimal voiding dysfunction; a total score of 13 or above is usually required to enroll patients in drug studies for the management of benign prostatic hyperplasia (BPH); and symptom scores above 23 suggest significant bladder outlet obstruction. Because similar symptoms can result from neurologic causes, the IPSS questionnaire cannot be used to make the diagnosis of prostatic hyperplasia but is only useful as an index of severity and of the response to treatment.

LOWER URINARY TRACT SYMPTOMS IN WOMEN Urethral obstruction is an uncommon cause of LUTS in women. A careful bimanual examination and passage of a urethral catheter are sufficient to exclude urethral stenosis, which is usually secondary to prior instrumentation or operative procedures, and urethral cancer. Urinary tract infection (cystitis) is more prevalent in women and must be excluded by urinalysis, and multiple sclerosis should be considered in middle-aged women presenting with frequency, urgency, or incontinence. In addition to many of the same disorders that produce voiding symptoms in men, estrogen deficiency, frequency-urgency syndrome, and interstitial cystitis (IC) with minimal pain must be considered. Cystocele and pelvic prolapse can cause urinary frequency secondary to impairment of bladder emptying.

EVALUATION Men and women with LUTS and concomitant neurologic disease should undergo a complete urodynamic evaluation. In the absence of neurologic disease, men with LUTS most commonly have prostatic hyperplasia. However, it is necessary to exclude prostate cancer, especially if there is a positive family history, an abnormal rectal examination, or an elevated level of prostate-specific antigen (PSA). In both sexes bladder cancer can also cause storage symptoms and is suggested by microscopic hematuria and/or abnormal urine cytology. Usually, a detailed genitourinary history, a symptom assessment, a careful neurologic examination including rectal examination and assessment of the bulbocavernosus reflex, measurements of urine flow and postvoid residual urine volume (by office bladder ultrasound), and limited laboratory evaluation (urinalysis, urine culture, PSA levels, urine cytology, urea/creatinine levels, as indicated) should be sufficient to direct therapy. More complex investigations of the lower urinary tract (cystoscopy, voiding cystography, urodynamics) and upper urinary tract (pyelogram or ultrasonography) are sometimes indicated.
→ *For therapy of BPH, see Chap. 97.*

INCONTINENCE

Incontinence is a condition where involuntary loss of urine is objectively demonstrated and is a social or hygienic problem. A common variant, *stress incontinence*, denotes involuntary loss of urine with physical exercise (coughing, sneezing, sports, sexual activity). *Urge incontinence* is an involuntary loss of urine associated with a strong desire to void, and *overflow incontinence* is an involuntary loss of urine when the elevation of intravesical pressure with bladder overfilling or distention exceeds the maximal urethral pressure. Loss of urine through channels other than the urethra is rare (ectopic ureter, fistulae) but causes total or continuous incontinence.

INCONTINENCE IN WOMEN Urinary incontinence affects approximately 20 million women in the United States. Among noninstitutionalized women 60 years of age and older, 25 to 30 percent have incontinence daily or weekly, and approximately half of the 1.5 million institutionalized women are incontinent more than once a day. The annual cost of caring for incontinent persons in the United States has been estimated at $10 billion.

Stress urinary incontinence (SUI) is secondary to urethral hypermobility or, less commonly (<10 percent), to intrinsic sphincteric deficiency (ISD). In the continent woman the bladder neck and proximal urethra are supported by the anterior vaginal wall and its lateral attachment to the levator muscles. Anterior vaginal wall relaxation causes urethral hypermobility, usually due to aging and/or estrogen deficiency or a prior traumatic delivery or pelvic surgery. Paradoxically, women can have clinical evidence of urethral hypermobility but no stress urinary incontinence.

Some women have an anatomically normal urethra and bladder neck but still have SUI due to damage to the internal sphincter (fixed, rigid, or "pipestem" urethra), due to prior anti-incontinence surgery, pelvic radiation or trauma, or neurologic disorders that cause denervation of the urethra. Urethral hypermobility and ISD can coexist in some patients and cause persistence (or rapid recurrence) of incontinence after a simple bladder neck suspension procedure that fixes the hypermobility but leaves the sphincter untreated.

Urge incontinence can be present alone or in association with SUI (mixed incontinence). The cause of the unsuppressible or uninhibited bladder contractions is usually idiopathic, but bacterial cystitis, bladder tumor, bladder outlet obstruction, and neurogenic bladder must be excluded. Overflow incontinence is due either to bladder outlet obstruction (rare in women), an acontractile bladder (diabetic neuropathy, multiple sclerosis), excessive smooth muscle relaxation from drugs (anticholinergic medications), or psychogenic retention.

INCONTINENCE IN MEN In men incontinence is less common than obstruction, but urgency and urge incontinence can occur as the result of bladder outlet obstruction (as from prostatic hyperplasia) that impairs detrusor smooth muscle function and leads to detrusor instability. Men with neurogenic bladders (diabetic neuropathy, multiple sclerosis, Parkinson's disease, stroke) can develop urge incontinence. Other causes such as bacterial cystitis or bladder tumor must be excluded. SUI in men is usually the result of distal sphincteric damage, for example, as the result of radical prostatectomy for prostate cancer.

INCONTINENCE IN THE ELDERLY Transient urinary incontinence is common in the elderly. A mnemonic devised by Resnick delineates its numerous causes, namely delirium, infection, atrophic urethritis, pharmacologic, psychological, excessive urine output (hyperglycemia, congestive heart failure), restricted mobility, and stool impaction (DIAPPERS). Urge incontinence is the next most common disorder in this age group and is attributed to the progressive loss of the modulating influence of the frontal lobes of the cortex on the micturition center in the brain stem.

EVALUATION The evaluation of urinary incontinence in women should include: history and quality-of-life assessment, voiding diary, physical examination including pelvic examination, urinalysis and urine culture, and measurement of postvoid residual urine volume. For patients with an unclear history or after prior pelvic or anti-incontinence procedures, evaluation may include cystoscopy, urodynamic evaluation, and imaging studies (lower and/or upper urinary tract). The history should define the onset, duration, evolution, and triggering events of leakage. Prior treatments with medications, frequent voiding schedules, and exercise regimens should be noted. Severity of incontinence is denoted by recording the type and number of pads used per day or at night and how the incontinence affects daily activities (incontinence-impact questionnaire). The amount and type of fluid consumed, sexual history (hormonal status, deliveries, venereal diseases), gastrointestinal function (fecal incontinence, constipation), and past urologic history (bed-wetting, surgeries) must also be documented. The physical examination should place special emphasis on the abdominal, genital, pelvic (associated prolapses), and neurologic systems. SUI must be demonstrated by asking the patient to cough, strain, or even stand or squat. While leakage during a cough confirms SUI, leakage after a cough is due to bladder instability (stress-induced instability). SUI in the absence of urethral hypermobility raises the suspicion of a sphincteric defect. More complex testing is needed to determine whether the urethral anatomy is normal (evaluation of urethral mobility, lateral view of the urethra on the voiding cystourethrogram, cystoscopy), whether urethral function is normal with adequate closure (leak point pressure, urethral profilometry, videourodynamics), or whether bladder function is normal (bladder volume based on home diary, filling cystometrogram).

℞ TREATMENT

Mild stress incontinence can be treated nonoperatively with medications, hormonal supplementation, or biofeedback techniques. Modalities such as urethral plugs and anterior vaginal wall prostheses are under investigation. Moderate to severe stress incontinence responds to surgical procedures aimed at supporting the anterior vaginal wall (vaginal, laparoscopic, or abdominal operations) or enhancing urethral closure when stress incontinence is secondary to internal sphincter deficiency (periurethral injection of teflon or collagen or insertion of an artificial urinary sphincter).

Urge incontinence responds to the management of its cause, for example, relief of outlet obstruction. When it is due to neurogenic or idiopathic causes, anticholinergic agents are partially effective, although side effects such as mouth dryness, blurring of vision, or constipation can limit their usefulness. Fluid restriction (which must be undertaken only with great caution) and bladder retraining with biofeedback may also be helpful. More aggressive intervention with bladder augmentation or urinary diversion are seldom necessary in the absence of neurologic disease.

BLADDER PAIN

Painful bladder disease is a general term for any bladder pathology that causes suprapubic, urethral, or pelvic pain. IC is the most common cause of bladder pain, but endometriosis, bacterial cystitis, and outlet obstruction that causes bladder instability can mimic the symptoms of IC.

INTERSTITIAL CYSTITIS IC is a severe, chronic bladder disorder that causes frequency, nocturia, and suprapubic pain. The disorder usually affects women and is rare in blacks. Routine urine culture is uniformly negative, and the symptoms do not respond to antibiotic therapy. The etiology is probably multifactorial (Table 48-1). Current hypotheses as to etiology include autoimmune reaction against bladder antigens, deficiency in the glycosaminoglycan layer of the bladder surface allowing presumed "toxins" to penetrate the mucosa, mast cell infiltration and activation leading to the histamine release, and local bladder wall damage from "cryptic" bacteria.

There are no universally accepted criteria to make the diagnosis, but the National Institutes of Health has established a series of criteria to define IC clinically (Table 48-2). The diagnosis is one of exclusion—infection, radiation cystitis, urethral diverticula, herpes simplex, and malignancy must be excluded. Cystoscopy under anesthesia may reveal

Table 48-1

CHAPTER 49
Fluid and Electrolyte Disturbances

265

Consensus Criteria for Diagnosis of Interstitial Cystitis

AUTOMATIC EXCLUSIONS

Less than 18 years old
Benign or malignant bladder tumors
Radiation cystitis
Bacterial cystitis
Vaginitis
Cyclophosphamide cystitis
Symptomatic urethral diverticulum
Uterine, cervical, vaginal, or urethral cancers
Active herpes
Bladder or lower urethral calculi
Waking frequency less than five times in 12 h
Nocturia less than twice nightly
Symptoms relieved by antibiotics, urinary antiseptics, urinary analgesics
 (e.g., phenazopyridine hydrochloride)
Duration less than 12 months
Involuntary bladder contractions (urodynamics)
Capacity greater than 400 mL, absence of sensory urgency

AUTOMATIC INCLUSIONS

Hunner's ulcer

POSITIVE FACTORS

Pain on bladder filling relieved by emptying
Pain (suprapubic, pelvic, urethral, vaginal, or perineal)
Glomerulations after hydrodistention on cystoscopy

---

glomerulations (submucosal vascular anomalies) or the infrequent Hunner's ulcer suggestive of IC; make it possible to estimate bladder capacity (an important guide to treatment); allow biopsy of the bladder wall when indicated; and, sometimes, provide therapeutic benefit with a reduction in pain level and urinary frequency up to 6 months, rarely longer.

EVALUATION Chronic urinary frequency and bladder pain affect the quality of life to an extreme degree, although most patients experience a waxing and waning evolution; only 10 percent of patients have a consistent progression in symptoms. Evaluation should include a detailed history; physical examination designed to exclude neurologic and gynecologic pathology; voiding cystogram to exclude urethral defects; and urodynamic testing to eliminate a neurogenic bladder, bladder instability, or outlet obstruction and to document sensory instability. Referral to specialists may be indicated to exclude adnexal pathology, endometriosis, or bowel dysfunction or to utilize modern pain management techniques to prevent drug addiction.

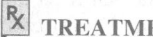
TREATMENT

Empiric treatments that have been used include oral medications (amitriptyline, hydroxyzine) and intravesical agents (dimethyl sulfoxide, chlorpactin, heparin). These measures may improve the urinary symptoms and occasionally reduce pain but do not modify the long-term course. Surgical intervention (augmentation cystoplasty,

---

Table 48-2

Possible Causes of Interstitial Cystitis

Infection
 Fastidious bacteria
 Latent viruses
Dysfunctional bladder epithelium
 Defective glycosaminoglycan layer
 Abnormal intercellular junctions
Toxic substances in urine
Allergic/immune/autoimmune causes
Neurogenic disturbances
Bladder mastocytosis
Psychosomatic
Others
 Food intolerance
 Endocrine causes

---

urinary diversion) is indicated in fewer than 5 percent of cases because this is a non-life-threatening, chronic disease with occasional spontaneous remissions. "Last-resort" interventions such as removal of the bladder and urethra are not a guarantee of success because some patients continue to experience pelvic pain afterwards.

BIBLIOGRAPHY

BARRY MJ et al: The American Urological Association symptom index for benign prostatic hyperplasia. The measurement committee of the American Urological Association. J Urol 148:1549, 1992
BERRY SJ et al: The development of human benign prostatic hyperplasia with age. J Urol 132:474, 1984
CHAI TB, STEERS WD: Neurophysiology of micturition and continence. Urol Clin North Am 23:221, 1996
DuBEAU CE: Interpreting the effect of common medical conditions on voiding dysfunction in the elderly. Urol Clin North Am 23:11, 1996
GILLENWATER JY, WEIN AJ: Summary of the National Institute of Arthritis, Diabetes, Digestive and Kidney Diseases Workshop on Interstitial Cystitis, National Institutes of Health, Bethesda, Maryland, August 28–29, 1987. J Urol 140:203, 1988
HURST RE et al: Urinary glycosaminoglycan excretion as a laboratory marker in the diagnosis of interstitial cystitis. J Urol 149:31, 1993
LEACH GE et al: Experience with 215 men with post-prostatectomy incontinence. J Urol 155:1256, 1996
McGUIRE EJ: Urodynamic evaluation of stress incontinence. Urol Clin North Am 22:551, 1995
RATLIFF TL et al: The etiology of interstitial cystitis. Urol Clin North Am 21:21, 1994
RESNICK N: Geriatric incontinence. Urol Clin North Am 23:55, 1996
RIVAS DA, CHANCELLOR MB: Neurogenic vesical dysfunction. Urol Clin North Am 22:579, 1995
ROMANZI LJ et al: Preliminary assessment of the incontinent woman. Urol Clin North Am 22:513, 1995
WEIN A: Neuromuscular dysfunction of the lower urinary tract, in *Campbell's Urology*, 6th ed, PC Walsh et al (eds). Philadelphia, Saunders, 1992, p 573

---

49   *Gary G. Singer, Barry M. Brenner*

FLUID AND ELECTROLYTE DISTURBANCES

SODIUM AND WATER

COMPOSITION OF BODY FLUIDS Water is the most abundant constituent in the body, comprising approximately 60 percent of body weight in men and 50 percent in women. This difference is attributable to differences in the relative proportions of adipose tissue in men and women. Total body water is distributed in two major compartments—55 to 75 percent is intracellular [intracellular fluid (ICF)], and 25 to 45 percent is extracellular [extracellular fluid (ECF)]. The ECF is further subdivided into intravascular (plasma water) and extravascular (interstitial) spaces in a ratio of 1:3.

The solute or particle concentration of a fluid is known as its osmolality and is expressed as milliosmoles per kilogram of water (mosmol/kg). Water crosses cell membranes to achieve osmotic equilibrium (ECF osmolality = ICF osmolality). The extracellular and intracellular solutes or osmoles are markedly different due to disparities in permeability, and the presence of transporters and active pumps. The major ECF particles are Na^+ and its accompanying anions Cl^- and HCO_3^-, whereas K^+ and organic phosphate esters (ATP, creatine phosphate, and phospholipids) are the predominant ICF osmoles. Solutes that are restricted to the ECF or the ICF determine the *effective osmolality* (or *tonicity*) of that compartment. Since Na^+ is largely restricted to the extracellular compartment, total body Na^+ content is a reflection of ECF volume. Likewise, K^+ and its attendant anions are predominantly limited to the ICF and are necessary for normal cell function. Therefore, the number of intracellular particles is relatively constant, and a change in ICF osmolality is usually due to a change in ICF water content. However, in certain situations, brain cells can vary the number of intracellular solutes in order to defend against large water shifts. This process of *osmotic adaptation* is important in the defense of cell volume and occurs in chronic hyponatremia and hypernatremia. This response is mediated initially by transcellular shifts of K^+ and Na^+, followed by synthesis, import, or export of organic solutes (so-called osmolytes) such as inositol, betaine, and glutamine. During chronic hyponatremia, brain cells lose solutes, thereby defending cell volume and diminishing neurologic symptoms. The converse occurs during chronic hypernatremia. Certain solutes, such as urea, do not contribute to water shift across cell membranes and are known as *ineffective osmoles*.

Fluid movement between the intravascular and interstitial spaces occurs across the capillary wall and is determined by the Starling forces—capillary hydraulic pressure and colloid osmotic pressure. The transcapillary hydraulic pressure gradient exceeds the corresponding oncotic pressure gradient, thereby favoring the movement of plasma ultrafiltrate into the extravascular space. The return of fluid into the intravascular compartment occurs via lymphatic flow.

WATER BALANCE (See also Chap. 269)   The normal plasma osmolality is 275 to 290 mosmol/kg and is kept within a narrow range by mechanisms capable of sensing a 1 to 2 percent change in tonicity. To maintain a steady state, water intake must equal water excretion. Disorders of water homeostasis result in hypo- or hypernatremia. Normal individuals have an obligate water loss consisting of urine, stool, and evaporation from the skin and respiratory tract. Gastrointestinal excretion is usually a minor component of total water output, except in patients with vomiting, diarrhea, or high enterostomy output states. Evaporative or insensitive water losses are important in the regulation of core body temperature. Obligatory renal water loss is mandated by the minimum solute excretion required to maintain a steady state. Normally, about 600 mosmols must be excreted per day, and since the maximal urine osmolality is 1200 mosmol/kg a minimum urine output of 500 mL/d is required for neutral solute balance.

Water Intake   The primary stimulus for water ingestion is *thirst*, mediated either by an increase in effective osmolality or a decrease in ECF volume or blood pressure. *Osmoreceptors*, located in the anterolateral *hypothalamus*, are stimulated by a rise in tonicity. Ineffective osmoles, such as urea and glucose, do not play a role in stimulating thirst. The average osmotic threshold for thirst is approximately 295 mosmol/kg and varies among individuals. Under normal circumstances, daily water intake exceeds physiologic requirements.

Water Excretion   In contrast to the ingestion of water, its excretion is tightly regulated by physiologic factors. The principal determinant of renal water excretion is *arginine vasopressin* (AVP; formerly antidiuretic hormone), a polypeptide synthesized in the supraoptic and paraventricular nuclei of the hypothalamus and secreted by the posterior pituitary gland. The binding of AVP to V_2 receptors on the basolateral membrane of principal cells in the collecting duct activates adenylyl cyclase and initiates a sequence of events that leads to the insertion of water channels into the luminal membrane. These water channels that are specifically activated by AVP are encoded by the *aquaporin-2* gene (Chap. 330). The net effect is passive water reabsorption along an osmotic gradient from the lumen of the collecting duct to the hypertonic medullary interstitium. The major stimulus for AVP secretion is hypertonicity. Since the major ECF solutes are Na^+ salts, effective osmolality is primarily determined by the plasma Na^+ concentration. An increase or decrease in tonicity is sensed by hypothalamic osmoreceptors as a decrease or increase in cell volume, respectively, leading to enhancement or suppression of AVP secretion. The osmotic threshold for AVP release is 280 to 290 mosmol/kg, and the system is sufficiently sensitive that plasma osmolality varies by no more than 1 to 2 percent.

Nonosmotic factors that regulate AVP secretion include *effective circulating* (arterial) *volume*, nausea, pain, stress, hypoglycemia, pregnancy, and numerous drugs. The hemodynamic response is mediated by baroreceptors in the carotid sinus. The sensitivity of these receptors is significantly lower than that of the osmoreceptors. In fact, depletion of blood volume sufficient to result in a decreased mean arterial pressure is necessary to stimulate AVP release, whereas small changes in effective circulating volume have little effect. In the setting of hypovolemia, the osmotic regulation of AVP remains intact. However, the osmotic threshold, or set point, for AVP release is decreased, and the sensitivity is increased.

To maintain homeostasis and a normal plasma Na^+ concentration, the ingestion of solute-free water must eventually lead to the loss of the same volume of electrolyte-free water. Three steps are required for the kidney to excrete a water load: (1) filtration and delivery of water (and electrolytes) to the diluting sites of the nephron; (2) active reabsorption of Na^+ and Cl^- without water in the thick ascending limb of the loop of Henle and, to a lesser extent, in the distal nephron; and (3) maintenance of a dilute urine due to impermeability of the collecting duct to water in the absence of AVP. Abnormalities of any of these steps can result in impaired free water excretion, and eventual hyponatremia.

SODIUM BALANCE   Sodium is actively pumped out of cells by the Na^+, K^+-ATPase pump. As a result, 85 to 90 percent of all Na^+ is extracellular, and the ECF volume is a reflection of total body Na^+ content. Normal volume regulatory mechanisms ensure that Na^+ loss balances Na^+ gain. If this does not occur, conditions of Na^+ excess or deficit ensue and are manifest as edematous or hypovolemic states, respectively. It is important to distinguish between disorders of osmoregulation and disorders of volume regulation since water and Na^+ balance are regulated independently. Changes in Na^+ concentration generally reflect disturbed water homeostasis, whereas alterations in Na^+ content are manifest as ECF volume contraction or expansion and imply abnormal Na^+ balance.

Sodium Intake   Individuals eating a typical western diet consume approximately 150 mmol of NaCl daily. This normally exceeds basal requirements. As noted above, sodium is the principal extracellular cation. Therefore, dietary intake of Na^+ results in ECF volume expansion which, in turn, promotes enhanced renal Na^+ excretion to maintain steady state Na^+ balance.

Sodium Excretion (See also Chap. 269)   The regulation of Na^+ excretion is multifactorial and is the major determinant of Na^+ balance. An Na^+ deficit or excess is manifest as a decreased or increased effective circulating volume, respectively. Changes in effective circulating volume tend to lead to parallel changes in glomerular filtration rate (GFR). However, tubule Na^+ reabsorption, and not GFR, is the major regulatory mechanism controlling Na^+ excretion. Almost two-thirds of filtered Na^+ is reabsorbed in the proximal convoluted tubule—this process is electroneutral and isoosmotic. Further reabsorption (25 to 30 percent) occurs in the thick ascending limb of the loop of Henle via the apical *Na^+-K^+-$2Cl^-$ cotransporter*—this is an active process and is also electroneutral. Distal convoluted tubule reabsorption of Na^+ (5 percent) is mediated by the *thiazide-sensitive Na^+-Cl^- cotransporter*. Final Na^+ reabsorption occurs in the cortical and medullary collecting ducts, the amount excreted being reasonably equivalent to the amount ingested per day (Chap. 269).

HYPOVOLEMIA

ETIOLOGY   True volume depletion, or hypovolemia, generally refers to a state of combined salt and water loss exceeding intake, leading to ECF volume contraction. The loss of Na^+ may be renal or extrarenal (see Table 49-1).

Renal   Many conditions are associated with excessive urinary NaCl and water losses, including diuretics. Pharmacologic diuretics inhibit specific pathways of Na^+ reabsorption along the nephron with a consequent increase in urinary Na^+ excretion. Enhanced filtration of non-reabsorbed solutes, such as glucose or urea, can also impair tubular reabsorption of Na^+ and water, leading to an osmotic or solute diuresis. This often occurs in poorly controlled diabetes mellitus and in patients receiving high-protein hyperalimentation. Mannitol is a diuretic that produces an osmotic diuresis because the renal tubule is impermeable to mannitol. Many tubule and interstitial renal disorders are associated with Na^+ wasting. Excessive renal losses of Na^+ and water may also occur during the diuretic phase of acute tubular necrosis (ATN) (Chap. 270) and following the relief of bilateral urinary tract obstruction. The natriuresis and water diuresis associated with these two conditions is often short-lived and an appropriate response to a state of ECF volume expansion that ensued as a result of prior oliguria. However, ongoing losses in the absence of adequate replacement fluids may eventually lead to a state of hypovolemia. Chronic renal insufficiency is associated with a diminished ability to regulate renal salt and water excretion appropriately (Chap. 271). Therefore, patients with a GFR of less than 25 mL/min have an obligatory renal Na^+ loss that may result in progressive ECF volume depletion if Na^+ intake is restricted. Finally, mineralocorticoid deficiency (hypoaldosteronism) causes salt wasting in the presence of normal intrinsic renal function.

Massive renal water excretion can also lead to hypovolemia. The ECF volume contraction is usually less severe since two-thirds of the volume lost is intracellular. Conditions associated with excessive urinary water loss include central and nephrogenic diabetes insipidus. These two disorders are due to impaired secretion of and renal unresponsiveness to AVP, respectively, and are discussed below.

Extrarenal Nonrenal causes of hypovolemia include fluid loss from the gastrointestinal tract, skin, and respiratory system and third space accumulations (burns, pancreatitis, peritonitis). Approximately 9 L of fluid enters the gastrointestinal tract daily, 2 L by ingestion and 7 L by secretion. Almost 98 percent of this volume is reabsorbed so that fecal fluid loss is only 100 to 200 mL/d. Impaired gastrointestinal reabsorption or enhanced secretion leads to volume depletion. Since gastric secretions have a low pH (high H^+ concentration), vomiting and diarrhea are often accompanied by metabolic alkalosis and acidosis, respectively.

Water evaporation from the skin and respiratory tract contributes to thermoregulation. These *insensible losses* amount to 500 mL/d. During febrile illnesses, prolonged heat exposure, or exercise, increased salt and water loss from skin, in the form of sweat, can be significant and lead to volume depletion. The Na^+ concentration of sweat is normally 20 to 50 mmol/L and decreases with profuse sweating due to the action of aldosterone. Since sweat is hypotonic, the loss of water exceeds that of Na^+. The water deficit is minimized by enhanced

Table 49-1

Causes of Hypovolemia

I. ECF volume contracted
  A. Extrarenal Na^+ loss
    1. Gastrointestinal
      (vomiting, nasogastric suction, drainage, fistula, diarrhea)
    2. Skin/respiratory
      (insensible losses, sweat, burns)
    3. Hemorrhage
  B. Renal Na^+ and water loss
    1. Diuretics
    2. Osmotic diuresis
    3. Hypoaldosteronism
    4. Salt-wasting nephropathies
  C. Renal water loss
    1. Diabetes insipidus (central or nephrogenic)
II. ECF volume normal or expanded
  A. Decreased cardiac output
    1. Myocardial, valvular, or pericardial disease
  B. Redistribution
    1. Hypoalbuminemia
      (hepatic cirrhosis, nephrotic syndrome)
    2. Capillary leak
      (acute pancreatitis, ischemic bowel, rhabdomyolysis)
  C. Increased venous capacitance
    1. Sepsis

thirst. Nevertheless, ongoing Na^+ loss is manifest as hypovolemia. Enhanced evaporative water loss from the respiratory tract may be associated with hyperventilation, especially in mechanically ventilated febrile patients.

Certain conditions lead to fluid sequestration in a *third space*. This compartment is extracellular but is not in equilibrium with either the ECF or the ICF. The fluid is effectively lost from the ECF and can result in hypovolemia. Examples include the bowel lumen in gastrointestinal obstruction, subcutaneous tissues in severe burns, retroperitoneal space in acute pancreatitis, and peritoneal cavity in peritonitis. Finally, severe hemorrhage from any source can result in volume depletion.

PATHOPHYSIOLOGY ECF volume contraction is manifest as a decreased plasma volume and hypotension. Hypotension is due to decreased venous return (preload) and diminished cardiac output; it triggers baroreceptors in the carotid sinus and aortic arch and leads to activation of the sympathetic nervous system and the renin-angiotensin system. The net effect is to maintain mean arterial pressure and cerebral and coronary perfusion. In contrast to the cardiovascular response, the renal response is aimed at restoring the ECF volume by decreasing the GFR and filtered load of Na^+ and, most importantly, by promoting tubular reabsorption of Na^+. Increased sympathetic tone increases proximal tubular Na^+ reabsorption and decreases GFR by causing preferential afferent arteriolar vasoconstriction. Sodium is also reabsorbed in the proximal convoluted tubule in response to increased angiotensin II and altered peritubular capillary hemodynamics (decreased hydraulic and increased oncotic pressure). Enhanced reabsorption of Na^+ by the collecting duct is an important component of the renal adaptation to ECF volume contraction. This occurs in response to increased *aldosterone* and AVP secretion, and suppressed *atrial natriuretic peptide* (ANP) secretion.

CLINICAL FEATURES A careful history is often helpful in determining the etiology of ECF volume contraction (e.g., vomiting, diarrhea, polyuria, diaphoresis). Most symptoms are nonspecific and secondary to electrolyte imbalances and tissue hypoperfusion and include fatigue, weakness, muscle cramps, thirst, and postural dizziness. More severe degrees of volume contraction can lead to end-organ ischemia manifest as oliguria, cyanosis, abdominal and chest pain, and confusion or obtundation. Diminished skin turgor and dry oral mucous membranes are poor markers of decreased interstitial fluid. Signs of intravascular volume contraction include decreased jugular venous pressure, postural hypotension, and postural tachycardia. Larger and more acute fluid losses lead to hypovolemic shock, manifest as hypotension, tachycardia, peripheral vasoconstriction, and hypoperfusion—cyanosis, cold and clammy extremities, oliguria, and altered mental status.

DIAGNOSIS A thorough history and physical examination are generally sufficient to diagnose the etiology of hypovolemia. Laboratory data usually confirm and support the clinical diagnosis. The blood urea nitrogen (BUN) and plasma creatinine concentrations tend to be elevated, reflecting a decreased GFR. Normally, the BUN:creatinine ratio is about 10:1. However, in *prerenal azotemia*, hypovolemia leads to increased urea reabsorption and a proportionately greater elevation in BUN than plasma creatinine, and a BUN:creatinine ratio of 20:1 or higher. An increased BUN (relative to creatinine) may also be due to increased urea production that occurs with hyperalimentation (high-protein), glucocorticoid therapy, and gastrointestinal bleeding.

Volume depletion may be associated with hyponatremia, hypernatremia, or a normal plasma Na^+ concentration, depending on the tonicity of the fluid lost, the presence of thirst, and the access to water. Hypokalemia is common in settings of increased renal or gastrointestinal K^+ loss, and hyperkalemia occurs in renal failure, adrenal insufficiency, and certain types of metabolic acidosis. Metabolic alkalosis occurs with diuretic-induced hypovolemia and in cases of vomiting or nasogastric suction. In contrast, metabolic acidosis is associated with renal failure, tubulointerstitial disorders, adrenal insufficiency, diarrhea, diabetic ketoacidosis, and lactic acid acidosis. Since albumin and erythrocytes are confined to the intravascular compartment, ECF volume contraction often leads to a relative elevation in hematocrit (hemoconcentration) and plasma albumin concentration.

The appropriate response to hypovolemia is enhanced renal Na^+ and water reabsorption, which is reflected in the urine composition. Therefore, the urine Na^+ concentration should usually be less than 20 mmol/L except in conditions associated with impaired Na^+ reabsorption, as in acute tubular necrosis (Chap. 270). Another exception is hypovolemia due to vomiting since the associated metabolic alkalosis and increased filtered HCO_3^- impair proximal Na^+ reabsorption. In this case, the urine Cl^- is low (less than 20 mmol/L). The urine osmolality and specific gravity in hypovolemic subjects are generally greater than 450 mosmol/kg and 1.015, respectively, reflecting the presence of enhanced AVP secretion. However, in hypovolemia due to diabetes insipidus, urine osmolality and specific gravity are indicative of inappropriately dilute urine.

℞ TREATMENT

The therapeutic goals are to restore normovolemia with fluid similar in composition to that lost and to replace ongoing losses. Symptoms and signs, including weight loss, can help estimate the degree of volume contraction and should also be monitored to assess response to treatment. Mild volume contraction can usually be corrected via the oral route. More severe hypovolemia requires intravenous therapy. Isotonic or normal saline (0.9% NaCl or 154 mmol/L Na^+) is the solution of choice in normonatremic and mildly hyponatremic individuals and should be administered initially in patients with hypotension or shock. Severe hyponatremia may require hypertonic saline (3.0% NaCl or 513 mmol/L Na^+). Hypernatremia reflects a proportionally greater deficit of water than Na^+, and its correction will therefore require a hypotonic solution such as half-normal saline (0.45% NaCl or 77 mmol/L Na^+) or 5% dextrose in water. Patients with significant hemorrhage, anemia, or intravascular volume depletion may require blood transfusion or colloid-containing solutions (albumin, dextran). Hypokalemia may be present initially or may ensue as a result of increased urinary K^+ excretion; it should be corrected by adding appropriate amounts of KCl to replacement solutions.

HYPONATREMIA

ETIOLOGY A plasma Na^+ concentration less than 135 mmol/L usually reflects a hypotonic state. However, plasma osmolality may be normal or increased in some cases of hyponatremia, referred to as *pseudohyponatremia*. Plasma is 93 percent water, the remaining 7 percent consisting of plasma proteins and lipids. Since Na^+ ions are dissolved in plasma water, increasing the nonaqueous phase artificially lowers the Na^+ concentration measured per liter of plasma (except when Na^+-sensitive glass electrodes are used). The plasma osmolality and the Na^+ concentration remain normal. This type of hyponatremia has little clinical significance, except to ascertain the cause of the hyperproteinemia or hyperlipidemia. Isotonic or slightly hypotonic hyponatremia may complicate transurethral resection of the prostate or bladder because large volumes of isoosmotic (mannitol) or hypoosmotic (sorbital or glycine) bladder irrigation solution can be absorbed and result in a dilutional hyponatremia. The metabolism of sorbitol and glycine to CO_2 and water may lead to hypotonicity if the accumulated fluid and solutes are not rapidly excreted. Hypertonic hyponatremia is usually due to hyperglycemia or, occasionally, intravenous administration of mannitol. Relative insulin deficiency causes myocytes to become impermeable to glucose. Therefore, during poorly controlled diabetes mellitus, glucose is an effective osmole and draws water from muscle cells, resulting in hyponatremia. Plasma Na^+ concentration falls by 1.4 mmol/L for every 100 mg/dL rise in the plasma glucose concentration.

Most causes of hyponatremia are associated with a low plasma osmolality (Table 49-2). In general hypotonic hyponatremia is due

either to a primary water gain (and secondary Na^+ loss) or a primary Na^+ loss (and secondary water gain). Hyponatremia in the absence of water retention is usually associated with hypovolemic shock. Contraction of the ECF volume stimulates thirst and AVP secretion. The increased water ingestion and impaired renal excretion result in hyponatremia. It is important to note that *diuretic-induced hyponatremia* is almost always due to thiazide diuretics. Loop diuretics decrease the tonicity of the medullary interstitium and impair maximal urinary concentrating capacity. This limits the ability of AVP to promote water retention. In contrast, thiazide diuretics lead to Na^+ and K^+ depletion, and AVP-mediated water retention. In the presence of a large K^+ deficit, transcellular ion exchange (K^+ exits and Na^+ enters cells) may contribute to hyponatremia.

Hyponatremia in the setting of ECF volume expansion is usually associated with edematous states, such as congestive heart failure, hepatic cirrhosis, and the nephrotic syndrome. These disorders all have in common a decreased effective circulating arterial volume, leading to increased thirst and increased AVP levels. Additional factors impairing the excretion of solute-free water include a reduced GFR, decreased delivery of ultrafiltrate to the diluting site (due to increased proximal fractional reabsorption of Na^+ and water), and diuretic therapy. The degree of hyponatremia often correlates with the severity of the underlying condition and is an important prognostic factor. Oliguric acute and chronic renal failure may be associated with hyponatremia if water intake exceeds the ability to excrete equivalent volumes.

Hyponatremia in the absence of ECF volume contraction, decreased effective circulating arterial volume, or renal insufficiency is usually due to increased AVP secretion resulting in impaired water excretion. Ingestion or administration of water is also required since high levels of AVP alone are usually insufficient to produce hyponatremia. This disorder, commonly termed the *syndrome of inappropriate antidiuretic hormone (ADH) secretion* (SIADH), is the most common cause of normovolemic hyponatremia and is due to the nonphysiologic release of AVP from the posterior pituitary or an ectopic source (Chap. 330). Renal free water excretion is impaired while the regulation of Na^+ balance is unaffected. The most common causes of SIADH include neuropsychiatric and pulmonary diseases, malignant tumors, major surgery (postoperative pain), and pharmacologic agents. Severe pain and nausea are physiologic stimuli of AVP secretion; these stimuli are inappropriate in the absence of hypovolemia or hyperosmolality.

Table 49-2

Causes of Hyponatremia

I. Pseudohyponatremia
  A. Normal plasma osmolality
    1. Hyperlipidemia
    2. Hyperproteinemia
    3. Posttransurethral resection of prostate/bladder tumor
  B. Increased plasma osmolality
    1. Hyperglycemia
    2. Mannitol
II. Hypoosmolal hyponatremia
  A. Primary Na^+ loss (secondary water gain)
    1. Integumentary loss: sweating, burns
    2. Gastrointestinal loss: vomiting, tube drainage, fistula, obstruction, diarrhea
    3. Renal loss: diuretics, osmotic diuresis, hypoaldosteronism, salt-wasting nephropathy, postobstructive diuresis, nonoliguric acute tubular necrosis
  B. Primary water gain (secondary Na^+ loss)
    1. Primary polydipsia
    2. Decreased solute intake (e.g., beer potomania)
    3. AVP release due to pain, nausea, drugs
    4. Syndrome of inappropriate AVP secretion
    5. Glucocorticoid deficiency
    6. Hypothyroidism
    7. Chronic renal insufficiency
  C. Primary Na^+ gain (exceeded by secondary water gain)
    1. Heart failure
    2. Hepatic cirrhosis
    3. Nephrotic syndrome

A variety of central nervous system disorders may be associated with SIADH, such as meningitis, encephalitis, hemorrhage, stroke, psychosis, primary and metastatic tumors, and acute porphyria. Pneumonia, empyema, tuberculosis, and acute respiratory failure can be complicated by hyponatremia secondary to SIADH. Hypoxemia, hypercarbia, and positive-pressure ventilation are all nonosmotic stimuli for AVP release. Various tumors, notably oat cell carcinoma of the lung, have been demonstrated to secrete AVP ectopically. Many drugs either stimulate AVP release or potentiate its actions on the kidney. The pattern of AVP secretion can be used to classify SIADH into four subtypes: (1) erratic autonomous AVP secretion (ectopic production); (2) normal regulation of AVP release around a lower osmolality set point or *reset osmostat* (cachexia, malnutrition); (3) normal AVP response to hypertonicity with failure to suppress completely at low osmolality (incomplete pituitary stalk section); and (4) normal AVP secretion with increased sensitivity to its actions or secretion of some other antidiuretic factor (rare).

Hormonal excess or deficiency may cause hyponatremia. Adrenal insufficiency (Chap. 332) and hypothyroidism (Chap. 331) may present with hyponatremia and should not be confused with SIADH. Although decreased mineralocorticoids may contribute to the hyponatremia of adrenal insufficiency, it is the cortisol deficiency that leads to hypersecretion of AVP both indirectly (secondary to volume depletion) and directly (cosecreted with corticotropin-releasing factor). The mechanisms by which hypothyroidism leads to hyponatremia include decreased cardiac output and GFR and increased AVP secretion in response to hemodynamic stimuli.

Finally, hyponatremia may occur in the absence of AVP or renal failure if the kidney is unable to excrete the dietary water load. In psychogenic or *primary polydipsia*, compulsive water consumption may overwhelm the normally large renal excretory capacity of 12 L/d (Chap. 330). These patients often have psychiatric illnesses and may be taking medications, such as phenothiazines, that enhance the sensation of thirst by causing a dry mouth. The maximal urine output is a function of the minimum urine osmolality achievable and the mandatory solute excretion. Metabolism of a normal diet generates about 600 mosmol/d, and the minimum urine osmolality in humans is 50 mosmol/kg. Therefore, the maximum daily urine output will be about 12 L (600 ÷ 50 = 12). A solute excretion rate of greater than ~750 mosmol/d is, by definition, an *osmotic diuresis*. A low-protein diet may yield as few as 250 mosmol/d, which translates into a maximal urine output of 5 L/d at a minimum urine tonicity of 50 mosmol/kg. Beer drinkers typically have a poor dietary intake of protein and electrolytes and consume large volumes (of beer), which may exceed the renal excretory capacity and result in hyponatremia. This phenomenon is referred to as *beer potomania*.

CLINICAL FEATURES   The clinical manifestations of hyponatremia are related to osmotic water shift leading to increased ICF volume, specifically brain cell swelling or cerebral edema. Therefore, the symptoms are primarily neurologic, and their severity is dependent on the rapidity of onset and absolute decrease in plasma Na^+ concentration. Patients may be asymptomatic, or complain of nausea and malaise. As the plasma Na^+ concentration falls, the symptoms progress to include headache, lethargy, confusion, and obtundation. Stupor, seizures, and coma do not usually occur unless the plasma Na^+ concentration falls acutely below 120 mmol/L or decreases rapidly. As described above, adaptive mechanisms designed to protect cell volume occur in chronic hyponatremia. Loss of Na^+ and K^+, followed by organic osmolytes, from brain cells decreases brain swelling due to secondary transcellular water shifts (from ICF to ECF). The net effect is to minimize cerebral edema and its symptoms.

DIAGNOSIS   Hyponatremia is not a disease but a manifestation of a variety of disorders. The underlying cause can often be ascertained from an accurate history and physical examination, including an assessment of ECF volume status and effective circulating arterial volume. The differential diagnosis of hyponatremia, an expanded ECF volume, and decreased effective circulating volume includes congestive heart failure, hepatic cirrhosis, and the nephrotic syndrome. Hypothyroidism and adrenal insufficiency tend to present with a near-normal ECF

volume and decreased effective circulating arterial volume. All of these diseases have characteristic signs and symptoms. Patients with SIADH are usually euvolemic.

Four laboratory findings often provide useful information and can narrow the differential diagnosis of hyponatremia: (1) the plasma osmolality, (2) the urine osmolality, (3) the urine Na^+ concentration, and (4) the urine K^+ concentration. Since ECF tonicity is determined primarily by the Na^+ concentration, most patients with hyponatremia have a decreased plasma osmolality. If the plasma osmolality is not low, pseudohyponatremia must be ruled out. The appropriate renal response to hypoosmolality is to excrete the maximum volume of dilute urine, i.e., urine osmolality and specific gravity of less than 100 mosmol/kg and 1.003, respectively. This occurs in patients with primary polydipsia. If this is not present, it suggests impaired free water excretion due to the action of AVP on the kidney. The secretion of AVP may be a physiologic response to hemodynamic stimuli or it may be inappropriate in the presence of hyponatremia and euvolemia. Since Na^+ is the major ECF cation and is largely restricted to this compartment, ECF volume contraction represents a deficit in total body Na^+ content. Therefore, volume depletion in patients with normal underlying renal function results in enhanced tubule Na^+ reabsorption and a urine Na^+ concentration less than 20 mmol/L. The finding of a urine Na^+ concentration greater than 20 mmol/L in hypovolemic hyponatremia implies a salt-wasting nephropathy, diuretic therapy, hypoaldosteronism, or occasionally vomiting. Both the urine osmolality and the urine Na^+ concentration can be followed serially when assessing response to therapy.

SIADH is characterized by hypoosmotic hyponatremia in the setting of an inappropriately concentrated urine (urine osmolality greater than 100 mosmol/kg). Patients are typically normovolemic and have normal Na^+ balance. They tend to be mildly volume expanded secondary to water retention and have a urine Na^+ excretion rate equal to intake (urine Na^+ concentration usually greater than 40 mmol/L). By definition, they have normal renal, adrenal, and thyroid function and usually have normal K^+ and acid-base balance. SIADH is often associated with hypouricemia due to the uricosuric state induced by volume expansion. In contrast, hypovolemic patients tend to be hyperuricemic secondary to increased proximal urate reabsorption.

CLINICAL APPROACH   See Fig. 49-1.

℞ **TREATMENT**

The goals of therapy are twofold: (1) to raise the plasma Na^+ concentration by restricting water intake and promoting water loss; and (2) to correct the underlying disorder. → *For further discussion, see Chap. 330.*

HYPERNATREMIA

ETIOLOGY   Hypernatremia is defined as a plasma Na^+ concentration greater than 145 mmol/L. Since Na^+ and its accompanying anions are the major effective ECF osmoles, hypernatremia is a state of hyperosmolality. As a result of the fixed number of ICF particles, maintenance of osmotic equilibrium in hypernatremia results in ICF volume contraction. Hypernatremia may be due to primary Na^+ gain or water deficit. The two components of an appropriate response to hypernatremia are increased water intake stimulated by thirst and the excretion of the minimum volume of maximally concentrated urine reflecting AVP secretion in response to an osmotic stimulus.

In practice, the majority of cases of hypernatremia result from the loss of water. Since water is distributed between the ICF and the ECF in a 2:1 ratio, a given amount of solute-free water loss will result in a twofold greater reduction in the ICF compartment than the ECF compartment. For example, consider three scenarios: the loss of 1 L of water, isotonic NaCl, or half-isotonic NaCl. If 1 L of water is lost, the ICF volume will decrease by 667 mL, whereas the ECF volume will fall by only 333 mL. Due to the fact that Na^+ is largely restricted to the ECF, this compartment will decrease by 1 L if the fluid lost is isoosmotic. One liter of half-isotonic NaCl is equivalent to 500 mL of water (one-third ECF, two-thirds ICF) plus 500 mL of isotonic saline (all ECF). Therefore, the loss of 1 L of half-isotonic saline decreases the ECF and ICF volumes by 667 mL and 333 mL, respectively.

The degree of hyperosmolality is typically mild unless the thirst mechanism is abnormal or access to water is limited. The latter occurs in infants, the physically handicapped, patients with impaired mental status, in the postoperative state, and in intubated patients in the intensive care unit. On rare occasions, impaired thirst may be due to *primary hypodipsia*. This usually occurs as a result of damage to the hypothalamic osmoreceptors that control thirst and tends to be associated with abnormal osmotic regulation of AVP secretion. Primary hypodipsia may be due to a variety of pathologic changes including granulomatous disease, vascular occlusion, and tumors. A subset of hypodipsic hypernatremia, referred to as *essential hypernatremia*, does not respond to forced water intake. This appears to be due to a specific osmoreceptor defect resulting in nonosmotic regulation of AVP release. Thus, the hemodynamic effects of water loading lead to AVP suppression and excretion of dilute urine.

The source of free water loss is either renal or extrarenal. Nonrenal loss of water may be due to evaporation from the skin and respiratory tract (insensible losses) or loss from the gastrointestinal tract. Insensible losses are increased with fever, exercise, heat exposure and severe burns and in mechanically ventilated patients. Furthermore, the Na^+ concentration of sweat decreases with profuse perspiration, thereby increasing solute-free water loss. Diarrhea is the most common gastrointestinal cause of hypernatremia. Specifically, osmotic diarrheas (induced by lactulose, sorbitol, or malabsorption of carbohydrate) and viral gastroenteritides result in water loss exceeding that of Na^+ and K^+. In contrast, secretory diarrheas (e.g., cholera, carcinoid, VIPoma) have a fecal osmolality (twice the sum of the concentrations of Na^+ and K^+) similar to that of plasma and present with ECF volume contraction and a normal plasma Na^+ concentration or hyponatremia.

Renal water loss is the most common cause of hypernatremia and is due to drug-induced or osmotic diuresis or diabetes insipidus (Chap. 330). Loop diuretics interfere with the countercurrent mechanism and produce an isoosmotic solute diuresis. This results in a decreased medullary interstitial tonicity and impaired renal concentrating ability. The presence of non-reabsorbed organic solutes in the tubule lumen impairs the osmotic reabsorption of water. This leads to water loss in excess of Na^+ and K^+, known as an osmotic diuresis. The most frequent cause of an osmotic diuresis is hyperglycemia and glucosuria in poorly controlled diabetes mellitus. Intravenous administration of mannitol and increased endogenous production of urea (high-protein diet) can also result in an osmotic diuresis. Hypernatremia secondary to nonosmotic urinary water loss is usually due to: (1) central or neurogenic diabetes insipidus characterized by impaired AVP secretion, or (2) nephrogenic diabetes insipidus resulting from end-organ (renal) resistance to the actions of AVP. The most common cause of *central diabetes insipidus* (CDI) is destruction of the neurohypophysis. This may occur as a result of trauma, neurosurgery, granulomatous disease, neoplasms, vascular accidents, or infection. In many cases, CDI is idiopathic and may occassionally be hereditary. The familial form of the disease is inherited in an autosomal dominant fashion and has been attributed to mutations in the propressophysin (AVP precursor) gene. *Nephrogenic diabetes insipidus* (NDI) may be either inherited or acquired. Congenital NDI is an X-linked recessive trait due to mutations in the V_2 receptor gene. Mutations in the autosomal aquaporin-2 gene may also result in NDI. The aquaporin-2 gene encodes the water channel protein whose membrane insertion is stimulated by AVP. The causes of sporadic NDI are numerous and include drugs (especially lithium), hypercalcemia, hypokalemia, and conditions that impair medullary hypertonicity (e.g., papillary necrosis or osmotic diuresis). Pregnant women, in the second or third trimester, may develop NDI as a result of excessive elaboration of vasopressinase by the placenta.

Finally, although infrequent, a primary Na^+ gain may cause hypernatremia. For example, inadvertent administration of hypertonic NaCl or $NaHCO_3$ or replacing sugar with salt in infant formula can produce this complication.

CLINICAL FEATURES   As a consequence of hypertonicity, water shifts out of cells, leading to a contracted ICF volume. A decreased brain cell volume is associated with an increased risk of subarachnoid or intracerebral hemorrhage. Hence, the major symptoms of hypernatremia are neurologic and include altered mental status, weakness, neuromuscular irritability, focal neurologic deficits, and occasionally coma or seizures. Patients may also complain of polyuria or thirst. For unknown reasons, patients with polydipsia from CDI tend to prefer ice-cold water. The signs and symptoms of volume depletion are often present in patients with a history of excessive sweating, diarrhea, or an osmotic diuresis. The mortality rate associated with a plasma Na^+ concentration greater than 180 mmol/L is very high. As with hyponatremia, the severity of the clinical manifestations is related to the acuity and magnitude of the rise in plasma Na^+ concentration. Chronic hypernatremia is generally less symptomatic as a result of adaptive mechanisms designed to defend cell volume. Brain cells initially take up Na^+ and K^+ salts, later followed by accumulation of organic osmolytes such as inositol. This serves to restore the brain ICF volume towards normal.

DIAGNOSIS   A complete history and physical examination will often provide clues as to the underlying cause of hypernatremia. Relevant symptoms and signs include the absence or presence of thirst, diaphoresis, diarrhea, polyuria, and the features of ECF volume contraction. The history should include a list of current and recent medications, and the physical examination is incomplete without a thorough mental status and neurologic assessment. Measurement of urine vol-

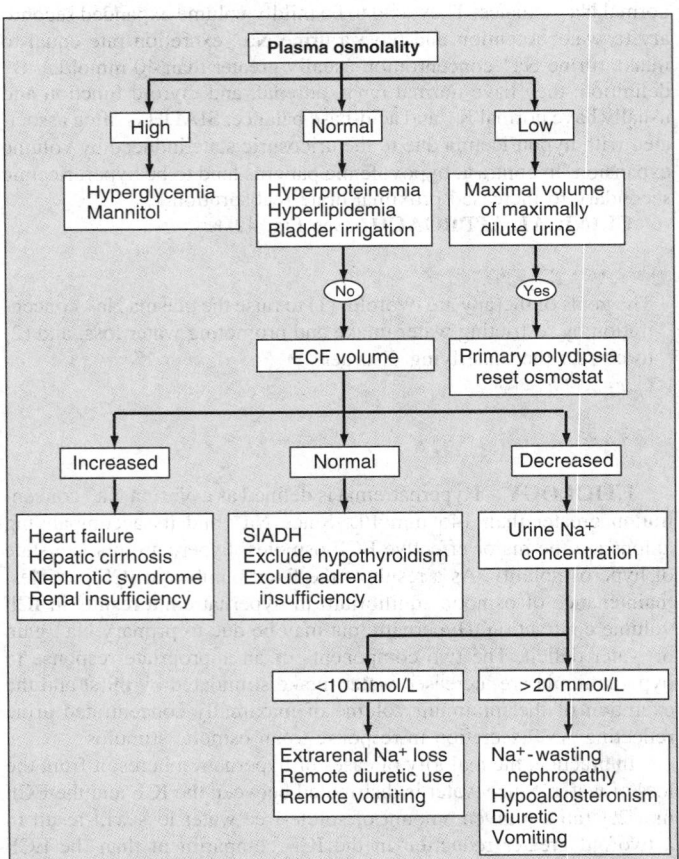

FIGURE 49-1   Algorithm depicting clinical approach to hyponatremia. ECF, extracellular fluid; SIADH, syndrome of inappropriate antidiuretic hormone secretion.

ume and osmolality are essential in the evaluation of hyperosmolality. The appropriate renal response to hypernatremia is the excretion of the minimum volume (500 mL/d) of maximally concentrated urine (urine osmolality greater than 800 mosmol/kg). These findings suggest extrarenal or remote renal water loss or administration of hypertonic Na^+ salt solutions. The presence of a primary Na^+ excess can be confirmed by the presence of ECF volume expansion and natriuresis (urine Na^+ concentration usually greater than 100 mmol/L). Many causes of hypernatremia are associated with polyuria and a submaximal urine osmolality. The product of the urine volume and osmolality, i.e., the solute excretion rate, is helpful in determining the basis of the polyuria (see above). To maintain a steady state, total solute excretion must equal solute production. As stated above, individuals eating a normal diet generate ~600 mosmol/d. Therefore, daily solute excretion in excess of 750 mosmol defines an osmotic diuresis. This can be confirmed by measuring the urine glucose and urea. In general, both CDI and NDI present with polyuria and hypotonic urine (urine osmolality less than 250 mosmol/kg). The degree of hypernatremia is usually mild unless there is an associated thirst abnormality. The clinical history, physical examination, and pertinent laboratory data can often rule out causes of acquired NDI. CDI and NDI can generally be distinguished by administering the AVP analogue desmopressin (10 μg intranasally) after careful water restriction. The urine osmolality should increase by at least 50 percent in CDI and will not change in NDI. Unfortunately, the diagnosis may sometimes be difficult due to partial defects in AVP secretion and action.

CLINICAL APPROACH   See Fig. 49-2.

Rx **TREATMENT**

The therapeutic goals are to stop ongoing water loss by treating the underlying cause and to correct the water deficit. The ECF volume should be restored in hypovolemic patients. The quantity of water required to correct the deficit can be calculated from the following equation:

$$\text{Water deficit} = \frac{\text{plasma } Na^+ \text{ concentration} - 140}{140} \times \text{total body water}$$

In hypernatremia due to water loss, total body water is approximately 50 and 40 percent of lean body weight in men and women, respectively. For example, a 50-kg woman with a plasma Na^+ concentration of 160 mmol/L has an estimated free water deficit of 2.9 L [(160 − 140) ÷ 140 × (0.4 × 50)]. As in hyponatremia, rapid correction of hypernatremia is potentially dangerous. In this case, a sudden decrease in osmolality could potentially cause a rapid shift of water into cells that have undergone osmotic adaptation. This would result in swollen brain cells and increase the risk of seizures or permanent neurologic damage. Therefore, the water deficit should be corrected slowly over at least 48 to 72 h. When calculating the rate of water replacement, ongoing losses should be taken into account, and the plasma Na^+ concentration should be lowered by 0.5 mmol/L per hour and by no more than 12 mmol/L over the first 24 h. The safest route of administration of water is by mouth or via a nasogastric tube (or other feeding tube). Alternatively, 5% dextrose in water or half-isotonic saline can be given intravenously. The appropriate treatment of CDI consists of administering desmopressin intranasally (Chap. 330). Other options for decreasing urine output include a low-salt diet in combination with low-dose thiazide diuretic therapy. In some patients with partial CDI, drugs which either stimulate AVP secretion or enhance its action on the kidney have been useful. These include chlorpropamide, clofibrate, carbamazepine, and nonsteroidal anti-inflammatory drugs (NSAIDs). The concentrating defect in NDI may be reversible by treating the underlying disorder or eliminating the offending drug. Symptomatic polyuria due to NDI can be treated with a low-Na^+ diet and thiazide diuretics as described above. This induces mild volume depletion, which leads to enhanced proximal reabsorption of salt and water and decreased delivery to the site of action of AVP, the collecting duct. By impairing renal prostaglandin synthesis, NSAIDs potentiate AVP action and thereby increase urine osmolality and decrease urine volume. Amiloride may be useful in patients with NDI who need to be on lithium. The nephrotoxicity of lithium requires the drug to be taken up into collecting duct cells via the amiloride-sensitive Na^+ channel.

POTASSIUM

POTASSIUM BALANCE   Potassium is the major intracellular cation. The normal plasma K^+ concentration is 3.5 to 5.0 mmol/L, whereas that inside cells is about 150 mmol/L. Therefore, the amount of K^+ in the ECF (30 to 70 mmol) constitutes less than 2 percent of the total body K^+ content (2500 to 4500 mmol). The ratio of ICF to ECF K^+ concentration (normally 38:1) is the principal result of the resting membrane potential and is crucial for normal neuromuscular function. The basolateral Na^+,K^+-ATPase pump actively transports K^+ in and Na^+ out of the cell in a 2:3 ratio, and the passive outward diffusion of K^+ is quantitatively the most important factor that generates the resting membrane potential. The activity of the electrogenic Na^+,K^+-ATPase pump may be stimulated as a result of an increased intracellular Na^+ concentration and inhibited in the setting of digoxin toxicity of chronic illness such as heart failure or renal failure.

The distribution of K^+ is also affected by several other factors, including hormones, acid-base balance, osmolality, and cell turnover. Insulin increases Na^+,K^+-ATPase activity indirectly and independent of its effect on glucose transport, leading to K^+ shift into muscle and liver cells. Conversely, insulin deficiency results in K^+ movement from the ICF to the ECF compartment. Catecholamines have variable effects on K^+ distribution—beta$_2$-adrenergic agonists promote whereas alpha-adrenergic agonists impair K^+ uptake by cells. The Na^+,K^+-ATPase pump as well as insulin secretion are stimulated by beta$_2$-adrenergic agonists. In contrast, alpha-adrenergic agonists have the opposite effect. The major action of aldosterone is to increase K^+ excretion (see below). The role of extracellular pH in K^+ balance relates to the underlying acid-base disorder. In metabolic acidosis, 60 percent of the H^+ load is buffered inside cells. To maintain electroneutrality, the H^+ ion must either be accompanied by an anion or ex-

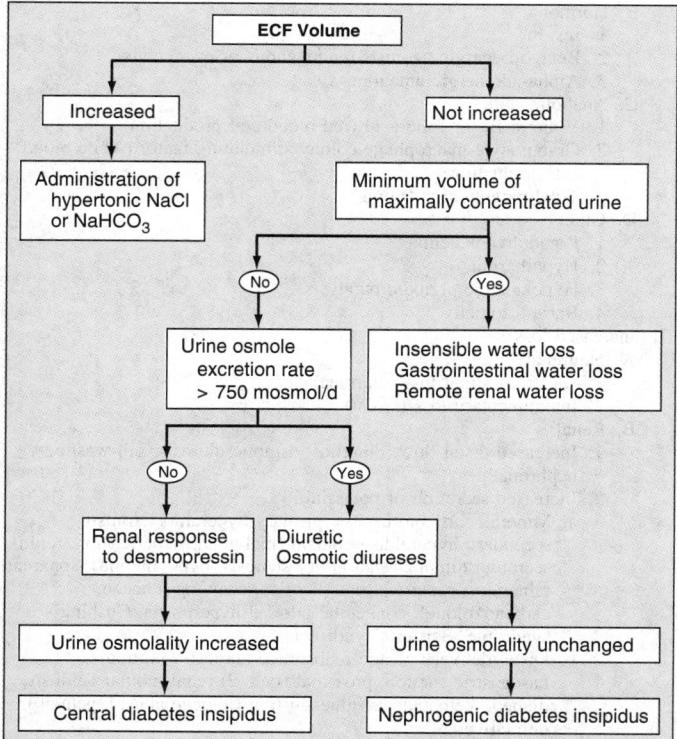

FIGURE 49-2   Algorithm depicting clinical approach to hypernatremia.

changed for intracellular K$^+$ (leading to hyperkalemia). Organic acidoses are not usually associated with a pH-related K$^+$ shift, since anions such as lactate and β-hydroxybutyrate can be readily taken up by the cell. The converse, movement of K$^+$ into cells, may be seen with metabolic alkalosis. However, this is less important due to diminished intracellular buffering. Primary respiratory disturbances in acid-base balance result in minimal transcellular K$^+$ shifts. In hyperosmolal states, K$^+$ diffuses out of cells along with water due to *solvent drag*. The concentration gradient favoring K$^+$ movement out of cells is also increased as a result of ICF water loss. Tissue destruction or breakdown results in the release of intracellular K$^+$, whereas the production of new cell shifts K$^+$ out of the ECF. Finally, moderate to severe exercise may be associatd with K$^+$ release from muscle, leading to glycogenolysis and local vasodilatation. This is usually transient but may affect the plasma K$^+$ concentration if patients repeatedly clench and unclench their fist prior to venipuncture.

The K$^+$ intake of individuals on an average western diet is 40 to 120 mmol/d or approximately 1 mmol/kg per day, 90 percent of which is absorbed by the gastrointestinal tract. Maintenance of the steady state necessitates matching K$^+$ ingestion with excretion. Initially, extrarenal adaptive mechanisms, followed later by urinary excretion, prevent a doubling of the plasma K$^+$ concentration that would occur if the dietary K$^+$ load remained in the ECF compartment. Immediately following a meal, most of the absorbed K$^+$ enters cells as a result of the initial elevation in the plasma K$^+$ concentration and facilitated by insulin release and basal catecholamine levels. Eventually, however, the excess K$^+$ is excreted in the urine (see below). The regulation of gastrointestinal K$^+$ handling is not well understood. The amount of K$^+$ lost in the stool can increase from 10 to 50 or 60 percent (of dietary intake) in chronic renal insufficiency. In addition, colonic secretion of K$^+$ is stimulated in patients with large volumes of diarrhea, resulting in potentially severe K$^+$ depletion.

POTASSIUM EXCRETION (See also Chap. 269) Renal excretion is the major route of elimination of dietary and other sources of excess K$^+$. The filtered load of K$^+$ (GFR $\times$ plasma K$^+$ concentration = 180 L/d $\times$ 4 mmol/L = 720 mmol/d is 10- to 20-fold greater than the ECF K$^+$ content. Ninety percent of filtered K$^+$ is reabsorbed by the proximal convoluted tubule and loop of Henle. Proximally, K$^+$ is reabsorbed passively with Na$^+$ and water, whereas the luminal Na$^+$-K$^+$-2Cl$^-$ cotransporter mediates K$^+$ uptake in the thick ascending limb of the loop of Henle. Therefore, K$^+$ delivery to the distal nephron (distal convoluted tubule and cortical collecting duct) approximates dietary intake. Net distal K$^+$ secretion or reabsorption occurs in the setting of K$^+$ excess or depletion, respectively. The cell responsible for K$^+$ secretion in the late distal convoluted tubule (or connecting tubule) and cortical collecting duct (CCD) is the principal cell. Virtually all regulation of renal K$^+$ excretion and total body K$^+$ balance occurs in the distal nephron. The driving force for K$^+$ secretion is a favorable electrochemical gradient across the luminal membrane of the principal cell. As a result of the action of the basolateral Na$^+$,K$^+$-ATPase pump, the intracellular K$^+$ concentration far exceeds that of the fluid in the lumen of the CCD. The electrical gradient is created by electrogenic Na$^+$ reabsorption leading to a lumen-negative transepithelial potential difference (TEPD), favoring K$^+$ secretion. The generation of a lumen-negative TEPD depends on the relative rates of reabsorption of Na$^+$ and its accompanying anion (primarily Cl$^-$). Equimolar reabsorption of Na$^+$ and Cl$^-$ at equivalent rates is electroneutral, whereas reabsorption of Na$^+$ in excess of Cl$^-$ is electrogenic. The cellular uptake of Na$^+$ by the principal cell occurs via an apical Na$^+$ channel and is driven by a low intracellular Na$^+$ concentration relative to that in the lumen of the CCD. The mechanism and regulation of distal nephron Cl$^-$ transport is less clear. Obviously, factors that impact on either Na$^+$ or Cl$^-$ reabsorption by the principal cell will influence the TEPD. Potassium secretion is regulated by two physiologic stimuli—aldosterone and hyperkalemia. Aldosterone is secreted by the zona glomerulosa cells of the adrenal cortex in response to high renin and angiotensin II or hyperkalemia. The actions of aldosterone on the principal cell include enhanced apical membrane Na$^+$ conductivity, stimulation of the basolateral Na$^+$,K$^+$-ATPase, and increased luminal K$^+$ channels. The plasma K$^+$ concentration, independent of aldosterone, can directly affect K$^+$ secretion. In addition to the K$^+$ concentration in the lumen of the CCD, renal K$^+$ loss depends on the urine flow rate, a function of daily solute excretion (see above). Since excretion is equal to the product of concentration and volume, increased distal flow rate can significantly enhance urinary K$^+$ output. Finally, in severe K$^+$ depletion, secretion of K$^+$ is reduced and reabsorption, via apical H$^+$,K$^+$-ATPase pumps in cortical and medullary collecting ducts, is upregulated.

HYPOKALEMIA

ETIOLOGY (See Table 49-3) Hypokalemia, defined as a plasma K$^+$ concentration less than 3.5 mmol/L, may result from one (or more) of the following: decreased net intake, shift into cells, or increased net loss. Diminished intake is seldom the sole cause of K$^+$ depletion since urinary excretion can be effectively decreased to less than 15 mmol/d as a result of net K$^+$ reabsorption in the distal nephron. With the exception of the urban poor and certain cultural groups, the amount of K$^+$ in the diet almost always exceeds that excreted in the urine. However, dietary K$^+$ restriction may exacerbate the hypokalemia secondary to increased gastrointestinal or renal loss. An unusual cause of decreased K$^+$ intake is ingestion of clay (geophagia), which binds dietary K$^+$ and iron. This custom was previously common among African-Americans in the American South.

Movement of K$^+$ into cells may transiently decrease the plasma K$^+$ concentration without altering total body K$^+$ content. For any

Table 49-3

Causes of Hypokalemia

I. Decreased intake
  A. Starvation
  B. Clay ingestion
II. Redistribution into cells
  A. Acid-base
    1. Metabolic alkalosis
  B. Hormonal
    1. Insulin
    2. Beta$_2$-adrenergic agonists (endogenous or exogenous)
    3. Alpha-adrenergic antagonists
  C. Anabolic state
    1. Vitamin B$_{12}$ or folic acid (red blood cell production)
    2. Granulocyte-macrophage colony stimulating factor (white blood cell production)
    3. Total parenteral nutrition
  D. Other
    1. Pseudohypokalemia
    2. Hypothermia
    3. Hypokalemic periodic paralysis
    4. Barium toxicity
III. Increased loss
  A. Nonrenal
    1. Gastrointestinal loss (diarrhea)
    2. Integumentary loss (sweat)
  B. Renal
    1. Increased distal flow: diuretics, osmotic diuresis, salt-wasting nephropathies
    2. Increased secretion of potassium
      a. Mineralocorticoid excess: primary hyperaldosteronism, secondary hyperaldosteronism (malignant hypertension, renin-secreting tumors, renal artery stenosis, hypovolemia), apparent mineralocorticoid excess (licorice, chewing tobacco, carbenoxolone), congenital adrenal hyperplasia, Cushing's syndrome, Bartter's syndrome
      b. Distal delivery of non-reabsorbed anions: vomiting, nasogastric suction, proximal (type 2) renal tubular acidosis, diabetic ketoacidosis, glue-sniffing (toluene abuse), penicillin derivatives
      c. Other: amphotericin B, Liddle's syndrome, hypomagnesemia

given cause, the magnitude of the change is relatively small, often less than 1 mmol/L. However, a combination of factors may lead to a significant fall in the plasma K^+ concentration and may amplify the hypokalemia due to K^+ wasting. Alkalosis, especially that due to a primary increase in plasma HCO_3^- (metabolic alkalosis), is often associated with hypokalemia. This occurs as a result of K^+ redistribution as well as excessive renal or gastrointestinal K^+ loss. Treatment of diabetic ketoacidosis with insulin may lead to hypokalemia due to stimulation of the Na^+-H^+ antiporter and (secondarily) the Na^+,K^+-ATPase pump. Furthermore, uncontrolled hyperglycemia often leads to K^+ depletion from an osmotic diuresis (see below). Stress-induced catecholamine release and administration of beta$_2$-adrenergic agonists directly induce cellular uptake of K^+ and promote insulin secretion by pancreatic islet β cells. *Hypokalemic periodic paralysis* is a rare condition characterized by recurrent episodic weakness or paralysis (Chap. 383). Since K^+ is the major ICF cation, anabolic states can potentially result in hypokalemia due to a K^+ shift into cells. This may occur following rapid cell growth seen in patients with pernicious anemia treated with vitamin B_{12} or with neutropenia after treatment with granulocyte-macrophage colony stimulating factor. Massive transfusion with thawed washed red blood cells (RBCs) could cause hypokalemia since frozen RBCs lose up to half of their K^+ during storage.

Excessive sweating may result in K^+ depletion from increased integumentary and renal K^+ loss. Hyperaldosteronism, secondary to ECF volume contraction, enhances K^+ excretion in the urine (Chap. 332). Normally, K^+ lost in the stool amounts to 5 to 10 mmol/d in a volume of 100 to 200 mL. Hypokalemia subsequent to increased gastrointestinal loss can occur in patients with profuse diarrhea (usually secretory), villous adenomas, VIPomas, or laxative abuse. However, the loss of gastric secretions does not account for the moderate to severe K^+ depletion often associated with vomiting of nasogastric suction. Since the K^+ concentration of gastric fluid is 5 to 10 mmol/L, it would take 30 to 80 L of vomitus to achieve a K^+ deficit of 300 to 400 mmol typically seen in these patients. In fact, the hypokalemia is primarily due to increased renal K^+ excretion. Loss of gastric contents results in volume depletion and metabolic alkalosis, both of which promote kaliuresis. Hypovolemia stimulates aldosterone release, which augments K^+ secretion by the principal cells. In addition, the filtered load of HCO_3^- exceeds the reabsorptive capacity of the proximal convoluted tubule, thereby increasing distal delivery of $NaHCO_3$ which enhances the electrochemical gradient favoring K^+ loss in the urine.

In general, most cases of chronic hypokalemia are due to renal K^+ wasting. This may be due to factors that increase the K^+ concentration in the lumen of the CCD or augment distal flow rate. As described above, distal nephron K^+ secretion is driven by a lumen-negative TEPD, affected by aldosterone and the relative rates of reabsorption of Na^+ and its accompanying anion(s). Mineralocorticoid excess commonly results in hypokalemia (Chap. 332). *Primary hyperaldosteronism* is due to dysregulated aldosterone secretion by an adrenal adenoma (Conn's syndrome) or carcinoma or to adrenocortical hyperplasia. In a rare subset of patients, the disorder is familial (autosomal dominant) and aldosterone levels can be suppressed by administering low doses of exogenous glucocorticoid. The molecular defect responsible for *glucocorticoid-remediable hyperaldosteronism* is a rearranged gene (due to a chromosomal crossover), containing the 5′-regulatory region of the 11β-hydroxylase gene and the coding sequence of the aldosterone synthase gene. Consequently, mineralocorticoid is synthesized in the zona fasciculata and regulated by corticotropin. A number of conditions associated with hyperreninemia result in secondary hyperaldosteronism and renal K^+ wasting. High renin levels are commonly seen in both renovascular and malignant hypertension. Renin-secreting tumors of the juxtaglomerular apparatus are a rare cause of hypokalemia. Other tumors that have been reported to produce renin include renal cell carcinoma, ovarian carcinoma, and Wilms' tumor. Hyperreninemia may also occur secondary to decreased effective circulating arterial volume.

In the absence of elevated renin or aldosterone levels, enhanced distal nephron secretion of K^+ may result from increased production of non-aldosterone mineralocorticoids in *congenital adrenal hyperplasia* (Chap. 332). Glucocorticoid-stimulated kaliuresis does not normally occur due to the conversion of cortisol to cortisone by 11β-hydroxysteroid dehydrogenase (11β-HSDH). Therefore, 11β-HSDH deficiency or suppression allows cortisol to bind to the aldosterone receptor and leads to the *syndrome of apparent mineralocorticoid excess*. Drugs that inhibit the activity of 11β-HSDH include glycyrrhetinic acid, present in licorice, chewing tobacco, and carbenoxolone. The presentation of Cushing's syndrome may include hypokalemia if the capacity of 11β-HSDH to inactivate cortisol is overwhelmed by persistently elevated glucocorticoid levels.

Liddle's Syndrome This is a rare familial (autosomal dominant) disease characterized by hypertension, hypokalemic metabolic alkalosis, renal K^+ wasting, and suppressed renin and aldosterone secretion (Chap. 332). This condition is caused by mutations in the β subunit of the principal cell apical Na^+ channel, resulting in increased conductivity. Appropriate therapy includes Na^+ restriction and treatment with amiloride, a specific inhibitor of the CCD luminal Na^+ channel. Increased distal delivery of Na^+ with a non-reabsorbable anion (not Cl^-) enhances the lumen-negative TEPD and K^+ secretion. Classically, this is seen with *proximal (type 2) renal tubular acidosis* (RTA) and vomiting, associated with bicarbonaturia. Diabetic ketoacidosis and toluene abuse (glue-sniffing) can lead to increased delivery of β-hydroxybutyrate and hippurate, respectively, to the CCD and to renal K^+ loss. High doses of penicillin derivatives administered to volume-depleted patients may likewise promote renal K^+ secretion as well as an osmotic diuresis. *Classic distal (type 1) RTA* is associated with hypokalemia due to increased renal K^+ loss, the mechanism of which is uncertain. Amphotericin B causes hypokalemia due to increased distal nephron permeability to Na^+ and K^+ and to renal K^+ wasting.

Bartter's Syndrome This is a disorder characterized by hypokalemia, metabolic alkalosis, hyperreninemic hyperaldosteronism secondary to ECF volume contraction, and juxtaglomerular apparatus hyperplasia (Chap. 332). The blood pressure is usually normal, and hypomagnesemia is often present as a result of renal Mg^{2+} wasting. The pathophysiology of Bartter's syndrome has yet to be elucidated. Proposed mechanisms include a defect in the Na^+-K^+-$2Cl^-$ cotransporter of the thick ascending limb of the loop of Henle, impaired distal Cl^- reabsorption, and excessive renal prostaglandin synthesis. Hypokalemia refractory to K^+ repletion is suggestive of Mg^{2+} depletion. Although the pathogenesis is unclear, hypomagnesemia may stimulate aldosterone secretion or decrease distal Cl^- transport. Finally, diuretic use and abuse are common causes of K^+ depletion. Carbonic anhydrase inhibitors, loop diuretics, and thiazides are all kaliuretic. The degree of hypokalemia tends to be greater with long-acting agents and is dose-dependent. Increased renal K^+ excretion is due primarily to increased distal solute delivery and secondary hyperaldosteronism (due to volume depletion).

CLINICAL FEATURES The clinical manifestations of K^+ depletion vary greatly between individual patients, and their severity depends on the degree of hypokalemia. Symptoms seldom occur unless the plasma K^+ concentration is less than 3 mmol/L. Fatigue, myalgia, and muscular weakness of the lower extremities are common complaints and are due to a lower (more negative) resting membrane potential. More severe hypokalemia may lead to progressive weakness, hypoventilation (due to respiratory muscle involvement), and eventually complete paralysis. Impaired muscle metabolism and the blunted hyperemic response to exercise associated with profound K^+ depletion increase the risk of rhabdomyolysis. Smooth-muscle function may also be affected and manifest as paralytic ileus.

The electrocardiographic changes of hypokalemia (Fig. 228-19) are due to delayed ventricular repolarization and do not correlate well with the plasma K^+ concentration. Early changes include flattening or inversion of the T wave, a prominent U wave, ST-segment depression, and a prolonged QU interval. Severe K^+ depletion may result in a prolonged PR interval, decreased voltage and widening of the QRS complex, and an increased risk of ventricular arrhythmias, especially in patients with myocardial ischemia or left ventricular hypertrophy. Hypokalemia may also predispose to digitalis toxicity. Epidemiologic studies have linked a low-K$^+$ diet with an increased prevalence of hypertension, particularly among African-Americans. Furthermore, in patients with essential hypertension, systemic blood pressure may be lowered by K$^+$ supplementation. The mechanism of the hypertensive effect of K$^+$ depletion is not certain but may relate to enhanced distal NaCl reabsorption.

Hypokalemia is often associated with acid-base disturbances related to the underlying disorder. In addition, K$^+$ depletion results in intracellular acidification and an increase in net acid excretion or new HCO$_3^-$ production. This is a consequence of enhanced proximal HCO$_3^-$ reabsorption, increased renal ammoniagenesis, and increased distal H$^+$ secretion. This contributes to the generation of metabolic alkalosis frequently present in hypokalemic patients. Nephrogenic diabetes insipidus (see above) is not uncommonly seen in K$^+$ depletion and is manifest as polydipsia and polyuria. Glucose intolerance may also occur with hypokalemia and has been attributed to either impaired insulin secretion or peripheral insulin resistance.

DIAGNOSIS In most cases, the etiology of K$^+$ depletion can be determined by a careful history. Diuretic and laxative abuse as well as surreptitious vomiting may be difficult to identify but should be excluded. Rarely, patients with a marked leukocytosis (e.g., acute myeloid leukemia) and normokalemia may have a low measured plasma K$^+$ concentration due to white blood cell uptake of K$^+$ at room temperature. This *pseudohypokalemia* can be avoided by storing the blood sample on ice or rapidly separating the plasma (or serum) from the cells. After eliminating decreased intake and intracellular shift as potential causes of hypokalemia, examination of the renal response can help to clarify the source of K$^+$ loss. The appropriate response to K$^+$ depletion is to excrete less than 15 mmol/d of K$^+$ in the urine, due to increased reabsorption and decreased distal secretion. Hypokalemia with minimal renal K$^+$ excretion suggests that K$^+$ was lost via the skin or gastrointestinal tract or that there is a remote history of vomiting or diuretic use. As described above, renal K$^+$ wasting may be due to factors that either increase the K$^+$ concentration in the CCD or increase the distal flow rate (or both). The ECF volume status, blood pressure, and associated acid-base disorder may help to differentiate the causes of excessive renal K$^+$ loss. A rapid and simple test designed to evaluate the driving force for net K$^+$ secretion is the *transtubular K$^+$ concentration gradient* (TTKG). The TTKG is the ratio of the K$^+$ concentration in the lumen of the CCD ([K$^+$]$_{CCD}$) to that in peritubular capillaries or plasma ([K$^+$]$_P$). The validity of this measurement depends on three assumptions: (1) few solutes are reabsorbed in the medullary collecting duct (MCD), (2) K$^+$ is neither secreted nor reabsorbed in the MCD, and (3) the osmolality of the fluid in the terminal CCD is known. In most situations, reabsorption of Na$^+$ salts in the MCD will have a small effect on the TTKG. Significant reabsorption or secretion of K$^+$ in the MCD seldom occurs, except in profound K$^+$ depletion or excess, respectively. When AVP is acting, the osmolality in the terminal CCD is the same as that of plasma, and the K$^+$ concentration in the lumen of the distal nephron can be estimated by dividing the urine K$^+$ concentration ([K$^+$]$_U$) by the ratio of the urine to plasma osmolality (OSM$_U$/OSM$_P$):

$$[K^+]_{CCD} = [K^+]_U \div (OSM_U/OSM_P)$$

$$TTKG = [K^+]_{CCD} \div [K^+]_P = \frac{[K^+]_U \div (OSM_U/OSM_P)}{[K^+]_P}$$

The urine osmolality must exceed that of plasma in order to calculate the TTKG. There is no normal range of values for the TTKG since it is dependent on the state of total body K$^+$ balance. Hypokalemia with a TTKG greater than 4 suggests renal K$^+$ loss due to increased distal K$^+$ secretion. Plasma renin and aldosterone levels are often helpful in differentiating the various causes of hyperaldosteronism.

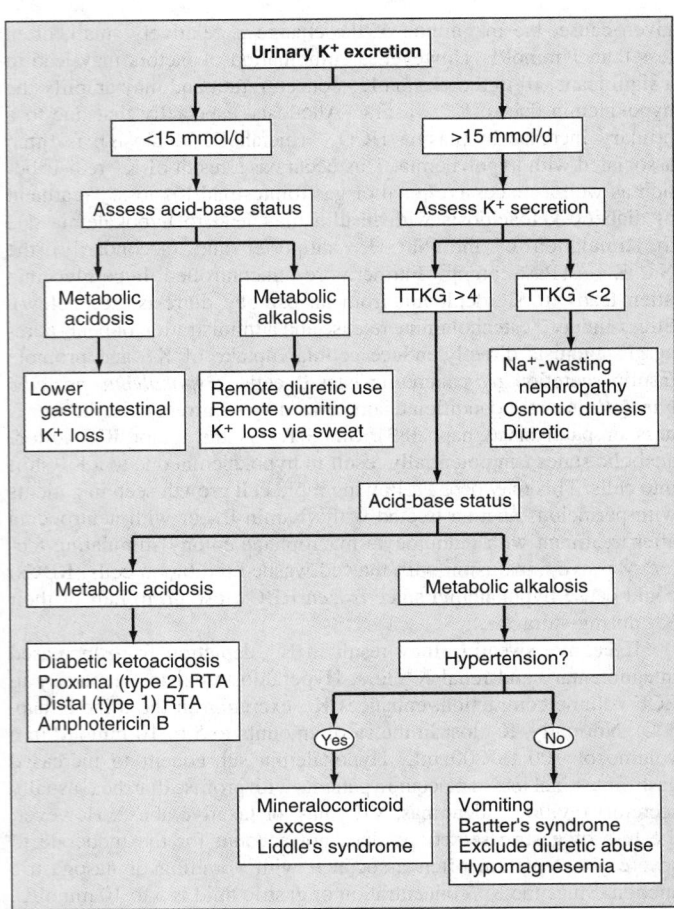

FIGURE 49-3 Algorithm depicting clinical approach to hypokalemia. RTA, renal tubular acidosis; TTKG, transtubular K$^+$ concentration gradient.

Bicarbonaturia and the presence of other non-reabsorbed anions also increase the TTKG and lead to renal K$^+$-wasting.

CLINICAL APPROACH See Fig. 49-3.

℞ **TREATMENT**

The therapeutic goals are to correct the K$^+$ deficit and to minimize ongoing losses. With the exception of periodic paralysis, hypokalemia resulting from transcellular shifts rarely requires intravenous K$^+$ supplementation, which can lead to rebound hyperkalemia. It is generally safer to correct hypokalemia via the oral route. The degree of K$^+$ depletion does not correlate well with the plasma K$^+$ concentration. A decrement of 1 mmol/L in the plasma K$^+$ concentration (from 4.0 to 3.0 mmol/L) may represent a total body K$^+$ deficit of 200 to 400 mmol, and patients with plasma levels under 3.0 mmol/L often require in excess of 600 mmol of K$^+$ to correct the deficit. Furthermore, factors promoting K$^+$ shift out of cells (e.g., insulin deficiency in diabetic ketoacidosis) may result in underestimation of the K$^+$ deficit. Therefore, the plasma K$^+$ concentration should be monitored frequently when assessing the response to treatment. Potassium chloride is usually the preparation of choice and will promote more rapid correction of hypokalemia and metabolic alkalosis. Potassium bicarbonate and citrate (metabolized to HCO$_3^-$) tend to alkalinize the patient and would be more appropriate for hypokalemia associated with chronic diarrhea or RTA.

Patients with severe hypokalemia or those unable to take anything by mouth require intravenous replacement therapy with KCl. The maximum concentration of administered K$^+$ should be no more than 40 mmol/L via a peripheral vein or 60 mmol/L via a central vein. The rate of infusion should not exceed 20 mmol/h unless paralysis or malignant ventricular arrhythmias are present. Ideally, KCl should be mixed in normal saline since dextrose solutions may initially exacerbate hypokalemia due to insulin-mediated movement of K^+ into cells. Rapid intravenous administration of K^+ should be used judiciously and requires close observation of the clinical manifestations of hypokalemia (electrocardiogram and neuromuscular examination).

HYPERKALEMIA

ETIOLOGY Hyperkalemia, defined as a plasma K^+ concentration greater than 5.0 mmol/L, occurs as a result of either K^+ release from cells or decreased renal loss. Increased K^+ intake is rarely the sole cause of hyperkalemia since the phenomenon of *potassium adaptation* ensures rapid K^+ excretion in response to increases in dietary consumption. Iatrogenic hyperkalemia may result from overzealous parenteral K^+ replacement or in patients with renal insufficiency. *Pseudohyperkalemia* represents an artificially elevated plasma K^+ concentration due to K^+ movement out of cells immediately prior to or following venipuncture. Contributing factors include prolonged use of a tourniquet with or without repeated fist clenching, hemolysis, and marked leukocytosis or thrombocytosis. The latter two result in an elevated serum K^+ concentration due to release of intracellular K^+ following clot formation. Pseudohyperkalemia should be suspected in an otherwise asymptomatic patient with no obvious underlying cause. If proper venipuncture technique is used and a plasma (not serum) K^+ concentration is measured, it should be normal. Intravascular hemolysis, tumor lysis syndrome, and rhabdomyolysis all lead to K^+ release from cells as a result of tissue breakdown. Metabolic acidoses, with the exception of those due to the accumulation of organic anions, can be associated with mild hyperkalemia resulting from intracellular buffering of H^+ (see above). As previously described (p. 271), insulin deficiency and hypertonicity (e.g., hyperglycemia) promote K^+ shift from the ICF to the ECF. The severity of exercise-induced hyperkalemia is related to the degree of exertion. It is due to release of K^+ from muscles and is usually rapidly reversible, often associated with rebound hypokalemia. Treatment with beta blockers rarely causes hyperkalemia but may contribute to the elevation in plasma K^+ concentration seen with other conditions. *Hyperkalemic periodic paralysis* (Chap. 383) is a rare autosomal dominant disorder characterized by episodic weakness or paralysis, precipitated by stimuli that normally lead to mild hyperkalemia (e.g., exercise). The genetic defect appears to be a single amino acid substitution due to a mutation in the gene for the skeletal muscle Na^+ channel. Hyperkalemia may occur with severe digitalis toxicity due to inhibition of the Na^+,K^+-ATPase pump. Depolarizing muscle relaxants such as succinylcholine can increase the plasma K^+ concentration, especially in patients with massive trauma, burns, or neuromuscular disease.

Chronic hyperkalemia is virtually always associated with decreased renal K^+ excretion due to either impaired secretion or diminished distal solute delivery (Table 49-4). The latter is seldom the only cause of impaired K^+ excretion but may significantly contribute to hyperkalemia in protein-malnourished (low urea excretion) and ECF

Table 49-4

Causes of Hyperkalemia

I. Renal failure
II. Decreased distal flow (i.e., decreased effective circulating arterial volume)
III. Decreased K^+ secretion
   A. Impaired Na^+ reabsorption
      1. Primary hypoaldosteronism: adrenal insufficiency, adrenal enzyme deficiency (21-hydroxylase, 3β-hydroxysteroid dehydrogenase, corticosterone methyl oxidase)
      2. Secondary hypoaldosteronism: hyporeninemia, drugs ACE inhibitors, NSAIDs, heparin)
      3. Resistance to aldosterone: pseudohypoaldosteronism, tubulointerstitial disease, drugs (K^+-sparing diuretics, trimethoprim, pentamidine)
   B. Enhanced Cl^- reabsorption (chloride shunt)
      1. Gordon's syndrome
      2. Cyclosporine

volume–contracted (decreased distal NaCl delivery) patients. Decreased K^+ secretion by the principal cells results from either impaired Na^+ reabsorption or increased Cl^- reabsorption, both of which give rise to a diminished (less lumen-negative) TEPD in the CCD. *Hyporeninemic hypoaldosteronism* is a syndrome characterized by euvolemia or ECF volume expansion and suppressed renin and aldosterone levels (Chaps. 332 and 334). This disorder is commonly seen in mild renal insufficiency, diabetic nephropathy, or chronic tubulointerstitial disease. Patients frequently have an impaired kaliuretic response to exogenous mineralocorticoid administration, suggesting that enhanced distal Cl^- reabsorption (electroneutral Na^+ reabsorption) may account for many of the findings of hyporeninemic hypoaldosteronism. NSAIDs inhibit renin secretion and the synthesis of vasodilatory renal prostaglandins. The resultant decrease in GFR and K^+ secretion is often manifest as hyperkalemia. As a rule, the degree of hyperkalemia due to hypoaldosteronism is mild in the absence of increased K^+ intake or renal dysfunction. Angiotensin-converting enzyme (ACE) inhibitors block the conversion of angiotensin I to angiotensin II, resulting in impaired aldosterone release. Patients at increased risk of ACE inhibitor–induced hyperkalemia include those with diabetes mellitus, renal insufficiency, decreased effective circulating arterial volume, bilateral renal artery stenosis, or concurrent use of K^+-sparing diuretics or NSAIDs.

Decreased aldosterone synthesis may be due to *primary adrenal insufficiency* (Addison's disease) or congenital adrenal enzyme deficiency (Chap. 332). Heparin (including low-molecular-weight heparin) inhibits production of aldosterone by the cells of the zona glomerulosa and can lead to severe hyperkalemia in a subset of patients with underlying renal disease; diabetes mellitus; or those receiving K^+-sparing diuretics, ACE inhibitors, or NSAIDs. *Pseudohypoaldosteronism* is a rare familial disorder characterized by hyperkalemia, metabolic acidosis, renal Na^+ wasting, hypotension, high renin and aldosterone levels, and end-organ resistance to aldosterone. The gene encoding the mineralocorticoid receptor is normal in these patients, and the electrolyte abnormalities can be reversed with suprapharmacologic doses of an exogenous mineralocorticoid (e.g., 9α-fludrocortisone) or an inhibitor of 11β-HSDH (e.g., carbenoxolone). The kaliuretic response to aldosterone is impaired by K^+-sparing diuretics. Spironolactone is a competitive mineralocorticoid antagonist, whereas amiloride and triamterene block the apical Na^+ channel of the principal cell. Two other drugs that impair K^+ secretion by blocking distal nephron Na^+ reabsorption are trimethoprim and pentamidine. These antimicrobial agents may contribute to the hyperkalemia often seen in patients infected with human immunodeficiency virus who are being treated for *Pneumocystis carinii* pneumonia.

Hyperkalemia frequently complicates acute oliguric renal failure due to increased K^+ release from cells (acidosis, catabolism) and decreased excretion. Increased distal flow rate and K^+ secretion per nephron compensate for decreased renal mass in chronic renal insufficiency. However, these adaptive mechanisms eventually fail to maintain K^+ balance when the GFR falls below 10 to 15 mL/min or oliguria ensues. Otherwise asymptomatic urinary tract obstruction is an often overlooked cause of hyperkalemia. Other nephropathies associated with impaired K^+ excretion include drug-induced interstitial nephritis, lupus nephritis, sickle cell disease, and diabetic nephropathy.

Gordon's Syndrome This is a rare condition characterized by hyperkalemia, metabolic acidosis, and a normal GFR. These patients are usually volume-expanded with suppressed renin and aldosterone levels as well as refractory to the kaliuretic effect of exogenous mineralocorticoids. It has been suggested that these findings can all be accounted for by increased distal Cl^- reabsorption (electroneutral Na^+ reabsorption), also referred to as a *Cl shunt*. A similar mechanism may be partially responsible for the hyperkalemia associated with cyclosporine nephrotoxicity. *Hyperkalemic distal (type 4) RTA* may be due to either hypoaldosteronism or a Cl^- shunt (aldosterone-resistant).

CLINICAL FEATURES Since the resting membrane potential is related to the ratio of the ICF to ECF K^+ concentration, hyperkalemia partially depolarizes the cell membrane. Prolonged depolarization impairs membrane excitability and is manifest as weakness, which may progress to flaccid paralysis and hypoventilation if the respiratory muscles are involved. Hyperkalemia also inhibits renal ammoniagenesis and reabsorption of NH_4^+ in the thick ascending limb of the loop of Henle. Thus, net acid excretion is impaired and results in metabolic acidosis, which may further exacerbate the hyperkalemia due to K^+ movement out of cells.

The most serious effect of hyperkalemia is cardiac toxicity, which does not correlate well with the plasma K^+ concentration. The earliest electrocardiographic changes include increased T-wave amplitude, or peaked T waves. More severe degrees of hyperkalemia result in a prolonged PR interval and QRS duration, atrioventricular conduction delay, and loss of P waves. Progressive widening of the QRS complex and merging with the T wave produces a sinewave pattern. The terminal event is usually ventricular fibrillation or asystole.

DIAGNOSIS   With rare exceptions, chronic hyperkalemia is always due to impaired K^+ excretion. If the etiology is not readily apparent and the patient is asymptomatic, pseudohyperkalemia should be excluded, as described above. Oliguric acute renal failure and severe chronic renal insufficiency should also be ruled out. The history should focus on medications that impair K^+ handling and potential sources of K^+ intake. Evaluation of the ECF compartment, effective circulating volume, and urine output are essential components of the physical examination. The severity of hyperkalemia is determined by the symptoms, plasma K^+ concentration, and electrocardiographic abnormalities.

The appropriate renal response to hyperkalemia is to excrete at least 200 mmol of K^+ daily. In most cases, diminished renal K^+ loss is due to impaired K^+ secretion, which can be assessed by measuring the TTKG (see above). A TTKG of less than 10 implies a decreased driving force for K^+ secretion due to either hypoaldosteronism or

resistance to the renal effects of mineralocorticoid. This can be determined by evaluating the kaliuretic response to administration of mineralocorticoid (e.g., 9α-fludrocortisone). Primary adrenal insufficiency can be differentiated from hyporeninemic hypoaldosteronism by examining the renin-aldosterone axis. Renin and aldosterone levels should be measured in the supine and upright positions, following three days of Na^+ restriction (Na^+ intake less than 10 mmol/d) in combination with a loop diuretic to induce mild volume contraction. Aldosterone-resistant hyperkalemia can result from the various causes of impaired distal Na^+ reabsorption or from a Cl^- shunt. The former leads to salt wasting, ECF volume contraction, and high renin and aldosterone levels. In contrast, enhanced distal Cl^- reabsorption is associated with volume expansion and suppressed renin and aldosterone secretion. As mentioned above, hypoaldosteronism seldom causes severe hypokalemia in the absence of increased dietary K^+ intake, renal insufficiency, transcellular K^+ shifts, or antikaliuretic drugs.

CLINICAL APPROACH   See Fig. 49-4.

℞ **TREATMENT**

The approach to therapy depends on the degree of hyperkalemia as determined by the plasma K^+ concentration, associated muscular weakness, and changes on the electrocardiogram. Potentially fatal hyperkalemia rarely occurs unless the plasma K^+ concentration exceeds 7.5 mmol/L and is usually associated with profound weakness and absent P waves, QRS widening, or ventricular arrhythmias on the electrocardiogram.

Severe hyperkalemia requires emergent treatment directed at minimizing membrane depolarization, shifting K^+ into cells, and promoting K^+ loss. In addition, exogenous K^+ intake and antikaliuretic drugs should be discontinued. Administration of calcium gluconate decreases membrane excitability. The usual dose is 10 mL of a 10% solution infused over 2 to 3 min. The effect begins within minutes but is short-lived (30 to 60 min), and the dose can be repeated if no change in the electrocardiogram is seen after 5 to 10 min. Insulin causes K^+ to shift into cells by mechanisms described previously and will temporarily lower the plasma K^+ concentration. Although glucose alone will stimulate insulin release from normal pancreatic β cells, a more rapid response generally occurs when exogenous insulin is administered (with glucose to prevent hypoglycemia). A commonly recommended combination is 10 to 20 units of regular insulin and 25 to 50 g of glucose. Obviously, hyperglycemic patients should not be given glucose. If effective, the plasma K^+ concentration will fall by 0.5 to 1.5 mmol/L in 15 to 30 min and the effect will last for several hours. Alkali therapy with intravenous $NaHCO_3$ can also shift K^+ into cells. This is safest when administered as an isotonic solution of 3 ampules per liter (134 mmol/L $NaHCO_3$) and ideally should be reserved for severe hyperkalemia associated with metabolic acidosis. Patients with end-stage renal disease seldom respond to this intervention and may not tolerate the Na^+ load and resultant volume expansion. When administered parenterally or in nebulized form, beta$_2$-adrenergic agonists promote cellular uptake of K^+ (see above). The onset of action is 30 min, lowering the plasma K^+ concentration by 0.5 to 1.5 mmol/L, and the effect lasts 2 to 4 h.

Removal of K^+ can be achieved using diuretics, cation-exchange resin, or dialysis. Loop and thiazide diuretics, often in combination, may enhance K^+ excretion if renal function is adequate. Sodium polystyrene sulfonate is a cation-exchange resin that promotes the exchange of Na^+ for K^+ in the gastrointestinal tract. Each gram binds 1 mmol of K^+ and releases 2 to 3 mmol of Na^+. When given by mouth, the usual dose is 25 to 50 g mixed with 100 mL of 20% sorbitol to prevent constipation. This will generally lower the plasma K^+ concentration by 0.5 to 1.0 mmol/L within 1 to 2 h and last for 4 to 6 h. Sodium polystyrene sulfonate can also be administered as a retention enema consisting of 50 g of resin and 50 mL of 70% sorbitol mixed in 150 mL of tap water. The sorbitol should be omitted from the enema in postoperative patients due to the increased incidence of sorbitol-induced colonic necrosis, especially following renal transplantation. The most rapid and effective way of lowering the plasma K^+ concentration is hemodialysis. This should be re-

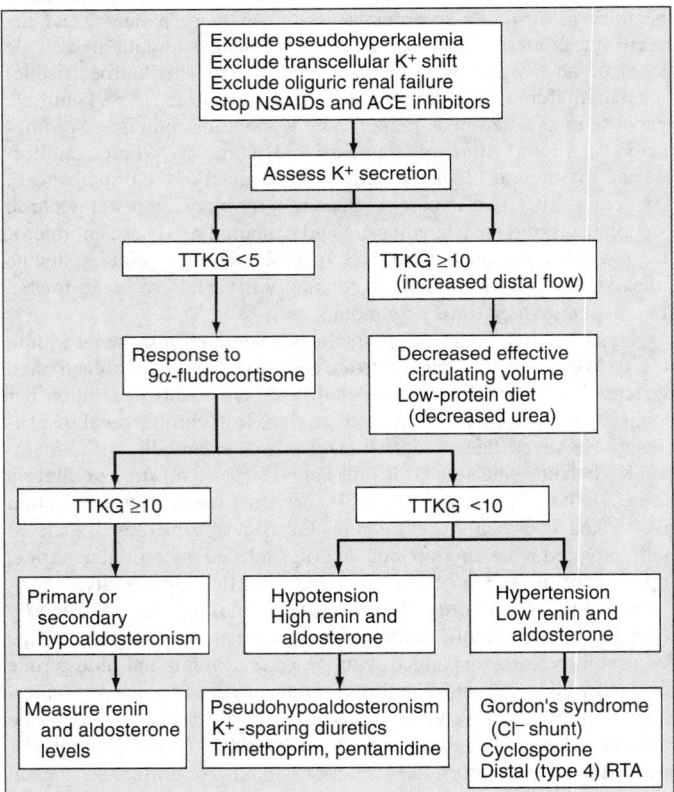

FIGURE 49-4   Algorithm depicting clinical approach to hyperkalemia. NSAID, nonsteroidal antiinflammatory drug; ACE, angiotensin converting enzyme; RTA, renal tubular acidosis; TTKG, transtubular K concentration gradient.

served for patients with renal failure and those with severe life-threatening hyperkalemia unresponsive to more conservative measures. Peritoneal dialysis also removes K^+ but is only 15 to 20 percent as effective as hemodialysis. Finally, the underlying cause of the hyperkalemia should be treated. This may involve dietary modification, correction of metabolic acidosis, cautious volume expansion, and administration of exogenous mineralocorticoid.

BIBLIOGRAPHY

WATER AND SODIUM

ABRAHAM WT, SCHRIER RW: Body fluid volume regulation in health and disease. Adv Intern Med 39:23, 1994

FUJIWARA TM et al: Molecular biology of diabetes insipidus. Ann Rev Med 46:331, 1995

GINES P et al: Vasopressin in pathophysiological states. Semin Nephrol 14:384, 1994

GULLANS SR, VERBALIS JG: Control of brain volume during hyperosmolar and hypoosmolar conditions. Ann Rev Med 44:289, 1993

KOVACS L, ROBERTSON GL: Syndrome of inappropriate antidiuretics. Endocrinol Metabol Clin North Am 21:859, 1992

NARINS RG, RILEY LJ: Polyuria: Simple and mixed disorders. Am J Kidney Dis 17:237, 1991

ROBERTSON GL: Disorders of thirst in man, in *Thirst: Physiological and Psychological Aspects*, DJ Ramsay, DA Booth (eds). London, Springer-Verlag, 1991, p 453

——, BERL T: Pathophysiology of water metabolism, in *The Kidney*, 5th ed, BM Brenner (ed). Philadelphia, Saunders, 1996, pp 873–928

STERNS RH et al: Neurologic sequelae after treatment of severe hyponatremia: A multicenter perspective. J Am Soc Nephrol 4:1522, 1994

——: Hyponatremia: Pathophysiology, diagnosis, and therapy, in *Clinical Disorders of Fluid and Electrolyte Metabolism*, 5th ed, RG Narins (ed). New York, McGraw-Hill, 1994, pp 583–615

POTASSIUM

BROWN RS: Extrarenal potassium homeostasis. Kidney Int 30:116, 1986

DEFRONZO RA, SMITH JD: Clinical disorders of hyperkalemia, in *Clinical Disorders of Fluid and Electrolyte Metabolism*, 5th ed, RG Narins (ed). New York, McGraw-Hill, 1994, pp 697–754

FIELD MJ et al: Regulation of renal potassium metabolism, in *Clinical Disorders of Fluid and Electrolyte Metabolism*, 5th ed, RG Narins (ed). New York, McGraw-Hill, 1994, pp 147–174

KAMEL KS et al: Disorders of potassium homeostasis: An approach based on pathophysiology. Am J Kidney Dis 24:597, 1994

—— et al: Disorders of potassium balance, in *The Kidney*, 5th ed, BM Brenner (ed). Philadelphia, Saunders, 1996, pp 999–1037

KNOCHEL JP: Neuromuscular manifestations of electrolyte disorders. Am J Med 72:521, 1982

KUPIN WL, NARINS RG: The hyperkalemia of renal failure: Pathophysiology, diagnosis, and therapy. Contrib Nephrol 102:1, 1993

STEIN JH: The pathogenetic spectrum of Bartter's syndrome. Kidney Int 28:85, 1985

TANNEN RL: Diuretic-induced hypokalemia. Kidney Int 28:988, 1985

WHITE PC: Disorders of aldosterone biosynthesis and action. N Engl J Med 331:250, 1994

| 50 | *Thomas D. DuBose, Jr.* |

ACIDOSIS AND ALKALOSIS

NORMAL ACID-BASE HOMEOSTASIS

Systemic arterial pH is maintained between 7.35 and 7.45 by extracellular and intracellular chemical buffering together with respiratory and renal regulatory mechanisms. The control of arterial CO_2 tension (Pa_{CO_2}) by the central nervous system and respiratory systems and the control of the plasma bicarbonate by the kidneys stabilize the arterial pH by excretion or retention of acid or alkali. The metabolic and respiratory components that regulate systemic pH are described by the Henderson-Hasselbalch equation:

$$pH = 6.1 + \log \frac{[HCO_3^-]}{Pa_{CO_2} \times 0.0301}$$

Under most circumstances, CO_2 production and excretion are matched, and the usual steady-state Pa_{CO_2} is maintained at 40 mmHg. Underexcretion of CO_2 produces hypercapnia, and overexcretion causes hypocapnia. Nevertheless, production and excretion are again matched at a new steady-state Pa_{CO_2}. Therefore, the Pa_{CO_2} is regulated primarily by neural respiratory factors (Chap. 263) and is not subject to regulation by the rate of CO_2 production. Hypercapnia is usually the result of hypoventilation rather than of increased CO_2 production. Increases or decreases in Pa_{CO_2} represent derangements of neural respiratory control or are due to compensatory changes in response to a primary alteration in the plasma $[HCO_3^-]$.

Primary changes in Pa_{CO_2} can cause acidosis or alkalosis, depending on whether Pa_{CO_2} is above or below the normal value of 40 mmHg (respiratory acidosis or alkalosis, respectively). Primary alteration of Pa_{CO_2} evokes cellular buffering and renal adaptation, a slow process that becomes more efficient with time. A *primary* change in the plasma $[HCO_3^-]$ as a result of metabolic or renal factors results in compensatory changes in ventilation that blunt the changes in blood pH that would occur otherwise. Such respiratory alterations are referred to as *secondary*, or compensatory, changes, since they occur in response to primary metabolic changes.

The kidneys regulate plasma $[HCO_3^-]$ through three main processes: (1) "reabsorption" of filtered HCO_3^-, (2) formation of titratable acid, and (3) excretion of NH_4^+ in the urine. The kidney filters approximately 4000 mmol of HCO_3^- per day. To reabsorb the filtered load of HCO_3^-, the renal tubules must therefore secrete 4000 mmol of hydrogen ions. Eighty to ninety percent of HCO_3^- is reabsorbed in the proximal tubule. The distal nephron reabsorbs the remainder and secretes protons, as generated from metabolism, to defend systemic pH. While this quantity of protons, 40 to 60 mmol/d, is small, it must be secreted to prevent chronic positive H^+ balance and metabolic acidosis. This quantity of secreted protons is represented in the urine as titratable acid and NH_4^+. Metabolic acidosis in the face of normal renal function increases NH_4^+ production and excretion. NH_4^+ production and excretion are impaired in chronic renal failure, hyperkalemia, and renal tubular acidosis.

In sum, these regulatory responses, including chemical buffering, the regulation of Pa_{CO_2} by the respiratory system, and of $[HCO_3^-]$ by the kidneys, act in concert to maintain a systemic arterial pH between 7.35 and 7.45.

DIAGNOSIS OF GENERAL TYPES OF DISTURBANCES

The most common clinical disturbances are *simple* acid-base disorders, i.e., metabolic acidosis or alkalosis or respiratory acidosis or alkalosis. Since compensation is not complete, the pH is abnormal in simple disturbances. More complicated clinical situations can give rise to mixed acid-base disturbances.

SIMPLE ACID-BASE DISORDERS Primary respiratory disturbances (primary changes in Pa_{CO_2}) invoke secondary metabolic responses (secondary changes in $[HCO_3^-]$), and primary metabolic disturbances elicit predictable respiratory responses. Physiologic compensation can be predicted from the relationships displayed in Table 50-1. Primary changes in Pa_{CO_2} or $[HCO_3^-]$ alter systemic pH and cause acidosis or alkalosis. To illustrate, metabolic acidosis due to an increase in endogenous acids (e.g., ketoacidosis) lowers extracellular fluid $[HCO_3^-]$ and decreases extracellular pH. As a result, the medullary chemoreceptors are stimulated to increase ventilation and to return the ratio of $[HCO_3^-]$ to Pa_{CO_2} and the subsequent pH toward normal. The degree of respiratory compensation expected in a simple form of metabolic acidosis can be predicted from the relationship: $Pa_{CO_2} = (1.5 \times [HCO_3^-]) + 8$, i.e., the Pa_{CO_2} is expected to decrease 1.25 mmHg for each mmol per liter decrease in $[HCO_3^-]$. Thus, a patient with metabolic acidosis and $[HCO_3^-]$ of 12 mmol/L would be expected to have a Pa_{CO_2} between 24 and 28 mmHg. Values for Pa_{CO_2} below 24

Table 50-1

Prediction of Compensatory Responses in Simple Acid-Base
Disturbances

Disorder	Prediction of Compensation
Metabolic acidosis	$Pa_{CO_2} = (1.5 \times [HCO_3^-]) + 8$
	or
	Pa_{CO_2} will $\downarrow$ 1.25 mmHg per mmol/L $\downarrow$ in $[HCO_3^-]$
Metabolic alkalosis	Pa_{CO_2} will $\uparrow$ 0.75 mmHg per mmol/L $\uparrow$ in $[HCO_3^-]$
	or
	Pa_{CO_2} will $\uparrow$ 6 mmHg per 10-mmol/L $\uparrow$ in $[HCO_3^-]$
	or
	$Pa_{CO_2} = [HCO_3^-] + 15$
Respiratory alkalosis	
Acute	$[HCO_3^-]$ will $\downarrow$ 2 mmol/L per 10-mmHg $\downarrow$ in Pa_{CO_2}
Chronic	$[HCO_3^-]$ will $\downarrow$ 4 mmol/L per 10-mmHg $\downarrow$ in Pa_{CO_2}
Respiratory acidosis	
Acute	$[HCO_3^-]$ will $\uparrow$ 1 mmol/L per 10-mmHg $\uparrow$ in Pa_{CO_2}
Chronic	$[HCO_3^-]$ will $\uparrow$ 4 mmol/L per 10-mmHg $\uparrow$ in Pa_{CO_2}

or greater than 28 mmHg define a mixed disturbance (metabolic acidosis and respiratory alkalosis or metabolic acidosis and respiratory acidosis, respectively). Another way to judge the appropriateness of the response in $[HCO_3^-]$ or Pa_{CO_2} is to use an acid-base nomogram (Fig. 50-1). While the shaded areas of the nomogram show the 95 percent confidence limits for normal compensation in simple disturbances, finding acid-base values within the shaded area does not necessarily rule out a mixed disturbance. Imposition of one disorder over another may result in values lying

within the area of a third. Thus, the nomogram, while convenient, is not a substitute for the equations in Table 50-1.

MIXED ACID-BASE DISORDERS Mixed acid-base disorders—defined as independently coexisting disorders, not merely compensatory responses—are often seen in patients in critical care units. As with simple acid-base disorders, the differential diagnosis associated with each of the mixed disturbances should be considered in light of the clinical context. Mixed respiratory and metabolic acidosis or mixed respiratory and metabolic alkalosis can lead to dangerous extremes of pH. A patient with diabetic ketoacidosis (metabolic acidosis) may develop an independent respiratory problem leading to respiratory acidosis or alkalosis. Patients with underlying pulmonary disease may not respond to metabolic acidosis with an appropriate ventilatory response because of insufficient respiratory reserve. Such imposition of respiratory acidosis on metabolic acidosis can lead to severe acidemia and a poor outcome. When metabolic acidosis and metabolic alkalosis coexist in the same patient, the pH may be normal or near normal. When the pH is normal, an elevated anion gap (see below) denotes the presence of a metabolic acidosis. A diabetic patient with ketoacidosis may have renal dysfunction resulting in simultaneous metabolic acidosis. Patients who have ingested an overdose of drug combinations such as sedatives and salicylates may have mixed disturbances as a result of the acid-base response to the individual drugs (metabolic acidosis mixed with respiratory acidosis or respiratory alkalosis, respectively). Even more complex are triple acid-base disturbances. For example, patients with metabolic acidosis due to alcoholic ketoacidosis may develop metabolic alkalosis due to vomiting and superimposed respiratory alkalosis due to the hyperventilation of hepatic dysfunction or alcohol withdrawal.

DIAGNOSIS OF ACID-BASE DISORDERS Care should be taken when measuring blood gases to obtain the arterial blood sample without using excessive heparin. In the determination of arterial blood gases by the clinical laboratory, both pH and Pa_{CO_2} are measured, and the $[HCO_3^-]$ is calculated from the Henderson-Hasselbalch equation. This calculated value should be compared with the measured $[HCO_3^-]$ (total CO_2) on the electrolyte panel. These two values should agree within 2 mmol/L. If they do not, the values may not have been drawn simultaneously, a laboratory error may be present, or an error could have been made in calculating the $[HCO_3^-]$. After verifying the blood acid-base values, one can then identify the precise acid-base disorder.

The most common causes of acid-base disorders should be kept in mind while probing the history for clues about the etiology. For example, established chronic renal failure is expected to cause a metabolic acidosis, and chronic vomiting frequently causes metabolic alkalosis. Patients with pneumonia, sepsis, or cardiac failure frequently have respiratory alkalosis, and patients with chronic obstructive pulmonary disease or a sedative drug overdose often display a respiratory acidosis. The drug history is important since loop or thiazide diuretics may cause metabolic alkalosis, and the carbonic anhydrase inhibitor, acetazolamide, can result in metabolic acidosis.

Blood for electrolytes and arterial blood gases should be drawn simultaneously prior to therapy, since an increase

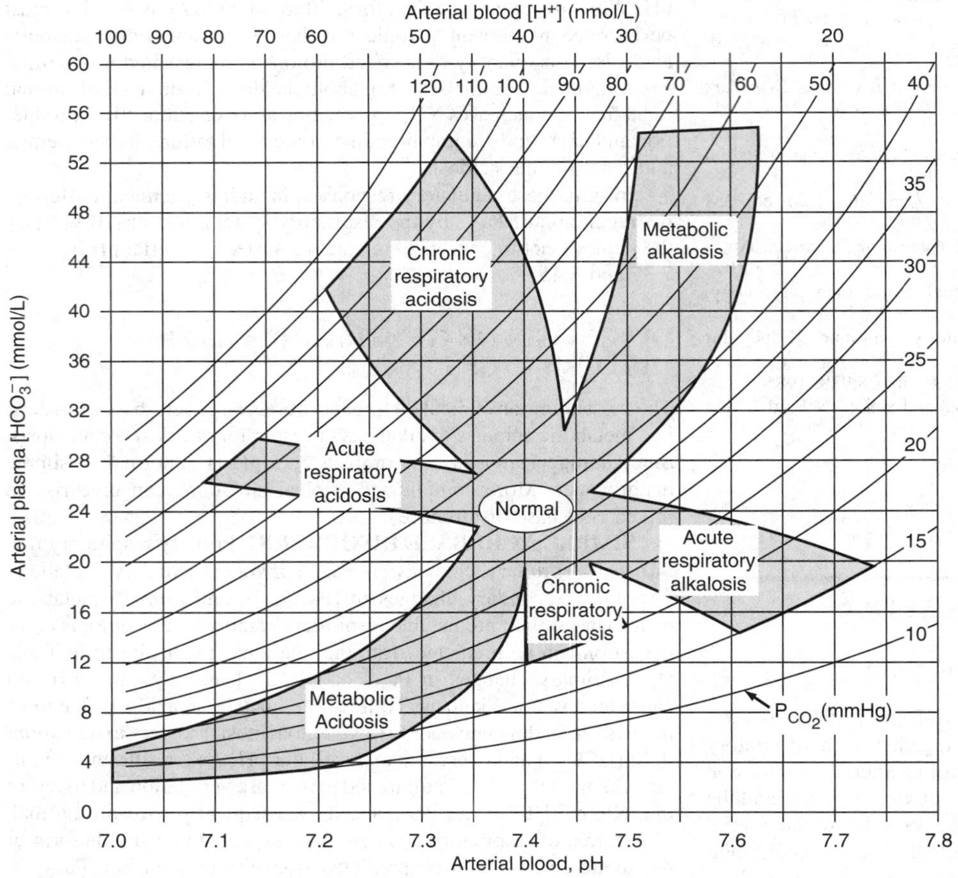

FIGURE 50-1 Acid-base nomogram. Shown are the 90 percent confidence limits of the normal respiratory and metabolic compensations for primary acid-base disturbances. [From TD DuBose et al: Acid-base disorders, in *The Kidney*, 5th ed, BM Brenner, FC Rector, Jr. (eds). Philadelphia, Saunders, 1996, pp. 929–998. Used with permission.]

in [HCO_3^-] occurs with metabolic alkalosis and respiratory acidosis. Conversely, a decrease in [HCO_3^-] occurs in metabolic acidosis and respiratory alkalosis.

Metabolic acidosis leads to hyperkalemia as a result of cellular shifts in which H^+ is exchanged for K^+ or Na^+. For each decrease in blood pH of 0.10, the plasma [K^+] should rise by 0.6 mmol/L. This relationship is not invariable. Diabetic ketoacidosis, lactic acidosis, diarrhea, and renal tubular acidosis are often associated with potassium depletion.

ANION GAP All evaluations of acid-base disorders should include a simple calculation of the anion gap (AG); it represents those unmeasured anions in plasma (normally 10 to 12 mmol/L) and is calculated as follows: $AG = [Na^+] - ([Cl^-] + [HCO_3^-])$. The unmeasured anions include anionic proteins, phosphate, sulfate, and organic anions. When acid anions, such as acetoacetate and lactate, accumulate in extracellular fluid, the AG increases, causing a high-AG acidosis. An *increase* in the AG may be due to a decrease in unmeasured cations (calcium, magnesium, potassium) or an increase in unmeasured anions. In addition, the AG may increase secondary to an increase in anionic albumin, either because of increased albumin concentration or alkalosis, which alters albumin charge. A *decrease* in the AG can be due to (1) an increase in unmeasured cations; (2) the addition to the blood of abnormal cations, such as lithium (lithium intoxication) or cationic immunoglobulins (plasma cell dyscrasias); (3) a reduction in the major plasma anion albumin concentration; (4) a decrease in the effective anionic charge on albumin by acidosis; or (5) hyperviscosity and severe hyperlipidemia, which can lead to an underestimation of sodium and chloride concentrations.

In the face of a normal serum albumin, a high AG is usually due to non-chloride-containing acids that contain inorganic (phosphate, sulfate), organic (ketoacids, lactate, uremic organic anions), exogenous (salicylate or ingested toxins with organic acid production), or unidentified anions. By definition, therefore, a *high-AG acidosis* has two identifying features: a low [HCO_3^-] and an elevated AG. The latter is present even if an additional acid-base disorder is superimposed to modify the [HCO_3^-] independently. Simultaneous metabolic acidosis of the high-AG variety plus either chronic respiratory acidosis or metabolic alkalosis represents such a situation in which [HCO_3^-] may be normal or even high. However, the AG is elevated, and [Cl^-] is depressed.

Similarly, normal values for [HCO_3^-], Pa_{CO_2}, and pH do not ensure the absence of an acid-base disturbance. For instance, an alcoholic who has been vomiting may develop a metabolic alkalosis with a pH of 7.55, Pa_{CO_2} of 48 mmHg, [HCO_3^-] of 40 mmol/L, [Na^+] of 135, [Cl^-] of 80, and [K^+] of 2.8. If such a patient were then to develop a superimposed alcoholic ketoacidosis with a β-hydroxybutyrate concentration of 15 mM, arterial pH would fall to 7.40, [HCO_3^-] to 25 mmol/L, and the Pa_{CO_2} to 40 mmHg. Although blood gases are normal, the AG is elevated at 26 mmol/L, indicating a mixed metabolic alkalosis and metabolic acidosis.

METABOLIC ACIDOSIS

Metabolic acidosis can occur because of an increase in endogenous acid production (such as lactate and ketoacids), loss of bicarbonate (as in diarrhea), or accumulation of endogenous acids (as in renal failure). Metabolic acidosis has profound effects on the respiratory, cardiac, and nervous systems. The fall in blood pH is accompanied by a characteristic increase in ventilation, especially tidal volume (Kussmaul respiration). Intrinsic cardiac contractility may be depressed, but inotropic function can be normal because of catecholamine release. Both peripheral arterial vasodilation and central venoconstriction can be present; the decrease in central and pulmonary vascular compliance predisposes to pulmonary edema with even minimal volume overload. Central nervous system function is depressed, with headache, lethargy, stupor, and, in some cases, even coma. Glucose intolerance may also occur.

 **TREATMENT**

It has been generally accepted that treatment of metabolic acidosis with alkali should be reserved for severe acidemia except when the patient has no "potential HCO_3^-" in plasma. Potential [HCO_3^-] can be estimated from the increment (Δ) in the anion gap (ΔAG = patient's AG − 10). It must be determined if the acid anion in plasma is metabolizable (i.e., β-hydroxybutyrate, acetoacetate, lactate) or nonmetabolizable (anions that accumulate in chronic renal failure and with toxin ingestion). The latter requires return of renal function to replenish the [HCO_3^-] deficit, a slow and often unpredictable process. Consequently, patients with no AG (hyperchloremic acidosis), a small AG (mixed hyperchloremic and AG acidosis), or an AG attributable to a nonmetabolizable anion in the face of renal failure should receive alkali therapy, either orally ($NaHCO_3$ or Shohl's solution) or intravenously ($NaHCO_3$), in an amount necessary to slowly increase the plasma [HCO_3^-] into the 20 to 22 mmol/L range.

Controversy exists, however, in regard to the use of alkali in patients with a pure AG acidosis owing to accumulation of a metabolizable organic acid anion (ketoacidosis or lactic acidosis). In general, severe acidosis (pH < 7.20) warrants the intravenous administration of 50 to 100 meq of $NaHCO_3$, over 30 to 45 min, during the initial 1 to 2 h of therapy. Provision of such modest quantities of alkali in this situation seems to provide an added measure of safety, but it is essential to monitor plasma electrolytes during the course of therapy, since the [K^+] may decline as pH rises.

As indicated above there are two major categories of clinical metabolic acidosis: (1) high-AG and (2) normal-AG, or hyperchloremic, acidosis (Tables 50-2 and 50-3).

HIGH-ANION-GAP ACIDOSES There are four principal causes of a high AG acidosis: (1) lactic acidosis, (2) ketoacidosis, (3) ingested toxins (Table 50-2), and (4) acute and chronic renal failure. Initial screening to differentiate the high AG acidoses should include: (1) a probe of the history for evidence of drug and toxin ingestion and measurement of arterial blood gas to detect coexistent respiratory alkalosis (salicylates); (2) determination of whether diabetes mellitus is present (diabetic ketoacidosis); (3) a search for evidence of alcoholism or increased levels of β-hydroxybutyrate (alcoholic ketoacidosis); (4) observation for clinical signs of uremia and determination of the blood urea nitrogen (BUN) and creatinine (uremic acidosis); (5) inspection of the urine for oxalate crystals (ethylene glycol); and (6) recognition of the numerous clinical settings in which lactate levels may be increased (hypotension, shock, cardiac failure, leukemia, cancer, and drug or toxin ingestion).

Lactic Acidosis Accumulation in plasma L-lactate may be secondary to obvious tissue hypoxia (type A)—circulatory insufficiency (shock, heart failure), severe anemia, cholera, mitochondrial enzyme defects, and inhibitors (carbon monoxide, cyanide)—or to more occult disorders (type B)—hypoglycemia (glycogen storage diseases), seizures, diabetes mellitus, ethanol, hepatic failure, malignancy, and

Table 50-2

Causes of High-Anion-Gap Metabolic Acidosis

Lactic acidosis (types A and B)
Ketoacidosis
    Diabetic
    Alcoholic
    Starvation
Toxins
    Ethylene glycol
    Methanol
    Salicylates
Renal failure (acute and chronic)

Table 50-3

Causes of Hyperchloremic Acidosis

I. Gastrointestinal bicarbonate loss
   A. Diarrhea
   B. External pancreatic or small-bowel drainage
   C. Urterosigmoidostomy, jejunal loop, ileal loop
   D. Drugs
      1. Calcium chloride (acidifying agent)
      2. Magnesium sulfate (diarrhea)
      3. Cholestyramine (bile acid diarrhea)
II. Renal acidosis
   A. Hypokalemia
      1. Proximal RTA (type II)
      2. Distal (classic) RTA (type I)
   B. Hyperkalemia
      1. Generalized distal nephron dysfunction (type IV RTA)
         a. Mineralocorticoid deficiency
         b. Mineralocorticoid resistance
         c. $\downarrow Na^+$ delivery to distal nephron
         d. Tubulointerstitial disease
         e. Ammonium excretion defect
   C. Normokalemia
      1. Early renal insufficiency
III. Drug-induced hyperkalemia (with renal insufficiency)
   A. Potassium-sparing diuretics (amiloride, triamterene, spironolactone)
   B. Trimethoprim
   C. Pentamidine
   D. Angiotensin-converting enzyme inhibitors
   E. Nonsteroidal anti-inflammatory drugs
   F. Cyclosporine
IV. Other
   A. Acid loads (ammonium chloride, hyperalimentation)
   B. Loss of potential bicarbonate: ketosis with ketone excretion
   C. Expansion acidosis (rapid saline administration)
   D. Hippurate
   E. Cation exchange resins

salicylates—in which overproduction and/or decreased hepatic removal of lactate can occur. Unrecognized bowel ischemia or infarction in a patient with severe atherosclerosis or cardiac decompensation receiving vasopressors is a common cause of lactic acidosis. D-Lactate acidosis, associated commonly with jejunoileal bypass or intestinal obstruction and due to formation by gut bacteria, may cause both an increased AG and hyperchloremia.

℞ TREATMENT

The underlying condition that disrupts lactate metabolism must first be corrected; tissue perfusion must be restored when it is inadequate. Vasoconstrictors should be avoided, if possible, since they may worsen tissue perfusion. Alkali therapy is generally advocated for acute, severe acidemia (pH < 7.1) to improve cardiac function and lactate utilization. However, $NaHCO_3$ therapy may paradoxically depress cardiac performance and exacerbate acidosis by enhancing lactate production (HCO_3^- stimulates phosphofructokinase). While the use of alkali in moderate lactic acidosis is controversial, it is generally agreed that attempts to return the pH or [HCO_3^-] to normal by administration of exogenous $NaHCO_3$ are deleterious. A reasonable approach is to infuse sufficient $NaHCO_3$ to raise the arterial pH to no more than 7.2 over 30 to 40 min.

$NaHCO_3$ therapy can cause fluid overload and hypertension because the amount required can be massive when accumulation of lactic acid is relentless. Fluid administration is poorly tolerated because of central venoconstriction, especially in the oliguric patient. If the underlying cause of the lactic acidosis can be remedied, blood lactate will be converted to HCO_3^- and may result in an overshoot alkalosis.

Ketoacidosis *Diabetic ketoacidosis* (See also Chap. 334) This condition is caused by increased fatty acid metabolism and the accumu-

lation of ketoacids (acetoacetate and β-hydroxybutyrate). Diabetic ketoacidosis usually occurs in insulin-dependent diabetes mellitus in association with cessation of insulin or an intercurrent illness, such as an infection, gastroenteritis, pancreatitis, or myocardial infarction, which increases insulin requirements temporarily and acutely. The accumulation of ketoacids accounts for the increment in the AG and is accompanied most often by hyperglycemia [glucose > 17 mmol/L (300 mg/dL)]. The management of this condition is described in Chap. 234. Here it should be noted that since insulin prevents production of ketones, bicarbonate therapy is rarely needed except with extreme acidemia (pH < 7.1), and then in only limited amounts (as discussed above for correction of lactic acidosis).

Alcoholic ketoacidosis Chronic alcoholics can develop ketoacidosis when alcohol consumption is abruptly curtailed; it is usually associated with vomiting, abdominal pain, starvation, and volume depletion. The glucose concentration is low or normal, and acidosis may be severe because of elevated ketones, predominantly β-hydroxybutyrate. Mild lactic acidosis may coexist because of alteration in the redox state. The nitroprusside ketone reaction (Acetest) can detect acetoacetic acid but not β-hydroxybutyrate, so that the degree of ketosis and ketonuria can be underestimated. Typically, insulin levels are low, and concentrations of triglyceride, cortisol, glucagon, and growth hormone are increased.

℞ TREATMENT

This consists of intravenous volume repletion and glucose administration (5% dextrose in 0.9% NaCl). Hypophosphatemia, hypokalemia, and hypomagnesemia may coexist and should be corrected. Hypophosphatemia usually emerges 12 to 24 h after admission, may be exacerbated by glucose infusion, and, if severe, may induce rhabdomyolysis. Upper gastrointestinal hemorrhage, pancreatitis, and pneumonia may accompany this disorder.

Drug- and Toxin-Induced Acidosis *Salicylates* Salicylate intoxication in adults causes a high-AG metabolic acidosis, in which only a portion of the AG is due to the salicylates. Lactic acid production is also often increased, partly as a direct effect of the drug and partly as a result of the central stimulation of the respiratory center induced by salicylate causing a decrease in Pa_{CO_2} (respiratory alkalosis). Mixed acid-base disturbances (metabolic acidosis concomitant with respiratory alkalosis) from salicylates is common in adults.

℞ TREATMENT

This should begin with vigorous gastric lavage with isotonic saline (not $NaHCO_3$) followed by administration of activated charcoal. To facilitate removal of salicylate, intravenous $NaHCO_3$ is administered in amounts adequate to alkalinize the urine and to maintain urine output (urine pH > 7.5). While this form of therapy is straightforward in acidotic patients, a respiratory alkalosis may make this approach hazardous. Acetazolamide may be administered when an alkaline diuresis cannot be achieved, but this drug can cause systemic metabolic acidosis if $NaHCO_3$ is not given concomitantly. The hypokalemia, which may be severe, is a result of the alkaline diuresis from $NaHCO_3$ or acetazolamide or of the respiratory alkalosis and should be treated promptly and aggressively. Glucose-containing fluids should be administered because of the danger of hypoglycemia. Excessive insensible fluid losses may cause severe volume depletion and hypernatremia. If renal failure prevents rapid clearance of salicylate, hemodialysis can be performed against a bicarbonate dialysate.

Alcohols Under most physiologic conditions, sodium, urea, and glucose generate the osmotic pressure of blood. Plasma osmolality is calculated according to the following expression: $P_{osm} = 2Na^+ + Glu + BUN$ (all in mmol/L), or, using conventional laboratory values in which glucose and BUN are expressed in mg per dL: $P_{osm} = 2Na^+ + Glu/18 + BUN/2.8$. The calculated and determined osmolality should agree within 10 to 15 mmol/kg H_2O. When the measured osmolality exceeds the calculated osmolality by more than 15 to 20 mmol/kg H_2O, one of two circumstances prevails. Either the serum sodium is spuriously low, as with hyperlipidemia or hyperproteinemia (pseudohyponatremia), or osmolytes other than sodium salts, glucose, or urea have accumulated in plasma. Examples include mannitol, radiocontrast media, isopropyl alcohol, ethylene glycol, ethanol, methanol, and acetone. In this situation, the difference between the calculated osmolality and the measured osmolality (osmolar gap) is proportional to the concentration of the unmeasured solute. With an appropriate clinical history and index of suspicion, identification of an osmolar gap is helpful in identifying the presence of poison-associated AG acidosis.

Ethylene glycol Ingestion of ethylene glycol (commonly used in antifreeze) leads to a metabolic acidosis and severe damage to the central nervous system, heart, lungs, and kidneys. The increased AG and osmolar gap are attributable to ethylene glycol and its metabolites, oxalic acid, glycolic acid, and other organic acids. Lactic acid production increases secondary to inhibition of the tricarboxylic acid cycle and altered intracellular redox state. Diagnosis is facilitated by recognizing oxalate crystals in the urine.

℞ **TREATMENT**

This includes the prompt institution of a saline or osmotic diuresis, thiamine and pyridoxine supplements, ethanol, and dialysis. The administration of ethanol intravenously to achieve a level of 22 mmol/L (100 mg/dL) serves to lessen toxicity because it competes with ethylene glycol for metabolism by alcohol dehydrogenase and alters the cellular redox state.

Methanol The ingestion of methanol (wood alcohol) causes metabolic acidosis, and its metabolites formaldehyde and formic acid cause severe optic nerve and cental nervous system damage. Lactic acid, ketoacids, and other unidentified organic acids may contribute to the acidosis. Due to its low molecular weight (32 Da), an osmolar gap is usually present.

℞ **TREATMENT**

This is similar to that for ethylene glycol intoxication, including general supportive measures, ethanol administration, and hemodialysis.

Renal Failure (See also Chaps. 270 and 271) The hyperchloremic acidosis of moderate renal insufficiency is eventually converted to the high-AG acidosis of advanced renal failure. Poor filtration and reabsorption of organic anions contribute to the pathogenesis. As renal disease progresses, the number of functioning nephrons eventually becomes insufficient to keep pace with net acid production. Uremic acidosis is characterized, therefore, by a reduced rate of NH_4^+ production, primarily due to decreased renal mass. $[HCO_3^-]$ rarely falls below 15 mmol/L, and the AG rarely exceeds 20 mmol/L. The acid retained in chronic renal disease is buffered by alkaline salts from bone. Despite significant retention of acid (up to 20 mmol/d), the serum $[HCO_3^-]$ does not decrease further, indicating participation of buffers outside the extracellular compartment. Chronic metabolic acidosis results in significant loss of bone mass due to reduction in bone calcium carbonate. Chronic acidosis also increases urinary calcium excretion, proportional to cumulative acid retention.

℞ **TREATMENT**

Both uremic acidosis and the hyperchloremic acidosis of renal failure require oral alkali replacement to maintain the $[HCO_3^-]$ between 20 and 24 mmol/L. This can be accomplished with relatively modest amounts of alkali (1.0 to 1.5 mmol/kg body weight per day). It is assumed that alkali replacement prevents the harmful effects of H^+ balance on bone. Sodium citrate (Shohl's solution) or $NaHCO_3$ tablets are equally effective alkalinizing salts. Citrate enhances the absorption of aluminum from the gastrointestinal tract and should never be given together with aluminum-containing antacids because of the risk of aluminum intoxication. When hyperkalemia is present, furosemide (60 to 80 mg/d) should be added.

HYPERCHLOREMIC METABOLIC ACIDOSES Alkali can be lost from the gastrointestinal tract in diarrhea or from the kidneys (renal tubular acidosis). In these disorders (Table 50-3), reciprocal changes in $[Cl^-]$ and $[HCO_3^-]$ result in a *normal* AG. In pure hyperchloremic acidosis, therefore, the increase in $[Cl^-]$ above the normal value equals the decrease in $[HCO_3^-]$. The absence of such a relationship suggests a mixed disturbance.

Diarrhea causes the loss of large quantities of HCO_3^- and decomposed HCO_3^-. Since diarrheal stools contain a higher $[HCO_3^-]$ and decomposed HCO_3^- than plasma, metabolic acidosis develops along with volume depletion. Instead of an acid urine pH (as anticipated with systemic acidosis), urine pH is usually around 6 because metabolic acidosis and hypokalemia increase renal synthesis and excretion of NH_4^+, thus providing a urinary buffer that increases urine pH. Metabolic acidosis due to gastrointestinal losses with a high urine pH can be differentiated from renal tubular acidosis (RTA) (Chap. 278), because urinary NH_4^+ excretion is typically low in RTA and high with diarrhea. Urinary NH_4^+ levels can be estimated by calculating the urine net charge (UNC): $UNC = [Na^+ + K^+]_u - [Cl^-]_u$. When $[Cl^-]_u > [Na^+ + K^+]$, the urine ammonium level is appropriately increased, suggesting an extrarenal cause of the acidosis. In addition to diarrhea (HCO_3^- loss from the gastrointestinal tract), another extrarenal cause of hyperchloremic metabolic acidosis is parenteral hyperalimentation with the Cl^- salts of basic amino acids and insufficient alkali (acetate). However, if urine $[NH_4^+]$ is low, the cause is likely to be RTA. Caution is urged since ketonuria or the presence of drug anions in the urine invalidates the net negative charge estimate.

Loss of functioning renal parenchyma by progressive renal disease leads to hyperchloremic acidosis when the glomerular filtration rate (GFR) is between 20 and 50 mL/min and to uremic acidosis with a high AG when the GFR falls to below <20 mL/min. Such a progression occurs commonly with tubulointerstitial forms of renal disease, but hyperchloremic metabolic acidosis can persist with advanced glomerular disease. In advanced renal failure, ammoniagenesis is reduced in proportion to the loss of functional renal mass, and ammonium accumulation and trapping in the outer medullary collecting tubule may also be impaired. Because of adaptive increases in K^+ secretion by the collecting duct and colon, the acidosis of chronic renal insufficiency is typically normokalemic.

Most *proximal* RTA (type 2 RTA) is due to generalized proximal tubular dysfunction, with glycosuria, generalized aminoaciduria, and phosphaturia (*Fanconi syndrome*). The urine is appropriately acidified (pH < 5.5), and there is either a low plasma $[HCO_3^-]$ or a high fractional excretion of $[HCO_3^-]$(>10 to 15 percent) with a near-normal serum HCO_3^- (>20 mmol/L). With proximal RTA, massive amounts of exogenous HCO_3^- are required, since HCO_3^- is not reabsorbed normally in the proximal tubule, resulting in enhanced renal potassium wasting and hypokalemia.

The typical findings in *classical distal* RTA (type 1 RTA) include hypokalemia, hyperchloremic acidosis, low urinary NH_4^- excretion (positive urine net charge), and inappropriately high urine pH (pH > 5.5). Such patients are unable to acidify the urine below pH = 5.5. These abnormalities suggest that one or both of the active proton pumps present in the collecting duct (the H^+-ATPase, or the H^+, K^+-ATPase) is defective. In addition, excretory rates of NH_4^+ are uniformly low when the degree of systemic acidosis is taken into account, indicating that the kidney is responsible for the metabolic acidosis. Ammonium excretion is low because of failure to trap NH_4^+ in the medullary collecting duct, as a result of higher than normal tubular fluid pH in this segment, and the urine pH is high because of impaired H^+ secretion. In amphotericin B poisoning, distal RTA is due to an inability to maintain a pH gradient across the collecting duct, whereas most other forms of distal RTA appear to be the result of deficient H^+ pump function or number.

Distal RTA usually occurs in association with a systemic illness, such as Sjögren's syndrome or multiple myeloma, and is referred to as "secondary" distal RTA. Conversely, distal RTA can occur as an inherited disorder unassociated with systemic disease. The RTA of renal transplantation can be either of the proximal or distal variety, but chronic rejection is usually associated with the distal type.

Although hyperchloremic metabolic acidosis and hyperkalemia occur with regularity in advanced renal insufficiency, in *type 4* RTA hyperkalemia is disproportionate to the reduction in GFR because of coexisting dysfunction of potassium and acid secretion. Urinary ammonium excretion is invariably depressed, and renal function may be compromised, for example, due to diabetic nephropathy, amyloidosis, or tubulointerstitial disease.

℞ **TREATMENT**

Chronic metabolic acidosis in classical distal RTA can usually be corrected by administration of sufficient oral alkali to neutralize the production of metabolic acids from the diet. In adult patients with distal RTA, this is usually equal to no more than 1 to 3 mmol/kg body weight per day in the form of Shohl's solution or $NaHCO_3$ tablets. Correction of acidosis reduces urinary potassium excretion, and hypokalemia and sodium depletion may resolve. Therefore, in most adult patients with distal RTA, potassium supplement is not necessary.

Hyporeninemic-Hypoaldosteronism (See also Chap. 332) This condition typically causes hyperchloremic metabolic acidosis, typically in older adults with diabetes mellitus or tubulointerstitial disease and renal insufficiency. Patients usually have mild to moderate renal insufficiency and acidosis with elevation in serum $[K^+]$ (5.2 to 6.0 mmol/L), concurrent hypertension, and congestive heart failure. Both the metabolic acidosis and the hyperkalemia are out of proportion to impairment in GFR. The nonsteroidal anti-inflammatory drugs also can cause hyperkalemia with hyperchloremic metabolic acidosis in patients with renal insufficiency. In hyporeninemic-hypoaldosteronism, plasma renin activity appears to be unresponsive to the usual physiologic stimuli, and aldosterone secretion is low as a result. Reduction in $[K^+]$ by administration of cation exchange resins may enhance renal ammoniagenesis and usually improves or corrects the metabolic acidosis and hyperkalemia. Mineralocorticoid replacement with fludrocortisone also improves net acid excretion but is contraindicated in the face of coexisting hypertension or congestive heart failure.

The combination of hyperchloremic metabolic acidosis, hyperkalemia, hypertension, undetectable plasma renin activity, and low aldosterone levels is termed *pseudohypoaldosteronism-type II*. This disorder is usually not associated with glomerular or tubulointerstitial disease. The acidosis is mild and can be accounted for by the hyperkalemia. Renin and aldosterone levels both increase if volume expansion is corrected by diuretics or salt restriction. Potassium excretion responds to sodium sulfate infusion. Mineralocorticoid resistance with salt wasting also causes hyperkalemic-hyperchloremic acidosis because of a decrease in mineralocorticoid effectiveness at the level of the cortical collecting tubule. Pseudohypoaldosteronism may occur with systemic lupus erythematosus, obstructive uropathy, sickle cell disease, drug-induced interstitial nephritis, cyclosporine therapy, or rejection of a kidney transplant.

℞ **TREATMENT**

Management of patients with metabolic acidosis and hyperkalemia with chronic renal insufficiency is not always necessary, and the decision to treat is often based on the severity of the hyperkalemia. Reduction in serum $[K^+]$ often improves the metabolic acidosis. Patients with hyporeninemic-hypoaldosteronism may respond to a cation-exchange resin (sodium polystyrene sulfonate), alkali therapy, or loop diuretics. Volume depletion should be avoided unless the patient is volume overexpanded or hypertensive. Supraphysiologic doses of mineralocorticoids may be necessary but should be administered in combination with a loop diuretic to avoid volume overexpan-

sion or aggravation of hypertension and to increase potassium excretion. Patients with pseudohypoaldosteronism-type II should receive thiazide diuretics coupled with dietary salt restriction.

METABOLIC ALKALOSIS

Metabolic alkalosis is manifested by an elevated arterial pH, an increase in the serum $[HCO_3^-]$, and an increase in Pa_{CO_2} as a result of compensatory alveolar hypoventilation. It is often accompanied by hypochloremia and hypokalemia. The patient with a high $[HCO_3^-]$ and a low $[Cl^-]$ has either metabolic alkalosis or chronic respiratory acidosis. As shown in Table 50-1, the Pa_{CO_2} increases 6 mmHg for each 10-mmol/L increase in the $[HCO_3^-]$ above normal. Stated differently, in the range of $[HCO_3^-]$ from 10 to 40 mmol/L, the predicted Pa_{CO_2} is approximately equal to the $[HCO_3^-]$ + 15. The arterial pH establishes the diagnosis, since it is increased in metabolic alkalosis and decreased or normal in respiratory acidosis. Metabolic alkalosis frequently occurs in association with other disorders such as respiratory acidosis or alkalosis or metabolic acidosis.

PATHOGENESIS Metabolic alkalosis occurs as a result of net gain of $[HCO_3^-]$ or loss of nonvolatile acid (usually HCl by vomiting) from the extracellular fluid. Since it is unusual for alkali to be added to the body, the disorder involves a *generative stage*, in which the loss of acid usually causes alkalosis, and a *maintenance stage*, in which the kidneys fail to compensate by excreting HCO_3^- because of volume contraction, a low GFR, or depletion of Cl^- or K^+.

Under normal circumstances, the kidneys have an impressive capacity to excrete HCO_3^-, and continuation of metabolic alkalosis represents a failure of the kidneys to eliminate HCO_3^- in the usual manner. For HCO_3^- to be added to the extracellular fluid, it must be administered exogenously or synthesized endogenously, in part or entirely by the kidneys. The kidneys will retain, rather than excrete, the excess alkali and maintain the alkalosis if one of two mechanisms is operative:

1. Cl^- deficiency (extracellular fluid contraction) existing concurrently with K^+ deficiency, reduced GFR, and/or enhanced proximal fraction HCO_3^- reabsorption. This combination of disorders evokes secondary hyperreninemic hyperaldosteronism and stimulates H^+ secretion by the collecting duct. The alkalosis is corrected by the administration of NaCl and KCl.
2. Hyperaldosteronism and hypokalemia are autonomous and unresponsive to increased extracellular fluid volume. The enhanced distal H^+ secretion is sufficient to reabsorb the increased filtered HCO_3^- load and to overcome the decreased proximal HCO_3^- reabsorption due to expansion of the extracellular fluid volume. To repair the alkalosis in this situation, it is necessary to inhibit the secretion or action of aldosterone or to surgically remove an aldosterone-secreting adrenal adenoma.

DIFFERENTIAL DIAGNOSIS To establish the cause of metabolic alkalosis (Table 50-4), it is necessary to assess the status of the extracellular volume (ECV), the recumbent and upright blood pressure, the serum K^+, and the renin-aldosterone system. For example, the presence of hypertension and hypokalemia in an alkalotic patient suggests either mineralocorticoid excess or a hypertensive patient receiving diuretics. Low plasma renin activity and normal urine $[Na^+]$ and $[Cl^-]$ in a patient who is not taking diuretics indicate a primary mineralocorticoid excess syndrome. The combination of hypokalemia and alkalosis in a normotensive, nonedematous patient can be due to Bartter's syndrome, magnesium deficiency, vomiting, exogenous alkali, or diuretic ingestion. Determination of urine electrolytes (especially the urine $[Cl^-]$) and screening of the urine for diuretics may be helpful. If the urine is alkaline, with elevated $[Na^+]$ and $[K^+]$ but low $[Cl^-]$, the diagnosis is usually either vomiting (overt or surreptitious) or alkali ingestion. If the urine is relatively acid and has low concentrations of Na^+, K^+, and Cl^-, the most likely possibilities are prior vomiting, the posthypercapnic state, or prior diuretic ingestion. If, on the other hand, neither the urine sodium, potassium, nor chloride concentrations are depressed, magnesium deficiency, Bartter's syndrome, or current diuretic ingestion should be considered.

Table 50-4

CHAPTER 50
Acidosis and Alkalosis   **283**

Causes of Metabolic Alkalosis

I. Exogenous HCO_3^- loads
  A. Acute alkali administration
  B. Milk-alkali syndrome
II. Effective ECFV contraction, normotension, K^+ deficiency, and
  secondary hyperreninemic hyperaldosteronism
  A. Gastrointestinal origin
    1. Vomiting
    2. Gastric aspiration
    3. Congenital chloridorrhea
    4. Villous adenoma
  B. Renal origin
    1. Diuretics
    2. Edematous states
    3. Posthypercapnic state
    4. Hypercalcemia/hypoparathyroidism
    5. Recovery from lactic acidosis or ketoacidosis
    6. Nonreabsorbable anions including penicillin, carbenicillin
    7. Mg^{2+} deficiency
    8. K^+ depletion
    9. Bartter's syndrome
  C. Gitelman's syndrome
III. ECFV expansion, hypertension, K^+ deficiency,
  and mineralocorticoid excess
  A. High renin
    1. Renal artery stenosis
    2. Accelerated hypertension
    3. Renin-secreting tumor
    4. Estrogen therapy
  B. Low renin
    1. Primary aldosteronism
      a. Adenoma
      b. Hyperplasia
      c. Carcinoma
    2. Adrenal enzyme defects
      a. 11β-Hydroxylase deficiency
      b. 17α-Hydroxylase deficiency
    3. Cushing's syndrome
      a. Ectopic corticotropin
      b. Adrenal adenoma
      c. Primary pituitary
    4. Other
      a. Licorice
      b. Carbenoxolone
      c. Chewer's tobacco
      d. Liddle's syndrome

NOTE: ECFV, extracellular fluid volume.

Alkali Administration   Chronic administration of alkali to individuals with normal renal function results in minimal, if any, alkalosis. However, in patients with chronic renal insufficiency, alkalosis can develop following alkali administration when the normal capacity to excrete HCO_3^- is exceeded or when coexistent hemodynamic disturbances cause enhanced fractional reabsorption of HCO_3^-. Such patients include those who receive oral or intravenous HCO_3^-, acetate loads (parenteral hyperalimentation solutions), citrate loads (transfusions), or antacids plus cation-exchange resins (aluminum hydroxide and sodium polystyrene sulfonate). A rare cause is long-standing ingestion of excessive milk and antacids. Both hypercalcemia and vitamin D excess may increase renal HCO_3^- reabsorption and cause nephrocalcinosis, renal insufficiency, or metabolic alkalosis. Discontinuation of alkali ingestion or administration is usually sufficient to repair the alkalosis.

METABOLIC ALKALOSIS ASSOCIATED WITH ECFV CONTRACTION, K^+ DEPLETION, AND SECONDARY HYPERRENINEMIC HYPERALDOSTERONISM

Gastrointestinal Origin   *Vomiting and gastric aspiration*   Gastrointestinal loss of H^+ results in retention of HCO_3^-. Increased H^+ loss through gastric secretions can be caused by vomiting, gastric aspiration, or a gastric fistula. The loss of fluid and NaCl in vomitus or nasogastric suction results in contraction of the extracellular fluid volume (ECFV) and an increase in the secretion of renin and aldosterone.

Volume contraction causes a reduction in GFR and an enhanced capacity of the renal tubule to reabsorb HCO_3^-. During active vomiting, there is continued addition of HCO_3^- to plasma in exchange for Cl^-, and the plasma $[HCO_3^-]$ exceeds the reabsorptive capacity of the proximal tubule. The excess $NaHCO_3$ reaches the distal tubule, where some Na^+ will be exchanged for K^+ by an aldosterone-mediated process. Because of contraction of the ECFV and hypochloremia, Cl^- is avidly conserved by the kidney. Upon cessation of vomiting, the plasma $[HCO_3^-]$ falls to the HCO_3^- threshold, which is elevated due to the combined effects of contraction of the ECFV, hypokalemia, and hyperaldosteronism. The alkalosis is less severe than during the phase of active vomiting, and the urine is relatively acidic with low concentrations of Na^+, Cl^-, and HCO_3^-. Correction of the contracted ECFV with NaCl may be sufficient to restore normal blood pH, even without repair of K^+ deficits. Good clinical practice, however, dictates K^+ repletion as well.

Villous adenoma   Metabolic alkalosis has been described in cases of villous adenoma and is most likely the result of potassium depletion.

Renal Origin   *Diuretics* (See also Chap. 233)   Drugs that induce chloruresis without bicarbonaturia, such as thiazides and loop diuretics (furosemide, bumetanide, torsemide, and ethracrynic acid), *acutely* diminish the ECFV without altering the total body bicarbonate content. The serum $[HCO_3^-]$ increases. The Pa_{CO_2} does not increase commensurately, and a "contraction" alkalosis results. The degree of alkalosis is usually small, owing to cellular and non-HCO_3^- buffering. The chronic administration of diuretics tends to generate an alkalosis by increasing distal salt delivery, so that K^+ and H^+ secretion are stimulated. Diuretics, by blocking Cl^- reabsorption in the distal tubule or by increasing proton pump activity, may also stimulate distal H^+ secretion, as evidenced by an increase in net acid excretion. The alkalosis is maintained by persistence of the contraction of the ECFV, secondary hyperaldosteronism, K^+ deficiency, and the direct effect of the diuretic (as long as diuretic administration continues). Repair of the alkalosis is achieved by providing isotonic saline to correct the ECFV deficit.

Posthypercapnia   Prolonged CO_2 retention with chronic respiratory acidosis enhances renal HCO_3^- absorption and the generation of new HCO_3^- (increased net acid excretion). If the Pa_{CO_2} is returned to normal, metabolic alkalosis results from the persistently elevated $[HCO_3^-]$. Alkalosis develops immediately if the elevated Pa_{CO_2} is abruptly returned toward normal by a change in mechanically controlled ventilation and the brisk bicarbonaturic response is proportional to the change in Pa_{CO_2}. The accompanying cation is predominantly K^+, especially if dietary K^+ is not limited, with natriuresis proportional to the salt intake. Secondary hyperaldosteronism in states of chronic hypercapnia may be responsible for this pattern of response. Associated ECFV contraction does not allow complete repair of the alkalosis by correction of the Pa_{CO_2} alone, and alkalosis persists until Cl^- supplementation is provided. Enhanced proximal acidification, the result of conditioning induced by the previous hypercapnic state, may also contribute to posthypercapnic alkalosis.

After treatment of lactic acidosis or ketoacidosis   When an underlying stimulus for the generation of lactic acid or ketoacid is removed rapidly, as with repair of circulatory insufficiency or with insulin therapy, the lactate or ketones are metabolized to yield an equivalent amount of HCO_3^-; H^+ is consumed by metabolism of the organic anions, with the liberation of an equivalent quantity of HCO_3^-. This process will regenerate HCO_3^- if the organic acids are metabolized to HCO_3^- before their renal excretion. This is partly offset by urinary loss of organic ions. Other sources of new HCO_3^- are additive with the original amount generated by organic anion metabolism to create a surfeit of HCO_3^-. Such sources include (1) new HCO_3^- added to the blood by the kidneys as a result of enhanced acid excretion during the preexisting period of acidosis, and (2) alkali therapy during the treatment phase of the acidosis. Acidosis-induced contraction of the ECFV and K^+ deficiency act to sustain the alkalosis.

Nonreabsorbable anions and magnesium deficiency Administration of large quantities of nonreabsorbable anions, such as penicillin or carbenicillin, can enhance distal acidification and K^+ secretion by increasing the luminal potential difference. Mg^{2+} deficiency results in hypokalemic alkalosis by enhancing distal acidification through stimulation of renin and hence aldosterone secretion.

Potassium depletion Pure K^+ depletion causes a modest metabolic alkalosis. K^+ depletion increases urinary acid excretion as NH_4^+ and enhances HCO_3^- reabsorption. Alkalosis is mild because K^+ depletion also causes positive NaCl balance with or without mineralocorticoid administration. The salt retention, in turn, minimizes the alkalosis. When access to both NaCl and K^+ is restricted, alkalosis is more severe. Alkalosis associated with severe K^+ depletion is resistant to salt administration, whereas repair of the K^+ deficiency corrects the alkalosis.

Bartter's syndrome → *See Chap. 278.*

METABOLIC ALKALOSIS ASSOCIATED WITH ECFV EXPANSION, HYPERTENSION, AND HYPERALDOSTERONISM Mineralocorticoid administration or excess production [primary aldosteronism of Cushing's syndrome and adrenal cortical enzyme defects (Chap. 332)] increases net acid excretion and may result in metabolic alkalosis, which may be worsened by associated K^+ deficiency. ECFV expansion from salt retention causes hypertension and antagonizes the reduction in GFR and/or increases tubule acidification induced by aldosterone and by K^+ deficiency. The kaliuresis persists and causes continued K^+ depletion with polydipsia, inability to concentrate the urine, and polyuria. Increased aldosterone levels may be the result of autonomous primary adrenal overproduction or of secondary aldosterone release due to renal overproduction of renin. In both situations, the normal feedback of ECFV on net aldosterone production is disrupted, and hypertension from volume retention can result.

Liddle's syndrome (Chap. 278) results from increased activity of collecting duct Na^+ channels and is a cause of volume expansion and hypokalemic alkalosis with normal aldosterone levels.

Symptoms These include changes in central and peripheral nervous system function similar to those of hypocalcemia; mental confusion, obtundation, and a predisposition to seizures, paresthesia, muscular cramping, tetany, aggravation of arrhythmias, and hypoxemia in chronic obstructive pulmonary disease. Related electrolyte abnormalities include hypokalemia and hypophosphatemia.

℞ **TREATMENT**

This is primarily directed at correcting the underlying stimulus for HCO_3^- generation. If primary aldosteronism is present, correction of the underlying cause will reverse the alkalosis. $[H^+]$ loss by the stomach or kidneys can be mitigated by the use of H_2 blockers or the discontinuation of diuretics, respectively. The second aspect of treatment is to remove the factors that sustain HCO_3^- reabsorption, such as ECFV contraction or K^+ deficiency. Although K^+ deficits should be repaired, NaCl therapy is usually sufficient to reverse the alkalosis if ECFV contraction is present, as indicated by a low urine $[Cl^-]$. Unusual cases, termed *saline-resistant*, are associated with marked K^+ deficits (>1000 mmol), Mg^{2+} deficiency, Bartter's syndrome, or primary autonomous hypermineralocorticoid states. Therapy in these cases must be directed toward the underlying pathophysiologic problem.

If associated conditions preclude infusion of saline, renal HCO_3^- loss can be accelerated by administration of acetazolamide, a carbonic anhydrase inhibitor, which is usually effective in patients with adequate renal function but can worsen K^+ losses. Dilute hydrochloric acid (0.1 *N* HCl) is also effective but can cause hemolysis. Infusion of amino acids such as arginine hydrochloride is safer and as effective. Acidification can also be achieved with oral NH_4Cl, which should be avoided in the presence of liver disease. Finally, hemodialysis against a dialysate low in $[HCO_3^-]$ and high in $[Cl^-]$ can be effective when renal function is impaired.

RESPIRATORY ACIDOSIS

Respiratory acidosis can be due to severe pulmonary disease, respiratory muscle fatigue, or abnormalities in ventilatory control and is due to the increase in Pa_{CO_2} (Table 50-5). In acute respiratory acidosis, there is an immediate compensatory elevation (due to cellular buffering mechanisms) in HCO_3^-, which increases 1 mmol/L for every 10-mmHg increase in Pa_{CO_2}. In chronic respiratory acidosis (>24 h), renal adaptation occurs and the HCO_3^- increases by 4 mmol/L for every 10-mmHg increase in Pa_{CO_2}. The serum HCO_3^- usually does not increase above 38 mmol/L. Renal compensation (increased reabsorption of HCO_3^-) begins within 12 to 24 h and is not complete for about 5 days.

The clinical features vary according to the severity and duration of the respiratory acidosis, the underlying disease, and whether there is accompanying hypoxemia. A rapid increase in Pa_{CO_2} may cause anxiety, dyspnea, confusion, psychosis, and hallucinations and may progress to coma. Lesser degrees of dysfunction in chronic hypercapnia include sleep disturbances, loss of memory, daytime somnolence, personality changes, impairment of coordination, and motor disturbances such as tremor, myoclonic jerks, and asterixis. Headaches and other signs that mimic raised intracranial pressure, such as papilledema, abnormal reflexes, and focal muscle weakness, are due to vasoconstriction secondary to loss of the vasodilator effects of CO_2.

Depression of the respiratory center by a variety of drugs, injury, or disease can produce respiratory acidosis. This may occur acutely with general anesthetics, sedatives, and head trauma or chronically with sedatives, alcohol, intracranial tumors, and the syndromes of sleep-disordered breathing, including the primary alveolar and obesity-hypoventilation syndromes (Chaps. 263 and 264). Abnormalities or disease in the motor neurons, neuromuscular junction, and skeletal muscle can cause hypoventilation via respiratory muscle fatigue. Mechanical ventilation, when not properly adjusted and supervised, may result in respiratory acidosis, particularly if CO_2 production suddenly rises (because of fever, agitation, sepsis, or overfeeding) or alveolar ventilation falls because of worsening pulmonary function. High levels of positive end-expiratory pressure in the presence of reduced cardiac output may cause hypercapnia as a result of large increases in alveolar dead space (Chap. 266).

Table 50-5

Respiratory Acid-Base Disorders

I. Alkalosis
   A. Central nervous system lesions
   B. Pregnancy
   C. Endotoxemia
   D. Salicylates
   E. Hepatic failure
   F. Hypoxemia
   G. Anxiety
   H. Pain
II. Acidosis
   A. Central
     1. Drugs (anesthetics, morphine, sedatives)
     2. Stroke
     3. Infection
   B. Airway
     1. Obstruction
     2. Asthma
   C. Parenchyma
     1. Emphysema
     2. Pneumoconiosis
     3. Bronchitis
     4. Adult respiratory distress syndrome
     5. Barotrauma
   D. Neuromuscular
     1. Poliomyelitis
     2. Kyphoscoliosis
     3. Myasthenia
     4. Muscular dystrophies
   E. Miscellaneous
     1. Obesity
     2. Hypoventilation

Acute hypercapnia follows sudden occlusion of the upper airway or generalized bronchospasm as in severe asthma, anaphylaxis, inhalational burn, or toxin injury. Chronic hypercapnia and respiratory acidosis occur in end-stage obstructive lung disease. Restrictive disorders involving both the chest wall and the lungs can cause respiratory acidosis because the high metabolic cost of respiration causes ventilatory muscle fatigue. Advanced stages of intrapulmonary and extrapulmonary restrictive defects present as chronic respiratory acidosis.

The diagnosis of respiratory acidosis requires, by definition, the measurement of Pa_{CO_2} and arterial pH. A detailed history and physical examination often indicate the cause. Pulmonary function studies (Chap. 250), including spirometry, diffusion capacity for carbon monoxide, lung volumes, and arterial Pa_{CO_2}, and O_2 saturation usually make it possible to determine if respiratory acidosis is secondary to lung disease. The workup for nonpulmonary causes should include a detailed drug history, measurement of hematocrit, and assessment of upper airway, chest wall, pleura, and neuromuscular function.

℞ TREATMENT

The management of respiratory acidosis depends on its severity and rate of onset. *Acute respiratory acidosis* can be life-threatening, and measures to reverse the underlying cause should be undertaken simultaneously with restoration of adequate alveolar ventilation. This may necessitate tracheal intubation and assisted mechanical ventilation. Oxygen administration should be titrated carefully in patients with severe obstructive pulmonary disease and chronic CO_2 retention who are breathing spontaneously (Chap. 258). When oxygen is used injudiciously, these patients may experience progression of the respiratory acidosis. Aggressive and rapid correction of hypercapnia should be avoided, because the falling Pa_{CO_2} may provoke the same complications noted with acute respiratory alkalosis (i.e., cardiac arrhythmias, reduced cerebral perfusion, and seizures). The Pa_{CO_2} should be lowered gradually in chronic respiratory acidosis, aiming to restore the Pa_{CO_2} to baseline levels and to provide sufficient Cl^- and K^+ to enhance the renal excretion of HCO_3^-.

Chronic respiratory acidosis is frequently difficult to correct, but measures aimed at improving lung function such as cessation of smoking, use of oxygen, bronchodilators, glucocorticoids, diuretics, and physiotherapy can help some patients and forestall further deterioration in most. The use of respiratory stimulants may be useful in selected patients, particularly if hypercapnia is out of proportion to the abnormality in lung function.

RESPIRATORY ALKALOSIS

Alveolar hyperventilation decreases Pa_{CO_2} and increases the HCO_3^-/Pa_{CO_2} ratio, thus increasing pH (Table 50-5). Nonbicarbonate cellular buffers respond by consuming HCO_3^-. Hypocapnia develops when a sufficiently strong ventilatory stimulus causes CO_2 output in the lungs to exceed its metabolic production by tissues. Plasma pH and $[HCO_3^-]$ appear to vary proportionately with Pa_{CO_2} over a range from 40 to 15 mmHg. The relationship between arterial hydrogen ion concentration and Pa_{CO_2} is about 0.7 mmol/L per mmHg (or 0.01 pH unit/mmHg), and that for plasma $[HCO_3^-]$ is 0.2 mmol/L per mmHg. Hypocapnia sustained longer than 2 to 6 h is further compensated by a decrease in renal ammonium and titrable acid excretion and a reduction in filtered HCO_3^- reabsorption. Full renal adaptation to respiratory alkalosis may take several days and requires normal volume status and renal function. The kidneys appear to respond directly to the lowered Pa_{CO_2} rather than to alkalosis per se. A 1-mmHg fall in Pa_{CO_2} causes a 0.4- to 0.5-mmol/L drop in HCO_3^- and a 0.3-mmol/L fall (or 0.003 rise in pH) in $[H^+]$.

The effects of respiratory alkalosis vary according to duration and severity but are primarily those of the underlying disease. Reduced cerebral blood flow as a consequence of a rapid decline in Pa_{CO_2} may cause dizziness, mental confusion, and seizures, even in the absence of hypoxemia. The cardiovascular effects of acute hypocapnia in the conscious human are generally minimal, but in the anesthetized or mechanically ventilated patient, cardiac output and blood pressure may fall because of the depressant effects of anesthesia and positive-

pressure ventilation on heart rate, systemic resistance, and venous return. Cardiac arrhythmias may occur in patients with heart disease as a result of changes in oxygen unloading by blood from a left shift in the hemoglobin-oxygen dissociation curve (Bohr effect). Acute respiratory alkalosis causes intracellular shifts of Na^+, K^+, and PO_4^- and reduces free $[Ca^{2+}]$ by increasing the protein-bound fraction. Hypocapnia-induced hypokalemia is usually minor.

Respiratory alkalosis is the most common acid-base disturbance in critically ill patients and, when severe, portends a poor prognosis. Many cardiopulmonary disorders manifest respiratory alkalosis in their early to intermediate stages, and the finding of normocapnia and hypoxemia in a patient with hyperventilation may herald the onset of rapid respiratory failure and should prompt an assessment to determine if the patient is becoming fatigued. Respiratory alkalosis is common during mechanical ventilation.

The hyperventilation syndrome may be disabling. Paresthesia, circumoral numbness, chest wall tightness or pain, dizziness, inability to take an adequate breath, and, rarely, tetany may themselves be sufficiently stressful to perpetuate the disorder. Arterial blood-gas analysis demonstrates an acute or chronic respiratory alkalosis, often with hypocapnia in the range of 15 to 30 mmHg and no hypoxemia. Central nervous system diseases or injury can produce several patterns of hyperventilation and sustained Pa_{CO_2} levels of 20 to 30 mmHg. Hyperthyroidism, high caloric loads, and exercise raise the basal metabolic rate, but ventilation usually rises in proportion so that arterial blood gases are unchanged and respiratory alkalosis does not develop. Salicylates are the most common cause of drug-induced respiratory alkalosis as a result of direct stimulation of the medullary chemoreceptor. The methylxanthines, theophylline, and aminophylline stimulate ventilation and increase the ventilatory response to CO_2. Progesterone increases ventilation and lowers arterial Pa_{CO_2} by as much as 5 to 10 mmHg. Therefore, chronic respiratory alkalosis is a common feature of pregnancy. Respiratory alkalosis is also prominent in liver failure, and the severity correlates with the degree of hepatic insufficiency. Respiratory alkalosis is often an early finding in gram-negative septicemia, before fever, hypoxemia, or hypotension develop.

The diagnosis of respiratory alkalosis depends on measurement of arterial pH and Pa_{CO_2}. The plasma $[K^+]$ is often reduced, and the $[Cl^-]$ increased. In the acute phase, respiratory alkalosis is not associated with increased renal HCO_3^- excretion, but within hours net acid excretion is reduced. In general, the HCO_3^- concentration falls by 2.0 mmol/L for each 10-mmHg decrease in Pa_{CO_2}. Chronic hypocapnia reduces the serum $[HCO_3^-]$ by 5.0 mmol/L for each 10-mmHg decrease in Pa_{CO_2}. It is unusual to observe a plasma $HCO_3^- < 12$ mmol/L as a result of a pure respiratory alkalosis.

When a diagnosis of respiratory alkalosis is made, its cause should be investigated. The diagnosis of hyperventilation syndrome is made by exclusion. In difficult cases, it may be important to rule out other conditions such as pulmonary embolism, coronary artery disease, and hyperthyroidism.

℞ TREATMENT

The management of respiratory alkalosis is directed toward alleviation of the underlying disorder. If respiratory alkalosis complicates ventilator management, changes in dead space, tidal volume, and frequency can minimize the hypocapnia. Patients with the hyperventilation syndrome may benefit from reassurance, rebreathing from a paper bag during symptomatic attacks, and attention to underlying psychological stress. Antidepressants and sedatives are not recommended, although beta-adrenergic blockers may ameliorate distressing peripheral manifestations of the hyperadrenergic state.

BIBLIOGRAPHY

ALPERN RJ et al: Metabolic alkalosis, in *The Kidney: Physiology and Pathophysiology*, 2d ed, DW Seldin, G Giebisch (eds). New York, Raven Press, 1992, pp 2733–2758

BIDANI A, DUBOSE TD JR: Cellular and whole body acid-base regulation, in *Fluid, Electrolyte, and Acid-Base Disorders*, 2d ed, AI Arieff, RA De-Fronzo (eds). New York, Churchill Livingstone, 1995, pp 69–104

COGAN MG: Diagnosis of acid-base disorders, in *Fluid and Electrolytes*, MG Cogan (ed). Norwalk, Appleton & Lange, 1991, pp 198–202

DUBOSE TD JR, ALPERN RJ: Renal tubular acidosis, in *The Metabolic and Molecular Bases of Inherited Disease*, 7th ed, CR Scriver et al (eds). New York, McGraw-Hill, 1995, pp 3655–3690

———— et al: Acid-base disorders, in *The Kidney*, 5th ed, BM Brenner (ed). Philadelphia, Saunders, 1996, pp 929–998

EMMETT M et al: Metabolic acidosis, in *The Kidney: Physiology and Pathophysiology*, 2d ed, DW Seldin, G Giebisch (eds). New York, Raven Press, 1992, pp 2759–2836

MADIAS NE, COHEN JJ: Respiratory alkalosis and acidosis, in *The Kidney: Physiology and Pathophysiology*, 2d ed, DW Seldin, G Giebisch (eds). New York, Raven Press, 1992, pp 2837–2872

SECTION 8

ALTERATIONS IN THE UROGENITAL TRACT

51   *John D. McConnell, Jean D. Wilson*

IMPOTENCE

A variety of endocrine, vascular, neurologic, and psychiatric diseases disrupt normal sexual and reproductive function in men. Furthermore, sexual dysfunction may be the presenting symptom of systemic disease.

NORMAL SEXUAL FUNCTION

Penile erection is initiated by neuropsychologic stimuli that ultimately produce vasodilation of the sinusoidal spaces and arteries within the paired corpora cavernosa. Erection is normally preceded by sexual desire (or libido), which is regulated in part by androgen-dependent psychological factors. Although nocturnal and diurnal spontaneous erections are suppressed in men with androgen deficiency, erections may continue for long periods in response to erotic stimuli. Thus, continuing action of testicular androgens appears to be required for normal libido but not for the erectile mechanism itself.

The penis is innervated by sympathetic, parasympathetic, and somatic fibers. Somatic fibers in the dorsal nerve of the penis form the afferent limb of the erectile reflex by transmitting sensory impulses from the penile skin and glans to the S2–S4 dorsal root ganglia via the pudendal nerve. Unlike the corpuscular-type endings in the penile shaft skin, most afferents in the glans terminate in free nerve endings. The efferent limb begins with parasympathetic preganglionic fibers from S2–S4 that pass in the pelvic nerves to the pelvic plexus. Sympathetic fibers emerging from the intermediolateral gray areas of T11–L2 travel through the paravertebral sympathetic chain ganglia, superior hypogastric plexus, and hypogastric nerves to enter the pelvic plexus along with parasympathetic fibers. Somatic efferent fibers from S3–S4 that travel in the pudendal nerve to the ischiocavernosus and bulbocavernosus muscles and postganglionic sympathetic fibers that innervate the smooth muscle of the epididymis, vas deferens, seminal vesicle, and internal sphincter of the bladder mediate rhythmic contraction of these structures at the time of ejaculation.

Autonomic nerve impulses, integrated in the pelvic plexus, project to the penis through the cavernous nerves that course along the postero-lateral aspect of the prostate before penetrating the pelvic floor muscles immediately lateral to the urethra. Distal to the membranous urethra, some fibers enter the corpus spongiosum, while the remainder enter the corpora cavernosa along with the terminal branches of the pudendal artery and exiting cavernous veins. If disruption of the cavernous nerves occurs following pelvic trauma or surgery, erectile impotence may ensue.

The brain exerts an important modulatory influence over spinal reflex pathways that control penile function. A variety of visual, auditory, olfactory, and imaginative stimuli elicit erectile responses that involve cortical, thalamic, rhinencephalic, and limbic input to the medial preoptic-anterior hypothalamic area, which acts as an integrating center. Other areas of the brain, such as the amygdaloid complex, may inhibit sexual function.

Although the parasympathetic nervous system is the primary effector of erection, the transformation of the penis to an erect organ is a vascular phenomenon. In the flaccid state the arteries, arterioles, and sinusoidal spaces within the corpora cavernosa are constricted due to sympathetic-mediated contraction of smooth muscle in the walls of these structures. The venules between the sinusoids and the dense tunica albuginea surrounding the cavernosa open freely to the emissary veins. Erection begins when relaxation of the sinusoidal smooth muscles leads to dilation of the sinusoids and a decrease in peripheral resistance, causing a rapid increase in arterial blood flow through internal pudendal and cavernosa arteries. Expansion of the sinusoidal system compresses the venules against the interior surface of the tunica albuginea, resulting in venous occlusion. The increase in intracorporeal pressure leads to rigidity; less than complete expansion of the sinusoidal spaces leads to less than complete rigidity.

Erection occurs when adrenergic-induced sinusoid tone is antagonized by sacral parasympathetic stimulation that produces sinusoidal relaxation primarily by synthesis and release of the nonadrenergic-noncholinergic (NANC) neurotransmitter nitric oxide (NO). The contribution of acetylcholine-dependent release of NO from the vascular endothelium is uncertain. In vitro electrical stimulation of isolated corpus cavernosum strips (with or without endothelium) produces sinusoidal relaxation by release of neurotransmitters within nerve terminals that is resistant to adrenergic and cholinergic blockers. Inhibitors of the synthesis of NO or of guanosine monophosphate (GMP), as well as nitric oxide scavengers, block sinusoidal relaxation. A variety of neuropeptides found in corporal tissues, including vasoactive intestinal peptide (VIP) and calcitonin gene–related peptide (CGRP), produce tumescence when injected into the penis but have uncertain physiologic roles. Norepinephrine plays an important role in the adrenergic mechanism of detumescence.

Seminal emission and ejaculation are under control of the sympathetic nervous system. Emission results from alpha-adrenergic–mediated contraction of the epididymis, vas deferens, seminal vesicles, and prostate which causes seminal fluid to enter the prostatic urethra. Concomitant closure of the bladder neck prevents retrograde flow of semen into the bladder, and antegrade ejaculation results from contraction of the muscles of the pelvic floor including the bulbocavernosus and ischiocavernosus muscles.

Orgasm is a psychosensory phenomenon in which the rhythmic contraction of the pelvic muscles is perceived as pleasurable. Orgasm can occur without either erection or ejaculation or in the presence of retrograde ejaculation.

Detumescence after orgasm and ejaculation is incompletely understood. Presumably, active tone in the vessels of the sinusoidal spaces is restored by contraction (probably adrenergic-mediated) of smooth muscles, which decreases the inflow of blood to the penis and promotes emptying of the erectile tissue. Following orgasm, there is a refractory period that varies in duration with age, physical condition, and psychic factors and during which erection and ejaculation are inhibited.

IMPOTENCE Simply defined, impotence is the failure to achieve erection, ejaculation, or both. Men with sexual dysfunction present with a variety of complaints, either singly, or in combination: loss of desire (libido), inability to initiate or maintain an erection, ejaculatory failure, premature ejaculation, or inability to achieve orgasm. Sexual dysfunction can be secondary to systemic disease or its treatment, to specific disorders of the urogenital or endocrine systems, or to psychological disturbance. It was previously thought that the majority of men with erectile impotency had a psychological etiology for the dysfunction, but it is now believed that most impotent men have a component of underlying organic disease. Since the selection and success of therapy depend upon the etiology, it is essential to evaluate all aspects of sexual function.

Loss of Desire A decrease in sexual desire, or libido, may be due to androgen deficiency (arising from either pituitary or testicular disease), psychological disturbance, or to some types of prescribed or habitually abused drugs. The possibility of androgen deficiency can be tested by measurement of plasma testosterone and gonadotropin. The minimal level of testosterone required for normal erectile function remains unknown. Hypogonadism may also result in the absence of emission, secondary to decreased secretion of ejaculate by the seminal vesicles and prostate.

Failure of Erection The organic causes of erectile impotence can be grouped into endocrine, drug, local, neurologic, and vascular causes (Table 51-1).

Decreased plasma testosterone secondary to testicular failure is an uncommon but easily recognized and treated disorder. A borderline decrease in plasma testosterone is not a cause of sexual dysfunction. However, hyperprolactinemia may cause impotence in some men with pituitary tumors and may not be obvious on physical examination; hyperprolactinemia suppresses the production of luteinizing hormone–releasing hormone (LHRH) and thus causes low or low-normal levels of plasma gonadotropin and testosterone. Bromocriptine, a dopamine agonist, may lower prolactin levels and reverse impotence in such patients.

Although many drugs are associated with impotence, antihypertensive agents, cimetidine, and monoamine oxidase inhibitors are more likely to lead to erectile dysfunction. Antihypertensive drugs with peripheral and central sympatholytic action or beta-adrenergic receptor blocking activity are the most frequently implicated. Angiotensin-converting enzyme inhibitors, calcium channel blockers, and peripheral vasodilators do not cause a significant incidence of sexual dysfunction. Histamine (H_2) receptor antagonists, such as cimetidine, have antiandrogenic properties in addition to increasing prolactin secretion. The 5α-reductase inhibitor, finasteride, used commonly for the treatment of benign prostatic hyperplasia, produces impotence, decreased libido, or impaired ejaculation in 10 to 12 percent of men. Monoamine oxidase inhibitors, antipsychotic drugs, and tricyclic depressants may impair sexual function via anticholinergic and sympatholytic actions.

Penile diseases including previous priapism, penile trauma, and Peyronie's disease can cause impotence due to fibrosis of the sinusoidal spaces of the corpora cavernosa, corporeal artery occlusion, or neurogenic mechanisms. Peyronie's disease is not rare; patients usually present with a painful plaque on the dorsum of the penis and may progress to development of penile curvature and decreased rigidity of erection.

Many types of neurologic disorders cause impotence, including lesions in the anterior temporal lobe, spinal cord disorders, insufficiency of sensory input as in tabes dorsalis, or damage to parasympathetic nerves, for example, following surgical procedures such as radical (total) prostatectomy or cystectomy. In contrast, transurethral prostatectomy does not cause organic impotence. Furthermore, the nerve supply to the penis (the cavernosal nerves) runs on the posterolateral surface of the prostate, and if the nerves are spared during radical prostate and bladder surgery, potency can be preserved in most men. If spinal cord injury is above the sacral region, reflex erections may occur, whereas diffuse injury of the sacral spinal cord results in total

Table 51-1

Some Organic Causes of Erectile Impotence in Men

I. Endocrine causes
   A. Testicular failure (primary or secondary)
   B. Hyperprolactinemia
II. Drugs
   A. Antiandrogens
      1. Histamine (H_2) blockers (e.g., cimetidine)
      2. Spironolactone
      3. Ketoconazole
      4. Finasteride
   B. Antihypertensives
      1. Central-acting sympatholytics (e.g., clonidine and methyldopa)
      2. Peripheral-acting sympatholytics (e.g., guanadrel)
      3. Beta blockers
      4. Thiazides
   C. Anticholinergics
   D. Antidepressants
      1. Monoamine oxidase inhibitors
      2. Tricyclic antidepressants
   E. Antipsychotics
   F. Central nervous system depressants
      1. Sedatives (e.g., barbiturates)
      2. Antianxiety drugs (e.g., diazepam)
   G. Drugs of habituation or addiction
      1. Alcohol
      2. Methadone
      3. Heroin
      4. Tobacco
III. Penile diseases
   A. Peyronie's disease
   B. Previous priapism
   C. Penile trauma
IV. Neurologic diseases
   A. Anterior temporal lobe lesions
   B. Diseases of the spinal cord
   C. Loss of sensory input
      1. Tabes dorsalis
      2. Disease of dorsal root ganglia
   D. Disease of nervi erigentes
      1. Radical prostatectomy and cystectomy
      2. Rectosigmoid operations
   E. Diabetic autonomic neuropathy and various polyneuropathies
V. Vascular disease
   A. Aortic occlusion (Leriche syndrome)
   B. Atherosclerotic occlusion or stenosis of the pudendal and/or cavernosa arteries
   C. Arterial damage from pelvic radiation
   D. Venous leak
   E. Disease of the sinusoidal spaces

impotence. As many as half of men with diabetes mellitus develop impotence within 6 years of the onset of diabetes, and impotence may be the first clinical manifestation of diabetic neuropathy. Vasculogenic dysfunction is a concomitant factor in most men with diabetic impotence. Several factors contribute to neuropathic impotence, including abnormalities in afferent sensory pathways, motor neuropathy in the cavernosa nerves (which carry the efferent pathways for vasodilation in the penis), and decreased level of neurotransmitters in the corpora cavernosa. In addition, denervation of the sinusoidal smooth muscle leads to a loss of contractile elements and fibrosis, which limits dilation of the spaces. Although the autonomic pathways in the penis can be tested by direct recording of electrical activity in the corporal smooth muscle, the test may not be necessary since most patients demonstrate other manifestations of autonomic neuropathy on careful examination. Many of the other polyneuropathies associated with impotence have similar effects.

Men with vasculogenic impotence may present with total erectile impotence, decreased penile rigidity, or loss of erection during intercourse. Vascular insufficiency may be due to aortic occlusion (Leriche syndrome) or to more distal atherosclerotic disease in the hypogastric, pudendal, and cavernosa arteries. The function of the sinusoidal tissue itself may be adversely affected by atherosclerosis and by the use of tobacco products, which contain a variety of vasocontractile agents. Significant disease in the pudendal and cavernosa arteries can occur in the absence of other clinical manifestations of peripheral vascular disease. The impotence commonly seen following pelvic radiation is probably due to vasculogenic causes. Together with neuropathy, vascular insufficiency contributes to the impotence in many men with diabetes mellitus.

Premature Ejaculation This disorder seldom has an organic cause. It is usually related to anxiety in the sexual situation, unreasonable expectations about performance, or emotional disorder. A variety of successful therapeutic modalities have been described, but behavioral therapy is most successful.

Absence of Emission This symptom may be produced by (1) retrograde ejaculation, (2) sympathetic denervation, (3) androgen deficiency, or (4) drugs. Retrograde ejaculation may occur following surgery on the bladder neck or develop spontaneously in diabetic men. Demonstration of sperm in a postcoital urine specimen establishes the diagnosis. Following sympathectomy or occasionally after extensive retroperitoneal surgery, the autonomic innervation of the prostate and seminal vesicles is lost, resulting in absence of smooth-muscle contraction at the time of ejaculation. Androgen deficiency results in a decrease in secretions of the prostate and seminal vesicles and in a decrease in the volume of ejaculate. Finally, drugs such as guanethidine, phenoxybenzamine, phentolamine, and sertraline primarily impair ejaculation rather than erection or libido.

Absence of Orgasm If libido and erectile function are normal, the absence of orgasm is almost always due to a psychiatric disorder.

Failure of Detumescence Priapism is a persistent painful erection, often unrelated to sexual activity. Priapism can be distinguished from a normal erection by the absence of tumescence of the glans penis. Priapism may be idiopathic but can be associated with sickle cell anemia, chronic granulocytic leukemia, spinal cord injury, or injection of vasodilator agents (such as alprostadil) into the penis. The disorder may be secondary to clotting of blood within the sinusoidal spaces of the penis or to abnormalities of the adrenergic-mediated mechanism for detumescence. Failure to treat priapism promptly usually results in fibrosis and subsequent loss of erectile function. In early phases, detumescence can sometimes be achieved by aspiration, irrigation of the corpora cavernosa, and injection of dilute vasoconstrictors. If this fails, surgical relief by shunting procedures may be necessary. In patients with priapism secondary to sickle cell anemia, conservative measures such as transfusion, oxygenation, and irrigation are generally preferred to shunting procedures.

EVALUATION OF IMPOTENCE The relative frequency of organic as opposed to psychogenic causes of erectile impotence is still debated. Nevertheless, anxiety and depressive states are common causes of impotence (see Chap. 385). Other psychological factors such as disinterest in the sexual partner, fear of sexual incompetence, marital discord, guilt about deviant sexual attitudes, worry, fatigue, and ill health often operate in various combinations to reduce sexual impulse. The central issue in the evaluation of impotence is to separate those instances due to psychological factors from those due to organic causes (Table 51-1). Often, the separation can be made on the basis of history. With the exception of severe depression, men with psychogenic impotence usually have normal nocturnal and early morning erections. From early childhood through the eighth decade, erections occur during normal sleep. This phenomenon, termed *nocturnal penile tumescence* (NPT), occurs during rapid eye movement sleep, and the total time of NPT averages 100 min per night. Consequently, if the impotent man gives a history of rigid erections under any circumstances (often when awakening in the morning), the efferent neurologic and circulatory systems that mediate erection are intact, and dysfunction is probably due to a psychiatric disorder. In these patients the workup should be limited. (Occasional patients with early sensory neuropathy may have nocturnal erections.)

If the history of nocturnal erections is questionable, measurements of NPT can be made formally with the use of a strain gauge in a sleep laboratory, or informally attached to a recorder, by snap gauge or home monitor. Although false-negative and false-positive results are possible, this procedure helps to differentiate psychogenic and organic impotence. Patients with vasculogenic impotence may have some degree of penile tumescence without the development of adequate rigidity, which may result in a false-positive NPT test. An alternative to NTP testing is the visual sexual stimulation test, which utilizes videotaped erotic material in a laboratory setting to monitor erection by strain gauge. Other features in favor of organic impotence include a slow, insidious onset not associated with any particular psychiatric symptomatology, a previous uninterrupted period of normal erectile function, and persistent sexual desire.

Having deduced an organic cause, the fundamental problem is the differential diagnosis of the etiology (Table 51-1). The history should be probed for indications of diabetes mellitus, manifestations of peripheral neuropathy or bladder dysfunction, symptoms referable to the vascular system such as intermittent claudication, and symptoms of penile disease such as a history of priapism or penile curvature (Peyronie's disease). A thorough drug history should be obtained, and inquiry made concerning past surgery that may have produced neurologic damage. Smoking is not only a risk factor for atherosclerotic disease but may inhibit sinusoidal relaxation directly.

Physical examination should include a detailed genital examination to identify abnormalities of the penis, especially Peyronie's disease, usually easily felt as a fibrotic plaque on the dorsum of the penis. The testes should be palpated for size, symmetry, and abnormal masses; if the length is less than 3.5 cm, hypogonadism should be considered. Evidence of feminization, such as gynecomastia and abnormal body hair distribution, should be sought. All pulses should be palpated, and the presence of bruits should be sought. Often, the pulse in the dorsal penile artery can be felt. If there is an indication from either history or physical examination of a vascular etiology, direct measurement of penile blood flow may be indicated.

With the advent of minimally invasive treatment options, extensive diagnostic testing is infrequently indicated. An initial discussion of treatment options should precede invasive diagnostic procedures. If the patient prefers nonsurgical therapy, further testing beyond history, physical examination, and measurement of plasma testosterone is unlikely to change management.

Pudendal arteriography provides the most accurate assessment of penile arterial disease, but it is expensive and invasive. Moreover, distal arterial lesions may not be identified unless the procedure is performed under conditions of chemical erection (e.g., alprostadil injection). The penile/brachial index can be used to estimate penile blood flow by dividing the penile systolic blood pressure, as determined by Doppler technique, by the simultaneously determined supine brachial systolic pressure. An index of less than 0.6 suggests vasculogenic impotence. However, the test only evaluates flow through the dorsal penile artery, which is not directly involved in the erectile process. Significant disease may be present in the cavernosa arteries despite normal flow through the dorsal artery. Pulsed Doppler analysis and high-resolution ultrasonography can be used in conjunction with intracorporeal injection of alprostadil to assess blood flow in the cavernosal arteries. Alternatively, dynamic infusion cavernosography, in which pressure is measured directly within the corpora, can be utilized to assess arterial inflow. Abnormalities in the venous occlusive mechanism of the penis can cause impotence due to "venous leak" but are usually the result of abnormalities in sinusoidal smooth muscle function or impaired arterial inflow rather than venous abnormalities. Moreover, surgical attempts to eradicate venous leakage seldom restore erectile function in the long term. Therefore, testing to identify venous leak is rarely indicated.

The neurologic examination should measure anal sphincter tone, perineal sensation, and the bulbocavernosus reflex. This reflex is elicited by squeezing the glans penis and noting the degree of anal sphincter constriction. An examination for peripheral neuropathy should include assessment of distal muscle function; the tendon reflexes in the legs; and vibratory, position, tactile, and pain sensation. In the presence of peripheral neuropathy, tests to evaluate penile neuropathy are seldom necessary. In cases with an uncertain neurogenic component, electromyographic sacral signal tracing of the bulbocavernosus reflex or direct electrical recording of the corpora cavernosa by needle or surface electrodes may be helpful. A specific test to document abnormalities in the penile autonomic efferent pathways is not available.

In the absence of hypogonadism or feminization, the serum testosterone is usually normal. Hyperprolactinemia, however, may not be suspected on the basis of history and physical examination. Although endocrine causes of erectile dysfunction are uncommon, measurement of serum prolactin and pooled serum testosterone and luteinizing hormone (see Chap. 336) is appropriate since abnormalities of these parameters are treatable.

℞ TREATMENT

Medical therapy with androgens offers little more than placebo benefit except in hypogonadal men, and empirical therapy may actually delay identification of organic etiologies. If a prolactin-secreting pituitary tumor is present, however, either surgical removal or treatment with bromocriptine usually results in return of potency. Yohimbine, an alpha$_2$-adrenergic antagonist, is widely prescribed but works only in psychogenic impotence by placebo effect. Surgical therapy may be useful in the treatment of decreased potency related to aortic obstruction; however, potency can be lost rather than improved after aortic surgery if the autonomic nerve supply to the penis is damaged. Penile revascularization is appropriate only in young men with traumatic arterial disease. Very few men with venous leak impotency benefit from venous ligation.

The injection of a variety of vasoactive substances into the corpora cavernosa can produce erection. Self-injection with prostaglandin E$_2$ (alprostadil) produces erection in more than 90 percent of men with psychogenic, neurogenic, and mild-to-moderate vasculogenic impotence. Side effects include occasional pain on injection, priapism (1 percent), and penile fibrosis (2 percent). Commercially available mechanical devices that utilize a vacuum to produce an erection and a rubber band to restrict venous return at the base of the penis provide a successful nonsurgical alternative in many patients, including those with diabetes mellitus and severe vascular disease.

Penile prostheses are a therapeutic alternative in impotent patients refractory to other forms of therapy. Malleable plastic rods implanted into the penis provide the simplest system and the lowest complication rates; however, the cosmetic and functional performance of the device is not uniformly satisfactory. Multicomponent, hydraulically operated prostheses offer the advantage of more physiologic erection and greater increase in penile diameter, but these devices are subject to mechanical failure.

Even in patients with organic impotence, psychotherapy is often beneficial in alleviating concomitant psychogenic factors that limit the success of medical and surgical therapy.

BIBLIOGRAPHY

ABRAMOWICZ M et al: Drugs that cause sexual dysfunction. Med Let 29:65, 1987
ALLEN RP et al: Comparison of duplex ultrasonography and nocturnal penis tumescence in evaluation of impotence. J Urol 151:1525, 1994
ANDERSSON KE: Pharmacology of lower urinary tract smooth muscles and penile erectile tissues. Pharmacol Rev 45:254, 1993
———, WAGNER G: Physiology of penile erection. Physiol Rev 75:191, 1995
BURNETT AL et al: Nitric oxide: A physiologic mediator of penile erection. Science 257:401, 1992
FISHMAN JF et al: Experience with inflatable penile prosthesis. Urology 23:86, 1984
GOLDSTEIN I et al: Radiation-associated impotence—a clinical study of its mechanism. JAMA 251:903, 1984
KAISER FE, KORENMAN SG: Impotence in diabetic men. Am J Med 85(Suppl 5A):147, 1988
KAPLAN HS: The combined use of sex therapy and intra penile injections in the treatment of impotence. J Sex Marital Ther 16:195, 1990

KIM N et al: A nitric-oxide like factor mediates nonadrenergic-noncholinergic neurogenic relaxation of penile corpus cavernosum smooth muscle. J Clin Invest 88:112, 1991
KNISPEL HH: Penile venous surgery in impotence: Results in highly selected cases. Urol Int 47:144, 1991
KOLODNY RC et al: Sexual function in diabetic men. Diabetes 23:306, 1974
KRANE RJ: Medical progress: Impotence. N Engl J Med 321:1648, 1989
KWAN M et al: The nature of androgen action on male sexuality: A combined laboratory–self-report study on hypogonadal men. J Clin Endocrinol Metab 57:557, 1983
LEVINE SB: Marital sexual dysfunction: Ejaculation disturbances. Ann Intern Med 84:575, 1976
LINET OL, OGRINC FG: Efficacy and safety of intracavernosal alprostadil in men with erectile dysfunction. The Alprostadil Study Group. N Engl J Med 334(14):873, 1996
LUE TF et al: Vasculogenic impotence evaluated by high-resolution ultrasonography and pulsed Doppler spectrum analysis. Radiology 155:777, 1985
——— et al: Functional evaluation of penile veins by cavernosography in papaverine-induced erection. J Urol 135:479, 1986
MEULEMAN EJ, DIEMONT WL: Investigation of erectile dysfunction. Urol Clin North Am 22:803, 1995
MONTAGUE DK et al: Infusion pharmacocavernosometry and normal penile tumescence findings in men with erectile dysfunction. J Urol 145:768, 1991
RAJFER J: Nitric oxide as a mediator of relaxation in response to non-adrenergic, non-cholinergic neurotransmission. N Engl J Med 326:90, 1992
SAYPOL DC et al: Impotence. Are the newer diagnostic methods a necessity? J Urol 130:260, 1983
TIEFER L, SCHUETZ-MUELLER D: Psychological issues in diagnosis and treatment of erectile disorders. Urol Clin North Am 22:767, 1995
VIRAG R et al: Intracavernous self-injection of vasoactive drugs in the treatment of impotence: 8-year experience with 615 cases. J Urol 145:287, 1991
WABEK AJ: Bulbocavernosus reflex testing in 100 consecutive cases of erectile dysfunction. Urology 25:495, 1985
WALSH PC et al: Impotence following radical prostatectomy: Insight into etiology and prevention. J Urol 128:492, 1982
WINTER CC: Priapism. Urol Surv 28:163, 1978
WITHERINGTON R: Vacuum constriction device for management of erectile impotence. J Urol 141:320, 1989

| 52 | *Bruce R. Carr, Karen D. Bradshaw* |

DISTURBANCES OF MENSTRUATION AND OTHER COMMON GYNECOLOGIC COMPLAINTS IN WOMEN

Complaints related to the female reproductive tract can be categorized as disorders of menstruation, pelvic pain, disturbances in sexual function, or infertility. However, a single disorder, e.g., leiomyoma of the uterus, can present with symptoms referable to any one or more of these categories. Furthermore, sexual dysfunction can interdigitate with other problems in several ways. On the one hand, in women with complaints related to other reproductive tract functions, the underlying problem may actually be severe sexual dysfunction or marital conflict. Alternatively, women with severe organic disorders of the pelvis, e.g., pelvic inflammatory disease, may present with sexual dysfunction such as dyspareunia that in fact is only a minor manifestation of the underlying disease.

Since normal reproductive function depends on the integrated action of the central nervous system, the endocrine glands, and the reproductive organs, menstrual cycle abnormalities, sexual dysfunction, and infertility may be the result of systemic and psychological disorders as well as of primary defects in the endocrine and reproductive organs. The endocrine and physiologic control—normal and abnormal—of puberty, reproductive life, and menopause are discussed in Chap. 337. The focus of this chapter is on the initial evaluation of women with disturbances of the reproductive tract.

DISTURBANCES IN MENSTRUATION Disorders of menstruation can be divided into abnormal uterine bleeding and amenorrhea.

Abnormal Uterine Bleeding The menstrual cycle is defined as the interval between the onset of one bleeding episode and the onset of the next. In normal women the cycle averages 28 ± 3 days, the mean duration of menstrual flow is 4 ± 2 days, and the average blood loss is 40 to 100 mL. Between menarche and menopause most women experience one or more episodes of abnormal uterine bleeding, here defined as any bleeding pattern outside the normal ranges of frequency, duration, and/or amount of blood loss. The decision to evaluate a patient depends on the severity and frequency of the abnormal bleeding pattern.

When vaginal bleeding occurs, it should first be determined whether the blood is derived from the uterine endometrium. Rectal, bladder, cervical, and vaginal sources of bleeding must be excluded. Once the bleeding is established to be uterine in origin, a pregnancy-related disorder (such as threatened or incomplete abortion or ectopic pregnancy) must be ruled out by physical examination and appropriate laboratory tests. It should also be remembered that uterine bleeding also may be the initial or principal manifestation of a generalized bleeding diathesis. The remaining causes of abnormal uterine bleeding can be divided into those associated with ovulatory or anovulatory cycles.

Ovulatory cycles Menstrual bleeding with ovulatory cycles is spontaneous, regular in onset, predictable in duration and amount of flow, and frequently associated with discomfort; it is the consequence of progesterone withdrawal at the end of the luteal (postovulatory) phase and requires prior estrogen priming of the endometrium during the follicular (preovulatory) phase of the cycle. When deviations from an established pattern of menstrual flow occur but the cycles are still regular, the usual cause is disease of the outflow tract. For example, regular, prolonged, excessive bleeding episodes can result from abnormalities of the uterus such as submucous leiomyomas, adenomyosis, or endometrial polyps. On the other hand, cyclic, predictable menstruation characterized by spotting or light bleeding suggests obstruction of the outflow tract as with uterine synechiae or scarring of the cervix. Intermittent bleeding between cyclic ovulatory menses is often due to cervical or endometrial lesions.

Anovulatory cycles Uterine bleeding that is irregular in occurrence, unpredictable as to amount and duration of flow, and usually painless is called *dysfunctional or anovulatory uterine bleeding*. This type of bleeding is the result of a failure of normal follicular maturation with consequent anovulation and may be either transient or chronic. Transient disruption of ovulatory cycles occurs most often in the early menarcheal years, during the perimenopausal period, or as the consequence of a variety of stresses and intercurrent illnesses. Persistent dysfunctional uterine bleeding during the reproductive years can occur in several organic diseases that affect ovarian function and is most often due to estrogen breakthrough bleeding. Estrogen breakthrough bleeding occurs when estrogen stimulation of the endometrium is continuous and is not interrupted by cyclic progesterone withdrawal, as can occur in polycystic ovarian disease.

Amenorrhea *Amenorrhea* is defined either as failure of menarche by age 16, regardless of the presence or absence of secondary sexual characteristics, or as the absence of menstruation for 6 months in a woman with previous periodic menses. Amenorrhea in a woman who has never menstruated is termed *primary*; cessation of menses is termed *secondary amenorrhea*. Because some disorders can cause both primary and secondary amenorrhea, we prefer a functional classification based on the nature of the underlying defect, namely, anatomic defects of the outflow tract (uterus, cervix, or vagina), ovarian failure, and chronic anovulation.

Anatomic defects of the outflow tract include congenital defects of the vagina, imperforate hymen, transverse vaginal septa, cervical stenosis, intrauterine adhesions (synechiae), absence of the vagina or

uterus, and uterine maldevelopment. The diagnosis of an anatomic defect is usually made by physical examination and confirmed by demonstrating failure of bleeding following administration of estrogen plus a progestagen for 21 days. Pelvic ultrasonography, magnetic resonance imaging, hysterosalpingogram, or hysteroscopy may be helpful in defining the defect.

Causes of *ovarian failure* include gonadal dysgenesis, deficiency of $P450_{17\alpha}$, resistant ovary syndrome, and premature ovarian failure. Ovarian failure encompasses disorders in which the ovary is deficient in germ cells and those in which the germ cells are resistant to follicle-stimulating hormone (FSH). The diagnosis of ovarian failure as the cause of amenorrhea is confirmed by an elevated plasma FSH level.

Women with *chronic anovulation* fail to ovulate spontaneously but have the capability of ovulating with appropriate therapy. In some women with chronic anovulation, total estrogen production is adequate, but it is not secreted in a cyclic fashion. In others, estrogen production is deficient.

Women who have adequate estrogen production and demonstrate withdrawal bleeding after progestagen challenge usually have polycystic ovarian disease (see Fig. 337-8). Other causes include hormone-secreting ovarian and adrenal tumors. Women with deficient or absent estrogen production, and therefore with absence of withdrawal bleeding after progestagen administration, usually have hypogonadotropic hypogonadism due to organic or functional disorders of the pituitary or central nervous system such as brain tumors, pituitary tumors (especially prolactin-secreting adenomas), primary hypopituitarism, or Sheehan's syndrome.

PELVIC PAIN Pelvic pain may originate in the pelvis or be referred from another region of the body. A pelvic source is suggested by the history (e.g., dysmenorrhea and dyspareunia) and physical findings, but a high index of suspicion must be entertained for extrapelvic disorders that refer to the pelvis, such as appendicitis, cholecystitis, intestinal obstruction, and urinary tract infections (see Chap. 14).

"Physiologic" Pelvic Pain *Pain associated with ovulation ("mittelschmerz")* Many women experience low abdominal discomfort with ovulation, typically a dull aching pain at midcycle in one lower quadrant lasting from minutes to hours. It is rarely severe or incapacitating. The pain may result from peritoneal irritation by follicular fluid released into the peritoneal cavity at ovulation. The onset at midcycle and short duration of pain are often diagnostic.

Premenstrual or menstrual pain In normal ovulatory women, somatic symptoms during the few days prior to menses may be insignificant or disabling. Such symptoms include edema, breast engorgement, and abdominal bloating or discomfort. A symptom complex of cyclic irritability, depression, and lethargy is known as the *premenstrual syndrome* (PMS). The cause of PMS is unknown, and there is no consensus about therapy.

Severe or incapacitating uterine cramping during ovulatory menses and in the absence of demonstrable disorders of the pelvis is termed *primary dysmenorrhea*. Primary dysmenorrhea is caused by prostaglandin-induced uterine ischemia and is treated with prostaglandin synthetase inhibitors or oral contraceptive agents.

Pelvic Pain due to Organic Causes Severe dysmenorrhea associated with disease of the pelvis is termed *secondary dysmenorrhea*. Organic causes of pelvic pain can be classified as (1) uterine, (2) adnexal, (3) vulvar or vaginal, and (4) pregnancy-associated.

Uterine pain Pain of uterine etiology is often chronic and continuous and increases in intensity during menstruation and intercourse. Causes include leiomyomas of the uterus (particularly submucous and degenerating leiomyomas), adenomyosis, and cervical stenosis. Infections of the uterus associated with intrauterine manipulation following dilatation and curettage or with intrauterine devices also can cause pelvic pain (see Chap. 337). Pelvic pain due to endometrial or cervical cancer is usually a late manifestation (see Chap. 337).

Adnexal pain The most common cause of pain in the adnexae (fallopian tubes and ovaries) is infection (see Chap. 130). Acute salpingo-oophoritis presents as low abdominal pain, fever, and chills; begins a few days after a menstrual period; and is usually due to chlamydial or gonococcal disease with or without a superimposed pyogenic infection. Chronic pelvic inflammatory disease results from either a single episode or multiple episodes of infection and may present as infertility associated with chronic pelvic pain that increases in intensity with menses and intercourse. On physical examination, the adnexae are tender, and adnexal thickening and/or masses may be present. Pelvic inflammatory disease may become a surgical emergency if peritonitis results from rupture of a tuboovarian abscess. Ovarian cysts or neoplasms may cause pelvic pain that becomes more severe with torsion or rupture of the mass, and ectopic pregnancy must be considered in the differential diagnosis (see below). Endometriosis involving fallopian tubes, ovaries, or peritoneum may cause both chronic low abdominal pain and infertility; the magnitude of tissue involvement does not always correlate with the severity of symptoms. Endometriosis pain typically increases with menstruation and, if the posterior ligaments of the uterus are involved, with intercourse.

Vulvar or vaginal pain Pain in these areas is most often due to infectious vaginitis caused by *Monilia*, *Trichomonas*, or bacteria and is characteristically associated with vaginal discharge and pruritus. Herpetic vulvitis, condyloma acuminatum, and cysts or abscesses of Bartholin's glands also may cause vulvar pain.

Pregnancy-associated disorders Pregnancy must be considered in the differential diagnosis of pelvic pain during the reproductive years. Threatened abortion or incomplete abortion often presents with uterine cramping, bleeding, or passage of tissue following a period of amenorrhea. Ectopic pregnancy may be insidious in presentation or result in abrupt intraperitoneal hemorrhage and maternal death.

Evaluation of Pelvic Pain The evaluation of pelvic pain requires a careful history and pelvic examination. This often leads to the correct diagnosis and institution of appropriate treatment. If the pain is severe and the diagnosis is unclear, the workup should follow that outlined for the acute abdomen (Chap. 14). A culdocentesis is indicated if a ruptured ectopic pregnancy is suspected. If there is a question of an adnexal mass or if the patient is so obese as to preclude a thorough pelvic examination, sonography may be useful. Serial human chorionic gonadotropin (hCG) measurements may help in establishing a diagnosis of tubal pregnancy. Finally, diagnostic laparoscopy and laparotomy may be indicated with pain of undetermined etiology.

SEXUAL DYSFUNCTION Some women with sexual dysfunction describe minor complaints related to the reproductive tract as a means of bringing sexual problems to the attention of the physician. Alternatively, sexual dysfunction may be thought to be the cause of low abdominal discomfort or dyspareunia when the actual etiology is organic. However, more and more women seek medical advice because of sexual problems that interface in provenance between medicine and sociology.

The normal sexual response begins with sexual arousal, which causes genital vasocongestion that results in vaginal lubrication in preparation for intromission. The lubrication is due to the formation of a transudate in the vagina and in conjunction with genital congestion produces the so-called orgasmic platform prior to orgasm. Sexual stimuli (visual, tactile, auditory, and olfactory) as well as healthy vaginal tissue are prerequisites for genital vasocongestion and vaginal lubrication. During the second stage of the sexual response, involuntary contractions of the muscles of the pelvis result in a pleasurable cortical sensory phenomenon known as orgasm. Direct or indirect stimulation of the clitoris is important in the production of the female orgasm. In simple terms, sexual dysfunction can be due to interference with the arousal or orgasmic phases of the sexual response. Either disorder can be due to an organic or functional cause or both.

Illnesses that impair neurologic function such as diabetes mellitus or multiple sclerosis can prevent normal sexual arousal. Local pelvic diseases such as vaginitis, endometriosis, and salpingo-oophoritis may preclude normal sexual response because of resulting dyspareunia. Debilitating systemic diseases such as cancer and cardiovascular diseases may inhibit normal sexual response indirectly.

More commonly, failure of a normal sexual response is due to psychological factors that impair sexual arousal. Such problems include misinformation, e.g., the perception of sexual satisfaction as bad, or feelings of guilt about previous psychologically traumatic

events such as incest, rape, or unwanted pregnancy. In addition, women who have had previous hysterectomy or mastectomy may perceive themselves as "incomplete." Stresses such as anxiety, depression, fatigue, and marital or interpersonal conflicts may lead to failure of the vasocongestive response and prevent normal vaginal lubrication. Women with such experiences may be unable to achieve normal sexual response unless they receive professional counseling. Such problems are approached by attempting to identify and reduce the causative stresses.

Failure to achieve orgasm is a specific form of sexual dysfunction. In the absence of orgasm many women enjoy sexual encounters to variable degrees because of the pleasure derived from closeness in a cherished relationship, particularly with a loving partner. However, for other women sexual relations with rare or absent orgasms are frustrating and unsatisfying. In many instances, failure of orgasm is due to insufficient clitoral stimulation and may be rectified by appropriate counseling and patient education.

A specific entity, "vaginismus," painful, involuntary contractions of the musculature surrounding the entrance to the vagina, is a rare cause of dyspareunia. It is a conditioned response to a previous real or imagined frightening or traumatic sexual experience. Treatment is directed to elimination of the conditioned response by progressive vaginal dilation by the patient in conjunction with marital therapy.

REPRODUCTION Infertility is discussed in detail in Chap. 337. The approach to infertile couples always involves evaluation of both the man and woman. The history should address the frequency of intercourse, the sexual responses of both, the use of contraceptives or lubricants, previous or past medical illnesses, and all medications taken.

Male-associated factors account for a third of infertility problems. Therefore, one of the first procedures in the workup of infertile couples should be a semen analysis (see Chap. 336). The initial evaluation of the woman includes documentation of normal ovulatory cycles. A history of regular, cyclic, predictable, spontaneous menses usually indicates ovulatory cycles, which may be confirmed by basal body temperature graphs, properly timed endometrial biopsies, or plasma progesterone measurements during the luteal phase of the cycle. Also, the diagnosis of luteal-phase dysfunction (low progesterone secretion during the luteal phase) can be established by these methods. Transvaginal ultrasonography is useful for evaluating follicular development. If the diagnosis is polycystic ovarian disease, attempts to induce ovulation can be undertaken by a variety of methods including administration of clomiphene, human menopausal gonadotropins, bromocriptine, or luteinizing hormone–releasing hormone (LHRH) agonists or by wedge resection of the ovaries (now usually done by laparoscopic cautery or laser drilling) (Chap. 337).

The most common cause of infertility in women is tubal disease, usually due to infection (pelvic inflammatory disease) or endometriosis. Tubal disease can be evaluated by obtaining a hysterosalpingogram or by diagnostic laparoscopy. Tubal diseases can usually be treated by laparoscopic tuboplasty and lysis of adhesions; in severe cases the infertility is treated by in vitro fertilization and embryo transfer.

A cervical factor as a cause of infertility is identified by a properly timed postcoital examination. During this examination, the sperm motility in cervical mucus is observed. Also, immunologic etiologies for infertility can be tested for by a variety of laboratory tests. The cause of infertility is unknown in 10 percent of couples. In many instances of infertility, it is now possible to use assisted reproductive technologies including in vitro fertilization and embryo transfer, gamete intrafallopian tube transfer, transfer of cryopreserved ova and embryos, and ovarian hyperstimulation with clomiphene citrate or gonadotropins followed by intrauterine insemination.

The desire for contraception is also a frequent cause for women to seek medical treatment or evaluation. The most widely used methods for fertility control include (1) rhythm and withdrawal techniques, (2) barrier methods, (3) intrauterine devices, (4) oral steroid contraceptives, (5) sterilization, and (6) abortion. These methods and their complications are discussed in Chap. 337.

BIBLIOGRAPHY

CARR BR, BLACKWELL RE: *Textbook of Reproductive Medicine.* Norwalk CT, Appleton & Lange, 1993

CUNNINGHAM FG et al: *Williams Obstetrics,* 19th ed. Norwalk, Appleton & Lange, 1993

HERBST AL et al: *Comprehensive Gynecology,* 2d ed. St. Louis, Mosby, 1992

FORDNEY DS: Dyspareunia and vaginismus. Clin Obstet Gynecol 21:205, 1978

HAMMOND DC: Screening for sexual dysfunction. Clin Obstet Gynecol 27:732, 1984

HATCHER RA et al: *Contraceptive Technology,* 16th ed. New York, Irvington, 1994

MASTERS W, JOHNSON V: *Human Sexual Response.* Boston, Little, Brown, 1966

ROSEN RJ et al: Prevention of sexual dysfunction in women. J Sex Med Ther 19:171, 1993

SPEROFF L et al: *Clinical Gynecologic Endocrinology and Infertility,* 4th ed. Baltimore, Williams & Wilkins, 1989

---

53 | *William J. Kovacs, Jean D. Wilson*

HIRSUTISM AND VIRILIZATION

Hirsutism, male pattern hair growth in women, is a common and perplexing problem. The distribution and growth of hair in normal persons is under complex genetic and endocrine control so that there is considerable variability in hair growth among normal men and women. As a consequence, abnormal hair growth is difficult to define: Some patients may seek medical attention because of what the physician may consider an insignificant cosmetic defect. Others, because of personal or cultural factors, may be undisturbed by significant degrees of hirsutism. The central issue in dealing with such patients is the separation of those infrequent instances in which hirsutism is a manifestation of a serious and remediable underlying disorder from the majority of hirsute women in whom excess hair is fundamentally a cosmetic problem.

CONTROL OF NORMAL HAIR GROWTH AND DISTRIBUTION Endocrine Control Androgens are the major determinants of hair distribution in both sexes. There are three principal circulating androgens in women—dehydroepiandrosterone, derived from the adrenal; androstenedione, which is derived equally from adrenal and ovary; and testosterone, which is both secreted by the ovary and adrenal and formed in extraglandular tissue from circulating dehydroepiandrosterone and androstenedione. The production of adrenal androgen is regulated primarily by adrenocorticotropin, while ovarian androgen secretion is regulated by luteinizing hormone (LH). These various androgens must be converted to testosterone (or dihydrotestosterone) before they can bind to the androgen receptor of target cells and induce an androgenic response. Thus, adrenal androgens virilize only in so far as they serve as precursors for testosterone and dihydrotestosterone.

Several types of relationships can be defined between hair growth and androgens in normal individuals. Eyebrows, eyelashes, and vellus hairs are not dependent on androgens. Axillary and lower pubic hair are sensitive to small amounts of androgen; hair growth in these areas begins at the time of adrenarche under the control of adrenal androgens and is approximately equal in men and women. In some areas such as the face, upper pubic triangle, chest, and ears, hair growth is more typical of males and appears to require the greater androgen levels produced by the testes. Finally, scalp hair exhibits androgen-mediated regression. The reason different body regions respond differently to

the same or similar androgen is unknown. The metabolism of androgens might differ in the various sites. The hair follicle, like some other androgen targets, requires conversion of testosterone to dihydrotestosterone for expression of androgen action, and hair follicles from all regions of the body perform this conversion. Moreover, the same receptor that is essential for androgen action in other cells (Chap. 336) mediates the effects of dihydrotestosterone in the hair follicle. Genetic disorders with normal testosterone production but absent androgen receptor have deficient or absent axillary, pubic, facial, truncal, and limb hair (Chap. 339). Regional differences in androgen responsiveness of hair in normal individuals could also be the consequence of regional differences in the amount of androgen receptor in hair follicles.

Genetic Factors Despite similar hormone levels, the distribution of hair varies among individuals and among different ethnic and racial groups. Dark-haired, darkly pigmented whites of either sex tend to be more hirsute than blond or fair-skinned persons. Asians, native Americans, and blacks on average are less hirsute than whites. Asians have scant facial and body hair except in the pubic and axillary regions, and native Americans, in addition, rarely develop baldness. Heterogeneity of hair patterns also exists within families. The inheritance of hair patterns is complex and probably polygenic in nature.

Other factors Aging is a prerequisite for some types of hair development. For example, in men hair on the trunk and extremities frequently increases for several years after maximal levels of plasma androgens have been reached. Conversely, loss of androgen may not result in diminution of normal hair growth in men or complete reversal of hirsutism in women. Women in the first trimester of pregnancy commonly have increased hairiness of the face, extremities, and breasts. Menopause is often associated with the loss of hair in the pubic area, axillae, and extremities, whereas growth of hair on the face increases in postmenopausal women. These changes cannot be explained solely by changes in androgen levels.

PATHOLOGIC HAIR GROWTH AND DISTRIBUTION A central consideration in the evaluation of women with hirsutism is whether evidence of virilization or defeminization is also present (Table 53-1) since such signs suggest profound androgen excess. In patients with overproduction of androgen, defeminizing signs, such as disturbances of menstruation, are more frequent than virilization. However, the presence or absence of overt virilization should be interpreted with caution for at least two reasons. First, signs of virilization (clitoromegaly, balding, coarsening of the hair, hirsutism) indicate androgen excess at some time in the patient's life but do not necessarily mean that active disease is present at the time of evaluation. It is necessary to measure plasma androgen levels and/or production rates to determine if androgen excess is ongoing. Second, severe overandrogenization may exist in the absence of marked virilization, i.e., at the same level of androgen production clitoromegaly may be present in one patient but not in another.

Diagnostic Considerations *Drugs* Excessive hair growth can be caused by drugs that exert their effects independent of androgens and do not produce defeminization or virilization. Such drugs include phenytoin, minoxidil, diazoxide, cyclosporine, and hexachlorobenzene; hair growth produced by these agents is usually vellus in character. Androgens produce hirsutism as well as virilization. Some synthetic progestagens have androgenic activity.

Table 53-1

Clinical Signs of Defeminization and Virilization

Signs of Defeminization	Signs of Virilization
Amenorrhea	Frontal balding
Decrease in breast size	Increase in size of shoulder girdle muscles
Loss of female body contours	Clitoromegaly
	Coarsening of the voice
	Acne

SOURCE: After L Karp, WL Herrmann, Diagnosis and treatment of hirsutism in women. Obstet Gynecol 41:283, 1973.

Tumors The rapid onset of hair growth with or without accompanying signs of frank virilization suggests a neoplastic source of androgen. Such tumors include adenomas and carcinomas of the adrenal and ovarian tumors such as arrhenoblastoma, which secrete androgens directly, and Krukenberg tumors of the ovary, which stimulate the surrounding ovarian stromal tissue to produce excess androgen.

Polycystic ovarian disease The most common cause of ovarian hyperandrogenism is polycystic ovarian disease. This disorder has a broad spectrum of manifestations that range from mild hirsutism to amenorrhea and virilization. The salient feature for the diagnosis is the pubertal onset of chronic anovulation and hirsutism. Enlarged cystic ovaries, obesity, and amenorrhea (i.e., the Stein-Leventhal syndrome) are present in half or fewer of women with this disorder and need not be present for the diagnosis (see Chap. 337). The fundamental abnormality in polycystic ovarian disease is not fully understood, but elevated levels of plasma LH cause enhanced androgen secretion by stromal and thecal cells of the ovary.

Attenuated forms of adrenal hyperplasia The adrenal can be the source of excess androgen in the absence of tumor. Heritable defects in adrenal steroidogenesis (congenital adrenal hyperplasia) such as deficiencies of 21-hydroxylase (P450$_{C21}$), 11β-hydroxylase (P450$_{C11B}$), and 3β-hydroxysteroid dehydrogenase isomerase (3β-HSD) can produce virilization, and each can occur in a "late-onset" form in which hirsutism or virilization and menstrual irregularities appear at the time of expected puberty or in adulthood (see Chap. 339). The clinical features in these cases resemble those in polycystic ovarian disease. Late-onset 21-hydroxylase deficiency is the most common attenuated form of congenital adrenal hyperplasia and has been studied extensively; its incidence in the general population of hirsute, oligomenorrheic women is on the order of 1 to 5 percent. The presence of elevated plasma levels of adrenal androgens (such as dehydroepiandrosterone sulfate) or of dexamethasone-suppressible hyperandrogenism does not necessarily imply that the overandrogenization is due to a specific adrenal steroidogenic defect, but these findings may be useful as a guide to therapy.

Idiopathic hirsutism In many women with hirsutism a specific diagnosis cannot be made. The term *idiopathic hirsutism* applies to those women with evidence of androgen excess but with normal menses, normal-sized ovaries, no evidence of tumors of the adrenal or ovary, and normal adrenal function. Slight elevations of plasma androstenedione and testosterone levels are common in such women, and testosterone production rates are increased, although to a lesser degree than in patients with polycystic ovarian disease.

Experience with the antiandrogens cyproterone acetate and flutamide indicates that this form of hirsutism is androgen-mediated, since therapy results in improvement. Women with idiopathic hirsutism might constitute the extreme end of a normal continuum of androgen production or represent a true pathologic subset. Some women with the tentative diagnosis of idiopathic hirsutism actually have mild or early polycystic ovarian disease, but in most, hirsutism is not accompanied by or followed by signs of ovarian dysfunction. If such women are merely extremes of the normal range of androgen production, then their hirsutism is fundamentally a cosmetic defect.

DIAGNOSTIC EVALUATION
The decision as to when to undertake a complex diagnostic evaluation depends on several factors. Such evaluation is appropriate in all women with hirsutism accompanied by virilization; whether it should be performed in women with iso-

lated hirsutism depends upon the severity, distribution, and rate of hair growth. An approach to the diagnostic evaluation of hirsute patients is shown in Fig. 53-1. The clinical history is taken with particular attention to drug ingestion and to the details of pubertal development and menstrual history and their relation to the onset of excessive hair growth. The physical examination is directed to the assessment of sites of growth of androgen-dependent hair (pubic, axillary, facial, truncal, and extremity) and evaluation for signs of virilization, which correlate with higher levels of androgen overproduction and raise the concern of androgen-producing neoplasms. Such signs include laryngeal enlargement (deepening of the voice), temporal balding, clitoromegaly, and increased muscle mass in the shoulder girdle. Signs of cortisol excess (plethora, centripetal obesity, striae, and enlarged dorsocervical and supraclavicular fat pads) should also be sought. Pelvic examination should include a search for palpable ovarian masses. Laboratory tests include measurement of serum androgens and, when indicated, radiologic imaging of ovaries and adrenal glands. Basal measurements of dehydroepiandrosterone sulfate greater than 22 μmol/L (8000 ng/mL) or of serum testosterone over 7 nmol/L (2 ng/mL) suggest neoplastic sources of androgen excess; plasma testosterone levels in the normal range are more difficult to interpret because total levels in women do not necessarily reflect the free or unbound levels of hormone under conditions when testosterone-binding globulin levels are either increased or decreased. Suspected Cushing's syndrome should be evaluated if a screening test (such as urinary free cortisol excretion or overnight dexamethasone suppression test) is abnormal. The diagnosis of polycystic ovarian disease is made from the history and clinical features in a woman with chronic anovulation. Women may be screened for delayed-onset adrenal hyperplasia by the short ACTH stimulation test and measurement of plasma 17-hydroxyprogesterone (see Chap. 332).

R/ **TREATMENT**

In the case of drug-induced hirsutism and neoplastic disease of the ovary or adrenals treatment is straightforward; administration of the drugs should be stopped, or the tumor should be removed. Adrenal steroidogenic defects are treated with glucocorticoids to suppress

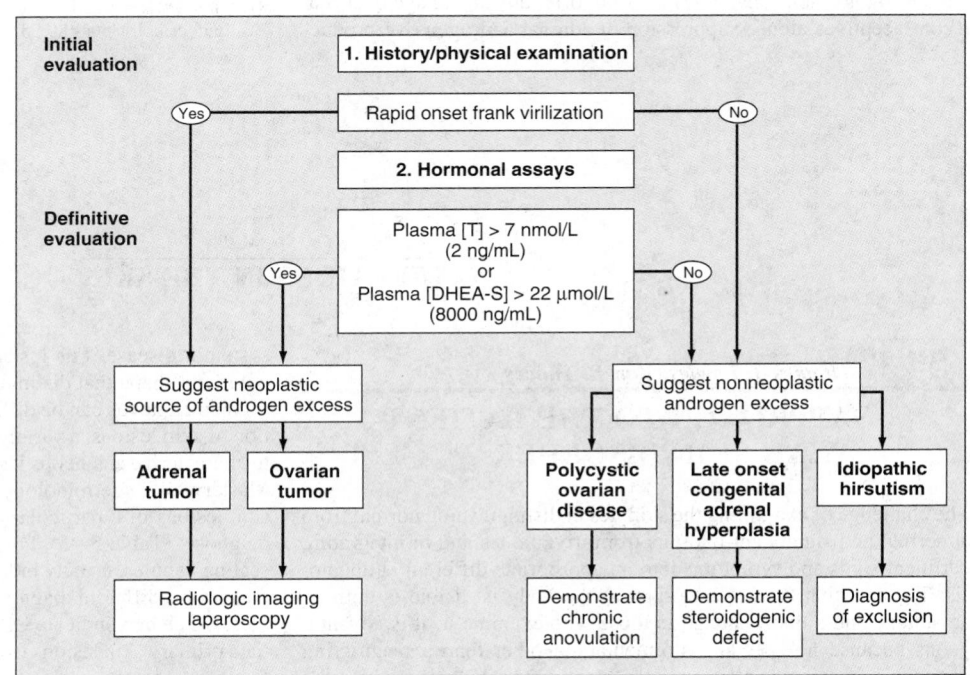

FIGURE 53-1 Diagnostic approach to the hirsute patient. T, testosterone; DHEA-S, dehydroepiandrosterone sulfate.

excess ACTH and inhibit adrenal androgen secretion. In most instances (polycystic ovarian disease as well as idiopathic hirsutism) both cosmetic treatment and suppression of androgen production or antagonism of its action at the receptor level need to be employed.

Cosmetic therapy is directed at the concealment or removal of hair from exposed skin areas. Small amounts of hair can be bleached with hydrogen peroxide. Methods for removal of hair are classified as depilatory (removal of hair from the surface of the skin) or epilatory (removal of the intact hair with the root). Depilatory techniques include shaving and chemical methods. Shaving does not have an adverse effect on hair growth rate or coarseness (although the blunt ends may feel coarse), but shaving of areas other than axillae or legs is unacceptable to most women. Chemical depilatories are effective for limited areas of hair removal and are generally safe if used properly. Most available depilatories are substituted mercaptans, such as thioglycollic acid, which reduce the disulfide bonds in the peptide chains of keratin. The hair fiber swells and softens to a consistency that can be washed from the skin. Care must be taken to avoid skin irritation because of the alkalinity of these preparations. Temporary epilation can be achieved by plucking (useful only for isolated hairs), wax treatment, or the use of epilatory devices. The waxes are melted and applied to the skin. When the wax cools and sets, it is stripped off, removing hair with it. The procedure is uncomfortable, and best results can be obtained by salon treatments. Permanent epilation can be achieved only by electrolysis. The treatments are expensive and time-consuming, and success depends on the skill of the electrologist.

While cosmetic treatment is undertaken, attempts to suppress androgen overproduction may also be appropriate. Treatment with combination oral contraceptives suppresses ovarian androgen secretion when restoration of fertility is not an objective. To minimize side effects oral contraceptives should contain progestagens with the least androgenic side effects (such as desogestrel or norgestimate) and the lowest effective dosage of estrogen. Women over 35 years of age, smokers, and those with hypertension, a history of thromboembolic disease, impaired liver function, or suspected estrogen-dependent neoplasm should not be treated with oral contraceptives. The combination of oral contraceptives and luteinizing hormone–releasing hormone analogues does not offer any advantage over oral contraceptives alone. Suppression of adrenal androgen overproduc-

tion can be achieved with small doses of dexamethasone and is most useful in late-onset 21-hydroxylase deficiency.

Antagonism of the effects of androgens at the hair follicle is the basis for treatment with antiandrogens. Cyproterone acetate has been used with success but is available in the United States only for compassionate use. The androgen receptor antagonist flutamide is also effective, but it can cause hepatic failure and probably should not be used for this purpose. Spironolactone has a dual action of blocking the androgen receptor and of inhibiting androgen production and is a useful alternative therapy. Cimetidine also binds to the androgen receptor and acts as an androgen antagonist but is not of general benefit in the treatment of hirsutism. The 5α-reductase inhibitor finasteride has been used successfully for this purpose but can cause toxic effects if it crosses the placenta.

If pharmacologic therapy is undertaken, the patient should be prepared to make a commitment of 6 months for an adequate trial of efficacy. Even when treatment is long-term, dramatic reversal of established hair growth is unlikely to be achieved by interference with androgen synthesis or action. Such hormonal manipulations can arrest or slow the rate of hair growth, but established hair must be dealt with by use of cosmetic treatment.

BIBLIOGRAPHY

CARR BR et al: Oral contraceptive pills, gonadotropin-releasing hormone agonists, or use in combination for treatment of hirsutism: A clinical research center study. J Clin Endocrinol Metab 80:1169, 1995

CUSAN L et al: Treatment of hirsutism with the pure antiandrogen flutamide. J Am Acad Dermatol 23:462, 1990

DERKSEN J et al: Identification of virilizing adrenal tumors in hirsute women. N Engl J Med 331:968, 1994

EHRMAN DA, ROSENFIELD RL: An endocrinologic approach to the patient with hirutism. J Clin Endocrinol Metab 71:1, 1990

FRUZZETTI F et al: Effects of finasteride, a 5alpha-reductase inhibitor, on circulating androgens and gonadotropin secretion in hirsute women. J Clin Endocrinol Metab 79:1115, 1994

KILLEEN AA et al: Prevalence of nonclassical congenital adrenal hyperplasia among women self-referred for treatment of hirsutism. Am J Med Genet 42:197, 1992

McKENNA TJ: Screening for sinister causes of hirsutism. N Engl J Med 331:1015, 1994

O'BRIEN RC et al: Comparison of sequential cyproterone acetate/estrogen versus spironolactone/oral contraceptive in the treatment of hirsutism. J Clin Endocrinol Metab 72:1008, 1991

RITTMASTER RS: Medical treatment of androgen-dependent hirsutism. J Clin Endocrinol Metab 80:2559, 1995

SECTION 9

ALTERATIONS IN THE SKIN

54

Thomas J. Lawley, Kim B. Yancey

APPROACH TO THE PATIENT WITH SKIN DISORDER

The challenge of examining the skin lies in distinguishing normal from abnormal and significant findings from trivial ones and in integrating pertinent signs and symptoms into an appropriate differential diagnosis. The fact that the largest organ in the body is visible is both an advantage and a disadvantage to those who examine it. It is advantageous because no special instrumentation, other than a magnifying glass, is necessary and because the skin can be biopsied with little morbidity. However, the casual observer can be overwhelmed by a variety of stimuli and overlook important, subtle signs of skin or

systemic disease. For instance, the sometimes minor differences in color and shape that distinguish a malignant melanoma from a benign pigmented nevus can be difficult to recognize. To aid in the interpretation of skin lesions, a variety of descriptive terms have been developed to characterize cutaneous lesions (Tables 54-1 and 54-2 and Fig. 54-1). Mastery of this terminology is important not only for categorizing the skin lesions of a particular case but also in formulating a differential diagnosis (Table 54-3). For instance, the finding of large numbers of scaling papules, usually indicative of a primary skin disease, places the patient in a different diagnostic category than would hemorrhagic papules, which may indicate vasculitis or sepsis. It is important to differentiate primary skin lesions from secondary skin changes. If the examiner focuses on linear erosions overlying an area of erythema and scaling, he or she may incorrectly assume that the erosion is the primary lesion and the redness and scale are secondary, while the correct interpretation

Table 54-1

CHAPTER 54
Approach to the Patient with Skin Disorder

295

Descriptions of Primary Skin Lesions

Macule: A flat, colored lesion, <2 cm in diameter, not raised above the surface of the surrounding skin. A "freckle," or ephelid, is a prototype pigmented macule.
Patch: A large (>2 cm), flat lesion with a color different from the surrounding skin. This differs from a macule only in size.
Papule: A small, solid lesion, <1 cm in diameter, raised above the surface of the surrounding skin and hence palpable (e.g., a closed comedone, or whitehead, in acne).
Nodule: A larger (1–5 cm), firm lesion raised above the surface of the surrounding skin. This differs from a papule only in size (e.g., dermal nevus).
Tumor: A solid, raised growth >5 cm in diameter.
Plaque: A large (>1 cm), flat-topped, raised lesion; edges may either be distinct (e.g., in psoriasis) or gradually blend with surrounding skin (e.g., in eczematous dermatitis).
Vesicle: A small, fluid-filled lesion, <1 cm in diameter, raised above the plane of surrounding skin. Fluid is often visible, and the lesions are often translucent [e.g., vesicles in allergic contact dermatitis caused by *Toxicodendron* (poison ivy)].
Pustule: A vesicle filled with leukocytes. Note: The presence of pustules does not necessarily signify the existence of an infection.
Bulla: A fluid-filled, raised, often translucent lesion >1 cm in diameter.
Cyst: A soft, raised, encapsulated lesion filled with semisolid or liquid contents.
Wheal: A raised, erythematous papule or plaque, usually representing short-lived dermal edema.
Telangiectasia: Dilated, superficial blood vessels.

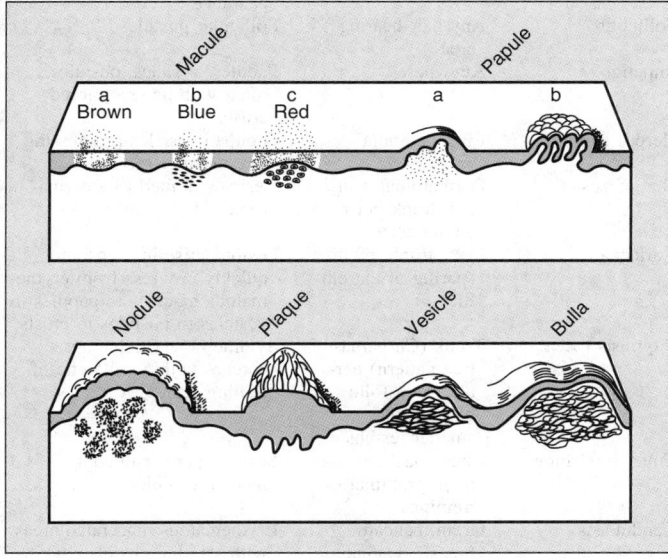

FIGURE 54-1 A schematic representation of several common primary skin lesions (see Table 54-1).

Table 54-2

Common Dermatologic Terms

Lichenification: A distinctive thickening of the skin that is characterized by accentuated skin-fold markings and that feels thick and firm on palpation.
Crust: Dried exudate of body fluids that may be either yellow (serous exudate) or red (hemorrhagic exudate).
Milia: Small, firm, white papules that are filled with keratin (and may in part resemble pustules).
Erosion: Epithelial deficit resulting in a superficial disruption of skin integrity.
Ulcer: Epithelial deficit resulting in a deep surface disruption.
Excoriations: Linear, angular erosions that may be covered by crust and are caused by scratching.
Atrophy: An acquired loss of substance. In the skin, this may appear as a depression with intact epidermis (i.e., loss of dermal or subcutaneous tissue) or as sites of shiny, delicate, wrinkled lesions (i.e., epidermal atrophy).
Scar: A change in the skin secondary to trauma or inflammation. Sites may be erythematous, hypopigmented, or hypertrophic depending on their age or character. Sites on hair-bearing areas may be characterized by destruction of hair follicles.

would be that the patient has a pruritic eczematous dermatitis and the erosions have been caused by scratching.

Approach to the Patient

In examining the skin it is usually advisable to assess the patient before taking a history. This way, the entire cutaneous surface is sure to be evaluated, and objective findings can be integrated with relevant historical data. Four basic features of any cutaneous lesion must be noted and considered in the examination of skin: the distribution of the eruption, the type(s) of primary lesion, the shape of individual lesions, and the arrangement of the lesions. In the initial examination it is important that the patient be disrobed as completely as possible. This will minimize chances of missing important individual skin lesions and make it possible to assess accurately the distribution of the eruption. The patient should first be viewed from a distance of about 1.5 to 2 m (4 to 6 ft) so that the general character of the skin and the distribution of lesions can be evaluated. Indeed, distribution of lesions often correlates highly with diagnosis (Fig. 54-2). For example, a hospitalized patient with a generalized erythematous exanthem is more likely to have a drug eruption than is a patient with a similar rash limited to the sun-exposed portions of the face. The presence or absence of lesions on mucosal surfaces also should be determined. Once the distribution of the lesions has been established, the nature of the primary lesion must be determined. Thus, when lesions are distributed on elbows, knees, and scalp, the most likely possibility based solely on distribution is psoriasis or dermatitis herpetiformis. The primary lesion in psoriasis is a scaly papule that soon forms erythematous plaques covered with a white scale, whereas that of dermatitis herpetiformis is an urticarial papule that quickly becomes a small vesicle. In this manner, identification of the primary lesion directs the examiner toward the proper diagnosis. Secondary changes in skin also can be quite helpful. For example, scale represents excessive epidermis, while crust is the result of an inadequate or inconsistent epithelial cell layer. Palpation of skin lesions also can yield insight into the character of an eruption. Thus red papules on the lower extremities that blanch with pressure can be a manifestation of many different diseases, but hemorrhagic red papules that do not blanch with pressure indicate palpable purpura characteristic of necrotizing vasculitis.

The shape of lesions is also an important feature. Flat, round, erythematous papules and plaques are common in many cutaneous diseases. However, target-shaped lesions that consist in part of erythematous plaques are specific for erythema multiforme. In the same way, the arrangement of individual lesions is important. Erythematous papules and vesicles can occur in many conditions, but their arrangement in a specific linear array suggests an external etiology such as allergic contact or primary irritant dermatitis. In contrast, lesions with a generalized arrangement are common and suggest a systemic etiology.

As in other branches of medicine, a complete history should be obtained to emphasize the following features:

1. Evolution of lesions
   a. Site of onset
   b. Manner in which eruption progressed or spread
   c. Duration
   d. Periods of resolution or improvement in chronic eruptions
2. Symptoms associated with the eruption
   a. Itching, burning, pain, numbness
   b. What, if anything, has relieved symptoms
   c. Time of day when symptoms are most severe
3. Current or recent medications (prescribed as well as over-the-counter)
4. Associated systemic symptoms (e.g., malaise, fever, arthralgias)
5. Ongoing or previous illnesses
6. History of allergies
7. Presence of photosensitivity
8. Review of systems

DIAGNOSTIC TECHNIQUES   Many skin diseases can be diagnosed on gross clinical appearance, but sometimes relatively simple diagnostic procedures can yield valuable information. In most instances, they can be performed at the bedside with a minimum of equipment.

Skin Biopsy   A skin biopsy is a straightforward minor surgical procedure; however, it is important to biopsy the anatomic site most likely to yield diagnostic findings. This decision may require expertise in skin diseases and knowledge of superficial anatomic structures in selected areas of the body. In this procedure, a small area of skin is anesthetized with 1% lidocaine with or without epinephrine. The skin lesion in question can be excised with a scalpel or removed by punch biopsy. In the latter technique, a punch is pressed against the surface of the skin and rotated with downward pressure until it penetrates to the subcutaneous tissue. The circular biopsy is then lifted with forceps, and the bottom is cut with iris scissors. Biopsy sites may or may not need suture closure depending on size and location.

KOH Preparation   A potassium hydroxide (KOH) preparation is performed on scaling skin lesions when a fungal etiology is suspected. The edge of such a lesion is scraped gently with a scalpel blade, and the removed scale is collected on a glass microscope slide and treated with 1 to 2 drops of a solution of 10 to 20% KOH. KOH dissolves keratin and allows easier visualization of fungal elements. Brief heating of the slide accelerates dissolution of keratin. When the preparation is viewed under the microscope, the refractile hyphae will be seen more easily when the light intensity is reduced. This technique can be utilized to identify hyphae in dermatophyte infections, pseudohyphae and budding yeast in *Candida* infections, and fragmented hyphae and spores in tinea versicolor. The same sampling technique can be used to obtain scale for culture of selected pathogenic organisms.

Table 54-3

Selected Common Dermatologic Conditions

Diagnosis	Common Distribution	Usual Morphology	Diagnosis	Common Distribution	Usual Morphology
Acne vulgaris	Face, upper back	Open and closed comedones, erythematous papules, pustules, cysts	Seborrheic keratosis	Trunk, face	Brown plaques with adherent, greasy scale; "stuck on" appearance
Rosacea	Blush area of cheeks, nose, forehead, chin	Erythema, telangiectasias, papules, pustules	Folliculitis	Any hair-bearing area	Follicular pustules
Seborrheic dermatitis	Scalp, eyebrows, perinasal	Erythema with greasy yellow-brown scale	Impetigo	Anywhere	Papules, vesicles, pustules, often with honey-colored crusts
Atopic dermatitis	Antecubital and popliteal fossae; may be widespread	Patches and plaques of erythema, scaling, and lichenification; pruritus	Herpes simplex	Lips, genitalia	Grouped vesicles progressing to crusted erosions
			Herpes zoster	Dermatomal, usually trunk but may be anywhere	Vesicles limited to a dermatome (often painful)
Stasis dermatitis	Ankles, lower legs	Patches of erythema and scaling on background of hyperpigmentation associated with signs of venous insufficiency	Varicella	Face, trunk, relative sparing of extremities	Lesions arise in crops and quickly progress from erythematous macules to papules to vesicles to pustules to crusts
Dyshidrotic eczema	Palms, soles, sides of fingers and toes	Deep vesicles	Pityriasis rosea	Trunk (Christmas tree pattern) herald patch followed by multiple smaller lesions	Symmetric erythematous patches with a collarette of trailing scale
Allergic contact dermatitis	Anywhere	Localized erythema, vesicles, scale, and pruritus, e.g., fingers, earlobes—nickel; dorsal aspect of foot—shoe dermatitis; exposed surfaces—poison ivy dermatitis; etc.	Tinea versicolor	Chest, back, abdomen, proximal extremities	Scaly hyper- or hypopigmented macules
Psoriasis	Elbows, knees, scalp, lower back, fingernails (may be generalized)	Papules and plaques covered with silvery scale; nails have pits	Candidiasis	Groin, beneath breasts, vagina, oral cavity	Erythematous macerated areas with satellite pustules; white, friable patches on mucous membranes
Lichen planus	Wrists, ankles, mouth (may be widespread)	Violaceous flat-topped papules and plaques	Dermatophytosis	Feet, groin, beard, or scalp	Varies with site, e.g., tinea corporis—scaly annular patch
Keratosis pilaris	Extensor surfaces of arms and thighs, buttocks	Keratotic follicular papules with surrounding erythema	Scabies	Groin, axillae, between fingers and toes, beneath breasts	Excoriated papules, burrows, pruritus
Melasma	Forehead, cheeks, temples, upper lip	Tan to brown patches	Insect bites	Anywhere	Erythematous papules with central puncta
Vitiligo	Periorificial, trunk, extensor surfaces of extremities, flexor wrists, axillae	Chalk-white macules	Cherry angioma	Trunk	Red, blood-filled papules
			Keloid	Anywhere (site of previous injury)	Firm tumor, pink, purple, or brown
			Dermatofibroma	Anywhere	Firm red to brown nodule that shows dimpling of overlying skin with lateral compression
Actinic keratosis	Sun-exposed areas	Skin-colored or red-brown macule or papule with dry, rough, adherent scale	Acrochordons (skin tags)	Groin, axilla, neck	Fleshy papules
Basal cell carcinoma	Face	Papule with pearly, telangiectatic border on sun-damaged skin	Urticaria	Anywhere	Wheals, sometimes with surrounding flare, pruritus
			Transient acantholytic dermatosis	Trunk, especially anterior chest	Erythematous papules
Squamous cell carcinoma	Face, especially lower lip, ears	Indurated and possibly hyperkaratotic lesions often showing ulceration and/or crusting	Xerosis	Extensor extremities, especially legs	Dry, erythematous, scaling patches, pruritus

Tzanck Smear A Tzanck smear, named after Arnault Tzanck, is a cytologic technique most often used in the diagnosis of herpesvirus infections (simplex or varicella-zoster). An early vesicle, not a pustule or crusted lesion, is unroofed, and the base of the lesion is scraped gently with a scalpel blade. The material is then placed on a glass slide, air-dried, and stained with Giemsa or Wright's stain. Multinucleated giant cells suggest the presence of herpes, but culture or immunofluorescence testing must be performed to identify the specific virus.

Diascopy Diascopy is designed to assess whether a skin lesion will blanch with pressure as, for example, in determining whether a red lesion is hemorrhagic or simply blood-filled. For instance, a hemangioma will blanch with pressure, whereas a purpuric lesion caused by necrotizing vasculitis will not. Diascopy is performed by pressing a microscope slide or magnifying lens against a specified lesion and noting the amount of blanching that occurs. Granulomas often have an "apple jelly" appearance on diascopy.

Wood's Light A Wood's lamp generates 360-nm ultraviolet (or "black") light that can be used to aid the evaluation of certain skin disorders. For example, a Wood's lamp will cause erythrasma (a superficial, intertriginous infection caused by *Corynebacterium minutissimum*) to show a characteristic coral red color, and wounds colo-

nized by *Pseudomonas* to appear pale blue. Tinea capitis caused by certain dermatophytes such as *Microsporum canis* or *M. audouini* exhibits a yellow fluorescence. Pigmented lesions of the epidermis such as freckles are accentuated, while dermal pigment such as post-inflammatory hyperpigmentation fades under a Wood's light. Vitiligo appears totally white under a Wood's lamp, and previously unsuspected areas of involvement often become apparent. A Wood's lamp also may aid in the demonstration of tinea versicolor and in recognition of ash leaf spots in patients with tuberous sclerosis.

Patch Tests Patch testing is designed to document sensitivity to a specific antigen. In this procedure, a battery of suspected allergens is applied to the patient's back under occlusive dressings and allowed to remain in contact with the skin for 48 h. The dressings are then removed, and the area is examined for evidence of delayed hypersensitivity reactions (e.g., erythema, edema, or papulovesicles). This test is best performed by physicians with special expertise in patch testing and is often helpful in the evaluation of patients with chronic dermatitis.

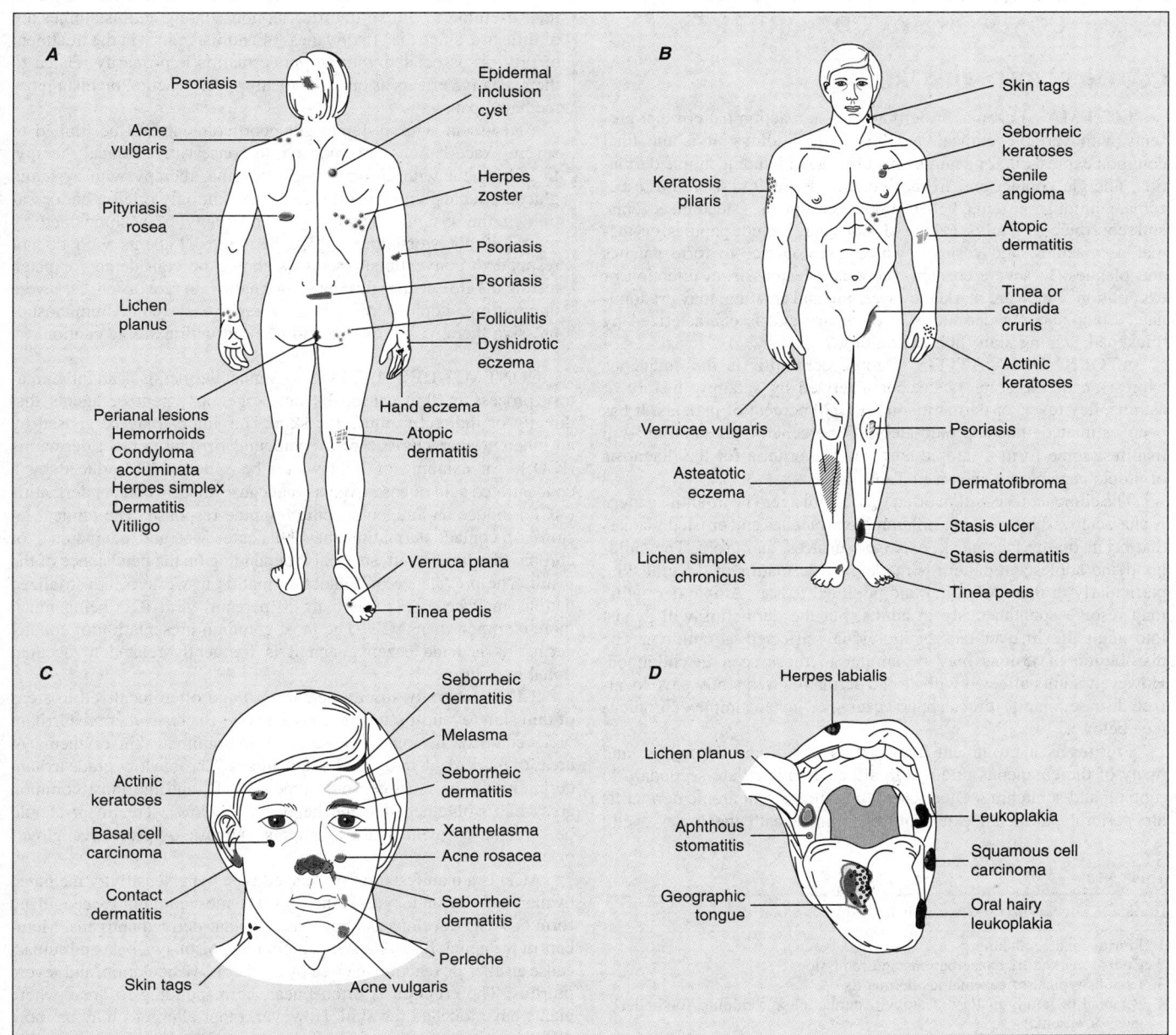

FIGURE 54-2 *A–D*. The distribution of some common dermatologic diseases and lesions.

BIBLIOGRAPHY

ARNDT KA et al (eds): *Cutaneous Medicine and Surgery, An Integrated Program in Dermatology.* Philadelphia, Saunders, 1996

ARNOLD HL et al (eds): *Andrew's Diseases of the Skin,* 8th ed. Philadelphia, Saunders, 1990

FITZPATRICK TB et al (eds): *Dermatology in General Medicine,* 4th ed. New York, McGraw-Hill, 1993

LOOKINGBILL DP, MARKS JG: *Principles of Dermatology.* Philadelphia, Saunders, 1986

ROOK A et al (eds): *Textbook of Dermatology,* 5th ed. Oxford, Blackwell Scientific, 1992

55   *Robert A. Swerlick, Thomas J. Lawley*

ECZEMA, PSORIASIS, CUTANEOUS INFECTIONS, ACNE, AND OTHER COMMON SKIN DISORDERS

COMMON SKIN DISORDERS

ECZEMA Eczema, or dermatitis, is a reaction pattern that presents with variable clinical and histologic findings; it is the final common expression for a number of disorders including atopic dermatitis, allergic contact and irritant contact dermatitis, dyshidrotic eczema, nummular eczema, lichen simplex chronicus, asteatotic eczema, and seborrheic dermatitis. Primary lesions may include papules, erythematous macules, and vesicles, which can coalesce to form patches and plaques. In severe eczema, secondary lesions from infection or excoriation, which are marked by weeping and crusting, may predominate. Long-standing dermatitis is often dry and is characterized by thickened, scaling skin (lichenification).

ATOPIC DERMATITIS Atopic dermatitis is the cutaneous expression of the atopic state, characterized by a family history of asthma, hay fever, or dermatitis in up to 70 percent of patients. It has been estimated that approximately 10 percent of all children will manifest some form of atopic eczema. The criteria for the diagnosis of atopic eczema are shown in Table 55-1.

The clinical presentation often varies with age. The infantile pattern is characterized by weeping inflammatory patches and crusted plaques that occur on the face, neck, extensor surfaces, and groin. The childhood and adolescent pattern is marked by dermatitis of flexural skin, particularly in the antecubital and popliteal fossae. Atopic dermatitis may resolve spontaneously in adults, but the dermatitis will persist into adult life in over half of individuals affected as children. The distribution of lesions may be similar to those seen in childhood. However, adults affected with atopic dermatitis frequently have localized disease, manifesting as hand eczema or lichen simplex chronicus (see below).

Pruritus is a prominent characteristic of atopic dermatitis, and many of the cutaneous findings in affected patients are secondary to rubbing and scratching. Other cutaneous stigmata of atopic dermatitis are perioral pallor, an extra fold of skin beneath the lower eyelid (Dennie's line), increased palmar markings, and increased incidence of cutaneous infections, particularly with *Staphylococcus aureus.* Atopic individuals often have dry, itchy skin, abnormalities in cutaneous vascular responses, and in some instances, elevated levels of serum IgE.

 TREATMENT Therapy of atopic dermatitis should be based on avoidance of cutaneous irritants, adequate cutaneous hydration, judicious use of low- or midpotency topical glucocorticoids, and prompt treatment of secondarily infected skin lesions. Patients should be instructed to bathe using warm, but not hot, water and to limit their use of soap. Immediately after bathing, the skin should be lubricated with a low- or midpotency topical glucocorticoid in a cream or ointment base. Crusted and weeping skin lesions should be treated with systemic antibiotics with activity against *Staph. aureus,* since secondary infection often exacerbates eczema. The role of dietary allergens in atopic dermatitis is controversial, but there is little evidence that they play any role outside of infancy.

Control of pruritus is essential for treatment, since atopic eczema often represents "an itch that rashes." Antihistamines are useful to control the pruritus that accompanies eczema, but sedation may limit their usefulness. Unlike in urticaria, nonsedating antihistamines are of little use, since the effectiveness of antihistamines in the treatment of pruritus associated with atopic dermatitis is primarily related to their sedative effects as opposed to any specific action on histamine-mediated pathways.

Treatment with systemic glucocorticoids should be limited to severe exacerbations unresponsive to conservative topical therapy. In the patient with chronic atopic eczema, therapy with systemic glucocorticoids will generally clear the skin only briefly, but cessation of the systemic therapy will invariably be accompanied by return, if not worsening, of the dermatitis. Patients who do not respond to conventional therapies should be considered for patch testing to rule out allergic contact dermatitis. In rare instances, severe unremitting atopic dermatitis may require systemic immunosuppressive therapy, but this should be used with extreme caution.

CONTACT DERMATITIS Contact dermatitis is an inflammatory process in skin caused by an exogenous agent or agents that directly or indirectly injure the skin. This injury may be caused by an inherent characteristic of a compound [irritant contact dermatitis (ICD)]. An example of ICD would be a dermatitis induced by a concentrated acid or base. Agents that cause allergic contact dermatitis (ACD) induce an antigen-specific immune response. The clinical lesions of contact dermatitis may be acute (wet and edematous) or chronic (dry, thickened, and scaly) depending on the persistence of the insult. The prevalence of contact dermatitis in western industrialized nations may be as high as 5 to 20 percent, with ICD being much more common than ACD. The most common presentation of contact dermatitis is hand eczema, and it is frequently related to occupational exposures.

ICD is generally strictly demarcated and often localized to areas of thin skin (eyelids, intertriginous areas) or to areas where the irritant was occluded. Lesions may range from minimal skin erythema to areas of marked edema, vesicles, and ulcers. Chronic low-grade irritant dermatitis is the most common type of ICD, and the most common areas of involvement are the hands (see below). Treatment should be directed to avoidance of irritants and use of protective gloves or clothing.

ACD is a manifestation of delayed type hypersensitivity mediated by memory T lymphocytes in the skin. The most commonly recognized form of ACD develops as a response to plant-derived antigens. Members of the genus *Toxicodendron,* including poison ivy, oak, and sumac, cause an allergic reaction marked by erythema, vesiculation, and severe pruritus. The eruption is often linear, corresponding to areas where plants have touched the skin. However, other allergens may be more difficult to identify, especially if the exposure is chronic and the skin becomes thickened and scaly.

Table 55-1

Clinical Criteria for the Diagnosis of Atopic Dermatitis

1. Pruritus and scratching
2. Course marked by exacerbations and remissions
3. Lesions typical of eczematous dermatitis
4. Personal or family history of atopy (asthma, allergic rhinitis, food allergies, or eczema)
5. Clinical course lasting longer than 6 weeks

If ACD is suspected and an offending agent is identified and removed, the eruption will resolve. Usually, treatment with a high-potency fluorinated topical glucocorticoid is enough to relieve symptoms while the ACD runs its course. Patients with particularly widespread disease, or disease involving the face or genitalia, may require treatment with oral glucocorticoids. Since the natural course of ACD is 2 to 3 weeks, therapy should be continued for that length of time. Treatment of ACD with very short, rapidly tapered courses of oral glucocorticoids is almost always accompanied by recurrence of skin lesions. Additionally, when systemic glucocorticoids are utilized, they are best given as single daily morning doses to limit potential side effects.

Identification of a contact allergen can be a difficult and time-consuming task. Patients with a dermatitis unresponsive to conventional therapy or with an unusual and patterned distribution should be suspected of having ACD. They should be questioned carefully regarding occupational exposures, topical medicaments, and oral medications. Common sensitizers include preservatives in topical preparations, nickel sulfate, potassium dichromate, neomycin sulfate, fragrances, formaldehyde, and rubber-curing agents. Patch testing is helpful in identifying these agents but should not be used on patients with widespread active dermatitis or on those taking systemic glucocorticoids.

HAND ECZEMA Hand eczema is a very common, chronic skin disorder. It represents the overwhelming majority of occupation-associated skin disease, which is responsible for a significant proportion of occupation-associated injury and time lost from work. It may be associated with other cutaneous disorders such as atopic dermatitis or may occur by itself. As with other forms of dermatitis, both exogenous and endogenous factors play important roles in the expression of hand dermatitis. Chronic, excessive exposure to water and detergents may initiate or aggravate this disorder. It may present with dryness and cracking of the skin of the hands, as well as with variable amounts of erythema and edema. Often the dermatitis will begin under rings where water and irritants are trapped. A variant of hand dermatitis, dyshidrotic eczema, presents with multiple, intensely pruritic, small papules and vesicles occurring on the thenar and hypothenar eminences and the sides of the fingers. Lesions tend to occur in crops that slowly form crusts and heal.

The evaluation of a patient with hand eczema should include an assessment of potential occupation-associated exposures. Predominant involvement of the dorsal surface of the hands with sparing of the palmar surface should suggest a possible contact dermatitis. The history should be directed to identifying possible irritant or allergen exposures. The use of rubber gloves to protect dermatitic skin is sometimes associated with the development of delayed type hypersensitivity reactions to agents used for cross-linking rubber. These delayed type hypersensitivity reactions can be detected by patch testing. Less commonly, patients may manifest hand dermatitis as a consequence of developing immediate type hypersensitivity reactions to latex. These reactions are of particular concern since these patients are at risk for anaphylactic reactions. The most sensitive method of detection is the use of scratch testing with latex extract. However, this should be done with extreme caution only in a setting where an anaphylactic reaction can be treated. A latex radioallergosorbent test (RAST) is avialable, but it is only about 60 percent sensitive.

TREATMENT

Therapy of hand dermatitis is directed toward avoidance of irritants, identification of possible contact allergens, treatment of coexistent infection, and application of topical glucocorticoids. Whenever possible, the hands should be protected by gloves, preferably vinyl. Most patients can be treated with cool moist compresses (dressings) to dry and debride acute inflammatory lesions and to decrease swelling, followed by application of a mid- to high-potency topical glucocorticoid in a cream or ointment base. As with atopic dermatitis,

treatment of secondary infection from staphylococci or streptococci is essential for good control. Additionally, patients with hand dermatitis should be examined for dermatophyte infection by potassium hydroxide (KOH) preparation and culture (see below).

NUMMULAR ECZEMA Nummular eczema is characterized by circular or oval "coinlike" lesions. Initially, this eruption consists of small edematous papules that become crusted and scaly. The most common locations are on the trunk or the extensor surfaces of the extremities, particularly on the pretibial areas or dorsum of the hands. It occurs more frequently in men and is most commonly seen in middle age. The etiology of nummular eczema is unknown. Whether nummular eczema represents a variant of atopic eczema is controversial. The treatment of nummular eczema is similar to that for other forms of dermatitis.

LICHEN SIMPLEX CHRONICUS Lichen simplex chronicus may represent the end stage of a variety of pruritic and eczematous disorders. It consists of a well-circumscribed plaque or plaques with lichenified or thickened skin due to chronic scratching or rubbing. Common areas involved include the posterior nuchal region, dorsum of the feet, or ankles. Treatment of lichen simplex chronicus centers around breaking the cycle of chronic itching and scratching, which often occur during sleep. High-potency topical glucocorticoids are helpful in alleviating pruritus in most cases, but in recalcitrant cases, application of topical glucocorticoids under occlusion or intralesional injection of glucocorticoids may be required. Oral antihistamines are useful as antipruritics primarily due to their sedating action and are particularly useful at bedtime.

ASTEATOTIC ECZEMA Asteatotic eczema, also known as xerotic eczema or "winter itch," is a mildly inflammatory variant of dermatitis that develops most commonly on the lower legs of elderly individuals during dry times of year. Fine cracks, with or without erythema, resembling cracks seen in china or porcelain characteristically develop on the anterior surface of the lower extremities. Pruritus is variable. Asteatotic eczema responds well to avoidance of irritants, rehydration of the skin, and application of topical emollients.

STASIS DERMATITIS AND STASIS ULCERATION Stasis dermatitis develops on the lower extremities secondary to venous incompetence and chronic edema. Early findings in stasis dermatitis may consist of mild erythema and scaling associated with pruritus. The typical initial site of involvement is over the medial aspect of the ankle, often over a distended vein. As the disorder progresses, the dematitis becomes progressively pigmented, due to chronic erythrocyte extravasation leading to cutaneous hemosiderin deposition. As with other forms of dermatitis, stasis dermatitis may become acutely inflamed, with crusting and exudate. Chronic stasis dermatitis is often associated with dermal fibrosis that clinically is recognized as brawny edema of the skin. Stasis dermatitis is often complicated by secondary infection and contact dermatitis. Severe stasis dermatitis may precede the development of stasis ulcers.

TREATMENT

Avoidance of irritants and use of emollients and/or midpotency topical glucocorticoids are the cornerstones of therapy for stasis dermatitis. Control of chronic edema is important to prevent leg ulcers. Patients should be encouraged to elevate the affected extremity whenever sitting. A compression stocking with a gradient of at least 30 to 40 mmHg is most effective for edema control and is much more effective for preventing chronic edema than antiembolism hose.

Stasis ulcers are difficult to treat, and resolution of these lesions is slow even under the best of circumstances. It is extremely important to elevate the affected limb as much as possible. The ulcer should be kept clear of necrotic material by gentle debridement and covered with a semipermeable dressing under pressure. Glucocorticoids should not be applied to ulcers, since they may retard healing. Secondarily infected lesions should be treated with appropriate oral antibiotics, but it should be noted that all ulcers will become colonized with bacteria, and the purpose of antibiotic therapy should not be to clear all bacterial growth. Some ulcers may take months to heal or require skin grafting.

SEBORRHEIC DERMATITIS Seborrheic dermatitis is a common, chronic disorder characterized by greasy scales overlying erythematous patches or plaques. The most common location is in the scalp, where it may be recognized as severe dandruff. On the face, seborrheic dermatitis affects the eyebrows, eyelids, glabella, nasolabial fold, or ears. Scaling within the external ear is often mistaken for a chronic fungal infection (otomycosis), and postauricular dermatitis often becomes macerated and tender. Additionally, seborrheic dermatitis may develop in the central chest, axilla, groin, submammary folds, and gluteal cleft. Rarely, it may cause a widespread generalized dermatitis. Seborrheic dermatitis is usually symptomatic, with patients complaining of itching or burning.

Seborrheic dermatitis may be evident within the first few weeks of life, and within this context it occurs in the scalp ("cradle cap"), face, or groin. It is rarely seen in children beyond infancy but becomes evident again during adult life. Although it is frequently seen in patients with Parkinson's disease, in those who have had cerebrovascular accidents, and in those with human immunodeficiency virus (HIV) infection, the overwhelming majority of individuals with seborrheic dermatitis have no underlying disorder.

℞ TREATMENT

Treatment with low-potency topical glucocorticoids in conjunction with shampoos containing coal tar and/or salicylic acid is generally sufficient to control activity of this disorder. High potency topical glucocorticoid solutions (betamethasone or fluocinonide) are effective for control of scalp involvement. Fluorinated topical glucocorticoids should not be used on the face since this is often associated with the development of rebound worsening and steroid induced rosacea or atrophy.

PAPULOSQUAMOUS DISORDERS (Table 55-2)

PSORIASIS Psoriasis is one of the most common dermatologic diseases, affecting up to 1 to 2 percent of the world's population. It is a chronic inflammatory skin disorder clinically characterized by erythematous, sharply demarcated papules and rounded plaques, covered by silvery micaceous scale. The skin lesions of psoriasis are variably pruritic. Traumatized areas often develop lesions of psoriasis (Koebner or isomorphic phenomenon). Additionally, other external factors may exacerbate psoriasis including infections, stress, and medications (lithium, beta blockers, and antimalarials).

The most common variety of psoriasis is called *plaque type*. Patients with plaque-type psoriasis will have stable, slowly growing plaques, which remain basically unchanged for long periods of time. The most common areas for plaque psoriasis to occur are the elbows, knees, gluteal cleft, and the scalp. Involvement tends to be symmetrical. *Inverse psoriasis* affects the intertriginous regions including the axilla, groin, submammary region, and navel, and it also tends to affect the scalp, palms, and soles. The individual lesions are sharply demarcated plaques but may be moist due to their location. Plaque-type psoriasis generally develops slowly and runs an indolent course. It rarely spontaneously remits.

Eruptive psoriasis (guttate psoriasis) is most common in children and young adults. It develops acutely in individuals without psoriasis or in those with chronic plaque psoriasis. Patients present with many small eythematous, scaling papules, frequently after upper respiratory tract infection with beta-hemolytic streptococci. The differential diagnosis should include pityriasis rosea and secondary syphilis. Patients with psoriasis may also develop pustular lesions. These may be localized to the palms and soles or may be generalized and associated with fever, malaise, diarrhea, and arthralgias.

About half of all patients with psoriasis have fingernail involvement, appearing as punctate pitting, nail thickening, or subungual hyperkeratosis. About 5 to 10 percent of patients with psoriasis have associated joint complaints, and these are most often found in patients with fingernail involvement. Although some have the coincident occurrence of classic rheumatoid arthritis (see Chap. 313), many have joint disease that falls into one of five types associated with psoriasis: (1) disease limited to a single or a few small joints (70 percent of cases); (2) a seronegative rheumatoid arthritis–like disease; (3) involvement of the distal interphalangeal joints; (4) severe destructive arthritis with the development of "arthritis mutilans"; and (5) disease limited to the spine.

The etiology of psoriasis is still poorly understood, but there is clearly a genetic component. Over 50 percent of patients with psoriasis report a positive family history, and twin studies report a 65 to 72 percent concordance among monozygotic twins. Evidence has accumulated clearly indicating a role for T cells in the pathophysiology of psoriasis. Psoriasis may become particularly severe in individuals who are HIV-infected (see Chap. 308). Stimulation of immune function with cytokines such as interleukin 2 has been associated with abrupt worsening of preexisting psoriasis, and bone marrow transplantation has resulted in clearance of disease. In addition, agents that inhibit activated T cell function are often effective for the treatment of severe psoriasis.

 TREATMENT

Treatment of psoriasis depends on the type, location, and extent of disease. All patients should be instructed to avoid excess drying or irritation of their skin and to maintain adequate cutaneous hydration.

Table 55-2

Papulosquamous Disorders

	Clinical Features	Other Notable Features	Histologic Features
Psoriasis	Sharply demarcated, erythematous plaques with mica-like scale; predominantly elbows, knees, and scalp; atypical forms may localize to intertriginous areas; eruptive forms may be associated with infection (Reiter's syndrome)	May be aggravated by certain drugs, infection; severe forms seen associated with HIV	Acanthosis, vascular proliferation
Lichen planus	Purple polygonal papules marked by severe pruritus; lacy white markings, especially associated with mucous membrane lesions	Certain drugs may induce: thiazides, antimalarial drugs	Interface dermatitis
Pityriasis rosea	Rash often preceded by herald patch; oval to round plaques with trailing scale; most often affects the trunk, and eruption lines up in skin folds give a "fir tree"-like appearance; generally spares palms and soles	Variable pruritus; self-limited resolving in 2–8 weeks; may be imitated by secondary syphilis	Pathologic features often nonspecific
Dermatophytosis	Polymorphous appearance depending on dermatophyte, body site, and host response; sharply defined to ill-demarcated scaly plaques with or without inflammation; may be associated with hair loss	KOH preparation may show branching hyphae; culture helpful	Hyphae and neutrophils in stratum corneum

Most patients with localized plaque-type psoriasis can be managed with midpotency topical glucocorticoids, although their long-term use is often accompanied by loss of effectiveness (tachyphylaxis). Crude coal tar (1 to 5% in an ointment base) is an old but useful method of treatment in conjunction with ultraviolet light therapy. A topical vitamin D analogue (calcipitriol) is also efficacious in the treatment of psoriasis.

Ultraviolet light is an effective therapy for patients with widespread psoriasis. The ultraviolet B (UV-B) spectrum is effective alone or may be combined with coal tar (Goeckerman regimen) or anthralin (Ingram regimen). Natural sunlight or an artificial light source can be used. The combination of the UV-A spectrum and either oral or topical psoralens (PUVA) is also extremely effective for the treatment of psoriasis, but long-term use may be associated with an increased incidence of squamous cell cancer of the skin.

Various other agents can be used for widespread psoriatic disease. Methotrexate is an effective agent, especially in patients with associated psoriatic arthritis. Liver toxicity from long-term use limits its use to patients with widespread disease not responsive to less aggressive modalities. The synthetic retinoid, etretinate, has been shown to be effective in some patients with severe psoriasis, but it is a potent teratogen with an extremely long tissue half-life, thus precluding its use in women with childbearing potential.

LICHEN PLANUS Lichen planus (LP) is a papulosquamous disorder in which the primary lesions are pruritic, polygonal, flat-topped, violaceous papules. Close examination of the surface of these papules will often reveal a network of gray lines (Wickham's striae). The skin lesions may occur anywhere, but they have a predilection for the wrists, shins, lower back, and genitalia. Involvement of the scalp may lead to hair loss. LP commonly involves mucous membranes, particularly the buccal mucosa, where it can present as a white netlike eruption. Its etiology is unknown, but cutaneous eruptions clinically resembling LP have been observed after administration of numerous drugs, including diuretics, gold, antimalarials, penicillamine, and phenothiazines, and in patients with skin lesions of chronic graft-versus-host disease. Additionally, LP associated with abnormal liver function has been correlated with viral hepatitis, particularly hepatitis C infection. The course of LP is variable, but most patients have spontaneous remissions 6 months to 2 years after the onset of disease. Topical glucocorticoids are the mainstay of therapy.

PITYRIASIS ROSEA Pityriasis rosea (PR) is a papulosquamous eruption of unknown etiology that occurs more commonly in the spring and fall. Its first manifestation is the development of a 2- to 6-cm annular lesion (the herald patch). This is followed in a few days to a few weeks by the appearance of many smaller annular or papular lesions with a predilection to occur on the trunk. The lesions are generally oval with their long axis parallel to the skin fold lines. The individual lesions may range in color from red to brown and have a trailing scale. PR shares many clinical features with the eruption of

secondary syphilis, but palm and sole lesions are extremely rare in PR and common in secondary syphilis. The eruption tends to be moderately pruritic and lasts 3 to 8 weeks. Treatment is generally directed at alleviating pruritus and consists of oral antihistamines, midpotency topical glucocorticoids, and, in some cases, the use of UV-B phototherapy.

CUTANEOUS INFECTIONS (Table 55-3)

IMPETIGO AND ECTHYMA Impetigo is a common superficial bacterial infection of skin caused by group A beta-hemolytic streptococci (see Chap. 143) or *Staph. aureus* (see Chap. 142). The primary lesion is a superficial pustule that ruptures and forms a characteristic yellow-brown "honey-colored" crust. Lesions caused by staphylococci may be tense, clear bullae, and this less common form of the disease is called *bullous impetigo*. Lesions may occur on normal skin or in areas already affected by another skin disease. Ecthyma is a variant of impetigo that generally occurs on the lower extremities and causes punched-out ulcerative lesions. Treatment of both ecthyma and impetigo involves gentle debridement of adherent crusts, which is facilitated by the use of soaks and topical antibiotics, in conjunction with appropriate oral antibiotics.

ERYSIPELAS AND CELLULITIS (See Chap. 133)

DERMATOPHYTOSIS Dermatophytes are fungi that infect skin, hair, and nails and include members of the genera *Trichophyton*, *Microsporum*, and *Epidermophyton*. Infection of the foot (tinea pedis) is most common and is often chronic; it is characterized by variable erythema and edema, scaling, pruritus, and occasionally vesiculation. Involvement may be widespread or localized, but almost invariably the web space between the fourth and fifth toes is affected. Infection of the nails (tinea unguium) occurs in many patients with tinea pedis and is characterized by opacified, thickened nails and subungual debris. The groin is the next most commonly involved area (tinea cruris), with males affected much more often than females. It presents as a scaling erythematous eruption that spares the scrotum. Microscopic examination of either untreated tinea pedis or tinea cruris scale after digestion with KOH preparation will generally demonstrate hyphae.

Dermatophyte infection of the scalp (tinea capitis) has returned in epidemic proportions, particularly in inner city clinics. The predominant organism is *T. tonsurans*. This organism can produce an inflammatory or relatively noninflammatory infection that may present with either well-defined or irregular, diffuse areas of mild scaling and hair loss. Tinea corporis, or widespread infection on non-hair-bearing skin, may have a variable appearance, depending on the extent of the associated inflammatory reaction. It may have the typical annular appearance

Table 55-3

Common Skin Infections

	Clinical Features	Etiologic Agent	Treatment
Impetigo	Honey-colored crusted papules, plaques, or bullae	Group A *Streptococcus* and *Staphylococcus aureus*	Systemic or topical anti-staphylococcal antibiotics
Dermatophytosis	Inflammatory or noninflammatory annular scaly plaques; may have hair loss; groin involvement spares scrotum; hyphae on KOH preparation	*Trichophyton*, *Epidermophyton*, or *Microsporum* sp.	Topical azoles, systemic griseofulvin, or azoles
Candidiasis	Inflammatory papules and plaques with satellite pustules, frequently in intertiginous areas; may involve scrotum; pseudohyphae on KOH preparation	*Candida albicans* and other *Candida* species	Topical nystatin or azoles; systemic azoles for resistant disease
Tinea versicolor	Hyperpigmented or hypopigmented scaly patches on the trunk; characteristic mixture of hyphae and spores on KOH preparation ("spaghetti and meatballs")	KOH preparation may show branching hyphae; culture helpful	Topical selenium sulfide lotion or azoles

of "ringworm" or appear as deep inflammatory nodules (on the scalp known as a *kerion*) or granulomas. KOH examination of scale or hair from patients with tinea capitis or inflammatory tinea corporis often does not reveal hyphae, and diagnosis may require culture or biopsy.

℞ **TREATMENT**

Both topical and systemic therapies may be used to treat dermatophyte infection. Treatment depends on the site involved and the type of infection. Topical therapy is generally effective for uncomplicated tinea corporis, tinea cruris, and tinea pedis. It is not effective as monotherapy for tinea capitis or tinea ungium. Topical imidazoles (miconazole, ketoconazole, econazole, clotrimazole, oxiconazole, and sulconazole), triazoles (terconazole), and allylamines (terbinafine and naftifine) may all be effective topical therapies for dermatophyte infections. Haloprogin, undecylenic acid, ciclopirox olamine, and tolnaftate are also effective, but nystatin is not active against dermatophytes. Treatment should continue until the patient is clear of infection by clinical examination and culture. Tinea pedis often requires longer treatment courses and is associated with very high relapse rates.

Griseofulvin is the drug of choice for dermatophyte infections requiring systemic therapy. A daily dose of 500 mg of microsized or 350 mg of ultramicrosized griseofulvin administered with a fatty meal is an adequate dose for most dermatophyte infections. Unresponsive infections may respond to doubling the dose. The most common side effects of griseofulvin are gastrointestinal distress and headache. It is also rarely associated with blood and liver function abnormalities, and patients on long-term therapy should be monitored at regular intervals.

For chronic noninflammatory tinea pedis, topical agents are useful to limit the pruritus and scaling but are rarely curative. Treatment with oral griseofulvin is effective for tinea pedis, but it may require months of therapy for cure. Even then, it is associated with a high relapse rate, particularly if the nails are involved. The therapy of tinea corporis depends on the extent of disease. Localized infection is best treated with topical imidazoles, but widespread disease, particularly in patients with decreased cellular immunity, requires systemic antifungal therapy. Dermatophyte infection of hair-bearing areas (such as tinea capitis) requires systemic antifungal therapy, and treatment should be continued for 6 to 8 weeks. The adjunctive use of topical antifungal agents in addition to systemic therapy may be useful, but topical therapy alone is not adequate. Markedly inflammatory tinea capitis may result in scarring and hair loss, and systemic or topical glucocorticoids may be helpful in preventing this sequela.

Systemic azoles are now available for oral administration. Ketoconazole was the first oral broad-spectrum azole available in the United States. Its use has been limited by idiosyncratic hepatic toxicity that has been estimated to occur in 1 in 10,000 patients. Both fluconazole and itraconazole are now available for systemic fungal infections, and studies are now underway examining their effectiveness for dermatophyte infections, particularly of the nails. These agents may ultimately replace griseofulvin as first-line therapy for dermatophyte infection.

TINEA VERSICOLOR Tinea versicolor is caused by a nondermatophyte dimorphic fungus, which is a normal inhabitant of the skin. As the yeast form *Pityrosporum orbiculare*, it generally does not cause disease (except for folliculitis in certain individuals). However, in some individuals, it converts to the hyphal form and causes characteristic lesions. The expression of infection is promoted by heat and humidity. The typical lesions consist of oval scaly macules, papules, and patches concentrated on the chest, shoulders, and back, but only rarely on the face or distal extremities. On dark skin, they often appear as hypopigmented areas, while on light skin, they are slightly hyperpigmented. In some darkly pigmented individuals, they may only appear as scaling patches. A KOH preparation from scaling lesions will dem-

onstrate a confluence of short hyphae and round spores (so-called spaghetti and meatballs). Solutions containing sulfur, salicylic acid, or selenium sulfide will clear the infection if used daily for a week, and then intermittently thereafter. Topical imidazoles are also effective.

CANDIDIASIS Candidiasis is a fungal infection caused by a related group of yeasts, whose manifestations may be localized to the skin or rarely may be systemic and life-threatening. The causative organism is usually *Candida albicans* but may also be *C. tropicalis*, *C. parapsilosis*, or *C. krusei*. These organisms are normal saprophytic inhabitants of the gastrointestinal tract but may overgrow (usually due to broad-spectrum antibiotic therapy) and cause disease at a number of cutaneous sites. Other predisposing factors include diabetes mellitus, chronic intertrigo, oral contraceptive use, and cellular immune deficiency. Candidiasis is a very common infection in HIV-infected individuals (see Chap. 308). The oral cavity is commonly involved. Lesions may occur on the tongue or buccal mucosa (thrush) and appear as white plaques. Microscopic examination of scrapings will demonstrate both pseudohyphae and yeast forms. Fissured, macerated lesions at the corners of the mouth (perlèche) are often seen in individuals with poorly fitting dentures and may also be associated with candidal infection. Additionally, candidal infections have an affinity for sites that are chronically wet and macerated and may occur around nails (onycholysis and paronychia) and in intertriginous areas. Intertriginous lesions are characteristically edematous, erythematous, and scaly, with scattered "satellite pustules." In males there is often involvement of the penis and scrotum as well as the inner aspect of the thighs. In contrast to dermatophyte infections, candidal infections are frequently accompanied by a marked inflammatory response. Diagnosis of candidal infection is based upon the clinical pattern and demonstration of yeast on KOH preparation, or culture.

℞ **TREATMENT**

Treatment routinely involves removing any predisposing factors such as antibiotic therapy or chronic wetness and the use of appropriate topical or systemic antifungal therapy. Effective topical agents include nystatin or topical azoles (miconazole, clotrimazole, econazole, or ketoconazole). These agents are generally effective in clearing mucous membrane or glabrous skin involvement in nonimmunosuppressed patients. The associated inflammatory response that often accompanies candidal infection on glabrous skin should be treated with a mild glucocorticoid lotion or cream (2.5% hydrocortisone) in a drying base. Systemic therapy is generally reserved for immunosuppressed patients or individuals with chronic or recurrent disease who fail to respond to or tolerate appropriate topical therpay. Vulvovaginal candidiasis may respond to treatment with a single dose of fluconazole (150 mg).

WARTS Warts are cutaneous neoplasms that are caused by papilloma viruses. Over 50 different human papilloma viruses (HPV) have been described, and this number will almost certainly continue to grow. Typical verruca vulgaris lesions are sessile, dome-shaped, usually about a centimeter in diameter, and their surface is made up of many small filamentous projections. The HPV that cause typical verruca vulgaris also cause typical plantar warts, flat warts (or verruca plana), and filiform warts in intertriginous areas. Plantar warts are endophytic and are covered by thick keratin. Paring of the wart will generally demonstrate a central core of keratinized debris and punctate bleeding points. Filiform warts are most commonly seen on the face, neck, and skin folds and present as papillomatous lesions on a narrow base. Flat warts are only slightly elevated and have a velvety, nonverrucous surface. They have a propensity for the face, arms, and legs and often are spread by shaving.

Multiple HPV types have been associated with genital tract lesions. They generally begin as small papillomas that may grow to form large fungating lesions. In women, they may involve either the labia, perineum, or perianal skin. Additionally, the mucosa of the vagina, urethra, and anus can be involved, as well as the cervical epithelium. In men, the lesions often occur initially in the coronal sulcus but may be seen on the shaft of the penis, the scrotum, perianal skin, or in the urethra.

Within the past decade, appreciable evidence has accumulated that suggests HPV plays a role in the development of neoplasia of the uterine cervix and external genitalia (see Chap. 99). HPV types 16 and 18 have been most intensely studied, while recent evidence also implicates other types. Lesions may initially appear as small, flat, velvety, hyperpigmented papules occurring on the genitalia or perianal skin. Histologic examination of biopsies from affected sites may reveal changes associated with typical warts and/or features typical of intra-epidermal carcinoma (Bowen's disease). Squamous cell carcinomas associated with papilloma virus infections have also been observed in extragenital skin (see Chap. 88). This is most commonly seen in patients immunosuppressed after organ transplantation.

℞ TREATMENT

There are many modalities available to treat warts, but no single therapy is universally effective. Perhaps the most useful and convenient method for treating warts in almost any location is cryotherapy with liquid nitrogen. Equally effective, but requiring much more patient compliance, is the use of keratolytic agents such as salicylic acid plasters or combinations of lactic acid and salicylic acid. For genital warts, application of podophyllin solution is moderately effective but may be associated with marked local reactions in certain individuals. Other topical agents used include trichloracetic acid or cantharidin. Electrodessication and curettage or carbon dioxide laser excision are also effective therapies but require local anesthesia. Recurrence of warts appears to be common to all these modalities because viral genomic material is present in normal-appearing skin adjacent to the clinical lesions. Treatment of warts should be tempered by the observation that an overwhelming majority of warts in normal individuals resolve spontaneously within 1 to 2 years. Also, only an extremely small proportion of warts are associated with neoplasia, and those are almost exclusively located on the genitalia or perianal skin.

HERPES SIMPLEX See Chap. 184
HERPES ZOSTER See Chap. 185

ACNE

ACNE VULGARIS Acne vulgaris is usually a self-limited disorder primarily of teenagers and young adults, although perhaps 10 to 20 percent of adults may continue to experience some form of the disorder. The permissive factor for the expression of the disease in adolescence is the increase in sebum release by sebaceous glands after puberty. Small cysts, called *comedones*, form in hair follicles due to blockage of the follicular orifice by retention of sebum and keratinous material. The activity of lipophilic yeast (*P. orbiculare*) and bacteria (*Proprionobacterium acnes*) within the comedones releases free fatty acids from sebum, causes inflammation within the cyst, and results in rupture of the cyst wall. An inflammatory foreign-body reaction develops as a result of extrusion of oily and keratinous debris from the cyst.

The clinical hallmark of acne vulgaris is the comedone, which may be closed (whitehead) or open (blackhead). Closed comedones appear as 1- to 2-mm pebbly white papules, which are accentuated when the skin is stretched. They are the precursors of inflammatory lesions of acne vulgaris. The contents of closed comedones are not easily expressed. Open comedones, which rarely result in inflammatory acne lesions, have a large dilated follicular orifice and are filled with easily expressible oxidized, darkened, oily debris. Comedones are usually accompanied by inflammatory lesions: papules, pustules, or nodules.

The earliest lesions seen in early adolescence are generally mildly inflamed or noninflammatory comedones on the forehead. Subsequently, more typical inflammatory lesions develop on the cheeks, nose, and chin. The most common location for acne is the face, but involvement of the chest and back is not uncommon. Most disease remains mild and does not lead to scarring. However, a small number of patients develop large inflammatory cysts and nodules, which may drain and result in significant scarring.

Exogenous and endogenous factors can alter the expression of acne vulgaris. Friction and trauma may rupture preexisting microcomedones

and elicit inflammatory acne lesions. This is commonly seen with headbands or chin straps of athletic helmets. Application of comedogenic topical agents in cosmetics or hair preparations or chronic topical exposure to certain industrial compounds that are comedogenic may elicit or aggravate acne. Glucocorticoids, applied topically or administered systemically in high doses, may also elicit acne. Other systemic medications such as lithium, isoniazid, halogens, phenytoin, and phenobarbital may produce acneiform eruptions, or aggravate preexisting acne.

℞ TREATMENT

Treatment of acne vulgaris is directed toward elimination of comedones, decreasing the population of lipophilic bacteria and yeast, and decreasing inflammation. Although areas affected with acne should be kept clean, there is little evidence to suggest that removal of surface oils plays an important role in therapy. Overly vigorous scrubbing may aggravate acne due to mechanical rupture of comedones. Oral tetracycline or erythromycin in doses of 250 to 1000 mg daily will decrease follicular colonization with some of the lipophilic organisms. They also appear to have an anti-inflammatory effect independent of their antibacterial effect. Topical agents such as retinoic acid, benzoyl peroxide, or salicylic acid may alter the pattern of epidermal desquamation, preventing the formation of comedones and aiding in the resolution of preexisting cysts. Topical antibacterial agents such as benzoyl peroxide, topical erythromycin, clindamycin, or tetracycline are also useful adjuncts to therapy. Severe nodulocystic acne not responsive to oral antibiotics and topical therapy may be treated with the synthetic retinoid isotretinin. It is used at doses of 0.5 to 2.0 mg/kg as a single daily dose for 15 to 20 weeks. The use of this drug is limited by its teratogenicity, and female patients must be screened for pregnancy prior to initiating therapy, maintain a method of birth control during therapy, and be screened for pregnancy during their treatment course. Patients receiving this medication develop extremely dry skin and cheilitis and must be followed for development of hypertriglyceridemia.

ACNE ROSACEA Acne rosacea is an inflammatory disorder predominantly affecting the central face. It is seen almost exclusively in adults, only rarely affecting patients under 30 years of age. Rosacea is seen more often in women, but those most severely affected are men. It is characterized by the presence of erythema, telangiectases, and superficial pustules but is not associated with the presence of comedones. Rosacea only rarely involves the chest or back.

There is a relationship between the tendency for pronounced facial flushing and the subsequent development of acne rosacea. Often, individuals with rosacea initially demonstrate a pronounced flushing reaction. This may be in response to heat, emotional stimuli, alcohol, hot drinks, or spicy foods. As the disease progresses, the flush persists longer and longer and may eventually become permanent. Papules, pustules, and telangiectases can become superimposed on the persistent flush. Rosacea of very long standing may lead to connective tissue overgrowth, particularly of the nose (rhinophyma). Rosacea may also be complicated by various inflammatory disorders of the eye, including keratitis, blepharitis, iritis, and recurrent chalazion. These ocular problems are potentially sight-threatening and warrant ophthalmologic evaluation.

℞ TREATMENT

Acne rosacea can generally be effectively treated with oral tetracycline in doses ranging from 250 to 1000 mg/daily. Topical metronidazole has also been shown to be effective. In addition, the use of low-potency, nonfluorinated topical glucocorticoids, particularly after cool soaks, is helpful in alleviating facial erythema. Fluorinated topical glucocorticoids should be avoided since chronic use of these preparations may actually elicit rosacea. Topical therapy is not effective treatment for ocular disease.

BIBLIOGRAPHY

ARNDT KA et al (eds): *Cutaneous Medicine and Surgery: An Integrated Program in Dermatology.* Philadelphia, Saunders, 1996

BATA-CSORGO Z et al: Intralesional T-lymphocyte activation as a mediator of psoriatic epidermal hyperplasia. J Invest Dermatol 105:89S, 1995

FITZPATRICK TB et al (eds): *Dermatology in General Medicine,* 4th ed. New York, McGraw-Hill, 1993

GOTTLIEB SL et al: Response of psoriasis to a lymphocyte-selective toxin (DAB389 IL-2) suggests a primary immune, but not keratinocyte, pathogenic basis. Nat Med 1:442, 1995

HANAFIN JM et al: Recombinant interferon gamma therapy for atopic dermatitis. J Am Acad Dermatol 28:189, 1993

MARKS JG JR, DELEO VA: *Contact and Occupational Dermatitis.* St. Louis, Mosby Year Book, 1992

MURPHY GF (ed): *Dermatopathology: A Practical Guide to Common Disorders.* Philadelphia, Saunders, 1995

PETO R, ZUR HAUSEN H: *Viral Etiology of Cervical Cancer. Banbury Report.* Cold Spring Harbor, NY, Cold Spring Harbor Laboratory, 1986

PLEWIG G, KLIGMAN AM: *Acne: Morphogenesis and Treatment.* New York, Springer, 1975

SOWDEN JM et al: Double-blind, controlled, cross-over study of cyclosporin in adults with severe refractory atopic dermatitis. Lancet 338:137, 1991

56	*Bruce U. Wintroub, Robert S. Stern*

CUTANEOUS DRUG REACTIONS

Cutaneous reactions are among the most frequent adverse reactions to drugs. Early in drug-induced illness, prompt therapeutic intervention may limit toxicity. This chapter focuses on adverse cutaneous reactions to drugs other than topical agents and reviews the incidence, patterns, and pathogenesis of cutaneous reactions to drugs and therapeutic agents.

USE OF PRESCRIPTION DRUGS IN THE UNITED STATES More than 1.5 billion prescriptions for 60,000 drug products, which include approximately 2000 different active agents, are dispensed each year in the United States. Hospital inpatients alone annually receive about 120 million courses of drug therapy, and half of adult Americans receive prescription drugs on a regular outpatient basis. As much as 15 percent of hospital days are devoted to treatment for drug toxicity.

INCIDENCE OF CUTANEOUS REACTIONS Although adverse drug reactions are common, it is difficult to ascertain their incidence, seriousness, and ultimate health effects. The fact that comprehensive information on these reactions is inadequate in part reflects the difficulty in establishing a system for postmarketing surveillance that is both economically feasible and capable of generating clinically useful data. Available information comes from evaluations of hospitalized patients, epidemiologic surveys, premarketing studies, and voluntary reporting.

In one study about 2 percent of medical inpatients had skin reactions consisting of rash, urticaria, or pruritus during hospitalization, and the overall reaction rate per course of drug therapy was 3:1000. Penicillins, sulfonamides, and blood products accounted for two-thirds of cutaneous reactions. Specific algorithmic estimates of drug-specific quantitative reaction rates for drugs commonly used in inpatients were calculated. Reaction rates for selected commonly used drugs are summarized in Table 56-1. This study showed that most cutaneous reactions occur within 1 week of exposure to the drug. Exceptions were semisynthetic penicillins and ampicillin; about half the reactions to these drugs occurred more than 1 week after initial administration. The risk of allergic reactions was not related to age, diagnosis, or blood level of urea nitrogen on admission. Skin reactions were more frequent among women.

Table 56-1

Rates (per 1000 Recipients) of Skin Reactions to Selected Medications

Drug	Reaction Rate
Amoxicillin	51
Trimethoprim-sulfamethoxazole	34
Ampicillin	33
Other penicillins	20
Blood	21
Allopurinol	8
Gentamycin	5
Barbiturates	4

SOURCE: Adapted from Bigby et al.

The distribution of morphologic patterns of drug eruptions cared for within a Finnish hospital dermatology department with a special interest in fixed drug eruptions included exanthematous reactions (32 percent), urticaria and/or angioedema (20 percent), fixed drug eruptions (34 percent), erythema multiforme (2 percent), Stevens-Johnson syndrome (1 percent), exfoliative dermatitis (1 percent), and photosensitivity reactions (3 percent).

Documenting the risk of the most serious forms of drug eruptions associated with specific drugs remains an important challenge. Based on successful population-based retrospective case registries of toxic epidermal necrolysis (TEN) and Stevens-Johnson syndrome in Germany and France, there are now prospective registries that serve as the basis for case-control studies in these and other countries. These data, together with data from health-maintenance organizations and Medicaid, suggest that the risk of these reactions is from 1 to 10 per million person-years. The drugs most often associated with these reactions include the sulfonamide antibiotics, the aminopenicillins, phenytoin and structurally related antiseizure medications, and some nonsteroidal anti-inflammatory drugs.

PATHOGENESIS OF DRUG REACTIONS

Untoward cutaneous responses to drugs can arise as a result of immunologic or nonimmunologic mechanisms. Immunologic reactions require activation of host immunologic pathways and are designated *drug allergy.* Drug reactions occurring through nonimmunologic mechanisms may be due to activation of effector pathways, overdosage, cumulative toxicity, side effects, ecologic disturbance, interactions between drugs, metabolic alterations, exacerbation of preexisting dermatologic conditions, or inherited protein or enzyme deficiencies. Nonimmunologic cutaneous reactions to drugs are more common, and immunologic reactions are unpredictable when they do occur. It is often not possible to specify the responsible drug or pathogenic mechanism because the skin responds to a variety of stimuli through a limited number of reaction patterns. The mechanism of many drug reactions is unknown.

IMMUNOLOGIC DRUG REACTIONS Drugs frequently elicit an immune response, but only a small number of individuals experience clinical hypersensitivity reactions. For example, most patients exposed to penicillin develop demonstrable antibodies to penicillin but do not manifest drug reactions when exposed to penicillin. Multiple factors determine the capacity of a drug to elicit an immune response, including the *molecular characteristics* of the drug and *host effects.*

Increases in *molecular* size and complexity are associated with increased immunogenicity, and macromolecular drugs such as protein or peptide hormones are highly antigenic. Most drugs are small organic molecules less than 1000 daltons in size, and the capacity of such small molecules to elicit an immune response depends on their ability to act as haptens, i.e., to form stable, usually covalent, bonds with tissue macromolecules. Fortunately, most drugs have little or no ability to form covalent bonds with tissue components, and clinical sensitization results from minor contaminants or conversion of the drugs themselves to reactive metabolic products.

Route of administration of a drug or simple chemical can influence the nature of the *host* immune response. For example, topical application of antigens tends to induce delayed hypersensitivity, and exposure to antigens via oral or nasal cavities stimulates production of secretory immunoglobins, IgA and IgE, and occasionally IgM. Some agents, such as pentadecacatechol, sensitize readily if applied to the skin but do so poorly if ingested orally or applied to a mucosal surface. Frequency of sensitization through intravenous administration of drugs varies, but anaphylaxis is a more likely clinical consequence with this route of exposure.

The degree of drug exposure and individual variability in absorption and metabolism of a given agent may alter immunogenic load. The variable degree of in vivo acetylation of hydralazine provides a clinical example of this phenomenon. Hydralazine produces a lupus-like syndrome associated with antinuclear antibody formation more frequently in patients who acetylate the drug slowly. Frequent high-dose and interrupted courses of therapy are also important risk factors for development of drug allergy.

Pathogenesis of Allergic Drug Reactions   Allergic drug reactions are most commonly IgE-dependent or immune-complex–dependent. Cytotoxicity and delayed hypersensitivity have not been shown to cause systemic cutaneous drug reactions.

IgE-dependent reactions   IgE-dependent drug reactions are usually manifest in the skin and gastrointestinal, respiratory, and cardiovascular systems (see Chap. 310). Primary symptoms and signs include pruritus, urticaria, nausea, vomiting, cramps, bronchospasm, and laryngeal edema and, on occasion, anaphylactic shock with hypotension and death. Immediate reactions may occur within minutes of drug exposure, and accelerated reactions occur hours or days after drug administration. Accelerated reactions are usually urticarial and may include laryngeal edema. IgE-dependent reactions are usually due to penicillins; manifestations are caused by release from sensitized tissue mast cells or circulating basophilic leukocytes of chemical mediators such as histamine, adenosine, leukotrienes, prostaglandins, platelet-activating factor, enzymes, and proteoglycans. Release is triggered when polyvalent drug protein conjugates cross-link IgE molecules fixed to sensitized cells. The clinical manifestations are determined by interaction of the released chemical mediator with its target organ, i.e., skin, respiratory, gastrointestinal, and/or cardiovascular systems. Certain routes of administration favor different clinical patterns (i.e., oral route: gastrointestinal effects; intravenous route: circulating effects).

Immune-complex–dependent reactions   Serum sickness is produced by circulating immune complexes and is characterized by fever, arthritis, nephritis, neuritis, edema, and an urticarial, papular, or pruritic rash (see Chap. 319). The syndrome requires an antigen that remains in the circulation for prolonged periods so that when antibody is synthesized, circulating antigen-antibody complexes are formed. Serum sickness was first described following administration of foreign sera, but drugs are now the usual cause. Drugs that produce serum sickness include the penicillins, sulfonamides, thiouracils, cholecystographic dyes, phenytoin, aminosalicylic acid, streptomycin, heparin, and antilymphocyte globulin. Symptoms develop 6 days or more after exposure to a drug, the latent period representing the time needed to synthesize antibody. The antibodies responsible for immune-complex–dependent drug reactions are largely of the IgG or IgM class.

NONIMMUNOLOGIC DRUG REACTIONS   While nonimmunologic mechanisms are responsible for the majority of drug reactions, only the most important mechanisms will be discussed.

Nonimmunologic Activation of Effector Pathways   Drug reactions may result from nonimmunologic activation of effector pathways by three mechanisms: First, drugs may release mediators directly from mast cells and basophils and present as anaphylaxis or as urticaria and/or angioedema. Urticarial anaphylactic reactions induced by opiates, polymyxin B, tubocurarine, radiocontrast media, and dextrans may occur by this mechanism. Second, drugs may activate complement in the absence of antibody. This is an additional mechanism through which radiocontrast media may act. Third, drugs such as aspirin and other nonsteroidal anti-inflammatory agents may alter pathways of arachidonic acid metabolism; such drugs inhibit the cyclooxygenase

that catalyzes the generation of prostaglandins from arachidonic acid in vitro.

Phototoxicity   Phototoxic reactions may be drug-induced or may occur in metabolic disorders in which an appropriate photosensitizing chemical is overproduced. In each case the phototoxic reaction occurs when enough chromophore (drug or metabolic product) absorbs sufficient radiation in reactive tissue. Drug-induced phototoxic reactions can occur on first exposure, and the incidence of phototoxicity is a direct function of the concentration of sensitizer and amount of light. At least three distinct photochemical mechanisms have been described: First, the reaction between the excited state of a phototoxic molecule and a biologic target may cause formation of a covalent photoaddition product. Second, the phototoxic molecule may absorb protons to form stable photoproducts that are toxic to biologic substrates. Third, radiation of a phototoxic molecule may result in transfer of energy to oxygen molecules and cause formation of toxic oxygen species, such as singlet oxygen, superoxide anion, or hydroxyl radical. Interaction of these species with biologic targets produces photooxidized molecules. Serum protein–dependent systems and circulating effector cells play a role in acute in vivo phototoxic tissue damage due to exogenous agents; normal numbers of polymorphonuclear leukocytes and an intact complement system are required for the full development of demeclocycline-induced phototoxic lesions.

Exacerbation of Preexisting Diseases   A variety of agents can exacerbate preexisting diseases. For example, lithium can exacerbate acne and psoriasis in a dose-dependent manner. Beta-blocking agents and lithium may induce a psoriasiform dermatitis, and withdrawal of glucocorticoids can exacerbate psoriasis or atopic dermatitis. Exacerbations of cutaneous lupus have been noted in association with cimetidine use. Vasodilators may exacerbate rosacea.

Inherited Enzyme or Protein Deficiencies   Specific genetically determined defects in the ability of an individual to detoxify toxic reactive drug metabolites may predispose such individuals to the development of severe drug reactions, especially hypersensitivity syndrome and TEN associated with use of sulfonamides and anticonvulsants.

Alterations of Immunologic Status   Alterations in patients' immunologic status also may modify the risk of cutaneous reactions. Bone marrow transplant patients often experience cutaneous reactions to drugs. These reactions may be very difficult to differentiate from acute graft-versus-host reactions even when skin biopsy is obtained.

Persons infected with human immunodeficiency virus (HIV) are about 5- to 10-fold more likely to develop cutaneous eruptions, and this increased risk is not accounted for merely by the higher number of drugs utilized by these patients (see Chap. 308). The risk of these reactions increases as immunologic function deteriorates. Skin reactions to trimethoprim-sulfamethoxazole are seen in about a third of HIV-infected users of this drug. Dapsone, trimethoprim alone, and amoxicillin-clavulanate are also frequent causes of drug eruptions in these patients. Some drugs result in specific problems in HIV-infected persons. For example, foscarnet causes a painful penile ulcer in a substantial fraction of users. HIV-infected persons are at higher risk of the most serious types of reactions, including TEN and Stevens-Johnson syndrome.

CHARACTERISTIC FEATURES OF CUTANEOUS DRUG REACTIONS

Cutaneous disorders induced by drugs by known mechanisms include urticaria, photosensitivity, disturbances of pigmentation, vasculitis, phenytoin hypersensitivity syndrome, and warfarin necrosis of skin. Reactions of uncertain mechanism include morbilliform reactions, erythema multiforme, fixed drug reactions, erythema nodosum, lichenoid reactions, bullous drug reaction, and TEN.

REACTIONS OF KNOWN CAUSE   Urticaria   *Urticaria* is a skin reaction characterized by pruritic, red wheals. Lesions may vary from a small point to a large area. Individual lesions rarely last more than 24 h. When deep dermal and subcutaneous tissues are also swollen, this reaction is known as *angioedema*. Angioedema may involve mucous membranes and may be part of a life-threatening anaphylactic reaction. Urticarial lesions, along with pruritus and morbilliform (or maculopapular) eruptions, are among the most frequent types of cutaneous reactions to drugs.

Drug-induced urticaria may be caused by three mechanisms: an IgE-dependent mechanism, circulating immune complexes (serum sickness), and nonimmunologic activation of effector pathways. IgE-dependent urticarial reactions usually occur within 36 h but can occur within minutes. Reactions occurring within minutes to hours of drug exposure are termed *immediate reactions*, whereas those which occur 12 to 36 h after drug exposure are designated *accelerated reactions*. Immune-complex–induced urticaria associated with serum sickness may occur from 4 to 12 days after challenge. In this syndrome, the urticarial eruption may be accompanied by fever, hematuria, arthralgias, hepatic dysfunction, and neurologic symptoms.

Certain drugs, such as nonsteroidal anti-inflammatory agents, the angiotensin-converting enzyme (ACE) inhibitors, and radiographic dyes, may induce urticarial reactions, angioedema, and anaphylaxis in the absence of drug-specific antibody. Although aspirin, penicillin, and blood products are the most frequent causes of urticarial eruptions, urticaria has been observed in association with nearly all drugs.

Drugs also may cause chronic urticaria, which lasts more than 6 weeks. The mechanisms of chronic urticaria are unclear. Aspirin frequently exacerbates this problem.

The treatment of urticaria or angioedema depends on the severity of the reaction and the rate at which it is evolving. In addition to drug withdrawal, for patients with only cutaneous symptoms and without symptoms of angioedema or anaphylaxis, oral antihistamines are usually sufficient. For patients with anaphylaxis, systemic glucocorticoids, sometimes intravenously administered, are helpful. In cases with severe respiratory or cardiovascular compromise, epinephrine is useful.

Photosensitivity Eruptions Photosensitivity eruptions are usually most marked in sun-exposed areas but may extend to sun-protected areas. Phototoxic reactions are more common than photoallergic reactions. Phototoxic reactions usually resemble sunburn, can occur with the first exposure to a drug, and are dose-related. The action spectrum for phototoxicity is similar to the ultraviolet absorption spectrum of the drug. No single test system seems to be a successful predictor of the photosensitivity potential for a given compound.

The mechanism for photoallergy to systemic medications is not well defined. Drug, immune response, and light are required to produce clinical photoallergy, and photoallergic reactions may be delayed hypersensitivity responses. Eruptions range from lichenoid papules to eczematous changes.

Orally administered drugs that cause photoallergic or phototoxic reactions include chlorpromazine, tetracycline, thiazides, two nonsteroidal anti-inflammatory agents (benoxaprofen and piroxicam), and the quinalone antibiotics. Based on test systems, the majority of the common photosensitizers seem to have action spectrums in the long-wave ultraviolet A (UV-A) range and are usually phototoxic. This is fortunate, since phototoxic reactions will abate with removal of either the drug or ultraviolet radiation, but some photoallergic reactions may persist after the drug is withdrawn. Because UV-A and visible light which trigger these reactions are not easily absorbed by nonopaque sunscreens, these reactions may be difficult to block.

Photosensitivity reactions are treated by avoiding exposure to ultraviolet light (sunlight) and treating the reaction as one would a sunburn. It should be remembered that individuals who have severe photosensitive reactions may react for some weeks after avoidance of sunlight as the drug may persist in the skin for some time. Occasionally, individuals develop persistent sensitivity to light, necessitating long-term avoidance of sun exposure.

Pigmentation Changes Drugs may cause a variety of pigmentary changes in the skin. Some drugs stimulate melanocytic activity and increase pigmentation. Drug deposition also can lead to pigmentation; this phenomenon occurs with heavy metals. Phenothiazines may be deposited in the skin and cause a slate-gray color. Antimalarial drugs may cause a slate-gray or yellow pigmentation. Long term minocycline use may cause slate-gray hyperpigmentation, especially in areas of chronic inflammation. Inorganic arsenic, once used to treat psoriasis, is associated with diffuse macular pigmentation. Other heavy metals that cause pigmentary changes include silver, gold, bismuth, and mercury. Long-term use of phenytoin can produce a chloasma-like pigmentation in women. Certain cytostatic agents also can cause pigmentary changes. Histologic examination is often diagnostic for drug deposition diseases.

Zidovudine (AZT) is a frequent cause of pigmentation, especially of the nails. Clofazimine, an aminophenazine dye used in the treatment of leprosy, causes a red skin color that is so marked that some patients discontinue therapy. Methysergide produces a red color in the skin and an orange-peel-like texture. Nicotinic acid in large doses may cause brown pigmentation. Oral contraceptives may produce chloasma, and adrenocorticotropin may cause a hypermelanosis similar to that of primary adrenal insufficiency. In addition, amiodarone may cause violaceous hyperpigmentation that is increased in sun-exposed skin. Drugs such as heavy metals, copper, antimalarial and arsenical agents, and ACTH also may discolor oral mucosa.

Vasculitis Cutaneous necrotizing vasculitis often presents as palpable purpuric lesions that may be generalized or limited to the lower extremities or other dependent areas (see Chap. 319). Urticarial lesions, ulcers, and hemorrhagic blisters also occur. Vasculitis may involve other organs, including the liver, kidney, brain, and joints. Drugs are only one cause of vasculitis. Immune-complex–dependent mechanisms are probably responsible for drug-induced vasculitis and/or serum sickness. Propylthiouracil induces a cutaneous vasculitis that is accompanied by leukopenia and splenomegaly. Direct immunofluorescent changes in these lesions suggest immune-complex deposition. Drugs implicated in vasculitic eruptions include allopurinol, thiazides, penicillin, and phenytoin.

Phenytoin (Anticonvulsant) Hypersensitivity Reaction The phenytoin hypersensitivity reaction, one of many phenytoin-induced cutaneous reactions, is an erythematous eruption that eventually becomes purpuric and is accompanied by fever, facial and periorbital edema, tender generalized lymphadenopathy, leukocytosis (often with atypical lymphocytes and eosinophils), hepatitis, and sometimes nephritis. The cutaneous reaction usually begins 1 to 3 weeks after phenytoin is begun and resolves rapidly with drug cessation and treatment with systemic glucocorticoids. The eruption recurs with rechallenge, and cross-reactions with other aromatic anticonvulsants, including carbamazepine and barbiturates, are frequent. This syndrome apparently results from an inherited deficiency of epoxide hydrolase, an enzyme required for metabolism of a toxic intermediate arene oxide that is formed during metabolism of phenytoin by the cytochrome P450 system. Although controlled studies are unavailable, systemic glucocorticoids (prednisone, 0.5 to 1.0 mg/kg) will reduce symptoms, signs, and laboratory evidence of severe anticonvulsant hypersensitivity reactions.

Warfarin Necrosis of the Skin This rare reaction occurs usually between the third and tenth days of therapy with warfarin derivatives, usually in women. Lesions are sharply demarcated, erythematous, indurated, and purpuric and may resolve or progress to formation of large, irregular, hemorrhagic bullae with eventual necrosis and slow-healing eschar formation.

Development of the syndrome is unrelated to drug dose or underlying condition. Favored sites are breasts, thighs, and buttocks. The course is not altered by discontinuation of the drug after onset of the eruption. Similar reactions have been associated with heparin. Warfarin reactions are associated with protein C deficiency. Protein C is a vitamin K–dependent protein with a shorter half-life than other clotting proteins and is in part responsible for control of fibrinolysis. Since warfarin inhibits synthesis of vitamin K–dependent coagulation factors, warfarin anticoagulation in heterozygotes for protein C deficiency causes a precipitous fall in circulating levels of protein C, permitting hypercoagulability and thrombosis in the cutaneous microvasculature, with consequent areas of necrosis. Heparin-induced necrosis may have clinically similar features but is probably due to heparin-induced platelet aggregation with subsequent occlusion of blood vessels.

Warfarin-induced cutaneous necrosis is treated with vitamin K and heparin. Vitamin K reverses the effects of warfarin, and heparin acts as an anticoagulant. Treatment with protein C concentrates may also be helpful in individuals with deficiencies of protein C, the predisposing factor for development of these reactions.

REACTIONS OF UNCERTAIN CAUSE **Morbilliform Reactions** *Morbilliform* or *maculopapular eruptions* may be the most common of all drug-induced reactions, often start on the trunk or areas of pressure or trauma, and consist of erythematous macules and papules that are frequently symmetric and may become confluent. Involvement of mucous membranes, palms, and soles is variable; the eruption may be associated with moderate to severe pruritus and fever.

The pathogenesis is unclear. A hypersensitivity mechanism has been suggested, although these reactions do not always recur following drug rechallenge. Diagnosis is rarely assisted by laboratory tests; differentiation from viral exanthem is the principal differential diagnostic consideration. While these reactions usually require discontinuation of drug, eruptions occasionally may decrease or fade with continued use of the responsible drug.

Morbilliform reactions usually develop within 1 week of initiation of therapy and last 1 to 2 weeks; however, reactions to some drugs, especially penicillin, may begin more than 2 weeks after therapy has begun and last as long as 2 weeks after therapy has ceased. These eruptions are common in patients receiving ampicillin, amoxicillin, or allopurinol; trimethoprim-sulfamethoxazole causes frequent reactions in AIDS patients.

Morbilliform eruptions are usually treated symptomatically. Oral antihistamines and soothing baths are useful for treatment of pruritus. Topical antihistamines may also have some useful effect as do emollients. Short courses of potent topical glucocorticoids can reduce inflammation and symptoms and are probably helpful. The beneficial effect of systemic glucocorticoids relative to risk is less clear for morbilliform eruptions.

Fixed Drug Reactions These reactions are characterized by one or more sharply demarcated, erythematous lesions in which hyperpigmentation results after resolution of the acute inflammation; with rechallenge, the lesion recurs in the same (i.e., "fixed") location. Lesions often involve the face, genitalia, and oral mucosa and cause burning. Fixed drug eruptions have been associated with phenolphthalein, sulfonamides, tetracycline, phenylbutazone, and barbiturates. Although cross-sensitivity appears to occur between different tetracycline compounds, cross-sensitivity was not elicited when different sulfonamide compounds were administered to patients as part of provocation testing.

Documentation of a characteristic papillary-dermal mononuclear cell infiltrate in close approximation to the dermoepidermal junction may confirm the clinical diagnosis. Extensive basal cell degeneration can lead to formation of bullae and pigment dispersion. Even when lesions are completely healed, melanin-laden macrophages are present in the dermis.

Erythema Nodosum *Erythema nodosum* is a panniculitis characterized by tender, subcutaneous, erythematous nodules, usually on the anterior portion of the legs. Drug hypersensitivity, frequently involving oral contraceptives, is one cause of this reaction. The mechanism is unknown.

Lichenoid Drug Eruptions A *lichenoid cutaneous reaction*, clinically and morphologically indistinguishable from lichen planus, is associated with a variety of drugs and chemicals. Eosinophils in lichen planus are more common when the reaction is drug-induced. Gold and antimalarials are most often associated with this eruption. Antihypertensive agents, including beta blockers and captopril, also have been reported to cause a lichenoid reaction.

Bullous Eruptions Blisters accompany a wide variety of cutaneous reactions, especially the severe morbilliform eruptions, and may be an integral part of phototoxic reactions, Stevens-Johnson syndrome, TEN, and fixed drug eruptions. Nalidixic acid and furosemide cause blistering eruptions indistinguishable from the primary bullous diseases. Other examples are a pemphigus foliaceus–like eruption seen with penicillamine and cicatricial pemphigoid that has been seen with clonidine.

Pustular Eruptions Active *pustular exanthemic eruptions* also are associated with exposure to drugs, most notably antibiotics. These eruptions can be distinguished from pustular psoriasis by more rapid onset of fever and pustulation and their rapid spontaneous resolution with drug withdrawal.

Erythema Multiforme *Erythema multiforme* is an acute, self-limited inflammatory disorder of skin and mucous membranes characterized by distinctive iris or target lesions, usually acrally distributed and often associated with sore throat and malaise. Many drugs, including sulfonamides, penicillin, phenytoin, and phenylbutazone, have been reported to cause erythema multiforme; long-acting sulfonamides are the best-studied. Erythema multiforme most often has nondrug causes, most commonly herpes simplex infection.

Stevens-Johnson Syndrome Stevens-Johnson syndrome (SJS) is a blistering disorder that is usually more severe than erythema multiforme. In addition to erosions of multiple mucous membranes, small blisters developing on dusky or purpuric macules or atypical target lesions characterize this eruption. Total percent of body surface area detachment is less than 10 percent. Overlap SJS/TEN shares characteristics of both SJS and TEN, with 10 to 30 percent of body surface area epidermal detachment. Fever and malaise also occur.

Toxic Epidermal Necrolysis TEN is the most serious cutaneous drug reaction and may be fatal. Drugs are the most frequent cause of TEN in adults. Onset is generally acute and is characterized by epidermal necrosis involving >30 percent of body area. This reaction is most often associated with sulfonamides, aminopenicillins, anticonvulsants, the oxicam nonsteroidal anti-inflammatory agents, and allopurinol.

DRUGS OF SPECIAL INTEREST

PENICILLIN The incidence of reactions to penicillin is about 1 percent. Not all adverse reactions are immunologic, as illustrated by ampicillin-induced morbilliform eruptions and central nervous system reactions to procaine penicillin.

IgG, IgM, and IgE antibodies can be produced; IgG and IgM anti-penicillin antibodies play a role in the development of hemolytic anemia, whereas anaphylaxis and serum sickness appear to be due to IgE antibodies in serum.

Since penicillin reactions often occur in patients without a prior history of penicillin allergy, the utility of accurate and easily administered tests for sensitization is apparent. Current practice is to perform skin testing with a commercially available penicilloyl determinant preparation (Pre-pen, Kremers-Urban) and with fresh penicillin and, if possible, with another source of minor (nonpenicilloyl) determinants such as aged or base-treated penicillin. Antibodies to minor determinants are common in patients experiencing anaphylaxis. Testing with major determinants alone detects most patients at risk for anaphylaxis.

Twenty-seven percent (10 to 36 percent) of patients with a positive history of penicillin allergy also have a positive skin test, while 6 percent (3 to 10 percent) with a negative history demonstrate a positive skin response to penicillin. Administering penicillin to those patients with a positive skin test produces reactions in a high proportion (50 to 100 percent); conversely, only a few patients (about 0.5 percent) with negative skin tests react to the drug, and reactions tend to be mild and to occur late. Since a negative skin test may occur during or just after an acute reaction, testing should be performed either prospectively or several months after a suspected reaction. As many as 80 percent of patients lose anaphylactic sensitivity and IgE antibody after several years. Radioallergosorbent test (RAST) and other in vitro tests offer no advantage over properly performed skin testing.

Some cross-reactivity exists between penicillin and nonpenicillin β-lactam antibiotics (e.g., cephalosporins). About half of patients who react to penicillin skin testing also react to cephalosporin skin testing; anaphylaxis from cephalosporins has occurred in patients testing positive to penicillin. The benefit of skin testing with penicillin derivatives and cephalosporins in addition to penicillin is uncertain; in one study, none of 120 patients with negative results to penicillin skin tests reacted to semisynthetic penicillinase-resistant agents.

In the face of a positive clinical history of penicillin reaction, another drug should be chosen. If this is not feasible or prudent (e.g., in a pregnant patient with syphilis; with enterococcal endocarditis), skin testing with penicillin is warranted. If skin tests are negative, cautious administration of penicillin is acceptable, although some recommend desensitization of such patients. In those with positive skin tests, desensitization is mandatory if therapeutic use of β-lactam antibiotics is to be undertaken. Various protocols are available, including oral and parenteral approaches. Oral desensitization appears to carry a lesser risk of serious anaphylactic reactions during desensitization. However, desensitization carries the risk of anaphylaxis regardless of how it is performed. After desensitization, many patients experience non-life-threatening IgE-mediated untoward reactions to penicillin during their course of therapy. Desensitization is not effective in those with exfoliative dermatitis or morbilliform reactions due to penicillin.

NONSTEROIDAL ANTI-INFLAMMATORY DRUGS Nonsteroidal anti-inflammatory drugs (NSAIDs), including aspirin (but not salicylates in general) and indomethacin (indometacin), cause two broad categories of allergic-like symptoms in susceptible individuals: (1) approximately 1 percent of persons experience urticaria or angioedema, and (2) about half as many (0.5 percent) experience rhinosinusitis and asthma; however, about 10 percent of adult asthmatics and one-third of individuals with nasal polyposis and sinusitis may respond adversely to aspirin.

Urticaria/angioedema may be delayed up to 24 h and may occur at any age. The rhinosinusitis-asthma syndrome generally develops within 1 h of drug administration. In young people, the reaction pattern often begins as watery rhinorrhea, which can be complicated by nasal and sinus infection, and polyposis, bloody discharge, and nasal eosinophilia. In many individuals with this syndrome, asthma eventually ensues that can be life-threatening whenever NSAIDs are subsequently ingested, and symptoms may persist despite avoidance of these drugs. Proof of the association of symptoms and NSAID use requires either clear-cut history of symptoms following drug ingestion or an oral challenge. For the latter to be performed with relative safety, (1) asthma must be under good control, (2) the procedure must be conducted in a hospital setting by experienced personnel capable of recognizing and treating acute respiratory responses, and (3) the challenge should begin with very low doses (i.e., <30 mg) of aspirin and increase every 1 to 2 h in doubling doses as tolerated to 650 mg. In a study of 50 consecutive patients with a positive history of aspirin-induced bronchospasm, 84 percent developed pulmonary or naso-ocular symptoms with aspirin, but 16 percent did not react; moreover, when subjects who initially tested positive to a challenge were reexposed to aspirin, the clinical reaction pattern was identical in only 60 percent.

While cross-reactivity between NSAIDs is common, it is not immunologic, and patients who are sensitive to NSAIDs cannot be identified by assessment of IgE antibody to aspirin, lymphocyte sensitization, or in vitro immunologic testing. All cross-reacting drugs are cyclooxygenase inhibitors, although salicylates also inhibit cyclooxygenase but (except for aspirin) do not cause the response.

"Desensitization" to the adverse effects of NSAIDs can be accomplished by the challenge procedure above, although repeated challenge at the initial provocation dose may be required. Desensitization works by unknown mechanisms, renders the subject tolerant to all NSAIDs yet studied, persists for at least 24 and up to 96 h, and is probably universal but does not have a positive effect on the underlying disorder.

RADIOCONTRAST MEDIA Large numbers of patients are exposed to radiocontrast agents, and 5 to 10 percent of patients receiving them develop some reaction: urticaria in 1 percent, dyspnea in 0.25 percent, and death in 0.01 percent. Reactions consisting of urticaria and angioedema, asthma, and hypotension mimicking anaphylaxis occur in fewer than 1 percent of radiocontrast procedures. About one-third of those with mild reactions to previous exposure rereact on reexposure.

There is no proof of an immunologic mechanism for radiocontrast media reactions. Elevations in plasma histamine levels occur in those with and without reaction and may be due to the hypertonicity of these media. In addition, complement activation by both classic and alternative pathways occurs in normal and reactive individuals. In short, the mechanism for these reactions is not understood, and no test identifies patients at risk for a radiocontrast medium reaction. Because repeat reactions are common, obtaining a thorough history is the best available technique for identifying those most likely to experience an adverse reaction. Several pretreatment regimens are claimed to decrease the repeat reaction rate to about 10 percent. One such regimen consists of 50 mg prednisone at 13, 7, and 1 h before the procedure and 50 mg diphenhydramine 1 h before the procedure.

HYDANTOINS Phenytoin and other hydantoins cause morbilliform eruptions, erythema multiforme, and TEN, as well as a hypersensitivity reaction (described above) and the pseudolymphoma syndrome. In one study, 5 percent of children treated with phenytoin developed a mild dose-dependent, maculopapular eruption lasting 3 to 5 days and occurring within 2 weeks of starting treatment.

The pseudolymphoma syndrome, consisting of lymphadenopathy and histopathologic lymph node atypia, is a more chronic form of the phenytoin hypersensitivity syndrome, and the cutaneous changes are less marked in this syndrome.

Use of phenytoin is frequently associated with gingival hyperplasia and rarely with a syndrome similar to systemic lupus erythematosus, severe exfoliative dermatitis, and polyarteritis nodosa. Because many hydantoin side effects may be dose-related, drugs that interfere with its elimination (e.g., chloramphenicol) effectively prolong those effects. Sulfasalazine, other sulfonamides, and allopurinol cause reactions that are indistinguishable from the phenytoin hypersensitivity syndrome.

THIAZIDES AND SULFONAMIDES Thiazides are among the most common causes of drug-induced urticaria and morbilliform eruptions; they also cause erythema multiforme, drug-induced cutaneous vasculitis, and lichenoid and photosensitivity eruptions. Because they are substituted sulfonamides, antibodies to these diuretics may cross-react with sulfonamide antibiotics and sulfonamide-based hypoglycemic agents. The combination of sulfamethoxazole and trimethoprim causes two distinct cutaneous reactions: (1) an urticarial eruption beginning in the first few days of treatment and (2) a morbilliform eruption often occurring more than 1 week after therapy has begun. The morbilliform reaction is frequent in patients with AIDS and is associated with pancytopenia in some patients. The eruption may have an intensely purpuric character, independent of the presence of vasculitis. One patient developed TEN and pancytopenia following administration of sulfamethoxazole-trimethoprim.

AGENTS USED IN CANCER CHEMOTHERAPY Since many agents used in cancer chemotherapy inhibit cell division, rapidly proliferating elements of the skin, including hair, mucous membranes, and appendages, are sensitive to their effects; as a result, stomatitis and alopecia are among the most frequent dose-dependent side effects of chemotherapy. Onychodystrophy (dystrophic changes in nails) is also seen with bleomycin, hydroxyurea (hydroxycarbamide), and 5-fluorouracil. Sterile cellulitis and phlebitis and ulceration of pressure areas occur with many of these agents. Urticaria, angioedema, exfoliative dermatitis, and erythema of the palms and soles also have been seen, as has local and diffuse hyperpigmentation. Diagnosis and treatment of these reactions are especially difficult because of the underlying malignancy.

TETRACYCLINES While urticaria and morbilliform eruptions are unusual, tetracyclines sometimes cause other cutaneous side effects, including a photosensitivity reaction (as a result of drug-induced phototoxicity) and onycholysis (sometimes with no apparent cutaneous photosensitivity). These reactions occur with demeclocycline, doxycycline, minocycline, tetracycline, and oxytetracycline. Tetracyclines also cause fixed drug and lichenoid eruptions. An acne-like, gram-negative folliculitis with long-term use of tetracycline is due to overgrowth of resistant bacteria.

Several pigmentary abnormalities have been noted. If used during pregnancy or early childhood, tetracycline stains the teeth, sometimes permanently. Minocycline also has been associated with a flulike syndrome (accompanied by headaches, malaise, and eosinophilia) that recurred with rechallenge.

GLUCOCORTICOIDS Both systemic and topical glucocorticoids cause a variety of skin changes, including acneiform eruptions, atrophy, striae, and other stigmata of Cushing's syndrome, and in sufficiently high doses can retard wound healing. Patients using glucocorticoids are at higher risk for bacterial, yeast, and fungal skin infections that may be misinterpreted as drug eruptions but are in fact drug side effects instead.

ANTIMALARIAL AGENTS Antimalarial agents are used as therapy for several skin diseases, including the skin manifestations of lupus and polymorphous light eruption, but they also can induce cutaneous reactions. In patients with asymptomatic porphyria cutanea tarda, chloroquine increases porphyrin levels and may exacerbate the disease.

Pigmentation disturbances, including black pigmentation of the face, mucous membranes, and pretibial and subungual areas, occur with antimalarials, and quinacrine (mepacrine) causes generalized, cutaneous yellow discoloration. Antimalarial agents may exacerbate psoriasis, and exfoliative dermatitis, fixed drug eruptions, lichenoid dermatitis, and erythema annulare centrifugum have all been reported with their use.

GOLD Chrysotherapy has been associated with a variety of dose-related dermatologic reactions (including maculopapular eruptions) that can develop as long as 2 years after initiation of therapy and require months to resolve. Erythema nodosum, psoriasiform dermatitis, vaginal pruritus, eruptions similar to pityriasis rosea, hyperpigmentation, and lichenoid eruptions resembling those seen with antimalarial agents have been reported. After a cutaneous reaction, it is sometimes possible to reinstitute gold therapy at lower doses without recurrence of the dermatitis.

DIAGNOSIS OF DRUG REACTIONS

Possible causes of an adverse reaction can be assessed as definite, probable, possible, or unlikely based on six variables: (1) previous experience with the drug in the general population, (2) alternative etiologic candidates, (3) timing of events, (4) drug levels or evidence of overdose, (5) patient reaction to drug discontinuation, and (6) patient reaction to rechallenge.

PREVIOUS EXPERIENCE Tables of relative reaction rates are available and are useful to assess the likelihood that a given drug is responsible for a given cutaneous reaction. The specific morphologic pattern of a drug reaction, however, may modify these reaction rates by increasing or decreasing the likelihood that a given drug is responsible for a given reaction. For example, since fixed eruptions due to drug are more often seen with barbiturates than with penicillin, a fixed drug reaction in a patient taking both types of agents is more likely to be due to the barbiturate, even though penicillins have a higher overall drug reaction rate.

ALTERNATIVE ETIOLOGIC CANDIDATES A cutaneous eruption may be due to exacerbation of preexisting disease or to development of new disease unrelated to drugs. For example, a patient with psoriasis may have a flare-up of disease coincidental with administration of penicillin for streptococcal infection; in this case, infection is a more likely cause for the flare-up than drug reaction.

TIMING OF EVENTS Since most drug reactions of the skin occur within 1 to 2 weeks of initiation of therapy, reactions beginning after 2 weeks are less likely to be due to drugs.

DRUG LEVELS Some cutaneous reactions are dependent on dosage or cumulative toxicity. For example, lichenoid dermatoses due to gold administration appear more often in patients taking high doses.

DISCONTINUATION Most adverse cutaneous reactions to drugs remit with discontinuation of the suspected agent. A reaction

Table 56-2

Clinical and Laboratory Findings Associated with More Serious Drug-Induced Cutaneous Clinical Findings

Cutaneous
  Confluent erythema
  Facial edema or central facial involvement
  Skin pain
  Palpable purpura
  Skin necrosis
  Blisters or epidermal detachment
  Positive Nikolsky's sign
  Mucous membrane erosions
  Urticaria
  Swelling of tongue

General
  High fever [temperature >40°C (>104°F)]
  Enlarged lymph nodes
  Arthralgias or arthritis
  Shortness of breath, wheezing, hypotension

Laboratory results
  Eosinophil count >1000/μL
  Lymphocytosis with atypical lymphocytes
  Abnormal liver function tests

SOURCE: Adapted from Roujeau and Stern.

is unlikely to be drug-related if improvement occurs while the drug is continued or if a patient fails to improve after stopping the drug and appropriate therapy.

RECHALLENGE Rechallenge provides the most definitive information concerning adverse cutaneous reactions to drugs, since a reaction failing to recur on rechallenge with a drug is unlikely to be due to that agent. Rechallenge is frequently impractical, however, because the need to ensure patient safety and comfort outweighs the value of the possible information derived from rechallenge.

Of special importance is the rapid recognition of reactions that may become serious or life-threatening. Table 56-2 lists clinical and laboratory features that, if present, suggest the reaction may be serious. Table 56-3 provides key features of the most serious adverse cutaneous reactions.

DIAGNOSIS OF DRUG ALLERGY

Tests for IgE responses include in vivo and in vitro methods, but such tests are available only for a limited number of drugs, including penicillins and cephalosporins, some peptide and protein drugs (insulin, xenogeneic sera), and some agents used for general anesthesia. In vivo testing is accomplished by prick puncture and/or by intradermal skin testing. A wheal-and-flare response 2×2 mm greater than that seen with a saline control within 20 min is considered indicative of IgE-mediated mast cell degranulation, provided (1) the patient is not dermographic, (2) the drug does not nonspecifically degranulate mast cells, (3) the drug concentration is not high enough to be irritating, and (4) the buffer itself does not cause wheal-and-flare responses.

Skin testing with major and minor determinants of penicillins or cephalosporins has proved useful for identifying patients at risk of anaphylactic reactions to these agents. However, skin tests themselves carry a small risk of anaphylaxis. Negative skin tests do not rule out IgE-mediated reactivity, and the risk of anaphylaxis in response to penicillin administration in patients with negative skin tests is about 1 percent; about two-thirds of patients with a positive skin test and history of a previous adverse reaction to penicillin experience an allergic response on rechallenge. Skin tests may be negative in allergic patients receiving antihistamines or in those whose allergy is to determinants not present in the test reagent. Although less well studied, similar techniques can identify patients who are sensitive to protein

Table 56-3

Clinical Features of Selected Severe Cutaneous Reactions Often Induced by Drugs

Diagnosis	Mucosal Lesions	Typical Skin Lesions	Frequent Signs and Symptoms	Alternative Causes not Related to Drugs
Stevens-Johnson syndrome	Erosions usually at ≥two sites	Small blisters on dusky purpuric macules or atypical targets; rare areas of confluence; detachment ≤10% of body surface area	10–30% of cases involve fever, lesions of the respiratory and gastrointestinal tracts	Postinfectious erythema multiforme major (especially in the case of infection with herpes simplex or mycoplasma)
Toxic epidermal necrolysis	Erosions usually at ≥two sites	Individual lesions like those seen in Stevens-Johnson syndrome; confluent erythema; outer layer of epidermis separates readily from basal layer with lateral pressure; large sheet of necrotic epidermis; total detachment of >30% of body surface area	Nearly all cases involve fever, "acute skin failure," leukopenia, lesions of the respiratory and gastrointestinal tracts	
Hypersensitivity syndrome	Infrequent	Severe exanthematous rash (may become purpuric), exfoliative dermatitis	30–50% of cases involve fever, lymphadenopathy, hepatitis, nephritis, carditis, eosinophilia, atypical lymphocytes	Cutaneous lymphoma
Small-vessel vasculitis	Infrequent	Palpable purpura, most often on the legs; nodules, ulcerations; urticaria	30–50% of cases involve the gastrointestinal tract, neuritis, fever, glomerulonephritis	Infection, rheumatic diseases, lymphomas
Serum sickness or reactions resembling serum sickness	Absent	Morbilliform lesions, sometimes with urticaria	Fever, arthralgias	Infection
Anticoagulant-induced necrosis	Infrequent	Erythema then purpura and necrosis, especially of fatty areas	Pain in affected areas	Disseminated intravascular coagulopathy, septicemia
Angioedema	Often involved	Urticaria or swelling of central part of face	Respiratory distress, cardiovascular collapse	Insect stings, foods

SOURCE: Adapted from Roujeau and Stern.

drugs and to agents such as gallamine and succinylcholine. Most other drugs are small molecules, and skin testing with them is unreliable.

In vitro testing for IgE may be done by assessing the ability of serum to bind to antigen and then to bind radiolabeled antibody to IgE (RAST test) or by assessing the ability of the drug to cause histamine release from basophils from drug-sensitive individuals. The RAST test is sensitive and specific but is not available for most drugs; even in the case of penicillin it is available for major determinants only. Similarly, basophil histamine release is a research technique that is not generally available.

There are no generally available and reliable tests for sensitivity to NSAIDs, to agents that directly degranulate mast cells, or to drugs that cause manifestations via immune-complex–mediated complement activation. Although it is possible to screen for the absence of IgA antibody, the utility of this maneuver in preventing transfusion-associated anaphylaxis in IgA-deficient individuals has not been documented.

BIBLIOGRAPHY

ALANKO K et al: Cutaneous drug reactions: Clinical types and causative agents. Five-year survey of inpatients (1981–1985). Acta Derm Venereol (Stockh) 69:223, 1989

BASTUJI-GARIN S et al: Clinical classification of cases of toxic epidermal necrolysis, Stevens-Johnson syndrome, and erythema multiforme. Arch Dermatol 129(1):92, 1993

BIELORY L et al: Human serum sickness: A prospective analysis of 35 inpatients treated with equine anti-thymocyte globulin for bone marrow failure. Medicine 67:40, 1988

BIGBY M et al: Drug-induced cutaneous reactions: A report from the Boston Collaborative Drug Surveillance Program on 15,438 consecutive inpatients, 1975–1982. JAMA 256:3358, 1986

CHAN HL et al: The incidence of erythema multiforme, Stevens-Johnson syndrome, and toxic epidermal necrolysis: A population-based study with particular reference to reactions caused by drugs among outpatients. Arch Dermatol 126:43, 1990

COOPMAN SA et al: Cutaneous disease and drug reactions in HIV infection. N Engl J Med 328(23):1670, 1993

JUNG AC, PAAUW DS: Management of adverse reactions to trimethoprim-sulfamethoxazole in human immunodeficiency virus-infected patients. Arch Intern Med 154(21):2402, 1994

KAUFMANN D et al: Severe episode of high fever with rash, lymphadenopathy, neutropenia, and eosinophilia after minocycline therapy for acne. Arch Intern Med 154(17):1983, 1994

ROUJEAU JC, STERN RS: Severe adverse cutaneous reactions to drugs. N Engl J Med 331(19):1272, 1994

———— et al: Acute generalized exanthematous pustulosis: Analysis of 63 cases. Arch Dermatol 127:1333, 1991

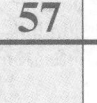

57 *Jean L. Bolognia, Irwin M. Braverman*

SKIN MANIFESTATIONS OF INTERNAL DISEASE

It is now a generally accepted concept in medicine that the skin can show signs of internal disease. Therefore, in textbooks of medicine one finds a chapter describing in detail the major systemic disorders that can be identified by cutaneous signs. The underlying assumption of such a chapter is that the clinician has been able to identify the disorder in the patient and needs only to read about it in the textbook.

In reality, concise differential diagnoses and the identification of these disorders are actually difficult for the nondermatologist because he or she is not well versed in the recognition of cutaneous lesions or their spectrum of presentations. Therefore, the authors of this chapter have decided to cover this particular topic of cutaneous medicine not by discussing individual disorders but by describing and discussing the various presenting clinical signs and symptoms that indicate the presence of these disorders. Concise differential diagnoses will be generated in which the significant diseases will be briefly discussed and distinguished from the more common disorders that have no significance for internal diseases. The latter disorders are reviewed in table form and always need to be excluded when considering the former. For a detailed description of individual diseases, the reader should consult a dermatologic text. The categories of skin lesions that are discussed include papulosquamous lesions, erythroderma, alopecia, figurate lesions, acne, pustules, telangiectasias, hypopigmentation, hyperpigmentation, vesicles/bullae, exanthems, urticaria, papulonodular lesions, purpura, and ulcers. In an attempt to determine the appropriate category for a particular lesion, it is important to examine carefully its surface qualities, shape, and color in addition to the location and distribution (see Chap. 54).

PAPULOSQUAMOUS SKIN LESIONS (Table 57-1) When an eruption is characterized by elevated lesions, papules (<1 cm) or plaques (>1 cm), in association with scale, it is referred to as *papulosquamous*. The most common papulosquamous diseases—*psoriasis*, *tinea*, *pityriasis rosea*, and *lichen planus*—are primary cutaneous disorders (Table 57-2). When psoriatic lesions are accompanied by arthritis, the possibility of psoriatic arthritis or *Reiter's disease* should be considered. A history of oral ulcers, conjunctivitis, uveitis, and/or urethritis points to the latter diagnosis. In *guttate psoriasis* there is an acute onset of small, widely scattered, uniform lesions, often in association with a streptococcal infection. Lithium, beta blockers, human immunodeficiency virus (HIV) infection, and a rapid taper of systemic glucocorticoids are also known to exacerbate psoriasis. Epidermal hyperproliferation and incomplete maturation are responsible for the plaque formation and scale that is characteristic of psoriasis. The papulosquamous diseases are discussed in detail in Chap. 55.

Whenever the diagnosis of pityriasis rosea or lichen planus is made, it is important to review the patient's medications because the

Table 57-1

Selected Causes of Papulosquamous Skin Lesions

1. Primary cutaneous disorders
   a. Psoriasis*
   b. Tinea*
   c. Pityriasis rosea*
   d. Lichen planus*
   e. Parapsoriasis
   f. Bowen's disease (squamous cell carcinoma in situ)†
2. Drugs
3. Systemic diseases
   a. Lupus erythematosus‡
   b. Cutaneous T cell lymphoma
   c. Secondary syphilis
   d. Reiter's disease

* Discussed in detail in Chap. 55.
† Associated with chronic sun exposure and exposure to arsenic.
‡ See also "Red Lesions" in "Papulonodular Skin Lesions."

eruption can be treated by simply discontinuing the offending agent. Pityriasis rosea–like drug eruptions are seen most commonly with beta blockers, captopril, gold, and metronidazole, while the drugs that can produce a lichenoid eruption include gold, antimalarials, thiazides, quinidine, phenothiazines, sulfonylureas, beta blockers, and captopril. Lichen planus–like lesions are also observed in chronic graft-versus-host disease.

Parapsoriasis is an intermediate disease, for it can remain solely as a primary cutaneous disease or it can progress to cutaneous T cell lymphoma (CTCL) after a latency period of as long as 40 years. There are several forms of parapsoriasis, including small plaque (0.5 to 5 cm), large plaque (>6 cm), and retiform. The lesions of both small plaque and large plaque parapsoriasis are thin and salmon-pink in color with fine white scale. In small plaque forms, the lesions are commonly on the trunk but can be widely scattered. In large plaque forms, the most common location is the "girdle" area, and fine wrinkling secondary to epidermal atrophy is often seen. Retiform parapsori-

Table 57-2

Papulosquamous Skin Diseases (Primary Cutaneous Disorders)*

	Characteristic Lesion	Location	Other Findings	Diagnostic Aids	Treatment†
Psoriasis	Pink-red, silvery scale; sharply demarcated	Elbows, knees, scalp, presacral area	Nail dystrophy: pitting, onycholysis, yellow discoloration Arthritis: primarily small joints (hands and feet)	Skin biopsy Culture for beta-hemolytic streptococci	Discontinue possible offending agents; topical glucocorticoids, keratolytics, tars, and vitamin D; UV-B‡; PUVA§; methotrexate
Tinea	Pink-red; central clearing common; active, scaling border	Inner thigh (tinea cruris), palms, soles, any area of body	Invasion of stratum corneum by dermatophytes	KOH and/or fungal culture of scale	Topical or systemic antifungals, e.g., imidazoles, triazoles, allylamines, griseofulvin
Pityriasis rosea	Salmon-pink; oval shape; long axis follows lines of cleavage in the skin, peripheral collarette of scale	Trunk, proximal extremities	Herald patch: initial lesion and usually the largest in size Spontaneous resolution over 2–3 months	Skin biopsy, VDRL to exclude secondary syphilis	Discontinue possible offending agents; antihistamines; topical glucocorticoids; UV-B‡ if widespread
Lichen planus	Violet-colored; polygonal, flat-topped, traversed by thin white lines (Wickham's striae)	Flexor wrists, ankles, presacral area, glans penis	Oral mucosa: lacelike white plaques and/or erosions Pruritus Nail dystrophy: pterygium, longitudinal ridging	Skin biopsy	Discontinue possible offending agents; topical glucocorticoids; PUVA§; oral glucocorticoids

* Discussed in detail in Chap. 55.
† When multiple treatments are listed, the treatments for mild to moderate disease are listed first, followed by those for severe involvement.
‡ UV-B, ultraviolet B.
§ PUVA, psoralens + ultraviolet A irradiation.

asis forms a netlike pattern, and the individual papules are red-brown and flat-topped. The latter two forms of parapsoriasis, large plaque and retiform, can progress to CTCL.

A clue to the development of *CTCL* within lesions of large plaque or retiform parapsoriasis is an increase in the palpable component of the plaque (increased infiltration). In its early stages, CTCL may be confused with ezcema or psoriasis, but it often fails to respond to the appropriate therapy for those inflammatory diseases. The diagnosis of CTCL is established by skin biopsy in which collections of atypical T lymphocytes are found in the epidermis and dermis. As the disease progresses, cutaneous tumors and lymph node involvement may appear.

In *secondary syphilis* there are scattered red-brown papules with thin scale. The eruption often involves the palms and soles, and it can resemble pityriasis rosea. Associated findings are helpful in making the diagnosis, and they include annular plaques on the face, nonscarring alopecia, condyloma lata (broad-based and moist), and mucous patches as well as lymphadenopathy, malaise, fever, headache, and myalgias. The interval between the primary chancre and the secondary stage is usually 4 to 8 weeks, and spontaneous resolution without appropriate therapy is seen.

ERYTHRODERMA (Table 57-3) *Erythroderma* is the term used when the majority of the skin surface is erythematous (red in color). There may be associated scale, erosions, or pustules as well as shedding of the hair and nails. Potential systemic manifestations include fever, chills, hypothermia, reactive lymphadenopathy, peripheral edema, hypoalbuminemia, and high-output cardiac failure. The major etiologies of erythroderma are (1) *cutaneous diseases* such as psoriasis and dermatitis (Table 57-4), (2) *drugs*, (3) *systemic diseases*, most commonly CTCL, and (4) *idiopathic*. In the first three groups, the location and description of the initial lesions, prior to the development of the erythroderma, aid in the diagnosis. For example, a history of red scaly plaques on the elbows and knees would point to psoriasis. It is also important to examine the skin carefully for a migration of the erythema and associated secondary changes such as pustules or erosions. Migratory waves of erythema studded with superficial pustules are seen in *pustular psoriasis*.

An erythroderma secondary to an underlying cutaneous disease is most commonly due to *psoriasis* or one of the various forms of *dermatitis* (eczema). Each type of dermatitis has its own distinguishing features, but they may be limited to the initial lesions (Table 57-4).

Drug-induced erythroderma (exfoliative dermatitis) may begin as a morbilliform eruption (Chap. 56), or it may arise as diffuse erythema. Fever and peripheral eosinophilia often accompany the eruption, and occasionally there is an associated allergic interstitial nephritis. A number of *drugs* can produce an erythroderma, including penicillins, sulfonamides, carbamazepine, phenytoin, gold, allopurinol, captopril, and granulocyte-macrophage colony stimulating factor. While reactions to anticonvulsants can lead to a pseudolymphoma syndrome, reactions to allopurinol may be accompanied by hepatitis, gastrointestinal bleeding, and nephropathy.

The most common malignancy that is associated with erythroderma is *CTCL*; in some series, up to 25 percent of the cases of erythroderma were due to CTCL. The patient may progress from isolated plaques and tumors, but more commonly the erythroderma is present throughout the course of the disease (Sézary syndrome). In the Sézary syndrome, there are circulating atypical T lymphocytes, pruritus, and lymphadenopathy. In cases of erythroderma where there is no apparent cause (idiopathic), longitudinal follow-up is mandatory to monitor for the possible development of CTCL. Other types of *lymphoma* can be associated with erythroderma, including Hodgkin's and non-Hodgkin's lymphoma, the former being more common. There also have been isolated case reports of erythroderma secondary to some solid tumors—lung, liver, prostate, thyroid, and colon—but it is usually in a late stage of the disease.

ALOPECIA (Table 57-5) The two major forms of *alopecia* are scarring and nonscarring. In *scarring alopecia* there is associated fibrosis, inflammation, and loss of hair follicles. A smooth scalp with a decreased number of follicular openings is usually observed clinically, but in some cases the changes are seen only in biopsy specimens from the affected areas. In *nonscarring alopecia* the hair shafts are gone, but the hair follicles are preserved, explaining the reversible nature of nonscarring alopecia.

Primary cutaneous disorders are the most common causes of nonscarring alopecia and they include *telogen effluvium, androgenetic alopecia, alopecia areata, tinea capitis,* and *traumatic alopecia* (Table 57-6). In women with androgenetic alopecia, an elevation in circulating levels of androgens may be seen as a result of ovarian or adrenal gland dysfunction. When there are signs of virilization, such as a deepened voice and enlarged clitoris, the possibility of an ovarian or adrenal gland tumor should be considered.

Exposure to various *drugs* also can cause diffuse hair loss, usually by inducing a telogen effluvium. An exception is the anagen effluvium observed with antimitotic agents such as daunorubicin. Alopecia is a side effect of the following drugs: warfarin, heparin, propylthiouracil, carbimazole, vitamin A, isotretinoin, etretinate, lithium, beta blockers, colchicine, amphetamines, and thallium. Fortunately, spontaneous regrowth usually follows discontinuation of the offending agent.

Less commonly, nonscarring alopecia is associated with *lupus erythematosus* and *secondary syphilis*. In systemic lupus there are two forms of alopecia—one is scarring secondary to discoid lesions (see below) and the other is nonscarring. The latter form may be diffuse and involve the entire scalp, or it may localized to the frontal scalp in the form of multiple short hairs ("lupus hairs"). Scattered, poorly circumscribed patches of alopecia with a "moth-eaten" appearance are a manifestation of the secondary stage of syphilis (see "Papulosquamous Skin Lesions"). Diffuse thinning of the hair is also associated with hypothyroidism, hyperthyroidism, hypopituitarism, HIV infection, and deficiencies of protein, iron, biotin, and zinc.

Scarring alopecia is more frequently the result of a primary cutaneous disorder such as *lichen planus, folliculitis decalvans, cutaneous lupus,* or *linear scleroderma (morphea)* than it is a sign of systemic disease. Although the scarring lesions of *discoid lupus* can be seen in patients with systemic lupus, in the majority of cases the disease process is limited to the skin. Less common causes of scarring alopecia include *sarcoidosis* (see "Papulonodular Skin Lesions") and cutaneous *metastases*.

In the early phases of discoid lupus, lichen planus, and folliculitis decalvans, there are circumscribed areas of alopecia. Fibrosis and subsequent loss of follicles are observed primarily in the center of the individual lesions, while the inflammatory process is most prominent at the periphery. The areas of active inflammation in *discoid lupus* are erythematous with scale, whereas the areas of previous inflammation are often hypopigmented with a rim of hyperpigmentation. In *lichen planus* the peripheral perifollicular macules are violet-colored, and postinflammatory hyperpigmentation is a characteristic finding. Complete examination of the skin and oral mucosa combined with a biopsy and direct immunofluorescence microscopy will aid in distinguishing these two entities. The peripheral active lesions in *folliculitis decalvans* are perifollicular pustules that routinely grow *Staphylococ-*

Table 57-3

Causes of Erythroderma

1. Primary cutaneous disorders
   a. Psoriasis*
   b. Dermatitis (atopic, stasis, contact, seborrheic)*
   c. Pityriasis rubra pilaris
2. Drugs
3. Systemic diseases
   a. Cutaneous T cell lymphoma
   b. Lymphoma
4. Idiopathic

* Discussed in detail in Chap. 55.

Table 57-4

Erythroderma (Primary Cutaneous Disorders)

	Initial Lesions	Location of Initial Lesions	Other Findings	Diagnostic Aids	Treatment
Psoriasis*	Pink-red, silvery scale, sharply demarcated	Elbows, knees, scalp, presacral area	Nail dystrophy, arthritis, pustules	Skin biopsy	Etretinate ± PUVA†; methotrexate
Dermatitis:*					
Atopic	Acute: Erythema, fine scale, crust, indistinct borders Chronic: Lichenification (increased skin markings)	Antecubital and popliteal fossae, neck, hands	Pruritus Family history of atopy, including asthma, allergic rhinitis or conjunctivitis, and atopic dermatitis Rule out secondary infection with *S. aureus* Rule out superimposed irritant contact dermatitis	Skin biopsy	Topical glucocorticoids, tar, and antipruritics; oral antihistamines; open wet dressings; UV-B‡ + UV-A§; PUVA; oral/IM** glucocorticoids Topical or oral antibiotics
Stasis	Erythema, crusting, excoriations	Lower extremities	Pruritus, lower extremity edema History of venous ulcers, thrombophlebitis, and/or cellulitis Rule out cellulitis Rule out superimposed contact dermatitis, e.g., topical neomycin	Skin biopsy	Topical glucocorticoids; open wet dressings; leg elevation; pressure stockings
Contact	Local: Erythema, crusting, vesicles, and bullae	Depends on offending agent	Irritant—onset often within hours Allergic—delayed-type hypersensitivity; lag time of 48 h	Patch testing	Remove irritant or allergen; topical glucocorticoids; oral antihistamines; oral/IM** glucocorticoids
Contact	Systemic: Erythema, fine scale, crust	Generalized	Patient has history of allergic contact dermatitis to topical agent and then receives systemic medication that is structurally related, e.g., ethylenediamine (topical) aminophylline (IV)	Patch testing	Same as local
Seborrheic	Pink-red, greasy scale	Scalp, nasolabial folds, eyebrows, intertriginous zones	Flares with stress, HIV infection Associated with Parkinson's disease	Skin biopsy	Topical glucocorticoids and imidazoles
Pityriasis rubra pilaris	Orange-red, perifollicular, papules	Generalized, but characteristic "skip" areas of normal skin	Wax-like keratoderma Rule out cutaneous T cell lymphoma	Skin biopsy	Isotretinoin or etretinate; methotrexate

* Discussed in detail in Chap. 55.
† PUVA, psoralens + ultraviolet A irradiation.
‡ UV-B, ultraviolet B.
§ UV-A, ultraviolet A.
** IM, intramuscular.

cus aureus or normal flora. These patients often have other forms of acne and folliculitis and can develop a reactive arthritis.

FIGURATE SKIN LESIONS (Table 57-7) In *figurate* eruptions, the lesions form rings and arcs that are usually erythematous but can be flesh-colored to brown. Most commonly, they are due to primary cutaneous diseases such as *tinea, urticaria, erythema annulare centrifugum*, and *granuloma annulare* (Table 57-8). An underlying systemic illness is found in a second, less common group of migratory annular erythemas. It includes *erythema gyratum repens, erythema migrans, erythema marginatum*, and *necrolytic migratory erythema*.

In *erythema gyratum repens*, one sees hundreds of mobile concentric arcs and wavefronts that resemble the grain in wood. A search for an underlying malignancy is mandatory in a patient with this eruption. *Erythema migrans* is the cutaneous manifestation of Lyme disease, which is caused by the spirochete *Borrelia burgdorferi*. In the initial stage (3 to 30 days after tick bite), a single annular lesion is usually seen, which can expand to ≥10 cm in diameter. Within several days, approximately half the patients develop multiple smaller erythematous lesions at sites distant from the bite. Associated symptoms include fever, headache, myalgias, photophobia, arthralgias, and malar rash. *Erythema marginatum* is seen in patients with rheumatic fever, primarily on the trunk. Lesions are pink-red in color, flat to mildly elevated, and transient.

There are additional cutaneous diseases that present as annular eruptions, but they lack an obvious migratory component. Examples include *CTCL, annular cutaneous lupus*, also referred to as *subacute*

lupus, secondary syphilis, and *sarcoidosis* (see "Papulonodular Skin Lesions").

ACNE (Table 57-9) *Acne vulgaris* and *acne rosacea* are the two major forms of acne (Table 57-10 and Chap. 55). Estrogens decrease sebaceous gland activity, whereas androgens enhance sebum production. Therefore, acne vulgaris in an adult, especially if it is of recent onset, may be a reflection of increased levels of circulating *androgens*. Dysfunction of the ovary or adrenal gland, e.g., polycystic ovary

Table 57-5

Causes of Alopecia

I. Nonscarring alopecia
  A. Primary cutaneous disorders
    1. Telogen effluvium
    2. Androgenetic alopecia
    3. Alopecia areata
    4. Tinea capitis
    5. Traumatic alopecia
  B. Drugs
  C. Systemic diseases
    1. Lupus erythematosus
    2. Secondary syphilis
    3. Hypothyroidism
    4. Hyperthyroidism
    5. Deficiencies of protein, iron, biotin, and zinc
    6. HIV infection

II. Scarring alopecia
  A. Primary cutaneous disorders
    1. Cutaneous lupus
    2. Lichen planus
    3. Folliculitis decalvans
    4. Linear scleroderma (morphea)
  B. Systemic diseases
    1. Lupus erythematosus
    2. Sarcoidosis
    3. Cutaneous metastases

Table 57-6

Nonscarring Alopecia (Primary Cutaneous Disorders)

	Clinical Characteristics	Pathogenesis	Treatment
Telogen effluvium	Diffuse shedding of normal hairs Follows either major stress (high fever, severe infection) or change in hormones (post partum) Reversible without treatment	Stress causes the normally asynchronous growth cycles of individual hairs to become synchronous; therefore, large numbers of growing (anagen) hairs simultaneously enter the dying (telogen) phase	Observation; discontinue any drugs that have alopecia as a side effect; check for underlying metabolic causes, e.g., hypothyroidism, hyperthyroidism
Androgenetic alopecia	Miniaturization of hairs along the midline of the scalp Recession of the anterior scalp line in men and some women	Increased sensitivity of affected hairs to the effects of testosterone Increased levels of circulating androgens (ovarian or adrenal source in women)	If no evidence of hyperandrogen state, then topical minoxidil ± tretinoin; hair transplant
Alopecia areata	Well-circumscribed, circular areas of hair loss, 2–5 cm in diameter In extensive cases, coalescence of lesions and/or involvement of other hair-bearing surfaces of the body Pitting of the nails	The germinative zones of the hair follicles are surrounded by T lymphocytes Occasional associated diseases: hyperthyroidism, hypothyroidism, vitiligo, Down's syndrome	Topical anthralin; intralesional glucocorticoids; topical contact sensitizers
Tinea	Varies from scaling with minimal hair loss to discrete patches with "black dots" (broken hairs) to boggy plaque with pustules (kerion)	Invasion of hairs by dermatophytes, most commonly *Trichophyton tonsurans*	Oral griseofulvin plus 2.5% selenium sulfide or ketoconazole shampoo; examine family members
Traumatic alopecia	Broken hairs Irregular outline	Traction with curlers, rubber bands, braiding Exposure to heat or chemicals Mechanical pulling (trichotillomania)	Discontinuation of offending hair style or chemical treatments; trichotillomania may require hair clipping and observation of shaved pila or biopsy for diagnosis followed by psychotherapy

Table 57-7

Causes of Figurate Skin Lesions

I. Primary cutaneous disorders
  A. Tinea
  B. Urticaria
  C. Erythema annulare centrifugum
  D. Granuloma annulare
II. Systemic diseases
  A. Migratory
    1. Erythema migrans
    2. Erythema gyratum repens
    3. Erythema marginatum
    4. Pustular psoriasis
    5. Necrolytic migratory erythema (glucagonoma syndrome)*
  B. Nonmigratory
    1. Sarcoidosis
    2. Subacute lupus erythematosus
    3. Secondary syphilis
    4. Cutaneous T cell lymphoma

* Migratory erythema with erosions; favors lower extremities and girdle area.

disease, Cushing's syndrome, or partial deficiency of the enzyme 21-hydroxylase, can lead to the hormonal imbalance. Examination of the patient for signs such as hirsutism, androgenetic alopecia, hypertension, and redistribution of subcutaneous fat will aid in the diagnosis.

Exacerbations of acne vulgaris follow the ingestion of several *drugs*, such as iodides, bromides, glucocorticoids, and lithium, as well as the application of oil-containing compounds. Acne-like lesions can be seen in patients with Behçet's disease (see "Ulcers"), and in immunocompromised hosts, disseminated *cryptococcosis* may present as an acneiform eruption.

Patients with the carcinoid syndrome have episodes of flushing of the head, neck, and sometimes the trunk. Resultant skin changes of the face, in particular telangiectasias, mimic the clinical appearance of acne rosacea. Suffusion of the face, as is seen in polycythemia vera, also can be confused with acne rosacea.

PUSTULAR LESIONS *Acneiform eruptions* (see "Acne") and *folliculitis* represent the most common pustular dermatoses. An important consideration in the evaluation of perifollicular pustules is a

Table 57-8

Figurate Eruptions (Primary Cutaneous Disorders)

	Clinical Characteristics	Pathogenesis	Treatment
Tinea	Active, scaling erythematous border with central clearing Expands slowly	Invasion of stratum corneum by dermatophytes	Topical or oral antifungals, e.g., imidazoles, allylamines
Urticaria	Central wheal with erythematous flare Transient and/or migratory Pruritic	Release of histamine from mast cells via immunologic (IgE, type 1 hypersensitivity) or nonimmunologic mechanisms (e.g., morphine)	Remove offending agent; antihistamines; if chronic, exclude urticarial vasculitis
Erythema annulare centrifugum	Enlarges slowly Erythematous, flat or slightly raised "Trailing scale"—scale on inner aspect of expanding ring Buttock, upper thighs	Not known Usually idiopathic Sometimes associated with tinea pedis, drug hypersensitivity Rarely, paraneoplastic	Observation; treat underlying fungal infection
Granuloma annulare	Border composed of flesh-colored to red-brown papules Extremities	Granulomatous process is limited to the skin Unknown etiology Disseminated form is associated with diabetes mellitus	Topical and intralesional glucocorticoids; niacinamide

Table 57-9

CHAPTER 57
Skin Manifestations of Internal Disease

315

Causes of Acneiform Eruptions

I. Primary cutaneous disorders
   A. Acne vulgaris
   B. Acne rosacea
II. Drugs
III. Systemic diseases
   A. Increased androgen production
      1. Adrenal origin, e.g., Cushing's disease, 21-hydroxylase deficiency
      2. Ovarian origin, e.g., polycystic ovary disease
   B. Cryptococcosis, disseminated
   C. Behçet's disease

determination of the associated pathogen, e.g., normal flora, *S. aureus, Pityrosperum.* Noninfectious forms of folliculitis include eosinophilic folliculitis and folliculitis secondary to drugs such as glucocorticoids and lithium. Eosinophilic folliculitis can be seen in HIV-infected individuals, and it is characterized by multiple pruritic lesions on the face and trunk. Administration of high-dose oral glucocorticoids can result in a widespread eruption of perifollicular pustules on the trunk, characterized by lesions in the same stage of development. With regard to underlying systemic diseases, pustules are a characteristic component of pustular psoriasis and can be seen in septic emboli of bacterial or fungal origin (see "Purpura"). For example, the cutaneous lesions of disseminated gonococcemia often have a halo of erythema surrounding a central pustule.

TELANGIECTASIAS (Table 57-11) In order to distinguish the various types of telangiectasias, it is important to examine the shape and configuration of the dilated blood vessels. *Linear telangiectasias* are seen on the face of patients with *actinically damaged skin* and *acne rosacea* and are found on the legs of patients with *venous hypertension* and *essential telangiectasia* (Table 57-12). Patients with an unusual form of *mastocytosis* (telangiectasia macularis eruptiva perstans), the *carcinoid* syndrome (see "Acne"), and *ataxia-telangiectasia* also have linear telangiectasias. In ataxia-telangiectasia, linear telangiectasias appear on the bulbar conjunctiva during childhood. Eventually, there is involvement of the ears, eyelids, cheeks, and/or flexural areas such as the antecubital and popliteal fossae. Lastly, linear telangiectasias are found in areas of cutaneous inflammation. For example, lesions of discoid lupus frequently have telangiectasias within them.

Poikiloderma is a term used to describe a patch of skin with (1) reticulated hypo- and hyperpigmentation, (2) wrinkling secondary to epidermal atrophy, and (3) telangiectasias. Poikiloderma does not imply a single disease entity—it is seen in skin damaged by *ionizing radiation*, in the disorders *poikiloderma vasculare atrophicans* (PVA) and *xeroderma pigmentosum*, as well as in patients with connective-tissue diseases, primarily *dermatomyositis* (DM). PVA is a precursor lesion of CTCL, and the areas of poikiloderma usually begin in the flexural areas of the axillae and groin.

In *scleroderma*, the dilated blood vessels have a unique configuration and are known as *mat telangiectasias*. The lesions are broad macules that usually measure 2 to 7 mm in diameter; occasionally, they are larger in size. Mats have a polygonal or oval shape, and their erythematous color may be uniform or the result of delicate telangiectasias. The most common locations for mat telangiectasias are the face, oral mucosa, and hands—peripheral sites that are prone to intermittent ischemia. The CREST (*c*alcinosis cutis, *R*aynaud's phenomenon, *e*sophageal dysmotility, *s*clerodactyly, and *t*elangiectasia) variant of scleroderma (see Chap. 314) is associated with a chronic course and anticentromere antibodies. Mat telangiectasias are an important clue to the diagnosis of the CREST syndrome as well as systemic scleroderma, for they may be the only cutaneous finding.

Periungual telangiectasias are pathognomonic signs of the three major connective tissue diseases—*lupus erythematosus, scleroderma,* and DM. They are easily visualized by the naked eye, and they occur in at least two-thirds of these patients. In both DM and lupus there is associated nailfold erythema, and in DM the erythema is often accompanied by "ragged" cuticles and fingertip tenderness. Under $10\times$ magnification, the blood vessels in the nailfolds of lupus patients are tortuous and resemble "glomeruli," whereas in scleroderma and DM there is a loss of capillary loops and those that remain are markedly dilated.

In *hereditary hemorrhagic telangiectasia* (Osler-Rendu-Weber disease), the lesions usually appear during adulthood and are most commonly seen on the mucous membranes, face, and distal extremities, including under the nails. They represent arteriovenous (AV) malformations of the dermal microvasculature, are dark red in color, and are usually slightly elevated. When the skin is stretched over an individual lesion, an eccentric punctum with radiating legs is seen. Although the degree of systemic involvement varies in this autosomal dominant disease, the major symptoms are recurrent epistaxis and gastrointestinal bleeding. The fact that these mucosal telangiectasias are actually AV communications helps to explain their tendency to bleed.

HYPOPIGMENTATION (Table 57-13) Disorders of hypopigmentation are classified as either diffuse or localized. The classic example of *diffuse* hypopigmentation is *oculocutaneous albinism* (OCA). The most common forms are due to mutations in the tyrosinase gene (type I) or the *P* gene (type II); some of the patients with type I OCA have a total lack of enzyme activity. At birth, different forms of OCA can appear similar—white hair, gray-blue eyes, and pink-white skin. However, the patients with no tyrosinase activity maintain this phenotype, whereas those with decreased activity or *P* gene mutations will acquire some pigmentation of the eyes, hair, and skin as they age. The degree of pigment formation is a function of their racial background, but a pigmentary dilution is readily apparent when they are compared to their first-degree relatives.

The ocular findings in OCA correlate with the degree of hypopigmentation and include decreased visual acuity, nystagmus, photophobia, and monocular vision. Generalized vitiligo, phenylketonuria, and homocystinuria are other unusual causes of diffuse pigmentary dilu-

Table 57-10

Acne (Primary Cutaneous Disorders)*

	Clinical Characteristics	Pathogenesis	Treatment
Acne vulgaris	Erythematous papules, pustules, open comedones (blackheads), closed comedones (whiteheads), and cysts	Epithelial hyperproliferation within the infundibulum of the hair follicle leads to comedone formation	Topical erythromycin, clindamycin, benzoyl peroxide, and tretinoin; oral antibiotics; if severe, isotretinoin
	Areas that contain sebaceous glands: face, neck, upper trunk	Additional factors: sebum-derived free fatty acids, *Propionibacterium acnes*	
Acne rosacea	Papules, pustules; central face	Unknown	Topical and oral antibiotics; topical metronidazole; avoidance of hot or spicy foods and alcohol
	Telangiectasias of nose and cheeks	No increased reactivity of cutaneous blood vessels to vasodilators	
	Facial erythema	Sebum production normal	
	Flushing reaction to hot foods and alcohol		
	Ocular involvement: conjunctivitis, blepharitis, keratitis		

* See Chap. 55.

Table 57-11

Causes of Telangiectasias

I. Primary cutaneous disorders
  A. Linear
    1. Acne rosacea
    2. Actinically damaged skin
    3. Venous hypertension
    4. Essential telangiectasia
  B. Poikiloderma
    1. Ionizing radiation
    2. Poikiloderma vasculare atrophicans
  C. Spider angioma
    1. Idiopathic
    1. Pregnancy

II. Systemic diseases
  A. Linear
    1. Carcinoid
    2. Ataxia-telangiectasia
    3. Mastocytosis
  B. Poikiloderma
    1. Dermatomyositis
    2. Xeroderma pigmentosum
    3. Cutaneous T cell lymphoma
  C. Mat
    1. Scleroderma
  D. Periungual
    1. Lupus erythematosus
    2. Scleroderma
    3. Dermatomyositis
  E. Papular
    1. Hereditary hermorrhagic telangiectasia
  F. Spider angioma
    1. Cirrhosis

Table 57-13

Causes of Hypopigmentation

I. Primary cutaneous disorders
  A. Diffuse
    1. Generalized vitiligo
  B. Localized
    1. Vitiligo
    2. Chemical leukoderma
    3. Piebaldism
    4. Nevus depigmentosus
    5. Postinflammatory
    6. Tinea versicolor

II. Systemic diseases
  A. Diffuse
    1. Oculocutaneous albinism
      a. Hermansky-Pudlak syndrome*
      b. Chédiak–Higashi syndrome†
  B. Localized
    1. Vogt-Koyanagi-Harada
    2. Scleroderma
    3. Melanoma-associated leukoderma
    4. Tuberous sclerosis
    5. Hypomelanosis of Ito/mosaicism
    6. Sarcoidosis
    7. Tuberculoid and indeterminate leprosy
    8. Cutaneous T cell lymphoma

* Platelet storage defect and restrictive lung disease secondary to deposits of ceroid-like material.
† Giant lysosomal granules and recurrent infections.

tion. In generalized vitiligo, melanocytes are not found in affected skin, whereas in OCA they are present but have decreased activity. Appropriate laboratory tests exclude the other disorders of metabolism.

The differential diagnosis of *localized* hypomelanosis includes the following primary cutaneous disorders: *vitiligo, chemical leukoderma, piebaldism, nevus depigmentosus* (see below), *postinflammatory hypomelanosis,* and *tinea versicolor* (Table 57-14). In this group of diseases, the areas of involvement are macules or patches with a decrease or absence of pigmentation, and in the first four disorders, secondary changes such as scale or crust are absent. Patients with vitiligo have an increased incidence of several autoimmune disorders, including hypothyroidism, Graves' disease, pernicious anemia, Addison's disease, uveitis, alopecia areata, chronic mucocutaneous candidiasis, and the polyglandular autoimmune syndromes (types I and II). Diseases of the thyroid gland are the most frequently associated disorders, occurring in up to 30 percent of patients with vitiligo. Circulating autoantibodies are often found, and the most common ones are antithyroglobulin, antimicrosomal, and antiparietal cell antibodies.

There are three systemic diseases that should be considered in a patient with skin findings suggestive of vitiligo—*Vogt-Koyanagi-Harada syndrome, scleroderma,* and *melanoma-associated leukoderma.* A history of aseptic meningitis, nontraumatic uveitis, tinnitus, hearing loss, and/or dysacousis points to the diagnosis of the Vogt-Koyanagi-Harada syndrome. In these patients, the face and scalp are the most common locations of pigment loss. The vitiligo-like leukoderma seen in patients with scleroderma has a clinical resemblance to idiopathic vitiligo that has begun to repigment as a result of treatment; that is, perifollicular macules of normal pigmentation are seen within areas of depigmentation. The basis of this leukoderma is unknown; there is no evidence of inflammation in areas of involvement, but it can resolve if the underlying connective-tissue disease becomes inactive. In contrast to idiopathic vitiligo, melanoma-associated leukoderma often begins on the trunk, and its appearance should prompt a search for metastatic disease. The possibility exists that the destruction of normal melanocytes is the result of an immune response against malignant melanocytes.

There are two systemic disorders that may have the cutaneous findings of piebaldism (see Table 57-14). They are *Hirschsprung's disease* and *Waardenburg's syndrome.* A possible explanation for both disorders is an abnormal embryonic migration or survival of two neural crest–derived elements, one of them being melanocytes and the other myenteric ganglion cells (Hirschsprung's disease) or auditory nerve cells (Waardenburg's syndrome). The latter syndrome is characterized by congenital sensorineural hearing loss, dystopia canthorum (lateral displacement of the inner canthi but normal interpupillary distance), heterochromic irises, and a broad nasal root, in addition to the piebaldism. Patients with Waardenburg's syndrome have been shown to have mutations in two genes that encode DNA-binding proteins,

Table 57-12

Telangiectasias (Primary Cutaneous Disorders)

Type	Associated Disorder	Clinical Characteristics	Pathogenesis	Treatment
Linear: Simple red or blue line that disappears with diascopy (pressure)	Acne rosacea	Face Associated with flushing, erythema, papulopustules, and rhinophyma	Vasodilatation	Laser, pulsed dye
	Actinically damaged skin	Face, arms, upper trunk Associated with hypopigmentation, hyperpigmentation, and keratoses	Damage to supportive connective tissue	Laser, pulsed dye
	Essential telangiectasia	Netlike sheets Begins on lower extremities May be widespread More common in women	Unknown	?Sclerotherapy
Spider angioma: Central pulsating punctum with radiating legs	Idiopathic Pregnancy	Upper half of the body Halo of pallor secondary to local steal phenomenon	Proliferation of blood vessels in association with increased circulating estrogens	Laser, pulsed dye

PAX-3 and *MITF*, while some patients with Hirschsprung's disease and white spotting have a mutation in one of the two endothelin receptors.

In *tuberous sclerosis*, the earliest cutaneous sign is an ash leaf spot. These lesions are often present at birth and are usually multiple; however, detection may require Wood's lamp examination, especially in fair-skinned individuals. The pigment within them is reduced but not absent. The average size is 1 to 3 cm, and the common shapes are oval, polygonal, and lance-ovate, whereas the less common shapes are dermatomal and confettilike. Examination of the patient for additional cutaneous signs such as adenoma sebaceum (multiple angiofibromas of the face), ungual and gingival fibromas, fibrous plaques of the forehead, and connective-tissue nevi (shagreen patches) is recommended. It is important to remember that an ash leaf spot on the scalp will result in *poliosis*, which is a circumscribed patch of gray-white hair. Internal manifestations include seizures, mental retardation, central nervous system (CNS) and retinal hamartomas, renal angiomyoli-

pomas, and cardiac rhabdomyomas. The latter can be detected in up to 60 percent of children (<18 years) with tuberous sclerosis by echocardiography.

Nevus depigmentosus is a stable, well-circumscribed hypomelanosis that is present at birth. There is usually a single circular or rectangular lesion, but occasionally the nevus has a dermatomal or whorled pattern. It is important to distinguish this entity from ash leaf spots especially when there are multiple lesions. In *hypomelanosis of Ito* (incontinentia pigmenti achromians), swirls and streaks of hypopigmentation run parallel to one another in a pattern that resembles a marble cake. Lesions may progress or regress with time, and in at least a third of patients, associated abnormalities are found including in the musculoskeletal system (asymmetry), the CNS (seizures and mental retardation), and the eyes (strabismus and hypertelorism). Chro-

Table 57-14

Hypopigmentation (Primary Cutaneous Disorders, Localized)

	Clinical Characteristics	Wood's Lamp Examination (UV-A; Peak = 365 nm)	Skin Biopsy Specimen	Pathogenesis	Treatment
Vitiligo	Acquired; progressive Symmetric areas of complete pigment loss Periorifical—around mouth, nose, eyes, nipples, umbilicus, anus Other areas—flexor wrists, extensor distal extremities Segmental form is less common—unilateral, dermatomal-like	More apparent Chalk-white	Absence of melanocytes Minimal inflammation	Possible autoimmune phenomenon that results in destruction of melanocytes—humoral and/or cellular Alternative hypothesis is self-destruction of melanocytes and circulating antibodies against melanocytes as a secondary phenomenon	Topical glucocorticoids; PUVA*; transplants; depigmentation if widespread
Chemical leukoderma	Similar appearance to vitiligo Often begins on hands Satellite lesions in areas not exposed to chemicals	More apparent Chalk-white	Decreased number or absence of melanocytes	Exposure to chemicals that selectively destroy melanocytes, in particular, phenols and catechols (germicides; rubber products) Release of cellular antigens and activation of circulating lymphocytes may explain satellite phenomenon	Avoid exposure to offending agent, then treat as vitiligo
Piebaldism	Autosomal dominant Congenital, stable White forelock Areas of hypomelanosis contain normally pigmented and hyperpigmented macules of various sizes Symmetric involvement of central forehead, ventral trunk, and mid regions of upper and lower extremities	Enhancement of leukoderma and hyperpigmented macules	Hypomelanotic areas—few to no melanocytes	Defect in migration of melanoblasts from neural crest to ventral skin or failure of melanoblasts to survive or differentiate in these areas Mutations within the *c-kit* proto-oncogene that encodes the tyrosine kinase receptor for mast/stem cell growth factor	None; occasionally transplants
Postinflammatory	Hypopigmentation can develop within active lesions, as in subacute lupus, or after the lesion fades, as in dermatitis	Depends on particular disease Usually less enhancement than in vitiligo	Type of inflammatory infiltrate depends on specific disease	Block in transfer of melanin from melanocytes to keratinocytes could be secondary to edema or decrease in contact time Destruction of melanocytes if inflammatory cells attack basal layer	Treat underlying inflammatory disease
Tinea versicolor	Common disorder Upper trunk and neck Shawl-like distribution Young adults Macules have fine white scale when scratched	Golden fluorescence	Hyphae and budding yeast in stratum corneum	Invasion of stratum corneum by the yeast *Pityrosporum* Yeast is lipophilic and produces C_9 and C_{11} dicarboxylic acids which in vitro inhibit tyrosinase	Selenium sulfide 2.5%; topical imidazoles; oral imidazoles or triazoles

* PUVA = psoralens + ultraviolet A irradiation

mosomal mosaicism and diploid/triploid mixoploidy have been reported in these patients; this lends support to the hypothesis that the pattern is the result of the migration of two clones of primordial melanocytes, each with a different pigment potential.

Localized areas of decreased pigmentation are commonly seen as a result of cutaneous inflammation (see Table 57-14) and have been observed in the skin overlying active lesions of *sarcoidosis* (see "Papulonodular Skin Lesions") as well as in *CTCL*. Cutaneous infections also present as disorders of hypopigmentation, and in *tuberculoid leprosy* there are a few asymmetric patches of hypomelanosis that have associated anesthesia, anhidrosis, and alopecia. Biopsy specimens of the palpable border show dermal granulomas that lack *Mycobacterium leprae* organisms.

HYPERPIGMENTATION (Table 57-15)   Disorders of hyperpigmentation are also divided into two groups—localized and diffuse. The *localized* forms are due to an epidermal alteration, a proliferation of melanocytes, or an increase in pigment production. Both *seborrheic keratoses* and *acanthosis nigricans* belong to the first group (Table 57-16). Seborrheic keratoses are common lesions, but in one clinical setting they are a sign of systemic disease, and that setting is the sudden appearance of multiple lesions, often with an inflammatory base and in association with acrochordons (skin tags) and acanthosis nigricans. This is termed the *sign of Leser-Trélat*, and it signifies an internal malignancy. *Acanthosis nigricans* also can be a reflection of an internal malignancy, most commonly of the gastrointestinal tract, and it appears as velvety hyperpigmentation (see Table 57-16). In the majority of patients, acanthosis nigricans is associated with obesity, but it may be a reflection of an endocrinopathy such as acromegaly, Cushing's syndrome, the Stein-Leventhal syndrome, or insulin-resistant diabetes mellitus (type A, type B, and lipoatrophic forms).

A proliferation of melanocytes results in the following pigmented lesions: *lentigo, melanocytic nevus,* and *melanoma* (see Table 57-16). In an adult, the majority of lentigines are related to sun exposure, which explains their distribution. However, in the Peutz-Jeghers and LEOPARD [*l*entigines; *E*CG abnormalities, primarily conduction defects, *o*cular hypertelorism; *p*ulmonary stenosis and subaortic valvular stenosis; *a*bnormal genitalia (cryptorchidism, hypospadias); *r*etardation of growth; and *d*eafness (sensorineural)] syndromes, lentigines do serve as a clue to systemic disease. In the multiple lentigines or *LEOPARD syndrome*, hundreds of lentigines develop during childhood and are scattered over the entire surface of the body. The lentigines in patients with *Peutz-Jeghers syndrome* are located primarily around the nose and mouth, on the hands and feet, and within the oral cavity. While the pigmented macules on the face may fade with age, the oral lesions persist. However, similar intraoral lesions are also seen in Addison's disease and as a normal finding in darkly pigmented individuals. Patients with this autosomal dominant syndrome have multiple benign polyps of the gastrointestinal tract, ovarian tumors, and an approximately 6 percent risk of developing a gastrointestinal malignancy when the polyps arise in the stomach, duodenum, or colon.

Lentigines are also seen in association with cardiac myxomas and have been described in two syndromes whose findings overlap: *LAMB* (*l*entigines, *a*trial myxomas, *m*ucocutaneous myxomas, and *b*lue nevi) *syndrome* and *NAME* [*n*evus, *a*trial myxoma, *m*yxoid neurofibroma, and *e*phelides (freckles)] *syndrome*. These patients also can have evidence of endocrine overactivity in the form of Cushing's syndrome, acromegaly, or sexual precocity.

The third type of localized hyperpigmentation is due to a local increase in pigment production, and it includes *ephelides* (see Table 57-16) and café au lait (CAL) spots. The latter are most commonly associated with two disorders—neurofibromatosis (NF) and Albright's syndrome. *CAL spots* are flat, uniformly light brown in color, and can vary in size from 0.5 to 12 cm. Approximately 80 percent of adult patients with *type I NF* will have six or more CAL spots measuring 1.5 cm or greater in diameter. Additional findings are discussed in the section on neurofibromas (see "Papulonodular Skin Lesions"). In

comparison with NF, the CAL spots in patients with *Albright's disease* [polyostotic fibrous dysplasia with precocious puberty in females due to mosaicism for a mutation in a G protein $(G_s\alpha)$] are usually larger, more irregular in outline, and respect the midline. CAL spots also have been associated with pulmonary stenosis (Watson syndrome), tuberous sclerosis, the LEOPARD syndrome, and ataxia telangiectasia, but a few such lesions can be found in normal individuals.

In incontinentia pigmenti, dyskeratosis congenita, and bleomycin pigmentation, the areas of localized hyperpigmentation form a pattern—swirled in the first, reticulated in the second, and flagellate in the third. Patients with the X-linked dominant disorder *incontinentia pigmenti* can have linear blisters and verrucous papules during infancy. During childhood, parallel swirls and streaks of hyperpigmentation appear on the trunk, and occasionally streaks of hypopigmentation appear on the extremities. Associated findings include seizures, mental retardation, strabismus, cataracts, and delayed or impaired dentition. Biopsy of the streaks will show pigment within dermal macrophages ("incontinent pigment"). In *dyskeratosis congenita*, atrophic reticulated hyperpigmentation is seen on the neck, thighs, and trunk, and it is accompanied by nail dystrophy, pancytopenia, and leukoplakia of the oral and anal mucosa. The latter often develops into squamous cell carcinoma. In addition to the flagellate pigmentation (linear

Table 57-15

Causes of Hyperpigmentation

I. Primary cutaneous disorders
  A. Localized
    1. Epidermal alteration
      a. Seborrheic keratosis
      b. Acanthosis nigricans (obesity)
      c. Pigmented actinic keratosis
    2. Proliferation of melanocytes
      a. Lentigo
      b. Nevus
      c. Melanoma
    3. Increased pigment production
      a. Ephelides (freckles)
      b. Café au lait spots
  B. Localized and diffuse
    1. Drugs
II. Systemic diseases
  A. Localized
    1. Epidermal alteration
      a. Seborrheic keratoses (sign of Leser-Trélat)
      b. Acanthosis nigricans (endocrine disorders, paraneoplastic)
    2. Proliferation of melanocytes
      a. Lentigines (Peutz-Jeghers, LEOPARD syndromes, xeroderma pigmentosum)
      b. Nevi [Carney complex (LAMB and NAME syndromes)]*
    3. Increased pigment production
      a. Café au lait spots (neurofibromatosis, Albright's syndrome)
      b. Urticaria pigmentosa (see "Papulonodular Skin Lesions")
    4. Dermal pigmentation
      a. Incontinentia pigmenti
      b. Dyskeratosis congenita
  B. Diffuse
    1. Endocrinopathies
      a. Addison's disease
      b. Nelson's syndrome
      c. Ectopic ACTH syndrome
    2. Metabolic
      a. Porphyria cutanea tarda
      b. Hemochromatosis
      c. Vitamin B_{12}, folate deficiency
      d. Pellagra
      e. Malabsorption, Whipple's disease
    3. Melanosis secondary to metastatic melanoma
    4. Autoimmune
      a. Biliary cirrhosis
      b. Scleroderma
      c. POEMS syndrome
      d. Eosinophilia-myalgia syndrome
    5. Drugs and metals

* Also lentigines.

streaks) on the trunk, patients receiving bleomycin often have hyperpigmentation on the elbows, knees, and small joints of the hand.

Localized hyperpigmentation is seen as a side effect of several other *systemic medications*, including those that produce fixed drug reactions (phenolphthalein, tetracyclines, sulfonamides, barbiturates, and analgesics) and those that can complex with melanin (antimalarials). Fixed drug eruptions recur in the same location as circular areas of erythema that can become bullous and then resolve as brown macules. The eruption usually appears within hours of administration of the offending agent, and common locations include the genitalia, extremities, and perioral region. Chloroquine and hydroxychloroquine produce gray-brown to blue-black discoloration of the shins, hard palate, and face, while blue macules can be seen on the lower extremities and in sites of inflammation with prolonged minocycline administration. Estrogen in oral contraceptives can induce melasma—symmetric brown patches on the face, especially the cheeks, upper lip, and forehead. Similar changes are seen in pregnancy, in patients receiving hydantoin, and in the adult form of Gaucher's disease. In the latter group there is also hyperpigmentation of the distal lower extremities.

In the *diffuse* forms of hyperpigmentation, the darkening of the skin may be of equal intensity over the entire body, or it may be accentuated in sun-exposed areas. The causes of diffuse hyperpigmentation can be divided into four groups—endocrine, metabolic, autoimmune, and drugs. The endocrinopathies that frequently have associated hyperpigmentation include *Addison's disease, Nelson's syndrome*, and *ectopic ACTH syndrome*. In these diseases, the increased pigmentation is diffuse, but it is accentuated in the palmar creases, sites of friction, scars, and the oral mucosa. An overproduction of any or all of the pituitary hormones α-MSH (melanocyte-stimulating hormone), ACTH, and β-lipotropin can lead to an increase in melanocyte activity. All these peptides are products of the proopiomelanocortin gene, and therefore, they exhibit homology; e.g., α-MSH and ACTH share 13 amino acids. A minority of the patients with Cushing's disease or hyperthyroidism have generalized hyperpigmentation.

The metabolic causes of hyperpigmentation include *porphyria cutanea tarda* (PCT), *hemochromatosis, vitamin B₁₂ deficiency, folic acid deficiency, pellagra, malabsorption*, and *Whipple's disease*. In patients with *PCT* (see "Vesicles/Bullae"), the skin darkening is seen in sun-exposed areas and is a reflection of the photoreactive properties of porphyrins. The increased level of iron in the skin of patients with *hemochromatosis* stimulates melanin pigment production and leads to the classic bronze color. Patients with *pellagra* have a brown discoloration of the skin, especially in sun-exposed areas, as a result of nicotinic acid (niacin) deficiency. In the areas of increased pigmentation, there is a thin varnishlike scale. These changes are also seen in patients who are vitamin B₆ deficient, have functioning carcinoid tumors (increased consumption of niacin), or take isoniazid. Approximately 50 percent of the patients with *Whipple's disease* have an associated generalized hyperpigmentation in association with diarrhea, weight loss, arthritis, and lymphadenopathy. A diffuse slate-blue color is seen in patients with melanosis secondary to *metastatic melanoma*. Although there is a debate as to whether the color is due to single-cell metastases in the dermis or to a widespread deposition of melanin resulting from the high concentration of circulating melanin precursors, there is more evidence to support the latter.

Of the autoimmune diseases associated with diffuse hyperpigmentation, *biliary cirrhosis* and *scleroderma* are the most common, and occasionally, both disorders are seen in the same patient. The skin is dark brown in color, especially in sun-exposed areas. In biliary cirrhosis the hyperpigmentation is accompanied by pruritus, jaundice, and xanthomas, whereas in scleroderma it is accompanied by sclerosis of the extremities, face, and, less commonly, the trunk. Additional clues to the diagnosis of scleroderma are telangiectasias, calcinosis cutis, Raynaud's phenomenon, and distal ulcerations (see "Telangiectasias"). The differential diagnosis of cutaneous sclerosis with hyperpigmentation includes the *POEMS syndrome* [polyneuropathy; organomegaly

Table 57-16

Hyperpigmentation (Primary Cutaneous Disorders, Localized)

	Clinical Characteristics	Histopathology	Treatment
Seborrheic keratosis	Tan to black papule Warty and/or greasy surface "Stuck on" appearance Trunk	Epidermal hyperplasia	Observation; if irritation or bleeding, removal
Acanthosis nigricans	Velvety surface Neck, axillae, groin Occasionally on dorsum of the hand, corners of mouth	Epidermal folds Increased pigment in basal layer	Topical tretinoin, α-hydroxy acids or keratolytics; weight loss if associated with obesity
Pigmented actinic keratosis	Brown macule, 3–10 mm Rough scale Sun-exposed areas, in particular face and dorsum of hand	Dysplasia of keratinocytes in lower third of epidermis Increased pigment in epidermis	Curettage or cryosurgery
Ephelides (freckles)	2–5-mm macule Tan color Sun-exposed surfaces Darkens following sun exposure	Increased pigment in epidermis	None
Lentigo	0.3–1.5 cm macule Tan to black Most commonly in sun-exposed areas Face, upper trunk, and extremities	Increased number of melanocytes in epidermis Increased pigment in epidermis	Observation; cryosurgery; lasers that target melanin
Nevus			
Junctional	Brown to black macule 2–6 mm	Nests of melanocytes at dermoepidermal junction	Observation for change
Compound	Tan to brown papule 2–8 mm	Nests of melanocytes in epidermis and dermis	Observation for change
Dermal	Flesh-colored papule	Nests of melanocytes in dermis	Observation
Melanoma	Variation in color—brown, black, blue, red, white Irregular outline and surface >5 mm in diameter Asymmetric	Malignant neoplasm of melanocytes	Excision, margins (0.5–2 + cm) dependent on Breslow depth*

* See Chap. 88.

(liver, spleen, lymph nodes); *endocrinopathies* (impotence, gynecomastia); *M-protein*; and *skin changes*]. The skin changes include hyperpigmentation, skin thickening, hypertrichosis, and angiomas.

Recently, an epidemic of the eosinophilia-myalgia syndrome was described that is presumably due to contaminated L-tryptophan preparations. In addition to maculopapular eruptions and alopecia, large areas of sclerodermalike induration are observed with overlying hyperpigmentation.

Diffuse hyperpigmentation that is due to *drugs* or *metals* can result from one of several mechanisms—induction of melanin pigment formation, complexing of the drug or its metabolites to melanin, and deposits of the drug in the dermis. Busulfan; cyclophosphamide; long-term, high-dose ACTH; and inorganic arsenic induce pigment production. Complexes containing melanin or hemosiderin plus the drug or its metabolites are seen in patients receiving chlorpromazine and minocycline. The sun-exposed skin as well as the conjunctivae of patients on long-term, high-dose chlorpromazine can become blue-gray in color. Patients taking minocycline may develop a diffuse blue-gray, muddy appearance in sun-exposed areas in addition to pigmentation of the mucous membranes, teeth, nails, bones, and thyroid. Administration of amiodarone can result in both a phototoxic eruption (exaggerated sunburn) and/or a brown or blue-gray discoloration of sun-exposed skin. Biopsy specimens of the latter show yellow-brown granules in dermal macrophages, which represent intralysosomal accumulations of lipids, amiodarone, and its metabolites. Actual deposits of a particular drug or metal in the skin are seen with silver (argyria), where the skin appears blue-gray in color; gold (chrysiasis), where the skin has a brown to blue-gray color; and clofazimine, where the skin appears reddish brown. The associated hyperpigmentation is accentuated in sun-exposed areas, and discoloration of the eye is seen with gold (sclerae) and clofazimine (conjunctivae).

VESICLES/BULLAE (Table 57-17)   Depending on their size, cutaneous blisters are referred to as *vesicles* (<0.5 cm) or *bullae* (>0.5 cm). The primary blistering disorders include *pemphigus vulgaris, pemphigus foliaceus, pemphigus erythematosus, bullous pemphigoid, herpes gestationis, cicatricial pemphigoid, epidermolysis bullosa acquisita, linear IgA disease,* and *dermatitis herpetiformis* (see Chap. 311).

Vesicles and bullae are also seen in *contact dermatitis*, both allergic and irritant forms (see Chap. 55). When there is a linear arrangement of vesicular lesions, an exogenous cause should be suspected. Bullous disease secondary to the ingestion of drugs can take one of several forms, including phototoxic eruptions, isolated bullae, toxic epidermal necrolysis, and erythema multiforme (Chap. 56). Clinically, phototoxic eruptions resemble an exaggerated sunburn with diffuse erythema and bullae in sun-exposed areas. The most commonly associated drugs are thiazides, tetracyclines, sulfonamides, phenothiazines, nonsteroidal anti-inflammatory drugs (NSAIDs), and psoralens. The development of a phototoxic eruption is dependent on the doses of both the drug and UV-A irradiation.

Toxic epidermal necrolysis (TEN) is characterized by bullae that arise on widespread areas of erythema and then slough. This results in large areas of denuded skin. The associated morbidity, such as sepsis, and mortality are relatively high, and they are a function of the extent of epidermal necrosis. In addition, these patients also may have involvement of the mucous membranes and intestinal tract. Drugs are the primary cause of TEN, and the most common offenders are phenytoin, barbiturates, sulfonamides, penicillins, and NSAIDs. Severe acute graft-versus-host disease (grade 4) also can resemble TEN.

In *erythema multiforme* (EM), the primary lesions are pink-red macules and edematous papules, the centers of which may become vesicular. The clue to the diagnosis of EM rather than of a drug-induced morbilliform exanthem is the development of a "dusky" violet color or petechiae in the center of the lesions. Target or iris lesions are also characteristic of EM, and they arise as a result of active centers and borders in combination with centrifugal spread. However,

iris lesions need not be present to make the diagnosis of EM. Preferred sites of involvement include the hands, extensor forearms, palms, soles, and mucous membranes (oral, nasal, ocular, and genital). Hemorrhagic crusts of the lips are characteristic of EM as well as of two other blistering disorders—pemphigus vulgaris and TEN. Fever, malaise, myalgias, sore throat, and cough may precede or accompany the eruption. The lesions of EM usually resolve over 3 to 6 weeks, but they may be recurrent.

Drugs can induce EM, in particular sulfonamides, phenytoin, barbiturates, penicillins, and carbamazepine, but they do not cause the majority of cases, especially in young adults. Infections with herpes simplex are the most common cause of EM in this age group, and the lesions appear 7 to 12 days after the viral eruption. Other infectious agents associated with EM include *Mycoplasma pneumoniae, Histoplasma capsulatum, Coccidioides immitis, Yersinia enterocolitica,* and several viruses (echovirus, coxsackievirus, Epstein-Barr, and influenza). EM also can follow vaccinations with BCG, poliomyelitis, or vaccinia viruses; radiation therapy; and exposure to environmental toxins.

In addition to primary blistering disorders and hypersensitivity reactions, bacterial and viral infections can lead to vesicles and bullae. The most common infectious agents are herpes simplex (see Chap. 184), herpes varicella-zoster (see Chap. 185), and staphylococci (see Chap. 142).

Staphylococcal scalded-skin syndrome (SSSS) and *bullous impetigo* are two blistering disorders associated with staphylococcal (phage group II) infection. In SSSS, the initial findings are redness and tenderness of the central face, neck, trunk, and intertriginous zones. This is followed by short-lived flaccid bullae and a slough or exfoliation of the superficial epidermis. Crusted areas then develop, characteristically around the mouth. SSSS is distinguished from TEN by the following features: younger age group, more superficial site of blister formation, no oral lesions, shorter course, less morbidity and mortality, and an association with staphylococcal exfoliative toxin ("exfoliatin"), not drugs. A rapid diagnosis of SSSS versus TEN can be made by a frozen section of the blister roof or exfoliative cytology of the blister contents. In SSSS the site of staphylococcal infection is usually extracutaneous (conjunctivitis, rhinorrhea, otitis media, pharyngitis, tonsillitis), and the cutaneous lesions are sterile, whereas in *bullous impetigo* the skin lesions are the site of infection. Impetigo is more localized than SSSS, and it usually presents with honey-colored crusts. Occasionally, superficial purulent blisters also form. *Cutaneous emboli* from gram-negative infections may present as isolated bullae, but the base of the lesion is purpuric or necrotic, and it may develop into an ulcer (see "Purpura").

Table 57-17

Causes of Vesicles/Bullae

I. Primary cutaneous diseases	II. Systemic diseases
A. Primary blistering diseases (autoimmune)	A. Autoimmune
1. Pemphigus*	1. Paraneoplastic pemphigus
2. Bullous pemphigoid†	B. Infections
3. Herpes gestationis†	1. Cutaneous emboli†
4. Cicatricial pemphigoid†	C. Metabolic
5. Dermatitis herpetiformis†	1. Diabetic bullae*†
6. Linear IgA disease†	2. Porphyria cutanea tarda†
7. Epidermolysis bullosa acquisita†	3. Porphyria variegata†
B. Secondary blistering diseases	4. Pseudoporphyria†
1. Contact*	5. Bullous dermatosis of hemodialysis†
2. Erythema multiforme*†	D. Ischemia
3. Toxic epidermal necrolysis*†	1. Coma bullae
C. Infections	
1. Varicella/zoster*‡	
2. Herpes simplex*‡	
3. Staphylococcal scalded-skin syndrome*	
4. Bullous impetigo*	

* Intraepidermal.   † Subepidermal.   ‡ Also systemic.

Several metabolic disorders are associated with blister formation, including diabetes mellitus, renal failure, and porphyria. Local hypoxia secondary to decreased cutaneous blood flow also can produce blisters, which explains the presence of bullae over pressure points in comatose patients (coma bullae). In *diabetes mellitus*, tense bullae with clear viscous fluid arise on normal skin. The lesions can be as large as 6 cm in diameter and are located on the distal extremities. There are several types of porphyria, but the most common form with cutaneous findings is *PCT*. In sun-exposed areas (primarily the face and hands), the skin is very fragile, and trauma leads to erosions and tense vesicles. These lesions then heal with scarring and formation of milia; the latter are firm, 2- to 3-mm white or yellow papules that represent epidermoid inclusion cysts. Associated findings can include hypertrichosis of the lateral malar region (males) or face (females) and, in sun-exposed areas, hyperpigmentation and firm sclerotic plaques. An elevated level of urinary uroporphyrins confirms the diagnosis and is due to a decrease in uroporphyrinogen decarboxylase activity. Precipitating agents include alcohol, iron, chlorinated hydrocarbons, and hepatitis C infection.

The differential diagnosis of PCT includes (1) *porphyria variegata*—the skin signs of PCT plus the systemic findings of acute intermittent porphyria; it has a diagnostic plasma porphyrin fluorescence emission at 626 nm; (2) *drug-induced bullous photosensitivity* (pseudoporphyria)—the clinical and histologic findings are similar to PCT, but porphyrins are normal; etiologic agents are furosemide, tetracycline, nalidixic acid, dapsone, naproxen, and pyridoxine; (3) *bullous dermatosis of hemodialysis*—the same appearance as PCT, but porphyrins are usually normal or occasionally borderline elevated; patients have chronic renal failure and are on hemodialysis; (4) PCT associated with hepatomas, hepatic carcinomas, and hemodialysis; and (5) *epidermolysis bullosa acquisita* (see Chap. 311).

EXANTHEMS (Table 57-18) Exanthems are characterized by an acute generalized eruption. The two most common presentations are erythematous macules and papules (morbilliform) and confluent blanching erythema (scarlatiniform). *Morbilliform* eruptions are usually due to either *drugs* or *viral infections*. For example, up to 5 percent of the patients receiving penicillins, sulfonamides, captopril, phenytoin, or gold will develop a maculopapular eruption. Accompanying signs may include pruritus, fever, eosinophilia, and transient lymphadenopathy. Similar maculopapular eruptions are seen in the classic childhood viral exanthems, including (1) *rubeola* (measles)—a prodrome of coryza, cough, and conjunctivitis followed by Koplik's spots on the buccal mucosa; the eruption begins behind the ears, at the hairline, and on the forehead and then spreads down the body, often becoming confluent; (2) *rubella*—it begins on the forehead and face and then spreads down the body; it resolves in the same order and is associated with retroauricular and suboccipital lymphadenopathy; and (3) *erythema infectiosum* (fifth disease)—erythema of the cheeks is followed by a reticulated pattern on extremities; it is secondary to a parvovirus infection, and an associated arthritis is seen in adults.

Both measles and rubella are seen in unvaccinated young adults, and an atypical form of measles is seen in adults immunized with either killed measles vaccine or killed vaccine followed in time by live vaccine. In contrast to classic measles, the eruption of atypical measles begins on the palms, soles, wrists, and knuckles, and the lesions may become purpuric. The patient with atypical measles can have pulmonary involvement and be quite ill. Rubelliform and roseoliform eruptions are also associated with *Epstein-Barr virus* (5 to 15 percent of patients), *echovirus, coxsackievirus,* and *adenovirus* infections. Detection of specific IgM antibodies or fourfold elevations in IgG antibodies allows the proper diagnosis. Occasionally, a maculopapular eruption is the result of a drug-viral interaction. For example, about 95 percent of the patients with infectious mononucleosis who are given ampicillin will develop a rash.

Of note, early in the course of infections with *Rickettsia* and *meningococcus*, prior to the development of purpura, the lesions may be erythematous macules and papules. This is also the case in chickenpox prior to the development of vesicles. Maculopapular eruptions

are associated with early *HIV infection*, early secondary *syphilis, typhoid fever,* and *acute graft-versus-host* disease. In the last, lesions frequently begin on the palms and soles; the macular rose spots of typhoid fever involve primarily the anterior trunk.

The prototypic *scarlatiniform* eruption is seen in *scarlet fever* and is due to an erythrotoxin produced by group A beta-hemolytic streptococcal infections, most commonly pharyngitis. This eruption is characterized by diffuse erythema, which begins on the neck and upper trunk, and red perifollicular puncta. Additional findings include a white strawberry tongue (white coating with red papillae) followed by a red strawberry tongue (red tongue with red papillae); petechiae of the palate; a facial flush with circumoral pallor; linear petechiae in the antecubital fossae; and desquamation of the involved skin, palms, and soles 5 to 20 days after onset of the eruption. A similar desquamation of the palms and soles is seen in toxic shock syndrome, Kawasaki's disease, and after severe febrile illnesses. Certain strains of staphylococci also produce an erythrotoxin that leads to the same clinical findings as in streptococcal scarlet fever, except that the antistreptolysin O titers are not elevated.

In *toxic shock syndrome* (TSS), staphylococcal (phage group I) infections produce an exotoxin (TSST-1) that causes the fever and rash, as well as enterotoxins. Initially, the majority of cases were reported in menstruating women who were using tampons. However, other sites of infection, including wounds and vaginitis, may produce TSS. The diagnosis of TSS is based on clinical criteria, and three of these involve mucocutaneous sites. The clinical criteria are (1) fever; (2) diffuse erythema of the skin; (3) desquamation of the palms and soles 1 to 2 weeks after onset of illness; (4) hypotension; and (5) involvement of three or more organ systems, including the gastrointestinal tract, muscles, kidney, liver, CNS, hematologic (thrombocytopenia), and mucous membranes. The latter is characterized by hyperemia of the vagina, oropharynx, or conjunctivae. Similar systemic findings have been described in *Streptococcal toxic shock–like syndrome* (Chap. 143), and although an exanthem is seen less often than in TSS due to a staphylococcal infection, the underlying infection is often in the soft tissue.

The cutaneous eruption in *Kawasaki's disease* (mucocutaneous lymph node syndrome) is polymorphous, but the two most common forms are morbilliform and scarlatiniform. The majority of cases are seen in children less than 5 years of age, but adult cases have been reported. The diagnosis is based on a fever lasting more than 5 days plus four of the five following criteria: (1) bilateral conjunctival injection; (2) exanthem; (3) cervical lymphadenopathy, usually unilateral; (4) erythema and edema of the hands and feet followed by desquamation; and (5) diffuse erythema of the oropharynx, red strawberry

Table 57-18

Causes of Exanthems

I. Morbilliform
   A. Drugs
   B. Viral
      1. Rubeola (measles)
      2. Rubella
      3. Erythema infectiosum
      4. Epstein-Barr, echovirus, coxsackievirus, and adenovirus
      5. Early HIV
   C. Bacterial
      1. Typhoid fever
      2. Early secondary syphilis
      3. Early *Rickettsia*
      4. Early meningococcus
   D. Acute graft-versus-host disease
II. Scarlatiniform
   A. Scarlet fever
   B. Toxic shock syndrome
   C. Kawasaki's disease

tongue, and erosions with crusting on the lips. This clinical picture can resemble TSS and scarlet fever, but clues to the diagnosis of Kawasaki's disease are the cervical lymphadenopathy, lip erosions, and increased platelets. The most serious associated systemic finding in this disease is coronary aneurysm secondary to arteritis. Aneurysms may lead to sudden death, primarily within the first 30 days of the illness. Scarlatiniform eruptions are also seen in the early phase of SSSS (see "Vesicles/Bullae") and as reactions to drugs.

URTICARIA (Table 57-19) *Urticaria* (hives) are transient lesions that are composed of a central wheal surrounded by an erythematous halo. Individual lesions are round, oval, or figurate, and they are often pruritic. *Acute* and *chronic* urticaria have a wide variety of allergic etiologies. Less common systemic causes of urticaria are mastocytosis (urticaria pigmentosa), hyperthyroidism, malignancy, and juvenile rheumatoid arthritis (JRA). In JRA, the lesions coincide with the fever spike and are transient but not migratory as in erythema marginatum.

The common *physical urticarias* include *dermographism, solar urticaria, cold urticaria,* and *cholinergic urticaria*. Patients with dermographism exhibit linear wheals following minor pressure or scratching of the skin. It is a common disorder, affecting approximately 5 percent of the population. Solar urticaria characteristically occur within minutes of sun exposure and are a skin sign of one systemic disease—erythropoietic protoporphyria. In addition to the urticaria, these patients have subtle pitted scarring of the nose and hands. Cold urticaria are precipitated by exposure to the cold, and therefore, exposed areas are usually affected. In some cases, the disease is associated with abnormal circulating proteins—more commonly cryoglobulins and cold hemolysins and less commonly cryofibrinogens and cold agglutinins. Additional systemic symptoms include wheezing and syncope, thus explaining the need for these patients to avoid swimming in cold water. Cholinergic urticaria are precipitated by heat, exercise, or emotion and are characterized by small wheals with relatively large flares. They are occasionally associated with wheezing.

Whereas urticaria are the result of dermal edema, subcutaneous edema leads to the clinical picture of *angioedema*. Sites of involvement include the eyelids, lips, tongue, larynx, and gastrointestinal tract as well as the subcutaneous tissue. Angioedema occurs alone or in combination with urticaria, including urticarial vasculitis and the physical urticarias. Both acquired and hereditary (autosomal dominant) forms of angioedema occur (see Chap. 310), and in the latter, urticaria is rarely seen.

Urticarial vasculitis is an immune complex disease that may be confused with simple urticaria. In contrast to simple urticaria, individual lesions tend to last longer than 24 h, and they usually develop central petechiae that can be observed even after the urticarial phase has resolved. The patient also may complain of burning rather than pruritus. On biopsy, there is a leukocytoclastic vasculitis of the small blood vessels. Although many cases of urticarial vasculitis are idiopathic in origin, it can be a reflection of an underlying systemic illness such as lupus erythematosus, Sjögren's syndrome, or hereditary complement deficiency. There is a spectrum of urticarial vasculitis that ranges from purely cutaneous to multisystem involvement. The most common systemic signs and symptoms are arthralgias and/or arthritis, nephritis, and crampy abdominal pain, with asthma and chronic obstructive lung disease seen less often. Hypocomplementemia occurs in one- to two-thirds of patients, even in the idiopathic cases. Similar cutaneous, joint, and renal findings can be seen in the prodrome of *hepatitis B infection, serum sickness,* and *serum sickness–like illnesses.*

PAPULONODULAR SKIN LESIONS (Table 57-20) In the *papulonodular diseases,* the lesions are elevated above the surface of the skin and may coalesce to form plaques. The location, consistency, and color of the lesions are the keys to their diagnosis. This section is organized on the basis of color, and the color groups are white, flesh, pink, yellow, red, red-brown, blue, violaceous, purple, and brown-black.

White Lesions In *calcinosis cutis* there are firm white to white-yellow papules with an irregular surface. When the contents are discharged, a chalky white material is seen. *Dystrophic* calcification is seen at sites of previous inflammation or damage to the skin. It develops in acne scars as well as on the distal extremities of patients with scleroderma and in the subcutaneous tissue and intermuscular fascial planes in DM. The latter is more extensive and is more commonly seen in children. An elevated calcium phosphate product, as in secondary hyperparathyroidism, can lead to nodules of *metastatic* calcinosis cutis, which tend to be subcutaneous and periarticular. This form is often accompanied by calcification of muscular arteries and subsequent ischemic necrosis (calciphylaxis).

Flesh-Colored Lesions There are several types of flesh-colored lesions, including epidermoid inclusion cysts, lipomas, rheumatoid nodules, neurofibromas, angiofibromas, neuromas, and adnexal tumors such as tricholemmomas. Both *epidermoid inclusion cysts* and *lipomas* are very common mobile subcutaneous nodules—the former are rubbery and compressible, and they drain cheeselike material (sebum and keratin) if incised. Lipomas are firm and somewhat lobulated on palpation. When extensive facial epidermoid inclusion cysts develop in childhood or there is a family history of such lesions, the patient should be examined for other signs of Gardner's syndrome, including osteomas and desmoid tumors. *Rheumatoid nodules* are firm, 0.5- to 4-cm nodules that tend to localize around pressure points, especially the elbows. They are seen in approximately 20 percent of patients with rheumatoid arthritis and 6 percent of patients with Still's disease. Biopsies of the nodules show palisading granulomas. Similar lesions that are smaller and shorter-lived are seen in rheumatic fever.

Neurofibromas (benign Schwann cell tumors) are soft papules or nodules that exhibit the "button-hole" sign, that is, they invaginate into the skin with pressure in a manner similar to a hernia. Single lesions are seen in normal individuals, but multiple neurofibromas, usually in combination with six or more CAL spots measuring >1.5 cm (see "Hyperpigmentation") and multiple Lisch nodules, are seen in von Recklinghausen's disease (NF type I). Lisch nodules are 1-mm yellow-brown spots within the iris that are best observed with slit-lamp examination. Additional manifestations include axillary freckling and peripheral and CNS tumors (see Chap. 375). In some patients the neurofibromas are localized and unilateral, whereas in others they are limited to the CNS.

Angiofibromas are firm, pink to flesh-colored papules that measure from 3 mm to several centimeters in diameter. When they are located on the central cheeks (adenoma sebaceum) or multiple fibromas are seen around the nails, the patient has tuberous sclerosis. It is an autosomal disorder, and the associated findings are discussed in the section on ash leaf spots as well as in Chap. 375.

Neuromas (benign proliferation of nerve fibers) are also firm, flesh-colored papules. They are more commonly found at sites of amputation and as rudimentary supernumerary digits. However, when there are multiple neuromas on the eyelids, lips, distal tongue, and/or oral mucosa, the patient should be investigated for other signs of the multiple

Table 57-19

Causes of Urticaria

I. Primary cutaneous disorders
  A. Acute and chronic urticaria
  B. Physical urticaria
    1. Dermatographism
    2. Solar urticaria*
    3. Cold urticaria*
    4. Cholinergic urticaria*
  C. Angioedema (hereditary and acquired)*
II. Systemic diseases
  A. Urticarial vasculitis
  B. Hepatitis B infection
  C. Serum sickness
  D. Angioedema (hereditary and acquired)

* Also systemic.

Table 57-20

CHAPTER 57
Skin Manifestations of Internal Disease

323

Papulonodular Skin Lesions According to Color Groups

I. White
  A. Calcinosis cutis
II. Flesh
  A. Rheumatoid nodule
  B. Neurofibromas (von Recklinghausen's disease)
  C. Angiofibromas (tuberous sclerosis)
  D. Neuromas (multiple endocrine neoplasia syndrome, type 2b)
  E. Adnexal tumors
    1. Basal cell epitheliomas (basal cell nevus syndrome)
    2. Tricholemmomas (Cowden's disease)
  F. Primary cutaneous disorders
    1. Epidermal inclusion cysts
    2. Lipomas
III. Pink/translucent
  A. Amyloidosis
  B. Papular mucinosis
IV. Yellow
  A. Xanthomas
  B. Tophi
  C. Necrobiosis lipoidica
  D. Pseudoxanthoma elasticum
  E. Sebaceous adenomas (Torre's syndrome)
V. Red
  A. Papules
    1. Angiokeratomas (Fabry's disease)
    2. Bacillary angiomatosis (primarily in AIDS)
  B. Papules/plaques
    1. Cutaneous lupus
    2. Lymphoma cutis
    3. Leukemia cutis

C. Nodules
  1. Panniculitis
  2. Cutaneous polyarteritis nodosa
  3. Systemic vasculitis
D. Primary cutaneous disorders
  1. Arthropod bites
  2. Cherry hemangiomas
  3. Infections, e.g., erysipelas, sporotrichosis
  4. Polymorphous light eruption
  5. Lymphocytoma cutis (pseudolymphoma)
VI. Red-brown
  A. Sarcoidosis
  B. Sweet's syndrome
  C. Urticaria pigmentosa
  D. Erythema elevatum diutinum (chronic leukocytoclastic vasculitis)
  E. Lupus vulgaris
VII. Blue
  A. Venous malformations (blue rubber bleb syndrome)
  B. Primary cutaneous disorders
    1. Venous lake
    2. Blue nevus
VIII. Violaceous
  A. Lupus pernio (sarcoidosis)
  B. Lymphoma cutis
  C. Cutaneous lupus
IX. Purple
  A. Kaposi's sarcoma
  B. Angiosarcoma
  C. Palpable purpura
X. Brown-black
  See "Hyperpigmentation"
XI. Any color
  A. Metastases

endocrine neoplasia syndrome, type 2b. Associated findings include marfanoid habitus, protuberant lips, intestinal ganglioneuromas, and medullary thyroid carcinoma (>75 percent of patients) (see Chap. 340).

Adnexal tumors are derived from pluripotential cells of the epidermis that can differentiate toward hair, sebaceous, apocrine, or eccrine glands or remain undifferentiated. *Basal cell epitheliomas* (BCEs) are examples of adnexal tumors that have little or no evidence of differentiation. Clinically, they are translucent papules with rolled borders, telangiectasias, and central erosion. BCEs commonly arise in sun-damaged skin of the head and neck. When a patient has multiple BCEs, especially prior to age 30, the possibility of the basal cell nevus syndrome should be raised. It is inherited as an autosomal dominant trait and is associated with jaw cysts, palmar and plantar pits, frontal bossing, rib anomalies, and calcification of the falx cerebri and diaphragma sellae. *Tricholemmomas* are also flesh-colored adnexal tumors, but they differentiate toward hair follicles and can have a wartlike appearance. The presence of multiple tricholemmomas on the face and oral mucosa points to the diagnosis of Cowden's disease (multiple hamartoma syndrome). The oral tricholemmomas are found primarily on the tongue and gingiva and give these areas a cobblestone appearance. Internal organ involvement (in decreasing order of frequency) includes fibrocystic disease and carcinoma of the breast, adenomas and carcinomas of the thyroid, and gastrointestinal polyposis. Keratoses of the palms, soles, and dorsa of the hands are also seen.

Pink Lesions The cutaneous lesions associated with primary systemic *amyloidosis* are pink in color and translucent. Common locations are the face, especially the periorbital and perioral regions, and flexural areas. On biopsy, homogeneous deposits of amyloid are seen

in the dermis and in the walls of blood vessels; the latter lead to an increase in vessel wall fragility. As a result, petechiae and purpura develop in clinically normal skin as well as in lesional skin following minor trauma, hence the term "pinch purpura." Amyloid deposits are also seen in the striated muscle of the tongue and result in macroglossia.

Even though specific mucocutaneous lesions are rarely seen in secondary amyloidosis and are present in only about 30 percent of the patients with primary amyloidosis, a rapid diagnosis of systemic amyloidosis can be made by an examination of abdominal subcutaneous fat. By special staining, deposits are seen around blood vessels or individual fat cells in 40 to 50 percent of patients. There are also three forms of amyloidosis that are limited to the skin and that should not be construed as cutaneous lesions of systemic amyloidosis. They are macular amyloid (upper back), lichenoid amyloidosis (usually lower extremities), and nodular amyloidosis. In macular and lichenoid amyloidosis, the deposits are composed of altered epidermal keratin. Recently, macular and lichenoid amyloidosis have been associated with multiple endocrine neoplasia syndrome, type 2a.

Patients with *multicentric reticulohistiocytosis* also have pink-colored papules and nodules on the face and mucous membranes as well as on the extensor surface of the hands and forearms. They have a polyarthritis that can mimic rheumatoid arthritis clinically. On histologic examination, the papules have characteristic giant cells that are not seen in biopsies of rheumatoid nodules. Pink to flesh-colored papules that are firm, 2 to 5 mm in diameter, and often in a linear arrangement are seen in patients with *papular mucinosis*. This disease is also referred to as *lichen myxedematosus* or *scleromyxedema*. The latter name comes from the brawny induration of the face and extremities that may accompany the papular eruption. Biopsy specimens of the papules show localized mucin deposition, and serum protein electrophoresis demonstrates a monoclonal spike of IgG, usually with a λ light chain.

Yellow Lesions Several systemic disorders are characterized by yellow-colored cutaneous papules or plaques—hyperlipidemia (xanthomas), gout (tophi), diabetes (necrobiosis lipoidica), pseudoxanthoma elasticum, and Torre's syndrome (sebaceous tumors). Eruptive xanthomas are the most common form of *xanthomas*, and they are associated with hypertriglyceridemia (types I, III, IV, and V). Crops of yellow papules with erythematous halos occur primarily on the extensor surfaces of the extremities and the buttocks in association with elevations of the circulating triglycerides. They spontaneously involute with a fall in serum lipids. Increased β-lipoproteins (primarily types II and III) result in one or more of the following types of xanthoma: xanthelasma, tendon xanthomas, and plane xanthomas. Xanthelasma are found on the eyelids, whereas tendon xanthomas are frequently associated with the Achilles and extensor finger tendons; plane xanthomas are flat and favor the palmar creases, face, upper trunk, and scars. Tuberous xanthomas are frequently associated with hypertriglyceridemia, but they are also seen in patients with hypercholesterolemia (type II) and are found most frequently over the large joints or hand. Biopsy specimens of xanthomas show collections of lipid-containing macrophages (foam cells).

Patients with several disorders, including biliary cirrhosis, can have a secondary form of hyperlipidemia with associated tuberous and planar xanthomas. However, patients with myeloma have *normolipemic* flat xanthomas. This latter form of xanthoma may be ≥12 cm in diameter and is most frequently seen on the upper trunk or side of the neck. It is also important to note that the most common setting for eruptive xanthomas is uncontrolled diabetes mellitus. The least specific sign for hyperlipidemia is xanthelasma because at least 50 percent of the patients with this finding have normal lipid profiles.

In *tophaceous gout* there are deposits of monosodium urate in the skin around the joints, particularly those of the hands and feet. Additional sites of *tophi* formation include the helix of the ear and the olecranon and prepatellar bursae. The lesions are firm, yellow in color, and occasionally discharge a chalky material. Their size varies from

1 mm to 7 cm, and the diagnosis can be established by polarization of the aspirated contents of a lesion. Lesions of *necrobiosis lipoidica* are found primarily on the shins (90 percent), and the majority of patients have diabetes mellitus or develop it subsequently. Characteristic findings include a central yellow color, atrophy (transparency), telangiectasias, and an erythematous border. Ulcerations also can develop within the plaques. Biopsy specimens show necrobiosis of collagen, granulomatous inflammation, and obliterative endarteritis.

In *pseudoxanthoma elasticum* (PXE) there is an abnormal deposition of calcium on the elastic fibers of the skin, eye, and blood vessels. In the skin, the flexural areas such as the neck, axillae, antecubital fossae, and inguinal area are the primary sites of involvement. Yellow papules coalesce to form reticulated plaques that have an appearance similar to that of plucked chicken skin. In severely affected skin, hanging, redundant folds develop. Some patients have a more subtle macular form of the disease, and careful inspection is required. Biopsy specimens of involved skin show swollen and irregularly clumped elastic fibers with deposits of calcium. In the eye, the calcium deposits in Bruch's membrane lead to angioid streaks and choroiditis; in the arteries of the heart, kidney, gastrointestinal tract, and extremities, the deposits lead to angina, hypertension, gastrointestinal bleeding, and claudication, respectively. Long-term administration of D-penicillamine can lead to PXE-like skin changes as well as elastic fiber alterations in internal organs.

Adnexal tumors that have differentiated toward sebaceous glands include sebaceous adenoma, sebaceous epithelioma, sebaceous carcinoma, and sebaceous hyperplasia. Except for sebaceous hyperplasia, which is commonly seen on the face, these tumors are fairly rare. Patients with Torre's syndrome have *sebaceous adenomas*, and in the majority of cases there are multiple such tumors. These patients also can have sebaceous carcinomas and sebaceous hyperplasia as well as keratoacanthomas. The internal manifestations of Torre's syndrome include *multiple* carcinomas of the gastrointestinal tract (primarily colon) as well as cancers of the larynx, genitourinary tract, ovary, and endometrium. Some patients also have a strong family history of cancer.

Red Lesions   Cutaneous lesions that are red in color have a wide variety of etiologies, and in an attempt to simplify their identification, they will be subdivided into papules, papules/plaques, and subcutaneous nodules. Common red papules include *arthropod bites* and *cherry hemangiomas*; the latter are small, bright-red, dome-shaped papules that represent benign proliferation of capillaries. In patients with AIDS, the development of multiple red hemangioma-like lesions points to bacillary angiomatosis, and biopsy specimens show clusters of bacilli that stain positive with the Warthin-Starry stain; the pathogens have been identified as *Rochalimaea henselae* and *Bartanella quintana*. Disseminated visceral disease is seen primarily in immunocompromised hosts but can occur in immunocompetent individuals.

Multiple *angiokeratomas* are seen in Fabry's disease, an X-linked recessive lysosomal storage disease that is due to a deficiency of α-galactosidase A. The lesions are red to red-blue in color and can be quite small in size (1 to 3 mm), with the most common location being the lower trunk. Associated findings include chronic renal failure, peripheral neuropathy, and corneal opacities (cornea verticillata). Electron photomicrographs of angiokeratomas and clinically normal skin demonstrate lamellar lipid deposits in fibroblasts, pericytes, and endothelial cells that are diagnostic of this disease. Widespread acute eruptions of erythematous papules are discussed in the section on exanthems.

There are several infectious diseases that present as erythematous papules or nodules in a sporotrichoid pattern, that is, in a linear arrangement along the lymphatic channels. The two most common etiologies are *Sporothrix schenckii* (sporotrichosis) and *Mycobacterium marinum* (atypical mycobacteria). The organisms are introduced as a result of trauma, and a primary inoculation site is often seen in addition to the lymphatic nodules. Additional causes include *Nocardia*, *Leishmania*,

and other dimorphic fungi; culture of lesional tissue will aid in the diagnosis.

The diseases that are characterized by erythematous plaques with scale are reviewed in the papulosquamous section, and the various forms of dermatitis are discussed in the section on erythroderma. Additional disorders in the differential diagnosis of red papules/plaques include *erysipelas*, *polymorphous light eruption* (PMLE), *lymphocytoma cutis*, *cutaneous lupus*, *lymphoma cutis*, and *leukemia cutis*. The first three diseases represent primary cutaneous disorders. PMLE is characterized by erythematous papules and plaques in a primarily sun-exposed distribution—dorsum of the hand, extensor forearm, and face. Lesions follow exposure to both UV-B and UV-A, and in northern latitudes PMLE is most severe in the late spring and early summer. A process referred to as "hardening" occurs with continued UV exposure, and the eruption fades, but in temperate climates it will recur in the spring. PMLE must be differentiated from cutaneous lupus, and this is accomplished by histologic examination and direct immunofluorescence of the lesions. Lymphocytoma cutis (pseudolymphoma) is a *benign* proliferation of lymphocytes in the skin that presents as infiltrated pink-red to red-purple papules and plaques. It must be distinguished from cutaneous lupus and lymphoma cutis.

Several types of red plaques are seen in patients with systemic *lupus*, including (1) erythematous urticarial plaques across the cheeks and nose in the classic butterfly rash; (2) erythematous discoid lesions with fine or "carpet-tack" scale, telangiectasias, central hypopigmentation, peripheral hyperpigmentation, follicular plugging, and atrophy located on the face, scalp, external ears, arms, and upper trunk; and (3) psoriasiform or annular lesions of subacute lupus with hypopigmented centers located on the face, extensor arms, and upper trunk. Additional cutaneous findings include (1) a violaceous flush on the face and vee of the neck; (2) urticarial vasculitis (see "Urticaria"); (3) lupus panniculitis (see below); (4) diffuse alopecia; (5) alopecia secondary to discoid lesions; (6) periungual telangiectasias and erythema; (7) erythema multiforme–like lesions that may become bullous; and (8) distal ulcerations secondary to Raynaud's phenomenon, vasculitis, or livedoid vasculitis. Patients with only discoid lesions usually have the form of lupus that is limited to the skin. However, 2 to 10 percent of these patients eventually develop systemic lupus. Direct immunofluorescence of involved skin shows deposits of IgG or IgM and C3 in a granular distribution along the dermal-epidermal junction.

In *lymphoma cutis* there is a proliferation of malignant lymphocytes or histiocytes in the skin, and the clinical appearance resembles that of lymphocytoma cutis—infiltrated pink-red to red-purple papules and plaques. Lymphoma cutis can occur anywhere on the surface of the skin, whereas the sites of predilection for lymphocytomas are the malar ridge, tip of the nose, earlobes, forearms, and scrotum. Patients with non-Hodgkin's lymphomas have specific cutaneous lesions more often than those with Hodgkin's disease, and occasionally, the skin nodules precede the development of extracutaneous non-Hodgkin's lymphoma. Arcuate lesions are sometimes seen in lymphoma and lymphocytoma cutis as well as in CTCL. *Leukemia cutis* has the same appearance as lymphoma cutis, and specific lesions are seen more commonly in monocytic leukemias than in lymphocytic or granulocytic leukemias. Cutaneous chloromas (granulocytic sarcomas) may precede the appearance of circulating blasts in acute nonlymphocytic leukemia and, as such, represent a form of aleukemic leukemia cutis.

Common causes of erythematous subcutaneous nodules include inflamed epidermoid inclusion cysts, acne cysts, and furuncles. *Panniculitis*, an inflammation of the fat, also presents as subcutaneous nodules and is frequently a sign of systemic disease. There are several forms of panniculitis, including erythema nodosum, erythema induratum, lupus profundus, Weber-Christian disease, α_1-antitrypsin deficiency, factitial, and fat necrosis secondary to pancreatic disease. In all these disorders, except for erythema nodosum, the lesions may break down and ulcerate or heal with a scar. The shin is the most common location for the nodules of erythema nodosum, whereas the calf is the most common location for lesions of erythema induratum. In erythema nodosum the nodules are initially red but then develop a blue color as they resolve. Patients with erythema nodosum and no underlying systemic illness can still have fever, malaise, leukocytosis, arthralgias and/or arthritis. However, the possibility of an underlying illness should be excluded, and the most common associations are streptococcal infections, upper respiratory infections, sarcoidosis, and inflammatory bowel disease. The less common associations include tuberculosis, histoplasmosis, coccidioidomycosis, psittacosis, drugs (oral contraceptives, sulfonamides, aspartame, bromides, iodides), cat-scratch fever, and infections with *Yersinia*, *Salmonella*, and *Chlamydia*.

In many patients, erythema induratum/nodular vasculitis is an idiopathic disease; however, in approximately 25 to 50 percent of patients, polymerase chain reaction (PCR) analysis will demonstrate *Mycobacterium tuberculosis* complex DNA. The lesions of lupus profundus are found primarily on the face, upper arms, and buttocks (sites of abundant fat) and are seen in both the cutaneous and systemic forms of lupus. The overlying skin may be normal, erythematous, or have the changes of discoid lupus. The subcutaneous fat necrosis that is associated with pancreatic disease is presumably secondary to circulating lipases and is seen in patients with pancreatic carcinoma as well as in patients with acute and chronic pancreatitis. In this disorder and in Weber-Christian disease there may be an associated arthritis, fever, and inflammation of visceral fat. Histologic examination of deep incisional biopsy specimens will aid in the diagnosis of the particular type of panniculitis.

Subcutaneous erythematous nodules are also seen in *cutaneous polyarteritis nodosa* (PAN) and as a manifestation of *systemic vasculitis*, e.g., systemic PAN, allergic granulomatosis, or Wegener's granulomatosis. Cutaneous PAN presents with painful subcutaneous nodules and ulcers within a red-purple, netlike pattern of livedo reticularis. The latter is due to slowed blood flow through the superficial horizontal venous plexus. The majority of lesions are found on the lower extremity, and while arthralgias and myalgias may accompany cutaneous PAN, there is no evidence of systemic involvement. In both the cutaneous and systemic forms of vasculitis, skin biopsy specimens of the associated nodules will show the changes characteristic of a vasculitis; the size of the vessel involved will depend on the particular disease.

Red-Brown Lesions The cutaneous lesions in *sarcoidosis* are classically red to red-brown in color, and with diascopy (pressure with a glass slide) a yellow-brown residual color is observed that is secondary to the granulomatous infiltrate. The waxy papules and plaques may be found anywhere on the skin, but the face is the most common location. Usually there are no surface changes, but occasionally the lesions will have scale. Biopsy specimens of the papules show "naked" granulomas in the dermis, i.e., granulomas surrounded by a minimal number of lymphocytes. Other cutaneous findings in sarcoidosis include annular lesions with an atrophic or scaly center, papules within scars, hypopigmented macules and papules, alopecia, acquired ichthyosis, erythema nodosum, and lupus pernio (see below). Additional physical findings are peripheral lymphadenopathy and parotid and lacrimal gland enlargement. When there is cutaneous involvement of the hands, radiographs often will show lytic lesions in the underlying bone.

The differential diagnosis of sarcoidosis includes foreign-body granulomas produced by chemicals such as beryllium and zirconium, late secondary syphilis, and *lupus vulgaris*. Lupus vulgaris is a form of cutaneous tuberculosis that is seen in previously infected and sensitized individuals. There is often underlying active tuberculosis elsewhere, usually in the lungs or lymph nodes. At least 90 percent of the lesions occur in the head and neck area and are red-brown plaques with a yellow-brown color on diascopy. Secondary scarring and squamous cell carcinoma can develop within the plaques. Cultures or PCR analysis of the lesions should be done because it is rare for the acid-fast stain to show bacilli within the dermal granulomas.

Sweet's syndrome is characterized by red to red-brown plaques and nodules that are frequently painful and occur primarily on the head, neck, and upper extremities. The patients also have fever, neutrophilia, and a dense dermal infiltrate of neutrophils in the lesions. In approximately 10 percent of the patients there is an associated malignancy, most commonly acute nonlymphocytic leukemia. Sweet's syndrome also has been reported with lymphoma, chronic leukemia, myeloma, myelodysplastic syndromes, and solid tumors (primarily of the genitourinary tract). Extracutaneous sites of involvement include joints, muscles, eye, kidney (proteinuria, occasionally glomerulonephritis), and lung (neutrophilic infiltrates). The idiopathic form of Sweet's syndrome is seen more often in women, following a respiratory tract infection.

A generalized distribution of red-brown macules and papules is seen in the form of mastocytosis known as *urticaria pigmentosa* (see Chap. 310). Each lesion represents a collection of mast cells in the dermis, with hyperpigmentation of the overlying epidermis. Stimuli such as rubbing and heat cause these mast cells to degranulate, and this leads to the formation of localized urticaria (Darier's sign). Additional symptoms can result from mast cell degranulation and include headache, flushing, diarrhea, and pruritus. Mast cells also infiltrate various organs such as the liver, spleen, and gastrointestinal tract in up to 30 to 50 percent of patients with urticaria pigmentosa, and accumulations of mast cells in the bones may produce either osteosclerotic or osteolytic shadows on radiographs. In the majority of these patients, however, the internal involvement remains fairly static. A subtype of chronic leukocytoclastic vasculitis, *erythema elevatum diutinum* (EED), also presents with papules that are red-brown in color. The papules coalesce into plaques on the extensor surfaces of knees, elbows, and the small joints of the hand. Flares of EED have been associated with streptococcal infections.

Blue Lesions Lesions that are blue in color are the result of either vascular ectasias and tumors or melanin pigment in the dermis. *Venous lakes* (ectasias) are compressible dark blue lesions that are found commonly in the head and neck region. *Venous malformations* are also compressible blue papules and nodules that can occur anywhere on the body, including the oral mucosa. When they are multiple rather than single congenital lesions, the patient may have the blue rubber bleb syndrome or Mafucci's syndrome. Patients with the blue rubber bleb syndrome also have vascular anomalies of the gastrointestinal tract that may bleed, whereas patients with Mafucci's syndrome have associated dyschondroplasia and osteochondromas. In the case of single hemangiomas that are relatively large in size, there can be associated platelet consumption (Kasabach-Merritt syndrome). *Blue nevi* (moles) are seen when there are collections of pigment-producing nevus cells in the dermis. These benign papular lesions are dome-shaped and occur most commonly on the dorsum of the hand and arm.

Violaceous Lesions Violaceous papules and plaques are seen in *lupus pernio, lymphoma cutis*, and *cutaneous lupus*. Lupus pernio is a particular type of sarcoidosis that involves the tip of the nose and the earlobes, with lesions that are violaceous in color rather than red-brown. This form of sarcoidosis is associated with involvement of the upper respiratory tract. The plaques of lymphoma cutis and cutaneous lupus may be red or violaceous in color and were discussed above.

Purple Lesions Purple-colored papules and plaques are seen in vascular tumors, such as *Kaposi's sarcoma* (see Chap. 308) and *angiosarcoma*, and when there is extravasation of red blood cells into the skin in association with inflammation, as in *palpable purpura* (see "Purpura"). Patients with congenital or acquired arteriovenous fistulas and venous hypertension can develop purple papules on the lower extremities that can resemble Kaposi's sarcoma clinically and histologically, and this condition is referred to as pseudo-Kaposi sarcoma (acral angiodermatitis). *Angiosarcoma* is found most commonly on the scalp and face of elderly patients or within areas of chronic lymphedema and presents as purple papules and plaques. In the head and neck region the tumor often extends beyond the clinically defined borders and may be accompanied by facial edema.

Brown and Black Lesions Brown- and black-colored papules are reviewed in "Hyperpigmentation."

Cutaneous Metastases These are discussed last because they can have a wide range of colors. Most commonly they present as either firm, flesh-colored subcutaneous nodules or firm, red to red-brown papulonodules. The lesions of lymphoma cutis range from pink-red to plum in color, whereas metastatic melanoma can be pink, blue, or black in color. Cutaneous metastases develop from hematogenous or lymphatic spread and are most often due to the following primary carcinomas: in men, lung, colon, melanoma, and oral cavity; and in women, breast, colon, and lung. These metastatic lesions may be the initial presentation of the carcinoma, especially when the primary site is the lung, kidney, or ovary.

PURPURA (Table 57-21) *Purpura* are seen when there is an extravasation of red blood cells into the dermis, and as a result, the lesions do not blanch with pressure. This is in contrast to those erythematous or violet-colored lesions that are due to localized vasodilatation—they do blanch with pressure. Purpura (≥3 mm) and petechiae (≤2 mm) are divided into two major groups, palpable and nonpalpable. The most frequent causes of *nonpalpable* petechiae and purpura are primary cutaneous disorders such as *trauma, solar purpura*, and *capillaritis*. Less common causes are *steroid purpura* and *livedoid vasculitis* (see "Ulcers"). Solar purpura are seen primarily on the extensor forearm, while glucocorticoid purpura secondary to potent topical steroids or endogenous or exogenous Cushing's syndrome can be more widespread. In both cases there is alteration of the supporting connective tissue that surrounds the dermal blood vessels. In contrast, the petechiae that result from capillaritis are found primarily on the lower extremities. In capillaritis there is an extravasation of erythrocytes as a result of perivascular lymphocytic inflammation. The petechiae are bright red, 1 to 2 mm in size, and scattered within annular or coin-shaped yellow-brown macules. The yellow-brown color is caused by hemosiderin deposits within the dermis.

Systemic causes of nonpalpable purpura fall into several categories, and those secondary to clotting disturbances and vascular fragility will be discussed first. The former group includes *thrombocytopenia* (see Chap. 117), *abnormal platelet function* as is seen in uremia, and *clotting factor defects*. The initial site of presentation for thrombocytopenia-induced petechiae is the distal lower extremity. Capillary fragility leads to nonpalpable purpura in patients with systemic *amyloidosis* (see "Papulonodular Skin Lesions"), disorders of collagen production such as *Ehlers-Danlos syndrome*, and *scurvy*. In scurvy there are flattened corkscrew hairs with surrounding hemorrhage on the lower extremities, in addition to gingivitis. Vitamin C is a cofactor for lysyl hydroxylase, an enzyme involved in the posttranslational modification of procollagen that is necessary for cross-link formation.

In contrast to the previous group of disorders, in which either capillary fragility or a clotting abnormality is responsible for the nonpalpable purpura, the purpura seen in the following group of diseases are associated with thrombi formation within vessels. It is important to note that these thrombi are demonstrable in skin biopsy specimens. This group of disorders includes *disseminated intravascular coagulation* (DIC), *monoclonal cryoglobulinemia*, *thrombotic thrombocytopenic purpura*, and *reactions to warfarin*. DIC is triggered by several types of infection (gram-negative, gram-positive, viral, and rickettsial) as well as by tissue injury and neoplasms. Widespread purpura and hemorrhagic infarcts of the distal extremities are seen. Similar lesions are found in purpura fulminans, which is a form of DIC associated with fever and hypotension that occurs more commonly in children following an infectious illness such as varicella, scarlet fever, or an upper respiratory tract infection. In both disorders, hemorrhagic bullae can develop in involved skin.

Monoclonal cryoglobulinemia is associated with multiple myeloma, Waldenström's macroglobulinemia, lymphocytic leukemia, and lymphoma. Purpura, primarily of the lower extremities, and hemorrhagic infarcts of the fingers and toes are seen in these patients. Exacerbations of disease activity can follow cold exposure or an increase in serum viscosity. Biopsy specimens show precipitates of the cryoglobulin within dermal vessels. Similar deposits have been found in the lung, brain, and renal glomeruli. Patients with *thrombotic throm-*

bocytopenic purpura also can have hemorrhagic infarcts as a result of intravascular thromboses. Additional signs include thrombocytopenic purpura, fever, and microangiopathic hemolytic anemia (see Chap. 109).

Administration of *warfarin* can result in painful areas of erythema that become purpuric and then necrotic with an adherent black eschar. This reaction is seen more often in women and in areas with abundant subcutaneous fat—breasts, abdomen, buttocks, thighs, and calves. The erythema and purpura develop between the third and tenth day of therapy, most likely as a result of a transient imbalance in the levels of anticoagulant and procoagulant vitamin K–dependent factors. Continued therapy does not exacerbate preexisting lesions, and patients with an inherited or acquired deficiency of protein C are at increased risk for this particular reaction as well as for purpura fulminans.

Purpura secondary to *cholesterol emboli* are usually seen on the lower extremities of patients with atherosclerotic vascular disease. They often follow anticoagulant therapy or an invasive vascular procedure such as an arteriogram but also occur spontaneously from disintegration of atheromatous plaques. Associated findings include livedo reticularis, gangrene, cyanosis, subcutaneous nodules, and ischemic ulcerations. Multiple step sections of the biopsy specimen may be necessary to demonstrate the cholesterol clefts with the vessels. Petechiae are also an important sign of *fat embolism* and occur primarily on the upper body 2 to 3 days after a major injury. By using special fixatives, the emboli can be demonstrated in biopsy specimens of the petechiae. Emboli of tumor or thrombus are seen in patients with atrial myxomas and marantic endocarditis.

In the *Gardner-Diamond syndrome* (autoerythrocyte sensitivity), female patients develop large ecchymoses within areas of painful, warm erythema. An episode of significant trauma frequently precedes the onset of this syndrome. Intradermal injections of autologous erythrocytes or phosphatidyl serine derived from the red cell membrane can reproduce the lesions in some patients; however, there are instances where a reaction is seen at an injection site of the forearm but not in the midback region. The latter has led some observers to view Gardner-Diamond syndrome as a cutaneous manifestation of severe emotional stress. *Waldenström's hypergammaglobulinemic purpura* is a chronic disorder characterized by petechiae on the lower extremities. There are circulating complexes of IgG–anti-IgG molecules, and exacerbations are associated with prolonged standing or walking.

Palpable purpura are further subdivided into vasculitic and embolic. In the group of vasculitic disorders, *leukocytoclastic vasculitis*

Table 57-21

Causes of Purpura

I. Primary cutaneous disorders	c. Thrombotic thrombocytopenic purpura
A. Nonpalpable	d. Warfarin reaction
1. Trauma	4. Emboli
2. Solar purpura	a. Cholesterol
3. Steroid purpura	b. Fat
4. Capillaritis	5. Possible immune complex
5. Livedoid vasculitis*	a. Gardner-Diamond syndrome (autoerythrocyte sensitization)
II. Systemic diseases	b. Waldenström's hypergammaglobulinemic purpura
A. Nonpalpable	B. Palpable
1. Clotting disturbances	1. Vasculitis
a. Thrombocytopenia (including ITP)	a. Leukocytoclastic vasculitis
b. Abnormal platelet function	b. Polyarteritis nodosa
c. Clotting factor defects	2. Emboli
2. Vascular fragility	a. Acute meningococcemia
a. Amyloidosis	b. Disseminated gonococcal infection
b. Ehlers-Danlos syndrome	c. Rocky Mountain spotted fever
c. Scurvy	d. Ecthyma gangrenosum
3. Thrombi	
a. Disseminated intravascular coagulation	
b. Monoclonal cryoglobulinemia	

* Also systemic.

(LCV), also known as *allergic vasculitis*, is the one most commonly associated with palpable purpura (see Chap. 319). *Henoch-Schönlein purpura* is a subtype of acute LCV that is seen primarily in children and adolescents following an upper respiratory infection. The majority of lesions are found on the lower extremities and buttocks. Systemic manifestations include fever, arthralgias (primarily of the knees and ankles), abdominal pain, gastrointestinal bleeding, and nephritis. Direct immunofluorescence examination shows deposits of IgA within dermal blood vessel walls. In *polyarteritis nodosa*, specific cutaneous lesions result from a vasculitis of arterial vessels rather than postcapillary venules as in LCV. The arteritis leads to ischemia of the skin, and this explains the irregular outline of the purpura (see below).

Several types of infectious emboli can give rise to palpable purpura. These embolic lesions are usually *irregular* in outline as opposed to the lesions of leukocytoclastic vasculitis, which are *circular* in outline. The irregular outline is indicative of a cutaneous infarct, and the size corresponds to the area of skin that received its blood supply from that particular arteriole or artery. The palpable purpura in LCV are circular because the erythrocytes simply diffuse out evenly from the postcapillary venules as a result of inflammation. Infectious emboli are most commonly due to gram-negative cocci (meningococcus, gonococcus), gram-negative rods (Enterobacteriaceae), and gram-positive cocci (staphylococcus). Additional causes include *Rickettsia* and, in immunocompromised patients, *Candida* and *Aspergillus*.

The embolic lesions in *acute meningococcemia* are found primarily on the trunk, lower extremities, and sites of pressure, and a gunmetal-gray color often develops within them. Their size varies from 1 mm to several centimeters, and the organisms can be cultured from the lesions. Associated findings include a preceding upper respiratory tract infection, fever, meningitis, DIC, and, in some patients, a deficiency of the terminal components of complement. In *disseminated gonococcal infection* (arthritis-dermatitis syndrome), a small number of papules and vesicopustules with central purpura or hemorrhagic necrosis are found over the joints of the distal extremities. Additional symptoms include arthralgias, tenosynovitis, and fever. To establish the diagnosis, a Gram stain of these lesions should be performed. *Rocky mountain spotted fever* is a tick-borne disease that is caused by *Rickettsia rickettsii*. A several-day history of fever, chills, severe headache, and photophobia precedes the onset of the cutaneous eruption. The initial lesions are erythematous macules and papules on the wrists, ankles, palms, and soles. With time, the lesions spread centripetally and become purpuric.

Lesions of *ecthyma gangrenosum* begin as edematous, erythematous papules or plaques and then develop central purpura and necrosis. Bullae formation also occurs in these lesions, and they are frequently found in the girdle region. The organism that is classically associated with ecthyma gangrenosum is *Pseudomonas aeruginosa*, but other gram-negative rods such as *Klebsiella*, *Escherichia coli*, and *Serratia* can produce similar lesions. In immunocompromised hosts, the list of potential pathogens is expanded to include *Candida* and *Aspergillus*.

ULCERS (Table 57-22) As an approach to the patient with a cutaneous ulcer, the etiologies are divided into two major groups: (1) primary cutaneous disorders and (2) underlying systemic diseases. Within the group of *primary cutaneous disorders*, there are three categories: vascular, tumor-associated, and infectious. The *peripheral vascular* group is the first to be discussed because it contains the most common cause of lower extremity ulcers in adults, *venous hypertension*. Stasis ulcers are characteristically painless and contain adequate granulation tissue. They are often found on the medial malleoli against a background of varicosities, stasis dermatitis, edema, and hemosiderin deposition (yellow-brown discoloration of the skin).

In contrast, lower extremity ulcers due to *arteriosclerosis obliterans* are often painful and are associated with cool, hairless, atrophic skin and dystrophic nails—all a reflection of a decrease in blood flow. The majority of patients are men, and they frequently have evidence of atherosclerosis in other large- and medium-sized arteries. *Thromboangiitis obliterans* (Buerger's disease) and *Mönckeberg's arteriosclerosis* are two less common arterial diseases that can lead to ulcers of the distal upper extremity as well as the lower extremity. The latter is found in patients with primary or secondary hyperparathyroidism,

and the calcification of the tunica media of involved muscular arteries is seen radiographically as a diffuse pipestem calcification. Buerger's disease occurs primarily in young men (ages 25 to 40) who smoke or have been smokers.

Livedoid vasculitis (atrophie blanche) represents a combination of a vasculopathy with intravascular thrombosis. Purpuric lesions and livedo reticularis are found in association with painful ulcerations of the lower extremities. These ulcers are often slow to heal, but when they do, irregularly shaped white scars are formed. The majority of cases are idiopathic in origin, but possible underlying illnesses include systemic lupus, the antiphospholipid syndrome, scleroderma, cryoglobulinemia, and cryofibrinogenemia. Patients with the antiphospholipid syndrome have anticardiolipin antibodies, biologic false-positive tests for syphilis, and prolonged activated partial thromboplastin times; the latter are due to a circulating lupus anticoagulant. These antiphospholipid antibodies are seen most commonly in patients with systemic lupus but are also associated with other connective tissue diseases. In addition to the lesions of livedoid vasculitis, patients with the antiphospholipid syndrome have recurrent venous thrombosis, arterial thrombosis (including cerebrovascular accidents), spontaneous abortions, and thrombocytopenia.

Several *carcinomas* can present as cutaneous ulcers, e.g., basal cell carcinoma, squamous cell carcinoma, and, less often, melanoma. When an ulcer on the lower extremity does not heal, despite appropriate treatment, it should be biopsied to rule out carcinoma, primarily squamous cell carcinoma. The same holds true for ulcers that develop within scars. Bacterial and viral *infections* also lead to cutaneous ulceration, and one of the more commonly isolated organisms is *Streptococcus*. The term *ecthyma* is used to describe the often widespread ulcerative lesions that are caused by this bacteria. Ecthyma is a primary cutaneous disorder and should not be confused with ecthyma gangrenosum, which is secondary to blood-borne emboli (see "Purpura"). In Meleney's ulcer, a gradually expanding ulcer begins at a site of trauma or surgery. The clinical appearance is similar to that of pyoderma gangrenosum, but the ulcer is due to a synergistic infection that usually includes anaerobic streptococci.

Table 57-22

Causes of Cutaneous Ulcers

I. Primary cutaneous disorders
  A. Peripheral vascular disease
    1. Venous
    2. Arterial
  B. Livedoid vasculitis*
  C. Squamous cell carcinoma, e.g., within scars
  D. Infections, e.g., ecthyma
II. Systemic diseases
  A. Legs
    1. Leukocytoclastic vasculitis
    2. Hemoglobinopathies
    3. Cryoglobulinemia, cryofibrinogenemia
    4. Cholesterol emboli
    5. Necrobiosis lipoidica
    6. Antiphospholipid syndrome
  B. Hands and feet
    1. Raynaud's phenomenon
  C. Generalized
    1. Pyoderma gangrenosum
    2. Infections, e.g., dimorphic fungi, chronic herpes varicella–zoster
    3. Lymphoma
  D. Mucosal
    1. Behçet's syndrome
    2. Erythema multiforme
    3. Primary blistering disorders
    4. Lupus erythematosus
    5. Inflammatory bowel disease

* Also systemic.

For one group of patients with cutaneous ulcers due to an underlying systemic disease, the lower extremity is the primary location for the lesions. In a young patient, ischemic cutaneous ulcers on the leg should raise the possibility of a *hemoglobinopathy* or *hereditary spherocytosis*. Intravascular thrombosis is the presumed cause of these ulcers as well as for the ulcers seen in patients with *monoclonal cryoglobulinemia* (see "Purpura"). Primary and secondary forms of *LCV* as well as *emboli of cholesterol* can result in cutaneous ulceration, again primarily on the lower extremities (see "Purpura"). For example, lower extremity ulcers in patients with rheumatoid arthritis are often due to vasculitis. In addition, the yellow atrophic plaques of *necrobiosis lipoidica* can break down centrally into an ulcer (see "Papulonodular Skin Lesions").

Vasospasm occurs in patients with *Raynaud's phenomenon* and can lead to ulcerations of the hands as well as the feet. Raynaud's phenomenon is defined as a triphasic reaction of pallor, cyanosis, and hyperemia in response to cold or emotional stress. Vasospasm is also seen in patients who receive systemic norepinephrine, vasopressin, ergot, and bleomycin. The patient with Raynaud's phenomenon and ulcerations on the tips of the digits should be examined carefully for periungual and mat telangiectasias, the subtle signs of scleroderma. Raynaud's phenomenon is also seen in patients with DM, systemic lupus, cryoglobulinemia, cervical rib and scalenus anticus syndromes, pneumatic hammer disease, and occupational acro-osteolysis (associated with the manufacture of polyvinyl chloride).

In *pyoderma gangrenosum*, the border of the ulcers has a characteristic appearance of an undermined necrotic bluish edge and a peripheral erythematous halo. The ulcers often begin as pustules that then expand rather rapidly to a size as large as 20 cm. Although these lesions are most commonly found on the lower extremities, they can arise anywhere on the surface of the body, including sites of trauma (pathergy). An estimated 30 to 50 percent of cases are idiopathic, and the most common associated disorders are ulcerative colitis and Crohn's disease. Less commonly, it is associated with chronic active hepatitis, seropositive rheumatoid arthritis, acute and chronic granulocytic leukemia, polycythemia vera, and myeloma. Additional findings in these patients, even those with idiopathic disease, are cutaneous anergy and a benign monoclonal gammopathy. Because the histology of pyoderma gangrenosum is nonspecific, the diagnosis is made clinically by excluding less common causes of similar-appearing ulcers such as necrotizing vasculitis, Meleney's ulcer (see above), dimorphic fungi, cutaneous amebiasis, spider bites, and factitial. In the myeloproliferative disorders, the ulcers may be more superficial with a pustulobullous border, and these lesions provide a connection between classic pyoderma gangrenosum and acute febrile neutrophilic dermatosis (Sweet's syndrome).

The clinical diagnosis of *Behçet's disease* (see Chap. 318) requires the presence of recurrent oral ulceration (at least three times in a 12-month period) in addition to two of the four following criteria: (1) recurrent genital ulcers, primarily of the vulva and scrotum; (2) eye lesions, either uveitis or retinal vasculitis; (3) skin lesions; and (4) a positive pathergy test. The oral ulcers are usually painful and well defined with an erythematous halo, whereas the genital ulcers tend to be deeper and heal with scarring. Erythema nodosum, "pseudofolliculitis," papulopustular lesions, *or* acneiform nodules in a postadolescent patient not on glucocorticoids are the entities included under the heading of skin lesions. The test for pathergy, which is defined as a reproduction of cutaneous lesions by trauma, is performed by injecting sterile saline into the dermis. Before the diagnosis of Behçet's disease can be made, the following disorders must be excluded: recurrent EM (see "Vesicles/Bullae"), herpes simplex, inflammatory bowel disease, systemic lupus, and primary blistering disorders.

FEVER AND RASH The major considerations in a patient with a fever and a rash are inflammatory diseases versus infectious diseases. In the hospital setting, the most common scenario is a patient who has a drug rash plus a fever secondary to an underlying infection.

However, it should be emphasized that a drug reaction can lead to both a cutaneous eruption and a fever ("drug fever"). Additional inflammatory diseases that are often associated with a fever include pustular psoriasis, erythroderma, and Sweet's syndrome. Lyme disease, secondary syphilis, and viral and bacterial exanthems (see "Exanthems") are examples of infectious diseases that produce a rash and a fever. Lastly, it is important to determine whether or not the cutaneous lesions represent septic emboli (see "Purpura"). Such lesions usually have evidence of ischemia in the form of purpura, necrosis, or impending necrosis (gunmetal-gray color). In the patient with thrombocytopenia, however, purpura can be seen in inflammatory reactions such as morbilliform drug eruptions and infectious lesions.

BIBLIOGRAPHY

ARNDT KA et al: *Cutaneous Medicine and Surgery*. Philadelphia, Saunders, 1995

BORK K: *Cutaneous Side Effects of Drugs*. Philadelphia, Saunders, 1988

BRAVERMAN IM: *Skin Signs of Systemic Disease*, 2d ed. Philadelphia, Saunders, 1981

CALLEN JP: *Dermatology Clinics*, vol 8, no 2: *Skin Signs of Internal Disease II*. Philadelphia, Saunders, 1990

———, JORIZZO JL: *Dermatology Clinics*, vol 7, no 3: *Skin Signs of Internal Disease*. Philadelphia, Saunders, 1989

CHAMPION RH et al (eds): *Textbook of Dermatology*, 5th ed. Oxford, Blackwell Scientific, 1992

LEVER WF, SCHAUMBURG-LEVER G: *Histopathology of the Skin*, 7th ed. Philadelphia, Lippincott, 1990

NOVICE FM et al: *Handbook of Genetic Skin Disorders*. Philadelphia, Saunders, 1994

ZURCHER K, KREBS A: *Cutaneous Drug Reactions*, 2d ed. Basel, Karger, 1992

58   *David R. Bickers*

PHOTOSENSITIVITY AND OTHER REACTIONS TO LIGHT

SOLAR RADIATION Sunlight is the most visible and obvious source of comfort in the environment. This natural proclivity for the sun has the beneficial results of warmth and vitamin D synthesis but also can produce pathologic consequences. Few effects of sun exposure beyond those on the skin have been identified, but cutaneous exposure to sunlight can evoke immunosuppressive responses and genetic changes that may be relevant to the pathogenesis of nonmelanoma skin cancer and perhaps infections such as herpes simplex.

The sun's energy encompasses a broad range from ultrashort ionizing radiation (10^{-2} μm) to ultralong radiowaves of very low photon energy (10^7 μm). Thus, the emission spectrum ranges over nine orders of magnitude, but that reaching the earth's surface is narrow and is limited to components of the ultraviolet (UV), visible light, and portions of the infrared. The cutoff at the short end of the UV is at approximately 290 nm, because stratospheric ozone is formed by ionizing radiation of wavelengths less than 100 nm and absorbs solar energy between 120 and 310 nm, thereby preventing penetration to the earth's surface of the shorter, more energetic, potentially more harmful wavelengths of solar radiation. Indeed, concern about destruction of the ozone layer by chlorofluorocarbons released into the atmosphere has led to international agreements to reduce production of these chemicals.

Measurements of solar flux indicate that there is a twentyfold regional variation in the amount of energy at 300 nm that reaches the earth's surface. This variability relates to seasonal effects, the path of sunlight transmission through ozone and air, the altitude (4 percent increase for each 300 m of elevation), the latitude (increasing intensity with decreasing latitude), and the amount of cloud cover, fog, and pollution.

The major components of the photobiologic action spectrum include the UV and visible wavelengths between 290 and 700 nm. In addition, the wavelengths beyond 700 nm in the infrared primarily evoke heat, but warming of the skin may enhance biologic responses to wavelengths in the UV and visible spectrum.

The UV spectrum is arbitrarily divided into three major segments: C, B, and A. This includes the wavelengths between 10 and 400 nm. Ultraviolet C (UV-C) consists of wavelengths between 10 and 290 nm and does not reach the earth because of its absorption by stratospheric ozone. These wavelengths are not a cause of photosensitivity except in occupational settings where artificial sources of this energy are employed, e.g., for germicidal effects. Ultraviolet B (UV-B) consists of wavelengths between 290 and 320 nm. This portion of the photobiologic action spectrum is the most efficient in producing redness or erythema in human skin and hence is sometimes known as the "sunburn spectrum." Ultraviolet A (UV-A) represents those wavelengths between 320 and 400 nm and is approximately 1000-fold less efficient in producing skin hyperemia than is UV-B. The UV-A has also been divided into two parts known as UV-A 1 (340 to 400 nm) and UV-A 2 (320 to 340 nm).

The visible wavelengths between 400 and 700 nm include the familiar white light which when directed through a prism can be shown to consist of various colors including violet, indigo, blue, green, yellow, orange, and red. The energy possessed by photons in the visible spectrum usually is not capable of damaging human skin in the absence of a photosensitizing chemical. The absorption of energy is critical to the development of photosensitivity. Thus the *absorption spectrum* of a molecule is defined as the range of wavelengths absorbed by it, whereas the *action spectrum* for an effect of incident radiation is defined as the range of wavelengths that evoke the response.

Photosensitivity occurs when a photon-absorbing chemical (chromophore) present in the skin absorbs incident energy, becomes excited, and transfers the absorbed energy to various structures or to oxygen. The absorbed energy must be dissipated by processes including heat, fluorescence, and phosphorescence. It is important to emphasize that absorption spectra and action spectra need not be superimposable, but there must be overlap at some point to produce photosensitization.

STRUCTURE AND FUNCTION OF SKIN The skin's exposure to sunlight permits the absorption of some wavelengths and the transmission of others. Essentially, human skin is a sandwich of two distinctive compartments, the epidermis and dermis, separated by a basement membrane. The outer epidermis is a stratified squamous epithelium comprising the surface stratum corneum (a protein- and lipid-rich compact membrane), the stratum granulosum, stratum spinosum, and the basal cell layer. The basal cell layer contains a heterogeneous population of cells, a subset of which migrate upward in the process of terminal differentiation that results in the expression of specific keratin genes and the formation of the stratum corneum. Epidermal cells include resident keratinocytes and melanocytes and immigrant cells, including the immunologically active Langerhans cells, lymphocytes, polymorphonuclear leukocytes, monocytes, and macrophages, making the epidermis a major component of the immune system. Branches of sensory nerve endings also reach into this compartment.

The second major component of skin is the dermis, which is relatively large and less densely populated with cells that include fibroblasts, endothelial cells within dermal vessels, and mast cells. Tissue macrophages and sparsely distributed inflammatory cells are also present. All these cells exist within an extracellular matrix of collagen, elastin, and glycosaminoglycans. In contrast to the epidermis, rich vascularization of the dermis allows it to play an important role in temperature regulation.

UV RADIATION (UVR) AND SKIN The epidermis and the dermis contain several chromophores capable of interacting with incident solar energy. These interactions include reflection, refraction, absorption, and transmission. The stratum corneum is a major impediment to the transmission of UV-B, and less than 10 percent of incident wavelengths in this region penetrate the basement membrane. Approximately 3 percent of radiation below 300 nm, 20 percent of radiation below 360 nm, and 33 percent of short visible radiation reaches the basal cell layer in untanned human skin. Proteins and nucleic acids absorb intensely in the short UV-B. In contrast, UV-A 1 and 2 penetrate

the epidermis efficiently to reach the dermis, where they likely produce changes in structural and matrix proteins that contribute to the aged appearance of chronically sun-exposed skin, particularly in individuals of light complexion.

One of the consequences of UV-B absorption by DNA is the production of pyrimidine dimers. These structural changes can be repaired by mechanisms that result in their recognition, excision, and the reestablishment of normal base sequences. The efficient repair of these structural aberrations is crucial, since individuals with defective DNA repair are at high risk for the development of cutaneous cancer. For example, patients with xeroderma pigmentosum, an autosomal recessive disorder, are characterized by variably decreased repair of UV-induced photoproducts, and their skin may develop the xerotic appearance of photoaging as well as basal cell and squamous cell carcinomas and melanoma in the first two decades of life. Studies in mice using knockout gene technology have verified the importance of genes regulating these repair pathways in preventing the development of UV-induced cancer.

Cutaneous Optics and Chromophores Chromophores are endogenous or exogenous chemical components that can absorb physical energy. Endogenous chromophores of skin are of two types: (1) chemicals that are normally present, including nucleic acids, proteins, lipids, and 7-dehydrocholesterol, the precursor of vitamin D; and (2) chemicals, such as porphyrins, synthesized elsewhere in the body that circulate in the bloodstream and diffuse into the skin. Normally, only trace amounts of porphyrins are present in the skin, but in the diseases known as the porphyrias, increased amounts are released into the circulation and are transported to the skin, where they absorb incident energy both in the Soret band around 400 nm (short visible) and to a lesser extent in the red portion of the visible spectrum (580 to 660 nm). This results in structural damage to the skin that may be manifest as erythema, edema, urticaria, or blister formation (see Chap. 343).

Acute Effects of Sun Exposure The immediate cutaneous consequences of sun exposure include sunburn and vitamin D synthesis.

Sunburn This very common affliction of human skin is caused by exposure to UVR. Generally speaking, the individual's ability to tolerate sunlight is inversely proportional to his or her melanin pigmentation. Melanin is a complex polymer of tyrosine that functions as an efficient neutral-density filter with broad absorbance within the UV portion of the solar spectrum. Melanin is synthesized in specialized epidermal dendritic cells termed *melanocytes* and is packaged into *melanosomes* that are transferred via dendritic processes into *keratinocytes*, where they provide photoprotection. Sun-induced melanogenesis is a consequence of increased tyrosinase activity in melanocytes that in turn may be due to a combination of eicosanoid and endothelin-1 release. Tolerance of sun exposure is a function of the efficiency of the epidermal-melanin unit and can usually be ascertained by asking an individual two questions: (1) Do you burn after sun exposure? and (2) Do you tan after sun exposure? By the answers to these questions, it is usually possible to divide the population into six skin types varying from type I (always burn, never tan) to type VI (never burn, always tan) (see Table 58-1).

There are two general theories about the pathogenesis of the sunburn response. First, the lag phase in time between skin exposure and

Table 58-1

Skin Type and Sunburn Sensitivity

Type	Description
I	Always burn, never tan
II	Always burn, sometimes tan
III	Sometimes burn, sometimes tan
IV	Sometimes burn, always tan
V	Never burn, sometimes tan
VI	Never burn, always tan

the development of visible redness (usually 4 to 12 h) suggests an epidermal chromophore that causes delayed production and/or release of vasoactive mediator(s), or cytokines, that diffuse to the dermal vasculature to evoke vasodilatation. Indeed UVR stimulates the release of numerous proinflammatory cytokines and nitric oxide by keratinocytes. Second, it is possible that the small amount of incident UV-B radiation (10 percent or less) that penetrates to the dermis can be absorbed directly by endothelial cells in the vasculature, thereby resulting in vasodilatation. The issue remains unresolved.

The action spectrum for sunburn erythema includes the UV-B and UV-A regions. Photons in the shorter UV-B are at least a 1000-fold more efficient than photons in the longer UV-B and the UV-A in evoking the response. However, UV-A may contribute to sunburn erythema at midday when much more UV-A than UV-B is present.

The mechanism of injury remains poorly defined, but the action spectrum for UV-B erythema closely resembles the absorption spectrum for DNA after adjusting for the absorbance of incident energy by the stratum corneum. Apoptotic keratinocytes (so-called sunburn cells) are visible histologically within an hour of exposure and are maximal within 24 h. UV-A is less effective than UV-B in producing sunburn cells. Mast cells may release inflammatory mediators after exposure to UV-B and UV-A. For example, erythema doses of both UV-B and UV-A increase histamine levels in suction blisters of human skin that return to normal after 24 h (before visible erythema has subsided). Prostaglandin E_2 increases to approximately 150 percent of control levels after 24 h and then diminishes. Since prostaglandins evoke both pain and redness when injected intradermally, their presence in suction blisters after UV-B exposure suggests a role in UV-B erythema. Age-related declines occur in the amount of inflammatory mediators detectable in human skin after UV-B irradiation. UV-A erythema results in few epidermal sunburn cells, but vascular endothelial injury is greater than with UV-B. In addition, there are increased levels of arachidonic acid and of prostaglandins D_2, E_2, and I_2 that peak within 5 to 9 h and then subside before peak redness occurs. Despite evidence for the role of prostaglandins in both UV-B- and UV-A-irradiated skin, administration of nonsteroidal anti-inflammatory drugs is more effective in reducing erythema evoked by UV-B than by UV-A. UV-B also induces cutaneous matrix-degrading metalloproteinases within hours of exposure.

Vitamin D photochemistry Cutaneous exposure to UV-B causes photolysis of epidermal previtamin D_3 (7-dehydrocholesterol) to previtamin D_3, which then undergoes a temperature-dependent isomerization to form the stable hormone vitamin D_3. This compound then diffuses to the dermal vasculature and circulates systemically where it is converted to the functional hormone 1,25-dihydroxy vitamin D_3 [$1,25(OH)_2D_3$]. Vitamin D metabolites from the circulation or those produced in the skin itself can augment epidermal differentiation signaling. Aging substantially decreases the ability of human skin to produce vitamin D_3. This, coupled with the widespread use of sunscreens that filter out UV-B, has led to concern that vitamin D deficiency may become a significant clinical problem in the elderly. Indeed, studies have shown that the use of sunscreens can prevent the production of vitamin D_3 in human skin.

Chronic Effects of Sun Exposure: Nonmalignant The clinical features of photodamaged sun-exposed skin consist of wrinkling, blotchiness, telangiectasia, and a roughened, irregular, "weatherbeaten" appearance. Whether these changes, which some refer to as *photoaging* or *dermatoheliosis*, represent accelerated chronologic aging or a separate and distinct process is not clear.

Within chronically sun-exposed epidermis there is thickening (acanthosis) and morphologic heterogeneity within the basal cell layer. Higher but irregular melanosome content may be present in some keratinocytes, indicating prolonged residence of the cells in the basal cell layer. These structural changes may help to explain the leathery texture and the blotchy discoloration of sun-damaged skin.

The dermis is the major site for sun-associated chronic damage, manifest as a massive increase in thickened irregular masses of tangled elastic fibers resulting from enhanced expression of elastin genes. Collagen fibers are also abnormally clumped in the deeper dermis. Fibroblasts are increased in number and show morphologic signs suggesting activation. Degraded mast cells may be present in the dermis, the relevance of which remains unclear.

These morphologic changes, both gross and microscopic, are features of chronically sun-exposed skin. The chromophore(s), the action spectra, and the specific biochemical events orchestrating these changes are unknown.

Chronic Effects of Sun Exposure: Malignant One of the major known consequences of chronic skin exposure to sunlight is nonmelanoma skin cancer. The two types of nonmelanoma skin cancer are basal cell and squamous cell carcinoma (see Chap. 88). There are three major steps for cancer induction: initiation, promotion, and progression. Chronic exposure of animal skin to artificial light sources that mimic solar UVR results in *initiation*, a step whereby structural (mutagenic) changes in DNA evoke an irreversible alteration in the target cell (keratinocyte) that begins the tumorigenic process. Exposure to a tumor initiator is believed to be a necessary but not sufficient step in the malignant process, since initiated skin cells not exposed to tumor promoters do not generally develop tumors. The second stage in tumor development is *promotion*, a multistep process whereby initiated cells are exposed to chemical and physical agents that evoke epigenetic changes that culminate in the clonal expansion of initiated cells and cause the development, over a period of weeks to months, of benign growths known as *papillomas*. Again, using transgenic animals, the importance of UV effects on the expression of additional oncogenes such as *fos* and *jun* in developing papillomas has been demonstrated. UV-B is a *complete carcinogen*, meaning that it can function as both an initiator and a promoter, leading to tumor induction. *Incomplete carcinogens* can initiate tumorigenesis but require additional skin exposure to tumor promoters to elicit tumors. The prototype tumor promoter is the phorbol ester 12-*O*-tetradecanoyl phorbol-13-acetate. Tumor promotion usually requires multiple exposures over time to evoke a neoplasm.

The final step in the malignant process is the conversion of benign precursors into malignant lesions, a process thought to require additional genetic alterations in already transformed cells. Indeed *ras* gene mutations have been detected in a minority of human nonmelanoma skin cancers. Mutations of the tumor suppressor gene p53 also occur in sun-damaged human skin.

Sun exposure is believed to cause nonmelanoma and melanoma cancers of the skin, although the evidence is far more direct for its role in nonmelanoma (basal cell and squamous cell carcinoma) than in melanoma. Approximately 80 percent of nonmelanoma skin cancers develop on exposed body area, including the face, the neck, and the hands. Men of fair complexion who work outdoors are twice as likely as women to develop these types of cancers. Whites of darker complexions (e.g., Hispanics) have one-tenth the risk of developing such cancers as do light-skinned individuals. Blacks are at lowest risk for all forms of skin cancer. Between 600,000 and 800,000 individuals in the United States develop nonmelanoma skin cancer annually, and the lifetime risk for a white individual to develop such a neoplasm is estimated at approximately 15 percent. A consensus exists that the incidence of nonmelanoma skin cancer in the population is rising for reasons that are unclear.

The relationship of sun exposure to melanoma is less clear-cut, but suggestive evidence supports an association. Melanomas occasionally develop by the teenage years, indicating that the latent period for tumor growth is less than that of nonmelanomas. Melanomas are among the most rapidly increasing of all human malignancies. Epidemiologic studies of immigrants of similar ethnic stock indicate that individuals born in one area or who migrated to the same locale before age 10 have higher age-specific melanoma rates than individuals arriving later. It is thus reasonable to conclude that life in a sunny climate from birth or early childhood increases the risk of melanoma. In general, risk does not correlate with cumulative sun exposure but may relate to sequelae of sun exposure in childhood. Thus a blistering sunburn is associated with a doubling of melanoma risk at the site of the reaction.

Immunologic Effects Exposure to solar radiation influences both local and systemic immune responses. UV-B appears to be most efficient in altering immune responses, likely related to the capacity of such energy to affect antigen presentation in skin by interacting with epidermal Langerhans cells. These bone marrow–derived dendritic cells possess surface markers characteristic of monocytes and macrophages. Following skin exposure to erythema doses of UV-B, Langerhans cells undergo both morphologic and functional changes that result in decreased contact allergic responses when haptens are applied to the irradiated site. This diminished capacity for sensitization is due to the induction of antigen-specific suppressor T lymphocytes. Indeed, while the immunosuppressive effect of irradiation is limited to haptens applied to the irradiated site, the net result is systemic immune suppression to that antigen because of the induction of suppressor T cells.

Higher doses of radiation evoke diminished immunologic responses to antigens introduced either epicutaneously or intracutaneously at sites distant from the irradiated site. These suppressed responses are also associated with the induction of antigen-specific suppressor T lymphocytes and may be mediated by as yet undefined factors that are released from epidermal cells at the irradiated site. The implications of this generalized immune suppression in terms of altered susceptibility to cutaneous cancer or to infection remain to be defined.

It is known that UV-induced tumors in murine skin are antigenic and are rapidly rejected when transplanted into normal syngeneic animals. If the tumors are transplanted into animals previously exposed to subcarcinogenic doses of UV-B, they are not rejected and instead grow progressively in the recipients. This failure of irradiated animals to reject the transplanted tumors is due to the development of T suppressor cells that prevent the rejection response. While the mechanism of suppression of tumor rejection is unknown, such a response might be a critical determinant of cancer risk in human skin.

PHOTOSENSITIVITY DISEASES The diagnosis of photosensitivity requires a careful history to define the duration of the signs and symptoms, the length of time between exposure to sunlight and the development of subjective complaints, and visible changes in the skin. The age of onset also can be a helpful clue; for example, the acute photosensitivity of erythropoietic protoporphyria almost always begins in childhood, whereas the chronic photosensitivity of porphyria cutanea tarda typically begins in the fourth and fifth decades. A history of exposure to topical and systemic drugs and chemicals may provide important information. Many classes of drugs can cause photosensitivity on the basis of either phototoxicity or photoallergy. Fragrances such as musk ambrette contained in numerous cosmetic products are also potent photosensitizers.

Examination of the skin also may offer important clues. Anatomic areas that are naturally protected from direct sunlight such as the hairy scalp, the upper eyelids, the retroauricular areas, and the infranasal and submental regions may be spared, whereas exposed areas show characteristic features of the pathologic process. These anatomic localization patterns are often helpful but not infallible in making the diagnosis. For example, airborne contact sensitizers that are blown onto the skin may produce dermatitis that can be difficult to distinguish from photosensitivity, despite the fact that such material may trigger skin reactivity in areas shielded from direct sunlight.

Many dermatologic conditions may be caused or aggravated by light (Table 58-2). The role of light in evoking these responses may be dependent on genetic abnormalities ranging from well-described defects in DNA repair that occur in xeroderma pigmentosum to the inherited abnormalities in heme synthesis that characterize the porphyrias. In certain photosensitivity diseases, the chromophore has been identified, whereas in the majority, the energy-absorbing agent is unknown.

Polymorphous Light Eruption After sunburn, the most common type of photosensitivity disease is *polymorphous light eruption*, the mechanism of which is unknown. Many affected individuals never seek medical attention because the condition is often transient, becoming manifest each spring with initial sun exposure but then subsiding spontaneously with continuing exposure, a phenomenon known as "hardening." The major manifestations of polymorphous light eruption include pruritic (often intensely so) erythematous papules that may coalesce into plaques on exposed areas of the face and arms or other areas as well, making the distribution spotty and uneven.

The diagnosis can be confirmed by skin biopsy and by performing phototest procedures in which skin is exposed to multiple erythema doses of UV-A and UV-B. The action spectrum for polymorphous light eruption is usually within these portions of the solar spectrum.

Treatment of this disease includes the induction of hardening by the cautious administration of UV light, either alone or in combination with photosensitizers such as the psoralens (see below).

Phototoxicity and Photoallergy These photosensitivity disorders are related to the topical or systemic administration of drugs and other chemicals. Both reactions require the absorption of energy by a drug or chemical resulting in the production of an excited-state photosensitizer that can transfer its absorbed energy to a bystander molecule or to molecular oxygen, thereby generating tissue-destructive chemical species.

Phototoxicity is a nonimmunologic reaction caused by drugs and chemicals, a few of which are listed in Table 58-3. The usual clinical manifestations include erythema resembling a sunburn that quickly desquamates or "peels" within several days. In addition, edema, vesicles, and bullae may occur.

Table 58-2

Classification of Photosensitivity Diseases	
Type	**Disease**
Genetic	Erythropoietic porphyria
	Erythropoietic protoporphyria
	Porphyria cutanea tarda—familial
	Variegate porphyria
	Hepatoerythropoietic porphyria
	Albinism
	Xeroderma pigmentosum
	Rothmund-Thompson disease
	Bloom's disease
	Cockayne's disease
	Phenylketonuria
Metabolic	Porphyria cutanea tarda—sporadic
	Hartnup disease
	Kwashiorkor
	Pellagra
	Carcinoid syndrome
	Pseudoporphyria
Phototoxic	
Internal	Drugs
External	Drugs, plants, food
Photoallergic	
Immediate	Solar urticaria
Delayed	Drug photoallergy
	Persistent light reaction/chronic actinic dermatitis
Neoplastic and degenerative	Photoaging
	Actinic keratoses
	Basal cell carcinoma
Idiopathic	Polymorphous light eruption
	Hydroa aestivale
	Actinic reticuloid
Photoaggravated	Lupus erythematosus
	Systemic
	Subacute cutaneous
	Dermatomyositis
	Pemphigus foliaceus
	Herpes simplex
	Lichen planus actinicus
	Acne vulgaris (aestivale)
	Transient acantholytic dermatosis

Photoallergy is distinct in that the immune system participates in the pathologic process. The excited-state photosensitizer may create highly unstable haptenic free radicals that bind covalently to macromolecules to form a functional antigen capable of evoking a delayed hypersensitivity response. Some of the drugs and chemicals that produce photoallergy are listed in Table 58-4. The clinical manifestations typically differ from those of phototoxicity in that an intensely pruritic eczematous dermatitis tends to predominate and evolves into lichenified, thickened, "leathery" changes in sun-exposed areas. A small subset (perhaps 5 to 10 percent) of patients with photoallergy may develop a persistent exquisite hypersensitivity to light even when the offending drug or chemical is identified and eliminated. Known as *persistent light reaction*, this may be incapacitating for years. Some have used the term *chronic actinic dermatitis* to encompass these chronic hyperresponsive states.

Diagnostic confirmation of phototoxicity and photoallergy often can be obtained using phototest procedures. In patients with suspected phototoxicity, determination of the minimal erythema dose (MED) while the patient is exposed to a suspected agent and then repeating the MED after discontinuation of the agent may provide a clue to the causative drug or chemical. Photopatch testing can be performed to confirm the diagnosis of photoallergy. This is a simple variant of ordinary patch testing in which a series of known photoallergens is applied to the skin in duplicate and one set is irradiated with a suberythema dose of UV-A. Development of eczematous changes at sites exposed to sensitizer and light is a positive result. The characteristic abnormality in patients with persistent light reaction is a diminished threshold to erythema evoked by UV-B. Patients with chronic actinic dermatitis may have a broad spectrum of UV hyperresponsiveness.

The management of drug photosensitivity is first and foremost to eliminate exposure to the chemical agents responsible for the reaction and to minimize sun exposure. The acute symptoms of phototoxicity may be ameliorated by cool, moist compresses, topical glucocorticoids, and systemically administered nonsteroidal anti-inflammatory agents. In severely affected individuals, a rapidly tapered course of systemic glucocorticoids may be useful. Judicious use of analgesics may be necessary.

Photoallergic reactions require similar management techniques. Furthermore, individuals suffering from persistent light reactivity must be meticulously protected against light exposure. In selected patients in whom chronic systemic high-dose glucocorticoids pose unacceptable risks, it may be necessary to employ cytotoxic agents such as azathioprine or cyclophosphamide.

Porphyria The porphyrias (see Chap. 343) are a group of diseases that have in common various derangements in the synthesis of heme. Heme is an iron-chelated tetrapyrrole or porphyrin, and the nonmetal chelated porphyrins are potent photosensitizers that absorb light intensely in both the short (400 to 410 nm) and the long (580 to 650 nm) portions of the visible spectrum.

Heme cannot be reutilized and must be continuously synthesized, and the two body compartments with the largest capacity for its production are the bone marrow and the liver. Accordingly, the porphyrias originate in one or the other of these organs, with the end result of excessive endogenous production of potent photosensitizing porphyrins. The porphyrins circulate in the bloodstream and diffuse into the skin, where they absorb solar energy, become photoexcited, and evoke cutaneous photosensitivity. The mechanism of porphyrin photosensitization is known to be photodynamic or oxygen-dependent and is mediated by reactive oxygen species such as superoxide anions.

Porphyria cutanea tarda is the most common type of human porphyria and is associated with decreased activity of the enzyme uroporphyrinogen decarboxylase associated with a number of gene mutations. There are two basic types of porphyria cutanea tarda: the sporadic or acquired type, generally seen in individuals ingesting ethanol or receiving estrogens, and the inherited type, in which there is autosomal dominant transmission of deficient enzyme activity. Both forms are associated with increased hepatic iron stores.

In both types of porphyria cutanea tarda, the predominant feature is a chronic photosensitivity characterized by increased fragility of sun-exposed skin, particularly areas subject to repeated trauma such as the dorsa of the hands, the forearms, the face, and the ears. The predominant skin lesions are vesicles and bullae that rupture, producing moist erosions often with a hemorrhagic base, and that heal slowly with crusting and purplish discoloration of the affected skin. Hypertrichosis,

Table 58-3

Phototoxic Drugs and Chemicals

	Topical	Systemic
COAL TAR DERIVATIVES		
Acridine	+	
Anthracene	+	
Phenanthrene	+	
DRUGS		
Amiodarone		+
Dacarbazine		+
Fluoroquinolones		+
5-Fluorouracil	+	+
Furosemide		+
Nalidixic acid		+
Phenothiazines		+
Psoralens	+	+
Retinoids	+	+
Sulfonamides		+
Sulfonylureas		+
Tetracyclines		+
Thiazides		+
Vinblastine		+
DYES		
Anthraquinone		+
Eosin		+
Methylene blue		+
Rose bengal		+

Table 58-4

Photoallergic Drugs and Chemicals

	Topical	Systemic
Antibiotics		
Sulfonamides		+
Antifungals		
Fenticlor	+	
Jadit	+	
Multifungin	+	
Diuretics		
Thiazides		+
Fragrances		
Musk ambrette	+	
6-Methylcoumarin	+	
Plant oleoresins	+	
Halogenated salicylanilides		
Bithionol	+	
Tetrachlorosalicylanilides	+	
Tribromosalicylanilide	+	
Nonsteroidal Anti-Inflammatory Agents		
Piroxicam	+	
Phenothiazines		
Chlorpromazine	+	
Promethazine	+	
Sulfonylureas		+
Sunscreens		
p-Aminobenzoic acid and esters	+	
Whitening Agents		
Stilbenes	+	

mottled pigmentary change, and scleroderma-like induration are associated features. Biochemical confirmation of the diagnosis can be obtained by measurement of urinary porphyrin excretion, plasma porphyrin assay, and by assay of uroporphyrinogen decarboxylase. Multiple mutations of the uroporphyrinogen decarboxylase gene have been identified in human populations including exon skipping and base substitutions.

Treatment consists of repeated phlebotomies to diminish the excessive hepatic iron stores and/or intermittent low doses of the antimalarial drugs chloroquine and hydroxychloroquine. Long-term remission of the disease can be achieved if the patient eliminates exposure to porphyrinogenic agents.

Erythropoietic protoporphyria originates in the bone marrow and is due to a decrease in the mitochondrial enzyme ferrochelatase secondary to a number of gene mutations. The major clinical features include an acute photosensitivity characterized by subjective burning and stinging of exposed skin that often develops during or just after exposure. There may be associated skin swelling and, after repeated episodes, a waxlike scarring.

The diagnosis is confirmed by demonstration of measurement of free elevated erythrocyte protoporphyrin. Detection of increased plasma protoporphyrin helps to differentiate lead poisoning and iron-deficiency anemia, in both of which elevated erythrocyte protoporphyrin occurs in the absence of cutaneous photosensitivity and of elevated plasma protoporphyrin.

Treatment consists of reducing sun exposure and the oral administration of the carotenoid β-carotene, which is an effective scavenger of free radicals. This drug increases tolerance to sun exposure in many affected individuals, although it has no effect on deficient ferrochelatase.

An algorithm for the approach to a patient with photosensitivity is illustrated in Fig. 58-1.

PHOTOPROTECTION Since photosensitivity of the skin results from exposure to sunlight, it follows that avoidance of the sun would eliminate these disorders. Unfortunately, social pressures make this an impractical alternative for most individuals, and this has led to a search for better approaches to photoprotection.

Natural photoprotection is provided by structural proteins in the epidermis, particularly keratins and melanin. The amount of melanin and its distribution in cells is genetically regulated, and individuals of darker complexion (skin types IV to VI) are at decreased risk for the development of cutaneous malignancy.

Other forms of photoprotection include clothing and sunscreens. Clothing constructed of tightly woven sun-protective fabrics, irrespective of color, affords substantial protection. Wide-brimmed hats, long sleeves, and trousers all reduce direct exposure. Sunscreens are of two major types—chemical and physical. Chemical sunscreens are chromophores that absorb energy in the UV-B and/or UV-A regions, thereby diminishing photon absorption by the skin (Table 58-5). Sunscreens are rated for their photoprotective effect by their *sun protective factor* (SPF). The SPF is simply a ratio of the time required to produce sunburn erythema with and without sunscreen application. SPF ratings of 15 or higher provide effective protection against UV-B and, to a lesser extent, UV-A. The major categories of chemical sunscreens include *p*-aminobenzoic acid and its esters, benzophenones, anthranilates, cinnamates, and salicylates. Physical sunscreens are light-opaque mixtures containing metal particles such as titanium oxide that scatter light, thereby reducing photon absorption by the skin.

In addition to light absorption, a critical determinant of the photoprotective effect of sunscreens is their ability to remain on the skin, a property known as *substantivity*. In general, the *p*-aminobenzoic acid esters formulated in moisturizing vehicles provide the greatest substantivity.

Photoprotection also can be achieved by limiting the time of exposure during the day. Since the majority of an individual's total lifetime sun exposure may occur by the age of 18, it is important to educate parents and young children about the hazards of sunlight. Simply eliminating exposure at midday will substantially reduce lifetime UV-B exposure.

PHOTOTHERAPY AND PHOTOCHEMOTHERAPY
UVR can also be used therapeutically. The administration of UV-B alone or in combination with topically applied agents can induce remissions of psoriasis and atopic dermatitis.

Photochemotherapy in which topically applied or systemically administered *psoralens* are combined with *UV-A* (PUVA) is also effective in treating psoriasis and in the early stages of cutaneous T cell lymphoma and vitiligo. Psoralens are tricyclic furocoumarins that, when intercalated into DNA and exposed to UV-A, form adducts with pyrimidine bases and eventually form DNA cross-links. These

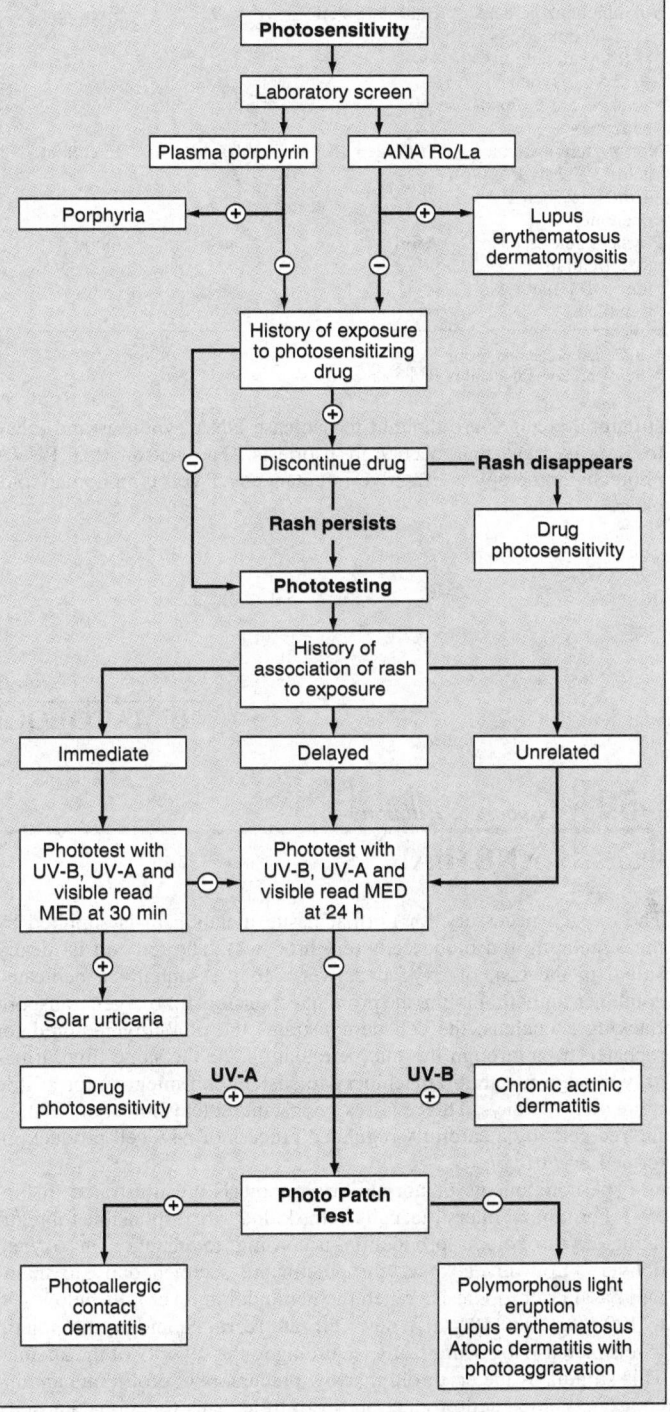

FIGURE 58-1 An algorithm for the diagnosis of a patient with photosensitivity.

Table 58-5

Properties of Selected Sunscreens

Ingredients	Trade Names	SPF* (Outdoors)	Substantivity†
p-Aminobenzoic acid (PABA) (5% in ethanol)	Pre-Sun-15	10–12	Excellent
p-Aminobenzoic acid esters (3.5% padimate A + 3.0% octyldimethyl PABA)	Original Eclipse	4–6	Fair
p-Aminobenzoic acid ester combinations (7.0% padimate O + 2.5% oxybenzone + 5.0% dioxybenzone)	Bain de Soleil	9	Excellent
Non-p-aminobenzoic acid (3% 2-hydroxy-4-methoxy benzophenone)	Ti-Screen-15	10–12	Excellent
Physical sunscreens (5% titanium dioxide + 5% methylanthranilate)	A-Fil	4–6	Good

* SPF, sun protective factor.
† Substantivity is the ability to remain on the skin.

structural changes are thought to decrease DNA synthesis and relate to improvement that occurs in psoriasis. The reason that PUVA photochemotherapy is effective in cutaneous T cell lymphoma is not clear.

In addition to its effects on DNA, PUVA photochemotherapy also stimulates melanin synthesis, and this provides the rationale for its use in the depigmenting disease vitiligo. Oral 8-methoxypsoralen and UV-A appear to be most effective in this regard, but as many as 100 treatments extending over 12 to 18 months may be required to promote satisfactory repigmentation.

The major side effects of UV-B phototherapy and PUVA photochemotherapy are due to the cumulative effects of photon absorption and include skin dryness, actinic keratoses, and an increased risk of nonmelanoma skin cancer. Despite these risks, the therapeutic index of these modalities is quite acceptable.

BIBLIOGRAPHY

FISHER GJ et al: Molecular basis of sun-induced premature skin aging and retinoid antagonism. Nature 379:335, 1996

GILCHREST BA et al: Mechanisms of ultraviolet light-induced pigmentation. Photochem Photobiol 63:1, 1996

GOULD JW et al: Cutaneous photosensitivity diseases induced by exogenous agents. J Am Acad Dermatol 33:551, 1995

HARBER LC, BICKERS DR: *Photosensitivity Diseases*, 2d ed. Toronto, Decker, 1989

HONIGSMANN H, STINGL G: *Therapeutic Photomedicine*. Basel, Karger, 1986

MAGNUS IA: *Dermatological Photobiology*. Oxford, Blackwell, 1976

PATHAK MA et al: Preventive treatment of sunburn, dermatoheliosis, and skin cancer with sun-protective agents, in *Dermatology in General Medicine*, 4th ed, TB Fitzpatrick et al (eds). New York, McGraw-Hill, 1993, Chap. 137

ZIEGLER A et al: Sunburn and p53 in the onset of skin cancer. Nature 372:773, 1994

SECTION 10
HEMATOLOGIC ALTERATIONS

59 *Robert S. Hillman*

ANEMIA

The oxygen necessary for normal tissue metabolism is supplied by the circulating red blood cells (erythrocytes). The red cell is ideally suited to the task of oxygen delivery. It is essentially a dedicated container for hemoglobin, the protein responsible for oxygen transport. Lacking a nucleus, the cell demonstrates the pliability required for repeated trips through the microcirculation. At the same time, it has only enough metabolic machinery to sustain cell integrity for a little more than 100 days. This requires a constant replenishment of circulating red cells by a carefully regulated process of new cell production, termed *erythropoiesis*.

The components of normal erythropoiesis are illustrated in Fig. 59-1. Peritubular interstitial cells of the kidney are responsible for regulating erythropoietin production according to changes in oxygen delivery. Low levels of erythropoietin are secreted daily to maintain basal erythropoiesis. When the hemoglobin level falls below 100 to 120 g/L (10 to 12 g/dL), new cells are recruited and erythropoietin levels increase logarithmically according to the severity of the anemia. This stimulates the erythroid marrow precursors to proliferate and increase red blood cell production severalfold. This functional capacity of the erythron requires normal renal function, a healthy marrow, and an adequate supply of key nutrients, especially iron. A defect in any one or several of the key components in erythropoiesis will result in anemia.

By definition, a patient has an anemia whenever the hemoglobin level or the number of circulating red blood cells is significantly reduced. From a laboratory standpoint, the presence and severity of an anemia are easily described based on the deviation of the patient's hemoglobin/hematocrit from a standard set of normal values. From a clinical perspective, however, the diagnosis of an anemia is more complex. If it were feasible, the most sensitive indicator of anemia would be a direct measure of the level of oxygen delivered to peripheral tissues. Lacking this, a clinically significant anemia is best detected and defined from observed changes in the normal process of erythropoiesis. Measurements of red blood cell production, maturation, morphology, and iron supply are used to identify and initially classify an anemia as a defect in either marrow production, erythroid precursor maturation, or adult red blood cell survival. This functional classification of anemia then serves to guide the selection of a number of clinical and laboratory studies to complete the differential diagnosis of individual disease states.

CLINICAL PRESENTATION

The presence of an anemia may be suspected based on the nature of the patient's illness. Severe hemorrhage will produce an acute blood loss anemia, while chronic blood loss can be expected to result in iron deficiency. On the other hand, a patient with a collagen vascular disease is likely to present with an autoimmune hemolytic anemia. The clinical signs and symptoms of anemia will depend on how rapidly it appears, its severity, and the age of the patient. A mild anemia is easily compensated for by the inate ability of the hemoglobin–oxygen dissociation curve to maintain oxygen delivery to tissues as the hemoglobin level falls (Fig. 107-2). However, the shift in the curve will progressively reduce the capacity of the red cells to respond to situations of increased demand. Patients will report a loss in stamina, a rapid heart rate, and shortness of breath with exercise. When the hemoglobin falls below 70 to 80 g/L (7 to 8 g/dL), exercise capacity is markedly reduced; any exertion is associated with dyspnea, palpitations, a pounding headache, and rapid exhaustion. Older individuals who suffer from cardiovascular disease can develop worsening angina, claudication, and heart failure.

The ability to compensate also depends on the cause and rate of onset of the anemia. Acute blood loss involves a sudden reduction in both the blood volume and the red blood cell mass. While the hemoglobin–oxygen dissociation curve adjustment to release more oxygen to the tissues can make up for a reduced number of circulating red cells (see Chap. 107), even a modest fall in the total blood volume interferes with the cardiovascular response. A patient with severe hemorrhage will demonstrate signs and symptoms of both tissue hypoxia and vascular collapse. This is not true for patients who develop a more chronic anemia where the total blood volume remains normal and changes in cardiac output and regional blood flow help compensate for the loss in oxygen-carrying capacity.

Approach to the Patient

A detailed history and physical examination are essential to the diagnosis and management of an anemia. Clues to the etiology may appear in any part of the history, present illness, past medical history, family history, or review of systems. Symptoms of an acute or chronic illness, information as to transfusion history, past blood count measurements, nutritional habits, drug or alcohol intake, and family history of anemia can all be valuable. Racial background is important since many of the red blood cell metabolic defects follow ethnic lines. Certain complaints provide clues to specific types of anemia. For example, the sickle cell anemia patient will describe a lifelong history of periodic, severe bone and joint pain. Patients with severe iron deficiency often report a sore mouth and difficulty swallowing or have a craving for ice or dirt (pica or picophagia).

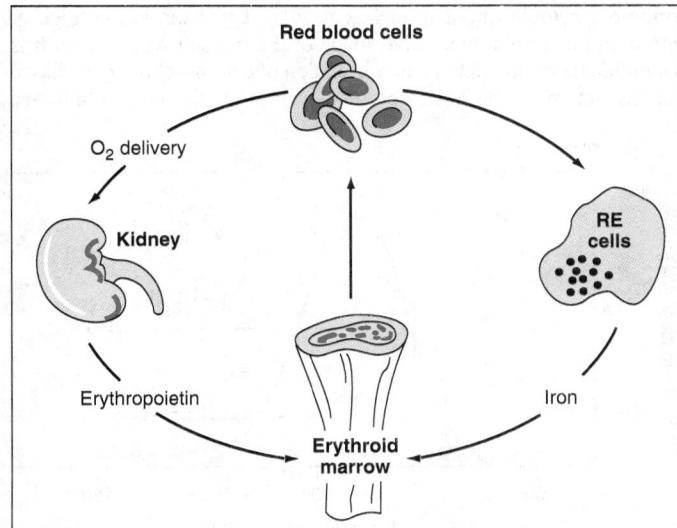

FIGURE 59-1 Components of normal erythropoiesis. The daily replacement of circulating red blood cells and the proliferative response to anemia is regulated by the kidney via release of erythropoietin. The response of the erythroid marrow to increasing levels of erythropoietin requires both a normal marrow and an adequate supply of iron from reticuloendothelial stores and oral intake.

The physical examination of a patient with anemia should emphasize the evaluation of tissue oxygen delivery. With acute blood loss, signs of hypovolemia and tissue hypoxia are the most reliable indicators of anemia severity. When more than 30 percent of the blood volume is suddenly lost, patients are unable to compensate with the usual mechanisms of venospasm and changes in regional blood flow. They will want to remain supine and will exhibit postural hypotension and tachycardia if mobilized. If the blood volume loss exceeds 40 percent (i.e., > 2000 mL in the average-sized adult), signs of hypovolemic shock including confusion, air hunger, diaphoresis, hypotension, and tachycardia will appear. Such patients are experiencing significant deficits in vital organ perfusion and require immediate volume replacement therapy.

When an anemia develops more gradually, hypovolemia is not a concern. In fact, a slight expansion of the blood volume and an increase in cardiac output are signs of effective compensation. The patient will exhibit a forceful apical impulse, strong peripheral pulses with a wide pulse pressure, and a mid- or holosystolic murmur secondary to increased blood flow and turbulence. Pallor of the skin and mucous membranes is another sign of severe anemia [a hemoglobin level < 80 to 100 g/L (8 to 10 g/dL)]. This is less reliable in patients with subcutaneous edema, marked reductions in skin blood flow, or deeply pigmented skin. Therefore, the examination should focus on areas where vessels are close to the surface, for example, the mucous membranes, nail beds, and palmar creases of the hand. When the palmar creases are lighter in color than the surrounding skin, the hemoglobin level is usually less than 80 g/L (8 g/dL).

Very mild anemias produce little in the way of clinical symptoms or signs. This is a tribute to the built-in mechanism of red cell compensation—the ability of the hemoglobin–oxygen dissociation curve to adjust oxygen delivery to tissues. Normally, only the topmost portion of the hemoglobin–oxygen dissociation curve is used, providing a considerable excess capacity for oxygen delivery for increased oxygen demands (see Fig. 107-2). In the case of acute anemia, slight changes in pH and CO_2 concentration at the periphery will instantaneously shift the curve to the right (Bohr effect), thereby increasing the release of oxygen to the tissues. With chronic anemia, the individual red blood cell maintains this shift by increasing the intracellular production of 2,3 bisphosphoglycerate. By itself, this mechanism of compensation is sufficient to maintain a normal delivery of oxygen to tissues despite hemoglobin falls of 20 to 30 g/L (2 to 3 g/dL). Because of this, a mild anemia is usually first detected from a screening measurement of hemoglobin or hematocrit, rather than from the history or physical examination.

Laboratory Evaluation   The clinical laboratory provides a number of tests useful in the diagnosis of anemia (Table 59-1). The most important of these are the complete blood count (CBC), reticulocyte count, and measurements of iron supply, including the serum iron, total iron-binding capacity, and serum ferritin. In patients with severe anemia and abnormalities in red blood cell morphology, a bone marrow aspirate and biopsy are important diagnostic tools. Other assays of value in the diagnosis of specific anemias are discussed in chapters on specific disease states.

COMPLETE BLOOD COUNT   Automated cell counters measure a number of parameters as a part of the CBC, including the hemoglobin, red blood cell count, red blood cell volume distribution, platelet count, and white blood cell count. The counter also calculates the hematocrit (based on the RBC count and volume), the mean cell volume (MCV) (based on volume distribution), mean cell hemoglobin (MCH) (hemoglobin divided by RBC count), mean cell hemoglobin concentration (MCHC) (hemoglobin divided by hematocrit), and the red cell distribution width (RDW). The red cell indices and RDW are used together with a direct inspection of the Wright-stained blood smear to evaluate red blood cell morphology.

The CBC provides a window into a number of the key components of erythropoiesis. The hemoglobin level and hematocrit are used inter-

Table 59-1

Laboratory Tests in Anemia Diagnosis

I. Complete blood count (CBC)
  A. Red blood cell count
    1. Hemoglobin
    2. Hematocrit
  B. Red blood cell indices
    1. Mean cell volume (MCV)
    2. Mean cell hemoglobin (MCH)
    3. Mean cell hemoglobin concentration (MCHC)
    4. Red cell distribution width (RDW)
  C. White blood cell count
    1. Cell differential
    2. Nuclear segmentation of neutrophils
  D. Platelet count
  E. Cell morphology
    1. Cell size
    2. Hemoglobin content
    3. Anisocytosis
    4. Poikilocytosis
    5. Polychromasia
II. Reticulocyte count
III. Iron supply studies
  A. Serum iron
  B. Total iron-binding capacity
  C. Serum ferritin, marrow iron stain
IV. Marrow examination
  A. Aspirate
    1. E/G ratio*
    2. Cell morphology
    3. Iron stain
  B. Biopsy
    1. Cellularity
    2. Morphology

* E/G ratio, ratio of erythroid to granulocytic precursors.

changeably to identify the presence and severity of an anemia according to a set of standard "normal" values (Table 59-2). Normal variations in the CBC with age are shown in the Appendix (Tables A-7 and A-8). Several physiologic and environmental factors can affect these normal values. The influences of age, sex, and pregnancy are recognized in Table 59-2. Higher normal values may be established for adult men and women who live at a high altitude or smoke more than 1 pack of cigarettes per day. This reflects a normal compensation for a decrease in arterial oxygen saturation. Heavy smokers can show an increase in the hemoglobin level of 5 to 10 g/L (0.5 to 1 g/dL) secondary to carbon monoxide binding to hemoglobin. It is also important to recognize that the range of normal values for the hemoglobin and hematocrit describe a Gaussian distribution around the normal mean. Therefore, the actual probability that a patient is anemic will depend on just how much lower the hemoglobin or hematocrit is from the reference value as well as the prevalence of various types of anemia in the population. A hemoglobin level < 100 g/L (< 10 g/dL) in an adult woman is definitely abnormal, while a value of 110 or 120 g/L (11 or 12 g/dL) may or may not indicate anemia.

Other components of the CBC can help in the detection and classification of an anemia. The red blood cell indices, especially the MCV,

Table 59-2

Normal Hemoglobin and Hematocrit Values

Age/Sex	Hemoglobin, g/L	Hematocrit, %
Adolescents	130	40
Adult men	160 (±20)*	47 (±6)*
Adult women	130 (±20)	40 (±6)
Adult women (postmenopausal)	140 (±20)	42 (±6)
Pregnancy (3rd trimester)	120 (±20)	37 (±6)

* ± 2 standard deviations.

Table 59-3

Normal Values for Red Cell Indices

Mean cell volume (MCV)	90 ± 9 fL
Mean cell hemoglobin (MCH)	32 ± 2 pg
Mean cell hemoglobin concentration (MCHC)	33 ± 3%
Red cell distribution width (RDW)	
RDW-CV	13 ± 1%
RDW-SD	42 ± 5 fL

will detect an increase (*macrocytosis*) or decrease (*microcytosis*) in red blood cell volume, while the MCH is sensitive to defects in hemoglobin production (*hypochromia*). The normal values for each of these measurements are listed in Table 59-3. Automated counters are quite precise in describing the red cell volume distribution (Fig. 59-2). The MCV that represents the peak of the distribution curve is not sensitive to the appearance of small populations of macrocytes or microcytes. Measurement errors can also be introduced by major distortions in red cell shape, red blood cell agglutination, or the presence of very high numbers of white blood cells. The technician or clinician can correct for these measurement errors by reviewing the actual red blood cell distribution curve produced by the counter and by direct inspection of the peripheral blood smear.

Automated counters also provide a numerical index of the distribution of red blood cell volumes, the RDW. As shown in Fig. 59-2, the RDW can be measured at two points on the red cell volume distribution curve. The RDW-CV is a ratio calculated as the width of the histogram at one standard deviation divided by the MCV, while the RDW-SD represents the width of the distribution curve at the 20 percent frequency level. Since it is a ratio, the RDW-CV will tend to magnify variations in cell size in patients with microcytic anemias. It is useful, therefore, in separating patients with early iron deficiency who have a mixed population of small and normal sized cells from the patient with thalassemia minor with more uniform microcytosis. At the same time, the RDW-CV is less sensitive to early macrocytosis. In contrast, the RDW-SD is very sensitive to the appearance of even small populations of microcytes or macrocytes.

PERIPHERAL BLOOD FILM Inspection of the peripheral blood film can provide important information as to the presence and nature of an erythropoietic defect. Careful preparation of the blood film is very important. Using glass slides or coverslips and a cytocentrifuge, a small drop of blood can be spread to create a monolayer of red blood cells. The well-dried blood film is then stained with Wright's stain to bring out cytoplasmic and nuclear details. If the film is too thick or too thin, the normal biconcave shape of the red cell will be lost. It is essential, therefore, that the interpretation of cell morphology be based on inspection of the best area of a well-prepared blood film. (**See**

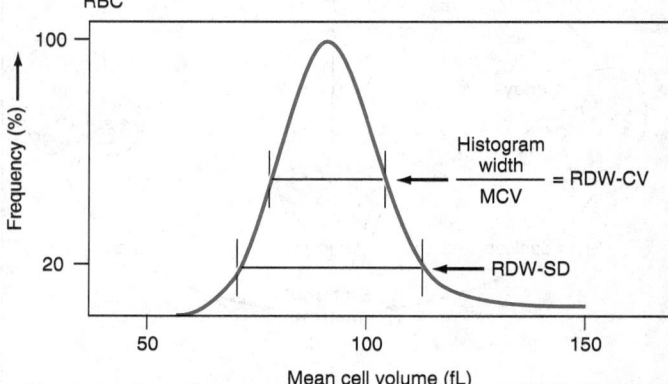

FIGURE 59-2 Automated cell counters display a distribution curve of the red blood cell volume and calculate two measurements of the width of the distribution curve. The RDW-CV is calculated as a ratio of the width of the curve at 1 standard deviation divided by the MCV. The RDW-SD is simply the width of the curve measured at the 20 percent frequency level (RDW, red cell distribution width). (From Hillman and Ault.)

Plate IV-1.) As a complement to the red cell indices, changes in individual cell diameter, shape, and hemoglobin content are looked for to identify microcytosis or macrocytosis even before there is a dramatic change in MCV, MCH, or RDW. The blood film is also important in describing variations in cell size (*anisocytosis*) and shape (*poikilocytosis*). The degree of anisocytosis usually correlates with increases in the RDW. Poikilocytosis suggests a defect in red blood cell precursor maturation or fragmentation hemolysis. The smear should also be inspected for *polychromasia*, that is, the presence of polychromatic macrocytes—cells that are slightly larger and grayish-blue in color. These are marrow reticulocytes containing residual amounts of RNA and ribosomes. They appear in the circulation in response to increased levels of erythropoietin stimulation and, therefore, can be used as a marker of the appropriateness of the erythropoietin response. Other individual cell abnormalities, including the appearance of nucleated red blood cells, Howell-Jolly bodies, targeting, sickle cells, etc., are clues to specific disease states.

RETICULOCYTE COUNT Like the CBC, an accurate measure of the reticulocyte count is key to the initial classification of any anemia. Reticulocytes are newborn red blood cells that contain sufficient residual RNA that they can be stained with a supravital dye and counted as a percent of the circulating red cell population. In the basal state, the normal reticulocyte count ranges from 1 to 2 percent according to the counting method. This correlates with the normal daily replacement of approximately 1 percent of the circulating red blood cell population. Increases in the reticulocyte count provide a reliable measure of the red blood cell production response to anemia.

To use the reticulocyte count as a production measure, it must first be corrected for changes in the patient's hematocrit and for the effect of erythropoietin on the early release of marrow reticulocytes into circulation. The hematocrit (Hct) correction converts the reticulocyte percentage to an absolute number:

$$\% \text{ Reticulocytes} \times \frac{\text{patient Hct}}{45\%} = \text{absolute \% reticulocytes}$$

The marrow reticulocyte ("shift") correction involves dividing the absolute percentage by a factor of 1.5 to 2.5 whenever there is prominent polychromasia on the peripheral blood smear (Fig. 59-3). The shift correction should always be applied to any patient with anemia and a very high reticulocyte count to provide a true index of effective red blood cell production. A normal patient will respond to a hematocrit less than 30 percent with a two- to threefold increase in the reticulocyte production index. Patients with severe, chronic hemolytic anemias can easily demonstrate a reticulocyte index of greater than five to six times normal. This measure alone, therefore, will confirm the fact that the patient has an appropriate erythropoietin response, a normal erythroid marrow, and sufficient iron supply to meet the challenge. When the reticulocyte index falls below 2, a defect in marrow proliferation or precursor maturation must be present.

TESTS OF IRON SUPPLY Standard measurements of iron supply include the serum iron, transferrin iron-binding capacity (TIBC), and the serum ferritin level. The normal serum iron ranges from 9 to 27 μmol/L (50 to 150 μg/dL), while the normal TIBC is 54 to 64 μmol/L (300 to 360 μg/dL). Therefore, in the basal state, only 30 to 50 percent of the transferrin in circulation is saturated with iron. Important information is provided by each measurement as well as the calculated percent saturation. The serum ferritin is used to evaluate body iron stores. Adult males have serum ferritin levels of between 50 and 150 μg/L, corresponding to iron stores of from 600 to 1000 mg. Adult females have lower serum ferritin levels (15 to 50 μg/L) and smaller iron stores (0 to 300 mg). Lower serum ferritin levels are observed as iron stores are depleted; levels below 15 μg/L indicate store exhaustion and iron deficiency. Iron overload (hemachromatosis and hemosiderosis) can produce levels in excess of 500 to 1000 μg/L.

BONE MARROW EXAMINATION A sample of bone marrow is readily obtained by needle aspirate or biopsy. It is of greatest value in patients who have a hypoproliferative anemia or a disorder of red blood cell maturation, providing valuable information as to marrow structure and cellularity, as well as precursor proliferation and maturation. The ratio of erythroid to granulocytic precursors (E/G ratio) is used to assess the proliferative capacity of erythroid precursors. A patient with a hypoproliferative anemia and a reticulocyte index < 2 will demonstrate an E/G ratio ≤ 1:3 or 1:2. In contrast, the hemolytic anemia patient with a production index ≥ 3 to 5 will have an E/G ratio > 1:1. Red cell precursor maturation defects are identified from the mismatch between the E/G ratio and reticulocyte production index. These individuals demonstrate an E/G ratio of greater than 1:1 together with a low reticulocyte index, typical of the ineffective erythropoiesis of a maturation disorder.

ADDITIONAL LABORATORY MEASUREMENTS There are a number of other laboratory tests that are of value in the diagnosis of specific disease states. Details as to the use of these tests are covered in the discussion of individual disorders. Normal values are listed in the "Appendix: Laboratory Values of Clinical Importance."

APPROACH TO ANEMIA DIAGNOSIS

The evaluation of anemia, whether a primary hematologic disorder or secondary to other illness, is common in clinical practice. Success will depend not only on the clinician's knowledge and understanding of causes of anemia but also on the speed and skill of the evaluation. As a rule, a significant anemia should be studied without delay, using a battery of laboratory tests so as to get a clear picture of the erythropoietic abnormality. This will help avoid the misinterpretation of a test because of a change in the patient's clinical status. For example, the ability to diagnose a nutritional anemia will be confounded as a patient changes diet or receives vitamin or mineral supplements. A blood transfusion given before the workup will, by reducing the erythropoietin response, change the red cell production measurements needed for diagnosis. It is also important never to assume a diagnostic relationship. Even when the cause of the anemia is suggested by the clinical presentation, a full laboratory evaluation is essential. Anemias are often the result of several contributing factors and not a single etiologic component.

INITIAL CLASSIFICATION OF ANEMIA The first step in anemia diagnosis is the classification according to the functional defect in erythropoiesis—whether there is a failure in red blood cell produc-

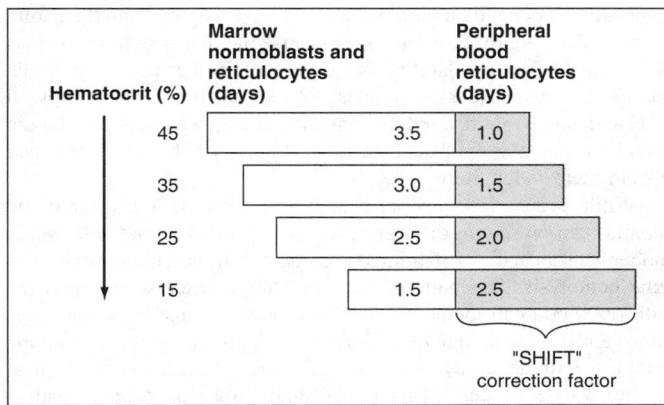

Hematocrit (%)	Marrow normoblasts and reticulocytes (days)	Peripheral blood reticulocytes (days)
45	3.5	1.0
35	3.0	1.5
25	2.5	2.0
15	1.5	2.5

"SHIFT" correction factor

FIGURE 59-3 Reticulocyte "shift" correction. As the level of erythropoietin stimulation increases with worsening anemia, marrow reticulocytes leave the marrow at an earlier point in their maturation. This effectively lengthens the maturation time in circulation and allows them to be counted for more than 1 day. This needs to be taken into account when interpreting the reticulocyte count. Whenever there is prominent polychromasia on the peripheral smear, the predicted delay in maturation of from 1.5 to 2.5 days should be used as a "shift" correction factor to calculate the true reticulocyte production index:

$$\frac{\text{Absolute \% reticulocytes}}{\text{"Shift" factor}} = \text{reticulocyte production index}$$

(From Hillman and Ault.)

tion, an abnormality in precursor maturation, or an increase in red blood cell destruction. In a patient with a moderate to severe anemia, the CBC and reticulocyte index are enough to make this distinction. As shown in Fig. 59-4, a defect in red cell production (hypoproliferative anemia) will show a low reticulocyte production index together with little or no change in red blood cell morphology, that is, a normocytic, normochromic anemia. Maturation disorders also demonstrate a low reticulocyte index but accompanied by either a macrocytic or microcytic morphology. Increased red blood cell destruction secondary to hemolysis or hemorrhage typically results in an increase in the reticulocyte index to levels greater than three times normal. Red blood cell morphology will depend on the specific disease state. The MCV is usually normal or slightly increased depending on the level of reticulocytosis. Inspection of the smear may reveal distinctive cell shapes that help make a specific diagnosis. Classifying an anemia according to the functional defect helps organize the subsequent use of laboratory studies.

HYPOPROLIFERATIVE ANEMIAS The majority of anemias seen in clinical practice are hypoproliferative, that is, they result from a failure in the appropriate erythroid marrow production response for the degree of anemia. As illustrated in Fig. 59-4, they can result from marrow damage (Chap. 110), iron deficiency, or a failure of the normal erythropoietin response to anemia (Chap. 106). The latter can reflect a suppression of erythropoietin release by inflammatory cytokines, a reduced metabolic need, or the permanent loss of peritubular interstitial cells as a part of end-stage renal disease. The laboratory measurements that help distinguish between these defects include the iron supply studies and bone marrow examination. Patients with the anemia of acute or chronic inflammation demonstrate a distinctive pattern of serum iron, TIBC, and serum ferritin. The same is true for iron loss leading to iron

deficiency. A primary failure in precursor proliferation due to marrow damage by a drug, leukemic change, or tumor infiltration can usually be diagnosed from the bone marrow morphology.

MATURATION DISORDERS Defects in erythroid precursor maturation are initially recognized from the combination of a low reticulocyte production index and a distinctive change in morphology. Patients present with either a macrocytic (MCV > 100 fL) or microcytic (MCV < 80 fL) anemia. The low reticulocyte index is a reflection of the ineffective erythropoiesis that results from the defect in precursor maturation. An examination of marrow morphology will show an increase in the E/G ratio to levels greater than 1:1, confirming the proliferation of the erythroid marrow. The reason for the failure in precursor development may also be apparent. A defect in nuclear maturation that produces a macrocytic anemia will demonstrate megaloblastic bone marrow morphology (Chap 108). Patients with cytoplasmic maturation defects will have poor hemoglobinization of the more mature erythroid precursors.

The most common causes of the nuclear and cytoplasmic maturation defects are listed in Fig. 59-4. Severe iron deficiency and the inherited defects in globin chain synthesis, the thalassemias, produce a moderate to marked microcytic, hypochromic anemia (Chap. 107). These disorders may be differentiated simply on the basis of blood smear morphology and the racial background of the patient. If not, measurements of iron supply will help make the diagnosis. Inherited or acquired abnormalities in mitochondrial function can result in either a microcytic or macrocytic anemia. Based on the distinctive finding of ringed sideroblasts on the marrow iron stain, they are initially classified as sideroblastic anemias (Chap. 106). Here again, iron supply studies are important to the differential diagnosis and management of the patient. Defects in nuclear maturation result from a deficiency in folic acid or vitamin B_{12}, exposure to a chemotherapeutic agent, and as a component of a myelodysplastic or preleukemic state (Chap. 110). As with the differential diagnosis of cytoplasmic defects, marrow morphology and iron studies are helpful in the differential diagnosis of the etiology of the disorder. Measurements of folic acid and vitamin B_{12} levels are of value in identifying a reversible vitamin deficiency.

INCREASED RED CELL DESTRUCTION This category of anemia is easily identified from the increase in the reticulocyte production index, together with normocytic or only slightly macrocytic red cell morphology (Fig. 59-4). This is a reflection of the capacity of the erythroid marrow to compensate for a blood loss or red cell hemolysis anemia with an increase in red blood cell production. The level of response will depend on both the severity of the anemia and the nature of the underlying disease process. Because the response to blood loss is limited by the availability of sources of iron supply, the initial reticulocyte response usually does not exceed three times the basal level and may be short-lived. In contrast, patients with acute or chronic hemolytic anemias will achieve much higher production levels and sustain them indefinitely.

While acute blood loss is usually clinically obvious, hemolytic anemias can present in different ways (Chap. 109). Some will appear suddenly as an acute, self-limited episode of intravascular or extravascular hemolysis. This pattern of presentation is often seen in patients with red blood cell metabolic defects or autoimmune hemolytic anemias. Patients with inherited defects of hemoglobin or membrane structure will generally describe a lifelong clinical history typical of the disease process. This is especially true for patients with a hemoglobinopathy such as sickle cell disease or combinations of sickle hemoglobin with other hemoglobinopathies (Chap. 107). Similarly, the patient with hereditary spherocytosis, a common membrane structural defect, will present with a complication stemming from their lifelong need to maintain a high level of red blood cell production, a hemolytic or aplastic crisis, symptomatic bilirubin gallstones, or significant splenomegaly (Chap. 109).

The differential diagnosis of the cause of an acute or chronic hemolytic anemia requires the careful integration of racial and family history data, the pattern of clinical presentation, and a number of targeted laboratory studies. Some of the more common congenital hemolytic anemias may be identified from the red blood cell morphol-

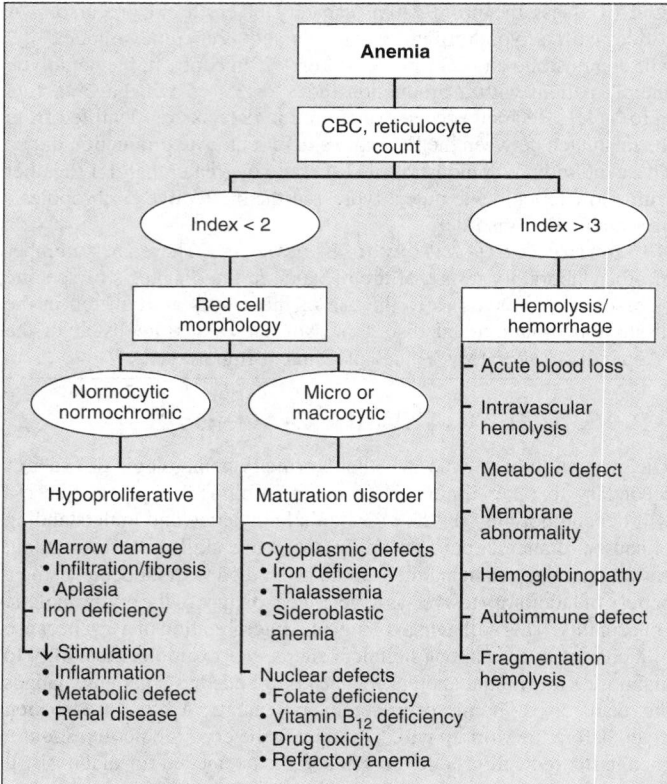

FIGURE 59-4 The classification of anemia. The complete blood count and reticulocyte index are used initially to classify an anemia as either hypoproliferative, a maturation disorder, or a hemolytic/hemorrhagic anemia. This provides a guide to the subsequent differential diagnosis of specific disease states within each category. The bone marrow examination and measurements of iron supply are very important in this differential.

ogy or a routine laboratory test such as the hemoglobin electrophoresis or an enzyme screening test. For example, the common β-chain hemoglobinopathies—sickle cell disease, hemoglobin SC disease, and sickle-thalassemia—have distinctive hemoglobin electrophoretic patterns. Glucose-6-phosphate dehydrogenase (G6PD) deficiency, a common red blood cell metabolic defect, can be easily screened for using a G6PD enzyme spot test. There are, however, a large number of other defects of red cell membrane, hemoglobin, and intracellular metabolism that can only be diagnosed with the help of an expert hematology reference laboratory.

℞ TREATMENT

The management of anemia begins at the time of evaluation. While it is important to perform a careful history, physical examination, and order a complete battery of laboratory tests without delay, it is equally important to quickly initiate any indicated treatment. When an anemia is so severe as to threaten the patient's survival, immediate steps must be taken to guarantee oxygen delivery to tissues. This will involve the appropriate infusion of electrolyte and colloid solutions to correct hypovolemia and red blood cell transfusions to guarantee tissue oxygen delivery. Administration of supplemental oxygen may be required. It may also involve the administration of an essential vitamin or chemotherapeutic drug(s) to address a specific disease process.

If the anemia is less severe, red cell transfusions and vitamin or mineral therapy should be withheld until the diagnosis is certain. "Shotgun" therapy where several vitamins and iron are administered simultaneously is never appropriate. The selection of the right therapy should be firmly based on the documented cause or causes of the anemia. Often, more than one etiologic component must be addressed in management. For example, a patient with the anemia of end-stage renal disease will require erythropoietin therapy to correct for the loss of erythropoietin-secreting cells. However, the effectiveness of recombinant erythropoietin will depend on the patient's iron status. If the patient lacks adequate reticuloendothelial iron stores, a failure in iron supply will prevent the erythroid marrow from proliferating in the face of erythropoietin therapy. It is important, therefore, to fully evaluate the patient's iron status before and during therapy.

The therapeutic options for the treatment of various anemias has expanded dramatically during the past two decades. Blood components are readily available and extremely safe. Effective therapies are now well established for the nutritional anemias, the hypoproliferative anemias associated with end-stage renal disease and chronic inflammation, severe aplastic anemia, and the hemolytic anemia associated with autoimmune diseases. Effective chemotherapy to help prevent sickle cell crises in sickle cell anemia patients has become available. In the future, it is anticipated that many of the congenital defects in hemoglobin structure and hemoglobin synthesis will be treated using the newer techniques of molecular engineering.

BIBLIOGRAPHY

Beutler E et al (eds): *Williams Hematology*, 5th ed. New York, McGraw-Hill, 1995, pp 3–22
Hillman RS, Ault KA: *Hematology in Clinical Practice*. New York, McGraw-Hill, 1995
———, Finch CA: *Red Cell Manual*, 7th ed. Philadelphia, FA Davis, 1996

60   *Robert I. Handin*

BLEEDING AND THROMBOSIS

Hemorrhage, intravascular thrombosis, and embolism are common clinical manifestations of many diseases. The normal hemostatic system limits blood loss by precisely regulated interactions between components of the vessel wall, circulating blood platelets, and plasma proteins. However, when disease or trauma damage large arteries and veins, excessive bleeding may occur, despite a normal hemostatic system. Less frequently, hemorrhage is caused by an inherited or acquired disorder of the hemostatic machinery itself. A large number of such bleeding disorders have now been identified.

In addition, unregulated activation of the hemostatic system may cause thrombosis and embolism, which can reduce blood flow to critical organs like the brain and myocardium. Although we understand less about the pathophysiology of thrombosis than of hemostatic failure, certain patient groups have been identified that are particularly prone to thrombosis and embolism. These include patients who (1) are immobilized after surgery, (2) have chronic congestive heart failure, (3) have atherosclerotic vascular disease, (4) have a malignancy, or (5) are pregnant. Most of these "thrombosis-prone" patients have no identifiable hemostatic disorder. However, there are certain patient groups who have inherited or acquired a "hypercoagulable" or "prethrombotic" state which predisposes them to recurrent thrombosis.

The cardinal manifestations of disordered hemostasis which cause bleeding or thrombosis are discussed below, along with the clinical approach to diagnosis and evaluation of these patients. Certain information in the patient's history, such as the mode of onset and sites of bleeding, a family bleeding tendency, and a record of drug ingestion help establish the correct diagnosis. Physical examination can identify bleeding in the skin or joint deformities due to previous hemarthroses. Ultimately, however, bleeding disorders are diagnosed by laboratory tests. General screening tests are used first, to document a systemic disorder, and are then supplemented by specific tests of coagulation protein or platelet function to arrive at an accurate diagnosis.

The hypercoagulable or prethrombotic patient can also be identified by a careful history. There are three important clues to this diagnosis: (1) repeated episodes of thromboembolism without an obvious predisposing condition; (2) a family history of thrombosis; and (3) well-documented thromboembolism in adolescents and young adults. Although several tests are being evaluated, there are, as yet, no clinically useful screening tests for the prethrombotic state. However, several of the inherited prethrombotic disorders can be diagnosed with specific immunologic and functional assays.

NORMAL HEMOSTASIS

Accurate diagnosis and treatment of patients with either bleeding or thrombosis requires some knowledge of the pathophysiology of hemostasis. The process can be divided into primary and secondary components and is initiated when trauma, surgery, or disease disrupt the vascular endothelial lining and blood is exposed to subendothelial connective tissue. *Primary hemostasis* is the name given to the process of platelet plug formation at sites of injury. It occurs within seconds of injury and is of prime importance in stopping blood loss from capillaries, small arterioles, and venules (Fig. 60-1). *Secondary hemostasis* consists of the reactions of the plasma coagulation system that result in fibrin formation. It requires several minutes for completion. The fibrin strands that are produced strengthen the primary hemostatic plug. This reaction is particularly important in larger vessels and prevents recurrent bleeding from occurring hours or days after the initial injury. Although presented here as separate events, primary and secondary hemostasis are closely linked. For example, activated platelets accelerate plasma coagulation, and products of the plasma coagulation reaction, such as thrombin, induce platelet activation.

Effective primary hemostasis requires three critical events—platelet adhesion, granule release, and platelet aggregation. Within a few seconds of injury, platelets adhere to collagen fibrils in vascular subendothelium via a specific platelet collagen receptor, glycoprotein Ia/IIa, which is a member of the integrin family. As shown in Fig. 60-2, this interaction is stabilized by the von Willebrand factor, an adhesive glycoprotein which allows platelets to remain attached to the vessel wall despite the high shear forces generated within the vascular lumen. The von Willebrand factor accomplishes this task by

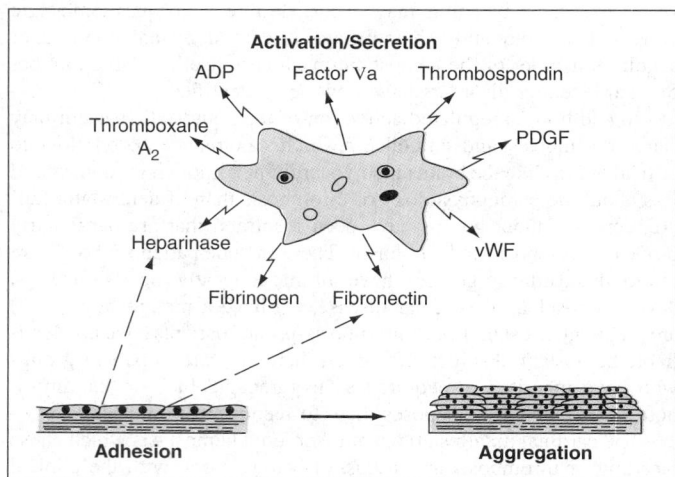

FIGURE 60-1 Schematic presentation of the major events in primary hemostasis. The first event is platelet adhesion, the interaction of platelets with a nonplatelet surface such as vascular subendothelium. This is followed by platelet activation and secretion. Some of the products secreted by platelets are depicted. Abbreviations: ADP, adenosine diphosphate; PDGF, platelet-derived growth factor; vWF, von Willebrand's factor. The final event is the binding of activated platelets to the adherent monolayer in the process of platelet aggregation.

forming a link between a platelet receptor site on glycoprotein Ib/IX and subendothelial collagen fibrils. The adherent platelets then release preformed granule constituents and generate de novo mediators like those depicted in Fig. 60-1.

As in other cells, platelet activation and secretion are regulated by changes in the level of cyclic nucleotides, the influx of calcium, hydrolysis of membrane phospholipids, and phosphorylation of critical intracellular proteins. The relevant pathways are depicted in Figs. 60-3 and 60-4. The binding of agonists such as epinephrine, collagen, or thrombin to platelet surface receptors activates two membrane enzymes—phospholipase C and phospholipase A$_2$. These enzymes catalyze the release of arachidonic acid from two of the major membrane phospholipids, phosphatidylinositol and phosphatidylcholine. Initially, a small quantity of the released arachidonic acid is converted to throm-

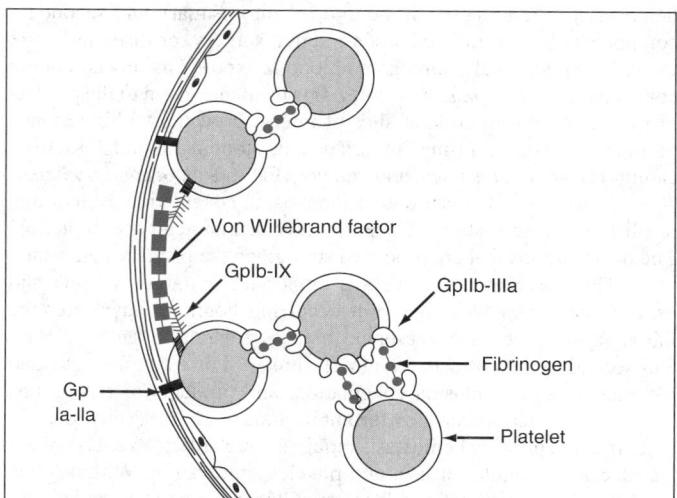

FIGURE 60-2 The molecular basis of platelet adhesion and aggregation. Adhesion of platelets to vascular subendothelium is facilitated by von Willebrand's factor, which forms a bridge between collagen fibrils in the vessel wall and receptors on platelet glycoprotein Ib/IX (GpIb–IX). In a similar manner, platelet aggregation is mediated by fibrinogen which links adjacent platelets via receptors on the platelet glycoprotein IIb and IIIa complex (GpIIb–IIIa).

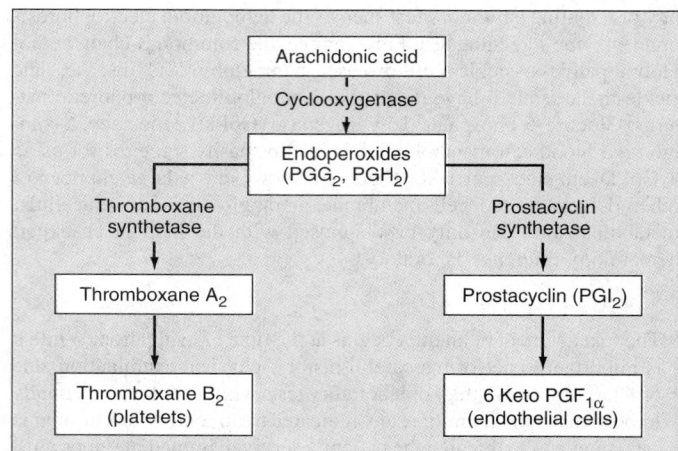

FIGURE 60-3 Generation of thromboxane A$_2$ in platelets and prostacyclin (PGI$_2$) in endothelial cells.

boxane A$_2$ (TXA$_2$), which, in turn, can activate phospholipase C. The formation of TXA$_2$ from arachidonic acid is mediated by the enzyme cyclooxygenase (see Fig. 60-3). This enzyme is inhibited by aspirin and nonsteroidal anti-inflammatory drugs. Inhibition of TXA$_2$ synthesis is a cause of mild bleeding in some patients, as well as the basis for the action of some antithrombotic drugs.

Hydrolysis of the membrane phospholipid phosphatidylinositol 4,5-bisphosphate (PIP$_2$) produces diacylglycerol (DAG) and inositol triphosphate (IP$_3$), both of which play critical roles in platelet metabolism. IP$_3$ mediates the movement of calcium into the platelet cytosol and stimulates the phosphorylation of myosin light chains. The latter interact with actin to facilitate granule movement and platelet shape

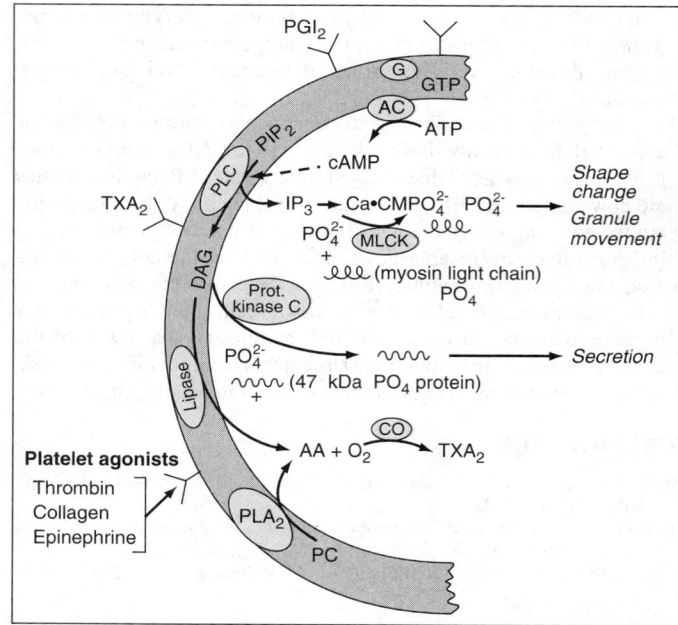

FIGURE 60-4 The biochemical basis of platelet activation and secretion. Binding of agonists such as thrombin, epinephrine, or collagen sets in motion a chain of events which hydrolyzes membrane phospholipids, inhibits adenylate cyclase, mobilizes intracellular calcium, and phosphorylates critical intracellular proteins. The net result is shape change, movement of granules to the canalicular system, generation of mediators like thromboxane A$_2$, and granule secretion. Abbreviations: AC, adenylate cyclase; G, guanine nucleotide–binding protein; PIP$_2$, phosphatidylinositol 4,5-bisphosphate; PLC, phospholipase C; DAG, diacylglycerol; PLA$_2$, phospholipase A$_2$; PC, phosphatidylcholine; AA, arachidonic acid; CO, cyclooxygenase; O$_2$, oxygen; IP$_3$, inositol triphosphate; cAMP, cyclic AMP; Ca-CM, calcium calmodulin complex; MLCK, myosin light chain kinase.

change. DAG activates protein kinase C which, in turn, phosphorylates several substrates, including myosin light chain kinase and a 47,000-Da protein (plekstrin). Phosphorylation of these or other proteins may regulate platelet granule secretion.

A finely balanced mechanism controls the rate and extent of platelet activation, illustrated in Fig. 60-3. TXA_2, a platelet product of arachidonic acid, stimulates platelet activation and secretion. In contrast, prostacyclin (PGI_2), an endothelial cell product of arachidonic acid metabolism, inhibits platelet activation by raising intraplatelet levels of cyclic adenosine monophosphate (cyclic AMP). Similar pathways to regulate activation and secretion occur in other cells.

Following activation, platelets secrete their granule contents into plasma. Endoglycosidases and a heparin-cleaving enzyme are released from lysosomes; calcium, serotonin, and adenosine diphosphate (ADP) are released from the dense granules; and several proteins, including the von Willebrand factor, fibronectin, thrombospondin, the platelet-derived growth factor (PDGF), and a heparin-neutralizing protein (platelet factor 4) are released from alpha granules. Released ADP binds to a specific purinergic receptor which, when activated, changes the conformation of the glycoprotein IIb/IIIa complex so that it binds fibrinogen, linking adjacent platelets into a hemostatic plug (Fig. 60-2). Released PDGF stimulates the growth and migration of fibroblasts and smooth muscle cells within the vessel wall, which is an important part of the repair process.

As the primary hemostatic plug is being formed, plasma coagulation proteins are activated to initiate secondary hemostasis. An overall picture of the coagulation scheme, including the role of various inhibitors, is shown in Fig. 60-5. The coagulation pathway can be broken down into a series of reactions (outlined in Fig. 60-6) which culminate in the production of sufficient thrombin to convert a small portion of plasma fibrinogen to fibrin. Each of the reactions requires the formation of a surface-bound complex and the conversion of inactive precursor proteins into active proteases by limited proteolysis, and each is regulated by both plasma and cellular cofactors and calcium.

In *reaction 1*, the intrinsic or contact phase of coagulation, three plasma proteins, Hageman factor (factor XII), high-molecular-weight kininogen (HMWK), and prekallikrein (PK) form a complex on vascular subendothelial collagen. After binding to HMWK, factor XII is slowly converted to an active protease (XIIa), which then converts both PK to kallikrein and factor XI to its active form (XIa). Kallikrein (K) in turn accelerates the conversion of XII to XIIa, while XIa participates in subsequent coagulation reactions. Although these interactions are well characterized in vitro, an alternative mechanism for the activation of factor XI may exist, as patients who are deficient in either factor XII, HMWK, or PK have apparently normal hemostasis and no clinical bleeding.

Reaction 2 provides a second pathway to initiate coagulation by converting factor VII to an active protease. In this extrinsic or tissue-factor-dependent pathway, a complex is formed between factor VII, calcium, and tissue factor, a ubiquitous lipoprotein present in cellular membranes which is exposed following cellular injury. There is increasing evidence that the tissue factor–VII pathway is continuously active and makes a major contribution to basal coagulation. Factor VII and three other coagulation proteins—factors II (prothrombin), IX, and X—require calcium and vitamin K for biologic activity. These proteins are synthesized in the liver, where a vitamin K–dependent carboxylase catalyzes a unique posttranslational modification which adds a second carboxyl group to certain glutamic acid residues. Pairs of these di-γ-carboxyglutamic acid (Gla) residues bind calcium, which anchors these proteins to negatively charged phospholipid surfaces and confers biologic activity. Inhibition of this posttranslational modification by vitamin K antagonists (e.g., warfarin) is the basis of one of the most common forms of anticoagulant therapy.

In *reaction 3*, factor X is activated by the proteases generated in the two previous reactions. In one reaction, a calcium- and lipid-dependent complex is formed between factors VIII, IX, and X. Within this complex, factor IX is first converted to IXa by factor XIa that was generated within the intrinsic pathway (reaction 1). Factor X is then activated by factor IXa in concert with factor VIII. Alternatively, both factors IX and X can be activated more directly by factor VIIa, which has been generated via the extrinsic pathway (reaction 2). Activation of factors IX and X provides an important link between the intrinsic and extrinsic coagulation pathways (see Fig. 60-5).

Reaction 4, the final step, converts prothrombin to thrombin in the presence of factor V, calcium, and phospholipid. Although prothrombin conversion can take place on various natural and artificial phospholipid-rich surfaces, it proceeds several thousand times faster on the surface of activated platelets. Thrombin, the product of this reaction, has multiple functions in hemostasis. Although its principal role in hemostasis is the conversion of fibrinogen to fibrin, it also activates factors V, VIII, and XIII and stimulates platelet aggregation and secretion. Following the release of fibrinopeptides A and B from the α and β chains of fibrinogen, the modified molecule, now called fibrin monomer, polymerizes into an insoluble gel. The fibrin polymer is then stabilized by the cross-linking of individual chains by factor XIIIa, a plasma transglutaminase (Fig. 60-5).

Although the classic view of coagulation outlined above had clinical utility, it left several important questions unanswered. These included the following: (1) Why does factor XII deficiency produce a dramatically prolonged partial thromboplastin time (PTT) but not cause bleeding? (2) Why is there heterogeneity in the bleeding symptoms of patients with factor XI deficiency? (3) Why do deficiencies in factors VIII or IX produce such dramatic bleeding even though the "extrinsic" pathway remains intact? It is now thought that factors IX and X activation by the tissue factor–VIIa complex plays a major role in the initiation of hemostasis. Once coagulation is initiated by this interaction, a recently discovered protein, the tissue factor pathway inhibitor (TFPI), blocks the pathway, and elements of the intrinsic pathway, particularly factors VIII and IX, become the dominant regulators of thrombin generation. This new step in the pathway would help to explain why factor XIII–deficient patients are asymptomatic and

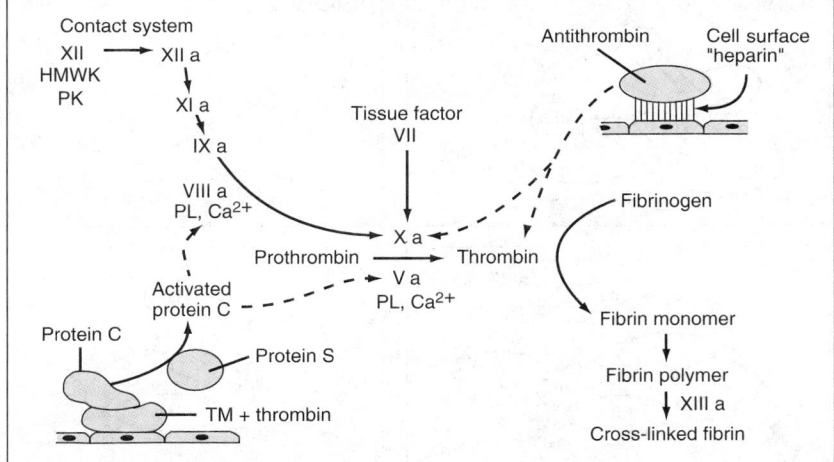

FIGURE 60-5 A schematic diagram of some of the clinically important coagulation reactions. The unactivated or precursor proteins are indicated by roman numerals, and the active form by the addition of a lowercase "a"—a standard convention. Other abbreviations: HMWK, high-molecular-weight kininogen; PK, prekallikrein; PL, phospholipid; TM, thrombomodulin; Ca^{2+}, calcium. There are two independent activation pathways, the contact system and the tissue factor–mediated or extrinsic system. They merge at the point of factor X activation and lead to the generation of thrombin, which converts fibrinogen into fibrin. These reactions are regulated by antithrombin, which forms complexes with all of the coagulation protein serine proteases except factor VII, and by the protein C–protein S system, which inactivates factors V and VIII.

why factor XI–deficient patients have a mild to moderate bleeding diathesis. This scheme is illustrated in Fig. 60-7.

Clot lysis and vessel repair begin immediately after the formation of the definitive hemostatic plug. There are three potential activators of the fibrinolytic system: Hageman factor fragments, urinary plasminogen activator (uPA) or urokinase (UK), and tissue plasminogen activator (tPA). The principal physiologic activators, tPA and uPA, diffuse from endothelial cells and convert plasminogen, adsorbed to the fibrin clot, into plasmin (Fig. 60-8). Plasmin then degrades fibrin polymer into small fragments, which are cleared by the monocyte-macrophage scavenger system. Although plasmin can also degrade fibrinogen, the reaction remains localized because (1) tPA and some forms of uPA activate plasminogen more effectively when it is adsorbed to fibrin clots, (2) any plasmin that enters the circulation is rapidly bound and neutralized by the α_2 plasmin inhibitor (the importance of this inhibitor is underscored by the fact that patients who lack it have unchecked fibrinolysis and bleed), and (3) endothelial cells release a plasminogen activator inhibitor (PAI-1), which directly blocks the action of tPA.

As noted above, the plasma coagulation system is tightly regulated so that only a small quantity of each coagulation enzyme is converted to its active form. As a consequence, the hemostatic plug does not propagate beyond the site of injury. Precise regulation is important, since there is enough clotting potential in a single milliliter of blood to clot all the fibrinogen in the body in 10 to 15 s. Blood fluidity is maintained by the flow of blood itself, which reduces the concentration of reactants; by the adsorption of coagulation factors to surfaces; and by the presence of multiple inhibitors in plasma. Antithrombin, proteins C and S, and TFPI are the most important inhibitors, collectively maintaining blood fluidity.

These inhibitors have distinct modes of action. Antithrombin forms complexes with all the serine protease coagulation factors except factor VII (see Fig. 60-5). Rates of complex formation are accelerated by heparin and heparin-like molecules on the surface of the endothelial cells. This ability of heparin to accelerate the activity of antithrombin is the basis for heparin's action as a potent anticoagulant. Protein C is converted to an active protease by thrombin after it is bound to an endothelial cell protein called thrombomodulin. Activated protein C

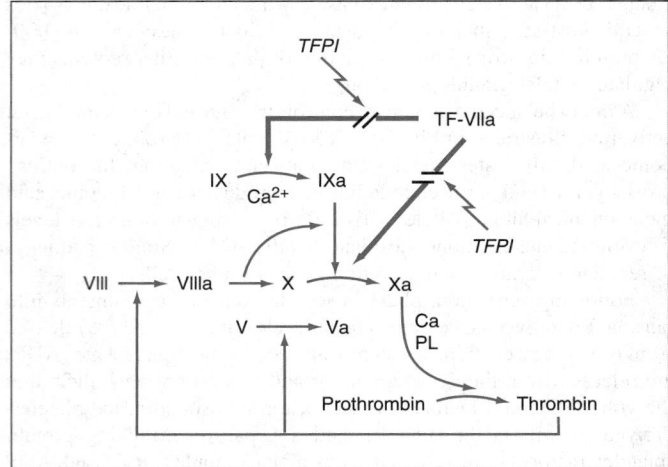

FIGURE 60-7 The contribution of the tissue factor–VIIa complex (TF-VIIa) and tissue factor pathway inhibitor (TFPI) to coagulation. Initial activation of factor IX by TF-VIIa compensates for deficiencies in the early factors, e.g. factors XII and XI. The subsequent inhibition of TF-VIIa by TFPI makes sustained activation of factor X by IXa and VIIIa critical for normal hemostasis. PL, phospholipid.

then inactivates the two plasma cofactors V and VIII by limited proteolysis, which slows down two critical coagulation reactions. Protein C may also stimulate the release of tissue plasminogen activator from endothelial cells. The inhibitory function of protein C is enhanced by protein S. As one might predict, reduced levels of antithrombin or proteins C and S, or dysfunctional forms of these molecules, result in a hypercoagulable or prethrombotic state. In addition, a particularly common heritable defect associated with a hypercoagulable state is the presence of a form of factor V (factor V Leiden) that is resistant to protein C inhibition. Twenty to fifty percent of patients with unexplained venous thromboembolism may have this defect.

The preceding description of blood coagulation implies that the process is uniform throughout the body. In fact, the process is not uniform, and the composition of the blood clot varies with the site of injury. Hemostatic plugs or thrombi that form in veins where blood flow is slow are rich in fibrin and trapped red blood cells and contain relatively few platelets. They are often called *red thrombi* because of their appearance in surgical and pathologic specimens. The friable ends of these red thrombi, which often form in leg veins, can break off and embolize to the pulmonary circulation. Conversely, clots that form in arteries under conditions of high flow are predominantly composed of platelets and have little fibrin. These *white thrombi* may readily dislodge from the arterial wall and embolize to distant sites, causing temporary or permanent ischemia. These clots are a particularly common cause of embolism in the cerebral and retinal circulation, where they may lead to transient neurologic dysfunction (transient ischemic attacks), including temporary monocular blindness (amaurosis fugax), or to strokes. In addition, most episodes of myocardial infarction are due to thrombi that form after the rupture of atherosclerotic plaques within diseased coronary arteries. It is important to remember that there is little difference between hemostatic plugs, which are a physiologic response to injury, and pathologic thrombi. To underscore the similarity, thrombosis has been described as coagulation occurring in the wrong place or at the wrong time.

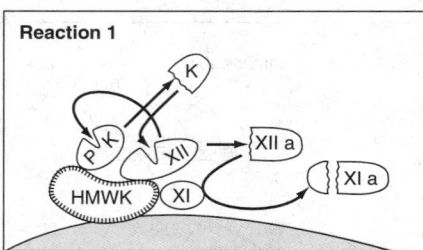

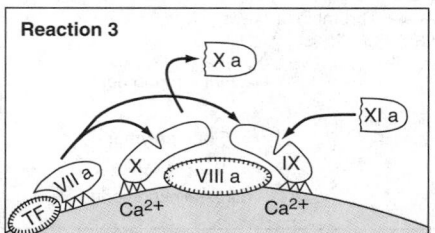

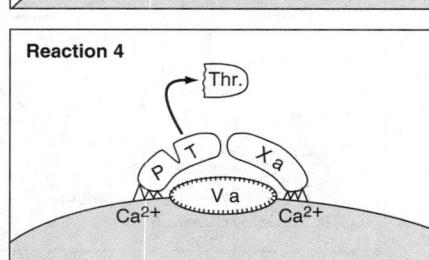

FIGURE 60-6 The major coagulation reactions are subdivided and depicted in schematic form to emphasize their similarity. They all rely on the formation of surface-bound enzyme-cofactor complexes. Abbreviations: PK, prekallikrein; K, kallikrein; HMWK, high-molecular-weight kininogen; TF, tissue factor; Ca²⁺, calcium; PT, prothrombin; Thr, thrombin. By convention, other coagulation factors are indicated by roman numerals, with a lowercase "a" appended to indicate their active form. The ∧∧∧ is used to indicate the Gla (di-γ-carboxyglutamic acid)–containing domains of factors VII, IX, X, Xa, and PT, which bind calcium and phospholipid. Hatching is used to indicate proteins that adhere to surfaces by hydrophobic interaction.

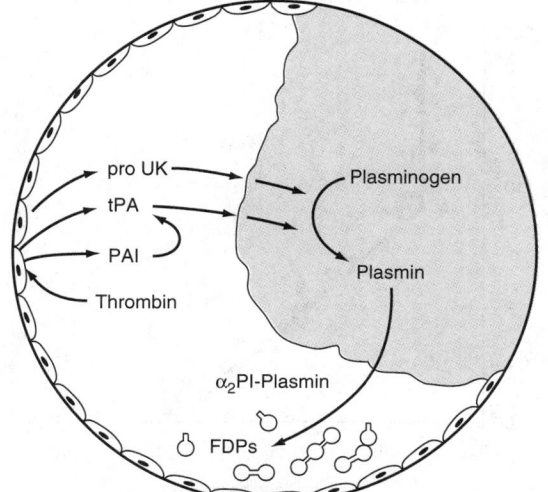

FIGURE 60-8 A schematic diagram of the fibrinolytic pathway. Tissue plasminogen activator (tPA) is released from endothelial cells, enters the fibrin clot, and activates plasminogen to plasmin. Any free plasmin is complexed with alpha$_2$ plasmin inhibitor (α_2PI). Fibrin is degraded to low-molecular-weight fragments, fibrin degradation products (FDPs).

CLINICAL EVALUATION

HISTORY Certain elements of the history are particularly useful in determining whether bleeding is caused by an underlying hemostatic disorder or by a local anatomic defect. One clue is a history of bleeding following common hemostatic stresses such as dental extraction, childbirth, or minor surgery. Bleeding that is sufficiently severe to require a blood transfusion merits special attention. A family history of bleeding and bleeding from multiple sites that cannot be linked to trauma or surgery also suggest a systemic disorder. Since bleeding can be mild, lack of a family history of bleeding does not exclude an inherited hemostatic disorder.

It may be possible to localize the defect to either the platelet or the plasma coagulation system (Table 60-1). Bleeding from a platelet disorder is usually localized to superficial sites such as the skin and mucous membranes, comes on immediately after trauma or surgery, and is readily controlled by local measures. In contrast, bleeding from secondary hemostatic or plasma coagulation defects occurs hours or days after injury and is unaffected by local therapy. Such bleeding most often occurs in deep subcutaneous tissues, muscles, joints, or body cavities. A careful and thorough history is probably the most important step in establishing the presence of a hemostatic disorder and in guiding initial laboratory testing.

Table 60-1

Differences in the Clinical Manifestations of Disorders of Primary and Secondary Hemostasis

Manifestations	Defects of Primary Hemostasis (Platelet Defects)	Defects of Secondary Hemostasis (Plasma Protein Defects)
Onset of bleeding after trauma	Immediate	Delayed—hours or days
Sites of bleeding	Superficial—skin, mucous membranes, nose, gastrointestinal and genitourinary tracts	Deep—joints, muscle, retroperitoneum
Physical findings	Petechiae, ecchymoses	Hematomas, hemarthroses
Family history	Autosomal dominant	Autosomal or X-linked recessive
Response to therapy	Immediate; local measures effective	Requires sustained systemic therapy

PHYSICAL EXAMINATION In conjunction with a careful history, physical examination can also be of help in evaluating patients with hemostatic disorders. The most common site to observe bleeding is in the skin and mucous membranes. Collections of blood in the skin are called *purpura* and may be subdivided on the basis of the site of bleeding in the skin. Small pinpoint hemorrhages into the dermis due to the leakage of red cells through capillaries are called *petechiae* and are characteristic of platelet disorders—in particular, severe thrombocytopenia. Larger subcutaneous collections of blood due to leakage of blood from small arterioles and venules are called *ecchymoses* (common bruises) or, if somewhat deeper and palpable, *hematomas*. They are also common in patients with platelet defects and result from minor trauma. There are other skin and mucous membrane lesions, like dilated capillaries or *telangiectasia*, that may cause bleeding without any hemostatic defect. In addition, the loss of connective tissue support for capillaries and small veins that accompanies aging increases the fragility of superficial vessels, such as those on the dorsum of the hand, leading to extravasation of blood into subcutaneous tissue—*senile purpura*. Menorrhagia is sometimes a serious problem in women with severe thrombocytopenia or platelet dysfunction. In addition, some patients with primary hemostatic defects, especially von Willebrand's disease, may have recurrent gastrointestinal hemorrhage.

As mentioned previously, bleeding into body cavities, the retroperitoneum, or joints is a common manifestation of plasma coagulation defects. Repeated joint bleeding may cause synovial thickening, chronic inflammation, and fluid collections and may erode articular cartilage and lead to chronic joint deformity and limited mobility. Such deformities are particularly common in deficiencies of factors VIII and IX, the two sex-linked coagulation disorders referred to as the *hemophilias*. For unclear reasons, hemarthroses are much less common in patients with other plasma coagulation defects. Blood collections in various body cavities or soft tissues can cause secondary necrosis of tissues or nerve compression. Retroperitoneal hematomas can cause femoral nerve compression, and large collections of poorly coagulated blood in soft tissues occasionally mimic malignant growths—the pseudotumor syndrome. Two of the most life-threatening sites of bleeding are in the oropharynx, where bleeding can compromise the airway, and in the central nervous system. Intracerebral hemorrhage is one of the leading causes of death in patients with severe coagulation disorders.

LABORATORY TESTS The most important screening tests of the primary hemostatic system are (1) a *bleeding time* (a sensitive measure of platelet function) and (2) a *platelet count*. The latter is particularly useful, as it is readily available and correlates well with the propensity to bleed. The normal platelet count is 150,000 to 450,000 platelets per microliter of blood. As long as the count is above 100,000/μL, however, patients usually are not symptomatic, and the bleeding time remains normal. Platelet counts of 50,000 to 100,000/μL cause mild prolongation of the bleeding time, so that bleeding occurs after severe trauma or other stress. Patients with platelet counts of less than 50,000/μL have easy bruising, which is manifested by skin purpura after minor trauma and bleeding after mucous membrane surgery. Patients with a platelet count below 20,000/μL have an appreciable incidence of spontaneous bleeding, usually have petechiae, and may have intracranial or other spontaneous internal bleeding. The major causes of thrombocytopenia are outlined in Table 60-2.

Patients with qualitative platelet abnormalities have a normal platelet count and a prolonged bleeding time (Table 60-3). The bleeding time is ascertained by making a small, superficial skin incision and timing the duration of blood flow from the wounded area. Although this is a rather crude "bioassay," by careful standardization it has become a reliable and sensitive test of platelet function. The most widely used technique uses a template or an automated scalpel to control the length and depth of the incision (usually 1 mm deep by 9 mm long) and a sphygmomanometer inflated to 40 mmHg to distend the capillary bed of the forearm uniformly. In order to be useful, the

Table 60-2

Causes of Thrombocytopenia

Decreased marrow production of megakaryocytes
  Marrow infiltration with tumor, fibrosis
  Marrow failure—aplastic, hypoplastic anemias, drug effects
Splenic sequestration of circulating platelets
  Splenic enlargement due to tumor infiltration
  Splenic congestion due to portal hypertension
Increased destruction of circulating platelets
  Nonimmune destruction
    Vascular prostheses, cardiac valves
    Disseminated intravascular coagulation
    Sepsis
    Vasculitis
  Immune destruction
    Autoantibodies to platelet antigens
    Drug-associated antibodies
    Circulating immune complexes (systemic lupus erythematosus, viral agents, bacterial sepsis)

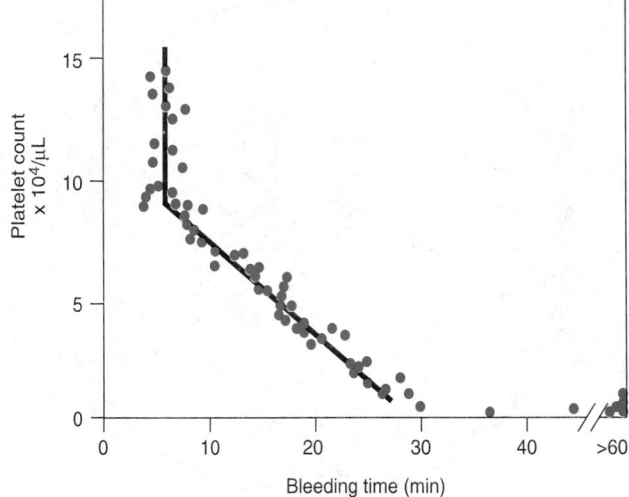

FIGURE 60-9   The relationship between the platelet count and the bleeding time. *(From LA Harker, Hemostasis Manual, 2d ed. Philadelphia, FA Davis Company, 1974.)*

bleeding time test must be performed by an experienced technician, as small differences in technique have a big effect on outcome. Although any patient with a bleeding time over 10 min has an increased risk of bleeding, the risk does not become great until the bleeding time exceeds 15 or 20 min. As shown in Fig. 60-9, there is a roughly linear relationship between the platelet count and the bleeding time. When a defect in primary hemostasis is uncovered, specialized testing is needed to determine the cause of the platelet dysfunction (Table 60-3). A precise diagnosis is important, since patients with bleeding due to a primary hemostatic disorder may need therapy with platelets, with one of several hormones (desmopressin, estrogen, glucocorticoids), or with plasma fractions, depending on the nature of the disorder. Occasional patients with a strong history of bleeding, particularly those with mild von Willebrand's disease, may have a normal bleeding time when initially tested, owing to cyclical variations in the level of the von Willebrand factor. Repeated testing may be necessary to establish an accurate diagnosis.

Plasma coagulation function is readily assessed with a few simple laboratory tests—the partial thromboplastin time (PTT), prothrombin time (PT), thrombin time (TT), and quantitative fibrinogen determination (Fig. 60-5, Table 60-4). The PTT screens the intrinsic limb of the coagulation system and tests for the adequacy of factors XII, HMWK, PK, XI, IX, and VIII. The PT screens the extrinsic or tissue factor–dependent pathway. Both tests also evaluate the common coagulation pathway involving all the reactions that occur after the activation of factor X. Prolongation of the PT and PTT that does not resolve

after the addition of normal plasma suggests a coagulation inhibitor. A specific test for the conversion of fibrinogen to fibrin is needed when both the PTT and PT are prolonged—either a TT or a clottable fibrinogen level can be employed. When abnormalities are noted in any of the screening tests, more specific coagulation factor assays can be ordered to determine the nature of the defect.

There are several rare coagulation abnormalities that may be missed as they do not perturb the results of the screening tests just discussed. They are factor XIII deficiency, α_2 plasmin inhibitor deficiency, PAI-1 deficiency (PAI-1 is the major inhibitor of plasminogen activators), and Scott's syndrome, a platelet coagulant defect. A test for factor XIII–dependent fibrin cross-linking, such as clot solubility in 5 M urea, should be ordered when the PT and PTT are both normal but there is a strong history of bleeding. The fibrinolytic system can be assessed by measuring the rate of clot lysis with the euglobulin lysis or whole blood clot lysis tests and by measuring the levels of α_2 plasmin inhibitor and PAI-1. Scott's syndrome can be detected by measuring the serum prothrombin time, which assesses the amount of residual prothrombin.

Table 60-3

Primary Hemostatic (Platelet) Disorders

Defects of platelet adhesion
  Von Willebrand's disease
  Bernard-Soulier syndrome (absence or dysfunction of GpIb/IX)
Defects of platelet aggregation
  Glanzmann's thrombasthenia (absence or dysfunction of GpIIb/IIIa)
Defects of platelet release
  Decreased cyclooxygenase activity
    Drug-induced—aspirin, nonsteroidal anti-inflammatory agents
    Congenital
  Granule storage pool defects
    Congenital
    Acquired
  Uremia
  Platelet coating (e.g., penicillin or paraproteins)
Defect of platelet coagulant activity
  Scott's syndrome

ABBREVIATION: Gp, glycoprotein.

Table 60-4

Relationship between Secondary Hemostatic Disorders and Coagulation Test Abnormalities

Prolonged partial thromboplastin time (PTT)
  No clinical bleeding—factors XII, HMWK, PK
  Mild or rare bleeding—factor XI
  Frequent, severe bleeding—factors VIII and IX
Prolonged prothrombin time (PT)
  Factor VII deficiency
  Vitamin K deficiency—early
  Warfarin anticoagulant ingestion
Prolonged PTT and PT
  Factor II, V, or X deficiency
  Vitamin K deficiency—late
  Warfarin anticoagulant ingestion
Prolonged thrombin time (TT)
  Mild or rare bleeding—afibrinogenemia
  Frequent, severe bleeding—dysfibrinogenemia
  Heparin-like inhibitors or heparin administration
Prolonged PT and/or PTT not corrected with normal plasma
  Specific or nonspecific inhibitor syndromes
Clot solubility in 5 M urea
  Factor XIII deficiency
  Inhibitors or defective cross-linking
Rapid clot lysis
  α_2 plasmin inhibitor

ABBREVIATIONS: HMWK, high-molecular-weight kininogen; PK, prekallikrein.

Table 60-5

CHAPTER 61
Enlargement of Lymph Nodes and Spleen **345**

Thrombotic Disorders

Inherited
  Defective inhibition of coagulation factors
    factor V Leiden (resistant to inhibition by activated protein C)
    antithrombin III deficiency
    protein C deficiency
    protein S deficiency
  Impaired clot lysis
    dysfibrinogenemia
    plasminogen deficiency
    tPA deficiency
    PAI-1 excess
  Uncertain mechanism
    homocystinuria
Acquired
  Diseases or syndromes
    lupus anticoagulant
    malignancy
    myeloproliferative disorder
    thrombotic thrombocytopenic purpura
    estrogen treatment
    hyperlipidemia
    diabetes mellitus
    hyperviscosity
    nephrotic syndrome
    congestive heart failure
    paroxysmal nocturnal hemoglobinuria
  Physiologic states
    pregnancy (especially postpartum)
    obesity
    postoperative state
    immobilization
    old age

Conditions associated with thrombosis are listed in Table 60-5. There are as yet no useful tests to screen patients suspected of having hypercoagulable or prethrombotic disorders. Tests have been developed in research laboratories which measure small peptides or enzyme-inhibitor complexes generated during coagulation. For example, radioimmunoassays have been developed for fibrinopeptides A and B, for the thrombin-antithrombin complex, and for prothrombin cleavage fragments. Elevated levels of these products have been reported in patients with prethrombotic disorders and in patients with thromboembolism. These tests require meticulous phlebotomy, special anticoagulants, and special handling of the blood and are not in general clinical use. At present, patients suspected of having a hypercoagulable state on the basis of clinical information should be tested with specific assays to screen for the small number of known defects (Table 60-5). Currently available tests can identify 10 to 20 percent of the cases of familial thrombosis, a small fraction of the many patients who present to physicians with thromboembolism.

Inhibitor syndromes or circulating anticoagulants are usually due to antibodies that impair coagulation factor activity. They are an infrequent cause of bleeding and require specialized diagnostic testing. Inhibitors are likely when screening test abnormalities cannot be reversed by adding normal plasma to patient plasma. Antibodies against specific coagulation factors may develop in (1) postpartum women, (2) patients with autoimmune disorders such as systemic lupus erythematosus, (3) patients taking drugs such as penicillin and streptomycin, and (4) otherwise healthy elderly individuals. In addition, between 10 and 20 percent of patients with severe hemophilia who have received multiple plasma infusions develop inhibitor antibodies. Some patients, especially those with systemic lupus erythematosus, may also have a nonspecific form of anticoagulant antibody which interferes with phospholipid binding of coagulation factors and prolongs the PT and PTT but does not cause clinical bleeding. The presence of the lupus anticoagulant may increase the risk of thromboembolism and may cause placental infarction and recurrent midtrimester abortion. Occasionally, patients develop inhibitors that are not antibodies. For example, several patients with clinical bleeding have been found to have circulating mucopolysaccharides that have heparin-like activity.

BIBLIOGRAPHY

Broze GJ: The role of tissue factor pathway inhibitor in a revised coagulation cascade. Blood 29:159, 1992
Colman RW et al (eds): *Hemostasis and Thrombosis: Basic Principles and Clinical Practice*, 4th ed. Philadelphia, Lippincott, 1996
Handin RI: Diseases of the platelet and vessel wall, in *Hematology of Infancy and Childhood*, 5th ed., DG Nathan et al (eds). Philadelphia, Saunders, 1997 (in press)
———— et al (eds): *Blood: Principles and Practice of Hematology and Hematologic Oncology*, 4th ed. Philadelphia, Lippincott, 1994
Lind SE: The bleeding time does not predict surgical bleeding. Blood 77:2547, 1991
Roberts HR, Lozier JN: New perspectives on the coagulation cascade. Hosp Pract Jan 1992, 97

 61   *Patrick H. Henry, Dan L. Longo*

ENLARGEMENT OF LYMPH NODES AND SPLEEN

This chapter is intended to serve as a guide to the evaluation of patients who present with enlargement of the lymph nodes (*lymphadenopathy*) or the spleen (*splenomegaly*). Lymphadenopathy is a rather common clinical finding in primary care settings, whereas palpable splenomegaly is less so.

LYMPHADENOPATHY

Lymphadenopathy may be an incidental finding in patients being examined for various reasons or it may be a presenting sign or symptom of the patient's illness. The physician must eventually decide whether the lymphadenopathy is a normal finding or one that requires further study, up to and including biopsy. Soft, flat, submandibular nodes (<1 cm) are often palpable in healthy children and young adults, and healthy adults may have palpable inguinal nodes of up to 2 cm, which are considered normal. Further evaluation of these normal nodes is not warranted. In contrast, if the physician believes the node(s) to be abnormal, then pursuit of a more precise diagnosis is needed.

Approach to the Patient

Lymphadenopathy may be a primary or secondary manifestation of numerous disorders, as shown in Table 61-1. Many of these disorders are infrequent causes of lymphadenopathy. Analysis of lymphadenopathy in primary care practice has shown that more than two-thirds of patients have nonspecific causes or upper respiratory illnesses (viral or bacterial), and fewer than 1 percent have a malignancy. In one study, researchers reported that 186 of 220 patients (84 percent) referred for evaluation of lymphadenopathy had a "benign" diagnosis. The remaining 34 patients (16 percent) had a malignancy (lymphoma or metastatic adenocarcinoma). Sixty-three percent (112) of the 186 patients with benign lymphadenopathy had a nonspecific or reactive etiology (no causative agent found), and the remainder had a specific cause demonstrated, most commonly infectious mononucleosis, toxoplasmosis, or tuberculosis. Thus, the vast majority of patients with lymphadenopathy will have a nonspecific etiology requiring few diagnostic tests.

Clinical Assessment   The physician will be aided in the pursuit of an explanation for the lymphadenopathy by a careful medical history, physical examination, selected laboratory tests, and perhaps an excisional lymph node biopsy.

The *medical history* should reveal the setting in which lymphadenopathy is occurring. Symptoms such as sore throat, cough, fever, night sweats, fatigue, weight loss, or pain in the nodes should be sought. The patient's age, sex, occupation, exposure to pets, sexual

Table 61-1

Diseases Associated with Lymphadenopathy

1. Infectious diseases
   a. Viral—infectious mononucleosis syndromes (EBV, CMV), infectious hepatitis, herpes simplex, herpesvirus-6, varicella-zoster virus, rubella, measles, adenovirus, HIV, epidemic keratoconjunctivitis, vaccinia
   b. Bacterial—streptococci, staphylococci, cat-scratch disease, brucellosis, tularemia, plague, chancroid, melioidosis, glanders, tuberculosis, atypical mycobacterial infection, primary and secondary syphilis, diphtheria, leprosy
   c. Fungal—histoplasmosis, coccidioidomycosis, paracoccidioidomycosis
   d. Chlamydial—lymphogranuloma venereum, trachoma
   e. Parasitic—toxoplasmosis, leishmaniasis, trypanosomiasis, filariasis
   f. Rickettsial—scrub typhus, rickettsialpox
2. Immunologic diseases
   a. Rheumatoid arthritis
   b. Juvenile rheumatoid arthritis
   c. Mixed connective tissue disease
   d. Systemic lupus erythematosus
   e. Dermatomyositis
   f. Sjögren's syndrome
   g. Serum sickness
   h. Drug hypersensitivity—diphenylhydantoin, hydralazine, allopurinol, primidone, gold, carbamazepine, etc.
   i. Angioimmunoblastic lymphadenopathy
   j. Primary biliary cirrhosis
   k. Graft-vs.-host disease
   l. Silicone-associated
3. Malignant diseases
   a. Hematologic—Hodgkin's disease, non-Hodgkin's lymphomas, acute or chronic lymphocytic leukemia, hairy cell leukemia, malignant histiocytosis, amyloidosis
   b. Metastatic—from numerous primary sites
4. Lipid storage diseases—Gaucher's, Niemann-Pick, Fabry, Tangier
5. Endocrine diseases—hyperthyroidism
6. Other disorders
   a. Castleman's disease (giant lymph node hyperplasia)
   b. Sarcoidosis
   c. Dermatopathic lymphadenitis
   d. Lymphomatoid granulomatosis
   e. Histiocytic necrotizing lymphadenitis (Kikuchi's disease)
   f. Sinus histiocytosis with massive lymphadenopathy (Rosai-Dorfman disease)
   g. Mucocutaneous lymph node syndrome (Kawasaki's disease)
   h. Histiocytosis X
   i. Familial mediterranean fever
   j. Severe hypertriglyceridemia
   k. Vascular transformation of sinuses
   l. Inflammatory pseudotumor of lymph node

behavior, and use of drugs such as diphenylhydantoin are other important historical points. For example, children and young adults usually have benign (i.e., nonmalignant) disorders, such as viral or bacterial upper respiratory infections, infectious mononucleosis, toxoplasmosis, and, in some countries, tuberculosis, which account for the observed lymphadenopathy. In contrast, after age 50 the incidence of malignant disorders increases and benign disorders decreases.

The *physical examination* can provide useful clues such as the extent of lymphadenopathy (localized or generalized), size of nodes, texture, presence or absence of nodal tenderness, signs of inflammation over the node, skin lesions, and splenomegaly. A thorough ear, nose, and throat (ENT) examination is indicated in adult patients with cervical adenopathy and a history of tobacco use. Localized or regional adenopathy implies involvement of a single anatomic area. Generalized adenopathy has been defined as involvement of three or more noncontiguous lymph node areas. Many of the causes of lymphadenopathy (Table 61-1) can produce localized *or* generalized adenopathy, so this distinction is of limited utility in the differential diagnosis. Nevertheless, generalized lymphadenopathy is frequently associated with non-

malignant disorders such as infectious mononucleosis [Epstein-Barr virus (EBV) or cytomegalovirus (CMV)], toxoplasmosis, AIDS, other viral infections, systemic lupus erythematosus (SLE), and mixed connective tissue disease. Acute and chronic lymphocytic leukemias and malignant lymphomas also produce generalized adenopathy in adults.

The site of localized or regional adenopathy may provide a useful clue about the cause. Occipital adenopathy often reflects an infection of the scalp, and preauricular adenopathy accompanies conjunctival infections and cat-scratch disease. The most frequent site of regional adenopathy is the neck, and most of the causes are benign—upper respiratory infections, oral and dental lesions, infectious mononucleosis, other viral illnesses. The chief malignant causes include metastatic cancer from head and neck, breast, lung, and thyroid primaries. Enlargement of supraclavicular and scalene nodes is always abnormal. Because these nodes drain regions of the lung and retroperitoneal space, they can reflect either lymphomas, other cancers, or infectious processes arising in these areas. Virchow's node is an enlarged left supraclavicular node infiltrated with metastatic cancer from a gastrointestinal primary. Metastases to supraclavicular nodes also occur from lung, breast, or genital cancers. Tuberculosis, sarcoidosis, and toxoplasmosis are (non-malignant) causes of supraclavicular adenopathy. Axillary adenopathy is usually due to injuries or localized infections of the ipsilateral upper extremity. Malignant causes include melanoma or lymphoma and, in women, breast cancer. Inguinal lymphadenopathy is usually secondary to infections or trauma of the lower extremities and may accompany sexually transmitted diseases such as lymphogranuloma venereum, primary syphilis, genital herpes, or chancroid. These nodes may also be involved by lymphomas and metastatic cancer from primary lesions of the rectum, genitalia, or lower extremities (melanoma).

The size and texture of the lymph node(s) and the presence of pain are useful parameters in evaluating a patient with lymphadenopathy. Nodes <1.0 cm² in area (1.0 × 1.0 cm or less) are almost always secondary to benign, nonspecific reactive causes. In one retrospective analysis of younger patients (9 to 25 years) who had a lymph node biopsy, a maximum diameter of >2 cm served as one discriminant for predicting that the biopsy would reveal malignant or granulomatous disease. Another study showed that a lymph node size of 2.25 cm² (1.5 cm × 1.5 cm) was the best discriminating limit for distinguishing malignant or granulomatous lymphadenopathy from other causes of lymphadenopathy. Patients with node(s) ≤1.0 cm² should be observed after excluding infectious mononucleosis and/or toxoplasmosis unless there are symptoms and signs of an underlying systemic illness.

The texture of lymph nodes may be described as soft, firm, rubbery, hard, discrete, matted, tender, movable, or fixed. Tenderness is found when the capsule is stretched during rapid enlargement, usually secondary to an inflammatory process. Some malignant diseases such as acute leukemia may produce rapid enlargement and pain in the nodes. Nodes involved by lymphoma tend to be large, discrete, symmetric, rubbery, firm, mobile, and nontender. Nodes containing metastatic cancer are often hard, nontender, and nonmovable because of fixation to surrounding tissues. The coexistence of splenomegaly in the patient with lymphadenopathy implies a systemic illness such as infectious mononucleosis, lymphoma, acute or chronic leukemia, SLE, sarcoidosis, toxoplasmosis, cat-scratch disease, or other less common hematologic disorders. The patient's story should provide helpful clues about the underlying systemic illness.

Nonsuperficial presentations (thoracic or abdominal) of adenopathy are usually detected as the result of a symptom-directed diagnostic workup. Thoracic adenopathy may be detected by routine chest roentgenography or during the workup for superficial adenopathy. It may also be found because the patient complains of a cough or wheezing from airway compression; hoarseness from recurrent laryngeal nerve involvement; dysphagia from esophageal compression; or swelling of the neck, face, or arms secondary to compression of the superior vena cava or subclavian vein. The differential diagnosis of mediastinal and hilar adenopathy includes primary lung disorders and systemic illnesses that characteristically involve mediastinal or hilar nodes. In the young, mediastinal adenopathy is associated with infectious

Enlarged intraabdominal or retroperitoneal nodes are usually malignant. Although tuberculosis may present as mesenteric lymphadenitis, these masses usually contain lymphomas or, in young men, germ cell tumors.

Laboratory Investigation   The laboratory investigation of patients with lymphadenopathy must be tailored to elucidate the etiology suspected from the patient's story and physical findings. One study from a family practice clinic evaluated 249 younger patients with "enlarged lymph nodes, not infected" or "lymphadenitis." The author found that 51 percent had no laboratory studies. When studies were performed, the most common were a complete blood count (33 percent), throat culture (16 percent), chest x-ray (12 percent), or monospot test (10 percent). Only eight patients (3 percent) had a node biopsy, and half of those were normal or reactive. The complete blood count can provide useful data for the diagnosis of acute or chronic leukemias, EBV or CMV mononucleosis, lymphoma with a leukemic component, pyogenic infections, or immune cytopenias in illnesses such as SLE. Serologic studies may demonstrate antibodies specific to components of EBV, CMV, human immunodeficiency virus (HIV), and other viruses; *Toxoplasma gondii*; *Brucella*; etc. If SLE is suspected, then antinuclear and anti-DNA antibody studies are warranted.

The chest x-ray is usually negative, but the presence of a pulmonary infiltrate or mediastinal lymphadenopathy would suggest tuberculosis, histoplasmosis, sarcoidosis, lymphoma, primary lung cancer, or metastatic cancer and demands further investigation.

The indications for lymph node biopsy are imprecise, yet it is a valuable diagnostic tool. The decision to biopsy may be made early in a patient's evaluation or delayed until a sufficient period (approximately 2 weeks) of observation has occurred. Prompt biopsy should occur if the patient's history and physical findings suggest a malignancy; examples include a solitary, hard, nontender cervical node in an older patient who is a chronic user of tobacco; supraclavicular adenopathy; and solitary or generalized adenopathy that is firm, movable, and suggestive of lymphoma. If a primary head and neck cancer is suspected as the basis of a solitary, hard cervical node, then a careful ENT examination should be performed. Any mucosal lesion that is suspicious for a primary neoplastic process should be biopsied first. If no mucosal lesion is detected, an excisional biopsy of the largest node should be performed. Fine-needle aspiration should not be performed as the first diagnostic procedure. Most diagnoses require more tissue than such aspiration can provide and it often delays a definitive diagnosis. Fine-needle aspiration should be reserved for thyroid nodules and for confirmation of relapse in patients whose primary diagnosis is known. If the primary physician is uncertain about whether to proceed to biopsy, consultation with a hematologist or medical oncologist should be helpful. In primary care practices, fewer than 5 percent of lymphadenopathy patients will require a biopsy. That percentage will be considerably larger in referral practices, i.e., hematology, oncology, or otolaryngology (ENT).

Two groups have reported algorithms that they claim will identify more precisely those lymphadenopathy patients who should have a biopsy. Both reports were retrospective analyses in referral practices. The first study involved patients age 9 to 25 years of age who had a node biopsy performed. Three variables were identified that predicted those young patients with peripheral lymphadenopathy who should undergo biopsy; lymph node size >2 cm in diameter and abnormal chest x-ray had positive predictive value, whereas recent ENT symptoms had negative predictive values. The second study evaluated 220 lymphadenopathy patients in a hematology unit and identified five variables [lymph node size, location (supraclavicular or non-supraclavicular), age (>40 years or <40 years), texture (nonhard or hard), and tenderness] that were utilized in a mathematical model to identify those patients requiring a biopsy. Positive predictive value was found

for age >40 years, supraclavicular location, node size >2.25 cm^2, hard texture, and lack of pain or tenderness. Negative predictive value was evident for age <40 years, node size <1.0 cm^2, nonhard texture, and tender or painful nodes. Ninety-one percent of those who required biopsy were correctly classified by this model. Since both of these studies were retrospective analyses and one was limited to young patients, it is not known how useful these models would be if applied prospectively in a primary care setting.

Most lymphadenopathy patients do not require a biopsy, and at least half require no laboratory studies. If the patient's history and physical findings point to a benign cause for lymphadenopathy, then careful follow-up at a 2- to 4-week interval can be employed. The patient should be instructed to return for reevaluation if the node(s) increase in size. Antibiotics are not indicated for lymphadenopathy unless there is strong evidence of a bacterial infection. Glucocorticoids should not be used to treat lymphadenopathy because their lympholytic effect obscures some diagnoses (lymphoma, leukemia, Castleman's disease) and they contribute to delayed healing or activation of underlying infections. An exception to this statement is the life-threatening pharyngeal obstruction by enlarged lymphoid tissue in Waldeyer's ring that is occasionally seen in infectious mononucleosis.

SPLENOMEGALY

STRUCTURE AND FUNCTION OF THE SPLEEN   The spleen is a reticuloendothelial organ that has its embryologic origin in the dorsal mesogastrium at about 5 weeks' gestation. It arises in a series of hillocks, migrates to its normal adult location in the left upper quadrant, and is attached to the stomach via the gastrolienal ligament and to the kidney via the lienorenal ligament. When the hillocks fail to unify into a single tissue mass, accessory spleens may develop in around 20 percent of persons. The function of the spleen has been elusive. Galen believed it was the source of "black bile" or melancholia, and the word *hypochondria* (literally, beneath the ribs) and the idiom "to vent one's spleen" attest to the beliefs that the spleen had an important influence on the psyche and emotions. Some but not all of its secrets have yielded to scientific inquiry. In humans, its normal physiologic roles seem to be the following:

1. Maintenance of quality control over erythrocytes in the red pulp by removal of senescent and defective red blood cells. The spleen accomplishes this function through a unique organization of its parenchyma and vasculature (Fig. 61-1).
2. Synthesis of antibodies in the white pulp.
3. The removal of antibody-coated bacteria and antibody-coated blood cells from the circulation.

An increase in these normal functions may result in splenomegaly with or without hypersplenism.

The spleen is composed of red pulp and white pulp, which are Malpighi's terms for the red blood–filled sinuses and reticuloendothelial cell–lined cords and the white lymphoid follicles arrayed within the red pulp matrix. The spleen is in the portal circulation. The reason for this is unknown but may relate to the fact that lower blood pressure allows less rapid flow and minimizes damage to normal erythrocytes. Blood flows into the spleen at a rate of about 150 mL/min through the splenic artery, which ultimately ramifies into central arterioles. Some blood goes from the arterioles to capillaries and then to splenic veins and out of the spleen, but the majority of blood from central arterioles flows into the macrophage-lined sinuses and cords. The blood entering the sinuses reenters the circulation through the splenic venules, but the blood entering the cords is subjected to an inspection of sorts. In order to return to the circulation, the blood cells in the cords must squeeze through slits in the cord lining to enter the sinuses that lead to the venules. Old and damaged erythrocytes are less deformable and are retained in the cords, where they are destroyed and

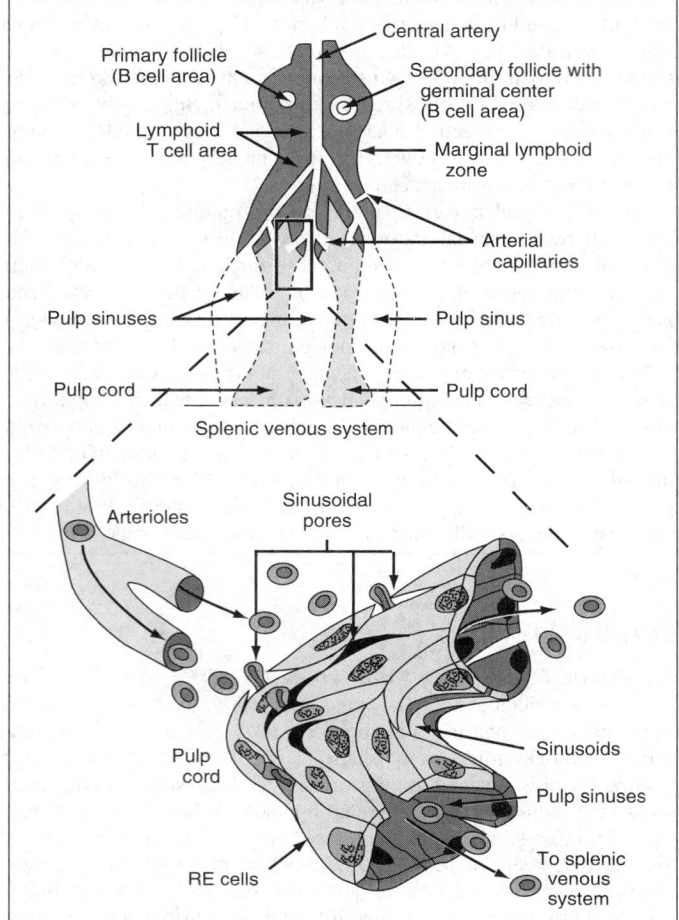

FIGURE 61-1 Schematic spleen structure. The spleen comprises many units of red and white pulp centered around small branches of the splenic artery, called central arteries. White pulp is lymphoid in nature and contains B cell follicles, a marginal zone around the follicles, and T cell–rich areas sheathing arterioles. The red pulp areas include pulp sinuses and pulp cords. The cords are dead ends. In order to regain access to the circulation, red blood cells must traverse tiny openings in the sinusoidal lining. Stiff, damaged, or old red cells cannot enter the sinuses. *(Bottom portion of figure from RS Hillman, KA Ault: Hematology in Clinical Practice. New York, McGraw-Hill, 1995.)*

their components recycled. Red cell inclusion bodies such as parasites, nuclear residua (Howell-Jolly bodies), or denatured hemoglobin (Heinz bodies) are pinched off in the process of passing through the slits, a process called *pitting*. The culling of dead and damaged cells and the pitting of cells with inclusions appear to occur without significant delay since the blood transit time through the spleen is only slightly slower than in other organs.

The spleen is also capable of assisting the host in adapting to its hostile environment. It has at least three adaptational functions: (1) clearance of bacteria and particulates from the blood, (2) the generation of immune responses to certain invading pathogens, and (3) the generation of cellular components of the blood under circumstances in which the marrow is unable to meet the needs (i.e., extramedullary hematopoiesis). The latter adaptation is a recapitulation of the blood-forming function the spleen plays during gestation. In some animals, the spleen also serves a role in the vascular adaptation to stress because it stores red blood cells (often hemoconcentrated to higher hematocrits than normal) under normal circumstances and contracts under the influence of beta-adrenergic stimulation to provide the animal with an autotransfusion and improved oxygen-carrying capacity. However, the normal

human spleen does not sequester or store red blood cells and does not contract in response to sympathetic stimuli. The normal human spleen contains approximately one-third of the total body platelets and a significant number of marginated neutrophils. These sequestered cells are available when needed to respond to bleeding or infection.

Approach to the Patient

Clinical Assessment The most common *symptoms* produced by diseases involving the spleen are pain and a heavy sensation in the left upper quadrant. Pain may result from acute swelling of the spleen with stretching of the capsule, infarction, or inflammation of the capsule. For many years, it was believed that splenic infarction was clinically silent, which at times is true. However, Soma Weiss, in his classic 1942 report of the self-observations by a Harvard medical student on the clinical course of subacute bacterial endocarditis, documented that severe left upper quadrant and pleuritic chest pain may accompany thromboembolic occlusion of splenic blood flow. Vascular occlusion, with infarction and pain, is commonly seen in children with sickle cell crises. Rupture of the spleen, either from trauma or infiltrative disease that breaks the capsule, may result in intraperitoneal bleeding, shock, and death. The rupture itself may be painless.

A palpable spleen is the major *physical sign* produced by diseases affecting the spleen and suggests enlargement of the organ. The normal spleen is said to weigh less than 250 g, decreases in size with age, normally lies entirely within the rib cage, has a maximum cephalocaudad diameter of 13 cm by ultrasonography or maximum length of 12 cm and/or width of 7 cm by radionuclide scan, and is usually not palpable. However, a palpable spleen was found in 3 percent of 2200 asymptomatic, male, freshman college students. Follow-up at 3 years revealed that 30 percent of those students still had a palpable spleen without any increase in disease prevalence. Ten-year follow-up found no evidence for lymphoid malignancies. Furthermore, in some tropical countries (e.g., New Guinea) the incidence of splenomegaly may reach 60 percent. Thus, the presence of a palpable spleen does not always equate with presence of disease. Even when disease is present, splenomegaly may not reflect the primary disease, but rather a reaction to it. For example, in patients with Hodgkin's disease, only two-thirds of the palpable spleens show involvement by the cancer.

Physical examination of the spleen utilizes primarily the techniques of palpation and percussion. Inspection may reveal a fullness in the left upper quadrant which descends on inspiration, a finding associated with a massively enlarged spleen. Auscultation may reveal a venous hum or a friction rub.

Palpation can be accomplished by bimanual palpation, ballotment, and palpation from above (Middleton maneuver). For bimanual palpation, which is at least as reliable as the other techniques, the patient is supine with flexed knees. The examiner's left hand is placed on the lower rib cage and pulls the skin toward the costal margin allowing the fingertips of the right hand to feel the tip of the spleen as it descends while the patient inspires slowly, smoothly, and deeply. Palpation is begun with the right hand in the left lower quadrant with gradual movement toward the left costal margin, thereby identifying the lower edge of a massively enlarged spleen. When the spleen tip is felt, the finding is recorded as centimeters below the left costal margin at some arbitrary point, i.e., 10 to 15 cm, from the midpoint of the umbilicus or the xiphisternal junction. This allows other examiners to compare findings or the initial examiner to determine changes in size over time. Bimanual palpation in the right lateral decubitus position adds nothing to the supine examination.

Percussion for splenic dullness is accomplished with any of three techniques described by Nixon, Castell, or Barkun:

1. *Nixon's method*: The patient is placed on the right side so that the spleen lies above the colon and stomach. Percussion begins at the lower level of pulmonary resonance in the posterior axillary line and proceeds diagonally along a perpendicular line toward the lower midanterior costal margin. The upper border of dullness is normally 6 to 8 cm above the costal margin. Dullness greater than 8 cm in an adult is presumed to indicate splenic enlargement.

2. *Castell's method*: With the patient supine, percussion in the lowest intercostal space in the anterior axillary line (8th or 9th) produces a resonant note if the spleen is normal in size. This is true during expiration or full inspiration. A dull percussion note on full inspiration suggests splenomegaly.

3. *Percussion of Traube's semilunar space*: The borders of Traube's space are the sixth rib superiorly, the left midaxillary line laterally, and the left costal margin inferiorly. The patient is supine with the left arm slightly abducted. During normal breathing, this space is percussed from medial to lateral margins, yielding a normal resonant sound. A dull percussion note suggests splenomegaly.

Studies comparing methods of percussion and palpation with a standard of ultrasonography or scintigraphy have revealed sensitivity of 56 to 71 percent for palpation and 59 to 82 percent for percussion. Reproducibility among examiners is better for palpation than percussion. Both techniques are less reliable in obese patients or patients who have just eaten. Thus, the physical examination techniques of palpation and percussion are imprecise at best. It has been suggested that the examiner perform percussion first and, if positive, proceed to palpation; if the spleen is palpable, then one can be reasonably confident that splenomegaly exists. However, not all left upper quadrant masses are enlarged spleens; gastric or colon tumors and pancreatic or renal cysts or tumors can mimic splenomegaly.

The presence of an enlarged spleen can be more precisely determined, if necessary, by liver-spleen radionuclide scan, computed tomography (CT), magnetic resonance imaging (MRI), or ultrasonography. The latter technique is the current procedure of choice for routine assessment of spleen size (normal = a maximum cephalocaudad diameter of 13 cm) because it has high sensitivity and specificity and is safe, noninvasive, quick, mobile, and less costly. Nuclear medicine scans are accurate, sensitive, and reliable but they are costly, require greater time to generate data, and utilize immobile equipment. They have the advantage of demonstrating accessory splenic tissue. CT and MRI provide accurate determination of spleen size, but the equipment is immobile and the procedures are expensive. MRI appears to offer no advantage over CT. Changes in spleen structure such as mass lesions, infarcts, inhomogeneous infiltrates, and cysts are more readily assessed by CT, MRI, or ultrasonography. None of these techniques is very reliable in the detection of patchy infiltration (e.g., Hodgkin's disease).

Differential Diagnosis Many of the diseases associated with splenomegaly are listed in Table 61-2. They are grouped according to the presumed basic mechanism responsible for organ enlargement:

1. Hyperplasia or hypertrophy related to a particular splenic function such as reticuloendothelial hyperplasia (work hypertrophy) in diseases such as hereditary spherocytosis or thalassemia syndromes that require removal of large numbers of defective red blood cells; immune hyperplasia in response to systemic infection (infectious mononucleosis, sub-

acute bacterial endocarditis) or to immunologic diseases (immune thrombocytopenia, SLE, Felty's syndrome).

2. Passive congestion due to decreased blood flow from the spleen in conditions that produce portal hypertension (cirrhosis, Budd-Chiari syndrome, congestive heart failure).

3. Infiltrative diseases of the spleen (lymphomas, metastatic cancer, amyloidosis, Gaucher's disease, myeloproliferative disorders with extramedullary hematopoiesis).

The differential diagnostic possibilities are much fewer when the spleen is "massively enlarged," that is, it is palpable more than 8 cm below the left costal margin or its drained weight is ≥ 1000 g (Table 61-3). The vast majority of such patients will have non-Hodgkin's lymphoma, chronic lymphocytic leukemia, hairy cell leukemia, chronic myelogenous leukemia, myelofibrosis with myeloid metaplasia, or polycythemia rubra vera.

Laboratory Assessment The major laboratory abnormalities accompanying splenomegaly are determined by the underlying systemic illness. Erythrocyte counts may be normal, decreased (thalassemia major syndromes, SLE, cirrhosis with portal hypertension), or increased (polycythemia rubra vera). Granulocyte counts may be normal, decreased (Felty's syndrome, congestive splenomegaly, leukemias),

Table 61-2

Diseases Associated with Splenomegaly Grouped by Pathogenic Mechanism

ENLARGEMENT DUE TO INCREASED DEMAND FOR SPLENIC FUNCTION	ENLARGEMENT DUE TO ABNORMAL SPLENIC OR PORTAL BLOOD FLOW
Reticuloendothelial system hyperplasia (for removal of defective erythrocytes)	Cirrhosis
Spherocytosis	Hepatic vein obstruction
Early sickle cell anemia	Portal vein obstruction, intrahepatic or extrahepatic
Ovalocytosis	Cavernous transformation of the portal vein
Thalassemia major	Splenic vein obstruction
Hemoglobinopathies	Splenic artery aneurysm
Paroxysmal nocturnal hemoglobinuria	Hepatic schistosomiasis
Nutritional anemias	Congestive heart failure
Immune hyperplasia	Hepatic echinococcosis
Response to infection (viral, bacterial, fungal, parasitic)	Portal hypertension (any cause including the above): "Banti's disease"
Infectious mononucleosis	
AIDS	**INFILTRATION OF THE SPLEEN**
Viral hepatitis	
Cytomegalovirus	*Intracellular or extracellular depositions*
Subacute bacterial endocarditis	Amyloidosis
Bacterial septicemia	Gaucher's disease
Congenital syphilis	Niemann-Pick disease
Splenic abscess	Tangier disease
Tuberculosis	Hurler's syndrome and other mucopolysaccharidoses
Histoplasmosis	Hyperlipidemias
Malaria	*Benign and malignant cellular infiltrations*
Leishmaniasis	Leukemias (acute, chronic, lymphoid, myeloid, monocytic)
Trypanosomiasis	Lymphomas
Disordered immunoregulation	Hodgkin's disease
Rheumatoid arthritis (Felty's syndrome)	Myeloproliferative syndromes (e.g., polycythemia vera)
Systemic lupus erythematosus	Angiosarcomas
Collagen vascular diseases	Metastatic tumors (melanoma is most common)
Serum sickness	Eosinophilic granuloma
Immune hemolytic anemias	Histiocytosis X
Immune thrombocytopenias	Hamartomas
Immune neutropenias	Hemangiomas, fibromas, lymphangiomas
Drug reactions	Splenic cysts
Angioimmunoblastic lymphadenopathy	
Sarcoidosis	**UNKNOWN ETIOLOGY**
Thyrotoxicosis (benign lymphoid hypertrophy)	
Extramedullary hematopoiesis	Idiopathic splenomegaly
Myelofibrosis	Berylliosis
Marrow damage by toxins, radiation, strontium	Iron-deficiency anemia
Marrow infiltration by tumors, leukemias, Gaucher's disease	

Table 61-3

Diseases Associated with Massive Splenomegaly*

Chronic myelogenous leukemia
Lymphomas
Hairy cell leukemia
Myelofibrosis with myeloid metaplasia
Polycythemia rubra vera
Gaucher's disease
Chronic lymphocytic leukemia
Sarcoidosis
Autoimmune hemolytic anemia
Diffuse splenic hemangiomatosis

* The spleen extends greater than 8 cm below left costal margin and/or weighs more than 1000 g.

or increased (infections or inflammatory disease, myeloproliferative disorders). In a similar manner the platelet count may be normal, decreased when there is enhanced sequestration or destruction of platelets in an enlarged spleen (congestive splenomegaly, Gaucher's disease, immune thrombocytopenia), or increased in the myeloproliferative disorders such as polycythemia rubra vera.

The complete blood count may reveal cytopenia of one or more blood cell types, which should suggest *hypersplenism*. This condition is characterized by splenomegaly, cytopenia(s), normal or hyperplastic bone marrow, and a response to splenectomy. The latter characteristic is less precise because reversal of cytopenia, particularly granulocytopenia, is sometimes not sustained after splenectomy. The cytopenias result from increased destruction of the cellular elements secondary to reduced flow of blood through enlarged and congested cords (congestive splenomegaly) or to immune-mediated mechanisms. In hypersplenism, various cell types usually have normal morphology on the peripheral blood smear, although the red cells may be spherocytic due to loss of surface area during their longer transit through the enlarged spleen. The increased marrow production of red cells should be reflected as an increased reticulocyte production index, although the value may be less than expected due to increased sequestration of reticulocytes in the spleen.

As mentioned earlier, the size of the spleen can be confirmed, if necessary, by ultrasound, radionuclide scan, CT, or MRI. The need for additional laboratory studies is dictated by the differential diagnosis of the underlying illness of which splenomegaly is merely a manifestation.

SPLENECTOMY Splenectomy is infrequently performed for diagnostic purposes, especially in the absence of clinical illness or other diagnostic tests that suggest underlying disease. More often splenectomy is performed for staging the extent of disease in patients with Hodgkin's disease, for symptom control in patients with massive splenomegaly, for disease control in patients with hairy cell leukemia or prolymphocytic leukemia, for bleeding control in patients with traumatic splenic rupture, or for correction of cytopenias in patients with hypersplenism or immune-mediated destruction of one or more cellular blood elements. Splenectomy is necessary for routine staging of patients with Hodgkin's disease only in patients with clinical stage I or II disease in whom radiation therapy is contemplated as the treatment. Noninvasive staging of the spleen in Hodgkin's disease is not a sufficiently reliable basis for treatment decisions because one-third of normal-sized spleens will be involved with Hodgkin's disease and one-third of enlarged spleens will be tumor-free. Although it has been clearly shown that splenectomy in chronic myelogenous leukemia does not affect the natural history of disease, removal of the massive spleen usually makes patients significantly more comfortable and simplifies their management by significantly reducing transfusion requirements. Splenectomy is an effective treatment for two chronic B cell leukemias, hairy cell leukemia and prolymphocytic leukemia, and for

the very rare splenic marginal zone lymphoma. Splenectomy in these diseases is associated with significant tumor regression in bone marrow and other sites of disease. Similar regressions of systemic disease have been noted after splenic irradiation in some types of lymphoproliferative disease, especially chronic lymphocytic leukemia. This has been termed the *abscopal effect*. Such systemic tumor responses to local therapy directed at the spleen suggest that there may be some hormone or growth factor produced by the spleen that affects tumor cell proliferation, but this conjecture is not yet substantiated. The most common indication for splenectomy is traumatic or iatrogenic splenic rupture. In a fraction of patients with splenic rupture, peritoneal seeding of splenic fragments can lead to splenosis—the presence of multiple rests of spleen tissue not connected to the portal circulation. This ectopic spleen tissue may cause pain or gastrointestinal obstruction, as in endometriosis. A large number of hematologic, immunologic, and congestive causes of splenomegaly can lead to destruction of one or more cellular blood elements. In the majority of such cases, splenectomy can correct the cytopenias, particularly anemia and thrombocytopenia. Perhaps the only contraindication to splenectomy is the presence of marrow failure, in which the enlarged spleen is the only source of hematopoietic tissue.

The absence of the spleen has minimal long-term effects on the hematologic profile. In the immediate postsplenectomy period, there may be some leukocytosis (up to $25,000/\mu L$) and thrombocytosis (up to $1 \times 10^6/\mu L$), but within 2 to 3 weeks, blood cell counts and survival of each cell lineage are usually normal. The chronic manifestations of splenectomy are marked variation in size and shape of erythrocytes (anisocytosis, poikilocytosis) and the presence of Howell-Jolly bodies (nuclear remnants), Heinz bodies (denatured hemoglobin), basophilic stippling, and an occasional nucleated erythrocyte in the peripheral blood. When such erythrocyte abnormalities appear in a patient whose spleen has not been removed, one should suspect splenic infiltration by tumor that has interfered with its normal culling and pitting function.

The most serious consequence of splenectomy is increased susceptibility to bacterial infections, particularly those with capsules such as *Streptococcus pneumoniae*, *Haemophilus influenzae*, and some gram-negative enteric organisms. Patients under age 20 years are particularly susceptible to overwhelming sepsis with *S. pneumoniae*, and the overall actuarial risk of sepsis in patients who have had their spleens removed is about 7 percent in 10 years. About 25 percent of such patients will develop a serious infection at some time in their life. The frequency is highest within the first 3 years after splenectomy. About 15 percent of the infections are polymicrobial, and lung, skin, and blood are the most common sites. There appears to be no increased risk of viral infection in patients who have no spleen. The susceptibility to bacterial infections relates to the inability to remove opsonized bacteria from the bloodstream and a defect in making antibodies to T cell–independent antigens such as the polysaccharide components of bacterial capsules. Pneumococcal vaccine may be prophylactic if administered before splenectomy, but there are no data supporting its use after splenectomy. In fact, because patients cannot make antibody to pneumococcal polysaccharide after splenectomy, administration of the vaccine may actually lower the titer of specific pneumococcal antibodies and, theoretically, could make patients more susceptible to infection. The vaccine to *H. influenzae* should also be given to patients in whom elective splenectomy is planned. No other vaccines are routinely recommended in this setting. Once the spleen has been removed, vaccines to T cell–dependent antigens are not contraindicated but those to T cell–independent antigens are ineffective.

In addition to an increased susceptibility to bacterial infections, splenectomized patients are also more susceptible to the parasitic disease babesiosis. The splenectomized patient should avoid areas where the parasite *Babesia* is endemic (e.g., Cape Cod, MA).

Surgical removal of the spleen is an obvious cause of *hyposplenism*. Patients with sickle cell disease often suffer from autosplenectomy as a result of splenic destruction by the numerous infarcts associated with sickle cell crises during childhood. Indeed, the presence of a palpable spleen in a patient with sickle cell disease after age 5 suggests a coexisting hemoglobinopathy, e.g., thalassemia or hemoglobin C.

In addition, patients who receive splenic irradiation for a neoplastic or autoimmune disease are also functionally hyposplenic. The term *hyposplenism* is preferred to *asplenism* in referring to the physiologic consequences of splenectomy because asplenia is a rare, specific, and fatal congenital abnormality in which there is a failure of the left side of the coelomic cavity (which includes the splenic anlagen) to develop normally. Infants with asplenia have no spleens, but that is the least of their problems. The right side of the developing embryo is duplicated on the left so there is liver where the spleen should be, there are two right lungs, and the heart comprises two right atria and two right ventricles.

BIBLIOGRAPHY

BARKUN AN et al: Splenic enlargement and Traube's space: How useful in percussion? Am J Med 87:562, 1989

―――― et al: The bedside assessment of splenic enlargement. Am J Med 91:512, 1991

CASTELL DO: The spleen percussion sign: A useful diagnostic technique. Ann Intern Med 67:1265, 1967

GRAVES SA et al: Does this patient have splenomegaly? JAMA 270:2218, 1993

KUBOTA T: The evaluation of peripheral adenopathy. Primary Care 7:461, 1980

MCINTYRE OR, EBAUGH FG JR: Palpable spleens: Ten year follow-up. Ann Intern Med 90:130, 1979

―――――, ―――――: Palpable spleens in college freshmen. Ann Intern Med 66:301, 1967

NIXON RK JR: The detection of splenomegaly by percussion. N Engl J Med 250:166, 1954

PANGALIS GA et al: Clinical approach to lymphadenopathy. Semin Oncol 20:570, 1993

SLAP GB et al: Validation of a model to identify young patients for lymph node biopsy. JAMA 255:2768, 1986

WEISS S: Self-observation and psychologic reactions of medical student A.S.R. to the onset and symptoms of subacute bacterial endocarditis. J Mt Sinai Hospital 8:1079, 1942

WILLIAMSON HA JR: Lymphadenopathy in a family practice: A descriptive study of 240 cases. J Fam Pract 20:449, 1985

ZUELZER W, KAPLAN J: The child with lymphadenopathy. Semin Hematol 12:323, 1975

| 62 | *Steven M. Holland, John I. Gallin* |

DISORDERS OF GRANULOCYTES AND MONOCYTES

Leukocytes are the major cellular components of inflammatory and immune responses and include neutrophils, T and B lymphocytes, natural killer (NK) cells, monocytes, eosinophils, and basophils. These cells have been assigned specific functions, such as antibody production by B lymphocytes or destruction of bacteria by neutrophils, but in no single infectious disease is the exact role of each of the cell types completely established. Thus, whereas neutrophils are classically thought to be critical to host defense against bacteria, there is increasing evidence that neutrophils play important roles in viral infections.

The blood is the most readily obtainable source of leukocytes and serves as the vehicle for their delivery to the various tissues from the bone marrow, where they are produced. Normal blood leukocyte counts are given in the Appendix (Tables A-7 and A-8). The various leukocytes are thought to derive from a common stem cell in the bone marrow. Three-fourths of the nucleated cells of bone marrow are committed to the production of leukocytes. Leukocyte maturation in the marrow is under the regulatory control of a number of different factors, known as colony stimulating factors and interleukins (see Chap. 105). Because an alteration in the number and type of leukocytes is a frequent association with disease processes, a total white blood count (WBC) (cells per microliter) and differential counts are obtained frequently. The lymphocytes and basophils are discussed in Chaps. 305 and 310, respectively. This chapter focuses on the neutrophils, monocytes, and eosinophils.

NEUTROPHILS

MATURATION Important events in the neutrophil life are summarized in Fig. 62-1. In normal humans, neutrophils are produced only in the bone marrow. Best estimates indicate that the appropriate number of stem cells necessary to support hematopoiesis is between 400 and 500. There is convincing evidence that human blood monocytes and tissue macrophages produce colony stimulating factors, hormones required for the growth of monocytes and neutrophils in the bone marrow. The hematopoietic system not only produces enough neutrophils (approximately 1.3×10^{11} cells per 80-kg person per day) to carry out physiologic functions but also has a large reserve stored in the marrow which can be mobilized in response to inflammation or infection. An increase in the number of blood neutrophils is called *neutrophilia*, and the presence of immature cells is termed a *shift to the left*. A diminution in the number of blood neutrophils is referred to as *neutropenia*.

Neutrophils and monocytes evolve from pluripotent stem cells under the influence of cytokines and colony stimulating factors (Fig. 62-2). The myeloblast is the first recognizable precursor cell and is followed by the *promyelocyte* (**Plate IV-15**). The promyelocyte evolves when the classic lysosomal granules, called the *primary* or *azurophil granules*, are produced. The primary granules contain hydrolases, elastase, myeloperoxidase, cationic proteins, and bactericidal/permeability-increasing (BPI) protein important for killing gram-negative bacteria. Azurophil granules also contain *defensins*, a family of cysteine-rich polypeptides with broad antimicrobial activity against bacteria, fungi, and certain enveloped viruses. The promyelocyte divides to produce the *myelocyte*, a cell responsible for the synthesis of the *specific* or *secondary granules* which contain unique (specific) constituents such as lactoferrin, vitamin B_{12}–binding proteins, membrane components of the nicotinamide-adenine dinucleotide phosphate (NADPH) oxidase required for hydrogen peroxide production, histaminase, and receptors for certain chemoattractants and adherence-promoting factors (CR3) as well as receptors for the connective tissue element laminin. The secondary granules do not contain acid hydrolases and therefore are not classic lysosomes. They are readily released extracellularly, and their mobilization is probably important in modulating inflammation. During the final stages of maturation there is no cell division, and the cell passes through the *metamyelocyte* stage and then to the *band* neutrophil with a sausage-shaped nucleus (**Plate IV-17**). As the band cell matures, the nucleus assumes a lobulated configuration. The nucleus of neutrophils normally contains up to four segments. Excessive segmentation (greater than five nuclear lobes) may be a manifestation of folate or vitamin B_{12} deficiency (**Plate IV-18**). The Pelger-Hüet anomaly (**Plate IV-19*B***), an infrequent dominant benign inherited trait, results in neutrophils with distinctive bilobed nuclei that must be distinguished from band forms. The physiologic role of the multilobed nucleus of neutrophils is unknown, but it may allow great deformation of neutrophils during migration into tissues at sites of inflammation.

In settings of severe acute bacterial infection, prominent neutrophil cytoplasmic granules called *toxic granulations* are occasionally seen (**Plate IV-16**). Toxic granulations are thought to be immature or abnormally staining azurophil granules. Cytoplasmic inclusions, also called *Döhle bodies* (**Plate IV-17**), can be seen during infection and probably represent fragments of ribosome-rich endoplasmic reticulum. Large neutrophil vacuoles are often present in acute bacterial infection and probably represent pinocytosed (internalized) membrane.

Neutrophils have long been thought to be a homogeneous population of cells. However, studies of neutrophil function have suggested that they are heterogeneous. Recently, monoclonal antibodies have been developed that recognize only a subset of mature neutrophils. The meaning of neutrophil heterogeneity is not known.

MARROW RELEASE AND CIRCULATING COMPARTMENTS Specific signals, including interleukin (IL) 1, tumor necro-

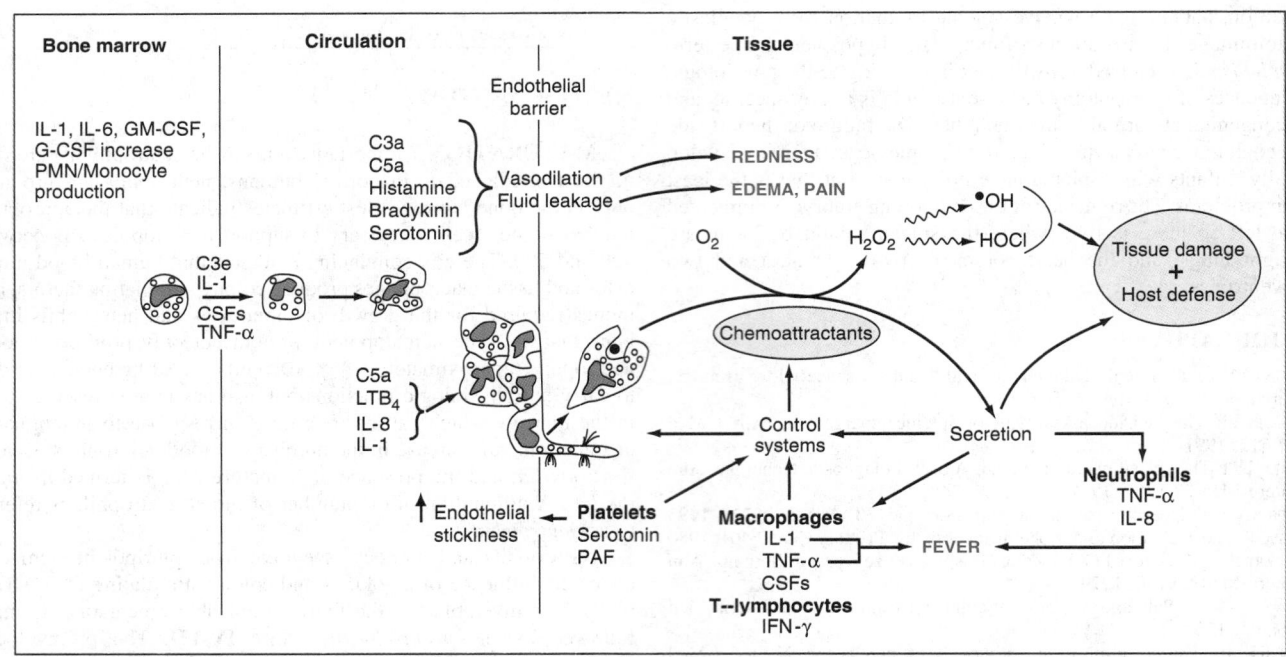

FIGURE 62-1 Events in inflammation. The four basic symptoms of inflammation are indicated by bold blue print.

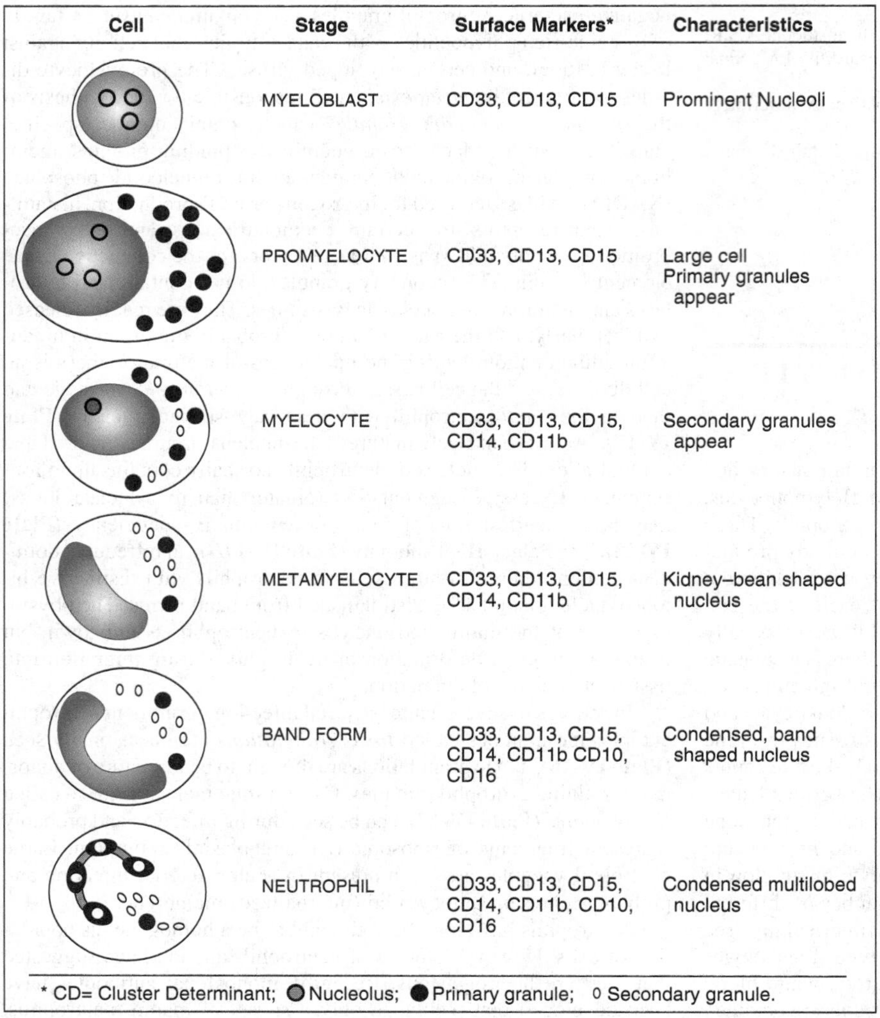

Cell	Stage	Surface Markers*	Characteristics
	MYELOBLAST	CD33, CD13, CD15	Prominent Nucleoli
	PROMYELOCYTE	CD33, CD13, CD15	Large cell Primary granules appear
	MYELOCYTE	CD33, CD13, CD15, CD14, CD11b	Secondary granules appear
	METAMYELOCYTE	CD33, CD13, CD15, CD14, CD11b	Kidney–bean shaped nucleus
	BAND FORM	CD33, CD13, CD15, CD14, CD11b CD10, CD16	Condensed, band shaped nucleus
	NEUTROPHIL	CD33, CD13, CD15, CD14, CD11b, CD10, CD16	Condensed multilobed nucleus

* CD= Cluster Determinant; ● Nucleolus; ● Primary granule; ○ Secondary granule.

FIGURE 62-2 Stages of neutrophil development are schematically shown. G-CSF and GM-CSF are critical to this process. Identifying cellular characteristics and specific cell-surface markers are listed for each maturational stage.

sis factor α (TNFα), the colony stimulating factors, the complement fragment C3e, and perhaps other cytokines mobilize leukocytes from the bone marrow and deliver them to the blood in an unstimulated state. Under normal conditions, about 90 percent of the neutrophil pool is in the bone marrow, 2 to 3 percent in the circulation, and the remainder in the tissues (Fig. 62-3).

The circulating pool exists in two dynamic compartments: freely flowing and marginated. The freely flowing pool is about one-half the neutrophils in the basal state and is composed of those cells that are in the blood and not in contact with the endothelium. Marginated leukocytes are those that are in close physical contact with the endothelium (Fig. 62-4). In the pulmonary circulation, where there is an extensive capillary bed (about 1000 capillaries per aleveolus), margination occurs because the capillaries are about the same size as a mature neutrophil. Therefore, neutrophil fluidity and deformability are necessary to make the transit through the pulmonary bed. Increased neutrophil rigidity and decreased deformability lead to augmented neutrophil trapping and margination in the lung. In contrast, in the systemic postcapillary venules, margination is mediated by the interaction of specific cell-surface molecules. *Selectins* are glycoproteins expressed on neutrophils and endothelial cells, among others, that cause a low-affinity interaction resulting in "rolling" of the neutrophil along the endothelial surface. On neutrophils, the molecule L-selectin [cluster determinant (CD) 62L] binds to glycosylated proteins on endothelial cells [e.g., glycosylation-dependent cell adhesion molecule (GlyCAM) 1 and CD34]. Glycoproteins on neutrophils, most importantly sialyl-Lewis^x (SLe^x, CD15s), are targets for binding of selectins expressed on endothelial cells [E-selectin (CD62E) and P-selectin (CD62P)] and other leukocytes. In response to

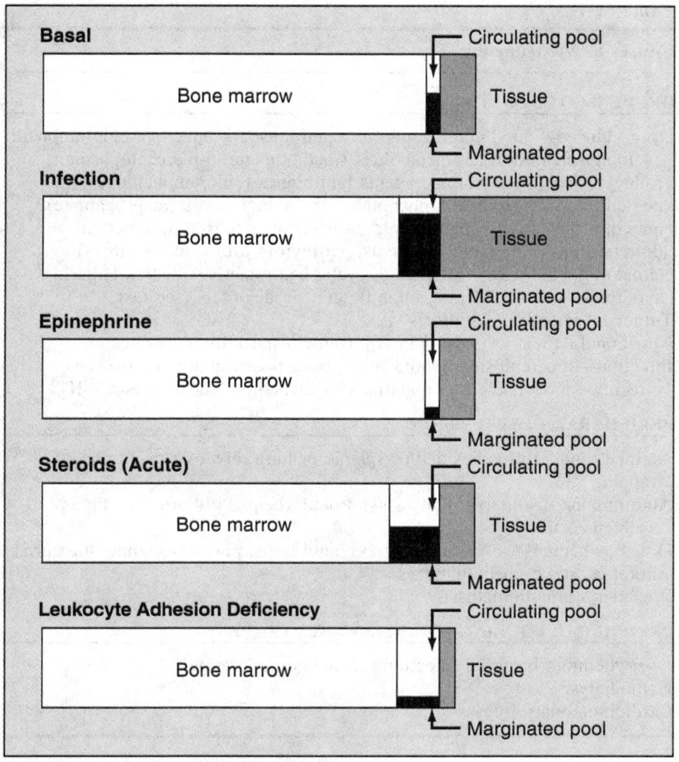

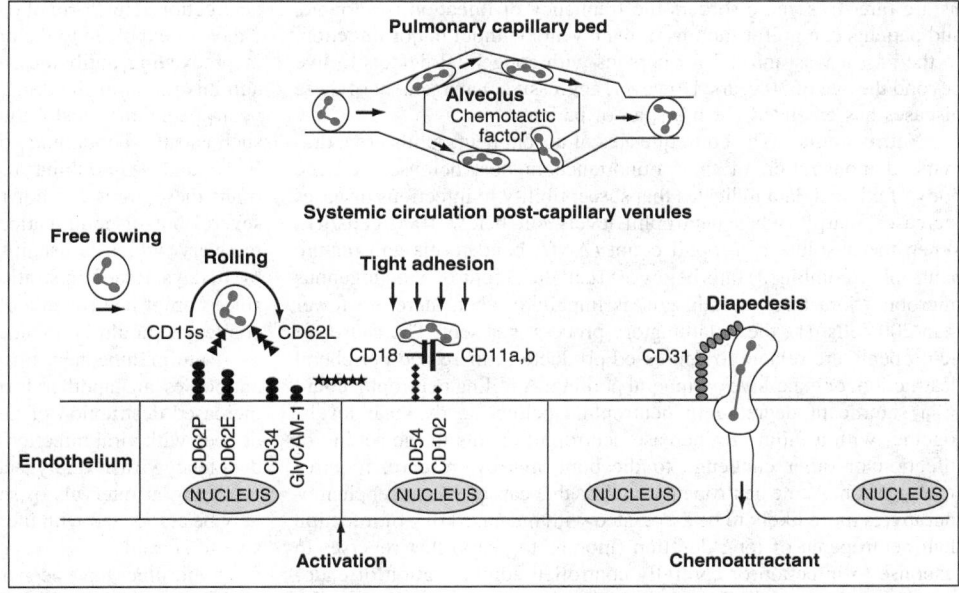

FIGURE 62-3 Schematic neutrophil distribution and kinetics between the different anatomic and functional pools.

chemotactic stimuli from injured tissues (e.g., the complement product C5a, the arachidonic acid derivative leukotriene B₄, the cytokine IL-8) or bacterial products [e.g., N-formylmethionylleucylphenylalanine (f-metleuphe)], neutrophil adhesiveness increases and they "stick" to the endothelium through *integrins*. The integrins are leukocyte glycoproteins that exist as complexes of a common CD18 β-chain with CD11a (LFA-1), CD11b (also called either Mac-1, CR3, or the C3bi receptor), and CD11c (p150,95). CD11a/CD18 and CD11b/CD18 mediate binding to specific endothelial receptors [intercellular adhesion molecules (ICAM)] 1 and 2.

Receptors for chemoattractants and opsonins are also mobilized; the phagocytes orient toward the chemoattractant source in the extravascular space, increase their motile activity (chemokinesis), and migrate with direction (chemotaxis) into tissues. The biochemistry and cell biology of these processes are rapidly unfolding (see "Bibliography"). The process of migration into tissues is called *diapedesis* and involves the crawling of neutrophils between postcapillary endothelial cells that open junctions between adjacent cells to permit leukocyte passage. Diapedesis involves platelet/endothelial cell adhesion molecule (PECAM) 1 (CD31), which is expressed on both the emigrating leukocyte and the endothelial cells. The endothelial responses (increased blood flow secondary to increased vasodilation and

permeability) are mediated by anaphylatoxins (e.g., complement products C3a and C5a) as well as vasodilators such as histamine, bradykinin, serotonin, and prostaglandins E and I. In the healthy adult, most neutrophils leave the body by migration through the mucous membrane of the gastrointestinal tract. Normally, neutrophils spend a relatively short time in the circulation, with a half-life of 6 to 7 h. Senescent neutrophils are cleared from the circulation by macrophages in the lung and spleen. Once in the tissues, neutrophils release enzymes such as collagenase and elastase, which may help establish abscess cavities. Neutrophils ingest (phagocytose) pathogenic materials that have been properly altered (opsonized) by substances such as IgG and the complement product C3b. Fibronectin and the tetrapeptide tuftsin facilitate the phagocytic process.

Concomitant with phagocytosis there is a burst of oxygen consumption and activation of the hexose-monophosphate shunt. A membrane-associated NADPH oxidase, consisting of membrane and cytosolic components, is assembled and catalyzes the reduction of oxygen to superoxide anion, which is then converted to hydrogen peroxide and other toxic oxygen products (e.g., hydrogen peroxide and hydroxyl radical). Hydrogen peroxide + chloride + neutrophil myeloperoxidase provide a particularly toxic system that generates hypochlorous acid (bleach), hypochlorite, and chlorine. These products oxidize and halogenate microorganisms and tumor cells and, when uncontrolled, can damage host tissue. Strongly cationic proteins and defensins also participate in microbial killing. Other enzymes, such as lysozyme and acid proteases, help digest microbial debris. After 1 to 4 days in tissues neutrophils die. Under certain conditions, such as in delayed-type hypersensitivity immunity, monocyte accumulation occurs within 6 to 12 h of initiation of inflammation. Neutrophils, monocytes, microorganisms in various states of digestion, and altered local tissue cells make up the inflammatory exudate, pus. Neutrophils shed their

FIGURE 62-4 Neutrophil travel through the pulmonary capillaries is dependent on neutrophil deformability. Neutrophil rigidity (e.g., caused by C5a) enhances pulmonary trapping and response to pulmonary pathogens in a way that is not so dependent upon cell-surface receptors. Intraalveolar chemotactic factors, such as those caused by certain bacteria (e.g., *Streptococcus pneumoniae*) lead to diapedesis of neutrophils from the pulmonary capillaries into the alveolar space. Neutrophil interaction with the endothelium of the systemic postcapillary venules is dependent on molecules of attachment. The neutrophil "rolls" along the endothelium using selectins: neutrophil CD15s (sialyl-Lewis^x) binds to CD62E (E-selectin) and CD62P (P-selectin) on endothelial cells; CD62L (L-selectin) on neutrophils binds to CD34 and other molecules (e.g., GlyCAM-1) expressed on endothelium. Chemokines or other activation factors stimulate integrin-mediated "tight adhesion": CD11a/CD18 (LFA-1) and CD11b/CD18 (Mac-1, CR3) bind to CD54 (ICAM-1) and CD102 (ICAM-2) on the endothelium. Diapedesis occurs between endothelial cells: CD31 (PECAM-1) expressed by the emigrating neutrophil interacts with CD31 expressed at the endothelial cell-cell junction.

L-selectin molecules into the circulation upon entry into inflammatory sites. Myeloperoxidase (previously called verdoperoxidase) confers the characteristic green color to pus and may participate in turning off the inflammatory process by inactivating chemoattractants and immobilizing phagocytic cells.

Neutrophils react to certain cytokines [interferon γ (IFNγ), granulocyte-macrophage colony stimulating factor (GM-CSF), IL-8] and produce cytokines [TNFα, IL-8, macrophage inflammatory protein (MIP) 1α] that modulate the inflammatory response. An expanding class of proinflammatory peptides important for neutrophil and monocyte recruitment and activation are the *chemokines* (*chemo*attractant *cytokines*). These small proteins are produced by many different cell types, including endothelial cells, fibroblasts, epithelial cells, neutrophils, and monocytes, and are necessary in the development of the inflammatory response. The chemokines transduce their signals through heterotrimeric G protein–linked receptors that have seven cell membrane–spanning domains, the same type of cell-surface receptor that mediates the response to the classical chemoattractants N-f-met-leuphe and C5a. There are two major structural and functional classes of chemokines: The α chemokines (e.g., IL-8) are mainly chemoattractant for neutrophils, whereas the β chemokines (e.g., MIP-1α) are more chemoattractant for monocytes and lymphocytes.

NEUTROPHIL ABNORMALITIES A defect anywhere in the neutrophil life cycle can lead to dysfunction and compromised host defenses. Inflammation is often depressed, and the clinical result is often recurrent and severe bacterial and fungal infections creating difficult management problems. Diagnosis of phagocytic cell disorders is suggested by clinical evaluation. Aphthous ulcers of mucous membranes (gray ulcers without pus) and gingivitis and periodontal disease are common. Patients with congenital phagocyte defects can have infections within the first few days of life. Skin, ear, upper and lower respiratory tract, and bone infections are common. Sepsis and meningitis are rare. In some disorders the frequency of infection is variable, and patients can go for months or even years without major infection. In the past it was unusual for persons with congenital defects to live beyond the age of 30 years. However, aggressive management of these diseases has extended the life span of patients.

Neutropenia The consequences of absent neutrophils are a dramatic demonstration of their importance in host defense. A large body of clinical data indicates that susceptibility to infectious diseases increases sharply when neutrophil levels fall below 1000 cells/μL. When the absolute neutrophil count (ANC; band forms and mature neutrophils combined) falls below 500 cells/μL, control of endogenous microbial flora (e.g., mouth, gut) is impaired; when there are fewer than 200 cells/μL, the inflammatory process is absent. The causes of neutropenia are related to depressed production, increased peripheral destruction, or excessive peripheral pooling. A falling neutrophil count or a significant decrease in neutrophils below steady state levels, together with a failure to increase neutrophil counts in the setting of infection or other challenge to the bone marrow reserve, requires investigation. Acute neutropenia, such as that caused by cancer chemotherapy, is more likely to be associated with increased risk of infection than neutropenia of long duration (months to years) that reverses in response to infection or carefully controlled administration of endotoxin (see "Laboratory Diagnosis," below).

Some causes of inherited and acquired neutropenia are listed in Table 62-1. The most common neutropenias are iatrogenic, resulting from the widespread use of cytotoxic or immunosuppressive therapies for malignancy or control of autoimmune disorders. These drugs cause neutropenia because they are toxic and result in decreased production of rapidly growing progenitor (stem) cells of the marrow. Cytotoxic chemotherapeutic agents fall into this category, but certain antibiotics such as chloramphenicol, trimethoprim-sulfamethoxazole, flucytosine, vidarabine, and the antiretroviral drug zidovudine may cause neutropenia by inhibiting proliferation of myeloid precursors. The marrow suppression is generally dose-related and dependent on continued

Table 62-1

Causes of Neutropenia

DECREASED PRODUCTION

Drug-induced—alkylating agents (nitrogen mustard, busulfan, chlorambucil, cyclophosphamide); antimetabolites (methotrexate, 6-mercaptopurine, 5-flucytosine); noncytotoxic agents [antibiotics (chloramphenicol, penicillins, sulfonamides), phenothiazines, tranquilizers (meprobamate), anticonvulsants (carbamazepine), antipsychotics (clozapine), certain diuretics, anti-inflammatory agents, antithyroid drugs, many others]
Hematologic diseases—idiopathic, cyclic neutropenia, Chédiak-Higashi syndrome, aplastic anemia, infantile genetic disorders (see text)
Tumor invasion, myelofibrosis
Nutritional deficiency—vitamin B_{12}, folate (especially alcoholics)
Infection—tuberculosis, typhoid fever, brucellosis, tularemia, measles, infectious mononucleosis, malaria, viral hepatitis, leishmaniasis, AIDS

PERIPHERAL DESTRUCTION

Antineutrophil antibodies and/or splenic or lung (alveolar macrophage) trapping
Autoimmune disorders—Felty's syndrome, rheumatoid arthritis, lupus erythematosus
Drugs as haptens—aminopyrine, α-methyl dopa, phenylbutazone, mercurial diuretics, some phenothiazines
Wegener's granulomatosis

PERIPHERAL POOLING (TRANSIENT NEUTROPENIA)

Overwhelming bacterial infection (acute endotoxemia)
Hemodialysis
Cardiopulmonary bypass

administration of the drug. Recombinant human granulocyte colony stimulating factor (G-CSF) is an important drug for reversing this form of neutropenia and is particularly useful in cancer chemotherapy.

Another important mechanism for iatrogenically induced neutropenia is the effect of drugs that serve as immune haptens and sensitize neutrophils or neutrophil precursors to immune-mediated peripheral destruction. This form of drug-induced neutropenia can be seen within 7 days of exposure to the drug; with previous drug exposure, resulting in preexisting antibodies, neutropenia may occur a few hours after administration of the drug. Although any drug can cause this form of neutropenia, the most frequent causes are commonly used antibiotics, such as sulfa-containing compounds, penicillins, and cephalosporins. Fever and eosinophilia also may be associated drug reactions, but often these signs are not present. Drug-induced neutropenia can be severe, but discontinuation of the sensitizing drug is sufficient for recovery, which is usually seen within 5 to 7 days and is complete by 10 days. Readministration of the sensitizing drug should be avoided, since abrupt neutropenia often will result. For this reason, diagnostic challenge should be avoided in most situations.

Autoimmune neutropenias caused by circulating antineutrophil antibodies are another form of acquired neutropenia that results in increased destruction of neutrophils. Acquired neutropenia also may be seen with viral infections, including those with the human immunodeficiency virus. Rarely, acquired neutropenia may be cyclic in nature, occurring at intervals of several weeks. Acquired cyclic neutropenia may be associated with increased natural NK cells and may be responsive to steroids.

Syndromes have been described in which expansion of large granular lymphocytes (LGL) is associated with neutropenia. Patients with LGL lymphocytosis may have moderate blood and bone marrow lymphocytosis, neutropenia, polyclonal hypergammaglobulinemia, splenomegaly, and absence of lymphadenopathy. Such patients may have a chronic and relatively stable course. Recurrent bacterial infections are frequent. There are both benign and malignant forms of this syndrome. In some patients, a spontaneous regression has occurred even after 11 years, suggesting an immunoregulatory defect as the basis for at least one form of the disorder.

Hereditary neutropenias are rare and may manifest in early childhood as a profound constant neutropenia or agranulocytosis. Examples of congenital forms of neutropenia include Kostmann's syndrome

Table 62-2

CHAPTER 62
Disorders of Granulocytes and Monocytes

355

Causes of Neutrophilia

INCREASED PRODUCTION

Idiopathic
Drug-induced—glucocorticoids
Infection—bacterial, fungal, rarely viral
Inflammation—thermal injury, tissue necrosis, myocardial and pulmonary infarction, hypersensitivity states, collagen vascular diseases
Myeloproliferative diseases—myelocytic leukemia, myeloid metaplasia, polycythemia vera

INCREASED MARROW MOBILIZATION

Glucocorticoids
Acute infection (endotoxin)
Inflammation—thermal injury

DEFECTIVE MARGINATION

Drugs—epinephrine, glucocorticoids, nonsteroidal anti-inflammatory agents
Stress, excitement, vigorous exercise
Leukocyte adhesion deficiency type 1 (integrin β chain, CD18), Leukocyte adhesion deficiency type 2 (selectin ligand, CD15s, sialyl-Lewis^x)

MISCELLANEOUS

Metabolic disorders—ketoacidosis, acute renal failure, eclampsia, acute poisoning
Drugs—lithium
Other—metastatic carcinoma, acute hemorrhage or hemolysis

(fewer than 100 neutrophils/μL), which is often fatal; more benign chronic idiopathic neutropenia (300 to 1500 neutrophils/μL); the hair-cartilage-hypoplasia syndrome; Shwachman syndrome associated with pancreatic insufficiency; and neutropenias associated with other immune defects (X-linked agammaglobulinemia, ataxia telangiectasia, IgA deficiency). Recently, forms of severe congenital neutropenia have been identified in which the G-CSF receptor encoded on chromosome 1 is mutated, leading to poor G-CSF responsiveness and apparently predisposing to development of myeloid malignancy. Hereditary cyclic neutropenia, an autosomal dominant trait, may occur in infancy and is characterized by a remarkably regular 3-week cycle. Hereditary cyclic neutropenia actually is cyclic hematopoiesis. Although the mechanism for hereditary cyclic neutropenia is not known, steroids and G-CSF blunt the cycling in some patients. Maternal factors can be associated with neutropenia in the newborn. Transplacental transfer of IgG directed against antigens on fetal neutrophils can result in peripheral destruction. Drugs (e.g., thiazide) ingested during pregnancy can cause neutropenia in the newborn by either depressed production or peripheral destruction.

The presence of immunoglobulin directed toward neutrophils is seen in Felty's syndrome (triad of rheumatoid arthritis, splenomegaly, and neutropenia; see Chap. 61). Patients with Felty's syndrome who respond to splenectomy with an increase in their neutrophil count also have lower postoperative serum neutrophil-binding IgG, a result suggesting that one beneficial effect of splenectomy is reduction in antibodies to neutrophils. Splenomegaly with peripheral trapping and destruction of neutrophils is also seen in lysosomal storage diseases and in portal hypertension.

Neutrophilia Neutrophilia results from increased neutrophil production, marrow release, or defective margination (Table 62-2). The most important acute cause of neutrophilia requiring prompt medical attention is infection. Neutrophilia from acute infection represents both increased production and increased marrow release. Increased production is also associated with chronic inflammation and certain myeloproliferative diseases. Increased marrow release and mobilization of the marginated leukocyte pool are induced by glucocorticoids. Release of epinephrine, as with vigorous exercise, excitement, or stress, will demarginate neutrophils in the spleen and lungs and double the neutrophil count. Leukocytosis with counts of 10,000 to 25,000 cells/μL occurs in response to infection and other forms of acute inflammation and results from both release of the marginated pool and mobilization of marrow reserves. Persistent neutrophilia of 30,000 to 50,000 cells/μL or greater is called a *leukemoid reaction*, a term often used to distinguish this degree of neutrophilia from leukemia. In a leukemoid reaction, the circulating neutrophils are usually mature and not clonally derived.

Abnormal Neutrophil Function The types of inherited and acquired abnormalities of phagocyte function are described in Table 62-3. The resulting diseases are best considered in terms of the functional defects of adherence, chemotaxis, and microbicidal activity. The distinguishing features of the important inherited disorders of phagocyte function are shown in Table 62-4, several of which are discussed below.

Two types of leukocyte adhesion deficiency (LAD) have been described: Both are autosomal recessive traits and result in the inability of neutrophils to exit the circulation to sites of infection, leading to constant leukocytosis and increased susceptibility to infection. Patients with LAD 1 have mutations in CD18, the common component of the integrins LFA-1, Mac-1, and p150,95, leading to a defect in tight adhesion between neutrophils and the endothelium. The heterodimer formed by CD18/CD11b (Mac-1) is also the receptor for the comple-

Table 62-3

Types of Granulocyte and Monocyte Disorders

Function	Cause of Indicated Dysfunction		
	Drug-Induced	Acquired	Inherited
Adherence-aggregation	Aspirin, colchicine, alcohol, glucocorticoids, ibuprofen, piroxicam	Neonatal state, hemodialysis	Leukoctye adhesion deficiency types 1 and 2
Deformability		Leukemia, neonatal state, diabetes mellitus, immature neutrophils	
Chemokinesis-chemotaxis	Glucocorticoids (high dose), auranofin, colchicine (weak effect), phenylbutazone, naproxen, indomethacin, interleukin 2	Thermal injury, malignancy, malnutrition, periodontal disease, neonatal state, systemic lupus erythematosus, rheumatoid arthritis, diabetes mellitus, sepsis, influenza virus infection, herpes simplex virus infection, acrodermatitis enteropathica, AIDS	Chédiak-Higashi syndrome, neutrophil-specific granule deficiency, hyper IgE–recurrent infection (Job's) syndrome (in some patients), Down syndrome, α-mannosidase deficiency, severe combined immunodeficiency, Wiskott-Aldrich syndrome
Microbicidal activity	Colchicine, cyclophosphamide, glucocorticoids (high dose)	Leukemia, aplastic anemia, certain neutropenias, tuftsin deficiency, thermal injury, sepsis, neonatal state, diabetes mellitus, malnutrition, AIDS	Chédiak-Higashi syndrome, neutrophil-specific granule deficiency, chronic granulomatous disease

ment-derived opsonin C3bi (CR3). The CD18 gene is located on distal chromosome 21q. Variable expression of the defect determines the magnitude of clinical disease. Complete lack of expression of the leukocyte adhesion proteins by resting neutrophils results in the severe phenotype in which inflammatory cytokines do not increase the expression of leukocyte adhesion proteins on neutrophils or activated T and B cells. The functional abnormalities are predictable because of the role these molecules play in normal leukocyte function. Neutrophils (and monocytes) from patients with LAD 1 adhere poorly to endothelial cells and protein-coated surfaces and exhibit defective spreading, aggregation, and chemotaxis. Patients with this syndrome have recurrent bacterial and fungal infections involving skin, oral and genital mucosa, and respiratory and intestinal tracts; persistent leukocytosis (15,000 to 20,000 neutrophils/μL) because cells do not marginate; and, in severe cases, a history of delayed separation of the umbilical stump. Infections, especially of the skin, tend to become necrotic with progressively enlarging borders, slow healing, and the development of dysplas-

tic scars. The most common bacteria are *Staphylococcus aureus* and enteric gram-negative bacteria. LAD 2 is caused by an abnormality of SLe^x (CD15s), the ligand on neutrophils that interacts with selectins on endothelial cells.

Abnormal neutrophil and monocyte chemotaxis occurs in the *hyperimmunoglobulin E–recurrent infection* (HIE) or *Job's syndrome*. The molecular basis for this syndrome is not known, but some cases appear to have autosomal dominant transmission. Patients with this syndrome have coarse facies; bone abnormalities including hyperostosis frontalis externa, hypertelorism, kyphoscoliosis, and osteoporosis; and eczema. They develop recurrent sinopulmonary and cutaneous infections that tend to be much less inflamed than appropriate for the degree of infection and have been referred to as "cold abscesses." A high degree of suspicion is required to diagnose infections in these patients, who may appear well despite extensive disease. For many years the cold abscesses were thought to be a reflection of impaired chemotaxis with too few phagocytes arriving too late, perhaps secondary to a lymphocyte factor inhibiting chemotaxis. However, it is now clear that the chemotactic defect in these patients is variable and the fundamental basis for the impaired defenses is complex and inadequately delineated.

Table 62-4

Inherited Disorders of Phagocyte Function: Differential Features

Clinical Manifestations	Cellular or Molecular Defects	Diagnosis
CHRONIC GRANULOMATOUS DISEASES OF CHILDHOOD (60% X-LINKED, 40% AUTOSOMAL RECESSIVE)		
Severe infections of skin, ears, lungs, liver, and bone with catalase-positive microorganisms such as *S. aureus*, *Burkholderia cepacia*, *Aspergillus* sp., *Chromobacterium violaceum*; often hard to culture organism; excessive inflammation with granulomas, frequent lymph node suppuration; granulomas can obstruct GI or GU tracts; gingivitis, aphthous ulcers, seborrheic dermatitis	Absent respiratory burst due to the lack of one of four NADPH oxidase subunits in neutrophils, monocytes, and eosinophils	NBT test; absent superoxide and H_2O_2 production by neutrophils; absent chemiluminescence; immunoblot for NADPH oxidase components
CHÉDIAK-HIGASHI SYNDROME (AUTOSOMAL RECESSIVE)		
Recurrent pyogenic infections, especially with *S. aureus*; many patients get lymphomatous-like illness during adolescence; periodontal disease; partial oculocutaneous albinism, nystagmus, progressive peripheral neuropathy, mental retardation in some patients	Reduced chemotaxis and phagolysosome fusion, increased respiratory burst activity, defective egress from marrow, abnormal skin window	Giant primary granules in neutrophils and other granule-bearing cells (Wright's stain)
SPECIFIC GRANULE DEFICIENCY (AUTOSOMAL RECESSIVE?)		
Recurrent infections of skin, ears, and sinopulmonary tract; delayed wound healing; decreased inflammation; bleeding diathesis	Abnormal chemotaxis, impaired respiratory burst and bacterial killing, failure to upregulate chemotactic and adhesion receptors with stimulation, defect in transcription of granule proteins	Lack of secondary (specific) granules in neutrophils (Wright's stain), absent neutrophil-specific granule contents (i.e., lactoferrin), absent defensins, platelet alpha granule abnormality
MYELOPEROXIDASE DEFICIENCY (AUTOSOMAL RECESSIVE)		
Clinically normal except in patients with underlying disease such as diabetes mellitus; then candidiasis or other fungal infections	Absent myeloperoxidase due to pre- and posttranslational defects	Absent peroxidase in neutrophils
LEUKOCYTE ADHESION DEFICIENCY (AUTOSOMAL RECESSIVE)		
Type 1 Delayed separation of umbilical cord, sustained granulocytosis, recurrent infections of skin and mucosa, gingivitis, periodontal disease	Impaired phagocyte adherence, aggregation, spreading, chemotaxis, phagocytosis of C3bi-coated particles; defective production of CD18 subunit common to leukocyte integrins	Reduced phagocyte surface expression of the CD18-containing integrins using monoclonal antibodies against LFA-1 (CD18/CD11a), Mac-1 or CR3 (CD18/CD11b), p150,95 (CD18/CD11c)
Type 2 Severe mental retardation, short stature, Bombay (hh) blood phenotype, recurrent infections, granulocytosis	Impaired phagocyte rolling along endothelium	Reduced phagocyte surface expression of Sialyl-Lewis^x, using monoclonal antibodies against CD15s
HYPER IgE–RECURRENT INFECTION SYNDROME (AUTOSOMAL) (JOB'S SYNDROME)		
Eczematoid or pruritic dermatitis, "cold" skin abscesses, recurrent pneumonias with *S. aureus* with bronchopleural fistulas and cyst formation, mild eosinophilia, mucocutaneous candidiasis, atopy, coarse facies, restrictive lung disease, scoliosis	Reduced chemotaxis in some patients, reduced suppressor T cell activity	Clinical features, serum IgE > 2000 IU/mL, high serum anti-*S. aureus* IgE, low or absent serum and salivary anti-*S. aureus* IgA

The most common neutrophil defect is *myeloperoxidase deficiency*, which is inherited as an autosomal recessive trait and may have an incidence as high as about 1 in 2000 persons. Isolated myeloperoxidase deficiency is not associated with clinically compromised defenses, because other defense systems such as hydrogen peroxide generation are accelerated. Microbicidal activity of neutrophils is delayed but not absent. However, if another underlying defect in host defense, such as poorly controlled diabetes mellitus, accompanies myeloperoxidase deficiency, then host defenses are likely to be significantly compromised. An acquired form of myeloperoxidase deficiency occurs in myelomonocytic leukemia and acute myeloblastic leukemia.

Chédiak-Higashi syndrome (CHS) is a rare disease with autosomal recessive inheritance. Neutrophils and all cells containing lysosomes from patients with CHS characteristically have large granules (**Plate IV-19A**). CHS patients have increased infections due to a multitude of infectious agents. CHS neutrophils and monocytes have impaired chemotaxis and abnormal rates of microbial killing due to slow rates of fusion of the lysosomal granules with phagosomes. Natural killer cell function is also impaired.

Chronic granulomatous disease (CGD) represents a group of disorders of granulocyte and monocyte oxidative metabolism. Although CGD is rare, currently estimated to occur once in 250,000 individuals, it is an important model of defective neutrophil oxidative metabolism. Most often CGD is inherited as an X-linked recessive pattern, although in about 40 percent of patients the disease is inherited with an autosomal recessive pattern. Mutations of four genes corresponding to four proteins that assemble at the plasma membrane account for all patients with CGD. Two proteins (a 91-kDa protein, abnormal in X-linked CGD, and a 22-kDa protein, absent in one form of autosomal recessive CGD) form the heterodimer cytochrome b-558 in the plasma membrane. Two other proteins (47 and 67 kDa, abnormal in the other autosomal recessive forms of CGD) are cytoplasmic in origin and interact with the cytochrome following cell activation to form NADPH oxidase, required for hydrogen peroxide production. Leukocytes from patients with CGD have severely diminished hydrogen peroxide production. The genes involved in each of the defects have been cloned and sequenced and the chromosome locations identified. Patients with CGD characteristically have increased infection with catalase-positive microorganisms (organisms that destroy their own hydrogen peroxide). When patients with CGD become infected, they often have extensive inflammatory reactions, and lymph node suppuration is common despite the administration of appropriate antibiotics. Aphthous ulcers and chronic inflammation of the nares are usually present. Granulomas are frequent and can obstruct the gastrointestinal or genitourinary tracts. The excessive inflammatory reactions probably reflect abnormal turnoff of inflammation by failure to degrade chemoattractants and failure to degrade antigens that cause persistent neutrophil accumulation. Impaired killing of intracellular microorganisms by macrophages may lead to persistent cell-mediated immunity and granuloma formation.

MONONUCLEAR PHAGOCYTES

The mononuclear phagocyte system is defined as a continuum linking monoblasts, promonocytes, and monocytes with the structurally diverse tissue macrophages that make up what was previously referred to as the reticuloendothelial system. Macrophages are long-lived phagocytic cells capable of many of the functions of neutrophils. In addition, they are important secretory cells that, through their receptors and secretory products, participate in many complex immunologic and inflammatory processes not attributed to neutrophils. Monocytes leave the circulation by diapedesis more slowly than neutrophils and have a half-life in the blood of 12 to 24 h.

After blood monocytes arrive in the tissues, they differentiate into macrophages ("big eaters") with specialized functions suited for specific anatomic locations. Macrophages are particularly abundant in capillary walls of the lung, spleen, liver, and bone marrow, where they function to remove microorganisms and other noxious elements from the blood. Alveolar macrophages, liver Kupffer cells, splenic macrophages, peritoneal macrophages, bone marrow macrophages, lymphatic macrophages, brain microglial cells, and dendritic macrophages all have specialized functions. Macrophage-secreted products include lysozyme, neutral proteases, acid hydrolases, arginase, numerous complement components, enzyme inhibitors (plasmin, α_2 macroglobulin), binding proteins (transferrin, fibronectin, transcobalamin II), nucleosides, and cytokines (TNFα, IL-1, -8, -12). Interleukin 1 (see Chaps. 17 and 305) has many important functions, including stimulating the hypothalamus to initiate fever, mobilizing leukocytes from the bone marrow, as well as activating lymphocytes and neutrophils. Tumor necrosis factor α (also called *cachectin*) is a pyrogen that duplicates many of the actions of IL-1 and plays an important role in the pathogenesis of gram-negative shock (see Chap. 124). It can stimulate vigorous production of hydrogen peroxide and related toxic oxygen species by macrophages and neutrophils. In addition, TNFα induces the catabolic responses of chronic inflammation, which contribute to the profound wasting (cachexia) associated with many chronic diseases.

Other macrophage-secreted products include reactive oxygen metabolites, bioactive lipids (arachidonate metabolites and platelet-activating factors), chemokines, bone marrow colony stimulating factors, and factors stimulating fibroblast and microvasculature proliferation. Macrophages help regulate the replication of lymphocytes and participate in the killing of tumors, viruses, and certain bacteria (*Mycobacterium tuberculosis* and *Listeria monocytogenes*). Macrophages are key effector cells in the elimination of intracellular microorganisms. Their ability to fuse to form giant cells that coalesce into granulomas in response to some inflammatory stimuli is important in the elimination of intracellular microbes and may be under the control of IFNγ.

Macrophages play an important role in the immune response (see Chap. 305). They process and present antigen to lymphocytes and secrete cytokines that modulate and direct lymphocyte development and function. Macrophages participate in autoimmune phenomena by removing immune complexes and other immunologically active substances from the circulation. Furthermore, they play a role in wound healing, in the disposal of senescent cells, and in the development of atheromas.

DISORDERS OF THE MONONUCLEAR PHAGOCYTE SYSTEM Many disorders of neutrophils extend to mononuclear phagocytes. Thus drugs that suppress neutrophil production in the bone marrow usually lead to monocytopenia. Transient monocytopenia also can be seen after stress or glucocorticoid administration. Monocytosis is associated with certain infections such as tuberculosis, brucellosis, subacute bacterial endocarditis, Rocky Mountain spotted fever, malaria, and visceral leishmaniasis (kala azar). Monocytosis is also seen in malignancies, leukemias, myeloproliferative syndromes, hemolytic anemias, chronic idiopathic neutropenias, and granulomatous diseases such as sarcoidosis, regional enteritis, and some collagen vascular diseases. Patients with LAD, HIE (Job's) syndrome, CHS, and chronic granulomatous diseases all have defects in the mononuclear phagocyte system. Impaired monocyte cytokine production has been found in some patients with disseminated nontuberculous mycobacterial infection who are not infected with the human immunodeficiency virus (HIV).

Certain viral infections impair mononuclear phagocyte function. For example, influenza virus infection is associated with abnormal monocyte chemotaxis. Mononuclear phagocytes can be infected by the HIV, and abnormal monocyte chemotaxis and abnormal clearance of IgG-coated erythrocytes (discussed below) by macrophages is also seen in AIDS (see Chap. 308). It is likely that the defects of the monocyte-macrophage system in AIDS contribute to the disordered immunoregulation and increased susceptibility to opportunistic infection due to intracellular microorganisms such as *Pneumocystis carinii* and *M. avium* complex. T lymphocytes produce IFNγ, which induces Fc-receptor expression and phagocytosis and stimulates hydrogen peroxide production by mononuclear phagocytes and neutrophils. In certain diseases, such as AIDS, IFNγ production may be deficient, while in other diseases, such as T cell lymphomas, excessive release of IFNγ is thought to cause erythrophagocytosis by splenic macrophages.

Specific defects of mononuclear phagocytes have been described in certain autoimmune diseases. Removal of IgG-coated radiolabeled autologous erythrocytes, presumably via the Fc receptor of splenic macrophages, is profoundly abnormal in patients with active systemic lupus erythematosus. Patients with other autoimmune diseases characterized by tissue deposition of immune complexes, as seen in Sjögren's syndrome, mixed cryoglobulinemia, dermatitis herpetiformis, and chronic progressive multiple sclerosis, also have defects in Fc-receptor function as judged by clearance of IgG-coated erythrocytes (see Chap. 311). Clinically, normal subjects with genetic haplotypes commonly associated with autoimmune disease (i.e., HLA-B8/DRw3) also have an increased incidence of defective Fc-receptor–specific functional activity, suggesting that this defect may predispose individuals with this genetic profile to immune-complex disease.

Monocytopenia occurs with acute infections, with stress, and following administration of glucocorticoids. Monocytopenia also occurs in aplastic anemia, hairy cell leukemia, and acute myelogenous leukemia and as a direct result of myelotoxic and immunosuppressive drugs.

EOSINOPHILS

Eosinophils and neutrophils share similar morphology, many lysosomal constituents, phagocytic capacity, and oxidative metabolism. Eosinophils express a specific chemoattractant receptor and respond to a specific chemokine, eotaxin. However, there are major differences between the two cell types, and little is known about the natural function of eosinophils. Eosinophils are much longer lived than neutrophils, and unlike neutrophils, tissue eosinophils can recirculate. During most infections, eosinophils do not appear to have any important function. However, in invasive helminthic infections, such as hookworm, schistosomiasis, strongyloidiasis, toxocariasis, trichinosis, filariasis, echinococcosis, and cysticercosis, the eosinophil likely plays a central role in host defense. Eosinophils are also associated with bronchial asthma, cutaneous allergic reactions, and other hypersensitivity states.

The characteristic red-staining eosinophil granules (Wright's stain) contain a number of unique constituents. The distinctive feature of the eosinophil granule is its crystalline core consisting of an arginine-rich protein (major basic protein) with histaminase activity, which is probably important in host defense against parasites. Eosinophil granules also contain a unique eosinophil peroxidase that catalyzes the oxidation of many substances by hydrogen peroxide and may facilitate killing of microorganisms.

Eosinophil peroxidase, in the presence of hydrogen peroxide and halide, initiates mast cell secretion in vitro and thereby may contribute to inflammation. Other substances found in eosinophils include cationic proteins, some of which bind to heparin and reduce its anticoagulant activity. Eosinophil cytoplasm contains Charcot-Leyden crystal protein, a hexagonal bipyramidal crystal first described in leukemia and then in sputum from asthma patients, which is lysophospholipase and may function to restrict the toxicity of certain lysophospholipids. Eosinophils also contain a powerful neurotoxin. Patients with hypereosinophilic syndrome and cerebral spinal fluid eosinophilia exhibit varied neurologic abnormalities.

Several factors enhance the eosinophil's function in host defense. For example, stimulated T cell–derived factors enhance the ability of eosinophils to kill parasites. Mast cell–derived eosinophil chemotactic factor of anaphylaxis (ECFa) increases the number of eosinophil complement receptors and enhances eosinophil killing of parasites. In addition, eosinophil colony stimulating factors (e.g., IL-5) produced by macrophages may not only increase eosinophil production in the bone marrow but also may activate eosinophils to kill parasites.

EOSINOPHILIA Eosinophilia is the presence of more than 500 eosinophils/μL of blood and is common in many settings besides parasite infection. Significant tissue eosinophilia can occur without an elevated blood count. The most common cause of eosinophilia is probably allergic reactions to drugs such as iodides, aspirin, sulfonamides, nitrofurantoin, penicillins, and cephalosporins. Allergies such as hay fever, asthma, eczema, serum sickness, allergic vasculitis, and pemphigus commonly are associated with eosinophilia. Eosinophilia is also seen in collagen vascular diseases (e.g., rheumatoid arthritis, eosinophilic fasciitis, allergic angiitis, and periarteritis nodosa) and malignancies (e.g., Hodgkin's disease, mycosis fungoides, chronic myelogenous leukemia, and cancer of the lung, stomach, pancreas, ovary, or uterus), as well as in rare diseases such as Job's syndrome and CGD; the mechanisms for the eosinophilia in these diseases are not known. Eosinophilia is commonly seen in the helminthic infections. Therapeutic administration of the cytokines IL-2 and GM-CSF frequently leads to transient eosinophilia. The most dramatic hypereosinophilic syndromes are Loeffler's syndrome, Loeffler's endocarditis, eosinophilic leukemia, and idiopathic hypereosinophilic syndrome (with counts as high as 50,000 to 100,000/μL).

The idiopathic hypereosinophilic syndrome represents a heterogeneous group of disorders with the common feature of prolonged eosinophilia of unknown cause and associated organ system dysfunction, including the heart, central nervous system, kidneys, lungs, gastrointestinal tract, and skin. The bone marrow is involved in all subjects, but the most severe complications involve the heart and central nervous system. Eosinophils are found in the involved tissues and are thought to cause tissue damage by local deposition of toxic eosinophil proteins such as eosinophil cationic protein and eosinophil major basic protein. In the heart, the pathologic changes lead to thrombosis, which may result in endocardial fibrosis and restrictive endomyocardiopathy. Similar pathologic changes are thought to contribute to the damage of tissues in other organ systems. Although the mechanism for the hypereosinophilia is not known, it has been shown that chemotherapy with glucocorticoids usually induces remission. In patients unresponsive to glucocorticoids, a cytotoxic agent such as hydroxyurea has been used successfully to lower the peripheral blood eosinophil counts and to improve markedly the prognosis. Interferon α also is effective in some patients, including those unresponsive to hydroxyurea. Aggressive medical and surgical approaches are employed for management of patients with cardiovascular complications.

The *eosinophilia-myalgia syndrome* is a multisystem disease with prominent cutaneous, hematologic, and visceral manifestations that frequently evolves into a chronic course and can occasionally be fatal. The syndrome is characterized by eosinophilia (greater than 1000 eosinophils/μL) and generalized disabling myalgias without other recognized causes. Eosinophil fasciitis, pneumonitis and myocarditis, neuropathy culminating in respiratory failure, and encephalopathy have been described. The association of the disease with ingestion of L-tryptophan–containing products originating from a single source has led to the identification and characterization of putative etiologic agents present as contaminants in these preparations. Although the accumulation of eosinophils, lymphocytes, macrophages, and fibroblasts in the affected tissues suggests that these cells play important roles in the pathogenesis of the eosinophilia-myalgia syndrome, the precise mechanism of their involvement has not been established. Several studies have demonstrated the activation of eosinophils and the deposition of eosinophil-derived toxic proteins in affected tissues. Fibroblast activation and increased expression of genes coding for various connective tissue molecules have been demonstrated. Furthermore, IL-5 and transforming growth factor β have been implicated as potential mediators. Treatment has included withdrawal of L-tryptophan–containing products and the administration of glucocorticoids. Most patients recover fully, remain stable, or show slow recovery, but in some patients (up to 5 percent) the disease can be fatal. This disease emphasizes the importance of chemical and environmental factors in the development of systemic disorders characterized by chronic inflammation and fibrosis.

EOSINOPENIA This occurs with stress, such as acute bacterial infection, and following administration of glucocorticoids. The mechanism of eosinopenia of acute bacterial infection is unknown but is independent of endogenous glucocorticoids, since it occurs in animals following total adrenalectomy. There is no known adverse effect of eosinopenia.

LABORATORY DIAGNOSIS AND MANAGEMENT

Initial studies of WBC and differential and often a bone marrow examination are followed by assessment of bone marrow reserves (steroid challenge test), marginated circulating pool of cells (epinephrine challenge test), and marginating ability (endotoxin challenge test) (see Fig. 62-3). In vivo assessment of inflammation is possible with a Rebuck skin window test or an in vivo blister assay, which measures the ability of leukocytes and inflammatory mediators to accumulate locally within the skin. In vivo clearance of IgG-coated erythrocytes provides a useful way to monitor the mononuclear phagocyte system. In vitro tests of phagocyte aggregation, adherence, chemotaxis, phagocytosis, degranulation, and microbicidal activity (for *Staph. aureus*) help pinpoint cellular or humoral lesions that can then be further characterized at the molecular level. Deficiencies of oxidative metabolism are screened with the nitroblue tetrazolium (NBT) dye test, which is based on the ability of products of oxidative metabolism to reduce yellow, soluble NBT to blue-black formazan, an insoluble material that precipitates intracellularly and can be seen microscopically. Further aspects of neutrophil oxidative metabolism are defined by studies of superoxide and hydrogen peroxide production.

The most important aspect of patient management is to appreciate that patients with leukopenias or leukocyte dysfunction often have delayed inflammatory responses. Therefore, clinical manifestations may be minimal despite overwhelming infection, and unusual infections must always be suspected. Early signs of infection demand prompt, aggressive culturing for microorganisms and use of antibiotics and surgical drainage of abscesses. Prolonged antibiotics are often required. Daily white blood cell transfusions (enriched for neutrophils) are controversial. In patients with CGD, prophylactic antibiotics trimethoprim-sulfamethoxazole) diminish the frequency of life-threatening infections. Surgery is required for thorough drainage of abscesses in lung, liver, and bones. Short courses of glucocorticoids have had dramatic effects in the management of the granulomas of CGD. For example, obstruction of the gastrointestinal or genitourinary tract in CGD can be diminished with a short course of steroids followed by a long one of a nonsteroidal anti-inflammatory agent. Recombinant human IFNγ, which nonspecifically stimulates phagocytic cell function, reduces the frequency of infections in CGD patients by 70 percent and reduces the severity of infection (hospital days for infection) as well. This effect of IFNγ in CGD is additive to the effect of prophylactic antibiotics. Interferon γ has been approved by the U.S. Food and Drug Administration for use in CGD at a recommended dose of 50 μL/m^2 of body surface area, subcutaneously three times weekly. Interferon γ also has been used successfully in the treatment of leprosy, nontuberculous mycobacteria, and visceral leishmaniasis.

Rigorous oral hygiene reduces but does not eliminate the discomfort of gingivitis, periodontal disease, and aphthous ulcers; chlorhexidine mouthwash and tooth brushing with a hydrogen peroxide–sodium bicarbonate paste helps many patients. Ketoconazole has caused dramatic improvement of mucocutaneous candidiasis in patients with Job's syndrome. Treatment to restore myelopoiesis in patients with

neutropenia due to impaired production has included use of androgens, glucocorticoids, lithium, and immunosuppressive therapy. Recombinant G-CSF is useful in the management of certain forms of neutropenia due to depressed production, especially that related to cancer chemotherapy. Patients with chronic neutropenia with evidence of a good bone marrow reserve should not receive prophylactic antibiotics.

Patients with constant or cyclic neutrophil counts below 500 cells/μL may benefit from prophylactic antibiotics and G-CSF during periods of neutropenia. Oral trimethoprim-sulfamethoxazole (160/800 mg) twice daily is commonly used to prevent infection, although concerns about its predisposing to fungal infections have been raised. Increased fungal infection is not seen in CGD patients on this regimen. Oral quinolones such as norfloxacin and ciprofloxacin have been suggested alternatives.

In the setting of cytotoxic chemotherapy with severe, persistent neutropenia, the proven effectiveness of trimethoprim-sulfamethoxazole in preventing *P. carinii* pneumonia may offer another incentive to use this form of prophylaxis. These patients, and patients with phagocytic cell dysfunction, should avoid heavy exposure to airborne soil, dust, or decaying matter (mulch, manure), which are often rich in spores of *Aspergillus* or other fungi. Restriction of activities or social contact probably makes little difference in risk of infection.

Cure of some congenital phagocyte defects is theoretically possible by bone marrow transplantation (see Chap. 116). However, complications of bone marrow transplantation are still serious, and with rigorous medical care many patients with phagocytic disorders can go for years without a life-threatening infection. The identification of specific gene defects in patients with LAD 1 and CGD has led to in vitro correction of B cells from these patients by gene transfer. Gene correction has been performed on peripheral blood progenitor cells from patients with CGD. This approach has been successful in vitro, leading to restoration of a functional NADPH oxidase. Initial experiments also have been carried out in humans, making gene therapy for CGD and other genetic disorders a likely emerging reality.

BIBLIOGRAPHY

Cassatella MA: The production of cytokines by polymorphonuclear neutrophils. Immunol Today 16:21, 1995

Dong F et al: Mutations in the gene for the granulocyte colony-stimulating factor receptor in patients with acute myeloid leukemia preceded by severe congenital neutropenia. New Engl J Med 333:487, 1995

Gallin JI et al: Interferon-γ in the management of infectious diseases. Ann Intern Med 123:216, 1995

Hogg JC, Doerschuk CM: Leukocyte traffic in the lung. Annu Rev Physiol 57:97, 1995

Holland SM, Gallin JI: Neutrophil disorders, in *Samter's Immunologic Diseases*, MM Frank et al (eds). Boston, Little, Brown, 1995, p 529

Kuhns DB et al: Increased circulating cytokines, cytokine antagonists, and E-selectin after intravenous administration of endotoxin in humans. J Infect Dis 171:145, 1995

Leto TL et al: Assembly of the phagocyte NADPH oxidase:binding of Src homology 3 domains to proline-rich targets. Proc Natl Acad Sci USA 91:10650, 1994

Lieschke GJ, Burgess AW: Granulocyte colony-stimulating factor and granulocyte-macrophage colony-stimulating factor. N Engl J Med 327:28, 99, 1992

Springer TA: Traffic signals for lymphocyte recirculation and leukocyte emigration: The multistep paradigm. Cell 76:301, 1994

Varga J et al: The cause and pathogenesis of the eosinophil-myalgia syndrome. Ann Intern Med 116:140, 1992

63 Daniel C. Ihde, Dan L. Longo

PRESENTATIONS OF THE PATIENT WITH CANCER: SOLID TUMORS IN ADULTS

THE MAGNITUDE OF THE PROBLEM

Cancer is a major cause of morbidity in the United States. In 1996, the American Cancer Society estimated that 1,359,150 people were diagnosed with a malignant neoplasm and 554,740 died from one of these diseases. Cancer is responsible for 23.9 percent of all American deaths and is exceeded only by heart disease as a cause of mortality (33.0 percent of deaths). Unfortunately, cancer mortality is increasing, while that from cardiac disease is declining, and sometime early in the next century cancer is expected to become the leading cause of death in this country, as it already is in Japan.

All cancers share the characteristic of disordered normal control over cell division, growth, and differentiation. Their initial clinical manifestations are extremely heterogeneous, however, since over 70 types of cancer arising in virtually every organ or tissue in the body are recognized. They may be entirely asymptomatic until late in the disease course. Symptoms related to cancerous cell growth generally fall into one of three categories: (1) local—pain or swelling that may be painful or painless in a site of tumor cell expansion; (2) regional—dysfunction in the organ of origin or in adjacent or distant organs, related to the local or metastatic growth of the tumor; and (3) systemic—remote effects of tumor related to production of hormones or cytokines by the tumor or the host reaction to the tumor (see Table 63-1). In addition to problems related to the tumor itself, there are also psychosocial manifestations related to the *diagnosis* of cancer. Psychological distress, anxiety, and depression may occur out of proportion to the prognosis in response to the diagnosis of cancer. → *The problems associated with the diagnosis of cancer are discussed in Chap. 81.*

Local effects may include pain without a mass or a painful or painless mass or swelling. Regional effects may include edema or effusion from obstruction of lymphatic drainage; organ dysfunction (e.g., liver function abnormality or myelophthisic anemia); obstruction of flow of air, blood, urine, cerebrospinal fluid, bile, stool, or lymph; nerve dysfunction from compression (e.g., hoarseness from laryngeal nerve compression); and breach of structural integrity (e.g., bone fracture, blood vessel rupture, or viscus perforation). → *The paraneoplastic effects of cancer are numerous and are discussed in greater detail in Chaps. 102 and 103.*

Nearly every cardinal manifestation of disease discussed in this book may be associated with cancer. However, certain manifestations are more likely to be found in the more common tumors. This chapter is therefore confined to discussing the more frequent presenting symptoms or findings that lead to the diagnosis of a malignant neoplasm in patients with the 10 most common solid tumors of both men and women, which are quantitatively by far the major causes of death from cancer. → *A similar discussion of diagnostic considerations in the evaluation of patients with hematopoietic neoplasia (leukemias and lymphomas) may be found in Chaps. 61 and 62.*

Table 63-2 illustrates that there is considerable overlap among the specific types of solid tumors that are most frequently diagnosed in men and women. Six of these cancers—those of the lung, colon and rectum, bladder, kidney, and pancreas and cutaneous melanoma—are among the 10 most common tumors in both genders. Four of the common cancers are gender-specific—endometrium, ovary, and cervix in women and prostate in men—and a fifth, breast cancer, occurs in women over 99 percent of the time. The remaining three, oropharyngeal/laryngeal, stomach, and brain, are among the 10 most common

cancers of men but are not rare in women. It is noteworthy that the number of cases of newly diagnosed cancer within the categories of the 10 most common solid tumors in each gender totals 1,090,100 individuals, 80.2 percent of all cancer patients diagnosed in 1996. Thus, knowledge of common symptoms and presentations in individuals who develop one of the 10 most common cancers in either men or women will be applicable to a substantial majority of all cancer patients.

CANCERS GROUPED BY ORGAN SYSTEM

UPPER AERODIGESTIVE TRACT CANCERS Oropharyngeal/Laryngeal Asymptomatic and symptomatic oral neoplasms, both precancerous and cancerous, are often first noted during dental examination. Leukoplakia, a whitish patch in the mouth that cannot be wiped away, and erythroplakia, a reddish, sometimes raised or velvety painless lesion, are sometimes precancerous lesions, especially when associated with dysplasia on biopsy. Squamous carcinoma is the most common persisting ulceration in the oral cavity. These lesions are often painless and exhibit both infiltrative (crater-like with raised borders) and whitish exophytic growth patterns. Unexplained oral ulcers that do not heal after several weeks should be biopsied.

Oropharyngeal, hypopharyngeal, and laryngeal tumors often present with nodal metastasis in the neck; excisional biopsy should always be considered for a persisting noninflammatory neck mass. Hoarseness is associated with laryngeal and oropharyngeal cancers, difficulty in swallowing with oropharyngeal lesions, and otalgia with hypopharyngeal tumors. These symptoms are often associated with more advanced disease. Malodorous breath and hemoptysis may also occur.

Lung A myriad of symptoms or signs can raise the first suspicion of lung cancer. Symptoms arising from the primary tumor include

Table 63-1

Manifestations of Malignant Disease

Local
  Pain
  Swelling
Regional and distant
  Pain
  Swelling
  Edema
  Organ dysfunction
  Obstruction of flow (air, blood, urine, CSF, bile, stool)
  Compression of nerves
  Weakening or breach of structural integrity (bone, blood vessels, bowel)
Paraneoplastic syndromes (see Chap. 102)
  Metabolic disorders
    Hypercalcemia
    Cachexia
    Fever
    Hyponatremia
  Ectopic hormone production
    ACTH
  Neuropathy and CNS abnormalities (see Chap. 103)
  Dermatologic conditions (see Chap. 57)
  Hematologic abnormalities, including clotting and bleeding
  Immunosuppression or autoimmunity
Psychosocial effects
  Anxiety
  Depression
  Loss of autonomy
  Fear of death and dying
  Fear of pain and altered body image
  Alienation

NOTE: CSF, cerebrospinal fluid; ACTH, adrenocorticotropic hormone; CNS, central nervous system.

postobstructive pneumonia, stridor, dyspnea from intrinsic or extrinsic tumor or a pleural effusion, hemoptysis, and cough. Regional intrathoracic symptoms vary and may include superior vena cava syndrome, diaphragmatic paralysis from phrenic nerve compression, hoarseness from recurrent laryngeal nerve compression by mediastinal nodes, dysphagia from esophageal compression, severe pain radiating down the arm from brachial nerve compression in Pancoast tumors, and pericardial tamponade.

The patient may first come to attention because of a distant tumor metastasis resulting in a seizure from brain or pain from bone or liver involvement. Paraneoplastic syndromes may include hypercalcemia or hypertrophic pulmonary osteoarthropathy in non-small cell lung cancer and Eaton-Lambert syndrome, inappropriate secretion of antidiuretic hormone, and ectopic Cushing's syndrome in small cell tumors. Decreased appetite and weight loss are not uncommon and are probably manifestations of a poorly characterized paraneoplastic syndrome. Among patients presenting with a carcinoma of unknown primary site, lung cancers are one of two tumors most often identified later. Discovery of a lung mass in an asymptomatic patient for whom a chest radiograph is ordered for another reason is not uncommon; these patients usually have a better prognosis.

BREAST CANCER Over the past decade, breast cancer is being diagnosed much earlier in the course of its natural history. The majority of patients now present with stage I disease (no evidence of lymph node involvement) or carcinoma in situ. Thus, a mammographic abnormality detected during a screening examination or a lump in the breast now constitute the most common presentations. → *A detailed discussion of evaluation of breast abnormalities is presented in Chap. 64.*

GASTROINTESTINAL CANCERS **Stomach Cancer** Few symptoms are associated with early gastric cancer, and most patients are diagnosed only after the disease is more advanced. The epigastric discomfort, anorexia, and minor weight loss that sometimes occur are relatively nonspecific. Unexplained anemia may lead to endoscopic evaluation and a diagnosis, but gastrointestinal bleeding infrequently occurs in more treatable early stage disease. Grave symptoms and signs such as early satiety from a diffusely infiltrating tumor, vomiting from pyloric obstruction, palpation of a left supraclavicular node or a rectal mass (Blumer's shelf), and ovarian metastases usually indicate incurable disease.

Pancreatic Cancer Most patients are incurable at the time of diagnosis. Severe pain radiating to the back, probably due to splanchnic nerve invasion, and weight loss are hallmarks of the disease. Obstructive jaundice, especially when not accompanied by pain and weight loss, is associated with tumors of the pancreatic head, which are more often surgically resectable. Tumors of the body do not cause obstruction and are usually not resectable when diagnosed. Gastric or duodenal obstruction by tumor is associated with disordered intestinal motility, possibly from infiltration of the splanchnic nerves.

Colorectal Cancer Colorectal cancer can be diagnosed in a patient with symptoms or as a result of a screening program with fecal occult blood tests or endoscopic examination. Patients with early, resectable disease are often asymptomatic or have only nonspecific symptoms; individuals shown not to have colorectal neoplasms also sometimes note changes in bowel habits, abdominal pain, and rectal bleeding.

Symptomatic patients with colorectal cancer usually have abdominal pain or nausea and vomiting due to obstruction; bleeding from the tumor, sometimes accompanied by anemia; or chronic or acute bowel perforation. In more advanced disease, hyperbilirubinemia or other biochemical abnormalities from liver metastases may be present.

Right colon tumors are more insidious and less likely to cause obstruction, because the bowel lumen is more ample and the stool more liquid. Malignant obstruction usually occurs in left-sided lesions, where the lumen diameter is smaller and the stool more solid. Rectal tumors more often present with hematochezia and tenesmus.

GYNECOLOGIC CANCERS **Ovarian Cancer** Some patients with ovarian cancer have nonspecific symptoms of nausea, dyspepsia, or a sensation of swelling or discomfort in the lower abdomen; others have no complaints at all. More striking symptoms, such as abdominal pain, distention or masses, and vaginal bleeding, are usually manifestations of advanced disease. At diagnosis, cancer has spread beyond the ovaries in 75 percent of patients and beyond the pelvis in 60 percent. All perimenopausal or postmenopausal women with pelvic or abdominal symptoms should have a pelvic and general physical examination. An adnexal mass in a postmenopausal woman should usually prompt exploratory laparotomy, since functional ovarian cysts should not occur in nonmenstruating women.

Endometrial Cancer Almost all women with carcinoma of the endometrium develop vaginal bleeding, either a serosanguinous discharge or frank bleeding. In the three-fourths of patients who are postmenopausal, this should be readily detectable. However, only about one-fifth of women with postmenopausal bleeding have endometrial cancer. Pelvic examination and endometrial biopsy should be obtained. Pyometria in a postmenopausal woman should also prompt pelvic examination and endometrial biopsy. Pain, vaginal discharge, weight loss, and urinary or gastrointestinal complaints usually occur only in the setting of more advanced disease.

Cervical Cancer Carcinoma in situ of the uterine cervix can be detected by Pap smear but is not associated with any symptoms. Early invasive cancer can be associated with vaginal discharge or bleeding, especially postcoital spotting. In more aggressive invasive cancer, serosanguinous or purulent vaginal discharge progressively increases. Intermenstrual bleeding becomes more pronounced. Pelvic pain and urinary and rectal symptoms can be associated with tumor necrosis or chronic inflammation. Low back or leg pain may indicate compression of lumbosacral nerves or ureteral obstruction. Urinary frequency or urgency, rectal tenesmus, and bleeding are consequences of direct bladder or rectal invasion.

Pap smears should be obtained during the pelvic examination of any woman but especially those with pelvic symptoms described above. Any visually abnormal findings should be followed up with colposcopy, endocervical curretage, and colposcopically directed cervical biopsies. If this examination reveals a positive endocervical curretage, unsatisfactory colposcopic visualization, or microinvasion or other abnormalities, a diagnostic cone biopsy is performed, which removes a conical portion of the cervix including the entire transformation zone and some of the endocervix.

Table 63-2

Ten Most Common Solid Tumors in Men and Women, 1996

	Men			Women	
Rank	Type	New Cases		Type	New Cases
1.	Prostate	317,100		Breast	184,300
2.	Lung	98,900		Lung	78,100
3.	Colorectal	67,600		Colorectal	65,900
4.	Bladder	38,300		Endometrial	34,000
5.	Oropharyngeal/laryngeal	29,300		Ovary	26,700
6.	Cutaneous melanoma	21,800		Cutaneous melanoma	16,500
7.	Kidney/upper urinary track	18,500		Cervix	15,700
8.	Stomach	14,000		Bladder	14,600
9.	Pancreas	12,400		Pancreas	13,900
10.	Brain/CNS	10,400		Kidney/upper urinary tract	12,100
	Total	628,300		Total	461,800

NOTE: CNS, central nervous system.
SOURCE: After Parker et al, with permission.

GENITOURINARY CANCERS   **Renal/Upper Urinary Tract Cancer**   The classic triad of pain, hematuria, and a flank mass occurs in fewer than 20 percent of patients with adenocarcinoma of the kidney (hypernephroma). About one-third of patients present with metastatic disease, one-quarter with locally advanced disease, and 45 percent with localized tumor. Systemic manifestations of disease include hypochromic anemia, fever, weight loss, and nonmetastatic abnormalities of liver function; the latter are associated with a poor prognosis but may be reversible if the primary tumor is removed. Up to 5 percent of patients have polycythemia or hypercalcemia.

Transitional cell carcinomas of both the renal pelvis and ureters are associated with cigarette abuse. These tumors are manifestations of a field defect in which patients with larger tumors and carcinoma in situ are at high risk of multifocal recurrences. Hematuria is the presenting symptom in most cases.

Bladder Cancer   Gross or microscopic hematuria, usually painless, is by far the most common presentation in patients with bladder cancer, occurring in approximately 75 percent. Intermittent microscopic hematuria may be the initial manifestation of cancer. Vesical irritation is present in about 30 percent of patients and is associated with carcinoma in situ. In patients with advanced bladder cancer, pelvic pain from an enlarging tumor mass or nerve root compression may be present. Flank pain is a prominent symptom in patients with ureteral obstruction. Lower extremity edema due to lymphatic or venous obstruction can also occur.

Prostate Cancer   Localized prostate cancer is often asymptomatic but can be detected by palpation of one or more nodules on digital rectal examination. Of the more than half of patients who present with locally advanced tumor or distant metastases, symptoms of urinary outlet obstruction or bone pain frequently occur. In the minority who present with more advanced disease, spinal cord compression, weight loss, anemia, and renal failure due to ureteral obstruction are sometimes observed.

More recently, early detection of prostate cancer by screening for elevated levels of prostate-specific antigen (PSA) in the serum has been achieved. Many patients who are diagnosed by this test have no palpable prostatic nodules, and cancer is documented by means of ultrasound-guided or blind biopsies. Such patients more frequently have lower stage disease, with tumors more often pathologically confined to the prostate, than patients whose tumors are detected because of clinical findings. Whether this earlier detection will result in reduced mortality from prostate cancer requires the results of controlled clinical trials of PSA-based screening programs and further follow-up.

CUTANEOUS MELANOMA   Malignant melanomas are deeply pigmented tumors of the skin, which may arise in any part of the body but are more common on women's legs and men's trunks. Variation in color, an irregular border with indentations, an irregular raised surface, and ulcerations on the surface of the lesions are typical features that lead to biopsy and diagnosis. Since melanomas can evolve into a variety of appearances, any pigmented lesion that changes in appearance should be biopsied.

People at greater risk of developing cutaneous melanoma include those with a tendency to severe sunburns, red or blond hair, fair skin, and more than 20 pigmented nevi. Individuals with dysplastic nevi or familial melanoma are at greatly increased risk and should have their entire skin surface examined frequently.

BRAIN TUMORS   Neoplasms of the brain in adults are more often metastases from cancer in other organs than from tumors that originate in the brain itself. The most common primary brain tumors in adults are astrocytomas, which comprise over half of all such tumors and arise from glial or supporting cells. They exhibit heterogeneous clinical behaviors, ranging from indolent growth rates in low-grade gliomas to a markedly aggressive course in glioblastoma multiforme. Headache, usually most prominent upon arising in the morning, is the most common presenting symptom of gliomas and usually results from increased intracranial pressure due to tumor mass. Seizures are the second most common manifestation of primary brain tumors in adults. Numerous symptoms are specific to the portion of the brain in which the tumor arises, for example, homonymous hemianopsia in occipital lobe lesions. Thorough neurologic examination and magnetic resonance imaging of the brain are indicated when a primary brain tumor is suspected.

CANCER'S SEVEN WARNING SIGNS

For many years, the American Cancer Society has publicized a list of seven warning signs of possible cancer to the general public. The presence of any of these signs should prompt examination by a physician.

1. Change in bowel or bladder habits. Development of diarrhea, constipation, difficulty passing the stool, and gray or black stools may indicate jaundice or gastrointestinal bleeding. Blood or pus in the urine, frequent painful urination, and sudden development of nocturia may indicate urinary tract bleeding or prostatic or other obstruction.
2. A sore on the skin that does not heal may indicate a skin cancer.
3. Unusual bleeding or discharge from the nose, mouth, skin, nipple, or vagina, although more often a sign of infection, may also be a manifestation of cancer.
4. A thickening or lump in the breast or elsewhere may be the first indication of a breast cancer or a sarcoma of the soft tissues.
5. Indigestion or difficulty in swallowing, although overwhelmingly due to benign causes such as a hiatal hernia, may be due to a tumor in the esophagus or stomach. If these symptoms persist or worsen, they should be brought to the attention of a physician.
6. Obvious changes in a wart or mole, such as increasing size, change in color, or change in shape, may be a sign of malignant melanoma. Medical attention should be sought.
7. Nagging cough, particularly if associated with expectoration of blood, and hoarseness, which may be due to compression of a nerve innervating the vocal cord, may both be signs of lung cancer, particularly if these symptoms occur in a cigarette smoker.

BIBLIOGRAPHY

BEATTIE EJ: Seven warning signs of cancer: A fuller explanation for patients. Prim Care Cancer September: 45, 1989
CONN RB (ed): *Current Diagnosis*, 8th ed. Philadelphia, Saunders, 1991
DEVITA VT et al (eds): *Cancer: Principles and Practice of Oncology*, 5th ed. Philadelphia, Lippincott, 1997
PARKER SL et al: Cancer statistics, 1996. CA Cancer J Clin 46:5, 1996

64   *Marc E. Lippman*

EVALUATION OF BREAST MASSES IN MEN AND WOMEN

Because the breasts are a common site of fatal disease in women and because they frequently provide clues to underlying systemic disease in both men and women, examination of the breasts is an essential part of the physical examination. Unfortunately, internists frequently do not examine the breasts in men and, in women, they are apt to refer this evaluation to gynecologists. Because of the association between early detection and improved outcome, it is the duty of every physician to distinguish breast abnormalities at the earliest possible stage and to institute a definitive diagnostic workup whenever appropriate. It is for this reason that all women should be trained in self-examination of the breasts. Although breast cancer in men is unusual, unilateral lesions should be evaluated in the same manner as in women, with the recognition that gynecomastia in men can sometimes begin unilaterally and is often asymmetric. Nevertheless, about as many suspicious breast lesions are now detected by screening mammography as by physical examination.

Virtually all breast cancer is diagnosed by biopsy of a nodule detected either on a mammogram or by palpation. A series of algorithms have been developed to enhance the likelihood of diagnosing breast cancer and to reduce the frequency of unnecessary biopsy.

THE PALPABLE BREAST MASS Women should be strongly encouraged to self-examine the breasts monthly. The minimum benefit of this practice is the greater likelihood of detecting a mass at a smaller size, when it can be treated with limited surgery. Breast examination by the physician should be performed in good light so as to see retractions and other skin changes. The nipple and areolae should be inspected, and an attempt should be made to elicit nipple discharge. All areas where regional lymph nodes are present should be examined, and any lesions should be measured. While lesions with certain features are more likely to be cancerous (hard, irregular, tethered or fixed, or painless lesions), physical examination alone cannot exclude malignancy. Furthermore, a negative mammogram in the presence of a persistent lump in the breast does not exclude malignancy.

In premenopausal women, lesions that are either equivocal or nonsuspicious on physical examination should be reexamined in 2 to 4 weeks, during the the follicular phase of the menstrual cycle. Days 5 to 7 of the cycle are the best time for breast examination. A dominant mass in a postmenopausal woman or a dominant mass that persists through a menstrual cycle in a premenopausal woman should be aspirated by fine needle biopsy or referred to a surgeon. If nonbloody fluid is aspirated and the lesion is thereby cured permanently, then diagnosis, therapy, and reassurance have all been accomplished at once. Solid lesions and persistent, recurrent, complex, or bloody cysts require mammography and biopsy, although in selected patients triple diagnostic techniques can be used to avoid biopsy (Figs. 64-1 to 64-3). Ultrasound can be used in place of fine needle aspiration to distinguish cysts from solid lesions. Not all solid masses are detected by ultrasound, however, so a palpable mass that is not visualized on ultrasound must be presumed to be solid.

Several points are essential in pursuing these management decision trees. First, risk factor analysis is not part of the decision structure. Second, fine needle aspiration should be used only in centers that have proven skill in obtaining such specimens *and* analyzing them cytopathologically. Although the likelihood of cancer is low in the setting of a "triple negative" (benign-feeling lump, negative mammo-

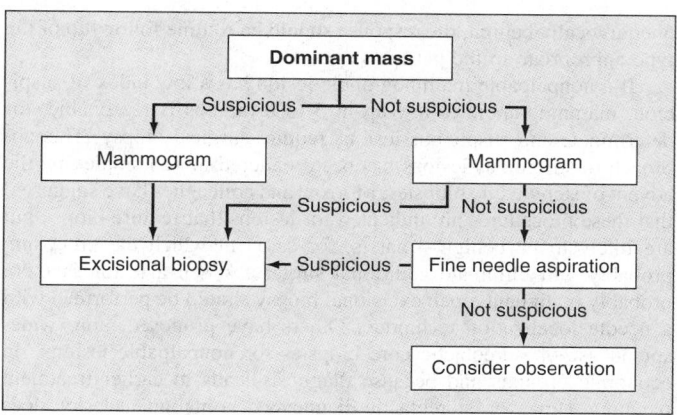

FIGURE 64-2 The "triple diagnosis technique."

gram, and negative fine-needle aspiration), it is not zero, and the patient and physician should be willing to assume about a 1 percent risk of false negativity. Third, additional technologies such as magnetic resonance imaging, ultrasound, and Sestamibi imaging cannot be used to exclude the need for biopsy, although in unusual circumstances they may provoke a biopsy.

THE ABNORMAL MAMMOGRAM Screening mammography has reduced the lethality of breast cancer by promoting detection at an earlier stage. The procedure is justified on an annual basis for women over age 50, and a meta-analysis suggests a benefit for women over age 40, but this is controversial.

Screening mammography should not be confused with diagnostic mammography which is performed after a palpable abnormality has been detected. Diagnostic mammography generally is aimed at evaluating the rest of the breast before biopsy is performed, or, occasionally, is part of the "triple test" strategy to exclude immediate biopsy.

Subtle abnormalities that are first detected by screening mammography should be evaluated carefully almost invariably by compression or magnified views. These abnormalities include clustered microcalcifications, densities (especially if spiculated), and new or enlarging architectural distortion. For some nonpalpable lesions, ultrasound may be helpful either to identify cysts or to guide biopsy. In general, the management of patients with findings of this type is straightforward. If there is no palpable lesion and detailed mammographic studies are

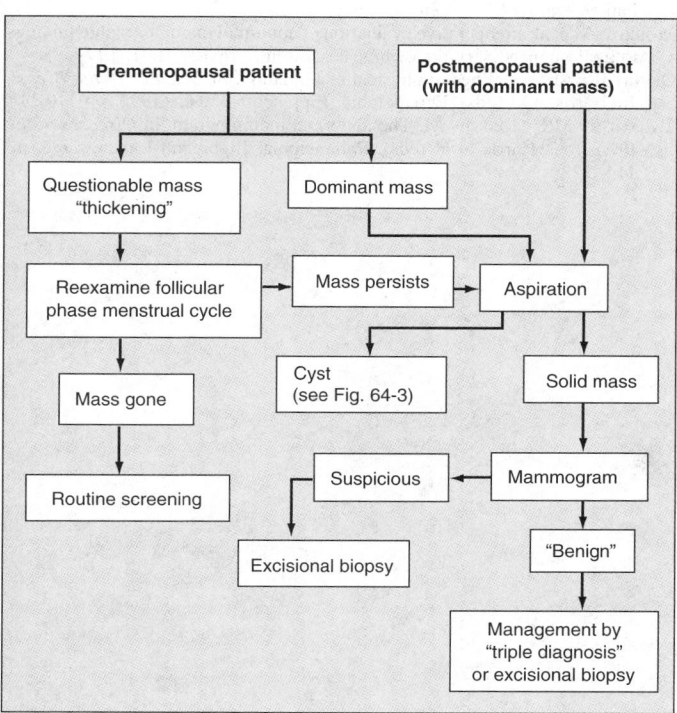

FIGURE 64-1 Approach to a palpable breast mass.

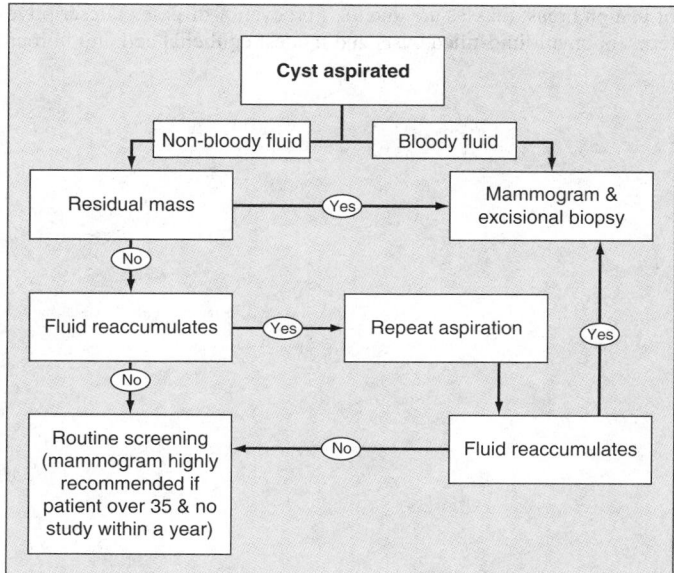

FIGURE 64-3 Management of a breast cyst.

unequivocally benign, the response should be routine follow-up of the type appropriate to the patient's age.

If a nonpalpable mammographic lesion has a low index of suspicion, mammographic follow-up in 3 to 6 months is reasonable. Indeterminate and suspicious lesions require surgical biopsy. This approach to suspicious lesions has been rendered more complex by the advent of stereotactic biopsies. Morrow and colleagues have suggested that these procedures are indicated for lesions that require biopsy but are likely to be benign—that is, for cases in which the procedure probably will eliminate additional surgery. When a lesion is more probably malignant, open excisional biopsy should be performed with a needle localization technique. Others have proposed more widespread use of stereotactic core biopsies for nonpalpable lesions, on economic grounds and because diagnosis leads to earlier treatment planning. However, stereotactic diagnosis of a malignant lesion does not eliminate the need for definitive surgical procedures, particularly if breast conservation is attempted. For example, after a breast biopsy with needle localization (i.e., local excision) of a stereotactically diagnosed malignancy, reexcision may still be necessary to remove the cancer with negative margins. To some extent, these issues are decided on the basis of referral pattern and the availability of the resources for stereotactic core biopsies. A reasonable approach is shown in Fig. 64-4.

Careful attention to these guidelines will greatly reduce the chance of failing to diagnose breast cancer.

BREAST MASSES IN THE PREGNANT OR LACTATING WOMAN   During pregnancy, the breast grows under the influence of estrogen, progesterone, prolactin, and human placental lactogen. Lactation is suppressed by estrogen and progesterone, which block the effects of prolactin. After delivery, lactation is promoted by the fall in estrogen and progesterone levels, which leaves the effects of prolactin unopposed. The development of a dominant mass during pregnancy or lactation should never be attributed to the hormonal changes, and biopsy should be performed under local anesthesia. Breast cancer develops in one in every 3000 to 4000 pregnancies. Stage for stage, breast cancer in pregnant patients is no different from premenopausal breast cancer in nonpregnant patients. However, pregnant women often have more advanced disease because a breast mass was ignored.

BENIGN BREAST MASSES   Only about one in every 5 to 10 patients who undergo a biopsy has a diagnosis of cancer, although the rate of positive biopsies varies in different countries. (These differences may be related to interpretation of mammograms.) The vast majority of benign breast masses are due to "fibrocystic" disease, a descriptive term for small fluid-filled cysts and modest epithelial cell and fibrous

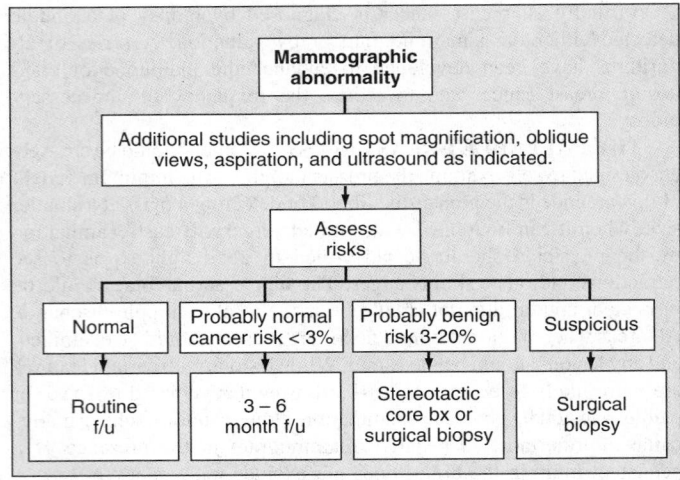

FIGURE 64-4   Approaches to abnormalities detected by mammogram.

tissue hyperplasia. However, fibrocystic disease is a histologic, not a clinical diagnosis, and women who have had a biopsy with benign findings are at a greater risk of developing breast cancer than those who have not had a biopsy. Indeed, the subset of women with ductal or lobular cell proliferation (about 30 percent of patients), particularly the small fraction (3 percent) with atypical hyperplasia, have a fourfold greater risk of developing breast cancer than unbiopsied women, and the increase in risk is about ninefold for women in this category who also have an affected first-degree relative. Thus, careful follow-up of these patients is required. By contrast, patients with a benign biopsy without atypical hyperplasia are at little risk and may be followed routinely.

→*The approach to the patient presenting with a nipple discharge or mastalgia is discussed in Chap. 338.*

BIBLIOGRAPHY

DONEGAN WL: Evaluation of a palpable breast mass. N Engl J Med 327:937, 1992

KERLIKOWSKE K et al: Efficacy of screening mammography. A meta-analysis. JAMA 273:149, 1995

LAYFIELD LJ et al: Fine needle aspiration in the management of breast masses. Pathol Annu 24:23, 1989

MORROW M et al: Preoperative evaluation of abnormal mammographic findings to avoid unnecessary breast biopsies. Arch Surg 129:1091, 1994

OSUCH JR: Abnormalities in physical examination, in *Diseases of the Breast*, JR Harris et al (eds). Philadelphia, Lippincott–Raven, 1996, pp 110-114

TALAMONT MS, MORROW M: The abnormal mammogram, in *Diseases of the Breast*, JR Harris et al (eds). Philadelphia, Lippincott-Raven, 1996, pp 114–122

PART THREE

GENETICS AND DISEASE

65 | Arthur L. Beaudet

GENETICS AND DISEASE

GENOMIC MEDICINE

Genomic medicine can be defined as the use of genotypic analysis (DNA testing) to enhance the quality of medical care, including presymptomatic identification of predisposition to disease, preventive intervention, selection of pharmacotherapy, and individual design of medical care based on genotype. The progress of the human genome project and research in molecular medicine have made genomic medicine an important strategy. Genotype can be deduced by analysis of protein (e.g., hemoglobin or α_1-antitrypsin), RNA, or DNA, but analysis of DNA is the usual method. It can be argued that there are no new principles or concepts involved in genomic medicine but that it will change the way medicine is practiced, particularly in regard to intervention for common diseases. Testing for predisposition to disease does have the potential for harm because it opens the possibility of various forms of discrimination, but it also has the potential of extraordinary benefits. Primary care physicians are in a pivotal position to provide the benefits and minimize the harm. Genotypic analysis is standard practice for diseases in which a single gene plays a prominent role, but the role of genetic testing in complex disease traits—where multiple genes and nongenetic factors are implicated—is less established. Nevertheless, genomic medicine has the potential of reducing the burden of these disorders. Genotypic information has two broad applications: first, to modify the medical care provided to the individual; and second, to make possible reproductive counseling to couples who wish to have children. It is important to distinguish those genotypic results that provide potential for benefit and/or intervention (e.g., hemochromatosis) as compared to those situations where no clear intervention is available (e.g., Alzheimer's or Huntington's disease), but most disorders fall in an intermediate category where opportunity for treatment or prevention is significant but limited.

The concept that it is good medical practice to screen the population to identify individuals with risks and to intervene to prevent disease processes in such persons is well established. For example, blood pressure and cholesterol are measured for screening purposes to identify individuals who are asymptomatic but have a predisposition to cardiovascular disease, and attempts are made to intervene in such individuals through pharmacology and changes in lifestyle. Although treatment is not always effective, there is frequent benefit to individuals and to society. Likewise, in perinatal medicine, population-based screening is used to identify individuals with particular genotypes who can benefit from prompt intervention, as exemplified by phenylketonuria. The rationales for routine mammography, screening for blood in the stool, measurement of prostate-specific antigen, and glaucoma screening are based on similar principles that early diagnosis can lead to beneficial intervention. Although some of these procedures test for disease rather than for predisposition to disease, all such strategies are based on the concept that early intervention can provide a medical benefit. The boundary between predisposition to disease and presymptomatic disease is not a clear one. Is hypertension a disease or a predisposition to a symptomatic event such as a stroke? Is a mutation in the breast and ovarian cancer gene BRCA1 a predisposition to breast cancer or an early phase of the disease process? As with any medical strategy, intervention based on genotypic information is valid only if the benefit to the individual outweighs the potential harm of genotypic analysis (see "Discrimination and Ethical Concerns," below). An example in which opportunities for genomic medicine have

been largely unutilized is population-based screening to identify individuals with predisposition to emphysema because of α_1-antitrypsin deficiency; such individuals can be identified by analysis of protein or DNA and should be counseled regarding the certainty of injury from smoking. The application and follow-up of widespread screening of this type may require major reorganization of medical care and its financing.

Recombinant DNA methods, the polymerase chain reaction (PCR), the human genome project, new technologies for analyzing DNA, and research in molecular medicine make it possible to obtain large amounts of genotypic information at very low cost using current and developing technologies but does not provide insight into which genotypic information can be used in a beneficial manner. As DNA information becomes routine, it should be incorporated into medical practice and into the medical record in the same way that blood pressure, cholesterol, and hemoglobin measurements are currently utilized. Proposals that DNA information be treated differently than other aspects of medical information reflect an exaggerated view of the predictive power of most DNA information. Indeed, many relatively public pieces of information such as obesity, alcohol intake, smoking, past medical conditions, and parental health history are likely to have greater predictive implications than most DNA analyses.

SINGLE-GENE DISORDERS Genotypic analysis is available for the diagnosis, counseling, and management of many so-called single-gene disorders in which one gene plays a predominant role in determining disease. The relevant genes have been cloned, and mutations have been identified for most common genetic disorders, including neurofibromatosis, Marfan's syndrome, familial hypercholesterolemia, osteogenesis imperfecta, myotonic dystrophy, achondroplasia, familial polyposis of the colon, Huntington's disease, adult polycystic kidney disease, cystic fibrosis, and globin disorders. For these disorders, genotypic analysis can confirm the diagnosis, determine the status of relatives at risk, sometimes predict severity, provide the option of presymptomatic diagnosis, and provide the basis for genetic counseling. An excellent example of the benefits of genotypic analysis is in multiple endocrine neoplasia type 2, where mutation analysis can eliminate the need for burdensome, expensive, and imprecise endocrine screening for large numbers of family members not carrying the mutation and makes possible improved preventive and therapeutic strategies for individuals found to have the mutant gene. Similar benefits attributable to precise diagnosis are now available for many genetic disorders. Single-gene mutations also can influence pharmacogenetic susceptibilities where administration of a particular drug may result in catastrophic side effects among a subgroup of patients with a susceptible genotype. Examples include glucose-6-phosphate dehydrogenase deficiency, suxamethonium sensitivity, malignant hyperthermia, 5-fluorouracil sensitivity, 6-mercaptopurine sensitivity, and others (see "Pharmacogenetics," below).

COMPLEX DISEASE TRAITS AND HETEROGENEITY In complex disease traits, also known as multifactorial diseases, multiple genes and nongenetic factors interact to contribute to the presence or absence of disease in a single individual. One example of a complex disease trait is type 1, or insulin-dependent, diabetes mellitus where familial clustering is believed to involve at least 10 genes, including the HLA region and the insulin gene. No one gene appears to contribute the major effect for type 1 diabetes. The situation where single genes have a predominant effect but in which the gene involved can vary from family to family is termed *genetic heterogeneity*. Examples of genetic heterogeneity include maturity onset diabetes of youth (MODY), where the causative gene may be the glucokinase gene or genes mapped to other chromosomes; hereditary breast cancer, which can be due to mutations in the BRCA1 gene on chromosome 17 or the BRCA2 gene on chromosome 13; and colon cancer, which can be caused by mutations in the gene for hereditary polyposis of the colon on chromosome 5 or by mutations in other genes that cause hereditary nonpolyposis colon cancer. Coronary artery disease (and perhaps most other common adult disorders) may involve either complex disease traits or genetic heterogeneity. Some individuals may have early onset coronary artery disease primarily due to mutations at a single locus, as for familial hypercholesterolemia or apolipoprotein E abnormalities, while most instances are thought to be due to interactions of nongenetic factors (e.g., smoking and diet) with variations in multiple genes, including apolipoprotein (a), apolipoprotein B, other apolipoproteins, lipoprotein receptors, lipoprotein lipase, angiotensin-converting enzyme, genes affecting homocysteine levels, genes affecting the clotting system, leukocyte and endothelial cell adhesion genes, and many others. Even when a single gene has a predominant effect, as in heterozygous familial hypercholesterolemia, other genes have secondary or modifier effects. The fact that there may be both major and minor effects in an individual disorder blurs the boundary between the concepts of complex disease traits and genetic heterogeneity.

Genetic heterogeneity is well documented for hypertension, with major single-gene effects involving the β or γ subunit of the renal amiloride-sensitive sodium channel, the enzyme 11β-hydroxysteroid dehydrogenase, dysregulated fusion genes (aldosterone synthase/11β-hydroxylase) leading to aldosterone synthesis under the control of ACTH, the renal thiazide-sensitive Na-Cl cotransporter, and many other loci. These disorders demonstrate dominant effects in some cases and recessive in others, considerable variation in findings even within a single family, and the need for different therapeutic intervention based on the specific defect. The extensive discoveries in the genetic basis of hypertension are shrinking the concept of "essential hypertension" and illustrate the potential for the practice of genomic medicine.

DISCRIMINATION AND ETHICAL CONCERNS There are widespread fears that discrimination in regard to employment, health care, and insurance underwriting will be based on the results of genetic testing. Such concerns are analogous to those related to other medical information including hypertension, hypercholesterolemia, family history of a specific genetic disorder such as Huntington's disease, or strong family history of breast cancer or coronary artery disease. It is imperative that individuals not be discriminated against based on genotype, and it is a challenge for society and for the medical profession to procure the benefits of genomic medicine and to prevent discrimination. Societal, governmental, and legal steps should be taken as needed to prohibit such discrimination (particularly based on genotype or predisposition) in the case of employment and health care. Many societies guarantee universal access to health care, and it is possible that genetic testing may increase the impetus in the United States for universal access to health care at standardized costs. The issues involved in this problem are complex, are not unique to genetics, and will continue to be debated. Anonymous genetic testing has been suggested as one option if individuals wish to obtain predictive information and minimize the risk of breach of confidentiality (e.g., anonymous testing for Huntington's disease or cancer susceptibility). Anonymous testing creates difficulties in assuring that individuals with burdensome results will be provided with proper interpretation, supportive counseling, and medical care, but there are some parallels to the experience with anonymous testing for human immunodeficiency virus.

MOLECULAR BASIS OF GENE EXPRESSION

The human genome is estimated to contain 50,000 to 100,000 genes, each of which is composed of a linear polymer of DNA. The genes are assembled into lengthy linear strands that, together with the proteins of chromatin, form the *chromosomes*. All normal nucleated human cells other than sperm or ova contain 46 chromosomes, arrayed in 23 pairs, one of each pair derived from each of the individual's parents.

The discovery that genes are not contiguous sequences of DNA but consist of coding sequences (exons) interrupted by intervening sequences (introns) led to a more complex view of gene expression.

Some approximations regarding the magnitude and organization of the human genome are presented in Fig. 65-1. The estimated 50,000 to 100,000 genes are encoded within the 3 billion base pairs (bp) of DNA that comprise a haploid genome. DNA length is ordinarily quantitated in kilobase (kb) units of 1000 bp or megabase (Mb) units of 1 million bp. Linkage studies indicate that the human genome is composed of approximately 3000 centimorgans (cM) in recombination distance. A centimorgan (1/100 of a Morgan) is a measure of genetic distance that reflects the probability of a crossover between two loci during meiosis. One centimorgan approximates a 1 percent chance of a crossover during meiosis. Thus, an average chromosome contains 2000 to 5000 genes within 130 million bp of DNA and is equivalent to about 130 cM of genetic material. A typical microband on a chromosome (stained at the 800 band level of resolution) should contain 3 to 5 million bp and 60 to 120 genes. This formulation oversimplifies many issues. Estimates of the total number of genes are imprecise, and although the average recombination distance is approximately 1 cM per million bp of DNA, there is wide variation in this rate over shorter distances and differences in recombination distance with sex. Genes range in size from small (1.5 kb for a globin gene) to large (about 2000 kb for the Duchenne muscular dystrophy locus). *Cis*-acting regulatory elements (i.e., on the contiguous DNA strand) may be a considerable distance from the coding region, e.g., 50 kb 5′ and 20 kb 3′ to the β-globin gene, thus extending the functional domains of genes and complicating the definition of boundaries. The human genome also contains numerous highly reiterated sequences of unknown function.

If one were to print *one copy* of *one strand* of the haploid human genome, it would fill a text 170 times the size of *Harrison's*. The analogy of the human genome to a large text can be carried further. The text can be envisioned as being bound into 23 separate volumes of various sizes, each the equivalent of one chromosome. Individuals would inherit one paternal set of 23 volumes and one maternal set of 23 volumes. The mutation that causes sickle cell anemia would be the equivalent of changing a single letter on one page of one volume

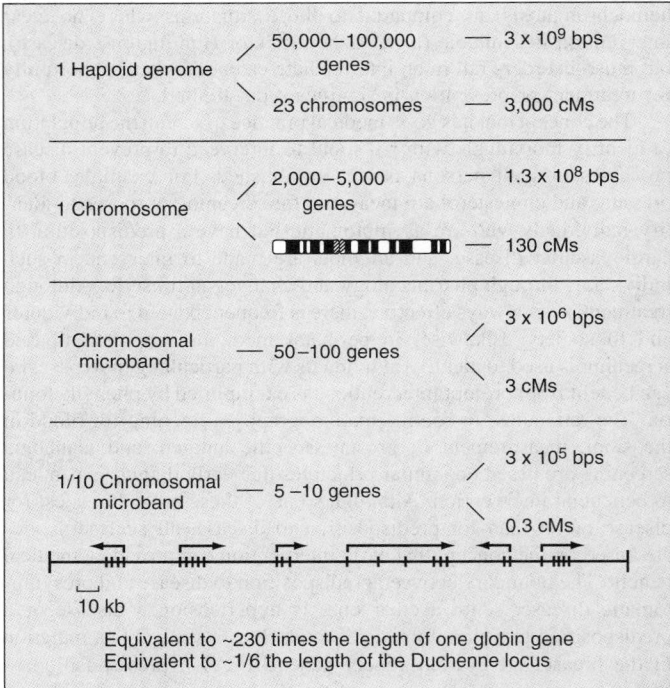

| 1 Haploid genome | 50,000–100,000 genes | — 3 x 10⁹ bps |
| | 23 chromosomes | — 3,000 cMs |

| 1 Chromosome | 2,000–5,000 genes | — 1.3 x 10⁸ bps |
| | | — 130 cMs |

| 1 Chromosomal microband | 50–100 genes | 3 x 10⁶ bps |
| | | 3 cMs |

| 1/10 Chromosomal microband | 5–10 genes | 3 x 10⁵ bps |
| | | 0.3 cMs |

10 kb

Equivalent to ~230 times the length of one globin gene
Equivalent to ~1/6 the length of the Duchenne locus

FIGURE 65-1 Perspectives on the amount of DNA, number of genes, and genetic distance in the human genome. The arrows in the lowest panel indicate hypothetical transcripts, with vertical lines indicating exons within genes. (*From Scriver et al, with permission.*)

from each of the sets, while deletion of the α-globin gene cluster in α-thalassemia would be equivalent to the loss of one or two pages of text in each set. This text can also be envisioned as having been copied over and over again for thousands of generations, with multiple errors or alterations (mutations) being introduced and passed to the progeny copies. Finally, to carry this analogy to the concept of crossing-over and linkage, each volume of each set can exchange parts with its corresponding partner at one to six sites per volume, so that a unique 23-volume text comprising mixed portions of the two available sets is passed to the next generation. This results in the unique genotype that is the basis of our genetic individuality.

THE MOLECULAR FLOW OF INFORMATION Much is known about how living organisms store, transmit, and utilize genetic information. Two excellent textbooks by Alberts et al. and by Darnell et al. provide a more systematic and comprehensive treatment of cellular and molecular biology, and the texts by Watson et al., 1987, and by Lewin provide a detailed view of molecular genetics.

The genetic information carried on chromosomes is transmitted to daughter cells under two different sets of circumstances. *Mitosis* occurs each time a somatic cell (i.e., a nongerm cell) divides and functions to transmit two identical copies of each gene to each daughter cell, thus maintaining a uniform genetic composition in all cells of a single organism. The other set of circumstances, *meiosis*, prevails when genetic information is to be transmitted from one individual to an offspring. In meiosis, the 46 chromosomes of an immature germ cell arrange themselves in 23 pairs at the center of the nucleus, each pair being composed of one chromosome derived from the mother and its homologous chromosome derived from the father. During the meiotic process, the two partner chromosomes separate, only one of each pair going into each gamete. Thus, meiosis reduces the number of chromosomes from 46 to 23, each gamete receiving one chromosome from each of the 23 pairs. The assortment of each pair of chromosomes is random, so that each gamete receives a different combination of maternal and paternal chromosomes. Fusion at fertilization of ovum and sperm cell, each of which has 23 chromosomes, produces an individual with 46 chromosomes.

The independent assortment of chromosomes into gametes during meiosis produces an enormous diversity among the possible genotypes of the progeny. For each 23 pairs of chromosomes, there are 2^{23} different combinations of chromosomes that could occur in a gamete, and the likelihood that one set of parents will produce two offspring with the identical complement of chromosomes is one in 2^{23} or one in 8.4 million (excepting monozygotic twins). Adding even further to the enormous genetic diversity in humans is the phenomenon of *genetic recombination* (see "The Genetic Map and the Principle of Genetic Linkage," below).

THE STRUCTURE OF DNA Most organisms store their genetic information in *deoxyribonucleic acid* (DNA). DNA is a linear polymer of four different monomeric units, collectively called *deoxyribonucleotides* or simply *nucleotides*, that are linked together in a chain by phosphodiester bonds. A typical DNA molecule consists of two interwound polynucleotide chains, each containing many thousand to several million bp. Each nucleotide in one chain is specifically linked by hydrogen bonds to a nucleotide in the other chain. Only two nucleotide pairings are found in DNA: deoxyadenosine monophosphate with thymidine monophosphate (A-T pairs) and deoxyguanosine monophosphate with deoxycytidine monophosphate (G-C pairs). Thus, the sequence of nucleotides of one chain fixes the sequence of the other, and the two chains are therefore said to be *complementary* to each other.

The sequence of the four nucleotides along a polynucleotide chain varies among the DNAs of unrelated organisms and indeed is the molecular basis of their genetic diversity. Because most genetic characteristics are stably transmitted from parent to progeny, the sequence of nucleotides in DNA must be faithfully copied or replicated as the organism reproduces itself. This occurs by unwinding of the two chains and polymerization of two daughter chains along the separated parental strands. The nucleotide sequence and the genetic information are conserved during this process because each nucleotide in the daughter chains is paired specifically with its complement in the parental or template chains before polymerization occurs.

The actual replication process is mechanically complex but conceptually simple. The two strands of DNA separate, and each is copied by a series of enzymes that inserts a complementary base opposite each base on the original strand of DNA. Thus, two identical double helices are generated from one.

THE GENETIC CODE The sequence of bases in a gene ultimately dictates the sequence of amino acids in a specific protein (Fig. 65-2). This colinearity between the DNA molecule and the protein sequence is achieved by means of the *genetic code*. The four types of bases in DNA are arranged in groups of three, each triplet forming a code word, or *codon*, that ultimately signifies a single amino acid. Triplet codons exist for each of the 20 amino acids that occur in proteins (Fig. 65-3); there are slight differences in the genetic code in mitochondria. Since 64 different triplets can be generated from the four bases and only 20 amino acids exist, the genetic code is said to be *degenerate*. That is, most amino acids are specified by more than one codon, each of which is completely specific. Thus, the double-stranded sequence adenine-adenine-adenine (or AAA) in the antisense [complementary to messenger RNA (mRNA)] strand and thymine-thymine-thymine (or TTT) in the sense (same sequence as mRNA) strand of DNA code for uridine-uridine-uridine (or UUU) in mRNA, which is translated to phenylalanine in protein (Fig. 65-2).

DNA → RNA → PROTEIN To translate its genetic information into a protein, a segment of DNA is first transcribed into mRNA. The mRNA contains a sequence of purine and pyrimidine bases that is complementary to the bases of the antisense strand of the DNA. By this mechanism each adenine of DNA becomes a uridine of RNA, each cytosine of DNA becomes a guanine of RNA, each thymine of DNA becomes an adenine of RNA, and each guanine of DNA becomes a cytosine of RNA. Thus, each DNA triplet codon is translated into a corresponding RNA triplet codon.

The mRNA for each gene is processed extensively within the cell nucleus including splicing to remove intronic sequences. It then crosses the nuclear membrane and enters the cytoplasm, where it serves as a template for the synthesis of a specific protein. To translate the mRNA

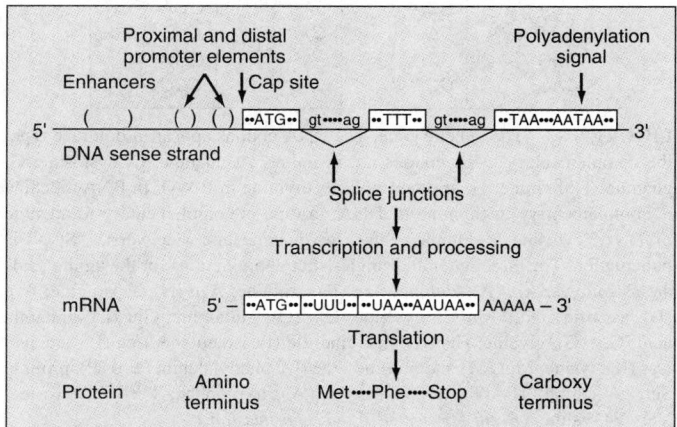

FIGURE 65-2 Prototypical eukaryotic gene. In schematic form, a cellular gene is depicted in which exons or coding regions (boxes) are separated by intervening sequences (introns). Introns begin with a dinucleotide GT and end with AG. A short motif of AATAA (or modified versions) direct endonucleolytic cleavage and polyadenylation of nascent RNAs. Promoter elements, shown as empty parentheses, lie upstream from the start of the gene and are often multiple in nature. Common promoter elements include motifs such as TATA and CCAAT (TATA and CAT boxes) GGCGGG (the Spl nuclear factor binding site). Additional sequences, known as enhancers, augment transcription and can lie either before, within, or downstream from the gene. After transcription, the RNA is processed to yield mature mRNA, which is translated to yield protein. (*From Scriver et al, with permission.*)

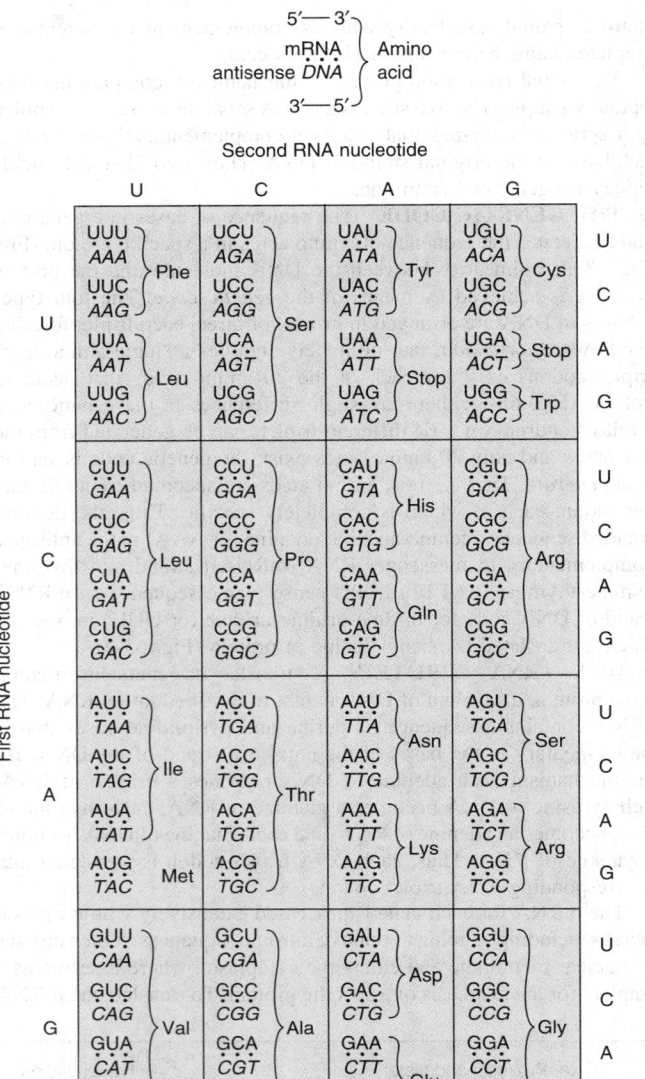

FIGURE 65-3 The genetic code. The RNA codons appear in boldface type; the complementary DNA codons are in italics. A, adenine; C, cystosine; G, guanine; T, thymine; U, uridine (replaces thymine in RNA). In RNA, adenine is complementary to thymine of DNA; uridine is complementary to adenine of DNA; cytosine is complementary to guanine and vice versa. "Stop" is punctuation. The three-letter and single-letter abbreviations for the amino acids are as follows: Ala (A), alanine; Arg (R), arginine; Asn (N), asparagine; Asp (D), aspartic acid; Cys (C), cysteine; Gln (Q), glutamine; Glu (E), glutamic acid; Gly (G), glycine; His (H), histidine; Ile (I), isoleucine; Leu (L), leucine; Lys (K), lysine; Met (M), methionine; Phe (F), phenylalanine; Pro (P), proline; Ser (S), serine; Thr (T), threonine; Trp (W), tryptophan; Tyr (Y), tyrosine; Val (V), valine. *(From Scriver et al, with permission.)*

code into a protein, the mRNA binds to a complex structure called a *ribosome*, which is composed of a different type of RNA [ribosomal RNA (rRNA)] and a large number of proteins. In order to be inserted into its proper place in the protein sequence, each of the 20 amino acids is attached in the cytoplasm to an additional type of RNA [transfer RNA (tRNA)]. Each tRNA contains an anticodon loop, which includes a sequence of three bases that is complementary to a specific codon in the corresponding mRNA. For example, phenylalanine is attached to a tRNA whose anticodon loop contains the sequence AAA, which is complementary to the mRNA codon UUU, which codes for phenylalanine.

Under the influence of cytoplasmic factors (initiation, elongation, and termination factors), peptide bonds are formed between the various amino acids that are aligned along the mRNA. Eventually, a terminator codon is reached, and the completed polypeptide is released from the ribosome. Since the primary sequence of bases in the coding regions of the DNA determines the sequence of amino acids in the protein, the gene and its protein are said to be *colinear*. This means that any alteration of the sequence of bases in the gene causes an alteration of the protein at a specific point in its sequence.

CONTROL OF GENE EXPRESSION The control of gene expression at a transcriptional level is complex. *Cis*-acting regulatory DNA sequences are part of the same duplex DNA molecule as the coding sequence, and *trans*-acting factors (usually proteins) are encoded by other genes. The *trans*-acting factors interact with the *cis* sequences to control the process of transcription. Many *cis*-acting transcriptional control elements are short distances upstream from the initiation site for transcription, but some occur at great distances (e.g., 5 to 50 kb) upstream and downstream from the initiation site for transcription.

The first described family of transcription factors was the helix-turn-helix proteins, and the homeodomain proteins contain a type of helix-turn-helix motif. Complex clusters of homeotic genes have been characterized in mouse and human; a number of these genes have been mutated in the mouse using gene-targeting methodology and an increasing number of human mutations are known. Another group of transcription factors contains "zinc finger" motifs such as the steroid receptors. Other families of transcription factors include proteins with "leucine zipper" motifs or helix-loop-helix motifs. Leucine zippers are characterized by heptad repeats of leucines, which promote dimer formation. The leucine zipper proteins can form various heterodimers that can activate or repress transcription. The helix-loop-helix proteins also appear to form dimers that can have positive or negative regulatory effects.

Regulation of gene expression also occurs at a posttranscriptional level, including regulation of export of mRNA from nucleus to cytoplasm, alternative splicing of transcripts, polyadenylation of transcripts, translation of mRNA, and stabilization of mRNA. There are numerous examples where gene function is regulated through alternative splicing, including control of immunoglobulin secretion, production of calcitonin or calcitonin gene–related peptide, and modulation of the structure and function of troponin-T.

MUTATION AS THE ORIGIN OF NORMAL VARIATION AND GENETIC DISEASE

Mutation was traditionally defined as a stable, heritable change in DNA, a definition that does not depend on the functional significance of the change. This definition implies a change in primary nucleotide sequence, and other changes such as those involving methylation are usually referred to as *epigenetic events*. Mutations in somatic cells may be relevant to cancer or aging and otherwise may be of less phenotypic significance. Mutations in germ cells have their impact on offspring of an individual. The concept that mutations are stable changes remains generally true, but the discovery of expanding triplet repeat mutations emphasizes that some mutations can be unstable either in somatic or in germ cells. Some mutations are genetically lethal and cannot be passed from one generation to the next, while others are less deleterious and are tolerated in the descendants. From the viewpoint of evolution, mutations provide sufficient genetic diversity to permit species to adapt to environmental changes through the mechanism of natural selection.

Mutations are quite diverse (Table 65-1) and can involve gross alterations (millions of base pairs) in the structure of a chromosome; these include duplications, deletions, and translocations of a portion of one chromosome to another (see Chap. 66). Mutations can even involve the entire genome (3 billion bp) as in triploidy, where there is a third copy of the whole chromosome constitution. On the other hand, mutations can be minute, involving deletion, insertion, or replacement of a single base. Single-base or very small mutations are

Table 65-1

CHAPTER 65
Genetics and Disease

369

Common Mechanisms of Mutation

Type	Usual Effect	Examples
LARGE MUTATION		
Deletions	Null*	Duchenne's dystrophy
		Contiguous gene
Insertions	Null	Hemophilia A/LINE repeat
Duplications	Null, gene disrupted	Duchenne's dystrophy
	Dosage, gene intact	Charcot-Marie-Tooth
Inversions	Null	Hemophilia A
Expanding triplet	Null	Fragile X
	?Gain of function	Huntington's disease
POINT MUTATION		
Silent (in or out of coding)	None	Cystic fibrosis
Missense or in-frame deletion	Null, hypomorphic, altered function, gain of function, benign	Globin Cystic fibrosis
Nonsense	Null	Cystic fibrosis
Frameshift	Null	Cystic fibrosis
Splicing (ag/gt)†	Null	Globin
Splicing (outside ag/gt)†	Hypomorphic	Globin
Regulatory (TATA, other)	Hypomorphic	Globin
Regulatory (poly A site)	Hypomorphic	Globin

* "Null" indicates no functional gene product.
† "ag/gt" indicates mutations in the almost absolutely canonical first two and last two base pairs of each intron, while "outside ag/gt" indicates splicing mutations in less canonical sequences of introns or exons.

called *point mutations*. If deletions or insertions of one or two bases occur in a coding region, they give rise to *frameshift mutations*, because they alter the reading frame of the triplet genetic code in the mRNA so that every codon distal to the mutation in the same gene is read in the wrong frame. Frameshift mutations alter the protein sequence and usually result in premature termination of the peptide chain because of the occurrence of a termination codon in the altered reading frame. Small deletions or insertions can also affect transcription, splicing, or RNA processing depending on their location.

When one base is replaced by another in the coding region, the point mutations may be of three types: (1) a *synonymous* or *silent mutation* (comprising about 23 percent of random base substitutions in coding regions), in which the base replacement does not lead to a change in the amino acid but only to the substitution of a different codon for the same amino acid (e.g., a replacement of a single base pair in the DNA so that a RNA codon for phenylalanine will be

transcribed into RNA not as UUU but as UUC, which still codes for phenylalanine); (2) a *missense mutation* (about 73 percent of base substitutions in coding regions), in which the base replacement changes the codon for one amino acid to another (e.g., the replacement of a base pair in DNA in the codon for phenylalanine such that it will be transcribed into RNA not as UUU but as UUA, which would change the codon to leucine); and (3) a *nonsense mutation* (about 4 percent of base substitutions in coding regions), in which the base replacement changes the codon to one of the termination codons (e.g., the replacement of a base pair in the codon for tyrosine such that it is transcribed into RNA not as UAU but as the stop codon UAA). Occasionally a base substitution in the coding region will alter RNA splicing either by creating a cryptic splice site or by interfering with function of a normal splice site. For missense mutations, the single letter amino acid code is often used to indicate substitutions, such that R560T indicates replacement of arginine (R) at position 560 in the protein by threonine (T).

Larger deletions may affect a portion of a gene, an entire gene, or a set of contiguous genes. Contiguous gene syndromes are discussed in Scriver et al. Such deletion mutations may interrupt or remove the coding region of a gene, causing the absence of its protein product. Alternatively, a deletion can bridge between the coding regions of two genes and produce a fusion, resulting in the production of a hybrid protein containing the initial sequence of one protein followed by the terminal sequence of another protein. This latter type of mutation may occur particularly by unequal crossing over between tandemly repeated homologous genes such as the globin genes. The range of mutations seen at the human β-globin locus provides a good perspective on the heterogeneity of possible mutations. More than 200 missense mutations cause amino acid substitutions in the β-globin locus, and various δβ and βδ fusions can occur. Numerous transcriptional, splicing, and RNA processing mutations cause β-thalassemia as depicted in Fig. 65-4. The reciprocal products of deletions caused by unequal crossover are duplications, and such duplications are the most common form of mutation causing type IA Charcot-Marie-Tooth disease. Insertions in genomic DNA also occur by retrotransposition as exemplified by the appearance of a repeat sequence in the factor VIII gene as a cause of hemophilia A. Inversion affecting the factor VIII gene is a common cause of severe hemophilia A.

Expanding triplet repeat mutations are known to cause fragile X mental retardation, myotonic dystrophy, spinobulbar muscular atrophy, Huntington's disease, spinocerebellar ataxia type I, and other disorders. These triplet repeat sequences can occur in the 5' untranslated, coding, intronic, or 3' untranslated regions. Longer repeat sequences are generally associated with a more severe and/or earlier onset phenotype, and repeat sequences slightly longer than normal

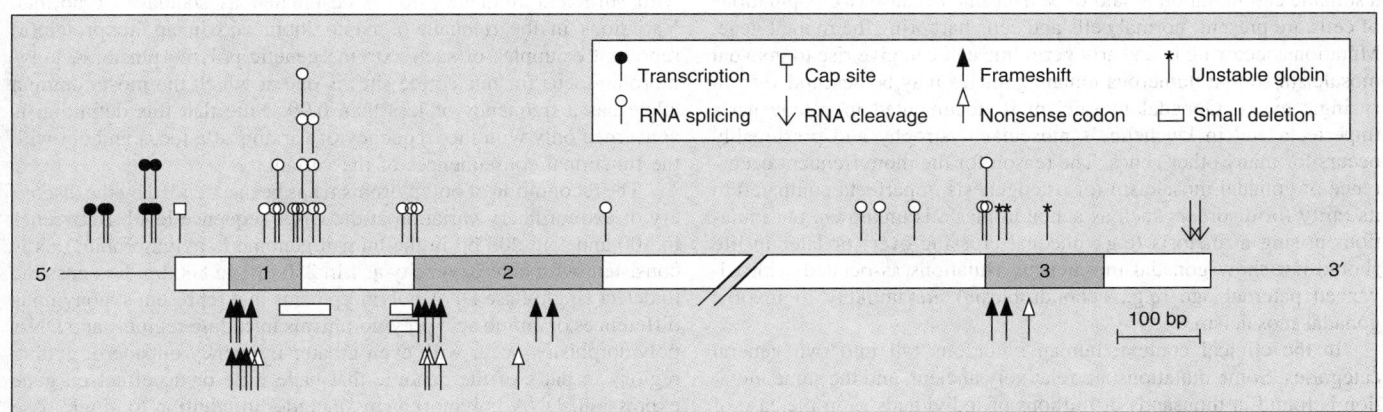

FIGURE 65-4 Point mutations in β thalassemia. The β-globin gene is shown with numbered hatched areas representing the coding regions of exons. Boxed open areas between the exons are introns, and boxed open areas at the 5' and 3' ends of the gene are untranslated regions that appear in the messenger RNA. The various types of mutations are depicted by different symbols. (*From HH Kazazian, Jr., CD Boehm, Blood 72:1107, 1988, with permission.*)

may function as premutations in asymptomatic individuals. The premutant and mutant expanded triplet repeats are unstable and may become more unstable when transmitted from females, as in the case of fragile X syndrome and myotonic dystrophy, or when transmitted from males as in Huntington's disease and spinocerebellar ataxia. For many of the neurodegenerative disorders (Huntington's disease, spinobulbar muscular atrophy, and spinocerebellar ataxia type I, and others), the expanded triplet repeat encodes a polyglutamine tract in the protein, but the mechanism by which this repeat causes neurodegeneration is not known. Expanding triplet repeat mutations are one mechanism underlying the phenomenon of *anticipation*, in which the phenotype of a disease may worsen over successive generations within a family.

The type and frequency of human mutations are complex topics (see Scriver et al.). Mutations that cause chromosomal aneuploidy occur at increasing frequency with advancing age of the mother. Some classes of mutations occur with increased frequency with advancing age of the father. Some loci such as those for Duchenne's muscular dystrophy and achondroplasia are subject to high rates of new mutation. In Duchenne's muscular dystrophy, this may be related in part to the unusually large size of the gene. The structure of a gene, its position within the genome, and the constraints on the gene product may contribute to the frequency of new mutations. The occurrence of 5-methylcytosine at the sites of CG base pairs provides sites of increased mutational frequency due to spontaneous deamination of 5-methylcytosine to yield a thymine base. This propensity leads to increased frequency of polymorphisms at CG sites in the genome and accounts for certain mutational hot spots; in achondroplasia one specific C-to-T base change is remarkably frequent, but similar alterations also occur for hemophilia A and B and many other disorders. The availability of recombinant DNA techniques makes possible the definition of the exact nature of mutations, determination of whether they arose from a maternal or paternal gamete, and analysis of whether the mutation is of recent or ancient origin. Mutations that are widespread in the population but are descended from a single event can be recognized by the occurrence of specific haplotypes of DNA polymorphisms surrounding the mutations; this has been well studied for thalassemia, phenylketonuria, and cystic fibrosis. A *haplotype* is a group of genetic markers linked together on a single chromosome, such as a group of close DNA polymorphisms or a group of human leukocyte antigen (HLA) alleles.

When mutations occur in germ cells, the altered expression of the mutant gene does not affect the phenotype of the individual in whom the mutation occurs but is manifest in subsequent generations. Usually such *new mutations* are sporadic events in human populations, but a mutation that occurs in somatic cells at an early developmental stage may affect the individual harboring the mutation and may or may not be passed to subsequent generations. The individual harboring such a somatic cell mutation is said to be a *mosaic* because two populations of cells are present: normal cells and cells harboring the mutant gene. Mutations occurring in an early germ line cell can give rise to gonadal mosaicism so that numerous mutant gametes may be descended from a single event. Gonadal mosaicism is documented in osteogenesis imperfecta and in Duchenne's muscular dystrophy and presumably occurs for many other genes. The reason for the more frequent occurrence of gonadal mosaicism for osteogenesis imperfecta compared to its rarity for disorders such as achondroplasia is unknown, but mutations arising at meiosis (e.g., unequal crossing-over) or later in life should not show gonadal mosaicism. Mutations associated with advanced paternal age (e.g., achondroplasia) are unlikely to involve gonadal mosaicism.

In the clinical context, human mutations fall into two general categories. Some mutations are relatively ancient, and the same mutation is found in thousands or millions of individuals as in the case of sickle cell anemia, the Z allele for α_1-antitrypsin deficiency, and the common mutation for cystic fibrosis. These ancient mutations either tend to be recessive so that the mutant allele persists in the population

through heterozygotes or are sufficiently benign as to permit reproduction. The presence of the same mutant allele in large numbers of individuals has implications for strategies in DNA diagnosis and screening (see "Analysis of Mutations," below). If genetic predisposition to common adult disorders were associated with ancient mutations, population screening with molecular methods would be feasible. Other human mutations are either recent or new to the first case diagnosed in a family. This circumstance is most common for autosomal dominant, deleterious mutations and for X-linked mutations that impair or prevent reproduction in males. These mutations tend to be heterogeneous with a different mutation in each family studied, with only rare recurrence of identical mutations. This scenario is typical for disorders such as Duchenne's muscular dystrophy, neurofibromatosis, retinoblastoma, and many other disorders that have an effect on reproductive fitness. New mutations are discussed further below (see "Dominant New Mutations" and "X-Linked New Mutations").

GENETIC DIVERSITY IN HUMANS: GARROD'S CHEMICAL INDIVIDUALITY AND THE CONCEPT OF POLYMORPHISM

In 1902, Garrod recognized that the aberrant metabolism seen in a condition such as alkaptonuria might imply far more extensive chemical individuality, and his concept of chemical individuality has found its explanation with the realization that the gene for a given protein frequently exists in different forms in different normal individuals and with the recognition that even more extensive variation exists in the DNA sequence of genomes among individuals. The widespread nature of genetic diversity was first apparent when it became possible to study enzymes by electrophoresis of cell extracts and thereby to detect structurally variant forms of enzymes without the necessity of purification. With the use of this technique, it was demonstrated that many proteins exist in two or more forms in the population. These multiple forms are due to the existence in the population of multiple variations of a gene (called *alleles*) at the same genetic locus coding for the same protein. For most loci, each individual possesses two alleles, one derived from each parent. If the two alleles are identical, the individual is said to be *homozygous*; if they differ, the individual is *heterozygous*. The various alleles have been derived from a single precursor allele by mutations during the evolution of the species; in general, they differ from each other only in the substitution of one base for another (missense mutations). In most cases, the proteins produced by both alleles at a given locus are equally functional, i.e., the amino acid difference is "neutral" or nearly so from the standpoint of natural selection.

At the level of protein sequence, many genetic loci (such as that for the β chain of hemoglobin) have a standard sequence/allele that accounts for the majority of alleles in the population, whereas the other alleles are rare. At other genetic loci, no single allele occurs with sufficient frequency to be designated as standard or normal. Variations in the α chain of haptoglobin and in apolipoprotein(a) represent examples of such extreme genetic polymorphism. A polymorphic locus (or nucleotide site) is one at which the most common allele has a frequency of less than 0.99. Note that this definition is concerned only with the frequency of variants at a locus and not with the functional consequences of the variant.

The recognition of polymorphism has been extended by the discovery of extraordinary variation at the DNA sequence level. Between 1 in 100 and 1 in 200 bp in the human genome is polymorphic; this is consistent with heterozygosity at 1 in 250 to 1 in 500 bp. It is possible to detect single-base DNA polymorphisms that represent synonymous differences or amino acid polymorphisms in coding regions, and DNA polymorphisms occur with even greater frequency outside of coding regions in parts of the genome that have little or no effect on gene expression. DNA polymorphisms include, in addition to single-base differences, insertions, deletions, and variation in numbers of tandemly repeated sequences. The latter are termed *variable number tandem repeats* (VNTR) if the repeats are long or *short tandem repeats* (STR) if the repeats are very short, e.g., tetra-, tri-, di-, or mononucleotide repeats.

With the recognition of the extent of DNA polymorphism (millions of nucleotide differences between two random haploid genomes), it is clear that the DNA of each individual contains millions of differences compared to the DNA of another individual, except in the case of identical twins. These DNA differences can be divided into four broad categories: (1) those with no phenotypic effect (e.g., DNA polymorphisms used for identity testing); (2) those causing phenotypic differences without affecting disease susceptibility (e.g., differences in height, hair color); (3) those making minor or modest contributions to disease processes (e.g., as for complex disease traits); and (4) those having a major role in causing a disease phenotype (e.g., as for single gene disorders).

METHODS FOR ANALYSIS OF HUMAN DNA

Molecular analyses of clinical relevance rely on multiple features and strategies, including: (1) the ability to clone genes and DNA fragments using recombinant methods, (2) determination of the sequence of DNA fragments, (3) the specificity of nucleic acid hybridization, (4) the specificity of recognition sites of restriction endonucleases, (5) the power of DNA amplification using the PCR, and (6) the ability to transcribe and translate DNA in vitro for analysis of the protein product. Various combinations of these approaches are used for diagnostic procedures, and some methods utilize mRNA rather than DNA as the starting material.

MOLECULAR CLONING AND SEQUENCING The size, complexity, and variability of the human genome constitute barriers to the analysis of individual traits and genes. The feasibility for such analysis was greatly enhanced by the development of recombinant DNA technology, which allows for isolation of small DNA fragments and production of unlimited amounts of the cloned material. Hundreds of human genes have been cloned, including the genes for cystic fibrosis, Marfan's syndrome, polyposis of the colon, neurofibromatosis, myotonic dystrophy, fragile X mental retardation, Huntington's disease, breast cancer (BRCA1), hereditary nonpolyposis colon cancer, and many other disorders. Once cloned, the various genes and gene products can be utilized for studies of gene structure and function in normal and disease states, with diagnostic, therapeutic, counseling, and research implications.

The cloning of DNA involves isolation of DNA fragments and their insertion into the nucleic acid from another biologic source (vector) for manipulation and propagation. These vectors can accommodate DNA fragments of tens to hundreds of kilobases in size. Various methods for DNA cloning are described in Watson et al., 1992.

Most genes are divided into coding exons and intervening introns in the genomic DNA. The mRNA from a gene is spliced to link the coding segments, and mRNA can be copied in vitro to synthesize cDNA (DNA complementary to mRNA) for analysis and cloning. Genomic DNA and cDNA clones have been isolated for hundreds of human genes, and for thousands of gene fragments and *anonymous* sequences. The anonymous genomic DNA regions represent unique sites in the genome and often are associated with polymorphic markers that map to that site. Complete cDNA clones or even fragments thereof can be deduced to encode protein sequences which may be homologous to known proteins. Radioactive, biotinylated, or otherwise modified copies of DNA can be prepared from any cloned fragment and can serve as a specific molecular *probe*. Radioactive probes can be detected by autoradiography, whereas biotinylated probes can be detected using avidin and secondary nonradioactive detection methods. Some of the

fruits of molecular cloning are the availability of probes for analytical procedures, the availability of DNA sequence data both to deduce protein sequence and to allow for DNA amplification (see "Polymerase Chain Reaction," below), and the ability to analyze for disease mutations.

NUCLEIC ACID HYBRIDIZATION Many of the steps in recombinant DNA analysis take advantage of the complementary nature of nucleic acid interaction, which is so essential for the synthesis of DNA and RNA. Linear pieces of double-stranded (native) DNA can be treated with heat or alkali to dissociate the two strands to yield single-stranded (denatured) DNA. The denatured DNA can be incubated under conditions that allow for nucleic acid hybridization, i.e., the recognition of two complementary strands and reformation of double-stranded molecules by base pairing. Nucleic acid hybridization is so sensitive that a single-stranded DNA molecule can be hybridized specifically to a complementary strand of RNA or DNA and detected if present at about 1 part in 10,000. It is possible to identify and distinguish fully homologous and partially homologous sequences. The specificity of nucleic acid hybridization, often in combination with fractionation or amplification procedures, allows detection of a single gene among tens of thousands or of nucleic acid from an infectious organism, which may be present at a frequency of less than one copy per human cell. The majority of hybridization probes have been prepared in radioactive form, but the use of nonradioactive detection methods is increasing.

A particularly useful variation of nucleic acid hybridization involves the use of allele-specific oligonucleotides (ASO). The ASO probe is a synthetic, single-stranded oligonucleotide, usually 15 to 20 bases in length. Two probes are synthesized usually differing at the mutation site by a single base, one perfectly matching the normal sequence and one perfectly matching the mutant sequence, with the variable nucleotide in the midportion of the oligonucleotide. Hybridization conditions are adjusted so that the oligonucleotide detects a perfectly matched sequence but fails to hybridize if there is a single base mismatch. ASO can be used in combination with Southern blotting but are now more widely used in combination with DNA amplification.

RESTRICTION ENDONUCLEASES The discovery in microorganisms of restriction endonucleases, commonly known as restriction enzymes, facilitated recombinant DNA manipulations. Each enzyme recognizes a specific short sequence in double-stranded DNA, typically 4 to 8 bp, and cleaves the DNA at this site. Hundreds of enzymes are known, each recognizing a unique DNA sequence (Fig. 65-5). For example, one enzyme (*Hae*III) that recognizes sequences only 4 bp in length cleaves the sequence 5'-GGCC-3'. The sequence specificity of restriction enzymes is a powerful tool in dissection of large genomes. When human DNA is digested with a particular restriction enzyme, hundreds of thousands of DNA fragments are reproducibly generated that vary from a few base pairs to several thousand base pairs in length, depending on the enzyme used. Restriction enzymes that recognize a sequence only 4 bp long cleave the DNA into smaller fragments than enzymes that recognize longer sequences, since shorter recognition sites occur more often. With the use of multiple restriction enzymes, it is possible to define a detailed map of restriction endonuclease cleavage sites for a particular segment of DNA. Such a map can span a region of from several hundred to tens of thousands of base pairs of DNA. Enzymes that cut the DNA infrequently can be used to prepare DNA maps over megabase dis-

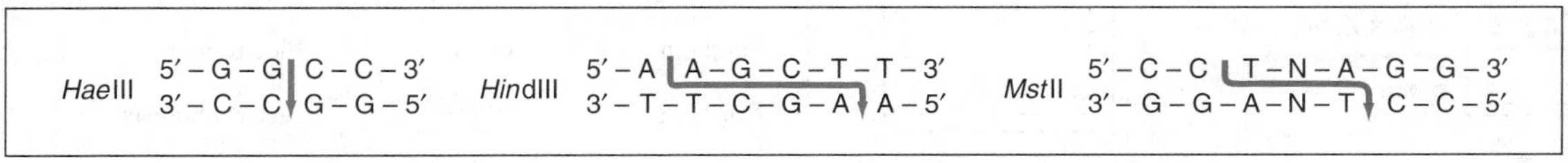

FIGURE 65-5 DNA sequence specificity and nuclease activity for three restriction endonucleases. *Hae*III leaves a blunt end, while the other enzymes leave single-stranded ends.

tances. As described below, variations in the sequences of cleavage sites may reveal polymorphisms or mutations in the human genome.

SOUTHERN BLOTTING Many analyses of the human genome utilize the blotting procedure developed by E. M. Southern, which involves hybridizing DNA in solution to DNA fixed on a membrane support. For clinical analysis, *Southern blotting* (Fig. 65-6) begins with the isolation of genomic DNA from sources such as peripheral leukocytes or fetal cells. The sensitivity of Southern blotting is achieved by cleaving the DNA into small segments, fractionating the fragments by electrophoresis on agarose gels, and applying a sensitive detection method to identify specific fragments (nucleic acid hybridization). Overall, this method can detect unique genomic DNA fragments that typically represent about 1 part in 1 million in the genome. The clinical power of Southern blotting resides in the capacity to analyze a specific small portion of the primary structure of human genomic DNA from an individual. The procedure is useful for detecting gross rearrangements in DNA and some point mutations, but most point mutations are not detected by routine Southern blotting.

An analogous procedure starting with RNA for analysis has been termed *northern blotting*—in contrast to Southern blotting. In this procedure, the presence or absence and approximate size of a particular mRNA can be determined. The term *immunoblotting*, or *western blot-*

ting, describes a procedure designed to analyze protein antigens. Proteins are separated by electrophoresis and transferred to a solid membrane through a blotting procedure. The membrane is analyzed by incubation with antibodies followed by a second step for enzymatic or radioactive detection of bound antibody. Thus, Southern blotting, northern blotting, and immunoblotting or western blotting each combines a fractionation and a detection method to provide a sensitive technique for the analysis of DNA, RNA, and protein, respectively (Table 65-2).

POLYMERASE CHAIN REACTION The technique of PCR for DNA amplification has had a revolutionary impact on molecular diagnosis. The technique is based on knowing the nucleic acid sequence for a region that, for a diagnostic application, is to be analyzed repeatedly from different individuals. Oligonucleotide primers are prepared that are complementary to opposite strands of the DNA and are separated by up to a few hundred base pairs (Fig. 65-7). The oligonucleotide primers are incubated with the target DNA to be amplified and with a DNA polymerase that synthesizes a complementary strand in a 5′-to-3′ direction. Considerable specificity is provided by the requirement that primers must lead to convergent synthesis for amplification to be effective. The reaction is subjected to a series of temperature variations including a denaturing temperature where double-stranded DNA is dissociated to single-stranded DNA, an annealing temperature where oligonucleotide primers hybridize to target DNA, and a polymerization temperature for the synthetic step. The reaction is usually carried out using a thermostable polymerase so that the polymerase remains active during the temperature cycles (usually ranging from 50 to 95°C). After a number of such cycles, typically 20 to 30 or more, hundreds of thousands of copies of the original target sequence are synthesized as depicted in Fig. 65-7. The bulk of the product is a double-stranded DNA fragment of specific length. The technique is so sensitive that it can be used to amplify and analyze DNA from a single human sperm that contains one duplex target DNA molecule. PCR is easily performed with minimal preparation of crude and even degraded samples, allowing analysis from whole blood, dried blood filters, mouthwash, old tissue sections, and other sources. PCR can be performed starting with genomic DNA as the template; alternatively, RNA can be reverse transcribed to yield cDNA for use as a template, a procedure known as reverse transcription-PCR (RT-PCR). Molecular diagnosis with PCR can include: (1) determining the presence or the absence of an amplified product, (2) digesting the amplified product with a restriction enzyme, (3) hybridizing the PCR product with allele-specific oligonucleotides, (4) direct sequencing of the PCR product, (5) analyzing the ratio of RNA from two alleles using RT-PCR, and (6) analysis for expression in vitro to search for truncation mutations. Variations and modifications include synthesis of single-stranded DNA by altering the ratio of the oligonucleotide primers, preparation of recombinant DNA constructs, mutagenesis of cloned DNA, detection of rare nucleotide sequences, and detection of nucleotide sequences of infectious agents. The PCR method offers extremely rapid analysis (single day), ease of automation, relative economy, and extraordinary specificity.

PROTEIN TRUNCATION TESTS Protein truncation tests (PTT) can be used to detect any mutation that results in premature termination of the peptide during protein synthesis; these are primarily nonsense, frameshift, and some splicing mutations (Fig. 65-8). In PTT,

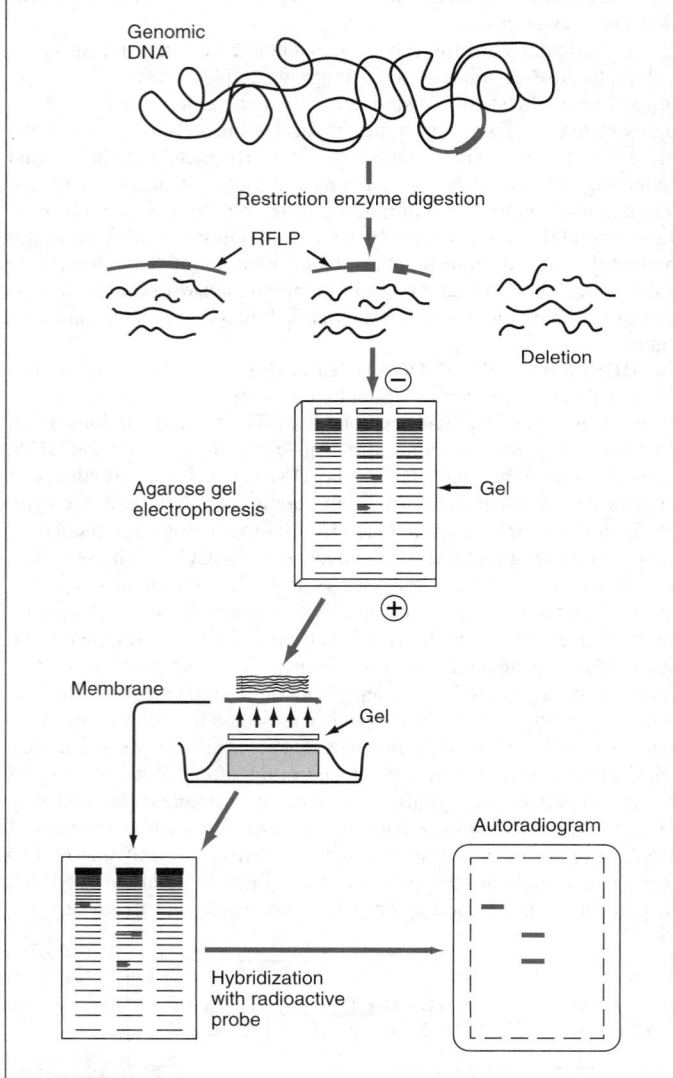

FIGURE 65-6 Southern blotting analysis of genomic DNA. RFLP, restriction fragment length polymorphism.

Genomic DNA

Restriction enzyme digestion

RFLP

Deletion

Agarose gel electrophoresis

Gel

Membrane

Gel

Autoradiogram

Hybridization with radioactive probe

Table 65-2

Analytical Blotting Procedures

Blot Method	Material Analyzed	Fractionation	Detection
Southern	DNA	Electrophoresis	Nucleic acid hybridization
Northern	RNA	Electrophoresis	Nucleic acid hybridization
Western or immunoblot	Protein	Electrophoresis	Immunologic

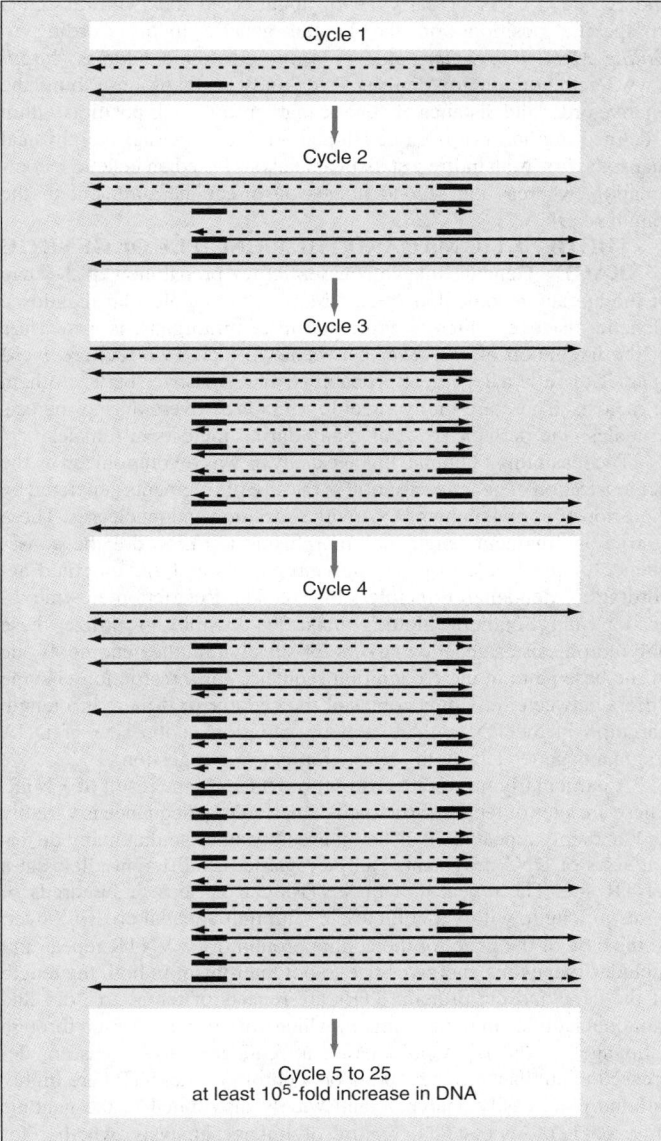

FIGURE 65-7 Polymerase chain reaction for amplification of DNA. The target DNA is shown as a solid line in cycle 1. Newly synthesized DNA is indicated by dotted lines in each cycle. Primer oligonucleotides are indicated by solid rectangles. Each DNA strand is marked with an arrow indicating 5′-to-3′ orientation.

the amplified genomic DNA encoding an exon or amplified cDNA is transcribed and translated in vitro, and the protein products are analyzed using gel electrophoresis to detect truncated proteins. PTT have been used mostly to detect heterozygous mutations in autosomal dominant disorders, but the method is generally applicable and is particularly suited for detection of loss-of-function mutations.

ANALYSIS OF MUTATIONS The challenge of detecting unknown mutations is different from diagnostic testing for the presence of known mutations. Large mutations are more easily detected, using Southern blotting or PCR to detect expansions of triplet repeats, deletions, insertions, and other rearrangements. RT-PCR is useful to detect absence of or major reduction in mRNA from a mutant allele; first, common polymorphisms are used to identify heterozygosity within an exon of genomic DNA, followed by analysis of the ratio of mRNA from the two alleles. This strategy will detect any mutation that profoundly reduces the level of mRNA. More discriminating methods are required for detection of point mutations. The best characterized methods for detection of unknown mutations include ribonuclease cleavage, denaturing gradient-gel electrophoresis, carbodiimide modi-

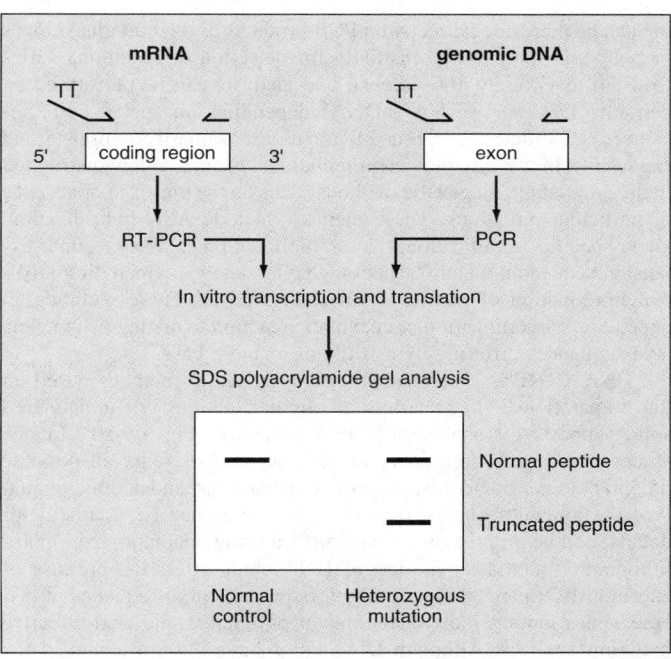

FIGURE 65-8 Protein truncation testing. Polymerase chain reaction (PCR) is performed starting with genomic DNA or reverse transcription-PCR (RT-PCR) is performed utilizing mRNA. Sequences for transcription and translation (TT) are introduced at the 5′ end of the coding segments. Mutations leading to truncation of a protein are detected by gel analysis.

fication, chemical cleavage of mismatches, single-strand conformation polymorphism analysis, heteroduplex analysis, and sequencing of DNA (Fig. 65-9). These methods involve chemical or enzymatic recognition of mismatches in nucleic acid duplexes, electrophoretic separation of single- or double-stranded DNA, or sequencing. DNA sequenc-

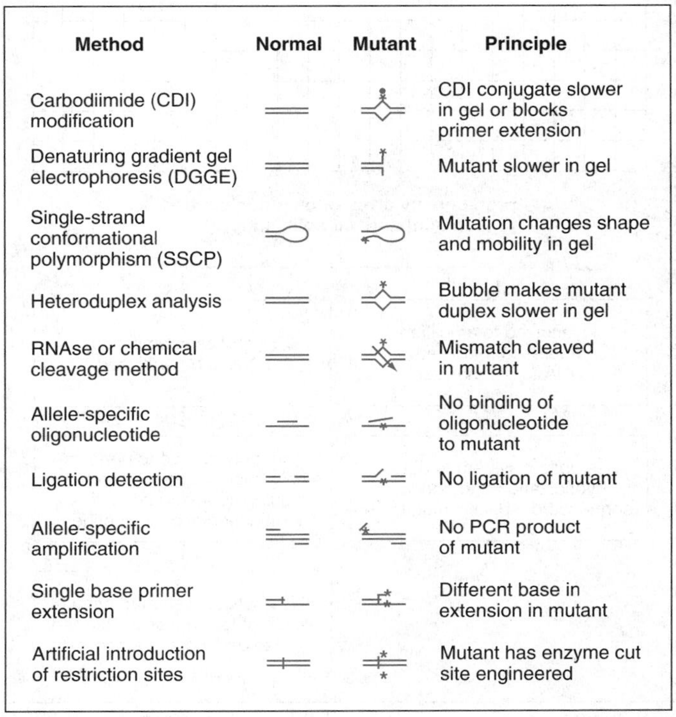

Method	Normal	Mutant	Principle
Carbodiimide (CDI) modification			CDI conjugate slower in gel or blocks primer extension
Denaturing gradient gel electrophoresis (DGGE)			Mutant slower in gel
Single-strand conformational polymorphism (SSCP)			Mutation changes shape and mobility in gel
Heteroduplex analysis			Bubble makes mutant duplex slower in gel
RNAse or chemical cleavage method			Mismatch cleaved in mutant
Allele-specific oligonucleotide			No binding of oligonucleotide to mutant
Ligation detection			No ligation of mutant
Allele-specific amplification			No PCR product of mutant
Single base primer extension			Different base in extension in mutant
Artificial introduction of restriction sites			Mutant has enzyme cut site engineered

FIGURE 65-9 Methods for detection of mutations. The asterisk represents the position of the mutation. PCR, polymerase chain reaction. (*Modified from Cotton, Hum Mutat 285:125, 1993, with permission.*)

ing can be performed directly on PCR products or on individual clones or pools of clones. The sensitivity for detection of mutations varies from 80 to virtually 100 percent, and analysis can be performed on genomic DNA or mRNA (cDNA) depending on specific circumstances. PTT detect a subset of mutations, primarily nonsense and frameshift. In the case of ancient mutations that are widely distributed in the population, diagnostic methods focus on the presence or absence of particular mutations. These methods include ASO hybridization, allele-specific amplification, ligase amplification or assay, primer extension sequencing, and restriction enzyme analysis (including artificial introduction of restriction sites; Fig. 65-9). These methods all depend on a hybridization or enzymatic reaction to distinguish nucleic acid sequences differing by as little as a single base.

DNA CHIPS The term *DNA chip* refers to methods based on the preparation of large arrays of oligonucleotides on miniaturized solid supports for analysis of DNA sequence (Fig. 65-10). In one strategy, a very large number of oligonucleotides (e.g., all possible 65,536 octomer nucleotides or each sequential decanucleotide to analyze the known sequence of a gene; see reference by Southern for details) can be arrayed on a small surface using adaptations of photolithographic methods. The use of DNA chips offers the promise of enormously expanded opportunity for comparison of sequence of disease genes among individuals and of automated and cost-effective mutation analysis. Although DNA chips have not yet achieved the status of practical application, these devices may become a key component of medical diagnosis in the future.

ANALYZING THE HUMAN GENOME

The topographic map of our genomic DNA can be divided into regions corresponding to the chromosomal bands visually identified by standard cytogenetic analysis of the 24 chromosomes (22 autosomes

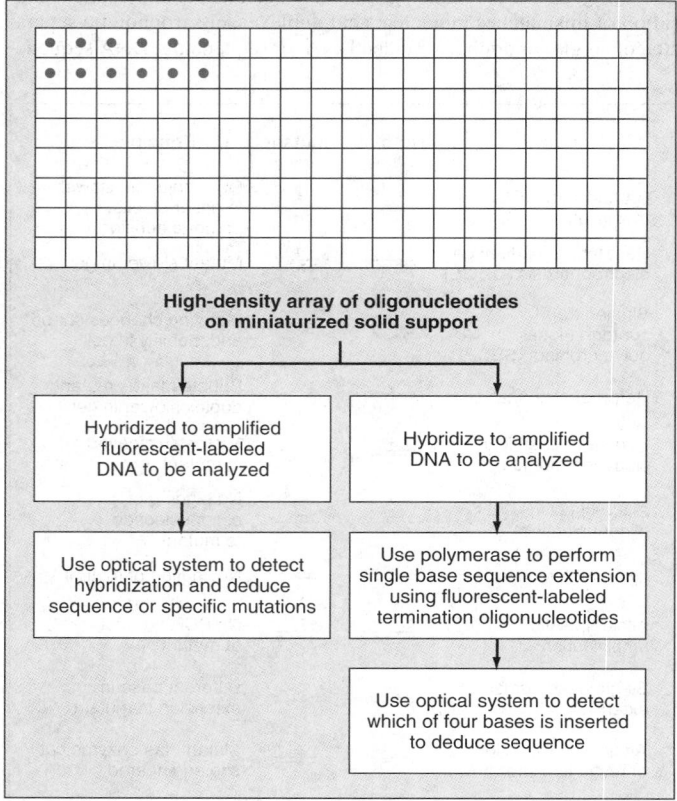

FIGURE 65-10 Use of DNA chips for molecular analysis. Large numbers of unique oligonucleotides are arrayed on a solid support and analyzed as indicated. See reference by Southern for detailed discussion.

and X and Y). As of early 1996, about 3700 loci were assigned to specific positions on the human genetic map according to *Online Mendelian Inheritance in Man* (electronic address: http://www3.ncbi.nlm.nih.gov/omin/). Two kinds of maps describing the relative order and distance of genetic markers and their position within a defined region have been developed—the genetic and the physical maps; the first is an indirect statistical analysis based on genetic recombination, whereas the second hinges on direct measurement of the length of DNA.

THE GENETIC MAP AND THE PRINCIPLE OF GENETIC LINKAGE Genetic linkage is essential for preparation of the map of the human genome and is used routinely for molecular diagnosis. Genetic distance, which is expressed in centimorgans, is a measure of the likelihood of crossover between two loci. Two loci are 1 cM apart if there is a 1 percent probability of a crossover between them at meiosis. There are on average 30 to 35 crossovers during meiosis in males, and perhaps twice as many during meiosis in females.

The feasibility of human linkage analysis was revolutionized by the demonstration of genetic variation in the size of fragments generated by digestion of normal human DNA with restriction endonucleases. These restriction fragment length polymorphisms (RFLPs) are the consequence of the DNA sequence polymorphisms and are inherited according to Mendelian principles (Fig. 65-11). Restriction enzyme digestion and Southern blotting make it possible to utilize these polymorphisms as genetic markers for sites within the genome. If one of the base pairs in the recognition sequence for a restriction enzyme differs between individual copies of the genome or if there is a length variation in the DNA, there will be variation in the size of DNA fragments generated by the restriction enzyme digestion.

A particularly informative subset of RFLPs is the result of VNTR. These are sites of length variation in which a DNA sequence is variably and tandemly repeated on different chromosomes so that many different sizes of DNA fragments can be regarded as different alleles at a VNTR site. The repeat unit in VNTRs can be tens or hundreds of bases in length, with variation arising through unequal crossing-over. In the case of the gene for the apolipoprotein (a), a VNTR repeat unit includes two exons and gives rise to polymorphism in both the length of the gene and the protein. STRs are repeats of tetra-, tri-, di-, and mononucleotides in the genome in which variation has arisen through "slippage" of the DNA polymerase at replication to increase or decrease the number of repeat units on a chromosome. STRs are highly polymorphic, easily analyzed, and widely distributed in the genome (Fig. 65-12). An essential feature of linkage analysis, whether for construction of the human gene map or for clinical diagnosis, is that DNA markers have different alleles at the marker locus of interest so that the two chromosomes of the individual can be distinguished.

Genetic linkage can be assessed between any group of markers, one of which may represent a mutation that causes a disease phenotype. For autosomal genes, each individual inherits one copy of each chro-

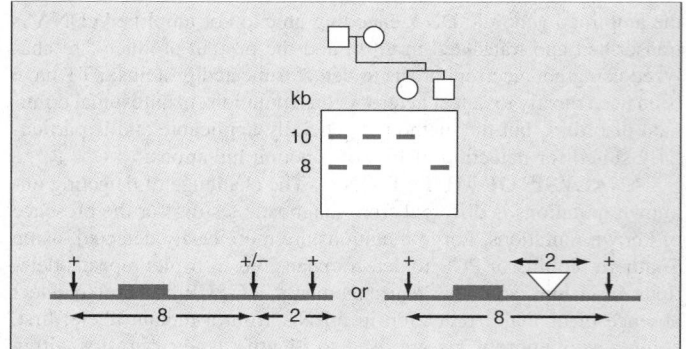

FIGURE 65-11 Example of restriction fragment length polymorphism (RFLP) in human DNA using Southern blotting. The solid blocks indicate segments of DNA used as probe. Parents are heterozygous and children are homozygous for the RFLP. Symbols above the arrows indicate cutting (+) or noncutting (−) by the restriction endonuclease. Numbers indicate DNA length in kilobases.

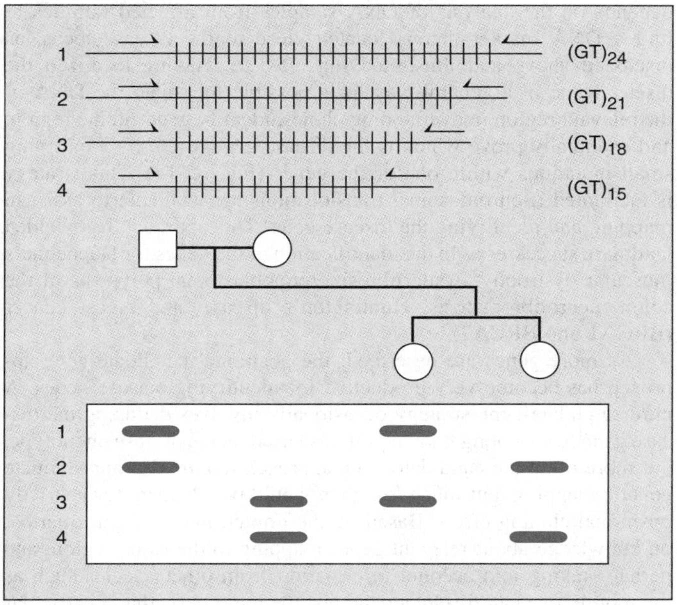

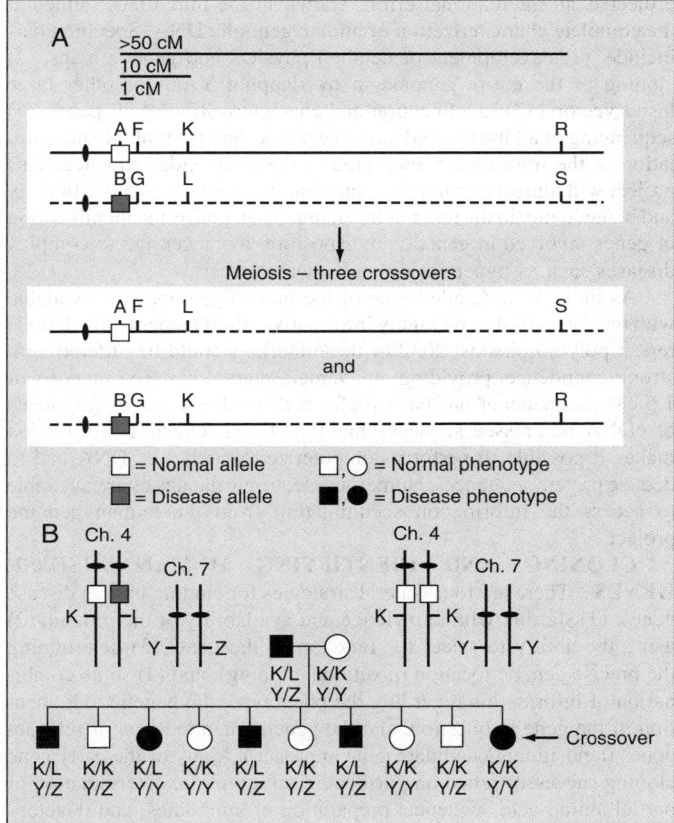

FIGURE 65-12 Depiction of a short tandem repeat polymorphism for a dinucleotide (GT)$_n$ repeat. Each repeat is separated by a vertical line. Sites for two primers for polymerase chain reaction (PCR) are indicated by arrows. Four alleles of 24, 21, 18, and 15 GT repeats are indicated. Inheritance of the alleles in a family as detected by PCR is shown below.

abundant DNA markers and the identification and cloning of the genes in a region.

Major strategies for physical mapping of the human genome include in situ hybridization, deletion mapping, long-range restriction mapping, and isolation of yeast artificial chromosome (YAC) or other large insert clones. With in situ hybridization, the direct hybridization of a DNA marker to a chromosome allows the assignment of the marker to a specific chromosomal band. With the advent of fluorescent in situ hybridization (FISH), it is now possible to use different colored probes for simultaneous mapping of more than one DNA marker, and hybridization to interphase nuclei allows determination of the order of markers within a particular chromosomal region. This technique is also very effective for the identification of chromosomal abnormalities (see Chap. 66).

Deletion mapping is based on the presence or absence of a particular region or locus in the DNA from patients with chromosomal abnormalities or from human/rodent somatic cell hybrids that contain defined segments of the human chromosomes. Deletion mapping is particularly useful for mapping of the X chromosome, because deletions of the X

mosome from each parent. Panel *A* of Fig. 65-13 depicts one pair of chromosomes ready to enter meiosis with one normal copy of a gene (open square) and one defective copy of the same gene (solid square). Four DNA markers, typically dinucleotide repeat polymorphisms, with A/B, F/G, K/L, and R/S alleles are depicted at 0, 1, 10, and >50 cM from the disease gene. After meiosis and three crossover events, gametes are formed containing one chromosome with various segments of the original chromosomes. Alleles A and F are at DNA markers within (A) or close to (F), the gene of interest, and remain on the chromosome with the normal copy of the gene. DNA markers further away have a greater probability to undergo crossing-over, and the L allele of one DNA marker is now on the chromosome with the normal copy of the defective copy of the gene. The greater the distance between markers and genes, the greater the probability of crossovers. Alleles for a gene and markers on different chromosomes are inherited in a completely independent fashion.

Panel *B* of Fig. 65-13 depicts the analysis of DNA markers in a family with an autosomal dominant disorder such as Huntington's disease. Data are shown for the K/L DNA marker that is 10 cM from the disease gene and for a Y/Z DNA marker on a different chromosome. A researcher trying to map a disease gene is likely to study many DNA markers, like the Y/Z marker, that show no correlation between which allele of the marker gene is inherited and whether the disease phenotype is inherited. Eventually a marker is discovered, such as K/L, that is close to the disease gene. Analysis of additional families can provide conclusive statistical evidence that a polymorphic DNA marker is near a disease gene and makes possible immediate application of the marker for diagnosis within a family such as that shown in Fig. 65-13 (see "Diagnosis by Linkage Analysis," below) and opens the way for positional cloning of the disease gene (see "Cloning and Identifying Human Disease Genes," below). The frequency of crossovers as shown for the last offspring in Fig. 65-13 is a measure of the genetic distance between the DNA marker and the disease gene. Once a linked DNA marker is found, closer DNA markers can be identified rapidly.

THE PHYSICAL MAP The physical map is based on direct DNA analysis and is not influenced by regional differences in recombination frequency. A physical map facilitates both the isolation of

FIGURE 65-13 Depiction of meiotic crossing-over and linkage analysis. *A.* Two copies of one chromosome (one in solid line and one in dashed line) from an individual before (above) and after (below) meiotic crossing-over. The individual is heterozygous for a disease locus with a normal allele (open square) and a disease allele (solid square) and is heterozygous for four DNA markers with alleles A/B, F/G, K/L, and R/S at 0, 1, 10, and >50 cM from the disease locus, respectively. *B.* Analysis in a family for an autosomal dominant disorder. The DNA marker with K/L alleles at 10 cM from the disease locus on chromosome 4 and another DNA marker with Y/Z alleles on chromosome 7 are depicted. The chromosomes 4 and 7 for each parent are shown, and the genotypes given for each family member. The disease phenotype is inherited from the father with the L allele for the DNA marker, except for the last child who represents a crossover of the type shown in A. See text for discussion.

chromosome frequently result in a disease phenotype in males and because the nullisomic regions can be defined without having to separate the abnormal chromosome in somatic cell hybrids. Deletion mapping is also useful in establishing relative orders of sets of markers in the genome, although it does not provide precise information as to the distance involved.

Information about physical distance is provided by long-range restriction mapping. In this technique, high-molecular-weight DNA is cut into large fragments (from 100 kb up to 4 Mb), using restriction enzymes that cut very rarely in the genome, and these fragments are separated by pulsed-field gel electrophoresis (PFGE) and hybridized to several DNA markers using Southern blotting procedures. If, for example, two DNA probes hybridize to the same 200-kb restriction fragment, it can be concluded that the maximum distance between the two loci is 200 kb.

Another strategy in physical mapping utilizes YAC clones, which carry large fragments of genomic DNA (from 50 kb to 1 or 2 Mb in length). These YAC vectors contain yeast telomeres and centromeres, and the clones are actually propagated as separate chromosomes in a yeast host.

THE HUMAN GENOME PROJECT The human genome project is an international effort, started in the mid 1980s, aimed at the complete characterization of human genomic DNA. Specific goals include: (1) development of detailed physical and genetic maps, (2) cloning of the entire genome in overlapping YACs or other large insert vectors, (3) identification and characterization of all genes, (4) sequencing of all the haploid human genome, and (5) biologic interpretation of the information encrypted in the nucleotide sequence. This project will almost certainly enhance knowledge both in basic biology and in medicine. In the latter field, an important goal is the identification of genes involved in genetic predisposition to cancer and to complex diseases such as hypertension and atherosclerosis.

As of 1996, a detailed map of the human genome was available with the analysis of 5264 highly informative, short tandem dinucleotide repeat polymorphisms; 2032 of these markers could be ordered with strong confidence, providing an average interval between markers of 1.6 cM. Sequencing has been performed for thousands of fragments of cDNA (expressed sequence tags), and this sequence information makes it possible to perform computerized searches of DNA and to deduce protein sequences. Numerous electronic databases are available to access the information accumulating from the human genome project.

CLONING AND IDENTIFYING HUMAN DISEASE GENES There are four general strategies for cloning human disease genes: (1) starting with knowledge and availability of the protein; (2) using the ability to select for function of the gene; (3) determining the precise genetic location (positional cloning); and (4) some combination of information regarding the phenotype, the genetic map location of the gene in question, and the genetic map location of relevant genes (a positional candidate gene approach). Many of the early gene cloning successes relied on purification of a protein, determination of partial amino acid sequence, preparation of antibodies, and development of enzymatic or other assays. Using this information, cDNA clones were isolated using approaches such as mRNA purification, hybridization screening with oligonucleotides based on available amino acid sequence, PCR amplification based on similar oligonucleotides, immunologic screening of expression cDNA libraries, and other related approaches. Currently, expressed DNA sequences can often be found in databases if minimal amino acid sequence is available. In some instances genes have been cloned based on a functional property, without knowing the protein or the genetic map location. For example, various genes involved in DNA repair disorders have been isolated using selection in tissue culture to identify clones that correct the cellular phenotype of defective DNA repair.

Positional cloning is the isolation of a disease gene based on its location in the genome with no knowledge of its function. This strategy depends on the analysis of DNA samples from affected families to find a DNA marker that is located close to the disease locus, as discussed above and illustrated Fig. 65-13*B*. Having localized the disease gene in a general way, it is possible to isolate the DNA of the relevant region in overlapping clones, identify genes in the region, and eventually prove which is the disease gene, often by identifying small mutations within one of the genes (Fig. 65-14). This strategy is facilitated if chromosomal translocations are available to assist in mapping and identifying the disease gene. This approach has yielded landmark successes as in the identification of the genes for Duchenne's muscular dystrophy, cystic fibrosis, retinoblastoma, polyposis of the colon, neurofibromatosis, Huntington's disease, and breast cancer (BRCA1 and BRCA2).

As more genes are described, the positional candidate-gene approach has become very productive for identifying disease genes. A pure candidate-gene strategy occasionally involves deducing the disease gene from among known proteins based on the disease phenotype, but more often the candidate-gene approach requires an approximate genetic mapping, but much less than would be adequate for a strictly positional cloning effort. Based on the limited mapping information, on knowledge about relevant genes mapping to the same region, and perhaps taking into account information from other species such as the mouse, one can formulate and test the hypothesis that a particular gene is mutated in a specific disease by amplification and/or cloning of the gene in question from affected patients to search for mutations. Such an approach led to the identification of mutations in the cardiac myosin heavy chain genes that cause familial hypertrophic cardiomyopathy, in the fibrillin gene in Marfan's syndrome, in the *RET* proto-oncogene in multiple endocrine neoplasia type 2, and in various mismatch DNA repair genes in hereditary nonpolyposis colon cancer. Use of information from the mouse led to the recognition that the *PAX3* gene is mutated in Waardenburg's syndrome. One variation on the candidate-gene approach involves the production of mice with targeted mutations and identifying candidate genes based on phenotypes in the mice that resemble a human phenotype. The map locations for many disorders are shown in Fig. 65-15, and the majority of these genes are cloned.

TRANSGENIC AND MUTANT MICE Gene structure and function are usually similar in mouse and human, and studies in the mouse can often be of value in understanding human disease (Fig. 65-16). After microinjection of cloned DNA sequences into the male pronucleus of fertilized mouse eggs, the injected DNA becomes integrated into the mouse chromosomal DNA in a fraction of the injected cells, including the germ cells, so that a series of descendant animals will express the transgene. Each site of integration of foreign DNA behaves as a single Mendelian trait, and heterozygous and homozygous animals can be bred. This strategy can be used to produce mouse models of human disease in the case of dominant negative or gain-of-function alleles, as has been done for osteogenesis imperfecta and spinocerebellar ataxia type 1.

Transgenic animals are particularly useful for the evaluation of *cis*-acting regulatory DNA sequences that control tissue-specific and temporal aspects of gene expression. Putative regulatory sequences are linked to a reporter gene that encodes an easily detectable product. Using this strategy, it has been shown that short DNA sequences provide exquisite tissue specificity for genes such as insulin and elas-

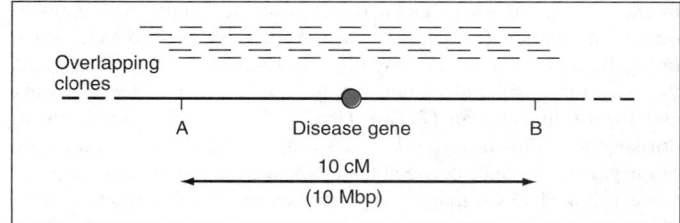

FIGURE 65-14 A positional cloning strategy. DNA markers at sites A and B are found to flank a disease gene. Overlapping DNA clones are isolated for the region, and the disease gene is identified within the region.

tase and that more complex and distant regulatory sequences control the expression of globin genes. The transgenic method has also been utilized to introduce viral or cellular oncogenes in animals to induce tumors, opening up approaches for the study of tumor biology. For example, a tissue-specific regulatory sequence linked to the SV40 T antigen produces tumors in specific cell types. Another transgenic mouse strategy involves linking of regulatory sequences to a toxin that will selectively kill cells that express the sequence. As an example, linking of insulin regulatory sequences to diphtheria toxin can generate mice with selective absence of pancreatic β cells. In yet another application, larger transgenic animals can be used for production of pharmaceuticals to be harvested from milk or blood.

It is also possible to induce mutations in mice, and treatment of male animals with ethylnitrosourea is quite effective in inducing small mutations. Since integration of transgenic DNA is relatively random, such insertions can on occasion interrupt normal mouse genes. Retroviruses can also be used to infect mouse embryonic cells to produce random insertional mutagenesis, and mutant phenotypes can then be ascertained in the resulting heterozygous or homozygous mice, including identification of defects that are benign in heterozygotes but are embryonic lethals in the homozygous state. Because the retrovirus inserts at the site of the affected gene, it is possible to identify many new mutations and to clone the relevant genes.

Homologous recombination with mouse embryonic stem (ES) cells provides additional opportunities. ES cells are totipotent cells that can be manipulated in culture and then reintroduced into mouse embryos. Using homologous recombination in ES cells, it is possible to target a specific gene for subtle mutation or inactivation ("knockout"). Altered ES cells are injected into recipient blastocysts and give rise to chimeric animals composed partially of mutant cells derived from the ES cell culture. The genetically altered cells are often represented in the sperm of the resulting chimeric animals, and mutant mice can be obtained and bred to study the gene in heterozygotes and homozygotes. The technique has allowed the production of mouse models of retinoblastoma, p53 oncogene deficiency (Li-Fraumeni familial cancer syndrome), cystic fibrosis, the Lesch-Nyhan syndrome, Gaucher's disease, apolipoprotein E deficiency, and others. In some instances there are phenotypic differences for the same mutation in mice and humans, providing an opportunity for important biologic insights, and in others, the phenotype in mice and humans is very similar, so that the animals are valuable for studies of pathogenesis and for therapeutic trials. Mutant mice of these types will be useful for unraveling the genetic factors in complex disease processes such as atherosclerosis and for analysis of neurologic functions. The ability to obtain mouse mutants for virtually any cloned gene provides an opportunity for analyzing the function of cloned genes whose biologic roles are not delineated.

CATEGORIES OF GENETIC DISORDERS

Genetic diseases generally fall into one of three categories: (1) *Chromosomal disorders* involve the lack, excess, or abnormal arrangement of one or more chromosomes, producing large amounts of excessive or deficient genetic material and affecting many genes. (2) *Mendelian* or *monogenic disorders* are determined primarily by a single mutant gene. These disorders display simple (Mendelian) inheritance patterns that can be classified into autosomal dominant, autosomal recessive, or X-linked types. (3) *Complex disease traits* are caused by an interaction of multiple genes and multiple exogenous or environmental factors. Although many of these complex traits, such as diabetes mellitus, gout, and cleft lip and palate, exhibit familial clustering, the inheritance pattern is complex, and the risk to relatives is less than in the single-gene disorders. Each of these categories of genetic disease presents different problems with respect to pathogenesis, prevention, diagnosis, genetic counseling, and treatment. Furthermore, this classification is in fact an oversimplification. For example, small chromosomal deletions can cause the simultaneous presence of multiple Mendelian or monogenic disorders, as exemplified by males with cytogenetically visible deletions in the short arm of the X chromosome in association with Duchenne's muscular dystrophy, chronic granulomatous disease, retinitis pigmentosa, and the McLeod phenotype. Deletions of the retinoblastoma locus on chromosome 13 may be visible or submicroscopic and may extend to nearby loci such as esterase D. Thus, these defects bridge the gap between chromosomal and monogenic disorders. The phenotype caused by chromosomal disorders obviously is due to the altered expression of single genes, within the abnormal region. Chromosomal translocations may interrupt single genes, as exemplified by some women with Duchenne's muscular dystrophy due to X/autosome translocations.

The phenotypes of many monogenic disorders are modified by the genes at other loci and by environmental factors. Indeed, a single locus *entirely* determines the disease phenotype in relatively few monogenic disorders. Examples of effects of nongenetic factors that influence monogenic disorders include drug exposure for glucose-6-phosphate dehydrogenase deficiency and acute intermittent porphyria, iron intake and blood loss for hemochromatosis, smoking for α_1-antitrypsin deficiency, and diet for lipoprotein lipase deficiency. Similarly, genes at other loci can modify the phenotype, as exemplified by the effect of the genotype at the α-globin cluster on sickle cell anemia. The border between monogenic disorders and complex traits is not a sharp one, since other genes frequently modify the phenotype of monogenic disorders and major genes often play a role in complex traits (e.g., HLA genotype and type 1 diabetes mellitus). Although monogenic disorders provide an excellent starting point for the study of human genetic disease, an even greater challenge is to understand the more common complex disease traits.

FREQUENCY OF GENETIC DISEASE In studies in Montreal, Baltimore, and Newcastle, 6 to 8 percent of diseases among hospitalized children were attributable to single-gene defects, and 0.4 to 2.5 percent were due to chromosomal abnormalities; another 22 to 31 percent were considered to be gene influenced. The overall frequency of monogenic disorders is about 1 percent, and about 5.3 percent of individuals below age 25 will have a disease with an important genetic component (single gene, chromosomal, or complex traits). If complex traits of late onset are included, about 60 percent of individuals have genetically influenced diseases at some time. Genetic factors contribute in a significant way to an even larger fraction of diseases in a population when common infectious disorders are controlled.

CHROMOSOMAL DISORDERS Chromosomal disorders involve the largest changes in DNA and can include an entire extra copy of the genome (triploidy), an extra chromosome (trisomy), deletions or duplications of portions of a chromosome, and other defects. Chromosomal abnormalities are frequent causes of spontaneous abortion, malformations, mental retardation, and tumors (Table 65-3). Chromosomal disorders are discussed in greater detail in Chap. 66.

MONOGENIC DISORDERS Although few phenotypes are entirely determined by a single locus, the concept of *monogenic disorders* is still valuable. Such disorders ordinarily exhibit one of three patterns of inheritance: (1) autosomal dominant, (2) autosomal recessive, or (3) X-linked. The overall population frequency of monogenic disorders is about 10 per 1000 live births, comprising about 7 in 1000 dominant, about 2.5 in 1000 recessive, and about 0.4 in 1000 X-linked conditions (excluding color blindness). Table 65-4 lists some of the more common Mendelian disorders in adults.

If a particular disease shows one of the three Mendelian patterns of inheritance, its pathogenesis, no matter how complex, must be due to an abnormality at a single site in the genome usually involving a single protein. For example, in sickle cell anemia, the entire clinical syndrome, including such seemingly unrelated disturbances as anemia, pain crises, nephropathy, and predisposition to pneumococcal infections, is the physiologic consequence of having a single base change at a specific site in the gene that codes for the β chain of hemoglobin, producing a substitution of a valine for a glutamic acid in the sixth amino acid position in the protein sequence. The mutant gene and

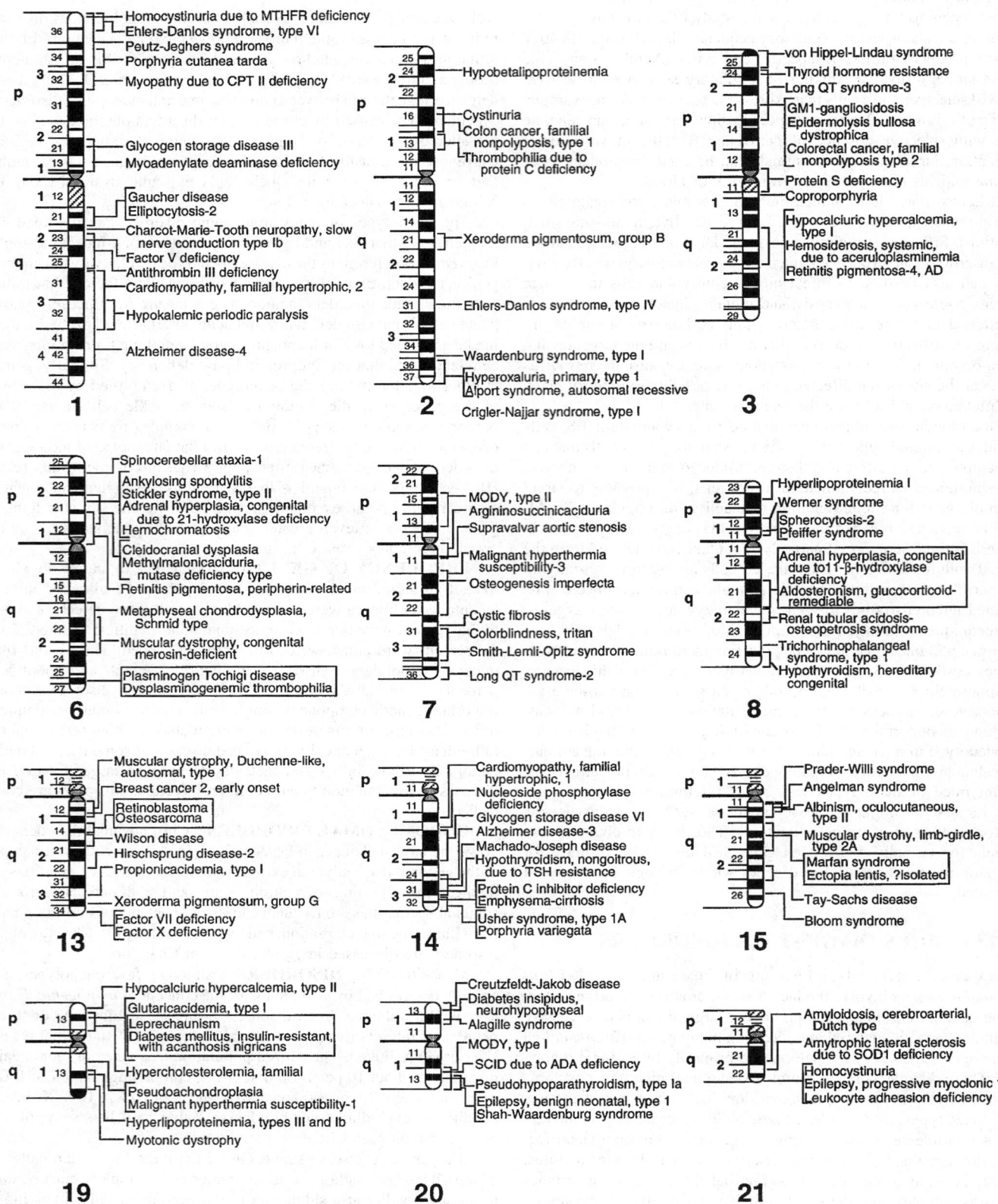

FIGURE 65-15 Morbid anatomy of the human genome adapted to emphasize disorders discussed in *Harrison's*.
(Courtesy of Joanna S. Amberger and Victor A. McKusick, M.D.)

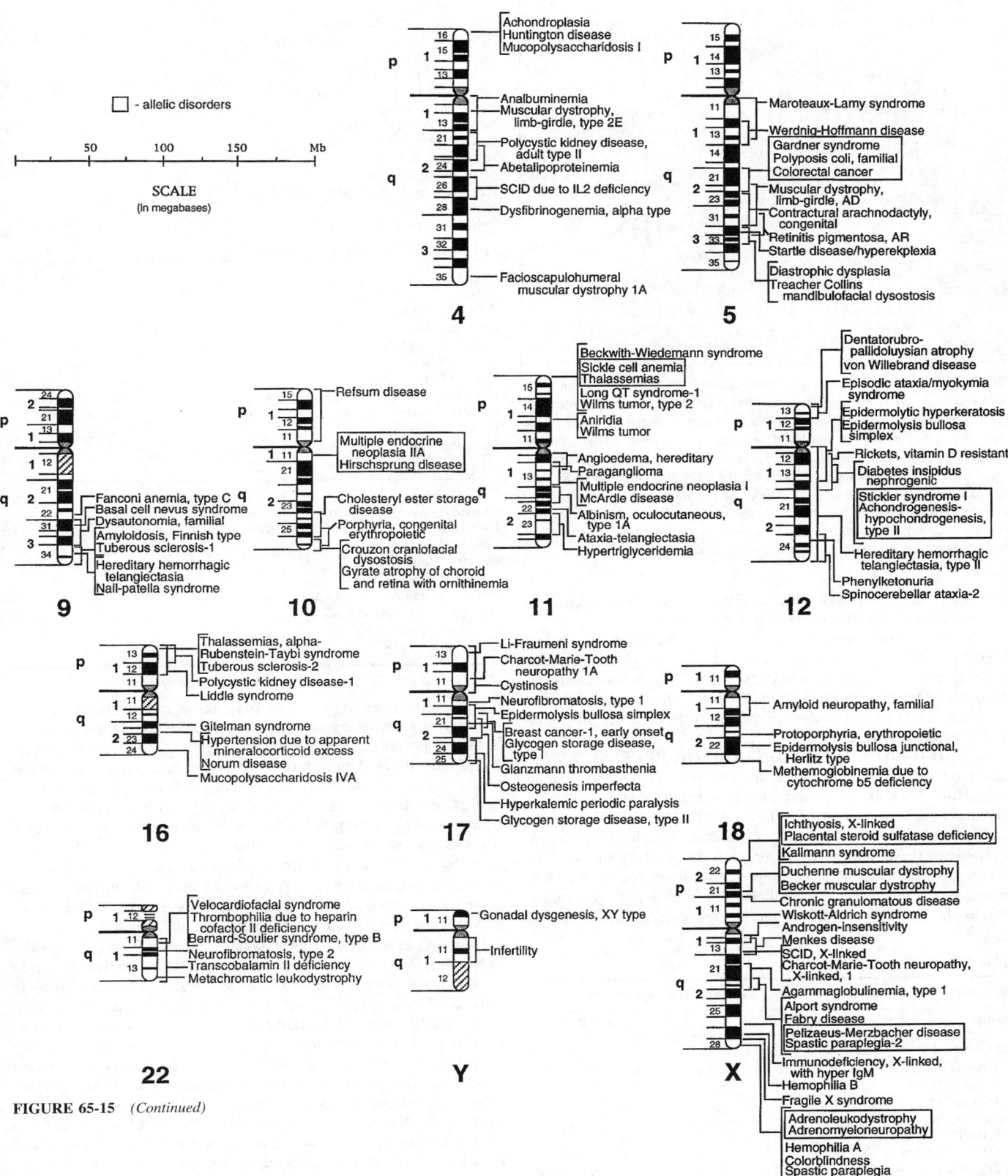

FIGURE 65-15 *(Continued)*

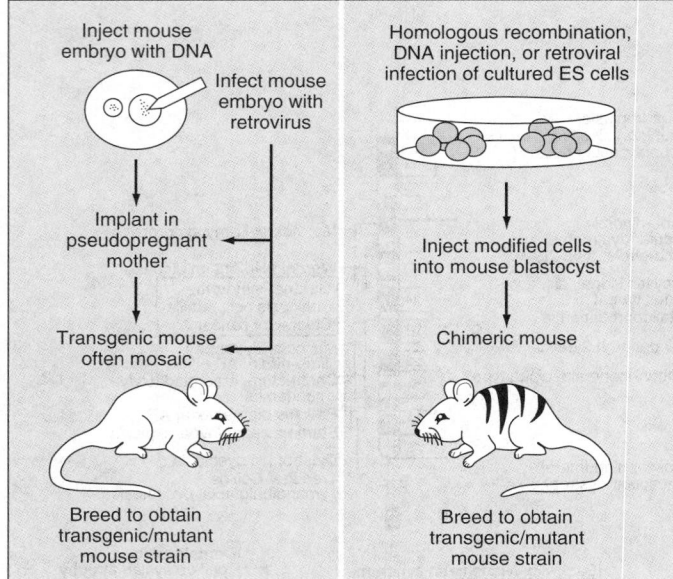

FIGURE 65-16 Various strategies for producing transgenic and mutant mice. DNA can be injected into the male pronucleus of fertilized mouse eggs followed by implantation in pseudopregnant mothers. Mouse embryos can be infected with retroviruses in vivo or in vitro. Transgenic mice may be mosaic, but the transgene can be recovered in nonmosaic form in the offspring of these mice. These strategies are depicted on the left. On the right, cultured embryonic stem (ES) cells can be modified by homologous or nonhomologous recombination or by retroviral infection. The modified cells can be selected and injected into a mouse blastocyst to produce a chimeric mouse, with subsequent recovery of the mutation in the germline of the offspring of the chimeric mouse.

protein for many common Mendelian disorders are known, even when the full pathogenesis of a disorder is not known.

The basic biochemical lesions in monogenic disorders involve defects in a wide variety of proteins, including enzymes, receptors, transport proteins, peptide hormones, immunoglobulins, collagens, transcription factors, and coagulation factors. Defects in genes that do not encode proteins (e.g., defects in genes for tRNA in the mitochondrial genome) are rare.

SIGNIFICANCE OF DOMINANCE OR RECESSIVENESS
Unless otherwise specified, the terms *dominant* and *recessive* refer to the clinical phenotype associated with a particular allele. This distinction is useful for clinical diagnosis, for linkage analysis, and for genetic counseling, but there are a number of complexities inherent in the use of these terms. The circumstance is relatively simple if the heterozygous individual is indistinguishable from one or the other homozygote. In this case, the dominant trait (disease) or allele (mutation) is the one that prevails in the heterozygote. In true recessive

Table 65-3

Frequency of Chromosomal Disorders Among Liveborn Infants

Disorders	Frequency
Autosomal abnormalities	
Trisomy 21 (Down's syndrome)	1 in 600
Trisomy 18	1 in 5000
Trisomy 13	1 in 15,000
Sex chromosome abnormalities	
Klinefelter syndrome (47,XXY)	1 in 700 males
XYY syndrome (47,XYY)	1 in 800 males
Triple-X syndrome (47,XXX)	1 in 1000 females
Turner syndrome (45,X or 45X/46XX or 45X/46,XY or isochromosome Xq)	1 in 1500 females

Table 65-4

Some Relatively Frequent Mendelian Disorders Affecting Adults

AUTOSOMAL DOMINANT DISORDERS

Familial hypercholesterolemia
Hereditary nonpolyposis colon cancer
Polyposis of the colon
BRCA1 and BRCA2 breast cancer
Hereditary hemorrhagic telangiectasia
Marfan's syndrome
Hereditary spherocytosis
Adult polycystic kidney disease
Huntington's chorea
Acute intermittent porphyria
Osteogenesis imperfecta tarda
von Willebrand's disease
Myotonic dystrophy
Familial hypertrophic cardiomyopathy
Neurofibromatosis
Tuberous sclerosis

AUTOSOMAL RECESSIVE DISORDERS

Deafness
Albinism
Wilson's disease
Hemochromatosis
Sickle cell anemia
β Thalassemia
Cystic fibrosis
Hereditary emphysema (α_1-antitrypsin deficiency)
Homocystinuria
Friedreich's ataxia
Phenylketonuria

X-LINKED DISORDERS

Hemophilia A
Glucose-6-phosphate dehydrogenase deficiency
Duchenne/Becker muscular dystrophy
Fabry's disease
Ocular albinism
Testicular feminization
Chronic granulomatous disease
Hypophosphatemic rickets
Fragile-X
Color blindness

disorders, the phenotype in heterozygotes is indistinguishable from normal, and in true dominant disorders, heterozygous individuals have a disease phenotype that is indistinguishable from homozygous affected individuals. Although many recessive medical disorders appear on the surface to qualify as true recessives, heterozygotes for many of these conditions exhibit subtle differences in phenotype that may be enhanced by environmental factors. Such subtle phenotypic consequences may be advantageous or disadvantageous. Even when clinically "normal," individuals who are heterozygous for recessive loss-of-function alleles often have demonstrable metabolic differences and always have demonstrable differences at the protein level. These complexities are exemplified by sickle cell anemia, which is clinically a recessive disorder in that heterozygotes are usually normal healthy individuals. Nevertheless, heterozygotes exhibit a selective advantage for resistance to malaria and have subtle physiologic abnormalities in renal concentrating ability and in cardiopulmonary function at high altitude. Subtle phenotypic effects in heterozygotes for recessive disorders may be more common than is generally recognized and may contribute to phenotypes usually considered to be complex disease traits. For example, heterozygotes for ataxia telangiectasia and other DNA repair disorders may be at increased risk of malignancy, heterozygosity for homocystinuria is probably a risk factor in vascular disease, and heterozygosity for α_1-antitrypsin deficiency may predispose to pulmonary disease. Heterozygosity for known recessive disorders makes a major contribution to biochemical and medical individuality.

The situation is different for dominant phenotypes; very few conditions qualify as true dominants, such as may be the case for Huntington's disease. Homozygotes for most dominant disorders are ascertained rarely, and, when recognized, the disease is usually more severe than in heterozygotes, indicating that most such disorders are actually semidominant (incompletely or partially dominant) traits (e.g., familial hypercholesterolemia and achondroplasia). The term *codominant* has relatively little clinical applicability and describes a situation such as the A and B blood group alleles in which the presence of one antigenic determinant does not affect the presence or absence of the other.

Additional complexities arise from the fact that the phenotypic consequences of heterozygosity may be inconsistent and cause uncertainty as to whether the disorder is dominant or recessive. Heterozygotes may display symptoms in only a very small fraction of cases, or heterozygotes may have subtle and mild symptoms that do not qualify as a disease diagnosis. Homozygotes for these traits typically have clear-cut disease manifestation. From a clinical and counseling vantage point, most medical disorders fall into the dominant or recessive category despite the fact that this classification is an arbitrary division of a continuum rather than a true biologic demarcation.

Although there is a tendency for a given disease locus to be considered as typically involving dominant or recessive mutations, the classification of a mutation or trait as dominant or recessive must be made on an allele-by-allele basis and not on a locus-by-locus basis, as in the case of osteogenesis imperfecta where different mutations in the same gene can have dominant or recessive effects. When two different mutant alleles are present at the same locus, patients are referred to as *compound heterozygotes* or *genetic compounds*. This is distinct from a double-heterozygote individual who is heterozygous at two different loci. Most compound heterozygous genotypes involve different recessive alleles at a locus, but phenotypic homozygotes for dominant traits (such as familial hypercholesterolemia) may be compound heterozygotes at a molecular level as well. Alternatively, compound heterozygotes may have one recessive allele and one dominant allele such that heterozygotes for the recessive allele are phenotypically normal, heterozygotes for the dominant allele have a disease process, and the compound heterozygote individuals have a disease process that is distinct (usually more severe) from the disease in heterozygotes for the dominant allele. Such instances are likely for osteogenesis imperfecta.

Mutant alleles may cause a total or partial loss of function (referred to as *null alleles* or *hypomorphic alleles*, respectively), may exhibit altered function, or may gain a novel function. In general, most loss-of-function alleles tend to be recessive, as in the case of the majority of enzyme deficiencies in humans and most null mutations produced in mice. However, some null alleles have phenotypic effects and cause human disease if a half-normal level of the encoded protein is insufficient for normal physiology. Whether a mutation generates a dominant or recessive disorder is determined by two factors: (1) the effect of the mutation on the function of the gene product, and (2) the tolerance of the biologic system to perturbation of that particular gene product. Mutations in tolerant systems tend to result in recessive phenotypes; mutations in less tolerant systems tend to result in dominant phenotypes. Loci that encode enzymes usually result in recessive phenotypes because of the catalytic nature of enzymes and because enzymes are usually present in excess of the quantity required to maintain relatively normal levels of substrates and products, so that a large change in enzyme activity can have a negligible effect on flux in many pathways. Examples where a heterozygous loss-of-function mutation causes a disease phenotype include several forms of porphyria, familial hypercholesterolemia, and osteogenesis imperfecta. In the case of recessive disorders, the presence of protein with residual function can result in mild forms of disorders, including disorders of amino acid metabolism and lysosomal storage diseases.

The term *dominant negative* is applied to mutant alleles in which a mutant protein interferes in one way or another with the function of normal protein being produced from the normal allele in a heterozygote. Dominant negative alleles occur when proteins are involved in subunit structures or when proteins interact with other proteins or nucleic acids. A dominant negative mechanism is often involved when a mutant allele causes a more severe phenotype in heterozygotes than

that caused by a null allele because of some adverse effect of the abnormal product on the function of the normal product. For example, in osteogenesis imperfecta, missense mutations can interfere with collagen fiber assembly and cause lethal osteogenesis imperfecta in heterozygotes, whereas null alleles cause a milder disease. In other instances, mutant alleles generate a novel biologic effect that cannot be described in terms of increased or decreased function of the normal allele; these are referred to as *gain-of-function alleles* or *neomorphic alleles*. In amyloidosis, the abnormal folding properties of the mutant protein lead to a harmful, extracellular deposition of material that appears unrelated to the normal function of the protein. The expanded polyglutamine tracts in the mutant alleles for Huntington's disease, spinocerebellar ataxia, and spinobulbar muscular atrophy may represent gain-of-function alleles, but the pathogenesis is not yet understood.

EXCEPTIONS TO THE RULES (UNSTABLE MUTATIONS, UNIPARENTAL DISOMY, IMPRINTED GENES, AND TRANSMISSION RATIO DISTORTION) The traditional formulation of single-gene disorders involved assumptions that are generally correct, including the stability of mutations, the inheritance of one allele from each parent for an autosomal locus, the equal expression of both alleles at an autosomal locus, and the random transmission of either allele to an offspring. Genetic counseling, linkage analysis, and interpretation of genetic data are based on these assumptions. However, examples of exceptions to these rules now abound.

As mentioned above, the clearest examples of unstable mutations involve the expanding triplet repeats that cause fragile X syndrome, myotonic dystrophy, Huntington's disease, spinobulbar muscular atrophy, spinocerebellar ataxia type 1, and other disorders. Previously, the significance of *anticipation* (defined as the worsening of a disease phenotype over generations within a family) was uncertain, and molecular documentation was lacking for the concept of premutation. Expanding triplet mutations have demonstrated that premutations can exist as modest expansions of triplet repeats (perhaps including minor sequence differences from stable alleles). These premutations do not themselves cause clear phenotypic effects but are prone to further expansion and causation of disease. The phenomenon of anticipation is due to increasing size of repeats, which causes earlier onset of disease or a more severe phenotype.

Recognition that individuals can inherit two copies of part or all of a chromosome from one parent and no copy from the other parent is also a rare departure from Mendelian inheritance. This phenomenon of *uniparental disomy* is relatively rare but contributes to the occurrence of the Prader-Willi and Angelman syndromes. The significance of uniparental disomy is in large part due to the existence of *imprinting*, whereby the maternal copy of a gene and the paternal copy of a gene are differentially expressed. The copies of the genes for insulin-like growth factor 2 (*IFG2*) and small nuclear ribonucleopolypeptide N (*SNRPN*) that are inherited from the father are expressed, while the copies inherited from the mother are repressed in mouse and human; in contrast, the maternal copy of the H19 gene is expressed, and the paternal copy is repressed in mouse and human. The gene(s) causing the Prader-Willi syndrome appear to be expressed from the paternal copy, while that causing Angelman's syndrome is expressed from the maternal copy. Patterns of inheritance for diseases involving mutations in imprinted genes deviate from usual Mendelian patterns (see "Disorders of Imprinted Genes," below).

Further deviations from simple Mendelian rules probably exist. *Transmission ratio distortion* (or meiotic drive) describes the circumstance where there is preferential transmission of an allele to the offspring from a heterozygous parent. This phenomenon is well documented for various alleles at the *T* locus in the mouse and may occur in humans.

AUTOSOMAL DOMINANT DISORDERS Dominant diseases are manifest in the heterozygous state, i.e., when only one abnormal gene (*mutant allele*) is present and the corresponding allele on the homologous chromosome is normal. By definition, the gene responsible for an autosomal dominant disorder must be located on one of the 22 autosomes; hence, both males and females can be affected. Since alleles segregate independently at meiosis, there is a 1 in 2 chance that the offspring of an affected heterozygote will inherit the mutant allele.

Figure 65-17 shows typical pedigrees involving an autosomal dominant trait: (1) each affected individual has an affected parent (unless the condition arose by a new mutation in the sperm or ovum that formed the individual or unless the mutant allele is present but without phenotypic effect in the affected parent as discussed under "Penetrance and Expressivity," below); (2) an affected individual has a 50 percent probability of passing the trait to each offspring; (3) normal children of an affected individual have only normal offspring; (4) males and females are affected in equal proportions except in sex-limited disorders; (5) each sex is equally likely to transmit the condition to male and female offspring, including male-to-male transmission; and (6) vertical transmission of the condition through successive generations occurs, when the trait does not impair reproductive capacity. Autosomal dominant disorders can be inherited in a sex-limited or sex-modified pattern, as exemplified by breast/ovarian cancer in women and by familial male precocious puberty in boys.

Dominant New Mutations   For autosomal dominant diseases, a certain proportion of cases are due to new mutations rather than to inherited mutations. Since a rough estimate of the frequency of mutation is 5×10^{-6} mutations per gene per generation and since there are two copies of each autosomal gene, one would expect that about 1 in 100,000 newborn persons possess a new mutation at any given genetic locus. Many of these mutations either do not impair the function of the gene product or involve a recessive effect, so that the mutation is clinically silent. Others, however, give rise to dominant traits. The parent in whose germ cells the mutation arose is clinically normal, and the sibs of the affected individual are usually normal since the mutation affects one or only a few germ cells. Given the nature of germ-cell proliferation, mutations are most likely to occur at one of the later cell divisions, but multiple mutant gametes may be descended from a single mutational event in some cases (gonadal mosaicism). Given these factors, and since humans have few offspring, the probability of a recurrence of the disorder among the siblings of an individual with a new mutation generally is quite low. The presence of the identical mutation in siblings when neither parent has the mutation in somatic cells can occur through gonadal mosaicism and will cause a higher recurrence risk in siblings, as has been well documented for osteogenesis imperfecta and Duchenne's muscular dystrophy. It is possible to assess the proportion of gonadal mosaicism by molecular analysis of sperm in some cases. Individuals affected with new dominant mutations are able to transmit the disease, and each offspring is at 50 percent risk for the condition.

The proportion of dominant disorders due to new mutations is inversely proportional to the effect on biologic fitness (Table 65-5).

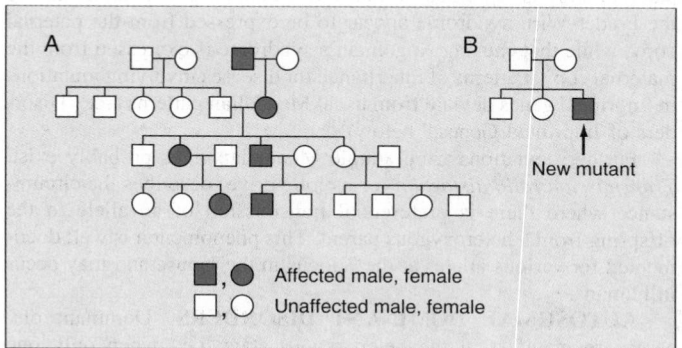

FIGURE 65-17   Pedigree pattern for an autosomal dominant trait. Note the *vertical* pattern of inheritance; compare new mutation and inherited pedigrees.

Table 65-5

Approximate Percentage of Patients Affected by New Germline Mutations in Some Autosomal Dominant Disorders

Disorder	Percentage
Achondroplasia	80
Tuberous sclerosis	80
Neurofibromatosis	40
Marfan's syndrome	30
Polyposis of the colon	30
Myotonic dystrophy	Anticipation*
Huntington's disease	Anticipation*
Adult polycystic kidney disease	1
Familial hypercholesterolemia	Very low
BRCA1 breast cancer	Very low

* Anticipation is intended to indicate a multistep process from wild type to premutation to mutation. A very high percentage of cases are inherited.

The term *biologic fitness* refers to the ability of an individual to produce children who survive to adult life and reproduce. In the extreme case, if a dominant mutation causes infertility, then all observed cases, of necessity, represent new mutations, and there would be no evidence of familial transmission. Thanatophoric dysplasia represents such a disorder. In moderately severe disorders, as in tuberous sclerosis, biologic fitness is about 20 percent of normal, and about 80 percent of cases are due to new mutations. In disorders such as familial hypercholesterolemia, in which there is little, if any, reduction in biologic fitness, almost all affected persons have a pedigree showing classic vertical transmission. The incidence of a dominant disorder is dependent both on the biologic fitness and on the mutation frequency for the locus, which is widely variable. Although the proportion of cases due to new mutation is directly related to biologic fitness, genetic counseling and reproductive planning now can alter this proportion.

Many new mutations occur in the germ cells of fathers who are of advanced age. For example, in Marfan's syndrome, the average age of fathers of sporadic or "new mutation" cases (37 years) is in excess of the age of fathers who transmit the disease as an inherited mutation (30 years). The paternal age effect is also prominent in achondroplasia. There is evidence that the mutations associated with advanced paternal age are frequently point mutations, often C to T transitions at CG dinucleotides. Differences in mutation rates for male and female gametes are discussed below under "X-linked New Mutations and Heterozygote Detection."

Before one concludes that a dominant disorder in a patient with unaffected parents is the result of a new mutation, it is important to consider two other possibilities: (1) the gene may be carried by one parent, in whom the mutant allele is not penetrant; and (2) nonpaternity may have occurred (i.e., the father is someone other than the putative father), as happens in 3 to 5 percent of randomly studied children in many cultures.

Penetrance and Expressivity   These terms are frequently the subject of confusion and slight variations in usage. In the medical context, *penetrance* is the proportion of individuals with a given genotype who present with *any* phenotypic features of the disorder (i.e., it is an all-or-none phenomenon). Although in one sense penetrance may vary with age, as in the case of Huntington's disease, variation in age of onset is most often considered as an aspect of variable expression. In some cases, penetrance depends on environmental exposure, as in glucose-6-phosphate dehydrogenase deficiency. In the autosomal dominant context, it is instructive to consider the concept of penetrance from a counseling perspective and in terms of molecular diagnosis. Penetrance is the question at issue when the apparently unaffected offspring of an individual with a dominant disorder wish to know if they carry the mutant gene and if they are at risk of having affected offspring. The mutant gene is not penetrant if an individual carrying the mutant gene shows absolutely no phenotypic effects. In molecular terms, the presence or absence of the mutant gene can be determined with appropriate diagnostic tests, and a person without the mutant gene can be distinguished from one carrying the impenetrant mutant gene. Clinically, definition of penetrance often depends on the quality of clinical methodologies; for example, magnetic resonance imaging might demonstrate findings not previously recognizable. In the medical context, the gene is usually considered penetrant if diagnostic abnormalities can be demonstrated even if the individual is asymptomatic. In the biologic context, the gene can be considered penetrant if it affects the function of the individual.

Expressivity, or *variability in clinical expression*, describes the range of phenotypic effects in individuals carrying a given mutation. This variability can include the type and severity of symptoms and the age of onset of symptoms. Variability in clinical expression is illustrated dramatically in multiple endocrine neoplasia, type 1. Patients in the same family with the same abnormal gene may have hyperplasia or neoplasia of one or all of a wide variety of endocrine tissues, including the pancreas, parathyroid glands, pituitary gland, or adipose tissue. The resulting manifestations are extremely diverse; different members of the same family may develop peptic ulcers, hypoglycemia, kidney stones, or pituitary tumors. In the case of some dominant disorders characterized by tumor formation, random second mutations in tumor suppressor genes may explain some of the clinical variability.

Variation in age of onset is seen in disorders such as Huntington's disease and adult polycystic kidney disease. These disorders often do not become symptomatic until adult life, even though the mutant gene is present throughout life. Whether variation in age of onset is considered as a form of variation in expression is somewhat arbitrary. In one sense, it cannot be said that the mutant gene was impenetrant in an individual until the person has had a complete evaluation and has died from other causes. Lack of penetrance can be considered as the absolute mildest end of the spectrum of expression so that no phenotypic effects are observed. In the counseling context, variation in expression, as distinct from penetrance, is the point in question when an individual with a dominant disorder wishes to know whether an offspring who carries the mutation would have mild or severe symptoms. In molecular terms, analysis of the single gene locus will not answer this question (i.e., predict variation in expression within a family) but can determine whether the mutant gene is present and not penetrant.

At least three factors underlie lack of penetrance and variability in expression: (1) the effects of genes at the same or other loci, (2) exogenous or environmental factors, and (3) stochastic factors. Effects within the same gene locus can be seen with mutations in α-spectrin, where a polymorphism in the level of gene expression affects the phenotype. The low-expression allele moderates the phenotype of hereditary elliptocytosis when in *cis* with the mutation but worsens the phenotype when in *trans* in a heterozygote for the mutation. In the case of cystic fibrosis, the phenotypic severity of the R117H mutation varies through a *cis* effect on the level of functional mRNA due to a splice junction polymorphism that influences skipping of an exon. The genotype at the α-globin locus that affects the sickle cell anemia phenotype and various loci that affect the monogenic hyperlipidemias are examples of effects by genes at other loci. The phenotypes in the monogenic hyperlipidemias, the porphyrias, and hemochromatosis can be affected by diet, alcohol use, smoking, and exercise. The effects of stochastic factors are exemplified by variability in the severity and distribution of lesions among identical twins with retinoblastoma, neurofibromatosis, or tuberous sclerosis. Other examples of stochastic events that can affect phenotypes are differences in random X chromosome inactivation among identical twin female heterozygotes for an X-linked disorder and somatic rearrangements and mutations associated with expression of immunoglobulins and T cell receptors. Although the issues of penetrance and expressivity are often defined in the context of autosomal dominant disorders, these principles are relevant to chromosomal disorders, autosomal recessive and X-linked disorders, and complex disease traits as well.

Biochemical Basis of Dominant Alleles The biochemical and/ or molecular defects causing dominant disorders such as familial hypercholesterolemia, amyloidosis, hereditary spherocytosis, osteogenesis imperfecta, hereditary retinoblastoma, neurofibromatosis, Marfan's syndrome, and Huntington's disease have been determined. A number

of mechanisms can account for an abnormal phenotype in the presence of one mutant gene. One mechanism is *haploinsufficiency*—meaning that a half-normal amount of gene product is insufficient to maintain a normal phenotype (i.e., the process is sensitive to reduced dosage). This is true, for example, when gene products regulate complex metabolic pathways, such as membrane receptors and rate-limiting enzymes in biosynthetic pathways under feedback control (e.g., familial hypercholesterolemia and dominant porphyrias). In other cases a dosage effect due to gene duplication can cause a dominant phenotype, as in the case of the common mutation in type 1A Charcot-Marie-Tooth disease where triploid dosage for the *PMP22* gene causes the condition. This means the organism is sensitive to 150 percent of the normal level of gene product. Another mechanism involves abnormalities of structural proteins where a complex network of direct protein interactions is involved (e.g., collagens in osteogenesis imperfecta and erythrocyte cytoskeleton proteins in spherocytosis and elliptocytosis). Dominant negative mutations are instances where the molecules of mutant gene product interfere with the function of the normal gene products. Many mutations involving structural proteins have a dominant negative component, and some missense mutations may be more deleterious than null mutations, as in the case of osteogenesis imperfecta. Dominant phenotypic effects can also occur when the remaining normal copy of a gene is mutated at a single-cell level so that both copies of the locus are inactivated (e.g., hereditary retinoblastoma). These defects may be considered dominant at the pedigree level and recessive at the single-cell level. Conceptually, it is useful to distinguish dominant mutations that generate products with new or neomorphic biologic properties and cause a harmful effect (e.g., amyloidosis) from those due to deficiency of normal gene product (e.g., familial hypercholesterolemia and porphyrias). In the former group, restoration of a normal level of gene product does not negate the effect of the mutant gene.

Disorders of Imprinted Genes If an autosomal locus is imprinted such that it is expressed from one allele and repressed from the other, there is no question of a dominant or recessive effect since the gene is functionally hemizygous. The familial pattern is more similar to dominant pedigrees since the disorder may occur over multiple generations (i.e., show vertical transmission; Fig. 65-18). There are good examples of large pedigrees with inherited phenotypes involving imprinted genes. Hereditary paragangliomas is a disorder in which the phenotype is expressed only when the mutant allele is inherited from the father (Fig. 65-18). In contrast, Angelman's syndrome is expressed only when the mutant allele is inherited from the mother (Fig. 65-18).

AUTOSOMAL RECESSIVE DISORDERS Autosomal recessive conditions are clinically apparent only in the homozygous or compound heterozygous state, i.e., when both alleles at a particular genetic locus are mutant. It is useful to distinguish phenotypic "homozygotes" (perhaps better referred to as affected individuals), in whom both copies of the gene are defective, from molecular homozygotes, in whom DNA analysis reveals identical mutations in both copies of the gene. By definition, the gene responsible for an autosomal recessive disorder must be located on one of the 22 autosomes so that both males and females can be affected.

Figure 65-19 shows two pedigrees for families with an autosomal recessive trait. Monoplex families (Fig. 65-19A) are the most common, but families with multiple affected individuals occur. The following features are characteristic: (1) the parents are clinically normal; (2) only sibs are affected, and vertical transmission usually does not occur; (3) males and females are affected in equal proportions, except for sex-limited effects; and (4) consanguinity can be a contributing factor.

The variety of recessive alleles and the requirement for two abnormal copies for clinical expression create special conditions for autosomal recessive inheritance: (1) the more infrequent the mutant gene in the population, the stronger the likelihood that affected individuals are the product of consanguineous matings (see "Consanguinity," below); (2) if both parents are carriers for the same autosomal recessive

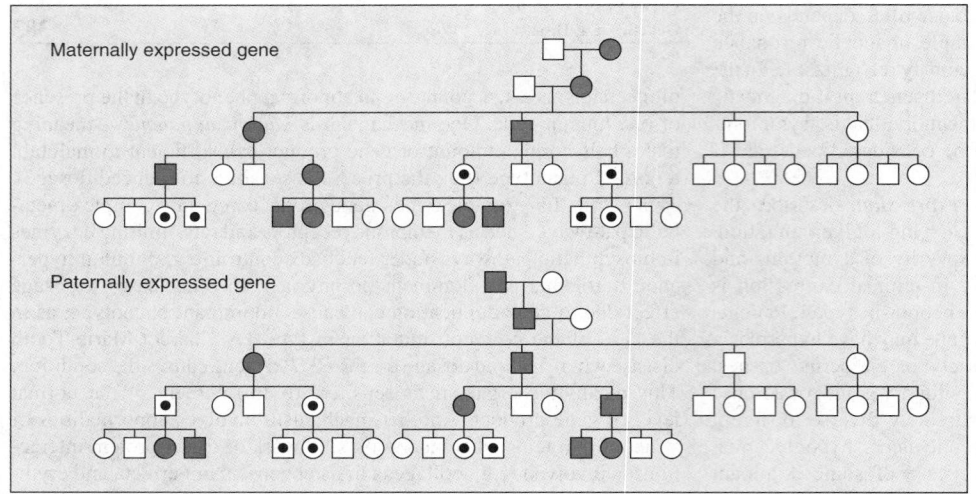

Maternally expressed gene

Paternally expressed gene

FIGURE 65-18 Idealized pedigrees for disorders involving imprinted genes. Filled symbols indicate individuals carrying the mutation and affected by the disorder. Symbols with a solid dot in the center indicate individuals who are asymptomatic but carry the mutation on the silenced allele. Open symbols indicate individuals who do not carry the mutation and are asymptomatic. The upper pedigree depicts a maternally expressed gene as in the case of Angelman's syndrome, while the lower pedigree depicts a paternally expressed gene as in the case of hereditary paragangliomas. *(Adapted from Sapienza and Hall, in Scriver et al, with permission.)*

gene, the probability for disease in offspring is 0.25, for a heterozygote (carrier) it is 0.50, and for a normal (noncarrier) offspring it is 0.25; (3) if an affected individual mates with a heterozygote, there is a 50 percent probability of disease for each child, and a pedigree simulating dominant inheritance may result; and (4) if two individuals with the same recessive disease mate, all the children will be affected.

The clinical features of autosomal recessive disorders tend to be more uniform than those of dominant diseases, and recessive disorders are more commonly diagnosed in children. Many autosomal recessive disorders present or cause major morbidity in adulthood, including hemochromatosis (see Chap. 342), α_1-antitrypsin deficiency, hemoglobinopathies, some forms of hyperlipidemia (see Chap. 341), and late-onset lysosomal storage diseases (see Chap. 346).

Since the probability is that only one in four individuals in a sibship will be affected, most cases of autosomal recessive disease may occur as isolated individuals, particularly when small families are common. Consider, for example, 16 families in which both parents are heterozygous for the same recessive disorder, such as cystic fibrosis. If each family has 2 children, the probability is that 9 of the 16 families will have no affected children, 6 will have 1 affected and 1 normal child, and only 1 of the 16 families will have 2 affected children. Because of the tendency toward small families, physicians usually see isolated cases of a recessive disease without an affected sib to alert them to the possibility of a genetic disorder. Fortunately, because of the relatively uniform manifestations of recessive disorders and because many conditions can be diagnosed directly by biochemical or molecular tests, the diagnosis of a genetic disease can frequently be made even when no other members of a family are clinically affected. Autosomal recessive disorders can be inherited in a sex-limited manner as exemplified by steroid 5α-reductase 2 deficiency, where only 46,XY males are phenotypically abnormal.

Biochemical Basis of Recessive Alleles The biochemical defects underlying many autosomal recessive disorders have been identified. Most alleles are complete or partial loss-of-function mutations, often involving enzymatic proteins. In these conditions, recessive inheritance occurs because a mutation that impairs the catalytic activity of an enzyme usually does not impair the health of a heterozygote. Regulatory mechanisms function to avert clinical consequences of this 50 percent deficiency, and so heterozygotes for enzyme defects usually are clinically normal as discussed above. On the other hand, when an individual inherits abnormal alleles at both loci specifying an enzyme, a disease results.

Many of the enzyme deficiencies in recessive diseases involve

enzymes in catabolic pathways, frequently enzymes that degrade organic molecules in the diet, such as galactose (galactosemia, see Chap. 349), phenylalanine (phenylketonuria, see Chap. 349), and phytanic acid (Refsum's syndrome). When deficiency affects an acid hydrolase (*lysosomal storage disorders*), the substrate, usually a complex lipid or polysaccharide, accumulates within swollen lysosomes. Examples of such lysosomal diseases include the mucopolysaccharidoses such as Hurler's syndrome (α-iduronidase deficiency) and the sphingolipidoses such as Gaucher's disease (glucocerebrosidase deficiency).

Population Genetics of Recessive Alleles In general, recessive diseases are rare because the reduced biologic fitness of homozygotes serves to remove the mutant gene from the population. A few lethal recessive disorders, such as cystic fibrosis, thalassemia, and sickle cell anemia are common. To explain this paradox, it has been postulated that the biologic fitness of heterozygotes is greater than that of noncarriers for these genes. In such a case, the frequency of the gene in the population depends on the balance between the increased fitness of the relatively numerous heterozygotes and the reduced fitness of the less common homozygotes. A small selective advantage of the heterozygote in terms of reproductive advantage results in a high gene frequency and hence a high birth frequency of homozygotes, even when the disease is lethal. Thus, about 1 in 25 Caucasians is heterozygous (a carrier) for the genetically lethal disease cystic fibrosis, and the disease occurs in about 1 in 2500 Caucasian births. To maintain such a high gene frequency, heterozygotes for cystic fibrosis may have a selective advantage over noncarriers, and this advantage may involve protection against death from childhood diarrhea. Alternatively, there could be a slight transmission ratio distortion (meiotic drive), i.e., gametes carrying the mutant gene could have a slightly greater probability of achieving fertilization compared to gametes with the normal gene, or disorders might achieve a high frequency without a selective advantage, i.e., by chance. Haplotype data indicate that chromosomes carrying the common ΔF508 allele for cystic fibrosis are descended from a single mutational event, but this does not explain why the mutant gene is so frequent. In sickle cell anemia, another recessive disorder with high frequency among certain populations, heterozygotes have increased resistance to falciparum malaria.

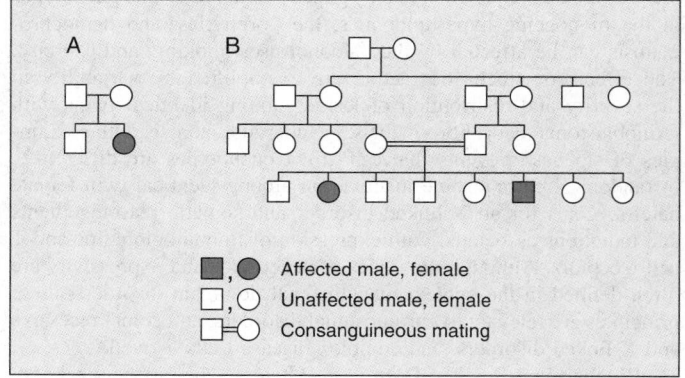

FIGURE 65-19 Pedigree pattern for an autosomal recessive trait. Note the *horizontal* pattern of inheritance and consanguinity in the multiplex pedigree (B) in comparison to the more common monoplex pedigree (A). *(From Scriver et al, with permission.)*

Consanguinity By definition, a recessive disease requires the inheritance of a mutant allele at the same genetic locus from each parent. When the genes are rare, the likelihood of unrelated parents being carriers for the same defect is small. If the parents have a common ancestor who carried a recessive gene, the likelihood that two of the descendants inherited the same allele is enhanced. The less frequent the recessive gene, the stronger the likelihood that an affected individual is the product of a consanguineous mating. On the other hand, when recessive genes are common in the population, the likelihood of two unrelated parents being carriers is great enough to minimize the role of consanguinity. For common traits such as sickle cell anemia, phenylketonuria, cystic fibrosis, and Tay-Sachs disease consanguinity is uncommon in the parents.

Recessive New Mutations New mutations for recessive disorders can rarely be identified because such mutations usually generate asymptomatic heterozygotes. Only generations later will the descendants of individuals with that mutation mate with other heterozygotes with a mutation at the same locus. The selective pressure to eliminate deleterious recessive traits from the population is low because these traits are easily passed on in heterozygous form. Most recessive diseases appear to be due to mutations that occurred many generations earlier, as indicated from haplotype analysis of mutations causing phenylketonuria, β-thalassemia, sickle cell anemia, Tay Sachs disease, cystic fibrosis, and other disorders.

X-LINKED DISORDERS The genes responsible for X-linked disorders are located on the X chromosome, and the clinical risks are different for the two sexes. Since a female has two X chromosomes, she may be either heterozygous or homozygous for a mutant gene, and the mutant allele may demonstrate either recessive or dominant expression. Expression in females is often variable and influenced by random X-chromosome inactivation. Males, on the other hand, have only one X chromosome, so they are more likely to display the full phenotype, regardless of whether the mutation produces a recessive or dominant allele in the female. Thus, the terms *X-linked dominant* or *X-linked recessive* refer only to the expression of the mutations in women.

The distinction of dominant and recessive X-linked disorders is complicated by the effect of X-chromosome inactivation. In both ornithine transcarbamoylase deficiency, often described as X-linked dominant, and Fabry's disease, often described as X-linked recessive, phenotypic abnormalities are relatively frequent in heterozygotes. Since there is no clear convention, it may be best to consider such disorders as simply X-linked without a dominant or recessive designation. The recessive or dominant descriptors are more useful for X-linked disorders in which heterozygotes are consistently asymptomatic (e.g., X-linked recessive Hunter's mucopolysaccharidosis) or consistently symptomatic in a manner similar to hemizygous males (e.g., X-linked dominant hypophosphatemic rickets).

An important feature of all X-linked inheritance is the absence of male-to-male (i.e., father-to-son) transmission of the trait. This follows because a male contributes his Y chromosome to his son and does not contribute an X chromosome. On the other hand, since a male contributes his sole X chromosome to each daughter, all daughters of a male with an X-linked disorder will inherit the mutant allele.

The pedigrees in Fig. 65-20 illustrate some of the characteristic features of X-linked inheritance. (1) In contrast to the vertical distribution in dominant traits (parents and children affected) and the horizontal distribution in autosomal recessive traits (sibs affected), the pedigree pattern in X-linked recessive traits tends to be oblique; that is, the trait occurs in the maternal uncles of affected males and in male cousins who are descended from the mother's sisters who are carriers (Fig. 65-20A). (2) Male offspring of carrier females have a 50 percent chance of being affected. (3) All female offspring of affected males are carriers, and affected males do not transmit the disease to their sons. (4) Unaffected males do not transmit the trait to any offspring. (5) Affected homozygous females occur only when an affected male mates with a carrier female.

Examples of X-linked recessive disorders in humans include the Lesch-Nyhan syndrome, glucose-6-phosphate dehydrogenase deficiency, testicular feminization, and Hunter's mucopolysaccharidosis.

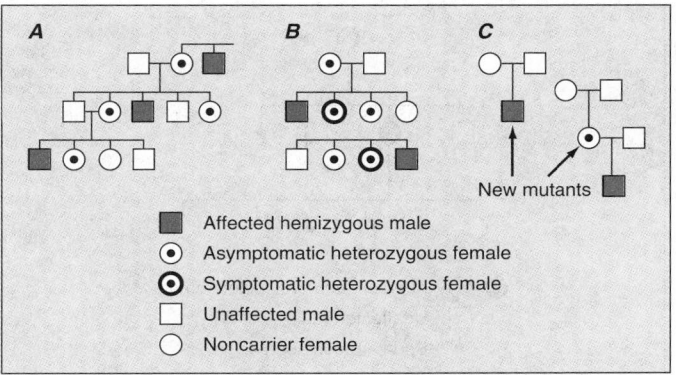

FIGURE 65-20 Pedigree pattern for an X-linked trait. *A.* Note the *oblique* pattern of inheritance. *B.* Note the occurrence of symptomatic and asymptomatic heterozygous females in the same pedigree. Heterozygotes are consistently asymptomatic in some disorders (recessive) and are variably symptomatic in other disorders (see text). *C.* New mutations can give rise to either affected males or heterozygous females. *(From Scriver et al, with permission.)*

Color blindness is a frequent X-linked recessive trait (occurring in about 8 percent of white males), so that the occurrence of homozygous color-blind females is no rarity. A pedigree for an X-linked disorder with variable symptomatology in females is depicted in Fig. 65-20*B*, and X-linked disease on the basis of new mutation is shown by the pedigrees in Fig. 65-20*C* (see "X-linked New Mutations and Heterozygote Detection," below).

X-linked dominant inheritance is illustrated by the pedigree in Fig. 65-21. (1) Females are affected about twice as often as males, (2) an affected female has a 50 percent probability of transmitting the disorder to her sons or daughters, (3) an affected male transmits the disorder to all of his daughters and to none of his sons, and (4) the phenotype may be more variable and less severe in heterozygous affected females than in hemizygous affected males. One common trait, the Xg (a+) blood group, is inherited as an X-linked dominant trait, as are a few diseases, such as hypophosphatemic rickets.

Some rare conditions may be inherited as X-linked dominant traits in which there is lethality in the hemizygous male (Fig. 65-22). (1) The disorder occurs only in females who are heterozygous for the mutant gene; (2) an affected mother has a 50 percent probability of transmitting the trait to her daughters; (3) an increased frequency of spontaneous abortions occurs in affected women, the abortions representing affected male fetuses. An example of a condition that is transmitted by this mode of inheritance is incontinentia pigmenti. Some X-linked disorders are lethal in utero in males and impair reproduction in females so that a condition occurs primarily or exclusively

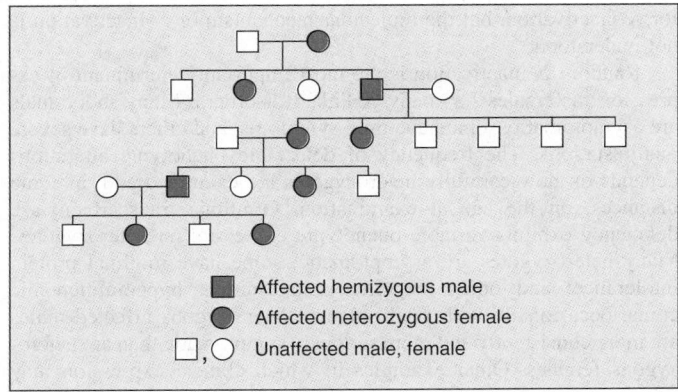

FIGURE 65-21 Pedigree pattern of an X-linked dominant trait. *(From Scriver et al, with permission.)*

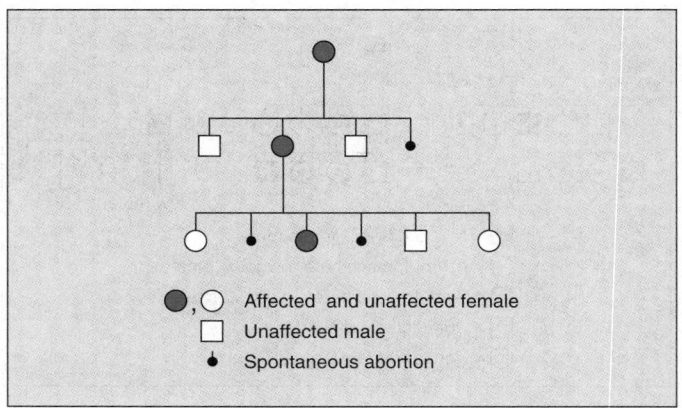

FIGURE 65-22   Pedigree pattern of an X-linked dominant trait lethal in the hemizygous male. *(From Scriver et al, with permission.)*

as a sporadic disorder in females due to new mutation. Aicardi's syndrome, Goltz's syndrome, and Rett's syndrome may represent such examples.

Genes in the pseudoautosomal region of the X chromosome have a homologous copy on the Y chromosome, and the pattern of inheritance of these genes is indistinguishable from autosomal circumstances, as the term implies.

X Inactivation   Phenotypic expression of X-linked traits in females is greatly influenced by the phenomenon of random X-chromosome inactivation. Early in embryonic development, one of the two X chromosomes in each somatic cell of a female is randomly inactivated so that for each cell there is an equal probability that the paternal or maternal X chromosome will be inactivated. The inactivation is stable so that all progeny of the initial cell inherit the same active and inactive X chromosomes. Thus, each female is a mosaic; on the average, half of the cells express the X chromosome of the father, and half express the X chromosome of the mother. If a mutation in a gene is carried on one of the X chromosomes, about one-half of the cells in each tissue will be normal and the other half will manifest the mutant phenotype. Chance or preferential survival of one clone of cells may alter these proportions in any given individual. Depending on the proportions of mutant and normal X chromosomes that are active in each tissue, a genetically heterozygous female may be clinically normal or have mild or severe manifestations of disease.

In each female cell the nonfunctional X chromosome can be identified as a condensed clump of chromatin—the Barr body. The inactive X chromosome is late replicating, and its DNA is more highly methylated. Methylation of DNA is thought to play a role in maintenance of X inactivation. The XIST gene [for X (inactive) specific transcripts] is transcribed exclusively from inactive X chromosomes and is required for X inactivation, but the molecular mechanism of X inactivation is not understood.

Random X inactivation is the most important determinant of expression in females for many X-linked disorders. Many individuals are asymptomatic, some have mild symptoms, and others have severe manifestations. The frequency of detectable phenotypic alterations depends on how carefully heterozygotes are examined and, in some instances, on the age at examination. Ornithine transcarbamylase deficiency exhibits variable phenotypic expression in heterozygotes. Many heterozygotes are asymptomatic; some have minimal protein intolerance; and others experience intermittent hyperammonemic coma, occasionally with fatal outcome. Hemizygous affected males are more consistently and more seriously symptomatic than are heterozygous females. Other examples in which clinical expression may occur in females include Duchenne's muscular dystrophy, hemophilia A, and Fabry's disease. In some cases the biochemical defect behaves in a cell autonomous fashion resulting in a mosaic tissue pattern, as

in choroideremia and certain forms of X-linked ocular albinism. If the defect involves a product that is secreted by cells, the phenotypic effect is an average for the relevant somatic tissues, as for factor VIII levels in hemophilia A. As already discussed under "X-Linked Disorders," it is preferable to describe these conditions as X-linked without applying the dominant or recessive descriptor since the literature is inconsistent.

X-Linked New Mutations and Heterozygote Detection   Identification of new mutations in X-linked genes is an important counseling issue in families ascertained because of an isolated affected male (monoplex families, Fig. 65-20C). In these families, the mother may be a noncarrier and may have contributed an egg with a new mutation. The father cannot contribute the new mutation, since he contributes a Y chromosome. Alternatively, the mother may be a carrier who received a gamete with a preexisting mutation from her mother or with a new mutation from either her father or her mother. If the new mutation rate for male gametes is greater than for female gametes, as is established in some instances, then a larger fraction of mothers of isolated male cases will be carriers. As formulated by Haldane, assuming that affected males do not reproduce, approximately two-thirds of mothers of isolated male cases are expected to be carriers, if the mutation rates for male and female gametes are identical. This proportion increases if the mutation rate for male gametes exceeds that for female gametes, a fact that is often ignored. Mutation rates for male and female gametes are similar for Duchenne's muscular dystrophy (a disorder predominantly due to large deletions), and the mutation rates for male gametes are higher for hemophilia A and B (disorders largely due to point mutations). Thus, a larger proportion of mothers of isolated hemophilia cases are carriers than are mothers of isolated Duchenne's muscular dystrophy cases.

Heterozygous females can sometimes be detected using biochemical methods, as in the Lesch-Nyhan syndrome, Fabry's disease, Hunter's syndrome, hemophilia A, hemophilia B, ornithine transcarbamylase deficiency, and Duchenne's muscular dystrophy. These biochemical methods are rarely completely accurate because random X inactivation may lead to a relatively normal biochemical result. Accuracy may be increased by sampling relatively clonal cells such as hair roots or cloned skin fibroblasts. Molecular methods can circumvent the problems of biochemical analysis of the gene product when the mutation can be detected directly.

Y-LINKED DISORDERS   Only a few genes are known on the Y chromosome, the gene encoding the sex-region determining Y (SRY) factor (also called the testis determining factor, TDF) being the most salient. Translocations between X and Y chromosomes can result in XY females where the Y chromosome is missing the SRY gene. The reciprocal situation exists in which XX males possess an X chromosome that carries a copy of the SRY gene. Point mutations that impair the function of the SRY factor can also result in XY females. For Y-linked genes, fathers pass the trait to all sons and to no daughters. The male phenotype is the most obvious Y-linked trait. The number of Y-linked disorders is likely to remain limited because of the small number of genes on the Y chromosome, but as many as 18 percent of men with severe oligospermia/azoospermia have microdeletions of the long arm of the Y chromosome that involve the azoospermia factor (AZF) gene.

MITOCHONDRIAL INHERITANCE   There are many genetic disorders affecting mitochondrial function. Mitochondria contain a 16.6-kb circular DNA genome that encodes the ribososomal RNAs and transfer RNAs for the distinct mitochondrial protein synthesis. This genome also encodes some of the proteins essential for oxidative phosphorylation, but many of the mitochondrial proteins are encoded in the nuclear genome, synthesized in the cytoplasm, and transported into mitochondria. Genetic disorders affecting mitochondria can be divided into two classes: mutations in the nuclear genome and those in the mitochondrial genome. For mutations in the nuclear genome, the inheritance is as for other nuclear genes, but mutations in the mitochondrial genome display a distinct pattern of inheritance.

There is wide variation in the number of mitochondria per cell and in the number of mitochondrial DNA genomes per mitochondrion (typically 2 to 10) so that each cell contains thousands of copies of mitochondrial DNA. Mitochondrial DNA is maternally inherited, with 200,000 to 300,000 copies per egg and insignificant contributions from sperm. This means that all individuals inherit their mitochondrial genome from their mothers. If a pathologic mutation is present in the mitochondrial genome, this typically affects some proportion of the mitochondrial genomes per cell, and this heterogeneity of mitochondrial DNA within a single cell and within an individual is referred to as *heteroplasmy*. If a woman carries a mutation in the mitochondrial genome, she will potentially transmit this mutation to all of her children, while a man with such a mutation will not transmit the trait to any of his children. This can give rise to a typical pattern of inheritance, with vertical transmission and the disease trait being passed to most or all of the offspring of affected women. The proportion of mutant to wild-type mitochondria may vary among individuals in a pedigree, leading to phenotypic heterogeneity. Disorders of the mitochondrial genome include chronic progressive external ophthalmoplegia, the Kearns-Sayre syndrome, Leber's hereditary optic neuropathy, myoclonic epilepsy, several forms of mitochondral myopathy, and other disorders (see Scriver et al.).

GENETIC HETEROGENEITY

Genetic heterogeneity can result from different mutations at a single locus (*allelic heterogeneity*) or from mutations at different genetic loci (*nonallelic* or *locus heterogeneity*). For example, Charcot-Marie-Tooth neurogenic atrophy, congenital sensorineural deafness, and retinitis pigmentosa all have autosomal dominant, autosomal recessive, and X-linked forms. Nonallelic heterogeneity is responsible in many cases, but allelic mutation also can account for dominant and recessive variation at a single locus. A similar bleeding disorder can be caused by mutations at either of two loci on the X chromosome, one causing deficiency of factor VIII (classic hemophilia, hemophilia A) and the other a deficiency of factor IX (Christmas disease, hemophilia B). Hereditary methemoglobinemia, once regarded as a homogeneous clinical entity, is the result of at least 10 different mutations at three distinct gene loci: two at the locus coding for the α chain of hemoglobin, three at the locus that encodes the β chain of hemoglobin, and at least five at the NADH dehydrogenase locus. Most hereditary diseases are genetically heterogeneous.

The extent of allelic heterogeneity is particularly impressive. Indeed, a large number of mutations have been characterized as causing hemoglobinopathies and thalassemias, cystic fibrosis, familial hypercholesterolemia, phenylketonuria, and breast cancer via the BRCA1 locus. A great deal of clinical heterogeneity is due to different mutations at a single locus. With detailed molecular characterization, many patients with autosomal recessive disorders are compound heterozygotes at a molecular level. Compound heterozygotes have different mutations in the mutant alleles, as exemplified by SC hemoglobinopathy or cystic fibrosis due to a ΔF508/G542X genotype. Exceptions to this generalization occur when a patient is the product of a consanguineous mating and when particular mutant alleles are present in high frequency in the population, e.g., sickle cell anemia with SS genotype or cystic fibrosis with a ΔF508/ΔF508 genotype.

Variation in manifestations due to allelic heterogeneity is particularly important. For example, Hurler's and Scheie's mucopolysaccharidoses were thought to be different genetic conditions based on the severe, lethal phenotype in Hurler's disease and the milder phenotype of bone and joint disease in Scheie's disease. In fact, these conditions are both due to deficiency of L-iduronidase. Similarly, the severe Duchenne's muscular dystrophy and milder Becker's muscular dystrophy are allelic disorders, each of which can be caused by gene deletions, most often out of frame for Duchenne's and in frame for Becker's. The classic and attenuated forms of adenomatous polyposis coli have about 15 years' difference in the age of onset, so that the attenuated disorder has minimal impact on reproduction, and unrecognized alleles of this type may be a significant contributor to the risk of colon cancer. Additional examples of different clinical manifestations due to allelic heterogeneity are found throughout genetics. In many instances a

classic phenotype occurs when no functional gene product is produced, and there is frequently a continuum of milder expression arising from mutations that partially impair the function of the gene product. Compound heterozygotes contribute to the complexity of the clinical continuum. At the mild end of the continuum, mutant alleles encode a product that leads to a nearly normal clinical phenotype or to a phenotype that is normal under most environmental circumstances. This continuum includes detectable biochemical variation that is ordinarily not associated with clinical effect. Obviously the amount of functional gene product required to prevent clinical symptoms depends on other genetic and environmental factors. As an example, an individual with "benign" methylmalonic acidemia is at risk during major catabolic disorders, so that the benign designation is merely conditional. This type of genetic heterogeneity forms a part of the border between monogenic disorders and multifactorial diseases.

COMPLEX DISEASE TRAITS

The common chronic diseases of adults (such as essential hypertension, gout, coronary heart disease, diabetes mellitus, peptic ulcer disease, and schizophrenia) and the common birth defects (such as cleft lip and palate, spina bifida, and congenital heart disease) have long been known to "run in families," indicating a genetic contribution to etiology. These disorders are *complex disease traits* or *multifactorial genetic diseases*. It is useful to recognize the heterogeneity of etiology of such disorders. For cleft lip and palate, some cases are due to single gene defects, some are due to chromosome abnormalities, and most appear to be due to multiple genetic and environmental factors. The concept of complex disease traits implies that in most instances multiple factors enter into the cause of a *single case*. Similarly, the etiology of coronary artery disease is heterogeneous; a small proportion of cases result from single gene defects (e.g., familial hypercholesterolemia), whereas most are multifactorial (i.e., multiple factors contribute to the etiology of individual cases). Complex disease traits imply the interaction of multiple genes and multiple environmental factors in the etiology of individual cases to cause familial aggregation without a simple Mendelian pattern of inheritance.

In complex disease traits, *constitutional (polygenic) components* consist of multiple genes at independent loci whose effects interact in a cumulative fashion. An individual who inherits a particular combination of these genes has a relative risk that may combine with an *environmental component* to cross a "threshold" of biologic significance so that the individual is affected with a disease. For another individual in the same family to express the same syndrome, a similar combination of genes would present similar risks. Since sibs share half of their genes, the probability of a sib inheriting the same combination of genes is $(\frac{1}{2})^n$, where n is the number of genes required to express the trait (assuming that none of the genes is linked).

The number of genes responsible for polygenic traits is unknown, and risk estimates are based on empiric risk figures (i.e., a direct tally of the proportion of affected relatives in previously reported families). In contrast to the monogenic disorders, in which 25 or 50 percent of the first-degree relatives of an affected proband are at genetic risk, complex disease traits usually affect no more than 5 to 10 percent of first-degree relatives. Moreover, the recurrence risk for these conditions varies from family to family and is influenced by two factors: The greater number of affected relatives and the more severe their disease, the higher the risk to other relatives. For example, the risk of cleft lip in the sibs of a child with unilateral cleft lip is about 2.5 percent, but if the lesion in the index case is bilateral, the risk in the sibs rises to 6 percent.

Multifactorial etiology is thought to be important for many diseases that develop after adolescence, and diseases with later age of onset have decreased heritability on average. For example, in nine multifactorial diseases a decline in the impact of the genes on disease was evident with increasing age.

The hypothesis of a polygenic component in the inheritance of multifactorial diseases is supported by the findings that at least 28 percent of all gene loci harbor polymorphic alleles. This variation in normal genes provides a substrate for variations in response to environmental factors. At present, the genetic loci most strikingly associated with predisposition to specific diseases are those that constitute the major histocompatibility or HLA gene complex located on the short arm of chromosome 6 and consisting of multiple closely linked but distinct loci (A, B, DR, DQ, and DP). The products of these genes are proteins on the surface of cells involved in cellular immune recognition. Each HLA locus in the population consists of multiple alleles, each of which produces an immunologically distinct protein. For example, an individual may inherit any 2 of more than 36 alleles at the HLA-B locus. The inheritance of certain alleles predisposes to the development of certain diseases when the individual is exposed to an environmental challenge (see Chap. 306).

Complex disease traits are heterogeneous in etiology in the sense that the relative contribution of genetic ("risk genes") and environmental factors varies from patient to patient. As discussed above, among common phenotypes that are largely multifactorial, some cases may be due to monogenic or chromosomal abnormalities. For example, although coronary heart disease is usually of complex etiology, about 5 percent of patients with premature myocardial infarctions are heterozygotes for familial hypercholesterolemia, a single-gene disorder that produces atherosclerosis in the absence of an extraordinary environmental factor (see Chap. 341). However, even in a single-gene disorder such as familial hypercholesterolemia, other loci [e.g., the genes for apolipoprotein B, apolipoprotein (a), lipoprotein lipase, and apolipoprotein E] and nongenetic factors (diet and smoking) can influence the phenotype. The complexity of the etiology for coronary artery disease is detailed further in Chap. 242. Multiple genetic and nongenetic factors affect the risk. An appreciation of this etiologic heterogeneity and careful investigation of each patient are necessary prerequisites for counseling families at risk for these disorders.

Methods for unraveling the molecular basis of multifactorial etiology include the analysis of candidate genes using association studies, sib-pair analysis, and other complex strategies. The advantages of focusing on molecular variations that are important in gene function has been emphasized. The complexity of these approaches is daunting, but major loci have been identified for a number of multifactorial

diseases, including hypertension (see "Complex Disease Traits," above) and insulin-dependent diabetes mellitus, in which several loci in addition to HLA are involved.

INTERACTION BETWEEN SINGLE GENETIC AND ENVIRONMENTAL FACTORS; PHARMACOGENETICS

In addition to polygenic states, many single-gene mutations can cause abnormal responses to environmental factors, as illustrated by disorders that produce major, often life-threatening idiosyncratic responses to drugs (Table 65-6). There is significant genetic variation is response to drugs such as isoniazid, some beta-adrenergic blockers, and tricyclic antidepressants. Other important interactions between genotype and drugs include glucose-6-phosphate dehydrogenase deficiency, acute intermittent porphyria, hemochromatosis, and muscle diseases with susceptibility to malignant hyperthermia.

Misinterpretation of adverse drug reactions can cause serious harm to patients, and unusual or idiosyncratic reactions should be considered to be genetically determined until proven otherwise. Fortunately, the pharmacogenetic disorders are a group of diseases for which therapy is straightforward: avoidance of the noxious drug by the patient and relatives at risk.

In addition to drugs, environmental factors may aggravate specific genetic traits. Cigarette smoke is particularly deleterious to persons homozygous (and possibly heterozygous) for α_1-antitrypsin deficiency, who are predisposed to the development of emphysema. Patients with xeroderma pigmentosum are sensitive to the ultraviolet exposure of sunlight. Avoidance of milk at an early age prevents the life-threatening complications of galactosemia, and diet is an important variable for most forms of hyperlipidemia. Unfortunately, a modern society is also subjected to an endless array of novel environmental exposures. The current widespread utilization of aspartame is an example of a special risk for persons with phenylketonuria.

TAKING THE FAMILY HISTORY

Recording a *family history* should be a routine part of primary care (Fig. 65-23) and should be performed with special care in patients with a likely genetic disorder. The first step is to obtain certain information on the *proband* or *index case* and on each of the *first-degree relatives* (i.e., the parents, siblings, and offspring of the proband). This information includes the given name, surname, maiden name, birth date

Table 65-6

Examples of Inherited Disorders Involving an Abnormal Response to Drugs

Disorder	Molecular Abnormality	Mode of Inheritance	Frequency	Clinical Effect	Drugs Producing Abnormal Response
Slow inactivation of isoniazid	Isoniazid acetylase in liver	Autosomal recessive	50% of U.S. population	Polyneuritis	Isoniazid, sulfamethazine, sulfamaprine, phenelzine, dapsone, hydralazine
Suxamethonium sensitivity	Pseudocholinesterase in plasma	Autosomal recessive	Several mutant alleles; most common affects 1 in 2500	Apnea	Suxamethonium, succinylcholine
Malignant hyperthermia	Ryanodine receptor	Autosomal dominant	1 in 20,000 anesthetized patients	Severe, hyperpyrexia, muscle rigidity, death	Such anesthetics as halothane, succinylcholine, methoxyflurane, ether, cyclopropane
Debrisoquine sensitivity	Cytochrome P450, CYP2D6	Autosomal recessive	5–10%; range 0–18% in ethnic groups	Toxicity of drugs, e.g., postural hypotension	Antiarrythmics, beta blockers, neuroleptics, tricyclic antidepressants
Glucose-6-phosphate dehydrogenase deficiency	Glucose-6-phosphate dehydrogenase in erythrocytes	X-linked recessive	$\sim 1 \times 10^8$ affected persons in world; common in persons of African, Mediterranean, Asiatic origin; multiple mutant alleles	Hemolysis	Analgesics, sulfonamides, antimalarials, nitrofurantoin, other drugs

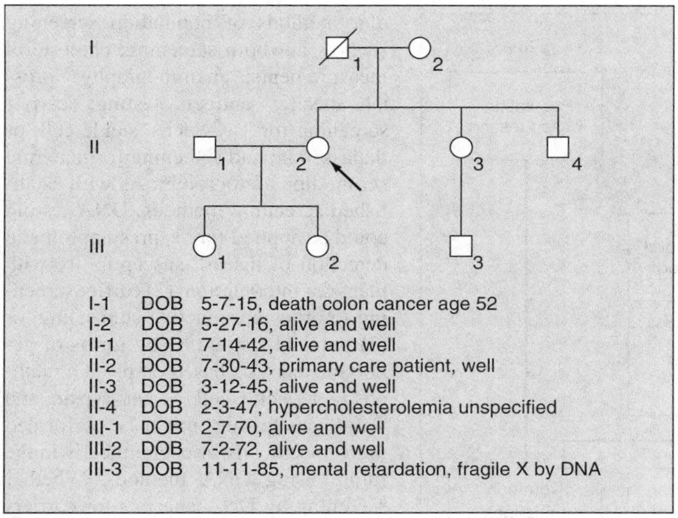

FIGURE 65-23 Suggested style for routine recording of family history. Individual II-2 is intended to represent a healthy individual (the patient) in a primary care setting.

I-1	DOB	5-7-15, death colon cancer age 52
I-2	DOB	5-27-16, alive and well
II-1	DOB	7-14-42, alive and well
II-2	DOB	7-30-43, primary care patient, well
II-3	DOB	3-12-45, alive and well
II-4	DOB	2-3-47, hypercholesterolemia unspecified
III-1	DOB	2-7-70, alive and well
III-2	DOB	7-2-72, alive and well
III-3	DOB	11-11-85, mental retardation, fragile X by DNA

or current age, age at death, cause of death, and name or description of any disease or defect. Similar information should be recorded on reproductive partners where appropriate. More distant relatives should be included for autosomal dominant disorders, X-linked disorders, and chromosomal translocations. For reproductive counseling, the reproductive plans for a couple should be recorded, including use of contraception or previous sterilization procedure. It is important to ask specifically about spontaneous abortions, stillbirths, and childhood deaths, since these are frequently omitted and may provide information of great relevance. Pedigrees should be drawn in a manner that distinguishes siblings and half siblings.

Direct inquiry regarding possible consanguinity should be a routine part of recording the family history and is of particular relevance to the occurrence of autosomal recessive disorders. Reproductive couples can be asked whether they may be related in any way, and this information should be supplemented by inquiries regarding surnames, ethnic status, and geographic origin of families. Cousin marriages are common in many societies and in isolated areas. Incest is an extreme form of consanguinity and may occur in the context of sexual abuse of children and teenagers. The risk of autosomal recessive disorders, including mental retardation, is high for incestuous matings.

Interpretation of the family history is aided by understanding the variation in expression in specific genetic disorders. Assuming that the family history is focused on the presence of a specific disorder within the family, meticulous questioning regarding possible manifestations in relatives is important. In addition to recording the general health status of all first-degree relatives, inquiry should be made about other genetically determined conditions in the family. This is often best done by asking whether any relatives have experienced genetic diseases, rare conditions, mental retardation, birth defects, childhood deaths, or occurrence of common adult disorders at a young age. The philosophy of the physician should be to identify any genetic issues of potential importance for all family members and to urge appropriate evaluation, education, counseling, and intervention as appropriate.

Ethnic and geographic origin of family members can be an important part of the family history, because monogenic and complex disease traits occur at different frequencies in different populations (Table 65-7). Screening for diabetes mellitus, hypertension, and hyperlipidemia is particularly important in high-risk populations (e.g., the high incidence of diabetes mellitus in some native North American populations), and different options for reproductive screening are offered to different ethnic groups (e.g., Tay Sachs testing for Ashkenazi Jews, thalassemia testing for Mediterranean populations, sickle cell testing for populations of African descent, and perhaps cystic fibrosis testing for populations of European descent).

Table 65-7

Examples of Simply Inherited Disorders that Occur with Increased Frequency in Specific Ethnic Groups

Ethnic Group	Simply Inherited Disorder
African blacks	Hemoglobinopathies, especially Hb S, Hb C, persistent Hb F, α and β thalassemia
	Glucose-6-phosphate dehydrogenase deficiency
Armenians	Familial Mediterranean fever
Ashkenazi Jews	Abetalipoproteinemia
	Bloom's syndrome
	Dystonia musculorum deformans (recessive form)
	Gaucher's disease (adult form)
	Tay-Sachs disease
	Breast ovarian cancer BRCA1 (specific mutation)
Chinese	α Thalassemia
	Glucose-6-phosphate dehydrogenase deficiency
	Adult lactase deficiency
Eskimos (Inuit)	Pseudocholinesterase deficiency
	Congenital adrenal hyperplasia
Finns	Congenital nephrosis
	Aspartylglucosaminuria
French Canadians	Tyrosinemia
	Familial hypercholesterolemia
Japanese	Acatalasemia
Lebanese	Familial hypercholesterolemia
Mediterranean peoples (Italians, Greeks, Sephardic Jews)	β Thalassemia
	Glucose-6-phosphate dehydrogenase deficiency
	Familial Mediterranean fever
	Glycogen storage disease, type III
Europeans	Cystic fibrosis
Scandinavians	α₁-antitrypsin deficiency
	LCAT (lecithin:cholesterol acyltransferase) deficiency
South African whites	Porphyria variegata
	Familial hypercholesterolemia

MOLECULAR STRATEGIES FOR ANALYSIS OF MENDELIAN DISORDERS

As for any form of clinical diagnosis, a detailed history, including family history, and clinical examination is the appropriate starting point. In some cases, the phenotype of the patient may be characteristic of a specific genetic disease, and the diagnostic information may be supplemented by the family history or by specific biochemical tests. A general scheme for utilization of molecular methods for diagnosis is depicted in Fig. 65-24. Although such techniques are powerful and provide precise information, the studies are often performed by research, academic, and commercial laboratories with variable levels of experience and attention to quality assurance. One report found 34 errors in a total of 360 tests analyzing for cystic fibrosis mutations in 40 laboratories. It is essential that clinicians be familiar with the quality of work in diagnostic laboratories and interpret data cautiously in the full context of the medical circumstance.

DEFINITE CLINICAL AND/OR BIOCHEMICAL GENETIC DIAGNOSIS In many cases, DNA analysis is undertaken to confirm a diagnosis already considered to be established. The goals in such cases may include genotype/phenotype correlation, i.e., predicting the severity of the disease based on the mutations. For example, some mutations cause nonneuronopathic Gaucher's disease, and others cause neuronopathic disease (see Chap. 346). Predicting the phenotype, future risks, and complications from the genotype is complex. Extensive studies are necessary, and great caution must be exercised to avoid overinterpretation or misinterpretation of molecular data. In principle, important therapeutic decisions can be based on genotypic data (e.g., α₁-antitrypsin deficiency or familial hypercholesterolemia), but exact predictions for individuals may be hazardous, due to variation in expression even when detailed molecular knowledge is available

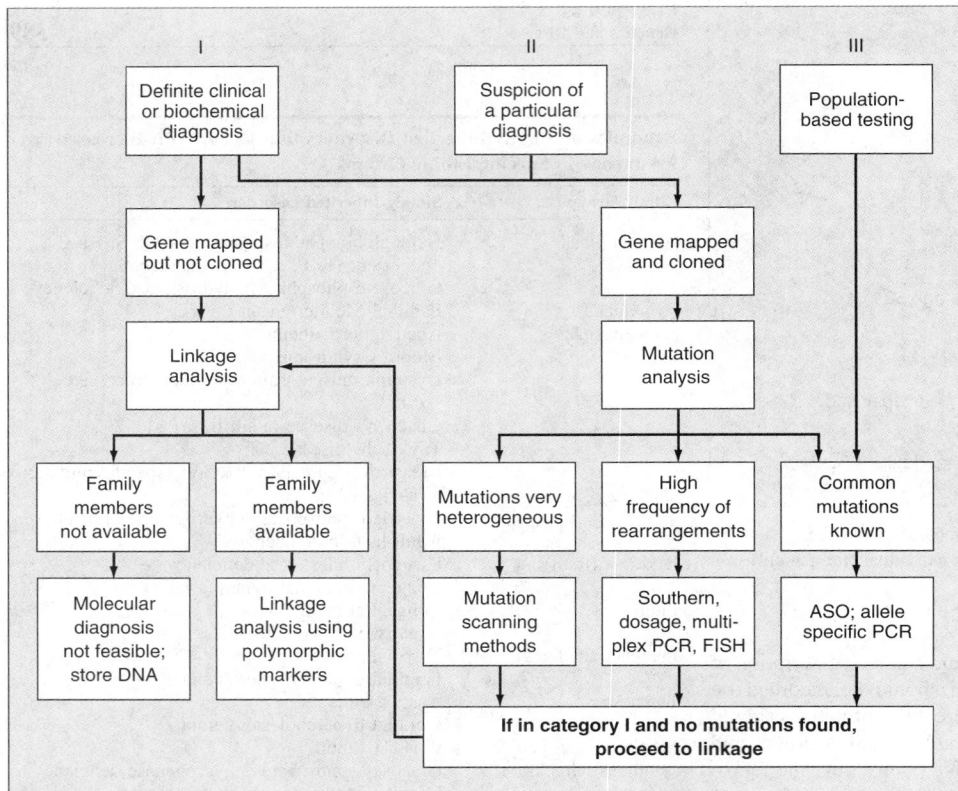

FIGURE 65-24 A scheme for utilization of DNA analysis for genetic diagnosis.

ular methods of population screening such as newborn screening; cholesterol measurements; mammography; prostate-specific antigen testing; carrier screening for Tay-Sachs, sickle-cell, or thalassemia; and screening for maternal serum alpha fetoprotein. As with established screening methods, DNA testing could be applied for (1) presymptomatic detection of disease susceptibility with plans for intervention, (2) carrier screening to offer reproductive counseling, or (3) prenatal testing. Many forms of genotypic analysis based on protein methods (e.g., sickle cell, α_1-antitrypsin, and Tay-Sachs testing) might be performed more specifically or economically in the future using DNA methods. Whether screening by DNA analysis for carriers of cystic fibrosis mutations should be offered routinely is being debated. With DNA variation of known or likely disease significance in apolipoprotein E, apolipoprotein(a), angiotensinogen, angiotensin-converting enzyme, α_1-antitrypsin, and many other genes, population-based DNA screening might become a powerful preventive approach by making possible pharmacologic and life-style interventions for individuals with high-risk genotypes. There is debate as to the appropriateness of population-based screening for disorders in which the definition of risk and potential for intervention are not fully known, as exemplified by BRCA1 mutations or mutations causing hereditary nonpolyposis colon cancer. Testing for disorders where specificity is low and/or there is no potential for intervention is generally discouraged (e.g., apolipoprotein E genotype and Alzheimer risk).

EXAMPLES OF MUTATION DETECTION As indicated in the section designated "Gene Mapped and Cloned" in Fig. 65-24, different methods of analysis will be employed for molecular diagnosis depending on the most common type of mutation for a particular disorder, whether the mutations are large rearrangements or point mutations, and whether the mutations are of predictable type from ancient origins or are more heterogeneous and more recent in origin (Table 65-8).

Examples of large molecular defects that can be detected by Southern blotting include α thalassemia, some forms of β thalassemia, and hereditary persistence of fetal hemoglobin (Fig. 65-25). For Duchenne/Becker muscular dystrophy, 60 to 70 percent of cases involve large deletions that are easily detected by Southern blotting (Fig. 65-26). If one considers Fig. 65-26 in the context of carrier detection for family members, a case such as lane 1 with a novel, junctional DNA fragment is optimal since the presence of this fragment will be absolutely diagnostic for carrier status for females in this family. For cases such as lane 3, heterozygote detection would depend on dosage analysis with one copy of the deleted fragments in carrier females, and two copies of the nondeleted fragments. Dosage analysis is more difficult and requires meticulous quantitation and attention to internal controls. For families of the type depicted in lane 2, where Southern blotting is normal and does not detect a presumed point mutation in the gene, this analysis would not be useful for carrier detection. Deletions such as those seen in Duchenne/Becker dystrophy can also be detected using PCR to test for the presence or absence of various regions in the gene (Fig. 65-27). Deleted segments are identified by the absence of particular PCR products in a multiplex reaction testing for the presence of various sites along the length of the gene.

Expanding triplet repeat mutations are the cause of myotonic dystrophy, fragile X mental retardation, Huntington's disease, X-linked

(i.e., triplet repeat length in Huntington's disease). Extensive studies are in progress for Marfan's syndrome and breast cancer due to BRCA1 mutations, but the power and the limitations of genotype/phenotype correlations have not been defined for many disorders. Genotype/phenotype correlation and confirmation of diagnosis rely on mutation analysis and generally cannot be based on linkage analysis. Additional applications of molecular diagnosis include heterozygote detection, presymptomatic diagnosis, and prenatal diagnosis. Family studies should be performed using mutation analysis if possible, reserving linkage analysis as a secondary option.

CLARIFICATION OF A POSSIBLE GENETIC DIAGNOSIS In some cases, there may be a suspicion of a particular genetic disease, but the findings may be inconclusive because it is too early in the clinical course or the findings are atypical in some way. This frequently occurs when it is possible to detect some mutations causing a disease, but when it is impractical to rule out the possibility of an undetected mutation. In the case of dominant disorders or X-linked diseases in males, a diagnosis may be established by demonstration of deletion, frameshift, or nonsense mutation; expanded triplet repeat; or unspecified truncation mutation. Failure to find a mutation does not rule out the diagnosis but makes it less likely if analysis is known to detect most disease mutations. Molecular analysis is particularly useful in the differential diagnosis of triplet repeat disorders, since virtually all clinically important expansions can be identified. Likewise, protein truncation testing can be helpful in evaluating possible cases of neurofibromatosis or hereditary breast cancer but will not detect all mutations. For autosomal recessive disorders, the situation may be complex (e.g., a phenotype of bronchiectasis possibly related to cystic fibrosis). Identification of pathologic mutations in both copies of the gene establishes a diagnosis, whereas identification of a pathologic mutation in one allele only increases the probability but does not prove that the suspect phenotype is related to mutation at this locus. Failure to identify any pathologic mutations lessens the likelihood that the disease is related to mutation at this locus but does not eliminate that possibility, since mutations can occur outside the coding sequence.

POPULATION-BASED DNA TESTING Utilization of DNA testing as a population-based screening method is similar to nonmolec-

spinobulbar muscular atrophy, and other neurodegenerative disorders. With fragile X mental retardation and myotonic dystrophy, severity of the disease increases as premutation progresses to mutation and mild mutation progresses to severe mutation, the phenomenon of anticipation. Depending on the size of the expanded triplet repeat, these mutations can be detected by Southern blotting and/or PCR analysis. An example of an expanded triplet repeat mutation with more severe disease in later generations is depicted in Fig. 65-28. Although the size of a triplet repeat expansion has potential information for genotype/phenotype correlations, experience and caution are needed to make phenotypic predictions.

For many disorders, typically including any autosomal recessive disorders and autosomal dominant and X-linked disorders with minimal effect on reproduction, mutations of ancient origin may be present in many people in the population, but even when common mutations exist, there may still be extensive molecular heterogeneity, as for β thalassemia (Fig. 65-4). Likewise in cystic fibrosis, the common ΔF508 mutation accounts for about 70 percent of mutations in most populations, but hundreds of different mutations have been identified among the remaining 30 percent of mutant chromosomes. Common mutations of this type are usually best tested using some allele-specific method such as hybridization with allele-specific oligonucleotides. Typically, such analysis for a single disease may require testing for only a few alleles as in α_1-antitrypsin deficiency or for 10 to 30 mutations in the case of β thalassemia or cystic fibrosis (Figs. 65-29 and 65-30).

In some cases, mutation analysis is difficult because most patients

Table 65-8

Examples of the Role of Molecular Analysis for Diagnosis of Genetic Disease

Disease	Mutation Detection*	Linkage Analysis	Comments
Sickle cell anemia	+ + + +		PCR with ASO
Other globin disorders	+ + + +	+	PCR with ASO
Hemophilia A & B	+ + +	+ +	Mutation scanning and sequencing
Phenylketonuria	+	+ +	PCR with ASO
α_1-Antitrypsin ZZ	+ + + +		PCR with ASO
Familial hypercholesterolemia	+ +	+ +	Mutation scanning and sequencing
Lesch-Nyhan syndrome	+ + + +	+	PCR and direct sequencing
Tay-Sachs disease	+ + +	+	PCR with ASO in Ashkenazim
Duchenne's muscular dystrophy	+ + +	+ +	Multiplex PCR, Southern
Retinoblastoma	+ + +	+	Mutation scanning and sequencing
Huntington's disease	+ + + +		Southern and PCR for expanding triplet
Myotonic dystrophy	+ + + +		Southern and PCR for expanding triplet
Adult polycystic kidney disease	+ +	+ +	Mutation scanning and sequencing
Fragile X syndrome	+ + + +		Southern and PCR for expanding triplet
Cystic fibrosis	+ + +	+	PCR with ASO
Neurofibromatosis 1	+ +	+ +	Mutation scanning and sequencing, PTT
BRCA1 breast cancer	+ + +	+	ASO for some and PTT
Polyposis of colon	+ +	+ +	Mutation scanning and sequencing, PTT
Marfan's syndrome	+ +	+ +	Mutation scanning and sequencing
Gaucher's disease	+ + + +	+	PCR with ASO in Ashkenazim
Glycogen storage disease, Ia	+ + +	+	PCR with ASO
Familial hypertrophic cardiomyopathy	+ + + +	+	Southern and mutation sequencing
Spinal muscular atrophy	+ + +	+	Southern and PCR for deletions
Charcot-Marie-Tooth disease IA	+ + + +	+	PFGE or FISH for duplication
Prader-Willi syndrome	+ + + +		FISH for deletion and STR for uniparental disomy
DiGeorge/Velo-Cardio-Facial syndromes	+ + + +		FISH for deletion

* Symbols of + to + + + + indicate relative importance of an approach as of 1996; the status for disorders could change rapidly.

NOTE: PCR, polymerase chain reactions; ASO, allele-specific oligonucleotide; PFGE, pulsed-field gel electrophoresis; STR, short tandem repeat; FISH, fluorescence in situ hybridization; PTT, protein truncation test.

carry heterogeneous point mutations, including autosomal dominant disorders that impair reproductive fitness and X-linked disorders that limit reproduction in males. The factors influencing the proportion of cases of autosomal dominant disorders due to new mutation are discussed above. In these cases of heterogeneous mutations, some method for analyzing the entire gene is needed. Sequencing all of the exons of a gene is feasible in a few cases if the coding region of the gene is small, and this approach is used for a few genes. However, full-length sequencing is expensive and impractical for most genes with current technology, and identification of mutations depends on a variety of procedures designed to detect small mutations in DNA as discussed above (see "Analysis of Mutations"). Protein truncation testing is useful for detecting certain classes of mutations and is quite useful for polyposis of the colon (Fig. 65-31) and breast cancer due to BRCA1 mutations. In many cases, searching for mutations is an activity for research laboratories and beyond the capacity of routine clinical service.

DIAGNOSIS BY LINKAGE ANALYSIS When a gene is cloned but it is not practical to identify the mutation or mutations in a given family, it is sometimes possible to perform molecular diagnosis using linkage analysis. In other cases, mutation analysis is impossible because the disease gene is not cloned, but informative DNA markers may be available. In such cases, linkage diagnosis can be performed with a negligible possibility of crossovers (see Fig. 65-13). For linkage analysis, some genetic marker near the disease locus must be *informative*, namely, key individuals in the pedigree must have two different alleles at the marker locus. Linkage analysis is appropriate when an individual carries one mutant gene and one normal gene and when the goal is to determine which has been transmitted to the next generation. Many such analyses are informative because highly polymorphic STR polymorphisms are frequently present within and near genes causing diseases.

A second requirement for linkage analysis is that of *phase* information between the marker locus and the disease locus for genetic analy-

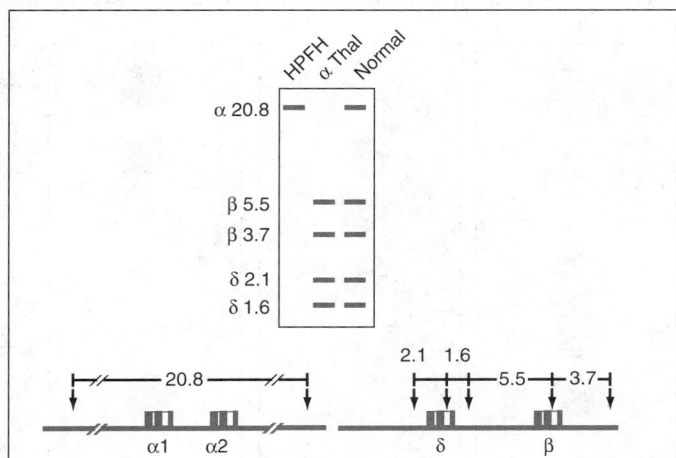

FIGURE 65-25 Depiction of Southern blot analysis of human globin genes. Above, DNA was isolated from a normal individual and from patients with homozygous hereditary persistence of fetal hemoglobin (HPFH) or homozygous α thalassemia. DNA was digested with the enzyme *Eco*RI. A mixed DNA probe was prepared by reverse transcription of reticulocyte globin mRNA. Below, arrows indicate *Eco*RI cut sites in the α- and β-globin regions, and numbers indicate DNA fragment sizes in kilobases. (*Adapted from YW Kan, AM Dozy, Proc Natl Acad Sci USA 75:5631, 1978, with permission.*)

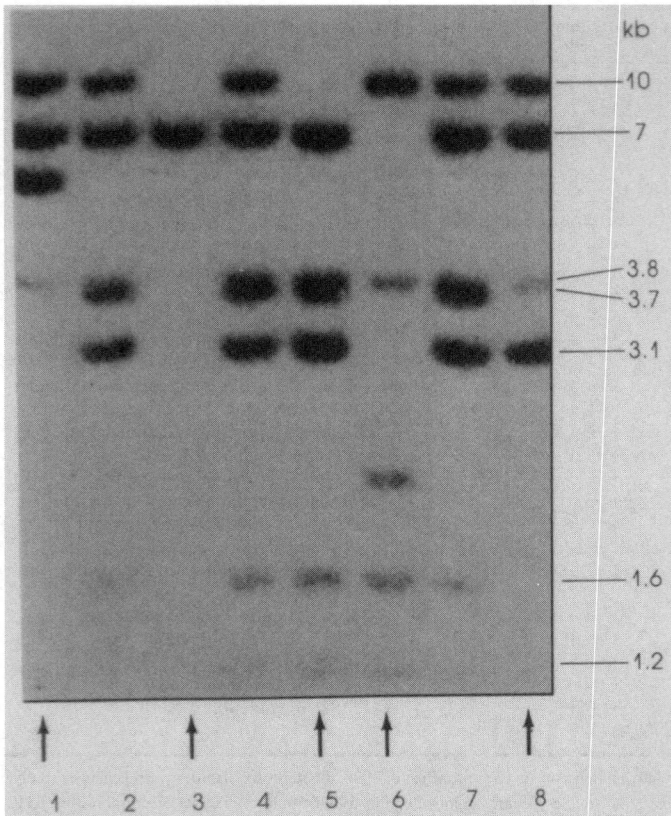

FIGURE 65-26 Detection of deletions in the DNA isolated from Duchenne's muscular dystrophy patients using a dystrophin cDNA probe. Southern blot analysis detects deletions (absence of fragments) in five of eight patients (arrows). A junction fragment is clearly demonstrated in patients 1 and 6. *(From M Koenig et al, Cell 50:509, 1987, with permission.)*

sis. If an individual is heterozygous for a marker that is tightly linked to a mutation, it must be determined which allele for the marker is on the chromosome with the disease allele and which is on the homologous chromosome with the normal allele. When the genetic marker is informative and the phase is known, genetic diagnosis can include heterozygote detection, presymptomatic diagnosis, detection of lack of penetrance, and prenatal diagnosis. When the DNA probe or marker is within the mutant gene, crossing-over between the genetic marker and the disease causing mutation usually is negligible. Duchenne's muscular dystrophy is an exception, since the responsible gene is extremely large, and crossing-over occurs at a detectable frequency within the gene.

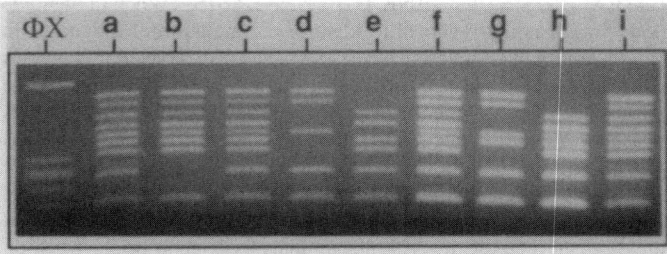

FIGURE 65-27 Multiplex amplification of DNA using polymerase chain reaction to detect deletions in the dystrophin gene. Nine amplifications detecting fragments of nine different exons are performed in a single tube and analyzed on an agarose gel. Deletions can be seen as missing fragments for the Duchenne's dystrophy patients shown in lanes b, d, e, g, and h, while no deletion is detected in lanes a, c, f, and i. φX indicates DNA markers. *(Used by permission, Multicenter Study Group, JAMA 267:2609, 1992.)*

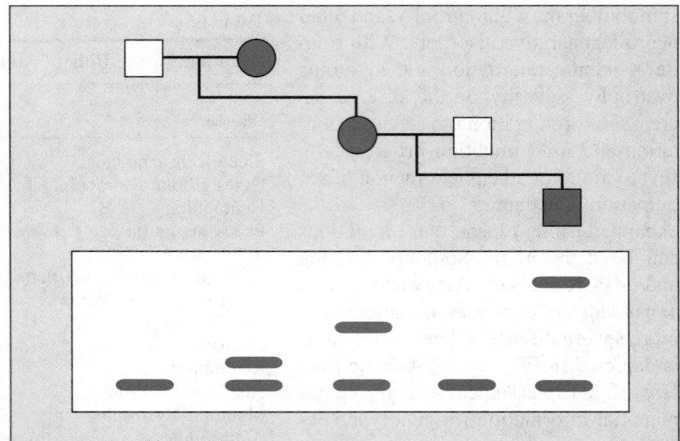

FIGURE 65-28 Diagramatic representation of Southern blot analysis revealing an expanding triplet mutation in a myotonic dystrophy family. A grandmother and mother with the adult form of the disease and a child with the infantile form of the disease are shown. The normal size genomic DNA fragment (lowest band) is present in homozygous form in the unaffected individuals and in heterozygous form in the affected family members. The larger mutant fragment is present in all affected individuals, with increasing size from grandmother, to mother, to child.

Examples of molecular diagnosis by linkage, when there is negligible recombination between the loci, are shown in Fig. 65-32. Genetic marker data are presented as letters that might represent simple marker alleles or haplotypes of markers. A *haplotype* is a cluster of tightly linked specific alleles on a chromosome. Phase can usually be determined from a single index case for autosomal recessive disorders (Fig. 65-32*A*). Fetuses of AC genotype are predicted to be affected in Fig. 65-32*A*, while fetuses of AA or BC genotype are predicted to be carriers and those of AB genotype to be noncarriers. In Fig. 65-32*B*, carrier detection is sought for the aunt and uncle of the affected. The data on the maternal side require analysis of the grandparents and predict that the aunt is a noncarrier. Although the paternal grandparents are deceased, it is still possible to conclude that the uncle is a noncarrier since he does not inherit the C haplotype that is linked to disease allele on the paternal side. For autosomal dominant disorders, linkage phase usually cannot be determined from a single affected individual (Fig. 65-32*C*). Exceptions occur in retinoblastoma, when analysis of tumor DNA may distinguish the allele on the abnormal chromosome

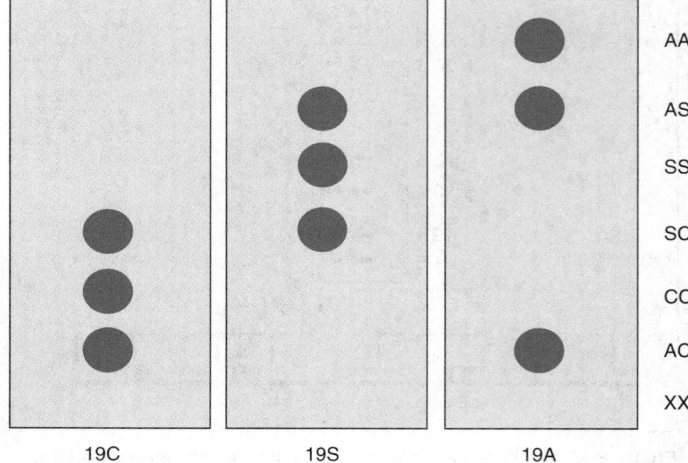

FIGURE 65-29 Genotype analysis of polymerase chain reaction amplified genomic DNA using allele-specific oligonucleotide (ASO) probes. DNA was extracted from the blood of individuals of β-globin genotypes AA, AS, SS, SC, CC, and AC and homozygous deletion (XX). The DNA was applied to replicate filters for hybridization with ASO as follows: β^A probe (19A), β^S probe (19S) or β^C probe (19C). *(From K Mullis et al, Cold Spring Harbor Symp Quant Biol 51:263, 1986, with permission.)*

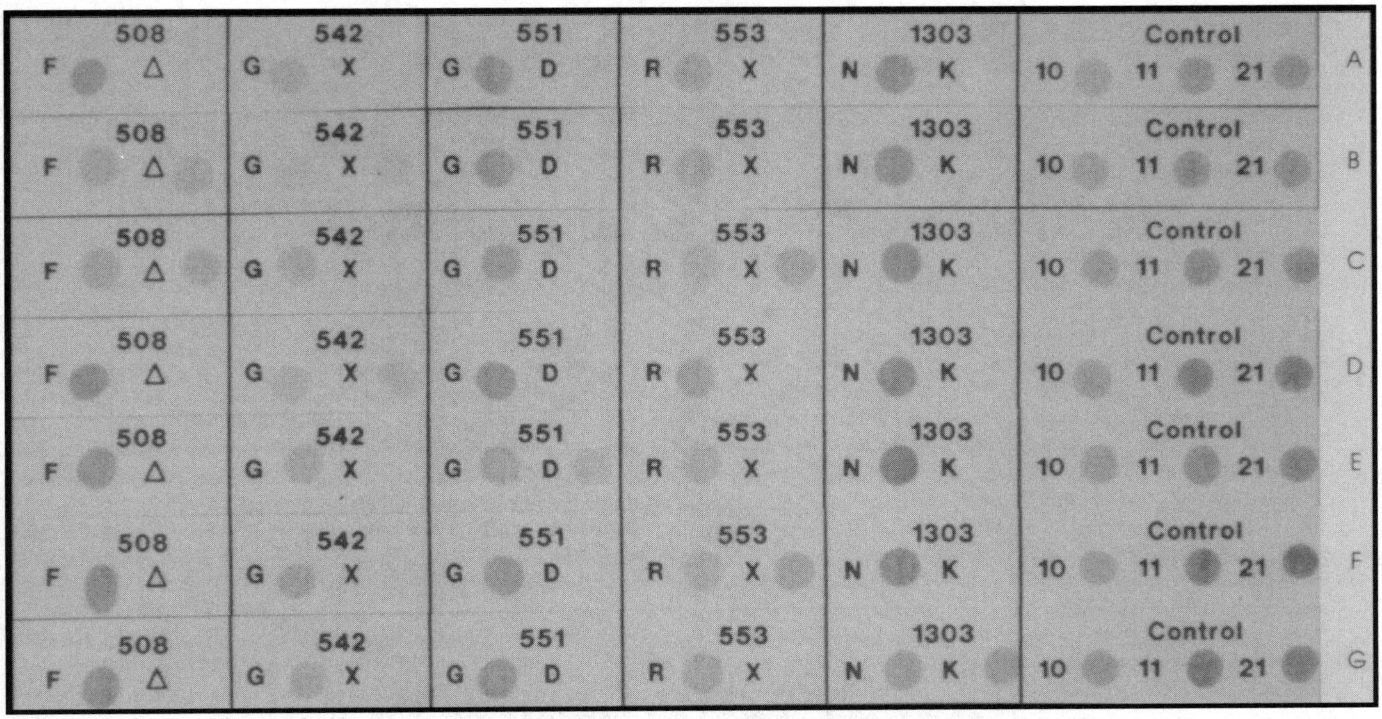

FIGURE 65-30 Reverse dot allele-specific oligonucleotide (ASO) analysis for various point mutations causing cystic fibrosis. For each mutation, the polymerase chain reaction product is hybridized to an ASO dot on the left for the normal allele and on the right for the mutant allele. The positions for each ASO are indicated as follows: F and Δ for the ΔF508 mutation, G and X for the G542X mutation, G and D for the G551D mutation, R and X for the R553X mutation, N and K for the N1303K mutation, and 10 or 11 or 21 under control for the ASO to detect the amplification of exons of those numbers. Mutations are designated by single-letter amino acid code (X, nonsense) with the normal amino acid followed by the position number followed by the substituted amino acid. Thus G551D is substitution of aspartic acid (D) for glycine (G) at position 551. ΔF508 is deletion of phenylalanine (F) at position 508. Letters at the right margin identify individuals of the following genotypes: A, no mutation; B, ΔF508/G542X compound heterozygote; C, ΔF508/R553X compound heterozygote; D, G542X heterozygote; E, G551D heterozygote; F, R553X heterozygote; G, N1303K heterozygote. *(Provided by H Erlich, Roche Molecular Systems.)*

(often retained in the tumor) from the allele on the normal chromosome (often lost in the tumor). Linkage phase for autosomal dominant disorders can be determined from two appropriate individuals, and it is not essential that both be affected if penetrance is complete. Fetuses of AA and AC genotype are predicted to be affected in Fig. 65-32D, while fetuses of AB and BC genotype are predicted to be affected in Fig. 65-32E. For X-linked disorders, phase information can be obtained from a single affected male individual (Fig. 65-32F). In general, although linkage information can predict the genotype of offspring of individuals of known genotype, it cannot be used consistently to determine the genotype of antecedents of individuals of known genotypes because of the possibility of new mutation from one generation to the next. This is exemplified by an X-linked disorder, where linkage information will not clarify whether or not the mother of an isolated affected male is a heterozygote (Fig. 65-32G). This limitation is an important difference between direct detection of a mutation and linkage analysis, but occasionally, linkage analysis can suggest the genotype of an antecedent. Note in Fig. 65-32G that the mutation arose on the chromosome from the unaffected maternal grandfather; it can be predicted that the maternal grandmother and the maternal aunt of the index case do not carry the mutation and that either the mother or the index case is the recipient of the new mutation. The situation is similar in Fig. 65-32H, except that the mutation is on the chromosome from the maternal grandmother, and the new mutation could go back further in the family. Still by linkage analysis, the maternal aunt is not a carrier of the mutation. The genotype of an antecedent also can be inferred when a woman has two sons with the same DNA marker, one son being affected and one son being unaffected with the X-linked disorder (Fig. 65-32I). In this instance, the mother is not a heterozygote for the X-linked disorder, although the possibility of gonadal mosaicism (i.e., some proportion of the maternal germ cells have the new mutation) is not eliminated.

Linkage analysis also can be performed with DNA markers that show detectable recombination with a disease locus, but this introduces probabilities of misdiagnosis due to recombination. Problems with recombination in linkage diagnosis become less common as innumerable highly informative markers are identified.

DIAGNOSIS AND PREVENTION OF GENETIC DISEASE

In the practice of medicine, it is important to recognize that many disease processes have a major contribution from a single gene. These single-gene disorders often go undiagnosed, or the genetic contribution to a disease process goes unrecognized unless the physician is well informed and has a high index of suspicion. Furthermore, partial genetic contribution to complex disease may be even more common. Primary care physicians should recognize the genetic contributions to disease and pursue the implications in regard to intervention and counseling. In many situations, genetic advice can be given by the primary physician once the relatively simple principles of medical genetics and genetic counseling are mastered. In other situations, the complexities may make referral to a genetic specialist necessary.

GENETIC COUNSELING WITH AN INDEX CASE The diagnosis of a single-gene disorder in an individual or family obliges the physician to provide appropriate genetic information and counseling. The first step is to establish the *correct diagnosis* with the maximum certainty, utilizing biochemical and/or molecular testing where possible. The certainty of the diagnosis is crucial for proper interpretation of the mode of genetic transmission and for calculating the risk of disease among relatives. Issues of new mutation, lack of penetrance, variation in expression, and genotype/phenotype correlations are frequently important. Family members should be counseled regarding

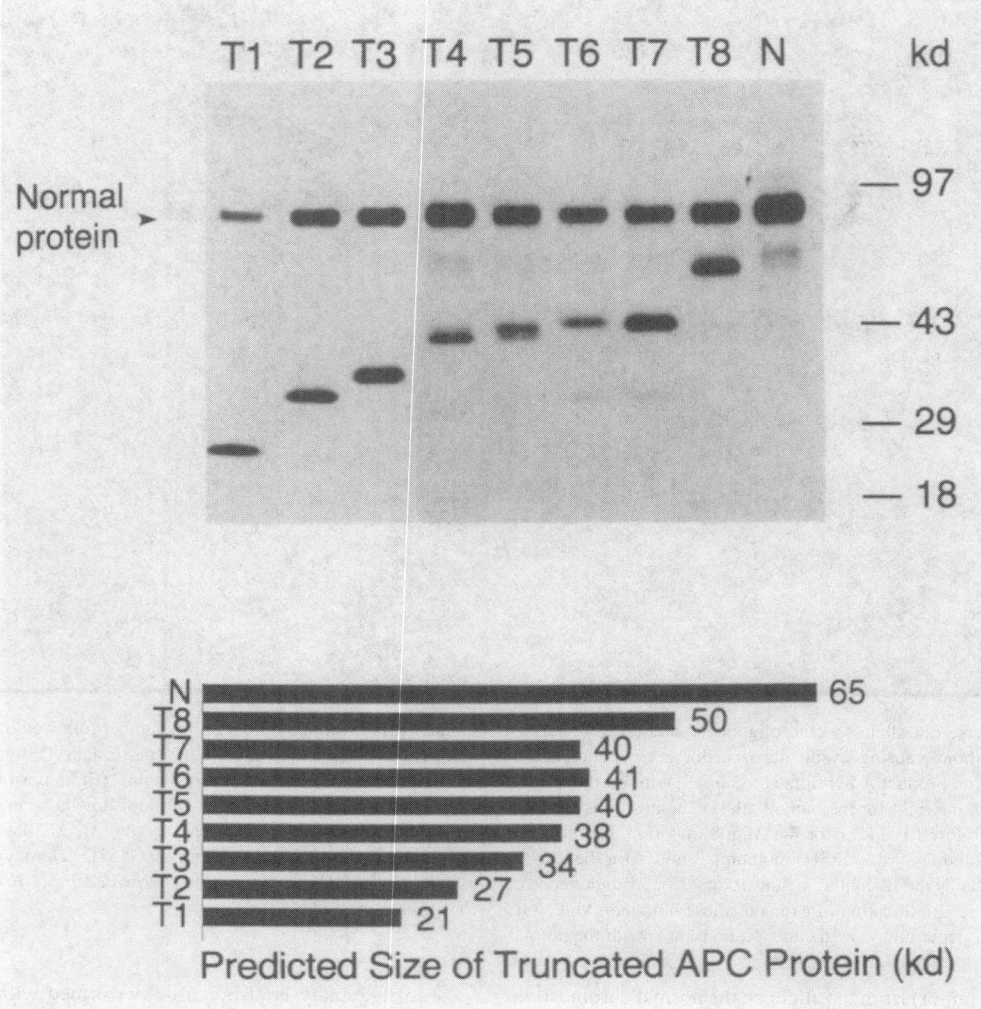

FIGURE 65-31 Protein assay for the detection of known truncating mutations causing familial polyposis. Representative samples of sporadic colorectal tumors (T1 through T8), known to have truncating mutations from sequence analysis, demonstrate the expected truncated APC (adenomatous polyposis coli) proteins. A substantial amount of normal, full-length APC protein is noted in the remaining normal alleles. A sample of normal tissue (N) is also shown. The numbers to the right of the horizontal bars indicate the predicted size of the truncated APC protein. (*From Powell et al, with permission.*)

options such as presymptomatic diagnosis, carrier testing, and availability of prenatal diagnosis.

REPRODUCTIVE COUNSELING, PRENATAL DIAGNOSIS, AND CARRIER SCREENING Prenatal diagnosis can be offered to couples with the known presence of a genetic disease in the family and in some routine pregnancies, as exemplified by cytogenetic testing in cases of advanced maternal age. Fetal samples obtained by amniocentesis or chorionic villus sampling (CVS) can be used for cytogenetic, biochemical, and molecular studies. Virtually all cytogenetic disorders can be detected using standard methods: fluorescent in situ hybridization can be used to detect subtle cytogenetic defects, most inborn errors of metabolism are detectable by biochemical methods, molecular methods can be used in many circumstances, and ultrasound methodology allows for detailed anatomic studies of the fetus.

Screening for genetic disorders and birth defects is a routine part of prenatal care, including analysis of maternal serum for alpha fetoprotein, human chorionic gonadotropin, and unconjugated estrol to screen for neural tube defects, trisomy, and other fetal pathology. Carrier testing for autosomal recessive disorders is an option for Tay Sachs disease and hemoglobinopathies in appropriate populations and may be used for disorders such as cystic fibrosis. Screening for serious X-linked disorders such as Duchenne's dystrophy and fragile X mental retardation is not routine at present.

POPULATION-BASED GENETIC SCREENING As discussed under "Genomic Medicine" at the beginning of this chapter, it may become practical to screen for genotypes that predispose to common adult diseases (hypertension, atherosclerosis, emphysema, hemochromatosis and various forms of cancer), although the pace at which such testing will become routine is difficult to predict. The usefulness of such testing is a function of the potential for medical intervention. Newborn screening for phenylketonuria is an example in which population-based screening for genetic disease in developed countries has provided extraordinary medical benefit. The future is likely to bring greater opportunity for medical benefit from population-based genetic testing.

ACKNOWLEDGMENTS This chapter represents the evolution of the cumulative contributions to chapters that have appeared in *Harrison's Principles of Internal Medicine* and in the *Metabolic and Molecular Bases of Inherited Disease*. Past contributors have included John B. Stanbury, James B. Wyngaarden, Donald S. Fredrickson, Joseph L. Goldstein, Michael S. Brown, Charles R. Scriver, William S. Sly, David Valle, and Andrea Ballabio. The author gratefully acknowledges the contributions of these predecessors and colleagues.

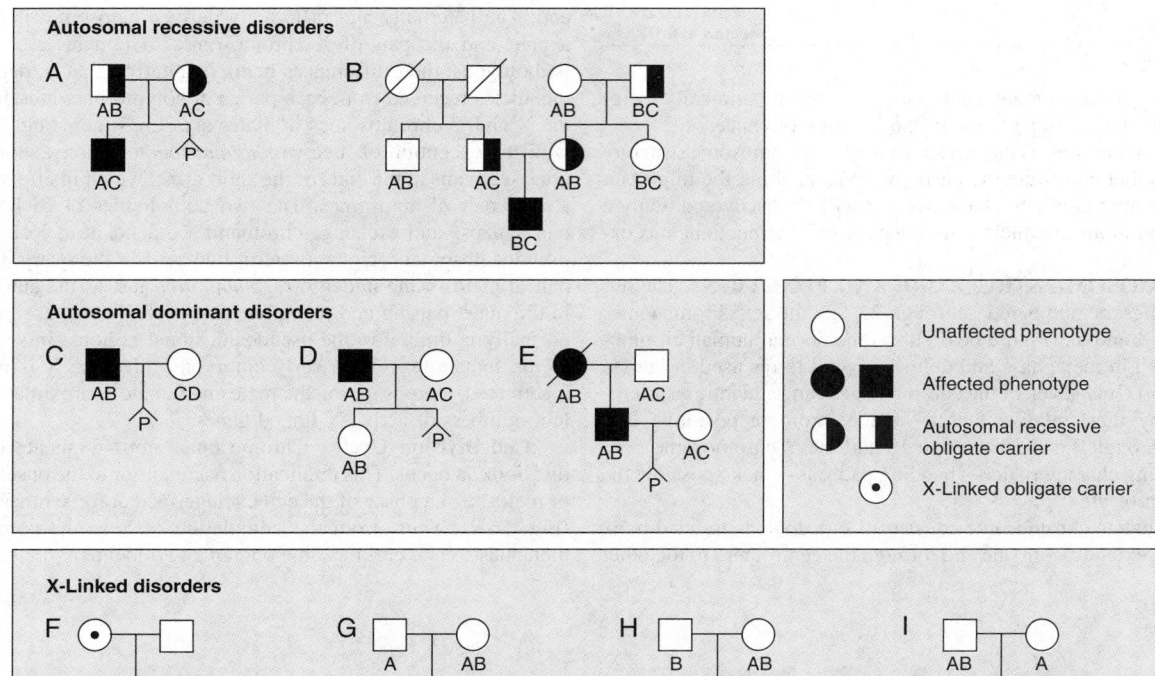

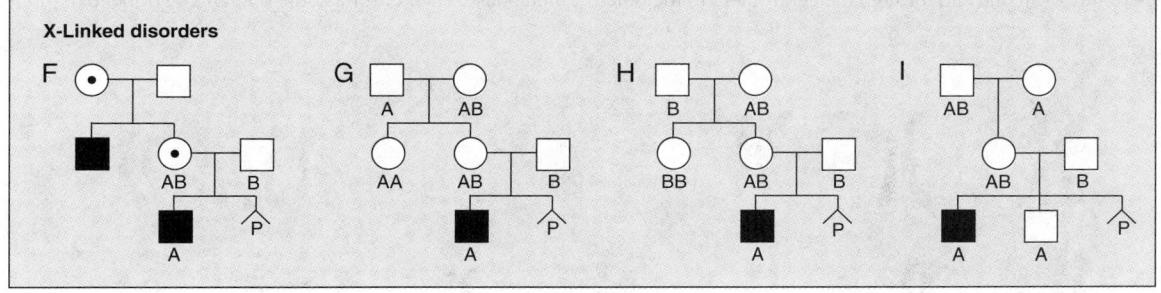

FIGURE 65-32 Examples of molecular diagnosis by genetic linkage with negligible recombination between the DNA probe and the disease locus. Letters below pedigree symbols indicate alleles for a DNA marker. Families *A* and *B* depict autosomal recessive disorders; *C* through *E* depict autosomal dominant disorders; and *F* through *I* depict X-linked disorders. Complete penetrance is assumed. See text for discussion.

BIBLIOGRAPHY

ALBERTS B et al: *Molecular Biology of the Cell*, 3d ed. New York, Garland Publishing, 1994

COLLINS FS: Positional cloning moves from perditional to traditional. Nat Genet 9:347, 1995

DARNELL J et al: *Molecular Cell Biology*, 3d ed. New York, Scientific American Books, 1995

HARPER PS: *Practical Genetic Counselling*, 4th ed. Stoneham, MA, Butterworth-Heinemann, 1993

LEWIN B: *Genes V*. New York, Oxford University Press, 1994

LIFTON RP: Molecular genetics of human blood pressure variation. Science 272:676, 1996

PATTERSON M, TODD JA: A complex issue. Trends Genet 11:592, 1995

POWELL SM et al: Molecular diagnosis of familial adenomatous polyposis. N Engl J Med 329:1982, 1993

RIMOIN DL et al: *Emery and Rimoin's Principles and Practice of Medical Genetics*, 3d ed. New York, Churchill and Livingstone, 1996

SCRIVER CR et al: *The Metabolic and Molecular Bases of Inherited Disease*, 7th ed. New York, McGraw-Hill, 1995

SIMPSON JL, ELIAS S: *Essentials of Prenatal Diagnosis*, vol I. New York, Churchill Livingstone, 1993

SOUTHERN EM: DNA chips: Analysing sequence by hybridization to oligonucleotides on a large scale. Trends Genet 12:110, 1996

THOMPSON MW et al: *Genetics in Medicine*, Philadephia, Saunders, 1993

VOGEL F, MOTULSKY AG: *Human Genetics: Problems and Approaches*, 3d ed. Berlin, Springer-Verlag, 1996

WATSON JD: *Molecular Biology of the Gene*, vols I and II, 4th ed. Menlo Park, CA, Benjamin/Cummings, 1987

———— et al: *Recombinant DNA*. New York, Freeman, 1992

66

James German

CYTOGENETIC ASPECTS OF HUMAN DISEASE

The chromosome complement is guarded carefully against change; most chromosome mutations, either structural or numerical, are deleterious. Only rarely is a structural rearrangement that results in neither deficiency nor duplication of chromosome segments introduced into the population and transmitted from generation to generation. As a rule, an abnormal number of autosomes results in early death, except for trisomy of the shortest chromosome. In contrast, an abnormal number of sex chromosomes is often tolerated reasonably well, although reproduction is usually impaired. Among human embryos, abnormalities in chromosome structure and number are the main known cause of fetal wastage. Not every fetus with an abnormal chromosome complement is aborted, however, and those that survive become the material of medical cytogenetics. Chromosome imbalances cause various features, including abnormal anatomic development, mental deficiency, behavioral disorders, and disturbances in growth and sexual development. Sometimes, apparently normal persons with abnormal chromosome complements are detected because of infertility, repeated abortion, or the birth of malformed children.

The chromosomal abnormalities just referred to affect tissues throughout the body. In addition, a change in the chromosome complement can occur in a single somatic tissue cell. Such a mutant cell may have a proliferative advantage over normal cells if the mutation affects certain growth-controlling loci, in which case a clone bearing the abnormal chromosome complement can develop among otherwise normal cells. Although many such mutant clones are clinically insignificant, some are of importance in the etiology of cancer.

This chapter addresses the aspects of normal chromosome structure and function that constitute the basis for understanding the important chromosome alterations that have been or will be discovered. Only a few such alterations and their consequences will be mentioned as examples.

CHROMOSOME STRUCTURE AND FUNCTION   The human autosomes are numbered 1 through 22, and the sex chromosomes are denoted X and Y. (Figure 66-1 shows the normal human chromosomes as seen in metaphase and defines several terms used in human cytogenetics.) Only seven of the chromosomes can be identified microscopically by their relative lengths and centromere positions (autosomes 1 through 3 and 16 through 18 and the Y chromosome), but unique staining characteristics—banding patterns—make possible the identification of all.

A mammalian chromosome consists of one double-stranded helix of DNA that extends from one end through the centromere to the other

end. The paternally and maternally derived autosomes that compose a pair, and the pair of X chromosomes in females are genetically homologous, their differences being qualitative, that is, dependent on the alleles received from each parent at polymorphic loci. In contrast, the X and Y chromosomes in males are almost completely different, with the exception of their *pseudoautosomal regions*, short homologous segments at the ends of the short arms, which in effect constitute a 24th pair of autosomes. The two homologues of each autosomal pair synapse and exchange chromatid segments at meiosis, as do the pseudoautosomal regions. In germ line cells in the ovary, the two Xs pair at meiosis and undergo *recombination* just as the autosomes do; in the male, pairing and recombination of the X and Y chromosomes normally is limited to the pseudoautosomal regions. In somatic cells of the female, except in early embryonic life, one X is extensively inactivated, thereby giving the male and female approximately equivalent numbers of active X-linked genes.

Cell-Division Cycle   Chromosomes must duplicate before cell division can occur. This duplication occurs prior to the onset of mitosis or meiosis, in a phase of the cell cycle termed *S*, for synthesis of DNA (Fig. 66-2). Thus, from the completion of S to the completion of metaphase, each chromosome contains two identical double-stranded

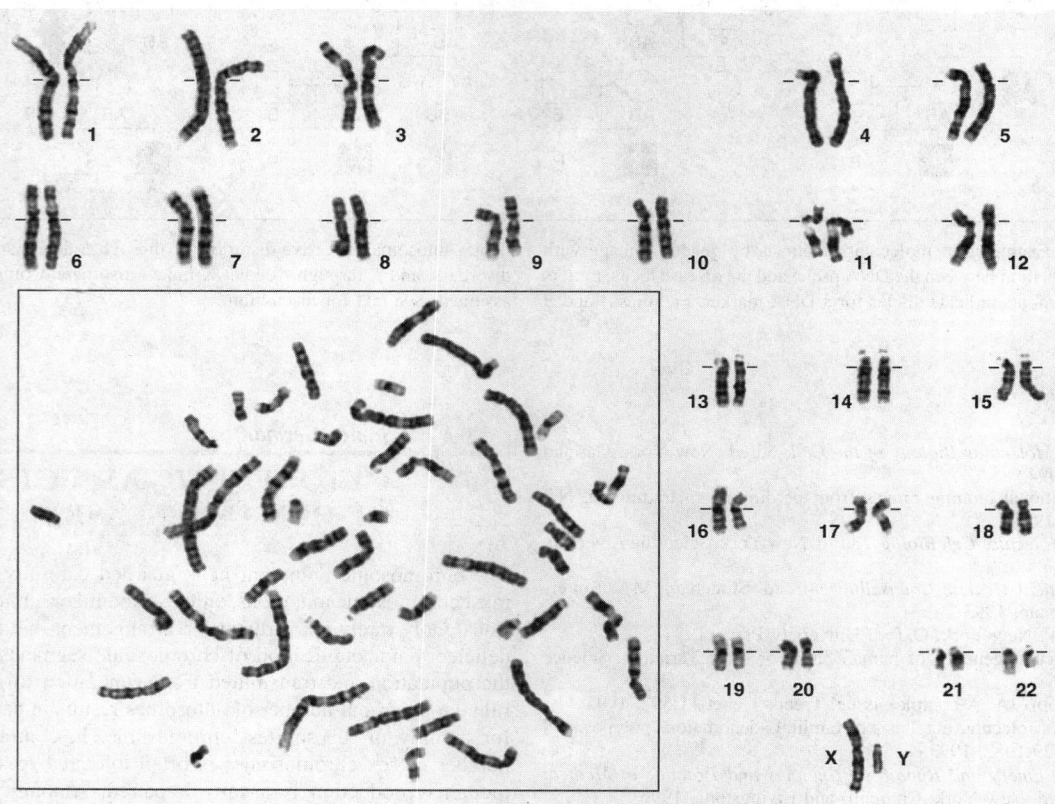

FIGURE 66-1   Normal human lymphocyte chromosomes arrested in metaphase and stained for G bands (G standing for Giemsa). The inset shows the arrangement of chromosomes in an intact cell, and the remainder of the figure shows them arranged into a karyotype. By the time mitosis begins, each chromosome consists of two identical parts called sister chromatids and is identified by its relative length, the location of its centromere (*short horizontal lines*), and a distinctive sequence of bands of varying lengths and depth of staining. The number of bands visible microscopically varies from cell to cell, depending on the degree of chromosome condensation. Approximately 500 bands can be seen in this cell, and with other techniques many of these bands could be resolved into subbands. Normally, the banding patterns of the two chromosomes of a homologous pair are alike, except in certain polymorphic regions. Examples of the latter are (1) the dark juxtacentromeric G band in chromosome 9 (located on the short arm in the chromosome on the right and in the usual position on the long arm in the chromosome on the left) and (2) the variant C bands shown in Fig. 66-3.

The centromere divides a chromosome into a short arm (p) and a long arm (q). Chromosomes 13 to 15, 21, 22, and Y are called *acrocentric* because of the nearly terminal position of their centromeres. The minute p arm of each acrocentric autosome bears a nucleolus-organizing region that often causes a secondary constriction in the metaphase chromosome (the primary constriction being the one at the centromere).

By standard nomenclature, the karyotype shown here is described as 46,XY, indicating that its chromosome number is 46 and its sex chromosomes are an X and a Y. The autosomes (the chromosomes other than the X and Y) number 44. The following examples show the general use of this nomenclature. A normal female karyotype is described as 46,XX. A female cell with an extra chromosome 18 (trisomic for 18) would be described as 47,XX, + 18. A cell with only one sex chromosome, an X, and with a deletion in the short arm of chromosome 5 would be described as 45,X,5p − . A male cell with a translocation between chromosomes 2 and 3, with breakpoints in band 13 of 2p and band 22 of 3p, would be described as 46,XY,t(2;3)(p13;p22). (See also footnote to Table 66-2.)

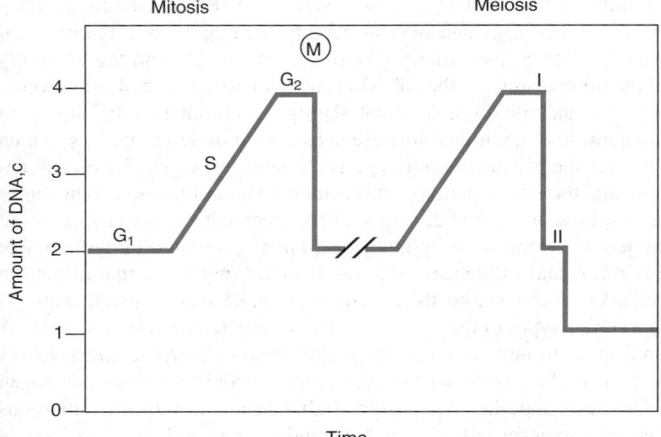

FIGURE 66-2 Schematic representation of the mitotic and meiotic cell-division cycles, as described in the text. G_1 and G_2 = time gaps before and after S, the period in which DNA replicates. Each of these intervals is several hours in duration; together they constitute interphase. M = mitosis; I and II = the two divisions of meiosis. The DNA content of the cycling cells is indicated on the vertical axis: 1c = the content in a gamete; 2c = that in either an egg immediately after fertilization or a somatic cell emerging from mitosis; 4c = the amount in a cell which has completed chromosome duplication and is ready to enter mitosis or meiosis.

DNA helices, and the nucleus contains four times as much DNA as a spermatozoon or ovum. During mitosis, chromosomes are condensed, and the two sister chromatids can be visualized by late prophase or early metaphase (Fig. 66-1). (Metaphase is the stage in the cell-division cycle ordinarily employed for cytogenetic analysis.)

At the onset of anaphase, the centromeric regions of each chromosome separate, and the two chromatids move quickly to opposite poles of the mitotic spindle. When the poles receive their full complements of chromatids (now called chromosomes), nuclear membranes assemble about each cluster to form the nuclei of the two sister cells that will emerge from mitosis. (The nuclear membrane is disassembled late in prophase.) The sister cells emerge in what is called the G_1 phase of the cell cycle, where they remain unreplicated unless another division is to be prepared for, in which case they enter S. Cells engaged in a differentiated function ordinarily remain unreplicated, in which case G_1 can be referred to as G_0.

Most normal cells in the human body are diploid; that is, they have twice the *haploid* number of chromosomes (the number in a gamete; in humans, the haploid number is 23, and the diploid number is 46). In the germ-cell lineage, the cells devoted to gamete formation, and destined eventually to differentiate into spermatozoa or ova, undergo mitotic cell cycling until they enter *meiosis*, a series of two specialized divisions unique to this lineage. In meiosis, homologous chromosomes pair up (the paternally derived chromosome 1 with the maternally derived chromosome 1, etc.), and genetic recombination occurs by a process called *crossing over*, an exchange of entire segments between paternal and maternal chromosomes by which the genetic constitution of each is altered qualitatively (see Chap. 65). In the first meiotic division, homologous chromosomes are segregated, and the diploid chromosome number is reduced to the haploid; that is, each daughter cell then contains one of each of the 22 (duplicated) autosomes plus one (duplicated) sex chromosome. No S phase takes place between the first and second meiotic divisions (Fig. 66-2, *right*), so that, at the second division, in which sister chromatids separate, the emerging cells maintain the haploid number of chromosomes but have reduced their DNA content to half that of diploid G_1 cells of somatic tissues. With fertilization, both the chromosome constitution and the DNA content of the zygote are restored to that of a G_1 somatic cell. An S period in the zygote then prepares the way for the regular cell-division cycles characteristic of somatic cells.

Chromosome Differentiation Chromosomes are differentiated along their length, and some aspects of this differentiation are resolv-

able microscopically. The DNA is complexed with a number of proteins in a highly specific way. The DNA-protein complex, together with some associated RNA, is called *chromatin*. The fine structure of chromatin, the manner in which the DNA is compacted and interacts with proteins, and the organization of chromatin in the interphase nucleus are thought to be involved in the control of RNA production and DNA replication and perhaps of cellular differentiation as well.

The sequences of DNA nucleotide bases that constitute the genes and can be transcribed into messenger RNA are distributed throughout the length of the various chromosomes. (These sequences are too short to be resolved microscopically.) Approximately 3000 genes have been assigned to specific chromosomes, in many cases to specific bands of a chromosome, where the order in which they are *linked* also has been determined.

Certain visible segments of at least 12 chromosomes vary in length among individuals. These can be delineated by their staining characteristics (for example, see Fig. 66-3). These variable segments consist of nontranscribed, highly repetitive nucleotide sequences of DNA and, like genes, are transmitted from parent to child in a straightforward Mendelian fashion. The techniques of molecular genetics also make possible the identification and molecular definition of innumerable heritable polymorphic segments of DNA that, like genes themselves, are submicroscopic. These noncoding segments are referred to as *restriction fragment length polymorphisms* (RFLPs), *variable number of tandem repeats* (VNTRs), or *polymorphic short tandem repeats of di- or tetranucleotides*. These normal variations in both microscopically visible and invisible segments usually are not associated with a detectable phenotypic effect. However, they serve as useful genetic markers in prenatal diagnosis when they are tightly linked to disease-associated loci (e.g., in Duchenne's muscular dystrophy) and in the determination of the zygosity of twins, paternity, and the survival of transplants. Also, these DNA markers, especially the short tandem repeats, which are highly polymorphic and are widely dispersed throughout the genome, are invaluable in the effort to map the human genome. In this undertaking, loci of importance in normal development and differentiated cell function, including those that, when mutant, result in human disease, are being assigned their correct order and interrelationships along the chromosomes.

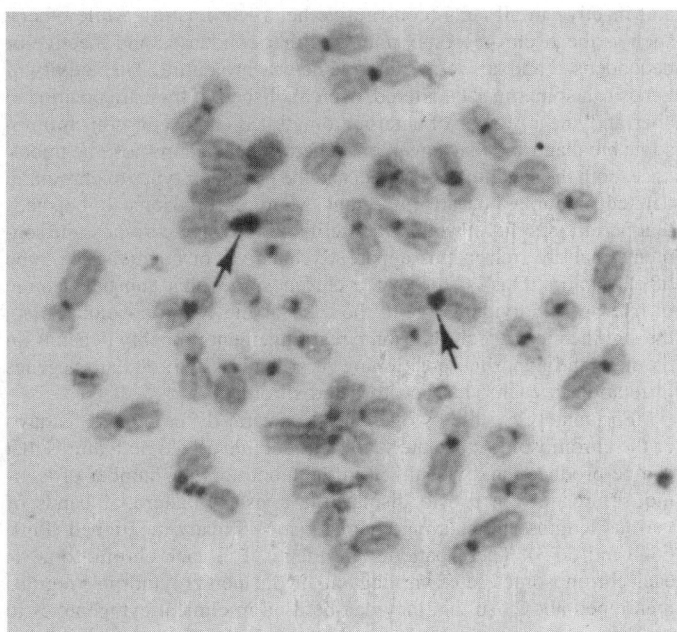

FIGURE 66-3 Metaphase chromosomes stained for C bands (C standing for centromeric or constitutive heterochromatin), showing inherited variation in lengths of the C bands in the chromosome 1 homologues (arrows).

Microscopically recognizable segments in the short arms of the acrocentric autosomes (see the legend to Fig. 66-1) are devoted to the production of ribosomal RNA and nucleoli. As mitosis progresses, these nucleolus-organizer regions remain relatively uncondensed. Consequently, at metaphase, they appear understained and demarcate condensed segments of chromatin distal to them on the chromosome arms—*satellites*. (The DNA of satellites contains no genes; they are examples of the polymorphic segments just mentioned.) Several other regions that remain relatively uncondensed at metaphase are recognizable in a low percentage of cells and are called *fragile sites* because they may undergo outright disruption ("breakage") in metaphase preparations. The only such region known to be of significance in relation to a human trait—the clinical condition called the *fragile X syndrome*—is one located near the distal end (the end away from the centromere) of the long arm of the X chromosome (see "Sex Chromosome Imbalance," below). Other examples of segmental specialization along the chromosome include *telomeres* and *centromeres*. Telomeres, the distal termini of each arm, have a relationship with the nuclear membrane and probably are important in the maintenance of order in the interphase nucleus and in the accurate pairing of homologues in meiosis; centromeric regions are sites of microtubule attachment at metaphase.

A further example of chromosome differentiation is the sequence by which various segments replicate during S; certain segments replicate early, others late. In general, late replication of a chromosome segment correlates with genetic inertness. This correlation is exemplified by one of the two X chromosomes in female cells; in one (either) X the entire chromosome, except for its terminal pseudoautosomal region and a few additional loci, is inactivated by a phenomenon referred to as the *Lyon effect* (see Chap. 65). The inactivated X is almost entirely late-replicating. During interphase it is tightly condensed and can be visualized microscopically as *sex chromatin* or the *Barr body*. The asynchrony of homologue replication that is best exemplified by the X chromosomes also occurs in short segments of some autosomes; its significance in autosomes is unknown but may be related to genomic imprinting (see below).

A little-understood type of chromatin is referred to as *heterochromatin*. It is tightly condensed, not just at metaphase but throughout interphase. Such condensation of chromatin correlates with genetic inactivity and also with late replication. Some regions are condensed and inactive in all cells (constitutive heterochromatin), while others, such as the X chromosome, may be either condensed and inactive or decondensed and active (facultative heterochromatin). The activity of genes can sometimes be altered, even abolished, if they are positioned aberrantly near regions of heterochromatin, as can occur with chromosome breakage and rearrangement. Therefore, in a chromosome imbalance, both the specific genetic loci and the particular types of chromatin deleted or duplicated are important. Many chromosome imbalances that permit viability beyond intrauterine life involve chromosome segments that are rich in this apparently inactive, or inactivatable, type of chromatin. This is true of the chromosomes that can be trisomic in live-born individuals or, in the case of the X, monosomic. Also, the significance of a chromosome rearrangement probably depends on the new and abnormal positioning of structural and regulatory genes in relation to each other and to heterochromatin.

Fortunately for the cytogeneticist, several differentiated features of the chromosome correlate with reproducible cytologic features that can be produced and visualized in the laboratory. A number of techniques are now in use to display the constant pattern of bands of various lengths and staining characteristics already mentioned (Figs. 66-1 and 66-3). These patterns are identical in each chromosome 1, each chromosome 2, etc., varying only in the inert polymorphic regions mentioned above, so that they can be used in clinical cytogenetics to identify chromosomes and to detect and define structural rearrangements.

Sources of Error A large number of genetic loci must be active to produce and regulate the enzymes and structural proteins required to initiate and complete a cell-division cycle. Precision and accuracy are demanded over and over in matters such as the passage of a cell from G_1 into S, the orderly progression of replication, the assembly of the mitotic spindle, the cohesion and then disjunction of the chromatids, and the spindle action that segregates chromatids at mitosis. In the germ line, additional loci are activated to undergo meiosis, which involves the pairing of homologous chromosomes, genetic recombination, and then the separation of recombined homologous chromosomes at anaphase of the first division. These mechanisms and processes are subject to errors, some spontaneous, others promoted by unfavorable environmental influences (Fig. 66-4) or by mutations that affect the cell cycle. Furthermore, the genetic material itself is subject to damage, and certain types of unrepaired or erroneously repaired lesions in DNA predispose to mutation, including chromosome rearrangement. Errors at many of these steps or errors introduced during the repair of damaged DNA must underlie chromosome imbalance. Chromosome mutations that arise in germ cells, during fertilization, or in early postfertilization divisions are important causes of embryonic maldevelopment and infertility; mutations in somatic cells are important causes of neoplasia.

CHROMOSOME ABNORMALITIES Mutations of a single base in a gene and deletions and duplications of chromosome segments involving even hundreds of base pairs are not visible microscopically. In fact, for the normal chromosome banding pattern to be detectably disturbed, a long segment of DNA, perhaps more than 3 million base pairs, must be deleted, duplicated, or transposed. However, the same environmental agents that produce point mutations (mutagens in the usual sense) also act as chromosome-breaking agents (clastogens), and vice versa. Thus, mutations form a spectrum extending from those visible to the cytogeneticist to mutations that must be defined by nucleotide sequencing. Visible mutations ordinarily exert a more widespread effect on development than do point mutations; ordinary genes—often many of them—as well as other specialized types of chromatin of unknown function and significance are involved in cytologically visible mutations.

If an entire chromosome is affected in an imbalance, the genome is said to be either *trisomic* or *monosomic* for the chromosome (e.g., trisomy 13, monosomy X). Genes and chromatin carried on the affected chromosome then are present in a triple or a single dose, respectively, rather than in the normal double—*disomic*—dose. An abnormal dosage affecting less than an entire chromosome (the result of chromosome breakage and rearrangement) is often termed *partial trisomy* or *partial*

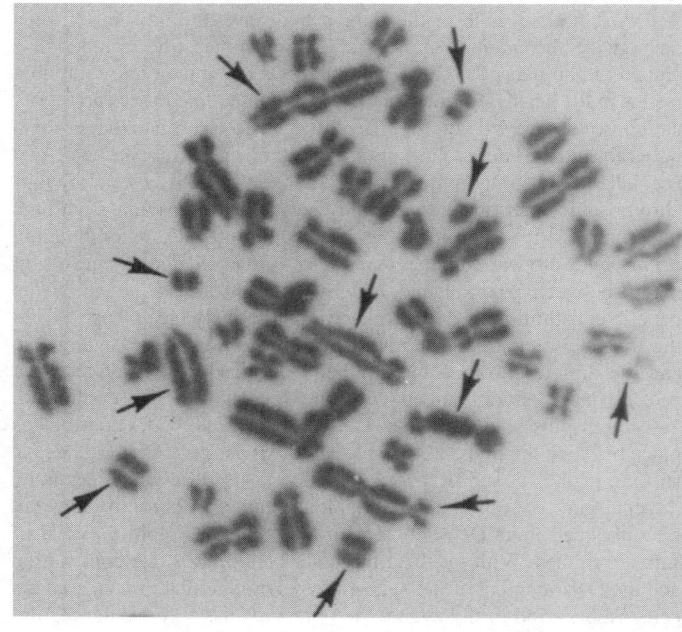

FIGURE 66-4 Breaks and rearrangements (*arrows*) in metaphase chromosomes of a blood lymphocyte that received ionizing irradiation before being stimulated by phytohemagglutinin to enter S and divide.

monosomy, to indicate that segments rather than entire chromosomes are involved (e.g., partial trisomy 13q, partial monosomy 4p). Some of the clinically important recurring chromosome imbalances, both numerical and structural, are listed in Table 66-1.

Uniparental disomy is the situation in which both chromosomes of a pair, or perhaps one of them plus a segment of the other, are erroneously inherited from a single parent. In such cases, the presence of a homozygous chromosome segment can have unfavorable effects on development. *Genomic imprinting* has critical effects on development (see "Autosome imbalance," below). In addition, the fact that the affected individual is homozygous at all the loci on the disomic chromosome (or segment) means that almost any deleterious recessive alleles that are present there may cause disease. The parent contributing the disomy would probably have been heterozygous at these loci and therefore healthy. (See also Chap. 65.)

Incidence The frequency with which chromosome imbalances are detectable depends on the population studied. At least 1 in 10 human conceptions has a chromosome abnormality, and chromosome imbalance is present in 5 to 6 percent of recognized pregnancies. In spontaneously aborted human embryos and fetuses, the incidence of chromosome imbalance peaks at 8 to 11 weeks of gestation. The contribution of chromosome imbalances to late abortion and stillbirth

is also significant. Surveys of more than 65,000 live-born babies examined in different laboratories found an incidence of approximately 1 in 200 for significant chromosome abnormalities, either numerical or structural. In such studies, at least 1 in 700 infants is trisomic for one of the autosomes 21, 18, or 13; about 1 in 350 newborn boys has the complement 47,XXY or 47,XYY. One in every several thousand newborns has monosomy X. One in 500 has some structural rearrangement, most of which are genetically balanced. Samplings of the general adult population reveal an occasional inherited balanced structural rearrangement as well as the expected number of XXY, XYY, and XXX complements; the inherited, apparently innocuous segmental polymorphisms (e.g., the chromosome 9 polymorphism shown in Fig. 66-1 and the C-band polymorphisms in Fig. 66-3) are found in abundance.

Of individuals with mental deficiency, 10 to 15 percent have a significant chromosome abnormality; the proportion is greater among individuals who also have anatomic malformations. In some groups of men with behavioral disorders or infertility, an increased incidence of individuals with an extra X or Y chromosome is found. Infertile

Table 66-1

Some Recurring Chromosome Imbalances that Result in Distinct Syndromes*

Class of Imbalance	Chromosome Affected	Karyotypes†	Clinical Features‡
Monosomy	X	45,X	Turner syndrome
Segmental deficiency ("partial monosomy")	X	46,X,Xp−; 46,X,Xq−; 46,X,r(X); 46,X,iso(Xp); 46,X,iso(Xq)	Turner syndrome or some features of it
	Y	46,X,Yp−; 46,X,Yq−; 46,X,r(Y); 46,X,iso(Yp); 46,X,iso(Yq)	Turner syndrome, or some features of it, sometimes with "mixed gonadal dysgenesis" when a 45,X cell line coexists (mosaicism)
	4	46,XY,4p−	Gr, Cf, Mi, Ey, Sk, Ge, Ht, Co, Me
	5	46,XY,5p−	5p− syndrome: Cr, Mi, Cf, Me
	8	46,XY,del(8)(q22q24)	Langer-Gideon syndrome
	11	46,XY,11p− or del(11)(p13)	WT, Ge, Me
	13	46,XY,13q−	RB, Cf, Me
	15	46,XY,15q− or del(15)(q11q13)	Prader-Willi or Angelman syndrome
	17	46,XY,del(17)(p13)	Miller-Dieker syndrome
	18	46,XY,18p−	Gr, Cf, Ea, Te, Po, Sk, Ht, Me
	18	46,XY,18q−	Cf, Hy, Sk, Ey
	21	46,XY,r(21)	Cf, Hp, Ea, Me
Trisomy	X	47,XXX	Se, Me (mild), Ps
	X	47,XXY	Klinefelter syndrome
	Y	47,XYY	Ta, Ac, Su, B; but often normal
	8	46,XY/47,XY,+8	Cf, Sk, Me (moderate)
	13	47,XY,+13	Trisomy 13 syndrome: Cp, Ey, Pd, Po, Ht, D, V, Sc, F, Ar, Me
	18	47,XY,+18	Trisomy 18 syndrome: Cf, Ea, V, F, Gr, D, He, Me
	21	47,XY,+21	Trisomy 21 (Down syndrome)
Segmental duplication ("partial trisomy")	Y	46,X,t(X;Y)§	XX male
	9	9p+†	Cf
	21	21q+(distal q)	Trisomy 21 syndrome
	22	22q+¶	Gr, Cf, Ea, Cp, Hy, Co
Chimerism	Entire complement	46,XY/46,XX	Pseudo- or true hermaphroditism; dimorphism of blood-cell-surface antigens
Triploidy	Entire complement	69,XXY	Hc, Me, Sy, Ht, Ge, D

* For complete listing, consult DeGrouchy and Turleau.

† The sex chromosome constitution might be either XY or XX, but in the example karyotypes given, XY arbitrarily is used in most.

‡ The clinical features given include only some of the more constant ones. Deficiency of one segment often is accompanied by duplication of another, and the phenotypic effect is the consequence of the combined imbalance. Abbreviations are defined below.

§ Translocation onto an X of a segment of the Y bearing the locus responsible for testicular differentiation.

¶ Brought about through any of several rearrangements.

Abbreviations: −, absence of a chromosome if placed in front of a number, or deletion from or of the chromosome arm indicated in placed after it; +, the opposite of the minus sign; Ac, acne; Ar, arrhinencephaly; B, behavior disorder; Cr, characteristically abnormal cry; Cf, characteristic craniofacial dysmorphism; Co, convulsions; Cp, cleft lip–palate; D, early death; del, deletion; Ea, characteristically abnormal ears; Ey, eye anomaly; F, characteristically flared, overlapping fingers; Ge, abnormality of external genitalia; Gr, severe growth deficiency; Hc, hydrocephaly; Hp, hypertonia; Ht, cardiac malformation; Hy, infantile hypotonia; iso, isochromosome of the chromosome arm indicated in round brackets; Me, intellectual deficit; Mi, microcephaly; Om, omphalocele; p, short arm of a chromosome; Po, characteristically abnormal posture; Pd, polydactyly; Ps, psychotic predisposition; q, long arm of a chromosome; r, a ring chromosome; RB, retinoblastoma; Sc, scalp defect; Se, secondary amenorrhea; Sk, skeletal anomalies; Su, subfertility; Sy, syndactyly; t, translocation of the chromosome placed in round brackets; Ta, tallness; Te, characteristically abnormal teeth; V, visceral anomalies; WT, Wilms's tumor with aniridia.

and subfertile women also include many individuals with missing or abnormal sex chromosomes. Approximately one-fourth of women with primary amenorrhea have some abnormality of the X chromosome. An appreciable number of infertile men and women have structural chromosome rearrangements.

Numerical Abnormalities Trisomy (47 chromosomes) is the most common chromosome imbalance in early spontaneous abortuses, followed by monosomy (45 chromosomes) and triploidy (69 chromosomes). The extra or missing chromosomes can be either paternal or maternal in origin, and the error in segregation of chromosomes can occur in the germ line, in the fertilized egg, or in the early embryo. Trisomy of every chromosome except chromosome 1 has been observed in spontaneous abortions, trisomy 16 being the most frequent. Most trisomic chromosomes are maternal in origin, and the incidence increases with maternal age. Triploidy is usually the result of dispermy (simultaneous fertilization of an egg by two sperms.)

Sex chromosome trisomies (XXY, XYY, and XXX) are compatible with intrauterine survival, whereas autosomal trisomies rarely permit survival to term. However, a small proportion of infants with autosomal trisomies are born alive. For practical purposes, the viable trisomies are those involving chromosome 21, 18, or 13, in order of decreasing frequency. Trisomies 18 and 13 usually cause death during infancy. Therefore, the only trisomies of significance in adults are trisomies 21, XXY, XXX, and XYY. A few other autosomal trisomies, such as trisomy 8, occur rarely, usually in mosaicism with a normal cellular component. (*Mosaicism* is the coexistence in one individual of multiple, genetically different populations of cells, all of which are derived from a single zygote.)

Autosomal monosomy is rare even in abortion material, whereas monosomy X (45,X) occurs in approximately 1.5 percent of conceptions. It is present in approximately 10 percent of spontaneously aborted human embryos and in one in every several thousand live-born babies. The reason for the failure of 45,X embryos and fetuses to survive is unknown, although cardiovascular and renal anomalies are common in the few that do survive. The cause of the lethality may be hemizygosity for some vital locus or loci of which normal individuals have two copies (the second copy being located on the Y chromosome in males and, in females, on one of the parts of the X chromosome that is not inactivated by the Lyon effect, such as the pseudoautosomal region). Occasional 45,X individuals may survive because of occult mosaicism—that is, mosaicism in which the normal cells, perhaps limited just to a few tissues, go undetected. In monosomy X, the missing sex chromosome can have been either a Y or an X and, if an X, either paternal or maternal in origin. Often the second sex chromosome is not completely absent but is replaced by a structurally rearranged Y or X. Mosaicism is often demonstrable in live-born infants with monosomy X; the nonmonosomic cells may have either a normal 46,XY or 46,XX complement or a complement in which the second sex chromosome is rearranged in some way.

The phenotypic effects of the autosomal trisomies, of 47,XXY, and of monosomy X (45,X) are characteristic and well defined, so their diagnosis usually is not difficult (see Chap. 339). The effects of the 47,XYY and 47,XXX constitutions are less striking, and these complements are underdiagnosed. In mosaicism, the phenotype may be indistinguishable from normal.

The mechanisms responsible for the numerical abnormalities are undefined and may be multiple. The extra chromosome is maternal in 95 percent of trisomy 21 cases and usually resulted from nonsegregation at the first meiotic division. There is a maternal age effect in trisomies 21, 18, 13, XXY, and XXX. Over a third of babies with trisomy 21 are born to women over 35, whereas only about a tenth of all births occur in this group. The frequency of trisomy 21 rises from 0.5 to 0.7 per 1000 live births between ages 21 and 23 to 3 per 1000 at age 35, 10 per 1000 at age 40, and 34 per 1000 at age 45. After a child with trisomy 21 is born, the risk of recurrence in future pregnancies is about 1 percent. As to the cause of monosomy X, the frequent association of the 45,X complement in mosaicism with normal cells and with cells with structural rearrangements of the X and Y suggests that it is due to a chromosome-breaking event in the zygote or very early embryo that only secondarily causes chromosome loss, rather than to a nondisjunctional event during meiosis as occurs in the trisomies.

Structural Abnormalities Some structural chromosome rearrangements are inherited, and others represent new mutations. The cause of the new rearrangements is unknown, although they are assumed to be partly spontaneous and partly the effect of environmental agents such as mutagenic chemicals or ionizing radiation (Fig. 66-4) acting on the germ line, zygote, or early embryo. Most de novo rearrangements are in paternally derived chromosomes.

Many chromosome rearrangements have been detected only once or a few times. Others are detected repeatedly in unrelated individuals and within families. For example, the most common translocation, which can either be inherited or arise by a de novo mutation, affects one chromosome 13 and one 14 at or near their centromeres. In this translocation, only inert chromatin or functional chromatin that is represented elsewhere in the genome—the nucleolus-organizing regions and satellites referred to earlier—is lost from the short arms. A similar recurring translocation affects chromosomes 14 and 21. The normal carriers of these abnormalities (so called Robertsonian translocations) have 45 rather than 46 chromosomes.

Chromosome complements bearing rearrangements can be genetically balanced—at least effectively so—and impart no unfavorable effect to their bearers; about two-thirds of rearrangements detected during surveys of live-born babies are balanced. Alternatively, the complement can be unbalanced and impair development, the usual case when rearrangements are detected in spontaneous abortuses or in individuals with multiple anomalies and mental deficiency.

Some balanced chromosome rearrangements are transmitted through multiple generations without producing clinical effects. In other cases, they cause the conception of embryos with unbalanced genomes. For example, inherited translocations involving chromosome 21 increase the chance of offspring with the trisomy 21 syndrome. Approximately 5 percent of live-born infants with that syndrome have a translocation, and in about a fifth of those it is detectable in one of the parents. Because most babies with trisomy 21 due to translocation are born to women under 30, a search should be made for a translocation when an affected child is born to young parents. Different translocations confer different risks of having offspring with unbalanced rearrangements (partial trisomies or partial monosomies). These risks frequently cannot be predicted on theoretical grounds. Empirical risk figures have been accumulated for the common translocations. In the case of the Robertsonian 14;21 translocation, for example, the risk of having a child with the trisomy 21 syndrome is 2 percent for a balanced male carrier and more than 10 percent for a female carrier.

Genetically Determined Chromosome Instability Many gene products interact with the chromosome in the course of DNA replication, transcription, recombination, and repair, including polymerases, helicases, topoisomerases, ligases, and deoxyribonucleases as well as gene products that regulate the cell cycle. Mutations in the genes that encode these proteins can have profound effects, including interference with the integrity of the chromosomes, as in DNA-repair defects, such as the one causing xeroderma pigmentosum, and chromosome breakage syndromes, such as Bloom's syndrome, ataxia-telangiectasia, Fanconi's anemia, and Werner's syndrome (see also Chap. 84). The chromosome breakage syndromes share two important features: a predisposition to cancer, and increased numbers of chromosome breaks and/or rearrangements in somatic cells. Bloom's syndrome is characterized by small body size, immunodeficiency, light-sensitive facial erythema, and a major predisposition to cancer. Ataxia-telangiectasia is associated with increased numbers of translocations, particularly involving the T cell receptor loci. Fanconi's anemia causes increased numbers of chromatid gaps and breaks, and Werner's syndrome is associated with translocations at various sites. As the genes mutated in these rare syndromes have been identified, the normal alleles of these genes have been found to play critical roles in genomic stability.

For example, the gene that is mutated in Bloom's syndrome codes for a DNA helicase that normally functions to guarantee the fidelity of chromosome replication. These rare syndromes are important models for the study of somatic mutational disorders.

Genomic imprinting can profoundly influence the developmental consequences of chromosome mutations. A few genetic loci are known to be subject to functional modulation that occurs presumably during passage through the germ line. The modulation differs depending on whether the genome passed through spermatogenesis or oogenesis. The parental source of a chromosome mutation that affects such an imprintable locus or loci can determine whether a developmental defect will arise and the nature of the defect. An example of imprinting concerns deletion of chromosome band 15q12; deletion of the region on the paternal chromosome (no paternal contribution) causes Prader-Willi syndrome, whereas deletion on the maternal chromosome causes the Angelman syndrome (Table 66-1). Because the disorders are due to lack of a contribution from a particular parent, uniparental disomy for chromosome 15 can also be responsible. For example, about one-fourth of Prader-Willi cases are due to maternal uniparental disomy; a smaller proportion of Angelman syndrome cases are due to paternal uniparental disomy. Chromosomes 7, 11, and 14 are also known to exert clinical effects by a uniparental disomy mechanism.

DISEASE ASSOCIATIONS   Various combinations of abnormalities in malformed and mentally defective individuals suggest chromosome abnormalities.

Autosome Imbalance   Of the three common autosomal trisomies found in live-born babies, only trisomy 21 is compatible with survival past infancy. The phenotype produced by an extra chromosome 21, formerly known as *mongolism* but now called the *Down syndrome* or *trisomy 21 syndrome*, is characteristic and easily diagnosed. Cardiac malformations lead to death in infancy in one-third of individuals, and other malformations may also cause early death. However, subjects who survive infancy often reach adulthood, and many reach old age. Early-onset Alzheimer's disease is common in adults with trisomy 21. Affected women occasionally become pregnant, and approximately half their children have trisomy 21.

Mosaicism of trisomy 21 with normal cells (46,XY/47,XY, + 21) may occur in normal individuals or people with modified features of the trisomy 21 syndrome. Children of persons with such a mosaicism have a higher than normal risk of having trisomy 21. Unfortunately, however, the abnormal cell population is usually detected only after the birth of an affected child.

Partial trisomy, partial monosomy, or a combination of the two affecting any of numerous chromosomal segments throughout the genome causes many instances of multiple developmental defects combined with mental deficiency. Sometimes a balanced autosomal translocation is detected in a normally developed adult who has repeated spontaneous abortions or subnormal fertility, with or without abnormal live-born children.

Although the phenotypic effects of many segmental chromosome imbalances are varied and nonspecific, the anomalies sometimes constitute recognizable clinical syndromes. Two examples are as follows. (1) Partial trisomy of the distal band of the long arm of chromosome 21 causes development of the full Down syndrome. (A triple dose of other segments of the long arm of chromosome 21 also produces adverse effects, but not the Down syndrome.) (2) Partial monosomy of a short segment in the short arm of chromosome 5 causes mental deficiency, a characteristic facies, and a characteristic cry during infancy. This group of signs is known as the *5p−*, or *cri-du-chat syndrome.*

Some additional syndromes produced by imbalance of chromosome segments are listed in Table 66-1, e.g., the 4p−, 9p partial trisomy, 13q−, and 18q− syndromes, to name a few. Furthermore, the application of high-resolution banding techniques and fluorescence in situ hybridization (FISH) (described below in the section "Technical Considerations") make possible identification of the exact band(s) that are deficient or duplicated. Molecular analysis employing a battery of techniques shows that unbalanced translocations and deletions too short to be detected by microscopy nevertheless can cause develop-

mental defects and mental deficiency. Additional rearrangements and their corresponding clinical syndromes still are being recognized. These syndromes may either be due to de novo chromosome rearrangement or to formation of a genetically unbalanced gamete in a developmentally normal person carrying a rearrangement affecting the relevant segment in a balanced state.

Many individuals with a chromosome imbalance, regardless of the segments affected, exhibit a degree of phenotypic similarity. These recurring, nonspecific features include mental deficiency; growth deficiency; dysmorphic ears, nose, and mouth; cardiac malformations of standard types; abnormalities of dermal ridges and creases; and dysmorphic digits. (As a rule, autosomal imbalance need not be considered in the etiology of anatomic defects not accompanied by mental deficiency.) Why similar abnormalities occur with so many different segmental imbalances is unknown, but when several such features are present, they constitute a valuable indication for cytogenetic analysis. Imbalances affecting certain segments also causes specific phenotypic changes, examples being the 5p− syndrome, retinoblastoma [mutation of a particular band of chromosome 13 (band 13q14.2)], the WAGR syndrome (Wilms's tumor, aniridia, genital anomalies, and mental deficiency) caused by deletion of band 11p13, and the Prader-Willi syndrome, which is often the consequence of deletion of a specific band near the centromere of chromosome 15 (band 15q12). Whereas the nonspecific changes serve to call attention to the possibility of some chromosome imbalance, the specific features or constellation of features can suggest the exact segment of the genome affected.

Certain constellations of features are referred to as *contiguous gene-deletion syndromes.* The WAGR syndrome mentioned above is an example; another is caused by deletions of segments of Xp that result in the loss of contiguous loci that, individually, are responsible for Duchenne's muscular dystrophy, chronic granulomatous disease, retinitis pigmentosa, and the MacLeod phenotype.

Apparently balanced translocations are also found at higher frequency in mentally subnormal persons. In these cases, the abnormalities presumably are due to small imbalances not detectable at the ordinary level of microscopic resolution or to alterations in gene positioning. The discovery of such a new translocation in prenatal diagnostic studies presents a difficult counseling issue; limited data suggest that such translocations impart a risk of about 7 percent for abnormality.

Sex Chromosome Imbalance (See also Chap. 339)   In contrast to autosomal trisomy, an extra sex chromosome causes relatively mild phenotypic effects. This is because X chromosomes beyond one in somatic cells are usually almost totally inactivated, because the pseudo-autosomal region is much shorter than any of the autosomes, and because the strictly sex-linked portions of the Y bear few genes. X-linked loci (in contrast to autosomal loci) function normally in a single dose. Females are functionally hemizygous for most loci on the X through the Lyon effect; males, with only one X chromosome, are hemizygous for X-linked genes, with the exception of loci clustered in the pseudoautosomal segment and a few scattered in the proximal Yp and Yq. The addition of an extra sex chromosome has a phenotypic effect, but not one that interferes with intrauterine survival. Since major anatomic defects are usually absent, men with the complements 47,XXY and 47,XYY and 47,XXX females often go unrecognized.

The *Klinefelter syndrome* (Chap. 339) typically consists of small testes, infertility, gynecomastia, and a variable degree of underandrogenization, sometimes with mild mental deficiency, antisocial behavior, or both. It is caused by the addition of an extra X to the male complement (47,XXY). The extra X interferes with the survival of germ cells and causes atrophy of the spermatogenic tubules and azoospermia. Sometimes the phenotypic effects are mild, with testicular atrophy being the noteworthy feature in an otherwise healthy man. 46,XY/47,XXY mosaicism sometimes occurs and may ameliorate the phenotypic effect of the extra X. More extreme phenotypic effects and mental deficiency result when more than one extra X chromosome is added to the normal male complement (48,XXXY or 49,XXXXY).

The phenotypic effect of 47,XYY is less well defined; although increased height, behavioral difficulties, and infertility are common, the extra Y is sometimes found in otherwise normal men. The rare complement 48,XXYY results in infertility. The phenotype associated with 47,XXX is also poorly defined; women with this complement may have mild mental deficiency, psychosis, and menstrual abnormalities or may be normal.

Loss of the Y or of the second X has drastic effects on development. If it does not cause abortion (as already discussed), it may be recognizable in the newborn girl because of the presence of loose nuchal skin folds and edema of the hands and feet with or without renal or cardiovascular anomalies. The *Turner syndrome* (gonadal dysgenesis) is the manifestation in subsequent life (Chap. 339): short stature, infantilism of the female external and internal genitalia, germ-cell-free gonads (referred to as *gonadal streaks*), and variable renal, cardiovascular, skeletal, and ectodermal anomalies.

The Turner syndrome is associated with several chromosome constitutions besides 45,X. Mosaicism and structural abnormalities of the second sex chromosome, either a Y or an X, cause a spectrum of disorders at both the clinical and cytogenetic levels. Common abnormalities of the Y and X include isochromosome formation (one arm deleted and the other duplicated) or deletion of part or all of one arm. Thus, all cells may have 46 chromosomes, but the sex chromosomes may consist of one normal X plus an abnormal Y or X; an example is 46,XXp−, in which there is deletion of a segment of the short arm of one of the X chromosomes. In other cases, a second or third cellular component is present as well, for example, 45,X/46,XX/46,XXp−. Various combinations of these karyotypes can cause the Turner phenotype if one of them is either monosomic or partially monosomic for the X. However, when Y-bearing cells coexist with the 45,X cells, for example, 45,X/46,XY, genital ambiguity often develops, and gonadal morphology ranges from streaks to functional testes (the syndrome of *mixed gonadal dysgenesis*); when a Y cell line is present, the risk of gonadal neoplasia is significant. When 46,XX cells coexist with 45,X cells, varying degrees of ovarian function may be maintained, including ovulation. Thus, the phenotype associated with monosomy X and structural abnormality of the Y or X ranges from male through the Turner syndrome to female.

X-Linked Mental Deficiency In the general population, more males than females are mentally deficient, and familial mental deficiency affects males preferentially. In some kindreds, mental deficiency segregates as an X-linked trait, and several such syndromes are now recognized. The most common of these, the *fragile X syndrome*, is characterized by mental deficiency, a characteristic facies, and macroorchia. The condition can be recognized by cytogenetic techniques. In a variable but usually small proportion of metaphases from affected persons, the abnormal X chromosome exhibits a so-called fragile site near the distal end of Xq. This site is responsible for the decondensed appearance of the region at metaphase, and its fragility is due to excess amplification of the trinucleotide sequence CGG. This base sequence is normally repeated 2 to 50 times at the fragile-X locus, whereas in affected individuals the number of repeats is expanded to more than 200. This amplification is believed to affect the normal functioning of neighboring genetic determinants and thereby to cause the abnormal phenotype. This disorder is now diagnosed by molecular techniques.

Chromosome Changes in Cancer Most human cancers have chromosome complements that are altered in a microscopically detectable way. Indeed, the cytogenetic findings in leukemias and solid tumors were some of the first evidence of the clonal nature of human cancer. Table 66-2 lists some of the alterations found with regularity in human malignancies. In the leukemias, lymphomas, and certain myeloproliferative disorders, the alterations are less extensive than in solid tumors and, therefore, easier to define. As examples, chromosome 14 is often found to have undergone structural rearrangement in certain lymphomas, with the breakpoint near or in the immunoglobulin heavy chain locus; the rearrangement translocates the *c-myc* locus from its

Table 66-2

Some Recurring Chromosome Abnormalities Encountered in Human Neoplasms*

Neoplasm	Aberration	Chromosome Region Affected
Leukemia		
Chronic granulocytic	Translocation	9q34 and 22q11
Acute nonlymphocytic		
M1	Translocation	9q34 and 22q11
M2	Translocation	8q22 and 21q22
M3	Translocation	15q22 and 17q11
Chronic lymphocytic	Trisomy	12
Acute lymphocytic		
L1–L2	Translocation	9q34 and 22q11
L3	Translocation	4q21 and 11q23
	Translocation	8q24 and 14q32
Lymphoma		
Burkitt's	Translocation	8q24 and 14q32
Follicular	Translocation	14q32 and 18q21
Solid tumors		
Benign		
Meningioma	Deletion or monosomy	22q
Leiomyoma, uterus	Translocation	2q13–15 and 14q23–24
Adenomas, salivary gland	Translocation	3p25 and 8q12
Malignant		
Ewing's sarcoma	Translocation	11q24 and 22q12
Rhabdomyosarcoma, alveolar	Translocation	2q35–37 and 13q14
Germ cell tumors, testis	Isochromosome	12p
Lung, small cell carcinoma	Deletion	3p13–23
Liposarcoma, myxoid	Translocation	12q13 and 16p11
Sarcoma, synovial	Translocation	Xp11 and 18q11
Neuroblastoma	Deletion	1p31 to 3p36
Ovary, cystadenocarcinoma	Translocation	6q21 and 14q24
Retinoblastoma	Deletion	13q14
Wilms's tumor	Deletion	11p13

* For more complete listing, see Solomon.

NOTE: The FAB (French-American-British) classification of leukemias is employed above. The chromosome breakpoint and band nomenclature is that of the Paris Conference (Birth Defects: Original Articles Series VIII (7):1–46, 1971). The chromosome and chromosome-arm designation (e.g., 9q means the long arm of chromosome 9) appears first and is followed by the chromosome region and band on that arm (e.g., 9q34 means the fourth band in the third region of the long arm of chromosome 9).

normal position on chromosome 8 to chromosome 14. Also, in over 95 percent of cases of chronic granulocytic leukemia, a translocation affecting chromosomes 9 and 22 (already mentioned) is detected, resulting in the Philadelphia (Ph[1]) chromosome, an abnormally short chromosome 22. If this leukemia progresses into a "blastic" phase, the already mutated karyotype evolves; certain new chromosome changes are added stepwise in a nonrandom sequence. In this and certain other leukemias, the chromosome changes, demonstrable either by conventional cytogenetic techniques and microscopy or by microscopy supplemented by molecular techniques, may have diagnostic utility as well as some value in prognosis and choice of therapy. Common carcinomas, such as those of the lung, breast, and colon, although more difficult to study by conventional cytogenetic techniques, also have specific chromosome mutations.

The chromosome mutations found with regularity in human neoplasms (Table 66–2) often affect loci that regulate growth in normal cells. In some cases, the chromosome breakpoints affect known cellular oncogenes, but analysis of cancer-associated breakpoints also has resulted in the identification of previously unrecognized important genes, including genes coding for factors that regulate transcription and loci concerned with the regulation of normal development. In some of the lymphoma examples given, *c-myc* in its new position on chromosome 14 is brought under the influence of the activating elements of the transcribing immunoglobulin locus in cells differentiated to synthesize antibodies. In follicular lymphoma, the translocation t(14;18)(q32;q21) results in activation of a locus that suppresses apoptosis and causes prolonged survival of lymphocytes. In the Ph[1] chromosome, the cellular oncogene *abl* is translocated from its normal position on chromosome 9 into a specific region on chromosome 22, thereby creating what is called a *fusion gene*; in myeloid cells, this mutant locus is transcribed, and the mRNA is translated into a novel protein that presumably helps to cause the growth of the neoplastic cell lineage that is recognized clinically as chronic granulocytic leukemia. Thus, chromosome mutations can cause activation of or de novo creation of growth-controlling genes.

Another process that appears to be important in the progression of some tumors is *gene amplification*. One particular chromosome segment is replicated selectively, sometimes to such a degree that the normal banding pattern at the chromosome region affected is visibly disturbed, a *homogeneously staining region* (HSR) appearing at the site. Sometimes the region amplified, rather than producing an HSR, is released from the chromosome, and multiple tiny centromereless bodies of DNA, known as *double minutes* (DMs), accumulate in the nucleus and can be seen at metaphase. Presumably, in both HSRs and DMs, amplification of the DNA of some particular locus is of selective value to the neoplastic cell, enhancing the neoplastic clone's progression or perhaps its resistance to chemotherapeutic agents.

Loss of a gene essential for the normal suppression of growth can also contribute to the initiation and progression of neoplasia. Such loss can occur from gene deletion or from disruption of a gene by a translocation breakpoint. Several such mutations are now recognized; they are considered to be recessive because the presence of a single wild type allele is sufficient to provide normal growth control. Such mutations can be inherited or arise de novo as new mutations; the chromosomal mechanisms by which normal genes can be lost in somatic cells include chromatid nondisjunction with loss of an entire chromosome, segmental deletion of a portion of a chromosome, and crossing over.

The consequence of hemi- or homozygosity at such a mutant locus is loss of normal growth control, that is, the acquisition of autonomous growth by the affected cell and its progeny. Such mutations were first recognized in the rare neoplasms retinoblastoma and Wilms's tumor, where the loci affected are on chromosomes 13 and 11, respectively. In some cases of retinoblastoma the original (recessive) mutation consisted of outright deletion of the locus; then, when somatic crossing-over occurred, homozygosity of the affected chromosome arm distal to the point of exchange was the consequence, and a cell and its progeny became *nullisomic* for the retinoblastoma locus. Transmission through the germ line of occult recessive mutations at such growth-suppressor loci explains why, in familial instances of those neoplasms, the pedigrees suggest dominant inheritance.

Thus, chromosome mutations of at least four types can serve as crucial steps in the initiation and progression of malignant neoplasia: (1) translocations that disturb the regulation of loci concerned with growth or that produce novel genes affecting growth; (2) deletion or mutation of recessive growth-controlling loci, such as the retinoblastoma locus just referred to (these mutations can either be inherited through the germ line or occur de novo in a somatic cell); (3) recombination yielding homozygosity for preexisting mutations affecting the last-mentioned type of locus; and (4) amplification of a locus that facilitates expansion of the neoplastic population. These mutations and their oncogenic consequences are the subject of intensive investigation. In turn, the breakpoints found in neoplasms help in identifying genetic determinants that regulate cellular proliferation and tissue growth.

TECHNICAL CONSIDERATIONS   Human metaphase chromosomes can be examined by light microscopy in any tissue in which sufficient cells are cycling. Preparations can therefore be made from almost any embryonic tissue and from adult bone marrow, lymphoid tissue, and malignant tissues. To identify mosaicism and chimerism, multiple tissues usually have to be studied. Some tissues unlikely to contain metaphase cells can be placed in culture, and chromosome preparations can be made from cells that reach mitosis in vitro. Blood T lymphocytes stimulated to enter cell division cycles by phytohemagglutinin are the standard material for diagnosing constitutional chromosome imbalances. In some myeloproliferative disorders and leukemias,

unstimulated circulating blood cells divide spontaneously after a few hours in culture. Amniotic fluid cells, which are fetal in origin, are widely used in the prenatal diagnosis of chromosome imbalances. Metaphase preparations also can be made from chorionic villus cells obtained by biopsy during the first trimester of pregnancy or from aborted fetal tissue. Fibroblasts can be cultured from minute skin biopsy samples or from fragments of many other tissues, although it takes longer to obtain cytogenetic preparations from this source. Meiotic chromosome preparations from testicular biopsy samples are sometimes useful in obscure cases of infertility, for identification of translocations and genetically determined disturbances of meiotic pairing.

Combining conventional techniques with recombinant DNA technology and fluorescence microscopy makes it possible to detect abnormalities such as trisomy, translocation, and segmental duplication or deficiency. Molecular probes for many specific marker loci whose map positions are known and that together blanket the genome can be used to identify rearrangements not detectable by banding techniques alone. By FISH, molecular probes specific for each chromosome can be used to "paint" a chromosome differentially throughout its length, revealing, for example, whether part of one chromosome has been translocated to another or whether a chromosome or chromosome segment is trisomic. FISH also makes possible the chromosomal localization of known DNA sequences, including specific genes, and the determination of their order. For certain questions, study of interphase nuclei using either painting (chromosome-specific) probes or cloned gene sequences circumvents the need to bring cells into metaphase for identification of mutations. The use of FISH along with microscopy, Southern blotting, and the polymerase chain reaction can provide minute definition of chromosome rearrangements, whether constitutional or occurring in a neoplastic clone.

Sometimes, metaphase or anaphase chromosomes are analyzed to determine whether damage to the genetic material has been induced by some environmental agent (radiation, a chemical, a virus) or to identify constitutional genomic instability. Cells that have proliferated in vivo and then been incubated briefly in vitro may be used in searching for evidence of damage to the genetic material of a person or population (see Fig. 66-4).

BIBLIOGRAPHY

COHEN MM et al: Human cytogenetics: A current overview. Am J Dis Child 147:1159, 1993
DE GROUCHY J, TURLEAU C: *Clinical Atlas of Human Chromosomes*, 2d ed. New York, Wiley, 1984
GARDNER RJM, SUTHERLAND GR: *Chromosome Abnormalities and Genetic Counseling*, 2nd ed. New York, Oxford University Press, 1996
GERMAN JL: Studying human chromosomes today. Am Sci 58:182, 1970
———: Bloom syndrome: A Mendelian prototype of somatic mutational disease. Medicine 72:393, 1993
GRUMBACH MM, CONTE FA: Disorders of sex differentiation, in *Williams Textbook of Endocrinology*, 8th ed, JD Wilson, DW Foster (eds). Philadelphia, Saunders, 1992, pp 853–951
SCHIZEL A: *Catalogue of Unbalanced Chromosome Aberrations*. Berlin, Walter de Gruyter, 1983.
SOLOMON E et al: Chromosome aberrations and cancer. Science 254:1153, 1991

67	*David Valle*

TREATMENT AND PREVENTION OF GENETIC DISEASE

Normal development and physiologic homeostasis depend on the coordinated interactions of the products of many genes working together in metabolic systems. These systems are adaptable within limits, allowing normal homeostasis to be maintained over a range of environmental conditions. For instance, the products of some 30 to 40 genes participate in blood glucose regulation; in concert they maintain a relatively constant blood glucose concentration despite intermittent and highly variable ingestion of glucose precursors. On a larger scale, developmental and homeostatic interactions of 10,000 or so gene products are believed to be necessary for normal development and function of the central nervous system. Mutations that reduce the adaptive capacity of these systems result in abnormalities that we recognize as genetic disease. The mutant gene may so compromise a particular developmental or homeostatic system that the system functions poorly or not at all under any circumstance, thereby producing a monogenic disorder. Alternatively, the mutant gene may have modest effects under ordinary conditions but in certain environments contribute to maldevelopment or dyshomeostasis that we recognize as a multifactorial disorder. Thus the role of the genes in health and disease is both central and complex. Consequently, treatment of genetic disease is both difficult and often less than completely effective.

℞ TREATMENT

Effective treatment of genetic disorders requires accurate diagnosis, early intervention prior to development of irreversible tissue damage, and an understanding of the abnormal biochemistry or metabolic pathophysiology. Progress in delineating the molecular basis of genetic disease has improved our capability for accurate diagnosis of monogenic disorders. Understanding of the metabolic pathophysiology is increasing at a slower rate, mainly because progress in this area often requires elucidation of integrative physiology by study of the intact organism. The development of noninvasive metabolic monitoring techniques such as positron emission tomography and topical magnetic resonance spectrometry, as well as new genetic technologies for the production of animal models of human genetic disease, offer great promise for progress in this area.

Approaches to treatment of genetic disease can be organized proceeding from the clinical phenotype through the abnormal metabolites and dysfunctional protein to the level of the defective gene (Table 67-1).

Treatment of the Clinical Phenotype Treatment of the clinical phenotype includes conventional medical practices such as patient education, pharmacologic interventions, and surgical procedures. It depends on a thorough understanding of the natural history of the particular disorder so that potential complications can be avoided or addressed early in the course to minimize the consequences. Although therapy at this level is not aimed at correcting the primary defect, it can markedly improve the quality of life. Examples include instruction to patients with albinism or xeroderma to limit sun exposure or to patients with glucose-6-phosphate dehydrogenase deficiency to avoid the offending drugs; administration of beta blockers to Marfan's syndrome patients to prevent or slow dilatation of the aortic root, anticonvulsants to patients with neurogenic disorders, or antihypertensive agents to patients with secondary hypertension; and a host of surgical interventions for patients with genetic malformations, skeletal dysplasias, and malignancies.

Treatment of the Metabolic Phenotype Treatment at the metabolite level involves nutritional or pharmacologic approaches and is dependent on understanding the biochemical pathophysiology (Fig. 67-1). Deficient function of a mutant protein may result in a disease phenotype for the following reasons: (1) a substrate accumulates to toxic levels (precursor toxicity); (2) the product of an alternative pathway is produced in excessive amounts (alternative pathway overflow); (3) formation of the reaction product or some downstream metabolite is reduced (product deficiency); or (4) there is some combination of these possibilities. Although this paradigm is most easily visualized for enzymes in a metabolic pathway, it holds for virtually all proteins. The pathophysiology may be *local* within the cell or tissue normally expressing the mutant protein, or it may

Table 67-1

Some Treatments for Monogenic Disorders

Level of Treatment and Method	Disorder(s)
CLINICAL PHENOTYPE	
Patient education	
Avoidance of aggravating agents (high carbohydrate diet, exposure to cold)	Periodic paralysis syndromes
Avoidance of certain drugs	Pharmacogenetic disorders, acute intermittent porphyria
Avoidance of sun exposure	Xeroderma pigmentosa, albinism
Avoidance of certain physical activity	Chondrodystrophies
Notify physician for rapid increase in size of mass or tinnitus	Neurofibromatosis
Pharmacologic	
Beta blockers	Marfan's syndrome
Anticonvulsants	Neurodegenerative disorders
Surgical	
Orthopedic reconstruction	Chondrodystrophies
Colectomy	Familial polyposis coli
Plastic reconstruction of facial malformations	Treacher-Collins syndrome, several monogenic cleft lip and/or palate syndromes
METABOLIC PHENOTYPE	
Metabolite alteration	
Substrate restriction	
Phenylalanine	Phenylketonuria
Branched-chain amino acids	Maple syrup urine disease
Galactose	Galactosemia
Fructose	Hereditary fructose intolerance
Lactose	Lactase deficiency
Phytanic acid	Refsum's disease
Alternative pathway utilization	
Benzoate and phenylacetate	Urea cycle disorders
Glycine	Isovaleric acidemia
Carnitine	Organic acidosis
Cysteamine	Cystinosis
Penicillamine	Wilson's disease
Metabolic inhibition	
Allopurinol	Gout
Mevinolin	Familial hypercholesterolemia
Replacement of deficient products	
Glucose polymers (cornstarch)	Glycogen storage disease, types I and III
Uridine	Hereditary orotic aciduria
Glucocorticoids	Congenital adrenal hyperplasia
Thyroxine	Familial goiter
Biotin	Biotinidase deficiency
Protein alteration	
Activation of the mutant protein	
Pyridoxine (vitamin B_6)	Homocystinuria
Thiamine	Maple syrup urine disease
Hydroxycobalamin (vitamin B_{12})	Some forms of methylmalonic acidemia
Replacement of the mutant protein	
Growth hormone	Growth hormone deficiency
Factor VIII	Classic hemophilia
α_1-Antitrypsin	α_1-Antitrypsin deficiency
Polyethylene glycol-adenosine deaminase	Adenosine deaminase deficiency
Mannose-terminated glucocerebrosidase	Gaucher's disease
Organ transplantation	
As a source for a specific protein	
Allogeneic bone marrow	Lysosomal storage diseases, β thalassemia
Liver	Glycogen storage disease, type I, familial hypercholesterolemia, ornithine transcarbamylase deficiency
As a protein source and replacement of damaged organ	
Liver	α_1-Antitrypsin deficiency, hepatorenal tyrosinemia
Kidney	Cystinosis

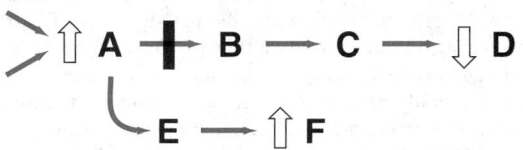

FIGURE 67-1 Pathophysiologic consequences of a genetic defect in a metabolic pathway. Substrate A is converted via a series of intermediates to a final product, D. The enzymes catalyzing these reactions are indicated by the horizontal arrows. A also is converted to F in an alternative pathway. Genetic deficiency of the enzyme converting A to B (indicated by the hatched rectangle) may have pathophysiologic consequences related to accumulation of A (precursor toxicity), overflow to F (alternative pathway overflow), reduced formation of D (product deficiency), or some combination of these possibilities.

involve *distant* biochemical effects as a consequence of perturbations of metabolite concentrations in the extracellular fluid. For example, the neurologic phenotype of Tay Sachs disease results from destruction of neurons caused by local deficiency of hexosaminidase A, whereas the mental retardation of untreated phenylketonuria due to deficiency of hepatic phenylalanine hydroxylase is a distant consequence of the systemic accumulation of phenylalanine.

PRECURSOR TOXICITY Correction of precursor toxicity frequently involves dietary restriction of a substrate whose major source is nutritional. Inborn errors of amino acid and carbohydrate metabolism are examples of this approach. A diet restricted in the branched-chain amino acids (leucine, isoleucine, valine) is effective in preventing the mental retardation associated with maple syrup urine disease caused by deficiency of branched-chain ketoacid decarboxylase (see Chap. 349). Such diets should be started soon after birth, continued for life, and monitored so that intake of these essential amino acids is just sufficient for normal growth. Illnesses that cause protein catabolism (e.g., those associated with intercurrent infections or trauma) periodically complicate this therapy by releasing large amounts of the offending amino acids from the breakdown of endogenous protein. These episodes may require hospitalization for administration of intravenous fluids or dialysis. Similarly, lifetime restriction of dietary galactose in patients with galactosemia due to deficiency of galactose-1-phosphate uridyl transferase corrects growth failure, prevents cataracts, and improves intellectual outcome (see Chap. 351).

ALTERNATIVE PATHWAY UTILIZATION For some disorders, alternative metabolic pathways may be utilized to remove toxic metabolites. The effectiveness of this approach is limited by the capacity of the alternative pathway and often must be combined with dietary restriction of the offending substrate. Administration of benzoate and phenylacetate to patients with inborn errors of urea metabolism is a good example of this approach. These compounds are conjugated with endogenous glycine and glutamine, forming hippurate and phenylacetylglutamine, respectively. When used in conjunction with restriction of dietary protein, this therapy reduces the accumulation of ammonia in patients with inborn errors of the urea cycle and organic acid metabolism. Similar approaches include the administration of carnitine, which conjugates with a variety of accumulated coenzyme A (CoA) esters, to patients with defects of organic acid metabolism; cysteamine, which helps to eliminate excess cystine in cystinosis; and penicillamine to reduce excessive stores of copper in Wilson's disease and iron in hemochromatosis.

INHIBITION OF AN OVERACTIVE PATHWAY For other disorders, particularly those in which alternative pathway overflow produces a toxic level of a particular metabolite, it may be possible to prevent the accumulation by inhibiting an enzyme in the affected pathway. This approach may lead to accumulation of upstream substrates that must be well tolerated if the treatment is to be successful. For instance, in gout and other disorders in which excessive purine degradation leads to uric acid accumulation, inhibition of xanthine oxidase by allopurinol reduces uric acid production and lowers the

incidence of uric acid nephropathy and gouty arthritis. Xanthine, which accumulates as a consequence, has greater aqueous solubility than uric acid and usually is well tolerated. In a similar fashion, hypercholesterolemic patients heterozygous for mutations of the low-density lipoprotein (LDL) receptor exhibit significant reductions in plasma cholesterol when treated with lovastatin, a drug that acts in part to inhibit hydroxymethylglutaryl CoA reductase that catalyzes an early, rate-limiting step in the synthesis of cholesterol (see Chap. 341).

PRODUCT DEFICIT For disorders in which the pathophysiology involves product deficit, nutritional or pharmacologic approaches to replenishing the product can be effective if the administered material reaches the appropriate physiologic compartment. For example, many of the inborn errors in hormone biosynthesis such as the various forms of congenital adrenal hyperplasia and hereditary defects in thyroid hormone biosynthesis respond well to pharmacologic replacement of the deficient hormones. By contrast, the administration of melanin to patients with albinism would not correct the pigment deficit in melanocytes.

Treatment Directed to the Protein Phenotype Therapy at the level of dysfunctional protein involves either activation or replacement of the mutant protein.

ACTIVATION OF THE MUTANT PROTEIN Activation may be possible if the protein requires a vitamin cofactor and the vitamin is one that is well tolerated in pharmacologic doses. Obviously, not all mutations of a gene encoding a vitamin-dependent protein will respond. Those that do are likely to be missense mutations that either decrease the affinity of an enzyme for its cofactor or destabilize a protein in a way that can be partially overcome by substantial increments in cofactor concentration. About one-third of the cases of homocystinuria due to deficiency of the pyridoxal phosphate–requiring enzyme cystathione-β-synthase exhibit a significant increment in the activity when treated with pharmacologic doses (50 to 500 mg/d) of pyridoxine (vitamin B_6). The actual increase in enzyme activity may be small, but it suffices to improve metabolic flux in the impaired pathway. Since activation of residual activity both reduces precursor accumulation and increases product formation, knowledge of the pathophysiologic mechanism is less critical for this form of treatment.

PROTEIN REPLACEMENT THERAPIES An alternative approach involves replacement with an exogenous supply of the protein. To be efficacious, the protein must be administered directly into or reach the appropriate physiologic compartment. Thus blood proteins or proteins that traverse the vascular compartment (e.g., peptide hormones) are candidates for this approach. Other considerations include the availability, stability, and immunogenicity of the protein. In some instances, the administered protein may be modified to enhance stability and/or targeting to the appropriate cell or tissue. For example, linkage of adenosine deaminase to polyethylene glycol increases stability, and partial deglycosylation of glucocerebrosidase exposes mannose residues on the surface of the protein that target it to macrophages via the mannose receptor. Recombinant DNA technology can frequently be utilized to supply sufficient amounts of the pure protein (e.g., human growth hormone, α_1-antitrypsin, and glucocerebrosidase). This advance ensures an adequate supply and avoids the risk of transmission of pathologic viruses contaminating protein purified from natural sources.

Organ Transplantation Organ transplantation is on the borderline between therapy at the level of the dysfunctional protein and gene therapy. On the one hand, a transplanted organ supplies a deficient protein; on the other, the transplant tissue also brings new genetic information which, in contrast to standard models of gene therapy, is not integrated into the recipient's genome. Kidney, liver, and bone marrow transplantation are utilized for a variety of genetic diseases. The development of more effective and specific immunosuppressants (cyclosporine and tacrolimus) and the inadequacy of many less invasive therapies account, in part, for the increased utilization of this form of treatment. In some instances, the goal of transplantation is to supply a tissue that can replace a mutant protein (e.g., liver transplant for deficiency of LDL receptor or one of the urea cycle enzymes). For other disorders (e.g., α_1-antitrypsin deficiency or hepatorenal tyrosinemia), the transplant both provides the protein and replaces a damaged organ. The pathophysiologic mechanism of the disease is relevant; the physician must consider if the newly supplied protein will only be used locally or, if not, will gain access to the involved tissue(s). The long-term efficacy and consequences of organ transplantation as treatment for genetic disorders remain to be determined.

Prospects for Gene Therapy Several methods are now available for introducing new genetic material into mammalian cells. These methods allow consideration of a more direct approach to treatment of genetic disease, namely, gene therapy or introduction of a functional gene to replace or supplement the activity of a resident defective gene. Typically, two strategies have been considered, germ-line and somatic cell gene therapy, which differ in the nature of the recipient cells. In the germ-line model, foreign DNA is introduced into the zygote or early embryo with the expectation that the newly introduced material will contribute to the germ line of the recipient, i.e., be passed on to the next generation. By contrast, in somatic gene therapy models, genetic material is introduced only into somatic cells and is not transmitted to the germ cells. A third approach to gene therapy involves activation of endogenous genes to augment or circumvent a defective gene. The use of hydroxyurea to increase fetal globulin synthesis for treatment of patients with β-hemoglobulinopathies is an excellent example of this strategy.

Much of the technology for germ-line gene therapy has been developed in transgenic mice. Fertilized mouse eggs are harvested from a superovulated female, microinjected with DNA molecules, and reimplanted in a pseudopregnant female. Several murine genetic diseases, including deficiency of growth hormone, myelin basic protein, and β-globin, have been "treated" in this fashion with the general result that the disease phenotype is markedly ameliorated.

These experiments have provided considerable information on the regulation of gene expression and the pathogenesis of genetic disease. However, the method is inefficient: Only 15 to 20 percent of injected eggs produce transgenic animals, and of these, only 20 to 30 percent actually express the introduced gene. Furthermore, there are appreciable risks, including damage to a resident gene by the random insertion of the foreign DNA (insertional mutagenesis), resulting in loss of function or aberrant regulation that can lead to cancer. For clinical medicine, availability of the molecular reagents necessary for attempting germ-line gene therapy would also make it possible to do prenatal diagnosis. The certainty of having an unaffected child as established by prenatal diagnosis is preferable to the uncertainty and risks of the transgenic approach. Thus, germ-line gene therapy is not applicable to human genetic disease.

In contrast, trials of somatic gene therapy for human genetic disease are underway. The methods for introducing the genetic material and the recipient cells vary, depending, in part, on the disease to be treated. The repertoire of delivery systems includes viral vectors (replication-deficient retrovirus, adenovirus, adeno-associated virus, herpes virus, and others) and nonviral systems such as liposomes, DNA-protein conjugates, and DNA-protein-defective virus conjugates. Delivery of the genetic material can be done ex vivo by introducing the genetic material into cultured cells that are then administered to the recipient. Alternatively, delivery can be done in vivo by transferring the gene and its vector directly to cells in the individual (Fig. 67-2). The latter method avoids problems of reintroducing adequate numbers of cells to a congenial and effective site in the patient. The former is still attractive for strategies that involve delivery to bone marrow stem cells and other cells that can be cultured ex vivo in large numbers. For both ex vivo and in vivo approaches it is important to consider the quantitative aspects of gene therapy. How much expression is required to ameliorate or correct the disease phenotype, and will the expression per transduced cell and number of transduced cells be adequate to achieve a therapeutic effect?

Viral vectors are being utilized for most trials of somatic gene therapy. Each has advantages and disadvantages. Replication-deficient retroviral vectors provide efficient integration of foreign DNA and permanent alteration of the recipient cell. However, they target

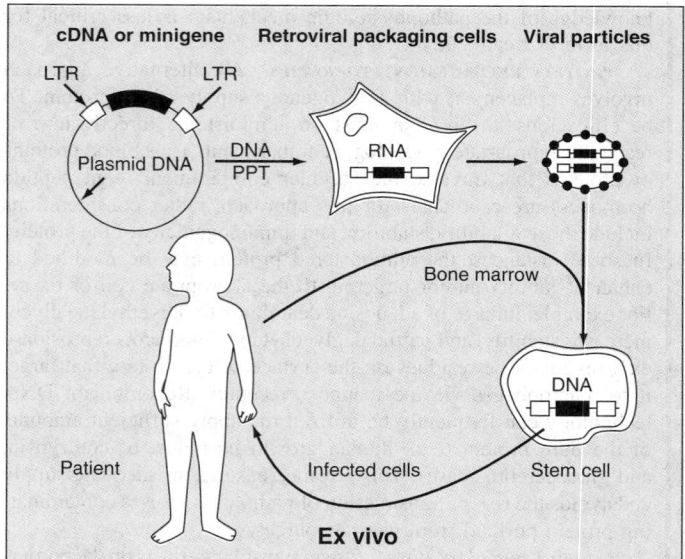

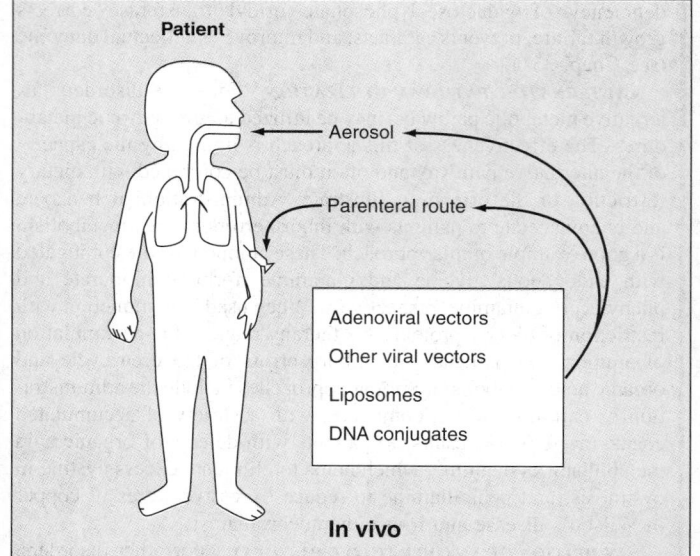

FIGURE 67-2 Comparison of ex vivo and in vivo strategies for somatic gene therapy. A procedure for ex vivo retroviral infection of bone marrow stem cells is shown on the left. On the right, this is compared to delivery by inhalation of aerosol for a disease such as cystic fibrosis or parenteral injection for targeting to organs such as liver or muscle using a variety of vectors or delivery systems. (*Courtesy of Arthur Beaudet, MD.*)

only dividing cells, have the risk of producing insertional mutations, and yield relatively low titers of recombinant virus, and the expression of the delivered gene often declines to unmeasurable levels over several months. Adenoviral vectors efficiently transfer genes to both dividing and nondividing cells, do not integrate and yield high titers of recombinant vector and high levels of expression of the introduced gene(s). However, the adenovirus vectors currently in use invoke nonspecific inflammation and antiviral cellular immunity responses, which limit expression to weeks or months. Thus, the viral vectors currently in use have major drawbacks. Considerable improvements in these and other vector systems will be necessary to make somatic gene therapy effective.

The number of candidate disorders for somatic gene therapy is expanding. The lessons learned from experience with conventional therapies will apply to gene therapy and should be considered for each candidate disorder. The importance of early intervention before the development of irreversible damage, consideration of the pathophysiologic mechanisms, and the need for regulated interactions of the product of the introduced gene with other members of the involved homeostatic system are all relevant. In addition to monogenic disorders, trials of somatic gene therapy are in progress for cancer, AIDS, and other disorders. The strategies under investigation for cancer include (1) alteration of cancer cells or other host cells to produce cytokines or other molecules to alter the host response to the malignancy; (2) expression of antigens (e.g., allogenic HLA proteins) on cancer cells to induce a host immune response; (3) insertion of tumor suppressor gene sequences or other sequences to slow cell growth; and (4) introduction of drug resistance genes into normal cells (e.g., bone marrow) to facilitate more aggressive chemotherapy. The first two immunomodulatory approaches are the basis of several current research protocols.

The ultimate contribution of somatic gene therapy to treatment of genetic disease and other disorders is unclear. After a detailed review of the field, it was concluded that the method has great promise but that considerable additional research is required to make gene therapy effective.

EVALUATION OF THERAPY FOR GENETIC DISEASE

Two general questions should be posed in an evaluation of therapy for a genetic disease. First, does the treatment provide therapeutic benefit? Second, does the treatment restore the patient to normality? These questions can be asked of any disease treatment but have special significance for genetic disorders that are predictable and preventable. In 1983 Costa, Scriver, and Childs evaluated the effect of therapy of 351 representative monogenic disorders on three basic variables: life span, reproductive capacity, and social adaptation; in their study, available therapies returned life span to normal in 15 percent, allowed reproductive capability in 11 percent, and improved social adaptation in 6 percent of the disorders. Slightly better outcomes were found with a subset of 65 diseases in which the basic defect is known. In a reexamination of the effect of treatment for the same 65 genetic diseases 10 years later, Treacy et al. found that therapy corrected all manifestations in 12 percent, was partially effective in 57 percent, and had no effect in 31 percent. Thus, the ability to treat genetic disease has improved but is still poor. It is hoped that increased understanding of the pathophysiology of specific diseases, in particular from study of disease models in "knockout" mice, and continued advances in gene therapy will result in substantial progress to treat genetic diseases in the future. Nevertheless, the slow rate of progress to date and recognition of the complexity of the problem make it clear that preventive measures for genetic disease should have high priority.

PREVENTION OF GENETIC DISEASE

Recognition of the limitation of therapy in genetic disease plus the predictability of the pattern of transmission of genes from one generation to the next have focused attention on prevention as the most reliable and effective means of dealing with hereditary disorders. The preventive approach includes genetic screening, counseling, and prenatal diagnosis.

GENETIC SCREENING There are two types of genetic screening programs for autosomal recessive disorders: Homozygote screening programs search for individuals who have the disorder; by contrast, heterozygote screening programs search for individuals who are carriers of a mutant gene and thus are at risk of having offspring with a particular disorder. Successful homozygote screening programs require an inexpensive and reliable test, the recognition of some benefit (treatment, counseling) of early diagnosis, and education of the individuals and/or families screened so that they understand the significance of the results. The best example of such programs are the newborn screening programs. The diseases screened vary from state to state but include phenylketonuria, homocystinuria, maple syrup urine disease, galactosemia, cystic fibrosis, hypothyroidism, and sickle cell disease. In each instance, the screening test allows early detection and the opportunity to initiate appropriate therapy prior to the onset of irreversible damage. Also, the parents of an affected individual are made aware of the risk to future offspring and have the option of prenatal diagnosis. Heterozygote screening programs are best exemplified by the program to detect carriers of Tay Sachs disease, a fatal autosomal recessive lysosomal storage disease for which there is no effective treatment. Heterozygote screening of defined subpopulations with an increased carrier frequency (e.g., Ashkenazi Jews, in whom the carrier frequency is approximately 1/25 as compared with approximately 1/200 in Anglo Saxons) identifies couples at risk in which both potential parents are heterozygotes with a 25 percent chance of having an affected child. Prenatal diagnosis is possible, and the procedure provides a means for the couple to have unaffected children.

GENETIC COUNSELING With the rapid growth in the general appreciation of the role of genes in disease, the demand for genetic counseling has increased. Individuals concerned about their own risk for a genetic disorder or about the risk of genetic disease in their offspring come to the physician with questions. Thus, all physicians should be familiar with the principles of medical genetics and use this knowledge to counsel patients. This effort may involve other professionals such as genetic counselors and medical geneticists who may perform the initial counseling with subsequent reinforcement and review provided by the personal physician.

Couples may be identified as being at increased risk for having a child with a genetic disease because of a previously affected child or other close relative. Alternatively, one or both parents may belong to a known high-risk group (e.g., identified as a carrier in a heterozygote screening test), or there may be advanced maternal age (35 years or greater at the time of delivery) with increased risk for an autosomal trisomy.

One aspect of genetic counseling involves determination of the risk for having an affected child and communication of this risk to the prospective parents so that they can make informed reproductive decisions. If a family member is affected with a genetic disease, the initial step is to assess the reliability of the diagnosis. This usually requires critical examination of existing medical data and/or additional evaluation of affected family member(s). The information is then assembled in the format of the family pedigree to determine the pattern of transmission within the family and to compare it with that expected for the diagnosed condition. Depending on the type of disease (monogenic, multifactorial, or chromosomal) and the reliability of the diagnosis, the risk to subsequent offspring may be predicted with a degree of certainty ranging from a rough estimate to nearly perfect. The reliability of the diagnosis will be influenced by whether multiple etiologies exist for a particular phenotype and the availability of specific diagnostic tests. Molecular tests that directly and unambiguously determine the parental genotype are sometimes available and allow precise prediction of the risk of recurrence and prenatal diagnosis for some monogenic disorders (see Chap. 65). For autosomal recessive and

X-linked disorders in which a primary biochemical defect is known, reliable diagnosis is possible by a functional test of the gene product (e.g., assay of enzyme activity). For many autosomal dominant disorders, the primary biochemical defect is not known, and the parental diagnosis is uncertain because of variable expressivity. Availability of linked molecular markers, e.g., restriction fragment length polymorphisms, and identification of the responsible genes greatly improves the reliability and precision of counseling for these conditions.

Counseling for many common multifactorial disorders (e.g., diabetes mellitus, hypertension, atherosclerosis, congenital malformations, and psychiatric disorders) is imperfect and will be so until we have a better understanding of the interactions of the various genes and environmental factors that produce these diseases. In some families the etiology may involve a major contribution of a single gene, and in others a mix of multiple genes and environmental factors is the cause. In the former the risk may be predicted by a monogenic model, while in the latter no simple model suffices. In these instances, the counselor must resort to empiric risk estimates derived from retrospectively assembled data based on the average outcome in many different families.

The risk, the prognosis, and the treatment of the disorder should be discussed, and the availability of prenatal diagnosis and carrier testing should be presented. Finally, the counselor must be sensitive to the emotional impact this information may have on those counseled.

During the counseling session, effective communication of the information depends on expressing the essentials in language understandable to those being counseled. Written notes and diagrams frequently are helpful and can be handed over at the end of the session. Finally, summary letters and reviews at subsequent visits help correct misconceptions and increase retention of the information. In this regard, the referring physician who has an established relationship with the family can reinforce information presented by a counselor who meets with the subjects on only one or two occasions.

PRENATAL DIAGNOSIS Following genetic counseling, the couple at risk for having a child with a genetic disease has several options depending, in part, on the type of disorder. They may feel reassured and proceed, despite the risk, without any subsequent monitoring. Or they may view the risks as too high and choose to have no additional children or to adopt. Alternatively, when both parents are heterozygous for an autosomal recessive disorder, they may choose to reduce the risk by utilizing artificial insemination by donor or donor eggs. The magnitude of the decrease in the risk provided by this option will depend on the carrier frequency for the particular disorder in the general population. For a couple with a 1 in 4, or 25 percent, chance of having a child with phenylketonuria, the risk with donor insemination will drop to 1 in 260 ($1 \times \frac{1}{65} \times \frac{1}{4}$), because the carrier frequency in the general population is 1 in 65. When mutant alleles for the gene in question are preferentially associated with particular linked markers (linkage disequilibrium) or if there is a prevalent mutant allele(s) in the population, it is possible to reduce the risk by prescreening the donors.

Finally, if the disorder can be detected antenatally, the couple may decide to proceed with reproduction and utilize prenatal diagnosis with elective abortion of affected fetuses. Because the risk of having an affected fetus ranges from a maximum of 50 percent for heterozygotes with autosomal dominant disorders to less than 10 percent for nearly all chromosomal and multifactorial disorders, the majority of pregnancies monitored by prenatal diagnosis have an unaffected fetus. This relatively low frequency of affected fetuses, together with an increase in reproductive activity which often results from the reassurance provided by the availability of prenatal diagnosis, leads to significant increases in the family size of at-risk couples. Thus, in contrast to some public misconceptions, availability of prenatal diagnosis actually results in increased numbers of offspring. Prenatal diagnosis is indicated when the risk of having an affected child is greater than the risk of the procedure (Table 67-2).

Table 67-2

Major Indications for Prenatal Diagnosis

Indication	Risk for Affected Fetus, %	Method of Detection
CHROMOSOMAL DISORDERS		
Advanced maternal age (≥ 35 y)	1–10 depending on maternal age	Chromosomal analysis of cells obtained by CVS* or amniocentesis
Parent with a balanced translocation	3–20 depending on the translocation	
Previous child with chromosomal abnormality	~1	
MONOGENIC DISORDERS		
Couple at risk for having a child with an autosomal recessive inborn error of metabolism	25	Biochemical and/or molecular analysis of cells obtained by CVS or amniocentesis
Couple at risk for having a child with a monogenic disorder for which molecular markers are available	25–50	Molecular analysis of DNA obtained from cells obtained by CVS or by amniocentesis
Couple at risk for having a child with a monogenic malformation syndrome without biochemical or molecular markers	25–50	Fetal imaging by ultrasound
MALFORMATION DISORDERS		
Couples at risk for having a child with a neural tube defect (anencephaly or meningomyelocele) or other multifactorial malformation syndrome	1–10	Fetal imaging by ultrasound and, for neural tube defects, measurement of alpha fetoprotein and other fetal markers in amniotic fluid obtained by amniocentesis

* CVS, chorionic villus sampling

Several methods for prenatal diagnosis are available (Table 67-3). Choice of a method depends on the disorder in question and on family preferences. Measurement of alpha fetoprotein (AFP) and other proteins in maternal serum is noninvasive and can be used to screen pregnancies for neural tube defects (increased maternal serum AFP) and for fetal aneuploidies (decreased maternal serum AFP). Ultrasonography can be used to visualize many fetal malformations and growth abnormalities and to monitor invasive fetal sampling techniques, with attendant reduction in the risks of the procedures. Second-trimester (15 to 16 weeks of gestation) fetal sampling by amniocentesis is widely used for obtaining fetal cells, and early amniocentesis at 12 to 14 weeks of gestation is available at some centers. Transcervical and transabdominal chorionic villus sampling (CVS) also provides fetal cells and can be performed at 10 to 12 weeks of gestation. CVS has the advantage of allowing the diagnosis to be made earlier, and if an abortion is chosen, it will take place at a stage of pregnancy when maternal-fetal bonding is less. Elective abortion at 12 weeks of gestation is a 2- to 3-h outpatient procedure, whereas a second-trimester elective abortion requires a 1- to 3-day hospitalization. The risks of CVS in experienced hands appear to compare well with those of amniocentesis, although in many centers the rate of miscarriages is slightly increased. The tissue obtained at CVS is fetal trophoblastic tissue, expresses nearly all enzymes found in amniocytes, and provides an excellent source of fetal DNA. Preimplantation prenatal diagnosis by molecular methods applied to a single cell removed from an 8-cell embryo produced by in vitro fertilization has been used successfully for a small number of monogenic disorders including cystic fibrosis and Tay Sachs disease. This method has the advantage that affected

Table 67-3

Methods of Prenatal Diagnosis

Method	Stage of Gestation, Weeks	Sample	Fetal Disorders	Risks
Maternal serum sampling	15–18	Alpha fetoprotein and other fetal proteins	Neural tube defects, aneuploidies	Negligible
Fetal ultrasonography	6–40	Image	Fetal dating, morphologic abnormalities, skeletal dysplasis	Negligible
Fetal sampling				
Chorionic villus sampling	9–12	Fetal trophoblastic tissue	Cytogenetic, biochemical, molecular	1–2% fetal loss
Amniocentesis	15–18	Amniotic fluid and cells	Cytogenetic, biochemical, molecular, neural tube defects	0.2–0.5% fetal loss
Fetal biopsy	18–20	Fetal skin	Dermatologic	~2% fetal loss
		Fetal liver	Liver-specific, enzyme deficiencies	2–5% fetal loss
		Umbilical cord, blood	Blood disorders	~2% fetal loss

embryos are not returned to the mother, obviating the need for abortion. However, the technique requires induction of ovulation and collection of eggs for in vitro fertilization and return of the normal embryos to the mother's uterus. These techniques are expensive and inefficient and require additional study to determine their reliability and risk.

BIBLIOGRAPHY

CHARACHE S et al: Effect of hydroxyurea on the frequency of painful crises in sickle cell anemia. N Engl J Med 332:1317, 1995

COSTA T et al: The effect of mendelian disease on human health: A measurement. Am J Hum Genet 21:231, 1985

CRYSTAL RG: Transfer of genes to humans: Early lessons and obstacles to success. Science 270:404, 1995

HARRISON MR et al: The Unborn Patient: Prenatal Diagnosis and Treatment, 2d ed. Philadelphia, Saunders, 1991

MARSHALL E: Gene therapy's growing pains. Science 269:1050, 1995

SCRIVER CR et al (eds): The Metabolic and Molecular Bases of Inherited Disease, 7th ed. New York, McGraw-Hill, 1995

TREACY E et al: Response to treatment in hereditary metabolic disease: 1993 survey and 10-year comparison. Am J Hum Genet 56:359, 1995

68   *John A. Oates, Grant R. Wilkinson*

PRINCIPLES OF
DRUG THERAPY

QUANTITATIVE DETERMINANTS
OF DRUG ACTION

Safe and effective drug therapy requires that drugs be delivered to their target tissues in concentrations within the range that yields efficacy without toxicity. Optimal precision in achieving concentrations of drug within this therapeutic "window" can be achieved with regimens that are based on the kinetics of the drug's availability to target sites. This chapter deals with the principles of drug elimination and distribution that form the basis for loading and maintenance regimens for the average patient and considers instances in which elimination of the drug is impaired (e.g., renal failure). The basis for optimal utilization of plasma level data is also discussed.

PLASMA LEVELS AFTER A SINGLE DOSE   The levels of lidocaine in plasma following intravenous administration decline in two phases, as illustrated in Fig. 68-1; such a biphasic decline is typical for many drugs. Immediately after rapid injection, essentially all of the drug is in the plasma or central compartment, and the high initial plasma level (Cp_0) reflects the confinement of the drug to this small volume. The drug is then transferred into an extravascular or peripheral compartment during a period called the *distribution phase*. For lidocaine, the distribution phase is virtually complete within 30 min. A phase of slower decline, the *equilibrium phase* or *elimination phase*, then occurs. During this phase, the drug levels in the plasma and in tissues change in parallel. Although this disposition profile is common to many drugs given intravenously, the characteristic parameters vary among drugs.

Distribution Phase   The pharmacologic events during the distribution phase depend on whether the level of drug at the receptor site is similar to that in the plasma. If that is the case, the pharmacologic effects, whether favorable or adverse, may be intense during this period because of the high initial levels in the plasma. For example, after a small bolus dose (50 mg) of lidocaine, antiarrhythmic effects may be evident during the early distribution phase, but they will disappear as levels fall below those which are minimally effective, even before equilibrium between plasma and tissue is reached. Thus, a larger single

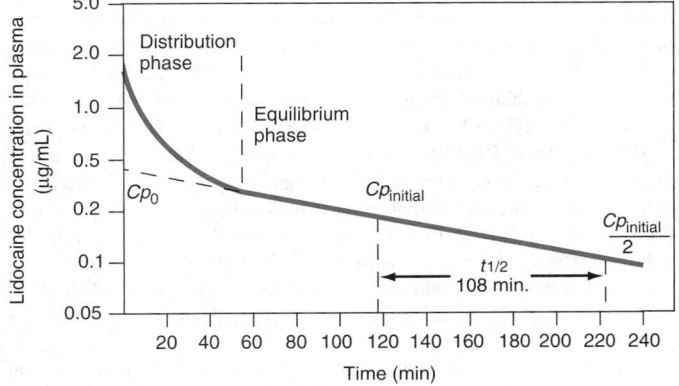

FIGURE 68-1   Concentrations of lidocaine in plasma following the administration of 50 mg intravenously. The half-life ($t_{1/2}$) of 108 min is computed as the time required for levels to fall from any given value during the equilibrium phase ($Cp_{initial}$) to one-half that level. Cp_0 is the hypothetical concentration of lidocaine in plasma at time zero if equilibrium had been achieved instantly.

dose or multiple small doses must be administered to achieve an effect that is sustained into the equilibrium phase. Toxicity resulting from high levels of some drugs during the distribution phase precludes administration of a single intravenous loading dose that will yield therapeutic levels during the equilibrium phase. For example, the administration of the entire loading dose of phenytoin as a single intravenous bolus can cause cardiovascular collapse due to the high levels during the distribution phase. If a loading dose of phenytoin is administered intravenously, it must be given in fractions at intervals sufficient to permit substantial distribution between doses (e.g., 100 mg every 3 to 5 min). For similar reasons, the intravenous loading dose of many potent drugs that equilibrate rapidly with their receptors either is divided into fractional doses given at intervals or administered by infusion over a similar period.

A dose given orally results in lower plasma levels during the initial period than an intravenous bolus dose that delivers the same amount of drug to the systemic circulation. Because the drug is not absorbed instantly after oral administration and is delivered into the systemic circulation more slowly, much of it has been distributed by the time absorption is complete. Thus, procainamide, which is almost totally absorbed after oral administration, can be given orally as a single 750-mg loading dose with little risk of hypotension; in contrast, loading of this drug by the intravenous route is more safely accomplished by giving the dose in fractions of about 100 mg at 5-min intervals or by slow infusion to avoid hypotension during the distribution phase.

In contrast, some drugs are distributed slowly to their sites of action during the distribution phase. For example, the level of digoxin at the receptor site (and the drug's pharmacologic effect) do not reflect plasma levels during the distribution phase. Digoxin is transported (or bound) to its cardiac receptors slowly by a process that proceeds throughout distribution. Thus, over the distribution phase of several hours, plasma levels fall while the level at the site of action and the pharmacologic effect increase. Only at the end of the distribution phase, when the drug has reached equilibrium with the receptor, does the concentration of digoxin in plasma reflect pharmacologic effect. For this reason, there should be a 6- to 8-h wait after administration before plasma levels of digoxin are measured as a guide to therapy.

Equilibrium Phase   After the concentration of drug in plasma has reached a dynamic equilibrium with that in the tissues, the levels in plasma and tissues fall in parallel as the drug is eliminated from the body. Thus, the *equilibrium phase* is also called the *elimination phase*. During this phase, drug concentrations measured in plasma provide the best index of drug levels in tissues.

Most drugs are eliminated as a first-order process. This means that the time required for the plasma level of the drug to fall to one-half the original value (the half-life, $t_{1/2}$) is the same regardless of the point on the plasma level curve at which measurement begins. Another characteristic of the first-order process is that a semilogarithmic plot of plasma concentration versus time is linear. From such a plot (Fig. 68-1), it can be seen that the half-life of lidocaine is 108 min.

If the half-life is known, one can calculate the amount of a dose remaining in the body at any time following administration. Table 68-1 shows how this amount changes over five successive half-lives. From a clinical standpoint, elimination is essentially complete when it has reached about 90 percent. Therefore, for practical purposes, *a first-order elimination process reaches completion after three to four half-lives.*

DRUG ACCUMULATION—LOADING AND MAINTE-NANCE DOSES   If a drug is given repeatedly at intervals shorter than the time required to eliminate a dose, both the amount of drug in the body and its pharmacologic effect increase with successive doses until they reach a plateau. Figure 68-2 shows the accumulation

Table 68-1

Amount of a Drug Dose Remaining in Body over Successive Half-Lives

No. of Elapsed Half-Lives	Amount of Dose Remaining in Body, %	Amount of Dose Eliminated, %
1	50	50
2	25	75
3	12.5	87.5
4	6.25	93.75
5	3.125	96.875

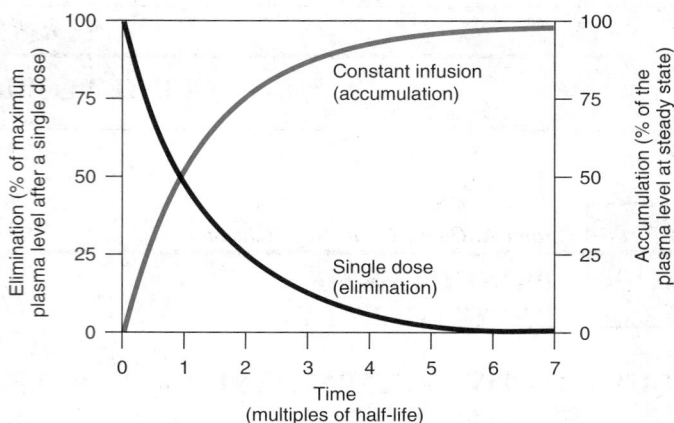

FIGURE 68-3 The time course of plasma levels of a drug following a single intravenous dose compared with those during a constant intravenous infusion. This relationship applies to all drugs that rapidly achieve equilibrium between plasma and tissues.

of digoxin administered in repeated maintenance doses (without a loading dose). Since the half-life of digoxin is about 1.6 days in a patient with normal renal function, 65 percent of a digoxin dose remains in the body at the end of 1 day. Thus, the second dose will raise the amount of digoxin in the body (and the average plasma level) to 165 percent of the level produced by the first dose. Each subsequent dose causes a further increase until a *steady state* is achieved. At that point, the drug intake per unit of time is the same as the rate of elimination, with the fluctuation between peak and trough plasma levels remaining constant. If the rate of drug delivery is then altered, a new steady state will be attained. Continuous infusion of a drug at constant rate also results in progressive accumulation to a predictable steady state (Fig. 68-3). In this case, the steady state plasma level (Cp_{ss}) is intermediate between the peak and trough levels produced by intermittent administration of the same amount of drug over the same period. For *all* drugs with first-order kinetics, the time required to achieve steady state levels can be predicted from the half-life, because accumulation is a first-order process with a half-life identical to that for elimination. Thus, accumulation reaches 90 percent of steady state levels at the end of three to four half-lives. This is true for either intermittent or continuous dosing (Fig. 68-3).

The time required to reach the steady state may be shortened by the administration of a *loading dose*—an amount of drug that will bring the equilibrium plasma concentration rapidly to the steady state level. The loading dose can be estimated if both the desired plasma level (Cp_{ss}) and the extent of the drug's extravascular distribution at equilibrium (the apparent volume of distribution V_d) are known:

$$\text{Loading dose} = \text{desired plasma level}$$
$$\times \text{ volume of distribution at steady state}$$
$$= Cp_{ss} \times V_d$$

Loading may be accomplished by the administration of a single loading dose or, if that would create a risk of toxicity, by the administration

of the loading amount in a series of fractions. The latter approach is appropriate for most drugs that have a low therapeutic index. (The *therapeutic index* is the ratio of the toxic dose to the therapeutic dose.) This approach permits better individualization of the loading amount and minimizes adverse effects.

The loading amount required to achieve steady state plasma levels also can be determined from the fraction of drug eliminated during the dosing interval and the maintenance dose (in the case of intermittent drug administration). For example, if the fraction of digoxin eliminated daily is 35 percent and the planned maintenance dose is 0.25 mg daily, then the loading dose to achieve steady state levels should be 100/35 times the maintenance dose, or approximately 0.75 mg. Thus,

$$\text{Loading dose} = \frac{100}{\substack{\% \text{ of drug eliminated} \\ \text{per dosage interval}}} \times \text{maintenance dose}$$

The fraction of drug eliminated during any dosing interval can be determined from a semilogarithmic graph in which the total amount in the body at time zero is set at 100 percent and the fraction remaining at the end of one half-life is 50 percent.[1]

To calculate a loading dose that will achieve the steady state plasma concentration of a known infusion rate,

$$\text{Loading dose} = \frac{\text{infusion rate}}{k}$$

where k is the fractional elimination constant that describes the rate of drug elimination.[1]

Regardless of the size of the loading dose, *after maintenance therapy has been given for three to four half-lives, the amount of drug in the body is determined by the maintenance dose.* The independence of the steady state plasma levels from the loading dose is illustrated in Fig. 68-3, which shows that the elimination of the loading dose would be practically complete after three to four half-lives.

DETERMINANTS OF PLASMA LEVELS DURING THE EQUILIBRIUM PHASE An important determinant of the level of drug in plasma during the equilibrium phase after a single dose is the extent to which the drug is distributed outside the plasma compartment. For example, if the distribution of a 3-mg dose of a large macromolecule is confined to a plasma volume of 3 L, then the concentration in plasma will be 1 mg/L. However, if a different drug is distributed so that 90 percent of it leaves the plasma compartment, then only 0.3

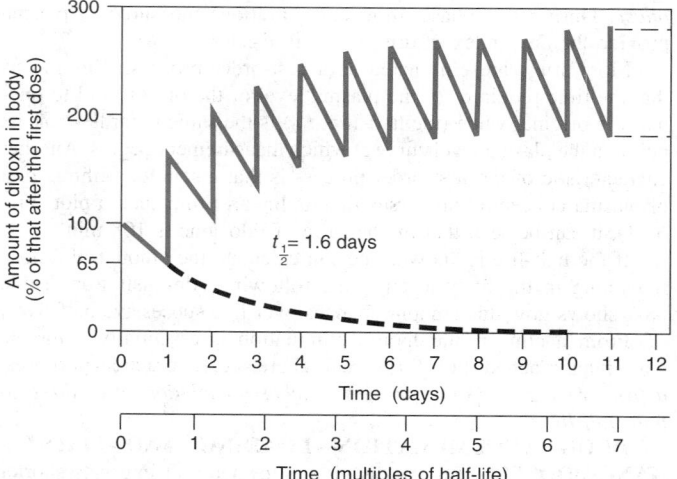

FIGURE 68-2 The time course of digoxin accumulation when a single daily maintenance dose is given without a loading dose. Note that accumulation is more than 90 percent complete by the end of four half-lives.

---

[1] Alternatively, the fraction of drug lost from the body during a dosage interval can be determined nongraphically from the following equation:

$$\text{Fraction of drug lost from body} = 1 - e^{-kt}$$

Values for e^{-kt} can be obtained from a table of natural exponential functions or by a calculator, where $k = (0.693/t_{1/2})$ is the fractional elimination constant (described in the next section) and t is the time interval after drug administration.

mg will remain in the 3-L plasma volume, and the concentration in plasma will be only 0.1 mg/L. The *apparent volume of distribution* V_d expresses the relationship between the amount of drug in the body and the plasma concentration at equilibrium:

$$V_d = \frac{\text{amount of drug in body}}{\text{plasma concentration}}$$

The amount of drug in the body is expressed as mass (e.g., milligrams), and the plasma concentration is expressed as mass per volume (e.g., milligrams per liter). Thus, V_d is a hypothetical volume into which a quantity of drug would distribute if its concentration in the entire volume were the same as that in plasma. Although it is not a real volume, it is an important concept because it determines the fraction of total drug in the plasma (central) compartment and therefore the fraction available to the organs of elimination. An approximation of V_d in the equilibrium phase can be obtained by estimating the concentration of drug in plasma at time zero (Cp_0) by back-extrapolation of the equilibrium-phase plot to zero time, as illustrated in Fig. 68-1. Then, after intravenous administration, when the amount in the body at time zero is the dose, we have

$$V_d = \text{dose}/Cp_0$$

For the administration of the large macromolecule mentioned above, the measured Cp_0 of 1 mg/L after a 3-mg dose indicates a V_d that is a real volume, the plasma volume. This is the exception, however, for the V_d of most drugs is larger than plasma volume; many drugs are so extensively taken up by cells that tissue levels exceed those in plasma. For such drugs, the hypothetical V_d is large, even greater than the volume of body water. For example, Fig. 68-1 indicates that the Cp_0 obtained by extrapolation after administration of 50 mg of lidocaine is 0.42 mg/L, yielding a V_d of 119 L.

Since elimination is performed largely by the kidneys and liver, it is useful to consider the elimination of drugs according to the *clearance* concept. For example, in the kidney, regardless of the extent to which removal of drug is determined by filtration, secretion, or reabsorption, the net result is a reduction of the concentration of drug in plasma as it passes through the organ. The extent of this reduction is expressed as the *extraction ratio*, E, which is constant as long as first-order elimination occurs.

$$E = C_a - C_v$$

where C_a = arterial plasma concentration and C_v = venous plasma concentration. If the extraction is complete, $E = 1$. If the total plasma flow to the kidneys is Q (mL/min), the total volume of plasma from which drug is completely removed in a unit of time (clearance, CL) is determined as

$$\text{CL}_{\text{renal}} = QE$$

If the renal extraction ratio of penicillin is 0.5 and renal plasma flow is 680 mL/min, then penicillin's renal clearance is 340 mL/min. If the extraction ratio is high, as is the case for renal extraction of aminohippurate or hepatic extraction of propranolol, then clearance is a function of organ blood flow.[2]

Clearance from the body (CL) is the sum of clearance from all organs of elimination and is the best measure of the efficiency of the elimination processes. If a drug is removed by both the kidney and liver, then

$$\text{CL} = \text{CL}_{\text{renal}} + \text{CL}_{\text{hepatic}}$$

Thus, if penicillin is eliminated by both renal clearance (340 mL/min) and hepatic clearance (36 mL/min) in a normal individual, the total clearance is 376 mL/min. If renal clearance is reduced by half, the total clearance is 170 + 36 or 206 mL/min. In anuria, total clearance equals hepatic clearance.

Only the drug in the vascular compartment can be cleared during each passage through an organ. To ascertain the effect of a given plasma clearance by one or more organs on the rate of removal of drug from the body, the clearance must be related to the volume of "plasma equivalents" to be cleared, that is, the volume of distribution.

If the volume of distribution is 10 L and clearance is 1 L/min, then one-tenth of the drug in the body is eliminated per minute. This fraction, CL/V_d, is known as a *fractional elimination constant* and is designated k:

$$k = \text{CL}/V_d$$

If the fraction k is multiplied by the total amount of drug in the body, the actual rate of elimination at any given time can be determined:

$$\text{Rate of elimination} = k \times \text{amount in body} = \text{CL} \cdot C_p$$

This is the general equation for all first-order processes and expresses the fact that rate is proportional to the declining quantity in a first-order process.

Since half-life is a temporal expression of the exponential first-order process, half-life ($t_{1/2}$) can be related to k as follows:

$$t_{1/2} = 0.693/k$$

Because

$$k = \text{CL}/V_d$$

then

$$t_{1/2} = 0.693V_d/\text{CL}$$

As shown in the section on drug dosage in renal failure ("Effects of Renal Disease," below), the linear relationship of k or CL to creatinine clearance makes k a useful parameter for the estimation of changes in drug elimination with reduction in creatinine clearance in renal insufficiency. By contrast, half-life is not linearly related to clearance.

The important relationship

$$t_{1/2} = 0.693V_d/\text{CL}$$

indicates clearly the dependence of half-life—a measure of rate of elimination—on the two physiologically independent variables of volume of distribution and clearance, the latter expressing the efficiency of elimination. For example, half-life is shortened when phenobarbital induces the enzymes responsible for hepatic clearance of a drug, and half-life is lengthened when a drug's renal clearance is attenuated in renal failure. Also, the half-life of some drugs is shortened when their volume of distribution is reduced. In treating patients after an overdose, the effects of hemodialysis on a drug's elimination depend on the drug's volume of distribution. When the volume of distribution is large, as with tricyclic antidepressants (the V_d of desipramine equals more than 1500 L), the removal of drug, even with a high-clearance dialyzer, proceeds slowly.

The extent to which a drug is bound to plasma proteins also determines the fraction extracted by the organ(s) of elimination. Altered binding changes the extraction ratio significantly, but only when elimination is limited to the unbound (free) drug in plasma. The extent to which binding influences elimination depends on the relative affinities of the drug for plasma binding and for the extraction process. The high affinity of the renal tubular anion transport system for many drugs leads to extraction of bound and unbound drug, and the efficient process by which the liver removes propranolol extracts most of this highly bound drug from blood. However, for drugs with low organ extraction ratios, only unbound drug is available for elimination.

STEADY STATE With a constant infusion of drug, the infusion rate equals elimination rate at steady state. Therefore,

$$\begin{array}{ccc} \text{Infusion rate} & = & Cp_{ss} & \times & \text{CL} \\ \text{(amt/unit time)} & & \text{(amt/vol)} & & \text{(vol/unit time)} \end{array}$$

when the units for amount, volume, and time are consistent.

Thus, if clearance (CL) is known, the infusion rate to achieve a given steady state plasma level can be calculated. Estimation of drug clearance is discussed in the section on renal disease.

When the dose is given intermittently instead of by infusion, the above relationship between plasma concentration and the dose administered at each dosage interval can be expressed as

$$\text{Dose} = Cp_{av} \times \text{CL} \times \text{dosage interval}$$

---

[2] When drug is present in the formed elements of blood and rapidly equilibrates with that in plasma, then it is more physiologically meaningful to calculate extraction and clearance from blood than from the plasma.

Because Cp_{av} is an average value, the actual plasma concentrations will be higher and lower at various points during the dosing interval, as shown in Fig. 68-2.

When a drug is given orally, the fraction F of the administered dose that reaches the systemic circulation is an expression of the drug's *bioavailability*. A reduction in bioavailability may reflect a poorly formulated dosage form that fails to disintegrate or dissolve in the gastrointestinal fluids. Regulatory standards have reduced the extent of this problem. Drug interactions also can impair absorption after oral dosing. Bioavailability also may be reduced by metabolism of the drug in the gastrointestinal tract and/or the liver during the absorption process, the *first-pass effect*. This is a particular problem for drugs that are extracted extensively by these organs, and there often is considerable interpatient variability in bioavailability. Lidocaine for the control of arrhythmias is not administered orally because of the first-pass effect. Drugs that are injected intramuscularly also may have low bioavailability, an example being phenytoin. An unexpected drug response should lead to consideration of bioavailability as a possible factor. The calculation of a dosage regimen may need to involve a correction for bioavailability:

$$\text{Oral dose} = \frac{Cp_{av} \times \text{CL} \times \text{dosage interval}}{F}$$

Localization of Drug Action Direct intraarterial administration of selected drugs may be considered as a means of achieving a pharmacologic effect that is targeted to a specific organ. For such a strategy to be beneficial, the drug must exert an efficacy in the target organ that is greater than oral or intravenous administration without increasing systemic adverse effects (i.e., a higher therapeutic ratio). To obtain a higher therapeutic ratio from intraarterial administration, a drug should be highly extracted by the organ during the first pass through its circulation. Furthermore, the local pharmacologic effect should be sustained for the duration required to achieve the therapeutic goal.

The intracoronary administration of nitroglycerin fulfills these criteria. Nitroglycerin is highly extracted during a single pass through an organ; it is a prodrug and its metabolism by the arterial wall to nitric oxide localizes its vasodilator action to the site of this metabolic activation. Experimentally, liposomes are being investigated as a means of targeted delivery of drugs, as they are highly extracted during the first circulatory passage through an organ. Evidence that a drug meets the criteria for achieving a higher therapeutic ratio by intraarterial administration should be strong enough to justify the risk of the required invasive procedure.

DRUG ELIMINATION THAT IS NOT FIRST-ORDER The elimination of some drugs, such as phenytoin, salicylate, propafenone, and theophylline, does not follow first-order kinetics when the amount of drug in the body is in the therapeutic range. For these drugs, the clearance changes as levels in the body fall during elimination or change after alterations in dose. This pattern of elimination is called *dose-dependent*. Accordingly, the time for the concentration to fall to one-half becomes less as plasma levels fall. (This halving time is not truly a half-life, because the term *half-life* applies to first-order kinetics and is a constant.) When a drug is eliminated by first-order kinetics, the plasma level at steady state is directly related to the amount of the maintenance dose, and a doubling of the dose should lead to doubling of the steady state plasma level. However, for drugs with dose-dependent kinetics, an increase in the dose may be accompanied by a disproportionate increase in the plasma level. Moreover, the magnitude of the increase is not predictable because of interpatient variability, in the extent to which elimination deviates from first order. Changes in dosage regimens for drugs with dose-dependent kinetics, such as phenytoin, theophylline, salicylates, and ethanol, should always be accompanied by surveillance for adverse effects and by measurement of the concentration of the drug in plasma after enough time has passed for a new steady state to be established. The mechanisms involved in dose-dependent kinetics may include the saturation of the rate-limiting step in metabolism or a feedback inhibition of the rate-limiting enzyme by a product of the reaction.

Optimal drug therapy requires administration of just the right amount of drug for the particular patient—too little and the drug is likely to be ineffective; too much and there is an increased risk of undesirable effects. When the desired response is a readily determined clinical effect, such as an alteration in blood pressure or coagulation time, then the optimal dosage can be achieved empirically. For potentially toxic drugs, however, changes in dosage should be modest (usually ≤50 percent of the existing dose) and should be made no more frequently than every two to three half-lives. In most cases, however, drug therapy must be guided by the concept of a "therapeutic window" in which drug concentrations must be maintained. If this therapeutic window is large—that is, if there is little dose-related toxicity—then maximal efficacy, should it be desired and achievable, may be obtained by administering a supraeffective dose. Such a strategy is often used for penicillins and many beta-adrenoceptor blocking agents. It is also possible to use this strategy to extend the duration of action of a drug, especially one that is eliminated rapidly from the body. Thus, 75 mg of captopril will result in reduced blood pressure for up to 12 h, even though the elimination half-life of this angiotensin converting enzyme inhibitor is about 2 h. The therapeutic window for most drugs, however, is much narrower, and in certain instances (see Table 68-5), as little as a twofold difference distinguishes the dose (concentration) of drug that produces the desired response from one that elicits an adverse effect. In these cases, the application of pharmacokinetic principles is critical to achieving the therapeutic objective.

During long-term therapy, the most important pharmacokinetic factor is the drug's clearance, since that determines the steady state plasma concentration. Thus, after an oral dose, and assuming that clearance is constant regardless of the dose (i.e., assuming first-order elimination),

$$Cp_{av} = \frac{\text{dosage rate}}{\text{clearance}} = \frac{F \times \text{oral dose}}{\text{CL} \times \text{dosage interval}}$$

Accordingly, steady state drug levels and, therefore, the intensity of response can be adjusted by modifying the dosing rate. In most cases, this is best achieved by changing the drug dose but not the dosing interval, for example, by giving 250 mg every 8 h instead of 200 mg every 8 h. A change of this type will cause a proportionate change in the average steady state drug level but will not alter the relative fluctuation between the maximum ($Cp_{max,SS}$) and minimum ($Cp_{min,SS}$) values. However, this approach is only acceptable if the resulting peak concentration is not toxic and the trough value does not fall below the minimum effective concentration for an undesirable length of time. Alternatively, the steady state may be changed by altering the frequency of intermittent dosing but not the size of each dose. In this case, the magnitude of the fluctuation around the average steady state level will change—the shorter the dosing interval, the smaller the difference between the peak and trough levels (Fig. 68-4).

EFFECTS OF RENAL DISEASE When urinary excretion is an important route of elimination, renal failure decreases the drug clearance and therefore slows the removal of the drug from the body, so that a given dosing schedule will produce a greater accumulation of drug in the body and thus an increased likelihood of toxicity. The goal in such cases is to modify the dosing schedule so that the profile of plasma drug concentration over time is as similar to the desired one as possible and so that the steady state is reached in about the same amount of time as in a patient with normal renal function. Careful modification of the dosing schedule is especially important for drugs with long half-lives and narrow therapeutic indexes (e.g., digoxin). Since

$$Cp_{av} = \frac{\text{dose}}{\text{dose interval}} \times \frac{F}{\text{CL}} = \frac{\text{dose}}{\text{dose interval}} \times \frac{F}{k \, V_d},$$

the Cp_{av} expected for a patient with normal renal function can be produced in a patient with renal impairment (and thus a decreased CL) by giving smaller doses, by lengthening the dosing interval, or by doing both. The modification factor for the dosing regimen depends on the ratio of the drug's clearance or rate of elimination in renal failure to that in uncompromised patients.

If the dose size alone is to be modified, then it is necessary to calculate the *fraction of the normal dose* to be given (at the usual dosing interval). This fraction can be determined from either the drug clearance (CL) or the fractional rate constant k, because both of these quantities are proportional to creatinine clearance (CL_{cr}). Creatinine clearance is best determined directly. However, serum creatinine (C_{cr}) may be used to estimate the value by the following equation (applicable to men):

$$CL_{cr} = \frac{(140 - age) \times weight\ (kg)}{72 \times C_{cr}\ (mg/dL)}\ (mL/min)$$

For women, the correct estimate is 85 percent of the value produced by this equation. This approach is not valid for patients with severe renal insufficiency ($C_{cr} > 5$ mg/dL) or when renal function is changing rapidly.

The Clearance Approach The most accurate basis for calculating drug dosage is the clearance of the drug. From data on the clearance of a drug, the dose in renal insufficiency ($Dose_{ri}$) may be calculated as follows:

$$Dose_{ri} = dose \times \frac{CL_{ri}}{CL}$$

where ri = renal insufficiency; CL = clearance from the whole body with normal renal function; CL_{ri} = clearance from the whole body with renal insufficiency; and Dose = maintenance dose with normal renal function ($CL_{cr} \approx 100$ mL/min).

The normal clearance and the clearance in renal impairment can be obtained by using the data in Table 68-2 in the following equations:

$$CL = CL_{renal} + CL_{nonrenal}$$

$$CL_{ri} = CL_{renal} \times \frac{measured\ CL_{cr}}{100\ mL/min} + CL_{nonrenal}$$

The CL_{renal} values in Table 68-2 are those found with $CL_{cr} = 100$ mL/min, and the renal clearance of drug in renal insufficiency is obtained by multiplying CL_{renal} by the ratio of measured CL_{cr} (in milliliters per minute) to 100 mL/min.

For gentamicin, which has a normal CL_{renal} of 78 mL/min and a $CL_{nonrenal}$ of 3 mL/min, the normal CL is 81 mL/min. Therefore, if the measured CL_{cr} in a patient with renal insufficiency is 12 mL/min, $CL_{ri} = 78 \times (12/100) + 3 = 12.4$ mL/min. If the dose of gentamicin for a given infection should be 4.5 mg/kg per day in the presence of normal renal function, and the dosing interval selected is 24 h, then

$$Dose_{ri} = \frac{4.5\ mg/kg}{24\ h} \times \frac{12.4\ mL/min}{81\ mL/min}$$
$$= 0.69\ mg/kg/24\ h$$

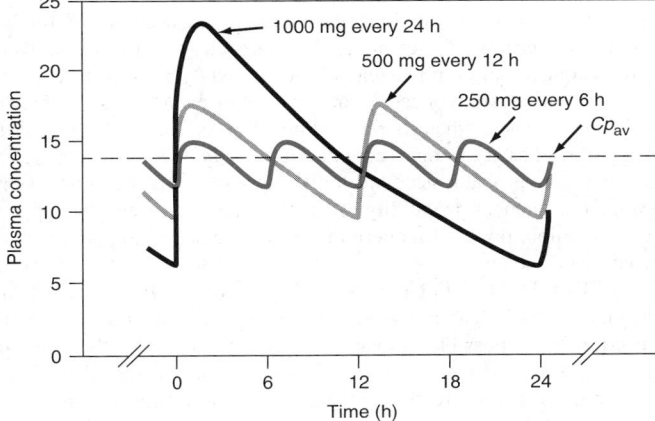

FIGURE 68-4 Plasma concentrations of a drug with an elimination half-life of 12 h during chronic therapy using different dosage regimens for a period sufficient to reach steady state. Proportionally reducing or increasing both the size of the maintenance dose and the interval between dosage changes the magnitude of the fluctuations in plasma levels but has no effect on the average steady state (Cp_{av}) value, since this depends on the ratio between D and τ.

Table 68-2

Clearance of Drugs

Drug	Renal Clearance,* mL/min	Nonrenal Clearance, mL/min
Ampicillin†	340	12
Carbenicillin	68	10
Digoxin†	110	36
Gentamicin	78	3
Kanamycin	60	0
Penicillin G‡	340	36

* The "normal" renal clearances are those associated with a clearance of creatinine of 100 mL/min.
† The fraction of digoxin absorbed after an oral dose (F) is approximately 0.75, and F for ampicillin is 0.5.
‡ One microgram of penicillin G = 1.6 units.

For a given dosing interval, the dose yielded by this calculation will produce the same average plasma level in the patient with renal insufficiency as the normal dose would produce in a patient with normal renal function. However, the difference between peak and trough levels will be smaller, the peak value could be below the therapeutic level and the trough level higher. To partially compensate for this flattening of the plasma concentration curve, the dosing interval for gentamicin in renal failure usually is adjusted, e.g., every 12 h for $CL_{cr} > 50$, every 24 h for $CL_{cr} = 10$ to 49 and every 48 h for $CL_{cr} < 10$ mL/min; the formula above would therefore be based on the appropriate dose for that dosing interval in a patient with normal renal function.

For some drugs, it is considered appropriate to modify only the dosing interval in renal failure, maintaining the same dose as with normal renal function:

$$Dosing\ interval \times \frac{CL}{CL_{ri}} = Dosing\ interval_{ri}$$

With this strategy, the potential that the plasma levels could be subtherapeutic for a deleterious period of time should be evaluated.

In some instances, it is desirable to calculate a dose that will yield a certain plasma level at steady state. This approach is most appropriate for constant intravenous infusions in which 100 percent of the dose is delivered to the systemic circulation. When the clearance of a drug in a patient with renal insufficiency is calculated as above, then

$$\begin{array}{ccc} Dose_{ri} & = & CL_{ri} & \times & Cp \\ (amt/unit\ time) & & (vol/unit\ time) & & (amt/vol) \end{array}$$

where the time, amount, and volume terms are uniform.

If a plasma concentration of carbenicillin of 100 μg/mL is the therapeutic objective in a patient with a creatinine clearance of 25 mL/min, the infusion rate is calculated as follows. Carbenicillin clearance is

$$CL_{ri} = \left(68 \times \frac{25}{100}\right) + 10 = 27\ mL/min$$

Therefore, carbenicillin should be infused at a rate of 2700 μg/min.

The Fractional Rate Constant (k) Approach For many drugs, clearance data in renal failure are not available. In these cases, the fraction of the normal dose that is required in a patient with renal failure can be approximated from the ratio of the fractional rate constant for elimination from the body in renal failure (k_{ri}) to that for normal renal function (k). This approach assumes that the distribution of the drug (V_d) is not affected by renal disease. The approach is the same as that employed with clearance data:

$$Dose_{ri} = dose \times \frac{k_{ri}}{k}$$

Since the ratio k_{ri}/k is the fraction of the usual dose employed in a given degree of renal insufficiency, it is termed the *dose fraction* and may be estimated from the information in Table 68-3 and the nomogram shown in Fig. 68-5. Table 68-3 gives the fraction of the usual

Table 68-3

Information for Estimation of Dose for Use in Patients with Renal Insufficiency

Drug	Dose fraction$_0$*	k (per hour)†
ANTIBIOTICS		
Amikacin	0.05	0.4
Amoxicillin	0.15	0.7
Ampicillin	0.1	0.6
Aztreonam	0.25	0.4
Carbenicillin	0.1	0.6
Cefazolin	0.06	0.35
Cefotaxime	0.3	0.7
Cefoxitin	0.1	0.8
Ceftazidime	0.1	0.4
Ceftriaxone‡	0.5	0.09
Cephalexin	0.04	0.7
Cephalothin	0.02	1.4
Chloramphenicol	0.8	0.3
Ciprofloxacin	0.33	0.2
Clindamycin	0.8	0.2
Cloxacillin	0.25	1.2
Dicloxacillin	0.5	1.2
Doxycycline	0.8	0.03
Erythromycin	0.7	0.5
Gentamicin	0.05	0.3
Imipenem	0.25	0.7
Isoniazid:		
Fast inactivators	0.8	0.5
Slow inactivators	0.5	0.25
Methicillin	0.12	1.4
Minocycline	0.9	0.06
Nafcillin	0.4	1.2
Norfloxacin	0.5	0.2
Ofloxacin	0.22	0.1
Oxacillin	0.25	1.4
Penicillin G	0.1	1.4
Piperacillin	0.33	0.5
Rifampin	1.0	0.25
Streptomycin	0.05	0.25
Sulfadiazine	0.45	0.7
Sulfamethoxazole	0.85	0.07
Tetracycline	0.12	0.08
Ticarcillin	0.1	0.6
Tobramycin	0.05	0.35
Trimethoprim	0.45	0.06
Vancomycin	0.03	0.12
MISCELLANEOUS DRUGS		
Chlorpropamide	0.4	0.02
Lidocaine	0.9	0.4
Sulfinpyrazone	0.55	0.3
CARDIAC GLYCOSIDES		
		k (per day)
Digitoxin	0.7	0.1
Digoxin	0.3	0.45

* Dose fraction$_0$, dose fraction for a patient with a creatinine clearance of zero.
† k, average overall fractional elimination rate constant for a patient with normal renal function.
‡ Extrarenal clearance also may be reduced in patients with renal failure who are uremic and/or ill.

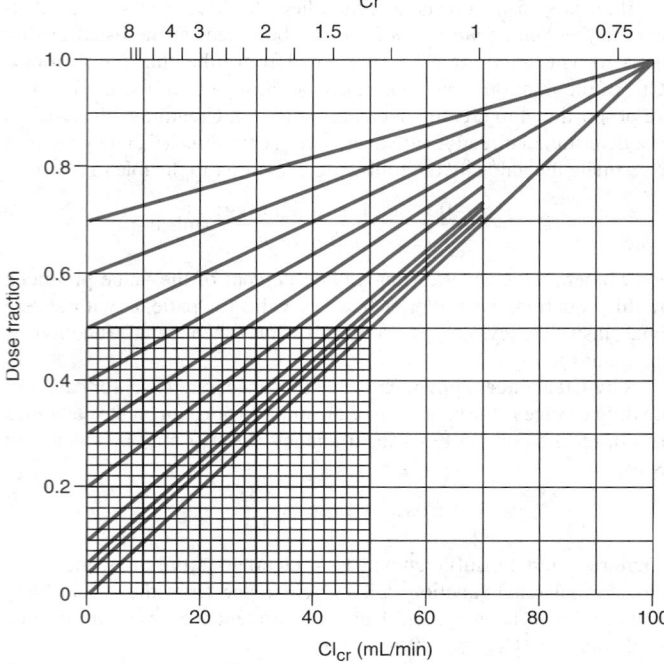

FIGURE 68-5 Nomogram for estimation of the dose fraction in patients with renal insufficiency. Cr, creatinine; CL$_{cr}$, creatinine clearance. (*From Dettli L: Drug dosage in renal disease. Clin Pharmacokinet 1:126, 1976.*)

measured creatinine clearance (on the lower abscissa) and this dose-fraction line is a coordinate for which the dose fraction (on the left ordinate) corresponds to the particular creatinine clearance.

The elimination of many drugs is sufficiently rapid in patients with normal renal function that the time required to reach steady state is not significant, and usually no loading dose is used. In renal failure, however, the prolonged half-life may cause this accumulation period to become unacceptably long. In these cases, a loading dose may be indicated; the size of the loading dose would be the same as in patients with normal renal function (see "Drug Accumulation—Loading and Maintenance Doses," above).

General Considerations for Determining Dosage in Renal Insufficiency Because of the differences between patients in volumes of distribution and rates of metabolism, calculations of drug dose in renal failure must be viewed as valuable approximations that prevent the use of doses that are grossly excessive or inadequate for most patients. However, *maintenance dosages are most accurate when plasma-level data are used to adjust the dose as necessary.*

Active or toxic metabolites of drugs also may accumulate in renal failure. Meperidine, for example, is cleared largely by metabolism, and its concentration in plasma is little altered by renal insufficiency. However, the plasma concentration of one of its metabolites, normeperidine, is increased when its renal elimination is impaired. Since normeperidine has a stronger convulsant activity than meperidine, its accumulation probably accounts for the signs of central nervous system excitation, such as irritability, twitching, and seizures, that appear when multiple doses of meperidine are administered to patients with renal insufficiency.

EFFECTS OF LIVER DISEASE In contrast to the predictable decline in renal clearance of drugs when glomerular filtration is reduced, it is not possible to make a general prediction of the effect of liver disease on hepatic biotransformation of drugs (see Chap. 291). Rather, the possible effects of hepatitis or cirrhosis range from impaired to increased drug clearance. Even in advanced hepatocellular disease, drug clearance usually is impaired only about two- to fivefold. The extent of such changes, however, cannot be predicted by the common tests of liver function. Consequently, even when it is suspected that drug elimination is altered in liver disease, there is no quantitative basis on which to adjust the dosage regimen other than assessment of clinical response and the concentration of the drug in plasma.

dose of a drug required at a creatinine clearance of zero (dose fraction$_0$). The nomogram presents the dose fraction as a linear function of creatinine clearance.

To calculate the dose fraction$_{ri}$, the dose fraction$_0$ is obtained from Table 68-3, plotted on the left ordinate of the nomogram, and connected by a straight line to the upper right-hand corner of the nomogram. This line describes the dose fraction over a range of creatinine clearances from 0 to 100 mL/min. The point of intersection between the

Under conditions of decreased
tissue perfusion, the cardiac output is redistributed to preserve blood
flow to the heart and brain at the expense of other tissues (Chap. 38).
As a result, the drug is distributed into a smaller volume of distribution,
higher drug concentrations are present in the plasma and the tissues
that are best perfused will be exposed to these higher concentrations.
If either the brain or heart is sensitive to the drug, an alteration in
response will occur.

Furthermore, the decreased perfusion of the kidney and liver may
impair drug clearance by these organs directly or indirectly. Thus, in
severe congestive heart failure, in hemorrhagic shock, and in cardiogenic shock, the response to the usual dose of drug may be excessive,
and dosage modification may be necessary. For example, the clearance
of lidocaine is reduced by about 50 percent in cardiac failure, and
therapeutic plasma levels are achieved at infusion rates only about
half those usually required. The volume of distribution of lidocaine
also is reduced, meaning that the correct loading dose will be smaller
than usual. Similar situations are thought to exist for procainamide,
theophylline, and possibly quinidine. Unfortunately, predictors of these
types of pharmacokinetic alterations are unavailable. Therefore, loading doses should be conservative, and continued therapy should be
monitored closely, following clinical indicators of toxicity and
plasma levels.

DISEASE-INDUCED CHANGES IN PLASMA BINDING
Many drugs circulate in the plasma partly bound to plasma proteins.
Since only the unbound (free) drug can distribute to the site of pharmacologic action, the therapeutic response should be related to the free
rather than the total circulating plasma drug concentration. In most
cases, the degree of binding is fairly constant across the therapeutic
concentration range, so that the total drug levels in plasma can be
used as a basis for adjusting dosage without resulting in significant
error. However, conditions such as hypoalbuminemia, liver disease,
and renal disease can decrease the extent of drug binding, particularly
of acidic and neutral drugs, so that at any total plasma level there is
a greater concentration of free drug than usual and thus a risk of
increased response and toxicity. By contrast, conditions that lead to
an increased plasma concentration of the acute-phase reactant alpha$_1$-
acid glycoprotein—such as myocardial infarction, surgery, neoplastic
disease, rheumatoid arthritis, and burns—cause an increase in drug
binding for the basic drugs that bind to this macromolecule, resulting
in an opposite set of effects. The drugs for which changes in binding
are important are those that are normally highly bound in the plasma
(>90 percent), because a small alteration in the extent of binding
produces a large change in the amount of unbound drug.

The consequences of these binding changes, particularly with respect to total drug levels, depend on whether clearance is determined
only by the unbound drug or by both forms of drug. For many drugs,
elimination and distribution are restricted largely to the unbound fraction, and, therefore, a decrease in binding leads to an increase in the
clearance and distribution of the drug. The relative magnitudes of
these changes are such that the net effect is a shortened half-life.

In the case of drugs bound to alpha$_1$-acid glycoprotein, a disease-
induced increase in binding has the opposite effects, reducing the
clearance and distribution of the total drug. For example, a constant-
rate infusion of lidocaine to control arrhythmias after myocardial infarction will lead to a greater accumulation of total drug.

VARIABLE ACTIONS OF DRUGS
CAUSED BY GENETIC DIFFERENCES
IN DRUG METABOLISM

ACETYLATION Isoniazid, hydralazine, procainamide, and a
number of other drugs are metabolized by acetylation of a hydrazino
or amino group. This reaction is catalyzed by N-acetyl transferase-2,
an enzyme in the liver cytosol that transfers an acetyl group from
acetyl coenzyme A to the drug. Individuals differ markedly in the rate
at which drugs are acetylated, and there is a bimodal distribution of
the population into "rapid acetylators" and "slow acetylators." The

rate of acetylation is under genetic control; slow acetylation is an
autosomal recessive trait.

Acetylation phenotype can be determined by measuring the ratio
of acetylated to nonacetylated dapsone or sulfamethazine in plasma
or urine following administration of a test dose of these acetylation
substrates. The ratio of monoacetyldapsone to dapsone in plasma at
6 h after dapsone administration is less than 0.30 for slow acetylators
and more than 0.35 for rapid acetylators. At 6 h after the administration
of sulfamethazine, the fraction of the drug in plasma that is in the
acetylated form is <25 percent in slow acetylators and >25 percent
in rapid acetylators; in the urine collected in the 5- to 6-h interval
after administration, the fraction of drug in the acetylated form is <70
percent in slow acetylators and >70 percent in rapid acetylators. More
recently, the acetylation of a metabolite of caffeine, possibly the most
widely consumed drug in the world because of its presence in a variety
of foods, has been used as an indicator of acetylator phenotype. In
this procedure, the urinary molar ratio of 5-acetylamino-6-amino-3-
methyluracil to methylxanthine after ingestion of a drink of coffee or
cola is determined. Antimodes of about 1.8 and 6.6 separate slow,
intermediate, and rapid acetylators; moreover, these three groups appear to correspond to the expected genotypes. The molecular bases
of impaired N-acetyltransferase activity have now been established at
the level of the gene, and several NAT-2 alleles have been characterized. As a result, it is now possible to identify a slow acetylator by
genotyping, using genomic DNA obtained from peripheral leukocytes.

METABOLISM BY MIXED-FUNCTION OXIDASES In
healthy individuals taking no other medications, the major determinant
of the rate of metabolism of drugs by the hepatic mixed-function
oxidases is genetic. Hepatic endoplasmic reticulum contains a family of
cytochrome P450 (CYP) isoforms with different substrate specificities.
Many drugs undergo oxidative metabolism by more than one isoform,
and the steady state concentrations of such drugs in the plasma is a
function of the sum of the activities of these and other metabolizing
enzymes. When a drug is metabolized by multiple pathways, the
catalytic activities of the participating enzymes are regulated by a
number of genes, so that the clearance rates and steady state concentrations of the drug tend to distribute unimodally within the population.
The range of activity may differ markedly (tenfold or more) between
different individuals, as is the case for chlorpromazine, and there is
no way to predict the rate before beginning therapy.

Certain metabolic pathways show a bimodal distribution of activity, suggesting control by a single gene, and several polymorphisms
have been identified. In these cases, two phenotypic populations are
usually present, as for N-acetylation (see above). Most individuals are
extensive metabolizers (the EM phenotype); a smaller group have a
lower ability to metabolize the drug (or no ability at all) and are called
poor metabolizers (the PM phenotype).

The cytochrome P450 isoform CYP2D6 is polymorphically distributed in the population, and about 8 to 10 percent of whites are
deficient in this enzyme. CYP2D6 represents the main metabolic pathway for a number of drugs, including antiarrhythmic agents (propafenone, flecainide), beta-adrenoceptor blockers (timolol, metoprolol, and
alprenolol), tricyclic antidepressants (nortriptyline, desipramine, imipramine, clomipramine), neuroleptic drugs (perphenazine, thioridazine,
and possibly haloperidol), selective serotonin reuptake inhibitors (fluoxetine and paroxetine), and certain opiates, such as codeine and
dextromethorphan. Thus, codeine has a much lower analgesic effect
in PM patients because of impaired production of the active metabolite,
morphine. Similarly, patients with the PM phenotype experience more
pronounced systemic beta-adrenoceptor blockade after the administration of timolol ophthalmic solution. The catalytic activity of CYP2D6
in humans may be assessed by using a test drug, debrisoquin, which
is eliminated almost entirely via hydroxylation by CYP2D6. A similar
situation occurs with the oxidative polymorphism that involves the
metabolism of mephenytoin by a different isoform, CYP2C19. This
enzyme is also involved in the metabolism of omeprazole, proguanil,

diazepam, and citalopram. The situation is further complicated by racial differences in the frequency of the polymorphisms. For example, impaired hydroxylation of mephenytoin is present in only 3 to 5 percent of whites, but the incidence is about 20 percent in individuals of Japanese and Chinese descent; likewise, the frequency of the PM phenotype for debrisoquin hydroxylation appears to decrease as one moves from Western (8 to 10 percent) to Eastern (0 to 1 percent) population groups.

Polymorphisms in drug-metabolizing ability may be associated with large differences in the disposition of a drug among individuals, especially when the involved pathway makes a major contribution to the elimination of the drug. For example, the clearance of mephenytoin given orally differs 100- to 200-fold between individuals of the EM and PM phenotypes. As a result, the peak plasma concentrations and bioavailability after oral administration may be much higher, and the rate of drug elimination much lower, in PM than in EM individuals. In PM individuals, the result is excessive drug accumulation and exaggerated pharmacologic responses, including toxicity, when usual drug dosages are administered. Inhibitory drug interactions involving compounds that are metabolized by CYP2D6 (e.g., certain selective serotonin reuptake inhibitors) or that noncompetitively inhibit the activity of the enzyme (e.g., quinidine), may be of considerable clinical importance in patients with the EM phenotype, as the concomitant administration of such agents often leads to impaired drug handling like that in the PM phenotype. Individualization of drug therapy is especially critical for drugs that exhibit polymorphic drug metabolism. As with the *NAT-2* polymorphism, the increasing availability of laboratory methods to identify the PM phenotype for CYP2D6 and CYP2C19 by genotyping should be useful for this purpose.

DRUG USE IN THE ELDERLY (See also Chap. 9)   The elderly (>65 years old) constitute about 12 percent of the U.S. population, and this fraction will increase to about 20 percent (50 to 60 million individuals) over the next 20 years. These patients use a disproportionate amount of prescription medications (30 percent). Also, 70 percent of the elderly regularly use over-the-counter drugs, compared with only 10 percent of the general adult population. Aging results in changes in organ function, especially of the organs involved in drug disposition, as well as alterations in body size and composition. Not surprisingly, therefore, pharmacokinetics are often different in elderly individuals than in younger adults. Unfortunately, few generalizations seem to be possible on the probable type, magnitude, or clinical importance of these age-related changes in an individual patient. Elderly patients often have multiple diseases and may therefore be taking a large number of drugs. Consequently, drug interactions as well as an increased vulnerability to morbidity and mortality, contribute to the higher incidence of adverse drug reactions in elderly patients. Increased sensitivity of target organs and impairment of physiologic control systems, such as those involved in the regulation of the circulation, also may be a factor. Accordingly, optimization of drug therapy in the elderly, particularly in frail patients, is often difficult, as a variety of factors (often poorly defined) accentuate the usual interindividual variability in drug response.

Although many individuals preserve good renal function into old age, elderly patients as a group have an increased likelihood of impaired renal excretion of drugs. Even in the absence of kidney disease, renal clearance is generally reduced by about 35 to 50 percent in elderly patients. Dosage adjustments analogous to those in patients with kidney dysfunction (see above) are therefore necessary for drugs that are eliminated mainly by the kidneys, such as digoxin, aminoglycosides, lithium, and other drugs listed in Table 68-3. In this regard, it is important to recognize that the reduced muscle mass of older individuals results in a reduced rate of creatinine production; thus, a normal serum creatinine concentration can be present even though creatinine clearance is impaired.

Aging also results in a decrease in the size of and blood flow to the liver and possibly in the activity of hepatic drug-metabolizing enzymes; accordingly, the hepatic clearance of some drugs is impaired in the elderly. Unfortunately, no consistent pattern of clinical application appears to be present. Moreover, the changes are often modest relative to the interindividual variability in these patients. However, even a small reduction in hepatic extraction may significantly increase the oral bioavailability of drugs with a high first-pass effect, such as propranolol and labetalol.

Impaired clearance and/or increased distribution may cause the elimination half-life of a drug to increase with aging. Thus, if a dosage modification in an elderly patient is required, it is often possible to accomplish it by decreasing the frequency of drug administration, possibly along with a reduction in dose.

Even if the pharmacokinetics of a drug are not altered, an elderly patient may require a smaller dosage because of an increase in pharmacodynamic sensitivity. Examples include increased analgesic effects of opioids, increased sedation from benzodiazepines and other central nervous system depressants, and increased risk of bleeding while receiving anticoagulant therapy, even when clotting parameters are well controlled. Exaggerated responses to cardiovascular drugs are also common because of the impaired responsiveness of normal homeostatic mechanisms. Such age-related changes require close monitoring of the patient's clinical response and appropriate dosage titration.

In general, when administering drug therapy to an elderly patient, one should be alert to the possibility of moderate reductions in drug clearance and the chance of exaggerated pharmacodynamic responsiveness.

INTERACTIONS BETWEEN DRUGS

The effect of some drugs can be altered markedly by the administration of other agents. Such interactions can sabotage therapy by adversely increasing or decreasing the action of a drug. Drug interactions must be considered in the differential diagnosis of unexpected responses to drugs, and it should be recognized that patients often come to the physician with a legacy of drugs acquired during previous medical experiences. A meticulous drug history will minimize such unknown elements. It should include examination of the patient's medications and, if necessary, calls to the pharmacist to identify prescriptions.

There are two principal types of interactions between drugs. In *pharmacokinetic interactions*, the delivery of a drug to its site of action is altered, whereas in *pharmacodynamic interactions*, the responsiveness of the target organ or system is modified.

An index of the drug interactions discussed in this chapter is provided in Table 68-4. The table includes interactions that have verified significance in patients, plus a few that are so potentially dangerous that cognizance should be taken of the experimental data or case reports suggesting they occur.

I. PHARMACOKINETIC INTERACTIONS CAUSING DIMINISHED DRUG DELIVERY

A. Impaired Gastrointestinal Absorption   Cholestyramine, an ion-exchange resin, binds thyroxine, triiodothyronine, and the cardiac glycosides sufficiently strongly to impair their absorption from the gastrointestinal tract. This resin probably also interferes with the absorption of other drugs, and it is safest not to give it within 2 h of their administration. Aluminum ions, present in antacids, form insoluble chelates with the tetracyclines, preventing absorption of these drugs. Ferrous ions similarly block tetracycline absorption. Kaolin-pectin suspensions bind digoxin, and when these substances are administered together, digoxin absorption is reduced by about one-half. However, when kaolin-pectin is administered 2 h after digoxin, digoxin absorption is unaffected.

Ketoconazole is a weak base that dissolves well only at acidic pH. Histamine H_2 receptor antagonists, such as ranitidine and cimetidine, reduce gastric acidity and thus impair the dissolution and absorption of ketoconazole. By contrast, the absorption of fluconazole is not impaired by an increase in gastric pH. Oral administration of aminosalicylate interferes with the absorption of rifampin by an unknown mechanism.

B. Induction of Hepatic Drug-Metabolizing Enzymes   When a drug is eliminated largely by metabolism, an increase in the rate of its metabolism reduces its availability to sites of action. Most drugs

Table 68-4

CHAPTER 68
Principles of Drug Therapy **419**

Drug Interaction Index

Drug	Section of Chapter Describing Interaction
Allopurinol	IIA
p-Aminosalicylate	IA
Amiloride	III
Amiodarone	IIA, IIC
Amphetamine	IC
Antidepressants, tricyclic (desipramine, nortriptyline, imipramine, doxepin, protriptyline, amitriptyline)	IC
Aspirin	IIB, III
Astemizole	IIA
Azathioprine	IIA
Barbiturates (class)	IB
Carbamazepine	IB, IIA
Chlorpromazine	IC, IIA
Cholestyramine	IA
Cimetidine	IA, IIA, IIB
Cisapride	IIA
Clofibrate	IIA
Clonidine	IC
Codeine	IIA
Cotrimoxazole	IIA
Cyclosporine	IB, IIA
Dexamethasone	IB
Digoxin	IA, IIC
Diltiazem	IIA
Diuretics	III
Erythromycin	IIA
Ephedrine	IC
Ethanol	IIA
Fluconazole	IIA
Fluoxetine	IIA
Guanadrel	IC
Guanethidine	IC
Haloperidol	IIA
Indomethacin	III
Isoniazid	IIA
Itraconazole	IB, IIA
Kaolin-pectin	IA
Ketoconazole	IA, IB, IIA
Lidocaine	IIA
Lovastatin	IIA
6-Mercaptopurine	IIA
Methadone	IB
Methotrexate	IIB
Methylprednisolone	IB, IIA
Metronidazole	IB, IIA
Metyrapone	IB
Mexiletine	IB
Nicardipine	IIA
Nifedipine	IIA
Nonsteroidal antiinflammatory drugs	III
Oral contraceptive steroids	IB
Phenobarbital	IB
Phenylbutazone	IIA, IIB
Phenytoin (diphenylhydantoin)	IB, IIA
Piroxicam	III
Potassium	III
Prednisone	IB
Probenecid	IIB
Procainamide	IIB
Propranolol	III
Quinidine	IB, IIA, IIC, III
Ranitidine	IA, IIA
Rifampin	IA, IB
Salicylate	IIB
Spironolactone	III
Terfenadine	IIA
Tetracycline	IA
Theophylline	IIA
Thiazide diuretics	III
Tolbutamide	IIA
Triamterene	III
Triazolam	IIA
Verapamil	IB, IIA, IIC
Warfarin	IB, IIA, III

are metabolized largely in the liver because of this organ's large mass, high blood flow, and high concentration of drug-metabolizing enzymes. The first step in the metabolism of many drugs is catalyzed by a group of cytochrome P450 mixed-function oxidases located in the endoplasmic reticulum (see "Metabolism by Mixed-Function Oxidases," above). These enzyme systems oxidize drug molecules by a variety of reactions, including aromatic hydroxylations, N-demethylations, O-demethylations, and sulfoxidations. The products of these reactions are usually more polar than the parent compound (and more readily excreted by the kidney).

The expression of some of the mixed-function oxidase (CYP) isoforms is regulated, and their content in the liver can be increased by a number of drugs. Phenobarbital is the prototype of these inducers, and all the barbiturates in clinical use increase CYP enzyme activity. Induction with phenobarbital can occur with doses of as little as 60 mg daily. Mixed-function oxidases also are induced by rifampin, carbamazepine, phenytoin, and glutethimide, and by smoking, exposure to chlorinated insecticides such as DDT, and chronic alcohol ingestion.

Phenobarbital, rifampin, and other inducers lower plasma levels of many drugs, including warfarin, quinidine, mexiletine, verapamil, ketoconazole, itraconazole, cyclosporine, dexamethasone, methylprednisolone, prednisolone (the active metabolite of prednisone), oral contraceptive steroids, methadone, metronidazole, and metyrapone. These interactions all have obvious clinical significance. In the case of the coumarin anticoagulants, the patient is placed at major risk if the appropriate level of anticoagulation is achieved when an inducer is also being administered and the inducer is later discontinued (for example, at discharge from the hospital). The plasma levels of the coumarin anticoagulant will rise as the induction effect wears off, leading to excessive anticoagulation.

There is considerable variation among individuals in the extent to which drug metabolism can be induced. In some patients, phenobarbital leads to marked acceleration in the rate of drug metabolism, whereas little induction is seen in others.

In addition to inducing certain of the CYP isoforms, phenobarbital has other effects on hepatic function. It increases liver blood flow, bile flow, and the hepatocellular transport of organic anions. The conjugation of drugs and bilirubin also may be enhanced by inducing agents.

C. Inhibition of Cellular Uptake or Binding The guanidinium antihypertensive agents guanethidine and guanadrel are transported to their site of action in adrenergic neurons by an energy-requiring membrane transport system for biogenic monoamines. Although the physiologic function of the transport system is reuptake of the adrenergic neurotransmitter, it also transports a variety of ring-substituted bases, including guanethidine and related guanidiniums, which it can import against a concentration gradient. Inhibitors of norepinephrine uptake prevent the uptake of the guanidinium antihypertensive agents into adrenergic neurons and thereby block their pharmacologic effects. The tricyclic antidepressants are potent inhibitors of norepinephrine uptake. Consequently, concomitant administration of clinical doses of tricyclic antidepressants, including desipramine, protriptyline, nortriptyline, and amitriptyline, almost totally abolishes the antihypertensive effects of guanethidine and guanadrel. Although they are less potent inhibitors of norepinephrine uptake, doxepin and chlorpromazine produce dose-related antagonism of the action of the guanidinium antihypertensives. Ephedrine, a component of many drug combinations used in asthma, also antagonizes the effect of guanethidine. In patients with severe hypertension, the loss of control of blood pressure from these drug interactions can lead to stroke and malignant hypertension.

The antihypertensive effect of clonidine is partially antagonized by tricyclic antidepressants. Clonidine lowers arterial pressure by reducing sympathetic outflow from the blood pressure–regulating centers in the hindbrain (Chap. 246). This central hypotensive action is antagonized by the tricyclic antidepressants.

II. PHARMACOKINETIC INTERACTIONS CAUSING INCREASED DRUG DELIVERY

A. Inhibition of Drug Metabolism If the active form of a drug is eliminated largely by biotransformation, inhibition of its metabolism leads to reduced clearance, prolonged half-life, and accumulation of the drug during maintenance therapy. Excessive accumulation due to inhibited metabolism can lead to adverse effects.

Cimetidine is a potent inhibitor of the oxidative metabolism of many drugs, including warfarin, quinidine, nifedipine, lidocaine, theophylline, and phenytoin. Adverse reactions, many of them severe, have resulted from the administration of these drugs in conjunction with cimetidine. Cimetidine is a more potent inhibitor of mixed-function oxidases than ranitidine, whereas ranitidine is more potent as a histamine H_2 receptor antagonist. Thus, ranitidine, when administered in doses of 150 mg twice daily, does not inhibit the oxidative metabolism of most drugs; where reduced drug elimination has been observed, the effects of ranitidine have been less than those of cimetidine and have not had appreciable pharmacodynamic consequences. Doses of ranitidine higher than 150 mg, however, may produce greater inhibition of drug oxidation. Famotidine and nizatidine are not known to produce clinically appreciable inhibition of drug metabolism.

Knowledge of the CYP isoforms that catalyze the main pathway of metabolism of a drug provides a basis for predicting and understanding drug interactions. For example, the CYP3A subfamily of isoforms catalyze the metabolism of many drugs for which blockage of metabolism results in toxicity. Drugs that depend on CYP3A as a major route of metabolism include cyclosporine, quinidine, lovastatin, warfarin, nifedipine, lidocaine, terfenadine, astemizole, cisapride, erythromycin, methylprednisolone, carbamazepine, midazolam, and triazolam.

Erythromycin, ketoconazole, and itraconazole are potent inhibitors of enzymes in the CYP3A family. When fluconazole levels are elevated as a result of higher doses and/or renal insufficiency, this drug also can inhibit CYP3A. Some of the calcium antagonists, diltiazem, nicardipine, and verapamil also can inhibit CYP3A, as can some of its other substrates, such as cyclosporine. Thus, cyclosporine can cause serious toxicity when its metabolism is inhibited by erythromycin, ketoconazole, diltiazem, nicardipine, or verapamil. Lovastatin causes severe myopathy with rhabdomyolysis when administered together with erythromycin or cyclosporine, and it is highly probable that other of the known inhibitors of CYP3A also can inhibit the disposition of lovastatin. Terfenadine, astemizole, and cisapride can cause polymorphic ventricular tachycardia (torsade de pointes) when their metabolism is blocked by inhibitors of CYP3A, such as ketoconazole, itraconazole, and erythromycin.

Whenever erythromycin, ketoconazole, or itraconazole is administered to a patient, the physician should be alert to the possibility of serious interactions with drugs that are metabolized by CYP3A.

The CYP2D6 isoform that catalyzes the polymorphic metabolism of debrisoquin is markedly inhibited by quinidine and also is blocked by a number of neuroleptic drugs, such as chlorpromazine and haloperidol, and by fluoxetine. The analgesic effect of codeine depends on its metabolism to morphine via CYP2D6 in individuals with the extensive metabolizer phenotype. Thus, quinidine reduces the analgesic efficacy of codeine in extensive metabolizers. Since desipramine is cleared largely by metabolism via CYP2D6 in extensive metabolizers, its levels are increased substantially by concurrent administration of quinidine, fluoxetine, or the neuroleptic drugs that inhibit CYP2D6.

Some drugs are inactivated by mechanisms other than the hepatic drug-metabolizing enzymes. Azathioprine is converted in the body to an active metabolite, 6-mercaptopurine, which in turn is oxidized by xanthine oxidase to 6-thiouric acid. When allopurinol, a potent inhibitor of xanthine oxidase, is administered concurrently with standard doses of azathioprine or 6-mercaptopurine, life-threatening toxicity (bone marrow suppression) can result.

Other drugs that inhibit biotransformation of pharmacologic compounds (with examples of drugs whose metabolism is blocked by the inhibitor listed in parenthesis) include:

- Amiodarone (warfarin, quinidine)
- Clofibrate (phenytoin, tolbutamide)
- Excessive ingestion of ethanol (warfarin)
- Isoniazid (phenytoin)
- Metronidazole, cotrimoxazole (warfarin)
- Phenylbutazone (warfarin, phenytoin, tolbutamide)

B. Inhibition of Renal Elimination A number of drugs are secreted by the renal tubular transport systems for organic anions. Inhibition of this tubular transport system can cause excessive accumulation of a drug. Phenylbutazone, probenecid, and salicylates competitively inhibit this transport system. Salicylate, for example, reduces the renal clearance of methotrexate, an interaction that may lead to methotrexate toxicity. Renal tubular secretion contributes substantially to the elimination of penicillin, which can be inhibited by probenecid.

Inhibition of the tubular cation transport system by cimetidine impedes the renal clearance of procainamide and its active metabolite N-acetylprocainamide.

C. Inhibition of Clearance at Multiple Sites The concentrations of digoxin in plasma are elevated by quinidine, owing largely to inhibition of renal elimination and in part to inhibition of biliary secretion. An increase in cardiac arrhythmia may occur when quinidine is given in conjunction with a cardiac glycoside.

Amiodarone, cyclosporine, itraconazole, and verapamil also inhibit the clearance of digoxin and increase the concentration of digoxin in plasma.

III. PHARMACODYNAMIC AND OTHER INTERACTIONS BETWEEN DRUGS

Therapeutically useful interactions occur in which the effect of two drugs in combination is greater than the sum of their effects when used individually. Favorable drug combinations are described in specific therapeutic sections in this text, and this section focuses on interactions that create unwanted effects. Two drugs may act on separate components of a common process to yield effects greater than either has alone. For example, although small doses of aspirin (less than 1 g daily) do not alter the prothrombin time appreciably in patients who are receiving warfarin therapy, aspirin nevertheless increases the risk of bleeding in these patients because it inhibits platelet aggregation. Thus the combination of impaired functions of platlets and the clotting system increases the potential for hemorrhagic complications in patients receiving warfarin therapy.

Nonsteroidal antiinflammatory drugs cause gastric and duodenal ulcers, and, in patients treated with warfarin, the risk of bleeding from a peptic ulcer is increased almost threefold by concomitant use of a nonsteroidal antiinflammatory drug. This clearly is a serious drug interaction.

Indomethacin, piroxicam, and probably other nonsteroidal antiinflammatory drugs antagonize the antihypertensive effects of beta-adrenergic receptor blockers, diuretics, converting-enzyme inhibitors, and other drugs. The resulting elevation in blood pressure ranges from trivial to severe. Aspirin and sulindac, however, do not elevate the blood pressure in treated hypertensive patients.

Polymorphic ventricular tachycardia (torsade de pointes) during quinidine administration occurs much more frequently in patients receiving diuretics, probably owing to potassium and/or magnesium depletion.

The administration of supplemental potassium leads to more frequent and more severe hyperkalemia when potassium elimination is reduced by concurrent treatment with angiotensin-converting enzyme inhibitors, spironolactone, amiloride, or triamterene.

CONCENTRATION OF DRUGS IN PLASMA AS A GUIDE TO THERAPY

In many cases, the plasma concentration of a drug is measured as a guide in the individualization of therapy. Genetic variation in elimination rates, interactions with other drugs, disease-induced alterations in elimination and distribution, and other factors combine to yield a wide range of plasma levels in patients given the same dose. Furthermore, the problem of noncompliance with prescribed regimens during continuing therapy is an endemic and elusive cause of therapeutic failure (see below). Clinical indicators assist in the titration of some drugs into the desired range, and no chemical determination is a substitute for careful observations of the response to treatment. However, the therapeutic and adverse effects are not precisely quantifiable for all drugs, and, in complex clinical situations, estimates of the action of a drug may be misleading. For example, previously existing neurologic disease may obscure the neurologic consequences of intoxication with phenytoin. Because clearance, half-life, accumulation, and steady state plasma levels are difficult to predict, the measurement of plasma levels is often useful as a guide to the optimal dose. This is particularly true when there is a narrow range between the plasma levels yielding therapeutic and adverse effects. For drugs having such characteristics—e.g., digoxin, theophylline, lidocaine, aminoglycosides, and anticonvulsants—dose optimization should involve modification of the standard dose on the basis of the pharmacokinetic principles described above. In certain instances, predictive nomograms and algorithms have been developed to facilitate the necessary modifications. However, the most flexible and accurate method for individualizing drug dosage appears to be a feedback approach using a small number of previously obtained plasma levels and Bayesian forecasting. In controlled studies, this type of computer-assisted dosing has been shown to improve patient care. However, the overall cost/benefit ratio of such methods in routine management still remains to be conclusively demonstrated.

For drugs with a narrow therapeutic window that exhibit first-order elimination, then, dosage adjustments may be made on the assumption that the average, maximum, and minimum steady state concentrations are related linearly to the dosing rate. Accordingly, the dose may be adjusted on the basis of the ratio between the desired and measured concentrations:

$$\frac{Cp_{SS} \text{ (desired)}}{Cp_{SS} \text{ (measured)}} = \frac{\text{dose (new)}}{\text{dose (previous)}}$$

For drugs that have dose-dependent kinetics (e.g., phenytoin and theophylline), plasma concentrations change disproportionately more than the alteration in the dosing rate. Not only should changes in dose be small to minimize the degree of unpredictability, but plasma concentration monitoring also is critical to ensure appropriate modification.

The variability among individual responses to given plasma levels must be recognized. This is illustrated by a hypothetical population concentration-response curve (Fig. 68-6) and its relationship to the

Table 68-5

Concentrations of Drugs in Plasma: Relation to Efficacy and Adverse Effects

Drug	Efficacy*	Adverse Effects†
Amikacin (peak)	20 μg/mL	40 μg/mL
Carbenicillin	100 μg/mL‡	300 μg/mL
Carbamazepine	3 μg/mL	10 μg/mL
Digitoxin	12 μg/mL	25–30 ng/mL
Digoxin	0.8 ng/mL	2.0 ng/mL
Ethosuximide	40 μg/mL	100 μg/mL
Gentamicin (peak)	5 μg/mL	10 μg/mL
Gentamicin (predose)		2.0 μg/mL
Lidocaine	1.5 μg/mL	5 μg/mL
Lithium	0.5 mEq/L	1.3 mEq/L
Penicillin G	1–25 μg/mL§	
Phenytoin (diphenylhydantoin)	10 μg/mL	20 μg/mL
Procainamide	4 μg/mL	10 μg/mL
Quinidine	2.5 μg/mL	6 μg/mL
Theophylline	8 μg/mL	20 μg/mL

* The therapeutic effect is infrequent or slight at levels below these.
† The frequency of adverse effects increases sharply when these levels are exceeded.
‡ Minimal inhibitory concentration (MIC) for most strains of *Pseudomonas aeruginosa*. MIC for other, more sensitive, organisms is less.
§ There is a wide range of MIC of penicillin for various organisms, and the MIC of all those for which penicillin is used is <20. "Massive" penicillin therapy with 20 million units daily achieves levels of 20 to 25 μg/mL in patients with clearance of creatinine of 100 mL/min.

therapeutic range or therapeutic window of desired plasma levels. The defined therapeutic window should include the levels at which the intended pharmacologic effect is achieved in most patients. However, a few persons, who are sensitive to the therapeutic effects, respond to lower levels, whereas others are refractory enough to require levels that may cause adverse effects. For example, a few patients with strong seizure foci require plasma levels of phenytoin exceeding 20 μg/mL to control seizures. Dosages to achieve this effect may be appropriate.

As also illustrated in Fig. 68-6, some patients are prone to adverse effects at levels that are tolerated by most of the population. Therefore, raising the plasma concentration of a drug to a level that has a high probability of being therapeutically effective may bring on unwanted actions in an occasional patient. Table 68-5 presents for a number of drugs the plasma concentrations that are associated with adverse and therapeutic effects in most patients. Use of this information according to the guidelines discussed should permit more effective and safer therapy for those patients who are not "average."

EFFECTIVE PARTICIPATION OF THE PATIENT IN THERAPY Measurement of the concentration of a drug in plasma is the most effective way to detect failure to take a drug. Such "noncompliance" is a frequent problem in the long-term treatment of diseases such as hypertension and epilepsy, occurring in 25 percent or more of patients in therapeutic environments in which no special effort is made to involve patients in the responsibility for their own health. Occasionally, noncompliance can be uncovered by sympathetic, nonincriminating questioning, but more often it is recognized only after determining that the concentration of drug in plasma is nil or is recurrently low. Because other factors can cause plasma levels to be lower than expected, comparison with levels obtained during inpatient treatment may be required to confirm that noncompliance has occurred. Once the physician is certain of noncompliance, a nonaccusatory discussion of the problem with the patient may clarify the reason for the noncompliance and serve as a basis for more effective cooperation on the part of the patient. Many approaches have been tried to make patients exercise more responsibility for their own treatment, most based on better communication regarding the nature of the disease and the chances of success or failure of the treatment. The patient is given a chance to discuss problems associated with treatment. The process may be improved by the involvement of nurses and other

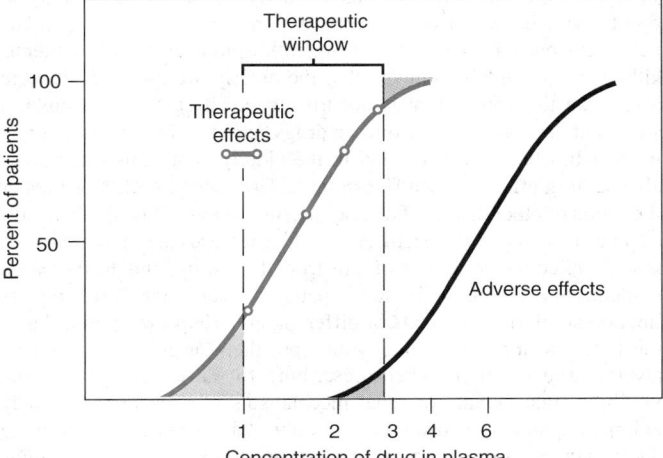

FIGURE 68-6 The cumulative percentage of patients responding to increasing levels of drug in plasma with both therapeutic and adverse effects. The therapeutic window defines the range of concentrations of drug that will achieve therapeutic effects in most patients with adverse effects in only a small percentage.

paramedical personnel. Minimizing the complexity of the regimen is helpful in terms of both the number of drugs and the frequency of administration. Educating patients to assume the principal role in their own health care requires a blend of the art and science of medicine.

BIBLIOGRAPHY

Benet LZ et al: Design and optimization of dosage regimens: Pharmacokinetic data, in *Goodman and Gilman's The Pharmacological Basis of Therapeutics*, 9th ed, JG Hardman et al (eds). New York, McGraw-Hill, 1995, Appendix II, p 1707

Bennett WM et al: *Drug Prescribing in Renal Failure: Dosing Guidelines for Adults*, 2d ed. Philadelphia, American College of Physicians, 1991

Brown GR et al: Drug concentration monitoring. An approach to rational use. Clin Pharmacokinet 24:187, 1993

Meyer UA: Drugs in special patient groups: Clinical importance of genetics in drug effects, in *Clinical Pharmacology: Basic Principles in Therapeutics*, 3d ed, KL Melmon et al (eds). New York, McGraw-Hill, 1992, p 875

Nebert DW et al: The P450 superfamily: Update on new sequences, gene mapping, accession numbers and nomenclature. Pharmacogenetics 6:1, 1996

Reynolds DJ, Aronson JK: ABCs of monitoring drug therapy. Making the most of plasma drug concentration measurements. BMJ 306:48, 1993

Tukey RH, Johnson EF: Molecular aspects of regulation and structure of drug metabolizing enzymes, in *Principles of Drug Action: The Basis of Pharmacology*, 3d ed, WB Pratt, P Taylor (eds). New York, Churchill Livingstone, 1990, p 423

69 *Alastair J. J. Wood*

ADVERSE REACTIONS TO DRUGS*

The beneficial effects of drugs are coupled with the inescapable risk of untoward effects. The morbidity and mortality from these untoward effects often present diagnostic problems because they can involve every organ and system of the body and are frequently mistaken for signs of underlying disease. Major advances in the investigation, development, and regulation of drugs ensure in most instances that they are uniform, effective, and relatively safe and that their recognized hazards are publicized. However, the large number and variety of drugs available over the counter (OTC) or by prescription make it impossible for patient or physician to obtain or retain the knowledge necessary to use all drugs well. It is understandable, therefore, that many OTC drugs are used unwisely by the public and that restricted drugs may be prescribed incorrectly by physicians.

Most physicians use no more than 50 drug products in their practice, gaining familiarity with their effectiveness and safety. Most patients probably use only a limited number of OTC drugs. Nevertheless, many patients receive care and drug prescriptions from more than one physician, and in any 30-day period, many patients consume more than three different OTC drug products containing nine or more different chemical agents.

Twenty-five to fifty percent of patients make errors in self-administration of prescribed medicines, and these errors can be responsible for adverse drug effects. Elderly patients are the group most likely to commit such errors, perhaps in part because they consume more medicines. One-third or more of patients also may not take their prescribed medications. Similarly, patients commit errors in taking OTC drugs by not reading or following the directions on the containers. Physicians must recognize that providing directions with prescriptions does not always guarantee compliance.

---

* John A. Oates was coauthor in the 12th edition, and this chapter represents a revision of that work.

Every drug can produce untoward consequences, even when used according to standard or recommended methods of administration. When used incorrectly, the effectiveness may be reduced, and adverse reactions can be expected to occur more frequently. Also, the administration of several drugs concurrently may result in adverse drug interactions (see Chap. 68). In the hospital, all drugs a patient is given should be under the control of a physician, and patient compliance is, in general, ensured. Errors may occur nevertheless—the wrong drug or dose may be given, or the drug may be given to the wrong patient—although improved drug distribution and administration systems have reduced this problem. On the other hand, there are no means for controlling how ambulatory patients take prescription or OTC drugs.

EPIDEMIOLOGY   Epidemiologic studies of adverse drug reactions have been helpful in evaluating the magnitude of the overall problem, in calculating the rate of reactions to individual drugs, and in characterizing some of the determinants of adverse drug effects.

Patients receive, on average, 10 different drugs during each hospitalization. The sicker the patient, the more drugs are given, and there is a corresponding increase in the likelihood of adverse drug reactions. When fewer than 6 different drugs are given to hospitalized patients, the probability of an adverse reaction is about 5 percent, but if more than 15 drugs are given, the probability is over 40 percent. Retrospective analyses of ambulatory patients have revealed adverse drug effects in 20 percent.

Thus, the magnitude of drug-induced disease is large. Of patients admitted to the medical and pediatric services of general hospitals, 2 to 5 percent are admitted because of illnesses attributed to drugs. The case/fatality ratio from drug-induced disease in hospitalized patients varies from 2 to 12 percent. Furthermore, some fetal or neonatal abnormalities are due to medicines taken by the mother during pregnancy or parturition.

A small group of widely used drugs accounts for a disproportionate number of reactions. Aspirin and other analgesics, digoxin, anticoagulants, diuretics, antimicrobials, steroids, antineoplastics, and hypoglycemic agents account for 90 percent of reactions, although the drugs involved differ between ambulatory and hospitalized patients. Estimates of the cost of drug-related morbidity and mortality in the ambulatory setting range from $30 billion to $130 billion.

ADVERSE DRUG REACTIONS IN THE ELDERLY (See also Chap. 9)   The elderly as a group have a greater burden of disease and receive a greater number of medications than other persons. Thus, it is not surprising that adverse drug reactions occur frequently in elderly patients. The issue of whether an elderly individual is more likely to develop an adverse drug reaction than a young person with a similar number of concurrent diseases and taking the same number of drugs has not been answered unequivocally. However, in population surveys of the noninstitutionalized elderly, as many as 10 percent report having had at least one adverse drug reaction in the last year. The incidence appears to be even greater in hospitalized elderly patients. Although it is widely believed that the elderly are more sensitive to drugs than the young, that is not true for all drugs. For example, a consistent decrease in sensitivity to drugs acting at the beta-adrenergic receptor has been demonstrated in the elderly. The consequences of adverse drug effects may differ in the elderly because of their greater likelihood of other disease. For example, use of long–half-life benzodiazepines is linked to the occurrence of hip fractures in elderly patients, perhaps reflecting both a risk of falls from these drugs and the increased incidence of osteoporosis in elderly patients. Even when a drug impairs function similarly in patients of different age groups, the poorer baseline function in elderly persons may put them at greater risk for an adverse drug reaction. When prescribing for an elderly patient, the possibility that hepatic or renal mechanisms of drug excretion may be impaired should be taken into account. Adverse drug effects in the elderly may be subtle and, as in all populations, the physician must be alert to the possibility that a patient's signs and symptoms reflect an adverse effect of medication.

ETIOLOGY   Most adverse drug reactions are preventable, and recent studies using a systems analysis approach suggest that the most common system failure associated with an adverse drug reaction is the failure to disseminate knowledge about drugs to individuals involved in prescribing and administering them. Most adverse reactions can be classified into two groups. The most frequent ones result from an exaggeration of a predicted pharmacologic action of the drug. Other adverse reactions ensue from toxic effects unrelated to the intended pharmacologic actions. The latter effects often are unpredictable, frequently are severe, and result from recognized as well as undiscovered mechanisms. Some mechanisms unrelated to the drug's primary pharmacologic activity include direct cytotoxicity, initiation of abnormal immune responses, and perturbation of metabolic processes in individuals with genetic enzymatic defects. Further understanding of interindividual differences in the expression of the enzymes responsible for drug metabolism has contributed to the understanding of adverse drug reactions that previously were thought to be idiosyncratic. For example, the hemotoxicity of dapsone, which includes hemolysis in patients with glucose-6-phosphate dehydrogenase (G6PD) deficiency as well as agranulocytosis, is thought to be due to the metabolism of dapsone to its hydroxylamine metabolite by specific cytochrome P450 enzymes. The extent to which dapsone is converted to this toxic metabolite depends on the activity of these cytochrome P450 enzymes in the individual, which thus determines the individual's susceptibility to the adverse effect. Conversely, an understanding of the enzymes responsible for producing the toxic metabolite may make it possible to coadminister specific enzyme inhibitors that will prevent the toxic effect.

Prior consideration of the factors known to modify drug action often make it possible to prevent adverse reactions of this type.

An abnormally high drug concentration at the receptor site (site of action) owing to pharmacokinetic variability is the usual cause of these reactions (see Chap. 68). For example, a reduction in the volume of distribution, in the rate of metabolism, or in the rate of excretion all result in higher than expected concentration of drug at the receptor site, with a consequent increase in the pharmacologic effect.

Recently, the specific cytochrome P450s involved in drug metabolism have been identified. Recognition of the polymorphic distribution of some of these enzyme activities within the population provides an explanation for interindividual variability in drug clearance. Also, as simple tests are developed to characterize an individual's specific cytochrome P450 activity, it should become possible to identify in advance individuals at particular risk for concentration-related adverse effects. For enzymes whose activity is polymorphically distributed a proportion of the population has little or no enzyme activity. In these individuals, the concentration of drugs achieved will be higher than normal and may produce toxicity. Conversely, where toxicity or efficacy is produced by a metabolite, poor metabolizers will have limited toxicity or efficacy. The polymorphic distribution of drug-metabolizing enzymes may explain some adverse drug effects previously labeled as idiosyncratic.

Alteration in the dose-response curve due to increased receptor sensitivity results in an increase in drug effect at a given drug concentration. An example is the excessive response of elderly persons to the anticoagulant warfarin at normal or lower than normal blood levels.

The shape of the dose-response curve also determines the likelihood of adverse drug reactions. Drugs with a steep dose-response curve or a narrow therapeutic index (see Chap. 68) are more likely to cause dose-related toxicity because a small increase in dose produces a large change in pharmacologic effect. An increase in the dose of drugs that exhibit nonlinear kinetics, such as phenytoin (see Chap. 68), may produce a proportionately greater increase in the blood level, resulting in toxicity.

Concurrent administration of other drugs may affect pharmacokinetics or pharmacodynamics. Pharmacokinetics may be affected by alterations in bioavailability, protein binding, or the rate of metabolism or excretion. Pharmacodynamics may be altered by another drug that competes for the same receptor sites, that prevents the drug from reaching its site of action, or that antagonizes or enhances the drug's pharmacologic effect. Inhibition of the metabolism of one drug by another may occur when both drugs bind to the same cytochrome P450. Therefore, as the specific cytochrome P450s responsible for the metabolism of individual drugs becomes known, prediction of drug interactions is put on a more rational scientific basis. An important recent example of such a mechanism is the inhibition of terfenadine's metabolism by inhibitors of Cyp3A, such as erythromycin and systemic antimycotics. Such inhibition has resulted in torsade de pointes and lethal cardiac arrhythmia (see Chap. 68).

TOXICITY UNRELATED TO A DRUG'S PRIMARY PHARMACOLOGIC ACTIVITY **Cytotoxic Reactions** The understanding of so-called idiosyncratic reactions has greatly improved with the recognition that many of them are due to irreversible binding of a drug or its metabolites to tissue macromolecules by covalent bonds. Some chemical carcinogens, such as the alkylating agents, combine directly with DNA. Usually, it is only after metabolic activation of a drug to reactive metabolites that covalent binding occurs. This activation usually occurs in the microsomal mixed-function oxidase system, the hepatic enzyme system responsible for the metabolism of many drugs (see Chap. 68). During the course of drug metabolism, reactive metabolites may covalently bind to tissue macromolecules, causing tissue damage. Because of the reactive nature of these metabolites, covalent binding often occurs close to the site of production. Typically that is the liver, but the mixed-function oxidase system is found in other tissues as well.

An example of this type of adverse drug reaction is the hepatotoxicity associated with isoniazid. This drug is metabolized principally by acetylation to acetylisoniazid, which is then hydrolyzed to acetylhydrazine. The further metabolism of acetylhydrazine by the mixed-function oxidase system liberates reactive metabolites that covalently bind to hepatic macromolecules, causing hepatic necrosis. The administration of drugs known to increase the activity of the mixed-function oxidase system, such as phenobarbital or rifampin, together with isoniazid results in the production of increased amounts of reactive metabolites, increased covalent binding, and a greater risk of hepatic damage.

The hepatic necrosis produced by overdosage of acetaminophen is also caused by reactive metabolites. Normally these metabolites are detoxified by combining with hepatic glutathione. When glutathione becomes exhausted, the metabolites bind instead to hepatic protein, with resultant hepatocyte damage. The hepatic necrosis produced by the ingestion of acetaminophen can be prevented, or at least attenuated, by the administration of substances such as *N*-acetylcysteine that reduce the binding of electrophilic metabolites to hepatic proteins. The risk of hepatic necrosis is increased in patients receiving drugs such as phenobarbital that increase the rate of drug metabolism and the rate of production of toxic metabolite(s).

It is likely, though as yet not proven, that other idiosyncratic reactions are caused by the covalent binding of reactive metabolites to tissue macromolecules, resulting either in direct cytotoxicity or in the initiation of an immune response.

Immunologic Mechanisms Most pharmacologic agents are poor immunogens because they are small molecules with molecular weights of less than 2000. Stimulation of antibody synthesis or sensitization of lymphocytes by a drug or one of its metabolites usually requires in vivo activation and covalent linkage to protein, carbohydrate, or nucleic acid.

Drug stimulation of antibody production may mediate tissue injury by one of several mechanisms. The antibody may attack the drug when the drug is covalently attached to a cell, and thereby destroy the cell. This mechanism occurs in penicillin-induced hemolytic anemia. Antibody-drug-antigen complexes may be passively adsorbed by a bystander cell, which is then destroyed by activation of complement; this occurs in quinine- and quinidine-induced thrombocytopenia. Drugs or their reactive metabolites may alter a host tissue, rendering it antigenic and eliciting autoantibodies. For example, hydralazine and procainamide can chemically alter nuclear material, stimulating the formation of anti-nuclear antibodies and occasionally causing lupus erythematosus. Autoantibodies can be elicited by drugs that neither interact with the host antigen nor have any chemical similarity to the host tissue; for example, α-methyldopa frequently stimulates the formation of antibodies to host erythrocytes, yet the drug neither attaches to the erythrocyte nor shares any chemical similarities with the antigenic determinants on the erythrocyte.

Drug-induced *pure red cell aplasia* (Chap. 110) is due to an immune-based drug reaction. Red cell formation in bone marrow cultures can be inhibited by phenytoin and purified IgG obtained from a patient with pure red cell aplasia associated with phenytoin.

Serum sickness (Chap. 310) results from the deposition of circulating drug-antibody complexes on endothelial surfaces. Complement activation occurs, chemotactic factors are generated locally, and an inflammatory response develops at the site of complex entrapment. Arthralgias, urticaria, lymphadenopathy, glomerulonephritis, or cerebritis may result. Penicillin is the most common cause of serum sickness today. Many drugs, particularly antimicrobial agents, induce production of IgE, which binds to mast cell membranes. Contact with a drug antigen initiates a series of biochemical events in the mast cell and results in the release of mediators that can produce the urticaria, wheezing, flushing, rhinorrhea, and (occasionally) hypotension characteristic of anaphylaxis.

Drugs also may excite cell-mediated immune responses. Topically administered substances may interact with sulfhydryl or amino groups in the skin and react with sensitized lymphocytes to produce the rash characteristic of contact dermatitis. Other types of rashes also may result from the interaction of serum factors, drugs, and sensitized lymphocytes. The role of drug-activated lymphocytes in the immune mechanisms governing destruction of visceral tissue is unknown.

Toxicity Associated with Genetically Determined Enzymatic Defects   In the porphyrias, drugs that increase the activity of enzymes proximal to the deficient enzyme in the biosynthetic pathway of porphyrins can increase the quantity of porphyrin precursors that accumulate proximal to the deficient enzyme (Chap. 343). These drugs are listed in Table 69-1.

Patients with a deficiency of G6PD develop hemolytic anemia in response to primaquine and a number of other drugs (Table 69-1) that do not cause hemolysis in patients with adequate quantities of this enzyme (Chap. 109).

DIAGNOSIS   The manifestations of drug-induced diseases frequently resemble those of other diseases, and a given set of manifestations may be produced by different and dissimilar drugs. Recognition of the role of a drug or drugs in an illness depends on appreciation of the possible adverse reactions to drugs in any disease, on identification of the temporal relationship between drug administration and development of the illness, and on familiarity with the common manifestations of the drugs. Many associations between particular drugs and specific reactions have been described, but there is always a "first time" for a novel association, and any drug should be suspected of causing an adverse effect if the clinical setting is appropriate.

Illness related to a drug's pharmacologic action often is more easily recognized than illness attributable to immune or other mechanisms. For example, side effects such as cardiac arrhythmias in patients receiving digitalis, hypoglycemia in patients given insulin, and bleeding in patients receiving anticoagulants are more readily related to a

Table 69-1

Clinical Manifestations of Adverse Reactions to Drugs

I. MULTISYSTEM MANIFESTATIONS

Anaphylaxis	Drug-induced lupus erythematosus	Fever	Serum sickness
ACE* inhibitors and dialysis	Acebutolol	Aminosalicylic acid	Aspirin
Cephalosporins	Asparaginase	Amphotericin B	β-lactams
Demeclocycline	Barbiturates	Antihistamines	Penicillins
Dextran	Bleomycin	Carbenicillin	Propylthiouracil
Insulin	Cephalosporins	Intravenous immune globulin	Streptokinase
Intravenous immune globulin	Hydralazine	Novobiocin	Streptomycin
Iodinated drugs or contrast media	Iodides	Pamidronate	Sulfonamides
Iron dextran	Isoniazid	Penicillins	Vasculitis
Lidocaine	Methyldopa	Streptokinase	Allopurinol
Penicillins	Phenolphthalein	Hyperpyrexia	Aminopenicillins
Procaine	Phenytoin	Antipsychotics	Hydantoins
Streptomycin	Procainamide	Neuroleptic malignant syndrome	Penicillin
Sulfobromophthalein	Quinidine	Antipsychotics	Propylthiouracil
Angioedema	Sulfonamides	Antidopaminergics	Sulfonamides
ACE* inhibitors	Thiouracil		Thiazides
Penicillin			

II. ENDOCRINE MANIFESTATIONS

Addisonian-like syndrome	Gynecomastia (*cont.*)	Sexual dysfunction	Thyroid dysfunction (*cont.*)
Busulfan	Isoniazid	Decreased libido and impotence	Colestipol and nicotinic acid
Etomidate	Methyldopa	(*cont.*)	Dimercaprol
Ketoconazole	Phenytoin	Methyldopa	Gold salts
Galactorrhea (may also cause	Reserpine	Oral contraceptives	Iodides
amenorrhea)	Spironolactone	Sedatives	Lithium
Domperidone	Testosterone	Impairment of spermatogenesis or	Oral contraceptives
Methyldopa	Sexual dysfunction	oogenesis	Phenindione
Metoclopramide	Impaired ejaculation	Cytotoxic agents	Phenothiazines (long-term)
Phenothiazines	Bethanidine	Priapism	Phenylbutazone
Reserpine	Debrisoquin	Trazodone	Phenytoin
Tricyclic antidepressants	Guanethidine	Thyroid dysfunction (disorders	Sulfonamides
Gynecomastia	Thioridazine	causing abnormal results on	Tolbutamide
Calcium channel antagonists	Decreased libido and impotence	thyroid function tests)	Vaginal carcinoma
Clomiphene	Beta blockers	Acetazolamide	Diethylstilbestrol (given to
Digitalis	Clonidine	Amiodarone	mother)
Estrogens	Diuretics	Bromsulfophthalein	
Ethionamide	Lithium	Chlorpropamide	
Griseofulvin	Major tranquilizers	Clofibrate	

(*continued*)

Table 69-1—(continued)

Clinical Manifestations of Adverse Reactions to Drugs

III. METABOLIC MANIFESTATIONS

Hyperbilirubinemia
  Novobiocin
  Rifampin
Hypercalcemia
  Antacids with absorbable alkali
  Calcitonin
  Thiazides
  Vitamin D
Hyperglycemia
  Asparaginase
  Chlorthalidone
  Diazoxide
  Encainide
  Ethacrynic acid
  Furosemide
  Glucocorticoids
  Growth hormone
  Niacin
  Oral contraceptives
  Phenytoin
  Pentamidine
  Thiazides
Hypoglycemia
  Insulin
  Octreotide
  Oral hypoglycemics
  Pentamidine
  Quinine

Hyperkalemia
  ACE* inhibitors
  Amiloride
  Cyclosporine
  Cytotoxics
  Digitalis overdose
  Heparin
  Lithium
  NSAIDs†
  Pentamidine
  Potassium preparations
    including salt substitute
  Potassium salts of drugs
  Spironolactone
  Succinylcholine
  Triamterene
  Trimethoprin
Hypokalemia
  Alkali-induced alkalosis
  Amphotericin B
  Carbenoxolone
  Corticosteroids
  Diuretics
  Gentamicin
  Insulin
  Laxatives (abused)
  Mineralocorticoids, some
    glucocorticoids

Hypokalemia (cont.)
  Osmotic diuretics
  Sympathomimetic agents
  Tetracycline (degraded)
  Theophylline
  Vitamin B₁₂
Hyperuricemia
  Aspirin (low dose)
  Chlorthalidone
  Cyclosporine
  Cytotoxics
  Ethacrynic acid
  Fructose (IV)
  Furosemide
  Hyperalimentation
  Pyrazinamide
  Thiazides
Hyponatremia
  Dilutional:
    Antipsychotics
    Carbamazepine
    Chlorpropamide
    Cyclophosphamide
    Desmopressin
    Diuretics
    Intravenous immune globulin
    Octreotide
    Vincristine

Hyponatremia (cont.)
  Salt-wasting:
    Diuretics
    Enemas
    Mannitol
Metabolic acidosis
  Acetazolamide
  Metformin
  Paraldehyde (degraded)
  Phenformin
  Salicylates
  Spironolactone
Porphyria exacerbation
  Barbiturates
  Chlordiazepoxide
  Chlorpropamide
  Estrogens
  Glutethimide
  Griseofulvin
  Meprobamate
  Oral contraceptives
  Phenytoin
  Rifampin
  Sulfonamides

IV. DERMATOLOGIC MANIFESTATIONS

Acne
  Anabolic and androgenic steroids
  Bromides
  Glucocorticoids
  Iodides
  Isoniazid
  Oral contraceptives
  Troxidone
Alopecia
  Beta blockers
  Colchicine
  Cytotoxics
  Ethionamide
  Fluconazole
  Heparin
  Interferon
  Lithium
  Oral contraceptives (withdrawal)
  Retinoids
Eczema
  Captopril
  Cream and lotion preservatives
  Lanolin
  Topical antihistamines
  Topical antimicrobials
  Topical local anesthetics
Erythema multiforme or Steven-
  Johnson syndrome/toxic epidermal
  necrolysis
  Allopurinol
  Aminopenicillins
  Barbiturates
  Carbamazepine
  Cephalosporins
  Chlorpropamide
  Codeine
  Ethosuximide

Erythema multiforme (cont.)
  Imidazoles
  Iodides
  Lamotrigine
  Nalidixic acid
  Penicillins
  Phenolphthalein
  Phenylbutazone
  Phenytoin
  Piroxicam
  Quinolones
  Salicylates
  Sulfonamides
  Sulfones
  Tetracyclines
  Thiazides
  Tocainide
  Valproic acid
Erythema nodosum
  Oral contraceptives
  Penicillins
  Sulfonamides
Exfoliative dermatitis
  Barbiturates
  Gold salts
  Penicillins
  Phenylbutazone
  Phenytoin
  Quinidine
  Sulfonamides
Fixed drug eruptions
  Barbiturates
  Captopril
  Foscarnet (penile ulceration)
  Phenolphthalein
  Phenylbutazone
  Quinine

Fixed drug eruptions (cont.)
  Salicylates
  Sulfonamides
Hyperpigmentation
  Bleomycin
  Busulfan
  Chloroquine and other
    antimalarials
  Corticotropin
  Cyclophosphamide
  Gold salts
  Oral contraceptives
  Phenothiazines
  Vitamin A (hypervitaminosis A)
Hypertrichosis
  Cyclosporin
  Minoxidil
  Phenytoin
Lichenoid eruptions
  Aminosalicylic acid
  Antimalarials
  Chlorpropamide
  Gold salts
  Methyldopa
  Phenothiazines
Nail changes
  Penicillamine
  Retinoids
  Tetracyclines
Photodermatitis
  Captopril
  Chlordiazepoxide
  Furosemide
  Griseofulvin
  Nalidixic acid
  NSAIDs†
  Oral contraceptives

Photodermatitis (cont.)
  Phenothiazines
  Sulfonamides
  Sulfonylureas
  Tetracyclines, particularly
    demeclocycline
  Thiazides
Purpura (see also
  thrombocytopenia)
  Aspirin
  Glucocorticoids
  Rashes (nonspecific)
  Allopurinol
  Ampicillin
  Barbiturates
  Indapamide
  Methyldopa
  Phenytoin
Raynaud's disease or digital
  necrosis
  Beta blockers
  Bleomycin
  Ergot alkaloids
Skin necrosis
  Warfarin
Urticaria
  Aspirin
  Barbiturates
  Captopril
  Enalapril
  Intravenous immune
    globulin
  Penicillins
  Sulfonamides

(continued)

Table 69-1—*(continued)*

Clinical Manifestations of Adverse Reactions to Drugs

V. HEMATOLOGIC MANIFESTATIONS

Agranulocytosis (see also
  pancytopenia)
  Aprindine
  Captopril
  Carbimazole
  Cefotaxime
  Chloramphenicol
  Clozapine
  Co-trimoxazole
  Cytotoxics
  Gold salts
  Indomethacin
  Methimazole
  Oxyphenbutazone
  Phenothiazines
  Phenylbutazone
  Propylthiouracil
  Sulfonamides
  Ticlopidine
  Tolbutamide
  Tricyclic antidepressants
Clotting and bleeding abnormalities/
  hypothrombinemia
  Cefamandole
  Cefoperazone
  Ketorolac
  Mezlocillin
  Moxalactam
  Piperacillin
  Valproic acid
Eosinophilia
  Aminosalicylic acid
  Chlorpropamide
  Erythromycin estolate
  Imipramine
  L-Tryptophan

Eosinophilia *(cont.)*
  Methotrexate
  Nitrofurantoin
  Procarbazine
  Sulfonamides
Hemolytic anemia
  Aminosalicylic acid
  Cephalosporins
  Chlorpromazine
  Dapsone
  Insulin
  Isoniazid
  Levodopa
  Mefenamic acid
  Melphalan
  Methyldopa
  Penicillins
  Phenacetin
  Procainamide
  Quinidine
  Rifampin
  Sulfonamides
Hemolytic anemia (in G6PD
  deficiency)
  Aminosalicylic acid
  Antimalarials, e.g., primaquine
  Aspirin
  Chloramphenicol
  Co-trimoxazole
  Dapsone
  Nalidixic acid
  Nitrofurantoin
  Phenacetin
  Probenecid
  Procainamide
  Quinidine

Hemolytic anemia *(cont.)*
  Sulfonamides
  Vitamin C
  Vitamin K
Leukocytosis
  Glucocorticoids
  Lithium
Lymphadenopathy
  Phenytoin
  Primidone
Megaloblastic anemia
  Co-trimoxazole
  Folate antagonists
  Nitrous oxide (repeated or
    prolonged exposure)
  Oral contraceptives
  Phenobarbital
  Phenytoin
  Primidone
  Triamterene
  Trimethoprim
Pancytopenia (aplastic anemia)
  Carbamazepine
  Carbimazole
  Chloramphenicol
  Cytotoxics
  Felbamate
  Gold salts
  Mepacrine
  Mephenytoin
  Oxyphenbutazone
  Phenylbutazone
  Phenytoin
  Potassium perchlorate
  Quinacrine
  Sulfonamides

Pancytopenia *(cont.)*
  Thiouracils
  Trimethadione
  Zidovudine (AZT)
Pure red cell aplasia
  Azathioprine
  Chlorpropamide
  Isoniazid
  Phenytoin
Thrombocytopenia (see also
  pancytopenia)
  Acetazolamine
  Aspirin
  Carbamazepine
  Carbenicillin
  Chlorpropamide
  Chlorthalidone
  Co-trimoxazole
  Digitoxin
  Furosemide
  Gold salts
  Heparin
  Indomethacin
  Isoniazid
  Methyldopa
  Moxalactam
  Novobiocin
  Oxyphenbutazone
  Phenylbutazone
  Phenytoin and other
    hydantoins
  Quinidine
  Quinine
  Thiazides
  Ticarcillin

VI. CARDIOVASCULAR MANIFESTATIONS

Acute chest pain (nonischemic)
  Bleomycin
Angina exacerbation
  Alpha blockers
  Beta-blocker withdrawal
  Ergotamine
  Excessive thyroxine
  Hydralazine
  Methysergide
  Minoxidil
  Nifedipine
  Oxytocin
  Sumatriptan
  Vasopressin
Arrhythmias
  Adriamycin
  Antiarrhythmic drugs
  Astemizole
  Atropine
  Anticholinesterases
  Beta blockers
  Cisapride
  Daunorubicin
  Digitalis
  Emetine
  Erythromycin
  Guanethidine

Arrhythmias *(cont.)*
  Ketanserin
  Lithium
  Papaverine
  Pentamidine
  Phenothiazines, particularly
    thioridazine
  Probucol
  Sympathomimetics
  Terfenadine
  Theophylline
  Thyroid hormone
  Tricyclic antidepressants
  Verapamil
AV block
  Clonidine
  Methyldopa
  Verapamil
Cardiomyopathy
  Adriamycin
  Daunorubicin
  Emetine
  Lithium
  Phenothiazines
  Sulfonamides
  Sympathomimetics

Fluid retention/congestive heart
  failure/edema
  Beta blockers
  Calcium blockers
  Carbenoxolone
  Diazoxide
  Estrogens
  Indomethacin
  Mannitol
  Minoxidil
  Phenylbutazone
  Steroids
  Verapamil
Hypotension (see also arrhythmias)
  Amiodarone (perioperative)
  Calcium channel blockers, e.g.,
    nifedipine
  Citrated blood
  Diuretics
  Interleukin 2
  Levodopa
  Morphine
  Nitroglycerin
  Phenothiazines
  Protamine
  Quinidine

Hypertension
  Clonidine withdrawal
  Corticotropin
  Cyclosporine
  Glucocorticoids
  Monoamine oxidase
    inhibitors with
    sympathomimetics
  NSAIDs (some)
  Oral contraceptives
  Sympathomimetics
  Tricyclic antidepressants
    with sympathomimetics
Pericarditis
  Emetine
  Hydralazine
  Methysergide
  Procainamide
Pericardial effusion
  Minoxidil
Thromboembolism
  Oral contraceptives

(continued)

Table 69-1—*(continued)*

Clinical Manifestations of Adverse Reactions to Drugs

VII. RESPIRATORY MANIFESTATIONS

Airway obstruction (bronchospasm, asthma; see also anaphylaxis)
  Adenosine
  Beta blockers
  Cephalosporins
  Cholinergic drugs
  NSAIDs, e.g., aspirin, indomethacin
  Penicillins
  Pentazocine
  Streptomycin
  Tartrazine (drugs with yellow dye)

Cough
  ACE inhibitors
Nasal congestion
  Decongestant abuse
  Guanethidine
  Isoproterenol
  Oral contraceptives
  Reserpine
Pulmonary edema
  Contrast media
  Heroin
  Hydrochlorthiazide
  Interleukin 2
  Methadone
  Propoxyphene

Pulmonary hypertension
  Fenfluramine
Pulmonary infiltrates
  Acyclovir
  Amiodarone
  Azothioprine
  Bleomycin
  Busulfan
  Carmustine (BCNU)
  Chlorambucil
  Cyclophosphamide
  Gold
  Melphalan
  Methotrexate

Pulmonary infiltrates *(cont.)*
  Methysergide
  Mitomycin C
  Nitrofurantoin
  Procarbazine
  Sulfonamides
Respiratory depression
  Aminoglycosides
  Hypnotics
  Opiates
  Polymyxins
  Sedatives
  Trimethaphan

VIII. GASTROINTESTINAL MANIFESTATIONS

Cholestatic hepatitis
  Acetohexamide
  Anabolic steroids
  Androgens
  Chlorpropamide
  Clavulanic acid/amoxicillin
  Cyclosporine
  Erythromycin estolate
  Flucloxacillin
  Gold salts
  Methimazole
  Nitrofurantoin
  Oral contraceptives
  Phenothiazines
Constipation or ileus
  Aluminum hydroxide
  Barium sulfate
  Calcium carbonate
  Ferrous sulfate
  Ganglionic blockers
  Ion exchange resins
  Opiates
  Phenothiazines
  Tricyclic antidepressants
  Verapamil
Diarrhea or colitis
  Antibiotics (broad-spectrum)
  Clindamycin
  Cocaine
  Colchicine
  Digitalis
  Guanethidine
  Lactose excipients
  Lincomycin
  Magnesium in antacids
  Methyldopa
  Misoprostol
  Oral contraceptives
  Purgatives
  Reserpine
  Ticlopidine

Diffuse hepatocellular damage
  Acetaminophen (paracetamol)
  Acebutolol
  Allopurinol
  Aminosalicylic acid
  Amiodarone
  Aprindine
  Carbenicillin
  Cyclophosphamide
  Dapsone
  Diclofenac
  Erythromycin estolate
  Ethionamide
  Felbamate
  Glyburide
  Halothane
  Isoniazid
  Ketoconazole
  Labetalol
  Lovastatin
  Methimazole
  Methotrexate
  Methoxyflurane
  Methyldopa
  Monoamine oxidase inhibitors
  Niacin
  Nifedipine
  Nitrofurantoin
  Oxyphenisatin
  Phenytoin and other hydantoins
  Propoxyphene
  Propylthiouracil
  Pyridium
  Quinidine
  Rifampin
  Salicylates
  Sodium valproate
  Sulfonamides
  Tacrine
  Tetracyclines
  Trazodone
  Verapamil
  Zidovudine (AZT)

Gallstones/biliary pseudolithiasis
  Ceftriaxone
Intestinal ulceration
  Solid KCl preparations
Malabsorption
  Aminosalicylic acid
  Antibiotics (broad-spectrum)
  Cholestyramine
  Colchicine
  Colestipol
  Cytotoxic agents
  Neomycin
  Phenobarbital
  Phenytoin
  Primidone
Nausea or vomiting
  Digitalis
  Estrogens
  Ferrous sulfate
  Levodopa
  Opiates
  Potassium chloride
  Tetracyclines
  Theophylline
Oral conditions
  Dental discoloration:
    Tetracycline
  Dry mouth:
    Anticholinergics
    Clonidine
    Levodopa
    Methyldopa
    Tricyclic antidepressants
  Gingival hyperplasia:
    Calcium antagonists
    Cyclosporine
    Phenytoin
  Salivary gland swelling:
    Bethanidine
    Bretylium
    Clonidine

Oral conditions
  Salivary gland swelling *(cont.)*
    Guanethidine
    Iodides
    Phenylbutazone
  Taste disturbances:
    Acetazolamide
    Biguanides
    Captopril
    Griseofulvin
    Lithium
    Metronidazole
    Penicillamine
    Rifampin
  Ulceration:
    Aspirin
    Cytotoxic agents
    Gentian violet
    Isoproterenol (sublingual)
  Pancreatin
Pancreatitis
  Asparaginase
  Azathioprine
  Didanosine
  Estrogens
  Ethacrynic acid
  Furosemide
  Glucocorticoids
  Mercaptopurine
  Opiates
  Oral contraceptives
  Pentamidine
  Sulfonamides
  Thiazides
  Valproic acid
Peptic ulceration or hemorrhage
  Aspirin
  Ethacrynic acid
  Glucocorticoids
  NSAIDs†
  Reserpine (large doses)

(continued)

Table 69-1—*(continued)*

Clinical Manifestations of Adverse Reactions to Drugs

IX. RENAL MANIFESTATIONS

Bladder dysfunction/incontinence
  Anticholinergics
  Disopyramide
  Monoamine oxidase inhibitors
  Prazosin
  Terazosin
  Tricyclic antidepressants
Calculi
  Acetazolamide
  Vitamin D
Concentrating defect with polyuria
  (or nephrogenic diabetes insipidus)
  Demeclocycline
  Lithium
  Methoxyflurane
  Vitamin D
Hemorrhage cystitis
  Cyclophosphamide

Interstitial nephritis
  Cephalosporins
  Ciprofloxacin
  Allopurinol
  Furosemide
  NSAIDs†
  Penicillins, esp. methicillin
  Phenindione
  Rifampin
  Sulfonamides
  Thiazides
Nephropathies
  Analgesics (e.g., phenacetin)
Nephrotic syndrome
  Captopril
  Gold salts
  Ketoprofen

Nephrotic syndrome *(cont.)*
  Penicillamine
  Phenindione
  Probenecid
Obstructive uropathy
  Extrarenal: methysergide
Intrarenal:
  Acyclovir
  Cytotoxic agents
  Methotrexate
  Metyrosine
Renal dysfunction
  ACE inhibitors
  Cyclosporine
  NSAIDs
  Pentamidine
  Triamterene

Renal tubular acidosis
  Acetazolamide
  Amphotericin B
  Degraded tetracycline
Tubular necrosis
  Aminoglycosides
  Amphotericin B
  Cephaloridine
  Colistin
  Cyclosporine
  Intravenous immune
    globulin
  Methoxyflurane
  Polymyxins
  Radioiodinated contrast
    medium
  Sulfonamides
  Tetracyclines

X. NEUROLOGIC MANIFESTATIONS

Aseptic meningitis
  Intravenous immune globulin
CNS/vasculitis/cerebral hemorrhage
  Phenylpropanolamine
Exacerbation of myasthenia
  Aminoglycosides
  D-Penicillamine
  Polymyxins
Extrapyramidal effects
  Butyrophenones, e.g., haloperidol
  Levodopa
  Methyldopa
  Metoclopramide
  Oral contraceptives
  Phenothiazines
  Reserpine
  Tricyclic antidepressants
Headache
  Bromides
  Ergotamine (withdrawal)
  Glyceryl trinitrate
  Hydralazine

Headache *(cont.)*
  Indomethacin
  Intravenous immune globulin
Peripheral neuropathy
  Amiodarone
  Chloramphenicol
  Chloroquine
  Chlorpropamide
  Cisplatin
  Clioquinol
  Clofibrate
  Demeclocycline
  Disopyramide
  Ethambutol
  Ethionamide
  Glutethimide
  Hydralazine
  Isoniazid
  Methysergide
  Metronidazole
  Mustine
  Nalidixic acid

Peripheral neuropathy *(cont.)*
  Nitrofurantoin
  Perhexiline
  Phenelzine
  Phenytoin
  Polymyxin, colistin
  Procarbazine
  Streptomycin
  Tolbutamide
  Tricyclic antidepressants
  Vincristine
Pseudotumor cerebri (or intracranial
  hypertension)
  Amiodarone
  Glucocorticoids,
    mineralocorticoids
  Vitamin A (hypervitaminosis A)
  Oral contraceptives
  Tetracyclines
Seizures
  Amphetamines
  Analeptics

Seizures *(cont.)*
  Imipenem
  Isoniazid
  Lidocaine
  Lithium
  Nalidixic acid
  Meperidine
  Penicillins
  Phenothiazines
  Physostigmine
  Theophylline
  Tricyclic antidepressants
  Vincristine
Sleep disorders
  Lovastatin
Stroke
  Cocaine
  Oral contraceptives
Tremor
  Beta-adrenergic agonists

XI. OCULAR MANIFESTATIONS

Cataracts
  Busulfan
  Chlorambucil
  Glucocorticoids
  Phenothiazines
Color vision alteration
  Barbiturates
  Digitalis
  Methaqualone
  Streptomycin
  Sulfonamides

Color vision alteration *(cont.)*
  Thiazides
  Troxidone
Corneal edema
  Oral contraceptives
Corneal opacities
  Chloroquine
  Indomethacin
  Mepacrine
  Vitamin D

Eye pain
  Nifedipine
Glaucoma
  Ipratropium bromide
  Mydriatics
  Sympathomimetics
Optic neuritis
  Aminosalicylic acid
  Chloramphenicol
  Clioquinol
  Ethambutol

Optic neuritis *(cont.)*
  Isoniazid
  Penicillamine
  Phenothiazines
  Phenylbutazone
  Quinine
  Streptomycin
Retinopathy
  Chloroquine
  Phenothiazines

XII. EAR MANIFESTATIONS

Deafness
  Aminoglycosides
  Aspirin
  Bleomycin
  Chloroquine
  Cisplatin
  Deferoxamine
  Erythromycin

Deafness *(cont.)*
  Ethacrynic acid
  Furosemide
  Interferon
  Mustine
  Nortriptyline
  Quinine

Vestibular disorders
  Aminoglycosides
  Mustine
  Quinine

(continued)

Table 69-1—(continued)

Clinical Manifestations of Adverse Reactions to Drugs

XIII. MUSCULOSKELETAL MANIFESTATIONS

Bone disorders	Myopathy or myalgia	Rhabdomyolysis
Osteoporosis:	Amphotericin B	Gemfibrozil
Glucocorticoids	Carbenoxolone	Lovastatin
Heparin	Chloroquine	Tendon rupture
Gout: see Hyperuricemia	Cimetidine	Quinolones
Osteomalacia:	Clofibrate	
Aluminum hydroxide	Glucocorticoids	
Anticonvulsants	Oral contraceptives	
Glutethimide	Zidovudine	

XIV. PSYCHIATRIC MANIFESTATIONS

Delirious or confusional states	Depression	Hallucinatory states	Memory loss
Amantadine	Amphetamine withdrawal	Amantadine	Triazolam
Aminophylline	Beta blockers	Beta blockers	Schizophrenic-like or paranoid
Anticholinergics	Centrally acting antihypertensives	Levodopa	reactions
Antidepressants	(reserpine, methyldopa,	Meperidine	Amphetamines
Bromides	clonidine)	Narcotics	Bromides
Cimetidine	Glucocorticoids	Pentazocine	Glucocorticoids
Digitalis	Levodopa	Tricyclic antidepressants	Levodopa
Glucocorticoids	Drowsiness	Hypomania, mania, or excited	Lysergic acid
Isoniazid	Antihistamines	reactions	Monoamine oxidase
Levodopa	Anxiolytic drugs	Glucocorticoids	inhibitors
Methyldopa	Clonidine	Levodopa	Tricyclic antidepressants
Penicillins	Major tranquilizers	MAO inhibitors	Sleep disturbances
Phenothiazines	Methyldopa	Sympathomimetics	Anorexiants
Ranitidine	Reserpine	Tricyclic antidepressants	Levodopa
Sedatives and hypnotics	Tricyclic antidepressants	Hypersexuality	Monoamine oxidase
Vigabatrin		Antiparkinsonian agents	inhibitors
			Sympathomimetics

* ACE, angiotensin converting enzyme
† NSAID, non–steroidal anti–inflammatory drug

specific drug than are symptoms such as fever or rash, which may be caused by many drugs or by other factors.

Once an adverse reaction is suspected, discontinuance of the suspected drug followed by disappearance of the reaction is presumptive evidence of a drug-induced illness. Confirming evidence may be sought by cautiously reintroducing the drug and seeing if the reaction reappears. However, that should be done only if confirmation would be useful in the future management of the patient and if the attempt would not entail undue risk. With concentration-dependent adverse reactions, lowering the dosage may cause the reaction to disappear, and raising it may cause the reaction to reappear. When the reaction is thought to be allergic, however, readministration of the drug may be hazardous, since anaphylactic shock may develop. Readministration is unwise under these conditions unless no alternative drugs are available and treatment is necessary.

If the patient is receiving many drugs when an adverse reaction is suspected, the drugs likeliest to be responsible can usually be identified. All drugs may be discontinued at once, or, if that is not practical, they should be discontinued one at a time, starting with the one that is most suspect, and the patient observed for signs of improvement. The time needed for a concentration-dependent adverse effect to disappear depends on the time required for the concentration to fall below the range associated with the adverse effect, and that, in turn, depends on the initial blood level and on the rate of elimination or metabolism of the drug. Adverse effects of drugs with long half-lives, such as phenobarbital, take a considerable time to disappear.

Drugs recognized as producing a number of reactions are listed in Table 69-1. This table includes both well-documented and some less well-documented reactions, focusing on those that are sufficiently devastating to require consideration. This information should be used to suggest the drug likely to be causing a reaction; the absence of a drug from the table does not mean that it cannot be responsible for the reaction, however.

Serum antibody has been demonstrated in some persons with drug allergies involving cellular blood elements, as in agranulocytosis, hemolytic anemia, and thrombocytopenia. For example, both quinine and quinidine can produce platelet agglutination in vitro in the presence of complement and the serum from a patient who has developed thrombocytopenia following use of this drug.

Eliciting a drug history from patients is important for diagnosis. Attention must be directed to OTC as well as prescription drugs. Each type can be responsible for adverse drug effects, and adverse interactions may occur between OTC drugs and prescribed drugs. In addition, it is common for patients to be cared for by several physicians, and duplicative, additive, counteractive, or synergistic drug combinations may therefore be administered if the physicians are not aware of the patients' drug histories. Every physician should determine what drugs a patient has been taking, at least during the preceding 30 days, before prescribing any medications. A frequently overlooked source of additional drug exposure is topical therapy; for example, a patient complaining of bronchospasm may not mention that an ophthalmic beta blocker is being used unless specifically asked. A history of previous adverse drug effects in patients is common. Since these patients have shown a predisposition to drug-induced illnesses, such a history should dictate added caution in prescribing drugs.

Patients with biochemical abnormalities such as erythrocyte G6PD deficiency can be identified. Most patients with the G6PD defect are blacks or of Mediterranean descent. Drug-induced hemolytic crisis can be avoided by testing for the enzyme defect before administering drugs that could cause the reaction. Similarly, persons with an abnormal serum pseudocholinesterase level may have abnormally prolonged apnea when given succinylcholine.

GENERAL COMMENTS No drug is completely without side effects, and a side effect in one patient may be the desired pharmacologic effect in another. Current drug regulations allow physicians to have considerable confidence in the purity, bioavailability, and effectiveness of the drugs they prescribe. However, physicians have to weigh potential toxicity against possible benefits. Toxicity that would be acceptable for an effective antineoplastic agent would not be permitted in an oral contraceptive, for example. Because of the necessarily small number of patients treated in premarketing studies, rare adverse reactions may not be identified, so the first responsibility for identifying and reporting these effects must rest with the practicing clinician through the use of the various national adverse reaction reporting systems, such as those operated by the Food and Drug Administration in the United States and the Committee on Safety of Medicines in Great Britain. The publication of a newly recognized adverse reaction can in a short time stimulate many similar such reports of reactions that previously had gone unrecognized.

The prevention of adverse drug reactions first involves a high index of suspicion that the development of a new symptom or sign may be drug-related. Reduction of the dose or discontinuation of the suspected agent usually clarifies the issue in concentration-dependent toxic reactions. Physicians should be familiar with the common adverse effects of the drugs they use and, when in doubt, should consult the literature.

BIBLIOGRAPHY

BRENNAN TA et al: Incidence of adverse events and negligence in hospitalized patients: Results of the Harvard Medical Practice Study I. N Engl J Med 324:370, 1991

DAVIES DM: *Textbook of Adverse Drug Reactions*, 4th ed. New York, Oxford University Press, 1991

FELDMANN U: Design and analysis of drug safety studies, with special reference to sporadic drug use and acute adverse reactions. J Clin Epidemiol 46:237, 1993

HALLAS J et al: Drug related admissions to medical wards: A population based survey. Br J Clin Pharmacol 33:61, 1992

HOIGNÉ R et al: Risk factors for adverse drug reactions: Epidemiological approaches. Eur J Clin Pharmacol 39:321, 1990

JOHNSON JA, BOOTMAN JL: Drug-related morbidity and mortality: A cost-of-illness model. Arch Intern Med 155:1949, 1995

LEAPE LL et al: The nature of adverse events in hospitalized patients. Results of the Harvard Medical Practice Study II. N Engl J Med 324:377, 1991

ROUJEAU J-C et al: Medication use and the risk of Stevens-Johnson syndrome or toxic epidermal necrolysis. N Engl J Med 333:1600, 1995

———, STERN RS: Severe adverse cutaneous reactions to drugs. N Engl J Med 331:1272, 1994

WALLER PC: Measuring the frequency of adverse drug reactions. Br J Clin Pharmacol 33:249, 1992

70 *Lewis Landsberg, James B. Young*

PHYSIOLOGY AND PHARMACOLOGY OF THE AUTONOMIC NERVOUS SYSTEM

FUNCTIONAL ORGANIZATION OF THE AUTONOMIC NERVOUS SYSTEM

The autonomic nervous system innervates vascular and visceral smooth muscle, exocrine and endocrine glands, and parenchymal cells throughout the various organ systems. Functioning below the conscious level, the autonomic nervous system responds rapidly and continuously to perturbations that threaten the constancy of the internal environment. The many functions governed by this system include the distribution of blood flow and the maintenance of tissue perfusion, the regulation of blood pressure, the regulation of the volume and composition of the extracellular fluid, the expenditure of metabolic energy and supply of substrate, and the control of visceral smooth muscle and glands.

ANATOMIC ORGANIZATION The autonomic neurons, located in ganglia outside the central nervous system, give rise to the postganglionic autonomic nerves that innervate organs and tissues throughout the body (Fig. 70-1). The activity of autonomic nerves is regulated by central neurons responsive to diverse afferent inputs. After central integration of afferent information, autonomic outflow is adjusted to permit the functioning of the major organ systems in accordance with the needs of the organism as a whole. Connections between the cerebral cortex and the autonomic centers in the brainstem coordinate autonomic outflow with higher mental functions.

The Sympathetic and Parasympathetic Divisions The preganglionic neurons of the parasympathetic nervous system leave the central nervous system in the third, seventh, ninth, and tenth cranial nerves and in the second and third sacral nerves, while the preganglionic neurons of the sympathetic nervous system exit the spinal cord between the first thoracic and the second lumbar segments (Fig. 70-1). Responses to sympathetic and parasympathetic stimulation are frequently antagonistic, as exemplified by their opposing effects on heart rate and gut motility. This antagonism reflects highly coordinated interactions within the central nervous system; the resultant changes in parasympathetic and sympathetic activity, often reciprocal, provide more precise control of autonomic responses than could be achieved by the modulation of a single system.

Neurotransmitters *Acetylcholine* (ACh) is the preganglionic neurotransmitter for both divisions of the autonomic nervous system as well as the postganglionic neurotransmitter of the parasympathetic

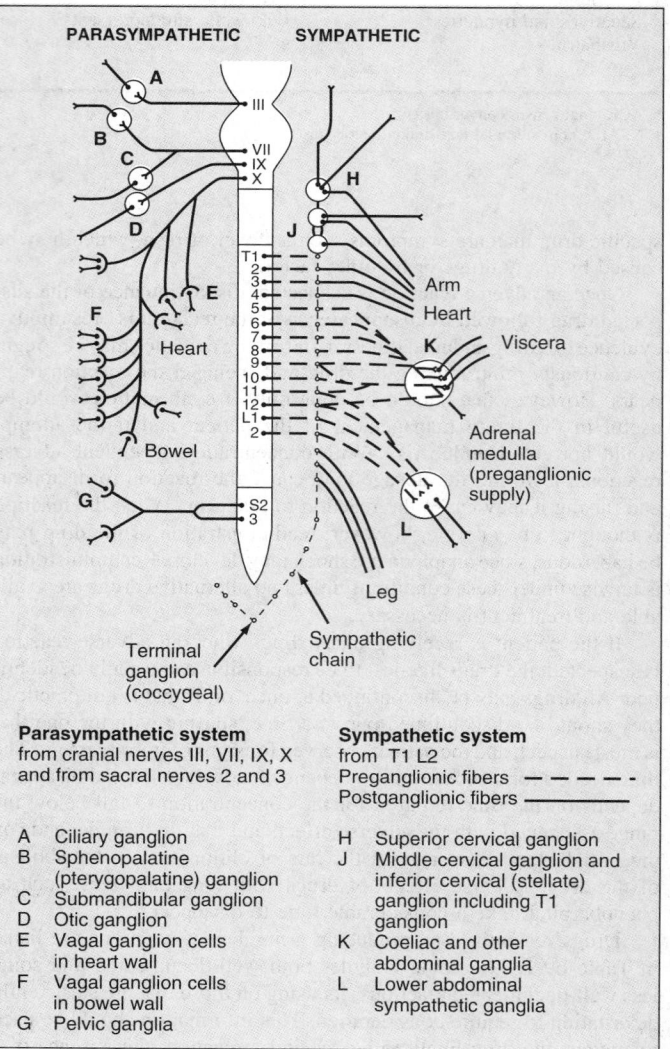

Parasympathetic system from cranial nerves III, VII, IX, X and from sacral nerves 2 and 3	**Sympathetic system** from T1 L2 Preganglionic fibers – – – – – Postganglionic fibers —————
A Ciliary ganglion	H Superior cervical ganglion
B Sphenopalatine (pterygopalatine) ganglion	J Middle cervical ganglion and inferior cervical (stellate) ganglion including T1 ganglion
C Submandibular ganglion	
D Otic ganglion	
E Vagal ganglion cells in heart wall	K Coeliac and other abdominal ganglia
F Vagal ganglion cells in bowel wall	L Lower abdominal sympathetic ganglia
G Pelvic ganglia	

FIGURE 70-1 Schematic representation of the autonomic nervous system. (*From Moskowitz M. Clin Endocrinol Metab 6:77, 1977.*)

neurons. Nerves that release ACh are said to be cholinergic. *Norepinephrine* (NE) is the neurotransmitter of the postganglionic sympathetic neurons; these nerves are said to be adrenergic. Within the sympathetic outflow, postganglionic neurons innervating the eccrine sweat glands (and perhaps some blood vessels supplying skeletal muscle) are of the cholinergic type.

THE SYMPATHETIC NERVOUS SYSTEM AND THE ADRENAL MEDULLA

CATECHOLAMINES   All three of the naturally occurring catecholamines, NE, *epinephrine* (E), and *dopamine*, function as neurotransmitters within the central nervous system. NE, the neurotransmitter of postganglionic sympathetic nerve endings, exerts its effects locally, in the immediate vicinity of its release. E, the circulating hormone of the adrenal medulla, influences processes throughout the body. A peripheral dopaminergic system also exists but has not been characterized in detail.

Biosynthesis (Fig. 70-2)   Catecholamines are synthesized from the amino acid tyrosine, which is sequentially hydroxylated to form dihydroxyphenylalanine (dopa), decarboxylated to form dopamine, and hydroxylated on the beta position of the side chain to form NE. The initial step, the hydroxylation of tyrosine, is rate-limiting and is regulated so that synthesis of dopa is coupled to NE release. This regulation is achieved by alterations in both the activity and the amount of tyrosine hydroxylase. In the adrenal medulla and in those central neurons utilizing E as neurotransmitter, NE is *N*-methylated to E by the enzyme phenylethanolamine-*N*-methyltransferase (PNMT).

Catecholamine Metabolism   The major metabolic transformations of catecholamines involve *O*-methylation at the meta-hydroxyl group and oxidative deamination. *O*-Methylation is catalyzed by the enzyme catechol-*O*-methyltransferase (COMT), and oxidative deamination is promoted by monoamine oxidase (MAO). COMT in liver and kidney is important in the metabolism of circulating catecholamines. MAO, a mitochondrial enzyme present in most tissues, including nerve endings, has a lesser role in the metabolism of circulating catecholamines but is important in regulating the catecholamine stores within the peripheral sympathetic nerve endings. The metanephrines and 4-hydroxy-3-methoxymandelic acid (VMA) are the major end products of E and NE metabolism. Homovanillic acid (HVA) is the end product of dopamine metabolism.

STORAGE AND RELEASE OF CATECHOLAMINES   In both the adrenal medulla and sympathetic nerve endings catecholamines are stored in subcellular granules and released by exocytosis. The large stores of catecholamines in these tissues provide an important physiologic reserve that maintains an adequate supply of catecholamines in the face of intense stimulation. A variety of substances may be stored along with catecholamines in sympathetic nerve endings and adrenal medulla and released with catecholamines during exocytosis. These substances, which may function as cotransmitters or neuromodulators, include peptides such as neuropeptide Y, substance P, and enkephalins; purines such as ATP and adenosine; and other amines such as serotonin. At the neuroeffector junction, coreleased neuromodulators modify the response to NE, while cotransmitters exert physiologic effects independent of those induced by NE.

Adrenal Medulla   The adrenal medullary chromaffin tissue in a pair of normal human adrenal glands weighs about 1 g and contains approximately 6 mg catecholamines, 85 percent of which is E.

Catecholamine secretion, stimulated by ACh from the preganglionic sympathetic nerves, occurs after calcium influx triggers fusion of the chromaffin granule membrane and cell membrane; obliteration of the cell membrane at the point of fusion and extrusion of the entire soluble contents of the granule into the extracellular space complete the process of exocytosis (Fig. 70-2). Although the molecular mechanisms involved in the exocytotic process are only partially understood, evidence has accumulated that specific calcium-binding proteins are involved. Once bound, calcium induces a conformational change in these proteins that induces fusion of granules and docking of granules at the cell membrane.

Peripheral Sympathetic Nerve Endings   The peripheral sympathetic nerve endings form a reticulum or ground plexus that brings the terminal fibers into close contact with effector cells. All the NE in peripheral tissues is in the sympathetic nerve endings, and heavily innervated tissues contain as much as 1 to 2 μg/g of tissue. NE stored in the nerve endings is in discrete subcellular particles analogous to the adrenal medullary chromaffin granules. MAO in the mitochondria of the nerve endings plays an important role in regulating the local concentration of NE (Fig. 70-2). Amines in storage vesicles are protected from oxidative deamination; amines within the cytoplasm, however, are deaminated to inactive metabolites. Release from the nerve ending occurs in response to action potentials propagated in terminal sympathetic fibers.

THE PERIPHERAL ADRENERGIC NEUROEFFECTOR JUNCTION   The peripheral sympathetic nerve endings possess an amine transport system that actively takes up amines from the extracellular fluid. Neuronal uptake or recapture of locally released NE terminates the action of the transmitter and contributes to the constancy of the NE stores.

A variety of factors alter the relationship between neuronal impulse traffic and NE release. Diminished temperature and acidosis, for example, both decrease the amount of NE released in response to sympathetic impulses. Several chemical mediators operate at the peripheral sympathetic nerve ending (referred to as *prejunctional* or *presynaptic sites*) to modify sympathetic neurotransmission by influencing the amount of NE released in response to nerve impulses. Prejunctional modulation may be either inhibitory or facilitatory.

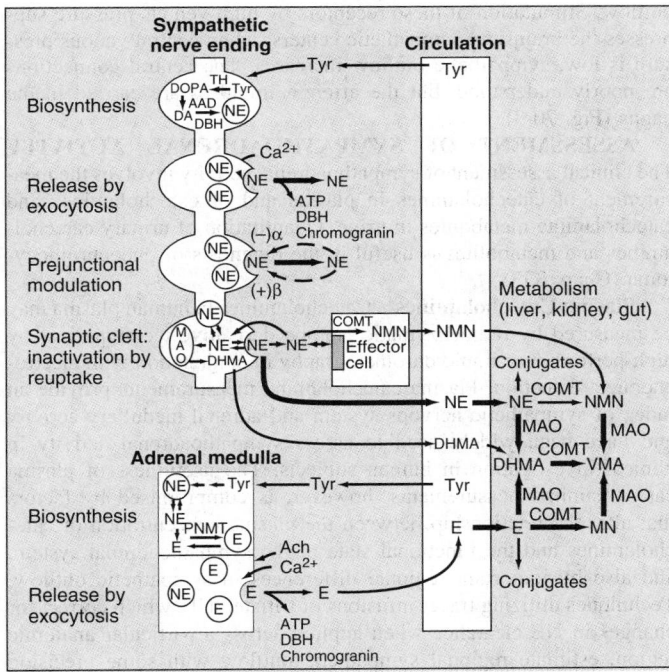

FIGURE 70-2   Catecholamine biosynthesis, release, and metabolism. Schematic representation of a peripheral sympathetic nerve ending is shown at the top; the bulbous areas on the terminal fiber represent varicosities identified by histochemical fluorescence techniques as areas of high neurotransmitter concentration. The processes of biosynthesis, release, modulation, and reuptake are shown sequentially for demonstration purposes only; in vivo they proceed concurrently. Adrenal medullary chromaffin cells are shown at the bottom of the diagram. (TH, tyrosine hydroxylase; AAD, aromatic-l-amino acid decarboxylase; DA, dopamine; DBH, dopamine-β-hydroxylase; NE, norepinephrine; PNMT, phenylethanolamine-*N*-methyltransferase; E, epinephrine; COMT, catechol-*O*-methyltransferase; NMN, normetanephrine; MAO, monoamine oxidase; DHMA, 3,4-dihydroxymandelic acid; VMA, 3-methoxy-4-hydroxymandelic acid.)

Certain modulators, such as catecholamines and ACh, may either inhibit or facilitate NE release, antagonistic effects that are mediated by different adrenergic or cholinergic receptors, respectively. Those compounds exerting an *inhibitory* effect on NE release at the prejunctional nerve ending include the following: catecholamines (alpha$_2$ receptor), ACh (muscarinic receptor), dopamine (D$_2$ receptor), histamine (H$_2$ receptor), serotonin, adenosine, enkephalins, and prostaglandins.

Catecholamines reduce NE release via prejunctional alpha receptors in a classic negative-feedback system. Feedback regulation is complicated by the fact that beta-receptor activation facilitates NE release.

Though both inhibitory and facilitatory effects of ACh on NE release have been described, the inhibitory effect of ACh, mediated by the muscarinic cholinergic receptor, occurs at lower ACh concentrations and is probably of greater physiologic significance.

CENTRAL REGULATION OF SYMPATHOADRENAL OUTFLOW Brainstem Sympathetic Centers Sympathetic outflow is initiated from the reticular formation of the medulla oblongata and pons and from centers in the hypothalamus. The rostral ventral portion of the medulla, particularly the area designated the rostral ventrolateral medulla (RVLM), appears to contain especially important sympathoexcitatory areas. Descending fibers originating from these centers synapse in the intermediolateral cell column of the spinal cord with the preganglionic sympathetic neurons. Changes in the physical and chemical properties of the extracellular fluid, including the circulating levels of hormones and substrates, also affect sympathetic nervous system outflow. The area postrema, in the floor of the fourth ventricle, along with other circumventricular organs lie outside the blood-brain barrier and may play an important role in this regard. Although the hallmark of intense sympathoadrenal stimulation is a global response (the fight-or-flight reaction of Cannon), discrete changes in sympathetic outflow to different organ systems continuously regulate many autonomic functions.

Relationship between the sympathetic nervous system and the adrenal medulla Sympathetic nervous system activity and adrenal medullary secretion are coordinated but not always congruent. During periods of intense sympathetic stimulation, such as cold exposure and exhaustive exercise, the adrenal medulla is progressively recruited, and circulating E reinforces the physiologic effects of sympathetic stimulation. In other situations, the sympathetic nervous system and the adrenal medulla are stimulated independently. The response to upright posture, for example, involves predominantly the sympathetic nervous system, while hypoglycemia stimulates only the adrenal medulla.

Sympathetic Regulation of the Cardiovascular System Stretch receptors in the systemic and pulmonary arteries and veins continuously monitor intravascular pressures; the resulting afferent impulses, after relay and integration in the brainstem, alter sympathetic activity in defense of blood pressure and blood flow to critical areas (Fig. 70-3).

Arterial baroreceptors An increase in blood pressure stimulates receptors in the carotid sinus and aortic arch. The ensuing afferent impulses, after relay within the nucleus of the solitary tract (NTS) in the brainstem, suppress the brainstem sympathetic centers (Fig. 70-3). This baroreceptor reflex arc forms a negative-feedback loop in which a rise in arterial pressure results in the inhibition of central sympathetic outflow. A brainstem noradrenergic pathway interacts with the NTS to participate in suppression of sympathetic outflow. This noradrenergic inhibitory pathway is stimulated by centrally acting alpha-adrenergic agonists and may be involved in the action of certain antihypertensive drugs, such as clonidine, that potentiate the baroreceptor-mediated vasodepressor response (Chap. 246). In the opposite manner, when the blood pressure falls, decreased afferent impulses diminish central inhibition, resulting in an increase in sympathetic outflow and a rise in arterial pressure.

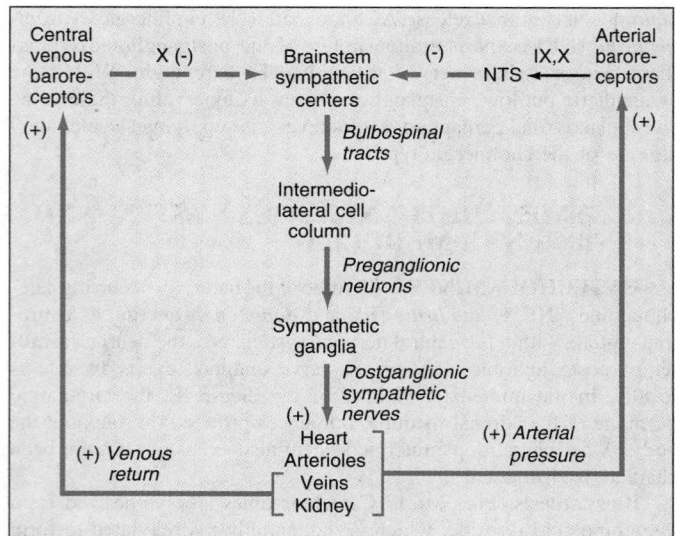

FIGURE 70-3 Sympathetic regulation of the circulation. Receptors in the venous and arterial circulations are stimulated by stretch, caused by an increase in pressure; afferent impulses from these receptors are carried to the central nervous system by the ninth (*IX*) and tenth (*X*) cranial nerves. The net result of these afferent impulses, after relay in the brainstem, is to inhibit central sympathetic outflow. The arterial baroreceptor reflex involves a relay in the nucleus of the tractus solitarius. (+, stimulation; −, inhibition.)

Central venous pressure Receptors in the walls of the great veins and within the atria are also involved in the regulation of sympathetic outflow. Stimulation of these receptors by high venous pressure suppresses the brainstem sympathetic centers; when central venous pressure is low, sympathetic outflow increases. The central connections are poorly understood, but the afferent impulses are carried in the vagus (Fig. 70-3).

ASSESSMENT OF SYMPATHOADRENAL ACTIVITY The clinical assessment of sympathoadrenal activity involves the measurement of catecholamines in plasma and of catecholamines and catecholamine metabolites in urine. Quantitation of urinary catecholamines and metabolites is useful in the diagnosis of pheochromocytoma (Chap. 333).

Plasma Catecholamines Catecholamines in human plasma may be measured by radioenzymatic isotope derivative techniques or by high-performance liquid chromatography in conjunction with electrochemical detection. Plasma catecholamine measurements provide an index of sympathetic nervous system and adrenal medullary activity and have been widely used to assess sympathoadrenal activity in clinical investigation in human subjects. The usefulness of plasma catecholamine measurements, however, is compromised by factors that alter the relationship between the plasma concentration of catecholamines and the functional state of the sympathoadrenal system, and also by important regional differences in sympathetic outflow. Techniques utilizing tracer infusions of triutiated NE, which correct for changes in NE clearance when applied across a particular anatomic region, estimate regional sympathetic outflow with some precision and have helped to define differentiated sympathetic nervous system activity in the investigational setting. The clinical usefulness of plasma catecholamine levels remains limited to the evaluation of patients with autonomic insufficiency and, on occasion, patients with suspected pheochromocytoma (Chap. 333).

Basal plasma NE concentrations are in the range of 0.09 to 1.8 nmol/L (150 to 350 pg/mL); basal E levels are about 135 to 270 pmol/L (25 to 50 pg/mL). The half-time of disappearance of NE from the circulation is approximately 2 min. The plasma NE level is markedly affected by a variety of factors, including posture; accordingly, the conditions under which blood is obtained for assay must be controlled. By convention, basal plasma NE levels are those obtained through an indwelling intravenous line after the patient has rested supine in a relaxed environment for 30 min.

Plasma NE response to upright posture The predictable increase in circulating NE concentration during upright posture provides a convenient test of sympathetic nervous system function. Five minutes of quiet standing results in a two- to threefold increase in plasma NE level. A normal response requires an intact afferent system, appropriate central nervous system relays, and an intact peripheral sympathetic nervous system; a defect of any of these components reduces the increment in circulating NE.

Plasma E levels are also dependent on the physical and mental state of the subject. Change in plasma E with upright posture is usually small. Hypoglycemia, strenuous exercise, and various types of mental stress, however, can cause large increases in the plasma E level.

PERIPHERAL DOPAMINERGIC SYSTEM

In addition to its role as neurotransmitter in the central nervous system, dopamine functions as an inhibitory transmitter in the carotid body and the sympathetic ganglia. A distinct peripheral dopaminergic system is also believed to exist. Dopamine elicits a variety of responses not attributable to stimulation of classic adrenergic receptors; it relaxes the lower esophageal sphincter, delays gastric emptying, causes vasodilation in the renal and mesenteric arterial circulation, suppresses aldosterone secretion, directly stimulates renal sodium excretion, and suppresses NE release at sympathetic nerve terminals by a presynaptic inhibitory mechanism. The mediation of these dopaminergic effects in vivo is poorly understood. Dopamine does not appear to be a circulating hormone.

ADRENERGIC RECEPTORS

Catecholamines influence effector cells by interacting with specific *receptors* on the cell surface. When stimulated by catecholamines, the adrenergic receptor initiates a series of membrane changes followed by a cascade of intracellular events that culminates in a measurable response.

Two major categories of response to catecholamines reflect the activation of two populations of adrenergic receptors, designated alpha and beta. Both alpha and beta receptors have been further divided into subtypes that serve different functions and are susceptible to differential stimulation and blockade.

ALPHA-ADRENERGIC RECEPTORS Alpha-adrenergic receptors mediate vasoconstriction, intestinal relaxation, and pupillary dilatation. E and NE are approximately equipotent as alpha-receptor agonists. Distinct $alpha_1$- and $alpha_2$-receptor subtypes are also recognized. Originally the postsynaptic or postjunctional alpha-adrenergic receptors on effector cells were designated $alpha_1$, while the prejunctional alpha-adrenergic receptors on the sympathetic nerve endings were designated $alpha_2$. It is now recognized that nonneuronal (postsynaptic) processes are mediated by the $alpha_2$ receptor as well. The $alpha_1$ receptor mediates the classic alpha effects, including vasoconstriction; phenylephrine and methoxamine are selective $alpha_1$ agonists, and prazosin is a selective $alpha_1$ antagonist. The $alpha_2$ receptor mediates presynaptic inhibition of NE release from adrenergic nerves and other responses, including inhibition of ACh release from cholinergic nerves, inhibition of lipolysis in adipocytes, inhibition of insulin secretion, stimulation of platelet aggregation, and vasoconstriction in some vascular beds. Specific $alpha_2$ agonists include clonidine and α-methylnorepinephrine; these agents, the latter derived from α-methyldopa in vivo, exert an antihypertensive effect by interacting with $alpha_2$ receptors within the brainstem sympathetic centers that regulate blood pressure. Yohimbine is a specific $alpha_2$ antagonist.

BETA-ADRENERGIC RECEPTORS Physiologic events associated with beta-adrenergic receptor responses include stimulation of heart rate and contractility, vasodilation, bronchodilation, and lipolysis. Beta-receptor responses also can be divided into two types. The $beta_1$ receptor responds equally to E and NE and mediates cardiac stimulation

and lipolysis. The $beta_2$ receptor is more responsive to E than to NE and mediates responses such as vasodilation and bronchodilation. Isoproterenol stimulates and propranolol blocks both $beta_1$ and $beta_2$ receptors. Other agonists and antagonists that have partial selectivity for the $beta_1$ or $beta_2$ receptors have been used therapeutically where the desired response involves predominantly one of the two subtypes.

Both pharmacologic and molecular genetic studies have demonstrated an additional distinct $beta_3$-adrenergic receptor that subserves lipolysis in white and brown adipose tissue as well as the stimulation of heat production in brown adipose tissue. The human $beta_3$-adrenergic receptor has been cloned, and a distinct polymorphism noted that may be associated with weight gain, insulin resistance, and type 2 diabetes mellitus. The $beta_3$-adrenergic receptor has a much greater affinity for NE than E and, unlike the $beta_1$ and $beta_2$ receptors, does not undergo desensitization. Synthetic agonists for the $beta_3$ receptor, currently under development, have a potential role in the treatment of obesity by increasing metabolic rate.

DOPAMINERGIC RECEPTORS Specific dopaminergic receptors, distinct from the classic alpha- and beta-adrenergic receptors, are present in the central and peripheral nervous system and in several nonneural tissues. Two types of dopaminergic receptors serve different functions and have different second messengers. Dopamine is a potent agonist of both types of receptors; the action of dopamine is antagonized by phenothiazines and thioxanthenes. The D_1 receptor mediates vasodilation in the renal, mesenteric, coronary, and cerebral vascular beds. Fenoldopam is an investigational agonist selective for the D_1 receptor. The D_2 receptor inhibits transmission in the sympathetic ganglia, inhibits NE release from sympathetic nerve endings by an effect on the presynaptic membrane (Fig. 70-2), inhibits prolactin release from the pituitary, and causes vomiting. Selective agonists of the D_2 receptor include bromocriptine, lergotrile, and apomorphine, while butyrophenones such as haloperidol (active within the central nervous system), domperidone (does not cross blood-brain barrier readily), and the benzamide sulpiride are relatively selective D_2 antagonists.

STRUCTURE AND FUNCTION OF ADRENERGIC RECEPTORS Adrenergic receptors belong to a superfamily of related membrane proteins, including the visual protein rhodopsin and the muscarinic acetylcholine receptors, that interacts with G proteins. These proteins share significant sequence homologies and, as deduced from the properties of the constituent amino acids, a similar topographic structure in the cell membrane. The postulated structure of this family of receptor proteins is shown schematically in Fig. 70-4. The characteristic features include seven membrane-spanning hydrophobic domains containing 20 to 28 amino acids each. The membrane-spanning domains, particularly M-7 (Fig. 70-4), appear to be important in determining the characteristic agonist binding.

Coupling of Receptor Occupancy with Cellular Response The major mediators of adrenergic (as well as many other) cellular responses are a family of regulatory proteins termed *G proteins* that, when activated, bind the nucleotide guanosine triphosphate (GTP). The best-characterized G proteins are those that stimulate or inhibit adenylyl cyclase, designated G_s or G_i, respectively (Fig. 70-5). The $beta_1$, $beta_2$, and D_1 receptors are coupled to G_s; receptor occupancy is therefore associated with stimulation of adenylyl cyclase and results in an increase in intracellular cyclic adenosine monophosphate (AMP), which in turn results in activation of protein kinase A and other cyclic AMP–dependent protein kinases. The resultant protein phosphorylation alters the activity of enzymes and the function of other proteins, culminating in a cellular response that is characteristic of the tissue being stimulated. The $alpha_2$, M_2 subtype of the muscarinic acetylcholine receptor and the D_2 receptor are coupled to G_i, resulting in diminished adenylyl cyclase activity and a fall in cyclic AMP. The subsequent alterations in enzyme activity and function of other proteins produce an alternate, frequently opposite, series of cellular responses. Although many

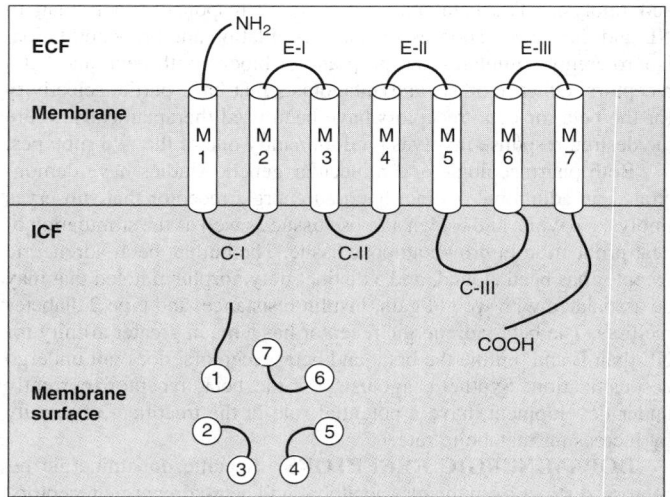

FIGURE 70-4 Proposed structure of adrenergic receptors as deduced from primary amino acid sequences. The single protein chain contains a hydrophilic N terminus (extracellular) and C terminus (intracellular) connected by seven lipophilic membrane-spanning regions (M-1 to M-7) which are interconnected by three extracellular loops (E-I to E-III) and three cytoplasmic loops (C-I to C-III). The $beta_1$-, $beta_2$-, $alpha_1$-, and $alpha_2$-adrenergic receptors have appreciable sequence homologies and are believed to fit the general structural model represented. Specificity of agonist binding may be conferred by the tertiary structure of several of the membrane-spanning domains while specificity of intracellular response may be related to the length and tertiary structure of the cytoplasmic loops and C terminus. The top portion of the figure is a longitudinal representation of the receptor protein in the cell membrane; shown below is a hypothetical, more compact arrangement seen from the membrane surface. (ECF, extracellular fluid; ICF, intracellular fluid.) (*From Landsberg and Young, 1992, with permission.*)

$alpha_2$ responses can be explained by inhibition of adenylyl cyclase, other mechanisms may be involved as well.

The $alpha_1$-adrenergic receptor (as well as the M_1 subtype of the acetylcholine receptor) appears to be coupled to a different G protein that activates phospholipase C; this G protein has not been as well characterized but is sometimes designated G_q. Receptor occupancy in this system stimulates phospholipase C, which catalyzes the breakdown of membrane-bound phospholipids, particularly phosphatidyl-inositol-4,5-bisphosphate (PIP_2) with the production of inositol-1,4,5-trisphosphate (IP_3) and 1,2-diacylglycerol (DAG), both of which act as second messengers (Fig. 70-5). IP_3 rapidly mobilizes calcium from intracellular stores within the endoplasmic reticulum, producing an

increase in free cytoplasmic calcium which by itself and via calcium-calmodulin–dependent protein kinases influences cellular processes appropriate to the stimulated cell. The transient rise in calcium induced by IP_3 from the intracellular stores is reinforced in the presence of continued agonist stimulation by alterations in membrane calcium flux that result eventually in net calcium uptake from the extracellular fluid by mechanisms that have been incompletely defined.

DAG, the other second messenger produced by the action of phospholipase C on PIP_2 (as well as other membrane phospholipids), remains associated with the cell membrane and activates protein kinase C, which has different substrates than the calcium-calmodulin kinases stimulated by IP_3. Protein phosphorylation stimulated by protein kinase C contributes to the tissue-specific response in ways that remain poorly understood. Increases in intracellular calcium also potentiate the activation of protein kinase C (Fig. 70-5).

REGULATION OF ADRENERGIC RECEPTORS Prolonged exposure to alpha- or beta-adrenergic agonists decreases the number of corresponding adrenergic receptors on effector cells. Although the biochemical mechanisms involved are obscure, internalization of the beta-adrenergic receptor within the cell occurs during agonist exposure in some systems, suggesting that internal translocation contributes to the decrease in receptor number under these circumstances.

Alteration in agonist concentration also may affect the affinity of the receptor for the agonist. Adrenergic receptors that utilize adenylyl cyclase for the second messenger (beta receptors, $alpha_2$ receptors) exist in high and low affinity states; exposure to agonist diminishes the proportion of receptors in the high-affinity state. Such alterations in adrenergic receptors induced by adrenergic agonists are termed *homologous regulation*. Agonist-induced alterations in adrenergic-receptor density and affinity are believed to contribute to the diminished physiologic response that occurs after prolonged exposure of an effector tissue to adrenergic agonist, a phenomenon known as *tachyphylaxis* or *desensitization*.

Adrenergic receptors are also influenced by factors other than adrenergic agonists, so-called *heterologous regulation*. Enhanced alpha-adrenergic-receptor affinity, for example, may underlie the potentiation of alpha-adrenergic responses that occur in response to lowered environmental temperatures. Thyroid hormones potentiate beta-receptor responses by alterations in beta-receptor number and in the efficiency of coupling receptor occupancy with physiologic response. Estrogen and progesterone alter the sensitivity of the myometrium to catecholamines by effects on alpha-adrenergic receptors. Glucocorticoids may influence adrenergic function by antagonizing agonist-induced decreases in adrenergic receptors, thereby counteracting tachyphylaxis in response to intense adrenergic stimulation.

Alterations in sensitivity to catecholamines also occur as a consequence of postreceptor changes, although the latter remain poorly characterized.

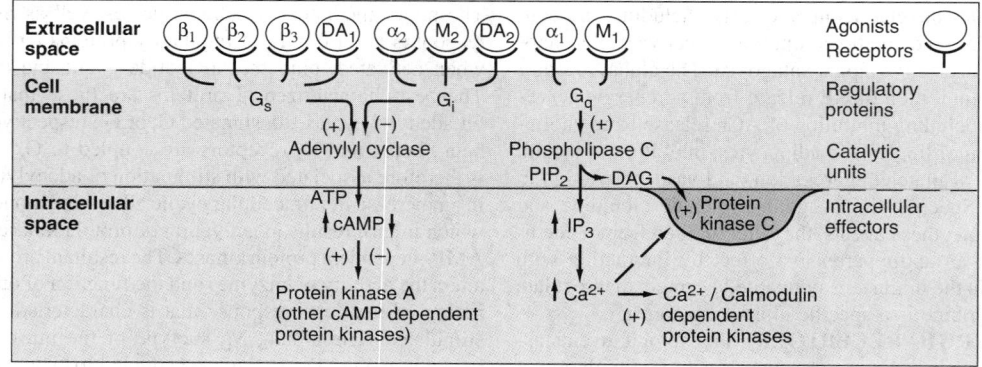

FIGURE 70-5 Interaction of autonomic agonists with membrane-bound regulatory proteins and cellular effector systems. The designations $alpha$ and $beta$ refer to adrenergic receptors, DA refers to dopaminergic receptors, and M, to muscarinic receptors. G designates the GTP-associated regulatory protein which may have a stimulatory (s) or inhibitory (i) effect on adenylyl cyclase or may stimulate phospholipase C (q). [(+) designates stimulation; (−) designates inhibition; PIP_2, phosphatidylinositol-4,5-bisphosphate; DAG, 1,2-diacylglycerol; IP_3, inositol-1,4,5-trisphosphate. See text for details.]

Catecholamines influence all of the major organ systems. The effects take place in seconds and may occur in anticipation of physiologic requirement. An increase in sympathoadrenal activity prior to strenuous exercise, for example, lessens the impact of exercise on the internal environment.

DIRECT EFFECTS OF CATECHOLAMINES   Cardiovascular system   Catecholamines stimulate vasoconstriction in the subcutaneous, mucosal, splanchnic, and renal vascular beds by alpha-receptor–mediated mechanisms. Although vasoconstriction was originally considered an alpha$_1$-receptor response, vascular tone appears to be more complexly regulated and, in many areas, involves alpha$_2$-mediated responses as well. The venous portion of the circulation, in particular, is endowed with alpha$_2$ receptors. Differential regulation of the two types of alpha receptors, under certain circumstances, contributes to an integrated physiologic response. Since vasoconstriction in the coronary and cerebral circulations is minimal, flow to these areas is maintained during sympathetic stimulation. Skeletal muscle vasculature contains beta receptors sensitive to low circulating levels of E so that skeletal muscle blood flow is augmented during adrenal medullary activation.

The effects of catecholamines on the heart are mediated by beta$_1$ receptors and include increase in heart rate, enhancement of cardiac contractility, and increase in conduction velocity. The increase in myocardial contractility is illustrated by a leftward and upward shift of the ventricular function curve (Fig. 232-6) that relates cardiac work to ventricular diastolic fiber length; at any initial fiber length, catecholamines increase cardiac work. Catecholamines also enhance cardiac output by stimulating venoconstriction, enhancing venous return, and increasing the force of atrial contraction, thereby augmenting diastolic volume and hence fiber length. The acceleration of conduction in the junctional tissues results in a more synchronous, and hence more effective, ventricular contraction. Cardiac stimulation increases myocardial oxygen consumption, a major factor in the pathogenesis and treatment of myocardial ischemia.

Metabolism   Catecholamines increase metabolic rate. In small mammals, mitochondrial respiration in brown adipose tissue is functionally uncoupled by NE. In a reaction unique to brown adipose tissue, NE stimulates the beta$_3$-adrenergic receptor that activates a specific mitochondrial uncoupling protein that dissipates the proton gradient between the inner mitochondrial matrix and the cytoplasm, thereby uncoupling substrate utilization and ATP synthesis. In humans, a functional role for brown adipose tissue has not been established with certainty, but increasing evidence suggests a potential role for this tissue in catecholamine-stimulated heat production in human beings.

Substrate mobilization   In a variety of tissues, catecholamines stimulate the breakdown of stored fuel with the production of substrate for local consumption; glycogenolysis in the heart, for example, provides substrate for immediate metabolism by the myocardium. Catecholamines also accelerate fuel mobilization in liver, adipose tissue, and skeletal muscle, liberating substrates (glucose, free fatty acids, lactate) into the circulation for use throughout the body.

Fluids and Electrolytes   By a direct action on the renal tubule, NE stimulates sodium reabsorption, thereby defending extracellular fluid volume. Dopamine, in contrast, promotes sodium excretion. NE and E also promote cellular uptake of potassium, thereby defending against the development of hyperkalemia.

Viscera   Catecholamines affect visceral function by actions on smooth muscle and glandular epithelium. Urinary bladder and intestinal smooth muscle are relaxed while the corresponding sphincters are stimulated. Gallbladder emptying also involves sympathetic mechanisms. Catecholamine-mediated smooth-muscle contraction in the female aids ovulation and ovum transport along the fallopian tubes, and in the male provides propulsive force for the seminal fluid during ejaculation. Inhibitory alpha$_2$ receptors on cholinergic neurons within the gut contribute to intestinal relaxation. Catecholamines induce bronchodilation by a beta$_2$-receptor mechanism.

INDIRECT EFFECTS OF CATECHOLAMINES   The ultimate physiologic response induced by catecholamines involves changes in hormone secretion and in blood flow distribution, both of which support and amplify the direct effects of catecholamines.

Endocrine System   Catecholamines influence the secretion of renin, insulin, glucagon, calcitonin, parathormone, thyroxine, gastrin, erythropoietin, progesterone, and, possibly, testosterone. Secretion of each of these hormones is governed by complex feedback loops. With the exception of thyroxine and the gonadal steroids, each is a polypeptide not under the direct control of the pituitary gland. Sympathoadrenal input into the secretion of these hormones provides a mechanism for regulation by the central nervous system and ensures a coordinated hormonal response in accord with the homeostatic needs of the organism.

Renin (See also Chap. 246)   Sympathetic stimulation increases renin release by a direct beta-receptor effect independent of vascular changes within the kidney. The renin response to volume depletion is sympathetically mediated and is initiated by a fall in central venous pressure. Since renin secretion activates the angiotensin-aldosterone system, angiotensin-induced vasoconstriction supports the direct effects of catecholamines on blood vessels, while aldosterone-mediated sodium reabsorption complements the direct increase in sodium reabsorption induced by sympathetic stimulation. Beta-receptor blocking agents suppress renin secretion.

Insulin and glucagon   Stimulation of pancreatic sympathetic nerves or an elevation in circulating catecholamines suppresses insulin and increases glucagon release. Inhibition of insulin secretion is mediated by the alpha$_2$ receptor, and stimulation of glucagon is mediated by the beta receptor. This combination of effects supports substrate mobilization, reinforcing the direct effects of catecholamines on hepatic glucose output and lipolysis. Although alpha-receptor–mediated suppression of insulin release usually predominates, a beta-receptor mechanism may augment insulin secretion under some circumstances.

SYMPATHOADRENAL FUNCTION IN SELECTED PHYSIOLOGIC AND PATHOPHYSIOLOGIC STATES   Support of the Circulation   The sympathetic nervous system functions to maintain an adequate circulation. During upright posture and volume depletion, reduction of afferent venous and arterial baroreceptor impulse traffic diminishes an inhibitory input to the vasomotor center, thereby increasing sympathetic activity (Fig. 70-3) and reducing efferent vagal tone. As a result, heart rate is increased, and cardiac output is diverted from the skin, subcutaneous tissues, mucosa, and viscera. Sympathetic stimulation of the kidney increases sodium reabsorption, and sympathetically mediated venoconstriction enhances venous return (Fig. 70-6). With pronounced hypotension, the adrenal medulla is recruited and E reinforces the effects of the sympathetic nervous system.

The intense sympathoadrenal stimulation that accompanies severe volume depletion may contribute to the development of ketoacidosis in alcoholics as well as to the ketoacidosis sometimes seen in association with hyperemesis gravidarum. Catecholamine-mediated suppression of insulin and stimulation of glucagon markedly potentiate ketogenesis in these disease states. Volume resuscitation and provision of adequate glucose promptly reverse the ketoacidosis in most cases.

Congestive heart failure   The sympathetic nervous system also provides circulatory support during congestive heart failure (Chap. 233). Venoconstriction and sympathetic stimulation of the heart increase cardiac output while peripheral vasoconstriction directs blood flow to the heart and brain. The afferent signals are less clear than in simple volume depletion because the venous pressure is usually elevated. In severe heart failure, depletion of cardiac NE may impair the effectiveness of sympathetic circulatory support. On the other hand, the possibility has been raised that intense sympathetic stimulation may further impair cardiac function, suggesting possible benefit from beta-adrenergic blockade. The use of beta blockers in the treatment of congestive heart failure, however, should be considered experimental and undertaken only with great caution.

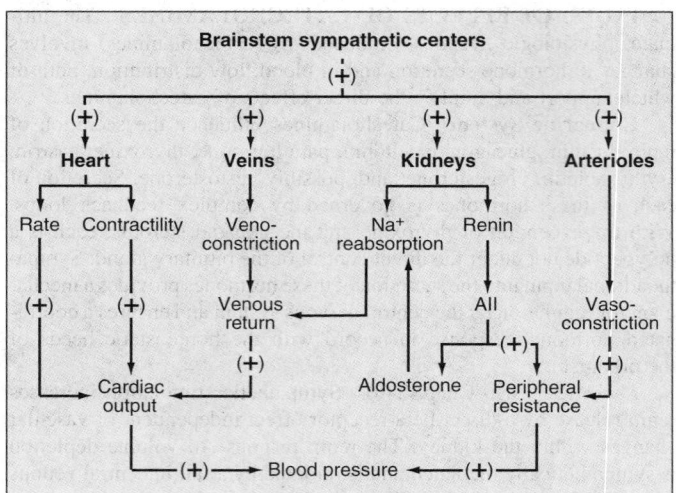

FIGURE 70-6 Sympathetic nervous system effects on blood pressure. Sympathetic stimulation (+) increases blood pressure by effects on the heart, the veins, the kidneys, and the arterioles. The net result of sympathetic stimulation is an increase in both cardiac output and peripheral resistance. AII = angiotensin II. [*From JB Young, L Landsberg, in P Sleight et al (eds), Scientific Foundations of Cardiology, London, Heinemann, 1981.*]

Trauma and shock In acute traumatic injury or shock, adrenal catecholamines support the circulation and mobilize substrates. In the chronic, reparative phase following injury, catecholamines also contribute to substrate mobilization and to the elevation in metabolic rate.

Exercise Sympathetic activation during exercise increases cardiac output and ensures sufficient substrate to meet the increased metabolic needs. Central neural factors, such as anticipation, and circulatory factors, such as fall in venous pressure, trigger the sympathetic response. Mild degrees of exercise stimulate the sympathetic nervous system alone; during more severe exertion the adrenal medulla is activated as well. Conditioning is associated with a decrease in sympathetic nervous system activity both at rest and during exercise, in comparison with the untrained state.

Hypoglycemia (See also Chap. 335) Hypoglycemia causes a marked increase in adrenal medullary E secretion. When glucose concentrations fall below overnight fasting levels, regulatory glucose-sensitive neurons in the central nervous system initiate a prompt increase in adrenal medullary secretion. The increase is especially intense at plasma glucose levels below 2.8 mmol/L (50 mg/dL), when plasma E levels increase 25 to 50 times above baseline, thereby increasing hepatic glucose output, providing alternative substrate in the form of free fatty acids, suppressing endogenous insulin release, and inhibiting insulin-mediated glucose utilization in muscle. Many clinical manifestations of hypoglycemia, such as tachycardia, palpitations, nervousness, tremor, and widened pulse pressure, are secondary to increased E secretion. These manifestations of E secretion constitute an "early warning" system in insulin-requiring diabetics. In patients with long-standing diabetes mellitus, however, the E response to hypoglycemia may be diminished or absent, leaving affected patients at greater risk to develop severe hypoglycemia.

Cold Exposure The sympathetic nervous system plays a critical role in the maintenance of normal body temperature during exposure to a cold environment. Receptors in the skin and central nervous system respond to a fall in temperature by activating hypothalamic and brainstem centers that increase sympathetic activity. Sympathetic stimulation leads to vasoconstriction in the superficial vascular beds, thereby diminishing heat loss. The sympathetic response involves a complex interaction between lowered environmental temperatures and alpha$_2$-adrenergic receptors. Acclimatization during chronic cold expo-

sure increases the capacity for metabolic heat production in response to sympathetic stimulation.

Dietary Intake Fasting suppresses and overfeeding stimulates the sympathetic nervous system. The reduction in sympathetic activity during fasting or starvation contributes to the decrease in metabolic rate, bradycardia, and hypotension in these states. Enhanced sympathetic activity during periods of increased caloric intake contributes to the elevation in metabolic rate associated with a chronic increase in dietary intake.

Hypoxia Chronic hypoxia is associated with stimulation of the sympathoadrenal system, and some of the cardiovascular changes attendant to hypoxia are dependent on catecholamines.

Orthostatic Hypotension The maintenance of arterial pressure during upright posture depends on an adequate blood volume, an unimpaired venous return, and an intact sympathetic nervous system. Significant postural hypotension, therefore, often reflects extracellular fluid volume depletion or dysfunction of the circulatory reflexes. Diseases of the nervous system, such as tabes dorsalis, syringomyelia, or diabetes mellitus, may disrupt these sympathetic reflexes with resultant orthostatic hypotension. Although any antiadrenergic agent may impair the postural sympathetic response, orthostatic hypotension is most prominent with drugs that block neurotransmission within the ganglia or adrenergic neurons.

The term *idiopathic orthostatic hypotension* refers to a group of degenerative diseases involving either the pre- or postganglionic sympathetic neurons (Chaps. 20 and 370).

Treatment of orthostatic hypotension is usually unsatisfactory except in the mildest cases. There is no way of reestablishing the normal relationship between fall in venous return and sympathetic neuronal activation. Volume expansion with fludrocortisone and a liberal salt diet in conjunction with fitted stockings to the waist, as well as elevation of the head of the bed to avoid recumbency, will maintain plasma volume and venous return and frequently provide symptomatic improvement.

PHARMACOLOGY OF THE SYMPATHOADRENAL SYSTEM

A variety of therapeutic agents affect sympathetic nervous system function or interact with adrenergic receptors, making it possible to stimulate or suppress effects mediated by catecholamines with some degree of specificity (Table 70-1).

SYMPATHOMIMETIC AMINES Sympathomimetic amines may directly activate adrenergic receptors (direct acting) or release NE from the sympathetic nerve endings (indirect acting). Many agents have both direct and indirect effects.

Epinephrine and Norepinephrine The naturally occurring catecholamines act predominantly by the direct stimulation of adrenergic receptors. NE is employed to support the circulation and elevate the blood pressure in hypotensive states (Chap. 38). Peripheral vasoconstriction is the major effect, although cardiac stimulation occurs as well. E, also employed as a pressor, has special usefulness in the treatment of allergic reactions, especially those associated with anaphylaxis. E antagonizes the effects of histamine and other mediators on vascular and visceral smooth muscle and is useful in the treatment of bronchospasm.

Dopamine *Dopamine* is used in treating hypotension, shock (Chap. 38), and certain forms of heart failure (Chap. 233). At low infusion rates it exerts a positive inotropic effect both by a direct action on the cardiac beta$_1$ receptors and by the indirect release of NE from sympathetic nerve endings in the heart. At low doses direct stimulation of dopaminergic receptors in the renal and mesenteric vasculature also results in vasodilation in the gut and kidney and facilitates sodium excretion. At higher infusion rates interaction with alpha-adrenergic receptors results in vasoconstriction, an increase in peripheral resistance, and an elevation of blood pressure.

Beta-Receptor Agonists *Isoproterenol*, a direct-acting beta-receptor agonist, stimulates the heart, decreases peripheral resistance, and relaxes bronchial smooth muscle. It raises the cardiac output and

Table 70-1

Some Commonly Used Autonomic Drugs[a,b,c]

Agent	Indication	Dose and Route	Comment
ADRENERGIC AGONISTS[d]			
Epinephrine	Anaphylaxis	300–500 µg SC or IM (0.3–0.5 mL of 1/1000 solution of hydrochloride salt); 25–50 µg IV (slowly) every 5–15 min; titrate as needed	Nonselective alpha and beta agonist; increases BP, heart rate Bronchodilation
Norepinephrine	Shock Hypotension	2–4 µg of NE base/min IV; titrate as needed	Alpha and beta$_1$ agonist Vasoconstriction predominates Extravasation causes tissue necrosis; infuse through IV cannula
Isoproterenol	Cardiogenic shock Bradyarrhythmias AV block	0.5–5.0 µg/min IV; titrate as needed	Nonselective beta agonist Increases cardiac rate and contractility (beta$_1$) Tachycardia limits usefulness
	Asthma	Inhalation	Dilates bronchi (beta$_2$); cardiac stimulation also occurs
Dobutamine	Refractory CHF Cardiogenic shock	2.5–25 (µg/kg)/min IV	Selective beta$_1$ agonist with greater effect on contractility than heart rate; a congener of dopamine but not a dopaminergic agonist
Phenylephrine	Hypotension	2–5 mg SC or IM 0.1–0.5 mg IV	Selective alpha$_1$ agonist; useful in antagonizing hypotension of spinal anesthesia
	Supraventricular tachycardia	150–800 µg slow IV push	Pressor effect induces vagotonic response; do not exceed 160 mmHg systolic BP
Terbutaline	Asthma	2.5–5.0 mg PO tid; 0.25–0.5 mg SC; inhalation every 4–5 h	Selective beta$_2$ agonist; beta$_1$ (cardiac) effects at higher doses (inhalation preferred route)
Bitolterol	Asthma	Inhalation every 4–6 h	Selective beta$_2$ agonist
Salmeterol	Asthma	Inhalation bid	Selective beta$_2$ agonist; long-acting agent for maintenance therapy
Albuterol	Asthma	2.0–4.0 mg PO tid or qid; 0.2 mg inhalation every 4–6 h	Selective beta$_2$ agonist; beta$_1$ effects (cardiac) at higher doses (inhalation preferred route)
Isoetharine	Asthma	Inhalation every 2–4 h	Selective beta$_2$ agonist; some beta$_1$ effects
Metaproterenol	Asthma	10–20 mg PO tid or qid; inhalation every 3–4 h	Selective beta$_2$ agonist; some beta$_1$ effects (inhalation preferred route)
Pirbuterol	Asthma	Inhalation every 4–6 h	Selective beta$_2$ agonist; some beta$_1$ effects
Ritodrine	Premature labor	50–350 µg/min IV	Selective beta$_2$ agonist; hypokalemia, hyperglycemia, hypotension, cardiac stimulation may occur Neonatal hypoglycemia, hypocalcemia reported
DOPAMINERGIC AGONISTS			
Dopamine	Shock	2–5 (µg/kg)/min IV (dopaminergic range) 5–10 (µg/kg)/min IV (dopaminergic and beta range) 10–20 (µg/kg)/min IV (beta range) 20–50 (µg/kg)/min IV (alpha range)	Pharmacologic effects are dose dependent: renal and mesenteric vasodilation predominate at lower doses; cardiac stimulation and vasoconstriction develop as the dose is increased
Bromocriptine	Amenorrhea-galactorrhea	2.5 mg PO bid or tid	Selective agonist of D$_2$ receptor; inhibits prolactin secretion
	Acromegaly	5–15 mg PO tid or qid	Lowers growth hormone in a minority of patients with acromegaly
INHIBITORS OF CENTRAL SYMPATHETIC OUTFLOW			
Clonidine	Hypertension	0.1–0.6 mg PO bid	Selective alpha$_2$ agonist; potentiates central baroreceptor depressor reflex Abrupt discontinuation may result in withdrawal syndrome with rebound hypertension
Methyldopa	Hypertension	250–500 mg PO every 6–8 h	Metabolized by decarboxylation and beta hydroxylation to α-methylnorepinephrine, a centrally active selective alpha$_2$ agonist
ADRENERGIC NEURON BLOCKING AGENTS			
Guanethidine	Hypertension	10–100 mg PO qd	Concentrated in sympathetic nerve endings; blocks release of NE in response to nerve impulses and depletes NE stores; prominent orthostatic hypotension
Bretylium	Ventricular fibrillation and tachycardia	150–300 mg IV 1–4 mg/min IV	In addition to blocking NE release, has direct effect on electrical properties of cardiac muscle

(continued)

Table 70-1—(continued)

Some Commonly Used Autonomic Drugs[a,b,c]

Agent	Indication	Dose and Route	Comment
BETA BLOCKING AGENTS[c]			
Propranolol	Hypertension	40–160 mg PO bid (or higher)	Lipophilic, nonselective Dosage highly variable
	Angina	10–40 mg PO tid or qid	
	Myocardial infarction	60–80 mg PO tid	Prolongs survival post MI
	Arrhythmias	10–30 mg PO tid or qid; 1–3 mg IV	
	Hypertrophic cardiomyopathy	20–40 mg PO tid or qid	
	Pheochromocytoma	10–20 mg PO tid or qid; 0.5–2.0 mg IV	After alpha blockade initiated
	Essential tremor	20–80 mg PO tid	
	Migraine	20–80 mg PO bid or tid	
	Hyperthyroidism	10–60 mg PO tid or qid	
Metoprolol	Hypertension	50–200 mg PO bid	Selective beta$_1$ (cardiac), lipophilic
	Myocardial infarction	100 mg PO bid	Prolongs survival post MI
Nadolol	Hypertension	80–320 mg PO qd	Hydrophilic, nonselective; lengthen dosage interval with renal failure
	Angina	80–240 mg PO qd	
Timolol	Hypertension	10–30 mg PO bid	Lipophilic, nonselective
	Myocardial infarction	10 mg PO bid	Prolongs survival post MI
Atenolol	Hypertension	50–100 mg PO qd	Selective beta$_1$, hydrophilic; lengthen dosage interval with renal failure
Pindolol	Hypertension	5–30 mg PO bid	Nonselective, lipophilic with partial agonist activity
	Angina	10 mg PO qid	
Acebutolol	Hypertension	200–800 mg qid	Selective beta$_1$, hydrophilic, partial agonist activity
	Arrhythmias	200–600 mg bid	
Penbutolol	Hypertension	20–40 mg PO qd	Nonselective
Betaxolol	Hypertension	15–20 mg PO qd	Selective β_1, hydrophilic
Carteolol	Hypertension	2.5–10 mg PO qd	Nonselective, partial agonist activity, hydrophilic; lengthen dosage interval with renal failure
Esmolol	Supraventricular tachycardia	50–200 (μg/kg)/min IV after loading dose of 500 μg/kg/min for 1 min	Selective beta$_1$, very short duration of action
Sotalol	Arrythmias	80–320 mg bid	Nonselective, hydrophilic
Bisoprolol	Hypertension	5–20 mg qd	Selective beta$_1$, lipophilic
ALPHA BLOCKING AGENTS			
Phenoxybenzamine	Pheochromocytoma	10–60 mg PO bid; titrate as needed	Noncompetitive, nonselective alpha blockade
Phentolamine	Pheochromocytoma	5 mg IV (after test dose of 0.5 mg)	Competitive, nonselective alpha blockade
Prazosin	Hypertension	1–5 mg PO bid or tid	Competitive, selective alpha$_1$ blockade
	CHF	2–7 mg PO qid	
Doxazosin	Hypertension	1–16 mg PO qd	Competitive selective alpha$_1$ blockade, long duration of action
	Prostatism		
Terazosin	Hypertension	1–5 mg PO qd	Competitive, selective alpha$_1$ blockade, long duration of action
	Prostatism		
COMBINED ALPHA-BETA BLOCKING AGENT			
Labetalol	Hypertension	100–1200 mg PO bid; titrate slowly as needed; 20–80 mg IV (by increments up to 300 mg); 2 mg/min by IV infusion	Competitive alpha and beta antagonist with relatively more activity against beta receptors
DOPAMINERGIC ANTAGONIST[f]			
Metoclopramide	Diabetic gastroparesis	10–15 mg PO qid	Competitive dopaminergic antagonist with prominent cholinergic agonist activity
	Gastroesophageal reflex	10–15 mg PO qid	
	Antiemetic (cancer chemotherapy)	10 mg IV	
GANGLIONIC BLOCKING AGENT			
Trimethaphan	Hypertensive crisis (aortic dissection)	0.5–5 mg/min IV	Competitive ganglionic blocker; some direct vasodilating effects; inhibits parasympathetic as well as sympathetic nervous system
CHOLINERGIC AGENT			
Bethanechol	Urinary retention (nonobstructive)	10–20 mg PO tid or qid; 2.5 mg SC	M$_2$ receptor agonist

(continued)

Table 70-1—*(continued)*

Some Commonly Used Autonomic Drugs[a,b,c]

Agent	Indication	Dose and Route	Comment
ANTICHOLINESTERASE AGENTS[g]			
Physostigmine	Central cholinergic blockade	1–2 mg IV (slow)	Tertiary amine; penetrates CNS well; may cause seizures; used to reverse central anticholinergic effects produced by overdose of atropine or tricyclic antidepressants
Edrophonium	Paroxysmal supraventricular tachycardia	5 mg IV (after 1.0-mg test dose)	Induces vagotonic response; rapid onset, short duration of action; effects reversed by atropine
CHOLINERGIC BLOCKING AGENTS[h]			
Atropine	Bradycardia and hypotension	0.4–1.0 mg IV every 1–2 h	Competitive inhibition of M_1 and M_2 receptor; blocks hemodynamic changes associated with increased vagal tone
Ipratropium	Asthma Chronic obstructive pulmonary disease	500 mg by inhalation (nebulizer) tid or qid	Anticholinergic bronchodilator

[a] Consult complete prescribing information. [b] Doses for children are not given. [c] Only the more common indications and routes of administration are listed.
[d] Dopaminergic agonists are listed separately although dopamine, at high doses, is an adrenergic agonist as well.
[e] Clinical efficacy of most beta blockers appears similar for major indications. Not all beta blockers are FDA approved for all indications listed in the table. When beta-blocking agents are discontinued, gradual dosage reduction is recommended. Both beta₁ selective and nonselective agents have cardioprotective effects after myocardial infarction.
[f] Neuroleptic and antipsychotic agents are also dopaminergic antagonists; these are not included in the table.
[g] A major use of cholinesterase inhibitors is in myasthenia gravis (Chap. 382). These agents, quaternary amines that do not penetrate the CNS, are not included here.
[h] A wide variety of synthetic atropine derivatives are available for the purpose of (1) diminishing GI tract motility and secretion and (2) increasing urinary bladder capacity. Their usefulness is limited by anticholinergic side effects. Some may be useful as adjuncts in the treatment of peptic ulcer disease.

accelerates atrioventricular conduction while increasing the automaticity of ventricular pacemakers. Isoproterenol is used in the treatment of heart block and bronchoconstriction. *Dobutamine*, a congener of dopamine with relative selectivity for the beta₁ receptor and with a greater effect on myocardial contractility than on heart rate, is also used in the treatment of congestive heart failure, often in combination with vasodilators (Chap. 233). In conjunction with radionuclide imaging or echocardiographic assessment of wall motion, dobutamine, as well as other investigational congeners that have a relatively greater effect on heart rate, is used in the diagnosis of demand-induced myocardial ischemia.

Selective beta₂-receptor agonists The cardiac stimulation caused by nonselective beta agonists, such as isoproterenol or epinephrine, is occasionally dangerous when these agents are used in the treatment of bronchoconstriction (see Chap. 252). Selective beta₂ agonists, administered by inhalation for bronchoconstriction, include agents with an intermediate duration of action (*metaproterenol, albuterol, terbutaline, pirbuterol, isoetharine,* and *bitolterol*) and the newer long-acting agents (*salmeterol* and *formoterol*); these drugs improve the therapeutic ratio by achieving bronchial dilatation with less activation of the cardiovascular system (see Chaps. 252 and 258). Although selectivity is relative and cardiac stimulation may occur with these agents at higher dose levels, inhaled agonists at the usual doses result in relatively little cardiac stimulation. Oral administration, which is no longer preferred, is associated with more systemic beta-agonist effects. *Ritodrine*, another selective beta₂ agonist, is used as a tocolytic agent (as is *terbutaline*) to relax the uterus and antagonize premature labor.

Alpha-Adrenergic Agonists *Phenylephrine* and *methoxamine* are direct-acting alpha agonists that elevate blood pressure by increasing peripheral vasoconstriction. They are used primarily in the treatment of hypotension and paroxysmal supraventricular tachycardia (Chap. 231), in the latter case by increasing cardiac vagal tone through reflex baroreceptor stimulation. Phenylephrine and a related proprietary compound, *phenylpropanolamine*, are common constituents of decongestant medications (often combined with antihistamines) for the treatment of allergic rhinitis and upper respiratory infections.

Miscellaneous Sympathomimetic Amines with Mixed Actions *Ephedrine* has both direct beta-receptor agonist properties and an indirect effect on sympathetic nerve endings, from which it releases NE, and is used primarily as a bronchodilator. *Sudephedrine*, a conge-

ner of ephedrine, is less potent at dilating bronchi and serves as a nasal decongestant. *Metaraminol* has both direct and indirect effects on sympathetic nerve endings and is employed in the treatment of hypotensive states.

Dopaminergic Agonists The D_2-receptor agonist *bromocriptine* is used to suppress prolactin secretion (Chap. 328). *Apomorphine*, another D_2-receptor agonist, is used to induce emesis.

ANTIADRENERGIC OR SYMPATHOLYTIC AGENTS (See also Chap. 246) **Agents Inhibiting Central Sympathetic Outflow** The antihypertensive agents *methyldopa, clonidine, guanabenz,* and *guanfacine* diminish central sympathetic outflow by stimulating a central alpha-adrenergic pathway (alpha₂ receptor) that diminishes vasomotor outflow. Central nervous system side effects such as sedation are common. When administration of clonidine is stopped abruptly, a withdrawal syndrome characterized by rebound hyperactivity of the sympathetic nervous system can produce a state resembling the crises of patients with pheochromocytoma. *Opiates* also may exert a central sympatholytic effect; the sympathetic excitation of morphine withdrawal responds to clonidine and vice versa. *Propranolol* and *reserpine* may exert some sympatholytic effects at the level of the central nervous system.

Ganglionic Blocking Agents Ganglionic transmission may be antagonized by drugs that block the (nicotinic) cholinergic synapse between the preganglionic and postganglionic autonomic nerves. These agents inhibit the parasympathetic as well as the sympathetic nervous system. Only *trimethaphan* is in general clinical use; its major application is in the treatment of hypertensive crises, particularly aortic dissection, when controlled hypotension and decreased myocardial contractility are desirable (Chap. 246).

Agents Acting at the Peripheral Sympathetic Nerve Endings Adrenergic neuron-blocking agents depress the function of the peripheral sympathetic nerves by decreasing the amount of neurotransmitter released. *Guanethidine*, the prototype of this class of drugs, is concentrated in the sympathetic nerve endings by the amine-uptake mechanism. Within the terminal it blocks the release of NE in response to nerve impulses and eventually depletes the nerve of NE by displacing it from the intraneuronal storage granules. The drug is occasionally useful in the management of severe hypertension, although orthostatic hypotension is a limiting side effect. *Bretylium*, an agent whose effects are similar to those of guanethidine, is employed in the treatment of ventricular fibrillation (Chap. 231). Both guanethidine and bretylium are antagonized by agents that affect the amine-uptake transport process such as sympathomimetic amines, tricyclic antidepressants, phenoxybenzamine, and phenothiazines. The antihypertensive action of guanethidine may be rapidly reversed by these drugs.

Reserpine depletes catecholamines from the peripheral sympathetic nerve endings, the brain, and the adrenal medulla. Its antihypertensive effect in humans is usually attributed to depletion of peripheral NE stores within sympathetic nerve endings. The sedation and occasionally morbid depression attending its use result from NE depletion within the central nervous system.

Adrenergic-Receptor Blocking Agents Adrenergic blocking agents antagonize the effects of catecholamines at the level of the peripheral tissue.

Alpha-adrenergic-receptor blocking agents Phenoxybenzamine and *phentolamine* are utilized principally in treating pheochromocytoma (Chap. 333). Phenoxybenzamine produces prolonged, noncompetitive alpha blockade, while phentolamine leads to reversible, competitive blockade. Because of its rapid action and short duration, phentolamine is commonly used in the treatment of acute hypertensive paroxysms secondary to catecholamine excess, such as occur with pheochromocytoma. Both phentolamine and phenoxybenzamine antagonize alpha$_1$ and alpha$_2$ receptors, although phenoxybenzamine is more potent at the alpha$_1$ receptor site. *Prazosin*, an alpha-adrenergic blocking agent with selectivity for the alpha$_1$ receptor, possesses properties that resemble those of primary vasodilators and has been used in the treatment of essential hypertension and as an afterload-reducing agent in congestive heart failure. *Doxazosin* and *terazosin*, long-acting selective alpha$_1$ blockers, are more useful in the treatment of essential hypertension because of better dosing schedule and less orthostatic hypotension. These agents also lower triglyceride levels and raise high-density lipoprotein (HDL) cholesterol levels. Selective alpha$_1$ blockers are potentially useful in the symptomatic treatment of urinary outflow track obstruction and prostatism because they antagonize contraction of the sphincter at the bladder trigone.

Beta-adrenergic-receptor blocking agents These drugs antagonize the effects of catecholamines on the heart and are useful in the treatment of angina pectoris, hypertension, and cardiac arrhythmias. The benefit of beta blockade in angina derives from the decrease in myocardial oxygen consumption following reduction in heart rate and myocardial contractility (Chap. 244). The hypotensive effect of beta blockade is not clearly understood (Chap. 246). Diminished cardiac output, decreased NE release at postganglionic sympathetic nerve endings, reduced renin secretion, and suppressed central sympathetic outflow are possible mechanisms. The efficacy of beta-blocking agents in the treatment of arrhythmias depends on reduction of the rate of spontaneous depolarization of pacemaker cells in the sinus node and junctional pacemakers and on slowing conduction within the atria and atrioventricular node. Beta blockade is also effective in the symptomatic management of hyperthyroidism and the control of tachycardia and arrhythmias in patients with pheochromocytoma. Beta-adrenergic blocking agents are also useful in the treatment of migraine, essential tremor, idiopathic hypertrophic subaortic stenosis, and aortic dissection. Several trials have demonstrated that beta-receptor blocking agents, administered long-term, diminish mortality following acute myocardial infarction. The mechanism of this cardioprotective effect may involve antiarrhythmic action, prevention of reinfarction, and reduction in infarct size (Chap. 243).

Pharmacologic properties of beta-receptor blocking agents Thirteen beta-blocking agents (atenolol, acebutolol, betaxolol, bisoprolol, carteolol, esmolol, metoprolol, nadolol, pindolol, penbutolol, propranolol, sotalol, and timolol) are available for use in the United States. Other agents (alprenolol, bevantolol, dilevalol, oxprenolol, etc.) are in use in other countries and investigational within the United States. The utility of these agents is derived predominantly from blockade of beta-adrenergic receptors. In general, the various agents have similar clinical efficacy.

Although much has been written about other pharmacologic properties, including cardioselectivity, membrane-stabilizing (local anesthetic) effects, intrinsic sympathomimetic (partial-agonist) activity, and lipid solubility, the clinical significance of these additional properties is small. Local anesthetic properties are most prominent with propranolol; however, membrane stabilization probably does not contribute substantially to the clinical utility. The various beta blockers do differ in their water and lipid solubility. The lipophilic agents (propranolol, metoprolol, oxprenolol, bisoprolol) are readily absorbed from the gastrointestinal tract, metabolized by the liver, have large volumes of distribution, and penetrate the central nervous system well; the hydrophilic agents (acebutolol, atenolol, betaxolol, carteolol, nadolol, sotalol) are less readily absorbed, not extensively metabolized, and have relatively long plasma half-lives. As a consequence, the hydrophilic agents may be administered once per day. Hepatic failure may prolong the plasma half-life of the lipophilic agents, whereas renal failure may prolong the action of the hydrophilic group. The degree of lipid solubility, therefore, provides a basis for choice of a particular agent in patients with hepatic or renal insufficiency. Although the hydrophilic agents penetrate the central nervous system less well, central nervous system side effects (sedation, depression, hallucinations) are well described with the hydrophilic as well as with the lipophilic agents.

Some beta-adrenergic blocking agents possess beta-agonist activity. This has been referred to as "intrinsic sympathomimetic activity" (ISA). Agents with partial agonist activity (pindolol, alprenolol, acebutolol, carteolol, dilevalol, oxprenolol) cause little or no depression of resting heart rate (partial agonist effect) while blocking the increase in heart rate that occurs in response to exercise or the administration of a beta agonist such as isoproterenol. The presence of partial agonist activity may be useful when bradycardia limits treatment in patients with slow resting heart rates. Pindolol also produces mild vasodilation, perhaps in part related to peripheral beta$_2$ stimulation. Agents with partial agonist activity cause less change in blood lipid levels than agents without agonist properties. On theoretical grounds, intrinsic sympathomimetic activity would be undesirable in the treatment of thyrotoxicosis, idiopathic hypertrophic subaortic stenosis, aortic dissection, and tachyarrhythmias.

Cardioselective (beta$_1$) adrenergic-receptor blocking agents Propranolol, the prototype of the nonselective beta-adrenergic blocking agent, induces a competitive blockade of both beta$_1$ and beta$_2$ receptors. Other nonselective beta-blocking agents include alprenolol, carteolol, dilevalol, nadolol, oxprenolol, penbutolol, pindolol, sotalol, and timolol. Metoprolol, esmolol, acebutolol, atenolol, and betaxolol possess relative selectivity for the beta$_1$ receptor. Although beta$_1$-(cardio-) selective agents have the theoretical advantage of producing less bronchoconstriction and less peripheral vasoconstriction, a clear-cut clinical advantage of the cardioselective agents has not been decisively demonstrated, since the beta$_1$ selectivity is only relative. Bronchoconstriction may occur when beta$_1$-selective agents are administered in full therapeutic doses.

Adverse effects of beta-receptor blocking agents Aside from the effects on the central nervous system, most adverse reactions to beta-blocking agents are consequences of beta-adrenergic blockade. These include the precipitation of heart failure in patients in whom cardiac compensation depends on enhanced sympathetic drive; the aggravation of bronchospasm in patients with asthma; predisposition to the development of hypoglycemia in insulin-requiring diabetics (blockade of catecholamine-mediated counterregulation and antagonism of the adrenergic warning signs of hypoglycemia); the development of hyperkalemia in diabetic or uremic patients with impaired potassium tolerance; the enhancement of coronary or peripheral arterial vasospasm; and elevation in triglycerides and depression of HDL levels. The lipid (and perhaps the peripheral vascular) effects are less (or absent) in agents with partial (beta$_2$) agonist activity.

Miscellaneous adrenergic blocking agents Labetalol, approved for use in the United States as an antihypertensive agent, is a competitive antagonist of both alpha- and beta-adrenergic receptors. Although labetalol induces relatively more beta- than alpha-receptor blockade, fall in peripheral resistance may be marked following acute administration of the drug. Vasodilation may be mediated in part by a partial agonist effect on the beta$_2$-adrenergic receptor; labetalol does not possess partial agonist activity for the beta$_1$ (cardiac) receptor.

Metoclopramide is a dopaminergic antagonist with cholinergic agonist properties. It enhances gastric emptying, increases the tone of the lower esophageal sphincter, increases prolactin and aldosterone secretion, and antagonizes emesis induced by apomorphine. It is useful clinically in enhancing gastric emptying (in the absence of organic obstruction such as in diabetic gastroparesis), in antagonizing gastroesophageal reflux, and as an antiemetic during cancer chemotherapy.

THE PARASYMPATHETIC NERVOUS SYSTEM

ACETYLCHOLINE   ACh serves as the neurotransmitter at all autonomic ganglia, at the postganglionic parasympathetic nerve endings, at the postganglionic sympathetic nerve endings innervating the eccrine sweat glands, and at the skeletal muscle end plate (neuromuscular junction). The enzyme choline acetyltransferase catalyzes the synthesis of ACh from acetyl coenzyme A (CoA) produced within the nerve ending and from choline, actively taken up from the extracellular fluid. Within the cholinergic nerve endings, ACh is stored in discrete synaptic vesicles and released in response to nerve impulses that depolarize the nerve terminals and increase calcium influx.

Cholinergic Receptors   Different receptors for ACh exist on the postganglionic neurons within the autonomic ganglia and at the postjunctional autonomic effector sites. Those within the autonomic ganglia and adrenal medulla are stimulated predominantly by nicotine (*nicotinic receptors*) and those on autonomic effector cells by the alkaloid muscarine (*muscarinic receptors*). Ganglionic blocking agents antagonize the nicotinic receptors, while atropine blocks the muscarinic receptors. The muscarinic (M) receptor, furthermore, has been recently subdivided into additional types. The M$_1$ receptor is localized to the central nervous system and perhaps parasympathetic ganglia; the M$_2$ receptor is the nonneuronal muscarinic receptor on smooth muscle, cardiac muscle, and glandular epithelium. Bethanechol is a selective agonist of the M$_2$ receptor; pirenzepine, an investigational agent, is a selective antagonist of the M$_1$ receptor that markedly reduces gastric acid secretion. The M$_2$ receptor inhibits adenylyl cyclase and utilizes the regulatory G$_i$ protein; the M$_1$ receptor interacts with G$_q$ and stimulates phospholipase C (Fig. 70-5). The M$_3$ receptor, present on smooth muscle and secretory glands, is antagonized by atropine and utilizes phospholipase C, IP$_3$, and DAG as second messengers. Other subtypes have been identified by molecular biologic techniques but have not yet been fully characterized.

Acetylcholinesterase   Hydrolysis of ACh by acetylcholinesterase inactivates the neurotransmitter at cholinergic synapses. This enzyme (also known as specific or true cholinesterase) is present within neurons and is distinct from butyrocholinesterase (serum cholinesterase or pseudocholinesterase). The latter enzyme is present in plasma and nonneuronal tissues and is not primarily involved in the termination of the effects of ACh at autonomic effector sites. The pharmacologic effects of anticholinesterase agents are due to inhibition of neuronal (true) acetylcholinesterase.

PHYSIOLOGY OF THE PARASYMPATHETIC NERVOUS SYSTEM   The parasympathetic nervous system participates in the regulation of the cardiovascular system, the gastrointestinal tract, and the genitourinary system. Tissues such as liver, kidney, pancreas, and thyroid also receive parasympathetic innervation, suggesting a role for the parasympathetic nervous system in metabolic regulation as well, although cholinergic effects on metabolism are not well characterized.

Cardiovascular System   Parasympathetic effects on the heart are mediated by the vagus nerve. ACh reduces the rate of spontaneous depolarization of the sinoatrial node and decreases heart rate. ACh also delays impulse conduction within the atrial musculature while shortening the effective refractory period, a combination of factors that may initiate or perpetuate atrial arrhythmias. At the atrioventricular

node, ACh reduces conduction velocity, increases the effective refractory period, and thus diminishes the ventricular response during atrial flutter or fibrillation (Chap. 231). The decrease in inotropy induced by ACh is related to a prejunctional inhibitory effect on sympathetic nerve endings as well as to a direct inhibitory effect on the atrial myocardium. The ventricular myocardium is not much affected since innervation by cholinergic fibers is minimal. A direct cholinergic contribution to the regulation of peripheral resistance appears unlikely since parasympathetic innervation of the vasculature is not extensive. The parasympathetic nervous system, however, may influence peripheral resistance indirectly by inhibiting NE release from sympathetic nerves.

Gastrointestinal Tract   Parasympathetic innervation of the gut is via the vagus nerve and the pelvic sacral nerves. The parasympathetic nervous system increases the tone of gastrointestinal smooth muscle, enhances peristaltic activity, and relaxes the gastrointestinal sphincters. ACh stimulates exocrine secretion from the glandular epithelium and enhances the secretion of gastrin, secretin, and insulin.

Genitourinary and Respiratory Systems   Sacral parasympathetic nerves supply the urinary bladder and genitalia. ACh increases ureteral peristalsis, contracts the urinary detrusor muscle, and relaxes the trigone and sphincter, thereby playing a critical role in the coordination of urination. The respiratory tract is innervated with parasympathetic fibers derived from the vagus nerve. ACh increases tracheobronchial secretions and stimulates bronchial constriction.

PHARMACOLOGY OF THE PARASYMPATHETIC NERVOUS SYSTEM   Cholinergic Agonists   ACh itself has no therapeutic role because of its widespread effects and short duration of action. Congeners of ACh are less susceptible to hydrolysis by cholinesterase and have a narrower range of physiologic effects. Bethanechol, the only systemic cholinergic agonist in general use, stimulates gastrointestinal and genitourinary smooth muscle with minimal effect on the cardiovascular system. It is used in the treatment of urinary retention in the absence of outflow tract obstruction and, less commonly, in gastrointestinal disorders such as postvagotomy gastric atony. Pilocarpine and carbachol are topical cholinergic agonists used in the treatment of glaucoma.

Acetylcholinesterase Inhibitors   Cholinesterase inhibitors enhance the effects of parasympathetic stimulation by diminishing the inactivation of ACh. The therapeutic application of reversible cholinesterase inhibitors depends on the role of ACh as neurotransmitter at the skeletal muscle neuroeffector junction and within the central nervous system and includes the treatment of myasthenia gravis (Chap. 382), the termination of neuromuscular blockade following general anesthesia, and the reversal of intoxication by agents with a central anticholinergic action. Physostigmine, a tertiary amine, penetrates the central nervous system well, while related quaternary amines (neostigmine, pyridostigmine, ambenonium, and edrophonium) do not. Organophosphorous cholinesterase inhibitors produce irreversible cholinesterase blockade; these agents are used principally as insecticides and are primarily of toxicologic interest. With regard to the autonomic nervous system, cholinesterase inhibitors are of limited use in the treatment of intestinal and bladder smooth-muscle dysfunction such as occurs in paralytic ileus and atonic urinary bladder. Cholinesterase inhibitors induce a vagotonic response in the heart and may be useful in terminating attacks of paroxysmal supraventricular tachycardia (Chap. 231).

Cholinergic-Receptor Blocking Agents   *Atropine* blocks muscarinic cholinergic receptors, with little effect on cholinergic transmission at the autonomic ganglia and the neuromuscular junctions. Many of the central nervous system actions of atropine and atropine-like drugs are attributable to blockade of central muscarinic synapses. The related alkaloid, *scopolamine*, is similar to atropine but causes drowsiness, euphoria, and amnesia, effects that make it suitable as a preanesthetic medication.

Atropine increases heart rate and enhances atrioventricular conduction, actions that may be useful in combating the bradycardia or heart block associated with heightened vagal tone. In addition, atropine reverses cholinergically mediated bronchoconstriction and diminishes respiratory tract secretions. These effects contribute to its utility as a preanesthetic medication.

Atropine also decreases gastrointestinal tract motility and secretion. Although various derivatives and congeners of atropine (such as *propantheline, isopropamide,* and *glycopyrrolate*) have been advocated in patients with peptic ulcer or with diarrheal syndromes, the chronic use of such agents is limited by other manifestations of parasympathetic inhibition such as dry mouth and urinary retention. The investigational selective M_1 inhibitor pirenzepine inhibits gastric secretion at doses that have minimal anticholinergic effects at other sites; this agent may be useful in the treatment of peptic ulcer. Atropine and its congener *ipratropium,* when given by inhalation, cause bronchodilation and have been used experimentally in the treatment of asthma.

BIBLIOGRAPHY

ARNER P: The β_3-adrenergic receptor—a cause and cure of obesity? N Engl J Med 333:382, 1995

CARON MG, LEFKOWITZ RJ: Catecholamine receptors: Structure, function and regulation. Recent Prog Horm Res 48:277, 1993

CHALMERS J, PILOWSKY P: Brainstem and bulbospinal neurotransmitter systems in the control of blood pressure. J Hypertens 9:675, 1991

CLÉMENT K et al: Genetic variation in the β_3-adrenergic receptor and an increased capacity to gain weight in patients with morbid obesity. N Engl J Med 333:352, 1995

ESLER M et al: Overflow of catecholamine neurotransmitters to the circulation: Source, fate, and functions. Physiol Rev 70:963, 1990

KUPFERMANN I: Functional studies of cotransmission. Physiol Rev 71(3):683, 1991

LANDSBERG L, YOUNG JB: Catecholamines and the adrenal medulla, in *Williams' Textbook of Endocrinology,* 8th ed, JD Wilson, DW Foster (eds). Philadelphia, Saunders, 1992, p 621

LOKHANDWALA MF, AMENTA F: Anatomical distribution and function of dopamine receptors in the kidney. FASEB J 5:3023, 1991

LOW PA: Autonomic nervous system function. J Clin Neurophysiol 10:14, 1993

MEISTER B, APERIA A: Molecular mechanisms involved in catecholamine regulation of sodium transport. Semin Nephrol 13:41, 1993

NELSON H: β-Andrenergic bronchodilators. N Engl J Med 333:499, 1995

PACHOLCZYK T et al: Expression cloning of a cocaine- and antidepressant-sensitive human noradrenaline transporter. Nature 350:350, 1991

RUFFOLO RR et al: Structure and function of α-adrenoceptors. Pharmacol Rev 43:475, 1991

VAN ZWIETEN PA et al: The parasympathetic system and its muscarinic receptors in hypertensive disease. J Hypertens 13:1079, 1995

WIDÉN E et al: Association of a polymorphism in the β_3-adrenergic-receptor gene with features of the insulin resistance syndrome in Finns. N Engl J Med 333:348, 1995

WILLIAMS JL et al: Area postrema: A unique regulator of cardiovascular function. News Physiol Sci 7:30, 1992

71 *Joseph Loscalzo*

NITRIC OXIDE: BIOLOGIC AND MEDICAL IMPLICATIONS

Nitric oxide (NO•) is a simple, heterodiatomic molecule with broad and diverse effects in human biology that have been recognized only recently. In 1980, Furchgott and Zawadzki reported that a product of the endothelial cell causes vasorelaxation, and this endothelium-derived relaxing factor (EDRF) was eventually shown to be NO•. NO• is now known to be produced by many cell types and to exert a wide range of biologic effects.

NO• is synthesized by a family of enzymes known as the nitric oxide synthases (NOSs) (Fig. 71-1). Three distinct isoforms have been identified, of which two are named after the cell types from which

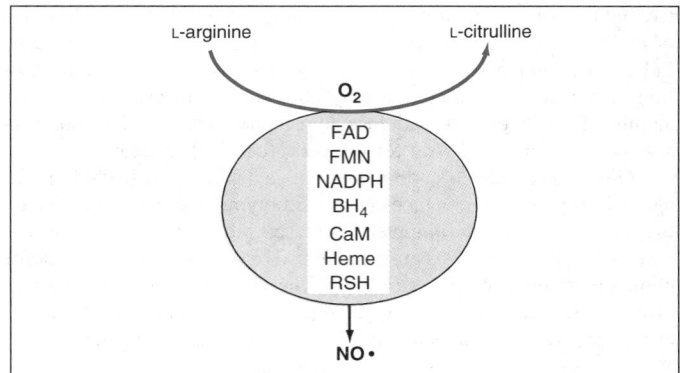

FIGURE 71-1 Nitric oxide synthases catalyze the five-electron oxidation of L-arginine to L-citrulline and nitric oxide. Cofactor requirements include flavin adenine dinucleotide (FAD), flavin mononucleotide (FMN), reduced β-nicotinamide adenine dinucleotide phosphate (NADPH), tetrahydrobiopterin (BH_4), calcium-calmodulin (CaM), a heme complex, and a thiol equivalent (RSH). (Adapted, with permission, from the Annual Review of Pharmacology and Toxicology, vol. 35, 1995, by Annual Reviews, Inc.)

they were first cloned: neuronal NOS (*nNOS, Nos1* gene product); inducible NOS (*iNOS, Nos2* gene product), present in monocytes/macrophages, smooth muscle cells, microvascular endothelial cells, fibroblasts, cardiomyocytes, hepatocytes, and megakaryocytes; and endothelial NOS (*eNOS, Nos3* gene product). As a free radical, NO• readily undergoes addition, substitution, redox, and chain-terminating reactions, which serve as the molecular basis for its biologic effects. NO• reacts with heme-bound iron to form a nitrosylated adduct. Reaction with the prosthetic heme group of guanylyl cyclase activates the enzyme; reaction with the heme group of hemoglobin traps NO•, making it biologically inactive and converting ferrous to ferric hemoglobin; reaction with the prosthetic heme groups of cytochromes uncouples oxidative phosphorylation.

PHYSIOLOGIC ACTIONS NO• is implicated in a wide variety of physiologic effects. The reaction of NO• with the heme group of guanylyl cyclase is the principal effector reaction of NO• in the cardiovascular system. This reaction leads to activation of guanylyl cyclase. In smooth muscle cells, the increase in cyclic guanosine 5′-monophosphate (cyclic GMP) leads to activation of cyclic GMP–dependent protein kinase, which, in turn, phosphorylates myosin light chain kinase. Phosphorylated myosin light chain kinase has a reduced affinity for the calcium-calmodulin complex and is less efficient at phosphorylating myosin light chain. Failure to phosphorylate the regulatory light chains of myosin stabilizes the inactive form of the enzyme and reduces smooth muscle contraction, thereby reducing vascular tone. Agonist–mediated increases in endothelial cell calcium activate *eNOS.* In addition, flow-mediated vasodilation with exercise depends in part on the flow-sensitive increase in endothelial cell calcium, which leads to an increase in *eNOS* activity.

Similar effects are exerted by NO• in smooth muscle cells of other organ systems. NO• relaxes gastrointestinal smooth muscle and leads to reduced motility, relaxation of the sphincter of Oddi, and relaxation of the lower esophageal sphincter. Relaxation of bronchial smooth muscle can be provoked by inhaled NO•, and endogenously produced NO• may contribute to the maintenance of basal bronchial and basal pulmonary arterial tone, as well.

Other effects of *eNOS* include maintenance of vascular integrity, impairment of leukocyte adhesion to the endothelium, and inhibition of smooth muscle migration and proliferation. Endothelial NO• also plays a critical role in hemostasis, making an important contribution to the normal inhibition of platelet function. Basal production of NO• by *eNOS* inhibits both adhesion and aggregation of platelets in the vasculature. Inhibition of platelet adhesion is a property of NO• not shared by the other principal antiplatelet product of the endothelium, prostacyclin.

Endothelial NO• is an important determinant of cerebral blood flow. *nNOS* in neuronal and glial cells contributes to the regulation of cerebrovascular tone and to memory and learning through its involvement in long-term potentiation in the central nervous system. NO• is a likely transmitter of nonadrenergic, noncholinergic neurons and may thereby participate in the regulation of myocardial contractility, heart rate, gastrointestinal motility, bronchial tone, and penile erection.

The production of NO• by *iNOS* in macrophages, lymphocytes, and neutrophils is an important determinant of immune and inflammatory responses. The bactericidal, fungicidal, viricidal, parasiticidal, and tumoricidal activities of macrophages are determined in part by the robust elaboration of NO• by *iNOS*. NO• also limits lymphocyte proliferation and attenuates the allogeneic immune response. Given the broad range of non-immune cell types shown to express *iNOS*, some investigators believe that NO• produced by this isoform is involved in nonspecific immunity, especially in the lung and liver. By a similar mechanism, NO• produced by *iNOS* may also be involved in apoptotic responses in a variety of cell types.

PATHOPHYSIOLOGIC EFFECTS OF NITRIC OXIDE
Both a deficiency and an excess of NO• are believed to be involved in several pathophysiologic states. NO• is a critical determinant of basal vascular tone, and a deficiency of NO• is associated with *hypertension*, as illustrated by recent observations in a murine model of *Nos3* gene inactivation by homologous recombination. Nevertheless, genetic linkage studies have thus far failed to suggest an association between the *Nos3* locus and essential hypertension. However, Deng and Rapp have demonstrated a clear linkage between the *Nos2* locus and salt-sensitive hypertension in the Dahl S rat. Also, the provision of L-arginine in the diet of these animals corrects the hypertensive response to dietary sodium chloride. In chronic renal failure, the plasma concentration of dimethylarginine, a naturally occurring derivative of L-arginine, is increased and competitively inhibits nitric oxide synthase activity, possibly contributing to the hypertension of chronic renal failure.

Common disorders that promote atherosclerosis, such as hypertension, hyperlipidemia, smoking, and diabetes, are all associated with abnormal endothelial function, one manifestation of which is a comparative deficiency of bioactive NO•. This deficiency, which represents either a true deficiency of the molecule or inactivation of it by reactive, oxygen-derived free radicals, is accompanied by increased vascular tone, reduced antithrombotic activity, decreased antiproliferative action, increased endothelial permeability, and enhanced susceptibility of low-density lipoprotein to oxidation. These many interrelated actions may promote atherosclerosis and its complications.

Expression of *iNOS* occurs in several disease states, the most prominent being *bacterial sepsis*. Induction of *Nos2* is induced by endotoxin and cytokines, and the elaboration of NO• in this setting accounts for the hypotension of septic shock states and contributes to the hemorrhagic diathesis of sepsis by profoundly inhibiting platelet function. The myocardial depression associated with septic shock may be explained in part by the inhibition of myocardial contractility by NO•. The cytokine-rich milieu that accompanies ischemia-reperfusion injury may also contribute to increased elaboration of NO• through increased expression of *iNOS* and the accompanying myocardial depression that follows successful coronary thrombolysis or revascularization.

A deficiency of NO•-producing neurons in the gastrointestinal tract is believed to be responsible for certain abnormalities in gastrointestinal motility, such as *Hirschsprung's disease*, *achalasia*, and *chronic intestinal pseudo-obstruction*. NO• is also believed to play an important role in gastric cytoprotection, possibly by way of increased mucosal blood flow and the modulation of gastric epithelial function.

Increased NO• production owing to the induction of *Nos2* in hepatocytes, fibroblasts, and endothelial cells is believed to underlie the hyperdynamic circulatory state of Laennec's cirrhosis. Also, NO• produced by hepatocyte *iNOS* plays a role in protection of these cells against a variety of hepatic toxins, including ethanol and acetaminophen. NO• inhibits protein synthesis in the hepatocyte at the posttranslational level and inhibits several mitochondrial enzymes involved in electron transport, including *cis*-aconitase, NADH-ubiquinone oxido-

reductase, and succinate-ubiquinone oxidoreductase. NO• also inhibits glyceraldehyde-3-phosphate dehydrogenase activity in hepatocytes, thereby influencing glucose metabolism. On exposure to an oxidizing hepatic toxin, NO• prevents the consumption of cell reducing equivalents (reduced glutathione). These several effects of NO• on hepatic function suggest that hepatoprotection results from a reduction in the metabolic activity of the cell, which conserves the cell's energy stores.

Cytotoxicity by NO• also appears to be important in the central nervous system. Following neuronal injury, large amounts of L-glutamate are released and elicit neurotoxicity by activation of *N*-methyl-D-asparate receptors. Activation of these receptors augments *nNOS* activity. While *nNOS*-containing neurons are resistant to the cytotoxic effects of receptor stimulation, NO• released from them is responsible for cytotoxicity in adjacent neurons. Interestingly, NO• may also be cytoprotective in the central nervous system, an effect that depends on the molecule's redox state: NO^+ reacts with the *N*-methyl-D-aspartate receptor and thereby limits entry of excessive Ca^{2+} into the cell cytosol; NO•, by contrast, promotes Ca^{2+} entry into the cell and thus cytotoxicity.

Impairment of NO• production by endothelial cells in disorders of endothelial dysfunction or following percutaneous angioplasty may help to facilitate smooth muscle proliferative responses in these settings. In addition, elevated NO• may contribute to cytotoxic mechanisms in *graft-versus-host disease* and in *transplant rejection*. The cytoprotective and cytotoxic effects of NO• are important and contrasting; the balance between them is determined by the local concentration of NO• in a given organ, the availability of other free radicals that can react with NO• to form other oxidative compounds (such as O_2•, which reacts with NO• to form $OONO^-$), and the susceptibility of the cell or organ to the toxic effects of oxidant stress.

THERAPEUTIC IMPLICATIONS
Therapeutic manipulation of NO• levels—by providing the compound or by inhibiting its production—has profound effects in many clinical settings. For over 100 years, congeners of NO•, the nitrovasodilators, have been used to provide exogenous NO• to dysfunctional coronary arteries. These agents, including nitroglycerin, isosorbide mononitrate and dinitrate, and nitroprusside, promote vasodilation and platelet inhibition and are metabolized to NO• (or NO^+) to achieve these effects. Inhibition of *iNOS* can be used to restore normal arterial pressures in the setting of *septic shock*; however, the risk of intravascular platelet thrombosis is increased by this approach in animals. Interestingly, glucocorticoids inhibit *Nos2* transcription, which may account for part of their protective effect in septic syndromes. Owing to the importance of NO• in penile erection, NO• donors may be useful for the treatment of *erectile impotence*. Recent data demonstrate that NO increases the oxygen affinity of sickle erythrocytes, suggesting a potential role for inhaled NO in the treatment of *sickle cell disease*.

Given the relative pulmonary selectivity of inhaled NO•, this gas may be useful at concentration of 10 to 40 ppm for the treatment of *persistent pulmonary hypertension of the newborn*, the pulmonary vasoconstriction that accompanies congenital diaphragmatic hernia, *primary pulmonary hypertension*, *high-altitude pulmonary edema*, and *adult respiratory distress syndrome*. Higher concentration of inhaled NO• may be toxic, owing to the reaction of NO• with oxygen to produce NO_2.

NO• may also be useful in the inhibition of proliferative responses following vascular injury. Local delivery of a long-acting NO^+ donor or gene therapy with *Nos3* or *Nos2* limits vascular smooth muscle proliferation following denuding endothelial injury, which suggests potentially useful therapies for limiting restenosis following angioplasty.

The simplicity of the NO• molecule belies its wide range of complex biologic, pathobiologic, and therapeutic effects. Our understanding of the biologic roles of this molecule and its potential therapeutic uses are in their infancy. With a clearer understanding of the organ-specific effects of NO•, its toxic and therapeutic potential in specific organ systems, and the mechanisms by which its actions may be inhibited or promoted, the full potential of this molecule as a therapeutic agent may be realized.

BIBLIOGRAPHY

HEAD CA et al: Low concentrations of nitric oxide increase oxygen affinity of sickle erythrocytes in vitro and in vivo. J Clin Invest 100:1193, 1997

IGNARRO LJ: Signal transduction mechanisms involving nitric oxide. Biochem Pharmacol 41:485, 1991

LOSCALZO J: Nitric oxide and vascular disease. N Engl J Med 333:251, 1995

———, WELCH G: Nitric oxide and its role in the cardiovascular system. Prog Cardiovasc Dis 38:87, 1995

MONCADA S, HIGGS EA: The L-arginine:nitric oxide pathway. N Engl J Med 329:2002, 1993

NATHAN C: Nitric oxide as a secretory product of mammalian cells. FASEB J 6:3051, 1992

SCHERRER U et al: Inhaled nitric oxide for high-altitude pulmonary edema. N Engl J Med 334:624, 1996

STAMLER JS et al: Biochemistry of nitric oxide and its redox-activated forms. Science 258:1898, 1992

ZHANG J, SYNDER SH: Nitric oxide in the nervous system. Annu Rev Pharmacol Toxicol 35:213, 1995

72 *Margo Denke, Jean D. Wilson*

NUTRITION AND NUTRITIONAL REQUIREMENTS

Adequate nutrition is essential for health and for the management of disease. Eating is intermittent, whereas energy needs are continuous. For example, it is essential to maintain a steady fuel supply to the brain, which requires about 5 g/h of glucose in both the fed and fasted states. To meet these needs, metabolic and hormonal controls promote the storage of nutrients during the absorptive state, largely in the form of glycogen and adipose tissue, and their retrieval in the postabsorptive period and during prolonged fasting. The stability of body weight requires that energy intake and expenditure be balanced over time. The internal signals that balance caloric intake with energy needs are poorly understood, but they do not operate on a meal-to-meal basis but rather over a period of days to make compensatory changes in the volume of food eaten. Long-term aberrations in these control factors can cause obesity on the one hand and anorexia on the other.

NUTRITIONAL REQUIREMENTS, ALLOWANCES, AND TOLERANCES The body contains thousands of types of molecules but requires for health the intake of only a small number of organic compounds—9 essential amino acids, 1 fatty acid, and 13 vitamins—in addition to sufficient energy, water, and minerals. The majority of organic compounds in food, although metabolized and assimilated by the body, are nonessential in the sense that their deletion from the diet does not cause illness. The simplicity of the nutritional requirements of the healthy individual, in contrast to the chemical complexity of the body, is the result of the remarkable capacity for endogenous synthesis of a vast number of organic molecules. The body tends to preserve its composition, and dietary factors modify body composition only to a limited degree; the vast majority of compounds ingested in food, including complex lipids, carbohydrates, waxes, and proteins, are broken down to their component parts, which are used for the de novo synthesis of fuels and body constituents.

In contrast, most inorganic molecules in food are nutritionally essential: calcium, phosphorus, potassium, sodium, chloride, and magnesium are major constituents of the body; moderate amounts of iron and zinc are required; and fluoride, copper, chromium, iodine, manganese, molybdenum, and selenium are required in trace amounts (less than 1 mg/d).

The requirement of an essential nutrient is defined as the smallest amount that maintains normal body mass, chemical composition, morphology, and physiologic function and prevents any clinical or chemical sign of the corresponding deficiency state. For most essential nutrients this value is exceedingly difficult to define even for healthy adults, and requirements may differ at different periods, as in the developing embryo, the growing child, and the lactating or pregnant women. Minimal requirements differ among normal individuals due to a variety of environmental, genetic, hormonal, and physiologic variables.

Consequently, at the clinical level the concept that nutritional standards should be based on absolute nutritional requirements has been replaced by that of the recommended dietary allowances (RDA), namely, the levels of intake of essential nutrients that, on the basis of scientific knowledge, are judged by the Food and Nutrition Board of the National Research Council to be adequate to meet the nutrient needs of healthy persons (Table 72-1). The RDAs have had a major impact on nutrition policy and on nutrition education; they are based on many types of evidence that vary in completeness and accuracy, including replacement studies in persons with nutrient deficiency, nutrient balance studies, biochemical assessments of function in relation to nutrient intake, the nutrient intakes of healthy people, epidemiologic studies of the relation between nutrient status and nutrient intake, and, in some cases, extrapolation of data from animal experiments. When data are insufficient for formulating a RDA, the category of *safe and adequate* is utilized by the Food and Nutrition Board, as in the case of biotin, copper, manganese, and molybdenum (Table 72-2). In principle, in formulating both the RDAs and the safe-and-adequate category, the minimal physiologic requirement is adjusted to encompass the variations in requirement and different efficiencies of utilization among individuals and differing bioavailability in different food sources. The aim of these recommendations (Tables 72-1 and 72-2) is to provide a safety factor appropriate to each nutrient by exceeding the actual requirements of most individuals. However, neither the RDA nor the safe-and-adequate category defines the level of a nutrient necessary for the optimal health of an individual.

Just as intake of any essential nutrient below a critical level causes disease, intake of many nutrients above a specific level disturbs body structure or function. Intake higher than the maximal daily tolerance can cause acute, progressive, or permanent disability. Obesity, fluorosis, atherosclerosis, hypervitaminosis A, and hypervitaminosis D are examples of the long-term consequences of excessive ingestion of nutrients; acute manifestations of dietary intolerances include nausea, abdominal cramps, vomiting, and diarrhea (excess food intake); arrhythmias (potassium intoxication); and hyponatremia (water intoxication). A healthy diet provides levels of nutrient intake between the two thresholds of minimal requirement and maximal tolerance. Recognition that tolerance for a nutrient can be exceeded is particularly important for parenteral nutrition, when the gastrointestinal mechanisms (fullness, emesis, incomplete absorption, diarrhea) that ordinarily help protect from the ill consequences of excess nutrient intake are bypassed. The maximal tolerance for many nutrients is uncertain. For example, it is not known whether very high intake of protein and/or amino acids by athletes and by food faddists is safe.

ALTERATIONS OF NUTRITIONAL REQUIREMENTS Both the RDA and maximal tolerance for each nutrient are influenced by a variety of factors: age, rate of growth, exercise, pregnancy and lactation, composition of the diet, concomitant diseases, and drugs. As the differences between requirement and tolerance narrow, the design of appropriate intake becomes more difficult, as in the appropriate protein intake for a cachectic patient with cirrhosis of the liver and hepatic encephalopathy.

Physiologic Factors Growth, strenuous exercise, pregnancy, and lactation (Tables 72-1 and 72-2) increase the requirements for energy and most essential nutrients. Under climatic extremes, nutritional requirements may either increase or decrease, depending on energy expenditure. In the elderly requirements for nutrients and energy per unit of lean body mass are the same as in younger individuals. However, because of decreased lean body mass and reduced activity in the very elderly, energy requirements usually decrease with age; for both social and medical reasons the elderly are particularly prone to the development of protein-energy malnutrition and to the deficiency of micronutrients such as ascorbic acid and folic acid.

Composition of the Diet Given diets with identical contents of nutrients, the biologic availability of the nutrients can vary. For example, all proteins do not have equal biologic value in terms of optimal amino acid content and the ability to support maximal linear growth in children; in particular, tryptophan content can vary widely among proteins. Protein in milk, eggs, and meat has high biologic value, whereas the proteins of corn (maize), soy flour, and wheat gluten have lower biologic value. Even when diets are adequate, individual factors

Table 72-1

Recommended Dietary Allowances[a]

Category	Age, years, or Condition	Weight[b], kg	(lb)	Height[b], cm	(in)	Protein (g)	Vitamin A, μg RE[c]	Vitamin D, μg[d]	Vitamin E, mg α-TE[e]	Vitamin K, μg
							Fat-Soluble Vitamins			
Infants	0.0–0.5	6	(13)	60	(24)	13	375	7.5	3	5
	0.5–1.0	9	(20)	71	(28)	14	375	10	4	10
Children	1–3	13	(29)	90	(35)	16	400	10	6	15
	4–6	20	(44)	112	(44)	24	500	10	7	20
	7–10	28	(62)	132	(52)	28	700	10	7	30
Males	11–14	45	(99)	157	(62)	45	1000	10	10	45
	15–18	66	(145)	176	(69)	59	1000	10	10	65
	19–24	72	(160)	177	(70)	58	1000	10	10	70
	25–50	79	(174)	176	(69)	63	1000	5	10	80
	51+	77	(170)	173	(68)	63	1000	5	10	80
Females	11–14	46	(101)	157	(62)	46	800	10	8	45
	15–18	55	(120)	163	(64)	44	800	10	8	55
	19–24	58	(128)	164	(65)	46	800	10	8	60
	25–50	63	(138)	163	(64)	50	800	5	8	65
	51+	65	(143)	160	(63)	50	800	5	8	65
Pregnant						60	800	10	10	65
Lactating	1st 6 months					65	1300	10	12	65
	2nd 6 months					62	1200	10	11	65

[a]The allowances, expressed as average daily intakes over time, are intended to provide for individual variations among most normal persons as they live in the United States under usual environmental stresses. Diets should be based on a variety of common foods in order to provide other nutrients for which human requirements have been less well defined.
[b]Weights and heights of Reference Adults are actual medians for the U.S. population of the designated age, as reported by National Health and Nutrition Examination Survey (NHANES) II.
[c]Retinol equivalents, 1 retinol equivalent = 1 μg retinol or 6 μg β-carotene.

can influence bioavailability, e.g., the absorption of calcium and magnesium may be impaired by phytates in the diet, and the absorption of nonheme iron is reduced in meals containing low amounts of ascorbic acid.

Route of Administration The nutrient recommendations in Tables 72-1 and 72-2 apply to food intake through the gastrointestinal tract. The absorption of ingested amino acids, carbohydrates, fats, sodium, chloride, and potassium is so efficient that the RDAs are the same for people on parenteral nutrition and on oral intake. However, for most minerals net absorption is only 50 percent or less, and the mineral requirements for parenteral nutrition are less than the oral requirements. Timing of administration can also be important. For example, since excess amino acids are not stored but are converted to fuel, all essential amino acids must be supplied simultaneously to support maximal protein synthesis.

Disease Disease can alter nutritional requirements and tolerances by a variety of mechanisms, including induction of anorexia (cancer, AIDS, gastrointestinal obstruction), increased utilization of nutrients (fever, infection, trauma, hemolysis, cancer, recovery from malnutrition), malabsorption (cystic fibrosis, sprue), impaired metabolism of nutrients (kidney and liver disease), nutrient wastage (burns, blood loss, nasogastric suction, diarrhea), hyperabsorption (hyperabsorptive hypercalciuria, hemochromatosis), impaired excretion (uremia), and drug therapy (cholestyramine, colestipol).

THE ESSENTIAL NUTRIENTS Water For practical purposes, 1 mL of water per kcal energy expenditure is appropriate for adults under average conditions. However, the risk of water intoxication is so remote that the suggested intake is often increased to 1.5 mL/kcal energy expenditure to allow for variations in activity level, sweating, and solute load. Normally, 50 to 100 mL/d of water is excreted in the feces, 500 to 1000 mL is lost by evaporation or exhalation, and 1000 mL or more is lost in urine. Water intake must equal these amounts to avoid under- or overhydration, particularly when external losses increase. Fecal losses may approach 5 L/d in severe diarrhea, and each degree Celsius of fever causes a daily loss of about 200 mL water. Provided renal function is normal and solute intake is adequate, most normal adults can safely excrete up to 18 L of urine per day because of the large capacity of the kidney to excrete free water.

Special attention must be given to the water needs of the elderly whose thirst sensation may be blunted. The increased water needs of

pregnancy only amount to about 30 mL/d, but during the first 6 months of lactation the additional water requirement approximates 1000 mL/d. Water requirements are increased in infants because of their larger surface area, the limited capacity of their kidneys to handle solute loads, and the limited ability to communicate their thirst.

Energy To maintain stable weight energy intake must equal energy output, namely, the energy expenditure required for basal energy expenditure (BEE), metabolism of food (specific dynamic action), and physical activity. The Harris-Benedict equations take into account weight (w, kg), height (h, cm), and age (a, years) in estimating BEE:

$$BEE_{women} = 655 + (9.5 \times w) + (1.8 \times h) - (4.7 \times a)$$
$$BEE_{men} = 666 + (13.7 \times w) + (5.0 \times h) - (6.8 \times a)$$

To this basal expenditure 30, 50, or 100 percent is added for sedentary, moderate, or strenuous activity. Nonstressed hospitalized patients usually require 120 percent of BEE, whereas catabolic patients require 150 to 200 percent of BEE to prevent tissue breakdown or allow anabolism. Energy expenditure is increased by fever (13 percent for each degree Celsius above normal), burns (40 to 100 percent), trauma (40 to 100 percent), and hyperthyroidism (10 to 100 percent). Patients with malabsorption may absorb as few as 25 percent of ingested calories, and it may be impossible to supply the increased energy needs of the sick by mouth if increased nutrient intake causes diarrhea. In such circumstances parenteral nutrition may be required to prevent progressive malnutrition. In hypometabolic states such as hypothyroidism or adrenal insufficiency, energy requirements are decreased. The hospitalized patient should be weighed daily, and energy intake should be adjusted appropriately.

Protein Dietary protein is a source of energy and supplies the mixture of amino acids for protein synthesis. Healthy adults require nine essential amino acids (threonine, valine, isoleucine, leucine, lysine, tryptophan, methionine-cystine, phenylalanine-tyrosine, and histidine) in amounts that vary from 250 to 1100 mg/d each. The requirement of dietary protein depends on the biologic value of the protein (determined primarily by the essential amino acid content). The biologic value of the major protein foods follows the general sequence: animal products > legumes > cereals (rice, wheat, corn) > roots. The adult RDA for protein (Table 72-1), about 0.6 g/kg body weight, assumes a high biologic value characteristic of animal protein; the lower the biologic value, the higher the protein requirement. The

Water-Soluble Vitamins							Minerals						
Vitamin C, mg	Thiamin, mg	Riboflavin, mg	Niacin, mg NE^f	Vitamin B$_6$, mg	Folate, μg	Vitamin B$_{12}$, μg	Calcium, mg	Phosphorus, mg	Magnesium, mg	Iron, mg	Zinc, mg	Iodine, μg	Selenium, μg
30	0.3	0.4	5	0.3	25	0.3	400	300	40	6	5	40	10
35	0.4	0.5	6	0.6	35	0.5	600	500	60	10	5	50	15
40	0.7	0.8	9	1.0	50	0.7	800	800	80	10	10	70	20
45	0.9	1.1	12	1.1	75	1.0	800	800	120	10	10	90	20
45	1.0	1.2	13	1.4	100	1.4	800	800	170	10	10	120	30
50	1.3	1.5	17	1.7	150	2.0	1200	1200	270	12	15	150	40
60	1.5	1.8	20	2.0	200	2.0	1200	1200	400	12	15	150	50
60	1.5	1.7	19	2.0	200	2.0	1200	1200	350	10	15	150	70
60	1.5	1.7	19	2.0	200	2.0	800	800	350	10	15	150	70
60	1.2	1.4	15	2.0	200	2.0	800	800	350	10	15	150	70
50	1.1	1.3	15	1.4	150	2.0	1200	1200	280	15	12	150	45
60	1.1	1.3	15	1.5	180	2.0	1200	1200	300	15	12	150	50
60	1.1	1.3	15	1.6	180	2.0	1200	1200	280	15	12	150	55
60	1.1	1.3	15	1.6	180	2.0	800	800	280	15	12	150	55
60	1.0	1.2	13	1.6	180	2.0	800	800	280	10	12	150	55
70	1.5	1.6	17	2.2	400	2.2	1200	1200	320	30	15	175	65
95	1.6	1.8	20	2.1	280	2.6	1200	1200	355	15	19	200	75
90	1.6	1.7	20	2.1	260	2.6	1200	1200	340	15	16	200	75

^{d}As cholecalciferol. 10 μg cholecalciferol = 400 IU of vitamin D.
^{e}α-Tocopherol equivalents. 1 mg d-α tocopherol = 1 α-TE.
^{f}1 NE (niacin equivalent) is equal to 1 mg of niacin or 60 mg of dietary tryptophan.
SOURCE: Recommended Dietary Allowances, 10th edition, National Academy Press, 1989.

Table 72-2

Estimated Safe and Adequate Daily Dietary Intakes of Selected Vitamins and Minerals

Category	Age, years	Trace Elements*					Vitamins	
		Copper, mg	Manganese, mg	Fluoride, mg	Chromium, μg	Molybdenum, μg	Biotin, μg	Pantothenic Acid, mg
Infants	0–0.5	0.4–0.6	0.3–0.6	0.1–0.5	10–40	15–30	10	2
	0.5–1	0.6–0.7	0.6–1.0	0.2–1.0	20–60	20–40	15	3
Children and adolescents	1–3	0.7–1.0	1.0–1.5	0.5–1.5	20–80	25–50	20	3
	4–6	1.0–1.5	1.5–2.0	1.0–2.5	30–120	30–75	25	3–4
	7–10	1.0–2.0	2.0–3.0	1.5–2.5	50–200	50–150	30	4–5
	11+	1.5–2.5	2.0–5.0	1.5–2.5	50–200	75–250	30–100	4–7
Adults		1.5–3.0	2.0–5.0	1.5–4.0	50–200	75–250	30–100	4–7

* Since the toxic levels for many trace elements may be only several times usual intakes, the upper levels for the trace elements given in this table should not be habitually exceeded.
SOURCE: Recommended Dietary Allowances, 10th edition, National Academy Press, 1989.

requirement for protein is also influenced by energy intake; when the energy requirement is met by nonprotein calories, ingested amino acids can be used for protein synthesis, but when energy intake is deficient, ingested amino acids tend to be diverted into the pathways of glucose synthesis and oxidation. Thus, energy undernutrition makes the individual more vulnerable to protein starvation, a phenomenon that accounts for the high prevalence of combined protein-energy malnutrition (see Chap. 74).

Protein requirements are increased by growth, pregnancy, lactation, and repletion after malnutrition and are decreased in liver failure and renal insufficiency. The decreased requirement in liver failure occurs because the catabolism of essential and nonessential amino acids is slowed and in renal failure is due to the fact that ammonia can be reutilized for the synthesis of nonessential amino acids. In both renal failure and liver disease, the tolerance for dietary protein is also decreased, and normal protein intake can precipitate encephalopathy in patients with cirrhosis of the liver and worsen the uremic state in those with renal failure.

Fat The absolute requirement for fat is only 1 g/d of linoleic acid (polyunsaturated fat) for prostaglandin synthesis. The typical American diet contains about 35 percent of the calories from fat, but to minimize the development of atherosclerosis it is recommended that no more than 30 percent of the calories should be from fat and that no more than a third of the fat intake should be saturated fat. In general carbohydrate is the nutrient that replaces fat. Diets devoid of

fat are less palatable and may result in protein-energy malnutrition if food selections are not made carefully.

Minerals and Vitamins The RDAs and safe daily intakes of the vitamins and minerals are listed in Tables 72-1 and 72-2, and the clinical disorders that result from their deficiencies are described in Chaps. 79, 80, and 354 to 357. It is critical to remember that the excessive intake of fat-soluble vitamins (Chap. 79), minerals (Chaps. 80, 354, 356, and 357), and electrolytes (fluorosis, hypertension, potassium toxicity) is particularly dangerous.

BIBLIOGRAPHY

ASKEW EW: Environmental and physical stress and nutrient requirements. Am J Clin Nutr 61(Suppl 3):631S, 1995

BEATON GH: Uses and limits of the use of the Recommended Dietary Allowances for evaluating dietary intake data. Am J Clin Nutr 41:155, 1985

ELIA M: Changing concepts of nutrient requirements in disease: Implications for artificial nutrition support. Lancet 345:1279, 1995

FOOD AND NUTRITION BOARD, COMMISSION ON LIFE SCIENCES, NATIONAL RESEARCH COUNCIL: Recommended Dietary Allowances, 10th ed. Washington DC, National Academy Press, 1989

KENDRICK ZV et al: Metabolic and nutritional considerations for exercising older adults. Compr Ther 20:558, 1994

REEDS PJ, HUTCHENS TW: Protein requirements: From nitrogen balance to functional impact. J Nutr 124(Suppl 9):1754S, 1994

ROSENBERG IH: Nutrient requirements for optimal health: What does that mean? J Nutr 124(Suppl 9):1777S, 1994

73 *Margo Denke, Jean D. Wilson*

ASSESSMENT OF
NUTRITIONAL STATUS

Nutritional deficiency is rare among healthy people who live in industrialized nations. High-quality dietary protein and other foods are abundant, virtually eliminating kwashiorkor and marasmus. Improved food preservation, packaging, and distribution have reduced seasonal variations in micronutrient intake. Fortification of foodstuffs with vitamins and essential minerals, such as iodine in salt, vitamin D in milk, and iron and B-complex vitamins in flour, has nearly eliminated once-common deficiency states such as iodine-deficient goiter, rickets, and folic acid deficiency. Indeed, in industrialized nations the prevalent nutritional disorder is obesity (see Chap. 75).

The success of these public health programs in preventing common dietary deficiencies has in some minds made the routine assessment of nutritional status obsolete, and nutritional diagnoses rarely appear in charts in workups or in progress notes. However, undernutrition makes a major contribution to morbidity and to mortality. Such deficiencies are often attributed to the underlying disease, but in many instances the compromise in nutritional status predates the development of disease, contributes to mortality, and impairs recovery. Routine assessment of the nutritional status is necessary to identify those situations in which nutritional intervention is essential for recovery.

The nutritional assessment is designed to evaluate three aspects of overall nutrition—energy, protein, and micronutrient balance—and has three components: the nutritional history, appropriate physical examination with simple anthropometric measurements, and laboratory studies.

THE NUTRITIONAL HISTORY Nutritional assessment should begin with a chronologic record of body weight and changes in body weight (Table 72-1). Inquiry as to the individual's weight at life milestones such as graduation from high school, college, or marriage can facilitate this assessment. Significant changes in weight should be investigated carefully. Did the weight change follow changes in physical activity, alterations in dietary intake, or changes in health status? Hip fracture is often preceded by weight loss, and hypertension, hyperlipidemia, and insulin resistance are often associated with weight gain. It should be kept in mind that change in weight can sometimes be ambiguous, particularly in the presence of edema. Furthermore, an initially obese individual can lose 15 kg because of a wasting illness and present with a normal body weight, despite shrinkage of lean body mass. In such circumstances estimation of muscle mass should be made by balance techniques as described below.

A healthy person consuming a variety of foods is unlikely to have a dietary deficiency, but not all individuals consume a varied diet. To evaluate dietary intake, the patient should be asked to list everything eaten in the past 24 h (breakfast, lunch, dinner, and snacks), and this information can be used to determine the variety and adequacy of food consumed (Table 73-1). In a typical day, does the patient consume several servings of different fruits and vegetables and calcium-containing foods? What food groups are missing? Is the portion size adequate, too large, or too small? Are meals prepared by the patient or someone else? Do social, medical, or dental problems restrict food choices?

Illness can affect weight by several mechanisms, including reduced dietary intake from anorexia or because energy intake does not increase sufficiently to meet the increased demands from fever, infection, or trauma. The diagnostic workup itself may contribute to weight loss by requiring fasting for testing or diagnostic procedures. Drug therapy may alter taste or reduce appetite, leading to weight loss. Not all illnesses cause weight loss; when the major effect on energy balance is a reduction in physical activity, weight gain can occur if energy intake remains unchanged or increases.

Acute and chronic illnesses increase the demands for energy, protein, and micronutrients. Protein requirements may triple in severe illnesses. Patients whose intake is restricted for any reason are at higher risk for nutritional deficiencies. When the initial assessment suggests dietary inadequacy, a formal assessment by a registered dietician is indicated.

In chronic illness, the duration, severity, and time course of weight loss or weight gain—steady, progressively worsening, waxing and waning—can provide a chronologic account of the course of the illness and of concomitant changes in appetite and physical activity. The nutritional history should encompass previous attempts to improve body weight and the presumed reasons for the success or failure of the attempts.

Nutrient Processing. Perhaps the most overlooked aspect of the nutritional history is the complex process by which nutrients and energy are absorbed (Table 73-2). The processing of food begins with appetite. Either anorexia or nausea can compromise the ability to maintain adequate intake. Do foods taste metallic or unpleasant? Are there mechanical difficulties with chewing such as poorly fitting dentures? Is there any difficulty swallowing? Is early satiety or a lack of satiety present? Is eating associated with gastrointestinal discomfort such as vomiting or diarrhea? Have there been changes in consistency, odor, and frequency of bowel movements? Queries regarding nutrient processing can uncover social problems, eating disorders, mechanical barriers to food ingestion, and malabsorption, any of which can alter nutritional status.

Associated Conditions That Increase Nutritional Demands Pregnancy, lactation, and, in children, periods of rapid growth increase metabolic demands and the requirements for specific nutrients. A series of acute illnesses, each in themselves self-limiting, can cumulatively compromise nutrition if adjustments are not made in food intake. A catalogue of these events and their duration and impact on general health status may help identify patients at risk.

Nutrient Supplements and Medication History Listing the amount and frequency of nutritional supplements together with both prescription and over-the-counter medications will provide insight as to whether intake of specific vitamins is excessive. Some medications alter nutrient bioavailability (see examples, Table 73-3), and use of these drugs should prompt inquiries regarding the intake of the nutrient affected.

PHYSICAL EXAMINATION Weight should be recorded at every outpatient visit. The presence and severity of edema or ascites should be noted, since these findings alter the interpretation of weight. Absolute body weight and changes in body weight have prognostic implications. Illness-associated weight loss of 10 to 20 percent over a period of 6 months or less can cause functional impairment of multiple organ systems. If weight loss exceeds 20 percent during illness, protein-energy malnutrition may be present.

Weight should be measured daily in the hospitalized patient. Total starvation causes a loss of approximately 0.4 kg/d of body weight; semi-starvation causes lesser degrees of weight loss. Most weight loss with starvation is initially from stored adipose tissue and then from catabolism of skeletal muscle protein and liver protein; other organ proteins are spared until wasting is extreme. Rapid increases in weight in the hospital setting are rarely due to increases in lean or fat mass. Hydration rapidly increases total body water and sodium, and renal compensation may be delayed. Rapid weight gain may occur when a starving patient is refed carbohydrate, replenishing glycogen stores and increasing hepatic water content.

Height should be measured annually and on every hospital admission. This measurement is of particular importance for detecting loss of height in subjects with metabolic bone disease and should be made with the patient standing straight and looking straight ahead. When loss in height is suspected or for individuals who cannot stand unassisted, maximal height can be estimated using knee height. Knee height is the distance between the sole of the foot to the anterior surface of the compressed thigh above the condyles of the femur and just proximal to the patella. It is measured with the patient in a sitting or recumbent position. Knee height is affected little by age or by changes in weight and can be calculated as follows:

$$\text{Height in men (cm)} = 64.19 - (0.04 \times \text{age}) + [2.2 \times \text{knee height (cm)}]$$

$$\text{Height in women (cm)} = 84.88 - (0.24 \times \text{age}) + [1.83 \times \text{knee height (cm)}]$$

Determination of *body mass index* (BMI) or *weight-for-frame size* provides insight as to whether the current weight is appropriate for the individual.

Body Mass Index Assessment of BMI (weight in kg divided by height in m²) has the advantage of simplicity and is useful for

Table 73-1

Nutritional Assessment

Ambulatory Patients	Acute Illness	Chronic Illness
ENERGY REQUIREMENTS		
Body weight and weight for height are indices of energy balance. Imbalance between energy intake and expenditure causes weight loss or weight gain. Track weight at life milestones (graduation, marriage, etc.). Are changes in weight voluntary or involuntary?	Acute illness affects both components of energy balance. Illness can reduce appetite and energy intake and increase energy demands because of fever, infection, and trauma or decrease energy demands because of reduced physical activity.	Chronic illness requires a long-term adaptation to changes in energy balance. The duration of compromise and previous attempts to correct energy balance may provide insight into the disturbances in energy balance.
PROTEIN REQUIREMENTS		
Most patients meet their protein requirements from a combination of foods and not a single food. For example, 0.5% by weight of cooked vegetables, 4% of milk, 23% of meat, and 10% of uncooked pasta is protein. 40 g of protein (sufficient for 50-kg person) is contained in any of the following: 200 g fish, poultry, red meat; 150 g tree nuts; 130 g peanuts or peanut butter; 200 g brick cheese; 7 eggs or 12 egg whites; 400 g cooked rice plus 470 g cooked beans; 500 g tofu; 1000 g milk. Normal daily protein requirements: 0.8–1.0 g/kg	Illness may increase protein demands through: 1. Higher metabolic rates 2. Protein losses from skin (burns, exfoliation), gastrointestinal tract (protein losing enteropathy), or kidney (proteinuria) Daily protein requirements 1. Moderately stressed: 1.0–2.0 g/kg (infection, fractures, surgery) 2. Severely stressed: 2.0–2.5 g/kg (burns, multiple fractures)	Chronic illness may increase the demand for dietary protein: Nephrotic syndrome: dietary protein intake must be increased to compensate for protein loss or protein depletion can occur Chronic infection: increased catabolism of protein for energy; protein requirements typically double to maintain adequate pool of amino acids for synthesis of new protein Hyperthyroidism: increased metabolic rate, leading to a higher rate of catabolism of protein for energy; protein requirements may double Psoriasis: increased protein loss from skin; dietary protein requirements increase proportional to losses
MICRONUTRIENT REQUIREMENTS		
By assessing the variety of intake, risk for vitamin deficiency can be assessed. This assessment is particularly important for patients with a fixed income or who live alone.	Acute illness is self-limited; micronutrients most likely to be affected are rapid-turn over B vitamins.	Chronic illness may alter absorption of micronutrients: Gastric resection: impairs calcium and iron absorption if duodenum is bypassed Resection of proximal small intestine: impairs absorption of calcium, folic acid, water-soluble vitamins Resection of distal small intestine: impairs absorption of B_{12} and bile salts

Vitamin A	Meat, milk, egg, leafy green and deep yellow vegetables
Thiamine	Meat, milk, egg, enriched flour
Riboflavin	Meat, milk, egg
Niacin	Meat, starchy vegetables and grains
Vitamin B_6	Meat, starchy vegetables
Vitamin B_{12}	Milk, meat, egg
Folic acid, pantothenic acid	Ubiquitous
Vitamin C	Vegetables, fruit, milk
Vitamin D	Fortified milk, meat
Vitamin E	Leafy green and deep yellow vegetables, meat, egg, fruit, milk
Iron	Meat, spinach, raisins, enriched flour, lentils
Calcium	Dairy products

Drugs may also alter micronutrient needs:
Chloroquine, levodopa, theophylline may induce a loss of appetite; propylthiouracil, rifampin change taste
Hydroxyzine, imipramine increase appetite
Ethanol excess may lead to a malabsorption of thiamine, B_{12}, and folate
Phenytoin, phenobarbital, primidone may reduce levels of folate, vitamin B_6, and vitamin B_{12} and increase vitamin D requirements
Methotrexate lowers folate levels by promoting folate excretion
Antimalarials (pyrimethamine and sulfadiazine) and the antibiotics (penicillins, sulfonamides) can reduce folate levels
Sodium bicarbonate may reduce folate absorption due to decreased jejunal pH
Salicylate may increase vitamin C and folate excretion and cause iron deficiency if gastrointestinal blood loss occurs
H_2 blockers impair B_{12} absorption, probably by reduced acid and pepsin production
Nonsteroidal anti-inflammatory agents may cause iron deficiency from gastrointestinal blood loss
Glucocorticoids increase calcium loss from bone

assessing both over- and undernutrition. A normal BMI is defined as 18.5 to 24.9 kg/m². Overweight is a BMI of 25.0 to 29.9 kg/m², obesity is a BMI of 30.0 to 39.9 kg/m², and morbid obesity is a BMI > 40 kg/m². Conversely, the risk for protein-energy malnutrition can be graded as mild: BMI = 17.0 to 18.4 kg/m²; moderate: BMI = 16.0 to 16.9 kg/m²; and severe: BMI < 16.0 kg/m². A BMI of 13 to 15 kg/m² suggests that the total body fat content is less than 5 percent of weight. The BMI is simple and is a widely used means of estimating energy balance, but it does not take into account differences in frame size.

Weight-for-Frame Size   Frame size is conventionally divided into three categories—small, medium, and large. Large skeletons require greater muscle mass for locomotion. Actuarial tables such as those of the Metropolitan Life Insurance Company classify ranges of weight associated with lower mortality in terms of frame size. Whereas some databases use wrist circumference as a measure of frame size, the breadth of the epicondyle of the humerus is a more accurate index of frame size (Table 73-4) because its measurement is less influenced by subcutaneous fat. On the basis of frame size, height, and gender, valuable insight can be obtained as to appropriate ideal weights for the individual and how far the actual weight deviates from this norm (Table 73-5). In patients with amputations, adjustments for the missing extremity should be made before this value can be interpreted. For example, 7.1 percent of body weight should be subtracted from the reference weight for an above-the-knee amputation, and 18.6 percent should be subtracted if the entire leg is amputated. Such tables have to be interpreted with caution in pregnant women, for whom special tables must be used.

In addition to weight, which provides assessment of overall energy balance, it is often useful to have insight into specific aspects of *body composition*, particularly into fat and muscle (protein or nitrogen) mass. Caliper measurements of skin-fold thickness provide a useful index of *fat mass*. The triceps skin thickness differs with frame size and height (Table 73-6). This assessment does not provide much information beyond the measurement of BMI or weight-for-frame size in evaluating the obese but is particularly useful in identifying those individuals whose fat stores are dangerously depleted. More direct techniques to measure percent body fat such as underwater weighing, x-ray absorptiometry, and nuclear magnetic resonance imaging can also be employed under some circumstances.

Muscle mass can either be assessed as a part of the laboratory evaluation or measured directly as part of the physical examination. Midarm circumference is a function of muscle mass, skin, subcutaneous fat,

Table 73-3

Body Mass Index* (kg/m²) by Gender for Blacks and Whites, Ages 18 to 50

	Blacks		Whites	
Percentile	Men	Women	Men	Women
5th	18.8	18.4	19.6	18.4
50th	22.2	25.8	25.0	22.9

* Based on data from the National Health and Nutrition Examination Survey I.

Table 73-4

Frame Size Defined by Elbow Breadth* (cm)

	Men			Women		
Age	Small†	Medium	Large†	Small	Medium	Large
18–24	≤ 6.6	6.6 to 7.7	≥ 7.7	≤ 5.6	5.6 to 6.5	≥ 6.5
25–34	≤ 6.7	6.7 to 7.9	≥ 7.9	≤ 5.7	5.7 to 6.8	≥ 6.8
35–44	≤ 6.7	6.7 to 8.0	≥ 8.0	≤ 5.7	5.7 to 7.1	≥ 7.1
45–54	≤ 6.7	6.7 to 8.1	≥ 8.1	≤ 5.7	5.7 to 7.2	≥ 7.2
55–64	≤ 6.7	6.7 to 8.1	≥ 8.1	≤ 5.8	5.8 to 7.2	≥ 7.2
65–74	≤ 6.7	6.7 to 8.1	≥ 8.1	≤ 5.8	5.8 to 7.2	≥ 7.2

* Based on data from the combined National Health and Nutrition Examination Surveys I and II.
† By definition, small frame and large frame each account for 15% of U.S. population.
SOURCE: AR Frisancho, Am J Clin Nutr 40:808, 1984.

bone, and the neurovascular bundle of the arm, and of these parameters the amounts of muscle, skin, and fat are determined by nutritional state. Skin and subcutaneous fat are corrected for by subtracting the triscapular skin-fold before calculating the area of muscle mass:

Midarm muscle area

$$= \frac{[\text{Arm circumference} - (\pi \times \text{triscapular skin fold})]^2}{4\pi}$$

where all measurements are in centimeters. This assessment is a valuable means of identifying protein malnutrition, a particular problem in the elderly. Table 73-7 contains midarm muscle values from the National Health and Nutrition Examination Surveys (NHANES) I and II. In comparing the observed with the controlled values, certain caveats should be noted. The midarm muscle circumference also measures the humerus and neurovascular structures, which do not decrease in size with weight loss, and in some tables the bone mass in the arm is corrected for by subtracting 10 cm² for men or 6.5 cm² for women as an estimate of the size of the humerus; since these values are constants this subtraction is clinically unimportant. Atrophic muscle has more water, total lipid, and collagen than normal muscle, and, as a consequence, the mass of functional muscle in deconditioned or cachectic patients is probably overestimated by this technique.

LABORATORY ASSESSMENT
Routine laboratory measurements do not provide a sensitive index of the level of nutrition because changes in the levels of serum proteins occur late in the course of malnutrition but can, under some circumstances, be useful for assessing the effectiveness of nutritional intervention. For the ambulatory patient, laboratory assessment should be focused on potential deficiencies identified by history and physical examination. However, insufficient dietary protein and energy intake is not the only cause of low serum protein levels in illness because serum protein levels can be influenced by many factors.

Table 73-2

Nutrient Processing

Ambulatory Patients	Acute Illness	Chronic Illness
All patients should be queried about the process of nutrient assimilation: Appetite Mastication Swallowing Bite size Meal size Meal frequency Satiety Heartburn Dyspepsia Belching Bloating Diarrhea Constipation Foul-smelling stools Light/dark-colored stools Flatulence	Are changes in nutrient processing: 1. Temporally related to disease? 2. Temporally related to treatment?	Same as acutely ill patient, *plus* ascertain previous attempts to address problems such as: 1. Reducing drug dosages that alter appetite 2. Improving denture fitting 3. Trial of special meals such as pureed foods, high-fiber diets, low-acid foods 4. Improved meal planning and delivery 5. Controlling gastrointestinal symptoms after eating

Table 73-5

5th and 50th Percentiles of Weight for Frame Size, Height, and Gender,* Ages 25 to 74

Height in cm (in Foam Slippers)	Weight in kg (in Examination Clothing)					
	Small		Medium		Large	
	5th	50th	5th	50th	5th	50th
MEN						
157	46	64	51	68	57	82
160	48	61	52	71	58	83
163	49	66	54	71	59	84
165	52	66	59	74	60	79
168	56	67	58	75	60	84
170	56	71	62	77	62	84
173	56	71	60	78	63	86
175	57	74	63	78	68	89
178	59	75	64	81	68	87
180	60	76	62	81	73	91
183	62	74	68	84	73	91
185	63	79	70	85	72	93
188	65	80	68	88	69	92
WOMEN						
147	37	52	41	60	56	86
150	42	53	47	66	56	78
152	42	53	47	60	55	87
155	44	54	47	61	54	81
157	44	55	49	61	59	81
160	46	55	49	62	58	83
163	49	57	50	62	59	79
165	50	60	52	63	59	81
168	46	58	52	63	55	75
170	47	59	54	65	58	80
173	48	62	58	67	51	76
175	49	63	49	68	50	79
178	50	64	50	70	50	76

* Based on data from the combined National Health and Nutrition Examination Surveys I and II.

This problem is illustrated by *serum albumin.* Dehydration can lead to concentration of all plasma components and cause apparent increase in albumin levels. Shifts from intra- to extravascular spaces with surgery or burn injuries lower serum albumin levels, whereas semi-starvation shifts albumin to the intravascular space and may increase albumin levels more than total protein levels. Albumin synthesis can decline during acute illness, as synthesis of acute phase reactants increases, and physiologic stress can increase albumin catabolism. Albumin concentrations can also fall as a result of accelerated losses from skin, kidney, or gastrointestinal tract. Whereas dehydration and shifts between the intra- and extravascular spaces cause early alterations in serum albumin levels, changes in synthesis and catabolism do not alter serum albumin concentrations for several days because the half-life of serum albumin is normally 18 to 20 days. Serum albumin concentrations usually reach a nadir 5 to 7 days after the onset of a self-limiting illness, and it is common for serum albumin to fall 5 g/L after elective surgery. Measurement of serum proteins with shorter half-lives can provide a more accurate assessment of protein status. *Transferrin* has a half-life of 8 to 9 days, and *prealbumin*

Table 73-6

Assessment of Body Fat as Indicated by the 5th and 50th Percentiles of Triceps Skin Fold Thickness by Frame Size and Gender, Ages 25 to 74

	Triceps Skin Fold, mm					
	Small Frame		Medium Frame		Large Frame	
	5th	50th	5th	50th	5th	50th
Men	5	10	5	12	6	14
Women	10	20	12	24	16	32

* Based on data from the combined National Health and Nutrition Examination Surveys I and II.

Table 73-7

Assessment of Muscle Mass as Indicated by the 5th and 50th Percentiles of Midarm Muscle Area by Frame Size and Gender*

Age	Midarm Muscle Area, cm²					
	Small Frame		Medium Frame		Large Frame	
	5th	50th	5th	50th	5th	50th
MEN						
25–54	42	55	49	65	56	72
55–74	37	55	46	62	51	66
WOMEN						
25–54	26	33	28	37	32	46
55–74	26	35	29	40	35	50

* Based on data from the combined National Health and Nutrition Examination Surveys I and II.

has a half-life of 2 to 3 days. Unfortunately, the levels of these proteins in serum are affected by the same factors that influence albumin level. Measurement of serum proteins can be helpful in predicting prognosis. Low serum albumin in the chronically ill is associated with longer hospital stays, frequent readmissions for poor wound healing and infection, and increased mortality. Laboratory assessment can also help monitor intervention. If dietary protein is responsible for low serum protein levels, serum prealbumin levels rapidly increase in response to increased dietary protein.

Measurement of 24-h urinary creatinine can provide a simple estimate of *lean body mass* by the following equation:

$$\text{Lean body mass (kg)} = 7.138 + 0.02908 \times \text{urine creatinine (mg)}$$

The ratio of 24-h urinary creatinine (mg) to height (cm) is another widely used index of muscle mass. In normal men ratios average 10.5 mg/cm, and ratios from 8.4 to 9.5 mg/cm, 7.4 to 8.4 mg/cm, and <7.4 mg/cm signify mild, moderate, and severe degrees of protein malnutrition, respectively. The usefulness of this measurement is tempered by the fact that urinary creatinine is impaired by renal failure and can be influenced by dietary protein intake, exercise, emotional stress, infection, fever, and trauma. As an index of response to replenishment regimens, a bedside estimate of daily nitrogen balance can be made as follows using daily measurements of protein intake and of 24-h urine urea nitrogen:

$$\text{N balance (g)} = \frac{\text{protein intake (g)}}{6.25} - [\text{urine urea nitrogen (g)} + 2.5\,\text{g}]$$

where 2.5 g is the approximate amount of fecal, integumental, and urinary nonurea nitrogen loss per day. This value provides an estimate of the change in protein mass during the period of observation but does not assess protein mass at the beginning or end of the intervention.

Regarding micronutrient adequacy, vitamin levels do not reflect vitamin stores with the exception of vitamin B_{12} (see Chap. 108), folate (see Chap. 108), and vitamin D (see Chaps. 354 and 355), and the diagnosis of vitamin deficiency is usually made on the basis of a high index of suspicion and documenting the response to specific replacement (see Chap. 79). Assessment of mineral status, particularly measurements of phosphorus, magnesium, calcium, potassium, and iron, is more useful clinically, although serum levels do not always change in parallel with body stores.

OVERALL ASSESSMENT The assessment of nutritional status is an important component of the history, physical examination, and laboratory evaluation. The intensity of the evaluation should match the severity of the illness and the degree of suspected malnutrition. For the ambulatory patient with adequate nutritional status, the focus should be on identifying potential factors that could produce future nutritional compromise, including change in weight, and guarding against impairment of nutrient processing.

For the hospitalized patient with acute or chronic illness, the most pressing issue is to identify that subset of patients with such severe nutritional compromise (fifth percentile or lower) that nutritional intervention is an essential component of acute management. For example, in a patient who cannot swallow because of a stroke it is appropriate to delay parenteral nutrition or assisted enteral nutrition for a week or 10 days if nutritional status is adequate, whereas delay of nutritional support might be disastrous in a cachectic individual. In most acute, self-limited disease, the focus should be on defining the interaction between the acute illness and the underlying nutritional state (weight, variety of dietary intake, and nutrient processing). The goal is to detect reversible factors that could influence the course of the disease and the risks for future complications. In chronic illness, the aim is to identify factors that contribute to nutritional compromise and to evaluate the effect of the nutritional compromise on the course of the illness. Anthropometric and laboratory measurements can be useful in this regard, but the basis of nutritional assessment rests on history and physical examination.

BIBLIOGRAPHY

GRANT A, DEHOOG S: Nutritional Assessment and Support, 1991. Anne Grant/Susan DeHoog, P.O. Box 75057 Northgate Station, Seattle, WA 98125

KERSTETTER JE et al: Malnutrition in the institutionalized older adult. *J Am Diet Assoc* 92:1109, 1992

LIPKIN EW, BELL S: Assessment of nutritional status. The clinician's perspective. *Clin Lab Med* 13:329, 1993

MANNING EM, SHENKIN A: Nutritional assessment in the critically ill. *Crit Care Clin* 11:603, 1995

MOWE M et al: Reduced nutritional status in an elderly population (>70 y) is probable before disease and possibly contributes to the development of disease. *Am J Clin Nutr* 59:317, 1994

OTTERY FD: Supportive nutrition to prevent cachexia and improve quality of life. *Semin Oncol* 22:98, 1995

SCHWENK A et al: Clinical risk factors for malnutrition in HIV-1-infected patients. *AIDS* 7:1213, 1993

SUITOR CW: Nutritional assessment of the pregnant woman. *Clin Obstet Gynecol* 37:501, 1994

74   *Margo Denke, Jean D. Wilson*

PROTEIN AND ENERGY MALNUTRITION

Insufficient consumption of protein and energy causes loss of both body mass and adipose tissue, although one or the other loss may predominate in a given individual. Protein-energy malnutrition (PEM) occurs primarily under two circumstances: in developing nations it may be present in endemic form, and under famine conditions the prevalence may approach 25 percent. The primary disorder occurs when socioeconomic factors limit the quantity and quality of food; it is a particular problem when vegetable proteins of low biologic value are major components of the diet and when the incidence of infectious diseases is high. The problem is accentuated when energy intake is insufficient so that dietary proteins are oxidized as fuel rather than utilized for the synthesis of body protein. In children of developing nations two syndromes of PEM have been distinguished: (1) *marasmus*, manifested by stunted growth, loss of adipose tissue, generalized wasting of protein mass, and no edema, is thought to be due to the combined effects of protein and energy malnutrition; and (2) *kwashiorkor*, manifested by growth failure, edema, hypoalbuminemia, fatty liver, and preservation of subcutaneous fat, is thought to be due to selective protein malnutrition. Mixed forms are common in both children and adults, and the distinction between pure protein malnutrition and PEM has little clinical significance.

In developed nations PEM occurs most commonly as a secondary disorder in people who were previously well nourished who develop the disorder in association with subacute or chronic illness. Predisposing features include anorexia, hypermetabolism, malabsorption, and drug and alcohol abuse, and, in the aged, depression, isolation, and low income may play a role. As many as half of the hospitalized elderly are malnourished at admission or develop nutritional deficits during hospitalization. Synergism between primary and secondary causes is common in that those individuals with scanty reserves of protein and energy develop clinical PEM more rapidly than well-nourished subjects when challenged by hypermetabolism, the anorexia of infection, or other catabolic illness.

EPIDEMIOLOGY   The prevalence among a given population can be assessed by measuring subcutaneous fat, midarm muscle area, or the ratio of 24-h urine creatinine to height (Chap. 73). The magnitude of the problem worldwide is immense. In 1983 the World Health Organization estimated that 300 million children had growth retardation secondary to malnutrition; the consequences for mortality, cognitive function, social organization, and economic development are dire but impossible to quantify. Preschool children in developing countries are particularly susceptible, because of their dependence on others for food, their higher protein and energy requirements, and their enhanced susceptibility to infection, especially under nonhygienic conditions. Gastrointestinal infections frequently precipitate clinical PEM because of the associated diarrhea, associated anorexia, vomiting, increased metabolic needs, and decreased intestinal absorption; parasitic infections play a major role in the problem in many parts of the world.

In the United States protein deficiency in adults tends to be mild and subclinical, but poor nutrition is not limited to the adult poor. In one survey that focused on low-income areas of the United States, 22 to 35 percent of children 2 to 6 years old were below the 15th percentile for weight, and in another survey 11 percent of low-income children had height-for-age measurements below the 5th percentile. In hospitalized patients, severe as well as mild deficiencies are even more common. Moreover, the nutritional status of patients frequently declines during hospitalization, and the occurrence of postoperative infections, time required for the healing of surgical wounds, and duration of hospitalization are increased in such individuals, a disturbing phenomenon since malnutrition is both preventable and reversible.

PATHOPHYSIOLOGY   When energy intake falls below the minimal requirements, the body responds with an orderly physiologic adaptation (Chap. 335), involving the hormones of energy metabolism, that causes mobilization of free fatty acids from adipose tissue and of amino acids from muscle to provide energy for the oxidative needs of the body and in particular of the brain. As amino acids are diverted into gluconeogenesis and oxidation, protein synthesis is curtailed, the metabolic rate declines, and lean body mass and adipose tissue contract. During the first week of starvation, 4 to 5 kg of body weight is lost, consisting of about 25 percent adipose tissue, 35 percent extracellular fluid, and 40 percent protein. During ensuing weeks, losses continue but at a slower pace. Different compartments contract at different rates: skeletal muscle faster than cardiac muscle; gastrointestinal tract and liver faster than kidney. Mobilization of amino acids from muscle supports the synthesis of some albumin so that hypoalbuminemia develops late.

The intake of protein can be more limiting than that of energy when proteins of low biologic value (chiefly vegetable proteins) are the major proteins of the diet or when glucose is the sole organic nutrient in the intravenous feeding of patients who cannot eat. The consequence in either case is to enhance insulin secretion, which in turn retards lipolysis of adipose tissue, preserves adipose tissue mass, and inhibits the mobilization of amino acids from muscle. Amino acid levels decline, and the synthesis of albumin and other proteins is impaired; hypoalbuminemia and edema are characteristic features, and fatty infiltration of the liver ensues. As stated above, these findings are typical of kwashiorkor.

Depletion of body minerals is in part due to contraction of body mass and extracellular fluid, but potassium and magnesium may be lost out of proportion to body mass due to shifts from intracellular stores. Deficiency of mineral intake (as in the patient in whom intravenous glucose is the sole energy source) and enhanced losses (diuresis, diarrhea, fistulas, etc.) may worsen mineral deficits.

Simple starvation, as described above, does not quickly lead to death but induces a gradual metabolic adaptation that involves the shift of the metabolism of the central nervous system to the oxidation of fatty acids and ketone bodies for energy and a profound reduction in the metabolic rate that conserves the residual protein stores. Starvation in the context of physical stress is considerably more deleterious. The extent to which the effects of stress are due to the direct metabolic consequences of inflammation, infection, fever, and wound healing as compared to the indirect consequences of the release of inflammatory cytokines such as tumor necrosis factor α, interleukin 2, and interleukin 6 is not clear, but the addition of stress to starvation increases the metabolic rate and accelerates the loss of weight and of nitrogen and micronutrients. It is for these reasons that severe PEM develops when both malnutrition and stress are present. It is of particular interest in this regard that PEM is a prominent feature of AIDS, where it is thought to be the consequence of anorexia (and diminished intake), fever, and diarrhea.

CLINICAL MANIFESTATIONS Mild to Moderate PEM Children fail to gain height and weight; adults generally lose weight, although edema may mask weight loss. Alternatively, if the individual was previously obese, loss of protoplasm can be hidden by a residue of fat. Triceps skin-fold thickness and midarm muscle area are reduced (see Tables 73-6 and 73-7). In the absence of renal disease the ratio of 24-h urine creatinine to height is a sensitive indicator of protein malnutrition and should be measured at weekly intervals. Levels of albumin, transferrin, and prealbumin in serum may be low. Serum triiodothyronine is decreased, the level of reverse triiodothyronine is increased, and the metabolic rate is low. Peripheral lymphopenia may be present, and glucose tolerance may be impaired. The heart size tends to be small.

Severe PEM Severe PEM is characterized by more profound abnormalities in body composition and in laboratory findings. Decrease in muscle mass is evident on physical examination, as indicated by excavation of the intercostal spaces and wasting of the temporal muscles and extremities, and subcutaneous adipose tissue is decreased or absent. Listlessness, easy fatigability, sensation of coldness, dry cracked skin, drawn facies, and dyspigmentation of the skin and hair are common. Decubiti and skin ulcers occur in advanced stages. Blood pressure is low, the pulse is decreased, and temperature may be low. There is a global impairment of organ system function.

Cardiovascular/renal/pulmonary The ventilatory response to hypoxia is blunted. During the course of malnutrition the heart and kidneys lose mass in proportion to the loss of lean body mass and the fall in metabolic rate, so that cardiac output and glomerular filtration rate are appropriate for body size and the metabolic state. However, congestive heart failure can occur during vigorous nutritional and volume repletion, with infection, and during other physical stresses.

Blood Blood volume, hematocrit, serum albumin, transferrin, and lymphocyte count are decreased. The anemia is normocytic and normochromic and is usually due to decreased red blood cell production, thought to reflect the general decrease in protein biosynthesis. Deficiencies of iron, folate, and pyridoxine may contribute to the anemia.

Metabolic rate In the absence of fever, basal metabolic rate falls and hypothermia is common, possibly the consequence of diminished levels of triiodothyronine and of the loss of the insulating protection of subcutaneous fat. Hypoglycemia may be a terminal event.

Gastrointestinal tract and pancreas Atrophy of the gastrointestinal tract involves the intestinal villi and both the exocrine and endocrine functions of the pancreas, and bacterial overgrowth may occur in the small intestine. Malabsorption and lactose intolerance may be present. The gastrointestinal manifestations may result, at least in part, from decreased oral feeding rather than starvation, since similar changes occur in individuals fully nourished by parenteral feeding.

Immune system Cell-mediated immunity is impaired, as indicated by all standard tests, whereas antibody responses are generally intact. Common infections and opportunistic infections can lead to increased morbidity and mortality. Pneumonia is common.

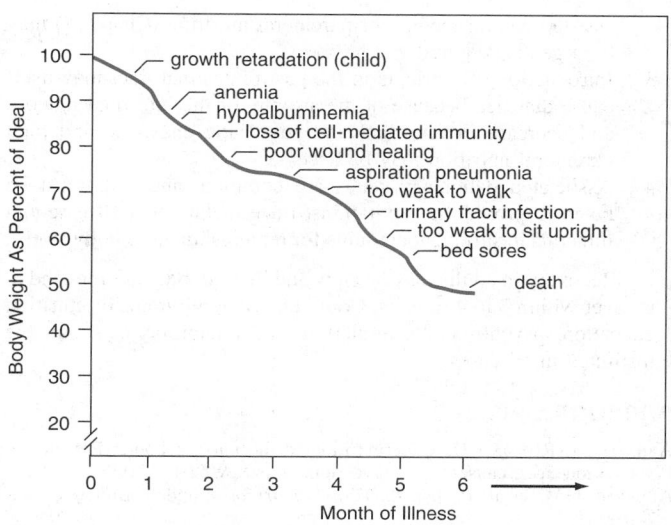

FIGURE 74-1 Hypothetical course of a typical patient with protein-energy malnutrition.

Wound healing All wounds and incisions heal more slowly in PEM. Wound dehiscence is common.

Reproduction Nearly every aspect of reproduction is impaired in the woman with PEM, including implantation, fetal growth, lactation, and parturition, and the infants are stunted in size and may have cognitive impairment if they survive.

COURSE A hypothetical course is illustrated in Fig. 74-1. In children slowing of growth is usually the first manifestation. Anemia, hypoalbuminemia, and amenorrhea follow, and loss of cell-mediated immunity predisposes to infection. The hypermetabolism and anorexia of infection accelerate the cachexia. In advanced PEM midarm fat below the fifth percentile and creatinine/height ratio less than 60 percent of the normal are associated with terminal infections.

RELATION TO OTHER DEFICIENCY STATES PEM rarely occurs as an isolated phenomenon. Common coexisting nutritional deficiencies include those for folic acid, thiamine, riboflavin, nicotinic acid, pyridoxine, and vitamin A; in children with PEM deficiency of vitamin A is a particular hazard. As PEM worsens and protoplasmic protein is consumed, the intracellular minerals potassium, phosphorous, and magnesium are excreted in parallel with nitrogen so that total-body deficits may become apparent upon refeeding.

℞ TREATMENT

In the case of mild to moderate PEM, any precipitating events must be addressed, and the intake of protein and energy (based on ideal weight) should be increased sufficiently to allow replenishment of deficits. It is appropriate to administer multivitamins to all such patients. It is also essential during repletion that the availability of all minerals and trace elements be adequate to prevent life-threatening hypokalemia, hypomagnesemia, hypophosphatemia, etc. from developing. Provided the patient can eat and swallow, most patients can be treated orally. However, if anorexia is a major problem or if the individual is edentulous, the diet may have to be supplemented with liquid formulas (Chap. 77) either by mouth or by assisted enteral feeding (Chap. 78).

Management of severe PEM is more emergent and more complicated for several reasons.

1. Precipitating illnesses tend to be more severe and difficult to manage, and it may not be possible to restore nitrogen balance until infection and fever are brought under control.
2. The degree of malnutrition itself may hamper recovery from associated life-threatening illness so that early intervention with

assisted enteral feeding or parenteral nutrition (Chap. 78) may be urgently required.

3. Introduction of nutrients in the gastrointestinal tract may itself cause diarrhea because of the atrophy of the intestinal mucosa and decrease in intestinal and pancreatic enzymes, and total parenteral nutrition may be necessary.

4. Associated deficiency states are common, and care must be taken to provide multivitamins, trace metals, and all essential minerals in sufficient amounts for replenishment of body stores.

Recovery in adults may be slow and limited, but children tend to recover within 3 to 4 months. Comprehensive programs of nutrition education, psychosocial stimulation, and rehabilitation should be instituted in all cases.

BIBLIOGRAPHY

ABBASI AA, RUDMAN D: Undernutrition in the nursing home: Prevalence, consequences, causes, and prevention. Nutr Rev 52:113, 1994

ALLEYNE GAO et al: *Protein-Energy Malnutrition*. London, Butler & Tanner, 1997

BECKER DJ: The endocrine responses to protein calorie malnutrition. Ann Rev Nutr 3:187, 1983

CAHILL GF: Starvation in man. N Engl J Med 200:220, 1970

HARDIN TC: Cytokine mediators of malnutrition: Clinical implications. Nutr Clin Pract 8:55, 1993

HEYMSFIELD SB et al: Nutritional assessment by anthropomorphic and biochemical methods, in *Modern Nutrition in Health and Disease*, 8th ed, ME Shils et al (eds). Philadelphia, Lea & Febiger, 1994, p 812

HOFFER LJ: Starvation, in *Modern Nutrition in Health and Disease*, 8th ed, ME Shils et al (eds). Philadelphia, Lea & Febiger, 1994, p 927

JAMES WP: The challenge of adult chronic energy deficiency. Eur J Clin Nutr 48(Suppl 3):S1, 1994

PARNES HL, AISNER J: Protein calorie malnutrition and cancer therapy. Drug Safety 7:404, 1992

POLLITT E: Functional significance of the covariance between protein energy malnutrition and iron deficiency anemia. J Nutr 125(Suppl 8):2272S, 1995

SULLIVAN DH: The role of nutrition in increased morbidity and mortality. Clin Geriatr Med 11:661, 1995

TORUM B, CHEW F: Protein-energy malnutrition, in *Modern Nutrition in Health and Disease*, 8th ed, ME Shils et al (eds). Philadelphia, Lea & Febiger, 1994, p 950

75 *George A. Bray*

OBESITY

Obesity is a chronic disease that is increasing in prevalence and that poses a serious risk for the development of diabetes mellitus, hypertension, heart disease, gall bladder disease, and certain forms of cancer. Obesity can be viewed as a consequence of the interaction between environmental forces and the individual genetic substrate, in particular with susceptibility genes. These genes enhance the storage of fat when food is limited and cause an increased risk of obesity when food is abundant and energy expenditure is reduced. The prevalence of obesity in the United States increased slowly after World War II and has increased 30 percent in the past decade. Against this environmental and genetic background, this chapter will define the problem, describe methods for measuring obesity, review the etiology and pathogenesis, consider the impact of differences in regional fatness as predictors of health risk, and summarize the available treatment options.

DEFINITION AND MEASUREMENT Both obesity and fat distribution are useful predictors of excess mortality and of the risks of diabetes mellitus, heart disease, hypertension, and gall bladder disease. *Obesity*, an increase in total body fat, is frequently used synonymously with *overweight* because the degree of overweight can readily be related to the risks assigned to obesity and direct measures of body fat are expensive. Regional fat distribution, or fat topography, also has a profound influence on health risks. For example, increased deposits of visceral or abdominal fat correlate with the risks for heart disease, diabetes mellitus, high blood pressure, gall bladder disease, and breast cancer.

Of the techniques for estimating or measuring total body fat (Table 75-1), height and weight can be measured with accuracy and reliability and provide valuable information. Dual energy x-ray absorptiometry, which was developed to evaluate bone density, provides the best assessment of total body fat. Regional fat can be measured accurately by magnetic resonance imaging or computed tomography scanning; for practical purposes, waist circumference or the sagittal diameter is the most useful parameter. The ratio of waist circumference to hip circumference is widely used to estimate regional fat but is not accurate.

Overweight can be defined from tables of height and weight and from estimates of percent overweight or relative weight (ratio of actual to desirable weight). However, the most widely used formula for relating height and weight is the body mass index (BMI), which is weight/(height)^2, where weight is in kilograms and height is in meters. A nomogram for estimating BMI is shown in Fig. 75-1. A BMI between 20 and 25 kg/m^2 is usually considered a good weight for most individuals. Overweight is defined as a BMI above 27 kg/m^2, and obesity is defined as a body mass index above 30 kg/m^2. Weight gain may confer increased health risks even if the BMI does not exceed 25 kg/m^2. In women a weight gain of more than 5 kg (11 lb) is associated with increased risks of diabetes and heart disease, and in men any weight gain after age 25 appears to carry increased health risks. At the practical level, determination of the BMI, estimation of abdominal girth (see below), and assessment of the presence of heart disease, diabetes mellitus, gall bladder disease, or hypertension in the family provide valuable information for evaluating the obese patient. Based on these considerations, a table of good weights for men and women has been developed (Table 75-2).

Body fat and fat distribution are affected by gender, age, degree of physical activity, and a number of drugs. In both men and women body fat increases with age. In lean young men, body fat is less than 20 percent and may rise in older men to more than 25 percent. In young women, body fat stores may be below 30 percent and increase gradually to more than 35 percent in older women. At all ages after puberty women are fatter than men.

Table 75-1

Methods of Estimating Body Fat and Its Distribution

Method	Cost	Ease of Use	Accuracy	Measures Regional Fat
Height and weight	$	Easy	High	No
Skin folds	$	Easy	Low	Yes
Circumferences	$	Easy	Moderate	Yes
Ultrasound	$$	Moderate	Moderate	Yes
Density				
Immersion	$	Moderate	High	No
Plethysmograph	$$$	Difficult	High	No
Heavy water				
Tritiated	$$	Moderate	High	No
Deuterium oxide, or heavy oxygen	$$$	Moderate	High	No
Potassium isotope (^{40}K)	$$$$	Difficult	High	No
Total-body electrical conductivity	$$$	Moderate	High	No
Bioelectric impedance	$$	Easy	High	No
Fat-soluble gas	$$	Difficult	High	No
Absorptiometry (dual energy x-ray absorptiometry; dual photon absorptiometry)	$$$	Easy	High	No
Computed tomography	$$$$	Difficult	High	Yes
Magnetic resonance imaging	$$$$	Difficult	High	Yes
Neutron activation	$$$$	Difficult	High	No

NOTE: $, low cost; $$, moderate cost; $$$, high cost; $$$$, very high cost.

PREVALENCE The prevalence of obesity depends upon the criteria for diagnosis. In most European countries obesity is defined as a BMI above 30 kg/m², and overweight is frequently defined as a BMI between 25 and 30 kg/m² or between 27 and 30 kg/m². The National Center for Health Statistics in the United States defines overweight as weights above the 85th percentile in men and women age 20 to 29 years. There has been a slow increase in the prevalence in both genders since surveys began more than 40 years ago, and between 1988 and 1991 there was an increase of more than 30 percent both in the United States and abroad (Fig. 75-2).

PATHOGENESIS Genetic Susceptibility Genetic determinants can either play a major role in the pathogenesis of obesity or enhance susceptibility to its development. The dysmorphic forms of human obesity in which genetics play a major role include the Prader-Willi syndrome, Ahlstrom's syndrome, the Laurence-Moon-Biedl syndrome, Cohen's syndrome, and Carpenter's syndrome (Table 75-3).

Four genes have been cloned in which mutations cause obesity in animals, and some of them appear to be important in human biology (Table 75-4). The leptin gene is expressed only in adipose tissue, and in the recessively inherited ob/ob obesity in mice, both copies of the gene are defective because of the presence of a stop codon that truncates the protein at amino acid 105. The leptin protein is normally secreted from fat cells, and the levels of leptin mRNA in fat cells and the circulating level of leptin are both increased in animal and human obesities. Treatment of obese mice with leptin reduces food intake and body fat. Splicing defects in the leptin receptor are responsible for the obesity in the db/db mouse, which is phenotypically similar to the ob/ob mouse. The gene defect called *tub* results from a defective phosphatase and causes retinitis pigmentosa and obesity in mice, making it similar to the Lawrence-Moon-Biedl syndrome in humans. Additional genes, including those for the beta₃-adrenergic receptor, tumor necrosis factor α, and lipoprotein lipase, have been implicated in the development of human obesity, but their contribution to the overall disorder is small.

Genetic susceptibility to obesity has been studied extensively, and between 30 and 50 percent of the variability in total-body fat stores is believed to be genetically determined. In animals that become obese when fed a high-fat diet, at least 12 chromosomal loci play an important role in the expression of this susceptibility, and the basis for genetic susceptibility to obesity in human beings is likely to be equally complex.

The Fat Cell and Obesity In addition to its role in fat storage, the fat cell is an important secretory organ. It produces lipoprotein lipase, which is involved in hydrolyzing the triglycerides of very low density lipoproteins (VLDL) and chylomicrons, and complements D (adipsin) and C3b. The adipocyte also produces cytokines such as tumor necrosis factor α, angiotensinogen, and leptin. The fat cell generates large quantities of lactate and metabolizes glucose to provide glycerol-3-phosphate for triglyceride synthesis. Under conditions of dietary surfeit, human fat cells synthesize long chain fatty acids.

Most forms of obesity are associated with enlarged fat cells and higher rates of basal lipolysis. Fat cells also serve as a reservoir for storage of fatty acids released during the clearance of chylomicrons and can in turn release these stored fatty acids by the intracellular hormone-sensitive lipase. In many forms of severe childhood-onset obesity, the total number of fat cells is increased.

Environmental Factors Environmental factors interact with genetic susceptibility in the pathogenesis of obesity. For example, hypothalamic injury from trauma or surgery and destructive lesions in the region of the ventromedial or the paraventricular nucleus in the hypothalamus can produce obesity. The two major factors in hypothalamic obesity are hyperphagia and a disturbance in the autonomic nervous system consisting of increased parasympathetic and reduced sympathetic nervous system activity. One explanation for this sequence of events may be altered secretion of neuropeptide Y (NPY). NPY is produced in the arcuate nucleus and acts in the hypothalamus to stimulate eating; it can also impair reproductive function, decrease sympathetic activity, and increase parasympathetic activity—other key features of hypothalamic obesity.

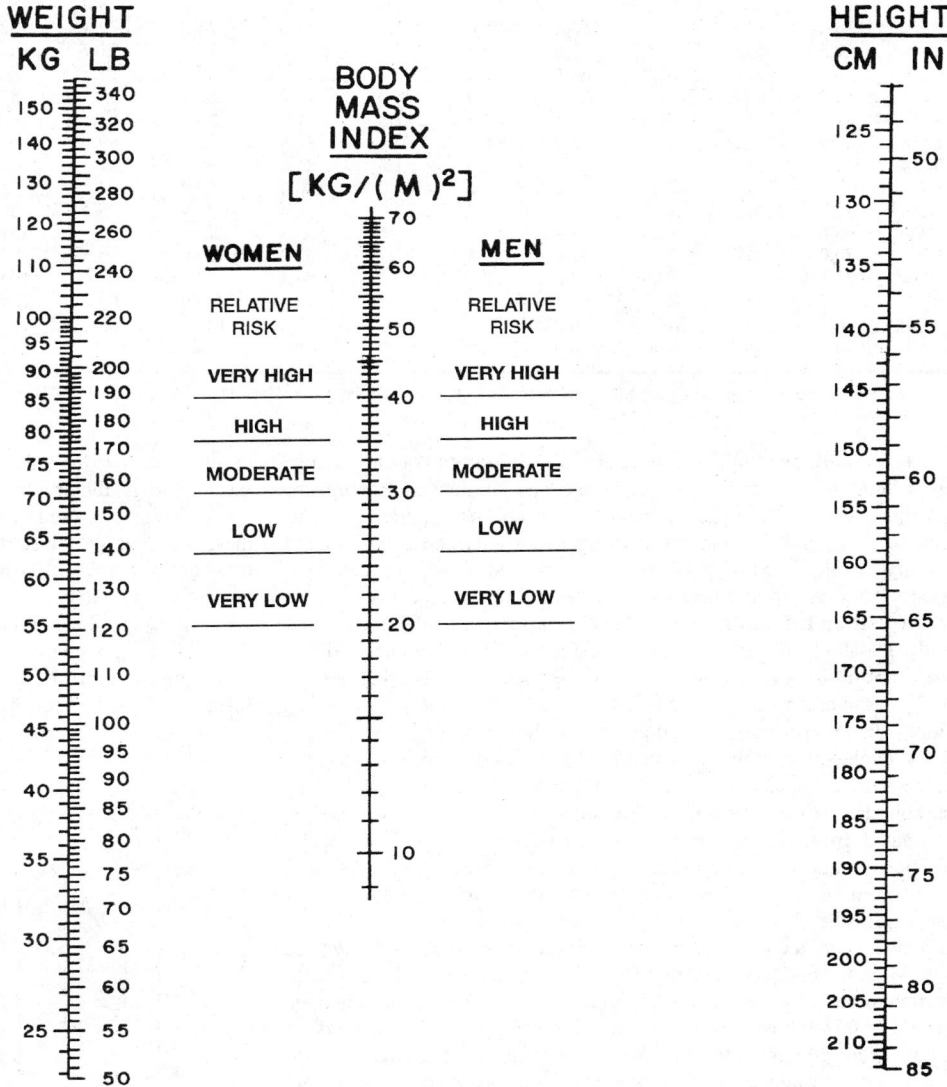

FIGURE 75-1 Nomogram for determining body mass index. To use this nomogram, place a ruler or other straight edge between the body weight (without clothes) in kilograms or pounds located on the left-hand line and the height (without shoes) in centimeters or in inches located on the right-hand line. The body mass index is read from the middle of the scale and is in metric units. (*Copyright 1978, George A. Bray. Used by permission.*)

Table 75-2

Chart to Find Body Mass Index (BMI) from Height and Weight, and Classification of Weight (Health Risk) According to BMI

Height	Good BMI						Borderline BMI		Increasing Risk BMI					
	19	20	21	22	23	24	25	26	27	28	29	30	35	40

Find your height on the left then move across the row to the weight which is closest to yours. Your BMI level is listed along the top.

HEIGHT IN CENTIMETERS, WEIGHT IN KILOGRAMS

Height	19	20	21	22	23	24	25	26	27	28	29	30	35	40
140.0	37.2	39.2	41.2	43.1	45.1	47.0	49.0	51.0	52.9	54.9	56.8	58.8	68.6	78.4
142.0	38.3	40.3	42.3	44.4	46.4	48.4	50.4	52.4	54.4	56.5	59.5	60.5	70.6	80.7
144.0	39.4	41.v5	43.5	45.6	47.7	49.8	51.8	53.9	56.0	58.1	60.1	62.2	72.6	82.9
146.0	40.5	42.6	44.8	46.9	49.0	51.2	53.3	55.4	57.6	59.7	61.8	63.9	74.6	85.3
148.0	41.6	43.8	46.0	48.2	50.4	52.6	54.8	57.0	59.1	61.3	63.5	65.7	76.7	87.6
150.0	42.8	45.0	47.3	49.5	51.8	54.0	56.3	58.5	60.8	63.0	65.3	67.5	78.8	90.0
152.0	43.9	46.2	48.5	50.8	53.1	55.4	57.8	60.1	62.4	64.7	67.0	69.3	80.9	92.4
154.0	45.1	47.4	49.8	52.2	54.5	56.9	59.3	61.7	64.0	66.4	68.8	71.1	83.0	94.9
156.0	46.2	48.7	51.1	53.5	56.0	58.4	60.8	63.3	65.7	68.1	70.6	73.0	85.2	97.3
158.0	47.4	49.9	52.4	54.9	57.4	59.9	62.4	64.9	67.4	69.9	72.4	74.9	87.4	99.9
160.0	48.6	51.2	53.8	56.3	58.9	61.4	64.0	66.6	69.1	71.7	74.2	76.8	89.6	102.4
162.0	49.9	52.5	55.1	57.7	60.4	63.0	65.6	68.2	70.9	73.5	76.1	78.7	91.9	105.0
164.0	51.1	53.8	56.5	59.2	61.9	64.6	67.2	69.9	72.6	75.3	78.0	80.7	94.1	107.6
166.0	52.4	55.1	57.9	60.6	63.4	66.1	68.9	71.6	74.4	77.2	79.9	82.7	96.4	110.2
168.0	53.6	56.4	59.3	62.1	64.9	67.7	70.6	73.4	76.2	79.0	81.8	84.7	98.8	112.9
170.0	54.9	57.8	60.7	63.6	66.5	69.4	72.3	75.1	78.0	80.9	83.8	86.7	101.2	115.6
172.0	56.2	59.2	62.1	65.1	68.0	71.0	74.0	76.9	79.9	82.8	85.8	88.8	103.5	118.3
174.0	57.5	60.6	63.6	66.6	69.6	72.7	75.7	78.7	81.7	84.8	87.8	90.8	106.0	121.1
176.0	58.9	62.0	65.0	68.1	71.2	74.3	77.4	80.5	83.6	86.7	89.8	92.9	108.4	123.9
178.0	60.2	63.4	66.5	69.7	72.9	76.0	79.2	82.4	85.5	88.7	91.9	95.1	110.9	126.7
180.0	61.6	64.8	68.0	71.3	74.5	77.8	81.0	84.2	87.5	90.7	94.0	97.2	113.4	129.6
182.0	62.9	66.2	69.6	72.9	76.2	79.5	82.8	86.1	89.4	92.7	96.1	99.4	115.9	132.5
184.0	64.3	67.7	71.1	74.5	77.9	81.3	84.6	88.0	91.4	94.8	98.2	101.6	118.5	135.4
186.0	65.7	69.2	72.7	76.1	79.6	83.0	86.5	89.9	93.4	96.9	100.3	103.8	121.1	138.4
188.0	67.2	70.7	74.2	77.8	81.3	84.8	88.4	91.9	95.4	99.0	102.5	106.0	123.7	141.4
190.0	68.6	72.2	75.8	79.4	83.0	86.6	90.3	93.9	97.5	101.1	104.7	108.3	126.4	144.4
192.0	70.0	73.7	77.4	81.1	84.8	88.5	92.2	95.8	99.5	103.2	106.9	110.6	129.0	147.5
194.0	71.5	75.3	79.0	82.8	86.6	90.3	94.1	97.9	101.6	105.4	109.1	112.9	131.7	150.5
196.0	73.0	76.8	80.7	84.5	88.4	92.2	96.0	99.9	103.7	107.6	111.4	115.2	134.5	153.7
198.0	74.5	78.4	82.3	86.2	90.2	94.1	98.0	101.9	105.9	109.8	113.7	117.6	137.2	156.8
200.0	76.0	80.0	84.0	88.0	92.0	96.0	100.0	104.0	108.0	112.0	116.0	120.0	140.0	160.0

NOTE: The health risk from any level of BMI is increased if you have gained more than 5 kg (11 lb) since age 25 or if you have a waist circumference above 40 in (100 cm) due to central fatness.

The syndrome of hypothalamic obesity is at one end of the genetic-environmental continuum. At the same end of this continuum are several endocrine diseases associated with obesity, including Cushing's disease and the polycystic ovary syndrome, and drug-induced obesity (Table 75-5). One of the drugs, megestrol acetate, has been used to increase food intake in the anorexia of cancer cachexia.

Nutrition Intake and Substrate Oxidation To maintain normal body fat stores dietary nutrients must be oxidized in the body in the proportion in which they occur in the diet. A typical distribution of macronutrients in a 2000-kcal diet and the fraction of body stores that these nutrients represent are shown in Fig. 75-3. Since daily intake of carbohydrate nearly equals body stores of glucose, carbohydrate stores are more vulnerable to changes in dietary carbohydrate than either fat or proteins. Oxidation of food can be estimated from the respiratory quotient (RQ) (the ratio of carbon dioxide produced to oxygen used). The corresponding ratio in food is referred to as the food quotient. As the percent of dietary fat increases, the RQ must decline if weight is to remain stable. If RQ does not decline, the body continues to oxidize carbohydrate stores and must replace these by eating more food to obtain carbohydrate or synthesize endogenous glucose from protein stores. Whether this adjustment occurs efficiently and readily appears to have strong genetic determinants. Physiologically, the adaptation to a high-fat, western-type diet requires a decrease in carbohydrate oxidation to preserve carbohydrate stores. If carbohydrate oxidation is reduced, the oxidation of fat increases to provide for nutrient needs and lower the RQ. If the body is unable to reduce carbohydrate oxidation, the compensatory mechanism is increased food intake to provide needed carbohydrate with increasing fat storage until a point is reached at which the oxidation of fatty acids increases to meet average dietary intake.

Whether measured from room calorimeters or doubly labeled water, there is a positive correlation between energy expenditure and fat-free mass or body weight. To maintain body weight, therefore, heavier individuals must on average ingest more food to provide the necessary energy. Obese persons tend to underreport food intake significantly (Fig. 75-4). Thus, a patient who says 'Doctor, I hardly eat anything' is not recording or reporting food intake accurately. Because of almost uniform unreliability, dietary histories should probably be abandoned for

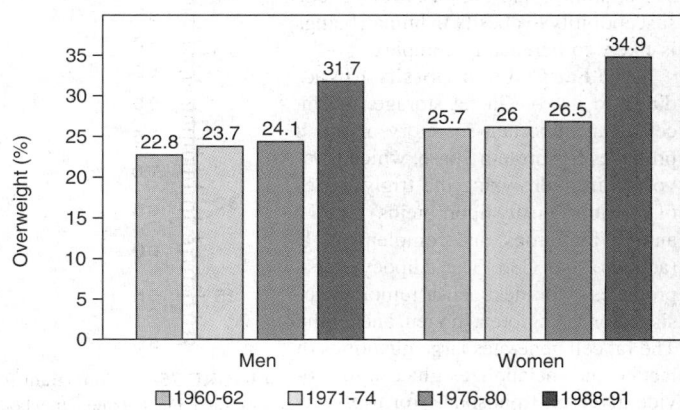

FIGURE 75-2 Prevalence of overweight status in four surveys. Data from the National Center for Health Statistics show the rise in prevalence of obesity over the past 30 years, particularly the past 10 years. (After Kuczmarski et al.)

Table 75-3

A Comparison of Syndromes of Obesity—Hypogonadism and Mental Retardation

| Feature | Syndrome | | | | |
	Prader-Willi	Laurence-Moon-Biedl	Ahlstrom	Cohen	Carpenter
Inheritance	Sporadic; two-thirds have defect	Autosomal recessive	Autosomal recessive	Probably autosomal recessive	Autosomal recessive
Stature	Short	Normal; infrequently short	Normal; infrequently short	Short or tall	Normal
Obesity	Generalized Moderate to severe Onset 1–3 yrs	Generalized Early onset, 1–2 yrs	Truncal Early onset, 2–5 years	Truncal Mid-childhood, age 5	Truncal, gluteal
Cranofacies	Narrow bifrontal diameter Almond-shaped eyes Strabismus V-shaped mouth High arched palate	Not distinctive	Not distinctive	High nasal bridge Arched palate Open mouth Short philtrum	Acrocephaly Flat nasal bridge High arched palate
Limbs	Small hands and feet Hypotonia	Polydactyly	No abnormalities	Hypotonia Narrow hands and feet	Polydactyly Syndactyly Genu valgum
Reproductive status	1° Hypogonadism	1° Hypogonadism	Hypogonadism in males but not in females	Normal gonadal function or hypogonadotrophic hypogonadism	2° Hypogonadism
Other features	Enamel hypoplasia Hyperphagia Temper tantrums Nasal speech			Dysplastic ears Delayed puberty	
Mental retardation	Mild to moderate		Normal intelligence	Mild	Slight

Table 75-4

Molecular Biology of Obesity

	Gene Symbol	Chromosome	Gene Defect	Mechanism
ANIMALS				
Yellow mouse	A^y; A^{vy}; A^{iy}	2	Overexpression of 133-amino-acid Agouti protein	Agouti protein competes with MSH receptors
Obese mouse	ob	6	1. Stop codon at 105 in the 167-amino-acid leptin protein 2. Nonsense mutation in the leptin protein	Absence of leptin (ob protein), which appears to modulate steroid superfamily expression
Diabetes	db	4	Splicing defects in leptin receptor	Receptor for leptin absent
Fatty rat (syntenic to db locus)	fa	5	Not identified	Receptor for leptin probably absent
Tub		7	Not identified	?
Fat		8	Carboxypeptidase E	Failure of cleavage for many peptides
HUMANS				
Prader Willi		15q 1.2		
Laurence-Moon-Biedl		3 and 16		

estimating energy needs. In our clinic, a reasonable guideline for energy expenditure (kcal) in the obese is to multiply body weight by 10. An alternative method (Table 75-6) takes into account height, weight, and age to estimate of basal energy expenditure.

Table 75-5

Drugs Associated with Increased Body Weight

Phenothiazines (chlorpromazine > thioridazine ≥ trifluoperazine > mesoridazine > promazine ≥ mepazine ≥ perphenazine ≥ prochlorperazine > haloperidol ≥ loxapine)
Antidepressants (amitriptyline > imipramine = doxepin = phenelzine > amoxapine = desipramine = trazodone = tranylcypromine)
Antiepileptics (valproate; carbamazepine)
Steroids (glucocorticoids; megestrol acetate)
Antihypertensives (terazosin)

There are three known predictors of future weight gain: a low metabolic rate; a high RQ, indicating carbohydrate oxidation and the need to eat to replace carbohydrate; and insulin resistance. The regulation of nutrient intake can be viewed as a feedback system with afferent and efferent signals (Fig. 75-5). Factors that increase hunger include a decrease in blood glucose, which precedes 60 percent or more of meals in animals and humans, and an increase in gastric contractions or abdominal uneasiness. These peripheral signals are integrated by neurotransmitters in the central nervous system to regulate food intake. Several neurotransmitters increase and a larger number decrease food intake. In addition, some neurotransmitters are specific modulators of the intake of one or another macronutrient (fat, carbohydrate, or protein). Thus, an increase or decrease in the intake of fat, carbohydrate, or protein can occur as major responses to specific neurotransmitters. These peptides and their monoamine substrates pro-

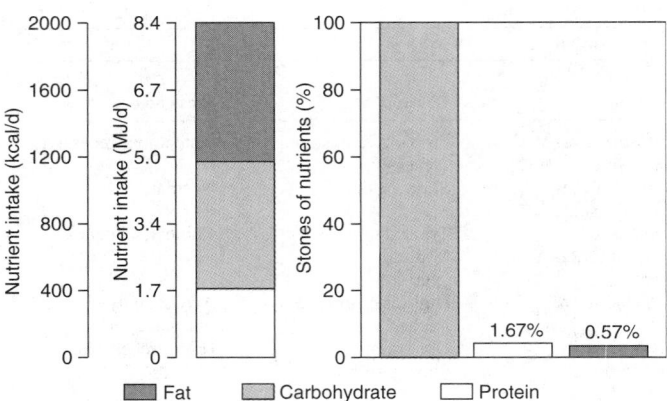

FIGURE 75-3 Nutrient intake versus stores. The daily intake of carbohydrate approximates body stores of carbohydrate. Intake of fat and protein are only a small fraction of the stored quantities of these nutrients.

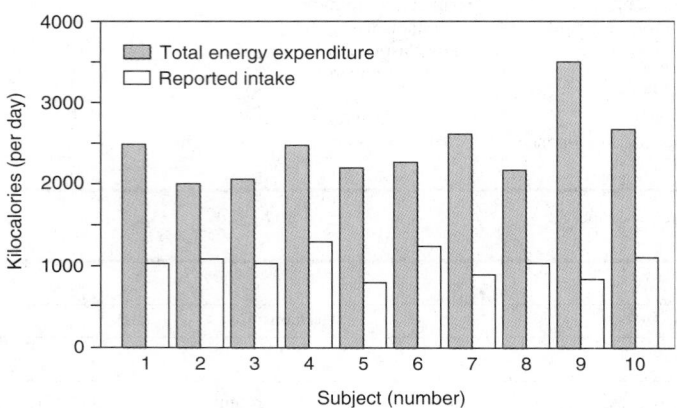

FIGURE 75-4 Comparison of energy expenditure and reported food intake in obese subjects. Total energy expenditure was determined by using doubly labeled water ($^2H^{18}O_2$). Food intake was determined from reported dietary intakes. The obese subjects consistently reported eating less than half the calories that were needed to maintain body weight.

Table 75-6

Estimating Energy Needs

EQUATIONS FOR ESTIMATING BASAL METABOLIC RATE (BMR)*

Men

18–30 years = (0.0630 × actual weight in kg + 2.8957) × 240 kcal/day

31–60 years = (0.0484 × actual weight in kg + 3.6534) × 240 kcal/day

Women

18–30 years = (0.0621 × actual weight in kg + 2.0357) × 240 kcal/day

31–60 years = (0.0342 × actual weight in kg + 3.5377) × 240 kcal/day

ESTIMATED TOTAL ENERGY NEEDS

Energy expenditure = BMR × activity factor

Activity level	Activity factor
Low (sedentary)	1.3
Intermediate (some regular exercise)	1.5
High (regular activity or demanding job)	1.7

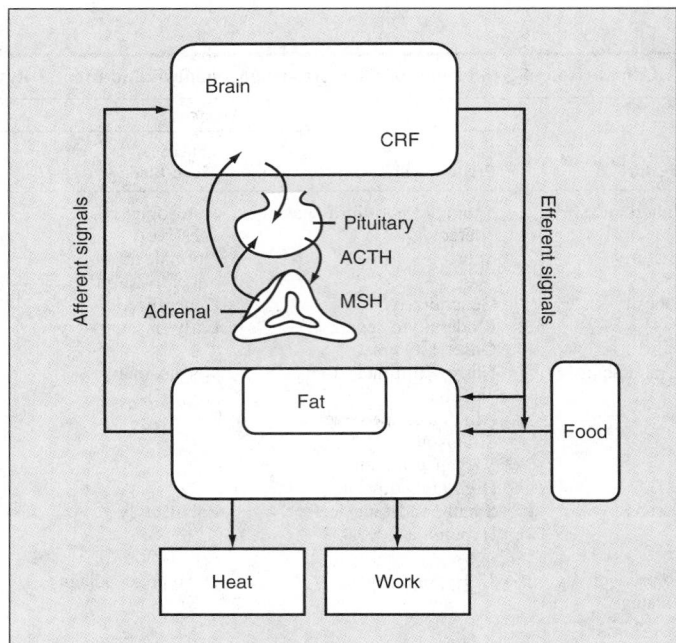

FIGURE 75-5 Model of a nutrient balance regulatory system for food intake. The afferent signals tell the brain about the state of nutrient stores and metabolism. This information is integrated in the central nervous system, which uses efferent endocrine and neural signals to modulate food intake and metabolism in the controlled system that digests, absorbs, metabolizes, or stores the ingested food.

vide a robust system for controlling the quantity and quality of food intake.

At least four processes are involved in the regulation of food intake: (1) olfactory and gustatory factors—these can stimulate intake when food is appetizing or inhibit intake when it is not; (2) gastrointestinal distention; (3) release of gastrointestinal hormones such as cholecystokinin and gastrin-releasing peptide; and (4) activation of a thermogenic component of the efferent sympathetic nervous system. These factors work together after food ingestion to induce satiety until the next glucose dip and increased gastric contractions produce a new arousal for seeking food.

OBESITY AND ITS ASSOCIATED RISKS The increased mortality associated with obesity results primarily from increased risks

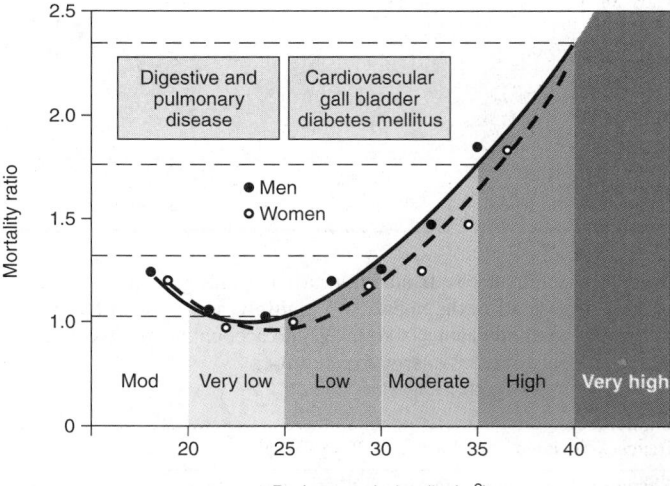

FIGURE 75-6 Mortality ratio and body mass index. Data from the American Cancer Society study are plotted for men and women to show relationship of body mass index (BMI) to overall mortality. At BMI < 20 kg/m² and > 25 kg/m² there is an increase in relative mortality. The major causes for this increased mortality are listed along with a division of BMI groupings into various levels of risk. (*Copyright 1987, George A. Bray. Used with permission.*)

for cardiovascular disease, high blood pressure, diabetes mellitus, and, possibly, some types of cancer (Fig. 75-6).

Cardiovascular System   In addition to the increased work load on the heart, obesity is also associated with an increased risk of sudden death, probably due to cardiac arrhythmias, and with an increased risk of atherosclerosis, probably a reflection of an abnormal lipid profile including decreased levels of high-density lipoprotein (HDL) cholesterol and increased levels of low-density lipoprotein cholesterol, particularly when these are in the form of small dense VLDL particles (B pattern). The prevalence of hypertension is also increased, the mechanism being unclear. One hypothesis suggests that hyperinsulinemia and insulin resistance enhance sodium reabsorption by the renal tubule and increase sympathetic outflow to promote arterial constriction.

Diabetes Mellitus   Type 2 diabetes mellitus [non-insulin-dependent diabetes mellitus (NIDDM)] is almost nonexistent in individuals with a BMI below 22 kg/m^2. In the Pima Indians the increased risk of diabetes with obesity has a strong familial tendency; when one or both Pima Indian parents is diabetic, 100 percent of the offspring will develop diabetes if they become sufficiently obese. If neither parent has diabetes, fewer than 20 percent of the obese offspring develop diabetes. In nonhuman primates that develop diabetes mellitus, obesity precedes the onset of diabetes by months to years. Among the earliest predictors of subsequent diabetes in obese monkeys is the development of insulin resistance. As with human beings, prevention of obesity in nonhuman primates prevents diabetes.

Cancer   The incidence of endometrial and postmenopausal breast cancers in women, prostate cancer in men, and colonorectal cancer in men and women is related to the degree of obesity. Visceral obesity increases the risk of postmenopausal breast cancer independent of the degree of obesity. One explanation for susceptibility to endometrial and breast cancer in obese women is the increased production of estrogen from the aromatization of circulating androstenedione in adipose tissue.

Gall Bladder Disease   Gall bladder disease increases with obesity and age, possibly related to increased excretion of biliary cholesterol. The amount of cholesterol synthesized by the body each day increases by about 20 mg for each kilogram of adipose tissue, so that a 10-kg increase in adipose tissue mass increases daily cholesterol production and excretion by an amount comparable to the cholesterol in one egg. Disturbances in nidation factors in the bile and alterations in the level of bile acids and phospholipids may promote precipitation of cholesterol stones.

Pulmonary Function   Moderate obesity in the absence of underlying pulmonary disease has little effect on respiratory function. Sleep apnea, however, can occur in severely obese individuals and poses a potentially serious problem. Obstructive sleep apnea is believed to occur because of local fat accumulation in the tracheopharyngeal area. The obstructive episodes of sleep apnea produce interrupted sleep associated with hypoxia and hypercapnia. If not corrected, this condition can lead to right heart failure. Continuous positive airway pressure can be administered at night to reduce or eliminate the episodes of sleep apnea. Weight loss is of particular value in remediating this problem.

Joint and Skin Problems   The increased incidence of osteoarthritis is no doubt partly due to the added trauma of increased weight bearing, but the fact that osteoarthritis also occurs in non-weight-bearing joints in such patients suggests that additional factors are involved. The prevalence of gout is also increased and may reflect impairment in urate clearance. Ketone bodies compete at the renal tubule for reabsorption of urate, and increased production of ketones from fat metabolism may increase urate levels.

Among the skin problems associated with obesity are acanthosis nigricans, manifested by darkening of the skinfolds on the neck, elbows, and dorsal interphalangeal spaces. Acanthosis nigricans is also associated with insulin resistance and NIDDM. Skin turgor and friability may also be increased in obesity, enhancing the risk of fungal and yeast infections in skinfolds. Finally, venous stasis is increased in the obese.

Endocrine System   Insulin resistance leading to hyperinsulinemia is a uniform feature and is directly related to the degree of obesity. Growth hormone secretion is reduced, but insulin-like growth

factor I levels are normal, suggesting that the level of growth hormone is sufficient to stimulate production of this important hormone.

Testosterone levels are decreased in men, but levels of free testosterone decline only with massive obesity. Obesity leads to an earlier onset of menarche, to a greater frequency of irregular and anovulatory cycles, and to earlier menopause. Distribution of body fat influences steroid metabolism in women. Women with central or visceral fat have a higher production of androgens such as testosterone, and women with gluteofemoral obesity have increased levels of estrone due to peripheral aromatization of circulating androgens.

Changes in thyroid hormone and its metabolism occur with changes in the level of nutrient intake. Triiodothyronine (T$_3$) can be increased by overfeeding and decreased by starvation. T$_3$ levels are also increased by high-carbohydrate diets and lowered by low-carbohydrate diets. In contrast, levels of thyroxine and thyrotropin (TSH) are unaffected by diet.

Obesity can sometimes be mistaken for Cushing's syndrome. The normal pattern of diurnal variation in plasma cortisol and the concentration of urinary free cortisol are normal in obesity but abnormal in Cushing's disease. If these patterns are equivocal, dynamic tests of adrenal function may be indicated.

Fat Topography   Regional distributions of body fat play an important role in the risk factors of obesity. To assess the distribution of body fat, the ratio of the circumference of the waist to the circumference of the hips has been a valuable tool for epidemiologic studies. For the individual patient, however, this ratio is not as useful as waist circumference itself. A waist circumference above 100 cm in men and above 90 cm in women is associated with increased levels of triglyceride and reduced levels of HDL cholesterol. Quantitative estimates of central fat distribution can be obtained from magnetic resonance imaging or computed tomographic scans of the abdomen (see Table 75-1).

Weight Cycling and Intentional Weight Loss   Regaining body weight after dieting is common and is referred to as *weight cycling*. Review of the literature concerning weight cycling does not reveal any convincing detrimental effects. To the contrary, intentional weight loss reduces health risks. Among 28,000 women aged 40 to 64 who had never smoked and who had no other health problems, a 9.1-kg (20-lb) intentional weight loss in the previous year resulted in a 25 percent reduction in all-cause, cardiovascular, and cancer mortality. In 15,069 women of the same age with coexisting health problems, any amount of intentional weight loss resulted in a 10 percent decrease in cardiovascular disease, a 20 percent reduction in all-cause mortality, a 30 to 40 percent decrease in mortality related to diabetes mellitus, and a 40 to 50 percent reduction in mortality from cancers of the breast and colon.

℞ TREATMENT

Treatment of obesity should be undertaken with a clear understanding of the realities of the problem and its outcome. First, obesity is a chronic disease that is increasing in prevalence. Second, the etiology is usually unknown, making a cure unlikely and palliation the therapeutic goal. Third, both obesity and increased visceral fat increase health risks even when total-body weight and fat are not markedly elevated. Fourth, obesity is a stigmatized condition in which the overweight subject is frequently viewed as responsible for the condition. Fifth, treatment of obesity with medication suffers from the negative "amphetamine halo." The introduction of amphetamines for the treatment of obesity more than 50 years ago was soon followed by a spate of addictions and gave a bad name to the use of drugs of this type. The various drugs of this class, called β-phenethylamines, work through diverse mechanisms. Amphetamine releases norepinephrine and dopamine, whereas other drugs in this class either affect serotonin metabolism, norepinephrine metabolism, or both without influencing dopamine metabolism. Sixth, recidivism, i.e., weight regain, is common in obesity. Seventh, drugs and other treatments for obesity do not work unless they are used; when

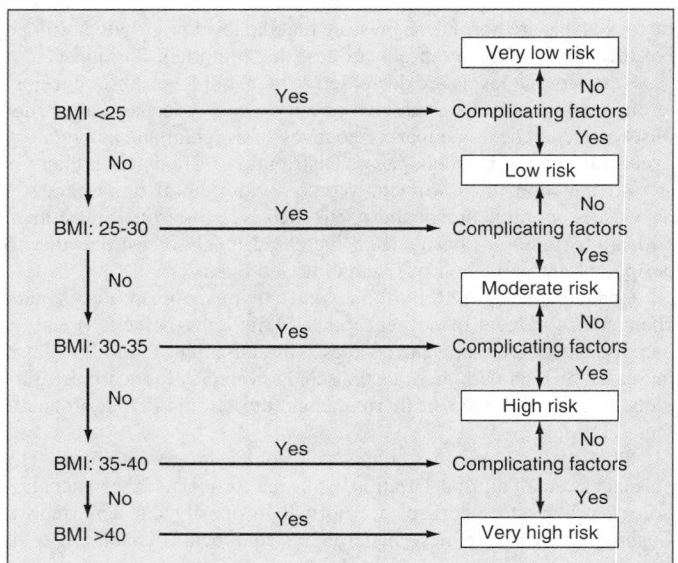

FIGURE 75-7 Risk classification algorithm. The patient is first placed into a category based on body mass index. The presence or absence of complicating factors determines the degree of health risk. Complicating factors include elevated abdominal-gluteal ratio (male: 0.95, female: 0.85), diabetes mellitus, hypertension, hyperlipidemia, male sex, and age < 40. (*Copyright 1987, George A. Bray. Used with permission.*)

appetite suppressing drugs are discontinued, patients regain weight, in keeping with the concept that the drugs do not cure obesity but only relieve its symptoms.

Selection of treatments can be made using the BMI as a guide and assessing the risks associated with obesity and central fat distribution (Fig. 75-7). Complicating factors include age; gender; comorbid conditions such as diabetes mellitus, hypertension, and hyperlipidemia; and a family history of hypertension, diabetes mellitus, or coronary heart disease. In young individuals under 40, especially men who have these risk factors or a positive family history, the need for treatment is more urgent.

Behavior Modification The principles of behavior modification provide the underpinnings for many current programs of weight reduction. The basic principles are those of operant conditioning and cognitive restructuring. Eating behavior is analyzed into its antecedents, the act of eating, and the consequences of eating by asking the patient to monitor and record these activities. The settings in which eating occurs, the eating event itself, and the use of rewards designed to change maladaptive behaviors are all monitored. Attempts are made to change thinking patterns from negative ones such as "I have just eaten that piece of cake, I am a bad person" into "I have just eaten a piece of cake, and now I need to go exercise" or other positive ways of solving the problem. Features of behavior modification of proven value in people who are successful in maintaining weight loss over an extended period of time include: (1) continued monitoring of food-related behaviors, (2) adoption of a low-fat diet, and (3) increased levels of physical activity.

Diet It is possible that increased dietary fat intake may be associated with increased risk of developing obesity in genetically susceptible subjects, and the prudent person should adopt a lower fat intake; the question is how low should this low-fat diet be? Extrapolation from experimental data suggests that a diet with fewer than 25 percent fat calories is a reasonable goal.

For anyone considering a weight-reducing diet, the quantity of food intake and the avoidance of settings in which excess quantities of high-fat food are eaten are equally important. Cafeterias and buffet meals are especially difficult. Controlling food intake is easier if the use of alcoholic beverages is reduced or eliminated, particularly since alcohol tends to blunt the ability to maintain other dietary controls. Increasing the frequency of eating is also a useful strategy. People who eat breakfast have a lower risk of developing obesity than individuals who do not. Ingestion of frequent small meals with relatively high carbohydrate and high fiber content is a way of decreasing fat intake and providing continued gastrointestinal fill.

Exercise Exercise is not good as a primary strategy for weight loss but is crucial in maintaining weight loss. Figure 75-8 illustrates the effect of adding exercise to a dietary program; of a group of men who completed an initial 8-week program, those who maintained an exercise program maintained the weight loss, whereas those who did not regained weight. This is clear demonstration of the importance of maintaining physical activity if body weight is to remain under control.

Use of Medication in the Management of Obesity Appetite-suppressing drugs may be useful but should be reserved for individuals with a BMI above 30 kg/m^2 or above 27 kg/m^2 if associated weight-related comorbid conditions are present. The options for pharmacologic intervention for obesity include several appetite-

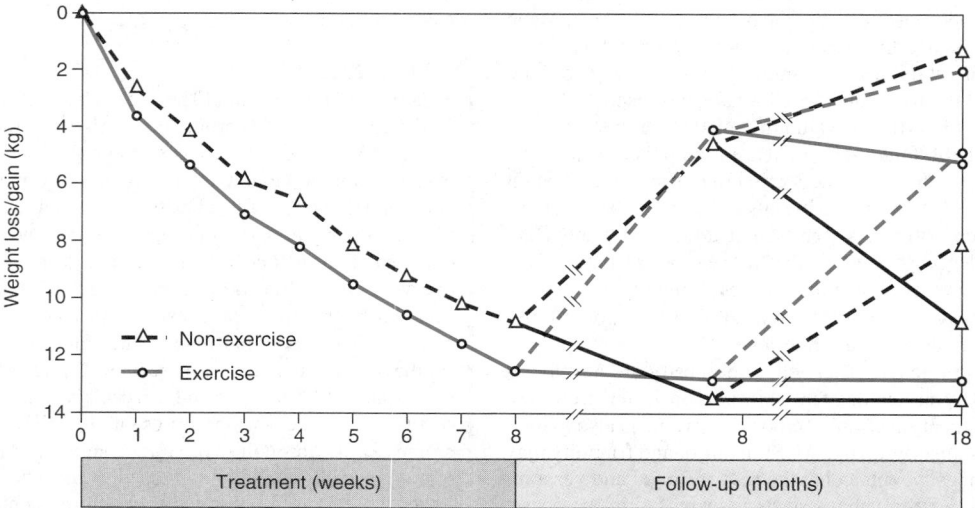

FIGURE 75-8 Weight loss and exercise. During the first 8 weeks, subjects were divided into two groups, one treated with diet and the other with diet plus exercise, with no difference in weight loss. Thereafter the subjects who exercised maintained better weight loss than those that did not. (*After Pavlou et al.*)

Table 75-7

Approved Appetite-Suppressing Drugs

	DEA Schedule	$t_{1/2}$, h	Tablet Size and Timing	Daily Dose Range, mg
NORADRENERGIC AGENTS				
Benzphetamine	III	6–12	25 or 50 mg before breakfast	25–50
Phendimetrazine	III	5–12	35 mg before meals or 105 mg (slow release) daily	17.5–105
Diethylpropion	IV	4–6	25 mg before meals;	25–75
			75 mg in A.M. (slow release)	75
Mazindol	IV	10	1 or 2 mg at noon	1–2
Phentermine HCI	IV	7–24	8 mg before meals	15–37.5
			15 or 37.5 mg before breakfast	
Phentermine resin	IV		15 or 30 mg resin before breakfast	15–30
Phenylpropanolamine	Not scheduled (OTC)		25 mg before meals	25–75
			75 mg (slow release) daily	
SEROTONERGIC AGENTS				
Dexfenfluramine	IV	11–30	15 mg bid	30
Fenfluramine	IV	11–30	20 mg before meals	60–120

NOTE: DEA, Drug Enforcement Agency; OTC, over the counter.

suppressing drugs. The drugs shown in Table 75-7 increase extraneuronal norepinephrine by enhancing its release (benzphetamine, phendimetrazine, phentermine, mazindol, and diethylpropion), or by blocking its uptake, by inhibiting alpha$_1$-adrenergic receptors (phenylpropanolamine), or by releasing serotonin and blocking its reuptake (fenfluramine). Data from the first 34 weeks of a 210-week trial of placebo versus a combination of fenfluramine and phentermine are shown in Fig. 75-9. The patients on the drug combination lost more than 15 percent of their initial body weight and maintained the loss for the first year of the study. Those initially on placebo who were switched to a drug at the end of 34 weeks also showed a drop in body weight. In some individuals weight did not decrease, indicating that some patients do not respond to this therapy.

The use of fenfluramine-phentermine combinations is associated with development of valvular heart disease, and fenfluramines, alone or in combination with other anorectic agents, can cause pulmonary hypertension. The possibility of neurotoxicity has not been excluded. Consequently, the only justifiable medical use of anorectic drugs is in seriously obese patients who have obesity-related illnesses such as coronary heart disease, diabetes mellitus, hypertension, and/or hyperlipidemia. Full disclosure of risks and benefits must be provided; patients must be monitored regularly with physical examinations and, when appropriate, echocardiography.

Surgery For individuals with a BMI above 35 kg/m^2 who have high risks for diabetes or family histories of early heart attacks and for individuals without these problems but with BMI above 40 kg/m^2, surgical manipulation of the gastrointestinal tract may be useful. A number of operative interventions have been used (Fig. 75-10). Data comparing different procedures suggest that the best long-term weight loss occurs with the gastric bypass operation in which a small upper pouch is attached by a Roux-en-Y anastomosis to the jejunum. Operative mortality is in the range of 0.1 to 0.5 percent. Weight regain and other problems are minimal with the Roux-en-Y operation and the vertically banded gastroplasty, the two recommended procedures.

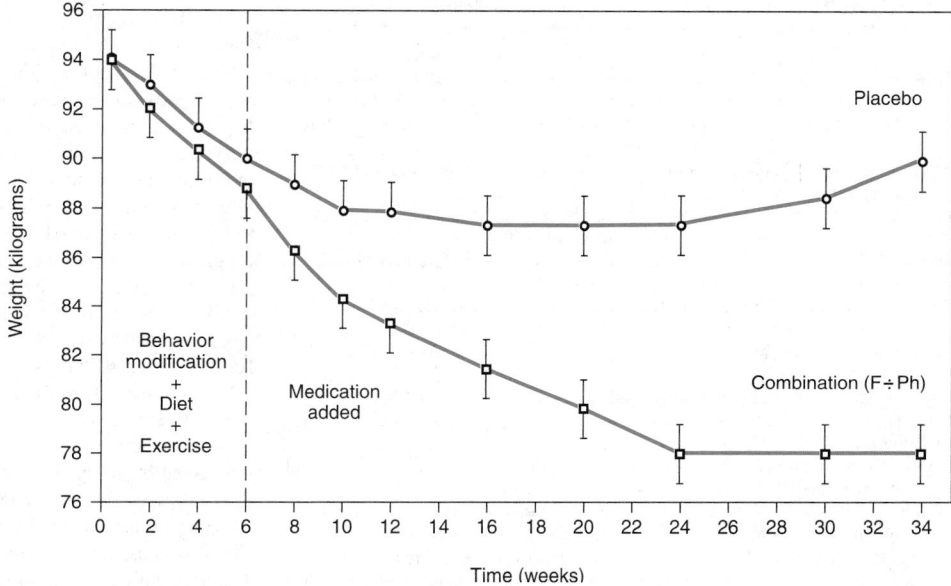

FIGURE 75-9 Double-blind randomized control comparison of placebo and combination drug therapy in treatment of obesity. During the first 6 weeks, both groups were given similar programs in behavior modification, diet, and exercise. At the end of this period, the double-blind period of drug treatment was begun. At the end of 34 weeks, the patients treated with the combination of fenfluramine (F) and phentermine (Ph) had lost significantly more weight than the placebo-treated controls. (*Weintraub M et al, reproduced with permission*).

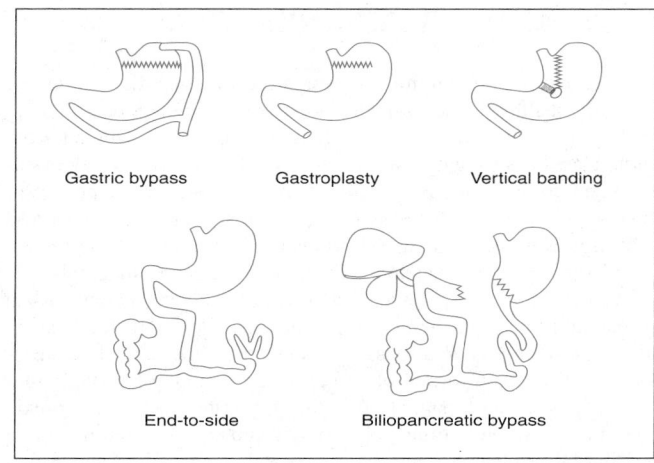

FIGURE 75-10 Examples of operative interventions used for surgical manipulation of the gastrointestinal tract.

BIBLIOGRAPHY

ANGEL A, BRAY GA: Synthesis of fatty acids and cholesterol by liver, adipose tissue and intestinal mucosa from obese and control patients. Eur J Clin Invest 9:355, 1979

ATKINSON RL et al: Weight cycling. JAMA 272:1196, 1994.

BALLOR DL, KEESEY RE: A meta-analysis of the factors affecting exercise-induced changes in body-mass, fat mass and fat-free mass in males and females. Int J Obes 15:717, 1991

BOUCHARD C (ed): *The Genetics of Obesity*. Boca Raton, FL, CRC Press, 1993

BRAY GA: Obesity, a disorder of nutrient partitioning: The MONA LISA hypothesis. J Nutr 121:1146, 1991

————: Evaluation of drugs for treating obesity. Obes Res 3:425S, 1995

CAMPFIELD LA et al: Mouse OB protein: Evidence for a peripheral signal linking adiposity and central neural networks. Science 269:546, 1995

CONNOLLY HM et al: Valvular heart disease associated with fenfluramine-phentermine. N Engl J Med 337:581, 1997

FOREYT JP et al: Psychological correlates of weight fluctuation. Int J Eating Dis 17:263, 1995

HALAAS JL et al: Weight-reducing effects of the plasma protein encoded by the obese gene. Science 269:543, 1995

KUCZMARSKI RJ et al: Increasing prevalence of overweight among US adults: The National Health and Nutrition Examination Surveys, 1960 to 1991. JAMA 272:205, 1994

LICHTMAN SW et al: Discrepancy between self-reported and actual caloric intake and exercise in obese subjects. N Engl J Med 327:1893, 1992

LISSNER L, HEITMANN BL: Dietary fat and obesity: Evidence from epidemiology. Eur J Clin Nutr 49:79, 1995

PAVLOU KN et al: Exercise as an adjunct to weight loss and maintenance in moderately obese subjects. Am J Clin Nutr 49:1115, 1989

PELLEYMOUNTER MA et al: Effects of the obese gene product on body weight regulation in ob/ob mice. Science 269:540, 1995

PORIES WJ et al: Surgical treatment of obesity and its effect on diabetes: 10-y follow-up. Am J Clin Nutr 55:S582, 1992

SCHAPIRA DV et al: Upper-body fat distribution and endometrial cancer risk. JAMA 266:1808, 1991

SJOSTROM LV: Morbidity of severely obese subjects. Am J Clin Nutr 55:508S, 1992

————: Mortality of severely obese subjects. Am J Clin Nutr 55:516S, 1992

WEINTRAUB M et al: Long term weight control study I (weeks 0–34). Clin Pharmacol Ther 31:486, 1992

WEST DB et al: Dietary obesity linked to genetic-loci on chromosome-9 and chromosome-15 in a polygenic mouse model. J Clin Invest 94:1410, 1994

WILLETT WC et al: Weight, weight change and coronary heart disease in women: Risk within the normal weight range. JAMA 273:461, 1995

WILLIAMSON DF et al: Prospective study of intentional weight-loss and mortality in never-smoking overweight US white women aged 40–64 years. Am J Epidemiol 141:1128, 1995

---

76   *Daniel W. Foster*

ANOREXIA NERVOSA AND BULIMIA NERVOSA

Anorexia nervosa and bulimia nervosa are eating disorders in young, previously healthy women who develop a paralyzing fear of becoming fat. The population at risk consists largely of white women from middle-class backgrounds. The disorders rarely occur in black or oriental women, in the poor, or in men. The driving force is the pursuit of thinness, all other aspects of life being secondary. In anorexia nervosa this aim is achieved primarily by radical restriction of food intake, the end result being emaciation. In bulimia massive binge eating is followed by vomiting and excessive use of laxatives. Weight loss in bulimic subjects is not great despite the obsession with food. Some authors consider the two disorders to be distinct illnesses, while others classify bulimia as a variant of anorexia nervosa. Overlap syndromes exist since emaciated patients fulfilling the criteria of true anorexia nervosa may exhibit bulimic behavior and subjects with bulimia often pass through a phase of anorexia. In this chapter it is assumed that the two disorders are different expressions of a psychological obsession with body weight.

PREVALENCE/INCIDENCE   The true prevalence and incidence of anorexia nervosa are not known. In high-risk populations, such as 16- to 18-year-old girls in private schools, the prevalence may be 1 percent, whereas public school girls of the same age have a prevalence of about 0.1 percent. In a study in Rochester, Minnesota, the prevalence was 0.2 percent in women and 0.02 percent in men. The probable prevalence is 0.2 to 1 percent in women and about one-tenth this level in men. The incidence rate (new case appearance), age- and sex-adjusted, was 7.3 per 100,000 population per year in the Rochester study.

The data for bulimia nervosa are even less satisfactory. A study in Ontario, Canada, suggested a lifetime prevalence in women of 1.1 percent and in men of 0.1 percent. All estimates of incidence are influenced by the cohort studied. For example, vomiting after eating occurs in up to 18 percent of women college students, a group in which incidence rates are high. Bulimia may now be more common than anorexia.

DIAGNOSIS   The diagnosis of both disorders is made on clinical grounds. The standards of the American Psychiatric Association have "softened" so that the diagnoses are now made more frequently. Criteria of the 1994 *Diagnostic and Statistical Manual of Mental Disorders* (DSM-IV) are given in Tables 76-1 and 76-2. The weight criterion for diagnosis is 85 percent or less than expected ideal weight. Although DSM-IV does not use the body mass index [weight in $kg/(height)^2$ in m], a body mass index of less than 18 is considered the threshold level for diagnosis. Amenorrhea is an invariable feature. Anorexia nervosa is thus the only psychiatric illness including a mandatory endocrine component. An expressed intense fear of gaining weight or becoming fat, even when underweight, and a disturbance of body image (the way the body is perceived by the patient) complete the diagnostic tetrad. Two subtypes of anorexia nervosa are specified: restricting and binge eating/purging. In the former, bulimic behavior is absent, while in the latter gorging and purging are components.

Diagnostic criteria for bulimia nervosa require that an amount of food be ingested that is greater than most people would eat in a similar period of time. The binge episodes must be accompanied by a feeling that eating is out of control and must occur at least twice a week for 3 months, and there must be evidence of compensatory behavior to keep weight down. Bulimic symptoms must not occur exclusively in the presence of anorexia nervosa, i.e., the patient is assigned to anorexia nervosa rather than bulimia nervosa if weight reduction is sustained. Finally, as in anorexia, distortion of body image is an essential feature. The two subtypes of bulimia nervosa are purging and nonpurging. Obsessive/compulsive behavior, self-mutilation, and antisocial behavior are not essential criteria although they occur more frequently in bulimia than in anorexia nervosa and in control populations.

Table 76-1

Diagnostic Criteria for Anorexia Nervosa

1. Refusal to maintain body weight at or above a minimally normal weight for age and height (e.g., weight loss leading to maintenance of body weight less than 85% of that expected; or failure to make expected weight gain during period of growth, leading to body weight less than 85% of that expected).
2. Intense fear of gaining weight or becoming fat, even though underweight.
3. Disturbance in the way in which one's body weight or shape is experienced, undue influence of body weight or shape on self-evaluation, or denial of the seriousness of the current body weight.
4. In postmenarchal females, amenorrhea, i.e., the absence of at least three consecutive menstrual cycles. [a woman is considered to have amenorrhea if her periods occur only following hormone (e.g., estrogen) administration.]

Specify type:

Restricting type: During the episode of anorexia nervosa the person does not regularly engage in binge-eating or purging behavior (i.e., self-induced vomiting or the misuse of laxatives, diuretics or enemas).

Binge eating/purging type: During the episode of anorexia nervosa, the person regularly engages in binge-eating or purging behavior (i.e., self-induced vomiting or the misuse of laxatives, diuretics or enemas).

SOURCE: From Diagnostic and Statistical Manual of Mental Disorders, 4th ed, Washington, DC, American Psychiatric Association, 1994.

Table 76-2

CHAPTER 76
Anorexia Nervosa and Bulimia Nervosa

463

Diagnostic Criteria for Bulimia Nervosa

1. Recurrent episodes of binge eating. An episode of binge eating is characterized by both of the following:
   a. Eating, in a discrete period of time (e.g., within any 2-h period), an amount of food that is definitely larger than most people would eat during a similar period of time and under similar circumstances.
   b. A sense of lack of control over eating during the episode (e.g., a feeling that one cannot stop eating or control what or how much one is eating).
2. Recurrent inappropriate compensatory behavior to prevent weight gain, such as self-induced vomiting, misuse of laxatives, diuretics, or other medications; fasting; or excessive exercise.
3. The binge eating and inappropriate compensatory behaviors both occur, on average, at least twice a week for 3 months.
4. Self-evaluation is unduly influenced by body shape and weight.
5. The disturbance does not occur exclusively during episodes of anorexia nervosa.

Specify type:
  Purging type: the person regularly engages in self-induced vomiting or the misuse of laxatives or diuretics.
  Nonpurging type: the person uses other inappropriate compensatory behaviors, such as fasting or excessive exercise, but does not regularly engage in self-induced vomiting or the misuse of laxatives or diuretics.

SOURCE: From Diagnostic and Statistical Manual of Mental Disorders, 4th ed, Washington, DC, American Psychiatric Association, 1994.

The diagnostic value of a disturbed perception of body image in patients with eating disorders has been questioned because many normal women evidence the same perceptual distortion. In practice a presumptive diagnosis of anorexia nervosa is justified if the following elements are present: (1) major weight loss; (2) absence of organic disease to account for weight loss; (3) absence of primary psychiatric illness that might account for failure to eat; (4) extreme restriction of food intake, with or without intermittent vomiting; (5) ritualized exercise; and (6) denial of hunger, fatigue, or emaciation. Late-onset disease is also now recognized, although usually symptoms begin in the teen years or early adulthood. While there is an emphasis on the absence of organic disease to cause weight loss, anorexia nervosa may coexist with other conditions that can cause loss of weight such as insulin-dependent diabetes mellitus.

The diagnosis of bulimia nervosa is secure if there is: (1) binge eating without major weight loss; (2) evidence of induced vomiting or regular use of laxatives or diuretics; (3) obsessive/compulsive behavior, antisocial activity or self-mutilation.

ETIOLOGY The cause of the eating disorders is unknown. Although primary dysfunction of the hypothalamus has been postulated, the recognized hypothalamic abnormalities revert to normal with weight gain and thus are secondary.

A psychiatric etiology is likely, but its nature is unclear. One view holds that the disorders begin in response to inadequate or destructive interpersonal relationships in families that are goal-oriented and highly achieving. Despite an outward normal appearance, interpersonal communications within such families tend to be inadequate, frequently following a pattern in which the father seeks success in work and the mother turns to the children for fulfillment and in the process becomes overdirective. Such families are said to be *enmeshed*, meaning that generational boundaries are blurred and that parents and children are deeply involved in each other's lives. Some investigators have suggested that sexual abuse plays a role, but this is controversial. Psychoanalytic interpretation tends to focus on anorexia as the mechanism whereby the patient reestablishes control of her own life independent of parental direction. It is not clear how this sequence might cause the intense fear of being fat that is central to both anorexia and bulimia. It is usually presumed that bulimia is a "backup" response in subjects at risk for anorexia but whose restrictive control fails.

The absence of serious psychiatric disease was previously required for the diagnosis of eating disorders, but depression and obsessive/compulsive behavior frequently accompany the disorders, especially bulimia. These abnormalities may be secondary or preexistent states that predispose to development of the eating disorder.

Some studies have suggested that a genetic component may be involved in the pathogenesis (e.g., increased prevalence of eating disorders in first-degree relatives of probands). Such a genetic component, if it exists, must be minor.

Cultural issues are important. The quest for health and slimness is a powerful force in modern society and may reinforce the fear of fatness in patients with an eating disorder or tip the borderline case into overt disease. Occupation may play a role. Dancers have a prevalence of anorexia nervosa 10 times that of the general population, and athletes, particularly runners, often seek to decrease body fat to very low levels (5 to 7 percent of body weight).

The defects that cause eating disorders remain obscure. There is some evidence of dysfunction in serotonin-mediated neurotransmission, thought to be a component of the satiety-signaling system. The peptide *leptin* (a product of the *ob* gene) is released into blood from adipose tissue and inhibits formation or release in the hypothalamus of neuropeptide Y, a powerful feeding signal. Serotonin may function as a neurotransmitter linking leptin and neuropeptide Y inhibition. Serotonin uptake inhibitors may be helpful in anorexia nervosa and in bulimia nervosa (see "Treatment"). Leptin levels have not been measured in either anorexia or bulimia.

CLINICAL FEATURES (Table 76-3). **Anorexia Nervosa** Anorexia nervosa usually begins before or shortly after puberty but may appear later (usually by the middle twenties). Many patients were overweight in childhood. Emaciation is similar to that in the concentration camp victims of World War II. Despite profound weight loss patients deny hunger, thinness, or fatigue. They are often physically active, and ritualized exercise is common. Frenzied calisthenics or running may follow food intake. There is preoccupation with food, and elaborate meals may be prepared for others. If social circumstances or binge eating causes more intake than usual, vomiting is induced as soon as possible, often in a public restroom. Constipation is common. Amenorrhea usually accompanies or follows weight loss but may appear prior to any physical change. Cold intolerance is presumably due to a defect in regulatory thermogenesis secondary to hypothalamic dysfunction.

In advanced cases bradycardia, hypothermia, and hypotension are present. Body fat is undetectable, and the bones protrude through the skin. Interestingly, breast tissue is often preserved. The skin may be

Table 76-3

The Eating Disorders

	Anorexia Nervosa	Bulimia
Predominant sex	Female	Female
Method of weight control	Restriction of intake	Vomiting
Binge eating	Uncommon	Invariant
Weight at diagnosis	Markedly decreased	Near normal
Ritualized exercise	Usual	Rare
Amenorrhea	100%	50%
Other endocrine changes	Common	Uncommon
Antisocial behavior	Rare	Frequent
Cardiovascular changes (bradycardia, hypotension)	Common	Uncommon
Skin changes (hirsutism, dryness, carotenemia)	Usual	Rare
Hypothermia	Usual	Rare
Edema	+/−	+/−
Medical complications	Hypokalemia, cardiac arrhythmias	Hypokalemia, cardiac arrhythmias, aspiration of gastric contents, esophageal or gastric rupture

NOTE: These features are characteristic of pure anorexia nervosa and pure bulimia. Overlap syndromes occur, and anorexia may evolve to bulimia. The bulimia→anorexia transformation is rare (see text).

dry and scaly and is often yellow due to carotenemia (particularly visible in the palms). Body hair is often increased and is usually of fine, lanugo quality, but frank hirsutism may occur. Parotid glands may be enlarged as in other forms of starvation. Mitral valve prolapse is due to valve–ventricular volume mismatch secondary to starvation-induced decrease in left ventricular volume. Edema in the absence of hypoalbuminemia is thought to be due to failure of extracellular fluid volume to contract proportionately with body mass during weight loss. Because of edema in the legs and parotid enlargement, which gives a fullness to the face, the true state of emaciation may be masked when the patient is dressed.

Laboratory abnormalities include anemia and leukopenia (with hypocellularity of the bone marrow), hypokalemia, and hypoalbuminemia. Serum β-carotene levels tend to be elevated. Vomiting and/or laxative use may cause prerenal azotemia with blood urea nitrogen levels as high as 21 to 25 mmol/L (60 to 70 mg/dL). Renal concentrating ability is impaired, possibly due to blunted responsiveness to vasopressin or diminished release of vasopressin in response to osmotic stimuli. Basal atrial natriuretic peptide levels are high and do not increase with saline infusion. Plasma cholesterol is occasionally high, but triglyceride levels are normal. Glucose tolerance is abnormal as in other forms of starvation. Additional abnormalities include low levels of IgG, IgM, and a variety of complement proteins. Despite these findings, immune function is generally preserved and serious infection is rare. Plasma iron and ceruloplasmin levels are normal, but iron-binding capacity is decreased. Serum zinc and copper are decreased, but levels of these metals are normal in hair. Serum amylase may be increased in the absence of pancreatitis.

Basal levels of luteinizing hormone (LH) and follicle stimulating hormone (FSH) are low when weight loss is severe, and the LH response to luteinizing hormone–releasing hormone (LHRH) is impaired. FSH response to LHRH is normal, although time to peak increase may be delayed. Studies of the 24-h circadian pattern of LH secretion show regression of the mature stage to the pattern characteristic of prepubertal or early pubertal girls, i.e., episodic LH release is missing or occurs only during sleep. These findings presumably account for the amenorrhea. Menses return with weight gain, although the weight required for reinitiation of menstruation may be somewhat higher (about 10 percent) than that needed for the original induction of menarche. Ovulatory menses may be induced in subjects with anorexia nervosa by appropriate treatment with LHRH agonists, suggesting that pituitary gonadotropin release is impaired because of hypothalamic dysfunction. Prolactin levels are normal. Plasma estradiol levels are low. Plasma testosterone is normal in women and low in men with anorexia nervosa.

Growth hormone (GH) may be normal or elevated in the basal state. A rise in GH occurs after injection of thyrotropin releasing hormone (TRH), as in other states with elevated basal levels of GH such as acromegaly, uremia, and protein-calorie malnutrition. Levels of insulin-like growth factor I are low and may contribute to growth hormone elevation via diminished negative feedback. Plasma cortisol levels are high due to increased secretion of corticotropin-releasing hormone from the hypothalamus because of impairment of negative feedback by cortisol. The suppression of plasma cortisol by dexamethasone and the stimulation of GH release by dexamethasone are both abnormal in many patients.

Levels of total thyroxine (T_4) and free T_4 are normal. Triiodothyronine (T_3) concentrations are reduced, while reverse T_3 (rT_3) levels are increased. Basal levels of thyroid stimulating hormone (TSH) and TSH response to TRH are normal. The primary defect in thyroid hormone metabolism is decreased activity of the $5'$-deiodinase that converts T_4 to T_3 and converts rT_3 to diiodothyronine in nonthyroidal tissues; these changes are characteristic of wasting diseases and are not specific for anorexia nervosa. Bone density is decreased; the mechanism has been thought to be estrogen deficiency, but estrogen replacement therapy does not restore bone density. Cortisol excess may contribute to bone loss. Plasma norepinephrine levels are decreased.

Bulimia Nervosa Bulimia, which means "ox-hunger," refers to the episodic, compulsive ingestion of large amounts of food, coupled with awareness that the eating is abnormal, a fear that eating cannot be stopped voluntarily, and feelings of depression at completion of the act. Bulimic patients have a morbid fear of becoming fat. While binge eating may occur in several types of emotional disorders, bulimic patients frequently give a history of overt or cryptic anorexia nervosa, suggesting that bulimia is a variant response to the same factors that cause anorexia nervosa. Episodes of binge eating are followed by induced vomiting, with or without the subsequent ingestion of laxatives. Initially vomiting is induced by placing a toothbrush or fingers in the throat or by ingestion of ipecac, but most patients learn to vomit reflexly. Bloating, flatulence, constipation, abdominal pain, borborygmi, and nausea are common.

Binge eating generally occurs daily; in one study the mean number of episodes per week was 12, ranging from 1 to 46, and the duration of the eating periods averaged 1.2 h but could last as long as 8 h. The amount of food ingested may be enormous, up to 200,000 kJ (50,000 kcal). High-carbohydrate foods are favored, and more than one food is usually eaten. The order of frequency in one report was: ice cream→bread→candy→doughnuts→soft drinks. The term *dietary chaos* describes the eating pattern. Because of the high-carbohydrate content of the diet, dental caries are frequent.

Secrecy about the eating-vomiting sequence is characteristic so that family and friends are often unaware. Stealing is common, and food is the item most often taken. There is a high rate of alcohol and drug abuse. Self-mutilation is not unusual and may be a manifestation of obsessive/compulsive disorder. Depression tends to be more severe than in anorexia nervosa, making suicide a definite risk. Hysterical behavior may occur. Families of patients with bulimia have a higher incidence of affective disorders, alcoholism, and illicit drug use than families of patients with anorexia nervosa.

Despite the close relationship with anorexia nervosa, a number of differences are noted. While many patients with bulimia are thin, weight is usually within 15 percent of the normal range as defined by ideal weight tables. Fluctuating weight is common, with cyclical gains and losses. Some patients are modestly overweight. In contrast to anorexia nervosa, many patients continue to menstruate and may become pregnant. Persistent menstruation probably reflects the absence of extreme weight loss. Sexual activity is greater in bulimic subjects than in those with anorexia.

The physical findings in bulimia nervosa are usually minimal. Scars from self-mutilation may be present and should be looked for in every patient.

The most common laboratory abnormality is hypokalemia secondary to vomiting and laxative use. Metabolic alkalosis may occur if potassium loss is significant. Endocrine changes are less prominent than in anorexia nervosa and may be absent. Some patients have deficient secretion of serotonin and cholecystokinin, the significance of which is unknown. Dexamethasone suppression of plasma cortisol is frequently abnormal. Unlike anorexia nervosa patients, some women with bulimia have low basal prolactin levels and an exaggerated prolactin response to TRH. Serum amylase may be elevated in the absence of pancreatitis in bulimia, as in anorexia nervosa.

COMPLICATIONS Patients with anorexia nervosa are vulnerable to sudden death from ventricular tachyarrhythmias. Electrocardiograms show prolonged QT intervals. The risk of death becomes high when weight declines 35 percent below ideal, probably because of protein deficiency. Complications of bulimia include aspiration, esophageal or gastric rupture, pneumomediastinum, hypokalemia with cardiac arrhythmias, pancreatitis, and ipecac-induced myopathy and/or cardiomyopathy.

PROGNOSIS The course of anorexia nervosa is variable. In long-term follow-up about half of patients achieve normal weight, 20 percent improve but remain underweight, 20 percent continue anorexic, 5 percent become obese, and 6 percent die. Even when weight gain occurs, binge eating, vomiting, and laxative use persist in up to two-thirds of patients. Death is usually due to starvation (cardiac arrhythmias primarily) or suicide. Poor prognostic signs include older age of onset, long duration of illness, bulimia or vomiting, extreme weight loss, and significant depression. Few long-term follow-up reports are available for bulimia. Because the psychiatric disturbance tends to be more severe (suicide occurs at high rates) and because of the medical dangers of gorging, prognosis is worse in bulimia than in anorexia. As many as 40 percent of treated patients remain bulimic after 18 months of treatment; relapse occurs in about two-thirds within a year of recovery. One study reported that about half of patients with bulimia still had an eating disorder after 5 years.

℞ TREATMENT

There is no specific treatment for anorexia nervosa or bulimia. The intense fear of becoming fat and the perceptual disturbance that causes overestimation of body size result in powerful resistance to therapy. The benefits of psychiatric intervention, behavior modification techniques, and group and family therapy are marginal. Supportive care by an understanding physician may accomplish as much as formal psychotherapy. The patient should be seen regularly for a review of weight change, diet, and exercise patterns. It is useful to establish a mutually agreeable explicit contract; for example, if the patient weighs 30 kg and ideal body weight is 52 kg, a goal of 40 kg might be set as a first stage. At every visit the patient should be reassured by the physician that "we will not let you get fat." A calm but realistic review of the dangers of starvation, including sudden death, should be given, coupled with statements like "my job is to help you deal with this illness so that you can have a normal life expectancy with reasonable happiness." The physician must be perceived not as an enemy or a parental surrogate but as an advisor and partner in the struggle.

A similar approach should also be used with bulimic patients. Even if the gorging-regurgitation cycle cannot be stopped, the lesser goals of limiting the load of food ingested (to minimize the chance of aspiration or gastric rupture) and decreasing the frequency of events may be achieved. Because depression and antisocial behavior are more common in bulimia, psychiatric therapy is sometimes required.

The issue of drug therapy is not settled. There is a general belief that antidepressants are helpful in bulimia nervosa but not anorexia nervosa. The serotonin uptake inhibitor fluoxetine may have an advantage over other antidepressants, and some reports suggest it is useful in anorexia as well. If used, a dose of 60 mg/d is suggested in adults instead of the usual dosages recommended for depression. Potassium supplementation may be necessary in vomiters or laxative users. Treatment of endocrine abnormalities is ordinarily not required since all revert if weight gain is achieved.

Hospitalization may be a lifesaving measure with severe anorexia nervosa. As noted above, sudden death may occur at weights more than 35 percent below ideal, particularly if weight loss has been rapid. Hypokalemia, hypotension, and prerenal azotemia due to volume depletion are other indications for hospitalization. A nasogastric tube may be required, but it is better to persuade the patient to eat. Total parenteral nutrition is rarely indicated. During initial hospitalization the patient should not be allowed to eat alone. Instruction about nutrition, occupational therapy, group therapy with the family, and individual psychotherapy may be useful. The "safety" of eating and assurances that obesity will not result should be emphasized repeatedly. Some specialists feel that all seriously affected anorexia patients benefit from initial hospitalization, but this view is not universal. Hospitalization for bulimic subjects is normally required only for medical complications (e.g., aspiration).

Treatment of the anorexia-bulimia syndromes is a long-term proposition, rife with failure, and requires perseverance by the patient, family, and physician.

BIBLIOGRAPHY

Foster DW: Eating disorders: Obesity, anorexia nervosa and bulimia nervosa in *Williams Textbook of Endocrinology*, 8th ed, JD Wilson, DW Foster (eds). Philadelphia, Saunders, 1992, p 1335

Garfinkel PE et al: Bulimia nervosa in a Canadian community sample: Prevalence and comparison of subgroups. Am J Psychiatry 152:1052, 1995
Herzog DB, Copeland PM: Eating disorders. N Engl J Med 313:295, 1985
——— et al: Outcome in anorexia nervosa and bulimia nervosa. A review of the literature. J Nerv Ment Dis 176:131, 1988
Isner JM et al: Anorexia nervosa and sudden death. Ann Intern Med 102:49, 1985
Kaye WH, Weltzin TE: Neurochemistry of bulimia nervosa. J Clin Psychiatry Suppl 52:21, 1991
Levy AB: Neuroendocrine profile in bulimia nervosa. Biol Psychiatry 25:98, 1989
Love L, Gold PW: The hypothalamic-pituitary-adrenal axis in anorexia nervosa and bulimia nervosa: Pathophysiologic implications. Adv Pediatr 38:287, 1991
Lucas ARE et al: Anorexia nervosa in Rochester, Minnesota: A 45-year study. Mayo Clin Proc 63:433, 1988
Mitchell JE et al: Medical complications and medical management of bulimia. Ann Intern Med 107:71, 1987
Newman MM, Halmi KA: The endocrinology of anorexia nervosa and bulimia nervosa. Endocrin Metab Clin North Am 7:195, 1988
Sullivan PF: Mortality in anorexia nervosa. Am J Pychiatry 152:1073, 1995
Thiel A et al: Obsessive-compulsive disorder among patients with anorexia nervosa and bulimia nervosa. Am J Psychiatry 152:72, 1995
Woodside DB: A review of anorexia nervosa and bulimia nervosa. Curr Probl Pediatr 25:67, 1995

---

77 | *Cheryl L. Rock, Ann M. Coulston, Mack T. Ruffin IV*

DIET THERAPY

Diet is an important component of health. Nutrition education and good eating patterns are essential for good health, nutritional problems contribute substantially to preventable illness and premature death, and alteration in food intake or dietary pattern is often an essential part of disease management. Nutritional requirements may be modified by disease, and dietary problems have an impact on the quality of life and the outcome of both acute and chronic diseases. For example, diet therapy plays a role both in the prevention of atherosclerosis and in the management of advanced coronary artery disease. Furthermore, major nutritional consequences can result from the treatment of disease, but nutrition and diet therapy are often of concern to the patient and the family, even when there is no solid evidence to support such therapy. In general, the usefulness of both new and traditional therapeutic diets deserves additional scientific scrutiny. As is true with all components of care, diet therapy should be soundly based and should be monitored to assess its impact on nutrition and health.

The first concept in diet therapy is that dietary intake or nutritional requirements may be altered as a result of disease or by the treatment (see Chap. 73), and the altered needs must be met by dietary modifications to prevent malnutrition. The second concept is that nutritional intervention can be critical for prevention, management, or treatment of disease. A complicating factor is that people eat food, rather than nutrients, so that the practical and psychosocial aspects of diet modification must be considered in making recommendations. Diet therapy is rarely an innocuous intervention, and adverse physical and psychological effects can result from inappropriate or ill-advised modification of the diet.

The aims of this chapter are to summarize the basic principles of diet therapy, to describe its application in common conditions, and to outline strategies for enhancing adherence to dietary recommendations.

BASIC DIETARY RECOMMENDATIONS

Variety, balance, and moderation are the basic components of dietary adequacy. The food guidance system developed by the U.S. Department of Agriculture and the Department of Health and Human Services is based on the "Dietary Guidelines for Americans," which emphasizes eating more grain products, vegetables, and fruits; eating less fat, saturated fat, and cholesterol; and choosing a diet moderate in sugars and sodium. By grouping foods into categories based on nutrient content, these guidelines can be translated into dietary prescriptions that meet nutritional requirements at different levels of energy intake (Table 77-1). The lower level of energy intake is usually appropriate for sedentary women and many older adults; the moderate level is for teenage girls, active women, and sedentary men; and the higher level is for teenage boys, many active men, and very active women. Alcohol contributes energy but little else nutritionally, and consumption should be no more than one to two drinks per day in adults who choose to drink.

Table 77-1

Sample Diets to Meet Daily Nutrient Requirements and Dietary Guidelines

Food Group Category	Level of Energy Intake		
	Low, 1600 kcal/d	Moderate, 2200 kcal/d	High, 2800 kcal/d
Bread/starch group servings 1 slice bread, 1 ounce ready-to-eat cereal, 1/2 cup cooked rice or pasta	6	9	11
Vegetable group servings 1 cup raw leafy vegetables, 1/2 cup other vegetables, cooked or chopped raw	3	4	5
Fruit group servings 1 medium piece, 1/2 cup chopped, cooked, or canned fruit	2	3	4
Milk group servings 1 cup milk or yogurt	2–3*	2–3*	2–3*
Meat or meat substitute group† (ounces)	5	6	7
Total fat‡ (grams)	53	73	93
Total added sugars§ (teaspoons)	6	12	18

* Women who are pregnant or breast feeding, teenagers, and young adults to age 24 need 3 servings.
† Meat group amounts are in total ounces. One egg, 1/2 cup cooked dry beans, or 2 tablespoons peanut butter are equivalent to 1 ounce cooked lean meat, poultry, or fish.
‡ Fats are mainly contributed by choices within the milk and meat groups and from added fats (1 teaspoon, considered one serving, provides 5 g fat).
§ Sugars are mainly contributed by choices within the bread, fruit, and milk groups and from added sugars.
SOURCE: Adapted from Human Nutrition Information Service, US Department of Agriculture, *The Food Guide Pyramid*, Hyattsville, MD US Dept of Agriculture, 1992

Table 77-2

Average Nutrient Values per Serving

Food Group	Energy, kcal	Carbohydrate, g	Protein, g	Fat, g
Bread/starch	80	15	3	1 or less
Vegetable	25	5	2	—
Fruit	60	15	—	—
Milk				
Skim	90	12	8	0–3
Low-fat	120	12	8	5
Whole	150	12	8	8
Meat and meat substitutes				
Very lean	35	—	7	0–1
Lean	55	—	7	3
Medium-fat	75	—	7	5
High-fat	100	—	7	8
Fat	45	—	—	5

SOURCE: Adapted from The American Diabetes Association, Inc, The American Dietetic Association, *Exchange Lists for Weight Management*, Chicago, American Dietetic Association, 1995

This food group system can also form the basis of meal planning in diet therapy because energy and macronutrient content can be estimated on the basis of standardized serving sizes (Table 77-2).

SPECIFIC DIET THERAPIES

CARDIOVASCULAR DISEASE (See also Chaps. 242 and 341) Atherosclerotic cardiovascular disease (CVD) has multiple etiologies and involves a variety of risk factors. Modifiable risk factors include smoking, hypertension, hyperlipidemia, glucose intolerance, obesity, and physical inactivity. Elevation of plasma cholesterol, especially of low-density lipoprotein (LDL) cholesterol, is a major risk factor that can be at least partially modified by dietary intervention. The National Cholesterol Education Program (NCEP) has identified low risk as a total serum cholesterol concentration <5.2 mmol/L (200 mg/dL), moderate risk as 5.2 to 6.2 mmol/L (200 to 239 mg/dL), and high risk as >6.2 mmol/L (240 mg/dL). Hypertriglyceridemia and low levels of high-density lipoprotein (HDL) cholesterol are also risk factors. The basic diet therapy for patients with elevations of LDL cholesterol involves reduction in the intake of total and saturated fat to <30 percent and <10 percent of total calories, respectively. Sources of saturated fat include animal fats (fatty meat, poultry skin, butterfat) and some vegetable fats (coconut oil, cocoa butter, and palm oil). Cholesterol, found only in foods of animal origin, is not as important a determinant of plasma cholesterol as is saturated fat. Nevertheless, dietary intake of cholesterol should be <300 mg/d. In patients whose serum cholesterol does not respond to this degree of diet modification, the NCEP step 2 diets, which involve a greater restriction of saturated fat and cholesterol intake, should be prescribed (Table 77-3).

Obesity is also a risk factor for CVD (see also Chap. 75). For every excess kilogram of body weight, endogenous cholesterol synthesis is increased by 20 mg/d, so that with 10 kg of excess weight, 200 mg of additional cholesterol enters the body pool daily to be catabolized, excreted, or stored. Obesity is also associated with hypertriglyceridemia, decreased HDL-cholesterol, increased production of LDL from very low density lipoproteins (VLDL), and increased hepatic synthesis of VLDL. The insulin resistance associated with obesity and the resulting hyperinsulinemia improve with even modest (5 to 10 kg) weight reduction.

In some patients restriction of total dietary fat lowers HDL cholesterol and raises serum triglyceride concentrations. A decrease in HDL cholesterol is a cause for concern, especially when the baseline level is low [<0.9 mmol/L (35 mg/dL)]; the phenomenon appears to be related primarily to increased intake of carbohydrate and possibly to increased polyunsaturated fats. Monounsaturated oils (e.g., canola, olive, peanut) maintain HDL cholesterol and lower LDL cholesterol concentration, and when saturated fat is reduced to <10 percent of calories and monounsaturated fats make up the remainder of fat, a significant reduction in total cholesterol can be achieved without decreasing the total fat intake or increasing the proportion of calories

Table 77-3

Dietary Modifications for Hypercholesterolemia

Dietary Component	Step 1 Diet	Step 2 Diet
Total fat	<30% of kcal	<30% of kcal
Saturated fat	8–10% of kcal	<7% of kcal
Polyunsaturated fat	<10% of kcal	<10% of kcal
Monounsaturated fat	10–15% of kcal	10–15% of kcal
Carbohydrate	50–60% of kcal	50–60% of kcal
Protein	10–20% of kcal	10–20% of kcal
Cholesterol	<300 mg/d	<200 mg/d
Total energy intake	To achieve and maintain desirable weight	To achieve and maintain desirable weight

SOURCE: Adapted from US Department of Health and Human Services, *Step by Step: Eating to Lower Your High Blood Cholesterol*, publication no. 94-2920, Bethesda, MD, National Heart, Lung, and Blood Institute, 1994

from carbohydrate. These patients should be advised to substitute monounsaturated for saturated fat.

It has been suggested that trans-fatty acids are a risk factor for CVD. Trans-fatty acids are formed when vegetable oils are hydrogenated to be solid at room temperature. Margarine is the most significant source of trans-fatty acids in the U.S. diet. Consumption of trans-fatty acids in amounts >7 percent of calories may cause a significant increase in total and LDL cholesterol levels and a decrease in HDL cholesterol. However, the effect is a graded one, and intakes typical of the United States (≤4 percent of calories as trans-fatty acids) do not appear to have a deleterious effect. Consequently, patients need not be concerned about this issue at present.

Fish oils with polyunsaturated fats of the omega-3 type have potent triglyceride-lowering effects but do not lower LDL cholesterol. Any antiatherogenic effects of fish and fish oil consumption are probably mediated through the antithrombotic and anti-inflammatory actions of omega-3 fatty acids. Omega-3 fatty acids are sometimes useful in the treatment of hypertriglyceridemia (see Chap. 341).

Effective diet therapy for CVD should not rely on a "good food versus bad food" approach but should aim to modify the eating habits to attain desirable body weight and to reduce intake of saturated fatty acids. There are approaches to fit most lifestyles and to enhance compliance to life-long dietary changes necessary to the achieve this goal. To prevent cardiovascular disease, diet therapy is the first line of intervention, and pharmacologic agents are only adjunctive therapy.

Hypertension (See also Chap. 246) Elevated blood pressure increases the risk for CVD and stroke. Although not all hypertensive patients are salt-sensitive, dietary sodium should be reduced to 2000 mg/d routinely. Even modest amounts of weight reduction in the obese may reduce elevated blood pressure.

Congestive Heart Failure (See also Chap. 233) Cardiac cachexia is a type of malnutrition that occurs in patients with congestive heart failure and is due to reduced cardiac output, small bowel changes that lead to malabsorption, anorexia, and hypermetabolism secondary to increased work of breathing. Dietary intake is limited because of fatigue and early satiety with eating. Diet therapy involves the provision of adequate calories, protein, and other nutrients and the restriction of fluid (to 1 to 1.5 L/d) and sodium (to 1000 to 2000 mg/d).

CANCER Dietary factors influence survival rates in patients with certain malignancies, such as breast cancer. A possible link between diet and the risk for cancer has also been suggested but has been difficult to prove for cancers of the breast, colon, and prostate. For example, dietary factors that may increase risk for cancer, such as fat, tend to vary inversely with potentially protective factors, such as carotenoids. In addition, people on high-fat diets usually eat fewer vegetables and fruits and thus consume less of the protective factors contributed by those foods. As another example, dietary fat appears to increase and fiber appears to decrease the risk for colon cancer, and these usually have inverse concentrations in foods. Table 77-4 summarizes dietary practices that may reduce risk for some cancers.

Weight loss with cancer has many causes. The metabolic and

energy requirements of the tumor may promote weight loss by the host. Circulating factors (e.g., cytokines) originating either in the host or tumor are also probably involved in weight loss, but decreased food intake, frequently associated with anorexia, plays a major role in most patients. Indeed, many cancer patients have manifestations of malnutrition at the time of initial diagnosis, as evidenced by weight loss, weakness, anemia, and abnormalities in protein, lipid, and carbohydrate metabolism. However, in some cancers (breast and prostate cancer, melanoma) weight loss occurs late in the course.

The effects of chemotherapy, immunotherapy, and radiotherapy on dietary intake and nutritional status include nausea and vomiting, diarrhea, constipation, change in taste, sore or dry mouth, and dental problems. Surgical interventions may cause difficulties in chewing and swallowing, dumping syndrome, or malabsorption. Anorexia is the most common problem in the cancer patient, and agents such as megestrol acetate, glucocorticoids, hydrazine sulfate, and dronabinol may enhance appetite to some degree. Individual patients sometimes have distinct circadian patterns of appetite and anorexia that are identifiable by careful evaluation of food preferences and eating patterns. Dietary strategies to increase appetite or intake include providing salty foods, nutrient-dense beverages such as fruit juice, and easy-to-eat snacks. Attractive meals and snacks should be provided when appetite is good, and liquid food supplements can be administered when appetite is poor.

Nausea and vomiting in cancer patients may be related to the primary tumor (i.e., obstruction), to metastatic disease (i.e., central nervous system involvement), or to chemotherapy. In patients with reduced capacity of the stomach, small frequent feedings may circumvent early satiety and improve nutrition. One strategy that reduces both food aversions and nausea during chemotherapy is the ingestion of a diet composed primarily of low-stimuli (i.e., odorless, colorless) foods served cold or at room temperature. Mucositis and stomatitis in patients with head and neck cancers may be managed with diets that minimize oral irritation and ease swallowing difficulties. Diarrhea can also be minimized with dietary modifications (discussed below).

Criteria for instituting nutrition support (see Chap. 78) in cancer patients are progressive weight loss or the threat of serious weight loss. Although some features of cancer cachexia may be improved by parenteral or enteral feeding, few studies document improvement in body composition or disease outcome. One exception may be in patients undergoing surgery for cancer because the risks for complications of surgery are increased in the malnourished.

DIABETES MELLITUS (See also Chap. 334) Diabetes mellitus results from an absolute or relative lack of insulin, which regulates key aspects of carbohydrate, protein, and lipid metabolism, and diabetes is associated with accelerated atherogenesis and a high incidence of CVD. About 10 percent of patients have type 1 diabetes, manifested by a profound deficiency of endogenous insulin, and most of the rest have type 2 diabetes, in which endogenous insulin is synthesized but is insufficient to overcome peripheral insulin resistance. All patients with diabetes require diet therapy in conjunction with medication and exercise to achieve optimal control of blood glucose and blood lipids. The aim of therapy is to prevent acute complications (primarily hypoglycemia and hyperglycemia) and reduce the risk of long-term complications such as ophthalmopathy, renal failure, cardiovascular disease, and neuropathy. The major nutritional issues are (1) the distribution of the calorie-containing nutrients, carbohydrate, protein, and fat; (2) the impact of dietary carbohydrate and fat on plasma glucose and lipid concentrations; and (3) achievement of a healthful body weight (which means weight reduction for many patients).

Diabetes control improves with even modest weight loss (4 to 9 kg) in patients who are overweight (body mass index >30 kg/m²). A moderate calorie restriction (250 to 500 kcal less than the daily energy requirement), coupled with an increase in physical activity, appears to be the best strategy. The improved metabolic control with such a regimen is probably due to a combination of decreased food intake,

---

Table 77-4

Dietary Recommendations that may Reduce Cancer Risk

1. Eat plenty of vegetables and fruits, especially cabbage family (cruciferous) vegetables, deeply pigmented fruits and vegetables containing β-carotene and other carotenoids, and fruits and vegetables rich in vitamin C. Aim for at least 5 servings of vegetables and fruits per day.
2. Eat plenty of high-fiber foods, such as whole grains, fruits, and vegetables, aiming for a daily fiber intake of 20–30 g/d.
3. Avoid obesity and aim for weight control through exercise and lower energy intake.
4. Decrease fat intake to 30% or less of total energy consumed.
5. Minimize consumption of salt-cured, smoked, and nitrite-cured foods, such as bacon, ham, and hot dogs.
6. Limit or eliminate alcohol intake.

SOURCE: Adapted from RR Butrum et al, Am J Clin Nutr 48:888, 1988; and Department of Health and Human Services, publication no. 95-3862, Bethesda, MD, National Cancer Institute, 1995

increased insulin sensitivity, and return of hepatic glucose production to normal, even when optimal body weight is not achieved.

For patients with diabetes, 10 to 20 percent of energy intake should consist of protein to ensure normal growth and development in children and maintain normal protein stores in adults. This intake is similar to the average protein intake in the United States of 14 to 18 percent of energy intake and is in accordance with the "recommended dietary allowance" of 0.8 g/kg body weight for adults. The intake of protein may accelerate the rate of renal failure, but a protein intake of 10 percent of caloric intake is tolerated by most diabetic patients. When nephropathy has progressed to end-stage renal disease, lower protein intakes (e.g., 0.6 g/kg body weight) may be necessary if patients are not on chronic dialysis (discussed below).

Carbohydrate and fat make up the remainder of the energy intake. Patients with diabetes have a dyslipidemia characterized by elevated total triglycerides and reduced HDL cholesterol concentrations. The hypertriglyceridemia is due to an increased hepatic production of triglyceride-rich VLDL and may be associated with increased circulating levels of small dense LDL. Because of the association of CVD with diabetes mellitus, dietary recommendations traditionally emphasized a low-fat (especially low saturated fat), high-carbohydrate intake, a diet that may enhance hypertriglyceridemia and lower HDL cholesterol. An alternative program is to replace saturated fat with monounsaturated fat, rather than with carbohydrate. This approach aims at adjusting dietary carbohydrate and fat to achieve the desired blood glucose and lipid concentrations, rather than to use a uniform, preconceived intake as a goal. Sugars and starches have the same effect on blood glucose, and the diet should contain both types of carbohydrate. Finally, diet therapy for patients with diabetes should be individualized according to lifestyle, cultural eating habits, and patient motivation (Table 77-5).

CHRONIC RENAL FAILURE (See also Chap. 271)   Diet therapy plays an essential role in the management of all stages of renal failure but is of particular importance in end-stage renal disease. Patients with chronic renal failure are particularly susceptible to malnutrition due to inadequate intake and altered nutrient metabolism. Without intervention, vitamin D deficiency may cause decreased calcium absorption, hyperparathyroidism, and osteodystrophy. Dialysis itself depletes nutrients, and dialysis patients are at risk for deficiencies of vitamin B_6, vitamin C, and folate; elevated plasma vitamin A levels and increased or decreased body stores of vitamin A; and abnormalities in carnitine metabolism.

Excess protein intake increases glomerular filtration and can accelerate loss of renal function; conversely, dietary protein restriction may retard the progression of renal disease. Energy intake must be adequate (35 kcal/kg per day) to spare the protein that is consumed and minimize endogenous protein catabolism and to reduce the risk of developing malnutrition. Patients with progressive renal failure may benefit from a diet providing 0.55 to 0.60 g protein/kg per day, including 0.35 g/kg per day of high-biological-value protein (animal proteins such as meat, eggs, and fish). If very low protein diets (0.28 g/kg per day of protein) are tried in patients with advanced renal failure, it is necessary to supplement them with amino acids or keto acids to prevent malnutrition. Reduced dietary phosphorus (5 to 10 mg/kg per day of phosphorus) is an inherent feature of a low-protein diet. More rigid dietary phosphorus restriction is necessary only if the serum phosphorus level is elevated. Restriction of dietary potassium is usually unnecessary for predialysis patients (unless hyperkalemia is present). Restriction of sodium intake to 1000 to 3000 mg/d is usually sufficient to control edema and hypertension of renal failure. Both nondialyzed and dialyzed patients with chronic renal failure often have elevated blood lipid levels. It is prudent to restrict dietary fat (<30 percent of energy), saturated fat (<10 percent energy), and cholesterol (<300 mg/d), although evidence that this strategy reduces lipid levels or mortality is limited.

Patients with end-stage renal disease on dialysis should be given increased dietary protein (1.0 to 1.4 g/kg per day for hemodialysis and 1.2 to 1.4 g/kg per day for peritoneal dialysis patients), along with adequate energy intake (approximately 35 kcal/kg per day) to compensate for the catabolic effects of dialysis. Indeed, hemodialysis patients consuming higher protein intakes (0.93 to 1.29 g/kg per day) may have lower mortality rates than those with lower intake (0.63 g/kg per day or less). Patients treated with continuous ambulatory or cycling peritoneal dialysis lose large amounts of protein in the dialysate, and glucose is absorbed from the peritoneal dialysate and must be included in calculations of energy intake.

Phosphorus retention with hyperphosphatemia occurs in end-stage renal disease, and management of patients on hemodialysis or peritoneal dialysis usually requires both phosphorus restriction (≤17 mg/kg per day) and administration of phosphorus-binding compounds. To maintain calcium balance, patients undergoing dialysis require 1400 to 1600 mg/d of calcium from the diet plus supplementation. To prevent hyperkalemia, potassium intake usually must be limited to 1500 to 2700 mg/d in patients treated with hemodialysis. Patients receiving peritoneal dialysis generally do not have elevated serum potassium levels, so that dietary potassium restriction is rarely necessary. Restrictions of sodium (1000 to 1500 mg/d) and fluids (700 to 1500 mL/d) are generally necessary for hemodialysis patients because they are usually oliguric or anuric, but achieving this degree of restriction is difficult for most patients. Higher intake of sodium and fluid (up to 6000 to 8000 mg/d of sodium and 3000 mL/d of fluids) is permitted for patients on peritoneal dialysis because the dialysate can be adjusted to remove the excess. Finally, supplementation with water-soluble vitamins and the active metabolite of vitamin D is necessary in end-stage renal disease, because of the likelihood of deficiency due to a restricted diet, excess losses, and metabolic abnormalities. Table 77-6 summarizes modifications of protein and minerals in the dietary management of chronic renal failure.

Table 77-5

Diet Therapy for Diabetes Mellitus

1. Maintain as near-normal levels of blood glucose as possible by balancing food intake with medications (insulin or oral agents) and activity.
2. Achieve optimal serum lipid levels.
3. Provide calories to maintain or achieve reasonable weight for adults or to promote recovery from catabolic illness. Promote weight loss in obese patients.
4. Aim for protein intake of 10–20% and saturated fat of <10% of daily calories.
5. Distribute the remaining 60–70% of daily calories between carbohydrate and fat based on treatment goals for blood glucose and lipid levels. Emphasize monounsaturated fats over polyunsaturated fats.
6. Sucrose and other "simple sugars" may be substituted for other carbohydrates.
7. As in the general population, aim for 20–35 g/d of dietary fiber.
8. If hypertension is present, limit sodium to <2400 mg/d.
9. Limit alcoholic beverages to <2/d.
10. Vitamin and mineral supplementation is unnecessary for most patients.

SOURCE: Adapted from The American Diabetes Association, Inc, The American Dietetic Association, J Am Diet Assoc 94:504, 1994

Table 77-6

Dietary Modifications for Chronic Renal Failure

Dietary Factor	Predialysis	Hemodialysis	Peritoneal Dialysis
Protein	0.55–0.60 g/kg per day (0.35 g/kg per day high biological value)	1.0–1.4 g/kg per day	1.2–1.4 g/kg per day
Calcium	1400–1600 mg/d	1400–1600 mg/d	1400–1600 mg/d
Phosphorus	5–10 mg/kg per day	≤17 mg/kg per day	≤17 mg/kg per day
Sodium	1000–3000 mg/d	1000–1500 mg/d	Remove excess with the dialysate
Potassium	Unnecessary unless hyperkalemic	1500–2700 mg/d	Rarely necessary

GASTROINTESTINAL DISORDERS Gastrointestinal disorders are nearly always associated with altered nutrient intake or utilization.

Lactose Intolerance (See also Chap. 285) About 25 percent of adults in the United States have lactose intolerance, as manifested by abdominal distention, flatulence, and diarrhea after the consumption of moderate to large amounts of lactose-containing foods. The disorder is managed by restricting the ingestion of these foods. Dairy products are the primary source of dietary lactose, but aged cheese (because of very low lactose content), yogurt with active cultures, and dairy products with added lactose-cleaving microbial enzymes are tolerated by most affected individuals. Indeed, most lactose-intolerant individuals have negligible symptoms when intake is limited to the equivalent of one cup of milk (approximately 12 g lactase) or less per day.

Diarrhea The symptomatic management of diarrhea involves volume repletion with isotonic saline, lactose restriction (<5 g per meal), and reduced intake of fat (<40 g/d) and fiber. Very restrictive diets, such as diets limited to bananas, rice, applesauce, and tea or toast, are not recommended because extreme dietary restriction may compromise recovery of gut mucosa. A cycle of malabsorption and diarrhea can result, especially in the immunologically compromised subject.

Constipation High-fiber diets, especially those with whole grain breads and cereals and bran products, are useful in the prevention and management of constipation. The typical U.S. diet provides <12 g/d of fiber, whereas a high-fiber diet provides 20 to 35 g/d of fiber from whole grain bread products, fruits, and vegetables. Very high intake of dietary fiber from supplements (>35 g/d) can cause gaseous distention, increase the risk for bowel obstruction, and cause malabsorption of micronutrients.

Gastroesophageal Reflux Dietary modifications may be useful in the management of gastroesophageal reflux. Because they decrease lower esophageal sphincter pressure, chocolate, fatty foods, and carminatives (e.g., spearmint, peppermint) should be avoided. Orange juice, tomato juice, and coffee should also be avoided because they are direct mucosal irritants. Weight loss for the obese, the use of drugs such as omeprozole (see Chap. 284), and allowing 3 h between meal ingestion and recumbency are other helpful strategies.

Irritable Bowel Syndrome Excessive intake of foods or beverages sweetened with fructose or sorbitol or of lactose-containing foods can produce symptoms suggestive of irritable bowel syndrome and may aggravate the syndrome if present. If constipation is present, a high-fiber diet may be useful, although studies evaluating the therapeutic effects of fiber (from the diet or from supplements) have yielded inconsistent results. Careful patient records of food intake in relation to symptoms make it possible to design individual diet therapy to control symptoms and ensure adequacy of nutrient intake (see Chap. 287).

Inflammatory Bowel Disease Weight loss is significant in 65 to 75 percent of patients with Crohn's disease and in 18 to 62 percent of patients with ulcerative colitis. Reduced dietary intake is a major cause of weight loss and is due to anorexia and pain with eating. Individual diet counseling may result in improved nutrition in these patients.

Protein-losing enteropathy and malabsorption of fat, fat-soluble vitamins, vitamin B_{12}, and minerals can also occur in patients with inflammatory bowel disease, in addition to intestinal losses of nutrients (such as zinc with diarrhea and iron with blood loss). Food-drug interactions are also of importance: for example, sulfasalazine is a competitive inhibitor of folate absorption, and glucocorticoids decrease calcium absorption, cause osteopenia, and promote protein catabolism.

Dietary modifications useful in the management of these disorders include reduced intake of lactose (if intolerance is suggested by history) and fat (<70 g/d or adjusted to patient tolerance, particularly if steatorrhea is present) and sufficient intake of energy and protein to promote tissue healing. Dietary fiber should not be restricted unless partial bowel obstruction is present. Formula diets that have been useful in patients with inflammatory bowel disease (see Chap. 78) contain proteins that have been predigested to amino acids, carbohydrates, and

essential nutrients. The rationale is to reduce the exposure of the damaged gut wall to intact proteins that would promote a secondary immune response and at the same time provide adequate energy and nutrients. In practice, the liquid diets that have been evaluated in these disorders include those containing short-chain peptides and moderate amounts of lipids, and blenderized foods may have some usefulness. Although a reduction in symptoms has been observed in some studies, enteral nutrition support is inferior to glucocorticoids in inducing remission in active Crohn's disease. Intolerance to the formulas, especially when delivered orally, further limits their usefulness in some patients.

LIVER DISEASE The liver plays a central role in carbohydrate, lipid, and protein metabolism. Liver failure causes both decreased protein synthesis and enhanced protein breakdown, which, together with anorexia and reduced food intake, can lead to severe protein-energy malnutrition and limit the capacity for regeneration and functional recovery of the liver. Generally, the more severe the malnutrition, the worse the prognosis. In patients with massive hepatic necrosis or portal hypertension, a large load of protein nitrogen in the diet may promote or exacerbate hepatic encephalopathy, but severe dietary restriction of protein intake should not be imposed unnecessarily.

Patients with stable disease or in early hepatic failure benefit by receiving at least 1 g/kg per day of protein with adequate energy for efficient use of protein sources (at least 30 kcal/kg per day). Diet counseling should be provided to patients with stable chronic liver disease so as to maintain adequate dietary intake and prevent nutritional depletion. With progression of liver failure, modification in dietary protein intake may be necessary because of encephalopathy. Plant proteins tend to be better tolerated than animal proteins, possibly because plants contain less nonprotein nitrogen. Studies of the effects of specialized formula diets enriched in branched-chain amino acids on amino acid and ammonia levels and on hepatic encephalopathy have yielded inconsistent results. When prescribing dietary protein, the best approach is to determine patient tolerance by monitoring neurologic status, using 1 g/kg per day of protein as a goal for intake. As a minimum, 0.50 to 0.75 g/kg per day of protein, or approximately 40 g/d, is suggested; more severe protein restriction may promote the catabolism of body protein (see Chaps. 298 and 299).

In some patients with liver disease, dietary fat restriction (<30 g/d) may also be necessary, because of malabsorption and steatorrhea. To improve energy intake, restriction of long-chain fatty acids can be combined with the use of medium-chain triglyceride preparations, which can be absorbed without bile salts. Water-miscible forms of fat-soluble vitamins and other essential micronutrients should be given. Sodium restriction (<2 g/d) is usually necessary due to edema and ascites, but very low levels (<1 g/d) are not well tolerated and limit food choices, thus increasing the risk of malnutrition. Regular bread products, dairy products, and all processed foods (unless special low-sodium products) must be severely restricted to achieve <1000 mg/d of sodium.

CHRONIC NEUROLOGIC DISORDERS **Parkinson's Disease** Patients with Parkinson's disease are at risk of nutritional problems because of the effects of this disease on the gastrointestinal tract. Varying degrees of dysphagia, with or without aspiration, and constipation contribute to nutritional depletion in these patients. Diet counseling is recommended to ensure that the diet is adequate in the early stages of the disease.

The decrease in clinical efficacy of levodopa, which occurs commonly in the course of Parkinson's disease and which results in motor fluctuations and increased disability, may be improved by changing the timing of protein intake. The interaction between protein intake and clinical response appears to be due to inhibition by neutral amino acids in plasma of the uptake of levodopa into the central nervous system. Therefore, daytime restriction of dietary protein (<7 g protein intake prior to the evening meal) reduces unpredictable motor-response fluctuations during the active and productive periods of the day. At the evening meal, increased amounts of protein-rich foods can supply the daily requirements. Motivated individuals who adhere to this regimen usually improve and have no adverse effects on nutrition status, but this strategy increases the risk of malnutrition when regular diets are only marginally adequate.

Alzheimer's Disease Patients with Alzheimer's disease have more risk factors and more indications of poor nutritional status than elderly control populations. Diminished olfactory function causes poor eating habits and increases the risk of eating spoiled food, and choking and food refusal are common. Agitation and wandering increase energy requirements. Use of semi-solid or other nutritional supplements is one means of increasing nutrient intake in these patients. During the later stages patients often become unable to feed themselves and require assistance in eating. Throughout the course, monitoring of dietary intake is necessary to prevent weight loss and worsening of cognitive and physiologic function due to malnutrition and to prevent dehydration, aspiration, and increased risk of infectious illness.

PULMONARY DISEASE Malnutrition is common in patients with chronic obstructive pulmonary disease (COPD). Diaphragmatic muscle mass and area are reduced in association with weight loss in malnourished COPD patients when compared with patients with COPD who are of normal weight. The reduced tidal volume, carbon dioxide production, and oxygen consumption of malnourished individuals may predispose to pulmonary infections. Patients with COPD and weight loss have a shorter survival than patients with stable weight. Limited evidence suggests that improved nutrition improves respiratory muscle strength and endurance, even over the short term.

Patients with COPD have a >10 percent increase in basal energy requirements, associated with the increased work of breathing due to both increased pulmonary resistance and reduced efficiency of respiratory muscles. However, inadvertent provision of excessive energy intake can result in more harm than good. Increased carbon dioxide production resulting from overfeeding with excess energy (1.5 to 2.25 times the resting energy expenditure), especially carbohydrate loads, can cause respiratory distress. The prescription of low-carbohydrate, high-fat diets and energy-dense enteral formulas (containing 2 kcal/L) has been useful. These diets, which provide 50 to 55 percent of energy from fat and 25 to 35 percent of energy from carbohydrate, promote improvement in pulmonary function as compared to high-carbohydrate, low-fat diets (e.g., 74 percent of energy from carbohydrate, 9 percent of energy from fat). A diet containing 1.2 times the estimated resting energy expenditure is a beginning point in the provision of adequate calories, with protein at a level of 1.2 to 1.5 g/kg per day. However, individual diet therapy is necessary to avoid under- or overfeeding of these patients.

TRANSITIONAL AND OTHER DIETS Modifications in the consistency and texture of the diet can be important (see Table 77-7), especially for the hospitalized patient. A *clear liquid diet* provides an oral source of fluids, energy, and nutrients; leaves minimal residue in the gastrointestinal tract; and is used to prepare for diagnostic procedures, as an initial feeding following surgery or intravenous feeding, or during acute gastrointestinal dysfunction. These diets are not nutritionally adequate without nutritional supplements and should not be used for more than 3 days. A *full liquid diet* is liquid or semiliquid at room temperature and is prescribed for patients with chewing difficulties or as an intermediate progression to solid foods after surgery or intravenous feeding; it also may not be nutritionally adequate without enteral nutritional supplements. A *pureed diet*, which includes strained, pureed, and liquid foods, is useful for patients who are edentulous or have other problems that limit the ability to chew foods. A *soft diet* consists of foods that can be chewed more easily than those in a regular diet and includes tender meat and soft solids, while omitting raw fruits and vegetables and coarse breads and cereals. Pureed and soft diets are nutritionally adequate provided a sufficient quantity and variety of the foods are consumed.

Diets that eliminate specific dietary constituents, such as oxalates (for management of hyperoxaluria), galactose (for management of galactosemia), and gluten (for management of celiac disease), have also been described. For more details of these and other specific diet therapies the reader is referred to the diet manuals listed in the Bibliography.

Drug-Nutrient Interactions Diet modifications may be necessary because of drug-nutrient interactions. Certain foods or meal patterns can alter drug effectiveness, and conversely, drugs can alter nutrient requirements. Drug absorption is generally slower when administered with food. The metabolism of drugs, especially those that are substrates for cytochrome P450 enzymes, can be affected by changes in protein intake and micronutrient status. Table 77-8 lists examples of important drug-nutrient interactions. Drugs can also enhance or reduce appetite and dietary intake by central and/or peripheral effects.

Table 77-7

Diets Modified in Consistency

Diet	Examples of Foods Included
Clear liquid diet	Fat-free broth, bouillon, coffee, tea, carbonated beverages, clear fruit juice, gelatin, residue-free liquid nutritional supplements
Full liquid diet	Cream soups, coffee, tea, carbonated beverages, milk, yogurt, strained cooked cereal, vegetable and fruit juice, gelatin, sherbet, ice cream, custard, liquid nutritional supplements
Pureed diet	All soups, all beverages, strained or pureed meat or poultry, blended cottage cheese, gravy, milk, yogurt, mashed potatoes, strained or pureed vegetables and fruits, ice cream, custard
Soft diet	All beverages, cooked cereal, canned fruit, tender meat, cooked vegetables, milk, potatoes, rice, bread or rolls, ice cream, pudding

Table 77-8

Examples of Drug-Nutrient Interactions

Effects of Diet on Drugs	Compound
Absorption reduced by food	Atenolol
	Captopril
	Cephalexin
	Penicillin and derivatives
	Tetracycline
Absorption delayed by food	Digoxin
	Glipizide
	Phenytoin
	Piroxicam
	Theophylline
Absorption increased by food	Diazepam
	Griseofulvin
	Lithium
	Propranolol
	Thiazide diuretics

Effects of Drugs on Nutrients	Drug (Nutrient Affected)
Reduced absorption	Cimetidine (vitamin B_{12})
	Cholestyramine (fat-soluble vitamins)
	Glucocorticoids (calcium)
	Phenytoin (calcium)
	Sulfasalazine (folate)
Impaired utilization	Coumarin anticoagulants (vitamin K)
	Isoniazid (vitamin B_6)
	Methotrexate (folate)
	Nitrous oxide (vitamin B_{12})
	Oral contraceptives (folate)
Increased losses	Gentamicin (magnesium)
	Aspirin and nonsteroidal anti-inflammatory drugs (iron)
	Loop diuretics (thiamin)
	Penicillamine (zinc)
	Thiazide diuretics (potassium)

ALTERNATIVE DIET THERAPIES

New or alternative diet therapies are promoted by the popular nutrition literature, which is produced by an array of practitioners who devise and recommend various diet therapies based on different rationales and varying supportive data. In addition, both practitioners and patients can have beliefs and attitudes classified as food faddism, food cultism, or food quackery. Food faddism is an exaggerated belief in the effects of specific aspects of nutrition on health and disease. Food cultism implies beliefs about food that contain a religious or philosophical component, often with the involvement of a charismatic authority figure. Food quackery carries the implication of fraud but also refers to people who are sincere in their beliefs but misguided in the promotion of questionable diet therapies.

Popular diets often focus on limiting or regulating specific foods, using either speculative information or half-truths to explain the rationale. Unusual foods, food combinations, or other rituals for eating may also be prescribed. Table 77-9 lists examples of popular diets in a few general categories. Unproven diet therapies exist for the treatment of chronic fatigue syndrome, premenstrual syndrome, arthritis, multiple sclerosis, and numerous other medical problems. Vegetarian diets are sometimes considered alternative diets, although nutritional needs can be met quite easily by adults who consume dairy products but avoid meat, poultry, and fish. A vegan diet, which means that all animal products are eliminated, can also be nutritionally adequate, although more thoughtful food choices and supplementation with fortified foods and vitamin B_{12} may be necessary.

Although a randomized clinical trial is the ultimate test of efficacy, popular theories about diet and disease are often derived from epidemiologic studies such as ecologic, case-control, and cohort studies. Such studies are useful for generating hypotheses, but the apparent associations between diets and disease may be confounded by uncontrolled factors and other potential determinants of health and disease. As in any other medical therapy, the use of diet therapies should be based on a scientific rationale and sound data, not on anecdotal experience.

Feelings of medical abandonment or a need or desire to exert some control over the management of illness can motivate patients to adopt fad or popular diets. Such diets may have particular appeal to those with chronic illness. Awareness of alternative diet therapies being promoted, exploring with patients the issues surrounding nutrition and diet in a noncritical manner, and addressing concerns with reassurance are strategies to mimimize the chance of fad diets becoming health risks.

A few general questions are central to the evaluation of popular or alternative diets. Is the diet nutritionally adequate and appropriate for the patient? Comparing the diet composition with the guidelines for nutritional adequacy addresses this concern. Is the rationale for the diet scientifically sound? A basic understanding of nutritional requirements (see Chap. 72) makes it possible to assess the safety of the diet. Will physical or psychological risks or hazards result from the diet therapy? Even if the diet appears to involve health risk, some patients will still choose such a regimen, and the patient's decision must be respected. Suggesting that the therapy be tried for a limited time only and that the patient then return for reassessment can be helpful. Continued monitoring for adverse effects, along with support and follow-up, reduce the likelihood that conventional treatment will be completely abandoned.

PROMOTING ADHERENCE TO DIET THERAPY

No diet therapy can be effective if it is not followed or is followed incorrectly. Many factors, such as the complexity and cost of the diet, environmental and social circumstances, the nature and quality of the patient-clinician interaction, and the techniques used to counsel and teach the patient, will influence adherence. Compliance with medical therapies of all types, including prescription medications and diets, is universally poor. Traditional approaches, such as providing the patient a set menu plan or a list of foods to avoid, are usually unsuccessful. Similarly, interacting in a manner that creates a power struggle between the physician and the patient is doomed to failure.

Large-scale clinical trials have demonstrated that adherence can be improved, even when the diet is complex, when diet therapy includes specific educational and behavioral strategies. Such strategies are based on contemporary behavioral theory and a self-management approach, particularly when dietary changes must be maintained throughout the paient's life and when the degree of modification may be extensive. A self-management approach means that the physician or diet counselor and the patient are partners in the process: for long-term adherence, patients need to learn problem-solving skills and to believe in their own capabilities.

A basic strategy to enhance adherence is to focus on positive behavior and appropriate food choices rather than on food restrictions. One technique is to begin with the baseline diet as described by the patient and to identify changes that the patient is willing and able to make. Building on achievable goals, patients can practice and develop skills through continued support from a guiding expert. Frequent contact with the physician or diet counselor, who encourages the patient and reinforces progress, also increases adherence and promotes sustained motivation. For almost all patients, the involvement and assistance of family members and social support are mandatory if diet therapy is to succeed. Individualized and tailored education and communication are also necessary, taking into consideration the sociocultural influences on food choices and eating patterns.

Success of diet therapy is enhanced by working with a health care practitioner trained in nutrition. To obtain credentials as a registered dietitian involves completing an approved program of academic training that includes both didactic and supervised practice components. Dietitians provide nutritional care in the hospital and in ambulatory clinics, physician practice groups, community-based programs, and public health departments. A dietitian can function as the guiding and supportive expert, translating nutritional and metabolic needs into specific food choices and developing strategies that enable patients to effect changes in dietary habits.

BIBLIOGRAPHY

AMERICAN DIETETIC ASSOCIATION: *Manual of Clinical Dietetics*, 2d ed. Chicago, American Dietetic Association, 1992

COMMITTEE ON DIET AND HEALTH, FOOD AND NUTRITION BOARD, NATIONAL RESEARCH COUNCIL: *Diet and Health: Implications for Reducing Chronic Disease Risk*. Washington, DC, National Academy Press, 1989

COUNCIL ON SCIENTIFIC AFFAIRS, AMERICAN MEDICAL ASSOCIATION: Report of the Council on Scientific Affairs. Diet and cancer: Where do matters stand? JAMA 153:50, 1993

Eating Hints for Cancer Patients, Publication No. 94-2079. Bethesda, MD, National Cancer Institute, 1994

EXPERT PANEL ON DETECTION, EVALUATION, AND TREATMENT OF HIGH BLOOD CHOLESTEROL IN ADULTS: Summary of the Second Report of the National Cholestrol Education Program (NCEP) Expert Panel on Detection, Evaluation, and Treatment of High Blood Cholesterol in Adults (Adult Treatment Panel II). JAMA 269:3015, 1993

Table 77-9

Examples of Popular Diets

Diet Type	Characteristics	Examples
Low carbohydrate	Causes ketosis if <100 g/d	Atkin's diet Scarsdale diet Stillman's diet The Zone diet
Very low fat	Limited bioavailability of micronutrients; provides limited protein and energy	Macrobiotic diet McDougall diet Pritikin diet Rice-fruit diet
Novel diets	Unusual food combinations; unscientific rationale	Fit for Life diet Beverly Hills diet Yeast-free diet for allergies

FRANZ MJ et al: Nutrition principles for the management of diabetes and related complications. Diabetes Care 17:490, 1994

KLAHR S et al: The effects of dietary protein restriction and blood-pressure control on the progression of chronic renal disease. N Engl J Med 330:877, 1994

NELSON JK et al (eds): *Mayo Clinic Diet Manual*, 7th ed. St. Louis, Mosby 1994

PENNINGTON JA: *Bowes & Church's Food Values of Portions Commonly Used*, 16th ed. Philadelphia, Lippincott, 1994

SHILS ME et al (eds): *Modern Nutrition in Health and Disease*, 8th ed. Philadelphia, Lea & Febiger, 1994

78 *Lyn Howard*

ENTERAL AND PARENTERAL NUTRITION THERAPY

Parenteral and enteral nutrition provide life-sustaining therapy for patients who cannot take adequate food by mouth and who consequently are at risk for malnutrition and its effects, including susceptibility to infection and weakness and immobility, which predispose in turn to aspiration pneumonia, pulmonary embolism, and pressure sores, all of which delay recovery from illness and increase mortality.

The term *enteral* refers to feeding via the gut and hence includes normal eating, but in the present context the term implies the infusion of formulas via a tube into the upper gastrointestinal tract. *Parenteral* refers to the infusion of nutrient solutions into the bloodstream. While these are different approaches to nutritional support, their goals are by and large the same. Where feasible, enteral nutrition is the preferred route because it sustains the digestive, absorptive, and immunologic barrier functions of the gastrointestinal tract. The cost of enteral tube feeding is about one-tenth the cost of parenteral feeding.

Several developments have made tube feeding easier and more acceptable to patients. Small-bore pliable tubes have largely replaced large-bore rubber tubes, and double-bore tubes are now available with a gastric suction arm and jejunal feeding arm for use when there is concern about gastric retention and aspiration. Enteral tubes can be inserted into the stomach or jejunum through the nose or, for long-term use, directly through the abdominal wall, using endoscopic, radiologic, or surgical techniques. Once the enterocutaneous tract is established, the protruding tube can be replaced by a "button" entry port flush with the abdominal wall.

Complete nutrition by vein with sufficient calories, amino acids, minerals, and vitamins to permit wound healing, restoration of normal body composition of a cachectic patient, or growth in children became feasible in the 1960s with the development of high-flow central vein catheters and is now available in all large hospitals and for some patients at home. Adequate calories and other nutrients can be delivered in the form of high-energy, isotonic intravenous fat solutions via a peripheral vein. However, peripheral veins usually cannot sustain such infusions indefinitely, and long-term support requires central venous access.

THE DECISION PROCESS FOR USING PARENTERAL OR ENTERAL NUTRITION The decision to use specialized nutrition support should be based on the likelihood that averting or redressing malnutrition will improve the quality of life or the ability to recover from a serious illness. Approximately 15 to 20 percent of hospitalized patients have evidence of malnutrition. Some malnourished patients benefit from specialized nutrition support, but for others wasting is an inevitable component of a terminal disease. Distinguishing between these possibilities requires knowledge of the potential benefits and risks of nutritional support, and the physician must inform the patient and family of these benefits and risks with awareness of the legal issues involved. Figure 78-1 is a flow diagram of the steps

involved in deciding whether specialized nutrition support should be undertaken and if so, how. Like all life-support measures, these therapies are difficult to withdraw once started.

The first step requires consideration of the nutritional implications of the disease process. Is the condition or its treatment likely to impair appetite or food ingestion and absorption for a prolonged period of time? Since prevention of malnutrition is easier than treatment, this issue must be considered in the initial evaluation. The second step is to determine whether the patient is already sufficiently malnourished that lean body mass is decreased and critical functions such as healing and ventilation will be impaired. The presence or absence of metabolic stress should be noted, since injury or infection can evoke the secretion of hormonal and cytokine factors that reduce the efficiency of nutrition repletion. The assessment of the nutritional status of patients is discussed in Chap. 73. Weight loss without physiologic impairment is probably of no consequence. Physiologic impairment usually becomes important when more that 20 percent of body protein is lost and is more likely if the relevant organ system is directly affected by disease. Once it is recognized that the patient is malnourished or at major risk, the question is whether specialized nutritional support will impact positively on the response to the disease and improve the quality of life. This issue involves risk-versus-benefit and ethical considerations. While the provision of food and water is part of basic medical care, nutrition support by enteral or parenteral means is associated with some risk and discomfort and should be recommended only when potential benefit exceeds risk and undertaken only with the consent of the patient.

If it is decided that preventing or treating malnutrition with specialized nutrition support would improve the prognosis and quality of life, the nutritional requirements must be determined and the route of nutrient delivery must be selected.

RISKS AND BENEFITS OF NUTRITION SUPPORT The risks are chiefly determined by the route required to deliver nutrition support. Providing nutritional requirements by special attention to oral intake of food or by adding oral liquid supplements together with monitoring food intake with frequent calorie counts is the best approach. It is also the most efficient metabolically because normal eating initiates the cephalic phase of digestion. Tube-fed infants grow better if the cephalic phase is stimulated by having the infant suck on a pacifier.

Anorexia, impairment of swallowing, or bowel disease may limit oral intake or the absorption of oral nutrients, in which case tube enteral nutrition is the next consideration. The bowel and its associated digestive organs derive 70 percent of their required nutrients directly from food in the lumen. In addition, glutamine, short-chain fatty acids, and nucleotides may have particular importance in maintaining gut integrity. Enteral feeding also supports gut function by stimulating splanchnic blood flow, neuronal activity, IgA antibody release, and secretion of gastrointestinal hormones such as epidermal growth factor that stimulate gut trophic activity. All these factors support the gut as an immunologic barrier against enteric pathogens.

For these reasons, some enteral nutrition should always be provided if possible, even when parenteral nutrition is required to provide most of the support. In the past, bowel rest through parenteral nutrition was thought to be the cornerstone of treatment of several severe gastrointestinal disorders, but the value of some enteral nutrition is now widely accepted and strict bowel rest is rarely advocated. Parenteral nutrition alone is still appropriate in the early phase of the extreme short bowel syndrome, severe hemorrhagic pancreatitis, necrotizing enterocolitis, prolonged ileus, and distal bowel obstruction.

Specialized nutrition support is expensive, accounting for over 1 percent of all health care dollars in 1992 (Table 78-1). Consequently, hard clinical endpoints such as rate of mortality, incidence of major complications, and duration of hospital stay are required of risk-benefit studies. Softer endpoints, such as better nitrogen balance, increased levels of serum albumin, and improved delayed hypersensitivity, are no longer acceptable.

Perioperative Nutrition While there is a clear-cut association between preoperative malnutrition and poor surgical outcome, it has

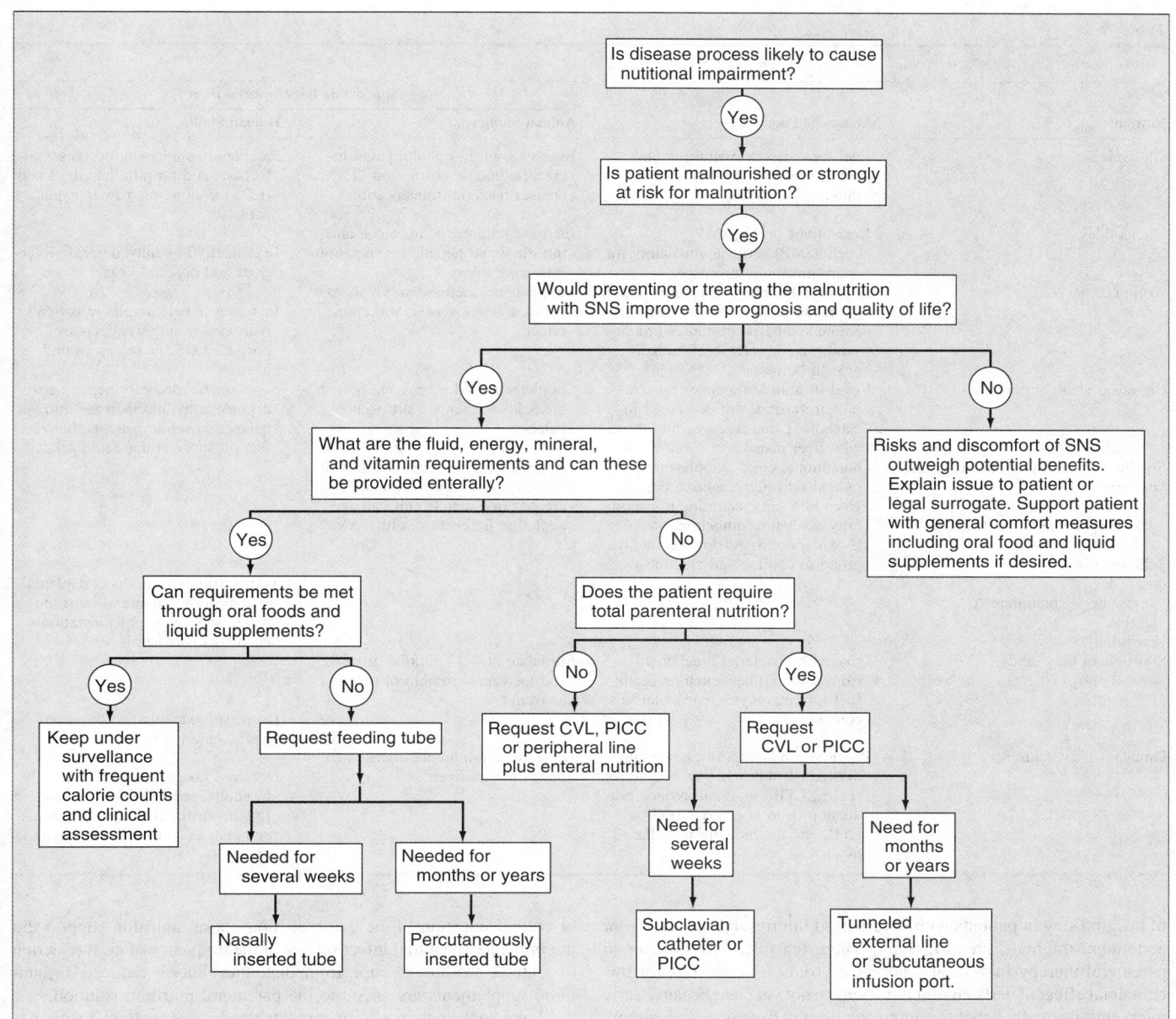

FIGURE 78-1 Should specialized nutrition support (SNS) be undertaken and if so, how? An algorithm. (PICC, Peripherally inserted, usually antecubital vein, central catheter; CVL, central venous line.)

been difficult to demonstrate the benefit of preoperative parenteral nutrition on the outcome of surgery in malnourished patients. However, a meta-analysis of 18 small studies and a large cooperative Veterans Administration study indicate that preoperative parenteral nutrition does improve the outcome of severely malnourished surgical patients.

Table 78-1

Estimate of Cost and Number of Persons Receiving Parenteral and Tube Enteral Nutrition in 1992 in the United States

Clinical Setting	Cost, $ Millions		Persons, Thousands	
	Parenteral	Enteral	Parenteral	Enteral
Hospital	6000	1200	500	1000
Home	780	357	40	152
Nursing home	6	410	<1	177
Dialysis center	20	<1	3	<1

SOURCE: Hospital estimate based on Anderson and Steinberg (data using quoted growth rates); nonhospital estimate based on Howard et al. (Medicare data and North American HPEN Registry information).

In treated patients, noninfectious complications (e.g., pulmonary emboli and delayed wound healing) are reduced in the postoperative period. In surgical patients with mild or moderate malnutrition, the risks of infection from preoperative parenteral therapy outweigh the benefits. These risks include line sepsis and infectious complications not directly related to the central line, such as pneumonia and wound infection. Effective preoperative restoration of nutrition by the parenteral route requires at least 7 to 14 days. Preoperative enteral nutrition, where feasible, is safe and more economical, especially if provided at home.

Immediate postoperative nutritional support is appropriate for patients who received preoperative support and for patients unlikely to resume oral feeding within 10 days. Commonly the parenteral route is used because of postoperative ileus or concern about disrupting a new bowel anastomosis. However, cautious jejunal feeding is often equally well tolerated. Specialized enteral formulas supplemented with a variety of conditionally essential nutrients may be particularly beneficial in debilitated and immunosuppressed postoperative patients (Table 78-2).

Critical Illness Very early nutrition support (within the first 48 h) improves survival, reduces infections, and reduces the length

Table 78-2

Conditionally Essential Nutrients

Nutrient	Metabolic Function	Supporting Experimental Data	
		Animal Studies	Human Studies
Glutamine	Fuel for enterocyte and immuno-cytes; preserves hepatic gluta-thione	Improves gut morphology and increases glucose absorption; decreases bacterial translocation	Parenteral supplement decreases infections and hospital length of stay (LOS) in bone marrow transplant patients
Nucleotides	Derivatives (cyclicAMP, cyclicGMP) serve as mediators for many metabolic processes	Increase immune competence and intestinal and hepatic regeneration following injury	In critically ill adults, decrease infections and hospital LOS
Arginine	Enhances lymphocyte cytotoxicity via nitric oxide; substrate for poly-amine synthesis; promotes protein synthesis via release of human growth hormone	Supplements increase survival from burns, trauma, sepsis; antitumor effect	Increases T helper cells in patients with cancer surgery; decreases hospital LOS; increases wound healing
Branched-chain amino acids	Level in muscle regulates muscle-protein breakdown; decreased in catabolic patients, especially those with liver disease	Supplements reduce muscle protein breakdown, increase nitrogen balance	Supplements decrease hepatic encephalopathy and increase nitrogen balance in septic patients, but effect on survival not demonstrated
Sulphur-containing amino acids [me-thionine ↓ S-adenosyl methionine (SAM) ↓ homocysteine ↓ cysteine→glutathione taurine carnitine]	Glutathione, chief cytoplasmic free radical scavenger; taurine conjugates bile salts; carnitine transports fatty acids into mitochondria for β-oxidation; SAM donates methyl group to choline and creatine	Decreased choline affects cell-wall fluidity; glutathione depletion increases free radicle cell damage; depletion is reversed with SAM	Transsulfuration products depleted in long-term parenteral nutrition patients; SAM supplementation decreases cholestasis
Short-chain fatty acids	Derived by bacterial breakdown from soluble fibers such as pectin; fuel for enterocytes, particularly colonocytes	Stimulate bowel epithilial growth and increases strength of colonic anastomoses	Decrease pouchitis and bypassed bowel enteritis
Omega-3 fatty acids	Promote production of prostaglandins and leukotrienes of N-3 series (PGE_3, LTB_5, etc.) and reduce production from N-6 series (PGE_2, LTB_4, etc.), which are proinflammatory	Decrease autoimmune disease and platelets adhesiveness	Decrease hospital LOS in critically ill adults; reduce blood pressure, IgA nephritis, rheumatoid arthritis, and platelet abnormalities in type 1 diabetes

of hospital stay in patients with severe head injuries, burns, and major abdominal trauma. Enteral therapy, where feasible, was superior to parenteral therapy in several randomized trials. The reasons for this beneficial effect of early enteral nutrition are not yet clear because early intervention equally benefits injured patients not overtly malnourished. Animal studies suggest that enteral feeding results in decreased systemic infections from gut bacteria and in reduction of the systemic catabolic response. These phenomena have not been substantiated in humans, but early enteral feeding may prevent bacterial overgrowth and decrease aspiration pneumonia.

The practical issue is obtaining jejunal access in a critically ill patient, who is not easily transferred for endoscopic or radiologic placement. Sometimes a nasal or percutaneous combined gastric suction and jejunal feeding tube can be inserted at the bedside. When a surgical laparatomy is indicated, a feeding tube can be placed simultaneously.

Most studies of enteral feeding in critically ill patients used either a general polymeric formula or one with hydrolyzed protein. Parenteral formulas enriched with large amounts of branched-chain amino acids (BCAA) improve nitrogen balance but do appear to affect clinical outcome.

Cancer Cachexia Early nonrandomized studies suggested that patients with cancer cachexia benefit from parenteral nutrition, but randomized trials demonstrated more risk than benefit for patients receiving chemotherapy or radiation. Severely malnourished cancer patients undergoing surgery do appear to benefit from preoperative parenteral nutrition, as do other malnourished patients.

In two randomized, prospective trials, patients undergoing bone marrow transplantation had better long-term survival after parenteral or enteral nutrition in the cytoreduction phase; nutrition support did not influence the initial infection rate or the frequency of graft rejection or graft-versus-host disease. Immediate morbidity is reduced if glutamine supplements are added to the parenteral nutrition solution.

For cancer patients with untreatable disease, enteral feeding is usually justified if it is desired by the patient and family. Parenteral feeding should be provided only if clinical improvement can be expected and when quality survival at home for several months is predicted.

Liver Failure Malnutrition is common in advanced liver disease. Patients with acute or chronic liver failure have decreased levels of BCAA and elevated levels of aromatic amino acids (AAA) in plasma and cerebrospinal fluid. Randomized, prospective trials with parenteral and enteral formulas high in BCAA and low in AAA have demonstrated better nitrogen balance and less risk of encephalopathy. One large multicenter study also reported improved survival. The BCAA-enriched formulas are expensive and should be used only in patients who have encephalopathy or who develop encephalopathy when fed a standard protein formula providing 0.8 g protein/kg per day.

Renal Failure Since renal failure is associated with impaired nitrogen excretion, it is rational to assume that protein restriction might benefit patients with chronic renal failure and that more complete protein restriction might improve the course of acute renal failure. However, the progression of renal impairment in patients on chronic dialysis is not slowed by low-protein oral diets. Patients with acute renal failure given parenteral calories and amino acids have fewer infectious complications and a better chance of leaving the hospital than similar patients given only calories. An early randomized study showed benefit when essential amino acids were the sole source of nitrogen, but in other studies standard solutions supplying both essential and nonessential amino acids provide similar advantage. Thus, the benefit of using expensive formulas containing only essential amino acids or their keto analogues is not established.

Fifteen to twenty percent of patients with chronic renal failure on dialysis have significant nutritional impairment, usually due to profound anorexia. The anorexia sometimes improves with stepped-up dialysis or treatment of gastritis but usually persists. The resulting growth impairment in younger patients has been treated with supplemental tube enteral nutrition. This approach has not been widely used in older patients, but parenteral nutrition that provides some extra calories and amino acids can be administered in the last 90 min of hemodialysis treatment and is said to improve appetite, serum protein levels, and body weight. No randomized studies have documented better survival, so that the appropriateness of this regimen is not established. Standard continuous ambulatory peritoneal dialysis uses glucose to provide an osmotic load, and some glucose calories are absorbed. Amino acids can be substituted for glucose and are also partly absorbed, offsetting the loss of endogenous amino acids into the dialysate. This approach also awaits a randomized study.

Pancreatitis   Parenteral nutrition does not improve the outcome of patients with mild or moderate pancreatitis. However, in severe pancreatitis survival decreases as malnutrition becomes more severe. When parenteral nutrition support was delayed beyond 72 h, patients with severe pancreatitis had a threefold higher complication and mortality rate, compared to similar patients treated earlier. In the absence of severe hyperlipidemia or thrombocytopenia, intravenous lipids appear safe and are especially useful if glucose intolerance is present. Several studies report successful enteral jejunal feeding in acute pancreatitis.

Inflammatory Bowel Disease (IBD)   Evidence of nutritional deficiencies such as weight loss, growth failure, anemia, and hypoalbuminenia are common in IBD, more so in Crohn's disease than in ulcerative colitis (see Chap. 286). Nutrition support plays a role in correcting these nutritional deficiencies, particularly prior to elective surgery. Since IBD often improves with diversion of the fecal stream, the question is whether bowel rest and parenteral nutrition have a role as primary treatment. However, randomized, prospective studies have shown no special benefit from bowel rest. Elemental diets can be used in place of steroids for inducing remission in acute Crohn's disease, but relapse is common when a regular diet is resumed. In controlled studies remissions are prolonged if the Crohn's patient does not return to a regular diet but instead eliminates from the diet those foods that induce gastrointestinal symptoms. For the majority of Crohn's patients this leads to avoidance of cereals, dairy products, and yeast.

Because of the possibility that diets high in omega 3 fatty acids have a beneficial effect in immune disorders by altering prostaglandin synthesis, their value in IBD is under investigation. Some studies suggest that high-fiber diets benefit IBD patients, but fiber can also cause obstruction in patients with bowel strictures.

Short Bowel Syndrome   Before the advent of parenteral nutrition, patients with acute short bowel syndrome from mesenteric vascular infarction or surgical resection seldom survived. Parenteral nutrition has allowed many patients to survive indefinitely with only a foot or two of small intestine. In some, the remaining bowel eventually adapts and allows the absorption of adequate calories and protein. However, fluid and electrolyte imbalance may persist so that some parenteral fluid and electrolyte support are required. Gradual increase of overnight tube enteral nutrition or constant sipping of an electrolyte solution may allow discontinuation of all parenteral support.

Pulmonary Disease   Weight loss in patients with advanced pulmonary disease is due to increased work of breathing and poor food intake. Patients with chronic pulmonary disease who are less than 90% percent of their ideal weight have a greater 5-year mortality, independent of pulmonary status. The recommended energy intake for these patients is 1.7 times their resting energy expenditure. In cystic fibrosis, malnutrition may hasten pulmonary deterioration, and enteral feeding via gastrostomy tubes enhances growth and stabilizes or improves pulmonary function, particularly in young children. The criteria for selection of patients and the psychological costs of such treatment have not been defined. The use of a low-carbohydrate formula is beneficial in the weaning of patients from ventilators, but the superiority of such formulas in ambulatory patients with chronic lung disease is not established.

Human Immunodeficiency Virus (HIV) Disease   The role of specialized nutritional support in weight loss associated with HIV disease is not established. Studies by Kotler have shown that parenteral nutrition repletes lean body mass when weight loss is due to inadequate oral intake, either because of oral problems or esophageal disease or because of inadequate absorption due to small-bowel disease. However, wasting associated with systemic infection and increased cytokine secretion is not effectively repaired by parenteral nutrition. In patients with systemic infections, any weight gain reflects increased fat and body water rather than protein mass. Slow tube enteral infusion is often tolerated, and its role in the early phase of HIV-related weight loss is under investigation.

Pregnancy   Severe hyperemesis gravidarum can make any oral or tube enteral nutrition impossible, and profound weight loss and ketosis may harm the developing fetus. The underlying mechanism of the disorder is not understood, but it is cured by abortion or delivery. Temporary parenteral nutrition usually results in a successful outcome in pregnancy complicated by severe hyperemesis, but nausea and vomiting tend to persist, despite bowel rest.

Home Parenteral and Enteral Nutrition   Some patients require long-term nutrition support and this can be administered at home. Table 78-3 summarizes the outcome for patients with severe intestinal disorders, 11 treated parenterally and 2 treated enterally. Nutritional support is not appropriate in terminal patients, but it is an option if a patient can be expected to survive for several months. Such therapy must make sense to the patient, and sufficient help must be available so that the treatment can be given at home without undue hazard. Both home therapies are relatively safe, with less than a 5 percent mortality.

THE DESIGN OF INDIVIDUAL REGIMENS   Fluid Requirements   These can be estimated by adding the normal daily requirement (120 mL/kg of body weight for infants, 35 mL/kg of body weight for adults) to any abnormal loss. If the patient is on parenteral therapy, any enteral intake should be subtracted from the estimate (see Table 78-4.) Since abnormal loss of enteric fluid implies significant mineral losses, extra amounts of these nutrients (Table 78-5) must be added to any standard parenteral formula.

Energy Requirements   These can be determined as outlined in Chap. 72. In the long run energy expenditure dictates energy requirements, but in the early phase of nutrition repletion, requirements may not reflect expenditure. For example, malnourished patients are hypometabolic and may expend only 85 kJ/kg (20 kcal/kg) per day, but more calories are needed for nutritional repletion because with refeeding the metabolic rate increases and extra calories are needed for tissue repair. Conversely, a highly stressed patient (burns, trauma) may expend 165 kJ/kg (40 kcal/kg) per day with a significant proportion of the calories coming from protein breakdown and gluconeogenesis and from catecholamine-induced lipolysis. Oxidation of exogenous glucose plateaus at 100 kJ/kg (25 kcal/kg) per day, and administering additional glucose induces hepatic steatosis. Furthermore, providing such patients with additional calories as exogenous fat does not suppress endogenous lipolysis. This is because the artificial chylomicrons of parenteral fat solutions, which are vegetable oils (soybean, safflower) emulsified with egg phospholipid, lack apoproteins and are are not metabolized like lipoproteins. For these reasons, modest hypocaloric glucose feeding with minimal parenteral fat is safer in the acutely stressed subject.

Parenteral lipid solutions are available as 10% or 20% isotonic solutions and can be infused separately from amino acids and glucose or as "three in one," obviating the need for an extra pump. However, three-in-one solutions are not as stable as the glucose and amino acid mix, and destabilized fat particles have the potential of coalescing into larger droplets and becoming fat emboli. To be safe, three-in-one solutions must be mixed by a pharmacist knowledgeable about the

Table 78-3

Summary of Outcome for Patients on Home Parenteral and Enteral Nutrition (HPEN)

Diagnosis	Number in Group	Age in Years	% Survival* on Therapy	Therapy Status, % at 1 year†‡			Rehabilitation‡§ Status, % in 1st year			Complications¶ per Patient-Year	
				Full Oral Nutrition	Continued on HPEN Rx	Died	C	P	M	HPEN‡	NonHPEN‡
HOME PARENTERAL NUTRITION											
Crohn's disease	562	36	96	70	25	2	60	38	2	0.9	1.1
Ischemic bowel disease	331	49	87	27	48	19	53	41	6	1.4	1.1
Motility disorder	299	45	87	31	44	21	49	39	12	1.3	1.1
Congenital bowel defect	172	5	94	42	47	9	63	27	11	2.1	1.0
Hyperemesis gravidarum	112	28	100	100	0	0	83	16	1	1.5	3.5
Chronic pancreatitis	156	42	90	82	10	5	60	38	2	1.2	2.5
Radiation enteritis	145	58	87	28	49	22	42	49	9	0.8	1.1
Chronic adhesive obstructions	120	53	83	47	34	13	23	68	10	1.7	1.4
Cystic fibrosis	51	17	50	38	13	36	24	66	16	0.8	3.7
Cancer	2122	44	20	26	8	63	29	57	14	1.1	3.3
AIDS	280	33	10	13	6	73	8	63	29	1.6	3.3
HOME ENTERAL NUTRITION											
Neurologic disorders of swallowing	1134	65	55	19	25	48	5	24	71	0.3	0.9
Cancer	1644	61	30	30	6	59	21	59	21	0.4	2.7

* Survival rates on therapy are values at 1 year, calculated by the life table method. This will differ from the percentage listed as died under Therapy Status, since all patients with known end points are considered in this latter measure. The ratio of observed versus expected deaths is equivalent to a Standard Mortality Ratio.

† Not shown are those patients who were back in hospital or who had changed therapy type by 12 months.

‡ Chi-square test, $P < .05$

§ Rehabilitation is designated complete (C), partial (P), or minimal (M), relative to the patient's ability to sustain normal age-related activity.

¶ Complications refer only to those complications that resulted in rehospitalization.

SOURCE: Derived from North American HPEN Registry.

appropriate mixing sequence of the ingredients and the amounts of divalent cations and trace elements that can be added. Patients who require parenteral iron and zinc must get these in non-lipid-containing parenteral solutions.

Polyunsaturated vegetable oils are used in most enteral formulas because they are better absorbed by the compromised gastrointestinal tract. The fat in parenteral and enteral formulas must supply the essential fatty acid requirement (1 to 4 percent of energy from linoleic and linolenic acid) (Table 78-6). In relatively stable patients the provision of 30 percent of energy as fat may reduce the problems that arise from providing glucose calories predominantly (e.g.,

hepatic steatosis). Substituting omega 3 polyunsaturated fish oils for ordinary polyunsaturated vegetable fats may reduce the catabolic response to burn injury, trauma, and radiation by reducing the synthesis of prostaglandins that enhance the inflammatory response (see Table 78-2).

Protein or Amino Acid Requirements The recommended dietary protein allowance of 0.8 g/kg per day is adequate for nonstressed patients, for example, a starved patient with a high-grade esophageal stricture. Catabolic patients, in contrast, may require up to 1.5 g/kg per day of protein to induce positive nitrogen balance and reconstitute normal body mass. Some studies suggest that nitrogen balance may be improved by giving human growth hormone, but it is not clear whether growth hormone increases muscle mass or enhances tissue healing. In a stable patient the adequacy of protein support can be assessed by analyzing protein balance:

Protein balance
= protein intake − protein loss

where protein loss = [(24-h urine urea nitrogen (g) + 4) × 6.25]. Over a long period, protein balance is assessed by documenting wound healing, restoration of normal body composition, or resumption of longitudinal growth.

In states of disturbed protein utilization (e.g., renal and hepatic failure), azotemia and abnormal plasma amino acid patterns develop. The benefit of special enteral and parenteral solutions that correct these aberrations is only established in hepatic encephalopathy (see "Risks and Benefits of Nutrition Support").

Table 78-4

Estimation of Daily Fluid Requirements

NORMAL 70-kg MAN

Intake
Normal requirement: 35 × 70 = ~2500 ml/d (derived from oral liquids of 1200 mL, or 5 glasses/cups per day and solid food providing 1300 mL, 1000 mL from water in food, 300 mL from water generated by metabolism of foods)

Output
Urine: 1600 mL/d
Insensible loss: 800 mL/d
Stool: 100 mL/d
[sweat loss can be up to 2 L/d; each degree of fever (C) = 200 mL/d]

TUBE ENTERAL PATIENT

58-kg woman recovering from total gastrectomy for gastric cancer and supported by jejunostomy feedings, taking nothing by mouth or intravenously but experiencing 600 mL of diarrheal losses/day:
Normal requirement 35 × 58 = ~2000 mL/d
Abnormal gastrointestinal loss 600 − 100 = 500 mL/d
Total per tube requirement = 2500 mL/d

PARENTERAL PATIENT

66-kg man with a high jejunostomy following massive bowel resection for Crohn's disease with oral intake of 2000 mL/day and jejunostomy loss of 4000 mL/day:
Normal requirement 35 × 66 = 2300 mL/d
Abnormal gastrointestinal loss (4000 − 100) minus oral intake (2000) = 1900 mL/d
Total parenteral requirement = 4200 mL/d

Table 78-5

CHAPTER 78
Enteral and Parenteral Nutrition Therapy   **477**

Enteric Fluid Volumes and Their Sodium, Potassium, Chloride, and Bicarbonate Content*

	L/d†	Na mmol/L	K‡ mmol/L	Cl mmol/L	HCO₃§ mmol/L
Oral intake	2–3				
Enteric secretions					
Saliva	1–2	10	30	10	30
Gastric juice	2	60	9	90	0
Bile	2–3	150	10	90	70
Small bowel	1	100	5	100	20
Colon	Variable	40	100	15	60

* Enteric secretions are also rich in divalent cations (Ca, Mg, Zn, Cu), and their loss is increased by steatorrhea, a high bowel fistula, or prolonged suction.

† Of the 9 L/d of oral and enteric fluid presented to the upper small bowel, normally 50 percent is absorbed in the jejunum, 40 percent in the ileum, and 10 percent in the colon. In short bowel patients, the colon can absorb greater amounts, up to 3 L/d.

‡ Potassium losses are small except in secretions distal to the ileocecal valve. The colon ion exchange is partly controlled by aldosterone, and therefore, Na⁺ depletion increases K⁺ loss in the stool.

§ Bicarbonate losses must be replaced in parenteral solutions as acetane or lactate because of potential precipitation of bicarbonate with ingredients such as calcium.

Certain organic compounds that can normally be synthesized endogenously become essential in severely ill patients when endogenous production or salvage pathways are impaired. This is true of glutamine, nucleotides, and the products of methionine metabolism (see Table 78-2). Glutamine, an important fuel for the enterocyte and lymphocyte, is fairly insoluble and is absent from standard parenteral formulas and present in low concentrations in most enteral formulas. Soluble glutamine-containing dipeptides are under investigation.

Nucleotides and their related metabolic products have beneficial effects on the immune system, growth of the small intestine, lipid metabolism, and hepatic function. Nucleotides can be synthesized de

Table 78-6

Daily Enteral (EN) and Parenteral (PN) Requirements of Essential Fatty Acids, Minerals, and Vitamins

Nutrient	Daily requirement, adult range	
	EN	PN
Essential fatty acids, % kcal	1–2	2–4
Calcium, g	0.8–1.2	0.2–0.4
Phosphorus, g	0.8–1.2	0.4–0.8
Potassium, g	2–5	3–4
Sodium, g	1–3	1–3
Chloride, g	2–5	3–4*
Magnesium, g	0.3	0.3
Iron, mg	10	1–2
Zinc, mg	15	3–12
Copper, mg	2–3	0.3–0.5
Iodine, mg	0.15	0.15
Manganese, mg	2–5	2–5
Chromium, μg	50–200	15–30
Molybdenum, μg	150–300	20–120
Selenium, μg	50–200	50–100
Ascorbic acid, mg	60	100
Thiamine, mg	1.4	3.0
Riboflavin, mg	1.6	3.6
Niacin, mg	18	40
Biotin, μg	60	60
Pantothenic acid, mg	5	15
Pyridoxine, mg	2.0	4.0
Folic acid, μg	400	400
Cobalamin, μg	3.0	5
Vitamin A, μg	1000	1000
Vitamin D, μg	10	5–10
Vitamin E, mg	8–10	10–15
Vitamin K, μg	70–140	200

* In addition to chloride anions there is a parenteral requirement for bicarbonate equivalents to protect normal acid-base balance. These are provided as 90 mmoL or more per day of acetate or lactate because of potential precipitation of bicarbonate with ingredients such as calcium.

novo in all cells only in small amounts, and the body therefore depends on dietary nucleotides or on salvage pathways that recycle nucleotides from purine and pyrimidine turnover. Nutritionally depleted patients benefit from formulas enriched in nucleotides.

When amino acids are infused systemically rather than via the more physiologic portal vein, methionine, the only sulfur-containing amino acid in most parenteral solutions, is transaminated in peripheral tissues rather than transulfurated in the liver. As a result, downstream sulfur products such as carnitine, taurine, and glutathione become relatively deficient. Preliminary studies suggest that the addition of an intermediate compound, *S*-adenosyl methionine, to parenteral solutions results in less cholestasis.

Mineral and Vitamin Requirements Parenteral and enteral mineral and vitamin requirements are summarized in Table 78-6. Electrolyte modifications are necessary if the patient has significant gastrointestinal losses (Table 78-5) or renal failure. Requirements of some minerals and vitamins may be higher when they are administered parenterally for several reasons. First, the micronutrients are delivered into the systemic rather than the portal circulation, partially bypassing the liver and being excreted into the urine. Second, patients with bowel disease may have enteric loss of sodium, potassium, chloride, and bicarbonate and malabsorption of divalent cations, fat soluble vitamins, and vitamin B₁₂. Third, nutrients may adhere to the tubing and delivery bags, and exposure to oxygen and light may destroy vitamins (particularly vitamin A).

PARENTERAL NUTRITION Infusion Technique and Patient Monitoring Partial and short-term total parenteral nutrition can be provided via a peripheral vein if the majority of the energy is supplied by isotonic fat solutions; long-term total parenteral nutrition using glucose as the chief energy source requires administration via a central vein catheter so that the hypertonic solution can be rapidly diluted in a high-flow system. The preferred site for central vein infusion is the superior vena cava, and the access and catheter choices are summarized in Table 78-7. Peripherally inserted central catheters are the most economical option for short-term parenteral nutrition. In one randomized study the number of catheter-related infections was the same with peripherally and centrally inserted catheters. Tunneled and implanted subcutaneous ports require operating room insertion and are more stable for long-term use. Central catheters should be changed when clinically indicated; routine changes are costly and hazardous. Chlorhexidine solution is a more effective local antiseptic than iodophor or alcohol. Although transparent dressings are helpful in stabilizing catheters and allow easy observation of the skin site, the incidence of catheter-related sepsis is higher than with traditional dry gauze dressings; newer transparent dressings that trap less moisture are under investigation. Catheters made from silastic material or polyurethane are associated with lower complications than polyvinylchloride catheters. Several types of needleless systems use hub valves; contamination rates for these devices are not yet known. Appropriate clinical and laboratory monitoring for patients on parenteral nutrition is summarized in Table 78-8.

Complications (See Table 78-9) *Mechanical* The insertion of a central venous catheter should be done only by trained personnel under aseptic techniques. Major mechanical complications include pneumothorax; hemothorax from laceration of the subclavian artery or vein; brachial plexus injury; and malpositioning of the catheter in a cerebral vein, the azygos vein, or the right ventricle. The correct catheter position must be confirmed by x-ray before hypertonic nutrient solution is infused. Catheters can subsequently back out of the vein, develop leaks, or become detached from the hub and embolize into the heart or pulmonary artery. Catheter thrombosis may occur, especially if the catheter is used for withdrawing blood samples, and extension of the thrombosis to the central vein is frequently coincident with infection. Thrombosed catheters can sometimes be unblocked by urokinase treatment. The addition of low-dose heparin (1000 units per liter) to limit thrombosis in parenteral catheters is controversial; no randomized, controlled studies dem-

Table 78-7

Central Venous Access for Parenteral Nutrition (PN)

Type of Catheters	Advantages	Disadvantages
Peripherally inserted central catheter (PICC) Single lumen Double lumen	Insertion cost low, can be done at bedside or by vascular radiology; especially advantageous for patients with neck wounds such as tracheostomies	High incidence of skin site irritation; tendency to break at hub; patient requires assistance with weekly dressing change
Centrally inserted externalized catheters (subclavian, jugular, femoral) Single lumen Triple lumen	Can be inserted at bedside; relatively low cost; can be changed over a guidewire if clinically indicated; catheter sepsis rate within subclavian < jugular < femoral vein	10% incidence of mechanical complication with insertion, higher if physician inexperienced; need dedicated PN line; multiple-lumen catheters have increased sepsis rate
Tunneled central catheters or subcutaneous ports	More stable for long-term use; when needle out, patients with ports have less disturbance of body image and can shower and swim without risk	More expensive device requiring operating room insertion; ports require needle stick.

onstrate benefit, and heparin can contribute to loss of bone mineral, which is already a problem with long-term parenteral nutrition.

Metabolic Fluid overload can cause congestive heart failure, particularly in elderly and debilitated patients. Glucose overload can cause an osmotic diuresis or stimulate insulin secretion, which in turn promotes extracellular to intracellular shifts of potassium and phosphorous. Such shifts are most dangerous in cachectic patients with depletion of potassium and phosphorus stores and can cause arrhythmias, cardiopulmonary dysfunction, and neurologic symptoms. To avoid these problems, parenteral nutrition should be started slowly and monitored carefully. Glucose content is increased gradually as the patient demonstrates tolerance of the high glucose load.

Late metabolic complications include cholestatic liver disease with bile sludging and gallstone formation. The exact cause of the liver disease is not understood, but lack of enteral stimulation of bile flow and defective sulfur amino acid metabolism appear to play a role. Cholestasis is less likely to occur if some enteral feeding is maintained. Parenteral nutrition induces hypercalcinuria, which can result in negative calcium balance and osteopenia. Hypercalcinuria may have several causes, including the high fixed-acid load of infused amino acids and the bisulfite preservative in the solutions. Earlier protein hydrolysates were contaminated with aluminum, which blocked bone mineralization, and aluminum is still a contaminant of some additives such as calcium gluconate. Once patients on long-term parenteral nutrition move from catabolic breakdown to sustained anabolism, deficiencies of micronutrients such as essential fatty acids, trace minerals, and vitamins may develop unless they are supplied in adequate amounts (see Table 78-6).

Infectious Infection of the access line rarely occurs in the first 72 h, and fever during this period is usually due to infection elsewhere or some other cause. Infection of the access line is likely if the fever defervesces when the infusion of the parenteral formula is tapered. Positive central line cultures suggests catheter sepsis, especially if no other infectious source is identified and if the organism is *Staphylococcus* or *Candida*. While removal of the central catheter may allow fungemia to clear spontaneously, antibiotic therapy is recommended for bacterial infections and the more invasive fungi. Catheter sepsis is equally likely with peripherally inserted central catheters, tunneled catheters, and single-lumen catheters dedicated exclusively to parenteral nutrition; multiple-lumen catheters are associated with a greater incidence of sepsis. While there is no evidence to support the use of prophylactic antibiotics, recurrent catheter sepsis may be avoided if cuffs are used around the catheter exit site or small amounts of an antibiotic solution are left in the line along with a heparin lock.

ENTERAL NUTRITION **Tube Placement and Patient Monitoring** The types of enteral feeding tubes, methods of insertion, their clinical uses, and potential complications are outlined in Table 78-10, and the various types of enteral formulas are listed in Table 78-11.

Table 78-8

Monitoring the Patient on Total Parenteral Nutrition

CLINICAL DATA MONITORED DAILY

Sense of well-being: symptoms suggesting fluid overload, high or low blood glucose, electrolyte imbalance, etc.
Strength as judged by graded activity: getting out of bed, walking, stair climbing.
Vital signs: temperature, blood pressure, pulse rate, and respiratory rate.
Fluid balance: weight; fluid input (intravenous +/− enteral) versus fluid output (urine, stool, gastric suction, etc.).
Delivery equipment for parenteral nutrition: composition of nutrient solution, tubing, pump, filter, catheter, dressing (skin checked for local infection at time of dressing change).

LABORATORY DATA

Plasma glucose	Four times daily until patient stable
Blood glucose Na⁺, K⁺, Cl⁻, HCO₃⁻ Blood urea nitrogen	Daily until glucose infusion load and patient stable, then twice weekly
Serum albumin, transferrin (or TIBC) Liver function studies Serum creatinine Ca^{2+}, PO_4^{2+}, Mg^{2+} Hb/Hct, WBC	Baseline, then twice weekly
Prothrombin time, partial thromboplastin time Micronutrient tests as indicated	Baseline, then weekly

Table 78-9

Complications of Total Parenteral Nutrition (TPN)

First 48 h	First 2 Weeks	3 Months Onward
MECHANICAL		
Complications from catheter insertion: Cephalad displacement Pneumothorax Hemothorax Detachment of line at catheter hub with blood loss or air embolism	Catheter coming out of vein, more common if Silastic Detachment of line at catheter hub with blood loss or air embolism	Detachment of line at catheter hub with blood loss or air embolism Fractures or tears in catheter
METABOLIC		
Fluid overload Hyperglycemia Hypophosphatemia Hypokalemia	Cardiopulmonary failure Hyperosmolar nonketotic hyperglycemic coma Acid-base imbalance Electrolyte imbalance	Essentially fatty acid deficiency Zinc, copper, chromium, selenium, molybdenum, deficiency Iron deficiency Vitamin deficiencies Refeeding edema TPN metabolic bone disease TPN liver disease
INFECTIOUS		
	Catheter-induced sepsis Exit site infection	Catheter-induced sepsis Tunnel infections Exit site infection

Table 78-10

Enteral Feeding Tubes

Type/Insertion Technique	Clinical Uses	Potential Complications
NASOGASTRIC TUBE		
External measurement, nostril, ear, xiphisternum; tube stiffened by ice water or stylet; position verified by injecting air and auscultating, aspirating gastric acid, or by x-ray	Short-term clinical situation (weeks) or longer periods with intermittent insertion; bolus feeding simpler, but continuous drip with pump better tolerated	Aspiration; ulceration of nasal and esophageal tissues, leading to stricture
NASOJEJUNAL TUBE		
External measurement: nostril, ear, anterior superior iliac spine (medical malleolus in infants); tube stiffened by stylet and passed through pylorus under fluoscopy or with endoscopic loop	Short-term clinical situations where gastric emptying impaired or proximal leak suspected; requires continuous drip with pump	Spontaneous pulling back into stomach (position reverified by aspirating content pH > 6); diarrhea common, fiber-containing formula may help
GASTROSTOMY TUBE		
Percutaneous placement endoscopically, radiologically, or surgically: after tract established, can be converted to a gastric "button"	Long-term clinical situations, swallowing disorders, or impaired small-bowel absorption requiring continuous drip	Aspiration; irritation around tube exit site; peritoneal leak; balloon migration and obstruction of pylorus
JEJUNOSTOMY TUBE		
Percutaneous placement endoscopically or radiologically via pylorus or surgically into jejunum sutured to abdominal wall using fine-bore tube or larger tube	Long-term clinical situations where gastric emptying impaired; requires continuous drip with pump	Clogging or displacement of tube; jejunal fistula if large-bore tube used; diarrhea
COMBINED GASTROJEJUNOSTOMY TUBE		
Percutaneous placement endoscopically, radiologically, or surgically; intragastric arm for continuous or intermittent gastric suction; jejunal arm for enteral feeding	Used for patients with impaired gastric emptying and at high risk for aspiration or patients with acute pancreatitis or proximal leaks	Clogging; irritation around tube exit site

Table 78-11

Enteral Formulas

Composition Characteristics	Clinical Indication
STANDARD ENTERAL FORMULA	

1. Complete dietary products (+)*
  a. Caloric density 1 kcal/mL
  b. Protein ~14% cals, caseinates, soy, lactalbumin
  c. Fat ~30% cals, corn, soy, safflower oils
  d. CHO ~60% cals, hydrolysed corn starch, maltodextrin, sucrose
  e. Recommended daily intake of all minerals and vitamins in ≥1500 kcal/d
  f. Osmolality (mosm/kg) ~300
	Suitable for most patients requiring tube feeding; flavors available for oral use

MODIFIED ENTERAL FORMULAS	
1. Caloric density 1.5–2 kcal/mL (+)	Fluid-restricted patients
2.	
a. High protein ~20% cals (+)	Protein malnutrition and ↓ wound healing
b. Hydrolysed protein to small peptides (+ +)	↓ Protein digestion/absorption or allergy
c. ↑ Glutamine, arginine, S-containing amino acids, nucleotides (+ + +)	Severely immunocompromised patients
d. Branch-chain amino acids, ↓ aromatic amino acids (+ + +)	Liver failure patients intolerant of 0.8 g/kg per day of regular protein
e. ↓ Protein, ↓ K, Mg, and P diets (+ +)	Renal failure patients
f. ↓ Protein, ↑ essential amino acids, ↓ minerals and vitamins (+ + +)	Renal failure patients not on dialysis
3.	
a. Low fat, partial MCT substitution (+)	Fat malabsorption
b. ↑ Fat >40% cals (+ +)	Pulmonary failure with ↑ P_{CO_2} on standard formulas
c. ↑ Fat from MUFA (+ +)	Poorly controlled diabetes mellitus
d. Fat ↑ in ω3 (fish oil) and ↓ ω6 (+ + +)	Immunocompromised and autoimmune disorder
4.	
a. Fiber provided as soy poly saccharide (+)	Diarrhea/constipation
b. Fiber provided as blenderized fruits and vegetables (+ +)	↓ Binding of dilantin
5. ↑ Minerals (Zn) and vitamins (A and C) (+ +)	Decubitus ulcers

* Cost: + inexpensive; + + moderately expensive; + + + very expensive.

NOTE: CHO, carbohydrate; MCT, medium chain triglyceride; MUFA, monunsaturated fatty acid, ω3 or ω6 polyunsatuated fat with first double bond at carbon 3 (fish oils) or carbon

Patients on enteral feeding are at risk for many of the same metabolic complications as those receiving parenteral nutrition and should be monitored in the same way (Table 78-8). Since small-bore tubes are easily displaced, tube position should be checked at intervals by aspirating and measuring the pH of the gut fluid (<4 in stomach, >6 in jejunum).

Complications *Aspiration* The debilitated patient with poor gastric emptying and impairment of the swallowing and cough mechanisms is at risk for aspiration; this is particularly so for those on respirators because tracheal suctioning induces coughing and gastric regurgitation and because the cuffs on the endotracheal tube or tracheostomy seldom provide protection against aspiration. Under these circumstances, it may be safer to use a large-bore feeding tube to allow for temporary removal of gastric contents during tracheal suction or to use jejunal feeding.

Constant gastric infusion of an enteral formula is better tolerated in sick patients than is intermittent bolus feeding. A continuous infusion is best achieved with a pump, especially when using fine-bore tubes that have a greater potential to clog. If long-term feeding is anticipated, endoscopic, radiologic, or surgical placement of a gastric tube is preferred by most patients. For long-term ambulatory patients, a gastrostomy tube can be converted to a gastric "button," an access device that is flush with the skin.

A nasojejunal tube reduces the risk of aspiration. However, fluoroscopic placement of fine bore tubes through the pylorus is time-consuming, and such tubes frequently pull back into the stomach. A large percutaneous gastric-suction and jejunal-feeding tube is more reliable. This can be placed radiologically, endoscopically, or surgically.

Diarrhea Enteral feeding often causes diarrhea, especially if bowel function is compromised by bowel disease or drugs. The diarrhea may be controlled by the use of continuous drip feeding or by the addition of bulking agents, such as psyllium hydrophilic mucilogs, or an anticholinergic medication in the formula. Diarrhea of enteral feeding does not necessarily imply inadequate absorption of nutrients, other than water and electrolytes. Furthermore, since luminal nutrients exert trophic effects on the gut mucosa and enhance the enteric immunologic barrier, it may be appropriate to persist, despite the diarrhea, even when this necessitates temporary supplemental parenteral fluid support.

THE COST OF NUTRITION SUPPORT As many as 25 percent of patients entering tertiary care hospitals have central catheters placed, and 20 to 30 percent of these catheters are used for parenteral nutrition. The incidence of catheter-related infection reflects the severity of the underlying medical conditions and varies from 2 to 30 per thousand catheter days, depending on the type of patients involved. In critically ill patients, catheter sepsis is associated with a 35 percent mortality rate and an attributable cost of about $40,000 per survivor. Most catheter-related complications derive from faulty insertion and management of the catheter rather than defects in the device. In large tertiary care hospitals, the insertion and management of these lines by specially trained teams can reduce complications by 80 percent, impacting significantly on outcome and costs.

The shift of focus of nutritional support of hospitalized patients from parenteral to enteral feeding also promises significant cost savings. Home parenteral nutrition costs approximately half as much as similar treatment in the hospital, and the cost of home enteral nutrition is one-tenth the cost of home parentral therapy.

BIBLIOGRAPHY

AMERICAN COLLEGE OF PHYSICIANS: Position paper: Parenteral nutrition in patients receiving cancer chemotherapy: A meta-analysis. Ann Intern Med 110:734, 1989

ANDERSON GF, STEINBERG EP: DRGs and specialized nutritional support: The need for reform. J Parenter Enter Nutr 10:3, 1986

BOWER RH et al: Early enteral administration of a formula (Impact) supplemented with arginine, nucleotides and fish oil in intensive care unit patients. Results of a multicenter, prospective, randomized, clinical trial. Crit Care Med 23:436, 1995

DALY JM et al: Enteral nutrition with supplemental arginine, RNA, and omega 3 fatty acids in patients after operation: Immunologic, metabolic and clinical outcome. Surgery 112:56, 1992

DETSKY AS et al: Perioperative parenteral nutrition: A meta-analysis. Ann Intern Med 107:195, 1987

FLYNN MB, LEIGHTTY FF: Preoperative outpatient nutritional support of patients with squamous cancer of the upper aerodigestive tract. Am J Surg 154:359, 1987

FREZZA M et al: Oral *S* adenosyl methionine in symptomatic treatment of intrahepatic cholestasis. Gastroenterology 99:211, 1990

GIAFFER MH et al: Controlled trial of polymeric versus elemental diet in treatment of active Crohn's disease. Lancet 335:816, 1990

GRAHM TW et al: The benefits of early jejunal hyperalimentation in the head-injured patient. Neurosurgery 25(5):729, 1989

GREENBERG GR et al: Controlled trial of bowel rest and nutritional support in the management of Crohn's disease. Gut 29:1309, 1988

HERNDON DN et al: Increased mortality with intravenous supplemental feeding in severely burned patients. J Burn Care Rehab 10:309, 1989

HILL GL: Body composition research: Implications for the practice of clinical nutrition. J Parenter Enter Nutr 16:197, 1992

HOWARD L et al: Current use and clinical outcome of home parenteral and enteral nutrition therapies in the United States. Gastroenterology 109:335, 1995

KALFARENTZOS FE et al: Total parenteral nutrition in severe acute pancreatitis. J Am Col Nutr 10(2):156, 1991

KUDSK KA et al: Enteral versus parenteral feeding: Effect on septic morbidity following blunt and penetrating trauma. Ann Surg 215(5):503, 1992

LIPMAN TO: Clinical trials of nutrition support in cancer. Hematol Oncol Clin North Am 5:91, 1991

McCANN RM et al: Comfort care for terminally ill patients. JAMA 272:1263, 1994

MOORE FA et al: TEN vs. TPN following major abdominal trauma—reduced septic morbidity. J Trauma 29:916, 1989

——— et al: Clinical benefits of an immune-enhancing diet for early post injury enteral feeding. J Trauma 37:607, 1994

NAYLOR CD et al: Parenteral nutrition with branched-chain amino acids in hepatic encephalopathy: A meta-analysis. Gastroenterology 97:1033, 1989

Perioperative total parenteral nutrition in surgical patients: Veterans Administration total parenteral nutrition cooperative study: N Engl J Med 325:525, 1991

RAAD II et al: Infectious complications of indwelling vascular catheters. Clin Infect Dis 15:197, 1992

RIORDAN AM et al: Treatment of active Crohn's disease by exclusion diet: East Anglian Multicenter Controlled Trial. Lancet 342:1131, 1993

SITZMANN JV et al: Statement on guidelines for total parenteral nutrition. Dig Dis Sci 34:489, 1989

WEINSIER RL et al: Cost containment: A contribution of aggressive nutrition support in burn patients. J Burn Care Rehabil 6:436, 1985

WEISDORF S et al: Influence of prophylactic total parenteral nutrition on long-term outcome of bone marrow transplantation. Transplantation 43:833, 1987

WOLFSON M: Use of nutritional supplements in dialysis patients. Semin Dialysis 5:285, 1992

ZIEGLER TR et al: Clinical and metabolic efficacy of glutamine-supplemented parenteral nutrition after bone marrow transplantation. Ann Intern Med 116:821, 1992

79 *Jean D. Wilson*

VITAMIN DEFICIENCY AND EXCESS

Vitamins play several roles in human disease. Deficiencies of single vitamins are now rarely endemic, even in developing nations, and are more likely to occur either as a component of general malnutrition, as a result of food faddism, as a complication of another disease such as malabsorption or alcoholism, as a consequence of therapy such as hemodialysis or total parenteral nutrition, or as the result of an inborn error of metabolism. Indeed, disorders of vitamin excess may now be

In considering vitamin physiology, several points are worth emphasis: (1) The fact that organic compounds cannot be synthesized within the body and are required constituents of the diet is the result of mutations, and the provision of vitamins in the diet is a form of therapy for an inborn error of metabolism. In some instances, such as the limited ability to synthesize thiamine, the requirement is common to many, if not all, animals, and the defect must have arisen early in evolution; in others, such as the single-gene defect that prevents ascorbic acid synthesis, humans share the defect with only a few species, such as the guinea pig. (2) Only small amounts of vitamins are required in the diet in contrast to the relatively large amounts of essential amino acids and essential fatty acids. This is a consequence of the fact that vitamins function not as building blocks of tissue mass or as substrates for energy production but as prosthetic groups for quantitatively minor tissue constituents or as catalytic cofactors for biologic reactions; like most catalysts, they are required only in small amounts. (3) Deficiency of some vitamins (e.g., pantothenic acid) has never been described in humans, implying that these vitamins either are so ubiquitous in food sources or are conserved so efficiently by the body that deficiency can become manifest, if at all, only in the context of a mixed nutritional and vitamin deficiency. (4) The fact that many vitamin deficiencies develop on the background of alcoholism is the consequence of several interlocking factors, including diminished vitamin intake, impairment of absorption and storage of vitamins, and, in some cases, predisposing genetic factors. (5) Biochemical means of proving vitamin deficiency, once suspected, are limited, and the role of vitamin deficiency in disease states is frequently not recognized because nonspecific vitamin therapy is a common part of standard supportive care. As a consequence, knowledge of the manifestations of vitamin deficiency and a high index of suspicion in the appropriate setting are essential for considering the diagnosis, and demonstration of a response to replacement therapy may be the most accurate way to confirm a diagnosis. (6) Excessive amounts of vitamins can be consumed either as the indirect consequence of dietary practice or, more commonly, as the result of deliberate ingestion. Syndromes of excess for the fat-soluble vitamins A and D are well characterized, whereas the toxicity syndromes produced by the water-soluble vitamins are inconsistent and less well understood.

DEFICIENCY STATES

NIACIN (PELLAGRA) **Biochemistry** *Niacin* is the generic term for nicotinic acid (pyridine-3-carboxylic acid) and derivatives that exhibit the nutritional activity of nicotinic acid (Fig. 79-1). In one sense, niacin is not a vitamin, since it can be formed from the essential amino acid tryptophan. In the human, an average of about 1 mg of niacin is formed from 60 mg of dietary tryptophan. Accordingly, estimates of the adequacy of dietary intake must take into account the content of both tryptophan and niacin. Many foodstuffs, especially cereals, contain bound forms of niacin from which the vitamin is not nutritionally available.

The vitamin is absorbed rapidly from the intestine by both active and passive transport mechanisms. The capacity to absorb niacin is approximately 3 to 4 g/d in the human. Approximately one-fifth of the vitamin is decarboxylated to nicotinuric acid, and the remainder is excreted in the urine as methylated products, largely *N*-methylnicotinamide (NMN) and *N*-methyl-2-pyridone-5-carboxamide.

Mechanism of Action Niacin is an essential component of nicotinamide adenine dinucleotide (NAD) and nicotinamide adenine dinucleotide phosphate (NADP), coenzymes for many oxidation-reduction reactions.

Requirements The requirements and recommended daily allowances for niacin and tryptophan are listed in Table 72-1. In contrast to most vitamins, the requirement for niacin does not appear to be increased during pregnancy.

Experimental Depletion After the institution of a diet deficient in niacin and tryptophan, the urinary excretion of niacin metabolites reaches minimal values (<1.5 mg/d) after 1 to 2 months. Clinical deficiency develops shortly thereafter and consists of dermatitis, glossitis, stomatitis, diarrhea, proctitis, mental depression, abdominal pain, vaginitis, dysphagia, and amenorrhea, findings similar to those in pellagra.

Clinical Deficiency Pellagra was previously an endemic disease in the American South and in many other parts of the world. The endemic disease is usually associated with a high intake of maize (American corn) or of millet (sorghum, jowar) and can be cured by the administration of niacin; nevertheless, the fact that large populations of people exist on a diet in which maize is the major source of protein but are free of endemic pellagra indicates that the relation between maize intake and the development of the disease is not straightforward. The niacin equivalent (available niacin and tryptophan) of maize, although low, is no lower than that of some cereals that are unassociated with endemic pellagra. As a consequence, the concept of the pathogenesis of pellagra has evolved from that of a pure vitamin deficiency or a mixed deficiency of tryptophan and available niacin in the diet to a more complicated etiology. The disorder may be due to an imbalance in dietary amino acids or to a complex deficiency state. Alternatively, the milling of maize influences the bioavailability of the niacin in the cereal. Treatment of maize with alkali in the preparation of foods in Latin America may serve to hydrolyze bound nicotinic acid and inactivate toxins that accumulate in stored grain contaminated with molds. In contrast, degermination of the cereal during the common milling process in the United States may inhibit the liberation of bound niacin. The effect of these treatments, respectively, would be to prevent or to predispose to the development of pellagra when maize is a major element of the diet.

Whatever the cause, endemic pellagra disappeared coincident with the improvement of nutritional education and the widespread supplementation of grain cereals with niacin but still occurs on occasion in epidemic form, for example, among refugees. Pellagra is also a rare manifestation of the carcinoid syndrome, in which up to 60 percent of tryptophan is catabolized by what is ordinarily a minor pathway (see Chap. 95), and Hartnup disease (see Chap. 349), an inherited disorder in which several amino acids including tryptophan are absorbed poorly from the diet. In both conditions, pellagra is due to diminished availability of effective niacin equivalents and can be cured by the administration of large amounts of the vitamin.

Pellagra is a chronic wasting disease typically associated with dermatitis, dementia, and diarrhea. The dermatitis is bilateral, symmetric, and present in sites exposed to sunlight and is due to photosensitivity. The mental changes are less discrete; fatigue, insomnia, and apathy may precede the development of an encephalopathy characterized by confusion, disorientation, hallucination, loss of memory, and eventually, organic psychosis. Paresthesias and polyneuritis may be the result of coexisting deficiencies of other vitamins. Diarrhea, when present, results from widespread inflammation of the mucous surfaces; other mucosal abnormalities include achlorhydria, glossitis, stomatitis, and vaginitis. The skin lesions are characterized by hyperkeratosis, hyperpigmentation, and desquamation. The course is progressive over a several-year period, and death is usually due to secondary complications. The relation between the coenzyme functions of NAD and NADP and the symptoms has not been defined. The mental changes in pellagra may be due to diminished conversion of tryptophan to serotonin.

No biochemical test is of diagnostic value, and diagnosis must be based on suspicion and response to replacement therapy. As predicted, urinary excretion of the metabolites of nicotinic acid and tryptophan is low but not lower than in patients with generalized malnutrition. Plasma tryptophan and erythrocyte NAD and NADP levels are also low.

The administration of small amounts of niacin (10 mg/d) in the face of adequate amounts of dietary tryptophan is sufficient to cure

Vitamin	Active derivative or cofactor form	Principal function
Niacin 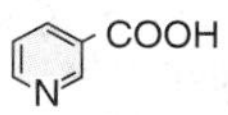 COOH (pyridine ring with N)	Nicotinamide adenine dinucleotide phosphate (NADP) and nicotine adenine dinucleotide (NAD)	Coenzymes for oxidations and reductions
Thiamine 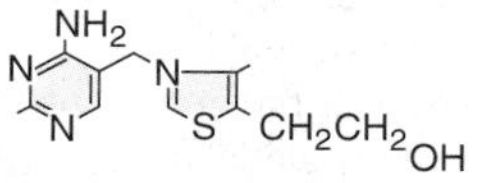 NH_2 ... CH_2CH_2OH	Thiamine diphosphate	Coenzyme for cleavage of carbon-carbon bonds
Pyridoxine 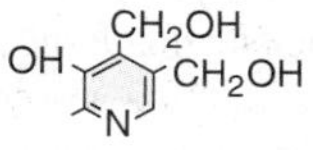 OH, CH_2OH, CH_2OH	Pyridoxal phosphate	Cofactor for enzymes of amino acid metabolism
Riboflavin 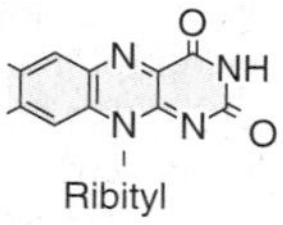 (Ribityl)	Flavin mononucleotide (FMN) and flavin adenine dinucleotide (FAD)	Cofactor for oxidation-reduction reactions and covalently attached prosthetic groups for some enzymes
Ascorbic acid 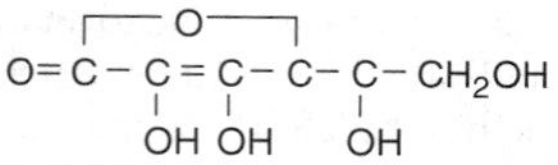 $O=C-C=C-C-C-CH_2OH$, OH OH OH	Ascorbic acid and dehydroascorbic acid	Participation as a redox ion in many biological oxidation reactions
Biotin 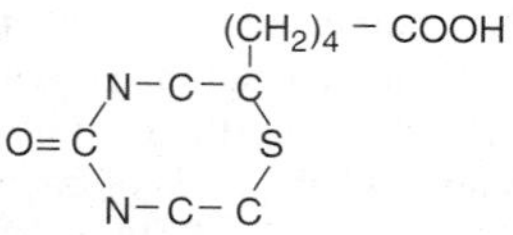 $(CH_2)_4-COOH$	Biotin	Apoenzyme for carboxylase enzymes
Vitamin A 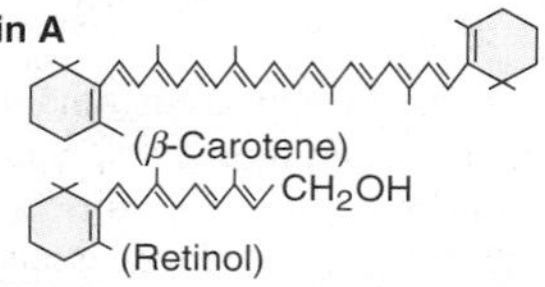 (β-Carotene) (Retinol) CH_2OH	Retinol, retinal, and retinoic acid	Formation of carotenoid proteins (vision) and glycoproteins (epithelial cell function)
Vitamin E 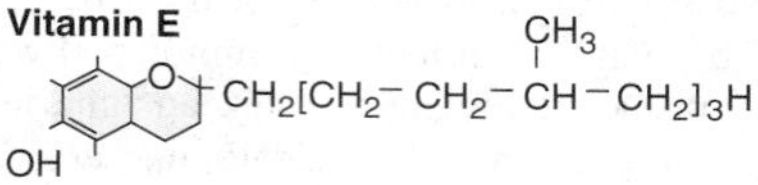 CH_3, $CH_2[CH_2-CH_2-CH-CH_2]_3H$, OH	Tocopherol	Antioxidant
Vitamin K 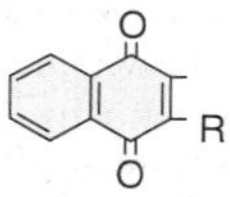 R	Menaquinone	Cofactor for post-translational carboxylation of many proteins including essential clotting factors

FIGURE 79-1 The structure and principal functions of some of the vitamins associated with human disorders.

endemic pellagra. Large amounts of niacin (40 to 200 mg/d) may be required in Hartnup disease and in the carcinoid syndrome.

THIAMINE (BERIBERI) Biochemistry Thiamine contains pyrimidine and thiazole moieties linked by a methylene bridge (see Fig. 79-1). The vitamin is synthesized by a variety of plants and microorganisms but not ordinarily by animals. However, rats and pigeons fed a thiamine-free diet can be protected from deficiency by large quantities of the pyrimidine and thiazole moieties, suggesting a small capacity to couple the subunits together. Small amounts may be synthesized by microorganisms in the gastrointestinal tract. Thiamine is absorbed both by an active-transport process and by passive diffusion. The capacity to absorb the vitamin in the human intestine is about 5 mg/d. Approximately 25 to 30 mg are stored in the body, 80 percent as thiamine diphosphate (pyrophosphate), 10 percent as thiamine triphosphate, and the remainder as thiamine monophosphate. Large amounts are present in skeletal muscles, heart, liver, kidneys, and brain. A number of thiaminase enzymes inactivate thiamine by splitting the vitamin into its two component parts. Several metabolites are excreted in the urine, principally thiamine itself (which is secreted by the renal tubules), an acetylated derivative, and derivatives of thiazole acetate and pyrimidine carboxylate.

Mechanism of Action Thiamine diphosphate acts as a coenzyme for several reactions that cleave carbon-carbon bonds—the oxidative decarboxylation of α-keto acids (pyruvate and α-ketoglutarate) and keto analogues of leucine, isoleucine, and valine and the transketolase reaction in the pentose phosphate pathway. Many features of thiamine deficiency are the result of inhibition of these enzymatic reactions and/or the accumulation of the proximal metabolites. Thiamine also may have a specific role in neurons independent of its function in general metabolism; thiamine and its esters are present in axonal membranes, and electrical stimulation of nerves effects the hydrolysis and release of thiamine diphosphate and triphosphate.

Requirements The recommended daily allowances for thiamine are given in Table 72-1. The vitamin has a widespread distribution in food and is absent only from oils, fats, cassava, and refined sugar. In vegetable products, the vitamin is largely in the form of thiamine. The outer layers of cereal grains are especially rich in the vitamin; hence machine-milled rice is a poor source. In animal tissues, thiamine is present largely in the form of phosphate esters. The esters are dephosphorylated by phosphatases in the intestine, and only the free vitamin is absorbed. A substantial loss of the vitamin takes place during cooking above 100°C.

Several factors influence the absorption and metabolism of the vitamin (and hence alter daily requirements). One is the presence of thiaminases in foods such as fresh fish, clams, shrimp, mussels, and some raw animal tissues and in microorganisms in the colon. Two, daily needs decrease when fat forms a large part of the diet and increase as carbohydrate intake increases. Requirements are increased by pregnancy, lactation, thyrotoxicosis, and fever. Accelerated loss of thiamine may occur with diuretic therapy, hemodialysis, peritoneal dialysis, and diarrhea. Defective absorption can occur in malabsorption states, alcoholism, chronic malnutrition, and folate deficiency.

Experimental Depletion Following the institution of a thiamine-free diet in control subjects, urinary thiamine excretion decreases to 5 percent of the control value after a week and is undetectable after 2 weeks. However, the excretion of the pyrimidine and thiazole catabolites remains unchanged for as long as a month, indicating that the body pool is slowly utilized when intake is low.

Within a week after the institution of a deficient diet, subjects develop a resting tachycardia, followed by the onset of weakness, decreased deep tendon reflexes, and (in some) sensory neuropathy. Symptoms include generalized malaise, headache, nausea, and aching of the muscles. Appearance of these symptoms is paralleled by a fall in red blood cell transketolase activity. Within a week of thiamine repletion (2 mg/d), all abnormal physical findings disappear, and the subjective symptoms clear after 2 weeks. (Experimental depletion in humans has not been carried to the point of development of severe manifestations.)

CHAPTER 79
Vitamin Deficiency and Excess

483

Clinical Deficiency In developed nations, thiamine deficiency occurs in alcoholics or food faddists and in special clinical situations, such as chronic peritoneal dialysis, hemodialysis, refeeding after starvation, after the administration of glucose to asymptomatic but thiamine-depleted patients, and in some studies in patients given large doses of diuretics chronically for congestive heart failure. In developing countries, the disorder is commonly due to the consumption of milled rice or foods containing thiaminases or (possibly) other antithiamine factors.

Development of thiamine deficiency in chronic alcoholics is due to low thiamine intake, impaired thiamine absorption and storage, accelerated destruction of thiamine diphosphate, and varying degrees of energy expenditure. However, clinical manifestations develop in only a fraction of alcoholics and other chronically malnourished persons. Genetic factors may be involved in susceptibility.

The two major manifestations of thiamine deficiency involve the cardiovascular (wet beriberi) and nervous systems (dry beriberi and the Wernicke-Korsakoff syndrome). The typical patient has mixed symptoms involving both the cardiovascular and nervous systems, but pure cardiovascular, neuropathic, and cerebral forms also occur. The relative preponderance of these manifestations is related in part to the duration and severity of deficiency, the degree of physical exertion, and the caloric intake. Severe physical exertion, high carbohydrate intake, and a moderate degree of chronic deficiency favor wet beriberi with little or no peripheral neuritis, whereas an equal deficiency with caloric restriction and relative inactivity favors the development of dry beriberi.

Beriberi heart disease comprises three major physiologic derangements: (1) peripheral vasodilatation leading to a high-output state, (2) retention of sodium and water leading to edema, and (3) biventricular myocardial failure. In the chronic form, peripheral vasodilatation leads to increased arteriovenous shunting of blood, rapid circulation time, tachycardia, increased cardiac output, and a venous congestive state characterized by elevated peripheral venous pressure, elevated right ventricular end-diastolic pressure, decreased arteriovenous extraction of oxygen, sodium retention, and edema. Decreased cerebral and renal blood flow and increased flow to muscles are common. Cardiac output increases so that notwithstanding the lowered peripheral vascular resistance, ventricular work, arterial blood pressure, and pulmonary wedge pressure tend to be elevated. Temporary appearance or worsening of hypertension may occur during thiamine repletion, presumably due to closing of arteriovenous shunts and temporary volume overload.

In acute fulminant cardiovascular (shoshin) beriberi, the myocardial lesion is the central feature of a course in which dyspnea, restlessness, and anxiety eventuate in acute cardiovascular collapse and death within hours to days. Physical findings include stocking-glove cyanosis, tachycardia, marked cardiomegaly, hepatomegaly, arterial bruits, and neck vein distention. The venous pressure is high, and the circulation time is rapid. Because of the fulminant course, edema may be minimal or absent. Administration of thiamine rapidly restores peripheral vascular resistance, but improvement in myocardial function may be delayed so that low-output failure supervenes during treatment.

Three types of nervous system involvement occur: peripheral neuropathy, Wernicke's encephalopathy (cerebral beriberi), and the Korsakoff syndrome. The neuropathy may or may not be painful and is characterized by a symmetric impairment of sensory, motor, and reflex function that affects predominantly the distal segments of limbs. The histologic lesion is a noninflammatory degeneration of myelin sheaths. No meaningful distinction can be made between this disorder and so-called alcoholic neuropathy on the basis of clinical criteria.

Wernicke's encephalopathy ordinarily develops in an orderly sequence and consists of vomiting, nystagmus (horizontal more commonly than vertical), palsies of the rectus muscles leading to unilateral or bilateral ophthalmoplegia (and decrease in the nystagmus), fever, ataxia, and progressive mental deterioration that eventuates in a global confusional state and may progress to coma and death. Improvement occurs after thiamine replacement, although Korsakoff's syndrome may supervene. Thus the eye palsies are corrected, the nystagmus improves in one-half, the ataxia improves or disappears in two-thirds, and the global confusional state disappears to be replaced by Korsakoff's syndrome. The latter consists of retrograde amnesia, impaired ability to learn, and (usually) confabulation. The patient is typically alert and responsive and exhibits no serious defect in behavior. Recovery (complete or partial) from Korsakoff's syndrome occurs only in one-half.

In summary, Wernicke's encephalopathy and the amnesic psychosis of Korsakoff's syndrome are not separate clinical events; instead, the changing ocular and ataxic signs, the transformation of the global confusional state into the amnesic-confabulatory syndrome, and the development of a nonconfabulatory amnesic state are successive stages in the recovery from a single process. → *Cerebral beriberi is discussed further in Chap. 380.*

Biochemical tests to detect thiamine deficiency include the measurement of blood thiamine, pyruvate, α-ketoglutarate, lactate, and glyoxylate; measurement of the urinary excretion of thiamine and thiamine metabolites; the thiamine-loading test; and measurement of urinary methylglyoxal. The most reliable is the measurement of whole-blood or erythrocyte transketolase activity. Any enhancement in enzymatic activity resulting from added thiamine diphosphate (TPP) is referred to as the *TPP effect* (expressed in percent). If the activity of the enzyme is increased more than 15 percent by the added thiamine diphosphate, then a deficiency state is probably present. Measurement of isolated transketolase levels is not useful, but demonstration of an increase in activity after treatment, coupled with a positive TPP test prior to treatment, suggests thiamine deficiency.

Another criterion for the diagnosis is the assessment of clinical response to thiamine administration. Clinical improvement may be dramatic in cardiovascular beriberi, with an increase in blood pressure and a decrease in heart rate within 12 h after start of therapy and diuresis and reduction in heart size within 1 to 2 days.

Prompt administration of thiamine is indicated when beriberi is diagnosed or suspected. Fifty milligrams per day should be given intramuscularly for several days, after which 2.5 to 5 mg/d can be administered by mouth. Larger amounts are usually not absorbed. All patients also should receive other water-soluble vitamins in therapeutic quantities.

Thiamine-Responsive Inborn Errors of Metabolism Thiamine-responsive inborn errors of metabolism, in which patients may respond to pharmacologic doses of thiamine, include thiamine-responsive megaloblastic anemia, which is due to decreased cellular transport of thiamine; thiamine-responsive lactic acidosis, which is due to low activity of the pyruvate dehydrogenase complex; thiamine-responsive branched-chain ketoaciduria, which is due to low activity of a branched chain α-keto acid dehydrogenase; and a subset of subjects with Leigh's encephalomyelopathy due to abnormality of the E1 alpha subunit of pyruvate dehydrogenase.

PYRIDOXINE (VITAMIN B$_6$) Biochemistry The biologic activity of the vitamin B$_6$ group is displayed by pyridoxine, pyridoxal, and pyridoxamine and their 5-phosphate esters (see Fig. 79-1). The coenzyme form is pyridoxal-5-phosphate, and the other compounds owe their activity to conversion to pyridoxal-5-phosphate. The vitamin is widely and uniformly distributed in all foods; muscle meats, liver, vegetables, and whole-grain cereals are among the best sources.

Mechanism of Action Pyridoxal phosphate acts as a cofactor for many enzymes involved in amino acid metabolism, including transaminases, synthetases, and hydroxylases. In humans, the vitamin is of particular importance in the metabolism of tryptophan, glycine, serine, glutamate, and the sulfur-containing amino acids. Pyridoxal phosphate is also required for the synthesis of the heme precursor δ-aminolevulinic acid. A large portion of body stores is in muscle phosphorylase, where it functions to stabilize the enzyme rather than as a catalyst. It also plays a poorly understood role in neuronal excitability, possibly as a result of its function in transsulfuration reactions or in γ-aminobutyric acid (GABA) metabolism.

Requirements The recommended daily allowances are given in Table 72-1. Even more than for most vitamins, the requirement is increased in pregnancy and by the administration of estrogens. Estrogens appear to inhibit the role of pyridoxal phosphate in tryptophan metabolism. Pyridoxine requirement also may be increased by high protein intake and by either chronic hemodialysis or peritoneal dialysis. The ethanol metabolite acetaldehyde displaces pyridoxal phosphate from proteins and thus enhances its degradation.

Experimental Depletion The feeding of pyridoxine-deficient diets leads to chemical evidence of deficiency (increased xanthurenic acid and decreased pyridoxine in urine) within a week. Electroencephalographic abnormalities occur within 3 weeks, and some subjects have grand mal seizures. Deficiency induced with the pyridoxine antagonist deoxypyridoxine causes, in addition, seborrheic dermatitis, cheilosis, glossitis, nausea, vomiting, weakness, and dizziness.

Clinical Deficiency The widespread occurrence of the vitamin in food is probably the reason that pure pyridoxine deficiency is rare except when the pyridoxine content of food is destroyed during processing, as has happened in some infant formulas. It is a paradox, therefore, that pyridoxine deficiency is now common because many drugs act as pyridoxine antagonists. Isoniazid, cycloserine, penicillamine, and carbonyl reagents in general form complexes with the aldehyde moiety of the vitamin and inhibit its function as a coenzyme. In each case abnormal tryptophan metabolism and convulsions can be prevented by supplementation with the vitamin.

Estimates of vitamin deficiency have been based on the correction of clinical signs of deficiency following administration of the vitamin, measurement of the excretion of tryptophan metabolites after tryptophan-loading tests, measurement of various amino acid transferase activities in blood, and measurement of the excretion of pyridoxine or its metabolites or of oxalate in urine. One index is the measurement of urinary tryptophan metabolites, particularly xanthurenic acid, following tryptophan loading. Alternatively, cystathionine can be assayed after administration of a methionine load. In vitro measurement of red blood cell glutamic pyruvic transaminase in the presence and absence of pyridoxal phosphate may be a better indicator of pyridoxine status than either loading test.

The appropriate management is prevention of deficiency. Supplementation of the diet with 30 mg pyridoxine returns tryptophan metabolism to normal in pregnancy, in users of oral contraceptives, and in patients taking isoniazid. Doses as high as 100 mg/d may be required in subjects taking penicillamine.

Pyridoxine-Responsive Diseases Several genetic disorders cause abnormalities in vitamin B$_6$ metabolism. In one group, infants develop convulsions and brain damage and die if not provided with large daily supplements of pyridoxine; the apoenzyme for glutamic acid decarboxylase in this disorder has a decreased binding affinity for pyridoxal phosphate. Consequently, these infants do not form normal amounts of GABA, a physiologic inhibitor of neurotransmission. Another group has pyridoxine-responsive sideroblastic anemia due to mutation in an erythrocyte-specific δ-aminolevulinate synthase; pyridoxine supplementation results in hematologic improvement but does not correct the morphologic abnormality in the erythrocytes.

The synthesis of cystathionine from homocystine and serine and its cleavage to cysteine and homoserine are catalyzed by two pyridoxal phosphate enzymes. Some patients with vitamin B$_6$-responsive xanthurenic aciduria or cystathioninuria have mutant apoenzymes that interact abnormally with pyridoxal phosphate, a defect that can be largely corrected by elevated concentrations of the cofactor. In contrast, the vitamin B$_6$ response in patients with homocystinuria due to cystathionine synthetase deficiency results from enhancement of the activity of the residual amount of normal enzyme present rather than from a restoration of the affected enzyme levels to normal.

RIBOFLAVIN Riboflavin in the form of the coenzymes flavin mononucleotide (FMN) and flavin adenine dinucleotide (FAD) (see Fig. 79-1) participates in a variety of oxidation-reduction reactions.

In addition, covalently attached flavins are essential to the structure of such enzymes as succinate dehydrogenase and monoamine oxidase. The vitamin is absorbed from the gastrointestinal tract either as free riboflavin or the 5'-phosphate by an active transport process. The recommended daily allowance is listed in Table 72-1. Covalently linked vitamin accounts for less than one-tenth of the tissue pool. The vitamin is excreted in urine predominantly in the free form, although a small fraction of the daily turnover is the result of catabolism by microorganisms in the gastrointestinal tract.

Riboflavin deficiency can be induced by feeding a riboflavin-deficient diet or by the administration of riboflavin antagonists such as galactoflavin. Deficiency is characterized by sore throat, hyperemia and edema of the oral mucous membranes, cheilosis, angular stomatitis, glossitis, seborrheic dermatitis, and normochromic, normocytic anemia due to red cell hypoplasia of the bone marrow. These features can be reversed by riboflavin administration. Thyroid hormones and adrenal steroids enhance FMN and FAD synthesis; phenothiazines and tricyclic antidepressants competitively inhibit flavin coenzyme biosynthesis, but these agents alone do not induce deficiency. Instead, riboflavin deficiency almost invariably occurs in combination with deficiencies of other water-soluble vitamins. Riboflavin requirements are increased in subjects on chronic hemodialysis or peritoneal dialysis.

VITAMIN C (SCURVY) Biochemistry In most animals, ascorbic acid (vitamin C) can be synthesized from glucose. However, humans, other primates, and the guinea pig are unable to synthesize L-ascorbic acid and require vitamin C in the diet (Fig 79-1). These species can perform the various reactions required for the biosynthesis of the vitamin from D-glucose except for one step, the conversion of L-gluconogammalactone to L-abscorbic acid. The enzyme that catalyzes this reaction (L-gluconolactone oxidase) is defective because of a mutation; thus the need for vitamin C in the diet is the result of an inborn error in carbohydrate metabolism.

Mechanism of Action L-Ascorbic acid readily undergoes reversible oxidation and reduction as follows:

$$\text{L-ascorbic acid} \rightleftharpoons \text{dehydro-L-ascorbic acid} + 2H^+ + 2e$$

This property of the vitamin is the key to understanding its role as a redox agent for biologic oxidation. However, ascorbic acid does not act as a conventional cofactor because its requirement can usually be replaced by other compounds with similar redox properties. The vitamin reduces the prosthetic metal ions in many enzymes and performs other antioxidant functions by removing free radicals. The best understood function is in the synthesis of collagen; absence of the vitamin leads to impairment of peptidyl hydroxylation of procollagen; nonhydroxylated collagen cannot form the triple helix required for normal tissue structure. In addition, the synthesis of both proteoglycan and collagen is decreased in ascorbic acid deficiency, possibly due to inhibition of insulin-like growth factor I. Many features of scurvy result from these defects in collagen synthesis, including the capillary fragility that underlies the hemorrhagic features, the poor healing of wounds, and (in part) the bony abnormalities of children. Collagens with the highest content of hydroxyproline are most severely affected, accounting for the early disruption of the adventitia, media, and basal laminae of blood vessels. Ascorbic acid also prevents oxidation of tetrahydrofolate and thus protects the active folic acid pool and regulates iron distribution and storage, probably by influencing the valence of stored iron and maintaining a normal ratio of ferritin to hemosiderin. Scorbutic patients excrete incompletely oxidized products of tyrosine metabolism, but the significance is not clear.

Requirements The recommended daily allowance for vitamin C is described in Table 72-1. The vitamin is present in milk and some meats (kidney, liver, fish) and is widely distributed in fruits and vegetables. A portion is lost after prolonged storage of unprocessed fruits and vegetables (e.g., potatoes), but it is partially preserved (half or greater) by most means of food processing (boiling, steaming, pressure cooking, preserving jams and jellies, freezing, dehydration, and canning). As a consequence, the recommended daily allowances can be met with even a modest intake of fruits and vegetables. Utilization of the vitamin is increased during pregnancy and lactation and in thyrotoxicosis, and absorption is decreased in diarrheal states and in achlorhydria.

Experimental Depletion   The total-body pool of vitamin C varies from 1.5 to 3 g. When a deficient diet is instituted, the pool is depleted at a rate that approximates 4 percent per day. In monkeys, the major catabolic pathway involves oxidation of the alcohol at carbon 6 to an aldehyde and then to an acid. Because of differences in initial pool size and rates of turnover, differences in the completeness of deficiency in various experimental diets, and variation among normal subjects at the cellular or enzymatic level, the time required for development of symptoms ranges from 1 to 3 months in different studies. Manifestations of deficiency correlate better with the total pool size than with plasma or blood levels. The first symptoms (petechial hemorrhages and ecchymoses) develop when the pool size is less than 0.5 g; with further depletion (pool size 0.1 to 0.5 g), manifestations include gum involvement, hyperkeratosis, congested hair follicles, arthralgias, coiled hairs, and joint effusions. When depletion is extreme (pool size <0.1 g), dyspnea, edema, oliguria, and neuropathy supervene. Progress of the disease may then be rapid.

Symptoms do not improve until the pool is repleted, and the larger the therapeutic dose, the more rapid is the repletion. However, with doses as small as 6.5 mg/d the body pool eventually returns to normal, and amelioration of symptoms follows.

Clinical Deficiency   Scurvy now occurs for the most part in areas of urban poverty. An increased incidence occurs at 6 to 12 months of age in infants whose processed milk formulas are unsupplemented with citrus fruit or vegetables as a result of maternal error or neglect. Another peak occurs in middle and old age; edentulous men who live alone and cook for themselves are particularly prone. Clinical scurvy is more severe than the experimental disease, doubtlessly because affected individuals usually have deficiencies of other dietary constituents as well and because the groups at risk (infants and the elderly) are especially vulnerable.

In adults, the features include perifollicular hyperkeratotic papules in which hairs become fragmented and buried; perifollicular hemorrhages; purpura beginning on the backs of the lower extremities coalescing to become ecchymoses (Fig. 79-2); hemorrhage into the muscles of the arms and legs with secondary phlebothromboses; hemorrhages into joints; splinter hemorrhages in the nail beds; gum involvement (only in people with teeth) that includes swelling, friability, bleeding, secondary infection, and loosening of the teeth; poor wound healing and breakdown of recently healed wounds; petechial hemorrhages in the viscera; and emotional changes. Symptoms resembling those of Sjögren's syndrome may occur. Terminally, icterus, edema, and fever are common, and convulsions, hypotension, and death may occur abruptly.

In infancy and childhood, hemorrhage into the periosteum of long bones causes painful swellings and may result in epiphyseal separation. The sternum may sink inward, leaving a sharp elevation at the rib margins (scorbutic rosary). Purpura and ecchymoses may develop in the skin, and gum lesions occur if the teeth have erupted. Retrobulbar, subarachnoid, and intracerebral hemorrhages rapidly culminate in death if treatment is delayed.

Normochromic, normocytic anemia is common and is due to bleeding into tissues. Anemia also may be macrocytic and/or megaloblastic (one-fifth of patients in one series). Many foods that contain vitamin C also contain folate, and diets that cause scurvy also may cause folate deficiency. However, ascorbic acid deficiency also results in an increased oxidation of formyl tetrahydrofolic acid to inactive folate metabolites and may cause a decrease in the active folate pool. Whether changes in iron distribution and storage are involved in the pathogenesis of the anemia is unclear. The anemia is corrected with replenishment of vitamin C and institution of a balanced diet.

In some hospitals, platelet ascorbic acid levels are useful in diagnosing scurvy and are usually less than one-fourth of the normal value. Plasma levels of the vitamin correlate less well with the clinical state. In infants, x-ray changes of the bones may be diagnostic. Bilirubin is frequently elevated. Capillary fragility is abnormal.

Scurvy is potentially fatal; if the diagnosis is suspected, blood

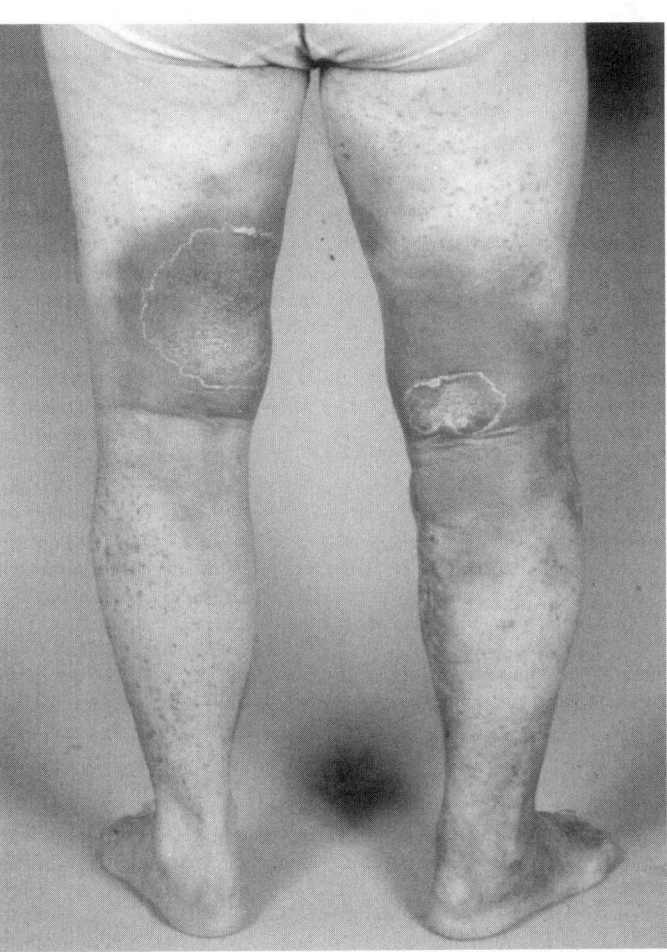

FIGURE 79-2   Hemorrhages and ecchymoses in a patient with scurvy. *(Photograph courtesy of Leonard L. Madison.)*

should be obtained, and ascorbic acid therapy should be instituted promptly. The usual dose in adults is 100 mg three to five times a day by mouth until 4 g has been administered, then 100 mg/d. In infants and children, administration of 10 to 25 mg three times a day is adequate. A diet rich in vitamin C should be initiated simultaneously. Spontaneous bleeding usually ceases within 24 h, muscle and bone pains subside quickly, and the gums begin to heal within 2 to 3 days. Even large ecchymoses and hematomas resolve in 10 to 12 days, although pigmentary changes in areas of hemorrhage may persist for months. Serum bilirubin becomes normal within 3 to 5 days, and the anemia is ordinarily corrected within 2 to 4 weeks.

BIOTIN   Biotin (see Fig. 79-1) functions as a cofactor in mammalian carboxylases. The vitamin is largely ingested in a form bound to protein, hydrolyzed by pancreatic biotinidase, and absorbed by what is probably an active transport process. The recommended daily allowance is given in Table 72-1. In cells, biotin is covalently attached to apocarboxylases to form four haloenzymes that catalyze the incorporation of bicarbonate into substrate, acetyl-CoA carboxylase, pyruvate carboxylase, methylcrotonyl CoA carboxylase, and propionyl CoA carboxylase. Biotin deficiency in the human occurs under at least four conditions: following the prolonged consumption of raw egg white (which binds biotin in the gut and prevents its absorption), after parenteral nutrition without biotin supplementation in patients with malabsorption, as a component of protein-energy malnutrition, and in subjects with multiple carboxylase deficiency due to abnormalities in holocarboxylase synthetase or biotinidase. In all these conditions the common manifestations of biotin deficiency resemble those of essential fatty acid deficiency and include perioral dermatitis, conjunctivitis, alopecia, ataxia, and, in children, developmental delay. In addition, serious neurologic defects and organic aciduria may occur in multiple carboxylase deficiency.

The diagnosis can be established by documenting reduced urinary excretion of biotin or by demonstrating resolution of the deficiency in response to supplementation with 100 μg/d.

VITAMIN A **Biochemistry** Vitamin A (retinol) can either be ingested or synthesized within the body from plant carotenes (see Fig. 79-1). The best sources of preformed vitamin A are liver, milk, and kidney, where it occurs largely in the form of fatty acid esters. The esters are hydrolyzed during digestion, absorbed in the free form, reesterified with fatty acids within the intestinal mucosa, and enter the circulation with lymph chylomicrons. The carotene substrates for synthesis of vitamin A, mainly β-carotenes, are widely distributed in plants. β-Carotene can either be absorbed intact or cleaved in the intestinal tract to form two molecules of retinaldehyde. Retinaldehyde is subsequently reduced by an aldehyde reductase to retinol. Retinol from whatever source is stored as retinyl esters in the liver. The normal body pool is 300 to 900 mg.

Prior to release from the liver, retinyl esters are hydrolyzed, and the free alcohol is bound to a specific transport protein, retinol-binding protein (RBP), for transport to peripheral tissues. In vitamin A deficiency, the release of RBP from the liver is inhibited, and the protein accumulates in liver; with repletion, RBP is rapidly released from preformed stores. Approximately equal amounts of retinol are excreted in the bile and urine.

Mechanism of Action The best-defined function of vitamin A is its role in vision; in the retina vitamin A constitutes the prosthetic group of carotenoid proteins that provide the molecular basis for visual excitation. In addition, vitamin A is required for growth, reproduction, and the maintenance of life. Retinol-phosphate-mannose glycolipid is present in a variety of cell membranes, and the vitamin plays a primary role in the synthesis of glycoproteins. The importance of glycoprotein to every cell implies that this is an equally important function of the vitamin. In all its functions, the vitamin is believed to act by binding to a transcription regulatory protein that controls gene expression (see Chap. 327).

Requirements The recommended daily allowance for vitamin A is listed in Table 72-1. The assumed utilization efficiency for the conversion of β-carotene to vitamin A in the human is one-sixth (0.167). Other carotenoids with provitamin A activity have, on average, about half the activity of β-carotene. Pregnancy and disease states that cause impaired absorption or storage, excessive utilization, or increased excretion of vitamin A may lead to increased requirements.

Experimental Depletion When experimental subjects are fed a diet deficient in both retinol and carotene, plasma levels fall, and the body pool shrinks to less than half the control value. Deficiency is manifested by follicular hyperkeratosis, impaired dark adaptation, and abnormalities of the electroretinogram. These changes are corrected after supplementation with 150 μg retinol or 300 μg β-carotene per day.

Clinical Deficiency Endemic deficiency results from inadequate amounts of the vitamin and provitamins in the diet and occurs in conjunction with deficiency of other nutrients or complicating diseases. In some developing countries, vitamin A deficiency is a major cause of blindness in the young as a consequence of failure to incorporate green leafy vegetables or other sources of the provitamin or vitamin into the diet. Vitamin A–deficient children appear to be particularly susceptible to the complications of measles. Vitamin A deficiency also may be a component of protein-calorie malnutrition. In developed countries, vitamin A deficiency is usually due either to intestinal malabsorption (as in sprue or after intestinal bypass surgery), abnormal storage (liver disease), or enhanced destruction or excretion of the vitamin (proteinuria). Vitamin A deficiency also has occurred in patients receiving total parenteral nutrition because of loss of vitamin A after prolonged storage of intravenous fluid.

Night blindness is the earliest symptom of deficiency, followed by degenerative changes in the retina. The bulbar conjunctiva becomes dry (xerosis), and small gray plaques with foamy surfaces develop (Bitôt's spots). These early lesions are reversible with administration of vitamin A. The more serious effects of deficiency are ulceration and necrosis of the cornea (keratomalacia), leading to perforation, endophthalmitis, and blindness. Dryness and hyperkeratosis of the skin may be present.

Vitamin A levels in plasma are not reliable for the assessment of stores in individual cases. Measurements of dark adaptation, rod scotometry, and electroretinography are useful indicators of vitamin A stores but require trained personnel and expensive equipment; consequently, the diagnosis is usually based on a high index of suspicion in malnourished children or in patients with predisposing factors for its development.

Night blindness and the milder conjunctival changes respond well to 30,000 IU of vitamin A daily for a week. Corneal damage constitutes a therapeutic emergency, and the usual treatment is 20,000 IU/kg of body weight per day for 5 days. Children who are at risk for vitamin A deficiency and who develop measles should be given 200,000 IU orally each day for 2 days.

VITAMIN E **Biochemistry** Eight naturally occurring tocopherols possess vitamin E activity. The structure of alpha tocopherol, the most widely distributed and most active of the tocopherols, is shown in Fig. 79-1. The vitamin is absorbed from the gastrointestinal tract and enters the circulation via the lymph, associated first with chylomicrons and then with plasma β-lipoproteins. Indeed, plasma levels correlate with plasma lipid levels. The vitamin is stored in all tissues, and the tissue stores can protect against vitamin deficiency for long periods. Approximately three-fourths of the vitamin is excreted in bile, and the balance is excreted as glucuronides in urine. Metabolites with quinone structures (including one similar to ubiquinone) are present in tissues.

Mechanism of Action The vitamin probably acts as an antioxidant rather than as a specific cofactor. In so acting it presumably inhibits oxidation of essential cellular constituents and prevents the formation of toxic oxidation products. Other antioxidants such as selenium, sulfur-containing amino acids, and the ubiquinone group can reverse the symptoms of vitamin E deficiency in animals.

Requirements The recommended daily requirement is 10 to 30 mg/d (see Table 72-1). Diets containing large amounts of polyunsaturated fatty acids increase and diets containing antioxidants decrease the requirement. The vitamin is widely distributed in food, so a primary deficiency state has never been recognized in otherwise healthy children or adults. Newborn infants have plasma concentrations about one-fifth that of maternal levels, implying poor placental transfer, but human milk (in contrast to cow's milk) has sufficient levels to meet the requirements in infants.

Experimental Depletion In long-term studies, vitamin E concentrations in plasma declined significantly only after months on a deficient diet. No manifestations of the depletion were detected in normal volunteers, making it difficult to establish that tocopherol is a human vitamin.

Clinical Deficiency Nevertheless, vitamin E deficiency may be associated with a discrete syndrome, as when deficiency is due to a selective malabsorption of the vitamin or when an autosomal recessive mutation causes vitamin E deficiency and ataxia. More commonly, intestinal fat malabsorption can cause deficiency of all fat-soluble vitamins including vitamin E, and children with abetalipoproteinemia or chronic cholestatic liver disease appear to be particularly susceptible. Measurement of the ratio of serum vitamin E to total-serum lipid is the preferred index for assessing vitamin E status. The manifestations of deficiency include areflexia, gait disturbance, decreased proprioceptive and vibratory sensation, and paresis of gaze and are associated with degeneration of the posterior columns of the spinal cord, selective loss of large-caliber, myelinated axons in peripheral nerves, and appearance of spheroids in the gracile and cuneate nuclei of the brain. Treatment (50 to 100 IU/d by mouth) is most effective when initiated early in the course of the disease.

VITAMIN K Vitamin K consists of a quinone ring attached to a side chain (labeled *R* in Fig. 79-1) that varies depending on the source of the vitamin. Vitamin K_1 (phylloquinone) is present in most edible vegetables, particularly in green leaves. Vitamin K_2 is produced by intestinal bacteria but not in sufficient amounts to supply daily requirements. The many compounds with vitamin K activity are structurally related to the simpler compound, 2-methyl-1,4-naphthoquinone (menadione). Menadione is formed in the gut by the removal of the side chain from the vitamin by intestinal bacteria. After absorption, menadione is converted in the body to the active menaquinone. The vitamin is a component of a specialized microsomal enzyme system that effects the posttranslational γ carboxylation of glutamic acid in proteins of the plasma, bone, kidney, and urine, including clotting factors II, VII, IX, and X, and the coagulation inhibitors proteins C and S. Death from hemorrhage in deficiency states ensues before deficiency of the other carboxylated proteins becomes manifest. The warfarin anticoagulant drugs induce hypoprothrombinemia by inhibiting the γ carboxylation of the precursor protein.

Under ordinary circumstances, about 80 percent of vitamin K is absorbed from the small bowel into the intestinal lymph. Deficiency can occur in association with diseases that interfere with fat absorption. In addition, long-term treatment with oral antibiotics may temporarily eliminate intestinal bacteria as a source for vitamin K and promote deficiency when the diet is marginal.

Newborn infants tend to be deficient in vitamin K and have low plasma levels of several coagulation factors in the prothrombin complex. Such deficiencies result from minimal stores of vitamin K at birth, lack of an established intestinal flora, and a limited dietary intake of the vitamin, but it is not clear whether all infants should be supplemented routinely.

Determination of prothrombin should be performed prior to surgical procedures or delivery. Subjects with levels below 70 percent of normal should receive therapy with vitamin K. Vitamin K deficiency can be separated from hypoprothrombinemia of liver disease by demonstration of the noncarboxylated prothrombin precursor that accumulates in plasma in the vitamin deficiency.

VITAMIN EXCESS

According to the National Health Interview Survey, more than 50 percent of adults in the United States use vitamin and/or mineral supplements, and in many instances ingestion is within a potentially toxic range. Multivitamins are the usual type ingested by children, whereas single vitamins are consumed commonly by adults. Supplement use is higher with the level of education and income and in those whose health is good.

Fat-soluble vitamins are stored to a variable extent in the body and hence are more likely to cause adverse effects when taken in excess; excess states for vitamins D (see Chap. 354) and A are well characterized. Water-soluble vitamins are readily excreted in the urine and stored only to a limited extent. Consequently, toxicity states for these vitamins only occur when very large amounts are taken.

VITAMIN A AND CAROTENES **Carotenemia** Carotenemia results from excessive intake of vitamin A precursors in foods, principally carrots. Excess carotene is not injurious apart from the cosmetic effect; the fact that carotenemia does not cause hypervitaminosis A indicates that the conversion of carotene to vitamin A must be regulated. Carotenemia is manifested by yellowing of the skin with greatest intensity on the palms and soles and by a corresponding yellowness of serum. The yellowing of the skin differs from jaundice in that the sclerae remain white. Hypothyroid patients are particularly susceptible. The omission of carrots from the diet leads to the rapid disappearance of the pigmentation. Discoloration of the skin also can result from the consumption of large amounts of other colored fruits and vegetables.

Vitamin A Toxicity Hypervitaminosis A can result from accidental overingestion by hunters or explorers (polar bear liver), as the result of food faddism (usually caused by overly solicitous parents),

or as a side effect of inappropriate therapy. Acute toxicity from a single massive dose consists of abdominal pain, nausea, vomiting, headache, dizziness, sluggishness, papilledema, and in infants a bulging fontanel followed within a few days by generalized desquamation of the skin and recovery. Chronic toxicity occurs after ingestion of 25,000 units or more daily for protracted periods and is characterized by bone and joint pain, hyperostoses, hair loss, dryness and fissures of the lips, anorexia, benign intracranial hypertension, low-grade fever, pruritus, weight loss, and hepatosplenomegaly. The only diagnostic laboratory finding is elevation of the vitamin in serum, chiefly in the form of retinyl esters. The concentration of retinol-binding protein is normal, and the excess vitamin A circulates in association with lipoprotein. Relief is usually prompt on discontinuation of the vitamin, but cirrhosis of the liver can develop as a late complication of overdosage.

VITAMIN E Relatively large doses of vitamin E have been taken by some for extended periods without apparent harm. In others, malaise, gastrointestinal complaint, headaches, and possibly hypertension have occurred. However, true toxicity appears to occur in two situations—in subjects receiving oral anticoagulants and in premature infants. In large amounts, vitamin E can antagonize vitamin K and prolong the prothrombin time; this phenomenon results in a potentiation of oral anticoagulants. Premature infants given parenteral vitamin E have developed ascites associated with hepatosplenomegaly, cholestatic jaundice, azotemia, and thrombocytopenia.

VITAMIN K Large amounts of vitamin K can block the effects of oral anticoagulants and when given to pregnant women can cause jaundice in the newborn.

PYRIDOXINE Most adults can consume up to 10 times the recommended daily allowance of 2 mg pyridoxine per day without adverse effects. However, severe peripheral neuropathies have developed after ingestion of several grams per day for prolonged periods; symptoms include ataxia, perioral numbness, and clumsiness of the hands and feet, and the findings include loss of position and vibration sense without impairment of reflexes or sensory function. Recovery is slow after ingestion ceases. Lower doses (25 mg/d) can antagonize the effects of levodopa in Parkinson's disease and decrease the anticonvulsant effects of phenytoin and barbiturates.

In women who consume vitamin supplements, the median dose of pyridoxine approaches the level of 120 mg/d found to cause paresthesia and muscle weakness in normal volunteers who consumed the vitamin for 6 months or greater.

VITAMIN C Vitamin C is consumed by 85 percent of all vitamin users because of the belief that large amounts of the vitamin (a gram or greater per day) prevent or minimize the symptoms of the common cold. However, in controlled studies, no significant differences in occurrence, severity, or duration of colds have been demonstrated in subjects treated with the vitamin. Use of the vitamin in this way is unwarranted and probably unwise. The long-term use of ascorbic acid in these doses can interfere with the absorption of vitamin B_{12}, enhance blood levels of estrogens in women on exogenous estrogens, cause uricosuria, and predispose to formation of oxalate kidney stones. In addition, large doses enhance the development of metabolizing enzymes in the fetus and may cause rebound scurvy in the offspring of mothers who have ingested large amounts of the vitamin during pregnancy. However, pharmacologic doses (200 mg daily) may correct leukocyte abnormalities in patients with the Chédiak-Higashi syndrome (see Chap. 62).

NIACIN Large doses of niacin are used for treatment of hypercholesterolemia (see Chap. 341) and occasionally for other purposes. The vitamin causes release of histamine, which in turn can cause severe flushing, pruritus, and gastrointestinal disturbances and may aggravate asthma. Acanthosis nigricans may occur. In doses of 3 g/d niacin can cause elevation of serum uric acid and of glucose. Large doses can also cause hepatic toxicity including cholestatic jaundice.

For further information, see Chap. 62, Water-soluble vitamins, and Chap. 63, Fat-soluble vitamins, in Goodman & Gilman's The Pharmacological Basis of Therepeutics, *9th ed. New York, McGraw-Hill, 1996.*

BIBLIOGRAPHY

GENERAL

BATES CJ: Vitamin undernutrition. Proc Nutr Soc 52:143, 1993

BROWN ML: *Present Knowledge in Nutrition.* Washington, International Life Science Institute, 1990

COMBS GF JR: *The Vitamins.* San Diego, Academic, 1992

ELSAS LJ, McCORMICK DB: Genetic defects in vitamin utilization. Part I: General aspects and fat-soluble vitamins. Vitam Horm 43:103, 1986

HOYUMPA AM: Mechanisms of vitamin deficiencies in alcoholism. Alcohol Clin Exp Res 10:573, 1986

LINDEN MC: *Nutritional Biochemistry and Metabolism.* New York, Elsevier, 1991

MUDD SH: Inborn errors of metabolism. Vitamin-responsive genetic disease. J Clin Pathol 27(Suppl) 8:38, 1974

RUDMAN D, WILLIAMS PJ: Nutrient deficiencies during total parenteral nutrition. Nutr Rev 43:1, 1984

NIACIN DEFICIENCY

CARPENTER KJ: The relationship of pellagra to corn and the low availability of niacin in cereals. Experientia(Suppl) 44:197, 1983

———, LEWIN WJ: A reexamination of the composition of diets associated with pellagra. J Nutr 115:543, 1985

CASTIELLO RJ, LYNCH PJ: Pellagra and the carcinoid syndrome. Arch Dermatol 105:574, 1972

FU CS et al: Biochemical markers for assessment of niacin status in young men. J Nutr 119:1949, 1989

GOLDSMITH GA: Experimental niacin deficiency. J Am Diet Assoc 32:312, 1956

HENDERSON LM: Niacin. Annu Rev Nutr 3:289, 1983

JUKES TH et al: The conquest of pellagra. Fed Proc 40:1519, 1980

LEVY HL: Hartnup disorder, in *The Metabolic Basis of Inherited Disease*, 7th ed, CR Scriver et al (eds). New York, McGraw-Hill, 1995, p 3629

MALFAIT P et al: An outbreak of pellagra related to changes in dietary niacin among Mozambican refugees in Malawi. Int J Epidemiol 22:504, 1993

OAKLEY A, WALLACE J: Hartnup disease presenting in an adult. Clin Exp Dermatol 19:407, 1994

THIAMINE DEFICIENCY

BETTENDORFF L: Thiamine in excitable tissues: Reflections on a non-cofactor role. Metab Brain Dis 9:183, 1994

BRADY JA, et al: Thiamine status, diuretic medications, and the management of congestive heart failure. J Am Diet Assoc 95:541, 1995

DE MEIRLEIR L et al: Aberrant splicing of exon 6 in the pyruvate dehydrogenase-E1 alpha mRNA linked to a silent mutation in a large family with Leigh's encephalomyelopathy. Pediatr Res 36:707, 1994

DURAN M, WADMAN SK: Thiamine-responsive inborn errors of metabolism. J Inherit Metab Dis 8(Suppl 1):70, 1985

DYCKNER T et al: Aggravation of thiamine deficiency by magnesium depletion. Acta Med Scand 218:129, 1985

ELLERINE NP et al: Thiamin-responsive maple syrup urine disease in a patient antigenically missing dihydrolipoamide acyltransferase. Biochem Med Met Biol 49:363, 1993

FINEGLAS PM: Thiamin. Int J Vit Nutr Res 63:270, 1993

HAAS RH: Thiamin and the brain. Annu Rev Nutr 8:483, 1988

HARPER CG et al: Clinical signs in the Wernicke-Korsakoff complex: A retrospective analysis of 131 cases diagnosed at necropsy. J Neurol Neurosurg Psychiatry 49:341, 1986

HOYUMPA AM: Mechanisms of thiamine deficiency in chronic alcoholism. Am J Clin Nutr 33:2750, 1980

KAWAI C et al: Reappearance of beriberi heart disease in Japan. Am J Med 69:383, 1980

KOZAM RL et al: Cardiovascular beriberi. Am J Cardiol 30:418, 1972

KURIYAMA M et al: Blood vitamin B_1, transketolase, and thiamine pyrophosphate (TPP) effect in beriberi patients. Clin Chim Acta 108:159, 1980

NAITO E et al: Molecular analysis of abnormal pyruvate dehydrogenase in a patient with thiamine-responsive congenital lactic acidemia. Pediatr Res 36:340, 1994

RINDI G et al: Further studies on erythrocyte thiamin transport and phosphorylation in seven patients with thiamin-responsive megaloblastic anaemia. J Inherit Metab Dis 17:667, 1994

SHIMON I et al: Improved left ventricular function after thiamine supplementa-

tion in patients with congestive heart failure receiving long term furosemide therapy. Am J Med 98:485, 1995

VICTOR M: Alcoholic dementia. Can J Neurol Sci 21:88, 1994

ZIPORIN ZZ et al: Excretion of thiamine and its metabolites in the urine of young adult males receiving restricted intakes of the vitamin. J Nutr 85:287, 1965

PYRIDOXINE DEFICIENCY

BASSIER KH: Megavitamin therapy with pyridoxine. Int J Vitam Nutr Res 58:105, 1988

BENDER DA: Novel functions of vitamin B_6. Proc Nutr Soc 53:625, 1994

BHAGAVAN HN, BRIN M: Drug–vitamin B_6 interaction. Curr Concepts Nutr 12:1, 1983

BITSCH R: Vitamin B_6. Int J Vit Nutr Res 63:278, 1993

COX TC et al: X-linked pyridoxine-responsive sideroblastic anemia due to a Thr388-to-Ser substitution in erythroid Δ-aminolevulinate synthase. N Engl J Med 330:675, 1994

GERSHOFF SN: Vitamin B_6, in *Nutrition Reviews' Present Knowledge in Nutrition*, 4th ed, DM Hegsted et al (eds). Washington, The Nutrition Foundation, 1976, p 149

GOSPE SM JR et al: Reduced GABA synthesis in pyridoxine-dependent seizures. Lancet 343:1133, 1994

GUILARTE TR: Vitamin B_6 and cognitive development: Recent research findings from human and animal studies. Nutr Rev 51:193, 1993

HU FL et al: Molecular basis of cystathionine beta-synthase deficiency in pyridoxine responsive and nonresponsive homocystinuria. Hum Mol Genet 2:1857, 1993

KRAUS JP, KOZICH V: Pyridoxine responsive and unresponsive homocystinuria. J Nutr Sci Vit Spec No: 589, 1992

KRETSCH MJ et al: Electroencephalographic changes and periodontal status during short-term vitamin B_6 depletion of young nonpregnant women. Am J Clin Nutr 53:1266, 1991

LUHBY AL et al: Vitamin B_6 metabolism in users of oral contraceptive agents: I. Abnormal urinary xanthurenic acid excretion and its correction by pyridoxine. Am J Clin Nutr 24:684, 1971

MYDLIK M et al: Vitamin B_6 requirements in chronic renal failure. Int Urol Nephrol 24:453, 1992

YOUNG RC, BASS JP: Iatrogenic nutritional deficiencies. Annu Rev Nutr 2:201, 1982

RIBOFLAVIN DEFICIENCY

BATES CJ: Human riboflavin requirements, and metabolic consequences of deficiency in man and animals. World Rev Nutr Diet 50:215, 1987

MERRILL AH JR et al: Formation and mode of action of flavoproteins. Annu Rev Nutr 1:281, 1981

PINTO JT, RIVLIN RS: Drugs that promote renal excretion of riboflavin. Drug Nutr Interact 5:143, 1987

——— et al: Mechanisms underlying the differential effects of ethanol on the bioavailability of riboflavin and flavin adenine dinucleotide. J Clin Invest 79:1343, 1987

ROE DA: Riboflavin deficiency: Mucocutaneous signs of acute and chronic deficiency. Semin Dermatol 10:293, 1991

ROSS NS, HANSEN TP: Riboflavin deficiency is associated with selective preservation of critical flavoenzyme-dependent metabolic pathways. Biofactors 3:185, 1992

ASCORBIC ACID DEFICIENCY

ADELMAN HM et al: Scurvy resembling cutaneous vasculitis. Cutis 54:111, 1994

BARNESS LA: Nutritional aspects of vegetarianism, health foods, and fad diets. Nutr Rev 59:153, 1977

BOXER LA et al: Correction of leucocyte function in Chédiak-Higashi syndrome by ascorbate. N Engl J Med 295:1041, 1971

BURNS JJ et al: *Third Conference on Vitamin C.* Ann NY Acad Sci Ser 498, 1987

ENGLAND S, SEIFTER S: The biochemical functions of ascorbic acid. Annu Rev Nutr 6:365, 1986

FRANCESCHI RT: The role of ascorbic acid in mesenchymal differentiation. Nutr Rev 50:65, 1992

HODGES RE et al: Clinical manifestations of ascorbic acid deficiency in man. Am J Clin Nutr 24:432, 1971

LEVINE M: New concepts in the biology and biochemistry of ascorbic acid. N Engl J Med 314:892, 1986

PADH H: Vitamin C: Newer insights into its biochemical functions. Nutr Rev 49:65, 1991

PETERKOFSKY B: Ascorbate requirement for hydroxylation and secretion of procollagen: Relationship to inhibition of collagen synthesis in scurvy. Am J Clin Nutr 54(Suppl 6):1135S, 1991

REULER JB et al: Adult scurvy. JAMA 253:805, 1985

SATO P, UNDENFRIEND S: Studies on ascorbic acid related to the genetic basis of scurvy, in *Vitamins and Hormones*, vol 36, P Munson et al (eds). New York, Academic, 1978, p 33

TOLBERT BM et al: New information on synthesis and metabolism of ascorbic acid. Nutr Rev 35:22, 1977

VILTER RW: Effects of ascorbic acid deficiency in man, in *The Vitamins*, WH Sebrell Jr et al (eds). New York, Academic, 1967, vol 1, p 457

WALLERSTEIN RO, WALLERSTEIN RO JR: Scurvy. Semin Hematol 13:211, 1976

BIOTIN

MARSHALL MM: The nutritional importance of biotin—an update. Nutr Today 22:26, 1987

MOCK DM: Skin manifestations of biotin deficiency. Semin Dermatol 10:296, 1991

SWEETMAN L, NYHAN WL: Inheritable biotin-treatable disorders and associated phenomena. Annu Rev Nutr 6:317, 1986

VELAZQUEZ A et al: Biotin supplementation affects lymphocyte carboxylases and plasma biotin in severe protein-energy malnutrition. Am J Clin Nutr 61:385, 1995

WOLF B: Disorders of biotin metabolism, *The Metabolic and Molecular Basis of Inherited Disease*, 7th ed, in Scriver CR et al (eds). New York, McGraw-Hill, 1995, p 3151

VITAMIN A DEFICIENCY

BATES CJ: Vitamin A. Lancet 345:31, 1995

DELUCA LM: The direct involvement of vitamin A in glycosyl transfer reactions of mammalian membranes, in *Vitamins and Hormones*, vol 35, PL Munson et al (eds). New York, Academic, 1977, p 1

FAWZI WW et al: Vitamin A supplementation and child mortality. A meta-analysis. JAMA 269:898, 1993

GIGUERE V et al: Identification of a receptor for the morphogen retinoic acid. Nature 330:624, 1987

GOODMAN DS: Vitamin A and retinoids in health and disease. N Engl J Med 310:1023, 1984

HOWARD L et al: Vitamin A deficiency from long-term parenteral nutrition. Ann Intern Med 93:576, 1980

OLSON JA: Hypovitaminosis A: Contemporary scientific issues. J Nutr 124(Suppl 8):1461S, 1994

SAUBERLICH HE et al: Vitamin A metabolism and requirements in the human studied with the use of labeled retinol, in *Vitamins and Hormones*, vol 32, RS Harris et al (eds). New York, Academic, 1974

SMITH FR, GOODMAN DS: Vitamin A transport in human vitamin A toxicity. N Engl J Med 294:805, 1976

SOMMER A: New imperatives for an old vitamin (A). J Nutr 119:96, 1989

TEE ES: Carotenoids and retinoids in human nutrition. Crit Rev Food Sci Nutr 31:103,1992

TIELSCH JM, SOMMER A: The epidemiology of vitamin A deficiency and xerophthalmia. Annu Rev Nutr 4:183, 1974

UNDERWOOD BA: The role of vitamin A in child growth, development and survival. Adv Exp Med Biol 352:201, 1994

VAHLQUIST A: Clinical use of vitamin A and its derivatives—physiological and pharmacological aspects. Clin Exp Dermatol 10:133, 1985

WALD G: Molecular basis of visual excitation. Science 162:230, 1968

VITAMIN E DEFICIENCY

BIERI JG et al: Medical uses of vitamin E. N Engl J Med 308:1063, 1983

DOERFLINGER N et al: Ataxia with vitamin E deficiency: Refinement of genetic localization and analysis of linkage disequilibrium by using new markers in 14 families. Am J Hum Genet 56:1116, 1995

KAYDEN HJ: The neurologic syndrome of vitamin E deficiency: A significant cause of ataxia. Neurology 43:2167, 1993

——, TRABER MG: Absorption, lipoprotein transport, and regulation of plasma concentrations of vitamin E in humans. J Lipid Res 34:343, 1993

LLOYD JK: The importance of vitamin E in human nutrition. Acta Paediatr Scand 79:6, 1990

MEYDANI M: Vitamin E. Lancet 345:170, 1995

MORRISSEY PA et al: Vitamin E. Int J Vitam Nutr Res 63:260, 1993

SITRIN MD et al: Vitamin E deficiency and neurologic disease in adults with cystic fibrosis. Ann Intern Med 107:51, 1987

SOKOL RJ et al: Isolated vitamin E deficiency in the absence of fat malabsorption—familial and sporadic cases: Characterization and investigation of causes. J Lab Clin Med 111:548, 1988

—— et al: Intestinal malabsorption of vitamin E in primary biliary cirrhosis. Gastroenterology 96:479, 1989

—— et al: Multicenter trial of D-alpha-tocopheryl polyethylene glycol 1000 succinate for treatment of vitamin E deficiency in children with chronic cholestasis. Gastroenterology 104:1717, 1993

TRABER MG et al: Lack of tocopherol in peripheral nerves of vitamin E–deficient patients with peripheral neuropathy. N Engl J Med 317:262, 1987

VITAMIN K DEFICIENCY

BERTINA RM et al: New method for the rapid detection of vitamin K deficiency. Clin Chim Acta 105:93, 1980

HUYSMAN MW, SAUER PJ: The vitamin K controversy. Curr Opin Pediatr 6:129, 1994

IBER FL et al: Vitamin K deficiency in chronic alcoholic males. Alcohol Clin Exp Res 10:679, 1986

LIPSKY JJ: Nutritional sources of vitamin K. Mayo Clin Proc 69:462, 1994

OLSON RE, SUTTIE JW: Vitamin K and γ-carboxyglutamate biosynthesis, in *Vitamins and Hormones*, vol 35, PL Munson et al (eds). New York, Academic, 1977, p 59

SHEARER MJ: Vitamin K. Lancet 345:229, 1995

SUTTIE JW: Vitamin K and human nutrition. J Am Diet Assoc 92:585, 1992

—— et al: Vitamin K deficiency from dietary vitamin K restriction in humans. Am J Clin Nutr 47:475, 1988

VITAMIN EXCESS

ALHADEFF L: Toxic effects of water-soluble vitamins. Nutr Rev 42:33, 1984

CHALMERS TC: Effects of ascorbic acid on the common cold. Am J Med 58:532, 1975

CORRIGAN JJ JR: The effect of vitamin E on warfarin-induced vitamin K deficiency. Ann NY Acad Sci 82:361, 1982

DALTON K, DALTON MJT: Characteristics of pyridoxine overdose neuropathy syndrome. Acta Neurol Scand 76:8, 1987

GEUBEL AP et al: Liver damage caused by therapeutic vitamin A administration: Estimate of dose-related toxicity in 41 cases. Gastroenterology 100:1701, 1991

JORENS PG et al: Vitamin A abuse: Development of cirrhosis despite cessation of vitamin A. A six-year clinical and histopathologic followup. Liver 12:381, 1992

LEMONS JA, MAISELS MJ: Vitamin E—how much is too much? Pediatrics 76:625, 1985

LOMBAERT A, CARTON H: Benign intracranial hypertension due to A-hypervitaminosis in adults and adolescents. Eur Neurol 14:340, 1976

LORCH V et al: Unusual syndrome with fatalities among premature infants: Association with a new intravenous vitamin E product. Morb Mort Week Rep 33:198, 1984

MOSS AJ et al: Use of vitamin and mineral supplements in the United States. Advance Data No. 174. Hyattsville, Md: National Center for Health Statistics, 1989

ROE DA: Assessment of risk factors for carotenodermia and cutaneous signs of hypervitaminosis A in college-aged populations. Semin Dermatol 10:303, 1991

SCHAUMBURG H et al: Sensory neuropathy from pyridoxine abuse: A new megavitamin syndrome. N Engl J Med 309:445, 1983

SHIN HB et al: Ascorbic acid–induced uricosuria: A consequence of megavitamin therapy. Ann Intern Med 84:385, 1976

Toxic effects of vitamin overdosage. Med Lett Drugs Ther 26:73, 1984

WOOLLISCROFT JO: Megavitamins: Fact and fancy. Dis Mon 24:1, 1983

80 | *Kenneth H. Falchuk*

DISTURBANCES IN TRACE ELEMENTS

CLASSIFICATION AND FUNCTIONS The *trace elements* comprise metals in biological fluids at concentrations <1 μg/g wet weight. Most are essential nutrients for humans (Table 80-1). Others (As, Ni, Sn, V, Si) are essential for some species and may be required by humans. The functions of trace elements and of more abundant metals (Na, K, Ca, Mg) are determined, in part, by their charges, mobilities, and binding constants to biological ligands. Some elements (Na, K) bind weakly to negatively charged ligands and cross cellular membranes without major impediment. They are used by living systems as charge carriers to conduct electric impulses along nerves, etc. Other elements (Mg, Ca) form moderately stable complexes with enzymes, nucleic acids, and other ligands. They act as "triggers," altering and/or controlling biological functions; for example, Ca affects muscle contraction and relaxation (Chap. 383). Those in a third group include Fe, Zn, Cu, and others that form strong static complexes with and become integral components of proteins and enzymes (Table 80-1).

METAL DEFICIENCY OR TOXICITY   Metals can cause disease through deficiency, imbalance, or toxicity. Deficiency usually results when dietary intake is inadequate or when intake is adequate but other conditioning factors come into play. Conditioned deficiencies can be caused by metal malabsorption in chronic diarrheal diseases, surgical resection of the small intestine, or formation within the gastrointestinal tract of metal complexes that are not readily absorbed, for example, between phytates and Zn. Deficiency can also result from increased losses through urine, pancreatic juice, or other exocrine secretions or from metabolic imbalances produced by antagonistic or synergistic interactions between metals. Large amounts of Ca, for example, decrease the absorption of Zn. Zinc supplements in excess of 10 times the recommended daily allowance cause a conditioned deficiency of copper including anemia. Similarly, Mo and Cu compete so that excessive Mo in cattle leads to Cu deficiency characterized by diarrhea and wasting. Trace element deficiencies in humans were previously rare but have been recognized more frequently with the use of total parenteral nutrition (TPN) (Chap. 78). Criteria for the recognition of deficiency states include decreases in metal content of whole blood, serum, hair, and/or other accessible fluids and tissues; changes in the activities of metalloenzymes, and characteristic signs and symptoms (Table 80-2).

Toxic effects depend on the chemical form, the amount ingested, the route of entry into the body, the biological ligands bound by the metal, the tissue distribution, the concentration achieved, and the excretion rate. Mechanisms of toxicity include inhibition of enzyme activity by binding to essential amino acid residues, alterations in nucleic acid function and structure, impairment of protein synthesis, altered membrane permeability, and impairment of phosphorylation, among others. Metal toxicity in patients undergoing chronic hemodial-

ysis can be severe and can involve several elements, e.g., Al, Zn, Cu, Ni, and Sn (Chap. 272). For example, even when present only in trace amounts in dialysis fluids, Al is readily absorbed into blood and accumulates in brain, bone, and erythroid tissues and can cause disabling neurologic, skeletal, and hematologic manifestations including malaise, memory loss, asterixis, dementia, twitches, and other manifestations of metabolic encephalopathy, including seizures and death. Osteomalacia unresponsive to vitamin D, fractures, muscular pain, weakness, and anemia may occur. The diagnosis is made by documenting increase in plasma Al concentration following deferoxamine administration.

DISORDERS OF METABOLISM OF SPECIFIC METALS
Zinc   The daily Zn requirement varies with age and growth state (Table 80-1); it is approximately 800 μg/day at 1 month of age, 3 to 10 mg/day between 1 and 10 years of age, and 10 to 15 mg/day in normal adults. During pregnancy, needs increase to 20 to 25 mg/day to provide Zn for the growing fetus. Absorption of Zn in the small intestine is decreased by fibers, phytate, phosphate, Ca, and Cu and increased by glucose, amino acids, peptides, iodoquinol, and other chelating agents. About 2 to 5 mg of Zn are excreted each day through secretions of the pancreas and intestine. Losses also occur through the renal proximal tubule ($\sim$500 to 800 μg/day) and from sweat glands ($\sim$500μg/day). Nearly 99 percent of total-body Zn (Table 80-1) is inside cells, the remainder is in plasma and extracellular fluids. The bplasma Zn concentration is approximately 100 μg/100 mL, 70 percent of which is bound to albumin and most of the rest is associated with α_2-macroglobulin, although a small amount is bound to uncharacterized proteins. Plasma Zn is the source of metal for cellular needs and its levels are fairly constant, with small diurnal variations. More significant changes take place under some circumstances. Plasma Zn levels are decreased in pregnancy and with the use of oral contraceptives, when intake or absorption is reduced (e.g., in regional enteritis), and when urinary losses are increased (e.g., in hypoalbuminemic states; with the administration of penicillamine or other chelating agents; in catabolic states such as trauma, burns, or surgery; and in hemolytic anemias and sickle cell disease). Plasma Zn levels also decrease with acute myocardial infarction, infections, malignancies, hepatitis, and

Table 80-1

Requirements and Functions of Trace Elements in Humans

Element	Requirements, mg/d*	Amount† Total, g/70 kg Body Wt	Serum μmol/L	Serum μ/dL	Selected Biochemical Functions	Enzyme and Protein Classes	Enzyme and Protein Examples
Fe	10–20	4.0	18	100	Oxygen transport	Oxidoreductases	Cytochrome oxidase
Zn	15–20	3.0	15	100	Nucleic acid and protein synthesis and degradation, alcohol metabolism	Transferases, hydrolases, lyases, isomerases, ligases, oxidoreductases, transcription factors	RNA polymerases, alcohol dehydrogenases, glucocorticoid receptor
Cu	2–6	0.25	16	100	Hemoglobin synthesis, connective tissue metabolism bone development	Oxidoreductases	Superoxide dismutase, ferroxidase (ceruloplasmin)
Co	0.0001	1.1	0.0001	0.0007	Methionine metabolism	Transferases	Homocysteine methyltransferase
Mn	2–5	0.02	0.001	0.06	Oxidative phosphorylation; fatty acid, mucopolysaccharide, and cholesterol metabolism	Oxidoreductases, hydrolases, ligases	Diamine oxidase, pyruvate carboxylase
Mo	0.15–0.5	0.07	0.007	0.07	Xanthine metabolism	Oxidoreductases	Xanthine oxidase
Se	0.05–0.2	(–)	1.6	13	Antioxidant	Oxidoreductases, transferases	Glutathione peroxidase
Ni	(–)	(–)	0.02	0.01	?Stabilizing RNA structure	Oxidoreductases, hydrolases	Urease
Cr	0.005–0.2	0.0006	0.004	0.02	?Binding of insulin to cells, glucose metabolism		

* Requirements may differ for different age groups and physiologic states, e.g., pregnancy.
† Reported normal values vary owing to differences in sample preparation, analytical instruments, and small quantities present in biologic materials.
NOTE: (–), Reported values variable or not available.

Table 80-2

CHAPTER 80
Disturbances in Trace Elements **491**

Disorders of Metal Metabolism in Humans

Element	Deficiency	Toxicity*
Fe	Anemia	Hepatic failure, diabetes, testicular atrophy, arthritis, cardiomyopathy, peripheral neuropathy, hyperpigmentation
Zn	Growth retardation, alopecia, dermatitis, diarrhea, immunologic dysfunction, failure to thrive, psychological disturbances, gonadal atrophy, impaired spermatogenesis, congenital malformations	Gastric ulcer, pancreatitis, lethargy, anemia, fever, nausea, vomiting, respiratory distress, pulmonary fibrosis
Cu	Anemia, growth retardation, defective keratinization and pigmentation of hair, hypothermia, degenerative changes in aortic elastin, mental deterioration, scurvy-like changes in skeleton	Hepatitis, cirrhosis, tremor, mental deterioration, *Kayser-Fleischer rings*, hemolytic anemia, renal dysfunction (*Fanconi-like* syndrome)
Mn	Bleeding disorder (increased prothrombin time)	Encephalitis-like syndrome, Parkinson-like syndrome, psychosis, pneumoconiosis
Co	Anemia (B$_{12}$ deficiency)	Cardiomyopathy, goiter
Mo	?Esophageal cancer	?Hyperuricemia
Cr	?Impairment of glucose tolerance	Renal failure, dermatitis (occupational), pulmonary cancer
Se	Cardiomyopathy, congestive heart failure, striated muscle degeneration	Alopecia, abnormal nails, emotional lability, lassitude, garlic odor to breath
Ni	?	Dermatitis (occupational), lung and nasal carcinomas, liver necrosis, pulmonary inflammation
Si	?Impaired early bone development	Pulmonary inflammation, granuloma, fibrosis
F	?Impaired bone and dental structure	Mottled dental enamel, nausea, abdominal pain, vomiting, diarrhea, tetany, cardiovascular collapse

* Symptoms are dependent on route of entry and tissue distribution (see text).

many other diseases. The decreases may be due to redistribution from plasma to tissues such as liver and are probably mediated by corticotropin, cortisol, and/or interleukins 2 and 6. Liver uptake is associated with concomitant entry of amino acids, iron, and other metal ions.

The functions of Zn in cells and tissues depend on those of the metalloproteins and enzymes with which it is associated (Table 80-1); systems influenced by Zn include the reproductive, neurologic, immune, dermatologic, and gastrointestinal systems. Testicular Zn is critical for normal spermatogenesis and for sperm physiology; it preserves genomic integrity in the sperm and stabilizes attachment of sperm head to tail. The function of Zn in mammalian eggs is poorly understood, but Zn is essential for normal embryoic development. Deficiency results in malformations of the brain, eyes, bones, heart, and other organs. The survival of the embryo is placed at risk when Zn intake is reduced even for a period of days, particularly in the first trimester. Steroid hormone action is zinc-dependent in that the receptors require Zn to bind to the genes they activate.

In the brain the highest amounts of Zn are in the hippocampus and cerebral cortex, particularly the giant boutons of the mossy fiber system. Zinc may function in these areas to inhibit binding of peptides and other ligands to their neuroreceptors (opioid, muscarinic, acetylcholine, γ-aminobutyric acid, *N*-methyl-D-aspartate) and to influence neurotransmission.

Zinc is essential for the formation and function of the immune system. With Zn deprivation, the thymus atrophies, and viable thymocytes are not formed. The functions of macrophages and T cells are impaired. The result is an inability to respond to antigens or defend the organism against infection. Zn also may play a role in the sense of taste and in wound healing.

Human Zn deficiency (Table 80-2) was reported first in adolescents who consumed a diet rich in phytic acid and devoid of any animal protein and who also ate dirt; it was described subsequently in patients who received TPN without supplemental Zn (see Chap. 78) and in patients with Wilson's disease after treatment with penicillamine. Some patients with chronic diarrheal disease and malabsorption, including cystic fibrosis, regional enteritis, celiac sprue, and disaccharide malabsorption, exhibit signs and symptoms of Zn deficiency (Table 80-2). In the autosomal recessive defect *acrodermatitis enteropathica*, Zn deficiency may be the consequence of a defect in Zn absorption; symptoms often begin when an affected infant is weaned from human to cow's milk and include psoriasiform dermatitis with epidermal hyperplasia, parakeratosis, edema, and focal necrosis; flattening of intestinal villi and mucosal ulcerations; ovoid or rhomboid lysosomal-like inclusion bodies within Paneth cells; and a hypoplastic thymus with decreased or absent germinal centers in lymph nodes and spleen and immature plasma cells in paracortical areas.

Zinc-deficient cells fail to divide and differentiate, with consequent growth impairment; tissues with a high rate of cellular turnover, including skin, gastrointestinal mucosa, chondrocytes, spermatogonia, and thymocytes, are affected (Table 80-2). Dermatologic manifestations include hyperkeratosis, parakeratosis, acrodermatitis, and *alopecia*. Keratotic lesions usually occur in areas that are readily traumatized (elbows, knees) but can develop in other areas as well. The keratotic lesions can become pustular or crusting, red, scaly plaques. Immunologic defects of T cell function impair the ability to mount an immunologic response to parasites and may cause superinfections with either fungi or bacteria.

Toxicity follows inhalation of Zn fumes (by welders), oral ingestion, or intravenous administration. Inhalation of zinc oxide fumes leads to *metal-fume fever* or *brass chills*, manifested by fever, chills, excessive salivation, headaches, cough, and leukocytosis. Dialysis fluids can be contaminated with Zn from the adhesive on the dialysis coils or from galvanized pipes. Toxicity with hemodialysis is characterized by anemia, fever, and central nervous system disturbances (Table 80-2) and may be due to impaired chemotaxis, phagocytosis, pinocytosis, and platelet aggregation.

Copper The liver, kidney, heart, and brain contain the highest amounts of Cu. Over 90 percent of plasma Cu is associated with ceruloplasmin, and 60 percent of that in red blood cells is bound to superoxide dismutase. The major excretory pathway is through the bile. Serum Cu levels are normally constant. Increases in patients with acute myocardial infarction, leukemia, solid tumors, infections, cirrhosis of the liver, hemochromatosis, thyrotoxicosis, and connective tissue disorders are of uncertain significance. Decreases occur in the nephrotic syndrome, *kwashiorkor*, the hepatolenticular degeneration of *Wilson's disease* (see Chap. 345), severe diarrheal diseases with malabsorption, and conditions associated with increased excretion or decreased synthesis of ceruloplasmin. Premature infants fed diets deficient in Cu develop decreased serum ceruloplasmin and Cu levels, anemia, osteopenia, skin and hair depigmentation, and psychomotor retardation. Cu deficiency in subjects receiving TPN is associated with anemia and neutropenia.

A complex disorder of Cu metabolism occurs in *Menkes' disease*, an X-linked recessive disorder (see also Chap. 350). Intestinal Cu uptake is normal. Cu levels are normal or high in intestine, kidney, and skin (fibroblast) cells and low in serum, liver, brain, and (likely) vascular cells. Ceruloplasmin content and the activities of some Cu enzymes (e.g., connective tissue amine oxidases) are decreased. The clinical picture is similar to that of Cu deficiency in animals except that anemia does not occur (Table 80-2). The patients have kinky hair, and decreased amounts of mature collagen and elastin cause dissecting aneurysms, sudden cardiac rupture, emphysema, and osteoporosis. Death usually occurs in the first 5 years of life.

Excessive oral intake of Cu or hemodialysis with water contaminated with Cu causes toxicity manifested by hemolytic anemia, nausea, vomiting, and diarrhea. The renal and hepatic failure and the central nervous system disorders that eventually develop (Table 80-2) are typical of the manifestations of Cu toxicity in Wilson's disease (see Chap. 345).

Cobalt   Co is a component of vitamin B$_{12}$, and deficiency syndromes are those associated with deficiency of the vitamin (see Chap. 108). Pharmacologic amounts of Co induce *erythropoiesis* and block iodine uptake by the thyroid, resulting in development of goiter.

Cardiomyopathy, congestive heart failure with pericardial effusions, polycythemia, thyroid enlargement, and neurologic abnormalities are manifestations of Co toxicity that occurred in drinkers of beer to which the metal had been added as a foam stabilizer. In the heart Co forms a complex with lipoic acid and interferes with decarboxylation reactions in pyruvate and fatty acid metabolism.

Manganese   Mn acts as an activator of enzymes and as a component of metalloenzymes (Table 80-1). Mn deficiency in animals causes skeletal, central nervous, and gonadal manifestations. Mn deficiency in humans is rare; increases in prothrombin time, unresponsive to vitamin K, have been noted. In serum, Mn is bound to transmanganin, and it is excreted primarily in bile and pancreatic secretions.

Serum Mn increases following myocardial infarction and is decreased in children with convulsive disorders. Miners who inhale large quantities of Mn dust over long periods of time develop asthenia, anorexia, apathy, headache, impotence, leg cramps, speech disturbances, and occasionally even more severe symptoms (Table 80-2).

Selenium   Se plays a critical role as a component of glutathione peroxidase in the control of oxygen metabolism, particularly in catalyzing the breakdown of H$_2$O$_2$. The metal is required for the growth of cells in tissue culture. Furthermore, Se cures or prevents *Keshan disease*, a syndrome characterized by multifocal myocardial necrosis and reduced serum Se content. The disorder is endemic to the Keshan Province in China, where the soil may be deficient in the metal. Manifestations vary from severe arrhythmias and cardiogenic shock to asymptomatic cardiac enlargement. Muscle degeneration causes peripheral myopathies (Table 80-2). Children and women of childbearing age are particularly susceptible. Se protects animals from a number of carcinogenic chemicals and viruses. Se binds Cd, Hg, and other metals and mitigates their toxic effects, even when tissue levels of the metals remain elevated. Se poisoning can occur after ingestion of water containing large amounts of the metal.

Other Trace Elements   *Silicon* is present in bone and skin and may play a role in the cross-linkage of collagen. Deficiency in animals results in decreased growth, abnormal bone development, and decreased hexosamine content of epiphyses and epiphyseal plates. Deficiency has not been described in humans. Inhalation of fine particles of SiO$_2$ causes granuloma formation and fibrosis (*silicosis*) of the lungs (see Chap. 254).

Fluoride is a constituent of teeth and bone. In appropriate doses it prevents dental caries and increases bone density in patients with osteoporosis (see Chap. 355). Complications of long-term toxicity include calcification of bony ligaments and tendons and fluorosis, characterized by weakness, weight loss, anemia, brittle bones, and mottling of teeth (if taken during stages of enamel formation). Acute ingestion of toxic amounts, as found in some insect poisons, causes severe abdominal pain, nausea, vomiting, diarrhea, hypocalcemia, tetany, and on occasion cardiorespiratory arrest occur.

Deficiencies of *arsenic*, *nickel*, *tin*, or *vanadium* cause pathologic manifestations in plants and some vertebrates. Their roles in human health are undefined.

BIBLIOGRAPHY

ALFREY AC: Aluminum toxicity in patients with chronic renal failure. Ther Drug Monit 15:593, 1993

BEDWARL RS, BAKUGUNA A: Zinc, copper, and selenium in reproduction. Experentia 50:626, 1994

FALCHUK KH: Effect of acute disease and ACTH on serum zinc proteins. N Engl J Med 296:1129, 1977

GE K, YANG C: The epidmiology selenium deficiency in the etiological study of endemic diseases in China. Am J Clin Nutr 47(2 Suppl):2595, 1993

KLEIN GL: Aluminum in parenteral solutions revisited: Again. Am J Clin Nutr 61:449, 1995

NIELSEN FH: Nutritional refinement for boron, vanadium, nickel and arsenic: Current knowledge and speculations. FASEB J 56:2661, 1991

SEGHIZZI P et al: Cobalt cardiomyopathy: A critical review of literature. Sci Total Environ 150:105, 1994

TING-KAI L, VALLEE BL: The biochemical and nutritional roles of other trace elements, in *Modern Nutrition in Health and Disease*, RS Goodhart and ME Shills (eds). Philadelphia, Lea and Febiger, 6th ed, 1980, p 408

TZAMALOUKAS AH: Diagnosis and management of bone disorders in chronic renal failure and dialyzed-patients. Med Clin North Am 74:961, 1990

VALLEE BL, FALCHUK KH: The biochemical and pathological basis of zinc physiology. Physiol Rev 73:79, 1993

YARZE JL et al: Wilson's disease: Current status. Am J Med 92:643, 1992

YOKEE RA: Aluminum chelation: Chemistry, clinical and experimental studies and the search for alternatives to desferroxamine. J Toxicol Environ Health 41:131, 1994

ZLOTKIN SH et al: Trace elements in nutrition for premature infants. Clin Perinatol 22:223, 1995

PART SIX

ONCOLOGY AND HEMATOLOGY

81

Dan L. Longo

APPROACH TO THE PATIENT WITH CANCER

The application of current treatment techniques (surgery, radiation therapy, chemotherapy, and biological therapy) results in the cure of over 50 percent of patients diagnosed with cancer. Nevertheless, patients experience the diagnosis of cancer as one of the most traumatic and revolutionary events that has ever happened to them. Independent of prognosis, the diagnosis brings with it a change in a person's self-image and in his or her role in the home and workplace. The prognosis of a person who has just been found to have pancreatic cancer is the same as the prognosis of the person with aortic stenosis who develops the first symptoms of congestive heart failure (median survival, about 8 months). However, the patient with heart disease may remain functional and maintain a view of himself or herself as a fully intact person with just a malfunctioning part, a diseased organ ("a bum ticker"). By contrast, the patient with pancreatic cancer has a completely altered self-image and is viewed differently by family and anyone who knows the diagnosis. He or she is being attacked and invaded by a disease that could be anywhere in the body. Every ache or pain takes on desperate significance. Cancer is an exception to the coordinated interaction among cells and organs. In general, the cells of a multicellular organism are programmed for collaboration. Many diseases occur because the specialized cells fail to perform their assigned task. Cancer takes this malfunction one step further. Not only is there a failure of the cancer cell to maintain the specialized function of its tissue of origin, but also the cancer cell strikes out on its own; the cancer cell competes to survive using natural mutability and natural selection to seek advantage over normal cells in a recapitulation of evolution. One consequence of the traitorous behavior of cancer cells is that the patient feels betrayed by his or her body. The cancer patient feels that he or she, and not just a body part, is diseased.

THE MAGNITUDE OF THE PROBLEM

There is no nationwide cancer registry; therefore, the incidence of cancer is estimated on the basis of the National Cancer Institute's Surveillance, Epidemiology, and End Results (SEER) database, which tabulates cancer incidence and death figures from nine sites accounting for about 10 percent of the U.S. population and from population data from the Bureau of the Census. In 1996, 1.36 million new cases of invasive cancer (765,000 men, 595,000 women) were diagnosed and 555,000 people (292,000 men, 263,000 women) died from cancer. The percent distribution of new cancer cases and cancer deaths by site for men and women are shown in Fig. 81-1.

The most significant risk factor for cancer overall is age; two-thirds of all cases were in people over age 65 years. Cancer incidence increases as the third, fourth, or fifth power of age in different sites. Thus, the probability of a person developing cancer is age-dependent: For the interval between birth and age 39 years, 1 in 58 men and 1 in 52 women will develop cancer; for the interval between ages 40 and 59 years, 1 in 13 men and 1 in 11 women will develop cancer; and for the interval between ages 60 and 79 years, 1 in 3 men and 1 in 4 women will develop cancer.

Cancer is the second leading cause of death behind heart disease. However, deaths from heart disease have declined 45 percent in the United States since 1950 and continue to decline, while cancer deaths are increasing (Fig. 81-2). Early in the next century, cancer is projected to be the leading cause of death. The five leading causes of cancer deaths are shown for various populations in Table 81-1. Along with the increase in incidence has come an increase in survival for cancer patients. The 5-year survival for white patients was 39 percent in 1960–1963 and 58 percent in 1986–1991. Cancers are more often deadly in blacks; the 5-year survival was 42 percent for the 1986–1991 interval. The basis for these racial differences in survival is unclear.

PATIENT MANAGEMENT

Important information is obtained from every portion of the routine history and physical examination. The duration of symptoms may reveal the chronicity of disease. The past medical history may alert the physician to the presence of underlying diseases that may affect the choice of therapy or the side effects of treatment. The social history

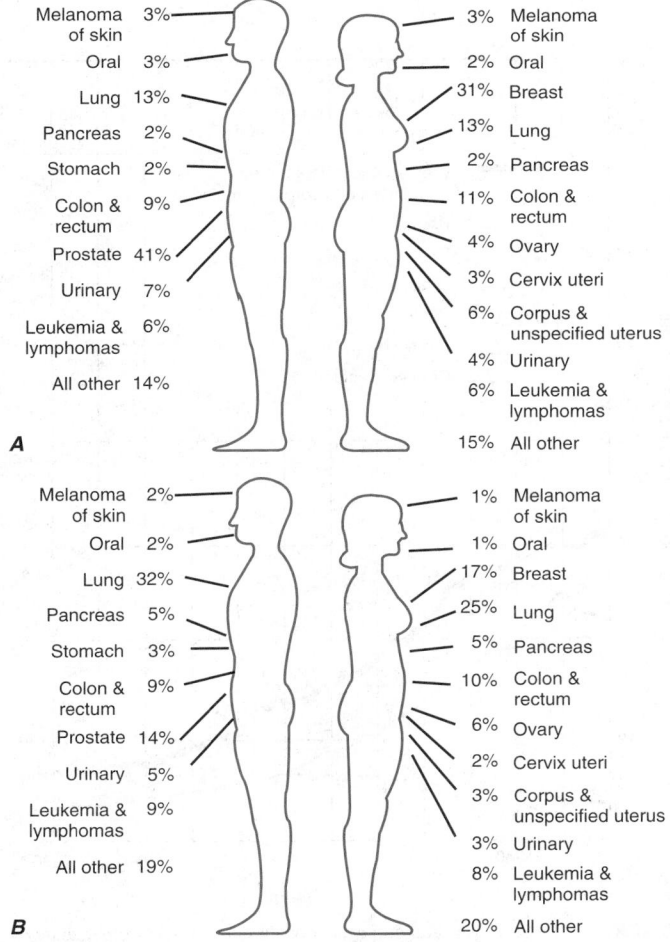

FIGURE 81-1 Distribution of (*A*) cancer incidence and (*B*) cancer deaths by sex for 1996. Data exclude basal and squamous cell skin cancers and carcinoma in situ except bladder. (*From Parker SL et al, CA Cancer J Clin 46:5, 1996.*)

may reveal occupational exposure to carcinogens, or habits, such as smoking or alcohol consumption, that may influence the course of disease and its treatment. The family history may suggest an underlying familial cancer predisposition and point out the need to begin surveillance or other preventive therapy for unaffected siblings of the patient. The review of systems may suggest early symptoms of metastatic disease or a paraneoplastic syndrome.

DIAGNOSIS The diagnosis of cancer relies most heavily on invasive tissue biopsy. The diagnosis should never be made without obtaining tissue; no noninvasive diagnostic test is sufficient to define a disease process as cancer. Although there are rare clinical settings (for example, thyroid nodules) where fine needle aspiration is an acceptable diagnostic procedure, in general, the diagnosis depends on removing from the patient adequate tissue to permit careful evaluation of the histology of the tumor, its grade, and its invasiveness and to yield further molecular diagnostic information, such as the expression of cell-surface markers or intracellular proteins that typify a particular cancer, or the presence of a molecular marker such as the t(8;14) translocation of Burkitt's lymphoma. Increasing evidence implicates the expression of certain genes with the prognosis and response to therapy (see Chaps. 83 and 84).

Occasionally a patient will present with a metastatic disease process that is defined as cancer on biopsy but has no apparent primary site of disease. Efforts should be made to define the primary site based on age, sex, sites of involvement, histology and tumor markers, and personal and family history. Particular attention should be focused on ruling out the most treatable causes (see Chap. 101).

Once the diagnosis of cancer is made, the management of the patient is best undertaken as a multidisciplinary collaboration among the primary care physician, medical oncologists, surgical oncologists, radiation oncologists, oncology nurse specialists, pharmacists, social workers, rehabilitation medicine specialists, and a number of other consulting professionals working closely with each other and with the patient and family.

DEFINING THE EXTENT OF DISEASE AND THE PROGNOSIS The first priority in patient management after the diagnosis of cancer is established and shared with the patient is to determine the extent of disease. The curability of a tumor usually is inversely proportional to the tumor burden. Ideally, the tumor will be diagnosed before symptoms develop (see Chaps. 63 and 64) or as a consequence of screening efforts (see Chap. 82). A very high proportion of such patients can be cured. However, most patients with cancer present with symptoms related to the cancer, caused either by mass effects of the tumor or by alterations associated with the production of cytokines or hormones from the tumor.

For most cancers, the extent of disease is evaluated by a variety of noninvasive and invasive diagnostic tests and procedures. This process is called *staging*. There are two types. *Clinical staging* is based on physical examination, radiographs, isotopic scans, computed tomography, and other imaging procedures; *pathologic staging* takes into account information obtained during a surgical procedure, which might include intraoperative palpation, resection of regional lymph nodes and/or tissue adjacent to the tumor, and inspection and biopsy of organs commonly involved in disease spread. Pathologic staging includes histologic examination of all tissues removed during the surgical procedure. Surgical procedures performed may include a simple lymph node biopsy or more extensive procedures such as thoracot-

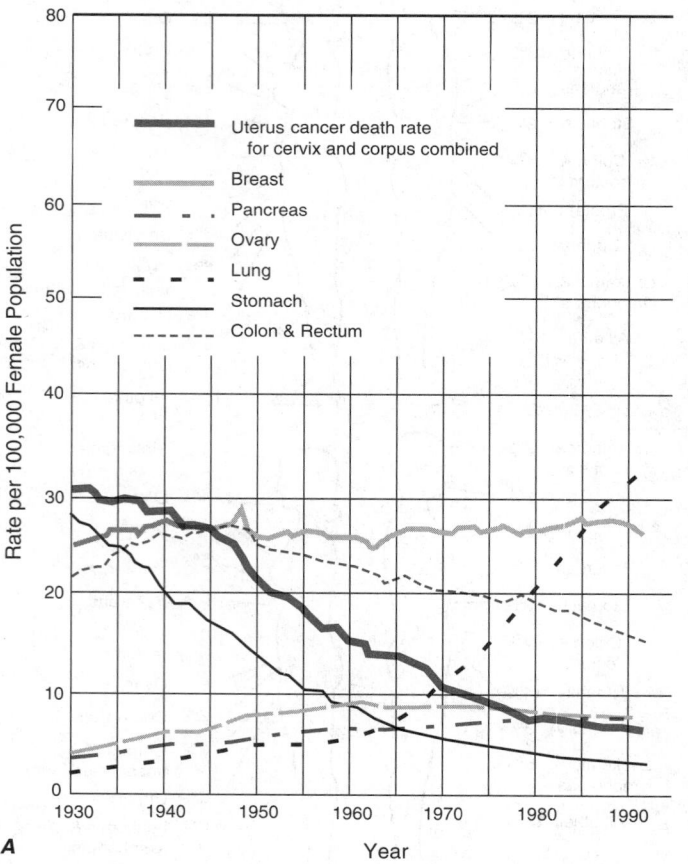

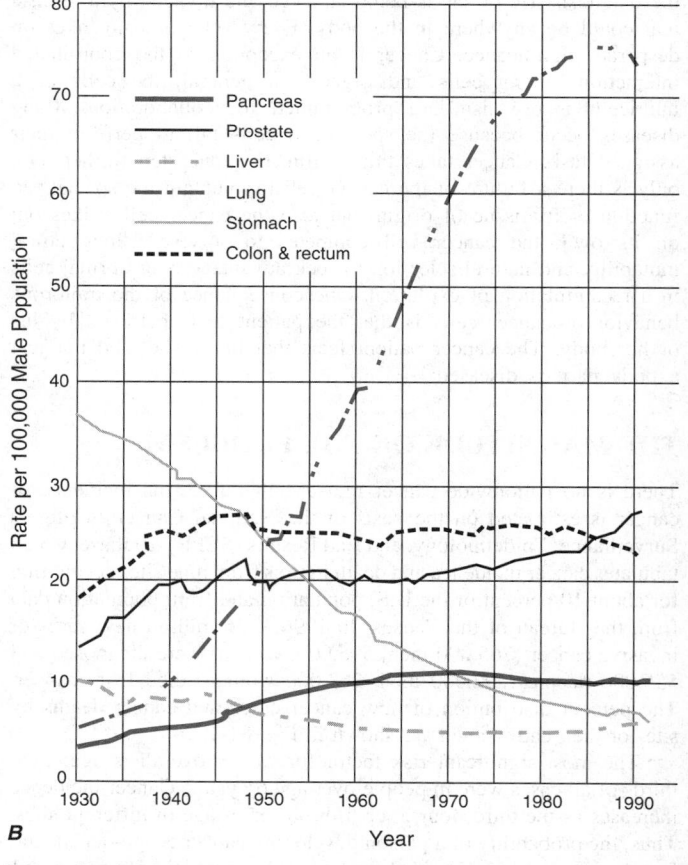

FIGURE 81-2 Sixty-year trend in cancer death rates for (*A*) women and (*B*) men, by site in the United States, 1930–1992. Rates are per 100,000 age-adjusted to the 1970 U.S. standard population. Note: Due to changes in the ICD coding, numerator information has changed over time. Rates for cancer of the liver are particularly affected by these coding changes. Denominator information for the years 1930–1967 and 1991–1992 is based on intercensal population estimates, while denominator information for the years 1968–1990 is based on postcensal recalculation of estimates. (*From Parker SL et al, CA Cancer J Clin 46:5, 1996.*)

Table 81-1

The Five Leading Primary Tumor Sites for Patients Dying of Cancer Based on Age, Sex, and Race

Rank	All Ages	Age					Race	
		Under 15	15–34	35–54	55–74	75+	White	Black
1	M: lung (94,400; 30-yr trend, +85%) F: lung (64,300; 30-yr trend, +438%)	M and F: leukemia	M: leukemia F: breast	M: lung F: breast	M and F: lung	M and F: lung	Lung	Lung
2	M: prostate (41,400; 30-yr trend, +29%) F: breast (44,300; 30-yr trend, +4%)	M and F: brain and CNS	M: lymphoma F: leukemia	M: colon, rectum F: lung	M: colon, rectum F: breast	M: prostate F: colon, rectum	Colon, rectum	Colon, rectum
3	M: colon, rectum (27,400; 30-yr trend, −9%) F: colon, rectum (27,500; 30-yr trend, −31%)	M and F: endocrine	M: brain and CNS F: cervix	M: lymphoma F: colon, rectum	M: prostate F: colon, rectum	M: colon, rectum F: breast	Breast	Prostate
4	M: pancreas (13,600; 30-yr trend, −5%) F: ovary (14,800; 30-yr trend, −8%)	M: lymphoma F: bone	M: skin F: brain and CNS	M: brain and CNS F: ovary	M: pancreas F: ovary	M and F: pancreas	Prostate	Breast
5	M: lymphoma (12,400; 30-yr trend, +30%) F: pancreas (14,200; 30-yr trend, +12%)	M and F: sarcoma	M: Hodgkin's F: lymphoma	M: pancreas F: cervix	M: lymphoma F: pancreas	M: leukemia F: ovary	Pancreas	Pancreas

ABBREVIATIONS: F, female; M, male.

omy, mediastinoscopy, or laparotomy. Surgical staging may occur in a separate procedure or may be done at the time of definitive surgical resection of the primary tumor.

Knowledge of the predilection of particular tumors for spread to adjacent or distant organs helps direct the staging evaluation. The sites of metastatic disease for common tumors are given in Table 85-1.

Information obtained from staging is used to define the extent of disease either as localized, as exhibiting spread outside of the organ of origin to regional but not distant sites, or as metastatic to distant sites. The most widely used system of staging is the TNM (tumor, node, metastasis) system codified by the International Union Against Cancer and the American Joint Committee on Cancer (AJCC).* The TNM classification is an anatomically based system that categorizes the tumor on the basis of the size of the primary tumor lesion (T1–4, where a higher value of the subscript indicates a tumor of larger size), the presence of nodal involvement (usually N0 and N1 for the absence and presence, respectively, of involved nodes, although some tumors have more elaborate systems of nodal grading), and the presence of metastatic disease (M0 and M1 for the absence and presence, respectively, of metastases). The various permutations of T, N, and M scores are then broken into stages, usually designated by the roman numerals I through IV. Tumor burden increases and curability decreases with increasing stage. Other anatomic staging systems are used for some tumors, for example, the Dukes classification for colorectal cancers, the International Federation of Gynecologists and Obstetricians (FIGO) classification for gynecologic cancers, and the Ann Arbor classification for Hodgkin's disease.

Certain tumors cannot be grouped appropriately on the basis of anatomic considerations. For example, hematopoietic tumors such as leukemia, myeloma, and lymphoma are often disseminated at presentation and do not spread in the fashion typical of solid tumors. For these tumors, other prognostic factors have been identified (see Chaps. 112, 113, and 114).

In addition to tumor burden, a second major determinant of treatment outcome is the physiologic reserve of the patient. Patients who are bedridden before developing cancer are likely to fare worse, stage for stage, than fully active patients. Physiologic reserve is a determinant of how a patient is likely to cope with the physiologic stresses imposed by the cancer and its treatment. This factor is difficult to assess directly. Instead, surrogate markers for physiologic reserve are used, such as

the patient's age or Karnofsky performance status (Table 81-2). Older patients and those with a Karnofsky performance status of less than 70 have a poor prognosis unless the poor performance is a reversible consequence of the tumor.

Increasingly, biologic features of the tumor are being related to prognosis. The expression of particular oncogenes, drug resistance genes, apoptosis-related genes, and genes involved in metastasis are being found to influence response to therapy and prognosis. The presence of selected cytogenetic abnormalities may influence survival. Tumors with higher growth fractions, as assessed by expression of proliferation-related markers such as proliferating cell nuclear antigen (PCNA), behave more aggressively than tumors with lower growth fractions. Information obtained from studying the tumor itself will increasingly be used to influence treatment decisions.

MAKING A TREATMENT PLAN From information on the extent of disease and the prognosis and in conjunction with the patient's wishes, it is possible to determine whether the treatment approach should be curative or palliative in intent. Cooperation among the various professionals involved in cancer treatment is of the utmost importance in treatment planning. For some cancers, chemotherapy or chemotherapy plus radiation therapy delivered before the use of

Table 81-2

Karnofsky Performance Index

Performance Status	Functional Capability of the Patient
100	Normal; no complaints; no evidence of disease
90	Able to carry on normal activity; minor signs or symptoms of disease
80	Normal activity with effort; some signs or symptoms of disease
70	Cares for self; unable to carry on normal activity or do active work
60	Requires occasional assistance but is able to care for most needs
50	Requires considerable assistance and frequent medical care
40	Disabled; requires special care and assistance
30	Severely disabled; hospitalization is indicated although death is not imminent
20	Very sick; hospitalization necessary; active supportive treatment is necessary
10	Moribund, fatal processes progressing rapidly
0	Dead

* The AJCC *Manual for Staging Cancer* can be obtained from the AJCC at 55 East Erie Street, Chicago, IL, 60611.

definitive surgical treatment (so-called neoadjuvant therapy) may improve the outcome, as seems to be the case for locally advanced breast cancer and head and neck cancers. In certain settings in which combined modality therapy is intended, coordination among the medical oncologist, radiation oncologist, and surgeon is crucial to achieving optimal results. Sometimes the chemotherapy and radiation therapy need to be delivered sequentially, and other times concurrently. Surgical procedures may precede or follow other treatment approaches. It is best for the treatment plan either to follow precisely a standard protocol or else to be part of an ongoing clinical research protocol evaluating new treatments. Ad hoc modifications of standard protocols are likely to compromise treatment results.

The choice of treatment approaches was formerly dominated by the local culture in both the university and the practice settings. However, it is now possible to gain access electronically to standard treatment protocols and to every approved clinical research study in North America through a personal computer interface with the Internet.*

The skilled physician also has much to offer the patient for whom curative therapy is no longer an option. Often a combination of guilt and frustration over the inability to cure the patient and the pressure of a busy schedule greatly limit the time a physician spends with a patient who is receiving only palliative care. Resist these forces. In addition to the medicines administered to alleviate symptoms (see below), it is important to remember the comfort that is provided by holding the patient's hand, continuing regular examinations, and taking time to talk.

MANAGEMENT OF DISEASE AND TREATMENT COMPLICATIONS Because cancer therapies are toxic (see Chap. 86), patient management involves addressing complications of both the disease and its treatment as well as the complex psychosocial problems associated with cancer. In the short term during a course of curative therapy, the patient's functional status may decline. Treatment-induced toxicity is less acceptable if the goal of therapy is palliation. The most common side effects of treatment are nausea and vomiting (see below), febrile neutropenia (see Chap. 87), and myelosuppression (see Chap. 105). Therapeutic tools are now available to minimize the acute toxicity of cancer treatment.

New symptoms developing in the course of cancer treatment should always be assumed to be reversible until proven otherwise. The fatalistic attribution of anorexia, weight loss, and jaundice to recurrent or progressive tumor could result in a patient dying from a reversible intercurrent cholecystitis. Intestinal obstruction may be due to reversible adhesions rather than progressive tumor. Systemic infections, sometimes with unusual pathogens, may be a consequence of the immunosuppression associated with cancer therapy. Some drugs used to treat cancer or its complications (e.g., nausea) may produce central nervous system symptoms that look like metastatic disease or may mimic paraneoplastic syndromes such as the syndrome of inappropriate antidiuretic hormone. A definitive diagnosis should be pursued and may even require a repeat biopsy.

A critical component of cancer management is assessing the response to treatment. In addition to a careful physical examination in which all sites of disease are physically measured and recorded in a flow chart by date, response assessment usually requires periodic repeating of imaging tests that were abnormal at the time of staging. If imaging tests have become normal, repeat biopsy of previously involved tissue is performed to document complete response by pathol-

ogy criteria. Biopsies are not usually required if there is macroscopic residual disease. Responses are graded as complete, if there has been disappearance of all evidence of disease, and partial, if there has been greater than 50 percent reduction in the sum of the products of the perpendicular diameters of all measureable lesions. Progressive disease is defined as the appearance of any new lesion or an increase of greater than 25 percent in the sum of the products of the perpendicular diameters of all measurable lesions. Tumor shrinkage or growth that does not meet any of these criteria is considered stable disease. Some sites of involvement (e.g., bone) or patterns of involvement (e.g., lymphangitic lung or diffuse pulmonary infiltrates) are considered unmeasurable. No response is complete without biopsy documentation of their resolution but partial responses may exclude their assessment unless clear objective (though unmeasurable) progression has occurred.

Tumor markers may be useful in patient management in certain tumors. Response to therapy may be difficult to gauge with certainty. However, some tumors produce or elicit the production of markers that can be measured in the serum or urine and, in a particular patient, rising and falling levels of the marker are usually associated with increasing or decreasing tumor burden, respectively. Some clinically useful tumor markers are shown in Table 81-3. Tumor markers are not in themselves specific enough to permit a diagnosis of malignancy to be made, but once a malignancy has been diagnosed and shown to be associated with elevated levels of a tumor marker, the marker can be used to assess response to treatment.

The recognition and treatment of depression is an important component of management. The incidence of depression in cancer patients is about 25 percent overall and may be greater in patients with greater debility. This diagnosis is likely in a patient with a depressed mood (dysphoria) and/or a loss of interest in pleasure (anhedonia) for at least 2 weeks. In addition, three or more of the following symptoms are usually present: appetite change, sleep problems, psychomotor retardation or agitation, fatigue, feelings of guilt or worthlessness, inability to concentrate, and suicidal ideation. Patients with these symptoms should receive therapy. Medical therapy with a serotonin reuptake inhibitor such as fluoxetine (10 to 20 mg/d), sertraline (50 to 150 mg/d), or paroxetine (10 to 20 mg/d) or a tricyclic antidepressant such as amitriptyline (50 to 100 mg/d) or desipramine (75 to 150 mg/d) should be tried allowing 4 to 6 weeks for response. Effective therapy should be continued at least 6 months after resolution of symptoms. If therapy is unsuccessful, other classes of antidepressants may be used. In addition to medication, psychosocial interventions such as support groups, psychotherapy, and guided imagery may be of benefit.

Many patients opt for unproven or unsound approaches to treatment when it appears that conventional medicine is unlikely to be curative. Those seeking such alternatives are often well educated and may be early in the course of their disease. Unsound approaches are usually hawked on the basis of unsubstantiated anecdotes and not only cannot help the patient but may be harmful. Physicians should strive to keep communications open and nonjudgmental, so that patients are more likely to discuss with the physician what they are actually doing. The appearance of unexpected toxicity may be an indication that a supplemental therapy is being taken.*

LONG-TERM FOLLOW-UP/LATE COMPLICATIONS At the completion of treatment, sites originally involved with tumor are reassessed, usually by radiography or imaging techniques, and any persistent abnormality is biopsied. If disease persists, the multidisciplinary team discusses a new salvage treatment plan. If the patient has been rendered disease-free by the original treatment, the patient is followed regularly for disease recurrence. The optimal guidelines for follow-up care are not known. For many years, a routine practice has been to follow the patient monthly for 6 to 12 months, then every other month for a year, every 3 months for a year, every 4 months

---

* The National Cancer Institute maintains a database called PDQ (Physician Data Query) that is accessible on the Internet under the name CancerNet at wwwicic.nci.nih.gov/health.htm. Information can be obtained through a facsimile machine using CancerFax by dialing 301-402-5874. Patient information is also provided by the National Cancer Institute in at least three formats: on the Internet via CancerNet at wwwicic.nci.nih.gov/patient.htm, through the CancerFax number listed above, or by calling 1-800-4-CANCER. The quality control for the information provided through these services is rigorous.

* Information about unsound methods may be obtained from the National Council Against Health Fraud, Box 1276, Loma Linda, CA 92354, or from the Center for Medical Consumers and Health Care Information, 237 Thompson Street, New York, NY 10012.

for a year, every 6 months for a year, and then annually. At each visit, a battery of laboratory and radiographic and imaging tests were obtained on the assumption that it is best to detect recurrent disease before it becomes symptomatic. However, where follow-up procedures have been examined, this assumption has been found to be untrue. Studies of breast cancer, melanoma, lung cancer, colon cancer, and lymphoma have all failed to support the notion that asymptomatic relapses are more readily cured by salvage therapy than symptomatic relapses. In view of the enormous cost of a full battery of diagnostic tests and their manifest lack of impact on survival, new guidelines are emerging for less frequent follow-up visits during which the history and physical examination are the major investigations performed.

As time passes, the likelihood of recurrence of the primary cancer diminishes. For many types of cancer, survival for 5 years without recurrence is tantamount to cure. However, there are important medical problems that occur in patients treated for cancer that must be examined. For some tumor types, such as breast cancer and head and neck cancer, second primary tumors are a feature of the disease. Secondary tumors may also be a consequence of the treatment approach. For example, chronic administration of alkylating agents is associated with secondary acute leukemia. Radiation therapy is associated with the occurrence of second solid tumors in the treatment field. The risk of a second tumor from radiation therapy is about 0.5 to 1 percent per year; second tumors involving some organs, such as the thyroid or breast, may not appear until 20 years or more after the initial treatment. Mediastinal irradiation may produce accelerated coronary atherosclerosis. Abdominal or pelvic surgery or irradiation may lead to adhesions and bowel obstruction. Radiation of the neck usually leads to thyroid insufficiency and can result in the loss of salivary secretion and poor dentition. Chemotherapy that includes alkylating agents usually leads to infertility. Other sexual problems may be very slow to resolve after cancer treatment. Pulmonary complications also may occur after both radiation therapy and chemotherapy. Endocrine ablation is a goal of therapy in some tumors, and its long-term consequences must be managed. There are many medical conditions that the alert physician should anticipate in a patient who has undergone curative cancer therapy.

Despite these concerns, most patients who are cured of cancer return to normal lives.

SUPPORTIVE CARE In many ways, the success of cancer therapy depends on the success of the supportive care. Failure to control the symptoms of cancer and its treatment may lead patients to abandon curative therapy. Of equal importance, supportive care is a major determinant of quality of life. Even when life cannot be prolonged, the physician must strive to preserve its quality. Quality of life measurements have become common end-points of clinical research studies. Furthermore, palliative care has been shown to be cost-effective when approached in an organized fashion. A credo for oncology could be to cure sometimes, to extend life often, and to comfort always.

Pain Pain occurs with variable frequency in the cancer patient: 25 to 50 percent of patients present with pain at diagnosis, 33 percent have pain associated with treatment, and 75 percent have pain with progressive disease. The pain may have several causes. In about 70 percent of cases, pain is caused by the tumor itself—by invasion of bone, nerves, blood vessels, or mucous membranes or obstruction of a hollow viscus or duct. In about 20 percent of cases, pain is related to a surgical or invasive medical procedure, to radiation injury (mucositis, enteritis, or plexus or spinal cord injury), or to chemotherapy injury (mucositis, peripheral neuropathy, phlebitis, steroid-induced aseptic necrosis of the femoral head). In 10 percent of cases, pain is unrelated to cancer or its treatment.

Assessment of pain requires the methodical investigation of the history of the pain, its location, character, temporal features, provocative and palliative factors, and intensity (see Chap. 12); a review of the oncologic history and past medical history as well as personal and social history; and a thorough physical examination. The patient should be given a 10-division visual analogue scale on which to indicate the severity of the pain. The clinical condition is often dynamic, making it necessary to reassess the patient frequently. Pain therapy should not be withheld while the cause of pain is being sought.

A variety of tools are available with which to address cancer pain. About 85 percent of patients will have pain relief from pharmacologic intervention. However, other modalities, including antitumor therapy (such as surgical relief of obstruction, radiation therapy, and strontium-89 treatment for bone pain), neurostimulatory techniques, regional analgesia, or neuroablative procedures are effective in an additional 12 percent or so. Thus, very few patients will have inadequate pain relief if appropriate measures are taken.

The World Health Organization (WHO) has devised a simple and effective method for the rational titration of oral analgesia, called the WHO ladder. The ladder has the following three steps. (1) For mild to moderate pain, one begins with acetaminophen (650 mg every 4 h or 975 mg every 6 h), aspirin (650 mg every 4 h or 975 mg every 6 h), or a nonsteroidal anti-inflammatory agent (NSAID; for example, ketoprofen, 25 to 60 mg every 6 h) with or without an adjuvant such as a glucocorticoid (dexamethasone) or an antidepressant (amitripty-

Table 81-3

Tumor Markers

Tumor Markers	Cancer	Non-Neoplastic Conditions
HORMONES		
Human chorionic gonadotropin	Gestational trophoblastic disease, gonadal germ cell tumor	Pregnancy
Calcitonin	Medullary cancer of the thyroid	
Catecholamines	Pheochromocytoma	
ONCOFETAL ANTIGENS		
Alphafetoprotein	Hepatocellular carcinoma, gonadal germ cell tumor	Cirrhosis, hepatitis
Carcinoembryonic antigen	Adenocarcinomas of the colon, pancreas, lung, breast, ovary	Pancreatitis, hepatitis, inflammatory bowel disease, smoking
ENZYMES		
Prostatic acid phosphatase	Prostate cancer	Prostatitis, prostatic hypertrophy
Neuron-specific enolase	Small cell cancer of the lung, neuroblastoma	
Lactate dehydrogenase	Lymphoma, Ewing's sarcoma	Hepatitis, hemolytic anemia, many others
TUMOR-ASSOCIATED PROTEINS		
Prostate-specific antigen	Prostate cancer	Prostatitis, prostatic hypertrophy
Monoclonal immunoglobulin	Myeloma	Infection, MGUS*
CA-125	Ovarian cancer, some lymphomas	Menstruation, peritonitis, pregnancy
CA 19-9	Colon, pancreatic, breast cancer	Pancreatitis, ulcerative colitis
CD30	Hodgkin's disease, anaplastic large cell lymphoma	—
CD25	Hairy cell leukemia, adult T-cell leukemia/lymphoma	—

* MGUS, monoclonal gammopathy of uncertain significance.

line). (2) When pain persists or increases, an opioid such as codeine or hydrocodone (30 mg every 3 to 4 h is roughly equivalent to 10 mg of intravenous morphine) should be added (not substituted); fixed combinations such as oxycodone/acetaminophen (Percocet) or oxycodone/aspirin (Percodan) are worth testing. (3) Pain that is persistent or that is moderate to severe at the outset should be treated by increasing the potency of the opioid or using higher dosages (for example, morphine, 15 to 30 mg every 3 to 4 h, or controlled-release morphine, 90 to 120 mg bid), and fixed opioid/NSAID combinations should be abandoned. Adjuvants may be used at all steps. The critical features of this approach are that the treatment is oral, should be given around the clock with supplemental doses as needed to control pain, and is tailored to the individual patient. Records of pain control should be a prominent component of the medical record. When opioids are used, the patient should be placed on a prophylactic regimen to prevent constipation.

Nausea Emesis in the cancer patient is usually caused by chemotherapy (see Chap. 86). Its severity can be predicted from the drugs used to treat the cancer. Three forms of emesis are recognized on the basis of their timing with regard to the noxious insult. *Acute emesis*, the most common variety, occurs within 24 h of treatment. *Delayed emesis* occurs 1 to 7 days after treatment; it is rare, but, when present, usually follows cisplatin administration. *Anticipatory emesis* occurs before administration of chemotherapy and represents a conditioned response to visual and olfactory stimuli previously associated with chemotherapy delivery.

Acute emesis is the best understood form. Stimuli that activate signals in the chemoreceptor trigger zone in the medulla, the cerebral cortex, and peripherally in the intestinal tract lead to stimulation of the vomiting center in the medulla, the motor center responsible for coordinating the secretory and muscle contraction activity that leads to emesis. Diverse receptor types participate in the process, including dopamine, serotonin, histamine, opioid, and acetylcholine receptors. The serotonin receptor antagonists ondansetron and granisetron are the most effective drugs against highly emetogenic agents, but they are expensive.

As with the analgesia ladder, emesis therapy should be tailored to the situation. For mildly and moderately emetogenic agents, prochlorperazine, 5 to 10 mg orally or 25 mg rectally, is effective. Its efficacy may be enhanced by administering the drug before the chemotherapy is delivered. Dexamethasone, 10 to 20 mg intravenously, is also effective and may enhance the efficacy of prochlorperazine. For highly emetogenic agents such as cisplatin, mechlorethamine, dacarbazine, and streptozocin, combinations of agents work best, and administration should begin 6 to 24 h before treatment. Ondansetron 8 mg orally every 6 h the day before therapy and intravenously on the day of therapy plus dexamethasone 20 mg intravenously before treatment is an effective regimen. Like pain, emesis is easier to prevent than to alleviate.

Delayed emesis may be related to bowel inflammation from the therapy and can be controlled with oral dexamethasone and oral metoclopramide, a dopamine receptor antagonist that also blocks serotonin receptors at high dosages. The best strategy for preventing anticipatory emesis is to control emesis in the early cycles of therapy to prevent the conditioning from taking place. If this is unsuccessful, prophylactic antiemetics the day before treatment may help. Experimental studies are evaluating behavior modification.

Effusions Fluid may accumulate abnormally in the pleural cavity, pericardium, or peritoneum. Asymptomatic malignant effusions may not require treatment. Symptomatic effusions occurring in tumors responsive to systemic therapy usually do not require local treatment but respond to the treatment for the underlying tumor. Symptomatic effusions occurring in tumors unresponsive to systemic therapy may require local treatment in patients with a life expectancy of at least 6 months.

Pleural effusions due to tumors may or may not contain malignant cells. Lung cancer, breast cancer, and lymphomas account for about 75 percent of malignant pleural effusions. Their exudative nature is usually gauged by an effusion/serum protein ratio of 0.5 or an effusion/serum lactate dehydrogenase ratio of 0.6. When the condition is symptomatic, thoracentesis is usually performed first. In most cases, symptomatic improvement occurs for less than 1 month. Chest tube drainage is required if symptoms recur within 2 weeks. Fluid is aspirated until the flow rate is less than 100 mL in 24 h. Then either 60 units of bleomycin or 1 g of doxycycline is infused into the chest tube in 50 mL of 5% dextrose in water; the tube is clamped; the patient is rotated on four sides, spending 15 min in each position; and, after 1 to 2 h, the tube is again attached to suction for another 24 h. The tube is then disconnected from suction and allowed to drain by gravity. If less than 100 mL drains over the next 24 h, the chest tube is pulled, and a radiograph taken 24 h later. If the chest tube continues to drain fluid at an unacceptably high rate, sclerosis can be repeated. Bleomycin may be somewhat more effective than doxycycline, but it is very expensive. Doxycycline is usually the drug of first choice. If neither doxycycline nor bleomycin is effective, talc can be used.

Symptomatic pericardial effusions are usually treated by creating a pericardial window or by stripping. If the patient's condition does not permit a surgical procedure, sclerosis can be attempted with doxycycline and/or bleomycin.

Malignant ascites is usually treated with repeated paracentesis of small volumes of fluid. If the underlying malignancy is unresponsive to systemic therapy, peritoneovenous shunts may be inserted. Despite the fear of disseminating tumor cells into the circulation, widespread metastases are an unusual complication. The major complications are occlusion, leakage, and fluid overload. Patients with severe liver disease may develop disseminated intravascular coagulation.

Nutrition Cancer and its treatment may lead to a decrease in nutrient intake of sufficient magnitude to cause weight loss and alteration of intermediary metabolism. The prevalence of this problem is difficult to estimate because of variations in the definition of cancer cachexia, but most patients with advanced cancer experience weight loss and decreased appetite. A variety of both tumor-derived factors (for example, bombesin, adrenocorticotropic hormone) and host-derived factors (for example, tumor necrosis factor, interleukins 1 and 6, growth hormone) contribute to the altered metabolism, and a vicious cycle is established in which protein catabolism, glucose intolerance, and lipolysis cannot be reversed by the provision of calories.

It remains controversial how to assess nutritional status and when and how to intervene. Efforts to make the assessment objective have included the use of a prognostic nutritional index based on albumin levels, triceps skin fold thickness, transferrin levels, and delayed-type hypersensitivity skin testing. However, a simpler approach has been to define the threshold for nutritional intervention as greater than 10 percent unexplained body weight loss, serum transferrin level less than 150 mg/dL, and serum albumin less than 3.4 g/dL.

The decision is important, because it appears that cancer therapy is substantially more toxic and less effective in the face of malnutrition. Nevertheless, it remains unclear whether nutritional intervention can alter the natural history. Unless there is some pathology affecting the absorptive function of the gastrointestinal tract, enteral nutrition provided orally or by tube feeding is preferred over parenteral supplementation. However, the risks associated with the tube may outweigh the benefits. Megestrol acetate, a progestational agent, has been advocated as a pharmacologic intervention to improve nutritional status. Research in this area may provide more tools in the future as cytokine-mediated mechanisms are further elucidated.

Psychosocial Support The psychosocial needs of patients vary with their situation. Patients undergoing treatment experience fear, anxiety, and depression. Self-image is often seriously compromised by deforming surgery and loss of hair. Women who receive cosmetic advice that enables them to look better also feel better. Loss of control over how one spends time can contribute to the sense of vulnerability. Juggling the demands of work and family with the demands of treatment may create enormous stresses. Sexual dysfunction is highly prevalent and needs to be discussed overtly with the patient. An empathetic health care team is sensitive to the individual patient's needs and permits negotiation where such flexibility will not adversely affect the course of treatment.

Cancer survivors have other sets of difficulties. Patients may have fears associated with the termination of a treatment they associate with their continued survival. Adjustments are required to physical losses and handicaps, real and perceived. Patients may be preoccupied with minor physical problems. They perceive a decline in their job mobility and view themselves as less desirable workers. They may be victims of job and/or insurance discrimination. Patients may experience difficulty reentering their normal past life. They may feel guilty for having survived and may carry a sense of vulnerability to colds and other illnesses. Perhaps the most pervasive and threatening concern is the ever-present fear of relapse (the Damocles syndrome).

Patients in whom therapy has been unsuccessful have other problems related to the end of life.

Death and Dying   The most common causes of death in patients with cancer are infection (leading to circulatory failure), respiratory failure, hepatic failure, and renal failure. Intestinal blockage may lead to inanition and starvation. Central nervous system disease may lead to seizures, coma, and central hypoventilation. About 70 percent of patients develop dyspnea preterminally. However, many months usually pass between the diagnosis of cancer and the occurrence of these complications, and during this period the patient is severely affected by the possibility of death. The path of unsuccessful cancer treatment usually occurs in three phases. First, there is optimism at the hope of cure; when the tumor recurs, there is the acknowledgment of an incurable disease, and the goal of palliative therapy is embraced in the hope of being able to live with disease; finally, at the disclosure of imminent death, another adjustment in outlook takes place. The patient imagines the worst in preparation for the end of life and may go through stages of adjustment to the diagnosis. These stages include denial, isolation, anger, bargaining, depression, acceptance, and hope. Of course, patients do not all progress through all the stages or proceed through them in the same order or at the same rate. Nevertheless, developing an understanding of how the patient has been affected by the diagnosis and is coping with it is an important goal of patient management.

It is best to speak frankly with the patient and the family regarding the likely course of disease. These discussions can be difficult for the physician as well as for the patient and family. The critical features of the interaction are to reassure the patient and family that everything that can be done to provide comfort will be done. They will not be abandoned. Many patients prefer to be cared for in their homes or in a hospice setting rather than a hospital. The American College of Physicians has published a book called *Home Care Guide for Cancer: How to Care for Family and Friends at Home* that teaches an approach to successful problem solving in home care. With appropriate planning, it should be possible to provide the patient with the necessary medical care as well as the psychological and spiritual support that will prevent the isolation and depersonalization that can attend in-hospital death.

The care of dying patients may take a toll on the physician. A "burnout" syndrome has been described that is characterized by fatigue, disengagement from patients and colleagues, and a loss of self-fulfillment. Efforts at stress reduction, maintenance of a balanced life, and setting realistic goals may combat this disorder.

End-of-Life Decisions   Unfortunately, a smooth transition in treatment goals from curative to palliative may not be possible in all cases because of the occurrence of serious treatment-related complications or rapid disease progression. Vigorous and invasive medical support for a reversible disease or treatment complication is assumed to be justified. However, if the reversibility of the condition is in doubt, the patient's wishes determine the level of medical care. These wishes should be elicited before the terminal phase of illness and reviewed periodically. This information can guide the physician should the patient be unable to speak for himself. The family cannot be expected to make such decisions without guidance from the patient and support from the physician when surrogate decisions are required. Advance directives such as the living will or the durable power of attorney for health care provide guidance for the health care team and the family regarding the patient's wishes and may protect the patient's assets from depletion on expensive but unwanted care.

Only about 15 percent of the population has implemented an advance directive. Physicians should take the initiative to speak with patients and family members about advance directives.*

BIBLIOGRAPHY

Clinical Practice Guideline Number 9, Management of Cancer Pain. U.S. Department of Health and Human Services, Agency for Health Care Policy and Research publication no. 94-0592, 1994
GRUNBERG SM, HESKETH PJ: Control of chemotherapy-induced emesis. N Engl J Med 329:1790, 1993
HOLLAND JC, ROWLAND JH (eds): *Handbook of Psycho-oncology: Psychological Care of the Patient with Cancer.* New York, Oxford University Press, 1989.
LEVY MH: Pharmacologic treatment of cancer pain. N Engl J Med 335:1124, 1996
PARKER SL et al: Cancer statistics, 1996. CA Cancer J Clin 46:5, 1996

* Information about them can be obtained from the American Association of Retired Persons, 601 E Street, N.W., Washington, DC 20049, 202-434-2277 or Choice in Dying, 250 West 57th Street, New York, NY 10107, 212-366-5540.

---

82   *Otis W. Brawley, Barnett S. Kramer*

PREVENTION AND EARLY DETECTION OF CANCER

The prevention and control of cancer is a burgeoning field because of advances in the understanding of the biology of carcinogenesis. The field has expanded beyond the identification and avoidance of carcinogens to include studies of specific interventions to lower cancer risk, as well as screening for early detection of cancer.

Central to the prevention and control of cancer is the concept that carcinogenesis is not an event but a process, a series of discrete cellular changes that result in progressively more autonomous cellular processes. *Primary prevention* consists in the identification and manipulation of the genetic, biologic, and environmental factors in the causal pathway. Smoking cessation, diet modification, and chemoprevention are primary prevention activities. *Secondary prevention* consists in the identification of asymptomatic neoplastic lesions combined with effective therapy. Screening is a form of secondary prevention.

EDUCATION AND HEALTHFUL HABITS   Public education on the avoidance of identified risk factors for cancer and the encouraging of healthy habits were among early efforts in cancer prevention and control. Many educational messages have come to the public through commercials in the print and electronic media and through school health courses. The physician is a potentially powerful messenger in this education campaign about the hazards of smoking, the benefits of a healthful diet, and sun avoidance.

Smoking Cessation   Cigarette smoking is the most avoidable risk factor for cardiovascular disease and cancer. There are clear correlations between lung cancer mortality rates and the number of cigarettes smoked per day as well as the degree of inhalation of cigarette smoke. Also, those who stop smoking have a lower lung cancer mortality rate than those who continue smoking. In addition to lung cancer, cigarette smoking has been associated as a causative agent in cancers of the larynx, oropharynx, esophagus, and bladder. Cessation and avoidance of smoking have the potential to save and extend more lives than any other public health activity. It is estimated that 400,000 Americans die prematurely every year because of cigarette smoking. A smoker has a one in three lifetime risk of dying of a cancer, cardiovascular, or pulmonary disease caused by cigarette smoking. Indeed, more human lives are lost owing to cardiovascular disease caused by smoking than from smoking-related cancer. The risk of tobacco smoke is not necessarily limited to the smoker. Epidemiologic studies suggest that environmental tobacco smoke may cause lung cancer and other pulmonary diseases in nonsmokers.

Nonsmoking persons should be encouraged not to start smoking, and persons who smoke should be encouraged to stop. In one sense, tobacco-related disease is a pediatric issue. Surveys show that over 80 percent of American smokers begin smoking before the age of 18. Indeed, nearly 20 percent of Americans aged 12 to 18 have smoked a cigarette in the past month. Counseling of adolescents and young adults is critical to prevention of smoking. Studies show that a physician's simple advice to not start smoking or to quit smoking can be of benefit.

Current approaches to smoking cessation recognize that smoking is an addiction (see Chap. 389). The smoker who is quitting goes through a process with identifiable stages that include contemplation of quitting, an action phase in which the smoker quits, and a maintenance phase. Smokers who quit completely are more likely to be successful than those who gradually reduce the number of cigarettes smoked or change to cigarettes lower in tar or nicotine. More than 90 percent of the Americans who have successfully quit smoking did so on their own without participation in an organized cessation program, but cessation programs are helpful for some smokers. The Community Intervention Trial for Smoking Cessation (COMMIT) was a community-based 4-year program sponsored by the National Cancer Institute and completed in 1994. One community of each of 11 matched community pairs was randomly assigned to intervention. The intervention included public education through the media and community-wide events, health care providers, worksites and other organizations, and cessation resources. COMMIT demonstrated that light smokers can benefit from simple cessation messages and cessation programs. The quit rate (fraction of the cohorts followed who achieved and maintained cessation at the end of the trial) was 30.6 percent in the intervention communities and 27.5 percent in the control communities. This finding is statistically significant, but it also shows that there was a trend toward a decrease in smoking even in the control communities. The COMMIT interventions were not successful for heavy smokers (>25 cigarettes per day). Experts believe heavy smokers generally need an intensive, broad-based cessation program that includes counseling, behavioral strategies, and pharmacologic adjuncts such as nicotine gum and nicotine patches.

Smokeless tobacco is the fastest growing part of the tobacco industry and represents a significant health risk. Chewing tobacco is a carcinogen linked to dental caries, gingivitis, oral leukoplakia, and oral cancer. The systemic effects of smokeless tobacco may increase risks for other cancers. Nitrosamines found in smokeless tobacco cause lung cancer in laboratory animals.

Diet Modification Dietary modification may have significant potential for lowering cancer risk in Western culture. Studies of international dietary patterns and animal studies suggest that diets high in fat increase the risk for cancers of the breast, colon, prostate, and endometrium. These cancers have their highest incidence and mortalities in Western countries, where fat makes up an average of 40 to 45 percent of the total calories consumed. In populations at low risk for these cancers, fat accounts for less than 20 percent of dietary calories.

Nonetheless, dietary fat has not been accepted by all as important in the etiology of cancers. Case-control and cohort epidemiologic studies give conflicting results. Some have argued that the relatively homogeneous fat intake levels in many of these studies could mask an effect. In addition, diet involves a complex exposure to many nutrients and chemicals. The protection against cancer apparently afforded by low-fat diets may in part reflect exposure to anticarcinogens found in vegetables, fruits, legumes, nuts, and grains. Substances found in these foods that may be protective include phenols, sulfur-containing compounds, flavones, and fiber.

Dietary fiber appears to afford protection against colonic polyps and invasive cancer of the colon. The mechanisms involved are complex and speculative. They include binding of oxidized bile acids, a decrease in bowel transit time, and generation of soluble fiber products, such as butyrate, that may have differentiating properties. The fiber in high-fiber diets may also protect against breast and prostate cancer by absorbing and inactivating dietary compounds that serve as cancer promoters through estrogenic and androgenic activity.

A simple way for an individual to decrease dietary fat and increase dietary fiber is to consume at least five to nine servings of fruits and vegetables per day. Although the effects of such a diet have not been fully assessed, it is likely to decrease the risk of colon cancer and possibly lower the risk for cancers of the breast, endometrium, and prostate. Such a diet may also lower the risk of cardiac disease.

The U.S. National Institutes of Health (NIH) Women's Health Initiative, launched in 1994, is a long-term clinical trial enrolling more than 100,000 women aged 45 to 69. It studies the potential cancer-preventing effects of a low-fat diet and vitamin supplementation. It must be stressed that the scientific evidence does not currently establish the anticarcinogenic value of vitamin, mineral, or nutritional supplements in amounts greater than that provided by a good diet.

Sun Avoidance Epidemiologic studies suggest that nonmelanoma skin cancers (basal cell and squamous cell) are induced by cumulative exposure to ultraviolet radiation. Intermittent acute sun exposure and sun damage have also been linked to melanoma. Sunburns, especially in childhood and adolescence, are associated with an increased risk of melanoma in adulthood. Reduction of sun exposure through use of protective clothing and changes in the pattern of outdoor activities has been advocated as a way of reducing skin cancer risk. Sunscreens may provide some protection, but how much has not been established.

Educational interventions to help persons accurately assess their risk of developing skin cancer have some impact. Self-examination for skin pigment characteristics associated with melanoma, such as freckling, may be useful in helping high-risk individuals identify themselves. Persons who recognize themselves as being at risk tend to comply better with sun-avoidance recommendations. Possible risk factors for melanoma include a propensity to sunburn, a large number of benign melanocytic nevi, and atypical nevi.

CANCER CHEMOPREVENTION Chemoprevention of cancer is a relatively new concept. It involves the use of specific natural or synthetic chemical agents to reverse, suppress, or prevent carcinogenesis before the development of invasive malignancy. While the concept that pharmacologic agents can prevent a cancer is relatively new, the idea that a compound can prevent chronic disease is not. Clinicians routinely prevent heart disease, kidney disease, and stroke by treating hypertension with pharmacologic agents. Lipid-lowering drugs are used to prevent coronary artery disease.

Improved understanding of the biology of cancer makes chemoprevention a real possibility. Cancer develops through an accumulation of genetic changes, which are potential points of intervention for preventing cancer. The initial genetic changes are termed *initiation*. Alterations of this type can be inherited or can be acquired through the action of physical, viral, or chemical carcinogens. Like most human diseases, cancer arises through an interaction between genetics and environmental exposures (Table 82-1). Influences that cause the initiated cell to progress through the carcinogenic process and to change phenotypically are termed *promoters*. Examples of promoters are hormones such as androgens, linked to prostate cancer, and estrogen, linked to breast and endometrial cancer. The distinction between an initiator and a promoter is sometimes arbitrary; some components of cigarette smoke are so-called complete carcinogens, acting as both initiators and promoters. Cancer can be prevented or controlled through interference with the factors that cause initiation, promotion, or progression. Compounds of interest in chemoprevention often have antimutagenic, antioxidant, or antiproliferative activity.

Cancer chemoprevention is not yet established in clinical practice, although it has attracted great interest. Before a chemoprevention strategy can become standard practice, evidence of benefit must be gathered from clinical trials. These trials are usually large, long-term, randomized, placebo-controlled, and double-blinded. They often allow for the study of drugs for prevention of multiple cancers and the study of end-points other than cancer, such as other chronic diseases. Several large clinical trials have been completed, and a number will be continuing into the twenty-first century.

Multiple Cancer Site Prevention Trials The Physicians' Health Trial is a study that began in 1982. It involves 22,071 American male physicians. Participants were randomly assigned to receive β-carotene, aspirin, and/or placebo in a 2×2 factorial design and followed. All major medical events were recorded. In 1988, the aspirin arm was unblinded after the trial demonstrated that aspirin therapy causes a significant reduction in cardiovascular mortality. The β-carotene arm of the study will continue until 1998, when an analysis for cancer end-points is planned.

The Women's Health Study, launched in 1992, is an 8-year trial involving 44,000 female nurses. Subjects are randomly assigned to β-carotene, alpha tocopherol, aspirin, and/or placebo in a factorial design yielding eight different treatment groups. The end-points being studied are total epithelial cancers, breast cancer, lung cancer, colon cancer, and vascular disease.

The Women's Health Initiative, described earlier, uses a partial factorial design that places women in 22 intervention groups. Participants can receive calcium and vitamin D supplementation, hormone replacement therapy, and counseling to increase exercise and cease smoking. This study promises to render findings about prevention of a number of cancers, cardiovascular disease, osteoporosis, and other diseases.

Prevention of Hormonally Driven Cancers Hormonal manipulation is being tested in the primary prevention of breast and prostate cancer. Tamoxifen is an antiestrogen that has partial estrogen agonistic activity in some tissues, such as endometrium and bone. One of its actions is to up-regulate transforming growth factor β, which decreases breast cell proliferation. In randomized placebo-controlled trials to assess tamoxifen as an adjuvant in breast cancer treatment, this drug reduced the number of new breast cancers in the uninvolved breast by more than a third. The primary prevention capabilities of tamoxifen are being tested further in a decade-long trial involving 16,000 women at high risk of developing breast cancer.

Finasteride is a 5α-reductase inhibitor. It inhibits the conversion of testosterone to dihydrotestosterone, which is a more potent stimulator of prostate cell proliferation than testosterone. In an F344 rat model of carcinogen-induced prostate cancer, finasteride has been shown to decrease the incidence of cancers. Finasteride is being tested as a preventive agent for prostate cancer in a 10-year study involving 18,000 men age 55 and older.

Chemoprevention of Cancers of the Upper Aerodigestive Tract Smoking causes diffuse epithelial injury in the head, neck, esophagus, and lung. Patients cured of squamous cell cancers of the lung, esophagus, head, and neck are at high risk of developing a second malignancy (a risk as high as 5 percent per year of a second cancer of the upper aerodigestive tract). Cessation of cigarette smoking does not markedly decrease the cured cancer patient's risk of second malignancy, even though it does lower the cancer risk in those who have never developed a malignancy. Smoking cessation may halt the early stages of the carcinogenic process (such as metaplasia), but it may have no effect on late

stages of carcinogenesis. This "field carcinogenesis" hypothesis for cancer of the upper aerodigestive tract has made "cured" patients an important population for chemoprevention of second malignancies. A randomized, placebo-controlled clinical trial has demonstrated that adjuvant isoretinoin (13 *cis*-retinoic acid) can reduce the incidence of second primary tumors in patients treated with local therapy for head and neck cancer.

Oral leukoplakia, a premalignant lesion commonly found in smokers, has been used as an intermediate marker allowing the demonstration of chemopreventive activity in smaller, shorter-duration, randomized, placebo-controlled trials. Response was associated with up-regulation of retinoic acid receptor β. Therapy with isoretinoin causes regression of oral leukoplakia. However, the lesions recur when the agent is withdrawn, suggesting the need for chronic administration of retinoids. Premalignant lesions in the oropharyngeal area have also responded to β-carotene, retinol, alpha tocopherol (vitamin E), and selenium. Further study to better define the activity of these drugs is ongoing. The ability of isoretinoin to prevent second malignancies in patients cured of low-stage non–small cell lung cancer is also being assessed.

Several large-scale trials have been launched to assess agents in the chemoprevention of lung cancer in patients at high risk. In the Alpha-Tocopherol/Beta-Carotene (ATBC) Lung Cancer Prevention Trial, participants were male smokers, aged 50 to 69 at entry. At entry, participants had smoked an average of one pack of cigarettes per day for 35.9 years. Participants received alpha tocopherol, β-carotene, and/or placebo in a randomized, 2×2 factorial design. Surprisingly, after a median follow-up of 6.1 years, there was a statistically significant *increase* in lung cancer incidence and mortality in those receiving β-carotene. Alpha tocopherol had no significant impact on lung cancer mortality, and there was no evidence of interaction between the two drugs. Patients receiving alpha tocopherol had a higher incidence of hemorrhagic stroke. The Beta-Carotene and Retinol Efficacy Trial (CARET) involved 17,000 American smokers and workers with asbestos exposure. Entrants were randomly assigned to one of four arms and received β-carotene, retinol, and/or placebo in a 2×2 factorial

Table 82-1

Carcinogens and Associated Cancers or Neoplasms

Carcinogens*	Associated Cancer or Neoplasm
Alkylating agents	Acute myelocytic leukemia, bladder cancer
Androgens	Prostate cancer
Aromatic amines (dyes)	Bladder cancer
Arsenic	Cancer of the lung, skin
Asbestos	Cancer of the lung, pleura, peritoneum
Benzene	Acute myelocytic leukemia
Chromium	Lung cancer
Diethylstilbestrol (Prenatal)	Vaginal cancer (clear cell)
Epstein-Barr virus	Burkitt's lymphoma, nasal T-cell lymphoma
Estrogens	Cancer of the endometrium, liver
Ethyl alcohol	Cancer of the liver, esophagus, head and neck
Helicobacter pylori	Gastric cancer
Hepatitis B or C virus	Liver cancer
Human immunodeficiency virus	Non-Hodgkin's lymphoma, Kaposi's sarcoma, squamous cell carcinoma
Human T-cell lymphotropic virus type I (HTLV-I)	Adult T-cell leukemia/lymphoma
Immunosuppressive agents (azathioprine, cyclosporine, corticosteriods)	Non-Hodgkin's lymphoma
Nitrogen mustard gas	Cancer of the lung, head and neck, nasal sinuses
Nickel dust	Cancer of the lung, nasal sinuses
Phenacetin	Cancer of the renal pelvis and bladder
Polycyclic hydrocarbons	Cancer of the lung, skin (especially squamous cell carcinoma of scrotal skin)
Schistosomiasis	Bladder cancer (squamous cell)
Sunlight (ultraviolet)	Skin cancer (squamous cell and melanoma)
Tobacco (including smokeless)	Cancer of the upper aerodigestive tract, bladder
Vinyl chloride	Liver cancer (angiosarcoma)

* Agents that are thought to act as cancer initiators and/or promoters.

design. This trial demonstrated a lung cancer rate of 5 per 1000 subjects per year for those taking placebo and of 6 per 1000 subjects per year for those taking β-carotene.

These ATBC and CARET results demonstrate the importance of testing chemoprevention hypotheses before implementing them widely, because the results stand in contrast to a number of observational epidemiologic studies. In the ATBC, participants taking alpha tocopherol had a one-third reduction in the incidence of prostate cancer, compared to those not taking alpha tocopherol. Investigation of this surprising trial result continues.

Chemoprevention of Colon Cancer Many of the current colon cancer prevention trials are based on the premise that most colorectal cancers develop from adenomatous polyps. These trials use adenoma recurrence or disappearance as a surrogate end-point to assess colon cancer prevention. Early clinical trial results suggest that nonsteroidal antiinflammatory drugs (NSAIDs), such as piroxicam, sulindac, and aspirin, may prevent adenoma formation or cause regression of adenomatous polyps. The mechanism of the antiproliferative action of NSAIDs is unknown, but they are presumed to work through the cyclooxygenase pathway. In the Physicians' Health Trial, described above, aspirin had no effect on colon cancer incidence, although the 6-year assessment period was not long enough to definitively evaluate this end-point.

Epidemiologic studies suggest that diets high in calcium lower colon cancer risk. Calcium binds bile and fatty acids, which cause hyperproliferation of colonic epithelium. It is hypothesized that this effect reduces intraluminal exposure to these compounds. Cancer chemoprevention trials using calcium-containing compounds and NSAIDs are under way.

Vaccines and Cancer Prevention A number of infectious agents have been linked to the development of cancer, leading to interest in development of vaccines to protect against these agents. The hepatitis B vaccine is quite effective in preventing hepatitis and, presumably, also hepatomas due to chronic hepatitis B infection. Public health officials are encouraging widespread administration of this vaccine, especially in Asia, where the disease is epidemic. In the future, human papilloma virus vaccines could be developed to prevent cervical cancer, and *Helicobacter pylori* vaccines may be developed to prevent gastric cancer.

CANCER SCREENING Screening is best defined as a means of detecting disease early, in asymptomatic individuals, with the goal of decreasing morbidity and mortality. Screening for cancer is intuitively appealing and has attracted great public interest as technology has generated a number of diagnostic tests and procedures that are safe, quick, and inexpensive. While screening can potentially save lives, and has been shown clearly to do so in the case of breast, cervical, and colon cancer, it is also subject to a number of biases, which can suggest a benefit when actually there is none, or even mask a net harm. Early detection does not in itself confer benefit. To be of value, screening must detect disease earlier, and treatment of earlier disease must yield a better outcome than treatment at the onset of symptoms.

Because screening is done on asymptomatic, healthy persons, it should offer substantial likelihood of benefit. A critical approach to screening is necessary to ensure that this condition is met. Screening tests and their appropriate use should be carefully evaluated before their use is widely encouraged in screening programs as a matter of public policy.

Generally, screening examinations, tests, or procedures are not diagnostic of cancer but instead indicate that a cancer may be present. The diagnosis is then made following a workup that generally includes a biopsy and pathologic confirmation.

A number of genes have been identified as predisposing the bearer to a disease, and many more will be identified in the near future. Testing for these genes can define a high-risk population. The ability to predict the development of a particular cancer may some day present therapeutic options as well as ethical dilemmas. It may eventually allow for early intervention to prevent a cancer or limit its severity. People at high risk will be ideal candidates for chemoprevention and screening; however, the efficacy of these interventions in the high-risk population should be investigated. Currently, persons at high risk for a particular cancer can engage in intensive screening. While this course is clinically prudent, it is not known if it saves lives in these populations.

The Accuracy of Screening Four indices are used to describe the accuracy, or ability to discriminate disease, of a screening test: sensitivity, specificity, positive predictive value, and negative predictive value (Table 82-2). *Sensitivity* is the proportion of people with the disease who test positive in the screen (i.e., the ability of the test to detect disease when it is present). *Specificity* is the proportion of people who do not have the disease and test negative in the screening test (i.e., the ability of a test to tell that the disease is not present). The *positive predictive value* is the proportion of persons who test positive and have the disease. Similarly, *negative predictive value* is the proportion who test negative and do not have the disease. The sensitivity and specificity of a test are relatively independent of the underlying prevalence (or risk) of the disease in the population screened, but the predictive values depend strongly on the prevalence of the disease (Table 82-3).

Table 82-2

Definition of Terms

Term	Definition
Sensitivity	The proportion of persons with the condition who test positive: $a/(a + c)$
Specificity	The proportion of persons without the condition who test negative: $d/(b + d)$
Positive predictive value	The proportion of persons with a positive test who have the condition: $a/(a + b)$
Negative predictive value	The proportion of persons with a negative test who do not have the condition: $d/(c + d)$

		Condition present	Condition absent
a = true positive			
b = false positive	Positive test	a	b
c = false negative			
d = true negative	Negative test	c	d

Table 82-3

Predictive Value Relationships*

Positive predictive value (PPV) is a function of sensitivity, specificity, and prevalence:

$$PPV = \frac{Prevalence \times Sensitivity}{(Prevalence \times Sensitivity) + (1 - Prevalence)(1 - Specificity)}$$

PPV values for a prevalence of 5 per 1000:

	PPV for a Sensitivity of	
Specificity	0.8	0.95
0.95	7%	9%
0.999	80%	83%

PPV values for a prevalence of 1 per 10,000:

	PPV for a Sensitivity of	
Specificity	0.8	0.95
0.95	0.2%	0.2%
0.999	7%	9%

* The positive predictive value is expressed as a percentage. It is influenced by the sensitivity and specificity of the screening test and the prevalence of the disease being screened for. As shown here, for relatively uncommon diseases, such as cancer, the positive predictive value is influenced particularly strongly by the specificity of the screening test at a given prevalence.

Screening is most beneficial, efficient, and economical when the target disease is common in the population being screened. To be valuable, the screening test should have a high specificity; sensitivity need not be very high, as demonstrated in Table 82-3.

Potential Biases of Screening Tests The common biases of screening are lead-time, length, and selection biases. These biases can make a screening test seem beneficial when actually it is not (or even causes net harm). Whether beneficial or not, screening can create the false impression of an epidemic by increasing the number of cancers diagnosed. It can also give the appearance of a shift in stage, thus improving survival statistics without reducing mortality (i.e., the number of deaths from a given cancer relative to the number of people at risk for the cancer). In such a case, the *apparent* duration of survival increases without lives being saved or life expectancy changing.

Lead-time bias occurs when a test does not lead to any change in the natural history of the disease; the patient is merely diagnosed at an earlier date. When lead time bias occurs, survival *appears* increased, but life is not really prolonged. The screening test only prolongs the time the subject is aware of the disease, which for cancer is not a benefit.

Length bias occurs when slow-growing, less aggressive, cancers are detected during screening. Cancers diagnosed owing to the onset of symptoms between scheduled screenings are on average more aggressive, and treatment outcomes are not as favorable. An extreme form of length bias is termed *overdiagnosis*, the detection of "pseudo-disease." The reservoir of some undetected slow-growing tumors is large. Many of these tumors fulfill the histologic criteria of cancer but will never become clinically significant or cause death. This problem is compounded by the fact that the most common cancers appear most frequently at ages when competing causes of death are more frequent.

Selection bias must be considered in assessing the results of any screening effort. The population most likely to seek screening may differ from the general population to which the screening test might be applied. The individuals screened may have volunteered because of a particular risk factor not found in the general population, such as a strong family history. In general, volunteers for studies may be more health conscious, and thus likely to have a better prognosis or lower mortality rate irrespective of the screening result. This is termed the "healthy volunteer effect."

Potential Drawbacks of Screening There are often risks associated with screening, including the risks of harm caused by the screening intervention itself, harm due to the further investigation of persons with positive test results (both true and false), and harm incident on the treatment of persons with a true-positive result, even if life is extended by treatment. The diagnosis and treatment of cancers that would never have caused medical problems can lead to the harm of unnecessary treatment and give patients the anxiety of a cancer diagnosis. The psychosocial impact of cancer screening, for persons with both positive and negative results, can also be substantial when applied to the entire population.

Assessment of Screening Tests Good clinical trial design can offset some biases of screening and demonstrate the relative risks and benefits of a screening test. A randomized, controlled screening trial with cause-specific mortality as the end-point provides the strongest support for a screening intervention. In a randomized trial, two like populations are randomly established. One is given the medical standard of care (which may be no screening at all), and the other receives the screening intervention being assessed. The two populations are compared over time. The efficacy of the test for the population studied is established when the group receiving the screening test has a better cause-specific mortality rate than the control group. Studies showing a reduction in the incidence of advanced-stage disease, an improved survival, or a stage shift are weaker evidence of benefit. These latter criteria are necessary but not sufficient to establish the value of a screening test.

Although a randomized, controlled screening trial provides the strongest evidence to support the usefulness of a screening test, it is not perfect. Unless the trial is population-based, it does not remove the issue of generalizability to the target population. Screening trials generally involve thousands of persons and last for years. Less defini-

tive study designs are therefore often used to estimate the effectiveness of screening practices. After a randomized controlled clinical trial, in descending order of strength, evidence may be derived from:

- The findings of internally controlled trials using intervention allocation methods other than randomization (e.g. allocation determined by birth date, date of clinic visit, etc.);
- The findings of cohort or case-control analytic observational studies;
- The results of multiple time series studies with or without the intervention;
- The opinions of respected authorities based on clinical experience, descriptive studies, or consensus reports of experts

The last of these forms of evidence is the weakest, because even experts can be misled by the biases described above.

Screening for Specific Cancers Studies have shown that widespread screening for breast, cervical, and colon cancer is beneficial for certain age groups. Special surveillance of those at high risk for a specific cancer because of a family history or a genetic risk factor may be prudent, but few studies have been carried out to assess the impact of this practice on mortality in specific high-risk populations. A number of organizations have considered whether or not to endorse routine use of certain screening tests. Because these groups have not used the same criteria to judge whether a screening test should be endorsed, they have arrived at different recommendations. The screening guidelines of the U.S. Preventive Services Task Force and those of the American Cancer Society are often quoted and show a range of recommendations (Table 82-4).

Breast cancer Breast self-examination, clinical breast examination by a care giver, and mammography have been advocated as useful screening tools. Only screening mammography alone and screening mammography with clinical exam have been evaluated in randomized controlled trials. In addition, there is an ongoing Canadian trial evaluating clinical breast exam with or without mammography in women aged 50 to 65, but final results have not yet been reported. A number of well-designed trials have demonstrated that annual or biennial screening with mammography or mammography plus clinical breast examination in women over the age of 50 saves lives. In these trials, the breast cancer mortality rate is decreased by about a third. These trials do not have enough statistical power to indicate definitively whether such screening is useful in normal-risk women younger than 50. Experts therefore disagree on whether average-risk women aged 40 to 49 should receive regular screening (see Table 82-4). An analysis of eight large randomized trials showed no benefit from mammographic screening for women aged 40 to 49 who were assessed 5 to 7 years after trial entry. However there may be a small benefit for women in these trials 10 to 12 years after study entry. What proportion of this possible benefit would be due to screening after these women turned 50 is not known but is an active area of study. While no study has shown breast self-examination to decrease mortality, it is recommended as prudent by many organizations.

Cervical cancer Cohort and case-control studies have shown that screening with Papanicolaou smears decreases cervical cancer mortality. The cervical cancer mortality rate has fallen significantly since the widespread use of the Pap smear, although this trend actually began earlier. Most screening guidelines recommend regular Pap testing for all women who are or have been sexually active or have reached the age of 18. With the onset of sexual activity comes the risk of sexual transmission of human papilloma virus, the most common etiologic factor for cervical cancer. The recommended interval for Pap screening varies from one to three years. It is not known whether there is an upper age limit at which screening ceases to be effective.

Colorectal cancer Fecal occult blood testing, rigid and flexible sigmoidoscopy, radiographic barium contrast studies, and colonoscopy have been considered for colorectal cancer screening. One randomized study indicates that annual fecal occult blood testing using hydrated specimens could reduce colorectal cancer mortality by a third. The sensitivity for fecal occult blood is increased if specimens are rehydrated before testing, but at the cost of lower specificity. The false-positive rate for rehydrated fecal occult blood testing is high; 1 to 5 percent of persons tested have a positive result. Approximately 10 percent of those with occult blood in the stool have cancer, and 20 to 30 percent have adenomas.

Two case-control studies suggest that regular screening of people over 50 with sigmoidoscopy decreases mortality. A quarter to a third of polyps can be discovered with the rigid sigmoidoscope; approximately half are found with a 35-cm flexible scope, and two-thirds to three-quarters are found with a 60-cm scope. Diagnosis of polyposis by sigmoidoscopy should lead to evaluation of the entire colon with colonoscopy and/or barium enema. The most efficient interval for screening sigmoidoscopy is unknown. Case-control studies suggest that testing at intervals of up to 9 years may confer benefit. Most authorities feel that full colonoscopy is too cumbersome and invasive for widespread use as a screening tool in standard-risk populations. It may be suitable for subjects at extremely high risk, however, such as members of families with a genetic predisposition to colorectal cancer. Likewise, barium contrast studies are often thought to be unsuitable for large-scale screening efforts.

Lung cancer Screening chest radiographs and sputum cytology have been evaluated as methods for lung cancer screening. No significant reduction in lung cancer mortality has been found in these studies, although all the controlled trials performed have had low statistical power. Even screening of high-risk subjects (smokers) has not been proved to be beneficial.

Ovarian cancer Adnexal palpation, transvaginal ultrasound, and serum CA-125 determination have been considered as methods for ovarian cancer screening. Adnexal palpation is considered by most to be far too insensitive to detect ovarian cancer at an early enough stage to substantially affect mortality. Neither transvaginal ultrasound nor CA-125 screening has been tested in a completed randomized prospective trial. Ovarian cancer screening can lead to an invasive diagnostic workup, which may include laparotomy. In a clinical study, 0.6 percent of 900 adult women had a serum CA-125 level greater than 35 U/ml. Thus, if 100,000 adult women were screened, 600 would be identified as having a high CA-125. The prevalence of ovarian cancer in the female adult population is approximately 20 per 100,000. Thus, the screening test would identify 600 women who would undergo further evaluation to identify 20 cases of ovarian cancer. Some of these 600

would only be inconvenienced by an ultrasound examination. Others would undergo an exploratory laparotomy. It should be noted that a large proportion of the 20 women identified as having ovarian cancer would have advanced, incurable disease and thus not benefit from screening. An NIH consensus conference in 1994 concluded that routine screening for ovarian cancer was not indicated for standard-risk women or for women with a single affected family member, but that it might be worthwhile in families with genetic ovarian cancer syndromes.

Prostate cancer The most common prostate cancer screening modalities are digital rectal examination and assays for serum prostate-specific antigen (PSA). Newer serum tests, such as measurement of the ratio of bound to free serum PSA, have yet to be fully evaluated. An emphasis on PSA screening has caused prostate cancer to become the most common nonskin cancer diagnosed in American males. Screening for this disease is very prone to lead time bias, length bias, and overdiagnosis, and there is substantial debate among experts as to whether it is effective. Some experts are concerned that prostate cancer screening, more than screening for other cancers, may cause net harm. Prostate cancer screening clearly detects many asymptomatic cancers, but the ability to distinguish tumors that are lethal but still curable from those that pose little or no threat to health is limited. Men over age 50 have a very high prevalence of indolent, clinically insignificant prostate cancers. No well-designed trial has been completed to test the true benefit of prostate cancer screening and treatment, but trials are in progress.

The effectiveness of radical prostatectomy, radiation therapy, and other treatments for low-stage prostate cancer is also under study in randomized trials. Definitive treatment of cancers detected by screening may cause morbidity for some men, such as impotence and urinary incontinence, and carries a low but finite risk of death. Pending the completion of ongoing randomized trials comparing usual care to prostate screening and comparing definitive therapy to "watchful waiting," organizations have provided conflicting recommendations on prostate cancer screening (Table 82-4). All agree, however, that a man should have a life expectancy of at least 10 years to be eligible for screening.

Skin cancer Visual examination of all skin surfaces by the patient or by a health care provider is used in screening for basal and squamous cell cancers and melanoma. No prospective randomized study has been performed to look for a mortality decrease. Observational epidemiologic evidence from Scotland and Australia suggest that screening programs have caused a stage shift in melanomas diagnosed. Screening may reinforce sun-avoidance and other skin cancer prevention behaviors.

Table 82-4

Screening Recommendations for Asymptomatic Subjects at Normal Risk*

Test or Procedure	USPSTF Recommendations	ACS Recommendations
Sigmoidoscopy	Over age 50: periodically Under age 50: not recommended	Ages 50 and over: every 3–5 years
Fecal occult blood testing	Ages 50 and over: every year	Ages 50 and over: every year
Digital rectal examination	No recommendation	Ages 40 and over: every year
Prostate-specific antigen determination	Recommended against	Men aged 50 and over: every year
Papanicolaou test	Women aged 18–65: every 1–3 years	Women over age 18: once yearly for 3 years; thereafter at physician's discretion
Pelvic examination	Not recommended; adnexal palpation should be performed during examination for other reasons	Women aged 18–40: every 1–3 years with Pap test; over age 40: every year
Endometrial tissue sampling	Not considered	At menopause if patient is obese or has a history of unopposed estrogen use
Breast self-examination	No recommendation	Women aged 20 and over: monthly
Clinical breast examination	Women over age 50: every year	Women aged 20–40: every 3 years; over age 40: yearly
Mammography	Women aged 50–75: every 1–2 years	Women aged 40–49: every 1–2 years; ages 50 and over: every year
Complete skin examination	Not recommended	Ages 20–39: every 3 years

* The above is a summary of the screening procedures recommended for the general population by the U.S. Preventive Services Task Force (USPSTF) and the American Cancer Society (ACS). These recommendations refer to asymptomatic persons who have no risk factors other than age or gender for the targeted condition.

BLOCK G et al: Fruit, vegetables, and cancer prevention: A review of the epidemiological evidence. Nutr Cancer 18:1, 1992

DOLL R, PETO R: The cause of cancer: Quantitative estimates of avoidable risks of cancer in the United States today. J Natl Cancer Inst 66:1191, 1981

FLETCHER SW et al: Report of the International Workshop on Screening for Breast Cancer. J Natl Cancer Inst 85:1644, 1993

GREENWALD P et al: Chemoprevention. CA Cancer J Clin 45:31, 1995

——— et al: *Cancer Prevention and Control.* New York, Marcel Dekker, 1995

LIPPMAN SM et al: Cancer chemoprevention. J Clin Oncol 12:851, 1994

SOX HC: Preventive health services in adults. N Engl J Med 330:1589, 1995

THE ALPHA-TOCOPHEROL, BETA CAROTENE CANCER PREVENTION STUDY GROUP: The effect of vitamin E and beta carotene on the incidence of lung cancer and other cancers in male smokers. N Engl J Med 330:1029, 1994

THE COMMIT RESEARCH GROUP: Community intervention trial for smoking cessation (COMMIT): I. Cohort results from a four-year community intervention. Am J Public Health 85:183, 1995

———: Community intervention trial for smoking cessation (COMMIT): II. Changes in adult cigarette smoking prevalence. Am J Public Health 85:193, 1995

U.S. PREVENTIVE SERVICES TASK FORCE: *Guide to Clinical Preventive Services,* 2nd ed: Washington D.C., Government Printing Office, 1996

WOOLF SH: Screening for prostate cancer with prostate-specific antigen. N Engl J Med 333:1401, 1995

83   *Robert G. Fenton, Dan L. Longo*

CELL BIOLOGY OF CANCER

Two characteristic features define a cancer: cell growth not regulated by external signals (i.e., autonomous) and the capacity to invade tissues and metastasize to and colonize distant sites (see Chap. 85). The first of these features, the uncontrolled growth of abnormal cells, is a property of all neoplasms, or new growths. A neoplasm may be benign or malignant. If invasion, the second cardinal feature of cancer, is present, the neoplasm is malignant. Cancer is a synonym for *malignant neoplasm.* Cancers of epithelial tissues are called *carcinomas*; cancers of nonepithelial (mesenchymal) tissues are called *sarcomas.*

Cancer is a genetic disease, but the level of its expression is the single cell. Although some forms of cancer are heritable, most mutations occur in somatic cells and are caused by intrinsic errors in DNA replication or are induced by carcinogen exposure. A single genetic lesion is usually not sufficient to induce neoplastic transformation of a cell. The malignant phenotype is acquired only after several (5 to 10) mutations (usually developing over many years) lead to derangements in a variety of gene products. Each genetic alteration may cause phenotypic changes typified by the progression in epithelial tissues from hyperplasia to adenoma to dysplasia to carcinoma in situ to invasive carcinoma. Resistance to neoplastic transformation is due to levels of control at every phase of cell function. Abnormalities in the function of one protein may be compensated by other proteins and pathways. An analogy can be drawn between the complex behavior of interacting signaling cascades and computer-based neural networks that can be adapted or trained to recognize patterns of complex inputs and respond to each pattern with a specific pattern of output.

The more than 200 discrete cell types in the body are not equally susceptible to developing cancer. Some cells, such as cardiac myocytes, sensory receptor cells for light and sound, and lens fibers, persist throughout life without dividing or being replaced. Neoplasia in such tissues is exceedingly rare. Most differentiated tissues undergo turnover characterized by cell death and replacement. When natural turnover rates are slow, fully differentiated cells may be induced to proliferate and produce fully differentiated daughter cells. For example, hepatocytes are capable of dividing to replace senescent, damaged, or surgically removed liver tissue.

In tissues with rapid turnover, such as skin, bone marrow, and gut, the differentiated function and the replacement function are carried out by different cell types. Under normal circumstances, an individual cell is on one of two largely mutually exclusive paths: division or differentiation. Cells capable of dividing are undifferentiated (stem cells), whereas terminally differentiated cells are unable to divide. Stem cells produce daughter cells that can either become new stem cells (thus replenishing the stem cell compartment) or undergo terminal differentiation, depending on the circumstances and the environmental signals. Stem cells are distinguished from differentiating cells by different patterns of gene expression. Gene expression is the product of the tissue-specific programming of gene expression interacting with environmental factors such as cell-to-cell contact; interactions with extracellular matrix; endocrine hormones; paracrine growth and differentiation factors; and stresses such as heat, oxidation, irradiation, and physical distortion or traction.

Cancer is most common in tissues with rapid turnover, especially those exposed to environmental carcinogens and whose proliferation is regulated by hormones. The most common genetic changes involve the activation of proto-oncogenes or the inactivation of tumor suppressor genes (see Chap. 84). Although genetic damage is nearly universal in human cancer, cells with neoplastic features can be generated in vitro without genetic damage. Removal and in vitro culture of cells from the epiblast of a murine embryo lead to the uncontrolled proliferation of the cells and the generation of a teratocarcinoma cell line capable of producing tumors when inoculated into animals. The removal of these normal embryonic cells from their normal environment leads to uncontrolled growth. However, if the teratocarcinoma cells are reinjected into an early embryo, under the inductive influence of their normal neighbors they can differentiate into normal organs and tissues appropriate for the location where they are injected.

Thus, environmental factors exert potent effects on the gene expression of target cells. The panoply of signals received by a particular cell leads to the activation of particular sets of transcription factors. The pattern of expression of transcription factors determines whether a cell will divide, differentiate, or die.

PRINCIPLES OF CELL CYCLE REGULATION

The mechanism of cell division is substantially the same in all dividing cells and has been conserved throughout evolution. The process assures that the cell accurately duplicates its contents, especially its chromosomes. The cell cycle is divided into four phases. During M phase, the replicated chromosomes are separated and packaged into two new nuclei by mitosis and the cytoplasm is divided between the two daughter cells by cytokinesis. The other three phases of the cell cycle are called *interphase*: G1 (gap 1), a period of growth during which the cell determines its readiness to commit to DNA synthesis; S (DNA synthesis), during which the genetic material is replicated and no re-replication is permitted; and G2 (gap 2), during which the fidelity of DNA replication is determined and errors are corrected.

During S phase, DNA synthesis begins with the unfolding of chromatin from the DNA and the addition of DNA helicase and single-strand binding proteins that help open the double helix. Replication origins are spaced roughly 100,000 nucleotide pairs apart throughout the genome. DNA polymerase and DNA primase attach to these sites and catalyze the polymerization of the DNA at a rate of about 50 nucleotides per second. Topoisomerases break and reseal DNA strands to prevent tangling. Although this system for replication is efficient and accurate, occasional mistakes are made, and these mistakes in the replicated sequences are repaired by a variety of mechanisms. In some cancers, the mismatch repair mechanisms are defective and errors are routinely passed along to daughter cells, increasing the development of new mutations. Once a DNA segment is replicated and the replication units reassembled, chromatin binds to the nascent DNA chain, assuring that each region is replicated only once. DNA polymerase is unable to replicate the end of a DNA chain completely. This problem has been solved by the addition of tandem repeats of a six-nucleotide sequence (GGGTTA) to the ends of each chromosome. These repeated sequences are called *telomeres* and are replicated through an RNA-dependent DNA polymerase called *telomerase*. Normal somatic cells do not express telomerase, presumably because they do not replicate or have a finite replication ability. Germ cells do express telomerase. The expression of telomerase in cancer cells is thought to be a component of the neoplastic process, assuring that the cell will be able to undergo many divisions without losing the information encoded near the ends of its chromosomes. Inhibition of telomerase activity in cancer cells could have antitumor effects.

The transitions between G1 and S and between G2 and M are tightly regulated to minimize errors in the replication process. Checkpoints in G1 and G2 that determine whether to enter S and M are regulated by protein kinases (cyclin-dependent kinases, or cdk) and kinase-associated proteins called *cyclins*. The enzymatic activity of the cdk is determined by their association with a cyclin and their phosphorylation state. There are at least seven cdk family members, each of which associates with a distinct cyclin molecule. The resulting complexes have characteristic substrate specificities, and are expressed in different phases of the cycle. Cyclin expression varies with the cell cycle, and the synthesis of these complexes is transcriptionally regulated and their degradation is mediated by ubiquitin-conjugation and destruction in proteasomes.

The cyclin B/cdc2 complex (also called *mitosis promoting factor*, or MPF) is the primary regulator of transition from G2 to M phase. It is activated by a cdk activating kinase (CAK) and a phosphatase (cdc25) that removes inhibitory phosphates. Some of the substrates of cyclinB/cdc2 are defined; its phosphorylation of histone H1, nuclear lamins, and microtubule-associated proteins facilitates chromosome condensation, nuclear membrane breakdown, and spindle formation, respectively.

The checkpoint regulating transition from G1 to S is frequently disrupted in cancer. The mechanism of the regulation is complex. Two cyclin/cdk complexes, cyclin D/cdk4 or -6 and cyclin E/cdk2, phosphorylate the retinoblastoma gene product, Rb, on 10 different sites and alter the ability of Rb to associate with cellular proteins. One such protein is E2F, a transcription factor that heterodimerizes with other transcription factors, such as DP1, and activates several genes required for S progression, including dihydrofolate reductase, thymidine kinase, DNA polymerase α, c-*myc*, c-*myb*, and cdc2 (Fig. 83-1). In addition to its role in promoting growth, Rb promotes differentiation through its association with transcription factors such as MyoD and activated transcription factor (ATF)/cyclic AMP response element binding (CREB) protein family members. Rb is the target of a number of transforming viruses including SV40 large T antigen, adenovirus E1A, and human papilloma virus E7.

The activity of cdk is also regulated by cdk inhibitors (cdki). These low-molecular-weight proteins either inhibit cdk activity broadly (p21$^{Cip1/Waf1}$, p27^{Kip1}, p57^{Kip2}) or selectively inhibit cyclin D/cdk4 or -6 complexes (p16^{INK4a}, p15^{INK4b}, p18). The first member of this family to be identified was p21, which inhibits both cdk and proliferating cell nuclear antigen (PCNA), a subunit of DNA polymerase δ. p21 is induced by DNA damage through transcriptional activation by p53 (see below) and inhibits cell cycle progression at several points, including G1 and S phases, and permits DNA repair to take place. If DNA damage is too great, a cell suicide pathway is induced to eliminate cells that may be dysfunctional (see below).

Cdki can be induced by growth inhibitors such as transforming growth factor (TGF) β and can be inhibited by positive growth factors such as interleukin (IL) 2. Genetic alterations in cdki, especially p16 and p15, occur with high frequency in certain tumors. Alterations at the p16 locus on chromosome 9p21 have been detected in 75 percent of pancreatic cancers; 40 to 70 percent of glioblastomas; 50 percent of esophageal cancers; and about 20 percent of non-small cell lung cancers, soft tissue sarcomas, and bladder cancers. Mutations in cdki often accompany cyclin D1 overexpression with the t(11;14) translocation in mantle cell lymphoma. Some tumors fail to express cdki because

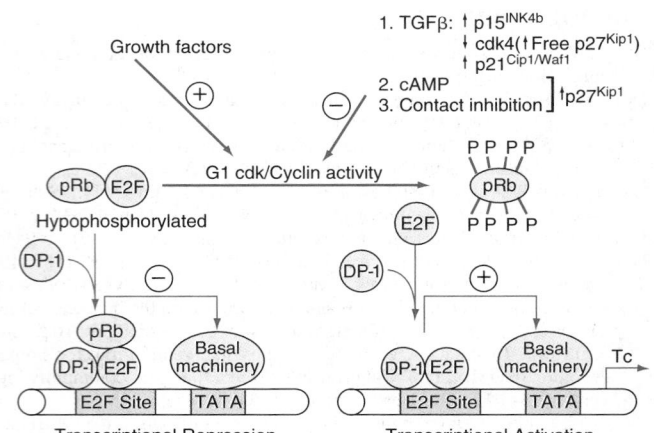

FIGURE 83-1 The retinoblastoma gene product, pRb, regulates cell cycle progression at the restriction point by sequestering the E2F transcription factor. Hypophosphorylated pRb forms an inactive complex with E2F preventing its association with DP-1, or by repressing the interaction of E2F/DP-1 with the basal transcription machinery. The kinase activities of *cdk*4/cyclin D and *cdk*2/cyclin E convert pRb to the hyperphosphorylated state with loss of binding pocket activity. G1 cdk activity is positively regulated by growth factors and inhibited by a variety of physiologic signals from the cell microenvironment. E2F is released and forms transcriptionally active complexes with DP-1, which initiate transcription from promoters containing E2F binding sites. Many of these genes are necessary for S phase progression.

the genes are methylated, an epigenetic mechanism for blocking transcription. Table 83-1 summarizes some of the changes in cell cycle regulators detected in human cancers.

Whereas Rb, cyclin D, cdk4, and p16 are commonly altered in cancer, E2F overexpression or p21 mutations have not yet been seen. Additional study may reveal why some components of the system are susceptible to alterations and other components are not.

p53 is known as the "guardian of the genome" and the "guardian of the G1 checkpoint." It is not usually called upon to act in the course of normal replication. However, with DNA damage, p53 influences transcription to either halt cell cycle progression (e.g., through induction of p21 expression to inhibit cdk kinase activity) to permit repair of the DNA or, if the damage is too great, to initiate cell suicide (*apoptosis*). p53 is the target of many tumor-causing viruses: human

Table 83-1

Cell Cycle Regulators in Human Cancers

Gene	Functional or Genetic Change*	Tumors
Retinoblastoma	Deletion Point mutation	Retinoblastomas, osteosarcoma, soft tissue sarcoma, small cell lung carcinoma, bladder and breast carcinomas
Cyclin D	Chromosome translocation Gene amplification	Parathyroid adenomas, mantle cell lymphomas; breast, head and neck, esophageal, and hepatocellular carcinomas
cdk4	Amplification Point mutation	Glioblastoma, sarcoma; melanoma
p16^{INK4a} (p15^{INK4b})	Deletion Point mutations Methylation	Pancreatic, esophageal, non-small cell lung carcinomas; glioblastoma, sarcoma, familial melanoma, familial pancreatic cancer

* Each of these genetic lesions results in loss of physiologic regulation of the phosphorylation state of pRb late in G1 at a checkpoint called the restriction point. Aberrant regulation of the restriction point permits dysregulated entry into S phase, and is thought to occur as an early step in the genesis of most, if not all, tumors. By understanding the pathophysiology of these molecular defects, therapies can be devised that reestablish normal restriction point control.

papillomavirus E6 protein decreases p53 half-life, and adenovirus E1B proteins and SV40 large T antigen interfere with p53 function, for example. Mutations in p53 are the most common genetic alteration found in human cancer (>50 percent). Usually one p53 allele on chromosome 17p is deleted and the other is mutated. The mutations often involve the region between codons 120 and 290, the portion of the gene specifying the site of p53 involved in transcription. Some environmental agents cause mutations at specific sites. In 81 percent of hepatomas from developing countries, codon 249 is mutated due to exposure to the carcinogen, aflatoxin. Codon 249 mutations occur in only 11 percent of hepatomas from industrialized countries where aflatoxin exposure is low.

Regardless of the pathogenesis of the tumor, most have some mechanism(s) to bypass the G1 checkpoint, avoid activation of cell suicide pathways, and propagate cells with damaged DNA. An overview of cell cycle regulation is shown in Fig. 83-2.

SIGNALING FROM OUTSIDE THE CELL TO THE NUCLEUS

The behavior of every cell in the body is tightly regulated by environmental signals. The ability of a cell to respond to a specific set of signals determines whether the cell will live or die, differentiate, proliferate, or remain quiescent. In normal cells and tissues, coordinated action such as wound healing or the inflammatory response is regulated by signaling pathways that convert extracellular signals into the performance of specialized action in the responding cells. In cancer cells, the process of invading and metastasizing is influenced by signal transduction pathways activated by paracrine and autocrine factors.

The coupling of extracellular signals to cell response varies for different receptor and signaling systems, but the binding of a growth factor [e.g., epidermal growth factor (EGF)] to its receptor on the cell surface produces measurable changes in the cell within seconds and elicits a sequence of events that may last for days. Important mechanisms have evolved for preventing overstimulation of cells. The growth factors and local mediators are produced in minute quantities and usually act over short distances. When the growth factor or local mediator binds to its receptor, it is usually internalized rapidly and destroyed rather than released to stimulate other cells. In addition, receptor desensitization to the stimulus can occur by several mechanisms, including downregulation of receptors such that fewer receptors are on the cell and the likelihood of activation is reduced, and biochemical desensitization of the receptor through phosphorylations or methylations that alter the affinity for the ligand or prevent receptor coupling to downstream substrates.

Glucocorticoids, thyroid hormone, and retinoids all induce signals by binding to a family of cytoplasmic receptors (intracellular receptor or steroid hormone receptor superfamily; see Chap. 327) that, in the presence of ligand, move to the nucleus and bind to specific DNA sequence motifs, known as *response elements*, located within transcriptional promoter or enhancer regions. These response elements are located in proximity to the genes under the control of the hormones, usually upstream of the TATA box (a short thymidine- and adenine-rich double helical DNA sequence) that signals transcription initiation. For most other families of transcription factors, there are many interme-

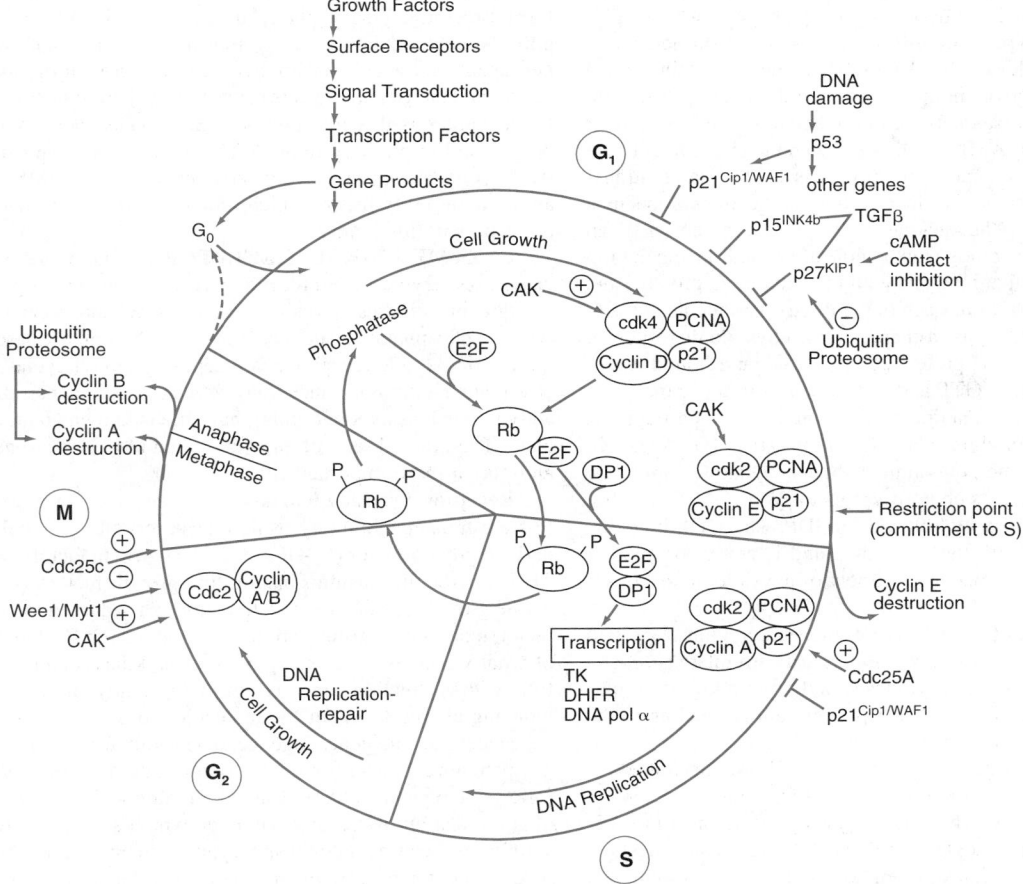

FIGURE 83-2 Integration of external stimuli with the mammalian cell cycle engine. Important checkpoint control mechanisms occur late in G1 near the restriction point and at the G2/M border. The phosphorylation of pRb by G1 cdk/cyclins releases E2F, which dimerizes with the transcription factor DP-1 and activates genes required for DNA synthesis. The cdk inhibitors p21, p15, and p27, induced in response to a variety of stimuli, block progression before the restriction point. External factors that positively or negatively influence the cycle are shown as impinging on the cycle. Cells in G1 may receive signals to halt proliferation and enter the G_0 state, as occurs during differentiation, or continue cycling if growth factors and other stimulatory signals are present.

diate biochemical steps between the signaling molecule and the transcription factors it activates.

Derangements in steroid hormone receptors occur in some human cancers. For example, the t(15;17) translocation in acute promyelocytic leukemia generates a chimeric retinoic acid receptor α that has an abnormal cellular distribution and is associated with a differentiation arrest of tumor cells at the promyelocytic stage of development. However, administration of pharmacologic doses of tretinoin (all-*trans* retinoic acid), a ligand for retinoic acid receptor α, results in normal nuclear localization of the receptor and induces terminal differentiation of the tumor cells.

Some differentiated cells such as endothelial cells and macrophages respond to specific environmental signals by the production of nitric oxide (NO) gas through the enzymatic breakdown of arginine. NO serves as a signaling molecule; it diffuses into the cell and stimulates guanylyl cyclase to produce cyclic GMP, which can activate a class of ion channels important in membrane depolarization. NO mediates a variety of physiologic responses, including blood vessel relaxation, and may serve as a neurotransmitter in the central nervous system (see Chap. 71). NO may be responsible for some of the toxic effects associated with the use of biologic agents such as IL-2 and interferon γ.

Many signaling molecules are hydrophilic and act on specific cell surface membrane receptors to initiate a signal transduction cascade that leads to transcription factor activation. There are three families of cell surface receptors: ion channel–linked receptors, G protein–linked receptors, and enzyme-linked receptors. Although ion channel–linked receptors are a component of growth-related activation in many cell types, they are primarily involved in neurotransmitter signal transduction and are somewhat less important in the pathogenesis of neoplasia than the other two types and will not be discussed further.

G PROTEIN–LINKED RECEPTORS The G protein–linked receptors do not induce covalent modification of their substrates, as do enzyme-linked receptors (see below), but generate second messenger molecules such as cyclic AMP, cyclic GMP, and calcium to activate downstream processes. Receptors of this class contain seven transmembrane segments that course in and out of the membrane in a serpentine fashion (thus, the nickname "serpentine receptors"), an extracellular domain that binds signal molecules, and an inner loop at the carboxyl terminal that interacts with the trimeric G proteins and regulates receptor sensitization. Each of the three components of the G protein complex (Table 83-2) has a characteristic physiologic response.

After association of the G protein complex to ligand-bound receptor, the Gα subunit binds to GTP and is released from the trimer. The GTP-α subunit mediates a function characteristic of the particular α subunit (G_s stimulates adenylyl cyclase; G_i inhibits adenylyl cyclase; G_s and G_o regulate calcium and potassium channels; G_q and G_{16} stimulate phospholipase Cβ; G_t couples photoreceptors to cyclic GMP phosphodiesterase) until the GTP is hydrolyzed to GDP. The GDP-bound α chain then reassociates with the βγ chains and is ready for another response. βγ Subunits also mediate a variety of physiologic responses (Table 83-2).

Cyclic AMP activates the cyclic AMP–dependent kinase (protein kinase A). The substrates of this enzyme primarily stimulate glycogen breakdown and inhibit glycogen synthesis, and protein kinase A activates transcription factors in the CREB protein family, leading to the transcription of a number of genes.

Perhaps the most important consequence of G protein–linked receptor activation is the elevation of intracellular calcium. G_q receptors activate phospholipase Cβ, which hydrolyses phosphoinositide 4,5-bisphosphate (PIP2) into diacylglycerol (DAG) and inositol triphosphate (IP3). DAG then activates protein kinase C (PKC), a family of serine threonine kinases that occur in a number of different forms with different substrates in different cell types. In many cells, PKC activates the MAP kinase cascade (see below) and phosphorylates IκB, an inhibitor molecule that keeps transcription factors of the *rel* family in the cytoplasm. A consequence of the activation of the MAP

Table 83-2

Heterotrimeric G Proteins

Subunits*	Effectors Regulated by α or βγ Subunits
Gα (16 genes, >20 proteins	
α_s (α_s, α_olf)	Stimulates or inhibits adenylycyclase
(choleratoxin-sensitive)	Regulates calcium and potassium channels
α_i (α_i 1–3, α_o, α_t, α_gust, α_z)	Activates cyclic AMP phosphodiesterase
(pertussis toxin–sensitive)	Activates PLCβ
α_q (α_q, α_11, α_14, α_15, α_16)	Regulates sodium/potassium exchanger
α_12 (α_12, α_13)	
Gβ (5 isoforms)	Stimulates or inhibits adenylycyclase
Gγ (6 isoforms)	Activates potassium channels
	Stimulates PLCβ
	Activates βARK
	Activates *ras*-MAP kinase pathway

* Multiple Gα and Gβγ subunits mediate a variety of physiologic responses. Cells often express multiple types of G proteins, so integration of signaling information is a complex task. Both Gα and Gβγ subunits mediate these signaling events.

NOTE: PLCβ, phospholipase Cβ; βARK, β-adrenergic receptor kinase; MAP, mitogen-activated protein.

kinase cascade is the generation of AP-1 transcription factor family members (usually heterodimeric proteins that include *fos* and *jun* family members). Phosphorylation of IκB leads to its release of *rel*/NFκB heterodimers and their translocation to the nucleus. The IP3 produced as a consequence of phospholipase C activity acts to release intracellular calcium stores, and the increase in intracellular calcium leads to the activation of a number of enzymes such as calcium/calmodulin-dependent protein kinases (CaM kinases).

The receptors for epinephrine, serotonin, chemotactic cytokines or chemokines (such as IL-8 and RANTES; see Chap. 305), and formyl-methionyl leucyl phenylalanine (f-met-leu-phe; a major neutrophil chemoattractant) are G protein linked. The bombesin family of neuropeptides, which are implicated in the growth of small cell lung cancer and breast and prostate cancers, use G protein–linked receptors. Point mutations that interfere with the GTPase activity of G_sα have been found in pituitary tumors. These mutations result in a constitutively activated G_s and overproduction of cyclic AMP. In addition, autocrine motility factor, which promotes tumor cell metastasis, uses a receptor in this family.

ENZYME-LINKED RECEPTORS There are at least five classes of enzyme-linked receptors: receptor guanylyl cyclases, receptor tyrosine kinases, tyrosine kinase–associated receptors, receptor tyrosine phosphatases, and receptor serine/threonine kinases. The atrial natriuretic peptide receptor is a receptor guanylyl cyclase. Some disease manifestations in cancer may be related to atrial natriuretic peptide activity (such as hyponatremia), but little is known about this receptor class. The other classes of enzyme-linked receptors are better defined and play a more important role in cancer.

Receptor Tyrosine Kinases The receptors for most growth factors are transmembrane tyrosine kinase receptors, including platelet-derived growth factor (PDGF), fibroblast growth factors (FGFs), EGF, TGFα, heregulin, insulin, insulin-like growth factors (IGF) I and II, nerve growth factor, stem cell factor, vascular endothelial growth factor, macrophage colony stimulating factors (CSF), and others. Much of what we know about receptor tyrosine kinases and the events that follow their ligation emerged from the study of the proliferation-inducing altered forms of the molecules (proto-oncogenes) that were the cancer-causing genes (oncogenes) in animal retroviruses. Although downstream events vary with the receptor, the activation of the receptor follows a typical pattern. Ligand binding induces dimerization or oligomerization of receptor subunits, which activates tyrosine kinase activity and causes autophosphorylation of the intracellular domains of the receptor chains. Finally, phosphorylated tyrosine residues on the receptors or on associated adaptor proteins form docking sights for other signal transduction molecules that contain one or more *src-homology region 2*, or SH2, domains, named because the sequence was first identified in the *src* nonreceptor tyrosine kinase. These associations via SH2 domains trigger subsequent events (Fig. 83-3).

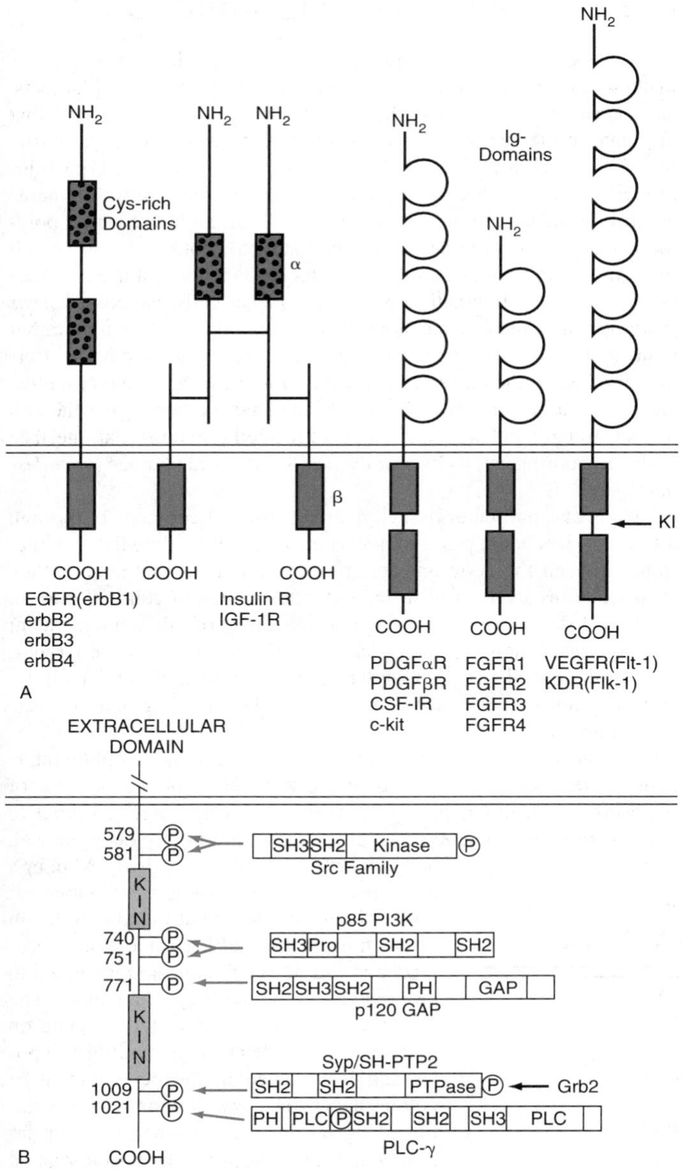

FIGURE 83-3 *A.* Structures of receptor tyrosine kinases activated by ligand-induced dimerization. Conserved extracellular domains, a single transmembrane spanning region, and a cytoplasmic domain encoding the tyrosine kinase characterize these receptors. The insulin and IGF-I receptors are disulfide-linked heterotetramers of α and β chains that undergo allosteric changes upon ligand binding. In the other cases shown, ligand binding induces homo- or heterodimerization within the subfamily followed by receptor autophosphorylation on tyrosine residues. Some kinase domains contain a kinase insert (KI). Flt-1 and Flk-1 are endothelial cell–specific receptors for vascular endothelial growth factor (VEGF) and are required for embryonic blood vessel differentiation and angiogenesis in the adult. Other members of the receptor kinase family are not shown but share structural similarities. *B.* Multiple tyrosine autophosphorylation sites on activated PDGF receptor β chains serve as docking sites for signal transduction molecules. These include enzymes that activate downstream substrates and docking proteins to provide SH2 or P-Tyr binding sites for other proteins. These interactions lead to the formation of a signal transduction complex whose structure determines the nature of the signal transduction pathways activated by a particular ligand. SH2, SH3, pleckstrin homology (PH), proline-rich (Pro), phospholipase C (PLC), phosphoinositol 3' kinase (PI3K), GTPase activating protein (GAP), and protein tyrosine phosphatase (PTPase) domains are shown.

The docking mechanisms of intracellular signaling molecules determine the specificity and kinetics of protein-protein interactions, and determine how a particular stimulus will lead to a characteristic response. The most common docking mechanisms are based on recog-

nition of particular protein sequences; the SH2 domains dock with phosphotyrosine-containing (P-Tyr) sequences, the SH3 domains dock with proline-rich sequences, and the pleckstrin homology domains (pleckstrin is a major PKC substrate in platelets) lead to associations by a mechanism not yet fully defined. Some molecules that do not have docking domains are brought into association with the receptors through the activity of adaptor proteins that are composed of docking domains only. Thus, the *ras* nucleotide exchange factor son of sevenless (SOS; named for its role in *Drosophila* eye development) is brought close to the membrane to activate *ras* through its association with the adaptor protein grb2 (identified because it "grabbed" phosphotyrosine-containing proteins).

Receptor tyrosine kinases in turn activate many signaling pathways including phospholipase C-γ, which stimulates calcium-dependent kinases and PKC; phosphoinositol 3'-kinase (PI3K), which activates protein kinase B and ribosomal S6 kinase (thus enhancing the efficiency of translation); and *src* family kinases, which leads to c-*myc* activation. Another consequence of receptor tyrosine kinase activation is stimulation of the *ras*/MAP kinase pathway that leads to activation of transcription factors in the *fos/jun*/AP-1 family. This pathway is frequently implicated in cancer cells.

ras is a 21-kDa member of a large family of proteins, including *rho*, *rac*, *rab*, and others, that regulate cytoskeletal changes, vesicular and nuclear transport, and proliferation and that share sequence homology with the Gα subunit of G protein–linked receptors. *ras* is attached to the inner cell membrane through an isoprenyl lipid group added by the enzyme farnesyl transferase. If the lipid group is not added, *ras* does not localize to the membrane and cannot function normally. In unstimulated cells, *ras* is bound to GDP and is inactive. Following activation of the receptor tyrosine kinase by its ligand, the guanine nucleotide exchange factor SOS is brought to the membrane by its association with grb2. SOS removes GDP from *ras* and adds GTP. GTP-bound *ras* then activates a cascade ending with MAP kinase, which migrates to the nucleus and phosphorylates (activates) a number of transcription factors (see Fig. 83-4).

About 30 percent of human cancers have mutated *ras*. The mutations usually involve codons 12, 13, or 61 and result in a *ras* that will not give up its GTP and is thus constitutively active. In the hereditary disorder, neurofibromatosis, a mutation in the gene that encodes neurofibromin, a GTPase activating protein (GAP), inhibits its ability to inactivate *ras* by converting the GTP to GDP. Some epithelial cancers overexpress one or more members of the receptor tyrosine kinase family. EGF receptors, IGF-I receptors, and HER-2/*neu* are overexpressed in lung, bladder, breast, head and neck, and ovarian cancers. Autocrine and paracrine sources of the relevant growth factors have been noted in some cases.

Tyrosine Kinase–Associated Receptors The receptors for growth hormone, prolactin, erythropoietin, IL-2, IL-3, IL-4, IL-6, IL-7, granulocyte CSF, granulocyte-macrophage CSF, interferon α, interferon γ, ciliary neurotrophic factor, and many other cytokines are members of the tyrosine kinase–associated receptor family. The receptors are often multisubunit receptors with each chain associating with a distinct set of signaling molecules via the docking mechanisms described above; however, the receptors themselves do not have tyrosine kinase activity. Three families of kinases are known to be associated with this class of receptors: *src* family (*src*, *yes*, *fgr*, *fyn*, *lck*, *lyn*, *hck*, *blk*, and counting), *syk* family (*syk*, ZAP-70), and Janus family (JAK1, JAK2, JAK3, Tyk2). The *src* family kinases can associate with receptor tyrosine kinases as well as tyrosine kinase–associated receptors, and, not surprisingly, signal transduction through either receptor class leads to the activation of similar signaling cascades. *myc* is one of the transcription factors activated as a consequence of *src* family activation. The *syk* family usually activates the *src* family member in the receptor complex. The Janus family leads to the phosphorylation and activation of a family of transcription factors called STATs (signal transduction and activation of transcription).

These receptors are often overexpressed on tumors of hematopoietic origin, and, similar to receptor tyrosine kinases, autocrine or paracrine stimulation may contribute to the neoplastic state of the tumor cell.

Serine/Threonine Kinase Receptors   These receptors recognize TGFβ, bone morphogenetic factors, and other activins as ligands. Ligand binding leads to activation of the receptor kinase activity, but downstream events are not well defined. Bone morphogenetic factors are important in bone formation and in determining ventral vs. dorsal orientation in the developing embryo. TGFβ induces fibroblast proliferation but inhibits the proliferation of most cell types, probably through the induction of cdki. Loss of expression or loss of function of TGFβ receptors occurs in several tumor types including colon cancer and lymphomas.

Tyrosine Phosphatase Receptors   The prototypical tyrosine phosphatase receptor is CD45; its ligand is unknown. CD45 plays a crucial role in T cell activation through its removal of phosphate from a negative regulatory site on the *src* family kinase, *lck*. This activates *lck* and permits signal transduction through the T cell antigen receptor. A role for CD45 in neoplasia has not been defined.

In addition to these known classes of receptors for soluble mediators and growth factors, some receptors bind and are triggered by components of the extracellular matrix (particular protein constituents or glycosaminoglycans) or by cell-cell adhesion. Integrins are the principal receptors involved in such interactions, and they influence the cytoskeleton of the cell through activation of kinases, such as focal adhesion kinase, and induce remodeling of actin filaments modulated through the *ras* family proteins, *rho* and *rac*. The intracellular pathway activated by these interactions is not well characterized.

CYTOSKELETON AND CELL ADHESION

The cytoskeleton, which controls the spatial organization of cells, is made up of three major types of fibers: microtubules, actin filaments, and intermediate filaments. Microtubules are polymers of tubulin that originate in the centrosome and terminate variably in the cytoplasm. Motor proteins use microtubules as "railways" to position organelles properly and transport some proteins to the nucleus. Actin filaments control the shape and movement of the cell; through directional polymerization and depolymerization, cell surface protrusions direct cell migration. Actin bundles are the main components of adhesion belts (special areas of interaction between adjacent cells, called *adherens junctions*) and focal contacts (adherens junctions with matrix rather than other cells). Intermediate filaments in different cells contain different proteins: epithelial cells use keratin, fibroblasts use vimentin, muscle cells use desmin, and so on. Intermediate filaments give the cell tensile strength and are components of the cell junctions that interface with neighboring cells (*desmosomes*) and with basal laminae (*hemidesmosomes*).

Cells of a particular tissue type maintain cell-cell contact through a calcium-dependent process involving cadherins that mediate interactions between the actin and intermediate filaments of the cells they join. Cells involved in host defense often maintain cell-cell contact between different cell types using one of a family of calcium-dependent carbohydrate-binding proteins called *selectins*. In some cell types, calcium-independent cell-cell interactions are mediated by intercellular adhesion molecules (ICAMs), members of the immunoglobulin supergene family.

In cancer, these highly organized mechanisms of intercellular interaction often become disrupted or are subsumed for the purpose of metastasizing (see Chap. 85). Individual cells no longer respond to signals from their neighbors, actin filaments are highly disorganized, and adherens junctions are lost. Although much less is known about how the cytoskeleton is disrupted than about the alterations in signal transduction, at least one example of a gene involved in cell adhesion is known to be involved in the etiology of a cancer. The adenomatous polyposis coli (APC) gene on chromosome 5 is defective in familial polyposis and is involved in the development of colon cancer. The *wnt* protein is a matrix-bound ligand that leads to the phosphorylation of the APC gene product. Phosphorylated APC binds to β-catenin and keeps levels of the protein low. The defective gene product cannot bind to β-catenin, and the free β-catenin disrupts adherens junctions and causes other cytoskeletal changes. Disruption of cell-cell communication is one of the many components of a multistep process leading to neoplastic transformation.

Drugs that attack the cytoskeleton, particularly tubulin (such as the vinca alkaloids and taxanes; see Chap. 86), are effective in a wide range of cancers.

REGULATION OF CELL DEATH

The homeostasis of adult organisms requires a balance between the generation of new cells and the death of old cells. Some cells die when their telomeres no longer protect the integrity of DNA replication. Some cells die when they have sustained sufficient hypoxic, heat, oxidative, or ultraviolet irradiation damage that cannot be repaired. A cell can be killed if it becomes infected with a virus or

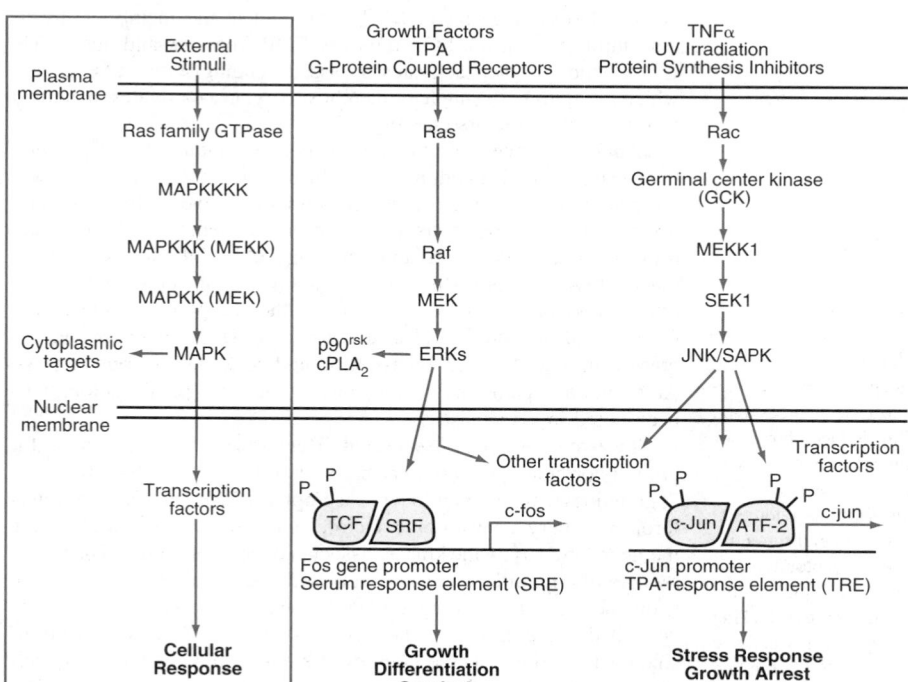

FIGURE 83-4   The MAP kinase cascades. MAP kinase signal transduction cascades link *ras* activation with the nucleus. The overall framework of the MAP kinase cascades is shown in the box at the left. A series of sequential serine/threonine kinase events results in the activation of MAP kinase which has cytoplasmic and nuclear targets. The nuclear targets of MAP kinase are transcription factors bound to their DNA recognition sites that require phosphorylation to induce transactivating functions. ERKs (extracellular signal response kinases) target the ternary complex factor (TCF), while JNK/SAPK targets c-*jun* and ATF-2. Transcription factors associated with other promoters also serve as targets for MAP kinases. Other MAP kinase cascades exist in the cell. Each pathway is activated by different stimuli and the pattern of gene expression induced by each pathway is characteristic of that pathway. Interactions between pathways permit an integrated response to diverse signals.

other intracellular pathogen that destroys the cell or is recognized by the host's lymphocytes, which kill the infected cell. Multicellular organisms are a model of cellular cooperation; some cells die to preserve the rest of the organism.

Apoptosis is a form of cell death initiated by extracellular or intracellular signals in which enzymes are activated to degrade nuclear DNA by making intranucleosomal cuts, causing the cell to shrink and finally break up. Extracellular signals through the tumor necrosis factor (TNF) receptor or a related receptor (called *fas*) or intracellular signals related to p53 detection of irreparable DNA damage lead to the activation of a series of cellular proteases in the IL-1-converting enzyme (ICE) family (IL-1 must be processed by this enzyme to be released from cells). Activated ICE family proteases cleave specific proteins at asparagine residues and activate the cell death pathway. In the immune system, this process is activated to delete autoreactive lymphocytes.

The *bcl2* family of genes was originally noted when *bcl2* was cloned from the chromosome 18q contribution to the t(14;18) translocation in follicular lymphoma. The gene did not transform cells but prolonged the life of cells destined to die in the lymphoid follicle. Members of the *bcl2* family fall into two groups: *bcl2* and *bcl*-X$_L$ prevent cell death, whereas *bax*, *bad*, *bak*, and others promote cell death. *bcl2* family members associate as homodimers or heterodimers; the combinatorial effects of the various dimers allow a fine level of control over cell survival. When any of the death promoters exist as homo- or heterodimers, the cell dies by apoptosis. When a death promoter heterodimerizes with either *bcl2* or *bcl*-X$_L$, cell death is prevented. Thus, the relative amounts of different *bcl2* family members determine whether a cell will survive potentially damaging insults. Furthermore, phosphorylation of *bcl2* family members by cellular kinases can alter the biologic activity of individual members, altering the balance in favor of death or survival.

In addition to its presumed role in the etiology of follicular lymphoma, *bcl2* is expressed in a number of cancers. It prevents the normal p53-mediated destruction of cells with damaged DNA and also appears to prevent the death of cells severely damaged by cancer chemotherapy. *bcl2* mediates drug resistance and contributes to neoplasia in a novel way, preventing the death that would normally eliminate the damaged cell, rather than promoting aberrant cell growth. Strategies to overcome *bcl2* function might well make available therapies more effective.

REGULATION OF GENE TRANSCRIPTION

Factors that regulate gene transcription recognize short stretches of double-helical DNA of a defined nucleotide sequence 6 to 12 bases in length. These recognition sites may be upstream or downstream of the transcription start site [the TATA box where the first subunit of the transcription machinery, transcription factor IID (TFIID) binds]. Transcription factors may affect transcription at sites remote from the start site by looping out large intervening DNA sequences.

Transcription factors contain specific amino acid sequences capable of recognizing the DNA sequence and usually form one of several structural motifs: helix-turn-helix, homeodomain, zinc finger, leucine zipper, and helix-loop-helix are all used as DNA-binding motifs or mediate dimerization of factors required for DNA binding. Transcription factors function in one or more of several ways. They can physically bend the DNA to permit the ordered addition of the components of the transcription machinery. They can facilitate the addition of those components. They can inhibit transcription by blocking binding of a positive transcription factor or preventing the assembly of a transcription complex. The complex interaction between positive and negative transcription factors dictates the level of gene transcription. Individual genes may have 20 or more sites for transcription factor binding.

Some growth factors and combinations of growth factors mediate different effects on different cell types. The receptors may be connected to a different combination of signaling pathways. Different combinations of transcription factors may be activated. Distinct patterns of chromatin condensation may make different regions of the genome available or unavailable for transcription. Some genes may be turned off in particular cell types by methylation of cytosine residues in critical cytosine- and guanosine-rich regions of the gene that prevent transcription. Most genes are regulated at multiple levels, though transcription initiation is the dominant control point. The von Hippel–Lindau gene on chromosome 3p (a tumor suppressor gene involved in the pathogenesis of renal cell cancer) appears to act by inhibiting the elongation of an RNA chain after transcription initiation. A message may be spliced alternatively and encode different proteins in different cells. Transport of the message from the nucleus to the cytoplasm may be altered. Messenger RNA turnover may be accelerated. Some proteins, such as apoferritin and thymidylate synthase, regulate the translation of their own messages (and perhaps other messages) by binding to mRNA and preventing initiation of protein synthesis. Thus, there are many levels at which gene expression may be influenced.

Some transcription factors were identified because of their transforming effects when their genes, usually in mutated form, were incorporated into animal retroviral genomes. *myc*, *rel*, *fos*, *jun*, and others are examples of proto-oncogene transcription factors that are overexpressed in certain cancers and that contribute to the malignant phenotype of tumor cells.

CELL BIOLOGY AND CANCER

For a cancer to arise, mutations must occur that affect a variety of pathways. Often the G1 cell cycle checkpoint is affected. The expression of telomerase is a common feature in cancers. Overexpression of growth factors and their receptors is frequently detected. Activation of the *ras* proto-oncogene or other changes leading to a constitutively active MAP kinase cascade are common. Changes in cytoskeleton and responsiveness to contact-mediated growth inhibition are frequent in cancer cells. Failure to induce expression of gene products required for apoptosis may be a component of the pathophysiology. Usually when a mutation occurs in one component of a signaling pathway, other mutations are seen in other pathways rather than in another component of the same pathway. The high level of mutability of cancer cells facilitates adaptation to the environment, including the development of resistance to anticancer drugs. As tumors progress, they acquire the ability to secrete proteases that aid in the escape from local barriers so that they may metastasize (see Chap. 85). Discrete steps in tumor progression lead to the production of factors by the tumor cells that permit neovascularization to supply nutrients to the growing tumor. Other mutations allow the tumor to escape immune surveillance mechanisms; for example, some tumors downregulate expression of class I major histocompatibility complex antigens so that they become invisible to T cells. The wide range of changes that must occur in a single cell to permit the behavior associated with a malignant neoplasm makes it clear why carcinogenesis is a multistep process and why human cancers may have 10 or more genetic lesions that account for the biology.

The characteristic of cancer cells that has dominated clinical thinking is their uncontrolled proliferation. However, the growth fraction of most human cancers is usually not higher than the growth fraction of normal gut epithelia or normal bone marrow, and most human tumor explants are difficult to propagate for long periods of time in culture. Cancer cell lines immortal in vitro may have additional genetic lesions that permit their growth in vitro. Naturally occurring tumors growing in vivo show a Gompertzian or exponential decline in their growth fraction because the daughter cells of a division are not uniformly capable of further division. The accumulation of genetic damage, poor oxygen or nutrient supply, and other unknown factors contribute to the senescence of some tumor cells, so that by the time a tumor becomes clinically apparent at a tumor burden of 10^8 to 10^9 cells, most of the proliferative capability of the tumor is finished. Often by this time, more malignant and highly selected clonal derivatives of the tumor have metastasized to other sites where new tumor deposits with more aggressive characteristics are formed. Thus, cancer cells can be viewed as having lost the altruism that usually characterizes cell behavior in multicellular organisms. Cancer cells operate under natural selection imposed by a hostile environment. Ironically, the more successful they are at achieving independence from environmental influences, the more assured is the destruction of their host and ultimately themselves.

Many potential therapeutic agents are in clinical development based on our concepts of tumor cell biology. They include the development of growth factor and growth factor receptor antagonists; inhibitors of phosphoryl transfer to block key kinases; selective inhibitors of PKC, phosphoinositol 3′ kinase, phospholipase C, and other targets; farnesyl transferase inhibitors that block the insertion of *ras* into the membrane; mutant versions of proteins such as *ras* and p53 that may make the cell vulnerable to immunologic attack if employed as a vaccine; inhibitors of angiogenesis or the steps in metastasis that may limit tumor growth and prevent its spread. However, it seems unlikely that a single target will be the highly sought after point of vulnerability. More likely, combinations of inhibitors will be required to improve antitumor effects. For example, the combination of chemotherapy and antibody to EGF receptors appears to produce greater antitumor effects than the sum of the effects produced individually.

BIBLIOGRAPHY

ALBERTS B et al: *Molecular Biology of the Cell*, 3d ed. New York, Garland, 1994
AMATI B, LAND H: Myc-Max, Mad: A transcription factor network controlling cell cycle progression, differentiation and death. Curr Opin Genet Dev 4:102, 1994
BERRIDGE MJ: Calcium signalling and cell proliferation. Bioessays 17:491, 1995
CANO E, MAHADEVAN LC: Parallel signal processing among mammalian MAP kinases. Trends Biochem Sci 20:117, 1995
COX LS, LANE DP: Tumor suppressors, kinases and clamps: How p53 regulates the cell cycle in response to DNA damage. Bioessays 17:501, 1995
HELDIN C-H: Dimerization of cell surface receptors in signal transduction. Cell 80:213, 1995
HILL CS, TREISMAN R: Transcriptional regulation by extracellular signals: Mechanisms and specificity. Cell 80:199, 1995
IHLE JN: Cytokine receptor signalling. Nature 377:591, 1995
WEINBERG RA: The retinoblastoma protein and cell cycle control. Cell 81:323, 1995

84	*Francis S. Collins, Jeffrey M. Trent*

CANCER GENETICS

THE CLONAL NATURE OF CANCER A critical feature of nearly all cancers is that they originate from a single cell. While multiple cumulative events are invariably required to move a cell from normal to the transformed phenotype (see below and Chap. 83), the origin of tumors from a single clone of cells is a critical discriminating feature between neoplasia and hyperplasia.

CANCER IS A GENETIC DISEASE Cancer arises because of alterations in DNA that result in unrestrained cellular proliferation. Most of these alterations involve actual sequence changes in the DNA (i.e., mutation). They may arise as a consequence of random replication errors, exposure to carcinogens (e.g., radiation), or faulty DNA repair processes.

While virtually all cancer is genetic, most cancer is not inherited. Certain individuals with cancer have inherited a germline mutation that predisposed them to the cancer, but even in that situation additional somatic mutations are required for a tumor to develop. In a truly sporadic cancer, *all* of the mutations responsible for the malignant

phenotype arise somatically. Such a cancer is caused by genetic alterations but has no hereditary implications.

RNA AND DNA TUMOR VIRUSES Many malignancies in animals are transmissible, and the etiologic agent is frequently a retrovirus, which possesses a single-stranded RNA genome. During the life cycle of the virus, the single-stranded RNA is converted to double-stranded DNA and is inserted at random into the host chromosome. On rare occasions, the virus can be remobilized, carrying along with it an adjacent segment of host DNA. Should this host DNA contain a growth-promoting gene, then the retrovirus is potentially transforming. Although efforts to identify retroviruses in human malignancies have mostly been fruitless, retroviruses are implicated in at least one human malignancy. Human T cell lymphotropic virus (HTLV) type I causes adult T cell lymphoma/leukemia, particularly in Japan and the Caribbean (see Chap. 192). Unlike animal retroviruses that induce neoplasia, HTLV-I does not contain a growth-promoting transforming oncogene. The tax protein, a 40-kDa molecule encoded in the pX region of the viral genome, induces the activation of a number of genes (including some promoting growth) through interactions with *rel* family and CREB (cyclic AMP response element binding protein) family transcription factors.

DNA tumor viruses are more commonly involved in human malignancy. Human papilloma viruses (especially types 16 and 18) cause cervical cancer (see Chap. 190), and both hepatitis B and hepatitis C viruses have been implicated in hepatocellular carcinoma (see Chap. 297). In addition, the Epstein-Barr virus, a herpesvirus that causes a mild illness in children but infectious mononucleosis in nonimmune adolescents and adults, causes Burkitt's lymphoma in Africa, nasopharyngeal carcinoma in the Orient, and lymphomas in the setting of immune deficiency (see Chap. 186).

GENERAL CLASSES OF CANCER GENES In 1914, Boveri hypothesized that cells become malignant either because of overactivation of a gene that promotes cell division or because of loss of function of a gene that normally restrains growth. This hypothesis is largely correct, although defects in DNA repair genes are also involved. Genes that promote normal cell growth are referred to as *proto-oncogenes*, and activation of such genes by point mutation, amplification, or dysregulation converts them to *oncogenes*.

Genes that normally restrain growth are called *tumor suppressors* (use of the alternative designation of anti-oncogenes is to be discouraged), and unregulated cell growth arises if their function is lost. The diploid nature of mammalian cells allows certain predictions about the consequences of somatic mutations of tumor suppressor genes. Loss of one allele is unlikely to have significant consequences in most instances, as the remaining normal allele is usually sufficient for normal function. Thus, most cells of an individual with an inherited loss of function of one tumor suppressor allele are functionally normal. Only the rare cell that loses or develops a mutation in the remaining normal copy will exhibit uncontrolled growth. This model correctly predicts that the inheritance pattern of cancer in a family with a tumor suppressor gene mutation will be expressed as an autosomal dominant trait, though the cellular mechanism is recessive.

The third category of genes that contribute to malignancy consists of the DNA repair genes. Every cell division involves the copying of 6 billion base pairs (bp) of DNA. DNA polymerase has a finite error rate, and many environmental influences can damage DNA; as a consequence, repair systems are essential to protect the integrity of the genome. When the repair systems themselves are faulty, either on the basis of inherited or acquired mutation, the rate of accumulation of mutations throughout the genome rises as cell divisions occur. To the extent that these mutations involve oncogenes and tumor suppressor genes, the likelihood of developing malignancy increases.

MENDELIAN CANCER SYNDROMES Roughly 100 syndromes of familial cancer have been reported, though many are rare. The majority are inherited as autosomal dominant traits, although some of those associated with DNA repair abnormalities (xeroderma pigmentosum, Fanconi anemia, ataxia telangiectasia) are autosomal recessives. Most of the genes responsible for the dominantly inherited cancer syndromes are tumor suppressor genes (Table 84-1). The hall-

Table 84-1

Selected Tumor Suppressor Genes Responsible for Familial Cancer Syndromes

Syndrome	Gene	Chromosome Location	Tumors
Basal cell nevus	PTC	9q22.3	Basal cell cancer, jaw cysts, medulloblastoma
Familial breast/ovarian cancer	BRCA1	17q21	Breast, ovarian, colon, prostate cancer
Familial breast cancer	BRCA2	13q12-13	Breast cancer, male breast cancer
Familial melanoma	p16	9p21	Melanoma, pancreatic cancer
Familial polyposis coli	APC	5q21	Intestinal polyposis, colorectal cancer
Familial retinoblastoma	RB	13q24	Retinoblastoma, osteosarcoma
Familial Wilms' tumor	WT1	11p13	Wilms' tumor, WAGR*
Hereditary multiple exostoses	EXT1	11p11-13	Exostoses, chondrosarcoma
Li-Fraumeni	p53	17q13	Sarcomas, breast cancer
Neurofibromatosis type 1	NF1	17q11.2	Neurofibroma, neurofibrosarcoma, brain tumor
Neurofibromatosis type 2	NF2	22q12	Acoustic neuroma, meningioma
Tuberous sclerosis	TSC2	16p13.3	Angiofibroma, renal angiomyolipoma
Von Hippel–Lindau	VHL	3p25-26	Renal cell cancer, pheochromocytoma, retinal angioma, hemangioblastoma

* WAGR, Wilms' tumor, aniridia, genitourinary abnormalities, and mental retardation.

marks of a tumor suppressor gene are as follows: (1) the germline mutation that affects one allele generally causes a loss of function, (2) tumors also show loss of the second normal allele as a result of a somatic mutation, and (3) often the *normal* function of the gene is to suppress unrestrained cellular growth or to promote differentiation.

The retinoblastoma (*RB*) gene is a paradigm of such a tumor suppressor gene. In a pedigree showing dominant inheritance of susceptibility to retinoblastoma, there is a loss-of-function germline mutation of one allele of the *RB* gene on chromosome 13. Analysis of the DNA from the tumors invariably shows that the wild-type allele has also been lost, by one of several possible mechanisms (Fig. 84-1). However, not all retinoblastoma tumors arise in the context of a strong family history. Sporadic retinoblastoma, which is usually unilateral and on average occurs at a slightly older age than familial retinoblastoma, is usually a consequence of somatic mutation in both alleles of the *RB* gene without any germline predisposition at all.

Another tumor suppressor gene is the p53 gene on chromosome 17p, which is frequently altered in solid tumors. p53 is somewhat unusual for a tumor suppressor gene in that missense mutations that produce a dominant negative protein product may also be growth promoting, so that not all alterations obliterate function. Given the role of p53 in a variety of tumors (mutations in p53 are found in nearly half of human tumors), it is not surprising that germline mutations in p53 have dramatic consequences, resulting in a phenotype known as the *Li-Fraumeni syndrome*, where affected individuals may develop a variety of sarcomas, brain tumors, and leukemia. Figure 84-2 illustrates a typical pedigree of this devastating disorder.

In many instances, the discovery of genes responsible for familial cancer syndromes has provided insight into the normal control of cell growth. For instance, in type I neurofibromatosis—one of the more common dominant disorders of humans—positional cloning efforts uncovered a previously unknown gene on chromosome 17q that, when mutated, produces a clinical phenotype of café au lait spots, neurofibromas, Lisch nodules of the iris, and a predisposition to neurofibrosarcoma and glioma. The responsible gene, which (like many of the genes in Table 84-1) has a close homo-

logue in yeast, is neurofibromin (*NF1*), a critical participant in the regulation of the proto-oncogene *ras*. As shown in Fig. 84-3, the NF1 protein is a GTPase-activating protein (GAP) that normally acts to convert *ras* from its active, growth-promoting, GTP-bound form to its inactive, GDP-bound form. Loss of both copies of *NF1* (one copy by inheritance, one by somatic mutation) thus renders a cell vulnerable to overgrowth, since *ras* is left in the "on" position.

While most autosomal dominant inherited cancer syndromes are due to mutations in tumor suppressor genes, there are a few interesting exceptions. Multiple endocrine neoplasia type II, a dominant disorder characterized by pituitary adenomas, medullary carcinoma of the thyroid, and (in some pedigrees) pheochromocytoma, is due to gain-of-function mutations in the proto-oncogene *ret* on chromosome 10. Interestingly, loss-of-function mutations in *ret* cause a totally different phenotype, namely Hirschsprung's disease (aganglionic megacolon) (see Chaps. 340 and 288).

Dominantly inherited colon cancer is sometimes associated with familial polyposis, which is usually due to mutations in the adenoma-

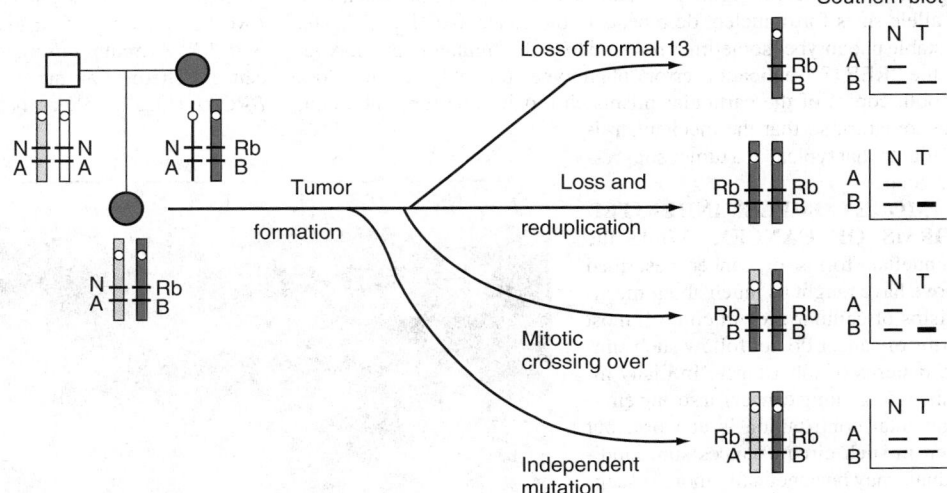

FIGURE 84-1 Diagram of possible mechanisms for tumor formation in an individual with familial retinoblastoma. On the left is shown the pedigree of an affected individual who has inherited the abnormal (RB) allele from her affected mother. The four chromosomes of her two parents are drawn to indicate their origin. Just below the retinoblastoma locus a polymorphic marker is also analyzed in this family. The patient is AB at this locus, like her mother, whereas her father is AA. Thus the B allele must be on the chromosome carrying the retinoblastoma disease gene. Tumor formation results when the normal allele (N), which this patient inherited from her father, is inactivated. On the right are shown four possible ways in which this could occur. In each case, the resulting chromosome 13 arrangement is shown, as well as the results of a Southern blot comparing normal tissue with tumor tissue. Note that in the first three situations the normal allele (A) has been lost in the tumor tissue, which is referred to as loss of heterozygosity. (*From TD Gelehrter and FS Collins, in Principles of Medical Genetics, Baltimore, Williams & Wilkins, 1990, with permission.*)

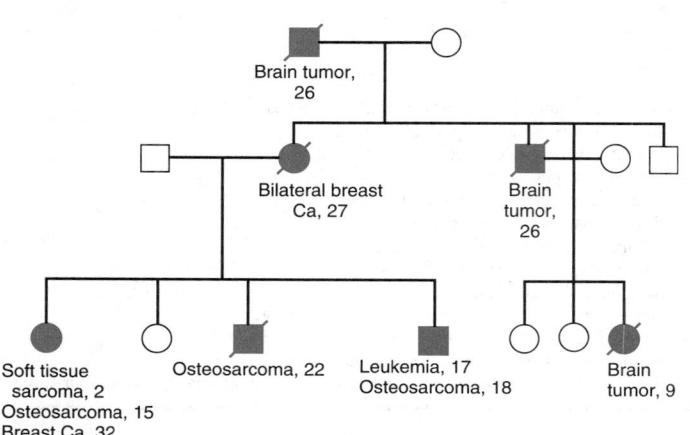

FIGURE 84-2 Pedigree of a family with the Li-Fraumeni syndrome. The affected individuals have developed sarcomas, brain tumors, leukemia, and breast cancer at an early age. All of the affected individuals were found to have a germline mutation in codon 252 of the p53 gene. *(After D Malkin, et al, Science 250:1233, 1990, with permission.)*

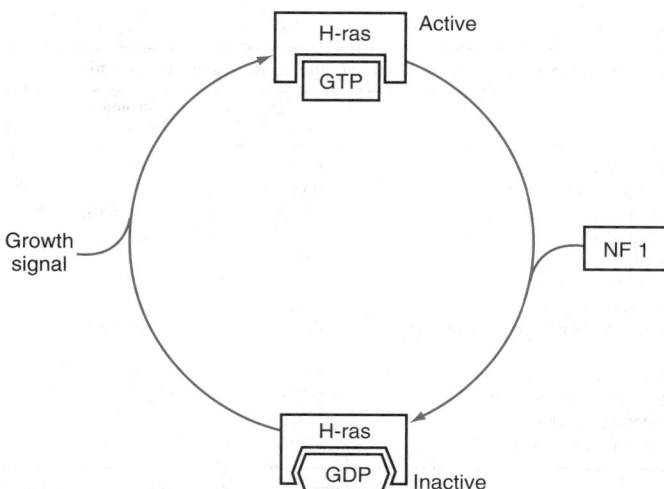

FIGURE 84-3 The *ras* pathway. The active form of the *ras* protein binds GTP and promotes cell division. The conversion to the inactive form, which binds GDP, is catalyzed by a number of proteins including the protein product of the neurofibromatosis type I (*NF1*) gene. Thus, loss of function of NF1 has the effect of leaving *ras* in the "on" position. Alternatively, mutations in the *ras* protein that block its inactivation also predispose to cancer.

tous polyposis coli (*APC*) tumor suppressor gene on chromosome 5 (Table 84-1). However, in most colon cancer families, affected individuals do not have familial polyposis, but instead the cancer arises from normal-appearing epithelium. Hereditary nonpolyposis colon cancer (HNPCC, or Lynch's syndrome) is commonly defined as the occurrence of colon cancer in at least three individuals over at least two generations and with at least one individual diagnosed under the age of 50. As many as 1 in 200 individuals in the general population may have HNPCC, although this number is somewhat controversial. Most HNPCC is due to mutations in one of four DNA mismatch repair genes (Table 84-2). All four of these genes are components of a repair system that is normally responsible for correcting errors in freshly copied DNA. Tumors in patients with HNPCC are characterized by profound genomic instability, especially for short repeated sequences called *microsatellites*. Figure 84-4 shows an example of the instability in allele sizes for dinucleotide repeats in the cancers in HNPCC. The unstable phenotype [sometimes referred to as the "mutator" phenotype, or the "RER⁺" (replication error) phenotype] probably requires loss of both copies of the particular mismatch repair gene (one inherited, one somatic), so that the mechanism is similar to that typical of a tumor suppressor gene.

MORE COMPLEX INHERITED FORMS OF CANCER While the Mendelian forms of cancer described above have taught us much about mechanisms of cellular growth control, most forms of cancer do not follow such simple patterns of inheritance. In many instances (e.g., lung cancer), a strong environmental contribution is at work, but even in such circumstances some individuals may be genetically more susceptible to developing cancer given the appropriate exposure.

In the case of breast and ovarian cancer, circumstantial evidence indicates that a subset of affected individuals (perhaps 5 to 10 percent) might be accounted for by dominantly inherited high-penetrance susceptibility genes, and two of these genes have been identified by positional cloning. *BRCA1*, located on chromosome 17, is capable

Table 84-2

Genetic Alterations in Kindreds With Hereditary Nonpolyposis Colon Cancer (HNPCC)

Gene	Percent of Cases
MSH2	31
MLH1	33
PMS1	2
PMS2	4

SOURCE: Liu B et al, Nature Med 2:169, 1996

when mutated of producing a high risk (perhaps as high as 85 percent lifelong) of breast cancer and also of ovarian cancer (perhaps 50 percent lifelong risk). Roughly 1 in 500 women carries a germline *BRCA1* mutation, often giving rise to a strong family history. Men with *BRCA1* mutations may have a modestly increased risk of prostate cancer. There is an array of mutational heterogeneity described for *BRCA1* (Fig. 84-5), as is often the case for genetic disorders. An

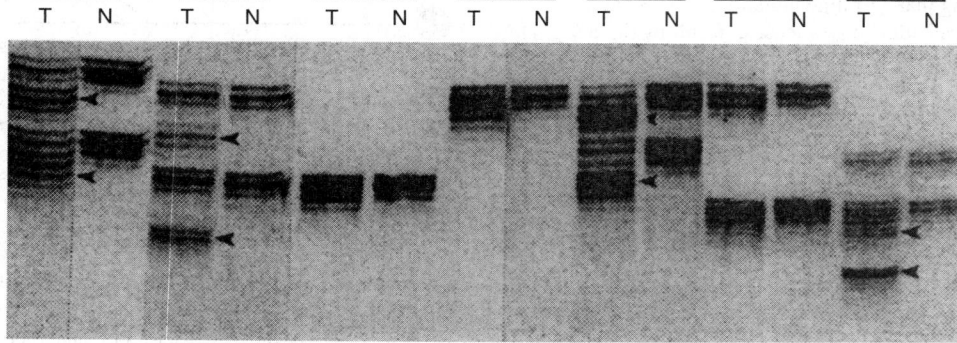

FIGURE 84-4 Demonstration of microsatellite instability in normal and tumor tissue from HNPCC (hereditary nonpolyposis colon cancer) patients. In each case the lane marked T contains DNA from a tumor, and the lane marked N contains DNA from normal tissue of the same patient. The marker (*D2S123*, located on chromosome 2) is a microsatellite composed of a tandem repeat of the dinucleotide CA, which varies in length from chromosome to chromosome. Normally, however, the length of the repeat is stable in somatic tissues. In this example, a polymerase chain reaction analysis has been applied to genomic DNA, and new alleles for the marker are apparent in tumors 1, 2, 5, and 7. Because the tumor tissue is defective in DNA mismatch repair, clonal abnormalities in copying of the CA repeat have arisen. Errors are also occurring in functional genes, eventually resulting in the malignant phenotype. *(From LA Aaltonen et al, Clues to the pathogenesis of familial colorectal cancer. Science 260:812, 1993, with permission.)*

exception is the Ashkenazi Jewish population, where 1 in 100 individuals carries a particular 2-bp deletion (denoted 185delAG) of *BRCA1,* apparently as a consequence of descent from a common ancestor.

Mutations in another gene on chromosome 13, *BRCA2,* also confer a high risk of breast cancer (and a somewhat lower risk of ovarian cancer), and men with *BRCA2* mutations are also prone to develop breast cancer. The frequency of *BRCA2* mutations is estimated to be about half that of *BRCA1.* About 1 percent of Ashkenazi Jews again have a common mutation: 6174delT.

What then of the 90 to 95 percent of breast cancers that arise in individuals without germline alterations in *BRCA1* or *BRCA2?* Hereditary factors may still contribute to a significant fraction of these, but those factors must be weaker and therefore more difficult to discern. One such factor may be the heterozygous state for mutations in the ataxia telangiectasia gene at 11q22. Such individuals have as much as a four- to fivefold increased risk of breast cancer and are likely to represent about 1 percent of the population.

GENETIC TESTING AND COUNSELING FOR CANCER SUSCEPTIBILITY The discovery of genes like *RB,* p53, *NF1, ret,* the HNPCC mismatch repair genes, *BRCA1,* and *BRCA2* raises the possibility of DNA analysis to predict risk of cancer. There are many complexities associated with such testing. First, one must know the sensitivity and specificity of the test; the mutational heterogeneity for each of these genes constitutes a considerable technical challenge, as it is often necessary to sample every nucleotide of the coding region, the splice junctions, and the promoter to identify most mutations. False-positive results, i.e., sequence alterations that turn out to be benign polymorphic variants (allelic variations) rather than disease-causing mutations, can present a thorny problem. Unless proven interventions are available and the test is sensitive, specific, and relatively inexpensive, it will be inappropriate to offer such tests to the general population, as the number of false-positive tests will exceed the number of true positives and a great deal of anxiety and expense will be incurred evaluating persons who are not at an increased risk. Generally, therefore, such testing is not considered except for individuals of higher-than-normal risk, usually on the basis of their family history. In deciding whether to offer such testing, it is critical to determine whether evidence exists for effective interventions to reduce the risk of cancer in those found to be at high risk. If such interventions do not exist (as is the case for Li-Fraumeni syndrome), then the value of the information is limited, and the major negative psychological consequences of this information must be seriously considered. For conditions such as colon and breast cancer, prophylactic measures exist (total colectomy and bilateral mastectomy, respectively), but these prophylactic measures are more radical and potentially disfiguring than the surgical procedures that would be used to treat the patient if the malignancies actually occurred (segmental bowel resection and

lumpectomy, respectively). Other potential negative consequences of a positive genetic test include insurance and employment discrimination. One can still argue, of course, that a close relative of an individual known to carry a mutation in a cancer-causing gene is already sensitized to their personal risk of cancer, and that a test that establishes that an individual at risk does *not* harbor the mutation can be quite useful. Testing should never be undertaken, however, without a full consideration of how the individual will handle a positive as well as a negative result.

Despite these caveats, there are some cancer syndromes for which genetic testing already appears to have greater benefits than risks, and in those situations it is reasonable to offer testing to individuals at high risk. This would include conditions such as multiple endocrine neoplasia type 2 (see Chap. 340) and von Hippel–Lindau disease (see Chap. 375). More in the gray zone, although potentially applicable to much larger numbers of individuals, are tests for *BRCA1, BRCA2,* and the HNPCC genes. More research is urgently needed in those situations to determine the effectiveness of various interventions (lifestyle, diet, surveillance, or surgery). Until those answers are available, such testing should be offered only as part of a research protocol. As more susceptibility genes are identified, better answers become available about the effectiveness of interventions, and health insurance discrimination is legislatively prohibited, genetic testing will move into the mainstream of medicine. Every physician of the future will need to have the skills of a genetic counselor.

ACQUIRED MUTATIONS IN CANCER The identification of mutations in the germline of patients with heritable cancers means that the alteration is present in every cell of the body. However, in most cancers, a normal cell becomes a malignant cell by a series of mutations that do not arise in the germline but in somatic cells. Usually mutations must occur in several genes to give rise to neoplasia. The underlying questions are "how many mutations cause a cancer?" and "what specific genes are affected?" rather than whether or not mutational events cause cancer.

While answers to these questions are not available for every human malignancy, advances in molecular and cellular biology and epidemiologic analyses of human and experimental cancers are providing insights in cancer causation. Table 84-3 summarizes evidence from several lines of investigation pointing to a mutational basis for cancer causation. One particularly striking feature is the fact that the overall incidence of cancer increases as the fourth to sixth power of age for most malignancies (Fig. 84-6A). For some tumors, the shape of the age-incidence curve suggests heterogeneity in molecular mechanisms. For example, Hodgkin's disease has a bimodal age distribution, sug-

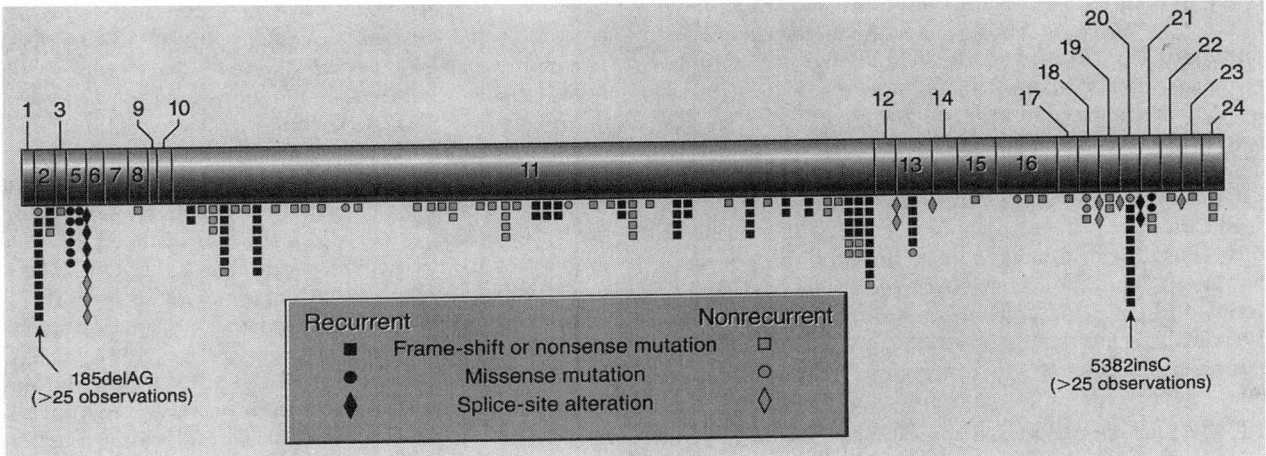

FIGURE 84-5 Germline mutations that have been reported in the *BRCA1* gene, primarily found in families with a high incidence of breast cancer, ovarian cancer, or both. The numbers refer to the exons of the gene; there is no exon 4. (*Information is provided courtesy of the Breast Cancer Information Core data base, which is accessible on the World Wide Web at http://www.nchgr.nih.gov/dir/lab_transfer/bic/.*)

Table 84-3

Table 84-3

Evidence That Mutations Cause Cancer

Malignant tumors are clonal in nature
Some cancers show a Mendelian pattern of inheritance
DNA from malignant cells can in some instances transform normal cells to
    a malignant phenotype
Most tumors contain somatic mutations in oncogenes and/or tumor
    suppressor genes
Recurring sites of chromosome change are observed in cancers at the sites
    of genes involved in cellular growth control
Most carcinogens are mutagens
Defects in DNA repair systems increase the probability of cancer

gesting that two etiologically (and therefore mutationally) distinct forms of this disease may exist (Fig. 84-6*B*).

MULTISTEP BASIS OF CANCER From 5 to 10 accumulated mutations are thought to be necessary for a cell to move from the normal to the fully malignant phenotype. At each step, the mutated cell may gain a slight growth advantage, so that it is increased in its representation relative to its neighbors. Figure 84-7, a representation of a lineage diagram hypothesized by Peter Nowell, illustrates how a single cell, afflicted with progressive alterations in tumor suppressor genes and proto-oncogenes, can develop into a clonal malignancy.

We are beginning to understand the precise nature of the genetic alterations responsible for some malignancies and to get a sense of the order in which they occur. Perhaps the best studied example is colon cancer, where an analysis of DNA from tissues extending from normal epithelium through adenoma to carcinoma have identified some of the genes mutated along the way (Fig. 84-8). However, the order of mutational events is far from uniform, and the diagram in Fig. 84-8 should be considered a generalization and not a rigorous depiction. Similar data are being accumulated for other malignancies.

MECHANISMS OF SOMATIC MUTATION OF ONCOGENES IN MALIGNANCY Cellular proto-oncogenes, their necessity and importance in normal cell growth, and their responsibility for transformation-associated change after removal of normal growth controls are discussed in Chap. 83. Mechanisms that upregulate (or activate) cellular proto-oncogenes can be grouped into three broad areas: point mutations, DNA amplification, and chromosome rearrangements.

Point Mutation A proto-oncogene that is commonly activated in solid tumors by point mutation is a member of the *ras* family of oncogenes; these were initially cloned from human bladder carcinoma cells and are critical regulators of normal and aberrant cell growth (Fig. 84-3). Mutations in one of the *ras* genes (H-*ras*, K-*ras*, or N-*ras*) are present in up to 15 percent of all human cancers. In studies of K-*ras* (particularly in lung and colon cancer), the mutational spectrum of this gene has been identified. Remarkably, and in contrast to the diversity of mutations observed in the *BRCA1* gene (Fig. 84-5), most of these activated genes contain point mutations in codons 12 or 61 (which convey resistance to the inactivating action of GAP). The specificity of this pattern of mutation means that it has potential value in diagnostic or prognostic studies of cancer. For K-*ras*, mutations may be a useful prognostic marker in lung cancer, but for most other cancers (including pancreas and colon cancer) no prognostic utility has been demonstrated. This is in part because *ras* mutations occur early in colon cancer (Fig. 84-8), being common in precancerous lesions of the bowel.

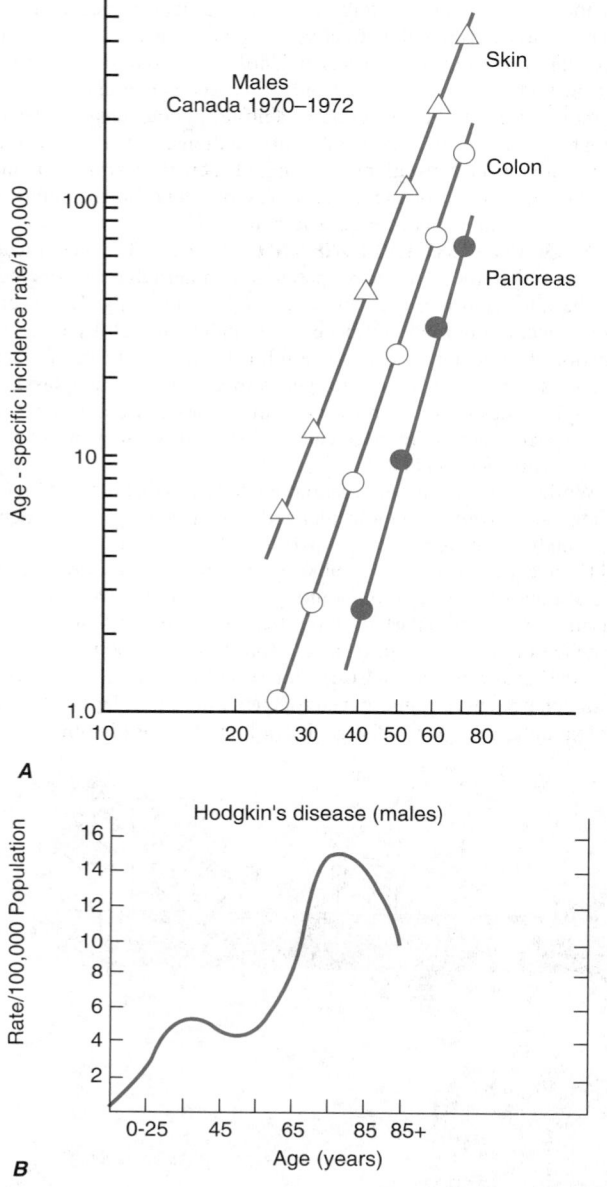

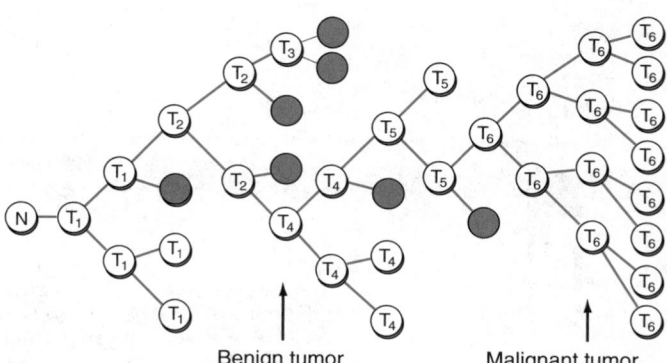

FIGURE 84-6 Relationship between age and cancer incidence. *A*. Age-specific incidence of skin, colon, and pancreas cancers in Canadian males. The curves appear as straight lines when plotted using logarithmic axes, fitting the multihit model of cancer (see text). *B*. For some tumor types (e.g., Hodgkin's disease), a bimodal age distribution is seen, perhaps indicative of a differing mutational basis (see text). (*From Tannock and Hall, with permission.*)

FIGURE 84-7 Multistep clonal development of malignancy. In this diagram, a series of five cumulative mutations (T1, T2, T4, T5, T6), each with a modest growth advantage acting alone, eventually results in a malignant tumor. Note that not all such alterations result in progression; for example, the T3 clone is a dead end. The actual number of cumulative mutations necessary to transform from the normal to the malignant state is unknown in most tumors. (*After P Nowell, Science 194:23, 1976, with permission.*)

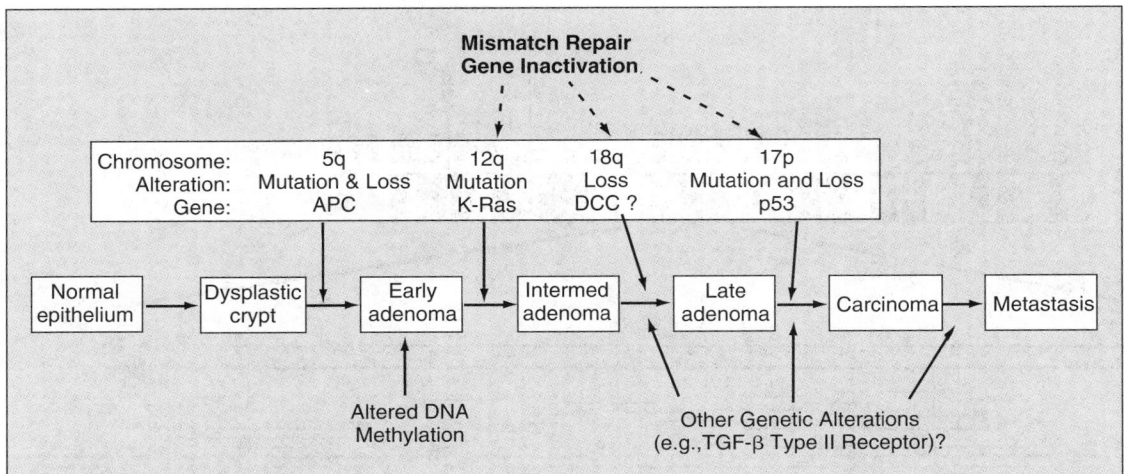

FIGURE 84-8 Progressive somatic mutational steps in the development of colon carcinoma. The accumulation of alterations in a number of different genes results in the progression from normal epithelium through early adenoma to full blown carcinoma. While the steps shown here do not always occur in this order, it is clear that an accumulation of somatic mutations is required before cancer develops. Patients with familial polyposis are already one step into this pathway, since they inherit a germline alteration of the *APC* gene.

DNA Amplification The second mechanism for activation of oncogene overexpression is DNA sequence amplification. This increase in DNA sequence copy number may cause cytologically recognizable chromosome alterations referred to as *homogeneous staining regions* (HSRs), if integrated within chromosomes, or *double minutes* (dmins), if extrachromosomal in nature (Fig. 84-9).

The recognition of DNA amplification was greatly facilitated by the development of a procedure based upon dual-color fluorescence in situ hybridization (FISH) called *comparative genomic hybridization* (CGH). DNA from tumor and normal cells is labeled with different fluorescent reporter molecules and then hybridized to normal metaphase chromosomes. Regions of duplications and deletions within tumor DNA are then demonstrated as quantifiable alterations in signal intensity at particular sites. With this technique, the entire genome can be surveyed for gains and losses of DNA sequences, thus pinpointing chromosomal regions likely to contain genes important in the development or progression of cancer.

Numerous genes are known to be amplified in human malignancies. Several genes including N-*myc* were identified because they were present within the amplified DNA sequences of a tumor and had homology to known oncogenes. Because the region amplified often extends to hundreds of thousands of base pairs, more than one oncogene may be amplified in some cancers (particularly sarcomas). Figure 84-10 illustrates the complex pattern of amplification observed in human sarcomas for a gene-dense region on human chromosome 12; genes simultaneously amplified in many cases include *MDM2*, *GLI*, *CDK4*, *SAS*, and others implicated in cellular growth control. The clinical implications of gene amplification have been explored for some cancers (most notably *ERBB2* in breast cancer and N-*myc* in neuroblastoma), and demonstration of amplification of a cellular gene is usually a predictor of poor prognosis. Once a patient has been exposed to the selective effects of chemotherapy, gene amplification may lead to drug resistance. Amplification of the dihydrofolate reductase gene may follow clinical exposure to methotrexate, a drug that inhibits the activity of the enzyme.

Chromosomal Alterations in Human Cancer Chromosomal alterations provide important clues as to the genetic changes in cancers. To date, most chromosome analyses have been performed on hematopoietic cancers, although solid tumors may also have translocations. The breakpoints of several recurring chromosome abnormalities often occur at the sites of cellular proto-oncogenes. Translocations are particularly common in lymphoid tumors, probably because these cell types normally rearrange DNA to generate antigen receptors. Indeed, antigen receptor genes are commonly involved in the translocations, implying that an imperfect regulation of receptor gene rearrangement may be involved in the pathogenesis. An example is Burkitt's lymphoma,

a B cell tumor characterized by a reciprocal translocation between chromosomes 8 and 14. Molecular analysis of Burkitt's lymphomas demonstrated that the breakpoints occurred within or near the *myc* locus on chromosome 8 and within the immunoglobulin heavy chain locus on chromosome 14, resulting in the transcriptional activation of

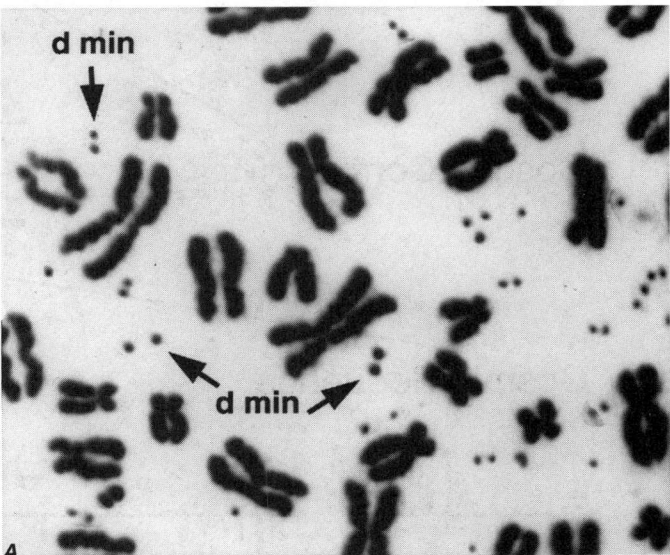

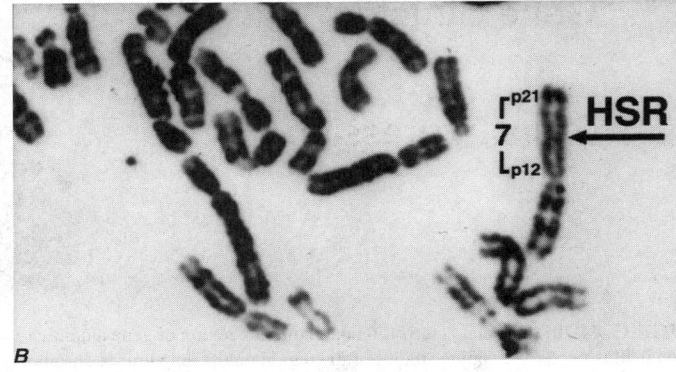

FIGURE 84-9 Representative examples of tumor cells containing cytogenetic evidence of gene amplification. *A.* Example of multiple copies of double minute (dmin) chromosomes from a patient with ovarian carcinoma. *B.* Example of a homogeneous staining region (HSR) on chromosome 7 from a patient with malignant melanoma.

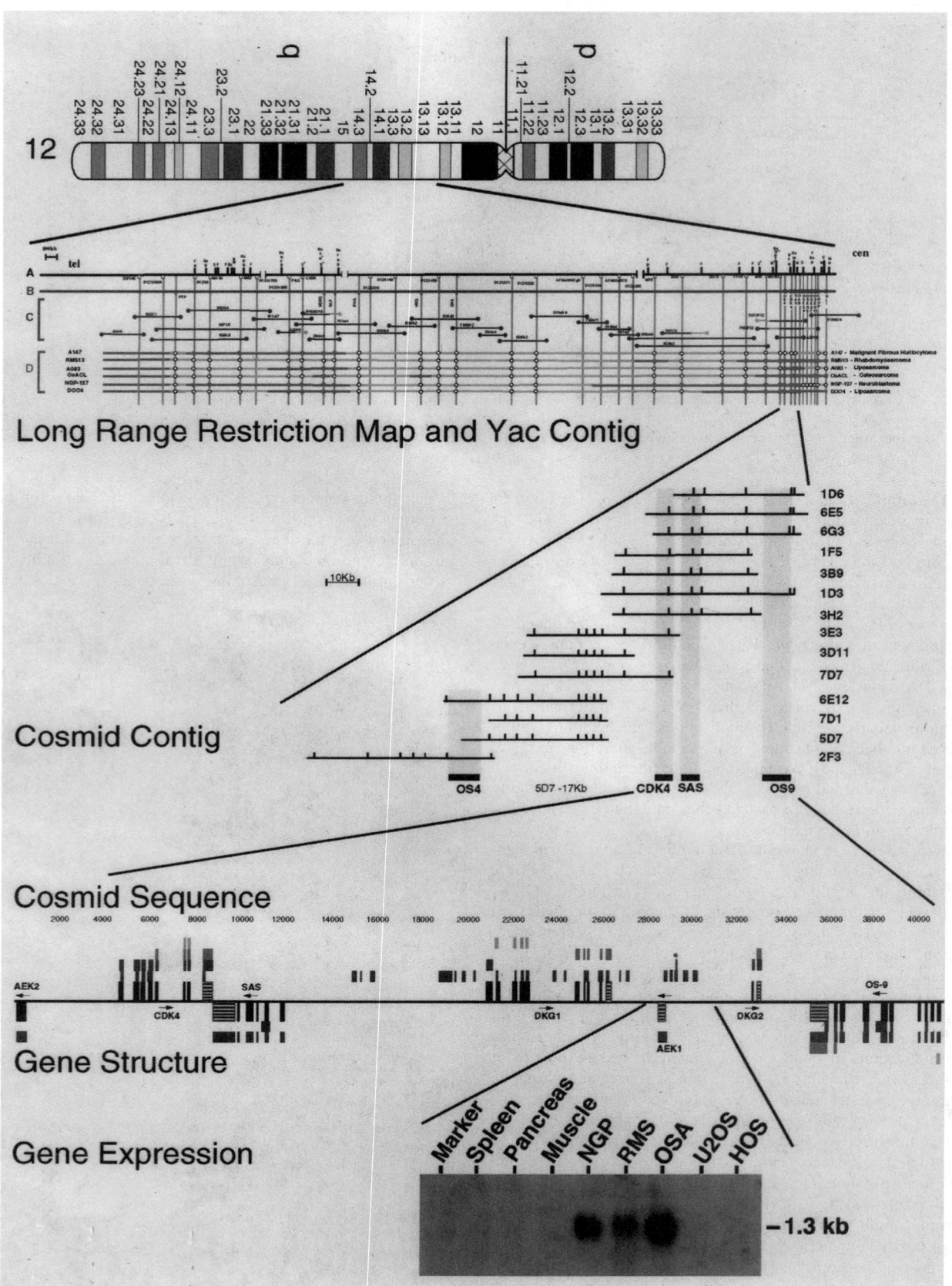

FIGURE 84-10 The characterization of a complex region of gene amplification is illustrated by mapping studies of the region on the long arm of chromosome 12 encoding the p53 regulator *MDM2* and the cyclin-dependent kinase *CDK4*. This region is frequently amplified in a subset of brain tumors and sarcomas. As shown at the top of the illustration, the amplicon is initially mapped at the relatively coarse level of the metaphase chromosome. Techniques of physical mapping are then used to define the segment(s) of the chromosome that contribute to the amplicon in various tumors. This defines the core region(s), which presumably contain the target gene(s). Higher resolution mapping and DNA sequencing are then applied to the core in order to localize genes within cosmids and their DNA sequence. Ultimately, the expression level of the genes identified in the amplification core is determined. (*Courtesy of AG Elkahloun and P Meltzer, NCHGR, NIH*).

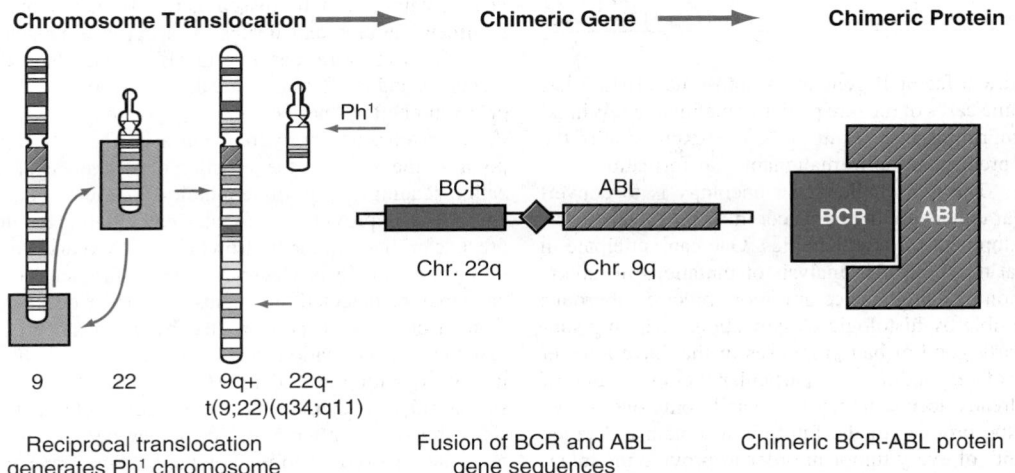

Chromosome Translocation ⟶ **Chimeric Gene** ⟶ **Chimeric Protein**

Ph¹

BCR   ABL   BCR   ABL

Chr. 22q   Chr. 9q

9   22   9q+   22q-
          t(9;22)(q34;q11)

Reciprocal translocation   Fusion of BCR and ABL   Chimeric BCR-ABL protein
generates Ph¹ chromosome   gene sequences

FIGURE 84-11 Specific translocation seen in chronic myelogenous leukemia (CML). The Philadelphia chromosome (Ph) is derived from a reciprocal translocation between chromosomes 9 and 22 with the breakpoint joining the sequences of the *ABL* oncogene with the *BCR* gene. The fusion of these DNA sequences allows the generation of an entirely novel fusion protein with modified function (see text). *(Courtesy of ER Fearon and KR Cho.)*

myc. Enhancer activation by translocation, although not universal, appears to play an important role in malignant progression.

Chromosome rearrangements can lead to the abnormal overexpression of a transcription factor that performs its normal function and turns on growth-related genes. The translocation may create a chimeric transcription factor that has altered function. For example, the t(15;17) of acute promyelocytic leukemia produces a retinoic acid receptor with an abnormal cell distribution that inhibits differentiation. Gene rearrangements most commonly involve transcription factors, but other components of signaling pathways may also be involved.

The first reproducible chromosome abnormality detected in human malignancy was the Philadelphia chromosome in chronic myelogenous leukemia (CML). This cytogenetic abnormality is generated by reciprocal translocation involving the *ABL* oncogene, a tyrosine kinase on chromosome 9 being placed in proximity to the *BCR* (breakpoint cluster region) on chromosome 22. Figure 84-11 illustrates the generation of the translocation and its protein product. The consequence of expression of the *BCR-ABL* gene product is the activation of signal transduction pathways, leading to cell growth independent of normal external growth factor signals.

In addition to transcription factors and signal transduction molecules, translocations may involve the overexpression of cell cycle regulatory proteins, such as cyclins, and of proteins that regulate cell death, such as bcl2. Table 84-4 lists representative examples of recurring chromosome alterations in malignancy and the associated gene(s) rearranged or dysregulated by the chromosomal change.

Technical obstacles have slowed the identification of recurring chromosome abnormalities in human solid tumors (particularly carcinomas) because of the complexity of chromosome alterations in such tumors, in contrast to the solitary, often reciprocal, nature of chromosome rearrangements in hematopoietic malignancies.

EPIGENETIC REGULATION OF GENE EXPRESSION AND CANCER   The term *epigenetic* refers to mechanisms of gene regulation independent of DNA sequence. The inactivation of the second X chromosome in female cells is an example of an epigenetic mechanism that prevents gene expression from the inactivated chromosome. During embryologic development, entire regions of chromosomes from one parent are silenced and gene expression proceeds from the chromosome of the other parent. For most genes, expression occurs from both parental alleles or randomly from one parent or the other. The preferential expression of a particular gene exclusively from the allele contributed by one parent is called *parental imprinting* and is thought to be regulated by the methylation of the silenced allele.

The role of epigenetic control mechanisms in the development of human cancer is unclear. However, a general decrease in the level of DNA methylation has been noted as a common change in cancers. In addition, the loss of imprinting of the normally silent maternal allele

Table 84-4

Representative Oncogenes at Chromosomal Translocations

Gene (Chromosome)	Translocation	Malignancy
ABL (9q34.1) *BCR* (22q11)	(9;22)(q34;q11)	Chronic myelogenous leukemia
AML1 (21q22) *EAP* (3q26) *EVI1* (3q26)	(3;21)(q26;q22)	Acute myelogenous leukemia, myelodysplasia
ATF1 (12q13) *EWS* (22q12)	(12;22)(q13;q12)	Malignant melanoma of soft parts (MMSP)
BCL1 (11q13.3) *IgH* (14q32)	(11;14)(q13;q32)	Mantle cell lymphoma
BCL2 (18q21.3) *IgH* (14q32)	(14;18)(q32;q21)	Follicular lymphoma
BCL3 (19q13.1) *IgH* (14q32)	(14;19)(q32;q13)	B cell chronic lymphocytic leukemia
ERG (21q22.3) *EWS* (22q12)	(22;21)(q12;q22)	Ewing's sarcoma
FLI1 (11q24) *EWS* (22q12)	(11;22)(q24;q12)	Ewing's sarcoma
LCK (1p34) *TCRB* (7q35)	(1;7)(p34;q35)	T cell acute lymphocytic leukemia (ALL)
MLL/ALL1/HRX (11q23)	(4;11)(q21;q23)	ALL
myc (8q24)	(8;14)(q24;q32)	Burkitt's lymphoma, B cell ALL
TAN1 (9q34) deletion	(7;9)(q34;q34)	T cell ALL
WT1 (11p13) *EWS* (22q12)	(11;22)(p13;q12)	Desmoplastic small round cell tumor (DSRCT)
TLS/FUS (16p11) *CHOP* (12q13)	(12;16)(q13;p11)	Myxoid liposarcoma
PAX3 (2q35) *FKHR/ALV* (13q14)	(2;13)(q35;q14)	Alveolar rhabdomyosarcoma
PAX7 (1p36) *KHR/ALV* (13q14)	(1;13)(p36;q14)	Alveolar rhabdomyosarcoma
ret (10q11.2)	(10;17)(q11.2;q23)	Papillary thyroid carcinomas

SOURCE: After Hesketh.

of the insulin-like growth factor II gene at chromosome 11p15.5 has been implicated in some cases of the rare pediatric malignancy, Wilms' tumor. The loss of imprinting may result in the overexpression of the growth factor and a predisposition to malignant transformation.

THE FUTURE The real challenge in oncology is to convert the growing molecular understanding of cancer into clinical advances, particularly the development of new therapies. One can anticipate in the coming years that the molecular analysis of mutations in tumors will allow stratification of malignancies into more precise subgroups than is currently possible by histologic classification, including subgroups with particularly good or bad prognoses or that have a lower or higher likelihood of responding to a particular therapy. Some of this information is already accumulating, but usually only one or two genes are assessed; the promise of the future is to obtain a detailed molecular "fingerprint" of every tumor in order to provide the maximum information about its biology and response to therapy.

Genetics will also influence cancer prevention and early detection. The ability to identify cancer susceptibility genes presages a new era of cancer prevention, if the potential risks of such testing can be surmounted. Currently, most cancer early detection strategies (such as mammography, stool occult blood testing, or digital rectal examination) are applied to population groups. The ability to identify the individuals at highest risk and to focus preventive medicine efforts accordingly may be both better received by patients and more cost effective. Early detection strategies will be even more effective if we can develop the ability to identify very small numbers of malignant or premalignant cells at a time when the risk of metastasis is still very low.

More importantly, detailed molecular information about the regulation of the cell cycle and the interplay of tumor suppressor genes and proto-oncogenes that control it may lead to new effective therapies, based on pathophysiology rather than empiricism. Whether such strategies will rely on drugs of the traditional types or will be based on more novel strategies such as gene therapy or immunotherapy is hard to predict.

BIBLIOGRAPHY

COLLINS FS: BRCA1—lots of mutations, lots of dilemmas. N Engl J Med 334:186, 1996

ELKAHLOUN AG et al: Molecular cytogenetic characterization and physical mapping of 12q13-15 amplification in human cancers. Genes Chromosomes Cancer 17:205, 1996

FEARON ER, CHO KR: The molecular biology of cancer, in *Principles and Practice of Medical Genetics,* AE Emery, DL Rimoin (eds). New York, Churchill Livingstone, 1996, chap 20.

HEIM S, MITELMAN F: *Cancer Cytogenetics,* 2d ed. New York, Wiley, 1995

HESKETH R: *The Oncogene Facts Book.* San Diego, Academic Press, 1995

PARK M: Oncogenes: Genetic abnormalities of cell growth, in *The Metabolic and Molecular Bases of Inherited Disease,* 7th ed, CR Scriver et al (eds). New York, McGraw-Hill, 1995, chap 10

TANNOCK I, HALL R: *The Basic Science of Oncology,* 2d ed. New York, McGraw-Hill, 1992

VOGELSTEIN B, KINZLER KW: The multistep nature of cancer. Trends Genet 9:138, 1993

85 *Elise C. Kohn, Lance A. Liotta*

INVASION AND METASTASIS

Unregulated cellular proliferation may produce a neoplastic growth, but the defining features of malignancy are invasion and metastasis. A malignant neoplasm is a new growth with the potential to invade locally and/or to metastasize to distant sites in the body. Malignant neoplasms are the second most common cause of death in the industrialized world, leading to more than 500,000 deaths in the United States

yearly, with metastatic dissemination primarily responsible for most treatment failures and deaths. Metastasis is present in an occult or overt form in more than two-thirds of patients at the time of initial diagnosis and is often multifocal, making localized surgery, radiation, or chemotherapy ineffective.

Invasion is necessary for metastasis. The critical pathologic turning point for the patient is the initiation of local invasion and neovascularization leading to the dissemination of tumor cells. Tumor-induced angiogenesis provides a vascular entry portal for dispersal that may precede primary tumor outgrowth by many years (Fig. 85-1A). Circulation of tumor cells is necessary but not sufficient, as circulating tumor cells may be detected in patients who never develop metastases. This clinical observation is supported by experimental studies indicating that metastasis initiation from circulating tumor cells is a low probability event, with fewer than 0.05 percent of circulating tumor cells successfully developing metastatic foci. Metastasis, like tumorigenesis, occurs only after a sufficient number of tumor cells with the requisite genotypic and phenotypic changes enter the circulation.

Invasion is the active translocation of neoplastic cells across tissue barriers and through host cellular and extracellular matrix barriers. It is not simply due to growth pressure but requires additional genetic and signaling dysregulation over that which caused malignant transformation. Invasion results from an imbalance and dysregulation of otherwise normal stimulatory and inhibitory events. Tightly controlled invasion occurs in many normal physiologic events, such as organ maintenance or remodeling, pregnancy and development, and wound healing. In cancer, this regulation is absent or attenuated so that malignant cells may not respond to signals originating from their environment and may rely on their own autocrine stimulation. In addition to invasion, metastasis requires angiogenesis and malignant cell proliferation. Successful metastasis requires that cells reach the secondary location, that they form colonies successfully at the secondary site, and that they avoid local and systemic host defenses. Thus, the process of invasion is a relatively individual process whereby the cell must be able to execute each of the required steps.

Historically, the changes occurring in the organization and integrity of the epithelial basement membrane have been considered by pathologists as the histologic markers of the transition from carcinoma in situ to invasive cancer (Fig. 85-1B). An early step that can be detected by simple histopathology is the interruption of basement membrane barriers in epithelial tumors. The basement membrane is a dense, acellular structure onto which epithelial or endothelial cells attach. It provides an infrastructure to support organ architecture or the vascular network. It is composed of a variety of glycoproteins and carbohydrates organized into a formidable barrier. The degradation of local basement membrane and surrounding interstitial stroma is necessary for invasion but is not sufficient for distant dissemination of malignant cells. The human breast provides an example of the progressive change from benign to malignant and invasive. Benign proliferative disorders of the human breast such as fibroadenoma, intraductal hyperplasia, and fibrocystic disease are all characterized by a continuous basement membrane separating the breast epithelium from its stroma. In contrast, multiple defects are found in the basement membrane of infiltrating malignancy. Defects in the basement membrane may also be observed adjacent or proximal to malignant cells in lymph nodes or at the site of parenchymal organ metastases.

Invasion and neovascularization may be very early events in cancer, frequently occurring even years before clinical detection. Invasion is required for advancement from in situ disease, and new blood vessel formation for adequate nutritional support for the growing tumors and as conduits for escape. Figure 85-1 shows a hypothetical time scale for the development of breast cancer. Note that invasion and angiogenesis occur several years before diagnosis, and that occult or overt metastases are present at the time of diagnosis. This is consistent with the data that in situ carcinoma of the breast is very infrequent.

Carcinomas can spread by both lymphatic and hematogenous routes, and metastases are found most commonly in organs fed by the downstream lymphatic and blood flow (Table 85-1). Sarcomas disseminate predominantly by vascular spread. In some cases, unusual

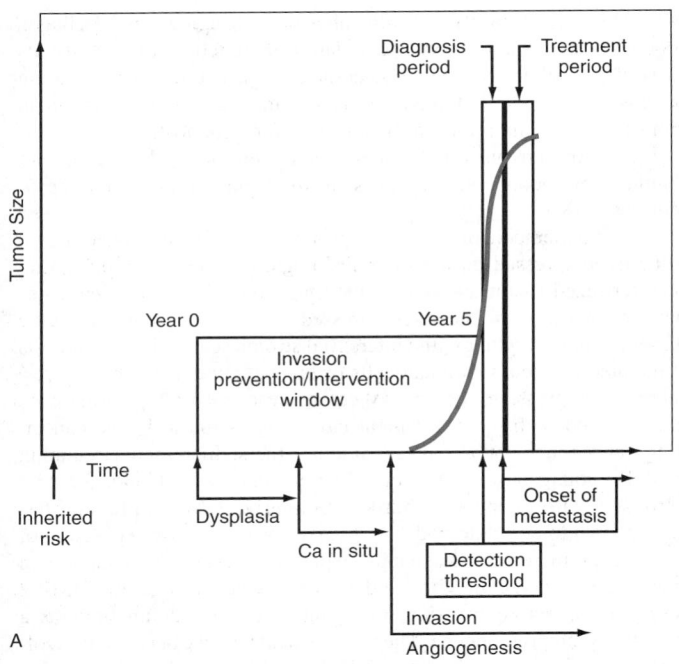

FIGURE 85-1 Cancer progression. *A.* Time course of cancer development and dissemination. This hypothetical time course shows the early initiation of angiogenesis and invasion in tumor progression. Diagnosis and treatment of cancer usually occur late in the disease course, when a high proportion of patients already have established occult or overt metastases. In contrast, progression through dysplasia to carcinoma in situ and the acquisition of the invasive and angiogenic phenotype may extend back over a period of years. This may define a window for therapeutic intervention before onset of metastasis. *B.* Progression to metastasis and associated genetic changes. Phenotypic progression from normal to hyperplastic, through carcinoma in situ to the initiation of invasion and angiogenesis, leads to metastatic dissemination. Through new techniques in molecular diagnostics, gene loss through mutation and deletion and increased expression through amplification can now be more readily defined. The processes of invasion, angiogenesis, and metastasis are associated with both metastasis-suppressor genes, such as *nm*23 and E-cadherin, and metastasis-promoting genes, such as matrix metalloproteinases and autotaxin. Chromosomal mapping and microdissection of tumor cells with their adjacent normal cells will allow for a more detailed analysis of the genetic changes involved in metastasis and lead to new targets for diagnostics and therapeutics.

sites of metastases have been documented and may be explained by a permissive environment.

ANGIOGENESIS Angiogenesis is the process of blood vessel formation. Under normal conditions in the adult, neovascularization is limited to menstruation, pregnancy, and wound healing. During angiogenesis, normally quiescent endothelial cells acquire an invasive phenotype, breaching their own basement membrane to invade into interstitial stroma during the development of new capillary buds. These cells return to a quiescent and noninvasive phenotype when the angiogenic stimulus ceases. These angiogenic stimuli may include tumor-derived growth factors, extracellular matrix components, and endothelial cell–derived factors. The development of new vessels has been found to be a critical component of tumor development, benign and malignant; it is required for nutrient delivery and is necessary for metastatic dissemination. Subpopulations of highly metastatic tumor cells may exist at a very early stage in the development of primary tumors. It has been calculated that metastases from breast carcinomas,

for example, may be initiated as early as the point at which the primary tumor becomes vascularized, at a size of less than 0.125 cm². Tumor dormancy, a phenomenon where late or delayed tumor dissemination is observed, may arise as a consequence of inadequate vascular supply.

The clinical importance of vascular development has been demonstrated in several ways. Assessment of tumor vessel number is correlated positively with risk and degree of dissemination in breast cancer (both lymph node–positive and –negative disease), prostate cancer, and ovarian cancer. In addition, several endothelial cell–derived cytokines that stimulate endothelial cell proliferation and migration have also been found to stimulate proliferation of malignant cells and in some cases to be secreted by malignant cells as autocrine and paracrine factors.

Normally endothelial cells are quiescent; however, they can show a 100-fold increase in proliferation during neovascularization. Several antiangiogenic agents have been identified where the primary or secondary targets are the endothelial cells or the process of neovascularization.

Table 85-1

Patterns of Metastasis: Most Common Sites of Spread

	Metastatic Site (% Involvement)							
Primary	Adrenal	Brain	Bone	Skin	Kidney	Lung	Liver	Nodes Local/Distant
Breast	31	23	62	20	17	66	40–60	60–80
Bladder	35	7	26	5	19			
Cervix	31	9	21	3	26			
Colorectum	31	11	27	5	13	16	44	53
Kidney	20	19	10	5	21	72	44	
Lung	35	37	56		16	8	73	83/29
Melanoma	48	48	48	44	27	60	63	58
Ovary	20	3	12	5	6	34	48	48/58
Prostate	17	2	67	3	11	49	36	68

SOURCE: Adapted from Weiss, L: Clin Exp Metastasis 10:191–199, 1992, references inclusive.

INVASION Cellular adhesion, local proteolysis, and locomotion constitute the triad of invasion. While each is necessary for successful metastasis, none is sufficient individually. The cells at the invasive front undergo a dynamic cycling through the steps of invasion, in which they reach out and attach anew to the basement membrane or interstitial stroma. By secretion of proteinases or induction of proteinase secretion by stromal cells, tumor cells create local access through which to migrate into the vasculature or secondary organ sites. The basement membrane may also be a storage depot for latent proteinases or cytokines, released and/or activated during invasion and to which tumor cells or endothelial cells may respond.

Adhesion The interaction of cells with their scaffolding, the extracellular matrix and basement membrane, involves adhesion through specific receptors. Several classes of adhesion molecules have been shown to have critical roles in tumorigenesis. There are several predominant classes of adhesion receptors. These include the extracellular matrix protein receptors, the integrins; transmembrane cell adhesion molecules, the CAMs; and cadherins, extracellular adhesion molecules. The presence of selected adhesion receptors, such as particular integrin subunits, has shown a positive correlation with invasive potential and metastatic dissemination.

There are several members of the cadherin family. Genetic and biochemical analysis has demonstrated marked similarities between family members despite anatomic segregation. E-cadherin, or epithelial cadherin, forms extracellular homotypic interactions creating a functional bond between epithelial cells. Special intracellular proteins, the catenins, are required to link the extracellular cell-cell bond with the cell cytoskeleton. The interaction is regulated at several levels through protein-protein interactions, tyrosine phosphorylation, and cell-cell communication. Mutation or loss at several points along this cell adhesion pathway has been shown to occur naturally in tumors including breast, bladder, endometrial, and lung cancers. Furthermore, mutation or reduced expression has been associated with a more metastatic phenotype. Intact cadherins and catenins suppress metastasis.

The integrin family of cell surface extracellular matrix protein receptors consists of heterodimeric proteins, many of which have promiscuous binding preferences for the glycoproteins of the basement membrane and extracellular matrix. This family of receptors contains members where loss (in cancers such as breast, prostate, and colon) or increased expression (in melanoma and squamous cell cancer of the head and neck) has been associated with a more aggressive phenotype. Integrin occupation and cell surface clustering are critical components of basement membrane remodeling during angiogenesis. Integrin stimulation is necessary to provide a survival stimulus in several settings. For example, ligation of integrin $\alpha v \beta 3$ by melanoma cells is required for survival in collagen matrices. Alternatively, loss of stimulation of integrins has been shown to stimulate apoptosis. Thus, the same signaling pathways necessary for cellular processing of integrin information for adhesion, migration, and metastasis can also, in a different setting, cause cell death. This suggests that integrins may function as a 'go–no go' switch to trigger such diverse functions as metastatic spread or programmed cell death. While adhesion alone may not be sufficient for invasion and distant dissemination, loss of normally signaled adhesion functions may result in more aggressive invasion or loss of metastatic potential.

Proteolysis Degradation of local basement membrane and surrounding interstitial stroma is necessary for invasion, but it alone, like adhesion and motility, is not sufficient for distant dissemination of malignant cells. Important structural components of the basement membrane and interstitial stroma are the collagens, triple helical proteins that help form the latticework of the acellular matrix architecture. The major barrier to invasion is collagen. The interstitial or stromal collagens are generally composed of type I and III collagen, whereas types IV and V are the predominant collagens in the basement membrane. Enzymatic cleavage of the collagens, necessary to provide an escape route for tumor cells, is carried out by matrix metalloproteinases

with substrate selectivity. As with adhesion and angiogenesis, collagen production and collagenolytic degradation are functions of normal cells as well as malignant cells. The collagenases, neutral metal-binding proteases, are a well-studied family of enzymes whose function in metastatic dissemination has been used for prognostic assessment; they are now targets for therapeutic intervention. Collagenases are regulated by endogenous inhibitors, the tissue inhibitors of metalloproteinases (TIMP).

Several members of the metalloproteinase family have been shown to be overexpressed during the physiologic invasion of implantation of a fertilized ovum and during menstruation. These same enzymes have been shown to be overexpressed in the milieu of metastatic dissemination, whether in the interstitial stroma secreted by fibroblasts stimulated by local malignant cells or by the cancer cells themselves. Increased expression of a type IV collagenase (MMP-2, gelatinase A) is associated with increased metastatic progression in breast cancer, lung cancer, and colon cancer, among others. Increased circulating type IV collagenase in the blood of patients with bladder cancer correlates with their tumor burden. Similarly, TIMP expression has been shown to correlate with the invasive process. Overexpression of TIMP-2 or increased exogenous expression results in reduction in invasive phenotype in vitro and in vivo, whereas loss of TIMP-2 results in increased invasion, implying that TIMP-2 functions as a metastasis-suppressor gene. There is a critical balance between proteolysis (e.g., collagenases) and physiologic inhibition (TIMP). In invasive cancer, there is frequently an immediate local imbalance in protease and inhibitor that may not be evident when one studies the organ or individual as a whole. Collagenase excess permits a cell to invade and cross membrane barriers.

Motility The ability to translocate through local rents in the body's structural barriers requires that individual cells have a capacity for locomotion. There is a precedent in normal, physiologic invasion for migration. The movement of endothelial cells during vessel formation requires that a leading cell migrate into the stroma to initiate vascular bud formation. In infection, circulating monocytes must migrate into the stroma to initiate vascular bud formation. Tumor cells, likewise, must be able to migrate from the primary mass to reach a vascular conduit, intravasate, be carried by blood flow to a distant capillary bed, extravasate, and migrate some distance to initiate colony formation. Tumor cell migration can be directed by soluble factors emanating from target host tissues or by factors bound to the extracellular matrix. Soluble factors include cytokines such as hepatocyte growth factor, produced by stromal cells, and autocrine motility stimulatory enzymes such as autotaxin, produced by the tumor cells themselves. The receptor for hepatocyte growth factor is the oncogene, *met*, a tyrosine kinase–containing transmembrane receptor. Overexpression of *met* induces a tumorigenic and metastatic phenotype. Activation of *met* results in induction of an invasive phenotype with increased collagenase production, increased invasive potential in vitro, and metastasis production in vivo. Autotaxin, an exokinase secreted and tethered on the extracellular side of the tumor cell, is an autocrine motility factor. Autotaxin can be clipped near its transmembrane domain to yield the soluble motility-stimulating factor component. Its receptor has autophosphorylation, phosphatase, and phosphodiesterase activity.

Solid-phase migration factors include components of the extracellular matrix and basement membrane. Matrix glycoproteins and collagens can stimulate migration in vitro both as solid-phase attractants and in solution. Fragments of matrix proteins have also been demonstrated to be strong attractants to tumor cells and to cells involved in wound healing, endothelial cells, and fibroblasts. These fragments are produced physiologically by local proteolytic cleavage by invasion-associated proteinases, such as the matrix metalloproteinases that cleave basement membrane and interstitial stromal collagens. Hence, motility, like adhesion and proteolysis, requires interaction with the local environment and is the net balance of the production and secretion of stimulatory factors, such as hepatocyte growth factor and autotaxin; the activation of receptors, such as phosphorylation of *met*; and the response of the tumor and stromal cells.

Other genes have been identified that are specifically related to the invasive and metastatic phenotype. Loss of *nm*23 expression is correlated with increased aggressiveness of breast cancer, both node-positive and -negative. Expression of *nm*23 has also been associated with reduced aggressiveness of ovarian cancer. Experimental reexpression of *nm*23 caused a reduction in metastatic potential and reduced locomotion in vitro. The data define *nm*23 as a metastasis-suppressor gene.

Since invasion and angiogenesis are very early events in the time line of cancer progression leading to metastatic dissemination (Fig. 85-1), they provide novel targets for anticancer drug design. Batimastat (BB-94) is an agent that inhibits the proteolytic activity of type IV collagenase. Intraperitoneal administration of batimastat to animals bearing human ovarian cancer xenografts resulted in marked reduction in the cellularity and quantity of ascites formed, with some reduction in the tumor mass. It has had minimal toxicity in early clinical trials. Endothelial cell replication or invasion has been targeted because of the rare neovascularization occurring under physiologic conditions in adults. New antiangiogenic agents in development include derivatives of the fungal product fumagillin, such as TNP-470, that also have direct antiproliferative effects on cancer cells in vitro and in xenograft models.

Select signal transduction pathways have also been targeted. While dysregulation is not unique to invasion and metastasis of cancer and may be found in many pathologic states, normal cells appear to have better ability to accommodate alteration in their signaling pathways. Signal transduction agents under study include inhibitors of calcium influx, protein kinase C activity, *ras* farnesylation, and tyrosine phosphorylation. Most inhibitors of angiogenesis, metastasis, and signaling have been predominantly cytostatic agents, and many have shown selective anti-invasive and antiangiogenic activity. The cytostatic activity and minimal toxicity observed with these classes of compounds make them ideal candidates as chemopreventive agents against the early development of angiogenesis and invasion.

CONCLUSIONS   The process of tumor invasion and metastasis is a complex cascade of biochemical and genetic events that are mediated by multiple signal transduction pathways and molecular systems. Simultaneously with an improved understanding of invasion and metastasis, new discoveries have yielded insight into the role of tumor heterogeneity, genetic progression, and the molecular events that modulate metastasis. Cellular and biochemical properties that are lost or augmented in metastatic cells will continue to be elucidated as research in this exciting field advances. In the future this knowledge will help identify new targets for diagnostic, therapeutic, and preventive modalities.

BIBLIOGRAPHY

Aaronson SA: Growth factors and cancer. Science 254:1146, 1991

Barsky SH et al: Loss of basement membrane components by invasive tumors but not their benign counterparts. Lab Invest 49:140, 1983

Folkman J: Seminars in medicine of the Beth Israel Hospital, Boston. Clinical applications of research on angiogenesis. N Engl J Med 333:1757, 1995

Kohn EC, Liotta LA: Molecular insights into cancer invasion: Strategies for prevention and intervention. Cancer Res 55:1856, 1995

Liotta LA et al: Quantitative relationships of intravascular tumor cells: Tumor vessels and pulmonary metastases following tumor implantation. Cancer Res 34:997, 1974

———— et al. Cancer metastasis and angiogenesis: An imbalance of positive and negative regulation. Cell 64:327, 1991

Montgomery AMP et al: Integrin alpha v-beta 3 rescues melanoma cells from apoptosis in three-dimensional dermal collagen. Proc Natl Acad Sci USA 91:8856, 1994

Stossel TP: On the crawling of cells. Science 260:1086, 1993

86

Christopher A. Slapak, Donald W. Kufe

PRINCIPLES OF CANCER THERAPY

The development of effective cancer therapy is a major focus of biomedical research. As a result of fundamental and applied research, certain previously lethal malignancies have become curable. Although progress in treating the most common epithelial-derived solid tumors has been slow, advances are leading to improvements in even these recalcitrant diseases. A further understanding of the process of malignant transformation has resulted in the identification of unique targets for therapeutic intervention. The discovery of biologic agents of potential clinical importance continues at a rapid pace. Tumor vaccine and gene transfer strategies are emerging from the laboratory and preclinical testing. New chemotherapeutic drugs, many with novel mechanisms of action, have entered clinical trials. The first differentiating agent effective in the treatment of a malignant disease has recently been approved for clinical use.

Cancer therapy is distributed among three interacting subspecialties. The role of the surgeon, the radiation oncologist, and the medical oncologist will continue to evolve as new agents become clinically available and a multimodality approach to cancer becomes the rule. The primary care physician will remain at the forefront of prevention and early detection of cancer. The further definition of cancer risk factors and the availability of more sensitive and specific screening procedures ensures that the internist will influence cancer morbidity and mortality. The approach to cancer therapy, whether it involves experimental therapeutics or standard therapy, must begin with an adequate data base. Each patient requires a proper histologic diagnosis of cancer. Every patient needs adequate staging and an appropriate plan of management.

DIAGNOSIS   The histologic diagnosis of cancer and the proper categorization of the tumor type are pivotal in planning further workup and in deciding among treatment options. Although a histologic diagnosis may frequently appear straightforward, the clinician must realize its limitations. Histologic subtyping with biochemical and immunologic tissue characterization has resulted in a level of distinction among diagnoses not previously possible. In addition to substantiating the diagnosis of malignancy, this subtyping provides information essential in guiding therapy. The distinction between histologically similar tumors is important, as therapeutic options may differ. For example, when histologic subtyping is not possible, the decision to obtain additional tissue must be made in consultation with an experienced oncologist to determine whether it could alter the approach to treatment.

STAGING   The extent of malignant disease is a prime determinant in planning appropriate therapy. Staging not only guides the selection of therapy but also provides important prognostic information and may help the clinician minimize morbid complications. The importance of staging has resulted in international attempts to adopt uniform criteria (see Chap. 81). No routine set of tests is appropriate for all patients. Understanding the natural history of the primary tumor, the pattern of spread to regional lymph nodes, and the possible sites of distant metastasis assists in the selection of tests. The risks to the patient from any study must be balanced against the benefits gained by having additional staging information.

MANAGEMENT   A plan of management must be developed after diagnosis and staging. The plan must reflect the biology and natural history of the tumor, the available treatment options and their appropriateness to the patient's clinical situation, and the patient's wishes. The clinician must establish the goals of any treatment plan, and these goals should be explicitly communicated to the patient. Treatment with curative intent is clearly most desirable. The level of aggressiveness frequently required, often with attendant serious complications, requires the physician to evaluate realistically the potential for disease eradication. Treatment to improve longevity without long-term disease-free survival requires that the physician consider carefully the risk-to-benefit ratios of each therapeutic option. The expected gain in survival must be weighed against hospitalization time, potential complications, and side effects of therapy. Finally, treatment for palliation should not subject the patient to any unwarranted side effects, unnecessary complications, or other additional discomforts. The goals of palliation—relief of symptoms, prevention of complications, and maximization of quality of life—must always be kept in mind.

PRINCIPLES OF SURGICAL THERAPY

Surgery was the first modality used successfully in the treatment of cancer. After the development of ether anesthesia in the 1840s and of the principles of antisepsis in the 1860s, advances in cancer surgery were pioneered by Billroth, Halsted, and others. During the first part of this century, surgery was the only cancer treatment widely available. It is still the only curative therapy for many common solid tumors. Advances in surgical techniques, as well as improved multimodality therapy, have dramatically altered the surgical approach to many cancers. Limited surgical resections that do not affect the outcome but minimize loss of normal organ function are now feasible for some tumor types. Surgery has a primary role in the diagnosis, staging, and treatment of many tumors; surgical oncologists play an integral part in the multimodality approach to cancer therapy. Surgery is also effective in cancer prevention.

DIAGNOSIS A significant role of surgery in the treatment of patients with cancer is in the obtaining of adequate tissue samples for a histologic diagnosis. Accurate diagnosis is a critical first step in planning cancer therapy. Once the diagnosis of cancer is entertained, it is essential to involve a surgeon experienced in the principles of oncologic diagnosis. An improperly performed biopsy may compromise subsequent surgical management and, ultimately, the outcome for the patient.

Several techniques are available for obtaining tissue specimens. An *aspiration biopsy* is generally performed by inserting a fine needle into the tissue of interest and aspirating material for cytologic examination. The availability of an experienced cytologist is essential for a proper interpretation. Superficial lesions are amenable to aspiration, as are internal sites when the aspiration is guided by sonography or computed tomography (CT). A definitive diagnosis of cancer may not be possible by cytology alone, however. A *needle biopsy* obtains a core of tissue using a specially designed cutting needle. Radiologic guidance may permit a percutaneous approach to internal structures, such as the lung, liver, pancreas, and kidney. However, with some tumors, particularly lymphomas and sarcomas, a larger amount of tissue is usually required for a definitive diagnosis. With either aspiration or needle biopsy, sampling errors are a significant problem, and a negative result usually does not eliminate malignancy from the differential diagnosis. *Incisional biopsy*—the removal of a section or wedge of tissue from a larger tumor—is performed when removal of the entire tumor is impossible, as during an endoscopic examination. It is often performed before major surgical extirpation, as may be necessary for a soft tissue or bony sarcoma. Sampling errors are still a problem, as the resected portion may not be representative of the tumor as a whole. An *excisional biopsy* removes the entire lesion with little margin of normal tissue and, when possible, is to be preferred to incisional biopsy. Excising the entire lesion ensures sufficient tissue for pathologic examination, lessens the risk of tumor dissemination, and eliminates sampling problems. The choice of the appropriate procedure is dictated by anatomic considerations, the biology of the presumed tumor type, and the requirements of the pathologist. For some tumors, obtaining sufficient tissue for specialized studies such as immunophenotyping, cytogenetics, electron microscopy, or estrogen receptor status, requires specialized handling and close interaction with the pathologist.

STAGING Surgery is a principal means in the staging of many neoplastic diseases. Exploratory laparotomy to detect intraabdominal

spread of Hodgkin's disease is often indicated when conservative therapy is planned. Axillary lymph node sampling in breast carcinoma provides important prognostic information that may guide further therapy. Intraoperative staging by the sampling of celiac lymph nodes will help establish the appropriateness of an esophagectomy in a patient with esophageal carcinoma.

THERAPY Surgery is an effective way to cure patients whose tumors are confined to particular anatomic sites. However, at presentation, fewer than half of patients have tumors that are amenable to surgical treatment alone. The challenge is to identify the subset of patients that can be successfully treated by surgery alone, thus avoiding unnecessary surgical morbidity in the majority who will ultimately relapse. The most important determinants of a successful surgical intervention are the absence of distant metastases and little or no local tumor infiltration. For most solid tumors, the spread of disease beyond local confines prohibits a curative resection.

Understanding the typical patterns of cancer dissemination guides the preoperative assessment of patients. Cancer spreads by four routes: (1) by direct extension to adjacent structures; (2) through lymphatics to regional lymph nodes; (3) via hematogenous dissemination after entering the vascular system by direct vessel invasion; and (4) along serous cavities after growth through the wall of an organ. An individual tumor often uses more than one mode of dissemination. Careful clinical staging after the history, physical examination, and laboratory and imaging studies have been done is a requisite for deciding on the appropriateness of surgery.

Once the decision to treat by surgery has been made, it is essential to have an experienced oncologic surgeon; the best and usually only chance for curative resection is the first operation. Standard oncologic surgical practices are directed toward minimizing the risk of local tumor seeding and preventing dissemination at the time of the procedure. Such techniques include strict isolation of the tumor with avoidance of contamination to the operating field, minimal manipulation of the tumor, and early ligation of the vascular pedicle.

Removal of most solid tumors requires en bloc resections of the tumor plus a wide margin of normal tissue. The tumor type is the main factor determining how wide an adequate margin must be. The initial resection plan may have to be altered during the procedure as the full extent of the tumor becomes evident. Microscopic invasion of surrounding normal tissue by tumor that is imperceptible to the surgeon may necessitate examination of multiple frozen biopsy samples to establish tumor-free margins. Resection or sampling of regional lymph nodes is usually indicated; however, extended resection of several involved nodal groups is generally not warranted, as this approach has not resulted in improved survival.

Surgical resection of metastatic disease with the intent to cure may be appropriate in special circumstances. Generally, this approach is reserved for patients with slowly growing tumors who have a localized metastasis occurring well after resection of the primary disease. The metastasis should be the only evidence of distant disease found by imaging and laboratory studies, and it should be resectable with low morbidity. Examples include pulmonary metastases in patients with osteogenic sarcoma and solitary liver metastases in patients with colorectal carcinoma. In a minority of patients, resection of these lesions can lead to long-term disease-free survival.

Surgery may be used for palliation in patients for whom cure is not possible. The selection of patients who will benefit from this approach requires considerable judgment and skill. Appropriate, judicious use of surgery in patients with metastatic disease may alleviate symptoms and improve the quality of life. Surgery may be indicated to relieve pain, stop hemorrhage, or alleviate obstruction. For example, the excision of an occluding colon carcinoma when metastatic disease is present may greatly palliate symptoms. However, overly aggressive surgical intervention in a palliative setting may lead to prolonged hospitalizations, unnecessary discomfort, and an additional financial burden on the patient or family.

Modern surgical oncology is one component of combined-modality therapy, the goals of which are to improve outcome and allow a decrease in the extent of surgery. The surgeon, the medical oncologist, and the radiation therapist develop an integrated plan to deliver the most effective coordinated treatment. Combined-modality approaches have led to the successful development of adjuvant therapies. Adjuvant therapy, usually chemotherapy, is administered after definitive surgical resection to a patient who has no clinical, radiologic, or pathologic evidence of residual malignant disease. Adjuvant therapy is used in this setting to eliminate undetectable micrometastatic disease. The term *neoadjuvant treatment* refers to the administration of chemotherapy before definitive surgery. A patient who responds to neoadjuvant chemotherapy may benefit from more conservative local therapy. An example of multimodality therapy is the treatment of early-stage breast carcinoma. Mastectomy with axillary lymph node dissection can often be replaced by lumpectomy with lymph node sampling together with local radiotherapy and, when indicated, systemic adjuvant chemotherapy.

The use of surgery to achieve cytoreduction when complete excision is not possible has a role in some diseases, if combined with other therapeutic modalities. This approach has been most successful in childhood tumors, as in the surgical debulking of Wilms's tumor before administration of chemotherapy. In adults, this approach has a limited role in the treatment of ovarian carcinoma or Burkitt's lymphoma. A consideration of tumor cell biology demonstrates the difficulties of this approach: Debulking a mass 10 cm in diameter, containing approximately 1×10^{12} tumor cells, to a mass with a 1 cm diameter reduces the tumor burden by three orders of magnitude, leaving 1×10^9 tumor cells remaining.

Reconstructive surgery after a definitive resection can improve function and appearance and be of significant psychological benefit to the patient. The use of myocutaneous flaps and improvements in microvascular anastomotic techniques has had a profound effect on the ability to restore new tissue to a previous surgical area. Reconstruction after primary radiation therapy has also helped to restore function to damaged tissues. Stabilization of weight-bearing bones weakened by metastatic tumor may avert significant problems.

PREVENTION   Surgery has a growing role in the prevention of cancer. Patients with conditions that predispose them to certain cancers or with genetic traits associated with cancer can have a normal life span with prophylactic surgery. Colectomy may be life-saving for patients with familial polyposis, nonpolyposis familial colon cancer, or ulcerative colitis. Women with multiple risk factors for breast cancer may benefit from prophylactic mastectomy. In light of the fact that the operation done for prophylaxis is more extensive than the operation done for control of the disease, most physicians would not recommend mastectomy unless the risk was more than 20 percent in 5 years. Oophorectomy is recommended for patients with familial ovarian cancer, and orchiectomy can prevent testicular cancer in men with undescended testes that have not been corrected before puberty. Orchiopexy can be preventive if performed early. Families with multiple endocrine neoplasia type II are at risk of developing medullary thyroid cancers. Thyroidectomy is prophylactic in this setting. Removal of premalignant skin lesions, such as dysplastic nevi and actinic keratoses, is the most common prophylactic surgery.

PRINCIPLES OF RADIATION THERAPY

Radiation therapy, like surgery, is a local modality used in the treatment of cancer. Its success depends on the inherent difference in radiosensitivity between the tumor and the adjacent normal tissues. Ideally, radiation therapy should destroy cancerous tissue while causing minimal disruption to surrounding normal structures. Other considerations are the ability of normal tissues to sustain and repair radiation-induced damage and for the patient to function adequately even if normal organ function is diminished.

PHYSICAL CHARACTERISTICS   Radiation therapy for most solid tumors involves the administration of ionizing radiation in the form of x-rays or gamma rays to a tumor site. The term *x-ray* denotes high-energy electromagnetic radiation (4 to 25 MeV) produced by electron-level transitions within the atom. X-rays are generated by instruments such as linear accelerators. *Gamma rays* are also high-energy radiation but are produced by radioactive isotope decay, typically from cobalt-60, cesium–137, or radium–226. Although there is no difference in the physical characteristics or biologic effects of x-rays and gamma rays, linear accelerators are more widely used and produce a more focused beam with a smaller penumbra. Megavoltage x-rays are commonly used to irradiate internal, deep-seated lesions, since high-energy, penetrating beams deliver a less intense superficial dose and spare the skin. Orthovoltage x-rays are of lesser energy and deliver a higher dose to superficial tissues; they can be used to treat skin cancers.

External beam therapy, or *teletherapy*, is radiation delivered from a source outside the body. Radiation delivered by sealed radioactive materials inserted in the body near or at the tumor site is called *brachytherapy*. Owing to the proximity of the radiation source to the tumor, the dose is more localized than with external beam therapy. Brachytherapy may consist of intracavitary inserts, used in the treatment of gynecologic malignancies such as cervical or vaginal carcinomas, or interstitial implants, such as those used for prostate carcinoma. Brachytherapy may also be used in conjunction with external beam therapy, for example in head and neck carcinoma, where the implants provide a high-intensity boost to the tumor bed.

Particle beam therapy, using neutron or proton beams, is available in specialized centers. This therapy has the advantage of more precise localization of energy release. The depth of particle penetration can be accurately controlled, with a resultant sparing of normal tissues. Electron beam therapy can be used to treat superficial tumors, such as skin cancers. The energy from these beams is rapidly absorbed, and, therefore, the dose to adjacent normal tissues is diminished.

BIOLOGIC CHARACTERISTICS   Radiation therapy is a means of imparting energy to tissues that ultimately results in biological damage. Radiation dose, measured in gray (Gy), is defined as an amount of absorbed energy: 1 Gy is the absorption of 1 J of energy per kilogram of tissue. The previously used unit, the rad, equals 0.01 Gy (1 Gy equals 100 rad). A given dose of radiation kills a constant percentage of cells, not a constant number. At high doses of radiation, cell survival decreases with first-order kinetics in proportion to increasing radiation dose. At lower radiation doses, a shoulder in the curve results from a decreased rate of cell death and may represent the presence of cellular repair mechanisms (see Chap. 396).

DNA is the primary target for radiation-induced cell death. Ionizing radiation generates free radicals and reactive oxygen intermediates that damage local cellular constituents, especially DNA. DNA double-stranded breaks appear to be the critical lesion that results in cell death. Cellular demise associated with DNA breaks may occur within several hours or may become apparent only after cellular division, a process called *mitotic cell death*. In either instance, the process of *programmed cell death*, or *apoptosis*, may ensue after radiation-induced cellular damage in normal and tumor cells. Apoptosis is a genetically encoded program that involves the activation of endogenous nucleases and results in fragmentation of genomic DNA, nuclear condensation, and subsequent loss of cellular membrane integrity. The tumor suppressor gene *p53* is a key regulator of apoptosis. In a high percentage of tumors, mutation or deletion of *p53* may affect the ability of tumor cells to undergo programmed cell death in response to ionizing radiation. Cells that do not undergo apoptosis may succumb to *necrosis*, a process whereby cellular membrane integrity is lost before DNA degradation.

Rapidly proliferating normal tissues such as intestinal mucosa, bone marrow, and skin are particularly susceptible to ionizing radiation and readily show evidence of cytotoxicity. With slowly proliferating tissues, radiation-induced damage may not be apparent until much later or may occur only after stress to the normal tissues. For example, an irradiated long bone may not cause symptoms, except during prolonged healing following a fracture.

The capacity and extent of cellular repair mechanisms determine in part the radiosensitivity of a given tumor or normal tissue. Cellular repair in normal tissues is usually complete within 4 to 6 h after radiation exposure. Oxygen concentration is also an important determinant of radiation sensitivity. Oxygen is important for generating and sustaining the free radicals produced by radiation. Hypoxic tissues are relatively resistant to the effects of radiation; it takes a dose of radiation two to three times higher to kill anoxic cells as oxygenated ones. Poorly vascularized central areas of larger tumor masses are likely to exhibit relative insensitivity to radiation.

THERAPY Radiation therapy is planned and performed by a team of nurses, dosimetrists, physicists, and radiation oncologists. Achieving the goal of radiation therapy—to uniformly irradiate the entire tumor volume while sparing adjacent normal tissues—depends on appropriate treatment planning, in which extensive use should be made of imaging studies, particularly CT and magnetic resonance imaging (MRI) scans. A course of radiation therapy is preceded by a simulation session in which low-energy beams are used to produce radiographic images that indicate the exact beam location. The positioning of the patient used in the simulation must be reproduced exactly for each treatment to ensure maximal tumor killing with minimal complications.

Radiation therapy is usually delivered in fractionated doses, such as 180 to 300 cGy per day, five times a week for a total course of 5 to 8 weeks. Clinical experience has demonstrated that fractional treatment schedules improve the therapeutic index and result in better tumor control. This better outcome may be related to several factors, including cellular repair of normal tissues, repopulation of destroyed tissues, and reoxygenation of relatively hypoxic tumor sites. Accelerated fractionation schedules increase the daily dose and reduce the overall treatment time. Although this approach may produce more acute toxicity, it may benefit patients with tumors that have a rapid doubling time, such as some head and neck tumors. Hyperfractionation delivers smaller individual doses several times a day and thereby increases the total number of treatments. In theory, hyperfractionation improves the therapeutic index for some tumors.

Radiation therapy is delivered from multiple external sites or fields which together focus on the tumor. This approach distributes the radiotherapy and lessens its toxicity to the normal tissues by minimizing the dose to vital structures. Increasing the number of fields may cause a larger volume of normal tissue to receive irradiation, but at more moderate doses.

Radiation therapy with curative intent as the sole treatment modality is employed in limited-stage Hodgkin's disease, some non-Hodgkin's lymphomas, certain head and neck carcinomas, limited-stage prostate carcinoma, gynecologic tumors, central nervous system neoplasms, and some skin cancers. Radiation therapy also is often an integral part of curative multimodality approaches. For example, radiation therapy combined with chemotherapy has largely replaced surgery as a curative treatment for squamous cell carcinoma of the anus. Radiation therapy is a central component of breast conservation in the multimodality treatment of breast carcinoma.

Radiation therapy is also used in the palliative management of many tumors. Irradiation of bony metastases may alleviate pain and stabilize weight-bearing structures in an attempt to prevent pathologic fractures. Brain metastases are often irradiated to provide symptomatic relief and prevent further neurologic complications. Palliative radiation therapy can also be employed to treat significant bleeding, refractory visceral pain, and vital organ obstruction. In general, the doses employed for palliative management are lower than those used for curative therapy and result in less acute toxicity and discomfort to the patient.

Radiation therapy may be required on an urgent basis for the treatment of complications of malignant disease. Impending spinal cord compression in a patient with metastatic carcinoma is usually best treated with radiotherapy to the involved area. Alleviation of an obstructed airway or superior vena cava is generally treated effectively by radiotherapy.

COMPLICATIONS Radiation therapy is associated with both acute toxicity and long-term sequelae. Acute reactions occur during or immediately after therapy and represent interruption of the repopulation of rapidly dividing tissues. They are self-limited and usually do not limit the amount of radiation therapy that can be administered. Common manifestations include systemic symptoms, such as fatigue, and local skin reactions that range from erythema to moist desquamation. Gastrointestinal toxicity, with nausea, vomiting, dysphagia, or diarrhea, is associated with treatment to the abdomen or pelvis. Irradiation of the head and neck results in oropharyngeal mucositis and xerostomia. Significant myelosuppression, with leukopenia, thrombocytopenia, or anemia, is unusual but can occur if large amounts of the proliferative bone marrow are irradiated. If symptoms become problematic during therapy, treatment may need to be temporarily halted to allow normal tissue repair.

Long-term sequelae are dose-limiting and occur many months or years after the completion of therapy. The frequency of long-term complications increases as normal tissue tolerances are approached. These complications tend to be progressive rather than self-limited. Their occurrence does not correlate with the appearance or severity of acute reactions. The mechanism of late complications is believed to be the disruption of vascular endothelium or the depletion of normal tissue stem cells. Table 86-1 lists the tissue tolerances of some common structures that exhibit late complications. The normal tissue tolerance is defined as the dose at which no more than 5 percent of patients will have the stated complication within 5 years.

Radiation therapy is known to be mutagenic, carcinogenic, and teratogenic and is associated with an increased risk of developing both secondary leukemias and solid tumors. The most complete data for these complications come from studies of patients who are long-term survivors after therapy for Hodgkin's disease. Although secondary leukemias may appear within the first few years after therapy, the median time to appearance of secondary solid tumors is greater than 10 years. The relative risk for developing secondary tumors in Hodgkin's disease is related to extent of treatment, age, use of combined-modality therapy, and sex. The risk is higher for women than for men owing to the development of secondary breast cancers in young patients who received mantle radiation.

RADIONUCLIDES For decades, radionuclides have been used systemically to treat malignant disorders. They are administered by specialists in nuclear medicine or radiation therapy.

Radioactive iodine in the form of ^{131}I is effective therapy for well-differentiated thyroid carcinomas. Iodine is selectively metabolized by thyroid tissue; other tissues are spared the detrimental effects of ^{131}I. In practice, uptake of ^{131}I by tumors is variable and is less than that of normal thyroid tissue.

Strontium-89 is used for the treatment of bony metastases. Strontium is an alkaline earth element in the same family as calcium and is metabolized by the same biochemical pathways as calcium. Strontium is accumulated in sites of active osteogenesis and becomes localized in bone mineral. ^{89}Sr will selectively irradiate blastic sites of primary and metastatic bone involvement and spare normal tissues. It is used in a palliative manner to relieve pain; its major toxic effect is myelosuppression.

Table 86-1

Tolerance of Normal Tissues for Radiation Therapy

Tissue	Dose (cGy)	Complications
Brain	6000	Necrosis
Spinal cord	4500	Myelitis
Heart	4500	Pericarditis, myocardial damage
Intestine	4500	Stenosis, perforation
Liver	3000	Hepatitis, hepatic vein thrombosis
Lung	2000	Pneumonitis, fibrosis
Kidney	2000	Nephropathy, renal failure
Bone marrow	250	Aplasia
Ovary	200	Sterilization
Testes	100	Sterilization

BACKGROUND Systemic chemotherapy is the main treatment available for disseminated malignant disease. Progress in drug therapy has resulted in the development of curative chemotherapy regimens for several tumors (Table 86-2). Chemotherapy also has a significant role in palliation, often with improved survival, in a variety of other tumors (Table 86-2). However, chemotherapy has only minor activity in several common solid tumors. One of the most important and still evolving roles for systemic chemotherapy is its use in the adjuvant setting. Table 86-2 lists tumors that can be treated effectively with adjuvant chemotherapy.

Chemotherapy, whether given with curative or palliative intent, usually requires multiple cycles of treatment. It is often desirable to assess the therapeutic efficacy of the treatment before completing the entire course. The discontinuation of an ineffective treatment may allow a different salvage regimen to be instituted or, at least, will spare the patient unnecessary toxicity. Response to therapy can be measured directly by palpating superficial tumor masses or by imaging internal lesions. Indirect measurements can be used but generally are less desirable in the evaluation of tumor response.

Uniform criteria for describing a response to therapy are widely accepted and make it possible to compare the efficacy of alternative treatments. A *complete response (complete remission)* is the disappearance of all detectable malignant disease. A *partial response* is a decrease by more than 50 percent in the sum of the products of the perpendicular diameters of all measurable lesions; also, there can be no increase in size of any lesion nor the appearance of any new lesions. *Stable disease* means that there is no change in measurable tumor dimensions. *Progressive disease* means an increase by at least 25 percent in the sum of the products of the perpendicular diameters of measurable lesions, or the appearance of new lesions.

The modern era of chemotherapy treatment for malignant disease began after the observation in World War II that exposure to mustard gas led to bone marrow and lymph node hypoplasia. The clinical use of nitrogen mustard was pioneered by Gilman at Yale in the 1940s in the treatment of lymphoma. Farber at Harvard, also in the 1940s, first induced remissions in childhood leukemia using aminopterin, a folate antagonist. In 1955, chemotherapy was first used to cure a solid tumor, gestational trophoblastic carcinoma. The subsequent development of multidrug regimens for childhood acute leukemia and Hodgkin's disease in the 1960s demonstrated that chemotherapy could consistently cure a high percentage of patients with certain chemoresponsive diseases. To appreciate more fully the development and application of modern chemotherapeutic regimens in the treatment of neoplastic diseases, it is necessary to understand the principles of cytokinetics and pharmacodynamics.

CYTOKINETICS A primary determinant of malignant transformation is uncontrolled growth. All somatic cells, whether normal or malignant, multiply by cell division through the mitotic cell cycle (see Chap. 83). Many chemotherapeutic agents, such as the antimetabolites and the alkylating agents, are cell-cycle–active; that is, they are cytotoxic mainly to actively cycling cells. In addition, some cycle-active agents are phase-specific; that is, they are cytotoxic to cells in a particular phase of the cell cycle. Other agents are capable of exerting cytotoxicity at any phase of cell cycle, including G0/G1, and are not considered cycle-active.

A model elucidating the effectiveness of chemotherapy in eliminating a tumor mass was proposed by Skipper and coworkers in the 1960s and is called the *log cell kill model*. According to this model, tumor growth is exponential with first-order kinetics and progresses at that rate until a lethal tumor burden is reached (Fig. 86-1*A*). The time required for a tumor to increase from 10^6 cells to 10^9 cells (a three-log or 1000-fold increase) is the same as the time for the tumor to increase from 10^9 to 10^{12} cells. A given chemotherapy dose will destroy a constant percentage of cells, not a constant number, regardless of the tumor burden. Thus, if a given dose kills 99 percent of the tumor cells (a two-log reduction) a tumor mass of 10^{11} cells will be reduced to 10^9 cells (Fig. 86-1*B*). Assuming no tumor regrowth, an additional cycle of chemotherapy will reduce the tumor to 10^7 cells, at which point it would no longer be clinically detectable, and the patient would have achieved a complete response. However, an additional four cycles of chemotherapy will be required to reduce the tumor burden to less than 1 cell to achieve a cure.

Most human solid tumors do not grow with a constant doubling rate. Instead, the rate of growth slows progressively with increasing tumor size, a pattern called *Gompertzian growth* (Fig. 86-2). As tumors enlarge, the growth rate slows, the growth fraction decreases, and tumor volume begins to plateau. Patients with large tumors often respond poorly to chemotherapy, primarily because of unfavorable tumor cytokinetics. Chemotherapy is usually most effective on a small tumor burden for which the growth fraction is maximal, as in the adjuvant setting, in which tumor size and cytokinetics favor a response.

PHARMOCODYNAMICS Chemotherapeutic agents exhibit a dose-response effect (Fig. 86-3). At sufficiently low concentrations, no cytotoxicity is observed. At increasing concentrations, cell kill is proportional to drug exposure. At high concentrations, the effect reaches a plateau. Normal cells also are susceptible to the cytotoxic effects of chemotherapeutic drugs and exhibit a dose-response effect, but the response curve is shifted relative to that of malignant cells (Fig. 86-3). This difference represents the therapeutic index; the usefulness of many chemotherapeutic drugs is limited by the fact that they have a narrow therapeutic index. The toxicity to normal tissue that limits further dose escalation is the *dose-limiting toxicity*. The dose just below this point is the *maximum tolerated dose*. Proliferative normal tissues such as the bone marrow and gastrointestinal mucosa are generally the most susceptible to chemotherapy-induced toxicity.

The concentration range over which the dose-response curve remains linear for a particular drug is an important consideration in designing dose-intensive regimens. Drugs such as the alkylating agents characteristically have steep dose-response curves: An increase in the drug concentration by an order of magnitude or more results in a proportional increase in tumor cell kill. By contrast, the dose-response curve of phase-specific agents, such as the antimetabolites, typically

Table 86-2

Response of Tumors to Chemotherapy

CURABLE BY CHEMOTHERAPY

Acute lymphoblastic leukemia	Non-Hodgkin's lymphoma
Acute myeloid leukemia	Burkitt's lymphoma
Ewing's sarcoma	Diffuse large cell lymphoma
Gestational trophoblastic carcinoma	Follicular mixed lymphoma
Hodgkin's disease	Lymphoblastic lymphoma
	Rhabdomyosarcoma
	Testicular carcinoma
	Wilms's tumor

CHEMOTHERAPY HAS SIGNIFICANT ACTIVITY

Anal carcinoma	Head and neck carcinoma
Bladder carcinoma	Lung (small cell) carcinoma
Breast carcinoma	Multiple myeloma
Chronic lymphocytic leukemia	Non-Hodgkin's lymphoma
Chronic myelogenous leukemia	Follicular lymphoma
Hairy cell leukemia	Ovarian carcinoma

CHEMOTHERAPY HAS MINOR ACTIVITY

Brain tumors (astrocytoma)	Lung (non-small-cell) carcinoma
Cervical carcinoma	Melanoma
Colorectal carcinoma	Pancreatic carcinoma
Hepatocellular carcinoma	Prostate carcinoma
Kaposi's sarcoma	Soft tissue sarcoma

ADJUVANT CHEMOTHERAPY IS EFFECTIVE

Breast carcinoma	Ovarian carcinoma (stage III)
Colorectal carcinoma (stage III)	Testicular carcinoma
Osteogenic sarcoma	

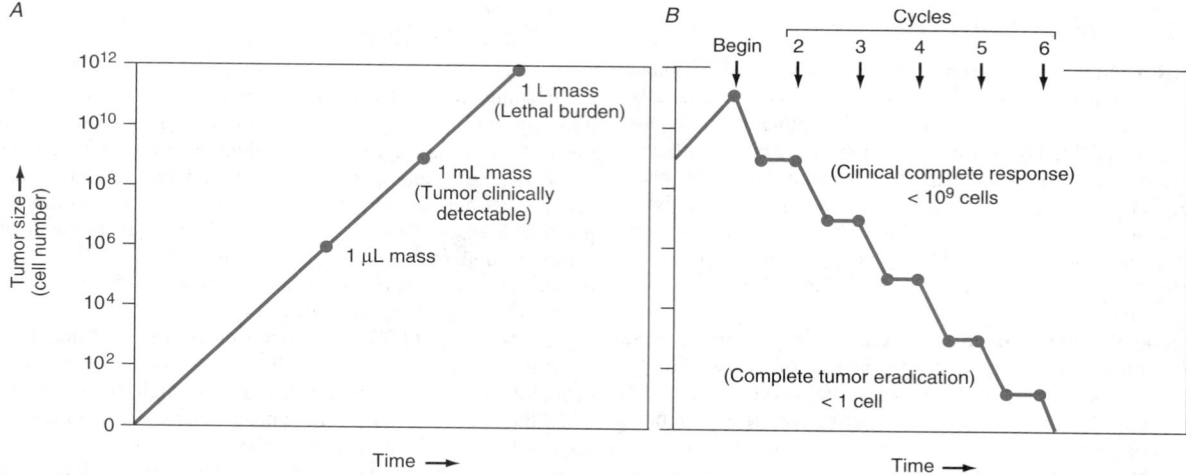

FIGURE 86-1 Model of logarithmic cell growth and cell killing. *A.* Tumor cell growth proceeds with first-order kinetics from a clinically undetectable mass to a lethal tumor burden. *B.* Tumor regression in response to chemotherapy also follows first-order kinetics. A given dose of chemotherapy kills a constant percentage of cells regardless of tumor size. In the case shown here, two cycles of chemotherapy will render the tumor clinically undetectable, but six cycles will be required for total tumor eradication.

is linear over only a narrow range. These agents are less suitable for dose escalation. However, increased tumor cell kill is observed after prolonged exposure to these agents. Increasing the exposure time means that a larger percentage of the tumor cells will enter the cell cycle and thus become susceptible to the cytotoxic effects of the drugs. These agents are often referred to as *schedule-dependent*.

The ability of chemotherapy to eradicate tumor cells without causing lethal host toxicity depends on drug selectivity. The basis for anticancer drug selectivity remains incompletely understood. Although cytokinetics are important, other differences between normal and tumor cells in cellular processes, such as metabolic pathways and susceptibility to programmed cell death, also contribute.

Most chemotherapeutic agents are inducers of programmed cell death. Drugs such as the alkylating agents, the purine/pyrimidine analogs, and the topoisomerase inhibitors result in DNA damage (see below). In response to genotoxic damage, cells can arrest at two identified checkpoints: the G1/S and G2/M boundaries. G1 arrest is mediated in part by the tumor suppressor p53 via activation of the expression of the cyclin-dependent kinase inhibitor p21. G1 arrest may allow the cell to repair damage before DNA replication, and G2 arrest permits repair prior to mitosis. If the DNA damage is irreparable, apoptosis may occur via p53-dependent or -independent pathways.

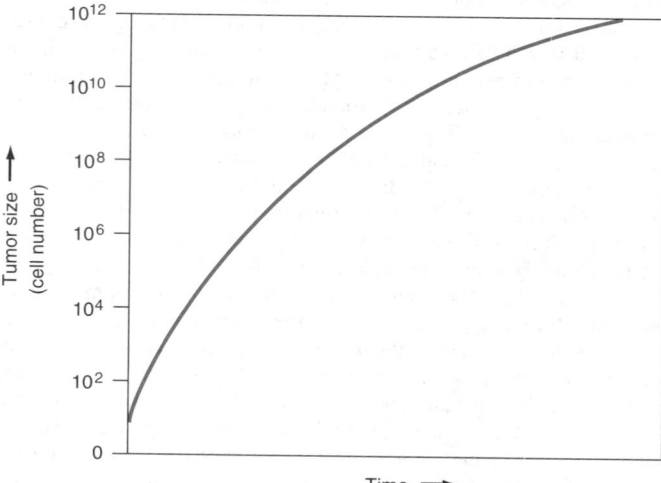

FIGURE 86-2 Model of Gompertzian growth. In Gompertzian growth, as the tumor size increases the growth rate slows and begins to plateau. Large tumors will be relatively insensitive to chemotherapy, owing primarily to unfavorable cytokinetics.

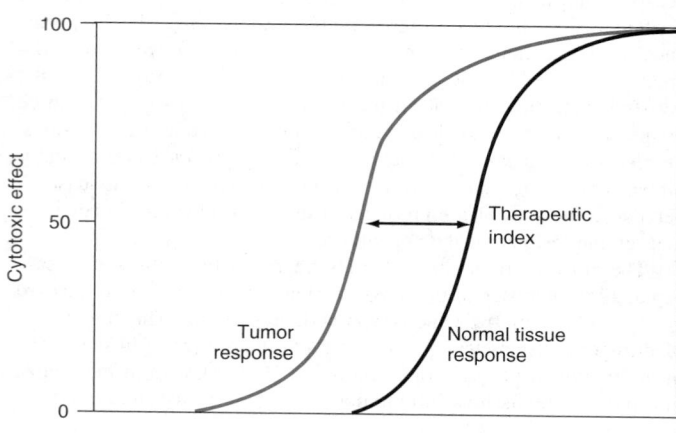

FIGURE 86-3 Dose-response effect. All cells, whether normal or malignant, demonstrate a dose-response effect when exposed to chemotherapeutic agents. The difference between the responses of the tumor and of normal tissue represents the therapeutic index.

CANCER CHEMOTHERAPY Most of the commonly used cytotoxic antitumor agents are discussed below. They should be administered only by physicians experienced in their use and expert at handling potentially serious side effects. The dose of most chemotherapeutic agents is based on a patient's body surface area (in square meters) calculated according to height and weight. The major diseases for which individual agents are commonly used are listed in Table 86-3.

Antimetabolites The antimetabolites induce cytotoxicity by serving as false substrates in biochemical pathways. They are cell-cycle–active and are specific mainly for the S phase. Many are nucleoside analogues that are incorporated into DNA or RNA and thereby inhibit nucleic acid synthesis. Other agents in this class inhibit enzymes involved in nucleotide biosynthesis.

Pyrimidine-Analogue Antimetabolites The fluorinated pyrimidine, *fluorouracil* (5-fluorouracil; 5FU), is activated intracellularly to one of several metabolites. Fluorodeoxyuridine monophosphate (FdUMP) is a potent inhibitor of thymidylate synthase, an enzyme necessary for the synthesis of dTTP and ultimately DNA; fluorouridine triphosphate (FUTP) is incorporated into RNA and interferes with its processing and function. Fluorodeoxyuridine triphosphate (FdUTP) is incorporated into DNA and eventually leads to DNA strand breakage. The interference of FdUMP with thymidylate synthesis requires the presence of reduced folates. Leucovorin, a folate analogue, has been administered with fluorouracil in an attempt to increase antitumor activity. Extensive first-pass hepatic metabolism for fluorouracil has led to direct hepatic artery infusions for the treatment of hepatic metastases. The fluorouracil analogue *floxuridine*, (FUDR) is also available for intrahepatic infusion.

Fluorouracil toxicity is schedule-dependent. With bolus infusion, bone marrow suppression predominates, whereas with continuous infusion, gastrointestinal toxicity may be more limiting. Fluorouracil has been associated infrequently with a myocardial ischemic syndrome. Neurologic symptoms, usually reversible, include headaches, cerebellar ataxia, and somnolence. Dermatologic complaints, such as dermatitis, hyperpigmentation, and skin atrophy, are not uncommon.

Cytarabine (ara-C) is the 2′ epimer of cytidine. After carrier-mediated uptake by the deoxycytidine transport system, this substance is phosphorylated sequentially to its active metabolite, ara-CTP, with deoxycytidine kinase activity being rate-limiting. Ara-CTP is incorporated into DNA and inhibits replication by acting as a chain terminator. Cytarabine can be degraded intracellularly to an inactive compound (ara-U) by cytidine deaminase. The net effects of cellular accumulation and of the balance between the activities of deoxycytidine kinase and cytidine deaminase ultimately determine the cellular toxicity of cytarabine.

Cytarabine is usually administered by continuous infusion and causes profound myelosuppression. Gastrointestinal toxicity, including oral mucositis, is frequently observed. High-dose regimens are associated with a syndrome of cholestatic jaundice, as well as cerebellar and cerebral toxicity. Patients with abnormal renal function, a greater than twofold elevation of alkaline phosphatase levels, or age greater than 40 are at increased risk for neurotoxicity. Conjunctivitis, preventable by ophthalmic corticosteroids, is common with high-dose regimens.

Gemcitabine is a difluorinated analogue of deoxycytidine. In a manner similar to cytarabine, it acts as a DNA chain terminator after carrier-mediated uptake and intracellular phosphorylation. However, gemcitabine appears to have better membrane permeability and greater affinity for deoxycytidine kinase. Once incorporated into DNA, it is more resistant to exonuclease excision than cytarabine. In addition, gemcitabine inhibits the enzyme ribonucleotide reductase and thereby leads to diminished pools of the competing natural compound, deoxycytidine. Myelosuppression is dose-limiting with gemcitabine. Other toxicities include lethargy and malaise.

Table 86-3

Antitumor Activities of Chemotherapeutic Agents

Agent	Tumors against which Agent Shows Activity*
ANTIMETABOLITES	
Pyrimidine analogs	
Cytarabine	Acute lymphoblastic leukemia, acute myeloid leukemia, non-Hodgkin's lymphoma
Fluorouracil (5FU)	Breast Ca, colorectal Ca, esophageal Ca, gastric Ca
Gemcitabine	Bladder Ca, non-small-cell lung Ca, pancreatic Ca
Purine analogues	
Cladribine	Hairy cell leukemia, follicular lymphoma
Fludarabine	Chronic lymphocytic leukemia, follicular lymphoma
Pentostatin	Hairy cell leukemia
Other	
Hydroxyurea	Chronic myelogenous leukemia, essential thrombocytosis
Methotrexate	Acute lymphoblastic leukemia, bladder Ca, breast Ca, gestational trophoblastic Ca, head/neck Ca, non-Hodgkin's lymphoma, osteogenic sarcoma
PLANT ALKALOIDS	
Taxanes	
Docetaxel	Breast Ca, ovarian Ca
Paclitaxel	Breast Ca, lung Ca, ovarian Ca
Vincas	
Vinblastine	Bladder Ca, breast Ca, Hodgkin's disease, lung Ca, non-Hodgkin's lymphoma, testicular Ca
Vincristine	Acute lymphoblastic leukemia, Hodgkin's disease, non-Hodgkin's lymphoma
Vinorelbine	Breast Ca, lung Ca
TOPOISOMERASE INHIBITORS	
Anthracyclines	
Daunorubicin	Acute lymphoblastic leukemia, acute myeloid leukemia
Doxorubicin	Bladder Ca, breast Ca, gastric Ca, hepatocellular Ca, Hodgkin's disease, lung Ca, non-Hodgkin's lymphoma, osteogenic sarcoma, soft tissue sarcoma
Idarubicin	Acute myeloid leukemia, non-Hodgkin's lymphoma
Epipodophyllotoxins	
Etoposide	Acute myeloid leukemia, lung Ca, non-Hodgkin's lymphoma, ovarian Ca, testicular Ca
Teniposide	Acute lymphoblastic leukemia, non-Hodgkin's lymphoma
Other	
Dactinomycin	Gestational trophoblastic Ca
Mitoxantrone	Acute myeloid leukemia, breast Ca, non-Hodgkin's lymphoma
ALKYLATING AGENTS	
Classic	
Busulfan	Chronic myelogenous leukemia
Chlorambucil	Chronic lymphocytic leukemia, Hodgkin's disease, non-Hodgkin's lymphoma
Cyclophosphamide	Bladder Ca, breast Ca, chronic lymphocytic leukemia, lung Ca, non-Hodgkin's lymphoma, ovarian Ca, soft tissue sarcoma
Ifosfamide	Breast Ca, non-Hodgkin's lymphoma, osteogenic sarcoma, testicular Ca
Mechlorethamine	Hodgkin's disease
Melphalan	Breast Ca, multiple myeloma, ovarian Ca
Thiotepa	Breast Ca, ovarian Ca
Nitrosoureas	
Carmustine	Astrocytoma, Hodgkin's disease, non-Hodgkin's lymphoma
Lomustine	Astrocytoma, Hodgkin's disease, non-Hodgkin's lymphoma
Platinum compounds	
Carboplatin	Bladder Ca, head/neck Ca, ovarian Ca
Cisplatin	Bladder Ca, esophageal Ca, head/neck Ca, lung Ca, osteogenic sarcoma, ovarian Ca, testicular Ca
ANTITUMOR ANTIBIOTICS	
Bleomycin	Hodgkin's disease, non-Hodgkin's lymphoma, testicular Ca
Mitomycin C	Breast Ca, colorectal Ca
MISCELLANEOUS AGENTS	
Dacarbazine	Hodgkin's disease, melanoma, soft tissue sarcoma
L-Asparaginase	Acute lymphoblastic leukemia
Procarbazine	Astrocytoma, Hodgkin's disease

* Ca, carcinoma.

Purine-Analogue Antimetabolites Three adenosine analogues have recently entered clinical practice. *Fludarabine* is a fluorinated derivative of the antiviral agent vidarabine (ara-A). Unlike vidarabine, it is resistant to intracellular deamination. Fludarabine is phosphorylated by deoxycytidine kinase before being incorporated into DNA and inhibiting DNA synthesis. A significant number (up to 20 percent) of patients experience mild, reversible neurotoxicity, although instances of severe, irreversible toxicity, including coma, have been reported. In addition to myelosuppression, fludarabine causes immunosuppression and episodes of opportunistic infection in some patients. *Cladribine* (chlorodeoxyadenosine) is also phosphorylated by deoxycytidine kinase before being incorporated into DNA and inhibiting DNA replication. Cladribine is myelosuppressive and immunosuppressive; other toxicities, such as gastrointestinal toxicity, are mild. *Pentostatin* (2′-deoxycoformycin) is an irreversible inhibitor of the enzyme adenosine deaminase, causing the toxic accumulation of deoxyadenosine nucleotides, particularly in lymphocytes. Pentostatin causes immunosuppression, especially of T-cell–mediated immunity. Myelosuppression, renal function impairment, central nervous system toxicity, and hepatoxicity have been attributed to treatment with this agent.

The thiopurine analogues *6-mercaptopurine* (6MP) and *6-thioguanine* (6TG) require modification by the enzyme hypoxanthine-guanine phosphoribosyltransferase (HGPRT) before they can inhibit purine biosynthesis. Patients receiving allopurinol require a 75 percent decrease in mercaptopurine dose size because elimination depends on the enzyme xanthine oxidase, the target for allopurinol inhibition. Cholestatic jaundice has been observed with both agents, although it is more common with 6MP. Both 6MP and 6TG produce myelosuppression and gastrointestinal toxicity, although the latter is usually mild.

Other Antimetabolites The antifolate *methotrexate* inhibits the enzyme dihydrofolate reductase. Dihydrofolate reductase activity is necessary to maintain intracellular pools of reduced tetrahydrofolates, which are required for the synthesis of purine nucleotides and thymidylate. After carrier-mediated cellular uptake, methotrexate is converted to a polyglutamate derivative that is more active than the parent drug. Administration of a reduced folate, such as leucovorin, bypasses the block created by methotrexate and can prevent severe gastrointestinal toxicity or marked bone marrow hypoplasia. It is generally used after administration of methotrexate at doses >100 mg/m². The accumulation of methotrexate in third-space fluids, such as pleural effusion or ascites, and the subsequent prolonged release of the agent can prolong drug elimination and lead to unusually severe toxicities.

Use of very high-dose methotrexate (>1000 mg/m²) requires the monitoring of serum methotrexate levels to adjust the dose and schedule of leucovorin rescue. Methotrexate is cleared mainly by renal excretion, and patients with impaired renal function require dosage adjustments. High-dose regimens have been associated with acute renal injury, which may be prevented by vigorous hydration and alkalinization of the urine. In the absence of normal renal function, there are no satisfactory methods (including hemodialysis) to eliminate methotrexate. Acute or chronic administration of methotrexate has been associated with hepatoxicity and an idiosyncratic pneumonitis.

Hydroxyurea inhibits the enzyme ribonucleotide reductase, which converts ribonucleotides to deoxyribonucleotides. Hydroxyurea produces a predictable leukopenia that is usually reversible within days of discontinuing therapy. Gastrointestinal toxicity is usually mild. Patients receiving long-term hydroxyurea therapy may develop mild dermatologic changes.

Plant Alkaloids The vinca alkaloids *vincristine* and *vinblastine* were originally isolated from the periwinkle plant, *Catharanthus roseus*. *Vinorelbine* is a newer semisynthetic derivative. The vinca alkaloids inhibit microtubule assembly by binding to tubulin and thus are cytotoxic predominately during the M phase of the cell cycle. *Paclitaxel* and *docetaxel* are members of the taxane family. Paclitaxel is isolated from the Pacific yew (*Taxus brevifolia*), whereas docetaxel

is synthesized from a noncytotoxic precursor isolated from the more readily accessible European yew (*Taxus baccata*). They function by stabilizing microtubules and preventing their disassembly.

Neurotoxicity is dose-limiting with vincristine and is manifested as peripheral sensory neuropathy and/or an autonomic neuropathy. With continued use of the agent, a motor neuropathy may develop. Mild neuropathy generally improves with discontinuation of treatment. Vincristine has been associated with inappropriate secretion of antidiuretic hormone. Although vincristine is essentially nonmyelosuppressive, bone marrow hypoplasia is dose-limiting with vinblastine and vinorelbine. Major neurotoxicity is less commonly observed with vinblastine and vinorelbine.

Paclitaxel and docetaxel infusions are associated with hypersensitivity reactions. The vehicle in which they are dissolved, cremophor EL or Tween 80, may contribute. Bradyarrhythmias (especially atrioventricular block), atypical chest pain, and, rarely, more severe cardiac problems have also been associated with paclitaxel. Myelosuppression is dose-limiting for both agents. Peripheral neuropathy and severe alopecia are also common with both. Glucocorticoids may prevent the hypersensitivity.

Topoisomerase Inhibitors During transcription and replication, DNA acquires conformational and topologic changes that must be relieved. The enzymes topoisomerase I and topoisomerase II perform this function by introducing and then repairing single- or double-stranded DNA breaks. Agents that interfere with this process have been found to have antitumor activity. *Camptothecin*, derived from the tree *Camptotheca accuminata*, is the prototypical inhibitor of topoisomerase I. The camptothecin analogues *9-aminocamptothecin*, *topotecan*, and *irinotecan* (CPT-11) are in clinical trials.

By contrast, topoisomerase II inhibitors, such the epipodophyllotoxins and anthracyclines, include some of the most widely used antitumor agents. These agents inhibit the DNA-rejoining activity of topoisomerase II, leading to DNA fragmentation and ultimately cell death. A serious complication first reported for the epipodophyllotoxins and now also recognized for the anthracyclines is the development of secondary leukemias. Epipodophyllotoxin-related acute myeloid leukemia appears to evolve within 3 years of treatment with the drug and has been associated with cytogenetic abnormalities involving chromosome 11q23. The incidence may exceed 5 percent and appears to be dose- and schedule-dependent. The incidence of secondary leukemia induced by anthracyclines is much lower.

The epipodophyllotoxins *etoposide* and *teniposide* are semisynthetic derivatives of the natural product podophyllotoxin, which is derived from the mandrake plant, *Podophyllum peltatum*. Leukopenia is the dose-limiting toxicity for etoposide and teniposide, with white cell counts reaching their nadir at approximately 14 days. Intravenous administration of either drug is associated with fever, hypotension, bronchospasm, and, rarely, anaphylaxis. The incidence of these symptoms can be minimized by administering the drugs over 1 h.

The anthracyclines include *doxorubicin*, *daunorubicin*, and *idarubicin*. In addition, *epirubicin* is available for clinical use outside the United States. Although the anthracyclines are topoisomerase II inhibitors, they also undergo one- and two-electron reductions with the generation of intracellular free radicals, particularly hydroxyl radicals, which are highly cytotoxic. The anthracyclines are myelosuppressive and cause gastrointestinal toxicity. They are severe vesicants, and extravasation during infusion may lead to local tissue necrosis. In extreme cases, skin grafting may be required. The anthracyclines are metabolized by the liver, and patients with elevations of serum bilirubin require dosage modifications. Long-term administration is limited by cumulative dose-dependent cardiotoxicity. Irreversible cardiomyopathy is a significant risk in patients who have received doses in excess of 500 to 550 mg/m² of doxorubicin or daunorubicin. Previous chest radiotherapy or concomitant cyclophosphamide therapy may lower the tolerable cumulative dose. *Dexrazoxane* is a chelating agent that may prevent anthracycline-induced cardiomyopathy. Although data are not yet definitive, it appears that dexrazoxane does not significantly decrease tumor response rates. It is recommended for patients who have already received 300 mg/m² of anthracycline.

Mitoxantrone, an anthracenedione, is structurally related to the anthracyclines. Although the incidence of cardiomyopathy with this agent is lower than for doxorubicin, patients are still at risk who have received lifetime doses greater than 125 mg/m². Mitoxantrone also causes marked myelosuppression. *Dactinomycin* currently has limited clinical use. It causes myelosuppression and gastrointestinal toxicity.

Alkylating Agents The alkylating agents are among the most widely used antitumor agents. Most alkylating agents are bifunctional and are efficient at cross-linking DNA, leading to strand breakage and ultimately cell death. Alkyl groups are preferentially added to N-7 or O-6 of guanine, as well as at other nitrogen or oxygen positions in adenine and cytidine. Although alkylation of DNA can occur at any phase of the cell cycle, cytotoxicity is greatest in cells that are progressing through the cell cycle. These agents are best regarded as cell-cycle–active but non-phase-specific. The covalent alkylation of DNA is mutagenic and carcinogenic and results in long-term serious complications, including detrimental effects on spermatogenesis and oogenesis as well as the development of secondary leukemias.

Azoospermia resulting from treatment with alkylating agents has been found in men receiving therapy for lymphoma and may be permanent. The severity of gonadal injury appears to be dose-dependent and in some men is reversible. Women who have received alkylating agents may experience amenorrhea and ovarian atrophy. The likelihood that normal menstrual cycles will resume is inversely related to the age of the patient and the cumulative dose received.

Another serious long-term complication of alkylating agent chemotherapy is the development of secondary leukemias. In patients who have received an alkylating agent as part of combination chemotherapy for Hodgkin's or non-Hodgkin's lymphoma, the incidence of secondary acute myeloid leukemia is about 2 percent. The incidence is augmented by the addition of radiation therapy. Secondary leukemias have also followed the use of alkylating agent therapy for multiple myeloma and ovarian carcinoma. Not all the alkylating agents are equally leukemogenic. Melphalan appears to be associated with a higher incidence of secondary acute leukemia than cyclophosphamide when used in the treatment of ovarian carcinoma.

The most common dose-limiting toxicity of the alkylating agents is myelosuppression. The severity and duration varies with the individual drugs. Most of the alkylating agents are quite emetogenic and require extensive premedication. Gastrointestinal epithelial damage, however, is not prominent.

Cyclophosphamide is one of the most widely used broad-spectrum antitumor agents. It is activated by microsomal liver metabolism to 4-hydroxycyclophosphamide and is further metabolized in peripheral tissues to phosphoramide mustard and to acrolein. Cyclophosphamide therapy may be complicated by hemorrhagic cystitis. This complication is due to the metabolite acrolein, which is excreted unchanged in the urine. Adequate hydration with standard-dose therapy, and administration of the bladder protectant *mesna* with high-dose therapy, can help prevent this complication. Chronic bladder inflammation as a result of cyclophosphamide therapy has been associated with the development of malignant bladder tumors. Cyclophosphamide administration is associated with a syndrome of inappropriate antidiuresis due to a distal renal tubular effect. Cyclophosphamide is also a potent immunosuppressive agent. In very high doses it has been associated rarely with acute myocardial necrosis.

Ifosfamide is an analogue of cyclophosphamide that is less myelosuppressive but more urotoxic. It is usually administered with the uroprotectant agent mesna. A reversible neurotoxicity, manifested primarily as altered mental status, has been observed with ifosfamide. *Melphalan* is a derivative of the amino acid phenylalanine, does not require hepatic activation, and does not cause hemorrhagic cystitis. Melphalan appears to be one of the most leukemogenic alkylating agents and has been associated rarely with the development of pulmonary fibrosis. *Busulfan* is toxic to myeloid stem cells and can cause prolonged bone marrow hypoplasia. Busulfan therapy is also associated rarely with interstitial pneumonitis and progressive pulmonary fibrosis. *Mechlorethamine* (nitrogen mustard), the first alkylating agent to be used widely, currently has limited use. Mechlorethamine is highly reactive in aqueous solution and is a severe vesicant. *Chlorambucil* is structurally related to mechlorethamine and is generally well tolerated. *Thiotepa* is a trivalent alkylating agent that currently has a limited clinical role.

Nitrosoureas The nitrosoureas *carmustine* (BCNU) and *lomustine* (CCNU) are a class of alkylating agents distinguished by high lipid solubility with excellent penetration into the central nervous system. The nitrosoureas produce a delayed myelosuppression lasting 4 to 6 weeks and appear to have a cumulative effect on the bone marrow. Moderate but reversible elevation of hepatic enzyme levels is common. A pulmonary fibrosis syndrome, similar to that seen with busulfan, has been reported. Prolonged treatment with the nitrosoureas can result in progressive renal insufficiency, even after cessation of therapy. Nitrosoureas are leukemogenic.

Platinum compounds The platinum compounds *cisplatin* and *carboplatin* are the only heavy metal compounds approved for use as antitumor agents. Although they are not true alkylating agents, they lead to the covalent cross-linking of DNA. Cisplatin is toxic to both proximal and distal renal tubule epithelial cells. Adequate intravenous hydration with saline diuresis, accompanied by administration of furosemide or mannitol, can decrease the incidence of nephrotoxicity. Nausea and vomiting are at times severe. Sensory neuropathy and high-frequency hearing loss after several cycles of therapy are not uncommon. Cisplatin produces modest myelosuppression. Carboplatin, a cisplatin analogue, is less nephrotoxic, less emetogenic, and less ototoxic, but more myelosuppressive.

Antitumor Antibiotics The antitumor antibiotics are isolated primarily from soil microorganisms. *Bleomycin* is a mixture of cytotoxic glycopeptides that interact with the ferrous iron ion (Fe^{2+}) and DNA simultaneously. This agent induces single- and double-stranded DNA breaks through free radical generation. It is cytotoxic mainly during the G2 and M phases of the cell cycle. Bleomycin has little myelosuppressive effect. Pulmonary toxicity manifested as a chronic interstitial pneumonitis is the most serious toxicity. The lifetime cumulative bleomycin dose should not exceed 200 U/m², and should be even less in patients with underlying pulmonary disease, previous chest radiotherapy, or advanced age. A test dose is often administered, because bleomycin infusion may be associated with hypersensitivity reactions.

Mitomycin C is activated intracellularly and then cross-links DNA. Mitomycin C exhibits delayed myelosuppression, with leukocyte and platelet counts reaching their nadir at 4 to 6 weeks. This agent can also precipitate progressive renal failure in association with a microangiopathic anemia (hemolytic-uremic syndrome).

Other Agents *Dacarbazine* appears to induce cytotoxicity by acting as an alkylating agent and damaging DNA after activation by hepatic microsomal enzymes. This agent produces moderate myelosuppression. Nausea and vomiting are often severe. *Procarbazine* is a monoamine oxidase inhibitor that, after oxidation by hepatic enzymes, functions like an alkylating agent, with methylation of nucleic acids. Procarbazine produces neurotoxicity manifested by peripheral sensory neuropathy and changes in mood and mental status. Nausea and vomiting may also be severe.

L-*Asparaginase*, the only enzyme used as an antitumor agent, results in depletion of extracellular pools of asparagine. Lymphocytes have a limited ability to synthesize the amino acid L-asparagine and are dependent on circulating pools. Asparaginase is associated with hypersensitivity reactions, and anaphylaxis may occur with the first dose. Hepatotoxicity, pancreatitis, and thromboses are occasionally observed.

COMBINATION CHEMOTHERAPY Most cancers are treated with multiagent chemotherapy. Although many regimens have been derived empirically, the principles that underlie most combinations of antitumor drugs can be summarized as follows. (1) Each of the agents in a regimen should have an independent activity against the specific tumor. Although unanticipated synergy may occur, adding an agent that by itself produces no response is likely to add toxicity without benefit. (2) Each drug should have a different mechanism of action. It is advantageous to target different steps along a biochemical pathway. Drugs that either inhibit the same enzyme or act by the same mechanism are less likely to have additive antitumor activity. (3) There should be no cross resistance among the agents used. A resistant tumor subpopulation selected by one drug is not likely to be cross-resistant to an agent that produces cytotoxicity through a different mechanism. (4) Each of the drugs should have a different dose-limiting toxicity. Administering two agents with the same toxicity profile at the maximum tolerated dose of each can produce unacceptable toxicity. Unfortunately, these principles are difficult to fulfill prospectively.

Bone marrow transplantation has been used to overcome severe myelosuppression after high-dose chemotherapy or chemoradiotherapy. The drugs most useful when transplantation is intended are generally the alkylating agents, such as busulfan and cyclophosphamide, which exhibit a linear response between drug dose and cell kill in vitro. Administering these drugs in myeloablative combination regimens results in higher tumor cytotoxicity. In autologous transplantation, the patient's bone marrow or peripheral blood stem cells are collected, cryopreserved, and then reinfused after delivery of systemic high-dose therapy. In allogeneic transplantation, bone marrow from a suitable donor is used to reconstitute the patient's hematopoietic system. Substantial evidence indicates that, in addition to the high-dose preparative regimens, immune effector mechanisms contribute to control of malignant disease after allogeneic bone marrow transplantation. The precise mediators of the so-called graft-versus-tumor effect remain to be elucidated. Transplantation has been most effective in treating tumors that are initially chemoresponsive, such as acute leukemia, Hodgkin's and non-Hodgkin's lymphoma, and testicular carcinoma. This approach has been ineffective, however, in treating common epithelial-derived malignancies, such as non-small cell lung carcinoma and colorectal carcinoma.

COMPLICATIONS Every chemotherapeutic regimen administered in adequate doses will have some deleterious side effect on normal tissues. Many complications can be anticipated, and considerable expertise has been gained in treating and preventing them. Myelosuppression, nausea and vomiting, stomatitis, and alopecia are the most frequently observed side effects.

Myelosuppression Chemotherapy-induced bone marrow suppression, manifested as leukopenia, thrombocytopenia, and anemia, is the most common dose-limiting toxicity. Blood counts usually reach their nadir between 10 and 14 days after treatment, with recovery noted by day 21 and a return to normal by day 28. Thus, most regimens are administered in cycles of 21 to 28 days. However, some agents, such as the nitrosoureas, involve a longer period of recovery and are usually administered every 6 weeks.

Neutropenia increases the risk of infectious complications. Fever is the hallmark of infection. Any patient with an absolute neutrophil count below 1.0×10^9/L and fever requires a prompt medical evaluation and subsequent administration of empirical, broad-spectrum parenteral antibiotics. Treatment with recombinant hematopoietic growth factors, particularly granulocyte colony stimulating factor and granulocyte-macrophage colony stimulating factor, can shorten the length of neutropenia associated with chemotherapy (see "Biologic Therapy," below).

Thrombocytopenia may occur in patients receiving chemotherapy but is less often dose-limiting than leukopenia. An increase in the bleeding time can be detected when the platelet count falls below 100×10^9/L, but most patients with platelet counts over 50×10^9/L are asymptomatic. The risk for a severe hemorrhagic complication, such as spontaneous intracranial bleeding, begins to increase when the platelet count falls below 20×10^9/L in patients with acute leukemia, or below 10×10^9/L in patients with solid tumors. Thrombocytopenia of this degree is usually observed only with very intense chemotherapeutic regimens, such as those used in the treatment of acute leukemia.

Some degree of anemia is to be anticipated with chemotherapy. However, except with dose-intensive regimens, transfusions usually are not required. In addition, there is no single hemoglobin level below which all patients should receive transfusions for chemotherapy-induced anemia. Rather, transfusions should be administered only after considering the long-term goals of therapy and weighing the risk-to-benefit ratio for each patient.

Nausea and Vomiting Nausea and vomiting are major side effects of cancer chemotherapy. Progress in preventing and treating chemotherapy-induced nausea and vomiting has resulted from the development of newer and more effective antiemetics, the completion of prospective clinical trials that addressed the problem, and the education of physicians regarding prevention and management.

Chemotherapy appears to induce nausea and vomiting through several pathways. Vomiting is controlled by two medullary centers, the vomiting center and the chemoreceptor trigger zone. The chemoreceptor trigger zone is stimulated directly by various toxins or drugs to release neurotransmitters, such as dopamine, which then interact with the vomiting center. The vomiting center coordinates the process of vomiting through multiple efferent tracts. Cerebral input, especially from visual or olfactory stimuli, can also stimulate the vomiting center.

Chemotherapeutic agents are not all equally emetogenic. Cisplatin consistently causes the most severe side effects. Dacarbazine, doxorubicin, and mechlorethamine are also highly emetogenic agents. However, many antimetabolites, such as methotrexate and fluorouracil, cause only minimal nausea and vomiting.

Prevention of nausea and vomiting should be a primary goal. Antiemetic regimens always should be given on a routine schedule, preferably beginning 24 h before chemotherapy administration. Treatment on an as-needed basis is generally inappropriate. Antiemetic regimens should err on the side of being too aggressive rather than insufficient, particularly for patients receiving chemotherapy for the first time. The treatment regimen should be commensurate with the emetogenic potential of the particular chemotherapy program.

The phenothiazines, such as *prochlorperazine* and *chlorpromazine*, are the most widely used antiemetic agents and appear to exert this effect through their antidopaminergic and antiserotoninergic activities. They are available in several formulations, making them useful for outpatient regimens. As single agents they are effective only for mildly emetogenic drugs, such as fluorouracil.

The benzamide *metoclopramide* appears to antagonize dopamine activity peripherally and centrally. When used parenterally in high doses (1 to 2 mg/kg every 2 to 4 h), it can effectively reduce the nausea and vomiting associated with the most emetogenic chemotherapeutic drugs. Metoclopramide used in high doses may cause extrapyramidal side effects and thus is often administered with an antihistamine (such as diphenhydramine) or a benzodiazepine (such as lorazepam).

The serotonin antagonists *ondansetron* and *granisetron* are the newest and among the most effective antiemetic agents. They selectively block the serotonin receptor 5-HT$_3$, which is present peripherally on the vagus nerve and centrally in the chemoreceptor trigger zone. They are effective in the treatment of nausea and vomiting due to cisplatin but are without the dystonic reactions that may accompany metoclopramide.

The cannabinoid *dronabinol* (Marinol) contains the principal psychoactive agent in marijuana, Δ-9-THC. It is available only in oral formulation and appears to be most effective against mild or moderately emetogenic chemotherapeutic regimens. It produces significant mood alterations, including dysphoria in some patients.

Other agents are frequently employed in combination antiemetic regimens. High-dose glucocorticoids, such as dexamethasone, may be used for brief intervals, particularly with metoclopramide. Benzodiazepines are useful as sedatives for patients with anticipatory nausea and vomiting and as amnestic agents. Antihistamines have modest antinausea properties but are useful to prevent dystonic reactions associated with phenothiazines or metoclopramide.

Stomatitis Stomatitis, an inflammation of the oral mucosa, is a major complication of cancer chemotherapy. Early signs of stomatitis are erythema and edema, which may progress to frank, painful ulcerátions that persist for from several days to a week or longer. The painful ulcers result in poor oral intake with subsequent dehydration and malnutrition. They also may become secondarily infected and further complicate patient management. Virtually all chemotherapeutic agents will cause stomatitis if given at a sufficient dose intensity. With the antimetabolites, the duration of exposure is probably a greater risk factor for developing stomatitis than the peak drug level.

Currently, there are no means to prevent stomatitis except to modify the doses of the offending chemotherapeutic agents. Meticulous oral hygiene will help to diminish pathogenic oral flora and decrease the risk of secondary infections. Treatment with topical oral anesthetics, such as viscous xylocaine, can relieve pain and help to maintain adequate oral intake. Capsaicin may help in symptom control.

Alopecia Chemotherapy-induced hair loss is one of the most distressing aspects of cancer treatment for some patients. It is due to the cytotoxic effects of antineoplastic agents on the hair follicle. The hair loss tends to be patchy and most severe on the scalp, and it is usually noticeable 1 to 2 weeks after the beginning of therapy. After the cessation of chemotherapy, the hair should eventually return to pretreatment levels, although it may be different in texture and color. Cyclophosphamide, dactinomycin, doxorubicin, paclitaxel, and vincristine generally cause the most profound alopecia. Scalp-cooling devices, which apparently decrease scalp perfusion, have been employed with mixed results.

DRUG RESISTANCE Tumor cell resistance to chemotherapeutic agents is a central problem in medical oncology. With improvements in supportive care, including a new generation of antimicrobials, treatment with multicomponent blood products and hematopoietic growth factors, specialized oncology nursing, and high-technology intensive care units, drug resistance is probably the single most important obstacle to achieving higher cure rates.

The problem of drug resistance can be divided into two types: de novo resistance and acquired resistance. In de novo resistance, tumor cells are unresponsive to chemotherapy from the start. Unfortunately, many of the most common solid tumors show de novo resistance. In acquired drug resistance, tumors that are initially responsive to chemotherapy develop resistance with continued therapy. Acquired resistance is a primary reason why only a small percentage of the many tumors that respond to chemotherapy can be cured with chemotherapy alone.

The appearance of resistant clones within a larger population of cells was addressed initially by Delbruck and Luria in studies on bacteria and later by Law and then Goldie and Coldman in tumor cells. Delbruck and Luria observed that populations of bacteria exhibited varying degrees of resistance to bacteriophage infection. They showed that resistant cells were present in the population owing to spontaneous mutations that existed before exposure to the phage. Development of resistance depended on mutation frequency and population size.

The Delbruck-Luria principles were extended to tumor cell biology and treatment. An important property of tumor cells is genomic instability. As a tumor grows from a single transformed cell to a clinically detectable 1-cm³ mass consisting of 10^9 cells, spontaneous mutations will give rise to a heterogeneous population of cells, some of which have mutated to a drug-resistant phenotype purely by chance. Treatment with chemotherapy will eliminate the most sensitive cells and leave the resistant subclones to grow. Clinically, this situation occurs in patients whose tumor has responded to therapy and entered a complete or partial remission, only to relapse and progress later in a drug-refractory form.

These concepts suggest important principles for maximizing the effectiveness of chemotherapy. Tumors are most likely to be responsive to chemotherapy when small in size, before multiple resistant subclones have developed. Regimens that are not effective against bulky tumors may be curative when used in the adjuvant setting. Effective treatment should consist of combination chemotherapy containing non-cross-resistant agents. The likelihood that a cell will undergo two simultaneous mutations affording resistance to two different classes of drugs is low (i.e., the product of two independent

probabilities). Thus, the greater the number of non-cross-resistant drugs administered at full dose, the greater the chance of eliminating the entire tumor population.

Although the principle of combination chemotherapy is useful, limitations exist. Many antitumor agents, such as the alkylating agents, the anthracyclines, and the epipodophyllotoxins, are mutagenic and thus can actively promote the appearance of drug-resistant mutant clones. Furthermore, resistance to certain antitumor drugs can be associated with cross-resistance to other agents that are structurally and mechanistically distinct.

Mechanisms of Single-Agent Drug Resistance Much of what is known about drug resistance is a result of in vitro studies. Cell lines have been selected for resistance to various chemotherapeutic agents by exposing them to gradually increasing concentrations of the drug. Comparison of resistant sublines to the parental cell lines can reveal the resistance mechanisms. Determining the clinical importance of these in vitro mechanisms has been difficult. Examples of specific resistance mechanisms for various agents are given in Table 86-4.

Mechanisms of Multiple Drug Resistance Clinical refractoriness to chemotherapy is often characterized by resistance to multiple drugs. The phenomenon of in vitro multiple drug resistance was first described in the 1970s by Biedler and by Ling. In multiple drug resistance, cells selected for resistance to one drug show cross-resistance to other, structurally and functionally unrelated compounds. The drugs that constitute the multidrug-resistance family broadly include the anthracyclines, the vinca alkaloids, the epipodophyllotoxins, and the taxanes. Multidrug-resistant cells demonstrate an energy-dependent outward efflux of cytotoxic drugs. The resistant cell lines overexpress a membrane glycoprotein of 170 kDa termed *P-glycoprotein* or a 190 kDa membrane protein termed the *multidrug resistance protein* (MRP). Both belong to the family of ATP-binding cassette proteins.

Efflux mediated by P-glycoprotein can be blocked and multiple drug resistance circumvented by various modulating agents. Existing modulating agents, such as verapamil, quinine, and cyclosporine, have produced unacceptable toxicity when used at doses required to inhibit P-glycoprotein activity. Newer analogues, such as *dexverapamil* and *PSC 833* (a cyclosporine derivative), have entered clinical trials attempting to overcome multiple drug resistance. Agents that modulate MRP activity have to date been more difficult to identify. Although P-glycoprotein and MRP expression are well-defined mechanisms of in vitro multiple drug resistance, their role in clinical drug resistance has yet to be defined fully. In a few tumors, particularly adult acute myeloid leukemia and childhood neuroblastoma, P-glycoprotein expression at presentation portends a worse prognosis.

Altered activity and/or expression of the enzyme topoisomerase II is associated with resistance to the anthracyclines and epipodophyllo-

Table 86-4

Mechanisms of Single-Agent Drug Resistance

Mechanism	Drugs	Target
Defective transport	Methotrexate	Folate transporter
	Cytarabine	Nucleoside transporter
	Mechlorethamine	Choline transporter
Decreased activating enzyme	Cytarabine	Deoxycytidine kinase
	Mercaptopurine	Hypoxanthine-guanine phosphoribosyl transferase
	Methotrexate	Folyl-polyglutamylate synthetase
Increased drug inactivation	Bleomycin	Bleomycin hydrolase
	Cyclophosphamide	Aldehyde dehydrogenase
	Cytarabine	Cytidine deaminase
Increased target enzyme	Fluorouracil	Thymidylate synthase
	Methotrexate	Dihydrofolate reductase
	Pentostatin	Adenosine deaminase
Alteration in target	Fluorouracil	Thymidylate synthase
	Hydroxyurea	Ribonucleotide reductase
	Vincristine	Tubulin

toxins. Altered topoisomerase activity may also exist in cells that simultaneously exhibit more than one mechanism of multiple drug resistance. The clinical significance of topoisomerase II–mediated resistance is unknown.

An enhanced reducing environment with increased activity of glutathione detoxification pathways and elevated cellular pools of reduced glutathione has been described. Resistance to alkylating agents, including the nitrogen mustard derivatives and the nitrosoureas as well as the anthracyclines, has been associated with increased glutathione detoxification. *Buthionine sulfoximine*, an agent that depletes cellular glutathione levels, has entered clinical trials as a chemosensitizing agent.

Failure to undergo programmed cell death in response to genotoxic stress may contribute to insensitivity to both chemotherapy and ionizing radiation. The Bcl-2 protein is a key modulator of apoptosis and can prevent p53-dependent and -independent pathways of apoptosis. Other homologous proteins, Bcl-X and Bax, are also involved in the regulation of apoptosis. Bcl-X is expressed in two forms by differential RNA splicing. Bcl-X_L acts like Bcl-2 in preventing apoptosis. However, Bcl-X_S and Bax appear to promote cell death unless their function is blocked by heterodimerization with Bcl-2. The clinical importance of this family of proteins in chemotherapy insensitivity is an area of active investigation.

NEW DRUG DEVELOPMENT   After the discovery in the 1940s of drugs with antitumor efficacy, the National Cancer Institute began a large-scale screening program. New compounds are tested against a panel of about 60 human cancer cell lines representing common solid tumors. Agents demonstrating in vitro antitumor activity are then tested against a panel of human tumor xenografts in nude mice. Compounds that are still promising then undergo further toxicology screening and formulation testing before beginning clinical trials. Antitumor agents proceed through a series of clinical trials marked by three distinct phases before they are accepted into widespread clinical use. It may take 10 years or longer for a compound to proceed from initial screening to approval by the Food and Drug Administration for a specific indication.

Phase I trials are performed to determine drug toxicity in humans. To be eligible, patients must have a cancer not responsive to available therapies. An initial dose is chosen on the basis of animal studies. Generally, small cohorts of patients are treated at a given dose before dose escalation, which proceeds sequentially until a dose-limiting toxicity is reached and the maximum tolerated dose is defined. Because phase I trials often involve a relatively small number of previously treated patients with diverse tumor types, lack of tumor response does not rule out ultimate clinical usefulness for the agent.

Phase II trials are designed to determine if a drug has activity for a particular tumor type. Generally, small groups of patients with advanced malignancies are treated according to a dose schedule determined from the phase I study. Patients must have measurable tumors, so that the efficacy of therapy can be assessed. A given compound may undergo several phase II studies against a broad array of tumor types. After the completion of phase II trials, a decision is made to proceed to phase III or to abandon further testing. Generally, compounds that induce responses in 20 percent or fewer of patients in phase II testing are not developed further.

Phase III studies are designed to test an agent against the standard existing therapy for a particular tumor. This testing usually requires a randomized, two-arm study. Patients generally have not received prior therapy at the time of treatment. Phase III trials require large numbers of patients and frequently are multi-institutional.

DIFFERENTIATING AGENTS   Models of malignant transformation include the concept of maturation arrest. The clinical observation of residual differentiated masses after treatment of germ cell tumors or neuroblastoma with cytotoxic chemotherapy suggested that therapy aimed at promoting tumor cell differentiation may be effective. Studies in vitro have demonstrated that a variety of compounds could induce tumor cells to differentiate and to display characteristics of a more mature phenotype. Agents such as retinoids, vitamin D, phorbol esters, and polar/planar compounds (such as dimethyl sulfoxide) have been extensively characterized for their effects on tumor cell lines.

Retinoids stimulate the growth of normal myeloid and erythroid progenitors in culture and the differentiation of myeloid leukemia cell lines in vitro. Clinical trials showed that all-*trans*-retinoic acid (ATRA; *tretinoin*) induced remissions in a high percentage of patients with acute promyelocytic leukemia, although the duration of remission was on average short (<6 months). Tretinoin commonly produces headache and dermatologic toxicity. A minority of patients, however, will experience a syndrome of fever, pulmonary infiltrates, and respiratory distress. Prompt treatment with glucocorticoids may prevent worsening of the capillary leak syndrome. Clinical evaluation of tretinoin, as well as other retinoids and differentiating agents, continues.

ENDOCRINE THERAPY   Endocrine therapy for hormone-responsive malignancies depends on the existence of underlying cellular growth control mechanisms derived from those of the normal tissues from which the tumor arose. For example, the presence of estrogen and progesterone receptors in breast carcinoma is predictive of a response to endocrine therapy. Many hormonal antitumor agents are functional agonists or antagonists of the steroid hormone family. Steroid hormones bind to specific intracellular receptors and induce a conformational change. The hormone-receptor complex interacts with DNA and functions as a transcription factor regulating gene expression.

Adrenocorticosteroids   Because the toxicities of glucocorticoids do not overlap with those of many chemotherapeutic agents, and in particular do not include myelosuppression, glucocorticoids are frequently used in combination regimens for the treatment of lymphocytic leukemias and lymphomas. They function by binding to glucocorticoid-specific receptors present in lymphoid cells and initiating programmed cell death. Although several synthetic glucocorticoids are available, the agents most often used in cancer therapy are *prednisone*, *methylprednisolone*, and *dexamethasone*.

Antiandrogens   The antiandrogen *flutamide* effectively blocks the binding of androgen to its receptor in peripheral tissues. Although serum testosterone levels may rise, levels in the target tissues are decreased. Flutamide is used in the treatment of disseminated prostate carcinoma and is often used with leuprolide. It has predictable antiandrogen side effects in men, including gynecomastia, decreased libido, and impotence. Elevation of hepatic transaminase levels has also been reported.

Estrogens   Estrogen therapy was once a mainstay in the palliative treatment of disseminated prostate carcinoma, where it appears to function as a potent antiandrogen. Estrogens are occasionally used in the palliative treatment of breast carcinoma. Two commonly used preparations are *diethylstilbesterol* (DES) and *ethinyl estradiol*. Estrogen therapy can exacerbate underlying ischemic heart disease, may predispose to thromboembolic phenomena, and may lead to fluid retention. Gynecomastia and impotence in men is common.

Antiestrogens   The antiestrogen *tamoxifen* is widely used in the therapy of breast carcinoma. It is employed in the adjuvant setting in postmenopausal women and as palliative therapy for metastatic disease in both premenopausal and postmenopausal women. Tamoxifen binds directly to the estrogen receptor and appears to function as a weak agonist/antagonist. It has a long plasma half-life and requires 4 weeks or longer to achieve steady state levels. Tamoxifen can cause amenorrhea, hot flashes, and, rarely, nausea and vomiting. It has been reported to modestly increase the risk of thromboembolic phenomenon. Chronic use is associated with a slightly increased risk of endometrial cancer. On the other hand, tamoxifen lowers the risk of death from cardiovascular disease and prevents osteoporosis.

Progestins   Progestational agents such as *medroxyprogesterone* and *megestrol acetate* are used in the treatment of endometrial carcinoma and breast carcinoma. Studies suggest they may disrupt the hypothalamic-pituitary-gonadal axis, alter expression of estrogen receptors, or have androgenic effects. Progestins frequently cause menstrual irregularities. Fluid retention, elevated levels of hepatic enzymes, and thromboembolic events have all been reported.

Aromatase Inhibitor *Aminoglutethimide* inhibits the enzymatic pathway responsible for the conversion of androgens to estrogens in the peripheral tissues. It also inhibits the conversion of cholesterol to pregnenolone, a key step in steroid hormone biosynthesis. Aminoglutethimide treatment functions as a medical adrenalectomy, and patients receiving relatively high doses may need maintenance hydrocortisone and/or mineralocorticoid. It is used in the palliative treatment of metastatic breast carcinoma. Toxicity includes mild neurologic and dermatologic symptoms. On rare occasions, reversible leukopenia and thrombocytopenia have been observed.

Gonadotropin-Releasing Hormone Agonists The gonadotropin-releasing hormone (GnRH) agonist *leuprolide* is used in the treatment of disseminated prostate carcinoma. Continuous stimulation of the pituitary by GnRH—as opposed to the normal pulsatile control—leads to eventual downregulation of luteinizing hormone (LH) and follicle-stimulating hormone (FSH) secretion, with subsequent diminution of androgen levels. During the first weeks of therapy, increased LH and FSH release may precipitate a worsening of symptoms, which may be avoided by instituting antiandrogen treatment. Antiandrogen effects, including gynecomastia, impotence, and hot flashes, are seen to a varying degree.

Somatostatin Analogues The somatostatin analogue *octreotide* is used in the symptomatic treatment of patients with metastatic carcinoid or vasoactive intestinal peptide–secreting tumors. Somatostatin analogues suppress the release of gastric and pancreatic peptides in addition to suppressing growth hormone release. Patients with functional endocrine tumors who are receiving octreotide experience a dramatic decrease in endocrine-related symptoms. The drug must be injected subcutaneously two or three times daily to maintain adequate relief of symptoms. Because somatostatin inhibits insulin secretion, patients must be monitored for hyperglycemia.

BIOLOGIC THERAPY

Most biologic agents act as *biologic response modifiers*, meaning that they function by altering the host response to cancer; however, some cause direct cytotoxicity. Assessing the clinical usefulness of these agents is at times difficult because the paradigms for cytotoxic chemotherapy may be inappropriate for biologic agents. Biologic agents usually demonstrate peak activity within a narrow concentration range; higher or lower concentrations may result in a suboptimal effect. Thus, the optimal clinical dose is the one that produces the maximum desired effect, which may not be the highest dose tolerated without unacceptable toxicity.

IMMUNOTHERAPY Manipulation of the host immune response to cancer is a major goal of biologic therapy. Animal studies have conclusively shown that the immune system can recognize and eliminate malignant tumors in vivo. Rejection of tumor cells in several animal models appears to be mediated primarily by cytotoxic lymphocytes, including cytotoxic T lymphocytes and natural killer cells. Other effector cells, such as helper T cells, B cells, and macrophages, may also participate. However, antitumor immune responses have been difficult to demonstrate in patients with cancer. Furthermore, immune recognition of malignant cells can occur without resulting in tumor rejection. Cancer immunotherapy seeks to evoke effective immune responses to human tumors. Approaches have included administration of monoclonal antibodies, immunomodulatory cytokines, autologous or allogeneic immunocompetent cells, and tumor vaccines.

Monoclonal Antibodies The ability to produce monoclonal antibodies to a specific antigenic determinant led to high expectations for their widespread use in cancer therapy. Although monoclonal antibodies are important tools in cancer diagnosis, their use in cancer therapy has remained investigational. Trials of unconjugated monoclonal antibodies as cytotoxic therapy have generally proved disappointing. Obstacles have included difficulty in defining tumor-specific antigens serologically, antigenic modulation by tumor cells, and the development of human anti-mouse antibodies. Efforts to improve the efficacy of this approach have led to ongoing trials of antibodies conjugated to drugs, radioisotopes, or toxins. Clinical studies are evaluating the use of monoclonal antibodies in purging harvested bone marrow of tumor cells before autologous transplantation.

The immunophenotyping of leukemias and lymphomas using monoclonal antibodies directed primarily against myeloid and lymphoid differentiation antigens has improved our understanding of the pathogenesis of these diseases and has facilitated diagnosis. It is now common to analyze the immunophenotype of all lymphoid and myeloid specimens. Monoclonal antibody–based serum assays are commonly used for monitoring disease progress in solid tumors. CA-125 can be used to monitor ovarian carcinoma, and the prostate-specific antigen (PSA) to monitor prostate cancer, although widespread use of PSA as a tool for screening is controversial.

Immunomodulatory Cytokines Cytokines are intercellular messenger proteins. They include the interferons and interleukins. Interferons α and β share a common cellular receptor and are referred to as type I interferons. *Interferon* α is the product of a multigene family of at least 20 members, whereas *interferon* β is the product of a single gene. Type I interferons have immunoregulatory and antiproliferative effects. Recombinant interferon α is approved for use in the treatment of chronic myeloid leukemia, hairy cell leukemia, and AIDS-related Kaposi's sarcoma; it is an effective adjuvant therapy for high-risk melanoma. In addition, interferon α has activity in low-grade non-Hodgkin's lymphoma, multiple myeloma, and renal cell carcinoma. *Interferon* γ, produced by lymphocytes, is referred to as type II interferon and has immunomodulatory properties distinct from those of type I interferons. It appears to have less single-agent antitumor activity than type I interferons. It is used in the treatment of chronic granulomatous disease but remains investigational as an antitumor agent. All interferons can produce a flu-like syndrome with fever, malaise, myalgias, and fatigue. Modest leukopenia is also common, and elevations in hepatic transaminase levels can be seen.

The interleukins are cytokines that function predominantly as leukocyte messengers. At least 17 interleukins have been identified, and several have entered clinical trials, but only recombinant *interleukin 2* is an approved anticancer agent. Interleukin (IL)-2, previously known as T-cell growth factor, is a key regulatory hormone in cell-mediated immunity. It stimulates the proliferation and cytolytic activity of T cells and natural killer cells. High-dose IL-2 therapy produces a response in a minority of patients with metastatic renal cell carcinoma and melanoma. A small percentage (5 to 10 percent) of patients achieve a complete response associated with long-term disease-free survival. However, cardiovascular complications, largely due to a vascular leak syndrome, may necessitate intensive care unit management. Other toxicities, which can involve virtually every organ system (particularly renal, hepatic, pulmonary, neurologic, hematopoietic, and dermatologic toxicities), are seen but are generally reversible. Trials of outpatient therapy using reduced doses, often administered by continuous infusion, have resulted in less acute toxicity. The optimal dose and schedule of IL-2 therapy have not been defined.

The other interleukins remain investigational agents for cancer therapy. *Interleukin 4* is produced primarily by T cells and mast cells and has diverse immunohematopoietic effects. Several phase I/II trials of IL-4 alone or in combination with IL-2 have been completed. Although IL-4 can be safely administered with only moderate toxicity, the low rates of tumor response have diminished enthusiasm for its ultimate role as an antitumor agent. *Interleukin 6* is a pleiotropic cytokine that has direct antiproliferative activity in a variety of tumor model systems, in addition to immunohematopoietic activity that directly affects B cells, T cells, and megakaryocytes. Clinical trials have begun to assess IL-6 as an antitumor agent and as a thrombopoietic agent. *Interleukin 12* stimulates the function of both T cells and natural killer cells. Phase I trials of IL-12 in patients with cancer and AIDS have been conducted, and additional clinical studies are in progress.

Tumor necrosis factor (TNF) plays a central role in the inflammatory response. TNF administration produces impressive antitumor responses in animal models. However, pronounced toxicity (mainly cardiovascular) in humans after systemic administration, combined with low tumor response rates, has limited its clinical development. The use of TNF for local and regional therapy, as in isolated limb perfusion, is under investigation.

Cellular Therapy Adoptive cellular therapy consists of transferring either autologous or allogeneic immune effector cells to a tumor-bearing host. Autologous effectors generally are activated and expanded ex vivo before administration. Lymphokine-activated killer (LAK) cells, generated by culturing peripheral blood lymphocytes with IL-2, can directly lyse freshly isolated solid tumor cells. However, administration of LAK cells generated ex vivo together with IL-2 does not appear to be better than administration of IL-2 alone. Tumor-infiltrating lymphocytes (TIL), isolated directly from solid tumors, can also be expanded ex vivo with IL-2. In experimental systems, TIL demonstrate significantly more antitumor efficacy than LAK cells. Although early clinical trials in patients with metastatic melanoma are promising, it is not known whether administration of TIL is more effective than IL-2 alone. Allogeneic immune effector cells have been used to treat patients who have relapsed after bone marrow transplantation. Clinical, cytogenetic, and molecular complete remissions have been induced in patients with chronic myeloid leukemia after infusion of donor-derived buffy coats. Complications have included graft-versus-host disease and myelosuppression (See Chap. 116).

Tumor Vaccines The search for cancer vaccines effective in humans was stimulated by animal models that demonstrated protection from tumor challenges after immunization with syngeneic tumors or their derivatives. However, rejection of previously established solid tumors in experimental systems has been generally possible only when combined with a reduction in tumor burden, as by surgery. Thus, tumor vaccines may prove most effective in humans when used as adjuvants or in a setting of minimal disease. The question of which are the optimal immunogens remains unresolved. The injection of autologous whole tumor cells (unmodified, modified, or with an adjuvant) has resulted in modest objective tumor responses in some patients with melanoma. However, the generally low response rates and short remission duration have prompted further investigations. Gene transfer techniques to induce the expression of immunomodulatory molecules, such as B7, IL-12, or granulocyte-macrophage colony stimulating factor (GM-CSF), may increase the immunogenicity of the autologous tumor.

HEMATOPOIETIC GROWTH FACTORS Hematopoietic growth and differentiation are under the regulation of cytokines known as colony stimulating factors (CSFs). These agents were initially defined by their ability to stimulate and support hematopoietic colony formation in vitro using a semisolid culture system. Thus, the classification of a cytokine as a CSF or an interleukin is primarily a historical artifact. The isolation and subsequent clinical development of hematopoietic growth factors has substantially changed the clinical care of patients receiving myelosuppressive chemotherapy. In particular, the two agents that support neutrophil maturation, *granulocyte-macrophage CSF* (GM-CSF) and *granulocyte CSF* (G-CSF), have received widespread acceptance despite the fact that their optimal clinical use is not defined. To better guide clinicians, both the American Society of Clinical Oncology (ASCO) and the European Consensus Conference assembled expert panels to review the clinical data and to issue guidelines for the use of colony stimulating factors. The ASCO guidelines are summarized in Table 86-5 (see also Chap. 105).

GM-CSF promotes the differentiation of committed myeloid progenitors into mature granulocytes, monocytes, and eosinophils. It also stimulates growth of the multilineage hematopoietic precursors. Recombinant GM-CSF hastens myeloid reconstitution after autologous bone marrow transplantation. GM-CSF administration is associated with constitutional symptoms (fevers, chills, myalgias, anorexia, lethargy) and bone pain. G-CSF stimulates the growth and differentiation of committed neutrophilic progenitor cells. Administration of G-CSF to patients can shorten the period of neutropenia associated with

Table 86-5

Use of Colony Stimulating Factors in Patients with Cancer

Circumstance	Recommendation
Primary administration (beginning with first cycle of chemotherapy)	Not recommended for routine use (unless febrile neutropenia is expected in ≥40% of patients or patient has a preexisting risk factor)
Secondary administration (after an episode of febrile neutropenia)	May be used, although reduction in chemotherapy dose should be considered as an alternative unless dose intensity is important
In afebrile neutropenic patients	Not recommended for routine use
In febrile neutropenic patients	May be used if factors predictive of deterioration are present (such as pneumonia, hypotension, sepsis, fungal infection)
To make possible an increase in the dose intensity of chemotherapy	Not recommended for routine use
To shorten the duration of neutropenia after bone marrow transplantation	May be routinely recommended to mobilize peripheral blood progenitor cells and to speed hematopoietic reconstitution
In patients with acute myeloid leukemia	May be used after induction chemotherapy in patients ≥55 years
In patients with myelodysplasia	May be used intermittently (if neutropenia and recurrent infection are present)

chemotherapy-induced myeloid suppression. Clinical experience suggests that G-CSF may be better tolerated than GM-CSF, but randomized studies comparing the two cytokines have not been reported. Bone pain is the most common side effect of G-CSF.

Interleukin 3 stimulates the growth and differentiation of multipotent hematopoietic progenitors as well as committed erythroid, myeloid, and megakaryocytic precursors. Clinical trial results have been disappointing.

Erythropoietin, the primary regulator of erythropoiesis, induces erythroid maturation in committed progenitor cells and increases the release of reticulocytes from the bone marrow. Erythropoietin is produced by the kidney and liver in response to hypoxia. Recombinant erythropoietin is clearly beneficial in treating deficiency states such as the anemia of chronic renal failure. Patients receiving myelosuppressive chemotherapy experience anemia to varying degrees, and clinical trials have demonstrated that erythropoietin is modestly effective in ameliorating this form of anemia after at least 2 months of use. However, many patients with cancer suffer from the anemia of chronic disease, which is associated with a blunted response to erythropoietin, and they are thus less likely to benefit from its use.

Thrombopoietin (previously known as the Mpl ligand) has been identified. It has been shown to support megakaryocyte maturation and platelet production and has entered clinical trials.

Cytokines that appear to be responsible for maintenance of the multipotent hematopoietic stem cell have also been identified. The *Flk2/Flt3 ligand* and *stem-cell* or *Steel factor* activate specific tyrosine kinase receptors that appear to be restricted to the earliest stem cells. They act synergistically with later-acting hematopoietic growth factors, such as IL-3 or GM-CSF, to cause proliferation and expansion of hematopoietic progenitors. They are just beginning to be tested in humans.

See Chap. 51, Antineoplastic agents, in Goodman & Gilman's The Pharmacological Basis of Therapeutics, 9th ed, JG Hardman, LE Limbird (eds), New York, McGraw-Hill, 1996, pp 1233–1287.

BIBLIOGRAPHY

AMERICAN SOCIETY OF CLINICAL ONCOLOGY UPDATE OF RECOMMENDATIONS FOR USE OF HEMATOPOIETIC COLONY-STIMULATING FACTORS: Evidence-based, clinical practice guidelines. J Clin Oncol 14:1957, 1996

BOOGAERTS M et al: Granulocyte growth factors: Achieving a consensus. Ann Oncol 6:237, 1995

CHABNER BA, LONGO DL: *Cancer Chemotherapy and Biotherapy: Principles and Practice.* Philadelphia, Lippincott, 1996

DEVITA VT et al (eds): *Biologic Therapy of Cancer*, 2d ed. Philadelphia, Lippincott, 1995

DRUGS OF CHOICE FOR CANCER CHEMOTHERAPY. Med Let 37:25, 1995

FISHER DE: Apoptosis in cancer therapy: Crossing the threshold. Cell 78:539, 1994

HOLLAND JF et al (eds): *Cancer Medicine*, 4th ed. Philadelphia, Lea & Febiger, 1996

PIZZO PH: Management of fever in patients with cancer and treatment-induced neutropenia. N Engl J Med 328:1323, 1993

87 *Robert Finberg*

INFECTIONS IN PATIENTS WITH CANCER

Infections are a common cause of death and an even more common cause of morbidity in patients with a wide variety of neoplasms. Autopsy studies show that most deaths from acute leukemia and half of deaths from lymphoma are caused directly by infection. With more intensive chemotherapy, patients with solid tumors have become more likely to die of infection rather than their underlying disease.

A physical predisposition to infection (Table 87-1) can be a result of the neoplasm's production of a break in the skin; for example, a squamous cell carcinoma may cause local invasion of the epidermis, which allows bacteria to gain access to the subcutaneous tissue and permits the development of cellulitis. The artificial closing of a normally patent orifice can also predispose to infection: Obstruction of a ureter by a tumor can cause urinary tract infection, and obstruction of the bile duct can cause cholangitis. Part of the host's normal defense against infection depends on the continuous emptying of a viscus; without emptying, a few bacteria present as a result of bacteremia or local transit can multiply and cause disease.

A similar problem can affect patients whose lymph node integrity has been disrupted by radical surgery, particularly patients who have had radical node dissections. A common clinical problem following radical mastectomy is the development of cellulitis (usually caused by streptococci or staphylococci) because of lymphedema and/or inadequate lymph drainage. In most cases, this problem can be addressed by local measures designed to prevent fluid accumulation and breaks in the skin, but antibiotic prophylaxis has been necessary in refractory cases.

A life-threatening problem common to many cancer patients is the loss of the reticuloendothelial capacity to clear microorganisms after splenectomy. Splenectomy is common in patients with Hodgkin's disease and in the management of hairy-cell leukemia, chronic lymphocytic leukemia (CLL), and refractory idiopathic thrombocytopenic purpura. Even after curative therapy for the underlying disease, the lack of a spleen predisposes such patients to rapidly fatal infections. The loss of the spleen through trauma similarly predisposes the normal host to overwhelming infection as long as 25 years after splenectomy. The splenectomized patient should be counseled about the risks of infection with certain organisms, such as the protozoan *Babesia* (Chap. 216) and *Capnocytophaga canimorsus* (formerly, dysgonic fermenter 2 or DF-2), a bacterium carried in the mouths of animals (Chap. 135). Since encapsulated bacteria (*Streptococcus pneumoniae, Haemophilus influenzae*, and *Neisseria meningitidis*) are the organisms most commonly associated with postsplenectomy sepsis, splenectomized persons should be vaccinated (and revaccinated; see Table 87-2) against the capsular polysaccharides of these organisms. Many clinicians recommend giving splenectomized patients a small supply of antibiotics effective against *S. pneumoniae, N. meningitidis*, and *H. influenzae* to avert rapid, overwhelming sepsis in the event that they cannot present for medical attention immediately after the onset of fever or other symptoms of bacterial infection.

The level of suspicion of infections with certain organisms should depend on the type of cancer diagnosed (Table 87-3). Diagnosis of multiple myeloma or CLL should prompt the measurement of immunoglobulin levels and the consideration of either antibody replacement or antibiotic prophylaxis. (In the case of CLL, antibiotic prophylaxis for likely pathogens has proven a cost-effective preventive measure.) Similarly, patients with acute lymphocytic leukemia (ALL), patients with non-Hodgkin's lymphoma, and all cancer patients treated with high-dose steroids (or steroid-containing chemotherapy regimens)

Table 87-1

Normal Barriers to Infections

Type of Defense	Specific Lesion	Cells Involved	Organisms	Cancer Association	Disease
Physical barrier	Breaks in skin	Skin epithelial cells	Staphylococci, streptococci	Head and neck, squamous cell carcinoma	Cellulitis, extensive skin infection
Emptying of fluid collections	Occlusion of orifices: ureters, bile duct, colon	Luminal epithelial cells	Gram-negative bacilli	Renal, ovarian, biliary tree, metastatic diseases of many cancers	Rapid, overwhelming bacteremia, urinary tract infection
Lymphatic disease	Node dissection	Lymph nodes	Staphylococci, streptococci	Breast cancer surgery	Cellulitis
Splenic clearance of microorganisms	Splenectomy	Splenic reticuloendothelial cells	*Streptococcus pneumoniae, Haemophilus influenzae, Neisseria meningitidis, Babesia, Capnocytophaga canimorsus*	Hodgkin's disease, leukemia, idiopathic thrombocytopenic purpura	Rapid, overwhelming sepsis
Phagocytosis	Lack of granulocytes	Granulocytes (neutrophils)	Staphylococci, streptococci, enteric organisms	Hairy-cell, acute myelocytic, and acute lymphocytic leukemias	Bacteremia
Humoral immunity	Lack of antibody	B cells	*S. pneumoniae, H. influenzae, N. meningitidis*	Chronic lymphocytic leukemia	Infections with encapsulated organisms, sinusitis, pneumonia
Cellular immunity	Lack of T cells	T cells and macrophages	*Mycobacterium tuberculosis, Listeria,* herpesviruses, fungi, other intracellular parasites	Hodgkin's disease, leukemia, T cell lymphoma	Infections with intracellular bacteria, fungi, parasites

should receive antibiotic prophylaxis for *Pneumocystis carinii* infection (Table 87-3).

In addition to their susceptibility to certain infectious organisms, patients with cancer are likely to manifest their infections in characteristic ways.

SYSTEM-SPECIFIC SYNDROMES

SKIN-SPECIFIC SYNDROMES (Plate ID-57) Skin lesions are common in cancer patients, and their appearance may permit the diagnosis of systemic bacterial or fungal infection. While cellulitis caused by skin organisms such as *Streptococcus* or *Staphylococcus* is common, neutropenic patients and those with impaired blood or lymphatic drainage may develop infections with unusual organisms. Innocent-looking macules or papules may be the first sign of bacterial or fungal sepsis in immunocompromised patients. In the neutropenic host, a macule progresses rapidly to ecthyma gangrenosum, a usually painless, round, necrotic lesion consisting of a central black or gray-black eschar with surrounding erythema. Ecthyma gangrenosum is located in nonpressure areas (as distinguished from necrotic lesions associated with lack of circulation) and is often associated with *Pseudomonas aeruginosa* bacteremia (Chap. 157) but may be caused by other bacteria.

Candidemia (Chap. 207) is also associated with a variety of skin conditions and commonly presents as a maculopapular rash. Punch biopsy of the skin may be the best method for diagnosis.

Cellulitis, an acute spreading inflammation of the skin, is most often caused by infection with group A *Streptococcus* or *Staphylococcus aureus*, virulent organisms normally found on the skin (Chap. 133). Although cellulitis tends to be circumscribed in normal hosts, it may spread rapidly in neutropenic patients [those with fewer than 500 functional polymorphonuclear leukocytes (PMNs) per cubic millimeter]. A tiny break in the skin may lead to spreading cellulitis, which is characterized by pain and erythema; in such patients, signs of infection (e.g., purulence) are often lacking. What might be a furuncle in a normal host may require amputation because of uncontrolled infection in a patient presenting with leukemia. A dramatic response to an infection that might be trivial in a normal host can mark the first sign of leukemia. Fortu-

nately, granulocytopenic patients are likely to be infected with certain types of organisms (Table 87-4); thus the selection of an antibiotic regimen is somewhat easier than it might otherwise be. (See discussion on the selection of antibiotics for use in neutropenic patients, below.) It is essential to recognize cellulitis early and to treat it aggressively. Patients who are neutropenic or have previously received antibiotics for other reasons may develop cellulitis with unusual organisms (e.g., *Escherichia coli*, *Pseudomonas*, or fungi). Early treatment, even of innocent-looking lesions, is essential to prevent necrosis and loss of tissue. Debridement to prevent spread may sometimes be necessary early in the course of disease, but it can often be performed after chemotherapy, when the PMN count increases.

Sweet's syndrome, or *febrile neutrophilic dermatosis*, was originally described in women with elevated white blood cell counts. The disease is characterized by the presence of leukocytes in the lower dermis, with edema of the papillary body. Ironically, this disease now is usually seen in patients with neutropenic cancer, most often in association with acute leukemia but also in association with a variety of other malignancies. Sweet's syndrome usually presents as red or bluish-red papules or nodules that may coalesce and form sharply bordered plaques. The edema may suggest vesicles, but on palpation the lesions are solid, and vesicles probably never arise in this disease. The lesions are most common on the face, neck, and arms. On the legs, they may be confused with erythema nodosum. The development of lesions is often accompanied by high fevers and an elevated erythrocyte sedimentation rate. Both the lesions and the temperature elevation respond dramatically to steroids. Treatment begins with high doses of steroids (60 mg of prednisone per day) followed by tapered doses over the next 2 to 3 weeks.

Recent data indicate that *erythema multiforme* with mucous membrane involvement is often associated with herpes simplex virus (HSV) infection and is distinct from Stevens-Johnson syndrome, which is associated with drugs and tends to have a more widespread distribution. Since cancer patients are both immunosuppressed (and therefore susceptible to herpes infections) and heavily treated with drugs (and therefore subject to Stevens-Johnson syndrome), both of these conditions are common in this population.

Cytokines, which are used as adjuvants or primary treatments for cancer, can themselves cause characteristic rashes, further complicating the differential diagnosis. This phenomenon is a particular problem in bone marrow transplant recipients (Chap. 136), who, in addition to having the usual chemotherapy-, antibiotic-, and cytokine-induced rashes, are plagued by graft-versus-host disease.

CATHETER-RELATED INFECTIONS Because intravenous catheters are commonly used in cancer chemotherapy and are prone to infection (Chap. 137), they pose a major problem in the care of patients with cancer. Recent reviews have emphasized that some infected catheters can be treated with antibiotics while others must be removed. If the patient has a "tunneled" catheter (which consists of an entrance site, a subcutaneous tunnel, and an exit site), a red streak over the subcutaneous part of the line (the tunnel) is grounds for immediate removal of the catheter. Failure to remove catheters under these circumstances may result in extensive cellulitis and tissue necrosis.

More common than tunnel infections are exit-site infections, often with erythema around the area where the line penetrates the skin. Most authorities (Chap. 142) recommend treatment (usually with vancomycin) for an exit-site

Table 87-2

Vaccination of Cancer Patients Receiving Chemotherapy

Vaccine	Use in Indicated Patients		
	Intensive Chemotherapy	Hodgkin's Disease	Bone Marrow Transplantation
Diphtheria-tetanus (diphtheria, pertussis, tetanus; DPT) for children <7 years old	Primary series and boosters as necessary	No special recommendation	12 and 24 months after transplantation
Poliomyelitis*	Complete primary series and boosters	No special recommendation	12 and 24 months after transplantation
Haemophilus influenzae type b	Primary series and booster for children	Immunization before treatment and booster 2 years afterward	12 and 24 months after transplantation
23-Valent pneumococcal	Every 6 years	Immunization before treatment and booster 2 years afterward	12 and 24 months after transplantation
4-Valent meningococcal	Every 6 years	Immunization before treatment and booster 2 years afterward	12 and 24 months after transplantation
Influenza	Seasonal immunization	Seasonal immunization	Seasonal immunization
Measles/mumps/rubella	Contraindicated	Contraindicated	After 24 months in patients without graft-versus-host disease
Varicella-zoster virus	Contraindicated†	Contraindicated	Contraindicated

* Live virus vaccine is contraindicated; inactivated vaccine should be used.
† Contact the manufacturer for more information on use in children with acute lymphocytic leukemia.

infection caused by a coagulase-negative *Staphylococcus*. Treatment of coagulase-positive staphylococcal infection is associated with a poorer outcome, and it is advisable to remove the catheter. Similarly, many clinicians remove catheters associated with infections due to *P. aeruginosa* and *Candida* species, since such infections are difficult to treat, and bloodstream infections with these organisms are likely to be deadly.

GASTROINTESTINAL TRACT–SPECIFIC SYNDROMES
Upper Gastrointestinal Tract Disease The oral cavity is rich in aerobic and anaerobic bacteria (Chap. 169) that normally live in a commensal relationship with the host. The antimetabolic effects of chemotherapy cause a breakdown of host defenses, leading to ulceration of the mouth and the potential for invasion by resident bacteria. Mouth ulcerations afflict most patients receiving chemotherapy and have been associated with viridans streptococcal bacteremia. A variety of topical rinses and elixirs have been proposed to treat these ulcerations. Although some may have a local anesthetic effect, the efficacy of any of these therapies in the prevention of disease is unproven. Similarly, the efficacy of mouthwashes in the prevention of esophagitis or invasive candidiasis is doubtful. Fluconazole, on the other hand, is clearly effective in the treatment of both local infections (thrush) and systemic infections (esophagitis) due to *Candida albicans*.

Noma (or *cancrum oris*), commonly seen in malnourished children, is a penetrating disease of the soft and hard tissues of the mouth and adjacent sites, with resulting necrosis and gangrene. It has a counterpart in immunocompromised patients and is thought to be due to invasion of the tissues by *Bacteroides*, *Fusobacterium*, and other normal inhabitants of the mouth. It is associated with debility, poor oral hygiene, and immunosuppression.

Viruses, particularly HSV, are a prominent cause of morbidity in immunocompromised patients, in whom they are associated with severe mucositis. The use of acyclovir, either prophylactically or therapeutically, is of value.

The differential diagnosis of esophagitis (usually presenting as substernal chest pain upon swallowing) includes herpes simplex and candidiasis, both of which are readily treatable.

Lower Gastrointestinal Tract Disease Hepatic candidiasis (Chap. 207) results from seeding of the liver (usually from a gastrointestinal source) in neutropenic patients. It is most common in patients being treated for acute leukemia and usually develops around the time the neutropenia resolves. The characteristic picture is that of persistent fever unresponsive to antibiotics; abdominal pain and tenderness or nausea; and elevated serum levels of alkaline phosphatase in a patient with hematologic malignancy who has recently recovered from neutropenia. The diagnosis of this disease (which may present in an indolent manner and persist for several months) is based on the finding of yeasts or pseudohyphae in granulomatous lesions. Hepatic ultrasound or computed tomography (CT) may reveal bull's-eye lesions. In some cases, magnetic resonance imaging (MRI) reveals small lesions not visible by other imaging modalities. The pathology (a granulomatous response) and the timing (with resolution of neutropenia and an elevation in granulocyte count) suggest that the host response to *Candida* is an important component of the manifestations of disease. In many cases, although organisms are visible, cultures of biopsied material may be negative. The designation *hepatosplenic candidiasis* or *hepatic candidiasis* is a misnomer because the disease often involves the kidneys and other tissues; the term *chronic disseminated candidiasis* may be more appropriate. Because of the risk of bleeding with liver biopsy, diagnosis is often based on radiographic abnormalities.

Amphotericin B is traditionally used for therapy (often for several months, until all manifestations of disease have disappeared), but fluconazole may be useful for outpatient therapy.

Typhlitis *Typhlitis*, sometimes referred to as necrotizing colitis, neutropenic colitis, necrotizing enteropathy, ileocecal syndrome, or cecitis, is a clinical syndrome of fever and right-lower-quadrant tenderness in an immunosuppressed host. This syndrome is almost always seen in neutropenic patients after chemotherapy with cytotoxic drugs. It may be more common among children than among adults and appears to be much more common among patients with acute myelocytic leukemia (AML) or ALL. Physical examination reveals right-lower-quadrant tenderness, with or without rebound tenderness. Associated diarrhea (often bloody) is common, and the diagnosis can be confirmed by the finding of a thickened cecal wall on CT or ultrasonography. Plain films may reveal a right-lower-quadrant mass, but CT with contrast or MRI is a much more sensitive means of making the diagnosis. Although surgery is sometimes attempted to avoid perforation from ischemia, most cases resolve with medical therapy alone. The disease is sometimes associated with positive blood cultures (usually for aerobic gram-negative bacilli), and therapy is recommended for a broad spectrum of bacteria (particularly gram-negative bacilli, likely bowel flora). Recurrence is rare, and most patients recover uneventfully.

***Clostridium difficile*–Induced Diarrhea** Cancer patients seem to be predisposed to the development of *C. difficile* diarrhea (Chap. 148) as a consequence of chemotherapy alone. Thus, they may have positive toxin tests before receiving antibiotics. Obviously, such patients are also subject to *C. difficile*–induced diarrhea as a result of antibiotic pressure. It is worth noting that toxins other than *C. difficile* may be associated with diarrhea; therefore, the detection of nonspecific toxins in the stool—without a specific neutralization test—does not prove that *C. difficile* infection is present. → *The treatment of* C. difficile *infection is discussed in Chap. 148.*

CENTRAL NERVOUS SYSTEM–SPECIFIC SYNDROMES
Meningitis While meningitis in immunocompetent adults is likely to be caused by *S. pneumoniae*, the same is not true in immunocompromised patients. As noted previously, splenectomized patients are susceptible to rapid overwhelming infection with encapsulated bacteria (including *S. pneumoniae*, *H. influenzae*, and *N. meningitidis*). Similarly, patients who are antibody deficient (such as patients with CLL, those who have received intensive chemotherapy, or those who have undergone bone marrow transplantation) are likely to have infections with these bacteria. Other cancer patients, however, because of their defective cellular immunity, are likely to be infected with other patho-

Table 87-3

Infections and Cancer

Cancer	Underlying Immune Abnormality	Organisms Causing Infection
Multiple myeloma	Hypogammaglobulinemia	*Streptococcus pneumoniae*, *Haemophilus influenzae*, *Neisseria meningitidis*
Chronic lymphocytic leukemia	Hypogammaglobulinemia	*S. pneumoniae*, *H. influenzae*, *N. meningitidis*
Acute myelocytic or lymphocytic leukemia	Granulocytopenia, skin and mucous-membrane lesions	Extracellular gram-positive and gram-negative bacteria, fungi
Hodgkin's disease	Abnormal T-cell function	Intracellular pathogens (*Mycobacterium tuberculosis*, *Listeria*, *Salmonella*, *Cryptococcus*, *Mycobacterium avium*)
Non-Hodgkin's lymphoma and acute lymphocytic leukemia	Steroid chemotherapy, T- and B-cell dysfunction	*Pneumocystis carinii*
Colon and rectal tumors	Local abnormalities*	*Streptococcus bovis* (bacteremia)
Hairy-cell leukemia	Abnormal T-cell function	Intracellular pathogens (*M. tuberculosis*, *Listeria*, *Cryptococcus*, *M. avium*)

* The reason for this association is not well defined.

Table 87-4

Organisms Likely to Cause Infections in Granulocytopenic Patients

Gram-positive cocci	*Enterobacter* species
Staphylococcus epidermidis	*Serratia* species
Staphylococcus aureus	*Acinetobacter* species*
Viridans *Streptococcus*	*Citrobacter* species
Enterococcus faecalis	Gram-positive bacilli
Streptococcus pneumoniae	Diphtheroids
Gram-negative bacilli	JK bacillus*
Escherichia coli	Fungi
Klebsiella species	*Candida* species
Pseudomonas aeruginosa	*Aspergillus* species
Non-*aeruginosa Pseudomonas* species*	

* Often associated with intravenous catheters.

gens (see Table 87-3). The presentation of meningitis in patients with lymphoma, patients receiving chemotherapy (particularly with steroids) for solid tumors, and patients who have received bone marrow transplants suggests a diagnosis of cryptococcal or listerial infection.

Encephalitis The spectrum of disease resulting from viral encephalitis is expanded in immunocompromised patients. Infection with varicella-zoster virus (VZV) has been associated with encephalitis that may be caused by VZV-related vasculitis. The slow viruses (e.g., Creutzfeldt-Jakob agent) may also be associated with dementia and encephalitic presentations, and a diagnosis of progressive multifocal leukoencephalopathy should be considered when a patient who has received chemotherapy presents with dementia. Other abnormalities of the central nervous system (CNS) that may be confused with infection include normal-pressure hydrocephalus and vasculitis resulting from CNS irradiation. It may be possible to differentiate these conditions by MRI.

Brain Abscess Brain abscesses in immunocompromised patients are likely to be due to *Cryptococcus* (particularly in patients with lymphoma or those receiving steroids), *Nocardia*, or *Aspergillus*. *Aspergillus* may enter via the lungs or—like *Mucor*—may invade the hard and soft palates to cause pneumonia (see below) with or without brain abscesses.

PULMONARY INFECTIONS Pneumonia (Chap. 255) in immunocompromised patients may be difficult to diagnose because conventional methods of diagnosis depend on the presence of neutrophils. Bacterial pneumonia in neutropenic patients may present without purulent sputum—or, in fact, without any sputum at all—and may not produce physical findings suggestive of chest consolidation (rales or egophony).

In granulocytopenic patients with persistent or recurrent fever, the chest x-ray pattern may help to localize an infection and thus to determine which investigative tests and procedures should be undertaken and which therapeutic options should be considered (Table 87-5). The difficulties encountered in the management of pulmonary infiltrates relate in part to the difficulties of performing diagnostic procedures on the patients involved. When platelet counts can be increased to adequate levels by transfusion, microscopic and microbiologic evaluation of the fluid obtained by endoscopic bronchial lavage is often diagnostic. Lavage fluid should be cultured for *Mycoplasma*, *Chlamydia*, *Legionella*, *Nocardia*, fungi, and more common bacterial pathogens. In addition, the possibility of *P. carinii* pneumonia should be considered, especially in patients with ALL or lymphoma who have not received prophylactic trimethoprim-sulfamethoxazole. The characteristics of the infiltrate may be helpful in decisions about further diagnostic and therapeutic maneuvers. Nodular infiltrates suggest fungal pneumonia (e.g., that caused by *Aspergillus* or *Mucor*).

Aspergillus species (Chap. 208) can colonize the skin and respiratory tract or cause fatal systemic illness. Although *Aspergillus* may cause aspergillomas in a previously existing cavity or may produce allergic bronchopulmonary aspergillosis, the major problem posed by this genus in neutropenic patients is invasive disease due to *Aspergillus*

fumigatus or *Aspergillus flavus*. The organisms enter the host through colonization of the respiratory tract, with subsequent invasion of the blood vessels. The disease is likely to present as a thrombotic or embolic event because of the ability of the organisms to invade blood vessels. The risk of infection with *Aspergillus* correlates directly with the duration of neutropenia. In prolonged neutropenia, positive surveillance cultures for colonization of the nasopharynx with *Aspergillus* may predict the development of disease.

Patients with *Aspergillus* infection often present with pleuritic chest pain and fever, which are sometimes accompanied by cough. Hemoptysis may be an ominous sign. Chest x-rays may reveal new focal infiltrates or nodules (Table 87-5). Chest CT may reveal a characteristic halo consisting of a mass-like infiltrate surrounded by an area of low attenuation. The presence of a "crescent sign" on a chest x-ray or a chest CT scan, in which the mass progresses to central cavitation, is characteristic of invasive *Aspergillus* infection but may develop only with the resolution of the lesions.

In addition to causing pulmonary presentations, *Aspergillus* may invade through the nose or palate, with deep sinus penetration. The appearance of a discolored area in the nasal passages or on the hard palate should prompt a search for invasive *Aspergillus*. This situation is likely to require surgical debridement. Treatment (Chap. 208) with high doses of amphotericin B has been successful in curing granulocytopenic patients of invasive *Aspergillus* infection after the return of granulocytes. Catheter infections with *Aspergillus* usually require both removal of the catheter and antifungal therapy.

Diffuse interstitial infiltrates suggest viral or parasitic pneumonia. If the patient has a diffuse interstitial pattern on chest x-ray, it may be reasonable to institute empirical treatment with trimethoprim-sulfamethoxazole (for *Pneumocystis*) and erythromycin (for *Chlamydia*, *Mycoplasma*, and *Legionella*) while considering invasive diagnostic procedures. Noninvasive procedures, such as staining of sputum smears for *Pneumocystis* and serum cryptococcal antigen tests, may be helpful on occasion. In transplant recipients who are seropositive for cytomegalovirus (CMV), culture of a nonpulmonary site for CMV may be worthwhile. Infections with viruses that cause only upper respiratory symptoms in immunocompetent hosts, such as respiratory syncytial, influenza, and parainfluenza viruses, may be associated with fatal pneumonitis in immunocompromised hosts. An attempt at early diagnosis by nasopharyngeal aspiration should be considered so that appropriate treatment can be instituted.

While bleomycin is the most common cause of chemotherapy-induced lung disease, other causes include alkylating agents (such as cyclophosphamide, chlorambucil, and melphalan), nitrosoureas [carmustine (BCNU), lomustine (CCNU), and methyl-CCNU], busulfan, procarbazine, methotrexate, and hydroxyurea. Both infectious and noninfectious (drug- and/or radiation-induced) pneumonitis can cause fever and abnormalities on chest x-ray; thus, the differential diagnosis of an infiltrate in a patient receiving chemotherapy encompasses a

Table 87-5

Differential Diagnosis of Chest Infiltrates in Immunocompromised Patients

	Cause of Pneumonia	
Infiltrate	Infectious	Noninfectious
Localized	Common bacterial pulmonary pathogens, *Legionella*, mycobacteria	Local hemorrhage or embolism, tumor
Nodular	Fungi (e.g., *Aspergillus* or *Mucor*), *Nocardia*	Recurrent tumor
Diffuse	Viruses (especially CMV), *Chlamydia*, *Pneumocystis carinii*, *Toxoplasma gondii*, mycobacteria	Congestive heart failure, radiation pneumonitis, drug-induced lung injury, diffuse alveolar hemorrhage (described after BMT)

ABBREVIATIONS: CMV, cytomegalovirus; BMT, bone marrow transplantation.

broad range of conditions (Table 87-5). Since the treatment of radiation pneumonitis (which may respond dramatically to glucocorticoids) or drug-induced pneumonitis is different from that of infectious pneumonia, a biopsy may be important in the diagnosis. Unfortunately, no definitive diagnosis can be made in approximately 30 percent of cases, even after bronchoscopy.

Open lung biopsy is the gold standard of diagnostic techniques. Biopsy via a visualized thoracostomy can replace an open procedure in many cases. When a biopsy cannot be performed, empirical treatment can be undertaken with erythromycin and trimethoprim-sulfamethoxazole (in the case of diffuse infiltrates) or with amphotericin B (in the case of nodular infiltrates). The risks should be weighed carefully in these cases. If inappropriate drugs are administered, empirical treatment may prove toxic or ineffective; either of these outcomes may be riskier than biopsy.

CARDIOVASCULAR INFECTIONS Patients with Hodgkin's disease are prone to persistent infections by *Salmonella*, sometimes (and particularly often in elderly patients) affecting a vascular site. The use of intravenous catheters deliberately lodged in the right atrium is associated with a high incidence of bacterial endocarditis (presumably related to valve damage followed by bacteremia). Nonbacterial thrombotic endocarditis has been described in association with a variety of malignancies (most often solid tumors) and reportedly follows bone marrow transplantation as well. The presentation of an embolic event with a new cardiac murmur suggests this diagnosis. Blood cultures are negative in this disease of unknown pathogenesis.

ENDOCRINE SYNDROMES In addition to infections of the skin, gastrointestinal tract, and pulmonary system, infections of the endocrine system have been described in immunocompromised patients. *Candida* infection of the thyroid during neutropenia can be defined by indium-labeled white-cell scans or gallium scans after neutrophil counts increase. CMV infection can cause adrenalitis with or without resulting adrenal insufficiency. The presentation of a sudden endocrine anomaly in an immunocompromised patient may be a sign of infection in the involved end organ.

MUSCULOSKELETAL INFECTIONS Infection that is a result of vascular compromise (resulting in gangrene) can occur when a tumor compromises the blood supply to muscles, bones, or joints. The process of diagnosis and treatment of such infection is similar to that in normal hosts, with the following caveats: (1) In terms of diagnosis, a lack of physical findings resulting from a lack of granulocytes in the granulocytopenic patient should make the clinician more aggressive in obtaining tissue rather than relying on physical signs. (2) In terms of therapy, aggressive debridement of infected tissues may be required, but it is usually difficult to operate on patients who have recently received chemotherapy, both because of a lack of platelets (which results in bleeding complications) and because of a lack of white blood cells (which may lead to secondary infection). A blood culture positive for *Clostridium perfringens* (an organism commonly associated with gas gangrene) can have a number of meanings (Chap. 148). Bloodstream infections with intestinal organisms like *Streptococcus bovis* and *C. perfringens* may arise spontaneously from lower gastrointestinal lesions (tumor or polyps); alternatively, these lesions may be harbingers of invasive disease. The clinical setting must be considered in order to define the appropriate treatment for each case.

RENAL AND URETERAL INFECTIONS Infections of the urinary tract are common among patients whose ureteral excretion is compromised (Table 87-1). *Candida*, which has a predilection for the kidney, can invade either from the bloodstream or in a retrograde manner (via the ureters or bladder) in immunocompromised patients. The presence of "fungus balls" or persistent candiduria suggests invasive disease. Persistent funguria (with *Aspergillus* as well as *Candida*) should prompt a search for a nidus of infection in the kidney.

Certain viruses are typically seen only in immunosuppression. BK virus (polyomavirus hominis 1) has been documented in the urine of bone marrow transplant recipients and, like adenovirus, may be associated with hemorrhagic cystitis. BK-induced cystitis usually remits with decreasing immunosuppression. Anecdotal reports have described the treatment of adenovirus with ribavirin in cases of severe hemorrhagic cystitis in immunocompromised patients.

ABNORMALITIES THAT PREDISPOSE TO INFECTION

THE LYMPHOID SYSTEM It is beyond the scope of this chapter to detail how all the immunologic abnormalities that result from cancer or from chemotherapy for cancer lead to infections. Disorders of the immune system are discussed in other sections of this book. As has been noted, patients with antibody deficiency are predisposed to overwhelming infection with encapsulated bacteria (including *S. pneumoniae*, *H. influenzae*, and *N. meningitidis*). Infections that result from the lack of a functional cellular immune system are described in the chapter on AIDS (Chap. 308). It is worth mentioning, however, that patients undergoing intensive chemotherapy for any form of cancer will have not only defects due to granulocytopenia but also lymphocyte dysfunction, which may be profound. Thus, these patients—especially those receiving steroid-containing regimens—should be given prophylaxis for *P. carinii* pneumonia.

THE HEMATOPOIETIC SYSTEM Initial studies in the 1960s revealed a dramatic increase in the incidence of infections (fatal and nonfatal) among cancer patients with a granulocyte count of $<500/\text{mm}^3$. Recent studies have cited a figure of 48.3 infections per 100 neutropenic patients (<1000 granulocytes per cubic millimeter) with hematologic malignancies and solid tumors, or 46.3 infections per 1000 days at risk.

Neutropenic patients are unusually susceptible to infection with a wide variety of bacteria; thus, antibiotic therapy should be initiated promptly to cover likely pathogens if infection is suspected. Indeed, early initiation of antibacterial agents is mandatory to prevent deaths. These patients are susceptible to gram-positive and gram-negative organisms found commonly on the skin and in the bowel (Table 87-4). Because treatment with narrow-spectrum agents leads to infection with organisms not covered by the antibiotics used, the initial regimen should target pathogens likely to be initial causes of bacterial infection in neutropenic hosts (Fig. 87-1).

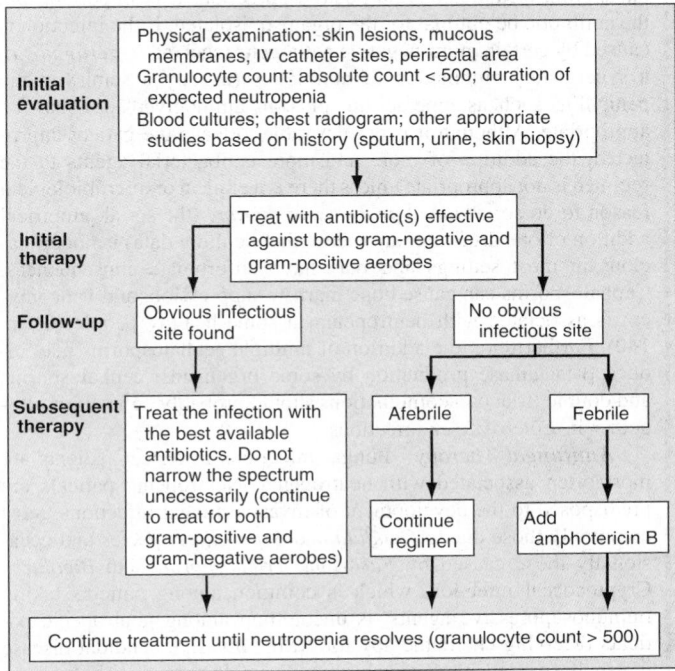

FIGURE 87-1 Diagnosis and treatment of febrile neutropenic patients: an algorithm.

℞ **TREATMENT**

Antibacterial Therapy Hundreds of antibacterial regimens have been tested for use in neutropenic patients with cancer. Many of the relevant studies involved small populations in which the outcomes were generally good, and most lacked the statistical power to detect differences among the regimens studied. Each febrile neutropenic patient should be approached as a unique problem, with particular attention given to previous infections and recent exposures to antibiotics. Several general guidelines are useful in the initial treatment of neutropenic patients with fever (Fig. 87-1):

1. It is necessary to use antibiotics active against both gram-negative and gram-positive bacteria (see Table 87-4) in the initial regimen.
2. An aminoglycoside or a quinolone (e.g., ciprofloxacin) alone is not adequate in this setting.
3. The agents used should reflect both the epidemiology and the antibiotic resistance pattern of the hospital. For example, in hospitals where there is gentamicin resistance, amikacin-containing regimens should be considered; in hospitals with frequent *P. aeruginosa* infections, a regimen with the highest level of activity against this pathogen (such as tobramycin plus a semisynthetic penicillin) would be reasonable for initial therapy.
4. A single third-generation cephalosporin constitutes an appropriate initial regimen in many hospitals (if the pattern of resistance justifies its use).
5. Most standard regimens are designed for patients who have not previously received prophylactic antibiotics. The development of fever in a patient receiving antibiotics affects the choice of subsequent therapy (which should target resistant organisms and organisms known to cause infections in patients being treated with the antibiotics already administered).

The initial antibacterial regimen should be refined on the basis of culture results (Fig. 87-1). Blood cultures are the most relevant cultures on which to base therapy; surface cultures of skin and mucous membranes may be misleading. In the case of gram-positive bacteremia or another gram-positive infection, it is important that the antibiotic be optimal for the organism isolated. If the infection is caused by certain gram-negative pathogens (such as *P. aeruginosa*), a synergistic combination of antibiotics (usually a semisynthetic penicillin, such as piperacillin, plus an aminoglycoside) may be appropriate. Although it is not desirable to leave the patient unprotected, the addition of more and more antibacterial agents to the regimen is not appropriate unless there is a clinical or microbiological reason to do so. *Planned progressive therapy* (the serial, empirical addition of one drug after another without culture data) is not efficacious in most settings and may have unfortunate consequences. Cephalosporins can cause bone marrow suppression, and vancomycin is associated with neutropenia in some healthy people (Chap. 140). Furthermore, the addition of multiple cephalosporins may induce β-lactamase production by some organisms; cephalosporins and double β-lactam combinations should probably be avoided altogether in *Enterobacter* infections.

Antifungal Therapy Fungal infections in cancer patients are most often associated with neutropenia. Neutropenic patients are predisposed to the development of invasive fungal infections, most commonly those due to *Candida* and *Aspergillus* species and occasionally those caused by *Fusarium*, *Trichosporon*, and *Bipolaris*. Cryptococcal infection, which is common among patients taking immunosuppressive agents, is uncommon among neutropenic patients receiving chemotherapy for AML. Invasive candidal disease is usually caused by *C. albicans* or *Candida tropicalis* but can be caused by *Candida krusei*, *Candida parapsilosis*, and *Candida glabrata*.

Most clinicians add amphotericin B to antifungal regimens if a neutropenic patient remains febrile despite 4 to 7 days of treatment with antibacterial agents. The rationale for the empirical addition of amphotericin B is that it is difficult to culture fungi before they cause disseminated disease and that mortality from disseminated fungal infections in granulocytopenic patients is high. The imidazoles (especially fluconazole) may have prophylactic efficacy in this regard, but their spectrum of activity is narrower than that of amphotericin B. Amphotericin B is the mainstay of therapy for disseminated *Candida* or *Aspergillus* infection in the neutropenic patient. The combined use of an imidazole and amphotericin B is controversial because of the theoretical antagonistic effects of these agents. The insolubility of amphotericin B has resulted in the marketing of several amphotericin B–lipid formulations. Most of these formulations appear to be less toxic than amphotericin B alone, but their therapeutic superiority has not yet been clearly proven in head-to-head trials. Thus, recommendations for their use as first-line therapy are problematic.

Other Therapeutic Modalities Another way to address the problems of the febrile neutropenic patient is to replenish the neutrophil population. Although granulocyte transfusions are efficacious in the treatment of refractory gram-negative bacteremia, they do not have a documented role in prophylaxis. Because of the expense, the risk of leukoagglutinin reactions (although this risk has probably been decreased by improved cell-separation procedures), and the risk of transmission of CMV from unscreened donors, granulocyte transfusion is reserved for patients unresponsive to antibiotics. This modality is efficacious for documented gram-negative bacteremia refractory to antibiotics, particularly in situations where granulocyte numbers will be depressed for only a short period.

A variety of cytokines, including granulocyte colony-stimulating factor and granulocyte-macrophage colony-stimulating factor, enhance granulocyte recovery after chemotherapy and consequently shorten the period of maximal vulnerability to fatal infections. The role of these cytokines in routine practice is still a matter of some debate. Most authorities recommend their use only when neutropenia is both severe and prolonged. The cytokines themselves may have adverse effects, including fever, hypoxemia, and pleural effusions or serositis in other areas. Since there is little evidence that their routine administration lessens the risk of death and since they are still expensive, the cytokines have not become the standard of care in all centers. The role of other cytokines (such as macrophage colony-stimulating factor for monocytes or interferon-γ) in preventing or treating infections in granulocytopenic patients is under investigation.

Once neutropenia has resolved, patients are not at high risk of infection. However, depending on what drugs they receive, patients who continue on chemotherapeutic protocols continue to be at high risk for certain diseases. Any patient receiving more than a maintenance dose of glucocorticoids (including many treatment regimens for diffuse lymphoma) should also receive prophylactic trimethoprim-sulfamethoxazole because of the risk of *P. carinii* infection; those with ALL should receive such prophylaxis for the duration of chemotherapy.

PREVENTION OF INFECTION IN CANCER PATIENTS

EFFECT OF THE ENVIRONMENT Outbreaks of fatal *Aspergillus* infection have been associated with construction and construction materials in several hospitals. The association between spore counts and risk of infection suggests the need for a high-efficiency air-handling system in hospitals that care for large numbers of neutropenic patients. The use of laminar-flow rooms and prophylactic antibiotics has decreased the number of infectious episodes in severely neutropenic patients. However, because of the expense of such a program and the failure to show that it dramatically affects mortality, most centers do not routinely use laminar flow to care for neutropenic patients. Some centers use "reverse isolation," in which health care providers and visitors to a patient who is neutropenic are dressed in gowns and gloves. Since most of the infections these patients develop are due to organisms that colonize the patients' own skin and bowel, the validity of such schemes is dubious, and limited clinical data do not support their use. Hand washing by all staff caring for neutropenic patients should be required to prevent the spread of resistant organisms.

The presence of large numbers of bacteria (particularly *P. aeruginosa*) in certain foods, especially fresh vegetables, has led some authorities to recommend a special "low-bacteria" diet. A diet consisting of cooked and canned food is satisfactory to most neutropenic patients and does not involve elaborate disinfection or sterilization protocols.

PHYSICAL MEASURES Although few studies address this issue, patients with cancer are predisposed to infections resulting from anatomic compromise (e.g., lymphedema resulting from node dissections after radical mastectomy). Surgeons who specialize in cancer surgery can provide specific guidelines for the care of such patients, and patients benefit from common-sense advice about how to prevent infections in vulnerable areas.

ANTIBIOTIC PROPHYLAXIS There is no consensus on the use of prophylactic antibiotics in neutropenic patients. The incidence of infection is lower among patients who receive broad-spectrum antibiotic prophylaxis than among those who do not. Because of the prolongation of neutropenia associated with the use of trimethoprim-sulfamethoxazole, some clinicians use broad-spectrum agents such as quinolones (e.g., ciprofloxacin). Either regimen can be given orally, and both have the advantage of inactivity against anaerobic organisms; thus, neither is unlikely to disrupt the bowel flora and permit colonization with new aerobes or *Candida*. However, both regimens have adverse effects and can lead to the selection of resistant organisms in a hospital. For these reasons, many clinicians reserve their use for patients with the longest periods of neutropenia (e.g., bone marrow transplant recipients). The same issues apply to the use of antifungal agents. While agents such as fluconazole may prevent infections with susceptible organisms (e.g., *C. albicans*), they can cause a concomitant increase in infections due to resistant fungi (e.g., *C. krusei*). Thus, the decision to use antifungal prophylaxis may vary with the fungi endemic in a given hospital. Prophylaxis for *P. carinii* is mandatory for patients with ALL and for all cancer patients receiving steroid-containing chemotherapy regimens.

VACCINATION OF CANCER PATIENTS In general, patients undergoing chemotherapy respond less well to vaccines than normal hosts. Their greater need for vaccines thus leads to a dilemma in their management. Purified proteins and inactivated vaccines are almost never contraindicated and should be given to patients even during chemotherapy. For example, all adults should receive diphtheria-tetanus toxoid boosters at the indicated times, as well as seasonal influenza vaccine. However, if possible, vaccination should not be undertaken concurrent with chemotherapy. If patients are expected to be receiving chemotherapy for several months and vaccination is indicated (for example, influenza vaccination in the fall), the vaccine should be given midcycle—as far as possible from the antimetabolic agents that will prevent an immune response. The meningococcal and pneumococcal polysaccharide vaccines should be given to patients before splenectomy, if possible. The Advisory Committee on Immunization Practices recommends reimmunization every 6 years for the pneumococcal vaccine; although no official stand has been taken, this recommendation seems reasonable for the meningococcal vaccine as well. The *H. influenzae* type b conjugate vaccine should be administered to all splenectomized patients; there is no current recommendation for reimmunization, but immunity appears to be much longer-lasting than that induced by polysaccharide vaccines.

In general, live virus (or live bacterial) vaccines should not be given to patients during intensive chemotherapy because of the risk of disseminated infection. Recommendations on vaccination are summarized in Table 87-2.

BIBLIOGRAPHY

AMBROSINO DM, MOLRINE DC: Critical appraisal of immunization strategies for prevention of infection in the compromised host. Hematol Oncol Clin North Am 7:1027, 1993

AMERICAN SOCIETY OF CLINICAL ONCOLOGY: Recommendations for the use of hematopoietic colony-stimulating factors: Evidence-based, clinical practice guidelines. J Clin Oncol 12:2471, 1994

CARLISLE PS et al: Nosocomial infections in neutropenic cancer patients. Infect Control Hosp Epidemiol 14:320, 1993

GREENE JN: Catheter-related complications of cancer therapy. Infect Dis Clin North Am 10:255, 1996

LEW MA et al: Ciprofloxacin versus trimethoprim/sulfamethoxazole for prophylaxis of bacterial infections in bone marrow transplant recipients: A randomized, controlled trial. J Clin Oncol 13:239, 1995

MAYORDOMO JI et al: Improving treatment of chemotherapy-induced neutropenic fever by administration of colony-stimulating factors. J Natl Cancer Inst 87:803, 1995

MOONEY BR et al: Infection control and bone marrow transplantation. Am J Infect Control 21:131, 1993

SEPKOWITZ KA et al: *Pneumocystis carinii* pneumonia among patients without AIDS at a cancer hospital. JAMA 267:832, 1992

SICKLES EA et al: Clinical presentation of infection in granulocytopenic patients. Arch Intern Med 135:715, 1975

| 88 | *Arthur J. Sober, Howard K. Koh, Nhu-Linh T. Tran, Carl V. Washington, Jr.* |

MELANOMA AND OTHER SKIN CANCERS

Pigmented skin lesions are among the most common findings on physical examination. The challenge is to distinguish cutaneous melanomas, which may be lethal, from the remainder, which with rare exceptions are benign. Cutaneous neoplasms are depicted in Section IB **(Plate IB-18 to 25)** of the Color Atlas; benign and malignant pigmented lesions are in Section IC **(Plate IC-26 to 31)**.

MELANOMA

Melanomas originate from melanocytes, pigment cells present normally in the epidermis and sometimes in the dermis. This tumor affects approximately 38,300 individuals per year in the United States, resulting in 7300 deaths. The tumor can affect adults of all ages, even young individuals (starting in the mid-teens); it has distinct clinical features that make it detectable at a time when cure by surgical excision is possible; and it is located on the skin surface, where it is visible. The incidence has increased dramatically (a 300 percent increase in the past 40 years). If the incidence continues to increase at the present rate, within a decade, lifetime risk of melanoma will approximate 1 percent or higher.

The reason for the increase in melanoma incidence is uncertain but may involve increased recreational sun exposure, especially early in life. Individuals of similar ethnic background who immigrate after childhood to areas of high sun exposure (e.g., Israel and Australia) have lower melanoma rates than individuals of similar age who were either born in those countries or immigrated before age 10. The individuals most susceptible to development of melanoma are those with fair complexions, red or blond hair, blue eyes, and freckles and who tan poorly and sunburn easily. In one literature survey, 9 of 11 studies linked increased melanoma risk to history of sunburn. Other factors associated with increased risk include a family history of melanoma (approximately 1 in 10 melanoma patients have a family member with melanoma); the presence of a clinically atypical mole (dysplastic nevus), a giant congenital melanocytic nevus, or a small to medium-sized congenital melanocytic nevus (see below); the presence of a higher than average number of ordinary melanocytic nevi; and immunosuppression (Table 88-1). A 64-fold increased risk for individuals with 50 or more moles ≥2 mm in size has been reported. About 30 percent of melanomas arise in a nevus. Melanoma is relatively rare in heavily pigmented peoples. Dark-skinned populations (such as those

Table 88-1

Risk Factors for Cutaneous Melanoma

High risk (>50-fold increase in risk)
    Persistently changing mole
    Clinically atypical moles in patient with two family members with mel-
        anoma
    Adulthood (vs. childhood)
    >50 nevi ≥2 mm in diameter
Intermediate risk (~10-fold increase in risk)
    Family history of melanoma
    Sporadic clinically atypical moles
    Congenital nevi (?)
    White ethnicity (vs. black or East Asian ethnicity)
    Personal history of prior melanoma
Low risk (2- to 4-fold increase in risk)
    Immunosuppression
    Sun sensitivity or excess exposure to sun

SOURCE: Adapted from Rhodes et al.

of India and Puerto Rico), blacks, and East Asians have rates 10 to 20 times lower than lighter-skinned whites. In keeping with the role of sun exposure, the incidence is inversely correlated with the latitude of residence; at any latitude, however, darker-skinned persons have the lowest incidence.

CLINICAL CHARACTERISTICS There are four types of cutaneous melanoma (Table 88-2). In three of these—superficial spreading melanoma, lentigo maligna melanoma, and acral lentiginous melanoma—the lesion has a period of superficial (so-called radial) growth during which it increases in size but does not penetrate deeply. It is during this period that the melanoma is most capable of being cured by surgical excision. The fourth type—nodular melanoma—does not have a recognizable radial growth phase and usually presents as a deeply invasive lesion, capable of early metastasis. When tumors begin to penetrate deeply into the skin, they are in the so-called vertical growth phase. Melanomas with a radial growth phase are characterized by irregular and sometimes notched borders, variation in pigment pattern, and variation in color. An increase in size or change in color is noted by the patient in 70 percent of early lesions. Bleeding, ulceration, and pain are late signs and are of little help in early recognition. Nodular melanomas are dark brown-black to blue-black nodules. Mela-nomas occasionally are amelanotic, in which case the diagnosis is established histologically after biopsy of a new or changing skin nodule. Lentigo maligna melanoma is usually confined to chronically sun-damaged, sun-exposed sites (face, neck, back of hands) in older individuals. Acral lentiginous melanoma occurs on the palms, soles, nail beds, and mucous membranes. While this type occurs in whites, it is most frequent (along with nodular melanoma) in blacks and East Asians. Superficial spreading melanoma is most frequent in whites. Melanomas arising in dysplastic nevi (see below) are usually of this type. The back is the most common site for melanoma in men. In women, the back and the lower leg (from knee to ankle) are frequent sites.

PROGNOSTIC FACTORS The most important prognostic factor is the stage at the time of presentation [see the discussion of revised American Joint Cancer Commission (AJCC) staging categories, below]. Five-year survival for clinical stages I and II (primary tumor; no clinical evidence of disease elsewhere) is about 85 percent. For clinical stage III (clinically palpable regional nodes that contain tumor), the 5-year survival is about 50 percent when only one node is involved and about 15 to 20 percent when four or more nodes are involved. The 5-year survival for clinical stage IV (disseminated disease) is less than 5 percent. Fortunately, most melanomas are diagnosed in clinical stages I and II. Within these stages, the prognosis depends on the thickness of the primary tumor (Table 88-3). This system is based on the rationale that the likelihood of metastasis should correlate with tumor volume, with thickness being the best single index of tumor volume. Melanomas less than 0.76 mm thick are usually cured by surgical removal (with 5-year survival rates of 96 to 99 percent). Approximately 40 percent of primary melanomas now fall in a low-risk category (thickness <1 mm). In low-risk patients who develop metastases, the primary tumors often exhibit either extensive microscopic features of regression or a vertical growth phase. Approximately 60 percent of individuals with melanomas ≥3.65 mm thick will develop metastatic disease and die of their melanoma. These thick tumors almost always are raised substantially above the plane of the skin. Two intermediate categories of thickness exist (Table 88-3). Certain anatomic sites affect the prognosis. The favorable sites appear to be the forearm and leg (excluding feet), while unfavorable sites include scalp, hands, feet, and mucous membranes. In general, women with stage I or II disease have a better survival than men, perhaps in part because of earlier diagnosis; women frequently have melanomas on the lower leg, where self-recognition is more likely and prognosis is better. Older individuals, in general, have poorer prognoses. This

Table 88-2

Clinical Features of Malignant Melanoma

Type	Site	Average Age at Diagnosis, Years	Duration of Known Existence, Years	Color
Lentigo maligna melanoma	Sun-exposed surfaces, particularly malar region of cheek and temple	70	5–20* or longer	In flat portions, shades of brown and tan predominant, but whitish gray occasionally present; in nodules, shades of reddish brown, bluish gray, bluish black
Superficial spreading melanoma	Any site (more common on upper back and, in women, on lower legs)	40–50	1–7	Shades of brown mixed with bluish red (violaceous), bluish black, reddish brown, and often whitish pink, and the border of lesion is at least in part visibly and/or palpably elevated
Nodular melanoma	Any site	40–50	Months to less than 5 years	Reddish blue (purple) or bluish black; either uniform in color or mixed with brown or black
Acral lentiginous melanoma	Palm, sole, nail bed, mucous membrane	60	1–10	In flat portions, dark brown predominantly; in raised lesions (plaques) brown-black or blue-black predominantly

* During much of this time, the precursor stage, lentigo maligna, is confined to the epidermis.
SOURCE: Adapted from AJ Sober, in *Pathophysiology of Dermatologic Diseases*, NA Soter, HP Baden (eds). New York, McGraw-Hill, 1984.

Table 88-3

CHAPTER 88
Melanoma and Other Skin Cancers
545

Prognosis of Melanoma by Thickness (Breslow) and AJCC Stages: 5-Year Survival Rates

AJCC Stage	Thickness Range, mm	% Overall Survival
IA (localized)	≤0.75	96
IB (localized)	0.76–1.50	87
IIA (localized)	1.5–2.49	75
	2.50–3.99	66
IIB (localized)	≥4.00	47
III (metastatic to regional nodes)		45 (one node)
		<20 (two nodes)
IV (metastatic to distant sites)		8–10*

* One-year survival

finding has been explained in part by a tendency toward later diagnosis (and thus thicker tumors) in men and by a higher proportion in men of acral melanomas (palmar-plantar), which have a poorer prognosis. Melanoma may recur after many years. About 10 to 15 percent of first-time recurrences develop more than 5 years after treatment of the original lesion. The time to recurrence varies inversely with tumor thickness. Other prognostic factors for stages I and II melanoma include the presence of an ulcer in the primary tumor, the mitotic rate, and the presence of microscopic tumor satellites (foci of tumor ≥0.05 mm in diameter in the reticular dermis or subcutaneous fat, distinct from the main body of the tumor). The presence of microscopic satellites is also predictive of microscopic metastases to the regional lymph nodes. An alternate prognostic scheme for clinical stages I and II melanoma, proposed by Clark, is based on the anatomic level of invasion in the skin. Level I is intraepidermal (in situ); level II penetrates the papillary dermis; level III spans the papillary dermis; level IV penetrates the reticular dermis; and level V penetrates into the subcutaneous fat. The 5-year survival for these stages averages 100, 95, 82, 71, and 49 percent, respectively.

NATURAL HISTORY Melanomas may spread by the lymphatic channels or the bloodstream. The earliest metastases are often to regional lymph nodes. Surgical lymphadenectomy usually controls regional disease. Liver, lung, bone, and brain are common sites of hematogenous spread, but unusual sites, such as the anterior chamber of the eye, also may be involved. Once widespread metastatic disease is established, the likelihood of cure is low.

MANAGEMENT The entire cutaneous surface, including the scalp and mucous membranes, should be examined in each patient. Bright room illumination is important, and a 7× to 10× hand lens is helpful for evaluating variation in pigment pattern. A history of relevant risk factors should be elicited. Any suspicious lesions should be biopsied, evaluated by a specialist, or recorded by chart and/or photography for follow-up. Examination of the lymph nodes and palpation of the abdominal viscera are part of the staging examination for suspected melanoma. The patient should be advised to have other family members screened if either melanoma or clinically atypical moles (dysplastic nevi) are present. The detection of early melanoma in relatives on screening has been reported. Melanoma prevention is based on protection from the sun. Routine use of a sunblock of SPF ≥15, use of protective clothing, and avoiding intense midday ultraviolet exposure should be recommended. The patient should be educated in the clinical features of melanoma and advised to report any growth or other change in a pigmented lesion. Patient education brochures are available from the American Cancer Society, the American Academy of Dermatology, the National Cancer Institute, and the Skin Cancer Foundation. Self-examination at 6- to 8-week intervals may enhance the likelihood of detecting change between follow-up visits. The importance of routine follow-up visits for melanoma patients and patients with clinically atypical moles (dysplastic nevi) should be emphasized, as these visits may facilitate early detection of new tumors.

Precursor Lesions Clinically atypical moles, also termed *dysplastic nevi*, occur in certain families affected by melanoma. In some families, melanomas occur nearly exclusively in the individuals with dysplastic nevi. These nevi appear to be transmitted as an autosomal dominant trait that involves chromosome 9p16. In other families, the nevi may not be present in all individuals with an increased risk of melanoma. The melanomas may arise in clinically atypical moles or in normal skin; (in the latter situation the mole acts as a marker of increased risk). Individuals with clinically atypical moles and two family members with melanoma have been reported to have a greater than 50 percent lifetime risk for developing melanoma. Table 88-4 lists the features that are characteristic of clinically atypical moles and that differentiate them from benign acquired nevi. The number of clinically atypical moles may vary from one to several hundred. Clinically atypical moles usually differ from each other in appearance. The borders are often hazy and indistinct, and the pigment pattern is more highly varied than that in benign acquired nevi. Of the 90 percent of melanoma patients whose disease is regarded as sporadic (i.e., who lack a family history of melanoma), about 40 percent have clinically atypical moles, as compared with an estimated 5 to 10 percent of the population at large. Further studies to determine the background frequency of clinically atypical moles are required, once greater unanimity exists regarding their clinical and histopathologic features. The observation that at least 20 percent of sporadic melanomas arise in association with a clinically atypical mole makes this nevus the most important precursor for melanoma.

Less frequent precursors include the giant congenital melanocytic nevus and the small congenital melanocytic nevus (although the latter relationship is disputed by some). Congenital melanocytic nevi are present at birth or appear in the neonatal period (tardive form). The giant melanocytic nevus, also called the bathing trunk, cape, or garment nevus, is a rare malformation that affects perhaps 1 in 30,000 to 1 in 100,000 individuals. These nevi are usually greater than 20 cm in diameter and may cover more than half the body surface. Giant nevi often occur in association with multiple small congenital nevi. The borders are sharp, and hair may be present. The lesions are usually dark brown and may have darker and lighter areas. Pigment is haphazardly

Table 88-4

Clinical Features Distinguishing Atypical Moles from Benign Acquired Nevi

Clinical Feature	Clinically Atypical Moles	Benign Acquired Nevi
Color	Variable mixtures of tan, brown, black, or red/pink within a single nevus; nevi may look very different from each other	Uniformly tan or brown
Shape	Irregular borders; pigment may fade off into surrounding skin; macular portion at the edge of the nevus	Round; sharp, clear-cut borders between the nevus and the surrounding skin; may be flat or elevated
Size	Usually more than 6 mm in diameter; may be more than 10 mm; occasionally smaller than 6 mm	Usually less than 6 mm in diameter
Number	Often very many (more than 100), but occasionally may be only one	In a typical adult, 10 to 40 are scattered over the body; perhaps 15% of patients have no nevi
Location	Sun-exposed areas; the back is the most common site, but dysplastic nevi may also be seen on the scalp, breasts, and buttocks	Generally on the sun-exposed surfaces of the skin above the waist; the scalp, breasts, and buttocks are rarely involved

SOURCE: Modified from Friedman et al, 1991b.

displayed. The surface is smooth to rugose or cerebriform and may vary from one portion of the lesion to another. A lifetime risk of melanoma development of 6 percent has been estimated. The risk is greatest before age 5 and next greatest between ages 5 and 10. Early detection of melanoma is difficult in these lesions because of the deep dermal or subcutaneous origin of primary melanoma and because of the large and varied surface of the nevus. Prophylactic excision early in life can be accomplished by staged removal with coverage by split-thickness skin grafts. The use of cultured keratinocytes for coverage appears promising. At present, there are no uniform management guidelines for giant congenital nevi.

The small- to medium-sized congenital melanocytic nevus, which affects approximately 1 percent of persons, presents usually as a raised dark- to medium-brown lesion with a smooth or papillomatous surface. The border is sharp, and lesions may be oriented along lines of skin cleavage. Follicular hyper- and hypopigmentation may coexist in a salt-and-pepper configuration. The lesion may have an excess of thick, coarse hairs. The risk of melanoma developing in these lesions is not known; however, melanomas can arise in these lesions. Considerations of body surface area suggest that the incidence of melanomas arising in small congenital melanocytic nevi is probably higher than would be expected by chance. The remnants of a nevus with histopathologic features of a congenital nevus have been observed in 2 to 6 percent of melanomas. The management of small- to medium-sized congenital melanocytic nevi remains controversial; prophylactic removal under local anesthesia in the early teen years is appropriate. Melanomas in small congenital melanocytic nevi appear to occur after this period of life.

Differential Diagnosis   The aim of differential diagnosis is to distinguish benign pigmented lesions from melanoma and its precursors. If melanoma is a consideration, then biopsy is appropriate. Some benign look-alikes may be removed in the process of trying to detect authentic melanoma. Table 88-5 summarizes the distinguishing features of benign lesions that may be confused with melanoma. Early detection of melanoma may be facilitated by applying the "ABCD rules": A—asymmetry, benign lesions are usually symmetric; B—border irregularity, most nevi have clear-cut borders; C—color variegation, benign lesions usually have uniform light or dark pigment; D—diameter >6 mm (the size of a pencil eraser).

Biopsy   Any pigmented cutaneous lesion that has changed in size or shape or has other features suggestive of malignant melanoma is a candidate for biopsy. The recommended technique is a full-thickness excisional biopsy, as that facilitates pathologic assessment of the lesion, permits accurate measurement of thickness if the lesion is melanoma, and constitutes treatment if the lesion is benign. Shave biopsy or curettage of a suspected melanoma is contraindicated. For large lesions or lesions on anatomic sites where excisional biopsy may not be feasible (such as the face, hands, or feet), an incisional biopsy through the most nodular or darkest area of the lesion is acceptable; this should include the vertical growth phase of the primary tumor, if present. Data from prospective studies do not indicate that an incisional biopsy facilitates the spread of melanoma.

Staging   Once the diagnosis of malignant melanoma has been confirmed, the tumor must be staged to determine prognosis and treatment. The history should probe for evidence of metastatic disease, such as malaise, weight loss, headaches, visual difficulty, or bone pain. The physical examination should be directed especially to the skin, regional draining lymph nodes, central nervous system, liver, and spleen. In the absence of signs or symptoms of metastasis, few laboratory or radiologic tests are indicated for staging purposes. Aside from a chest radiograph and, possibly, liver function tests, no other tests or scans are routinely indicated unless the history or physical examination suggests metastasis to a specific organ. Specifically, liver-spleen scans and computed tomography have a low yield and are not cost-effective. However, once signs of metastasis exist, favored sites of spread, such as the liver, lungs, bone, and brain, should be scanned.

Table 88-5

Pigmented Lesions That Must Be Distinguished from Cutaneous Melanoma and Its Precursors

Lesion	Description
Blue nevus	Gunmetal or cerulean blue, blue-gray. Stable over time. One-half occur on dorsa of hand and feet. Lesions are usually single, small, 3 mm to <1 cm. Must be distinguished from nodular melanoma.
Compound nevus	Round or oval shape, well-demarcated, smooth-bordered. May be dome-shaped or papillomatous; colors range from flesh colored to very dark brown, with individual nevi being relatively homogeneous in color.
Hemangioma	Dome-shaped reddish, purple, blue nodule. Compression with a glass microscope slide may result in blanching. Must be distinguished from nodular melanoma.
Junctional nevus	Flat to barely raised brown lesion. Sharp border. Fine pigmentary stippling visible, especially upon magnification.

Lentigo
  Juvenile
  Solar
	Flat, uniformly medium or dark brown lesion with sharp border. Solar lentigines are acquired lesions on sites of chronic solar exposure (face and backs of hands). Lesions are 2 mm to ≥1 cm. Solar lentigines have reticulate pigmentation upon magnification.

Pigmented basal cell carcinoma	Papular border. May have central ulceration. Usually on a sun-exposed surface in an older patient. Patient usually has dark brown eyes and dark brown or black hair.
Pigmented dermatofibroma	Lesion is not well demarcated visually, is firm, and dimples downward when compressed laterally. Usually on extremities. Usually <6 mm.
Seborrheic keratosis	Rough, sharp-bordered lesions that feel waxy and "stuck on"; range in color from flesh to tan, to dark brown. Presence of keratin plugs in surface is helpful for discriminating especially dark lesions from melanoma.
Subungual hematoma	Maroon (red-brown) coloration. As lesion grows out from nail fold, a curving clear area is seen.
Tattoo (medical or traumatic)	In medical tattoo, lesions are small pigmentary dots, often blue or green, which make a regular pattern (rectangle). Traumatic tattoos are irregular, and pigmentation may appear black.

Appropriate evaluations place patients into four clinical stages (see Table 88-3).

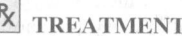 **TREATMENT**

Surgical Management   For a newly diagnosed cutaneous melanoma, wide surgical excision of the lesion with a margin of normal skin is necessary to remove all malignant cells and minimize local recurrence. The appropriate width of the margin is a source of controversy. A World Health Organization trial prospectively randomized between 1- and 3-cm margins in 612 patients with thin malignant melanomas (≤2 mm thick) reported that the narrower margin resulted in higher rates of local recurrence but no difference in rates of nodal or distant metastases, disease-free survival, or overall survival after 7.5 years of follow-up. Another large randomized trial comparing 2- or 4-cm surgical margins for intermediate-thickness lesions (1 to 4 mm thick) also found no significant differences in overall survival. The following margins can be recommended for primary melanoma: in situ: 0.5 cm; invasive up to 1 mm thick: 1.0 cm; 1 to 4 mm thick: 2.0 cm; >4 mm thick: 2.5 to 3.0 cm. For lesions on the face, hands, and feet, strict adherence to these margins must give way to individual considerations about the constraints of surgery and minimization of morbidity. In all instances, however, inclusion of subcutaneous fat in the surgical specimen facilitates adequate thickness measurement and assessment of surgical margins by the pathologist.

Elective Regional Node Dissection Elective regional node dissection in AJCC stage II disease (without palpable adenopathy) has been advocated, based on the hypothesis that melanoma metastasizes in an orderly fashion from the skin to regional lymph nodes and finally to distant sites. If that is the case, surgical excision of nodal micrometastases could theoretically provide definitive treatment at a time of relatively low tumor burden and perhaps improve survival. The efficacy of this procedure remains controversial; while some retrospective series suggest a survival benefit, two randomized studies examining this question in patients with limb melanomas and clinical stage I disease showed no survival advantage for wide local excision followed by immediate elective regional node dissection compared with wide local excision followed by delayed dissection (only if nodes became palpable). Furthermore, the procedure has associated morbidity, and some lesions, especially those on the trunk, have ambiguous nodal draining sites, making it difficult to decide which area to dissect. Results of biopsy of the first drainage node—the so-called sentinel node—predicts the likelihood of metastases in higher nodes. Sentinel nodes can be identified by injecting a blue dye or radioactive isotope around the primary tumor site. A negative biopsy result appears to obviate the need for elective regional nodal dissection. Patients with lesions <0.75 mm thick have an excellent prognosis and need no node dissection; at the other extreme, patients with lesions >3.50 mm thick have such a high risk for distant metastases that elective node dissection may not alter the ultimate clinical outcome. A subset of patients with AJCC stage II lesions of intermediate thickness may benefit from elective regional node dissection, but there is no consensus about which patients should undergo this procedure. An ongoing randomized surgical trial may resolve this issue.

Adjuvant Therapy For patients who are free of disease but at high risk for metastases, adjuvant therapy that complements surgery is needed to destroy occult micrometastases, prolong disease-free survival, and improve the cure rate. Many strategies have been tried unsuccessfully. However, adjuvant interferon α (either 2a or 2b) is capable of improving disease-free and overall survival significantly, particularly in patients with nodal metastases (stage III disease). The FDA has recently approved a high dose interferon adjuvant protocol consisting of 20 million units per square meter intravenously 5 days a week for 4 weeks followed by 10 million units per square meter subcutaneously three times a week for 11 months. Ongoing studies are attempting to define the minimal effective dose, because, in nearly half of patients, these doses of interferon are associated with severe toxicity, including flu-like illness and decline in performance status. The toxicity reverses promptly with lower doses and when therapy is stopped.

Treatment of Metastatic Disease Melanoma can metastasize to any organ, the brain being a particularly common site. Metastatic melanoma generally is incurable, with survival in patients with visceral metastases generally less than 1 year. Thus, the goal of treatment is usually palliation. Patients with soft-tissue and node metastases fare better than those with liver and brain metastases. Metastases limited to regional nodes (AJCC stage III disease) warrant a therapeutic lymph node dissection. Surgical excision of a single metastasis to the lung or to a surgically accessible brain site can prolong survival. Trials of stereotactic radiosurgery will determine its future role in the treatment of brain metastases. More often, however, patients have multiple brain metastases that require radiation therapy and glucocorticoids. Radiation therapy can provide local palliation for recurrent tumors or metastases. Patients who have advanced regional disease limited to a limb may benefit from hyperthermic limb perfusion with melphalan and tumor necrosis factor. Complete response rates greater than 90 percent have been reported; responses are associated with significant palliation of symptoms.

A number of drugs and biologicals have minimal antitumor activity (15 to 20 percent partial response rates) in metastatic melanoma, including dacarbazine (DTIC), the nitrosoureas carmustine (BCNU), lomustine (CCNU), and semustine (methyl-CCNU), platinum analogues such as cisplatin and carboplatin, vinca alkyloids such as vincristine, vinblastine, and vindesine, the taxanes paclitaxel (taxol) and docetaxel, interferon α, and interleukin 2 (IL-2). Single-agent dacarbazine is considered the standard treatment. This agent has been given at a number of different doses and schedules; 250 mg/m² intravenously every day for 5 days every 3 weeks is a standard schedule. There is increasing evidence that dacarbazine-based combination regimens are probably more effective. Ongoing trials are attempting to define superior combinations. Interferon and IL-2 produce response rates similar to those seen with cytotoxic agents; however, at active doses, they usually cause greater toxicity than chemotherapy.

Considerable evidence suggests that melanomas can express cell surface antigens that may be recognized by host immune cells. A number of melanoma-associated antigens have been discovered. Melanoma antigens (MAGEs)-1, -2, and -3 (endogenous proteins controlled by genes on the X chromosome; there may be up to 12 of these genes), and tyrosinase, an enzyme involved in melanin synthesis, are antigens that are processed into peptides and presented to T cells via HLA-A antigens on the tumor, particularly the HLA-A1 and A2 alleles, which are expressed in about 85 percent of patients with melanoma. In addition, there is a melanoma antigen called MART that is recognized in the context of class II MHC antigens. These melanoma-associated antigens alone or in combination may make it possible to develop vaccination strategies against melanoma. Such strategies include the use of purified proteins as immunogens and the use of genetically altered tumor cells to elicit a T-cell response. Alternative experimental approaches include efforts to expand tumor-specific T cells (obtained either from the tumor as tumor-infiltrating lymphocytes or harvested from the peripheral blood after vaccination) in vitro and transfer them into patients in large numbers. In addition, monoclonal antibodies to tumor antigens are being tested, with some early indication of efficacy in around 15 percent of patients. All of these experimental approaches will need considerable further development before being applicable on a wide scale. However, once an approach that appears to be active in metastatic disease is found, it is possible that it will prove most useful when administered as an adjuvant.

The absence of curative therapy for patients with metastatic melanoma underscores the importance of early detection and prevention as strategies to decrease melanoma mortality.

NONMELANOMA SKIN CANCER

Nonmelanoma skin cancer is the most common cancer in the United States, with an estimated annual incidence of more than 800,000 cases. Basal cell carcinomas (BCCs) account for 70 to 80 percent of nonmelanoma skin cancers. Squamous cell carcinomas (SCCs), while representing only about 20 percent of nonmelanoma skin cancers, are more significant because of their ability to metastasize; they account for most of the 2300 deaths annually. Incidence rates have risen dramatically over the past decade.

ETIOLOGY The cause of BCC and SCC is multifactorial. Cumulative exposure to sunlight, principally the ultraviolet B (UV-B) spectrum, is the most significant factor. Other factors associated with a higher incidence of skin cancer are male sex, older age, Celtic descent, a fair complexion, a tendency to sunburn easily, and an outdoor occupation. The incidence of these tumors increases with decreasing latitude. Most tumors develop on sun-exposed areas of the head and neck. Tumors are more common on the left side of the body in the United States but on the right side in England, presumably owing to asymmetric exposure during driving. As the earth's protective ozone shield continues to thin, further increases in the incidence of skin cancer can be anticipated. In certain geographic areas, exposure to arsenic in well water or from industrial sources may significantly increase the risk of BCC and SCC. Skin cancer in affected individuals may be seen with or without other cutaneous markers of chronic arsenism (e.g., arsenical keratoses). Less common is exposure to the cyclic aromatic hydrocarbons in tar, soot, or shale. The risk of lip or oral SCC is increased with cigarette smoking. Human papillomaviruses and UV-B light may act as cocarcinogens.

Host factors associated with a high risk of skin cancer include immunosuppression induced by disease or drugs. Transplant recipients receiving chronic immunosuppressive therapy are particularly prone to SCC. The frequency of skin cancer is proportional to the duration of immunosuppression and the extent of sun exposure. Skin cancer is a not uncommon finding in patients infected with the human immunodeficiency virus (HIV), and it may be more aggressive in this setting. As the life span of HIV-infected persons increases, skin cancer may become a greater problem. Other factors include ionizing radiation, thermal burns, and certain scars and chronic ulcerations. Several heritable conditions have been associated with skin cancer (e.g., albinism, xeroderma pigmentosum, and BCC nevus syndrome).

CLINICAL PRESENTATION Nonmelanoma skin cancers are often asymptomatic, but nonhealing ulceration, bleeding, or pain can occur.

Basal Cell Carcinoma BCC is a malignancy arising from epidermal basal cells. There are several clinical types of BCC. The most common is *noduloulcerative BCC*, which begins as a small, pearly nodule, often with small telangiectatic vessels on its surface. The nodule grows slowly and may undergo central ulceration. Various amounts of melanin may be present in the tumor; tumors with a heavier accumulation are referred to as *pigmented BCC*. While clinically no more aggressive than the noduloulcerative variant, the latter may be mistaken for malignant melanoma. *Superficial BCC* consists of one or several erythematous, scaling plaques that slowly enlarge. Although they are more commonly found on the trunk and extremities, the head and neck also can be affected. The lesions may be confused with benign inflammatory dermatoses, especially nummular eczema and psoriasis. *Morpheaform (fibrosing) BCC* manifests itself as a solitary, flat or slightly depressed, indurated, whitish or yellowish plaque. Borders are typically indistinct, a feature associated with a greater potential for extensive subclinical spread.

Squamous Cell Carcinoma Primary cutaneous SCC is a malignant neoplasm of keratinizing epidermal cells. Unlike BCC, which has a very low metastatic potential, SCC can metastasize and grow rapidly. The clinical features of SCC vary widely. Commonly, SCC appears as an ulcerated nodule or a superficial erosion on the skin or lower lip, but it may present as a verrucous papule or plaque. Unlike BCC, overlying telangiectasias are uncommon. The margins of this tumor may be ill-defined, and fixation to underlying structures may occur. Cutaneous SCC may develop anywhere on the body, but it usually arises on sun-damaged skin. A related neoplasm, keratoacanthoma, typically appears as a dome-shaped papule with a central keratotic crater, expands rapidly, and commonly regresses without therapy. This lesion can be difficult to differentiate from SCC.

SCC has several premalignant forms (actinic keratosis, actinic cheilitis, and some cutaneous horns) and in situ forms (e.g., Bowen's disease) that are confined to the epidermis. Actinic keratoses and cheilitis are hyperkeratotic papules and plaques that occur on sun-exposed areas. While the potential for malignant degeneration is low in any individual lesion, the risk of SCC increases with larger numbers of lesions. Bowen's disease presents as a scaling, erythematous plaque, which may develop into invasive SCC in up to 20 percent of cases. Controversy exists regarding the association of Bowen's disease with internal malignancy; however, recent evidence suggests that there is no significant relationship when other predisposing factors (e.g., arse-nic) are absent. Treatment of premalignant and in situ lesions reduces the subsequent risk of invasive disease.

NATURAL HISTORY **Basal Cell Carcinoma** The natural history of BCC is that of a slowly enlarging, locally invasive neoplasm. The degree of local destruction and risk of recurrence vary with the size, duration, and location of the tumor, the histologic subtype, the presence of recurrent disease, and various patient characteristics. Location on the central face (e.g., the nose, the nasolabial fold, or the periorbital or perioral area), the ears, or the scalp may portend a higher risk. Small nodular, pigmented, cystic, or superficial BCCs respond well to most treatments. Large nodular, noduloulcerative, and especially morpheaform BCCs are usually more aggressive. The metastatic potential of BCC has been estimated to be 0.0028 to 0.1 percent. Persons with either BCC or SCC have an increased risk of developing subsequent skin cancers.

Squamous Cell Carcinoma The natural history of SCC depends on both tumor and host characteristics. Tumors arising on actinically damaged skin have a lower metastatic potential than those on protected surfaces. The metastatic frequency of cutaneous SCC, reported at 0.3 to 3.7 percent, is lower than that of mucosal SCC. Tumors occurring on the lower lip and ear have metastatic potential approaching 13 and 11 percent, respectively. The metastatic potential of SCC arising in burn scars, chronic ulcerations, or the genitalia is higher. The overall metastatic rate for recurrent tumors may approach 30 percent. Poorly differentiated, deep tumors with perineural or lymphatic invasion often behave aggressively. Multiple tumors with rapid growth and aggressive behavior can be a therapeutic challenge in immunosuppressed patients. Regional lymph nodes are the most common site of metastasis. In patients with metastatic disease, the 5-year survival rate may be low.

℞ **TREATMENT**

Basal Cell Carcinoma The treatment modalities used for BCC include electrodesiccation and curettage (ED&C), excision, cryosurgery, radiation therapy, Mohs micrographic surgery (MMS), and others. The mode of therapy chosen depends on tumor characteristics, on the age, medical status, and preferences of the patient, and on other factors. ED&C remains the method most commonly employed by dermatologists. This method is selected for low-risk tumors (e.g., a small primary tumor of a less aggressive subtype in a favorable location). Excision, which offers the advantage of histologic control, is usually selected for more aggressive tumors or those in high-risk locations, or, in many instances, for aesthetic reasons. Cryosurgery using liquid nitrogen may be used in certain low-risk tumors, but it requires specialized equipment (cryoprobes) to be effective for advanced neoplasms. Radiation therapy, while not employed as often as surgical modalities, offers an excellent chance for cure in many cases of BCC. It is useful in patients not considered surgical candidates and as a surgical adjunct in high-risk tumors. Younger patients may not be good candidates for radiation therapy because of the risks of long-term carcinogenesis and radiodermatitis. MMS is a specialized type of surgical excision which permits the ultimate in histologic control and preservation of uninvolved tissue. It is preferred for lesions that are recurrent, in a high-risk location, or large and ill-defined, and where maximal tissue conservation is critical (e.g., the eyelids). Topical chemotherapy with 5-fluorouracil (5FU) cream has limited usefulness in the management of BCC and should be used only for treating superficial BCC. Intralesional 5FU is being investigated as a treatment modality for BCC. Intralesional interferon is effective in certain primary tumors. Photodynamic therapy, which employs selective activation of a photoactive drug by visible light, may be useful in patients with numerous tumors, but further investigation is needed. Lasers also have been used for the treatment of skin cancer.

Squamous Cell Carcinoma The therapy of cutaneous SCC should be based on an analysis of risk factors influencing the biologic behavior of the tumor. These include the size, location, and degree of histologic differentiation of the tumor and the age and physical condition of the patient. Surgical excision, MMS, and radiation are standard methods of treatment. Cryosurgery and ED&C have been used successfully for small primary tumors. Metastases are treated with lymph node dissection, irradiation, or both. 13-*Cis*-retinoic acid (1 mg orally every day) plus interferon α (3 million units subcutaneously or intramuscularly every day) may produce a partial response in most patients. Systemic chemotherapy combinations that include cisplatin may also be palliative in some patients.

PREVENTION Since the vast majority of skin cancers are related to chronic UV-B exposure, patient and physician education could dramatically reduce their incidence. Emphasis should be placed on preventive measures beginning early in life. Patients must understand that damage from UV-B begins early, despite the fact that cancers develop years later. Regular use of sunscreens and protective clothing should be encouraged. Avoidance of tanning salons and sun exposure during midday (10 A.M. to 2 P.M.) is recommended. Precancerous and in situ lesions should be treated early. Early detection of small tumors affords simpler treatment modalities with higher cure rates and lower morbidity. In patients with a history of skin cancer, long-term follow-up for the detection of recurrence, metastasis, and new skin cancers should be emphasized. Chemoprophylaxis using synthetic retinoids is useful in controlling new lesions in some patients with multiple tumors.

OTHER TYPES OF CUTANEOUS CANCER

Neoplasms of cutaneous adnexa, and sarcomas of fibrous, mesenchymal, fatty, and vascular tissues make up 1 to 2 percent of nonmelanoma skin cancers. The recent rapid rise in the incidence of Kaposi's sarcoma is attributed to HIV infection and immunosuppressive therapy. Epidemiologic patterns suggest infectious agents as possible etiologic factors. A novel herpesvirus, human herpesvirus 8, is a potential cause of several types of Kaposi's sarcoma. Current therapy is palliative and depends on the symptoms and sites of involvement. Treatment modalities include cryosurgery, intralesional vinblastine, excision, radiation, interferon α, and systemic combination chemotherapy. As further etiologic factors are identified, safer and more effective therapy may be devised (see Chap. 308).

BIBLIOGRAPHY

ALBERT L et al: Dysplastic melanocytic nevi and cutaneous melanoma: Markers of increased melanoma risk for affected individuals and blood relatives. J Am Acad Dermatol 7:69, 1990

ARMSTRONG BK: Epidemiology of malignant melanoma: Intermittent or total accumulated exposure to the sun. J Dermatol Surg Oncol 14:835, 1988

BALCH CM et al (eds): *Cutaneous Melanoma: Clinical Management and Treatment Results Worldwide*, 2d ed. Philadelphia, Lippincott, 1992

———— et al: Efficacy of 2-cm surgical margins for intermediate-thickness melanomas (1–4 mm). Ann Surg 218:262, 1993

BOON T: Tumor antigens recognized by cytolytic T lymphocytes present perspectives for specific immunotherapy. Int J Cancer 54:177, 1993

CLARK WH JR et al: The histogenesis and biologic behavior of primary human malignant melanoma of the skin. Cancer Res 29:705, 1969

CREAGAN ET et al: Randomized surgical adjuvant clinical trial of recombinant interferon-alfa-2a in selected patients with malignant melanoma. J Clin Oncol 13:2776, 1995

DRAKE LA et al: Guidelines of care of basal cell carcinoma. J Am Acad Dermatol 26:117, 1992

———— et al: Guidelines of care for cutaneous squamous cell carcinoma. J Am Acad Dermatol 28:628, 1993

FRIEDMAN RJ et al: Malignant melanoma in the 1990s: The continued importance of early detection and the role of physician examination and self-examination of the skin. CA 41:201, 1991

———— et al (eds): *Cancer of the Skin*. Philadelphia, Saunders, 1991, pp 27–94

JOHNSON TM et al: Current therapy for cutaneous melanoma. J Am Acad Dermatol 32:689, 1995

KWA RE: Biology of cutaneous squamous cell carcinoma. J Am Acad Dermatol 26:1, 1992

KOH HK: Cutaneous melanoma. N Engl J Med 325:171, 1991

MARKS R: An overview of skin cancers. Incidence and causation. Cancer 75(Suppl):607, 1995

PRESTON DS et al: Nonmelanoma cancer of the skin. N Engl J Med 327:1649, 1992

LIPPMAN SM et al: 13cis-retinoic acid and interferon-α2a: Effective combination therapy for advanced squamous cell carcinoma of the skin. J Natl Cancer Inst 84:235, 1992

RHODES AR: Neoplasms: Benign neoplasias, hyperplasias, and dysplasias of melanocytes, in *Dermatology in General Medicine*, 4th ed, TB Fitzpatrick et al (eds). New York, McGraw-Hill, 1993, pp 996–1097

———— et al: Risk factors for cutaneous melanoma. JAMA 258:3146, 1987

RIGEL DS et al: Dysplastic nevi. Markers for increased risk for melanoma. Cancer 63:386, 1989

ROSENBERG SA: The immunotherapy and gene therapy of cancer. J Clin Oncol 10:180, 1992

VERONESI U et al: Delayed regional lymph node dissection in stage 1 melanoma of the skin of the lower extremities. Cancer 49:2420, 1982

————, CASCINELLI N: Narrow excision (1 cm margin), a safe procedure for thin cutaneous melanoma. Arch Surg 126:438, 1991

89 *Everett E. Vokes*

HEAD AND NECK CANCER

Epithelial carcinomas of the head and neck arise from the mucosal surfaces in the head and neck area and typically are squamous-cell in origin. This category includes tumors of the paranasal sinuses, the oral cavity, and the nasopharynx, oropharynx, hypopharynx, and larynx. Tumors of the salivary glands are discussed also in this chapter, although they differ from the more common carcinomas of the head and neck in etiology, histopathology, clinical presentation, and therapy. → *Thyroid malignancies are described in Chap. 331.*

INCIDENCE AND EPIDEMIOLOGY The annual number of new cases of head and neck cancers in the United States is approximately 40,000, accounting for about 5 percent of adult malignancies. Head and neck cancers are more common in some other countries, and the worldwide incidence probably exceeds half a million cases annually. In North America and Europe, the tumors usually arise from the oral cavity, oropharynx, or larynx, whereas nasopharyngeal cancer is more common in the Mediterranean countries and in the Far East.

ETIOLOGY AND GENETICS Alcohol and tobacco use are the most common risk factors for head and neck carcinogenesis in the United States, and the combination of alcohol and tobacco exposure is the most potent carcinogen. Even smokeless tobacco may be an etiologic agent for oral cancers. Other potential carcinogens include marijuana and occupational exposures such as nickel refining, exposure to textile fibers, and woodworking.

Dietary factors may contribute. There may be an inverse association between the consumption of fruits and vegetables and the incidence of head and neck cancer. Certain vitamins, including dietary carotenoids, may be protective; this relationship may provide a strategy for the prevention of head and neck cancers.

Some head and neck cancers may have a viral etiology. The DNA of human papilloma virus has been detected in the tissue of larynx and tonsil cancers, and there is an association with Epstein-Barr virus (EBV) infection and nasopharyngeal cancer. EBV DNA is present in nasopharyngeal cancers, and elevated antibody titers are present in most patients with nasopharyngeal cancer. The DNA of EBV has also been detected in premalignant lesions of the nasopharynx, further supporting a role for EBV in the pathogenesis. Nasopharyngeal cancer occurs endemically in some countries of the Mediterranean and Far East, where EBV antibody titers can be measured to screen high-risk populations. Nasopharyngeal cancer has also been associated with other environmental factors, such as consumption of salted fish.

No specific risk factors or environmental carcinogens have been identified for salivary gland tumors. Radiation exposure in early life is a risk factor for thyroid malignancies.

HISTOPATHOLOGY, CARCINOGENESIS, AND MOLECULAR BIOLOGY The head and neck carcinomas of squamous cell origin can be divided into well-differentiated, moderately well-differentiated, and poorly differentiated categories. Patients with poorly differentiated tumors are believed to have a worse prognosis than those with well-differentiated tumors. In Mediterranean countries and the Far East, the less common differentiated squamous cell carcinoma is distinguished from nonkeratinizing and undifferentiated carcinoma (lymphoepithelioma) that contains infiltrating (bystander) lymphocytes.

Salivary gland tumors can arise from the major (parotid, submandibular, sublingual) or minor salivary glands (the latter located in the submucosa of the upper aerodigestive tract). Most parotid tumors are benign, but half of submandibular and sublingual gland tumors, and most minor salivary gland tumors, are malignant. Malignant tumors include mucoepidermoid and adenoidcystic carcinomas and adenocarcinomas.

The mucosal surface of the entire pharynx is exposed to alcohol and tobacco-related carcinogens and is at risk for the development of a premalignant or malignant lesion, such as erythroplakia or leukoplakia (hyperplasia, dysplasia), that can progress to invasive carcinoma. Alternatively, multiple synchronous or metachronous cancers can develop. In fact, patients with early-stage head and neck cancer are at greater risk of dying of a second malignancy than of dying from a recurrence of the primary disease.

Unlike the second malignancies that develop after combined-modality therapy for malignant lymphomas, second head and neck malignancies are not therapy-induced but, instead, reflect the exposure of the upper aerodigestive mucosa to the same carcinogens that caused the first cancer. These second primaries can develop in the head and neck area, the lung, or the esophagus.

Chromosomal deletions and other alterations, most frequently involving chromosomes 3p, 9p, 17p, and 13q, have been identified in both premalignant and malignant head and neck lesions as have been mutations in tumor suppressor genes, commonly the *p53* gene. Amplification of oncogenes is less common, but overexpression of PRAD-1/bcl-1 (cyclin D1) and the epidermal growth factor receptor have been described. The latter finding correlates positively with tumor size and poor outcome.

Attempts have been made to use this information in therapy. Resected tumor specimens with histopathologically negative margins ("complete resection") can have histopathologically undetectable residual tumor cells with persistent *p53* mutations at the margins. Thus, a tumor-specific *p53* mutation can be detected in some phenotypically "normal" surgical margins, indicating residual disease. Early data suggest that patients with such submicroscopic marginal involvement have a worse prognosis than patients with negative margins. It may also prove possible to use molecular techniques for the early diagnosis or screening of malignant or premalignant lesions in high-risk populations (smokers and drinkers).

CLINICAL PRESENTATION AND DIFFERENTIAL DIAGNOSIS Most head and neck cancers occur after age 50, although these cancers can appear in younger patients, including those without known risk factors. The manifestations vary according to the stage and primary site of the tumor. A high index of suspicion is warranted for patients with nonspecific signs and symptoms in the head and neck area, particularly if the symptoms persist longer than 2 to 4 weeks.

Cancer of the nasopharynx typically does not cause early symptoms. However, on occasion it may cause unilateral serous otitis media due to obstruction of the eustachian tube, unilateral or bilateral nasal obstruction, or epistaxis. Advanced nasopharyngeal carcinoma causes neuropathies of the cranial nerves.

Carcinomas of the oral cavity present as nonhealing ulcers, changes in the fit of dentures, or painful lesions. Tumors of the tongue base or oropharynx can cause decreased tongue mobility and alterations in speech. Cancers of the oropharynx or hypopharynx rarely cause early symptoms, but they may cause sore throat and/or otalgia.

Hoarseness may be an early symptom of laryngeal cancer, and persistent hoarseness requires referral to an otorhinolaryngologist for indirect laryngoscopy and/or radiographic studies. If a head and neck lesion treated initially with antibiotics does not resolve in a short period, further workup is indicated; to simply continue the antibiotic treatment may be to lose the chance of early diagnosis of a malignancy.

Advanced head and neck cancers in any location can cause severe pain, otalgia, airway obstruction, cranial neuropathies, trismus, odynophagia, dysphagia, decreased tongue mobility, fistulas, skin involvement, and massive cervical lymphadenopathy, which may be unilateral or bilateral. Some patients have enlarged lymph nodes even though no primary lesion can be detected by endoscopy or biopsy; these patients are considered to have carcinoma of unknown primary. If the enlarged nodes are located in the upper neck and the tumor cells are of squamous cell histology, the malignancy probably arose from a mucosal surface in the head or neck. Tumor cells in supraclavicular lymph nodes may also arise from a primary site in the chest or abdomen, however.

The physical examination should include scrutiny of all visible mucosal surfaces and palpation of the floor of mouth and tongue and of the neck. In addition to tumors themselves, leukoplakia—a white mucosal patch—or erythroplakia—a red mucosal patch—may be observed; these "premalignant" lesions can represent hyperplasia, dysplasia, or carcinoma in situ. Biopsy of all visible lesions is recommended. Further examination should be performed by the otorhinolaryngologist. Additional staging procedures include computed tomography of the head and neck to identify the extent of the disease. Patients with lymph node involvement should also undergo screening for distant metastases, including chest radiography and a bone scan. The definitive staging procedure is an endoscopic examination under anesthesia, which may include laryngoscopy, esophagoscopy, and bronchoscopy; during this procedure, multiple biopsy samples are obtained to establish a primary diagnosis, to define the extent of primary disease, and to identify any additional premalignant lesions or second primaries.

Head and neck tumors are classified according to the TNM system of the American Joint Committee on Cancer. This classification varies according to the specific anatomic subsite (Table 89-1); generally, T1 through T3 describe the size of the primary lesion, and T4 indicates involvement of a vital structure in the head and neck, such as the tongue base, a cranial nerve, or the thyroid cartilage. The lymph nodes are staged uniformly for head and neck cancers of all sites (Table 89-1). Distant metastases are found in less than 10 percent of patients at initial diagnosis, but in autopsy series, microscopic involvement of the lungs, bones, or liver is more common, particularly in patients with advanced neck lymph node disease.

In patients with lymph node involvement and no visible primary, the diagnosis should be made by lymph node excision. If the results indicate squamous cell carcinoma, a panendoscopy should be performed, with biopsy of all suspicious-appearing areas and directed biopsies of common primary sites, such as the nasopharynx, tonsil, tongue base, and pyriform sinus.

℞ **TREATMENT**

Generally, patients with head and neck cancer can be categorized into three clinical groups: those with localized disease, those with locally or regionally advanced disease, and those with recurrent and/or metastatic disease.

Localized Disease Approximately one-third of patients have localized disease; that is, T1 or T2 (stage I or stage II) lesions without detectable lymph node involvement or distant metastases. These lesions are treated with curative intent by surgery or radiation. The choice of modality differs according to institutional expertise. Generally, radiation therapy is preferred for laryngeal cancer to preserve voice function, and surgery is preferred for small lesions in the oral cavity to avoid the long-term complications of radiation, such as xerostomia and dental decay.

Locally Advanced Disease Locally or regionally advanced disease—that is, disease with a large primary tumor and/or lymph node metastases—can also be treated with curative intent. This treatment usually consists of extensive surgery followed by postoperative radiation therapy. However, unresectable lesions, such as cancers of the nasopharynx or tongue base, are treated solely with radiotherapy. Even with the use of this two-modality approach, most cancers recur in the head and neck region, usually within 2 years of therapy, and cause death. This fact reflects the inability of surgery and radiation to eliminate all microscopic disease. To improve the outcome, chemotherapy has been added, along two major investigational lines referred to as induction chemotherapy and concomitant chemoradiotherapy.

INDUCTION CHEMOTHERAPY In this strategy, patients with advanced disease receive chemotherapy before surgery and radiotherapy. The most common combination is cisplatin and fluorouracil (5FU). Most patients who receive three cycles of this combination show tumor reduction, and the response is clinically complete in up to half of these patients. It is not clear whether this "sequential" multimodality therapy cures more patients than surgery plus radiation therapy alone. Large, randomized studies comparing surgery and radiotherapy with chemotherapy followed by surgery and radiotherapy suggest that there is no benefit in terms of survival.

Nevertheless, induction chemotherapy allows for organ preservation. For example, one study comparing surgery and radiation therapy with chemotherapy and radiation therapy found no difference in survival (50 percent at 2 years) for patients with advanced larynx cancer; however, the use of chemotherapy allowed the preservation of the larynx in two-thirds of patients. Another study found similar results for patients with hypopharyngeal cancer. Thus, chemotherapy plus radiotherapy should be considered in this group of patients in place of laryngectomy plus radiotherapy.

Induction chemotherapy has also been studied in patients with nasopharyngeal cancer (who frequently present with advanced lymph node involvement). Preliminary results indicate a longer time to recurrence for chemotherapy and radiation therapy than for radiation therapy alone. Chemotherapy may also improve survival.

CONCOMITANT CHEMORADIOTHERAPY With the concomitant strategy, chemotherapy and radiation therapy are given simultaneously rather than sequentially. Because most patients with head and neck cancer develop recurrent disease in the head and neck area, this approach is aimed at killing radiation-resistant cancer cells with chemotherapy. Indeed, some chemotherapy agents appear to increase the cytotoxicity of radiation. Three studies in patients with unresectable disease have suggested that radiation therapy plus concomitant 5FU gives better survival than radiation therapy alone. However, because the survival benefit in all three studies was small and because toxicity (mucositis) was increased with concomitant chemoradiotherapy, this treatment is not widely used. The use of radiation therapy together with cisplatin has produced markedly improved survival in patients with nasopharyngeal cancer.

Recurrent and/or Metastatic Disease Patients with recurrent and/or metastatic disease are, with few exceptions, treated with palliative intent. Some patients may require local or regional radiotherapy for pain control, but most are given chemotherapy. Response rates to chemotherapy average only 30 to 50 percent, the duration of response averages only 3 months, and the median survival time is 6 months. Therefore, chemotherapy provides transient symptomatic

---

Table 89-1

TNM Classification for Head and Neck Cancer

	Primary Tumor Site					
T Grade	Lip	Oral Cavity	Oropharynx	Hypopharynx	Nasopharynx	Larynx
TX			Primary tumor cannot be assessed			
T0			No evidence of primary tumor			
Tis			Carcinoma in situ			
T1	0–2 cm	0–2 cm	0–2 cm	1 site	1 site	1 site or limited to vocal cords
T2	2.1–4 cm	2.1–4 cm	2.1–4 cm	>1 site, no vocal cord fixation	>1 site	>1 site or impaired cord mobility
T3	>4 cm	>4 cm	>4 cm	vocal cord paralysis	Extension to nasal cavity or oropharynx	Vocal cord paralysis
T4	>4 cm with massive invasion		Massive soft tissue, bone, or cartilage invasion			

REGIONAL LYMPH NODES (N)

NX	Regional lymph nodes cannot be assessed
N0	No regional lymph node metastasis
N1	Metastasis in a single ipsilateral lymph node, 3 cm or less in greatest dimension
N2	Metastasis in a single ipsilateral lymph node, more than 3 cm but not more than 6 cm in greatest dimension; or in multiple ipsilateral lymph nodes, none more than 6 cm in greatest dimension; or in bilateral or contralateral lymph nodes, none more than 6 cm in greatest dimension
	N2a Metastasis in single ipsilateral lymph node more than 3 cm but more than 6 cm in greatest dimension
	N2b Metastasis in multiple ipsilateral lymph nodes, none more than 6 cm in greatest dimension
	N2c Metastasis in bilateral or contralateral lymph nodes, none more than 6 cm in greatest dimension
	N3 Metastasis in a lymph node more than 6 cm in greatest dimension

DISTANT METASTASIS (M)

MX	Presence of distant metastasis cannot be assessed
M0	No distant metastasis
M1	Distant metastasis

STAGE GROUPING

Stage 0	Tis	N0	M0	Stage IV	T4	N0	M0
Stage I	T1	N0	M0		T4	N1	M0
Stage II	T2	N0	M0		Any T	N2	M0
Stage III	T3	N0	M0		Any T	N3	M0
	T1	N1	M0		Any T	Any N	M1
	T2	N1	M0				
	T3	N1	M0				

benefit. Drugs with single-agent activity in this setting include methotrexate, 5FU, cisplatin, and paclitaxel. Combinations of cisplatin and 5FU, carboplatin and 5FU, and cisplatin and paclitaxel are also used.

CHEMOPREVENTION Another line of clinical research is aimed at preventing the transformation of premalignant disease into invasive carcinoma. β-Carotene and *cis*-retinoic acid can lead to the regression of leukoplakia. In addition, the use of *cis*-retinoic acid may reduce the incidence of second primaries. Large confirmatory randomized studies are under way to determine the effectiveness of this approach.

TREATMENT COMPLICATIONS Complications of the treatment of head and neck cancer are usually related to the extent of surgery. Several attempts have been made to limit the extent of surgery or to replace it with chemotherapy and radiation therapy. Acute complications of radiation include mucositis and dysphagia, and long-term complications include xerostomia, loss of taste, decreased tongue mobility, second malignancies, and dysphagia and neck fibrosis. The complications of chemotherapy vary with the regimen used but usually include myelosuppression, mucositis, nausea and vomiting, and nephrotoxicity (with cisplatin).

SALIVARY GLAND TUMORS Most benign salivary gland tumors are treated with surgical excision, and patients with invasive salivary gland tumors are treated with surgery and radiation. Neutron radiation may be particularly effective. These tumors may recur regionally; adenoidcystic carcinoma has a tendency to recur along the nerve tracks. Distant metastases may occur as late as 10 to 20 years after the initial diagnosis. For metastatic disease, therapy is given with palliative intent, usually chemotherapy with doxorubicin and/or cisplatin.

BIBLIOGRAPHY

ADELSTEIN DJ: The community approach to salvage therapy for advanced head and neck cancer. Semin Oncol 21(Suppl 7):52, 1994

BRENNAN JA et al: Molecular assessment of histopathological staging in squamous-cell carcinoma of the head and neck. N Engl J Med 332:429, 1995

BROWMAN GP, CRONIN L: Standard chemotherapy in squamous cell head and neck cancer: What we have learned from randomized trials. Semin Oncol 21:311, 1994

———— et al: Placebo-controlled randomized trial of infusional fluorouracil during standard radiotherapy in locally advanced head and neck cancer. J Clin Oncol 12:2648, 1994

FANDI A, et al: Nasopharyngeal cancer: Epidemiology, staging, and treatment. Semin Oncol 21:382, 1994

LIPPMAN SM, et al: Comparison of low-dose isotretinoin with beta carotene to prevent oral carcinogenesis. N Engl J Med 328:15, 1993

THE DEPARTMENT OF VETERANS AFFAIRS LARYNGEAL CANCER STUDY GROUP: Induction chemotherapy plus radiation compared with surgery plus radiation in patients with advanced laryngeal cancer. N Engl J Med 324:1685, 1991

VOKES EE, ATHANASIADIS I: Chemotherapy for squamous cell carcinoma of head and neck: The future is now. Ann Oncol 7:15, 1996

————, WEICHSELBAUM RR: Concomitant chemoradiotherapy: Rationale and clinical experience in patients with solid tumors. J Clin Oncol 8:911, 1990

———— et al: Head and neck cancer. N Engl J Med 328:184, 1993

90   *John D. Minna*

NEOPLASMS OF THE LUNG

Each year, primary carcinoma of the lung affects 99,000 males and 78,000 females in the United States, 86 percent of whom die within 5 years of diagnosis, making it the leading cause of cancer death in both men and women. The incidence of lung cancer peaks between ages 55 and 65 years. Lung cancer accounts for 32 percent of all cancer deaths in men and for 25 percent of all cancer deaths in women.

The effects of smoking cessation efforts begun 20 years ago have finally started to be seen in a slowing of the rate of age-adjusted cancer death from lung cancer in white males (57 per 100,000 male population), while, unfortunately, the rate in females is still increasing (26 per 100,000 female population). Lung cancer is the leading cancer killer in all racial groups in the United States. At the time of diagnosis, only 15 percent of all lung cancer patients will have local disease, while ~25 percent will have disease spread to regional lymph nodes, and >55 percent will have distant metastatic cancer. Even in the patients with localized disease, the 5-year survival is only 48 percent, while survival is 18 percent for patients with regional disease and 14 percent overall. Of clinical significance, the 5-year overall lung cancer survival rate has increased steadily from 8 percent in the 1960s to 14 percent in the 1990s. These increases have been seen in both whites and African Americans. The main cause of these changes appears to be advances in combined-modality treatment with surgery, radiotherapy, and chemotherapy. Thus, primary carcinoma of the lung is a major health problem with a generally grim prognosis. However, an orderly approach to diagnosis, staging, and treatment based on knowledge of the clinical behavior of lung cancer allows selection of the best therapy for either potential cure or optimal palliation of individual patients. This approach should be multidisciplinary, involving interaction of internists, chest physicians, medical, radiation, and surgical oncologists, pathologists, and supportive care personnel.

PATHOLOGY

The histologic classification of primary lung neoplasms recommended by the World Health Organization in 1981 should be used. The term *lung cancer* is usually reserved for tumors arising from the respiratory epithelium (bronchi, bronchioles, and alveoli). Mesotheliomas, lymphomas, and stromal tumors (sarcomas) usually are given a pathologic diagnosis distinct from epithelial lung cancer. Four major cell types make up 88 percent of all primary lung neoplasms (Table 90-1). These are *squamous* or *epidermoid carcinoma*, *small cell* (also called *oat cell*) *carcinoma*, *adenocarcinoma* (including bronchioloalveolar), and *large cell* (also called *large cell anaplastic*) *carcinoma*. The remainder include undifferentiated carcinomas, carcinoids, bronchial gland tumors (including adenoid cystic carcinomas and mucoepidermoid tumors), and rarer tumor types. The various cell types have different natural histories and responses to therapy, and thus a correct histologic diagnosis by an experienced pathologist is the first step to correct treatment. In the past 20 years, for unknown reasons, adenocarcinoma has replaced squamous cell carcinoma as the most frequent histologic subtype for all sexes and races combined (Table 90-1).

Major treatment decisions are made on the basis of whether a tumor is classified histologically as a small cell carcinoma or as one of the non-small cell varieties (which include epidermoid, adenocarcinoma, large cell carcinoma, bronchioloalveolar carcinoma—a subtype of adenocarcinoma—and mixed versions of these). Some of these distinctions are summarized in Tables 90-1 and 90-2. In general, small cell carcinomas have already spread at the time of presentation beyond the bounds where surgery with curative intent could be undertaken, and they are managed primarily by chemotherapy with or without radiotherapy. In contrast, non-small cell cancers that are found to be localized at the time of presentation should be considered for curative treatment with either surgery or radiotherapy. Further, the response of non-small cell cancers to chemotherapy usually is not dramatic, making such therapy less important in metastatic disease than it is in cases of small cell lung cancer.

Ninety percent of patients with lung cancer of all histologic types are current or former cigarette smokers. Currently, ~50,000 of the annual 177,000 new cases of lung cancer develop in former smokers. With increased success in smoking cessation efforts, this number will grow, and such former smokers will be important candidates for future early detection and chemoprevention efforts. By far the most common form of lung cancer arising in lifetime nonsmokers, in women, and in young patients (<45 years old) is adenocarcinoma. However, in nonsmokers with adenocarcinoma involving the lung, the possibility of other primary sites should be considered. Epidermoid and small cell cancers usually present as central masses with endobronchial growth, while adenocarcinomas and large cell cancers tend to present as peripheral nodules or masses, frequently with pleural involvement. Epidermoid and large cell cancers cavitate in approximately 10 to 20 percent of cases. Bronchioloalveolar carcinoma, a special form of adenocarcinoma arising from peripheral airways, can present as a single mass, as a diffuse, multinodular lesion, or as a fluffy infiltrate.

ETIOLOGY

The large majority of lung cancers are caused by carcinogens and tumor promoters ingested via cigarette smoking. The prevalence of smoking in the United States is 28 percent for males and 25 percent for females, 18 years old or older. Overall, the relative risk of developing lung cancer is increased about 13-fold by active smoking and about 1.5-fold by long-term passive exposure to cigarette smoke. Probably there is a cocarcinogenic effect of smoking and industrial or environmental pollutants such as radon gas from natural sources in the ground. There is a dose-response relationship between the lung cancer death rate and the total amount (often expressed in "cigarette pack-years") of cigarettes smoked, such that the risk is increased 60- to 70-fold for a man smoking two packs a day for 20 years as compared with a nonsmoker. Conversely, the chance of developing lung cancer decreases with cessation of smoking but may never return to the nonsmoker level. The increase in lung cancer rate in women is also associated with a rise in cigarette smoking. However, of great importance, women with lung cancer are more likely to have never smoked than men. Also, the dose-response odds ratio of developing lung cancer over cumulative exposure to cigarette smoking was ~1.5 higher in women than men for all histologic types. This gender difference is likely due to a higher susceptibility to tobacco carcinogens in women. As a preventive measure, efforts to get persons to stop smoking are mandatory. However, smoking cessation is extremely difficult, because the smoking habit represents a powerful addiction to nicotine (see Chap. 389). Therefore, it is of vital importance to prevent people from starting to smoke. This goal requires new efforts targeted at children, since addiction to cigarettes usually has occurred by the late teen years.

The poor prognosis for most patients with lung cancer requires the continued performance of well-designed clinical trials—trials of combinations of chemotherapy with surgery or radiotherapy and of the relative effectiveness of using chemotherapy and radiotherapy in an adjuvant (after surgery) and a neoadjuvant (before surgery) fashion; tests of biologic response modifiers, oncopeptide vaccines, and gene therapy; prospective testing of tumor sensitivity in vitro to drugs, radiation therapy, and biologic response modifiers; and tests of the application of newer methods for early detection and chemoprevention. The key intervention remains prevention, and broad efforts to help persons to stop smoking and to prevent persons from starting smoking must continue. Initial reports suggest that retinoids have a significant ability to prevent the development of second aerodigestive tract malignancies. Work in this area will expand rapidly in the immediate future, particularly in relation to former smokers. The detection of genetic lesions predisposing to malignancy in airway epithelial cells would be a major step forward in focusing preventive efforts, providing intermediate end-points and molecular means of early diagnosis, and eventually targeting therapy at the products of the lesions that make lung cancer cells malignant.

While human lung cancer is not thought of as a genetic disease, a variety of molecular genetic studies have shown that lung cancer cells have acquired a number of genetic lesions, including activation of dominant oncogenes and inactivation of tumor suppressor or recessive oncogenes (Chaps. 83 and 84). In fact, lung cancer cells may have to accumulate a large number (perhaps 10 or more) of such lesions. For the dominant oncogenes, these include point mutations in the coding regions of the *ras* family of oncogenes (particularly in the K-*ras* gene in adenocarcinoma of the lung); amplification, rearrangement, and/or loss of transcriptional control of *myc* family oncogenes (c-, N-, and L-*myc*; changes in c-*myc* are found in non-small cell cancers, while changes in all *myc* family members are found in small cell lung cancer); and overexpression of *bcl-2*, *Her-2/neu*, and the telomerase gene (Table 90-2). Tumor mutations in *ras* genes are associated with a poor prognosis in non-small cell lung cancer, while tumor amplification of c-*myc* is associated with a poor prognosis in small cell lung cancer.

For the recessive oncogenes (*tumor suppressor genes*), cytogenetic and allelotyping analyses have shown deletions (allele loss) involving chromosome regions 1p, 1q, 3p12-13, 3p14 (*FHIT* gene region), 3p21, 3p24-25, 3q, 5q, 8p, 9p (*p16/CDKN2*, *p15* gene cluster), 11p13, 11p15, 13q14 (retinoblastoma, *rb*, gene), 16q, and 17p13 (*p53* gene), as well as other sites. There appear to be several candidate recessive oncogenes on chromosome 3p that are involved in nearly all lung cancers. The *p53* and *rb* genes are both mutated in more than 90 percent of small cell lung cancers, while *p53* is mutated in more than 50 percent and *rb* in 20 percent of non-small cell lung cancers. *p16/CDKN2* is abnormal in ~10 percent of small cell and >50 percent of non-small cell lung cancers. Rb and *p16/CDKN2* appear to be part of the same G1-to-S cell cycle regulatory pathway. Either one or the other of these elements appears to be mutated or to have its expression turned off (e.g., by hypermethylation) in the large majority of lung cancers. The large number of genetic lesions in clinically evident cancer has prompted a search for these mutations in lung tissue before classic cytopathologic evidence of malignancy can be found, to provide for molecular early diagnosis and as intermediate end-points in prevention efforts, including chemoprevention treatment. Histologically identifiable preneoplastic lesions found in the respiratory epithelium of lung cancer patients and smokers include hyperplasia, dysplasia (progressively severe), and carcinoma in situ. 3p allele loss (hyperplasia) followed by 9p (*p16/CDKN2*) allele loss (hyperplasia) are the earliest events; 17p (*p53*) abnormalities and then *ras* mutations usually are only found in carcinoma in situ and invasive cancer. Thus, molecular changes involving allele loss and microsatellite alteration can be found in the earliest preneoplastic lesions and potentially even before any histologic changes are noted. Clinical trials of early diagnosis will be needed to prove the usefulness of these molecular

Table 90-1

Frequency, Age-Adjusted Incidence, and Survival Rates for Different Histologic Types of Lung Cancer (All Races, Both Sexes, and All Stages)*

Histologic Type of Thoracic Malignancy	Frequency, %	Age-Adjusted Rate	5-year Survival Rate (All Stages)
Adenocarcinoma (and all subtypes)	32	17	17
Bronchioloalveolar carcinoma	3	1.4	42
Squamous cell (epidermoid) carcinoma	29	15	15
Small cell carcinoma	18	9	5
Large cell carcinoma	9	5	11
Carcinoid	1.0	0.5	83
Mucoepidermoid carcinoma	0.1	<0.1	39
Adenoid cystic carcinoma	<0.1	<0.1	48
Sarcoma and other soft tissue tumors	0.1	0.1	30
All others and unspecified carcinomas	11.0	6	NA
Total	100	52	14

* Data on histology frequency and age-adjusted incidence rates per 100,000 U.S. population are from 60,514 cases of invasive lung cancer involving all races and both sexes obtained from the data for 1983–1987 of the Surveillance, Epidemiology, and End Results (SEER) Program of the National Cancer Institute; 5-year relative survival rates for all stages, all races, and both sexes are from the SEER data on 87,128 carcinomas, 1978–1986. NA, not available.

SOURCE: Summarized from Travis et al.

markers in the identification of very early lung cancer and in the monitoring of treatment and chemoprevention.

The large number of lesions shows that lung cancer, like other common epithelial malignancies, is a multistep process that is likely to involve both carcinogens and tumor promoters. Prevention can be directed at both processes. Cell-biologic studies have shown that lung cancer cells both produce a large number of peptide hormones and express receptors for these hormones, which thereby can act to stimulate tumor cell growth in an "autocrine" fashion. Nicotine may play a very central role in lung cancer pathogenesis. Highly carcinogenic derivatives of nicotine are formed in cigarette smoke. Smoking is tied to nicotine addiction, and nicotine gum and patches are now widely used to help persons to stop smoking. Lung cancer cells of all histologic types express receptors for nicotine that are very similar to nicotinic acetylcholine receptors. Thus, it is possible that nicotine itself could be directly involved in lung cancer pathogenesis.

While lung cancer does not have a clear pattern of Mendelian inheritance, there are several indications of a potential for familial association. These include inherited mutations in *rb* (patients with retinoblastomas living to adulthood) and *p53* (Li-Fraumeni syndrome)

genes; studies that show that first-degree relatives of lung cancer probands have a two- to threefold excess risk of lung cancer or other cancers, many of which are not smoking-related; and a strong risk of developing lung cancer linked with the development of chronic obstructive pulmonary disease. Finally, genetic epidemiologic studies have proposed an association between the P450 enzyme or chromosome fragility (*mutagen sensitivity*) genotypes and the development of lung cancer. The genetic identification of persons at very high risk of developing lung cancer would be very important in early detection and prevention efforts.

CLINICAL MANIFESTATIONS AND MODE OF PRESENTATION

Lung cancer gives rise to signs and symptoms caused by local tumor growth, invasion or obstruction of adjacent structures, growth in regional nodes via lymphatic spread, growth in distant metastatic sites after hematogenous dissemination, or remote effects (paraneoplastic syndrome). The latter usually result from peptide hormone secretion by the tumor or immunologic cross-reaction between tumor and normal tissue antigens (Chap. 102).

Although 5 to 15 percent of patients are detected while asymptomatic, usually on a routine chest radiograph, the vast majority of patients

Table 90-2

Comparison Between Small Cell and Non-Small Cell Lung Cancers

	Small Cell	Non-Small Cell
Histology	Scant cytoplasm; small, hyperchromatic nuclei with fine chromatin pattern; nucleoli indistinct; diffuse sheets of cells	Abundant cytoplasm; pleomorphic nuclei with coarse chromatin pattern; nucleoli often prominent; glandular or squamous architecture
General neuroendocrine properties		
Dense-core granules	Present	Absent*
L-Dopa decarboxylase activity	High	Absent
Chromogranin	Present	Absent
Synaptophysin	Present	Absent
Neuron-specific enolase	High	Low
Creatine kinase BB isozyme	High	Low
CD56 and CD57 antigens	Present	Absent
Peptide hormone production		
Gastrin-releasing peptide gene products	Present	Absent
Other neuropeptides	ACTH, AVP, calcitonin, ANF	PTH
Other markers		
HLA, β₂-microglobulin	Absent/low	Present
Intermediate filament pattern	"SCLC"	"Non-SCLC"
Neurofilaments	Present	Absent
Opioid receptors	Present	Present
Nicotine receptors	Present	Present
EGF receptors	Low or absent	Present
Mucin	Absent	Present in adenocarcinomas
Surfactant-associated proteins	Absent	Often present
Carcinoembryonic antigen	Present	Present
Recessive oncogene (tumor suppressor gene) and allelotype abnormalities		
3p deletions	>90%	>80%
rb mutations	~90%	~20%
p16/CDKN2 mutations	~10%	~50%
p53 mutations	>90%	>50%
5q, 8p, 11p and other allele losses	Present	Present
Microsatellite alterations	Present	Present
Dominant oncogene abnormalities		
ras mutations	<1%	~30%
myc family overexpression	>50%	>50%
bcl-2 overexpression	>75%	>50%
Her-2/neu overexpression	<10%	~30%
Telomerase overexpression	>90%	>90%
Response to radiotherapy	Objective shrinkage in 80–90%; often complete response	Objective shrinkage in 30–50%; response uncommonly complete
Response to combination chemotherapy		
Overall regression rate	90%	30–40%
Rate of complete regression	50%	5%

* Ten percent of non-small cell lung cancers have populations of cells expressing neuroendocrine markers, and these are best demonstrated by immunohistochemical stains.

Abbreviations: ACTH, adrenocorticotropic hormone; ANF, atrial natriuretic factor; AVP, arginine vasopressin; CD56, neural cell adhesion molecule (NCAM)-1; CD57, Leu-7 or HNK-1; HLA, human leukocyte antigen; PTH, parathormone; SCLC, small cell lung cancer.

present with some sign or symptom. Signs and symptoms secondary to central or endobronchial growth of the primary tumor include cough, hemoptysis, wheeze and stridor, dyspnea, and postobstructive pneumonitis (fever and productive cough). Signs and symptoms secondary to the peripheral growth of the primary tumor include pain from pleural or chest wall involvement, cough, dyspnea on a restrictive basis, and symptoms of lung abscess resulting from tumor cavitation. Signs and symptoms related to the regional spread of tumor in the thorax (by contiguous growth or by metastasis to regional lymph nodes) include tracheal obstruction, esophageal compression with dysphagia, recurrent laryngeal nerve paralysis with hoarseness, phrenic nerve paralysis with elevation of the hemidiaphragm and dyspnea, and sympathetic nerve paralysis with Horner's syndrome (enophthalmos, ptosis, miosis, and ipsilateral loss of sweating). *Pancoast's* (or *superior sulcus tumor*) *syndrome* results from local extension of a tumor (usually epidermoid) growing in the apex of the lung with involvement of the eighth cervical and first and second thoracic nerves, with shoulder pain which characteristically radiates in the ulnar distribution of the arm, often with radiologic destruction of the first and second ribs. Often Horner's syndrome and Pancoast's syndrome coexist. Other problems of regional spread include *superior vena cava syndrome* from vascular obstruction; pericardial and cardiac extension with resultant tamponade, arrhythmia, or cardiac failure; lymphatic obstruction with resultant pleural effusion; and lymphangitic spread through the lungs with hypoxemia and dyspnea. In addition, bronchioloalveolar carcinoma can spread transbronchially, producing tumor growing along multiple alveolar surfaces with resultant impairment of oxygen transfer, respiratory insufficiency, dyspnea, hypoxemia, and production of large amounts of sputum.

Extrathoracic metastatic disease is found at autopsy in over 50 percent of patients with epidermoid carcinoma, 80 percent of patients with adenocarcinoma and large cell carcinoma, and over 95 percent of patients with small cell cancer. These autopsy studies have found lung cancer metastases in virtually every organ system. Thus, the majority of lung cancer patients eventually need therapy to palliate symptoms. Common clinical problems related to metastatic lung cancer include brain metastases with neurologic deficits; bone metastases with pain and pathologic fractures; bone marrow invasion with cytopenias or leukoerythroblastosis; liver metastases causing biochemical liver dysfunction, biliary obstruction, and pain; lymph node metastases in the supraclavicular region and occasionally in the axilla and groin; and spinal cord compression syndromes from epidural or bone metastases.

Paraneoplastic syndromes are common in lung cancer patients and may be the presenting finding or first sign of recurrence. In addition, paraneoplastic syndromes may mimic metastatic disease and, unless detected, lead to inappropriate palliative rather than curative treatment. Often the paraneoplastic syndrome may be relieved with successful treatment of the tumor, and tumor treatment is the basis for correcting such syndromes. In some cases, the pathophysiology of the paraneoplastic syndrome is known, particularly when a hormone with biologic activity is secreted by a tumor (Chap. 102). However, in many cases the pathophysiology is unknown. *Systemic symptoms* of anorexia, cachexia, weight loss (seen in 30 percent of patients), fever, and suppressed immunity are paraneoplastic syndromes of unknown etiology. *Endocrine syndromes* are seen in 12 percent of patients and have the best understood pathophysiology, including hypercalcemia and hypophosphatemia resulting from the ectopic production by epidermoid tumors of parathyroid hormone (PTH) or PTH-related peptide production, hyponatremia with the syndrome of inappropriate secretion of antidiuretic hormone or possibly atrial natriuretic factor by small cell cancer, and ectopic secretion by small cell cancer of adrenocorticotropic hormone (ACTH). ACTH secretion usually results in additional electrolyte disturbances, especially hypokalemia, rather than in the changes in body habitus seen in Cushing's syndrome from a pituitary adenoma.

Skeletal–connective tissue syndromes include clubbing in 30 percent of cases (usually non-small cell carcinomas) and hypertrophic pulmonary osteoarthropathy in 1 to 10 percent of cases (usually adenocarcinomas) with periostitis and clubbing giving pain, tenderness, and swelling over the affected bones and a positive bone scan. *Neurologic–*

myopathic syndromes are seen in only 1 percent of patients but are dramatic and include the myasthenic *Eaton-Lambert syndrome* and retinal blindness with small cell cancer, while peripheral neuropathies, subacute cerebellar degeneration, cortical degeneration, and polymyositis are seen with all lung cancer types. Many of these are caused by autoimmune responses such as the development of anti-voltage-gated calcium channel antibodies in the Eaton-Lambert syndrome (Chap. 103). *Coagulation, thrombotic, or other hematologic manifestations* occur in 1 to 8 percent of patients and include migratory venous thrombophlebitis (*Trousseau's syndrome*), nonbacterial thrombotic (marantic) endocarditis with arterial emboli, disseminated intravascular coagulation with hemorrhage, and anemia, granulocytosis, and leukoerythroblastosis. *Cutaneous manifestations* such as dermatomyositis and acanthosis nigricans are uncommon (1 percent or less), as are the *renal manifestations* of nephrotic syndrome or glomerulonephritis (1 percent or less).

DIAGNOSIS AND STAGING

EARLY DIAGNOSIS The screening of asymptomatic persons at high risk (men over 45 years of age who smoke 40 or more cigarettes per day) for lung cancer by means of sputum cytology and chest radiographs has not been proved effective. Studies using these screening procedures found a prevalence of lung cancer of 4 to 8 cases per 1000 persons. With follow-up screening every 4 months, four new cases of lung cancer are found per 1000 persons followed per year. These lung cancers are detected 72 percent of the time by radiographs alone and 20 percent by cytology alone, while 6 percent are detected by both methods. In contrast to nonscreened patients, 90 percent of these screened patients who develop lung cancer are asymptomatic, 62 percent have resectable lung cancer, and 53 percent of all the new cases are postoperative stage I (see below) with a 5-year survival probability of 45 percent. However, there was no difference in the survival rate between the screened and nonscreened groups of smoking males 45 years of age or older. The reason for this poor survival was the development of clinically silent and undetected metastases in the majority of patients even when primary tumors were detected at a very early stage. Newer screening methods involving fluorescent bronchoscopy and molecular analysis will be analyzed in clinical trials in the hope of improving the detection of lung cancer before metastases develop.

ESTABLISHING A TISSUE DIAGNOSIS OF LUNG CANCER Once signs, symptoms, or screening studies suggest lung cancer, it is necessary to establish a tissue diagnosis of malignancy, to determine the histologic cell type, and to stage the patient for appropriate treatment. In the initial evaluation of each patient, tumor tissue should be obtained so that a histologic diagnosis of cancer and tumor cell type can be made. Tumor tissue can be obtained by a bronchial or transbronchial biopsy during fiberoptic bronchoscopy; by node biopsy during mediastinoscopy; from the operative specimen at the time of definitive surgical resection; by percutaneous biopsy of an enlarged lymph node, soft tissue mass, lytic bone lesion, bone marrow, or pleural lesion; by fine-needle aspiration of thoracic or extrathoracic tumor masses using computed tomography (CT) guidance; or from an adequate cell block obtained from a malignant pleural effusion. In the vast majority of cases, the pathologist should be able to definitely make a diagnosis of epithelial malignancy and make the crucial distinction of small cell from non-small cell lung cancer.

STAGING PATIENTS WITH LUNG CANCER Lung cancer staging consists of two parts: first, a determination of the location of tumor (anatomic staging) and, second, an assessment of a patient's ability to withstand various antitumor treatments (physiologic staging). For example, in a patient with non-small cell lung cancer, it is crucial to determine both whether the tumor could be resected by a standard surgical procedure such as a lobectomy or pneumonectomy (determination of *resectability*), which depends on the anatomic stage of the tumor, and whether the patient could tolerate such a surgical procedure (determination of *operability*), which depends on the cardiopulmonary condition of the patient.

Non-Small Cell Lung Cancer The TNM international staging system (ISS), which was developed by the American Joint Committee (AJC) on End Results Reporting and modified by an international commission, should be used for cases of non-small cell lung cancer, particularly in preparing patients for curative attempts with surgery or radiotherapy (Table 90-3). The various T (tumor size), N (regional node involvement), and M (presence or absence of distant metastasis) factors are combined to form different stage groups (stages I, II, IIIA, IIIB, and IV) (Table 90-3). At presentation, approximately one-third of patients will have disease localized enough for a curative attempt with surgery or radiotherapy (patients with stage I or II disease and some with stage IIIA disease), one-third will have distant metastatic disease (stage IV disease), and the remaining one-third will have local or regional disease that may or may not be amenable to a curative attempt (some patients with stage IIIA disease and patients with stage IIIB disease) (see below). This staging system provides useful prognostic information.

Small Cell Lung Cancer A simple two-stage system is used. In this system, *limited-stage disease* (representing about 30 percent of all small cell cancer patients) is defined as disease confined to one hemithorax and regional lymph nodes (including mediastinal, contralateral hilar, and usually ipsilateral supraclavicular nodes), while *extensive-stage disease* (representing about 70 percent of all patients) is defined as disease exceeding those boundaries. Employed in staging are clinical studies such as physical examination, x-rays, scans, and bone marrow examination. In part, the definition of limited-stage disease relates to whether the known tumor can be encompassed within a tolerable radiation therapy port. Thus, contralateral supraclavicular nodes, recurrent laryngeal nerve involvement, and superior vena caval obstruction can all be part of limited-stage disease. However, cardiac

tamponade, malignant pleural effusion, and bilateral pulmonary parenchymal involvement generally qualify disease as extensive-stage because of the size of the radiation therapy port required to cover all known disease.

GENERAL STAGING PROCEDURES (See Table 90-4) All lung cancer patients should have a complete history and physical examination, with evaluation of all other medical problems and a determination of performance status and weight loss, both of which have great prognostic value. An ear, nose, and throat examination is also necessary because of the frequent occurrence of second cancers in this area. While not done in every patient, fiberoptic bronchoscopy remains a cornerstone of lung cancer staging and follow-up, providing material for pathologic examination as well as information on tumor size, location, degree of bronchial obstruction, and recurrence.

Table 90-4

Pretreatment Staging Procedures for Lung Cancer Patients

ALL PATIENTS

Complete history & physical examination
    Determination of performance status and weight loss
    Ear, nose, and throat examination
Complete blood count with platelet determination
Measurement of serum electrolytes, glucose, calcium, and phosphorus; renal and liver function tests
Electrocardiogram
Skin test for tuberculosis
Chest x-ray
Computed tomography scan of brain, chest, and abdomen, and radionuclide scan of bone if any of the above studies suggest the presence of tumor metastasis in these organs
X-rays of suspicious bony lesions detected by scan or symptom
Barium-swallow radiographic examination if esophageal symptoms exist
Pulmonary function studies and arterial blood gas measurements if signs or symptoms of respiratory insufficiency are present
Biopsy of accessible lesions suspicious for cancer if a histologic diagnosis is not yet made or if treatment or staging decisions would be based on whether or not a lesion contained cancer

PATIENTS WITH NON-SMALL CELL LUNG CANCER WHO HAVE NO OBVIOUS CONTRAINDICATION TO CURATIVE SURGERY OR RADIOTHERAPY

All the above procedures, plus the following:
    Fiberoptic bronchoscopy with washings, brushings, and biopsy of suspicious areas
    Pulmonary function tests and arterial blood gas measurements
    Coagulation tests
    Computed tomographic scans of brain, chest, and abdomen
    If surgical resection is planned: surgical evaluation of the mediastinum at mediastinoscopy or at thoracotomy
    If the patient is a poor surgical risk or a candidate for curative radiotherapy: transthoracic fine-needle aspiration biopsy or transbronchial forceps biopsy of peripheral lesions if material from routine fiberoptic bronchoscopy is negative

PATIENTS PRESENTING WITH SMALL CELL OR NON-SMALL CELL LUNG CANCER THAT IS NOT CURABLE BY EITHER SURGERY OR RADIOTHERAPY ALONE*

For proven small cell lung cancer, all the procedures under "All Patients," plus the following:
    Fiberoptic bronchoscopy with washings and biopsy
    Chest, abdomen, and brain CT scans
    Bone marrow aspiration and biopsy
For non-small cell lung cancer or cancer of unknown histology, all the procedures under "All Patients," plus the following:
    Fiberoptic bronchoscopy if indicated by hemoptysis, obstruction, pneumonitis, or no histologic diagnosis of cancer
    Biopsy of accessible lesions suspicious for tumor to obtain a histologic diagnosis or if therapy would be altered by finding of tumor
    Transthoracic fine-needle aspiration biopsy or transbronchial forceps biopsy of peripheral lesions if fiberoptic bronchoscopy is negative and no other material exists for a histologic diagnosis
    Diagnostic and therapeutic thoracentesis if a pleural effusion is present

---

* Patients with non-small cell lung cancer and extrathoracic metastatic disease, malignant pleural effusion, or intrathoracic disease beyond the bounds of a tolerable radiotherapy port.

Table 90-3

International TNM (Tumor, Node, Metastasis) Staging System for Lung Cancer

Stage	TNM Descriptors	5-Year Survival (%)
I	T1–T2 N0 M0	60–80
II	T1–T2 N1 M0	25–50
IIIA	T3 N0–1 M0	25–40
	T1–3 N2 M0	10–30
IIIB	Any T4 or any N3 M0	<5
IV	Any M1	<5

TUMOR (T) STATUS DESCRIPTOR

T0	No evidence of a primary tumor
TX	Malignant cells found by cytologic examination but no lesion seen on x-ray or fiberoptic bronchoscopy
TIS	Carcinoma in situ
T1	Tumor <3 cm diameter
T2	Tumor >3 cm diameter or has distal atelectasis extending to hilum
T3	Tumor extends directly into pleura, chest wall, diaphragm, or pericardium, is <2 cm from carina, or causes total atelectasis
T4	Tumor invades mediastinum (heart, great vessels, trachea, esophagus, vertebral body, carina), or malignant pleural effusion is present

LYMPH NODE (N) INVOLVEMENT DESCRIPTOR

N0	No lymph node involvement
N1	Metastasis in bronchopulmonary or ipsilateral hilar lymph nodes
N2	Metastasis in ipsilateral mediastinal or subcarinal lymph nodes
N3	Metastasis to contralateral mediastinal or hilar lymph nodes or to any scalene or supraclavicular lymph nodes

DISTANT METASTASIS (M) DESCRIPTOR

M0	No known distant metastasis
M1	Distant metastasis present with site specified (e.g., brain)

SOURCE: Adapted from CF Mountain et al, Chest 96:475, 1989, and from Ginsberg et al.

Chest radiographs are needed to evaluate tumor size and nodal involvement, and it is very useful to obtain old x-ray films for comparison. CT scans are of use in the preoperative staging of non-small cell lung cancer to detect mediastinal nodes and pleural extension and occult abdominal disease (e.g., of the liver and adrenal glands), as well as in the planning of curative radiation therapy to allow the design of fields to encompass all the known tumor while avoiding as much normal tissue as possible. However, mediastinal nodal involvement should be documented histologically. Thus, sampling of lymph nodes via mediastinoscopy or thoracotomy to establish the presence or absence of N2 or N3 nodal involvement is of vital importance in considering or rejecting a curative surgical approach for non-small cell lung cancer patients with clinical stage I, II, or III disease. This is particularly true for patients with modest nodal abnormalities on chest CT scans. Likewise, unless the CT-detected abnormalities are unequivocal, malignancy of suspicious abdominal lesions should be confirmed by procedures such as fine-needle aspiration if the patient would otherwise be considered for curative treatment. In small cell lung cancer, CT scans are used in the planning of chest radiation treatment and in the assessment of the response to chemotherapy and radiation therapy. In following patients after surgery or radiotherapy—procedures that can make interpretation of conventional chest x-rays difficult—CT scans can provide good evidence of tumor recurrence.

If signs or symptoms suggest organ involvement by tumor, appropriate CT or radionuclide scans (e.g., of brain, liver, or bone) are performed, as well as radiography of any suspicious bony lesions. Any accessible lesions suspicious for cancer should be biopsied if a histologic diagnosis has not already been made or if treatment decisions would be based on whether or not the lesion contained cancer.

In patients presenting with a mass lesion on chest x-ray and no obvious contraindications to a curative approach with surgery or radiotherapy after the initial evaluation, the mediastinum must be investigated. Approaches vary between different centers and include performing chest CT scan and mediastinoscopy (for right-sided tumors) or lateral mediastinotomy (for left-sided lesions) on all patients and proceeding directly to thoracotomy for staging of the mediastinum. In patients presenting with disease that is confined to the chest but not resectable, and who thus are candidates for neoadjuvant chemotherapy plus surgery or for curative radiotherapy, other tests are done as indicated to evaluate specific symptoms. In patients presenting with non-small cell cancer that is not curable by surgery, radiotherapy, or a combination of either with chemotherapy, all the general staging procedures are done, plus fiberoptic bronchoscopy as indicated to evaluate hemoptysis, obstruction, or pneumonitis, as well as thoracentesis with cytologic examination (and chest tube drainage as indicated) if fluid is present. As a rule, a radiographic finding of an isolated lesion (such as an enlarged adrenal gland) should be confirmed as cancer by fine-needle aspiration before a curative attempt is rejected.

STAGING OF SMALL CELL LUNG CANCER Pretreatment staging for patients with histologically documented small cell lung cancer includes the initial general lung cancer evaluation as well as fiberoptic bronchoscopy with washings and biopsies to determine the tumor extent before therapy; brain CT scan, since 10 percent of patients have metastases; bone marrow biopsy and aspiration, since 20 to 30 percent of patients have tumor in the bone marrow; and CT (liver) and radionuclide scans (bone) if symptoms or other findings are suggestive of disease involvement in these areas. Chest and abdominal CT scans are very useful to evaluate and follow tumor response to therapy, and chest CT scans are helpful in planning chest radiotherapy ports.

If signs or symptoms of spinal cord compression or leptomeningitis develop at any time in lung cancer patients with disease of any histologic type, a CT scan or magnetic resonance scan and examination of the cerebrospinal fluid cytology are performed to determine the need for local therapy to the site of compression (usually with radiotherapy) and for intrathecal chemotherapy (usually with methotrexate) if malignant cells are detected. In addition, a brain CT scan is performed to search for brain metastases, which often are associated with spinal cord or leptomeningeal metastases.

DETERMINATION OF RESECTABILITY AND OPERABILITY In patients with non-small cell lung cancer, the following are major contraindications to curative surgery or radiotherapy alone: extrathoracic distant metastases; superior vena cava syndrome; vocal cord and, in most cases, phrenic nerve paralysis; malignant pleural effusion; cardiac tamponade; tumor within 2 cm of the carina (not curable by surgery but potentially curable by radiotherapy); metastasis to the contralateral lung; bilateral endobronchial tumor (potentially curable by radiotherapy); metastasis to the supraclavicular lymph nodes; lymph node metastasis in the contralateral mediastinum (potentially curable by radiotherapy); and involvement of the main stem pulmonary artery. While a histologic diagnosis of small cell lung cancer is usually highly correlated with other findings of unresectability, if all other findings suggest the potential for resection, that option should be considered. This situation is usually encountered in cases of small peripheral small cell lung cancer lesions (see below).

PHYSIOLOGIC STAGING Patients with lung cancer often have cardiopulmonary and other problems related to chronic obstructive pulmonary disease as well as other medical problems. To improve their preoperative condition, correctable problems (e.g., anemia, electrolyte and fluid disorders, infections, and arrhythmias) should be addressed, smoking stopped, and appropriate chest therapy instituted. Since it is not always possible to predict whether a lobectomy or pneumonectomy will be required until the time of operation, a conservative approach is to restrict resectional surgery to patients who could potentially tolerate a pneumonectomy. In addition to nonambulatory performance status, a myocardial infarction within the past 3 months is a contraindication to thoracic surgery because 20 percent of patients will die of reinfarction alone, while an infarction in the past 6 months is a relative contraindication. Other major contraindications include uncontrolled major arrhythmias, a maximum breathing capacity less than 40 percent of the predicted value, an FEV$_1$ (forced expiratory volume in 1 s) of less than 1 L, CO$_2$ retention (which is more serious than hypoxemia), and severe pulmonary hypertension. Recommending surgery when the FEV$_1$ is 1.1 to 2.4 L requires careful judgment, while an FEV$_1$ of over 2.5 L will usually permit a pneumonectomy. In patients with borderline pulmonary status or a question of pulmonary hypertension, split pulmonary function testing by ventilation-perfusion lung scans can define physiologic operability. The activity from quantitative scans is summed for each lung in the anterior and posterior views, and the ratio of the normal to total lung activity is multiplied by the FEV$_1$. Pneumonectomy usually is physiologically tolerable if this predicted value is greater than 1 L.

TREATMENT

After a histologic diagnosis is obtained and appropriate anatomic and physiologic staging studies are completed, the overall treatment approach to patients with lung cancer may be formulated (Table 90-5). Even after the diagnosis is made, patients should be encouraged to stop smoking. Those who do fare better than those who continue to smoke.

Non-Small Cell Lung Cancer: Localized Disease SURGERY In patients with non-small cell lung cancer of stages I and II (see Table 90-3) who can tolerate operation, the treatment of choice is pulmonary resection. In stage IIIA cases where the patient's age and cardiopulmonary function and the anatomy are favorable, resection also should be considered. If a complete resection is possible, the 5-year survival rate for N1 disease is about 50 percent, while it is about 20 percent for N2 disease. However, only 20 percent of all cases of N2 disease are technically resectable, and most of these resectable cases are discovered to be N2 only at thoracotomy. Surgery for N2 disease is the most controversial area in the surgical management of lung cancer. In this regard, it is useful to divide N2 disease into "minimal" disease (involvement of only one node with microscopic foci, usually discovered at thoracotomy or mediastinoscopy); and the more common "advanced," bulky disease, clinically

Table 90-5

Summary of Treatment Approach to Lung Cancer Patients

NON-SMALL CELL LUNG CANCER

Stages I and II, some IIIA:
  Surgical resection for stages I, II
  Surgical resection with complete mediastinal lymph node dissection and
    consideration of neoadjuvant CT for stage IIIA disease with "minimal
    N2 involvement" (discovered at thoracotomy or mediastinoscopy)
  Postoperative RT for patients found to have N2 disease if no neoadjuvant
    therapy given
  Curative potential RT for "nonoperable" patients
Stage IIIA with selected types of stage T3 tumors:
  Tumors with chest wall invasion (T3): en bloc resection of tumor with in-
    volved chest wall and consideration of postoperative radiotherapy.
  Superior sulcus (Pancoast's) (T3) tumors: preoperative radiotherapy
    (3000–4500 cGy) followed by en bloc resection of involved lung and
    chest wall with consideration of postoperative radiotherapy or intraopera-
    tive brachytherapy.
  Proximal airway involvement (<2 cm from carina) without mediastinal
    nodes: sleeve resection if possible preserving distal normal lung or pneu-
    monectomy
Stages IIIA "advanced, bulky, clinically evident N2 disease" (discovered
  preoperatively) and IIIB disease that can be included in a tolerable radio-
  therapy port:
  Curative potential RT + CT if performance status is reasonable; other-
    wise, RT alone
  Consider neoadjuvant chemotherapy and surgical resection for IIIA dis-
    ease with advanced N2 involvement
Stage IIIB disease with carinal invasion (T4) but without N2 involvement:
  consider pneumonectomy with tracheal sleeve resection with direct reanas-
  tomosis to contralateral mainstem bronchus.
Stage IV and more advanced IIIB disease:
  RT to symptomatic local sites
  CT for patients with good performance status and evaluable lesions
  Chest tube drainage of large malignant pleural effusions
  Consider resection of primary tumor and metastasis for isolated brain or
    adrenal metastases

SMALL CELL LUNG CANCER

Limited stage (good performance status): combination chemotherapy +
  chest RT
Extensive stage (good performance status): combination chemotherapy
Complete tumor responders (all stages): prophylactic cranial RT
Poor-performance-status patients (all stages):
  Modified-dose combination chemotherapy
  Palliative RT

ALL PATIENTS

Radiotherapy for brain metastases, spinal cord compression, weight-bearing
  lytic bony lesions, symptomatic local lesions (nerve paralyses, obstructed
  airway, hemoptysis in non-small cell lung cancer and in small cell cancer
  not responding to chemotherapy)
Appropriate diagnosis and treatment of other medical problems and supportive care during chemotherapy
Encouragement to stop smoking
Entrance into clinical trial, if eligible

Abbreviations: CT, chemotherapy; RT, radiotherapy.

obvious on CT scans and discovered preoperatively. Patients with contralateral or bilateral positive mediastinal (N3) nodes, extracapsular nodal involvement, or fixed nodes are not considered resectable. New approaches that may make resection possible in situations where currently it is not include chest wall resection for direct extension of tumor, tracheal sleeve pneumonectomy, and sleeve lobectomy for lesions near the carina. Neoadjuvant (preoperative) chemotherapy gives tumor response rates of 50 to 60 percent and causes unresectable disease to become resectable in many responding patients. Video-assisted thoracic surgery (VATS) via thoracoscopy is being evaluated but is not a generally accepted approach for curative lung cancer resection.

The extent of resection is a matter of surgical judgment based on findings at exploration. In general, conservative resection that encompasses all known tumor gives survival equal to that obtained with more extensive procedures. However, lobectomy is superior to wedge resection in terms of reducing the rate of local recurrence. Thus, lobectomy is preferred to pneumonectomy and wedge resection, while wedge resection and segmentectomy are reserved for patients with poor pulmonary reserve and small peripheral lesions. Approximately 43 percent of all lung cancer patients will undergo thoracotomy. Of these, 76 percent will have a definitive resection, 12 percent will only be explored for disease extent, and 12 percent will have a palliative procedure with known disease left behind. The fraction of long-term survivors following definitive surgical therapy is remarkably consistent for all the major centers performing lung cancer surgery in the United States (Table 90-3). Approximately 30 percent of all patients treated with resection for cure survive 5 years, and 15 percent survive 10 years. The 30-day hospital mortality following pulmonary resection at major centers is also very consistent, being 3 percent for lobectomy and 6 percent for pneumonectomy. Thus, most patients who initially may be thought to have a "curative" resection ultimately die of metastatic disease (usually within 5 years of surgery).

MANAGEMENT OF OCCULT AND STAGE 0 CARCINOMAS In the uncommon situation where malignant cells are identified in a sputum or bronchial washing specimen but the chest radiograph appears normal (TX tumor stage), the lesion must be localized. Over 90 percent can be localized by meticulous examination of the bronchial tree with a fiberoptic bronchoscope under general anesthesia and collection of a series of differential brushings and biopsies. Often, carcinoma in situ or multicentric lesions are found in these patients. Current recommendations are for the most conservative surgical resection, allowing removal of the cancer and conservation of lung parenchyma, even if the bronchial margins are positive for carcinoma in situ. The 5-year overall survival for these occult cancers is approximately 60 percent. Close follow-up of these patients is indicated because of the high incidence of second primary lung cancers (approximately 5 percent per patient per year). A new approach to in situ or multicentric lesions uses systemically administered hematoporphyrin (which localizes to tumors and sensitizes them to light) followed by bronchoscopic phototherapy.

SOLITARY PULMONARY NODULE When a patient presents with an asymptomatic, solitary pulmonary nodule (defined as an x-ray density completely surrounded by normal aerated lung, with circumscribed margins, of any shape, usually 1 to 6 cm in greatest diameter), a decision to resect or follow the nodule must be made. Approximately 35 percent of all such lesions in adults will be malignant, most being primary lung cancer, while less than 1 percent are malignant in nonsmoking patients under 35 years of age. A complete history, including a smoking history, physical examination, routine laboratory tests, fiberoptic bronchoscopy, and old chest x-rays is obtained. If no diagnosis is immediately apparent, the following risk factors would all argue strongly in favor of proceeding with resection to establish a histologic diagnosis: a history of cigarette smoking; age 35 years or older; a relatively large lesion; lack of calcification; chest symptoms; associated atelectasis, pneumonitis, or adenopathy; and growth of the lesion revealed by comparison with old x-rays. At present, only two radiographic criteria are reliable predictors of the benign nature of a solitary pulmonary nodule: lack of growth over a period greater than 2 years and certain characteristic patterns of calcification. Calcification alone does not exclude malignancy. However, a dense central nidus, multiple punctate foci, and "bull's eye" (granuloma) and "popcorn ball" (hamartoma) calcifications are all highly suggestive of a benign lesion.

When old x-rays are not available and the characteristic calcification patterns are absent, the following approach is reasonable: Nonsmoking patients under 35 years can be followed with serial chest x-rays every 3 months for 1 year and then yearly. If any significant growth is found, a histologic diagnosis is needed. For patients over age 35 and all patients with a smoking history, a histologic diagnosis must be made. The sample for histologic diagnosis can be obtained either at the time of nodule resection or, if the patient is a poor operative risk, via transthoracic fine-needle biopsy. Some institutions would use preoperative fine-needle aspiration on all such lesions; however, all positive lesions will have to be resected, and negative cytologic findings will in most cases have to be confirmed by histology on a resected specimen. While much has been made of sparing patients an operation, the high probability of finding a malignancy (particularly in smokers over age 35) and the excellent chance for surgical cure when the tumor is small both suggest an aggressive approach to these lesions.

RADIOTHERAPY WITH CURATIVE INTENT   Patients with stage III disease, as well as patients with stage I or II disease who refuse surgery or appear not to be candidates for pulmonary resection for medical reasons, should be considered for radiation therapy with curative intent. The decision to administer high-dose and potentially curative radiotherapy is based on the extent of disease and the volume of the chest that requires irradiation. Patients with distant metastases, positive supraclavicular nodes, pleural effusion, or cardiac involvement are generally not considered for such curative radiation treatment. The median survival for patients with unresectable non-small cell lung cancer localized to the chest who undergo primary radiotherapy with curative intent is less than 1 year. However, 6 percent of these patients are alive at 5 years and are cured by radiotherapy alone. In addition to being potentially curative, radiotherapy, by controlling the primary tumor, may increase the quality and length of life of noncured patients. Treatment usually involves midplane doses of 55 to 60 Gy (5500 to 6000 rad), and the major concern is the amount of lung parenchyma and other organs in the thorax included in the treatment plan, including the spinal cord, heart, and esophagus. In patients with a major degree of underlying pulmonary disease, the treatment plan may have to be compromised because of the deleterious effect of radiation on pulmonary function. Recent studies suggest that continuous-fraction radiotherapy be given. The development of radiation pneumonitis is proportional to the dose of radiation and the volume of lung in the radiation field. The full clinical syndrome (dyspnea, fever, and radiographic infiltrate corresponding to the treatment port) occurs in 5 percent of cases. Acute radiation esophagitis occurs during treatment but usually is self-limited, while spinal cord injury should be avoided by careful treatment planning. Twice-daily fractionated chest radiotherapy may achieve high doses and avoid toxicity. This approach has been used primarily for small cell lung cancer. In addition, brachytherapy (local radiotherapy delivered by placing radioactive "seeds" in a catheter in the tumor bed) provides a way to give a high local dose while sparing surrounding normal tissue.

COMBINED-MODALITY THERAPY WITH CURATIVE INTENT   Many centers give high-dose postoperative radiation therapy if N1 or N2 nodal disease is found at operation, and postoperative radiation therapy currently is considered standard for N2 disease. However, a randomized trial of postoperative radiotherapy, while showing improved local tumor control, did not show a survival benefit.

As a special case, carcinomas of the superior pulmonary sulcus producing *Pancoast's syndrome* are usually treated with combined radiotherapy and surgery. These patients should have the usual preoperative staging procedures, including mediastinoscopy and CT scans to determine tumor extent and a neurologic examination (and sometimes nerve conduction studies) to document neurologic findings. Often a histologic diagnosis is not made, but the combination of tumor location and pain distribution permit a diagnostic accuracy for cancer of better than 90 percent. If mediastinoscopy is negative, two curative approaches may be used in treating a Pancoast's syndrome tumor. In the first, preoperative irradiation [30 Gy (3000 rad) in 10 treatments] is given to the area, followed by an en bloc resection of the tumor and involved chest wall 3 to 6 weeks later. At 3 years, survival figures of 42 percent for epidermoid and 21 percent for adeno- and large cell carcinomas have been reported. The second approach involves radiotherapy alone in curative doses and standard fractionation, which leads to survival rates similar to those from

combined-modality therapy. Although small cell lung cancer responds to chemotherapy, this modality is not so effective for non-small cell lung cancer. While gratifying responses sometimes occur in patients with non-small cell lung cancer, substantial toxicities are associated with treatment and palliation, and survival benefits may be small. Because the toxicities, inconvenience, and expense of chemotherapy are borne alike by patients with responding and nonresponding disease and because the absolute survival benefits observed for chemotherapy of non-small cell lung cancer are relatively small, data from large numbers of patients participating in randomized clinical trials are needed to evaluate the clinical utility of chemotherapy in this setting.

A meta-analysis concerning the benefits of chemotherapy in non-small cell lung cancer was performed using updated data on 9,387 individual patients from 52 randomized trials, both published and unpublished, with the main outcome measure being survival. Overall, the results for modern regimens containing cisplatin favored chemotherapy in all comparisons. Trials in early-stage disease comparing surgery with surgery plus chemotherapy gave a hazard ratio of 0.87 (13 percent reduction in risk of death at 5 years) in favor of including chemotherapy. Trials in locally advanced disease comparing radical radiotherapy with radiotherapy plus chemotherapy also gave a hazard ratio of 0.87 (13 percent reduction in risk of death at 2 years) in favor of including chemotherapy.

While these results are statistically significant overall, the clinical benefits they show are only modest. This is particularly true for stage IV disease, where survival is increased by only a few months. The most clinically significant benefits were found when chemotherapy was added to radiotherapy for locally advanced disease (stage IIIB and some stage IIIA disease) and when chemotherapy was given preoperatively in a neoadjuvant fashion in stage IIIA disease. Thus, provided the risk:benefit ratio of using chemotherapy is discussed appropriately with patients, such therapy can be administered in a noninvestigational setting. While there are data supporting a benefit of chemotherapy as an adjuvant to surgery for early-stage disease, the confidence limits of these data are wide, and adjuvant chemotherapy cannot yet be recommended as standard therapy. In contrast to the beneficial results from trials using cisplatin, older trials using alkylating agents (not currently used for non-small cell lung cancer) tended to show a detrimental effect of chemotherapy. Randomized clinical trials also are needed to evaluate the usefulness of the new agents with activity against non-small cell lung cancer, including the taxanes (paclitaxel and docetaxel), vinorelbine, gemcitabine, and camptothecins (topotecan and CPT-11).

Disseminated Non-Small Cell Lung Cancer   The 70 percent of patients who have unresectable non-small cell cancer have a poor prognosis. For example, median survival times of 34, 25, 17, 8, and 4 weeks are seen for such patients with performance status scores of 0 (asymptomatic), 1 (symptomatic, fully ambulatory), 2 (in bed <50 percent of the time), 3 (in bed >50 percent of the time), and 4 (bedridden), respectively. Standard medical management, the judicious use of pain medications, and the appropriate use of radiotherapy form the cornerstone of management. Patients whose primary tumor is causing symptoms such as bronchial obstruction with pneumonitis, hemoptysis, or upper airway or superior vena cava (SVC) obstruction should, in general, have radiotherapy to the primary tumor. The case for prophylactic treatment of the asymptomatic patient is to prevent major symptoms from occurring within the thorax. However, if the patient can be followed closely, it is appropriate to defer treatment until symptoms develop. Usually a course of 30 to 40 Gy (3000 to 4000 rad) over 2 to 4 weeks is given to the tumor. Radiation therapy provides relief of intrathoracic symptoms with the following frequencies: hemoptysis, 84 percent; SVC syndrome, 80 percent; dyspnea, 60 percent; cough, 60 percent; atelectasis, 23 percent; and vocal cord paralysis, 6 percent. Other symptoms of metastatic disease treated with radiotherapy include cardiac-tamponade (treated with pericardiocentesis and radiation therapy to the entire cardiac silhouette), painful bony metastases (with relief in 66 percent of cases), brain or spinal cord compression, and brachial plexus involvement. Usually, with brain and cord compression, dexamethasone (25 to 100 mg per day in four divided doses) is also given and then rapidly tapered to the lowest dosage that relieves symptoms.

Brain metastases often are noted as isolated sites of relapse in patients with adenocarcinoma of the lung otherwise controlled by surgery or radiotherapy. However, there is no proven value for prophylactic cranial irradiation or for CT scans of the head in asymptomatic patients.

The key to effective palliation of lung cancer is to detect complications and begin radiotherapy as early as possible. Pleural effusions are common and are usually treated with thoracentesis as needed but not with radiotherapy. If they recur and are symptomatic, chest tube drainage with a sclerosing agent such as intrapleural doxycycline is used. First, the chest cavity is completely drained. Xylocaine 1% is instilled (15 mL), followed by 50 mL normal saline. Then 500 to 750 mg doxycycline HCl is dissolved in 100 mL normal saline, and this is injected via the chest tube. The chest tube is clamped for 4 h if tolerated, and the patient is rotated onto different sides to distribute the sclerosing agent. The chest tube is removed 24 to 48 h later, after drainage has become slight (usually less than 100 mL per 24 h). Recently, video-assisted thoracoscopy has been used to drain and treat large malignant effusions. Symptomatic endobronchial lesions that recur after surgery or radiotherapy or that develop in patients with severely compromised pulmonary function are difficult to treat with conventional therapy. There are several approaches to this problem. Neodynium-YAG (yttrium-aluminum-garnet) laser therapy administered via a flexible fiberoptic bronchoscope (usually under general anesthesia) can provide palliation in 80 to 90 percent of patients even when the tumor has relapsed after radiotherapy. Local radiotherapy delivered by brachytherapy, photodynamic therapy using a photosensitizing agent, and endobronchial stents are other measures that can relieve airway obstruction from tumor.

CHEMOTHERAPY The use of chemotherapy for non-small cell lung cancer requires careful judgment to balance potential benefits and toxicity. However, modest survival benefits (of 1 to 2 months) may accrue from such combination chemotherapy. From the large meta-analysis cited above, randomized trials in advanced disease comparing supportive care with supportive care plus chemotherapy gave a hazard ratio of 0.73 (27 percent reduction in risk of death at one year) in favor of including chemotherapy. Approximately 30 to 40 percent of patients will have objective tumor response to combination chemotherapy. However, a complete clinical regression of tumor (a *complete response*) occurs in less than 5 percent of cases. Those patients whose tumors respond to chemotherapy have significantly longer survival times (around 30 to 40 weeks median survival) than patients who do not respond to therapy (10 to 20 weeks median survival). The problem is that the responding patients also have better prognostic features (such as good performance status), and it is difficult to separate the effect of these features on survival from that of chemotherapy. However, in patients with good performance status, response to chemotherapy is also associated with prolonged survival and, in some cases, relief of symptoms. Thus, in patients with non-small cell lung cancer who desire chemotherapy, it is reasonable to give chemotherapy if the patient is fully ambulatory, has an evaluable tumor mass (so that the response to therapy can be followed), has not received prior chemotherapy, and is able to understand and accept the potential benefits and toxicities from such therapy. The chemotherapy should be delivered by a medical oncologist, who should use one of the published standard regimens, such as etoposide + cisplatin and also administer appropriate antiemetics and supportive care. New drugs with proven activity in non-small cell lung cancer include paclitaxel, vinorelbine, and gem-

citabine. Finally, all eligible patients should be encouraged to enter clinical studies that are designed to determine the benefits and toxicities of these new treatments.

Small Cell Lung Cancer Untreated patients with small cell lung cancer have median survivals of only 6 to 17 weeks, while patients treated with combination chemotherapy have median survivals of 40 to 70 weeks. Thus, the correct use of chemotherapy with or without radiotherapy or surgery is the cornerstone of the treatment of small cell cancer. The goal of treatment is to achieve a complete clinical regression of tumor documented by repeating the initial positive staging procedures, particularly fiberoptic bronchoscopy with washings and biopsy. The initial response, determined 6 to 12 weeks after the start of therapy, predicts both the median and long-term survival and the potential for cure. Patients who achieve a complete clinical regression survive longer than patients with only partial regression (shrinkage of the visible tumor by more than 50 percent with no sign of tumor progression elsewhere), who in turn survive longer than patients with no response. In addition, all long-term (>3-year) survivors come from the complete response group.

Following initial staging, patients are classified as having limited or extensive disease and as being physiologically able or not able to tolerate combination chemotherapy or combined-modality chemo-radiotherapy. The overall mortality rate from initial combination chemotherapy even in these selected patients is about 5 percent at major centers. This figure is comparable with the operative mortality rate for pulmonary resection and indicates the need for physiologic staging of patients before chemotherapy. Such therapy should be reserved for ambulatory patients with no prior chemotherapy or radiotherapy, no other major medical problems, and adequate heart, liver, renal, and bone marrow function. The arterial P_{O_2} on room air should be above 6.6 kPa (50 mmHg), and there should be no CO_2 retention. For patients with limitations in any of these areas, the initial combined-modality therapy or chemotherapy must be modified to prevent undue toxicity. In all patients, these treatments must be coupled with supportive care for infectious, hemorrhagic, and other medical complications. This induction period is best supervised by a medical oncologist. Meticulous attention to the details of therapy and to the day-to-day management of the patient through the initial 6 to 12 weeks of treatment is essential if therapy-related mortality and morbidity are to be kept low.

CHEMOTHERAPY A variety of effective combination chemotherapy regimens have been reported for small cell lung cancer. At present, the combination most widely used is etoposide plus cisplatin, given every 3 weeks on an outpatient basis. Appropriate supportive care (antiemetic therapy, administration of fluid and saline boluses with cisplatin, monitoring of blood counts and blood chemistries, monitoring for signs of bleeding or infection, and, as required, administration of erythropoietin and granulocyte colony-stimulating factor) and adjustment of chemotherapy doses on the basis of nadir granulocyte counts are essential. The initial combination chemotherapy may result in moderate to severe granulocytopenia (e.g., granulocyte counts of less than 500 to 1500/μL) and thrombocytopenia (platelet counts of less than 50,000 to 100,000/μL). After the initial six to eight cycles of therapy, patients should be restaged to determine if they have entered a *complete clinical remission*, indicated by complete disappearance of all clinically evident lesions and paraneoplastic syndromes, or a *partial remission*, or have *no response* or tumor progression (seen in 10 percent or fewer of patients). Chemotherapy is then stopped in responding patients. More prolonged chemotherapy has not been shown to be of value. Patients whose tumors are progressing or not responding should be switched to a new chemotherapy regimen, preferably one involving a combination of agents that will not show cross-resistance with the previous combination, in an attempt to get an objective tumor response. Oral etoposide, as a single agent, has been shown to produce a clinical benefit in the initial treatment of patients who are elderly or have a very poor performance status.

RADIOTHERAPY High-dose [40 Gy (4000 rad)] radiotherapy to the whole brain should be given to patients with documented brain metastases. Prophylactic cranial irradiation (PCI) may be given to patients with complete responses, since it will significantly decrease the development of brain metastases (which occur in 60 to 80 percent of patients living 2 or more years who do not receive such prophylactic radiotherapy), but such prophylactic therapy has not been shown to prolong survival. Because some studies indicate possible deficits in cognitive ability that could be related to PCI, the long-term quality of life after PCI needs to be further studied. In the case of symptomatic, progressive lesions in the chest or at other critical sites, if radiotherapy has not yet been given to these areas, it may be administered in full doses [e.g., 40 Gy (4000 rad) to the chest tumor mass].

COMBINED-MODALITY THERAPY Most patients with limited-stage small cell lung cancer should receive combined-modality therapy with etoposide plus cisplatin and concurrent radiotherapy. There are definite toxicities of both an acute and chronic nature that should be expected with combined-modality chemoradiotherapy, particularly when the chemotherapy and radiotherapy are given concurrently. However, retrospective analyses of long-term survivors and analyses of local failures in the chest following chemotherapy alone suggest that chest radiotherapy is of benefit, and thus it is currently recommended for limited-stage patients. Patients should be selected (limited-stage disease and a performance status of 0 to 1 and initial good pulmonary function) such that radiotherapy can be given in full doses and in a manner that will not sacrifice too much lung function. The radiation oncologist must be prepared to deliver tailored radiotherapy with shaping of fields during treatment, much as is done for Hodgkin's disease. Several centers that give twice-daily radiotherapy concurrently with chemotherapy using etoposide plus cisplatin have reported improved local tumor control and acceptable toxicity. For extensive-stage disease, chest radiotherapy usually is not advocated. However, in favorable patients (e.g., those with a performance status of 0 to 1, good pulmonary function, and only one site of extensive disease), the addition of chest radiotherapy to chemotherapy can be considered. In all patients, if chemotherapy is inadequate to relieve local tumor symptoms, a course of radiotherapy can be added.

Several centers around the world have reported potential cure rates of 15 to 25 percent for limited-stage disease and of 1 to 5 percent for extensive-stage disease. Overall, approximately 50 percent of patients with limited-stage and 30 percent of patients with extensive-stage disease will enter a complete remission, and 90 to 95 percent of all patients will have some objective tumor shrinkage (complete or partial response). These responses increase the median survival to 10 to 12 months for patients with extensive-stage disease and 14 to 18 months for patients with limited-stage disease, as compared with 2 to 4 months for untreated patients. In addition, most patients have relief of their tumor-related symptoms and improvement of performance status. However, the maintenance of good performance status in a patient receiving outpatient chemotherapy requires judgment and skill on the part of the medical oncologist delivering the chemotherapy to avoid undue therapeutic toxicity. New treatments, such as new drug combinations, very intensive initial or "reinduction" therapy with autologous bone marrow infusion, and novel ways of combining chemotherapy, radiotherapy, and surgery, should all be given only in the context of an approved clinical protocol.

While surgical resection is not routinely recommended for small cell lung cancer, occasional patients with this cancer meet the usual requirements for resectability (stage I or II disease with negative mediastinal nodes). Also, in some patients, this histologic diagnosis is made only on review of the resected surgical specimen. Such patients have been reported to have high cure rates (above 25 percent) if adjuvant combination chemotherapy is used.

BENIGN LUNG NEOPLASMS

The benign neoplasms of the lung, representing less than 5 percent of all primary tumors, include bronchial adenomas and hamartomas (90 percent of such lesions) and a group of very uncommon neoplasms

(chondromas, fibromas, lipomas, hemangiomas, leiomyomas, teratomas, pseudolymphomas, and endometriosis). The diagnostic and primary-treatment approach is basically the same for all these neoplasms. They can present as central masses causing airway obstruction, cough, hemoptysis, and pneumonitis. The masses may or may not be visible on radiographs but usually are accessible to fiberoptic bronchoscopy. Alternatively, they can present without symptoms as solitary pulmonary nodules and thus will be evaluated as part of a solitary pulmonary nodule workup. In all cases, the extent of surgery must be determined at operation, and a conservative procedure with appropriate reconstructions is usually performed.

BRONCHIAL ADENOMAS Bronchial adenomas (80 percent of which are central) are slow-growing, endobronchial lesions; they represent 50 percent of all benign pulmonary neoplasms. A total of 80 to 90 percent are carcinoids, 10 to 15 percent are adenocystic tumors (or cylindromas), and 2 to 3 percent are mucoepidermoid tumors. Adenomas present in patients 15 to 60 years old (average age, 45) as endobronchial lesions and are often symptomatic for several years. Patients may have a chronic cough, recurrent hemoptysis, or obstruction with atelectasis, lobar collapse, or pneumonitis and abscess formation. Bronchial carcinoids, which usually follow a benign course, and small cell lung cancers, which are highly malignant, are both derived from the same normal bronchial epithelial component, the Kulchitsky cell. This cell is part of the amine precursor uptake and decarboxylation (APUD) system. Carcinoids, like small cell lung cancers, may secrete other hormones, such as ACTH or arginine vasopressin, and thus can cause paraneoplastic syndromes that resolve upon resection. In addition, bronchial carcinoid metastases (usually to the liver) may produce the carcinoid syndrome, with cutaneous flush, bronchoconstriction, diarrhea, and cardiac valvular lesions (see Chap. 95), which small cell lung cancer does not. Occasionally, pathologists may have difficulty in distinguishing carcinoids from small cell lung cancers. Carcinoid tumors that have an unusually aggressive histologic appearance (referred to as *atypical carcinoids*) metastasize in 70 percent of cases to regional nodes, liver, or bone, compared with only a 5 percent rate of metastasis for carcinoids with typical histology.

Bronchial adenomas of all types, because of their endobronchial and often central location, are usually visible by fiberoptic bronchoscopy, and tissue for histologic diagnosis is obtained in this manner. Because they are hypervascular, they can bleed profusely after bronchoscopic biopsy, and this problem should be anticipated. Bronchial adenomas must be dealt with as potentially malignant and thus require removal not only for symptom relief but also because they can be locally invasive or recurrent, potentially can metastasize, and may produce paraneoplastic syndromes. Surgical excision is the primary treatment for all types of bronchial adenomas. The extent of surgery is determined at operation and should be as conservative as possible. Often bronchotomy with local excision, sleeve resection, segmental resection, or lobectomy is sufficient. Five-year survival rates following surgical resection are 95 percent, decreasing to 70 percent if regional nodes are involved. The treatment of metastatic pulmonary carcinoids is currently unclear because they can either be indolent, growing slowly over several years, or behave more like small cell lung carcinoma. Assessment of the tempo and histology of the disease in the individual patient is necessary to determine if and when chemotherapy or radiotherapy is indicated.

HAMARTOMAS Pulmonary hamartomas have a peak incidence at age 60 and are more frequent in men than in women. Histologically, they contain normal pulmonary tissue components (smooth muscle and collagen) in a disorganized fashion. They are usually peripheral, clinically silent, and benign in their behavior. While it would be advantageous to avoid thoracotomy in these older patients, unless the radiographic findings are pathognomonic for hamartoma, with "popcorn" calcification, the lesions will usually have to be resected for diagnosis, particularly if the patient is a smoker.

METASTATIC PULMONARY TUMORS

The lung is a frequent site of metastases from primary cancers outside the lung. Usually such metastatic disease is considered incurable. However, two special situations should be borne in mind. The first is the development of a solitary pulmonary shadow on a chest x-ray in a patient known to have an extrathoracic neoplasm. This shadow may represent a metastasis or a new primary lung cancer. Because the natural history of lung cancer is worse than that of most other primary tumors, it is wise to approach a single pulmonary nodule in a patient with a known extrathoracic tumor as though the nodule is a primary lung cancer, particularly if the patient is over 35 years of age and a smoker. This means a vigorous evaluation looking for other sites of active cancer and, if none are found, surgical resection of the nodule. Second, in some cases, multiple pulmonary nodules can be resected with curative intent. This tactic is usually recommended if, after careful staging, it is decided that (1) the patient can tolerate the contemplated pulmonary resection, (2) the primary tumor has been definitively and successfully treated, and (3) all known metastatic disease can be encompassed by the projected pulmonary resection. The key is selection and screening of patients to exclude those with uncontrolled primary tumors and extrapulmonary metastases. Primary tumors whose pulmonary metastases have been successfully resected for cure include osteogenic and soft tissue sarcomas; colon, rectal, uterine, cervix, and corpus tumors; head and neck, breast, testis, and salivary gland cancer; melanoma; and bladder and kidney tumors. Five-year survival rates of 20 to 30 percent have been found in carefully selected patients, and the most dramatic results have been seen in osteogenic sarcomas, where resection of pulmonary metastases (sometimes requiring several thoracotomies) is becoming a standard curative treatment approach.

BIBLIOGRAPHY

BENOWITZ N: Pharmacologic aspects of cigarette smoking and nicotine addiction. N Engl J Med 319:1318, 1988

GAZDAR AF et al: Molecular genetic changes found in human lung cancer and its precursor lesions. Cold Spring Harbor Symp Quant Biol 59:565, 1994

GINSBERG RJ et al: Non-small cell lung cancer, in *Cancer: Principles and Practice of Oncology,* 5th ed, VT DeVita Jr et al (eds). Philadelphia, Lippincott-Raven, 1997, pp 858–911

IHDE DC et al: Small cell lung cancer, in *Cancer: Principles and Practice of Oncology,* 5th ed, VT DeVita Jr et al (eds). Philadelphia, Lippincott-Raven, 1997, pp 911–949

LIPPMAN SM et al: Epidemiology, biology, and chemoprevention of aerodigestive cancer. Cancer 74(Suppl 9):2719, 1994

MINNA JD et al: Molecular biology of lung cancer, in *Cancer: Principles and Practice of Oncology,* 5th ed, VT DeVita Jr et al (eds). Philadelphia, Lippincott-Raven, 1997, pp 849–857

MITCHELL JB et al: *Lung Cancer: Principles and Practice.* Philadelphia, Lippincott-Raven, 1996

NON-SMALL CELL LUNG CANCER COLLABORATIVE GROUP: Chemotherapy in non-small cell lung cancer: A meta-analysis using updated data on individual patients from 52 randomised clinical trials. BMJ 311:899, 1996

PARKER SL et al: Cancer statistics, 1996. CA Cancer J Clin 46(1):5, 1996

TRAVIS WD et al: Lung cancer. Cancer 75:191, 1995

ZANG EA, WYNDER EL: Differences in lung cancer risk between men and women: Examination of the evidence. J Natl Cancer Inst 88:183, 1996

91   *Marc E. Lippman*

BREAST CANCER

DEFINITION   Breast cancer represents a malignant proliferation of epithelial cells lining the ducts or lobules of the breast. In 1996, there were approximately 185,000 cases of invasive breast cancer and 46,000 deaths in the United States. Breast cancer is the most common cancer in women (excluding skin cancer), although it is quite rare in men. This chapter will not consider rare malignancies of the breast, including sarcomas and lymphomas. Human breast cancer is a clonal disease. That is, a single transformed cell—the end result of a series of somatic (acquired) or germline (inherited) mutations—is able to express full malignant potential, in a series of events that occur in a sequential and stochastic manner. Thus, breast cancer may exist for a long period as either a noninvasive disease or an invasive but nonmetastatic disease. This fact makes the need for timely diagnosis and appropriate management more urgent.

GENETICS   Probably only about 10 percent of human breast cancers can be linked directly to germline mutations. This area has undergone remarkable evolution with the identification of several genes responsible for the familial cases. The first to be identified were germline mutations in the tumor suppressor gene *p53.* In the disorder caused by these mutations—called the Li-Fraumeni syndrome—inherited mutations in *p53* lead to an increased incidence of breast cancer, osteogenic sarcomas, and other malignancies.

Another putative tumor suppressor gene, *BRCA-1,* has been identified at the chromosomal locus 17q21; this gene encodes a zinc finger protein, and the product therefore may function as a transcription factor. Women who inherit a mutated allele of this gene from either parent have an approximately 85 to 90 percent lifetime chance of developing breast cancer, as well as about a 33 percent chance of developing ovarian cancer. Men who carry a mutant allele of the gene have an increased incidence of prostate cancer but usually not of breast cancer. A third gene, termed *BRCA-2,* which has been localized to chromosome 11, is associated with an increased incidence of breast cancer in men and women.

The ataxia-telangiectasia gene is associated with remarkable radiation sensitivity even in the heterozygous state, which occurs in the population at a frequency of 1 to 2 percent. Because of their susceptibility to radiation-induced cancer, heterozygous carriers of this gene may be at risk from such procedures as screening mammography.

Even more important than the role these genes play in inherited forms of breast cancer susceptibility may be their role in sporadic breast cancer. For example, the *p53* mutation is present in approximately 40 percent of human breast cancers as an acquired defect. Thus far, evidence for *BRCA-1* mutation in primary breast cancer has not been reported. However, in a small series of sporadic breast cancers, decreased expression of BRCA-1 mRNA occurs. An abnormal cellular location of the BRCA-1 protein has also been found in some breast cancers, and BRCA-1 therefore may play a role in their pathogenesis. In addition, as evidenced by loss of heterozygosity, other types of tumor-suppressor activity appear to be lost in sporadic cases of human breast cancer. Finally, one dominant oncogene plays a role in about a quarter of human breast cancer cases. The product of this gene, a member of the EGF receptor superfamily called erbB2 (HER-2, neu), is overexpressed in these breast cancers owing to gene amplification, and this overexpression can transform human breast epithelium.

While restoration gene therapy is not a clinical reality yet, several approaches aimed at dealing with overexpressed genes are under clinical trial. The eventual hope for breast cancer is to alter the course of the disease by directly targeting the genes responsible for the malignant process.

EPIDEMIOLOGY   Breast cancer is a hormone-dependent disease. Women without functioning ovaries who never receive estrogen replacement do not develop breast cancer. The female-to-male ratio for the disease is about 150 to 1. A host of findings indicate that hormones play a critical role as promoters of the disease. For most epithelial malignancies, a log-log plot of incidence versus age shows a straight-line increase with every year of life. A similar plot for breast cancer shows the same straight line increase, but with a decrease in slope beginning at the age of menopause. The three dates in a woman's life that have a major impact on breast cancer incidence are age of menarche, age at first full-term pregnancy, and age of menopause. Women who experience menarche at age 16 have only 50 to 60 percent of the lifetime breast cancer risk of women who experience menarche at age 12. Similarly, menopause occurring 10 years before the median age (52 years), whether natural or surgically induced, reduces lifetime breast cancer risk by about 35 percent. Compared with nulliparous women, women who have a first full-term pregnancy by age 18 have 30 to 40 percent the risk of breast cancer. Thus, length of menstrual life—particularly the fraction occurring before the first full-term pregnancy—is a substantial component of the total risk of breast cancer. This factor can account for 70 to 80 percent of the variation in breast cancer frequency in different countries.

International variation has provided some of the most important clues on hormonal carcinogenesis. A woman living to age 80 in North America has 1 chance in 9 of developing invasive breast cancer. Asian women have one-fifth to one-tenth the risk of breast cancer of women in North America or Western Europe. Asian women have substantially lower concentrations of estrogens and progesterone. These differences cannot be explained on a genetic basis, because Asian women living in a Western environment have a risk identical to that of their Western counterparts. These women also differ markedly in height and weight from Asian women in Asia; height and weight are critical regulators of age of menarche and have substantial effects on plasma concentrations of estrogens.

The role of diet in breast cancer etiology is controversial. While there are associative links between total caloric intake and breast cancer risk, the strongest link is with high dietary fat intake. However, within the range of dietary fat intake common in Western cultures, there is no convincing evidence that variations in dietary fat alter breast cancer risk. However, there is a risk associated with moderate alcohol intake; the mechanism is unknown. Recommendations favoring abstinence from alcohol must be weighed against other social pressures and the possible cardioprotective effect of moderate alcohol intake.

The potential role of exogenous hormones in breast cancer is of extraordinary importance, because millions of American women regularly use oral contraceptives. The most credible meta-analyses of oral contraceptive use suggest that these agents cause little if any increased risk of breast cancer. When the very substantial protective effect that oral contraceptives offer against ovarian epithelial tumors and endometrial cancers is considered, the data suggest that the use of oral contraceptives is highly protective against malignancy in general, with little impact on breast cancer. Far more controversial are the data surrounding hormone replacement therapy (HRT) in hypogonadal and/or menopausal women. First, HRT with estrogens alone, usually in the form of equine conjugated estrogens, provides less than the physiologic equivalent of premenopausal estrogens but is associated with an increased risk of endometrial cancer, a reduction in the symptoms of estrogen deprivation, a reduction in osteoporosis and resultant hip fractures, and a reduction by about one-third in the incidence of deaths due to cardiovascular disease. Meta-analyses suggest a small increase in breast cancer incidence, particularly with high dosages and a long duration of treatment. For the average woman, the negative effect on the breast is far outweighed by the protective effects on the bones and heart. Preliminary data suggest that there is a reduction in the risk of colon cancer as well.

The addition of progestogens to HRT regimens drastically reduces the risk of endometrial cancer. It is not clear whether the protective effects against cardiovascular and osteoporotic bone diseases are altered. However, progestogens are copromoters of breast cancer in model systems, and an increased risk of breast cancer is possible.

Whether a history of previous biopsy findings of atypical hyperplasia or in situ carcinoma or a strong family history of breast cancer alter the risk-to-benefit ratios for HRT is unknown. It is likely that the average woman benefits from HRT.

In addition to the other factors, radiation may be a risk factor in younger women. Women who have been exposed before age 30 to radiation in the form of multiple fluoroscopies (200 to 300 cGy) or treatment for Hodgkin's disease (>3600 cGy) have a substantially increased risk of breast cancer, whereas radiation exposure after age 30 appears to have a minimal carcinogenic effect on the breast.

DIAGNOSIS   The diagnosis of breast cancer was described in Chap. 64. Suffice it to say that no combination of risk factors can be used to define a group of women who have no risk of breast cancer. However, identification of the *BRCA-1* gene makes it possible to identify women who face an 85 to 90 percent lifetime likelihood of

developing breast cancer (with a 70 percent risk of breast cancer by age 60). Breast cancer is virtually unique among epithelial tumors in adults in that screening (in the form of annual mammography) improves survival. Meta-analysis examining outcomes from every randomized trial of mammography conclusively shows a 25 to 30 percent reduction in the chance of dying from breast cancer with annual screening after age 50; the data for women between ages 40 and 50 are almost as positive. Although this remains an area of some controversy, it seems prudent to recommend annual mammography routinely for women past the age of 40. While the benefit of this practice may be debatable, for the vast majority of women it likely carries no risk. It should also be pointed out that no randomized study of breast self-examination has ever shown any improvement in survival. While breast self-examination should be encouraged, its major benefit appears to be identification of tumors appropriate for conservative local therapy, rather than a major increase in survival. It is hoped that better mammographic technology, including digitized radiography, routine use of magnified views, and greater skill in interpretation, combined with newer diagnostic techniques (magnetic resonance imaging, magnetic resonance spectroscopy, positron emission tomography, etc.) will make it possible to identify breast cancers yet more reliably and earlier.

STAGING   Correct staging of breast cancer patients is of extraordinary importance. Not only does it permit an accurate prognosis, but in many cases therapeutic decision making is based largely on the TNM classification (Table 91-1). Comparison with historical series should be undertaken with caution, as the staging has changed in the past 10 years.

Table 91-1

Staging of Breast Cancer*

Primary Tumor (T)	
T0	No evidence of primary tumor
Tis	Carcinoma in situ
T1	Tumor ≤2 cm
T2	Tumor >2 cm but ≤5 cm
T3	Tumor >5 cm
T4	Extension to chest wall, inflammation

Regional Lymph Nodes (N)	
N0	No tumor in regional lymph nodes
N1	Metastasis to movable ipsilateral nodes
N2	Metastasis to matted or fixed ipsilateral nodes
N3	Metastasis to ipsilateral internal mammary nodes

Distant Metastasis (M)	
M0	No distant metastasis
M1	Distant metastasis (includes spread to ipsilateral supraclavicular nodes)

Stage Grouping			
Stage 0	TIS	N0	M0
Stage 1	T1	N0	M0
Stage IIA	T0	N1	M0
	T1	N1	M0
	T2	N0	M0
Stage IIB	T2	N1	M0
	T3	N0	M0
Stage IIIA	T0	N2	M0
	T1	N2	M0
	T2	N2	M0
	T3	N1, N2	M0
Stage IIIB	T4	Any N	M0
	Any T	N3	M0
Stage IV	Any T	Any N	M1

* Modified from the TNM classification proposed by the American Joint Committee on Cancer, 1992.

Rx **TREATMENT**

Primary Breast Cancer The management of breast cancer that is apparently localized to the breast or regional lymph nodes has changed since 1985. A series of randomized clinical trials both in the United States and abroad have shown that breast-conserving treatments, consisting of the removal of the primary tumor by some form of lumpectomy with or without irradiation to the breast, results in a survival that is as good as that after extensive procedures, such as mastectomy or modified radical mastectomy, with or without further irradiation. While breast conservation is associated with a possibility of recurrence in the breast, the 10-year survival is still as good as that after more radical surgery. Similarly, multiple studies have shown that the addition of radiotherapy to any form of mastectomy does not improve survival. However, radiation therapy can reduce the rate of local or regional recurrence, and, for women with high-risk primary tumors (i.e., T2 in size, positive margins, positive nodes), it may be considered following mastectomy. At present, approximately one-third of women with breast cancer in the United States are managed by lumpectomy. Breast-conserving surgery is not suitable for all patients, however. For example, it is not suitable for tumors larger than 7 cm (or for smaller tumors if the breast is small), for tumors involving the nipple areolar complex, for tumors with extensive intraductal disease involving multiple quadrants of the breast, for women with a history of collagen-vascular disease, and for women who either do not have the motivation for breast conservation or do not have convenient access to radiotherapy. However, these groups probably do not account for more than one-third of patients. The implication is that a great many women who undergo mastectomy could safely avoid this procedure.

An extensive intraductal component is a predictor of recurrence in the breast, and so are several clinical variables. Axillary lymph node involvement and involvement of vascular or lymphatic channels by metastatic tumor in the breast are associated with a higher risk of relapse in the breast but are not contraindications to breast-conserving treatment. When these patients are excluded, and when lumpectomy with negative tumor margins is achieved, breast conservation is associated with a recurrence rate in the breast of approximately 10 percent. The survival of patients who have recurrence in the breast is somewhat worse than that of women who do not. Thus, recurrence in the breast is a negative prognostic variable for long-term survival. However, recurrence in the breast is not the *cause* of distant metastasis. This conclusion is based on the fact that survival is the same for patients treated with breast-conserving therapy and patients treated with mastectomy. If recurrence in the breast caused metastatic disease, then women treated with lumpectomy, who have a higher rate of recurrence in the breast, should have a lower survival. Most patients should consult with a radiation oncologist before making a final decision concerning local therapy. However, a multimodality clinic approach in which the surgeon, radiation oncologist, medical oncologist, and other care givers cooperate to evaluate the patient and develop a treatment plan has gained widespread acceptance and is usually considered a major advantage by patients.

ADJUVANT THERAPY One of the significant advances in the treatment of solid tumors of adults has been the improved survival resulting from the use of systemic therapy after local management of breast cancer. While this therapy is imperfect in terms of effectiveness, toxicity, and patient selection, more than one-quarter of the women who would otherwise die of metastatic breast cancer remain disease-free when treated with the appropriate systemic regimen. In this section we will review patient selection, treatment regimens, and toxicities.

PROGNOSTIC VARIABLES At the time of local therapy, it is critical to identify patients at a substantial risk of eventual relapse. For patients likely to be cured by local therapy, systemic treatment offers no further benefit and involves a needless hazard. Furthermore, as

therapies become increasingly specific, identification of variables associated with disease relapse may make it possible to choose the best therapy for the individual patient.

The most important prognostic variables are provided by *tumor staging*. The size of the tumor and the status of the axillary lymph nodes provide reasonably accurate information on the likelihood of tumor relapse. The relation of pathologic stage to 5-year survival is shown in Table 91-2. For most women, the need for adjuvant therapy can be readily defined on this basis alone. In the absence of lymph node involvement, involvement of microvessels (either capillaries or lymphatic channels) in tumors is considered by many as nearly equivalent to lymph node involvement. The greatest controversy concerns women with intermediate prognoses. Obviously, *there is no justification for adjuvant chemotherapy in women with tumors less than 1 cm in size whose axillary lymph nodes are negative.*

A large number of analyses have been performed to try to identify other significant prognostic variables. For each of these variables, differences in the methods of analysis and the populations studied, as well as the effects of chance, have resulted in discordant results. However, for several variables, the association with disease-free survival and overall survival seems clear. What is less clear is whether or not they add to the information from pathologic staging.

Estrogen and progesterone receptor status are of prognostic significance. Tumors that lack either or both of these receptors are more likely to recur than tumors that have them.

Several *measures of tumor growth rate* correlate with early relapse. S-phase analysis using flow cytometry is the most accurate measure, and indirect S-phase assessments using antigens associated with the cell cycle, such as PCNA and Ki67, are also valuable. Several studies suggest that tumors with a high proportion (more than the median) of cells in the S phase pose a greater risk of relapse and that chemotherapy offers the greatest survival benefit for these tumors. For this reason, some clinicians use S-phase assessment as a deciding factor for instituting adjuvant therapy when other pathologic features are unclear. Assessment of DNA content in the form of ploidy is of modest value, with nondiploid tumors having a somewhat worse prognosis.

Histologic classification of the tumor has also been used as a prognostic factor. Tumors with a poor nuclear grade have a higher degree of recurrence than tumors with a good nuclear grade. The reproducibility of this measurement is reasonable when semiquantitative measures such as Elston score are employed.

Molecular changes in the tumor are also useful. For example, tumors that overexpress the epidermal growth factor receptor erbB2 or that have a mutated *p53* gene have a bad prognosis. Particular interest has centered on erbB2 overexpression as measured by histochemistry. A cooperative group study suggests that tumors that overexpress erbB2 are more likely to respond to higher doses of doxorubicin-containing regimens. For this reason, erbB2 expression is usually worth measuring as a means of deciding on therapy.

To grow, a tumor must generate a neovasculature (see Chap. 85). On the basis of a semiquantitative scoring system, the presence of more microvessels in tumors has been shown by several groups to be associated with a worse prognosis.

Table 91-2

5-Year Survival Rate for Breast Cancer by Stage*

Stage	5-Year Survival (Percent of Patients)
0	99
I	92
IIA	82
IIB	65
IIIA	47
IIIB	44
IV	14

* Modified from data of the National Cancer Institute—Surveillance, Epidemiology, and End Results (SEER).

Other variables that have also been used to evaluate prognosis include proteins associated with invasiveness, such as type IV collagenase, cathepsin D, plasminogen activator, plasminogen activator receptor, and the metastasis suppressor gene *nm23*. None of these has been widely accepted as a prognostic variable for therapeutic decision-making.

One problem in interpreting these prognostic variables is that most of them have not been examined in a study using a substantial cohort of patients. For example, what should be done for a patient who has a 1-cm tumor with negative lymph nodes but has one or more bad prognostic variables? We aren't sure.

ADJUVANT REGIMENS Selection of appropriate adjuvant chemotherapy or hormone therapy regimens is a highly controversial issue in some situations. Meta-analyses have helped to define broad limits for therapy but do not help in choosing optimal regimens or in choosing a regimen for certain subgroups of patients. A general summary of recommendations is shown in Table 91-3. In general, premenopausal women for whom any form of adjuvant systemic therapy is indicated should receive chemotherapy. The effect on survival of adjuvant anti-estrogen (tamoxifen) therapy in premenopausal patients with any lymph node status is minimal, and this therapy should probably not be administered alone. The benefit of adding tamoxifen to chemotherapy in premenopausal women who are to be treated has not been well established, although it is common practice to follow chemotherapy with tamoxifen in premenopausal women whose tumors are positive for the estrogen receptor. Prophylactic castration may also be associated with a substantial survival benefit (primarily in estrogen receptor–positive patients), but this treatment has not been widely used in this country.

Data on postmenopausal women are also controversial. The impact of adjuvant chemotherapy is less clear-cut than in premenopausal patients, although some survival advantage has been shown. In general, the first decision is whether chemotherapy or tamoxifen should be used. While adjuvant tamoxifen improves survival regardless of axillary lymph node status, the improvement is modest for patients in whom multiple lymph nodes are involved. For this reason, it is usual to give chemotherapy to postmenopausal patients who have no medical contraindications and who have more than one positive lymph node; tamoxifen is commonly given simultaneously or subsequently. For postmenopausal women for whom systemic therapy is warranted but who have a more favorable prognosis, tamoxifen may be used as a single agent.

There is little agreement about optimal chemotherapy regimens. In fact, most comparisons of adjuvant chemotherapy regimens show little difference among them. However, dose-intensive doxorubicin-containing regimens appear to be better than lower-dose regimens of the same drugs. Whether this finding represents a threshold effect or a dose-response curve (in which case effectiveness would increase with even higher doses) is under examination. Combinations of very high drug doses and either stem cell or autologous bone marrow support for poor-prognosis stage II patients will be discussed in a separate section.

One approach—so-called neoadjuvant chemotherapy—involves the administration of adjuvant therapy before definitive surgery and radiation therapy. Because the objective response rates of patients with breast cancer to systemic therapy in this setting exceed 75 percent, many patients will be "down-staged" and may thus become candidates for breast-conserving therapy. Whether survival is improved by such approaches is unknown.

Other adjuvant treatments under trial include the use of new drugs, such as paclitaxel, and therapy based on alternative kinetic and biologic models. In such approaches, high doses of single agents are used separately in relatively dose-intensive cycling regimens. One randomized trial suggests that patients treated intensively with one drug combination followed by a second drug combination have better survival than patients given the same drugs in an alternating format. It would not be surprising if different uses of available drugs improved long-term survival. Regrettably, trials require a reasonably large number of homogeneous patients and prolonged follow-up.

Systemic Therapy for Metastatic Disease Unfortunately, after varying periods of disease-free survival, nearly half of patients treated for apparently localized breast cancer develop metastatic disease. Although some of these patients can be salvaged by combinations of systemic and local therapy, most eventually succumb. Soft tissue, bony, and visceral (lung and liver) metastases each account for approximately one-third of initial relapses. However, by the time of death, most patients will have bony involvement. Recurrences can appear at any time after primary therapy. In fact, half of all initial breast cancer recurrences occur more than 5 years after initial therapy.

Biopsy must be performed to demonstrate the presence of metastatic disease, because this diagnosis alters the outlook for the patient so drastically that it should not be made without certainty. Every oncologist has seen patients with tuberculosis, gallstones, primary hyperparathyroidism, or another nonmalignant disease misdiagnosed and treated as metastatic breast cancer. This is a catastrophic mistake and justifies biopsy for virtually every patient at the time of presentation of metastatic disease.

The choice of optimal therapy requires consideration of local therapy needs, of the overall medical condition of the patient, and of the hormone receptor status of the tumor, as well as the exercise of clinical judgment. Because therapy of systemic disease is palliative, the potential toxicities of therapies should be balanced against the response rates. Several variables influence the response to systemic therapy. For example, the presence of estrogen and progesterone receptors are strong indications for endocrine therapy, since the response rates for tumors that express both receptors may approach 70 percent. On the other hand, patients with short disease-free inter-

Table 91-3

Suggested Approaches to Adjuvant Therapy for Women

Age Group	Lymph Node Status*	Endocrine Receptor Status	Tumor	Recommendation	Comment
Premenopausal	Positive†	Any	Any	Multidrug chemotherapy	
Premenopausal	Negative	Any	>2 cm, or 1–2 cm with other poor prognostic variables	Multidrug chemotherapy	Role of tamoxifen not clear
Postmenopausal	Positive†	Negative	Any	Multidrug chemotherapy	
Postmenopausal	Positive†	Positive	Any	Tamoxifen with or without chemotherapy	
Postmenopausal	Negative	Positive	>2 cm, or 1–2 cm with other poor prognostic variables	Tamoxifen	
Postmenopausal	Negative	Negative	>2 cm, or 1–2 cm with other poor prognostic variables	Consider multidrug chemotherapy	

* As determined by pathologic examination.
† For patients with 6 or more positive nodes, consider enrollment in high dose chemotherapy trials.

vals, rapidly progressive visceral disease, lymphangitic pulmonary disease, or intracranial disease are unlikely to respond to endocrine therapy.

In many cases, systemic therapy can be withheld while the patient is treated with appropriate local therapy. The effectiveness of radiation therapy and occasionally of surgery for relieving the symptoms of metastatic disease, particularly when bony sites are involved, cannot be overemphasized. Many patients with bone-only or bone-dominant disease have a relatively indolent course. Under such circumstances, systemic chemotherapy has a modest effect, whereas radiation therapy may be effective for long periods. Other systemic treatments, such as strontium-89 and/or bisphosphonates, may provide a palliative benefit without inducing an objective response. Since the goal of therapy is to maintain well-being for as long as possible, emphasis should be placed on avoiding the most hazardous complications of metastatic disease, including pathologic fracture of the axial skeleton and spinal cord compression. New back pain in patients with cancer should be explored aggressively on an emergent basis; to wait for neurologic symptoms can be catastrophic. Also, metastatic involvement of endocrine organs can cause profound dysfunction, including adrenal insufficiency and hypopituitarism. Similarly, obstruction of the biliary tree or other impairment of organ function may be better managed with a local therapy than with a systemic approach.

ENDOCRINE THERAPY Normal breast tissue is estrogen-dependent. Both primary breast cancer and metastatic breast cancer may retain this phenotype. The best means of ascertaining whether a breast cancer is hormone-dependent is through analyses of estrogen and progesterone receptor levels. Tumors that are positive for the estrogen receptor and negative for the progesterone receptor have a response rate of approximately 30 percent. Tumors that have both receptors have a response rate approaching 70 percent. If neither receptor is present, the objective response rates are less than 10 percent. In general, receptor analyses provide information as to the correct ordering of endocrine therapies. Because of the lack of toxicity and because some patients whose receptor analyses are reported as negative respond to endocrine therapy, an endocrine treatment should be attempted at some point in every patient with metastatic breast cancer. Potential endocrine therapies are summarized in Table 91-4. Little information suggests that any of these endocrine therapies is superior to another. The choice of endocrine therapy is usually determined by toxicity profile and availability. In most patients, the initial endocrine therapy is the antiestrogen tamoxifen. Newer antiestrogens that are free of agonistic effects are in clinical trial. Cases in which tumors shrank in response to tamoxifen withdrawal (as well as withdrawal of pharmacologic doses of estrogens) have been reported. Endogenous estrogen formation may be blocked by aromatase inhibitors or analogues of luteinizing hormone–releasing hormone (LHRH). Additive endocrine therapies, including treatment with progestogens, estrogens, and androgens, may also be tried in patients who respond to initial endocrine therapy; the mechanism of action of these latter therapies is unknown. However, patients who respond to one endocrine therapy have at least a 50 percent chance of responding to a second endocrine therapy. It is not uncommon for patients to respond to two or three sequential endocrine therapies; however, combination endocrine therapies do not appear to be superior to individual agents, and combinations of chemotherapy with endocrine therapy are not useful. The median survival of patients with metastatic disease is approximately 2 years, and many patients, particularly older persons and those with hormone-dependent disease, respond to endocrine therapy for 3 to 5 years or longer.

CHEMOTHERAPY Unlike other epithelial malignancies, breast cancer responds to several chemotherapeutic agents, including anthracyclines, alkylating agents, taxanes, and antimetabolites. Multiple combinations of these agents have been found to improve response rates somewhat, but they have had little impact on duration of response or survival. As previously mentioned, the median survival from diagnosis of metastatic disease to death is approximately 2 years. The choice among multidrug combinations frequently depends on whether adjuvant chemotherapy was administered and, if so, what type. While patients treated with adjuvant regimens of cyclophosphamide, methotrexate, and fluorouracil (CMF regimens) may subsequently respond to the same combination in the metastatic disease setting, most oncologists use drugs to which the patients have not been previously exposed. Once patients have progressed after combination drug therapy, it is most common to treat them with single agents. Given the significant toxicity of most drugs, the use of a single effective agent will minimize toxicity by sparing the patient exposure to drugs that would be of little value. Unfortunately, no form of in vitro drug sensitivity testing to select the drugs most efficacious for a given patient has been demonstrated to be useful.

Most oncologists use either an anthracycline or paclitaxel following failure with the initial regimen. However, the choice has to be balanced with individual needs.

HIGH-DOSE CHEMOTHERAPY INCLUDING AUTOLOGOUS BONE MARROW TRANSPLANTATION Autologous bone marrow transplantation combined with high doses of single agents can produce improvement even in heavily pretreated patients. However, such responses are rarely, if ever, durable and are unlikely to substantially alter the clinical course for most patients with advanced metastatic disease. However, given the success of such regimens in chronic myelogenous leukemia and Hodgkin's disease, this approach has been tried in patients who have poor-prognosis breast cancer but a relatively small disease burden. These have included patients who have multiple axillary lymph node involvement at primary presentation, patients with stage III breast cancer, and patients with stage IV breast cancer who either have been rendered free of disease by localized therapy (that is, who had an apparently single metastasis and in whom surgical or radiation therapy resulted in disappearance of all objective disease) or showed a nearly complete response to conventional-dose systemic treatment. Several thousand patients in the United States have been treated with these regimens, but it is difficult to assess the success of the regimens because of the problem of comparing the results with historical controls. Nevertheless, the toxicity of these approaches has been reduced by the use of cytokine support and antibiotic prophylaxis, so that these therapies are more widely available. Some oncologists believe that this approach offers a significant advantage for patients.

Stage III Breast Cancer Between 10 and 25 percent of patients have so-called locally advanced or stage III breast cancer at diagnosis. Many of these cancers are technically operable, whereas others, particularly cancers with chest wall involvement, inflammatory breast cancers, or cancers with large matted axillary lymph nodes, cannot be managed with surgery initially. Although no randomized

Table 91-4

Endocrine Therapies for Breast Cancer

Therapy	Comments
Castration	For premenopausal women
Surgical	
LHRH agonists	
Antiestrogens	
Tamoxifen	Useful in pre- and postmenopausal women
"Pure" antiestrogens	Promising early clinical data
High-dose progestogens	Common second-line choice
Adrenalectomy	
Surgical	Rarely employed second-line choice
"Medical" adrenalectomy	Probably works to decrease the formation of estrogen precursors (aromatase inhibitor)
Aromatase inhibitors	Promising early clinical trials in postmenopausal women
Hypophysectomy	Rarely used
Additive androgens or estrogens	Plausible third-line therapies; potentially toxic

trials have proved the efficacy of induction chemotherapy, this approach has gained widespread use. More than 90 percent of patients with locally advanced breast cancer show a partial or better response to multidrug chemotherapy regimens that include an anthracycline. Early administration of this treatment reduces the bulk of the disease and frequently makes the patient a suitable candidate for salvage surgery and/or radiation therapy. These patients should be managed in multimodality clinics if possible to coordinate surgery, radiationtherapy, and systemic chemotherapy. Most published series suggest that such approaches produce a long-term disease-free survival in about 30 to 50 percent of patients. It is difficult to make direct comparisons between the various reports because of differences in patient selection and drug regimens.

Breast Cancer Prevention   The endocrine promotion of breast cancer has been reviewed in this chapter. Studies of hormone-dependent rodent models of breast cancer suggest that the endocrine milieu has a significant impact on the long-term risk of breast cancer.

Because tamoxifen is effective and relatively safe in both the advanced and adjuvant disease setting, the agent has been tried as a breast cancer preventive. Women who have one breast cancer are at risk of developing a contralateral breast cancer at a rate of approximately 0.5 percent per year. When adjuvant tamoxifen is administered to these patients, the rate of development of contralateral breast cancers is reduced. In other tissues of the body, tamoxifen has estrogen-like effects that are potentially beneficial. These include preservation of bone mineral density and long-term lowering of cholesterol. However, tamoxifen has estrogen-like effects on the uterus, leading to an increased risk of uterine cancer. Consequently, tamoxifen cannot at this time be regarded as a safe agent for prevention of breast cancer. Large-scale prevention trials are being carried out, however. Antiestrogens without estrogen-like effects are now in early clinical trials and may be even more effective in this regard.

Noninvasive Breast Cancer   Breast cancer develops as a series of molecular changes in epithelial cells that lead to ever more malignant behavior. Increased use of mammography and better mammographic diagnosis have led to more frequent diagnosis of noninvasive breast cancer. These lesions fall into two groups: ductal carcinoma in situ (DCIS) and lobular carcinoma in situ (lobular neoplasia). The management of both entities is controversial, and careful consideration should be given to their treatment.

DUCTAL CARCINOMA IN SITU   Proliferation of cytologically malignant breast epithelial cells within the ducts is termed DCIS. Significant pathologic disagreement can occur in differentiating atypical hyperplasia from DCIS. At least one-third of cases of untreated DCIS progress within 5 years to invasive breast cancer, and therefore appropriate therapy is warranted. For many years, the standard treatment for this disease was mastectomy. However, since treatment of this condition by lumpectomy and radiation therapy gives survival that is as good as the survival for invasive breast cancer treated by mastectomy, it appears paradoxical to recommend more aggressive therapy for a "less malignant" disease. Although both wide excision and wide excision plus radiation therapy are used for this disease in some centers, few randomized studies have compared different therapies; therefore, the optimal treatment is unclear. In one randomized trial, the combination of wide excision plus irradiation for DCIS caused a substantial reduction in the local recurrence rate as compared to wide excision alone with negative margins. Thus far, survival is identical in the two arms. Unfortunately, no studies have compared either of these regimens to mastectomy. Several prognostic features may help to identify patients at high risk for local recurrence after either lumpectomy alone or lumpectomy with radiation therapy. These include extensive disease, age less than 40, and cytologic features such as necrosis, poor nuclear grade, and comedo subtype with overexpression of erbB2. Some data suggest that adequate excision with careful determination of pathologically clear margins is associated with a low recurrence rate. When such surgery is combined with radiation therapy, recurrence (which is usually in the same quadrant) occurs with a frequency of 10 percent or less. Given the fact that half of these recurrences are invasive, about

5 percent will eventually develop into invasive breast cancer. A reasonable expectation of mortality for these patients is about 1 percent, a figure that approximates the mortality rate for DCIS managed by mastectomy. Although this train of reasoning has not formally been proved valid, it is reasonable at present to recommend that patients who desire breast preservation and in whom DCIS appears to be reasonably localized be managed by adequate surgery, with meticulous pathologic evaluation, followed by breast irradiation. The role of subsequent adjuvant tamoxifen in this setting is now being explored. For patients with localized DCIS, there is no need for axillary lymph node dissection. More controversial is the question of what management is optimal when there is any degree of invasion. Because of a significant likelihood (10 to 15 percent) of axillary lymph node involvement even when the primary lesion shows only microscopic invasion, it is prudent to do at least a level 1 and 2 axillary lymph node dissection for all patients with any degree of invasion. Management is dictated by the presence of nodal spread.

LOBULAR NEOPLASIA   The management of patients with proliferation of cytologically malignant cells within the lobules (lobular neoplasia) is controversial. From historical data, it appears that approximately 30 percent of patients who have had adequate local excision of the lesion develop invasive breast cancer (usually infiltrating ductal cell carcinoma) over the next 15 to 20 years. Ipsilateral and contralateral disease are about equally common. Therefore, lobular neoplasia may be a premalignant lesion that suggests an elevated risk of subsequent breast cancer, rather than a form of malignancy itself, and aggressive local management seems unreasonable. Most patients should be followed with careful annual mammography and semiannual physical exams; whether they should receive tamoxifen is unknown. Additional molecular analysis of these lesions may make it possible to discriminate between patients who are at risk of further progression and require additional therapy and those in whom simple follow-up is adequate.

Breast Cancer in Men   Breast cancer is about 1/150th as frequent in men as in women. It usually presents as a unilateral lump in the breast and is frequently not diagnosed promptly. Given the smaller amount of soft tissue and the unexpected nature of the problem, locally advanced presentations are somewhat more common. When male breast cancer is matched to female breast cancer by age and stage, its overall prognosis is identical. Although gynecomastia may initially be unilateral or asymmetrical, any unilateral mass in a man over the age of 40 should receive a careful workup all the way through biopsy. On the other hand, bilateral symmetrical breast development rarely represents breast cancer and is almost invariably due to endocrine disease or a drug effect. It should be kept in mind, nevertheless, that the risk of cancer is much greater in men with gynecomastia; in such men, gross asymmetry of the breasts should arouse suspicion of cancer. Male breast cancer is best managed by mastectomy and axillary lymph node dissection (modified radical mastectomy). Patients with locally advanced disease should also be treated with irradiation. Approximately 90 percent of male breast cancers have the estrogen receptor, and approximately 60 percent of cases with metastatic disease respond to endocrine therapy. There are no randomized studies exploring adjuvant therapy for male breast cancer. Two historical experiences suggest that the disease responds well to adjuvant systemic therapy, and, if not medically contraindicated, the same criteria for the use of adjuvant therapy in women should be applied to men.

The sites of relapse and spectrum of response to chemotherapeutic drugs are virtually identical for breast cancers in the two sexes.

Experimental Therapy   Experimental approaches to the treatment of breast cancer include attempts to block the cell surface receptor erbB2, antiangiogenic therapies, and agents aimed at blocking cell-surface–receptor tyrosine kinases and other signal transduction pathways. An effort should be made to offer such experimental approaches to patients with breast cancer, given the relative lack of success of conventional therapies in prolonging the survival of patients with metastatic disease. Advances during the past 10 to 15 years have added to the quality of life for patients with breast cancer (breast-conserving surgery, more effective reconstructive surgery, the availability of cytokines to ameliorate toxicity, and less toxic endocrine therapies). It is hoped that the next generation of trials will have even greater impact on the long-term outlook for this disease.

BIBLIOGRAPHY

BYERS T: Nutritional risk factors for breast cancer. Cancer 74:288, 1994

DICKSON RB, LIPPMAN ME: Growth factors in breast cancer. Endocr Rev 16:559, 1995

EARLY BREAST CANCER TRIALISTS' COLLABORATIVE GROUP: Systemic treatment of early breast cancer by hormonal, cytotoxic, or immune therapy. Lancet 1:71, 1992

FISHER B et al: Ten-year results of a randomized clinical trial comparing radical mastectomy and total mastectomy with or without radiation. N Engl J Med 312:674, 1985

FRIEDMAN LS et al: The search for *BRCA1*. Cancer Res 54:6374, 1994

HARRIS J et al: Breast cancer: Recent trends and progress and future prospects. Parts I, II, III. N Engl J Med 327:319, 390, 473, 1992

———— et al (eds): *Diseases of the Breast*. Philadelphia, Lippincott-Raven, 1995

SANTEN RJ et al: Endocrine treatment of breast cancer in women. Endocr Rev 11:221, 1990

SHAPIRO S: Screening: Assessment of current studies. Cancer 74(Suppl):231, 1994

92   *Robert J. Mayer*

GASTROINTESTINAL TRACT CANCER

After the prostate, the gastrointestinal tract is the second most common noncutaneous site for cancer in the United States. Cancer of the alimentary tract is the second major cause of cancer-related mortality in the American population, following respiratory tract cancer.

ESOPHAGEAL CANCER

INCIDENCE AND ETIOLOGY In the United States, cancer of the esophagus is a relatively uncommon but extremely lethal malignant condition. It is estimated that the diagnosis was made in 12,300 Americans in 1996, leading to 11,200 deaths. Worldwide, the incidence of esophageal cancer varies strikingly. It occurs frequently within a so-called Asian esophageal cancer belt extending from the southern shore of the Caspian Sea on the west to northern China on the east and encompassing parts of Iran, Central Asia, Afghanistan, Siberia, and Mongolia. High-incidence "pockets" of the disease also are present in such disparate locations as Finland, Iceland, Curaçao, southeastern Africa, and northwestern France. In North America and western Europe, the disease is far more common in blacks than whites, is more common in males than females, appears most often after age 50, and seems to be associated with a lower socioeconomic status.

A variety of causative factors have been implicated in the development of the disease (Table 92-1). In the United States, most esophageal cancer cases are believed to be attributable to excess consumption of alcohol and/or a long-standing history of cigarette smoking. The relative risk increases with the amount of tobacco smoked or alcohol consumed. The consumption of whiskey seems to be linked to a higher incidence than the consumption of wine or beer. The development of esophageal cancer has also been associated with the ingestion of other carcinogens such as nitrites, smoked opiates, and fungal toxins in pickled vegetables, as well as with mucosal damage caused by such

Table 92-1

Some Etiologic Factors Believed to Be Associated with Esophageal Cancer

Excess alcohol consumption
Cigarette smoking
Other ingested carcinogens
   Nitrates (converted to nitrites)
   Smoked opiates
   Fungal toxins in pickled vegetables
Mucosal damage from physical agents
   Hot tea
   Lye ingestion
   Radiation-induced strictures
   Chronic achalasia
Host susceptibility
   Esophageal web with glossitis and iron deficiency (i.e., Plummer-Vinson or Paterson-Kelly syndrome)
   Congenital hyperkeratosis and pitting of the palms and soles (i.e., tylosis palmaris et plantaris)
? Dietary deficiencies molybdenum, zinc, vitamin A
? Celiac sprue
Chronic gastric reflux (i.e., Barrett's esophagus) for adenocarcinoma

physical insults as long-term exposure to extremely hot tea, the ingestion of lye, radiation-induced strictures, and chronic achalasia. The presence of an esophageal web in association with glossitis and iron deficiency (i.e., Plummer-Vinson or Paterson-Kelly syndrome) and congenital hyperkeratosis and pitting of the palms and soles (i.e., tylosis palmaris et plantaris) have each been linked with esophageal cancer, as have dietary deficiencies of molybdenum, zinc, and vitamin A. The risk for esophageal cancer may be slightly greater in individuals with celiac sprue and is definitely increased in the presence of chronic gastric reflux (i.e., Barrett's esophagus). In contrast to other esophageal cancers, neoplasms arising from Barrett's esophagus afflict whites far more often than blacks.

CLINICAL FEATURES Approximately 15 percent of esophageal cancers occur in the upper third of the esophagus (cervical esophagus), 45 percent in the middle third, and 40 percent in the lower third. In the past, more than 75 percent of esophageal tumors were squamous cell carcinomas, arising from the squamous epithelium that lines the lumen of the esophagus. Adenocarcinomas, while less common, more often develop from columnar epithelium, which may appear dysplastic in the distal esophagus in association with chronic gastric reflux (i.e., Barrett's esophagus). Such dysplastic epithelium frequently contains cells with an abnormal DNA content (aneuploidy) and mutations in the *p53* tumor suppressor gene. These adenocarcinomas have the biologic behavior of gastric rather than esophageal cancers. The incidence of adenocarcinoma has risen steadily, while the number of cases of squamous cell carcinomas has remained relatively stable. Attempts at endoscopic and cytologic screening for carcinoma in patients with Barrett's esophagus, while effective as a means of detecting high-grade dysplasia, have not yet been shown to improve the prognosis in individuals found to have a carcinoma. Squamous cell carcinomas are more common in blacks than whites, while adenocarcinomas are more common in whites than blacks. Squamous cell carcinomas and adenocarcinomas of the esophagus cannot be distinguished radiographically or endoscopically.

Progressive dysphagia and weight loss of short duration are the initial symptoms in the vast majority of patients. Dysphagia initially occurs with solid foods and gradually progresses to include semisolids and liquids. By the time these symptoms develop, the disease is usually incurable, since difficulty in swallowing does not occur until 60 percent or more of the esophageal circumference is infiltrated with cancer. Dysphagia may be associated with pain on swallowing (odynophagia), pain radiating to the chest and/or back, regurgitation or vomiting, and aspiration pneumonia. The disease most commonly spreads to adjacent and supraclavicular lymph nodes, liver, lungs, and pleura. Tracheoesophageal fistulas may develop as the disease advances, leading to severe suffering. As with other squamous cell carcinomas, hypercalcemia occasionally may occur in the absence of osseous metastases. It is believed to result from parathormone-related peptide secreted by tumor cells (see Chap. 102).

DIAGNOSIS Routine contrast radiographs effectively identify esophageal lesions large enough to cause symptoms. In contrast to benign esophageal leiomyomas, which result in esophageal narrowing with preservation of a normal mucosal pattern, esophageal carcinomas characteristically cause ragged, ulcerating changes in the mucosa in association with deeper infiltration, producing a picture resembling achalasia. Smaller, potentially resectable tumors are often poorly visualized despite technically adequate esophagograms. Because of this, esophagoscopy should be performed in all patients suspected of having an esophageal abnormality, to visualize the tumor and to obtain histopathologic confirmation of the diagnosis. Because the population of persons at risk for squamous cell carcinoma of the esophagus (i.e., smokers and drinkers) also has a high rate of cancers of the lung and the head and neck region, endoscopic inspection of the larynx, trachea, and bronchi also should be done. A thorough examination of the fundus of the stomach (by retroflexing the endoscope) is imperative as well. Endoscopic biopsies of esophageal tumors fail to recover malignant tissue in one-third of cases because the biopsy forceps cannot penetrate deeply enough through normal mucosa pushed in front of the carcinoma. Cytologic examination of tumor brushings frequently complements standard biopsies and should be performed routinely. The extent of tumor spread to the mediastinum and paraaortic lymph nodes should also be assessed by computed tomography (CT) scans of the chest and abdomen.

℞ **TREATMENT**
The prognosis for patients with esophageal carcinoma is poor. Fewer than 5 percent of patients are alive 5 years after the initial diagnosis, leading many physicians to focus management efforts solely on symptomatic control. Surgical resection of all gross tumor (i.e., total resection) is feasible in only 40 percent of cases, with residual tumor cells frequently present at the resection margins. Such esophagectomies have been associated in the past with a postoperative mortality rate in excess of 20 percent due to anastomotic fistulas, subphrenic abscesses, and respiratory complications; more recent reports suggest far better tolerance and diminished morbidity from these surgical procedures. Fewer than 20 percent of patients who survive a total resection can be expected to be alive after 5 years. The therapeutic outcome following the administration of primary radiation therapy (5500 to 6000 cGy) is not dissimilar to that of radical surgery, sparing patients perioperative morbidity but often resulting in less satisfactory palliation of obstructive symptoms. The evaluation of chemotherapeutic agents in patients with esophageal carcinoma has been hampered by ambiguity in the definition of "response" (i.e., benefit) and the debilitated physical condition of many treated individuals. Nonetheless, significant reductions in the size of measurable tumor masses have been reported in 15 to 25 percent of patients given single-agent treatment and in 30 to 60 percent of patients treated with drug combinations that include cisplatin. Combination chemotherapy and radiation therapy as the initial therapeutic approach, either alone or followed by an attempt at operative resection, may be of benefit. When administered along with radiation therapy, chemotherapy produces a better survival outcome than radiation therapy alone. The use of preoperative chemotherapy and radiation therapy followed by esophageal resection appears to prolong survival as compared with historical controls and has been shown to be superior to surgery alone in at least one small randomized clinical trial.

For the incurable, surgically unresectable patient with esophageal cancer, dysphagia, malnutrition, and the management of tracheoesophageal fistulas loom as major issues. Approaches to palliation of these cancer-related complications include repeated endoscopic dilatation, the surgical placement of a gastrostomy or jejunostomy for hydration and feeding, and endoscopic placement of an expansive metal stent to bypass the tumor. Endoscopic fulguration of the obstructing tumor with lasers appears to be the most promising of these techniques.

TUMORS OF THE STOMACH

GASTRIC ADENOCARCINOMA **Incidence and Epidemiology** For unclear reasons, the incidence and mortality rates for gastric cancer have decreased markedly during the past 60 years. In 1930, gastric cancer was the leading cause of cancer-related deaths among American men by a factor of two, while in women the disease ranked just behind tumors of the uterine cervix and breast. During the ensuing years, the mortality rate from gastric cancer in the United States has dropped in men from 28 to 5.0 per 100,000 population, while in women, the rate has decreased from 27 to 2.3 per 100,000. Nonetheless, it was estimated in 1996 that 22,800 new cases of stomach cancer were diagnosed in the United States and that 14,000 Americans died of the disease. The decreased incidence in gastric cancer in the United States is also reflected worldwide. The incidence of gastric cancer varies widely among different countries, being comparatively high in Japan, China, Chile, and Ireland; however, a decrease in both incidence and mortality has occurred in these areas as well.

Epidemiologic surveys have suggested the risk of gastric cancer to be greater among lower socioeconomic classes. Furthermore, migrants from high- to low-incidence nations appear to maintain their susceptibility to gastric cancer, while the risk for their offspring more closely approximates that of the new homeland. These findings suggest that an environmental exposure, probably beginning early in life, is related to the development of gastric cancer, with dietary carcinogens considered the most likely factor(s).

Pathology Approximately 85 percent of stomach cancers are adenocarcinomas, with 15 percent due to non-Hodgkin's lymphomas and leiomyosarcomas. Gastric adenocarcinomas may be subdivided into two categories: a *diffuse type* in which cell cohesion is absent, so that individual cells infiltrate and thicken the stomach wall without forming a discrete mass; and an *intestinal type* characterized by cohesive neoplastic cells that form glandlike tubular structures. The diffuse carcinomas occur more often in younger patients, develop throughout the stomach, including the cardia, result in a loss of distensibility of the gastric wall (so-called linitis plastica or "leather bottle" appearance), and carry a far more ominous prognosis. Intestinal-type lesions are frequently ulcerative, more commonly appear in the antrum and lesser curvature of the stomach, and are often preceded by a prolonged precancerous process. While the incidence of diffuse carcinomas is similar in most populations, the intestinal type tends to predominate in the high-risk geographic regions mentioned earlier and is less likely to be found in areas where the frequency of gastric cancer is declining. Thus, different etiologic factor(s) may be involved in these two subtypes. In the United States, the distal stomach is the site of origin of about 30 percent of gastric cancers. Approximately 20 percent of these tumors arise in the midportion of the stomach, while upwards of 37 percent of gastric tumors now originate in the proximal third of the stomach. The remaining 13 percent of gastric carcinomas involve the entire stomach.

Etiology The relationship between dietary patterns and the development of gastric carcinoma has been investigated extensively. The long-term ingestion of high concentrations of nitrates in dried, smoked, and salted foods appears to be associated with a higher risk. The nitrates are thought to be converted to carcinogenic nitrites by bacteria (Table 92-2). Such bacteria may be introduced exogenously through the ingestion of partially decayed foods, which are consumed in abundance worldwide by the lower socioeconomic classes. Bacteria such as *Helicobacter pylori* may also contribute to this effect. Loss of gastric acidity may permit bacterial growth in the stomach. Loss of acidity may occur when acid-producing cells of the gastric antrum were removed surgically 15 to 20 years earlier in a partial gastrectomy performed to control benign peptic ulcer disease or when achlorhydria, atrophic gastritis, and even pernicious anemia develop in the elderly. Serial endoscopic examinations of the stomach in patients with atrophic gastritis have documented replacement of the usual gastric mucosa

Table 92-2

Nitrate-Converting Bacteria as a Factor in the Causation
of Gastric Carcinoma*

Exogenous sources of nitrate-converting bacteria:
  Bacterially contaminated food (common in lower socioeconomic classes,
    who have a higher incidence of the disease; diminished by improved
    food preservation and refrigeration)
  ? *Helicobacter pylori* infection
Endogenous factors favoring growth of nitrate-converting bacteria in the
  stomach:
  Decreased gastric acidity
  Prior gastric surgery (antrectomy) (15 to 20 year latency period)
  Atrophic gastritis and/or pernicious anemia
  ? Prolonged exposure to histamine H_2-receptor antagonists

* Hypothesis: Dietary nitrates are converted to carcinogenic nitrites by bacteria.

by intestinal-type cells. This process of intestinal metaplasia may lead
to cellular atypia and eventual neoplasia. Since the declining incidence
of gastric cancer in the United States primarily reflects a decline in
distal, ulcerating, intestinal-type lesions, it is conceivable that better
food preservation and the availability of refrigeration to all socioeconomic classes have decreased the dietary ingestion of exogenous bacteria. It remains uncertain whether the iatrogenic achlorhydria induced
by the widespread, prolonged use of histamine antagonists will result
in a future increase in intestinal-type gastric cancer.

Several additional etiologic factors have been associated with gastric carcinoma. Gastric ulcers and adenomatous polyps have occasionally been so linked, but data regarding a cause-and-effect relationship
are unconvincing. The inadequate clinical distinction between benign
gastric ulcers and small ulcerating carcinomas may, in part, account
for this presumed association. The presence of extreme hypertrophy
of gastric rugal folds (i.e., Menetrier's disease), giving the impression
of polypoid lesions, has been associated with a striking frequency
of malignant transformation; such hypertrophy, however, does not
represent the presence of true adenomatous polyps. Individuals with
blood group A have been reported to have a higher incidence of
gastric cancer than persons with blood group O; it is possible that this
observation is related to differences in the mucous secretion of the
various ABO blood groups, thereby leading to greater or lesser mucosal
protection from carcinogens. No association has been identified between duodenal ulcers and gastric cancer.

Clinical Features   Gastric cancers, when superficial and surgically curable, usually produce no symptoms. As the tumor becomes
more extensive, patients may complain of an insidious upper abdominal discomfort varying in intensity from a vague, postprandial fullness
to a severe, steady pain. Anorexia, often with slight nausea, is very
common but is not the usual presenting complaint. Weight loss may
eventually be observed, and nausea and vomiting are particularly
prominent with tumors of the pylorus; dysphagia may be the major
symptom caused by lesions of the cardia. There are no early physical
signs of the disease, and the finding of a palpable abdominal mass
generally indicates long-standing growth and regional extension.

Gastric carcinomas spread by direct extension through the gastric
wall to the perigastric tissues, occasionally adhering to adjacent organs
such as the pancreas, colon, or liver. The disease also spreads via
lymphatics or by seeding of peritoneal surfaces. Metastases to intraabdominal and supraclavicular lymph nodes occur frequently, as do
metastatic nodules to the ovary (Krukenberg's tumor), periumbilical
region ("Sister Mary Joseph node") or peritoneal cul-de-sac (Blumer's
shelf palpable on rectal or vaginal exam); malignant ascites may also
develop. The liver is the most common site for hematogenous spread
of tumor.

The presence of iron-deficiency anemia in men and of occult blood
in the stool in both sexes should mandate a search for an occult lesion
in the gastrointestinal tract. Such a careful assessment is of particular

importance in patients having atrophic gastritis or pernicious anemia.
Unusual clinical features associated with gastric adenocarcinomas include migratory thrombophlebitis, microangiopathic hemolytic anemia, and acanthosis nigricans.

Diagnosis   A double-contrast radiographic examination is the
simplest diagnostic procedure for the evaluation of a patient with
epigastric complaints. The use of double-contrast techniques helps to
detect small lesions by improving mucosal detail. The stomach should
be distended at some time during every radiographic examination,
since decreased distensibility may be the only indication of a diffuse
infiltrative carcinoma. Although gastric ulcers can be detected fairly
early, it may be impossible to distinguish benign from malignant
lesions. The anatomic location of an ulcer is not in itself an indication
of the presence or absence of a cancer.

Gastric ulcers that appear benign by radiography present special
problems. Some physicians believe that gastroscopy is not mandatory
if the radiographic features are typically benign, if complete healing
can be visualized by x-ray within 6 weeks, and if a follow-up contrast
radiograph obtained several months later shows a normal appearance.
However, we recommend gastroscopic biopsy and brush cytology for
all patients with a gastric ulcer in order to exclude a malignancy. It
is crucial to identify malignant gastric ulcers before they penetrate
into surrounding tissues, because the rate of cure of early lesions
limited to the mucosa or submucosa is greater than 80 percent. Since
gastric carcinomas are difficult to distinguish clinically or radiographically from gastric lymphomas, endoscopic biopsies should be
made as deep as possible, due to the submucosal location of lymphoid
tumors.

The staging system for gastric carcinoma is shown in Table 92-3.

 TREATMENT
Surgical removal of the complete tumor with resection of adjacent
lymph nodes offers the only chance for cure. However, this is possible in fewer than one-third of patients. In general, a subtotal gastrectomy is the treatment of choice for patients with distal carcinomas,
while total or near-total gastrectomies are required for more proximal
tumors. The prognosis following complete surgical resection depends on the degree of tumor penetration into the stomach wall and
is also adversely influenced by regional lymph node involvement,
vascular invasion, and abnormal DNA content (i.e., aneuploidy),
characteristics found in the vast majority of American patients. As
a result, the probability of survival after 5 years for the 25 to 30
percent of patients in the United States able to undergo a complete
resection of a gastric cancer is approximately 20 percent for distal
tumors and less than 10 percent for proximal tumors, with recurrences continuing to occur for at least 8 years after surgery. In the
absence of ascites or extensive hepatic or peritoneal metastases,
however, even patients whose disease is believed to be incurable
by surgery should be offered an attempt at resection of the primary
lesion, since reduction of tumor bulk is the best form of palliation
and may enhance the probability of benefit if chemotherapy and/or
radiation therapy are administered.

Gastric adenocarcinoma is a relatively radioresistant tumor, and
adequate control of the primary tumor requires doses of external
beam irradiation that exceed the tolerance of surrounding structures,
such as bowel mucosa and spinal cord. As a result, the major role
of radiation therapy in patients with gastric cancer has been limited
to palliation of pain. Radiation therapy alone after a complete resection does not prolong survival. In the setting of surgically unresectable disease limited to the epigastrium, patients treated with 3500
to 4000 cGy did not live longer than similar patients not receiving radiotherapy; however, survival was prolonged slightly when
5-fluorouracil (5-FU) was given in combination with radiation therapy. In this clinical setting, the 5-FU may well be functioning as
a radiosensitizer.

The administration of combinations of cytotoxic drugs to patients
with advanced gastric carcinoma has been associated with reductions
of greater than 50 percent in measurable tumor mass ("partial responses") in 30 to 50 percent of cases, providing significant benefit

to individuals who respond to treatment. Such drug combinations have generally included 5-FU and doxorubicin together with mitomycin-C, cisplatin, or high doses of methotrexate. Despite this encouraging response rate for a malignant condition once thought untreatable, complete disappearances of tumor masses remain uncommon; the partial responses are transient; and the overall impact of such multidrug therapy on survival has been a source of debate. The use of prophylactic (i.e., adjuvant) chemotherapy following the complete resection of a gastric cancer as a means of eradicating clinically undetectable micrometastases and improving the potential for cure has generally proven to be unsuccessful. The role of such adjuvant treatment as well as of preoperative ("neoadjuvant") chemotherapy should be considered investigational.

PRIMARY GASTRIC LYMPHOMA Primary lymphoma of the stomach is relatively uncommon, accounting for fewer than 15 percent of gastric malignancies and about 2 percent of all lymphomas. The stomach is, however, the most frequent extranodal location for lymphoma, and gastric lymphoma has appeared with increased frequency during the past 20 years. The disease is difficult to distinguish clinically from gastric adenocarcinoma; both tumors are most often detected during the sixth decade of life; present with epigastric pain, early satiety, and generalized fatigue; and are usually characterized by ulcerations with a ragged, thickened mucosal pattern demonstrated by contrast radiographs. The diagnosis of lymphoma of the stomach may occasionally be made through cytologic brushings of the gastric mucosa, but usually it requires a biopsy at the time of gastroscopy or laparotomy. Failure of gastroscopic biopsies to detect lymphoma in a given case should not be interpreted as being conclusive, since superficial biopsies may miss the deeper lymphoid infiltrate. The macroscopic pathology of gastric lymphoma may also mimic that of adenocarcinoma, consisting of either a bulky ulcerated lesion localized in the corpus or antrum or a diffuse process spreading throughout the entire gastric submucosa and even extending into the duodenum. Microscopically, the vast majority of gastric lymphoid tumors are non-Hodgkin's lymphomas of B cell origin; Hodgkin's disease involving the stomach is extremely uncommon. Histologically, these tumors may range from well-differentiated, superficial processes [mucosa-associated lymphoid tissue (MALT)] to high-grade, large cell lymphomas. Infection with *H. pylori*, the same bacterium associated with the development of gastric adenocarcinoma, appears to increase the risk for gastric lymphoma in general and MALT lymphomas in particular. Gastric lymphomas spread initially to regional lymph nodes (often to Waldeyer's ring) and may then disseminate. Gastric lymphomas are staged like other lymphomas (Chap. 113).

Previous concerns that the rapid destruction of lymphoma masses by chemotherapy might lead to life-threatening hemorrhage seem to have been eased by the results of clinical trials. Although radiation therapy to the abdomen has been employed in the past following surgical resection, this practice also has been questioned, because most recurrences develop at sites distant from the epigastrium and, consequently, outside the radiation treatment fields. If widespread disease is discovered at the time of laparotomy, combination chemotherapy should be used.

GASTRIC (NONLYMPHOID) SARCOMA Leiomyosarcomas are the most common of this group of gastric malignancies and make up approximately 1 to 3 percent of all gastric neoplasms. They most frequently involve the anterior and posterior walls of the gastric fundus and often ulcerate and bleed. Even those lesions that appear benign on histologic examination may behave in a malignant fashion. Leiomyosarcomas rarely invade adjacent viscera and characteristically do not metastasize to lymph nodes, but they may spread to the liver and lungs. The treatment of choice is surgical resection. Combination chemotherapy should be reserved for patients with metastatic disease.

COLORECTAL CANCER

INCIDENCE Cancer of the large bowel is second only to lung cancer as a cause of cancer death in the United States. Approximately 133,500 new cases occurred in 1996, resulting in 54,900 deaths. The incidence rate for this extremely common malignant condition has not changed substantially during the past 40 years, although, for some reason, the mortality rate has decreased in recent years, particularly in females. Colorectal cancer generally occurs in individuals 50 years of age or older.

POLYPS AND MOLECULAR PATHOGENESIS Most colorectal cancers, regardless of etiology, are believed to arise from adenomatous polyps. A polyp is a grossly visible protrusion from the mucosal surface and may be classified pathologically as a nonneoplastic hamartoma (*juvenile polyp*), a hyperplastic mucosal proliferation (*hyperplastic polyp*), or an adenomatous polyp. Only adenomas are clearly premalignant, and only a minority of such lesions ever develop into cancer. Population-screening studies and autopsy surveys have revealed that adenomatous polyps may be found in the colons of about 30 percent of middle-aged or elderly people. Based on this prevalence and the known incidence of colorectal cancers, it appears that fewer

℞ **TREATMENT**

Primary gastric lymphoma is a far more treatable disease than adenocarcinoma of the stomach, a fact that underscores the need for making the correct diagnosis. Antibiotic treatment to eradicate *H. pylori* infection has led to regression of about half of gastric MALT lymphomas and should be considered before surgery, radiation therapy, or chemotherapy are undertaken in patients having such tumors. Subtotal gastrectomy, usually followed by combination chemotherapy, has led to 5-year survival rates of 40 to 60 percent in patients with localized high-grade lymphomas. The need for this major surgical procedure has been questioned, particularly in patients with preoperative radiographic evidence of nodal involvement, for whom chemotherapy alone has been proposed as a substitution for resection.

Table 92-3

Staging System for Gastric Carcinoma

Stage	TNM	Features	Data from American College of Surgeons	
			Number of Cases, %	5-Year Survival, %
0	TisN0M0	Node negative; limited to mucosa	1	90
IA	T1N0M0	Node negative; invasion of lamina propria or submucosa	7	59
IB	T2N0M0	Node negative; invasion of muscularis propria	10	44
II	T1N2M0 T2N1M0	Node positive; invasion beyond mucosa but within wall *or*	17	29
	T3N0M0	Node negative; extension through wall		
IIIA	T2N2M0 T3N1-2M0	Node positive; invasion of muscularis propria or through wall	21	15
IIIB	T4N0-1M0	Node negative; adherence to surrounding tissue	14	9
IV	T4N2M0	Node positive; adherence to surrounding tissue *or*	30	3
	T1-4N0-2M1	Distant metastases		

than 1 percent of polyps ever become malignant. Most polyps produce no symptoms and remain clinically undetected. Occult blood in the stool may be found in fewer than 5 percent of patients with such lesions.

A number of molecular changes have been described in DNA obtained from adenomatous polyps, dysplastic lesions, and polyps containing microscopic foci of tumor cells (carcinoma in situ), which are thought to represent a multistep process in the evolution of normal colonic mucosa to life-threatening invasive carcinoma. These developmental steps towards carcinogenesis include point mutations in the K-ras proto-oncogene; hypomethylation of DNA, leading to gene activation; loss of DNA ("allelic loss") at the site of a tumor suppressor gene [the adenomatous polyposis coli (APC) gene] located on the long arm of chromosome 5 (5q21); allelic loss at the site of a tumor suppressor gene located on chromosome 18q [so-called the deleted in colorectal cancer (DCC) gene]; and allelic loss at chromosome 17p, associated with mutations in the p53 tumor suppressor gene (see Chap. 84). Thus, the altered proliferative pattern of the colonic mucosa, which results in progression to a polyp and then to carcinoma, may involve the mutational activation of an oncogene followed by and coupled with the loss of genes that normally suppress tumorigenesis. While the present model includes five such molecular alterations, others are likely involved in the carcinogenic process. It remains uncertain whether the genetic aberrations always occur in a defined order. Based on this model, however, it is believed that neoplasia develops only in those polyps in which all of these mutational events take place.

Clinically, the probability of an adenomatous polyp becoming a cancer depends on the gross appearance of the lesion, its histologic features, and its size. Adenomatous polyps may be pedunculated (stalked) or sessile (flat-based). Cancers develop more frequently in sessile polyps. Histologically, adenomatous polyps may be tubular, villous (i.e., papillary), or tubulovillous. Villous adenomas, most of which are sessile, become malignant more than three times as often as tubular adenomas. The likelihood that any polypoid lesion in the large bowel contains invasive cancer is related to the size of the polyp, being negligible (<2 percent) in lesions smaller than 1.5 cm, intermediate (2 to 10 percent) in lesions 1.5 to 2.5 cm in size, and substantial (10 percent) in lesions larger than 2.5 cm.

Following the detection of an adenomatous polyp, the entire large bowel should be visualized endoscopically or radiographically, since synchronous lesions are present in approximately one-third of cases. Colonoscopy should then be repeated periodically, even in the absence of a previously documented malignancy, since such patients have a 30 to 50 percent probability of developing another adenoma and are at a higher-than-average risk for developing a colorectal carcinoma. Adenomatous polyps are thought to require more than 5 years of growth before becoming clinically significant; the results of a randomized trial conducted by the National Polyp Study have indicated that colonoscopy need not be carried out more frequently than every 3 years.

ETIOLOGY AND RISK FACTORS Risk factors for the development of colorectal cancer are listed in Table 92-4.

Diet The etiology for most cases of large-bowel cancer appears to be related to environmental factors. The disease occurs more often in upper socioeconomic populations who live in urban areas. Epidemiologic studies in various countries have documented a direct correlation between mortality from colorectal cancer and per capita consumption of calories, meat protein, and dietary fat and oil as well as elevations in the serum cholesterol concentration and mortality from coronary artery disease. Any geographic variations in incidence do not appear to be related to genetic differences, since migrant groups tend to assume the large-bowel cancer incidence rates of their adopted countries. Furthermore, population groups such as Mormons and Seventh Day Adventists, whose lifestyle and dietary habits differ somewhat from those of their neighbors, have incidence and mortality rates for colorectal cancer that are significantly lower than expected, while the appearance of colorectal cancer has increased in Japan since that nation

Table 92-4

Risk Factors for the Development of Colorectal Cancer

Diet
   Animal fat
   ? Fiber
Hereditary syndromes (autosomal dominant inheritance)
   Polyposis coli
   Nonpolyposis syndrome (Lynch syndrome)
Inflammatory bowel disease
Streptococcus bovis bacteremia
Ureterosigmoidostomy
? Tobacco use

has adopted a more "western" diet. It is therefore assumed that dietary patterns influence the development of colorectal cancer. At least two hypotheses have been proposed to explain this relationship, neither of which is fully satisfactory.

Animal fats Based on the association of colorectal cancer with hypercholesterolemia and coronary artery disease as well as the increased incidence of large-bowel tumors in geographic areas where meat is a dietary staple, it has been suggested that the ingestion of animal fats leads to an increased proportion of anaerobes in the gut microflora, resulting in the conversion of normal bile acids into carcinogens. This provocative hypothesis is supported by several reports of increased amounts of fecal anaerobes in the stools of patients with colorectal cancer. Moreover, prospective cohort and case control studies in large numbers of people have revealed a consistently enhanced risk for the development of colorectal adenomas and carcinomas in association with elevated serum cholesterol levels and diets high in animal (but not vegetable) fat.

Fiber The observation that South African Bantus ingest a diet far higher in roughage, produce more frequent, bulkier stools, and have a lower incidence of large-bowel cancer than their American and European counterparts led to the proposal that the higher rate of colorectal cancer in western society is in large part the result of a low intake of dietary fiber. This theory suggests that dietary fiber accelerates intestinal transit time, thereby reducing the exposure of colonic mucosa to potential carcinogens and diluting these carcinogens because of enhanced fecal bulk. Such a proposition appears somewhat simplistic when subjected to careful scrutiny. Although an enhanced fiber intake increases fecal bulk, there has been no consistent evidence that a higher fiber intake consistently shortens the transit time of stool. In addition, despite the generally higher fiber intake in low-incidence countries, the environmental differences between developing and industrialized nations are myriad and include such other important dietary variables as meat and fat consumption. Finally, a diet low in fiber may lead to chronic constipation and such associated conditions as diverticulosis. If a low-fiber diet alone were a significant factor in colorectal cancer, individuals having diverticulosis should be at higher risk for the development of large-bowel tumors; this does not appear to be the case.

Thus, the weight of epidemiologic evidence clearly implicates diet as being the major etiologic factor for colorectal cancer. The available data strongly associate a high intake of animal fat with the development of large-bowel cancer.

HEREDITARY FACTORS AND SYNDROMES As many as 25 percent of patients with colorectal cancer may have a family history of the disease, suggesting a hereditary predisposition. Such inherited large-bowel cancers can be divided into two main groups: the well-studied but uncommon polyposis syndromes and the increasingly well-defined, more common nonpolyposis syndromes (Table 92-5).

Polyposis Coli Polyposis coli (familial polyposis of the colon) is a rare condition characterized by the appearance of thousands of adenomatous polyps throughout the large bowel. It is transmitted in an autosomal dominant manner; the occasional patients with no family history are thought to have developed the condition due to a spontaneous mutation. Molecular studies have associated polyposis coli with a deletion in the long arm of chromosome 5 (including the APC gene) in both neoplastic (somatic mutation) and normal (germline mutation) cells. It has been hypothesized that the loss of this genetic material (i.e., allelic loss) results in the absence of tumor suppressor genes whose protein products would normally inhibit neoplastic growth. The presence of soft tissue and bony tumors and of ampullary cancers in addition to the colonic polyps characterizes a subset of polyposis coli known as *Gardner's syndrome*, while the appearance of malignant tumors of the central nervous system accompanying polyposis coli defines *Turcot's syndrome*. The colonic polyps in all these conditions are rarely present before puberty but are generally evident in affected individuals by age 25. If the polyposis is not treated surgically, colorectal cancer will develop in almost all patients before age 40. Polyposis coli has been studied intensively and appears to result from a defect in the colonic mucosa leading to an abnormal proliferative pattern and an impaired ability for cellular repair following exposure to radiation or ultraviolet light. Once the multiple polyps that constitute polyposis coli are detected, patients should undergo a total colectomy. In the past it was unclear whether the optimal operative approach in such a clinical setting was to resect the entire colon and rectum, leaving a young patient with a permanent ileostomy, or to perform an ileoproctostomy. While the latter procedure retained the distal rectum and anal sphincter, it placed the patient at continued risk for the development of cancer in the rectal remnant and necessitated semiannual or annual proctoscopic surveillance. The development of the ileoanal anastomotic technique allows removal of the entire bowel while retaining the anal sphincter; this appears to be the best treatment. Medical therapy with nonsteroidal anti-inflammatory drugs such as sulindac has been reported to decrease the number and size of polyps in patients with polyposis coli; however, this effect on polyps is only temporary. Colectomy remains the primary therapy for patients with polyposis coli. The offspring of patients with polyposis coli, who often are prepubertal when the diagnosis is made in the parent, have a 50 percent risk for the eventual development of this premalignant disorder and should be carefully screened by annual flexible sigmoidoscopy until age 35. Such proctosigmoidoscopy is a sufficient screening procedure because polyps tend to be evenly distributed from cecum to anus, making more invasive and expensive techniques such as colonoscopy or barium enema unnecessary. Testing for occult blood in the stool is an inadequate screening maneuver. An alternative and still experimental method for identifying carriers of this inherited trait is testing DNA from peripheral blood mononuclear cells for the presence of a mutated APC gene. The detection of such a germline mutation can lead to a definitive diagnosis before the development of polyps.

Hereditary Nonpolyposis Colon Cancer Hereditary nonpolyposis colon cancer (HNPCC), also known as Lynch syndrome, is another condition inherited in an autosomal dominant manner. It has the following characteristics: the presence of three or more relatives with histologically documented colorectal cancer, one of whom is a first-degree relative of the other two; one or more cases of colorectal cancer diagnosed before age 50 in the family; and colorectal cancer involving at least two generations. In contrast to polyposis coli, HNPCC is associated with an unusually high frequency of cancer arising in the proximal large bowel. The median age for the appearance of an adenocarcinoma is under 50 years, which is 10 to 15 years younger than the median age for the general population. Families with HNPCC often include individuals with multiple primary cancers; the association of colorectal cancer with either ovarian or endometrial carcinomas is especially strong in women. It has been recommended that members of such families undergo biennial colonoscopy beginning at age 25 years with in-

termittent pelvic ultrasonography and endometrial biopsy offered to potentially afflicted women; such a screening strategy has not yet been validated. HNPCC is associated with germline mutations of several genes, particularly *hMSH2* on chromosome 2 and *hMLH1* on chromosome 3. These mutations lead to errors in DNA replication and are thought to result in DNA instability because of defective repair of DNA mismatches, resulting in abnormal cell growth and tumor development.

INFLAMMATORY BOWEL DISEASE (See also Chap. 286) Large-bowel cancer represents a not infrequent complication in patients with long-standing inflammatory bowel disease. Neoplasms appear to develop more commonly in patients with ulcerative colitis than in those with granulomatous colitis, but this impression may result in part from the occasional difficulty of differentiating these two conditions. The risk of colorectal cancer in a patient with inflammatory bowel disease is relatively small during the initial 10 years of the disease, but then it appears to increase at a rate of approximately 0.5 to 1.0 percent per year. Actuarially derived cumulative cancer rates in such symptomatic patients have ranged from 8 to 30 percent after 25 years. The risk is generally considered to be higher in younger patients with pancolitis.

Cancer surveillance in patients with inflammatory bowel disease is unsatisfactory. Symptoms such as bloody diarrhea, abdominal cramping, and obstruction, which may signal the appearance of a tumor, are similar to the complaints caused by a flare-up of the underlying disease. In patients with a history of inflammatory bowel disease lasting 15 years or more who continue to experience exacerbations, the surgical removal of the colon can significantly reduce the risk for cancer and also eliminate the target organ for the underlying chronic gastrointestinal disorder. The value of such surveillance techniques as colonoscopy with mucosal biopsies and brushings for less symptomatic individuals with chronic inflammatory bowel disease is uncertain. The purpose of such procedures has been the identification of premalignant mucosal dysplasia, thereby justifying surgical intervention. The lack of uniformity regarding the pathologic criteria that characterize dysplasia and the absence of data that such surveillance reduces the development of lethal cancers, however, has made this costly practice an area of controversy.

OTHER HIGH-RISK CONDITIONS *Streptococcus bovis Bacteremia* For unknown reasons, individuals who develop endocarditis or septicemia from this fecal bacteria seem to have a high incidence of occult colorectal tumors and, possibly, upper gastrointestinal cancers as well. Endoscopic or radiographic screening appears advisable.

Table 92-5

Hereditable (Autosomal Dominant) Gastrointestinal Polyposis Syndromes

Syndrome	Distribution of Polyps	Histologic Type	Malignant Potential	Associated Lesions
Familial colonic polyposis	Large intestine	Adenoma	Common	None
Gardner's syndrome	Large and small intestine	Adenoma	Common	Osteomas, fibromas, lipomas, epidermoid cysts, ampullary cancers
Turcot's syndrome	Large intestine	Adenoma	Common	Brain tumors
Nonpolyposis syndrome (Lynch syndrome)	Large intestine (often proximal)	Adenoma	Common	Endometrial and ovarian tumors
Peutz-Jeghers syndrome	Small and large intestines, stomach	Hamartoma	Rare	Mucocutaneous pigmentation; tumors of the ovary, breast, pancreas, endometrium
Juvenile polyposis	Large and small intestines, stomach	Hamartoma, rarely progressing to adenoma	Rare	Various congenital abnormalities

Ureterosigmoidostomy There is a 5 to 10 percent incidence of colon cancer 15 to 30 years after ureterosigmoidostomy to correct congenital extrophy of the bladder. Neoplasms characteristically are found at a site distal to the ureteral implant where colonic mucosa is chronically exposed to both urine and feces.

Tobacco Use Prospective cohort studies have linked cigarette smoking to the development of colorectal adenomas, particularly after more than 35 years of tobacco use. No biologic explanation for this association has yet been proposed.

PRIMARY PREVENTION Several orally administered synthetic and naturally occurring materials have been assessed as possible inhibitors of colon cancer. The most effective class of these chemopreventive agents is aspirin and other nonsteroidal anti-inflammatory drugs, which are thought to suppress cell proliferation by inhibiting prostaglandin synthesis. Case-control studies have indicated that regular aspirin use reduces the risk for colonic adenomas and carcinomas as well as for death from large-bowel cancer; this inhibiting effect on colonic carcinogenesis appears to increase with the duration of drug use. While antioxidant vitamins such as ascorbic acid, tocopherols, and β-carotene are present in diets rich in fruits and vegetables, which have been associated with lower rates of colorectal cancer, they have been found to be ineffective in a prospectively randomized trial as a means of reducing the incidence of subsequent adenomas in patients who had undergone the removal of a colonic adenoma. Estrogen replacement therapy has been associated in prospective cohort studies with a reduction in the risk of colorectal cancer in women, conceivably by an effect on bile acid synthesis and composition. Possibly the otherwise unexplained reduction in colorectal cancer mortality in women may be a result of the widespread use of estrogen replacement in postmenopausal individuals. Oral calcium supplements have also been noted to inhibit colon epithelial cell proliferation, but efficacy in cancer prevention has not been proven.

SCREENING The rationale for colorectal cancer screening programs is that the earlier detection of localized, superficial neoplasms in asymptomatic individuals will increase the surgical cure rate. Such screening programs appear to be especially indicated for individuals having a family history of the disease in first-degree relatives. The relative risk for developing colorectal cancer increases to 1.75 in such people and may be even higher if the relative was afflicted before 60 years of age. Screening strategies have been based on the assumption that more than 60 percent of early lesions are located in the rectosigmoid, making them accessible to rigid proctosigmoidoscopy. For unexplained reasons, however, there has been a consistent decrease during the past several decades in the proportion of large-bowel cancers arising in the rectum, with a corresponding increase in the proportion of cancers in the more proximal descending colon. As such, the potential for rigid proctosigmoidoscopy to detect a sufficient number of occult neoplasms to make the procedure cost-effective has been questioned. Nonetheless, in support of periodic rigid proctosigmoidoscopic examination is a case-control study reporting a reduction in mortality from distal large bowel cancer in individuals who had undergone such screening. The availability of flexible, fiberoptic sigmoidoscopes, permitting trained operators to visualize the colon for up to 60 cm, should further enhance cancer detection and resolve this issue.

Most programs directed at the early detection of colorectal cancers have focused on digital rectal examinations and testing stool for the presence of occult blood. The digital examination should be part of any routine physical evaluation in adults older than age 40, serving as a screening test for prostate cancer in men, a component of the pelvic examination in women, and an inexpensive maneuver for the detection of masses in the rectum. The development of the Hemoccult test has greatly facilitated the detection of occult fecal blood. Unfortunately, even when performed optimally, the Hemoccult test has major limitations as a screening technique. Approximately 50 percent of patients with documented colorectal cancers have a negative fecal Hemoccult test, consistent with the intermittent bleeding pattern of these tumors. When random cohorts of asymptomatic persons have been tested, 2 to 4 percent have Hemoccult-positive stools. Colorectal cancers have been found in only 5 to 10 percent of these "test-positive" cases, with benign polyps being detected in an additional 20 to 30 percent. Consequently, a colorectal neoplasm will not be found in most asymptomatic individuals with occult blood in their stool. Nonetheless, persons found to have Hemoccult-positive stool routinely undergo further medical evaluation, which includes sigmoidoscopy, barium enema, and/or colonoscopy—procedures that not only are uncomfortable and expensive but also are associated with a low but finite risk for significant complications. The added cost of these studies would appear justifiable if the small number of patients found to have occult neoplasms because of Hemoccult screening could be shown to have an improved prognosis and prolonged survival. Prospectively controlled trials addressing this issue are in progress. One of these studies, conducted at the University of Minnesota and involving more than 46,000 participants, reported a statistically significant reduction in mortality from colorectal cancer for individuals undergoing annual screening. However, this benefit only emerged after more than 13 years of follow-up and was extremely expensive to achieve, since all positive tests (most of which were false-positive) were followed by colonoscopy. Moreover, these colonoscopic examinations may have represented "chance selection" for more effective endoscopic screening and may also have provided the opportunity for cancer prevention through the removal of potentially premalignant adenomatous polyps.

Screening techniques for large-bowel cancer in asymptomatic persons remain unsatisfactory. Recommendations from governmental and private agencies are conflicting. At present, the American Cancer Society suggests annual digital rectal examinations beginning at age 40, annual fecal Hemoccult screening beginning at age 50, and sigmoidoscopy (preferably flexible) every 3 to 5 years beginning at age 50 for asymptomatic individuals having none of the high-risk factors for colorectal cancer. The use of colonscopy for screening has not yet been systematically examined. More effective techniques for screening are needed, perhaps taking advantage of the molecular changes that have been described in these tumors. An analysis for specific *ras* proto-oncogene mutations from DNA recovered from stool in patients with a history of colorectal cancer represents an initial step in this direction.

CLINICAL FEATURES **Presenting Symptoms** Symptoms vary with the anatomic location of the tumor.

Since stool is relatively liquid as it passes through the ileocecal valve into the right colon, neoplasms arising in the cecum and ascending colon may become quite large, significantly narrowing the bowel lumen, without resulting in any obstructive symptoms or noticeable alterations in bowel habits. Lesions of the right colon commonly ulcerate, leading to chronic, insidious blood loss without a change in the appearance of the stool. Consequently, patients with tumors of the ascending colon often present with symptoms such as fatigue, palpitations, and even angina pectoris and are found to have a hypochromic, microcytic anemia indicative of iron deficiency. Since the cancer may bleed intermittently, however, a random test for the presence of occult blood in the stool may be negative. As a result, the unexplained presence of iron-deficiency anemia in any adult (with the possible exception of a premenopausal, multiparous woman) mandates a thorough endoscopic and/or radiographic visualization of the entire large bowel (Fig. 92-1). For unknown reasons, blacks have a higher incidence of right colon lesions than do whites.

Since stool becomes more concentrated as it passes into the transverse and descending colon, tumors arising there tend to impede the passage of stool, resulting in the development of abdominal cramping, occasional obstruction, and even perforation. Radiographs of the abdomen often reveal characteristic annular, constricting lesions ("apple-core" or "napkin-ring") (Fig. 92-2).

Neoplasms arising in the rectosigmoid often are associated with hematochezia, tenesmus, and narrowing of the caliber of stool; nonetheless, anemia is an infrequent finding. While these symptoms may lead patients and their physicians to suspect the presence of hemorrhoids, the development of rectal bleeding and/or altered bowel habits

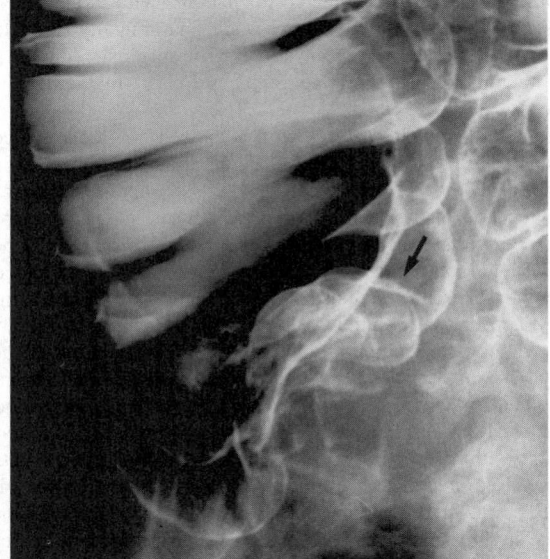

FIGURE 92-1 Double-contrast air-barium enema revealing a sessile tumor of the cecum in a patient with iron-deficiency anemia and guaiac-positive stool. The lesion at surgery was a stage B adenocarcinoma.

demands a prompt digital rectal examination and proctosigmoidoscopy.

Staging, Prognostic Factors, and Patterns of Spread The prognosis for individuals having colorectal cancer is closely related to the depth of tumor penetration into the bowel wall and the presence of both regional lymph node involvement and distant metastases. These variables are incorporated into the staging system introduced by Dukes and recently applied to a TNM classification method, in which T represents the depth of tumor penetration, N the presence of lymph

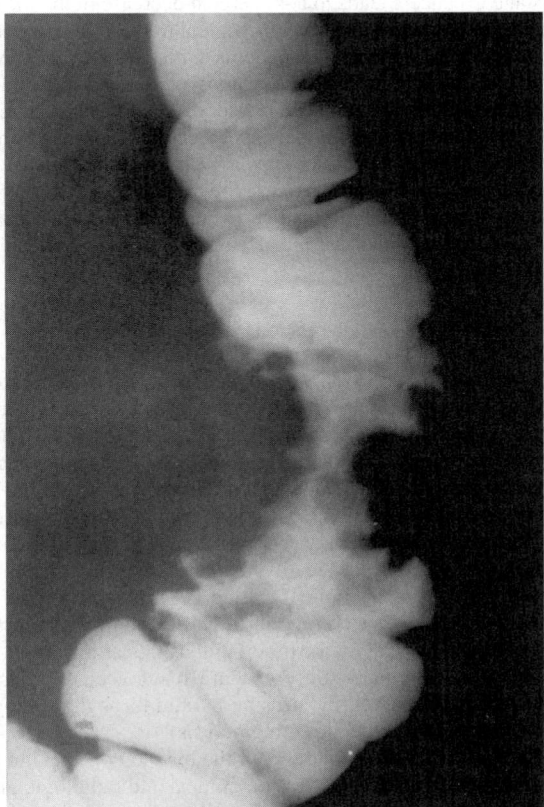

FIGURE 92-2 Annular, constricting adenocarcinoma of the descending colon. This radiographic appearance is referred to as an "apple-core" lesion and is always highly suggestive of malignancy.

node involvement, and M the presence or absence of distant metastases (Table 92-6). Patients with superficial lesions that do not penetrate into the muscularis or involve regional lymph nodes are designated as having *stage A* (T1N0M0) disease; patients whose tumors have penetrated more deeply but have not spread to lymph nodes have *stage B* disease [subclassified as *stage B₁* (T2N0M0) if lesions are restricted to the muscularis and as *stage B₂* (T3N0M0) if lesions involve or penetrate the serosa]; regional lymph node involvement defines *stage C* (TxN1M0) disease; and metastatic spread to sites such as liver, lung, or bone indicates *stage D* (TxNxM1) disease. Unless gross evidence of metastatic disease is present, it is impossible to accurately determine disease stage before surgical resection and pathologic analysis of the operative specimens.

Most recurrences after a surgical resection of a large-bowel cancer occur within the first 4 postoperative years, making the 5-year mark a fairly reliable indicator of cure. The likelihood for 5-year survival in patients with colorectal cancer is closely associated with their stage (Table 92-6). That likelihood has appeared to improve during the past several decades when similar surgical stages have been compared. The most plausible explanation for this improvement appears to be more thorough intraoperative and pathologic staging. In particular, more exacting attention to pathologic detail has revealed that the prognosis following the resection of a colorectal cancer is not related merely to the presence or absence of regional lymph node involvement but may be more precisely assessed by the number of involved lymph nodes (one to four lymph nodes versus five or more lymph nodes). Other predictors of a poor prognosis after a total surgical resection include tumor penetration through the bowel wall into pericolic fat, poorly differentiated histology, perforation and/or tumor adherence to adjacent organs (increasing the risk for an anatomically adjacent recurrence), and venous invasion by tumor (Table 92-7). Regardless of the clinicopathologic stage, a preoperative elevation of the plasma carcinoembryonic antigen (CEA) titer is suggestive of eventual tumor recurrence. The presence of an abnormal DNA content (i.e., aneuploidy) and specific chromosomal deletions, such as allelic loss in chromosome 18q (involving the DCC gene) in tumor cells, appears to predict a higher risk for metastatic spread, particularly in patients with stage B₂ (T3N0M0) disease. In contrast to most other carcinomas and sarcomas, the prognosis in individuals with colorectal cancer is not influenced by the size of the primary lesion when adjusted for nodal involvement and histologic differentiation.

Cancers of the large bowel generally spread to regional lymph nodes or to the liver via the portal venous circulation. The liver represents the most frequent visceral site of metastatic dissemination; it is the initial site of distant spread in one-third of recurring colorectal cancers and has become involved in more than two-thirds of such patients at the time of death. In general, colorectal cancer rarely metastasizes to the lungs, supraclavicular lymph nodes, bone, or brain without prior spread to the liver. A major exception to this rule occurs in

Table 92-6

Staging of and Prognosis for Colorectal Cancer

| Stage | | | | Approximate 5-Year |
Dukes	TNM	Numerical	Pathologic Description	Survival, %
A	T1N0M0	I	Cancer limited to mucosa and submucosa	>90
B₁	T2N0M0	II	Cancer extends into muscularis	85
B₂	T3N0M0	II	Cancer extends into or through serosa	70–80
C	TxN1M0	III	Cancer involves regional lymph nodes	35–65
D	TxNxM1	IV	Distant metastases (i.e. liver, lung, etc.)	5

Table 92-7

Predictors of Poor Outcome Following Total Surgical Resection
of Colorectal Cancer

Tumor spread to regional lymph nodes
Number of regional lymph nodes involved
Tumor penetration through the bowel wall
Poorly differentiated histology
Perforation
Tumor adherence to adjacent organs
Venous invasion
Preoperative elevation of CEA titer (>5.0 ng/mL)
Aneuploidy
Specific chromosomal deletion (e.g., allelic loss on chromosome 18q)

patients having primary tumors in the distal rectum, from which tumor cells may spread through the paravertebral venous plexus, escaping the portal venous system and thereby reaching the lungs or supraclavicular lymph nodes without hepatic involvement. The median survival after the detection of distant metastases may range from 6 to 9 months (hepatomegaly, liver abnormalities) to 24 to 30 months (small liver nodule initially identified by elevated CEA level and subsequent CT scan).

℞ TREATMENT

Total resection of tumor is the optimal treatment when a malignant lesion is detected endoscopically or radiographically in the large bowel. An evaluation for the presence of metastatic disease, including a thorough physical examination, a chest radiograph, biochemical assessment of liver function, and measurement of the plasma CEA level, should be performed before surgery. When possible, a colonoscopy of the entire large bowel should be performed to identify synchronous neoplasms and/or polyps. The detection of metastases should not preclude surgery in patients with tumor-related symptoms such as gastrointestinal bleeding or obstruction, but it often prompts the use of a less radical operative procedure. At the time of laparotomy, the entire peritoneal cavity should be examined, with thorough inspection of the liver, pelvis, and hemidiaphragm and careful palpation of the full length of the large bowel. Following recovery from a complete resection, patients should be observed carefully for 5 years by semiannual physical examinations and yearly blood chemistry measurements. If a complete colonoscopy was not performed preoperatively, it should be carried out within the first several postoperative months. Some authorities favor measuring plasma CEA levels at 3-month intervals because of the sensitivity of this test as a marker for otherwise undetectable tumor recurrence. Subsequent endoscopic or radiographic surveillance of the large bowel, probably at triennial intervals, is indicated, since patients who have been cured of one colorectal cancer have a 3 to 5 percent probability of developing an additional bowel cancer during their lifetime and a risk in excess of 15 percent for the development of adenomatous polyps. Anastomotic ("suture-line") recurrences are infrequent in colorectal cancer patients provided the surgical resection margins were adequate and free of tumor.

Radiation therapy to the pelvis is generally recommended for patients with rectal cancer because of the 30 to 40 percent probability of regional recurrences following complete surgical resection of stage B or C tumors, especially if they have penetrated through the serosa. This alarmingly high rate of local disease recurrence is believed to be due to the fact that the contained anatomic space within the pelvis limits the extent of the resection and because the rich lymphatic network of the pelvic side wall immediately adjacent to the rectum facilitates the early spread of malignant cells into surgically inaccessible tissue. The prophylactic use of radiation therapy, either pre- or postoperatively, reduces the likelihood of pelvic recurrences but does not appear to prolong survival. Preoperative

radiotherapy is clearly indicated for patients with large, potentially unresectable rectal cancers, since such anatomically fixed lesions may shrink enough to permit subsequent surgical removal. Radiation therapy is not effective in the primary treatment of colon cancer.

Chemotherapy in patients with advanced colorectal cancer has proven to be of only marginal benefit. Since its introduction into clinical trials more than 30 years ago, 5-FU remains the most effective agent for this disease. It is as useful when given alone as when combined with other drugs, but its use has only a 15 to 20 percent likelihood of reducing measurable tumor mass by 50 percent or more (i.e., a partial response). While the probability of tumor response appears to be somewhat greater for patients with liver metastases when such chemotherapy is infused directly into the hepatic artery as compared to a peripheral vein, intraarterial treatment is costly and toxic and does not appear to prolong survival. The concomitant administration of folinic acid (also known as leucovorin or citrovorum factor) improves the efficacy of 5-FU in patients with advanced colorectal cancer, presumably by enhancing the binding of 5-FU to its target enzyme, thymidylate synthase, thereby increasing the suppression of DNA synthesis and accompanying cytotoxicity. A threefold improvement in the likelihood of partial response is noted when folinic acid is combined with 5-FU; however, the effect on survival appears to be marginal and the optimal dose schedule remains to be defined.

Patients with solitary hepatic metastases without clinical or radiographic evidence of additional tumor involvement should be considered for partial liver resection, because such procedures are associated with 5-year survival rates of 25 to 30 percent when performed on selected individuals by experienced surgeons.

The value of postoperative chemotherapy and/or radiation therapy has been assessed in patients with stage B or C cancers as a means of eradicating clinically undetectable micrometastases and thereby increasing the probability of cure. The administration of adjuvant 5-FU with the anthelmintic agent levamisole to patients with stage C cancers leads to a 40 percent decrease in the likelihood of recurrence and to a modest improvement in survival. No statistical benefit has been observed in patients with stage B_2 tumors. The levamisole is thought to act as a nonspecific immunomodulator. Comparisons of 5-FU and levamisole with 5-FU and folinic acid are in progress. In rectal cancer, postoperative radiation therapy, when combined with chemotherapy, appears to reduce the likelihood of regional recurrences and increase the chance of cure. The chemotherapy acts as a radiation sensitizer when given to individuals who have been operated on for rectal cancer, enhancing the biologic effect of the radiotherapy.

TUMORS OF THE SMALL INTESTINE

Small-bowel tumors make up only 3 to 6 percent of gastrointestinal neoplasms. Because of their rarity, a correct diagnosis is often delayed. Abdominal symptoms are usually vague and poorly defined, and conventional radiographic studies of the upper and lower intestinal tract often appear normal. Small-bowel tumors should be considered in the differential diagnosis in the following situations: (1) recurrent, unexplained episodes of crampy abdominal pain; (2) intermittent bouts of intestinal obstruction, especially in the absence of inflammatory bowel disease or prior abdominal surgery; (3) intussusception in the adult; and (4) evidence of chronic intestinal bleeding in the presence of negative conventional contrast radiographs. A careful small-bowel barium study is the diagnostic procedure of choice; the diagnostic accuracy may be improved by infusing barium through a nasogastric tube placed into the duodenum (enteroclysis).

BENIGN TUMORS In general, the histology of benign small-bowel tumors is difficult to predict on clinical and radiologic grounds alone. The symptomatology of benign tumors is not distinctive, with pain, obstruction, and hemorrhage being the most frequent symptoms. These tumors are usually discovered during the fifth and sixth decades of life, more often in the distal rather than the proximal small intestine.

The most common benign tumors are adenomas, leiomyomas, lipomas, and angiomas.

Adenomas These tumors include those of the islet cells and Brunner's glands as well as polypoid adenomas. *Islet cell adenomas* are occasionally located outside the pancreas; the associated syndromes are discussed in Chap. 95. *Brunner's gland adenomas* are not truly neoplastic but represent a hypertrophy or hyperplasia of submucosal duodenal glands. These appear as small nodules in the duodenal mucosa that secrete a highly viscous alkaline mucus. Most often, this is an incidental radiographic finding not associated with any specific clinical disorder.

Polypoid Adenomas Approximately 25 percent of benign small-bowel tumors are polypoid adenomas (see Table 92-5). They may present as single polypoid lesions or, less commonly, as papillary villous adenomas. As in the colon, the sessile or papillary form of the tumor is sometimes associated with a coexisting carcinoma. Occasionally, patients with Gardner's syndrome (a variant of polyposis coli) develop premalignant adenomas in the small bowel; such lesions are generally in the duodenum. Multiple polypoid tumors may occur throughout the small bowel (and occasionally the stomach and colorectum) in the Peutz-Jeghers syndrome. The polyps are usually hamartomas (juvenile polyps) having a low potential for malignant degeneration. Mucocutaneous melanin deposits as well as tumors of the ovary, breast, pancreas, and endometrium are also associated with this autosomal dominant condition.

Leiomyomas These neoplasms arise from smooth-muscle components of the intestine and are usually intramural, affecting the overlying mucosa. Ulceration of the mucosa may cause gastrointestinal hemorrhage of varying severity. Cramping, intermittent abdominal pain is frequently encountered.

Lipomas These tumors occur with greatest frequency in the distal ileum and at the ileocecal valve. They have a characteristic radiolucent appearance, are usually intramural and asymptomatic, but on occasion are associated with bleeding.

Angiomas While not true neoplasms, these lesions are important because they frequently cause intestinal bleeding. They may take the form of telangiectasia or hemangiomas. Multiple intestinal telangiectasias occur in a nonhereditary form confined to the gastrointestinal tract or as part of the hereditary Osler-Rendu-Weber syndrome. Vascular tumors may also take the form of isolated hemangiomas, most commonly in the jejunum. Angiography, especially during bleeding, is the procedure of choice in the evaluation of these lesions.

MALIGNANT TUMORS While rare, small-bowel malignancies occur in patients with long-standing regional enteritis and celiac sprue as well as in individuals with AIDS. In contrast to benign tumors, malignant tumors of the small bowel are frequently associated with fever, weight loss, anorexia, bleeding, and a palpable abdominal mass. After ampullary carcinomas (many of which arise from biliary or pancreatic ducts), the most frequently occurring small-bowel malignancies are adenocarcinomas, lymphomas, carcinoid tumors, and leiomyosarcomas.

Adenocarcinomas The most common primary cancers of the small bowel are adenocarcinomas, which account for about 50 percent of the malignant tumors. These neoplasms occur most often in the distal duodenum and proximal jejunum, where they tend to ulcerate and cause hemorrhage or obstruction. Radiologically, they may be confused with chronic duodenal ulcer disease or with Crohn's disease if the patient has long-standing regional enteritis. The diagnosis is best made by endoscopy and biopsy under direct vision. Surgical resection is the treatment of choice.

Lymphomas Lymphomatous involvement of the small bowel may be primary or secondary. A diagnosis of a primary intestinal lymphoma requires histologic confirmation in a clinical setting in which palpable adenopathy and hepatosplenomegaly are absent and there is no evidence of lymphoma on a chest radiograph, CT scan, or peripheral blood smear or on bone marrow aspiration and biopsy. In general, symptoms referable to the small bowel are present, usually accompanied by an anatomically discernible lesion. Secondary lymphoma of the small bowel consists of involvement of the intestine by

a lymphoid malignancy extending from involved retroperitoneal or mesenteric lymph nodes and hence is a manifestation of a generalized systemic neoplasm (see Chap. 113).

Primary intestinal lymphoma accounts for about 20 percent of malignancies of the small bowel. Essentially all these neoplasms are non-Hodgkin's lymphomas; they usually have a diffuse, large cell histology and usually are of T cell origin. Intestinal lymphoma involves the ileum more frequently than the jejunum, which, in turn, is more commonly affected than the duodenum, a pattern that mirrors the relative amount of normal lymphoid cells in these anatomic areas. The risk of small-bowel lymphoma is increased in patients with a prior history of malabsorptive conditions (e.g., celiac sprue), regional enteritis, and depressed immune function due to congenital immunodeficiency syndromes, prior organ transplantation, autoimmune disorders, or AIDS.

The development of localized or nodular masses that narrow the lumen results in periumbilical pain (made worse by eating) as well as weight loss, vomiting, and occasional intestinal obstruction. The diagnosis of small-bowel lymphoma may be suspected from the appearance on contrast radiographs of patterns such as infiltration and thickening of mucosal folds, mucosal nodules, areas of irregular ulceration, or stasis of contrast material. The diagnosis can be confirmed by surgical exploration and resection of involved segments. Intestinal lymphoma occasionally can be diagnosed by peroral intestinal mucosal biopsy, but since the disease mainly involves the lamina propria, full-thickness surgical biopsies are usually required.

Resection of the tumor constitutes the initial treatment modality. While postoperative radiation therapy has been given to some patients following such a total resection, most authorities favor short-term systemic treatment with combination chemotherapy. The frequent presence of widespread intraabdominal disease at the time of diagnosis and the occasional multicentricity of the tumor often make a total resection impossible. The probability of sustained remission or cure is approximately 75 percent in patients with localized disease but is 25 percent or less in individuals with unresectable lymphoma. In patients whose tumors are not resected, chemotherapy may lead to bowel perforation.

A unique form of small-bowel lymphoma, diffusely involving the entire intestine, was first described in oriental Jews and Arabs and is referred to as *immunoproliferative small intestinal disease* (IPSID), *Mediterranean lymphoma,* or *α-heavy chain disease*. This is a B cell tumor. The typical presentation includes chronic diarrhea and steatorrhea associated with vomiting and abdominal cramps; clubbing of the digits may be observed as well. A curious feature in many patients with IPSID is the presence in the blood and intestinal secretions of an abnormal IgA that contains a shortened α-heavy chain and is devoid of light chains. It is suspected that the abnormal α chains are produced by plasma cells infiltrating the small bowel. The clinical course of patients with IPSID is generally one of exacerbations and remissions, with death frequently resulting from either progressive malnutrition and wasting or the development of an aggressive lymphoma. The use of oral antibiotics such as tetracycline appears to be beneficial in the early phases of the disorder, suggesting a possible infectious etiology. Combination chemotherapy has been administered during later stages of the disease, with variable results. Results are better when antibiotics and chemotherapy are combined.

Carcinoid Tumors Among the more common epithelial tumors of the small intestine are carcinoid tumors. They arise from argentaffin cells of the crypts of Lieberkühn and are found from the distal duodenum to the ascending colon, areas embryologically derived from the midgut. More than 50 percent of intestinal carcinoids are found in the distal ileum, with most congregating close to the ileocecal valve. Most intestinal carcinoids are asymptomatic and of low malignant potential, but invasion and metastases may occur, leading to the carcinoid syndrome (Chap. 95).

Leiomyosarcomas Large, bulky tumors, leiomyosarcomas often are more than 5 cm in diameter and may be palpable on abdominal examination. Bleeding, obstruction, and perforation are common.

CANCERS OF THE ANUS

Cancers of the anus account for 1 to 2 percent of the malignant tumors of the large bowel. Most such lesions arise in the anal canal, which is defined as the anatomic area extending from the anorectal ring to a zone approximately halfway between the pectinate (or dentate) line and the anal verge. Carcinomas arising proximal to the pectinate line (i.e., in the transitional zone between the glandular mucosa of the rectum and the squamous epithelium of the distal anus) are known as basaloid, cuboidal, or cloacogenic tumors; approximately one-third of anal cancers have this histologic pattern. Malignancies arising distal to the pectinate line have a squamous cell histology, ulcerate more frequently, and constitute approximately 55 percent of anal cancers. The prognosis for patients with basaloid and squamous cell cancers of the anus is identical when corrected for tumor size and the presence or absence of nodal spread.

Anal cancers occur most commonly in individuals with a prior history of chronic anal irritation. Such irritation may result from condylomata accuminata (viral lesions thought to be caused by papillomavirus infection), perianal fissures and/or fistulas, chronic hemorrhoids, and leukoplakia. The risk for anal cancer appears to be increased among homosexual males, presumably relating to trauma from anal intercourse. The likelihood of developing anal cancers is also enhanced in both men and women with AIDS, possibly because their immunocompromised condition makes them more susceptible to papillomavirus infection. Anal cancers occur most commonly in middle-aged individuals, develop more frequently in women than men, and at the time of diagnosis are most often associated with bleeding, pain, the sensation of a perianal mass, and perianal pruritus.

Until recently, radical surgery (abdominal-perineal resection with lymph node sampling and a permanent colostomy) was the treatment of choice for this tumor type. The 5-year survival rate after such a procedure ranged from 55 to 70 percent in the absence of spread to regional lymph nodes and was less than 20 percent if nodal involvement was present. However, an alternative therapeutic approach combining external beam radiation therapy with concomitant chemotherapy has resulted in biopsy-proven disappearance of all tumor in more than 80 percent of patients whose initial lesion was less than 3 cm in size. Tumor has recurred in fewer than 10 percent of these patients. Thus, it appears that approximately 70 percent of patients with anal cancers can be cured with nonoperative treatment and that disfiguring surgery should be reserved for the minority of individuals who are found to have residual tumor after being managed initially with radiation therapy combined with chemotherapy.

BIBLIOGRAPHY

BLOT WJ: Esophageal cancer trends and risk factors. Semin Oncol 21:403, 1994

FLAM M et al: Role of mitomycin in combination with fluorouracil and radiotherapy, and of salvage chemoradiation in the definitive nonsurgical treatment of epidermoid carcinoma of the anal canal: Results of a phase III randomized intergroup study. J Clin Oncol 14:2527, 1996

FUCHS CS et al: A prospective study of family history and the risk of colorectal cancer. N Engl J Med 331:1669, 1994

———, MAYER RJ: Gastric carcinoma. N Engl J Med 333:32, 1995.

HAMILTON SR: The molecular genetics of colorectal neoplasia. Gastroenterology 105:3, 1993

HANSSON LE et al: The risk of stomach cancer in patients with gastric or duodenal ulcer disease. N Engl J Med 335:242, 1996

LYNCH HT, SMYRK T: Hereditary nonpolyposis colorectal cancer (Lynch syndrome). An updated review. Cancer 78:1149, 1996

MELBYE M et al: High incidence of anal cancer among AIDS patients. Lancet 343:636, 1994

MOERTEL CG et al: Fluorouracil plus levamisole as effective adjuvant therapy after resection of stage III colon carcinoma: A final report. Ann Intern Med 122:321, 1995

TORIBARA NW, SLEISENGER MH: Screening for colorectal cancer. N Engl J Med 332:861, 1995

WALSH TN et al: A comparison of multimodal therapy and surgery for esophageal carcinoma. N Engl J Med 335:462, 1996

WOTHERSPOON AC et al: Regression of primary low-grade B-cell gastric lymphoma of mucosa-associated lymphoid tissue after eradication of *Helicobacter pylori*. Lancet 342:575, 1993

---

93   *Kurt J. Isselbacher, Jules L. Dienstag*

TUMORS OF THE LIVER AND BILIARY TRACT

BENIGN LIVER TUMORS

HEPATOCELLULAR ADENOMAS Hepatocellular adenomas are benign tumors of the liver found predominantly in women in their third and fourth decades. Their preponderance in women suggests a hormonal influence in their pathogenesis, and oral contraceptives have been implicated. There has been a striking increase in these adenomas since oral contraceptives were introduced, and most patients with those tumors have used these hormonal agents. Multiple hepatic adenomas have been associated with glycogen storage disease type I.

Hepatic adenomas occur predominantly in the right lobe of the liver, may be multiple, and are often quite large (>10 cm). Microscopically, they consist of normal or slightly atypical hepatocytes. These cells have an increased amount of glycogen, making them appear paler and larger than normal. Clinical features include pain and the presence of a palpable mass or features of intratumor hemorrhage (pain and circulatory collapse). The diagnosis is usually made by a combination of techniques: sonography, computed tomography (CT), magnetic resonance imaging (MRI), selective hepatic arteriography, and radionuclide scans. The angiographic appearance is typically hypervascular, but often also includes hypovascular regions. Technetium 99m scans usually show a defect, because phagocytosing Kupffer cells are absent. There is a risk of malignant change in the range of 10 percent; the risk is higher for large (>10 cm) and multiple adenomas.

As far as management is concerned, a patient taking oral contraceptives should stop doing so. If the lesion is large (8 to 10 cm), near the surface, and resectable, surgery is appropriate. Because of the risk of rupture, pregnancy should be avoided.

FOCAL NODULAR HYPERPLASIA Focal nodular hyperplasia is a benign tumor often identified incidentally on imaging studies or at laparoscopy done for other reasons. Like hepatic adenomas, it occurs predominantly in women; however, oral contraceptives do not appear to be implicated, and hemorrhage and necrosis are rare. The risk of hemorrhage, however, appears to be higher in women taking oral contraceptives. Typically, the lesion is a solid tumor, often in the right lobe, with a fibrous core and stellate projections. The fibrous projections contain atypical hepatocytes, biliary epithelium, Kupffer cells, and inflammatory cells. A radionuclide technetium scan will usually show a hot spot because of the presence of Kupffer cells. The lesion appears vascular on angiography, and septations may be detectable. If the lesion is asymptomatic, surgery is not indicated.

HEMANGIOMA AND OTHER BENIGN TUMORS *Hemangiomas* are probably the most common benign liver tumors, occurring predominantly in women and usually detected when abdominal imaging is done for unrelated symptoms, or unexpectedly at surgery. The prevalence in the general population is in the range of 0.5 to 7.0 percent. These vascular lesions are usually asymptomatic and can be identified by MRI, contrast-enhanced CT, labeled red blood cell nuclide scans, or hepatic angiography. They do not need to be removed unless they are large and are producing a mass effect. Hemorrhage is rare, and malignant change does not occur.

Nodular regenerative hyperplasia consists of multiple hepatic nodules resulting from periportal hepatocyte regeneration with surrounding atrophy. It may be associated with an underlying condition such as malignancy or connective tissue disease. Portal hypertension (in the absence of cirrhosis) is the most common clinical manifestation. Other, less common benign hepatic lesions include *bile duct adenomas* and *cystadenomas. Juvenile hemangioendotheliomas* occur in children in association with congestive heart failure and cutaneous hemangiomas.

CARCINOMAS OF THE LIVER

HEPATOCELLULAR CARCINOMA Epidemiology and Etiology Primary hepatocellular carcinoma is one of the most common tumors in the world. It is especially prevalent in regions of Asia and sub-Saharan Africa, where the annual incidence is up to 500 cases per 100,000 population. In the United States and western Europe, it is much less common, accounting for only 1 to 2 percent of malignant tumors at autopsy. Hepatocellular carcinoma is up to four times more common in men than in women and usually arises in a cirrhotic liver. The incidence peaks in the fifth to sixth decades of life in western countries but one to two decades earlier in regions of Asia and Africa with a high prevalence of liver carcinoma.

The principal reason for the high incidence of hepatocellular carcinoma in parts of Asia and Africa is the frequency of chronic infection with *hepatitis B virus* (HBV) and *hepatitis C virus* (HCV). These chronic infections frequently lead to cirrhosis, which itself is an important risk factor for hepatocellular carcinoma (the risk of liver cancer in a cirrhotic liver is ~3 percent per year); 60 to 90 percent of these tumors occur in patients with macronodular cirrhosis. The role of HBV as a factor has been fairly convincingly demonstrated. Studies in regions of Asia where hepatocellular carcinoma and HBV infection are prevalent have shown that the incidence over time of this cancer is about 100-fold higher in individuals with evidence of HBV infection than in noninfected controls. In China, the lifetime risk of developing hepatocellular carcinoma in patients with chronic hepatitis B approaches 40 percent. In patients with HBV infection and hepatocellular carcinoma, HBV DNA may be integrated into host genomic DNA, both in the tumor cells and in adjacent, uninvolved hepatocytes. In addition, there can be modifications of cellular gene expression by insertional mutagenesis, chromosomal rearrangements, or the transcriptional transactivating activity of the X and the pre-S2 regions of the HBV genome. These alterations probably occur during the process of liver cell injury and repair.

Since the discovery of hepatitis C virus as the agent responsible for most cases of non-A, non-B hepatitis, an increasing body of evidence has implicated HCV in hepatocellular carcinoma. In fact, in Europe and Japan HCV appears to be substantially more prevalent than HBV in cases of hepatocellular carcinoma. Both HBV and HCV can be demonstrated in some patients, but the clinical course of liver malignancy in these patients does not appear to differ from that when only one virus is implicated. One distinction in high-prevalence areas between hepatocellular carcinoma associated with HBV infection and with HCV infection is in the timing of onset. In Asia, HBV is acquired at birth via perinatal transmission, while HCV infection is acquired primarily during adulthood from transfused blood. Correspondingly, the onset of liver carcinoma occurs one to two decades earlier in those with lifelong hepatitis B than in persons with adult-acquired hepatitis C. Retrospective analysis indicates that hepatocellular carcinoma occurs on average approximately 30 years after HCV infection and almost exclusively in patients with cirrhosis.

Any agent or factor that contributes to chronic, low-grade liver cell damage and mitosis makes hepatocyte DNA more susceptible to genetic alterations. Thus, as indicated above, *chronic liver disease* of any type is a risk factor and predisposes to the development of liver cell carcinoma. These conditions include alcoholic liver disease, α_1-antitrypsin deficiency, hemochromatosis, and tyrosinemia. In Africa and southern China, *aflatoxin B1* is an important public health hazard. This mycotoxin appears to induce a very specific mutation at codon 249 in the tumor suppressor gene *p53*.

The loss, inactivation, or mutation of the *p53* gene has been implicated in tumorigenesis and is the most common genetic derangement present in human cancers. Thus HBV and aflatoxin B_1 have been implicated in the pathogenesis of hepatocellular carcinoma in regions of Africa and southern China where both agents are prevalent.

In view of the male predominance of liver cancer, hormonal factors also may play a role. Hepatocellular tumors may occur with long-term androgenic steroid administration, with exposure to thorium dioxide or vinyl chloride (see below), and possibly with exposure to estrogens in the form of oral contraceptives.

Clinical and Laboratory Features Cancers of the liver initially may escape clinical recognition because they often occur in patients with underlying cirrhosis, and the symptoms and signs may suggest progression of the underlying disease. The most common presenting features are abdominal *pain* with detection of an abdominal mass in the right upper quadrant. There may be a *friction rub* or *bruit* over the liver. Blood-tinged ascites occurs in about 20 percent of cases. Jaundice is rare, unless there is significant deterioration of liver function or mechanical obstruction of the bile ducts. Serum elevations of alkaline phosphatase and alpha fetoprotein (AFP) are common (see below). An abnormal type of prothrombin, des-γ-carboxy prothrombin, is also detectable and in general correlates with AFP elevations.

A small percentage of patients with hepatocellular carcinoma have evidence of *paraneoplastic syndrome*; erythrocytosis may result from erythropoietin-like activity produced by the tumor; hypercalcemia may result from secretion of a parathyroid-like hormone. Other manifestations may include hypercholesterolemia, hypoglycemia, acquired porphyria, dysfibrinogenemia, and cryofibrinogenemia.

Imaging procedures used to detect liver tumors include ultrasound, CT, MRI, hepatic artery angiography (see Chap. 281), and radionuclide scans with technetium 99m. Ultrasound is frequently used to screen high-risk populations and should be the first procedure if hepatocellular carcinoma is suspected; it is less costly than scanning procedures, is relatively sensitive, and can detect most tumors larger than 3 cm. MRI, however, is being used with increasing frequency.

AFP levels greater than 500 µg/L are found in about 70 to 80 percent of patients with hepatocellular carcinoma. Lower levels may be found in patients with large metastases from gastric or colonic tumors and in some patients with acute or chronic hepatitis. The presence and persistence of high levels of serum AFP (over 500 to 1000 µg/L) in an adult with liver disease and without an obvious gastrointestinal tumor strongly suggest hepatocellular carcinoma. A rising level suggests progression of the tumor or recurrence after hepatic resection or therapeutic approaches such as chemotherapy or chemoembolization (see below).

Percutaneous *liver biopsy* can be diagnostic if the sample is taken from an area localized by ultrasound or CT. Because these tumors tend to be vascular, percutaneous biopsies should be done with caution. Cytologic examination of ascitic fluid is invariably negative for tumor cells. Occasionally, *laparoscopy* or *minilaparotomy*, to permit liver biopsy under direct vision, may be used. This approach has the additional advantage of sometimes identifying patients who have a localized resectable tumor suitable for partial hepatectomy.

℞ TREATMENT

The course of clinically apparent disease is rapid; if untreated, most patients die within 3 to 6 months of diagnosis. When hepatocellular carcinoma is detected very early by serial screening of AFP and ultrasound, survival of 1 to 2 years is possible, as is resection. In selected cases, therapy may prolong life. *Surgical resection* offers the only chance for cure; however, few patients have a resectable tumor at the time of presentation, because of underlying cirrhosis, involvement of both hepatic lobes, or distant metastases (common sites are lung, brain, bone, and adrenal), and the 5-year survival is low. In patients at high risk for the development of hepatocellular carcinoma, such as patients positive for the hepatitis B surface antigen (HBsAg) and patients with cirrhosis (including that caused by chronic hepatitis C), screening programs have been initiated to identify small tumors when they are still resectable. Because 20 to 30 percent of patients with early hepatocellular carcinoma do not have elevated levels of circulating AFP, ultrasonographic screening is recommended as well as AFP determination. In a study in the Far East, HBsAg-positive persons, with or without liver disease, were screened serially; a number of patients with small, subclinical tumors were identified, and surgical resection undertaken. Follow-up observation revealed a 5-year survival rate in this group of 70 percent and a 10-year survival rate of 50 percent. These Asian patients, however, were unusual in that they had minimal or no liver disease and their tumors tended to be unifocal or encapsulated. The findings are in contrast to a study in a large population of Italian patients with cirrhosis, associated in most cases with chronic HBV and/or HCV infections; screening every 3 to 12 months permitted the detection of a 3 percent annual incidence of cancer in this cohort, but in most cases failed to achieve the goal of early detection of surgically treatable disease.

Liver transplantation may be considered as a therapeutic option, but recurrence of tumor or metastases after transplantation have limited its usefulness (see Chap. 301). Other approaches include (1) hepatic artery embolization with chemotherapy (chemoembolization), (2) alcohol ablation via ultrasound-guided percutaneous injection, (3) ultrasound-guided cryoablation, (4) immunotherapy with monoclonal antibodies tagged with cytotoxic agents, and (5) gene therapy with retroviral vectors containing genes expressing cytotoxic agents.

Prevention is the preferred strategy. Hepatitis B vaccine can prevent infection and its sequelae. Treatment with interferon α lowers the risk of development of liver cancer in patients with hepatitis C–related chronic active hepatitis and cirrhosis (see Chap. 297).

OTHER MALIGNANT LIVER TUMORS

Fibrolamellar carcinoma differs from the typical hepatocellular carcinoma in that it tends to occur in young adults without underlying cirrhosis. This tumor is nonencapsulated but well circumscribed and contains fibrous lamellae; it grows slowly and is associated with a longer survival if treated. Surgical resection has resulted in 5-year survivals exceeding 50 percent; if the lesion is nonresectable, liver transplantation is an option, and the outcome far exceeds that observed in the nonfibrolamellar variety of liver cancer. *Hepatoblastoma* is a tumor of infancy that typically is associated with very high serum AFP levels. The lesions are usually solitary, may be resectable, and have a better 5-year survival than that of hepatocellular carcinoma. *Angiosarcoma* consists of vascular spaces lined by malignant endothelial cells. Etiologic factors include prior exposure to thorium dioxide (Thorotrast), polyvinyl chloride, arsenic, and androgenic anabolic steroids. *Epithelioid hemangioendothelioma* is of borderline malignancy; most cases are benign, but metastases occur. This tumor occurs in early adulthood, presents with right upper quadrant pain, is heterogeneous on sonography, hypodense on CT, and without neovascularity on angiography. Immunohistochemical staining reveals expression of factor VIII antigen. In the absence of extrahepatic metastases, these lesions can be treated by surgical resection or liver transplantation.

METASTATIC TUMORS Metastatic tumors of the liver are common, ranking second only to cirrhosis as a cause of fatal liver disease. In the United States, the incidence of clinically significant metastatic carcinoma is at least 20 times greater than that of primary carcinoma. At autopsy, hepatic metastases occur in 30 to 50 percent of patients dying from malignant disease.

Pathogenesis The liver is uniquely vulnerable to invasion by tumor cells. Its size, high rate of blood flow, double perfusion by the hepatic artery and portal vein, and its Kupffer cell filtration function combine to make it the next most common site of metastases after the

lymph nodes. In addition, local tissue factors or endothelial membrane characteristics appear to enhance metastatic implants. Virtually all types of neoplasms except those primary in the brain may metastasize to the liver. The most common primary tumors are those of the gastrointestinal tract, lung, and breast, as well as melanomas. Less common are metastases from tumors of the thyroid, prostate, and skin.

Clinical Features Most patients with metastases to the liver present with symptoms referable only to the primary tumor, and the asymptomatic hepatic involvement is discovered in the course of clinical evaluation. Sometimes hepatic involvement is reflected by nonspecific symptoms of weakness, weight loss, fever, sweating, and loss of appetite. Rarely, features indicating active hepatic disease, especially abdominal pain, hepatomegaly, or ascites, are present. Patients with widespread metastatic liver involvement usually have suggestive clinical signs of cancer and hepatic enlargement. Some have localized induration or tenderness, and, occasionally, a friction rub may be found over tender areas of the liver.

Results of liver biochemical tests are often abnormal, but the elevations in marker levels often are only mild and nonspecific. These signs reflect the effects of fever and wasting as well as those of the infiltrating neoplastic process itself. An increase in serum alkaline phosphatase is the most common and frequently the only abnormality. Hypoalbuminemia, anemia, and occasionally a mild elevation of aminotransferase levels also may be found with more widespread disease. Substantially elevated serum levels of carcinoembryonic antigen are usually found when the metastases are from primary malignancies in the gastrointestinal tract, breast, or lung.

Diagnosis Evidence of metastatic invasion of the liver should be sought actively in any patient with a primary malignancy, especially of the lung, gastrointestinal tract, or breast, before resection of the primary lesion. An elevated level of alkaline phosphatase or a mass apparent on ultrasound, CT, or MRI examination of the liver may provide a presumptive diagnosis. Blind percutaneous needle biopsy of the liver will result in a positive diagnosis of metastatic disease in only 60 to 80 percent of cases with hepatomegaly and elevated alkaline phosphatase levels. Serial sectioning of specimens, two or three repeated biopsies, or cytologic examination of biopsy smears may increase the diagnostic yield by 10 to 15 percent. The yield is greatly increased when biopsies are directed by ultrasound or CT or obtained during laparoscopy.

℞ TREATMENT

Most metastatic carcinomas respond poorly to all forms of treatment, which is usually only palliative. On rare occasions, a single, large metastasis can be removed surgically. Systemic chemotherapy may slow tumor growth briefly and reduce symptoms, but it does not significantly alter the prognosis. Chemoembolization, intrahepatic chemotherapy, and alcohol ablation may provide palliation. It remains to be determined whether newer drugs, combination chemotherapy, or novel strategies (including immunologic targeting) will eventually prove to be more effective.

CHOLANGIOCARCINOMA Benign tumors of the extrahepatic bile ducts are extremely rare causes of mechanical biliary obstruction. Most of these are papillomas, adenomas, or cystadenomas and present with obstructive jaundice or hemobilia. Adenocarcinoma of the extrahepatic ducts is more common. There is a slight male preponderance (60 percent), and the incidence peaks in the fifth to seventh decades. Apparent predisposing factors include (1) some chronic hepatobiliary parasitic infestations, (2) congenital anomalies with ectatic ducts, (3) sclerosing cholangitis and chronic ulcerative colitis, and (4) occupational exposure to possible biliary tract carcinogens (employment in rubber or automotive plants). Cholelithiasis is not clearly a predisposing factor for cholangiocarcinoma. The lesions of cholangiocarcinoma may be diffuse or nodular; lesions of the latter type often arise at the bifurcation of the common bile duct (Klatskin tumors). This tumor is usually associated with a *collapsed gallbladder*, and that finding mandates that the proximal hepatic ducts be visualized by cholangiography.

Patients with cholangiocarcinoma usually present with biliary obstruction, painless jaundice, pruritus, weight loss, and acholic stools. A deep-seated, vaguely localized right upper quadrant pain may be an associated complaint. Hepatomegaly and a palpable, distended gallbladder (unless the lesion is high in the duct) are frequent accompanying signs. Fever is unusual unless associated with ascending cholangitis. Because the obstructing process is gradual, the cholangiocarcinoma is often far advanced by the time it presents clinically. The diagnosis is most frequently made by cholangiography following ultrasound demonstration of dilated intrahepatic bile ducts. Any focal strictures of the bile ducts should probably be considered malignant until proved otherwise. Survival of 1 to 2 years is possible in some cases with palliative drainage (stenting) of the biliary tree.

CARCINOMA OF THE PAPILLA OF VATER The ampulla of Vater may be involved by extension of tumor arising elsewhere in the duodenum or may itself be the site of origin of a sarcoma, carcinoid tumor, or adenocarcinoma. Papillary adenocarcinomas are associated with slow growth and a more favorable clinical prognosis than diffuse, infiltrative cancers of the ampulla, which are more frequently widely invasive. The presenting clinical manifestation is usually obstructive jaundice. Endoscopic retrograde cannulation of the pancreatic duct (ERCP) is probably the preferred diagnostic technique when ampullary carcinoma is suspected, because it allows for direct endoscopic inspection and biopsy of the ampulla as well as for performance of pancreatography to exclude a diagnosis of pancreatic malignancy. Cancer of the papilla is usually treated by wide, often radical, surgical excision. Lymph node or other metastases are present at the time of surgery in approximately 20 percent of cases, and the 5-year survival rate following surgical therapy in this group is only 5 to 10 percent. In the absence of metastases, however, radical pancreaticoduodenectomy (the Whipple procedure) is associated with 5-year survival rates as high as 40 percent, and several long-term survivors have been reported.

CANCER OF THE GALLBLADDER Most cancers of the gallbladder develop in conjunction with stones rather than polyps. In patients with gallstones, the risk for developing gallbladder cancer, while increased, is still quite low. In one study, gallbladder cancer developed in only 5 of 2583 patients with gallstones followed for a median of 13 years. In the United States, adenocarcinomas make up the vast majority of the estimated 6500 new cases of gallbladder cancer diagnosed each year. The female/male ratio is 4:1, and the mean age at diagnosis is approximately 70 years. The clinical presentation is most often one of unremitting right upper quadrant pain associated with weight loss, jaundice, and a palpable right upper quadrant mass. Cholangitis may supervene. The preoperative diagnosis of the condition has been facilitated by ultrasound and CT. CT is also useful in guiding fine needle aspiration and biopsy.

Once symptoms have appeared, spread of the tumor outside the gallbladder by direct extension or by lymphatic or hematogenous routes is almost invariable. Over 75 percent of gallbladder carcinomas are unresectable at the time of surgery, the exceptions being tumors discovered incidentally at laparotomy. The 1-year mortality rate for unresectable disease is approximately 95 percent, and only 5 percent of patients survive 5 years or more from the time of diagnosis. Radical operative resection does not appear to improve survival. Trials of radiation and chemotherapy in patients with primary gallbladder cancer also have been disappointing.

BIBLIOGRAPHY

DE BAC C et al: Pathogenic factors in cirrhosis with and without hepatocellular carcinoma: A multicenter Italian study. Hepatology 20:1225, 1994
FATTOVICH G et al: Occurrence of hepatocellular carcinoma and decompensation in western European patients with cirrhosis type B. Hepatology 21:77, 1995
GROUPE D'ETUDE ET DE TRAITEMENT DU CARCINOMA HEPATOCELLULAIRE: A comparison of lipiodol chemoembolization and conservative treatment for unresectable hepatocellular carcinoma. N Engl J Med 332:1256, 1995
LIANG TJ et al: Viral pathogenesis of hepatocellular carcinoma in the United States. Hepatology 18:1326, 1993

OKA H et al: Prospective study of α-fetoprotein in cirrhotic patients monitored for development of hepatocellular carcinoma. Hepatology 19:61, 1994
OKUDA K: Hepatocellular carcinoma: Recent progress. Hepatology 15:948, 1992
SHEINER PA et al: Treatment of metastatic cancer to the liver. Semin Liver Dis 14:169, 1994
TAKANO S et al: Incidence of hepatocellular carcinoma in chronic hepatitis B and C: Prospective study of 251 patients. Hepatology 21:650, 1995
TAO LC: Oral contraceptive–associated liver cell adenoma and hepatocellular carcinoma: Cytomorphology and malignant transformation. Cancer 68:341, 1991
TSUKUMA H et al: Risk factors for hepatocellular carcinoma among patients with chronic liver disease. N Engl J Med 328:1797, 1993
VAUTHEY J-N et al: Recent advances in management of cholangiocarcinomas. Semin Liver Dis 14:109, 1994
WEITZ IC et al: Des-γ-carboxy (abnormal) prothrombin and hepatocellular carcinoma: A critical review. Hepatology 18:990, 1993

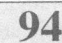

94   *Robert J. Mayer*

PANCREATIC CANCER

INCIDENCE AND ETIOLOGY The incidence of pancreatic carcinoma in the United States has increased significantly as the median life expectancy of the American population has lengthened. The tumor results in the death of more than 98 percent of afflicted patients. Approximately 27,800 individuals died of pancreatic cancer in 1996, making it the fifth most common cause of cancer-related mortality. The disease appears to be somewhat more common in males than in females and in blacks than in whites. It rarely develops before the age of 50.

Little is known about the causes of pancreatic cancer. Cigarette smoking is the most consistently observed risk factor for the development of the tumor, with the disease being two to three times more common in heavy smokers than in nonsmokers. It is uncertain whether this apparent association reflects a direct carcinogenic effect of metabolites of cigarette smoking on the pancreas or whether an as yet undefined exposure that occurs more frequently in cigarette smokers is responsible for the enhanced risk. A large case-control study has correlated chronic pancreatitis with an increased risk of pancreatic cancer. A meta-analysis of 20 case-control and cohort studies has also shown a higher frequency of pancreatic cancer in persons with long-standing diabetes mellitus. There are no convincing data to link such epidemiologic factors as alcohol abuse or cholelithiasis with the development of pancreatic cancer. Furthermore, the weight of clinical data has failed to support any association between coffee consumption and pancreatic cancer. Mutations in K-*ras* genes have been found in more than 85 percent of specimens of human pancreatic cancer. The development of pancreatic cancer has also been associated with a mutation of the *p16^{INK4}* gene located on chromosome 9p21, a gene also implicated in the pathogenesis of cutaneous malignant melanoma.

CLINICAL FEATURES More than 90 percent of pancreatic cancers are ductal adenocarcinomas, with islet cell tumors constituting the remaining 5 to 10 percent. Pancreatic cancers occur twice as frequently in the pancreatic head (about 70 percent of cases) as in the body (about 20 percent) or tail (about 10 percent) of the gland.

With the exception of jaundice, the initial symptoms associated with pancreatic cancer are often insidious and usually are present for more than 2 months before the cancer is diagnosed (Table 94-1). Pain and weight loss are present in more than 75 percent of patients. The pain typically has a gnawing, visceral quality, occasionally radiating from the epigastrium to the back. It generally is a more severe problem in lesions arising in the body or tail of the gland, as such tumors may become quite large before being detected. Characteristically, the pain improves somewhat when the patient bends forward.

Table 94-1

Presenting Signs and Symptoms of Pancreatic Carcinoma

Frequent
   Abdominal pain
   Weight loss
   Jaundice (lesions of pancreatic head only)
Infrequent
   Glucose intolerance
   Palpable gallbladder
   Migratory thrombophlebitis
   Gastrointestinal hemorrhage
   Splenomegaly

The development of significant pain is suggestive of retroperitoneal invasion and infiltration of the splanchnic nerves, indicating that the primary lesion is far advanced and is not surgically resectable. Rarely, such pain may be transient and associated with hyperamylasemia, indicative of acute pancreatitis caused by ductal obstruction by tumor. The weight loss observed in most patients having pancreatic carcinoma is primarily the result of anorexia, although in the initial period of the disease, subclinical malabsorption may also be a contributing factor.

Jaundice due to biliary obstruction is found in more than 80 percent of patients having tumors in the pancreatic head and is typically accompanied by darkening of urine, a claylike appearance of stool, and pruritus. In contrast to the "painless jaundice" sometimes observed in patients having carcinomas of the bile ducts, duodenum, or periampullary regions, most icteric individuals having ductal carcinomas of the pancreatic head will complain of significant abdominal discomfort. Although the gallbladder is usually enlarged in patients with carcinoma of the head of the pancreas, it is palpable in less than 50 percent of cases (Courvoisier's sign). However, the presence of an enlarged gallbladder in a jaundiced patient without biliary colic should suggest malignant obstruction of the extrahepatic biliary tree.

Glucose intolerance, presumably a direct consequence of the tumor, often develops within 2 years of the clinical diagnosis. Other initial manifestations include venous thrombosis and migratory thrombophlebitis, gastrointestinal hemorrhage resulting from varices due to compression of the portal venous system by tumor, and splenomegaly caused by cancerous encasement of the splenic vein.

DIAGNOSTIC PROCEDURES (Fig. 94-1)   Despite the availability of serologic tests for tumor-associated antigens, such as the carcinoembryonic antigen (CEA) and CA 19-9, and noninvasive imaging techniques, such as computed tomography (CT) and ultrasonography, the early diagnosis of a potentially resectable pancreatic carcinoma remains extremely difficult. The nonspecificity of the initial symptoms and the poor sensitivity of both serologic assays and noninvasive techniques have frustrated the development of effective screening procedures. When the disease is clinically suspected in a patient having vague, persistent abdominal complaints, ultrasound should be performed to visualize the gallbladder and the pancreas, as well as upper gastrointestinal contrast radiographs to rule out a hiatal hernia or a peptic ulcer. If these studies fail to provide an explanation for the symptoms, a CT scan should be considered. It should encompass not only the pancreas but also the liver, retroperitoneal lymph nodes, and pelvis, as pancreatic cancer frequently spreads within the abdomen. While more costly than ultrasonography, CT is technically simpler, more reproducible, provides better definition of the body and tail of the pancreas, and requires less interpretive skill. CT generally detects a malignant pancreatic lesion in over 80 percent of cases; in 5 to 15 percent of patients with proven pancreatic carcinoma, the CT scan shows only generalized pancreatic enlargement suggestive of pancreatitis rather than malignancy. False-positive results have also been reported in about 5 to 10 percent of cases where no tumor was found on laparotomy. Magnetic resonance imaging (MRI) has not been shown to be better than CT in the evaluation of pancreatic lesions. In selected situations in which clinical circumstances dictate additional diagnostic evaluation, endoscopic retrograde cholangiopancreatography (ERCP) may clarify the cause of ambiguous CT or ultrasound findings. The characteristic findings are stenosis or obstruction of either the pancreatic or the common bile duct; both duct systems are abnormal in over half the cases. It can be quite difficult to distinguish between carcinoma and chronic pancreatitis by ERCP, particularly if both diseases are present. False-negative results with ERCP are quite infrequent (less than 5 percent) and usually occur in the setting of islet cell, rather than ductal, carcinomas.

Selective and superselective angiography may be of value in some patients. Angiography is an effective means of detecting carcinomas in the body and tail of the pancreas by the demonstration of vascular narrowing, displacement, or occlusion by tumor. Angiography is also useful in assessing whether encasement of peripancreatic vessels is present; this

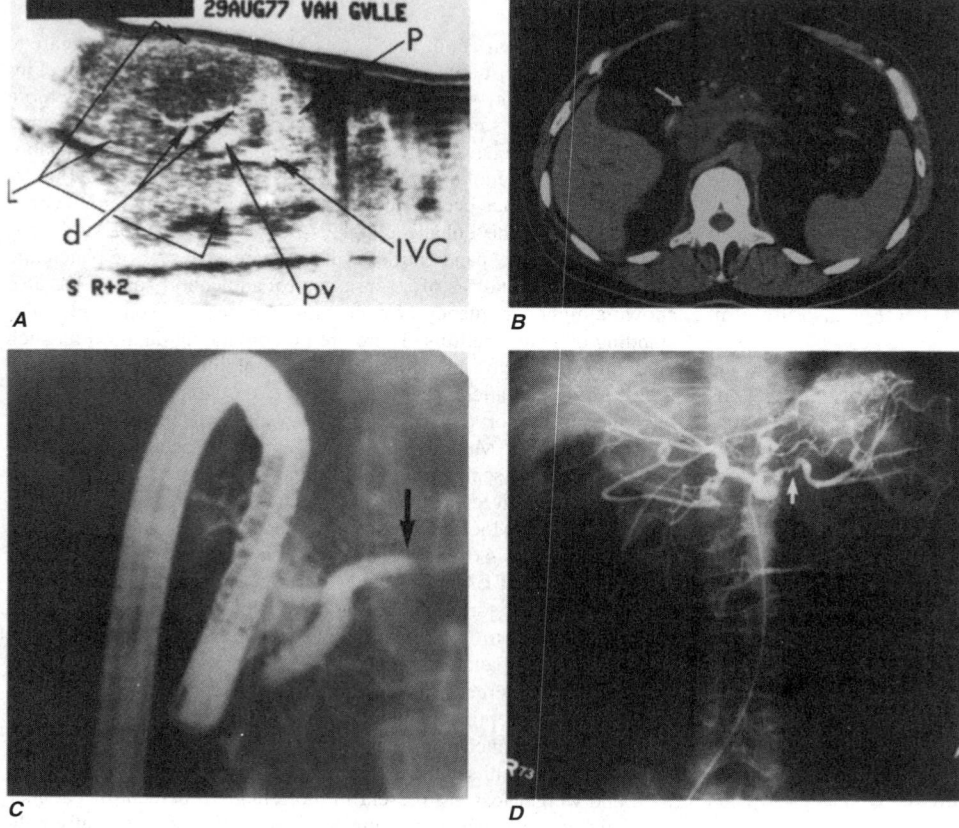

FIGURE 94-1   Carcinoma of the pancreas. *A.* Sonogram showing pancreatic carcinoma (P), dilated intrahepatic bile ducts (d), dilated portal vein (pv), and inferior vena cava (IVC). *B.* CT scan showing pancreatic carcinoma (*arrow*). *C.* ERCP showing abrupt cutoff of the duct of Wirsung (*arrow*). *D.* Arteriogram showing sheathing of splenic artery by tumor encasement (*arrow*).

assessment is of less importance in determining the potential for surgical resection.

Regardless of the results of the above diagnostic studies, a histologic confirmation of a presumed pancreatic cancer is mandatory to be absolutely certain that malignancy exists and to rule out the presence of such other neoplasms as islet cell tumor or lymphoma, for which the therapeutic approach and prognosis differ significantly from those for ductal carcinoma. Such tissue confirmation may be obtained through a percutaneous needle aspiration biopsy of the pancreas with CT or ultrasonographic guidance, thereby obviating surgical exploration.

Patients with carcinoma of the pancreas may undergo several months of investigation before a diagnosis is established. In the past, this period of diagnostic delay and accompanying emotional uncertainty led to the erroneous impression that the pain and weight loss might not have an organic cause, resulting in an association of pancreatic cancer and depression. The availability of CT scans has resulted in more prompt diagnosis and dispelled this incorrect notion. Unfortunately, however, even laparotomy may not provide a definitive diagnosis, because chronic pancreatitis may also produce a hard mass in the head of the pancreas indistinguishable from carcinoma by palpation. Furthermore, a superficial biopsy of such a mass may not show neoplastic tissue, revealing only evidence of pancreatitis, as the cancer is often surrounded by edematous, inflamed, and fibrotic tissue (i.e., chronic pancreatitis).

℞ TREATMENT

Complete surgical resection of pancreatic tumors offers the only effective treatment for this disease. Unfortunately, such "curative" operations are only possible in 10 to 15 percent of patients with pancreatic cancer, usually those individuals with a tumor in the pancreatic head in whom jaundice was the initial symptom. Patients considered for such a procedure should have no evidence of metastatic spread on a chest radiograph and abdominal-pelvic CT scan and should be operated on by an experienced surgeon, as mortality rates of greater than 15 percent have been associated with this procedure. Although the potential for cure in patients with pancreatic cancer is restricted to the few who are able to undergo a complete surgical resection, the 5-year survival rate following such operations is only 10 percent. Nonetheless, the procedure is worth attempting, particularly for lesions in the pancreatic head, since ductal carcinomas often cannot be distinguished preoperatively from ampullary, duodenal, and distal bile duct tumors or pancreatic cyst adenocarcinomas, all of which have far higher rates of resectability and cure. Furthermore, patients who undergo resection and eventually experience disease recurrence survive three to four times longer than those whose tumor is not excised, indicating that such operations have a palliative effect. The risk for tumor recurrence is not affected by the type of operative procedure—i.e., total pancreatectomy versus pancreaticoduodenectomy ("Whipple resection")—but it is increased by the presence of lymph node metastases or tumor invasion into adjacent viscera. As a rule, pancreaticoduodenectomy or distal pancreatectomy seems preferable to total pancreatectomy because of the retention of exocrine function and avoidance of brittle diabetes.

The median survival for patients whose pancreatic cancers are surgically unresectable is approximately 6 months. Management of such individuals should be directed at palliation of symptoms. Ambulatory patients having tumors in the pancreatic head should be considered for surgical diversion of the biliary system. If jaundice has already developed, therapeutic options include either nonoperative biliary decompression by endoscopic or percutaneous, transhepatic biliary drainage or surgical biliary bypass. External beam radiation in patients with unresectable tumors that have not spread beyond the pancreas does not appear to prolong survival, although a sufficient reduction in tumor size may lead to palliation of pain. However,

the addition of chemotherapy with fluorouracil (5-FU) to external beam irradiation has increased the survival time for these patients, perhaps because 5-FU acts as a radiosensitizing agent. In a small patient population, a similar combination of radiation therapy and 5-FU appears to have prolonged the survival and increased the cure rate as compared to a prospectively randomized nontreatment control group of patients who had a complete surgical resection of their pancreatic cancer. This observation needs to be confirmed before it can be accepted. The possibility of administering such chemoradiation therapy at diagnosis and before surgery ("neoadjuvant" treatment), as a means of increasing the potential for resectability, is under investigation. Intraoperative radiation therapy has the potential to deliver higher doses of radiation to the tumor while sparing neighboring tissues. However, this strategy has not been shown to give better results than external beam treatment.

The experience of using chemotherapy in the management of patients with widely metastatic pancreatic cancer has been disappointing. Gemcitabine, a deoxycytidine analogue, has been shown to produce improvement in the quality of life for patients with advanced pancreatic cancer. However, duration of survival is only moderately improved. Newer forms of treatment, including therapies directed at specific molecular targets, such as K-*ras*, must be developed and should constitute the initial treatment for consenting, ambulatory patients. → *Pancreatic endocrine tumors are discussed in Chap. 95.*

BIBLIOGRAPHY

CANCER OF THE PANCREAS TASK FORCE: Staging of cancer of the pancreas. Cancer 47:1631, 1981

CONNOLLY MM et al: Survival in 1001 patients with carcinoma of the pancreas. Ann Surg 206:366, 1987

EVERHART J, WRIGHT D: Diabetes mellitus as a risk factor for pancreatic cancer. A meta-analysis. JAMA 273:1605, 1995

GASTROINTESTINAL TUMOR STUDY GROUP: Pancreatic cancer. Adjuvant combined radiation and chemotherapy following curative resection. Arch Surg 120:899, 1985

GOLDSTEIN AM et al: Increased risk of pancreatic cancer in melanoma-prone kindreds with p16^{INK4} mutations. N Engl J Med 333:970, 1995

GULLO L et al: Diabetes and the risk of pancreatic cancer. N Engl J Med 331:81, 1994

JANES RH JR et al: National patterns of care for pancreatic cancer: Results of a survey by the Commission on Cancer. Ann Surg 223:261, 1996

LIN A, FELLER ER: Pancreatic carcinoma as a cause of unexplained pancreatitis: Report of ten cases. Ann Intern Med 113:166, 1990

LOWENFELS AB et al: Pancreatitis and the risk of pancreatic cancer. N Engl J Med 328:1433, 1993

MOERTEL CT et al: Therapy of locally unresectable pancreatic adenocarcinoma: A randomized comparison of high dose (6,000 rads) radiation alone, moderate dose radiation (4,000 rads) + 5-fluorouracil, and high dose radiation + 5-fluorouracil. The Gastrointestinal Tumor Study Group. Cancer 48:1705, 1981

MOORE M et al: A randomized trial of gemcitabine (GEM) versus 5-FU as first-line therapy in advanced pancreatic cancer. Proc Am Soc Clin Oncol 14:199, 1995

MOOSSA AR, LEVIN B: The diagnosis of "early" pancreatic cancer: The University of Chicago experience. Cancer 47:1688, 1981

SCHNALL S, MACDONALD JS: Chemotherapy of adenocarcinoma of the pancreas. Semin Oncol 23:220, 1996

SILVERMAN DT et al: Cigarette smoking and pancreas cancer: A case-control study based on direct interview. J Natl Cancer Inst 86:1510, 1994

SPEER AG et al: Randomized trial of endoscopic versus percutaneous stent insertion in malignant obstructive jaundice. Lancet 2:57, 1987

STEINBERG WM et al: Comparison of the sensitivity and specificity of the CA 19-9 and carcinoembryonic antigen assays in detecting cancer of the pancreas. Gastroenterology 90:343, 1986

WADE TP et al: The Whipple resection for cancer in U.S. Department of Veterans Affairs hospitals. Ann Surg 221:241, 1995

WARSHAW AL, FERNANDO-DEL CASTILLO C: Pancreatic carcinoma. N Engl J Med 326:455, 1992

95   *Lee M. Kaplan*

ENDOCRINE TUMORS OF THE GASTROINTESTINAL TRACT AND PANCREAS

Tumors arising from neuroendocrine cells of the gastrointestinal tract and pancreas present special challenges in diagnosis and therapy. Unlike other gastrointestinal neoplasms, these tumors often cause symptoms from excess hormone secretion rather than from growth, invasion, or local anatomic effects. Frequently slow growing, they may nonetheless be life-threatening because of uncontrolled release of specific hormones and neurotransmitters. These neoplasms arise from within the gastrointestinal mucosa and pancreatic islets in cells that normally secrete regulatory monoamines and peptide hormones. For example, gastrin-secreting G cells within the gastric and duodenal mucosa regulate gastric acid secretion, and insulin-secreting β cells within the pancreatic islets have a crucial role in the homeostatic control of glucose metabolism. Overall, more than 30 distinct secretory products have been identified within neuroendocrine cells of the gut.

BIOLOGIC CONSIDERATIONS A striking feature of neuroendocrine tumors is the preservation of highly differentiated cell function. Tumor cells contain secretory granules and maintain the capacity for *a*mine *p*recursor *u*ptake and *d*ecarboxylation (APUD), a process essential for the production of monoamine neurotransmitters such as serotonin, dopamine, and histamine. This characteristic has fostered the term *APUDomas* for neoplasms derived from these cells, which can be located in the thyroid (C cells), adrenal medulla, lung (neuroendocrine cells), skin (melanocytes), and nervous system (glial cells and neuroblasts), as well as the gastrointestinal tract and pancreas. These cells also synthesize and secrete *peptide* hormones by a separate mechanism. Several of the known APUDomas are listed in Table 95-1. It was postulated that this specialized capability implies a common embryologic origin for these diverse cells, but in fact, cells of *varied* heritage can acquire the APUD phenotype during differentiation.

Studies of neuroendocrine cell physiology have revealed several important characteristics of secretory cells and the clinical syndromes caused by their humoral products:

1. Cellular phenotype does not predict the nature of the secreted product. Thus, neurons may secrete peptide "hormones" into the synaptic cleft, and endocrine cells may secrete monoamines previously classified as neurotransmitters. Individual cells have the capacity to synthesize and secrete both peptide and monoamine transmitters, which may coexist in individual secretory granules. Many symptoms of enterochromaffin cell tumors (carcinoid tumors) appear to arise from the combined actions of monoamine and peptide products.
2. Transmitter secretion by neuroendocrine cells is frequently episodic or pulsatile. Although the regulation of secretion is incompletely understood, the temporal pattern of hormone release may vary depending on the hormonal milieu, physiologic state, or stage

of development. Thus, symptoms produced by abnormal secretion of hormones from neuroendocrine tumors may be intermittent, especially in early stages when tumor cells may behave more like their normal counterparts.

3. Individual cells have the *potential* to secrete a wide array of transmitters. This feature is particularly evident for the peptide hormones. Depending on the stage of development, cellular environment, and other as yet unidentified factors, neuroendocrine cells can change secretory profiles dramatically. For example, in cell culture, clonal populations may suddenly change from the secretion of insulin to secretion of cholecystokinin, gastrin, or even glucagon. Endocrine tumors may contain heterogeneous populations of cells, so that within individual tumors, a single cell type may predominate, or there may be multiple cell types in varying proportions. In addition, the secretory profile of a tumor may vary with time, producing a dramatic alteration of symptoms. Individual metastatic implants also can display different phenotypes from the primary tumor and from each other.
4. Individual hormones and transmitters secreted by neuroendocrine cells may regulate physiologic activity (e.g., secretion, absorption, or contractility), stimulate or inhibit growth, or affect the development of target cells. Thus, the humoral activity of gut neuroendocrine tumors can cause a wide variety of effects, including gastric acid hypersecretion, abnormal intestinal motility, gastric epithelial hyperplasia, gallstone formation, mesenteric and cardiac fibrosis, and necrosis of the skin.
5. Hormone production by neuroendocrine cells is tightly regulated at many levels, including RNA transcription, precursor peptide processing, and secretion. These cells, in addition, may be subject to control by neighboring secretory cells (*paracrine regulation*). Thus, multiple cell types may act in concert to control the growth, secretory characteristics, and thus the clinical manifestations of individual tumors. Abnormal secretion by the tumors themselves may disrupt the normal regulated function of neighboring neuroendocrine cells, and neoplastic transformation may disturb hormone secretion by these cells. Cells may secrete partially processed hormone precursors, leading to unpredictable effects, or display altered susceptibility to regulation by exogenous stimuli. Occasionally, such characteristics can be exploited to permit specific diagnostic tests for individual tumors.

Neuroendocrine tumors of the gastrointestinal tract can be classified by cell type, major hormone secreted, and site of origin. These characteristics, alone or in combination, correlate well with the observed clinical syndromes. Table 95-2 lists the important tumors in this category, along with their clinical presentations, major secreted products, cells of origin, and biologic behavior.

DIAGNOSTIC CONSIDERATIONS Several distinct syndromes of hormone excess have been described in which symptoms may suggest the presence of an endocrine tumor of the gastrointestinal tract or pancreas. Moreover, these tumors may present as part of the type 1 multiple endocrine neoplasia (MEN 1) syndrome (see Chap. 340). MEN 1 patients frequently develop parathyroid and pituitary adenomas that may produce symptoms of hypercalcemia, hyperprolactinemia, hyperthyroidism, or growth hormone excess. Diagnosis is suggested by history, physical findings, elevated blood levels of the relevant peptide hormone(s), or elevated urinary levels of the major metabolites of monoamine transmitters. Further confirmation of hormone-producing tumors may be provided by provocative tests that reveal abnormalities in the regulation of hormone secretion. For example, tolbutamide may enhance somatostatin secretion from somatostatinoma cells. Normal somatostatin-secreting D cells do not show this effect. Other examples of *abnormal* regulation in tumor cells include enhancement by secretin of gastrin secretion in gastrinomas and pentagastrin stimulation of calcitonin secretion in medullary thyroid (C cell) tumors.

Anatomic definition for pancreatic tumors should be sought by computed tomography (CT) and/or endoscopic ultrasonography, and endoscopic visualization with ultrasonography or barium contrast studies should be obtained for suspected mucosal and submucosal tumors.

Table 95-1

Distribution of APUD Tumors

Origin	Tumors
Gastrointestinal tract	Carcinoid tumor
Pancreas	Islet cell carcinoma
Central nervous system	Ganglioneuroblastoma, neuroblastoma, chemodactoma, paraganglionoma
Thyroid	Medullary thyroid carcinoma
Skin	Melanoma
Adrenal medulla	Pheochromocytoma
Lung	Carcinoid tumor, small cell carcinoma

Table 95-2

Gastrointestinal Endocrine Tumor Syndromes

Syndrome	Cell Type	Clinical Features	Percentage Malignant	Major Products
Carcinoid syndrome	Enterochromaffin, enterochromaffin-like	Flushing, diarrhea, wheezing, hypotension	~100	Serotonin, histamine, miscellaneous peptides
Zollinger-Ellison, gastrinoma	Non-β islet cell, duodenal G cell	Peptic ulcers, diarrhea	~70	Gastrin
Insulinoma	Islet β cell	Hypoglycemia	~10	Insulin
VIPoma (Verner-Morrison, WDHA)	Islet D_1 cell	Diarrhea, hypokalemia, hypochlorhydria	~60	Vasoactive intestinal peptide
Glucagonoma	Islet A cell	Mild diabetes mellitus, erythema necrolytica migrans, glossitis	>75	Glucagon
Somatostatinoma	Islet D cell	Diabetes mellitus, diarrhea, steatorrhea, gallstones	~70	Somatostatin
GRFoma	Non-β islet cell	Acromegaly	—	Growth hormone–releasing hormone (GRF)
CRFoma	Non-β islet cell	Cushing's syndrome	—	Corticotropin-releasing hormone (CRF)
PPoma	Islet PP cell	Rare necrolytic erythema	—	Pancreatic polypeptide (PP)
Neurotensinoma	Non-β islet cell	Mild diarrhea	—	Neurotensin
Miscellaneous tumors	Non-β islet cell	Hypercalcemia, SIADH, hyperpigmentation	—	Parathyroid hormone, vasopressin, melanocyte-stimulating hormone

ABBREVIATION: SIADH, syndrome of inappropriate antidiuretic hormone secretion.

In cases where tumors are too small to be visualized by these noninvasive methods, angiography or selective venous sampling for hormone determination may provide anatomic localization. CT and magnetic resonance imaging (MRI) are the preferred means of assessing metastatic spread, since the liver and lymph nodes are the initial sites of tumor metastasis.

THERAPEUTIC CONSIDERATIONS Therapy of endocrine tumors has two goals: (1) to decrease or reverse the growth and spread of the tumor and (2) to relieve the symptoms of hormone overproduction. When the tumor is localized, both goals may be accomplished by surgical excision. However, most of these tumors are malignant and have spread by the time of diagnosis, and control of growth in such malignant tumors has proven difficult. Thus far, the greatest benefit has been seen with chemotherapeutic regimens that include streptozocin, alone or in combination with fluorouracil or doxorubicin. Interferon-alpha at high doses may also limit tumor growth. Control of hepatic metastases has been achieved with surgical resection of isolated lesions, hepatic artery embolization, or direct injection with cytotoxic agents (e.g., ethanol), although these approaches are palliative rather than curative.

Several approaches are used to control the effects of excess hormone production by these tumors. The most common is to block the function of the target tissue. For example, gastric acid hypersecretion induced by gastrin-producing tumors may be reversed by medications that inhibit acid secretion (e.g., H_2 receptor blockers or proton pump inhibitors) or by surgical resection of the stomach. Diazoxide is used to help reverse the effects of hyperinsulinemia, and hypomotility agents and inhibitors of intestinal chloride secretion may ameliorate the diarrhea caused by hypersecretion of vasoactive intestinal peptide (VIP), gastrin, somatostatin, neurotensin, or serotonin.

A second approach is to block release of the transmitter from the tumor cells. The success of this approach depends on the continued ability of the tumor cells to respond to such physiologic or pharmacologic stimuli. Initial trials used somatostatin, a peptide hormone that inhibits the release of numerous hormones and amine transmitters. While somatostatin controls the symptoms of many of these tumors, it has a short half-life and must be given intravenously. These limitations have been largely overcome by the use of octreotide, a longer-acting analogue of somatostatin with similar actions that can be administered subcutaneously. The chemical structures of somatostatin and octreotide are shown in Fig. 95-1 (see also Chap. 328). Octreotide frequently relieves the symptoms of several endocrine tumors that are inadequately controlled by tumor resection or ablation. In addition, tumor regression has oc-

curred in occasional patients, suggesting that the hormone agonist may have some growth-inhibiting effects. The major known side effects of octreotide are dose-dependent and are similar to symptoms of somatostatin excess, including steatorrhea, mild hyperglycemia, nausea, and abdominal pain. Patients on long-term therapy with this agent have an increased tendency to develop gallstones. The clinical disorders that respond to therapy with octreotide are summarized in Table 95-3.

CARCINOID TUMORS

Carcinoid tumors are the most protean and the most common gastrointestinal endocrine tumors, accounting for approximately 75 percent of such neoplasms. The incidence of carcinoid tumors in the United States is approximately 15 per 1 million population per year. They may present with gastrointestinal bleeding, abdominal pain, obstruction from tumor growth or tumor-induced mesenteric fibrosis, or symptoms arising from tumor-secreted hormones. The name *carcinoid* was applied to these tumors because slow growth and the homogeneous appearance of tumor cells led early investigators to underestimate their malignant potential. They pursue an indolent course, and the interval

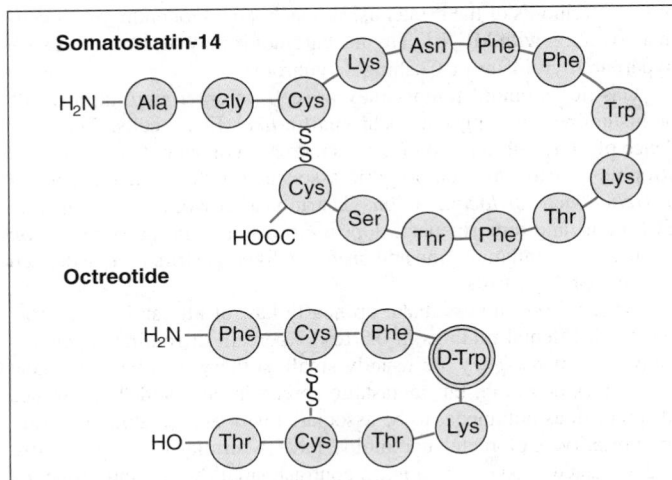

FIGURE 95-1 Structures of somatostatin-14 and octreotide. The double circle denotes the substitution of D-tryptophan for the naturally occurring L-tryptophan. This substitution inhibits peptide degradation and prolongs serum half-life.

Table 95-3

Clinical Uses of Octreotide in Gastrointestinal Disease

Disease	Effect
Hormone-secreting tumors	
Carcinoid tumor	Inhibits cutaneous flushing, controls diarrhea, reverses hypotension, aids perioperative management, ?inhibits growth
VIPoma	Controls diarrhea
Insulinoma	Controls hypoglycemia acutely, aids perioperative management
Gastrinoma	Aids perioperative management, ?controls diarrhea
Glucagonoma	Controls necrolytic erythema
Dumping syndrome	Controls diarrhea, vasomotor symptoms
Diarrhea	Inhibits intestinal secretion, motility
Short-bowel syndrome	
Ileostomy	
Diabetic neuropathy	
AIDS	
Fistulas	Inhibits fluid and enzyme secretion, promotes healing
Pancreatic	
Enteric	
Crohn's disease	
Gastrointestinal bleeding	
Portal hypertensive gastropathy	Reduces portal pressure, splanchnic blood flow
Esophageal and gastric varices	Reduces portal pressure, splanchnic blood flow

between onset of symptoms and diagnosis averages 4.5 years. Carcinoid tumors arise from neuroendocrine cells throughout the body but are most prevalent in the gastrointestinal tract, pancreas, and pulmonary bronchi. Ninety percent of these tumors arise in the enterochromaffin, or Kulchitsky, cells within the gastrointestinal tract. The tumors can be found anywhere from the stomach to the rectum and are most common in the appendix, ileum, and rectum. In the small intestine, carcinoid tumors are one of the two most common malignancies, along with adenocarcinoma. Gastrointestinal carcinoids frequently cause abdominal pain, bleeding, or intestinal obstruction. Although they are rarely large, the tumors may become the leading point for intussusception. In addition, mesenteric and peritoneal spread stimulates a local fibrous reaction, causing intestinal kinking, obstruction, and vascular compromise. Rare sites of carcinoid tumors include the thymus, esophagus, biliary duct, Meckel's diverticulum, breast, and ovary. No risk factors have been clearly defined for these enterochromaffin cell tumors. Carcinoids of the bronchus, stomach, and duodenum may occur in association with MEN 1. Thymic carcinoids may be associated with hyperparathyroidism or Cushing's syndrome.

Gastric carcinoid tumors may arise from enterochromaffin cells or histamine-secreting enterochromaffin-*like* (ECL) cells. The incidence of ECL cell-derived tumors is increased in patients with chronic atrophic gastritis and achlorhydria associated with pernicious anemia or *Helicobacter pylori* infection. Gastrin is a growth factor for gastric ECL cells, and tumorigenesis appears to result from the *combination* of the chronic inflammation and profound hypergastrinemia associated with atrophic gastritis.

Appendiceal tumors make up nearly half of all carcinoid tumors and are incidental findings in 0.3 to 0.7 percent of routine appendectomy specimens. They are usually small, solitary, and benign. Local invasion is common, but metastatic spread is rare, and the presence of tumor does not appear to be associated with appreciable morbidity or mortality. Colorectal carcinoids have a similarly benign course and are usually asymptomatic. In contrast, small-bowel and bronchial carcinoids have a more malignant course. Local transmural invasion, early metastasis to lymph nodes and liver, and symptoms from hormone secretion are common. Other sites of metastatic spread include bone and, less commonly, heart, breast, and eye. The risk of metastatic

spread is dependent on tumor size. Metastases are found in fewer than 2 percent of tumors less than 1 cm in diameter but in nearly 100 percent of tumors greater than 2 cm. Additional primary tumor implants within the gastrointestinal tract are found in 40 percent of patients.

CARCINOID SYNDROME Enterochromaffin cells secrete a variety of hormones and are embryologically related to thyroid C cells, adrenal medullary cells, and melanocytes. Tumors of each of these cell types may produce syndromes of hormone excess. Hormone secretion by carcinoid cells can cause distinctive and debilitating effects (carcinoid syndrome) long before local growth or metastatic spread is otherwise apparent. Manifestations of the carcinoid syndrome include the "classic" triad of cutaneous flushing, diarrhea, and valvular heart disease and, less commonly, telangiectasias, wheezing, and paroxysmal *hypo*tension. Flushing, which is present in approximately 85 percent of patients with carcinoid syndrome, is also seen with many other conditions, including menopause, autonomic nervous system dysfunction, ethanol ingestion, disulfiram treatment, drug withdrawal, and a variety of hormone-secreting tumors, including pheochromocytoma, medullary thyroid carcinoma, VIPoma, and mastocytosis. It is estimated that approximately 5 percent of individuals presenting with the new onset of flushing will be found to have the carcinoid syndrome. Early in the course, symptoms are usually episodic and may be provoked by stress, catecholamines, and ingestion of food or alcohol. During acute paroxysms, systolic blood pressure typically falls 20 to 30 mmHg. Diarrhea may result from several mechanisms. The most common type is mixed secretory and hypermotility-induced, producing watery stools unresponsive to fasting. Other causes include partial mechanical obstruction from tumor or fibrosis and mesenteric vascular insufficiency from local fibrosis. Endocardial fibrosis can cause valvular heart disease, usually affecting the proximal side of the tricuspid and pulmonary valves and leading to tricuspid insufficiency, pulmonary stenosis, and secondary right-sided heart failure. Left-sided valvular disease may occur in association with bronchial carcinoids, presumably because venous effluent from these tumors passes directly into the pulmonary veins, evading inactivation of the hormone mediators in the lung.

Approximately 5 percent of all patients with carcinoid tumors experience one or more symptoms of the carcinoid syndrome. The likelihood that symptoms will develop depends strongly on the origin and behavior of the tumor. While 30 to 60 percent of small-bowel carcinoids are associated with systemic manifestations, only 3.5 percent of lung, 1 percent of appendix, and virtually no rectal carcinoids produce the syndrome. In patients with intestinal carcinoids, the humoral symptoms only develop in the setting of metastatic disease to the liver. Bronchial and other extraintestinal carcinoids, whose hormone products are not immediately cleared by the liver, may produce the carcinoid syndrome in the absence of metastasis.

Carcinoid tumors may be classified on the basis of embryonic origin (Table 95-4). Clinical features, secreted hormones, diagnostic evaluation, and prognosis vary according to whether a carcinoid arises in foregut, midgut, or hindgut structures. For example, carcinoid syndrome is less common in patients with foregut carcinoids than with midgut tumors, but the syndrome, when it occurs, is more likely to include wheezing. Patients with foregut carcinoid syndrome more often have dramatic cutaneous flushing involving the whole body than those with tumors of midgut or hindgut organs. The flush of bronchial carcinoids may be prolonged (lasting hours to days); may be associated with excessive lacrimation, salivation, and facial edema; and occasionally produces significant hypotension. The cutaneous manifestations of gastric enterochromaffin cell carcinoids, though lasting only minutes, are frequently well-circumscribed and associated with wheals, pruritus, and high levels of histamine secretion. In contrast, gastric ECL cell carcinoid tumors are rarely associated with carcinoid syndrome.

Midgut carcinoids commonly cause the carcinoid syndrome. Acute episodes of flushing tend to be less severe than those associated with foregut tumors, but facial telangiectasias may develop late in the course. Midgut tumors are more frequently associated with cardiac manifestations and peritoneal fibrosis. Hindgut tumors rarely cause the carcinoid syndrome. A rare variant syndrome associated with ovarian carcinoids causes severe peritoneal fibrosis.

Table 95-4

Characteristics of Carcinoid Tumors

Embryonic Origin	Site of Primary Tumor	Carcinoid Syndrome			Monoamines
		Frequency, %	Characteristics		
Foregut	Bronchus	3.5	Intense flush, lasting up to several hours; associated lacrimation, salivation, facial edema; wheezing; diarrhea; left- and right-sided cardiac lesions		5-HT, ± histamine
	Stomach	~5	Intense, patchy, whole-body flush, with defined borders, wheals, usually lasting several minutes; pruritus; wheezing; diarrhea		5-HTP, histamine, ± 5-HT
	Duodenum, jejunum	~40	Diarrhea		5-HT
	Pancreas, gallbladder	Rare	Occasional necrolytic erythema		5-HT, ± histamine
		~40	Facial flush, usually lasting seconds to minutes; telangiectasias; cardiac lesions; peritoneal fibrosis; diarrhea		
Midgut	Ileum	~1			
	Appendix				
	Colon	Rare	Mild facial flush		5-HT
Hindgut	Rectum	0	Diarrhea		

ABBREVIATIONS: 5-HT, 5-hydroxytryptamine (serotonin); 5-HTP, 5-hydroxytryptophan.

Serotonin (5-hydroxytryptamine, 5-HT) is the most common secretory product of carcinoid tumors. As shown in Fig. 95-2, carcinoid tumors synthesize serotonin by enzymatic modification of circulating tryptophan. Up to 50 percent of the dietary intake of tryptophan can be converted to serotonin by these cells, which may leave inadequate substrate for incorporation into proteins and conversion to niacin. As a result, patients with widely metastatic carcinoid tumors may suffer symptoms of protein malnutrition (see Chap. 74) or mild pellagra (see Chap. 79). Serotonin induces intestinal secretion, inhibits intestinal absorption, and stimulates intestinal motility. High serotonin levels are likely the cause of diarrhea in most cases of carcinoid syndrome. Serotonin also stimulates fibroblast growth and fibrogenesis and thus may mediate or accelerate the peritoneal and cardiac valvular fibrosis in this disease. Excess serotonin secretion alone does not account for cutaneous flushing. Multiple monoamine and peptide factors contribute to the vasomotor changes; the relative contributions of each mediator may vary from patient to patient.

Carcinoid tumors elaborate multiple monoamines and peptide hormones, including histamine, catecholamines, bradykinins, tachykinins, enkephalins and endorphins, vasopressin, gastrin, adrenocorticotrophin, and prostaglandins (Table 95-5). Many secrete somatostatin, neurotensin, substance P, neurokinin A, TRH-like peptide (EEP-NH$_2$) and motilin. The elevated circulating levels of these substances mediate many of the pathophysiologic changes of carcinoid syndrome, although the relative contributions of each remain to be identified.

DIAGNOSIS The diagnosis of carcinoid tumors is influenced by the presenting features of the tumor. Patients with nonfunctional tumors (i.e., without the carcinoid *syndrome*) usually present with symptoms due to the direct effects of the tumor in the gastrointestinal tract, including abdominal pain or tenderness, nausea, malaise, weight loss, intestinal or biliary obstruction, or gastrointestinal bleeding. Depending on the location of the tumor and on whether metastases are present, endoscopy, barium studies, or CT may allow anatomic localization. Radiographic studies should include small-bowel follow-through or direct instillation of radiographic contrast material into the small bowel (enteroclysis) to identify tumors in the jejunum and ileum. Despite the improved detection of tumors, however, their pathologic identity is usually not suspected before resection or liver biopsy.

Evaluation of patients with clinical features of carcinoid syndrome is based on the observation that serotonin is synthesized and secreted by the large majority of functional carcinoid tumors. As shown in Fig. 95-2, serotonin is metabolized in the blood to 5-hydroxyindoleacetic acid (5-HIAA), which is cleared by the kidneys. Plasma and platelet serotonin and urinary 5-HIAA levels are usually elevated in the setting of carcinoid syndrome. Measurement of urinary 5-HIAA excretion is the most useful diagnostic test, and approximately 75 percent of pa-

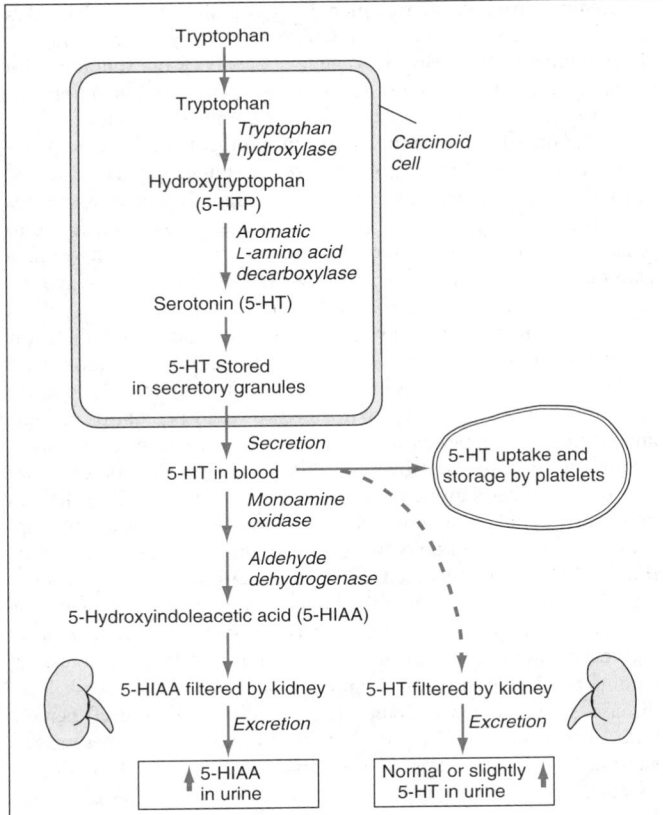

FIGURE 95-2 Metabolic pathway of serotonin in the carcinoid syndrome.

Table 95-5

Hormone Mediators of Carcinoid Syndrome

Clinical Feature	Frequency, %	Candidate Mediators
Diarrhea	78	5-HT, histamine, prostaglandins, VIP, glucagon, gastrin, calcitonin
Cutaneous flushing	94	5-HT, 5-HTP, kallikrein, NKA, histamine, SK, SP, prostaglandins
Telangiectasia	25	Unknown
Wheezing	18	5-HT, histamine
Abdominal pain	51	Tumor, hepatic enlargment, bowel ischemia (fibrosis)
Heart disease		5-HT
Right-sided	40	
Left-sided	13	
Pellagra dermatosis	7	Tryptophan depletion (5-HT synthesis)

ABBREVIATIONS: 5-HT, 5-hydroxytryptamine (serotonin): 5-HTP, 5-hydroxytryptophan; NKA, neurokinin A; SK, substance K; SP, substance P; VIP, vasoactive intestinal peptide.

SOURCE: After W Creutzfeldt and F Stockmann, Am J Med 82:4, 1987.

tients excrete more than 80 µmol/d (15 mg/d). The specificity of this test approaches 100 percent after exclusion of ingested substances known to elevate 5-HIAA levels; these include bananas, plantain, pineapple, kiwi fruit, walnuts, plums, pecans, avocados, guaifenesin, and acetaminophen. Conversely, aspirin and levodopa ingestion can cause a falsely depressed 5-HIAA level. In some patients with carcinoid syndrome and normal urinary 5-HIAA, documentation of elevated plasma or platelet serotonin concentrations may establish the diagnosis. However, many foregut carcinoid tumors lack aromatic L-amino acid decarboxylase and convert 5-hydroxytryptophan (5-HTP) to serotonin with low efficiency. Since 5-HTP is not metabolized to 5-HIAA, urinary studies may be misleading. These patients may have elevated urinary serotonin levels, since renal cells contain aromatic L-amino acid decarboxylase. Diagnosis in these cases may be confirmed by demonstrating elevated plasma 5-HTP, histamine, or peptide hormone levels, although it frequently rests on the anatomic detection of the tumor itself. Attempts to provoke cutaneous flushing are helpful for documenting flushing in cases when the clinical history is equivocal. Ethanol, pentagastrin, or *micro*gram quantities of epinephrine can be used for this purpose. CT, MRI, and selective angiography are the most sensitive tests for detecting metastatic disease in the liver. Since most patients with the humoral syndrome have metastases, liver biopsy is the most common access to histologic diagnosis. Additional information about bone metastases and cardiac sequelae may be obtained with bone scans and echocardiography, respectively. In patients in whom a tumor cannot be detected, scintigraphic imaging with radiolabeled octreotide is often helpful. Octreotide binds tightly to type 2 somatostatin receptors, which are expressed in large numbers by most carcinoid tumor cells. Octreotide scintigraphy identifies the sites of primary and metastatic tumor in approximately two-thirds of patients with carcinoid syndrome. The sensitivity of this method is improved with high doses ($\geq$200 MBq) of radionuclide and single photon emission CT (SPECT) imaging. It is far more sensitive than scintigraphy with metaiodobenzyl guanidine (MIBG), which was previously used for this purpose.

℞ TREATMENT

Effective treatment of the carcinoid syndrome may require more than one approach. Therapy should be selected according to the severity of symptoms. Since nearly all patients with carcinoid syndrome have metastatic disease, resection is rarely curative. Mild diarrhea may be controlled with hypomotility agents such as loperamide or diphenoxylate/atropine. In patients who have undergone ileal resection, diarrhea can be exacerbated by bile salt malabsorption and frequently responds to cholestyramine. Flushing, if rare and mild, may not require therapy. Combination therapy with histamine H_1 and H_2 receptor antagonists (e.g., diphenhydramine and ranitidine) can inhibit the cutaneous flush associated with foregut carcinoids. Phenoxybenzamine may provide additional benefit by inhibiting the release of bradykinin. Methylxanthine bronchodilators and glucocorticoids are helpful in relieving the dyspnea and wheezing associated with bronchial carcinoids. Beta-adrenergic agonists should be avoided because they may provoke acute exacerbations. Serotonin antagonists, including cyproheptadine and methysergide, have been used to provide relief of diarrhea. Unfortunately, these agents have little effect on flushing and other vasomotor symptoms, and methysergide can induce fibrosis similar to that caused by the carcinoid itself.

Octreotide is a potent inhibitor of hormone secretion by carcinoid cells. At doses of 150 to 1500 µg/d, this agent provides effective control of diarrhea, flushing, and wheezing in more than 75 percent of cases. Octreotide is effective in the management of acute, life-threatening manifestations of the carcinoid syndrome, such as hypotension or resulting angina, as well as of the transient exacerbation of symptoms caused by hepatic artery embolization or the induction of general anesthesia. Octreotide must be administered in two or three subcutaneous injections each day. The development of long-acting preparations of other somatostatin analogues, such as lanreotide, should provide even more convenient therapy. It is not yet known whether octreotide can prevent the observed cardiac (or mesenteric) fibrosis. Established valvular heart disease is not reversed by any form of medical therapy.

Surgery, hepatic artery embolization, and chemotherapy have been used to reduce the burden of tumor tissue. Surgery is the treatment of choice for small (<2 cm diameter) carcinoid tumors of the appendix or large bowel, as well as for the anatomic effects of these tumors (e.g., intestinal obstruction, ischemia, or bleeding). Curative resection also may be effective in patients with carcinoid syndrome from isolated bronchial or other extraintestinal carcinoids. Most patients with carcinoid syndrome, however, have gross metastatic disease. Hepatic resection generally provides only transient amelioration of symptoms and no improvement in survival. In isolated cases, however, long-term palliation has been achieved by resection of a *single* hepatic metastasis after removal of the primary tumor. Orthotopic liver transplantation for hepatic metastases has not provided long-term benefit. Several less invasive approaches have been tried to limit the hepatic tumor burden and control humoral symptoms, including local irradiation, selective hepatic artery infusion of chemotherapy, CT-guided instillation of ethanol into metastatic implants, CT-guided cryoablation, and hepatic arterial chemoembolization. Carcinoid tumors are generally radioresistant, although radiotherapy may provide transient relief of pain from bone metastases; they respond poorly to chemotherapy. Arterial occlusion by Gelfoam embolization provides rapid relief of symptoms for up to 1 year in approximately 90 percent of patients. Its success derives in part from the fact that the hepatic artery supplies less than half the blood supply of normal liver tissue but nearly all the blood supply of the tumor. Side effects of therapy include abdominal pain, fever, and occasional synthetic liver dysfunction. The effectiveness of therapy can be monitored by means of serum transaminase levels, which should rise substantially over the first 24 to 48 h after embolization. Patients undergoing embolization may experience acute exacerbation of carcinoid symptoms provoked by the sudden release of hormones from the tumor. Although such effects are rarely life-threatening, prophylactic treatment with histamine receptor blockers and octreotide is recommended. Combination therapy with hepatic arterial infusion of cytotoxic agents (usually 5-fluorouracil with streptozocin or doxorubicin), followed by arterial embolization, appears to offer no additional benefit over embolization alone.

Several systemic chemotherapeutic protocols have been evaluated. Various combinations of streptozocin, fluorouracil, cyclophosphamide, dacarbazine, and doxorubicin induce objective responses in approximately one-third of patients with metastatic disease. Combination therapy with streptozocin and doxorubicin appears to provide the best response, inducing tumor regression in approximately 40 percent of patients and a small but significant increase in patient survival. Chemotherapy is generally reserved for patients with debilitating symptoms inadequately controlled by octreotide or those with carcinoid cardiac disease or impaired liver function. Interferon-alpha decreases tumor size in approximately 10 to 20 percent of patients and decreases symptoms and urinary 5-HIAA excretion in up to two-thirds of patients. However, this immunomodulator does not improve survival significantly and does not enhance the effect of more standard chemotherapeutic regimens. Although octreotide appears to have induced objective responses in a few cases, controlled trials have not demonstrated a significant effect.

The prognosis of carcinoid tumor is highly dependent on the site and stage of the disease at diagnosis. As noted above, appendiceal and rectal carcinoids rarely affect survival. For other gastrointestinal carcinoids, 5-year survival is approximately 95 percent with local disease, 65 percent with lymph node involvement, and 20 percent with liver metastases. In patients with carcinoid syndrome, median survival is 2.5 years after the first episode of flushing. Prognosis is inversely correlated with the degree of urinary 5-HIAA elevation. Despite attempts at therapy, patients excreting >800 µmol/d (>150 mg/d) have a median survival of only 1 year.

The endocrine functions of the pancreas are mediated by the islets of Langerhans, which are distributed throughout the pancreatic parenchyma. Each mature islet is composed of four major classes of secretory cells: A cells, whose major secreted product is glucagon; B (or β) cells, which secrete insulin; D cells, which secrete somatostatin; and PP cells, which secrete pancreatic polypeptide. Each of these cells secretes additional regulatory peptides in lower concentrations. During development of the islets, precursors are transiently formed that secrete several additional regulatory peptides, including gastrin, VIP, adrenocorticotropin (ACTH), and others. Pancreatic islet cell tumors can arise from any of these cell populations. These tumors may therefore secrete one or more biologically active peptides, giving rise to a number of recognizable humoral syndromes (see Table 95-2).

GASTRINOMA (ZOLLINGER-ELLISON SYNDROME)
(See also Chap. 284) In 1955, Zollinger and Ellison reported the association of severe peptic ulcer disease and gastrin-secreting tumors of the pancreas. These gastrinomas generate high serum gastrin levels, leading to hypersecretion of gastric acid and consequent duodenal and jejunal ulcers. Gastrinomas are the most common of the hormone-secreting tumors of the pancreatic islets, constituting nearly one-tenth of gastroenteropancreatic endocrine tumors and occurring with a frequency of approximately 4 in 10 million in an unselected population in Ireland. Zollinger-Ellison syndrome may account for up to 0.1 percent of patients with duodenal ulcer disease in the United States. Ulcer disease develops in almost all patients with gastrinoma and is the presenting problem in approximately 70 percent. More than half of patients experience diarrhea (either watery stools or steatorrhea), and approximately 30 percent present with diarrhea alone. Radiologic and endoscopic examinations frequently reveal increased gastric fluid and thickened rugal folds. The age distribution of patients with gastrinoma is similar to that in ordinary acid peptic disease, with a broad peak in the fifth to eighth decades. Gastrinoma should be considered in all patients with recurrent or refractory ulcer disease, ulcers associated with gastric hypertrophy, ulcers in the distal duodenum or jejunum, ulcers in association with diarrhea, kidney stones, hypercalcemia, or pituitary disease, or a strong family history of duodenal ulcer disease or endocrine tumors.

Between one-fourth and one-half of gastrinomas occur in association with the MEN 1 syndrome (see Chap. 340). Hyperparathyroidism is the most common component of MEN 1 and occurs in about 80 percent of patients with this form of Zollinger-Ellison syndrome. All gastrinoma patients should be screened for possible MEN 1 by measurement of serum calcium, phosphorus, cortisol, and prolactin levels and imaging of the sella turcica. First-degree relatives of patients with MEN 1 should be similarly screened.

Approximately 80 percent of gastrin-secreting tumors arise in pancreatic islets, including nearly all those associated with MEN 1, and most are located in the pancreatic head. Another 10 to 15 percent arise from G cells in the duodenum, and the remainder are scattered in the distal small bowel, stomach, spleen, liver, lymph nodes, and ovary (mucinous cystadenoma). The tumors are usually small and are frequently multifocal, especially when associated with MEN 1. The biologic behavior may be variable. In most reported series, one-half to two-thirds of these tumors are malignant, with metastases to lymph nodes and liver and less frequently to bone. However, the prevalence of metastatic disease at the time of diagnosis appears to have decreased, perhaps owing to the more widespread consideration and earlier detection of these tumors. Such observations have important therapeutic implications, since isolated tumors are more likely to be cured by resection. Gastrinomas, like most other islet cell tumors, are generally slow-growing, but growth patterns vary widely, and metastases may be more aggressive than the primary tumor itself.

℞ **TREATMENT**
Treatment of Zollinger-Ellison syndrome is directed at the sequelae of excess gastrin secretion and at the tumor itself. The availability of potent inhibitors of gastric acid secretion, including H_2 receptor blockers and the H^+,K^+-ATPase inhibitors omeprazole and lansoprazole, has reduced the need for gastric surgery in these patients. The rare patient who fails to respond to medical therapy should be treated surgically. However, patients with coexistent hyperparathyroidism should undergo parathyroid resection before a decision is made about gastric surgery, since resolution of hypercalcemia may permit better medical control of gastric acid secretion.

Because of the effective control of hormone-mediated symptoms, morbidity and mortality from gastrinoma are increasingly related to the growth and spread of the tumor itself. Curative resection of the gastrinoma is possible in 15 to 20 percent of cases and is favored by an extrapancreatic location and by small tumor size. Gastrinomas in association with MEN 1 syndrome are not amenable to surgical cure, although these tumors generally have a benign natural history. A variety of imaging studies are used preoperatively to identify the primary tumor mass and exclude metastases. More than 90 percent of gastrinomas can be identified using a combination of CT, endoscopic ultrasonography, and octreotide scintigraphy. Each of these tests alone has a sensitivity of between 38 and 70 percent for detecting primary gastrinomas. (Transabdominal ultrasonography detects only 10 to 20 percent of these primary tumors, but it can identify approximately 50 percent of liver metastases.) In cases where these approaches fail to identify the tumor, angiography, selective venous hormone sampling, intraoperative palpation, and intraoperative ultrasonography are frequently effective. *Intraoperative* octreotide scintigraphy provides no additional diagnostic advantage.

Treatment of unresectable gastrinoma includes chemotherapy, hormonal therapy, and hepatic artery embolization. Chemotherapeutic regimens including streptozocin and fluorouracil, with or without doxorubicin, commonly induce partial responses. Interferon-alpha also may cause an objective response, but octreotide does not appear to be effective. Hepatic artery embolization may decrease hepatic tumor burden and ameliorate pain. Unfortunately, none of these approaches prolongs survival of patients with metastatic disease, which approximates 25 percent at 10 years.

INSULINOMA (β CELL TUMOR)
The hallmark of pancreatic β cell tumors is the development of symptomatic hypoglycemia from unregulated insulin hypersection (see also Chap. 335). Insulinomas are the second most common functioning islet cell tumors and have a reported prevalence of approximately 8 in 10 million in an unselected Irish population. They arise most frequently in the fifth to seventh decades, although cases have been reported at all ages. In infants and children, insulinoma must be distinguished from diffuse β cell adenomatosis and nesidioblastosis. Whipple's triad, the classic presentation of insulinoma, consists of fasting hypoglycemia, *symptoms* of hypoglycemia, and immediate relief after intravenous glucose administration. Weight gain may result from increased food ingested to combat symptoms of hypoglycemia. In the current era, the diagnosis of insulinoma is made by demonstrating fasting hypoglycemia in the presence of normal or elevated plasma insulin levels. Symptoms related to the hypoglycemia include headache, slurred speech, psychological alterations, visual disturbances, confusion, and, ultimately, coma and death. Hypoglycemia also induces the secondary release of catecholamines, leading to tremulousness, diaphoresis, pallor, palpitations, cardiac arrhythmias, and behavioral irritability. Because of the episodic release of insulin, symptoms early in the course may be intermittent or occur only after somewhat prolonged periods of fasting. However, symptoms do develop early, so that tumors are usually small and solitary at the time of diagnosis. Multiple primary tumors are found in approximately 10 percent of patients. An additional 10 percent of patients have malignant disease, with spread to the local lymph nodes and the liver. As with gastrinomas, insulinomas are frequently associated with MEN 1 (see Chaps. 335 and 340), and such tumors are more likely to be multifocal. Extrapancreatic insulin-

secreting tumors are rare and usually arise in ectopic pancreatic tissue.

Diagnosis is made by demonstrating fasting hypoglycemia and an inadequate response of insulin to the hypoglycemia (see Chap. 335 for details). Patients are fasted under close supervision for up to 72 h, followed, if necessary, by an exercise tolerance test. Most patients with insulinoma develop hypoglycemia within 24 h, as evidenced by a serum glucose level of less than 2.8 mmol/L (50 mg/dL) in men or 2.5 mmol/L (45 mg/dL) in women. However, there is no absolute glucose level that defines hypoglycemia, so the diagnosis of insulinoma depends on the demonstration of inadequate insulin suppression in the face of falling glucose levels. Documentation of rising cortisol levels excludes hypoglycemia secondary to hypothalamic-pituitary-adrenal dysfunction. It is also necessary to exclude other causes of fasting hypoglycemia, including administration of exogenous insulin, sulfonylurea ingestion, severe liver failure, and tumors that secrete insulinlike growth factors (e.g., fibrosarcoma, mesothelioma, and hemangiopericytoma). Exogenous insulin administration can be excluded by measuring levels of the C peptide of proinsulin, which normally vary in parallel with the plasma insulin concentrations. Since insulin administration suppresses endogenous insulin secretion, detection of normal or elevated C-peptide levels is inconsistent with insulin abuse. In addition, because insulinoma cells often process proinsulin incompletely, the serum often has an increased ratio of proinsulin to insulin. A ratio greater than 20 percent in the appropriate clinical setting is suggestive of insulinoma. Serum levels of sulfonylureas should be elevated if hyperinsulinemic hypoglycemia is caused by these agents. Normal glucose/insulin ratios exclude liver failure and tumors that secrete insulin-like growth factors.

Rx **TREATMENT**

Once a diagnosis of insulinemia is established, acute treatment is supportive, with intravenous glucose infusion as required to maintain plasma levels within the normal range. Hyperglycemic agents, including diazoxide, beta-adrenergic receptor blockers, and phenytoin, can be used to support serum glucose levels, but their effects are variable and may last only a short time. Octreotide frequently inhibits insulin secretion by these tumors and may be an effective agent for acute management. Definitive therapy is accomplished by surgical resection. Because insulinomas are usually small (most are <2 cm in diameter), only half are detected by CT. Two-phase (arterial and parenchymal) contrast techniques improve the sensitivity of CT somewhat. In contrast, endoscopic ultrasonography detects 80 to 90 percent of tumors. Angiography with selective venous sampling for insulin levels is also about 80 percent sensitive, as is palpation during surgery. At surgery, all detectable tumors should be resected. The effectiveness of intervention is monitored by determination of intraoperative blood glucose levels. In cases where no tumors are detected by any of these methods, stepwise distal pancreatectomy is performed until frozen sections of resected specimens and/or blood glucose measurements indicate that all tumor has been removed. If no tumor is found, or if multiple tumors are present, pancreatectomy is limited to 70 to 80 percent to preserve digestive and endocrine pancreatic function.

Patients with metastatic disease and those whose insulinomas are not removed by partial pancreatectomy can frequently be managed with hyperglycemic agents such as diazoxide or octreotide. In one study, all seven patients with metastatic insulinoma showed a response to octreotide, although the degree of response varied. However, hypoglycemia may be worsened by octreotide administration, perhaps owing to inhibition of glucagon or growth hormone by this agent. Diazoxide, though frequently effective, can cause troubling side effects, including salt and fluid retention, hypertrichosis, and gastrointestinal upset. The combination of streptozocin and doxorubicin is the mainstay of chemotherapy for metastatic disease; it is superior to streptozocin-fluorouracil. These agents in

duce objective remission in approximately half of patients and are associated with a modest but significant increase in survival. Patients with residual tumor should be followed carefully for changes in secretory profile which may affect therapy. Such changes may include development of hyperglycemia as a result of glucagon-secreting metastases.

VIPOMA [VERNER-MORRISON SYNDROME; WATERY DIARRHEA, HYPOKALEMIA, ACHLORHYDRIA (WDHA) SYNDROME] Verner and Morrison described a syndrome of watery diarrhea, hypokalemia, and renal failure in association with non-β-cell tumors of the pancreatic islets. The clinical features of this syndrome are caused by the high levels of VIP secreted by the tumors. VIPomas comprise approximately 2 percent of gastroenteropancreatic tumors and have a prevalence of approximately 1 in 10 million in the Irish population studied. The manifestations of VIPoma include secretory diarrhea, profound weakness, hypokalemia, and hypochlorhydria. Stool volume is greater than 3 L/d in most patients, and non-anion-gap acidosis usually occurs as a result of bicarbonate losses in the stool. Other electrolyte abnormalities include hypercalcemia (in approximately two-thirds of patients) and hypophosphatemia. Approximately half of patients develop hyperglycemia, which results from hypokalemia- and VIP-induced glycogenolysis in the liver, and a fifth of patients experience cutaneous flushing. Although most symptoms can be reproduced by infusion of exogenous VIP, these tumors also contain other peptide hormones, including the VIP-related peptide histidine-methionine (PHM), somatostatin, helodermin, and neurotensin, each of which may contribute to clinical features exhibited by individual patients. Diagnosis rests on the demonstration of high plasma VIP levels in the setting of a stool volume of at least 1 L/d. Lesser increases in VIP levels occur in patients with hepatic failure and intestinal ischemia.

VIPomas are most commonly pancreatic tumors. Unlike gastrinomas and insulinomas, however, VIPomas frequently grow to a large size before becoming clinically apparent. On average, the size of these tumors at the time of diagnosis is second only to that of nonfunctioning pancreatic islet cell tumors. Although they are slow-growing, these tumors are usually malignant. Approximately three-fifths are metastatic at the time of diagnosis. Most VIPomas are located in the body or tail of the pancreas. A few cases have been seen in association when MEN 1; however, there is no constant relation between the two syndromes. Between 10 and 15 percent of VIP-secreting tumors arise from neuroendocrine cells in the intestinal mucosa, and a few are ganglioneuroblastomas, mastocytomas, pheochromocytomas, or small cell carcinomas of the lung.

Rx **TREATMENT**

Treatment is surgical extirpation whenever possible. However, metastases may preclude this approach. Preoperative evaluation should include CT or MRI to localize the tumor and any metastases. In addition to supportive therapy with fluids and electrolytes, prednisone is frequently effective in reducing the volume of diarrhea, despite its inability to alter serum VIP levels. Octreotide inhibits the secretion of VIP and ameliorates symptoms in most patients, although most patients eventually become refractory to this agent. VIPomas often produce symptoms related to the large size of the tumor itself. Surgery may be indicated to relieve local effects or to remove a single large primary tumor. For patients with symptomatic metastatic disease, chemotherapy and hepatic artery embolization have the greatest benefit on tumor burden. Regimens combining streptozocin and doxorubicin or streptozocin-fluorouracil are the most effective chemotherapy, inducing objective partial remission in up to 90 percent of cases.

GLUCAGONOMA In 1966, McGovern described a rare syndrome of diabetes mellitus and necrolytic migratory erythema in association with a pancreatic islet cell tumor. The observation that these tumors secrete high levels of glucagon suggested a cause for the diabetes and the possibility that the peptide may have a role in the other clinical features. Although these tumors frequently synthesize and secrete additional peptides, including pancreatic polypeptide, somatostatin, insulin, and gastrin, the common link is hyperglucagonemia. Glucagonomas are characteristically single, large, and slow-growing. More than 75 percent have metastasized at the time of diagnosis, most commonly to the liver and bones. Glucagonoma has been reported in association with MEN 1 (see Chap. 340). A fasting plasma glucagon level of >1000 ng/L (>1000 pg/mL) establishes the diagnosis. More modest elevations of plasma glucagon levels may occur in diabetic ketoacidosis, renal failure, hepatic failure, sepsis, prolonged fasting, and gluten-sensitive enteropathy. Hypocholesterolemia and hypoaminoacidemia are common, with alanine, glycine, and serine levels usually less than 25 percent of normal. Glucagonoma may be distinguished from other hyperglucagonemic syndromes by the failure of glucose to suppress and the failure of arginine to increase serum glucagon concentrations.

The characteristic glucagonoma skin rash (necrolytic migratory erythema) is erythematous, raised, scaly, sometimes bullous, sometimes psoriatic, and ultimately crusted. It is located primarily on the face, abdomen, perineum, and distal extremities. After resolution, the regions of the acute eruption usually remain indurated and hyperpigmented. Patients also may experience glossitis, stomatitis, angular cheilitis, dystrophic nails, and hair thinning. The diabetes is usually mild or asymptomatic and may appear only as an abnormality on an oral glucose tolerance test. Ketoacidosis has not been reported. Weight loss, hypoaminoacidemia, anemia, and thromboembolic disease also occur in association with this syndrome. A causal association between hyperglucagonemia and skin disease has been difficult to prove, leading to speculation that the rash may result from nutritional deficiency. In some patients, the rash responds to oral zinc or to infusions of amino acids or essential fatty acids. Octreotide therapy also has yielded good results. However, dermatologic symptoms frequently recur after each of these therapies.

Because the primary tumor is usually large and found only in the pancreas, it is easily identified by CT, ultrasound, or angiography. Surgical therapy is curative in approximately 30 percent of patients. Resection is more frequently aimed at decreasing tumor burden. Despite occasional objective responses, attempts at chemotherapy with combinations of streptozocin, fluorouracil, doxorubicin, dacarbazine, octreotide, and interferon-alpha have little impact. As for other tumors described in this chapter, hepatic artery embolization, chemoembolization, cryotherapy, and direct instillation of ethanol can provide relief of symptoms. Fortunately, the slow-growing nature of the tumor allows for prolonged survival even in many cases of metastatic disease.

SOMATOSTATINOMA Somatostatin-secreting tumors are the most recent group to be identified with a defined clinical syndrome. The classic triad of somatostatinoma consists of diabetes mellitus, steatorrhea, and cholelithiasis. These symptoms derive from the widespread inhibitory actions of somatostatin, including inhibition of insulin release, pancreatic enzyme and bicarbonate secretion, and gallbladder motility, respectively. The diabetes is usually mild, and, in a few cases, *hypo*glycemia has been seen, perhaps from the concurrent secretion of other peptides. Individual somatostatinomas have been shown to secrete insulin, calcitonin, gastrin, VIP, ACTH, prostaglandins, substance P, motilin, and glucagon. Patients with somatostatinomas also may develop hypochlorhydria, weight loss, and paroxysmal hypertension.

Approximately 60 percent of reported somatostatinomas are located in the pancreas. The second most common site is in the small intestine, although intestinal tumors are associated with lower plasma somatostatin levels and are more commonly asymptomatic. Like glucagonomas and VIPomas, these tumors are usually single, large, and metastatic at the time of diagnosis. Somatostatinomas have not been reported in association with MEN 1. Curiously, the occasional coincidence of pheochromocytoma, café au lait spots, and neurofibromatosis suggests a possible association with MEN type 2b (see Chap. 340). Small cell lung carcinomas, medullary thyroid carcinomas, pheochromocytomas, and paragangliomas that secrete somatostatin also have been described.

MISCELLANEOUS FUNCTIONAL ISLET CELL TUMORS In addition to the diseases described above, islet cell tumors have been associated with several other syndromes of hormone excess, including acromegaly (growth hormone or growth hormone–releasing hormone), hypercalcemia (parathyroid hormone–related peptide), diarrhea and diabetes mellitus (neurotensin), and Cushing's syndrome (corticotropin-releasing factor or ACTH). Secretion by islet cell tumors of ACTH, alone or in combination with other peptides, appears to be a marker of more aggressive disease.

NONFUNCTIONING ISLET CELL TUMORS (See also Chap. 94) More than 15 percent of pancreatic islet cell tumors are not associated with any definable hormone-mediated syndrome. Nonetheless, many of these nonfunctioning islet cell tumors synthesize and secrete one or more regulatory peptides, including pancreatic polypeptide, substance P, and motilin. With increasing availability of radioimmunoassay and immunohistochemical reagents, protein products will probably be defined for more and more of these tumors. Nonetheless, most of these tumors behave in a similar fashion. They arise most commonly in the head or tail of the pancreas and are frequently large (5 to 10 cm in diameter) at the time of diagnosis. The most common clinical manifestations are abdominal pain, jaundice, a palpable mass, malaise, and bleeding esophageal or gastric varices (from splenic vein compression). Though slow-growing, at least half of these tumors present with metastases to the liver or lymph nodes. Surgical cure is achieved in approximately 20 percent. The remainder are poorly responsive to chemotherapy. Streptozocin with or without fluorouracil induces objective responses in approximately 60 percent of patients. Five-year survival for patients with these tumors is approximately 40 percent, with many long-term survivors despite known metastatic disease.

BIBLIOGRAPHY

CARCINOID TUMORS AND SYNDROME

ERICKSSON B, OBERG K: Peptide hormones as tumor markers in neuroendocrine gastrointestinal tumors. Acta Oncol 30:477, 1991

GODWIN JD: Carcinoid tumors: An analysis of 2837 cases. Cancer 36:560, 1975

JOENSUU H et al: Treatment of metastatic carcinoid tumor with recombinant interferon-alpha. Eur J Cancer 28A:1650, 1992

KVOLS LK et al: Treatment of the malignant carcinoid syndrome: Evaluation of a long-acting somatostatin analogue. N Engl J Med 315:663, 1986

MOERTEL CG et al: Carcinoid tumor of the appendix: Treatment and prognosis. N Engl J Med 317:1699, 1987

NORHEIM I et al: Malignant carcinoid tumors: An analysis of 103 patients with regard to tumor localization, hormone production, and survival. Ann Surg 206:115, 1987

PERRY RR, VINIK AI: Endocrine tumors of the gastrointestinal tract. Annu Rev Med 47:57, 1996

RUSNIEWSKI P et al: Treatment of the carcinoid syndrome with the long-acting somatostatin analogue lanreotide. Gut 39:279, 1996

SAINI A, WAXMAN J: Management of carcinoid syndrome. Postgrad Med 67:506, 1991

THORSON A et al: Malignant carcinoid of the small intestine with metastases to the liver, valvular disease of the right side of the heart, peripheral vasomotor symptoms, bronchoconstriction, and an unusual type of cyanosis: A clinical and pathologic syndrome. Am Heart J 47:795, 1954

ISLET CELL TUMORS

BIESMA B et al: Recombinant interferon alpha-2b in patients with metastatic apudomas: Effect on tumors and tumor markers. Br J Cancer 66:850, 1992

BLOOM SR, POLAK JM: Glucagonoma syndrome. Am J Med 82(Suppl 5B):25, 1987

BOSTWICK DG et al: Expression of opioid peptides in tumors. N Engl J Med 317:1439, 1987

GIBRIL F et al: Somatostatin receptor scintigraphy—its sensitivity compared with that of other imaging methods in detecting primary and metastatic gastrinomas. A prospective study. Ann Intern Med 125:26, 1996

GORDEN P et al: Somatostatin and somatostatin analogue (SMS 201-995) in treatment of hormone-secreting tumors of the pituitary and gastrointestinal tract and nonneoplastic diseases of the gut. Ann Intern Med 110:35, 1989

KLEIN S et al: In vivo assessment of the metabolic alterations in glucagonoma syndrome. Metabolism 41:1171, 1992

KREIS GJ: VIPoma syndrome. Am J Med 82(Suppl 5B):37, 1987

KVOLS LK et al: Treatment of metastatic islet cell carcinomas with a somatostatin analogue (SMS 201-995). Ann Intern Med 107:162, 1987

MOERTEL CG et al: Streptozocin-doxorubicin, streptozocin-fluorouracil or chlorozocin in the treatment of advanced islet cell carcinoma. N Engl J Med 326:519, 1992

OBERG K: Neuroendocrine gastrointestinal tumours. Ann Oncol 7:453, 1996

VINIK AI et al: Somatostatinomas, PPomas, neurotensinomas. Semin Oncol 14:263, 1987

WYNICK D et al: Symptomatic secondary hormone syndromes in patients with established malignant pancreatic endocrine tumors. N Engl J Med 319:605, 1988

96   *Howard I. Scher, Robert J. Motzer*

BLADDER AND RENAL CELL CANCER

BLADDER CANCER

Transitional epithelium lines the urinary tract starting at the renal pelvis and extending through the ureter, the urinary bladder, and the proximal two-thirds of the urethra. In the distal third of the urethra, a squamous epithelium is predominant. Carcinomas occur in all four sites, 90 percent developing in the bladder, 8 percent in the renal pelvis, and 2 percent in the ureter or urethra. Once diagnosed, these tumors tend to recur, and serial monitoring of the urothelial tract with cystoscopy and/or urinary cytology is essential. Bladder cancer is the fourth most common cancer in men and the ninth in women, with an estimated 52,900 new cases (38,300 in males and 14,600 in females) and 11,700 deaths (7800 males and 3900 females) predicted for 1996. The median age at diagnosis is 65 years.

EPIDEMIOLOGY   The long latency period between exposure to putative carcinogens and the development of the clinical disease makes the establishment of causative links difficult. Nevertheless, estimates are that 25 percent of the cancers in men are related to occupational exposure, and 50 percent to cigarette smoking. Smoking duration is a key element in determining risk, which persists for up to 10 years after smoking cessation. The primary chemical compounds associated with increased risk are the polycyclic aromatic hydrocarbons such as 2-naphthylamine, 4-aminobiphenyl, and benzidine. They are detoxified by acetylation, and slow acetylators have a higher risk of bladder cancer. Individuals involved in the manufacture of aluminum and polychlorinated biphenyls and those who work as chimney sweeps and dry cleaners are also at increased risk. Dietary factors include a high consumption of fried meats and fats, while vitamin A supplements are protective. Chronic cyclophosphamide exposure increases the risk ninefold, while *Schistosoma haematobium* exposure is associated with an increased risk of squamous (70 percent) and transitional cell carcinomas (30 percent).

CLINICAL PRESENTATION, DIAGNOSIS, AND STAGING   Hematuria is the first sign of bladder cancer in 80 to 90 percent of patients, followed by urinary frequency or irritative symptoms. Depending on the location of the tumor, ureteral obstruction may result in flank pain or discomfort. Less commonly, symptoms of metastatic disease occur. Screening of asymptomatic subjects for hematuria increases the likelihood that tumors will be diagnosed at an early stage but has not been shown to influence survival. The bladder is the most common source of gross hematuria (~40 percent), but benign cystitis (22 percent) is a more common cause than bladder cancer (15 percent) (see Chap. 48). Microscopic hematuria is more commonly of prostatic origin (25 percent); bladder cancer accounts for this sign in only 2 percent of cases. The evaluation of hematuria or of a suspected bladder

tumor requires a urinary cytologic evaluation, visualization of the urothelial tract by sonography or an intravenous pyelogram, and cystoscopy. The endoscopic evaluation involves an examination under anesthesia to determine whether a palpable mass is present. A flexible endoscope is then inserted into the bladder, and the bladder is irrigated to evaluate for the presence of malignant cells. Visualized abnormal areas are biopsied, and an attempt is made to resect all visible tumors. Removal of all tumor is essential for both diagnostic and therapeutic purposes, and a portion of the muscle layer should be included to permit assessment of the depth of invasion of a tumor. As the endoscope is withdrawn, the urethra is inspected. Selective catheterization of the ureters with retrograde examination is used to evaluate for upper tract disease.

Computed tomography (CT) and magnetic resonance imaging (MRI) may assist in distinguishing tumors that extend to the perivesical fat (T3b) or to adjacent structures such as the prostate or vagina (T4) from those that do not (T3a) and in determining whether regional lymph nodes are involved (N +). Neither procedure accurately predicts the depth of invasion within the bladder wall. The presence of distant metastases is assessed by CT of the abdomen, chest x-rays, or radionuclide imaging of the skeleton. The need for these studies is based in part on the local extent of the lesion.

Staging follows the TNM (tumor, nodes, metastasis) staging system, which accounts for growth patterns observed clinically (Fig. 96-1). In general, tumors of stage T1 or below are managed by endoscopic means initially, while for those that invade muscle, surgical removal of the bladder is considered standard therapy.

PATHOLOGY   In North America, 90 to 95 percent of bladder tumors are transitional; pure squamous tumors (with keratinization) make up 3 percent; adenocarcinomas, 2 percent; and small cell tumors (with paraneoplastic syndromes), <1 percent. Adenocarcinomas develop in the dome of the bladder in the urachal remnant or in the periurethral tissues. Some assume a signet cell histology. Lymphomas or melanomas are rare. Overall, 75 percent of tumors present as superficial lesions, 20 percent have muscle invasion, and in 5 percent there is metastatic disease. Among superficial lesions, the most frequent histologic subtype of transitional cell tumors is a low-grade papillary lesion that grows on a central stalk. These lesions are very friable, have a tendency to bleed, and have a high risk of recurrence. They rarely progress to the more lethal invasive variety. In contrast, carcinoma in situ (CIS) is a high-grade tumor and is believed to be the precursor of muscle-invasive disease. In other cases, the tumor invades directly and assumes a solid growth pattern.

Histologic grade provides prognostic information. Grade I lesions (highly differentiated tumors) rarely progress to a higher stage. In contrast, a Ta grade III tumor has a higher risk of progression to a more advanced stage. The risk of recurrence in the primary and distant sites correlates with lesion size, number of lesions, growth pattern, the presence of disease in the prostatic urethra or of carcinoma in situ in other sites, and the presence of hydronephrosis.

PATHOGENESIS   Molecular genetic analyses of tumors of defined stage and grade have shown a number of *primary chromosomal aberrations* that are associated with tumor *development*, and *secondary abnormalities* that are related to *progression* to a more advanced stage. Evolving data suggest that superficial tumors that tend to recur but not invade and those that tend to invade and to metastasize result from distinct genetic defects (Table 96-1). Alterations on the long arm of chromosome 13, including those that affect the retinoblastoma gene locus on 13q14, occur more often in muscle-invasive than in non-muscle-invading tumors. Deletions of 17p (the *p53* locus), 18q (the *DCC* locus), and the *RB* gene are more frequent in invasive lesions, while 9q deletions appear to be an early event, given their high frequency in Ta and T1 recurring lesions. 3p and 5q deletions are more prevalent in invasive tumors but absent in superficial lesions. Patients with invasive disease whose tumors lack the *RB* gene have a poorer survival than those with *RB*-positive lesions. Similarly, *p53* overexpression is associated with a higher frequency of progression to a more advanced stage and a higher rate of death from bladder cancer for patients with Ta, T1, and CIS disease. In addition to the functional loss of tumor suppressor genes, bladder cancers often overexpress the epidermal growth factor receptor and the related receptor tyrosine kinase, HER-2/neu. Activating mutations of oncogenes (e.g., *ras*) are rare.

℞ TREATMENT

The choice of treatment is based on disease extent: superficial, invasive, or metastatic. Superficial tumors are treated by endoscopic resection with or without intravesical therapy. Once invasive disease is documented, the standard treatment is surgical removal of the bladder. Based on pathologic findings at surgery, systemic chemotherapy may or may not be advised. Combination chemotherapy is used to treat metastatic disease.

Superficial Disease Intravesical therapy is used to eliminate existing disease or more commonly as an adjuvant or as prophylaxis to prevent recurrence following endoscopic resection. Although transurethral resection is effective at completely eradicating disease in 80 percent of cases, 30 to 80 percent of patients develop recurrent disease, and grade and stage progression occurs in up to 30 percent. Indications for intravesical therapy vary, but treatment is generally advised for patients with four or more recurrences in a given year, involvement of more than 40 percent of the bladder surface by tumor, diffuse CIS, or T1 disease. Administration of the immune adjuvant bacillus Calmette-Guérin (BCG) is considered the standard therapy, but efficacy has also been observed for several chemotherapeutic agents including doxorubicin and mitomycin C. BCG reduces recurrence rates by 40 to 45 percent, compared to 8 to 18 percent for drug instillation. The most frequent symptoms of toxicity associated with intravesical therapy include bladder irritation, frequency, dysuria, and contact dermatitis (from mitomycin C). In rare cases, BCG treatment can result in a systemic infection that requires antituberculin therapy. Significant BCG toxicities occur in fewer than 6 percent of patients.

After an initial course of treatment, the patient is reevaluated at 3-month intervals to ensure that no recurrence has developed. Those with persistent or new tumors may be considered for more aggressive management including cystectomy. Recurrence may also occur in extravesical sites along the urothelial tract, including the distal ureter and/or urethra, supporting the concept of a "field change" in bladder carcinogenesis.

Muscle-Infiltrating Tumors Once a tumor involves muscle, the standard treatment is surgical removal of the entire organ by radical cystectomy. In 5 to 10 percent of cases, the tumor occurs in a location where only a partial cystectomy is required. Rarely, a transurethral resection alone is used. In males, radical cystectomy involves the removal of the bladder, prostate, seminal vesicles, proximal vas deferens, and proximal urethra, with a margin of adipose tissue and peritoneum. If the nervi erigentes, which are responsible for erectile capacity, are preserved, erectile function can be recovered. In females, the resection includes removal of the bladder, urethra, uterus, fallopian tubes, ovaries, anterior vaginal wall, and surrounding fascia. Grossly abnormal lymph nodes are sampled by frozen section. If spread is confirmed, the cystectomy is aborted unless a urinary diversion is required to relieve symptoms. This operation constitutes major surgery, and appropriate medical clearance is required.

Urinary flow is directed through a conduit diversion to the skin (Bricker procedure), or a low-pressure internal reservoir is created using a detubularized bowel segment and anastamosed to the skin

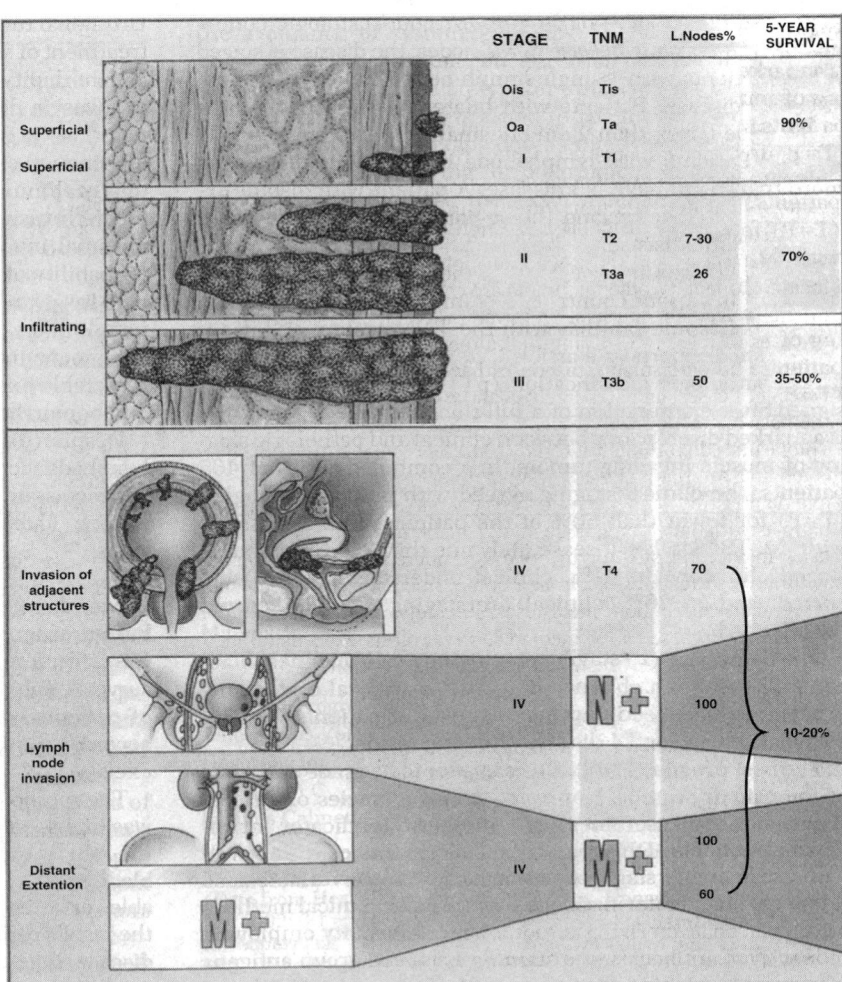

FIGURE 96-1 Clinical classification of the bladder. [Modified from WR Fair et al, Cancer of the bladder, in *Cancer: Principles and Practice of Oncology,* 4th ed, VT DeVita, Jr., et al (eds): Philadelphia, Lippincott, 1993].

(Koch pouch) or the urethra (Mainz or Indiana pouch). When an anastomosis to the urethra is created, the patient can void in a normal fashion. Reservoirs attached to the skin require intermittent catheterization. Contraindications to a continent reservoir include the presence of carcinoma in the prostatic urethra. An ileal conduit is the most widely used. A syndrome characterized by hypochloremic acidosis, hyperkalemia, hyponatremia, and uremia has been described when a segment of jejunum is used. Concurrent diseases in the bowel, such as ulcerative colitis or Crohn's disease, preclude the use of resected bowel.

The 5-year survival rate varies inversely with the depth of invasion and lymph node status. The 5-year survival rate is 70 percent for those with T2/3a (stage II) disease and 50 percent for those with T3b disease with no positive nodes, up to 35 percent for those with one node positive, and 10 percent for those with six or more positive

Table 96-1

Molecular Genetic Defects in Bladder Cancer

Chromosome Abnormality	Frequency, %	Phenotype
Loss of part or all of chromosome 9	55	Superficial recurrent
17p deletion ($\pm p53$ mutation)	40	Invasive
11p deletion	40	Invasive
13q deletion	20	Invasive

SOURCE: From Gordon-Cardo et al, with permission.

nodes. The influence of depth of invasion on survival after surgery is shown in Table 96-2. In some countries, external-beam radiation therapy is standard, but in the United States it is generalaly reserved for patients who are not suitable candidates for cystectomy. The 5-year survival after treatment with 5000 to 7000 cGy is 30 to 45 percent.

Metastatic Disease This cohort includes patients who present with metastases and those who develop metastases after definitive local treatment. Urothelial tumors are chemosensitive, and a number of single agents result in short-term regressions in 20 to 30 percent of cases (Table 96-3). Using multidrug combinations, in particular those based on cisplatin, responses have been observed in up to 70 percent of cases, and 20 percent of these responses are complete. On the basis of randomized trials, the M-VAC regimen [methotrexate, vinblastine, doxorubicin (Adriamycin), and cisplatin] is considered standard. Alternatively, a CMV regimen (cisplatin, methotrexate, and vinblastine) can be used. In general, a higher proportion of patients with only lymph node involvement than patients with metastases to visceral sites or to bone is rendered tumor-free. Patients with adverse features, such as a compromised performance status, visceral disease, or bone metastases, are rarely cured with chemotherapy alone. In these cases, median survival rarely exceeds 6 months, and the toxicities of treatment are significant. Long-term survival has been reported in 10 to 15 percent of patients with metastatic disease and in 20 to 25 percent of patients with unresectable nodal disease at presentation. Approximately 20 to 40 percent of patients develop neutropenic fever due to hematologic toxicity. Mucositis occurs in 10 to 20 percent, and a decrease in renal and auditory function as well as a peripheral neuropathy may be seen. Alopecia is universal; fatigue can be dose-limiting in some cases. For patients who relapse after first-line chemotherapy, activity has been seen with gallium nitrate, ifosfamide, gemcitabine, 5-fluorouracil-based combination regimens, and the taxanes. A number of groups are also exploring combinations of these agents (VIG—vinblastine, ifosfamide, and gallium nitrate—or ITP—ifosfamide, paclitaxel, and cisplatin) as initial treatment.

Chemotherapy for Invasive Disease Chemotherapy has also been integrated into the management of invasive bladder tumors either before (neoadjuvant) or after (adjuvant) definitive local therapy for patients with a high risk of metastases. It has also been used either alone or as part of combined-modality treatment with radiation therapy, with the aim of bladder preservation. Nonrandomized phase II trials have shown that the proportion of bladders rendered free of tumor varies inversely with T stage, with cumulative proportions in the range of 20 to 25 percent when the bladder is removed and examined pathologically. No survival benefit has been proved yet using a neoadjuvant approach.

An alternative approach preferred by many physicians is the removal of the bladder followed by a decision to use or omit chemotherapy based on the pathologic findings at surgery. Indications for chemotherapy include a finding of nodal disease, extravesical tumor extension, or vascular invasion in the resected specimen. Several trials, both nonrandomized and randomized, suggest a survival benefit using this approach. Most compare a policy of surgery followed by immediate chemotherapy (usually four cycles) with surgery followed by chemotherapy at the time of recurrence. None is definitive, however, because not enough patients have been enrolled and treated.

Table 96-2

Survival Relative to Pathologic Stage

	5-Year Survival, %, for Stage:		
P2	P3a	P3b	N+
62–83	50–74	15–57	4–35

SOURCE: Modified from H Scher et al, *Principles and Practice of Oncology*, 5th ed, VT DeVita et al (eds). Philadelphia, Lippincott, 1997.

Table 96-3

Selected Single Agents with Activity in Urothelial Tract Malignancies

Agent	No. Responding/ No. Treated	Percent Responding	95% Confidence Interval, %
Cisplatin	200/706	28	26–32
Methotrexate	8/236	45	37–50
Doxorubicin	47/274	17	13–22
Vinblastine	6/38	16	4–28
Ifosfamide	28/101	28	19–37
Gallium nitrate	9/29	29	13–45
Paclitaxel	11/26	42	23–61

Bladder Preservation Several groups are investigating bladder-sparing strategies. Most use a treatment policy that includes an aggressive transurethral resection followed by systemic chemotherapy either alone or in combination with external beam radiation therapy. The decision to leave the bladder in situ is based on the posttherapy assessment of response. A trial performed by Kaufman and colleagues involved giving two cycles of CMV and 4000 cGy of external beam radiation therapy with concurrent cisplatin. Patients with nonresponsive tumors were referred for cystectomy. After 4 years of follow-up, 45 percent of patients were alive with no evidence of disease. While these results, and those of others, show that bladder preservation is feasible in selected cases, any bladder left in situ must be monitored continuously for the development of new tumors. This approach should be undertaken with the caveat that survival equivalent to that achieved with the standard approach has not yet been proved. Quality of life is better with bladder preservation.

RENAL CELL CARCINOMA

Renal cell carcinoma accounts for 90 to 95 percent of malignant neoplasms arising from the kidney. Notable features include refractoriness to cytotoxic agents, infrequent but reproducible responses to biologic response modifiers such as interferon α and interleukin (IL) 2, and a variable clinical course for patients with metastatic disease, including anecdotal reports of spontaneous regression.

EPIDEMIOLOGY AND ETIOLOGY The incidence of renal cell carcinoma in the United States in 1996 was 30,600 cases (18,500 male; 12,100 female); the disease caused 12,000 deaths. The incidence peaks between the ages of 50 and 70, although this malignancy may be diagnosed at any age. Many environmental factors have been investigated as possible causal factors. The strongest associations are with cigarette smoking (accounting for as many as 20 to 30 percent of cases) and obesity. The risk of renal cell carcinoma is increased in patients who have acquired cystic disease of the kidney associated with end-stage renal disease.

Most cases are sporadic, although two familial forms have been reported: a rare form with autosomal dominant inheritance, and a form associated with von Hippel-Lindau syndrome. Nearly 35 percent of patients with von Hippel-Lindau disease develop renal cell cancers. An increased incidence has also been reported in patients with tuberous sclerosis and polycystic kidney disease.

Most of these cancers arise from the epithelical cells of the proximal tubules. A number of genetic alterations have been described, of which abnormalities on chromosome 3 are most frequent. A 3;8 translocation was first described in a pedigree of patients with the familial form of the disease, while deletions in 3p21-26 have been identified in familial as well as sporadic tumors. More recently, the gene for von Hippel-Lindau disease on chromosome 3p was cloned, and von Hippel-Lindau mutations can be identified in nearly 60 percent of sporadic, nonpapillary renal cell cancers and associated cell lines.

PATHOLOGY AND GENETICS In the past, renal cell cancers were grouped by cell type (clear, granular, oncocytic, and spindle) and growth pattern (acinar, sarcomatoid, and tubulopapillary). This

Table 96-4

CHAPTER 96
Bladder and Renal Cell Cancer

595

Signs and Symptoms in Patients with Renal Cell Cancer

Presenting Sign or Symptom	Incidence, %
Classic triad: hematuria, flank pain, flank mass	10–20
Hematuria	40
Flank pain	40
Palpable mass	25
Weight loss	33
Anemia	33
Fever	20
Hypertension	20
Abnormal liver function	15
Hypercalcemia	5
Erythrocytosis	3
Neuromyopathy	3
Amyloidosis	2
Increased erythrocyte sedimentation rate	55

diograph, as it will detect significantly smaller lesions, and their presence may influence the approach to the primary tumor. MRI is useful in evaluating the status of the inferior vena cava in cases of suspected tumor involvement or invasion by thrombus, as well as for patients in whom iodinated contrast cannot be administered owing to either allergy or renal dysfunction. In clinical practice, any solid renal mass should be considered malignant until proven otherwise and requires a definitive diagnosis. If no metastases are demonstrated, surgery is indicated, even if there is invasion of the renal vein. The differential diagnosis of a renal mass includes cysts, benign neoplasms (adenoma, angiomyolipoma, oncocytoma), inflammatory lesions (pyelonephritis or abscesses), and other primary or metastatic malignant neoplasms. Other malignancies that may involve the kidney include transitional cell carcinoma of the renal pelvis, sarcoma, lymphoma, Wilms's tumor, and metastatic disease, especially from melanoma primaries. All of these are less common as kidney malignancies than is renal cell carcinoma.

STAGING AND PROGNOSIS The most widely used staging system in the United States is that developed by Robson. In this schema, stage I tumors are confined to the kidney; stage II tumors extend through the renal capsule but are confined by Gerota's fascia; stage III tumors involve the renal vein or vena cava (stage IIIA) or the hilar lymph nodes (stage IIIB); and stage IV disease includes tumors that are locally invasive to adjacent organs (excluding the adrenal gland) or distant metastases. Five-year survival varies by stage: 66 percent for stage I, 64 percent for stage II, 42 percent for stage

schema has been abandoned because most tumors proved to contain mixtures of cell types and patterns. A current classification scheme based on the results of immunohistochemical and genetic studies consists of five variants: clear cell tumors, representing 75 percent of cases; chromophilic tumors (15 percent); chromophobic tumors (5 percent); oncocytic tumors (3 percent); and collecting duct or Bellini duct tumors (2 percent). Clear cell tumors are characterized by tumor cells with clear cytoplasm, which consistently show a 3p deletion. Chromophilic tumors, previously termed *tubulopapillary*, tend to be bilateral and multifocal. Trisomy 7 and/or trisomy 17 are the most frequent genetic abnormalities. Chromophobic tumors are characterized by multiple chromosomal losses but do not exhibit 3p deletions and have a more indolent clinical course. Similarly, oncocytomas have a characteristic morphology including a deeply eosinophilic cytoplasm, do not exhibit 3p deletions or trisomy 7 or 17, and rarely metastasize. In contrast, Bellini duct carcinomas are very rare and are believed to arise from the collecting ducts in the renal medulla. They tend to affect younger patients and have a very aggressive clinical course.

CLINICAL PRESENTATION The presenting signs and symptoms include hematuria, abdominal pain, and a flank or abdominal mass. This classic triad occurs in 10 to 20 percent of patients. Other symptoms are fever, weight loss, anemia, and a varicocele; the tumor may also be found incidentally on a radiograph. A spectrum of paraneoplastic syndromes has been associated with these malignancies, including erythrocytosis, hypercalcemia, nonmetastatic hepatic dysfunction (Stauffers' syndrome), and acquired dysfibrinogenemia. Erythrocytosis is present at presentation in only about 3 percent of patients. More frequently, anemia, a sign of advanced disease, is reported (Table 96-4).

The standard evaluation of patients with suspected renal cell tumors includes an intravenous pyelogram (IVP), ultrasonography, CT of the abdomen and pelvis, a chest radiograph, urine analysis, and urine cytology (Fig. 96-2). CT of the chest is warranted if metastatic disease is suspected from the chest ra-

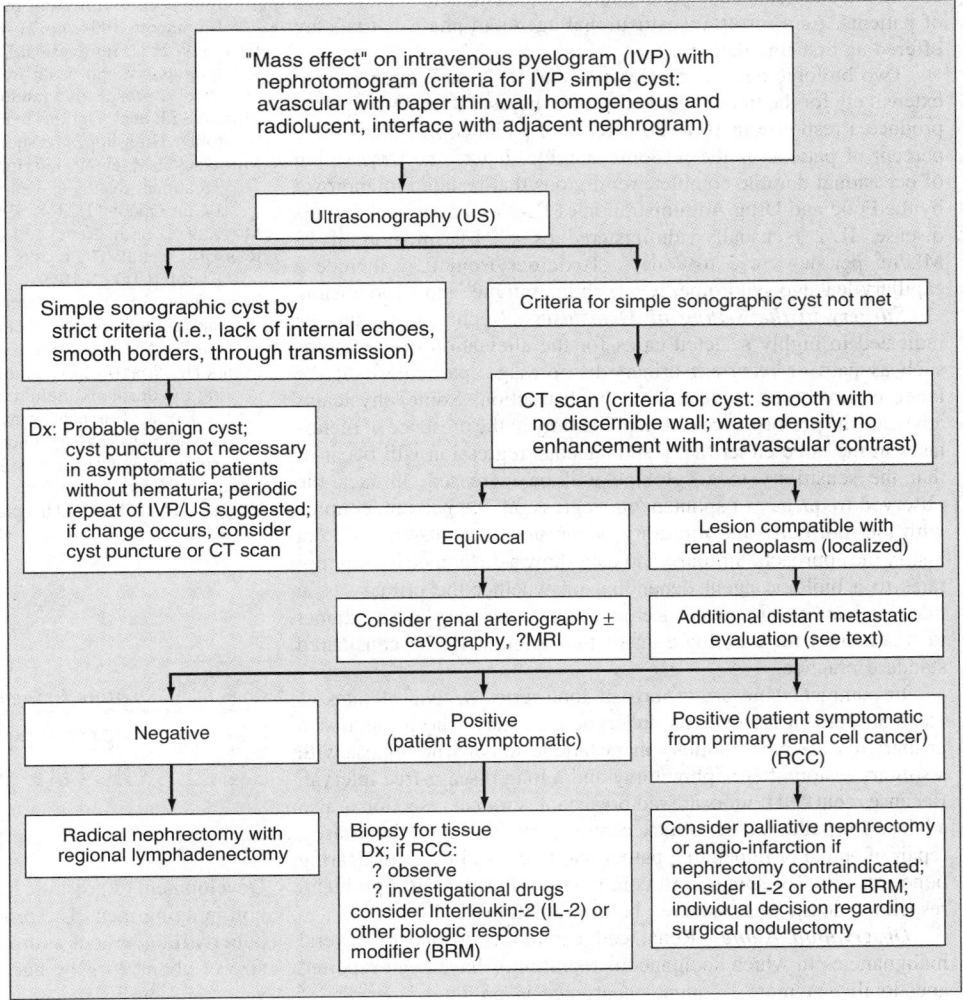

FIGURE 96-2 Standard evaluation of patients with suspected renal cell tumors. (Redrawn from MB Garnick, BM Brenner, Tumors in urinary tract, Fig. 247-1, in *HPIM*, 13th edition.)

III, and 11 percent for stage IV. The prognosis for stage IIIA lesions is similar to that for stage I or II disease, whereas the 5-year survival for stage IIIB lesions is only 20 percent, closer to that for stage IV tumors.

 TREATMENT

Localized Disease The standard management for stage I or II tumors and selected cases of stage III disease is radical nephrectomy. This procedure involves en bloc removal of Gerota's fascia and its contents, including the kidney, the ipsilateral adrenal gland, and adjacent hilar lymph nodes. The role of a regional lymphadenectomy is controversial. For patients with stage IIIA disease, the tumor should be resected from the renal vein or vena cava.

In selected patients who have only one kidney, and depending on the size and location of the lesion, a partial nephrectomy may be performed. Partial nephrectomy may also be performed in patients with bilateral tumors, accompanied by a radical nephrectomy on the opposite side. There is no proven role for adjuvant chemotherapy, immunotherapy, or radiation therapy following successful surgical removal of the tumor, even in cases with a poor prognosis.

Advanced Disease Metastatic renal cell carcinoma, for which there is no effective therapy, is associated with a dismal survival. A number of options have been explored, including hormonal therapy, chemotherapy (with cytotoxic agents), and immunotherapy. Responses to hormonal therapy (progestins) are rare (1 to 2 percent) and of short duration. No chemotherapy agent has been shown consistently to produce objective tumor regressions in >20 percent of patients. As a result, investigational agents in phase II trials are offered as first-line therapy.

Two biologic agents, interferon α and IL-2, have been studied extensively for the treatment of advanced disease. Both reproducibly produce a response in 10 to 20 percent of patients; in fewer than 5 percent of patients is the response durable. It was the observation of occasional durable complete remissions that resulted in approval by the Food and Drug Administration of IL-2 as a treatment for this disease. IL-2 is usually administered as a 24-h infusion of 18 MU/m^2 per day for 5 to 7 days. Toxicities from IL-2 include a capillary leakage syndrome, fever, chills, fatigue, and hypotension.

Surgery in the Setting of Metastases Nephrectomy may be indicated in highly selected cases for the alleviation of symptoms such as pain or recurrent urinary hemorrhage, particularly if the latter is severe or associated with obstruction. Some physicians advocate the performance of a nephrectomy in the presence of metastases in the hope either that a spontaneous regression will occur or that the sensitivity to a cytokine will be increased. In fact, the observed frequency of spontaneous regression, 0.8 percent, coupled with the morbidity and mortality of the procedure itself, does not justify the approach. Similarly, no data show a difference in response rates to a biologic agent depending on whether the primary is in place or has been removed. Removal of the primary as an adjunct to treatment with a biologic agent thus should not be considered standard practice.

In contrast, there are reports of long-term survival at rates of 15 to 50 percent for patients undergoing surgery who present with primary disease plus a solitary metastatic lesion or who relapse with a solitary lesion after nephrectomy and a long disease-free interval. Because renal cell tumors are radioresistant, surgical resection is also advised for palliation of solitary central nervous system metastases, repair of actual or impending pathologic fractures in weight-bearing bones, or relief of spinal cord compression. For the latter problem, resection should be considered before radiation.

Observation Alone Renal cell carcinoma is one of several malignancies in which spontaneous regressions have been reported anecdotally. A more frequent occurrence is prolonged periods of stable disease; up to 10 percent of patients with metastatic disease may show no progression for >12 months. Because responses to systemic therapy are uncommon and all systemic therapies are associated with treatment-related toxicity, an option for management in asymptomatic patients with metastases is close observation until disease progression or symptoms occur, at which time appropriate therapy is initiated.

CARCINOMA OF THE RENAL PELVIS AND URETER

About 500 cases of renal pelvis and ureter cancer occur each year, and over 90 percent are transitional cell carcinomas similar to bladder cancer in appearance. Smoking is a risk factor, as is chemical and hydrocarbon exposure. This tumor is also associated with chronic phenacetin abuse and with Balkan nephropathy, a chronic interstitial nephritis endemic in Bulgaria, Greece, Bosnia-Herzegovina, and Romania.

The most common symptom is painless gross hematuria, and the disease usually is detected on IVP during the workup for hematuria. Patterns of spread are like those in bladder cancer. For disease localized to the renal pelvis and ureter, nephroureterectomy (including excision of the distal ureter with a portion of the bladder) is associated with a 5-year survival rate of 80 to 90 percent for low-grade lesions. More invasive or histologically less well differentiated tumors are more likely to recur locally and metastasize. Metastatic disease is treated with M-VAC or CMV chemotherapy. The outcome is similar to that for metastatic transitional cell carcinoma of bladder origin.

BIBLIOGRAPHY

CORDON-CARDO C et al: Genetic alterations associated with bladder cancer, in *Important Advances in Oncology*, DeVita VT et al (eds). Philadelphia, Lippincott, 1994, pp 71–84

HERR HW et al: Intravesical Bacillus Calmette-Guerin therapy prevents tumor progression and death from superficial bladder cancer: Ten-year follow-up of a prospective randomized trial. J Clin Oncol 13:1404, 1995

MARTINS FE et al: Options in replacement cystoplasty following radical cystectomy: High hopes or successful reality. J Urol 153:1363, 1995

MINASIAN LM et al: Interferon alfa-2a in advanced renal cell carcinoma: Treatment results and survival in 159 patients with long-term follow-up. J Clin Oncol 11:1368, 1993

MOTZER RJ et al: Renal cell carcinoma. N Engl J Med 335:865, 1996

ROBSON CJ et al: The results of radical nephrectomy for renal cell carcinoma. J Urol 101:297, 1969

ROSENBERG SA et al: Treatment of 283 consecutive patients with metastatic melanoma or renal cell cancer using high dose bolus intravenous interleukin-2. JAMA 271:907, 1994

SCHER HI, NORTON L: Chemotherapy for urothelial tract malignancies: Breaking the deadlock. Semin Surg Oncol 8:316, 1992

SHUIN T et al: Frequent somatic mutations and loss of heterozygosity of the von Hippel-Lindau tumor suppressor gene in primary human renal cell carcinomas. Cancer Res 54:2852, 1994

STADLER W, VOGELZANG N (eds): Bladder cancer. Semin Oncol 23:533, 1996

VINEIS P et al: Molecular epidemiology of bladder cancer: Known chemical causes of bladder cancer: Occupation and smoking. Urol Oncol 1:137, 1995

97 *Arthur I. Sagalowsky, Jean D. Wilson*

HYPERPLASIA AND CARCINOMA OF THE PROSTATE

PROSTATIC HYPERPLASIA

Development of prostatic hyperplasia is an almost universal phenomenon in aging men. The prostate weighs only a few grams at birth; at puberty it undergoes androgen-mediated growth and reaches the adult size of about 20 g by age 20. It remains stable in size for about 25 years, and during the fifth decade a second growth spurt commences in the majority of men. Consequently, the disorder affects men over the age of 45 and increases in frequency with age so that by the eighth

autopsy. Because of the development of effective therapies the disorder is not a major cause of death, but it continues to be a leading cause of morbidity in elderly men. The prostate surrounds the urethra, and prostatic hyperplasia is the most common cause of obstruction to urinary outflow in men. The disorder occurs in all populations but may be less common in the Orient. The mean age for development of symptomatic disease is about 65 years for whites and about 60 years for blacks. It is not clear whether prostatic hyperplasia predisposes to the development of prostatic cancer.

PATHOGENESIS Unlike the pubertal growth spurt which involves the gland diffusely, prostatic hyperplasia begins in the periurethral region as a localized proliferation and progresses to compress the remaining normal gland. Histologically, the hyperplastic tissue is nodular and composed of varying amounts of glandular epithelium, stroma, and smooth muscle. The hyperplasia can compress and obstruct the urethra; the hyperplastic gland can also grow posteriorly to obstruct the rectum and cause constipation.

The pathogenesis is not well understood, but two necessary features for the process are aging and the presence of testes; whether the testes play a direct or permissive role is not known, but the active androgen that mediates prostatic growth at all ages is dihydrotestosterone, which is formed within the prostate from plasma testosterone (see Chap. 336). In the castrated dog, hormone replacement that increases dihydrotestosterone levels in the prostate causes prostatic enlargement comparable with that seen in spontaneous canine prostatic hyperplasia. Estradiol levels in men increase with age (absolutely or relative to testosterone levels), and in dogs estrogen acts synergistically with dihydrotestosterone to induce prostatic growth by enhancing the amount of androgen receptor protein in the tissue. Consequently, the role of aging in human prostatic hyperplasia might be due, at least in part, to the augmentation of dihydrotestosterone action by estrogen.

DIAGNOSIS Urethral obstruction results from the elongation, tortuosity, and compression of the posterior urethra, but there is no straightforward relationship between obstruction and prostate size or between symptoms and obstruction. Indeed, severe obstruction can occur when the hyperplasia has not yet caused an increase in the size of the normal gland, and some men with very large prostates are asymptomatic. Early symptoms can be minimal because compensatory hypertrophy of the detrusor musculature of the bladder can compensate for the resistance to urine flow. With increasing obstruction, diminution in the caliber and force of the urinary stream, hesitancy in initiating voiding, postvoiding dribbling, the sensation of incomplete emptying,

and on occasion urinary retention supervene. These *obstructive* symptoms must be distinguished from *irritative* symptoms such as dysuria, frequency, and urgency that also can result from inflammatory, infectious, or neoplastic causes. As the amount of residual urine increases, nocturia, overflow urinary incontinence, and a palpable bladder may be present. Eventually, the manifestations of chronic urinary retention and obstruction supervene, or acute urinary retention can be precipitated by infection, tranquilizing drugs, antihistamines, or alcohol. On occasion, profound obstruction can be compensated to the extent that symptoms are minimal or absent, and patients present with obstructive uropathy.

The natural history of this disorder is poorly understood, but it is clear that the majority of men with prostatic enlargement never develop significant obstruction and that in many men minor irritative and/or obstructive symptoms do not progress or progress very slowly. Consequently, it is not always clear when in the course to intervene, but increased size alone is not a valid reason to treat.

In the evaluation of the patient with prostatism a detailed *history* should focus on the urinary tract to identify other causes of voiding dysfunction. For quantification of symptoms the preferred questionnaire is the self-administered *AUA Symptom Index* in which the symptoms can be classified as mild, moderate, or severe on the basis of seven questions (Table 97-1). This index is useful in planning and in follow-up. On *digital rectal examination* (DRE), the prostate should be characterized with regard to size, consistency, and shape. Hyperplasia commonly produces a smooth, firm, elastic enlargement, but obstruction can occur in the absence of abnormalities on DRE. The measurement of prostate-specific antigen (PSA) is useful for excluding the diagnosis of advanced prostatic cancer, but the test does not discriminate between prostatic hyperplasia and early prostate cancer (see below). Several additional diagnostic tests are available, but it is not established whether any of them is of value in predicting the results of treatment. Such tests include *uroflowmetry*, which can identify those patients whose maximum flows are normal and who are unlikely to benefit from treatment; measurement of *postvoid residual urine volume*, which, although poorly reproducible in an individual patient, identifies those patients with a greater likelihood of failing a watchful-waiting strategy; *pressure-flow studies*, which are particularly helpful in patients at risk for primary bladder dysfunction; and *urethrocystoscopy*, which is of use in some patients before invasive treatment and

Table 97-1

AUA Symptom Index

Questions To Be Answered	AUA Symptom Score (Circle 1 Number on Each Line)					
	Not at All	Less Than 1 Time in 5	Less Than Half the Time	About Half the Time	More Than Half the Time	Almost Always
Over the past month, how often have you had a sensation of not emptying your bladder completely after you finished urinating?	0	1	2	3	4	5
Over the past month, how often have you had to urinate again less than 2 h after you finished urinating?	0	1	2	3	4	5
Over the past month, how often have you found you stopped and started again several times when you urinated?	0	1	2	3	4	5
Over the past month, how often have you found it difficult to postpone urination?	0	1	2	3	4	5
Over the past month, how often have you had a weak urinary stream?	0	1	2	3	4	5
Over the past month, how often have you had to push or strain to begin urination?	0	1	2	3	4	5
Over the past month, how many times did you most typically get up to urinate from the time you went to bed at night until the time you got up in the morning?	0 (None)	1 (1 time)	2 (2 times)	3 (3 times)	4 (4 times)	5 (5 times or more)

Sum of 7 circled numbers (AUA Symptom Score): _____

SOURCE: Barry, Fowler, O'Leary, et al. The American Urological Association symptom index for benign prostatic hyperplasia. J Urol 148:1549, 1992. Used with permission.

when there is some specific indication such as hematuria. Imaging of the upper urinary tract by ultrasonography or intravenous pyelography should be reserved for patients with indications such as hematuria, a history of stones, or prior urinary tract problems.

 TREATMENT

Asymptomatic patients with prostate enlargement generally do not require treatment. Those patients with specific complications of prostatic hyperplasia (inability to urinate, renal insufficiency, urinary tract infection, hematuria, or bladder stones) are clear candidates for prostate surgery. All other patients should, in consultation with their physician, decide on treatment based on the degree of incapacity and/or discomfort present and a consideration of the likely outcome of each potential treatment strategy. A variety of decision diagrams have been proposed for aiding physicians and patients in making decisions about the most appropriate management strategy, but ultimately the decision depends on the severity of symptoms and the patient's expectations and acceptance of the risks of treatment.

Watchful Waiting Watchful waiting is appropriate for most patients because the probability of disease progression or the development of complications is unknown. These patients should be monitored at least annually by reassessment of symptoms and clinical manifestations.

Medical Therapy Finasteride, a competitive inhibitor of the 5α-reductase enzyme, blocks the conversion of testosterone to dihydrotestosterone, the principal androgen in the prostate. In a dose of 5 mg/d by mouth the drug causes an average decrease in prostate size of around 24 percent, an increase in urine flow rates, and, in some, improvement in symptoms. Long-term efficacy has not been documented, but improvement is known to be sustained for as long as 3 years provided the therapy is continued. Patients who respond to this regimen may elect to continue indefinitely, and those whose symptoms are bothersome and do not improve or worsen are appropriate candidates for surgery. What is not clear is how to manage the half of patients whose symptoms do not change; indirect evidence suggests that the therapy halts the progression of the disease, but this is not proven. Alpha$_1$-adrenergic blockers such as terazosin relax smooth muscle of the bladder neck and cause an increase in peak urinary flow rate and a perceptible reduction in symptoms. However, there is no reason to expect that such agents will influence the progression of the disease.

Surgery Prostate surgery offers the best chance for improvement in symptoms but also has the highest rate of significant complications. Transurethral resection of the prostate is the most common surgical procedure. Transurethral incision of the prostate is of similar efficacy in men with relatively small prostates and can be performed in ambulatory settings. Open prostatectomy is usually reserved for men with massive prostates and may employ retropubic, suprapubic, or perineal approaches. Given proper patient selection, benefits are probably equivalent with each procedure, but complication rates differ. Open prostatectomy has a greater incisional morbidity and longer recovery time and a greater risk for impotence. Transurethral incision has the lowest morbidity and lowest rates of ejaculatory disturbances. Surgery is the appropriate initial therapy in many patients and appropriate as the second line of therapy for others who fail to respond to medical treatment or worsen with watchful waiting, but it should not be recommended on the grounds that surgical risk will increase with age. New technologies under evaluation include laser therapy, coils, stents, thermal therapy, and hyperthermia.

PROSTATIC CARCINOMA

Cancer of the prostate is the most common malignancy in men in the United States and the third most common cause of cancer death in men above age 55 (after carcinomas of the lung and colon). In the United States there are approximately 317,000 newly diagnosed cases

and more than 41,000 deaths from the disorder each year. Only about a third of cases identified at autopsy are manifest clinically. The disease is rare before age 50, and the incidence increases with age. The frequency varies in different parts of the world. The United States has 14 deaths per 100,000 men per year, compared with 22 for Sweden and 2 for Japan. However, Japanese immigrants to the United States develop prostatic cancer at a frequency similar to other men in this country, suggesting that environmental factors are the principal cause for population differences. The disease is more common among American blacks than whites; the reason for this difference is not known.

CLASSIFICATION Some carcinomas of the prostate are slow-growing and may persist for long periods without causing significant symptoms, whereas others behave aggressively. It is not known whether tumors can become more malignant with time. Insight into the natural history of a given tumor is provided by careful histopathologic grading, surgical evaluation of the pelvic lymph nodes, and measurement of the primary lesion, a size less than 1.5 mL in volume carrying a good prognosis.

Histologic Grading Over 95 percent of prostatic cancers are adenocarcinomas that arise in the prostatic acini. Adenocarcinoma may begin anywhere in the prostate but, in contrast to hyperplasia, has a predilection for the periphery. The tumors are frequently multifocal. Variability in cellular size, nuclear and nucleolar shape, glandular differentiation, and the content of acid phosphatase and mucin may occur within a single specimen, but the most poorly differentiated area of tumor (i.e., the area with the highest histologic grade) appears to determine its biologic behavior. In the Gleason grading scheme, the dominant and secondary glandular histologic patterns are independently assigned numbers from 1 to 5 (best to least differentiated), and these numbers are summed to give a total score of 2 to 10 for each tumor. Such grading is reproducible and correlates with the course of the disease and with patient survival.

The remaining prostatic cancers are divided among squamous cell and transitional cell carcinomas that arise in the prostatic ducts, carcinoma of the prostatic utricle (a müllerian duct remnant), carcinosarcomas that arise in the mesenchymal elements of the gland, and occasional metastatic tumors (usually carcinoma of the lung, melanoma, or lymphoma). These tumors will not be considered further.

DIAGNOSIS Symptoms and Signs Both early and advanced carcinoma of the prostate may be asymptomatic at the time of diagnosis, and in the past more than 80 percent of patients had locally advanced or metastatic disease at the time of diagnosis (see below). In symptomatic subjects, common presenting complaints (in descending order) include dysuria, difficulty in voiding, increased urinary frequency, complete urinary retention, back or hip pain, and hematuria. A high index of suspicion should be entertained in all men over age 40 with dysuria, frequency, or difficulty in voiding in the absence of mechanical urethral obstruction. Additional complications of advanced disease may include spinal cord compression from intradural metastases, deep venous thrombosis and pulmonary emboli, and myelophthisis.

Digital Rectal Examination Palpation of the prostate is an essential test for optimal detection of all stages of disease other than stage T1 (see "Staging and Assessment of Metastatic Disease"). Indeed, the importance of the DRE in the routine physical examination of men cannot be stressed too strongly. The posterior surfaces of the lateral lobes, where carcinoma begins most often, are easily palpable on DRE. Carcinoma characteristically is hard, nodular, and irregular, but induration also may be due to fibrous areas in benign prostatic hyperplasia, to focal infarcts, or to calculi as well as to tumor. The midline furrow between the lateral lobes may be obscured by either benign or malignant enlargement. Local extraprostatic extension of tumor into the seminal vesicles can often be detected by rectal examination. Scrotal and/or lower extremity lymphedema secondary to infiltration of pelvic lymph nodes indicates extensive disease.

Biochemical Markers The serum PSA level is the most sensitive test for early detection of prostatic cancer and is elevated in approximately 65 percent of cases. This antigen is an imperfect tumor marker because of insensitivity (approximate 35 percent false-negative rate) and lack of specificity (elevations can occur with benign prostatic hyper-

and in men with prostatic hyperplasia. For these reasons, the value of routine screening is not established. However, the combined use of serum PSA measurements and DRE allows detection of more than 60 percent of cases of prostatic cancer while it is still localized. An approach to the use of DRE and PSA measurements for evaluating men at risk is shown in Fig. 97-1. If the DRE is abnormal or if the PSA level is >10 ng/mL, transrectal biopsy of the prostate under sonography should be performed; if the DRE is negative and the PSA level is <4 ng/mL, annual follow-up is appropriate. The issue of what to do if the DRE is negative and the PSA level is equivocal (4.1 to 10 ng/mL) is not clear; some surgeons biopsy all such patients, some biopsy only if the transrectal ultrasound is abnormal, and some utilize refinements of the PSA assay to determine the need for biopsy. Refinements in PSA testing that may improve the diagnostic accuracy and are under investigation include correlating absolute PSA levels with prostate volume (PSA density) or patient age (age-specific reference ranges); analysis of the rate of rise in PSA level with time (PSA velocity); and quantifying free and protein-bound forms of serum PSA. In patients with known prostatic cancer, PSA measurements are useful in staging (see below), in assessing response to therapy, and in detecting early relapse. Nevertheless, the correct management of patients with isolated PSA relapse is not clear.

Imaging With the use of transrectal prostatic sonography, carcinoma is revealed as hypoechoic densities within the peripheral zone. The procedure is a sensitive means of identifying prostate cancer but is not specific enough for use as a screening test. Ultrasonography is most useful for directing needle biopsy to assure uniform sampling of the prostate and for documenting the degree of extension of the tumor into the bladder and seminal vesicles. Magnetic resonance imaging (MRI) and to a lesser degree computed tomography (CT) of the prostate also may be helpful in defining the extent of tumor and locating nodes for aspiration needle biopsy. Transrectal prostatic sonography is recommended if either the DRE is positive or the PSA level is elevated. The findings on sonography, the amount of PSA elevation relative to prostate size, and the index of suspicion for carcinoma by history all affect the decision of whether or not to perform a biopsy. The combined use of these modalities allows early detection of large numbers of prostatic cancers and an increased proportion of localized and curable lesions. The biologic significance of individual lesions remains to be defined. Whether early diagnosis leads to improved survival and decreased morbidity from prostate cancer requires further study.

Biopsy Biopsy of the prostate is essential for establishing the diagnosis and is indicated when an abnormality is detected by palpation or measurement of serum PSA level and/or by imaging or when lower urinary tract symptoms occur in men who have no known cause of obstruction. Core-needle biopsy may be performed transperineally or transrectally, with less risk of bacterial contamination with the former and more precise sampling with the latter. Transrectal prostatic biopsy with a rapid-fire spring-loaded needle under sonography provides the most accurate sampling of the index lesion and the remainder of the gland and is the preferred technique. Fine-needle aspiration cytology offers immediate diagnosis with minimal patient discomfort and morbidity. Open perineal biopsy is performed infrequently because it carries the risk of at least temporary impotence and is a more extensive surgical procedure. Transurethral biopsy is also used infrequently because most early lesions are in the peripheral regions of the gland.

Staging and Assessment of Metastatic Disease Adenocarcinoma of the prostate may spread by three routes: direct extension, the lymphatics, and the bloodstream. The prostatic capsule is a natural boundary against growth of tumor into adjacent structures, but direct extension occurs upward into the seminal vesicles and bladder floor. Lymphatic spread can best be assessed by surgical exploration; the frequency with which it occurs correlates with the size and histologic grade of the tumor and with the level of serum PSA. Only about one-tenth of tumors with a grade of less than 5 have lymph node involvement, while more than 70 percent of tumors with a Gleason grade of 9 or 10 have coexisting lymphatic invasion at the time of diagnosis. Lymphatic metastases are present in fewer than 10 percent of patients in whom the serum PSA level is <10 ng/mL. The route of lymphatic spread (in decreasing order) is to obturator, internal iliac, common iliac, presacral, and paraaortic nodes. Hematogenous metastases occur to bone (pelvis > lumbar vertebrae > thoracic vertebrae > ribs) more frequently than to viscera (lung > liver > adrenal gland). Diffuse pulmonary involvement is infrequent.

The TNM staging scheme involving assessment of primary *t*umor, *n*odes, and *m*etastases has replaced the Whitmore-Jewett system (Table 97-2). Stage T1 represents cancer not detectable by DRE and is subdivided into three groups. Stages T1a and T1b represent small but increasing amounts of well-differentiated tumor found in a surgical specimen removed at autopsy or during operation for prostatic hyperplasia, and stage T1c comprises the large number of nonpalpable tumors diagnosed by biopsy that was performed because of an elevated serum PSA level. Stage T2 disease is palpable but confined to the prostate. Stage T2a disease is a single nodule involving only one lobe and surrounded by tissue that is normal to palpation; stage T2b involves the majority of one lobe; and stage T2c involves both lobes of the gland. In stage T3 palpable tumor extends beyond the prostate, but there are no distant metastases. In all T stages, the presence of metastatic disease is designated M+. Stage M1-2 means that only pelvic nodes are involved with no other metastases, whereas the M2+ category means that metastatic disease is more widespread. Any of the primary stages (T1, T2, T3) may progress directly to stage M+. In the past, failure to include pelvic lymphadenectomy in the staging process resulted in marked underestimation of the frequency of lymph node metastases; for example, about one-fifth of tumors tentatively classified as T1b solely on the basis of prostate pathology were shown to be stage M+ disease when appropriate surgical staging was performed. The need for routine staging lymphadenectomy is being reassessed because large numbers of small-volume stage T1c tumors are being detected, and lymphatic metastases are rare in such patients with levels of serum PSA <10 ng/mL and with tumors of Gleason score <5. The frequency with which early hematogenous metastases are missed with the current staging procedures is uncertain. Utilizing a reverse transcriptase polymerase chain reaction to amplify PSA messenger RNA, it is now possible to detect small numbers of prostate cancer cells in the circulation, but the clinical significance of detecting such cells is not clear at present.

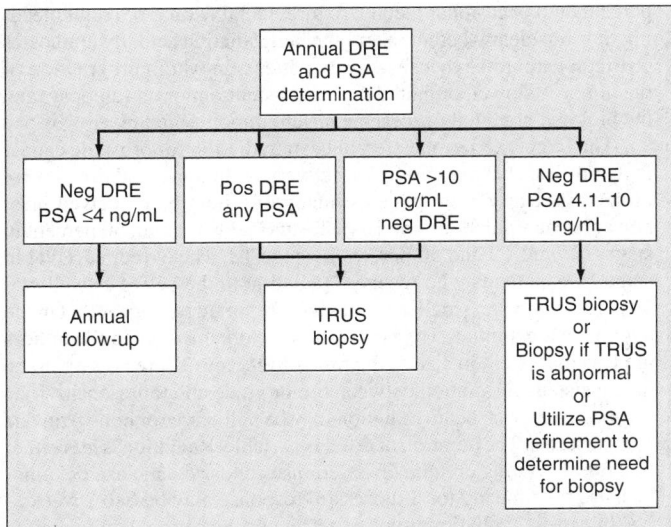

FIGURE 97-1 The use of the annual digital rectal examination (DRE) and measurement of prostate-specific antigen (PSA) as guides for deciding which men should have transrectal prostate biopsy under sonography (TRUS). There are at least three schools of thought about what to do if the DRE is negative and the PSA is equivocal (4.1 to 10 ng/mL).

Table 97-2

Comparison of Clinical Stage by the TNM Classification System and the Whitmore-Jewett Staging System

TNM Stage	Description	Whitmore-Jewett Stage	Description
T1a	Nonpalpable, with 5% or less of resected tissue with cancer	A1	Well differentiated tumor on few chips from 1 lobe
T1b	Nonpalpable, with >5% of resected tissue with cancer	A2	Involvement more diffuse
T1c	Nonpalpable, detected due to elevated serum PSA		
T2a	Palpable, half of one lobe or less	BIN	Palpable, < one lobe, surrounded by normal tissue
T2b	Palpable, > half of one lobe but not both lobes	B1	Palpable, < one lobes
T2c	Palpable, involves both lobes	B2	Palpable, one entire lobe or both lobes
T3a	Palpable, unilateral extracapsular extension	C1	Palpable, outside capsule, not into seminal vesicles
T3b	Palpable, bilateral extracapsular extension		
T3c	Tumor invades seminal vesicle(s)	C2	Palpable, seminal vesicle involved
MI	Distant metastases	D	Metastatic disease

SOURCE: Adapted from FF Schroder et al: TNM classification of prostate cancer. Prostate (Suppl) 4:129, 1992; and American Joint Committee on Cancer, 1992.

Bony metastases from prostatic carcinoma usually contain both osteoblastic and osteolytic components. The bony pelvis and lumbar vertebrae are involved most often, and metastases also occur in thoracic vertebrae, ribs, skull, and long bones. Skeletal survey has a low sensitivity of detection because a significant portion of bone must be involved to permit detection on a routine x-ray. Bone scans using radionuclides such as technetium 99 are more sensitive but not specific because positive scans may occur in any metabolically hyperactive bone; this includes sites of inflammation, healing fractures, osteoarthritis, and Paget's disease. Therefore, when a positive radionuclide scan is obtained during an initial survey for bone metastases, the presence of other lesions must be excluded by conventional radiography or biopsy of the affected site. Radionuclide bone scans are also useful for monitoring progression and response to therapy. Bone metastases are rare if the serum PSA level is <10 ng/mL. Consequently, bone scans are not necessary in initial staging or for the follow-up of every patient.

Surgical staging is still a common modality for assessing lymph node involvement and determining therapy. The procedure usually includes removal of the external iliac, internal iliac, and obturator lymph node chains and is either performed by open surgery or at laparoscopy. Pelvic lymphadenectomy may be performed by itself or in conjunction with prostatic surgery or implantation of radioactive beads. In patients at high risk for metastases and with a medical contraindication to lymphadenectomy, a pelvic CT scan or lymphangiogram can be obtained, followed when positive by confirmatory thin-needle biopsy of the affected lymph nodes.

℞ TREATMENT

Surgery Total prostatoseminovesiculectomy is the oldest treatment for carcinoma of the prostate. Radical perineal prostatectomy allows an easier vesicourethral anastomosis and less bleeding, while radical retropubic prostatectomy affords access to the pelvic lymph nodes. In experienced hands, both procedures have a low risk of major urinary incontinence. Formerly, both operations caused impo-

tence in most patients, but improvements in surgical technique, particularly for the retropubic procedure, protect the neurovascular supply to the corpora cavernosa and preserve potency in most patients below age 60 without compromising the thoroughness of the operation.

Radical prostatectomy is not required for some stage T1a and T1c cancer, since the disease may be cured definitively by the simple prostatectomy at which the diagnosis is made. PSA determinations and sonographic biopsy of residual prostatic tissue aid in identifying those stage T1a and T1c patients with additional tumor who may require further therapy. True stage T1b disease in which pelvic nodes show no evidence of metastases may behave aggressively and be benefited by radical surgery, particularly when the neoplasm has a Gleason score ≥5. Indeed, 5- and 10-year survivals equivalent to those of age-matched controls have been reported following such treatment for stage T1b disease.

Radical prostatectomy has its clearest indication in stage T2 disease. Nearly all the apparent surgical cures in this stage are in men who have 1- to 2-cm nodules involving only one lobe of the prostate (i.e., stages T2a and T2b). Improvements in early diagnosis (see above) have increased the number of such patients diagnosed. In addition, subjects with stage T2c disease also may be candidates for radical prostatectomy.

The effectiveness of radical prostatectomy is less certain for locally advanced disease (stages T3 and M1). Clinical staging by DRE underestimates stage T2 and overestimates stage T3 disease in 40 to 50 percent of cases. Lymphadenectomy alone has no therapeutic benefit, but diminished surgical morbidity and renewed interest in early and total androgen ablation (see below) have spurred a reassessment of a role for radical prostatectomy in locally advanced disease. Morbidity rates from local pelvic symptoms, bladder outlet obstruction, hematuria, and ureteral obstruction may be decreased by radical prostatectomy in stage T3 and M1 disease, but controlled studies comparing morbidity rates after surgery with those following other therapies are lacking.

Radiation Radiation therapy was developed as a primary treatment in prostatic carcinoma because of a desire to avoid the impotence and occasional incontinence that may follow radical prostatectomy. The standard regimen is the administration of approximately 60 to 70 Gy (6000 to 7000 rad) to the prostate over 6 weeks by a variety of delivery patterns. Pelvic nodes may or may not be radiated. Acute proctitis and urethritis are common side effects but are usually controllable by local measures and adjustments in delivery pattern. Chronic complications after full courses of external beam radiation include impotence in 30 to 60 percent, chronic proctitis in 10 to 15 percent, and occasional rectal stricture, rectal fistula, or rectal bleeding. It is not clear whether external beam radiation actually eradicates prostatic carcinoma, because many patients in whom progression of the tumor is slowed or halted have persistent tumor on rebiopsy, and the biologic potential of these persistent tumors is not clear.

The largest series on external beam radiation for prostatic cancer is that of Bagshaw; a variety of delivery techniques and doses were utilized in nearly 1300 patients, many of whom had received prior hormone manipulation. The 10-year survival was about 50 percent in stages T1 and T2 and 30 percent in stage T3. The 5-year survival in stage M+ patients who received radiation to the pelvis as well was 58 percent. Several smaller studies have reported responses that in the aggregate are similar. The best results are obtained when the tumors are less than 2 cm in size at the time of therapy. There appears to be no consistent correlation between tumor grade and radiosensitivity.

Focal external beam radiation may be palliative for bone pain due to metastases. The duration of relief is variable. Radiation is less effective for alleviating ureteral obstruction secondary to metastatic tumor because the time lag for a successful response may be 6 to 8 weeks.

Interstitial radiation involves retropubic or perineal implantation of seeds of ^{125}I, ^{198}Au, ^{103}Pa, or ^{192}Ir. This treatment avoids major extirpative surgery and provides a concentrated delivery of radiation to the target tissue. Successful seed implantation requires a well-defined primary tumor with a diameter less than 5 cm, a tumor volume less than 30 to 40 mL, and uniform distribution of seeds throughout the prostate. In the initial reports, 5-year survival following staging pelvic lymphadenectomy and retropubic implantation of ^{125}I or ^{198}Au seeds was comparable with survival rates after other forms of treatment, but the incidence of tumor progression is higher. Potency is preserved in more than 90 percent, and early complications are fewer and less severe than after external beam radiation. Interstitial irradiation with seeds of palladium or iridium provides a higher radiation dose and a shorter half-life and may improve efficacy and decrease complications. Improvements in three-dimensional imaging of the prostate make it possible to distribute the seeds more evenly in the gland.

The efficacy and complication rates of several experimental therapies for the primary tumor, including hyperthermia, cryosurgery, and high-intensity focused ultrasound are under investigation.

In summary, except for impotence following external beam radiation, serious morbidity is infrequent following either form of radiation therapy. Practical considerations make ^{125}I or ^{198}Au seed implantation most suited to stage T2a disease. The long-term efficacy of either form of radiation as compared with radical prostatectomy for the treatment of localized carcinomas (stages T1 and T2) is not clear, but current data suggest that radiotherapy may be less curative than radical prostatectomy.

Androgen Deprivation Because growth of the normal prostate is dependent on testicular androgens (see Chap. 336), it was logical to try androgen deprivation for treatment of advanced prostatic cancer. Androgen deprivation can be achieved in four ways: (1) surgical extirpation of the glands that synthesize androgens (castration and adrenalectomy); (2) inhibition of pituitary gonadotropin [and/or adrenocorticotropin (ACTH)] production [estrogen therapy, hypophysectomy, or treatment with luteinizing hormone–releasing hormone (LHRH) analogues such as leuprolide or buserelin]; (3) inhibition of androgen synthesis by the testes and adrenals (aminoglutethimide); and (4) inhibition of the binding of androgen to its receptor protein (cyproterone, flutamide, or bicalutamide).

Since testicular secretion accounts for more than 95 percent of testosterone production, bilateral orchiectomy results in a 90 percent decline of plasma levels. Estrogens such as diethylstilbestrol are potent inhibitors of the release from the pituitary gland of luteinizing hormone (LH), the gonadotropin that regulates testosterone production, and consequently, estrogen administration also causes a fall in plasma testosterone to castration levels. Maximum depression of plasma testosterone is achieved with 3 mg/d diethylstilbestrol. Other estrogens (conjugated estrogens, ethinyl estradiol, diethylstilbestrol diphosphate) are no more effective in the lowering of plasma testosterone level than is diethylstilbestrol.

Androgen deprivation by means of bilateral orchiectomy, diethylstilbestrol therapy, or combined orchiectomy plus diethylstilbestrol was a standard form of treatment for carcinoma of the prostate for many years, based largely on comparison of treatment groups with historical controls. Subsequently, in prospective control studies, the effectiveness of high-dose diethylstilbestrol or orchiectomy, alone or in combination, in enhancing survival in any stage of prostatic cancer was not clear-cut. Furthermore, death from cardiovascular disease was more frequent in patients treated with large doses of diethylstilbestrol. LHRH analogues have largely replaced estrogen therapy because of their safer cardiovascular profile. These analogues inhibit LH secretion and lower plasma testosterone levels.

Each of the above forms of androgen ablation still leaves a small amount of circulating adrenal androgen that may be detrimental in the control of advanced prostate cancer. Androgen depletion beyond that achieved by surgical castration, LHRH analogues, or estrogen administration can be accomplished by adrenalectomy or hypophysectomy. Adrenalectomy can be accomplished either by surgical ablation or by medical therapy with exogenous glucocorticoids, which inhibit ACTH secretion and the synthesis of adrenal androgen, or antiandrogens such as flutamide or nilutamide, which inhibit the binding of androgen to its cytoplasmic receptor protein. Extensive clinical trials in patients with metastatic disease comparing early androgen ablation alone with various forms of LHRH analogue

therapy versus androgen ablation with orchiectomy or LHRH analogues combined with antiandrogens have yielded inconsistent results. However, in most trials combination therapy resulted in a small but significant prolongation in both disease-free survival and overall survival; patients with the least amount of disease had the greatest degree of improvement with combination therapy. The modest improvement in outcomes in subsets of patients must be balanced against the added cost and the side effects of combination therapy. Although the appropriate time for initiating therapy remains controversial, the current trend is for early androgen ablation and, frequently, combination androgen ablation therapy in advanced prostatic cancer.

Even when there is no beneficial effect on survival, however, androgen deprivation decreases bone pain in two-thirds of symptomatic stage M+ patients and hence constitutes a major adjunctive therapy in the disease. Once the decision is made to institute such therapy, the choice must be made as to which form of androgen deprivation is appropriate. When acceptable to the patient, orchiectomy is safe and inexpensive and circumvents compliance problems. Diethylstilbestrol is also inexpensive and is usually safe in dosages of 3 mg/d or less in men who do not have preexisting cardiovascular disease. In men at risk for cardiovascular complications, LHRH analogues have similar response rates and fewer cardiovascular complications than diethylstilbestrol. The roles of intermittent androgen deprivation and of androgen blockers such as flutamide and bicalutamide in combination with each of the preceding means of establishing androgen deprivation are under study. In one study preoperative androgen deprivation in clinically localized prostate cancer resulted in a lower number of surgical specimens with positive margins. Whether such therapy improves rates of recurrence or survival is not clear.

As many as half of prostate cancers that have escaped from androgen ablation therapy have somatic mutations in the gene that encodes the androgen receptor in the prostate cancer cells. Many of these mutations cause amino acid substitutions in the hormone-binding domain of the protein that cause the loss of specificity for ligand, so that the receptor can respond to hormones such as progesterone that it would not ordinarily recognize or even to antiandrogens. The role of these mutations in the relentless progression of the disease is not established. Many prostate cancers express bcl 2 when they become androgen-independent.

Chemotherapy Chemotherapy is reserved for hormone-unresponsive disease and is used for palliation. The age group at greatest risk for prostatic cancer has poor tolerance for chemotherapy. This feature, coupled with the variable course and long doubling time of the disease, makes it difficult to determine the effectiveness of such therapy. However, several comprehensive trials utilizing chemotherapy have been undertaken in stage M+ disease following relapse after hormonal treatment, a situation in which mean survival time is only 7 to 8 months. The agents studied most extensively are estramustine phosphate, prednimustine, and cisplatin; more limited trials have been conducted with 5-fluorouracil, melphalan, and hydroxyurea. Complete response is rare, and only one-tenth of stage M+ patients have an objective partial response. In other trials, combinations of chemotherapeutic agents have been tested in stage M+ disease, most commonly estramustine phosphate plus prednimustine and cisplatin; more limited trials have been conducted with 5-fluorouracil, melphalan, and hydroxyurea. Complete response is again rare, and only one-fourth of patients or fewer show any objective improvement. For progressive, symptomatic stage M+ prostatic cancer, endocrine ablation therapy should be undertaken first, but chemotherapeutic agents may provide some benefit when such patients relapse. Development of new forms of therapy for disease refractory to androgen deprivation is an urgent need in the management of prostatic carcinoma.

Palliation of Bone Metastases Diffuse spread of metastases to bone limits the usefulness of external beam radiation therapy for relief of bone pain, which is a major cause of morbidity in the late phases of the disease when it is no longer responsive to androgen deprivation. Bone-seeking radiopharmaceuticals such as ^{89}Sr or diphosphonates unlabeled or labeled with samarium ([153]Sm) can be of benefit in the control of pain even in the absence of objective response of the tumor.

BIBLIOGRAPHY

BENIGN PROSTATIC HYPERPLASIA

LEPOR H et al: The efficacy and safety of terazosin for the treatment of symptomatic BPH. Prostate 18:345, 1991

McCONNELL JD et al: *Clinical Practice Guideline Number 8: Benign Prostatic Hyperplasia: Diagnosis and Treatment.* US Dept of Health and Human Services AHCPR publication No. 94-0582. Rockville, MD, 1994

STONER E et al: Maintenance of clinical efficacy with finasteride therapy for 24 months in patients with benign prostatic hyperplasia. Arch Intern Med 154:83, 1994

WALSH PC: Benign prostatic hyperplasia, in *Campbell's Urology*, 6th ed, PC Walsh et al (eds). Philadelphia, Saunders, 1992, p 1007

WILSON JD: The pathogenesis of prostatic hyperplasia. Am J Med 68:745, 1980

CARCINOMA OF THE PROSTATE

ALBERTSON PC et al: Long-term survival among men with conservatively treated localized prostate cancer. JAMA 274:626, 1995

BAGSHAW MA: External radiation therapy of carcinoma of the prostate. Cancer 45:1912, 1980

BYAR DP, CORLE DK: VACURG randomized trial of radical prostatectomy for stages I and II prostate cancer. Urology 17(Suppl 4):7, 1981

CATALONA WJ: Screening for prostate cancer. JAMA 273:1174, 1995

———, BIGG SW: Nerve-sparing radical prostatectomy: Evaluation of results after 250 patients. J Urol 143:538, 1990

COONER WH et al: Prostate cancer detection in a clinical urological practice by ultrasonography, digital rectal examination and prostate specific antigen. J Urol 143:1146, 1990

CRAWFORD ED et al: A controlled trial of leuprolide with and without flutamide in prostatic carcinoma. N Engl J Med 321:419, 1989

EISENBERGER MA et al: A critical assessment of the role of chemotherapy for endocrine resistant prostatic carcinoma. AUA Update Series Lesson 28, vol 7, 1988

HENNRICKSSON P, JOHANSSON S-E: Prediction of cardiovascular complication in patients with prostatic cancer treated with estrogen. Am J Epidemiol 125:970, 1987

HERR HW: Iodine 125 implantation in the management of localized prostatic carcinoma. Urol Clin North Am 7:605, 1980

HUGOSSON J et al: Prostate cancer mortality in patients surviving more than 10 years after diagnosis. J Urol 154:2115, 1995

ISRAELI RS et al: Sensitive detection of prostatic hematogenous tumor cell dissemination using prostate specific antigen and prostate specific membrane-derived primers in the polymerase chain reaction. J Urol 153:573, 1995

JEWETT HJ: Radical perineal prostatectomy for palpable clinically localized, non-obstructive cancer: Experience at the Johns Hopkins Hospital, 1909–1963. J Urol 124:492, 1980

KATZ A et al: Enhanced reverse transcriptase-polymerase chain reaction for prostate specific antigen as an indicator of true pathologic stage in patients with prostate cancer. Cancer 75:1642, 1995

LAING AH et al: Strontium-89 chloride for pain palliation in prostatic skeletal malignancy. Br J Radiol 64:816, 1991

MORGAN TO et al: Age-specific reference ranges for serum prostate-specific antigen in black men. N Engl J Med 336:304, 1996

NATIONAL INSTITUTES OF HEALTH CONSENSUS DEVELOPMENT CONFERENCE: The management of clinically localized prostate cancer. J Urol 138:1369, 1987

OESTERLING JE et al: Free, complexed and total serum prostate specific antigen: The establishment of appropriate reference ranges for their concentrations and ratios. J Urol 154:1090, 1995

STAMEY TA, McNEAL JE: Adenocarcinoma of the prostate, in *Campbell's Urology*, 6th ed, PC Walsh et al (eds). Philadelphia, Saunders, 1992, p 1159

TAPLIN ME et al: Mutations of the androgen receptor gene in metastatic androgen-independent prostate cancer. N Engl J Med 332:1393, 1995

TYRRELL CJ et al: A multicenter randomized trial comparing the luteinizing hormone–releasing hormone analogue goserelin acetate alone and with flutamide in the treatment of advanced prostate cancer. J Urol 146:1321, 1991

98   *Robert J. Motzer, George J. Bosl*

TESTICULAR CANCER

TESTICULAR CANCER (GERM CELL TUMORS)

Primary germ cell tumors (GCTs) of the testis, arising by the malignant transformation of primordial germ cells, constitute 95 percent of all testicular neoplasms. Infrequently, GCTs arise from an extragonadal site, including the mediastinum, retroperitoneum and, very rarely, the pineal gland. This disease is notable for the young age of the afflicted patients, the totipotent capacity for differentiation of the tumor cells, and its curability; more than 90 percent of all newly diagnosed patients will be cured, and, since the advent of cisplatin-based chemotherapy, about 70 to 80 percent of patients with metastatic disease are cured.

INCIDENCE AND EPIDEMIOLOGY In 1996, approximately 7400 new cases of testicular GCT were diagnosed in the United States; the incidence of this malignancy has increased slowly over the past 40 years. The tumor occurs most frequently between the ages of 20 and 40. A testicular mass in a man aged 50 years or greater should be regarded as a lymphoma until proved otherwise. GCT is at least four to five times more common in white than in African-American males, and a higher incidence has been observed in Scandinavia and New Zealand than in the United States.

ETIOLOGY AND GENETICS Cryptorchidism is associated with a severalfold higher risk of GCT. Abdominal cryptorchid testes are at a higher risk than inguinal cryptorchid testes. Orchiopexy should be performed before puberty if possible. The protective effect of orchiopexy is difficult to quantify, but most studies suggest that early orchiopexy reduces the risk of GCT and improves the ability to save the testis. If an abdominal cryptorchid testis cannot be brought into the scrotum, it should be removed. Approximately 2 percent of men with GCTs of one testis will develop a primary tumor in the other testis. Testicular feminization syndromes increase the risk of testicular GCT, and Klinefelter's syndrome is associated with mediastinal GCT.

CLINICAL PRESENTATION A painless testicular mass is pathognomonic for a testicular malignancy. More commonly, patients present with testicular discomfort or swelling suggestive of epididymitis and/or orchitis. In this circumstance, a trial of antibiotics is reasonable. However, if symptoms persist or a residual abnormality remains, then testicular ultrasound examination is indicated. Back pain from retroperitoneal metastases is common and must be distinguished from musculoskeletal pain. Dyspnea from pulmonary metastases occurs infrequently. Patients with increased serum levels of human chorionic gonadotropin (hCG) may present with gynecomastia. A delay in diagnosis is associated with a more advanced stage and possibly worse survival.

Ultrasound examination of the testis is indicated whenever a testicular malignancy is considered and for persistent or painful testicular swelling. If this examination shows an intratesticular mass, a radical inguinal orchiectomy should be performed. Because the testis develops originally from the gonadal ridge in the peritoneal cavity, its blood supply and lymphatic drainage originate intraabdominally and descend with the testis into the scrotum. Cutting through the skin of the scrotum to remove the testis by a scrotal orchiectomy may breach anatomic barriers and permit tumor cells to spread by additional pathways; for this reason, the scrotal approach is discouraged. The staging evaluation for GCT includes a determination of serum levels of alpha fetoprotein (AFP) and hCG. Following orchiectomy, a chest radiograph and a computed tomography (CT) scan of the abdomen and pelvis should be performed. A chest CT scan is required if mediastinal or hilar disease is suspected. *Stage I disease* is defined as disease limited to the testis, epididymis, or spermatic cord. *Stage II disease* is defined as disease limited to retroperitoneal (regional) lymph nodes. *Stage III disease* is defined as disease outside the retroperitoneum, involving supradiaphragmatic nodal sites or viscera. The staging may be "clinical"—defined solely by physical examination, blood marker evaluation, and radiographs—or "pathologic"—defined by an operative procedure.

CHAPTER 98
Testicular Cancer   **603**

The regional draining lymph nodes for the testis are in the retroperitoneum, and the vascular supply originates from the great vessels (for the right testis) or the renal vessels (for the left testis). As a result, the lymph nodes that are involved first by a right testicular tumor are the interaortocaval lymph nodes just below the renal vessels. For a left testicular tumor, the first involved lymph nodes are lateral to the aorta (para-aortic) and below the left renal vessels. In both cases, further nodal spread is inferior and contralateral and, less commonly, above the renal hilum. Lymphatic involvement can extend cephalad to the retrocrural, posterior mediastinal, and supraclavicular lymph nodes. Treatment is determined by tumor histology (seminoma versus nonseminoma) and clinical stage (Table 98-1).

PATHOLOGY GCTs are divided into nonseminoma and seminoma subtypes. Nonseminomatous GCTs are most frequent in the third decade of life and can display the full spectrum of embryonic and adult cellular differentiation. This entity comprises four histologies: embryonal carcinoma, teratoma, choriocarcinoma, and endodermal sinus (yolk sac) tumor. Choriocarcinoma, consisting of both cytotrophoblasts and syncytiophoblasts, represents malignant trophoblastic differentiation and is invariably associated with secretion of hCG. Endodermal sinus tumor is the malignant counterpart of the fetal yolk sac and is associated with secretion of AFP. Pure embryonal carcinoma may secrete AFP, or hCG, or both; this pattern is biochemical evidence of differentiation. Teratoma is composed of somatic cell types derived from two or more germ layers (ectoderm, mesoderm, or endoderm). Each of these histologies may be present alone or in combination with others. Nonseminomatous GCTs tend to metastasize early to sites such as the retroperitoneal lymph nodes and lung parenchyma. Approximately one-third of patients present with disease limited to the testis (stage I), one-third with retroperitoneal metastases (stage II), and one-third with more extensive supradiaphragmatic nodal or visceral metastases (stage III).

Seminoma represents about 50 percent of all GCTs, has a median age in the fourth decade, and generally follows a more indolent clinical course. Most patients (70 percent) present with stage I disease, about 20 percent with stage II disease, and 10 percent with stage III disease; lung or other visceral metastases are rare. Seminoma is radiosensitive, and radiotherapy is the treatment of choice in patients with stage I disease and stage II disease where the nodes are <5 cm in maximum diameter. When a tumor contains both seminoma and nonseminoma components, patient management is directed by the more aggressive nonseminoma component.

An isochromosome of the short arm of chromosome 12 [i(12p)] is a chromosomal marker specific for GCT. It has been found in all histologic types and has diagnostic and possibly prognostic significance. One clinical application of this marker is in the diagnosis of patients with midline tumors of uncertain histogenesis (see below).

TUMOR MARKERS Careful monitoring of the serum tumor markers AFP and hCG is essential in the management of patients with GCT, as these markers are important for diagnosis, as prognostic indicators, in monitoring treatment response, and in the detection of early relapse. Approximately 70 percent of patients presenting with disseminated nonseminomatous GCT have increased serum concentrations of AFP and/or hCG. While hCG concentrations may be increased in patients with either nonseminoma or seminoma histology, AFP is increased only in patients with nonseminoma histology. The finding of an increased AFP level in a patient whose tumor showed only seminoma indicates that an occult nonseminomatous component is present, and that the patient should be treated according to guidelines for a nonseminomatous GCT. The serum lactate dehydrogenase (LDH) level serves as an additional marker of all GCTs, but it is not as specific as either AFP or hCG. LDH levels will be increased in 50 to 60 percent of cases of metastatic nonseminoma and up to 80 percent of cases of advanced seminoma.

Determination of AFP, hCG, and LDH levels should be done before and after orchiectomy. Increased serum AFP and hCG concentrations decay according to first-order kinetics; the half-life is 24 to 36 h for hCG and 5 to 7 days for AFP. AFP and hCG should be assayed serially during and after treatment. Either reappearance of hCG and/or AFP or failure of these markers to decline according to the predicted half-life are indicators of persistent or recurrent tumor.

℞ TREATMENT

Stage I Nonseminoma If, after an orchiectomy (for clinical stage I disease), radiographs and physical examination show no evidence of disease, and serum AFP and hCG concentrations either are normal or are declining to normal according to the known half-life, patients may be managed by either a nerve-sparing retroperitoneal lymph node dissection (RPLND) or surveillance. The retroperitoneal lymph nodes will be pathologically involved by GCT (pathologic stage II) in 20 to 50 percent of these patients. The decision between surveillance or RPLND is based on the pathology of the primary tumor. If the primary tumor shows no pathologic evidence for lymphatic or vascular invasion *and* is limited to the testis (T1), then either option is reasonable. If lymphatic or vascular invasion is present *or* the tumor extends into the tunica, spermatic cord, or scrotum (T2 through T4), then surveillance should not be offered. Either approach should cure more than 95 percent of patients.

A RPLND is the standard operation for removal of the regional lymph nodes of the testis (the retroperitoneal nodes). The operation removes the lymph nodes ipsilateral to the primary site and the nodal groups adjacent to the primary landing zone. The standard (modified bilateral) RPLND removes all node-bearing tissue down to the bifurcation of the great vessels, including the ipsilateral iliac nodes. The major long-term effect of this operation is retrograde ejaculation and infertility. A nerve-sparing RPLND, usually accomplished by identification and dissection of individual nerve fibers, avoids injury to the sympathetic nerves responsible for ejaculation. Normal ejaculation is preserved in approximately 90 percent of patients. Patients with pathologic stage I disease are observed, and only the 10 percent who relapse require additional therapy. If retroperitoneal nodes are found to be involved at RPLND, then a decision regarding adjuvant chemotherapy is made on the basis of the extent of retroperitoneal disease (see below).

Table 98-1

Germ Cell Tumor Staging System and Treatment

		Treatment	
Stage	**Extent of Disease**	**Seminoma**	**Nonseminoma**
I	Testis only, T1, no vascular/lymphatic invasion	Radiation therapy	RPLND or observation
	T2–4 or vascular/lymphatic invasion present	Radiation therapy	RPLND
IIA	Nodes <2 cm	Radiation therapy	RPLND
IIB	Nodes 2–5 cm	Radiation therapy	RPLND +/− adjuvant chemotherapy or chemotherapy followed by RPLND
IIC	Nodes >5 cm	Chemotherapy	Chemotherapy followed by RPLND
III	Distant metastases	Chemotherapy	Chemotherapy, often followed by surgery (biopsy or resection)

RPLND, retroperitoneal lymph node dissection

Surveillance is an option in the management of clinical stage I disease when no vascular/lymphatic invasion is found and the primary tumor is classified as T1. In this situation, only 20 to 30 percent of patients will have pathologic stage II disease, implying that most RPLNDs in this situation are not therapeutic. Although surveillance has not been compared to RPLND in a randomized trial, all large studies show that surveillance and RPLND lead to equivalent long-term survival. Patient compliance is essential if surveillance is to be successful. Patients must be carefully followed with periodic chest radiography, physical examination, CT scan of the abdomen, and serum tumor marker determinations. The median time to relapse is about seven months, and late relapses (later than 2 years) are rare. The 70 to 80 percent of patients who do not relapse require no intervention after orchiectomy; treatment is reserved for those who do relapse. When the primary tumor is classified as T2 through T4 *or* lymphatic/vascular invasion is identified, nerve-sparing RPLND is preferred. About 50 percent of these patients will have pathologic stage II disease and are destined to relapse.

Stage II Nonseminoma GCT Patients with limited, ipsilateral retroperitoneal adenopathy (nodes usually 3 cm in greatest diameter or smaller) generally undergo a modified bilateral RPLND as primary management. Nearly all patients with pathologic stage II disease whose disease is completely resected by RPLND are cured. The in-field recurrence rate after a properly performed RPLND is very low. Depending on the extent of disease, the postoperative management options include either surveillance or two cycles of adjuvant chemotherapy. Surveillance is the preferred approach for patients with resected "low-volume" metastases (all nodes with metastatic tumor are ≤2 cm in diameter, *and* fewer than six nodes are involved) because the probability of relapse is one-third or less. Because relapse occurs in 50 percent or more of patients with "high-volume" metastasis (fewer than six nodes involved, *or* any involved node >2 cm in largest diameter, *or* extranodal tumor extension), two cycles of adjuvant chemotherapy should be considered, as it results in cure in ≥98 percent of patients. Regimens consisting of etoposide (100 mg/m^2 daily on days 1 through 5) plus cisplatin (20 mg/m^2 daily on days 1 through 5) with or without bleomycin (30 units per day on days 2, 9, and 16) given at 3-week intervals are effective and well tolerated.

Stages I and II Seminoma Inguinal orchiectomy followed by retroperitoneal radiation therapy cures about 98 percent of patients with stage I seminoma. The dose of radiotherapy (2500 to 3000 cGy) is low and well tolerated, and the in-field recurrence rate is negligible. About 2 percent of patients will relapse with supradiaphragmatic or systemic disease. Surveillance has been proposed as an option, and studies have shown that there is an approximately 15 percent probability of relapse. The median time to relapse is 12 to 15 months, and late relapses during surveillance (>5 years) may be more frequent than with nonseminoma tumors. Chemotherapy is usually required to treat the relapse. Surveillance for clinical stage I seminoma is generally not recommended in the United States.

Nonbulky retroperitoneal disease (stage IIA and IIB) is also treated with radiotherapy alone. Prophylactic supradiaphragmatic radiotherapy is not indicated. Relapses in the anterior mediastinum are unusual, and the cumulative effect of infradiaphragmatic plus supradiaphragmatic radiotherapy causes extremely severe hematologic toxicity when chemotherapy is needed at relapse. The proportion of patients who achieve relapse-free survival with retroperitoneal masses <5 cm in diameter is about 90 percent. Because at least one-third of patients with bulkier disease relapse, initial chemotherapy is preferred for stage IIC disease.

Chemotherapy for Advanced GCT Regardless of histology, patients with stage IIC and stage III GCT are treated with chemotherapy. Combination chemotherapy programs developed in the 1970s and 1980s, based on bleomycin and cisplatin at doses of 100 to 120 mg/m^2 per cycle plus etoposide, showed that 70 percent and 80

percent, respectively, of such patients will be cured. Complete response (the complete disappearance of all clinical evidence of tumor on physical examination and radiography plus normal serum levels of AFP and hCG for 1 month or more) occurs after chemotherapy alone in about 60 percent of patients, and another 10 to 20 percent are rendered free of disease with surgical resection of all sites of residual disease. Randomized clinical trials have shown that lower doses of cisplatin result in inferior survival.

The toxicity of four cycles of the cisplatin/bleomycin/etoposide (BEP) regimen is substantial. Nausea, vomiting, and hair loss occur in most patients, although nausea and vomiting have been markedly ameliorated by modern antiemetic regimens. Myelosuppression is frequent, and symptomatic bleomycin pulmonary toxicity occurs in about 5 percent of patients. Treatment-induced mortality due to neutropenia with septicemia or bleomycin-induced pulmonary failure occurs in 1 to 3 percent of patients. Dose reductions for myelosuppression are rarely indicated. Long-term permanent toxicities include nephrotoxicity (reduced glomerular filtration and persistent magnesium wasting), ototoxicity, and peripheral neuropathy. When bleomycin is administered by weekly bolus injection, Raynaud's phenomenon appears in 5 to 10 percent of treated patients. Less often, other evidence of small blood vessel damage has been reported, including transient ischemic attacks and myocardial infarction.

Because not all patients are cured and significant treatment-related toxicities are known, it became necessary to stratify patients into "good-risk" and "poor-risk" groups. For good-risk patients, the goal is to achieve maximum efficacy with minimal toxicity. For poor-risk patients, the goal is to identify more effective therapy with tolerable toxicity. In general, good-risk patients have tumor of smaller extent with metastases limited to the retroperitoneum and lung and low serum levels of tumor markers. The presence of a primary mediastinal nonseminoma, high serum concentrations of hCG, and/or nonpulmonary visceral metastases indicate poor-risk disease (i.e., disease unlikely to be cured with standard therapy).

For patients with good-risk GCTs, four cycles of etoposide plus cisplatin (EP) or three cycles of BEP will result in a durable, complete response in about 90 percent of patients, with minimal acute and chronic toxicity. With these regimens, pulmonary toxicity is absent when bleomycin is not used and is rare when therapy is limited to 9 weeks; myelosuppression with neutropenic fever is less frequent; and treatment mortality is negligible. Randomized trials have shown that carboplatin, a less toxic analogue of cisplatin, is less effective than cisplatin. Bleomycin should not be deleted when treatment is limited to three cycles.

Only 35 to 50 percent of patients with poor-risk GCT are cured. No regimen has been found to be better than four cycles of BEP, a fact that emphasizes the need for more effective therapy. Randomized clinical trials have shown that the substitution of ifosfamide for etoposide and the use of higher doses of cisplatin (200 mg/m^2 per cycle) do not improve survival. Chemotherapy using a dose-intensive regimen of carboplatin, etoposide, and either cyclophosphamide or ifosfamide followed by hematopoietic stem cell rescue improves overall survival, and a randomized trial is in progress to test this hypothesis. If possible, patients with poor-risk GCT should be referred to centers and treated on clinical trials.

Postchemotherapy Surgery Resection of residual metastases after the completion of chemotherapy is an integral part of therapy. If the initial histology is nonseminoma and the marker values have normalized, all sites of residual disease should be resected. In general, residual retroperitoneal disease requires a modified bilateral RPLND, which is associated with retrograde ejaculation. Thoracotomy (unilateral or bilateral) and neck dissection are less frequently required to remove residual mediastinal, pulmonary parenchymal, or cervical nodal disease. Viable tumor (seminoma, embryonal carcinoma, yolk sac tumor or choriocarcinoma), mature teratoma, or necrotic debris and fibrosis will be present in about 15 percent, 40 percent, and 45 percent of resected specimens respectively. The frequency of teratoma or viable disease is highest in residual mediastinal tumors. If necrotic debris or mature teratoma is present, no further chemotherapy is necessary. If viable tumor is present but is completely excised, then two additional cycles of chemotherapy are needed.

If the initial histology is pure seminoma, mature teratoma is rarely present and the most frequent finding is necrotic debris. For residual retroperitoneal disease, a complete RPLND is technically difficult owing to extensive postchemotherapy fibrosis. Close observation is recommended when no radiographic abnormality exists or a residual mass smaller than 3 cm is present. Controversy exists over what to do when the residual mass exceeds 3 cm in diameter. About 25 percent of such masses will contain viable GCT. Some investigators prefer excision or biopsy, but radiotherapy or surveillance are alternatives.

Salvage Chemotherapy Of patients with advanced GCT, 20 to 30 percent fail to achieve a durable complete response to first-line chemotherapy. A combination of cisplatin, ifosfamide and, vinblastine (VeIP) will induce a durable complete response in 25 percent of patients as a second-line therapy. Patients are more likely to achieve a durable complete response to VeIP if they had a testicular primary tumor and have relapsed from a prior complete remission to first-line cisplatin-containing chemotherapy. In contrast, if the patient failed to achieve a complete response or has a primary mediastinal nonseminoma, then VeIP is rarely beneficial. Those patients are candidates for dose-intensive treatment.

Chemotherapy consisting of dose-intensive, high-dose carboplatin (≥ 1500 mg/m^2) plus etoposide (≥ 1200 mg/m^2), with or without cyclophosphamide or ifosfamide, with peripheral blood- or bone marrow–derived stem cell support will induce a complete response in 25 to 40 percent of patients who have failed ifosfamide-containing salvage chemotherapy. About one-half of the complete responses will be durable. High-dose therapy is the treatment of choice and standard of care for this patient population. Paclitaxel is active in previously treated patients. It is being studied as a new component in dose-intensive therapy.

EXTRAGONADAL GCT AND MIDLINE CARCINOMA OF UNCERTAIN HISTOGENESIS The prognosis and management of patients with extragonadal GCTs depends on the tumor histology and site of origin. All patients with a diagnosis of extragonadal GCT should have a testicular ultrasound examination. Nearly all patients with retroperitoneal or mediastinal seminoma achieve a durable complete response to BEP or EP. The clinical features of patients with primary retroperitoneal nonseminoma GCT are similar to those of patients with a primary of testis origin, and careful evaluation will find evidence of a primary testicular GCT in about two-thirds of cases. In contrast, a primary mediastinal nonseminomatous GCT is associated with a poor prognosis, with no more than one-third of patients being cured with standard therapy (four cycles of BEP). Patients with newly diagnosed mediastinal nonseminoma are considered to have poor-risk disease and should be considered for clinical trials testing regimens of possibly greater efficacy. In addition, mediastinal nonseminoma is associated with hematologic disorders, including acute myelogenous leukemia, myelodysplastic syndrome, and essential thrombocytosis unrelated to previous chemotherapy. An i(12p) isochromosome has been identified in both the primary GCT and leukemic cells, indicating a common clonal origin. These hematologic disorders are very refractory to treatment.

A group of patients with poorly differentiated tumors of unknown histogenesis has been reported. These tumors are most common in males, are midline in distribution, and are not associated with secretion of AFP or hCG; a minority of patients (10 to 20 percent) are cured by standard cisplatin-containing chemotherapy. Recently, conventional and molecular cytogenetic studies have shown that i(12p) is present in about 25 percent of such tumors, confirming their origin from primitive germ cells. This finding is also predictive of response to cisplatin-based chemotherapy and resulting long-term survival. Genetic analysis of these tumors has also identified other histologies, including neuroepithelial tumors and lymphoma, demonstrating the heterogeneity of this group of tumors.

FERTILITY Infertility is an important consequence of the treatment of GCTs. In addition, preexisting infertility or impaired fertility is often present. Azoospermia and/or oligospermia are present at diagnosis in at least 50 percent of patients with testicular GCTs. Ejaculatory dysfunction is associated with RPLND, and germ cell damage may result from cisplatin-containing chemotherapy. Nerve-sparing techniques to preserve the retroperitoneal sympathetic nerves have made retrograde ejaculation less likely in patient subgroups that are candidates for this operation. Spermatogenesis does recover in some patients after chemotherapy. However, because there is a significant risk of impaired reproductive capacity due either to a preexisting condition or to treatment, semen analysis and cryopreservation of sperm (in a "sperm bank") should be recommended to all patients before radiotherapy, chemotherapy, or RPLND.

BIBLIOGRAPHY

BAJORIN DF et al: Current perspectives on the role of adjunctive surgery in combined modality treatment for patients with germ cell tumors. Semin Oncol 19:148, 1992

———— et al: Randomized trial of etoposide and cisplatin versus etoposide and carboplatin in patients with good-risk germ cell tumors: A multiinstitutional study. J Clin Oncol 11:598, 1993

BOSL GJ et al: Clinical relevance of the i(12p) marker chromosome in germ cell tumors. J Natl Cancer Inst 86:349, 1994

———— et al: Cancer of the Testis, in *Cancer: Principles and Practice of Oncology*, 5th ed, VT DeVita, S Hellman, SA Rosenberg (eds). Lippincott, Philadelphia, 1997, pp 1397–1425

EINHORN LH et al: Evaluation of optimal duration of chemotherapy in favorable-prognosis disseminated germ cell tumors: A Southeastern Cancer Study Group protocol. J Clin Oncol 7:387, 1989

FELDMAN S et al: Low-risk metastatic gestational trophoblastic disease. Semin Oncol 22:166, 1995

MOTZER RJ, BOSL GJ: High-dose chemotherapy for resistant germ cell tumors: Recent advances and future directions. J Natl Cancer Inst 84:1703, 1992

99   *Robert C. Young*

GYNECOLOGIC MALIGNANCIES

OVARIAN CANCER

Incidence and Epidemiology Epithelial ovarian cancer is the leading cause of death from gynecologic cancer in the United States. In 1996 there were 26,700 new cases diagnosed and 14,800 deaths. The disease accounts for 5 percent of all cancer deaths in women in the United States; more women die of this disease than from cervical and endometrial cancer combined.

The age-specific incidence of the common epithelial type of ovarian cancer increases progressively and peaks in the eighth decade. It is uncommon before the age of 40. Epidemiologic studies suggest higher incidences in industrialized nations and an association with disordered ovarian function, including infertility, nulliparity, frequent miscarriages, and use of ovulation-inducing drugs such as clomiphene. Each pregnancy reduces the ovarian cancer risk by about 10 percent, and breast feeding and tubal ligation also appear to reduce the risk. Oral contraceptives reduce the risk of ovarian cancer in patients with a familial history of cancer and in the general population. Many of these risk reductions support the "incessant ovulation" hypothesis for ovarian cancer etiology, which implies that an aberrant repair process of the surface epithelium is central to ovarian cancer development. Estrogen replacement after menopause does not appear to increase the risk of ovarian cancer, although one study showed a modest increase in risk with more than 11 years of use.

Familial cases account for about 5 percent of all ovarian cancer, and a family history of ovarian cancer is a major risk factor. Compared to a life-time risk of 1.6 percent in the general population, women with one affected first-degree relative have a 5 percent risk. In families with two or more affected first-degree relatives, the risk may exceed 50 percent. Three types of autosomal dominant familial cancer are recognized: (1) site-specific in which only ovarian cancer is seen, (2) families with cancer of the ovary and breast, and (3) the Lynch type II cancer family syndrome with nonpolyposis colorectal cancer, endometrial cancer, and ovarian cancer.

Etiology and Genetics   In women with hereditary breast-ovarian cancer, the susceptibility locus, BRCA-1, is located on chromosome 17q12-21. It is likely that BRCA-1 is a tumor suppressor gene and that its protein product acts as a negative regulator of tumor growth. A large number of mutations of BRCA-1 have now been described; most are frameshift or nonsense mutations, and 86 percent produce truncated protein products. The exact implications of the myriad of other mutations including many missense mutations are not known. Men in such families have an increased risk of prostate cancer.

Cytogenetic analysis of sporadic epithelial ovarian cancers generally reveals complex karyotypic rearrangements. Structural abnormalities frequently appear on chromosomes 1 and 11, and loss of heterozygosity (LOH) is common on 3q, 6q, 11q, 13q, and 17. Abnormalities of oncogenes are frequently found in ovarian cancer and include c-*myc*, H-*ras*, K-*ras*, and *neu*.

Ovarian tumors (usually not epithelial) are sometimes components of complex genetic syndromes. Peutz-Jeghers syndrome (mucocutaneous pigmentation and intestinal polyps) is associated with ovarian sex cord stromal tumors and Sertoli cell tumors in men. Patients with gonadal dysgenesis (46XY genotype or mosaic for Y-containing cell lines) develop gonadoblastomas, and women with nevoid basal cell carcinomas have an increased risk of ovarian fibromas.

Clinical Presentation and Differential Diagnosis   Most patients with ovarian cancer are first diagnosed when the disease has already spread beyond the true pelvis. The occurrence of abdominal pain, bloating, and urinary symptoms usually indicates advanced disease. Localized ovarian cancer is generally asymptomatic. However, progressive enlargement of a localized ovarian tumor can produce urinary frequency or constipation, and rarely torsion of an ovarian mass causes acute abdominal pain or a surgical abdomen. In contrast to cervical or endometrial cancer, vaginal bleeding or discharge is rarely seen with early ovarian cancer. The diagnosis of early disease usually occurs with palpation of an asymptomatic adnexal mass during routine pelvic examination. However, most ovarian enlargements discovered this way are benign functional cysts that characteristically resolve over one to three menstrual cycles. Adnexal masses in premenarchal or postmenopausal women are more likely to be pathologic, and exploratory surgery is usually required. Other causes of adnexal masses include pedunculated uterine fibroids, endometriosis, benign ovarian neoplasms, and inflammatory lesions of the bowel.

Evaluation of patients with suspected ovarian cancer should include measurement of serum levels of the tumor marker CA-125. CA-125 determinants are glycoproteins with molecular masses from 220 to 1000 kDa, and a radioimmunoassay is used to determine circulating CA-125 antigen levels. Between 80 and 85 percent of patients with epithelial ovarian cancer have levels of CA-125 ≥ 35 U/mL. Other malignant tumors can also elevate CA-125 levels, including cancers of the endometrium, cervix, fallopian tubes, pancreas, breast, lung, and colon. Certain nonmalignant conditions that can elevate CA-125 levels include pregnancy, endometriosis, pelvic inflammatory disease, and uterine fibroids. One percent of normal females have serum CA-125 levels >35 U/mL. However, in postmenopausal women with an asymptomatic pelvic mass and CA-125 levels ≥ 65 U/mL, the test has a sensitivity of 97 percent and a specificity of 78 percent.

Screening   In contrast to patients who present with advanced disease, patients with early ovarian cancers (stages I and II) are commonly curable with conventional therapy. For this reason, effective screening procedures would improve the cure rate in this disease. Although pelvic

examination can occasionally detect early disease, it is a relatively insensitive screening procedure. Transvaginal sonography has replaced the slower and less sensitive abdominal sonography, but there are significant false-positive results, particularly in premenopausal women. In one study, 67 laparotomies were required to diagnose 1 primary ovarian cancer. Doppler flow imaging coupled with transvaginal ultrasound may improve accuracy and reduce the high rate of false positives.

CA-125 has been studied as a screening tool. Unfortunately, half of women with stages I and II ovarian cancer have CA-125 levels <65 U/mL. Other nonmalignant disorders can elevate the CA-125 level, and both false-negative and -positive results have been reported in most screening studies.

Attempts have been made to improve the sensitivity and specificity by combinations of procedures, commonly transvaginal ultrasound and CA-125 levels. In a screening study of 22,000 women, 42 had a positive screen and 11 had ovarian cancer (7 with advanced disease). In addition, eight women with a negative screen developed ovarian cancer. Thus, while screening can detect early ovarian cancer in asymptomatic women, the false-positive rate would lead to a large number of unnecessary (i.e., negative) laparotomies if each positive screen resulted in a surgical exploration. The National Institutes of Health Consensus Conference recommended against screening for ovarian cancer among the general population without known risk factors for the disease.

Pathology   Common epithelial tumors comprise most (85 percent) of the ovarian neoplasms. These may be benign (50 percent), frankly malignant (33 percent), or tumors of low malignant potential (16 percent), or so-called tumors of borderline malignancy. Epithelial tumors of low malignant potential have the cytologic features of malignancy but do not invade the ovarian stroma. More than 75 percent present in early stage and generally occur in younger women. They have a natural history that is much better than their malignant counterpart.

There are five major subtypes of common epithelial tumors: serous (50 percent), mucinous (25 percent), endometroid (15 percent), clear cell (5 percent), and Brenner tumors (1 percent), the latter derived from the urothelial epithelium. Benign common epithelial tumors are almost always serous or mucinous and develop in women ages 20 to 60. They are frequently large (20 to 30 cm), bilateral, and typically cystic.

Malignant epithelial tumors are usually seen in women over 40. They present as solid masses, with areas of necrosis and hemorrhage. Masses larger than 10 to 15 cm have usually already spread into the intraabdominal space. Spread eventually results in intraabdominal carcinomatosis, which leads to bowel and renal obstruction and cachexia.

Although most ovarian tumors are epithelial, two other important ovarian tumor types exist—stromal and germ cell tumors. These tumors are distinct in their cell of origin but also have different clinical presentations and natural histories and are often managed differently (see below).

Metastasis to the ovary can occur from breast, colon, gastric, and pancreatic cancers, and the Krukenberg tumor was classically described as bilateral ovarian masses from metastatic mucin-secreting gastrointestinal cancers.

Staging and Prognostic Factors   Although laparotomy is often the primary procedure used to establish the diagnosis, less invasive studies can often aid in defining the extent of spread. These include chest x-rays, abdominal computed tomography scans, and abdominal and pelvic sonography. If the woman has specific gastrointestinal symptoms, a barium enema or gastrointestinal series can be performed. Symptoms of bladder or renal dysfunction can be evaluated by cystoscopy or intravenous pyelography.

A careful staging laparotomy will establish the stage and extent of disease and allow for the cytoreduction of tumor masses in patients with advanced disease. Proper laparotomy requires a vertical incision of sufficient length to ensure adequate examination of the abdominal contents. The presence, amount, and cytology of any ascites fluid should be noted. The primary tumor should be evaluated for rupture, excrescences, or dense adherence. Careful visual and manual inspection of the diaphragm and peritoneal surfaces is required. In addition to total abdominal hysterectomy and bilateral salpingo-oophorectomy, a partial omentectomy should be performed and the paracolic gutters inspected. Pelvic lymph nodes as well as para-aortic nodes in the region

CHAPTER 99
Gynecologic Malignancies

607

of the renal hilus should be biopsied. Since this surgical procedure defines stage, establishes prognosis, and determines the necessity for subsequent therapy, it should be performed by a surgeon with special expertise in ovarian cancer staging. Studies have shown that patients operated upon by gynecologic oncologists were properly staged 97 percent of the time, compared to 52 and 35 percent of cases staged by obstetricians/gynecologists and general surgeons respectively. At the end of staging, 23 percent of women have stage I disease (cancer confined to the ovary or ovaries); 13 percent have stage II (disease confined to the true pelvis); 47 percent have stage III (disease spread into but confined to the abdomen); and 16 percent have stage IV disease (spread outside the pelvis and abdomen). The 5-year survival correlates with stage of disease: stage I—90 percent, stage II—70 percent, stage III—15 to 20 percent, and stage IV—1 to 5 percent (see Table 99-1).

Prognosis in ovarian cancer is dependent not only upon stage but on the extent of residual disease and histologic grade. Patients presenting with advanced disease but left without significant residual disease after surgery have a median survival of 39 months, compared to 17 months for those with suboptimal tumor resection.

Prognosis of epithelial tumors is also highly influenced by histologic grade but less so by histologic type. Some studies in early stage disease have suggested a better survival for mucinous adenocarcinoma than endometrial and serous types, and a worse prognosis for clear cell carcinomas. Although grading systems differ among pathologists, all grading systems show a better prognosis for well- or moderately differentiated tumors and a poorer prognosis for poorly differentiated histologies. Typical 5-year survivals for patients with all stages of disease are: well differentiated—88 percent, moderately differentiated—58 percent, poorly differentiated—27 percent.

The prognostic significance of pre- and postoperative CA-125 levels is uncertain. Serum levels generally reflect volume of disease, and high levels usually indicate unresectability and a poorer survival. Postoperative levels, if elevated, usually indicate residual disease. Nevertheless, on multivariate analysis, CA-125 is not an independent prognostic factor because of the association with volume of disease. The rate of decline of CA-125 levels during initial therapy or the absolute level after one to three cycles of chemotherapy correlates with prognosis but is not sufficiently accurate to guide individual treatment decisions. Even when the CA-125 level falls to normal after surgery or chemotherapy, "second-look" laparotomy identifies residual disease in 60 percent of women. Other more quantitative approaches to define prognosis include ploidy analysis and image cytometry (automated analysis of cell morphology), but, while promising, they remain investigational.

Genetic and biologic factors may influence prognosis. Increased tumor levels of p53 are associated with a worse prognosis in advanced disease. Epidermal growth factor receptors in ovarian cancer are associated with a high risk of progression, but the increased expression of HER-2/neu has given conflicting prognostic results, and expression of Mdr-1 has not been of prognostic value.

℞ TREATMENT

The selection of therapy for patients with epithelial ovarian cancer depends upon the stage, extent of residual tumor, and histologic grade. In general, patients are considered in three separate treatment groups: (1) those with early (stages I and II) ovarian cancer and microscopic or no residual disease; (2) patients with advanced (stage III) disease but minimal residual tumor (<1 cm) after initial surgery; and (3) patients with bulky residual tumor and advanced (stage III or IV) disease.

Patients with stage I disease, no residual tumor, and well or moderately differentiated tumors need no adjuvant therapy after definitive surgery and have a 5-year survival in excess of 95 percent. For all other patients with early disease and those stage I patients with poor prognosis histologic grade, adjuvant therapy is probably warranted, and total-abdominal irradiation, single-agent cisplatin, or drug combinations used in advanced disease are appropriate. Five-year survival for this group exceeds 80 percent.

For the patients with advanced (stage III) disease but with limited or no residual disease after definitive cytoreductive surgery (about 50 percent of all stage III patients), the primary therapy is combination chemotherapy. Approximately 70 percent of women respond to initial combination chemotherapy, and 40 to 50 percent have a complete regression of disease. Only about half of these patients are free of disease if surgically restaged. Although a variety of combinations are active, a randomized prospective trial of paclitaxel and cisplatin compared to cyclophosphamide and cisplatin in patients with more advanced disease demonstrated better results for the paclitaxel-cisplatin combination (response rate 77 versus 64 percent, complete remission rate 54 versus 33 percent, median survival 37.5 versus 24.4 months). This regimen of paclitaxel, 135 mg/m^2 body surface area over 24 h by infusion, followed by cisplatin, 75 mg/m^2, is now the standard therapy for advanced disease. Current trials are exploring the potential for reduction of cisplatin toxicity with substitution of carboplatin dosed to an AUC (area under the curve) of 7.5. The efficacy of this substitution and the appropriateness of alterations in the duration of paclitaxel infusion time have not been established through large randomized trials.

Patients with advanced disease (stages III and IV) and bulky residual tumor are generally treated with a paclitaxel-platinum combination regimen as well and, while the overall prognosis is poorer, 5-year survival may reach 10 to 15 percent. In some instances, cytoreductive surgery can be performed after initial response to chemotherapy, and a multicenter European trial demonstrated that this strategy led to a significant improvement in progression-free interval and survival.

Historically, patients who have had an excellent initial response to chemotherapy and have no clinical evidence of disease have had a second-look laparotomy. For patients with stage I ovarian cancer or for germ cell tumors, the operation rarely detects residual tumor and has been largely abandoned. For those with stages II and III epithelial tumors, the procedure can be appropriate in the context of a clinical trial or if unique therapy for minimal-residual disease is contemplated. However, there is no evidence that the second-look

Table 99-1

Staging and Survival in Gynecologic Malignancies

Stage	Ovarian	5-Year Survival, %	Endometrial	5-Year Survival, %	Cervix	5-Year Survival, %
0	—		—		Carcinoma in situ	100
I	Confined to ovary	90	Confined to corpus	89	Confined to uterus	85
II	Confined to pelvis	70	Involves corpus and cervix	80	Invades beyond uterus but not to pelvic wall	60
III	Intraabdominal spread	15–20	Extends outside the uterus but not outside the true pelvis	30	Extends to pelvic wall and/or lower third of vagina, or hydronephrosis	33
IV	Spread outside abdomen	1–5	Extends outside the true pelvis or involves the bladder or rectum	9	Invades mucosa of bladder or rectum or extends beyond the true pelvis	7

surgical procedure itself prolongs overall survival. The routine use of second-look laparotomy cannot be recommended. There is also no evidence that any form of maintenance therapy is beneficial in preventing recurrences in patients in complete remission.

Patients with advanced disease whose disease recurs after initial treatment are usually not curable but may benefit significantly from limited surgery to relieve intestinal obstruction, localized radiation therapy to relieve pressure or pain from mass lesions or metastasis, or palliative chemotherapy. The selection of chemotherapy for palliation depends upon the initial regimen used for treatment and evidence of drug resistance. Often patients who have a complete regression of disease that lasts 6 months or more respond to reinduction with the same agents. Patients relapsing within the first 6 months of initial therapy rarely do. Chemotherapeutic agents with ~20 percent activity in patients relapsing after initial combination chemotherapy include carboplatin, ifosfamide, hexamethylmelamine, and etoposide, and intraperitoneal chemotherapy may be used if a small residual volume (<1 cm^3) of tumor exists. Progestational agents and antiestrogens produce responses in 5 to 15 percent of patients and have minimal side effects. Experimental approaches with some promise include the agents gemcitabine and topotecan and high-dose chemotherapy with hematopoietic stem cell support.

OVARIAN GERM CELL TUMORS Fewer than 5 percent of all ovarian tumors are germ cell in origin. They include teratomas, dysgerminoma, endodermal sinus tumor, and embryonal carcinoma. Germ cell tumors of the ovary generally occur in younger women (75 percent of ovarian malignancies in women under 30), display an unusually aggressive natural history, were often fatal before the combination chemotherapy era, and now are commonly cured with less extensive nonsterilizing surgery and chemotherapy. There are now many reports of normal children born to women cured of these malignancies.

These neoplasms can be divided into three major groups: (1) benign tumors (usually dermoid cysts); (2) malignant tumors that arise from dermoid cysts; and (3) primitive malignant germ cell tumors including dysgerminoma, yolk sac tumors, immature teratomas, embryonal carcinomas, and choriocarcinoma.

Dermoid cysts are teratomatous cysts usually lined by epidermis and skin appendages. They often contain hair and calcified bone or teeth can sometimes be seen on conventional pelvic x-ray. They are almost always curable by surgical resection. Approximately 1 percent of these tumors have malignant elements, usually squamous cell carcinoma.

Malignant germ cell tumors are usually large (median—16 cm). Bilateral disease is rare except in dysgerminoma (10 to 15 percent bilaterality). Abdominal or pelvic pain in young women are the usual presenting symptoms. Serum human chorionic gonadoptropin (hCG) and alpha fetoprotein (αFP) levels are useful in the diagnosis and management of these patients. Before the advent of chemotherapy, extensive surgery was routine but has now been replaced by careful evaluation of extent of spread followed by resection of bulky disease and preservation of one ovary, uterus, and cervix if feasible. This allows many affected women to preserve fertility. After surgical staging 60 to 75 percent of women have stage I disease and 25 to 30 percent have stage III disease. Stages II and IV are infrequent.

Most of the malignant germ cell tumors are managed with chemotherapy after surgery. VAC (vincristine, actinomycin-D, cyclophosphamide) produces 70 to 90 percent cures in stage I disease but fewer than 50 percent for stage III disease. Regimens used in testicular cancer like PVB (cisplatin, vinblastine, bleomycin) and BEP (bleomycin 30 units IV weekly, etoposide 100 mg/m^2 days 1 to 5, and cisplatin 20 mg/m^2 days 1 to 5) with three or four courses given at 21-day intervals have produced excellent results. Postoperative chemotherapy with BEP in 93 patients (stages I to III) has achieved a 95 percent long-term survival (median follow-up >38 months). This regimen is the treatment of choice for all malignant germ cell tumors except grade I, stage I immature teratoma, where surgery alone is adequate, and per-

haps early stage dysgerminoma, where surgery and radiation therapy are used.

Dysgerminoma is the ovarian counterpart of testicular seminoma. The tumor has commonly been treated with radiation therapy and is very radiosensitive. Results in early disease are excellent (5-year disease-free survival—100 percent) but less so in stage III disease (5-year disease-free survival—61 percent). Unfortunately, the use of radiation therapy makes many patients infertile. BEP chemotherapy is equally or more effective and does not cause infertility. In incompletely resected patients with dysgerminoma, the 2-year disease-free survival was 95 percent and infertility was not observed. These data have led most physicians to replace postoperative radiation therapy with combination chemotherapy (BEP) in women with ovarian dysgerminoma.

OVARIAN STROMAL TUMORS Stromal tumors make up fewer than 10 percent of ovarian tumors. They are named for the stromal tissue involved: granulosa, theca, Sertoli, Leydig, and collagen-producing stromal cells. The granulosa and theca cell stromal cell tumors occur most frequently in the first three decades of life. Granulosa cell tumors frequently produce estrogen and cause menstrual abnormalities, bleeding, and precocious puberty. Endometrial carcinoma can be seen in 5 percent of these women, perhaps related to the persistent hyperestrogenism. Sertoli and Leydig cell tumors, when functional, produce androgens with resultant virilization or hirsutism. Seventy-five percent of these stromal cell tumors present in stage I and can be cured with total abdominal hysterectomy and bilateral salpingo-oophorectomy. Stromal tumors generally grow slowly, and recurrences can occur 5 to 10 years after initial surgery. Neither radiation therapy nor chemotherapy have been documented to be consistently effective, and surgical management remains the primary treatment.

CARCINOMA OF THE FALLOPIAN TUBE

The fallopian tube is the least common site of cancer in the female genital tract although its epithelial surface far exceeds that of the ovary, where epithelial cancer is 20 times more common. There are approximately 300 new cases yearly; 90 percent are papillary serous adenocarcinomas, with the remainder being mixed mesodermal, endometroid, and transitional cell tumors. The gross and microscopic characteristics and the spread of the tumor are similar to those of ovarian cancer but can be distinguished if the tumor arises from the endosalpinx, the tubal epithelium shows a transition between benign and malignant, and the ovaries and endometrium are normal or minimally involved. The differential diagnosis includes primary or metastatic ovarian cancer, chronic salpingitis, tuberculous salpingitis, salpingitis isthmica nodosa, and cautery artifact.

Unlike ovarian cancer, patients frequently present with early symptoms, usually postmenopausal vaginal bleeding, pain, and leukorrhea. Surgical staging is similar to that used for ovarian cancer, and prognosis is related to stage and extent of residual disease. Patients with stages I and II disease are generally treated with surgery alone or with surgery and pelvic radiation therapy, although there is no clear evidence for improved 5-year survival with irradiation (5-year survival stage I—74 versus 75 percent, stage II—43 versus 48 percent). Patients with stages III and IV disease are treated with the same chemotherapy regimens used in advanced ovarian carcinoma, and 5-year survival is similar (stage III—20 percent, stage IV—5 percent).

UTERINE CANCER

Carcinoma of the endometrium is the most common female pelvic malignancy. Approximately 34,000 new cases are diagnosed yearly, although in most (75 percent) tumor is confined to the uterine corpus at diagnosis and therefore most can be cured. The 6000 deaths yearly make uterine cancer only the seventh leading cause of death from malignancy in females. It is primarily a disease of postmenopausal women, although 25 percent of cases occur in women below age 50 and 5 percent below age 40. The disease is common in Eastern Europe and the United States and uncommon in Asia.

Phenotypic characteristics and risk factors common in patients with endometrial cancer include obesity, altered menstruation, low fertility index, late menopause, anovulation, and postmenopausal bleeding. Many of these features suggest that exposure to unopposed estrogen from either endogenous or exogenous sources may play a central etiologic role. Women taking tamoxifen for breast cancer treatment or prevention are also at somewhat increased risk.

Endometrial carcinoma occurs most often in the sixth and seventh decades of life. Symptoms often include abnormal vaginal discharge (90 percent), abnormal bleeding (80 percent), which is usually postmenopausal, and leukorrhea (10 percent). Initial evaluation of patients suspected of endometrial cancer should include a history and physical and pelvic examination followed by an endometrial biopsy or a fractional dilation and curettage. Outpatient procedures such as endometrial biopsy or aspiration curettage can be used but are definitive only when positive.

Between 75 and 80 percent of all endometrial carcinomas are adenocarcinomas, and the prognosis depends upon stage, histologic grade, and extent of myometrial invasion. Grade I tumors are highly differentiated adenocarcinomas, grade II contain some solid areas, and grade III tumors are largely solid or undifferentiated. Adenocarcinoma with squamous differentiation is seen in 10 percent of patients; the most differentiated form is known as *adenoacanthoma*, and the poorly differentiated form is called *adenosquamous carcinoma*. Other less common pathologies include mucinous carcinoma (5 percent) and papillary serous carcinoma (<10 percent). This latter type has a natural history indistinguishable from ovarian carcinoma. Rarer histologies include secretory (2 percent), ciliated, clear cell, and undifferentiated carcinomas.

The staging of endometrial cancer requires surgery to establish the extent of disease and the depth of myometrial invasion. Peritoneal fluid should be sampled; the abdomen and pelvis explored; and pelvic and para-aortic lymphadenectomy performed depending upon the histology, grade, and depth of invasion in the uterine specimen on frozen section. After evaluation and staging, 74 percent of patients are stage I, 13 percent are stage II, 9 percent are stage III, and 3 percent are found to be stage IV. Five-year survival by stage is as follows: stage I—89 percent, stage II—80 percent, stage III—30 percent, and stage IV—9 percent (see Table 99-1).

Patients with uncomplicated endometrial carcinoma are effectively managed with total abdominal hysterectomy and bilateral salpingo-oophorectomy. Pre- or postoperative irradiation has been used, and although vaginal cuff recurrence is reduced, survival is not altered. In women with poor histologic grade, deep myometrial invasion, or extensive involvement of the lower uterine segment or cervix, intracavitary or external beam irradiation is warranted.

About 15 percent of women have endometrial carcinoma with extension to the cervix only (stage II), and management depends upon the extent of cervical invasion. Superficial cervical invasion can be managed like stage I disease, but extensive cervical invasion requires radical hysterectomy or preoperative radiotherapy followed by extrafascial hysterectomy. Once disease is outside the uterus but still confined to the true pelvis (stage III), management generally includes surgery and irradiation. Patients who have involvement only of the ovary or fallopian tubes generally do well with such therapy, and 5-year survivals of 80 percent have been reported. Other stage III patients with disease extending beyond the adnexa or those with serous carcinomas of the endometrium have a significantly poorer prognosis (5-year survival of 15 percent).

Patients with stage IV disease (outside the abdomen or invading the bladder or rectum) are generally treated symptomatically with irradiation, surgery, and/or progestational agents. Progestational agents are the most commonly used systemic treatment and produce responses in about 25 percent of patients. Well-differentiated tumors respond most frequently, and responses can be correlated with the level of progesterone-receptor expression in the tumor. The commonly used progestational agents hydroxyprogesterone (Dilalutin), megastrol (Megace), and deoxyprogesterone (Provera) all produce similar response rates, and the antiestrogen tamoxifen (Nolvadex) produces responses in 10 to 25 percent of patients in a salvage setting.

Chemotherapy is not very successful in advanced endometrial carcinoma. The most active single agents with consistent response rates of 20 percent or more include cisplatin, carboplatin, doxorubicin, epirubicin, and paclitaxel. Combinations of drugs with or without progestational agents have generally produced response rates similar to single agents.

CERVIX CANCER

Carcinoma of the cervix was once the most common cause of cancer death in women, but over the past 30 years, the mortality rate has decreased by 50 percent. Now, cervix cancer trails breast, lung, colorectal, endometrium, and ovarian cancers in incidence. In 1996, there were approximately 15,700 new cases of invasive cervix cancer, and more than 50,000 cases of carcinoma in situ. There were 4,900 deaths from the disease, and of those patients, approximately 85 percent had never had a Pap smear at any time in their lives. The disease remains the major gynecologic cancer in underdeveloped countries. It is more common in lower socioeconomic groups, women with early initial sexual activity, multiple sexual partners, and in smokers. Many of these factors suggest a venereal transmission. It appears that human papilloma virus (HPV) has an important etiologic role. Over 66 types of human papilloma viruses have been isolated, and many are associated with genital warts. Those types associated with cervical carcinoma are 16, 18, 31, 45, and 51 to 53. These, along with many other types, are also associated with cervical intraepithelial neoplasia (CIN). Of particular interest, the protein product of HPV-16, the E7 protein, binds and inactivates the tumor suppressor gene Rb, and the E6 protein of HPV-18 has sequence homology to the SV40 large T antigen and has the capacity to bind and inactivate the tumor suppressor gene p53. E6 and E7 are both necessary and sufficient to cause cell transformation in vitro. These binding and inactivation events may explain the carcinogenic effects of the viruses (see Chap. 190).

Uncomplicated HPV lower genital tract infection and condylomatous atypia of the cervix can progress to CIN. This lesion precedes invasive cervical carcinoma and is classified as low-grade squamous intraepithelial lesion (SIL), high-grade SIL, and carcinoma in situ. Carcinoma in situ demonstrates cytologic evidence of neoplasia without invasion through the basement membrane, can persist unchanged for 10 to 20 years, but eventually progresses to invasive carcinoma.

The Papanicolaou smear is 90 to 95 percent accurate in detecting early lesions such as CIN but is less sensitive in detecting cancer when frankly invasive cancer or fungating masses are present. Inflammation, necrosis, and hemorrhage may produce false-positive smears, and colposcopic-directed biopsy is required when any lesion is visible on the cervix, regardless of Pap smear findings. The American Cancer Society recommends that women after onset of sexual activity, or over age 20, have two consecutive yearly smears. If negative, smears should be repeated every 3 years. The American College of Obstetrics and Gynecology recommends yearly Pap smears with routine annual pelvic and breast examinations. Women with suspicious or abnormal Pap smears should have colposcopic-directed cervical biopsy. Colposcopy is a technique using a binocular microscope and 3% acetic acid applied to the cervix in which abnormal areas appear white and can be directly biopsied. This procedure has reduced the need for cone biopsy, which is still required when endocervical tumor is suspected, colposcopy is inadequate, the diagnosis of microinvasive carcinoma is made on biopsy, or when there is a discrepancy between the Pap smear and the colposcopic findings. Cone biopsy alone is therapeutic for CIN in many patients, although a less radical electrocautery excision may be sufficient.

Approximately 80 percent of invasive cervix carcinomas are squamous cell tumors; 10 to 15 percent are adenocarcinomas; 2 to 5 percent are adenosquamous with epithelial and glandular structures; and 1 to 2 percent are clear cell mesonephric tumors.

Patients with cervix cancer generally present with abnormal bleeding or postcoital spotting that may increase to intermenstrual or prominent menstrual bleeding. Yellowish vaginal discharge, lumbosacral back pain, and urinary symptoms can also be seen.

The staging of cervical carcinoma is clinical and generally completed with a pelvic examination under anesthesia with cystoscopy and proctoscopy. Chest x-rays, intravenous pyelograms, and computed tomography are generally required, and magnetic resonance imaging (MRI) may be used to assess extracervical extension. Stage 0 is carcinoma in situ; stage I is disease confined to the cervix; stage II disease invades beyond the cervix but not to the pelvic wall or lower third of the vagina; stage III disease extends to the pelvic wall or lower third of the vagina or causes hydronephrosis; stage IV is present when the tumor invades the mucosa of bladder or rectum or extends beyond the true pelvis. Five-year survivals are as follows: stage I—85 percent, stage II—60 percent, stage III—33 percent, and stage IV—7 percent (see Table 99-1).

Carcinoma in situ (stage 0) can generally be successfully managed by cone biopsy or by abdominal hysterectomy. For stage I disease, results appear equivalent for either radical hysterectomy or radiation therapy. Patients with stages II to IV disease are primarily managed with radical radiation therapy. Retroperitoneal lymphadenectomy is being investigated in clinical trials, but its benefit is unproven. Pelvic exenterations, although uncommon, are performed for centrally recurrent or persistent disease. Significant advances have been made in the reconstruction of the vagina, bladder, and rectum following this operation.

The majority of patients can be managed with either surgery, radiation therapy, or combinations of the two. Chemotherapy has been investigated in patients with unresectable advanced disease, recurrent disease, and as a radiation sensitizer. Active agents with ≥20 percent response rates include cisplatin, 5-fluorouracil (5-FU), hexamethylmelamine, and vincristine. Combination chemotherapy has been studied actively, but no combination has been proved better than single agents. Intraarterial chemotherapy has been studied, either pre- or postoperatively, but is associated with substantial local toxicity and response rates of approximately 20 percent. Recent interest has centered on the use of chemotherapy as a radiosensitizer. Active agents include hydroxyurea, 5-FU, and cisplatin. Although definitive randomized trials have not been completed, concomitant chemoradiation is feasible, and response and survival rates appear to be better than in similar groups treated with radiation alone.

GESTATIONAL TROPHOBLASTIC NEOPLASIA

While gestational choriocarcinoma accounts for fewer than 1 percent of female gynecologic malignancies, it is important because it is cured with appropriate chemotherapy and represents one of the triumphs of modern cancer management. Before the use of chemotherapy, fewer than 10 percent of patients survived, but now with appropriate management, deaths from this disease have become rare in the United States. The spectrum of disease ranges from benign hydatidiform mole to trophoblastic malignancy (placental-site trophoblastic tumor and choriocarcinoma).

Epidemiology In the United States, the incidence is about 1 per 1000 pregnancies; in Asia, 2 per 1000 pregnancies. Maternal age greater than 45 years is a risk factor for hydatidiform mole. A prior history of molar pregnancy is also a risk factor. Choriocarcinoma occurs approximately once in 25,000 pregnancies or once in 20,000 live births. Prior history of hydatidiform mole is a risk factor for choriocarcinoma. A woman with a molar pregnancy is 1000 times more likely to develop choriocarcinoma than a woman with a prior normal-term pregnancy.

Pathology and Etiology The trophoblastic neoplasms have been divided by morphology into complete or partial hydatidiform mole, invasive mole, placental-site trophoblastomas, and choriocarcinomas. Hydatidiform moles contain clusters of villi with hydropic changes, hyperplasia of the trophoblast, and the absence of fetal vessels. Invasive moles differ only by invasion into the uterine myometrium. Placental-site trophoblastic tumors are predominately made up of cytotrophoblast

cells arising from the placental implantation site. Choriocarcinomas consist of anaplastic trophoblastic tissue with both cytotrophoblastic and syncytiotrophoblastic elements and no identifiable villi.

Complete moles result from uniparental disomy in which loss of the maternal genes (23 autosomes plus X) occurs by unknown mechanisms and is followed by duplication of the paternal haploid genome (23 autosomes plus X). Uncommonly (5 percent), moles result from dispermic fertilization of an empty egg, resulting in either 46XY or 46XX genotype. Partial moles result from dispermic fertilization of an egg with retention of the maternal haploid set of chromosomes, resulting in diandric triploidy (see Chap. 65).

Clinical Presentation Molar pregnancies are generally associated with first-trimester bleeding, ectopic pregnancies, or threatened abortions. The uterus is inappropriately large for the length of gestation, and hCG levels are higher than expected. Fetal parts and heart sounds are not present. The diagnosis is generally made by the passage of grapelike clusters from the uterus, but ultrasound demonstration of the hydropic mole can be diagnostic. Patients suspected of a molar pregnancy require a chest film, careful pelvic examinations, and weekly serial monitoring of hCG levels.

℞ TREATMENT

Patients with hydatidiform moles require surgical evacuation coupled with postevacuation monitoring of hCG levels. In most women (80 percent), the hCG titer progressively declines within 8 to 10 days of evacuation (serum half-life is 24 to 36 h). Patients should be monitored on a monthly basis and should not become pregnant for at least a year. Patients found to have invasive mole at curettage are generally treated with hysterectomy and chemotherapy. Approximately half of patients with choriocarcinoma develop the malignancy after a molar pregnancy, and the other half develop the malignancy after abortion, ectopic pregnancy, or occasionally after a normal full-term pregnancy.

Chemotherapy is generally used for gestational trophoblastic neoplasia and is often used in hydatidiform mole if hCG levels rise or plateau or if metastases develop. Patients with invasive mole or choriocarcinoma require chemotherapy. Several regimens are effective, including methotrexate at 30 mg/m^2 intramuscularly on a weekly basis until hCG titers are normal. However, methotrexate (1 mg/kg) given every other day for 4 days followed by leukovorin (0.1 mg/kg) given intravenously 24 h after methotrexate is associated with a cure rate of ≥90 percent and low toxicity. Intermittent courses are generally continued until the hCG titer becomes undetectable for 3 consecutive weeks, and then patients are monitored monthly for a year.

Patients with high-risk tumors (high hCG levels, disease presenting ≥4 months after antecedent pregnancy, brain or liver metastasis, or failure of single-agent methotrexate) are initially treated with combination chemotherapy. MAC chemotherapy with methotrexate, actinomycin-D, and cyclophosphamide has been the most commonly used regimen, with cycles of therapy given every 3 weeks until complete remission. Other effective regimens include EMA-CO (a cyclic noncross-resistant combination of etoposide, methotrexate, and dactinomycin alternating with cyclophosphamide and vincristine); cisplatin, bleomycin, and vinblastine; and cisplatin, etoposide, and bleomycin. EMA-CO is now the regimen of choice for patients with high-risk disease because of excellent survival rates (>80 percent) and less toxicity than MAC. Patients with brain or liver metastasis are usually treated with local irradiation to metastatic sites in conjunction with chemotherapy. Long-term studies of patients cured of trophoblastic disease have not demonstrated an increased risk of maternal complications or fetal abnormalities with subsequent pregnancies.

BIBLIOGRAPHY

BARAKAT RR et al: Corpus epithelial tumors, in *Principles and Practice of Gynecologic Oncology*, 2d ed, WJ Hoskins et al (eds). Philadelphia, Lippincott, 1996, pp 859–896

BOLIS G et al: EMA/CO regimen in high-risk gestational trophoblastic tumor (GTT). Gynecol Oncol 31:439, 1988

CRESSMAN WT, DISAIA PJ: Screening in ovarian cancer. Am J Obstet Gynecol 165:7, 1991

GOLDSTEIN DP: Gestational trophoblastic neoplasia in the 1990's. Yale J Biol Med 64:639, 1991

HACKER NF: Uterine cancer, in *Practical Gynecologic Oncology*, 2d ed, JS Berek, NF Hacker (eds). Baltimore, Williams & Wilkins, 1994, pp 285–326.

MCGUIRE WP et al: Cyclophosphamide and cisplatin compared with paclitaxel and cisplatin in patients with stage III and stage IV ovarian cancer. N Engl J Med 334:1, 1996

OZOLS RF et al: Epithelial ovarian cancer, in *Principles and Practice of Gynecologic Oncology*, 2d ed, WJ Hoskins et al (eds). Philadelphia, Lippincott, 1996, pp 919–986

SOPER VT: Identification and management of high-risk gestational trophoblastic disease. Semin Oncol 22:172, 1995

STEHMAN FB et al: Uterine cervix, in *Principles and Practice of Gynecologic Oncology*, 2d ed, WJ Hoskins et al (eds). Philadelphia, Lippincott, 1996, pp 785–857

VANDERBURG ME et al: Intervention debulking surgery does improve survival in advanced epithelial ovarian cancer. N Engl J Med 332:629, 1995

WILLIAMS S et al: Adjuvant therapy of ovarian germ cell tumors with cisplatin, etoposide and bleomycin: A trial of the Gynecologic Oncology Group. J Clin Oncol 12:701, 1994

YOUNG RC et al: Adjuvant therapy in stage I and stage II epithelial ovarian cancer. Results of two prospective trials. N Engl J Med 327:1021, 1990

100 Shreyaskumar R. Patel, Robert S. Benjamin

SARCOMAS OF SOFT TISSUE AND BONE

Sarcomas are rare mesenchymal neoplasms that arise in bone and soft tissues. They constitute less than 1 percent of all malignancies. Most of these tumors are mesodermal in origin, although a few are derived from neuroectoderm, and they are biologically distinct from the more common epithelial malignancies. Sarcomas affect all age groups; 15 percent are found in children younger than age 15, and 40 percent occur after age 55. Sarcomas are one of the most common solid tumors of childhood and are the fifth most common cause of cancer deaths in children. Sarcomas may be divided into two groups, those derived from bone and those derived from soft tissues.

SOFT TISSUE SARCOMAS

Soft tissues include muscles, tendons, fat, fibrous tissue, synovial tissue, vessels, and nerves. Approximately 60 percent of soft-tissue sarcomas arise in the extremities, with the lower extremities involved three times as often as the upper extremities. Thirty percent arise in the trunk, the retroperitoneum accounting for 40 percent of all trunk lesions. The remaining 10 percent arise in the head and neck.

INCIDENCE Approximately 6400 new cases of soft tissue sarcomas occurred in the United States in 1996. The annual age-adjusted incidence is approximately 2 per 100,000 population, but the incidence varies with age and with the types of neoplasms included in the definition. Soft tissue sarcomas constitute 0.7 percent of all cancers in the general population and 6.5 percent of all malignancies in children.

EPIDEMIOLOGY Malignant transformation of a benign soft tissue tumor is extremely rare, with the exception that malignant peripheral nerve sheath tumors (neurofibrosarcoma, malignant schwannoma) can arise from neurofibromas in patients with neurofibromatosis. Several etiologic factors have been implicated in the pathogenesis of soft tissue sarcomas.

Environmental Factors Trauma or previous injury is rarely involved, but sarcomas can arise in scar tissue resulting from a prior operation, burn, fracture, or foreign body implantation. Chemical carcinogens such as polycyclic hydrocarbons, asbestos, and dioxin may be involved in the pathogenesis.

Iatrogenic Factors Sarcomas in bone or soft tissues occur in cancer patients who are treated with radiation and survive at least 5 years. The tumor nearly always arises in the irradiated field. The risk increases with time.

Viruses The association of Kaposi's sarcoma (KS) with human immunodeficiency virus (HIV) type 1 has led to studies of the role of viruses in the pathogenesis of KS. Herpesvirus-like DNA sequences have been documented in AIDS-associated KS, classic KS, and KS in HIV-negative homosexual men, leading to the hypothesis that this new herpes virus [human herpes virus (HHV8)] may be the common etiologic factor for all three variants of KS.

Immunologic Factors Congenital or acquired immunodeficiency, including therapeutic immunosuppression, is associated with or influences sarcoma development.

Genetic Factors Li-Fraumeni syndrome is a familial cancer syndrome in which affected individuals have germ-line abnormalities of the tumor suppressor gene *p53* and an increased incidence of soft tissue sarcomas and other malignancies, including breast cancer, osteosarcoma, brain tumors, leukemia, and adrenal carcinoma (Chap. 84). Neurofibromatosis 1 (NF-1, peripheral form, von Recklinghausen's disease) is characterized by multiple neurofibromas and café au lait spots. Neurofibromas occasionally undergo malignant degeneration to become malignant peripheral nerve sheath tumors. The gene for NF-1 is located in the pericentromeric region of chromosome 17 and encodes neurofibromin, a tumor suppressor protein with GTPase-activating activity that inhibits Ras function (Chap. 375). Germ-line mutation of the *Rb-1* locus (chromosome 13q14) in patients with inherited retinoblastoma is associated with the development of osteosarcoma in those who survive the retinoblastoma and of soft tissue sarcomas unrelated to radiation therapy. Other soft tissue tumors, including desmoid tumors, lipomas, leiomyomas, neuroblastomas, and paragangliomas, occasionally show a familial predisposition.

Insulin-like growth factor (IGF) type 2 is produced by some sarcomas and is thought to act both as an autocrine growth factor and as a motility factor that promotes metastatic spread. Antibodies to IGF-1 receptors block the stimulation of growth by IGF-2 in vitro but do not affect IGF-2–induced motility. If secreted in large amounts, IGF-2 may produce hypoglycemia (see Chaps. 102 and 335).

CLASSIFICATION Approximately 20 different types of sarcomas are recognized on the basis of the pattern of differentiation toward normal tissue. For example, rhabdomyosarcoma shows evidence of skeletal muscle fibers with cross-striations; leiomyosarcomas contain interlacing fascicles of spindle cells representing smooth muscle features; liposarcomas contain adipocytes; and angiosarcomas contain a rich network of blood vessels. When precise characterization of the type is not possible, the tumors are called *unclassified sarcomas*. All of the primary bone sarcomas also can arise from soft tissues (e.g., extraskeletal osteosarcoma, extraskeletal Ewing's sarcoma, and extraskeletal chondrosarcoma). The entity *malignant fibrous histiocytoma* includes a large number of tumors previously classified as fibrosarcomas or as pleiomorphic variants of other sarcomas and is characterized by a mixture of spindle (fibrous) cells and round (histiocytic) cells arranged in a storiform pattern with frequent giant cells and areas of pleiomorphism.

For purposes of treatment, most soft tissue sarcomas can be lumped together, with the choice of treatment depending mainly on the stage of disease. However, some aspects of the natural history require that specific histologic diagnoses be considered in planning treatment and follow-up. For example, the term *liposarcoma* indicates histogenesis from adipose tissue but gives no indication of biologic behavior. Pleiomorphic liposarcomas and dedifferentiated liposarcomas behave like other high-grade sarcomas; in contrast, well-differentiated liposarcomas (better termed *atypical lipomatous tumors*) lack metastatic potential, and myxoid liposarcomas metastasize infrequently but, when they do, have a predilection for unusual metastatic sites containing fat, such as the retroperitoneum, mediastinum, and subcutaneous tissue. Rhabdomyosarcomas, Ewing's sarcoma, and other small cell sarcomas tend to be more aggressive, even when small, and are more responsive to chemotherapeutic agents than the more typical soft tissue sarcomas.

DIAGNOSIS The most common presentation is an asymptomatic mass. Mechanical symptoms referable to pressure, traction, or entrapment of nerves or muscles may be present, especially with large tumors. All new and persistent or growing masses should be biopsied, either by a cutting needle (core-needle biopsy) or preferably by a small incision, placed so that it can be encompassed in the subsequent excision without compromising a definitive resection. Sarcomas tend to metastasize through the blood rather than the lymphatic system. Consequently, the incidence of lymph node metastases is low (5 percent) for most of these tumors, although it is higher (17 percent) for certain tumors—e.g., synovial and epithelioid sarcomas, clear-cell sarcoma (melanoma of the soft parts), angiosarcoma, and rhabdomyosarcoma. The pulmonary parenchyma is the most common site of metastases in the vast majority of sarcomas. Exceptions are leiomyosarcomas arising in the gastrointestinal tract, which metastasize to the liver; myxoid liposarcomas, which seek fatty tissue: and clear-cell sarcomas, which may metastasize to bones. Central nervous system metastases are rare, except in the case of alveolar soft tissue sarcoma.

Radiographic Evaluation   Imaging of the primary tumor is best accomplished by plain radiographs and magnetic resonance imaging (MRI) for tumors of the extremities or head and neck and by computed tomography (CT) for tumors of the chest, abdomen, or retroperitoneal cavity. A radiograph and CT scan of the chest are important for the detection of lung metastases. Other imaging studies may be indicated, depending on the symptoms, signs, or histology.

STAGING SYSTEMS   The histologic grade and size of the primary tumor are the most important prognostic factors. Tumors are staged according to two systems, the American Joint Commission on Cancer (AJCC) staging system and the Musculoskeletal Tumor Society staging system.

AJCC Staging System   The primary determinant of stage is *tumor histologic grade*. Grade 1 (well-differentiated) tumors are stage I; grade 2 (moderately well differentiated) tumors are stage II; and grade 3 (poorly differentiated) tumors are stage III. These stage designations are qualified further on the basis of tumor size as either A (tumor diameter <5 cm) or B (tumor diameter ≥5 cm). Tumors with lymph node metastases are stage IVA, and those with distant metastases are stage IVB.

Musculoskeletal Tumor Society Staging System   This system is based on grade and compartmental localization. A Roman numeral reflects the tumor grade: stage I is low-grade, stage II is high-grade, and stage III includes tumors of any grade that have lymph node or distant metastases. In addition, the tumor is given a letter reflecting its compartmental localization. Tumors designated A are intracompartmental (i.e., confined to the same soft tissue compartment as the initial tumor), and tumors designated B are extracompartmental (i.e. extending into the adjacent soft tissue compartment or into bone). Thus, a stage IA tumor is a low-grade tumor confined to its compartment of origin, whereas a stage IB tumor is a low-grade tumor that extends outside its original compartment.

PROGNOSIS   Prognosis is related to the stage, with 5-year survival rates averaging 75 percent for AJCC stage I, 55 percent for stage II, and 29 percent for stage III. The 5-year survival rate for stage IV disease is <20 percent, but a small number of patients in this category can be cured. Most patients with stage IV disease die within 6–12 months, but there is great variability in survival, and patients may live with slowly progressive disease for many years.

℞ **TREATMENT**

Surgery   Soft tissue sarcomas tend to grow along fascial planes in the path of least resistance. As a result, the surrounding soft tissues are compressed to form a pseudocapsule that gives the sarcoma the appearance of a well-encapsulated lesion. This is invariably deceptive, because "shelling out" or marginal excision of such lesions results in a 50 to 90 percent probability of local recurrence. Radical excision with a negative margin, incorporating the biopsy site, is the standard surgical procedure for local disease. The adjuvant use of radiation therapy and/or chemotherapy improves the local control rate and per-

mits the use of limb-sparing surgery with a local control rate comparable to that achieved by radical excisions and amputations. The National Institutes of Health consensus conference in 1984 recommended limb-sparing surgery in conjunction with adjuvant irradiation and/or chemotherapy as effective therapy for local control except when negative margins are not obtainable, when the risks of radiation are prohibitive, or when neurovascular structures are involved so that resection will result in serious functional consequences to the limb. When appropriately performed, conservative limb-sparing procedures result in local failure rates of only 10 to 15 percent.

Radiation Therapy   External beam radiation therapy is an adjuvant to limb-sparing surgery for improved local control. Preoperative administration of radiation therapy allows the use of smaller fields and smaller doses but results in a higher rate of wound complications. When radiation therapy is given postoperatively, the field of radiation must be larger, as the entire surgical bed must be encompassed, and the dose must be higher to compensate for hypoxia in the operated field. Brachytherapy or interstitial therapy, in which the radiation source is inserted into the tumor bed, is thought to be comparable in efficacy and also less time consuming and less expensive. Intraoperative irradiation has not been studied thoroughly.

Adjuvant Chemotherapy   The role of adjuvant chemotherapy is controversial except for Ewing's sarcoma and rhabdomyosarcoma, where it is standard. Doxorubicin-based combination chemotherapy improves disease-free survival but has less effect on overall survival. Nevertheless, meta-analysis indicates that there is a significant decrease in the risk of disease recurrence (either local or distant) and death for patients with high-grade extremity sarcomas who are treated with adjuvant chemotherapy. This approach is considered reasonable for high-risk primary tumors. An alternative approach is to treat such patients preoperatively with chemotherapy; the subset of patients who respond continue adjuvant therapy postoperatively, and the nonresponders can be spared the toxicity of systemic therapy to which they are unlikely to respond. Neither strategy has been proved superior.

Advanced Disease   Metastatic soft tissue sarcomas are largely incurable, but up to 20 percent of patients who are rendered free of clinical evidence of disease become long-term survivors. The therapeutic intent, therefore, is to produce a complete remission with chemotherapy and/or surgery. Surgical resection of metastases, whenever possible, is an integral part of the management. Some patients benefit from repeated surgical excision of metastases. Despite their histologic heterogeneity, the sensitivity to chemotherapy of most soft tissue sarcomas is poor. The two most active chemotherapeutic agents are doxorubicin and ifosfamide, an analogue of cyclophosphamide. There is a steep dose-response relationship for these drugs in sarcomas. Dacarbazine (DTIC) has modest activity as a single agent but has better activity in combination with doxorubicin. Vincristine, etoposide, and dactinomycin are effective in Ewing's sarcoma and rhabdomyosarcoma, especially in children. Chondrosarcomas and leiomyosarcomas arising from the gastrointestinal tract are unresponsive to standard chemotherapeutic drugs.

Dose-intensive regimens (i.e., ones involving higher and more frequent doses) of doxorubicin and ifosfamide-based combinations, with growth factor support to ameliorate myelosuppression, may improve the rates of complete and partial response. Myeloablative doses of chemotherapy in combination with bone marrow transplantation have not been successful.

BONE SARCOMAS

INCIDENCE AND EPIDEMIOLOGY   Bone sarcomas are rarer than soft tissue sarcomas; they accounted for only 0.2 percent of all new malignancies and approximately 2500 new cases in the United States in 1996. Several benign bone lesions have the potential for malignant transformation. Enchondromas and osteochondromas can transform into chondrosarcoma; and fibrous dysplasia, bone infarcts, and Paget's disease of bone can transform into either malignant fibrous histiocytoma or osteosarcoma.

CLASSIFICATION **Benign Tumors** The common benign bone tumors include enchondroma, osteochondroma, chondroblastoma, and chondromyxoid fibroma, all of cartilaginous origin; osteoid osteoma and osteoblastoma, of bone origin; fibroma and desmoplastic fibroma, of fibrous tissue origin; hemangioma, of vascular origin; and giant cell tumor, of unknown origin.

Malignant Tumors The most common malignant tumors of bone are plasma cell tumors (see Chap. 114). The four most common malignant tumors of nonhematopoietic origin are osteosarcoma, chondrosarcoma, Ewing's sarcoma, and malignant fibrous histiocytoma. Rare malignant tumors include chordoma (of notochordal origin), malignant giant cell tumor and adamantinoma (of unknown origin), and hemangioendothelioma (of vascular origin). Sarcomas of bone are staged according to the Musculoskeletal Tumor Society staging system outlined above.

OSTEOSARCOMA Osteosarcoma, accounting for almost 45 percent of all bone sarcomas, is a spindle cell neoplasm that produces osteoid (unmineralized bone) or bone. About 60 percent of all osteosarcomas occur in children and adolescents in the second decade of life, and about 10 percent occur in the third decade of life. Osteosarcomas in the fifth and sixth decades of life are frequently secondary to either radiation therapy or transformation in a preexisting benign condition, such as Paget's disease. Males are affected 1.5 to 2 times as often as females. Osteosarcoma has a predilection for metaphyses of long bones, and the most common sites of involvement are the distal femur, proximal tibia, and proximal humerus. The classification of osteosarcoma is complex, but 75 percent of osteosarcomas fall in the "conventional or classic" category, which include osteoblastic, chondroblastic, and fibroblastic osteosarcomas. The remaining 25 percent are classified as "variants" on the basis of (1) clinical characteristics, as in the case of osteosarcoma of the jaw, postradiation osteosarcoma, or Paget's osteosarcoma; (2) morphologic characteristics, as in the case of telangiectatic osteosarcoma, small cell osteosarcoma, or malignant fibrous histiocytoma; or (3) location, as in parosteal or periosteal osteosarcoma. Diagnosis usually requires a synthesis of clinical, radiologic, and pathologic features. Patients typically present with pain and swelling of the affected area. A plain radiograph reveals a destructive lesion with a moth-eaten appearance, a spiculated periosteal reaction (sunburst appearance), and a cuff of periosteal new bone formation at the margin of the soft tissue mass (Codman's triangle). A CT scan of the primary tumor is best for defining bone destruction and the pattern of calcification, whereas MRI is better for defining intramedullary and soft tissue extension. A chest radiograph and CT scan are used to detect lung metastases. Metastases to the bony skeleton should be imaged by a bone scan. Almost all osteosarcomas are hypervascular. Angiography is not helpful for diagnosis, but it is the most sensitive test for assessing the response to preoperative chemotherapy. Pathologic diagnosis is established either with a core-needle biopsy, where feasible, or with an open biopsy with an appropriately placed incision that does not compromise future limb-sparing resection. Most osteosarcomas are high-grade. The most important prognostic factor for long-term survival is response to chemotherapy. The 2-year survival of historical controls treated with surgery alone is <20 percent. The efficacy of adjuvant chemotherapy is better defined in osteosarcoma than in soft tissue sarcoma. Prospective, randomized trials have shown that adjuvant chemotherapy improves survival. The current state of the art, therefore, is preoperative chemotherapy followed by limb-sparing surgery (which can be accomplished in >80 percent of patients) followed by postoperative chemotherapy. The effective drugs are doxorubicin, ifosfamide, cisplatin, and high-dose methotrexate with leucovorin rescue. The various combinations of these agents that have been used have all been about equally successful. With the current management strategy, long-term survival rates in extremity osteosarcoma range from 60 to 70 percent. Osteosarcoma is radioresistant; radiation therapy has no role in the routine management. Malignant fibrous histiocytoma is considered a part of the spectrum of osteosarcoma and is managed similarly.

CHONDROSARCOMA Chondrosarcoma, which constitutes approximately 20 to 25 percent of all bone sarcomas, is a tumor of adulthood and old age with a peak incidence in the fourth to sixth decades of life. It has a predilection for the flat bones, especially the shoulder and pelvic girdles, but can also affect the diaphyseal portions of long bones. Chondrosarcomas can arise de novo or as a malignant transformation of an enchondroma or, rarely, of the cartilaginous cap of an osteochondroma. Chondrosarcomas have an indolent natural history and typically present as pain and swelling. Radiographically, the lesion may have a lobular appearance with mottled or punctate or annular calcification of the cartilaginous matrix. It is difficult to distinguish low-grade chondrosarcoma from benign lesions by x-ray or histologic examination. The diagnosis is therefore influenced by clinical history and physical examination. A new onset of pain, signs of inflammation, and progressive increase in the size of the mass suggest malignancy. The histologic classification is complex, but most tumors fall within the conventional or classic category. Like other bone sarcomas, high-grade chondrosarcomas spread to the lungs. Most chondrosarcomas are resistant to standard sarcoma chemotherapy, and surgical resection of primary or recurrent tumors, including pulmonary metastases, is the mainstay of therapy. There are two histologic variants for which this rule does not hold, however. Dedifferentiated chondrosarcoma is a low-grade tumor that dedifferentiates into a high-grade osteosarcoma or a malignant fibrous histiocytoma, a tumor that responds to chemotherapy. Mesenchymal chondrosarcoma, a rare variant composed of a small-cell element, also is responsive to systemic chemotherapy and is treated like Ewing's sarcoma.

EWING'S SARCOMA Ewing's sarcoma, which constitutes approximately 10 to 15 percent of all bone sarcomas, is common in adolescence and has a peak incidence in the second decade of life. It typically involves the diaphyseal region of long bones and also has an affinity for flat bones. The plain radiograph may show a characteristic "onion-peel" periosteal reaction with a generous soft tissue mass, which is better demonstrated by CT or MRI. This mass is composed of sheets of monotonous, small, round, blue cells and can be confused with lymphoma, embryonal rhabdomyosarcoma, and small cell carcinoma. The product of the *mic-2* gene (which is called p30/32) maps to the pseudoautosomal region of the X and Y chromosomes and is a cell-surface marker for Ewing's sarcoma [and other members of a family of tumors called *peripheral primitive neuroectodermal tumors* (PNETs)]. Most PNETs arise in soft tissues; they include peripheral neuroepithelioma, Askin's tumor (chest wall), and esthesioneuroblastoma. Glycogen-filled cytoplasm detected by immunohistochemical staining with periodic acid–Schiff is also characteristic of Ewing's sarcoma cells. The classic cytogenetic abnormality associated with this disease (and other PNETs) is a reciprocal translocation of the long arms of chromosomes 11 and 22, t(11;22), which creates a chimeric gene product of unknown function with components from the *fli-1* gene on chromosome 11 and *ews* on 22. This disease is very aggressive, and it is therefore considered a systemic disease. Common sites of metastases are lung, bones, and bone marrow. Systemic chemotherapy is the mainstay of therapy, often being used before surgery. Several chemotherapeutic drugs are active, including doxorubicin, cyclophosphamide or ifosfamide, etoposide, vincristine, and dactinomycin. Local treatment for the primary tumor includes surgical resection, usually with limb salvage or radiation therapy. Patients with lesions below the elbow and below the mid-calf have a 5-year survival of 80 percent with effective treatment. Ewing's sarcoma is a curable tumor, even in the presence of obvious metastatic disease, especially in children less than 11 years old. High-dose chemotherapy with hematopoietic support can cure a substantial fraction of patients with metastatic disease.

TUMORS METASTATIC TO BONE

Bone is a common site of metastasis for carcinomas of the prostate, breast, lung, kidney, bladder, and thyroid and for lymphomas and sarcomas. Prostate, breast and lung primaries account for 80 percent of all bone metastases. Metastatic tumors of bone are more common than primary bone tumors. Tumors usually spread to bone hematogenously, but local invasion from soft tissue masses also occurs. In descending order of frequency, the sites most often involved are the vertebrae, proximal femur, pelvis, ribs, sternum, proximal humerus, and skull. Bone metastases may be asymptomatic or may produce pain, swelling, symptoms of encroachment on a nerve root or the spinal cord, pathologic fracture, or myelophthisis (replacement of the marrow). Symptoms of hypercalcemia may be noted in cases of bony destruction.

Pain is the most frequent symptom. It usually develops gradually over weeks, is usually localized, and often is more severe at night. When patients with back pain develop neurologic signs or symptoms, emergency evaluation for spinal cord compression is indicated (see Chap. 104). Bone metastases exert a major adverse effect on quality of life in cancer patients.

Cancer in the bone may produce osteolysis, osteogenesis, or both. Osteolytic lesions result when the tumor produces substances that can directly elicit bone resorption (vitamin D–like steroids, prostaglandins, or parathyroid hormone–related peptide) or cytokines that can induce the formation of osteoclasts (interleukin 1 and tumor necrosis factor). Osteoblastic lesions result when the tumor produces cytokines that activate osteoblasts. In general, purely osteolytic lesions are best detected by plain radiography, but they may not be apparent until they are larger than 1 cm. These lesions are more commonly associated with hypercalcemia and with the excretion of hydroxyproline-containing peptides indicative of matrix destruction. When osteoblastic activity is prominent, the lesions may be readily detected using radionuclide bone scanning (which is sensitive to new bone formation), and the radiographic appearance may show increased bone density or sclerosis. Osteoblastic lesions are associated with higher serum levels of alkaline phosphatase, and, if extensive, may produce hypocalcemia. Although some tumors may produce mainly osteolytic lesions (e.g., kidney cancer) and others mainly osteoblastic lesions (e.g., prostate cancer), most metastatic lesions produce both types of lesion and may go through stages where one or the other predominates.

In older patients, particularly women, it may be necessary to distinguish metastatic disease of the spine from osteoporosis. In osteoporosis, the cortical bone may be preserved, whereas cortical bone destruction is usually noted with metastatic cancer.

Treatment of metastatic bone disease depends on the underlying malignancy and the symptoms. Some metastatic bone tumors are curable (lymphoma, Hodgkin's disease), and others are treated with palliative intent. Pain may be relieved by local radiation therapy. Hormonally responsive tumors are responsive to hormone inhibition (antiandrogens for prostate cancer, antiestrogens for breast cancer). Strontium 89 is a bone-seeking radionuclide that can exert antitumor effects and relieve symptoms. Bisphosphonates such as pamidronate may relieve pain and inhibit bone resorption. When the integrity of a weight-bearing bone is threatened by an expanding metastatic lesion that is refractory to radiation therapy, prophylactic internal fixation is indicated. Overall survival is related to the prognosis of the underlying tumor. Bone pain at the end of life is particularly common; an adequate pain relief regimen including sufficient amounts of narcotic analgesics is required.
→ *The management of hypercalcemia is discussed in Chap. 354.*

BIBLIOGRAPHY

BRENNAN MF, et al: The role of multi-modality therapy in soft tissue sarcoma. Ann Surg 214:328, 1991

———: Soft tissue sarcoma, in *Cancer: Principles and Practice of Oncology*, 5th ed, VT DeVita et al (eds). Philadelphia, Lippincott, 1997, pp 1738–1788

BURGERT EO et al: Multimodal therapy for the management of nonpelvic localized Ewing's sarcoma of bone: IESS II. J Clin Oncol 8:1514, 1990

CANGIR A et al: Ewing's sarcoma metastatic at diagnosis—Results and comparisons of two intergroup studies. Cancer 66:887, 1990

EVANS RG et al: Multimodal therapy for the management of localized Ewing's sarcoma of pelvic and sacral bones: A report from the second intergroup study. J Clin Oncol 9:1173, 1991

JABLONS D, et al: Metastasectomy for soft tissue sarcoma—further evidence for efficacy and prognostic indicators. J Thorac Cardiovasc Surg 97:695, 1989

LINDBERG RD, et al: Conservative surgery and post-operative radiotherapy in 300 adults with soft tissue sarcomas. Cancer 47:2391, 1981

LINK MP et al: The effect of adjuvant chemotherapy on relapse-free survival in patients with osteosarcoma of the extremity. N Engl J Med 314:1600, 1986

MALAWER MM et al: Sarcomas of bone, in *Cancer: Principles and Practice of Oncology*, 5th ed, VT DeVita et al (eds). Philadelphia, Lippincott, 1997, pp 1789–1852

PATEL SR, BENJAMIN RS: The role of chemotherapy in soft-tissue sarcomas. Cancer Control 1:599, 1994

———, ——— (eds): Sarcomas. Part I. Hematol Oncol Clin North Am 9:513, 1995

———, ——— (eds): Sarcomas. Part II. Hematol Oncol Clin North Am 9:707, 1995

NIH Consensus Development Panel on Limb Sparing Treatment of Adult Soft Tissue Sarcomas and Osteosarcomas. JAMA, 254:1791, 1985

ROTH JA: Resection of pulmonary metastases from osteogenic sarcoma. Cancer Bull 42:244, 1990

101   *Richard M. Stone*

METASTATIC CANCER OF UNKNOWN PRIMARY SITE

INCIDENCE AND EPIDEMIOLOGY The presenting findings in a patient with a newly discovered malignancy may not definitively reveal the site of origin of the neoplasm. Patients with cancer of unknown primary site (CUPS) present difficult diagnostic and therapeutic dilemmas. First, since the additional studies that could be ordered may be many, costly, and/or uncomfortable for the patient, the strategy used in searching for the primary must take into account what, if any, result the precise identification of the site of origin would have on the patient's treatment and length of survival. Second, while individuals with CUPS fare poorly overall (median survival is approximately 6 to 9 months), certain subgroups of patients are more likely to benefit from treatment and, in some cases, to enjoy long intervals without evidence of disease. The literature is a poor guide for the care of such patients, owing to the largely retrospective nature of the reports, the heterogeneity of the tumors, the selection bias in small, individual retrospective studies, and the variability in both the definition of the syndrome and the thoroughness of the evaluation performed to identify a primary site.

While there is no universally accepted definition of the CUPS syndrome, a truly occult neoplasm should fulfill all of the following criteria: (1) biopsy-proven malignancy, (2) unrevealing history, physical examination, chest film, abdominal and pelvic computed tomography (CT) scans, complete blood counts, chemistry survey, mammography (women), β human chorionic gonadotropin (βhCG) levels (men), alpha fetoprotein (AFP) levels (men), and prostate-specific antigen (PSA) levels (men), (3) histologic evaluation not consistent with a primary tumor at the biopsy site, and (4) failure of additional diagnostic studies (based only on findings from the laboratory and pathologic review) to identify the primary site. Such additional diagnostic tests could include, for example, colonoscopy in a patient whose rectal examination discloses guaiac-positive stool or a meticulous otolaryngologic examination in a patient who presents with squamous cell carcinoma in a cervical node. With increased understanding of the natural history of certain tumors and with the routine use of CT as well as detailed pathologic studies, there are many cases that fulfill the definition of CUPS but for which there is a reasonable suspicion that a given organ is the probable site of origin. Epidemiologic data suggest that the incidence of cancers for which the primary site is classified as unknown is decreasing. CUPS probably accounts for 2 to 3 percent of all cancer diagnoses currently, whereas it has been estimated that 10 to 15 percent of all cancers fell in this category in the last decade. Most patients with CUPS are over age 60.

BIOLOGIC CONSIDERATIONS The biologic behavior of CUPS is unique compared with that of other nonhematopoietic neoplasms. Such cancers as breast and prostate are relatively uncommon causes of CUPS. Breast primaries, for example, almost always are identified either before or simultaneously with their metastatic disease. Moreover, cancers presenting as CUPS often display unusual patterns of metastatic spread (e.g., pancreatic cancer presenting with bony metastases). The fact that more tumor bulk is present at distant sites than in the tissue of origin suggests that the genetic lesions underlying cases of CUPS produce a distinctly aggressive phenotype. Frequently, biopsy of an involved site will reveal a poorly differentiated histology, which is the morphologic correlate of this biologic behavior. The propensity of CUPS tumors to grow in distant locations also implies that the malignant cells can proliferate in the absence of the specific host factors (e.g., growth-promoting proteins, a vascular supply) that are important in the development of more typical cancers. Although physiologic and genetic data that might account for the distinctive natural history of CUPS neoplasms are scant, cell lines derived from such tumors may have abnormalities of chromosome 1, a finding generally associated with advanced malignancy.

CLINICAL PRESENTATION, DIAGNOSTIC EVALUATION, AND PATHOLOGY **History and Physical Examination** Patients present with a variety of symptoms and signs, including fatigue, weight loss, and other systemic symptoms, pain, abnormal bleeding, abdominal swelling, subcutaneous masses, and lymphadenopathy. Once it has been determined that metastatic cancer is present but that no primary site is obvious, the physician's approach must involve reasonable efforts to identify the primary site or to determine the histology or subcategory of the metastatic tumor to decide on the optimal therapy. Though usually unrevealing, a thorough history and physical examination should be carried out to elicit easily obtainable clues regarding the primary site. The patient should be questioned concerning epigastric pain, which, if present, would mandate careful exclusion of pancreatic carcinoma as well as other gastrointestinal malignancies. Symptoms referable to a given location (e.g., new cough, hematochezia, hemoptysis, change in bowel habits, unusual vaginal bleeding, nipple discharge) should prompt an aggressive specific diagnostic approach. Occupational exposure to asbestos, for example, would raise the suspicion of mesothelioma. The absence of prior smoking reduces the likelihood of lung cancer but does not exclude it. A history of fulguration of a skin lesion, colonic polypectomy, dilatation and curettage, or prostate biopsy should prompt a review of the original histology. Other than inferences drawn from the location of the involved area (see below), the physical examination will probably be unrevealing unless a thorough pelvic and rectal examination has not been performed previously.

Pathology Review The most important aspect of the workup of a patient with CUPS is the evaluation of the tissue obtained at biopsy. Vital clues pertaining to the primary site and the patient's management can be obtained by careful review of light-microscopic, immunohistochemical, ultrastructural, immunologic, karyotypic, and molecular biologic findings. First, if the original biopsy sample may be inadequate for either confirmation of malignancy or the performance of additional specialized studies, rebiopsy is mandatory. The clinician must have a close working relationship with a pathologist skilled in the evaluation of tumor specimens, especially when the organ of origin is uncertain. On either the initial or subsequent biopsy, plans may be made to process the tissue for (1) routine fixation for light-microscopic, histochemical, and immunohistochemical analysis, (2) freezing for DNA isolation or for additional immunologic evaluation (certain antibody-based detection methods, for example, cannot be applied to fixed, paraffin-embedded tissue), and (3) fixation, usually in glutaraldehyde, for ultrastructural analysis. Fresh tissue may be disaggregated into a single-cell suspension for short-term culture for purposes of cytogenetic analysis.

If routine histologic analysis fails to suggest the tissue of origin (e.g., gland formation in adenocarcinoma, psammoma bodies in ovarian or thyroid cancer, or spindle architecture in sarcomas), special histochemical studies may be helpful. For example, mucin positivity is helpful in recognizing a poorly differentiated adenocarcinoma. Light-microscopic review including histochemical analysis will show approximately 60 percent of CUPS tumors to be adenocarcinomas and 10 to 20 percent to be squamous cell carcinomas, usually of head and neck or lung origin. In the remaining poorly differentiated neoplasms, immunohistochemical, cytogenetic, and molecular biologic studies can be extremely useful in identifying sarcomas, germ cell carcinomas, lymphomas, neuroendocrine neoplasms (including melanoma), and other tumors whose diagnosis would suggest a more specific therapeutic approach.

Immunohistochemical Analysis Antibodies to specific cell components and the ability to detect binding by sensitive visualization methods such as peroxidase or streptavidin-biotin make it possible to characterize tumors that are not identified by standard techniques. Since in most situations no single antibody is specific enough to identify the primary site with certainty, a battery of such reagents must be employed. Table 101-1 provides a list of antigens that may be assessed by immunohistochemical analysis in undifferentiated or poorly differentiated specimens. It is particularly important to exclude the diagnosis of lymphoma by employing antibodies reactive to the leukocyte common antigen (LCA, CD45). The presence of LCA suggests that the patient has a lymphoid neoplasm and has the same chances of responding to therapy as if there were no diagnostic ambiguity. About half of patients with aggressive-histology lymphoma can be cured with combination chemotherapy (see Chap. 113). The immunohistochemical detection of specific types of filament proteins is helpful in the identification of carcinomas and sarcomas. The presence of keratin suggests carcinoma, since essentially all epithelial tumors contain this protein. However, certain sarcomas, mesotheliomas, and germ cell tumors are also keratin-positive, emphasizing the need for the judicious use of a battery of immunohistochemical markers. Sarcomas may react with antibodies to desmin. Prostate, breast, and thyroid carcinomas are suggested, respectively, by a reaction with antibodies to PSA or prostatic alkaline phosphatase, gross cystic fluid protein, or thyroglobulin. Immunohistochemistry may also identify sarcoma subgroups, including rhabdomyosarcoma (myoglobin) and angiosarcoma or Kaposi's sarcoma (factor VIII). The finding of AFP, βhCG, or placental alkaline phosphatase staining is very helpful in assigning a germ cell origin. The S-100 protein is present in virtually all primary and metastatic melanomas, including the amelanotic variety, the latter being difficult to classify by routine techniques. However, S-100 positivity is also found in many other tumors of neuroendocrine origin (e.g., small cell lung cancer, carcinoid, neuroepithelioma); a more specific marker for melanomas is the HMB45 (human melanoma black) antigen.

Other Diagnostic Approaches Ultrastructural analysis with electron microscopy can identify cell junctions (i.e., desmosomes, typical of epithelial cancers), neuroendocrine granules, melanosomes, and muscle filaments, which can be very helpful in identifying the tissue of origin. Cytogenetic analysis of solid tumors is a means of classifying neoplasms associated with specific chromosomal translocations or other genetic abnormalities and is used increasingly (Table 101-1). Cytogenetic abnormalities can also be determined by fluorescence in situ hybridization with chromosome-specific probes, a technique that does not require cells to divide, as is the case with traditional karyotype analysis. Fresh tissue may be required for detection of estrogen or progesterone receptors where breast cancer is a possibility or of antigens that are not fixation-resistant (such as those found on certain T cells). In addition to immunologic analysis, lymphomas can be diagnosed by using molecular approaches on DNA isolated from tumor tissue to detect lymphoid-specific gene rearrangements such as those of immunoglobulin, T-cell receptor, or *bcl*-2 genes. Since minimal amounts of template DNA are required for amplification by the polymerase chain reaction, paraffin-embedded tissue blocks may yield sufficient diagnostic material. As additional tumors are found to have specific acquired chromosomal rearrangements or mutations in genes controlling

Table 101-1

Possible Pathologic Evaluation of Biopsy Specimens from Patients with Metastatic Cancer of Unknown Primary Site

Evaluation/Findings	Suggested Primary Site or Neoplasm
HISTOLOGY (HEMATOXYLIN AND EOSIN STAINING)	
Psammoma bodies, papillary configuration	Ovary, thyroid
Signet ring cells	Stomach
IMMUNOHISTOLOGY	
Leukocyte common antigen (LCA, CD45)	Lymphoid neoplasm
Leu-M1	Hodgkin's disease
Epithelial membrane antigen	Carcinoma
Cytokeratin intermediate filaments	Carcinoma
CEA	Carcinoma
HMB45	Melanoma
Desmin	Sarcoma
Thyroglobulin	Thyroid carcinoma
Calcitonin	Medullary carcinoma of the thyroid
Myoglobin	Rhabdomyosarcoma
PSA/prostatic acid phosphatase	Prostate
AFP	Liver, stomach, germ cell
Placental alkaline phosphatase	Germ cell
B, T cell markers	Lymphoid neoplasm
S-100 protein	Neuroendocrine tumor, melanoma
Gross cystic fluid protein	Breast, sweat gland
Factor VIII	Kaposi's sarcoma, angiosarcoma
FLOW CYTOMETRY	
B, T cell markers	Lymphoid neoplasm
ULTRASTRUCTURE	
Actin-myosin filaments	Rhabdomyosarcoma
Secretory granules	Neuroendocrine tumors
Desmosomes	Carcinoma
Premelanosomes	Melanoma
CYTOGENETICS	
Isochromosome 12p; 12q($-$)	Germ cell
t(11;22)	Ewing's sarcoma, primitive neuroectodermal tumor
t(8;14)*	Lymphoid neoplasm
3p($-$)	Small cell lung carcinoma; renal cell carcinoma, mesothelioma
t(X;18)	Synovial sarcoma
t(12;16)	Myxoid liposarcoma
t(12;22)	Clear cell sarcoma (melanoma of soft parts)
t(2;13)	Alveolar rhabdomyosarcoma
1p($-$)	Neuroblastoma
RECEPTOR ANALYSIS	
Estrogen/progesterone receptor	Breast
MOLECULAR BIOLOGIC STUDIES	
Immunoglobulin, *bcl*-2, T-cell receptor gene rearrangement	Lymphoid neoplasm

* Or any other rearrangement involving an antigen-receptor gene

growth and differentiation, the detection of altered DNA and/or altered gene products will become increasingly useful in diagnosis.

Additional Studies If the pathology review fails to disclose a histology likely to be responsive to chemotherapy, it is unlikely that additional expensive diagnostic tests will benefit the patient, so they must be ordered only judiciously. In females with metastatic adenocarcinoma or poorly differentiated carcinoma, mammography should be performed, although the diagnostic yield will be quite low except in

patients with axillary metastases. The use of abdominal/pelvic CT scans leads to the identification of the primary site in as many as 35 percent of patients and will certainly reduce the number of cases of pancreatic cancer in which the primary site is obscure before death. Whether or not to measure routinely serum tumor markers such as AFP, βhCG, carcinoembryonic antigen (CEA), CA-125 (associated with ovarian cancer), and PSA is controversial. Many different adenocarcinomas elaborate CEA, CA-125, or both; these markers are useful for following the response to therapy rather than for identifying a primary site. Moreover, poorly differentiated colonic tumors frequently fail to produce CEA, and patients with benign prostate hypertrophy may have modestly elevated PSA levels, reducing the reliability of these markers in defining the primary site in a patient with metastatic cancer. Numerous studies have shown a lack of benefit of contrast studies (upper gastrointestinal series, barium enema or intravenous pyelogram) in patients with metastatic cancer of unknown primary who have no specific symptoms and no findings referable to the gastrointestinal or urinary tract. Moreover, autopsy series reveal that the most likely primary site of origin includes epithelial tissues such as lung, stomach, colon, and kidney, which give rise to tumors that respond poorly to chemotherapy, minimizing the therapeutic impact of such a diagnosis. Additional invasive diagnostic studies are indicated if the presentation strongly suggests a particular primary site. For example, radiographic evidence of lung or mediastinal involvement would mandate fiberoptic bronchoscopy to exclude lung cancer. In the relatively unusual case of metastatic squamous cell cancer presenting in an inguinal lymph node, anoscopy and colposcopy should be performed to detect carcinoma of the vulva, cervix, vagina, penis, or anus, all of which may be cured even with lymph node spread. A summary of a reasonable diagnostic approach is found in Table 101-2.

℞ TREATMENT

Prognostic Subgroups Regardless of patient age, the exclusion of treatable and potentially curable neoplasms is important. Patients with squamous cell carcinoma have a somewhat longer median survival (9 months) than do those with adenocarcinoma or unclassifiable neoplasms (4 to 6 months). If laboratory studies indicate a significant likelihood that the neoplasm is a lymphoma, germ cell tumor, sarcoma, neuroendocrine tumor, or breast or prostate cancer, then disease-appropriate therapy should be administered. Patients with lymphoma or a germ cell neoplasm may be cured with combination chemotherapy. In other malignancies, effective palliative chemotherapy (for sarcoma or a breast or neuroendocrine tumor) or hormonal therapy (for breast or prostate cancer) should be strongly considered. Although often requiring electron microscopy for diagnosis, neuroendocrine tumors (especially if anaplastic) are expected to respond to cisplatin-based chemotherapy.

Patients in whom the primary site can be identified fare somewhat better than those in whom it remains undefined. Generally favorable prognostic factors identified by multivariate analysis of large series of patients with CUPS include limited sites of involvement (especially if lymphadenopathy is present) and neuroendocrine histology. Patients often may be categorized as having one of several clinical features or syndromes suggesting a specific form of potentially beneficial therapy (Table 101-3).

Table 101-2

Suggested Clinical Evaluation of Patients with Metastatic Cancer of Unknown Primary Site

History: smoking history, asbestos exposure, abdominal pain
Physical examination: lymph nodes, thyroid, skin;
  Men: prostate
  Women: breasts, pelvic examination
Laboratory evaluation: stool evaluation for occult blood; urinalysis; complete blood count; liver function tests; measurement of serum levels of PSA, βhCG, AFP, CEA, and CA-125 (women); chest x-ray; abdominal and pelvic CT; mammography
Pathologic evaluation: see Table 101-1

Table 101-3

CHAPTER 101
Metastatic Cancer of Unknown Primary Site **617**

Presentations That Dictate Specific Therapies in Patients with CUPS

Clinicopathologic Features	Suspected Primary Site	Suggested Therapy
Squamous cell carcinoma, cervical node	Head and neck cancer	Radical neck dissection; radiotherapy ± chemotherapy
Carcinoma, axillary nodes (female)	Breast cancer	Breast radiotherapy or mastectomy, systemic adjuvant therapy
Peritoneal carcinomatosis (female)	Ovarian cancer	Debulking surgery, cisplatin-based chemotherapy
Poorly differentiated cancer, age <50, lung or retroperitoneal or mediastinal mass or lymph nodes, elevated serum βhCG or AFP levels	Germ cell tumor (extragonadal)	Cisplatin/VP-16-based chemotherapy
Bony metastases (male)	Prostate cancer	Androgen blockade (leuprolide plus flutamide)
Adenocarcinoma, liver metastases, elevated CEA level	Gastrointestinal malignancy	Colonoscopy with resection (if appropriate) of detected tumors; 5-fluorouracil/leucovorin

SYNDROME OF UNRECOGNIZED EXTRAGONADAL GERM CELL CANCER A subset of patients with poorly differentiated carcinoma of unknown primary site are extremely responsive to chemotherapy. These patients display one or more of the following features: age less than 50; tumor involving midline structures, lung parenchyma, or lymph nodes; an elevated serum AFP or βhCG level; evidence of rapid tumor growth; or tumor responsiveness to previously administered radiotherapy or chemotherapy. Cisplatin-based chemotherapy has led to long-term survival in a sizable fraction of patients with these features, especially those who have a favorable performance status at diagnosis, suggesting that their tumors behaved like germ cell neoplasms. If all patients with poorly differentiated carcinoma (including poorly differentiated adenocarcinoma) are treated with a chemotherapy regimen designed for those with germ cell cancer (e.g., cisplatin plus etoposide or vinblastine, often also with bleomycin) (see Chap. 98), about one-quarter will respond completely and one-third will experience a partial response. Patients whose disease does not respond to two cycles of therapy should not be committed to longer treatment. Approximately one in six patients is likely to survive more than 5 years without evidence of disease. Individuals with poorly differentiated carcinoma are more likely to respond to combination chemotherapy than those whose tumors display somewhat more mature features. Patients with poorly differentiated carcinoma or adenocarcinoma whose tumors have abnormalities of chromosome 12 similar to those described in patients with proven germ cell cancer are more likely to respond to platinum-based chemotherapy than are patients with a similar presentation whose tumors lack this cytogenetic abnormality.

PERITONEAL CARCINOMATOSIS IN WOMEN Women who present with increased abdominal girth and a pelvic mass or pain and who are found to have adenocarcinoma throughout the peritoneal cavity but without a clear site of origin also may benefit from platinum-based chemotherapy. This syndrome has been termed *primary peritoneal papillary serous carcinoma* or *multifocal extraovarian serous carcinoma*. While breast cancer or a gastrointestinal malignancy can produce these findings, peritoneal carcinomatosis is most commonly ascribed to ovarian cancer, even in patients with apparently normal ovaries at the time of laparotomy. Especially if psammoma bodies or a papillary configuration is noted in the pathology examination or if the CA-125 level is elevated, women with adenocarcinoma of the peritoneal cavity without a defined primary should receive maximum surgical cytoreduction followed by cisplatin-based ther-

apy. The stage-specific response to such therapy appears to be comparable to that for patients with proven ovarian cancer. Approximately 10 percent of patients who present in this fashion may remain free of disease 2 years after diagnosis.

CARCINOMA IN AN AXILLARY LYMPH NODE IN A FEMALE Women with an axillary mass proved to be adenocarcinoma or poorly differentiated carcinoma should receive treatment appropriate for stage II breast cancer whether or not a careful breast examination or mammography suggests the diagnosis of primary breast cancer and whether or not estrogen or progesterone receptors are detectable in the node. Even if no lesion is found in the breast, a breast recurrence will develop in one-half of these patients if no mastectomy is performed. Appropriate therapy generally includes either modified radical mastectomy or breast irradiation to reduce the risk of local recurrence. In addition, adjuvant systemic therapy (chemotherapy and/or tamoxifen, depending on menopausal status and whether or not estrogen receptor protein was found in the axillary tumor) to reduce the risk of developing evident metastatic breast cancer should be considered (see Chap. 91). Adjuvant systemic therapy may be administered before definitive local radiation treatment. Women with axillary metastases without an obvious breast primary appear to have the same likelihood of prolonged disease-free survival as patients with typical stage II breast cancer.

BONE METASTASES IN MALES Particularly if the lesions are osteoblastic, the serum PSA concentration should be measured, since the probability of prostate carcinoma is high in these patients. Empirical hormonal therapy (e.g., leuprolide and flutamide) should be strongly considered.

CERVICAL LYMPH NODE METASTASES Patients who present with a neck mass should be considered to have a primary tumor of the upper aerodigestive tract (usually termed *head and neck cancer*) until a different source is proven. Especially if the pathology analysis suggests a squamous histology and the node is located in a high or midcervical area, a careful ear, nose, and throat examination including direct laryngoscopy, nasopharyngoscopy, and random blind biopsies should be undertaken. A thyroid examination and scan also must be performed to rule out a primary thyroid tumor, especially if the histology is not definitely squamous. Particularly for patients in whom a primary site is discovered in the head or neck, definitive local therapy (external beam radiation or radical neck dissection) combined with platinum-based chemotherapy may lead to prolonged survival (see Chap. 89).

ADENOCARCINOMA AND LIVER METASTASES Although the entity of liver metastases proved to be adenocarcinoma is not as well characterized as the unrecognized germ cell cancer syndrome (nor as responsive to therapy), there is a significant likelihood of a primary stomach, biliary, or colorectal tumor. An elevated serum CEA level in this setting would be further evidence suggesting a gastrointestinal malignancy. It may be reasonable to perform a flexible sigmoidoscopy or colonoscopy to rule out a potentially obstructive colonic lesion. If a tumor is found, resection may be beneficial, depending on the tumor's size; even if none is found, treatment with a combination of 5-fluorouracil plus leucovorin is palliative for some patients with presumed metastatic gastrointestinal malignancy. Given both the severe and even life-threatening diarrhea that may be a consequence of this regimen and the relative resistance of gastrointestinal tumors to chemotherapy, patients should be made aware of the risks before embarking on such therapy.

Patients not falling into one of the preceding categories should be treated palliatively. In some patients, observation is appropriate. For example, individuals without evidence of additional metastatic disease who have undergone resection of a solitary pulmonary nodule containing malignant cells may actually have undergone definitive therapy for a small primary lung tumor. Radiation therapy is indicated in patients with local disease causing bony pain or neurologic compromise. The largest and most poorly responsive subgroup are those with moderate to well differentiated adenocarcinomas. Combination chemotherapy is frequently employed in such patients; however, response rates to "all-purpose" regimens [e.g., FAM (5-fluorouracil, doxorubicin, mitomycin C), FACP (5-fluorouracil, doxorubicin, cyclophosphamide, cisplatin)], or to ICE (ifosfamide, carboplatin, etoposide) are generally well under 50 percent, especially if patients with poorly differentiated adenocarcinoma, who have a higher response rate, are excluded; complete responses are rare. Regimens containing mitomycin C are associated with the risk of hemolytic uremic syndrome. In some series, patients with a good performance status whose disease is limited to soft tissue sites or extends only above the diaphragm have shown a better rate of response to therapy. While patients whose disease responds to treatment seem to have better survival than those whose disease does not respond, the difference may be related to inherent characteristics of the tumor rather than to a beneficial effect of chemotherapy.

Before combination chemotherapy is attempted in a patient with CUPS, the potential benefits must be weighed carefully against the certainty of toxicity. While some randomized studies have reported a benefit of one form of therapy over another, these reports are generally plagued by small numbers of patients and inadequate control of potential prognostic variables. Depending on motivation, eligibility, and availability, patients with CUPS may be candidates for evaluation of new (phase I) therapies.

BIBLIOGRAPHY

ABBRUZZESE JL et al: Analysis of a diagnostic strategy for patients with suspected tumors of unknown origin. J Clin Oncol 13:2094, 1995
———— et al: Unknown primary carcinoma: Natural history and prognostic factors in 657 consecutive patients. J Clin Oncol 12:1272, 1994
DE BRAUD F, AL-SERRAF M: Diagnosis and management of squamous cell carcinoma of unknown primary tumor site of the neck. Semin Oncol 20:273, 1993
ELLERBROEK N et al: Treatment of patients with isolated axillary nodal metastases from an occult primary carcinoma consistent with breast origin. Cancer 66:1461, 1990
FLETCHER JA et al: Diagnostic relevance of clonal cytogenetics in malignant soft tissue tumors. N Engl J Med 324:436, 1991
HAINSWORTH JD, GRECO FA: Treatment of patients with cancer of an unknown primary site. N Engl J Med 329:257, 1993
HORNING SJ et al: Lymphomas presenting as histologically unclassified neoplasms: Characteristics and response to treatment. J Clin Oncol 17:1281, 1989
MOERTEL CG et al: Treatment of neuroendocrine carcinomas with combined etoposide and cisplatin: Evidence of major therapeutic activity in the anaplastic variety of these neoplasms. Cancer 68:227, 1991
MOTZER RJ et al: Molecular and cytogenetic studies in the diagnosis of patients with poorly differentiated carcinomas of unknown primary site. J Clin Oncol 13:274, 1995
MUGGIA FM, BARANDA J: Management of peritoneal carcinomatosis of unknown primary tumor site. Semin Oncol 20:268, 1993
SPORN JR, GREENBERG BR: Empirical chemotherapy for adenocarcinoma of unknown primary tumor site. Semin Oncol 20:261, 1993

102 *Bruce E. Johnson*

PARANEOPLASTIC SYNDROMES

ENDOCRINE SYNDROMES

There are three major classes of hormones: steroids, monoamines, and peptides/proteins. Production of steroid hormones by malignant tumors is rare; lymphomas may produce 1,25-dihydroxyvitamin D from circulating 1-hydroxyvitamin D, but most other steroid-producing tumors are benign tumors of the glands that normally secrete the steroid.

Monoamines such as norepinephrine and epinephrine are secreted by pheochromocytomas (see Chap. 333), but they are not secreted ectopically by malignant tumor cells.

Most hormonal syndromes in patients with cancer are related to the production of peptide or protein hormones. The most common of these endocrine syndromes are listed in Table 102-1, together with the protein hormones that mediate them and the tumors that most commonly produce the hormones. A peptide hormone generally is encoded by an mRNA that is translated into a larger prohormone molecule, which undergoes a number of posttranslational modifications, including cleavage, glycosylation, and/or other steps. For example, pro-opiomelanocortin can be cleaved to yield adrenocorticotropin (ACTH), lipotropin, endorphin, melanocyte-stimulating hormone, and/or enkephalin, with different cell types producing different products. In addition, some cells use alternatively spliced forms of the message to produce different proteins (e.g., calcitonin vs. calcitonin gene–related peptide).

Tumor cells of nonendocrine organs often lack certain components of the pathway that leads from prohormone to biologically active hormone to secreted product. As a result of defects in protein processing or post-translational changes, generally, tumor cells may produce proteins that are structurally related to but biologically less active than the normal hormones. Thus, cancer patients may have elevated levels of immunoreactive hormones in plasma in the absence of clinical syndromes of hormone excess.

The severity of paraneoplastic endocrine syndromes often parallels the clinical course of the cancer. However, with some benign or slowly growing tumors, the hormone syndrome can be the major cause of morbidity. Despite their production by tumor cells, hormones are not very good tumor markers. Human chorionic gonadotropin (hCG) is a reliable tumor marker in some forms of testicular cancer, but no other hormone is used to quantitate tumor mass.

Most endocrine cancer syndromes occur with tumors derived from neuroendocrine or neural crest tissue (small cell lung cancer, carcinoid tumors). The genetic mechanisms that account for the production of a hormone by a cell that does not usually produce it are not clear. Oncogenes may activate other cellular genes (including genes that encode hormones) that normally are silent. Alternatively, demethylation of normally methylated inactive genes may permit expression in rapidly dividing cells.

HYPERCALCEMIA OF MALIGNANCY Hypercalcemia of malignancy, the most common paraneoplastic endocrine syndrome, is responsible for approximately 40 percent of all hypercalcemia (see Chap. 354). Hypercalcemia with cancer is classified as humoral hypercalcemia of malignancy (HHM), which is caused by circulating hormones, or local osteolytic hypercalcemia (LOH), which is caused by local paracrine factors secreted by cancers within bone. Parathyroid hormone–related peptide (PTHrP) causes nearly all cases of humoral hypercalcemia of malignancy, while the mediators of LOH in bone are heterogeneous.

Pathogenesis Eighty percent of patients with hypercalcemia of malignancy have HHM. PTHrP is composed of 139 to 173 amino acids, and 8 of the first 13 amino acids at the amino-terminal end are identical to the amino-terminal portion of parathyroid hormone (PTH). PTHrP binds to PTH receptors in the bone and kidney and causes increased bone resorption, decreased bone formation, increased renal tubular reabsorption of calcium, increased phosphaturia, and increased urinary levels of cyclic adenosine monophosphate, leading to hypercalcemia. PTHrP is detected in the plasma in approximately 80 percent of cancer patients with hypercalcemia. Rare patients have been reported to have hypercalcemia caused by ectopically produced authentic PTH. HHM in lymphoma may be caused by the production of 1,25-dihydroxyvitamin D by the tumor.

Twenty percent of patients with hypercalcemia have LOH in which hypercalcemia is caused by the local production of hormones or cytokines by cancers that have spread to the bone or bone marrow; such factors increase bone resorption in the area around the cancer. The ectopically produced hormones that may play a role in LOH include transforming growth factors α and β, interleukin (IL) 1, IL-6, prostaglandins, and tumor necrosis factor.

Clinical Manifestations The initial symptoms and signs of hypercalcemia (calcium level ≥ 2.6 mmol/L)[1] include malaise, fatigue, confusion, anorexia, bone pain, polyuria, polydipsia, weakness, constipation, nausea, and vomiting. Neurologic symptoms and signs in profound hypercalcemia (>3.5 mmol/L) include confusion, lethargy, coma, and death. The cancers responsible for HHM in patients are non-small cell lung cancer and cancers of the breast, kidney, head and neck, and bladder. HHM is particularly common in patients with cancers of squamous cell histology. Hypercalcemia is uncommon at presentation (<1 percent of patients) with these tumors but becomes more common as the cancer progresses and is present in 10 to 20 percent of patients near the time of death. LOH is responsible for hypercalcemia in patients with breast cancer, myeloma, lymphoma, and leukemia. Among hypercalcemic patients with breast cancer, approximately half have HHM and half LOH.

Table 102-1

Common Paraneoplastic Endocrine Syndromes

Syndrome	Proteins	Tumors Typically Associated with Syndrome
Hypercalcemia of malignancy	Parathyroid hormone-related peptide (PTHrP) Parathyroid hormone (PTH)	Non-small cell lung cancer Breast cancer Renal cell carcinoma Head and neck cancer Bladder cancer Myeloma
Syndrome of inappropriate vasopressin secretion (SIADH)	Arginine vasopressin (AVP) Atrial natriuretic peptide	Small cell lung cancer Head and neck cancer Non-small cell lung cancer
Cushing's syndrome	Adrenocorticotropic hormone (ACTH) Corticotropin-releasing hormone (CRH)	Small cell lung cancer Carcinoid tumors
Acromegaly	Growth hormone–releasing hormone (GHRH) Growth hormone (GH)	Carcinoid Small cell lung cancer Pancreatic islet cell tumors
Gynecomastia	Human chorionic gonadotropin (hCG)	Testicular cancer Lung cancer Carcinoid tumors of the lung and gastrointestinal tract
Non-islet cell tumor hypoglycemia	Insulin-like growth factor-2 (IGF-2)	Sarcomas

Diagnosis The patient with cancer who develops hypercalcemia should be evaluated for other causes of hypercalcemia, including use of thiazide diuretics, vitamin D, or lithium, hyperthyroidism, and sarcoidosis. Elevation of serum PTH as measured by immunoassay suggests primary hyperparathyroidism, which may be responsible for as many as 10 percent of cases of cancer and which should be treated like other cases of hyperparathyroidism (see Chap. 356), if the underlying cancer is controlled. A normal PTH level and a low serum phosphorus level in the absence of bone metastases support the diagnosis of HHM, while a normal PTHrP level and normal phosphorus in a patient with bone metastases suggest LOH.

℞ **TREATMENT**

The median survival of patients with hypercalcemia of malignancy is only 1 to 3 months. Intervention to reverse hypercalcemia should be undertaken when the cancer is likely to be controlled with appropriate systemic or local treatment.

The treatment of HHM and LOH is similar (see Chap. 354). Patients with mild to moderate hypercalcemia (2.65 to 3.5 mmol/L) can be treated with 2 to 4 L of saline hydration per day and furosemide to prevent intravascular volume overload. The bisphosphonate pamidronate (60 to 90 mg intravenously) decreases osteoclastic bone resorption. Combined administration of diuretics and pamidronate reduces the serum calcium to normal values in 80 percent of patients within 7 days. Doses may be repeated as needed. In patients with LOH, glucocorticoids may inhibit the production of cytokines that promote bone resorption. Severe hypercalcemia [>3.50 mmol/L (>14 mg/dL)] with alteration of mental status can be treated with all of the above plus salmon calcitonin, 4 to 8 U/kg, administered intramuscularly or subcutaneously every 12 h. Calcitonin administration will decrease the serum calcium within 24 h, and its hypocalcemic effect can be prolonged in patients with LOH by adding glucocorticoids. If these agents are not effective in reducing the serum calcium, plicamycin and gallium nitrate may be added.

HYPONATREMIA OF MALIGNANCY Hyponatremia of malignancy (Na^+ level < 130 mmol/L) is usually due to the inappropriate secretion of arginine vasopressin (AVP) and is termed the *syndrome of inappropriate antidiuretic hormone secretion* (SIADH). In rare cases, atrial natriuretic peptide produces hyponatremia.

Pathogenesis Small cell lung cancer is the malignancy chiefly responsible for producing ectopic AVP. AVP mRNA is expressed and translated, and the product is processed into the nonapeptide AVP, which is secreted into the circulation. The ectopically produced AVP binds to receptors in the kidney, causing retention of free water with resulting hypoosmolality in the plasma and hyperosmolality in urine (see Chap. 330).

About 15 percent of cancer patients with SIADH do not have evidence of ectopic production of AVP. In some of these patients, tumors secrete atrial natriuretic peptide. This hormone inhibits sodium reabsorption in the proximal tubule and inhibits release of renin and aldosterone. It is not yet clear how atrial natriuretic peptide leads to hyponatremia.

Clinical Manifestations SIADH is commonly recognized as asymptomatic hyponatremia on routine serum chemistry examination. It is present at the time of diagnosis in 15 percent of patients with small cell lung cancer, 3 percent of patients with head and neck cancer, and <1 percent of patients with non-small cell lung cancer. Hyponatremia may also occur with primary brain tumors, hematologic malignancies, melanoma, sarcoma, and gynecologic, gastrointestinal, breast, prostate, and bladder cancer. The symptoms of mild hyponatremia (>120 mmol/L) include difficulty focusing attention, fatigue, nausea, vomiting, anorexia, weakness, and headache. Profound hyponatremia (<120 mmol/L) can cause confusion, lethargy, coma, seizures, and death.

Diagnosis (See Chap. 330) SIADH is suspected in patients with hyponatremia (serum sodium < 130 mmol/L) and a concentrated urine (osmolality > 300 mmol/kg). Patients are euvolemic, are not using diuretics, and have normal thyroid and adrenal function. Polydipsia is excluded by the urine osmolality. Pseudohyponatremia can be present if serum glucose, triglyceride, or protein levels are high. Conditions other than cancer that can cause the SIADH include central nervous system disorders, pulmonary infections, positive-pressure breathing, pneumothorax, asthma, and a wide array of drugs, including chemotherapeutic agents (vincristine, vinblastine, cisplatin, cyclophosphamide, melphalan, levamisole), thiazide diuretics, carbamazepine, antidepressants, nicotine, and narcotics.

℞ **TREATMENT**

The treatment should be directed at the underlying cancer. Patients whose tumors have not been or cannot be controlled are candidates

---

[1] Calcium measurements given in millimoles per liter can be multiplied by 4 to convert to milligrams per deciliter or by 2 to convert to milliequivalents per liter.

for restriction of fluid intake to 500 mL/d. Such restriction corrects hyponatremia within 7 days in most patients, but it is difficult and uncomfortable for patients to maintain fluid restriction for extended periods. Oral demeclocycline (600 to 1200 mg/d) may be useful in blocking the effects of AVP but can cause renal insufficiency. Other agents that may be used for the treatment of hyponatremia include dilantin and lithium.

Rare patients develop profound hyponatremia and altered mental status. These patients should be treated with 0.9 percent saline hydration and furosemide diuresis. If that is not effective, 3 percent saline can be administered via a central line together with furosemide diuresis to prevent hypervolemia. Hypertonic saline is rarely required and must be given slowly; fluid balance and electrolytes should be monitored several times per day, and the increase in sodium should be limited to 0.5 mmol/L per hour to prevent pontine lysis (see Chap. 330).

ECTOPIC ACTH SYNDROME   Ectopic production of ACTH by cancer cells is responsible for approximately 15 percent of all cases of Cushing's syndrome and for most cases of Cushing's syndrome that occur in cancer patients (see Chaps. 328 and 332). In rare patients, Cushing's syndrome is caused by ectopically produced corticotropin-releasing hormone (CRH), which in turn stimulates pituitary ACTH release.

Pathogenesis   When pro-opiomelanocortin mRNA is expressed in cancer cells, the 241-amino-acid prohormone is translated and processed into a variety of molecules, including, in some cases, the 39-amino-acid hormone ACTH, which can be secreted into the circulation. The ectopically produced ACTH causes excessive secretion of glucocorticoids and mineralocorticoids by the adrenals.

Clinical Manifestations   Women make up 50 percent of patients with ectopic ACTH syndrome and 90 percent of patients with pituitary Cushing's disease. Therefore, Cushing's syndrome in men is more likely to be caused by ectopic ACTH than by a pituitary tumor. Because of mineralocorticoid excess, patients with ectopic Cushing's syndrome usually have hypokalemic alkalosis at presentation, a rare finding in patients with Cushing's disease. Other common manifestations of ectopic ACTH syndrome include weakness, hypertension, and hyperglycemia. Ectopic ACTH syndrome in patients with slow-growing cancers (e.g., carcinoids) may develop typical features of central obesity, moon facies, hyperpigmentation, and hirsutism in addition to the metabolic abnormalities.

Ectopic ACTH syndrome is most commonly due to small cell lung cancer (50 percent of cases), bronchial carcinoid tumors (10 percent), thymic carcinoid tumors or thymomas (10 percent), pancreatic islet cell tumors (10 percent), pheochromocytoma or other neural crest tumors (5 percent), or medullary carcinoma of the thyroid (5 percent). About 2 percent of patients with small cell lung cancer and bronchial carcinoids have the ectopic ACTH syndrome at the time of diagnosis. Patients with small cell lung cancer and ectopic ACTH syndrome have shorter survival than patients without the syndrome and are more likely to develop opportunistic infections.

Diagnosis   (See Chaps. 328 and 332)   Ectopic ACTH syndrome is usually characterized by elevated levels of urinary free cortisol that do not decrease after administration of high doses of dexamethasone (8 mg/d). However, in one-third of patients with carcinoid tumors, urinary cortisol levels decrease by more than 50 percent after administration of high-dose dexamethasone. The plasma levels of ACTH are markedly elevated in more than half of patients. If these tests do not provide definitive evidence of ectopic ACTH syndrome, bilateral inferior petrosal vein sampling will show an elevated ACTH level in petrosal vein blood that does not increase after administration of CRH.

℞ **TREATMENT**

Treatment of the ectopic ACTH syndrome should be directed at the underlying cancer: chemotherapy for small cell lung cancer; surgical resection or radiation therapy for carcinoids. Some patients with ectopic Cushing's syndrome have no evidence of tumor after extensive evaluation. These patients should be treated symptomatically and followed closely with periodic imaging studies, because they may have slow-growing tumors amenable to surgical resection.

Agents that inhibit steroidogenesis in the adrenal gland include ketoconazole (400 to 1200 mg/d), which reduces urinary cortisol excretion by more than half in two-thirds of patients, and metyrapone (1 to 4 g/d), which also reduces urinary cortisol excretion. Patients who are in good condition and whose manifestations are not controlled by drugs may be considered for adrenalectomy.

ECTOPIC ACROMEGALY   Ectopic production of growth hormone-releasing hormone (GHRH) is the predominant cause of ectopic acromegaly (see Chap. 328).

Pathogenesis   GHRH is processed into 40- and 44-amino-acid peptides and binds to receptors in the pituitary, causing them to increase production of growth hormone. Rare cases of ectopic acromegaly are due to ectopic production of growth hormone itself by tumors.

Clinical Manifestations   The symptoms and signs of ectopic acromegaly develop over several years and include increasing glove and shoe size, facial disfigurement, arthralgias, amenorrhea-galactorrhea or impotence, hypertension, muscle weakness, and diabetes mellitus. Ectopic acromegaly has been reported in fewer than 100 patients and accounts for 1 percent or less of all cases of acromegaly. The cancers associated with ectopic acromegaly include carcinoid tumors of the bronchus, pancreatic islet cell tumors, and cancers of the lung, breast, colon, and adrenal glands.

Diagnosis   If a clinical diagnosis of acromegaly is suspected in a patient with cancer, the serum levels of GHRH and insulin-like growth factor (IGF)-1 and the glucose-suppressed growth hormone (GH) serum level should be measured (see Chap. 328). Patients with elevated GHRH levels and acromegaly have ectopic acromegaly. Patients without evidence of cancer who have elevated GHRH levels should undergo imaging of the central nervous system, chest, and abdomen to look for an occult cancer. Patients with cancer, low GHRH levels, high GH levels, and elevated IGF-1 levels should undergo magnetic resonance imaging (MRI) of the pituitary and hypothalamus. If no pituitary tumor is detected, GH may be secreted directly by the known tumor. Not all GH-secreting tumors of the pituitary are demonstrable by imaging techniques, however.

℞ **TREATMENT**

The therapy of ectopic acromegaly should be directed at the underlying cancer and should consist of surgical resection or radiation therapy for patients with carcinoid and islet cell tumors. Agents for medical control of ectopic acromegaly include bromocriptine (20 to 60 mg/d) and octreotide (100 to 200 μg every 8 h), both of which can inhibit secretion of growth hormone by the pituitary. These agents produce symptomatic improvement in approximately half of patients.

GYNECOMASTIA   Ectopic production of hCG or estrogens by tumors such as cancers of the lung and testis is responsible for approximately 3 percent of cases of gynecomastia detected in men (see Chap. 338). Ectopic production of hCG is the most common cause of paraneoplastic gynecomastia; the hCG acts by stimulating the Leydig cells of the testis to produce increased amounts of estrogen. Alternatively, on rare occasions, a tumor (such as a hepatoma or a germ cell tumor with choriocarcinoma elements) contains aromatase enzyme activity that converts circulating androgens to estrogen. Leydig cell or Sertoli cell tumors may also secrete estradiol. In all cases, the increased ratio of estrogen to testosterone leads to the proliferation of breast tissue and gynecomastia. Other tumors rarely associated with ectopic gynecomastia include carcinoid tumors of the bronchus, intestine, and small cell lung cancer.

The clinical manifestations of gynecomastia are described in Chap. 338. About 5 percent of men with testicular choriocarcinoma present with an enlarging breast mass. In the absence of an obvious cancer, men presenting with gynecomastia should have a careful examination of the testes and measurement of serum hCG. Patients with a testicular mass should undergo an inguinal orchiectomy for diagnosis and treatment. If no testicular mass is found by physical examination, the testes should be examined with ultrasound. Patients with an elevated hCG level and no testicular mass should undergo a workup for an extragonadal germ cell tumor.

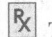 **TREATMENT**

The therapy of tumor-associated gynecomastia should be directed at the underlying cancer: Chemotherapy is used for testicular cancers, and surgical resection or radiation therapy for carcinoids and islet cell tumors. In patients with testicular cancer, gynecomastia completely resolves in three-fourths of cases.

NON-ISLET CELL TUMOR HYPOGLYCEMIA Hypoglycemia that is not caused by the ectopic production of insulin (as in patients with islet cell tumors of the pancreas) can occur with large, slow-growing sarcomas (see Chap. 335). Ectopic production of IGF-2 is responsible for hypoglycemia in most patients with non-islet cell tumors. The ectopically produced IGF-2 inhibits glycogenolysis and gluconeogenesis in the liver, suppresses lipolysis, and increases peripheral glucose utilization, thereby causing hypoglycemia. IGF-2 may also act as an autocrine growth factor for the tumor.

Patients with large sarcomas (1 to 10 kg) may develop hypoglycemia, particularly with fasting. Headache, fatigue, confusion, or seizures may occur. Patients with a large sarcoma and hypoglycemia are likely to have non-islet cell tumor hypoglycemia. Although IGF-2 protein or mRNA is detectable in tumor tissue, the diagnosis is usually made on clinical grounds, because the plasma levels of IGF-2 are typically not elevated. Levels of IGF binding proteins may be increased.

 TREATMENT

The therapy of non-islet cell hypoglycemia should be directed at the underlying cancer and should consist of surgical resection or radiation therapy. Patients whose tumor cannot be successfully resected or irradiated can be treated with frequent oral feedings or constant intravenous administration of glucose.

HEMATOLOGIC SYNDROMES

The elevation of granulocyte, platelet, and eosinophil counts in most patients with myeloproliferative disorders is caused by the proliferation of the myeloid elements due to the underlying disease rather than by a paraneoplastic syndrome. The paraneoplastic hematologic syndromes in patients with solid tumors are less well characterized than the endocrine syndromes, because the ectopic hormone(s) or cytokines responsible have not been identified in most of these tumors (Table 102-2). The severity of the paraneoplastic syndromes parallels the course of the cancer.

ERYTHROCYTOSIS Ectopic production of erythropoietin by cancer cells causes most paraneoplastic erythrocytosis. The ectopically produced erythropoietin stimulates the production of red blood cells in the bone marrow and raises the hematocrit. Other lymphokines and hormones produced by cancer cells may stimulate erythropoietin release but have not been proven to cause erythrocytosis.

Most patients with erythrocytosis have an elevated hematocrit (>52 percent in men and >48 percent in women) that is detected on a routine blood count. Approximately 3 percent of patients with renal cell cancers, 10 percent of patients with hepatocarcinomas, and 15 percent of patients with cerebellar hemangioblastomas have erythrocytosis. In most cases the erythrocytosis is asymptomatic.

Patients with erythrocytosis due to a renal cell cancer, hepatocarcinoma, or central nervous system cancer should have measurement of red cell mass. If the red cell mass is elevated, the serum erythropoietin level should be measured. Patients with an appropriate cancer, elevated erythropoietin levels, and no other explanation for erythrocytosis (e.g., a hemoglobinopathy that causes increased O_2 affinity, see Chap. 107) have the paraneoplastic syndrome.

Table 102-2

Paraneoplastic Hematologic Syndromes

Syndrome	Proteins	Cancers Typically Associated with Syndrome
Erythrocytosis	Erythropoietin	Renal cancers
		Hepatocarcinoma
		Cerebellar hemangioblastomas
Granulocytosis	G-CSF	Lung cancer
	GM-CSF	Gastrointestinal cancer
	IL-6	Ovarian cancer
		Genitourinary cancer
Thrombocytosis	IL-6	Lung cancer
		Gastrointestinal cancer
		Breast cancer
		Ovarian cancer
		Lymphoma
Eosinophilia	IL-5	Lymphoma
		Leukemia
		Lung cancer
Thrombophlebitis	Unknown	Lung cancer
		Pancreatic cancer
		Gastrointestinal cancer
		Breast cancer
		Genitourinary cancer
		Ovarian cancer
		Prostate cancer
		Lymphoma

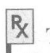 **TREATMENT**

Successful resection of the cancer usually causes the erythrocytosis to resolve. If the tumor neither can be resected nor treated effectively with radiation therapy or chemotherapy, phlebotomy may control any symptoms related to erythrocytosis.

GRANULOCYTOSIS Approximately 30 percent of patients with solid tumors have granulocytosis (granulocyte count > 8000/μL). In about half of patients with granulocytosis and cancer, the granulocytosis has an identifiable nonparaneoplastic etiology (infection, tumor necrosis, glucocorticoid administration, etc.). The other patients have proteins in urine and serum that stimulate the growth of bone marrow cells. A few tumors and tumor cell lines from patients with lung and bladder cancer have been documented to produce granulocyte colony stimulating factor (G-CSF), granulocyte-macrophage colony stimulating factor (GM-CSF), and/or IL-6. However, the etiology of granulocytosis has not been characterized in most patients.

Patients with granulocytosis are nearly all asymptomatic, and the differential white blood cell count does not have a shift to immature forms of neutrophils. Granulocytosis occurs in 40 percent of patients with lung and gastrointestinal cancers, 20 percent of patients with breast cancer, 30 percent of patients with brain tumors and ovarian cancers, and 10 percent of patients with renal cell carcinoma. Patients with advanced-stage disease are more likely to have granulocytosis than those with early-stage disease.

Paraneoplastic granulocytosis does not require treatment. The granulocytosis resolves when the underlying cancer is successfully treated.

THROMBOCYTOSIS Thirty-five percent of patients with thrombocytosis (platelet count > 400,000/μL) have an underlying diagnosis of cancer. IL-6, a candidate molecule for the etiology of paraneoplastic thrombocytosis, stimulates the production of platelets in vitro and in vivo. Some patients with cancer and thrombocytosis have elevated levels of IL-6 in plasma. Another candidate molecule is thrombopoietin, a peptide hormone that stimulates megakaryocyte proliferation and platelet production. The etiology of thrombocytosis has not been established in most cases.

Patients with thrombocytosis are nearly all asymptomatic. There is no clear link between thrombocytosis and thrombosis in patients with cancer. Thrombocytosis is present in 40 percent of patients with lung and gastrointestinal cancers, 20 percent of patients with breast and ovarian cancers, and 10 percent of patients with lymphoma and is most likely to be present in advanced-stage disease. Paraneoplastic thrombocytosis does not require treatment.

EOSINOPHILIA Eosinophilia is present in approximately 1 percent of patients with cancer. Tumors and tumor cell lines from patients with lymphomas or leukemia may produce IL-5, which stimulates eosinophil growth. Activation of IL-5 transcription in lymphomas and leukemias may involve translocation of the long arm of chromosome 5, to which the genes for IL-5 and other cytokines map.

Patients with eosinophilia are typically asymptomatic. Eosinophilia is present in 10 percent of patients with lymphoma, 3 percent of patients with lung cancer, and occasional patients with cervical, gastrointestinal, renal, and breast cancer. Patients with markedly elevated eosinophil counts ($>5000/\mu L$) can develop shortness of breath and wheezing. A chest radiograph may reveal diffuse pulmonary infiltrates from eosinophil infiltration and activation in the lungs.

℞ TREATMENT

Definitive treatment is directed at the underlying malignancy: Tumors should be resected or treated with radiation or chemotherapy. In most patients who develop shortness of breath related to eosinophilia, symptoms resolve with the use of oral or inhaled glucocorticoids.

THROMBOPHLEBITIS Approximately 15 percent of patients who develop deep venous thrombosis or pulmonary embolism have a diagnosis of cancer (see Chap. 118). The coexistence of peripheral venous thrombosis with visceral carcinoma, particularly pancreatic cancer, is called *Trousseau's syndrome*.

Pathogenesis Patients with cancer are predisposed to thromboembolism because they are often at bedrest or immobilized. In addition, clotting may be promoted by release of procoagulants or cytokines from tumor cells or associated inflammatory cells, or by platelet adhesion or aggregation. The specific molecules that mediate the increased risk of thromboembolism have not been identified.

Clinical Manifestations Patients with cancer who develop deep venous thrombosis usually develop swelling or pain in the leg, and physical examination reveals tenderness, warmth, and redness. Patients who present with pulmonary embolism develop dyspnea, chest pain, and syncope, and physical examination shows tachycardia, cyanosis, and hypotension. Approximately 5 percent of patients with no history of cancer who have a diagnosis of deep venous thrombosis or pulmonary embolism will have a diagnosis of cancer within 1 year. The most common cancers associated with thromboembolic episodes include lung, pancreatic, gastrointestinal, breast, ovarian, and genitourinary cancers, lymphomas, and brain tumors. Patients with cancer who undergo surgical procedures requiring general anesthesia have a 20 to 30 percent risk of deep venous thrombosis.

Diagnosis The diagnosis of deep venous thrombosis in patients with cancer is made by an evaluation with impedance plethysmography. If this evaluation suggests the presence of a clot in the vein, venography and/or Doppler ultrasound can confirm the diagnosis. Patients with symptoms and signs suggesting a pulmonary embolism should be evaluated with a chest radiograph, electrocardiogram, arterial blood gas analysis, and ventilation–perfusion scan. Patients with equivocal ventilation–perfusion findings should be considered for a pulmonary angiogram.

Patients without a diagnosis of cancer who present with an initial episode of thrombophlebitis or pulmonary embolus need no additional tests for cancer other than a careful history and physical exam. In light of the many possible primary sites, diagnostic testing in asymptomatic patients is wasteful. However, if the clot is refractory to standard treatment or is in an unusual site, or if the thrombophlebitis is migratory or recurrent, additional efforts to find an underlying cancer are indicated.

℞ TREATMENT

Patients with cancer and a diagnosis of deep venous thrombosis or pulmonary embolism should be treated initially with intravenous heparin. Patients with proximal deep venous thrombosis and a relative contraindication to heparin anticoagulation (brain metastases or pericardial effusion) should be considered for placement of a filter in the inferior vena cava (Greenfield filter) to prevent pulmonary embolism. Coumadin should be administered for 3 to 6 months. Patients with cancer who undergo a major surgical procedure should be considered for heparin prophylaxis or pneumatic boots. Breast cancer patients undergoing chemotherapy and patients with implanted catheters should be considered for prophylaxis (1 mg coumadin per day).

→ *Cutaneous paraneoplastic syndromes are discussed in Chap. 57. Neurologic paraneoplastic syndromes are discussed in Chap. 103. More extensive discussion of functional endocrine tumors is given in Chap. 95.*

BIBLIOGRAPHY

BARTTER F, SCHWARTZ W: The syndrome of inappropriate secretion of antidiuretic hormone. Am J Med 42:790, 1967

BECKER M, ARON DC: Ectopic ACTH syndrome and CRH-mediated Cushing's syndrome. Endocrinol Metab Clin North Am 23:585, 1994

BRAUNSTEIN GD: Gynecomastia. N Engl J Med 328:490, 1993

FAGLIA G et al: Ectopic acromegaly. Endocrinol Metab Clin North Am 21:575, 1992

GROSS AJ et al: Atrial natriuretic factor and arginine vasopressin production in tumor cell lines from patients with lung cancer and their relationship to serum sodium. Cancer Res 53:67, 1993

KAUSHANSKY K: Thrombopoietin: The primary regulator of platelet production. Blood 86:419, 1995

PRANDONI P et al: Deep-vein thrombosis and the incidence of subsequent symptomatic cancer. N Engl J Med 327:1128, 1992

RAUE F, PECHERSTORFER M: Drug therapy of hypercalcemia due to malignancy. Recent Results Cancer Res 137:138, 1994

SORENSEN JB et al: Syndrome of inappropriate secretion of antidiuretic hormone (SIADH) in malignant disease. J Intern Med 238:97, 1995

WINQUIST EW et al: Ketoconazole in the management of paraneoplastic Cushing's syndrome secondary to ectopic adrenocorticotropin production. J Clin Oncol 13:157, 1995

103

Robert H. Brown

PARANEOPLASTIC NEUROLOGIC SYNDROMES

Neoplasia can alter neurologic function in numerous ways, as outlined in Table 103-1. Several neurologic syndromes have been delineated that are a consequence of a remotely located neoplasm but do not arise from direct involvement of the nervous system by metastasis or from a known secondary complication of cancer or its therapy (e.g., malnutrition, opportunistic infection, drug-induced neuropathy). These paraneoplastic syndromes, outlined in Table 103-2, share several characteristics. They are clinically dramatic, arising subacutely in weeks or even days to produce neurologic symptoms that may be profoundly disabling. They may precede detection of the neoplasm by months or even years; their recognition should prompt a timely search for carcinoma. More than one syndrome may arise with a given neoplasm. In general, as outlined in Table 103-2, certain syndromes are associated with particular types of tumors. The diagnosis of a paraneoplastic neurologic disorder depends primarily on (1) the presence of a recognized clinical syndrome; (2) careful exclusion of other cancer-related

Table 103-1

CHAPTER 103
Paraneoplastic Neurologic Syndromes **623**

Effects of Malignancy on the Nervous System

Direct invasion
Metastatic invasion
  Parenchymatous
  Vascular (neoplastic angioendotheliosis)
  Meningeal (meningeal carcinomatosis)
Opportunistic infections
  Bacterial (e.g., listeriosis)
  Nonbacterial
    Typical and atypical viral (e.g., progressive multifocal
      leukoencephalopathy)
    Fungal (e.g., cryptococcosis)
Complications of antineoplastic therapy
  Complications of radiation therapy (e.g., radiation necrosis)
  Complications of chemotherapy (e.g., vincristine neuropathy)
Metabolic complications
  Nutritional deficiency
  Ectopic hormone production
Paraneoplastic syndromes

disorders, as in Table 103-1; and (3) in some instances, confirmatory laboratory studies, including measurement of serum or cerebrospinal fluid (CSF) antibodies with specific patterns of reactivity (Table 103-3) or electromyographic studies to detect findings typical of myasthenia gravis or myasthenic syndrome. CSF often shows protein elevation and a mild lymphocytic pleocytosis.

INCIDENCE Studies of the incidence of these syndromes are problematic because the syndromes are rare and because classifications vary among studies. In one series, these syndromes were detected in 7 percent of nearly 1500 patients with tumors, although recent studies suggest that the true incidence may be lower. Tumors that are most often associated with paraneoplastic neurologic syndromes are cancers of the lung (47 percent), stomach (12 percent), breast (12 percent), ovary (9 percent), and colon (6 percent). Paraneoplastic neurologic syndromes are encountered in one-sixth of all cases of ovarian tumors, one-seventh of lung tumor cases, and less frequently in cases of stomach, prostate, or breast cancer.

PATHOLOGIC CHANGES One group of paraneoplastic syndromes is characterized by *encephalomyelitis*, in which perivascular lymphocytosis, microglial proliferation, and loss of neurons occur. While these changes may be diffuse throughout the neuraxis, they often predominate in a specific anatomic location that dictates the resulting clinical abnormalities. Thus, as outlined below, the manifestations of limbic encephalitis may differ from those of brainstem encephalitis. Inflammatory destruction of the sensory neuronal cell bodies (*neuronopathy*) in the dorsal root ganglia results in wallerian degeneration of axons in peripheral nerves and corresponding ascending long tracts (posterior columns of the spinal cord).

In a second pathologic form of paraneoplastic disease, severe degeneration or loss of neurons occurs without inflammation. This is exemplified by the selective loss of Purkinje neurons in the cerebellum in subacute cortical cerebellar degeneration. This disorder may occur in isolation or concurrently with encephalomyelitis; thus, in cortical cerebellar degeneration there may be some accompanying cerebellar inflammation. In other paraneoplastic syndromes, the associated pathologic changes occur in the peripheral nervous system and consist of multifocal demyelination, myonecrosis, or ultrastructural changes in the neuromuscular junction.

PATHOGENESIS Several mechanisms have been invoked to explain these disorders, including release by the tumor of neurotoxic substances, viral or retroviral infections of tumor, and/or neural tissues, and an autoimmune response directed against common antigenic determinants expressed by the tumor and the affected neural cells. Some paraneoplastic disorders are characterized by serum and CSF antibodies with highly specific patterns of reactivity with neural tissue or muscle. These are exemplified by the Lambert-Eaton myasthenic syndrome and myasthenia gravis, in which circulating antibodies react with pre- and postsynaptic proteins, respectively. Both syndromes have

been reproduced in animals by passive administration of fractionated immunoglobulins. In some cases of paraneoplastic cerebellar degeneration, serum and spinal fluid antibodies react specifically with cerebellar cytoplasmic antigens. In some instances, immunoglobulins from patients with different paraneoplastic neurologic syndromes may produce similar patterns of reactivity against neural tissue. Thus, antibodies recognizing neuronal nuclear antigens are common in patients with small cell carcinoma of the lung (SCLC), which may be associated with paraneoplastic encephalomyelitis or subacute sensory neuronopathy. In these cases, it appears that one or more pathogenic antibodies, possibly cross-reacting with antigens on the tumor, may provoke autoimmune neural injury in more than one region of the neuraxis. Detection of such antibodies may confirm that an evolving neurologic disorder is of paraneoplastic origin even though the antibodies are not diagnostic of a specific neurologic syndrome.

In general, treatment of the paraneoplastic disorders is difficult and is often unsuccessful. Resection of the underlying tumor is surprisingly ineffective, although there are isolated reports of symptomatic improvement following tumor removal. Immunosuppression is also of little benefit for most paraneoplastic disorders. Plasma exchange or immunosuppression may ameliorate some disorders such as Lambert-Eaton syndrome (see below). Otherwise, therapy is largely symptomatic.

The following is an outline of the salient features of the major paraneoplastic neurologic syndromes.

BRAIN, CEREBELLUM, AND SPINAL CORD Visual Paraneoplastic Syndromes Patients with carcinoma of the lung (and, rarely, of the breast, cervix, or endometrium) may develop progressive, painless loss of vision with photosensitivity due to loss of retinal photoreceptors. Lymphocytic inflammation of the retina accompanies loss of rods and cones. The electroretinogram is typically abnormal, and cells may be present in the spinal fluid. This cancer-associated retinopathy (CAR) is commonly associated with high titers of serum antibodies to one or more CAR antigens, including the 23-kDa photoreceptor protein recoverin, which is implicated in photoreceptor signal transduction.

Paraneoplastic Encephalomyelitis SCLC may precipitate an encephalomyelitis of variable distribution and, in consequence, variable but often overlapping clinical presentations. In addition, it is often accompanied by an inflammatory paraneoplastic sensory neuronopathy (see below). Serum and CSF from patients with paraneoplastic encephalomyelitis and neuropathy demonstrate antibodies to neuronal nuclear antigens. These antibodies recognize at least three closely homologous 35- to 40-kDa proteins (HuD, HuC, and Hel-N1) believed to be neuronal RNA-binding proteins required for normal neuronal differentiation.

Limbic Encephalitis In some cases, the encephalitis is most extensive in limbic structures such as the hippocampus and amygdala, producing affective changes in personality (anxiety and agitated depression), selective early memory loss suggestive of Korsakoff's psychosis, or confusion and hallucinations. In some cases, the initial presentation is an amnesic syndrome. The affective disorder often prompts psychiatric evaluation. Abnormalities of the electroencephalogram or overt seizures may be present early in the syndrome. While cognition may be spared initially, dementia is common as the disease progresses; symptoms referable to encephalitic involvement in other regions are often superimposed.

Brainstem Encephalitis Symptoms of brainstem encephalitis relate directly to the distribution of the inflammation. The predominant symptoms are due to medullary involvement producing nausea, vomiting, nystagmus, vertigo, and ataxia. A syndrome suggestive of progressive bulbar palsy with marked dysarthria and dysphagia is associated with pontine involvement. Mesencephalic inflammation and neuronal loss result in nuclear or internuclear eye movement abnormalities; diplopia and oscillopsia may be disabling. Rostral midbrain and nigral involvement may cause rigidity.

Cerebellar Encephalitis Inflammatory changes are rare in the cerebellar cortex but may be severe in deep cerebellar nuclei such as the dentate nucleus, causing myoclonus.

Table 103-2

Paraneoplastic Neurologic Syndromes

Site	Evolution	Clinical Features*	Cancer	Pathology
BRAIN AND CEREBELLUM				
Photoreceptor, retinal degeneration	Weeks to months	Painless visual loss progressing to blindness[1]	SCLC, rarely cervical cancer	Loss of rods and cones, infiltration of retina with mononuclear cells
Limbic encephalitis	Weeks to months	Agitated, confusional state, memory loss followed by dementia[2]	SCLC	Neuronal loss in medial temporal lobe and elsewhere in the limbic system, perivascular and meningeal lymphocytic infiltration
Brainstem encephalitis	Days to weeks	Nystagmus, diplopia, vertigo, ataxia, dysarthria, dysphagia[2]	SCLC	Neuronal loss in brainstem, inflammatory changes as above
Subacute cortical cerebellar degeneration	Weeks to months	Cerebellar ataxia, dysarthria[2,3]	SCLC, ovarian and breast cancer, Hodgkin's disease	Loss of Purkinje cells
Opsoclonus-myoclonus	Weeks	Dancing eyes and feet, cerebellar ataxia, and possibly encephalopathy in adults[2,4]	Neuroblastoma, bronchial carcinoma	In adults, degeneration of dentate nuclei
SPINAL CORD				
Necrotizing myelopathy	Hours, days, or weeks	Para- or quadriplegia with areflexia, sensory loss and bladder dysfunction	SCLC, lymphoma	Severe necrosis of gray and white matter
Subacute motor neuronopathy	Weeks or months	Flaccid weakness and muscle atrophy; legs affected more than arms	Non-Hodgkin's lymphoma	Inflammation of ventral horns, loss of anterior horn cells
PERIPHERAL NERVE				
Acute demyelinating polyneuropathy (Guillain Barré syndrome)	Hours to days	Ascending paralysis, areflexia, possibly ascending sensory loss, high spinal fluid protein level	Hodgkin's disease	Segmental demyelination, inflammation of peripheral nerves
Chronic demyelinating polyneuropathy	Weeks to months	Chronic progressive or relapsing weakness with sensory loss, high spinal fluid protein level	Rarely lung, breast, or gastric cancer; lymphoma, myeloma	As in acute demyelinating polyneuropathy
Neuropathy with paraproteinemia	Weeks to months	Chronic; may be predominantly sensory or motor[2,5]	Myeloma, osteosclerotic myeloma	As in chronic demyelinating polyneuropathy
Subacute sensory neuronopathy	Weeks to months	Severe sensory loss with areflexia and ataxia; paresthesias, pain[2]	SCLC and other lung tumors	Inflammation and neuronal degeneration in dorsal root ganglia; secondary axon loss
Sensorimotor neuropathy	Weeks to months	Distal motor and sensory loss[2]	SCLC and other tumors	Axonopathy, some segmental loss of myelin
NEUROMUSCULAR JUNCTION				
Lambert-Eaton myasthenic syndrome	Weeks to months	Proximal weakness, fatigability, dry mouth, possibly ptosis[6]	SCLC; cancers of the breast, prostate, stomach	Disruption of active zones on presynaptic terminals
Myasthenia gravis	Weeks to months	Weakness, fatigability, ptosis, diplopia[7]	Thymoma	Disruption of postsynaptic junctional membrane folds
MUSCLE				
Polymyositis	Months to years	Proximal weakness, myalgias, cardiomyopathy, high creatine phosphokinase level	Possible association with breast, ovary, lung tumors; lymphoma	Lymphocytic inflammation of muscle interstitium; myofiber necrosis, phagocytosis
Necrotizing myopathy	Days to weeks	Rapidly progressive proximal weakness, possibly dysphagia, dyspnea	Bronchial carcinoma, SCLC	Severe myonecrosis with minimal inflammation or phagocytosis

* Superscripts denote possible immunoglobulin reactivity as in Table 103-3.

Myelitis In paraneoplastic myelitis, the gray matter of the cord is diffusely infiltrated with leukocytes, leading to profound neuronal degeneration. The myelitis may be widespread through the cord or restricted to a few segmental levels. Anterior horn cell destruction typically produces muscle weakness and neurogenic atrophy, which is often asymmetric. There may be selective involvement of the neck and upper extremities or lower extremities alone. Corticospinal findings (hyperreflexia, weakness, Babinski signs) result from involvement

Table 103-3
CHAPTER 103
Paraneoplastic Neurologic Syndromes
625

Defined Antibodies Associated with Paraneoplastic Neurologic Syndromes*

Antibody†	Paraneoplastic Syndrome	Tumor	Antigen
[1]Anti-CAR	Retinopathy	SCLC	Recoverin, 25-kDa cone Ca^{2+} binding protein
[2]Anti-Hu	Encephalomyelitis, sensory neuronopathy	Mainly SCLC	35- to 40-kDa nuclear RNA-binding proteins
[3]Anti-Yo	Cerebellar degeneration	Gynecologic tumors, breast cancer	34- and 62-kDa leucine zipper proteins
[4]Anti-Ri	Opsoclonus-myoclonus	Breast cancer	55-kDa RNA-binding protein in motor system neurons
[5]Anti-MAG	Demyelinating neuropathy	Myeloma	Myelin-associated glycoprotein
[6]LEMS Ab	Lambert-Eaton myasthenic syndrome	SCLC	Voltage-sensitive calcium channel and associated proteins
[7]MG Ab	Myasthenia gravis	Thymoma	Acetylcholine receptor subunit

* Other patterns of reactivity have also been described for some of these antigens.
† Superscripts correspond to the antibody activities noted in Table 103-2.

of this tract in the cord or brainstem. The corticospinal tract dysfunction (and in some cases motor neuronopathy) should not be confused with motor neuron disease; typical amyotrophic lateral sclerosis does not appear to arise on a paraneoplastic basis. The presence of sensory signs with cancer denotes either dorsal root ganglioradiculitis or inflammation of the posterior horns.

Necrotizing Myelopathy This is a rare complication of malignancy, presenting clinically as a subacute, transverse myelitis, often in a thoracic location. It can be distinguished from the less fulminant encephalomyelitis described above by the evolution of an intensely necrotic, central thoracic cord lesion which tails off rostrally and caudally over several segmental levels. In some instances, there are multiple necrotic foci within the cord. Clinical findings include leg (and possibly arm) plegia, sensory loss, and loss of sphincter control. The lesion frequently is asymmetrical initially, mimicking a Brown-Séquard syndrome. In severe cases, the protein concentration and cell count in the CSF are increased, and myelography demonstrates focal cord swelling. Although not all cases are associated with tumor, lung cancers, lymphoma, and leukemia are known to occur in such patients.

Opsoclonus-Myoclonus A syndrome of opsoclonus, myoclonus, and ataxia ("dancing eyes–dancing feet") occurs in both children and adults. About one-half of affected children have differentiated neuroblastomas, usually in the thorax. In adults, the syndrome may be associated with solid tumors such as bronchial carcinoma. The onset is subacute, and in some instances the syndrome lasts for months and is followed by permanent encephalopathy or retardation. Pathologic findings in adults include prominent neuronal degeneration in the dentate nucleus of the cerebellum, suggesting a relationship to cortical cerebellar degeneration. Occasionally there is diffuse lymphocytic cuffing in the central nervous system and cerebrospinal fluid pleocytosis. In some individuals, this syndrome responds to glucocorticoids or treatment of the cancer. A subgroup of women developing opsoclonus with breast cancer have an antibody (anti-Ri) directed against a 55-kDa RNA-binding protein present in the nuclei of neurons and of the associated tumors.

Subacute Cortical Cerebellar Degeneration Subacute cortical cerebellar degeneration (SCCD) is a subacutely progressive cerebellar disorder characterized by profound truncal and appendicular ataxia arising in association with gynecologic tumors (ovarian in 50 percent of cases; breast in 25 percent), SCLC, or Hodgkin's disease. Symptoms referable to the brainstem include vertigo, dysarthria, diplopia and nystagmus, and corticospinal signs. As a rule, any nonfamilial ataxia arising in a patient over the age of 45 should raise the suspicion of this entity. By contrast with paraneoplastic encephalomyelitis, described above, the predominant pathologic finding in SCCD is widespread loss of cerebellar Purkinje cell neurons with astrogliosis and secondary loss of Purkinje cell axons. Many cases are associated with dementia for which an anatomic basis has not been well established. The CSF commonly reveals a mild pleocytosis; cerebellar atrophy may be evident on magnetic resonance imaging or computed tomography scans.

Several types of anti-Purkinje cell antibodies have been detected in sera of patients with subacute cerebellar degeneration. Women with cancer of the breast or ovary and SCCD demonstrate antibodies (anti-Yo) recognizing a family of 34-kDa cytoplasmic leucine zipper proteins expressed in Purkinje cell neurons and in the gynecologic tumors. About a third of patients with Hodgkin's disease have anti-Purkinje cell antibodies that recognize an antigen distinct from that detected by anti-Yo antisera. A different cytoplasmic antigen is recognized by immunoglobulins from patients with SCCD and adenocarcinoma of the lung. In some patients with SCLC and SCCD, anti-Hu antibodies (see above) are present. Finally, a small subset of patients with SCCD and SCLC do not have anti-Hu or anti-Purkinje cell antibodies; in these patients, SCCD may coexist with Lambert-Eaton myasthenic syndrome (below).

PERIPHERAL NERVES A number of clinical syndromes affecting the peripheral nerves occur in association with malignancy. Paraneoplastic *subacute sensory neuropathy*, arguably the most clinically distinctive of these syndromes, is a ganglioradiculitis which may arise with other manifestations of encephalomyelitis. Other paraneoplastic neuropathies are difficult to distinguish from noncarcinomatous neuropathies. However, their recognition is important, as they are relatively common and their manifestations often precede diagnosis of the underlying neoplasia. By electrodiagnostic criteria, neuropathy may be evident in as many as 50 percent of patients with lung cancer. In evaluating a possible paracarcinomatous neuropathy, it is particularly helpful to ascertain whether the neuropathy (1) affects motor fibers, sensory fibers, or both; (2) predominantly involves axons or myelin, or (3) occurs with an abnormal serum paraprotein.

Subacute Sensory Neuronopathy This disorder primarily affects axons, with relative sparing of myelin. The typical pathology is a ganglioradiculitis, as noted earlier. Clinically, the onset is characterized by the subacute development of paresthesias and pain (sometimes severe) in the distal limbs and associated truncal sensory ataxia. The sensory ataxia may be profoundly disabling. Although often initially restricted only to arms and legs, the symptoms eventually affect all four extremities. In most cases, symptoms of the neuronopathy precede the diagnosis of the underlying malignancy by more than a year. The serum of some patients contains anti-Hu antibodies.

Acute Demyelinating Polyneuropathy Acute inflammatory demyelinating polyneuropathy (Guillain-Barré syndrome), discussed in detail elsewhere (Chap. 381), is characterized by subacutely ascending paralysis, sensory loss which is often mild by comparison with the motor deficits, areflexia, and a characteristic elevation of spinal fluid protein concentration without pleocytosis. Histopathology reveals lymphocytic infiltration of nerves, segmental demyelination, and relative axonal sparing. This disorder is associated with Hodgkin's disease.

Chronic Demyelinating Polyneuropathy Chronic demyelinating polyneuropathy includes a group of chronic progressive or relapsing, inflammatory demyelinating peripheral neuropathies that are distinguished from acute polyneuritis by their time course, more prominent involvement of sensory nerves, lack of involvement of autonomic nerves, and responsiveness to immunotherapy. As in acute demyelinating polyneuropathy, the demyelinating nature of these neuropathies is manifested physiologically by abnormalities such as slowed nerve conduction velocities or dispersion of compound muscle action potentials; the pathologic hallmark of both conditions is segmental loss of myelin with relative preservation of axons. In some cases, physiologic studies reveal only marginal slowing of conduction, while the biopsy clearly demonstrates selective myelin loss. Sural nerve biopsy may fail to reveal any alterations when the demyelination is proximal (and therefore detectable only with electrophysiologic methods). Elevation of the spinal fluid protein concentration helps confirm the diagnosis.

Chronic demyelinating polyneuropathy usually is not associated with neoplasia. Rarely, however, it occurs in association with solid tumors of the lung, breast, and stomach. It also occurs with Waldenstrom's macroglobulinemia, gamma heavy chain disease, and lymphoma. In many instances, the paraneoplastic form is characterized by the presence of a serum paraprotein, typically a monoclonal immunoglobulin ("M component"). As many as 10 to 15 percent of patients with monoclonal gammopathies of undetermined significance develop significant hematologic disease, including myeloma.

Two chronic demyelinating neuropathies are distinctive in this context. The first is associated with a monoclonal IgM that reacts with a myelin-associated glycoprotein (MAG) in peripheral nerve myelin. This pattern of reactivity occurs in about half of patients with an IgM gammopathy and neuropathy. This IgM anti-MAG neuropathy is more sensory than motor; it is only slowly progressive, as compared to the subacute sensory neuropathy (below). It remains to be established whether the anti-MAG antibody is a cause or consequence of the demyelination. The second distinctive subtype of chronic demyelinating polyneuropathy occurs with osteosclerotic myeloma and monoclonal IgG or IgA antibodies that do not react with MAG. This polyneuropathy is predominantly motor and often quite indolent, although it may eventually produce severe limb wasting. Sensory and autonomic findings are unusual. A related group of patients develop polyneuropathy, organomegaly, endocrinopathy, the M protein, and skin changes (POEMS syndrome); one-half have osteosclerotic myeloma and IgG or IgA M proteins with lambda light chains. Some patients with demyelinating neuropathies and IgM M proteins respond well to immunosuppressive therapy. Those with osteosclerotic myeloma may improve after treatment of the underlying plasmacytoma, particularly if it is solitary.

Sensorimotor Neuropathy This category of mixed sensory and motor axonopathy is perhaps the most common paraneoplastic neuropathy. Symptoms depend on the severity of the neuropathy and may include muscle wasting and weakness, distal limb paresthesias, and sometimes pain. Pathologically there is noninflammatory degeneration of axons and mild myelin loss, presumably secondary to the axonopathy. Paraneoplastic sensorimotor neuropathy has been reported with several types of tumors (SCLC, breast, stomach) and hematologic malignancies (Hodgkin's disease, lymphoma, multiple myeloma). In amyloidosis, itself often associated with myeloma, there may be an axonal neuropathy with intraneural deposition of amyloid fibrils derived from immunoglobulin light chains. Axonal neuropathy has been reported as a manifestation of occult insulinoma, possibly as a consequence of hypoglycemia. Infrequently, these neuropathies remit spontaneously; often they progress even with aggressive treatment of the underlying malignancy.

Subacute Motor Neuronopathy Another striking paracarcinomatous disorder of peripheral nerves is a subacutely progressive motor neuropathy that causes slowly evolving weakness of the legs heralding an otherwise occult lymphoma. Pathologic changes include loss of motorneurons in the anterolateral gray matter of the spinal cord, gliosis, loss of myelin in ventral roots, and some Schwann cell proliferation. Although there is no clearly effective treatment for this condition, many patients seem to improve following immunosuppressive therapy for the malignancy. In other patients, progression of the weakness may cease independently of the status of the lymphoma.

NEUROMUSCULAR JUNCTION Lambert-Eaton Myasthenic Syndrome (See also Chap. 382) Lambert-Eaton myasthenic syndrome (LEMS) occurs in association with either a malignancy or with other manifestations of autoimmune disease. It is characterized by weakness, myalgias, and fatigability, often most severe in the lower extremities and in the proximal muscles. Ptosis may be seen. Dysautonomic features are common and may include dryness of the mouth and eyes, impotence, diminished sweating, and orthostatic symptoms. The disorder afflicts men more often than women. The incidence of associated malignancy is 70 percent in men and 25 percent in women. In most cases the tumor is SCLC. The predominant clinical finding is a striking reduction in strength at rest with transient improvement in power on repetitive maximal exertion. Edrophonium chloride (Tensilon) has no effect or may marginally improve strength. Electromyography demonstrates motor unit potentials whose amplitude is low at rest but increases with exercise or tetanic stimulation; this contrasts with the electromyographic findings in myasthenia gravis. Electron microscopy of the presynaptic motor nerve terminals at the neuromuscular junction reveals a decrease in the number of active zones, which are believed to correspond to voltage-sensitive calcium channels. LEMS is believed to be an autoimmune disorder associated with diminished quantal release of acetylcholine. It is associated with other autoimmune disorders and appears to be HLA-linked (B8 and DRw3 antigens). In paraneoplastic LEMS, physiologic data incriminate antibodies directed against voltage-dependent calcium channels that are present both on tumor cells and on distal motor nerve terminals. Antibody activity has also been detected against the β subunits of these channels and against presynaptic proteins such as synaptotagmin. As noted, LEMS may arise concurrently with other paraneoplastic neurologic syndromes such as SCCD or sensory neuropathy. Treatment is directed toward the underlying neoplasm or autoimmune disease or toward augmenting acetylcholine release with drugs that prolong presynaptic depolarization and thereby enhance calcium influx. Guanidine hydrochloride and 3,4-diaminopyridine may be beneficial in either autoimmune or paraneoplastic LEMS; plasma exchange and immunosuppression may also be effective.

Myasthenia Gravis This disorder, discussed elsewhere in detail (Chap. 382), is characterized by exercise-induced muscle weakness caused by an antibody-mediated reduction in the numbers of acetylcholine receptors at the postsynaptic junction. About 15 percent of cases are associated with thymoma; other autoimmune disorders may coexist.

MUSCLE Polymyositis-Dermatomyositis This subject is discussed in Chap. 315. An increased incidence of malignancy exists in elderly patients with dermatomyositis.

Necrotizing Myopathy Carcinoma of the bronchus is associated rarely with a fatal, subacute, widespread, necrotizing myopathy that involves all muscles, including bulbar and diaphragmatic muscles. Intrafusal muscle fibers are also involved. Deep tendon reflexes are preserved. The muscle undergoes degeneration without phagocytosis or a significant inflammatory response. The cause of the necrotizing process is unknown.

OTHER Several other neurologic syndromes have been reported to be paraneoplastic but are less well characterized than the ones described above. *Stiff-man syndrome*—diffuse hypertonia with painful spasms due to loss of inhibitory spinal interneurons—may arise in association with carcinoma. In the nonneoplastic stiff-man syndrome, autoantibodies have been detected that react with glutamic acid decarboxylase (GAD). This enzyme is essential for the synthesis of gamma-aminobutyric acid, a central nervous system inhibitory neurotransmitter. Similar autoantibodies are present in the serum of patients with insulin-dependent diabetes mellitus, although in stiff-man syndrome the antibodies are present in higher titer and react against different epitopes of GAD. Patients with stiff-man syndrome associated with breast cancer may also have antibodies against the synaptic vesicle–associated protein amphiphysin. Although paraneoplastic syndromes are rare with prostate cancer, a syndrome of *impaired horizontal gaze and orofacial spasm* has been associated with this tumor. Nonfamilial *subacute chorea* and *dystonia* occur with SCLC. *Optic neuritis* may develop as a paraneoplastic disorder, but it is difficult to exclude direct involvement of the optic nerve or chiasm by cancer cells or indirect effects of the underlying malignancy, as outlined in Table 103-1. Among the most striking autoimmune disorders of the nervous system is Rasmussen's encephalitis, a disorder characterized by slowly evolving focal encephalitis; some patients with this disorder have antibodies directed against a glutamate receptor subunit (GluR3). Cases of Rasmussen's disorder with neoplasia have not been reported, although focal, progressive limbic encephalitis (see above) is well documented to be a remote effect of cancer, and patients with paraneoplastic syndromes have been shown recently to possess antibodies against other glutamate receptor subunits (GluR1, GluR4, GluR5/6).

BIBLIOGRAPHY

BUCKANOVICH RJ et al: Nova, the paraneoplastic Ri antigen, is homologous to an RNA-binding protein and is specifically expressed in developing motor system. Neuron 11:657, 1993

DALMAU J, POSNER JB: Neurologic paraneoplastic antibodies (anti-Yo; anti-Hu; anti-Ri): The case for a nomenclature based on antibody and antigen specificity. Neurology 44:2241, 1994

DARNELL RB: Onconeural antigens and the paraneoplastic neurological disorders: At the intersection of cancer, immunity, and the brain. Proc Natl Acad Sci USA 93:4529, 1996

DECAMILLI P et al: The synaptic vesicle-associated protein amphiphysin is the 128-kD autoantigen of stiff-man syndrome with breast cancer. J Exp Med 178:2219, 1993

FURNEAUX HM et al: Characterization of a cDNA encoding a 34-kDa Purkinje neuron protein recognized by sera from patients with paraneoplastic cerebellar degeneration. Proc Natl Acad Sci USA 86:2873, 1989

GAHRING LC et al: Autoantibodies to neuronal glutamate receptors in patients with paraneoplastic neurodegenerative syndrome enhance receptor activation. Mol Med 1:245, 1995

HORMIGO A et al: Immunological and pathological study of anti-Ri-associated encephalopathy. Ann Neurol 36:896, 1994

KIM J et al: Higher autoantibody levels and recognition of a linear NH_2-terminal epitope in the autoantigen GAD_{65} distinguish stiff-man syndrome from insulin-dependent diabetes mellitus. J Exp Med 180:595, 1994

MARTIN-MOUTOT N et al: Synaptotagmin: A Lambert-Eaton myasthenic syndrome antigen that associates with presynaptic calcium channels. J Physiol 87:37, 1993

POLANS AS et al: Recoverin, a photoreceptor-specific calcium-binding protein, expressed by the tumor of a patient with cancer-associated retinopathy. Proc Natl Acad Sci USA 92:9176, 1995

POSNER JB, DALMAU J: Clinical enigmas of paraneoplastic neurologic disorders. Clin Neurol Neurosurg 97:61, 1995

---

104   *Rasim Gucalp, Janice Dutcher*

ONCOLOGIC EMERGENCIES

Emergencies in patients with cancer may be related directly to the underlying cancer or may result from its treatment. They can be classified into three groups: pressure or obstruction caused by a space-occupying lesion, metabolic or hormonal problems (paraneoplastic syndromes, see Chap. 102), and complications arising from the effects of treatment.

STRUCTURAL-OBSTRUCTIVE ONCOLOGIC EMERGENCIES

SUPERIOR VENA CAVA SYNDROME   Superior vena cava syndrome (SVCS) is the clinical manifestation of obstruction of the superior vena cava (SVC), with severe reduction in venous return from the head, neck, and upper extremities. Malignant tumors, such as lung cancer, lymphoma, and metastatic tumors, are responsible for more than 90 percent of all SVCS cases. Lung cancer, particularly of small-cell and squamous-cell histologies, accounts for approximately 85 percent of all cases of malignant origin. Metastatic cancers to the mediastinum, such as testicular and breast carcinomas, account for a small proportion of cases. Other causes include benign tumors, aortic aneurysm, thyroid enlargement, thrombosis, and fibrosing mediastinitis caused by prior irradiation or histoplasmosis.

Patients with SVCS usually present with complaints of neck and facial swelling (especially around the eyes), dyspnea, and cough. Other symptoms include hoarseness, tongue swelling, headaches, nasal congestion, epistaxis, hemoptysis, dysphagia, pain, dizziness, syncope, and lethargy. Bending forward or lying down may aggravate the symptoms. The characteristic physical findings are dilated neck veins, an increased number of collateral veins covering the anterior chest wall, cyanosis, and edema of the face, arms, and chest. More severe cases include proptosis, glossal and laryngeal edema, and mental obtundation. The clinical picture is milder if the obstruction is located above the azygos vein.

Obstruction of recent onset is likeliest to be malignant in origin, whereas a longstanding obstruction is more likely to be of nonmalignant origin. The exception to this rule is SVC thrombosis due to a central venous line, in which the development of clinical symptoms and signs is rapid. The diagnosis of SVCS is essentially a clinical one. The most significant chest radiographic finding is widening of the superior mediastinum, most commonly on the right side. Pleural effusion occurs in only 25 percent of cases, often on the right side. However, a normal chest radiograph is still compatible with the diagnosis if other characteristic findings are present. Computed tomography (CT) provides the most reliable view of the mediastinal anatomy. The diagnosis of SVC syndrome requires diminished or absent opacification of central venous structures with prominent collateral venous circulation. Magnetic resonance imaging (MRI) has no advantages over CT. Invasive procedures, including bronchoscopy, percutaneous needle biopsy, mediastinoscopy, and even thoracotomy can be performed by a skilled clinician without any major risk of bleeding. For patients with a known malignancy, a detailed workup usually is not necessary, and appropriate treatment may be started after obtaining a CT scan of the thorax. For those with no history of malignancy, a detailed evaluation is absolutely necessary to rule out benign causes and also to determine a specific tumor histology to direct the appropriate therapy. This should be obtained before initiation of glucocorticoid or radiation therapy to obtain accurate diagnosis, since in rapidly responding tumors like lymphomas, delay in diagnostic procedures may result in inability to make an exact diagnosis.

℞ **TREATMENT**

The one potentially life-threatening complication of a superior mediastinal mass is tracheal obstruction. Upper airway obstruction demands emergent therapy. Diuretics with a low salt diet, head elevation, and oxygen may produce temporary symptomatic relief.

Radiation therapy is the primary treatment for SVC syndrome caused by non-small cell lung cancer and other metastatic solid tumors. Chemotherapy has been found to be an effective modality for the management of SVC syndrome with underlying malignancies such as small cell carcinoma of the lung or lymphoma. Because these tumors have a tendency to recur locally in areas of bulky disease, radiation therapy is recommended in addition. Surgery may provide immediate relief for patients in whom a benign process is causing obstruction of the SVC.

Clinical improvement occurs in most patients, although this improvement may be due to the development of adequate collateral circulation. The mortality associated with SVCS does not relate to caval obstruction, but rather to the underlying cause.

SVCS and Central Venous Catheters in Adults   The use of long-term central venous catheters has become common practice in patients with cancer. Major vessel thrombosis may occur. In these cases, catheter removal should be combined with anticoagulation to prevent embolization. SVCS in this setting, if detected early, can be treated successfully by fibrinolytic therapy without sacrificing the catheter. Monthly urokinase flushing may reduce the occlusive and infectious complications related to these catheters.

PERICARDIAL EFFUSION/TAMPONADE   Malignant pericardial disease is found at autopsy in 5 to 10 percent of patients with cancer, most frequently in patients with lung cancer, breast cancer, leukemias, and lymphomas. However, cardiac tamponade as the initial presentation of extrathoracic malignancy is rare. The origin is not malignancy in about 50 percent of cancer patients with symptomatic pericardial disease, but instead may be related to irradiation, drug-induced pericarditis, hypothyroidism, idiopathic pericarditis, infection, or autoimmune diseases. Two types of radiation pericarditis have been described: an acute inflammatory, effusive pericarditis occurring within months of irradiation, which usually resolves spontaneously, and a chronic effusive pericarditis that may appear up to 20 years after radiotherapy and is accompanied by a thickened pericardium.

Most patients with pericardial metastasis are asymptomatic. However, the common symptoms are dyspnea, cough, chest pain, orthopnea, and weakness. Pleural effusion, sinus tachycardia, jugular venous distension, hepatomegaly, peripheral edema, and cyanosis are the most frequent physical findings. Relatively specific diagnostic findings, such as paradoxical pulse, diminished heart sounds, pulsus alternans (pulse waves alternating in amplitude between those of greater and lesser volume with successive beats), and friction rub are less common than with nonmalignant pericardial involvement. Chest radiographs and electrocardiography reveal abnormalities in 90 percent of cases, but half of these abnormalities are nonspecific. Echocardiography is the most helpful diagnostic test. Pericardial fluid may be serous, serosanguineous, or hemorrhagic, and cytologic examination of pericardial fluid is diagnostic in most patients. False negative cytology may occur in patients with lymphoma and mesothelioma.

℞ TREATMENT

The treatment of malignant pericardial effusions includes pericardiocentesis with or without the introduction of sclerosing agents, the creation of a pericardial window, complete pericardial stripping, cardiac irradiation, or systemic chemotherapy. Acute pericardial tamponade with life-threatening hemodynamic instability requires immediate drainage of fluid. This can be quickly achieved by pericardiocentesis. Alternatively, subxyphoid pericardiotomy can be performed in 45 min under local anesthesia.

INTESTINAL OBSTRUCTION   Intestinal obstruction and reobstruction is a common problem in patients with advanced cancer, particularly colorectal or ovarian carcinoma. However, other cancers, such as lung or breast cancer and melanoma, can metastasize within the abdomen, leading to intestinal obstruction. Intestinal pseudoobstruction is caused by infiltration of the mesentery or bowel muscle by tumor, involvement of the celiac plexus, or paraneoplastic neuropathy in patients with small cell lung cancer. Paraneoplastic neuropathy is associated with IgG antibodies reactive to neurons of the myenteric and submucosal plexuses of the jejunum and stomach. Ovarian cancer can lead either to authentic luminal obstruction or to pseudoobstruction that results when circumferential invasion of a bowel segment arrests the forward progression of peristaltic contractions.

The onset of obstruction is usually insidious. Pain is the most common symptom and is usually colicky in nature. Pain can also be due to abdominal distension, tumor masses, or hepatomegaly. Vomiting can be intermittent or continuous. Patients with complete obstruction usually have constipation. Physical examination may reveal abdominal distension with tympany, ascites, visible peristalsis, high-pitched bowel sounds, and tumor masses. Erect plain abdominal films may reveal multiple air-fluid levels and dilation of the small or large bowel. Acute cecal dilation to more than 12 to 14 cm is considered a surgical emergency because of the high likelihood of rupture. The overall prognosis for the cancer patient who develops intestinal obstruction is poor, with the median survival being about 3 to 4 months. About one-fourth to one-third of cases are found to have intestinal obstruction due to causes other than cancer. Adhesions from previous operations are a particularly common benign cause. Ileus induced by vincristine is another reversible cause of obstruction.

℞ TREATMENT

The management of intestinal obstruction in patients with advanced malignancy depends on the individual case. The extent of the underlying malignancy and the functional status of the major organs should be determined before decisions are made. The initial management should include surgical evaluation. Operation is not always successful and may lead to further complications with a substantial mortality rate (10 to 20 percent). Patients known to have advanced intraabdominal malignancy should receive a prolonged course of conservative management, including nasogastric decompression. Treatment with antiemetics, antispasmodics, and analgesics may allow patients to remain outside the hospital. The somatostatin analogue octreotide has been used successfully in the management of intestinal obstruction in cancer patients. The inhibitory effect of octreotide on gastrointestinal secretion reduces vomiting and pain.

URINARY OBSTRUCTION   Urinary obstruction may occur in patients with prostatic or gynecologic malignancies, particularly cervical carcinoma, or metastatic disease from a variety of primary sites. Radiation therapy to pelvic tumors may cause fibrosis and subsequent ureteral obstruction. Bladder outlet obstruction is usually due to prostate and cervical cancers and may lead to bilateral hydronephrosis and subsequent renal failure.

Flank pain is the most common symptom. Persistent urinary tract infection, persistent proteinuria, or hematuria in patients with a cancer should alert the physician to the possibility of ureteral obstruction. Total anuria and/or anuria alternating with polyuria may occur. A slow, continuous rise in the serum creatinine value necessitates immediate evaluation in patients with cancer. Renal ultrasound examination is the safest and least expensive way to identify hydronephrosis. The function of an obstructed kidney can be evaluated by a nuclear scan. CT can be helpful in identifying a retroperitoneal mass or retroperitoneal adenopathy.

℞ TREATMENT

Bilateral ureteral or bladder outlet obstruction requires immediate attention. Obstruction associated with flank pain, sepsis, or fistula formation is an indication for palliative urinary diversion. There are many newer techniques by which internal ureteral stents can be placed under local anesthesia. Percutaneous nephrostomy offers an alternative approach for drainage. In the case of bladder outlet obstruction due to malignancy, a suprapubic cystostomy can be used for urinary drainage.

MALIGNANT BILIARY OBSTRUCTION   This common clinical problem can be caused by a primary carcinoma arising in the pancreas, ampulla of Vater, bile duct, or liver or by metastatic disease to the periductal lymph nodes or liver parenchyma. The most common metastatic tumors causing biliary obstruction are gastric, colon, breast, and lung cancers. Jaundice, light-colored stools, dark urine, pruritus, and weight loss due to malabsorption are usual symptoms. Pain and secondary infection are uncommon in malignant biliary obstruction. Ultrasound, CT, or percutaneous transhepatic or endoscopic retrograde cholangiography will identify the site and nature of the biliary obstruction.

℞ TREATMENT

Palliative intervention is indicated only in patients with disabling pruritus resistant to medical treatment, severe malabsorption, or infection. Therapeutic intervention by stenting under radiographic control, surgical bypass, or radiation therapy with or without chemotherapy may alleviate the obstruction. The choice of modality should be based on the site of obstruction (proximal versus distal), the type of tumor (sensitive to radiotherapy, chemotherapy, or neither), and the general condition of the patient. In the absence of pruritus, biliary obstruction may be a largely asymptomatic cause of death.

SPINAL CORD COMPRESSION   Spinal cord compression occurs in 5 to 10 percent of patients with cancer. Epidural tumor is the first manifestation of malignancy in about 10 percent of patients. In most of these cases, the underlying cancer is identified during the initial evaluation; lung cancer is most commonly the primary malignancy.

Metastatic tumor involves the vertebral column more often than any other part of the bony skeleton. Lung, breast, and prostate cancer are the most frequent offenders. Multiple myeloma also has a high incidence of spine involvement. The thoracic spine is the most common site (70 percent), followed by the lumbosacral spine (20 percent) and the cervical spine (10 percent). Involvement of multiple sites is most frequent in patients with breast and prostatic carcinoma. By contrast, carcinoma of the lung almost invariably produces a single site of vertebral involvement. Cord injury develops when metastases to the vertebral body or pedicle enlarge and compress the underlying dura. Another cause of cord compression is direct extension of a paravertebral lesion through the intervertebral foramen. These cases usually involve a lymphoma, myeloma, or pediatric neoplasm. Parenchymal spinal cord metastasis due to hematogenous spread occurs in rare cases.

The most common initial symptom in patients with spinal cord compression is localized back pain and tenderness due to involvement of vertebrae by tumor. Pain is usually present for days or months before other neurologic findings appear. It is exacerbated by movement and by coughing or sneezing. It can be differentiated from the pain of disc disease by the fact that it worsens when the patient lies supine. Radicular pain is less common than localized back pain and usually develops later. Radicular pain in the cervical or lumbosacral areas may be unilateral or bilateral. Radicular pain from the thoracic roots is often bilateral and is described by patients as a feeling of tight, band-like constriction around the thorax and abdomen. Typical cervical radicular pain radiates down the arm; in the lumbar region, the radiation is down the legs. Loss of bowel or bladder control may be the presenting symptom.

On physical examination, pain induced by straight leg raising, neck flexion, or vertebral percussion may help to determine the level of cord compression. Patients develop numbness and paresthesias in the extremities or trunk. Loss of sensibility to pinprick is as common as loss of sensibility to vibration or position. The upper limit of the zone of sensory loss is often one or two vertebrae below the site of compression. Motor findings include weakness, spasticity, and abnormal muscle stretching. The presence of an extensor plantar reflex reflects significant compression. Deep tendon reflexes may be brisk. Motor and sensory loss usually precede sphincter disturbance. Patients with autonomic dysfunction may present with decreased anal tonus, decreased perineal sensibility, and a distended bladder. The absence of the anal wink reflex or the bulbocavernosus reflex confirms cord (conus or cauda equina) involvement. In doubtful cases, evaluation of post-voiding urinary residual volume can be helpful. A residual volume of more than 150 mL suggests bladder dysfunction. Autonomic dysfunction is an unfavorable prognostic factor. Patients with progressive neurologic symptoms should have frequent neurologic examinations and rapid therapeutic intervention.

Patients with known cancer who develop back pain should be evaluated for spinal cord compression as quickly as possible (Fig. 104-1). Treatment is more often successful in patients who are ambulatory and still have sphincter control at the time treatment is initiated. Patients should have a neurologic examination and plain films of the spine. Those whose physical examination suggests cord compression should receive dexamethasone (6 mg per os every 6 h), starting immediately. There is no specific upper limit to the dexamethasone dose. If neurologic function improves in response to 24 mg a day but examination still shows abnormalities, doubling the dose may lead to further improvement.

Erosion of the pedicles (the "winking owl" sign) is the earliest radiologic finding of vertebral tumor. Other radiographic changes include increased intrapedicular distance, vertebral destruction, lytic or sclerotic lesions, scalloped vertebral bodies, and vertebral body collapse. Vertebral collapse is not a reliable indicator of the presence of tumor; about 20 percent of cases of vertebral collapse, particularly those in older patients and postmenopausal women, are not due to

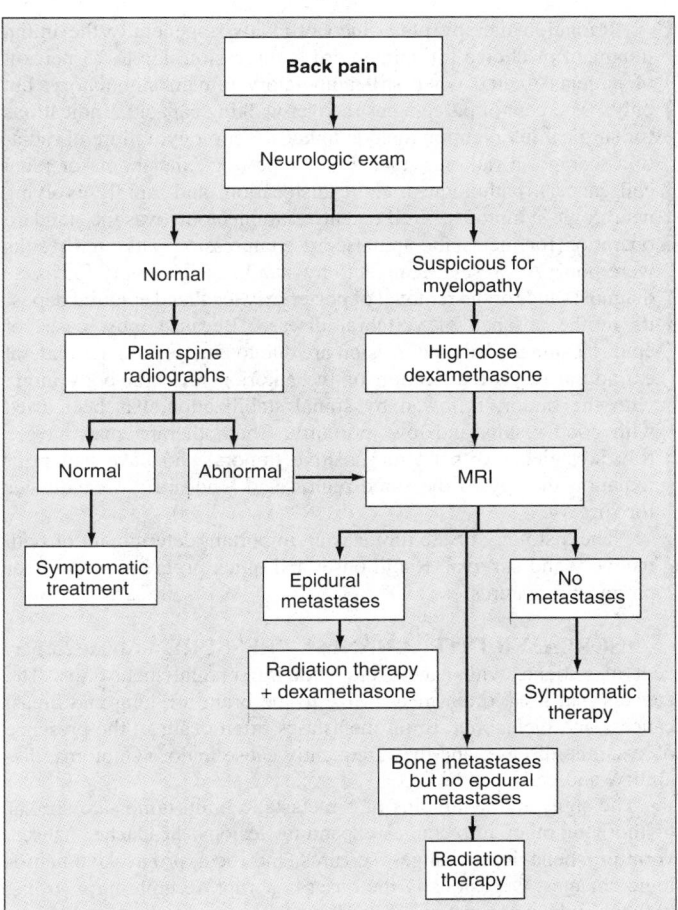

FIGURE 104-1 Management of cancer patients with back pain.

cancer. Also, a normal appearance on plain films of the spine does not exclude the diagnosis of cancer. The role of bone scans in the detection of cord compression is not clear. This method is sensitive, but it is less specific than spinal radiography.

The full-length image of the cord provided by MRI may be useful in the workup of patients with spinal cord compression. On T1-weighted images, there is good contrast between the cord, cerebrospinal fluid, and extradural lesions. Owing to their sensitivity in demonstrating the replacement of bone marrow by tumor, these MR images can show which parts of a vertebra are involved by tumor (the body, pedicle, lamina, spinous process, etc.). These images also visualize intraspinal extradural masses compressing the cord. T2-weighted images are most useful for the demonstration of intramedullary pathology. Gadolinium-enhanced MRI can help to characterize and delineate intramedullary disease. Comparative studies have shown that MRI is as good as or better than myelography plus postmyelogram CT in detecting metastatic epidural disease with cord compression. Myelography should be reserved for patients who have poor MR images or who cannot undergo MRI promptly. CT in conjunction with myelography clearly enhances the detection of small areas of spinal destruction.

In patients with spinal cord compression and an unknown primary tumor, a simple workup including chest radiography, mammography, measurement of prostate-specific antigen, and abdominal CT will usually reveal the underlying malignancy.

℞ TREATMENT

The treatment of patients with spinal cord compression is directed toward relief of pain and restoration of neurologic function (Fig. 104-1).

Radiation therapy plus glucocorticoids is generally the initial treatment of choice for spinal cord compression. Up to 75 percent of patients treated when still ambulatory remain ambulatory, but only 10 percent of paraplegics recover walking capacity. Indications for surgical intervention include unknown etiology, failure of radiation therapy, a radioresistant tumor type (e.g., melanoma or renal cell cancer), pathologic fracture dislocation, and rapidly evolving neurologic symptoms. Until recently, laminectomy was the standard operation for metastatic spinal cord compression, although results were poor. At present, laminectomy should be used only for tissue diagnosis and for the removal of posteriorly localized epidural deposits in the absence of vertebral disease. Because most cases of epidural spinal cord compression are due to anterior or anterolateral extradural disease, resection of the anterior vertebral body along with the tumor, followed by spinal stabilization, has been tried with good results and low mortality. Chemotherapy may have a role in patients with chemosensitive tumors who have had prior radiation therapy to the same region and who are not candidates for surgery.

The histology of the tumor is an important determinant of both recovery and survival. Rapid onset and quick progression are poor prognostic features.

INCREASED INTRACRANIAL PRESSURE About 25 percent of patients with cancer die with intracranial metastases. The cancers that most often metastasize to the brain are lung and breast cancers and melanoma. Brain metastases often occur in the presence of systemic disease, and they frequently cause major symptoms, disability, and early death.

The signs and symptoms of a metastatic brain tumor are similar to those of other intracranial expanding lesions: headache, nausea, vomiting, behavioral changes, seizures, and focal, progressive neurologic changes. Occasionally the onset is abrupt, resembling a stroke, with the sudden appearance of headache, nausea, vomiting, and neurologic deficits. This picture is usually due to hemorrhage into the metastasis. Of the metastatic tumors, melanoma, germ cell tumors, and renal cell cancers have a particularly high incidence of intracranial bleeding. The tumor mass and surrounding edema may cause obstruction of the circulation of cerebrospinal fluid, with resulting hydrocephalus. Patients with increased intracranial pressure may have papilledema with visual disturbances and neck stiffness. As the mass enlarges, brain tissue may be displaced through the fixed cranial openings, producing various herniation syndromes.

CT and MRI are equally effective in the diagnosis of brain metastases. CT with contrast should be used as a screening procedure. The CT scan shows brain metastases as multiple enhancing lesions of various sizes with surrounding areas of low-density edema. If there is a single lesion or if no metastases are visualized by contrast-enhanced CT, MRI of the brain should be performed. Gadolinium-enhanced MRI is more sensitive than CT at revealing small lesions, particularly in the brainstem or cerebellum.

℞ TREATMENT

If signs and symptoms of brain herniation (particularly headache, drowsiness, and papilledema) are present, the patient should be intubated and hyperventilated to maintain P_{CO_2} between 25 and 30 mmHg and should receive infusions of mannitol (1 to 1.5 g/kg) every 6 h. Dexamethasone is the best initial treatment for all symptomatic patients with brain metastases (see above). Patients with multiple lesions should receive whole-brain radiation therapy. Patients with a single brain metastasis and with controlled extracranial disease may be treated with surgical excision followed by whole-brain radiation therapy, especially if they are younger than 60 years. Radioresistant tumors should be resected if possible. Some patients with increased intracranial pressure associated with hydrocephalus may benefit from neurosurgical intervention.

SEIZURES Seizures occurring in a cancer patient can be caused by the tumor itself, by metabolic disturbances, by radiation injury, by cerebral infarctions, by chemotherapy-related encephalopathies, or by central nervous system infections. Metastatic disease to the central nervous system is the most common cause of seizures in cancer patients. The frequency with which seizures are a presenting symptom of intracranial metastasis ranges from 6 to 29 percent in published series. Approximately 10 percent of patients with intracranial metastasis eventually develop seizures. The presence of frontal lesions correlates with early seizures, and the presence of hemispheric symptomatology increases the risk for late seizures. Both early and late seizures are uncommon in patients with primarily posterior fossa lesions. Seizures are also common in patients with intracranial metastases from melanoma. Very rarely, cytotoxic drugs such as etoposide, busulfan, and chlorambucil cause seizures.

℞ TREATMENT

Patients in whom seizures due to intracranial metastases have been demonstrated should receive anticonvulsive treatment with diphenylhydantoin. Prophylactic anticonvulsant therapy is not recommended unless the patient is at a high risk for late seizures. In those cases, serum diphenylhydantoin levels should be monitored closely and the dosage adjusted accordingly.

INTRACEREBRAL LEUKOCYTOSTASIS Intracerebral leukocytostasis (Ball's disease) is a potentially fatal complication of acute leukemia (particularly myelogenous leukemia) that can occur when the peripheral blast cell count is greater than $100,000/\mu L$. At such high blast cell counts, blood viscosity is increased and blood flow is slowed, and the primitive leukemic cells are capable of invading through endothelium and causing hemorrhage into the brain. Patients may experience stupor, dizziness, visual disturbances, ataxia, coma, or sudden death. Administration of 600cGy of whole-brain irradiation can protect against this complication and can be followed by rapid institution of antileukemic therapy. This complication is not a feature of the high white cell counts associated with chronic lymphocytic leukemia or chronic myelogenous leukemia.

HEMOPTYSIS While hemoptysis is usually caused by nonmalignant conditions, it may develop in older patients with lung cancer or lung metastases who have coagulation defects or thrombocytopenia. The volume of bleeding is often difficult to gauge. When respiratory difficulty occurs, hemoptysis should be treated emergently. Often patients can tell where the bleeding is occurring. They should be placed bleeding side down, given supplemental oxygen, and subjected to emergency bronchoscopy. If the site of the lesion is detected, either the patient undergoes a definitive surgical procedure or the lesion is treated with a neodymium:yttrium-aluminum-garnet (Nd:YAG) laser, endobronchial tamponade, or bronchial artery catheterization and embolization. The surgical option is preferred; the other procedures are less effective in the face of brisk bleeding, and complications are common with tamponade and embolization procedures. The thrombocytopenia and coagulation defects should be corrected, if possible.

AIRWAY OBSTRUCTION Generally, *airway obstruction* refers to a blockage at the level of the mainstem bronchi or above. It may result either from intraluminal tumor growth or from extrinsic compression of the airway. If the obstruction is proximal to the larynx, a tracheostomy may be life-saving. For more distal obstructions, surgery is preferred. However, radiation therapy (either external-beam irradiation or brachytherapy) given together with glucocorticoids may also open the airway. For intrinsic lesions, particularly incomplete centrally obstructing lesions, Nd:YAG laser treatment or photodynamic therapy (photosensitizers plus light) can be effective. Photodynamic therapy has the advantage of being suitable for use in patients who are not surgical candidates.

METABOLIC EMERGENCIES

HYPERCALCEMIA Hypercalcemia is the most common paraneoplastic syndrome (see Chaps. 102 and 353), occurring in about 10 percent of patients with advanced cancer. It is associated most often with cancers of the lung, breast, head and neck, and kidney and with multiple myeloma.

Increased release of calcium from bone is the main factor leading to hypercalcemia. Bone resorption is increased dramatically through stimulation of the proliferation and activity of osteoclasts, and bone formation is not stimulated in parallel. The kidney may play an important role through an increase in the reabsorption of calcium in the distal tubule. Parathormone-related protein (PTHrP) produced by tumors has a central role as a mediator of hypercalcemia in cancer. PTHrP shares 80 percent homology with the first 13 amino acids of parathormone (PTH), which are in the region responsible for binding to the PTH receptor. PTHrP acts via the PTH hormone receptors on osteoblasts and renal tubular cells to stimulate bone resorption and renal calcium conservation, leading to hypercalcemia. Elevated plasma PTHrP levels are also found in most hypercalcemic patients with bone metastases, in whom hypercalcemia has traditionally been explained by local osteolysis due to the production of osteolytic factors by tumors. Transforming growth factors, cytokines (interleukins 1 and 6), and other unknown factors could play a contributory role. True "ectopic" PTH production by malignant tumors is rare. In lymphoma, a vitamin D–related product of the tumor may also increase calcium absorption in the gut.

The clinical features of hypercalcemia in cancer patients are nonspecific and include fatigue, anorexia, constipation, polydipsia, muscle weakness, nausea, and vomiting. They may easily be attributed to the malignancy itself or to its treatment. Laboratory assessment should include measurement of serum electrolytes, calcium, phosphate, and albumin. Hypoalbuminemia is common in malignancy and, if present, will affect the total serum concentration of calcium. If ionized calcium level cannot be obtained, then corrected serum calcium concentration should be calculated using the following formula:

$$\text{Corrected serum calcium} = \text{measured serum calcium} + 0.8 \ (4.0 - \text{measured serum albumin})$$

Most patients with hypercalcemia of malignancy have obvious evidence of malignancy, and their serum PTH levels are suppressed. Measurements of PTHrP and serum 1,25-dihydroxyvitamin D should be confined to research studies in patients with advanced cancer. The results of routine serum chemistry evaluations are not reliable alone for distinguishing between malignant and nonmalignant causes of hypercalcemia.

℞ TREATMENT

Not all patients with moderate to severe hypercalcemia (corrected calcium ≥12 mg/dL) should be treated. The decision of whether or not to treat will depend on the patient's quality of life, the current symptoms, and the prospect for further treatment. Treatment directed at hypercalcemia only extends life in patients for whom effective cancer treatment is available. Nonetheless, corrective therapy may be indicated on a palliative basis to improve symptoms and the quality of life. Treatment of symptomatic hypercalcemia begins with intravenous saline to restore the depleted intravascular volume, which may be 4 to 8 L below normal at presentation. However, rehydration usually has little effect on calcium levels, producing a median effective decrease of only 1 mg/dL. Antiresorptive agents are essential to decrease osteoclastic activity and control hypercalcemia. Bisphosphonates, which are potent inhibitors of bone resorption, have essentially replaced traditional agents such as calcitonin and mithramycin and have changed the therapeutic approach to this frequent complication of advancing cancer. Bisphosphonate therapy is easy to administer, is virtually free of side effects, and is rapidly effective in lowering serum calcium. Pamidronate is the most effective of the commercially available bisphosphonates. The recommended dose of pamidronate is 60 mg for moderate hypercalcemia (corrected calcium 12 to 13.5 mg/dL) and 90 mg for severe hypercalcemia (corrected calcium >13.5 mg/dL). The dose is given as a single infusion over 4 or 24 h.

Gallium nitrate inhibits osteoclast function, thus reducing serum calcium. Clinical use of this agent has been limited by the risk of nephrotoxicity and the inconvenient method of administration (200 mg/m² per day as a 5-day continuous intravenous infusion).

SYNDROME OF INAPPROPRIATE SECRETION OF ANTIDIURETIC HORMONE (SIADH) SIADH is attributed to production of arginine vasopressin by the tumor cells and is characterized by hyponatremia, urine osmolarity inappropriately higher than plasma osmolarity, and high urinary sodium excretion in the absence of volume depletion. Renal, adrenal, and thyroid insufficiency must be excluded, because these disorders can also present with hyponatremia and impaired urinary dilution. Low serum levels of urea and uric acid are useful in distinguishing SIADH from conditions associated with renal hypoperfusion (see Chaps. 102 and 330).

A broad spectrum of malignant tumors have been reported to cause SIADH. Ectopic vasopressin secretion may occur in some 38 percent of small cell carcinomas of the lung; often there is cosecretion of adrenocorticotropic hormone. The presence of hyponatremia in patients with small cell lung cancer confers a poor prognosis. SIADH may also be caused by various other conditions, such as central nervous system and pulmonary disorders and some surgical procedures. A variety of drugs have also been shown to produce SIADH, including cytotoxic drugs such as vincristine, ifosfamide, cyclophosphamide, cisplatin, levamisole, and melphalan.

Most patients with SIADH are asymptomatic. The severity of symptoms and signs is related to the degree of hyponatremia and the rapidity with which it develops. Early changes include anorexia, depression, lethargy, irritability, confusion, muscle weakness, and marked personality changes. When the plasma sodium level falls below 110 mEq/L, extensor plantar responses, areflexia, and pseudobulbar palsy may be noted, and further reductions may cause coma, convulsions, and death.

℞ TREATMENT

The optimal therapy for SIADH is to treat the underlying malignancy. If that is not possible, other therapeutic approaches are available, such as water restriction or the administration of demeclocycline (900 to 1200 mg per os bid), urea, or lithium carbonate (300 mg per os tid). Demeclocycline is usually used first. It inhibits the effects of vasopressin on the distal renal tubule. Patients with seizure or coma from hyponatremia may require normal saline infusion plus furosemide to enhance free water clearance. The rate of sodium correction should be slow [0.5 to 1 (mEq/L)/h] to prevent rapid fluid shifts and central pontine myelinolysis. Serum calcium should be monitored closely to avoid hypocalcemia.

LACTIC ACIDOSIS This is a rare and potentially fatal metabolic complication of cancer. Lactic acidosis associated with sepsis and circulatory failure is a common preterminal event in many malignancies. Lactic acidosis in the absence of hypoxemia may occur in patients with leukemia, lymphoma, or solid tumors. Extensive involvement of the liver by tumor is present in most cases. Alteration of liver function may be responsible for the lactate accumulation. Tachypnea, tachycardia, change of mental status, and hepatomegaly may be seen. The serum level of lactic acid may reach 10 to 20 mEq/L (90 to 180 mg/dL). Treatment is aimed at the underlying disease. The danger from lactic acidosis is from the acidosis, not the lactate. Sodium bicarbonate should be added if acidosis is very severe or if hydrogen ion production is very rapid and uncontrolled. The prognosis is poor.

HYPOGLYCEMIA Persistent hypoglycemia occasionally is associated with tumors other than pancreatic islet cell tumors. Usually these tumors are large, and often they are of mesenchymal origin or are hepatomas or adrenocortical tumors. Mesenchymal tumors are usually located in the retroperitoneum or thorax. In these patients, obtundation, confusion, and behavioral aberrations occur in the postabsorptive period and may precede the diagnosis of the tumor. Hypoglycemia is due to unregulated overproduction of the insulin-like growth factors by a tumor or to the induction of autoantibodies to the insulin receptor. Treatment of the hypoglycemia has generally been symptomatic, relying on the administration of glucose.

ADRENAL INSUFFICIENCY In cancer patients, adrenal insufficiency may go unrecognized because the symptoms, such as nausea, vomiting, anorexia, and orthostatic hypotension, are nonspecific and may be mistakenly attributed to progressive cancer or to cancer therapy. In the cancer patient, primary adrenal insufficiency may develop owing to replacement of both glands by metastases (of lung, breast, colon, or kidney cancer) or infiltrating lymphoma, to removal of both glands, or to hemorrhagic necrosis in association with sepsis or anticoagulation. Impaired adrenal steroid synthesis occurs in patients being treated for cancer with mitotane, aminoglutethimide, ketoconazole, or the investigational agent suramin or undergoing rapid reduction in glucocorticoid therapy. Rarely, metastatic replacement will cause primary adrenal insufficiency as the first manifestation of an occult malignancy. Metastasis to the pituitary or hypothalamus is found at autopsy in up to 5 percent of patients with cancer, but associated secondary adrenal insufficiency is rare.

Acute adrenal insufficiency is potentially lethal. Treatment of suspected adrenal crisis is initiated after sampling serum cortisol and ACTH levels (see Chap. 332).

TREATMENT-RELATED EMERGENCIES

TUMOR LYSIS SYNDROME This is a well-recognized clinical entity that is characterized by various combinations of hyperuricemia, hyperkalemia, hyperphosphatemia, lactic acidosis, and hypocalcemia and is caused by the mass destruction of a large number of rapidly proliferating neoplastic cells. Frequently, acute renal failure develops as a result of tumor lysis syndrome.

Tumor lysis syndrome is most frequently associated with the treatment of Burkitt's lymphoma, acute lymphoblastic leukemia, and other high-grade lymphomas, but it also may be seen with chronic leukemias and, rarely, with solid tumors. This syndrome has been seen in patients with chronic lymphocytic leukemia after treatment with fludarabine. Tumor lysis syndrome usually occurs during or shortly (1 to 5 days) after chemotherapy. Rarely, spontaneous necrosis of malignancies causes tumor lysis syndrome.

Hyperuricemia may be present at the time of chemotherapy. Effective treatment accelerates the destruction of malignant cells and leads to increased serum uric acid levels from the turnover of nucleic acids. Owing to the acidic local environment, uric acid can precipitate in the tubules, medulla, and collecting ducts of the kidney, leading to renal failure. Lactic acidosis and dehydration may contribute to the precipitation of uric acid in the renal tubules. The finding of uric acid crystals in the urine is strong evidence for uric acid nephropathy. The ratio by weight of urinary uric acid to urinary creatinine is >1 in patients with acute hyperuricemic nephropathy and <1 in patients with renal failure due to other causes.

Hyperphosphatemia, which can be caused by the release of intracellular phosphate pools by tumor cell lysis, produces a reciprocal depression in serum calcium, which causes severe neuromuscular irritability and tetany. Deposition of calcium phosphate in the kidney and hyperphosphatemia may cause renal failure. Potassium is the principal intracellular cation, and massive destruction of malignant cells may lead to hyperkalemia. Hyperkalemia in patients with renal failure may rapidly become life-threatening. Hyperkalemia can cause ventricular arrhythmias and sudden death.

The likelihood that the tumor lysis syndrome will occur in patients with Burkitt's lymphoma is related to the tumor burden and renal function. Hyperuricemia and high serum levels of lactate dehydrogenase LDH (>1500 units per liter), both of which correlate with total tumor burden, also correlate with the risk of posttreatment tumor lysis

syndrome. In patients at risk for tumor lysis, pretreatment evaluations should include a complete blood count, serum chemistry evaluation, and urine analysis. High leukocyte and platelet counts may artificially elevate potassium levels ("pseudohyperkalemia") due to lysis of these cells after the blood is drawn. In these cases, plasma potassium instead of serum potassium should be followed. In pseudohyperkalemia, no electrocardiographic abnormalities will be present. In patients with abnormal baseline renal function, the kidneys and retroperitoneal area should be evaluated by sonography and/or CT. Urine output should be watched closely.

Recognition of risk and prevention are the most important steps in the management of this syndrome (Fig. 104-2). Despite aggressive pretherapy management, tumor lysis syndrome and/or oliguric or anuric renal failure may occur. Dialysis is often necessary and should be considered early in the course. Hemodialysis is preferred. The prognosis is excellent, and renal function recovers after the uric acid level is lowered by dialysis to less than 10 to 20 mg/dL.

HEMOLYTIC-UREMIC SYNDROME Hemolytic-uremic syndrome (HUS) and, less commonly, thrombotic thrombocytopenic purpura (TTP) occurring after treatment with antineoplastic drugs have been described. Mitomycin is by far the most common agent causing this peculiar syndrome. Other chemotherapeutic agents, particularly cisplatin and bleomycin, have also been reported to be associated with this syndrome. This syndrome occurs most often in patients with gastric, colorectal, and breast carcinoma. In one series, 35 percent of patients were without evident cancer at the time of the development of this syndrome. Secondary HUS/TTP has also been reported as a rare but sometimes fatal complication of bone marrow transplantation.

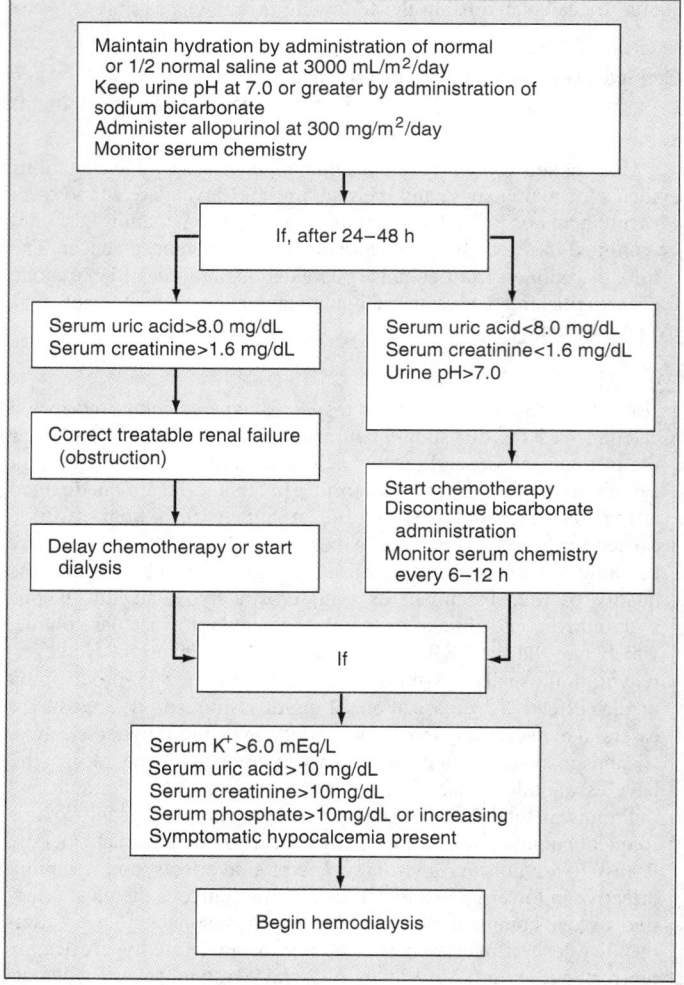

FIGURE 104-2 Management of patients at high risk for the tumor lysis syndrome.

HUS usually has its onset 4 to 8 weeks after the last dose of chemotherapy, but it is not rare to detect it several months later. HUS is characterized by microangiopathic hemolytic anemia, thrombocytopenia, and renal failure. Dyspnea, weakness, fatigue, oliguria, and purpura are also common initial symptoms and findings. Systemic hypertension and pulmonary edema commonly occur. Severe hypertension, pulmonary edema, and rapid worsening of hemolysis and renal function may occur after a blood transfusion. Cardiac findings include atrial arrhythmias, pericardial friction rub, and pericardial effusion. Raynaud's phenomenon has been reported as part of the syndrome in patients treated with bleomycin.

Laboratory findings include severe to moderate anemia associated with red cell fragmentation and numerous schistocytes on peripheral smear. Reticulocytosis, decreased plasma haptoglobin, and an elevated LDH level provide additional evidence of hemolysis. The serum bilirubin level is usually normal or slightly elevated. The Coombs test is negative. The white cell count is usually normal, and thrombocytopenia ($<100,000/\mu L$) is almost always present. Most patients have a normal coagulation profile, although some have mild elevations in thrombin time and in level of fibrin degradation products. The serum creatinine level is elevated at presentation and shows a pattern of subacute worsening within weeks of the initial azotemia. The urinalysis reveals hematuria, proteinuria, and granular or hyaline casts, and circulating immune complexes may be present.

The basic pathologic lesion appears to be deposition of fibrin in the walls of capillaries and arterioles, and these deposits are similar to those seen in HUS due to other causes. These microvascular abnormalities involve mainly the kidneys and rarely occur in other organs. The pathogenesis of chemotherapy-related HUS is unknown. Immune complexes have been proposed but not confirmed to be etiologic.

The case fatality rate is high, most patients dying within a few months. Plasmapheresis and plasma exchange may normalize the hematologic abnormalities, but renal failure is not reversed in most patients. Immunoperfusion over a staphylococcal protein A column is the most successful treatment. About half of the patients treated with immunoperfusion respond with resolution of thrombocytopenia, improvement in anemia, and stabilization of renal failure. Treatment is well tolerated. It is not clear how the treatment works.

NEUTROPENIA AND INFECTION These remain the most common serious complications of cancer therapy. → *They are covered in detail in Chap. 87.*

PULMONARY INFILTRATES Patients with cancer may present with dyspnea associated with diffuse interstitial infiltrates on chest radiographs. Such infiltrates may be due to progression of the underlying malignancy, to treatment-related toxicities, to infection, and/or to unrelated diseases. The cause may be multifactorial; however, most commonly they occur as a consequence of treatment. Infiltration of the lung by malignancy has been described in cases of leukemia, lymphoma, and breast and other solid cancers. Pulmonary lymphatics may be involved diffusely by neoplasm (pulmonary lymphangitic carcinomatosis), resulting in a diffuse increase in interstitial markings on chest radiographs. The patient is often mildly dyspneic at the onset, but pulmonary failure develops rapidly over a period of weeks. In some patients, dyspnea precedes changes on the chest radiographs and is accompanied by a nonproductive cough. This syndrome is characteristic of solid tumors. In leukemic patients, diffuse microscopic neoplastic peribronchial and peribronchiolar infiltration is frequent but may be asymptomatic. However, some patients present with diffuse interstitial infiltrates, an alveolar capillary block syndrome, and respiratory distress. In these situations, glucocorticoids can provide symptomatic relief, but specific chemotherapy should always be started promptly.

In addition, accumulation of leukemic blasts in the pulmonary capillary system may cause pulmonary distress and failure in patients with acute myelogenous leukemia. This complication is strongly related to high peripheral blast counts (more than $100,000/\mu L$) and a short tumor cell doubling time. Some patients with pulmonary leukostasis may have nodular and/or floccular, diffuse infiltrates on chest radiographs. In addition to dyspnea, patients may develop dizziness, confusion, tinnitus, ataxia, visual blurring, and retinal abnormalities due to leukostasis in cerebral vessels. Leukapheresis and/or chemotherapy should be started without delay. Pulmonary irradiation may reduce symptoms.

Several cytotoxic agents, such as bleomycin, methotrexate, busulfan, and the nitrosoureas, may cause pulmonary damage. The most frequent presentations are interstitial pneumonitis, alveolitis, and pulmonary fibrosis. Some cytotoxic agents, including methotrexate and procarbazine, may cause an acute hypersensitivity reaction. Cytosine arabinoside has been associated with noncardiogenic pulmonary edema. Administration of multiple cytotoxic drugs, as well as radiation therapy and preexisting lung disease, may potentiate the pulmonary toxicity. Supplemental oxygen may potentiate the effects of drugs and radiation injury. Patients should always be managed with the lowest F_{IO_2} that is sufficient to maintain hemoglobin saturation.

The onset of symptoms may be insidious, with symptoms including dyspnea, nonproductive cough, and tachycardia. Patients may have bibasilar crepitant rales, end-inspiratory crackles, fever, and cyanosis. The chest radiograph generally shows an interstitial and sometimes an intraalveolar pattern that is strongest at the lung bases and may be symmetric. A small effusion may occur. Hypoxemia with decreased carbon monoxide diffusing capacity is always present. Glucocorticoids may be helpful in patients in whom pulmonary toxicity is related to radiation therapy or to chemotherapy with mitomycin C, busulfan, methotrexate, or procarbazine. Treatment is otherwise supportive.

Radiation pneumonitis and/or fibrosis is a relatively frequent side effect of thoracic radiation therapy when the dosage exceeds 40 Gy and may be acute or chronic. It has its onset usually from 2 to 6 months after completion of radiation therapy. The clinical syndrome, which varies in severity, consists of dyspnea, cough with scanty sputum, low-grade fever, and an initial hazy infiltrate on chest radiographs. The infiltrate and tissue damage generally are confined to the radiation field. The patients subsequently may develop a patchy alveolar infiltrate and air bronchograms, which may progress to acute respiratory failure, sometimes fatal. A lung biopsy may be necessary to make the diagnosis. Asymptomatic infiltrates found incidentally after radiation therapy need not be treated. However, prednisone should be administered to patients with fever or other symptoms. The dosage should be tapered slowly after the resolution of radiation pneumonitis, as abrupt withdrawal of glucocorticoids may cause an exacerbation of pneumonia. Delayed radiation fibrosis may occur years after radiation therapy and is signaled by dyspnea on exertion. Often it is mild, but it can progress to chronic respiratory failure. Therapy is supportive.

Pneumonia is a common problem in patients undergoing treatment for cancer. Bacterial pneumonia typically causes a localized infiltrate on chest radiographs. Therapy is tailored to the causative organism. When diffuse interstitial infiltrates appear in a febrile patient, the differential diagnosis is extensive and includes pneumonia due to infection with *Pneumocystis carinii,* cytomegalovirus, or intracellular pathogens such as mycoplasma and *Legionella;* effects of drugs or radiation; tumor progression; nonspecific pneumonitis; and fungal disease. However, studies have shown that empirical intervention with trimethoprim-sulfamethoxazole plus erythromycin in nonneutropenic patients, with these antibiotics plus ceftazidime in neutropenic patients, covers nearly every treatable diagnosis (except tumor progression) and gives as good overall survival as a strategy based on early invasive intervention with bronchoalveolar lavage or open lung biopsy. If the patient does not improve in 4 days, open lung biopsy is the procedure of choice. Bronchoscopy with bronchoalveolar lavage may be used in patients who are poor candidates for surgery.

In patients with pulmonary infiltrates who are afebrile, heart failure and multiple pulmonary emboli form part of the differential diagnosis.

TYPHLITIS Typhlitis is the necrosis of the cecum and adjacent colon that may complicate the treatment of acute leukemia. The patient develops right lower quadrant abdominal pain, often with rebound tenderness and a tense, distended abdomen, in a setting of fever and neutropenia. Watery diarrhea and bacteremia are common, and bleeding may occur. Rapid institution of broad-spectrum antibiotic coverage and nasogastric suction may reverse the disease. Surgical intervention should be considered if there is no improvement by 24 h after the start of antibiotic treatment. If the localized abdominal findings become diffuse, the prognosis is poor.

HEMORRHAGIC CYSTITIS This condition can develop in patients receiving cyclophosphamide or ifosfamide. Both drugs are metabolized to acrolein, which is a strong chemical irritant that is excreted in the urine. Prolonged contact or high concentrations may lead to bladder irritation and hemorrhage. The best management is prevention. Maintaining a high rate of urine flow minimizes exposure. In addition, 2-mercaptoethanesulfonate (mesna) detoxifies the metabolites and can be coadministered with the instigating drugs. Mesna usually is given three times on the day of ifosfamide administration in doses that are each 20 percent of the total ifosfamide dose. If hemorrhagic cystitis develops, the maintenance of a high urine flow may be sufficient supportive care. If conservative management is not effective, irrigation of the bladder with an 0.37 to 0.74 percent formalin solution for 10 min stops the bleeding in most cases. *N*-acetylcysteine may also be an effective irrigant. In extreme cases, cystectomy may be necessary.

TREATMENT OF ACUTE PROMYELOCYTIC LEUKE-MIA Therapy for this malignancy can produce two life-threatening syndromes. Chemotherapy acts by killing leukemic cells, and the dying cells release procoagulants from their cytoplasmic granules that can produce disseminated intravascular coagulation (see Chap 119). Heparin therapy may reverse this process. Cryoprecipitate and fresh-frozen plasma are used to replace depleted clotting factors. By contrast, treatment with all-*trans*-retinoic acid (ATRA, tretinoin) induces the leukemic cells to differentiate. This approach avoids bleeding complications but creates problems related to high white blood cell counts. The so-called ATRA syndrome includes fever, dyspnea, pleural and pericardial effusion, and hypotension. Leukocytosis and the ATRA syndrome can be prevented by chemotherapy. The syndromes caused by treatment with either chemotherapy alone or ATRA alone each may cause death in about 15 to 20 percent of patients. The use of chemotherapy and tretinoin together may reduce the mortality by preventing both syndromes.

In summary, the diagnosis of cancer and its treatment carry risk of a multitude of medical problems. Knowledge of both the disease process and the potential hazards of the treatment is required to anticipate and treat these emergent complications.

BIBLIOGRAPHY

AHMANN FR: A reassessment of the clinical implications of the superior vena caval syndrome. J Clin Oncol 2:961, 1984

BOOGERD W et al: Diagnosis and treatment of spinal cord compression in malignant disease. Cancer Treat Rev 19:129, 1993

BROWNE MJ et al: A randomized trial of open lung biopsy versus empiric antimicrobial therapy in cancer patients with diffuse interstitial infiltrates. J Clin Oncol 8:222, 1990

GUCALP R et al: Treatment of cancer-associated hypercalcemia: Double blind comparison of rapid and slow intravenous infusion regimens of pamidronate and saline alone. Arch Intern Med 154:1935, 1994

IHDE JK et al: Adrenal insufficiency in the cancer patient: Implications for the surgeon. Br J Surg 77:1335, 1990

JONES DP et al: Tumor lysis syndrome: Pathogenesis and management. Pediatr Nephrol 9:206, 1995

LOKICH J et al: Biliary tract obstruction secondary to cancer: Management guidelines and selected literature review. J Clin Oncol 5:969, 1987

RIPAMONOTI C: Management of bowel obstruction in advanced cancer. Curr Opin Oncol 6:351, 1994

SNYDER HW et al: Treatment of cancer chemotherapy–associated thrombotic thrombocytopenic/hemolytic uremic syndrome by protein A immunoadsorption of plasma. Cancer 71:1882, 1993

SORENSON JB et al: Syndrome of inappropriate secretion of antidiuretic hormone (SIADH) in malignant disease. J Intern Med 238:97, 1995

VAITKUS PT et al: Treatment of malignant pericardial effusion. JAMA 272:59, 1994

SECTION 2

DISORDERS OF HEMATOPOIESIS

105 *Francis W. Ruscetti, Jonathan R. Keller, Dan L. Longo*

HEMATOPOIESIS

Hematopoiesis is the formation of blood cells. The cellular elements of the peripheral blood play a critical role in oxygen delivery to the tissues, hemostasis, and host defense. The turnover of differentiated hematopoietic cells in an adult weighing 70 kg (154 lbs) is over 0.5 trillion cells per day including 200 billion red blood cells (RBC) and 70 billion neutrophilic leukocytes. Under physiologic conditions, production and turnover are coordinated. The average RBC lives about 120 days; the average granulocyte lives 6 to 8 h; the average platelet survives 7 to 10 days. Lymphocytes may be very long-lived, indeed some may survive for many years. However, lymphopoiesis is marked by inefficiency. Many cells are generated but few (5 percent or so) survive to be selected from the marrow or the thymus into the periphery. Under conditions of stress, the production of one or more lineages must be increased to meet increased demand. Thus, the maintenance of normal numbers of peripheral blood components requires essentially continuous production of new cells. This continuous blood cell formation is supported by a small number of cells (0.01 percent) in the bone marrow termed hematopoietic stem cells (HSC), from which all the blood cells arise. When the marrow fails, clinical manifestations of the failure appear as a function of the turnover of the normal cellular endproduct. Thus, patients with marrow failure initially lose granulocytes, which may lead to susceptibility to infection, followed by bleeding related to decreased platelets. Generally pallor, weakness, and dyspnea on exertion related to decreased RBC mass are the last to appear.

The anatomy and physiology of the hematopoietic organs regulating this remarkable process are complex. However, the understanding of blood cell formation, or hematopoiesis, has been enhanced by recent advances in cell culture techniques and applications of recombinant DNA technology.

HEMATOPOIETIC STEM CELLS HSC are capable of restoring normal hematopoiesis in irradiated animals (radioprotection); long-term multilineage reconstitution (LTRC), and formation of spleen colony forming units [day 12 colony forming units spleen (CFU-S)] that give rise to colonies containing granulocytic, monocytic, erythroid, megakaryocytic, and lymphoid lineages. These three assays have become endpoints for purifying stem cells. Stem cell purification techniques have exploited differences in physical properties (density centrifugation, countercurrent elutriation), cell surface antigen expression detected by monoclonal antibodies, and cell cycle status [Hoechst 33342, a DNA-binding dye, and Rhodamine 123 (Rh123), a mitochondrial-binding dye].

HETEROGENEITY OF STEM CELLS Using these purification methods, it has become clear that both LTRC and short-term repopulating cells (STRC) exist. STRC have radioprotective ability but not long-term persistence. Experiments using bone marrow cells (BMC) distinguishable by alloenyzme or retroviral integration showed that early after bone marrow transplant (BMT), numerous clones actively contributed to hematopoiesis only to be replaced by a few long-lived clones after 3 to 4 months. Using highly enriched Thy 1.1[lo], Sca-1 +, and lineage-specific marker-negative (lin −) BMC, it was shown that cells that stain brightly for Rh123 have STRC activity and lower proliferative potential, and cells that stain poorly for Rh123 are enriched for cells with LTRC and have higher growth potential. This suggests that repopulating cells are part of a continuum of HSC with different abilities to provide long- and short-term reconstitution. This is further supported by studies in which serially transplanted marrow was eventually depleted of LTRC, leaving only STRC. The loss of LTRC activity is likely a consequence of the pressure to produce differentiated progeny in a transplant setting, suggesting that rapidly dividing HSC have an advantage in competitive repopulation, but with reduced clonal longevity.

It is generally accepted that most stem cells are quiescent and only a few stem cells supply all the blood cells at a given time. Stem cell factor is a cytokine capable of promoting stem cell proliferation. Its receptor is c-kit (see Table 305-3). Separation of stem cells by elutriation was combined with separation into c-kit^{pos} and c-kit^{neg} fractions. While both cell types had LTRC, only the c-kit^{pos} cells proliferated in response to multiple cytokines in vitro, formed day 12 CFU-S in vivo, and could protect mice from radiation-induced death when transplanted in vivo. While c-kit^{neg} cells do not have primary day 12 CFU-S activity, transplantation of BMC from the primary recipient mice into secondary recipients gives rise to CFU-S. Thus, deeply quiescent c-kit^{neg} cells are pluripotent stem cells that can give rise to cells with CFU-S activity but require growth and differentiation in vivo, further subdividing the stem cell compartment (Fig. 105-1).

THE HEMATOPOIETIC MICROENVIRONMENT Bone marrow has an organized and structured architecture in which close relationships exist between a regulatory microenvironment and primitive hematopoietic cells. The more rapidly proliferating CFU-S are near the bone surface, while the more primitive, slowly cycling CFU-S are near the central axis. Thus, it is reasonable to conclude that specific positional effects exist and they are maintained and regulated by products of the microenvironment. Components of the microenvironment include adipocytes, fibroblastoid cells, and reticular-endothelioid cells as well as macrophages and T lymphocytes (Fig. 105-2). The role or even the presence of each cell type in the microenvironment in vivo is not clear.

The main evidence that stem cells bind to the stroma comes from in vitro long-term bone marrow cultures where data show that maturing precursors and terminally differentiated cells are present as nonadherent cells, while stem cells and primitive precursors bind tightly to the stroma. Similarly, aggregates of stroma and hematopoietic cells isolated from freshly explanted marrow are enriched in primitive hematopoietic cells. The differential expression of cell adhesion molecules plays a major role in cell-cell contact between hematopoietic cells and stroma. Antibodies to murine CD44 abrogate lympho- and myelopoiesis in long-term bone marrow cultures without any apparent effect on stroma formation. Similarly, antibodies to either vascular cell adhesion molecule 1 expressed on stromal cells or its ligand VLA-4 expressed on stem cells interfere with cell-cell interaction and cause the release of stem cells from stroma. Other adhesive interactions are mediated by cytokine receptors that specifically bind membrane-associated cytokines, such as stem cell factor, or extracellular matrix–bound ligands [proteoglycans can bind

granulocyte-macrophage (GM) colony stimulating factor (CSF); fibronectin can bind transforming growth factor β (TGFβ)]. Components of extracellular matrix include numerous types of collagen, laminin, fibronectin, hemonectin, and many proteoglycans. Extracellular matrix proteins can also serve as adhesion molecules. The multitude of these adhesive interactions suggests that they are physiologically important in the regulation of hematopoiesis. The processes by which stem cells remain quiescent, self-renew, or commit to lineage-specific differentiation are not well understood. It is likely that both intrinsic and extrinsic events contribute to these processes.

CYTOKINE REGULATION OF HEMATOPOIETIC PROGENITOR CELLS Progenitor cell production is regulated by combinations of cytokines. Dormant stem cells that have differentiated into a state capable of cycling can be purified by flow cytometry based on cell surface phenotype, blast morphology, and metabolic markers. While these cells show no proliferation to single cytokines, their maximal growth is promoted by combinations of factors that include, for example, one member of each of the following groups: (1) either stem cell factor or flt3 ligand; (2) interleukin (IL) 6, IL-11, IL-12, thrombopoietin (Tpo), or granulocyte (G) colony stimulating factor (G-CSF); and (3) IL-3, IL-4, or GM-CSF. These synergistic effects are direct (being observed in single cell assays). Synergy can be due to induction of cycling in resting cells and/or enhanced proliferative rate. The most primitive cells have the highest proliferative potential, eventually giving rise to multipotential colony forming cells; these give rise to mixed-lineage differentiated progeny but have little capacity for self-replicative divisions. Synergistic effects on progenitor cell colony formation were found to be consistently preceded by increased CSF receptor expression on enriched progenitor cells, which was not detectable on unfractionated marrow. The maximum upregulation of CSF receptor expression was observed by 24 h and occurred in a dose- and time-dependent manner.

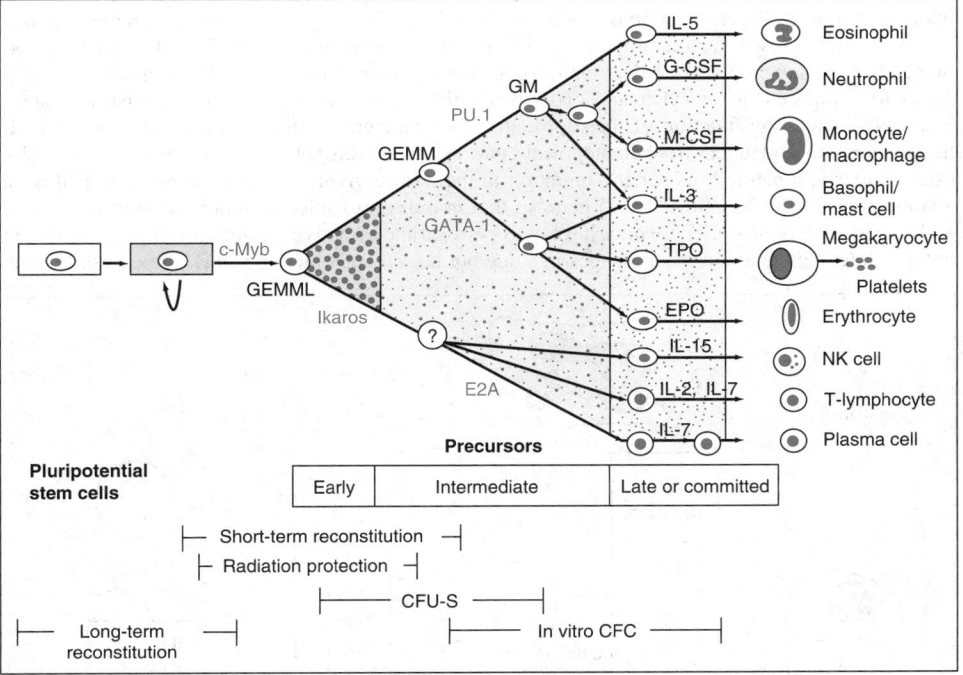

FIGURE 105-1 Cellular basis of hematopoiesis. Mature cells are derived from a common multipotent progenitor. Lineage development appears to occur as a consequence of the ordered expression of transcription factors (in blue). Thus, mice in which PU.1 expression has been blocked develop normal erythrocytes and megakaryocytes, but no other cell lineages. Once lineage commitment occurs, cytokines and colony-stimulating factors (in black) regulate development, again through the induction of transcription factors. Abbreviations: HSC, hematopoietic stem cell; GEMML, cell giving rise to granulocyte, erythroid, monocyte, megakaryocyte, and lymphoid cells; GEMM, cell giving rise to granulocytic, erythroid, monocyte, and megakaryocytic cells; GM, cell giving rise to granulocytic and monocyte cells.

MATURING CELLS—LATE-ACTING LINEAGE-SPECIFIC FACTORS The final proliferation cycles of the differentiated cells as they mature to become fully functional blood cells are stimulated by a number of factors that act in a lineage-specific manner (Fig. 105-1). For example, erythropoietin (Epo) and Tpo are the physiologic regulators for erythrocyte and megakaryocyte differentiation, respectively; however, both can also act on bipotent progenitors capable of differentiating into either lineage. IL-3, IL-5, and G-CSF drive basophilic, eosinophilic, and neutrophilic leukocyte maturation, respectively. IL-3 and G-CSF can also act on earlier cells. These mature cells exit the marrow environment via the central venous sinus and enter the peripheral circulation. The cells perform many functions (see Chap. 305). Also, many cell types are responsive to a variety of stress situations during which they perform their specialized functions.

PHYSIOLOGIC SOURCES OF HEMATOPOIETIC GROWTH FACTORS

Hematopoietic growth factors orchestrate the body's response to infection and other stresses (Fig. 105-2). In response to bacteria, several cytokines such as macrophage (M) colony stimulating factor (M-CSF or CSF-1), GM-CSF, and G-CSF are produced and secreted into the circulation. Furthermore, the inflammatory cytokines, IL-1, IL-6, and tumor necrosis factor α (TNFα) are released from a broad range of cells in the stroma (Fig. 105-2). Not only do they have direct effects on hematopoietic progenitors but they also initiate a cascade of cytokine production that stimulates the production of other cytokines. In addition, neuroendocrine hormones such as growth hormone and prolactin have growth-promoting activities on hematopoiesis that allow for improved myeloid recovery after BMT. The mechanism is partially direct and partially indirect through the stimulation of other growth factors like insulin-like growth factor-1. Another group of cytokines [IL-2, IL-3, IL-4, IL-5, and interferon (IFN) α] are made by T lymphocytes upon activation by foreign antigens.

Only a few growth factors are known to function in maintenance of steady state hematopoiesis. Mice homozygous for mutations in the genes for stem cell factor (Sl locus) or its receptor c-kit (at the W locus) that affect the function of these proteins have deficiencies in the development and function of hematopoiesis, particularly erythropoiesis. Similarly, a naturally occurring mutation in the mouse involves a stop codon in the M-CSF (CSF-1) gene so that homozygous mice make no M-CSF (CSF-1). These mice have osteopetrosis and a relative, not absolute, deficiency in macrophages in some but not all anatomic sites. In addition, mice with either flt3 or IL-7 genes disrupted (so-called gene knockout mice) show deficiencies in development of lymphocyte lineages.

The steady-state regulation of erythropoietin is essential to the regulation of erythropoiesis. The primary site of Epo production after birth is the kidney, likely in peritubular interstitial cells located in the inner cortex and outer medulla. In response to sensing a lower oxygen pressure (hypoxia), Epo gene transcription increases, regulated by hypoxia responsive regions in 5′ and 3′ enhancers of the Epo gene. It is not known how cells detect changes in P_{O_2}. Evidence has been presented that a heme-carrying protein, cytochrome b_{559} in carotid bodies, might regulate superoxide ions that mediate sensing P_{O_2} changes. In hematopoietic tissues, elevated Epo results in increased erythroid cell production. This results in an increase in the oxygen-carrying capacity of the blood, thereby alleviating the hypoxic stimulus and providing a negative feedback loop shutting off Epo production. In patients with normal renal function, serum erythropoietin levels are inversely proportional to the hemoglobin concentration.

HEMATOPOIETIC CELL GROWTH INHIBITORS The growth and differentiation of hematopoietic cells have been shown to be negatively regulated both in vitro and in vivo by IFNα, -β and -γ, TNFα, macrophage inflammatory protein 1α, and several other chemokines as well as other agents such as prostaglandins, lactoferrin, and the heavy subunits of ferritin (H ferritin). It has been proposed that constitutive hematopoiesis is regulated, in part, by the balance of both positive and negative growth signals. The TGFβ family of proteins has potent hematopoietic regulatory properties, ranging from inhibitory effects on the growth of primitive stem cells to the differentiated functions of mature cells. TGFβ can have both inhibitory and stimulatory actions on these systems, depending on the differentiation state of the target cell and the other cytokines interacting with the cell. TGFβ has direct effects on cell surface expression of many cytokine receptors, suggesting that it is part of the mechanism of action of TGFβ. The major biologic effect of TGFβ on hematopoietic cell growth is the reversible inhibition of entry into the cell cycle. The in vivo injection of TGFβ mimics the in vitro effects, and the presence of increased myeloid cells and in some cases myeloid hyperplasia in TGFβ1 knockout mice supports the antiproliferative role of TGFβ in vivo.

There exists a balance between positive and negative growth regulation in hematopoiesis. For example, IL-3 and stem cell factor optimally stimulate Lin − Thy-1 + murine progenitor cell growth in single cell assays, and TGFβ inhibits more than 90 percent of this growth. While the addition of a cocktail of five additional stimulatory cytokines does not increase the number of responding progenitors, the effect of TGFβ is reversed. In contrast, TNFα and IFNγ cooperate with TGFβ to reverse the growth-promoting effects of these multiple growth factors. Thus, the overall biologic effect is determined by the contrasting effects and relative abundance of various cytokines.

GENERALITIES ABOUT CYTOKINE REGULATION Every cytokine (including hematopoietic growth factors and interleukins) has multiple biologic effects. Different cytokines may exert the same biologic effects, producing a system with redundancies. Cytokines are capable of both direct and indirect stimulatory (or inhibitory) effects. Cytokine action is often amplified by other factors. Cytokines that act on early lineage progenitors often act also on more mature lineage cells, though their effects may be different on cells at different stages of maturation. Cytokines work best in combinations. Cytokines and cytokine receptors each share certain structural features and signal

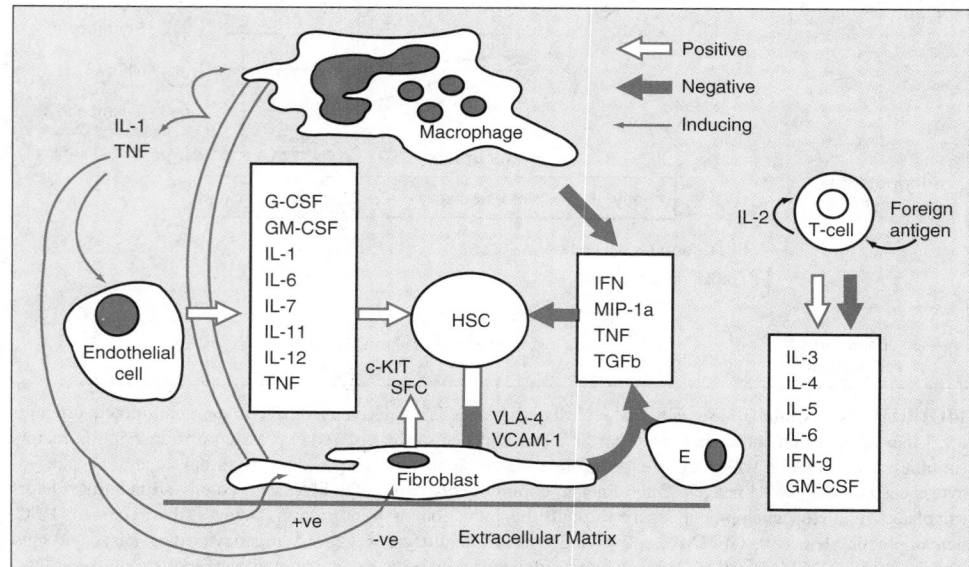

FIGURE 105-2 The cellular and humoral influences on hematopoietic stem/progenitor cells.

transduction pathways. In some instances cytokines share receptor components. Genetic alterations in cytokine or cytokine receptor genes can lead to dysregulation of hematopoiesis.

CLINICAL IMPLICATIONS OF STEM CELL BIOLOGY

PATHOGENESIS OF MARROW DISORDERS Marrow stem cell organization provides excess production capacity to respond to increases in demand for blood elements imposed by stressful situations throughout the lifespan. However, marrow disease states can lead to pathologic hematopoiesis. The two major manifestations of hematopoietic stem cell disorders are aplasia, cytopenia of one or many cell lineages (see Chap. 110) or neoplasia, clonal expansion of one or many cell lineages (Chaps. 111 to 114). Aplasia may be polyclonal, as when the immune system suppresses or a toxin kills the stem cells, or clonal, as in paroxysmal nocturnal hemoglobinuria where the abnormal clone interferes with normal stem cells. Neoplasia is always clonal in origin, with genetic defects accumulating over time in the progenitors of a single cell (Fig. 105-1). The spectrum of genetic alterations and the lineage and stage of differentiation of the neoplastic progenitor influence the clinical manifestations of a hematologic malignancy. For example, normal promyelocytes have granules containing procoagulants. Thus, clotting abnormalities are a prominent feature of acute promyelocytic leukemia. Specific genetic lesions may lead to differentiation arrest, autonomous or unregulated growth, or defective cell turnover or apoptosis.

The clonal nature of a hematologic malignancy only rarely needs to be demonstrated. Some cellular infiltrates may resemble neoplasms, but are found to be polyclonal on genetic analysis. Neoplasms often contain characteristic chromosomal translocations detectable by cytogenetic examination (Chap. 66). In addition, amplification of particular genes by the polymerase chain reaction can permit the detection of clonal translocations not visible on cytogenetics and can identify clonal rearrangements of immunoglobulin or T-cell receptor genes to assist in defining the lineage of a tumor. The most common clinical use of such data is in assessing the presence of residual disease after treatment.

BONE MARROW TRANSPLANTATION The ability of HSC to protect animals from death due to radiation-induced marrow failure has directly led to the use of high doses of both radiation and chemotherapy with BMT for the treatment of malignant disease (see Chap. 116). BMT has become the treatment of choice for several hematologic malignancies and is in use as a means of delivering dose-intensive therapy to patients with a variety of solid tumors, particularly those with poor prognosis.

In patients undergoing autologous BMT, the infused bone marrow may contain residual tumor cells. By using labeled cells, it has been demonstrated that these reinfused tumor cells are in some cases responsible for the subsequent disease relapse. The use of purified stem cell preparations in this setting of autologous BMT has the potential to reduce the rate of relapse secondary to the presence of tumor cells in the marrow.

In patients undergoing allogeneic BMT, the infusion of alloreactive donor cells is associated with two clinically important immunologic phenomena: (1) graft-versus-host disease (GVHD), caused by an immune response of donor T cells against host tissues (a major cause of both morbidity and mortality), and (2) the graft-versus-tumor (GVT) effect caused by the presence of either donor T cells or natural killer cells and responsible for the reduced risk of relapse of patients with leukemia and lymphoma.

Depleting the marrow of T cells to reduce the severity of GVHD in patients receiving an allograft has also increased the number of graft failures and reduced the GVT effects. Presumably the T cells play a role in producing important CSFs needed for marrow engraftment, or perhaps they inhibit the production of growth inhibitory cytokines that act to prevent engraftment. The use of positively selected purified stem cell populations devoid of alloreactive T cells may circumvent the development of GVHD. The addition back to the graft of T cell subsets that mediate the GVT effect (but not GVHD) could decrease the incidence

of tumor recurrence and graft rejection. Addition of T cells cytotoxic to Epstein-Barr virus–infected cells to BMT has proven beneficial in reducing the development of Epstein-Barr virus–mediated lymphoma. The efficacy of this approach might be enhanced by vaccinating the marrow donor against the recipient's tumor in a specific fashion.

The treatment of patients with either chemotherapy or hematopoietic growth factors produces a dramatic mobilization of stem cell activity into the peripheral blood. Apheresis of peripheral blood mononuclear cells following growth factor mobilization yields cell preparations that provide engraftment as (or more) rapidly as (than) conventional BMT. The use of peripheral blood stem cells offers several potential advantages over bone marrow. Collection of these cells involves less invasive procedures than bone marrow harvest. Patients who are not candidates for a bone marrow harvest can now be transplanted with autologous peripheral blood–derived stem cells. In a variety of diseases, such as breast cancer and certain subtypes of lymphoma, significant contamination of the bone marrow by tumor cells may be avoided by using peripheral blood stem cells.

GENE THERAPY A variety of germ line mutations result in the development of a wide spectrum of hematologic diseases. A single nucleotide base substitution gives rise to hemoglobin S and produces sickle cell anemia (see Chap. 107). Similarly, the inheritance of impaired cellular and humoral immunity in many instances is attributable to mutations in a single gene, as in the case of adenosine deaminase deficiency.

Tissue-specific patterns of gene expression in these inherited hematologic diseases provide a clinical setting in which the transfer of genes into somatic cells could correct the underlying defect. The introduction of genes encoding enzymes critical for cellular immune function, such as adenosine deaminase, into HSCs should permit the development of functional T and B lymphocytes. However, at present several problems, including unsustained low levels of tissue-specific gene expression, prevent the broader application of this technology to inherited hematologic diseases.

THERAPEUTIC USE OF HEMATOPOIETIC GROWTH FACTORS—ERYTHROPOIETIN AND THROMBOPOIETIN If iron status is normal, erythropoietin (Epo) is a useful treatment in patients with erythropoietin-deficiency anemias, which occur mainly in the setting of renal failure. Anemias accompanying chronic renal failure and myeloma are usually responsive to Epo. AIDS patients with anemia related to zidovudine may improve with Epo. Weekly administration of Epo to patients several weeks before they undergo elective surgical procedures can decrease the need for RBC transfusions postoperatively. Epo has become a drug of abuse among certain athletes. Its ability to increase RBC mass leads to enhanced oxygen carrying capacity and enhanced performance. Epo use is difficult to detect. In clinical trials in cancer patients, 32 to 85 percent of patients respond with a significant increase in hematocrit after 2 months of therapy. Epo is well tolerated, producing symptoms of hypertension or venous thrombosis only if given to patients with an elevated RBC mass. The starting dose is generally 50 units per kilogram of body weight subcutaneously three times weekly. Patients whose serum ferritin level is less than 400 µg/L (400 ng/mL) or whose serum Epo level is 100 units per liter or higher at the start of therapy are much less likely to respond. If the hemoglobin has not increased by at least 5 g/L (0.5 g/dL) after 2 weeks of therapy, the iron status should be checked. If the patient is not iron-deficient, Epo is unlikely to lead to improvement.

Tpo increased megakaryopoiesis and platelet production manyfold in both normal and myelosuppressed monkeys. Also red cell recovery was markedly enhanced in Tpo treated animals. Tpo is just entering clinical trials.

G-CSF AND GM-CSF The myeloid growth factors G-CSF and GM-CSF have been shown to stimulate neutrophil production in various clinical settings, but they are not universally effective. In cancer patients undergoing intensive cytotoxic chemotherapy, G-CSF stimulation of granulopoiesis translated into decreased incidence of neutropenia-associated fever and infection in patients with a high likelihood

PREVENTIVE USES

With the first cycle of chemotherapy (so-called primary CSF administration)
  Not needed on a routine basis
  Use if the probability of febrile neutropenia is 40% or greater
  Use if patient has preexisting neutropenia or active infection
With subsequent cycles if febrile neutropenia has previously occurred (so-called secondary CSF administration)
  Not needed after short duration neutropenia without fever
  Use if patient had febrile neutropenia in previous cycle
  Use if prolonged neutropenia (even without fever) delays therapy

THERAPEUTIC USES

Afebrile neutropenic patients
  No evidence of benefit
Febrile neutropenic patients
  No evidence of benefit
  May feel compelled to use in the face of clinical deterioration from sepsis, pneumonia, or fungal infection, but benefit unclear
To augment dose-intensity of chemotherapy in patients with curable malignancies
  No evidence of benefit to date
In bone marrow or peripheral blood stem cell transplantation
  Use to mobilize stem cells from marrow
  Use to hasten myeloid recovery
In acute myeloid leukemia
  No evidence of benefit and may be harmful
In myelodysplastic syndromes
  Not routinely beneficial
  Use intermittently in subset with neutropenia and recurrent infection

WHAT DOSE AND SCHEDULE SHOULD BE USED?

G-CSF: 5 µg/kg per day subcutaneously
GM-CSF: 250 µg/m^2 per day subcutaneously

WHEN SHOULD CSF THERAPY START AND END?

When indicated, start 24–72 h after chemotherapy
Continue until absolute neutrophil count is 10,000/µL
Do not use concomitantly with chemotherapy or radiation therapy

---

of developing granulocytopenia (Table 105-1). G-CSF has also been studied in patients with AIDS, congenital and cyclic neutropenia, myelodysplastic syndromes, and aplastic anemia; it increases the neutrophil count in many patients with these disorders. In neutropenic patients, G-CSF often increases the neutrophil count enough to decrease the frequency and severity of infection. G-CSF has been generally well tolerated, with no apparent dose-limiting toxicity. GM-CSF has been used in settings similar to those in which G-CSF was used. Although GM-CSF has proliferative effects on a broader range of hematopoietic progenitors in vitro, its primary clinical benefit in vivo has been on granulopoiesis. GM-CSF increases myeloid recovery following autologous BMT for lymphoid neoplasias and in patients who have undergone allogeneic or autologous BMT in whom engraftment has failed or is delayed. GM-CSF is more toxic than G-CSF, with bone pain, rash, fevers, fatigue, anorexia, phlebitis, thrombosis, and, at high doses, capillary leak syndrome with pleural and pericardial effusions and edema observed.

G-CSF-mobilized stem/progenitor cells collected by leukapheresis can be reinfused along with growth factors following intensive chemotherapy. In this setting, recovery of all blood lineages can be accelerated to 8 to 9 days rather than the 14 to 17 days seen with autologous marrow. These biologic effects will allow peripheral blood stem cell transplantation to be used more widely and safely.

IL-3, IL-6, IL-1 AND Pixy-321 IL-3 has been tested clinically in the hope that its effects on earlier progenitors might lead to beneficial effects on platelets as well as granulocytes. Clinical results have been disappointing. IL-3 has no significant effects on platelet recovery and is not more effective than G-CSF in its effects on granulocytes, but it is toxic. IL-6 was also predicted to exert significant effects on

platelets. However, its diverse biologic effects produce toxicity at doses that appear to have no effect on platelets.

IL-1 has been shown to have significant effects on both granulocyte and platelet recovery after cytotoxic chemotherapy. However, when it is given intravenously, it may produce hypotension and atrial arrhythmias at the biologically active doses. By contrast, subcutaneous administration preserves the beneficial effects on platelets and granulocytes and prevents the adverse side effects.

Pixy-321 is not a molecule found in nature. It is a chimeric fusion protein made in the laboratory and composed of active components of both IL-3 and GM-CSF. Although it appears to exert synergistic biologic effects on some cell types in vitro, clinical trials demonstrated only minor effects on granulocytes. In addition, its beneficial effects were restricted to the first cycle of administration because it elicits a potent neutralizing antibody response.

The future of hematopoietic growth factor therapy is difficult to predict. There is reason to hope that combinations of factors would be more effective than single agents. However, the tight physiologic regulation of hematopoiesis by both positive and negative growth regulators may make it difficult to achieve substantial beneficial effects. Hyperstimulation may simply lead to an amplification of inhibitory circuits. Some combination of stimulation plus inhibition of inhibitory pathways may be more successful. Even if such manipulations are successful, it is possible that the increase in proliferative demand on the stem cell population induced by repeated cycles of stem cell recruitment and chemotherapy could result in stem cell depletion and marrow aplasia or myelodysplasia.

Acknowledgment

The authors wish to acknowledge Dr. Mark A. Goldberg and Dr. H. Franklin Bunn, authors of the chapter on Molecular and Cellular Hematopoiesis in the 13th edition of this book, for some of the text we retained in this edition.

BIBLIOGRAPHY

AMERICAN SOCIETY OF CLINICAL ONCOLOGY: Guidelines for the use of colony-stimulating factors. J Clin Oncol 12:2471, 1994
APPELBAUM FR: Allogeneic bone marrow transplantation and the use of hematopoietic growth factors. Stem Cells (Dayt) 13:344, 1995
BECKER AJ et al: Cytological demonstration of the clonal nature of spleen colonies derived from transplanted mouse marrow cells. Nature 197:452, 1963
CHEN S-J et al: Acute promyelocytic leukemia: From clinic to molecular biology. Stem Cells (Dayt)13:22, 1995
CROSS AR et al: Involvement of NAD(P)H oxidase as a P_{O_2} sensor protein in the rat carotid body. Biochem J 272:743, 1990
ESCHBACH JW et al: Treatment of the anemia of progressive renal failure with recombinant human erythropoietin. N Engl J Med 321:158, 1989
FARESE AM et al: Recombinant human megakaryocytic growth and differentiation factor stimulates thrombocytopoiesis in normal nonhuman primates. Blood 86:54, 1995
JACOBSEN SEW et al: Growth response of hematopoietic progenitors to cytokines is determined by the balance between the synergy of multiple stimulators and negative cooperation of multiple inhibitors. Exp Hematol 22:985, 1994
JONES RJ et al: Separation of pluripotent hematopoietic stem cells from spleen-colony forming cells. Nature 347:188, 1990
SPANGRUDE GJ et al: Purification and characterization of mouse hematopoietic stem cells. Science 241:58, 1988

---

106 *Robert S. Hillman*

IRON DEFICIENCY AND OTHER HYPOPROLIFERATIVE ANEMIAS

Normal erythropoiesis, including the expected proliferative response of the erythroid marrow to anemia, involves both the appropriate erythropoietin stimulation of a healthy erythroid marrow and an adequate supply of iron. A defect in one of these components results in a hypoproliferative or iron-deficiency anemia. This is a common and important mechanism of disease in clinical medicine. Hypoproliferative anemias are seen frequently in patients with renal insufficiency, marrow damage, iron deficiency, and acute and chronic inflammatory states. Furthermore, the pattern of the anemia can be of considerable value in diagnosis and management. Changes in red blood cell morphology and measurements of iron supply help in the differential diagnosis of the etiology of a hypoproliferative state. Effective management of patients with hypoproliferative anemias with hematinics and recombinant erythropoietin depends on a careful analysis of the defects involved.

CONTROL OF NORMAL ERYTHROPOIESIS

The pathophysiology of a hypoproliferative or iron-deficiency anemia is essentially a disruption of the control of normal erythropoiesis. The proliferative response of the erythron is a function of anemia severity and iron supply. Peritubular interstitial cells of the kidney produce erythropoietin in response to lower oxygen delivery. As the hemoglobin level falls below 100 g/L (10 g/dL), erythropoietin levels increase logarithmically, stimulating the erythroid marrow to proliferate and increase red blood cell production severalfold. The level of response can generally be predicted for the clinical situation. Blood-loss anemia in a patient with a healthy marrow and normal iron stores will usually generate a 2- to 3-fold increase in red cell production within 7 to 10 days. Higher levels of production are observed in patients with hemolytic anemias as the erythroid marrow expands within the marrow cavity. In fact, production levels in excess of five to six times normal can be observed in patients with congenital hemolytic anemias and inherited defects in hemoglobin synthesis.

Iron supply plays a key role in this production response. The bulk of the iron required for basal erythropoiesis is recycled from senescent red cells by the reticuloendothelial system (Fig. 106-1). This iron is transported through the plasma by transferrin, a plasma glycoprotein that binds two atoms of iron. The majority of iron-laden transferrin molecules are destined to bind to specific receptors on the surface of erythroid precursors and are subsequently internalized. The iron is then released, and the transferrin-receptor complex returns to the cell surface where transferrin molecules are released back to the circulation to complete the transport cycle. The erythroid precursor uses the delivered iron for the synthesis of hemoglobin, storing any excess as ferritin. A smaller amount of iron is taken up by other cells in the body, especially the liver parenchymal cells, for incorporation into heme enzymes and for ferritin storage.

The amount of iron delivered to and accepted by the marrow is determined by several factors, including the level of iron stores, the amount of iron bound to transferrin, the blood flow to the marrow, the number of erythroid marrow precursors, and the expression of unoccupied transferrin receptor sites. The number of precursors and the expression of transferrin receptors on the cell surface are directly influenced by the level of erythropoietin stimulation. On the delivery side, the amount of iron available for transport is a function of available sources of iron supply, including the amount of reticuloendothelial iron stores, the level of food iron intake, and the rate of red blood cell turnover. To achieve a maximum proliferative response, iron supply and erythropoietin stimulation must be balanced. If iron delivery is suboptimal, the proliferative response of the marrow to erythropoietin is inhibited and normal hemoglobin synthesis is disrupted. The result is a hypoproliferative marrow response and, in situations of severe iron-supply deficiency, a microcytic, hypochromic anemia.

IRON-DEFICIENCY ANEMIA

While iron-deficiency anemia has traditionally been defined as a microcytic, hypochromic anemia secondary to a total-body iron deficit, a more sensitive definition of iron deficiency has to include the concepts of negative iron balance and iron-deficient erythropoiesis. By definition, iron-store depletion refers to an imbalance between normal physiologic demands such as body growth, menstrual blood loss, and pregnancy and the level of dietary iron intake. Iron-deficient erythropoiesis goes a step further and indicates a limitation in red blood cell production. Iron-deficiency anemia with microcytic, hypochromic red blood cell morphology indicates a prolonged period of negative iron balance and anemia severe enough to stimulate the production of poorly hemoglobinized cells. The incidence of each of these clinical states in any population depends on several variables, including the amount and character of dietary iron supply, the efficiency of iron absorption, and the incidence of disease states that result in iron loss.

NUTRITIONAL IRON BALANCE The amount of iron absorbed from the diet is a function of the kinds of foods eaten, the daily caloric intake, and the absorptive capacity of the small intestine. A key element is the heme iron content of the diet. Inorganic iron is toxic and not readily absorbed. Heme iron is much more available for absorption than inorganic forms of iron. Meat-eating individuals ingest more heme-containing myoglobin than do vegetarians. Populations existing on diets made up of primarily vegetables and grains are at a further disadvantage in maintaining iron homeostasis, because these foods contain certain compounds, such as phosphates and phytates, that inhibit iron absorption. In contrast, the ascorbic acid present in citrus fruits can promote iron absorption.

An adult male on a balanced diet containing both meat and vegetable products will ingest approximately 15 to 20 mg of iron each day, while the adult female will ingest 10 to 15 mg/d. In the male, only 1 to 2 mg needs to be absorbed to replace the iron lost from desquamation of skin and mucosal cells. The adult premenopausal female needs to absorb more from the diet to make up for menstrual blood loss. The same is true for the frequent blood donor. Infants, children, and adolescents may be unable to maintain normal iron balance because of the increased demands of body growth and much lower dietary intakes of iron. This is also true for the pregnant woman. During the last two trimesters of pregnancy, the daily iron requirement increases to 5 to 6 mg, a level that cannot be supported unless the diet is rich in heme iron or the woman receives an iron supplement. Some countries have taken to supplementing foods, such as bread, cereals, and bakery products, to help prevent negative iron balance in target populations. Multivitamins containing iron are recommended for patients at high risk, including adolescents, pregnant women, and regular blood donors.

Iron absorption by the proximal small intestine is a carefully regulated process that is tuned to the level of body iron stores and

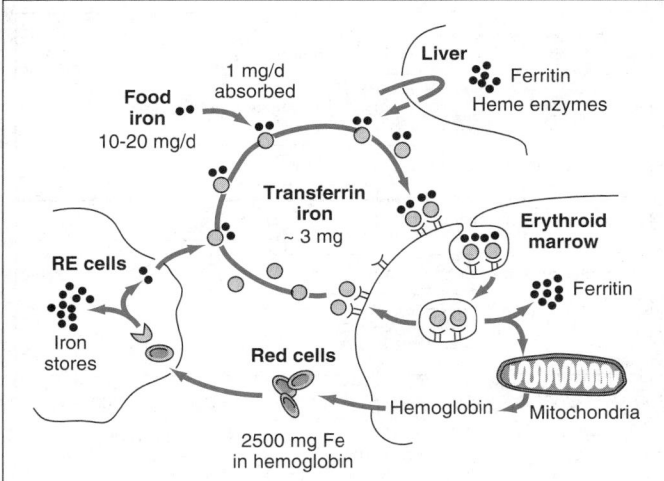

FIGURE 106-1 Normal iron transport pathways. Iron recovered from senescent red cells and absorbed from food is bound to transferrin and transported to the erythroid marrow and other tissues. Iron-laden transferrin binds to transferrin receptors on the surface of erythroid precursors and is internalized. Once the iron is harvested for hemoglobin production, the transferrin–transferrin receptor complex returns to the cell surface, and the transferrin is released to complete the cycle. Males lose about 1 mg/d of iron and have iron stores in ferritin of about 1000 mg. Females may lose up to 2 mg/d of iron (particularly in menstruation) and have iron stores of 100 to 400 mg. (From Hillman and Ault, with permission.)

the demands of erythropoiesis. It becomes more efficient as body iron stores are depleted. Patients with certain types of anemias, especially those with high levels of ineffective erythropoiesis, have a tendency to absorb excess amounts of iron. In some cases, this can lead to iron overload and tissue iron damage. The normal individual, however, is capable of markedly reducing iron absorption in situations of excessive intake of either food or medicinal iron. This provides a considerable margin of safety when iron supplements are administered over a long period of time. Individuals at special risk of absorbing too much iron are those with idiopathic hemochromatosis, an inherited disorder where the normal regulation of iron absorption is defective (see Chap. 342).

Similar to the normal "range" of values for hemoglobin/hematocrit according to age and sex (Chap. 59), the distribution of body iron pools will depend on the patient's age, sex, and dietary content of iron (Table 106-1). The iron sequestered in red cells and in tissues as myoglobin or enzyme iron correlates with the patient's red blood cell mass and body size. The level of reticuloendothelial iron stores will reflect the balance between dietary intake and iron losses. An adult male will have from 600 to 1000 mg of reticuloendothelial iron stores, while women and adolescents generally have less than 300 mg of stores. Younger children, pregnant women, and women with very heavy menses will have little or no iron in their reticuloendothelial cells.

CLINICAL PRESENTATION   There are situations where iron deficiency can be anticipated (Table 106-2). The delicate balance between iron intake and natural requirements means that any decreased intake or increased loss of iron may lead to deficiency. Significant chronic blood loss from any cause will deplete iron stores and exceed the capacity to absorb iron from the diet. Patients with severe malabsorption can also present with an iron-deficiency anemia regardless of the adequacy of their iron intake. The symptoms and signs of severe iron deficiency largely reflect the severity of the patient's anemia and include fatigue, pallor, and a decreased exercise capacity. When iron deficiency is severe and prolonged, the patient may complain of mouth soreness, difficulty swallowing, and a softening and curling of the nails called *spooning*. However, these findings are not very sensitive or specific; the diagnosis of an iron-deficiency state is basically a laboratory exercise.

LABORATORY IRON STUDIES   The principal measurements of iron supply used in clinical diagnosis are the serum iron (SI), the transferrin iron-binding capacity (TIBC), and the serum ferritin level. Other useful studies include the inspection of the marrow aspirate or biopsy for reticuloendothelial iron stores and sideroblasts and red blood cell protoporphyrin and serum transferrin receptor levels. Measurements of plasma iron turnover and iron absorption are possible using tracer amounts of radioactive iron. From a research standpoint, such studies have been very important in defining the distribution of iron stores and the patterns of abnormal erythropoiesis. They do not play a significant role in clinical diagnosis.

Serum Iron Studies   The SI is a measure of the amount of iron bound to transferrin, while the TIBC is a measure of the total binding capacity of transferrin. The normal SI falls between 9 and 27 μmol/L (50 and 150 μg/dL); the normal TIBC between 54 and 64 μmol/L (300 and 360 μg/dL). It is also routine to calculate the percent saturation of transferrin (SI $\div$ TIBC = percent saturation). A normal

Table 106-1

Body Iron Distribution

	Iron Content, mg	
	Adult Male (80 kg)	**Adult Female (60 kg)**
Hemoglobin	2500	1700
Myoglobin/enzymes	500	300
Transferrin iron	3	3
Iron stores	600–1000	0–300

Table 106-2

Causes of Iron Depletion/Deficiency

Iron-Store Depletion	Iron-Deficient Erythropoiesis	Iron-Deficiency Anemia
Rapid growth	Blood loss	Blood loss
Infancy	Excessive menses or	GI hemorrhage
Adolescence	donation	Intravascular
Menstrual blood loss	Hemodialysis	hemolysis
Inadequate diet	GI hemorrhage	Surgical blood loss
Blood donation	Pregnancy	Hookworm
	Malabsorption	infestation
	Polycythemia vera treated	Severe malabsorption
	with phlebotomy	Gastrectomy
		Sprue
		Inflammatory bowel
		disease

NOTE: GI, gastrointestinal.

individual has a percent saturation of between 30 and 50 percent. Iron-deficiency states are associated with saturation levels below 20 percent, while clinically dangerous iron overload occurs if the saturation exceeds 50 to 60 percent (Fig. 106-2).

Serum Ferritin Level   Iron is stored as ferritin or hemosiderin. The protein, apoferritin, binds to free ferrous ion and stores it as ferric ion. Iron plus apoferritin is ferritin. Apoferritin mRNA is present in the cell with a molecule of the protein bound to the message, which inhibits translation. Free iron leads to removal of the protein from the message, increased translation of apoferritin mRNA, and increased protein levels. When ferritin is taken up by cells in the reticuloendothelial system, it can be catabolized to hemosiderin. Iron in ferritin can be extracted for the synthesis of heme, whereas that in hemosiderin is less reliably available for metabolic needs. Ferritin found in the circulation is in equilibrium with tissue ferritins. The serum measurement correlates with the level of total-body iron stores. The normal value for a serum ferritin level will, therefore, vary according to the age and sex of the individual. The adult male has a serum ferritin level of 50 to 150 μg/L, while most adult women demonstrate levels between 15 and 50 μg/L. Once iron stores are depleted, the serum ferritin level declines to levels below 15 μg/L. This reduction correlates with a decrease in the intracellular synthesis of apoferritin protein because the free apoferritin binds again to its mRNA.

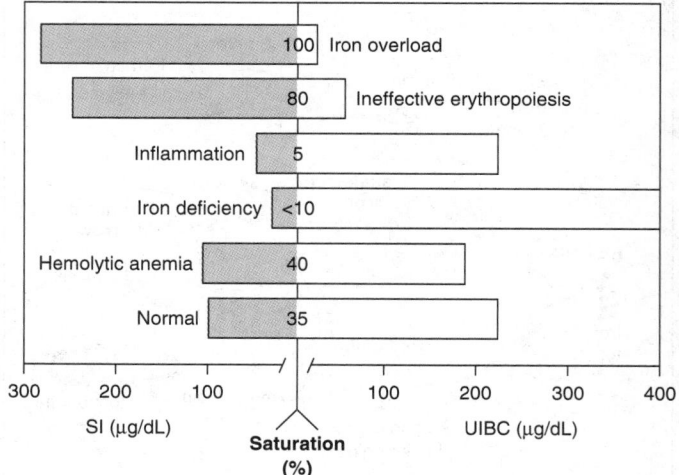

FIGURE 106-2   The patterns of serum iron (SI) and total iron-binding capacity [TIBC = unsaturated iron-binding capacity (UIBC) + SI] vary with different types of anemia. Normal individuals and patients with hemolytic anemias have SIs in the normal range of 50 to 150 μg/dL (9 to 27 μmol/L), and normal TIBCs. In contrast, iron-deficient patients have very low serum irons with TIBCs greater than 360 μg/dL (64 μmol/L). Inflammatory anemia patients have low SIs and low TIBCs. Finally, patients with ineffective erythropoiesis and iron overload have fully saturated iron-binding capacities. (From Hillman and Finch, with permission.)

Marrow Iron Stores Reticuloendothelial cell iron stores can be estimated from the Prussian blue stain of a marrow aspirate or a biopsy specimen. By convention, the stores are graded on a scale of 0 to 4+. While this is not quantitative, the visual grading of stores correlates fairly well with the ferritin and hemosiderin iron present in reticuloendothelial cells and available for erythropoiesis (Table 106-3). In situations of iron overload, the marrow iron stain is not as good as the serum ferritin level, which also reflects the level of iron sequestered in hepatocytes and other tissue cells. The marrow iron stain does provide information as to the delivery of iron to erythroid precursors. In a normal male, 50 to 60 percent of the more mature erythroid precursors will have a few visible ferritin iron granules in their cytoplasm. This represents excess iron not needed for hemoglobin formation. In disease states such as the sideroblastic anemias, the number and pattern of iron granules in marrow normoblasts is distinctly abnormal. In the case of ringed sideroblastic anemia, iron-encrusted mitochondria form a collar or ring of iron granules immediately around the nucleus (see Chap 110).

Red Cell Protoporphyrin Level Protoporphyrin is the molecule made in mitochondria to which iron is added to form heme (see Chap. 343). The level of red cell protoporphyrin is another sensitive indicator of iron-deficient erythropoiesis. Higher-than-normal levels indicate an inadequate iron supply to erythroid precursors to support the formation of heme. The assay can be performed on very small amounts of blood. Normal values fall below 0.53 μmol/L (30 μg/dL) of red blood cells, while iron-deficient individuals have values in excess of 1.77 μmol/L (100 μg/dL). Protoporphyrin levels also rise in children exposed to lead. This reflects the inhibition of heme synthetase, the enzyme required for the formation of heme (see Chap. 397).

Serum Transferrin Receptor Serum levels of serum transferrin receptor correlate with the level of erythroid precursor proliferation and the adequacy of iron supply to the marrow. Normal levels are 4 to 9 μg/L by immunoassay. Levels increase rapidly in patients with iron-deficient erythropoiesis and/or a proliferative marrow, including states of ineffective erythropoiesis. This test is not commonly employed.

STAGES OF IRON DEFICIENCY The several stages of iron deficiency, including iron-store depletion, iron-deficient erythropoiesis, and iron-deficiency anemia, can be distinguished using these measurements of iron supply (Fig. 106-3).

Iron-Store Depletion This is identified using the serum ferritin level and marrow iron stain. A ferritin level less than 20 μg/L and visible iron stores of only 0 to 1+ suggest usable iron stores of less than 100 to 300 mg. As long as some stores are still available, the SI, TIBC, and red cell protoporphyrin levels are within normal limits. Moreover, the patient is not anemic, and red blood cell morphology is normal.

Iron-Deficient Erythropoiesis This can be distinguished based on further changes in the serum ferritin level and marrow iron stain and abnormalities of the plasma iron, TIBC, and red cell protoporphyrin. By definition, marrow iron stores are no longer visible, and the serum ferritin level falls to levels below 15 μg/L. The SI also falls to levels below 11 μmol/L (60 μg/dL), while the TIBC increases, resulting in a percent saturation of less than 20 percent. The protoporphyrin level increases to greater than 1.77 μmol/L (100 μg/dL) of red blood cells. These abnormalities in iron supply are still not accompanied by a change in red blood cell morphology. There is, however,

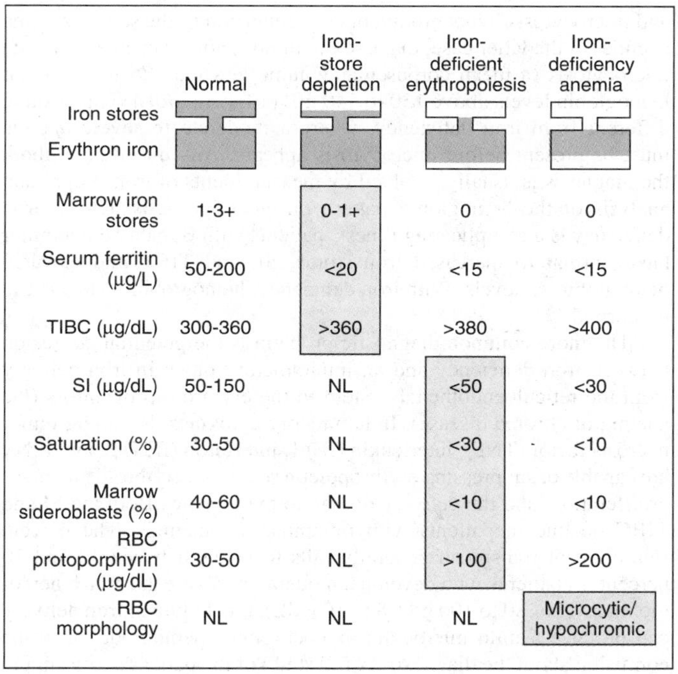

FIGURE 106-3 Laboratory studies in the evolution of iron deficiency. Measurements of marrow iron stores, serum ferritin, and TIBC are sensitive to early iron-store depletion. Iron-deficient erythropoiesis is recognized from additional abnormalities in the SI, percent saturation of transferrin, the pattern of marrow sideroblasts, and the red blood cell protoporphyrin level. Finally, patients with iron-deficiency anemia demonstrate all of these same abnormalities plus an anemia characterized by microcytic hypochromic morphology. (From Hillman and Finch, with permission.)

an impairment of the proliferative capacity of the marrow resulting in a mild normocytic, normochromic anemia, with hemoglobin levels of 100 to 120 g/L (10 to 12 g/dL).

Iron-Deficiency Anemia This is recognized from the combination of abnormal iron-supply studies and microcytic, hypochromic red blood cell morphology. The SI falls to very low levels [<4 μmol/L (<30 μg/dL)], while the TIBC increases, resulting in a percent saturation of less than 10 percent. The ferritin level is always less than 15 μg/L. Once the patient's hemoglobin level falls below 100 to 110 g/L (10 to 11 g/dL), poorly hemoglobinized cells begin to enter the circulation. When the anemia is only of moderate severity, the cells tend to be microcytic but not hypochromic. At lower hemoglobin levels, both microcytosis and hypochromia become more pronounced. Furthermore, red blood cell production becomes increasingly ineffective, resulting in greater degrees of aniso- and poikilocytosis. With very severe iron-deficiency anemia, cigar- or pencil-shaped red blood cells may be observed. As a rule, target cells are not seen with iron deficiency. When present, they suggest a globin chain production defect, one of the thalassemias. They may also be seen in the presence of liver disease.

Only a few diseases need to be considered in the differential diagnosis of an iron-deficiency anemia. Both α and β thalassemia are associated with microcytosis, hypochromia, and anemia of varying severity. The racial background and family history of the patient may be clues to the presence of thalassemia. However, this does not exclude the possibility of iron deficiency either alone or in combination with a globin production defect. Therefore, a full laboratory assessment is important (see Chap. 107). This should permit an accurate diagnosis of the cause of the microcytosis and hypochromia, whether a single or combined defect (Table 106-4). Morphologic clues that point to the diagnosis of thalassemia include the presence of target cells, a normal red cell distribution width indicating a uniform microcytosis,

Table 106-3

Iron Store Measurements

Iron Stores	Marrow Iron Stain, 0–4+	Serum Ferritin, μg/L
0	0	<15
1–300 mg	Trace to 1+	15–30
300–800 mg	2+	30–60
800–1000 mg	3+	60–150
1–2 g	4+	>150
Iron overload	—	>500–1000

and microcytosis/hypochromia out of proportion to the severity of the anemia. In the latter case, thalassemia minor patients can demonstrate microcytosis (a mean corpuscular volume less than 75 to 80 fL) at hemoglobin levels above 130 to 140 g/L (13 to 14 g/dL). This is quite different from iron deficiency, where a moderate to severe anemia must be present before microcytosis appears. Any uncertainty about the diagnosis is usually resolved by measurements of iron supply and analysis of the hemoglobin pattern on electrophoresis. Unless iron deficiency is a complicating illness, patients with β thalassemia minor have normal to increased iron stores, SI, and TIBC and elevated hemoglobin A_2 levels. With iron deficiency, hemoglobin A_2 levels can be normal.

The more common diagnostic problem is the potential confusion between iron deficiency and an inflammatory block in iron delivery from the reticuloendothelial system to the erythroid progenitors (the anemia of chronic disease). Inflammatory cytokines, including tumor necrosis factor (TNF), interleukin (IL) 1, interferon (IFN) β, and IFNγ are capable of suppressing erythropoietin secretion, erythroid precursor proliferation, and the delivery of iron to the marrow. Both the SI and TIBC decline in patients with inflammatory anemias. The percent saturation of transferrin generally falls to levels between 10 and 20 percent. In patients who develop a moderately severe anemia, a hemoglobin level of 80 to 100 g/L (8 to 10 g/dL), this failure in iron delivery can produce a mild microcytic, hypochromic anemia, adding to the confusion about the diagnosis. A full study of the patient's iron supply should distinguish between the two conditions (Table 106-5). Inflammatory anemia patients typically show a low SI, low TIBC, a normal to high serum ferritin level, and, if a marrow aspiration is performed, normal to increased iron stores together with a hypoproliferative marrow morphology. The serum transferrin receptor assay can also distinguish between the two conditions. Transferrin receptor levels tend not to increase with inflammation as compared to a two- to four-fold increase seen with true iron deficiency.

Patients with a defect in mitochondrial function resulting in a sideroblastic anemia can also present with a microcytic, hypochromic anemia. Hereditary sideroblastic anemia is a rare condition that presents in childhood either as an X-linked or autosomally inherited condition. Red blood cell morphology is typically dimorphic, and measurements of iron supply make the distinction from iron deficiency quite easy (see Table 106-4). Patients who develop an acquired ringed sideroblastic anemia typically exhibit excessive iron accumulation, even to the point of tissue iron overload. Their red blood cell morphology can be quite variable, while marrow morphology demonstrates the pathognomonic finding of ringed sideroblasts. In children, lead poisoning can produce anemia with impaired hemoglobin formation and ringed sideroblasts. Lead poisoning makes the diagnosis of iron deficiency in children more difficult, because the inhibition of mitochondrial heme synthetase by lead results in very high red cell protoporphyrin levels. This must be kept in mind whenever the red cell protoporphyrin assay is used to screen for iron-deficient erythropoiesis.

℞ TREATMENT

The management of a patient with iron deficiency will be governed by the etiology of the deficiency state and the severity of the anemia (see Table 106-3). The ability of the patient to tolerate oral iron preparations will also be a factor. Higher dosages of oral iron result in significant gastrointestinal side effects. This can interfere with patient compliance and prevent a full and rapid recovery.

Situations of negative iron balance secondary to increased physiologic needs are readily corrected by dietary supplementation. Treatment of iron deficiency secondary to blood loss or malabsorption requires accurate diagnosis and effective control of the primary disease state. Continued blood loss can easily exceed the capacity of iron therapy to replenish iron supplies. In patients with gastrointestinal malabsorption, oral iron therapy will be ineffective. Response to iron therapy will also depend on the level of erythropoietin response and the health of the erythroid marrow. Patients with end-stage renal disease, a complicating inflammatory illness, or a damaged marrow will demonstrate a less than optimal response to treatment. In each of these situations, the clinician must decide between the judicious use of red blood cell transfusion and treatment with oral or parenteral iron therapy. Moreover, when the response to iron therapy is delayed or inadequate, a careful reevaluation of the patient is required to look for continued bleeding, the presence of an inflammatory disorder, or a defect in iron absorption.

Oral Iron Preparations Standard oral preparations of iron in tablet and elixir form are listed in Table 106-6. While the various preparations contain different amounts of ferrous iron, they are all readily absorbed and, therefore, quite effective in the treatment of iron-deficiency anemia. A number of other compoundings of iron are sold on the market. Some contain "absorption-enhancing" substances, such as amino acids and ascorbic acid. Others are advertised as delayed-release formulations aimed at prolonging iron absorption over several hours. All of these preparations tend to be more expensive. Moreover, attempts to enhance absorption can increase the incidence of gastrointestinal side effects.

To maximize the response to iron in an adult patient with a moderate to severe iron-deficiency anemia, a standard oral iron preparation such as ferrous sulfate should be given in tablet or elixir form, one tablet (325 mg) or 5 mL (300 mg) three to four times a day between meals. Patients who are achlorhydric or who have had gastric surgery should be treated with iron elixir, because the removal of the tablet coat depends on normal stomach acidity. A fourth dose of iron at bedtime will help maintain iron delivery to the marrow during late evening and night hours. Otherwise, the serum iron can decline to iron-deficient levels during the night, thereby dampening the marrow's proliferative response.

Three to four ferrous sulfate tablets should provide 200 to 250 mg of elemental iron per day, that is, 2 to 3 mg/kg in the average-sized adult. From this, the iron-deficient patient will absorb 40 to 60 mg of iron. This will support a red blood cell production level of up to three times normal in the patient with a normal erythroid marrow and a full erythropoietin response for the anemia. However, as the hemoglobin level rises, iron absorption declines and the rate of red blood cell production falls, regardless of the oral iron intake. Therefore, the dosage can be reduced as the hemoglobin rises to levels above 110 to 120 g/L (11 to 12 g/dL). This will help guarantee patient compliance for a therapy that must continue for several months. More than a quarter of individuals experience gastrointestinal distress, either abdominal pain, nausea, vomiting, constipation, or diarrhea, with the full treatment dose of three to four iron tablets per day. This will improve with smaller doses, although some patients have difficulty tolerating even one or two tablets a day. This can be a significant barrier in management, especially in reestablishing adequate iron stores. At least 6 months of iron supplementation is required in a normal adult to rebuild reticuloendothelial iron stores.

Usually the reticulocyte count increases 3 to 4 days after the initiation of therapy and reaches a peak at about 10 days. If a response does not occur, there are a number of possible explanations: patient noncompliance (common) or abnormal iron absorption (rare), persistent blood loss exceeding intake, and incorrect diagnosis or an additional diagnosis such as marrow damage or chronic inflammation. In any of the first three possibilities, it may be necessary (among other things) to increase iron delivery with a parenteral iron preparation.

Parenteral Iron Therapy Iron can be administered parenterally in patients who are unable to tolerate oral iron or who suffer from gastrointestinal malabsorption. Parenteral iron has also been used in the treatment of patients receiving recombinant erythropoietin to guarantee adequate iron delivery to support erythroid precursor proliferation. Iron for injection is formulated as ferric hydroxide–dextran compound and marketed as iron dextran injection, InFe (Schein). Two preparations are available: one containing 0.5% phenol for intramuscular use and a second that is phenol-free for intramuscular or intravenous use. The phenol-containing compound should never be used for intravenous administration because it can produce phlebitis.

Small amounts of iron dextran can be administered by intramuscular injection, but care must be taken to prevent skin staining. The injection track should follow a Z pattern and no more than 2 mL (100 mg) of the iron dextran compound injected in each buttock site. For the treatment of an iron-deficiency anemia, the preferred method of administration is a bolus intravenous injection of the total dose required to correct the deficiency state. The amount of iron needed can be calculated as follows:

Body weight (kg) $\times$ 2.3 $\times$ (15 $-$ patient's hemoglobin, g/dL) + 500 to 1000 mg (for stores) = Total dose (mg)

When administering intravenous iron dextran, care must be taken to anticipate and avoid an immediate anaphylactic-like reaction. If the patient gives a history of a past reaction to iron dextran, either an anaphylactic or a late serum sickness–like reaction with malaise, fever, arthralgias, skin rash, or lymphadenopathy, further exposure to iron dextran therapy should be avoided. When iron dextran is administered as a large intravenous bolus, it is best diluted in 100 to 250 mL of 0.9% sodium chloride solution and administered over 30 to 90 min. At the beginning of the infusion, a small test dose—less than 0.5 mL of the iron dextran solution—should be infused over 5 to 10 min while observing for any complaints of itching, shortness of breath, or chest or back pain. The blood pressure should be monitored during the test dose and throughout the period of administration. If the patient becomes hypotensive, the infusion should be stopped immediately. Dialysis patients on long-term erythropoietin therapy may require repeated injections of iron dextran to keep up with their iron needs. For this purpose, monthly intravenous injections of 100 to 200 mg of iron dextran will prevent iron deficiency and guarantee a steady supply of iron to the erythroid marrow.

OTHER HYPOPROLIFERATIVE ANEMIAS

Hypoproliferative anemias are common in patients with acute and chronic inflammatory disorders, end-stage renal disease, severe hypothyroidism, and other hormone deficiencies. In each case, the failure in the marrow proliferative response is primarily the result of a reduced erythropoietin response for the degree of anemia. With acute or chronic inflammatory disease, inhibition of iron delivery and erythroid precursor growth also contribute. However, the anemias of renal disease and chronic inflammation (the anemia of chronic disease) can usually be corrected with recombinant erythropoietin therapy if adequate iron stores are available. This reinforces the concept that the failure in erythropoietin stimulation is the most important factor.

INFLAMMATORY ANEMIAS The anemia associated with acute infections and chronic inflammatory diseases results from the release of inflammatory cytokines. TNF, IL-1, IFNβ, IFNγ, and neopterin all have suppressive effects on erythropoiesis. TNF and IFNβ are mediators in patients with bacterial infections and neoplasms, while IL-1 and IFNγ are involved in patients with chronic inflammatory states (the anemia of chronic disease). In both situations, these cytokines are capable of inhibiting the proliferative capacity of erythroid precursors, erythropoietin release by the kidney, and the delivery of iron from reticuloendothelial cells (Fig. 106-4). The impact is rapid and dramatic. With acute bacterial infections, a mild anemia [hemoglobin 100 to 120 g/L (10 to 12 g/dL)] can appear within 24 to 48 h. The initial drop

in hemoglobin is the result of a self-limited hemolytic event, where the oldest red blood cells in circulation are rapidly removed by the reticuloendothelial system. The persistence of the anemia over the next several days or weeks reflects the cytokine suppression of erythropoiesis.

With chronic inflammatory states, the nature of the primary disease will tend to determine the severity and pattern of the anemia. While a majority of patients demonstrate a normocytic, normochromic anemia, some will appear to have a more severe defect in iron supply and will develop a mild microcytosis and hypochromia. Patients with severe lupus erythematosus and rheumatoid arthritis can exhibit more severe hemolysis secondary to autoantibodies and a cytokine/T cell driven suppression of granulocytopoiesis (Felty syndrome).

Clinical and Laboratory Findings The inflammatory anemia associated with acute infection is generally of mild to moderate severity and, therefore, asymptomatic. However, this may not be true for older patients, in whom a modest anemia can provoke symptoms and signs of cardiovascular disease. It is usually first detected on the routine complete blood count as a normocytic, normochromic anemia [hemoglobin of 100 to 120 g/L (10 to 12 g/dL)], with a reticulocyte index of less than 2. The full erythropoietic profile that distinguishes this type of anemia from iron deficiency, renal disease, or a hypometabolic state is illustrated in Table 106-5. Iron-supply studies are the key to the diagnosis. They show an SI of less than 9 μmol/L (50 μg/dL) and a TIBC of less than 54 μmol/L (300 μg/dL), giving a percent saturation of 10 to 20%. This characteristic decline in both the SI and the TIBC is accompanied by an increase in the serum ferritin level. For adult males, the serum ferritin will increase to levels of between 150 and 350 μg/L, while females show a less impressive rise according to their basal serum ferritin level. This pattern is distinctly different from that seen with other hypoproliferative anemias. If a ferritin level is not available or there is confusion regarding the patient's iron status, a bone marrow examination can be used to document the presence of reticuloendothelial cell iron stores. A patient with an iron-deficiency anemia will have no visible stores, while inflammatory disease patients have normal to increased iron stores. Furthermore, with chronic inflammatory diseases, extra large hemosiderin granules form within the reticuloendothelial cells.

Direct measurements of inflammatory cytokines, serum erythropoietin, and levels of serum transferrin receptor, while feasible, are not

Table 106-4

Diagnosis of Microcytic Anemia

Tests	Iron Deficiency	Thalassemia	Sideroblastic Anemia
Smear	Micro/hypo	Micro/hypo with targeting	Variable
SI	Low	Normal to high	Normal to high
TIBC	High	Normal	Normal
Percent saturation	<10	30–80	30–80
Ferritin (μg/L)	<15	50–300	50–300
Hemoglobin pattern	Normal	Abnormal	Normal

Table 106-5

Diagnosis of Hypoproliferative Anemias

Tests	Iron Deficiency	Inflammation	Renal Disease	Hypometabolic States
Anemia	Mild to severe	Mild	Mild to severe	Mild
MCV (fL)	70–90	80–90	90	90
Morphology	Normo-microcytic	Normocytic	Normocytic	Normocytic
SI	<30	<50	Normal	Normal
TIBC	>360	<300	Normal	Normal
Saturation (%)	<10	10–20	Normal	Normal
Serum ferritin (μg/L)	<15	30–200	115–150	Normal
Iron stores	0	2–4 +	1–4 +	Normal

NOTE: MCV, mean corpuscular volume.

Table 106-6

Oral Iron Preparations

Generic Name	Tablet (Iron Content), mg	Elixir (Iron Content), mg in 5 mL
Ferrous sulfate	325 (65)	300 (60)
	195 (39)	90 (18)
Extended release	525 (105)	
Ferrous fumarate	325 (107)	
	195 (64)	100 (33)
Ferrous gluconate	325 (39)	300 (35)
Polysaccharide iron	150 (150)	100 (100)
	50 (50)	

necessary for the clinical diagnosis and differential diagnosis of an inflammatory anemia. One exception to this is the evaluation of anemia in patients with AIDS. With disease progression, AIDS patients develop a moderate to severe hypoproliferative anemia because of complicating infections and/or marrow damage secondary to involvement with human immunodeficiency virus or drug toxicity. Marrow damage may be suspected because of the appearance of a marked pancytopenia. However, a measurement of the serum erythropoietin level can help distinguish between marrow damage and an inflammatory anemia. The finding of a low serum erythropoietin level predicts a significant inflammatory component to the anemia. It is this type of patient who will respond to treatment with recombinant erythropoietin.

THE ANEMIA OF RENAL DISEASE Renal disease with progressive renal failure is almost always accompanied by a moderate to severe hypoproliferative anemia. In general, the severity of the anemia correlates with the severity of the renal failure. As the blood urea nitrogen (BUN) approaches 36 mmol/L (100 mg/dL) and creatinine is above 265 to 442 μmol/L (3 to 5 mg/dL), the hemoglobin will fall to levels below 70 g/L (7 g/dL). This reflects a combination of a significant reduction in circulating red blood cell life span secondary to the uremia and a failure of the erythropoietin response because of the kidney damage. There are certain situations of acute renal failure where the loss of renal function and the erythropoietin response do not correlate. For example, patients with hemolytic-uremic syndrome demonstrate a marked increase in red blood cell production in response to their hemolysis despite renal failure sufficient to require dialysis.

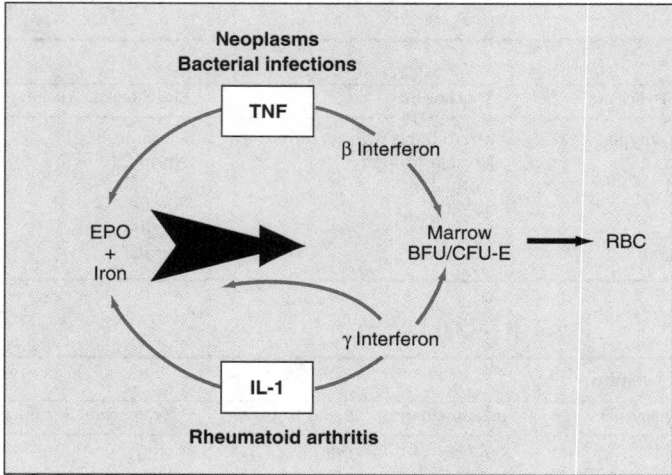

FIGURE 106-4 Suppression of erythropoiesis by inflammatory cytokines. Neoplasms and bacterial infections through the release of tumor necrosis factor (TNF) and interferon β suppress erythropoietin production, the release of iron from reticuloendothelial stores, and the proliferation of erythroid progenitors (BFU/CFU-E). The mediators in patients with vasculitis and rheumatoid arthritis include IL-1 and interferon γ. The blue arrows indicate sites of inflammatory cytokine inhibitory effects.

Polycystic renal disease is another situation where erythropoietin production can be preserved in the face of progressive renal failure. In contrast, patients with diabetes mellitus can demonstrate a more severe anemia than would be predicted from their BUN and creatinine, suggesting an early defect in erythropoietin production.

Clinical and Laboratory Findings Similar to other hypoproliferative anemias, the anemia of renal disease is typically a normocytic, normochromic anemia with a low reticulocyte production index. Moreover, there are no diagnostic clues provided by the red cell morphology. Exceptions to this rule include the appearance of burr cells (echinocytes) with liver disease and fragmented red cells in patients with vasculitic syndromes, especially hemolytic-uremic syndrome and thrombotic thrombocytopenic purpura (see Chap. 109).

Iron-supply studies provide the key to the diagnosis and successful management of the renal disease anemia patient. At presentation, the SI, TIBC, and serum ferritin levels should all be within the normal range, a pattern that is distinctly different from that seen with iron-deficiency or an inflammatory anemia (see Table 106-5). Subsequently, the pattern of iron studies will vary according to the clinical course. Patients maintained on chronic hemodialysis can become iron deficient secondary to procedural blood losses. Therefore, repeated iron studies are important in planning management, especially the use of recombinant erythropoietin to ameliorate the anemia. As with the other hypoproliferative states, a direct measurement of serum erythropoietin levels is not clinically useful. Measurable levels of serum erythropoietin are observed even in anephric patients. The underlying defect is not a total loss of erythropoietin production but a failure in the appropriate response for the degree of anemia.

HYPOMETABOLIC STATES A mild to moderate hypoproliferative anemia may be observed in patients who are hypometabolic secondary to protein starvation or hypothyroidism. The reduced erythropoietin response causing the anemia reflects a reduced oxygen requirement. It would appear that the sensor cells of the kidney are capable of assessing oxygen delivery according to their metabolic level.

Endocrine Deficiency States The measurable difference in hemoglobin levels between males and females is attributable to the effect of androgen and estrogen hormones on erythropoiesis. Testosterone and anabolic steroids enhance the erythropoietin stimulation of erythroid precursors, resulting in a mean hemoglobin level in adult males that is 10 to 30 g/L (1 to 3 g/dL) higher. Castration or estrogen administration will reduce the hemoglobin level in males by as much as 20 g/L (2 g/dL). Pituitary and thyroid function play an even more important role. Most patients who are clinically hypothyroid demonstrate a modest anemia, with a hemoglobin of 110 to 120 g/L (11 to 12 g/dL). Marked myxedema can be accompanied by a more severe anemia. In addition to the defect in erythropoietin stimulation, these patients can show abnormalities in iron and folic acid absorption as well as an overall reduction in dietary intake. This may result in a clinical presentation that is somewhat confusing, because one or another of the nutritional deficiencies may dominate. It is unlikely, however, that the anemia will resolve unless the hypometabolic state is corrected with appropriate thyroid replacement, reflecting the underlying impairment in erythropoietin response.

Addison's disease patients may present with a mild to moderate anemia, depending on the levels of impairment of thyroid function and androgen hormone production. When a patient presents in Addisonian crisis, shifts in plasma volume and total blood volume may obscure the anemia. In this situation, a rapid fall in the hemoglobin level will be observed as the patient receives cortisol and volume replacement. A mild hypoproliferative anemia has also been observed in patients with hyperparathyroidism. While the mechanism is not fully defined, it has been suggested that it is related either to an inhibition of erythroid progenitors or a defect in erythropoietin production secondary to renal calcification.

Protein Deprivation A very mild hypoproliferative anemia, with hemoglobin reduction of 10 to 30 g/L (1 to 3 g/dL), can result from protein deprivation. This has been suggested to play a role in elderly individuals on restricted diets. A more impressive reduction in red blood cell mass is observed with severe starvation. Marasmic individuals, who are both protein and calorie deprived, exhibit a reduced erythropoietin response that correlates with their reduced basal metabolism, although the severity of the red cell mass reduction may not be revealed until the patient is refed. With the recovery of albumin production and reconstitution of the plasma volume, the hemoglobin level will fall. The pattern of anemia in these patients is typically normocytic, normochromic with the low reticulocyte index of a hypoproliferative anemia. In situations of prolonged starvation, iron and vitamin deficiencies must also be considered. They may not be obvious from the pattern of anemia or the initial studies of iron supply. Therefore, the patient should be carefully monitored with repeated iron studies and measurements of folic acid and vitamin B_{12}.

Anemia in Liver Disease   Patients with chronic liver disease from nearly any cause often develop a mild normocytic anemia. Patients with impaired lecithin cholesterol acyltransferase may accumulate excess cholesterol in the red blood cell membrane, leading to burr cells and stomatocytes. This may shorten red cell survival, but the marrow does not adequately compensate for the decreased life span of the cells. This form of anemia rarely requires treatment.

In alcoholic liver disease, this pathophysiology may be complicated by toxic effects of alcohol on bone marrow cells, nutritional folate deficiency, and iron deficiency related both to decreased dietary intake and increased blood loss.

℞ TREATMENT

The management of any hypoproliferative anemia must be tailored to the individual patient and the primary disease process. This makes accurate diagnosis very important. It also requires a careful evaluation of the mechanisms underlying the defect in erythropoiesis. A patient with an acute infection and a mild hypoproliferative anemia can be expected to recover spontaneously as the infection is treated. The same is true for a patient with chronic inflammatory anemia, unless the patient is elderly with cardiovascular disease. In this case, judicious transfusion therapy may be necessary to maintain the patient's exercise tolerance and well being. Patients with end-stage renal disease and severe anemia generally require therapy, either chronic transfusion or recombinant erythropoietin therapy. Selected AIDS patients can also benefit from treatment with erythropoietin. However, in both of these situations, careful monitoring of the patient's iron status is essential.

Transfusion Therapy   Red blood cell transfusion should be reserved for those patients with anemia severe enough to result in cardiovascular compromise. Because younger individuals can easily tolerate hemoglobin levels as low as 70 to 80 g/L (7 to 8 g/dL), most acute and chronic inflammatory anemias in this age group should not be transfused. In elderly patients who experience worsening angina or congestive failure or who demonstrate a marked reduction in exercise tolerance, transfusion may be necessary to maintain a hemoglobin level above 110 to 120 g/L (11 to 12 g/dL). The amount of blood required will obviously depend on the severity of the initial anemia and the patient's red blood cell production level. A unit of packed red blood cells will increase the hemoglobin by approximately 10 g/L (1 g/dL). In general, a transfusion of 2 to 3 units of packed red cells will sustain the patient for several weeks to a month or longer as the patient adapts physiologically to lower hemoglobin levels. Repeat transfusions of red blood cells does run a small risk of transmission of infectious agents and alloimmunization (see Chap. 115). If a large number of red cell transfusions are given, the patient is at risk of iron overload.

Erythropoietin Therapy   Recombinant erythropoietin therapy has proven to be very effective in the treatment of severe anemia in patients with end-stage renal disease. A majority of dialysis-dependent patients given a dose of erythropoietin of 50 to 150 U/kg three times a week by subcutaneous or intravenous injection will show a gradual increase in their hemoglobin to levels of 100 to 120 g/L (10 to 12 g/dL). The speed and level of response will depend on the individual patient and the level of iron supply. Hemodialysis patients are at risk for the development of iron deficiency secondary to procedural blood losses. They need to be monitored with iron

studies and continuously supplemented with either oral or parenteral iron to maximize iron delivery and guarantee a full production response. Once treatment has begun for patients with end-stage renal disease, they must be treated chronically with recombinant erythropoietin to sustain their hemoglobin in a range of 100 to 120 g/L (10 to 12 g/dL). The average maintenance dose is around 75 U/kg three times per week. However, individual patient requirements can be as little as 10 to more than 300 U/kg. Furthermore, any complicating inflammatory illness will interfere with the erythropoietin response. This needs to be recognized in the long-term care of a renal disease patient. While a higher dose of erythropoietin may overcome the impact of inflammatory cytokines on red blood cell production, it may make more sense to discontinue erythropoietin therapy during periods of acute inflammatory illness and maintain the patient's hemoglobin level with red blood cell transfusions. An increasing erythropoietin requirement or apparent refractoriness to treatment can also occur with aluminum toxicity or hyperparathyroidism. Here again, a return to transfusion therapy may be necessary.

See Chap. 53, Hematopoietic agents: Growth factors, minerals, and vitamins, in Goodman and Gilman's The Pharmacological Basis of Therapeutics, *9th ed, New York, McGraw Hill, 1996.*

BIBLIOGRAPHY

COOK JD, SKIKNE BS: Iron deficiency: Definition and diagnosis. J Intern Med 226:349, 1989
——— et al: Serum transferrin receptor. Annu Rev Med 44:63, 1993
FINCH CA, HUEBERS H: Perspectives in iron metabolism. N Engl J Med 306:1520, 1982
GUYATT GH et al: Laboratory diagnosis of iron-deficiency anemia. An overview. J Gen Intern Med 7:145, 1992
HILLMAN RS, AULT KA: *Hematology in Clinical Practice.* New York, McGraw-Hill, 1995
———, FINCH CA: *Red Cell Manual,* 7th ed. Philadelphia, Davis, 1996
MASSEY AC: Microcytic anemia. Differential diagnosis and management of iron deficiency anemia. Med Clin North Am 76:549, 1992
MEANS RT, KRANTZ SB: Progress in understanding the pathogenesis of the anemia of chronic disease. Blood 30:1639, 1992
NISSENSON AR et al: Recombinant human erythropoietin and renal anemia: Molecular biology, clinical efficacy, and nervous system effects. Ann Intern Med 114:402, 1991

107   *Ernest Beutler*

DISORDERS OF HEMOGLOBIN

In general, microcytic anemias result from abnormalities in hemoglobin production. The production of hemoglobin requires a supply of iron, synthesis of heme, and synthesis of globin. Problems with iron supply are discussed in Chap. 106, defects in heme synthesis are discussed in Chap. 343, and defects in globin synthesis will be discussed here. Lead interferes with heme synthesis (among other enzymatic processes), and lead intoxication is discussed in Chap. 397. When globin synthesis is defective, as in the thalassemias, the resulting red cells are microcytic. However, some abnormalities of hemoglobin do not produce microcytic anemia but lead to hemolysis, while others may not even cause anemia.

Hereditary disorders that result in a structurally abnormal hemoglobin (the hemoglobinopathies) or an insufficient quantity of hemoglobin (the thalassemias) are the most common genetic diseases of humans. Hemoglobin is not only essential for normal oxygen delivery by erythrocytes, but as the major component of these cells it also influences their shape, size, and deformability. Genetic and acquired alterations in hemoglobin structure can impair oxygen delivery and oxygen-carrying capacity, shorten cell life span, and impede passage through the microvasculature. Hemolytic anemia and localized tissue ischemia result. Because many changes in the hemoglobin molecule are compatible with life, and even with normal health, the physician encounters many disorders that are due to hereditary or acquired abnormalities of hemoglobin. Moreover, because of the ready availability of hemoglobin, it has been a favorite tool of the basic scientist, particularly in physiology, biochemistry, and genetics. Sickle cell disease was the first human disorder to be understood at the amino acid level, and the β-globin gene was the first human gene to be cloned.

STRUCTURE AND FUNCTION OF HEMOGLOBIN

Most of the hemoglobin in the red cells of adults exists as a tetramer of two α chains, each with 141 amino acids, and two β chains, each with 146 amino acids. Imbedded in each globin chain is one heme molecule; oxygen is carried by the iron of the heme. The iron must be in the ferrous state to bind oxygen. The α and β chains can undergo a change in conformation, both individually and in relation to one another, so that the molecule can exist in a series of forms with different oxygen affinities. The oxygen affinity of the oxygen-free molecule is low, and its affinity for additional oxygen molecules increases as oxygen begins to bind to heme. The result of this "cooperative interaction" is the well-known sigmoid oxygen association curve (Fig. 107-1). The position of this curve is affected by the pH (the Bohr effect); the CO_2 tension; the level of the metabolic intermediate 2,3-bisphosphoglycerate (2,3-BPG; formerly designated 2,3-DPG) and ATP; the temperature; and by mutations that may affect the globin chains.

The α- and β-globin chains are the products of a family of closely related genes. These genes exist as clusters of α-like genes on chromosome 16 and of β-like genes on chromosome 11 (Fig. 107-2). Normally, hemoglobins contain two α-like chains (α or ζ) and two β-like chains (β, δ, ε, or γ). During ontogeny, different globin genes are successively expressed so that the predominant hemoglobin changes during development. At birth, for example, very few β chains are expressed, and the predominant β-like chain is the γ chain, which complexes to α chains to form fetal hemoglobin ($\alpha_2\gamma_2$). As will be

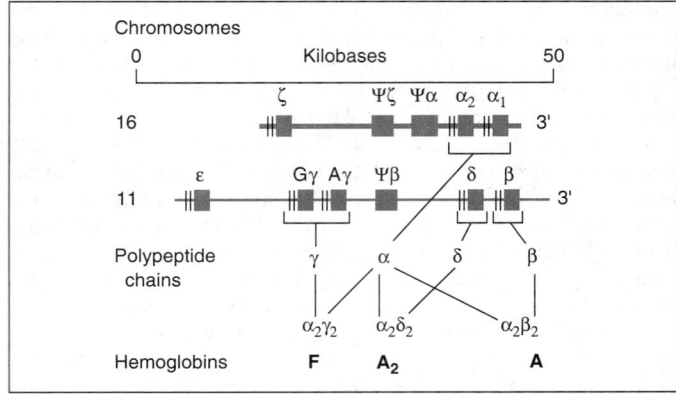

FIGURE 107-2 The globin genes. The α-like genes (α,ζ) are encoded on chromosome 16; the β-like genes (β,γ,δ,ε) are encoded on chromosome 11.

noted below, this normal pattern of activation of globin chains is altered in some disease states and may therefore be of diagnostic importance. Homotetramers of β-like chains can also exist: the γ-chain tetramer is designated *hemoglobin Barts*, and the β-chain tetramer *hemoglobin H*. Because these homotetramers are found in substantial quantities only in disorders in which insufficient α-like chains are produced (α thalassemias), their presence is of diagnostic importance.

REGULATION OF HEMOGLOBIN PRODUCTION

Despite their great importance in the understanding and treatment of the hemoglobinopathies, the mechanisms by which the appropriate globin genes are successively activated at the right moment in ontogenesis are not understood. A powerful upstream enhancer, designated the locus control region, apparently plays an important role and is required for the high level of globin synthesis needed during the development of red cells. When a globin gene is activated, its promoter binds factors necessary for transcription of DNA into the primary mRNA. Globin genes contain three exons and two introns. The introns are spliced from the primary messenger to provide the template for translation into the globin. Defects that prevent normal transcription of the gene, splicing of the messenger, or its translation into protein all have been identified as causes of thalassemias.

CLASSIFICATION, DEFINITIONS, AND NOMENCLATURE

A classification of hereditary or acquired disorders due to abnormal hemoglobins is presented in Table 107-1. Changes in the amino acid sequence of one of the globin chains give rise to what are usually designated *hemoglobinopathies*. Abnormalities in which there are no abnormal globin chains but rather a decrease in the quantity of normal globin chains produced are usually designated *thalassemias*. However, the thalassemic state is often also defined as a clinical syndrome, one that consists of a hereditary anemia characterized by small and poorly hemoglobinized (i.e., microcytic hypochromic) red cells. The distinction between hemoglobinopathies and thalassemias is not, in reality, an absolute one. Thalassemic clinical manifestations may also result from amino acid substi-

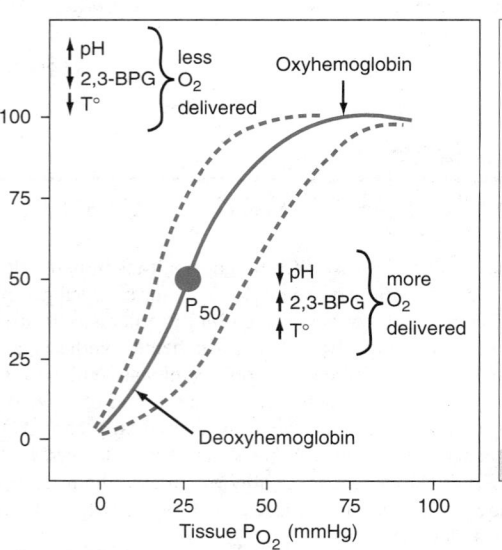

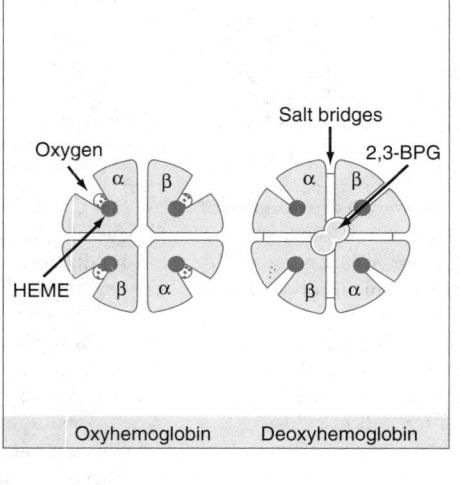

FIGURE 107-1 Hemoglobin-oxygen dissociation curve. The hemoglobin tetramer can bind up to four molecules of oxygen in the iron-containing sites of the heme molecules. As oxygen is bound, 2,3-BPG and CO_2 are expelled. Salt bridges are broken, and each of the globin molecules changes its conformation to facilitate oxygen binding. Oxygen release to the tissues is the reverse process, salt bridges being formed and 2,3-BPG and CO_2 bound. Deoxyhemoglobin does not bind oxygen efficiently until the cell returns to conditions of higher pH, the most important modulator of O_2 affinity (Bohr effect). When acid is produced in the tissues, the dissociation curve shifts to the right facilitating oxygen release and CO_2 binding. Alkalosis has the opposite effect, reducing oxygen delivery.

Table 107-1

CHAPTER 107
Disorders of Hemoglobin

647

A Classification of Disorders due to Hemoglobin Abnormalities

I. Hereditary
  A. Abnormal hemoglobins (hemoglobinopathies)
    1. Sickling and related disorders
    2. Unstable hemoglobins
    3. Hemoglobins with abnormal oxygen affinities
    4. Methemoglobins (hemoglobins M)
  B. Thalassemias
    1. α Thalassemias
    2. β Thalassemias, including hereditary persistence of fetal hemoglobin
  C. Methemoglobinemia due to NADH diaphorase (methemoglobin reductase) deficiency
II. Acquired
    1. Toxic sulfhemoglobinemia
    2. Toxic methemoglobinemia
    3. Toxic carboxyhemoglobinemia

tutions such as in the unstable hemoglobins; in read-through mutations such as hemoglobin Constant Spring (which produces a longer-than-normal globin chain because a stop codon is lost); and in the hemoglobins Lepore, in which a fusion gene composed of a portion of the δ- and a portion of the β-chain gene forms very little globin. In hemoglobin E disease, abnormal mRNA splicing occurs as a consequence of the very same mutation that produces an amino acid substitution.

Globin chains are represented by Greek letters, and mutations are shown as superscripts. The superscript A is used for normal hemoglobin, and for a common abnormal hemoglobin such as sickle hemoglobin (hemoglobin S), the designation β^S is commonly employed. More generally, however, the amino acid change is used, so that the mutation of hemoglobin S could also be designated $\beta^{6Glu \rightarrow Val}$. β Thalassemia mutations are usually categorized as β^0 thalassemia for those in which no β chains are made or β^+ when some β chains are produced. δβ Thalassemias are those in which the formation of δ chains as well as β chains is compromised, so that hemoglobin A_2 (i.e., $\alpha_2\delta_2$) levels are not increased in heterozygotes. In the α thalassemias the designation α^0 has been used for the deletion of both α loci, while a single deletion has been designated α^+. Alternatively, the double deletion is sometimes shown as $--$ and a single deletion as $-\alpha$.

The inheritance of abnormal hemoglobins follows Mendelian genetics. Heterozygotes for abnormal hemoglobins or thalassemia have the *trait* corresponding to the homozygous disorder. Thus, a person with one normal β-globin gene and one sickle β-globin gene (genotype = β^A/β^S) has sickle trait, one who has the β^A/β^C genotype has hemoglobin C trait, and a heterozygote for β thalassemia has thalassemia trait. Those who are homozygous for abnormal hemoglobins have the *disease*. For example, one who has the β^C/β^C genotype has hemoglobin C disease. The thalassemias are divided clinically into thalassemia trait (thalassemia minor) and thalassemia major, based on disease severity. Patients with the trait are usually heterozygotes, while more severely affected patients are homozygotes or compound heterozygotes (that is, they have inherited different mutant alleles from each parent). Hereditary persistence of fetal hemoglobin may be considered as a subset of β thalassemia in which few β chains are synthesized, but the thalassemic features are mild or absent, and fetal hemoglobin represents much of the circulating hemoglobin.

Abnormal amounts of chemically altered hemoglobin molecules may appear in the circulating red cells after certain environmental stresses, resulting in syndromes known by the name of the abnormal pigment that accumulates. These include *methemoglobinemia* (oxidized hemoglobin with ferric rather than ferrous iron), *sulfhemoglobinemia* (sulfur is present in the porphyrin ring and alters its ability to bind oxygen), and *carboxyhemoglobinemia* (carbon monoxide bound to the heme iron). Methemoglobinemia may also occur as a hereditary disorder, either as a hemoglobinopathy in which oxidized hemoglobin resists reduction or as an enzyme defect (e.g., methemoglobin reductase or NADH diaphorase) in which the pathway for the reduction of hemoglobin is defective.

POPULATION GENETICS

The frequency of different hemoglobinopathies varies greatly among different populations. Common mutations, such as those of hemoglobin S, C, and E, and many of the mutations that cause thalassemia represent "balanced polymorphisms." Such mutations are concentrated in certain populations in which they have conferred a selective advantage upon the carrier. This advantage is generally resistance to infection with malaria, which counterbalances the deleterious effect of the homozygous state. In contrast, mutations that occur randomly are panethnic in their distribution and are each relatively rare.

Among African Americans, approximately 7.8 percent are carriers of the sickle mutation, i.e., they have sickle cell trait; 2.3 percent have hemoglobin C trait; and 0.8 percent have β-thalassemia trait. The predicted frequency of the homozygous state for sickle hemoglobin is approximately 1:650; for hemoglobin SC disease it is 1:1100, and for sickle-thalassemia it is 1:3200. In southeast Asia the incidence of hemoglobin E trait is as high as 30 percent in some areas, and that of β thalassemia is also very high in this region. β Thalassemias are very common in many parts of southern Europe. In Sardinia, for example, 12 percent of the population have thalassemia trait. Until the 1970s, 1 in every 250 newborns had thalassemia major, but, as indicated below, the birth incidence has been decreased considerably by organized genetic counseling.

There are many genetically neutral polymorphic sites throughout the genome, and when a new mutation occurs in an individual, it occurs in the context of other polymorphic sites in that region. Such an array of polymorphic sites has been termed a *haplotype*. Because rearrangements of nearby sites by crossing over during meiosis occur only very slowly, genes that have originated relatively recently in evolution (e.g., within 5000 years) are found in the context of the same haplotype in most or all of the descendants of the individual in whom the mutation first occurred. Haplotype identification may be important in several respects. It provides information regarding the number of times a mutation has arisen independently. The sickle mutation is found in five distinct haplotypes, four in Africa, designated Senegal, Benin, Central African Republic, and Cameroon, and one in India. This suggests that the sickle mutation arose independently at least five times. The severity of manifestations of the sickle gene is in part associated with the haplotype in which the mutation is found (see below). Because of the stable linkage between polymorphic sites and disease-producing mutations, haplotypes are also useful in prenatal diagnosis, even when the precise mutation itself is not, as may occur in the thalassemias; all affected children will have the same haplotype.

THE HEMOGLOBINOPATHIES

Mutations of the globin genes may produce abnormal protein molecules by a variety of mechanisms. The most common of these is a single base-pair change in the DNA code resulting in an amino acid substitution. Several hundred such mutations are now known. About half of the variants are clinically silent. Those that are not clinically silent generally either produce a change in oxygen affinity or a physically unstable hemoglobin molecule. The clinical manifestations observed are a function of which globin chain is affected and the consequence of the mutation on protein structure and function. Mutations of one of the α genes tend to have relatively mild clinical consequences because four copies of the α chain exist in the normal genome. β-Globin gene mutations tend to have more severe consequences because in the homozygous state all of the β chains will be abnormal. Mutations of embryonic ζ- and fetal γ-globin chains are of no clinical importance in adult medicine.

Mutations that decrease the stability of hemoglobin produce *Heinz body anemias*. The sickle cell mutation (see below) alters solubility of the deoxy form of hemoglobin and results in distortion of the

Table 107-2

Some Abnormal Hemoglobins

Designation	Mutation	Population	Main Clinical Effects
Sickle or S	$\beta^{6Glu\rightarrow Val}$	African	Anemia, ischemic infarcts
C	$\beta^{6Glu\rightarrow Lys}$	African	Mild anemia
E	$\beta^{26Glu\rightarrow Lys}$	Southeast Asian	Microcytic anemia, splenomegaly
Köln	$\beta^{98Val\rightarrow Met}$	Sporadic	Hemolytic anemia, Heinz bodies when splenectomized
Yakima	$\beta^{99Asp\rightarrow His}$	Sporadic	Polycythemia
Kansas	$\beta^{102Asn\rightarrow Lys}$	Sporadic	Mild anemia

erythrocytes when they are deoxygenated. Mutations that raise the oxygen affinity of hemoglobin result in hereditary polycythemia; those that lower oxygen affinity result in anemia. Hemoglobin mutants (hemoglobins M) that cannot be reduced by red cell enzymes result in methemoglobinemia.

SICKLE CELL DISORDERS **Definitions** *Sickle cell disorders* include all states in which a sickle gene has been inherited, but *sickle diseases* refer to states in which a morbid condition ensues, such as hemoglobin SC disease and hemoglobin S-β-thalassemia. The term *sickle cell anemia* is usually reserved for the homozygous state for hemoglobin S.

Pathophysiology Hemoglobin S is characterized by the substitution of a valine for glutamic acid as the sixth amino acid in the β-globin chain, resulting from a DNA substitution of thymine for adenine (Table 107-2). The diminished solubility of the deoxy form of this hemoglobin results in the formation of a gelatinous network of fibrous polymers, called *tactoids*, that stiffen and distort the cell, producing rigid, misshapen erythrocytes that traverse small blood vessels with great difficulty or not at all. After repeated episodes of sickling and unsickling, irreversible sickle cells may be formed. The removal of abnormal cells from the circulation at a rate that exceeds the capacity of the marrow to replace them results in a hemolytic anemia. The obstruction of small vessels by sickle cells results in repeated infarctions, leading to gradual involvement of all organ systems, most notably spleen, lungs, kidney, and brain. The obstruction of small blood vessels by sickle cells is not due entirely to their altered shape and rigidity. There are also membrane changes that may play an important role. Sickle cells adhere to endothelium.

The sickling of red cells containing sickle hemoglobin depends not only upon the degree of oxygenation of the hemoglobin in the cell but also upon the concentration of sickle hemoglobin in the cell, the pH, and the temperature. Moreover, the formation of the characteristic tubules that result when sickle hemoglobin molecules aggregate is not instantaneous; the time that has elapsed since conditions favoring sickling were achieved is of importance. Some hemoglobins interfere more with the sickling process than do others. Thus, fetal hemoglobin interferes with sickling more than does hemoglobin A. Hemoglobin C interacts so effectively with hemoglobin S that hemoglobin SC disease is clinically very similar and often indistinguishable from homozygous sickle cell disease.

Clinical Manifestations Patients with sickle cell disease manifest the signs and symptoms of chronic anemia with pallor of the mucous membranes, fatigue, and decreased exercise tolerance. Because most patients with sickle cell disease are of African origin, pallor is more readily appreciated on examining the mucus membranes than the skin, but the skin may have a grayish cast. Because of the chronic hemolysis, jaundice is commonly present and patients are prone to gallstone formation.

In addition to these general manifestations of anemia, symptoms and signs related more to the rheologic abnormalities than to the anemia are common. These include leg ulcers, priapism, repeated episodes of pulmonary infarction, and "acute chest syndrome" characterized by fever, chest pain, and pulmonary infiltrates. Damage to the pulmonary vasculature can produce pulmonary hypertension, heart failure, and death. Retinal vessel obstruction may result in hemorrhage, scarring, retinal detachment, and blindness. Renal papillary necrosis with hematuria occurs in sickle cell diseases and is one of the few clinical manifestations of the sickle cell trait. The hypertonic milieu in the renal medulla draws water out of the red blood cell and promotes sickling. Although the spleen may be enlarged in small children with sickle cell disease, repeated episodes of splenic infarction cause the spleen to be reduced to a small calcified remnant, a phenomenon that has been termed "autosplenectomy." As a result of the functional asplenic state, and for other poorly understood reasons, patients with sickle cell disease have an increased susceptibility to infection. Salmonella osteomyelitis is one such infection that is rarely seen in patients without sickling disorders. Stroke is a serious complication of sickle cell disease and may occur in very young children, leaving them permanently disabled. Progressive renal and pulmonary failure are of great importance in the fourth and fifth decades of life in patients with sickle diseases and are a common cause of death in these patients. Aseptic necrosis of the femoral head may occur, occasionally even in patients with sickle trait (see Table 107-3).

In addition to these chronic manifestations of sickle cell diseases, three types of acute episodes, termed *crises*, occur. By far the most common of these is the *infarctive or painful crisis*. This type of crisis is characterized by severe skeletal pain, which may persist for several days or even weeks. Fever is commonly present, but there is usually no change in the hemoglobin concentration of the blood. *Sequestration crises* are largely limited to infants and young children, although occasionally they may occur in the few adults who have splenomegaly. In this type of crisis, there is sudden massive pooling of red cells in

Table 107-3

Clinical Features of Sickle Hemoglobinopathies

Condition	Clinical Abnormalities	Hemoglobin Level, g/L (g/dL)	Mean Corpuscular Volume, fL	Hemoglobin Electrophoresis
Sickle cell trait	None; rare painless hematuria	Normal	Normal	Hb S/A:40/60
Sickle cell anemia	Vasoocclusive crises with infarction of spleen, brain, marrow, kidney, lung; aseptic necrosis of bone; gallstones; priapism; ankle ulcers	70–100 (7–10)	80–100	Hb S/A:100/0 Hb F:2–25%
S/β° thalassemia	Vasoocclusive crises; aseptic necrosis of bone	70–100 (7–10)	60–80	Hb S/A:100/0 Hb F:1–10%
S/β⁺ thalassemia	Rare crises and aseptic necrosis	100–140 (10–14)	70–80	Hb S/A:60/40
Hemoglobin SC	Rare crises and aseptic necrosis; painless hematuria	100–140 (10–14)	80–100	Hb S/A:50/0 Hb C:50%

the spleen with an acute fall in the hemoglobin concentration of the blood. It is not uncommon for such crises to have a fatal outcome. *Hemolytic crises* are uncommon and are characterized by a fall in the hemoglobin concentration of the blood with marked increase in jaundice. Crises may last a few hours or a few days.

Sickle trait, which occurs in nearly 8 percent of African Americans, is unaccompanied by anemia and is almost always clinically silent. Individuals with the trait have an impaired ability to concentrate urine and rarely may develop clinical signs under conditions of severe anoxia. For example, splenic infarction has occurred occasionally during unpressurized ascent to high altitudes.

Factors Influencing the Severity of Sickle Cell Disease Different genotypes can give rise to sickle cell disease. The classic form of the disease may be considered to be the homozygous state for hemoglobin S, i.e., SS disease or sickle cell anemia. However, the manifestations of SC disease, sickle cell β thalassemia, and hemoglobin SD disease are very similar. While, on the average, sickle cell anemia has the most severe clinical course and splenomegaly may be more likely to occur in hemoglobin SC disease and S thalassemia than in SS disease, there is a great deal of overlap between the severity and clinical manifestations of these disorders. The principal importance of the distinctions between different sickle disease genotypes is in their diagnosis and in genetic counseling.

A number of factors influence the course of sickle cell disease and may be important in precipitating crises. These include infection and fever, dehydration, and exposure to low oxygen tension. Even apart from these factors, the severity of the clinical manifestations of sickle cell disease varies greatly from patient to patient, not only in the degree to which they are affected but also with respect to which of the morbid manifestations predominate. Thus, some may suffer chiefly from anemia with few, if any, painful episodes, while others experience many painful crises but have hemoglobin levels that are nearly normal. In still other patients, strokes may be the predominant clinical events, and occasional patients have virtually no manifestations of the disease. The causes of this variability are unknown. Yet it is of great practical importance because of the high risk of some therapeutic measures that may be contemplated, particularly allogeneic bone marrow transplantation. There is a statistically significant association between the haplotype in which the sickle gene exists (Central African Republic is worst and Senegal is best) and the severity of disease. Concurrent α thalassemia seems to protect on the average against the clinical manifestations of sickle disease, and high levels of fetal hemoglobin are also protective. However, each of these predictors, individually or collectively, is weak, and good predictors of prognosis that can be applied to young children are badly needed.

Survival, though difficult to predict for an individual, correlates with the frequency of crises; the median age at death for those with more than three crises per year is 35 years, whereas those with fewer crises per year may live into their 50s.

Diagnosis The presence of sickle hemoglobin can be established by demonstrating that the red cells assume their characteristic morphologic form when the hemoglobin is deoxygenated, as by treatment with a reducing agent such as sodium metabisulfite. The classic sickling procedure does not distinguish between the different sickling disorders and is less well suited for large scale screening of blood samples than is electrophoretic separation of the hemoglobins. Electrophoresis of hemoglobins readily identifies the presence of the slow-moving hemoglobin S, but routine electrophoretic methods do not distinguish it from some other slow-moving hemoglobins such as hemoglobin D. Thus, the identity of the hemoglobin as hemoglobin S must be confirmed, usually by the use of a sickling or a solubility test. Quantitation of the different hemoglobins by electrophoresis also provides information regarding the genotype of the patient. If there is more hemoglobin A than hemoglobin S, then the patient has sickle cell trait. If hemoglobins S and A are present but hemoglobin S predominates, then the patient has sickle β⁺ thalassemia disease. When hemoglobin C is present with hemoglobin S, the patient has SC disease (Table 107-3).

Diagnosis of the genetic status of the unborn child is much more difficult than is postnatal diagnosis, both because of the difficulty and risk attendant upon obtaining fetal blood and because there is very meager expression of the β-globin locus during fetal life. DNA analysis is thus of principal value in prenatal diagnosis. DNA obtained either on chorionic villus biopsy or amniocentesis can be amplified by the polymerase chain reaction, and the sickle mutation readily ascertained.

TREATMENT

Symptomatic Management The mainstays of management of patients with sickle disease are the avoidance of complications and their treatment when they do arise. Patients with sickle cell disease should be counseled to avoid high altitudes, to maintain an adequate fluid intake, and to treat infections promptly when they occur. They should be given folic acid—1 mg/day. *Haemophilus influenzae* type b vaccine and pneumococcal and meningococcal polysaccharide vaccines are recommended early (before spleen damage), and children with sickle cell disease should receive penicillin prophylaxis until the age of 6 years.

Leg ulcers may respond to prolonged bed rest and to surgical grafting. Priapism may be managed with pain medication and nifedipine. Priapism persisting for more than a day is usually managed surgically, and impotence is the common outcome in sexually mature males.

The management of painful crises is one of the most frequent and difficult challenges faced by the treating physician. Therapy consists of hydration, keeping the patient warm, and possibly the use of oxygen. Because of the renal papillary necrosis, patients have difficulty reabsorbing water from the urine and are particularly susceptible to dehydration. The use of analgesics in the treatment of painful crises represents a particularly difficult problem because of the propensity of patients with sickle cell disease, in common with patients with any type of chronic or recurrent pain, to become addicted to narcotics. Continuous infusions of morphine should be employed to keep the pain under control. Younger patients may require higher doses. Chronic transfusion therapy has been used to decrease the frequency of crises and may be useful in some severely affected patients. However, over the long term, this approach may lead to iron overload.

Patients with the acute chest syndrome require broad-spectrum antibiotics (ceftriaxone and erythromycin for *Mycoplasma*) in addition to hydration and O₂. In the face of respiratory insufficiency (Pa$_{O_2}$ < 60 mmHg), exchange transfusion may be necessary.

A relatively high rate of fetal loss occurs during pregnancy. Maternal mortality was once about 33 percent but has declined to an average of 1.6 percent in areas where good prenatal care is available. The patient should be apprised of these risks. Chronic transfusion therapy has been attempted as a means of decreasing maternal and fetal mortality in sickle cell disease, but without success.

Specific Measures Many different antisickling agents have been tested therapeutically, but of these the only one that has proven to be clinically beneficial in controlled trials is hydroxyurea. This drug interferes with normal erythropoiesis in such a way as to increase the production of γ chains. The increased fetal hemoglobin levels interfere with the sickling process and decrease the incidence of crises. Its effects may be enhanced with the concomitant use of erythropoietin. Hydroxyurea administration should be limited to more severely affected patients with sickle cell disease.

Allogeneic bone marrow transplantation is the only currently available treatment that can cure sickle cell disease. Its use remains uncommon. Because the short- and intermediate-term mortality from bone marrow transplantation is 5 to 10 percent, the selection of patients to undergo this treatment is particularly difficult. Clearly, the risk is justified in patients who are destined to suffer the most severe manifestations of the disease, particularly strokes. Yet, as pointed out above, criteria for clearly identifying such patients do not yet exist.

Gene transfer therapy has the potential to provide marked improvement in or cure of patients with sickle cell disease while avoiding some of the risks of allogeneic transplantation. There was considerable optimism about this approach in the early 1980s. However, it is now apparent that for several reasons the difficulties in implementing gene therapy for sickle cell disease are much greater than those encountered in the treatment of enzyme defects such as adenosine deaminase deficiency, where gene transfer has been performed with some modest success. In sickle cell disease, the clinical manifestations are caused by the functioning of the abnormal gene, and merely placing a normal gene into the hematopoietic stem cell does not prevent the formation of sickle hemoglobin. Moreover, to be effective it is necessary for the transduced gene not only to function but to function at a very high level. The rate at which hemoglobin is normally synthesized is several orders of magnitude higher than that of most other proteins. Finally, it has been difficult to maintain continuing expression of genes transduced into primate hematopoietic stem cells. Prolonged activity would be essential for gene transfer therapy to be successful in sickle cell disease.

HEMOGLOBIN C DISORDERS   The most important clinical consequence of the hemoglobin C mutation is its interaction with the sickle mutation to cause hemoglobin SC disease, a form of sickle cell disease, as discussed above. Hemoglobin C trait is asymptomatic, and hemoglobin CC disease, the homozygous state, causes a mild anemia characterized by target-shaped, flattened, and sometimes folded erythrocytes. Characteristic intraerythrocytic crystals can sometimes be found, but the diagnosis of this disorder depends upon hemoglobin electrophoresis. A patient with manifestations of sickle cell disease who has splenomegaly and whose erythrocytes are target cells is likely to have SC disease.

HEMOGLOBIN E DISORDERS   The hemoglobin E mutation produces an amino acid substitution, 26Glu→Lys, through a G→A mutation in the 79th nucleotide of the coding sequence of the cDNA. It is unusual in that some of the mRNA bearing this mutation is spliced abnormally because of the substitution, and because the abnormally spliced message cannot be translated into globin, there is a marked β-globin deficiency. As a result, the hemoglobin E mutations cause a thalassemia-like state. Hemoglobin E trait is characterized by the presence of target cells, hypochromia, microcytosis, and mild anemia. The homozygous state for hemoglobin E is also clinically mild, with striking microcytosis usually without splenomegaly. The β thalassemia/hemoglobin E compound heterozygote has a somewhat more severe presentation than homozygous hemoglobin E disease; splenomegaly is usually present.

UNSTABLE HEMOGLOBINS   Some mutations cause the formation of unstable hemoglobin molecules that precipitate in vivo, causing hemolytic anemia. Most of these mutations affect the binding of heme by globin or the intermolecular contacts between the globin chain in the tetramer. A single copy of a gene for an unstable hemoglobin is sufficient to cause hemolytic disease, and thus these hemoglobinopathies are inherited as autosomal dominant disorders. Hemoglobins Geneva and Köln are examples. Hemolysis varies greatly in severity and may be accentuated by the ingestion of "oxidative" drugs, such as those that cause hemolysis in patients with glucose-6-phosphate dehydrogenase (G6PD) deficiency (see Chap. 109). Sulfonamides have been the chief offending agents. Heinz bodies, particles of denatured protein adhering to the cell membrane, are usually seen in patients who have been splenectomized.

Although unstable hemoglobins may be electrophoretically abnormal, they are best detected by the isopropanol stability test. In recent years a thalassemia-like state inherited as a dominant disorder and designated as a *hyperunstable hemoglobin syndrome* has been delineated. Here, the hemoglobin is so unstable that none of it can be detected

in red cells. Instead, the diagnosis must be established by showing a defect in the globin gene by DNA analysis. Even though only one of the copies of the β chain is abnormal, the very unstable hemoglobin apparently damages the erythrocytes sufficiently that severe hemolytic anemia occurs.

HEMOGLOBINS WITH ABNORMAL OXYGEN AFFINITY   The steady-state level of hemoglobin is presumably maintained by an as yet uncharacterized oxygen sensor. When an abnormal hemoglobin binds oxygen too tightly (i.e., has an increased oxygen affinity), the sensor causes more erythropoietin to be released. Consequently, the red cell mass increases. Patients with such mutations may become sufficiently polycythemic so as to require periodic phlebotomies. High-affinity hemoglobins are commonly also unstable, so that a compensated hemolytic state with a normal hemoglobin level results. Hemoglobins Zürich and Yakima are examples. Conversely, mutant hemoglobins with a decreased oxygen affinity cause a mild, usually asymptomatic anemia. Hemoglobin Kansas is an example.

These hemoglobinopathies are diagnosed by determining the oxygen dissociation of the hemoglobin freed of 2,3-BPG. This compound must be removed to distinguish high- and low-affinity hemoglobins from hereditary metabolic disorders of the red cell such as phosphofructokinase deficiency, which causes polycythemia by lowering the 2,3-BPG level, or pyruvate kinase deficiency, which increases the red cell 2,3-BPG level. Like the hemoglobinopathies caused by the unstable hemoglobins, the clinical syndromes caused by these mutant hemoglobins are inherited in an autosomal dominant fashion.

THE THALASSEMIAS

The thalassemias are divided into the α thalassemias, in which it is the production of α globin that is deficient, and the β thalassemias, in which β globin production is defective.

THE α THALASSEMIAS   Pathophysiology   α Thalassemias result in an excess production of β chains in adults and children and γ chains in newborns. The β chains that accumulate form tetramers—hemoglobin Barts (γ_4) in infants and hemoglobin H (β_4) in adults. These tetramers are abnormal hemoglobins with marked instability, a left-shifted oxygen dissociation curve with a lack of cooperativity, i.e., the normal sigmoid shape. The hematologic manifestations of the α thalassemias are a function principally of the extent to which these abnormal tetramers accumulate. This, in turn, depends upon how many of the four α loci have been deleted or inactivated by a mutation, as indicated below.

Clinical Manifestations (Table 107-4)   *Deletion or mutation of all four α loci*   Deletion of all of the α-globin genes is the most catastrophic form of α thalassemia. It is incompatible with extrauterine life, and the infants are either dead at birth with hydrops fetalis or die shortly after birth. They are severely edematous and have little circulating hemoglobin, which is almost entirely hemoglobin Barts.

Deletion or mutation of three of the four α loci   Hemoglobin H disease results from deletion of all but one of the α-globin genes. The disorder resembles an unstable hemoglobinopathy, because both hemoglobin Barts and hemoglobin H are, in fact, unstable hemoglobins. Patients have a microcytic hypochromic anemia with target cells and Heinz bodies on the blood smear. Onset may be apparent during childhood, but in milder cases it is often not until adult life. Hemolytic anemia with marked splenomegaly is the characteristic presentation. Reticulocytes are increased.

Deletion or mutation of two of the four α loci   Two α loci are sufficient for nearly normal erythropoiesis. This state has been called α-*thalassemia trait* and is characterized by mild anemia and moderate microcytosis and hypochromia. The hemoglobin concentration is usually within 10 or 20 g/L (1 or 2 g/dL) of normal, and the mean corpuscular volume (MCV) is in the 70 to 80 fL range. Because of the extraordinarily high prevalence (~30 percent) of deletion of one of the two α-globin loci on chromosomes of people of African origin, the inheritance of two such chromosomes is very common. This condition is very commonly mistaken for iron deficiency and treated inappropriately with iron.

Deletion or mutation of one of the four α loci Three α-globin loci are sufficient for essentially normal function. Anemia and hypochromia do not occur in these persons. They have been designated *silent carriers*.

Diagnosis The diagnosis of the severe forms (three and four gene deletions) of α thalassemia is readily made by demonstrating the presence of the rapidly moving hemoglobin Barts in infants and hemoglobin H in adults. The erythrocytes show typical inclusions after incubation with an oxidant dye such as brilliant cresyl blue. Diagnosis of the milder forms is much more difficult, because the amounts of hemoglobins Barts and H are too small to detect reliably. Diagnosis is most reliably established by measuring the ratio of synthesis of α- to β-globin chain in isolated peripheral blood reticulocytes, a test that is, unfortunately, not widely available. Because most α thalassemias are due to deletions, Southern blotting of endonuclease-digested genomic DNA can be very useful but may be difficult to interpret in patients with the αα/− − genotype, in whom a normal pattern is seen.

℞ **TREATMENT**

There is currently no treatment for hydrops fetalis. However, the disease can be prevented by properly establishing the genotypes of parents. Only when two parents have a chromosome with the two-locus deletion, i.e., either αα/− − or α −/− −, is it possible to bear a child with no α-globin genes. The diagnosis can be established prenatally by examining DNA from a chorionic villus or from amniotic fluid cells.

Splenectomy is sometimes helpful in the treatment of patients with hemoglobin H disease, either when the anemia is quite severe or when massive splenomegaly is troublesome for the patient.

No treatment is required for deletions of only one or two α-globin loci.

THE β THALASSEMIAS **Pathophysiology** The excess α chains that are formed in β thalassemia do not self-associate to form tetramers but instead are bound to the red cell membrane, producing membrane damage. The severity of the β-thalassemic defect varies with different mutations. Some mutations (β°) prevent the formation of any β chains at all; others (β⁺) allow some β-chain formation to occur. Thus, depending on which two mutations are inherited, a broad range of compromise of β-chain formation can be encountered.

Hereditary persistence of fetal hemoglobin is a heterogeneous, clinically benign disorder characterized by elevated fetal hemoglobin levels. Both deletions and point mutations may cause this disorder, and exactly why some mutations produce this relatively innocuous disorder rather than thalassemia is not fully understood.

Clinical Manifestations When both β-globin genes bear a thalassemic mutation, a severe anemia is generally present, associated, in the untreated patient, with bone changes due to expansion of the marrow space and often growth retardation. This increase in erythropoiesis produces a characteristic "chipmunk" facies. The skin may be a peculiar copper color from pallor, icterus, and melanin deposition. Hepatosplenomegaly may be massive. Many such patients with β thalassemia major (Cooley's anemia) are transfusion-dependent, and these patients, in particular, generally develop iron overload. In untreated patients this usually leads to death in the second decade.

β-Thalassemia trait β *thalassemia minor* presents as a modest anemia with striking microcytosis. The hemoglobin may be as much as 30 g/L (3 g/dL) below normal, and the MCV is often less than 70 fL. Patients with this trait sometimes complain of weakness and tiredness, which they are inclined to blame on their anemia, but it is by no means certain that such symptoms are more common in patients with β-thalassemia trait than in the general population.

Diagnosis Most patients with β-thalassemia trait have twofold elevated levels of hemoglobin A₂ (α₂δ₂) (∼5 percent of total). Exceptions are patients with concurrent iron deficiency and those with a less common form of thalassemia, δβ thalassemia, in which δ-chain as well as β-chain production is compromised. In about one-third of patients with β-thalassemia trait, hemoglobin F is elevated (1 to 3 percent), and in δβ thalassemia, hemoglobin F may account for 5 to 15 percent of the total hemoglobin. Measurement of globin chain synthetic ratios is a definitive method of diagnosis; however, it is difficult to perform and therefore not readily available. In β thalassemia major, greatly elevated levels of fetal hemoglobin, comprising nearly all of the pigment, are present.

℞ **TREATMENT**

Untreated severe β thalassemia is uniformly fatal in childhood. Life can be prolonged by periodic transfusions, and if the hemoglobin level of the blood is maintained adequately, the bone changes and growth impairment can be largely prevented. When the spleen is greatly enlarged splenectomy may produce a clinically significant decrease in the transfusion requirement. Iron overload then becomes a serious problem that can be ameliorated by treatment with regular intravenous or subcutaneous infusions of desferrioxamine at 50 mg per kilogram body weight. The drug may cause skin reactions at the injection site or neurologic side effects, particularly visual and auditory, but these effects are dose-related. Cure of the disease can be achieved with marrow transplantation. Although this carries some risk of death due to the procedure itself, and in some patients the thalassemic cells regrow, displacing the graft, marrow transplantation has an important place in the treatment of patients with this very serious disease (Fig. 107-3).

Heterozygotes for β-thalassemic mutations do not need to be treated, but in regions in which the incidence of these mutations is very high, as in Sardinia, screening for β thalassemia combined with skillful counseling has played an important role in greatly decreasing the incidence of the disease. Only a generation ago, the incidence of thalassemia was 1:250; now its occurrence is rare.

Table 107-4

The α Thalassemias

Condition	Hemoglobin A, %	Hemoglobin H (β⁴), %	Hemoglobin level, g/L (g/dL)	MCV, fL
Normal	97	0	150 (15)	90
Silent thalassemia: − α/αα	98–100	0	150 (15)	90
Thalassemia trait: − α/− α homozygous α-thal-2* or − −/αα heterozygous α-thal-1*	85–95	Rare red blood cell inclusions	120–130 (12–13)	70–80
Hemoglobin H disease: − −/− α heterozygous α-thal-1/α-thal-2	70–95	5–30	60–100 (6–10)	60–70
Hydrops fetalis: − −/− − homozygous α-thal-1	0	5–10†	Fatal in utero or at birth	

* When both α alleles on one chromosome are deleted, the locus is called α-thal-1; when only a single α allele on one chromosome is deleted, the locus is called α-thal-2.
† 90–95% of the hemoglobin is hemoglobin Barts (tetramers of γ chains).

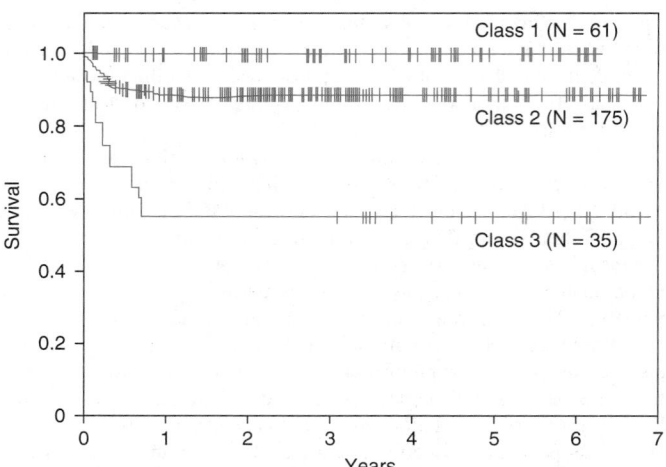

FIGURE 107-3 The probability of survival for 271 thalassemic patients under 17 years of age. The patients received marrow transplantation from HLA-identical family members after conditioning with busulfan and cyclophosphamide. The degree of hepatomegaly and the presence of portal fibrosis was used to assign patients to risk classes. (*From G. Lucarelli and RA Clift, in SJ Forman et al (eds), Bone Marrow Transplantation, Boston, Blackwell Scientific, 1994, with permission.*)

COMPOUND HEMOGLOBINOPATHIES

HEMOGLOBIN E/THALASSEMIA   Hemoglobin E (lysine for glutamic acid at position 26 of the β chain) results in a defect in mRNA processing and the production of an unstable hemoglobin. Both heterozygotes and homozygotes show microcytosis and hypochromia, but heterozygotes are not anemic. This form of hemoglobin is common in Cambodia and Thailand (30 to 40 percent). Patients who are compound heterozygotes for hemoglobin E and β thalassemia have the clinical features of β thalassemia major including severe hemolytic anemia and splenomegaly, require chronic transfusion, and suffer iron overload.

HEMOGLOBIN S/THALASSEMIA   Compound heterozygotes of hemoglobin S and β thalassemia are most commonly seen in African and Mediterranean populations. They develop a clinical picture consistent with sickle cell anemia except that splenomegaly is usually present. Therapy consists of raising hemoglobin F levels with hydroxyurea.

HEMOGLOBIN C/THALASSEMIA   Also noted in Mediterranean and African populations, hemoglobin C/β° thalassemia is associated with a moderately severe hemolytic anemia, splenomegaly, target cells, and a hypochromic microcytic peripheral blood smear. In blacks, hemoglobin C may occur with β⁺ thalassemia, which produces a milder disease.

OTHER ACQUIRED AND INHERITED HEMOGLOBIN ABNORMALITIES

The most common cause of cyanosis is reduced arterial oxygen tension related to lung disease or right-to-left cardiac shunts. Hemoglobin can on rare occasions account for cyanosis either through mutations producing molecules with decreased oxygen affinity (e.g., hemoglobin Kansas-$\beta^{102Asn \to Thr}$) or through the accumulation of methemoglobin or sulfhemoglobin.

METHEMOGLOBINEMIA AND SULFHEMOGLOBINE-MIA   Accumulation of large amounts of the brown, reversibly oxidized methemoglobin in red cells can occur for three reasons: (1) a dominantly inherited abnormality in hemoglobin, one of the hemoglo-bins M, in which the structural lesion prevents the reduction of methemoglobin to hemoglobin; (2) a recessively inherited deficiency in the enzyme methemoglobin reductase; and (3) exposure to hemoglobin-oxidizing chemicals or drugs such as nitrites, xylocaine, or benzene derivatives. Differentiation of these forms of methemoglobinemia from each other depends upon the clinical history; the pattern of transmission in the family; examination of the optical spectrum of the hemoglobin, which is abnormal in the hemoglobins M; and assay of the erythrocyte methemoglobin reductase.

The irreversible formation of another hemoglobin pigment with distinctively abnormal spectral properties, sulfhemoglobin, results from the administration of drugs, particularly sulfonamides. It produces marked cyanosis but disappears spontaneously as the cells containing the abnormal pigment are gradually removed from the circulation.

Methemoglobinemia induced by drugs or chemicals is spontaneously reversible when the agent is withdrawn. However, high levels of the pigment amounting to more than 30 to 40 percent of the total pigment can be life-threatening and are best treated by the infusion of methylene blue, 1 to 2 mg per kilogram body weight. This dye links the highly efficient NADP-linked methemoglobin-reducing system to methemoglobin and thus will result in rapid reduction of methemoglobin to hemoglobin in all but G6PD-deficient patients. Although methemoglobinemia due to methemoglobin reductase deficiency also responds to methylene blue treatment, this chronic disorder is best treated by the daily oral administration of 1 to 2 g ascorbic acid. Cyanosis due to hemoglobin M does not respond to treatment but is ordinarily a benign condition.

CARBOXYHEMOGLOBINEMIA   Hemoglobin has an affinity for carbon monoxide (CO) that is about 200 times higher than its affinity for oxygen. The displacement of even one oxygen molecule by CO greatly increases the strength with which remaining oxygen molecules are bound. The left shift produced in the oxygen dissociation curve impairs delivery of oxygen to the tissues to an extent that is much greater than would otherwise occur from the decrease in the amount of oxygen carried by the blood. In contrast to methemoglobin, carboxyhemoglobin is cherry red in color and its presence may not be suspected by gross examination of the blood. Carbon monoxide poisoning may be caused by combustion of hydrocarbons such as by faulty heaters in poorly ventilated areas, in industrial accidents, and in fires. Smokers of cigarettes or cigar smokers who inhale the smoke may have carboxyhemoglobin levels as high as 20 percent. Displacement of more than 50 percent of the oxygen by CO can be fatal. Oxygen will gradually displace the CO from hemoglobin, so that in mildly affected patients administration of oxygen or no treatment at all may be sufficient. In severely compromised patients blood transfusions may be necessary.

BIBLIOGRAPHY

BEUTLER E: The sickle cell diseases and related disorders, in *Williams' Hematology*, 5th ed, E Beutler et al (eds). New York, McGraw-Hill, 1995, pp 616–654

————, SULLIVAN KM: Bone marrow transplantation for sickle cell disease, in *Bone Marrow Transplantation*, SJ Forman et al (eds). Boston, Blackwell Scientific, 1994, pp. 840–848

CAO A: 1993 William Allan Award address. Am J Hum Genet 54:397, 1994

CHARACHE S et al: Hydroxyurea: Effects on hemoglobin F production in patients with sickle cell anemia. Blood 79:2555, 1992

EHLERS KH et al: Prolonged survival in patients with beta-thalassemia major treated with deferoxamine. J Pediatr 118:540, 1991

EMBURY SH et al (eds): *Sickle Cell Disease: Basic Principles and Clinical Practice*. Hagerstown, MD, Lippincott-Raven, 1994

THEIN SL: Dominant beta thalassaemia: Molecular basis and pathophysiology. Br J Haematol 80:273, 1992

WALTERS MC et al: Bone marrow transplantation for sickle cell disease. N Engl J Med 335:369, 1996

WEATHERALL DJ: The thalassemias, in *Williams' Hematology*, 5th ed, E Beutler et al (eds). New York, McGraw-Hill, 1995, pp 581–615

WINTERBOURN CC: Oxidative denaturation in congenital hemolytic anemias: The unstable hemoglobins. Semin Hematol 27:41, 1990

MEGALOBLASTIC ANEMIAS

The megaloblastic anemias are disorders caused by impaired DNA synthesis. Cells primarily affected are those having relatively rapid turnover, especially hematopoietic precursors and gastrointestinal epithelial cells. Cell division is sluggish, but cytoplasmic development progresses normally, so megaloblastic cells tend to be large, with an increased ratio of RNA to DNA. Megaloblastic erythroid cells tend to be destroyed in the marrow. Thus, marrow cellularity is often increased but production of red blood cells (RBC) is decreased, an abnormality termed *ineffective erythropoiesis* (see Chap. 59).

Most megaloblastic anemias are due to a deficiency of cobalamin (vitamin B_{12}) and/or folic acid. The various clinical entities associated with megaloblastic anemia are listed in Table 108-1. This classification is easier to comprehend if the physiologic and biochemical principles discussed below are kept in mind.

PHYSIOLOGIC CONSIDERATIONS

FOLIC ACID Folic acid is the common name for pteroylmonoglutamic acid. It is synthesized by many different plants and bacteria. Fruits and vegetables constitute the primary dietary source of the vitamin. Some forms of dietary folic acid are labile and may be destroyed by cooking. The minimum daily requirement is normally about 50μg, but this may be increased severalfold during periods of enhanced metabolic demand such as pregnancy.

The assimilation of adequate amounts of folic acid is dependent on the nature of the diet and its means of preparation. Folates in various foodstuffs are largely conjugated to a chain of glutamic acid residues. This highly polar side chain impairs the intestinal absorption of the vitamin. However, conjugases (γ-glutamyl carboxypeptidases) in the lumen of the gut convert polyglutamates to mono- and diglutamates, which are readily absorbed in the proximal jejunum.

Plasma folate is primarily in the form of N^5-methyltetrahydrofolate, a monoglutamate. N^5-Methyltetrahydrofolate is transported into cells by a carrier that is specific for the tetrahydro forms of the vitamin. Once in the cell, the N^5-methyl group is removed in a cobalamin-requiring reaction (see below), and the folate is then reconverted to the polyglutamate form. The polyglutamate form may be useful for retention of folate by the cell.

A folate-binding protein occurs in plasma, milk, and other body fluids. The function of this folate binder and its membrane-bound precursor is unknown. Neither the binder nor its precursor is related to the tetrahydrofolate carrier.

Normal individuals have about 5 to 20 mg folic acid in various body stores, half in the liver. In light of the minimum daily requirement, it is not surprising that a deficiency will occur within months if dietary intake or intestinal absorption is curtailed.

COBALAMIN This vitamin is a complex organometallic compound in which a cobalt atom is situated within a corrin ring, a structure similar to the porphyrin from which heme is formed. Unlike heme, however, cobalamin cannot be synthesized in the human body and must be supplied in the diet. The only dietary source of cobalamin is animal products: meat and dairy foods. The minimum daily requirement for cobalamin is about 2.5 μg.

During gastric digestion, cobalamin in food is released and forms a stable complex with gastric R binder, one of a closely related group of glycoproteins of unknown function that are found in secretions (e.g., saliva, milk, gastric juice, bile), phagocytes, and plasma. On entering the duodenum, the cobalamin–R binder complex is digested, releasing the cobalamin, which then binds to intrinsic factor (IF). This 50-kDa glycoprotein is produced by the parietal cells of the stomach. The secretion of intrinsic factor generally parallels that of hydrochloric acid. The cobalamin-IF complex is resistant to proteolytic digestion and travels to the distal ileum, where specific receptors on the mucosal brush border bind the cobalamin-IF complex, thereby enabling the

Table 108-1

Classification of the Megaloblastic Anemias

COBALAMIN DEFICIENCY

  I. Inadequate intake: vegetarians (rare)
 II. Malabsorption
     A. Inadequate production of intrinsic factor (IF)
        1. Pernicious anemia
        2. Gastrectomy
        3. Congenital absence or functional abnormality of IF (rare)
     B. Disorders of terminal ileum
        1. Tropical sprue
        2. Nontropical sprue
        3. Regional enteritis
        4. Intestinal resection
        5. Neoplasms and granulomatous disorders (rare)
        6. Selective cobalamin malabsorption (Imerslund's syndrome) (rare)
     C. Competition for cobalamin
        1. Fish tapeworm
        2. Bacteria: "blind loop" syndrome
     D. Drugs: *p*-aminosalicylic acid, colchicine, neomycin
III. Other
     A. Nitrous oxide
     B. Transcobalamin II deficiency (rare)

FOLIC ACID DEFICIENCY

  I. Inadequate intake: unbalanced diet (common in alcoholics, teenagers, some infants)
 II. Increased requirements
     A. Pregnancy
     B. Infancy
     C. Malignancy
     D. Increased hematopoiesis (chronic hemolytic anemias)
     E. Chronic exfoliative skin disorders
     F. Hemodialysis
III. Malabsorption
     A. Tropical sprue
     B. Nontropical sprue
     C. Drugs: Phenytoin, barbiturates, (?) ethanol
 IV. Impaired metabolism
     A. Inhibitors of dihydrofolate reductase: methotrexate, pyrimethamine, triamterene, pentamidine, trimethoprim
     B. Alcohol
     C. Rare enzyme deficiencies: dihydrofolate reductase, others

OTHER CAUSES

  I. Drugs that impair DNA metabolism
     A. Purine antagonists: 6-mercaptopurine, azathioprine, etc.
     B. Pyrimidine antagonists: 5-fluorouracil, cytosine arabinoside, etc.
     C. Others: procarbazine, hydroxyurea, acyclovir, zidovudine
 II. Metabolic disorders (rare)
     A. Hereditary orotic aciduria
     B. Others
III. Megaloblastic anemia of unknown etiology
     A. Refractory megaloblastic anemia
     B. Di Guglielmo's syndrome*
     C. Congenital dyserythropoietic anemia

* A form of acute nonlymphocytic leukemia with atypical, dysplastic changes in erythroid series.

vitamin to be absorbed. Thus intrinsic factor, like transferrin for iron, serves as a cell-directed carrier protein. The receptor-bound cobalamin-IF complex is taken into the ileal mucosal cell, where the IF is destroyed and the cobalamin is transferred to another transport protein, transcobalamin (TC) II. The cobalamin–TC II complex is then secreted into the circulation, from which it is rapidly taken up by the liver, bone marrow, and other cells. The pathway of cobalamin absorption is shown in Fig. 108-1. Normally, about 2 mg cobalamin is stored in the liver, and another 2 mg is stored elsewhere in the body. In view of the minimum daily requirement, about 3 to 6 years would be required for a normal individual to become deficient in cobalamin if absorption were to cease abruptly.

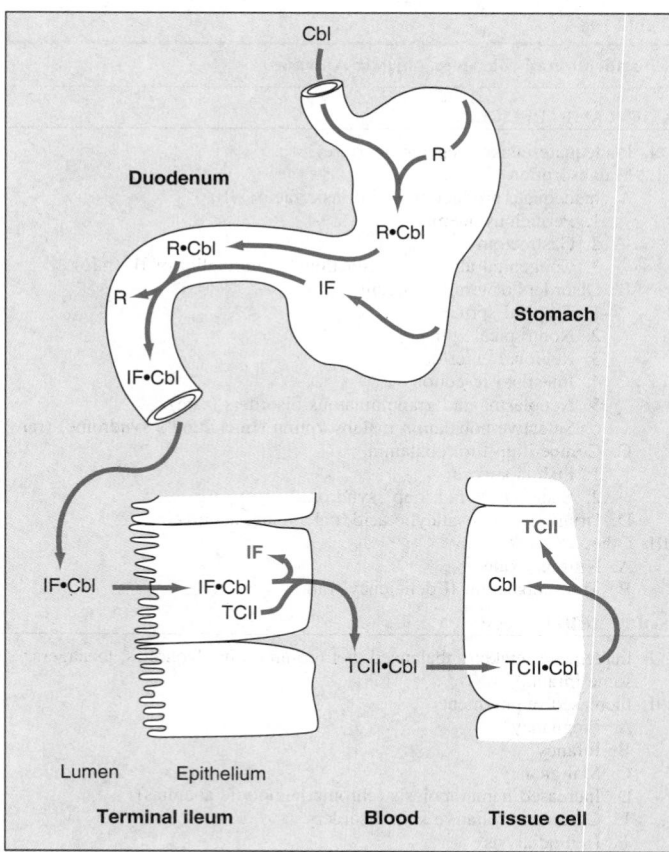

FIGURE 108-1 The assimilation of cobalamin. On entering the stomach, dietary cobalamin (Cbl) forms a complex with R binding protein. As this protein is digested, cobalamin is transferred to intrinsic factor (IF). This complex passes through the intestine until it reaches specific receptors on the mucosa of the distal ileum. The internalized Cbl is then transferred to transcobalamin II (TC II), which circulates in the plasma until it binds to receptors on cells throughout the body and is internalized.

Although TC II is the acceptor for newly absorbed cobalamin, most circulating cobalamin is bound to TC I, a glycoprotein closely related to gastric R binder. TC I appears to be derived in part from leukocytes. The paradox that most circulating cobalamin is bound to TC I rather than TC II, even though TC II initially carries all the cobalamin that is absorbed by the intestine, is explained by the fact that cobalamin bound to TC II is rapidly cleared from the blood ($t_{1/2}$ about 1 h), while clearance of cobalamin bound to TC I requires many days. The function of TC I is unknown.

BIOCHEMICAL CONSIDERATIONS

FOLATE The prime function of this vitamin is to transfer 1-carbon moieties such as methyl and formyl groups to various organic compounds (see Fig. 108-2). The source of these 1-carbon moieties is usually serine, which reacts with tetrahydrofolate to produce glycine and $N^{5,10}$-methylenetetrahydrofolate. An alternative source is formiminoglutamic acid, an intermediate in histidine catabolism, which gives up its formimino group to tetrahydrofolate to yield N^5-formiminotetrahydrofolate and glutamic acid. These derivatives provide entry into an interconvertible donor pool consisting of tetrahydrofolate derivatives carrying various 1-carbon moieties. The constituents of this pool can donate their 1-carbon moieties to appropriate acceptor compounds to form metabolic intermediates, which are ultimately converted to building blocks used in the synthesis of biologic macromolecules. The most important building blocks are (1) purines, in which the C-2 and

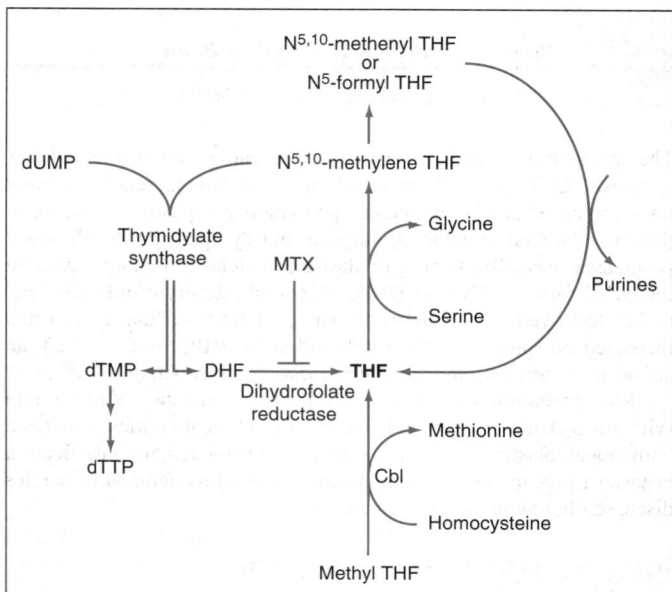

FIGURE 108-2 Folate metabolism. Folate is essential for the de novo synthesis of purines, deoxythymidylate monophosphate (dTMP) and methionine, serving as an intermediate carrier of 1-carbon fragments used in the biosynthesis of these compounds. Its active form is tetrahydrofolate (THF). THF acquires the 1-carbon fragment principally from serine, which is converted to glycine in the course of the reaction. For purine synthesis, the 1-carbon fragment is first oxidized to the level of formic acid, then transferred to substrate. For methionine synthesis, a cobalamin-requiring reaction, the 1-carbon fragment is first reduced to the level of a methyl group, then transferred to homocysteine. In these reactions the cofactor is released as THF, which can immediately participate in another 1-carbon transfer cycle. During the production of dTMP from dUMP, however, the 1-carbon fragment is reduced from formaldehyde to a methyl group in the course of the transfer reaction. The hydrogen atoms used for this reduction come from the cofactor, which is therefore released, not as THF, but as dihydrofolate (DHF). To participate further in the 1-carbon transfer cycle, the DHF has to be re-reduced to THF, a reaction catalyzed by dihydrofolate reductase.

The anemia of cobalamin deficiency is really due to tissue folate deficiency. This deficiency results from an impairment in the cobalamin-dependent transfer of the methyl group from N^5-methylTHF to homocysteine, leading to a delay in the attachment of a polyglutamate chain to the folate molecule (a process known as conjugation) and the leakage of the unconjugated folate out of the cell. Folate therefore corrects the anemia of cobalamin deficiency. The neurologic defects of cobalamin deficiency, however, are thought to result from inadequate methionine synthesis, leading to a deficiency of the methylating agent S-adenosylmethionine and an abnormality in the production of methylated phospholipids such as phosphatidylcholine. Folate does not correct the neurologic defects seen in cobalamin deficiency.

C-8 atoms are introduced in folate-dependent reactions, (2) deoxythymidylate monophosphate (dTMP), synthesized from $N^{5,10}$-methylenetetrahydrofolate and deoxyuridylate monophosphate (dUMP), and (3) methionine, formed by the transfer of a methyl group from N^5-methyltetrahydrofolate to homocysteine (two of these three reactions are shown in Fig. 108-2).

In all but one of the 1-carbon transfer reactions, tetrahydrofolate is produced. It can immediately accept a 1-carbon moiety and reenter the donor pool. The single exception is the thymidylate synthase reaction (dUMP → dTMP), in which dihydrofolate is the product (Fig. 108-2). This must be reduced to tetrahydrofolate by the enzyme dihydrofolate reductase before it can reenter the donor pool. A number of drugs are able to inhibit dihydrofolate reductase (Table 108-1), thereby diverting folate from the donor pool and producing what amounts to a state of folate deficiency in the face of normal tissue folate concentrations.

COBALAMIN In humans there are two metabolically active forms of cobalamin, identified by the alkyl group attached to the sixth coordination position of the cobalt atom: methylcobalamin and adenosylcobalamin. The vitamin preparation that is used therapeutically is cyanocobalamin (also called vitamin B_{12}). Cyanocobalamin has no known physiologic role and must be converted to a biologically active form before it can be used by tissues.

Methylcobalamin is an essential cofactor in the conversion of homocysteine to methionine (Fig. 108-2). When this reaction is impaired, folate metabolism is deranged, and it is this derangement that is thought to underlie the defect in DNA synthesis and the megaloblastic maturation pattern in patients who are deficient in cobalamin. In cobalamin deficiency, the unconjugated N^5-methyltetrahydrofolate newly taken from the bloodstream cannot be converted to other forms of tetrahydrofolate by methyl transfer. This is the so-called folate trap hypothesis. Because N^5-methyltetrahydrofolate is a poor substrate for the conjugating enzyme, it largely remains in the unconjugated form and slowly leaks from the cell. Tissue folate deficiency therefore develops, and this results in megaloblastic hematopoiesis. This hypothesis explains why tissue folate stores in cobalamin deficiency are substantially reduced, with a disproportionate reduction in conjugated as compared with unconjugated folates, despite normal or supranormal serum folate levels. It also explains why large doses of folate can produce a partial hematologic remission in patients with cobalamin deficiency.

Plasma homocysteine levels are elevated in both folate and cobalamin deficiency, and high levels of plasma homocysteine appear to be a risk factor for thrombosis on both the venous and arterial side. It is not yet known, however, if hyperhomocysteinemia due to folate or cobalamin deficiency predisposes to thrombosis or alters its response to treatment.

Impairment in the conversion of homocysteine to methionine also may be partly responsible for the neurologic complications of cobalamin deficiency (see below). The methionine formed in this reaction is needed for the production of choline and choline-containing phospholipids. Nervous system damage is postulated to result at least in part from interference with these processes due to decreased methionine production in cobalamin deficiency.

Adenosylcobalamin is required for the conversion of methylmalonyl coenzyme A (CoA) to succinyl CoA. Lack of this cofactor leads to large increases in the tissue levels of methylmalonyl CoA and its precursor, propionyl CoA. As a consequence, nonphysiologic fatty acids containing an odd number of carbon atoms are synthesized and incorporated into neuronal lipids. This biochemical abnormality also may contribute to the neurologic complications of cobalamin deficiency (see below).

CLINICAL DISORDERS

CLASSIFICATION OF MEGALOBLASTIC ANEMIAS (See Table 108-1) The cause of megaloblastic anemia varies in different parts of the world. In temperate zones, folate deficiency in alcoholics and pernicious anemia are the common types of megaloblastic anemias. In certain areas close to the equator, tropical sprue is endemic and an important cause of megaloblastic anemia, while in Scandinavia, it is occasionally secondary to infestations by the fish tapeworm, *Diphyllobothrium latum*.

The dietary intake of cobalamin is more than adequate for the body's requirements, except in true vegetarians (individuals who live on a purely vegetable diet) and their breast-fed infants. Thus deficiency of cobalamin is almost always due to malabsorption. As noted above, the absorption of cobalamin depends on a specific binding protein produced in the stomach and uptake by a specific receptor in the mucosa of the distal ileum. Accordingly, several steps in this process can go awry and lead to malabsorption. In contrast, the dietary intake of folic acid is marginal in many parts of the world. Furthermore, because the body's stores of folate are relatively low, folic acid deficiency can arise rather suddenly during periods of decreased dietary intake or increased metabolic demand. Finally, folic acid deficiency may be due to malabsorption. Often two or more of these factors coexist in a given patient.

Combined deficiencies of cobalamin and folic acid are not uncommon. Patients with tropical sprue are often deficient in both vitamins. The biochemical lesion that results in megaloblastic maturation of bone marrow cells also causes structural and functional abnormalities of the rapidly proliferating epithelial cells of the intestinal mucosa. Thus severe deficiency of one vitamin can lead to malabsorption of the other. Furthermore, as discussed above, a deficiency of cobalamin causes a secondary reduction in cellular folic acid.

Finally, megaloblastic anemias may occasionally be induced by factors unrelated to a vitamin deficiency. Most such cases are caused by one or more of the many drugs that interfere with DNA synthesis. Less commonly, megaloblastic maturation is encountered in certain acquired defects of hematopoietic stem cells. Rarest of all are specific congenital enzyme deficiencies.

COBALAMIN DEFICIENCY There are many conditions in which cobalamin deficiency may develop. Although each has its own characteristic manifestations, certain clinical features are common to all. These clinical features involve the blood, the gastrointestinal tract, and the nervous system.

The hematologic manifestations are almost entirely the result of anemia, although very rarely purpura may appear, due to thrombocytopenia. Symptoms of anemia may include weakness, light-headedness, vertigo, and tinnitus, as well as palpitations, angina, and the symptoms of congestive failure. On physical examination, the patient with florid cobalamin deficiency is pale, with slightly icteric skin and eyes. Elevated bilirubin levels are related to high RBC turnover in the marrow. The pulse is rapid, and the heart may be enlarged; auscultation will usually reveal a systolic flow murmur.

The gastrointestinal manifestations reflect the effect of cobalamin deficiency on the rapidly proliferating gastrointestinal epithelium. The patient sometimes complains of a sore tongue, which on inspection will be smooth and beefy red. Anorexia with moderate weight loss also may be evident, possibly accompanied by diarrhea and other gastrointestinal symptoms. These latter manifestations may be in part caused by megaloblastosis of the small-intestinal epithelium, which results in malabsorption.

The neurologic manifestations often fail to remit fully on treatment. They begin pathologically with demyelination, followed by axonal degeneration and eventual neuronal death; the final stage, of course, is irreversible. Sites of involvement include peripheral nerves; the spinal cord, where the posterior and lateral columns undergo demyelination; and the cerebrum itself. Signs and symptoms include numbness and paresthesias in the extremities (the earliest neurologic manifestations), weakness, and ataxia. There may be sphincter disturbances. Reflexes may be diminished or increased. The Romberg and Babinski signs may be positive, and position and vibration senses are usually diminished. Disturbances of mentation will vary from mild irritability and forgetfulness to severe dementia or frank psychosis. It should be emphasized that *neurologic disease may occur in a patient with a normal hematocrit* and normal RBC indexes.

In the classical patient, in whom hematologic problems predominate, the blood and bone marrow show characteristic megaloblastic changes (described under "Diagnosis" below). The anemia may be very severe—hematocrits of 15 to 20 are not infrequent—but is surprisingly well tolerated by the patient because it develops so slowly.

Pernicious Anemia The most common cause of cobalamin deficiency in temperate climates is pernicious anemia, in which intrinsic factor secretion ceases owing to atrophy of the gastric mucosa. It is most frequently seen in individuals of northern European descent and African-Americans and is much less common in southern Europeans and Asians. Men and women are equally affected. It is a disease of the elderly, the average patient presenting near age 60; it is rare under age 30, although typical pernicious anemia can be seen in children under age 10 (juvenile pernicious anemia). Inherited conditions in which a histologically normal stomach secretes either an abnormal intrinsic factor or none at all will induce cobalamin deficiency in infancy or early childhood.

There is considerable evidence for immunologic abnormalities in pernicious anemia. The incidence of pernicious anemia is substantially increased in patients with other diseases thought to be of immunologic origin, including Graves' disease, myxedema, thyroiditis, idiopathic adrenocortical insufficiency, vitiligo, and hypoparathyroidism. Patients with pernicious anemia also have abnormal circulating antibodies related to their disease: 90 percent have antiparietal cell antibody, while 60 percent have anti-intrinsic factor antibody. Antiparietal cell antibody is also found in 50 percent of patients with gastric atrophy without pernicious anemia, as well as in 10 to 15 percent of an unselected patient population, but anti-intrinsic factor antibody is usually absent from these patients. Relatives of patients with pernicious anemia have an increased incidence of the disease, and even clinically unaffected relatives may have anti-intrinsic factor antibody in their serum. Finally, treatment with glucocorticoids has been reported to reverse the disease both pathologically and clinically.

The destruction of parietal cells in pernicious anemia is thought to be mediated by complement-fixing antibodies against the parietal cell surface. The observation that pernicious anemia is unusually common in patients with agammaglobulinemia, however, suggests that the cellular immune system also may play a role in its pathogenesis. In contrast, *Helicobacter pylori* has little to do with parietal cell destruction in pernicious anemia.

Pathologically, the most characteristic finding in pernicious anemia is gastric atrophy affecting the acid- and pepsin-secreting portion of the stomach; the antrum is spared. Other pathologic changes are secondary to the deficiency of cobalamin; these include megaloblastoid alterations in the gastric and intestinal epithelium and the neurologic changes described above. The abnormalities in the gastric epithelium appear as cellular atypia in gastric cytology specimens, a finding that must be carefully distinguished from the cytologic abnormalities seen in gastric malignancy.

The *clinical manifestations* are primarily those of cobalamin deficiency, as described above. The disease is of insidious onset and progresses slowly. Laboratory examination will reveal hypergastrinemia and pentagastrin-fast achlorhydria as well as the hematologic and other laboratory abnormalities discussed under "Diagnosis."

Through appropriate replacement therapy, patients with pernicious anemia should experience complete and lifelong correction of all abnormalities that are due to cobalamin deficiency, except to the extent that irreversible changes in the nervous system may have occurred before treatment. These patients, however, are unusually subject to gastric polyps and have about twice the normal incidence of cancer of the stomach. Thus, patients should be followed with frequent stool guaiac examinations together with further diagnostic studies when indicated.

Postgastrectomy Following total gastrectomy or extensive damage to gastric mucosa as, for example, by ingestion of corrosive agents, megaloblastic anemia may develop because the source of intrinsic factor has been removed. In such patients, the absorption of orally administered cobalamin is impaired. Megaloblastic anemia also may follow partial gastrectomy, but the incidence is lower than after total gastrectomy, in which cobalamin malabsorption occurs in 100 percent of patients. The cause of cobalamin deficiency after partial gastrectomy may be intestinal overgrowth of bacteria, but it does not always respond to antibiotics.

Intestinal organisms Megaloblastic anemia may occur with intestinal stasis due to anatomic lesions (strictures, diverticula, anastomoses, "blind loops") or pseudoobstruction (diabetes mellitus, scleroderma, amyloid). This anemia is caused by colonization of the small intestine by large masses of bacteria that divert cobalamin from the host. Steatorrhea also may be seen under these circumstances, because bile salt metabolism is disturbed when the intestine is heavily colonized with bacteria. Hematologic responses have been observed after administration of oral antibiotics such as tetracycline and ampicillin.

Megaloblastic anemia is seen, in Scandinavia especially, in persons harboring the fish tapeworm, *D. latum*. The anemia has been attributed to competition by the worm for cobalamin. Destruction of the worm eliminates the problem.

Ileal Abnormalities Cobalamin deficiency is commonly found in tropical sprue, while it is an unusual complication of nontropical sprue (gluten-sensitive enteropathy; see Chap. 285). Virtually any disorder that compromises the absorptive capacity of the distal ileum can result in cobalamin deficiency. Specific entities include regional enteritis, Whipple's disease, and tuberculosis. Segmental involvement of the distal ileum by disease can cause megaloblastic anemia without any other manifestations of intestinal malabsorption such as steatorrhea. Cobalamin malabsorption is also seen after ileal resection. The Zollinger-Ellison syndrome (intense gastric hyperacidity due to a gastrin-secreting tumor) may cause cobalamin malabsorption by acidifying the small intestine. This will retard the transfer of the vitamin from R binder to intrinsic factor and will impair the binding of the cobalamin-IF complex to the ileal receptors. Chronic pancreatitis also may cause cobalamin malabsorption by impairing the transfer of the vitamin from R binder to intrinsic factor. This abnormality can be detected by tests of cobalamin absorption (see below, Schilling test), but it is invariably mild and never causes clinical cobalamin deficiency. Finally, there is a rare congenital disorder, Imerslund-Gräsbeck disease, in which a selective defect in cobalamin absorption is accompanied by proteinuria.

FOLIC ACID DEFICIENCY Patients with folic acid deficiency are more apt to be malnourished than those with cobalamin deficiency. Accordingly, they are likely to appear wasted. The gastrointestinal manifestations are similar to but may be more widespread and more severe than those of pernicious anemia. Diarrhea is often present, and cheilosis and glossitis are also encountered. However, in contrast to cobalamin deficiency, neurologic abnormalities do not occur.

The hematologic manifestations of folic acid deficiency are the same as those of cobalamin deficiency. Folic acid deficiency can generally be attributed to one or more of the following factors: inadequate intake, increased demand, and malabsorption.

Inadequate Intake Folic acid malnutrition is commonly encountered among a number of groups. Alcoholics frequently become folate deficient because their main source of caloric intake is alcoholic beverages. Distilled spirits are virtually devoid of folic acid, while beer and wine do not contain enough of the vitamin to satisfy the daily requirement. In addition, alcohol may interfere with folate metabolism. Narcotic addicts are also prone to become folate deficient because of malnutrition. Many indigent and elderly individuals who subsist primarily on canned foods or "tea and toast" and occasional teenagers whose diet consists of "junk food" develop folate deficiency.

Increased Demand Tissues with a relatively high rate of cell division such as the bone marrow or gut mucosa have a large requirement for folate. Therefore, patients with chronic hemolytic anemias or other causes of very active erythropoiesis may become deficient if their high folate requirement is not met by dietary intake. Likewise, a pregnant woman may become deficient in folic acid because of the high demand of the developing fetus. Deficiency in pregnancy can cause neural tube defects in newborns. Thus, pregnant women should receive oral folate supplementation. Folate deficiency also may occur during the growth spurts of infancy and adolescence. Patients on chronic hemodialysis may require supplementary folate to replace that lost in the dialysate.

Malabsorption Folic acid deficiency is a common accompaniment of tropical sprue. Both the gastrointestinal symptoms and malabsorption are improved by the administration of either folic acid or antibiotics by mouth. Patients with nontropical sprue (gluten-sensitive enteropathy) also may develop significant folic acid deficiency which parallels other parameters of malabsorption. Similarly, folate deficiency in alcoholics may be due in part to malabsorption. In addition, other primary small-bowel disorders are sometimes associated with vitamin deficiency. These entities are all discussed in Chap. 285.

DRUGS Next to deficiency of folate or cobalamin, the most common cause of megaloblastic anemia is drug ingestion. Drugs that cause megaloblastic anemia do so by interfering with DNA synthesis, either directly or by antagonizing the action of folate. They can be classified as follows:

1. *Direct inhibitors of DNA synthesis.* They include purine analogues (6-thioguanine, azathioprine, 6-mercaptopurine), pyrimidine analogues (5-fluorouracil, cytosine arabinoside), and other drugs that interfere with DNA synthesis by a variety of mechanisms (hydroxyurea, procarbazine). The antiviral agent zidovudine (AZT), used for treating the human immunodeficiency virus (HIV), often causes severe megaloblastic anemia.

2. *Folate antagonists.* The most toxic of these is methotrexate, an exceedingly powerful inhibitor of dihydrofolate reductase which is used in the treatment of certain malignancies. Much less toxic but still capable of inducing a megaloblastic anemia are several weak dihydrofolate reductase inhibitors that are used to treat a variety of nonmalignant conditions. These include pentamidine, trimethoprim, triamterene, and pyrimethamine.

The megaloblastic changes in methotrexate poisoning appear to result from a buildup of dUMP owing to impaired methylation to dTMP. The excess dUMP is partially phosphorylated to deoxyuridine triphosphate (dUTP), which accumulates in the cell and is incorporated into newly synthesized DNA. As a result, defective strands of DNA are produced in which T is partly replaced by U. U-rich DNA is also present in folate and cobalamin deficiency, suggesting a similar abnormality in DNA synthesis in the nutritional megaloblastic anemias.

3. *Nitrous oxide.* Nitrous oxide inhalation causes the destruction of endogenous cobalamin. As ordinarily used, this anesthetic does not destroy enough cobalamin to cause clinical manifestations. Repeated or protracted exposure, however, may lead to a megaloblastic anemia. Fatal megaloblastic anemia has been reported in patients with tetanus who were given nitrous oxide continuously for weeks.

4. *Others.* A number of drugs antagonize folate by mechanisms that are poorly understood but are thought to involve an effect on absorption of the vitamin by the intestine. In this category are the anticonvulsants phenytoin (Dilantin) and primidone (Mysoline) and phenobarbital (Luminal). Megaloblastic anemia induced by these agents is mild.

OTHER Hereditary Megaloblastic anemia may be seen in several hereditary disorders. It is a regular feature of orotic aciduria, a deficiency of orotidylic decarboxylase and phosphorylase, leading to a defect in pyrimidine metabolism and characterized by retarded growth and development as well as by the excretion of large amounts of orotic acid. Megaloblastic anemia has been reported in a single case of the Lesch-Nyhan syndrome, a condition resulting from a deficiency of hypoxanthine-guanine phosphoribosyltransferase whose clinical manifestations include gout, mental retardation, and self-mutilation. It also has been described in methylmalonic aciduria due to a combined defect in the biosynthesis of methyl and adenosyl cobalamins, although it is not seen in methylmalonic aciduria due to methylmalonyl CoA mutase deficiency. Congenital folate malabsorption causes megaloblastic anemia, accompanied by ataxia and mental retardation. Megaloblastic anemia has been reported to accompany the congenital deficiency of two other folate-metabolizing enzymes: dihydrofolate reductase and N^5-methyltetrahydrofolate:homocysteine methyltransferase. These deficiencies are less well documented than is congenital folate malabsorption. A thiamine-responsive megaloblastic anemia accompanied by nerve deafness and diabetes mellitus has been reported in several children. Megaloblastic changes as well as multinuclearity of red blood cell precursors are seen in the marrow of certain patients with congenital dyserythropoietic anemia, a group of inherited disorders characterized by mild to moderate anemia presenting at any age and pursuing a benign course.

Transcobalamin II deficiency, like the congenital abnormalities in cobalamin absorption described previously, causes pronounced deficiency in cobalamin in infancy or early childhood, with all the accompanying manifestations. Megaloblastic anemia is not seen in hereditary TC I deficiency.

Refractory Megaloblastic Anemia This is a form of myelodysplasia in which megaloblastic erythropoiesis may sometimes be seen. Megaloblastic changes are restricted to the RBC series; large granulocyte precursors and giant metamyelocytes are not seen (see below). As with other forms of myelodysplasia, refractory megaloblastic anemia is associated with an increased incidence of acute leukemia.

Megaloblastic changes are seen in erythremic myelosis and acute erythroleukemia (di Guglielmo), where RBC precursors are prominently involved. Here, the marrow is characterized by bizarre erythroid maturation, with multinuclearity and multipolar mitotic figures in the RBC precursors. Erythroleukemia is discussed further in Chap. 112.

MEGALOBLASTIC DISEASE WITHOUT ANEMIA Megaloblastic disease is easily overlooked in non-anemic patients. It can present in one of two ways.

Acute Megaloblastic Anemia Occasionally, a full-blown megaloblastic state can develop over the course of just a few days. This is usually seen following nitrous oxide anesthesia but may occur in any patient with a serious illness requiring intensive care, especially a patient receiving multiple transfusions, dialysis, or total parenteral nutrition. An acute megaloblastic state also can be precipitated by the administration of a weak antifolate (e.g., trimethoprim) to a patient with marginal tissue folate stores.

The condition resembles an immune cytopenia, with a rapidly developing thrombocytopenia and/or leukopenia in the absence of anemia. The blood smear may be completely normal, but the marrow is always floridly megaloblastic. Acute megaloblastic anemia responds rapidly to treatment with folate plus cobalamin in the usual therapeutic doses.

Cobalamin Deficiency without Anemia Cobalamin deficiency without hematologic abnormalities is surprisingly common, especially in the elderly. These patients may present with neuropsychiatric abnormalities, including peripheral neuropathies, gait disturbance, memory loss, and psychiatric symptoms, sometimes with abnormal evoked potentials. Serum cobalamin levels may be normal or low, but serum levels of methylmalonic acid are almost invariably increased due to a deficiency of cobalamin at the tissue level. The neuropsychiatric abnormalities tend to improve and serum methylmalonic acid levels generally return to normal after treatment with cobalamin.

DIAGNOSIS The finding of significant macrocytosis [mean corpuscular volume (MCV) > 100 fL] suggests the presence of a megaloblastic anemia. Other causes of macrocytosis include hemolysis, liver disease, alcoholism, hypothyroidism, and aplastic anemia. If the macrocytosis is marked (MCV > 110 fL), the patient is much more likely to have a megaloblastic anemia. Macrocytosis is less marked with concurrent iron deficiency or thalassemia. The reticulocyte count is low, and the leukocyte and platelet count also may be decreased, particularly in severely anemic patients. The blood smear **(see Plate IV-2)** demonstrates marked anisocytosis and poikilocytosis, together with macroovalocytes, which are large, oval, fully hemoglobinized erythrocytes typical of megaloblastic anemias. There is some basophilic stippling, and an occasional nucleated RBC may be seen. In the white blood cell series, the neutrophils show hypersegmentation of the nucleus. This is such a characteristic finding that a single cell with a nucleus of six lobes or more should raise the immediate suspicion of a megaloblastic anemia. A rare myelocyte also may be seen. Bizarre, misshapen platelets are also observed. The bone marrow examination is very helpful in the diagnosis of megaloblastic anemia. The marrow is hypercellular with a decreased myeloid/erythroid ratio and abundant stainable iron. RBC precursors are abnormally large and have nuclei that appear much less mature than would be expected from the development of the cytoplasm (nuclear-cytoplasmic asynchrony). The nuclear chromatin is more dispersed than it should be and consequently stains less intensely than normal. To the extent that it is aggregated, it condenses in a peculiar fenestrated pattern that is very characteristic of megaloblastic erythropoiesis. Abnormal mitoses may be seen. Granulocyte precursors are also affected, many being larger than normal, including giant bands and metamyelocytes. Megakaryocytes are decreased and show abnormal morphology.

Megaloblastic anemias are characterized by ineffective erythropoiesis (Chap. 59). In a severely megaloblastic patient, as many as 90 percent of the RBC precursors may be destroyed before they are released into the bloodstream, compared with 10 to 15 percent in the normal subject. Enhanced intramedullary destruction of erythroblasts results in an increase in unconjugated bilirubin and lactic acid dehydrogenase (isoenzyme 1) in plasma. Abnormalities in iron kinetics also attest to the presence of ineffective erythropoiesis, with increased iron turnover but low incorporation of labeled iron into circulating RBC.

In evaluating a patient with megaloblastic anemia, it is important to determine whether there is a specific vitamin deficiency by measuring serum cobalamin and folate levels. The normal range of cobalamin in serum is 200 to 900 pg/mL; values less than 100 pg/mL indicate clinically significant deficiency. The normal serum concentration of folic acid ranges from 6 to 20 ng/mL; values of 4 ng/mL or less are generally considered to be diagnostic of folate deficiency. Unlike serum cobalamin, serum folate levels may reflect recent alterations in dietary intake. Measurement of RBC folate level provides useful information because it is not subject to short-term fluctuations in folate intake and is, therefore, better than serum folate as an index of folate stores.

Once cobalamin deficiency has been established, its pathogenesis can be delineated by means of a Schilling test. A patient is given radioactive cobalamin by mouth, followed shortly thereafter by an intramuscular injection of unlabeled cobalamin. The proportion of the administered radioactivity excreted in the urine during the next 24 h provides an accurate measure of absorption of cobalamin, assuming that a complete urine sample has been collected. Because cobalamin deficiency is almost always due to malabsorption (see Table 108-1), this first stage of the Schilling test should be abnormal (i.e., small amounts of radioactivity in the urine). The patient is then given labeled cobalamin bound to intrinsic factor. Absorption of the vitamin will now approach normal if the patient has pernicious anemia or some other type of intrinsic factor deficiency. If cobalamin absorption is still decreased, the patient may have bacterial overgrowth (blind loop syndrome) or ileal disease (including an ileal absorptive defect secondary to the cobalamin deficiency itself). Cobalamin malabsorption due to bacterial overgrowth can frequently be corrected by the administration of antibiotics. The Schilling test can provide equally reliable information after the patient has had adequate therapy with parenteral cobalamin.

A normal Schilling test in a patient with documented cobalamin deficiency may indicate poor absorption of the vitamin when mixed with food. This can be established by repeating the Schilling test with radioactive cobalamin scrambled with an egg.

Serum methylmalonic acid and homocysteine are useful in the diagnosis of megaloblastic anemias. Levels of both are elevated in cobalamin deficiency, while elevated levels of homocysteine but not methylmalonic acid are seen in folate deficiency. These tests measure tissue vitamin stores and may demonstrate a deficiency even when the more traditional but less reliable folate and cobalamin levels are normal. Patients (particularly older patients) with normal serum cobalamin levels but elevated levels of serum methylmalonic acid may develop neuropsychiatric abnormalities. Treatment of patients with this "subtle" cobalamin deficiency may result in improvement.

℞ TREATMENT

Cobalamin Deficiency Apart from specific therapy related to the underlying disorder (e.g., antibiotics for intestinal overgrowth with bacteria), the mainstay of treatment for cobalamin deficiency is replacement therapy. Because the defect often is one of absorption, replacement should be administered parenterally, specifically in the form of intramuscular cyanocobalamin. (If intramuscular administration is contraindicated or refused, cobalamin deficiency can be managed by oral replacement therapy, but at doses of 300 to 1000 μg daily, it is an expensive mode of treatment that requires very close

medical supervision to avoid relapse.) Treatment should be started with 100 μg cobalamin per day for a week. The frequency of administration of the vitamin may then be decreased, the goal being to give a total of 2000 μg during the first 6 weeks. The patient may then be placed on 100 μg cyanocobalamin intramuscularly every month, a regimen that must be maintained for the rest of the patient's life. If necessary, larger doses may be given at less frequent intervals (e.g., 1 mg every 2 to 4 months), but the risk of relapse is substantially greater than if the vitamin is given monthly.

The response to treatment is gratifying. Shortly after treatment is begun, and several days before a hematologic response is evident in the peripheral blood, the patient will experience an increase in strength and an improved sense of well-being. Marrow morphology begins to revert toward normal within a few hours after treatment is initiated. Reticulocytosis begins 4 to 5 days after therapy is started and peaks at about day 7 (Fig. 108-3), with subsequent remission of the anemia over the next several weeks. If a reticulocytosis does not occur, or if it is less brisk than expected from the level of the hematocrit, a search should be made for other factors contributing to the anemia (e.g., infection, coexisting folate deficiency, or hypothyroidism). Hypokalemia and salt retention may occur early in the course of therapy. Thrombocytosis may also be seen.

In most cases, replacement therapy is all that is needed for the treatment of cobalamin deficiency. Occasionally, however, a patient with a severe anemia will have such a precarious cardiovascular status that emergency transfusion is necessary. This must be done with great care, because it is very easy to precipitate florid congestive failure in such patients by fluid overload. Blood must be administered slowly in the form of packed cells, with very close observation, giving as an initial dose no more than 100 mL. This small volume will frequently be enough to ameliorate the cardiovascular problems sufficiently that further therapy can be restricted to cobalamin replacement. If necessary, blood may be administered by exchanging patient blood (mostly plasma) for packed cells.

With lifelong treatment, patients should experience no further manifestations of cobalamin deficiency. As previously stated, neurologic symptoms may not be fully corrected even by optimal therapy. The potential for late development of gastric carcinoma in pernicious anemia necessitates careful follow-up of the patient.

Folate Deficiency As for cobalamin deficiency, folate deficiency is treated by replacement therapy. The usual dose of folate is 1 mg/d, by mouth, but higher doses (up to 5 mg/d) may be required for folate deficiency due to malabsorption. Parenteral folate is rarely necessary. The hematologic response is similar to that seen after replacement therapy for cobalamin deficiency—that is, a brisk reticulocytosis after about 4 days, followed by correction of the anemia over the next 1 to 2 months. The duration of therapy depends on the basis of the deficiency state. Patients with a continuously increased requirement (such as patients with hemolytic anemia) or those with malabsorption or chronic malnutrition should continue to receive oral

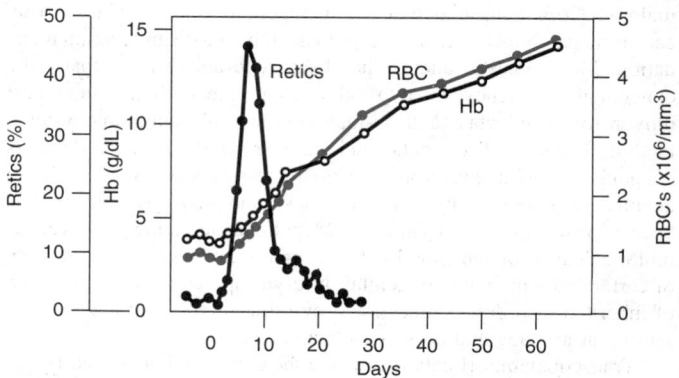

FIGURE 108-3 Hematologic response of a patient with pernicious anemia to an intramuscular injection of 100 μg cobalamin on day 0. (From A Erslev, TG Gabuzda, *Pathophysiology of Blood,* Philadelphia, Saunders, 1975, with permission.)

folic acid indefinitely. In addition, the patient should be encouraged to maintain an optimal diet containing adequate amounts of folate.

Folate, particularly in large doses, can correct the megaloblastic anemia of cobalamin deficiency without altering the neurologic abnormalities. The neurologic manifestations may even be aggravated by folate therapy. Cobalamin deficiency can thus be masked in patients who for one reason or another are taking large doses of folate. For this reason, a hematologic response to folate must never be used to rule out cobalamin deficiency in a given patient; cobalamin deficiency can be excluded only by appropriate laboratory evaluation.

Other Causes of Megaloblastic Anemia Megaloblastic anemia due to drugs can be treated, if necessary, by reducing the dose of the drug or eliminating it altogether. The effects of folate antagonists that inhibit dihydrofolate reductase can be counteracted by folinic acid [5-formyl tetrahydrofolate (THF)] in a dose of 100 to 200 mg/d (Fig. 108-2). It circumvents the block in folate metabolism imposed by dihydrofolate reductase inhibitors, replenishing the tissues with a form of folate that can directly enter the 1-carbon donor pool. Certain of the congenital megaloblastic anemia–producing enzyme deficiencies can be treated by appropriate specific therapeutic regimens. For the megaloblastic forms of sideroblastic anemia, pyridoxine in pharmacologic doses (as high as 300 mg/d) should be tried. Pyridoxalphosphate may also work presumably in part through promoting the conversion of THF to 5,10-methylene THF. A few patients will respond to one or the other vitamin B_6 congener. Simple supportive measures are all that appear to be in order for treatment of refractory megaloblastic anemia. Acute erythroleukemia (di Guglielmo's disease) is usually treated like other types of acute nonlymphocytic leukemia (see Chap. 112).

See Chap. 53, Hematopoietic agents: Growth factors, minerals, and vitamins, in Goodman & Gilman's The Pharmacological Basis of Therapeutics, 9th ed, New York, McGraw-Hill, 1996.

BIBLIOGRAPHY

ALLEN RH et al: Metabolic abnormalities in cobalamin [vitamin B_{12}] and folate deficiencies. FASEB J 7:1344, 1993

BABIOR BM: The megaloblastic anemias, in *Williams' Hematology*, 5th ed, E Beutler et al (eds). New York, McGraw-Hill, 1995, p 471

CARMEL R et al: The frequently low cobalamin levels in dementia usually signify treatable metabolic, neurologic and electrophysiologic abnormalities. Eur J Haematol 54:245, 1995

COOPER TR, ROSENBLATT DS: Inherited defects of vitamin B_{12} metabolism. Annu Rev Nutr 7:291, 1987

DICKINSON CJ: Does folic acid harm people with vitamin B_{12} deficiency? QJM 88:357, 1995

HSING AW et al: Pernicious anemia and subsequent cancer. Cancer 71:745, 1993

KAPADIA CR, DONALDSON RM: Disorders of cobalamin (vitamin B_{12}) absorption and transport. Annu Rev Med 36:93, 1985

LINDENBAUM J et al: Neuropsychiatric disorders caused by cobalamin deficiency in the absence of anemia or macrocytosis. N Engl J Med 318:1720, 1988

SAVAGE DG et al: Sensitivity of serum methylmalonic acid and total homocysteine determinations for diagnosing cobalamin and folate deficiencies. Am J Med 96:239, 1994

SCHILLING RF, WILLIAMS WJ: Vitamin B_{12} deficiency: Underdiagnosed, overtreated? Hosp Prac (Off Ed) 30:47, 1995

STABLER SP et al: Clinical spectrum and diagnosis of cobalamin deficiency. Blood 75:871, 1990

WATERS HM et al: High incidence of type II autoantibodies in pernicious anemia. J Clin Pathol 46:45, 1993

109 *Wendell Rosse, H. Franklin Bunn*

HEMOLYTIC ANEMIAS AND ACUTE BLOOD LOSS

Anemia may be caused by the loss of red cells either through hemorrhage or, less commonly, through premature destruction of the red cells (hemolysis) by a number of mechanisms. Hemolysis or blood loss will lead to an increase in red cell production, which is clinically manifested by an increase in the reticulocyte production index to greater than three times normal.

HEMOLYTIC ANEMIAS

Red blood cells (RBC) normally survive 90 to 120 days in the circulation. Red cell life span may be shortened in a number of disorders, often resulting in anemia if the bone marrow is not able to replenish adequately the prematurely destroyed red cells. The disorders associated with hemolytic anemias are generally identified by the abnormality that brings about the premature destruction of the red cells. In this chapter, we shall describe the general attributes of this important group of anemias, the diagnostic procedures useful in identifying the causes of the accelerated red cell breakdown, and the pathogenesis and management of specific hemolytic disorders.

In all patients with hemolytic anemia, a careful history and physical examination are important in the diagnosis. The patient may complain of fatigue and other symptoms of anemia (see Chap. 59). Less commonly, jaundice and even red-brown urine (hemoglobinuria) are reported. A complete drug and toxin exposure history and the family history are important in the diagnosis. The physical examination may show icterus and jaundice of skin and mucosae. The cardiac signs of anemia (flow murmurs, etc.) may be present. Splenomegaly is encountered in a variety of hemolytic anemias. As discussed in detail in this chapter, a wide array of other historical and physical findings is associated with specific hemolytic anemias.

Laboratory tests may be used initially to demonstrate the presence of hemolysis (Table 109-1) and then to demonstrate the cause of hemolysis. Elevation of the reticulocyte count in the anemic patient is the most useful indicator of hemolysis, reflecting erythroid hyperplasia of the bone marrow; biopsy of the bone marrow is often unnecessary. Reticulocytes are also elevated in patients with active blood loss, those with myelophthisis, and those who are recovering from suppression of erythropoiesis (see Chap. 59). The morphology of the red cells as seen on the peripheral blood film is often abnormal and may provide evidence both of hemolysis and of its cause; the characteristic abnormalities and their associated causes and syndromes are listed in Table 109-2. While the peripheral blood smear alone is rarely if ever truly pathognomonic, in many cases it is a low-cost, important clue to the presence of hemolysis and to diagnosis.

Red blood cells may be prematurely removed from the circulation by macrophages, particularly those of the spleen and liver (extravascular lysis), or less commonly by disruption of their membranes during their circulation (intravascular hemolysis). Both mechanisms result in increased heme catabolism and enhanced formation of the tetrapyrrole

Table 109-1

Laboratory Evaluation of Hemolysis

	Extravascular	Intravascular
HEMATOLOGIC		
Routine blood film	Polychromatophilia	Polychromatophilia
Reticulocyte count	↑	↑
Bone marrow examination	Erythroid hyperplasia	Erythroid hyperplasia
PLASMA OR SERUM		
Bilirubin	↑ Unconjugated	↑ Unconjugated
Haptoglobin	↓, Absent	Absent
Plasma hemoglobin	N−↑	↑↑
Lactate dehydrogenase	↑ (Variable)	↑↑ (Variable)
URINE		
Bilirubin	0	0
Hemosiderin	0	+
Hemoglobin	0	+ in severe cases

Table 109-2

The Value of Red Blood Cell Morphology in Diagnosis
of Hemolytic Anemia

Morphology	Cause	Syndromes
Spherocytes	Loss of membrane	Hereditary spherocytosis, autoimmune hemolytic anemia
Target cells	Increased ratio of RBC surface area to volume	Hemoglobin disorders: thalassemias, hemoglobin S, C, etc.; liver disease
Schistocytes	Traumatic disruption of membrane	Microangiopathic conditions, intravascular prostheses
Sickled cells	Polymerization of hemoglobin S	Sickle cell syndromes
Acanthocytes	?Abnormal membrane lipids	Severe liver disease (spur cell anemias)
Agglutinated cells	Presence of IgM antibody	Cold agglutinin disease
Heinz bodies	Precipitated hemoglobin	Unstable hemoglobin, oxidant stress

unconjugated bilirubin, which is normally metabolized by the liver by conjugation and subsequent excretion. The plasma level of unconjugated bilirubin may be high enough to produce readily apparent jaundice. The unconjugated (indirect) bilirubin level can be further elevated by a commonly encountered defect in transport of bilirubin (Gilbert's syndrome) (see Chap. 294). In patients with hemolysis, the level of unconjugated bilirubin never exceeds 70 to 85 μmol/L (4 to 5 mg/dL), unless liver function is impaired.

Other serum tests are also useful in the assessment of hemolysis. *Haptoglobin* is an alpha globulin that is present in high concentration (~1.0 g/L) in the plasma (and serum). It binds specifically and tightly to the protein (globin) in hemoglobin. The hemoglobin-haptoglobin complex is cleared within minutes by the mononuclear phagocyte system. Thus patients with significant hemolysis, either intravascular or extravascular, have low or absent levels of serum haptoglobin. Haptoglobin synthesis is decreased in patients with hepatocellular disease. Conversely, synthesis is enhanced in inflammatory states. These facts must be considered in the interpretation of serum haptoglobin. Intravascular hemolysis (which is relatively uncommon) results in the release of hemoglobin into the plasma. In these cases, plasma hemoglobin is increased in proportion to the degree of hemolysis but may be falsely elevated due to lysis of red cells in vitro. If the haptoglobin-binding capacity of the plasma is exceeded, free hemoglobin passes through renal glomeruli. This filtered hemoglobin is reabsorbed by the proximal tubule, where it is catabolized in situ, and the heme iron is incorporated into storage proteins (ferritin and hemosiderin). The presence of hemosiderin in the urine, detected by staining the sediment with Prussian blue, indicates that a significant amount of circulating free hemoglobin has been filtered by the kidneys. Hemosiderin appears 3 to 4 days after the onset of hemoglobinuria and may persist for weeks after its cessation. When the absorptive capacity of the tubular cells is exceeded, hemoglobinuria results. The presence of hemoglobinuria indicates severe intravascular hemolysis. Hemoglobinuria must be distinguished from hematuria (in which case red cells are seen in the examination of a fresh specimen of urine) and from myoglobin due to rhabdomyolysis; in all three cases, the urine will be positive with the benzidine reaction, commonly used in analysis of urine. The distinction between hemoglobinuria and myoglobinuria can best be made by specific tests that exploit immunologic differences or differences in solubility. After centrifugation of an anticoagulated specimen, the plasma of patients with hemoglobinuria has a reddish-brown color, whereas that of patients with myoglobinuria is normal in color. Because of its higher molecular weight, hemoglobin has

lower glomerular permeability than myoglobin and is less rapidly cleared by the kidneys.

CLASSIFICATION The hemolytic anemias can be conveniently grouped in three different ways, shown in Table 109-3. From an anatomic vantage point, the cause of accelerated red cell destruction can be regarded as either (1) a molecular defect (hemoglobinopathy or enzymopathy) inside the red cell, (2) an abnormality in membrane structure and function, or (3) an environmental factor such as mechanical trauma or an autoantibody. In *intracorpuscular types* of hemolysis, the patient's red cells have an abnormally short life span in a normal recipient (with a compatible blood type), while compatible normal red cells survive normally in the patient. The opposite is true in *extracorpuscular types* of hemolysis. Finally, as exemplified in the organization of the remainder of this chapter, hemolytic disorders can be conveniently classified as either inherited or acquired.

INHERITED HEMOLYTIC ANEMIAS The inherited hemolytic anemias are due to inborn defects in one of three main components of red cells: the membrane, the enzymes, or hemoglobin. With the advent of biochemical genetics, these defects are often known at the genomic level, but for the most part we still rely on the clinical and usual laboratory manifestations for their identification.

Red Cell Membrane Disorders These are usually readily detected by morphologic abnormalities of the red cells on examination of the blood film. There are three types of inherited abnormalities of the red cell membrane: hereditary spherocytosis, hereditary elliptocytosis (including hereditary pyropoikilocytosis), and hereditary stomatocytosis.

Hereditary spherocytosis This condition is characterized by spherical red cells due to a molecular defect in one of the proteins in the cytoskeleton of the red cell membrane, leading to a loss of membrane and hence decreased ratio of surface area to volume and consequently spherocytosis. This disorder usually has an autosomal dominant inheritance pattern and an incidence of approximately 1:1000 to 1:4500. In 20 percent of patients, the absence of hematologic abnormalities in family members suggests either autosomal recessive inheritance or, less commonly, a spontaneous mutation. The disorder is sometimes clinically apparent in early infancy but often escapes detection until adult life.

CLINICAL MANIFESTATIONS The major clinical features of hereditary spherocytosis are anemia, splenomegaly, and jaundice. The prominence of the last finding accounts for its prior designation as "congenital hemolytic jaundice" and is due to an increased concentration of unconjugated (indirect-reacting) bilirubin in plasma. Jaundice may be intermittent and tends to be less pronounced in early childhood. Because of the increased bile pigment production, gallstones of pigment type are common, even in childhood. Compensatory erythroid hyperplasia of the bone marrow occurs, with the extension of red marrow into the midshafts of long bones and occasionally with extramedullary erythropoiesis, at times leading to the formation of paravertebral masses visible on chest x-ray. Because the bone marrow's capacity to increase erythropoiesis by six- to eightfold exceeds the usual rate of hemolysis in this disease, anemia is usually mild or moderate and

Table 109-3

Classifications of Hemolytic Anemias

Intracorpuscular	1. Abnormalities of RBC interior a. Enzyme defects b. Hemoglobinopathies (Chap. 107) 2. RBC membrane abnormalities a. Hereditary spherocytosis etc. b. Paroxysmal nocturnal hemoglobinuria c. Spur cell anemia	Hereditary
Extracorpuscular	3. Extrinsic factors a. Hypersplenism b. Antibody: immune hemolysis c. Microangiopathic hemolysis d. Infections, toxins, etc.	Acquired

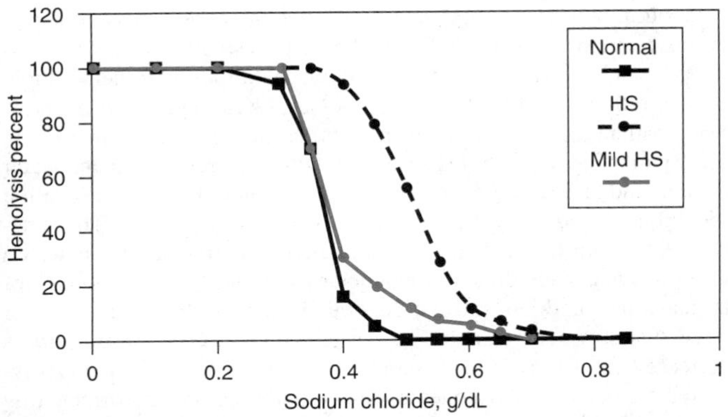

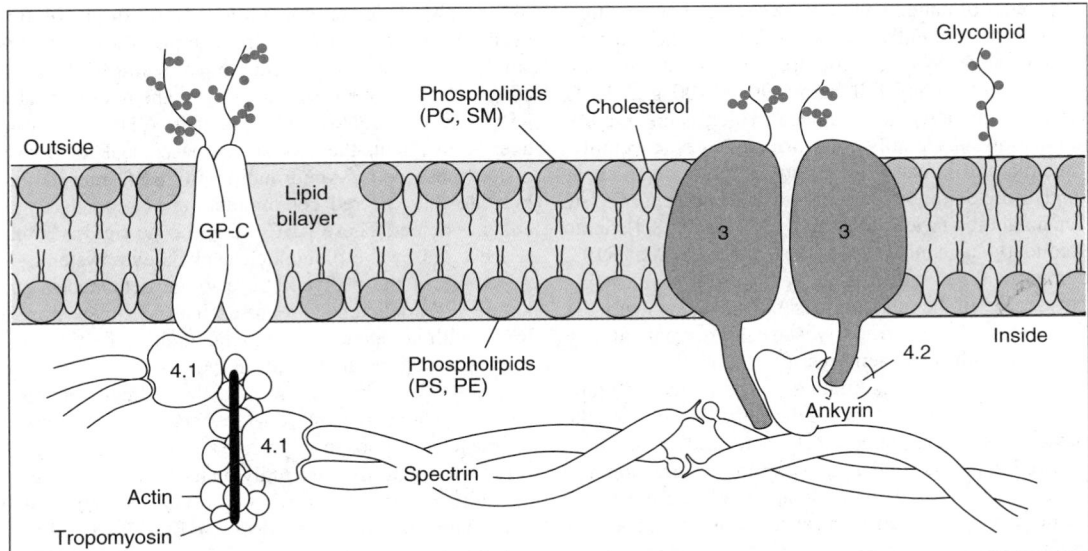

FIGURE 109-1 Osmotic fragility of red blood cells in hereditary spherocytosis (HS). The cells of two patients are compared to normal red cells.

may even be absent in an otherwise healthy individual. Compensation may be temporarily interrupted by episodes of erythroid hypoplasia precipitated by infections, particularly parvovirus. Splenomegaly is a very common finding in hereditary spherocytosis. The hemolytic rate may increase transiently during systemic infections, which induce further splenic enlargement. Chronic leg ulcers, similar to those observed in sickle cell anemia, occur occasionally.

The characteristic erythrocyte abnormality is the spherocyte (**Plate IV-10**). The mean corpuscular volume (MCV) is usually normal or slightly decreased, and the mean corpuscular hemoglobin concentration (MCHC) is increased to 350 to 400 g/L. Spheroidicity may be quantitatively assessed by measurement of the osmotic fragility of the red cells upon exposure to hypoosmotic solutions causing a net influx of water (Fig. 109-1). Because spherocytes have a decreased surface area per unit volume, they are able to take in less water and hence lyse at a higher concentration of saline than normal cells. On microscopic examination, spherocytes are usually detected as small cells without central pallor. They will ordinarily not influence the osmotic fragility test unless they constitute more than 1 or 2 percent of the total cell population. An increase in the osmotic fragility of RBC following sterile incubation of whole blood for 24 h at 37°C is also characteristic of hereditary spherocytosis. The autohemolysis test which measures the amount of spontaneous hemolysis occurring after 48 h of sterile incubation is also useful. In hereditary spherocytosis, about 10 to 50

percent of the RBC are lysed (versus fewer than 4 percent of normal red blood cells). Autohemolysis of these RBC is largely prevented by the addition of glucose prior to incubation.

PATHOGENESIS The molecular abnormality in hereditary spherocytosis involves the proteins of the underlying cytoskeleton, primarily those responsible for tethering the lipid bilayer to the underlying cytoskeletal network. Nearly all patients have a significant deficiency of spectrin, which is sometimes secondary to an inherited molecular defect in that protein. About 50 percent of patients have a defect in ankyrin, the protein that forms a bridge between protein 3 and spectrin (Fig. 109-2). Those who have a recessive inheritance pattern for ankyrin deficiency have more severe anemia than those with the more common dominant form. About 25 percent of patients have a mutation of protein 3, resulting in a deficiency of that protein and mild anemia with dominant inheritance. Most of the remaining 25 percent have mutations of spectrin, leading to impaired synthesis or self-association; β-spectrin deficiency is generally mild, with dominant inheritance, while α-spectrin deficiency is severe, with a recessive inheritance pattern. Because the lipid bilayer is not well anchored when these proteins are defective, part of it is lost by vesiculation, resulting in a more spherical and less deformable cell. Because of their shape and rigidity, spherocytes cannot traverse the interstices of the spleen, especially those in the lining of the splenic venous sinuses, and they are exposed to an environment in which their increased metabolic rate cannot be sustained, causing a further loss of surface membrane. This "conditioning" produces a subpopulation of hyperspheroidal RBC in the peripheral blood.

DIAGNOSIS Hereditary spherocytosis must be distinguished primarily from the spherocytic hemolytic anemias associated with RBC antibodies. The family history of anemia and/or splenectomy is helpful, when present. The diagnosis of immune spherocytosis is usually readily established by a positive direct Coombs test (see below). Spherocytes are also seen in association with hemolysis induced by splenomegaly in patients with cirrhosis, in clostridial infections, and in certain snake envenomations (due to the action of phospholipases on the membrane). A few spherocytes are seen in the course of a wide variety of hemolytic disorders, particularly glucose-6-phosphate dehydrogenase (G6PD) deficiency.

FIGURE 109-2 Diagram of a cross section of the red blood cell membrane. Spectrin, actin, tropomyosin, and protein 4.1 form a meshwork that laminates the inner surface of the membrane. In contrast, other proteins such as the glycophorins (GP) and protein 3 (anion transport channel) traverse the lipid bilayer. Long polysaccharide chains are covalently attached to these proteins on the outer surface of the cell and also to glycolipid. Ankyrin and protein 4.2 form a bridge between spectrin and a fraction of the anion transport proteins. Protein 4.1 binds to GP. Phospholipids in the lipd bilayer include phosphatidylcholine (PC) and sphingomyelin (SM), which are located primarily on the outer surface of the membrane, and phosphatidylserine (PS) and phosphatidylethanolamine (PE), which are located primarily on the inner surface of the membrane.

℞ TREATMENT

Splenectomy reliably corrects the anemia, although the RBC defect and its consequent morphology persist. The operative risk is low. RBC survival after splenectomy is normal or nearly so; if it is not, an accessory spleen or another diagnosis should be sought. Because of the potential for gallstones and for episodes of bone marrow hypoplasia or hemolytic crises, splenectomy should be performed in individuals in whom the disease causes symptoms; cholecystectomy should not be performed without splenectomy, as intrahepatic gallstones may result. Splenectomy in children should be postponed until age 4, if possible, in order to minimize the risk of severe infections with gram-positive encapsulated organisms. Polyvalent pneumococcal vaccine should be administered to all patients before they undergo splenectomy. In patients with hemolysis, folic acid (1 mg/d) should be administered prophylactically.

Hereditary elliptocytosis and hereditary pyropoikilocytosis   Red blood cells of oval or elliptic shape are normally found in birds, reptiles, camels, and llamas; however, they occur in appreciable numbers in humans only in *hereditary elliptocytosis*, a disorder that is transmitted as an autosomal dominant trait and affects 1 per 4000 to 5000 of the population, a frequency similar to that of hereditary spherocytosis (rarely, patients with myelodysplastic disorders of the bone marrow may have acquired elliptocytosis). The elliptic shape is acquired as the cell deforms to traverse the microcirculation but does not spring back to its initial biconcave shape. In most affected individuals, this is due to a structural abnormality of erythrocyte spectrin that leads to impaired assembly of the cytoskeleton. In some families, affected individuals have a deficiency of erythrocyte membrane protein 4.1, which is important in stabilizing the interaction of spectrin and actin in the cytoskeleton (see Fig. 109-2); homozygotes with total absence of this protein have more marked hemolysis. In Southeast Asia there is a high incidence of hereditary ovalocytosis, in which a small internal deletion of protein 3 makes the membrane rigid and confers resistance against malaria.

The great majority of patients manifest only mild hemolysis, with hemoglobin levels above 120 g/L, reticulocytes less than 4 percent, depressed haptoglobin levels, and RBC survivals just under the normal range. In 10 to 15 percent of patients with more severe abnormalities, the rate of hemolysis is substantially increased, with median survival times of RBC as short as 5 days and reticulocytes ranging up to 20 percent. Hemoglobin levels rarely fall below 90 to 100 g/L. RBC destruction occurs predominantly in the spleen, which is enlarged in patients with overt hemolysis. Hemolysis is corrected by splenectomy.

In both the anemic and nonanemic varieties of this disorder, at least 25 percent and, more commonly, greater than 75 percent of RBC are elliptic, with an axial ratio (width/length) of less than 0.78. Patients with hemolysis frequently have microovalocytes, bizarre-shaped RBC, and red cell fragments, all of which increase in number following splenectomy. The degree of hemolysis does not correlate with the percentage of elliptocytes. Osmotic fragility is usually normal but may be increased in patients with overt hemolysis.

Hereditary pyropoikilocytosis is related to hereditary elliptocytosis, since both have been encountered in the same family. Hereditary pyropoikilocytosis is a rare disorder characterized by bizarre-shaped, microcytic red cells that undergo disruption at temperatures of 44 to 45°C (in contrast, normal red cells are stable up to 49°C). This results from a deficiency of spectrin and an abnormality of spectrin self-assembly. Hemolysis, which is usually severe, is recognized in childhood and is partially responsive to splenectomy.

Hereditary stomatocytosis   Stomatocytes are RBC that are concave on one face and convex on the other. This results in a slitlike central zone of pallor on dried smears. The syndrome of hereditary hemolytic anemia and stomatocytic RBC is inherited in an autosomal dominant pattern. RBC have an increased permeability to sodium and

potassium, which is compensated for by an increased active transport of these cations. In some patients, the RBC is swollen with an excess of ions and water and a decreased mean corpuscular hemoglobin concentration (overhydrated stomatocytes, "hydrocytosis"); many of these patients lack the red cell membrane protein 7.2 (stomatin). In other patients, the red cell is shrunken, with a decreased ion and water content and an increased mean corpuscular hemoglobin concentration (dehydrated stomatocytes, "desiccytosis" or "xerocytosis"). Those patients in whom the RBC are overhydrated have true stomatocytes on dried smears. Dehydrated stomatocytes assume the morphology of target cells on dried smears. In both instances, RBC are cup- or bowl-shaped when examined in wet preparation. Osmotic fragility is increased in overhydrated stomatocytes and decreased in underhydrated stomatocytes. Autohemolysis is increased and is corrected by glucose. Red cells lacking Rh proteins (Rh_{null} cells) are stomatocytic and have a shortened life span.

Most patients have splenomegaly and mild anemia. Splenectomy decreases but does not totally correct the hemolytic process; the indications for it are similar to those for hereditary spherocytosis.

Red Cell Enzyme Defects   During its maturation, the RBC loses its nucleus, ribosomes, and mitochondria and thus its capability for protein synthesis and oxidative phosphorylation. The mature circulating RBC has a relatively simple pattern of intermediary metabolism (Fig. 109-3) in keeping with its modest metabolic obligations. ATP must be generated from the Embden-Meyerhof pathway to drive the cation pump which maintains the ionic milieu within the RBC. Smaller amounts of energy are needed for the preservation of hemoglobin iron in the ferrous (Fe^{2+}) state and perhaps for the renewal of the lipids in the RBC membrane. About 10 percent of the glucose consumed by the RBC is metabolized via the hexose-monophosphate shunt (Fig. 109-3). This pathway protects both hemoglobin and the membrane from exogenous oxidants, including certain drugs.

Studies of RBC enzyme defects have provided valuable information on the metabolic control of normal erythrocytes. In Fig. 109-3 is shown a large number of recognized specific enzyme deficiency states affecting the glycolytic pathway or the hexose-monophosphate shunt. Many of these enzyme abnormalities appear to be restricted to RBC. The long life span of the RBC and its inability to synthesize proteins pose a challenge to the stability of its enzymes. Therefore, a mutation resulting in decreased stability will be detected more readily in RBC compared with other tissues capable of renewing unstable enzymes.

Defects in the Embden-Meyerhof pathway   Deficiencies of most of the enzymes of the Embden-Meyerhof (or glycolytic) pathway have been reported (Fig. 109-3). In general, all these enzymopathies have similar pathophysiologic and clinical features. Patients present with a congenital nonspherocytic hemolytic anemia of variable severity. The RBC are often relatively deficient in ATP, considering their young age. As a result, there is an increased leak of potassium ion from inside these cells. Abnormalities in RBC morphology (see below) indicate that the red cell membrane is secondarily affected by the enzyme defect. These RBC are apt to be rigid and thus more readily sequestered by the mononuclear phagocyte system.

Some of these glycolytic enzyme deficiencies such as pyruvate kinase (PK) deficiency and hexokinase deficiency are localized to the RBC, with no apparent metabolic abnormality in leukocytes or other cells that have been studied; in the case of PK deficiency, this is due to specific isozymes confined to the red cell. In other disorders, the enzyme deficiency is more widespread. Glucose phosphate isomerase deficiency and phosphoglycerate kinase deficiency also involve leukocytes, although affected individuals have no apparent abnormalities of white blood cell function. Individuals with deficiency of triose phosphate isomerase have decreased levels of enzyme in leukocytes, muscle cells, and cerebrospinal fluid. Furthermore, they have a progressive neurologic disorder. Some patients with phosphofructokinase deficiency have a myopathy.

Among the reported defects of glycolytic enzymes, about 95 percent are due to PK deficiency and about 4 percent are due to glucose phosphate isomerase deficiency. The remainder, shown in Fig. 109-3, are extremely rare. Most have been encountered in isolated families.

A number of different nucleotide substitutions and hence amino acid replacements result in PK deficiency. Some of these result in decreased reaction with substrate (phosphoenolpyruvate), an enhancing molecule (fructose 1,6 diphosphate), or ADP. Thus, there is considerable variability in the clinical manifestations and laboratory findings among individuals reported as having PK deficiency. Most of these patients are compound heterozygotes who have inherited a different defective enzyme from each parent. The clinical manifestations of the other less common glycolytic enzyme defects are also quite variable.

Most of the glycolytic enzyme defects are inherited in an autosomal recessive pattern. Thus, the parents of affected patients are heterozygotes. Heterozygotes generally possess half-normal levels of enzyme activity, which are more than adequate for normal metabolic function. Thus, these individuals are entirely asymptomatic. Since the gene frequency for this group of enzymopathies is low, it is not surprising that true homozygotes are often the offspring of a consanguineous mating. More often, affected individuals are compound heterozygotes. Phosphoglycerate kinase deficiency is inherited as a sex-linked disorder. Affected males have a severe hemolytic anemia, while female carriers may have a mild hemolytic process.

CLINICAL MANIFESTATIONS   Patients with severe hemolysis usually present during early childhood with anemia, icterus, and splenomegaly. Other stigmata of chronic hemolysis are occasionally seen.

LABORATORY FINDINGS   Patients have a normocytic (or slightly macrocytic), normochromic anemia with reticulocytosis. In those with PK deficiency, bizarre erythrocytes, including spiculated cells, are noted on the peripheral smear. Spherocytes are usually infrequent or absent. Hence the term *congenital nonspherocytic hemolytic anemia* has been applied to these disorders. Unlike hereditary spherocytosis, the osmotic fragility of freshly drawn blood is usually normal. Incubation brings out an osmotically fragile population of RBC, and this abnormality is not corrected by the addition of glucose.

The diagnosis of this group of anemias depends on specific enzymatic assays; care must be taken to provide an appropriate concentration of substrate so as to detect those variants with a low affinity for substrate or enhancing molecule. An abnormality in enzyme kinetics, differences in electrophoretic mobility, pH optimum, or heat stability may be found useful in documenting heterogeneity among enzyme variants.

℞ **TREATMENT**

Most patients do not require therapy. Those with severe hemolysis should be given a daily supplement of folic acid (1 mg/d). Blood transfusions may be necessary during a hypoplastic crisis. Women with PK deficiency may become very anemic during pregnancy, sometimes leading to the diagnosis for the first time.

Because of their enzymatic defect, the younger cells (reticulocytes) depend on mitochondrial respiration rather than glycolysis for maintenance of ATP. However, in the hypoxic environment of the spleen, aerobic metabolism is curtailed and the ATP-depleted cells are destroyed in situ. Reticulocytes are normally retained in the spleen for 24 to 48 h. Patients with PK deficiency may benefit from splenectomy as they may have a marked increase in circulating reticulocytes. Patients with deficiency of glucose phosphate isomerase also may improve after splenectomy. There is not sufficient information to indicate whether this operation would help individuals with other glycolytic enzymopathies.

Defects in the hexose-monophosphate shunt   The normal RBC is well endowed to protect itself against oxidant stress. Upon exposure to a drug or toxin that results in the generation of oxygen radicals, the amount of glucose that is metabolized via the hexose-monophosphate shunt is normally increased severalfold. In this way reduced glutathione is regenerated, protecting the sulfhydryl groups of hemoglobin and the RBC membrane from oxidation. Individuals with an inherited defect in the hexose-monophosphate shunt are unable to maintain an adequate level of reduced glutathione in their RBC. As a result, hemoglobin sulfhydryl groups become oxidized, and the hemoglobin tends to precipitate within the RBC, forming Heinz bodies.

Among the congenital shunt defects, by far the most common is *G6PD deficiency*. It affects more than 200 million people throughout the world; like hemoglobin S, it probably partially protects the patient from malaria by providing a defective home for the merozoite. As with the glycolytic enzymopathies, there is considerable genetic heterogeneity among affected individuals, and over 400 variants of G6PD have been described. Abnormalities in primary DNA or protein sequence have been established in a number of the G6PD variants; in almost all cases, the alteration is one or more base substitutions, leading to an amino acid replacement and not a deletion in the protein. Evidence

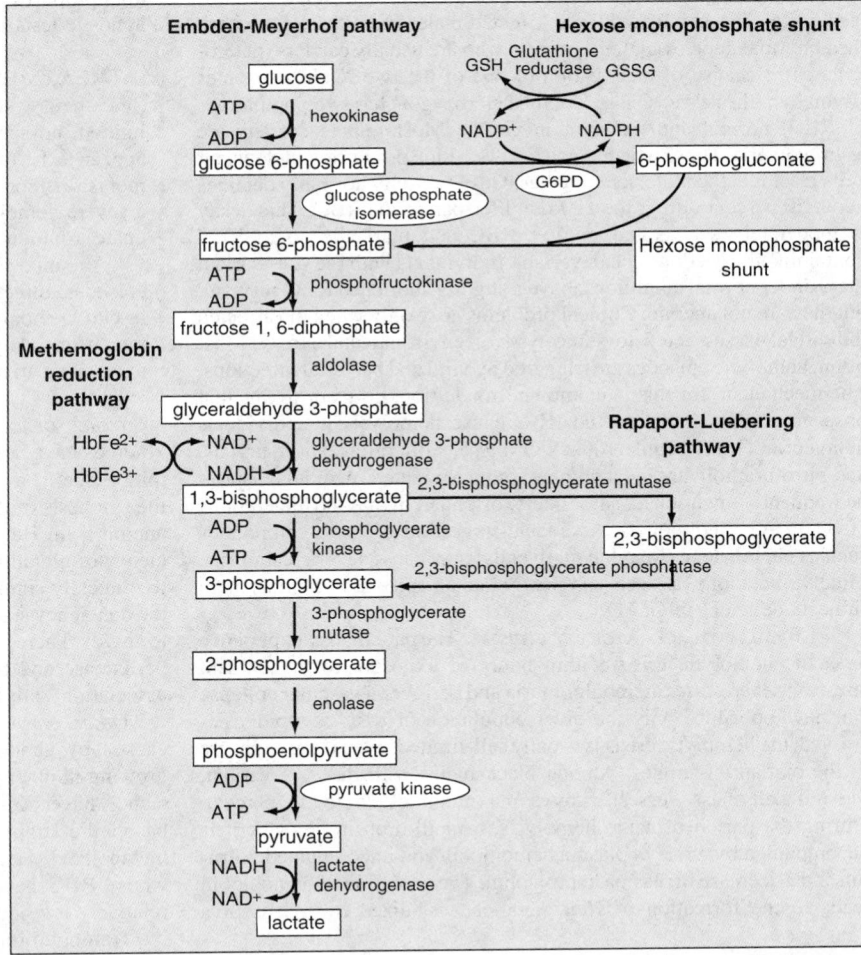

FIGURE 109-3   Red blood cell metabolic pathways. Four metabolic pathways maintain hemoglobin function and membrane integrity. The Embden-Meyerhof pathway (glycolysis) generates ATP for energy and membrane maintenance. The methemoglobin reduction pathway maintains hemoglobin in a reduced state. The hexose monophosphate shunt generates NADPH that is used to reduce glutathione, which protects the red cell against oxidant stress. The Rapaport-Luebering pathway controls the oxygen affinity of hemoglobin by regulating 2,3-bisphosphoglycerate levels. Enzyme deficiency states in order of prevalence: glucose-6-phosphate dehydrogenase (G6PD)>>>pyruvate kinase>glucose-6-phosphate isomerase>rare deficiencies of other enzymes in the pathway. The more common enzyme deficiencies are encircled.

of the abnormality in structure is seen in the differences in electrophoretic mobility, enzyme kinetics, pH optimum, and heat stability. These differences result in great variation of clinical severity, ranging from nonspherocytic hemolytic anemia without demonstrable oxidant stress (particularly shortly after birth), through hemolytic anemia only when stimulated by marked to mild oxidant stress, to no clinically detectable abnormality. The normal G6PD is designated as type B. About 20 percent of individuals of African descent have a G6PD (designated A+) that differs by a single amino acid and is electrophoretically distinguishable but functionally normal. Among the clinically significant G6PD variants, the most common, the so-called A− type, is due to two base substitutions and is encountered primarily in individuals with ancestral origins in central Africa. The A− G6PD has the same electrophoretic mobility as the A+ type, but it is unstable and has abnormal kinetic properties. This variant is found in about 11 percent of African-descended males in the United States. A second relatively common G6PD variant is encountered among peoples of the Mediterranean circumlittoral, particularly Sardinians and Sephardic Jews; this variant is more severe than the A− variant and may result in nonspherocytic hemolytic anemia. A third relatively common and slightly less severe variant occurs in southern Chinese populations.

The G6PD gene is located on the X chromosome. Thus the deficiency state is a sex-linked trait. Affected males (hemizygotes) inherit the abnormal gene from their mothers who are usually carriers (heterozygotes). Because of inactivation of one of the two X chromosomes (Lyon hypothesis: see Chap. 65), the heterozygote has two populations of RBC: normal and deficient in G6PD. Most female carriers are asymptomatic. Those who happen to have a high proportion of deficient cells resemble the male hemizygotes. G6PD activity normally declines about 50 percent during the 120-day life span of the RBC. This decay is moderately accelerated in A− RBC and markedly so in RBC containing the Mediterranean variant. Individuals with the A− variant may, under normal conditions, have a slightly shortened RBC survival, but they are not anemic. Clinical problems arise only when the affected individual is subjected to some type of environmental stress. Most often, hemolytic episodes are triggered by viral and bacterial infections. The mechanism for this is unknown. In addition, drugs or toxins that pose an oxidant threat to the RBC cause hemolysis in individuals deficient in G6PD (Table 109-4). Of these, sulfa drugs, antimalarials, and nitrofurantoin are most commonly incriminated. Although aspirin is frequently mentioned as a likely offender, it has no deleterious effect in A− individuals. Accidental ingestion of toxic compounds such as naphthalene (found in moth balls) may cause severe hemolysis. Finally, metabolic acidosis can precipitate an episode of hemolysis in subjects deficient in G6PD.

CLINICAL AND LABORATORY FEATURES The patient may experience an acute hemolytic crisis within hours of exposure to the oxidant stress. In severe cases, hemoglobinuria and peripheral vascular collapse can develop. Since only the older population of RBC is rapidly destroyed, the hemolytic crisis is usually self-limited, even if the exposure to the oxidant continues. Among black males with the A− variant, the red cell mass decreases by a maximum of 25 to 30 percent. During the period of acute hemolysis, a rapid drop in hematocrit is accompanied by a rise in plasma hemoglobin and unconjugated bilirubin and a decrease in plasma haptoglobin. The oxidation of hemoglobin leads to the formation of Heinz bodies, visualized by means of a

Table 109-4

Drugs Causing Hemolysis in Subjects Deficient in G6PD

Antimalarials: Primaquine, pamaquine, dapsone
Sulfonamides: Sulfamethoxazole
Nitrofurantoin
Analgesics: Acetanilid
Miscellaneous: Vitamin K (water-soluble form), doxorubicin, methylene blue, nalidixic acid, furazolidone, niridazole, phenazopyridine

supravital stain such as crystal violet. However, Heinz bodies are usually not seen after the first day or so, since these inclusions are readily removed by the spleen. Their removal leads to the formation of "bite cells," red cells that have lost a peripheral portion of the cell. Multiple bites cause the formation of fragments. Small numbers of spherocytes also may be present. Individuals with the Mediterranean type G6PD have a more unstable enzyme and, therefore, a much lower overall enzyme activity than individuals with the A− variant. As a result, they have more severe clinical manifestations. Some have a chronic hemolytic anemia, even in the absence of any exposure to oxidants. A minority of patients are exquisitely sensitive to fava beans and will develop a fulminant hemolytic crisis following exposure. The oxidants in *Vicia fava* are two β-glycosides whose aglycones, when autooxidized, produce free radicals of oxygen. The incidence of favism is highly variable; this may be due to variations in concentration, in absorption, or in metabolism of the aglycones. Favism is not encountered in individuals with the A− variant.

The *diagnosis* of G6PD deficiency should be considered in any individual, particularly a male of African or Mediterranean descent, who experiences an acute hemolytic episode. The patient should be thoroughly questioned about possible exposure to oxidant agents. A number of screening tests are available to establish the diagnosis. However, since the deficiency occurs primarily in older RBC, a false-negative test may be seen during a hemolytic episode when there is a high proportion of young RBC. It may be necessary to repeat these diagnostic tests after the patient has recovered.

℞ **TREATMENT**

Since hemolysis in patients deficient in A− G6PD is usually self-limited, no specific treatment is necessary. Splenectomy does not appear to be of benefit to Mediterranean patients with chronic hemolysis. Blood transfusions are rarely indicated. If a patient develops a severe hemolytic episode with hemoglobinuria, maintaining adequate urine output is important.

Attention should be directed toward the *prevention* of hemolytic episodes. Infections ought to be treated promptly. Subjects deficient in G6PD should be warned about risks posed by oxidant drugs and fava beans. Any patient of African or Mediterranean ancestry about to be given an oxidant drug should be screened for G6PD deficiency.

OTHER DEFECTS OF THE HEXOSE-MONOPHOSPHATE SHUNT A few kindreds have been found to have congenital deficiency in RBC glutathione due to a defect in either of the two enzymes responsible for the synthesis of this tripeptide. Affected individuals have a hemolytic anemia with Heinz bodies that is aggravated by oxidant drugs. Deficiency of glutathione reductase has been reported, but its relationship to clinically significant hemolysis is not well established. Sometimes the deficiency state can be corrected by the administration of riboflavin (5 mg/d). There are also isolated reports of deficiencies of glutathione peroxidase and 6-phosphogluconate dehydrogenase, but again, their association with hemolysis is uncertain.

Other enzyme defects Hemolytic anemia may sometimes be caused by abnormalities in enzymes of nucleotide metabolism. A growing number of individuals with pyrimidine 5′-nucleotidase deficiency have been encountered. Their red cells have marked coarse basophilic stippling because the mRNA of the cell is not properly metabolized. Hemolytic anemia also has been noted in individuals whose RBC have supranormal levels of adenosine deaminase and relatively low levels of ATP.

Hemoglobinopathies The sickling disorders constitute an important form of congenital hemolytic anemia. Less commonly, hemolysis may be due to the inheritance of an unstable hemoglobin variant. In β-thalassemia major or intermedia, anemia is due to a combination of ineffective erythropoiesis and hemolysis of circulating cells. → *For further discussion, see Chap. 107.*

ACQUIRED HEMOLYTIC ANEMIAS In most patients with acquired hemolytic anemia, red cells are made normally but are prematurely destroyed because of damage acquired in the circulation. (The exceptions are rare disorders characterized by acquired dysplasia of the cells of the bone marrow and the production of structurally and functionally abnormal red cells.) The damage that occurs may be mediated by antibodies or toxins that mark the cell for premature death or may be due to vicissitudes encountered during the circulation, including an overactive mononuclear phagocyte system or traumatic lysis by natural or artificial impediments to smooth circulation. The acquired hemolytic anemias can be classified into five categories (see Table 109-5).

Hypersplenism The spleen is particularly efficient in trapping and destroying RBC that have minimal defects, often so mild as to be undetectable by in vitro techniques. This unique ability of the spleen to filter mildly damaged RBC results from its unusual vascular anatomy (see Chap. 61). Almost all the blood circulating through the spleen flows rapidly from arterioles in the white pulp to sinuses in the spleen's red pulp and then into the venous system. In contrast, a small portion of splenic blood flow (normally 1 to 2 percent) passes into the "marginal zone" of the lymphatic white pulp. Although the cells that occupy this zone are not phagocytic, they serve as a mechanical filter that hinders the progress of severely damaged blood cells. As RBC leave this zone and enter the red pulp, they flow into narrow cords, rich in macrophages, that end blindly but communicate with sinuses through small openings between the lining cells of the sinuses. These openings, averaging 3 μm in diameter, test the ability of RBC (4.5 μm in diameter) to undergo a deformation of shape. RBC that do not pass the stringent test imposed on them by the spleen filter are engulfed by phagocytic cells and destroyed (see Fig. 61-1).

The normal spleen retains reticulocytes for 1 to 2 days but otherwise poses no difficulties to normal RBC until they become senescent. However, the situation is different when splenomegaly exists. Splenomegaly is usually due to infiltrative diseases such as myeloproliferative disorders (Chap. 111), lymphomas (Chap. 113), and storage diseases such as Gaucher's disease (Chap. 346) as well as to systemic inflammatory diseases leading to splenic hypertrophy or diseases that cause congestive splenomegaly, particularly cirrhosis of the liver and thrombosis of the splenic, portal, or hepatic veins. Splenomegaly, therefore, may result in increased destruction of the cells of the blood, including the red cells. This is in part due to pooling of the blood in an environment relatively deprived of nutrients and full of phagocytic cells. Hemolysis is least predictable in infiltrative diseases of the spleen, where substantial splenomegaly may exist with no apparent hemolysis, whereas inflammatory and congestive splenomegaly is commonly associated with modest shortening of RBC survival, along with more marked granulocytopenia and thrombocytopenia (hypersplenism). Patients with cytopenia(s) sufficient to produce symptoms generally benefit from splenectomy.

Immunologic Causes of Hemolysis Immune hemolysis in the adult is usually induced by IgG or IgM antibodies with specificity for antigens associated with the patient's red cells (often called "autoantibodies") (Table 109-6); rarely, transfused red cells may be hemolyzed by alloantibodies directed against foreign antigens on those cells (Chap. 115).

The Coombs antiglobulin test is the major tool for diagnosing autoimmune hemolysis. This test relies on the ability of antibodies specific for immunoglobulins (especially IgG) or complement components (especially C3) to agglutinate RBC when these human serum immunoproteins are present on the RBC surface. In the *direct Coombs test*, the ability of anti-IgG or anti-C3 antisera to agglutinate the patient's RBC is determined. The presence or absence of IgG and/or C3 may give important information about the origin of the immune hemolytic anemia (see Table 109-6). Rarely, neither IgG nor complement may be found on the red cells of the patient (Coombs-negative immune hemolytic anemia).

At times, it may be important to demonstrate antibody in the serum of the patient by reacting the serum with normal red cells bearing the antigen. IgM antibodies (usually cold-reacting) may be detected by agglutination of normal or fetal red cells. IgG antibodies may be detected by the *indirect Coombs test*, in which the serum of the patient is incubated with normal red cells and antibody is detected with anti-IgG, as in the direct Coombs test.

"Warm" antibodies Antibodies that react with protein antigens usually are IgG and react at body temperature; occasionally, they are IgA and rarely IgM. This acquired syndrome is frequently designated *autoimmune hemolytic (or immunohemolytic) anemia, warm antibody type.*

CLINICAL MANIFESTATIONS Immunohemolytic anemia of the warm antibody type is induced by IgG antibody and occurs at all ages but is more common in adults, particularly women. In approximately one-fourth of patients this disorder occurs as a complication of an underlying disease affecting the immune system, especially neoplasms of the immune system (chronic lymphocytic leukemia, non-Hodgkin's and Hodgkin's lymphoma); collagen vascular diseases, especially systemic lupus erythematosus (SLE); and congenital immunodeficiency diseases (Table 109-7). The presentation and course of IgG immunohemolytic anemia are quite variable. In its mildest form, the only manifestation is a positive direct Coombs test. In this instance, insufficient antibody is present on the RBC surface to permit the reticuloendothelial system to recognize the cell as abnormal.

Most symptomatic patients have a moderate to severe anemia [hemoglobin levels of 60 to 100 g/L and reticulocyte counts of 10 to 30 percent (200 to 600 × 10³/μL)], spherocytosis (**Plate IV-11**), and splenomegaly.

In its most severe form, immunohemolytic anemia presents with fulminant, overwhelming hemolysis associated with hemoglobinemia, hemoglobinuria, and shock; this syndrome may be rapidly fatal unless aggressively treated.

Table 109-5

Causes of Acquired Hemolytic Anemia

I. Entrapment
II. Immune
  A. Warm-reactive (IgG) antibody
  B. Cold-reactive IgM antibody (cold agglutinin disease)
  C. Cold-reactive IgG antibody (paroxysmal cold hemoglobinuria)
  D. Drug-dependent antibody
    1. Autoimmune
    2. Haptene
III. Traumatic hemolytic anemia
  A. Impact hemolysis
  B. Macrovascular defects—prostheses
  C. Microvascular causes
    1. Thrombotic thrombocytopenic purpura/hemolytic-uremic syndrome
    2. Other causes of microvascular abnormalities
    3. Disseminated intravascular hemolysis
IV. Hemolytic anemia due to toxic effects on the membrane
  A. Spur cell hemolytic anemia
  B. External toxins
    1. Animal or spider bites
    2. Metals (e.g., copper)
    3. Organic compounds
V. Paroxysmal nocturnal hemoglobinuria

Table 109-6

Use of the Direct Coombs Test in Diagnosing the Cause of Autoimmune Hemolytic Anemia

Reaction with		Causes
Anti-IgG	**Anti-C3**	
Yes	No	Antibodies to Rh proteins, hemolysis caused by α-methyldopa or penicillin; not seen in SLE
Yes	Yes	Antibodies to glycoprotein antigens, SLE
No	Yes	Cold-reacting antibodies (agglutinins or Donath-Landsteiner antibody), most drug-related antibodies, IgM antibodies, IgG antibodies of low affinity, activation of complement by immune complexes

Table 109-7

Hemolysis due to Antibodies

WARM-ANTIBODY IMMUNOHEMOLYTIC ANEMIA

1. Idiopathic
2. Lymphomas: Chronic lymphocytic leukemia, non-Hodgkin's lymphomas, Hodgkin's disease (infrequent)
3. SLE and other collagen-vascular diseases
4. Drugs
    a. α-Methyldopa type (autoantibody to Rh antigens)
    b. Penicillin type (stable hapten)
    c. Quinidine type (unstable hapten)
5. Postviral infections
6. Other tumors (rare)

COLD-ANTIBODY IMMUNOHEMOLYTIC ANEMIA

1. Cold agglutinin disease
    a. Acute: *Mycoplasma* infection, infectious mononucleosis
    b. Chronic: Idiopathic, lymphoma
2. Paroxysmal cold hemoglobinuria

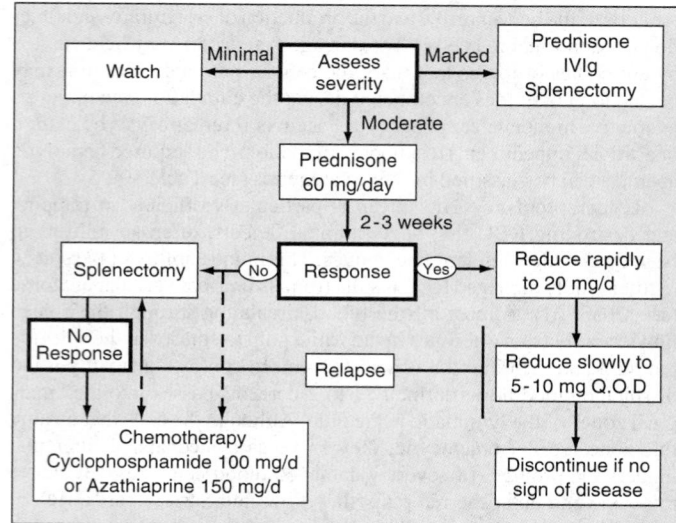

FIGURE 109-4   Algorithm for the treatment of patients with IgG-mediated immune hemolytic anemia. The patient with minimal disease may be watched carefully. The patient with very severe disease may need all modalities of treatment applied at once. The more common patient with moderate disease may be treated with prednisone at a high dose; if no response is seen, then either splenectomy or chemotherapy is given. If a response is seen, the dose of prednisone is reduced over time. If relapse occurs during this process, splenectomy or chemotherapy may be needed.

The direct Coombs test is positive in more than 98 percent of patients; usually IgG is detected with or without C3. Rarely, the cells may be agglutinated by the antibody, causing difficulty in analysis by flow cytometry.

Immune thrombocytopenia also may be present (*Evans's syndrome*), a disorder in which separate antibodies are directed against platelets and RBC. Occasionally, venous thrombosis occurs.

PATHOGENESIS   IgG antibodies bring about the destruction of the cells by two mechanisms: (1) immune adherence of red cells to destructive cells of the immune system mediated by the antibody itself and by complement components that become fixed to the membrane (by far the more important mechanism of destruction), and (2) completion of the complement sequence, resulting in rupture of the membrane. In IgG-mediated immune adherence, the affixed antibody reacts with Fc receptors on macrophages; this binds the target to the destroyer and activates phagocytic processes that internalize the target, destroying it. If internalization is only partial, membrane is preferentially removed, resulting in the formation of spherocytes. These spherocytes are not able to pass through the fenestrations in the wall of the splenic sinus and thus accumulate in the spleen, where they are destroyed. Complement-mediated immune adherence involves the interaction of C3b and C4b with a series of receptors on the macrophage; this is much less likely to lead to destruction of the target by itself but markedly increases the immune adherence due to IgG. Immune adherence, particularly that due to the IgG antibody, is also enhanced by the transit of red cells into the cords and sinuses of the spleen, which brings cells into intimate contact with phagocytic cells. Significant lysis by the direct action of complement does not commonly occur.

℞ **TREATMENT**

In the initial evaluation of the patient, it is important to be sure that drugs that are known to cause immunohemolytic anemia are not involved (see below).

Patients having a mild degree of hemolysis usually do not require therapy. In those with clinically significant hemolysis, initial therapy consists of glucocorticoids (e.g., prednisone, 1.0 mg/kg per day). A rise in hemoglobin is frequently noted within 3 or 4 days and occurs in most patients within 1 to 2 weeks. Prednisone at this dosage is continued until the hemoglobin level has risen to normal values, and thereafter it is tapered rapidly to about 20 mg/d, then slowly over the course of several months. An algorithm for this tapering process is given in Fig. 109-4. For chronic therapy with prednisone, alternate-day administration is preferred. More than 75 percent of patients will achieve an initial significant and sustained reduction in hemolysis; however, in half these patients the disease will relapse, either during the period of steroid tapering or following the cessation of steroid therapy. Steroids appear to have two modes of action: an immediate effect due to inhibition of the clearance of IgG-coated RBC by the mononuclear phagocyte system and a later effect due to steroid-induced inhibition of antibody synthesis. Splenectomy is the second line of therapy in immune hemolytic anemia due to IgG antibodies. It is recommended for patients who cannot tolerate or fail to respond to steroid therapy. Care must be taken that remnants of splenic tissue do not remain to cause trouble later.

Patients who have been refractory to steroid therapy and to splenectomy are treated with immunosuppressive drugs such as azathioprine and cyclophosphamide. A success rate of about 50 percent has been reported with each. Intravenous gamma globulin may be used when rapid cessation of hemolysis is required; however, it is not nearly as effective in this disorder as it is in immune thrombocytopenia.

Patients with severe anemia may require blood transfusions. Because the antibody in this disease is usually a "panagglutinin," reacting with nearly all normal donor cells, the usual compatibility tests (e.g., cross matching) are impossible. The goal in selecting blood for transfusion is to avoid administering red cells with antigens to which the patient may have *allo*antibodies. A common procedure is to adsorb the panagglutinin present in patient's serum using the patient's own red cells from which antibody has been previously eluted. Serum freed of autoantibody in this way can then be tested for the presence of alloantibody to specific donor blood groups. ABO-compatible red cells matched in this fashion are administered slowly, with attention paid to the possibility of an immediate-type hemolytic transfusion reaction.

PROGNOSIS   In the majority of patients, this disease is controlled by steroid therapy alone, by splenectomy, or by a combination. In most of the remaining patients, a partial degree of control is achieved. Fatalities occur among three subsets of patients: (1) rare patients with overwhelming hemolysis in whom death is directly attributable to anemia; (2) those whose host defenses are impaired by glucocorticoids, splenectomy, and/or immunosuppressive agents; and (3) rarely, those with major thrombotic events coincident with active hemolysis.

In patients in whom immunohemolysis develops as a complication of an underlying disorder, the prognosis is often dominated by that of the primary disease.

Immunohemolytic anemia secondary to drugs Drugs that have been directly implicated in immunohemolytic anemia are of two kinds, as distinguished by their mechanisms of action: (1) drugs, such as α-methyldopa (an antihypertensive; Chap. 246), that induce a disorder identical almost in every respect to the warm-antibody immunohemolytic anemia described above, and (2) drugs that can become associated as haptenes with the RBC surface and induce the formation of an antibody directed against the RBC-drug complex. The association of drug and membrane protein may be relatively tight, as in the case of penicillin, or relatively loose, as in the case of quinidine and most other drugs.

A positive direct Coombs test is observed in up to 10 percent of patients receiving α-methyldopa therapy in doses of 2.0 g/d or higher. A small minority of these patients develop spherocytosis and hemolysis, which may be of severe degree. This "autoimmune" disorder is probably due to the fact that α-methyldopa alters the protein(s) of the Rh complex so that the protein becomes immunogenic; the resulting antibodies cross-react with the normal Rh protein. Thus the antibody does not react with the drug, and the indirect Coombs test is positive in almost all patients even when the drug is not added to the test. The red cells are coated with IgG but not C3. Hemolysis decreases over the course of several weeks after cessation of drug therapy, although the direct Coombs test may remain positive for more than 1 year.

In most other cases, when a drug induces an immune hemolytic reaction, the antibody is directed against the combination of the drug and the membrane glycoprotein to which it is attached. The hemolytic reaction in vivo is dependent on the presence of the drug and usually ceases shortly after the drug has been discontinued. Penicillin and its congeners may cause this type of reaction if the drug is given in very high doses (10 million units per day or more). In this case, the drug adheres relatively firmly to the protein of the red cell membrane. Complement is not usually fixed, and the hemolysis in vivo is usually not severe. Since the antibody is usually IgG, spherocytosis and splenic destruction may occur. Most other drugs (such as quinine, quinidine, sulfonamides, sulfonureas, phenacetin, stibophen, and dipyrone) do not adhere as tightly to their glycoproteins, and they and the antibodies that they have generated are removed during the washing steps of the direct and indirect Coombs reactions. Most of these antibodies are able to fix complement (especially those that are IgM), and these components remain on the red cell surface; thus the direct Coombs test is positive with anti-C3 but not anti-IgG. The antibody is detected in the *indirect* Coombs test only when the drug is added to the incubation mixture. Hemolysis may be quite severe, sometimes resulting in signs of intravascular hemolysis; resolution is usually prompt after the drug is discontinued.

Immune hemolysis due to cold-reactive antibodies Antibodies that react with polysaccharide antigens are usually IgM and react better at temperatures lower than 37°C, hence the name *cold-reactive antibodies*. Uncommonly, the antibody is IgG (the Donath-Landsteiner antibody of paroxysmal cold hemoglobinuria).

Cold agglutinins arise in two clinical settings: (1) monoclonal antibodies as the product of lymphocytic neoplasia or paraneoplasia and (2) polyclonal antibodies in response to infection. In many elderly patients, the "neoplasm" is benign monoclonal gammopathy, and, although chronic, it does not progress and the protein product remains its only manifestations. In a few patients, the lymphoma may be aggressive. Occasionally, cold agglutinins are found in patients with nonlymphocytic neoplasms.

Transient cold agglutinins occur commonly in two infections: *Mycoplasma pneumoniae* infection and infectious mononucleosis. In both, the titer of antibody is usually too low to cause clinical symptoms, but its presence is of diagnostic value; only occasionally is hemolysis present. Cold agglutinins are less frequently encountered in a number of other viral infections. Their manifestations are usually benign.

The specificity of the antibody may be of diagnostic value. Cold agglutinins reacting more strongly with adult cells than fetal (cord) cells are called *anti-I*; these antibodies are seen in benign lymphoproliferation (chronic cold agglutinin monoclonal gammopathy) and in *Mycoplasma* infections. Those reacting more strongly with cord cells

are called *anti-i*; these antibodies are seen in aggressive lymphomas and in infectious mononucleosis. Rarely, the antibody may react with other antigens that are equally expressed on adult and cord cells. The clinical manifestations elicited by the antibody upon exposure to cold are of two sorts: intravascular agglutination (acrocyanosis) and hemolysis. Acrocyanosis is the marked purpling of the extremities, ears, and nose when the blood becomes cold enough to agglutinate in the veins; it clears on warming and does not have the vasospastic characteristics of Raynaud's phenomenon (see Chap. 248). Patients may also have symptoms from the same cause when swallowing cold food or drinks.

The hemolysis is usually not severe and is manifest by a mild reticulocytosis, agglutination on the blood film, and agglutination during analysis of the blood by particle analysis (giving rise to a falsely high mean corpuscular volume). The degree of hemolysis depends on several variables.

1. *Antibody titer.* In general, the titer in symptomatic patients is above 1:2000 dilution of serum and may range to as high as 1:50,000. When collecting samples for testing the titer, great care must be taken that the serum is separated from the cells while maintaining the sample at 37°C so that the antibody will not adsorb onto the patient's own cells.

2. *Thermal amplitude of the antibody* (the highest temperature at which the antibody will react with the red cell). For most antibodies, this is 23 to 30°C. Those with a higher thermal amplitude (up to 37°C) will be more hemolytic, since it is more likely that these temperatures will be encountered during the circulation of the cells.

3. *Environmental temperature.* Since the reaction can only occur at temperatures below body temperature, frequency and degree of exposure to cold are major determinants of the rate of hemolysis.

The hemolysis that occurs is due primarily to the hemolytic action of complement, since there are no functional Fc receptors for the IgM antibody. Complement is readily fixed, since a single molecule of antibody is enough to effect binding of C1 and initiate the sequence of reactions. However, the normal human red cell is remarkably resistant to the hemolytic action of complement because of several defense mechanisms. Therefore, severe hemolysis with hemoglobinuria will occur only with massive activation of the antibody, such as by sudden chilling. The activation of complement is always marked by the accumulation of a degradation product of C3, C3dg, on the surface; this is what is detected with appropriate antisera in the direct Coombs test in all patients with significant cold agglutinin disease. The cutaneous manifestations of this disorder are best treated by maintaining the patient in a warm environment. This will also reduce hemolysis.

Splenectomy is usually not of value in this disorder. Glucocorticoids are of limited value, although patients with the panthermal variety of cold agglutinin disease may respond favorably to this therapy. Chlorambucil and cyclophosphamide are the most commonly employed agents in those patients with benign monoclonal gammopathy in whom therapy is indicated. Although some patients have experienced a dramatic improvement, the effectiveness of this therapy is usually marginal. Appropriate therapy of a malignant neoplasm responsible for the cold agglutinin will often reduce the titer of antibody and the severity of the hemolysis.

Chronic cold agglutinin disease tends to be unremitting. The overall prognosis is dominated by the underlying lymphoproliferative disease, if present. In those patients in whom cold agglutinin disease appears to arise spontaneously, malignant lymphoproliferative disease may become apparent after several years.

Paroxysmal cold hemoglobinuria (PCH) Now a rare disorder, PCH was more frequent at a time when tertiary syphilis was prevalent; now, most cases are either secondary to a viral infection or are autoimmune. It results from the formation of the Donath-Landsteiner antibody, an IgG antibody that is directed against the P antigen (see Chap.

115) and that can induce complement-mediated lysis. Attacks are precipitated by exposure to cold and are associated with hemoglobinemia and hemoglobinuria; chills and fever; back, leg, and abdominal pain; headache; and malaise. Recovery from the acute episode is prompt, and between episodes patients are usually asymptomatic. When this syndrome accompanies acute viral infections (e.g., measles and mumps in children), it is self-limited but may be severe. Although the direct Coombs test may show complement to be present (seldom IgG), this test may be completely negative. The diagnosis is made by demonstrating cold-reacting IgG antibodies either by lytic tests (when the titer is very high) or by special antiglobulin tests. When PCH is secondary to syphilis, it responds favorably to specific therapy for this disorder. Chronic autoimmune PCH may respond to prednisone or cytotoxic therapy (azathioprine or cyclophosphamide) but does not respond to splenectomy. Despite the severity of individual episodes, the natural history of this disease often extends over many years.

Hemolysis due to Trauma in the Circulation Red cells may be fragmented by mechanical trauma as they circulate; this invariably leads to intravascular hemolysis and in most cases to red cell fragments called *schistocytes*. Schistocytes are identified by the sharp points that result from the faulty resealing of the fractured membrane (**Plate IV-7**). Such mechanical trauma leading to hemolysis occurs in three clinical settings: (1) when RBC flow through small vessels over the surface of bony prominences and are subject to external impact during various physical activities, (2) when they flow across a pressure gradient created by an abnormal heart valve or valve prosthesis and are disrupted by a shear stress (macrovascular), and (3) when the deposition of fibrin in the microvasculature exposes them to a physical impediment that fragments them (microvascular) (Table 109-8).

External impact Hemoglobinemia and hemoglobinuria have been observed in a small proportion of individuals who have undergone a prolonged march or a prolonged jog, most typically on a hard surface and while wearing thin-soled shoes. The role of direct external trauma in this process has been demonstrated by the fact that hemolysis can be prevented by the insertion of a soft inner sole in the runner's shoes. Similar types of hemolysis have been described following karate and the playing of bongo drums. No abnormality of RBC morphology has been demonstrated, even during the acute episode, and no underlying RBC abnormality has been uncovered. Susceptible individuals will develop hemoglobinemia and hemoglobinuria when exposed to the conditions described above. As a result of muscle damage during some of these activities, myoglobinuria also may occur, but renal function is preserved. No specific therapy is required except to obtain better running shoes.

Macrovascular fragmentation hemolysis Hemolysis associated with fragmented red blood cells (**Plate IV-7**) occurs in approximately 10 percent of patients with artificial aortic valve prostheses. This

incidence is somewhat greater with valves having stellite rather than Silastic occluders, greater with small valves as compared with larger valves, and greater when valves are cloth-covered or when there is a paravalvular leak. Traumatic hemolysis is rare in recipients of porcine valves. Severe hemolysis may occur after repair of ostium primum or endocardial cushion defects with a prosthetic patch. Mitral valve prostheses also have been associated with hemolysis, but since the pressure gradient across these valves is lower than across aortic prostheses, the incidence is lower. A moderately shortened RBC survival with little or no anemia occurs in some patients with severe calcific aortic stenosis. Indeed, almost any intracardiac lesion that alters hemodynamics may lead to some shortening of RBC survival. In addition, traumatic hemolysis has been observed in patients who have undergone aortofemoral bypass.

CLINICAL MANIFESTATIONS In severe cases, hemoglobin levels fall to 50 to 70 g/L with reticulocytosis, fragmented RBC in the peripheral blood, depressed haptoglobin, elevated serum lactate dehydrogenase (LDH), and hemoglobinemia and hemoglobinuria. Iron loss (as hemoglobin or hemosiderin) in the urine may lead to iron deficiency. The direct Coombs test may rarely become positive.

PATHOGENESIS A number of factors combine to cause the fragmentation of RBC by prostheses: (1) the shear stress resulting from turbulent blood flow, particularly when blood is forced through a small aperture by high pressure (e.g., a paravalvular leak around an aortic valve); (2) direct mechanical trauma of RBC at the time of seating of the occluder of the prosthetic valve; and (3) the deposition of fibrin across disrupted attachment points.

℞ TREATMENT

Iron deficiency should be corrected by the administration of oral iron. The elevated hemoglobin that results may permit a decrease in the cardiac output and a slowing of the hemolytic rate. Limitation in physical activity also lessens the hemolytic rate. When these measures fail, any paravalvular leak must be repaired or the prosthetic valve replaced.

Microvascular causes of traumatic hemolysis If fibrin is deposited in arteriolar sites, red cells may be trapped on the meshwork and fragmented by the force of the blood pressure. This may occur due to localized intravascular coagulation at sites of arteriolar wall injury, as in thrombotic thrombocytopenic purpura and the hemolytic-uremic syndrome, and in other disorders, such as malignant hypertension, eclampsia, rejection of a renal allograft, disseminated cancer, hemangiomas, or disseminated intravascular coagulation (DIC).

Abnormalities of the vessel wall The degree of hemolysis induced by this family of disorders is usually quite mild, although the number of fragments in the peripheral blood may be striking. In some patients, thrombocytopenia may be severe. In each case, therapy is best directed at the primary disease. Thus reversal of renal graft rejection, treatment of malignant hypertension and eclampsia, control of cancer, etc., lead to a cessation of the hemolytic process. The relative importance of the primary vascular abnormality and of the deposition of fibrin in causing hemolysis is unclear.

Thrombotic thrombocytopenia purpura (TTP) This disorder is characterized by arteriolar lesions in various organs that contain platelets and fibrin. This results in thrombocytopenia and hemolytic anemia due to fragmentation of the red cells. The tissue hypoxia resulting from the occlusion may cause organ dysfunction, most frequently manifest in the nervous system or the kidney. It affects individuals of all ages but primarily young adults, more often women.

CLINICAL MANIFESTATIONS The classic pentad of TTP includes hemo-

Table 109-8

Disturbances of the Formed Elements of Blood Secondary to Intravascular Trauma

Etiology	Fragments	Hemolysis	Thrombocytopenia
Impact: march hemoglobinuria, etc.	0	+	0
Cardiac (turbulence):			
Aortic valve prosthesis	+ + + +	+ + + +	0
Mitral valve prosthesis	+ +	+ +	0
Calcific aortic stenosis	+	±	0
Vessel disease*	+ + +	+	+
Thrombotic thrombocytopenic purpura	+ + + +	+ + + +	+ + + +
Hemolytic-uremic syndrome	+ + + +	+ + + +	+ + + +
Adenocarcinoma	+ + + +	+ + + +	+ + + +
Disseminated intravascular coagulation	+ +	±	+ + + +

* Malignant hypertension, eclampsia, renal graft rejection, hemangiomas, immune disease (scleroderma).

lytic anemia with fragmentation of erythrocytes and signs of intravascular hemolysis, thrombocytopenia, diffuse and nonfocal neurologic findings, decreased renal function, and fever. These signs and symptoms occur variably, depending upon the number and sites of the arteriolar lesions. The anemia may be very mild to very severe, and the thrombocytopenia in general parallels it. The neurologic and renal symptoms are usually seen only when the platelet count is very significantly diminished (<20 to $30 \times 10^3/\mu L$). Fever is not reliably present. TTP may be very acute in onset, but its course spans days to weeks in most patients and occasionally continues for months. If the brain and kidneys are involved, their dysfunction is frequently the ultimate cause of death. Proteinuria and a moderate elevation of blood urea nitrogen may be found on initial presentation, and there can be a continued rise in blood urea nitrogen and a fall in urine output if the patient develops renal failure. Neurologic symptoms develop in more than 90 percent of patients whose disease terminates in death. Initially, there may be changes in mental status such as confusion, delirium, or altered states of consciousness. Focal findings include seizures, hemiparesis, aphasia, and visual field defects. These neurologic symptoms may fluctuate and terminate in coma. Involvement of myocardial blood vessels may be a cause of sudden death in some patients. The severity of the disorder can be estimated from the degree of anemia and thrombocytopenia as well as the serum LDH level, which is elevated as a result of the intravascular hemolysis. Tests of coagulation, such as the prothrombin time, partial thromboplastin time, fibrinogen concentration, and the level of fibrin split products are usually normal or only mildly abnormal. If the coagulation tests indicate a major consumption of procoagulants, the diagnosis of TTP is doubtful. A positive antinuclear antibody (ANA) determination is obtained in approximately 20 percent of patients.

PATHOGENESIS   The cause of TTP is unknown, but the manifestations can be explained by *localized* platelet thrombi and fibrin deposition. Arterioles are filled with hyalin material, presumably fibrin and platelets, and similar material may be seen beneath the endothelium of otherwise uninvolved vessels. Immunofluorescence studies have shown the presence of immunoglobulin and complement in arterioles. Microaneurysms of arterioles are often present. An association with pregnancy, AIDS, SLE, scleroderma, and Sjögren's syndrome suggests an immunologic origin.

DIAGNOSIS   The combination of hemolytic anemia with fragmented RBC, thrombocytopenia, normal coagulation tests, fever, neurologic disorders, and renal dysfunction is virtually pathognomonic of TTP. Although they are not usually required for diagnosis, biopsies of skin and muscle, gingiva, lymph node, or bone marrow may demonstrate the arteriolar abnormalities described above. TTP must be distinguished from idiopathic thrombocytopenic purpura or Evans's syndrome (the former plus immunohemolytic anemia) by the finding of fragmented but not spherocytic red blood cells in the peripheral blood and a negative direct Coombs test.

℞ TREATMENT

Until recently, this disease was almost universally fatal, but with the availability of plasmapheresis, more than 90 percent of patients can survive if therapy is promptly and aggressively instituted. Many patients require daily or even twice daily plasmapheresis with plasma replacement. If a response is obtained (as indicated by increasing platelet count and decreasing plasma LDH and fragmented red cells), plasmapheresis may be given progressively less frequently but often must be continued for several weeks to months. Most patients also receive high doses of glucocorticoids and may receive platelet-active agents (dipyridamole, sulfinpyrazone, dextran, aspirin), but the efficacy of these is not known. Immunosuppression with vincristine or cyclophosphamide as well as splenectomy has been used in patients who do not respond to plasmapheresis. Even deep coma is not a contraindication to therapy, since full neurologic recovery is the rule in patients responding to therapy. Relapses have been noted in approximately 10 percent of patients but are usually responsive to therapeutic intervention. Platelet transfusions should not be given because they can precipitate thrombotic events.

Hemolytic-uremic syndrome   This disorder is similar to TTP and is characterized by the same arteriolar lesions, which may be confined to the kidney, and by similar laboratory findings. It is usually encountered in young children. Often the patient has a prodrome of a gastroenteritic bloody diarrhea caused by *Escherichia coli* 0157:H7, and the lesions are thought to be due to the elaboration of Shiga-like verotoxins that bind to the renal vascular endothelial cells and inhibit ribosomal activity. Several outbreaks of the disorder associated with undercooked meat have been reported. Very rarely, the disorder appears to be familial. Patients present with acute hemolytic anemia, thrombocytopenic purpura, and acute oliguric renal failure. Most patients have either hemoglobinuria or anuria. Unlike TTP, neurologic manifestations are uncommon. The peripheral blood findings and coagulation tests are usually indistinguishable from those of TTP.

Patients are treated with plasmapheresis, dialysis, and transfusions. The efficacy of glucocorticoids, dextran, and heparin is uncertain. The mortality in children ranges from 5 to 20 percent but is considerably higher in adults. A disorder resembling the hemolytic-uremic syndrome has been described in adults treated with the antineoplastic drug mitomycin C, usually in combination with other drugs. It may also occur in patients receiving high-dose chemotherapy with autologous stem cell transplantation.

Disseminated intravascular coagulation   When the coagulation system is inappropriately activated in the plasma, the resulting accumulations of fibrin in small vessels may result in RBC fragmentation in the microvasculature (microangiopathic hemolytic anemia). This occurs in about one-fourth of patients with DIC (Chap. 118). The degree of hemolysis is much less in DIC than in either TTP or the hemolytic-uremic syndrome, and anemia with reticulocytosis and nucleated RBC is distinctly rare.

Environmental Alteration of the Red Cell Membrane by "Toxic" Effects   Changes in the red cell membrane by external influences (chemical, bacterial, etc.) may result in hemolysis. A variety of infections may be associated with severe hemolysis. The microorganisms in bartonellosis (Chap. 165), malaria (Chap. 216), and babesiosis (Chap. 216) directly parasitize RBC. Other infectious organisms exert their damaging effects on RBC indirectly. The most striking is that resulting from septicemia with *Clostridium welchii* (Chap. 148). The phospholipase produced by this organism is capable of cleaving the phosphoryl bond of lecithin, thereby lysing human RBC. A mild, transient hemolysis frequently accompanies bacteremia with diverse organisms such as pneumococci, staphylococci, and *E. coli*.

Hemolysis may result from the direct action of snake and spider venoms on the RBC. Although cobra venom is directly lytic in vitro, the clinical disease induced by the bite of the cobra is one of moderate hemolysis associated with spherocytosis. Spider bites, particularly that of the brown recluse spider, are known to induce acute intravascular hemolysis associated with spherocytosis. The hemolytic disease continues for several days up to 1 week.

Copper has a direct hemolytic effect on RBC. Hemolysis has been observed following exposure of individuals to copper salts (such as during hemodialysis). In addition, the transient episodes of hemolysis observed in patients with Wilson's disease are probably due to copper toxicity.

The RBC membrane is unstable at temperatures above 49°C due to denaturation of the cytoskeletal protein spectrin. When studied in vitro, the RBC undergoes a process of budding, cleavage, and resealing above this temperature. The same process is observed in individuals who have suffered extensive burns. These patients have prominent spherocytosis as well as hemoglobinemia and sometimes hemoglobinuria.

Spur Cell Anemia   Hemolytic anemia with bizarre-shaped RBC occurs in some patients with severe hepatocellular disease, usually advanced Laennec's cirrhosis.

It is observed in approximately 5 percent of patients with manifestations of severe cirrhosis and is a very poor prognostic sign. It has also been reported in neonatal hepatitis.

Clinical manifestations Anemia is more severe than is observed in otherwise uncomplicated cirrhosis. Hematocrit levels range between 16 and 30 percent. Splenomegaly is always present and is greater than in patients who have cirrhosis but who do not have spur cell anemia. Jaundice may be severe because of the hemolysis and liver dysfunction, and hepatic encephalopathy is common. The characteristic RBC are irregularly shaped with multiple spicules, and a small number of bizarre-shaped fragments are commonly seen on peripheral blood smears (**Plate IV-8**). Reticulocytosis and other signs of hemolysis are present. The tests of liver function are similar to values obtained in most patients with severe cirrhosis.

RBC half-life is decreased to as short as 6 days (normal being 26 to 32 days), and red cell destruction is localized to the spleen. Normal transfused RBC acquire the defect and have a survival similar to that of the patient's own RBC.

Pathogenesis The surface membrane of a spur cell contains 50 to 70 percent excess cholesterol, but its total phospholipid content is normal; this is distinct from the pattern seen in the more usual target RBC in liver disease, which possesses an excess of both cholesterol and phospholipid. This results from the presence in serum of an abnormal low-density lipoprotein with an increased mole ratio of free (unesterified) cholesterol to phospholipid. Cholesterol out of proportion to phospholipid decreases the fluidity of the spur cell membrane, and cell deformability is decreased.

These rigid, cholesterol-laden RBC cannot pass through the filtering system of the spleen, further impeded by congestive splenomegaly in cirrhosis.

Diagnosis Spur cell anemia is characterized by evidence of hemolysis and the cells with the specific morphologic abnormality. Increasing anemia in a patient with chronic cirrhosis most commonly results from blood loss, folic acid deficiency, or iron deficiency.

RBC of similar morphologic appearance are seen in patients with abetalipoproteinemia. However, these individuals have a minimal amount of hemolysis.

Spur cells and acanthocytes must be distinguished from regularly scalloped, crenated red blood cells (echinocytes). These are a frequent artifact on blood smears, and they are present in some patients with uremia ("burr cells") (**Plate IV-9**). Small, dense crenated spheres (spheroechinocytes) are sometimes seen in congenital nonspherocytic hemolytic anemia due to enzyme deficiencies in the Embden-Meyerhof pathway (see above).

℞ TREATMENT

Since normal RBC acquire the spur abnormality when transfused into patients with this form of anemia, transfusion therapy is of limited benefit. Attempts to influence RBC cholesterol by the use of various lipid-lowering agents have been unsuccessful. Splenectomy has been reported to prevent both the conditioning of RBC in the spleen and their premature destruction. However, splenectomy carries a high risk in patients with severe liver disease complicated by portal hypertension and coagulation defects, and it must be reserved for selected patients in whom hemolysis is a major clinical problem and who appear to be relatively good surgical risks.

Prognosis In most patients, spur cell anemia occurs during the late stages of cirrhosis, and more than 90 percent of patients succumb to their underlying liver disease within 1 year of the diagnosis of spur cell anemia.

Paroxysmal Nocturnal Hemoglobinuria (PNH) This condition is distinctive among hemolytic disorders because it is an intracorpuscular defect acquired at the stem cell level.

Clinical manifestations There are three common manifestations of PNH: hemolytic anemia, venous thrombosis, and deficient hematopoiesis. Anemia is of exceedingly variable degree, with hematocrit values of 20 percent and lower in occasional patients and normal values in others.

RBC are normochromic and normocytic unless iron deficiency has occurred owing to the chronic loss of iron in the urine.

Mild granulocytopenia and thrombocytopenia are commonly present and are manifestations of deficient hematopoiesis. Clinical hemoglobinuria is present only intermittently in most patients and never occurs in some, but hemosiderinuria is usually present in all patients. The lack of two proteins, decay-accelerating factor (DAF, CD55) and a membrane inhibitor of reactive lysis (MIRL, CD59) (see below) make the red cells more sensitive to the lytic effect of complement.

DAF normally disrupts the enzyme complexes from either the classical (antibody-driven) pathway or the alternative pathway that activate C3 and C5; CD59 inhibits the conversion of C9 by the membrane attack complex C5b-8 to a polymeric complex capable of penetrating the membrane.

The platelets also lack these proteins; however, the life span of the platelet is normal. On the other hand, the activation of complement indirectly stimulates platelet aggregation and hypercoagulability; this is probably responsible for the tendency to thrombosis seen in PNH.

Venous thrombosis is a common complication, affecting about 40 percent of patients at one time or another. It occurs primarily in intraabdominal veins (hepatic, portal, mesenteric, etc.) and results in the Budd-Chiari syndrome, congestive splenomegaly, and abdominal pain. It may occur in cerebral venous sinuses and is a common cause of death in patients with PNH. The deficit in hematopoiesis may not be clinically manifest by examination of the bone marrow cellularity but is evident in all patients when the growth of marrow progenitors is examined. About 15 to 30 percent of long-term survivors of aplastic anemia will have PNH cells manifest at some time or other; in some patients, the manifestations of PNH become dominant. Patients with PNH may have aplastic periods lasting from weeks to years. PNH may be seen in association with other stem cell disorders, including myelofibrosis, and (rarely) other myelodysplastic or myeloproliferative disorders.

Pathogenesis PNH is an acquired clonal disease, probably arising from an inactivating somatic mutation in a single abnormal stem cell of a gene on the X-chromosome (*pig-A*) important for the biosynthesis of the glycosylphosphatidylinositol (GPI) anchor. This anchor is necessary for the attachment of a number of proteins to the external membrane surface, and its partial or complete absence results in the absence of those proteins; to date, about 20 proteins have been found to be missing on the blood cells of patients with PNH. The normal clone of stem cells and its descendants do not completely disappear, and the proportion of cells that are abnormal varies from patient to patient and from time to time in a single patient.

Diagnosis PNH should be suspected in anyone with otherwise unexplained hemolytic anemia, especially with leukopenia and/or thrombocytopenia and with evidence of intravascular hemolysis (hemoglobinemia, hemoglobinuria, hemosiderinuria, elevated LDH of the erythrocyte type). Anyone recovering from aplastic anemia should be examined at intervals for the appearance of the diagnostic cells. The diagnosis is often delayed because (1) it is not considered, (2) hemoglobinuria is confused with hematuria, (3) elevation of the LDH is confused with that seen in liver disease, and (4) the tests commonly used (Ham's test and the sucrose lysis test) are not reliable.

Ham's test is performed by incubating the patient's RBC with normal serum acidified to a pH of 6.2. Complement is activated under these conditions, and the defective PNH cells are lysed but not normal cells (including the normal cells of the patient). The sensitivity of the test is increased by optimizing the Mg^{2+} concentration and by using sera of normal donors known to be potent in this test. The test may miss small populations of abnormal cells but is falsely positive only in a rare form of congenital dyserythropoietic anemia, which can be readily distinguished on clinical grounds. The sucrose lysis test, in which complement is activated by reduction of the ionic strength of the incubation medium, is more sensitive but less specific. The most sensitive and specific test is determination of the absence of the GPI-linked proteins on erythrocytes and granulocytes by flow cytometry (e.g., CD59, DAF).

Table 109-9

TREATMENT

Transfusion therapy is useful in PNH not only for raising the hemoglobin level but also for suppressing the marrow production of RBC during episodes of sustained hemoglobinuria. Whole blood transfusions infrequently cause an exacerbation of the hemolytic process. This can be prevented by using washed RBC rather than whole blood. Therapy with androgens frequently results in a rise in hemoglobin level. Glucocorticoids also may be effective in reducing the rate of hemolysis but should be given in moderate doses (15 to 30 mg prednisone) *only on alternate days.*

Because of iron loss in the urine, iron deficiency is common. An exacerbation of hemolysis often follows the administration of iron because of the formation of a large number of young RBC, many of which are sensitive to complement. This may be minimized by giving prednisone (60 mg/d) or by suppressing the bone marrow with transfusions.

Acute thrombosis in PNH, particularly the Budd-Chiari syndrome and cerebral thrombosis, should be treated aggressively with thrombolytic agents. Heparin therapy should be instituted rapidly and maintained for several days before changing to coumadin therapy. Antithymoctye globulin is often of use in treating marrow hypoplasia, as it is in the related disease, aplastic anemia. A total dose of 150 mg/kg is given over 4 to 10 days; large doses of prednisone are usually needed to counteract the immune-complex disease that results from the administration of this foreign protein.

In patients, especially the younger ones, with either hypoplasia or thrombosis who have an appropriate sibling donor, marrow transplantation should be considered early in the course of the disease. The usual conditioning programs are sufficient to eradicate the aberrant clone.

ANEMIA OF ACUTE BLOOD LOSS

The normal capacity to compensate for acute blood loss involves cardiovascular mechanisms, an adjustment in the oxygen affinity of hemoglobin, and an increase in erythropoiesis in the marrow. The signs and symptoms of blood loss relate to the volume of the blood loss and the time frame over which the hemorrhage occurs (see Table 109-9). Blood losses of up to 20 percent of the blood volume are normally tolerated by redistribution of blood flow mediated by reflex venospasm, but the presence of fever or pain may interfere with this compensation. With larger blood losses, blood volume redistribution is not adequate to maintain normal blood pressure: initially, changes are only seen on standing, but with greater losses progressively greater problems are encountered maintaining blood pressure in sitting or supine positions. If the blood loss is more gradual, plasma volume may increase, but albumin production usually lags behind the fluid shifts. It may take 2 to 3 days for the liver to generate the albumin lost in a 1500-mL bleed.

The most rapid hematologic adjustment to acute blood loss is an increase in oxygen delivery to the tissues. This is first mediated by the Bohr effect, where the more acidic milieu of the hypoperfused tissues shifts the hemoglobin oxygen dissociation curve to the right. Over several hours the red cells increase their production of 2,3-bisphosphoglycerate, which also enhances the unloading of oxygen to tissues. These two mechanisms can nearly double the capacity of each red cell to deliver oxygen to the tissues.

The marrow response to hemorrhage is related to the generation of erythropoietin in the kidney in response to decreased oxygen tensions. A normal response depends upon the production of erythropoietin, the presence of normal erythroid progenitors in the marrow, and an adequate supply of iron. If these three elements are normal, reticulo-

Table 109-9

Signs and Symptoms of Blood Loss

Percent Blood Loss	Volume of Loss, mL*	Symptoms	Signs
<20	<1000	Restlessness	+/− Vasovagal reaction
20–30	1000–1500	Anxiety, DOE	Orthostatic hypotension, tachycardia on exertion
30–40	1500–2000	Syncope on sitting or standing	Orthostatic hypotension, tachycardia at rest
>40	>2000	Confusion, shortness of breath	Shock, poor perfusion

* Based on an estimated total blood volume of 5000 mL (70-kg adult).

cytes begin to increase in number in the first 2 days based upon early release of reticulocytes from the marrow. However, it takes 3 to 6 days for erythroid hyperplasia to appear and 7 to 10 days before the erythropoietic response is maximal, producing reticulocyte counts up to 20 to 30 percent, a reticulocyte index of 3 or greater, and a marked increase in the marrow erythoid/granulocytic ratio.

DIAGNOSIS Usually it is clear that a patient is bleeding; however, in some cases, large volumes of blood loss can occur internally from the gastrointestinal tract (esophageal varicies, cancer in the stomach or colon), a ruptured spleen, fractures and other trauma, or other lesions that can cause massive hemorrhage into the peritoneal cavity, pleural cavity, or the retroperitoneal space. Patients who have bled sufficiently to develop hypotension generally develop anemia, but this is only apparent after volume replacement. The granulocyte count may increase to 20,000 cells/μL or more and include immature cell types such as metamyelocytes and myelocytes. Epinephrine-induced demargination of peripheral granulocytes and release of cells from the marrow may account for this change. Nucleated RBC may appear in the circulation, and platelet counts may exceed $1 \times 10^6/\mu$L. The basis for the increased platelet count is unclear. Hemorrhage within an internal cavity is accompanied by a rise in unconjugated bilirubin and a fall in serum haptoglobin.

TREATMENT

Treatment of the underlying cause of the hemorrhage is of paramount importance. If the patient is severely anemic or sufficiently hypovolemic, packed red cells should be transfused. In less severe cases, if the patient has normal kidneys (and presumably a normal erythropoietin response to anemia), normal bone marrow function, and an adequate supply of iron, no specific therapy for the anemia is required.

BIBLIOGRAPHY

Amidon TM et al: Mitral and aortic paravalvular leaks with hemolytic anemia. Am Heart J 125:266, 1993

Becker PS, Lux SE: Disorders of the red cell membrane, in *Hematology of Infancy and Childhood*, DG Nathan, FA Oski (eds). Philadelphia, Saunders, 1992, pp 529–633

Beutler E: Study of glucose-6-phosphatedehydrogenase: History and molecular biology. Am J Hematol 42:53, 1993

Hirono A et al: Enzymatic diagnosis in non-spherocytic hemolytic anemia. Medicine 67:110, 1988

Miwa S, Fujii H: Molecular basis of erythroenzymopathies associated with hemolytic anemia: Tabulation of mutant enzymes. Am J Hematol 51:122, 1996

Palek J, Sahr SE: Mutations of the red blood cell membrane proteins: From clinical evaluation to detection of the underlying genetic defect. Blood 80:308, 1992

Robson WL et al: Hemolytic-uremic syndrome. Curr Probl Pediatr 23:16, 1993

Rose M et al: The changing course of thrombotic thrombocytopenic purpura and modern therapy. Blood Rev 7:94, 1993

Rosse WF: *Clinical Immunohematology.* Cambridge, Blackwell Scientific, 1990

———, Ware RE: The molecular basis of paroxysmal nocturnal hemoglobinuria. Blood 86:3277, 1995

Thompson CE et al: Thrombotic microangiopathies in the 1980s: Clinical features. Blood 80:1890, 1992

110

Hugo Castro-Malaspina, Richard J. O'Reilly

APLASTIC ANEMIA AND MYELODYSPLASTIC SYNDROMES

The anemias discussed in this chapter are usually normochromic and normocytic and associated with a low reticulocyte count. The hypoproliferative anemias associated with marrow damage include aplastic anemia, pure red cell aplasia, myelodysplastic syndromes, and myelophthisis (Fig. 59-4).

APLASTIC ANEMIA

Aplastic anemia is a disorder of hematopoiesis characterized by marked reduction or absence of erythroid, granulocytic, and megakaryocytic cells in the bone marrow with resultant pancytopenia. Hematopoiesis is markedly decreased, as shown by the marrow histology as well as the absent or reduced numbers of CD34+ cells and colony forming cells (**see Plate IV-33**). Hematopoietic stem cells in aplastic anemia are unable to proliferate and differentiate to give rise to mature blood cells and their precursors. The stem cell failure results in most cases from an acquired intrinsic stem cell defect and/or from an immune mechanism. Other potential mechanisms, such as growth factor deficiency and microenvironment defects, are rare and not well documented.

The overall incidence of aplastic anemia in Western countries has been estimated as 5 to 10 cases per million persons per year; about 1000 new cases are diagnosed every year in the United States. The disease can occur at any age, but is most common in young adults (15 to 30 years old) and elderly patients (>60 years old), with about the same incidence in males and females. The disease is more frequent in Asia than in North America and Europe, particularly in younger adults.

ETIOLOGY Most cases of aplastic anemia are acquired, but the disease may also occur as the result of inherited abnormalities, such as Fanconi's anemia. For acquired forms of aplastic anemia, a variety of causative factors, including certain drugs, viruses, organic compounds, and radiation, have been implicated (Table 110-1). However, for over half of patients, no cause can be determined (so-called idiopathic aplastic anemia). Even for patients in whom a well-defined association between exposure (e.g., to chloramphenicol) and subsequent development of aplastic anemia has been established, it remains unclear why only a small proportion of those exposed to a given agent develop the disease. Furthermore, the mechanisms by which certain agents or classes of agents (e.g., viruses, drugs) cause aplastic anemia are still poorly understood.

Table 110-1

Etiology of Aplastic Anemia

Acquired
  Drugs: antimetabolites, antimitotic agents, gold, chloramphenicol, phenylbutazone, sulfonamides (see Table 110-2)
  Radiation
  Chemicals: benzene, solvents, insecticides
  Viruses: non-A, non-B, non-C hepatitis, human immunodeficiency virus, Epstein-Barr virus*
  Paroxysmal nocturnal hemoglobinuria
  Miscellaneous: pregnancy, connective tissue disorders, graft-versus-host disease
Hereditary
  Fanconi's anemia
  Dyskeratosis congenita
  Shwachman syndrome
Idiopathic: 50–65% of cases

* Parvovirus B19 may also produce transient aplastic crisis, but pure red cell aplasia is the more common manifestation.

Table 110-2

Drugs Associated with Aplastic Anemia

Antineoplastic drugs
  Antimetabolites: fluorouracil, mercaptopurine, methotrexate
  Alkylating agents: busulfan, cyclophosphamide, nitrogen mustard, melphalan
  Cytotoxic antibiotics: daunorubicin, doxorubicin, mitoxantrone
Antimicrobial drugs
  Antibacterials: chloramphenicol, dapsone, β-lactam antibiotics
  Antifungals: amphotericin, flucytosine
  Antiprotozoals: quinacrine, chloroquine, pyrimethamine, mepacrine
Anti-inflammatory drugs: phenylbutazone, oxyphenbutazone, indomethacin, ibuprofen, naproxen, sulindac
Antiarthritic drugs: gold salts, colchicine
Anticonvulsant drugs: carbamazepine, phenytoin, ethosuximide, primidone
Analgesic drugs: phenacetin, salicylamide, aspirin
Antiarrhythmic drugs: quinidine, tocainamide
Antithyroid drugs: carbimazole, methimazole, methylthiouracil, potassium perchlorate, propylthiouracil, sodium thiocyanate
Sulfonamides and derivatives
  Antibacterials: sulfonamides
  Diuretics: acetazolamide, chlorothiazide, furosemide
  Hypoglycemics: chlorpropamide, tolbutamide
Antihypertensive drugs: captopril, methyldopa, enalapril
Antihistamine drugs: chlorpheniramine, pyrilamine, tripelennamine
Sedatives: chlordiazepoxide, chlorpromazine, lithium, meprobamate
Antiplatelet drugs: ticlopidine

Drugs Population-based case-control studies have shown an association between certain drugs and aplastic anemia. Drug-induced aplastic anemia may be dose-related or idiosyncratic. Table 110-2 shows some of the medications linked to aplastic anemia. The major classes of myelotoxic drugs are anticonvulsants, antibacterials, hypoglycemic and diuretic sulfonamides, antimetabolites, antimitotic agents, and synthetic antithyroid drugs. Certain classes of agents, such as antineoplastic drugs, antimetabolites, and sulfonamides, have a direct dose-dependent myelotoxic activity. However, for the other agents commonly associated with aplastic anemia, particularly chloramphenicol, phenylbutazone and oxyphenbutazone, indomethacin, and gold salts, aplasias are idiosyncratic and not dose related. The mechanisms contributing to aplasia are unclear. For instance, chloramphenicol produces a dose-related reversible suppression of erythropoiesis during treatment and an idiosyncratic, dose-independent global marrow suppression many weeks or months after cessation of therapy. Many other drugs have been linked to the development of aplastic anemia. For some of them, the incidence of aplastic anemia in exposed patients seems to be high enough to suggest an etiologic role, whereas with other drugs there is only a sporadic occurrence, and the causal relationship is difficult to establish.

Radiation Acute exposure causes a dose-related transient marrow suppression, which is reversible at low doses but is permanent and life-threatening at high doses. Chronic exposure to low-dose and localized radiation may cause late permanent marrow failure. For instance, patients irradiated for ankylosing spondylitis have a higher incidence of aplastic anemia. However, the incidence of aplastic anemia has been reported not to be increased in long-term survivors of the atomic bombings.

Benzene and Insecticides Benzene was the first organic solvent linked to aplastic anemia. There is a dose-effect relationship between exposure to benzene and the incidence of development of cytopenias. Chronic exposure has been associated with the development of aplastic anemia and leukemias. Benzene and related aryl hydrocarbons may generate catabolites that are directly toxic to stem cells. However, they may also induce formation of haptens that may stimulate immune responses. Benzene-induced aplasia in rabbits can be reversed following immunosuppression with antithymocyte globulin. DDT and lindane, well-recognized etiologic agents, are now outlawed as insecticides in the United States.

Viruses Viral illnesses are a precipitating event in some patients with aplastic anemia. The most common viral infection associated with aplastic anemia is viral hepatitis. Other viruses implicated in aplastic anemia include the Epstein-Barr virus, parvovirus B19, human immunodeficiency virus (HIV), and others. Approximately 1 to 5 percent of cases of aplastic anemia follow an overt hepatitis. Although hepatitis A, B, and C have been implicated in aplastic anemia in a small number of cases, most cases are not related to these viruses. Hepatitis G virus may be the major infection associated with marrow failure. Hepatitis preceding aplastic anemia is not usually severe, but posthepatitis aplastic anemia is commonly severe. While hepatitis viruses may induce lytic infection of primitive hematopoietic stem cells, the remissions of aplasia induced by immunosuppressive therapies in some cases of posthepatitis aplasia have suggested that immune responses induced by infection may also play a major role.

Parvovirus B19, the etiologic agent of erythema infectiosum (see Chap. 189), can cause transient erythroid aplasia in patients with underlying spherocytic anemias and hemoglobinopathies, and it can cause chronic marrow failure in immunodeficient patients. This virus infects and lyses hematopoietic stem cells. Persistent infection results from the inability to mount an adequate antibody response and is associated with pure red-cell aplasia. Epstein-Barr virus–induced infectious mononucleosis is rarely associated with aplastic anemia; blood counts usually recover spontaneously. Cytomegalovirus (CMV) has also been associated with marrow failure, particularly in marrow transplant recipients. Certain strains of CMV may infect the marrow stromal cells that support hematopoietic cell growth, thereby inducing secondary aplasia.

Pregnancy   Women may develop aplastic anemia during pregnancy. In a proportion of cases, aplasia has resolved with natural or premature termination of pregnancy, but it has sometimes recurred with a subsequent pregnancy. The pathogenesis and causal relationship between pregnancy and aplastic anemia is unknown.

Paroxysmal Nocturnal Hemoglobinuria   Paroxysmal nocturnal hemoglobinuria (PNH) is a clonal hemopathy caused by a defect in the *PIG-A* gene and is characterized by partial or complete inability to construct a glycosylphosphatidylinositol (GPI) anchor for the attachment of membrane proteins such as CD55, CD59, and others (see Chap. 109). Aplastic anemia can be the initial hematologic manifestation of this disease. PNH can also develop months to years after the diagnosis of aplastic anemia. The mechanisms whereby PNH induces aplastic anemia are unknown. The PNH clone may inhibit the growth of normal marrow progenitors. Alternatively, PNH clones may be less sensitive than normal counterparts to injury induced by viruses or toxins or the immune responses they elicit. A history of thrombosis and evidence of hemolysis in a patient with an aplastic anemia suggests the diagnosis of PNH. The diagnosis may be difficult to make, because the proportion of PNH cells in the blood may be too small to be detected by the Ham test (acidification of serum to pH 6.2 activates complement and lyses PNH cells). Flow cytometry using antibodies against cell-surface proteins, such as CD55 and CD59, which are lacking in this disease, are helpful in establishing this diagnosis. Aplastic patients with a positive Ham test may respond to anti-T-cell therapies such as cyclosporine and antithymocyte globulin.

Other Acquired Causes   Eosinophilic fasciitis, a rare connective tissue disease characterized by painful swelling and induration of the skin and subcutaneous tissue (see Chap. 383), has been associated with aplastic anemia. Myelosuppression is thought to be antibody-mediated. A similar mechanism has been implicated in systemic lupus erythematosus (SLE). However, patients with SLE and other autoimmune diseases are often treated with anti-inflammatory drugs and gold salts, which have been linked to aplastic anemia. Graft-versus-host disease may cause severe marrow suppression. Certain disorders of the immune system, including thymoma, X-linked lymphoproliferative disorder, and T-gamma lymphocyte proliferation have also been associated with marrow failure. Aplastic anemia also, in rare instances, precedes acute leukemia. The hypocellular variant of myelodysplastic syndrome (MDS) may present clinical and pathologic features difficult to distinguish from those of aplastic anemia.

Congenital Disorders   Fanconi's anemia (FA) is an autosomal recessive disorder characterized by a progressive pancytopenia, diverse congenital abnormalities, an increased predisposition to malignancy,

and increased chromosomal fragility or cellular hypersensitivity to mutagenic chemicals. The features of FA include short stature, café-au-lait spots, kidney and urinary tract abnormalities, microphthalmia, mental retardation, and skeletal abnormalities, most often affecting the thumb and radius. Cells from FA patients are uniquely hypersensitive to the damaging effects of DNA-modifying agents such as diepoxybutane (DEB) and cyclophosphamide. Complementation analyses suggest that at least five different genetic defects may induce Fanconi's anemia. One genetic variant of this disease, type C, is due to a mutation of the *FACC* gene, which is involved in the cellular response to DNA damage.

Aplastic anemia also may occur as the result of other inherited disorders, such as Shwachman-Diamond syndrome and dyskeratosis congenita. Patients with Shwachman syndrome have pancreatic insufficiency, malabsorption, neutropenia, and an increased risk of aplastic anemia. Dyskeratosis congenita is a rare X-chromosome dermatologic syndrome characterized by reticular hyperpigmentation, mucous membrane leukoplakia, and dystrophic nails. About half of patients with this disease develop aplastic anemia.

PATHOGENESIS   The pathogenesis of this disease is complex and only partially understood. Acquired aplastic anemia results from two main pathogenic mechanisms: an acquired intrinsic stem cell defect and/or an immune suppressive mechanism. The fact that 40 to 50 percent of recipients of syngeneic transplants for aplastic anemia can achieve hematologic reconstitution without pretransplant immunosuppression suggests that a stem cell defect is responsible for the marrow failure in a significant proportion of patients. In the other 50 to 60 percent of recipients of syngeneic grafts, the donor marrow fails to engraft. However, use of immunosuppression before a second transplant can lead to prolonged hematologic recovery. Thus, in some cases, an immune mechanism contributes to the disease. The contribution of the immune system to the pathogenesis of aplastic anemia has been further supported by documentation of autologous recovery in patients receiving allogeneic bone marrow transplants after immunosuppressive conditioning and in patients with aplastic anemia who have achieved remission of disease following treatment with antithymocyte globulin and/or cyclosporine without transplantation. Activated cytotoxic T cells derived from the blood and the marrow of a significant proportion of patients with aplastic anemia overproduce cytokines such as interferon γ and tumor necrosis factor β (lymphotoxin) that suppress hematopoietic progenitors.

Approximately 25 percent of patients with aplastic anemia are cured by immunosuppressive therapy. However, 20 to 50 percent of patients with aplastic anemia who achieve a partial or, less commonly, a complete reconstitution of hematopoiesis following treatment with antithymocyte globulin develop myelodysplastic syndromes months to years after completion of immunosuppressive therapy. This high frequency has suggested the possibility that these patients develop aplastic anemia as a manifestation of an immune response directed against preexisting abnormal hematopoietic stem cells, or that these abnormal hematopoietic stem cells preferentially recover following immunosuppressive therapy. Whether stem cells in patients with aplastic anemia are normal or abnormal is under study.

CLINICAL MANIFESTATIONS   The onset of aplastic anemia is usually insidious. The most common presenting symptoms are those secondary to anemia and thrombocytopenia and include progressive weakness and fatigue and bleeding from the skin, nose, gums, vagina, or gastrointestinal tract. Although the patient may be severely neutropenic, infection is rarely the presenting symptom. The most frequent physical findings are cutaneous and conjunctival pallor and hemorrhages (petechiae, ecchymoses, and gum bleeding). If anemia is severe, tachycardia and murmurs associated with high-flow states may be present. Hepatosplenomegaly and lymphadenopathy are notably absent.

DIAGNOSIS   The diagnosis of aplastic anemia should be considered if a pancytopenic patient has a normochromic, normocytic (or slightly macrocytic) anemia, a low reticulocyte count (reticulocyte index < 2) indicative of a hypoproliferative mechanism, thrombocytopenia with normal-sized platelets, neutropenia, and the absence of abnormal cells in the leukocyte differential. Confirmation requires morphologic and cytogenetic evaluation of the bone marrow.

The bone marrow aspirate typically shows numerous spicules with empty fatty spaces and few hematopoietic cells. The hypocellularity is secondary to a marked decrease in megakaryocytes, granulocytes, and erythroid cells. Although sometimes the erythroid cells exhibit megaloblastic changes, the morphology of marrow elements is usually normal. The presence of overt dysplasia favors the diagnosis of hypocellular MDS. Lymphocytes, plasma cells, and mast cells are relatively increased and, in severe cases, constitute over 65 percent of the cells. Sometimes the cellularity appears normal because of isolated foci (hot spots) of hematopoiesis. The marrow biopsy allows a better assessment of the cellularity and permits evaluation for the presence of tumor cells, hairy cells, and fibrosis. Marrow cytogenetic studies distinguish aplastic anemia from MDS and Fanconi's anemia. The presence of clonal chromosomal abnormalities favors the diagnosis of MDS. However, a normal karyotype does not rule out this diagnosis. Assessment of clonality based on X chromosome inactivation in females suggests that stem cell abnormalities may be more frequent than originally suspected.

Serum levels of lactate dehydrogenase (LDH) and haptoglobin, Ham's test, and flow-cytometric analysis of peripheral blood cells using antibodies against the GPI-linked proteins are useful to establish or to rule out the diagnosis of PNH. In younger patients, the cytogenetics of marrow cells in the presence or absence of diepoxybutane may be diagnostic of FA, since patients with FA may not have a family history or other clinical findings of the disease.

CLASSIFICATION The International Aplastic Anemia Study Group distinguished severe and moderate forms of aplastic anemia. Aplasia is defined as *severe* when two or more of the following criteria are met: neutrophil count <500/μL, platelet count <20,000/μL, and reticulocyte count <20,000/μL. A new form with a worse prognosis characterized by a neutrophil count of <200/μL has been termed *super-severe* or *very severe*, aplastic anemia. This form has a lower response rate to and a poorer survival rate following immunosuppressive therapy.

DIFFERENTIAL DIAGNOSIS Patients with *hypocellular myelodysplastic syndrome* also have pancytopenia and a hypocellular bone marrow. However, the review of blood smears may show the presence of immature granulocytes or nucleated red cells. The few myeloid elements in the marrow have dysplastic changes, and the marrow karyotype may show a clonal abnormality. The differential diagnosis may be difficult when the dysplastic changes are subtle. *Hypocellular acute leukemia* can be misdiagnosed as aplastic anemia when the few mononuclear cells present in the bone marrow are not identified as blasts. Although *hairy cell leukemia* usually presents with splenomegaly and a hypercellular marrow, occasionally it presents without these features. The diagnosis is established by recognizing the few hairy cells by their typical morphology, as well as their cytochemical (tartrate-resistant acid phosphatase) and phenotypic (CD25+ monoclonal B cells) characteristics (see Chap. 113).

COURSE OF THE DISEASE AND PROGNOSIS The pancytopenia of aplastic anemia is progressive and life-threatening. With transfusion support alone, up to 80 percent of patients with severe aplastic anemia succumb to the disease within 18 to 24 months. Prognosis at diagnosis is closely correlated with the neutrophil count. The risk of infection, mainly bacterial and fungal, and associated mortality is high in patients with super-severe aplastic anemia. Before the advent of immunosuppressive therapy and allogeneic bone marrow transplantation, more than 25 percent of patients with severe aplastic anemia died within 4 months of diagnosis, and half died within one year. Treatment with androgens or glucocorticoids did not affect outcome.

Two therapeutic approaches, allogeneic bone marrow transplantation and immunosuppressive therapy, have radically improved the prognosis of patients with severe forms of aplastic anemia. Currently, treatment with a human leukocyte antigen (HLA)-matched related marrow transplant is curative in 60 to 90 percent of patients. However, a proportion of long-term survivors suffer from chronic graft-versus-host disease. The success of bone marrow transplant correlates with age and degree of matching. The upper age limit for marrow transplantation continues to increase as better approaches are developed to prevent or treat transplant-related complications (see Chap. 116). Immunosuppressive therapy with antithymocyte or anti-thoracic duct lymphocyte globulin and/or cyclosporine can induce at least partial remission of disease in 60 to 80 percent of patients. However, about one-third of these responders relapse, and about 20 to 50 percent develop myelodysplastic syndromes. Patients who do not respond to immunosuppression can be maintained with supportive therapy, but their prognosis is poor. HLA-mismatched family member or unrelated donor marrow transplantation is an option for these patients.

℞ **TREATMENT**

Withdrawal of the etiologic agent is the most direct approach to the treatment of aplastic anemia. Discontinuation of a suspected drug, thymectomy in patients with thymoma, or delivery or therapeutic abortion in patients with pregnancy-associated aplastic anemia may result in recovery of blood counts. Unfortunately, these cases account for a very small proportion of patients.

Once the diagnosis of aplastic anemia is established, family HLA typing should be done as soon as possible, particularly in younger patients (<45 years), since these patients are most likely to benefit from bone marrow transplantation from a histocompatible sibling. Transfusions of blood products from family members should be avoided in transplant candidates to prevent sensitization to minor histocompatibility antigens, which increases the risk of graft rejection after transplantation. Whenever possible, only CMV-negative blood products should be given to CMV-seronegative potential transplant candidates to reduce the incidence of CMV infection in the post-transplant period. Immunosuppressive therapy is the treatment of choice for patients without a histocompatible sibling.

Supportive Therapy Blood and platelet transfusions should be used with caution because of short-term and long-term complications. The risk of bleeding should be carefully assessed, and platelet transfusions should be given only when the platelet count is less than 10,000/μL or if there is active bleeding with a higher platelet count. Pooled-donor platelets are usually used until sensitization occurs, as manifested by a failure of the transfusion to boost the platelet count. Ideally, single-donor platelets should be used from the beginning to minimize the risk of sensitization, but in practice, this alternative is difficult to carry out. Refractoriness to platelet transfusion is a major problem with long-term transfusion support. Refractory patients may need HLA-compatible platelet transfusions in case of severe hemorrhage.

Packed red cells also should be transfused when the hemoglobin concentration is <7 g/dL (70 g/L). Younger patients may tolerate lower values, whereas a higher threshold may be indicated in older patients. Packed red cells should be filtered to remove leukocytes and platelets to reduce sensitization. Chronic administration of red-cell transfusions results in secondary hemochromatosis, as each unit has approximately 200 to 250 mg of iron. Serum ferritin values should be monitored, and chelation therapy with deferoxamine should be given to reduce iron overload (see Chap. 342).

Patients with aplastic anemia who develop sepsis or other severe bacterial infections require intensive treatment with parenteral antibiotics. Leukocyte transfusions are likely only indicated in severely neutropenic (neutrophil count <200/μL) aplastic anemia patients with a documented fungal infection unresponsive to amphotericin, or bacterial infections with organisms that are resistant to most antibiotics. The modest benefits of such infusions should be weighed against the risks of sensitization and transmission of infectious agents, particularly CMV, which may compromise subsequent therapies (e.g., transplantation). Prophylactic use of antibiotics in afebrile neutropenic patients has no benefits and favors the emergence of resistant strains. *Staphylococcus epidermidis* is a common pathogen in patients with indwelling catheters. Neutropenic precautions should be used in patients who are hospitalized and have a neutrophil count of <500/μL. Menstruating females should be given suppressive doses of birth control pills to avoid severe blood losses.

Immunosuppressive Agents   Several agents, including antithymocyte globulin (ATG) and cyclosporine (alone or in combination), glucocorticoids, and cyclophosphamide, have been used in aplastic anemia patients who do not qualify for transplantation because of their age or lack of a compatible donor. The licensed ATG preparations contain purified and concentrated gamma globulins, primarily monomeric IgG from hyperimmune serum of horses (also rabbits or goats) immunized with human thymocytes or thoracic duct lymphocytes. Several studies have recorded response rates to ATG treatment ranging from 50 to 70 percent. Of these responders, 20 to 30 percent achieve a complete and durable recovery of blood counts. The other 70 to 80 percent achieve a partial response and will be transfusion independent with platelet counts exceeding 20,000/μL and neutrophil counts exceeding 1000/μL.

The basis for the effects of ATG is unclear. Although ATG is an immunosuppressant, responses usually occur 8 to 12 weeks after its administration, long after the immunosuppressive effects of ATG have resolved. The response to ATG correlates with severity of the disease. Patients with the super-severe form have a lower response rate. Also, children have lower response rates than adults. The post-treatment survival is correlated with the severity of neutropenia and the level of response. Not surprisingly, complete responders have a better survival. Relapse occurs in approximately one-third of patients, particularly in those who achieve only a partial response. A second course of immunosuppressive therapy can induce a second response in a proportion of cases. The major long-term complication of therapy with ATG is the development of overt myelodysplastic syndrome or paroxysmal nocturnal hemoglobinuria in 30 to 60 percent of patients many months to years after therapy. These late complications are more frequent in patients who achieve a partial response. ATG is also associated with a higher incidence of secondary solid tumors, similar to that observed in aplastic anemia patients prepared for allogeneic bone marrow transplantation with regimens involving radiation therapy.

The experience with cyclosporine is less mature. Cyclosporine and ATG induce similar response rates. Combined therapy with ATG and cyclosporine induces higher and earlier response rates as compared to ATG alone, particularly in patients with the super-severe forms of aplasia. However, this combination has not significantly improved long-term survival. The impact of combined immunosuppressive therapy on the incidence of long-term complications is not known yet. Very-high-dose glucocorticoid treatment (prednisone at 10 to 20 mg/kg) can induce responses in a small proportion of patients with aplastic anemia, but glucocorticoids are no longer used as single agents because of their side effects and the better response rates achieved with other agents.

In one trial, therapy with cyclophosphamide alone was shown to induce complete responses in 7 of 10 patients with aplastic anemia. Strikingly, no MDS cases have been observed in long-term follow-up of this series, which contrasts with the 30 to 60 percent rates of MDS in patients treated with ATG. This treatment is not only immunosuppressive but also cytotoxic, and it may eliminate abnormal stem cell clones that give rise to MDS, thus favoring the expansion of suppressed normal stem cells.

Hematopoietic Growth Factors   Recombinant hematopoietic growth factors have been explored as a first-line therapy for aplastic anemia and in the treatment of aplasia refractory to immunosuppressive therapy. Erythropoietin, granulocyte colony-stimulating factor (G-CSF), granulocyte-macrophage colony-stimulating factor (GM-CSF), interleukins (ILs) 1, 3, and 6, and stem cell factor can improve the blood counts, particularly the neutrophil counts, in only a small proportion of patients. Unfortunately, these increments are entirely dependent on the presence of residual normal hematopoietic progenitors. Patients with no neutrophils or very severe neutropenia (neutrophil count <200/μL) do not respond to growth factors. In patients who respond, blood counts drop to pretreatment values following discontinuation of the growth factor.

A common drawback to immunosuppressive treatments is that the response usually takes up to 12 weeks to appear, and, as a result, significant early mortality occurs, due in most cases to infections. The use of hematopoietic growth factors, particularly G-CSF, following intensive immunosuppression with ATG and cyclosporine, has resulted not only in a reduced frequency of infections because of rapid correction of neutropenia but also in a higher response rate. However, generalization of this approach awaits the results of randomized trials and long-term follow-up studies.

Data from randomized trials suggest that androgens are not beneficial in aplastic anemia; yet occasional patients who have failed other therapies respond to androgens.

Bone Marrow Transplantation   Transplantation from an HLA-compatible sibling is a curative treatment for aplastic anemia. Unfortunately, this approach is only applicable to a minority of patients because the proportion of patients who have an HLA-matched sibling is about 25 to 30 percent. Current survival rates achievable with transplant (70 to 90 percent) reflect improvements in the management of transplant-related complications, particularly graft failure and graft-versus-host disease (GVHD). Early studies recorded a 20 to 30 percent incidence of graft failure in multiply transfused patients who were prepared for transplantation with cyclophosphamide alone. In contrast, the risk of graft failure in patients who had not been transfused was <5 percent. Subsequently, several approaches incorporating total-body or total-lymphoid irradiation in addition to cyclophosphamide administration were explored in an attempt to reduce the incidence of graft failure in sensitized patients. Although these treatments reduced the incidence of graft failure, long-term survival was not improved, because of the added transplant-related morbidity and mortality associated with these regimens. High-dose cyclophosphamide with ATG for pretransplant immunosuppression and cyclosporine prophylaxis for GVHD after transplantation has markedly reduced the incidence of graft failure and GVHD and has significantly improved the long-term survival (90 percent at 2 years after transplantation in one series).

What can be done for patients lacking sibling donors? Extended family searches, particularly in patients inheriting common HLA haplotypes, have led to the identification of donors who are HLA-matched or are mismatched in only a single HLA allele in a small proportion of cases (<5 percent). Transplants from such donors are associated with a higher incidence of acute and chronic GVHD. However, long-term survival is only slightly inferior to that achieved with matched related donor grafts. With the development of the National Marrow Donor Program and the European donor banks, over 2 million volunteer donors are now available for transplantation. Searches for donors in these pools has led to the identification of matched unrelated donors for up to 20 percent of patients. Matched unrelated donor transplants show a high incidence of acute and chronic GVHD. In addition, when the preparative regimen omitted total body irradiation, graft failure was common, and survival rates were only about 30 percent. Unrelated transplants should only be considered for patients who have failed immunosuppressive therapies and remain severely pancytopenic, particularly those who are affected with repeated infections and are refractory to platelet transfusions.

PURE RED CELL APLASIA

The selective absence of erythroid progenitors in an otherwise normal marrow is pure red cell aplasia (PRCA). Hereditary PRCA is the Diamond-Blackfan syndrome; anemia is detected within the first year of life, and other physical anomalies are present in about 30 percent of cases. The differential diagnosis includes in utero parvovirus infection and transient erythroblastopenia of childhood. PRCA in adults is usually an acquired disease. It may be idiopathic or associated with other medical problems such as thymoma, lymphoid malignancies, solid tumors, immunologic diseases like SLE and rheumatoid arthritis, or infections [especially viral; HIV, parvovirus, Epstein-Barr, hepatitis viruses, human T-lymphotropic virus type I (HTLV-I)]. Many of the drugs that may cause aplastic anemia (Table 110-2) may also cause PRCA, especially phenytoin, azathioprine, chloramphenicol, procainamide, and isoniazid. PRCA may complicate pregnancy. In some cases, immunoglobulin molecules directed at erythropoietin, at erythropoietin-responsive erythroid precursor cells, or at erythroblasts themselves may block the effects of erythropoietin or destroy erythroid cells. T-cell cytokines made by the tumor cells may block the response of erythroid precursors to erythropoietin in T-cell chronic lymphocytic leukemia and T-gamma lymphoproliferative disease. Parvovirus B19 may cause aplastic anemia acutely and transiently in people with underlying hemolytic anemia. The virus has a tropism for erythroid precursors and lyses them. In people who cannot mount an antibody response against the virus, the infection and destruction of erythroid progenitors persists, leading to PRCA. Parvoviral PRCA is usually detectable by the presence of giant pronormoblasts in the bone marrow, which are cells that are infected with parvovirus and are destined to die.

℞ TREATMENT

All medications should be stopped. A chest radiograph should be obtained to evaluate the presence of thymoma. Resection of thymoma usually reverses PRCA. Thymoma may be present in up to one-third of cases of PRCA. In the presence of evidence for persistent parvovirus infection (giant pronormoblasts, underlying immunosuppression), intravenous immunoglobulin is usually successful at treating the infection. PRCA that has been shown not to be due to thymoma, drugs, infection, or cancer is usually caused by an autoimmune mechanism and requires immunosuppressive therapy. Prednisone alone or with ATG, cyclosporine, azathioprine, or cyclophosphamide will successfully treat two-thirds of patients. Relapses may occur, but responses to a second or subsequent course of the same or alternative therapy are common. Progression to leukemia is rare (<5 percent).

MYELODYSPLASTIC SYNDROMES

Myelodysplastic syndromes, also referred to as preleukemic disorders, oligoblastic leukemia, or smoldering leukemia, are a group of acquired blood disorders that often progress to acute leukemia and are characterized by pancytopenias and low reticulocyte counts associated with a bone marrow that is typically normocellular or hypercellular with cells displaying overt morphologic abnormalities or dysplastic changes (alterations in size, shape, and organization of cells). Hematopoiesis in MDS is ineffective and, as a result, patients are pancytopenic in spite of having a cellular marrow.

In Western developed countries, MDSs are diagnosed in about 1 to 10 per 100,000 people every year; approximately 3000 new cases are expected each year in the United States. The rising incidence in recent years probably reflects increased awareness, better diagnostic criteria, and perhaps increased exposure to agents such as drugs or chemicals contributing to its etiology. Primary (or idiopathic) MDS may occur at any age, but is more common in elderly patients and is rare in children and young adults. The median age is usually between 70 and 80. Primary MDS is more common in males. The annual incidence is about 25 per 100,000 after age 70 years, comparable to that for chronic lymphocytic leukemia. The incidence of therapy-related (or secondary) MDS, particularly in younger patients, is increasing as more tumors are cured with radiation therapy and chemotherapy.

ETIOLOGY Although the causes of MDS are not well understood, certain factors are known to be contributory, including certain genetic and congenital anomalies, as well as exposure to radiation and to mutagenic chemicals.

Genetic and Congenital Factors Children with Down's syndrome have an increased risk of developing MDS and other forms of leukemia. Other genetic disorders prominently associated with MDS include Fanconi's anemia and von Recklinghausen's disease (neurofibromatosis).

Radiation Epidemiologic studies have linked MDS with exposure to high or repeated doses of ionizing radiation (x-rays and gamma rays). Atomic bomb survivors had 20- to 25-fold increase in the incidence of leukemia and MDS. Similarly, patients with cancers treated with high-dose radiation therapy, such as Hodgkin's disease and breast cancer, have a higher incidence of *therapy-related MDS*.

Chemicals and Drugs Individuals exposed over long periods to benzene have an increased higher incidence of MDS and other leukemias. Alkylating agents used in chemotherapy are known to induce therapy-related MDS.

Aplastic Anemia Of patients with aplastic anemia who are treated with immunosuppressive agents, 30 to 60 percent develop morphologic changes in the marrow cells and/or chromosome abnormalities consistent with the diagnosis of MDS, many years after the diagnosis of aplastic anemia. Similarly, a proportion of children with congenital neutropenia treated chronically with G-CSF develop this disorder.

PATHOGENESIS MDSs are clonal acquired disorders affecting the hematopoietic stem cells. Clonality has been demonstrated not only by the presence of clonal chromosome abnormalities but also through the study of glucose-6-phosphate dehydrogenase isoenzyme patterns and analysis of DNA polymorphism at X chromosome–linked loci. These studies have shown that MDS results from neoplastic transformation of the pluripotent stem cell with involvement of myeloid and, much less commonly, of lymphoid cell lineages.

The myeloid cells in MDS have not lost their ability to proliferate and differentiate, but they do undergo an abortive maturation resulting in an inadequate production of mature blood cells. As a result, most MDS patients have a cellular marrow but have low blood cell counts. Ineffective hematopoiesis is a hallmark of MDS. The ineffectiveness of the marrow cell production results from extensive intramedullary apoptotic cell death of myeloid precursors. The molecular basis of this phenomenon is not known.

CLINICAL MANIFESTATIONS MDSs are difficult to diagnose early in the course of the disease. The major difficulty in detecting MDS in its early stages is that patients are often asymptomatic. It is not uncommon for the disease to be discovered accidentally during a routine physical examination or a blood test. When symptoms do appear, they usually manifest in very subtle and varied forms of general malaise. Most common are complaints attributable to anemia, namely weakness, fatigue, palpitations, dizziness, headaches, and irritability. Thrombocytopenia may be manifested by excessive bleeding after a minor injury or surgical procedure, or by abnormal or unexplained skin bruises. Women may also present with heavy menstrual periods. Infections as a presenting symptom are less common and are usually associated with very severe neutropenia (neutrophil count <200/μL). A small proportion of patients present with a chronic or recurrent vasculitic skin rash.

The physical examination in patients with MDS is usually remarkable for anemia-related findings, such as pallor and tachycardia. Hepatosplenomegaly is rare and, if present, is usually moderate, except in patients with chronic myelomonocytic leukemia (CMML). Lymphadenopathy and purpura are uncommon.

DIAGNOSIS Since the symptoms outlined above are similar to those of other bone marrow failure syndromes, acute and chronic leukemia, and many other serious diseases, the diagnosis of MDS in patients with unexplained cytopenias requires careful morphologic evaluation of the blood and bone marrow cells.

Peripheral Blood The blood of a patient with MDS exhibits cytopenias involving one or multiple lineages. The reticulocyte count is low, indicating that the anemia is secondary to defective marrow production. Substantial anisocytosis with normocytic or mildly macrocytic indices is present. Some red blood cells may be macrocytic with a mean corpuscular volume of over 100 fL and exhibit abnormalities such as Howell-Jolly bodies, Abbott rings, and basophilic stippling. Nucleated red blood cells are not uncommon, and often they exhibit dysplastic changes. Mature neutrophils may have hypolobulated nuclei (pseudo Pelger-Huet anomaly) and very few or absent intracytoplasmic granules. In addition, immature granulocytes can be seen in the peripheral blood. A peculiar feature of MDS is an increase in the number of monocytes. Monocytosis is a distinctive feature of the CMML variant. Platelets in blood smears are often large and agranular. Rarely, micromegakaryocytes can be seen in peripheral blood.

Bone Marrow   The confirmation of the diagnosis of MDS requires the morphologic examination of marrow elements. The bone marrow samples are analyzed for three important features: the cellularity, the number of blasts and ringed sideroblasts, and the presence of dysplastic changes. The marrow cellularity in MDS is typically normal or hypercellular. However, some cases present with a hypocellular marrow. The blast count and the number of ringed sideroblasts are important for defining the MDS subtype. The marrow cells of most patients with MDS exhibit dysplastic changes. Dyserythropoietic changes include nuclear abnormalities (multinuclearity, nuclear fragmentation, bizarre nuclear shape, abnormal mitosis, internuclear bridging, and abnormally dense chromatin), cytoplasmic abnormalities (Howell-Jolly bodies, defective hemoglobinization, and ringed sideroblasts), as well as nuclear-cytoplasmic asynchrony (dense chromatin nucleus with poorly hemoglobinized cytoplasm). The most common dysgranulopoietic changes are hypogranulation and hyposegmentation. The most frequent dysmegakaryopoietic changes are micromegakaryocytosis, megakaryocytes with multiple small nuclei, and hypolobulation. Sometimes dysplasia is subtle, requiring evaluation by an experienced hematologist.

Cytogenetic Studies   Cytogenetic analysis of the marrow is an important diagnostic tool. Approximately half of patients with primary MDS and about 75 percent of patients with therapy-related MDS have chromosomal abnormalities. There is no single distinguishing chromosomal abnormality associated with MDS, but there are abnormalities that are more frequent, such as monosomy 7, 5q−, and trisomy 8. A variety of translocations are also common.

Molecular studies have also demonstrated an increased incidence of mutations involving the *ras, cFms* [monocyte colony-stimulating factor (M-CSF) receptor], *p53* and *RB* oncogenes in the hematopoietic cells of patients with MDS, and have identified some of the genes involved in specific chromosome deletions and translocations, such as loss of the interferon regulatory factor (IRF-1) gene in the 5q− abnormality, and the generation of a tel-PDGF-beta fusion gene in the t(5,12) translocation associated with CMML. The loss of a tumor suppressor gene such as *IRF-1* has been hypothesized to play a role in the pathogenesis of the disease.

CLASSIFICATION   In 1976 and 1982, a group of hematologists from France, America, and Britain (FAB) published criteria providing a standardized and uniform basis for the diagnosis of MDS and a definition of subtypes. The FAB criteria are based on morphologic characteristics, including the blood and marrow blast count, the monocyte count, the presence of ringed sideroblasts, and the presence of Auer rods. There are five well-defined subtypes: *refractory anemia* (RA), *refractory anemia with ringed sideroblasts* (RARS), *refractory anemia with excess blasts* (RAEB), *refractory anemia with excess*

blasts in transformation (RAEB-t), and *chronic myelomonocytic leukemia* (CMML). The criteria used to distinguish the MDS subtypes are shown in Table 110-3.

In addition to these subtypes, there are less common variants of MDS, such as *hypocellular MDS* and *myelofibrotic MDS*, that are not included in this international classification. In contrast to most cases of MDS, the bone marrow of hypocellular MDS exhibits decreased cellularity, and the few remaining cells exhibit dysplasia. Myelofibrotic MDS is characterized by pancytopenia, minimal organomegaly, and a hypercellular bone marrow with fibrosis, trilineage dysplasia, and atypical megakaryocytic proliferation.

DIFFERENTIAL DIAGNOSIS   Although the diagnosis of MDS is based on morphologic changes seen in the peripheral blood and bone marrow, none of these changes is specific for MDS. However, if these changes are associated with a clonal chromosomal abnormality, the diagnosis of MDS can be safely established. Cytopenias and dysplastic changes can also result from other etiologies, such as drugs, infections, toxic exposure, rheumatologic disorders, hypersplenism, vitamin deficiencies, tumors infiltrating the bone marrow, acute leukemia, and aplastic anemia.

Vitamin Deficiency   Deficiencies of vitamins B_{12}, folic acid, and particularly vitamin B_6 can induce a hematologic picture similar to that of MDS. Therefore, serum levels of these vitamins should be measured, and attention should be paid to other symptoms that are associated with vitamin deficiency, e.g., neurologic symptoms in B_{12} deficiency.

Aplastic Anemia   The blood and marrow picture of aplastic anemia and hypocellular MDS are very similar. Hypocellular MDS is sometimes difficult to distinguish from aplastic anemia, particularly when the dysplastic changes in the few remaining cells are subtle and there are no chromosomal abnormalities.

Paroxysmal Nocturnal Hemoglobinuria   Although PNH more often presents with a picture of aplastic anemia, the blood and marrow picture is sometimes indistinguishable from that of MDS. Flow cytometry detects the absence of GPI-linked proteins.

Aleukemic Acute Leukemia   Some patients with acute leukemia can present with pancytopenia without circulating blasts. The FAB has established that the diagnosis of acute leukemia should be made if the marrow blast count is >30 percent.

Acute and Chronic Myelofibrosis   In acute myelofibrosis, the marrow is fibrotic, and the cells are mostly blasts, which in most instances are megakaryoblasts. In chronic myelofibrosis, organomegaly is prominent.

Other: Myelophthisic Anemia, Cirrhosis   Metastasis of certain malignancies to the marrow may induce cytopenias with circulating immature marrow cells suggestive of MDS. The differential diagnosis of marrow metastasis from MDS requires a marrow biopsy study. Additional studies are usually necessary to exclude other pathologies.

COURSE OF THE DISEASE AND PROGNOSIS   The course of MDS is closely related to two main factors: the severity of the cytopenia and the number of blasts. Patients with low-risk MDS (<5 percent blasts), which includes RA and RARS, usually have a long

Table 110-3

French-American-British (FAB) Classification of Myelodysplastic Syndromes

Fab Type	% of Cases	% Blasts Marrow	% Blasts Blood	% Ringed Sideroblasts*	Monocytes	Dyspoiesis	Auer Rods
RA	28	<5	<1	<15	Rare	+	Absent
RARS	24	<5	<1	>15	Rare	+	Absent
RAEB	23	5–20	<5	<15	Rare	+ +	Absent
CMML	16	1–20	<5	<15	$>1 \times 10^9/L$	+ +	Absent
RAEB-t	9	20–30	>5	<15	Variable	+ +	+/−

* A ringed sideroblast is shown in **Plate IV-39**.

ABBREVIATIONS: RA, refractory anemia; RARS, refractory anemia with ringed sideroblasts; RAEB, refractory anemia with excess blasts; CMML, chronic myelomonocytic leukemia; RAEB-t, refractory anemia with excess blasts in transformation.

chronic phase with progressive worsening of the pancytopenia. Many patients succumb to complications associated with the pancytopenia or to the measures taken to treat them. For instance, patients who have received multiple red cell transfusions develop progressive hemochromatosis. Some of the low risk MDS patients eventually develop acute leukemia and die of its complications.

Patients with high-risk MDS usually have more severe cytopenias and a higher frequency of transformation to acute leukemia, which correlates with the number of blasts. However, many patients may die of complications associated with neutropenia, thrombocytopenia, and, less frequently, secondary hemochromatosis.

The prognosis for patients with MDS is shown in Table 110-4. Patients with RAEB and RAEB-t generally have a higher rate of progression to acute leukemia and a shorter survival. In contrast, patients with RA and RARS have a better prognosis. Patients with CMML have an intermediate prognosis. In addition to the FAB classification, the presence of chromosomal abnormalities has been shown the have a significant prognostic value. Patients with no chromosomal abnormalities have a lower chance of developing leukemia and a higher chance of longer survival. More refined prognostic scoring systems are based on the age, the number of blasts, the severity of pancytopenia, and the presence of chromosomal abnormalities.

℞ TREATMENT

Allogeneic bone marrow transplantation (BMT) is the only curative treatment for MDS. Unfortunately, this treatment is only applied to the minority of MDS patients who are under 55 years of age and have histocompatible donors. For all other patients, supportive therapy is the mainstay of the management. The results achieved with other approaches, such as chemotherapy, have not altered the natural history of the disease.

Supportive Therapy   Red cell and platelet transfusions and the use of antibiotics to treat infection constitute the most common therapies used in MDS patients. Although patients can receive many red cell and platelet transfusions, secondary hemochromatosis and alloimmunization limit repeated and prolonged use of these treatments. In heavily transfused patients, iron chelation with deferoxamine may prevent or delay the complications associated with hemochromatosis.

Hematopoietic Growth Factors   Hematopoietic growth factors can induce improvements in targeted cell counts in a relatively small proportion of patients. Those patients who do respond require continuous administration of growth factor to maintain the response. In some patients, progression to acute leukemia may be facilitated by chronic administration of cytokines. Erythropoietin and G-CSF are the most beneficial in MDS. Erythropoietin is effective in improving red cell production only in patients with low serum erythropoietin levels. G-CSF is beneficial in MDS patients who are neutropenic and have an infection. The increase in neutrophil counts in these cases can be lifesaving. The prophylactic use of G-CSF is not recommended unless the neutrophil count is $<200/\mu L$.

Vitamin Therapy, Steroid Hormones, and Immunosuppressive Agents   Certain vitamins, such as B_6, B_{12}, and folic acid, may be of help in some patients with MDS, since the increased but ineffective production of blood cells may deplete the body of these vitamins. Vitamin deficiency can worsen the pancytopenia. Glucocorticoids are of limited benefit in most patients with MDS, and their prolonged use can cause serious side effects. Androgens improve the blood counts of only a small proportion of patients with MDS. Administration of immunosuppressive agents, specifically antithymocyte globulin and/or cyclosporine, improves the blood counts of some patients with hypocellular MDS. These agents have not been systematically evaluated in patients with the other variants of MDS.

Differentiation Therapy   A prominent feature of MDS is the inability of the transformed marrow cells to fully differentiate to functional cells. Retinoic acids, vitamin D_3, and interferon α can induce the differentiation of immature malignant cell lines in vitro. Unfortunately, the use of these differentiation agents in the treatment of MDS has been disappointing. Most trials have demonstrated only a limited benefit in a very small proportion of patients.

Low-Dose Chemotherapy   Cytosine arabinoside, azacytidine, and topotecan, when given at low doses, can induce responses in some patients with MDS. These agents do not induce differentiation. They suppress the growth of the leukemic clone and allow the few remaining normal clones to repopulate the bone marrow and give rise to normal blood cells. Unfortunately, these responses are transient and are achieved in only a minority of patients.

Intensive (High-Dose) Chemotherapy   Chemotherapeutic agents given at high doses, as in the treatment of acute leukemia, can also induce remission in 40 to 60 percent of MDS patients. Such remissions are short-lived. Intensive chemotherapy often induces serious side effects, but it can be of some benefit in high-risk MDS patients who are candidates for BMT. Intensive chemotherapy is usually employed in patients with advanced forms of MDS, and it should not be used in older patients, since toxic side effects can be fatal in this age group.

Bone Marrow Transplantation   A bone marrow transplant from a histocompatible sibling can be curative in up to 60 percent of patients with MDS. The problems that have limited the success of BMT in MDS are mainly the transplant-related complications and recurrence of the disease in the post-transplant period. In MDS, GVHD is a common transplant-related complication, since the majority of MDS patients are older adults, in whom GVHD is more frequent. Post-transplant disease relapse is a major complication for those patients who have an excess of blasts at the time of transplantation. Of patients with RAEB and RAEB-t, 25 to 50 percent relapse within the first 2 years after the transplantation, versus <1 percent for patients with RA or RARS. Two approaches are being used to overcome this limitation. The first invokes intensive myeloablative treatments immediately before transplant in an attempt to eradicate the MDS. The higher intensity of these regimens is associated with a higher morbidity and mortality. Another approach invokes treatment of the patient with conventional induction chemotherapy to achieve remission or a phase of MDS without excess blasts and then perform BMT. Unfortunately, HLA-matched sibling donors are identified in no more than 25 to 30 percent of patients with MDS. Transplants from matched unrelated donors or partially mismatched related donors are associated with complications; particularly severe acute and chronic GVHD and infections have limited their success.

MYELOPHTHISIC ANEMIA

Replacement of the marrow with fibrosis (see Plate IV-34), often accompanied by a leukoerythroblastic response (neutrophilia, immature granulocytes, nucleated red cells, teardrop-shaped red cells) in the peripheral blood (see Plate IV-12), can occur as a primary hematologic disease called myeloid metaplasia or myelofibrosis (see Chap. 111) or as a secondary process called myelophthisis. The obliteration of the marrow space by fibrosis may be a reaction to invading tumor cells, infectious agents, particularly *Mycobacterium tuberculosis* or fungi, lipid storage diseases such as Gaucher's disease, or granulomas (e.g., sarcoidosis). In addition, in a rare congenital bone disease, osteopetrosis, the failure of osteoclasts to remodel bone can lead to

Table 110-4

Survival and Leukemic Transformation in Myelodysplastic Syndrome

Syndrome	Median Survival in Months (Range)	% Leukemic Transformation (Range)
RA	37 (19–64)	11 (0–20)
RARS	49 (21–76)	5 (0–15)
CMML	22 (8–60+)	20 (3–55)
RAEB	9 (7–15)	23 (11–50)
RAEB-t	6 (5–12)	48 (11–75)

obliteration of the marrow space with bone and fibrous tissue. The tumors associated with marrow fibrosis are both hematopoietic (hairy cell leukemia, acute and chronic leukemia, lymphoma, Hodgkin's disease, myeloma) and epithelial (especially breast, lung, prostate, stomach) in origin. Many cytokines produced by tumor cells, during a chronic inflammatory response, or by cells resident in the bone marrow may stimulate fibroblast expansion including transforming growth factor β and platelet-derived growth factor. However, the cause of myelophthisis is usually not defined. Patients usually have normocytic, normochromic anemia with characteristic teardrop red cells suggesting membrane damage done by collagen fibers, low reticulocyte count, and circulating normoblasts. Platelet counts are reduced but granulocyte counts are normal or increased initially. The marrow fibrosis is often associated with extramedullary hematopoiesis (and sometimes hepatosplenomegaly) that maintains neutrophil production but fails to generate adequate red cells and platelets. Marrow may be difficult to aspirate ("dry tap"), but biopsy reveals fibrosis and usually the primary process—tumor or granuloma—is apparent. Therapy is aimed at the primary process. Some of the cancers that produce myelophthisis are more treatable than others. It is crucial to rule out tuberculosis and fungal infections that may be treatable.

BIBLIOGRAPHY

APLASTIC ANEMIA

BACIGALUPO A et al: Antithymocyte globulin, cyclosporine, and granulocyte colony-stimulating factor in patients with acquired severe aplastic anemia: A pilot study of the EBMT working party. Blood 85:1348, 1995

GLUCKMAN E et al: Marrow transplantation for severe aplastic anemia: Influence of conditioning and graft-versus-host disease prophylaxis regimens on outcome. Blood 79:269, 1992

MARSH JCW et al: Haemopoietic growth factors in aplastic anemia: A cautionary note. Lancet 344:172, 1994

STORB R et al: Cyclophosphamide combined with anti-thymocyte globulin in preparation for allogenic marrow transplants in patients with aplastic anemia. Blood 84:941, 1994

YOUNG N et al: The treatment of severe aplastic anemia. Blood 85:3367, 1995

MYELODYSPLASTIC SYNDROMES

ANDERSON JE et al: Allogeneic bone marrow transplantation for 93 patients with myelodysplastic syndromes. Blood 82:677, 1993

BENNETT JM et al: Proposals for the classification of the myelodysplastic syndromes. Br J Haematol 51:189, 1982

MOREL P et al: Cytogenetic analysis has strong independent prognostic value in the novo myelodysplastic syndromes and can be incorporated in a new scoring system: A report of 408 cases. Leukemia 7:1315, 1993

RAZA A et al: Apoptosis in bone marrow biopsy samples involving stromal and hematopoietic cells in 50 patients with myelodysplastic syndromes. Blood 86:268, 1995

SAN MIGUEL JF et al: Myelodysplastic syndromes. Crit Rev Oncol Hematol 23:57, 1996

SANZ GF et al: Two regression models and a scoring system for predicting survival and planning treatment in myelodysplastic syndromes: A multivariate analysis of prognostic factors in 370 patients. Blood 74:395, 1989

111   *Jerry L. Spivak*

POLYCYTHEMIA VERA AND OTHER MYELOPROLIFERATIVE DISEASES

Polycythemia vera, idiopathic myelofibrosis, essential thrombocytosis, and chronic myelogenous leukemia are commonly classified together under the rubric *the chronic myeloproliferative disorders*, because their pathophysiology involves the clonal expansion of a multipotent hematopoietic progenitor cell with the overproduction of one or more of the formed elements of the blood. These entities may transform into acute leukemia naturally or as a consequence of mutagenic treatment. However, while polycythemia vera, idiopathic myelofibrosis, essential thrombocytosis, and chronic myelogenous leukemia share similar phenotypic characteristics, chronic myelogenous leukemia is genotypically distinct from the other three disorders because it alone is associated with translocation of genetic material between the long arms of chromosomes 9 and 22, resulting in the production of the unique fusion protein, bcr-abl. Furthermore, in contrast to the other chronic myeloproliferative disorders, based on its natural history, chronic myelogenous leukemia is more appropriately considered as a form of leukemia. → *This is discussed in Chap. 112 with the leukemias.*

POLYCYTHEMIA VERA

Polycythemia vera is a clonal disorder involving a multipotent hematopoietic progenitor cell in which there is overproduction of phenotypically normal red cells, granulocytes, and platelets in the absence of a recognizable physiologic stimulus. Polycythemia vera is the most common of the chronic myeloproliferative disorders, with a frequency as high as 29 per 100,000. It spares no age group amongst adults. In several families, vertical transmission has been documented, establishing a genetic basis for the disorder. Although a slight overall male predominance has been observed, our experience suggests female predominance within the reproductive age range.

ETIOLOGY   The etiology of polycythemia vera is unknown. Although nonrandom chromosome abnormalities such as 20q-, trisomy 8 or 9 have been documented in a small percentage of untreated polycythemia vera patients, no consistent cytogenetic abnormality has been associated with the disorder and no specific genetic defect has yet been identified. In contrast to normal erythroid progenitor cells, polycythemia vera erythroid progenitor cells can grow in vitro in the absence of erythropoietin. However, this phenotypic abnormality is not specific for polycythemia vera and has been documented in essential thrombocytosis as well as in patients with erythrocytosis of undefined etiology in the presence of a normal or high serum erythropoietin level. Polycythemia vera erythroid progenitor cells are more resistant to apoptosis induced by erythropoietin deprivation, but the biochemical basis for this is unknown. Additionally, the transformed hematopoietic progenitor cells in polycythemia vera, as in other myeloproliferative disorders, exhibit clonal dominance and by an unknown mechanism suppress the proliferation of normal hematopoietic progenitor cells. As a consequence, eventually the circulating formed elements of the blood represent only progeny of the transformed clone.

CLINICAL FEATURES   Although massive splenomegaly may be the initial presenting sign in polycythemia vera, most often the disorder is first recognized by the discovery of a high hemoglobin or hematocrit, and with the exception of aquagenic pruritus, no symptoms distinguish polycythemia vera from other causes of erythrocytosis.

Uncontrolled erythrocytosis can, of course, lead to neurologic symptoms such as vertigo, tinnitus, headache, and visual disturbances. Systolic hypertension also accompanies an elevated red cell mass. In some patients venous or arterial thrombosis may be the presenting manifestation of polycythemia vera. Intraabdominal venous thrombosis is particularly common and may be catastrophic when there is sudden compromise of the hepatic vein. Indeed, polycythemia vera should be suspected in any patient who develops the Budd-Chiari syndrome. Digital ischemia may also occur. Easy bruising, epistaxis, or gastrointestinal hemorrhage may be observed, and given the overactive hematopoietic system, polycythemia vera patients are frequently hypermetabolic. Because isolated erythrocytosis is a common initial presentation for polycythemia vera but no clonal marker is available for the disease, the first task of the physician is to distinguish this autonomous clonal form of erythrocytosis from the many other types of erythrocytosis, most of which are correctable (Table 111-1). It is helpful in this regard to understand the physiology of erythropoietin, the primary regulator of erythropoiesis.

Table 111-1

Causes of Absolute Erythrocytosis

Hypoxia
    Carbon monoxide intoxication
    High altitude
    Pulmonary disease
    High-affinity hemoglobin
    Sleep-apnea syndrome
    Respiratory center dysfunction
    Supine hypoventilation
    Right-to-left cardiac shunts
Renal disease
    Renal cysts
    Hydronephrosis
    Renal artery stenosis
    Focal glomerulonephritis
    Renal transplantation
Tumors
    Hypernephroma
    Hepatoma
    Cerebellar hemangioblastoma
    Adrenal adenoma
    Pheochromocytoma
    Meningioma
    Uterine fibromyoma
Familial (with normal hemoglobin function)
Bartter's syndrome
Androgen therapy
Recombinant erythropoietin therapy
Polycythemia vera

Under normal circumstances, erythropoiesis is regulated by the glycoprotein hormone erythropoietin. Erythropoietin, which in adults is produced primarily in the kidneys and to a small extent in the liver, promotes the proliferation of erythroid progenitor cells, maintains their survival, and facilitates their differentiation. Because erythropoietin acts as a survival factor, it is constitutively produced and, like the red cell mass, its level in a given individual is constant as long as tissue oxygenation is adequate. The plasma erythropoietin level, like the red cell mass, does differ amongst individuals but in adults is not affected by either age or gender. Erythropoietin production is regulated at the level of gene transcription. Hypoxia is the only physiologic stimulus that increases the number of cells producing erythropoietin, and as a corollary, the production and metabolism of erythropoietin are independent of its plasma level. Thus, in the absence of renal or hepatic disease, plasma erythropoietin levels reflect erythropoietin production, and because there is only one form of erythropoietin in the circulation, the assay for plasma erythropoietin provides a measure of renal erythropoietin production and, therefore, a surrogate assay for tissue hypoxia. There is a caveat to this, however. Erythropoietin is a potent hormone, active at the picomolar level, and its production is tightly regulated. Thus, until the hemoglobin level falls below 105 g/L, the plasma erythropoietin level does not rise outside the normal range. This is not meant to imply that an increase in erythropoietin production does not occur as the hemoglobin level falls below normal, but because the normal range for plasma erythropoietin is wide (4 to 26 mU/mL), unless the patient's baseline level is known, any increase will not be recognized until the hemoglobin falls below 105 g/L. Thereafter, there is a log-linear inverse correlation between the levels of plasma erythropoietin and hemoglobin. With erythrocytosis, erythropoietin production is suppressed; this suppression reflects not only the increase in tissue oxygen transport associated with the increase in red cell number but also an additional negative-feedback mechanism that is independent of oxygen transport but is related to the erythrocytosis-induced increase in blood viscosity alone. The summation of both these mechanisms accounts for the paradoxical observation that many patients with hypoxic erythrocytosis due to cyanotic congenital heart disease or obstructive lung disease have a "normal" plasma erythropoietin

Table 111-2

Effect of Sampling Time on the Determination of the Red Cell Mass by Isotope Dilution

Time after Injection of ^{51}C-labeled Erythrocytes, min	Red Cell Mass, mL/kg
60	54
90	62
180	68
240	71

level. Of course, normal is relative in this circumstance because the normal range is so wide. Nevertheless, the plasma erythropoietin level is a useful diagnostic test in patients with isolated erythrocytosis, because an elevated level essentially excludes polycythemia vera as the cause for the erythrocytosis.

DIAGNOSIS When confronted with an elevated hemoglobin or hematocrit level, it is important to obtain previous values to determine the duration of this laboratory abnormality. Because the hemoglobin or hematocrit level is affected by the plasma volume, and there is not a linear correlation between hematocrit and red cell mass, a red cell mass determination must also be performed to distinguish absolute erythrocytosis from relative erythrocytosis due to a reduction in plasma volume alone (also known as *stress* or *spurious erythrocytosis* or *Gaisböck's syndrome*). The importance of red cell mass determination cannot be overemphasized because in polycythemia vera, in contrast to erythropoietin-driven erythrocytosis, the plasma volume is frequently elevated, not only masking the true extent of red cell mass expansion but often its presence. Indeed, a significant proportion of patients with polycythemia vera with a hematocrit within the normal range actually have an elevated red cell mass, and this is particularly true in patients with a substantial splenomegaly. Failure to recognize this phenomenon is undoubtedly the basis for many of the reported instances of hepatic or portal vein thrombosis in patients with a so-called undefined myeloproliferative disorder.

The only reliable method for determining the red cell mass is by isotope dilution using the patient's ^{51}C-tagged red cells; extrapolations made by determining directly only the plasma volume are unacceptable. Furthermore, to allow ample time for equilibration of the labeled red cells, measurements should be made over a period of no less than 90 min. Only in this manner can an adequate assessment of red cell mass be obtained (Table 111-2).

Once the presence of erythrocytosis has been established, its cause must be determined. An elevated plasma erythropoietin level suggests either an hypoxic cause for erythrocytosis or autonomous erythropoietin production, in which case assessment of pulmonary function and an abdominal computed tomography scan to evaluate renal and hepatic anatomy are appropriate. As mentioned above, a normal erythropoietin level does not exclude an hypoxic cause for erythrocytosis. In polycythemia vera, in contrast to hypoxic erythrocytosis, the arterial oxygen saturation is normal. However, a normal oxygen saturation does not exclude a high-affinity hemoglobin as a cause for erythrocytosis, and it is here that documentation of previous hemoglobin levels and a family study become important. Because there is no clonal marker for polycythemia vera, clinical guidelines have been proposed to define the disease. A modified version is provided in Table 111-3. However, it must be strongly emphasized that these are only guidelines; they do not establish clonality, and in some patients only with time will the

Table 111-3

Suggested Criteria for the Clinical Diagnosis of Polycythemia Vera*

Elevated red cell mass
Normal arterial oxygen saturation
Splenomegaly
In the absence of splenomegaly:
    Leukocytosis and thrombocytosis
Plasma erythropoietin level less than 4 mU/mL

* It must be emphasized that these criteria do not establish clonality.

underlying disorder become apparent. Diagnostic ambiguity, however, does not preclude the initiation of therapy as described below.

Other laboratory studies that may prove useful diagnostically include the red cell count, mean corpuscular volume, and red cell distribution width (RDW). Only three situations cause microcytic erythrocytosis: β-thalassemia trait, hypoxic erythrocytosis, and polycythemia vera. However, with β-thalassemia trait the RDW is normal, whereas with hypoxic erythrocytosis and polycythemia vera, the RDW is usually elevated. A properly made blood smear from a patient with erythrocytosis will be virtually unreadable due to the marked elevation in red cell count, but as mentioned above, there are no specific histologic abnormalities of the leukocytes or platelets in polycythemia vera. However, when these are also elevated the diagnosis is assured. In many patients, the leukocyte alkaline phosphatase is also increased, as is the uric acid. Elevated serum vitamin B_{12} or B_{12}-binding capacity may be present.

Although much has been written about bone marrow histology in polycythemia vera, a bone marrow aspirate and biopsy will provide no specific diagnostic information, and unless there is a need to establish the presence of myelofibrosis or exclude some other disorder, these procedures cannot be routinely recommended. The presence of a cytogenetic abnormality such as trisomy 8 or 9 or 20q- in the setting of an expansion of the red cell mass of course supports the existence of a clonal etiology for this expansion. However, as mentioned above, there is no specific cytogenetic abnormality associated with polycythemia vera, and the absence of a cytogenetic marker does not exclude the diagnosis.

COMPLICATIONS The major clinical complications of polycythemia vera relate directly to the increase in blood viscosity associated with elevation of the red cell mass and indirectly to the increased turnover of red cells, leukocytes, and platelets and the attendant increase in uric acid and histamine production. The latter appears to be responsible for the increase in peptic ulcer disease seen in patients with polycythemia vera and also for the pruritus associated with this disorder, although little formal proof for this has been obtained. A sudden massive increase in spleen size is another problem and can be associated with splenic infarction or progressive cachexia. Myelofibrosis and myeloid metaplasia can also develop with transfusion-dependent anemia, but the frequency with which these occur has never been established in a prospective study. Although acute nonlymphocytic leukemia is reported to have a higher incidence in polycythemia vera, the incidence of acute leukemia in untreated patients is low and there is no correlation between the development of leukemia and disease duration, suggesting that other factors such as the type of treatment employed may be more important in this regard than the disease itself.

Erythromelalgia is a curious syndrome of unknown etiology involving primarily the lower extremities and manifested usually by erythema, warmth, and pain of the affected appendage and occasionally digital infarction. It occurs with a variable frequency in patients with a myeloproliferative disorder and is usually responsive to salicylates. It is not unlikely that some of the central nervous system symptoms observed in patients with polycythemia vera represent a variant of erythromelalgia.

As mentioned earlier, if left uncontrolled, erythrocytosis can lead to intravascular thrombosis that frequently involves vital organs such as the liver, heart, brain, or lungs. Patients with massive splenomegaly are particularly prone to thrombotic events because the associated increase in plasma volume masks the true extent of the red cell mass elevation as measured by the hematocrit or hemoglobin level. A "normal" hematocrit or hemoglobin level in a polycythemia vera patient with massive splenomegaly should be considered as indicative of an elevated red cell mass until proven otherwise.

℞ **TREATMENT**
Polycythemia vera is generally an indolent disorder whose clinical course can run many decades, and its medical management should reflect the tempo of the disorder. Maintenance of the hemoglobin level at 140 g/L or less in men and 120 g/L or less in women is mandatory to avoid the thrombotic complications associated with an elevated red cell mass. It cannot be emphasized too strongly that thrombosis due to erythrocytosis is the most significant complication of this disorder. Statements to the effect that the erythrocytosis of polycythemia vera cannot be controlled by phlebotomy alone, or that phlebotomy-induced iron deficiency is detrimental metabolically as well as contributing to the hyperviscosity observed in this disorder, unfortunately reflect a total misunderstanding of the pathophysiology of polycythemia vera and its treatment. Phlebotomy serves initially to reduce hyperviscosity by bringing the red cell mass into the normal range. Periodic phlebotomies thereafter serve to maintain the red cell mass within the range of normal and to induce a state of iron deficiency, which prevents an accelerated reexpansion of the red cell mass. In most polycythemia vera patients, once an iron-deficient state is achieved, phlebotomy is usually required only at 3-month intervals. Although both phlebotomy and iron deficiency, in addition to the disease itself, tend to increase the platelet count, it cannot be emphasized enough that there is no correlation between thrombocytosis and thrombosis in polycythemia vera, in contrast to the strong correlation between erythrocytosis and thrombosis in this disease. Indeed, the use of salicylates as a tonic against thrombosis in polycythemia vera patients is potentially harmful, and salicylates should be employed only to treat erythromelalgia. There is also no routine indication for the use of oral anticoagulants, which may be difficult to employ owing to the artifactual imbalance between the test tube anticoagulant and plasma that occurs when blood from these patients is assayed for prothrombin or partial thromboplastin activity. Asymptomatic hyperuricemia requires no therapy, but allopurinol should be administered to avoid further elevation of the uric acid when chemotherapy is employed to reduce splenomegaly or leukocytosis-associated pruritus. Generalized pruritus intractable to antihistamines can be a major problem in polycythemia vera, and both hydroxyurea and psoralens with ultraviolet light in the A range (PUVA) therapy have been used effectively in this situation. Asymptomatic thrombocytosis requires no therapy. When it is necessary to lower the platelet count or reduce splenomegaly, hydroxyurea or recombinant interferon α have been useful, although each can be associated with significant side effects and neither is totally effective. Anagrelide, a quinazolin derivative and platelet antiaggregant that also lowers the platelet count, is currently under investigation for the treatment of thrombocytosis, but attention to the platelet count should not be allowed to divert attention from the important issues in polycythemia vera. A reduction in platelet number may be necessary in the treatment of erythromelalgia if salicylates are not effective, or if the thrombocytosis is associated with migraine-like symptoms, but any therapeutic decision in this regard should be made only after the red cell mass has been reduced to normal. Alkylating agents and ^{32}P are leukemogenic in polycythemia vera, and their use should be avoided. In some patients, massive splenomegaly unresponsive to reduction by hydroxyurea or interferon α therapy and associated with intractable weight loss will require splenectomy.

When approached from this perspective, patients with polycythemia vera can be expected to live long and useful lives, and reports of limited life expectancy due to thrombotic events appear to be primarily a consequence of inadequate control of the red cell mass, which in turn reflects a lack of understanding of the basic pathophysiology of this unique disorder. Furthermore, in those patients with isolated erythrocytosis for which the cause is not clear, potentially harmful treatment can be avoided because chemotherapy is never indicated to control the red cell mass unless venous access is impossible.

IDIOPATHIC MYELOFIBROSIS

Idiopathic myelofibrosis (other designations include *agnogenic myeloid metaplasia* or *myelofibrosis with myeloid metaplasia*) is a clonal disorder of a multipotent hematopoietic progenitor cell of unknown etiology characterized by marrow fibrosis, myeloid metaplasia with extramedullary hematopoiesis, and splenomegaly. Idiopathic myelofibrosis is uncommon, and in the absence of a specific clonal marker, establishing this diagnosis is difficult because myelofibrosis and myeloid metaplasia with splenomegaly are also features of both polycythemia vera and chronic myelogenous leukemia. Furthermore, myelofibrosis and splenomegaly occur in a variety of benign and malignant disorders (Table 111-4), many of which are amenable to specific therapies not effective in idiopathic myelofibrosis. In contrast to the other chronic myeloproliferative disorders and so-called acute or malignant myelofibrosis, which can occur at any age, idiopathic myelofibrosis primarily afflicts individuals in their sixth decade or later.

ETIOLOGY The etiology of idiopathic myelofibrosis is unknown. Although nonrandom chromosome abnormalities such as 20q-, 13q-, and trisomy 21 are not uncommon, no specific cytogenetic abnormality has been identified. There is also no correlation between the degree of myelofibrosis and the extent of extramedullary hematopoiesis. Analysis of collagen synthesis in this disorder has revealed overproduction of type III collagen, and this notion has been hypothetically linked to overproduction of platelet-derived growth factor or transforming growth factor β, but no biochemical substantiation for this notion has been forthcoming. Importantly, fibroblasts in idiopathic myelofibrosis are not part of the neoplastic clone, while the nature of collagen synthesis in other disorders complicated by myelofibrosis (Table 111-4) has not been evaluated to the same extent.

CLINICAL FEATURES There are no specific signs or symptoms associated with idiopathic myelofibrosis. Early in the course of the disease, most patients are asymptomatic and are usually detected by the discovery of splenic enlargement during a routine examination. Evaluation of a blood smear reveals the characteristic features of extramedullary hematopoiesis: teardrop-shaped red cells, nucleated red cells, myelocytes, and promyelocytes; myeloblasts may also be present but have no prognostic significance. Anemia, usually mild initially, is the rule, while the leukocyte and platelet counts are either normal or increased but either can be depressed. Mild hepatomegaly may accompany the splenomegaly, and both the LDH and serum alkaline phosphatase can be elevated. The leukocyte alkaline phosphatase can be low, normal, or elevated. Marrow may be unaspirable due to the myelofibrosis, and bone x-rays may reveal osteosclerosis. If it is exuberant, extramedullary hematopoiesis can cause ascites, pulmonary hypertension, intestinal or ureteral obstruction, intracranial hypertension, pericardial tamponade, spinal cord compression, or skin nodules. Splenic enlargement can be sufficiently rapid to cause splenic infarctions with fever and pleuritic chest pain. Hyperuricemia and secondary gout may ensue.

DIAGNOSIS While the clinical picture described above is characteristic of idiopathic myelofibrosis, it cannot be emphasized too strongly that all of the clinical features described can be observed in polycythemia vera or chronic myelogenous leukemia. Indeed, massive

Table 111-4

Causes of Myelofibrosis

Carcinoma metastatic to the marrow
Infection
Lymphoma
Hodgkin's disease
Acute leukemia (lymphocytic or myelocytic)
Hairy cell leukemia
Multiple myeloma
Chronic myelogenous leukemia
Polycythemia vera
Idiopathic myelofibrosis
Systemic mastocytosis
Thorium dioxide (Thorotrast) exposure
Systemic lupus erythematosus
Renal osteodystrophy

splenomegaly commonly masks erythrocytosis in polycythemia vera, and reports of intraabdominal thromboses in idiopathic myelofibrosis undoubtedly represent instances of unrecognized polycythemia vera. Furthermore, as mentioned above, many other disorders have features that overlap with idiopathic myelofibrosis but respond to distinctly different therapies. Therefore, the diagnosis of idiopathic myelofibrosis is one of exclusion, which requires that the disorders listed in Table 111-4 be ruled out.

The presence of teardrop-shaped red cells, nucleated red cells, myelocytes, and promyelocytes establishes the presence of extramedullary hematopoiesis; the presence of leukocytosis, thrombocytosis with large and bizarre platelets, as well as circulating myeloblasts suggests the presence of a myeloproliferative disorder as opposed to a secondary form of myelofibrosis (Table 111-4). Marrow is usually not aspirable due to increased marrow reticulin, but marrow biopsy will reveal a hypercellular marrow with trilineage hyperplasia and, in particular, increased megakaryocytes, but there are no characteristic morphologic abnormalities that distinguish idiopathic myelofibrosis from the other chronic myeloproliferative disorders. Splenomegaly due to extramedullary hematopoiesis may be sufficiently massive to cause portal hypertension and variceal formation. In some patients, as mentioned above, exuberant extramedullary hematopoiesis can dominate the clinical picture. An intriguing feature of idiopathic myelofibrosis is the occurrence of autoimmune abnormalities such as immune complexes, antinuclear antibodies, rheumatoid factor, or a positive Coombs' test. Whether these represent a host reaction to the disorder or are involved in its pathogenesis is unknown. Cytogenetic analysis, of either blood or marrow, if aspirable, is useful both to exclude chronic myelogenous leukemia and for prognostic purposes, because complex karyotype abnormalities portend a poor prognosis in idiopathic myelofibrosis.

COMPLICATIONS Idiopathic myelofibrosis is a chronic disorder but with a median survival of only 5 years, a duration much shorter than for polycythemia vera or essential thrombocytosis. The natural history of idiopathic myelofibrosis is one of inexorable marrow failure with transfusion-dependent anemia and increasing organomegaly. Patients with this disorder are prone to deep-seated tissue infections, particularly of the lungs. As with chronic myelogenous leukemia, idiopathic myelofibrosis can evolve from a chronic phase to an accelerated phase with constitutional symptoms and increasing marrow failure. In approximately 10 percent of patients, the disorder terminates in a rapidly progressive form of acute leukemia for which therapy is usually ineffective. Important prognostic factors with respect to disease acceleration include anemia, thrombocytopenia, age, the presence of complex cytogenetic abnormalities, and constitutional symptoms such as unexplained fever, night sweats, or weight loss. Any nonrandom cytogenetic abnormality is associated with a shortened life span, and the presence or development of multiple cytogenetic abnormalities is highly indicative of disease acceleration.

℞ **TREATMENT**

There is no specific therapy for idiopathic myelofibrosis. Anemia may be exacerbated by deficiency of folic acid or iron, and in rare instances, pyridoxine therapy has been effective. However, anemia is more often due to ineffective erythropoiesis not compensated for by the extramedullary hematopoiesis in the spleen and liver, and neither therapy with androgens nor recombinant erythropoietin has been consistently effective. A red cell splenic sequestration study can be useful in establishing the presence of hypersplenism, for which splenectomy is indicated. Splenectomy may also be necessary if splenomegaly impairs alimentation and should be performed before cachexia sets in. In this situation, splenectomy should not be avoided because of concern over rebound thrombocytosis, loss of hematopoietic capacity, or compensatory hepatomegaly. Such concerns have no clinical foundation. Allopurinol should be used to control significant hyperuricemia and hydroxyurea has proved useful in some patients for controlling organomegaly. The role of recombinant interferon α is still undefined, and its side effects are more pronounced in the older individuals who are affected with this disorder.

ESSENTIAL THROMBOCYTOSIS

Essential thrombocytosis (other designations include *essential thrombocythemia*, *idiopathic thrombocytosis*, *primary thrombocytosis*, *hemorrhagic thrombocythemia*) is a clonal disorder of unknown etiology involving a multipotent hematopoietic progenitor cell and is manifested clinically by the overproduction of platelets in the absence of a definable cause. Essential thrombocytosis is an uncommon disorder, but its frequency is unknown because there is no clinically applicable clonal marker with which to distinguish it from the more common nonclonal, reactive forms of thrombocytosis (Table 111-5). The epidemiology of essential thrombocytosis is also not well defined, not only because of the lack of a clonal marker but also because clinical recognition of thrombocytosis is unlikely in the largely asymptomatic persons affected by this disorder. As a consequence, essential thrombocytosis was formerly considered to be a disease of the elderly and to be responsible for significant morbidity due to hemorrhage or thrombosis. However, with the advent of electronic particle counters and the widespread application of platelet counting, it is now clear that not only can essential thrombocytosis occur at any age in adults but also in the absence of symptoms or disturbances of hemostasis. Furthermore, there is an unexplained female predominance, in contrast to the reactive forms of thrombocytosis where no gender bias exists. Because thrombocytosis is often a prominent feature of the other chronic myeloproliferative disorders, the treatment and prognosis of which differ from essential thrombocytosis, and because, as noted above, no clonal marker is available for the disorder, clinical criteria have been proposed to distinguish it from the other chronic myeloproliferative disorders (Table 111-6). It cannot be emphasized too strongly, however, that these criteria do not establish clonality; therefore, they are truly useful only in identifying disorders such as chronic myelogenous leukemia, polycythemia vera, or myelodysplasia, which can masquerade as essential thrombocytosis, as opposed to establishing the presence of essential thrombocytosis. Furthermore, it has not been sufficiently emphasized that, as with "primary" erythrocytosis, there may exist nonclonal, benign forms of thrombocytosis that have not been recognized simply because we currently lack the diagnostic tools to do so.

ETIOLOGY Megakaryocytopoiesis and platelet production are still incompletely defined processes, but with the identification and molecular cloning of the genes for thrombopoietin and its receptor, the c-Mpl proto-oncogene, the physiology of thrombopoiesis should soon be clarified. As in the case of early erythroid and myeloid progenitor cells, early megakaryocytic progenitors require the presence of interleukin 3 and stem cell factor for optimal proliferation, and their subsequent development is enhanced by interleukins 6 and 11. However, megakaryocyte maturation and terminal differentiation still require the presence of thrombopoietin.

Table 111-5

Causes of Thrombocytosis

Iron-deficiency anemia
Hyposplenism
Postsplenectomy*
Malignancy
Collagen vascular disease
Inflammatory bowel disease
Infection
Hemolysis
Hemorrhage
Polycythemia vera
Idiopathic myelofibrosis
Essential thrombocytosis
Chronic myelogenous leukemia
Idiopathic sideroblastic anemia
Myelodysplasia (5q- syndrome)
Postsurgery
Rebound (cessation of ethanol intake, correction of vitamin B_{12}
  or folate deficiency)

* If the platelet count is greater than $2 \times 10^6/\mu L$, the etiology is most likely a myeloproliferative disorder.

Table 111-6

Suggested Criteria for the Clinical Diagnosis of Essential Thrombocytosis*

Platelet count $\geq 500,000/\mu L$
Absence of a known cause of reactive thrombocytosis (see Table 111-5)
Absence of the Ph chromosome and the bcr-abl gene rearrangement
Normal red cell mass
Presence of marrow iron
Absence of myelofibrosis
Absence of myelodysplasia clinically and by cytogenetic analysis
Splenomegaly

* The concept that a platelet count greater than $1 \times 10^6/\mu L$ distinguishes essential thrombocytosis from other causes of thrombocytosis has no clinical validity.

Megakaryocytes are unique amongst hematopoietic progenitor cells because they undergo endomitotic as opposed to mitotic reduplication of their genome. In the absence of thrombopoietin, endomitotic megakaryocytic reduplication and, by extension, the cytoplasmic development necessary for platelet production are impaired. Like erythropoietin, thrombopoietin is produced in both the liver and the kidneys, and an inverse correlation between the platelet count and plasma thrombopoietic activity has been observed. However, whether thrombopoietin, like erythropoietin, behaves like a hormone and whether it acts as a mitogen, a survival factor, or both is unknown. In contrast to erythropoietin, but like its myeloid counterparts granulocyte and granulocyte-macrophage colony stimulating factors, thrombopoietin not only enhances the proliferation of its target cells but also activates their end-stage product, in this case the platelet. Whether thrombopoietin has a role in essential thrombocytosis or whether its production, like that of erythropoietin in polycythemia vera, is suppressed is also unknown.

The clonality of essential thrombocytosis has been established by the use of the isoenzymes of glucose-6-phosphate dehydrogenase in patients who are hemizygous for this gene, by the use of X-linked DNA polymorphisms, and by the identification of nonrandom, although variable cytogenetic abnormalities. Such studies together with in vivo clonal assays for hematopoietic progenitor cells have shown that the multipotent hematopoietic progenitor cell involved in this disorder can vary; in some patients lymphocytes contained the same clonal marker as the megakaryocytes, erythrocytes, and myeloid cells, whereas in others the lymphocytes were not involved. Similar observations have been made in polycythemia vera. Furthermore, a number of families have been described in which essential thrombocytosis was inherited, in one instance as an autosomal dominant trait. In one kindred, in addition to essential thrombocytosis, idiopathic myelofibrosis and polycythemia vera were also individually documented.

CLINICAL FEATURES Clinically, essential thrombocytosis is most often identified incidentally when a platelet count is obtained during the course of a routine or diagnostic evaluation. Occasionally, review of previous platelet counts will reveal that an elevation was present but overlooked. There are no symptoms or signs specific for essential thrombocytosis, but these patients do have hemorrhagic and thrombotic tendencies expressed as easy bruising for the former or microvascular occlusions for the latter, which may be manifested by erythromelalgia, migraine, or transient ischemic attacks. Physical examination is generally unremarkable except for the presence of mild splenomegaly. Massive splenomegaly is more characteristic of the other myeloproliferative disorders, particularly polycythemia vera or idiopathic myelofibrosis.

Anemia is unusual, but a mild neutrophilic leukocytosis is not. The blood smear, however, is most remarkable for the number of platelets present, some of which may be very large. The leukocyte alkaline phosphatase score is either normal or elevated. The large mass of circulating platelets may prevent the accurate measurement of serum potassium due to the release of platelet potassium upon blood clotting. This hyperkalemia is a laboratory artifact and is not associated with any ECG abnormalities. Similarly, arterial oxygen measurements can be rendered inaccurate unless the blood is collected on ice. The prothrombin and partial thromboplastic times are normal, while abnormalities of platelet function such as a prolonged bleeding time and impaired platelet aggregation can be present. However, in spite of much study, there are neither characteristic nor consistent platelet function abnormalities associated with essential thrombocytosis, and there is no correlation between any platelet function test and the presence of clinically significant bleeding or thrombosis.

The elevated platelet count may hinder the collection of a marrow aspirate, but marrow biopsy usually reveals both megakaryocyte hyperplasia and hypertrophy, as well as an overall increase in marrow cellularity. An increase in marrow reticulin may be present, but if extensive, another diagnosis should be considered. The absence of stainable iron demands an explanation, because iron deficiency alone can cause thrombocytosis and absent marrow iron is a feature of polycythemia vera.

While nonrandom cytogenetic abnormalities have been identified in essential thrombocytosis, there is no consistently identifiable abnormality and, in particular, none involving chromosomes 3 and 1 where the genes for thrombopoietin and its receptor c-Mpl, respectively, are located.

DIAGNOSIS Given the important role for certain cytokines in megakaryocytopoiesis, it is not surprising that thrombocytosis is encountered in a variety of clinical disorders (Table 111-5) in which production of these cytokines is increased. Thus, the first obligation of the physician when confronted with a high platelet count is to determine if it is a consequence of another disorder. In this regard, a cytogenetic evaluation is mandatory to determine if the thrombocytosis is due to chronic myelogenous leukemia or a myelodysplastic disorder such as the 5q- syndrome. Because the bcr-abl translocation can be present in the absence of the Ph chromosome, it has been suggested that gene rearrangement studies should be performed in all patients with thrombocytosis in whom a cytogenetic study is normal. Anemia and ringed sideroblasts are not features of essential thrombocytosis, but they are features of idiopathic refractory sideroblastic anemia, in which thrombocytosis can also occur. The presence of massive splenomegaly should suggest the possibility of another myeloproliferative disorder, and in this setting a red cell mass determination is mandatory because substantial splenomegaly can mask the presence of erythrocytosis. In this regard, it should be noted that essential thrombocytosis can evolve into polycythemia vera and that often only the passage of time will resolve the true nature of the underlying myeloproliferative disorder.

COMPLICATIONS Perhaps no other situation in clinical medicine has caused otherwise astute physicians to intervene inappropriately more often than thrombocytosis, particularly if the platelet count is greater than 1×10^6 per microliter. It is commonly believed that a high platelet count must cause intravascular stasis and thrombosis; however, no controlled clinical study has ever established either association.

Indeed, quite to the contrary, very high platelet counts are associated primarily with hemorrhage, while platelet counts of less than a million are more often associated with thrombosis. In this regard, the role of platelet mass as opposed to platelet number has never been resolved. This is not meant to imply that an elevated platelet count cannot cause symptoms in a patient with essential thrombocytosis, but rather that the focus should be on the patient, not the platelet count. For example, some of the most dramatic neurologic problems in essential thrombocytosis are migraine-related but may respond only to lowering of the platelet count; other symptoms may be a manifestation of erythromelalgia and respond simply to platelet cyclooxygenase inhibitors such as aspirin, without resorting to a reduction in platelet number. Still others may represent an interaction between an atherosclerotic vascular system and a high platelet count, and others may have no

relationship to the platelet count whatsoever. A fundamental problem in this area is that the existing literature is largely uncritical and evolved in an era when not only was essential thrombocytosis often not distinguished from polycythemia vera but other causes for hypercoagulability, such as the lupus anticoagulant or factor V Leiden, were not yet appreciated.

℞ TREATMENT

An elevated platelet count per se in an asymptomatic patient requires no therapy, and before any therapy is initiated in a patient with thrombocytosis, the cause of symptoms must be clearly identified to be a consequence of the elevated platelet count. Although the literature is replete with extreme measures, such as plasmapheresis and cytotoxic therapy for reducing the platelet count in symptomatic patients with thrombocytosis, none of these measures has ever been documented to be more than anecdotally efficacious and none can be recommended. Furthermore, the development of acute leukemia in patients with essential thrombocytosis treated with ^{32}P or alkylating agents without any proof of benefit from such therapy should be a strong caution to their use. If platelet reduction is deemed necessary on the basis of neurologic symptoms refractory to salicylates, the physician currently has the choice of hydroxyurea, a mutagen, or recombinant interferon α, an immunosuppressive agent with substantial side effects. Anagrelide, a quinazolin derivative, can reduce the platelet count and is currently undergoing clinical trials, but it is neither uniformly effective nor without significant side effects. Bleeding associated with thrombocytosis usually responds to ε-aminocaproic acid, which can be given prophylactically before and after elective surgery. As more clinical experience is acquired, it appears that essential thrombocytosis is more benign than previously thought, and that evolution to acute leukemia is more likely to be a consequence of prior chemotherapy than of the disease itself. In managing patients with thrombocytosis, the physician's first obligation is to do no harm.

BIBLIOGRAPHY

ADAMSON JW et al: Polycythemia vera: Stem cell and probable clonal origin of the disease. N Engl J Med 295:913, 1976

BUSS DH et al: The incidence of thrombotic and hemorrhagic disorders in association with extreme thrombocytosis: An analysis of 129 cases. Am J Hematol 20:365, 1985

JACOBSON RJ et al: Agnogenic myeloid metaplasia: A clonal proliferation of hematopoietic stem cells with secondary myelofibrosis. Blood 51:189, 1978

MERTENS F et al: Karyotypic patterns in chronic myeloproliferative disorders: Report on 74 cases and review of the literature. Leukemia 5:214, 1990

SCHAFER AI: Bleeding and thrombosis in the myeloproliferative disorders. Blood 64:1, 1984

————: Essential thrombocythemia. Prog Hemost Thromb 10:69, 1991

VARKI A et al: The syndrome of idiopathic myelofibrosis: A clinicopathologic review with emphasis on the prognostic variables predicting survival. Medicine 62:353, 1983

112 *Meir Wetzler, Clara D. Bloomfield*

ACUTE AND CHRONIC MYELOID LEUKEMIA

The myeloid leukemias are a heterogeneous group of diseases characterized by infiltration of the blood, bone marrow, and other tissues by neoplastic cells of the hematopoietic system. In 1996, the estimated number of new myeloid leukemia cases in the United States was 12,800. These leukemias comprise a spectrum of malignancies that, untreated, range from among the most rapidly fatal to ones that are slowly growing. Based on their untreated course, the myeloid leukemias have traditionally been designated *acute* or *chronic*.

INCIDENCE The incidence of acute myeloid leukemia (AML) is approximately 2.3 per 100,000 people per year, and the age-adjusted incidence is higher in men than in women (2.9 versus 1.9). There has been no significant change in AML incidence over the past 20 years. The incidence of AML increases with age; under 65 years the incidence is 1.3, and above 65 the incidence is 12.2.

ETIOLOGY Heredity, radiation, chemical and other occupational exposures, and drugs have been implicated in the development of AML. There is no direct evidence of a viral etiology in AML.

Heredity Certain syndromes with somatic cell chromosome aneuploidy, e.g., Down (trisomy of chromosome 21), Klinefelter (XXY and variants), and Patau (trisomy of chromosome 13), are associated with an increased incidence of AML. Inherited diseases with excessive chromatin fragility, e.g., Fanconi anemia, Bloom syndrome, ataxia telangiectasia, and Kostmann syndrome, are also associated with an increased incidence of AML.

Radiation Survivors of the atomic bomb explosions in Japan during World War II had an increased incidence of myeloid leukemias that peaked 5 to 7 years following exposure. Therapeutic radiation alone seems to add little risk of acute leukemia but can increase the risk in people exposed to alkylating agents (see below).

Chemical and Other Exposures Benzene, used as a solvent in the chemical, plastic, rubber, and pharmaceutical industries, has been associated with an increased incidence of AML. Smoking and exposure to petroleum products, paint, embalming fluids, ethylene oxide, herbicides, pesticides, and electromagnetic fields have also been associated with an increased risk of AML.

Drugs Antineoplastic drugs are the leading cause of drug-related (or treatment-associated) AML. Alkylating agent–associated leukemias occur on average 48 to 72 months after exposure and demonstrate aberrations in chromosomes 5 and 7. Topoisomerase II inhibitor–associated leukemias occur 1 to 3 years after exposure and usually have aberrations involving chromosome band 11q23. Similarly, chloramphenicol, phenylbutazone, and less commonly chloroquine and methoxypsoralen have been reported to result in bone marrow failure that may evolve into AML.

CLASSIFICATION The categorization of acute leukemia into biologically distinct groups is based on morphology, cytochemistry, and immunophenotype as well as cytogenetic and molecular techniques.

Morphologic and Cytochemical Classification The diagnosis of AML is established by the presence of at least 30 percent myeloblasts in blood and/or bone marrow. Myeloblasts have nuclear chromatin that is uniformly fine or lacelike in appearance and large nucleoli (two to five per cell). If specific cytoplasmic granules, Auer rods, or the nuclear folding and clefting characteristic of monocytoid cells are not present, the morphologic features observed under light microscopy may not be sufficient to clarify the diagnosis.

AML is classified based on morphology and cytochemistry according to the French, American, and British (FAB) schema, which includes eight major subtypes, M0 to M7 (Table 112-1). In AML of the M1 variety, a positive myeloperoxidase reaction (i.e., presence of myeloperoxidase in 3 percent or more of the blast cells) may be the only distinguishing characteristic separating it from L2 acute lymphoblastic

Table 112-1

The French-American-British (FAB) Classification of AML

FAB subtype	% of Cases	Morphology	Cytochemistry[a] Peroxidase/ Sudan Black	Nonspecific Esterase[b]	Flow Cytometry[c]	Cytogenetic Association[d]
M0: Minimally differentiated leukemia	2–3	Immature morphology	−	−	CD13 or 33	
M1: Myeloblastic leukemia without maturation	20	Few blasts with azurophilic granules, Auer rods, or both	3% or more	−	CD13, 33, 34, HLA-DR +	
M2: Myeloblastic leukemia with maturation	25–30	Azurophilic granules, Auer rods are often present Variant: M2Baso: blasts with basophil granules	+	−	CD13, 15, 33, 34, HLA-DR +	t(8;21) (q22;q22)[e]
M3: Hypergranular promyelocytic leukemia	8–15	Hypergranular promyelocytes with multiple Auer rods Variant: hypogranular	+	−	CD13, 15, 33, HLA-DR −	t(15;17) (q22;q11-12)
M4: Myelomonocytic leukemia	20–25	Granulocytic and monocytic blasts Variant: M4Eo: increase in abnormal marrow eosinophils	+/−	+	CD11b, 13, 14[f], 15, 33, HLA-DR +	M4Eo: inv(16) (p13q22)
M5: Monocytic leukemia	20–25	M5a undifferentiated M5b differentiated	−	+	CD11b, 13, 14[f], 15, 33, HLA-DR +	11q23 translocations
M6: Erythroleukemia (Di Guglielmo's disease)	5	Erythroblasts >50% of nucleated cells, myeloblasts >30% of nonerythroid cells	+/−	−	CD33, HLA-DR +	
M7: Megakaryoblastic leukemia	1–2	Megakaryoblasts >30% of all nucleated cells	−	−	CD33, 41	

[a] Periodic acid Schiff staining is characteristic of the neoplastic erythroid precursors of M6.
[b] With fluoride inhibition.
[c] The antigens listed are the most commonly expressed in the given FAB subtype.
[d] A subset of M2 and M5 demonstrate the listed cytogenetic abnormality.
[e] CD19 positivity is characteristically associated with t(8;21).
[f] CD14, if present denotes monocytic lineage.

SOURCE: JM Bennett et al, Ann Intern Med 103:620, 1985; BD Cheson et al, J Clin Oncol 8:813, 1990.

leukemia (ALL). The M2 and M3 types are most strongly peroxidase positive, while M4 exhibits less intense activity, and the peroxidase reaction occurs to a limited extent or not at all in M5 and M7 subtypes. Other cytochemical stains useful in diagnosis are shown in Table 112-1.

Immunophenotypic Classification The phenotype of human myeloid leukemia cells can be studied by multiparameter flow cytometry following labeling with monoclonal antibodies to cell-surface antigens. Results are useful both for diagnosis and prognosis. For example, M0, which is characterized by immature morphology and no lineage-specific cytochemical reactions, is diagnosed by flow cytometric demonstration of the myeloid-specific antigens cluster designation (CD) 13 or 33. Similarly, M7 can often be diagnosed only by expression of the platelet-specific antigen CD41 or by electron-microscopic demonstration of myeloperoxidase. An example of the use of immunophenotyping for prognosis is the poor outcome shown in patients whose leukemic cells coexpress CD13, CD14, and CD34. In addition, the use of multiparameter flow cytometry to detect residual disease following therapy in AML is under investigation by several groups.

Chromosomal Classification Chromosomal analysis of the leukemic cell currently provides the most important pretreatment prognostic information in AML. Only two cytogenetic abnormalities have been invariably associated with a specific FAB group: t(15;17)(q22;q11-12) with M3 and inv(16)(p13q22) with M4Eo. However, many chromosomal abnormalities have been associated primarily with one FAB group, including t(8;21)(q22;q22) with M2, and t(9;11)(p22;q23), and other translocations involving 11q23, with M5. Many of the recurring chromosomal abnormalities in AML have been associated with specific clinical characteristics. More commonly associated with younger age are t(8;21) and t(15;17), and with older age, del(5q) and del(7q). Lymphadenopathy is associated with inv(16); chloromas with t(8;21); disseminated intravascular coagulation (DIC) with t(15;17); central nervous system involvement with inv(16); and diabetes insipidus, fever, and infection, all with monosomy 7. The reasons for most associations of chromosomal abnormalities with specific clinical features are unknown.

Molecular Classification The many recurring cytogenetic abnormalities led to molecular studies, which have revealed several genes that may play a causative role in leukemogenesis. The 15;17 translocation, characteristic of M3 leukemia, encodes a chimeric protein, Pml/Rarα, which is formed by the fusion of the retinoic acid receptor α (RARα) gene from chromosome 17 and the promyelocytic leukemia (PML) gene from chromosome 15. The RARα gene encodes a member of the steroid/thyroid hormone receptor family of transcription factors. After binding retinoic acid, Rarα can bind to specific DNA sequences in the promoters of a variety of genes. The 15;17 translocation juxtaposes PML with RARα in a head-to-tail configuration that is under the transcriptional control of PML. There are three different breakpoints within the PML gene leading to various fusion proteins, which may correlate with remission duration. The molecular data are intriguing given the excellent clinical response of M3 patients with t(15;17) to tretinoin (all-*trans*-retinoic acid or ATRA). In a rare form of M3 which has a related translocation, t(11;17)(q23;q21), the RARα gene is juxtaposed to the promyelocytic leukemia zinc finger gene from chromosome 11, resulting in a chimeric gene that renders the cells unresponsive to ATRA.

The inv(16), characteristic of M4Eo, results in a fusion of the core-binding factor β (CBFB) gene on the q arm and the myosin heavy chain (MYH11) gene on the p arm. The CBFB gene encodes a subunit of the transcription factor complex core-binding factor, also known as polyomavirus enhancer binding protein 2 gene. This gene is involved in the determination of differentiation-dependent and cell type–specific expression of the polyomavirus enhancer. Interestingly, Cbf proteins are composed of an α subunit, the Aml1 protein, and a β subunit, the Pebp2 protein. The 8;21 translocation involves the core-binding factor α (CBFA) gene on chromosome 21, more commonly

designated as the AML1 gene, which encodes a transcription factor that regulates myeloid cell differentiation. Unraveling the interactions between CBFA and CBFB may explain the differences and the similarities between inv(16)- and t(8;21)-associated leukemia.

Most translocations that involve 11q23 rearrange the ALL1 gene (also known as myeloid-lymphoid or mixed-lineage leukemia gene). The ALL1 gene has two regions that encompass multiple zinc fingers, and has at least two additional potential DNA-binding motifs. Abnormalities in the ALL1 gene are relatively common in patients with AML who do not have 11q23 rearrangements cytogenetically.

These various molecular aberrations are increasingly being used for diagnosis and detection of residual disease following treatment. At this point, the molecular information is useful for therapy only for M3 leukemia. However, antisense techniques to block translation of the specific transcripts are being developed for gene-directed therapy.

CLINICAL PRESENTATION **Symptoms** Patients with AML most often present with nonspecific symptoms that begin gradually or abruptly and are the consequence of anemia, leukocytosis, leukopenia or leukocyte dysfunction, or thrombocytopenia. Nearly half have had symptoms for 3 months or more before the leukemia is diagnosed.

Half mention fatigue as the first symptom, but most complain of fatigue or weakness at the time of diagnosis. Other nonspecific complaints, such as anorexia and weight loss, are common. Fever, with or without an identifiable infection, is the initial symptom in approximately 10 percent of patients. Similarly, signs of abnormal hemostasis (bleeding, easy bruising) are noted first in 5 percent of all cases. On occasion, bone pain, lymphadenopathy, nonspecific cough, headache, or diaphoresis are the presenting symptoms.

Rarely patients may present with symptoms from a mass lesion located in the soft tissues, breast, uterus, ovary, cranial or spinal dura, gastrointestinal tract, lung, mediastinum, prostate, bone, or other organs. The mass lesion represents a tumor of leukemic cells and is called a *granulocytic sarcoma*, or *chloroma*. Typical AML may occur simultaneously, later, or not at all in these patients. This rare presentation is more common in patients with t(8;21) translocations.

Physical Findings Fever, splenomegaly, hepatomegaly, lymphadenopathy, sternal tenderness, and evidence of infection and hemorrhagic tendencies are often found at diagnosis. Significant gastrointestinal bleeding, intrapulmonary hemorrhage, or intracranial hemorrhage occur most often in M3 leukemia. Bleeding associated with coagulopathies may also occur in M5 leukemia and with extreme degrees of leukocytosis or thrombocytopenia in other FAB subtypes. Retinal hemorrhages are detected in 15 percent of patients. Infiltration of the gingivae, skin, soft tissues, or the meninges with leukemic blasts at diagnosis is characteristic of the monocytic subtypes (M4 and M5).

Hematologic Findings Anemia is usually present at diagnosis and can be severe. The degree varies considerably irrespective of other hematologic findings, splenomegaly, or the duration of symptoms. The anemia is usually normochromic normocytic. Decreased erythropoiesis often results in a reduced reticulocyte count, and erythrocyte survival is decreased by accelerated destruction. Active blood loss also contributes to the anemia.

The median presenting leukocyte count is about 15,000/μL. Twenty-five to 40 percent of patients will have counts less than 5000/μL, and 20 percent will have counts greater than 100,000/μL. Fewer than 5 percent will have no detectable leukemic cells in the blood. There can be poor neutrophil function, demonstrated functionally by impaired phagocytosis and migration and morphologically by abnormal lobulation and deficient granulation.

Platelet counts under 100,000/μL are found at diagnosis in about 75 percent of patients, and about 25 percent of patients will have counts less than 25,000/μL. Both morphologic and functional platelet abnormalities can be observed. These include, for example, large and bizarre shapes with abnormal granulation and inability of platelets to aggregate or adhere normally to one another.

Pretreatment Evaluation Once the diagnosis of AML is suspected, a rapid evaluation and initiation of appropriate therapy should follow (Table 112-2). In addition to clarifying the subtype of leukemia,

Table 112-2

CHAPTER 112
Acute and Chronic Myeloid Leukemia 687

Diagnostic Evaluation of Patients with AML

History and physical examination
Hemoglobin level, leukocyte count (differential), platelet count
Bone marrow aspirate and biopsy
   Morphology
   Cytochemistry
   Cell membrane immunophenotyping
   Cytogenetics
   Molecular studies
   Cryopreservation of viable cells
Blood chemistries
   Hepatic enzymes, creatinine, serum electrolytes, lactic dehydrogenase, uric acid, calcium, phosphorus, lysozyme
Coagulation profile
   Prothrombin time, partial thromboplastin time, thrombin time, fibrinogen, fibrin split products
Chest roentgenogram
Electrocardiogram and evaluation of left ventricular ejection fraction
Blood type and HLA determination (also evaluate family members as potential blood component and allogeneic bone marrow donors)
Lumbar puncture (in symptomatic patients only)

initial studies should evaluate the overall functional integrity of the major organ systems, including the cardiovascular, pulmonary, hepatic, and renal systems. Factors that have prognostic significance, either for achieving complete remission (CR) or for predicting the duration of CR, should also be assessed before initiating treatment. Leukemic cells should be obtained from all patients and cryopreserved for future use as new tests become available. All patients should be evaluated for overt or inapparent infection.

The majority of patients are anemic and thrombocytopenic at presentation. Immediately after results of the initial studies are known, prompt replacement of the appropriate blood components, if necessary, should begin. Because qualitative platelet dysfunction or the presence of an infection may increase the likelihood of bleeding, evidence of hemorrhage justifies the immediate use of platelet transfusion, even if the platelet count is only moderately decreased.

Liver function tests will be abnormal in approximately 20 percent of patients at diagnosis. Because some chemotherapeutic agents are detoxified and excreted by the liver, drug dosages in patients with hepatic dysfunction may require modification. Some drugs, such as purine analogues and anthracyclines, can also be hepatotoxic and aggravate underlying liver disease.

Approximately 50 percent of patients will have a mild to moderate elevation of serum uric acid at presentation. Only 10 percent have marked elevations, but renal precipitation of uric acid and the nephropathy that may result are serious potential complications. The initiation of chemotherapy may aggravate hyperuricemia, and patients are usually immediately started on allopurinol and bicarbonate at diagnosis. Finally, lysozyme, a marker for monocytic differentiation, when present in high concentrations may be etiologic in renal tubular dysfunction, which could intensify other renal problems that often arise during the initial phases of the therapy.

PROGNOSTIC FACTORS The single most important factor related to an improved survival is attainment of CR. CR is defined following examination of both blood and bone marrow and should last ≥4 weeks. For a patient to be considered to have achieved CR, the blood neutrophil count must be ≥1500/μL and the platelet count ≥100,000/μL. Neither hemoglobin concentration nor hematocrit are considered in determining CR. Circulating blasts should not be present. While a rare blast may be detected in the blood during marrow regeneration, they should disappear on successive studies. Bone marrow cellularity should be >20 percent with trilineage maturation. The bone marrow should contain <5 percent blasts, and Auer rods should not be detected. Extramedullary leukemia should not be present. For patients in CR, reverse transcriptase polymerase chain reaction (RT-PCR) to detect AML-associated molecular abnormalities, and fluorescence in situ hybridization (FISH) to detect AML-associated cytogenetic aberrations are currently employed to detect residual disease. Although further study is needed, such detection of minimal residual disease may become a reliable discriminator between patients in CR who do or do not require additional and/or alternative therapies.

Many factors have been identified that influence the likelihood of entering CR. More recently, factors specifically related to the length of CR and curability have been determined. It is important to remember that prognostic factors are highly dependent on the treatment used. Age at diagnosis remains among the most important pretreatment risk factors, with advanced age (>60 years) being associated with a poorer prognosis primarily because of its influence on the patient's ability to survive induction therapy and thus achieve a CR. Chronic and intercurrent diseases impair tolerance to rigorous therapy; acute medical problems at diagnosis negatively influence the likelihood of survival. Performance status, independent of age, also influences ability to survive induction therapy and thus respond to treatment. Age may also influence outcome because AML in older patients may differ biologically. The leukemic cells in elderly patients more commonly express CD34 and the mdr1 efflux pump that conveys resistance to natural product-derived agents such as the anthracyclines (see below). Data also suggest that with each successive decade of age, a greater proportion of patients will have more resistant disease.

Chromosome findings at diagnosis are another important independent prognostic factor. Patients with t(8;21) and inv(16) have extremely good prognoses, while those with no cytogenetic abnormality or with t(15;17) have moderately favorable outcomes with high-dose cytarabine. Patients with del(5q), -7, and abnormalities involving 12p have a very poor prognosis. Patients with certain abnormalities, such as inv(3), do not achieve CR with standard induction chemotherapy.

A prolonged symptomatic interval preceding diagnosis is another pretreatment clinical feature that remains strongly associated with a lower CR rate and shorter survival. The duration of symptoms before diagnosis and the documented presence of an antecedent hematologic disorder before the emergence of leukemia are related factors. The CR rate has been lower in patients who have had anemia, leukopenia, and/or thrombocytopenia for more than 1 month before the diagnosis of acute leukemia when compared to those without such a history. In fact, responsiveness to chemotherapy appears to decline steadily as the duration of the antecedent disorder(s) increases. In addition, secondary AML developing following treatment with cytotoxic agents and/or irradiation for other malignancies has proved extremely difficult to treat successfully.

A number of prognostic factors have been reported in some series but not in others. An inverse relationship between the duration of CR and the presenting leukocyte count or absolute circulating myeloblast count has been reported. Among patients with hyperleukocytosis (>100,000/μL), those who are older or have pulmonary leukostasis, hepatomegaly, hyperbilirubinemia or hypofibrinogenemia, have been reported to be at a greater risk for early death during induction.

Although the FAB classification has not usually been found to be an independent prognostic factor, other characteristics of the leukemic cell have been reported, in some studies, to have prognostic significance. These include Auer rods, ultrastructural features, in vitro and in vivo growth characteristics and chemotherapeutic sensitivity, and immunophenotype. Recently, the importance of the multidrug resistance gene 1 has been suggested in several studies. This gene encodes a protein that actively pumps out a variety of lipophilic compounds (e.g., anthracyclines) from the cell. Patients whose leukemic cells express multidrug resistance gene 1 have had lower CR rates and decreased CR duration.

In addition to pretreatment variables, several treatment factors have been reported to correlate with prognosis in AML, in particular with CR duration. One is the rapidity with which the blast cells disappear from the blood following the institution of therapy. In addition, patients who achieve CR following one induction cycle have longer CR than those requiring multiple cycles. Patients whose marrow at the time of CR has fewer than 1 percent blasts also fare better.

℞ **TREATMENT**

Treatment of the newly diagnosed patient with AML is usually divided into two phases, induction and postremission management (Fig. 112-1). The initial goal in treatment is to eradicate the leukemia quickly and induce CR. Once CR is obtained, further strategies must be applied to prolong survival and establish cure.

Induction Chemotherapy The most commonly used CR induction regimens (for patients with all FAB subtypes except M3) consist of combination chemotherapy with cytarabine (cytosine arabinoside) and an anthracycline. Cytarabine is a cell cycle S-phase-specific antimetabolite that becomes phosphorylated to an active triphosphate form that interferes with DNA synthesis. Anthracyclines are DNA intercalaters. Their primary mode of action is considered to be interaction with topoisomerase II, leading to breakage of DNA. Cytarabine is usually administered as a continuous intravenous infusion at 100 to 200 mg/m² per day for 7 days. Anthracycline therapy generally consists of daunorubicin, 45 mg/m² intravenously on days 1, 2, and 3 of cytarabine given as above (*the 7 and 3 regimen*). Treatment with idarubicin, a new anthracycline, at 12 or 13 mg/m² per day for 3 days in conjunction with cytarabine by 7-day continuous infusion is at least as effective and may be superior to daunorubicin, according to several randomized trials.

Following induction chemotherapy, the bone marrow is examined when the blood counts reach normal levels or plateau to determine CR or residual leukemia. CR is usually achieved within 4 weeks of initiation of chemotherapy. If there is unequivocal persistent or recurrent leukemia in the bone marrow on day 14 or subsequently,

the patient has traditionally been retreated with cytarabine and an anthracycline in doses similar to those given initially but for 5 and 2 days, respectively. Our recommendation, however, is to change therapy in this setting. We prefer to give high-dose cytarabine (3 g/m² over 1 h every 12 h for a total of 12 doses, with a reduction to 1.5 g/m² for patients over 50 years of age) and an anthracycline (e.g., idarubicin 12 mg/m² daily for 3 days) as a second course of induction therapy for patients with clear-cut persistent or recurrent leukemia in a cellular marrow after one cycle of standard dose cytarabine and daunorubicin therapy. We also recommend consideration of bone marrow transplantation (BMT) early in the management of these patients.

With the 7 and 3 cytarabine/daunorubicin regimen outlined above, CR is achieved in 65 to 75 percent of adults with de novo AML. Two-thirds achieve CR after a single course of therapy, and one-third require two courses. Approximately 50 percent of patients who do not achieve a CR have a leukemia that is resistant to the therapy administered, and 50 percent do not achieve CR because of fatal complications of bone marrow aplasia or impaired recovery of normal stem cells.

High-dose cytarabine–based regimens have been used as initial remission-induction therapy in several single-arm clinical trials with very high CR rates reported following a single cycle of therapy. When given in high doses, more cytarabine may enter the cells, saturate the cytarabine-inactivating enzymes, and increase the intracellular levels of 1-β-D-arabinofuranylcytosine-triphosphate, the active metabolite incorporated into the DNA. Thus higher doses of cytarabine may increase the inhibition of DNA synthesis and thereby overcome resistance to standard-dose cytarabine. In two randomized studies, one by the Southwest Oncology Group (SWOG) and one by the Australian Leukemia Study Group (ALSG), high-dose cytarabine with an anthracycline produced CR rates similar to those seen with standard 7 and 3 regimens. However, the ALSG demonstrated that the CR duration was much longer following high-dose cytarabine as compared to standard-dose cytarabine. Another approach to using high-dose cytarabine would be as induction therapy in patients whose leukemic cells contain the inv(16), t(8;21), or RAS (named after the rat sarcoma virus) mutations, because these groups appear particularly likely to benefit from it.

The hematologic toxicity of high-dose cytarabine–based induction regimens has typically been greater than that associated with 7 and 3 regimens. A current trial at Roswell Park Cancer Institute suggests that administration of recombinant human granulocyte colony stimulating factor (G-CSF) beginning 12 h following completion of chemotherapy accelerates count recovery following high-dose cytarabine and anthracycline chemotherapy, such that hematologic toxicity does not exceed and is often less than that associated with 7 and 3 regimens without growth factor. When high-dose cytarabine regimens are used for patients over 50 years old, the cytarabine dose must be reduced (maximum dose 1.5 to 2 g/m²) because of the higher risk of cerebellar toxicity in older patients. All patients treated with high-dose cytarabine must be closely monitored for cerebellar toxicity. Full cerebellar testing should be performed before each dose, and further high-dose cytarabine should be withheld if evidence of cerebellar toxicity develops. For treatment-associated AML, the high-dose cytarabine and anthracycline combination has yielded better results than 7 and 3 in some, but not all, studies.

Because of the synergy between cytarabine and etoposide, etoposide was added to the 7 and 3 induction regimen in a randomized trial by the ALSG. Etoposide interacts with topoisomerase II, an enzyme that binds to DNA, producing temporary double strand breaks to control the degree of supercoiling. Etoposide stabilizes the DNA/topoisomerase II complex leading to permanent double strand DNA breaks. The results showed improved CR duration but no change in overall survival.

Supportive Care Measures geared to supporting patients through several weeks of granulocytopenia and thrombocytopenia are critical to the success of AML therapy. Patients with AML should be treated in centers expert in providing supportive measures for their management.

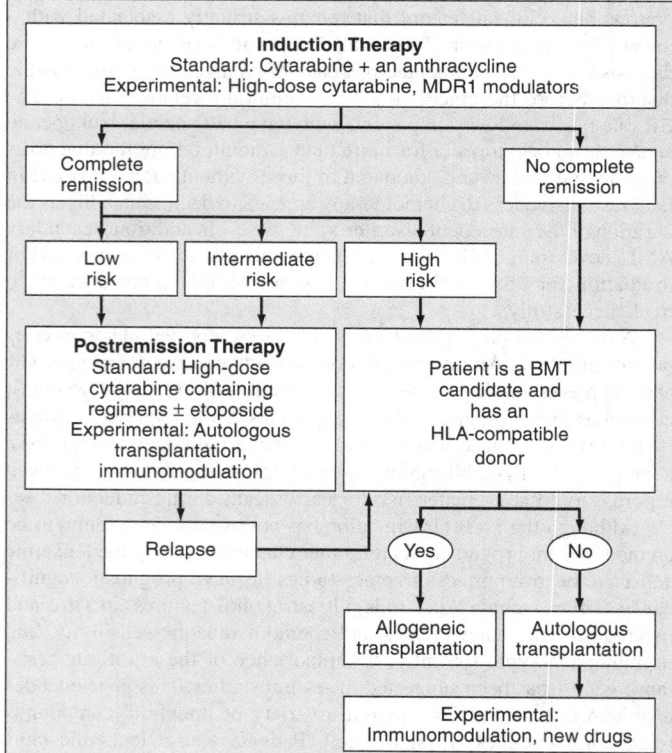

FIGURE 112-1 Flow chart for the therapy of newly diagnosed AML. For all forms of AML except M3, standard therapy includes a 7-day continuous infusion of cytarabine (100–200 mg/m² per day) and a 3-day course of daunorubicin (45 mg/m² per day) or idarubicin (12–13 mg/m² per day). Patients who achieve complete remission undergo some form of maintenance therapy with either high-dose cytarabine or high-dose combination chemotherapy with allogeneic marrow transplantation. Patients with AML M3 usually receive tretinoin together with combination chemotherapy for remission induction.

Recombinant hematopoietic growth factors have been incorporated into clinical trials in AML. These trials have been designed either to lower the infection rate after chemotherapy, to sensitize (prime) the leukemic blasts to chemotherapy, or to achieve both goals. Both G-CSF and granulocyte-macrophage colony stimulating factor (GM-CSF) have reduced the median time to neutrophil recovery by an average of 5 to 7 days. This accelerated rate of neutrophil recovery, however, has not always translated into significant reductions in infection rates. A randomized study from 22 centers in Europe demonstrated a higher CR rate, especially in patients with unfavorable cytogenetics, with G-CSF, as compared to placebo, used following completion of induction chemotherapy. A placebo-controlled, randomized study from the Eastern Cooperative Oncology Group has demonstrated longer median survival in patients treated with GM-CSF following induction therapy. The positive effects on CR rate and survival reported could reflect either reduced fatal infection rates or changes in leukemic cell proliferation. Effects on disease-free survival are not significant. The priming hypothesis is based on in vitro data showing enhanced sensitivity to cell cycle–specific chemotherapeutic agents by increasing the number of cells in S-phase. The use of growth factors for a short time (1 to 2 days) before and/or during chemotherapy has not supported this hypothesis. We favor the use of growth factors following chemotherapy for AML only in the setting of clinical trials, so that long-term follow-up data can be obtained to monitor for late adverse effects.

Megakaryocyte growth and development factor, thrombopoietin, may have a beneficial effect on treatment outcome by shortening the duration of thrombocytopenia. Clinical trials are ongoing.

Multilumen right atrial catheters should be inserted through a subcutaneous tunnel as soon as patients with newly diagnosed AML have been stabilized. They should be used thereafter for administration of intravenous medications and transfusions, as well as for blood drawing. The separation between the vascular access site and the exit site and the presence of a Dacron cuff in the subcutaneous channel reduce the risk of infectious complications. With meticulous attention to sterile technique in catheter placement and maintenance, catheters may often be left in place for months.

Adequate and prompt blood bank support is critical to therapy of AML. Platelet transfusions should be given as needed to maintain a platelet count above 20,000/μL. We believe that the platelet count should be kept at higher levels in febrile patients and during episodes of active bleeding or DIC. Measures that may be used in patients with poor posttransfusion platelet count increments include administration of platelets from human leukocyte antigen (HLA)-matched donors and intravenous immunoglobulin therapy. Red blood cell transfusions should be administered to keep the hemoglobin above 85 g/L (8.5 g/dL). Blood products leukodepleted by filtration should be used to avert or delay alloimmunization as well as febrile reactions. Blood products should also be irradiated to prevent graft-versus-host disease (GVHD). Cytomegalovirus (CMV)-negative blood products should be used for CMV-seronegative patients who are potential candidates for allogeneic BMT. Leukodepleted products are also effective for these patients if CMV-negative products are not available.

Infectious complications remain the major cause of morbidity and of death during induction and postremission chemotherapy for AML. Prophylactic administration of antibacterial antibiotics in the absence of fever is controversial. Oral nystatin or clotrimazole are recommended to prevent localized candidiasis. For patients who are herpes simplex virus–positive, acyclovir prophylaxis is effective in preventing reactivation of latent herpes infections.

Fever develops in the vast majority of AML patients, but infections are documented in only half of febrile patients. Early initiation of empiric broad-spectrum antibacterial and antifungal antibiotics has significantly reduced the number of patients dying of infectious complications (see Chap. 87). A combination of antibiotics adequate to treat both gram-negative and -positive organisms should be instituted at the onset of fever in a granulocytopenic patient, following clinical evaluation and procurement of cultures and roentgenograms aimed at documenting the source of fever. Specific antibiotic regimens should be based on antibiotic sensitivity data obtained from the institution at which the patient is being treated. We prefer to use imipenem-cilastatin with vancomycin as first-line therapy. Other acceptable regimens include an antipseudomonal semisynthetic penicillin (e.g., piperacillin) combined with an aminoglycoside, a third-generation cephalosporin with antipseudomonal activity (i.e., ceftazidine) or double β-lactam combinations (ceftazidine and piperacillin), with or without vancomycin. Aminoglycosides should be avoided if possible in patients with renal insufficiency. For patients with known immediate type hypersensitivity reactions to penicillin, aztreonam may be substituted for β-lactams. Aztreonam should be combined with an aminoglycoside rather than used alone. Empiric amphotericin B therapy should be initiated in neutropenic patients who remain febrile without a known source for 7 days or who develop new fever while on broad-spectrum antibacterial antibiotics. Antibacterial and antifungal antibiotics should be continued until patients are no longer neutropenic, regardless of whether a specific source has been found for the fever.

Treatment of M3 Leukemia Daily oral ATRA during induction has been shown to improve outcome in patients with t(15;17). The cells in this subtype are induced to differentiate, and complications of cytotoxic therapy (e.g., DIC) are usually averted. However, retinoic acid syndrome may develop within the first 3 weeks of therapy. The syndrome includes fever, chest pain, dyspnea, pulmonary infiltrates, and progressive hypoxemia. Unless reversed, it can rapidly be fatal. It must be aggressively managed with early initiation of glucocorticoid therapy, oxygen, and supportive care measures. Patients with elevated leukocyte counts are at particular risk for this syndrome, but it may also develop in the setting of low white blood cell counts. Some investigators advocate the addition of chemotherapy if the leukocyte count rises above 10,000/μL. It is important that patients induced into CR with ATRA receive consolidation chemotherapy, as essentially all patients treated with ATRA alone relapse.

In M3 leukemia patients treated with 7 and 3, a second course of chemotherapy should be withheld despite persistence of leukemic promyelocytes in the bone marrow on days 14 to 28, as CR frequently follows one course of standard 7 and 3 therapy in this subtype of AML, despite persistence of leukemic cells in the bone marrow during the initial weeks of therapy.

The importance of ATRA for M3 leukemia was demonstrated in a National Cancer Institute–sponsored intergroup study, where patients were randomized to receive either ATRA or standard 7 and 3 for induction. This was followed by one cycle of standard 7 and 3 therapy and one cycle of high-dose cytarabine and daunorubicin for all patients and a second randomization for the maintenance phase between ATRA or observation. Although the follow-up is relatively short, almost all patients who received chemotherapy alone followed by observation have relapsed. Patients receiving ATRA mostly remain in CR. This study demonstrates the importance of ATRA therapy in patients with t(15;17), although the best time for administering it is still not clear.

The clinical relevance of RT-PCR in detecting residual disease in M3 leukemia has been shown by several groups. With current assays, the complete and sustained disappearance of the PML-RARα transcript by RT-PCR is associated with a high probability of maintaining disease-free survival. Persistence of the RT-PCR product predicts for relapse, suggesting that the disease was not eradicated, and further therapy is indicated.

Postremission Therapy Induction of a durable first CR is critical to long-term disease-free survival in AML. Once relapse has occurred, AML is generally curable only by BMT.

Postremission therapy is designed to eradicate any residual leukemic cells. Therefore it should prevent relapse and prolong survival.

Approaches to postremission therapy in AML include intensive chemotherapy and allogeneic or autologous BMT. Initial postinduction chemotherapy studies demonstrated a dose-response effect for cytarabine, and randomized studies have substantiated the superiority of high-dose over standard-dose cytarabine. The Cancer and Leukemia Group B, for example, compared the duration of CR in patients randomized to four cycles of either high (3 g/m² every 12 h on days 1, 3, and 5), intermediate (400 mg/m² for 5 days by continuous infusion), or standard (100 mg/m² per day for 5 days by continuous infusion) doses of cytarabine postremission. A dose-response effect for cytarabine in patients with AML who were 60 years of age or younger was demonstrated. High-dose cytarabine significantly prolonged CR and increased the fraction cured in patients with favorable [t(8;21) and inv(16)] and normal cytogenetics but had no significant effect on patients with other abnormal karyotypes.

Allogeneic BMT in first CR, in patients under age 65 years without major organ dysfunction (e.g., renal, pulmonary, cardiac, or hepatic damage) who have an HLA-compatible related bone marrow donor or in those under age 55 years with an HLA-compatible unrelated donor, results in cure in 40 to 60 percent of patients. However, toxicity is relatively high with treatment-related complications, including venoocclusive disease, GVHD, and infections. To test whether allogeneic BMT is superior to postremission intensive chemotherapy in first CR, several groups have prospectively studied AML patients at diagnosis for an HLA-compatible sibling and genetically randomized them between the two treatment options. Patients with an HLA-compatible sibling have been offered an allogeneic BMT as early as possible after CR achievement, and patients without an HLA-compatible sibling have received high-dose intensive chemotherapy. Attempts have been made to minimize biases related to patient selection, transplantation center referral, and time delay between CR achievement and BMT. Although there is a tendency toward a lower risk of relapse in the BMT arm of these studies, no significant differences have generally been detected in overall survival rate between the treatment approaches. This may be because (1) some patients with a compatible donor do not undergo BMT, (2) there is a higher incidence of treatment-related complications after BMT, and (3) the availability of better salvage therapy for patients who relapse after intensive chemotherapy (i.e., allogeneic BMT) as compared to patients who relapse after BMT. The use of predictive models based on prognostic factors may help to select patients for whom BMT is recommended in first CR.

Autologous BMT for postinduction therapy uses the same high-dose chemotherapy as in allogeneic BMT, except that the patients subsequently receive their own cells, collected while in remission and temporarily stored. In a study from the European Organization for Research and Treatment of Cancer and the Gruppo Italiano Malattie Ematologiche Maligne dell'Adulto, in which patients without an HLA-identical related donor were randomly assigned to undergo autologous BMT with unpurged marrow or a second course of high-dose cytarabine and daunorubicin, the projected rate of disease-free survival at 4 years was 48 percent and 30 percent, respectively. The overall survival, using an intent-to-treat analysis, was not different between the two groups. Stratifying patients according to risk groups and the development of more sensitive methods to detect minimal residual disease might help to discern a population more likely to benefit from autologous BMT.

For autologous BMT, ex vivo purged marrow has been used in an attempt to avoid reinfusing residual viable leukemic cells. However, this method results in a significantly higher risk, for a prolonged time, of infection and bleeding. In some patients, blood stem cells that do not appear to contain the malignant clone, even when sensitive molecular techniques such as RT-PCR are used, can be harvested early in the recovery period following dose-intensive chemotherapy and can be used to restore normal hematopoiesis after myeloablative therapy. Because stem cells collected from the blood during the recovery phase after chemotherapy (mobilization) appear to be enriched for normal CD34+ cells, they also may be better starting material than bone marrow for subsequent selection of CD34+ subsets or other ex vivo manipulation designed to eliminate leukemic cells that may remain after mobilization. Studies in first CR of this and other approaches to decrease the incidence of relapse, such as the ex vivo use of monoclonal antibodies (against the leukemic cells) with or without chemotherapy to purge the chemotherapy-mobilized stem cells, are ongoing.

A major focus of current research is detection of residual leukemic cells in the bone marrow of CR patients using techniques such as RT-PCR, FISH, and multiparameter flow cytometry. The availability of sensitive and specific methods for detection of occult residual leukemia cells during CR would allow optimization of postinduction management for individual patients. The use of immune modulation postremission is another experimental approach. It is based on the following observations: (1) natural killer cells are defective in patients with leukemia, (2) allogeneic transplant recipients who develop significant GVHD have a decreased risk of leukemic relapse compared with patients in whom GVHD does not develop, and (3) infusions of donor leukocytes alone (without prior conditioning or GVHD prophylaxis) for relapse after allogeneic BMT induces CR. These have led to speculation that an adoptive immune response, termed *graft-versus-leukemia* (GVL), mediated by cytotoxic T cells, and possibly natural or lymphokine-activated killer cells, may be the reason for the enhanced antileukemia effect seen in unmanipulated allografts as compared to T cell–depleted allografts. Thus stimulation of a GVL or immunologic effect in patients with AML in remission may lead to a decreased relapse rate. The hypothesis from these observations is that the immune system is an important element in the cure of AML. Several approaches are under investigation that attempt to stimulate the immune system postremission. One such approach is the use of low-dose (1.2 × 10⁶ units/m²) interleukin (IL) 2,[1] administered subcutaneously for 10 days, to induce natural killer cell expansion, followed by continuous infusion IL-2 (3 × 10⁶ units/m²) to induce natural killer cell cytotoxicity.

Another postremission approach being used by several groups has emerged from the findings on the role of the multidrug resistance gene in AML. Modulators (e.g., cyclosporine) that can block drug efflux are being administered along with postremission chemotherapy.

Relapse Once relapse occurs following the standard induction and postremission chemotherapy approach described above and outlined in Fig. 112-1, patients are rarely cured with further standard-dose chemotherapy. Patients eligible for allogeneic or autologous BMT should be expeditiously transplanted at the first sign of relapse. Long-term disease-free survival is approximately the same (30 percent) using allogeneic BMT in first relapse or in second remission. The most important factors predicting response at relapse are the length of the previous CR, whether initial CR was achieved with one or two courses of chemotherapy, and the type of postremission therapy. Because of the poor outcome of patients in early (<6 months) first relapse, it is justified (for patients without HLA-compatible donors) to explore innovative approaches, such as new drugs. Patients with longer (>12 months) first CR generally relapse with drug-sensitive disease and may achieve a second remission with the original induction regimen. However, for these patients too, long-term disease-free survival requires treatment with additional agents, not previously received, or BMT. Salvage regimens used for relapsed disease, as well as for initially refractory disease, include high-dose cytarabine with an anthracycline or mitoxantrone (for patients who have not received high-dose cytarabine in induction or postremission) and high-dose etoposide in conjunction with high-dose cyclophosphamide.

---

[1] This drug has not been approved for this purpose by the Food and Drug Administration at the time of publication.

CHRONIC MYELOID LEUKEMIA

INCIDENCE The incidence of chronic myeloid leukemia (CML) is approximately 1.3 per 100,000 people per year, and the age-adjusted incidence is higher in men than in women (1.7 versus 1.0). There was a slight decrease in the incidence of CML between 1973 and 1991 (1.5 versus 1.3). The incidence of CML increases slowly with age until the middle forties, when the incidence starts to rise rapidly.

DEFINITION The diagnosis of CML is established by identifying cytogenetically or molecularly a clonal expansion of a hematopoietic stem cell possessing a reciprocal translocation between chromosomes 9 and 22. This translocation results in the head-to-tail fusion of the breakpoint cluster region (BCR) gene on chromosome 22 at band q11 with the ABL (named after the abelson murine leukemia virus) gene located on chromosome 9 at band q34. The disease is characterized by the inevitable transition from a chronic phase to an accelerated phase and on to blast crisis.

ETIOLOGY No clear correlation with exposure to cytotoxic drugs, such as alkylating agents, has been found, and there is no direct evidence of a viral etiology. Cigarette smoking has been shown to accelerate the progression to blast crisis and therefore has an adverse effect on survival in CML. The effect of radiation was demonstrated in the study of the atomic bomb survivors, where it has been estimated that the development of a CML cell mass of $10,000/\mu L$ takes 6.3 years. The Chernobyl nuclear facility accident and the availability of more sensitive techniques to detect the product of the t(9;22) may teach us more about initiation events in the pathogenesis of CML.

PATHOPHYSIOLOGY The product of the fusion gene resulting from the t(9;22) is believed to play a central role in the initial development of CML. This chimeric gene is transcribed into a hybrid BCR-ABL mRNA in which exon 1 of ABL is replaced by variable numbers of 5′ BCR exons. Bcr-Abl fusion proteins, $p210^{BCR-ABL}$, are produced that contain NH_2-terminal domains of Bcr and the COOH-terminal domains of Abl. The oncogenic potential of the Bcr-Abl fusion proteins has been validated by their ability to transform hematopoietic progenitor cells in vitro. Furthermore, there is a model where reconstituting lethally irradiated mice with bone marrow cells infected with retrovirus carrying the gene encoding the $p210^{BCR-ABL}$ leads to the development of a myeloproliferative syndrome resembling CML in 50 percent of the experimental animals. Another approach that supports a role for Bcr-Abl in the growth of t(9;22)-positive leukemic cells involves the use of specific antisense oligomers to the BCR-ABL junctions. After exposure to BCR-ABL antisense, suppression of leukemia colony formation was detected, whereas granulocyte-macrophage colony formation from normal marrow progenitors was unaffected. Taken together, these data provide cogent evidence for BCR-ABL gene participation in leukemogenesis.

The mechanism(s) by which $p210^{BCR-ABL}$ promotes the transition from the benign state to the fully malignant one is still unclear. However, attachment of the BCR sequences to ABL results in three critical functional changes: (1) the Abl protein becomes constitutively active as a tyrosine kinase enzyme, (2) the DNA protein–binding activity of Abl is attenuated, and (3) the binding of Abl to cytoskeletal actin microfilaments is enhanced.

Disease Progression The events associated with transition to the acute phase are poorly understood. Chromosomal instability of the malignant clone, resulting, for example, in the acquisition of an additional t(9;22), trisomy 8, or 17p-, is a fundamental characteristic of CML. It is generally believed that acquisition of resultant genetic and/or molecular abnormalities are critical to the phenotypic transformation. Several groups have reported that the site of the breakpoint within the BCR gene predicts the time to development of blast crisis, but these results have been refuted by others. Heterogeneous structural alterations of the p53 gene, as well as structural alterations and lack of protein production of the retinoblastoma gene, have been associated with disease progression in a subset of patients. Similarly, several reports have demonstrated rare cases with alterations in the RAS gene. Sporadic reports also exist indicating the presence of an altered MYC (named after the myelocytomatosis virus) gene or the appearance of

$p190^{BCR-ABL}$, the protein commonly found in adult ALL and occasionally in AML, during the clinical evolution of small numbers of patients with CML. Progressive de novo DNA methylation at the BCR-ABL locus has also been shown to herald blastic transformation. Finally, IL-1β may be involved in the progression of CML to the blastic phase. In summary, multiple pathways to disease transformation exist, although the exact timing and the relevance of each of these remains unclear.

CLINICAL PRESENTATION **Symptoms** The clinical onset of the chronic phase is generally insidious. Accordingly, some patients are diagnosed while still asymptomatic, during health screening tests; other patients present with fatigue, malaise, and weight loss or have symptoms resulting from splenic enlargement, such as early satiety and left upper quadrant pain or mass. Less common are features related to granulocyte or platelet dysfunction, such as infections, thrombosis, or bleeding. Occasionally, patients present with leukostatic manifestations due to severe leukocytosis or thrombosis such as vasoocclusive disease, cerebrovascular accidents, myocardial infarction, venous thrombosis, priapism, visual disturbances, and pulmonary insufficiency.

Progression of CML is associated with worsening symptoms. Unexplained fever, significant weight loss, increasing dose requirement of the drugs controlling the disease, bone and joint pain, bleeding, thrombosis, and infections suggest transformation into accelerated or blastic phases. Presentation with accelerated disease or with de novo blastic phase CML represents fewer than 10 to 15 percent of newly diagnosed cases.

Physical Findings In most patients the abnormal finding on physical examination at diagnosis is minimal to moderate splenomegaly; mild hepatomegaly is found occasionally. Persistent splenomegaly despite continued therapy is a sign of disease acceleration. Lymphadenopathy and extramedullary leukemic deposition (chloromas) are unusual except late in the course of the disease, and when present, the prognosis is poor.

Hematologic Findings Elevated white blood cell counts, with various degrees of immaturity of the granulocytic series, are observed at diagnosis. Usually there are fewer than 5 percent circulating blasts and fewer than 10 percent blasts and promyelocytes. Cycling of the counts may be observed when following patients without treatment. Platelet counts are almost always elevated at diagnosis, and a mild degree of normochromic normocytic anemia is present. Leukocyte alkaline phosphatase is characteristically low in CML cells. Serum levels of vitamin B_{12} and vitamin B_{12}–binding proteins are generally elevated. Phagocytic functions are usually normal at diagnosis and remain normal during the chronic phase. Increased histamine production secondary to basophilia occurs in later stages, causing diarrhea and flushing.

At diagnosis, increased bone marrow cellularity, primarily of the myeloid and megakaryocytic lineages, with a greatly altered myeloid to erythroid ratio, is found in almost all CML patients. The marrow blast percentage is generally normal or slightly elevated. Marrow or blood basophilia, eosinophilia, and monocytosis may be observed. While collagen fibrosis in the marrow is unusual at presentation, significant degrees of reticulin stain–measured fibrosis are noted in about half of the patients.

Disease acceleration is defined by the development of increasing degrees of anemia unaccounted for by bleeding or chemotherapy, cytogenetic clonal evolution, blood or marrow blasts ≥ 15 percent but < 30 percent, blood or marrow blasts and promyelocytes ≥ 30 percent, blood or marrow basophils ≥ 20 percent, or platelet count $< 100,000/\mu L$. *Blast crisis* is defined as acute leukemia, with blood or marrow blasts ≥ 30 percent. Hyposegmented neutrophils may appear (Pelger-Huët anomaly). Blast cells can be classified as myeloid, lymphoid, erythroid, or undifferentiated, based on morphologic, cytochemical, and immunologic features. About half of the cases are acute myeloid leukemia, one-third are acute lymphoid leukemia, 10 percent are acute erythroleukemia, and the rest are undifferentiated.

Chromosomal Findings The cytogenetic hallmark of CML, found in 90 to 95 percent of the cases, is the t(9;22)(q34;q11). Originally, this was recognized by the presence of a shortened chromosome 22 (22q-), designated as the *Philadelphia chromosome*, that arises from the reciprocal 9;22 translocation. Some patients may have complex translocations (designated as *variant translocations*) involving three, four, or five chromosomes (usually including chromosomes 9 and 22). However, the molecular consequences of these chromosomal changes appear similar to those resulting from the typical t(9;22).

PROGNOSTIC FACTORS The clinical outcome of patients with CML is variable. Death is expected in 10 percent of patients within 2 years and in somewhat fewer than 20 percent yearly thereafter. The median survival is about 4 years. Therefore, several prognostic models that identify different risk groups in CML have been developed. The most commonly used staging systems have been derived from multivariate analyses of prognostic factors. The Sokal index identified percentage of circulating blasts, spleen size, platelet count, cytogenetic clonal evolution, and age as the most important prognostic indicators. Two models, that of Tura and the combined model of Kantarjian, divide patients according to the number of negative prognostic factors. Age ≥60, spleen ≥10 cm below the costal margin, blasts ≥3 percent in blood or ≥5 percent in marrow, basophils ≥7 percent in blood or ≥3 percent in marrow, platelets ≥700,000/mL, or any of the characteristics of accelerated disease are associated with a very poor short-term prognosis and a threefold higher hazard rate, or risk of death per unit of time, in the first year.

℞ **TREATMENT**

The goal of therapy in CML is to achieve prolonged, durable, nonneoplastic nonclonal hematopoiesis, which entails the eradication of any residual cells containing the BCR-ABL transcript. Hence the goal is complete molecular remission and cure (Table 112-3). A proposed treatment plan for the newly diagnosed CML patient is presented in Fig. 112-2.

Allogeneic BMT Allogeneic BMT is the only curative therapy for CML and, when feasible, is the treatment of choice. However, it is complicated by a high early mortality rate owing to the transplant procedure. When the outcome of all patients undergoing allogeneic BMT reported to the International Bone Marrow Transplant Registry was compared to the outcome of all patients treated with hydroxyurea or interferon (IFN) α by the German CML Study Group, the survival for the former group was statistically better, but only starting 5 years from the time of transplant. When only low-risk patients (by Sokal's criteria) were evaluated, the benefit in survival for allogeneic BMT was seen after 6 years. Outcome of BMT depends on multiple factors

Table 112-3

Response Criteria in CML

Hematologic	
Complete response*	White blood cell count <10,000/μL, normal morphology
	Normal hemoglobin and platelet counts
Incomplete response	White blood cell count ≥10,000/μL
Cytogenetic	Percentage of bone marrow metaphases with t(9;22)
Complete response	0
Partial response	≤35
Minor response	36–85†
No response	85–100
Molecular	Presence of BCR-ABL transcript by RT-PCR
Complete response	None
Incomplete response	Any

* Complete hematologic response requires the disappearance of splenomegaly.
† Up to 15% normal metaphases are occasionally seen at diagnosis (when 30 metaphases are analyzed).

NOTE: RT-PCR, reverse transcriptase polymerase chain reaction.

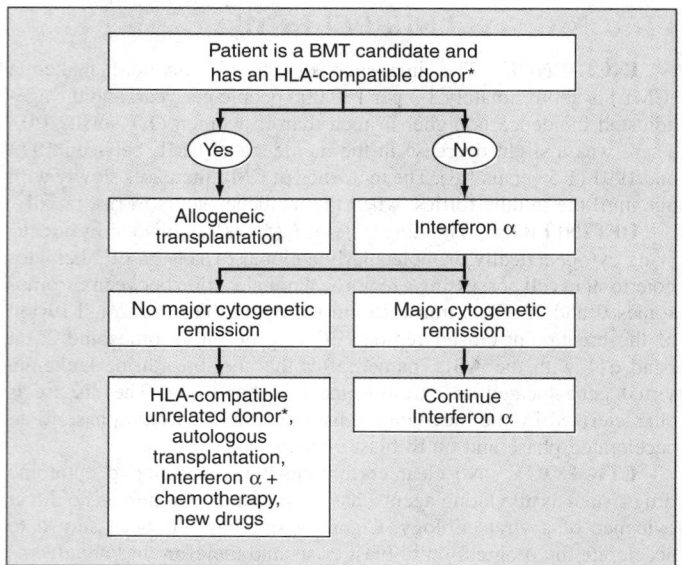

FIGURE 112-2 Flow chart for the therapy of newly diagnosed CML. Patients with an HLA-compatible donor often receive high-dose therapy plus an allogeneic marrow transplant as initial therapy. The asterisk denotes that some centers employ allogeneic marrow transplant only if interferon-α fails to induce a response. Most data suggest that treatment outcome is superior if marrow transplantation is performed earlier rather than later in the course of disease.

including: (1) the patient (i.e., age and phase of disease); (2) the type of donor [i.e., syngeneic (monozygotic twins) or HLA-compatible allogeneic, related or unrelated]; (3) the preparative regimen; (4) GVHD; and (5) posttransplantation treatment.

THE PATIENT As experience has been gained, and safety and efficacy established, it has become clear that patients should be relatively young (<65 years) and have a healthy and histocompatible donor. Furthermore, survival following BMT in the accelerated and blastic phases of the disease is significantly worse and is associated with a very high rate of relapse. The Seattle data demonstrate that transplantation early in the chronic phase (1 to 2 years from diagnosis) is superior to later transplant. It has been shown that the overall survival, disease-free survival, incidence and severity of acute and chronic GVHD, and relapse rates are not influenced by prior IFNα treatment.

THE DONOR Transplantation from a family donor, who is either fully matched or mismatched at only one HLA locus, should be considered standard therapy for any CML patient who is a candidate for an HLA-related sibling transplant. Syngeneic transplantation in chronic phase CML patients has been reported from the Seattle group to result in 7-year disease-free survival in 55 percent, with a 30 percent relapse rate. With HLA-identical sibling transplantation in the chronic phase, many groups have reported 5-year disease-free survival in 40 to 70 percent of patients, with a 25 percent relapse rate. Transplantation from an HLA-matched unrelated donor has been reported by the Seattle group to result in a 74 percent probability of surviving 3 years for patients who are in chronic phase, less than 1 year from diagnosis, and younger than 50 years old. A 2-year actuarial incidence of disease-free (based on hematologic analyses) survival of 45 percent (±21 percent) for unrelated transplants, matched or mismatched at only one locus, transplanted less than 1 year from diagnosis was reported by the National Marrow Donor Program. Patients in the age group of 40 to 50 fared poorly (15 of 55 survived). The probability of 2-year disease-free (based on cytogenetic analyses) survival in a report on unrelated transplants from the Medical College of Wisconsin, using a standardized conditioning regimen and T cell depletion, was 52 percent for patients transplanted in chronic phase (regardless of the time from diagnosis). Unrelated transplants have higher rates of graft failure and acute and chronic GVHD and prolonged convalescence following treatment, compared to related allogeneic transplants. Peripheral blood is now being studied as a source of allogeneic hematopoietic progenitor cells; it may offer rapid engraftment and less risk for the donor.

PREPARATIVE REGIMENS These have been studied by several groups. A randomized study from the Seattle group compared cyclophosphamide and total-body irradiation with busulphan and cyclophosphamide. They found no significant differences in the 3-year probabilities of survival, relapse, event-free survival, speed of engraftment, or incidence of venoocclusive disease of the liver. Significantly more patients in the total-body irradiation arm experienced major creatinine elevations, acute GVHD, longer periods of fever, positive blood cultures, hospital admissions, and longer inpatient hospital stays. These data suggest that the combination of busulphan and cyclophosphamide is the preferred regimen. Other preparative regimens are being tested with the primary goal of reducing the relapse rate.

THE DEVELOPMENT AND TYPE OF GVHD Development of grade I GVHD, as compared to no GVHD, has been shown by The European Group for Blood and Marrow Transplantation to decrease the incidence of relapse. A lower relapse rate was observed also in patients with grade II GVHD but was accompanied by a substantially higher transplant-related mortality. The decreased relapse rate may be caused by a GVL effect. Depletion of T lymphocytes from donor marrow can prevent GVHD but results in an increased risk of relapse, which exceeds the relapse rate following syngeneic BMT. Thus, T lymphocytes from the donor marrow mediate a significant antileukemic, or GVL, effect, and even syngeneic marrow may exhibit limited GVL activity in CML.

POSTTRANSPLANTATION TREATMENT Further support for the existence of an immunologically mediated GVL effect comes from the observation that donor leukocyte infusions (without prior conditioning or GVHD prophylaxis) can induce hematologic and cytogenetic remissions in CML patients who have relapsed after allogeneic BMT.

The activity of IFNα in patients with early chronic-phase CML was the basis for the use of IFNα after BMT, either to induce cytogenetic remissions in relapsed patients or to prevent relapse after BMT for high-risk patients. The main concern about IFNα use after allogeneic BMT has been the development or worsening of GVHD, because IFNα is known to act as an immunomodulator. However, in published reports comprising 52 allogeneic recipients who were free of GVHD and were either at high risk for relapse or had already relapsed, only 6 subsequently developed GVHD after IFNα therapy was initiated. IFNα has also been combined with mononuclear cells obtained from donor blood to induce cytogenetic remissions in relapsed patients. Cytogenetic remissions have been achieved, but the exact role of IFNα as opposed to the mononuclear cells is unclear. IL-2, with or without IFNα, is also being evaluated for its ability to restore complete cytogenetic remission in patients relapsing following BMT.

IFNα has also been used following BMT to prevent relapse in patients with advanced disease at time of transplant (patients at high risk for relapse). Maintenance of cytogenetic CR as long as 2 years posttransplantation in patients with blast crisis or second chronic phase has been reported in small numbers of patients. Similarly, IL-2 (2.5×10^6 to 6×10^6 units/m² per day) has been given following T cell–depleted allogeneic BMT in an effort to induce GVL without GVHD, and thus prevent relapse. Preliminary data suggest that, compared with historical controls, patients treated with IL-2 have a lower risk of disease relapse. A randomized trial is warranted.

Interferons When allogeneic BMT is not feasible, IFNα therapy is the treatment of choice. The interferons are a complex group of naturally occurring proteins produced by eukaryotic cells in response to viruses, antigens, and mitogens. Three distinct groups of IFN species have been identified: IFNα, -β, and -γ. Although a variety of interferons have become available for clinical investigation, the most data have been generated using IFNα preparations.

Interferons have potent, pleiotropic biological effects, spanning a spectrum of antiviral, microbicidal, immunomodulatory, and anti-

proliferative properties. While interferons have been shown to downregulate the expression of several oncogenes and cytokines, they also upregulate the expression of interferon regulatory factor-1 (a transcriptional activator with antioncogenic activity), adhesion molecules, and the histocompatibility genes. Interferons have also been shown to inhibit angiogenesis and to induce a cellular immune response. Although bench research has revealed a diverse array of possibilities for interferons, a clear knowledge of their mode(s) of action is still lacking.

The initial studies of IFNα in the treatment of CML were singleagent, single-arm trials that attempted to determine an effective dose, the patient population that would benefit from the treatment, and toxicity. An association between IFNα dose and the quality of response became clear from these studies. The effective dose was found to be 5 million units subcutaneously daily. Treatment with IFNα was found to be effective only when initiated within the first year of diagnosis. Experience with IFNα suggests that segregation of patients into IFNα-sensitive and -resistant subgroups correlates strongly with time from diagnosis and prognosis at diagnosis.

Patients develop both acute and chronic side effects from IFNα therapy. Acute side effects (flulike symptoms) appear early in the course of the treatment. Most flulike symptoms respond to acetaminophen, and tachyphylaxis develops within 1 to 2 weeks. Chronic reactions, such as fatigue and lethargy, weight loss, myalgias, and arthralgias, occur in approximately half of the patients and may require dose reduction. Patients also report cough, postnasal drip, and dryness of the skin. Infrequently, immune-mediated thrombocytopenia and anemia develop. In addition, long-term therapy has been associated with late autoimmune side effects, such as hypothyroidism and occasionally generalized autoimmune phenomena.

The most important persistent side effects in CML patients treated with IFNα are neurologic. All IFNα-treated patients are subject to some neurologic toxicity, the most common symptom being lethargy. Up to 20 percent of patients have neurologic side effects that are associated with compromised quality of life and reduction in their ability to carry out their regular activity, such as full-time work. In addition, at the required doses, impotence in men is not infrequent. In an effort to modify the side effects, the role of antidepressant agents such as amitriptyline hydrochloride is currently being tested. Furthermore, because IFNα has been shown to have opioid-like effects, and the opioid antagonist naloxone modifies IFNα-induced changes both in vitro and in vivo, a trial with naltrexone (an opioid antagonist) has been initiated at the M.D. Anderson Cancer Center.

Hematologic remissions are generally achieved within 1 to 2 months of starting IFNα. However, some patients show a cyclic response pattern with progressively lower peak and nadir counts over a period of months. The increase in counts during the cycling that occurs in the first few months of therapy should not be confused with resistance. Cytogenetic responses generally start at 3 to 12 months, and complete cytogenetic responses may require 6 months to 4 years of therapy. However, most complete cytogenetic responses are achieved within 12 to 18 months, and in single-agent, singlearm studies they have been seen in up to 26 percent of patients.

Randomized trials of IFNα versus chemotherapy have found that both treatment modalities are effective in achieving hematologic remissions. The incidence of IFNα-induced hematologic and cytogenetic responses have been considerably lower in the randomized trials than in the single-arm studies. These results are probably explained by lower IFNα doses, patient population heterogeneity (some studies have included high-risk patients, as defined by Sokal's criteria), multicenter participation without a unified policy on dose modification, and premature discontinuation of treatment.

Three randomized studies (those of the Italian Cooperative Study Group, the United Kingdom Medical Research Council, and the Kouseisho Leukemia Study Group) have demonstrated an association between IFNα therapy and improved survival. Interestingly, in the first two of these studies, a survival advantage for achieving a cytogenetic response in the IFNα-treated groups was seen, but this advantage was unrelated to the degree of that response. A fourth trial, by the German CML Study Group, did not show an increase in survival for IFNα-treated patients. These results probably differ from those of the previous studies because of the inclusion of patients with more advanced CML.

Chemotherapy Initial management of patients with chemotherapy is currently reserved for rapid lowering of white blood cell counts, reduction of symptoms, and reversal of symptomatic splenomegaly. Hydroxyurea, a ribonucleotide reductase inhibitor, induces rapid disease control. The initial dose is 1 to 4 g/d, and the dose should be reduced by half with each 50 percent reduction of the leukocyte count. Unfortunately, cytogenetic remissions with hydroxyurea are uncommon. Busulphan, an alkylating agent that acts on early progenitor cells, has a more prolonged effect. However, we do not recommend its use because of its serious side effects. These include unexpected, and occasionally fatal, myelosuppression in 5 to 10 percent of patients; pulmonary, endocardial, and marrow fibrosis; and an Addison-like wasting syndrome.

Intensive combination chemotherapy has also been used in chronic phase CML, with 30 to 50 percent of patients achieving complete cytogenetic responses. However these cytogenetic remissions have been short lived. Consequently, intensive combination chemotherapy regimens are being used today only to mobilize normal progenitors in the blood in order to collect circulating stem cells for autologous transplantation. Another role for chemotherapy (e.g., homoharringtonine or low-dose cytarabine) is in combination with IFNα. An M.D. Anderson Cancer Center trial has shown an improved survival for CML patients who were more than 1 year from diagnosis and who were treated with low-dose cytarabine and IFNα, as compared to a historical control population treated with IFNα alone.

Autologous BMT Autologous hematopoietic stem cell transplantation could potentially cure CML if a means to select the residual normal progenitors, which are known to coexist with their malignant counterparts, could be developed. As a source of autologous hematopoietic stem cells for transplantation, blood offers certain advantages over marrow (e.g., faster engraftment and no general anesthesia). Normal hematopoietic stem cells appear with increased frequency in the blood of patients with CML during the recovery phase after chemotherapy and G-CSF.

A retrospective analysis of over 200 autologous progenitor cell transplants performed for CML at eight centers worldwide suggests that autologous transplantation prolongs survival in chronic- or accelerated-phase patients when compared retrospectively with conventional therapy. Disease phase at transplant included 93 patients in chronic phase, 25 in accelerated phase, and 114 in blast crisis or second chronic phase. Patients received autologous bone marrow and/or blood hematopoietic stem cells. In 42 cases the hematopoietic progenitors were subjected to ex vivo manipulation, either by long-term bone marrow culture, by incubation with recombinant IFNγ, or by chemotherapy. In 49 cases the hematopoietic progenitors were harvested during the recovery phase following various chemotherapy regimens. Following autologous stem cell transplantation, 29 of 93 (31 percent) patients in first chronic phase achieved complete cytogenetic remissions. The median duration of cytogenetic remission was 14 months, with a range of 2 to 68 months. Approaches to treat minimal residual disease following autologous transplantation, such as immune modulation, are currently being investigated.

Leukapheresis and Splenectomy Intensive leukapheresis may control the blood counts in chronic phase CML; however, it is expensive and cumbersome. It is useful in emergencies where leukostasis-related complications such as pulmonary failure or cerebrovascular accidents are likely. It may also have a role in pregnant women in whom it is important to avoid potentially teratogenic drugs.

Splenectomy was used in CML in the past because of the suggestion that evolution to the acute phase might occur in the spleen. However, this does not appear to be the case, and splenectomy is now reserved for symptomatic relief of painful splenomegaly unresponsive to chemotherapy or for significant anemia or thrombocytopenia associated with hypersplenism. Splenic radiation is used on rare occasions to reduce the size of the spleen.

Minimal Residual Disease The correlation between residual cells with the t(9;22) and disease recurrence is not completely understood. Initial studies using RT-PCR to predict disease recurrence following IFNα therapy found residual disease in all samples tested from patients with complete cytogenetic remissions. Later studies demonstrated the elimination of the BCR-ABL mRNA transcript after more prolonged IFNα treatment in some cases. It is now possible to quantify transcripts, and longer follow-up may indicate whether quantitation of the BCR-ABL transcript is useful for predicting cytogenetic and clinical relapse.

The nature of the complete molecular remission after IFNα therapy was studied at the M.D. Anderson Cancer Center. Blood, bone marrow, and individually plucked soft agar colonies were simultaneously analyzed for the presence of the BCR-ABL transcript in patients with complete cytogenetic and molecular responses. The RT-PCR-amplified BCR-ABL transcripts were detected only in myeloid or erythroid colonies. These observations demonstrate that residual disease resides in myeloid or erythroid colony forming cells; whether they have the potential to repopulate the bone marrow and thus induce a relapse is unknown. It is possible that IFNα induces tumor dormancy in CML.

Following allogeneic BMT, RT-PCR analysis may be positive for residual disease during the first 6 months in patients who subsequently achieve a long-lasting remission. However, late persistence of RT-PCR positivity appears to indicate a reduced probability of cure. RT-PCR positivity at any single time point is not predictive of imminent relapse. Patients are often divided according to RT-PCR results following allogeneic BMT into one of three groups: (1) persistently positive, (2) intermittently negative, and (3) persistently negative. These three groups have a low, intermediate, and high probability of maintaining remission and disease free-survival, respectively. This suggests that patients who are persistently RT-PCR positive more than 6 months following allogeneic BMT need additional therapeutic interventions. Further, in patients who do not have any evidence for GVHD and are intermittently RT-PCR negative, GVL may be induced by alloreactive donor cells (without the side effects of GVHD) to suppress the proliferation of the leukemic cells.

Future Directions The use of BCR-ABL antisense oligonucleotides to purge residual leukemic cells from autologous hematopoietic progenitors before reinfusion, as well as approaches to induce GVL in the setting of minimal residual disease without inducing GVHD, are underway.

Treatment of Blast Crisis The treatment for all forms of blast crisis is generally ineffective. Treatment is tailored to the phenotype of the blast cell. Myeloid crises are treated as for AML, but remissions occur in only a minority of cases and are generally short lived. Patients may present without having had a chronic phase. AML with a t(9;22) is probably blast crisis of CML and carries a poor prognosis. Erythroid blast crisis is treated like AML and also has a poor outcome.

Lymphoid blast crisis is treated like ALL (Chap. 113) with vincristine (1.4 mg/m² weekly) plus prednisone (60 mg/m² PO qd) induction therapy. About one-third of patients will reenter chronic phase after 2 to 3 weeks of treatment, but the remissions last only a median of about 4 months. Even marrow transplantation is poorly effective during blast crises. Novel treatment approaches are needed.

BIBLIOGRAPHY

APPELBAUM FR et al: Bone marrow transplantation for chronic myelogenous leukemia. Semin Oncol 22:405, 1995

BLOOMFIELD CD, HERZIG GP (eds): Advances in the management of acute leukemia. Hematol Oncol Clin North Am 7:1, 1993

DEGOS L et al: All-trans-retinoic acid as a differentiation agent in the treatment of acute promyelocytic leukemia. Blood 85:2643, 1995

KHOURI I et al: Chronic myeloid leukemia, in *Clinical Oncology*, MD Abeloff et al (eds). New York, Churchill Livingstone, 1995, pp 2035–2051

STONE RM, MAYER RJ: Acute myeloid leukemia in adults, in *Clinical Oncology*, MD Abeloff et al (eds). New York, Churchill Livingstone, 1995, pp 1959–1976

WETZLER M et al: Interferon-α therapy for chronic myelogenous leukemia. Am J Med 99:402, 1995

113 Arnold S. Freedman, Lee M. Nadler

MALIGNANCIES OF LYMPHOID CELLS

DEFINITION Lymphoid leukemias and malignant lymphomas are malignant counterparts of normal lymphoid cells at distinct stages of differentiation. The precursor B and T cell lymphoblastic leukemias correspond to normal pre-B and pre-T cells, respectively. Consequently, these malignant cells originate in the bone marrow, where their normal cellular counterparts reside. In contrast, malignant lymphomas are neoplastic transformations of cells that reside predominantly in lymphoid tissues. Although both leukemias and lymphomas involve reticuloendothelial organs, they are biologically and clinically distinct (Table 113-1).

CELLULAR AND DEVELOPMENTAL ASPECTS OF MALIGNANCIES OF LYMPHOCYTES Lymphoid leukemias, non-Hodgkin's lymphomas, and Hodgkin's disease are classified morphologically (as shown in Tables 113-2, 113-3, and 113-4). Multiple classification schemes have been employed over the past 30 years. The most widely used have been the FAB (French-American-British) classification for acute leukemias, the "Working Formulation" or the Kiel classification for lymphomas, and the Rye classification for Hodgkin's disease.

A classification known as the Revised European-American Classification of Lymphoid Neoplasms (R.E.A.L.) has been created that encompasses all of the lymphoid malignancies. The R.E.A.L. classification has included clinical and pathologic entities that were not included in the other schemes and utilizes detailed immunologic studies and cytogenetics to further characterize various diseases. Since it is hypothesized that acute and chronic lymphoid leukemias and non-Hodgkin's lymphomas represent neoplastic counterparts of normal populations of cells that reside in lymphoid tissues and the bone marrow, it is within the context of normal B and T cell [and natural killer (NK) cell] differentiation (see Chap. 305) that the R.E.A.L. classification has subgrouped the various pathologic entities. In this chapter the R.E.A.L. classification will be presented within a clinical context. General aspects of lymphocytic leukemias and lymphomas will be presented, followed by specific discussions of chronic leukemias/lymphomas, non-Hodgkin's lymphoma with detailed discussion of the indolent and aggressive forms, acute lymphoblastic leukemias/lymphomas, and Hodgkin's disease.

Leukemias and Lymphomas of B Cell Origin Some 80 percent of lymphoblastic leukemias and 90 percent of non-Hodgkin's lymphomas are of B cell derivation, based upon the expression of B lineage–restricted antigens and clonal rearrangements of immunoglobulin heavy and light chain genes. These tumors correspond to major and minor subpopulations of pre-B and mature B cells (Fig. 113-1). Within the context of lineage derivation of these diseases, it is important that they be viewed within a clinically meaningful perspective. For this reason, the lymphoid leukemias and non-Hodgkin's lymphomas will be discussed as being clinically indolent or aggressive in behavior.

Indolent B cell malignancies Chronic lymphocytic leukemia (CLL) is the most common type of indolent leukemia. The malignant cells correspond to a minor subpopulation of B cells that express cell surface immunoglobulins IgM/D and the T cell–associated antigen CD5. Small lymphocytic lymphoma, like B cell CLL, appears to correspond to a unique subpopulation of B cells that express pan-B cell antigens, surface IgM/D, CD23, and CD5. In contrast to CLL, small lymphocytic lymphomas express the adhesion molecule CD11a/CD18, which may account for the differences in anatomic sites of involvement of the two diseases. Hairy cell leukemia is a rare disorder with characteristics of activated B cells, with expression of interleukin (IL) 2 receptors (CD25) and specific adhesion molecules involved in localizing cells to the spleen and marrow. Prolymphocytic leukemias have morphologic and phenotypic characteristics of transformed B cells and have stronger expression of sIg than do CLL cells. The majority of indolent lymphomas are the follicular lymphomas. Follicular lymphomas include the grade I (small cleaved cell), grade II (mixed small cleaved and large cell), and grade III (large cell) subtypes. Follicular large cell lymphoma has a more rapid natural history and is grouped with the aggressive B cell lymphomas. Follicular lymphomas are thought to correspond to germinal center B cells, which express pan-B cell antigens, surface immunoglobulin (IgM, 60 percent; IgG, 40 percent), and CD10. Consistent with their ability to disseminate widely, these tumors express the molecules that are involved in lymphocyte homing and recirculation—CD44 and L-selectin.

Lymphoplasmacytoid lymphoma/Waldenström's macroglobulinemia is an indolent lymphoma in which cells have characteristics of B cells that are differentiating toward plasma cells. The marginal zone lymphomas, which are hypothesized to be lymphomas of the memory B cell compartment, lack surface IgD and can occur in the following locations: lymph nodes, where they are known as monocytoid B-cell lymphoma; extranodal tissues, where they are referred to as lymphomas of mucosal-associated lymphoid tissues (MALT); and the spleen (splenic lymphoma with or without villous lymphocytes).

Aggressive B cell malignancies Diffuse large cell lymphoma is the most common histologic type of aggressive lymphoma. These tumors express pan-B cell antigens and several B cell activation antigens and resemble transformed activated B cells. Within this category there are patients who present with predominantly mediastinal tumors, which are thought to arise from thymic B cells. From a clinical point of view the follicular large cell (grade III) lymphomas are considered aggressive diseases. Like grade I follicular lymphoma, follicular large cells express pan-B cell antigens, variable surface Ig, and CD10,

Table 113-1

Lymphoid Leukemias and Lymphomas

	Lymphoblastic Leukemia	Non-Hodgkin's	Hodgkin's
Cellular derivation	80% B	90% B	Unresolved
	20% T	10% T	
Sites of disease			
Localized	Uncommon	Uncommon	Common
Nodal spread	Common	Discontiguous	Contiguous
Extranodal	Common	Common	Uncommon
Mediastinal	Common (T cell)	Uncommon	Common
Abdominal	Uncommon	Common	Uncommon
Bone marrow	Always	Common	Uncommon
B symptoms	Common	Uncommon	Common
Chromosomal abnormalities	Common (translocations, deletions)	Common (translocations, deletions)	Common (aneuploidy)
Curability	40–60%	30–40%	75–85%

whereas B cell diffuse large cell lymphomas are generally CD5 − and CD10 − . Mantle cell lymphomas, which include many cases of "diffuse small cleaved cell lymphoma," express surface IgM/D and CD5, characteristics of normal B cells that reside in the mantle zone of

lymphoid follicles. Burkitt's lymphomas are related to normal germinal center B cells and follicular lymphomas in that they express pan-B cell antigens, B cell activation antigens, and CD10. The endemic (African) Burkitt's lymphoma cells, which have the Epstein-Barr virus (EBV) genome present in the tumor cells, express the EBV receptor CD21, whereas the nonendemic (American) variant cells do not. The aggressive Burkitt-like lymphomas are similar to Burkitt's lymphoma

Table 113-2

Histologic Classification of Lymphoid Leukemias and Non-Hodgkin's Lymphoma

R.E.A.L. Classification	Working Formulation	Kiel Classification	Rappaport Terminology	Cellular Lineage, %	Chromosomal Abnormalities
INDOLENT					
B cell CLL, small lymphocytic, prolymphocytic leukemia	A: Small lymphocytic	Lymphocytic (CLL), pro-lymphocytic leukemia	Diffuse well-differentiated lymphocytic (DWDL)	B	Trisomy 12; t(11;14), t(14;19), t(9;14)
T cell CLL, prolymphocytic leukemia	A: Small lymphocytic E: Diffuse small cleaved cell	Lymphocytic (CLL), pro-lymphocytic leukemia	DWDL, diffuse poorly differentiated lymphocytic (DPDL)	T	
Large granular lymphocyte leukemia	A: Small lymphocytic E: Diffuse small cleaved cell	Lymphocytic (CLL), pro-lymphocytic leukemia	DWDL, DPDL	T	
Hairy cell leukemia		Hairy cell leukemia		B	
Follicular center (grade I)	B: Follicular, predominantly small cleaved cell	Centroblastic/ centrocytic	Nodular poorly differentiated lymphocytic (NPDL)	B	t(14;18); del(6)
Follicular center (grade II)	C: Follicular mixed, small cleaved and large cell	Centroblastic/ centrocytic	Nodular mixed lymphocytic histiocytic (NM)	B	t(14;18); del(2) Trisomy 8
Marginal zone B cell (nodal/extranodal-MALT)		Monocytoid/ immunocytoma (nodal/extranodal)		B	
Mycosis fungoides		Small cell cerebriform (mycosis fungoides)		T	
AGGRESSIVE					
Follicular center (grade III)	D: Follicular, predominantly large cell	Centroblastic (follicular)	Nodular histiocytic (NH)	B	t(14;18); Trisomy 7
Mantle cell	E: Diffuse small cleaved cell	Centrocytic	DPDL	B	t(11;14)
Diffuse large B cell	F: Diffuse mixed, small and large cell G: Diffuse large cell H: Large cell immunoblastic	Centroblastic	Diffuse mixed lymphocytic-histiocytic (DM); diffuse histiocytic (DH)	B	t(14;18)/IgH-*bcl* 2 t(3;22)/*bcl* 6 t(3;14) t(2;3); Trisomy 4, 7, 21; del(6), (8), (13)
Primary mediastinal (thymic) B cell	G: Diffuse large cell	Large cell, sclerosing B cell lymphoma of mediastinum	DH	B	
Peripheral T cell	F: Diffuse mixed, small and large cell G: Diffuse large cell H: Large cell immunoblastic	Lymphoepithelioid, pleiomorphic (small, medium, or large cell)	DM, DH	T	t(14;14)(q11;q32)/ TCR-tcl 1 inv (14)(q11;q32) t(8;14)(q24;q11) t(10;14)(q24;q11)
Angioimmunoblastic T cell		Angioimmunoblastic		T	
Adult T cell lymphoma/ leukemia		Pleiomorphic (small, medium, or large cell HTLV +)		T	
Angiocentric			DH	T	
Intestinal T cell		Pleiomorphic (small, medium, or large cell)		T	
Anaplastic large cell	H: Large cell immunoblastic	Large cell anaplastic (Ki-1 +)		T (70) Null (30)	t(2;5)
Precursor T/B cell lymphoblastic lymphoma	I: Lymphoblastic	T lymphoblastic, lymphoblastic	Diffuse lymphoblastic (LL)	T (90) B (10)	
Precursor T/B cell lymphoblastic leukemia				B (80) T (20)	pre-B: t(9;22), t(4;11), t(1;19) T cell: 14q11 or 7q34 B cell: t(8;14), t(2;8), t(8;22)
Burkitt's	J: Small noncleaved cell; Burkitt's	Burkitt's	Diffuse undifferentiated (DUL)	B (95) T (5)	t(8;14), t(2;8), t(8;22)

Table 113-3

Classification of Acute Lymphoblastic Leukemia (ALL)

Immunologic Subtype	% of Cases	FAB Subtype	Cytogenetic Abnormalities
Pre-B ALL	75	L1, L2	t(9;22), t(4;11), t(1;19)
T cell ALL	20	L1, L2	14q11 or 7q34
B cell ALL	5	L3	t(8;14), t(8;22), t(2;8)

NOTE: FAB, French-American-British classification.

Table 113-4

Rye Classification of Hodgkin's Disease

Histologic Subgroup	Incidence, %	Pathology	
		Reed-Sternberg Cell	Other
Lymphocyte-predominant	2–10	Rare	Predominance of normal-appearing lymphocytes
Nodular sclerosis	40–80	Frequent "lacunar variants"	Lymphoid nodules, collagen bands
Mixed cellularity	20–40	Numerous	Pleiomorphic infiltrate
Lymphocyte-depleted	2–15	Numerous, often bizarre	Lymphocytes, pleiomorphic fibrosis

(BL) except they lack surface Ig and probably correspond to an activated peripheral B cell. The vast majority of acute lymphoblastic leukemias (ALL) in the R.E.A.L. classification are pre-B lymphoblastic leukemias, which express characteristics of pre-B cells. Pre-B cell (L1, L2) ALL express CD19 and in most cases CD10 (Fig. 113-1; Table 113-3). Approximately 50 percent of pre-B ALL also express CD20. The B cell (L3) surface Ig+ ALL are morphologically and phenotypically identical to Burkitt's lymphoma cells. Approximately 20 to 30 percent of adult ALL express myeloid antigens (CD13 and or CD33), which are associated with a worse prognosis in some studies.

Leukemias and Lymphomas of T Cell Origin The most widely expressed T cell antigens that define lineage are CD2 and CD7. As depicted in Fig. 113-2, T cell malignancies reflect distinct stages of T cell ontogeny.

Indolent T cell malignancies The indolent-behaving T cell lymphoproliferative disorders include T cell CLL, T cell prolymphocytic leukemia (PLL) and the large granular lymphocytic (LGL) leukemias (T and NK types), and the cutaneous T cell lymphomas. Fewer than 5 percent of CLL and about 20 percent of PLL are of T cell origin. Most cases of T-CLL and T-PLL have mature T helper cell phenotypes (CD2+, CD3+, CD4+, CD5+, CD7+, CD11a+), with occasional cases having cells coexpressing CD4 and CD8. LGL leukemias are clonal expansions of either CD3+/CD8+ cytotoxic T cells or CD3− NK, cells which express other characteristic antigens of NK cells, including CD16 (Fcγ receptor) and CD56. The cutaneous T cell lymphomas express a mature activated T helper cell phenotype: CD2, CD3, CD4, CD5, CD7, CD25 (IL-2 receptor), and CD71 (transferrin receptor).

Aggressive T cell malignancies Nearly all T cell lymphomas are considered aggressive diseases. Peripheral T cell lymphomas have been previously classified within the Working Formulation as diffuse small cleaved cell, diffuse mixed small and large cell, and diffuse large cell.

The tumor cells variably express the mature T cell antigens CD2, CD3, CD5, CD6, and CD7. Most express CD4, with a small fraction expressing CD8. Within this category are other specific histologic subtypes with unique clinical presentations, including the following: angioimmunoblastic T cell lymphoma and angiocentric lymphoma (nasal T cell/NK type and pulmonary angiocentric lymphoma-lymphomatoid granulomatosis), which are EBV-related diseases; intestinal T cell lymphoma (± gluten enteropathy-associated); hepatosplenic γδ T cell lymphoma; and subcutaneous panniculitis-like T cell lymphoma. The adult T cell lymphomas associated with human T cell leukemia/lymphoma virus (HTLV) I are similar to the cutaneous T cell lymphomas in that they express CD2, CD3, CD4, CD5, CD7, and CD25. The anaplastic large cell lymphomas characteristically involve the sinusoids of lymph nodes. These tumors express the CD30 (Ki-1) antigen and generally express the phenotype of mature activated T cells (HLA-DR, CD25), although a minor subset have no clear T or B cell lineage by immunophenotyping. Lymphoblastic lymphomas correspond to stage II thymocytes, and the majority express CD1, CD2, CD4, CD7, and CD8. Rarely, lymphoblastic lymphomas will have an immature B cell phenotype. Approximately 20 percent of adult lymphoblastic leukemias are of T cell lineage. Precursor T cell leukemias, although heterogeneous, have immunophenotypic characteristics of early thymocytes, expressing CD2 along with CD5 and CD7, with expression of cytoplasmic CD3, which is associated with the T cell antigen receptor complex. In contrast to T cell lymphoblastic lymphoma, T cell ALL are often CD4− and CD8−.

LYMPHOCYTIC LEUKEMIAS AND NON-HODGKIN'S LYMPHOMA— GENERAL ASPECTS

EPIDEMIOLOGY AND ETIOLOGY The majority of patients with ALL are children and young adults. The incidence in adults is about 1/100,000 persons per year. ALL is more common in males than females and in whites more than in blacks. In contrast to ALL, CLL is the most common adult leukemia in western countries. The

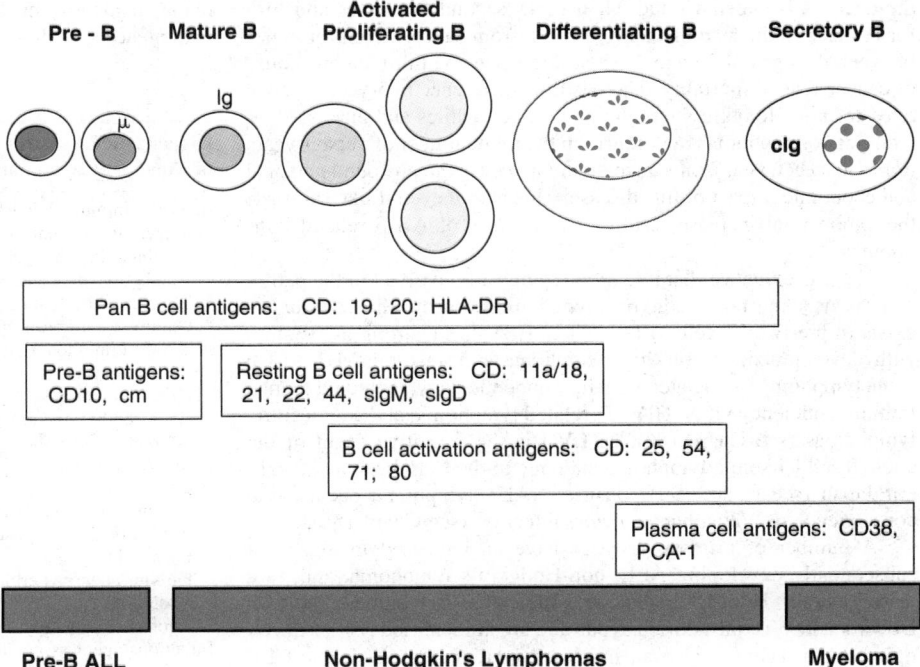

FIGURE 113-1 Correlation of B cell differentiation and B cell malignancies.

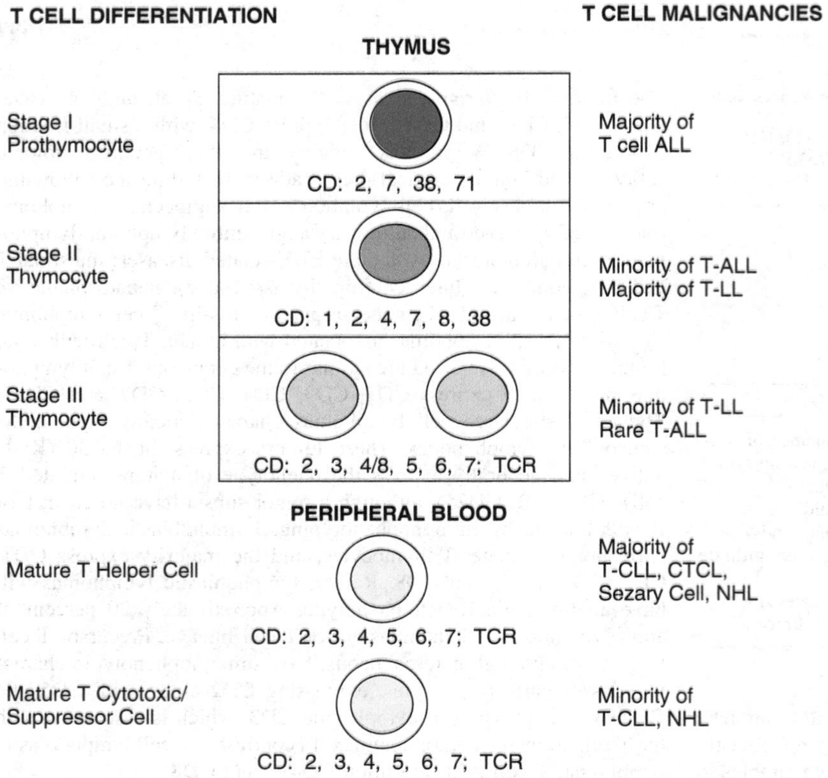

FIGURE 113-2 Correlation of T cell differentiation and T cell malignancies.

Non-Hodgkin's lymphomas occur in the context of drug-induced immunosuppression and acquired or congenital immunodeficiency. Non-Hodgkin's lymphomas develop in up to 30 percent of HIV-1 infected individuals and between 40 and 50 percent are EBV-associated. EBV is also present in virtually all the primary central nervous system (CNS) lymphomas seen in HIV-1 patients. The association between immunosuppression and induction of non-Hodgkin's lymphomas appears to be compelling; if the immunosuppression can be reversed (e.g., by discontinuing immunosuppressive agents following organ transplantation), a percentage of these lymphomas regress spontaneously. The incidence of lymphoma in iatrogenic immune suppression, HIV-1 infection, and autoimmune disease argues strongly for the contribution of immune dysregulation to the development of lymphoma. It is controversial as to whether certain chemical exposures including dioxin, phenoxyherbicides, pesticides, and hair dyes are involved in the pathogenesis of non-Hodgkin's lymphoma. Other potential environmental associations include exposure to arsenic, phenoxyacetic acids, chlorophenols, organic solvents, halomethane, lead, vinyl chloride, or asbestos. Occupational exposures associated with an increased risk include farming, welding, and work in the lumber industry. There is an increased incidence of ALL and non-Hodgkin's lymphoma in survivors of nuclear explosions or reactor accidents and of other radiation exposures. Moreover, non-Hodgkin's lymphoma has been observed as a late complication of prior chemotherapy and/or radiation therapy. Specifically, patients with Hodgkin's disease treated with radiation therapy and chemotherapy exhibit an increased risk of developing secondary large cell lymphomas. Lymphoma-like syndromes have also been found in patients treated with phenytoin. Although in most cases this disease regresses when the drug is stopped, a significant number of patients still develop malignant lymphomas.

MOLECULAR GENETICS Although limited progress has been made in identifying agents that might be involved in inducing ALL and non-Hodgkin's lymphomas, exciting advances have been made in identifying those genes that appear to be involved in the pathogenesis of these diseases. Cytogenetic abnormalities have been

incidence of CLL is over 10/100,000 for persons over 70 but less than 1/100,000 for those under 50. CLL is also more common in males and in whites.

About 45,000 new cases of non-Hodgkin's lymphoma occur each year in the United States, and this number is increasing. Although the total number of patients is relatively small compared to some of the more common solid tumors, non-Hodgkin's lymphoma ranks as the sixth most common cause of cancer-related death in the United States. For males, non-Hodgkin's lymphoma ranks as the fourth leading cause of cancer mortality for individuals under the age of 15. In the decades between 15 and 34, it ranks second for males and fifth for females as the leading cause of death from cancer. Even for males between the ages of 35 and 54, it still ranks as the third leading cause of cancer-related mortality. There is little difference in 5-year survival rates for non-Hodgkin's lymphoma between whites and blacks. Non-Hodgkin's lymphomas rank fourth in the total number of person-years of life lost each year from cancer, demonstrating the profound personal and economic impact of this disease. This is true even if one subtracts the exponential increase resulting from cases of AIDS-related lymphomas.

There is evidence that infectious agents are involved in the pathogenesis of some non-Hodgkin's lymphomas, but no direct evidence exists in pre-B or T cell ALL or CLL. EBV has a strong association with development of Burkitt's lymphoma and leukemia (L3 ALL); some lymphomas associated with immunodeficiency, including human immunodeficiency virus (HIV) 1–related lymphoma; and angiocentric lymphomas (see Chap. 186). HTLV-I is the causative agent of the adult T cell leukemia/lymphoma endemic to the Caribbean and southern Japan (see Chap. 192). Gastric MALT lymphoma occurs as a consequence of *Helicobacter pylori* infection (see Chap. 156).

A number of primary diseases have an increased incidence of subsequently developing ALL, non-Hodgkin's lymphoma, and, to a lesser extent, Hodgkin's disease (Table 113-5). Individuals with Down's and Wiskott-Aldrich syndrome are at increased risk of developing ALL. There is also an increased incidence of ALL and CLL among family members who have these diseases. Diseases of inherited and acquired immunodeficiency as well as autoimmune diseases are associated with an increased incidence of lymphoma (Table 113-5).

Table 113-5

Diseases or Exposures Associated with Increased Risk of Development of Malignant Lymphoma

Inherited immunodeficiency disease
　Klinefelter's syndrome
　Chédiak-Higashi syndrome
　Ataxia telangiectasia syndrome
　Wiscott-Aldrich syndrome
　Common variable immunodeficiency disease
Acquired immunodeficiency diseases
　Iatrogenic immunosuppression
　HIV-1 infection
　Acquired hypogammaglobulinemia
Autoimmune disease
　Sjögren's syndrome
　Celiac sprue
　Rheumatoid arthritis and systemic lupus erythematosus
Chemical or drug exposures
　Phenytoin
　Dioxin, phenoxyherbicides
　Radiation
　Prior chemotherapy and radiation therapy
Infectious agent association (other than HIV)
　Epstein-Barr virus
　Human T cell leukemia/lymphoma virus-I
　Helicobacter pylori

well documented in a number of non-Hodgkin's lymphomas and ALL (Tables 113-2, 113-3). DNA sequence analysis of several of these chromosomal translocations has demonstrated that genes that normally regulate heavy and light chain immunoglobulin synthesis have been juxtaposed to genes that regulate normal cellular activation and proliferation. It is postulated that these transforming genes, or *oncogenes*, have come under the control of those regulatory elements that normally control B cell proliferation and differentiation. The best-studied example is the t(8;14) or variant t(2;8) or t(8;22) translocations of Burkitt's lymphoma present in over 90 percent of Burkitt's lymphomas and a subgroup of pre-B cell ALL. In this disease, the c-*myc* oncogene on chromosome 8 is joined to either the immunoglobulin heavy chain locus on chromosome 14, the κ light chain locus on chromosome 2, or the λ light chain locus on chromosome 22, leading to activation and overexpression of the c-*myc* gene product. Another example is the t(14;18) translocation, which is seen in approximately 85 percent of patients with follicular lymphomas and 25 percent of patients with diffuse lymphomas. In t(14;18), the gene *bcl*-2 (chromosome 18) is juxtaposed to the immunoglobulin heavy chain locus (chromosome 14). The *bcl*-2 gene product prevents programmed cell death, or *apoptosis*. By blocking apoptosis, the overexpression of the *bcl*-2 protein can lead to prolonged cell survival, and additional genetic changes are more likely to occur. Moreover, transgenic mice which overexpress the *bcl*-2 gene in their B cells develop a unique benign polyclonal lymphoproliferative syndrome. It is hypothesized that this alteration in *bcl*-2 expression is involved in the pathogenesis of the follicular lymphomas. Two other genes on chromosomes 11 and 3, when joined to immunoglobulin gene loci on chromosome 14, are associated with certain non-Hodgkin's lymphomas. On chromosome 11q13 a number of breakpoints have been identified, and one of the sequences has been identified as the *bcl*-1 gene. This translocation, seen in mantle cell lymphoma, leads to dysregulated expression of the gene that encodes for cyclin D1, which is involved in cell cycle regulation. More recently, a candidate oncogene, termed *bcl*-6, has been identified at the 3q27 breakpoint in a subset of diffuse large B cell non-Hodgkin's lymphomas. The protein encoded by this gene is homologous to zinc finger transcription factors and may be involved in activating certain growth-promoting genes. The t(2;5) in anaplastic large cell lymphoma produces a fusion protein consisting of the nucleophosmin (NPM) nucleolar phosphoprotein gene on chromosome 5q35 fused to a protein tyrosine kinase gene, ALK (for anaplastic large cell lymphoma kinase) on chromosome 2p23.

The t(9;22) BCR-ABL rearrangement leading to the formation of the abnormal tyrosine kinase (p190 or p210 BCR-ABL) is seen in about 30 percent of adult pre-B cell ALL. Chromosomal translocations involving 11q23 (MLL, HRX, ALL-1 gene) are seen in about 5 percent of adult pre-B ALL. These translocations lead to the development of abnormal DNA binding proteins, consequently to abnormal gene transcription. Translocations involving 11q23 are also involved in predominantly acute myeloid leukemias following epipodophyllotoxin exposures. Other translocations include t(1;19) in a subset of pre-B ALL and translocations involving the T cell antigen receptor genes (14q11, 7q34) in about half of the cases of T cell ALL. Analogous to those involving immunoglobulin genes, these T cell antigen receptor translocations lead to abnormal expression of certain transcription factors.

CHRONIC LEUKEMIAS/LYMPHOMAS

CLINICAL FEATURES AND NATURAL HISTORY
Chronic Lymphocytic Leukemia/Small Lymphocytic Lymphoma The most common chronic leukemia/lymphoma is B cell CLL, which presents with asymptomatic lymphocytosis in patients with a median age of 60. A reactive lymphocytosis, which is usually of normal T cells, is the major diagnosis that must be excluded. Approximately 40 percent of patients with B cell CLL have only lymphocytosis, with no anemia, thrombocytopenia, lymphadenopathy, or organomegaly. Constitutional symptoms are uncommon unless there is intercurrent infection, very extensive bulky disease, or histologic transformation

to a more aggressive lymphoma, usually diffuse large B cell lymphoma (Richter's syndrome). In Richter's syndrome, which occurs in ~5% of cases, patients also have rapidly growing nodal and extranodal masses. With more extensive marrow compromise and/or splenic involvement, patients with B cell CLL can develop cytopenias or immunosuppression, which can lead to symptoms. The white cell count usually ranges between 10 and 200 × 10^9/L with 70 to 95 percent small lymphocytes. The minimum lymphocytosis to make the diagnosis of CLL is 5 × 10^9/L. The absolute neutrophil count is usually normal, and red cell and platelet counts mildly decreased. The marrow is universally involved, and the extent of involvement influences survival, with a nodular infiltration being more favorable than diffuse involvement. Most patients have depressed serum immunoglobulin levels, which worsen with disease progression. Autoimmune phenomena can occur in up to 20 percent of patients, most commonly hemolytic anemia and less frequently thrombocytopenia or pure red cell aplasia. In B cell CLL the clinical staging of patients is of prognostic importance (Table 113-6). Other prognostic factors that predict for a shorter survival include a lymphocyte doubling time of <12 months, initial absolute lymphocyte count >50,000/μL, and an abnormal karyotype, most commonly trisomy 12.

Small lymphocytic lymphoma is the lymphomatous presentation of CLL and therefore occurs in middle-aged and older patients. Patients usually present with asymptomatic generalized lymphadenopathy. Unlike in CLL, the peripheral blood may appear normal or reveal only a mild lymphocytosis (60 percent will have absolute lymphocytosis of >4000/μL at diagnosis). In contrast, the bone marrow is involved in 75 to 95 percent of patients. A serum paraprotein is found in about 20 percent of patients, and hypogammaglobulinemia is also common. These patients can often be observed without treatment for 3 to 4 years; median survival is 8 to 10 years.

Other Chronic Leukemias There are other chronic leukemias that can present with lymphocytosis, including T cell CLL, PLL, LGL leukemia, hairy cell leukemia, splenic lymphoma with villous lymphocytes, and non-Hodgkin's lymphoma in leukemic phase. These "other" chronic leukemias are rare disorders. Patients with T cell CLL often present with prominent splenomegaly and extensive skin lesions and can have a rapidly progressive course. PLL can be of T or B cell lineage, with malignant cells that are larger than those in CLL and with prominent nucleoli. In contrast to CLL, patients with PLL present with higher levels of lymphocytosis, splenomegaly with minimal adenopathy, and a poor response to treatment. The LGL leukemias consist of two distinct clinical and pathologic entities. Patients with T cell LGL have a median age of 55 and present with recurrent bacterial infections due to severe neutropenia. Patients will have marrow involvement and splenomegaly. About one-third of patients will have rheumatoid arthritis resembling patients with Felty's syndrome. Most patients have a more indolent disease, with 60 percent alive more than 2 years from diagnosis. In contrast, patients with NK cell LGL leukemia have a median age of 39 and often present with fever in

Table 113-6

Staging of B Cell CLL and Relation to Survival

Stage	Clinical Features	Median Survival, years
RAI		
0	Lymphocytosis	12
I	Lymphocytosis + adenopathy	9
II	Lymphocytosis + splenomegaly	7
III	Anemia	1–2
IV	Thrombocytopenia	1–2
BINET		
A	No anemia/thrombocytopenia, <3 involved sites	>10
B	No anemia/thrombocytopenia, >3 involved sites	5
C	Anemia and/or thrombocytopenia	2

the absence of infection and no signs or symptoms of rheumatoid arthritis. These patients have significant hepatosplenomegaly as well as marrow involvement. Neutropenia is less severe than in T cell LGL leukemia, but anemia and thrombocytopenia are more pronounced. NK cell LGL leukemia is a very aggressive disease with a poor response to therapy.

Hairy cell leukemia is a rare disease occurring predominantly in males over age 40; it presents with cytopenias, splenomegaly, and large malignant B cells with characteristic morphologic and immunologic features. The presentation of patients can range from asymptomatic lymphocytosis to profound granulocytopenia, and some patients have vasculitis-like syndromes. The bone marrow biopsy is usually hyperplastic, with fibrosis common. An indolent course is commonly seen, with a median survival of over 4 years. The indications for treatment include pancytopenia, recurrent infections (including bacterial and opportunistic pathogens), and symptomatic splenomegaly.

℞ TREATMENT

The approach to patients with B cell CLL is very similar to that for patients with indolent non-Hodgkin's lymphoma, such as follicular lymphoma (see below). Since most patients are asymptomatic at presentation, with a disease that can have a very long natural history without treatment, initial observation is generally recommended. Randomized trials in very early stage patients (Binet A, Rai 0, I, II) involving no therapy versus initial treatment with an alkylating agent (chlorambucil) with prednisone suggested no benefit for early treatment. The indications for treating patients include symptomatic lymphadenopathy or organ involvement, cytopenia due to progressive disease or autoimmune phenomena, or systemic symptoms. The choices for initial therapy are many but generally involve alkylating agents given daily or in pulse fashion, with or without prednisone. Randomized trials suggest that chlorambucil is equivalent to combination therapy with cyclophosphamide, vincristine, and prednisone (CVP) in terms of complete response (CR) rate (25 percent), response duration (2 years), and median survival (4 years). Although controversial, some trials have demonstrated that in Binet stage B patients, more aggressive combination chemotherapy with cyclophosphamide, doxorubicin, vincristine, and prednisone (CHOP) was superior to CVP.

The nucleoside analogues fludarabine, pentostatin, and cladribine are very active in CLL. In previously treated patients, the response rate to fludarabine is around 50 percent [15 percent CR, including "nodular CRs" in the marrow; 40 percent partial response (PR)]. In previously untreated patients, the CR rates are over 30 percent, with 45 percent PRs. When one takes into account "nodular CRs" with residual "normal" nodules in the marrow, the CR rates are even higher. This has led to a randomized trial comparing fludarabine to alkylating agent–based treatment. Early analysis shows superiority for fludarabine in previously treated patients, but results are presently not clear for previously untreated patients. The toxicities of fludarabine and other purine analogues can be profound, with marked immunosuppression, depression of CD4+ T cells, opportunistic infections, and myelosuppression. Although not as extensively studied, results with cladribine are similar to fludarabine, while responses to pentostatin appear inferior to fludarabine. It is unlikely that patients who are resistant to fludarabine will respond to cladribine.

Intravenous immunoglobulin has been given to patients who are hypogammaglobulinemic. In these studies there is a significant decrease in serious infections; however, the treatment is costly. High-dose therapy and bone marrow transplantation (BMT) are being investigated in CLL using both purged autologous as well as allogeneic marrow. Early results are encouraging, but the follow-up is relatively short. There are several scenarios in which splenectomy is indicated in patients with CLL, including marked cytopenias often with symptomatic splenomegaly. Patients can have dramatic improvement in anemia and thrombocytopenia that can last for years

(median survival of responders >3 years). Splenectomy has also been used in the 25 percent of patients with autoimmune hemolytic anemia or thrombocytopenia that has not responded to glucocorticoids or intravenous immunoglobulin. Palliative radiation therapy to the spleen can be of limited benefit to some patients, as can radiation of bulky nodal masses.

The treatment of the other chronic leukemias with the exception of hairy cell leukemia has been largely unsuccessful. PLL and the NK and T cell LGL leukemias are generally resistant to combination chemotherapy. The standard treatment for cytopenias due to hairy cell leukemia used to be splenectomy, with a median duration of response of 8 months. The treatment of hairy cell leukemia has been revolutionized by the purine analogues, specifically cladribine. Cladribine induces a high CR rate (>80 percent) often with one course of treatment, with long clinical remissions, many in excess of 3 years. Cladribine is very active in patients previously treated with pentostatin or interferon α. It remains unknown if these patients will be cured, since minimal residual disease can be detected in patients in long clinical remissions.

NON-HODGKIN'S LYMPHOMA— GENERAL CONSIDERATIONS

CLINICAL PRESENTATION AND DIFFERENTIAL DIAGNOSIS More than two-thirds of patients with non-Hodgkin's lymphoma present with persistent, painless peripheral lymphadenopathy (see Chap. 61). At the time of presentation, the differential diagnosis of generalized lymphadenopathy necessitates the exclusion of infectious etiologies including bacteria, viruses (e.g., infectious mononucleosis, cytomegalovirus, and HIV), and parasites (toxoplasmosis). It is generally agreed that a firm lymph node larger than 1 cm that is not associated with a documentable infection and that persists longer than 4 weeks should be considered for biopsy. However, lymph nodes in several histopathologic subtypes of non-Hodgkin's lymphomas frequently wax and wane. Therefore, incomplete regression does not exclude a diagnosis of non-Hodgkin's lymphoma. In teenagers and young adults, infectious mononucleosis and Hodgkin's disease should be placed high in the differential diagnosis. A number of clinical features are suggestive of the diagnosis of non-Hodgkin's lymphoma. Involvement of Waldeyer's ring, epitrochlear, and mesenteric nodes are more frequently observed in patients with non-Hodgkin's lymphoma than with Hodgkin's disease. Unlike patients with Hodgkin's disease who present with weight loss, fever, or night sweats, fewer than 20 percent of patients with non-Hodgkin's lymphoma present with systemic complaints. Systemic symptoms are more common in patients with diffuse aggressive histologies, especially in those with hepatic and extranodal involvement. Less frequent presenting symptoms include fatigue, malaise, and pruritus, occurring in fewer than 10 percent of patients.

Non-Hodgkin's lymphomas also present with thoracic, abdominal, and/or extranodal symptoms. Although much less common than with Hodgkin's disease, approximately 20 percent of patients with non-Hodgkin's lymphoma present with mediastinal adenopathy. These patients most frequently present with persistent cough or chest discomfort or without clinical symptoms but having an abnormal chest x-ray. Occasionally, a superior vena caval syndrome is noted at presentation. Differential diagnosis of mediastinal presentation includes infections (e.g., histoplasmosis, tuberculosis, infectious mononucleosis), sarcoidosis, Hodgkin's disease, and other neoplasms. Involvement of retroperitoneal, mesenteric, and pelvic nodes is common in most histologic subtypes of non-Hodgkin's lymphoma. Unless massive or leading to obstruction, nodal enlargement in these sites usually does not produce symptoms. In contrast, patients who come to medical attention because of an abdominal mass, massive splenomegaly, or primary gastrointestinal lymphoma present with complaints similar to those caused by other abdominal space-occupying lesions. These complaints include chronic pain, abdominal fullness, early satiety, symptoms associated with visceral obstruction, or even acute perforation and gastrointestinal hemorrhage. Symptoms due to extralymphatic disease are common in some subtypes of aggressive non-Hodgkin's lymphoma but are uncommon in indolent lymphomas. Rarely, patients present with symptoms of unexplained anemia. Those with aggressive non-Hodgkin's lymphomas can present with primary cutaneous lesions, testicular masses, acute spinal cord compression, solitary bone lesions, and, rarely, lymphomatous meningitis. Primary non-Hodgkin's lymphoma of the CNS constitutes only 1 percent of all non-Hodgkin's lymphomas. However, with increasing incidence of HIV-1 infection, as well as increasing use of high-dose immunosuppressive therapy, primary CNS lymphoma has become as common as glioblastoma multiforme.

When non-Hodgkin's lymphoma is present in an extranodal site, the differential diagnosis is more difficult. Patients with non-Hodgkin's lymphoma uncommonly present with bronchovascular-lymphangitic, nodular, or alveolar patterns of involvement in the lung. In contrast, hepatic infiltration is common, although frequently not clinically evident. Between 25 and 50 percent of patients with non-Hodgkin's lymphoma present with hepatic infiltration, although relatively few present with large hepatic masses. Nearly 75 percent of patients with advanced-stage indolent lymphomas have microscopic hepatic infiltration at presentation. In contrast, primary hepatic lymphoma is extremely rare and is nearly always an aggressive histology tumor. Another extranodal presentation occurring in fewer than 5 percent of patients is primary lymphoma of bone. This is virtually always diffuse large B cell lymphoma, which presents as a painful bony site. Most frequently, lytic lesions are observed on bone x-ray. The most common sites of primary lymphoma of bone include femur, pelvis, and vertebrae. Approximately 5 percent of non-Hodgkin's lymphomas occur as primary gastrointestinal lymphoma. These patients present with hemorrhage, pain, or obstruction since the stomach is most frequently infiltrated, followed by small intestine and colon, respectively. Most gastrointestinal lymphomas have diffuse aggressive histologies, with a subset being low-grade non-Hodgkin's lymphoma (MALT lymphoma). An uncommon presentation of non-Hodgkin's lymphoma is renal infiltration, and even less common is localized presentation in the prostate, testis, or ovary. Localized skin infiltration by lymphoma is another uncommon site of presentation, usually of aggressive histology lymphoma. CNS presentation is relatively uncommon, although primary spinal cord and brain lymphomas are the most frequent areas of involvement. Primary CNS symptoms include headache, lethargy, focal neurologic symptoms, seizures, or paralysis. Rare sites of primary lymphoma include the orbit, heart, breast, salivary glands, thyroid, and adrenal gland.

STAGING AND DISEASE DETECTION The Ann Arbor staging system developed for Hodgkin's disease has also been used in staging non-Hodgkin's lymphomas. This staging system focuses on the number of tumor sites (nodal and extranodal), location, and the presence or absence of systemic symptoms. Table 113-7 summarizes this staging system. In stages I and II, sites of disease are on the same side of the diaphragm. Stage III disease involves both sides of the diaphragm, whereas stage IV is defined as extranodal lymphomatous involvement, most frequently of the bone marrow and liver. Systemic symptoms (fever, weight loss of >10 percent of body weight, and night sweats; i.e., B symptoms) are less common in non-Hodgkin's lymphomas (about 20 percent of cases) than in Hodgkin's disease. This staging scheme was specifically developed for Hodgkin's

disease, which disseminates by contiguous lymphatic extension and to a much lesser extent hematogenously. Since non-Hodgkin's lymphomas most frequently disseminate hematogenously, this staging system has proven to be less useful in this type of lymphoma.

The concept of staging has a small impact on treatment strategy in patients with non-Hodgkin's lymphomas. Only 10 percent of patients with follicular lymphoma have localized disease and are candidates for local radiation therapy. For the diffuse aggressive lymphomas, even patients with localized disease now receive systemic treatment. Therefore, staging is undertaken in non-Hodgkin's lymphomas to identify those small numbers of patients who can be treated with local therapy and to identify prognostic subgroups within histologic subtypes.

Staging Procedures after Biopsy Diagnosis Staging must be undertaken in the context of histology. A suggested staging workup for patients with non-Hodgkin's lymphoma is summarized in Table 113-8. After the initial excisional biopsy and documentation of the pathologic and immunologic subtype of disease, blood tests should be obtained, including complete blood count, routine chemistries, liver function tests including lactic dehydrogenase (LDH), serum protein electrophoresis to document the presence of circulating monoclonal paraprotein, and serum β_2-microglobulin, which has been shown to predict prognosis in both indolent and aggressive lymphomas. Waldeyer's ring involvement is often associated with intestinal involvement, and gastrointestinal contrast studies or endoscopy are indicated if the patient appears to have localized disease. Chest radiography is used to exclude mediastinal and hilar adenopathy, pleural effusions, and pulmonary parenchymal infiltration. Computed tomography (CT)

Table 113-8

Staging Evaluation for Non-Hodgkin's Lymphoma

Essential
1. Pathologic documentation by hematopathologist
2. Physical examination
3. Documentation of B symptoms
4. Laboratory evaluation
    a. Complete blood counts
    b. Liver function tests including LDH
    c. Renal function tests
    d. Uric acid
    e. Calcium
    f. Serum protein electrophoresis
    g. Serum β_2-microglobulin
5. Chest radiograph
6. CT scan of abdomen and pelvis
7. Bone marrow biopsy

Essential Under Certain Circumstances
1. Chest CT scan
2. Head CT scan
3. Lumbar puncture
4. Barium studies of gastrointestinal tract
5. Endoscopic examination
6. Cytologic examination of effusion
7. Gallium scan (planar or SPECT)

Useful But Not Essential Tests
1. Cell surface marker phenotypic analysis
2. Cytogenetic analysis
3. Gene rearrangement analysis
4. Polymerase chain reaction analysis of minimal residual disease
5. Flow cytometry for DNA analysis
6. Liver scan
7. Liver biopsy
8. Bone scan
9. Thallium scan
10. Lymphangiography
11. Ultrasonography
12. Magnetic resonance imaging
13. Echocardiogram
14. Laparotomy

Table 113-7

Ann Arbor Staging System

Stage I	Involvement in single lymph node region or single extralymphatic site
Stage II	Involvement of two or more lymph node regions on the same side of diaphragm
	Localized contiguous involvement of only one extralymphatic site and lymph node region (stage IIE)
Stage III	Involvement of lymph node regions on both sides of diaphragm; may include spleen
Stage IV	Disseminated involvement of one or more extralymphatic organs with or without lymph node involvement

scan of the chest is used to assess the extent of disease more precisely and is strongly recommended for patients with abnormal chest radiographs. It is not indicated if the chest x-ray is normal. However, abdominal/pelvic CT scan is essential for accurate staging to assess lymphadenopathy in retroperitoneal, mesenteric, and retrocrural areas. Lymphangiography is less useful than in Hodgkin's disease, since common sites of disease in non-Hodgkin's lymphoma include nodes in the mesentery, hilum of liver, spleen, or kidneys as well as nodes in the deep bony pelvis, none of which are detected by this procedure. The major advantage of lymphangiography over abdominal/pelvic CT is its ability to detect infiltrated but normal-sized retroperitoneal nodes and the ability to monitor the progress of treatment cheaply with a plain abdominal film. The primary indication for lymphangiography in non-Hodgkin's lymphoma is for patients with localized inguinal disease who may be candidates for local radiotherapy, where CT scanning for intraabdominal disease may be falsely negative. Bilateral percutaneous bone marrow biopsies must be performed, since the likelihood of lymphomatous involvement of the marrow is relatively high, especially in low-grade lymphoma, where marrow involvement occurs in up to 70 percent of cases. With any indication of hepatic abnormalities on blood tests or on liver scan, a percutaneous liver biopsy may be indicated in patients who would otherwise have stage I disease. In patients with aggressive lymphomas with marrow, bone, testicular, or paranasal sinus involvement, or if clinically indicated, examination of the cerebrospinal fluid by lumbar puncture should be performed.

More invasive tests are reserved for the uncommon presentation with stage I or II non-Hodgkin's lymphoma. While staging laparotomy may be performed in Hodgkin's disease, this is not so in the non-Hodgkin's lymphomas. In the aggressive non-Hodgkin's lymphomas, all stages can be considered to reflect disseminated disease and are therefore usually treated with chemotherapy. In contrast, only stages I and II indolent-histology lymphoma will be considered as localized and treated with radiation alone. Therefore, for most patients with non-Hodgkin's lymphoma it is less critical to ascertain the precise pathologic stage of disease. Moreover, it is common for these patients to exhibit disseminated disease after routine staging tests (e.g., bone marrow or liver biopsy). For example, within follicular lymphomas (grades I and II), following clinical staging and bone marrow biopsy, more than 85 percent of these patients will have stage III or stage IV disease. Thus, surgical staging should never be considered a routine procedure in patients with non-Hodgkin's lymphoma.

A number of other tests are becoming more important both in staging and in advancing our knowledge of the biology of non-Hodgkin's lymphoma. Gallium radionuclide scans appear to have clinical utility. Gallium scans are positive in virtually all intermediate- and high-grade lymphomas and in about 50 percent of low-grade lymphomas. Gallium scans, with high doses of isotope which permit delayed imaging, combined with single photon emission computed tomography (SPECT) are very sensitive in detecting tumor infiltration. These tests are also very useful in monitoring response to therapy. Magnetic resonance imaging appears to be most valuable for detecting occult marrow involvement and for evaluation of the brain and spinal cord. Thallium scanning may be a useful diagnostic modality to assess tumor infiltration by low-grade follicular lymphomas. There is little, if any, thallium uptake by high- or intermediate-grade lymphomas. Immunologic and molecular biologic studies are proving increasingly useful in confirming diagnosis. For example, in cases with difficult histopathologic patterns, cell-surface markers can distinguish between non-Hodgkin's lymphoma and carcinoma (leukocyte common antigen, CD45, is specific for lymphoid cells). Similarly, monoclonal antibodies directed against lineage-restricted antigens and detection of rearrangement of immunoglobulin or T cell receptor genes are useful in identifying lymphoid tumors. The delineation of the cell-surface phenotype is becoming important because an increasing number of treatment approaches employ monoclonal antibodies for purging of autologous stem cells for support of high-dose therapy and as part of investigational antibody-based treatments. Definition of a specific chromosomal abnormality in some studies appears to be of prognostic significance in certain histologic subtypes.

Sensitive Techniques to Detect Minimal Residual Disease The development of molecular techniques to define immunoglobulin and T cell receptor gene rearrangements has resulted in very sensitive tools with which to assess tumor cell infiltration more accurately. The most common and accessible tissues to be tested include peripheral blood and bone marrow. Whereas conventional histologic analysis of the bone marrow can detect 1 lymphoma cell infiltrating 20 normal cells, immunologic flow cytometric and Southern blot analysis each improve this level of detection to 1 lymphoma cell in approximately 100 normal cells. Similarly, flow cytometry has been used to detect "clonal excess" in the blood of patients with B cell non-Hodgkin's lymphoma. More recently, molecular biologic techniques have demonstrated that minimal disease detection can be markedly improved. For those non-Hodgkin's lymphomas with a known chromosomal translocation, it is now possible to identify a unique chromosomal "breakpoint." This has been most elegantly accomplished for the t(14;18) translocation present in the majority of follicular lymphomas and in about 25 percent of diffuse lymphomas. Based on DNA sequence, it is possible to amplify this unique stretch of DNA using specific oligonucleotide primers and the polymerase chain reaction (PCR). For those cases where a classic translocation is not known, PCR analysis of the IgH chain CDRIII region may be used. With this approach, 1 tumor cell in 10^5 to 10^6 normal cells can be detected. Thus, while other tests may be negative, PCR may demonstrate that the blood or bone marrow is contaminated by lymphoma cells. These techniques are presently being compared to more conventional staging methods. Considering their sensitivity, they may be useful in assessing complete remission more accurately and, more importantly, in determining whether treatment should be prolonged, truncated, or intensified. On the other hand, the presence of cells bearing the t(14;18) may not imply impending disease relapse or progression. Some normal people without a history of lymphoma have cells bearing t(14;18), and even patients with lymphoma in remission for many years may have such cells. Additional data are needed to assess the meaning of PCR-detected clonal cells.

PATHOLOGIC CLASSIFICATION The histologic classification of the non-Hodgkin's lymphomas is based on assessment of the overall pattern of lymph node architecture as well as on the cytologic classification of the neoplastic cell. It is clear that immunophenotype, genetic analysis, and cytogenetic analysis can, in many cases, refine the diagnosis. As the diagnostic techniques are improved, an increasing number of discrete clinicopathologic entities have been defined. Many of the entities are very rare. Thus, it has become necessary to group certain lymphomas together based on their likely natural history. Over time, it is anticipated that specialized treatment approaches will be developed for each disease entity. Table 113-2 compares the R.E.A.L., Working Formulation, modified Kiel, and the Rappaport classifications. In current clinical practice these classification schemes are frequently used interchangeably. However, disease entities are not necessarily easily translated from one to the other. For example, mantle cell lymphoma may be classified in five different Working Formulation categories. The crucial attributes of a pathologic diagnosis are accuracy and reproducibility, for it has been found that the histologic diagnosis provides critical predictors of clinical pattern of disease, response to treatment, and prognosis.

INDOLENT LYMPHOMAS Clinical Features and Natural History *Follicular center lymphoma* Follicular lymphomas account for approximately 50 percent of the non-Hodgkin's lymphomas; the grade I (small cleaved cell) type is the most common. Patients usually present with painless peripheral adenopathy in cervical, axillary, inguinal, and femoral regions. Patients frequently note that lymph node enlargement has been present for long periods of time, often years, and the nodes have "waxed and waned." Less typically, there is enlargement of Waldeyer's ring and epitrochlear nodes. Some patients present with asymptomatic large abdominal and retroperitoneal masses, with or without evidence of gastrointestinal and/or renal obstruction. Although patients may present with one or more sites of nodal disease, noninvasive workup usually demonstrates widely disseminated disease with involvement of spleen and bone marrow in over 80 percent of patients. Bone marrow involvement in follicular lymphoma reveals a unique pattern of paratrabecular infiltration. Peripheral blood involvement is seen in about 20 percent of patients, and CNS disease is rare, although epidural disease can be seen. In contrast to aggressive lymphomas, about 20 percent of patients present with extramedullary extranodal disease, and fewer than 10 percent present with B symptoms. The course of this disease is quite variable. The conventional approach for most patients is that they can be observed with waxing and waning disease for an average of 3 years without the need for therapy. In patients with stage I or limited stage II disease, local radiation therapy may provide long-term remissions or possible cure. Some patients demonstrate more disseminated and rapid growth and require treatment because massive nodal or organ enlargement leads to pain, lymphatic obstruction, organ obstruction, or, more rarely, neurologic symptoms. At the time of increasing generalized disease or rapid growth at a single site, involved nodes should be considered for rebiopsy. A significant number of rapidly progressing patients will demonstrate a "conversion" or "transformation" to a more aggressive histologic pattern, often diffuse large cell. This conversion is associated with acquisition of additional genetic abnormalities and occurs in about 7 percent of patients per year. Nearly all patients with follicular lymphoma who die of lymphoma have undergone histologic progression. Histologic conversion is associated with infiltration of extranodal sites, the development of systemic symptoms, and a poor prognosis since the tumor is much less responsive to treatment. Historically, both disease-free and overall survivals of patients with follicular lymphoma have not improved despite many different therapeutic approaches. Although 40 to 80 percent of patients achieve complete remissions (noninvasively staged) with conventional single-agent or aggressive combination chemotherapy, the median duration of remission is between 2 and 3 years. Following relapse, patients can be observed or retreated; however, the median survival after first relapse is 5 years. Patients with follicular non-Hodgkin's lymphoma survive long periods of time, with median overall survivals for patients with stages III and IV disease approaching 7 to 9 years. The grade II (mixed small and large cell) type can have a slightly different clinical presentation. Bone marrow infiltration at diagnosis is less frequent than in grade I (small cell) type, but large abdominal masses are more commonly seen. Since these patients generally progress faster if not treated and some studies suggest that a subset of these patients may be cured with conventional therapy, these patients are generally not observed but are treated soon after diagnosis with combination chemotherapy.

Marginal zone lymphomas These lymphomas present in nodal or extranodal sites and are then referred to as monocytoid B cell lymphomas or MALT lymphomas, respectively. A third related disease, splenic lymphoma ($\pm$ circulating villous lymphocytes), presents as splenomegaly. Many patients with marginal zone lymphomas present with stage I or II disease. There is no age predilection for the extranodal tumors, which can involve the gastrointestinal tract, respiratory tract, lacrimal and salivary glands, thyroid, breast, or lung but usually not peripheral blood and marrow. Patients can present with peptic ulcer disease, abdominal pain, and sicca syndrome (Sjögren's syndrome). The clinical behavior of this disease is similar to that of the indolent follicular lymphomas.

Mycosis fungoides The cutaneous T cell lymphomas are diseases of middle-aged adults, with a slight male predominance. Major variants include mycosis fungoides and the Sézary syndrome, characterized by peripheral blood involvement. These diseases present with cutaneous manifestations and lymphadenopathy and follow an indolent course. Later, patients will develop hepatic, splenic, gastrointestinal tract, pulmonary, and renal involvement. Infiltration of the bone marrow and circulating leukemia cells (Sézary cells), usually in the presence of generalized erythroderma, are also frequent late manifestations. The median survival from diagnosis is about 10 years, with infection being the most common cause of death.

℞ TREATMENT

The majority of patients with indolent non-Hodgkin's lymphomas present with advanced disease, with fewer than 10 percent having pathologic stage I/II. Early-stage patients treated with radiotherapy have 5-year relapse-free survival of 60 to 80 percent, with overall 5-year survivals approaching 100 percent. In early-stage disease, chemotherapy alone has rarely been used due to the radioresponsiveness of these tumors, and there is no significant advantage of combined modality over local radiotherapy.

The long natural history of indolent non-Hodgkin's lymphomas and the lack of symptoms in the majority of patients at diagnosis have led to close observation as the initial approach to some of these patients. The advantages of this approach include a prolonged period free of treatment during which tumor cells will not be selected for drug resistance by continuous exposure to drugs. Moreover, spontaneous remissions of longer than 1 year have been reported to occur in 23 percent of patients. When treatment is started, these diseases are very sensitive to both single-agent and combination chemotherapy. The complete response rates of previously untreated patients to single alkylating agents such as cyclophosphamide or chlorambucil range between 30 and 60 percent, with a median duration of remission of about 2 years. More aggressive chemotherapy regimens have produced more rapid and higher percentages of complete remissions but unfortunately have not clearly changed the overall survival of patients with these diseases. Attempts to treat patients for prolonged periods of time with single-agent therapy or the addition of long-term "maintenance" treatment also have not improved survival. Following relapse, most patients can be successfully retreated; however, the ability to achieve third and subsequent remissions becomes more difficult, and the duration of those remissions is usually shorter. The implications on prognosis of conversion from indolent to aggressive histology continues to be controversial. Although most patients do poorly when treated with combination chemotherapy, the subset of patients with sensitive disease who achieve a CR may experience prolonged remission and survival. In addition to its curative potential in stage I patients, radiotherapy is frequently used in conjunction with systemic therapy to treat sites of bulk disease and to palliate sites of symptomatic disease. However, it remains controversial whether the addition of radiotherapy increases the overall disease-free survival. A subset of patients with follicular center lymphoma, grade II (mixed small cleaved and large cell lymphoma), are reported to experience long-term remissions and possible cure following treatment with combination chemotherapy; however, this remains controversial. The combinations used are either cyclophosphamide, Oncovin (vincristine), prednisone, and procarbazine (C-MOPP) or CHOP.

The subtype of indolent lymphoma that is associated with MALT, known as *extranodal marginal zone lymphoma*, is often treated surgically with or without local radiotherapy. Since these diseases tend to remain localized for long periods of time before systemic spread, surgery remains a highly effective approach. For patients with advanced disease, the use of chemotherapy with alkylating agents for MALT lymphomas has received limited attention but appears to be effective at inducing remissions. Primary gastric MALT lymphomas associated with *H. pylori* gastritis respond to omeprazole and amoxycillin, suggesting that eradication of infection induces regression of lymphoma. Unfortunately, for most sites of disease, the stimulating antigen, if any, has not been defined.

Local and systemic therapy are used in the treatment of mycosis fungoides. Patients with disease limited to the skin may be cured with electron beam radiation therapy. Topical treatment of skin lesions with chemotherapeutic agents such as nitrogen mustard can induce remissions in up to 90 percent of patients with disseminated disease. Systemic therapy with either drugs alone or combined modality therapy can induce high response rates (up to 80 percent), but few long-term remissions are seen in advanced-stage patients. Oral psoralens combined with ultraviolet light often induce PR. Interferon α is one effective second-line palliative therapy. Monoclonal antibodies (unconjugated and conjugated to toxins or radioisotopes), extracorporeal phototherapy, and the adenosine deaminase inhibitor pentostatin remain investigational. Fludarabine and cladribine may also be active.

Several new agents have been examined in advanced-stage follicular lymphomas. Interferon α is an active agent. Several prospective randomized trials have examined the role of interferon when added to combination chemotherapy in patients with advanced-stage disease and have found a significant prolongation of remission duration. However, a prolongation of survival was seen in only one trial. The purine analogues cladribine and fludarabine induced responses in 40 to 50 percent of previously treated patients. A humanized anti-CD20 antibody appears to induce PR in 50 percent and CR in 5 to 10 percent of patients, with little or no toxicity.

If these diseases are to be cured, either more aggressive high-dose chemotherapy regimens must be evaluated or new therapeutic modalities must be employed. Patients with advanced-stage follicular lymphomas are being treated earlier in the course of their disease with aggressive chemotherapy combined with total nodal irradiation or high-dose chemoradiotherapy and autologous stem cell transplantation. These studies suggest that high CR rates in the range of 80 percent or greater are possible. However, the impact of these studies on long-term disease-free survival and overall survival remain uncertain due to limited follow-up.

AGGRESSIVE LYMPHOMAS Clinical Features and Natural History *Follicular center lymphoma (large cell)* Although the follicular architecture of these tumors is preserved, this disease behaves much more like diffuse large B cell lymphoma. In contrast to other follicular lymphomas, this histologic variant has less frequent infiltration of the marrow and liver and presents with large masses and, frequently, extranodal disease. A finite cure rate has been reported in selected series. Follicular large cell lymphomas often evolve into diffuse large B cell lymphoma.

Mantle cell lymphoma This entity has also been called *diffuse intermediate lymphocytic lymphoma* and *centrocytic lymphoma*. However, it does not develop from centrocytes and no "intermediate" stage of differentiation has been defined. Typical sites of involvement include lymph nodes, spleen, liver, gastrointestinal tract, and bone marrow. Peripheral blood involvement has been reported in approximately 25 percent of patients at presentation, and systemic B symptoms are observed in approximately one-third of patients. Mantle cell lymphoma can involve any region of the gastrointestinal tract, occasionally presenting as multiple intestinal polyposis. Lymphomas with a mantle zone pattern, pseudoproliferation centers, and low growth fraction (Ki-67 expression) are reported to have a better prognosis, whereas those with a more diffuse form and higher proliferation index are thought to have a poorer prognosis. However, median survival is about 3 years.

Diffuse large B cell lymphoma Patients, who are generally middle-aged or older, present with either nodal enlargement (especially in the neck or abdomen) or extranodal disease (in the gastrointestinal tract, testes, bone, thyroid, salivary glands, skin, or brain). During the course of the disease, the liver, kidneys, and lung may be involved. Diffuse large B cell lymphoma is highly invasive, with local compression of vessels or airways, involvement of peripheral nerves, and destruction of bone. Although bone marrow involvement is found in only 10 to 20 percent of patients initially, its detection is important because of its strong correlation with later spread to the CNS. Later in the disease, some patients demonstrate both extensive bone marrow infiltration and peripheral blood involvement. A subset of patients present with predominantly mediastinal disease, known as *primary mediastinal (thymic) B cell lymphoma*. Mediastinal B cell lymphoma affects young females predominantly and is locally aggressive.

Aggressive T cell lymphomas These diseases are rare and consist of a number of distinct pathologic and clinical entities. *Peripheral T cell lymphomas*, so called because of their shared immunophenotype with peripheral blood T cells, clinically resemble diffuse large B cell lymphomas. *Angioimmunoblastic T cell lymphoma* is a disease of older adults, presenting with the acute onset of generalized lymphadenopathy, rash, hepatosplenomegaly, and B symptoms. Immunologic abnormalities are common and include plasmacytosis, polyclonal hypergammaglobulinemia, and a positive Coombs' test. This disease is progressive and frequently fatal, with median survival of 30 months. Angiocentric lymphomas clinically present as two entities: (1) *nasal T cell lymphoma*, probably associated with EBV and previously known as lethal midline granuloma; and (2) *pulmonary angiocentric lymphoma*, previously in the spectrum of lymphomatoid granulomatosis. The nasal lymphomas tend to be locally aggressive and recur locally after therapy. Patients with gluten-sensitive enteropathy are at risk of developing *intestinal T cell lymphomas*. They involve the ileum predominantly. These diseases present with abdominal pain, obstruction, and perforation, and surgical debulking is often indicated in their management. The *anaplastic large cell lymphomas* are either of T cell or null cell lineage. These diseases present with extranodal disease, often skin, and at nodal sites as well. Clinically these patients present with symptoms similar to those with aggressive diffuse large B cell lymphoma.

AIDS-related lymphomas Although not a separate pathologic entity, non-Hodgkin's lymphoma occurs in 10 to 30 percent of patients with AIDS. Virtually all cases are diffuse large B cell or Burkitt's type. In these cases extranodal involvement is common, with CNS, bone marrow, liver, and gastrointestinal tract the most frequent sites. Most patients present with widespread disease, rapid nodal enlargement, and B symptoms. A subset present with an effusion, without a mass. Primary CNS lymphoma—a disease with a short survival—is common in advanced AIDS patients. When treated with the most aggressive combinations of chemotherapy, results have been poor, largely due to the high death rate from intercurrent infections associated with severe immunodeficiency.

℞ TREATMENT

To decide the appropriate treatment regimen, the clinician must know the histology and extent of disease. Most patients with aggressive-histology lymphoma should be treated initially with curative intent. Choice of therapy may be influenced by age and the presence of comorbid diseases (cardiac, renal, pulmonary, hepatic), which might significantly affect end-organ toxicity.

The treatment of diffuse large B cell lymphoma is one of the major success stories of modern chemotherapy. The first successful regimen for this disease was C-MOPP, which induced complete remissions in approximately 45 percent of patients and with long-term disease-free survival for about one-third of patients. The CHOP regimen achieves complete remissions in about 50 percent of patients, with long-term disease-free survival of 35 percent. Success with this and subsequent regimens requires attention to administering full doses and adhering to schedules as strictly as possible. Over the past 15 years, attempts have been made to improve the percentage of complete remissions and overall cure rate. Additional agents have been added to those in CHOP including bleomycin, methotrexate, procarbazine, nitrogen mustard, cytosine arabinoside, and etoposide (e.g., M-BACOD, m-BACOD, ProMACE-MOPP, COP-BLAM, MACOP-B, ProMACE/CytaBOM). With these approaches, the complete remission rate now approaches 80 percent for the most aggressive regimens. However, toxicities have also increased (e.g., infections as well as cardiac and pulmonary complications). Within individual institutional studies, the results with some of these third-generation regimens has been far superior to CHOP, with approximately 70 percent of patients appearing to be cured. However, a multi-institutional randomized trial comparing CHOP to m-BACOD, ProMACE/CytaBOM, or MACOP-B found no difference in the overall survival, response rate, or time to treatment failure between the four treatment arms. Confidence in this trial is undermined by the 30 percent lower than expected CR rates obtained with MACOP-B and ProMACE-CytaBOM. Prolonged "maintenance" therapy has not improved overall survival. A significant proportion of patients with diffuse aggressive lymphoma are over age 60, and the outcome for patients over age 60 is worse than for younger patients. The reasons for these differences may be related to less intensive treatment delivered as well as to the presence of comorbid diseases. In some studies, increased deaths unrelated to lymphoma or its treatment have been reported, whereas in others, an increased treatment-related mortality has been reported. Attempts to modify regimens and improve supportive care may improve the treatment of aggressive lymphomas in elderly patients. Selected patients with localized aggressive diffuse large B cell lymphomas have been treated in the past with local radiation therapy, with 50 to 60 percent attaining long-term disease-free survival; however, the use of four cycles of chemotherapy with local radiation results in cure of 85 to 90 percent of such patients. Local radiation therapy may also improve the effect of chemotherapy on the aggressive nasal T cell lymphomas, which have a high propensity to recur locally. However, for the vast majority of patients with aggressive lymphoma, radiation therapy is of no proven benefit.

AIDS-related lymphomas are among the most aggressive of the non-Hodgkin's lymphomas. Initial studies with aggressive regimens yielded dismal results, with only one-third of patients achieving complete remission, and a high frequency of CNS relapse and fatal opportunistic infection. Subsequent studies using modified doses of chemotherapy and CNS prophylaxis have given CR rates of 50 percent, with a median survival of 15 months for those patients in complete remission. Since neutropenia was a major problem even in modified-dose therapy, the addition of the hematopoietic growth factors has permitted tolerable escalation of chemotherapy doses. Response rates appear to be related to clinical factors, including history of AIDS, CD4 T cell counts, and performance status. For patients who do not respond or who relapse, the results of salvage treatment are very poor, with short survival.

Prognostic Factors CLINICAL PROGNOSTIC FACTORS Without question, the response to treatment is one of the most important prognostic indicators, particularly in patients with aggressive non-Hodgkin's lymphoma. Patients with aggressive non-Hodgkin's lymphoma who do not respond to first-line therapy generally have very short survival. In contrast, patients with diffuse large B cell lymphoma who rapidly attain a clinical complete remission have a 70 to 80 percent likelihood of having long-term disease-free survival.

Analysis of a large group (2031) of patients with aggressive non-Hodgkin's lymphomas, largely diffuse large B cell lymphomas, has led to the establishment of a prognostic factor model that appears to apply to both indolent and aggressive lymphomas. A large number of factors were examined for all patients studied: age (≤60 vs. >60), serum LDH (normal vs. >1 × normal), performance status (0 or 1 vs. 2 to 4), stage (I or II vs. III or IV), and extranodal involvement (≤1 site vs. >1 site) were independently prognostic for overall survival. For the patients age 60 or less, only stage, LDH, and performance status were of prognostic significance. For relapse-free survival, age, stage, and performance status were significant parameters for predicting outcome. These data permitted the identification of four risk groups based on the number of risk factors: low risk with no or one factor; low-intermediate with two factors; high-intermediate with three factors; and high with four or five factors (Table 113-9).

LABORATORY PROGNOSTIC FACTORS Markers of proliferating cells such as expression of specific proteins (Ki-67, PCNA) and thymidine uptake have been associated with decreased survival. Similarly, it remains unclear whether the expression of certain cell surface markers such as adhesion molecules or T or B cell antigens is associated with clinical presentation or outcome. High serum levels of β_2-microglobulin are associated with poor prognosis.

A number of chromosomal abnormalities have been reported to influence prognosis: absence of normal metaphase cells, complexity of the karyotype, the presence of specific chromosomal abnormalities such as t(8;14), abnormality of the short arm of chromosome 1,

Table 113-9

The International Index and Prognosis in Diffuse Aggressive Non-Hodgkin's Lymphoma

Risk Group (Patients of All Ages)	Risk Factors*	Distribution of Cases, %	Complete Response Rate, %	5-Year Survival Rate, %
Low	0, 1	35	87	73
Low-intermediate	2	27	67	51
High-intermediate	3	22	55	43
High	4, 5	16	44	26

* Age (≤60 vs. >60); serum LDH (normal vs. >1 × normal); performance status (0 or 1 vs. 2–4); stage (I or II vs. III or IV); and extranodal involvement (≤1 site vs. >1 site)
SOURCE: Adapted from Shipp.

trisomy 7, trisomy 18, deletions of chromosome 6, and the presence of abnormalities of chromosome 17. Rearrangement of the *bcl*-6 gene, present in approximately one-third of diffuse large B cell lymphomas, may be a favorable independent prognostic variable.

SIGNIFICANCE OF MINIMAL RESIDUAL DISEASE Following aggressive therapy of patients with follicular lymphoma using high-dose ablative therapy and autologous BMT, those patients who consistently lack a *bcl*-2 translocation in the bone marrow and the peripheral blood have a significantly better disease-free survival than patients with PCR-detectable disease. The presence of abnormal cells after therapy of aggressive lymphoma may also predict relapse. The meaning of a "molecular" complete response as compared to the usual clinical criteria for complete response is being assessed. Currently, molecular assessment of remission is a research tool.

Salvage Chemotherapy The prognosis for patients with intermediate- and high-grade non-Hodgkin's lymphoma who fail to achieve a complete remission or who relapse following aggressive therapy is very poor. Salvage chemotherapy employing drugs such as cytosine arabinoside, cisplatin, etoposide, ifosfamide, given as single agents or in combination, have been used to induce remissions. Depending upon the histology and regimen, approximately 20 to 30 percent of patients attain a complete remission after conventional dose salvage therapy, with partial remissions in another 30 percent. Unfortunately, these remissions tend to be short-lived (approximately 2 to 6 months), with fewer than 3 percent of patients in remission beyond 2 years.

Stem Cell Transplantation (BMT) Patients with disease resistant to conventional or salvage therapeutic regimens can still be induced into a complete remission with very high doses of chemotherapy or the combination of high-dose chemotherapy and radiotherapy. A steep dose-response curve persists in non-Hodgkin's lymphomas, even after relapse. This treatment approach is complicated by very significant and prolonged myelosuppression. Bone marrow as a source of hematopoietic stem cells can be infused from an identical twin (syngeneic), an HLA-matched relative (allogeneic), or from the patient (autologous). Alternatively, hematopoietic stem cells can be isolated from peripheral blood. The vast majority of transplants for patients with lymphoma have employed autologous stem cells. Stem cell transplantation has become widespread in the treatment of patients with refractory or relapsed non-Hodgkin's lymphoma. Patients whose disease has never responded to primary therapy are presently not salvaged by this approach. Following relapse from remission, fewer than 15 percent of patients whose disease is resistant to all forms of salvage therapy have long-term disease-free survival. In contrast, approximately 40 percent of those patients whose disease is still responsive to therapy have long-term disease-free survival with high-dose therapy and BMT. High-dose therapy and autologous BMT are superior to conventional-dose salvage therapy with DHAP (cisplatin, cytarabine, dexamethasone) in relapsed patients with diffuse large B cell lymphoma. While the majority of patients undergoing BMT have intermediate- and high-grade non-Hodgkin's lymphoma, studies in those with low-grade lymphomas suggest that a subset of patients experience long-term disease-free survival. Early studies with BMT reported treatment-related deaths in the range of 20 to 30 percent; however, as patients with no associated comorbid disease are treated, this mortality has significantly decreased to less than 5 percent. The use of recombinant hematopoietic growth factors to hasten myeloid cell recovery has also significantly reduced morbidity and length of hospitalization following high-dose therapy and stem cell transplantation.

Lower treatment-related mortality has led some groups to use high-dose therapy as consolidation therapy in patients with poor prognosis non-Hodgkin's lymphomas in first remission. Patients who are at high risk for relapse following conventional therapy have a significantly better disease-free survival with consolidation autologous BMT than with conventional treatment alone. Although this modality is capable of curing some patients with relapsed non-Hodgkin's lymphomas, many issues still remain, including optimal therapeutic regimen, timing of transplantation, source of hematopoietic stem cells, the need to purge autologous marrow, and methods to minimize morbidity and mortality.

New Therapeutic Approaches Although great strides have been made in the treatment of non-Hodgkin's lymphoma with conventional, salvage, and high-dose ablative therapy, many patients are not cured. However, unlike most other cancers, many patients can achieve a complete remission. This suggests that the major obstacle to cure is subpopulations of resistant neoplastic cells. There are a number of newer approaches to the treatment of non-Hodgkin's lymphomas that may overcome resistance. There are a growing number of cytokines that may be either cytostatic or cytotoxic to neoplastic cells. Monoclonal antibodies (unconjugated, conjugated to toxins, or conjugated to a radionuclide) are being used to treat patients with non-Hodgkin's lymphomas. Anti-B cell (anti-CD20) monoclonal antibodies conjugated to ^{131}I have shown promising results with limited follow-up. Endogenously or exogenously activated lymphocytes or NK cells can be used to attack lymphoma cells specifically. Infusion of cytokines (such as IL-12) that augment antitumor immunity are in clinical trials and may well have a role in the minimal disease state. Vaccination studies are underway using the tumor Ig idiotype to induce specific immunity against residual tumor cells. Another approach is to modify the tumor cells to make them more immunogenic and more susceptible to endogenous effector mechanisms.

ACUTE LEUKEMIA/LYMPHOMA

CLINICAL FEATURES AND NATURAL HISTORY **Lymphoblastic Leukemia** Patients with lymphoblastic leukemia present with signs and symptoms of marrow failure. These include pallor and fatigue, bleeding and bruising, and fever and infection—due to anemia, thrombocytopenia, and neutropenia, respectively. The risk of bleeding increases with platelet counts less than $20 \times 10^5/\mu L$ and often involves skin and mucosal sites. With platelet transfusions, hemorrhage is no longer a major cause of death, although alloimmunization can limit optimal platelet support of patients, particularly when patients have been heavily transfused. The increased risk of infection occurs with absolute neutrophil counts less than $500/\mu L$ and is the leading cause of death. Febrile patients should be promptly treated with broad-spectrum antibiotics, and these should be continued until neutropenia is resolved. Infections commonly involve mucosal sites such as the pharynx and perianal area as well as the lungs and skin (particularly intravenous line sites). The most common bacterial organisms are *Staphylococcus* spp. and gram-negative organisms. Patients in relapse or under treatment, particularly when on broad-spectrum antibiotics, are susceptible to opportunistic organisms such as anaerobic bacteria, yeast (*Candida* spp.), fungi (*Aspergillus, Mucor, Pneumocystis*), and viruses (such as herpesviruses).

Patients with ALL can present with infiltration of spleen, lymph nodes, liver, skin, or CNS (particularly as a site of relapse). Patients with leukemic meningitis generally present with headache, nausea, and cranial nerve palsies. Involvement of the testis as an extramedullary site of relapse is not uncommon. A mediastinal mass is a frequent presentation of T cell lymphoblastic leukemia/lymphoma (see below). Bone pain, particularly sternal tenderness, is seen in many patients with lymphoblastic leukemia.

Several metabolic abnormalities are seen in patients with ALL. Uric acid nephropathy is caused by the rapid turnover of acute leukemia cells. This is aggravated by dehydration, acidosis, and therapy leading to tumor cell lysis. The use of hydration, alkalinization of the urine, and allopurinol can prevent urate nephropathy. Both hypokalemia and hyperkalemia can occur in patients with ALL. The cause of the hypokalemia is unknown in ALL but is caused by an unknown renal tubular defect. Hyperkalemia is seen along with hypocalcemia and hyperphosphatemia as part of the tumor lysis syndrome following initiation of therapy (see Chap. 104). This syndrome is most commonly seen in L3 ALL/Burkitt's lymphoma and is aggravated by renal failure.

In order to make a diagnosis of acute leukemia, the marrow must be involved, with >30 percent lymphoblasts, although a similar number of blasts in the peripheral blood also makes the diagnosis. There is some relationship between immunophenotype with subtype of ALL and clinical findings. Patients with pre-B ALL (French-American-British L1, L2), the "classic" childhood ALL, often have splenomegaly and rarely have white blood counts over $25,000/\mu L$. T cell ALL (L1, L2) has a male predominance and CNS and mediastinal disease. B cell ALL (L3) often has extramedullary presentation with metabolic abnormalities. The distribution of subtypes of ALL differs between adults and children. In contrast to childhood ALL, where L1 morphology is most common, L2 is the most common subtype in adults. T cell phenotype is also more common in adults (20 percent of cases) than in children. Finally, t(9;22) is seen in about 20 percent of adults but is rare in childhood ALL.

Precursor T Cell/B Cell Lymphoblastic Lymphoma Although lymphoblastic lymphomas represent a major subgroup of childhood non-Hodgkin's lymphomas, they are much less common in adults (fewer than 5 percent of adult non-Hodgkin's lymphomas). Such patients are usually males in their twenties and thirties who present with lymphadenopathy in cervical, supraclavicular, and axillary regions (50 percent) or with a mediastinal mass (50 to 70 percent). In most patients the mediastinal mass is anterior, >10 cm, is symptomatic often with superior vena cava syndrome, and is associated with pleural effusions. Less commonly, patients present with extranodal disease (e.g., skin, testicular, or bony involvement). More than 90 percent of patients present with stage III or stage IV disease, and half have B symptoms. Although the bone marrow can be normal at presentation, approximately 60 percent of patients develop bone marrow infiltration and a subsequent leukemic phase indistinguishable from T cell ALL. Before current aggressive acute leukemia–like therapy, this disease was rapidly fatal.

Burkitt's Lymphoma Burkitt's lymphoma is a childhood tumor that has two major clinical presentations. The endemic (African) form generally presents as a jaw or abdominal tumor that spreads to extranodal sites, especially to the bone marrow and meninges. The nonendemic (American) form has an abdominal presentation with massive disease; ascites; and skin, bone, and peripheral node involvement. Like the African form, it also spreads to the bone marrow and CNS (although less than in the African form). Before aggressive therapeutic programs, all children died rapidly. These tumors are now treated with very aggressive chemotherapeutic programs with more gratifying results. Burkitt's lymphoma is uncommon in adults but is occasionally seen in patients up to age 35. In contrast, the high-grade Burkitt-like lymphomas are heterogeneous and aggressive and frequently present like diffuse large B cell lymphoma in extranodal sites. Burkitt-like lymphoma behaves more like diffuse large cell lymphoma.

Adult T Cell Leukemia/Lymphoma This entity has been observed in southwestern Japan, the Caribbean, and in blacks in the southeastern United States and is associated with the HTLV-I retrovi-

Adult T cell leukemia/lymphoma (ATLL) presents with generalized lymphadenopathy, hepatosplenomegaly, cutaneous infiltration,
hypercalcemia, lytic bone lesions, elevated LDH, and a leukemia
characterized by pleomorphic CD4+ T cells. The skin lesions can
vary from papules to plaques to tumors to ulcerations. Marrow involvement is not marked, and anemia and thrombocytopenia are not common. This disease has a fulminant course, and its natural history
has been minimally altered by aggressive combination chemotherapy.
Although 50 to 70 percent of patients will achieve a complete remission, the median duration of remission is about 12 months. The incidence of infection, often opportunistic, is very high in patients with
ATLL because of an underlying immunodeficiency in these HTLV-
I-infected patients. A chronic form has also been described with skin
lesions, mild lymphocytosis without significant numbers of circulating
blasts, and absence of hepatosplenomegaly or lymphadenopathy. These
patients can survive for years before converting to the more aggressive
form of the disease.

℞ **TREATMENT**

Although the clinical distinction between lymphoblastic leukemia
and lymphoma is based upon the percentage of marrow involvement,
both diseases require similar aggressive therapy with induction, consolidation, CNS prophylaxis, and maintenance therapy. With this
approach, 40 percent or more of patients are cured. Optimum induction therapy for adults with ALL must include an anthracycline
in addition to vincristine and prednisone ($\pm$L-asparaginase). This
improves the CR rate from 50 percent to as high as 85 percent in
some series. The use of more intensive induction regimens has added
no significant benefit to date. Once CR is achieved, postremission
therapy (which in some studies is very intensive) is critical to improving the duration of CR in patients with ALL. CNS prophylaxis is
more optimally given early rather than late during postremission
therapy. Cranial radiation with intrathecal methotrexate or intrathecal
and high-dose systemic methotrexate are effective methods of prophylaxis. Maintenance therapy lasting about 2 years, similar to that
given to children, generally includes methotrexate, 6-mercaptopu-
rine, vincristine, and prednisone. However, the optimal duration and
intensity of maintenence therapy in adults are unclear.

Precursor T cell or B cell lymphoblastic lymphoma in adults
has been treated with some success, although inferior to that seen
in children. When treated with regimens initially developed for
childhood ALL with intrathecal therapy, about 40 percent of adults
are reported to survive at 5 years. CNS prophylaxis is critical in
treating these diseases since the CNS is a sanctuary site for recurrence. Similarly, Burkitt's lymphoma in adults has been treated with
regimens designed for the pediatric populations, which involve the
use of high doses of cyclophosphamide, cytosine arabinoside, and
CNS prophylaxis with methotrexate. The cure rate is about 60 percent
in experienced centers.

Prognostic Factors As is the case in non-Hodgkin's lymphoma, age remains an independent prognostic variable in ALL,
with older adults (>35) having a worse prognosis. Other adverse
factors include delay in achieving CR; B cell phenotype (L3 or
Burkitt's morphology); high white cell count at presentation
(>50,000/μL); and presence of certain cytogenetic abnormalities,
specifically t(9;22), t(8;14), t(1;19), and t(4;11). T cell phenotype
was previously thought to be a poor prognostic factor, although with
more intensive induction regimens the prognosis for patients with
T cell ALL is no worse than for B cell ALL. With the identification
of these prognostic factors, distinct treatment approaches have
evolved for patients with poor-prognosis subtypes of ALL. The
major focus has been on myeloablative therapy for patients with
suitable marrow donors.

Treatment of Recurrent ALL and the Role of BMT Despite
postremission therapy and CNS prophylaxis, remission duration in
adults with ALL is shorter than in children. The prognosis of patients
who fail to achieve remission or who relapse on therapy is very
poor. Although second remissions can be obtained, they are usually
of very short duration. Patients who relapse after maintenance have

a greater likelihood of attaining a second CR, but virtually all relapse.
Patients who have isolated extramedullary relapses, such as in the
CNS or testis, are treated with radiation, and intrathecal therapy, or
radiation, respectively, but they should also receive reinduction to
prevent systemic relapse. In general, due to the poor prognosis of
patients with relapsed adult ALL, consideration should be made
for BMT. For selected patients in second remission, the long-term
leukemia-free survival following BMT from a matched sibling donor
is 20 to 30 percent.

The role of allogeneic BMT in adults with ALL in first remission
is unclear. It appears from retrospective and prospective studies that
the 3-year disease-free survivals are similar after chemotherapy and
allogeneic BMT—around 45 percent. However, patient selection,
high transplant-related mortality, and late relapses after chemotherapy alone have contributed to the failure to define the need for
transplantation. Patients with unfavorable cytogenetics, L3 morphology, and very high presenting white cell counts should be considered
for allogeneic transplantation in first remission. For example, patients
with t(9;22) ALL (a disease that has evolved from Ph' CML), who
have a dismal prognosis with chemotherapy alone, have a disease-
free survival of 38 percent with BMT. Similar results are reported
with patients with t(4;11) ALL. For patients without suitable allogeneic or matched unrelated donors, high-dose therapy with either
purged or unpurged autologous marrow has been performed. In
highly selected patients, the long-term leukemia-free survival with
autologous BMT in second remission is approximately 30 percent.
Although the treatment-related mortality in these studies is significantly lower than in allogeneic transplants, a high relapse rate remains in patients undergoing autologous transplantation, related in
part to the absence of a graft-vs.-tumor effect.

HODGKIN'S DISEASE

**CELLULAR ORIGIN OF THE REED-STERNBERG CELL
OF HODGKIN'S DISEASE** Reed-Sternberg (RS) cells, in the appropriate cytoarchitectural milieu, are required for the diagnosis of
Hodgkin's disease. In Hodgkin's disease tissues, the majority of cells
are small lymphocytes with a mature T cell phenotype (CD2, CD3,
CD4 > CD8, CD5) together with a variable number of B cells. RS
cells and their variants may be immunologically distinguished from
the neoplastic cells of most non-Hodgkin's lymphomas by their lack
of a characteristic pattern of expression of T and B cell–associated
antigens. The exception is lymphocyte-predominant Hodgkin's disease; the malignant cells in this subset express B cell markers. RS
cells of lymphocyte-predominant Hodgkin's disease also express the
leukocyte common antigen (CD45RB), whereas RS cells in other
subtypes of Hodgkin's disease are CD45RB negative.

Two antigens expressed on the RS cell have proven to be diagnostically useful. The first is CD15 (identified by monoclonal antibody
Leu M1), which is the Lewis X blood group antigen and functions as
an adhesion receptor. CD15 is expressed on RS cells in all subtypes
of Hodgkin's disease except for the lymphocyte-predominant variant.
The second antigen is the CD30 antigen (Ki-1), which is present on
virtually all RS cells. The CD30 antigen also is expressed on some
activated B cells, activated T cells, dendritic cells, EBV-transformed
cell lines, and tumor cells isolated from some patients with anaplastic
large cell lymphomas.

Molecular studies of RS-enriched populations and in situ hybridization studies have provided conflicting results about the origin of
these cells. RS cells may have monoclonal or polyclonal immunoglobulin gene rearrangements. In some cases, T cell receptor β-chain
rearrangements have been demonstrated. Sensitive in situ hybridization
studies have identified a clonal form of the EBV genome in RS cells
in about 30 percent of cases examined. This supports a role for EBV
in some cases of Hodgkin's disease, usually the mixed cellularity
subtype. RS cells are certainly of hematopoietic lineage, but specific

lineage assignment is difficult. Hodgkin's disease is a heterogeneous disease, derived from subpopulations of activated lymphohematopoietic cells. The distinct biologic and clinical behaviors (Table 113-1) of Hodgkin's and non-Hodgkin's lymphomas may be a reflection of their divergent cellular origins.

EPIDEMIOLOGY AND ETIOLOGY Approximately 7500 new cases of Hodgkin's disease are diagnosed annually in the United States. In non-Hodgkin's lymphomas, there is a linear increase in incidence with age. In contrast, in Hodgkin's disease the age-specific incidence curve is characteristically bimodal, with an initial peak in young adults (15 to 35 years) and a second peak after age 50. However, in Japan, there is an absence of the early peak, and in some third world countries, there is a shift of the first peak into childhood as well as a shift of histology from nodular sclerosis to mixed cellularity and lymphocyte predominant. Hodgkin's disease is more prevalent in males, and when the age-specific incidence curve is compared to the sex distribution of the patients, the increased male prevalence is most prominent in young adults. A disproportionate number of patients in the first modal peak exhibit nodular sclerosis histology. In childhood Hodgkin's disease, this male predominance is even more striking, with over 80 percent of patients being male. This has led some investigators to hypothesize a sex-linked genetic or hormonally related increase in susceptibility.

Hodgkin's disease is 99-fold more common in an identical twin of an affected case than in the general population, fueling suspicion of a genetic contribution.

Although controversial, clustering of patients with Hodgkin's disease has been reported. Increased risk has been associated with decreased number of siblings, single family dwellings, decreased number of playmates, early birth order, a sibling with Hodgkin's disease, tonsillectomy, and certain HLA antigens. These findings have been used to suggest that Hodgkin's disease is caused by a virus possessing low oncogenic potential that increases with age from the time of infection. However, exhaustive search has yielded nothing. There is strong evidence for a role of EBV in the pathogenesis of a subset of cases. The EBV genome is present and is monoclonal in some cases, dependent upon histologic subtype: 60 percent of mixed cellularity, 30 percent of nodular sclerosis and lymphocyte-depleted subtypes. As in non-Hodgkin's lymphomas, there is an increased risk of Hodgkin's disease in patients with immunodeficiencies and autoimmune diseases (Table 113-5). In contrast to non-Hodgkin's lymphoma, where chromosomal deletions and translocations are common, cytogenetic studies have uncommonly found clonal hyperdiploid abnormalities in the neoplastic Hodgkin's disease CD30 + cells, though aneuploidy is common.

CLINICAL FEATURES AND DIFFERENTIAL DIAGNOSIS Hodgkin's disease usually presents as a localized disease and subsequently spreads to contiguous lymphoid structures; ultimately, it disseminates to nonlymphoid tissues, with a potentially fatal outcome. Hodgkin's disease commonly presents with a newly detected mass or group of lymph nodes that are firm, freely moveable, and usually nontender. Approximately half of patients present with adenopathy in the neck or supraclavicular area, and over 70 percent of patients present with superficial lymph node enlargement. Because these are frequently not painful, detection by the patient may be delayed until the lymph nodes are quite large. Approximately 60 percent of patients present with mediastinal adenopathy. This is sometimes first detected on a routine chest x-ray. Nodes involved by Hodgkin's disease tend to be centripetal or axial, in contrast to non-Hodgkin's lymphomas, which have a tendency to be centrifugal and involve epitrochlear, Waldeyer's Ring, and abdominal nodes. In 2 to 5 percent of patients, lymph nodes or other tissues involved with Hodgkin's disease can become painful after the ingestion of alcoholic beverages. The growth of lymph nodes may be quite variable; some lesions can remain stable for long periods of time, while spontaneous and temporary regression of some nodes may also occur.

The majority of patients presenting with Hodgkin's disease have few or no symptoms related to their disease. However, 25 to 30 percent of patients have some constitutional symptoms; the most common is low-grade fever, which can be associated with recurrent night sweats. For some patients, night sweats may be the sole complaint. A small number of patients may have high fluctuating fevers accompanied by drenching night sweats. These fevers can persist for several weeks followed by afebrile intervals (Pel-Epstein fevers). Fevers and night sweats are more commonly seen in older patients and in those with more advanced stage disease. Some patients with extensive abdominal but limited peripheral adenopathy are first evaluated for fever and night sweats. They undergo a workup for fever of unknown origin and usually are found to have mixed cellularity or lymphocyte-depleted Hodgkin's disease. Another important presenting symptom is unexplained weight loss of greater than 10 percent over 6 months or less. Other frequent symptoms include fatigue, malaise, and weakness. Pruritus occurs in approximately 10 percent of patients at initial diagnosis; it is usually generalized, may be associated with a skin rash, and rarely may be the only disease manifestation. It is not a B symptom. Mediastinal, pulmonary, pleural, or pericardial involvement may be associated with cough, chest pain, shortness of breath, or hypertrophic osteoarthropathy; bone involvement may be associated with bone pain. Occasionally a patient will present with obstruction of the superior vena cava as the first symptom. Sudden spinal cord compression can be a presenting complaint but is usually a complication of advanced progressive disease. Headache or visual disturbances may be seen in the very rare patient with intracranial Hodgkin's disease, and abdominal involvement may result in abdominal pain, bowel disturbances, and even ascites.

The differential diagnosis is similar to that described for non-Hodgkin's lymphoma. In patients with cervical adenopathy, infections including bacterial or viral pharyngitis, infectious mononucleosis, and toxoplasmosis must be excluded. Other malignancies such as non-Hodgkin's lymphomas, nasopharyngeal cancers, and thyroid cancers can also present with localized cervical adenopathy. Axillary adenopathy must be differentiated from non-Hodgkin's lymphoma and breast cancer. Mediastinal adenopathy must be distinguished from infections, sarcoid, and other tumors. In older patients, the differential diagnosis includes tumors of the lung and mediastinum, specifically small cell and non-small cell carcinomas. Reactive mediastinitis and hilar adenopathy from histoplasmosis can be confused with lymphoma since it occurs in otherwise asymptomatic people. Primary abdominal disease with hepatomegaly, splenomegaly, and massive adenopathy is uncommon, and other neoplastic diseases, especially non-Hodgkin's lymphoma, must be excluded under these circumstances.

DIAGNOSIS AND PATHOLOGIC CLASSIFICATION The diagnosis of Hodgkin's disease requires a biopsy that contains sufficient tissue to permit an accurate microscopic diagnosis. Biopsy specimens are usually from lymph nodes but may occasionally be from other tissues. Needle aspirations or needle biopsies are not adequate for the primary histologic diagnosis of Hodgkin's disease or any other lymphoma.

The criteria for the diagnosis and classification of Hodgkin's disease have remained unchanged since 1966 when the Rye classification was adopted (Table 113-4). Central to the diagnosis is the presence of the RS cell, a large cell with a bilobed or multilobulated nucleus with prominent inclusion-like nucleoli. (**See Plate IV-25.**) There are several morphologic variants of RS cells, and it is the frequency of these variants as well as the cellular and stromal background of the node that help to establish the histologic subtypes of Hodgkin's disease. RS cells may occasionally be found in other conditions such as infectious mononucleosis and non-Hodgkin's lymphomas. Thus, an accurate diagnosis of Hodgkin's disease depends on additional cellular and architectural features of the tissue.

Hodgkin's disease is subdivided into four types: (1) lymphocyte predominant, (2) nodular sclerosis, (3) mixed cellularity, and (4) lymphocyte depleted. The R.E.A.L. classification includes these four major subtypes. Treatment and prognosis in Hodgkin's disease is dependent on the stage of disease, whereas in non-Hodgkin's lymphoma, treatment is largely based on histologic subtype.

STAGING AND OTHER LABORATORY ABNORMALITIES **Ann Arbor Classification** Following biopsy and histopathologic classification of Hodgkin's disease, one must define the extent of the disease (i.e., staging), which is essential for the selection of optimal therapy. In the Ann Arbor staging classification (Table 113-7), the patient receives both a clinical and a pathologic stage. The clinical stage is defined by the extent of disease based on physical examination and other noninvasive studies. The pathologic stage is defined by data obtained from invasive tests including biopsy specimens obtained from different sites, usually during a staging laparotomy. The presence of localized extralymphatic disease is designated by the suffix *E*. Such extralymphatic involvement may include solitary involvement of lung or bone. Multifocal involvement in these organs usually is defined as disseminated disease. Bone involvement must be separated from bone marrow involvement, since bone marrow and liver involvement are always defined as stage IV disseminated disease.

The presence of systemic symptoms (fever, night sweats, weight loss) is designated by the suffix *B* and their absence by the suffix *A*. The presence of both fevers and weight loss results in a less favorable prognosis, while night sweats are currently thought to be of no independent prognostic importance. Patients with early-stage disease, such as pathologic stage IA or IIA, are treated effectively with radiotherapy alone; patients with more disseminated disease, such as pathologic stage III, IVA, or IVB, are most effectively treated with combination chemotherapy alone. Patients of any stage with a very large mediastinal mass are usually treated with combined modality therapy.

Staging Procedures After Biopsy Diagnosis The diagnostic studies recommended for complete staging are outlined in Table 113-10. Detailed physical examination with attention to documentation of all sites of nodal involvement and splenomegaly is essential. The chest radiograph is usually sufficient to exclude mediastinal, hilar, pleural, and parenchymal involvement. However, in patients with demonstrable thoracic disease, chest CT more accurately defines the extent of disease. CT of the abdomen and pelvis may assess certain groups of nodes but is not sensitive for detecting splenic and hepatic disease or node involvement that does not produce enlargement. CT scanning can detect the exact location and extent of all enlarged nodes including iliac, mesenteric, and retrocrural nodal areas. A lymphangiogram evaluates the paraaortic and common internal and external iliac nodes and is essential if radiation therapy alone is a treatment option.

Radiation therapy is a local treatment. Disease not within a treatment portal is not eradicated. For this reason, a number of more invasive diagnostic tests are required if patients are clinically stage I, II, or IIIA and radiation therapy is a treatment option. Lymphangiograms are more sensitive than abdominal/pelvic CT scans. Moreover, lymphangiograms are useful before staging laparotomy to direct the surgeon to the nodes to be biopsied. However, the accuracy of this procedure is highly dependent on the experience of the radiologist. If a staging laparotomy is considered, patients should undergo bilateral bone marrow biopsies to exclude stage IV disease. The frequency of a positive bone marrow biopsy in clinical stage IA or IIA disease is low, but if present, makes laparotomy unnecessary. Staging laparotomy includes biopsy of selected lymph nodes in the retroperitoneum, splenectomy, and several needle and wedge biopsies of the liver. Traditionally, all patients without obvious stage IV disease underwent laparotomy, and nearly one-third had their initial clinical stage changed as a result of the procedure. For example, one-third of patients with normal-sized spleens had demonstrable tumor infiltration at laparotomy, whereas 35 percent of patients with clinical splenomegaly had no histologic evidence of disease. Liver involvement is more common in patients with positive lymphangiograms and enlarged spleens. Laparotomy should be utilized in patients whose clinical stages make them candidates for treatment with radiation therapy alone and in whom evidence of unsuspected abdominal disease will significantly change treatment. Approximately one-third of patients with clinical stage I or II (with or without B symptoms) will have occult upper abdominal or spleen disease not dectected by noninvasive studies. A staging laparotomy should not be performed in patients who are to receive chemotherapy based upon the presence of bulky chest disease, more than four nodal sites, bulky abdominal involvement, or clinical stage III or stage IV disease. A staging laparotomy with splenectomy should be performed by a surgeon who is skilled in this procedure after careful review of clinical, laboratory, pathologic, and radiologic studies. Finally, a number of ancillary studies may be very useful in selected patients and are listed in Table 113-10. Gallium scintigraphy is most useful in following response to treatment and to detect early recurrences; it is not useful at the time of initial staging.

Laboratory Abnormalities Routine blood counts, liver function tests, and renal function tests are all necessary parts of the medical workup but do not provide information about the extent of Hodgkin's disease or of specific organ involvement. A moderate, normochromic, normocytic anemia associated with low serum iron and low iron-binding capacity, but with normal or increased iron stores in the bone marrow, may be present in patients with Hodgkin's disease as well as in other neoplastic and chronic diseases. This reflects a cytokine-mediated inhibition of iron reutilization. A moderate to marked leukemoid reaction is common, particularly in symptomatic patients and usually disappears with treatment. Mild peripheral absolute eosinophilia is not uncommon, especially in patients with pruritus. Absolute monocytosis is also observed. Absolute lymphocytopenia (<1000 cells/μL) usually occurs in patients with more advanced disease. Many tests have been evaluated as indicators of disease activity. To date, the erythrocyte sedimentation rate still is the best monitor, but it suffers from its lack of specificity and can return to normal when residual disease is still demonstrable. Other abnormal tests include increased serum levels of copper, calcium, lactic acid, alkaline phosphatase, lysozyme, globulins, C-reactive protein, and other acute-phase reactants. Soluble CD30, soluble CD25, and soluble CD4 have been suggested as tumor markers.

Immunologic Abnormalities Hodgkin's disease is associated with a well-described but poorly understood immunologic defect. Untreated patients, including those with limited disease, have defective cellular immunity characterized by anergy to routine skin tests. They also have a reversal of the CD4:CD8 ratio, suggesting that this anergy may be due to increased numbers of suppressor T cells as well as decreased numbers of CD4+ cells. T cells from patients with Hodgkin's disease have defects in signal transduction, including decreased T cell receptor ζ chain and decreased tyrosine kinase activation. In

---

Table 113-10

Staging Evaluation for Hodgkin's Disease

Essential
1. Pathologic documentation by hematopathologist
2. Physical examination
3. Documentation of B symptoms
4. Laboratory evaluation
   a. Complete blood counts
   b. Liver function tests
   c. Renal function tests
   d. Uric acid
   e. Erythrocyte sedimentation rate
5. Chest radiograph
6. CT scan of chest, abdomen, and pelvis
7. Bone marrow biopsy

Essential Under Certain Circumstances
1. Liver biopsy
2. Bipedal lymphangiogram
3. Gallium scan
4. Staging laparatomy
5. Bone scan
6. Bone radiographs

Useful But Not Essential Tests
1. Cell-surface marker phenotypic analysis
2. Gene rearrangement analysis
3. Ultrasonography
4. Magnetic resonance imaging
5. Delayed-hypersensitivity skin tests

several studies, decreased immune reactivity correlates with both advanced stages of disease and the presence of systemic symptoms. However, anergy to recall and neoantigens appears to have no prognostic significance. Following successful therapy, anergy to recall antigens reverses but is still present in some patients to neoantigens. In addition to anergy, other tests of T cell function, including responses to mitogens and suppressor cell function, suggest a defect in immune function before and following treatment. Humoral immunity with antibody production to soluble antigens is normal in untreated patients. Thus, patients who undergo staging laparotomy and splenectomy will develop humoral immunity to pneumococcal antigens if immunized with the pneumococcal vaccine before splenectomy, but not after. The clinical impact of these immune defects is limited. Except for a higher than normal incidence of herpes zoster and development of warts, these patients are not plagued by opportunistic infections.

NATURAL HISTORY ACCORDING TO HISTOLOGIC SUBTYPE Patients with lymphocyte-predominant Hodgkin's disease are usually asymptomatic at presentation and tend to have localized disease. These patients are usually young, rarely have systemic symptoms or mediastinal mass, and are predominantly males. Nodular sclerosis Hodgkin's disease is found most frequently in adolescents and young adults who usually have localized disease; a preponderance are young women who present with a large mediastinal mass. Lymphocyte-depleted Hodgkin's disease is usually disseminated at the time of diagnosis and occurs in older patients who frequently have systemic symptoms. The mixed cellularity type occurs in all age groups and stages and is only slightly more common in males. There is a tendency toward an older age peak (30 to 40 years) than with nodular sclerosis, and approximately half of these patients have advanced disease. Patients with lymphocyte-predominant and nodular sclerosis Hodgkin's disease, if untreated, have a more indolent disease associated with a longer survival and are more likely to be cured with radiotherapy.

℞ TREATMENT

With appropriate treatment, about 85 percent of patients with Hodgkin's disease are curable. Radiotherapy may cure over 80 percent of patients with localized Hodgkin's disease, and chemotherapy over 70 percent of those with disseminated disease. Nearly half of those not cured with primary treatment are cured with salvage therapy. The choice of treatment is dependent on stage of disease. As with all neoplasms, the therapy of Hodgkin's disease is constantly being reevaluated to improve disease-free survival and decrease toxicity.

Treatment of Early-Stage Disease The mainstay of therapy for early-stage (I and II) Hodgkin's disease has been radiation therapy. With the knowledge that Hodgkin's disease spreads by lymphatic contiguity, three radiation fields were devised to cover likely sites of disease—the mantle field, paraaortic field, and the pelvic field. The mantle field includes the submandibular, cervical, supraclavicular, infraclavicular, axillary, mediastinal, and hilar lymph nodes. The paraaortic field covers the transverse processes of the abdominal vertebral bodies and the spleen, if it has not been removed. Pelvic irradiation includes the common iliac, hypogastric, external iliac, and inguinal nodes. When there is gross pelvic nodal involvement, the femoral nodes are also treated. Sometimes the pelvic and paraaortic fields are treated as one unit, which is commonly called the "inverted-Y" field. The use of pelvic irradiation has been recently reduced since stages I and II supradiaphragmatic Hodgkin's disease can be treated without pelvic irradiation. Patients now receive mantle and paraaortic irradiation and only rarely total nodal irradiation (i.e., all three fields). Patients receive doses of 3000 to 3600 cGy with an additional "cone down" dose for a total of 4000 cGy to areas of bulk disease.

Patients with localized nodal Hodgkin's disease (pathologic stages IA and IIA) treated with mantle or paraaortic radiation therapy have nearly an 80 percent long-term disease-free survival beyond 10 years, with less than a 10 percent mortality from Hodgkin's

disease. Randomized trials comparing radiation therapy to combination chemotherapy plus radiation show a relapse-free survival advantage for combined-modality treatment but no survival advantage. Although the disease-free survival is somewhat higher, salvage therapy after relapse from radiation is very efficacious and overall survival is not improved. Patients with stages IB and IIB have a slightly reduced disease-free survival (70 percent); however, most patients who relapse can be successfully treated with combination chemotherapy.

The very high rate of radiation therapy–related fatal complications, including second malignancies (0.5 to 1 percent risk per year up to at least 30 years after treatment) and a greater than threefold increased risk of fatal myocardial infarction (see below), has led to consideration of using primary combination chemotherapy in patients with early-stage Hodgkin's disease after clinical staging. The success of this approach is at least equal to using radiation therapy and spares the patient the unpleasant consequences of splenectomy for staging (i.e., infectious risk) and radiation therapy.

Treatment of Advanced-Stage Disease Chemotherapy with the combination of mechlorethamine (nitrogen mustard), vincristine (Oncovin), procarbazine, and prednisone (MOPP) produces CR in 85 to 90 percent of patients; about two-thirds of the CR are durable. MOPP therapy has been associated with significant toxicity. Nearly all patients experience some degree of nausea and vomiting and bone marrow suppression. About 2 percent of patients treated with MOPP develop myelodysplasia and/or acute leukemia 4 to 6 years after treatment. However, those who survive 10 years or more without developing leukemia are unlikely to do so. Infertility is another important toxicity.

Other multiple-drug regimens have been developed for the treatment of advanced Hodgkin's disease. However, none of the "MOPP-derived combinations" have been superior to the original MOPP administered at optimal dose and schedule. Substitution of chlorambucil for mechlorethamine and vinblastine for vincristine (ChlVPP) yields a regimen that is associated with less gastrointestinal and neurotoxicity with similar efficacy. Several regimens have been developed to treat MOPP-resistant patients. The best known of these is Adryamicin (doxorubicin), bleomycin, vinblastine, and dacarbazine (ABVD). ABVD has some efficacy in MOPP treatment failures and is comparable to MOPP in activity in previously untreated patients. Several randomized trials have attempted to determine optimum initial therapy, comparing MOPP, ABVD, and combinations of MOPP/ABVD. MOPP alternating with ABVD appears to be superior to a modified version of MOPP, achieving a higher CR rate (89 percent vs. 74 percent) as well as improved disease-free survival (68 percent vs. 46 percent) and overall survival (69 percent vs. 58 percent). However, alternating MOPP/ABVD gave similar results to ABVD alone. Studies that have compared a combination including all the MOPP/ABVD drugs into each cycle (hybrid) rather than alternating each monthly regimen have found no difference in response rate or duration or survival. ABVD has the advantage of sparing fertility but the disadvantage of a 3 percent risk of fatal pulmonary toxicity. The seven- (MOPP/ABV) or eight-drug (MOPP/ABVD) regimens produce no risk of acute leukemia or fatal pulmonary fibrosis but induce infertility in half the men and in 25 percent of the women. Thus, the choice of therapy involves trade-offs of toxicity risk. If fertility is the overriding issue, ABVD is the treatment of choice. If minimizing the risk of fatal toxicity is overriding, MOPP/ABV hybrid or MOPP/ABVD is the treatment of choice.

Prognostic Factors Prognostic factors have been identified that alter therapy for early-stage patients. Early-stage patients with large mediastinal involvement appear to have a higher risk of relapse after radiation therapy alone (disease-free survival of 40 to 55 percent) compared to patients with minimal or no mediastinal disease; they should be managed with chemotherapy followed by involved-field or mantle irradiation. Patients over age 40 also have a decreased survival. Finally, patients with pathologic stage IB or IIB and who have fevers and weight loss (but not night sweats) and are treated with radiation alone have a decreased disease-free and overall survival. They might best be treated with combination chemotherapy. Prognostic variables have been identified for patients who are clinical stages I and II. The factors that adversely affect outcome include male sex, multiple sites, high erythrocyte sedimentation rate, bulky mediastinal disease, mixed cellularity and lymphocyte-depleted histologies, and treatment with involved-field radiation. In advanced-stage patients who would be treated with combination chemotherapy, several clinical and laboratory parameters are independently significant for an unfavorable survival. These include stage IV disease, B symptoms, inguinal node involvement, large mediastinal mass, male gender, bulky disease, leukocytosis, lymphocytosis, and anemia. Even placing all of these factors together, the group with the worst prognosis has a 5-year survival of 54 percent. Thus, there is no single group of patients who are obvious candidates for primary high-dose therapy with hematopoietic support. Using these parameters, clinical investigations are focused on minimizing or intensifying therapy in appropriate patients.

Salvage Therapy After proper restaging, further radiotherapy can be delivered (if technically feasible) to a subset of patients with early-stage disease who have relapsed outside of a radiation field or following combination chemotherapy. In patients not achieving a complete remission or relapsing after MOPP, second-line non-cross-resistant regimens are available. If patients relapse more than 12 months after the completion of primary chemotherapy, they can be retreated with the original treatment regimen; if they relapse in less than 12 months, they should be treated with an alternative salvage regimen, such as ABVD for MOPP, MOPP for ABVD, and mini BEAM (carmustine, etoposide, cytarabine, and melphalan) for MOPP/ABVD or MOPP/ABV. Conventional-dose salvage regimens will produce complete response in 30 to 40 percent of patients and long-term survival in 10 to 25 percent. Poor prognostic variables for salvage include stage IV disease at diagnosis, B symptoms at relapse, poor performance status, or remission lasting <12 months. Various salvage regimens containing combinations of cisplatin, etoposide, and ifosfamide have been used for patients who have failed two regimens such as MOPP and ABVD, with good responses that unfortunately are not durable. As is the case with non-Hodgkin's lymphoma, autologous or allogeneic BMT or peripheral blood stem transplantation is an effective salvage treatment for many relapsed patients. Hodgkin's disease patients whose disease remains sensitive to chemotherapeutic agents are more likely to experience long-term disease-free survival in the range of 50 percent, while resistant patients have disease-free survivals of 15 to 25 percent. In contrast to non-Hodgkin's lymphoma, total body irradiation has limited value, and virtually all ablative regimens include high-dose chemotherapy. The acute lethal pulmonary and hepatic toxicity from these high-dose regimens, however, can be as high as 25 percent in patients previously treated with radiation therapy, although with better patient selection and supportive care, mortality is now less than 5 percent. Any patient with a short initial remission should have high-dose therapy as a component of their salvage treatment.

Complications of Treatment Radiation therapy can lead to acute and late complications. Acute side effects of mantle irradiation include transient xerostomia, pharyngitis, fatigue, and weight loss. Within several months of mantle irradiation, approximately 15 percent of patients develop paresthesia in the lower extremities upon flexion of the neck or thighs (Lhermitte's syndrome). This syndrome usually resolves spontaneously; there is no correlation between this syndrome and irreversible spinal injury. Other long-term side effects include radiation pneumonitis (severe in fewer than 5 percent of patients) and symptomatic pulmonary fibrosis (<1 percent). Late complications of mantle radiation include cardiac damage such as pericardial effusion and myocardial damage. Cardiac irradiation accelerates coronary artery disease and induces a greater than threefold risk of fatal myocardial infarctions. Anthracycline cardiomyopathy can occur but usually not with the doses administered with the ABVD or MOPP/ABVD regimens. It remains unclear whether long-term cardiac toxicity will occur in patients treated with combined-modality therapy that includes doxorubicin. Hypothyroidism may

occur in up to 30 percent of patients following mantle irradiation. Paraaortic irradiation is rarely associated with significant side effects. Pelvic irradiation acutely induces transient diarrhea and bladder irritation associated with frequency. Chronic effects include potential long-term bone marrow suppression and sterility; therefore, pelvic irradiation is infrequently employed. Gonadal dysfunction is also a significant problem in patients treated with MOPP or other regimens containing alkylating agents. Infertility is about one-half as frequent in patients who received MOPP/ABVD and is rare in patients treated with ABVD alone. Increasing numbers of secondary tumors are being observed in patients treated for Hodgkin's disease. In 15-year survivors with Hodgkin's disease treated with radiation therapy, a cumulative risk of development of second tumors 2.8 fold higher than expected has been observed. MOPP chemotherapy has not been associated with the development of second solid tumors. The most common cancers involve breast, thyroid, lung (in smokers), stomach, and skin as well as sarcomas and primary bone tumors. Secondary acute nonlymphocytic leukemia (usually seen between 5 and 10 years later) occurs in about 2 percent of MOPP-treated patients and in 8 percent of patients treated with MOPP plus radiation therapy. These leukemias usually have an antecedent myelodysplastic syndrome characterized by chromosomal deletions involving 5q and 7q. Leukemias associated with epipodophyllotoxins are seen rarely, but with a shorter latent period. High-grade non-Hodgkin's lymphomas are also seen with increased frequency, independent of the type of therapy. This complication may be related to the underlying immune defect in Hodgkin's disease patients.

Therapeutic Recommendation by Stage STAGES IA AND IIA, *NONBULKY DISEASE* Following staging laparotomy in patients with supradiaphragmatic disease, mantle or mantle and paraaortic irradiation is the treatment of choice. In patients with subdiaphragmatic lymphoma, radiotherapy is delivered to an inverted-Y field including the splenic pedicle in stage I disease and through total nodal irradiation in stage II disease. Some studies suggest that treatment with involved-field radiotherapy combined with chemotherapy produces comparable results, but most do not consider this the best treatment choice. For patients with subdiaphragmatic stage II disease of paraaortic nodes, chemotherapy is recommended. Chemotherapy alone is an appropriate treatment for patients who are clinically staged.

STAGES IB AND IIB, *NONBULKY DISEASE* The therapy is the same as for stages IA and IIA Hodgkin's disease; however, the relapse rate is higher (20 percent). Relapse can usually be salvaged with chemotherapy. Subtotal or combination chemotherapy with involved-field irradiation remains an alternative treatment for these patients. Chemotherapy alone is an appropriate treatment for patients who are clinically staged.

STAGE II, *BULKY DISEASE* Stage II disease with bulky mediastinal/hilar adenopathy should be managed with combined-modality therapy. This should include six cycles of combination chemotherapy and radiotherapy (usually a mantle field) to sites of bulk disease.

STAGES IIIA, IIIB, AND IV Combination chemotherapy is recommended, consisting of two cycles beyond achieving complete remission. For most patients, six cycles of therapy are adequate; 15 percent of patients may require eight cycles. Although only 10 to 15 percent of patients fail to achieve a CR with combination chemotherapy, about half of the partial responders may be converted to CR with the addition of involved-field radiation therapy.

BIBLIOGRAPHY

BHATIA S et al: Breast cancer and other second neoplasms after childhood Hodgkin's disease. N Engl J Med 334:745, 1996

BIERMAN P et al: Autologous transplantation for Hodgkin's disease. Blood 83:1161, 1994

CANELLOS GP et al: Chemotherapy of advanced Hodgkin's disease with MOPP, ABVD, or MOPP alternating with ABVD. N Engl J Med 327:1478, 1992

COPELAN EA, McGUIRE EA: The biology and treatment of acute lymphoblastic leukemia in adults. Blood 85:1151, 1995

FREEDMAN AS, NADLER LM: Immunologic markers in non-Hodgkin's lympho-
    mas. Hematol Oncol Clin North Am 5:871, 1991

HARRIS N et al: A revised European-American classification of lymphoid neo-
    plasms: A proposal from the International Lymphoma Study Group. Blood
    84:1361, 1994

KAPLAN HS: *Hodgkin's Disease*, 2d ed. Cambridge, MA, Harvard University
    Press, 1980

LEVINE AM: Acquired immunodeficiency syndrome–related lymphomas.
    Blood 80:8, 1992

LONGO DL: What's the deal with follicular lymphomas? J Clin Oncol
    11:202, 1993

O'BRIEN S et al: Advances in the biology and treatment of B-cell chronic
    lymphocytic leukemia. Blood 85:307, 1995

SHIPP MA: Prognostic factors in aggressive non-Hodgkin's lymphoma: Who
    has "high risk" disease? Blood 83:1165, 1994

URBA WJ, LONGO DL: Hodgkin's disease. N Engl J Med 326:678, 1992

---

114 | Dan L. Longo

PLASMA CELL DISORDERS

GENERAL PRINCIPLES The *plasma cell disorders* are monoclonal neoplasms related to each other by virtue of their development from common progenitors in the B lymphocyte lineage. Multiple myeloma, Waldenström's macroglobulinemia, primary amyloidosis (see Chap. 309), and the heavy chain diseases comprise this group and may be designated by a variety of synonyms such as *monoclonal gammopathies, paraproteinemias, plasma cell dyscrasias,* and *dysproteinemias*. Normal development of B lymphocytes is discussed in Chap. 305. Mature B lymphocytes destined to produce IgG bear surface immunoglobulin molecules of both M and G heavy chain isotypes with both isotypes having identical idiotypes (variable regions). Under normal circumstances, maturation to antibody-secreting plasma cells is stimulated by exposure to the antigen for which the surface immunoglobulin is specific; however, in the plasma cell disorders the control over this process is lost. The clinical manifestations of all the plasma cell disorders relate to the expansion of the neoplastic cells, to the secretion of cell products (immunoglobulin molecules or subunits, lymphokines), and to some extent to the host's response to the tumor.

There are three categories of structural variation among immunoglobulin molecules that form antigenic determinants, and these are used to classify immunoglobulins (Chap. 305). *Isotypes* are those determinants that distinguish among the main classes of antibodies of a given species and are the same in all normal individuals of that species. Therefore, isotypic determinants are, by definition, recognized by antibodies from a distinct species (heterologous sera) but not by antibodies from the same species (homologous sera). There are five heavy chain isotypes (M, G, A, D, E) and two light chain isotypes (kappa, lambda). *Allotypes* are distinct determinants that reflect regular small differences between individuals of the same species in the amino acid sequences of otherwise similar immunoglobulins. These differences are determined by allelic genes, and by definition, they are detected by antibodies made in the same species. *Idiotypes* are the third category of antigenic determinants. They are unique to the molecules produced by a given clone of antibody-producing cells. Idiotypes are formed by the unique structure of the antigen-binding portion of the molecule.

Antibody molecules (see Fig. 305-8) are composed of two heavy chains (mol wt ~50,000) and two light chains (mol wt ~25,000). Each chain has a constant portion (limited amino acid sequence variability) and a variable region (extensive sequence variability). The light and heavy chains are linked by disulfide bonds and are aligned so that their variable regions are adjacent to one another. This variable region forms the antigen recognition site of the antibody molecule; its unique structural features form a particular set of determinants, or idiotypes, that are reliable markers for a particular clone of cells because each antibody is formed and secreted by a single clone. Each chain is specified by distinct genes, synthesized separately, and assembled into an intact antibody molecule after translation (see Fig. 114-1). Because of the mechanics of the gene rearrangements necessary to specify the immunoglobulin variable regions (VDJ joining for the heavy chain, VJ joining for the light chain; see Fig. 114-1), a particular clone rearranges only one of the two chromosomes to produce an immunoglobulin molecule of only one light chain isotype and only one allotype (allelic exclusion). After exposure to antigen, the variable region may become associated with a new heavy chain isotype (class switch). Each clone of cells performs these sequential gene arrangements in a unique way. This results in each clone producing a unique immunoglobulin molecule. In most cells, light chains are synthesized in slight excess, are secreted as free light chains by plasma cells, and are cleared by the kidney, but less than 10 mg of such light chains is excreted per day.

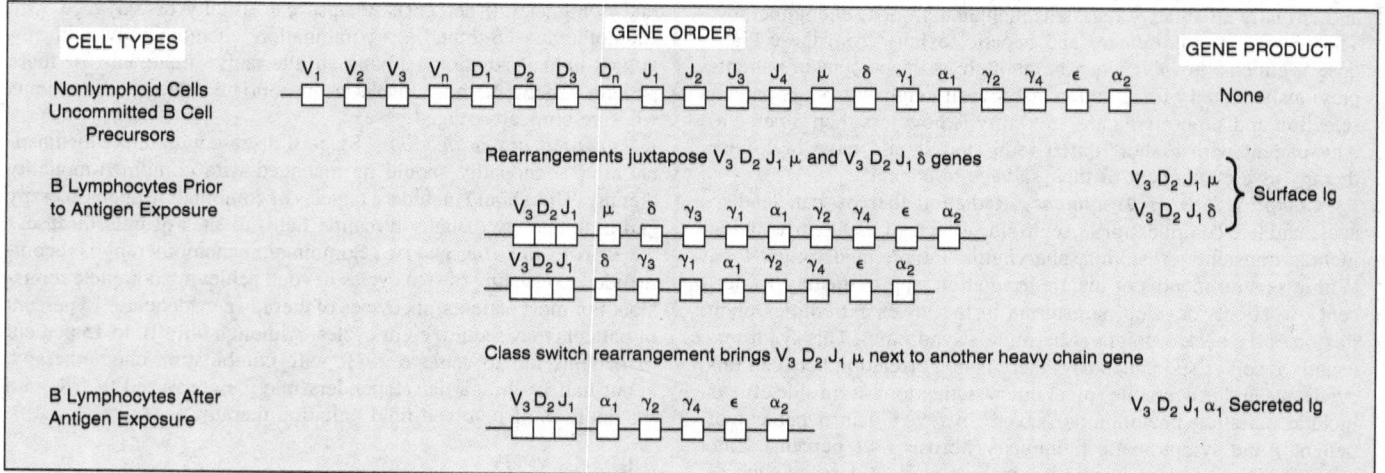

FIGURE 114-1 Immunoglobulin heavy chains are encoded by four distinct genetic elements, variable (Igh-V), diversity (Igh-D), joining (Igh-J), and constant (Igh-C) genes. The variable region of the immunoglobulin heavy chain is encoded by the V, D, and J genes. The same variable region may be associated with any of the 10 heavy chain constant region genes. In the germline genome (all cells except B cells) the V, D, and J genes are widely separated and exist in numerous forms. Once a cell becomes committed to B cell differentiation, a single V gene and a single D gene translocate to a single J gene, and the intervening genetic material is excised (VDJ joining). The newly formed VDJ gene is transcribed into a single message along with either an M or D isotype C gene. Upon exposure to antigen, another rearrangement may occur so that the VDJ gene may be associated with a G, A, or E isotype C gene. In light chain genes there appear to be no D genes, and thus light chain variable regions are formed by VJ joining.

Electrophoretic analysis of components of the serum proteins permits determination of the amount of immunoglobulin in the serum (Fig. 114-2). The variety of immunoglobulins move heterogeneously in an electric field and form a broad peak in the gamma region. The gamma globulin region of the electrophoretic pattern is usually increased in the sera of patients and animals with plasma cell tumors. There is a sharp spike in this region called an *M component* (M for monoclonal). Less commonly, the M component may appear in the beta₂ or alpha₂ globulin region. The antibody must be present at a concentration of at least 5 g/L (0.5 g/dL) to be detectable by this method. This corresponds to approximately 10^9 cells producing the antibody. Confirmation that such an M component is truly monoclonal relies on the use of immunoelectrophoresis that shows a single light and heavy chain type. Hence immunoelectrophoresis and electrophoresis provide qualitative and quantitative assessment of the M component, respectively. Once the presence of an M component has been confirmed, electrophoresis provides the more practical information for managing patients with monoclonal gammopathies. In a given patient, the amount of M component in the serum is a reliable measure of the tumor burden. This makes the M component an excellent tumor marker, yet it is not specific enough to be used to screen asymptomatic patients. In addition to the plasma cell disorders, M components may be detected in other lymphoid neoplasms such as chronic lymphocytic leukemia and lymphomas of B or T cell origin; nonlymphoid neoplasms such as chronic myelogenous leukemia, breast and colon cancer; a variety of nonneoplastic conditions such as cirrhosis, sarcoidosis, parasitic diseases, Gaucher's disease, and pyoderma gangrenosum; and a number of autoimmune conditions, including rheumatoid arthritis, myasthenia gravis, and cold agglutinin disease. A very rare skin disease known as lichen myxedematosus or papular mucinosis is associated with a monoclonal gammopathy. Highly cationic IgGλ is deposited in the dermis of patients with this disease. It is unclear whether this organ specificity reflects the specificity of the antibody for some antigenic component of the dermis.

The nature of the M component is variable in plasma cell disorders. It may be an intact antibody molecule of any heavy chain subclass, or it may be an altered antibody or fragment. Isolated light or heavy chains may be produced. In some plasma cell tumors such as extramedullary or solitary bone plasmacytomas, less than a third of patients will have an M component. In about 20 percent of myelomas, only light chains are produced and in most cases are secreted in the urine

as Bence Jones proteins. The frequency of myelomas of a particular heavy chain class is roughly proportional to the serum concentration, and therefore IgG myelomas are more common than IgA and IgD myelomas.

MULTIPLE MYELOMA **Definition** Multiple myeloma represents a malignant proliferation of plasma cells derived from a single clone. The terms *multiple myeloma* and *myeloma* may be used interchangeably. The tumor, its products, and the host response to it result in a number of organ dysfunctions and symptoms of bone pain or fracture, renal failure, susceptibility to infection, anemia, hypercalcemia, and occasionally clotting abnormalities, neurologic symptoms, and vascular manifestations of hyperviscosity.

Etiology The cause of myeloma is not known. Myeloma occurred with increased frequency in those exposed to the radiation of nuclear warheads in World War II after a 20-year latency. In contrast to most other B cell tumors, consistent chromosomal alterations have not been found in patients with myeloma, though cytogenetic abnormalities are noted in a substantial fraction of cases. Overexpression of *myc* or *ras* genes has been noted in some cases. Mutations in p53 and Rb-1 have also been described, but no common molecular pathogenesis has yet emerged. The murine plasmacytoma models suggest that the induction of plasmacytomas (e.g., with mineral oil injection) may require exposure to foreign antigens as well as a cellular event. Thus chronic antigenic stimulation may play a role in the transformation of a particular B cell clone. This is supported by evidence that M proteins from different persons sometimes share idiotypes. There is also some evidence for a genetic predisposition to myeloma in humans. Myeloma has been seen more commonly than expected among farmers, wood workers, leather workers, and those exposed to petroleum products. The neoplastic event in myeloma may involve cells earlier in B cell differentiation than the plasma cell. Circulating B cells bearing surface immunoglobulin that share the idiotype of the M component are present in myeloma patients. It is possible that the malignant clone escapes normal control mechanisms at a pre-plasma cell stage of differentiation and the chronic exposure to a particular antigenic stimulus drives the cell to terminal differentiation. Interleukin (IL) 6 may play a role in driving myeloma cell proliferation; a large fraction of myeloma cells exposed to IL-6 in vitro respond by proliferating. It remains difficult to distinguish benign from malignant plasma cells on the basis of morphologic criteria in all but a few cases. **(See Plate IV-27)**

Incidence and Prevalence About 14,400 cases of myeloma were diagnosed in 1996, and 10,400 people died from the disease. Myeloma increases in incidence with age. The median age at diagnosis is 68 years. It is rare under age 40. The yearly incidence is around 4 per 100,000 and remarkably similar in countries throughout the world. Males are slightly more commonly affected than females, and blacks have nearly twice the incidence of whites. In the age group over 25 the incidence is 30 per 100,000. Myeloma accounts for about 1 percent of all malignancies in whites and 2 percent in blacks; 13 percent of all hematologic cancers in whites and 33 percent in blacks.

Pathogenesis and Clinical Manifestations (Table 114-1) Bone pain is the most common symptom in myeloma, affecting nearly 70 percent of patients. The pain usually involves the back and ribs, and unlike the pain of metastatic carcinoma, which often is worse at night, the pain of myeloma is precipitated by movement. Persistent localized pain in a patient with myeloma usually signifies a pathologic fracture. The bone lesions of myeloma are caused by the proliferation of the tumor cells and the activation of osteoclasts that destroy the bone. The osteoclasts respond to osteoclast activating factors (OAF) made by the myeloma cells [OAF activity can be mediated by several cytokines, including IL-1, lymphotoxin, and tumor necrosis factor (TNF)]. However, production of these factors stops following administration of glucocorticoids or interferon (IFN)-γ. The bone lesions are lytic in nature and are rarely associated with osteoblastic new bone formation; therefore, radioisotopic bone scanning is less useful in diagnosis than

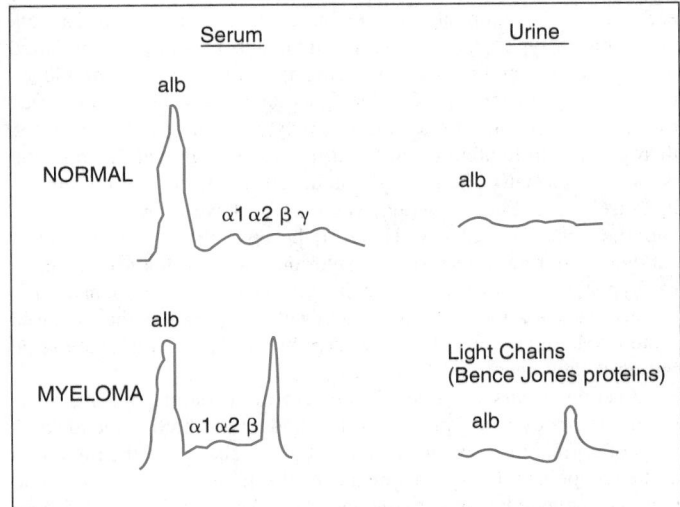

FIGURE 114-2 Representative electrophoretic patterns of serum and urine. The upper panel illustrates the normal pattern of serum and urine protein on electrophoresis. Since there are many different immunoglobulins in the serum, their differing mobilities in an electric field produce a broad peak. The lower panel illustrates the patterns of serum and urine proteins in a patient with myeloma. The predominance of a product of a single cell is reflected by a "church spire" sharp peak. The presence of free light chains in the urine is reflected in a peak as well.

Table 114-1

Pathogenesis and Clinical Manifestations of Multiple Myeloma

Clinical Finding	Underlying Cause	Pathogenic Mechanism
Hypercalcemia, pathologic fractures, cord compression, lytic bone lesions, osteoporosis, bone pain	Skeletal destruction	Tumor expansion; production of osteoclast activating factors (OAF) by tumor cells
Renal failure	Light chain proteinuria, hypercalcemia, urate nephropathy, amyloid glomerulopathy (rare) Pyelonephritis	Toxic effects of tumor products, light chains, OAF, DNA breakdown products Hypogammaglobulinemia
Anemia	Myelophthisis, decreased production, increased destruction	Tumor expansion; production of inhibitory factors and autoantibodies by tumor cells
Infection	Hypogammaglobulinemia, decreased neutrophil migration	Decreased production due to tumor-induced suppression; increased IgG catabolism
Neurologic symptoms	Hyperviscosity, cryoglobulins, amyloid deposits Hypercalcemia, cord compression	Products of tumor; properties of M component; light chains OAF
Bleeding	Interference with clotting factors, amyloid damage of endothelium, platelet dysfunction	Products of tumor; antibodies to clotting factors; light chains; antibody coating of platelets
Mass lesions		Tumor expansion

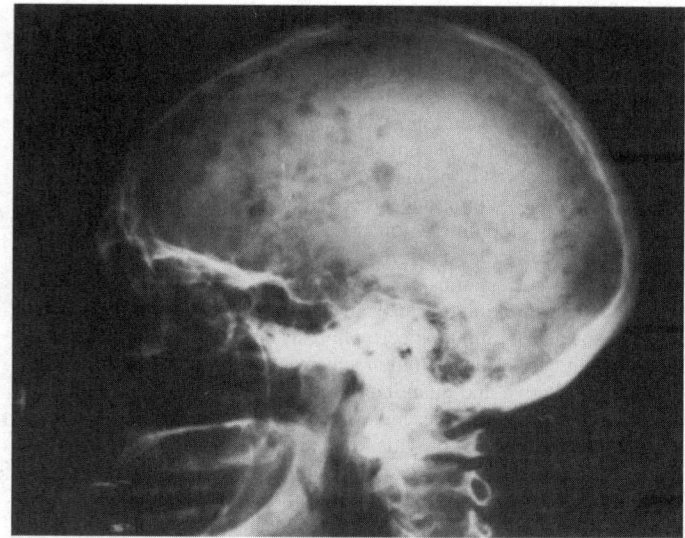

FIGURE 114-3   Bony lesions in multiple myeloma. The skull demonstrates the typical "punched out" lesions characteristic of multiple myeloma. The lesion represents a purely osteolytic lesion with little or no osteoblastic activity. (*Courtesy of Dr. Geraldine Schechter.*)

plain radiography. The bony lysis results in substantial mobilization of calcium from bone, and serious acute and chronic complications of hypercalcemia may dominate the clinical picture (see below). Localized bone lesions may expand to the point that mass lesions may be palpated, especially on the skull (Fig. 114-3), clavicles, and sternum, and the collapse of vertebrae may lead to symptoms of spinal cord compression.

The next most common clinical problem in patients with myeloma is susceptibility to bacterial infections. The most common infections are pneumonias and pyelonephritis, and the most frequent pathogens are *Streptococcus pneumoniae*, *Staphylococcus aureus*, and *Klebsiella pneumoniae* in the lungs and *Escherichia coli* and other gram-negative organisms in the urinary tract. In about 25 percent of patients, recurrent infections are the presenting features, and over 75 percent of patients will have a serious infection at some time in their course. The susceptibility to infection has several contributing causes. First, patients with myeloma have diffuse hypogammaglobulinemia if the M component is excluded. The hypogammaglobulinemia is related to both decreased production and increased destruction of normal antibodies. Moreover, some patients generate a population of circulating regulatory cells in response to their myeloma that can suppress normal antibody synthesis. In the case of IgG myeloma, normal IgG antibodies are broken down more rapidly than normal because the catabolic rate for IgG antibodies varies directly with the serum concentration. The large M component results in fractional catabolic rates of 8 to 16 percent instead of the normal 2 percent. These patients have very poor antibody responses, especially to polysaccharide antigens such as those on bacterial cell walls. Such responses are normally T cell–independent. Most measures of T cell function in myeloma are normal, but a subset of CD4+ cells may be decreased. Granulocyte lysozyme content is low, and granulocyte migration is not as rapid as normal in patients with my-

eloma, probably the result of a product of the tumor. There are also a variety of abnormalities in complement functions in myeloma patients. All these factors contribute to the immune deficiency of these patients.

Renal failure occurs in nearly 25 percent of myeloma patients, and some renal pathology is noted in over half. There are many contributing factors. Hypercalcemia is the most common cause of renal failure. Glomerular deposits of amyloid, hyperuricemia, recurrent infections, and occasional infiltration of the kidney by myeloma cells all may contribute to renal dysfunction. However, tubular damage associated with the excretion of light chains is almost always present. Normally, light chains are filtered, reabsorbed in the tubules, and catabolized. With the increase in amount of light chains presented to the tubule, the tubular cells become overloaded with these proteins, and tubular damage results either directly from light chain toxic effects or indirectly from the release of intracellular lysosomal enzymes. The earliest manifestation of this tubular damage is the adult Fanconi syndrome (a type 2 proximal renal tubular acidosis) with increased loss of glucose, amino acids, and defects in the ability of the kidney to acidify and concentrate the urine. The proteinuria is not accompanied by hypertension, and the protein is nearly all light chains. Generally, there is very little albumin in the urine because glomerular function is usually normal. When the glomeruli are involved, the proteinuria is nonselective. Patients with myeloma also have a decreased anion gap [i.e., $Na^+ - (Cl^- + HCO_3^-)$] because the M component is cationic, resulting in retention of chloride. This is often accompanied by hyponatremia that is felt to be artificial (pseudohyponatremia) because each volume of serum has less water as a result of the increased protein. Myeloma patients are susceptible to developing acute renal failure if they become dehydrated.

Anemia occurs in about 80 percent of myeloma patients. It is usually normocytic and normochromic and related both to the replacement of normal marrow by expanding tumor cells and to the inhibition of hematopoiesis by factors made by the tumor. In addition, mild hemolysis may contribute to the anemia. A larger than expected fraction of patients may have megaloblastic anemia due to either folate or vitamin B12 deficiency. Granulocytopenia and thrombocytopenia are very rare. Clotting abnormalities may be seen due to the failure of antibody-coated platelets to function properly or to the interaction of the M component with clotting factors I, II, V, VII, or VIII. Raynaud's phenomenon and impaired circulation may result if the M component forms cryoglobulins, and hyperviscosity syndromes may develop depending on the physical properties of the M component (most common with IgM, IgG3, and IgA paraproteins). Hyperviscosity is defined on the basis of the relative viscosity of serum as compared with water. Normal relative serum viscosity is 1.8 (i.e., serum is normally almost twice as viscous as water). Symptoms of hyperviscosity occur at a level of 5 to 6, a level usually reached at paraprotein concentrations of around 40 g/L (4 g/dL) for IgM, 50 g/L (5 g/dL) for IgG3, and 70 g/L (7 g/dL) for IgA.

Although neurologic symptoms occur in a minority of patients, they may have many causes. Hypercalcemia may produce lethargy, weakness, depression, and confusion. Hyperviscosity may lead to headache, fatigue, visual disturbances, and retinopathy. Bony damage and collapse may lead to cord compression, radicular pain, and loss of bowel and bladder control. Infiltration of peripheral nerves by amyloid can be a cause of carpal tunnel syndrome and other sensorimotor mono- and polyneuropathies.

Many of the clinical features of myeloma, e.g., cord compression, pathologic fractures, hyperviscosity, sepsis, and hypercalcemia, can present as medical emergencies. Despite the widespread distribution of plasma cells in the body, tumor expansion is dominantly within bone and bone marrow and, for reasons unknown, rarely causes enlargement of spleen, lymph nodes, or gut-associated lymphatic tissue.

Diagnosis and Staging The classic triad of myeloma is marrow plasmacytosis (>10 percent), lytic bone lesions, and a serum and/or urine M component. The diagnosis may be made in the absence of bone lesions if the plasmacytosis is associated with a progressive increase in the M component over time or if extramedullary mass lesions develop. There are two important variants of myeloma, solitary bone plasmacytoma and extramedullary plasmacytoma. These lesions are associated with an M component in fewer than 30 percent of the cases, they may affect younger individuals, and both are associated with median survivals of 10 or more years. Solitary bone plasmacytoma is a single lytic bone lesion without marrow plasmacytosis. Extramedullary plasmacytomas usually involve the submucosal lymphoid tissue of the nasopharynx or paranasal sinuses without marrow plasmacytosis. Both tumors are highly responsive to local radiation therapy. If an M component is present, it should disappear after treatment. Solitary bone plasmacytomas may recur in other bony sites or evolve into myeloma. Extramedullary plasmacytomas rarely recur or progress.

The most difficult differential diagnosis in patients with myeloma involves their separation from individuals with benign monoclonal gammopathies or monoclonal gammopathies of uncertain significance (MGUS). MGUS are vastly more common than myeloma, occurring in 1 percent of the population over age 50 and in up to 10 percent over age 75. Patients with MGUS usually have <10 percent bone marrow plasma cells; <30 g/L (3 g/dL) of M components; no urinary Bence Jones protein; and no anemia, renal failure, lytic bone lesions, or hypercalcemia. When bone marrow cells are exposed to radioactive thymidine in order to quantitate dividing cells, patients with MGUS always have a labeling index <1 percent and patients with myeloma always have a labeling index >1 percent. Other discriminators include plasma cell acid phosphatase and β-glucuronidase, both of which are low in MGUS patients, and the salmon calcitonin stimulation test, which is positive only in patients with active ongoing bone destruction. With long-term follow-up, about 25 percent of patients with MGUS go on to develop myeloma. Typically, patients with MGUS require no therapy. Their survival is about 2 years shorter than age-matched controls without MGUS.

The clinical evaluation of patients with myeloma includes a careful physical examination searching for tender bones and masses. It is paradoxical that only a small minority of patients have an enlargement of the spleen and lymph nodes, the physiologic sites of antibody production. Chest and bone radiographs may reveal lytic lesions or diffuse osteopenia. A complete blood count with differential may reveal anemia. Erythrocyte sedimentation rate is elevated. Very rare patients (~2 percent) may have plasma cell leukemia with more than 2000 plasma cells per microliter. This may be seen in disproportionate frequency in IgD (~12 percent) and IgE (~25 percent) myelomas. Serum calcium, urea nitrogen, creatinine, and uric acid levels may be elevated. Protein electrophoresis and measurement of serum immuno-globulins are useful for detecting and characterizing M spikes, supplemented by immunoelectrophoresis, which is especially sensitive for identifying low concentrations of M components not detectable by protein electrophoresis. A 24-h urine specimen is necessary to quantitate protein excretion, and a concentrated aliquot is used for electrophoresis and immunologic typing of any M component. Serum alkaline phosphatase is usually normal even with extensive bone involvement because of the absence of osteoblastic activity. It is also important to quantitate serum β_2-microglobulin (see below). Serum-soluble IL-6 receptor levels and C-reactive protein may reflect physiologic IL-6 levels in the patient.

The serum M component will be IgG in 53 percent of patients, IgA in 25 percent, and IgD in 1 percent, and 20 percent of patients will have only light chains in serum and urine. Dipsticks for detecting proteinuria are not reliable at identifying light chains, and the heat test for detecting Bence Jones protein is falsely negative in about 50 percent of patients with light chain myeloma. Fewer than 1 percent of patients have no identifiable M component, and these patients usually have light chain myelomas in which renal catabolism has made the light chains undetectable in the urine. IgD myeloma may also present as light chain myeloma. About two-thirds of patients with serum M components also have urinary light chains. The light chain isotype may have an impact on survival. Patients secreting lambda light chains have a significantly shorter overall survival than those secreting kappa light chains. It is not clear whether this is due to some genetically important determinant of cell proliferation or because lambda light chains are more likely to cause renal damage and form amyloid than are kappa light chains. The heavy chain isotype may have an impact on patient management as well. About half of patients with IgM paraproteins develop hyperviscosity compared with only 2 to 4 percent of patients with IgA and IgG M components. Among IgG myelomas, it is the IgG3 subclass that has the highest tendency to form both concentration- and temperature-dependent aggregates, leading to hyperviscosity and cold agglutination at lower serum concentrations.

The staging system for patients with myeloma is a functional system for predicting survival and is based on a variety of clinical and laboratory tests, unlike the anatomic staging systems for solid tumors. Details of the staging system are given in Table 114-2. Based on the hemoglobin, calcium, M component, and degree of skeletal involvement, the total-body tumor burden is estimated to be low (stage I, $<0.6 \times 10^{12}$ cells per square meter), intermediate (stage II, 0.6 to 1.2×10^{12} cells per square meter), or high (stage III, $>1.2 \times 10^{12}$ cells per square meter), and the stages are further subdivided on the basis of renal function [A if serum creatinine < 177 μmol/L (<2 mg/dL), B if > 177 (>2)]. Patients in stage IA have a median survival of more than 5 years and those in stage IIIB about 15 months. β_2-Microglobulin is a protein of 11,000 mol wt with homologies with the constant region of immunoglobulins that is the light chain of the class I major histocompatibility antigens (HLA-A, -B, -C) on the surface of every cell. Serum β_2-microglobulin is the single most powerful predictor of survival and can substitute for staging. Patients with β_2-microglobulin levels less than 0.004 g/L have a median survival of 43 months and those with levels higher than 0.004 g/L only 12 months. It is also felt that once the diagnosis of myeloma is firm, histologic features of atypia may also exert an influence on prognosis. IL-6 may be an autocrine and/or paracrine growth factor for myeloma cells; elevated levels are associated with more aggressive disease. High labeling index and high levels of lactate dehydrogenase and thymidine kinase are also associated with poor prognosis.

℞ **TREATMENT**

About 10 percent of patients with myeloma will have an indolent course demonstrating only very slow progression of disease over many years. Such patients only require antitumor therapy when the serum myeloma protein level rises above 50 g/L (5 g/dL) or

Table 114-2

Myeloma Staging System

Stage	Criteria	Estimated Tumor Burden, $\times 10^{12}$ cells/m^2

I	All the following:
	1. Hemoglobin >100 g/L (>10 g/dL)
	2. Serum calcium <3 mmol/L (<12 mg/dL)
	3. Normal bone x-ray or solitary lesion
	4. Low M-component production
	  a. IgG level <50 g/L (<5 g/dL)
	  b. IgA level <30 g/L (<3 g/dL)
	  c. Urine light chain <4 g/24 h
		<0.6 (low)

II	Fitting neither I nor III	0.6–1.20 (intermediate)

III	One or more of the following:
	1. Hemoglobin <85 g/L (<8.5 g/dL)
	2. Serum calcium >3 mmol/L (>12 mg/dL)
	3. Advanced lytic bone lesions
	4. High M-component production
	  a. IgG level >70 g/L (>7 g/dL)
	  b. IgA level >50 g/L (>5 g/dL)
	  c. Urine light chains >12 g/24 h
		>1.20 (high)

SUBCLASSIFICATION BASED ON SERUM CREATININE LEVELS

Level	Stage	Median Survival, Months
A < 177 mmol/L (<2 mg/dL)	IA	61
B > 177 mmol/L (≧2 mg/dL)	IIA,B	55
	IIIA	30
	IIIB	15

STAGING BASED ON SERUM β_2-MICROGLOBULIN LEVELS

Level	Stage	Median Survival, Months
<0.004 g/L (<4 mg/mL)	I	43
>0.004 g/L (≧4 mg/mL)	II	12

progressive bone lesions develop. Patients with solitary bone plasmacytomas and extramedullary plasmacytomas may be expected to enjoy prolonged disease-free survival after local radiation therapy to a dose of around 40 Gy. There is a low incidence of occult marrow involvement in patients with solitary bone plasmacytoma. Such patients are usually detected because their serum M component falls slowly or disappears initially only to return after a few months. These patients respond well to systemic chemotherapy.

The vast majority of patients with myeloma require therapeutic intervention. In general, such therapy is of two sorts: systemic chemotherapy to control the progression of myeloma, and symptomatic supportive care to prevent serious morbidity from the complications of the disease. All patients with stage II or III disease and stage I patients exhibiting Bence Jones proteinuria, progressive lytic bone lesions, vertebral compression fractures, recurrent infections, or rising serum M component should be treated with systemic combination chemotherapy. Therapy can prolong and improve the quality of life for myeloma patients.

The standard treatment has consisted of intermittent pulses of an alkylating agent [L-phenylalanine mustard (L-PAM, melphalan), cyclophosphamide, or chlorambucil] and prednisone administered for 4 to 7 days every 4 to 6 weeks. The alkylating agents appear to be roughly equally active, but resistance to one agent is often accompanied by resistance to the others. The usual doses are as follows: melphalan, 8 mg/m^2 of body surface area per day; cyclophosphamide, 200 mg/m^2 per day; chlorambucil, 8 mg/m^2 per day; prednisone, 25 to 60 mg/m^2 per day. Melphalan is used most commonly, but because of their near equivalence in antitumor efficacy,

we favor cyclophosphamide as the alkylating agent because it is less toxic to the marrow stem cell compartment and results in a lower incidence of acute myelodysplastic syndromes than do the other alkylating agents. Doses may need adjustment based on marrow tolerance. However, there are few constraints on the dose of the steroid pulse, and it appears that more is better. Patients responding to therapy generally have a prompt and gratifying reduction in bone pain, hypercalcemia, and anemia and often have fewer infections. The serum M component lags substantially behind the symptomatic improvement, often taking 4 to 6 weeks to fall. This fall depends on the rate of tumor kill and the fractional catabolic rate of immunoglobulin, which in turn depends on the serum concentration (for IgG). Light chain excretion, with a functional half-life of approximately 6 h, may fall within the first week of treatment. However, since urine light chain levels may relate to renal tubular function, they are not a reliable measure of tumor cell kill. Calculations of tumor cell kill are made by extrapolation of the serum M component level and rely heavily on the assumption that every tumor cell produces immunoglobulin at a constant rate. About 60 percent of patients will achieve at least a 75 percent reduction in serum M component level and tumor cell mass in response to an alkylating agent and prednisone. Although this is a tumor reduction of less than one log, clinical responses may last many months. The important feature of the level of the M protein is not how far or how fast it falls, but the rate of its increase after therapy. Efforts to improve the fraction of patients responding and the degree of response have involved adding other active chemotherapeutic agents to the treatment program. Patients with more advanced disease may benefit most from such an approach. High-dose therapy with hematopoietic support is also being tested in younger patients. Sequential treatment with combination chemotherapy regimens followed by two successive high-dose melphalan treatments, each supported with peripheral blood stem cell transplants, have achieved complete responses in 50 percent of patients treated within a year of diagnosis. Complete responses are rare (<10 percent) with standard therapy. Long-term follow-up is not yet available. Allogeneic transplants may also produce high response rates, but treatment-related mortality may be as high as 40 percent.

The ideal duration of therapy has not been determined. Most physicians treat every 4 to 6 weeks for 1 or 2 years. Cessation of therapy is followed by relapse, usually within a year. Retreatment may be associated with a second response in up to 80 percent of patients. Maintenance therapy (e.g., with IFNα) may prolong the duration of response, but this therapy is toxic and has generally not prolonged survival. The regrowth rate of the tumor during relapse accelerates with each relapse. This observation suggests that kinetic resistance to therapy (i.e., increase in cycling cells) is perhaps more important than drug resistance controlled by mdr-1 expression. Patients often respond to treatment, but the length of the response progressively shortens. Patients primarily resistant to initial therapy have a median survival of less than a year. High-dose pulsed steroids used alone (200 mg prednisone every other day or 1 g/m^2 per day methylprednisolone for 5 days) or VAD combination chemotherapy (vincristine, 0.4 mg/d in a 4-day continuous infusion; doxorubicin, 9 mg/m^2 per day in a 4-day continuous infusion; dexamethasone, 40 mg/d for 4 days per week for 3 weeks) may offer useful palliation in patients resistant to primary therapy.

About 15 percent of patients die within the first 3 months after diagnosis, and subsequently, the death rate is about 15 percent per year. The disease usually follows a chronic course for 2 to 5 years before developing an acute terminal phase, usually marked by the development of pancytopenia with a cellular marrow that is refractory to treatment. Widespread organ infiltration by myeloma cells occurs, and survival is less than 6 months. About 46 percent of patients die in the chronic phase of disease from progressive myeloma (16 percent) and renal failure (10 percent), sepsis (14 percent), or both (6 percent). Death in the acute terminal phase (26 percent) is chiefly from progressive myeloma (13 percent) and sepsis (9 percent). Five percent of patients die of acute leukemia, myeloblastic or monocytic, and although it has been debated that this is related to the primary disease, it appears more likely to be the result of chronic therapy with alkylating agents. Nearly 23 percent of patients die of myocardial infarction, chronic lung disease, diabetes, or stroke, all intercurrent illnesses related more to the age of the patient group than to the tumor.

Supportive care directed at the anticipated complications of the disease may be as important as primary antitumor therapy. The hypercalcemia generally responds well to glucocorticoid therapy, hydration, and natriuresis. Calcitonin may add to the inhibitory effects of steroids on bone resorption. Bisphosphonates (e.g., pamidronate 90 mg once a month) reduce osteoclastic bone resorption and preserve performance status and quality of life. Treatments aimed at strengthening the skeleton, such as fluorides, calcium, and vitamin D, with or without androgens, have been suggested but are not of proven efficacy. Iatrogenic worsening of renal function may be prevented by the use of allopurinol during chemotherapy to avoid urate nephropathy and by maintaining a high fluid intake to prevent dehydration and to help excrete light chains and calcium. In the event of acute renal failure, plasmapheresis is approximately 10 times more effective at clearing light chains than peritoneal dialysis, and acutely reducing the protein load may result in functional improvement. Urinary tract infections should be watched for and treated early. Chronic dialysis probably should not be initiated in patients who have failed to respond to antitumor therapy. Plasmapheresis may be the treatment of choice for hyperviscosity syndromes. Although the pneumococcus is a dreaded pathogen in myeloma patients, pneumococcal polysaccharide vaccines may not elicit an antibody response. The advent of intravenous gamma globulin preparations raises some hope that prophylactic administration may prevent some serious infections, but this has not been tested. Chronic oral antibiotic prophylaxis is probably not warranted. Patients developing neurologic symptoms in the lower extremities, severe localized back pain, or problems with bowel and bladder control may need emergency myelography and radiation therapy for palliation. Most bone lesions respond to analgesics and chemotherapy, but certain painful lesions may respond most promptly to localized radiation. The chronic anemia may respond to hematinics (iron, folate, cobalamin), and some have responded to androgens. The pathogenesis of the anemia should be established and specific therapy instituted, where possible.

WALDENSTRÖM'S MACROGLOBULINEMIA In 1948, Waldenström described a malignancy of lymphoplasmacytoid cells that secreted IgM. In contrast to myeloma, the disease was associated with lymphadenopathy and hepatosplenomegaly, but the major clinical manifestation was the hyperviscosity syndrome. The disease resembles the related diseases chronic lymphocytic leukemia, myeloma, and lymphocytic lymphoma. Waldenström's macroglobulinemia and IgM myeloma both follow a similar clinical course. The diagnosis of IgM myeloma is usually reserved for patients with lytic bone lesions and is important only because of the hazard of pathologic fractures.

The cause of macroglobulinemia is unknown. The disease is similar to myeloma in being slightly more common in men and occurring with increased incidence with age (median 64 years). There have been reports that the IgM in some patients with macroglobulinemia may have specificity for myelin-associated glycoprotein (MAG), a protein that has been associated with demyelinating disease of the peripheral nervous system and may be lost earlier and to a greater extent than the better known myelin basic protein in patients with multiple sclerosis. Sometimes patients with macroglobulinemia develop a peripheral neuropathy before the appearance of the neoplasm. There is speculation that the whole process begins with a viral infection that may elicit an antibody response that cross-reacts with a normal tissue component.

Like myeloma, the disease involves the bone marrow, but unlike myeloma, it does not cause bone lesions or hypercalcemia. Like myeloma, a serum M component is present in the serum in excess of 30 g/L (3 g/dL), but unlike myeloma, the size of the IgM paraprotein results in little renal excretion and only around 20 percent of patients excrete light chains. Therefore, renal disease is not common. The light chain isotype is kappa in 80 percent of the cases. Patients present with weakness, fatigue, and recurrent infections, similar to myeloma patients, but epistaxis, visual disturbances, and neurologic symptoms such as peripheral neuropathy, dizziness, headache, and transient paresis are much more common in macroglobulinemia. Physical examination reveals adenopathy and hepatosplenomegaly, and ophthalmoscopic examination may reveal vascular segmentation and dilatation of the retinal veins characteristic of hyperviscosity states. Patients may have a normocytic, normochromic anemia, but rouleaux formation and a positive Coombs' test are much more common than in myeloma. Malignant lymphocytes are usually present in the peripheral blood. About 10 percent of macroglobulins are cryoglobulins. These are pure M components and are not the mixed cryoglobulins seen in rheumatoid arthritis and other autoimmune diseases. Mixed cryoglobulins are composed of IgM or IgA complexed with IgG, for which they are specific. In both cases, Raynaud's phenomenon and serious vascular symptoms precipitated by the cold may occur, but mixed cryoglobulins are not commonly associated with malignancy. Patients suspected of having a cryoglobulin based on history and physical examination should have their blood drawn into a warm syringe and delivered to the laboratory in a container of warm water to avoid errors in quantitating the cryoglobulin.

℞ TREATMENT

Control of serious hyperviscosity symptoms such as an altered state of consciousness or paresis can be achieved acutely by plasmapheresis because 80 percent of the IgM paraprotein is intravascular. Fludarabine (25 mg/m² per day for 5 days every 4 weeks) or cladribine (0.1 mg/kg per day for 7 days every 4 weeks) are highly effective single agents. About 80 percent of patients respond to chemotherapy, and their median survival is over 3 years. The absence of other serious organ toxicities results in a longer life span of patients with macroglobulinemia compared with those with myeloma.

POEMS SYNDROME The features of this syndrome are *p*olyneuropathy, *o*rganomegaly, *e*ndocrinopathy, *m*ultiple myeloma, and *s*kin changes (POEMS). Patients usually have a severe, progressive sensorimotor polyneuropathy associated with sclerotic bone lesions from myeloma. Polyneuropathy occurs in about 1.4 percent of myelomas, but the POEMS syndrome is only a rare subset of that group. Unlike typical myeloma, hepatomegaly and lymphadenopathy occur in about two-thirds of patients and splenomegaly is seen in one-third. The lymphadenopathy frequently resembles Castleman's disease histologically, a condition that has been linked to IL-6 overproduction. The endocrine manifestations include amenorrhea in women and impotence and gynecomastia in men. Hyperprolactinemia due to loss of normal inhibitory control by the hypothalamus may be associated with other central nervous system manifestations such as papilledema and elevated cerebrospinal fluid pressure and protein. Type 2 diabetes mellitus occurs in about one-third of patients. Hypothyroidism and adrenal insufficiency are occasionally noted. Skin changes are diverse: hyperpigmentation, hypertrichosis, skin thickening, and digital clubbing. Other manifestations include peripheral edema, ascites, pleural effusions, fever, and thrombocytosis.

The pathogenesis of the disease is unclear, but high circulating levels of the proinflammatory cytokines IL-1β, IL-6, and TNFα have been documented and levels of the inhibitory cytokine transforming growth factor β (TGFβ) are lower than expected. Treatment of the myeloma may result in an improvement in the other disease manifestations.

HEAVY CHAIN DISEASES The heavy chain diseases are rare lymphoplasmacytic malignancies. Their clinical manifestations vary with the heavy chain isotype. Patients secrete a defective heavy chain that usually has an intact Fc fragment and a deletion in the Fd region. Gamma, alpha, and mu heavy chain diseases have been described, but no reports of delta or epsilon heavy chain diseases have appeared. Molecular biologic analysis of these tumors has revealed structural genetic defects that may account for the aberrant chain secreted.

Gamma Heavy Chain Disease (Franklin's Disease)   This disease affects people of widely different age groups and countries of origin. It is characterized by lymphadenopathy, fever, anemia, malaise, hepatosplenomegaly, and weakness. Its most distinctive symptom is palatal edema, resulting from node involvement of Waldeyer's ring, and this may progress to produce respiratory compromise. The diagnosis depends on the demonstration of an anomalous serum M component [often <20 g/L (<2 g/dL)] that reacts with anti-IgG but not anti-light chain reagents. *The M component is typically present in both serum and urine.* Most of the paraproteins have been of the gamma$_1$ subclass, but other subclasses have been seen. The patients may have thrombocytopenia, eosinophilia, and nondiagnostic bone marrow. Patients usually have a rapid downhill course and die of infection; however, some patients have survived 5 years with chemotherapy.

Alpha Heavy Chain Disease (Seligmann's Disease)   This is the most common of the heavy chain diseases. It is closely related to a malignancy known as *Mediterranean lymphoma*, a disease that affects young people in parts of the world such as the Mediterranean, Asia, and South America in which intestinal parasites are common. The disease is characterized by an infiltration of the lamina propria of the small intestine with lymphoplasmacytoid cells that secrete truncated alpha chains. Demonstrating alpha heavy chains is difficult because the alpha chains tend to polymerize and appear as a smear instead of a sharp peak on electrophoretic profiles. Despite the polymerization, hyperviscosity is not a common problem in alpha heavy chain disease. Without J chain–facilitated dimerization, viscosity does not increase dramatically. Light chains are absent from serum and urine. The patients present with chronic diarrhea, weight loss, and malabsorption and have extensive mesenteric and paraaortic adenopathy. Respiratory tract involvement occurs rarely. Patients may vary widely in their clinical course. Some may develop diffuse aggressive histologies of malignant lymphoma. Chemotherapy may produce long-term remissions. Rare patients appear to have responded to antibiotic therapy, raising the question of the etiologic role of antigenic stimulation perhaps by some chronic intestinal infection. Chemotherapy plus antibiotics may be more effective than chemotherapy alone.

Mu Heavy Chain Disease   The secretion of isolated mu heavy chains into the serum appears to occur in a very rare subset of patients with chronic lymphocytic leukemia. The only features that may distinguish patients with mu heavy chain disease are the presence of vacuoles in the malignant lymphocytes and the excretion of kappa light chains in the urine. The diagnosis requires ultracentrifugation or gel filtration to confirm the nonreactivity of the paraprotein with the light chain reagents because some intact macroglobulins fail to interact with these serums. The tumor cells seem to have a defect in the assembly of light and heavy chains because they appear to contain both in their cytoplasm. There is no evidence that such patients should be treated differently from other patients with chronic lymphocytic leukemia (see Chap. 113).

BIBLIOGRAPHY

ALEXANIAN R, DIMOPOULOS M: The treatment of multiple myeloma. N Engl J Med 330:484, 1994

ATTAL M et al: A prospective, randomized trial of autologous bone marrow transplantation and chemotherapy in multiple myeloma. N Engl J Med 335:91, 1996

BERENSON JR et al: Efficacy of pamidronate in reducing skeletal events in patients with advanced multiple myeloma. N Engl J Med 334:488, 1996

DIMOPOULOS MA, ALEXANIAN R: Waldenström's macroglobulinemia. Blood 83:1452, 1994

GHERARDI RK et al: Overproduction of proinflammatory cytokines imbalanced by their antagonists in POEMS syndrome. Blood 87:1458, 1996

GREGORY WM et al: Combination chemotherapy versus melphalan and prednisone in the treatment of multiple myeloma: An overview of published trials. J Clin Oncol 10:334, 1992

GRIEPP PR: Prognosis in myeloma. Mayo Clin Proc 69:895, 1994

HOLLAND J et al: Plasmacytoma. Treatment results and conversion to myeloma. Cancer 69:1513, 1992

KYLE RA: "Benign" monoclonal gammopathy—after 20–35 years of follow-up. Mayo Clin Proc 68:26, 1993

——— (ed): Myeloma and related disorders, in *Neoplastic Diseases of the Blood*. New York, Churchill Livingstone, 1996, pp 411–705

LUST JA: Role of cytokines in the pathogenesis of monoclonal gammopathies. Mayo Clin Proc 69:691, 1994

NORDIC MYELOMA STUDY GROUP: Interferon-α2b added to melphalan-prednisone for initial and maintenance therapy in multiple myeloma. A randomized, controlled trial. Ann Intern Med 124:212, 1996

VESOLE DH et al: High-dose therapy for refractory multiple myeloma: Improved prognosis with better supportive care and double transplants. Blood 85:950, 1994

---

115   *Jeffery S. Dzieczkowski, Kenneth C. Anderson*

TRANSFUSION BIOLOGY AND THERAPY

BLOOD GROUP ANTIGENS AND ANTIBODIES

The study of red blood cell (RBC) antigens and antibodies reactive with them forms the foundation of transfusion medicine. Serologic studies initially characterized these antigens, but now the molecular composition and structure of many are known. These antigens are assigned to blood group systems based upon the structure and the similarity of the determinant epitopes. The composition of antigens may be carbohydrate or protein. Other cellular blood elements and plasma proteins are also antigenic and can result in *alloimmunization*, the production of antibodies directed against the blood group antigens of another individual. These antibodies are called *alloantibodies*.

Antibodies directed against RBC antigens may result from "natural" exposure, particularly to carbohydrates that mimic some blood group antigens. Those antibodies that occur via natural stimuli are usually produced by a T cell–independent response (thus, generating no memory) and are IgM isotype. *Autoantibodies* (antibodies against autologous blood group antigens) arise spontaneously or as the result of infectious sequelae (e.g., from *Mycoplasma pneumoniae*) and are also often IgM. These antibodies are often clinically insignificant due to their low affinity for antigen at body temperature. However, IgM antibodies can activate the complement cascade and result in hemolysis. Antibodies that result from allogeneic exposure, such as transfusion or pregnancy, are usually IgG. IgG antibodies commonly bind to antigen at warmer temperatures and may hemolyze RBCs. Unlike IgM antibodies, IgG antibodies can cross the placenta and bind fetal erythrocytes bearing the corresponding antigen, resulting in hemolytic disease of the newborn, or *hydrops fetalis*.

Alloimmunization to leukocytes, platelets, and plasma proteins may also result in transfusion complications such as fevers and urticaria but generally does not cause hemolysis. Assay for these other alloantibodies is not routinely performed; however, they may be detected using special assays.

ABO ANTIGENS AND ANTIBODIES   The first blood group antigen system, recognized in 1900, was ABO, the most important in transfusion medicine. The major blood groups of this system are A, B, AB, and O. The latter includes red cells that lack A or B antigens. These antigens are carbohydrates attached to a precursor backbone, may be found on the cellular membrane either as glycosphingolipids or glycoproteins, and are secreted into plasma and body fluids as glycoproteins. H substance is the immediate precursor upon which the A and B antigens are added. This H substance is formed by the addition of fucose to the glycolipid or glycoprotein backbone. The subsequent addition of *N*-acetylgalactosamine creates the A antigen, while the addition of galactose produces the B antigen.

The genes that determine the A and B phenotypes are found on chromosome 9p and are expressed in a Mendelian codominant manner. The gene products are glycosyl transferases, which confer the enzymatic capability of attaching the specific antigenic carbohydrate. Individuals who lack the "A" and "B" transferases are phenotypically type

"O," while those who inherit both transferases are type "AB." Rare individuals lack the H gene, which codes for fucose transferase, and cannot form H substance. These individuals are homozygous for the silent h allele (hh) and have Bombay phenotype (O_h).

The ABO blood group system is important because essentially all individuals produce antibodies to the ABH carbohydrate antigen that they lack. The naturally occurring anti-A and anti-B antibodies are termed *isoagglutinins*. Thus, type A individuals produce anti-B, while type B individuals make anti-A. Neither isoagglutinin is found in type AB individuals, while type O individuals produce both anti-A and anti-B. Thus, persons with type AB are "universal recipients" because they do not have antibodies against any ABO phenotype, while persons with type O blood can donate to essentially all recipients because their cells are not recognized by any ABO isoagglutinins. The rare individuals with Bombay phenotype produce antibodies to H substance (which is present on all red cells except those of hh phenotype) as well as to both A and B antigens and are therefore compatible only with other hh donors.

In most people, A and B antigens are secreted by the cells and are present in the circulation. Nonsecretors are susceptible to a variety of infections (e.g., *Candida albicans*, *Neisseria meningitidis*, *Streptococcus pneumoniae*, *Haemophilus influenzae*). Many organisms may bind to polysaccharides on cells; soluble blood group antigens may block this binding.

Rh SYSTEM   The Rh system is the second most important blood group system in pretransfusion testing. The Rh antigens are found on a 30- to 32-kDa RBC membrane protein, which has no defined function. Although more than 40 different antigens in the Rh system have been described, five determinants account for the vast majority of phenotypes. The presence of the D antigen confers Rh "positivity," while people who lack the D antigen are Rh negative. Two allelic antigen pairs, E/e and C/c, are also found on the Rh protein. The three Rh genes, E/e, D, and C/c, are arranged in tandem on chromosome 1 and inherited as a haplotype, i.e., cDE or Cde. Two haplotypes can result in the phenotypic expression of two to five Rh antigens.

The D antigen is a potent alloantigen. About 15 percent of people lack this antigen. Exposure of these Rh-negative people to even small amounts of Rh-positive cells, by either transfusion or pregnancy, can result in the production of anti-D alloantibody.

OTHER BLOOD GROUP SYSTEMS AND ALLOANTIBODIES   There are more than 100 recognized blood group systems, composed of more than 500 antigens. The presence or absence of certain antigens has been associated with various diseases and anomalies; antigens also act as receptors for infectious agents. Alloantibodies of importance in routine clinical practice, and their respective antigens, are listed in Table 115-1.

Antibodies to *Lewis system* carbohydrate antigens are the most common cause of incompatibility during pretransfusion screening. The Lewis gene product is a fucosyl transferase and maps to chromosome 19. The antigen is not an integral membrane structure but is adsorbed to the RBC membrane from the plasma. Antibodies to Lewis antigens are usually IgM and cannot cross the placenta. Lewis antigens may be adsorbed onto tumor cells and may be targets of therapy.

I system antigens are also oligosaccharides related to H, A, B, and Le. I and i are not allelic pairs but are carbohydrate antigens that differ only in the extent of branching. The i antigen is an unbranched chain that is converted by the I gene product, a glycosyltransferase, into a branched chain. The branching process affects all the ABH antigens, which become progressively more branched in the first 2 years of life. Some patients with cold agglutinin disease or lymphoma can produce anti-I autoantibodies that cause RBC destruction. Occasional patients with mononucleosis or *Mycoplasma* pneumonia may develop cold agglutinins of either anti-I or anti-i specificity. Most adults lack i expression; thus, finding a donor for patients with anti-i is not difficult. Even though most adults express I antigen, binding is generally low at body temperature. Thus, administration of warm blood prevents isoagglutination.

The *P system* is another group of carbohydrate antigens controlled by specific glycosyltransferases. Its clinical significance is in rare cases of syphilis and viral infection that lead to paroxysmal cold hemoglobinuria. In these cases, an unusual autoantibody to P is produced that binds to RBCs in the cold and fixes complement upon warming. Antibodies with these biphasic properties are called *Donath-Landsteiner antibodies*. The P antigen is also expressed on urothelial cells and may be a receptor for *Escherichia coli* binding.

The *MNSsU system* is regulated by genes on chromosome 4. M and N are determinants on glycophorin A, an RBC membrane protein, and S and s are determinants on glycophorin B. Anti-S and anti-s IgG antibodies may develop after pregnancy or transfusion and lead to hemolysis. Anti-U antibodies are rare but create a situation in which virtually every donor is incompatible because nearly all persons express U.

The *Kell* protein is very large (720 amino acids) and its secondary structure contains many different antigens. The immunogenicity of Kell is third behind the ABO and Rh systems. The absence of the Kell precursor protein (controlled by a gene on X) is associated with acanthocytosis, shortened RBC survival, and a progressive form of muscular dystrophy that includes cardiac defects. This rare condition is called the *McLeod phenotype*. The K_x gene is linked to the 91-kDa component of the NADPH-oxidase on the X chromosome, deletion or mutation of which accounts for about 60 percent of cases of chronic granulomatous disease.

The *Duffy* antigens are codominant alleles, Fy^a and Fy^b, that also serve as receptors for *Plasmodium vivax*. More than 70 percent of persons in malaria-endemic areas lack these antigens, probably as a result of selective influences of the infection on the population.

The *Kidd* antigens, Jk^a and Jk^b, may elicit antibodies transiently. A delayed hemolytic transfusion reaction that occurs with blood tested as compatible is often related to delayed appearance of anti-Jk^a.

PRETRANSFUSION TESTING

Pretransfusion testing of a potential recipient consists of the "type and screen." The "forward type" determines the ABO and Rh phenotype of the recipient by using reagent antisera directed against the A, B, and D antigens. The "reverse type" detects isoagglutinins in the patient's serum and should correlate with the ABO phenotype, or forward type.

The alloantibody screen identifies antibodies directed against other RBC antigens. The detection and characterization of alloantibodies before transfusion is important to ensure the selection of antigen-negative red cell components. The alloantibody screen is performed by mixing patient serum with type O RBC that contain the major antigens of most blood group systems and whose extended phenotype is known. The specificity of the alloantibody is identified by correlating the presence or absence of antigen with the results of the agglutination.

Cross matching is ordered when there is a high probability that the patient will require a packed RBC transfusion. Blood selected for cross matching must be ABO compatible and lack antigens for which

Table 115-1

RBC Blood Group Systems and Alloantigens

Blood Group System	Antigen	Alloantibody	Clinical Significance
Rh (D, C/c, E/e)	RBC protein	IgG	HTR, HDN
Lewis (Le^a, Le^b)	Oligosaccharide	IgM/IgG	Rare HTR
Kell (K/k)	RBC protein	IgG	HTR, HDN
Duffy (Fy^a/Fy^b)	RBC protein	IgG	HTR, HDN
Kidd (Jk^a/Jk^b)	RBC protein	IgG	HTR (often delayed), HDN (mild)
I/i	Carbohydrate	IgM	None
MNSsU	RBC protein	IgM/IgG	Anti-M rare HDN, anti-S, -s, and -U HDN, HTR

NOTE: RBC, red blood cell; HDN, hemolytic disease of the newborn; HTR, hemolytic transfusion reaction.

the patient has clinically significant alloantibodies. Nonreactive cross matching confirms the absence of any major incompatibility and reserves that unit for the patient.

In the case of Rh-negative patients, every attempt must be made to provide Rh-negative blood components to prevent alloimmunization to the D antigen. In an emergency, Rh-positive blood can be safely transfused to a Rh-negative patient who lacks anti-D; however, the recipient is then at risk for becoming alloimmunized and producing anti-D. Rh-negative women with child-bearing potential who are inadvertently transfused with products containing Rh-positive RBCs should receive passive immunization with anti-D (RhoGam or WinRho) to reduce or prevent sensitization.

BLOOD COMPONENTS

Blood products intended for transfusion are routinely collected as whole blood (450 mL) in various anticoagulants. Most donated blood is processed into components: packed red blood cells (PRBC), platelets, and fresh frozen plasma (FFP) or cryoprecipitate (Table 115-2). Whole blood is first separated into PRBC and platelet-rich plasma by slow centrifugation. The platelet-rich plasma is then centrifuged at high speed to yield one unit of random donor (RD) platelets and one unit of FFP. Cryoprecipitate is produced from FFP by slowly thawing to precipitate the plasma proteins, which are then separated by centrifugation.

Apheresis technology, in addition to its therapeutic applications, is used for the collection of multiple units of platelets from a single donor. These single-donor apheresis platelets (SDAP) contain the equivalent of at least six units of RD units and often have fewer contaminating leukocytes than pooled RD platelets.

Plasma may also be collected by apheresis. Plasma derivatives such as albumin, intravenous immunoglobulin, antithrombin 3, and coagulation factor concentrates are prepared from very large plasma pools (~20,000 donors per pool) but are unlikely to transmit infections because of the use of various methods of postcollection sterilization.

WHOLE BLOOD Whole blood provides both oxygen-carrying capacity and volume expansion. It is the ideal component for patients who have sustained acute hemorrhage of 25 percent or greater total blood volume loss. Whole blood is stored at 4°C to maintain erythrocyte viability, but platelet dysfunction and degradation of some coagulation factors occurs. In addition, 2,3-BPG levels fall over time, leading to an increase in the oxygen affinity of the hemoglobin and a decreased capacity to deliver oxygen to the tissues, a problem with all red cell storage. Whole blood is not readily available because of the need to process blood into components that can be used for different recipients.

PACKED RED BLOOD CELLS This product increases oxygen-carrying capacity in the anemic patient. Adequate oxygenation can be maintained with a hemoglobin content of 70 g/L in the well-perfused patient (normovolemic, able to increase cardiac output); however, comorbid factors often necessitate transfusion at a higher threshold. The decision to transfuse should be guided by the clinical situation and not by an arbitrary laboratory value.

PRBC may be modified to prevent or reduce the incidence of certain adverse reactions. Contaminating donor leukocytes are responsible for inducing fevers in the recipient and causing alloimmunization to HLA antigens. Contaminating leukocytes can be removed by several methods, with varying degrees of success. These methods include filtration and centrifugation. Although bedside filtration is the most popular method of leukocyte depletion and removes 99.9 percent of donor leukocytes, recent studies suggest it may not be effective in avoiding reactions or alloimmunization. Due to the difficulty of quality control of bedside filtration and the evolving role of cytokines that accumulate during storage of cellular blood components in mediating transfusion reactions, leukoreduction is more commonly being done in the blood bank before storage of cellular components.

Donor plasma may cause transfusion complications such as allergic reactions. Plasma can be removed from cellular blood components by washing.

PLATELETS Thrombocytopenia is a risk factor for hemorrhage, and platelet transfusion has been shown to reduce the incidence of bleeding. While the threshold for prophylactic platelet transfusion remains controversial, 10,000 to 20,000/μL has been widely used. Recently, 5000/μL has been suggested as sufficient to prevent spontaneous hemorrhage. However, 50,000/μL platelets is the usual minimum target level for hemostasis during invasive procedures.

Platelets are given either as pools prepared from five to eight RD or as SDAP from a single donor. In an unsensitized patient without increased platelet consumption [splenomegaly, fever, disseminated intravascular coagulation (DIC)], six to eight units of RD platelets are pooled and transfused, and each unit is anticipated to increase the platelet count 5000 to 10,000/μL. Patients who have received multiple transfusions are exposed to many HLA- and platelet-specific antigens, which may result in alloimmunization. These sensitized patients often have little or no increase in their posttransfusion platelet counts and are thus considered to be refractory. Patients who are anticipated to require multiple transfusions are best served by receiving SDAP and leukocyte-reduced components to lower the risk of alloimmunization.

Refractoriness to platelet transfusion may be evaluated using the corrected count increment (CCI):

$$CCI = \frac{\text{posttransfusion count} - \text{pretransfusion count}}{\text{number of platelets transfused} \times 10^{11}} \times BSA$$

where BSA is body surface area measured in square metres. The posttransfusion count performed 1 h after the transfusion is acceptable if the CCI is 10×10^9/mL, and after 18 to 24 h an increment of 7.5×10^9/mL is expected. Patients who have suboptimal responses are likely to have received multiple transfusions and have antibodies directed against class I HLA antigens. Refractoriness can be investigated by detecting anti-HLA antibodies in the recipient's serum. Patients who are sensitized will often react with 100 percent of the lymphocytes used for the HLA-antibody screen, and HLA-matched SDAP should be considered for those patients who require transfusion. Although ABO-identical HLA-matched SDAP provide the best chance for increasing the platelet count, locating these products is difficult. Additional clinical causes for a low platelet CCI should be considered, such as fever, bleeding, splenomegaly, DIC, or medications in the recipient.

FRESH FROZEN PLASMA FFP contains stable coagulation factors and plasma proteins: fibrinogen, antithrom-

Table 115-2

Characteristics of Selected Blood Components

Component	Volume, mL	Content	Clinical Response
PRBC	180–200	RBCs with variable leukocyte content and small amount of plasma	Increase hemoglobin 10 g/L and hematocrit 3%
Platelets	50–70	5.5×10^{10}/RD unit	Increase platelet count 5000–10,000/μL
	200–400	$\geq 3.0 \times 10^{11}$/SDAP product	CCI $\geq 10 \times 10^9$/L within 1 h and $\geq 7.5 \times 10^9$/L within 24 h posttransfusion
FFP	200–250	Plasma proteins—coagulation factors, proteins C and S, antithrombin	Increases coagulation factors about 2%
Cryoprecipitate	10–15	Cold-insoluble plasma proteins, fibrinogen, factor VIII, vWF	Topical fibrin glue, also 80 IU factor VIII

NOTE: PRBC, packed red blood cells; RBC, red blood cell; CCI, corrected count increment; FFP, fresh frozen plasma; vWF, von Willebrand factor.

bin, albumin, as well as proteins C and S. Indications for FFP transfusion include correction of coagulopathies, including the rapid reversal of coumadin; supplying deficient plasma proteins; and treatment of thrombotic thrombocytopenic purpura. Although FFP is an excellent volume expander, it should not be routinely used in this role. FFP is an acellular component and therefore does not transmit intracellular infections, i.e., cytomegalovirus (CMV). Patients who are IgA-deficient and require plasma support should receive FFP collected from IgA-deficient donors because the risk of anaphylaxis is increased with normal donors (see below).

CRYOPRECIPITATE Cryoprecipitate is a source of fibrinogen, factor VIII, and von Willebrand factor (vWF). It is ideal for supplying fibrinogen to the volume-sensitive patient. Cryoprecipitate is also used as a source of fibrinogen to create fibrin glue, a topical hemostatic sealant used in the surgical setting. When factor VIII concentrates are not available, cyroprecipitate is an option since each unit contains approximately 80 units of factor VIII. vWF may also be supplied to patients with dysfunctional vWF multimers (type II von Willebrand disease) and those who lack the capacity to generate vWF altogether (type III).

PLASMA DERIVATIVES Plasma from thousands of donors may be pooled to derive specific protein concentrates. These products include albumin, intravenous immunoglobulin, antithrombin, and coagulation factor concentrates. In addition, donors who have high titer antibodies to specific agents or antigens provide hyperimmune globulins, such as anti-D (RhoGam, WinRho), and antisera to hepatitis B virus (HBV), varicella-zoster virus, CMV, and a number of other infectious agents.

ADVERSE REACTIONS TO BLOOD TRANSFUSION

Adverse reactions to transfused blood components occur despite multiple tests, inspections, and checks. Fortunately, the most common reactions are not life-threatening, although serious reactions can present with mild symptoms and signs. Some reactions can be reduced or prevented by modified (filtered, washed, or irradiated) blood components. When an adverse reaction is suspected, the transfusion should be stopped and reported to the blood bank for investigation.

Transfusion reactions may result from immune and nonimmune mechanisms. Immune-mediated reactions are often due to preformed donor or recipient antibody; however, cellular elements may also cause adverse effects. Nonimmune causes of reactions are due to the chemical and physical properties of the stored blood component and its additives.

Infectious complications of transfusion have become less frequent, although fear of these complications remains the primary concern of both patients and clinicians. The incidence of transfusion-related infections has been reduced substantially due to improved donor screening and testing of collected blood. Infections, like any adverse transfusion reaction, must be brought to the attention of the blood bank for appropriate "look-back" studies (Table 115-3).

IMMUNE-MEDIATED REACTIONS Acute Hemolytic Transfusion Reactions Immune-mediated hemolysis occurs when the recipient has preformed antibodies that bind and lyse donor erythrocytes. The ABO isoagglutinins are responsible for the majority of these reactions, although alloantibodies directed against other red blood cell antigens, i.e., Rh, Kell, and Duffy, may result in intravascular hemolysis.

Acute hemolytic reactions may present with hypotension, tachypnea, tachycardia, fever, chills, hemoglobinemia, hemoglobinuria, chest and/or flank pain, and discomfort at the catheter or infusion site. Monitoring the patient's vital signs before and during the transfusion is important to identify these reactions promptly. When acute hemolysis is suspected, the transfusion must be immediately stopped, intravenous access maintained, and the reaction reported to the blood bank. A correctly labeled posttransfusion blood sample and any untransfused blood should be sent to the blood transfusion service for investigation. The laboratory evaluation for hemolysis includes the measurement of haptoglobin, lactate dehydrogenase (LDH), and indirect bilirubin levels in the recipient's serum.

Table 115-3

Risks of Transfusion Complications

	Frequency, Episodes : Unit
Reactions	
Febrile (FNHTR)	1–4:100
Allergic	1–4:100
Delayed hemolytic	1:1,500
Acute hemolytic	1:12,000
Fatal hemolytic	1:100,000
Anaphylactic	1:150,000
Infections*	
Hepatitis C	1:103,000
Hepatitis B	1:200,000
HIV-1	1:490,000
HIV-2	None reported
HTLV-I (II)	1:641,000
Malaria	1:4,000,000
Other complications	
RBC allosensitization	1:100
HLA allosensitization	1:10
Graft-versus-host disease	Rare
Hypervolemia	NQ†
Iron overload	NQ
Hypothermia	NQ

* Infectious agents rarely associated with transfusion or theoretically possible, unknown risk include parvovirus B-19, *Babesia microti* (babesiosis), *Borrelia burgdorferi* (Lyme disease), *Trypanosma cruzi* (Chagas' disease), and *Treponema pallidum.*
† NQ, not quantified.
NOTE: FNHTR, febrile nonhemolytic transfusion reaction; HIV, human immunodeficiency virus; HTLV, human T lymphotropic virus; RBC, red blood cell.

The immune complexes that result in RBC lysis can cause renal compromise and failure. Diuresis should be induced, using furosemide or mannitol with intravenous fluids, to prevent or minimize this complication. Tissue factor released from the lysed erythrocytes may initiate DIC. Coagulation studies including prothrombin time (PT), activated partial thromboplastin time (aPTT), fibrinogen, and platelet count should be monitored in patients with hemolytic reactions.

Errors at the patient's bedside, such as mislabeling the sample or transfusing an incorrect patient, are responsible for the majority of these reactions. The blood bank investigation of these reactions includes examination of the pre- and posttransfusion samples for hemolysis, repeat typing of the patient samples; direct antiglobulin test (DAT), sometimes called the direct Coombs test, of the posttransfusion sample; repeating the cross matching of the blood component; and checking all clerical records for errors. DAT detects the presence of antibody or complement bound to RBCs in vivo. In addition to confirming whether an immune hemolytic reaction has taken place, detecting or preventing the reciprocal error, i.e., patient A received blood intended for patient B and vice versa, is important.

Delayed Hemolytic and Serologic Transfusion Reactions Delayed hemolytic transfusion reactions (DHTR) are not completely preventable. A good transfusion history by the clinician can lower the risk. If the patient has had past transfusion or cross matching difficulties, the blood bank may be able to trace the problem. These reactions occur in patients previously sensitized to RBC alloantigens who have a negative alloantibody screen due to low antibody levels. When the patient is transfused with antigen-positive blood, an anamnestic response results in the early production of alloantibody that binds donor RBCs. The alloantibody is detectable 1 to 2 weeks following the transfusion, and the posttransfusion DAT may become positive due to circulating donor RBCs coated with antibody or complement. The transfused, alloantibody-coated erythrocytes are removed by the reticuloendothelial system, resulting in their extravascular clearance. Most commonly these reactions are detected in the blood bank when a subsequent patient sample, often there for additional cross matching, reveals a positive alloantibody screen or a new alloantibody in a recently transfused recipient.

No specific therapy is usually required, although additional RBC transfusions may be necessary to treat the falling hematocrit. Delayed serologic transfusion reactions (DSTR) are similar to DHTR, as the DAT is positive and alloantibody is detected; however, there is no evidence of RBC clearance.

Febrile Nonhemolytic Transfusion Reaction The most frequent reaction associated with the transfusion of cellular blood components is a febrile nonhemolytic transfusion reaction (FNHTR). These reactions are characterized by chills and rigors and a 1°C or greater rise in temperature. Since FNHTR is primarily a diagnosis of exclusion, it is important to rule out other causes of fever in the transfused patient. Classically, antibodies directed against donor leukocyte and HLA antigens have been proposed to mediate these reactions, and multiply transfused patients and multiparous women therefore are felt to be at increased risk. Although it is sometimes possible to demonstrate the offending antibodies in the recipient's serum, this is not necessary because of the mild nature of most FNHTR. The use of leukocyte-reduced blood products may prevent or delay sensitization to leukocyte antigens and thereby reduce the incidence of these febrile episodes. Of note, cytokines that accumulate within stored cellular blood components may mediate FNHTR, suggesting the utility of leukoreduction before storage to prevent these reactions. The incidence and severity of these reactions can be decreased by premedicating the patient with acetaminophen or other antipyretic agents, but this should be reserved only for patients with recurrent reactions.

Allergic Reactions Urticarial reactions, characterized by a pruritic rash, edema, headache, and dizziness, are related to plasma proteins found in transfused components. Mild reactions may be treated symptomatically by temporarily stopping the transfusion and administering antihistamines (diphenhydramine, 50 mg by mouth or intramuscularly). The transfusion may be completed after the signs and/or symptoms resolve. Patients with a history of allergic transfusion reaction should be premedicated with an antihistamine. Cellular components can be washed to remove residual plasma for the extremely sensitized patient.

Anaphylactic Reaction This severe reaction presents after transfusion of only a few milliliters of the blood component. Symptoms and signs include difficulty breathing, coughing, nausea and vomiting, hypotension, bronchospasm, respiratory arrest, shock, and loss of consciousness. Treatment includes stopping the transfusion, maintaining vascular access, and administering epinephrine (0.5 to 1.0 mL of 1:1000 dilution SQ). Glucocorticoids may be required in severe cases.

Patients who are IgA-deficient may be sensitized to this Ig class and are at risk for anaphylactic reactions associated with plasma transfusion. Individuals with severe IgA deficiency should therefore receive only IgA-deficient plasma and washed cellular blood components. Patients who have anaphylactic or repeated allergic reactions to blood components should be tested for IgA deficiency.

Graft-Versus-Host Disease Graft-versus-host disease (GVHD) is a frequent complication of allogeneic bone marrow transplantation, in which setting viable lymphocytes derived from donor marrow cannot be eliminated by an immunodeficient host. Transfusion-related GVHD is mediated by donor T lymphocytes that recognize host HLA antigens as foreign and mount an immune response, which is manifested clinically by the development of fever, a characteristic cutaneous eruption, diarrhea, and liver function abnormalities. GVHD can also occur when blood components that contain viable T lymphocytes are transfused to immunodeficient recipients or to immunocompetent recipients who share HLA antigens with the donor. In addition to the aforementioned clinical features, transfusion-associated (TA-GVHD) GVHD is further characterized by marrow aplasia and pancytopenia. In contrast to GVHD that develops in the setting of allogeneic marrow transplantation, TA-GVHD is notoriously resistant to treatment with immunosuppressive therapies, including glucocorticoids, cyclosporine, antithymocyte globulin, and ablative therapy followed by allogeneic bone marrow transplantation. Clinical manifestations appear at 8 to 10 days,

and death occurs at 3 to 4 weeks posttransfusion. The resistance to treatment and fatal outcome highlight the need for identification of patient groups at risk for TA-GVHD and use of methods for its prevention.

TA-GVHD can be prevented by irradiation of cellular components (minimum of 2500 cGy) before transfusion to patients at risk. At present, patients at risk for TA-GVHD include fetuses receiving intrauterine transfusions, selected immunocompetent (e.g., lymphoma patients) or immunocompromised recipients, recipients of donor units known to be from a blood relative, and recipients who have undergone marrow transplantation. Directed donations by family members should be discouraged (they are not less likely to transmit infection); lacking other options, the blood products from family members should always be irradiated.

Transfusion-Related Acute Lung Injury This uncommon reaction results from the transfusion of donor plasma that contains high titer anti-HLA antibodies that bind the corresponding antigens on recipient leukocytes. The leukocytes are thought to aggregate in the pulmonary vasculature and release mediators that increase capillary permeability. The recipient develops symptoms of respiratory compromise and signs of noncardiogenic pulmonary edema, including bilateral interstitial infiltrates on chest x-ray. Treatment is supportive, and patients usually recover without sequelae. Testing the donor's plasma for anti-HLA antibodies can support this diagnosis. The implicated donors are frequently multiparous women, and transfusion of their plasma component should be avoided.

Posttransfusion Purpura This reaction presents as thrombocytopenia 7 to 10 days after platelet transfusion and occurs predominantly in women. Platelet-specific antibodies are found in the recipient's serum, and the most frequently recognized antigen is HPA-1a found on the platelet glycoprotein IIIa receptor. The delayed thrombocytopenia is due to the production of antibodies that react to both donor and recipient platelets. Additional platelet transfusions can worsen the thrombocytopenia and should be avoided. Treatment with intravenous immunoglobulin may neutralize the offending antibodies, or plasmapheresis can be used to remove the antibodies should therapy be required.

Alloimmunization Cellular blood elements and plasma proteins bear a number of antigens to which the recipient may become alloimmunized. Alloantibodies to RBC antigens are detected during pretransfusion testing, and their presence may delay finding antigen-negative crossmatch-compatible products for transfusion. Women of child-bearing age who are sensitized to certain RBC antigens (i.e., D, c, E, Kell, or Duffy) are at risk for bearing a fetus with hemolytic disease of the newborn. Matching for D antigen is the only pretransfusion selection test to prevent RBC alloimmunization.

Alloimmunization to antigens on leukocytes and platelets can result in refractoriness to platelet transfusions. Once alloimmunization has developed, identifying and supplying HLA-compatible platelets from donors who share similar antigens with the recipient may be time-consuming and often futile. Hence, prudent transfusion practice is directed at preventing sensitization through the use of leukocyte-reduced cellular components, as well as limiting antigenic exposure by the judicious use of transfusions and transfusion of SDAP.

NONIMMUNOLOGIC REACTIONS **Fluid Overload** Blood components are excellent volume expanders, and transfusion may quickly lead to volume overload. Monitoring the rate and volume of the transfusion, along with the use of a diuretic, can minimize this problem.

Hypothermia Blood components stored either refrigerated (4°C) or frozen (−18°C or below) can result in hypothermia when rapidly infused. Particular attention is required when transfusing via a central venous catheter, because cardiac dysrhythmias can result from exposing the sinoatrial node to cold fluid. Use of an in-line warmer will prevent this complication.

Electrolyte Toxicity RBC leakage during storage increases the plasma concentration of potassium in the unit. Neonates and patients in renal failure are at risk for hyperkalemia. Measuring the recipient's serum potassium level or noting electrocardiographic changes characteristic of hyperkalemia is diagnostic. Preventive measures, such as using fresh or washed RBCs, are warranted for neonatal transfusions because this complication can be fatal.

Citrate, commonly used to anticoagulate blood components, chelates calcium and thereby inhibits the coagulation cascade. Hypocalcemia, manifested by circumoral numbness and/or tingling sensation of the fingers and toes, may result from multiple rapid transfusions. Because citrate is quickly metabolized to bicarbonate, calcium supplementation is seldom required in this setting. If calcium or any other intravenous infusion is necessary, it must be given through a separate intravenous line or site.

Iron Overload   Each unit of RBCs contains 200 to 250 mg of iron. The transfused iron is added to the normal body store of 1 to 3 g, because excretion mechanisms are inadequate for the iron excess. Symptoms and signs of iron overload affecting endocrine, hepatic, and cardiac function are common after 100 units of RBCs have been transfused (total body iron load of 20 g). Preventing this complication by using alternative therapies (i.e., erythropoietin) and judicious transfusion is preferable and cost effective. Deferoxamine and other chelating agents are available, but the response is often suboptimal.

INFECTIOUS COMPLICATIONS   Viral Infections   *Hepatitis C virus* (HCV)   The major etiologic agent of what was previously termed non-A non-B hepatitis remains the most common cause of transfusion-associated viral hepatitis. Testing donated blood for the presence of antibodies to HCV, using the first-generation assay, reduced the incidence of posttransfusion HCV infection to 3 in 10,000 transfusion episodes. Since the implementation of an improved screening assay for HCV antibodies, this risk has been lowered further (1 in 103,000). Infection with HCV may be asymptomatic or lead to chronic active hepatitis, cirrhosis, and liver failure.

Hepatitis B virus   Increased and improved donor selection and screening, along with increased vaccination of the donor and recipient population, has markedly reduced the incidence of this transfusion-associated infection. Vaccination of individuals who require long-term transfusion therapy can prevent this complication.

Human immunodeficiency virus (HIV) type 1   Intensive donor screening and testing has dramatically reduced the risk of HIV-1 infection via blood transfusion. The risk of HIV-1 infection per transfusion episode is 1 in 490,000. The use of donor testing for HIV-1 p24 antigen may further reduce this risk. HIV-2 may also be transmitted via blood; accordingly, in 1992 a specific assay to detect antibodies to HIV-2 was added to the serologic tests performed on donated blood. There have been no reported cases of HIV-2 infection related to transfusion in the United States, and to date only two donors have tested positive for HIV-2 antibodies.

Cytomegalovirus   This ubiquitous virus infects 50 percent or more of the general population and is transmitted by the infected "passenger" white blood cells found in transfused PRBC or platelet components. Donated blood is not routinely tested for serologic evidence of donor exposure. Classically, blood components harvested from CMV-seronegative donors have been utilized to avoid transfusion-related infection, but more recently, cellular components that are leukocytye-reduced have been shown to have a decreased risk of transmitting CMV, regardless of the serologic status of the donor. Groups at risk for CMV infectious complications include immunosuppressed patients, CMV-seronegative transplant recipients, and neonates; these patients should receive seronegative or leukoreduced components.

Human T lymphotropic virus (HTLV) type I   This virus is associated with adult T cell leukemia/lymphoma and tropical spastic paraparesis in a small percentage of infected persons (see Chap. 192). The reported risk of HTLV-I infection via transfusion is 1 in 641,000 transfusion episodes. HTLV-II may also be transmitted by blood products, although to date it is unclear what diseases may be associated with the virus.

Parvovirus B-19   Blood components and products derived from pooled plasma can transmit this virus, the etiologic agent of erythema infectiosum, or fifth disease, in children. Parvovirus B-19 shows tropism for erythroid precursors and inhibits both erythrocyte production

and maturation. Pure red cell aplasia, presenting either as acute aplastic crisis or chronic anemia with shortened RBC survival, may occur in individuals with an underlying hematologic disease, such as sickle cell disease or thalassemia. The fetus of a seronegative woman is at risk for developing hydrops if infected with this virus.

Bacterial Contamination   Blood components may be contaminated with bacteria (1) at the time of donation due to inadequate skin cleansing before venipuncture, (2) during component processing, or (3) from the bacteremic donor. Because most bacteria do not grow well at cold temperatures, packed RBCs and frozen plasma are not common sources of bacterial contamination. However, some gram-negative bacteria, notably *Yersinia* and *Pseudomonas* species, can grow at 1 to 6°C. Platelet concentrates, which are stored at room temperature, are more likely to be contaminated with skin contaminants such as gram-positive organisms, including coagulase-negative staphylococci.

Recipients of transfusions contaminated with bacteria may develop fever and chills, which can progress to septic shock and DIC. These reactions may occur abruptly, within minutes of initiating the transfusion, or after several hours. Characteristically the onset of symptoms and signs is sudden and fulminant, which will aid in differentiating bacterial contamination from a FNHTR. The reactions, particularly those related to gram-negative contaminants, are the result of infused endotoxins formed within the contaminated stored component.

When contaminated transfusions are suspected (i.e., when there is sudden development of shock), the transfusion must be stopped immediately. Therapy is directed at supporting the recipient's blood pressure, cardiac output, oxygenation, and renal function. The laboratory investigation should include cultures of any untransfused component, along with the routine blood bank clerical checks and serologic studies. Broad-spectrum antibiotic coverage should be started immediately and may be adjusted after the culture and sensitivity reports are available.

Parasites   Various parasites including those causing malaria, babesiosis, and Chagas' disease have been or potentially can be transmitted by blood transfusion. Geographical migration and travel of donors can shift the incidence of these rare infections. Because these infections can prove fatal, they should be considered in the transfused patient in the appropriate clinical setting.

ALTERNATIVES TO TRANSFUSION

There is much interest in finding alternatives to allogeneic blood transfusions and thereby avoiding homologous donor exposures with attendant immunologic and infectious risks. When transfusion support is required, autologous blood is the best available option. However, the benefit-to-cost ratio of autologous transfusion has been challenged. No transfusion is a zero-risk event, and even with autologous transfusions clerical errors and bacterial contamination remain potential complications. Additional methods of autologous transfusion in the surgical patient include preoperative hemodilution, recovery of shed blood from sterile surgical sites, and postoperative drainage collection. Directed or designated donation, from friends and family of the potential recipient, has not proven to reduce the risk of transfusion-related infection below that of volunteer donor component transfusions. Such directed donations may in fact place the recipient at higher risk for complications, such as GVHD and alloimmunization.

Oxygen-carrying blood substitutes, such as perfluorocarbons and aggregated hemoglobin solution, are presently in various stages of clinical trials. Granulocyte- and granulocyte-macrophage colony stimulating factor (G- or GM-CSF) are clinically useful to hasten leukocyte recovery in patients with leukopenia related to high-dose chemotherapy. Erythropoietin stimulates erythrocyte production in patients with anemia of chronic renal failure and other conditions, thus avoiding or reducing the need for transfusion. This hormone can also stimulate erythropoiesis in the autologous donor to enable additional donation.

Thrombopoietin, the hormonal stimulus for megakaryocyte proliferation and maturation, is anticipated to play a similar role in stimulating thrombopoiesis in thrombocytopenic patients, thereby avoiding homologous platelet transfusion.

Finally, synthetic products, such as DDAVP (a vasopressin analogue) and recombinant factor VIII, provide therapeutic options that also avoid homologous donor exposure for patients with coagulopathies.

BIBLIOGRAPHY

AGRE P, CARTRON JP: Molecular biology of the Rh antigens. Blood 78:551, 1991

ANDERSON KC, NESS PM (eds): *Scientific Basis of Transfusion Medicine, Implications for Clinical Practice.* Philadelphia, Saunders, 1994

DZIECZKOWSKI JS et al: Characterization of reactions after exclusive transfusion of white cell–reduced cellular blood components. Transfusion 35:20, 1995

ETCHSON J et al: The cost effectiveness of preoperative autologous blood donations. N Engl J Med 332:719, 1995

KAUSHANSKY K: Thrombopoietin: The primary regulator of platelet production. Blood 86:419, 1995

PISCIOTTO PT et al: Prophylactic versus therapeutic platelet transfusion practices in hematology and/or oncology patients. Transfusion 35:498, 1995

SCHREIBER GB et al: The risk of transfusion-transmitted viral infections. N Engl J Med 334:1685, 1996

SHULMAN IA: Parasitic infections and their impact on blood donor selection and testing. Arch Pathol Lab Med 118:366, 1994

WALKER RR et al: *The Technical Manual,* 11th ed. Arlington, VA, American Association of Blood Banks, 1993

YAMAMOTO F et al: Molecular genetic basis of the histo-blood group ABO system. Nature 345:229, 1990

116 *James O. Armitage*

BONE MARROW TRANSPLANTATION

Hematopoietic stem cell transplantation is usually carried out for one of two reasons: (1) to replace an abnormal but not malignant marrow that has been purposefully destroyed with either radiation or chemotherapy, or (2) to allow for the administration of higher than usual doses of myelotoxic chemotherapy and/or radiation therapy to treat a malignancy. The types of bone marrow abnormalities treated with this procedure include both congenital and acquired diseases; the malignancies treated with hematopoietic support include acute leukemias and lymphomas, as well as solid tumors that appear to have a dose-response curve to chemotherapy (Table 116-1). The source of hematopoietic stem cells may be the bone marrow, peripheral blood, cord blood, or fetal liver of another individual, generally one who is immunologically matched at the major histocompatibility complex (see Chap. 306). Cord blood is usually available in too small a volume to reconstitute an adult; thus, cord blood transplants are performed nearly exclusively in children. Fetal liver between 10 and 14 weeks of gestation is a rich source of hematopoietic stem cells, but such transplants are rare because of the scarcity of material. When another individual is the stem cell donor, the transplantation is termed *allogeneic*. Autologous bone marrow and peripheral blood may also be stored before marrow ablation for reinfusion after myeloablative therapy. Such transplants are termed *autologous*. In the special case where the donor is an identical twin, i.e., genetically identical to the recipient, the transplantation is termed *syngeneic*. In all these types of transplants, hematopoietic stem cells are infused into a peripheral vein of the recipient and the stem cells home to the marrow to reestablish hematopoiesis.

The beginning of modern bone marrow transplantation can be traced to animal experiments in which mice were saved from a lethal dose of whole-body irradiation by shielding of the spleen. It was subsequently shown that intravenous infusion of bone marrow could also rescue such lethally irradiated animals. Allogeneic bone marrow transplantation was first performed successfully in the late 1960s and was gradually accepted as a legitimate therapy in the 1970s. Autologous bone marrow transplantation was first successfully employed to cure patients with lymphoma in the late 1970s, and its use became widespread in the 1980s. The annual number of autologous transplants now surpasses that of allogeneic transplants.

ALLOGENEIC AND SYNGENEIC BONE MARROW TRANSPLANTATION

Allogeneic bone marrow transplantation is usually restricted to persons less than 60 years of age. The results tend to be poorer in older patients because of increased complications associated with graft-versus-host disease (GVHD) in this population. However, the patient's general health is also very important, and many transplantation groups make decisions about intervening on the basis of the patient's physiologic rather than chronologic age.

For patients without a twin, an HLA-matched sibling donor is the best choice for an allogeneic bone marrow transplantation. The genes for the HLA antigens are found on chromosome 6. One would expect that the HLA type would follow the rules of mendelian genetics, namely, that any two siblings would have one chance in four of sharing the same HLA type. Except for an approximate 1 percent chance of crossover (a switch in genetic material between chromosomes during meiosis), this is in fact the case, forming the basis for HLA family

Table 116-1

Diseases Treated with Hematopoietic Stem Cell Transplantation

	Allogeneic	Autologous
MALIGNANCIES		
Acute leukemia (lymphoblastic or myelogenous)	+	+
Chronic myelogenous leukemia	+	+
Myelodysplastic syndrome	+	−
Lymphoma	+	+
Hodgkin's disease	+	+
Multiple myeloma	+	+
Chronic lymphocytic leukemia	+	+
Myelofibrosis	+	−
Breast cancer	−	+
Testicular cancer	−	+
Ovarian cancer	−	+
Neuroblastoma	+	+
Peripheral neuroepithelial tumors	−	+
Wilms's tumor	−	+
Ewing's sarcoma	−	+
NONMALIGNANT CONDITIONS		
Aplastic anemia	+	−
Pure red cell aplasia	+	−
Paroxysmal nocturnal hemoglobinuria	+	−
Fanconi's anemia	+	−
Sickle cell anemia	+	−
Thalassemia	+	−
Severe combined immunodeficiency	+	−
Leukocyte adhesion defects	+	−
Glanzmann's thrombasthenia	+	−
Gaucher's disease	+	−
Chronic granulomatous disease	+	−
Chédiak-Higashi syndrome	+	−
Hurler's syndrome	+	−
Hunter's syndrome	+	−
Metachromatic leukodystrophy	+	−
Adrenoleukodystrophy	+	−
Lesch-Nyhan syndrome	+	−
Type IIa glycogen storage disease	+	−
Osteopetrosis	+	−
Radiation accidents	+	−
Others	+	−

typing. Because of the relatively small size of American families, only about 30 percent of Americans have an HLA-identical sibling. The formula for calculating the chance that a particular person has an HLA-matched sibling is $1 - (0.75)^n$, where n denotes the number of potential sibling donors.

For patients who may benefit from an allogeneic bone marrow transplant but lack an HLA-matched sibling donor, there are two possible solutions. One is to identify an unrelated but closely HLA-matched person willing to donate marrow or peripheral blood, and the other is to use marrow from a related donor who is less than perfectly matched. The extremely large number of possible HLA phenotypes (the number of theoretical possibilities is larger than the total world population) makes the search for an unrelated donor a difficult undertaking. Fortunately, in patients with a similar genetic background, certain HLA phenotypes occur more frequently than might be expected based upon random population genetics.

For example, for a person of European ancestry, it has been estimated that a registry of 200,000 potential donors also of European ancestry would provide a 40 to 50 percent chance of containing an HLA-matched donor. The National Marrow Donor Program has been developed to facilitate the search for unrelated donors in the United States. Because of the imprecision of traditional serologic studies, HLA typing at the molecular level has been widely adopted as a technique for identifying HLA-matched unrelated donors.

Bone marrow transplantation using unrelated donors has become a widely applied therapy. While the results remain somewhat inferior to those seen when using an HLA-matched sibling donor, treatment outcomes with this approach have been improving as the techniques to manage GVHD and graft rejection have been refined (see below).

An alternative approach is to identify a related individual who shares most, but not all, of the patient's HLA antigens. Successful allogeneic transplantation can be performed using marrow from such donors, but the risk of graft rejection and GVHD increases with the level of mismatch. Long-term survival for recipients of marrow with one antigen mismatched is about the same as that for recipients of HLA-identical marrow. There is a somewhat higher rate of death from GVHD, but there is a somewhat lower rate of death from tumor relapse because the mismatched marrow exerts a greater graft-versus-tumor effect. However, with more than one gene mismatched, more serious complications are encountered; results deteriorate substantially with two or three antigen mismatched marrow.

Once a donor has been identified, the actual transplantation procedure begins. It consists of three phases: preparation for transplant, transplant, and management after transplant.

PREPARATION FOR TRANSPLANT High doses of chemotherapy with or without radiation therapy are delivered to the recipient with two main goals: destruction of the residual malignant or dysfunctional cells and destruction of the immune system of sufficient degree to avoid rejection of the allograft by residual, immunoglogically active cells in the host. In some cases, this therapy also serves to create space in the marrow for the new cells to engraft, but this is debated.

The choice of drugs for the preparative regimen is somewhat limited because higher doses of myelotoxic drugs often cause other serious organ toxicities. For example, doses of doxorubicin cannot be significantly increased because of cardiac toxicity. Most preparative regimens include alkylating agents such as cyclophosphamide, ifosfamide, busulfan, or melphalan; topoisomerase II inhibitors such as etoposide; antimetabolites such as cytarabine; and nitrosoureas such as carmustine. Even high doses of combinations of these agents may not be myeloablative. When allogeneic transplants are performed using T cell–depleted donor marrow to lower the risk of GVHD (Table 116-2), engraftment is not as efficient. Many such patients develop so-called mixed chimerism in which cells of both donor and host origin are present, indicating survival of host hematopoietic cells. No single preparative regimen has been proven superior to others.

THE TRANSPLANTATION PROCEDURE Collection of bone marrow from a donor is referred to as *harvesting*. Marrow is usually harvested by repeated aspiration from the posterior iliac crest until an adequate number of cells has been removed. If a sufficient

Table 116-2

Prevention of Acute Graft-versus-Host Disease

Histocompatibility matching of donor and recipient
Sterile environment
In vivo prophylaxis
    Cyclosporine ± methotrexate ± prednisone
    Antithymocyte globulin
    FK-506
In vitro marrow T cell depletion
    Antibodies ± complement
    Immunotoxins
    E-rosette depletion
    Lectin treatment
    Immunoadsorbent column separation
    Elutriation

number of cells cannot be obtained from the posterior iliac crest, marrow can also be harvested from the anterior iliac crest and sternum. If peripheral blood stem cells are being harvested, the donor may receive a colony stimulating factor (CSF) to augment the number of circulating stem cells and then will undergo repetitive apheresis procedures lasting several hours on consecutive days. The risk to the donor is very slight and predominantly associated with the risk of the anesthesia used. The procedure is usually accomplished on an outpatient basis, and donors usually return promptly to their usual activities, requiring only oral analgesia.

The smallest number of nucleated marrow cells required for long-term hematopoietic repopulation in humans is not precisely known. Operationally, the number of marrow cells harvested is usually 1 to 3×10^8 per kilogram of recipient body weight. 10^8 marrow cells usually contain 1 to 3×10^6 CD34+ stem cells. When peripheral blood cells are used, 5 to 8×10^8 cells/kg are infused, which corresponds to 1 to 3×10^6 CD34+ cells/kg. For a number of conditions, it appears that the more marrow cells given, the better the outcome. In nonmalignant hematologic disorders, a larger number of donor cells may be compensating for the use of a somewhat less intensive preparative regimen. A larger number of donor cells is also required when the donor marrow is depleted of T cells or when the donor and host are HLA-mismatched.

Marrow is sometimes treated in vitro to remove unwanted cells before being administered to the patient. When the donor and patient have a major ABO red cell incompatibility, it is necessary to remove the mature erythrocytes from the graft to avoid a hemolytic transfusion reaction. Alternatively, one may avoid a hemolytic transfusion reaction by performing a plasma exchange and removing anti-A or anti-B antibodies from the recipient's circulation. While this may seem more drastic than depleting red cells from the donor marrow, all manipulations of the marrow result in a loss of stem cells. In settings where the number of marrow cells is low and may be limiting, the plasma exchange approach is sometimes taken. The removal of T cells from an allograft can reduce the incidence and severity of GVHD, but this has never been shown to translate into better long-term survival, probably because T cell depletion also increases the risk of graft rejection and tumor relapse.

MANAGEMENT AFTER TRANSPLANT All patients undergoing bone marrow transplantation require intense supportive care between the time that the hematopoietic progenitor cells are infused and when they are able to produce adequate numbers of granulocytes, platelets, and erythrocytes. Early after the transplant, therapy is focused on prophylaxis against infection, bleeding, and GVHD. Acute GVHD prophylaxis measures are shown in Table 116-2. Beyond careful HLA matching, some combination of methotrexate, cyclosporine, and prednisone appears to be the most effective prophylactic drug regimen. In addition, supportive care usually includes blood components as needed to keep the platelet count above 20,000/µL and the hemoglobin above 80 g/L (8 g/dL), protective isolation, and broad-spectrum antibiotics (see Table 116-3). Blood components should be irradiated to avoid inducing GVHD mediated by lymphocytes from an HLA-incompatible donor. The average time to recovery of granulocyte counts greater than 500/μL is 10 to 20 days. Platelets are usually the slowest to recover. Platelet recovery is measured as time to independence from platelet transfusions, but a normal platelet count may not be achieved until day 100 or later. In some centers, patients routinely receive parenteral hyperalimentation and almost all patients receive CSFs. Despite intensive efforts to prevent complications, patients undergoing transplantation may develop serious medical problems (see Table 116-4 and Fig. 116-1).

Acute Graft-versus-Host Disease Even when the donor and host are completely matched at the HLA loci, there are usually differences between the donor and the host at minor histocompatibility loci. The infusion of functional lymphocytes from the donor into the host, whose cells express antigens perceived as foreign by the donor lymphocytes, results in the stimulation of an immune response in which donor CD4 + and CD8 + T cells and natural killer cells participate. The activated T cells and natural killer cells produce cytokines such as interferon γ and tumor necrosis factor α that are thought to mediate the tissue destruction associated with acute GVHD. The disease is manifested by a skin rash, liver function test abnormalities, and diarrhea. Histologically, the skin disease is a lichenoid reaction, the liver shows bile duct inflammation, and the gastrointestinal tract shows inflammation of crypts and mucosal inflammation and sloughing. The onset of the disease is usually within the first 2 months post transplant. The severity of the disease is graded based upon the organ dysfunction. It is not clear why some organs are spared damage in this systemic immune response. In addition to the damage to the affected end organs, florid acute GVHD is associated with immunosuppression and susceptibility to infection.

This complication is more frequent and more rapid in onset when the donor and host are mismatched at two or more HLA loci. With appropriate prophylaxis, GVHD of grades II to IV occurs in fewer than 40 percent of patients. The frequency is increased when marrow from an alloimmunized female (e.g., a woman who has given birth) is given to a male recipient. In addition, those receiving transplants from donors with cytotoxic T cell precursors that respond to recipient type cells are at greater risk. When acute GVHD develops, it is usually treated with high doses of methylprednisolone. Antibodies to T cells may be a useful second-line treatment. Experimental agents aimed at counteracting the cytokine effects (such as pentoxyfylline and thalidomide) have not yet been proven useful.

Paradoxically, despite our efforts to prevent acute GVHD, it appears that some low-grade disease may actually be beneficial through the mediation of a graft-versus-tumor effect. Reduction in the incidence and grade of GVHD is associated with higher rates of tumor relapse.

Chronic GVHD Although chronic GVHD may occasionally develop in the absence of acute GVHD, it is clear that the diseases are largely related. Chronic GVHD usually develops more than 3 months after transplant. It is characterized by skin rash, sclerodermatitis, alopecia, hepatic dysfunction, oral lichenoid lesions, and a sicca complex (dry eyes and mouth) and may involve obliterative bronchiolitis and gastrointestinal motility disorders. The disease is mediated by donor T cells, most of which are recognizing minor histocompatibility complex differences in the host. In addition, there may be autoreactive donor T cells that recognize a self-antigen shared by the donor and host, especially when there is tissue damage. The activated T cells produce a variety of cytokines, including interleukin (IL) 4, which has been suggested as a primary mediator of the disease. Apparently newly developed T cells in the adoptive host do not undergo normal negative selection to delete autoreactive cells and induce self-tolerance. Patients who had grade II or greater acute GVHD and those who are older are at increased risk. For the majority of patients, the disease is self-limited. Treatment is with immunosuppressive agents. By 3 years after transplant, very few patients have persistent chronic GVHD and can be tapered off their chronic immunosupression. The basis for this late development of self-tolerance is not understood. The greatest threat to life from chronic GVHD is opportunistic infection related both to the underlying autoimmune disease and its treatment. Patients produce few antibodies to carbohydrates and are susceptible to bacterial infections. Prophylactic cotrimoxazole and intravenous immunoglobulin may reduce serious infectious sequelae. Thrombocytopenia and hyperbilirubinemia are adverse prognostic factors.

Infections Infections that complicate allogeneic bone marrow transplantation are discussed in Chap. 136.

Delayed Immune Recovery After bone marrow transplantation, donor stem cells attempt to recapitulate the ontogeny of the immune

Table 116-4

Complications of Allogeneic Bone Marrow Transplantation

EARLY COMPLICATIONS

Regimen-related toxicity	Venoocclusive disease of the liver
Cystitis	Idiopathic pneumonia syndrome
Mucositis	Graft failure
Pulmonary complications	Infection
Renal toxicity	Immunodeficiency
Neurologic toxicity	Acute graft-vs.-host disease
	Bleeding

LATE COMPLICATIONS

Regimen-related toxicity	Immunodeficiency
Cataracts	Infection
Neurologic toxicity	Chronic graft-vs.-host disease
Gonadal toxicity	Relapse of primary tumor
Endocrine toxicity	Second malignancy
Abnormal growth and development	

Table 116-3

Antimicrobial Prophylaxis in Allogeneic Marrow Transplantation

Pathogen	Prophylaxis	Timing
Bacteria	Variable	By onset of neutropenia until engraftment
Fungi	Fluconazole, 100 mg PO qd	Day −7 to engraftment
Pneumocystis carinii	Bactrim-DS, 2 PO twice weekly	Engraftment to day 180*
Viruses		
Herpes simplex	Acyclovir, 250 mg/m² IV q 8 h	Day −1 to engraftment
Cytomegalovirus†	Ganciclovir, 5 mg/kg twice weekly	Engraftment to day 100

* Or until immunosuppressive therapy is stopped.
† In seropositive patients or recipients of seropositive marrow; it is best to use seronegative blood products in seronegative patients or to filter white cells from seropositive donors.

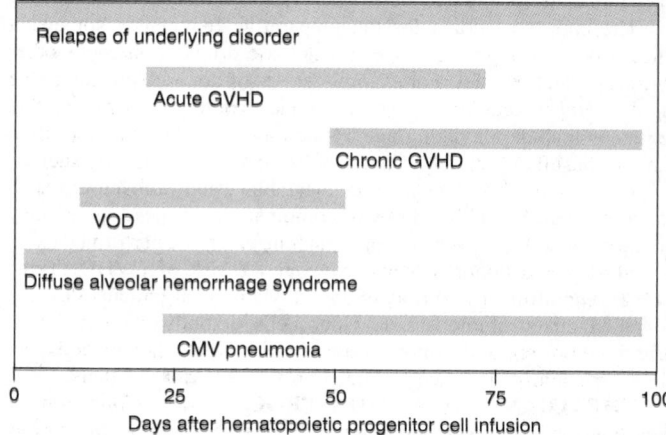

FIGURE 116-1 Timing of major complications of bone marrow transplantation.

system. However, in adults, thymic involution often leads to inadequate generation of new T cells. The T cell function of the transplant recipient is dependent upon peripheral expansion of the relatively few T cells transferred with the marrow graft. T cell recovery after transplantation may take 18 months or more. The initial T cells detected in the peripheral blood are not fully functional, often failing to produce IL-2 upon stimulation. With time, normal T cell responses may develop; however, the use of live viral vaccines is to be avoided.

Regimen-Related Toxicities The toxicities associated with chemotherapy and radiation therapy are discussed in Chap. 86.

Graft Rejection Rejection of a bone marrow graft in most cases represents destruction of the graft by functional host lymphocytes that survived the preparative regimen. This complication is most frequent in patients with aplastic anemia who do not receive total-body radiation therapy. Predisposing factors include previous blood transfusions (which sensitize the host), less intensive preparative regimens (which fail to kill host lymphocytes), and the removal of T cells from the allograft (donor T cells produce CSFs and may interfere with host cell rejection). Graft rejection is less likely to occur when patients undergo transplantation before any blood products are transfused, but this is often not practical. Infusion of buffy coat preparations from the donor in the days following the transplant reduces the frequency of graft rejection but increases the frequency of severe acute GVHD. The primary approach to the prevention of graft rejection is the use of more immunosuppressive preparative regimens. CSFs are not useful in preventing graft rejection.

Tumor Recurrence In general, tumor recurrence is an authentic recurrence of malignant cells of host origin. Although several approaches to this problem may be taken, the infusion of large numbers of donor T cells, obtained by leukapheresis or aspiration of buffy coat of donor blood, often induces complete remission in relapsed leukemia, particularly chronic granulocytic leukemia. Such donor T cells may also worsen GVHD. Experimental efforts to further improve the efficacy of donor T cells include the administration of IL-2 after transplant and immunizing the donor against the tumor before the transplant.

Pulmonary Complications After transplantation, between 5 percent and 10 percent of patients develop a nonbacterial, nonfungal interstitial pneumonitis characterized by fever, interstitial infiltrates, hypoxia, and the adult respiratory distress syndrome. Cytomegalovirus (CMV) is the most common pathogen, and the pneumonitis occurs more commonly in the setting of GVHD in the second month or later after transplantation. In CMV-seropositive patients, the prophylactic use of ganciclovir can reduce the risk of developing CMV pneumonia. In CMV-seronegative patients, scrupulous use of blood products only from CMV-seronegative donors will minimize the risk. If only CMV-seropositive donor blood is available, leukocyte filters to remove donor leukocytes will usually prevent transmission. Some cases may be caused by the human herpesvirus 6. When this syndrome occurs early (within the first 2 weeks) and an infectious etiology is not defined, the idiopathic pneumonia syndrome may be related to the use of pulmonary toxins in the preparative regimen. It has a mortality rate of 50 percent or greater. Pathologically, the lesion is diffuse alveolar hemorrhage. Frequently beneficial results may be obtained with high-dose glucocorticoids.

Venoocclusive Disease of the Liver Up to 50 percent of patients undergoing transplantation may develop two of the three primary symptoms of hepatic venoocclusive disease (jaundice, tender hepatomegaly, and ascites or unexplained weight gain) within the first few weeks following transplant. The disease is caused by damage to the hepatocytes, endothelial cells, and sinusoids surrounding the central vein of the liver mediated by radiation or chemotherapy. About 70 percent of patients recover, but the disease can be fatal, especially in patients who develop the hemolytic-uremic syndrome. Thrombolytic therapy with tissue plasminogen activator appears to reduce the fatality rate of established disease. Criteria for intervening are not yet clear.

Psychosocial Complications The great majority of patients who survive bone marrow transplantation, who do not develop significant chronic GVHD and do not experience disease recurrence return to full activity and resume a normal life. Full recovery may take more than 1 year. The most common persisting abnormalities are infertility and sexual dysfunction.

AUTOLOGOUS BONE MARROW TRANSPLANTATION

Autologous bone marrow transplantation involves the use of the patient's own hematopoietic progenitor cells to reestablish hematopoietic cell function after the administration of high-dose chemotherapy and/or radiation therapy. The reinfused hematopoetic progenitors may come from the patient's bone marrow or peripheral blood. When the latter source is used, the procedure is called peripheral blood stem cell transplantation. Generally, before peripheral stem cell harvest, the stem cell content of the blood is augmented by treating the patient with chemotherapy and CSFs, especially granulocyte CSF, a manipulation that results in marrow stem cells being released into the peripheral blood.

Autologous bone marrow transplantation differs from allogeneic transplantation in several ways. Although many of the complications are similar to those encountered in allogeneic transplants, usually the incidence is lower and there are no complications related to GVHD. The early clinical problems arise mainly from regimen-related toxicity. Interstitial pneumonitis may occur in 10 to 15 percent of patients but is more likely to be idiopathic than CMV-related. In addition, hematopoietic reconstitution is often more rapid than in allogeneic transplants (granulocyte recovery in 8 to 14 days, platelet recovery in 14 to 21 days). CSFs are essentially always used in autologous transplants. Because of this more favorable toxicity profile, autologous transplantation may be employed safely in older patients.

Increasingly, autologous stem cell transplantation is being performed on an outpatient basis. Patients are treated with prophylactic antibiotics and see the physician in clinic daily. The development of neutropenic fever or overt infection is the stimulus to admission.

A concern related specifically to autologous transplantation is the possible presence of contaminating tumor cells in the graft. A number of approaches have been employed to rid the graft of tumor cells, including purging tumor cells with antibody plus complement, an immunotoxin, and incubating the marrow with chemotherapeutic agents. In addition, positive selection methods have been employed to enrich for CD34+ stem cells. It has also been observed that the act of freezing the marrow and thawing it for delivery to the patient may preferentially kill tumor cells. Despite all this concern, there is little evidence that purging techniques influence disease-free survival. When relapses occur, they are generally at previous sites of disease rather than widely disseminated, as might be expected by hematogenous distribution. Nevertheless, three pieces of data support the concern that the graft may be a source of tumor. Retrospective analysis has suggested that purging leads to a reduced rate of relapse in patients with acute myeloid leukemia or malignant lymphoma. When tumor cells can be cultured from histologically negative marrow in patients with lymphoma, leukemia, or breast cancer, those patients have a higher rate of relapse than those with negative cultures. Finally, early attempts to introduce genetic markers into stem cells (contaminated with tumor cells) in vitro and trace their fate in vivo have suggested that some patients relapse with cells from the graft. However, purging techniques are not generally employed.

DISEASES TREATED BY BONE MARROW TRANSPLANTATION

Interpretation of the results of trials of bone marrow transplantation is always complicated by the problem of patient selection. The efficacy of transplantation can be underestimated if only patients with the worst prognosis are studied and overestimated if only those with the best prognosis are studied. Randomized trials, which might help resolve problems in interpretation, have been very difficult to conduct. Even with imperfect data, however, it is necessary to make the best possible recommendations to patients.

NONMALIGNANT DISEASES Aplastic Anemia, Thalassemia, and Sickle Cell Anemia Allogeneic bone marrow transplantation leads to disease-free survival in up to 85 to 90 percent of patients with severe aplastic anemia. As compared with immunosuppression induced by antithymocyte globulin with or without cyclosporine, allogeneic transplantation is more likely to produce a complete hematologic remission. However, many centers recommend a trial of immunosuppressive therapy before proceeding to bone marrow transplantation in older patients (i.e., 40 to 55 years of age) and in patients with only moderately severe disease. Allogeneic bone marrow transplantation is effective in the treatment of all forms of aplastic anemia, including that following paroxysmal nocturnal hemoglobinuria. However, Fanconi's anemia poses special problems, and patients with this disorder require modified preparative regimens because of an increase in the toxic effects of treatment to liver and lungs.

The effectiveness of allogeneic bone marrow transplantation in patients with thalassemia was demonstrated more than a decade ago. Busulfan and cyclophosphamide are most often used as a preparative regimen, rather than total-body radiotherapy and cyclophosphamide, in an attempt to avoid long-term complications. Treatment-related deaths are unusual when transplantation is performed before severe complications related to iron overload develop. Disease-free survival is approximately 75 percent. Adverse prognostic factors include hepatomegaly and portal fibrosis—complications presumably related to previous transfusions.

Sickle cell anemia is another serious hematologic disorder that is potentially curable with allogeneic bone marrow transplantation. Available reports suggest that allogeneic transplantation can establish normal hematopoiesis and alleviate the symptoms of the disorder; it is especially useful in patients with frequent crises who do not respond to hydroxyurea.

Immunodeficiency Disorders Allogeneic bone marrow transplantation was first successfully utilized in treating children with life-threatening immunodeficiency disorders. The procedure can replace defective stem cells with normal cells in patients with severe combined immunodeficiency, Wiskott-Aldrich syndrome, and Chédiak-Higashi syndrome. When an HLA-identical sibling is available as a donor for a child recognized to have any of these lethal disorders, allogeneic bone marrow transplantation is the treatment of choice. Unfortunately, such donors are often not available, but transplants are often attempted with less than perfectly matched family donors.

Other Genetic Disorders In principle, allogeneic bone marrow transplantation should be a successful therapy for any genetic disorder involving the immunologic or hematopoietic system. Examples of its application include the reversal of infantile malignant osteopetrosis, Gaucher's disease, infantile metachromatic leukodystrophy, and X-linked adrenoleukodystrophy. One lesson learned from the experience with these disorders is that damage to the extramedullary organs, once inflicted, sometimes cannot be reversed by replacing hematopoietic stem cells, and transplantation may therefore have to be performed very early in the course of the disease.

MALIGNANT DISEASES Well over 90 percent of all bone marrow transplants are performed for the treatment of malignant disease. Table 116-1 identifies those disorders in which bone marrow transplantation has been shown to be curative or to prolong survival.

Leukemia Acute myeloid leukemia was one of the first disorders to be shown to be curable with allogeneic bone marrow transplantation. In patients with end-stage, refractory leukemia, cure rates of approximately 10 percent are possible. When patients are treated in second or subsequent remission, 20 to 40 percent cure rates are achievable, and patients transplanted in their first complete remission can be cured 40 to 70 percent of the time. However, because some patients can be cured with standard chemotherapy regimens alone, the relative advantages of transplanting all patients who have matched donors and

are in first complete remission versus only transplanting those patients who eventually relapse are still debated. Autologous bone marrow transplantation has also been used in patients with acute myeloid leukemia but has been associated with a higher relapse rate and, in most series, a lower cure rate.

Myelodysplastic syndrome frequently develops into acute myeloid leukemia. This disorder is more common in elderly patients but is occasionally seen in younger adults. When an HLA-identical sibling donor is available, allogeneic bone marrow transplantation offers a potentially curative therapy.

Acute lymphoblastic leukemia can also be cured with allogeneic bone marrow transplantation. Results of standard intensive chemotherapy in children with this disorder are sufficiently good so that bone marrow transplantation should be reserved only for those with very high risk cytogenetic abnormalities—for example, Philadelphia chromosome–positive acute lymphoblastic leukemia. However, children who have early relapse after a standard chemotherapy regimen should undergo allogeneic bone marrow transplantation if they have a donor. Adults with acute lymphoblastic leukemia have poorer results with standard chemotherapy than do children. However, use of bone marrow transplantation in first complete remission has not been shown to improve treatment outcome. Autologous transplantation has been performed in acute lymphoblastic leukemia, but, as in acute myeloid leukemia, the relapse rate is higher than with allogeneic transplantation, although long-term disease-free survival can be achieved in some patients.

Chronic myelogenous leukemia is the most common indication for allogeneic bone marrow transplantation. In a patient of appropriate age who has an HLA-matched sibling donor, allogeneic bone marrow transplantation should be performed within the first year of diagnosis. If an HLA-matched sibling donor is not available, transplants using unrelated donors are frequently used, but with somewhat poorer results. Autologous transplantation has also been used in patients unable to undergo allogeneic bone marrow transplantation with some positive results.

Chronic lymphocytic leukemia rarely occurs in young patients who might be candidates for bone marrow transplantation. However, allogeneic bone marrow transplantation has been demonstrated to produce complete remissions in some patients. It will take many years to determine whether bone marrow transplantation can be curative in this type of leukemia because of the indolent natural history of the disorder.

Lymphoma and Myeloma The most common diseases treated by autologous transplantation are non-Hodgkin's lymphoma and Hodgkin's disease. Long-term disease-free survival and cure can be achieved in patients with aggressive non-Hodgkin's lymphoma and Hodgkin's disease. The chances for cure are related to the timing of the transplantation. Patients with end-stage, refractory disease are cured infrequently, while patients with chemotherapy-sensitive disease at relapse are cured 30 to 50 percent of the time. Autologous transplantation has been shown in a randomized trial to be superior to chemotherapy at standard doses for patients with relapsed aggressive non-Hodgkin's lymphoma (Fig. 116-2). Currently, studies are under way testing the utility of bone marrow transplantation as part of the primary therapy of these disorders. At the present time, transplantation is the treatment of choice for patients with aggressive non-Hodgkin's lymphoma and Hodgkin's disease who relapse after an effective chemotherapy regimen.

The use of bone marrow transplantation to treat patients with low-grade non-Hodgkin's lymphoma is a more recent development. Studies using either purged bone marrow or peripheral blood progenitor cells in patients with first relapse of low-grade follicular lymphoma has demonstrated a 40 to 50 percent disease-free survival 5 years after treatment. Because late relapses tend to occur in these disorders, a very long follow-up will be necessary to determine whether transplantation is curative.

Allogeneic bone marrow transplantation is also performed for patients with non-Hodgkin's lymphoma and Hodgkin's disease. In general, allogeneic bone marrow transplants have been selected in younger patients and those in whom blood and marrow involvement by the lymphoma make collection of uncontaminated hematopoietic progenitors difficult or impossible. Also, certain patients who have

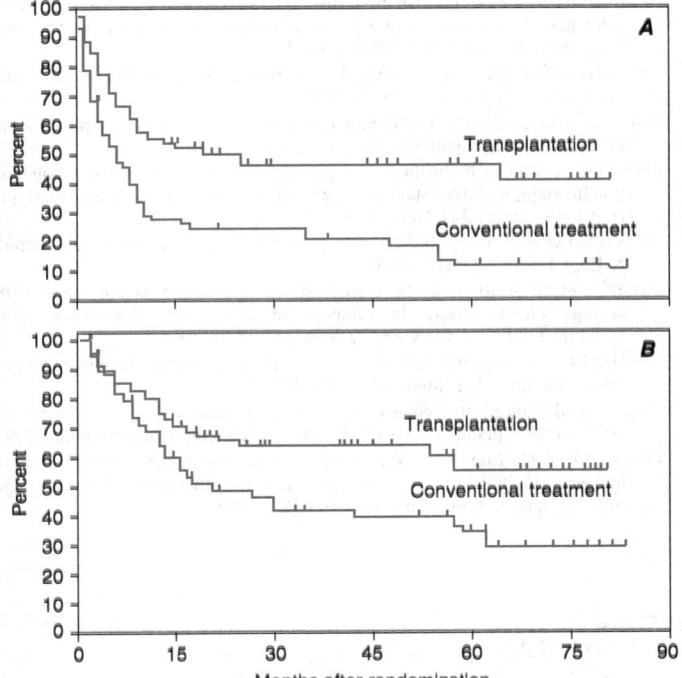

FIGURE 116-2 The curves depict the treatment outcome for patients with chemotherapy sensitive, relapsed aggressive non-Hodgkin's lymphoma randomly assigned to continue standard dose therapy or undergo autologous bone marrow transplantation. *A.* Event-free survival, $p = .001$. *B.* Overall survival, $p = .038$.

developed myelodysplasia from their initial therapy for their lymphoma are also candidates for allogeneic bone marrow transplantation.

Both allogeneic and autologous bone marrow transplantation have been performed for the treatment of multiple myeloma. Few patients with multiple myeloma are young enough to be good candidates for allogeneic bone marrow transplantation. However, for those few patients, long-term disease-free survival might be possible. Autologous bone marrow transplantation incorporated into the primary treatment of patients with multiple myeloma has been tested in a randomized trial. This study showed prolonged survival for the patients undergoing autologous transplantation as compared to further standard therapy.

Solid Tumors Breast cancer has become the individual disease most frequently treated by autologous transplantation in the United States. The use of this treatment has been controversial. At the present time, autologous bone marrow transplantation as adjuvant treatment for patients with high-risk breast cancer is undergoing randomized clinical trials measured against standard-dose therapy. One randomized trial has been completed comparing autologous bone marrow transplantation with standard-dose chemotherapy in patients with metastatic breast cancer. Although it was unclear if patients in either group were cured, the median survival was approximately doubled with autologous bone marrow transplantation.

Neuroblastoma in children has often been treated with allogeneic and autologous bone marrow transplantation. Disease-free survival rates as high as 40 percent at 2 years for patients with stage IV disease have been reported. However, the occurrence of late relapses and improved results of chemotherapy not requiring bone marrow transplantation have raised questions about the role of transplantation in the treatment of this disorder.

Autologous bone marrow transplantation has been used in patients with testicular cancer who were not able to be cured with platinum-based chemotherapy regimens. Approximately 10 to 20 percent of such patients with advanced, refractory disease can be cured when transplanted. This is similar to the outcome reported for patients with lymphoma.

Autologous bone marrow transplantation has been used to treat patients with malignant melanoma, soft tissue sarcoma, ovarian or

uterine cancer, brain tumors, small cell lung cancer, and colon cancer. For the treatment of malignant melanoma, colon cancer, and small cell lung cancer, the results of transplantation have been discouraging. For gynecologic cancers, soft tissue sarcoma, and brain tumors, however, transplantation has had more positive results, stimulating further trials.

PATIENT FOLLOW-UP AFTER BONE MARROW TRANSPLANTATION

While only a few physicians actually perform bone marrow transplantation, many physicians are involved in the care of these patients after a successful transplant. Usually the referring physician expects to accept a major part of the patient's care by 3 months after a patient has undergone bone marrow transplantation. By this time most patients will have recovered normal hematopoietic function, although a few patients will demonstrate chronic marrow injury—usually with low platelet counts. A significant proportion of patients undergoing allogeneic bone marrow transplantation will still be receiving therapy for chronic GVHD.

The most important long-term complications that need to be monitored are infection and the development of relapse of the underlying disorder. In patients treated for malignant disease, recurrence of the malignancy is the major cause of death after autologous bone marrow transplantation and an important cause of death after allogeneic bone marrow transplantation. Late infections, particularly herpes zoster, are not infrequent. Patients with chronic GVHD sometimes have functional asplenia and are at risk for overwhelming infection by encapsulated bacteria. Patients who receive radiotherapy as part of their primary treatment or as part of the transplant regimen are at risk for the development of hypothyroidism. This diagnosis can be difficult and requires an alert physician. Patients who have total-body radiotherapy as part of their preparative regimen need to be monitored for cataracts. Most patients who undergo bone marrow transplantation will be infertile. However, this is not always the case, and patients sometimes recover fertility following transplantation. Fertility is most likely to return in patients who did not have extensive alkylating agent therapy before coming to transplantation, those who did not receive total-body radiotherapy as part of their preparative regimen, and those who came to transplantation at a younger age. Women seem more likely to recover fertility than men. It is important to make patients aware of this possibility.

Patients exposed to alkylating agents, etoposide, and radiotherapy are at increased risk to develop second malignancies. Acute leukemia seems to be a risk for patients who undergo autologous transplantation for Hodgkin's disease or non-Hodgkin's lymphoma—particularly if they receive total body radiotherapy as part of their preparative regimen. All patients who have been irradiated as part of their primary treatment or as part of the bone marrow transplant preparative regimen are at risk for the development of late solid tumors. This increased risk should lead to early institution of appropriate screening maneuvers, such as regular mammography in young women who received radiotherapy to the mediastinum that included the breast. It is useful to know that Pap smears done early after bone marrow transplantation will often be abnormal because of dysplastic cells induced by the high-dose chemotherapy/radiotherapy. This should not be overinterpreted.

CONCLUSIONS

Allogeneic bone marrow transplantation is likely to remain an important treatment of leukemia, aplastic anemia, and certain genetic disorders for many years to come. Autologous bone marrow transplantation as a treatment for malignant disease might be avoided in some patients as effective new chemotherapeutic agents are developed and/

or new generations of hematopoietic growth factors become available. The most important improvement today in the use of autologous bone marrow transplantation could come from identifying those patients at high risk for treatment failure with standard therapies and the early institution of this treatment. If genetic manipulation of hematopoietic progenitor cells becomes practical, autologous bone marrow transplantation might become a common treatment for a variety of nonmalignant disorders.

BIBLIOGRAPHY

CHAO NJ et al: Cycolosporine, methotrexate and prednisone compared with cyclosporine and prednisone for prophylaxis of acute graft-vs-host disease. N Engl J Med 329:1225, 1993

CLIFT RA et al: Allogeneic marrow transplantation during untreated first relapse of acute myeloid leukemia. J Clin Oncol 10:1723, 1992

DAVIES SM et al: Unrelated donor bone marrow transplantation: Influence of HLA A and B incompatibility on outcome. Blood 86:1636, 1995

GLUCKMAN E et al: Bone marrow transplantation for severe aplastic anemia: Influence of conditioning and graft-versus-host disease prophylaxis regimens on outcome. Blood 79:269, 1992

KENNEDY MJ: High-dose chemotherapy of breast cancer: Is the question answered? J Clin Oncol 13:2477, 1995

KOLB HJ et al: Graft-versus-leukemia effect of donor lymphocyte transfusions in marrow grafted patients. Blood 86:2041, 1995

LINCH DC et al: Dose intensification with autologous bone marrow transplantation in relapsed and resistant Hodgkin's disease: Results of a BNLI randomized trial. Lancet 341:1051, 1993

LUCARELLI G et al: Bone-marrow transplantation in patients with thalassemia. N Engl J Med 322:417, 1990

PHILIP T et al: Autologous bone marrow transplantation as compared with salvage chemotherapy in relapses of chemotherapy-sensitive non-Hodgkin's lymphoma. N Engl J Med 333:1540, 1995

THOMAS ED et al: Marrow transplantation for the treatment of chronic myelogenous leukemia. Ann Intern Med 104:155, 1986

VOSE J et al: Long-term sequelae of autologous bone marrow of peripheral stem cell transplantation for lymphoid malignancies. Cancer 69:784, 1992

ZHANG M et al: Long-term follow-up of adults with acute lymphoblastic leukemia in first remission treated with chemotherapy or bone marrow transplantation. Ann Intern Med 123:428, 1995

SECTION 3

DISORDERS OF HEMOSTASIS

| 117 | *Robert I. Handin* |

DISORDERS OF THE PLATELET AND VESSEL WALL

Patients with platelet or vessel wall disorders usually bleed into superficial sites such as the skin, mucous membranes, or genitourinary or gastrointestinal tract. Bleeding begins immediately after trauma and either responds to simple measures such as pressure and packing or requires systemic therapy with glucocorticoids, plasma fractions, or platelet concentrates. The most common platelet/vessel wall disorders are (1) various forms of thrombocytopenia, (2) von Willebrand's disease (vWD), and (3) drug-induced platelet dysfunction. This chapter reviews the diagnosis and treatment of quantitative and qualitative platelet disorders as well as vessel wall defects that cause bleeding. The physiology of normal hemostasis and the cardinal manifestations of bleeding arising from hemostatic disorders have been reviewed in Chap. 60.

PLATELET DISORDERS

Platelets arise from the fragmentation of megakaryocytes, which are very large, polyploid bone marrow cells produced by the process of endomitosis. They undergo from three to five cycles of chromosomal duplication without cytoplasmic division. After leaving the marrow space, approximately one-third of the platelets are sequestered in the spleen, while the other two-thirds circulate for 7 to 10 days. Normally, only a small fraction of the platelet mass is consumed in the process of hemostasis, so most platelets circulate until they become senescent and are removed by phagocytic cells. The normal blood platelet count is maintained between 150,000 and 450,000 per microliter. A decrease in platelet mass stimulates an increase in the number, size, and ploidy of megakaryocytes, releasing additional platelets into the circulation. This process is regulated by thrombopoietin (TPO) binding to its megakaryocyte receptor, a proto-oncogene called c-mpl. TPO, also called the c-mpl ligand, is secreted continuously at a low level and binds tightly to circulating platelets. A reduction in platelet mass increases the level of free TPO and thereby stimulates megakaryocyte and platelet production. Recombinant TPO is being tested in clinical trials as a means to prevent or reduce thrombocytopenia in patients receiving cytotoxic chemotherapy.

The platelet count varies during the menstrual cycle, rising following ovulation and falling at the onset of menses. It is also influenced by the patient's nutritional state and can be decreased in severe iron, folic acid, or vitamin B_{12} deficiency. Platelets are *acute-phase reactants*, and patients with systemic inflammation, tumors, bleeding, and mild iron deficiency may have an increased platelet count, a benign condition called *secondary* or *reactive thrombocytosis*. The cytokines interleukin (IL)-3, IL-6, and IL-11 may stimulate platelet production in acute inflammation. In contrast, the increase in platelet count that is characteristic of the myeloproliferative disorders such as polycythemia vera, chronic myelogenous leukemia, myeloid metaplasia, and essential thrombocytosis can cause either severe bleeding or thrombosis. In these patients, unregulated platelet production is secondary to a clonal stem cell abnormality affecting all the bone marrow progenitors.

THROMBOCYTOPENIA Thrombocytopenia is caused by one of three mechanisms—decreased bone marrow production, increased splenic sequestration, or accelerated destruction of platelets. In order to determine the etiology of thrombocytopenia, each patient should have a careful examination of the peripheral blood film, an assessment of marrow morphology by examination of an aspirate or biopsy, and an estimate of splenic size by bedside palpation supplemented, if necessary, by ultrasonography or computed tomographic (CT) scan. Occasional patients have "pseudothrombocytopenia," a benign condition in which platelets agglutinate or adhere to leukocytes when blood is collected with EDTA as anticoagulant. This is a laboratory artifact, and the actual platelet count in vivo is normal. A scheme for classifying patients with thrombocytopenia based on these clinical observations and laboratory tests is outlined in Fig. 117-1.

Impaired Production Disorders that injure stem cells or prevent their proliferation in marrow frequently cause thrombocytopenia. They usually affect multiple hematopoietic cell lines so that thrombocytopenia is accompanied by varying degrees of anemia and leukopenia. Diagnosis of a platelet production defect is readily established by examination of a bone marrow aspirate or biopsy, which should show a reduced number of megakaryocytes. The most common causes of decreased platelet production are marrow aplasia, fibrosis, or infiltration with malignant cells, all of which produce highly characteristic marrow abnormalities. Occasionally, thrombocytopenia is the presenting laboratory abnormality in these disorders. Cytotoxic drugs, which are frequently used in cancer chemotherapy, impair megakaryocyte proliferation and maturation and frequently cause thrombocytopenia. There are also rare marrow disorders such as congenital amegakaryocytic hypoplasia and *t*hrombocytopenia with *a*bsent *r*adii (TAR syndrome), which selectively decrease megakaryocyte production.

Splenic Sequestration Since one-third of the platelet mass is normally sequestered in the spleen, splenectomy will increase the platelet count by 30 percent. Postsplenectomy thrombocytosis is a benign self-limited condition that does not require specific therapy. In contrast, when the spleen enlarges, the fraction of sequestered platelets increases, lowering the platelet count. The most common causes of splenomegaly are portal hypertension secondary to liver disease and splenic infiltration with tumor cells in myeloproliferative or lymphoproliferative disorders or with macrophages in storage disorders such as Gaucher's disease. Isolated splenomegaly is rare, and in most patients, splenomegaly is accompanied by other clinical manifestations of an underlying disease. Many patients with leukemia, lymphoma, or a myeloproliferative syndrome have both marrow infiltration and splenomegaly and develop thrombocytopenia from a combination of impaired marrow production and splenic sequestration of platelets.

Accelerated Destruction Abnormal vessels, fibrin thrombi, and intravascular prostheses can all shorten platelet survival and cause *nonimmunologic thrombocytopenia*. For example, thrombocytopenia is common in patients with vasculitis, the hemolytic uremic syndrome (HUS), thrombotic thrombocytopenic purpura (TTP), as one manifestation of disseminated intravascular coagulation (DIC), and in patients with prosthetic cardiac valves. In addition, platelets coated with antibody, immune complexes, or complement are rapidly cleared by mononuclear phagocytes in the spleen or other tissues inducing *immunologic thrombocytopenia*. The most common causes of immunologic thrombocytopenia are viral or bacterial infections, drugs, and a chronic autoimmune disorder referred to as *idiopathic thrombocytopenic purpura* (ITP). Patients with immunologic thrombocytopenia do not usually have splenomegaly and have an active bone marrow with an increased number of megakaryocytes.

DRUG-INDUCED THROMBOCYTOPENIA Many common drugs can cause thrombocytopenia (Table 117-1). As previously mentioned, many chemotherapeutic agents are cytotoxic and depress megakaryocyte production. Ingestion of large quantities of alcohol has a similar marrow-depressing effect leading to transient thrombocytopenia. The syndrome is particularly common in binge drinkers. Thiazide diuretics, which are used commonly to treat hypertension or congestive heart failure, impair megakaryocyte production and can produce mild thrombocytopenia (50,000 to 100,000/μL), which may persist for several months after the drug is discontinued.

Most drugs induce thrombocytopenia by eliciting an immune response in which the platelet is an innocent bystander. The platelet is damaged by complement activation following the formation of drug-antibody complexes. Current laboratory tests can identify the causative agent in 10 percent of patients with clinical evidence of drug-induced thrombocytopenia. The best proof of a drug-induced etiology is a prompt rise in the platelet count when the suspected drug is discontinued. Patients with drug-induced platelet destruction also may have a secondary increase in megakaryocyte number without other marrow abnormalities.

Although most patients recover within 7 to 10 days and do not require therapy, occasional patients with platelet counts below 10,000 to 20,000/μL have severe hemorrhage and may require temporary support with glucocorticoids, plasmapheresis, or platelet transfusions while waiting for the platelet count to rise. A patient who has recovered from drug-induced immunologic thrombocytopenia should be in-structed to avoid the offending drug in the future, since only minute amounts of drug are needed to set up subsequent immune reactions. Certain drugs such as phenytoin and gold salts may induce prolonged thrombocytopenia, since the drugs are cleared from body storage depots quite slowly. Heparin deserves special mention because it is a common cause of thrombocytopenia in hospitalized patients. It is estimated that 10 to 15 percent of patients receiving therapeutic doses of heparin develop thrombocytopenia and, occasionally, may have severe bleeding or intravascular platelet aggregation and paradoxical thrombosis. Heparin-induced thrombosis, sometimes called the "white clot syndrome," can be fatal unless recognized promptly. Most cases of heparin thrombocytopenia are due to drug-antibody binding to platelets, although some may be secondary to direct platelet agglutination by heparin. The offending antigen is a complex formed between heparin and the platelet-derived heparin neutralizing protein, platelet factor four. Prompt cessation of heparin will reverse both thrombocyto-

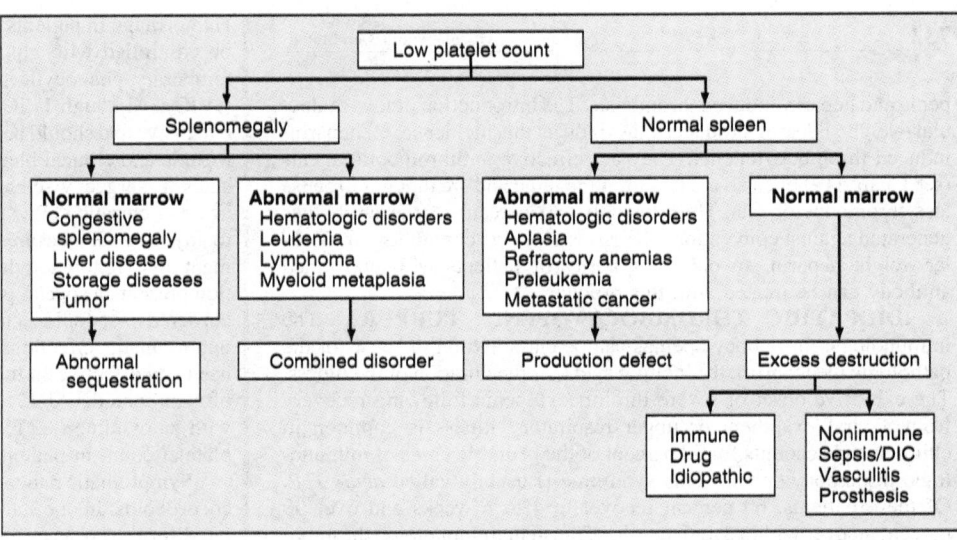

FIGURE 117-1 Clinical evaluation of patients with thrombocytopenia. [*Modified from RI Handin, in W Beck (ed), Hematology, 4th ed, Cambridge, MA, MIT Press, 1985.*]

Table 117-1

Drugs Implicated in Thrombocytopenia

SUPPRESSION OF PLATELET PRODUCTION

Myelosuppressive drugs
  Severe: cytosine arabinoside, daunorubicin
  Moderate: cyclophosphamide, busulfan, methotrexate, 6-mercaptopurine
  Mild: vinca alkaloids
Thiazide diuretics
Ethanol
Estrogens

IMMUNOLOGIC PLATELET DESTRUCTION

Clinical suspicion plus convincing experimental evidence
  Antibiotics: sulfathiazole, novobiocin, *p*-aminosalicylate
  Cinchona alkaloids: quinidine, quinine
  Foods: beans
  Sedatives, hypnotics, anticonvulsants: apronalide, carbamazepine
  Arsenical drugs used to treat syphilis
  Digitoxin
  Methyldopa
  Stibophen
Clinical suspicion (major drugs implicated)
  Aspirin
  Chlorpropamide
  Chloroquine
  Chlorothiazide and hydrochlorothiazide
  Gold salts
  Insecticides
  Sulfadiazine, sulfisoxazole, sulfamerazine, sulfamethazine, sulfamethoxypyridazine, sulfamethoxazole, sulfatolamide

penia and heparin-induced thrombosis. The introduction of low-molecular-weight heparin products may reduce the incidence of heparin-induced thrombocytopenia. They are effective antithrombotic agents (see Chap. 119) but also are less immunogenic and are thought to cause less thrombocytopenia. Unfortunately, 80 percent of the antibodies generated against conventional heparins cross-react with low-molecular-weight heparin, so only a minority of patients with preformed antibody can be treated with this product.

IDIOPATHIC THROMBOCYTOPENIC PURPURA The immunologic thrombocytopenias can be classified on the basis of the pathologic mechanism, the inciting agent, or the duration of the illness. The explosive onset of severe thrombocytopenia following recovery from a viral exanthem or upper respiratory illness is common in children and accounts for 90 percent of the pediatric cases of immunologic thrombocytopenia. This syndrome is usually called *acute ITP*. Of these patients, 60 percent recover in 4 to 6 weeks and over 90 percent recover within 3 to 6 months. Transient immunologic thrombocytopenia also complicates some cases of infectious mononucleosis, acute toxoplasmosis, or cytomegalovirus infection and can be part of the prodromal phase of viral hepatitis and infection with the human immunodeficiency virus (HIV). Acute ITP is rare in adults and accounts for fewer than 10 percent of postpubertal patients with immune thrombocytopenia. Acute ITP is caused by immune complexes containing viral antigens that bind to platelet Fc receptors or by antibodies produced against viral antigens that cross-react with the platelet. In addition to the viral disorders described above, the differential diagnosis should include atypical presentations of aplastic anemia, acute leukemias, or metastatic tumor. A bone marrow examination is essential to exclude these disorders, which can occasionally mimic acute ITP.

Most adults present with a more indolent form of thrombocytopenia that may persist for many years and is referred to as *chronic ITP*. Women aged 20 to 40 are afflicted most commonly and outnumber men by a ratio of 3:1. They may present with an abrupt fall in platelet count and bleeding similar to patients with acute ITP. More often they have a prior history of easy bruising or menometrorrhagia. These patients have an autoimmune disorder with antibodies directed against target antigens on the glycoprotein IIb-IIIa or glycoprotein Ib-IX complex (see Fig. 60-2). Although most antibodies function as opsonins and accelerate platelet clearance by phagocytic cells, occasional antibodies bind to epitopes on critical regions of these glycoproteins and impair platelet function. A number of tests have been introduced to measure platelet-associated IgG. Although the tests are quite sensitive, their specificity is a problem. First, there is a high "background" level of IgG on normal platelets. Second, an elevation in plasma immunoglobulin levels or in circulating immune complexes will nonspecifically increase platelet-associated IgG.

Since a low platelet count may be the initial manifestation of systemic lupus erythematosus (SLE) or the first sign of a primary hematologic disorder, all patients with chronic ITP should have a bone marrow examination and an antinuclear antibody determination. In addition, patients with hepatic or splenic enlargement, lymphadenopathy, or atypical lymphocytes should have serologic studies for hepatitis, cytomegalovirus, Epstein-Barr virus, toxoplasma, and HIV. HIV infection has rapidly become a common cause of immunologic thrombocytopenia and should be considered in the differential diagnosis of thrombocytopenia, especially in high-risk groups—homosexuals, hemophiliacs, intravenous drug abusers, and heterosexual individuals with multiple partners. Thrombocytopenia can be the initial symptom of HIV infection or a complication of fully developed clinical AIDS.

℞ **TREATMENT**

Treatment of patients with ITP must take into account the age of the patient, the severity of the illness, and the anticipated natural history. Although adults have a higher incidence of intracranial bleeding than children, specific therapy may not be necessary unless the platelet count is under 20,000/μL or there is extensive bleeding.

Hemorrhage in patients with either acute or chronic ITP usually can be controlled with glucocorticoids but, in rare cases, may require temporary phagocytic blockade with intravenous immunoglobulin (IVIG). Although IVIG is an effective form of therapy, it is quite expensive and should be reserved for patients with severe thrombocytopenia and clinical bleeding who have not responded to other measures. Emergency splenectomy is usually reserved for patients with acute or chronic ITP who are desperately ill and have not responded to any medical measures designed to improve hemostasis. The treatment of symptomatic thrombocytopenia in patients with HIV infection presents a special problem because the administration of glucocorticoids or splenectomy may increase susceptibility to the opportunistic infections that threaten these patients. Splenectomy has been effective in the course of HIV infection prior to the onset of symptomatic AIDS. There is increasing evidence that treatment with zidovudine (AZT) and other antiviral agents can improve the platelet count in patients with HIV-induced thrombocytopenia.

Symptomatic patients with chronic ITP are usually placed on glucocorticoids. In one standard regimen, 60 mg prednisone is administered for 4 to 6 weeks and then decreased slowly over another few weeks. Approximately 50 percent of patients with chronic ITP will normalize their platelet count on high doses of prednisone. However, the majority will have a fall in platelet count following steroid withdrawal. Patients with chronic ITP who fail to maintain a normal platelet count after a course of steroids are eligible for elective splenectomy. These steroid-responsive but steroid-dependent patients are very likely to respond to splenectomy, and 70 percent will have a normal platelet count within 1 week after surgery. Some patients who do not respond to glucocorticoids may still respond to splenectomy. Occasionally, patients may fail to respond to splenectomy because of the failure to remove an accessory spleen. In other patients, a small inactive accessory spleen may grow or new splenic foci may develop from splenic cells shed at the time of surgery and cause the late onset of thrombocytopenia. In either case, the presence of splenic tissue can be diagnosed by examination of the blood smear for Howell-Jolly bodies that appear in the red cells of asplenic individuals. Persistent splenic tissue can be confirmed by a radionuclide scan.

Patients who are still thrombocytopenic after steroid therapy or splenectomy or who relapse months to years after initial therapy have received a variety of immunosuppressive drugs including azathioprine, cyclophosphamide, vincristine, and vinblastine. Danazol has also been used with some success. Although each of these drugs may be beneficial, it is important to use some restraint because they have serious side effects. IVIG has become a popular therapy, although it is only transiently effective and quite expensive. It should be used to temporarily raise the platelet count and to support patients before surgery or labor and delivery. Anti-RhD therapy appears to be equally effective and is now available commercially as WinPro. If a patient is not bleeding and maintains a platelet count over 20,000/μL, consideration should be given to withholding therapy, since there are many patients with severe chronic thrombocytopenia who have lived with their disease for two or three decades.

FUNCTIONAL PLATELET DISORDERS As described in Chap. 60, normal hemostasis requires three critical platelet reactions—adhesion, aggregation, and granule release. Clinical bleeding can result from a failure of any of these important functions. Table 117-2 provides an outline of the major functional platelet disorders discussed below. Table 117-3 discusses the methods to assess platelet function.

Von Willebrand's Disease vWD is the most common inherited bleeding disorder, occurring in as many as 1 in 800 to 1000 individuals. The von Willebrand factor (vWF) is a heterogeneous multimeric plasma glycoprotein with two major functions. It facilitates platelet adhesion under conditions of high shear stress by linking platelet membrane receptors to vascular subendothelium; it also serves as the plasma carrier for factor VIII, the antihemophilic factor, a critical blood coagulation protein. Discrete domains in each vWF subunit mediate each of these important functions. The normal plasma vWF level is 10 mg/L. The vWF activity is distributed among a series of

Table 117-2

CHAPTER 117
Disorders of the Platelet and Vessel Wall   **733**

Classification of Functional Platelet Disorders

I. Disorders of adhesion
  A. Inherited
    1. Bernard-Soulier syndrome
    2. von Willebrand's disease (vWD)
  B. Acquired
    1. Uremia
    2. Acquired vWD
II. Disorders of aggregation
  A. Inherited
    1. Glanzmann's thrombasthenia
    2. Afibrinogenemia
  B. Acquired
    1. Fibrin degradation product inhibition
    2. Dysproteinemias
    3. Drug ingestion—e.g., ticlopidine, anti-IIb/IIIa antibodies
      (RheoPro)
III. Disorders of granule release
  A. Inherited
    1. Oculocutaneous albinism (Hermansky-Pudlak syndrome)
    2. Chédiak-Higashi syndrome
    3. Isolated dense (δ) granule deficiency
    4. Gray-platelet syndrome—combined α and δ granule deficiency
  B. Acquired
    1. Cardiopulmonary bypass
    2. Myeloproliferative disorders
    3. Drugs—aspirin and other nonsteroidal anti-inflammatory agents

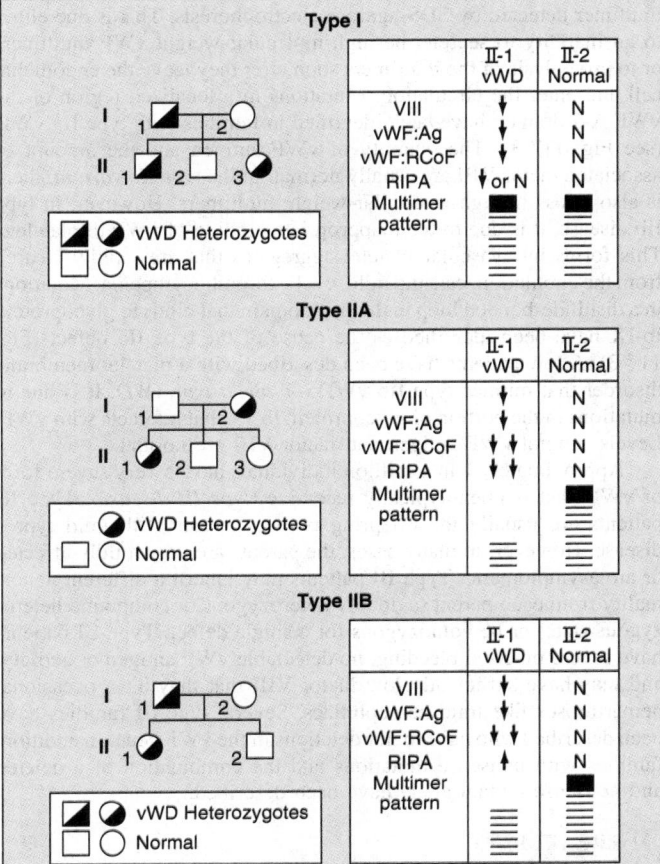

FIGURE 117-2 Pattern of inheritance and laboratory findings in von Willebrand's disease. The assays of platelet function include a coagulation assay of factor VIII bound and carried by von Willebrand factor (vWF), abbreviated as VIII; immunoassay of total vWF protein, abbreviated vWF:Ag; bioassay of the ability of patient plasma to support ristocetin-induced agglutination of normal platelets, abbreviated vWF:RCoF; and ristocetin-induced aggregation of patient platelets abbreviated RIPA. The multimer pattern illustrates the protein bonds present when plasma is electrophoresed in a polyacrylamide gel. The II-1 and II-2 columns refer to the phenotypes of the second generation offspring.

plasma multimers with estimated molecular weights ranging from 400,000 to over 20 million. A single large vWF precursor subunit is synthesized in endothelial cells and megakaryocytes, where it is cleaved and assembled into the disulfide-linked multimers present in plasma, platelets, and vascular subendothelium. A modest reduction in plasma vWF concentration or a selective loss in the high-molecular-weight multimers decreases platelet adhesion and causes clinical bleeding.

Although vWD is heterogeneous, there are certain clinical features that are common to all the syndromes. With one exception (type III disease), all forms are inherited as autosomal dominant traits, and affected patients are heterozygous with one normal and one abnormal vWF allele. In mild cases, bleeding occurs only after surgery or trauma. More severely affected patients have spontaneous epistaxis or oral mucosal, gastrointestinal, or genitourinary bleeding. The laboratory findings are variable. The most diagnostic pattern is the combination of (1) a prolonged bleeding time, (2) a reduction in plasma vWF concentration, (3) a parallel reduction in biologic activity as measured with the ristocetin cofactor assay, and (4) reduced factor VIII activity.

Table 117-3

Evaluation of Platelet Function

Bleeding time
  Modified Ivy method
  Skin incision—time to stop bleeding
  Global screen of platelet role in hemostasis
von Willebrand factor assays
  vWF Ag—immunoassay of total vWF protein
  vWF R:Cof—bioassay of vWF that measures ability of patient plasma to
    support agglutination of normal platelets in the presence of ristocetin
  Factor VIII—coagulation assay of factor VIII bound and carried by
    plasma vWF
Platelet aggregometry
  Measures platelet aggregation in response to a panel of agonists, usually
    ADP, collagen, arachidonic acid, and epinephrine
Membrane glycoproteins
  Presence of glycoproteins Ib-IX and IIb-IIIa can be measured using
    monoclonal antibodies and flow cytometry
Platelet granule content
  Dense granules—electron microscopy or uptake and retention of
    radiolabeled serotonin
  Alpha granules—electron microscopy and/or immunoassays for platelet-
    associated proteins—vWF, fibrinogen, platelet factor four

NOTE: vWF, von Willebrand factor; ADP, adenosine diphosphate; Ag, antigen; R:Cof, ristocetin cofactor.

The variability in laboratory tests is related to both the heterogeneous nature of the defects in vWD and the fact that plasma levels are influenced by ABO blood group type, central nervous system disorders, systemic inflammation, and pregnancy. Since vWD is an autosomal dominant disorder, some vWF is produced by the remaining normal allele. Thus patients with mild defects may have laboratory values that fluctuate over time and may occasionally be within the normal range.

There are three major types of vWD. Their mode of inheritance and laboratory findings are summarized in Fig. 117-2. Patients with *type I disease*, the most common abnormality, have a mild to moderate decrease in plasma vWF. In the milder cases, although hemostasis is clearly impaired, the vWF level is just below the lower limit of normal (50 percent activity, or 5 mg/L). In type I disease, there is a parallel decrease in vWF antigen, factor VIII activity, and ristocetin cofactor activity, with a normal spectrum of multimers detected by sodium dodecyl sulfate (SDS)–agarose gel electrophoresis. Cultured endothelial cells derived from the umbilical cords of patients with vWD synthesize and secrete reduced quantities of vWF multimer and have a two- to fourfold reduction in vWF mRNA.

The variant forms of vWD (*type II disease*), which are much less common, are characterized by normal or near-normal levels of a dysfunctional protein. Patients with the *type IIa variant* of vWD have a deficiency in the high- and medium-molecular-weight forms of vWF multimer detected by SDS-agarose electrophoresis. This is due either to an inability to secrete the high-molecular-weight vWF multimers or to proteolysis of the multimers soon after they leave the endothelial cell and enter the circulation. Mutations in a localized region of the vWF A-2 domain have been identified in families with type IIa vWD (see Fig. 117-3). The quantity of vWF antigen and the amount of associated factor VIII are usually normal. In the *type IIb variant*, there is also a loss in high-molecular-weight multimers. However, in type IIb disease, it is due to the inappropriate binding of vWF to platelets. This forms intravascular platelet aggregates that are rapidly cleared from the circulation, causing mild, cyclic thrombocytopenia. Mutations in a disulfide-bonded loop in the A-1 domain that binds to glycoprotein Ib-IX have been identified as the cause of the type IIb defect (Fig. 117-3). A few patients have been described with a platelet membrane disorder that mimics type IIb vWD—*platelet-type vWD*. It is due to mutations in the portion of glycoprotein Ib-IX that interacts with vWF. Levels of total vWF antigen and factor VIII are normal.

Approximately 1 in 1 million individuals have a very severe form of vWD that is phenotypically recessive (*type III disease*). Type III patients are usually the offspring of two parents with mild type I disease. However, in many cases, the parents are very mildly affected or are asymptomatic. Type III patients may inherit a different abnormality from each parent (a doubly heterozygous or compound heterozygous state) or be homozygous for a single defect. Type III patients have severe mucosal bleeding, no detectable vWF antigen or activity, and may have sufficiently low factor VIII that they have occasional hemarthroses like mild hemophiliacs. Several type III families have been described who have major deletions in the vWF gene. In addition, families with nonsense mutations and the combination of a deleted and nonsense mutant allele have been described.

℞ TREATMENT

Appropriate therapy of vWD depends on the symptoms and the underlying type of disease. There are two therapeutic options. One involves the use of cryoprecipitate, a plasma fraction enriched in vWF, or factor VIII concentrates, which retain high-molecular-weight vWF multimers (Humate-P, Koate HS). The factor VIII concentrates are highly purified and heat-treated to destroy HIV and are appropriate treatments for all the inherited forms of vWD. During surgery or after major trauma, patients should receive cryoprecipitate or factor VIII concentrate twice daily. This regimen should be continued for 48 to 72 h to ensure optimal hemostasis. Minor bleeding episodes such as prolonged epistaxis or severe menorrhagia may respond to a single infusion. Recurrent menorrhagia, a major problem for women with severe vWD, can be treated effectively with oral contraceptive agents that suppress menses.

A second therapeutic option, which avoids the use of plasma, is the use of 1-desamino-8-D-arginine vasopressin (DDAVP) or desmopressin, a vasopressin analogue that has minimal blood pressure–elevating and fluid-retaining properties and raises the plasma vWF level in both normal individuals and patients with mild vWD. Patients with type I disease are the best candidates for DDAVP therapy. However, they must be tested for an adequate response before anticipated surgery, and vWF levels must be monitored closely during therapy, since the patient may develop tachyphylaxis when therapy is continued for more than 48 h. DDAVP should not be given to patients with variant forms of vWD without prior testing, since it may not improve multimer pattern or hemostasis in type IIa patients and it may actually worsen the defect by depleting high-molecular-weight multimers, inducing intravascular platelet aggregation, and lowering the platelet count in type IIb patients. It is also ineffective therapy for patients with the severe (type III) form of vWD.

Acquired vWD   Although most cases of vWD are inherited, there are also acquired forms of vWD caused by antibodies that inhibit vWF function or by lymphoid or other tumors that selectively adsorb vWF multimers onto their surfaces. Anti-vWF antibodies have developed in patients with severe vWD following multiple transfusions, as well as in patients with autoimmune and lymphoproliferative disorders. Adsorption of vWF to tumor surfaces has been documented in patients with Waldenström's macroglobulinemia and Wilms' tumor and inferred in other patients with lymphoma. Treatment of acquired vWD should focus on controlling the underlying disease, since plasma derivatives and DDAVP are often not effective and the disorder can be fatal.

Platelet Membrane Defects   Receptors that modulate platelet adhesion and aggregation are located on the two major platelet surface glycoproteins. As previously discussed (see Chap. 60), vWF facilitates platelet adhesion by binding to glycoprotein Ib-IX, while fibrinogen links platelets into aggregates via sites on the glycoprotein IIb-IIIa complex. There are two rare but well-defined platelet defects characterized by a loss of or a defect in these glycoprotein receptors. Patients with the *Bernard-Soulier syndrome* have markedly reduced platelet adhesion and cannot bind vWF to their platelets owing to deficiency or dysfunction of the glycoprotein Ib-IX complex. They also have reduced levels of several other membrane proteins, mild thrombocytopenia, and extremely large, lymphocytoid platelets. Platelets from patients with *Glanzmann's disease* or *thrombasthenia* are deficient in or have a defect in the glycoprotein IIb-IIIa complex. Their platelets do not bind fibrinogen and cannot form aggregates, although the platelets undergo shape change and secretion and are of normal size.

Both these disorders are inherited as autosomal recessive traits and are characterized by markedly impaired hemostasis and recurrent episodes of severe mucosal hemorrhage. In keeping with the selective nature of the defects, Bernard-Soulier platelets react normally to all stimuli except ristocetin. In contrast, thrombasthenic platelets adhere normally and will agglutinate with ristocetin but will not aggregate with any of the agonists that require fibrinogen binding, such as adenosine diphosphate (ADP), thrombin, or epinephrine.

The only effective therapy for hemorrhagic episodes in these two disorders is transfusion with normal platelets. This is usually effective, although alloimmunization will eventually limit the life span of infused platelets. In addition, a few patients have developed inhibitor antibodies with specificity for the missing protein. These antibodies bind to the protein that is expressed on the transfused normal platelets and impair their function.

Platelet Release Defects   The most common mild bleeding disorders arise from the ingestion of aspirin and

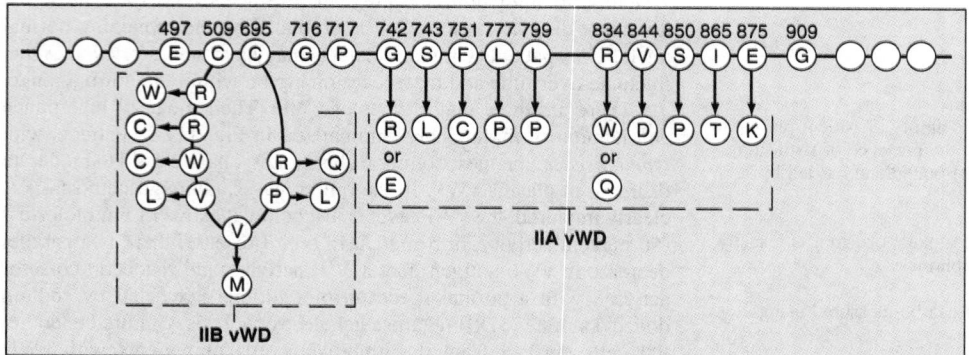

FIGURE 117-3   Location of mutations in types IIa and IIb von Willebrand's disease. Mutations in the region of the protein between amino acids 742 and 875 have been identified in patients with type IIa disease. These result in a deficiency in high- and medium-molecular-weight multimers either due to failure to secrete high-molecular-weight forms of vWF or to their proteolytic degradation in the circulation. In type IIb disease, there is also a decrease in high-molecular-weight vWF, but the defect is due to the failure of vWF with mutations in the A-1 domain of the protein (amino acids 509–695) to bind properly to platelet glycoprotein Ib-IX.

other nonsteroidal anti-inflammatory drugs (NSAIDs) that inhibit platelet production of thromboxane A_2, an important mediator of platelet secretion and aggregation (see Figs. 60-3 and 60-4). These drugs are inhibitors of the enzyme cyclooxygenase, which converts arachidonic acid to a labile endoperoxide intermediate that is critical for thromboxane formation. Aspirin is the most potent agent, since it irreversibly acetylates the platelet enzyme so that a single dose impairs hemostasis for 5 to 7 days. The other agents are competitive and reversible inhibitors with more transient effects. Blocking thromboxane A_2 synthesis partially inhibits platelet release and aggregation with weak agonists such as ADP and epinephrine and produces a mild hemostatic defect. The administration of high doses of certain antibiotics, particularly penicillin, can coat the platelet surface, block platelet release, and impair hemostasis.

Patients generally have minimal symptoms such as easy bruising, and bleeding is usually confined to the skin. Occasional patients will have prolonged oozing after surgery, particularly with procedures involving mucous membranes such as periodontal, oral, or reconstructive plastic surgery. Not surprisingly, the antiplatelet effect of drugs such as aspirin is more dramatic when they are administered to patients with underlying defects like vWD or hemophilia. Patients with drug-induced cyclooxygenase deficiency often but not always have a mildly prolonged bleeding time, and their platelets fail to aggregate when incubated with arachidonic acid, epinephrine, or low doses of ADP. Since the bleeding time is not entirely reliable, if patients have taken aspirin, they should be treated as if they have a mild hemostatic defect for the next 5 to 7 days. Platelet responses to collagen and thrombin are impaired at low doses but normal at higher doses. Symptomatic patients should be encouraged to use drugs such as acetaminophen that do not impair platelet function. Although most cases of cyclooxygenase deficiency are drug-induced, occasional patients have inherited disorders in platelet cyclooxygenase activity that impair thromboxane production or receptor level defects that prevent platelets from responding to thromboxane A_2.

Although a number of metabolic disorders can perturb hemostasis, uremic platelet dysfunction is clinically the most important. The mechanism by which uremia impairs platelet function is not well understood, and retention of phenolic and guanidinosuccinic acids, excess prostacyclin production, or impaired vWF-platelet interactions have all been implicated. There is a good correlation between the degree of uremia and bleeding symptoms and the degree of anemia and bleeding. Bleeding can usually be reversed by dialysis and often improves after red cell transfusion or treatment with erythropoietin. In addition, the administration of cryoprecipitate or DDAVP, which raise plasma vWF levels, can also improve hemostasis. Conjugated estrogens improve hemostasis and can be used as long-term therapy.

Storage Pool Defects Platelet granules have considerable amounts of adenine nucleotides, calcium, and adhesive glycoproteins such as thrombospondin, fibronectin, and vWF, all of which promote platelet adhesion and aggregation. Thus, it is not surprising that patients with defective platelet granules have a mild bleeding disorder. Platelet storage pool defects may be inherited as an isolated disorder or be part of systemic granule packaging defects such as oculocutaneous albinism or the Hermansky-Pudlak or Chédiak-Higashi syndromes. Clinically, these patients cannot be distinguished from those with other functional platelet disorders, since they all have easy bruising, mucosal bleeding, and a prolonged bleeding time. They can be differentiated from patients with the cyclooxygenase defects because their platelets will usually aggregate in response to arachidonic acid. In addition, their platelets have decreased levels of specific granule constituents such as ADP and serotonin and abnormalities in granule morphology that are best visualized by electron microscopy.

Occasionally, patients with acute or chronic leukemia or one of the myeloproliferative disorders develop an acquired storage pool disorder due to dysplastic megakaryocyte development. In addition, patients with liver disease and some patients with SLE or other immune-complex–mediated disorders may have circulating platelets that have degranulated prematurely. Platelet degranulation and a transient storage pool disorder also have been described following prolonged cardiopulmonary bypass. Fortunately, most patients with storage pool defects have only mildly impaired hemostasis. They can be treated with platelet transfusions. Occasional patients have responded to DDAVP.

VESSEL WALL DISORDERS

Bleeding from vascular disorders (nonthrombocytopenic purpura) is usually mild and confined to the skin and mucous membranes. The pathogenesis of bleeding is poorly defined in many of the syndromes, and classical tests of hemostasis, including the bleeding time and tests of platelet function, are usually normal. Vascular purpura arises from damage to capillary endothelium, abnormalities in the vascular subendothelial matrix or extravascular connective tissues that support blood vessels, or from the formation of abnormal blood vessels. There are also several idiopathic disorders that involve the vessel wall and can cause more severe bleeding and organ dysfunction.

THROMBOTIC THROMBOCYTOPENIC PURPURA TTP is a fulminant, often lethal disorder that may be initiated by endothelial injury and subsequent release of vWF and other procoagulant materials from the endothelial cell. Causes include pregnancy, metastatic cancer, mitomycin C, and high-dose chemotherapy. Characteristic findings include the microvascular deposition of hyaline thrombi that stain for fibrin, thrombocytopenia, microangiopathic hemolytic anemia, fever, renal failure, fluctuating levels of consciousness, and evanescent focal neurologic deficits. The presence of hyaline thrombi in arterioles, capillaries, and venules without any inflammatory changes in the vessel wall is diagnostic. Gingival biopsies are positive in 30 to 40 percent of patients, and marrow biopsies are occasionally helpful. The presence of a severe Coombs-negative hemolytic anemia with schistocytes or fragmented red blood cells in the peripheral blood smear, coupled with thrombocytopenia, and minimal activation of the coagulation system help to confirm the clinical suspicion of TTP. This disorder should be distinguished from vasculitis and SLE, which can predispose patients to TTP. Levels of platelet-associated IgG and complement are usually normal in TTP.

The treatment of acute TTP has changed radically in the past few years. Steroids and heparin or emergency splenectomy have been abandoned, and the enthusiasm for antiplatelet therapy has diminished. Increasingly, treatment has focused on the use of exchange transfusion or intensive plasmapheresis coupled with infusion of fresh frozen plasma. With this therapeutic approach, the overall mortality has been markedly reduced, and the majority of patients with TTP are recovering from this formerly fatal disorder. Most patients surviving the acute illness recover completely with no residual renal or neurologic disease. Occasional patients with a chronic, relapsing form of TTP require maintenance plasmapheresis and plasma infusion, and a few patients are only controlled with glucocorticoids.

HEMOLYTIC-UREMIC SYNDROME HUS is a disease of infancy and early childhood that closely resembles TTP. Patients present with fever, thrombocytopenia, microangiopathic hemolytic anemia, hypertension, and varying degrees of acute renal failure. In many cases, onset is preceded by a minor febrile or viral illness, and an infectious or immune-complex–mediated cause has been proposed. As in TTP, there is no evidence of disseminated intravascular coagulation. In contrast to TTP, the disorder remains localized to the kidney, where hyaline thrombi are seen in the afferent arterioles and glomerular capillaries. Such thrombi are not present in other vessels, and neurologic symptoms, other than those associated with uremia, are uncommon. There is no effective therapy; however, with dialysis for acute renal failure, the initial mortality is only 5 percent. Between 10 and 50 percent of patients are left with some chronic renal impairment.

HENOCH-SCHÖNLEIN PURPURA Henoch-Schönlein or anaphylactoid purpura is a distinct, self-limited type of vasculitis that occurs in children and young adults. Patients have an acute inflammatory reaction in capillaries, mesangial tissues, and small arterioles that leads to increased vascular permeability, exudation, and hemorrhage. Vessel lesions contain IgA and complement components. The syndrome may be preceded by an upper respiratory infection or streptococcal pharyngitis or be associated with food or drug allergies. Patients develop a purpuric or urticarial rash on the extensor surfaces of the arms and legs and on the buttocks; they also have polyarthralgias or arthritis, colicky abdominal pain, and hematuria from focal glomerulonephritis. Despite the hemorrhagic features, all coagulation tests are normal. A small number of patients may develop fatal acute renal failure, and 5 to 10 percent develop chronic nephritis. Glucocorticoids provide symptomatic relief of the joint and abdominal pains but do not alter the course of the illness.

METABOLIC AND INFLAMMATORY DISORDERS A number of acute febrile illnesses cause capillary fragility and skin bleeding. Immune complexes containing viral antigens or the viruses themselves may damage endothelial cells. In addition, certain pathogens such as the rickettsiae that cause Rocky Mountain spotted fever replicate in endothelial cells and damage them. Thrombocytopenia is also a frequent finding in acute infectious disorders and may contribute to skin bleeding. In addition, whenever the platelet count falls below 10,000 per microliter, gaps that develop between endothelial cells allow the diapedesis of red cells into the dermis, leading to the formation of petechiae. Drugs such as the sulfonamides, penicillin, and allopurinol may cause vascular inflammation resulting in maculopapular or urticarial rashes. Some of these mechanisms are additive, and drug reactions in thrombocytopenic individuals cause an intensely hemorrhagic rash.

Occasionally, patients with diffuse polyclonal hyperglobulinemia will develop purpuric lesions on the lower limbs—a benign condition referred to as *hyperglobulinemic purpura*. Vascular purpura may occur in patients with various monoclonal plasma protein abnormalities, including Waldenström's macroglobulinemia, multiple myeloma, and cryoglobulinemia. These proteins markedly increase serum viscosity and may impair blood flow through capillaries. Thus retinal hemorrhage, central nervous system dysfunction, and skin necrosis have all been described in these syndromes due to the marked elevation in viscosity. In addition, the globulins may impair platelet aggregation and adhesion and interfere with fibrin polymerization. Patients with mixed cryoglobulinemia develop a more extensive maculopapular lesion due to immune-complex–mediated damage to the vessel wall. The mixed cryoglobulinemia (usually IgG and anti-IgG) may be associated with arthralgias, diffuse weakness, and unexplained nephritis. Plasmapheresis will temporarily lower the level of globulins, remove immune complexes, and improve symptoms in these patients. However, long-term management must include control of the underlying disease that produces the abnormal globulins or immune complexes.

Patients with *scurvy* (vitamin C deficiency) develop painful episodes of perifollicular skin bleeding as well as bleeding into muscles and, occasionally, into the gastrointestinal and genitourinary tracts. The diagnosis is confirmed by the presence of hyperkeratosis of skin, gum swelling, and low levels of the vitamin in leukocytes. Vitamin C–deficient patients have markedly defective collagen synthesis, since ascorbic acid is needed to synthesize hydroxyproline, an essential constituent of collagen. Patients with *Cushing's syndrome*, which is characterized by excess production of glucocorticoids, or patients on large doses of glucocorticoids develop generalized protein wasting and may show skin bleeding or easy bruising due to atrophy of the supporting connective tissue around blood vessels. Aging causes a similar atrophy of perivascular connective tissue on the extensor surfaces of the hands and arms, leading to "senile purpura." These individuals develop dark purple, irregularly shaped hemorrhagic areas due to abnormal skin mobility that tears small blood vessels.

Patients with inherited disorders of the connective tissue matrix such as *Marfan's syndrome*, *Ehlers-Danlos syndrome*, and *pseudoxanthoma elasticum* also have easy bruising. In addition to having fragile skin vessels and easy bruising, patients with Ehlers-Danlos syndrome

may develop aneurysms in intraabdominal vessels and apoplectic rupture and hemorrhage due to defects in the vascular collagen network. Primary vascular abnormalities also can lead to bleeding. Patients with *Osler-Weber-Rendu disease* (hereditary hemorrhagic telangiectasia), an inherited autosomal dominant disorder, have frequent episodes of nasal and gastrointestinal bleeding from abnormal telangiectatic capillaries; patients with *angiodysplasia* of the colon have increased incidence of gastrointestinal bleeding. In the *Kasabach-Merritt syndrome*, patients may have very extensive and progressively enlarging vascular malformations that may involve large portions of their extremities. Bleeding is secondary to disseminated intravascular coagulation triggered by stagnant blood flow through the tortuous abnormal vessels.

BIBLIOGRAPHY

EWENSTEIN BM, HANDIN RI: von Willebrand's disease, in *Blood: Principles and Practice of Hematology*, RI Handin et al (eds). Philadelphia, Lippincott, 1994, pp 1069–1094

WARKENTON TE, KELTON J: The platelet life cycle: Quantitative disorders in blood, in *Blood: Principles and Practice of Hematology*, RI Handin et al (eds). Philadelphia, Lippincott, 1994 pp 973–1049

118	*Robert I. Handin*

DISORDERS OF COAGULATION AND THROMBOSIS

Patients with congenital plasma coagulation defects characteristically bleed into muscles, joints, and body cavities hours or days after an injury. Most of the *inherited* plasma coagulation disorders are due to defects in single coagulation proteins, with the two X-linked disorders, factors VIII and IX deficiency, accounting for the majority of the congenital coagulation disorders. These patients merit special attention because they may have severe bleeding and chronic disability and require specialized medical therapy. With rare exceptions, the known disorders prolong either the prothrombin time (PT), partial thromboplastin time (PTT), or both of these important laboratory screening tests. If they are abnormal, quantitative assays of specific coagulation proteins are then carried out using the PT or PTT tests with plasma from congenitally deficient individuals as substrate. The corrective effect of varying concentrations of patient plasma is measured and expressed as a percentage of a normal pooled plasma standard. The interval range for most coagulation factors is from 50 to 150 percent of this average value, and the minimal level of most individual factors needed for adequate hemostasis is 25 percent.

Acquired coagulation disorders are both more frequent and more complex, arising from deficiencies of multiple coagulation proteins and simultaneously affecting both primary and secondary hemostasis. The most common acquired hemorrhagic disorders are (1) disseminated intravascular coagulation (DIC), (2) the hemorrhagic diathesis of liver disease, and (3) vitamin K deficiency and complications of anticoagulant therapy.

Although congenital and acquired bleeding disorders are relatively rare, venous and arterial thrombosis and embolism are common medical disorders that have been recognized for over 100 years. Although risk factors such as atherosclerotic vascular disease, congestive heart failure, malignancy, and immobility predispose patients to thrombosis, specific coagulation defects have not yet been identified in most patients with thromboembolism. Several inherited coagulation abnormalities have now been described that induce a hypercoagulable or prethrombotic state and predispose patients to thrombosis. These disorders merit special attention because they affect young people, cause recurrent episodes of thromboembolism, and may involve multiple members of a single family. An understanding of the biochemical basis of thromboembolism is also important because anticoagulant and antithrombotic regimens are based on the premise that modifying critical coagulation reactions will reduce the incidence of thrombosis. This chapter will review the diagnosis, natural history, and therapy of congenital and acquired plasma coagulation disorders, as well as the inherited prethrombotic disorders. → *The physiology of normal hemostasis and the cardinal manifestations of the hemorrhagic and thrombotic disorders are described in Chap. 60.*

FACTOR VIII DEFICIENCY—HEMOPHILIA A Pathogenesis and Clinical Manifestations

The antihemophilic factor (AHF), or factor VIII coagulant protein, is a large (265-kDa), single-chain protein that regulates the activation of factor X by proteases generated in the intrinsic coagulation pathway (see Figs. 60-5 and 60-6). It is synthesized in liver parenchymal cells and circulates complexed to the von Willebrand factor (vWF) protein. Previous efforts to purify and characterize the factor VIII molecule were limited by its low concentration (10 μg/L) and susceptibility to proteolysis. However, the cloning and sequencing of complementary DNA (cDNA) encoding the factor VIII molecule and the mapping of the factor VIII gene on the X chromosome have provided a detailed picture of its structure and have led to improved methods for carrier detection and prenatal diagnosis of hemophilia A.

One in 10,000 males is born with deficiency or dysfunction of the factor VIII molecule. The resulting disorder, hemophilia A, is characterized by bleeding into soft tissues, muscles, and weight-bearing joints. Although normal hemostasis requires at least 25 percent factor VIII activity, symptomatic patients usually have factor VIII levels below 5 percent, with a close correlation between the clinical severity of hemophilia and plasma AHF level. Patients with <1 percent factor VIII activity have *severe* disease; they bleed frequently even without discernible trauma. Patients with levels between 1 and 5 percent have *moderate* disease with less frequent bleeding episodes. Those with levels over 5 percent have *mild* disease with infrequent bleeding that is usually secondary to trauma. Occasional patients with factor VIII levels as high as 25 percent are discovered when they bleed after major trauma or surgery. The majority of patients with hemophilia A have factor VIII levels below 5 percent.

Hemophilic bleeding occurs hours or days after injury, can involve any organ, and, if untreated, may continue for days or weeks. This can result in large collections of partially clotted blood putting pressure on adjacent normal tissues and can cause necrosis of muscle (compartment syndromes), venous congestion (pseudophlebitis), or ischemic damage to nerves. For example, hemophiliacs often develop femoral neuropathy due to pressure from an unsuspected retroperitoneal hematoma. They also can develop large calcified masses of blood and inflammatory tissue that are mistaken for soft tissue sarcomas (pseudotumor syndrome).

Patients with severe hemophilia are usually diagnosed shortly after birth because of an extensive cephalhematoma or profuse bleeding at circumcision. However, young children with moderate disease may not bleed until they begin to walk or crawl, and individuals with mild hemophilia may not be diagnosed until they are adolescents or young adults. Typically, a hemophiliac patient presents with pain followed by swelling in a weight-bearing joint, such as the hip, knee, or ankle. The presence of blood in the joint (hemarthrosis) causes synovial inflammation, and repetitive bleeding erodes articular cartilage and causes osteoarthritis, articular fibrosis, joint ankylosis, and eventually muscle atrophy. Although bleeding may occur into any joint, after a joint has been damaged, it may become a site for subsequent bleeding episodes.

Hematuria, in the absence of any genitourinary pathology, is also common. It is usually self-limited and may not require specific therapy. The most feared complications of hemophilia are oropharyngeal and central nervous system bleeding. Patients with oropharyngeal bleeding may require emergency intubation to maintain an adequate airway. Central nervous system bleeding can occur without antecedent trauma or without evidence of a specific lesion.

Patients suspected of having hemophilia should have screening tests of hemostasis, including a platelet count, bleeding time, PT, and PTT. Typically, the patient will have a prolonged PTT with all other tests normal. Because of the clinical similarity of factor VIII deficiency and factor IX deficiency, any male with an appropriate bleeding history and a prolonged PTT should have specific assays for factor VIII and factor IX.

℞ TREATMENT

There are several tenets regarding the treatment of bleeding in hemophiliac patients: (1) Symptoms often precede objective evidence of bleeding. (2) Signs of bleeding may not appear until several days after well-documented trauma. Physicians caring for these patients have learned to rely on their patients to inform them of early symptoms, usually pain, and to begin treatment at that time. Early treatment is more effective, less costly, and can be lifesaving. (3) It is critical to avoid the use of aspirin or aspirin-containing drugs, which impair platelet function and may cause severe hemorrhage.

Plasma products enriched in factor VIII have revolutionized the care of hemophilia patients, reduced the degree of orthopedic deformity, and permitted virtually any form of elective and emergency surgery. The widespread use of factor VIII concentrates also has produced serious complications, including viral hepatitis, chronic liver disease, and AIDS. *Cryoprecipitate*, which contains about half the factor VIII activity of fresh frozen plasma in one-tenth the original volume, is simple to prepare and is produced in hospital or regional blood banks. It must be stored frozen and is thawed and pooled before administration. Partially purified *factor VIII concentrate*, which is prepared from multiple donors and supplied as a lyophilized powder, can be refrigerated and reconstituted just before use.

Three developments have increased the safety of factor VIII therapy and have changed medical practice. First, heating of lyophilized factor VIII concentrates under carefully controlled conditions can inactivate human immunodeficiency virus (HIV) without destroying factor VIII coagulant activity. Second, highly purified factor VIII can be produced by adsorbing and eluting factor VIII from monoclonal antibody columns. Third, recombinant factor VIII is now available. Patients with hemophilia should receive either monoclonal purified or recombinant factor VIII to minimize viral infections and exposure to irrelevant proteins.

It has been determined empirically that each unit of factor VIII infused, defined as the amount present in 1 mL normal plasma, will raise the plasma level of the recipient by 2 percent per kilogram of body weight. Factor VIII has a half-life of 8 to 12 h, making it necessary to infuse it continuously or at least twice daily to sustain a chosen factor VIII level. In patients with mild hemophilia, an alternative to the use of plasma products is desmopressin (DDAVP), which transiently increases the factor VIII level. Desmopressin, in general, will increase the factor level two- to threefold. Although generally safe, it occasionally causes hyponatremia or may precipitate thrombosis in elderly patients.

An uncomplicated episode of soft tissue bleeding or an early hemarthrosis can be treated with one infusion of sufficient factor VIII concentrate to raise the factor VIII level to 15 or 20 percent. A more extensive hemarthrosis or retroperitoneal bleeding requires twice-daily or continuous infusions in order to keep the factor VIII level between 25 and 50 percent for at least 72 h. Life-threatening bleeding into the central nervous system or major surgery may require therapy for 2 weeks with levels kept at a minimum of 50 percent of normal. In addition to the prompt infusion of factor VIII–enriched plasma products, patients need skilled orthopedic care with immobilization of inflamed joints to promote healing and to prevent contractures and physical therapy to strengthen muscles and maintain joint mobility. Before surgery, every patient should be screened for the presence of an inhibitor to factor VIII.

Patients with hemophilia who do not have an inhibitor should receive factor VIII infusions just before surgery and will require daily monitoring so that the factor VIII level is maintained above 50 percent for 10 to 14 days after surgery. When patients undergo joint replacement or other major orthopedic surgery, therapy should be continued for 3 weeks. This permits adequate wound healing and the institution of necessary joint mobilization and physical therapy.

Hemophiliacs also require treatment before dental procedures. Filling of a carious tooth can be managed by a single infusion of cryoprecipitate or factor VIII concentrate coupled with the administration of 4 to 6 g of ε-aminocaproic acid (EACA) four times daily for 72 to 96 h after the dental procedure. EACA is a potent antifibrinolytic agent that will inhibit plasminogen activators present in oral secretions and stabilize clot formation in oral tissue. Alternatives include tranexamic acid, a longer-acting antifibrinolytic. EACA is also effective when used as a mouthwash. For major oral and periodontal surgery and extractions of permanent teeth, patients should probably be hospitalized briefly and also treated with factor VIII concentrates. Therapy should begin just before surgery and be continued for a minimum of 48 to 72 h.

Many centers have organized home care programs so that patients can administer their own factor VIII infusions with the onset of symptoms. Occasional patients with very frequent bleeding receive regularly scheduled infusions. However, the expense and inconvenience usually limit the use of "prophylactic" infusions. Concern regarding transmission of AIDS has complicated therapy of hemophilia, and some patients are reluctant to treat themselves, despite the fact that current blood products carry a very low or no risk of transmitting HIV.

Complications Most hemophiliac patients have had multiple episodes of hepatitis, and a majority have elevated hepatocellular enzyme levels and abnormalities on liver biopsy. Between 10 and 20 percent of patients also have hepatosplenomegaly, and a small number develop chronic active or persistent hepatitis or cirrhosis. A few patients with hemophilia and end-stage liver disease have received liver transplants with cure of both diseases. Along with homosexuals and intravenous drug abusers, hemophiliacs are at high risk for AIDS because they frequently receive blood products. Hemophiliacs also can present with the full range of AIDS-related syndromes, including diffuse lymphadenopathy and immune thrombocytopenia. Although as many as 80 percent of multiply transfused hemophiliacs are HIV-positive and some have clinical AIDS, the advances in factor VIII concentrate technology discussed previously should prevent future HIV infection.

Despite frequent bleeding, severe iron-deficiency anemia is uncommon because most of the bleeding is internal and iron is effectively recycled. Mild iron deficiency from chronic epistaxis or gastrointestinal bleeding has been noted in some patients. In addition, after receiving large doses of the partially purified factor VIII concentrates, some patients have developed a mild Coombs-positive hemolytic anemia due to small amounts of anti-A and anti-B antibody that are present in commercial concentrates.

Following multiple transfusions, between 10 and 20 percent of patients with severe hemophilia develop inhibitors to factor VIII. Inhibitors are, generally, IgG antibodies that rapidly neutralize factor VIII activity. There are two types of inhibitors which have different biologic characteristics and lead to different clinical presentations. Patients with type I inhibitors have a typical anamnestic response and raise their antibody titer following exposure to factor VIII. Patients with a type II inhibitor have a low antibody titer that cannot be stimulated by factor VIII infusion. Patients with the type I inhibitor should not receive factor VIII. Control of bleeding may require the infusion of either porcine factor VIII concentrates, which may not cross-react with inhibitors, or prothrombin complex concentrates, which contain trace quantities of activated coagulation factors and can bypass the block in coagulation produced by the inhibitor. Patients with low-titer type II antibodies may respond to higher than normal doses of factor VIII.

Genetic Counseling and Carrier Detection Carrier detection formerly required biologic and immunologic assays that compared the

ratio of factor VIII to vWF protein and were predictive in only 70 to 80 percent of cases. It is now possible to trace the defective allele in some families by examining the inheritance of restriction fragment length polymorphisms (RFLP) linked to the factor VIII gene. In addition, in families in which a specific mutation has been defined in the factor VIII gene, it can be readily detected by gene amplification and allele-specific oligonucleotide hybridization. For example, 45 percent of patients with severe hemophilia A have a chromosomal inversion arising from recombination between homologous sequences in intron 22 and an upstream gene. The inversion is readily detected by polymerase chain reaction (PCR) or Southern blotting. Previously, prenatal diagnosis required sampling fetal blood for coagulant activity. Now, in families with an identifiable RFLP linked to the gene or a known mutation, precise diagnosis is possible early in pregnancy from either chorionic villus biopsy or amniocentesis. The amount of material required for diagnosis has decreased, and the rapidity of diagnosis has increased with the introduction of PCR to amplify desired segments of genes.

Female carriers of hemophilia, who are heterozygotes, usually produce sufficient factor VIII from the factor VIII allele on their normal X chromosome for normal hemostasis. However, occasional hemophilia carriers will have factor VIII levels far below 50 percent due to random inactivation of normal X chromosomes in tissue producing factor VIII. These symptomatic carriers may bleed with major surgery or bleed occasionally with menses. Rarely, true female hemophiliacs arise from consanguinity within families with hemophilia or from concomitant Turner's syndrome or XO mosaicism in a carrier female.

FACTOR IX DEFICIENCY—HEMOPHILIA B Factor IX is a single-chain, 55-kDa proenzyme that is converted to an active protease (IXa) by factor XIa or by the tissue factor–VIIa complex. Factor IXa then activates factor X in conjunction with activated factor VIII. Factor IX is one of a group of six proteins synthesized in the liver that require vitamin K for biologic activity. As previously discussed (see Chap. 60), vitamin K is a cofactor for a unique posttranslational modification that inserts a second carboxyl group onto certain glutamic acid residues on factor IX. This modification permits calcium binding and adsorption onto phospholipid surfaces. Factor IX cDNA has been cloned and the gene locus mapped to the X chromosome. Many patients with deletions and mutations in the IX gene have now been described.

Factor IX deficiency or dysfunction (hemophilia B, Christmas disease) occurs in 1 in 100,000 male births. Accurate laboratory diagnosis is critical, since it is indistinguishable clinically from factor VIII deficiency (hemophilia A) but requires treatment with a different plasma fraction. Either fresh frozen plasma or a plasma fraction enriched in the prothrombin complex proteins is used. Monoclonally purified or recombinant factor IX preparations are undergoing clinical trials. In addition to the expected complications of hepatitis, chronic liver disease, and AIDS, the therapy of factor IX deficiency has a special hazard. Trace quantities of activated coagulation factors in prothrombin complex concentrates may activate the coagulation system and cause thrombosis and embolism. This is particularly common in immobilized surgical patients and patients with liver disease. As a result, some centers have returned to fresh frozen plasma for factor IX–deficient surgical patients, while others have recommended the addition of small doses of heparin to the concentrate to activate antithrombin III during the infusion and reduce hypercoagulability. The recombinant or monoclonally purified products are unlikely to be thrombogenic.

FACTOR XI DEFICIENCY Factor XI is a 160-kDa dimeric protein that is activated via the intrinsic coagulation pathway. It is converted to an active protease (XIa) by factor XIIa, in conjunction with high-molecular-weight kininogen and kallikrein (see Figs. 60-5 and 60-6). Factor XI deficiency is inherited as an autosomal recessive trait and is especially common in Ashkenazi Jews. In contrast to factors VIII and IX deficiency, the correlation between factor level and propensity to bleed is not as precise, there is less spontaneous bleeding, and hemarthroses are rare. Many patients with factor XI deficiency present with posttraumatic bleeding or with bleeding in the perioperative period, and occasional factor XI–deficient women have menorrhagia. Daily infusions of fresh frozen plasma are sufficient, since the half-life of factor XI is approximately 24 h. The majority of defective factor XI alleles were accounted for by a limited number of mutations in one large study.

OTHER FACTOR DEFICIENCIES Deficiencies in factors V, VII, X, and prothrombin (factor II) are all exceedingly rare autosomal recessive disorders. Although spontaneous or posttraumatic musculoskeletal bleeding or menorrhagia can occur with these deficiencies, hemarthroses are uncommon. Fresh frozen plasma is the appropriate therapy, although prothrombin concentrates may be employed for patients with severe prothrombin or factors VII and X deficiency as long as the risks of hepatitis and thrombosis are recognized.

Defects in the contact activation pathway involving Hageman factor (factor XII), high-molecular-weight kininogen, and prekallikrein cause laboratory abnormalities but no clinical bleeding. Despite dramatic prolongation of the PTT, which is often greater than 100 s, deficient individuals have normal hemostasis and can undergo major surgery without plasma replacement therapy. It is important to recognize and diagnose these disorders because the patients should neither be treated inappropriately with plasma nor denied indicated surgery on the basis of these laboratory abnormalities. As discussed in Chap. 60, direct activation of factor IX by the tissue factor–VIIa complex may bypass this defective step in coagulation (Fig. 60-7).

AFIBRINOGENEMIA AND DYSFIBRINOGENEMIA Fibrinogen is a 340-kDa dimeric molecule made up of two sets of three covalently linked polypeptide chains. Thrombin sequentially cleaves fibrinopeptides A and B from the Aα and Bβ chains of fibrinogen to produce fibrin monomer, which then polymerizes to form a fibrin clot. Although fibrinogen is needed for platelet aggregation and fibrin formation, severe fibrinogen deficiency, paradoxically, does not usually cause serious bleeding except after surgery. Patients with afibrinogenemia, who have no detectable fibrinogen in plasma or platelets, may have infrequent, mild bleeding episodes. Preliminary genetic analyses do not show any gross deletion or structural changes in the genes encoding the α, β, and γ chains of fibrinogen despite the total absence of plasma fibrinogen.

Fibrinogen is an abundant plasma protein (2.5 g/L) that has been very well characterized. Mutations have been identified that alter the release of fibrinopeptides from the Aα and Bβ chains of fibrinogen, the rate of polymerization of fibrin monomers, and the sites for fibrin cross-linking. These dysfibrinogenemias are almost always inherited as autosomal dominant traits, so patients have approximately equal concentrations of normal and mutant fibrinogen in their plasma. Patients with dysfibrinogenemia have a slightly prolonged PT and PTT, a prolonged thrombin time, and a disparity between the quantity of fibrinogen measured with functional and immunologic assays. Despite these abnormalities, most patients have no symptoms, while other patients have moderate bleeding. A few dysfibrinogenemias induce a hypercoagulable state and increase the risk of thrombosis, and others have been associated with an increased incidence of abortion (see Chap. 119). Some patients with liver disease, AIDS, and lymphoproliferative disorders developed an acquired form of dysfibrinogenemia.

FACTOR XIII DEFICIENCY AND DEFECTIVE FIBRIN CROSS-LINKING Factor XIII is a transglutaminase that stabilizes fibrin clots by forming ε-amino–γ-glutamyl cross-links between adjacent α and γ chains of fibrin. Factor XIII deficiency is an extremely rare inherited syndrome with only a few hundred documented cases. Patients usually bleed in the neonatal period from their umbilical stump or circumcision. In addition to hemorrhage, these patients may have poor wound healing, a high incidence of infertility among males and abortion among affected females, and a high incidence of intracerebral hemorrhage. These observations suggest that the enzyme may be important in other physiologic and pathologic processes beyond hemostasis, including placental implantation, spermatogenesis, and wound healing. Several drugs, including isoniazid, may bind to cross-linking sites on fibrinogen and mimic factor XIII deficiency by blocking enzyme activity. Normal hemostasis requires only 1 percent of normal enzyme activity, which can be achieved with a single infusion of fresh frozen plasma or a purified factor XIII-rich product

derived from human placenta called Fibrogammin. Factor XIII has a 14 day half-life.

VITAMIN K DEFICIENCY Vitamin K is a fat-soluble vitamin that plays a critical role in hemostasis. Dietary vitamin K is absorbed in the small intestine and stored in the liver. The vitamin is also synthesized by endogenous bacterial flora resident in the small intestine and colon; however, there is controversy regarding the quantity of endogenous vitamin K that is absorbed from the large intestine. Following absorption and transport, vitamin K is converted to an active epoxide in liver microsomes and serves as a cofactor in the enzymatic carboxylation of glutamic acid residues on prothrombin complex proteins (Fig. 118-1).

There are three major causes of vitamin K deficiency—inadequate dietary intake, intestinal malabsorption, and loss of storage sites due to hepatocellular disease. Neonatal vitamin K deficiency, which causes hemorrhagic disease of the newborn, has disappeared from western countries with the routine administration of vitamin K to all newborn infants. Although there is, theoretically, a 30-day store of vitamin K in the normal liver, acutely ill patients can become deficient within 7 to 10 days. Acute vitamin K deficiency is particularly common in patients recovering from biliary tract surgery who have no dietary intake of vitamin K, have T-tube drainage of bile, and are on broad-spectrum antibiotics. Vitamin K deficiency is also seen in chronic liver disease, particularly primary biliary cirrhosis, and in some malabsorption states (see Chaps. 285 and 298). The cephalosporin antibiotics induce vitamin K deficiency in a manner analogous to the coumarin anticoagulants—they inhibit the reduction and recycling of vitamin K.

With the onset of vitamin K deficiency, plasma levels of all the prothrombin complex proteins (factors II, VII, IX, X; protein C and protein S) decrease. Factor VII and protein C, which have the shortest half-lives, decrease first. Because of the rapid fall in factor VII, patients with mild vitamin K deficiency may have a prolonged PT and a normal PTT. Later, as the levels of the other factors fall, the PTT also will become prolonged. Parenteral administration of 10 mg vitamin K rapidly restores vitamin K levels in the liver and permits normal production of prothrombin complex proteins within 8 to 10 h. Severe hemorrhage can be treated with fresh frozen plasma, which immediately corrects the hemostatic defect. If the cause of vitamin K deficiency cannot be eliminated, patients may need monthly injections. Purified prothrombin complex concentrates should be avoided because they contain trace quantities of activated forms of the prothrombin complex proteins and can cause thrombosis in patients with liver disease. They also will expose patients to an increased risk of hepatitis.

DISSEMINATED INTRAVASCULAR COAGULATION DIC can be either an explosive and life-threatening bleeding disorder or a relatively mild or subclinical disorder. Although there is a long list of diseases complicated by DIC, it is most frequently associated with obstetrical catastrophes, metastatic malignancy, massive trauma,

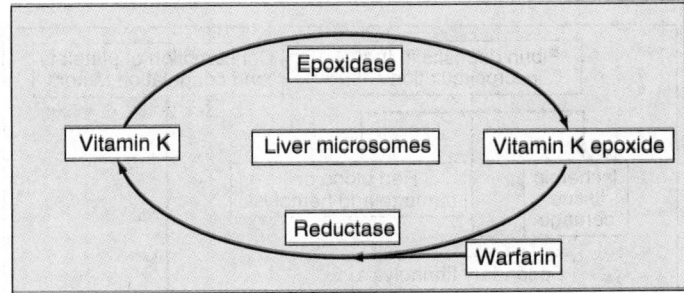

FIGURE 118-1 The mechanism of action of vitamin K, a cofactor in the formation of di-γ-carboxyglutamic acid residues on coagulation proteins, is depicted. Vitamin K is converted to an epoxide in liver microsomes. The epoxide is the active form and is reduced back to vitamin K by a liver membrane reductase. Warfarin blocks the action of the reductase and competitively inhibits the effects of vitamin K.

Table 118-1

Etiologic Factors and Disorders Causing Disseminated Intravascular Coagulation

Liberation of tissue factors	Obstetrical syndromes—abruptio placentae, amniotic fluid embolism, retained dead fetus, second trimester abortion
	Hemolysis
	Neoplasms, particularly mucinous adenocarcinomas, acute promyelocytic leukemia
	Intravascular hemolysis
	Fat embolism
	Tissue damage—burns, frostbite, head injury, gunshot wounds
Endothelial damage	Aortic aneurysm
	Hemolytic uremic syndrome
	Acute glomerulonephritis
	Rocky Mountain spotted fever
Vascular malformation and decreased blood flow	Kasabach-Merritt syndrome
Infections	Bacterial: staphylococci, streptococci, pneumococci, meningococci, gram-negative bacilli
	Viral: arboviruses, varicella, variola, rubella
	Parasitic: malaria, kala-azar
	Rickettsial: Rocky Mountain spotted fever
	Mycotic: acute histoplasmosis

SOURCE: Modified from RI Handin, RD Rosenberg, in *Hematology*, 4th ed, WS Beck (ed), Cambridge, MA, MIT Press, 1985.

and bacterial sepsis (Table 118-1). In each case, a tentative triggering mechanism has been identified. For example, tumors and traumatized or necrotic tissue release tissue factor into the circulation, while endotoxin from gram-negative bacteria activates several steps in the coagulation cascade. In addition to a direct effect on the activation of Hageman factor (factor XII), endotoxin induces the expression of tissue factor on the surface of monocytes and endothelial cells. These activated cell surfaces then accelerate coagulation reactions. These potent thrombogenic stimuli cause the deposition of small thrombi and emboli throughout the microvasculature. This early thrombotic phase of DIC is then followed by a phase of procoagulant consumption and secondary fibrinolysis. Continued fibrin formation and fibrinolysis lead to hemorrhage from the depletion of coagulation proteins and platelets and the antihemostatic effects of fibrin degradation products (Fig. 118-2).

The clinical presentation varies with the stage and severity of the syndrome. Most patients have extensive skin and mucous membrane bleeding and hemorrhage from multiple sites—usually surgical incisions or venipuncture or catheter sites. Less often, patients present with peripheral acrocyanosis, thrombosis, and pregangrenous changes in digits, genitalia, and nose—areas where blood flow is markedly

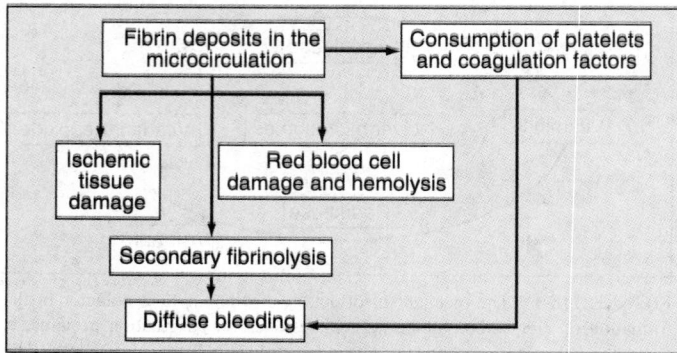

FIGURE 118-2 The pathophysiology of disseminated intravascular coagulation (DIC). Shown are the interactions between coagulation and fibrinolytic pathways that result in bleeding in patients with DIC.

reduced by vasospasm or microthrombi. Some patients, particularly those with chronic DIC secondary to malignancy, have laboratory abnormalities without any evidence of thrombosis or hemorrhage.

The laboratory manifestations include thrombocytopenia and the presence of schistocytes or fragmented red blood cells that arise from cell trapping and damage within fibrin thrombi; prolonged PT and PTT and thrombin time and a reduced fibrinogen level from depletion of coagulation proteins; and elevated fibrin degradation products (FDP) from intense secondary fibrinolysis. The D dimer immunoassay, which specifically measures cross-linked fibrin derivatives, is a more specific FDP assay. The cardinal manifestation of DIC which correlates most closely with bleeding is the plasma fibrinogen level; low fibrinogen levels are associated with more bleeding.

℞ TREATMENT

DIC, although sometimes indolent, can cause life-threatening hemorrhage and may require emergency treatment. This should include (1) an attempt to correct any reversible cause of DIC; (2) measures to control the major symptom, either bleeding or thrombosis; and (3) a prophylactic regimen to prevent recurrence in cases of chronic DIC. Treatment will vary with the clinical presentation. In patients with an obstetric complication such as abruptio placentae or acute bacterial sepsis, the underlying disorder is easy to correct, and prompt delivery of the fetus and placenta or treatment with appropriate antibiotics will reverse the DIC syndrome. In patients with metastatic tumor causing DIC, control of the primary disease may not be possible, and long-term prophylaxis may be necessary.

Patients with bleeding as a major symptom should receive fresh frozen plasma to replace depleted clotting factors and platelet concentrates to correct thrombocytopenia. Those with acrocyanosis and incipient gangrene or other thrombotic problems need immediate anticoagulation with intravenous heparin. The use of heparin in the treatment of bleeding is still controversial. Although it is a logical way to reduce thrombin generation and prevent further consumption of clotting proteins, it should be reserved for patients with thrombosis or those who continue to bleed despite vigorous treatment with plasma and platelets.

Patients who initially have mild DIC and may not be symptomatic may begin to bleed following surgery or chemotherapy. For example, mild DIC, without clinical bleeding, has been documented during saline- or prostaglandin-induced midtrimester abortions. Prophylactic treatment of patients with heparin may prevent progression of a mild DIC syndrome and has been used in the treatment of patients with acute promyelocytic leukemia and in some patients with a retained dead fetus who require surgical extraction. However, most patients with low-grade DIC can be managed simply with plasma and platelet replacement and do not require heparin. Chronic DIC does not respond to oral warfarin anticoagulants, but it can be controlled with long-term heparin infusion. Occasional patients with indolent tumors and severe DIC have been maintained on heparin administered by intermittent subcutaneous injection or continuous infusion with portable pumps.

Despite our detailed understanding of the pathophysiology of DIC and a vigorous approach to therapy, there is little evidence that its treatment will change the natural history of the underlying disorder. Therapy will only stabilize the patient, prevent exsanguination or massive thrombosis, and permit institution of definitive therapy.

COAGULATION DISORDERS IN LIVER DISEASE Since the liver plays a central role in the synthesis and metabolism of coagulation proteins, liver dysfunction is frequently accompanied by a hemostatic defect. The major causes of hemorrhage in patients with liver disease are outlined in Table 118-2. It is important to recognize that bleeding is usually due to an anatomic lesion, which can then be exacerbated by a hemostatic defect. Most patients bleed from complications of portal hypertension such as esophageal varices or from gastritis and peptic ulceration of the gastrointestinal tract. Portal hypertension also causes splenomegaly, with splenic sequestration of plate-

Table 118-2

CHAPTER 118
Disorders of Coagulation and Thrombosis 741

Causes of Bleeding in Liver Disease

ANATOMIC FACTORS

Portal hypertension
  Varices
  Splenomegaly and secondary thrombocytopenia
Peptic ulceration
Gastritis

HEPATIC FUNCTION ABNORMALITIES

Decreased synthesis of procoagulant proteins: fibrinogen, prothrombin,
  factors V, VII, IX, X, XI
Decreased synthesis of coagulation inhibitors: protein C, protein S,
  antithrombin III
Impaired absorption and metabolism of vitamin K
Failure to clear activated coagulation proteins leading to:
  Disseminated intravascular coagulation
  Systemic fibrinolysis

COMPLICATIONS OF THERAPY

Dilution of platelets and coagulation proteins from massive transfusions
Infusion of activated coagulation proteins in prothrombin complex
  concentrates
Bleeding from heparin; thrombosis from ε-aminocaproic acid (EACA)

lets and thrombocytopenia, which contributes to the hemostatic defect (see Chap. 298).

Patients with hepatocellular liver disease cannot store vitamin K optimally and may have some degree of vitamin K deficiency. Cholestasis, which is a frequent feature of liver disease, impairs vitamin K absorption and further decreases liver vitamin K stores. Abnormalities in the gamma carboxylation of prothrombin complex proteins independent of vitamin K and the production of abnormal proteins also have been described. Patients also may have decreased production of other coagulation proteins, including fibrinogen and factor V. The liver also produces inhibitors of coagulation such as antithrombin III and proteins C and S and is the clearance site for activated coagulation factors and fibrinolytic enzymes. Thus patients with liver disease are also "hypercoagulable" and predisposed to developing DIC or systemic fibrinolysis. For these reasons, coagulation defects in advanced liver failure are often difficult to distinguish from those of DIC.

Each patient with hemorrhage and liver disease should have a PT, PTT, platelet count, and fibrinogen determination, although it is not always possible to determine the major hemostatic abnormality from a single set of laboratory values. It is helpful to have previous laboratory data available for patients with chronic liver disease who develop an acute complication. There is a good correlation between the degree of prolongation of the PT and the risk of bleeding. Most patients present with moderate prolongation of the PT and PTT, mild thrombocytopenia, and a normal fibrinogen level. However, they also may present with a more complex defect combining defective synthesis, abnormal clearance, and active consumption of coagulation proteins. Since vitamin K deficiency is so common, it is advisable to administer a single parenteral dose of vitamin K after initial laboratory studies have been obtained, even though this may only partially correct the laboratory abnormalities. The presence of severe thrombocytopenia or a low fibrinogen level suggests the additional complication of DIC and may require further studies and therapy.

The safest replacement therapy for a patient with liver disease is fresh frozen plasma, since it supplies all known coagulation factors. However, even this form of therapy has drawbacks, since large quantities of plasma may precipitate hepatic encephalopathy and cause fluid and sodium overload. Prothrombin complex concentrates should be avoided because they only replace the vitamin K–dependent factors, may be contaminated with hepatitis and AIDS virus, and contain trace quantities of activated coagulation proteins. Similarly, fibrinogen concentrates (or cryoprecipitate) which are rich in factor VIII and fibrinogen should not be used without additional fresh frozen plasma. Anticoagulation with heparin has been advocated to control DIC, but this is particu-

larly hazardous and not recommended in cirrhosis because heparin is metabolized erratically and may thus lead to severe bleeding.

FIBRINOLYTIC DEFECTS Bleeding also can occur from defects in the fibrinolytic system. Patients with alpha$_2$ plasmin inhibitor deficiency or plasminogen activator inhibitor (PAI)1 have rapid fibrinolysis following fibrin deposition after trauma or surgery and so may experience recurrent hemorrhage. Similarly, patients with cirrhosis have an impaired clearance of tissue plasminogen activator (tPA) and systemic fibrinolysis that may contribute to their hemorrhagic defect. Rarely, patients with tumors such as metastatic prostatic carcinoma may develop diffuse bleeding from primary fibrinolysis rather than DIC. Clues to the diagnosis include a disproportionately low fibrinogen level with a relatively normal PT and PTT and the presence of a normal or nearly normal platelet count. Although there are some exceptions, patients with primary fibrinolysis should have an elevated titer of FDP but a normal D dimer level. However, it is sometimes difficult or impossible to differentiate primary fibrinolysis from the secondary fibrinolysis accompanying DIC. Patients with clearly established primary fibrinolysis should not receive heparin; they do require plasma therapy and, occasionally, fibrinolytic inhibitors such as EACA. However, EACA should not be given to patients suspected of having DIC unless they are also receiving heparin, since EACA can cause massive, often fatal, thrombosis in a patient with DIC.

CIRCULATING ANTICOAGULANTS Circulating anticoagulants, or inhibitors, are usually IgG antibodies that interfere with coagulation reactions. Specific inhibitors inactivate individual coagulation proteins and may cause severe hemorrhage. As previously discussed, they arise in 15 to 20 percent of patients with factor VIII or factor IX deficiency who have received plasma infusions. *Specific* inhibitors also occur in previously normal individuals. Although the most common target protein is factor VIII, inhibitors have been described with specificity for each of the coagulation proteins. In addition to hemophiliacs, anti-factor VIII antibodies are seen in postpartum females, in patients on various drugs, as part of the spectrum of autoantibodies in systemic lupus erythematosus (SLE) patients, and in normal elderly individuals. Circulating anticoagulants also have been reported in patients with AIDS.

Nonspecific (lupus-like) inhibitors prolong coagulation tests by binding to phospholipids. They are assayed by their anticoagulant effect [lupus anticoagulant (LA) activity] or their ability to bind to the complex phospholipid cardiolipin [anticardiolipin antibody (ACLA) activity]. While they are most often encountered in patients with SLE, these nonspecific inhibitors have also been noted in patients with many other disorders and also in otherwise normal individuals.

The critical laboratory feature, which identifies the presence of either type of inhibitor, is the failure of normal plasma to correct a prolonged PT, PTT, or both. Plasma from patients with a specific inhibitor will progressively inactivate a coagulation protein and thus prolong whichever of these screening tests requires the participation of that clotting factor. This effect persists after dilution. Nonspecific inhibitors immediately prolong the PT and PTT and, at low dilution, block multiple coagulation reactions. However, these effects can be overcome by altering the quantity or type of phospholipid or by diluting the plasma.

Hemorrhage in patients with specific inhibitors may require treatment with massive plasma or concentrate infusion, the use of activated prothrombin complex concentrates to bypass the antibodies against factors VIII or IX, and plasmapheresis or exchange transfusion to lower antibody titer. Chronic immunosuppressive regimens have been sometimes employed and have been particularly useful in otherwise normal individuals with an acquired factor VIII antibody. Many patients lose their antibody and recover within 6 to 12 months, although the acute mortality rate from uncontrollable bleeding may approach 10 percent.

Patients with LA activity have normal hemostasis and will not bleed unless they have concomitant thrombocytopenia or prothrombin deficiency. Both thrombocytopenia and hypoprothrombinemia are secondary to autoantibodies that bind either to platelets or the prothrombin molecule. While these antibodies have no effect on function, they accelerate clearance of the coated platelets or the antibody-prothrombin complexes.

There is increasing evidence that the presence of LA activity may predispose patients to thromboembolism and may cause midtrimester abortions. However, it is difficult to make firm predictions about the risk of thrombosis and the appropriate therapy for individual patients. First, tests for either LA or ACLA activity are not well standardized, and results vary among patients and can vary with serial measurements. The best predictor is a consistent prolongation of more than one coagulation test coupled with a high titer of ACLA activity. Second, the risk of thrombosis is increased in patients who have SLE compared with those with idiopathic LA or ACLA activity. There is little evidence that prophylactic therapy is beneficial or that treatments aimed at reducing the titer of antibody are superior to conventional antithrombotic therapy.

Although therapy should be individualized, the following general guidelines may be helpful. They are based on personal experience and review of a rapidly expanding and changing literature. Patients with SLE and either LA or ACLA activity who have had a thrombotic episode are at high risk for a recurrence and should receive long-term anticoagulant therapy. Women who have had more than one midtrimester abortion, especially those with SLE, should have a trial of anticoagulant therapy. Patients with a single thrombotic episode and no other risk factor except LA or ACLA activity may be treated, but the evidence for efficacy in this setting is minimal. Asymptomatic patients with laboratory abnormalities only should not be treated. Glucocorticoids should only be administered in conjunction with antithrombotic agents and are not of proven efficacy.

INHERITED PRETHROMBOTIC DISORDERS As previously discussed (see Chap. 60), coagulation is carefully regulated by a series of inhibitors that limit thrombin generation and fibrin formation and by the fibrinolytic system which effectively removes fibrin thrombi (see Figs. 60-5 and 60-6). Inherited defects in the natural coagulation inhibitors (i.e., antithrombin, protein C, and protein S), abnormalities in the fibrinolytic system, and certain dysfibrinogenemias predispose patients to thrombosis (see Table 60-5). A single point mutation in the factor V gene (factor V Leiden), which converts arginine 506 to glutamine and makes the molecule resistant to degradation by activated protein C, may account for 25 percent of inherited prethrombotic states. Antithrombin, protein C, and protein S defects are all autosomal dominant traits, so heterozygous individuals, who have a 50 percent reduction in protein concentration or a mixture of mutant and normal molecules, will have an increased risk of thrombosis. The effect of inheriting one or two factor V Leiden alleles is discussed in detail below. The patients all have similar clinical presentations with a strong family history of thrombosis, episodes of recurrent venous thromboembolism, and symptoms by their early twenties. Any patient with this distinctive history should be tested for the molecule abnormalities described below.

ANTITHROMBIN DEFICIENCY Antithrombin complexes with activated coagulation proteins and blocks their biologic activity (see Fig. 60-5). The rate of this reaction is enhanced by heparin-like molecules within the vessel wall or on endothelial cells. Plasma antithrombin III content varies from 5 to 15 mg/L (50 to 150 percent), with values only slightly below normal increasing the risk of thrombosis. For optimal screening, it is important to assess both the antithrombin III concentration by immunoassay and the plasma antithrombin and heparin cofactor activity with functional assays. The most common defect is mild (heterozygous) antithrombin deficiency, which occurs in 1 in 2000 individuals. In addition, dysfunctional antithrombin molecules, with mutations affecting either the serine protease–binding site or the heparin-binding site, or activation of inhibitor by heparin have been described.

Patients with antithrombin deficiency who develop acute thrombosis or embolism can be treated with intravenous heparin, since there is usually sufficient normal antithrombin to act as a heparin cofactor. Following their first episode of thromboembolism, patients should be placed on oral anticoagulants for life to prevent recurrent thrombosis. Family studies should be conducted when an antithrombin-deficient individual is discovered, since up to half the members of a kindred may be affected. Asymptomatic individuals with antithrombin deficiency should receive prophylactic anticoagulation with heparin or plasma infusions to raise their antithrombin level before medical or surgical procedures that may increase their risk of thrombosis. Chronic oral anticoagulation is not recommended until individuals at risk have a clinical thrombotic episode.

DEFICIENCIES OF PROTEINS C AND S Protein C is a vitamin K–dependent hepatic protein that binds to the endothelial cell surface protein thrombomodulin and is converted to an active protease by thrombin (see Fig. 60-5). Activated protein C, in conjunction with protein S, proteolyzes factors Va and VIIIa, which shuts off fibrin formation. Activated protein C also may stimulate fibrinolysis and accelerate clot lysis. Deficiencies of proteins C and S are usually autosomal dominant disorders, and deficiencies in the two proteins cause an identical syndrome of recurrent venous thrombosis and pulmonary embolism. Dysfunctional molecules also have been definitely identified in some patients with thrombosis. In addition, rare patients with homozygous protein C deficiency have fulminant neonatal intravascular coagulation and require prompt diagnosis and treatment.

The correlation between protein C and S levels and the risk of thrombosis is not as precise as for antithrombin III deficiency. In fact, as large surveys have been completed, asymptomatic individuals with protein C "deficiency" have been discovered. Protein C levels in these individuals overlap those with recurrent thromboembolism. In addition, in some well-studied protein C–deficient kindreds, asymptomatic individuals may have protein C levels as low as or lower than relatives with recurrent thrombosis. These observations raise the possibility that an as yet undiscovered comorbid condition is present in symptomatic patients. Finally, since a fraction of the available protein S is bound to C4b-binding protein and is unavailable for coagulation reactions, it may be important to measure both free and total protein S or to have a concomitant measurement of C4b-binding protein for maximum accuracy.

Heterozygous patients with protein C or S deficiencies who develop acute thrombosis should be heparinized and then placed on oral anticoagulants. There are, however, two potential problems with the use of coumarin anticoagulants in these patients. First, these vitamin K antagonists (see Fig. 118-1 and Fig. 60-5), which lower the level of the procoagulant factors II, VII, IX, and X, also may reduce the concentration of proteins C and S sufficiently to nullify the desired antithrombotic effect. In addition, there are patients with coumarin-induced skin necrosis who are protein C–deficient, suggesting that this defect may predispose patients to a rare but serious complication of oral anticoagulants. Patients with homozygous protein C deficiency require periodic plasma infusions rather than oral anticoagulants to prevent recurrent intravascular coagulation and thrombosis.

RESISTANCE TO ACTIVATED PROTEIN C AND THE FACTOR V LEIDEN MUTATION Several years ago there was an intriguing clinical observation that some patients with familial or recurrent venous thromboembolism did not prolong their PTT when activated protein C was added to their plasma. It has subsequently been shown that these patients all have an identical mutation in which arginine 506 in factor V is converted to glutamine. This amino acid substitution abolishes a protein C cleavage site in factor V and, thus, prolongs the thrombogenic effect of factor V activation. Approximately 3 percent of the population worldwide is heterozygous for this mutation, and presence of this mutation may account for 25 percent of patients with recurrent deep venous thrombosis or pulmonary embolism.

There is a clear relationship between inheritance of this defect and other thrombogenic stimuli. For example, heterozygosity at this allele increases an individual's lifetime risk of venous thromboembolism sevenfold. The risk also rises steadily with age. A homozygote has a 20-fold increased risk of thrombosis. In addition, heterozygosity coupled with ingestion of oral contraceptives or pregnancy increases the risk at least 15-fold. Coinheritance of factor V Leiden and another low-penetrance defect such as protein C or S deficiency are also additive. Many previous studies of risk factors predisposing patients to venous thromboembolism are being reevaluated to take into account this common mutation.

Approach to the Patient

With Venous Thromboembolism The following approach is suggested for the evaluation of patients who present with deep venous thrombosis or pulmonary embolism. Patients who develop venous thromboembolism without a clear predisposing factor, have a strong family history, present under the age of 30, or have more than one episode should definitely have studies sent for antithrombin III, proteins C and S, and factor V Leiden. Patients who present with deep venous thrombosis or pulmonary embolism during pregnancy or while using oral contraceptives have a 30 percent chance of having factor V Leiden and probably also deserve screening upon presentation.

Recommendations regarding treatment of patients with the inherited prethrombotic disorders are more controversial. All patients should receive standard initial therapy with heparin, either conventional or low dose (see Chap. 119), followed by 3 months of an oral anticoagulant such as warfarin. This regimen should allow for maximal healing and reendothelialization of the thrombosed vessels and minimize recurrence in the damaged vascular beds. There is not yet general agreement about which patients should go on to receive long-term (perhaps lifelong) anticoagulation, a judgment that depends on a careful balancing of the risk/benefit ratio.

The following approach is recommended based on current information about the natural history of these disorders. Patients with antithrombin III deficiency who become symptomatic have a high likelihood of recurrent events and should be placed on lifelong anticoagulation. Patients with protein C or S deficiency or heterozygous factor V Leiden patients have a lower likelihood of recurrent disease and do not need long-term anticoagulation until their second or subsequent episode of thromboembolism. Homozygous factor V Leiden patients should be placed on long-term anticoagulation after their initial episode, and all patients should receive replacement therapy or receive heparin prophylaxis during surgery or after trauma; women with these defects should avoid the use of oral contraceptives. The asymptomatic relatives of patients who are shown to have these disorders should receive appropriate prophylaxis but not start anticoagulation until they are symptomatic. In the absence of a congenital defect predisposing a patient to thrombosis, recurring or migratory thrombophlebitis may indicate an underlying malignancy.

DYSFIBRINOGENEMIAS AND FIBRINOLYTIC DEFECTS Several families have now been described with recurrent venous thrombosis and embolism due to defects in fibrinogen or plasminogen or with decreased synthesis or release of tPA. While the majority of dysfibrinogenemias cause bleeding, several variants are characterized by excessively rapid release of fibrinopeptides and recurrent thromboembolism. Patients with this disorder as well as those with an abnormal plasminogen that resists activation by streptokinase and urokinase have been treated successfully with heparin and oral anticoagulants. Defects in tPA content or release have not been completely characterized. One group of patients with recurrent venous thrombosis and embolism failed to increase venous blood fibrinolytic activity when challenged with local ischemia or physical exercise. The other group had impaired fibrinolytic activity in extracts prepared from biopsied veins. The cloning of cDNA for tPA coupled with the availability of immunoassays for tPA should facilitate more detailed studies of this class of defects. There is also evidence that young

patients with acute myocardial infarction may have impaired fibrinolysis due to increased plasma levels of PAI, a serine protease inhibitor that binds to tPA and is derived from endothelial cells.

In addition to the inherited disorders that predispose patients to thromboembolism, many common illnesses are associated with an increased risk of thrombosis (see Table 60-5). These patients are said to have a "hypercoagulable" or "prethrombotic" state. This increased risk is seen in patients with chronic congestive heart failure and metastatic malignancy and in patients undergoing major surgery. In these patients, the generation of tissue factor activity in damaged or ischemic tissue or metastatic tumor, coupled with venous stasis and endothelial injury, induces the formation of venous and, more rarely, arterial thrombi. There are also several hematologic disorders including paroxysmal nocturnal hemoglobinuria, essential thrombocythemia, and polycythemia vera in which poorly defined abnormalities in circulating leukocytes and platelets or changes in blood flow and viscosity predispose patients to venous and arterial thrombosis. Diseases that affect the endothelial cell, such as Behçet's syndrome, Kawasaki's disease, and homocystinuria, or the administration of drugs such as the oral contraceptives, which lower antithrombin III levels, or L-asparaginase, which inhibits production of multiple coagulation factors, also may predispose patients to thrombosis. Infusion of granulocyte-macrophage colony stimulating factor (GM-CSF) has been associated with thrombosis as well.

There is increasing interest in the relationship between plasma homocysteine levels and the risk of both venous and arterial thromboembolism. It is well recognized that individuals with the congenital homocystinuria syndrome have, in addition to their Marfanoid habitus, an increased incidence of strokes and coronary artery disease. These patients have well-recognized enzyme defects (see Chap. 349), excrete homocysteine in their urine, and have very high plasma levels of the amino acid. There are also patients with early-onset cerebral vascular events who have mild homocystinuria that can be brought out by a methionine loading test. Epidemiologic studies show a relationship between homocysteine levels that are nearer to the normal range and coronary arterial disease. Although this correlation is not yet definitive, the relationship remains intriguing and of potential clinical relevance.

BIBLIOGRAPHY

ANTONARAKIS SE: The molecular genetics of hemophilia A and B in man. Factor III and factor IX deficiency. Adv Hum Genet 17:17, 1988

DESTEFANO V et al: Inherited thrombophilia: Pathogenesis, clinical syndromes and management. Blood 87:3531, 1996

FEINSTEIN DI: Lupus anticoagulant, anticardiolipin antibodies, fetal loss and systemic lupus erythematosus. Blood 80:859, 1992

GIDDINGS JC, PEAKE IR: Laboratory support in the diagnosis of coagulation disorders. Clin Haematol 14:571, 1985

GINSBURG KJ et al: Anticardiolipin antibodies and the risk for ischemic stroke and venous thrombosis. Ann Intern Med 117:997, 1992

KANE WH, DAVIE EW: Blood coagulation factors V and VIII: Structural and functional similarities and their relationship to hemorrhagic and thrombotic disorders. Blood 71:539, 1988

KASPER CK, DIETRICH SL: Comprehensive management of haemophilia. Clin Haematol 14:489, 1985

LAKICH D et al: Inversions disrupting the factor VIII gene are a common cause of servere hemophilia A. Nat Genet 5:226, 1993

LAWN R: The molecular genetics of hemophilia. Sci Am 254:48, 1986

LUSHER JM et al: Recombinant factor VIII for the treatment of untreated patients with hemophilia A: Safety, efficacy and development of inhibitors. N Engl J Med 328:453, 1993

MAMMEN E: Congenital coagulation disorders. Semin Thromb Hemost 9:1, 1983

PIERCE GF et al: The use of purified clotting factor concentrates in hemophilia. Influence of viral safety, cost and supply on therapy. JAMA 261:3434, 1989

WHITE GC, SHOEMAKER CB: Factor VIII gene and hemophilia A. Blood 73:1, 1989

119 *Robert I. Handin*

ANTICOAGULANT, FIBRINOLYTIC, AND ANTIPLATELET THERAPY

ANTICOAGULANT AND FIBRINOLYTIC THERAPY

Anticoagulation with heparin, followed by treatment with oral vitamin K antagonists, is the standard treatment for acute venous thrombosis and pulmonary embolism. In addition, chronic oral anticoagulation is used to prevent cerebral arterial embolism from cardiac sources such as ventricular mural thrombi, atrial thrombi, or from an atherosclerotic, partially stenosed carotid or vertebral artery. Anticoagulants are also used, less successfully, to treat peripheral or mesenteric arterial thrombosis. These agents retard fibrin deposition on established thrombi and prevent the formation of new thrombi. The induction of a fibrinolytic state by the infusion of plasminogen activators such as recombinant tissue plasminogen activator (rtPA), streptokinase (SK), or urokinase (UK) has become an accepted mode of therapy for some thromboembolic disorders. Fibrinolytic therapy has been proposed for patients with massive pulmonary embolism and systemic hypotension and to restore the patency of acutely occluded peripheral and coronary arteries. Prompt fibrinolytic therapy can reduce both myocardial damage and mortality following acute coronary occlusion (see Chap. 243). Fibrinolytic therapy may also be effective in acute thrombotic strokes and in venoocclusive disease of the liver.

ACUTE ANTICOAGULATION WITH HEPARIN Heparin is a naturally occurring mucopolysaccharide polymer with tetrasaccharide sequences that bind to and activate antithrombin III. It is an extremely potent anticoagulant that can dramatically reduce thrombin generation and fibrin formation in patients with acute venous and arterial thrombosis or embolism (Table 119-1). Heparin is administered to patients with acute thrombosis or embolism by continuous intravenous infusion at a rate sufficient to raise the activated partial thromboplastin time (APTT) to 1.5 to 2 times the patient's preheparin APTT. This requires infusion of approximately 1000 U.S.P. units per hour and is continued while patients are begun on oral anticoagulants and achieve appropriate prolongation of the prothrombin time. The usual duration of combined heparin-warfarin therapy is 5 to 7 days. Heparin is then discontinued, and the patient is maintained on warfarin. Alternatives to a continuous infusion include the administration of 5000 U.S.P. units of heparin four times a day either subcutaneously or intravenously. Commercial heparin preparations are heterogeneous, with only 20 percent of the product biologically active. In addition, active heparin fractions may vary considerably in molecular weight.

Table 119-1

Anticoagulant Therapy with Heparin

Clinical Indication	Dose, U.S.P. Units	Route
Prophylaxis in general surgery	5000 q 12 h	SC
Prophylaxis in medical patients with congestive heart failure, cardiomyopathy, or myocardial infarction	10,000 q 12 h	SC
Venous thromboembolism (acute)	5000 (bolus), then 1000 qh	IV
Venous thromboembolism (prophylaxis in pregnancy, warfarin failures, or chronic disseminated intravascular coagulation)	1000 qh	SC pump

ABBREVIATION: SC, subcutaneous

Biologically active, low-molecular-weight heparin preparations, while more expensive than unfractionated heparin, have several advantages: (1) they can be administered subcutaneously once or twice daily, (2) their pharmacokinetics are so predictable that APTT monitoring is not necessary, and (3) they are less immunogenic and less likely to cause thrombocytopenia. Many patients with deep venous thrombosis, a frequent cause for hospitalization, can be given low-molecular-weight heparin as outpatients. Given their other advantages and equivalent efficacy, low-molecule-weight heparin preparations may replace unfractionated heparin.

Long-term heparin administration via portable external or implantable pumps is occasionally needed for patients with recurrent thromboembolism that is refractory to oral anticoagulants, for pregnant women with thromboembolism, and for patients with chronic disseminated intravascular coagulation (DIC). Lower doses of heparin (5000 U.S.P. units every 12 h) have also been used to prevent deep venous thrombosis in high-risk surgical and medical patients. Patients with congestive heart failure, myocardial infarction, or cardiomyopathy may require 10,000 U.S.P. units every 12 h for similar protection.

The major complication of heparin therapy is bleeding—especially from surgical sites and into the retroperitoneum. Aspirin or aspirin-containing drugs impair platelet function. Thus, intramuscular injections in patients on both heparin and an antiplatelet drug may cause significant bleeding. Heparin's anticoagulant effect can be rapidly reversed by the administration of protamine sulfate. However, this is usually not necessary, since reduction or omission of a heparin dose usually improves hemostasis and stops bleeding. Thrombocytopenia occurs in about 10 percent of heparin recipients and is usually mild, with the platelet count falling to 50,000 to 100,000/μL. Thrombocytopenia is more common in patients receiving heparin derived from beef lung as opposed to porcine intestinal mucosa. Thus, porcine heparin is the preferred agent. As previously discussed, low-molecular-weight heparin is less likely to cause thrombocytopenia. Unfortunately, the majority of the antibodies arising from exposure to unfractionated heparin cross-react, so low-molecular-weight heparin cannot usually be used to treat patients with established thrombocytopenia. Occasionally, thrombocytopenia can be severe and may be accompanied by intravascular platelet agglutination and arterial thrombosis. Recognition of the rare complication of thrombocytopenia and paradoxical thrombosis is critical, since discontinuing heparin can promptly reverse the syndrome and may be lifesaving. Heparin administration for longer than 5 months also carries a risk of osteoporosis, perhaps through its activation of osteoclasts.

CHRONIC ORAL ANTICOAGULATION The coumarin anticoagulants, which include warfarin and dicumarol (dicoumarol), prevent the reduction of vitamin K epoxides in liver microsomes and induce a state analogous to vitamin K deficiency (see Fig. 118-1). They slow thrombin generation and clot formation by impairing the biologic activity of the prothrombin complex proteins and are used to prevent the recurrence of venous thrombosis and pulmonary embolism. Although regimens employing loading doses of drug have been advocated, the simplest way to induce anticoagulation is to administer a single dose of a coumarin compound and monitor the prothrombin time (PT) until the desired prolongation is achieved. For example, treatment can be initiated with 5 to 10 mg/d of warfarin or equivalent, with the goal of prolonging the PT to 1.5 to 2 times the control value. Although the PT may reach this value after a few days of therapy, effective anticoagulation, with stable reduction of all the prothrombin complex proteins, requires at least 1 week of warfarin administration. Most patients require a daily maintenance dose of 2.5 to 7.5 mg of warfarin to remain anticoagulated. As discussed above, patients should remain on heparin until the appropriate dose of a coumarin anticoagulant, such as warfarin, is established.

There is increasing concern that a more precise method is needed to assess the intensity of anticoagulation with warfarin. Commercial thromboplastins have different potencies and markedly affect the resulting PT. The International Normalized Ratio (INR) method has been adopted by most hospital laboratories and clinicians. In this reporting method, the ratio of the patient's PT is compared to the

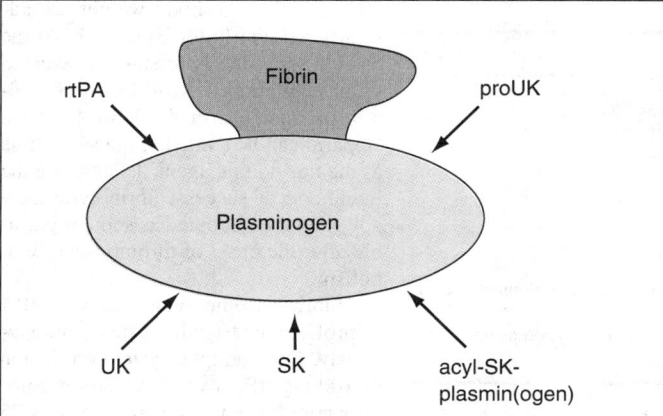

FIGURE 119-1   The mechanism of action of various plasminogen activators used for thrombolytic therapy. Recombinant tissue plasminogen activator (rtPA) and pro-urokinase (proUK) preferentially activate plasminogen bound to fibrin and are called "fibrin-specific" activators. Urokinase (UK), streptokinase (SK), and acylated streptokinase-plasminogen conjugates activate both free and fibrin-bound plasminogen.

mean PT for a group of normal individuals. The ratio is adjusted for the sensitivity of the laboratory's thromboplastin determined by the International Sensitivity Index (ISI). Thus, INR = $(PT_{patient}/PT_{normal})^{ISI}$. Use of the INR permits physicians to obtain the appropriate level of anticoagulation independent of laboratory reagents and to follow published recommendations for intensity of anticoagulation. The intensity of anticoagulation may be varied somewhat depending on the clinical indication. For example, the goal for anticoagulation in patients with venous thrombosis is to achieve an INR of 2 to 3. Patients with paroxysmal atrial fibrillation or a porcine bioprosthetic valve, who are taking a warfarin anticoagulant as a prophylactic measure, may be protected with an INR of 1.5 to 2. In contrast, patients with lupus-like anticoagulants and thromboembolism or those patients with mechanical cardiac valves require more intense anticoagulation. Satisfactory control requires an INR of 3 to 4. Patients with chronic indwelling venous catheters may be maintained on 1 mg/d of warfarin to prevent clot formation at the catheter tip; such a dose has no effect on the PT.

Although warfarin anticoagulants reduce the recurrence of deep venous thrombosis and pulmonary or cerebral embolism, they may also cause bleeding. Any patient who takes oral anticoagulants requires frequent monitoring of the PT. Despite the most careful management, fluctuations in PT can occur. Various drugs that alter liver microsomal metabolism of coumarins or compete for albumin-binding sites can increase or decrease the potency of these drugs (Table 119-2).

There is a direct relation between the duration of anticoagulation and the risk of recurrent thrombosis. Although recommendations vary somewhat, most patients with a single uncomplicated thromboembolic event have maximal benefit after 3 to 6 months of anticoagulation. About 10 percent of patients on an oral anticoagulant for 1 year have a serious complication requiring medical supervision, and 0.5 to 1 percent have a fatal hemorrhagic event despite careful medical management. The anticoagulant effects of coumarins can be reversed by infusion of fresh frozen plasma or by the administration of vitamin K. In many cases, reduction or omission of several doses improves hemostasis and stops hemorrhage. Despite the risk of bleeding, patients with prosthetic heart valves, severe mitral stenosis, cardiomyopathy, chronic congestive heart failure, recurrent or persistent atrial fibrillation, or an inherited "prethrombotic" disorder may require lifelong anticoagulation.

One devastating complication of oral anticoagulation is hemorrhagic skin necrosis. Some patients with this complication are deficient in protein C, a natural anticoagulant protein whose activity is reduced by vitamin K antagonists. Patients with suspected protein C deficiency should not begin oral anticoagulant therapy unless they simultaneously

Table 119-2

Effect of Drugs and Metabolic Changes on Oral Anticoagulant Potency

I. Factors leading to enhanced potency and increased prothrombin time
  A. Reduced coumarin clearance
    1. Disulfiram
    2. Metronidazole
    3. Trimethoprim-sulfamethoxazole
  B. Reduced albumin binding
    Phenylbutazone
  C. Additive hemostatic effect of certain drugs or disorders
    1. Aspirin
    2. Heparin
    3. Liver disease
    4. Thrombocytopenia
    5. Vitamin K deficiency
  D. Increased turnover of vitamin K
    1. Clofibrate
    2. Hypermetabolism (e.g., hyperthyroidism)
II. Factors leading to diminished potency and decreased prothrombin time
  A. Accelerated coumarin clearance—induction of hepatic metabolizing enzymes
    1. Barbiturates
    2. Rifampin
  B. Reduced absorption
    Cholestyramine
  C. Impaired metabolism
    Genetic coumarin resistance

receive heparin or plasma infusions to restore protein C levels to normal. Patients with an inherited trait that causes coumarin resistance may require extremely high doses to get an anticoagulant effect. Psychologically disturbed patients may surreptitiously ingest coumarin and present with unexplained bleeding and a prolonged PT. Plasma coumarin levels can be measured to confirm such ingestion.

FIBRINOLYTIC THERAPY   Fibrinolysis, an important part of the normal hemostatic process, is initiated by the release of either tissue plasminogen activator (tPA) or pro-urokinase (proUK) from endothelial cells. These agents preferentially activate plasminogen, which is adsorbed onto fibrin clots. This serves to direct and localize the lytic process to sites that contain fibrin thrombi. Although fibrinolysis begins immediately after vascular injury, clot lysis and vessel recanalization may not be complete for 7 to 10 days. As previously discussed (see Chap. 60), the fibrinolytic pathway is important in normal hemostasis, as defects can predispose patients to either hemorrhage or recurrent thrombosis (see Chap. 118). Activators of the fibrinolytic system are frequently used to accelerate clot lysis in patients with thromboembolism (see Fig. 119-1, Table 119-3).

The pharmacologic agents being used to accelerate clot lysis are either derived from natural products or are chemically modified derivatives. They differ with respect to fibrin specificity and some types of complications (see Table 119-3). For example, many individuals have antistreptococcal antibodies that react with streptokinase and reduce its potency and cause febrile reactions. All fibrinolytic agents cause hemorrhage. tPA, proUK, and several other agents are relatively "fibrin-specific" and preferentially activate plasminogen in the presence of fibrin. Although this makes it theoretically possible to achieve selective clot lysis, in practice there is little difference in either the efficacy or toxicity of the "specific" and "nonspecific" fibrinolytic agents. There is, however, a substantial difference in cost, with equivalent doses of rtPA costing ten times that of SK.

It is important to remember that there is always some systemic fibrinolysis after the infusion of clinically effective doses of fibrin-specific agents. In fact, the fibrinogen level falls approximately 25 percent after infusion of lytic doses of rtPA. In addition, both the fibrin-specific and -nonspecific agents can cause hemorrhage as they cannot differentiate between vital hemostatic plugs and pathologic thrombi. To minimize the risk of bleeding, systemic lytic therapy is

Table 119-3

Fibrinolytic Activators

Product	Source	Molecular Weight	Fibrin	Complications
Recombinant tissue plasminogen activator (rtPA)	Recombinant	70,000	+	Bleeding
Pro-urokinase (proUK)	Melanoma cell cultures	55,000	+	Bleeding
Urokinase (UK)	Renal tubular cell cultures	33,000	+	Bleeding
Streptokinase (SK)	β-Hemolytic streptococci	47,000	−	Immune reactions—hypotension, fever Bleeding
Acyl-SK-plasmin(ogen)	Chemical synthesis	139,000	+/−	Immune reactions—hypotension, fever Bleeding

not recommended for patients with recent surgery or a history of neurologic lesions, gastrointestinal bleeding, or hypertension.

The current indications for fibrinolytic therapy are listed in Table 119-4. Fibrinolytic agents have been given to patients with pulmonary embolism for over 30 years. Such therapy is currently recommended for patients with massive pulmonary embolism that is complicated by hypotension, hypoxemia, and right heart strain. It is also used for selected patients with peripheral arterial embolism or occlusion and for patients with extensive iliofemoral thrombophlebitis. While lytic therapy may hasten the resolution of venous thrombi, the long-term benefit still remains unproven, and there is no firm evidence that lytic therapy reduces postphlebitic complications. In contrast, fibrinolytic therapy may be of distinct benefit in patients with axillary vein thrombosis, a condition that does not usually respond to conventional anticoagulation. Fibrinolytic agents are also used to restore the patency of occluded venous catheters and dialysis shunts. For this indication the agents are instilled locally. The extensive literature on the use of fibrinolytic agents to treat patients with coronary artery disease and myocardial infarction is reviewed in Chap. 243. When given within a few hours of infarction, fibrinolytic therapy reduces mortality and myocardial damage.

Although the doses and mode of administration may differ slightly, the general principles and complications are the same for all the fibrinolytic agents. SK and UK are the oldest and most extensively studied fibrinolytic agents. SK is a bacterial enzyme, and UK is a product of renal tubular epithelial cells. SK is an indirect plasminogen activator that interacts with circulating plasminogen to form an equimolar complex with proteolytic activity. The SK-plasminogen complex then activates additional plasminogen molecules that initiate fibrinolysis. In contrast, UK has intrinsic proteolytic activity and can activate plasminogen directly.

In the case of SK, a loading dose of 250,000 units is usually given irrespective of body weight. Since patients may have antistreptococcal antibodies, the loading dose may need to be repeated. In addition, patients may develop acute allergic symptoms including urticaria and, occasionally, serum sickness reactions. With UK, a loading dose of 4400 units per kilogram body weight is administered over 10 to 30 min. Both regimens induce an intense lytic state as evidenced by a drop in fibrinogen, prolongation of the thrombin time, and a prolongation of the euglobulin lysis time—an in vitro measure of fibrinolytic activity. After the initial loading dose, 100,000 units of SK or 4400 units of

Table 119-4

Indications for Fibrinolytic Therapy

Acute coronary occlusion/infarction
Acute peripheral arterial occlusion
Massive pulmonary embolism
Axillary vein thrombosis
Massive iliofemoral vein thrombosis
Occluded arteriovenous shunt
Arterial or venous cannulae
Venoocclusive disease of the liver

UK per kilogram body weight are administered hourly for 24 to 72 h. At the desired time, the lytic state is reversed by discontinuing UK or SK and by administering heparin for 7 to 10 days. Heparin can be started at the same time as the fibrinolytic agent. To enhance the likelihood of success, fibrinolytic therapy should be initiated as soon as possible after the onset of thrombosis or embolism.

Fibrin-specific agents such as rtPA or proUK are also administered intravenously. For example, systemic infusion of 100 mg rtPA over 6 h restores coronary artery patency in approximately 75 percent of patients. Patients are then maintained on heparin for several days. ProUK given in a similar manner has almost identical effects.

ANTIPLATELET DRUG THERAPY

Antiplatelet drugs have a role to play in the management of patients with arterial vascular disease and thromboembolism (see Table 119-5). Aspirin is the most widely studied of these drugs because of its unique pharmacology. A single dose of aspirin irreversibly acetylates and inactivates the enzyme cyclooxygenase and thereby inhibits platelet production of thromboxane A_2. Although aspirin may also inactivate cyclooxygenase in some tissues, including endothelial cells, such cells recover rapidly by synthesizing new enzyme. Platelets, which are anucleate, cannot synthesize new enzyme and remain inactive for the rest of their life span. As little as one 160-mg tablet of aspirin daily or a 325-mg tablet every other day inhibits platelet thromboxane production and aggregation.

Patients with coronary artery disease who have unstable angina are at high risk for myocardial infarction (Chap. 243). In two large clinical trials, the prompt administration of aspirin dramatically reduced progression to myocardial infarction in this group, although aspirin had no effect on the frequency, intensity, or duration of chronic angina. Aspirin also reduces the incidence of second infarction by 25 percent when administered to men who have had a myocardial infarct. In a large study of male physicians, daily aspirin therapy also reduced the incidence of first infarcts and is now widely used for prevention of myocardial infarction. The preliminary results of large-scale clinical and epidemiologic studies carried out in women suggest that the same beneficial effects of aspirin may be expected. The combination of aspirin and dipyridamole, when begun before surgery, may also increase the patency of coronary bypass grafts, and the same combination reduces the incidence of cerebral emboli in patients on warfarin who have prosthetic intracardiac valves. Although dipyridamole has been a popular antithrombotic agent, it has little efficacy when given alone. There is abundant evidence that aspirin is probably the only active agent in the combination aspirin-dipyridamole trials. Thus, dipyridamole can be eliminated in favor of aspirin alone.

Table 119-5

Indications for Antiplatelet Drug Therapy

A. Cerebrovascular disease
  1. Transient ischemic attacks
  2. Secondary prevention of cerebrovascular accidents
B. Cardiovascular disease
  1. Unstable angina pectoris
  2. Primary prevention of myocardial infarction
  3. Secondary prevention of myocardial infarction
  4. Following coronary bypass grafting
  5. Following insertion of a prosthetic valve
C. Renal disease
  1. To maintain the patency of arteriovenous cannulas
  2. ? To slow the progression of glomerular disease

Aspirin also reduces the frequency of transient ischemic attacks in patients with occlusive cerebrovascular disease. It has largely supplanted anticoagulation with the coumarin compounds in patients with transient ischemia. Aspirin also reduces the incidence of a second stroke by 25 percent when administered to men following the first cerebrovascular accident. Aspirin is also effective in maintaining the patency of arteriovenous cannulas inserted into patients with renal failure who require hemodialysis. Aspirin plus dipyridamole may also slow the progression of some forms of glomerulonephritis, although these drugs are not widely used in the treatment of renal disease. However, aspirin appears not to be effective in maintaining the patency of vessels following percutaneous angioplasty.

Although aspirin is clearly the most efficacious antiplatelet agent in clinical use today, there are a large number of new drugs being tested that may soon supplement aspirin therapy. Ticlopidine, which is a potent inhibitor of platelet function, has shown efficacy in several clinical trials. It is being used as an alternative to aspirin in patients with cerebrovascular disease and is superior to aspirin or warfarin-type anticoagulants in maintaining coronary stent patency. Monoclonal antibodies and both recombinant and chemically synthesized peptides that block either platelet adhesion or aggregation are being tested in clinical trials. A monoclonal antibody that blocks fibrinogen binding to platelet GpIIb/IIIa and thereby inhibits platelet aggregation (RheoPro) has been thoroughly tested and is now licensed for use in patients with coronary artery disease who undergo angioplasty. RheoPro is also being evaluated in other settings, e.g., as an adjunct to fibrinolytic therapy in patients with an acute myocardial infarction. There are also several orally active GpIIb/IIIa inhibitors in clinical trials that could be used chronically in patients with various coronary artery syndromes.

See Chap. 54, Anticoagulant, thrombolytic and antiplatelet drugs, in Goodman & Gilman's The Pharmacological Basis of Therapeutics 9th ed, New York, McGraw-Hill, 1996, pp 1341–1359.

BIBLIOGRAPHY

AMERICAN COLLEGE OF CHEST PHYSICIANS: Fourth Consensus Conference on Antithrombotic Therapy. Chest 108(Suppl): 2255, 1995

COLLER BS: Platelets and thrombolytic therapy. N Engl J Med 322:33, 1990

LEVINE MN, HIRSH J: Hemorrhagic complications of anticoagulation therapy. Semin Thromb Hemost 12L:39, 1986

SAOUR JN et al: Trial of different intensities of anticoagulation in patients with prosthetic heart valves. N Engl J Med 322:428, 1990

SCHWARTZ L, SEIDELIN PH: Antithrombotic and thrombolytic therapy in patients undergoing coronary artery intervention: A review. Prog Cardiovasc Dis 38:67, 1995

120 *Lawrence C. Madoff, Dennis L. Kasper*

INTRODUCTION TO INFECTIOUS DISEASES: HOST-PARASITE INTERACTION

Despite decades of dramatic progress in their treatment and prevention, infectious diseases remain a major cause of death and debility and are responsible for worsening the living conditions of many millions of people around the world. Infections frequently challenge the physician's diagnostic skill and must be considered in the differential diagnoses of syndromes affecting a multitude of organ systems.

With the advent of antimicrobial agents, some medical leaders believed that infectious diseases would soon be eliminated and become of historic interest only. Indeed, the hundreds of chemotherapeutic agents developed since World War II, most of which are potent and safe, include drugs effective not only against bacteria but also against viruses, fungi, and parasites. Nevertheless, we now realize that, as we developed antimicrobial agents, microbes developed the ability to elude our best weapons and to counterattack with new survival strategies. Antibiotic resistance occurs at an alarming rate among all classes of mammalian pathogens. Diseases once thought to have been nearly eradicated from the developed world—tuberculosis, cholera, and rheumatic fever, for example—have rebounded with renewed ferocity. Newly discovered and emerging infectious agents appear to have been brought into contact with humans by changes in the environment and movements of populations. Many of these agents have been discovered only in recent decades. Ebola virus, hantavirus, the agent of human granulocytic ehrlichiosis, and retroviruses such as human immunodeficiency virus (HIV) humble us despite our deepening understanding of pathogenesis at the most basic molecular level. Even in developed countries, infectious diseases have made a resurgence. Between 1980 and 1992, age-adjusted mortality from infectious diseases in the United States increased by 39 percent. The role of infectious agents in the etiology of diseases once believed to be noninfectious is being increasingly recognized. For example, it is now widely accepted that *Helicobacter pylori* is the causative agent of peptic ulcer disease and perhaps of gastric malignancy. Human papillomavirus is likely to be the most important cause of invasive cervical cancer. A new human herpesvirus (HHV-8) is believed to be the cause of most cases of Kaposi's sarcoma. Epstein-Barr virus is a likely cause of certain lymphomas and may play a role in the genesis of Hodgkin's disease. The possibility certainly exists that other diseases of unknown cause, such as rheumatoid arthritis, sarcoidosis, or inflammatory bowel disease, have infectious etiologies.

Medical advances over infectious diseases have been hindered by changes in the patient population. Immunocompromised hosts now constitute a significant proportion of the seriously infected population. Physicians immunosuppress their patients to prevent the rejection of transplants and to treat neoplastic and inflammatory diseases. Some infections, most notably that caused by HIV, immunocompromise the host in and of themselves. Lesser degrees of immunosuppression are associated with other infections, such as influenza and syphilis. Infectious agents that coexist peacefully with immunocompetent hosts wreak havoc in those who lack a complete immune system. AIDS has brought to prominence once-obscure organisms such as *Pneumocystis carinii*, *Cryptosporidium parvum*, and *Mycobacterium avium*.

For any infectious process to occur, the parasite and the host must first encounter each other. Factors such as geography, environment, and behavior thus influence the likelihood of infection. Though the initial encounter between a susceptible host and a virulent organism frequently results in disease, some organisms can be harbored in the host for years before disease becomes clinically evident. For a complete view, individual patients must be considered in the context of the population. Infectious diseases often do not occur in isolation; rather, they spread through a group exposed from a point source (e.g., a contaminated water supply) or from individual to individual (e.g., via respiratory droplets). Thus, the clinician must be alert to infections prevalent in the community as a whole. A detailed history, including information on travel, behavioral factors, exposures to animals or potentially contaminated environments, and living and occupational conditions, must be elicited. For example, the likelihood of infection by *Plasmodium falciparum* can be significantly affected by altitude, climate, terrain, season, and even time of day. Antibiotic-resistant strains are localized to specific geographic regions, and a seemingly minor alteration in a travel itinerary can dramatically influence the likelihood of acquiring chloroquine-resistant malaria. If such important details in the history are overlooked, inappropriate treatment may result in the death of the patient. Likewise, the chance of acquiring a sexually transmitted disease can be greatly affected by relatively minor variation in sexual practices, such as the method used for birth control. Knowledge of the relationship between specific risk factors and disease allows the physician to influence a patient's health even before the development of infection by modification of these risk factors and—when a vaccine is available—by immunization.

Many specific host factors influence the likelihood of acquiring an infectious disease. Age, immunization history, prior illnesses, level of nutrition, pregnancy, coexisting illness, and perhaps emotional state all have some impact on the risk of infection after exposure to a potential pathogen. The importance of individual host defense mechanisms, either specific or nonspecific, becomes apparent in their absence, and our understanding of these immune mechanisms is enhanced by studies of clinical syndromes developing in immunodeficient patients (Table 120-1). For example, the frequent occurrence of meningococcal disease in people with deficiencies in specific complement proteins of the "membrane attack complex" underscores the importance of an intact complement system in the prevention of meningococcal infection.

Medical care itself increases the patient's risk of acquiring an infection in several ways: (1) through contact with pathogens during hospitalization; (2) through breaching of the skin (with intravenous devices or surgical incisions) or mucosal surfaces (with endotracheal tubes or bladder catheters); (3) through introduction of foreign bodies; (4) through alteration of the natural flora with antibiotics; and (5) through treatment with immunosuppressive drugs.

Infection involves complicated interactions of parasite and host and inevitably affects both. In most cases, a pathogenic process consisting of several steps is required for the development of infections. Since the competent host has a complex series of barricades in place to prevent infection, the successful parasite must utilize specific strategies at each of these steps. The specific strategies used by bacteria (see Chap. 139), viruses (see Chap. 182), and parasites have some remarkable conceptual similarities, but the strategic details are unique not only for each class of organism but also for individual species within a class.

Table 120-1

Infections Associated with Common Defects in Inflammatory or Immunologic Response

Host Defect	Disease or Therapy Associated with Defect	Common Etiologic Agent of Infection
NONSPECIFIC IMMUNITY		
Impaired cough	Rib fracture, neuromuscular dysfunction	Bacteria causing pneumonia, aerobic and anaerobic oral flora
Loss of gastric acidity	Achlorhydria, histamine blockade	*Salmonella* spp., enteric pathogens
Loss of cutaneous integrity	Penetrating trauma, athlete's foot	*Staphylococcus* spp., *Streptococcus* spp.
	Burn	*Pseudomonas aeruginosa*
	Intravenous catheter	*Staphylococcus* spp., *Streptococcus* spp., gram-negative rods, coagulase-negative staphylococci
Implantable device	Heart valve	*Streptococcus* spp., coagulase-negative staphylococci, *Staphylococcus aureus*
	Artificial joint	*Staphylococcus* spp., *Streptococcus* spp., gram-negative rods
Loss of normal bacterial flora	Antibiotic use	*Clostridium difficile*, *Candida* spp.
Impaired clearance		
Poor drainage	Urinary tract infection	*Escherichia coli*
Abnormal secretions	Cystic fibrosis	Chronic pulmonary infection with *P. aeruginosa*
INFLAMMATORY RESPONSE		
Neutropenia	Hematologic malignancy, cytotoxic chemotherapy, aplastic anemia, HIV infection	Gram-negative enteric bacilli, *Pseudomonas* spp., *Staphylococcus* spp., *Candida* spp.
Chemotaxis	Chédiak-Higashi syndrome, Job's syndrome, protein-calorie malnutrition	*S. aureus*, *Streptococcus pyogenes*, *Haemophilus influenzae*, gram-negative bacilli
Phagocytosis (cellular)	Systemic lupus erythematosus, chronic myelogenous leukemia, megaloblastic anemia	*Streptococcus pneumoniae*, *H. influenzae*
Splenectomy	—	*H. influenzae*, *S. pneumoniae*, other streptococci, *Capnocytophaga* spp., *Babesia microti*, *Salmonella* spp.
Microbicidal defect	Chronic granulomatous disease	Catalase-positive bacteria and fungi: staphylococci, *E. coli*, *Klebsiella* spp., *P. aeruginosa*, *Aspergillus* spp., *Nocardia* spp.
	Chédiak-Higashi syndrome	*S. aureus*, *S. pyogenes*
	Interferon γ-receptor defect	*Mycobacterium* spp., *Salmonella* spp.
COMPLEMENT SYSTEM		
C3	Congenital liver disease, systemic lupus erythematosus, nephrotic syndrome	*S. aureus*, *S. pneumoniae*, *Pseudomonas* spp., *Proteus* spp.
C5	Congenital	*Neisseria* spp., gram-negative rods
C6, C7, C8	Congenital, systemic lupus erythematosus	*Neisseria meningitidis*, *Neisseria gonorrhoeae*
Alternative pathway	Sickle cell disease	*S. pneumoniae*, *Salmonella* spp.
IMMUNE RESPONSE		
T lymphocyte deficiency/ dysfunction	Thymic aplasia, thymic hypoplasia, Hodgkin's disease, sarcoidosis, lepromatous leprosy	*Listeria monocytogenes*, *Mycobacterium* spp., *Candida* spp., *Aspergillus* spp., *Cryptococcus neoformans*, herpes simplex virus, varicella-zoster virus
	AIDS	*Pneumocystis carinii*, cytomegalovirus, herpes simplex virus, *Mycobacterium avium-intracellulare*, *C. neoformans*, *Candida* spp.
	Mucocutaneous candidiasis	*Candida* spp.
	Purine nucleoside phosphorylase deficiency	Fungi, viruses
B cell deficiency/dysfunction	Bruton's X-linked agammaglobulinemia	*S. pneumoniae*, other streptococci
	Agammaglobulinemia, chronic lymphocytic leukemia, multiple myeloma, dysglobulinemia	*H. influenzae*, *N. meningitidis*, *S. aureus*, *Klebsiella pneumoniae*, *E. coli*, *Giardia lamblia*, *P. carinii*, enteroviruses
	Selective IgM deficiency	*S. pneumoniae*, *H. influenzae*, *E. coli*
	Selective IgA deficiency	*G. lamblia*, hepatitis virus, *S. pneumoniae*, *H. influenzae*
Mixed T and B cell deficiency/ dysfunction	Common variable hypogammaglobulinemia	*P. carinii*, cytomegalovirus, *S. pneumoniae*, *H. influenzae*, various other bacteria
	Ataxia-telangiectasia	*S. pneumoniae*, *H. influenzae*, *S. aureus*, rubella virus, *G. lamblia*
	Severe combined immunodeficiency	*S. aureus*, *S. pneumoniae*, *H. influenzae*, *Candida albicans*, *P. carinii*, varicella-zoster virus, rubella virus, cytomegalovirus
	Wiskott-Aldrich syndrome	Agents of infections associated with T and B cell abnormalities

SOURCE: Adapted from H Masur and A Fauci, in *Harrison's Principles of Internal Medicine,* 13th ed, KJ Isselbacher et al (eds), New York, McGraw-Hill, 1994.

SURFACE CONTACT Most often, the first contact between host and parasite is at a mucosal or cutaneous surface. In order to prevent the initiation of the infectious process during such contact, the host has developed highly effective defense mechanisms operating at the body's interface with the outside world. Many of these initial mechanisms of host defense are not specifically directed at individual species of organisms. Mechanical barriers, for example, including the tough cornified epithelium of the skin and the flow of secretions from glands, tend to prevent infection by any potential pathogen. Chemical barriers, such as the acidic environment of the stomach and urinary bladder, represent hostile environments for most microorganisms. The

CHAPTER 120
Introduction to Infectious Diseases: Host-Parasite Interaction

751

bladder, represent hostile environments for most microorganisms. The normal microflora, composed of nonpathogenic organisms that inhabit mucosal surfaces, makes colonization by pathogens more difficult by competing for environmental resources. Behavioral and neurologic mechanisms, such as gagging and coughing, help prevent infection of the lower respiratory tract.

We recognize the importance of these mechanisms by the diseases that arise when they are impaired (Table 120-1). Patients with a suppressed cough (e.g., due to pain associated with a fractured rib) are very susceptible to pneumonia. Achlorhydric individuals are particularly likely to develop salmonellosis after the ingestion of contaminated food or drink because a lower inoculum is required for organisms to reach the intestine. The abnormal bronchial secretions in patients with cystic fibrosis usually permit chronic pulmonary infection with *Pseudomonas aeruginosa*. A break in the skin resulting from an animal or insect bite, a burn, a scratch, trauma, or surgery allows the entry of pathogenic or opportunistic agents. The eradication of the normal bowel flora by antibiotics may render organisms such as *Clostridium difficile* pathogenic.

The host has also evolved an organism-specific immune system that functions at mucosal surfaces. Specialized macrophages and lymphocytes, which play a role in the specific defense system, reside in the epithelium of the gut, in the nasal and vaginal mucosae, and at other sites that interface with the environment. This mucosa-associated lymphoid tissue appears to play a role in trapping antigens and allowing them to be presented to lymphocytes at the mucosal surface. In certain areas, these tissues become anatomically distinct; examples include the oropharyngeal tonsil and—in the gastrointestinal tract—Peyer's patches and the appendix. Central to this defense system is the elaboration of surface immunoglobulins, particularly secretory IgA, which prevents adherence and penetration of organisms.

Pathogens have evolved an array of methods for breaching this well-developed boundary between the host and the outside world. In order to invade, most pathogens must first attach. Many microorganisms have developed a highly specialized apparatus for binding to the surface of the host. For example, pili of uropathogenic *Escherichia coli* recognize certain host glycoproteins that serve as sites for bacterial attachment to epithelial cells. The binding of Epstein-Barr virus to a specific complement receptor (CR2) on B lymphocytes allows the subsequent internalization of the virus. HIV binds to the CD4 complex present in certain human T lymphocytes. Many bacterial pathogens produce enzymes or surface components that bind to or inactivate secretory IgA. Other organism factors impair ciliary motility, thus hindering clearance.

Some potentially pathogenic organisms are capable of living symbiotically with the host, colonizing but not infecting for extended periods. It is important for the astute clinician to distinguish colonization from infection. *E. coli* is normally present in large numbers in the colon, where it contributes to the synthesis of vitamin K and induces natural immunity to other bacteria. It is only when *E. coli* penetrates the mucosal barriers and enters normally sterile sites that it becomes an opportunistic pathogen. The penetration of *E. coli* into the peritoneum through a mechanical breach in the bowel wall, its entry into the urinary bladder, and its invasion of the bloodstream are events associated with infection and disease. Some virulent pathogens, such as group A streptococci and *Neisseria meningitidis*, are able to colonize most individuals for prolonged intervals without untoward effects. In these cases, the individuals involved may already have developed specific immunity following colonization with antigenically similar nonpathogenic organisms, or invasion may be prevented by nonspecific host defenses while specific immunity is being stimulated. Certain viruses (e.g., herpesviruses) inhabit tissue for the life of the host, causing little harm as long as the host's immune system is intact but inducing severe symptomatic disease if the immune status is altered.

INVASION Microorganisms attached to a mucosal surface use specific mechanisms to invade deeper host structures. Meningococci and gonococci penetrate and traverse mucosal epithelial cells by transcytotic mechanisms. *Haemophilus influenzae* enters the vascular system by squeezing through the junction between epithelial cells. Salmo-

nellae induce their own phagocytosis by the host's gastrointestinal macrophages (i.e., in Peyer's patches); these bacteria then resist killing by the phagolysosome of the unactivated macrophage and subsequently proliferate, spilling into the bloodstream. Schistosomal cercariae penetrate the epidermis of the host in contaminated fresh water and are able to uncoat, mature, and enter the circulation. Other pathogens, including bacteria (e.g., *Rickettsia rickettsii* and *Yersinia pestis*), viruses (e.g., dengue and eastern equine encephalitis virus), and parasites (e.g., *Plasmodium* and *Trypanosoma*), may enlist the aid of an insect vector to breach the protective skin and enter the circulation.

Infection has a substantial impact on the microorganism as well as the host. It is increasingly recognized that the invading microbe senses and adapts to changes in its environment through complex regulatory mechanisms, "turning on" the virulence factors necessary for invasion and survival in the host. For example, *Yersinia* spp., *Shigella* spp., and *Bordetella pertussis* all express virulence factors in response to exposure to the 37°C temperature likely to be encountered at the time of infection. Other virulence determinants—the Shiga-like toxin of enterohemorrhagic *E. coli*, for example—are expressed in response to low levels of free iron that exist in the host, where iron is tightly bound by transferrin and other proteins. Many such bacterial virulence factors are controlled by two-component regulatory systems: one protein component senses environmental changes and then signals (often by phosphorylation) a second protein that coordinately regulates the expression of a group of genes whose products facilitate survival in the host milieu.

TROPISM In order to infect a host successfully, many pathogens occupy highly specific niches within the host and thus are tropic to a particular body site or cell type. This tropism has many implications for the life cycle of the pathogen, for the immune system of the host, and for the disease process. Malaria sporozoites, for example, are rapidly cleared from the blood into hepatocytes, where they undergo maturation and release into the circulation; trophozoites, in turn, can infect only the erythrocyte. The bacterial pathogen *H. pylori* produces the enzyme urease, which, by cleaving urea to form ammonium ion, may allow the organism to inhabit a neutral microenvironment within the highly acidic gastric mucosa. Many viruses are tropic for specific tissues; for example, the hepatitis viruses are tropic for hepatocytes, HIV is tropic for CD4-bearing T lymphocytes, herpesviruses are tropic for neural tissues, and rhinoviruses are tropic for the nasal epithelium.

The central nervous system (CNS) is uniquely protected from perturbations in the environment by a blood-brain barrier—a system of tight junctions in capillaries of the CNS that resists the entry of inflammatory cells, pathogens, and even macromolecules into the subarachnoid space. Certain pathogens have devised highly specialized, and as yet poorly understood, mechanisms for breaching this barricade. One strategy employed by organisms such as rabies virus and herpes simplex virus in humans and by reovirus in experimental animals is to travel within peripheral nerves into the CNS. Other organisms, such as certain highly encapsulated bacteria and fungi, enter from the bloodstream and possess surface components that allow them to traverse the capillary tight junctions. The degree of specialization required for this mechanism is demonstrated by the predilection of certain serotypes of organisms within a species to cause meningitis. Type III strains account for the vast majority of cases of neonatal meningitis caused by group B *Streptococcus*, even though other serotypes cause much of the invasive disease outside the CNS. This disparity appears to be due solely to the arrangement of the component sugars of the capsular polysaccharide: other serotypes of group B *Streptococcus* rarely cause neonatal meningitis even though their capsules possess the same four component sugars in different structural arrangements.

MICROBIAL VIRULENCE STRATEGIES Microbes have developed a variety of strategies for escaping host immunity. Many bacteria are encapsulated with polysaccharides that allow them to evade complement deposition in the absence of specific antibodies. These organisms proliferate freely until the host is able to generate capsule-specific antibodies. Several species of gram-positive bacteria possess surface proteins that bind immunoglobulins, thereby perhaps interfering with immune recognition. Other organisms even employ the host's immune response as a survival strategy. *Schistosoma mansoni* recognizes the host cytokine tumor necrosis factor (TNF) and responds to it by depositing eggs. Some pathogenic organisms elaborate toxins and enzymes that facilitate invasion of the host and are often responsible for the disease state. Pathogenic strains of *Vibrio cholerae* (Chap. 161) elaborate a potent and well-characterized toxin that enters the host's enterocytes via a specific receptor (the monosialyl GM_1 ganglioside) and then enzymatically activates the host cell's adenylate cyclase system. This event in turn leads to the copious electrolyte and fluid secretion by the enterocyte and the voluminous watery diarrhea that are characteristic of cholera. *Staphylococcus aureus* expresses a large number of extracellular proteins that contribute to the variety of disease states associated with this bacterium (Chap. 142). Enterotoxins cause staphylococcal food poisoning, even though viable organisms may never enter the host. Toxic shock syndrome toxin 1 (TSST-1) is responsible for the many systemic effects of toxic shock syndrome, even though the organism is confined to a mucosal surface or a wound. Toxin-mediated damage to mucosal surfaces sometimes permits proliferation of a pathogen at a mucosal site, whether or not the organism invades. Pertussis toxin impairs the ability of ciliated epithelium to clear the pathogen from the host's bronchial tree. Enteropathogenic *E. coli* and *V. cholerae* are examples of toxin-producing bacteria that normally do not invade. In contrast, other toxins are clearly capable of promoting invasion and spread. The extracellular enzymes of *Streptococcus pyogenes*, such as hyaluronidase, facilitate movement through tissue planes, and streptolysins O and S disrupt leukocyte membranes and thus impair the host's defense.

Integral components of pathogens are often responsible for much of the disease process that results from infection. Lipopolysaccharides of gram-negative bacteria act as a potent endotoxin (*endo-* in this case indicating that the lipopolysaccharides are part of the bacterial membrane, not a secreted product) that is the proximate cause of the sepsis syndrome. The cell walls of gram-positive bacteria appear to elicit a similar host inflammatory response. The anaerobic pathogen *Bacteroides fragilis* possesses a capsular polysaccharide that promotes abscess formation by the host.

IMMUNE RESPONSE   Once in the bloodstream or a normally sterile body site, the microorganism faces the host's tightly integrated cellular and humoral immune systems. Cellular immunity (Chap. 305), comprising T lymphocytes, macrophages, and natural killer cells, primarily recognizes and combats pathogens that proliferate intracellularly. Cellular immune mechanisms are important in immunity to all classes of infectious agents, including most viruses and many bacteria (e.g., *Mycoplasma*, *Chlamydia*, *Listeria*, *Salmonella*, *Mycobacterium*), parasites (e.g., *Trypanosoma*, *Toxoplasma*, *Leishmania*), and fungi (e.g., *Histoplasma*, *Cryptococcus*, and *Coccidioides*). Usually, T lymphocytes are activated by macrophages and B lymphocytes, which present foreign antigens along with the host's own major histocompatibility complex antigen. Activated T cells may then act in several ways to fight infection. Cytotoxic T cells may directly attack and lyse host cells that express foreign antigens. Helper T cells stimulate the proliferation of B cells and the production of immunoglobulins. T cells elaborate cytokines (e.g., interferon), which directly inhibit the growth of pathogens or stimulate killing by host macrophages and cytotoxic cells. Cytokines also augment the host's immunity by stimulating the inflammatory response (fever, the production of acute-phase serum components, and the proliferation of leukocytes). Cytokine stimulation does not always result in a favorable response in the host; septic shock (see Chap. 124) and toxic shock syndrome (see Chaps. 142 and 143) are among the conditions that are mediated by these inflammatory substances.

The reticuloendothelial system comprises monocyte-derived phagocytic cells that are located in the liver (Kupffer cells), lung (alveolar macrophages), spleen, kidney (mesangial cells), brain (micro-

glia), and lymph nodes and that clear circulating microorganisms. Although these tissue macrophages and polymorphonuclear leukocytes (PMNs) are capable of killing microorganisms without help, they function much more efficiently when pathogens are first *opsonized* (from the Greek for "to prepare for eating") by components of the complement system such as C3b and/or by antibodies.

Extracellular pathogens, including most encapsulated bacteria, are attacked by the humoral immune system, which includes antibodies, the complement cascade, and phagocytic cells. Antibodies are complex glycoproteins (also called immunoglobulins) that are produced by mature B lymphocytes, circulate in body fluids, and are secreted on mucosal surfaces. Antibodies specifically recognize and bind to foreign antigens. One of the most impressive features of the immune system is the ability to generate an incredible diversity of antibodies capable of recognizing virtually every foreign antigen yet not reacting with self. In addition to being exquisitely specific for antigens, antibodies come in different structural and functional classes: IgG predominates in the circulation and persists for many years after exposure; IgM is the earliest specific antibody to appear in response to infection; secretory IgA is important in immunity at mucosal surfaces, while monomeric IgA appears in the serum; and IgE is important in allergic and parasitic diseases. Antibodies may act by directly impeding the function of an invading organism, by neutralizing secreted toxins and enzymes, or by facilitating the removal of the antigen (invading organism) by phagocytic cells. Immunoglobulins participate in cell-mediated immunity by promoting the antibody-dependent cellular cytotoxicity functions of certain T lymphocytes. Antibodies also promote the deposition of complement components on the surface of the invader.

The complement system (see Chap. 305) consists of a group of serum proteins that function as a cooperative, self-regulating cascade of enzymes that adhere to—and in some cases disrupt—the surface of invading organisms. Some of these surface-adherent proteins (e.g., C3b) can then act as opsonins for destruction of microbes by phagocytes. The later, "terminal" components (C7, C8, and C9) can directly kill some bacterial invaders (notably, many of the neisseriae) by forming a "membrane attack complex" and disrupting the integrity of the bacterial membrane, thus causing bacteriolysis. Other complement components, such as C5a, act as chemoattractants for PMNs. Complement activation and deposition occur by either or both of two pathways: the classic pathway is activated primarily by immune complexes (i.e., antibody bound to antigen), and the alternative pathway is activated by microbial components, frequently in the absence of antibody. PMNs have receptors for both antibody and C3b, and antibody and complement function together to aid in the clearance of infectious agents.

PMNs, short-lived white blood cells that engulf and kill invading microbes, are first attracted to inflammatory sites by chemoattractants such as C5a, which is a product of complement activation at the site of infection. PMNs localize to the site of infection by adhering to cellular adhesion molecules expressed by endothelial cells. Endothelial cells express these receptors, called *selectins* (CD-62, ELAM-1), in response to inflammatory cytokines such as TNFα and interleukin 1. The binding of these selectin molecules to specific receptors on PMNs results in the adherence of the PMN to the endothelium. Cytokine-mediated upregulation and expression of intercellular adhesion molecule 1 (ICAM 1) on endothelial cells then take place, and this latter receptor binds to β_2 integrins on the PMN, thereby facilitating diapedesis into the extravascular compartment. Once the PMNs are in the extravascular compartment, various molecules such as arachidonic acids further enhance the inflammatory process.

Approach to the Patient

The clinical manifestations of infectious diseases at presentation are myriad, varying from fulminant life-threatening processes to brief and self-limited conditions to indolent chronic maladies. The clinician must use all the skills of medicine to diagnose the infection and prescribe appropriate treatment. First, a careful history is essential and must include details on underlying chronic diseases; medications; occupation; travel; and risk factors for exposure to certain types of pathogens, such as those associated with sexual contacts, family illnesses, illicit drug use, particular animals, blood transfusions, ingestion of contaminated liquids or foods, or bites of insect vectors. Since infectious diseases may involve many organ systems, a careful review of systems may elicit important clues as to the disease process. The physical examination must be thorough, and attention must be paid to seemingly minor details: a soft heart murmur that might indicate bacterial endocarditis; an evanescent skin rash that suggests rheumatic fever; or a retinal lesion that suggests disseminated candidiasis or cytomegalovirus (CMV) infection.

LABORATORY INVESTIGATIONS Laboratory studies must be carefully considered and directed toward establishing an etiologic diagnosis in the shortest possible time, at the lowest possible cost, and with the least possible discomfort to the patient. Cultures must be performed in a manner that minimizes the likelihood of contamination with normal flora while maximizing the yield. A sputum sample is far more likely to be valuable when elicited with careful coaching by the clinician than when collected in a container simply left at the bedside with cursory instruction. Gram's stains of specimens should be interpreted carefully, and the quality of the specimen assessed. The findings on Gram's staining should correspond to the results of culture; a discrepancy may suggest diagnostic possibilities such as infection due to fastidious or anaerobic bacteria.

The microbiology laboratory must be an ally in the diagnostic endeavor (see Chap. 121). Astute laboratory personnel will suggest optimal culture and transport conditions or alternative tests to facilitate diagnosis. If informed about specific potential pathogens, an alert laboratory staff will allow sufficient time for these organisms to become evident in culture, even when present in small numbers or when slow-growing. The parasitology technician who is attuned to the specific diagnostic considerations relevant to a particular case may be able to detect the rare, otherwise-elusive egg or cyst in a stool specimen. In cases where a diagnosis appears difficult, serum should be stored during the early acute phase of the illness so that a diagnostic rise in titer of antibody to a specific pathogen can be detected later. Bacterial and fungal antigens can sometimes be detected in body fluids, even when cultures are negative or are rendered sterile by antibiotic therapy. Techniques such as the polymerase chain reaction allow the amplification of specific DNA sequences so that minute quantities of foreign nucleic acids can be recognized in host specimens.

℞ **TREATMENT**
Optimal therapy for infectious diseases requires a broad knowledge of medicine and careful clinical judgment. Life-threatening infections such as bacterial meningitis or sepsis, viral encephalitis, or falciparum malaria must be treated immediately, often before a specific causative organism is identified. Antimicrobial agents must be chosen empirically and must be active against the range of potential infectious agents consistent with the clinical scenario. In contrast, good clinical judgment sometimes dictates withholding of antimicrobials in a self-limited process or until a specific diagnosis is made. The dictum *primum non nocere* should be adhered to, and it should be remembered that all antimicrobials carry a risk (and a cost) to the patient. Direct toxicity may be encountered—e.g., ototoxicity due to aminoglycosides, bone marrow toxicity due to zidovudine, and hepatotoxicity due to antituberculous agents such as isoniazid and rifampin. Allergic reactions are common and can be serious. Since superinfection sometimes follows the eradication of the normal flora and colonization by a resistant organism, one invariable principle is that infectious disease therapy should be directed toward as narrow a spectrum of infectious agents as possible. Treatment specific for the pathogen should result in as little perturbation as possible of the host's microflora. With few exceptions, abscesses require surgical or percutaneous drainage for cure. Foreign bodies, including medical devices, must generally be removed in order to eliminate an infection of the device or of the adjacent tissue. Other infections, such as necrotizing fasciitis, peritonitis due to a perforated organ, gas gangrene, and chronic osteomyelitis, require surgery as the primary

means of cure; in these conditions, antibiotics play only an adjunctive role.

Recently, the role of immunomodulators in the management of infectious diseases has received increasing attention. Glucocorticoids have been shown to be of benefit in the treatment of *H. influenzae* meningitis in children and in therapy for *P. carinii* pneumonia in patients with AIDS. The use of these agents in other infectious processes remains less clear and in some cases (in cerebral malaria and septic shock, for example) is detrimental. Other agents that modulate the immune response include prostaglandin inhibitors, specific lymphokines, and TNF inhibitors. Specific antibody therapy has been shown to play a role in the treatment and prevention of many diseases. Specific immunoglobulins have long been known to prevent the development of symptomatic rabies and tetanus. More recently, CMV immune globulin has been recognized as important not only in preventing the transmission of the virus during organ transplantation but also in treating CMV pneumonia in bone marrow transplant recipients. There is a strong need for well-designed clinical trials to evaluate each new interventional modality.

PERSPECTIVE The genetic simplicity of many infectious agents allows them to undergo rapid evolution and to develop selective advantages that result in constant variation in the clinical manifestations of infection. Moreover, changes in the environment and the host can predispose new populations to a particular infection. An epidemic of lethal respiratory failure—later identified as hantavirus pulmonary syndrome—on a Navajo reservation in the southwestern United States in 1993 caused nationwide alarm exemplifying the fear that new plagues induce in the human psyche. The potential for infectious agents to emerge in novel and unexpected ways requires that physicians and public health officials be knowledgeable, vigilant, and open-minded in their approach to the consideration of unexplained illness. The emergence of antimicrobial-resistant pathogens (e.g., enterococci that are resistant to all known antimicrobial agents and cause infections that are essentially untreatable) has led some to conclude that we are entering the "postantibiotic era." Others have held to the perception that infectious diseases no longer represent as serious a concern to world health as they once did. The progress that science, medicine, and society as a whole have made in combating these maladies is impressive, and it is ironic that, as we stand on the threshold of an understanding of the most basic biology of the microbe, infectious diseases are posing renewed problems. We are threatened by the appearance of new diseases such as AIDS, hepatitis C, and Ebola virus infection and by the reemergence of old foes like tuberculosis, cholera, plague, and *S. pyogenes* infection. True students of infectious diseases were perhaps less surprised than anyone else by these developments. Those who know pathogens are aware of their incredible adaptability and diversity. As ingenious and successful as therapeutic approaches may be, our ability to develop methods to counter infectious agents so far has not matched the myriad strategies employed by the sea of microbes that surrounds us. Their sheer numbers and the rate at which they can evolve are daunting. Moreover, environmental changes, rapid global travel, population movements, and medicine itself—through its use of antibiotics and immunosuppressive agents—all increase the impact of infectious diseases. Although new vaccines, new antibiotics, improved global communication, and new modalities for treating and preventing infection will be developed, pathogenic microbes will continue to develop new strategies of their own, presenting us with an unending and dynamic challenge.

BIBLIOGRAPHY

BERKELMAN RL, HUGHES JM: The conquest of infectious diseases: Who are we kidding? Ann Intern Med 119:426, 1993

BUCKLEY RH: Immunodeficiency diseases. JAMA 268:2797, 1992

FIELDS BN: Pathogenesis of viral infections, in *Virology*, BN Fields (ed). New York, Raven, 1996, pp 191–239

MAHMOUD A: Parasitic protozoa and helminths. Science 246:1015, 1989

NEWPORT MJ et al: A mutation in the interferon-γ-receptor gene and susceptibility to mycobacterial infection. N Engl J Med 335:1941, 1996

NICAS TI, EISENSTEIN BI: Introduction to bacterial diseases, in *Principles and Practice of Infectious Diseases*, 4th ed, GL Mandell et al (eds). New York, Wiley, 1995, pp 1484–1489

PINNER RW et al: Trends in infectious diseases mortality in the United States. JAMA 275:189, 1996

QUAGLIARELLO V, SCHELD MW: Bacterial meningitis: Pathogenesis, pathophysiology, and progress. N Engl J Med 327:864, 1992

Report of the Task Force on Microbiology and Infectious Diseases. NIH Publication No. 92-3320. Bethesda, MD: National Institute of Allergy and Infectious Diseases, April 1992

121 *Andrew B. Onderdonk*

LABORATORY DIAGNOSIS OF INFECTIOUS DISEASES

The laboratory diagnosis of infection requires the demonstration, either direct or indirect, of viral, bacterial, mycotic, or parasitic agents in tissues, fluids, or excreta of the host. Clinical microbiology laboratories are responsible for processing these specimens and also for determining the antibiotic susceptibility of bacterial pathogens. Traditionally, detection of pathogenic agents largely relies on either the microscopic visualization of pathogens in clinical material or the growth of microorganisms in the laboratory. Identification is generally based on phenotypic characteristics, such as fermentation profiles for bacteria, cytopathic effects in tissue culture for viral agents, and microscopic morphology for fungi and parasites. These techniques are reliable but are often time-consuming.

DETECTION METHODS Reappraisal of the methods employed in the clinical microbiology laboratory has led to the development of strategies for detecting pathogenic agents through nonvisual biologic signal detection systems. Much of this methodology is based on computerization of detection systems with relatively inexpensive but sophisticated computers. In this chapter, both the methods currently available and those under development will be discussed. → *Chapter 213 discusses the detection of parasitic agents.*

Biologic Signals A *biologic signal* is a material that can be reproducibly differentiated from other substances present in the same physical environment. Key issues in the use of biologic (and electronic) signals are distinguishing the signal from background "noise" and translating it into meaningful information. Examples of biologic signals applicable to clinical microbiology include structural components of bacteria, fungi, and viruses; specific antigens; metabolic end products; unique DNA or RNA base sequences; enzymes; toxins or other proteins; and surface polysaccharides.

Detection Systems A detector is used to sense (or detect) a signal and to discriminate between the signal and background noise. Detection systems range from the trained eyes of a technologist assessing morphologic variations to sensitive electronic instruments, such as gas-liquid chromatographs coupled to computer systems for signal analysis. The sensitivity with which signals can be detected varies widely. It is essential to use a detection system that discerns small amounts of signal even when biologic background noise is present—i.e., a system that is both sensitive and specific. Some common detection systems used in microbiology are immunofluorescence, the detection of substrate utilization or end-product formation as color changes, the detection of enzyme activity as a change in light absorbance, chemiluminescence for DNA/RNA probes, flame ionization detection of short- or long-chain fatty acids, and the detection of turbidity changes, cytopathic effects in cell lines, and agglutination of particles.

Amplification Amplification of weak signals enhances the sensitivity with which the signals can be detected. The most common microbiologic amplification technique is growth of a single bacterium into a discrete colony on an agar plate or into a suspension containing many identical organisms. The advantage of growth as an amplification method is that it requires nothing but an appropriate medium; the disadvantage is the amount of time required for amplification. More rapid, specific amplification of biologic signals can be achieved with techniques such as polymerase (ligase) chain reactions (for DNA/RNA), enzyme immunoassays (EIAs, for antigens and antibodies), electronic amplification (for gas-liquid chromatography assays), antibody capture methods for concentration and/or separation, and selective filtration or centrifugation.

Although a variety of methods are available for the amplification and detection of biologic signals on a research basis, thorough testing is required before they are validated as diagnostic assays.

DIRECT DETECTION Microscopy The field of microbiology has been defined largely by the development and use of the microscope. The examination of specimens by microscopic methods often provides useful diagnostic information rapidly. Staining techniques permit organisms to be seen more clearly.

The simplest method for microscopic evaluation is the wet mount, which is used, for example, to examine cerebrospinal fluid (CSF) for the presence of *Cryptococcus neoformans*, with India ink as a background against which to visualize large-capsuled yeast cells. Wet mounts with dark-field illumination are also used to detect spirochetes from genital lesions. Skin scrapings and hair samples can be examined with use of either 10% KOH wet-mount preparations or the calcofluor white method and ultraviolet (UV) illumination to detect fungal elements as fluorescing structures. Staining of wet mounts—for example, with lactophenol cotton blue stain for fungal elements—is often used for morphologic identification. These techniques enhance signal detection and decrease the background by making it easier to identify specific fungal structures.

Staining *Gram's stain* Without staining, bacteria are difficult to see at the magnifications (400 to 1000×) usually used for their detection. Although simple one-step stains can be used, differential stains are more common. Gram's stain differentiates between those organisms with thick peptidoglycan cell walls (gram-positive) and those whose outer membranes can be dissolved with alcohol or acetone (gram-negative).

Gram's stain is particularly useful for examining sputum for the presence of polymorphonuclear leukocytes (PMNs) and bacteria. Sputum specimens with 25 or more PMNs and fewer than 10 epithelial cells per low-power field often provide clinically useful information. However, the presence in "sputum" samples of more than 10 epithelial cells per low-power field and of multiple bacterial types suggests contamination with oral microflora. Despite the difficulty of discriminating between normal microflora and pathogens, Gram's stain may prove useful for specimens from areas with a large resident microflora if a useful biologic marker (signal) is available. Gram's staining of vaginal swab specimens is useful for detecting epithelial cells covered with gram-positive bacteria, which are regarded as a sign of bacterial vaginosis. Similarly, examination of stained stool specimens for the presence of leukocytes is useful as a screening procedure before testing for *Clostridium difficile* toxin or other enteric pathogens.

The examination of CSF and joint, pleural, or peritoneal fluid with Gram's stain is useful for determining whether bacteria and/or PMNs are present. The sensitivity is such that $>10^4$ bacteria per milliliter should be detected. Centrifugation is often performed before staining to concentrate specimens suspected of containing low numbers of organisms. The pellet is then examined after staining. This simple method is particularly useful for examination of CSF for bacteria and white blood cells or of sputum for acid-fast bacilli.

Acid-fast stain The acid-fast stain identifies organisms capable of retaining carbol fuchsin dye after acid/organic solvent disruption (e.g., *Mycobacterium* species). Modifications of this procedure also allow the differentiation of *Actinomyces* from *Nocardia* or other weakly acid-fast organisms. The acid-fast stain is employed for sputum, gastric aspirates, other fluids, or tissue samples when acid-fast bacilli (AFB; e.g., *Mycobacterium* species) are suspected. The identification of the pink/red AFB against the blue background of the counterstain requires a trained eye, since few AFB may be detected in an entire smear, even when the specimen has been concentrated by centrifugation. An alternative method is the auramine-rhodamine combination fluorescent dye technique.

Fluorochrome stains   Fluorochrome stains, such as acridine orange, are used to identify white blood cells, yeasts, and bacteria in body fluids. Other specialized stains, such as Dappe's stain, may be used in the detection of *Mycoplasma* in cell cultures designated for this purpose. Capsular, flagellar, and spore stains are also used for identification or demonstration of characteristic structures.

Immunofluorescent stains   The direct immunofluorescent antibody (DFA) technique uses antibody that is coupled to a fluorescing compound, such as fluorescein, and directed at a specific antigenic target to visualize organisms or subcellular structures. When samples are examined under appropriate conditions, the fluorescing compound absorbs the UV light and reemits light at a higher (visible) wavelength that can be detected by the human eye. In the indirect immunofluorescent antibody (IFA) technique, an unlabeled (target) antibody binds a specific antigen. The specimen is then stained with labeled polyclonal antibody directed at the target antibody. Because each unlabeled target antibody attached to the appropriate antigen has multiple sites for attachment of the second antibody, the visual signal can be intensified (i.e., amplified). This form of staining is called *indirect* because a two-antibody system is used to generate the signal for detection of the antigen. Both direct and indirect fluorescence methods can be used to detect viruses such as cytomegalovirus and herpes simplex virus within cultured cells as well as many difficult-to-grow bacterial agents (e.g., *Legionella pneumophila*) directly in clinical specimens.

Macroscopic Antigen Detection   Latex agglutination assays and EIAs are rapid and inexpensive methods for identifying organisms or extracellular toxins and viral agents by means of protein and polysaccharide antigens. Such assays may be performed directly on clinical samples or after growth of organisms on agar plates or in viral cell cultures. The biologic signal in each case is the antigen to be detected. Monoclonal or polyclonal antibodies are used.

Techniques such as direct agglutination of bacterial cells with specific antibody are simple but relatively insensitive, while latex agglutination procedures and EIAs are more sensitive. Some cell-associated antigens, such as capsular polysaccharides, lipopolysaccharides, and other surface-expressed antigens, can be detected by agglutination of a suspension of bacterial cells when antibody is added, a method useful for typing of the somatic antigens of *Shigella* and *Salmonella*. In systems such as EIAs, which employ monoclonal antibodies coupled to an enzyme, an antigen-antibody reaction results in the conversion of a colorless substrate to a colored product. Because the coupling of an enzyme to the monoclonal antibody can amplify a weak biologic signal, the sensitivity of such assays is often high. In each instance, the basis for antigen detection is antigen-antibody binding, with the detection system changed to accommodate the biologic signal. Most such assays provide information as to whether antigen is present but do not quantify the antigen. EIAs have also proved to be useful for detecting the presence of bacterial toxins. For instance, this technique is commonly employed for detecting *C. difficile* toxin in stool, as the presence of the organism alone is not diagnostic for toxin-mediated disease.

DETECTION OF PATHOGENIC AGENTS BY CULTURE
Specimen Collection and Transport   To culture bacterial, mycotic, or viral pathogens, an appropriate sample must be placed into the proper medium for growth (amplification). The success or failure of efforts to identify a specific microbial pathogen often depends on the collection and transport process. Appendix B lists procedures for collection and transport of common specimens. Because there are many pathogen-specific paradigms for these procedures, it is important to seek advice from the microbiology laboratory when in doubt about a particular situation.

Isolation of Bacterial Pathogens   The isolation of the suspect pathogen(s) from clinical material relies on the use of artificial media designed to support the growth of bacteria in vitro. Such media are composed of agar, which is not metabolized by bacteria, and nutrients to support the growth of the microbial species of interest, often in combination with substances to inhibit the growth of other bacteria. Broth for growth (amplification) of organisms is employed for specimens with low numbers of bacteria, such as peritoneal dialysis fluid, CSF, or samples in which anaerobes may be present. Two basic strategies are used to isolate pathogenic bacteria. The first is to employ enriched media for the growth of any bacteria that may be present in a sample such as blood or CSF. Since bacteria are not present in such fluids under normal conditions, the finding of organisms is usually significant. Broths that allow the growth of small numbers of organisms may be subcultured to solid media when growth is detected. The second strategy is to isolate (amplify) specific bacterial species from stool, genital tract secretions, or sputum—sites that contain large numbers of bacteria under normal conditions. For this purpose, antimicrobial agents or other inhibitory substances are incorporated into the agar medium to inhibit growth of all but the bacteria of interest. After incubation, organisms that grow on such media are further characterized to determine whether they are pathogens. Selection for organisms that may be pathogens from the normal microflora shortens the time required to make the diagnosis.

Isolation of Viral Agents   (See Chap. 182)   Pathogenic viral agents often are cultured when the presence of serum antibody is not a criterion of active infection or when an increase in serum antibody may not be detected during infection. The biologic signal, virus, is thus amplified to a level at which detection is possible. Although a number of techniques are available, the essential elements include a monolayer of cultured mammalian cells sensitive to infection with the suspected viral pathogen. These cells serve as the amplification system by allowing the proliferation of viral particles. Virus may be detected by direct observation of the cultured cells for cytopathic effects or by immunofluorescent detection of viral antigens following incubation. Culture methods are particularly useful for detection of rapidly propagated agents, such as cytomegalovirus or herpes simplex virus.

IDENTIFICATION METHODS   Once bacteria are isolated, traditional methods of phenotypic characterization are often used for the identification of specific isolates. Phenotypic characteristics include the traits of the organism that are readily detectable after growth on agar media (colony size, color, hemolytic reactions, odor), use by the organism of specific substrates and carbon sources (such as carbohydrates), formation of specific end products during growth, and microscopic appearance. Broth tubes containing specific substrates are commonly employed for such characterization procedures.

Classic Phenotyping   Automated systems allow identification of bacterial pathogens on the basis of phenotypic characteristics in a matter of hours. Most such systems are based on biotyping techniques, in which isolates are grown in multiple substrates and the pattern of reactions is compared with known patterns for various bacterial species. This procedure is relatively fast, and commercially available systems include a coding system to simplify recording of results, probability calculations for the most likely candidate pathogens, and miniaturized fermentation methods. If the biotyping approach is automated and the reading process is coupled to computer-based data analysis, rapidly growing organisms, such as the Enterobacteriaceae, can be identified within hours of detection on agar plates.

Several systems use preformed enzymes for speedier identification (within 2 to 3 h). Such systems do not rely on bacterial growth per se to determine whether a substrate has been used or not. They employ a heavy inoculum in which enzymes are present in sufficient quantity to convert substrate to product rapidly. In addition, some systems use fluorogenic substrate/end-product detection methods to increase sensitivity (through signal amplification).

Gas-Liquid Chromatography   Gas-liquid chromatography is used for the detection of metabolic end products of bacterial fermentations. A common application of this technique is identification of the short-chain fatty acids produced by obligate anaerobes during the fermentation of glucose. Because the types of volatile acids and their relative concentrations differ among the various genera and species that make up this group of organisms, such information serves as a metabolic "fingerprint" for a particular isolate.

Gas-liquid chromatography can be coupled to a sophisticated signal-analysis computer software system for identification and quantitation of long-chain fatty acids (LCFAs) in the outer membranes and cell walls of bacteria and fungi. For any given species, the types and relative concentrations of LCFAs are different enough to allow identification of even closely related species. An organism may be identified definitively within a few hours after the start of growth on appropriate media. LCFA analysis is one of the most advanced procedures currently available for phenotypic characterization.

Nucleic Acid Probes   In recent years, techniques for the detection of specific DNA and RNA base sequences in clinical specimens have become powerful tools for the diagnosis of bacterial, viral, parasitic, and fungal infections. The basic strategy is to detect a relatively short sequence of bases specific for a particular pathogen on single-stranded DNA or RNA by hybridization of a complementary sequence of bases (probe) coupled to a "reporter" molecule that serves as the signal for detection. Detection of an organism by nucleic acid probes does not depend on its viability. Thus, this approach offers a decided advantage over culture methods for difficult-to-grow organisms. Current technology encompasses a wide array of methods for amplification and signal detection, some of which have been approved by the Food and Drug Administration for clinical diagnosis.

Use of nucleic acid probes generally involves lysis of intact cells and denaturation of the DNA or RNA to render it single-stranded. The probe may be hybridized to the target sequence in a solution or on a solid support, depending on the system employed. In situ hybridization of a probe to a target is also possible and allows the use of probes with agents that are present in tissue specimens. Once the probe has been hybridized to the target (biologic signal), a variety of strategies may be employed to amplify and/or detect the target-probe complex (Fig. 121-1).

Probes for direct detection of pathogens in clinical specimens Nucleic acid probes for the direct detection in clinical specimens of various bacterial pathogens (including *L. pneumophila*, *Chlamydia trachomatis*, *Neisseria gonorrhoeae*, group A *Streptococcus*, and *Gardnerella vaginalis*) are available commercially. In addition, probes for the direct detection of human papillomavirus, *Candida* spp., and *Trichomonas vaginalis* have been approved for use. An assortment of probes for confirming the identity of cultured pathogens, such as *Mycobacterium* and *Salmonella* spp., are also available. Probes for the direct detection of bacterial pathogens are often directed at highly conserved 16S ribosomal RNA sequences, because there are many more copies of the ribosomal RNA sequence than there are of any single genomic DNA sequence in a bacterial cell. The sensitivity and specificity of probe assays for direct detection are comparable to those of more traditional assays, including EIA and culture methods. Many laboratories have developed their own probes for the detection of microbial and viral pathogens; however, unless a method-validation protocol for diagnostic use has been performed, the use of such probes is restricted to research by federal law.

Nucleic acid probe amplification strategies   In theory, a single target nucleic acid sequence can be amplified to detectable levels. There are several strategies for target and/or probe amplification, including the polymerase chain reaction (PCR), the ligase chain reaction, strand displacement amplification, and self-sustaining sequence replication. In each case, a target sequence or hybridized probe is amplified exponentially to obtain a signal that can be detected, usually by the attachment of chemiluminescent reporter groups. The PCR strategy requires repeated heating of the DNA or RNA to separate the two complementary strands of the double helix, hybridization of the primer sequence to the appropriate target sequence, target amplification using the PCR for complementary strand extension, and signal detection via a labeled probe. The sensitivity of such assays is far greater than that of traditional assay methods such as cul-

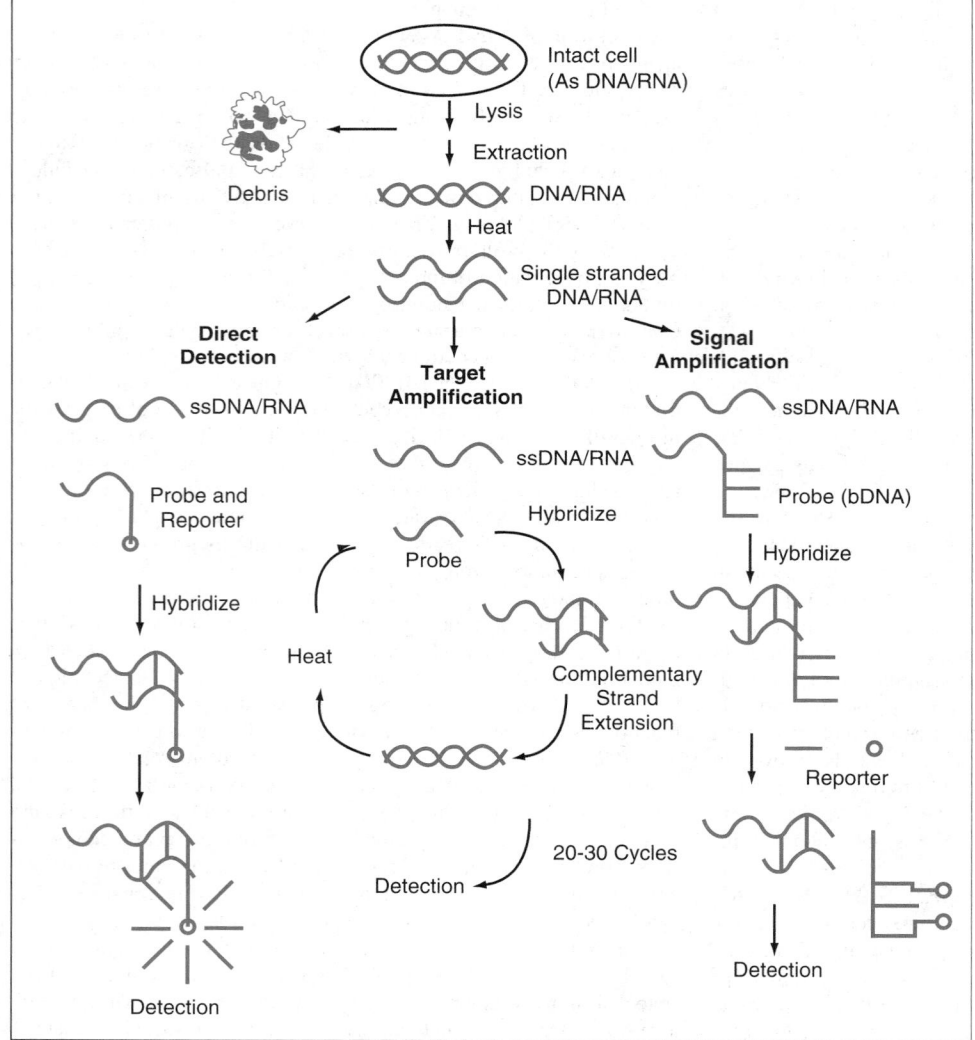

FIGURE 121-1   Strategies for amplification and/or detection of a target-probe complex. DNA or RNA extracted from microorganisms is heated to create single-stranded (ss) DNA/RNA containing appropriate target sequences. These target sequences may be hybridized directly (direct detection) with probes attached to reporter molecules; they may be amplified by repetitive cycles of complementary strand extension (polymerase chain reaction) before attachment of a reporter probe; or the original target-probe signal may be amplified via hybridization with an additional probe containing multiple copies of a secondary reporter target sequence (branched-chain DNA, or bDNA).

ture. However, the care with which the assays are performed is important, because cross-contamination of clinical material with DNA or RNA from other sources (even at low levels) can cause false-positive results. At present, amplification assays for the detection of *Mycobacterium tuberculosis* and *C. trachomatis* are available. As is the case for direct detection probes, many laboratories have used commercially available heat-stable *taq* polymerase, probe sequences, and reagents to develop "in-house" assays for diagnostic use. Issues related to quality control, interpretation of results, sample processing, and regulatory requirements have slowed the commercial development of diagnostic assay kits.

In other systems, probes attached to complementary target sequences are amplified by the attachment of a second probe and an amplification multimer to the original probe. One such system, termed *branched-chain DNA* (bDNA)-*based amplification*, attaches bDNA to a site different from the target-binding sequence of the original probe. Enzyme-labeled oligonucleotides can then bind to multiple repeating sequences on the bDNA. The amplified bDNA signal is detected by chemiluminescence. The advantage of this system over PCR is that only a single step is required to hybridize the target-binding probe to the target sequence.

Application of nucleic acid probe technology   Nucleic acid probe technology is currently being applied to the identification of difficult-to-grow bacterial pathogens such as *Mycobacterium* spp. Further applications of these techniques in the clinical microbiology laboratory will likely include the replacement of culture methods for the identification of many pathogens in clinical material, the detection of antibiotic resistance markers, and the detection of a variety of difficult-to-cultivate or noncultivable pathogens, such as *Ehrlichia*, *Rickettsia*, *Babesia*, *Borrelia*, and *Rochalimaea*. Probe technology also has the potential to detect viral pathogens faster than is possible with current culture techniques. However, if clinical microbiology laboratories are to take full advantage of probe technology, the cost of reagents and automation of the assays must be competitive with the cost and automation of existing methodology. At present, the detection of agents such as *C. trachomatis* or *N. gonorrhoeae* by probe technology is more expensive for most laboratories than detection by traditional culture or EIA methods. Moreover, because automated processing equipment has not yet been designed for clinical use, PCR methods are both more labor-intensive and more expensive than other detection systems. In the absence of clear documentation of clinical utility, many laboratories continue to wait for approval of commercially available DNA probe assays rather than validating in-house assays.

SUSCEPTIBILITY TESTING   One of the principal responsibilities of the clinical laboratory is to determine which antimicrobial agents are inhibitory for a specific bacterial isolate. Two approaches are useful for this purpose. The first is to use a qualitative assessment of susceptibility, categorizing responses as susceptible, resistant, or intermediate. This qualitative approach can involve either the placement of paper disks containing antibiotics on an agar surface inoculated with the bacterial strain to be tested (Kirby-Bauer or disk/agar-diffusion method) or the use of broth tubes containing a set concentration of antibiotic (breakpoint method). These methods have been carefully calibrated against quantitative methods and clinical experience with each antibiotic.

The second approach is to inoculate the test strain of bacteria into a series of broth tubes (or agar plates) with increasing concentrations of antibiotic. The lowest concentration of antibiotic that inhibits microbial growth in this test system is known as the *minimum inhibitory concentration* (MIC). If tubes in which no growth occurs are subcultured, the minimum concentration of antibiotic required to kill the starting inoculum can also be determined. This measurement is called the *minimum bactericidal concentration* (MBC). Quantitative susceptibility testing using the *microbroth dilution technique*, a miniaturized version of the macrobroth dilution technique using microwell plates, lends itself to automation and is used commonly in larger clinical laboratories.

A novel version of the disk/agar-diffusion method employs a quantitative diffusion gradient, or epsilometer (E-test), and uses an absorbent strip with a known gradient of antibiotic concentrations along its length. When the strip is placed on the surface of an agar plate seeded with a bacterial strain to be tested, antibiotic diffuses into the medium, and bacterial growth is inhibited. The MIC is estimated by determining the lowest concentration on the gradient strip that inhibits microbial growth.

AUTOMATION OF MICROBIAL DETECTION IN BLOOD   The detection of microbial growth in blood is difficult because the numbers of organisms present in the sample are often low and because the integrity of the organisms and their ability to replicate may be damaged by humoral defense mechanisms or antimicrobial agents. Over the years, systems that rely on the detection of CO_2 produced by the organisms in blood culture bottles have allowed the automation of the detection procedure. The most common system involves inserting a sampling device into each bottle at periodic intervals and drawing off the head-space gas of the bottle. An infrared monitor is used to determine the CO_2 level. The system interprets levels exceeding a set concentration as indicative of microbial growth. Such methods are no more sensitive than the human eye in detecting a positive culture, but because the bottles in an automated system are generally monitored more frequently, a positive culture is often detected more rapidly than by manual techniques, and important information, including the results of Gram's stain and preliminary susceptibility assays, can be obtained sooner.

One technique for automated blood-culture monitoring uses reflectance optics consisting of a photodiode and a light-emitting diode to monitor the amount of CO_2 produced in each blood-culture bottle every 10 min through a self-contained sensor that is part of each bottle. Each reflectance measurement is then stored in computer memory. When an appropriate change in reflectance occurs, the system alerts the clinical laboratory to the presence of a positive culture via audible and visible alarms. The continuous scanning of bottles used in this system shortens detection times and permits early reporting of positive cultures. In addition, the noninvasive monitoring procedure decreases the likelihood of laboratory contamination.

Automated systems also have been applied to the detection of microbial growth from specimens other than blood, such as peritoneal and other normally sterile fluids. *Mycobacterium* spp. can be detected in certain automated systems if appropriate media are used for culture.

DETECTION OF PATHOGENIC AGENTS BY SERO-LOGIC METHODS   Measurement of serum antibody provides an indirect marker for past or current infection with a specific viral agent or with other pathogens, including *Brucella*, *Legionella*, *Rickettsia*, and *Chlamydia*. The biologic signal is usually either IgM or IgG antibody directed at surface-expressed antigen(s). The detection systems include those used for bacterial antigens (agglutination reactions, immunofluorescence, and EIA) and unique systems such as hemolysis inhibition and complement fixation. Serologic methods generally fall into two categories: those that determine protective antibody levels and those that measure changing antibody titers to detect current infection. Determination of an antibody response as a measure of current immunity is important for viral agents such as rubella virus or varicella-zoster virus; assays for this purpose normally use one or two dilutions of serum for a qualitative determination of protective antibody levels. Quantitative serologic assays to detect increases in antibody titers most often employ paired serum samples obtained 10 to 14 days apart (i.e., acute- and convalescent-phase samples). Since the incubation period before symptoms are noted may be long enough for an antibody response to occur, the demonstration of acute-phase antibody alone is often not enough to establish the diagnosis of active infection as opposed to past exposure. In such circumstances, the finding of IgM may be useful as a measure of an early, acute-phase antibody response. A fourfold increase in total antibody titer or in EIA activity between the acute- and convalescent-phase samples is also regarded as evidence for active infection.

For certain viral agents, such as Epstein-Barr virus, the antibodies produced may be directed at different antigens during different phases of the infection. For this reason, most laboratories test for antibody directed at both viral capsid antigens and antigens associated with recently infected host cells to determine the stage of infection.

BIBLIOGRAPHY

COLLINS ML et al: Preparation and characterization of RNA standards for use in quantitative branched DNA hybridization assays. Anal Biochem 226:120, 1995

HALONNEN P et al: Detection of enteroviruses and rhinoviruses in clinical specimens by PCR and liquid-phase hybridization. J Clin Microbiol 33:648, 1995

HERMANN JE: Immunoassays for the diagnosis of infectious diseases, in *Manual of Clinical Microbiology*, 6th ed, P Murray et al (eds). Washington, American Society for Microbiology, 1995

MILLER JM et al: Specimen collection, transport and storage, in *Manual of Clinical Microbiology*, 6th ed, B Murray et al (eds). Washington, American Society for Microbiology, 1995

PFYFFER GE et al: Diagnostic performance of amplified *Mycobacterium tuberculosis* direct test with cerebrospinal fluid, other nonrespiratory and respiratory specimens. J Clin Microbiol 34:834, 1996

PODZORSKI RP et al: Molecular detection and identification of microorganisms, in *Manual of Clinical Microbiology*, 6th ed, P Murray et al (eds). Washington, Americal Society for Microbiology, 1995

SCHOCHETMAN G et al: Polymerase chain reaction. J Infect Dis 158:1154, 1988

WILSON ML: General principles of specimen collection and transport. Clin Infect Dis 22:766, 1996

122   Gerald T. Keusch, Kenneth J. Bart

IMMUNIZATION PRINCIPLES AND VACCINE USE

Most humans live their lives ignoring the certainty of their own mortality. Perhaps this fact explains why the adage "an ounce of prevention is worth a pound of cure" has so little effect on their everyday behavior. Even when it comes to acting to protect their young, parents are capable of ignoring the potential for mortality among their children (in the developed world) and of accepting the certainty of childhood deaths (in the developing world). In both settings, parents all too often fail to seek out and demand the best preventive measures available. Unless mandated by the law in the former setting or provided by benevolent organizations or governments in the latter, universal immunization has invariably remained an unattained goal. Compulsion and benevolence, it seems, are two essential components of immunization.

However, the integration of immunization practices (a major component of primary disease prevention) into routine health care services has provided caregivers with control over a substantial proportion of the disease and mortality that plagued the United States during the first half of the twentieth century (Table 122-1). For society today, immunization represents one of the most cost-effective means of preventing infectious disease. For every dollar spent, diphtheria/tetanus/pertussis (DTP) vaccine saves $29, measles/mumps/rubella (MMR) vaccine saves $21, trivalent oral poliovirus vaccine (OPV) saves $6, varicella vaccine saves $5, and *Haemophilus influenzae* type b (Hib) vaccine saves $2. At present, more than 50 biologic products are licensed in the United States, and 6 vaccines (12 antigens) are used for routine immunization in the young, including diphtheria/tetanus/acellular pertussis vaccine (DTaP), OPV, MMR, Hib vaccine, hepatitis B virus (HBV) vaccine, and varicella vaccine. Five vaccines are designed for routine use in adults, including tetanus/diphtheria (Td) toxoids, adsorbed, for adult use; HBV vaccine; influenza virus vaccine; polyvalent pneumococcal polysaccharide vaccine; and varicella vaccine. Some preparations are designated as special-use vaccines (e.g., hepatitis A vaccine for travelers). Unfortunately, vaccines for eukaryotic pathogens (protozoa and helminths), which affect a large proportion of the world's population, have been difficult to develop and remain only a hope for the future.

Table 122-1

Changes in the Incidence of Vaccine-Preventable Diseases in the United States

Disease	Peak Incidence Year	Peak Incidence No. of Cases	No. of Cases in 1995[a]	Decrease from Maximum as of 1995, %
Diphtheria	1921	206,939	0	100.00
Measles	1941	894,134	288	99.97
Mumps	1968	152,209	840	99.45
Pertussis	1934	265,269	4315	98.37
Poliomyelitis (paralytic)	1952	21,269	0[b]	100.00
Rubella	1969	57,686	146	99.75
Congenital rubella syndrome	1965	20,000[c]	7	99.97
Tetanus[d]	1923	1560	43	97.24
Haemophilus influenzae type b[e]	—	20,000[f]	270	98.65

[a] Provisional.
[b] Projected to be 5 to 10 vaccine-associated cases.
[c] Estimated.
[d] All ages.
[e] Invasive disease, children <5 years old.
[f] Not notifiable before 1991; estimated prevaccine-era annual incidence, all ages.
SOURCE: Centers for Disease Control and Prevention.

IMPACT OF IMMUNIZATION The epidemiologically appropriate use of vaccines has resulted in the global eradication of smallpox; the elimination of poliomyelitis in the Americas; the virtual elimination of congenital rubella syndrome, tetanus, and diphtheria in the United States; and a dramatic reduction in pertussis, rubella, measles, and mumps in the United States. Figure 122-1 shows the effect of vaccines on the incidence of Hib meningitis. The Hib conjugate vaccines in particular have exerted a remarkable influence on invasive *Haemophilus* infections, presumably because they reduce nasopharyngeal carriage of Hib and induce protection before the period of greatest vulnerability in infancy.

DEFINITIONS *Vaccination* and *immunization* are often used as interchangeable terms. However, the former denotes only the administration of a vaccine or toxoid, whereas the latter describes the process of inducing or providing immunity by any means, whether active or

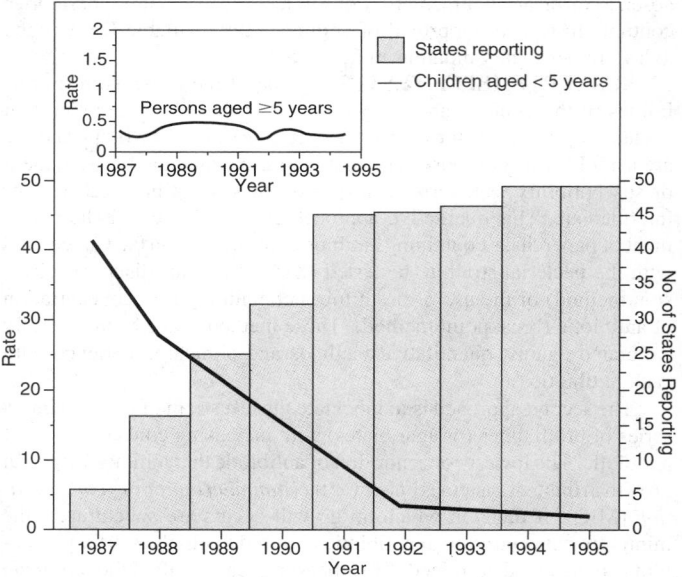

FIGURE 122-1   Incidence rate of invasive *Haemophilus influenzae* disease per 100,000 children <5 years of age and number of states reporting to the CDC *H. influenzae* surveillance system. The insert shows the incidence rate among persons ≥5 years of age. Because of the low number of states reporting surveillance data during 1987–1990, rates for those years were race-adjusted on the basis of the 1990 U.S. population. (*From the Centers for Disease Control and Prevention.*)

passive. Thus, vaccination does not guarantee immunization. *Active immunization* refers to the induction of immune defenses by the administration of antigens in appropriate forms, whereas *passive immunization* involves the provision of temporary protection by the administration of exogenously produced immune substances. Immunizing agents thus include vaccines, toxoids, and antibody-containing immunoglobulin preparations from human or animal donors (Table 122-2).

PRINCIPLES OF IMMUNIZATION Artificial induction of immunity closely follows two well-tested principles of nature. The first, active immunization, can be traced at least as far back as Thucydides, who noted that people surviving epidemics of plague in Athens were spared during later outbreaks of the same disease. The second, passive immunization, is a natural process as well and is exemplified by the transplacental transmission of maternal antibodies to the fetus to provide protection against several diseases during the first months of life. Use of the two measures together may produce a complementary effect (as with HBV vaccine plus hepatitis B immune globulin) or may actually interfere with the development of immunity (as when measles vaccine is administered within 6 weeks of immunoglobulin). Depending on whether there are multiple species or serotypes of an organism and—if so—whether there are common, cross-reactive, protective antigens, a specific vaccine may induce protection against all representative forms of an infectious agent or against the immunizing strain only. One of the intrinsic virtues of whole-organism vaccines is that they potentially contain all protective antigens of the organism. However, this virtue is counterbalanced by an inherent problem with such vaccines: the possibility of adverse responses to reactive but nonprotective antigens present in the mix. Because the immune response to specific antigens is controlled genetically, all individuals cannot be expected to respond identically to the same vaccine.

APPROACHES TO ACTIVE IMMUNIZATION The two principal approaches to active immunization are (1) the use of live, generally attenuated, infectious agents (e.g., measles virus) and (2) the use of inactivated agents, detoxified extracts or toxins from these agents, or specific antigens obtained by genetic recombination (e.g., HBV). For many diseases (e.g., poliomyelitis, influenza), both approaches have been employed. Live attenuated vaccines are believed to induce an immunologic response more nearly like that resulting from natural infection than the response induced by killed vaccines. Currently available inactivated or killed vaccines consist of inactivated whole organisms (e.g., plague vaccine); detoxified protein exotoxins (e.g., tetanus toxoid); recombinant protein antigens (e.g., HBV vaccine); or carbohydrate antigens, either present as soluble purified capsular material (e.g., *Streptococcus pneumoniae* polysaccharides) or conjugated to a protein carrier (e.g., Hib polysaccharide conjugated to diphtheria or tetanus toxoids).

APPROACHES TO PASSIVE IMMUNIZATION Passive immunization is generally used to provide temporary immunity in an unimmunized subject exposed to an infectious disease when active immunization either is unavailable (e.g., for cytomegalovirus infection) or has not been implemented before exposure (e.g., for rabies). Passive immunization is used in the treatment of certain disorders associated with toxins (e.g., diphtheria), in certain bites (those of snakes and spiders), and as a specific or nonspecific immunosuppressant [Rho(D) immune globulin and antilymphocyte globulin, respectively].

Three types of preparations are used in passive immunization: (1) standard human immune serum globulin for general use (e.g., gamma globulin), administered intramuscularly or intravenously; (2) special immune serum globulins with a known content of antibody for specific agents (e.g., HBV or varicella-zoster immune globulin); and (3) animal sera and antitoxins.

ROUTE OF ADMINISTRATION The route of administration in part determines the rapidity and nature of the immune responses to vaccines. Vaccines can be administered orally, intranasally, intradermally, subcutaneously, or intramuscularly. Parenterally administered vaccine may not induce mucosal secretory IgA, and mucosal immunization may not induce good systemic responses. Vaccines must be administered by the licensed route to ensure immunogenicity and safety. For example, administration of HBV vaccine into the gluteal rather than the deltoid muscle often fails to induce an adequate immune response, while subcutaneous rather than intramuscular administration of DTP increases the risk of reactions.

AGE The age of the individual influences the response to vaccines. Therefore, recommended schedules for immunization are based on age-dependent responses determined empirically from clinical trials. The presence of high levels of maternal antibody and/or the immaturity of the immune system in the early months of life impairs the initial immune response to some antigens (e.g., measles vaccine but not HBV vaccine). In the elderly, vaccine responses may be diminished because of natural waning of the immune system. Hence, larger amounts of an antigen may be required to produce the desired response (e.g., in vaccination against influenza).

ADJUVANT POTENTIATION The immune response to some antigens is potentiated by the addition of adjuvants such as aluminum salts or, in the case of polysaccharides (e.g., the polyribose phosphate oligosaccharide of Hib), by conjugation to a peptide. Adjuvants, nonspecific boosters of immune responses, are used with inactivated products such as diphtheria and tetanus toxoids, acellular pertussis (aP) vaccine, and HBV vaccine. The mechanism for adjuvant enhancement of antigenicity is not well defined but relates in part to the rendering of soluble antigens into a particulate form, the mobilization of phagocytes to the site of antigen deposition, and the slowing down of the release of antigens, which prolongs stimulation of the immune response.

THE IMMUNE RESPONSE Although many constituents of infectious microorganisms and their products, such as exotoxins, are or can be made to be antigenic, only a limited number stimulate a protective immune response. The immune system is complex, and antigen composition and presentation are critical for stimulation of the desired immune responses.

The Primary Response In the primary response to a vaccine antigen, an apparent latent period of several days precedes the detection of humoral and cell-mediated immunity, although the immune response is turned on by contact with the antigen and the immune system. Circulating antibodies do not appear for 7 to 10 days. The immunoglobulin class of the response also changes over time. Early-appearing IgM antibodies generally exhibit only low affinity for the antigen, whereas later-appearing IgG antibodies display high affinity. For "thymus-dependent" antigens, T helper lymphocytes control the switch from IgM to IgG. Some individuals do not respond, even when presented repeatedly with a vaccine antigen, perhaps because they lack the major histocompatibility complex determinants required to recognize the antigen. This situation is known as *primary vaccine failure*.

The Secondary Response Heightened humoral or cell-mediated responses are elicited by a second exposure to the same antigen. These secondary responses occur rapidly, usually within 4 or 5 days, and

Table 122-2

Definitions of Immunizing Agents

Term	Definition
Vaccine	A suspension of attenuated live or killed microorganisms or antigenic portions of these agents presented to a potential host to induce immunity and prevent disease
Toxoid	A modified bacterial toxin that has been made nontoxic but retains the capacity to stimulate the formation of antitoxin
Immune globulin	An antibody-containing solution derived from human blood by cold ethanol fractionation of large pools of plasma and used primarily for maintenance of the immunity of immunodeficient persons or for passive immunization; intramuscular and intravenous preparations available
Antitoxin	An antibody derived from the serum of animals after stimulation with specific antigens and used to provide passive immunity

result in increased titers of IgG antibody. The secondary response depends on immunologic memory after the first exposure and is characterized by a marked proliferation of antibody-producing B lymphocytes and/or effector T cells. Polysaccharide vaccines, such as that for *S. pneumoniae*, evoke immune responses that are independent of T cells and are not enhanced by repeated administration. Linking of polysaccharides to proteins converts the former to T cell–dependent antigens that induce immunologic memory and secondary responses to revaccination. Although levels of vaccine-induced antibodies may decline over time (*secondary vaccine failure*), revaccination or exposure to the organism may elicit a rapid protective secondary response consisting of IgG antibodies with little or no detectable IgM. This *anamnestic response* indicates that immunity has persisted. The lack of measurable antibody does not necessarily mean that the individual is unprotected. Furthermore, the mere presence of detectable antibodies after the administration of some vaccines and toxoids does not ensure clinical protection. A minimal circulating level of antibody is known to be required for protection from some diseases (e.g., 0.01 IU/mL for tetanus antitoxin).

Hypersensitivity Reactions Independent of antibody production, the stimulation of the immune system by vaccination may elicit unanticipated responses, especially hypersensitivity reactions. In the past, killed measles vaccine induced incomplete humoral immunity and cell-mediated hypersensitivity, resulting in the development of a syndrome of atypical measles in some children after subsequent exposure; thus this type of vaccine is no longer in use.

Mucosal Immunity Some pathogens are confined to and replicate only at mucosal surfaces (e.g., *Vibrio cholerae*), while others are able to penetrate the mucosa and replicate (e.g., poliovirus, rubella virus, and influenza virus). At the mucosal site, these organisms induce secretory IgA. The induction of secretory IgA by vaccines may be an efficient way to block the essential first steps in pathogenesis, whether the organism is restricted to mucosal surfaces or systemically invades the host across mucosal surfaces.

Measurement of the Immune Response Immune responses to vaccines are often gauged by the concentration of specific antibody in serum. While seroconversion serves as a dependable indicator of an immune response, it measures only one immunologic parameter and does not necessarily indicate protection. The development of circulating antibodies after immunization often correlates directly with clinical protection (e.g., against measles or rubella). Some responses may not in themselves confer immunity but may be sufficiently associated with protection that they remain useful proxy measures of protective immunity (e.g., vibriocidal serum antibodies in cholera).

HERD IMMUNITY It is not necessary to immunize every person in order to stop transmission of an infectious agent through a population. For those organisms dependent on person-to-person transmission, there may be a definable prevalence of immunity in the population above which it becomes difficult for the organism to circulate and reach new susceptibles. This prevalence is called *herd immunity*. When herd immunity is operative, the goals of immunization are converted from the immunization of every person in the community to the immunization of a specified minimum percentage of persons at risk. Herd immunity may be lost when immunity wanes (as in diphtheria in the new independent states of the former Soviet Union) or when a sufficient percentage of individuals refuse to be immunized. The latter situation developed with regard to pertusis in the United Kingdom and Japan in the 1970s because concern about infrequent—albeit severe—vaccine reactions came to exceed the fear of the disease itself. In both situations, loss of herd immunity has led to renewed increases in the circulation of the organism and susceptibility to infection, with subsequent large outbreaks.

TARGET POPULATIONS AND TIMING OF IMMUNIZATION For common and highly communicable childhood diseases like measles, the target population is the universe of susceptible individuals, and the time to immunize is as early in life as is feasible.

Epidemiologic differences in measles in different settings, however, dictate different strategies of immunization. In the industrialized world, immunization with live-virus vaccine at 12 to 15 months of age has been the norm because the vaccine protects more than 95 percent of those immunized at this age and there is little measles morbidity/mortality among very young infants. In contrast, in the developing world, measles accounts for a significant proportion of deaths of young infants. Thus it is desirable to immunize children during the first few months of life in order to narrow the window of vulnerability between the rapid decline of maternal antibody after 4 to 6 months and the development of vaccine-induced active immunity.

Hib causes meningitis, epiglottitis, and pneumonia in early childhood. As in measles, the majority of cases of severe Hib disease occur in this age group, with rates rising sharply after the disappearance of maternally derived antibody. However, the first Hib vaccines were subject to primary failure when administered during infancy; this failure was due mainly to an age-related inability to respond to polysaccharide antigens. To overcome this problem, the protective polysaccharide was coupled to protein and was thereby converted to a T cell–dependent antigen to which young infants could respond.

In contrast to measles and Hib infection, rubella is primarily a threat to the fetus; young infants and children are not at risk of serious illness. Given the risk to the fetus, immunization of all women of reproductive age before pregnancy would be an ideal strategy. However, it is difficult to systematically vaccinate adolescent and young-adult females. Thus, to assure the protection of as many women as possible, the rubella component is included in a combination vaccine with mumps and measles (MMR) that is administered during infancy.

Some vaccines are now used primarily for adults. For example, influenza virus and polyvalent pneumococcal polysaccharide vaccines are used to prevent pneumonia deaths in the elderly. Unfortunately, these vaccines are underutilized, in part because physicians and otherwise healthy individuals in the target group ignore the indications and in part because there is still a tendency to think about disease prevention with vaccines as a strategy for children. Pneumococcal polysaccharide vaccine is also recommended for children over 2 years of age who are at risk of severe or even life-threatening pneumococcal infection, such as those with sickle cell disease, asplenia (whether functional or anatomic), renal failure with nephrotic syndrome, cerebrospinal fluid leak, and human immunodeficiency virus (HIV) infection or other immunosuppressive disease states.

THE DEVELOPMENT OF VACCINES

BIOLOGIC IMPEDIMENTS There are often major technical problems to overcome in vaccine development. Influenza virus, characterized biologically by its antigenic drift, periodically emerges in a new antigenic version capable of causing a global pandemic for which a new vaccine must be rapidly devised, produced, and distributed. In contrast to the circulation of one major antigenic type of influenza A virus at any one time is the circulation of many prevalent pneumococcal polysaccharide serotypes at all times. However, because immunity to the pneumococcus is serotype specific, an individual is susceptible to all serotypes against which he or she lacks antibody. Serotype-specific protection made it more difficult to develop an effective pneumococcal vaccine than it was to develop a vaccine against *H. influenzae*, of which one capsular serotype (type b) is associated with a significant portion of cases of severe disease. To overcome this problem, pneumococcal vaccine currently includes 23 polysaccharides that represent approximately 80 percent of the virulent serotypes commonly encountered in the United States. Unfortunately, some serotypes are poorly immunogenic, and immunized individuals remain susceptible to the serotypes not included in the vaccine.

STRATEGY FOR VACCINE DEVELOPMENT Vaccine development depends on the systematic application of a four-phase strategy: (1) studies in animals to identify protective antigen, (2) determination of how to present this antigen effectively to the immune system, (3) assessment of the safety and immunogenicity of the preparation in small and then in large human populations at various ages, and (4) evaluation of safety and efficacy in the target population. Each of these steps is simple in concept but difficult in execution, not least because of the clinical trials necessary to assess safety and efficacy; failure at any level stops the process. Thus, in 1995, more than 190 candidate vaccines were under investigation, but just 5 new products were licensed in the United States. Progress in immunology has taught us much about the organization and function of the immune system (see Chap. 305); it has also taught us that the immune system is complicated and that details of antigen composition and presentation are critical for stimulating desired immune responses.

In the development of vaccines, initial studies are typically carried out in animal models, if available, to demonstrate the production of immune responses, an ability to protect the host, and relative safety. Ultimately, vaccines for humans must be tested in humans. When initial in vitro and animal data look promising, graded doses of vaccine are given to small numbers of humans to assess immune responses, optimal dosage, and safety. Human clinical trials of vaccine efficacy are then performed with a larger group, often consisting of informed volunteers who are challenged with a virulent strain. After clinical trials in the community, typically involving 1000 to 10,000 vaccinees, licensure may be sought. Because of their limited size, however, these trials cannot be expected to detect rare adverse effects. Thus, licensing does not guarantee that a new vaccine is completely safe, and post-licensing monitoring is needed to ensure effectiveness and to document the occurrence of adverse events of low frequency.

The development of vaccines goes beyond technology and proof of principle to issues such as development costs, manufacturers' liability and indemnity, perceived public health needs, and the likelihood that a product will be used or sold. Given the complex science required, the costs of vaccine development are high and success is uncertain, adding risk to the development decision. It is unfortunate that the one sure implication of uncertainty in vaccine development is increased cost. In addition, a rational assignment of costs for development between the public and private sectors in the United States has never been achieved.

VACCINE FORMULATIONS Studies of clinical immunology have shown that living and dead antigens do not necessarily induce the same immune responses and that the requirements for the development of protective immunity differ with the organism. These insights, together with the refinement of epidemiologic concepts surrounding immunization, have changed the strategy of vaccine development. The goal is not only to select the correct antigens but also to ensure that the vaccines will result in the type of immune response needed for protection, whether the T cell–mediated activation of macrophages or the generation of cytotoxic T cells, B cell–mediated secretory IgA, or a particular IgG subtype response to a specific polysaccharide epitope.

Live vaccines consist of selected or genetically altered organisms that are avirulent or dramatically attenuated yet remain immunogenic. These agents are expected to cause a subclinical illness that mimics natural infection except for the lack of clinically significant disease. They offer the advantage of replication in vivo, which increases the antigenic load presented to the host's immune system; they are believed to confer lifelong protection with one dose; they present a diversity of antigens, thus overcoming immunogenetic restrictions in some hosts; they may reach the local sites most relevant to the induction of protective immunity; and they may produce important protective antigens in vivo that are not efficiently expressed in vitro.

In contrast, with nonviable vaccines, what is presented to the host in terms of antigen load and specific antigenic determinants defines the ultimate response. Nonviable preparations may fail to elicit mucosal IgA-mediated immunity, as they lack a delivery system that will transport them to local antigen-processing cells as effectively as living organisms are conveyed. Moreover, except for pure polysaccharide antigens, these preparations must almost always be given in multiple doses to induce effective responses. However, killed vaccines can be extremely effective. For example, the nonviable hepatitis A vaccine formulation appears to be close to 100 percent effective in inducing protective immunity.

In spite of their advantages, live vaccines are not always to be preferred. For example, live OPV is contraindicated for use in children with immune-deficiency diseases and in their adult contacts. In addition, even though killed poliovirus vaccine does not completely immunize the gut and can neither reduce the circulation of wild-type poliovirus nor immunize contacts of vaccine recipients, this vaccine is preferred for the immunization of adults when urgency of protection is not an issue because of the greater risk of vaccine-associated polio posed by live OPV. In some countries (e.g., Denmark and Israel), a combination schedule of killed and live poliovirus vaccine has been recommended.

To create a deliverable vaccine, constituents other than the antigens are required (Table 122-3). These constituents can affect the immunogenicity, efficacy, and safety of a vaccine and can render one formulation superior to another.

PRODUCTION OF VACCINES As products to be given to healthy individuals to prevent disease, vaccines not only must be efficacious but also must lack the capacity to cause harm. In the United States, quality assurance is the responsibility of vaccine manufacturers. Standards of manufacture of biologics [known as good manufacturing practices (GMPs)] are regulated and supervised by the Food and Drug Administration (FDA). Proof of the safety, efficacy, sterility, and purity of products is required before licensure, and sterility and purity are continually monitored for all lots of vaccine after licensure. Post-marketing studies of safety (phase IV studies) are part of routine regulatory control. On rare occasions, either GMP or quality assurance is inadequate; for example, the release of incompletely killed Salk polio vaccine in 1955 caused an outbreak of poliomyelitis in nearly 200 vaccine recipients and their contacts. Unregulated and uncontrolled manufacture of vaccines in developing countries has sometimes led to the release and use of inactive products that fail to provide the expected protective immunity.

Another problem in the production of vaccines has unexpectedly cropped up in the past decade. For various reasons, including the high costs of vaccine development and the prospect of much higher profitability from investments in other products, the number of vaccine manufacturers in the United States has declined and the cost of some basic childhood vaccines has increased. Concern therefore exists about the future availability of these essential biologics for national use. Furthermore, pricing decisions made within the private-sector pharmaceutical industry can have a major impact on vaccine use. This situation has stimulated an initiative toward increased public involvement in the supplying of vaccine to individuals for whom price is an issue (as in the Vaccines for Children Program discussed below) as well as in oversight of the vaccine supply and of price negotiations with the industry.

ADMINISTRATION OF VACCINES Health care workers administering vaccines must take the precautions necessary to minimize the risk of spreading disease. They should be immunized against hepatitis B, measles, rubella, influenza, and varicella, and they should wash their hands before seeing each new patient. The syringes and

Table 122-3

Constituents of Vaccines

Constituent(s)	Examples/Purpose
Preservatives, stabilizers, antibiotics	These components are used to prevent the vaccine's deterioration before use, to inhibit or prevent bacterial growth, or to stabilize the antigen. Any of these additives may elicit allergic reactions.
Adjuvants	An aluminum salt is used in some vaccines (e.g., toxoids, hepatitis B vaccine) to enhance the immune response.
Suspending fluid	The suspending fluid can be sterile water, saline, buffer, or more complex fluids derived from the growth medium or biologic system in which the agent is produced (e.g., egg antigens, cell culture ingredients, serum proteins).

needles they use for injection must be sterile and preferably disposable to minimize the risk of contamination. Different vaccines should not be mixed in the same syringe unless such a practice is specifically endorsed by licensure. Disposable needles and syringes should be discarded in labeled, puncture-proof containers to prevent inadvertent needlestick injury or reuse.

The recent addition of new, individually injectable vaccines to the immunization schedule has heightened parental concerns about the administration of up to four injections at a single clinic visit. The development and use of combinations of vaccines are intended to mitigate these concerns. Even when multiple injections are required, providers must make every effort to administer all indicated vaccines at each visit.

Wherever effective primary health care systems ensure access to medical services for the majority and the population is educated about the need for and efficacy of vaccines, coverage rates for basic immunization are usually high, regardless of the route of vaccine administration or the number of doses necessary. However, without systematic attention to the completion of multiple-dose vaccine schedules, coverage rates for second, third, and booster doses may drop off significantly.

USE OF VACCINES

Until recently, recommendations for vaccine use in the United States were developed by several different groups. In order to establish a single childhood immunization schedule, the American Academy of Pediatrics (AAP) and the Advisory Committee on Immunization Practices (ACIP) have unified their vaccine recommendations, and this unified version has been approved by the American Academy of Family Practice (AAFP). These recommendations are the result of a collaborative process among the recommending groups, the pharmaceutical industry, and the FDA.

Vaccines recommended in 1996 for routine administration to infants, children, and adults are shown in Table 122-4; vaccines recommended for special use are shown in Table 122-5; and schedules for immunization of children and adults are shown in Fig. 122-2 and Table 122-6, respectively. The recommendations on route, site, and dosages for vaccination are derived from theoretical considerations, experimental trials, and clinical experience; deviation from these recommendations can result in inadequate protection. The administration of doses at intervals longer than those recommended does not diminish the ultimate protective response but merely delays it. It is not necessary to restart an interrupted series from the beginning or to add an extra dose. In contrast, giving vaccines at shorter-than-recommended intervals may result in poor responses.

RECORDING AND REPORTING REQUIREMENTS   Certain aspects of vaccine use are regulated by the National Childhood Vaccine Injury Act (NCVIA) of 1986 (modified in 1995). The act requires that all mandated childhood vaccinations be recorded by health care providers in the child's permanent medical record, including date of administration, manufacturer and lot number, and name of the provider administering the vaccine. State-based immunization information systems and registries are being developed to help public and private providers manage their immunization activities and particularly to address the problem of assessing immunization coverage when an individual's records are divided among multiple medical facilities.

Parents should maintain an up-to-date immunization record on their children. The NCVIA requires that the potential for reactions to vaccines and the benefits of vaccination to the child be explained to parents. Educational materials providing the required information are available from the AAP or the Centers for Disease Control and Prevention (CDC).

VACCINES FOR ROUTINE USE   Infants and Children Recommended routine-use vaccines and schedules for their administration to infants and children are shown in Table 122-4 and Fig. 122-2, respectively. It is current practice for all children in the United States to receive DTaP, poliovirus, MMR, Hib, HBV, and varicella vaccines

Table 122-4

Routinely Recommended Vaccines for Infants, Children, and Adults

Vaccine	Year Licensed	Type of Immunizing Agent	Protective Antibody	Route of Administration	Efficacy, %	Adverse Events
DT	1949	Toxoid	Diphtheria and tetanus neutralizing antitoxins, ≥0.1 IU/mL each	IM	D: 95	Local reactions
Td	1955				T: 95	Hypersensitivity to tetanus toxoid
aP	1993	Inactivated bacterial antigen	Not known	IM	80–90	Reduced local reactions compared with whole-cell vaccines; no serious reactions reported
	1996	Acellular (DTaP)				
Hib	1987	Bacterial polysaccharide-protein conjugate	Antibody to capsular polysaccharide, 0.15 μg/mL	IM	90	Few local, no serious reactions
HBV	1981	Inactivated serum-derived viral antigen	Antibody to surface antigen, 10 mIU/mL	IM	80–95	Few (? Guillain-Barré syndrome)
	1987	Recombinant antigen				
Influenza	1945	Inactivated virus or viral components	Neutralizing antibody	IM	40–60	? Guillain-Barré syndrome with swine influenza vaccine
MMR	1971	Live viruses	Neutralizing measles antibody, ≥200 mIU/mL; not known for mumps or rubella	SC	M: 95	Acute encephalopathy (measles)
					Mu: 90	Rare parotitis or orchitis (mumps)
					R: 95	Arthralgia and rare arthropathy (rubella)
Pneumococcus	1983	Bacterial polysaccharide of 23 types	Antibody to capsular polysaccharide	IM or SC	60–80	Local reactions; rare anaphylaxis
Poliomyelitis	1963	OPV, live virus of 3 serotypes	Neutralizing antibody at any detectable titer	Oral	95*	Rare vaccine-associated polio
	1967	IPV-e, inactivated virus of 3 serotypes		SC	95	No significant reactions

* In developing countries, OPV efficacy is only 70 to 90 percent, presumably because of interfering enteroviruses in the intestinal tract.

NOTE: DT, diphtheria and tetanus toxoids, adsorbed; Td, tetanus and diphtheria toxoids, adsorbed, for adult use; aP, acellular pertussis; Hib, *Haemophilus influenzae* type b; HBV, hepatitis B virus; MMR, measles-mumps-rubella; OPV, trivalent oral poliovirus vaccine; IPV-e, inactivated poliovirus vaccine, enhanced; IM, intramuscular; SC, subcutaneous.

SOURCE: Recommendations of the Advisory Committee on Immunization Practices, the American Academy of Pediatrics, and the American College of Physicians.

unless there are specific contraindications. A four-dose schedule of DTaP and *either* a four-dose poliovirus vaccine schedule consisting of two doses of inactivated poliovirus vaccine, enhanced (IPV-e), followed by two doses of OPV *or* a four-dose schedule of either OPV or IPV-e, including a booster dose at 4 to 6 years of age, constitute the full series. The combined IPV-e/OPV schedule is intended to reduce the incidence of vaccine-associated poliomyelitis. DTaP (Connaught, Tripedia) was first licensed in 1996 for primary immunization of infants. DTaP is now the preferred vaccine, although DTP may still be used. A booster dose is recommended at 4 to 6 years of age. Adult-formulation Td boosters are recommended every 10 years thereafter. One dose of MMR vaccine along with varicella vaccine is recommended at 15 months. MMR is given again at school entry or in middle school. DTaP, MMR, varicella, poliovirus, and Hib vaccines may be given simultaneously at 15 months of age without increasing rates of adverse reactions or impairing the immune response. Unvaccinated children who lack a reliable history of chickenpox should receive varicella vaccine before the teenage years.

Adults (See Table 122-6)   All adults should be immune to diphtheria and tetanus. If not previously immunized, adults require a primary immunizing course of three doses of Td, with the second dose 4 to 8 weeks after the first, the third dose at 12 months, and boosters every 10 years thereafter. Many individuals remain immune to tetanus into adulthood because they have received tetanus toxoid rather than Td after injuries, but they are commonly at risk of diphtheria because of the decline in titer of diphtheria antitoxin and the lack of boosting against diphtheria. Routine immunization against polio is not recommended for adults unless they are at particular risk of exposure (e.g., through travel to endemic regions, as discussed below) or are the parents or guardians of a child with an immunodeficiency disorder. Adults should be protected from measles, mumps, and rubella; they should be vaccinated unless they are known to have received vaccine on or after their first birthday or to have had physician-diagnosed disease. Rubella vaccine should be given to all women of childbearing age unless they have documentary proof of immunization after their first birthday or laboratory evidence of immunity. An unsupported history of rubella disease is unreliable and should not be accepted. Adults without a clear history of chickenpox should receive varicella vaccine.

Table 122-5

Special-Use Vaccines

Vaccine	Year Licensed in United States	Type of Immunizing Agent	Route of Administration	Indications	Efficacy	Adverse Events
Anthrax	1970	Inactivated avirulent bacteria	SC (6 doses primary; annual booster)	For high risk of exposure (i.e., persons in contact with or involved in manufacture of animal hides, furs, bone meal, wool, goat hair)	90% antibody response but efficacy uncertain	No serious adverse effects known
Tuberculosis (BCG)	1950	Living bacteria (attenuated *Mycobacterium bovis*)	ID	PPD-negative individuals in prolonged contact with active TB patient	Controversial; reduces disseminated disease in children (0–80% protection against pulmonary TB; 75–86% protection against miliary and meningitic TB)	Regional adenitis, disseminated BCG infection, osteitis
Hepatitis A	1995	Killed virus antigen	IM	Travelers or persons living in high-risk areas	94%	Local reactions
Cholera	1914	Inactivated bacteria	SC or IM	Not recommended for public health use	50% (short-lived)	Frequent fever, local pain, swelling
Meningococcus A, C, Y, W135	1981	Bacterial polysaccharide of 4 serotypes	SC	Military personnel; principally travelers to epidemic areas	90% for 2- to 3-year-olds	Rare
Plague	1911	Inactivated bacteria	IM	Laboratory workers; foresters in endemic areas; travelers	90% antibody response but efficacy uncertain	10% local reactions; rare sterile abscesses and hypersensitivity
Rabies (human diploid)	1980	Inactivated virus	IM or ID	Travelers; laboratory workers; veterinarians	Virtually 100%	25% local reactions; 6% arthropathy, arthritis, angioedema
Yellow fever	1953	Live virus	SC	Laboratory workers; travelers	High	Encephalitis; encephalopathy
Japanese encephalitis	1993	Inactivated virus	SC	Travelers	80–90%	Anaphylactic/severe delayed allergic reactions common; recipient should be observed for 10 days
Typhoid						
Phenol and heat-killed	1952	Killed whole bacteria	IM	Not routinely recommended in U.S.; used for travelers, contacts of carriers	50–70% (short-lived)	Frequent fever, local swelling, pain
Ty$_{21a}$	1992	Live mutant bacteria	Oral	Travelers, contacts of carriers	50–70%	None
Vi	1995	Vi capsular polysaccharide	IM	Travelers	70–75%	Local reactions

NOTE: SC, subcutaneous; BCG, bacille Calmette-Guérin; ID, intradermal; PPD, purified protein derivative; TB, tuberculosis; IM, intramuscular.

SOURCE: Recommendations of the Advisory Committee on Immunization Practices, the American Academy of Pediatrics, and the American College of Physicians.

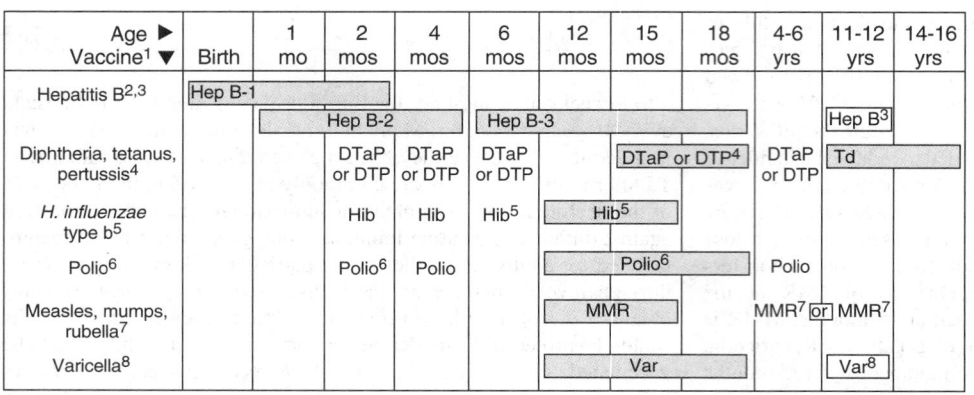

Age ▶ Vaccine[1] ▼	Birth	1 mo	2 mos	4 mos	6 mos	12 mos	15 mos	18 mos	4-6 yrs	11-12 yrs	14-16 yrs
Hepatitis B[2,3]	Hep B-1										
		Hep B-2			Hep B-3					Hep B[3]	
Diphtheria, tetanus, pertussis[4]			DTaP or DTP	DTaP or DTP	DTaP or DTP		DTaP or DTP[4]		DTaP or DTP	Td	
H. influenzae type b[5]			Hib	Hib	Hib[5]	Hib[5]					
Polio[6]			Polio[6]	Polio		Polio[6]			Polio		
Measles, mumps, rubella[7]						MMR			MMR[7] or MMR[7]		
Varicella[8]						Var				Var[8]	

FIGURE 122-2 Recommended childhood immunization schedule in the United States for January through December 1997. Vaccines are listed under the routinely recommended ages. Shaded bars indicate a range of acceptable ages for vaccination; clear bars indicate timing of catch-up vaccination: at 11 or 12 years of age, hepatitis B vaccine should be administered to children not previously vaccinated, and varicella vaccine should be administered to children not previously vaccinated who lack a reliable history of chickenpox. Vaccine abbreviations: Hep B, hepatitis B; DTaP, diphtheria/tetanus/acellular pertussis; DTP, diphtheria/tetanus/pertussis; Hib, *Haemophilus influenzae* type b; Td, tetanus/diphtheria toxoids, adsorbed; MMR, measles/mumps/rubella; Var, varicella-zoster. **Key to footnotes:** [1] *This schedule indicates the recommended age* for routine administration of currently licensed childhood vaccines. Some combination vaccines are available and may be used whenever administration of all components of the vaccine is indicated. Providers should consult the manufacturers' package insert for detailed recommendations. [2] *The hepatitis B surface antigen (HBsAg) status of pregnant women,* if not known, should be determined as soon as possible during pregnancy. *Infants born to HBsAg-negative mothers* should receive 2.5 μg of Recombivax HB (Merck, Sharpe and Dohme) or 10 μg of Engerix-B (Smith-Kline Beecham) at birth or within the first 2 months of life. The second dose should be administered ≥1 month after the first dose. In this setting a *combination Hep B/Hib vaccine (Comvax, Merck) released in January 1997 may be used* and may be given along with other recommended pediatric vaccines. *Infants born to HBsAg-positive mothers* should receive immunoprophylaxis with 0.5 mL of hepatitis B immune globulin along with 5 μg of Recombivax or 10 μg of Engerix-B within 12 h of birth. The second dose of vaccine is recommended at 1 to 2 months of age and the third dose at 6 months of age. *Infants born to mothers whose HBsAg status remains unknown at delivery* should receive either 5 μg of Recombivax or 10 μg of Engerix-B within 12 h of birth. The second dose of vaccine is recommended at 1 month of age and the third dose at 6 months of age. Blood should be drawn at the time of delivery to determine the mother's HBsAg status; if it is positive, the infant should receive hepatitis B immune globulin as soon as possible and no later than 1 week of age. The size and timing of subsequent vaccine doses are based on the mother's HBsAg status. [3] *Adolescents who have not previously received three doses of Hep B vaccine* should have the series initiated or completed at 11 or 12 years of age. The second dose should be administered at least 1 month after the first dose, and the third dose should be administered at least 4 months after the first dose and 2 months after the second dose. [4] *DTaP is the preferred vaccine for all doses,* including completion of the series in children who have received ≥1 dose of whole-cell DTP. Whole-cell DTP is an acceptable alternative to DTaP. The fourth dose of DTaP may be administered at 12 months, provided that 6 months have elapsed since the third dose, and if the child is unlikely to return at 15 to 18 months of age. A booster dose of DTaP (or DTP) is given at 4 to 6 years. Td is recommended at 11 or 12 years of age if at least 5 years have elapsed since the last dose of DTaP, DTP, or DT. [5] *Three Hib conjugate vaccines* are licensed for infant use. If PRP-OMP (PedVaxHIB [Merck]) is administered at 2 and 4 months of age, no dose is required at 6 months. After completion of the primary series, any Hib conjugate vaccine may be used as a booster. [6] *Two poliovirus vaccines are currently licensed in the United States:* enhanced inactivated poliovirus vaccine (IPV-e) and oral poliovirus vaccine (OPV). Three schedules are acceptable, and parents and providers may choose among them: (1) IPV-e at 2 and 4 months; OPV at 12 to 18 months and 4 to 6 years; (2) IPV-e for all four doses; (3) OPV for all four doses. IPV is the only poliovirus vaccine recommended for persons with a congenital or acquired immunodeficiency disease or an altered immune status resulting from disease or immunosuppressive therapy and for their household contacts. [7] *The second dose of MMR vaccine* is routinely recommended at 4 to 6 years of age or at 11 or 12 years of age but may be administered at any visit, provided that at least 1 month has elapsed since receipt of the first dose. [8] *Varicella-zoster virus vaccine* can be administered to susceptible children at any time after 12 months of age. Unvaccinated children who lack a reliable history of chickenpox should be vaccinated at 11 to 12 years of age. *(From the Advisory Committee on Immunization Practices, the American Academy of Pediatrics, and the American Academy of Family Practice in conjunction with the Food and Drug Administration and the pharmaceutical industry.)*

Adverse Events Modern vaccines, while safe and effective, are associated with adverse effects that range from infrequent and very mild to rare and life-threatening. The decision to use a vaccine involves an assessment of the risks of disease, the benefits of vaccination, and the risks associated with vaccination. Because these factors may change over time, continued assessment is essential. Table 122-7 lists valid and invalid contraindications to immunization and describes appropriate precautions in the use of specific vaccines.

Vaccine components, including protective antigens, animal proteins introduced during vaccine production, and antibiotics or other preservatives or stabilizers, can cause allergic reactions in some recipients. These reactions may be local or systemic and may include urticaria and serious anaphylaxis. The most common extraneous allergen is egg protein introduced when vaccines such as those for measles, mumps, influenza, and yellow fever are prepared in embryonated eggs. Local or systemic reactions can result from too-frequent administration of vaccines such as Td, diphtheria/tetanus (DT), or rabies; these reactions are probably due to antigen-antibody complexes. In addition, live-virus vaccines can interfere with tuberculin test responses. When a tuberculin skin test is indicated, it should be done either on the day of immunization or 6 weeks later.

All detected adverse events temporally related to vaccination are expected to be reported to both the local health department and the vaccine manufacturer. The NCVIA requires health care providers to report certain suspected adverse events following the receipt of a mandated vaccine to the FDA's Vaccine Adverse Events Reporting System (Table 122-8). Although a temporal relationship does not establish cause and effect, this surveillance system remains the only mechanism for collecting the data needed to form conclusions and make decisions.

USE OF VACCINES IN SPECIAL CIRCUMSTANCES **Pregnancy** Because of theoretical risk to the fetus and real risk of litigation to the practitioner, routine immunization of pregnant women is best avoided. However, wherever hygienic conditions during delivery cannot be guaranteed, it is essen-

Current recommendations also include influenza vaccine for routine annual administration to adults ≥65 years of age and to individuals with chronic illness at any age. Polyvalent pneumococcal polysaccharide vaccine is similarly recommended for the elderly or chronically ill. HBV vaccine is recommended for individuals at high risk of exposure, including health care workers exposed to potentially infected blood or blood products, homosexuals, injection drug users, individuals living and working in institutions for the mentally retarded, and household contacts of known carriers of hepatitis B surface antigen.

tial to ensure that pregnant women are immune to tetanus: the transfer of maternal antitoxin is an important means of preventing neonatal tetanus, and pregnant women can safely receive tetanus as well as diphtheria toxoids. Although live-virus vaccines in general should be withheld during pregnancy, polio and yellow fever vaccines are exceptions and may be administered if the risk of exposure to disease is great. If indicated, some inactivated-virus vaccines (e.g., HBV, influenza, and pneumococcal vaccines) are safe for pregnant women. Known pregnancy is considered a contraindication to the receipt of rubella, measles, mumps, and varicella vaccines. Although of theoreti-

Table 122-6

CHAPTER 122
Immunization Principles and Vaccine Use
765

Adult Immunization Schedule

Vaccine	Timing of Immunization
Hepatitis A*	Two doses are recommended for individuals requiring long-term protection, with the second dose 6–12 months after the first.
Hepatitis B*	Three doses are given, with the second dose 1 month after the first and the third dose 5 months after the second.
Measles/mumps/ rubella	One dose is given to adults born in 1957 or later **and not previously immunized.** A second dose may be required in some work or school settings.
Tetanus/diphtheria toxoids, adsorbed	A three-dose schedule applies for individuals who **have not received an initial immunization series in childhood.** The second dose is given 1 month after the first and the third dose 6 months after the second. Boosters are then given every 10 years.
Varicella	Two doses are given to individuals ≥13 years of age who have not had chickenpox. The second dose is given 1–2 months after the first.
Influenza	Vaccine is administered yearly to individuals ≥65 years of age; to younger people with chronic medical problems, such as heart disease and diabetes; and to those who work or live with high-risk persons.
Streptococcus pneumoniae	Vaccine is usually given once to individuals ≥65 years of age. A repeat dose may be given 5 years later for those at highest risk. Immunization is also recommended for younger people with chronic medical problems, such as heart disease, diabetes, renal failure, and sickle cell anemia, and for those who work or live with high-risk persons.

* For individuals at risk.
SOURCE: National Coalition for Adult Immunization.

cal concern, no cases of congenital rubella syndrome or abnormalities attributable to rubella vaccine virus have been observed in infants born to susceptible mothers who received rubella vaccine during pregnancy. A registry for susceptible women who have inadvertently received varicella vaccine during pregnancy has been established for the purpose of data collection.

Breast Feeding Neither killed nor live vaccine affects the safety of breast feeding for either mother or infant. Breast-fed infants can be immunized on a normal schedule. Breast feeding does not adversely affect the immune response and is not a contraindication for any vaccine. Although live vaccine viruses multiply within the mother's body, most are not excreted in breast milk. Mothers may therefore receive OPV or yellow fever vaccine without interrupting breast feeding. Rubella vaccine virus may be transmitted in breast milk; however, the virus usually does not infect the infant, and if it does the infection is well tolerated.

Occupational Exposure Immunization recommendations for most occupational groups remain to be developed. Specific practices are now mandated by the Occupational Safety and Health Administration for the immunization of health care workers against hepatitis B in the United States. Those at particular risk of exposure to hepatitis B, such as surgeons and health care workers dealing with blood products, must be immunized. Many medical institutions now give HBV vaccine to all health care workers and to all medical, dental, and nursing students. Rubella is transmitted to and from health care workers in medical facilities, particularly in pediatric practice. Health care workers who might transmit rubella to pregnant patients should be immune to rubella; it is prudent to screen these employees for antibodies to rubella virus and to immunize susceptible individuals. Persons providing health care are also at greater risk from measles and varicella than the general public, and those who are likely to come into contact with measles- and varicella-infected patients should be immune. Persons employed in caring for patients with chronic diseases can transmit influenza; such workers should be vaccinated annually. Unfortunately, these recommendations often are not fully implemented, even in academic institutions.

HIV Infection and Other Immunocompromised States Limited studies in HIV-infected individuals have found no increase in the risk of adverse events from live or inactivated vaccines. However, immune responses may not be as vigorous in immunocompromised individuals as in subjects with a normal immune system. Persons known to be infected with HIV should be immunized with recommended vaccines—except for poliovirus vaccine—in the same manner as individuals with a normal immune system and as early in the course of their disease as possible, before immune function becomes significantly impaired. Live attenuated MMR vaccine can be administered to this group, but OPV cannot (Table 122-9). IPV-e should be used when vaccination against polio is indicated because the risk of vaccine-associated poliomyelitis is too great with OPV. Household contacts of immunocompromised individuals should be immune to polio; when vaccinated, they should receive IPV-e and not OPV. In practice, it is not necessary to test for HIV before making decisions about the immunization of asymptomatic individuals from known HIV risk groups.

Live attenuated vaccines are normally contraindicated in immunocompromised patients, including those with congenital immunodeficiency syndromes and those receiving immunosuppressive therapy. Passive immunization with immunoglobulin preparations or antitoxins can be considered in individual cases, either as postexposure prophylaxis or as part of the treatment of established infection.

Postexposure Immunization For certain infections, active or passive immunization soon after exposure prevents or attenuates disease expression. The immune globulins and antitoxins currently available in the United States are listed in Table 122-10, and the recommended postexposure immunization regimens are compiled in Table 122-11. Measles immune globulins given within 6 days of exposure may prevent or modify infection, and measles vaccine given within the first few days after exposure may prevent symptomatic infection. Although clinical manifestations of rubella in pregnant women are minimized by postexposure passive immunization, this approach may not prevent maternal viremia, fetal infection, and congenital rubella syndrome. Therefore, the administration of immune globulin is recommended only for women developing rubella during pregnancy who will not consider abortion under any circumstances. Tetanus immune globulin can be used in patients with tetanus. Survivors with no history of tetanus immunization should receive a primary series of toxoid injections since disease does not result in the development of protective levels of antitoxin. Administration of rabies immune globulin plus rabies vaccine in the immediate postexposure period is highly effective in preventing disease. Similarly, for persons who have not been actively immunized, the use of immune globulin within 2 weeks of exposure to hepatitis A is likely to prevent clinical illness. Good data indicate the efficacy of human hepatitis B immune globulin in preventing disease after exposure. While no high-titer preparation is available for postexposure protection against non-A, non-B hepatitis, standard human immune serum globulin is efficacious.

Simultaneous Administration of Multiple Vaccines The simultaneous administration of the most widely used live and inactivated vaccines has not resulted in impaired antibody responses or in increased rates of adverse reactions. Simultaneous administration of vaccines is advantageous in that it increases the probability that a child will ultimately be fully immunized; it is also useful in any age group when the potential exists for exposure to multiple infectious diseases during travel to endemic countries. Inactivated vaccines can often be given together in a single injection or at separate sites at the same time. Administration of the combined MMR vaccine yields results comparable to those obtained with the administration of the individual vaccines at different sites; combined administration has greatly facilitated effective immunization for the three infections with little increase in cost. Although recent administration of OPV is not a contraindication to the use of MMR, other live-virus vaccines not given together on the same day should generally be administered at least 30 days apart.

Neither the response to OPV nor that to yellow fever vaccine is altered by the administration of immune globulins. In contrast, since high doses of immune globulin may inhibit the efficacy of measles and rubella vaccines, an interval of at least 3 months is recommended between the administration of immune globulin and that of MMR or its components. Postpartum vaccination of rubella-susceptible women should not be delayed because of the administration of anti-Rho(D) immune globulin or any other blood product during the last trimester or at delivery. Should administration of an immune globulin preparation become necessary after vaccination, it should be postponed, if possible, for at least 14 days to allow time for vaccine-virus replication and

development of immunity. In general, there is little interaction of immune globulin with inactivated vaccines, and postexposure passive prophylaxis can be given together with HBV vaccine or tetanus toxoid, resulting in both immediate and long-lasting protection.

Travel The International Sanitary Regulations allow countries to impose requirements for yellow fever and killed cholera vaccines as a condition for admission, even though the latter is not an effective public health tool. Travelers should know whether these vaccines are required for entry into the countries on their itinerary to avoid being turned back or immunized on the spot. Infants, children, and adults should have all routine immunizations updated before traveling, with

Table 122-7

Immunization Contraindications and Precautions

Vaccine	Contraindication or Precaution[a] Valid	Invalid
General[b]	Anaphylactic reaction to vaccine (contraindication to further doses of that vaccine) Anaphylactic reaction to vaccine constituent (contraindication to use of vaccines containing that substance) Moderate or severe illnesses, with or without fever	Mild to moderate local reaction (soreness, redness, swelling) following dose of injectable antigen Mild acute illness, with or without low-grade fever Current antimicrobial therapy Convalescent phase of illness Prematurity (same dosage and indications as for normal, full-term infants) Recent exposure to an infectious disease History of penicillin or other nonspecific allergies or family history of such allergies
DTaP/DTP	Encephalopathy within 72 h after dose Fever of ≥40.5°C (105°F) within 48 h after dose (P) Collapse or shocklike state (hypotonic-hyporesponsive episode) within 48 h after dose (P) Seizures within 3 days after dose (P) Persistent, inconsolable crying lasting ≥3 h within 48 h after dose (P)	Temperature of <40.5°C (105°F) after dose Family history of convulsions[c] Family history of an adverse event following vaccination Family history of sudden infant death syndrome
OPV[d]	Infection with HIV or a household contact infected with HIV Known immunodeficiency (hematologic and solid tumors, congenital immunodeficiency, and long-term immunosuppressive therapy) Immunodeficient household contact Pregnancy[e] (P)	Breast feeding Current antimicrobial therapy Diarrhea
IPV/IPV-e	Anaphylactic reactions to neomycin or streptomycin Pregnancy[e]	—
MMR	Anaphylactic reactions to eggs or to neomycin[f] Pregnancy Known immunodeficiency (hematologic and solid tumors, congenital immunodeficiency syndrome, and long-term immunosuppressive therapy) Recent IG administration (P)	Tuberculosis or positive PPD test Simultaneous TB skin testing[g] Breast feeding Pregnancy of mother of recipient Immunodeficient family member or household contact Infection with HIV Nonanaphylactic reactions to eggs or neomycin
Hib	None identified	History of Hib disease
HBV	None identified	Pregnancy
Influenza	First trimester of pregnancy (vaccination avoided on theoretical grounds) Anaphylactic reactions to eggs	—
Pneumococcus	Has not been evaluated in pregnancy	—
Varicella	Primary acquired immunodeficiency History of anaphylactic reaction to neomycin Pregnancy	Contact dermatitis in response to neomycin

[a] Precautions are followed by "(P)." The events or conditions listed as precautions, although not contraindications, should be carefully reviewed. The benefits and risks of administering a specific vaccine to an individual under the circumstances should be considered. If the risks are believed to outweigh the benefits, the vaccine should be withheld; if the benefits are believed to outweigh the risks (for example, during an outbreak or foreign travel), the vaccine should be administered. Whether and when to administer DTaP to children with proven or suspected underlying neurologic disorders should be decided on an individual basis.

[b] For DTP/DTaP, OPV, IPV/IPV-e, MMR, Hib, HBV, influenza, pneumococcus, and varicella.

[c] If a child has a precaution to the receipt of a subsequent dose of whole-cell DTP, the child should not routinely receive DTaP. If a child has a contraindication to the receipt of a subsequent dose of whole-cell DTP, the child should not receive DTaP. Acetaminophen given before DTaP and thereafter every 4 h for 24 h should be considered for children with a personal or family (sibling or parent) history of convulsions.

[d] No data exist to substantiate the theoretical risk of a suboptimal immune response when OPV and MMR are given within 30 days of each other.

[e] It is prudent on theoretical grounds to avoid vaccinating pregnant women. However, if immediate protection against poliomyelitis is needed, OPV is preferred, although IPV may be considered if vaccination can be completed before the anticipated imminent exposure.

[f] Persons with a history of anaphylactic reactions following egg ingestion should be vaccinated only with caution. Protocols have been developed for vaccinating such persons and should be consulted (J Pediatr 102:196, 1983; J Pediatr 113:504, 1988).

[g] Measles vaccination may temporarily suppress tuberculin reactivity. If skin testing cannot be done on the day of MMR vaccination, the test should be postponed for 4 to 6 weeks.

NOTE: IPV, inactivated polio vaccine; PPD, purified protein derivative; TB, tuberculosis; IG, immunoglobulin.

SOURCES: Standards for Pediatric Immunization Practices, Centers for Disease Control and Prevention; ACIP: Morb Mort Week Rep 38:73, 1989; ACIP: Morb Mort Week Rep 42:1, 1993. This information is based on the recommendations of the Advisory Committee on Immunization Practices (ACIP) and those of the Committee on Infectious Diseases (Red Book Committee) of the American Academy of Pediatrics (AAP). Sometimes these recommendations vary from those contained in the manufacturers' package inserts. For more detailed information, providers should consult the published recommendations of the ACIP and the AAP as well as the manufacturers' package inserts.

Table 122-8

CHAPTER 122
Immunization Principles and Vaccine Use **767**

Reportable Events Following Vaccination, as Required by the National Childhood Vaccine Injury Act of 1986 (Modified in 1995)*

Vaccine/Toxoid	Event	Interval from Vaccination
DTaP; P; DTP-Hib; DT; Td or TT	Anaphylaxis	4 h
	Encephalopathy (or encephalitis)	72 h
MMR, MR, or M	Anaphylaxis	4 h
	Encephalopathy (or encephalitis)	5–15 days
	Residual seizure disorder	5–15 days
Rubella-containing vaccines (MMR, MR, R)	Chronic arthritis	42 days
	Anaphylaxis	4 h
	Encephalopathy (or encephalitis)	5–15 days
	Residual seizure disorder	5–15 days
OPV	Paralytic poliomyelitis	
	In an immunocompetent recipient	30 days
	In an immunocompromised recipient	6 months
	In a vaccine-associated community case	No limits
Inactivated polio vaccine	Anaphylaxis	4 h

* Compensation (under the NCVIA) is effective for claims filed on or after March 10, 1995. Any acute complications or sequelae of an illness, disability, injury, or condition that arose within the prescribed period (including deaths) are also covered.

NOTE: P, pertussis; TT, tetanus toxoid; MR, measles/rubella; M, measles; R, rubella.

particular attention to polio, measles, and DTP/DTaP or Td vaccines. The use of hepatitis A vaccine or pooled human gamma globulin may be advisable for travelers to some locales. Special-use vaccines (Table 122-5), including rabies, meningococcal A and C polysaccharide, typhoid (oral live or Vi polysaccharide), Japanese encephalitis, and plague vaccines, should be considered for those individuals who expect to go beyond the usual tourist routes or to spend extended periods in rural areas in disease-endemic regions. Most U.S. cities have at least one travel clinic that maintains up-to-date epidemiologic information and can provide the appropriate vaccines. Military personnel, some laboratory personnel, and some individuals subject to occupational hazards (e.g., veterinarians) may receive special-use vaccines when indicated.

DELIVERY OF VACCINES   Over the past 20 years, considerable progress has been made to ensure that every child in the United States is fully immunized by the time of school entry. All 50 states now require immunization for school entry, and most have laws addressing attendance at preschools and day-care centers. Survey data (collected before the widespread use of Hib conjugate vaccine and HBV vaccine) indicated that up to 98 percent of all children were immunized against five vaccine-preventable diseases by the time they entered school. The impact of immunization and of other improvements in the health care provided to the American population on the incidence of vaccine-preventable illness is shown in Table 122-1 and Fig. 122-1.

By the mid-1980s, however, it was recognized that large numbers of preschool children were not fully immunized by 15 months of age. Only 37 to 56 percent of preschoolers in the United States had been completely immunized,[1] and this rate was as low as 10 percent in some communities. The failure to vaccinate preschool children was largely responsible for the resurgence of measles between 1989 and 1991, with 55,467 cases, more than 11,200 admissions to the hospital, more than 44,100 days of hospitalization, and more than 130 measles-related deaths. The number of cases of congenital rubella syndrome increased from 6 in 1988 to 47 in 1991. Outbreaks of pertussis and mumps were on the rise for the same reason: low immunization rates among preschool children.

ACCESS TO IMMUNIZATION   Four major barriers to infant and childhood immunization have been identified within the health care system: (1) low public awareness and lack of public demand for immunization, (2) inadequate access to immunization services, (3) missed opportunities to administer vaccines, and (4) inadequate resources for public health and preventive programs. These problems are sources of public concern, and their solution is a priority for national health policy in the United States. In response, the Children's Immunization Initiative was begun in 1990. At the national level, this program includes outreach and educational campaigns to promote parental awareness of the value of vaccination and to encourage health care providers to use every opportunity to vaccinate the children in their care. At the state and local levels, community and business groups, religious and service groups, schools, and the media have joined together in community-based networks. A National Immunization Week each April has been established to focus attention on the vaccination needs of infants and children. To improve the quality and quantity of vaccination services, expanded immunization-clinic hours and computerization of immunization records are being implemented as well.

One of the national health objectives for the millennium established under the Healthy People 2000 plan—a set of national health promotion and disease prevention objectives for the year 2000—is to achieve full coverage with the recommended vaccines for 90 percent of children under 2 years of age. By 1995, the National Immunization Survey showed vaccination coverage estimates to be at an all-time high (Table 122-12), while vaccine-preventable childhood diseases were at an all-time low (Table 122-13). Despite this success, about 25 percent of toddlers in the United States (or almost 1.4 million children from 19 to 35 months of age) still lacked one or more doses of the 4 DTP/3 polio/1 MMR series.

[1] By the second birthday, a fully immunized child will have received four doses of DTP/DTaP, three or four doses of a poliovirus vaccine (IPV-e and/or OPV), one dose of MMR, three doses of HBV vaccine, one dose of varicella vaccine, and three or four doses of a suitable Hib conjugate vaccine.

Table 122-9

Recommendations for Routine Immunization of HIV-Infected Persons in the United States

Vaccine	HIV Clinical Status Asymptomatic	Symptomatic	Comments
DTaP/Td	Yes	Yes	No change in usual immunization schedule
OPV	No	No	Increased risk of vaccine virus proliferation and paralytic polio; IPV-e used for household contacts of HIV-infected persons
IPV-e	Yes	Yes	Antibody response potentially impaired in symptomatic patients
MMR	Yes	Yes	No change in usual immunization schedule; with high risk of exposure to measles, first dose given at 6–11 months of age, second dose at >12 months of age; with documented infection, measles immune globulin potentially administered (see Table 122-11)
Hib conjugate	Yes	Yes	No change in usual immunization schedule
HBV	Yes	Yes	Antibody response potentially impaired; higher-dose vaccine available, but no data address optimal dose; possibly wise to check antibody titer after immunization and give additional doses if titer is inadequate
Pneumococcus	Yes	Yes	Should be given to all ≥2 years old
Influenza	Yes	Yes	Antibody response potentially impaired in symptomatic patients
Varicella	No	No	Vaccine use in asymptomatic HIV persons not studied

SOURCE: Centers for Disease Control and Prevention.

There has been only modest progress towards the goals for adult immunization in the United States promulgated under Healthy People 2000. Adult-immunization goals are important: as many as 60,000 adults die each year of vaccine-preventable diseases for which effective vaccines are not being optimally used. As few as 41 percent of persons ≥65 years of age receive influenza vaccine each year, and fewer than 30 percent of this group have ever received pneumococcal vaccine (Table 122-14). Health care providers more often miss vaccination opportunities with adults than with infants and children. Sixty to 90 percent of adults hospitalized for or dying of influenza-associated respiratory disease have received medical care during the previous year and could have been immunized at that time. Medicare reimbursement for excess hospitalization during influenza epidemics ranges from $750 million to $1 billion. Additional efforts are required to ensure that adults receive pneumococcal, Td, and HBV vaccines as well.

Financing Immunization Many private health insurance policies do not provide adequate coverage for immunization, and physicians and other health care providers pass these costs directly on to patients. In 1994, as a part of the Children's Immunization Initiative, the Vaccines for Children Program was implemented to remove critical barriers to protection against nine vaccine-preventable diseases. The program is designed to reach more children with free vaccine at public clinics and at the offices of their primary care providers. Moreover, states can buy vaccines at reduced prices from the Federal government. Thus, cost is no longer a barrier for the poorest children, and free vaccines are available from the provider of choice.

In contrast, gaps for immunization of adults exist under Medicare. Medicare coverage includes the cost of influenza and pneumococcal vaccines and their administration to all enrolled individuals; it also includes HBV vaccine for those at high risk of exposure (i.e., renal dialysis patients). However, reimbursement is not adequate to encourage vaccine use among providers, and the program does not cover other vaccines, such as Td.

STANDARDS FOR IMMUNIZATION PRACTICES National standards of immunization for adult and pediatric practice have been established to define common policies and practices for public health clinics and in physicians' private offices (Table 122-15). These guidelines highlight the need to distinguish between valid contraindications and conditions that are often considered but are not in fact contraindications (Table 122-7). Among the valid contraindications applicable to all vaccines are a history of anaphylaxis or other serious allergic reactions to a vaccine or vaccine component and the presence of a moderate or severe illness, with or without fever. Infants who develop encephalopathy within 72 h of a dose of DTP or DTaP should not receive further doses; those who develop a "precaution" (Table 122-7) should not normally receive further doses. Because of theoretical risks to the fetus, pregnant women should not receive MMR or varicella vaccine. Diarrhea, minor respiratory ill-

Table 122-10

Immune Globulins and Antitoxins* Available in the United States and Indications for Their Use, 1996

Immunobiologic Preparation	Indication(s)
Botulinum antitoxin (equine)	Treatment of botulism
Cytomegalovirus immune globulin, intravenous	Prophylaxis for liver, kidney, and possibly bone marrow transplant recipients
Diphtheria antitoxin (equine)	Treatment of respiratory diphtheria
Immune globulin	Hepatitis A pre- and postexposure prophylaxis; measles postexposure prophylaxis
Intravenous immune globulin	Replacement therapy for antibody deficiency disorders; immune thrombocytopenic purpura; hypogammaglobulinemia in chronic lymphocytic leukemia; Kawasaki disease
Hepatitis B immune globulin	Hepatitis B postexposure prophylaxis
Rabies immune globulin†	Rabies postexposure management of persons not previously immunized
Tetanus immune globulin	Tetanus treatment; postexposure prophylaxis for persons not adequately immunized with tetanus toxoid
Vaccinia immune globulin	Treatment of eczema vaccinatum, vaccinia necrosum, and ocular vaccinia
Varicella-zoster immune globulin	Postexposure prophylaxis of susceptible immunocompromised persons, certain susceptible pregnant women, and perinatally exposed newborns

* Immune globulins and antitoxins are administered intramuscularly unless indicated otherwise.
† Rabies immune globulin is administered around the wound in addition to being injected intramuscularly.

Table 122-11

Recommended Postexposure Immunization with Immunoglobulin Preparations in the United States

Disease	Indicated	Comments
Measles	Yes	Standard human immune globulin is recommended for exposed infants and adults with normal immunocompetence (but with a contraindication to measles vaccine) and for immunocompromised patients exposed to measles (regardless of immunization status). Patients should be immunized 3–6 months after immunoglobulin administration. Recommended dose: 0.25–0.5 mL/kg (40–80 mg of IgG/kg) IM; 80 mg of IgG/kg for immunocompromised contact; maximum, 15 mL.
Rubella	No	Efficacy is unreliable; therefore, standard human immune globulin is recommended for administration only to antibody-negative pregnant women in the first trimester who have a documented rubella exposure and who will not consider terminating the pregnancy. Recommended dose: 0.55 mL/kg (90 mg of IgG/kg) IM.
Tetanus	Yes	Human tetanus immune globulin (TIG) has replaced equine tetanus antitoxin because of the risk of serum sickness with equine serum. Recommended dose for postexposure prophylaxis: 250–500 units of TIG (10–20 mg of IgG/kg) IM. Recommended dose for treatment of tetanus: 500–3000 units of TIG IM.
Rabies	Yes	Human rabies immune globulin (RIG) is preferred over equine rabies antiserum because of the risk of serum sickness. RIG or antiserum is recommended for nonimmunized individuals with animal bites in which rabies cannot be ruled out and with other exposures to known rabid animals. Recommended dose of RIG: 20 IU/kg (22 mg of IgG/kg). Recommended dose of antiserum: 40 IU/kg. Rabies vaccine is given as well at 0, 3, 7, 14, and 28 days.
Hepatitis A	Yes	Standard immune serum globulin is given in a single dose of 0.02–0.04 mL/kg or (for continuous exposure) in a dose of up to 0.06 mL/kg every 5 months. Postexposure treatment with hepatitis A immune globulin has not been studied.
Hepatitis B	Yes	Standard immune serum globulin is not reliably effective. Special human hepatitis B immune globulin is useful and is recommended for neonates born to an infected mother and after mucous-membrane or parenteral contact with infected persons or infected blood or serum. Recommended dose for neonates: 0.5 mL IM within 12 h of birth. Recommended dose for percutaneous or mucosal exposure: 0.06 mL/kg (10 mg of IgG/kg) IM.
Non-A, non-B hepatitis	Yes	Standard immune serum globulin may be valuable. Recommended dose: 0.12 mL/kg (10 mg of IgG/kg) IM, up to 10 mL.

SOURCES: Advisory Committee on Immunization Practices (ACIP), Morb Mort Week Rep 42(RR-4):1, 1993; ACIP, 1991b; ACIP, Morb Mort Week Rep 40(RR-3):1, 1991; ACIP, 1991c; ACIP, Morb Mort Week Rep 39(RR-15):1, 1990.

Table 122-12

CHAPTER 122
Immunization Principles and Vaccine Use   **769**

Vaccination Levels Among Children Aged 19 to 35 Months, by Vaccine—National Immunization Survey, United States, April 1994 through March 1995

Vaccine/Dose	1996 Goal, %	Year 2000 Objective, %	Coverage in April 1994–March 1995 (95% confidence interval)
DTP/DT			
≥3 doses	90	90	94 (±0.6%)
≥4 doses	—	90	77 (±1.0%)
Poliovirus, ≥3 doses	90	90	84 (±0.9%)
Hib, ≥3 doses	90	90	90 (±0.7%)
MMR, ≥1 dose	90	90	89 (±0.8%)
HBV, ≥3 doses	70	90	42 (±1.2%)
19–24 months			58 (±1.4%)
25–30 months			41 (±1.4%)
31–35 months			24 (±1.3%)
Combined series			
4 DTP/3 polio/1 MMR	—	90	75 (±1.0%)
4 DTP/3 polio/1 MMR/3 Hib	—	90	72 (±1.1%)

SOURCE: Centers for Disease Control and Prevention.

ness with or without fever, mild to moderate local reactions to a previous dose of vaccine, the concurrent or recent use of antimicrobial agents, mild to moderate malnutrition, or the convalescent phase of an acute illness are not valid contraindications to routine immunization. Failure to vaccinate children because of these conditions is increasingly being viewed as a missed opportunity for immunization.

THE ROLE OF INDUSTRY Except in the states of Michigan and Massachusetts, which manufacture certain vaccines and immune globulin preparations, the American public is entirely dependent upon the willingness of the commercial sector to make and market vaccines. This willingness has declined over the past two decades, and many manufacturers no longer produce vaccines. There are currently just one or two U.S.-based commercial sources for most childhood vaccines.

THE NATIONAL VACCINE INJURY COMPENSATION PROGRAM The use of mandated vaccines benefits society as a whole by reducing morbidity and the cost of care for preventable diseases and by reducing childhood mortality. Thus, in the United States, society has assumed the obligation to care for those injured by the administration of mandated vaccines. The NCVIA of 1986 (modified in 1995) is the instrument in use to ensure fairness to injured persons as well as protection for Federal, state, and local immunization programs; private immunization providers; and vaccine manufacturers. The act was designed to implement two vital public policies: (1) to provide prompt and fair compensation to the families of children who have died or have been injured as a result of routine mandated immunization; and (2) to reduce the adverse impact of the tort system

Table 122-13

Vaccine-Preventable Disease Targets

Disease	1987 Baseline	1995	2000 Target
Diphtheria among people aged 25 and younger	1	0	0
Tetanus among people aged 25 and younger	3	5	0
Polio (wild-type virus)	0	0	0
Measles	3058	288	0
Rubella	225	146	0
Congenital rubella syndrome	6	7	0
Mumps	4866	840	<500
Pertussis	3450	4315	<1000
Haemophilus influenzae type b	20,000*	1164	0

* Not notifiable before 1991; estimated prevaccine-era annual incidence.

SOURCE: *Healthy People 2000: National Health Promotion and Disease Prevention Objectives,* Washington, DC, Department of Health and Human Services, 1990.

on vaccine supply, cost, and innovation/development. The success of immunization programs in the United States depends upon the continued viability of the National Vaccine Injury Compensation Program.

CONTROL OF VACCINE-PREVENTABLE DISEASE

A continuing task of public health practice is to maintain individual and herd immunity. The job is not over once a population is fully vaccinated; rather, it is imperative to immunize each subsequent generation as long as the threat of the disease persists. Ongoing surveillance and prompt reporting of disease to local or state health departments are essential to this goal, ensuring a continuing awareness of the possibility of vaccine-preventable illness. Nearly all vaccine-preventable diseases are now notifiable, and individual case data are routinely forwarded to the CDC. These data are used to detect outbreaks or other unusual events that require investigation and to evaluate prevention and control policies, practices, and strategies.

As a direct consequence of successes in immunization, vaccine-preventable diseases have become less visible; ironically, this situation may foster complacency among parents and health care providers about routine immunization of children. Even among the affluent and educated, immunization levels may be low, reflecting a misunderstanding of the continuing threat of disease with which parents and health care providers have limited experience or perhaps an unjustifiably greater fear of adverse reactions to vaccination than of the potential for illness and death due to vaccine-preventable diseases. Health care workers play an essential role in influencing the attitudes of patients regarding appropriate immunization; therefore, it is essential that these professionals continually update their own knowledge about vaccines and about the epidemiology of vaccine-preventable illnesses.

RESEARCH ON VACCINES AND IMMUNIZATION

To accomplish the preventive goals of Healthy People 2000, current immunization recommendations in the United States call for every child to receive 10 different vaccines (many at the same time and most requiring more than one dose) between birth and entry into kindergarten. This agenda requires at least five visits to a health care provider by age 2, with an additional visit before entry into school. This is a formidable task, particularly for persons with limited access to health care, and compliance can be expected to become more difficult as new vaccines are licensed.

THE CHILDREN'S VACCINE INITIATIVE The potential to eradicate selected diseases and to build sustainable immunization programs that reach every child is not being fulfilled with existing vaccines and delivery technology. New vaccines or new formulations that will not only improve protective responses but also simplify the

Table 122-14

Estimates of Vaccine Coverage or Immunity Among Adults

Vaccine	Percent
Influenza (age 65+)	41*
Pneumococcus (age 65+)	28†
Hepatitis B (age 65+)	1–60‡
Tetanus	16–59§
Diphtheria	34–51§
Measles	85–95§
Rubella	80–90‡
Mumps	91‡
Varicella	93

* Year 2000 target is 60%.   ‡ Varies by risk group.
† Year 2000 target is 60%.   § Varies by study.

SOURCE: Centers for Disease Control and Prevention.

Table 122-15

Standards for Immunization Practices

Standard Number	Standard

PEDIATRIC PRACTICE

1. Immunization services are readily available.
2. There are no barriers to or unnecessary prerequisites for the receipt of vaccines.
3. Immunization services are available free or for a minimal fee.
4. Providers use all clinical encounters to screen and, when indicated, immunize children.
5. Providers educate parents and guardians about immunization in general terms.
6. Providers question parents or guardians about contraindications and, before immunizing a child, inform them in specific terms about the risks and benefits of the immunizations their child is to receive.
7. Providers follow only true contraindications.
8. Providers administer simultaneously all vaccine doses for which a child is eligible at the time of each visit.
9. Providers use accurate and complete recording procedures.
10. Providers coschedule immunization appointments in conjunction with appointments for other child health services.
11. Providers report adverse events following immunization promptly, accurately, and completely.
12. Providers operate a tracking system.
13. Providers adhere to appropriate procedures for vaccine management.
14. Providers conduct semiannual audits to assess immunization coverage levels and to review immunization records for the patient populations they serve.
15. Providers maintain up-to-date, easily retrievable medical protocols at all locations where vaccines are administered.
16. Providers operate with patient-oriented and community-based approaches.
17. Vaccines are administered by properly trained individuals.
18. Providers receive ongoing education and training on current immunization recommendations.

ADULT PRACTICE

1. Appropriate vaccine use is promoted through information campaigns for health care practitioners and trainees, employers, and the public about the benefits of immunizations.
2. Providers are completely immunized to protect themselves and prevent transmission to patients.
3. Providers routinely determine the immunization status of their adult patients, offer vaccines to those for whom they are indicated, and maintain complete immunization records.
4. Providers identify high-risk patients in need of influenza vaccine and develop a system to recall them for annual immunization.
5. Providers and institutions identify high-risk adult patients in hospitals and other treatment centers and ensure that appropriate vaccination is considered either before discharge or as part of discharge planning.
6. Licensing/accreditation agencies support the development by health care institutions of comprehensive immunization programs for staff, trainees, volunteer workers, inpatients, and outpatients.
7. States establish preenrollment immunization requirements for colleges and other institutions of higher education.
8. Institutions that train health care professionals, deliver health care, or provide laboratory or other medical support services require appropriate immunizations for persons at risk of contracting or transmitting vaccine-preventable illnesses.
9. Health care benefit programs, third-party payers, and government health care programs provide coverage for adult immunization services.
10. A standard personal and institutional immunization record is adopted as a means of verifying the immunization status of patients and staff.

SOURCE: For pediatric standards: Ad Hoc Working Group for the Development of Standards for Pediatric Immunization Practices. JAMA 269:1817, 1993; for adult standards: The National Coalition for Adult Immunization.

immunization schedule are needed. The Children's Vaccine Initiative is an international effort to attain these ends. The ideal is to develop vaccines that can be administered orally early in life, that provide lifelong protection against multiple infections, that can be given as one or only a few doses, and that are less reactive and more heat stable than current vaccines. To attain these ambitious goals may take years or decades, but progress is already being made in the development of new combinations of current vaccines to facilitate complete immunization. Strategies for research directed toward improved vaccine delivery are listed in Table 122-16. The results will be applicable to immunization programs in both developed and developing countries.

REEMERGENCE OF CONTROLLED DISEASE AND EMERGENCE OF NEW DISEASE The emergence of new pathogens is fostered by the genetic potential of microbes to evolve as well as by rapid changes in human demographics and behavior and in a global ecology that creates new or more favorable hosts. Proof of the need for continuing vaccine research is found in the emergence of new infectious diseases such as HIV infection, Lyme borreliosis, hantavirus pulmonary syndrome, and hepatitis C; the appearance of a new epidemic cholera strain (serotype O139 Bengal) that exhibits no cross-immunity with the traditional O1 serotype; and the increase in global incidence and in drug resistance of familiar diseases that were once considered under control, such as tuberculosis and malaria. In addition, some common illnesses without a previously known etiology, such as peptic ulcer disease and cervical and nasopharyngeal cancer, have now been epidemiologically linked to specific infectious agents and have thus become potentially vaccine-preventable conditions.

DEVELOPMENT OF NEW VACCINES For many serious or even life-threatening infectious diseases, no effective vaccines are available. Although many new vaccines are undergoing human trials (Table 122-17), the task of developing vaccines is proving very complex. Priorities for the United States currently include research on the following vaccines: HIV, pneumococcus (conjugate), group B *Streptococcus*, respiratory syncytial virus, rotavirus, *Mycobacterium tuberculosis*, herpes simplex virus, influenza A and B viruses, and hepatitis C virus. Also of high priority are vaccines for two virus-associated tumors: cervical cancer (human papillomavirus) and nasopharyngeal cancer (Epstein-Barr virus).

INTERNATIONAL CONSIDERATIONS

Since the establishment of the World Health Organization's Expanded Programme on Immunization in 1981, levels of coverage for the recommended basic children's vaccines (bacille Calmette-Guérin, polio, DTP, measles, and hepatitis B) have risen from 5 percent to approximately 80 percent worldwide. Each year, at least 2.7 million deaths from measles, neonatal tetanus, and pertussis and 200,000 cases of paralysis due to polio are prevented by immunization. Despite the successes of this program, many vaccine-preventable diseases remain prevalent in the developing world. Measles, for example, continues to kill an estimated 1.5 million children each year, and cases of diphtheria, whooping cough, polio, and neonatal tetanus still occur at unacceptably high rates. It is estimated that between 20 and 35 percent of all deaths of children under the age of 5 years are still associated with vaccine-preventable diseases.

In addition to the antigens included in the Expanded Programme for routine use in the developing world, others (Hib, Japanese B encephalitis, yellow fever, group A meningococcus, mumps, and rubella) are used regionally, depending on disease epidemiology and resources. Polio has been targeted for eradication by the year 2000; this disease has already been eliminated in the Americas and is close to elimination in the Western Pacific.

Because infectious diseases know no geographic or political boundaries, uncontrolled disease anywhere in the world poses a threat to the United States. Vaccines offer the opportunity to control and even eradicate some diseases, and eradication means that vaccines are no longer needed. The experience with smallpox has shown that the eradication of disease is a remarkably good economic investment.

Table 122-16

Examples of Scientific Research Directed Toward Improved Vaccine Delivery

Delivery System Change Desired	Scientific Input	Products in Process
Decrease number of visits required for full immunization	Development of new combination vaccines	MMRV; DTaP-Hib
	Research on recombinant live multiantigen vaccines	Canarypox-measles, Canarypox-RSV, vaccinia-rabies, vaccinia-influenza, *Salmonella*-BCG
Decrease number of doses	Development of time-release products	Microencapsulated forms of tetanus toxoid, hepatitis B, pertussis, influenza
Decrease number of injections	Research on oral vaccines	Pertussis
	Research on mucosal immunity	Cholera
	Research on antigen presentation	Influenza
Immunize as early in life as possible	Research on maternal immunization	Hib, meningococcus, pneumococcus
	Research on neonatal immunity	Group B *Streptococcus*, measles
Decrease rates of adverse events	Research on mechanisms of adverse events	Pertussis, OPV
Increase protection	Research on more immunogenic antigens	Group B *Streptococcus*
	Development of conjugate vaccines	Meningococcus, pneumococcus
	Research on adjuvants	Typhoid, influenza
Increase thermal stability	Research on stabilizers	Chemical stabilizers, freeze drying
Immunize by the oral route	Development of oral delivery systems	Iscoms, liposomes, polylactic and polyglycolic acid polymers, etc.

NOTE: MMRV, measles/mumps/rubella/varicella; RSV, respiratory syncytial virus; BCG, bacille Calmette-Guérin.

Table 122-17

Vaccines Undergoing Human Trials

Bacterial	Viral
Vibrio cholerae	Respiratory syncytial
Mycobacterium leprae	Dengue
Salmonella typhi	Rotavirus
Salmonella paratyphi	Japanese B encephalitis
Neisseria meningitidis	Influenza A and B
Streptococcus pneumoniae	Parainfluenza
Group B *Streptococcus*	Measles
Shigella spp.	Cytomegalovirus
Enterotoxigenic *Escherichia coli*	Rabies
Enterohemorrhagic *E. coli*	Junin
Borrelia burgdorferi	Chikungunya
Fungal	Rift Valley fever
Cryptococcus neoformans	Herpes simplex
Parasitic	Yellow fever
Plasmodium spp.	

The entire sum that the United States spent for the global smallpox eradication campaign has been recouped, in 1968 dollars, every 2.5 months since 1971. The global eradication of polio will save the United States over $300 million a year in vaccine and associated delivery costs and will save over $1.5 billion a year worldwide.

SOURCES OF INFORMATION ON IMMUNIZATION

- Official vaccine package circulars
- Report of the Committee on Infectious Diseases of the American Academy of Pediatrics ("Red Book")
- Recommendations of the Advisory Committee on Immunization Practices (ACIP), Centers for Disease Control and Prevention
- Guide for Adult Immunization, American College of Physicians
- Health Information for International Travel (published yearly) and Advisory Memoranda on Travel (published periodically), Centers for Disease Control and Prevention
- Control of Communicable Diseases in Man, American Public Health Association
- Technical Bulletin of the College of Obstetrics and Gynecology

BIBLIOGRAPHY

ADVISORY COMMITTEE ON IMMUNIZATION PRACTICES: General recommendations on immunization: Recommendations of the Immunization Practices Advisory Committee (ACIP). Morb Mort Week Rep 38:205, 1989

————: Diphtheria, tetanus, and pertussis: Recommendations for vaccine use and other preventive measures. Immunization Practices Advisory Committee (ACIP). Morb Mort Week Rep 40:1, 1991a

————: Update on adult immunization. Recommendations of the Immunization Practices Advisory Committee (ACIP). Morb Mort Week Rep 40(RR-12):1, 1991b

————: Hepatitis B virus: A comprehensive strategy for elimination of transmission in the United States through universal childhood vaccination. Recommendations of the Immunization Practices Advisory Committee (ACIP). Morb Mort Week Rep 40(RR-13):1, 1991c

————: Pertussis vaccination: Acellular pertussis vaccine for the fourth and fifth doses of the DTP series: Update to the supplementary ACIP statement: Recommendations of the Advisory Committee on Immunization Practices. Morb Mort Week Rep 41(RR-15):1, 1992

————: Recommendations for use of *Haemophilus* b conjugate vaccines and a combined diphtheria, tetanus, pertussis, and *Haemophilus* b vaccine. Morb Mort Week Rep 42(RR-13):1, 1993

————: General recommendations on immunization: Recommendation of the Advisory Committee on Immunization Practices (ACIP). Morb Mort Week Rep 1995;44(RR-5):1, 1995

————: Recommended childhood immunization schedule—United States, January 1995. Morb Mort Week Rep 43:959, 1995

————: National, state and urban area vaccination coverage levels among children 19–35 months—United States, April 1994–March 1995. Morb Mort Week Rep 45:145, 1996

AMERICAN ACADEMY OF PEDIATRICS: *Report of the Committee on Infectious Diseases ("Red Book"),* 22d ed, G Peter et al (eds). Elk Grove Village, IL, 1994

AMERICAN COLLEGE OF PHYSICIANS: *Guide for Adult Immunization,* 2d ed. Philadelphia, American College of Physicians, 1994

AMERICAN PUBLIC HEALTH ASSOCIATION: *Control of Communicable Diseases in Man,* 16th ed, AS Benenson (ed). Washington, DC, American Public Health Association, 1995

BRICKMAN HF et al: The timing of tuberculin tests in relation to immunization with live viral vaccines. Pediatrics 55:392, 1975

CHANDER J, SUBRAHMANYAN S: Mass polio vaccination. Eradication by 2000 is a realistic goal. BMJ 312:1178, 1996

DE QUADROS CA et al: Measles elimination in the Americas. Evolving strategies. JAMA 275:224, 1996

KING GE, HADLER SC: Simultaneous administration of childhood vaccines: An important public health policy that is safe and efficacious. Pediatr Infect Dis J 13:394, 1994

NINANE J et al: Disseminated BCG in HIV infection. Arch Dis Child 63:1268, 1988

SIBER GR et al: Interference of immune globulin with measles and rubella immunization. J Pediatr 122:204, 1993

SOMANI J, LARSON RA: Reimmunization after allogeneic bone marrow transplantation. Am J Med 98:389, 1995

VETTER RT, JOHNSON GM: Vaccination update. Hib, hepatitis, polio, varicella, influenza, pneumococcal and meningococcal disease. Postgrad Med 98:141, 1995

WATSON BM et al: Safety and immunogenicity of a combined live attenuated measles, mumps, rubella, and varicella vaccine (MMR$_{II}$V) in healthy children. J Infect Dis 173:731, 1996

WHITE CJ: Clinical trials of varicella vaccine in healthy children. Infect Dis Clin North Am 10:595, 1996

123 *J.S. Keystone, P.E. Kozarsky*

HEALTH RISKS TO TRAVELERS

In 1991, the World Health Organization estimated that more than 30 million persons traveled from industrialized countries to the developing world. Studies show that between 50 and 75 percent of short-term travelers to the tropics or subtropics report some health impairment. Most of these health problems are minor, with only 5 percent requiring medical attention and fewer than 1 percent requiring hospitalization.

Although infectious agents contribute substantially to morbidity in travelers, these pathogens account for only about 1 percent of deaths among this population. Cardiovascular disease and injuries are the most frequent causes of death among travelers from the United States, accounting for 49 and 22 percent of deaths, respectively. Age-specific rates of mortality due to cardiovascular disease are similar to those among nontravelers. In contrast, rates of death due to injury—the majority from motor vehicle, drowning, or aircraft accidents—are several times higher among travelers. Figure 123-1 summarizes the monthly incidence of health problems during travel in developing countries.

TRAVELER'S DIARRHEA Diarrhea is the leading cause of illness in travelers (see Chap. 128) and is usually a short-lived, self-limited condition; however, 40 percent of affected individuals need to alter their scheduled activities, and another 20 percent are confined to bed. The most important determinant of risk is the destination of the traveler. Incidence rates per 2-week stay have been reported to be as low as 8 percent in industrialized countries and as high as 55 percent in parts of Africa, Central and South America, and Southeast Asia. Infants and young adults are at particularly high risk. The incidence of diarrhea is proportional to the number of dietary indiscretions. Studies of U.S. students in Mexico showed that eating meals in restaurants and cafeterias or consuming food from street vendors was associated with increased risk.

The most frequently identified pathogen causing traveler's diarrhea is toxigenic *Escherichia coli*, although in some parts of the world (notably North Africa and Southeast Asia), *Campylobacter* infections appear to predominate. Other common causative organisms include *Salmonella*, *Shigella*, rotavirus, and the Norwalk agent. Except for

giardiasis, parasitic infections are uncommon causes of traveler's diarrhea. A growing problem for travelers is the development of antibiotic resistance in many bacterial pathogens; examples include strains of *Campylobacter* resistant to quinolones and strains of *E. coli*, *Shigella*, and *Salmonella* resistant to trimethoprim-sulfamethoxazole.

Although extremely common, acute traveler's diarrhea is usually self-limited or amenable to antibiotic therapy. Travelers who have chronic bowel problems after their return home are more likely to seek medical attention from a specialist, because the etiology of this problem is less well defined. Infectious agents appear to be responsible for only a small proportion of cases with chronic bowel symptoms; of the pathogens detected in these instances, *Giardia intestinalis* (also called *Giardia lamblia*; see Chap. 220) is by far the most common, whereas *Cyclospora cayetanensis*, *Cryptosporidium* species, and *Entamoeba histolytica* are rare. By far the most frequent causes of chronic diarrhea after travel are postinfectious sequelae, such as lactose intolerance or an irritable bowel syndrome. When no infectious etiology can be identified, a trial of metronidazole therapy for presumed giardiasis, a strict lactose-free diet for 1 week, or a several-week trial of high-dose hydrophilic mucilloid relieves the symptoms of many patients.

MALARIA It is estimated that more than 30,000 American and European travelers develop malaria each year (see Chap. 216). The risk of malaria is highest in sub-Saharan Africa and Oceania (1:50 to 1:1000) and during the past decade has increased more than fivefold for travelers to Kenya. The risk is intermediate (1:1000 to 1:12,000) for travelers to Haiti and the Indian subcontinent and is low (less than 1:50,000) for travelers to Asia and to Central and South America. Of the 1000 cases of malaria reported annually in the United States, 90 percent of those due to *Plasmodium falciparum* occur in travelers returning or immigrating from Africa and Oceania. With the worldwide increase in chloroquine- and multidrug-resistant falciparum malaria, decisions about chemoprophylaxis have become more difficult. In addition, the spread of malaria due to primaquine- and chloroquine-resistant strains of *Plasmodium vivax* has added to the complexity of treatment. The case-fatality rate of falciparum malaria in the United States is 4 percent; however, in only one-third of patients who die is the diagnosis of malaria considered before death. Compliance with antimalarial chemoprophylaxis regimens and use of personal protection measures to prevent mosquito bites are keys to the prevention of malaria. Several recent studies indicate that fewer than 50 percent of travelers adhere to basic recommendations for malaria prevention.

VACCINE-PREVENTABLE DISEASES **Immunizations of Worldwide Importance** *Diphtheria, tetanus, and polio* Diphtheria continues to be a problem worldwide, with recent large outbreaks in the new independent states formerly encompassed by the Soviet Union (see Chap. 144). Serosurveys now show that tetanus antitoxin is lacking in many North Americans, especially those over the age of 50 (see Chap. 146). Although the risk of polio to the international traveler is extremely low, studies in the United States have found varying levels of immunity in the general population, and recent data indicate that 12 percent of adult American travelers are unprotected against at least one serogroup (see Chap. 195). Foreign travel is an ideal opportunity to have these immunizations updated (see Chap. 122).

Measles Measles (rubeola) continues to be a major cause of morbidity and mortality in the developing world (see Chap. 196). Several outbreaks of measles in the United States have been linked to imported cases. The group at highest risk consists of persons born after 1956 and vaccinated before 1980, in many of whom primary vaccination failed. Travelers in this group should be reimmunized.

Influenza Influenza occurs year-round in the tropics and during the summer months in the Southern Hemisphere (i.e., the winter months in the Northern Hemisphere). Vaccination should be considered for all travelers to these regions, particularly those who are elderly or chronically ill (see Chap. 193).

Special Immunizations for Travelers *Hepatitis A and B* Hepatitis A (see Chap. 295) is the most frequent vaccine-preventable infection of travelers; the incidence of symptomatic infection during a 1-month stay in a developing country ranges from 3 to 6 cases per 1000. The risk is six times greater for those who stray from the usual

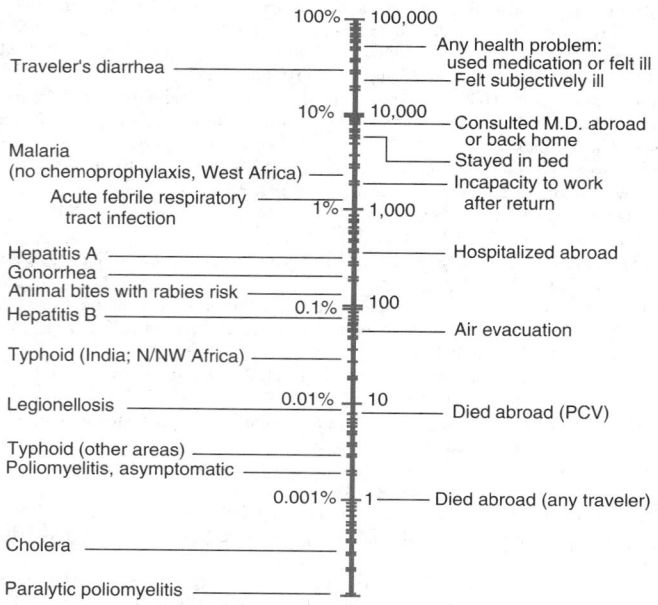

FIGURE 123-1 Incidence rate, per month, of health problems during a stay in developing countries. PCV, Peace Corps volunteer. (*From Steffen and Lobel*, with permission from Chapman and Hall, New York.)

tourist routes. The monthly incidence of hepatitis B infection, both symptomatic and asymptomatic, is 80 to 240 cases per 100,000. For reasons that are not entirely clear, long-stay overseas workers are at considerable risk for hepatitis B infection.

Typhoid and cholera The attack rate for typhoid fever is 1 case per 30,000 per month of travel to the developing world (see Chap. 158). However, the rates in India, Senegal, and North Africa are 10-fold higher, and, within these areas, rates are especially high among travelers to more remote destinations and among persons who are returning to their homeland to visit and stay with relatives or friends. These same groups, because they are more likely than other travelers to commit dietary indiscretions, are at higher risk for cholera as well. Overall, the risk of cholera to travelers is extremely low: approximately 1 case per 500,000 journeys to endemic areas (see Chap. 161). Cholera vaccine is not indicated for most travelers.

Miscellaneous infections The incidence of yellow fever among travelers is extremely low, probably because the vaccine is highly efficacious and is required by health authorities for entry into most countries of sub-Saharan Africa and South America in which this infection exists (see Chap. 200). Many cases of rabies have been reported in travelers, but there are no data on the risk of infection. Domestic animals are the major transmitters of rabies in developing countries (see Chap. 199). Countries where canine rabies is highly endemic include Mexico, the Philippines, Sri Lanka, India, Thailand, and Vietnam. Almost half of the cases of rabies reported in the United States in recent years have been acquired outside of the country. The risk of Japanese encephalitis, an infection transmitted by mosquitoes in rural Asia and Southeast Asia, is approximately 1:5000 per month of stay in an endemic area (see Chap. 200). Most symptomatic infections in U.S. residents have been in military personnel or their families. Although the risk of meningococcal disease in travelers has not been quantified, it appears to be highest among travelers who live with the indigenous population in overcrowded conditions (see Chap. 149).

PREGNANCY AND TRAVEL A woman's medical history and itinerary, the quality of medical care at her destinations, and her degree of flexibility determine whether travel is wise during pregnancy. According to the American College of Obstetrics and Gynecology, the safest part of pregnancy in which to travel is the second trimester (between 18 and 24 weeks), when there is the least danger of spontaneous abortion or premature labor. Some obstetricians prefer that women stay within a few hundred miles of home after the 28th week of pregnancy in case problems arise; in general, however, healthy women may be advised that it is acceptable to travel.

Despite this general recommendation, there are some relative contraindications to international travel during pregnancy, including certain obstetrical risk factors: a history of miscarriage, premature labor, incompetent cervix, or toxemia. General medical problems such as diabetes, heart failure, severe anemia, or a history of thromboembolic disease should also prompt the pregnant woman to postpone her travels. Finally, regions in which the pregnant woman and her fetus may be at excessive risk (e.g., those at high altitudes and those where live-virus vaccines are required or where multidrug-resistant malaria is endemic) are not ideal destinations during any trimester.

Malaria Malaria during pregnancy carries a significant risk of morbidity and death. Levels of parasitemia are highest and failure to clear the parasites after chloroquine treatment are most frequent among primigravidae. Severe disease, with complications such as cerebral malaria, massive hemolysis, and renal failure, is especially likely in pregnancy. Fetal sequelae include spontaneous abortion, stillbirth, preterm delivery, and congenital infection.

Traveler's Diarrhea Because dehydration due to traveler's diarrhea can lead to inadequate placental blood flow, pregnant travelers must be extremely cautious regarding their food and beverage intake. The exclusive consumption of bottled (carbonated) or boiled drinks without ice, the eating of well-cooked meats and pasteurized dairy products, and the avoidance of pre-prepared salad items should help protect against traveler's diarrhea due to the usual causes as well as against infections such as toxoplasmosis and listeriosis, which can have serious sequelae in pregnancy.

The mainstay of therapy for traveler's diarrhea is rehydration. Kaolin-pectin combinations and loperamide may be used if necessary, but many of the usual antibiotics (e.g., quinolones) are contraindicated during pregnancy. Ampicillin alone or with clavulanic acid may be used, but many strains of *E. coli* and other organisms implicated in traveler's diarrhea are resistant. An oral third-generation cephalosporin may be the best option.

Because of the major problems encountered when infants are given local foods and beverages, women are strongly encouraged to breast-feed when traveling with a neonate. A nursing mother with traveler's diarrhea should not stop breast-feeding but should increase her fluid intake.

Air Travel and High-Altitude Destinations Commercial air travel is not a risk to the healthy pregnant woman or to the fetus. Fetal oxygenation is not adversely affected by the decreased cabin pressures because of the fetal hemoglobin dissociation curve; the higher radiation levels reported at altitudes of more than 35,000 feet should pose no problem to the healthy traveler. Since each airline has a policy regarding pregnancy and flying, it is best to check with the specific carrier when booking reservations. Domestic air travel is usually permitted until the 36th week, whereas international air travel is generally curtailed after the 32d week.

There are no known risks for pregnant women who travel to high-altitude destinations and stay for short periods. However, there are likewise no data on the safety of pregnant women at altitudes of greater than 15,000 feet. Because of the harsh conditions usually associated with such trips, they are generally contraindicated for other reasons.

THE HIV-INFECTED TRAVELER The traveler infected with human immunodeficiency virus (HIV) is at special risk of serious infections due to a number of pathogens that may be more prevalent at travel destinations than at home. However, the degree of risk depends primarily on the state of the immune system at the time of travel. For persons whose CD4+ cell counts are normal or above 500/μL, no data suggest a greater risk during travel than for persons without HIV infection. Individuals with AIDS (CD4+ counts of <200/μL) and others who are symptomatic need special counseling and should visit their primary care physician before traveling, especially to the developing world.

Several countries now deny routine entry to HIV-positive individuals, even though no data show that these restrictions decrease rates of transmission of the virus. In general, HIV testing is required of those individuals who wish to stay abroad longer than 3 months or who intend to work or study abroad. Some countries will accept an HIV serologic test done within 6 months of departure, whereas others will not accept a blood test done at any time in the traveler's home country. In addition, border officials often have the authority to make inquiries of individuals entering a country and to check the medications they are carrying. If a drug such as zidovudine is identified, the person may be barred from entering the country. Information on testing requirements for specific countries is available from consular offices but is subject to frequent change.

Health insurance policies should be checked to make sure they are valid for care in other countries. The HIV-positive traveler should strongly consider obtaining trip cancellation insurance and evacuation insurance in case of illness. It is ideal to have the name of a physician at the travel destination who is familiar with the treatment of patients with AIDS, as the clinical findings associated with infection may be atypical in a patient with AIDS, and several infections may exist simultaneously. The traveler should be encouraged to visit the physician promptly if problems arise.

Immunizations All of the HIV-infected traveler's routine immunizations should be up to date (see Chap. 122). The response to immunization may be impaired at CD4+ cell counts of <200/μL (and in some cases at even higher counts). However, when the risk of illness is high or the sequelae of illness are serious, immunization is recommended. In certain circumstances, it may be prudent to check the adequacy of the serum antibody response before departure (e.g., yellow fever neutralization if exposure is unavoidable).

Because of the increased risk of infections due to *Streptococcus pneumoniae* and other bacterial pathogens that cause pneumonia following influenza, pneumococcal polysaccharide and influenza vaccines should be administered. The estimated rates of response to influenza vaccine are more than 80 percent among persons with asymptomatic HIV infection and less than 50 percent among those with AIDS.

In general, live attenuated vaccines are contraindicated for persons with immune dysfunction. Live oral polio vaccine should not be given to HIV-infected patients or to members of their households. Instead, inactivated polio vaccine (eIPV) should be used; most HIV-infected individuals without AIDS will develop protective antibody levels in response to this vaccine.

Because measles (rubeola) can be a severe and lethal infection in HIV-positive patients, the measles vaccine (or the combination measles-mumps-rubella vaccine) should be given to these individuals. Although this is a live vaccine, there have been no reports of serious complications in this population. Between 18 and 58 percent of symptomatic HIV-infected vaccinees develop adequate antibody titers, and between 50 and 100 percent of those who are infected but asymptomatic seroconvert.

The decision of whether or not to administer any of the special vaccines to an HIV-infected traveler should be based on the individual's risk. Inactivated vaccines can be administered without concern for safety but with concern about adequate protection. For example, data suggest that HIV-infected persons do not have as strong an antibody response to the meningococcal meningitis vaccine as do uninfected persons. Moreover, few data are available on the efficacy of many of the other vaccines (e.g., those for hepatitis A, typhoid, and cholera).

It is recommended that live yellow-fever vaccine not be given to HIV-infected travelers. Nevertheless, when inadvertently administered to HIV-positive military personnel, this vaccine elicited no adverse reactions. Therefore, if the traveler's CD4+ count is >200/μL and travel in an endemic area is absolutely necessary, the vaccine can probably be administered safely. HIV-infected persons whose CD4+ count is <200/μL should be discouraged from traveling to these regions. If the traveler is passing through or traveling to an area where the vaccine is required but the disease risk is low, a physician's waiver should be issued. Bacille Calmette-Guérin vaccine should not be given because of reports of disseminated infection in HIV-infected persons.

A transient (days to weeks) burst of viremia has been demonstrated in HIV-infected individuals following immunization with vaccines for such diseases as influenza, pneumococcal infection, and tetanus (see Chap. 308). However, at this point, there is no evidence that this transient increase in viremia is detrimental over time. Furthermore, it is likely that immune activation associated with infection with the live organisms in question would result in increases in viremia of greater magnitude and duration than those associated with vaccination. Therefore, the vaccination recommendations discussed above need not be modified at this time.

Gastrointestinal Illness   Decreased levels of gastric acid, abnormal gastrointestinal mucosal immunity, and other complications of HIV infection, as well as medications taken by HIV-infected patients, make traveler's diarrhea especially problematic in these individuals. Traveler's diarrhea is likely to occur more frequently, be more severe, and be more difficult to treat in association with HIV infection. *Salmonella, Shigella,* and *Campylobacter* infections also are more protracted and more often accompanied by bacteremia in HIV-infected persons.

Cryptosporidium (see Chap. 220), a common cause of diarrhea in tropical countries, produces severe chronic diarrhea and cholecystitis with increased mortality among patients with AIDS. *Isospora belli* also causes infections at high rates among AIDS patients in the developing world. This infection is associated with malabsorption, weight loss,

and relapses after treatment. Persistent diarrhea due to microsporidiosis has also been reported.

Because of these potential problems, the HIV-infected traveler needs to be careful to consume only appropriately prepared foods and beverages. In addition, this group of individuals may benefit from prophylaxis for traveler's diarrhea, using bismuth subsalicylate or a daily antibiotic (ideally a quinolone derivative) for short-term travel to the developing world. If the traveler is already taking a sulfonamide preparation for prophylaxis of *Pneumocystis* pneumonia, a regimen of self-treatment with a quinolone would be appropriate.

Other Travel-Related Infections   Data are lacking on the severity of vector-borne diseases in HIV-infected individuals. Malaria is more severe in asplenic and certain immunocompromised hosts, although increased severity has not been demonstrated in AIDS. *Babesia* infection is known to cause serious illness and to recur in HIV-infected patients; this tick-transmitted illness occurs in parts of the United States but is not known to be a widespread problem.

Visceral leishmaniasis (see Chap. 217) has been reported in numerous HIV-infected travelers. Because the usual signs—splenomegaly and hyperglobulinemia—are nonspecific and may even be lacking, the diagnosis is difficult to make. In addition, serological results are often negative. This infection is hard to treat, and its associated mortality is high. Even short-term travelers to southern Europe have developed the illness; thus, the avoidance of sandfly bites is critical.

Certain respiratory illnesses, such as histoplasmosis and coccidioidomycosis, cause greater morbidity and mortality among patients with AIDS than in the general population. Though tuberculosis is common among HIV-infected persons (especially in developing countries), the acquisition of this infection by the short-term traveler is not a major concern. The possibility of acquiring *Legionella* infections from spas should be considered, although no data confirm an increase in the severity of such infections in AIDS.

Finally, the HIV-infected traveler should always be cautioned about safe sexual practices, which may help prevent both the transmission of HIV to others and the acquisition by the traveler of other sexually transmitted diseases that may be drug resistant or may result in serious sequelae (e.g., syphilis).

Medications   Adverse events due to medications and drug interactions are common and raise complex issues for HIV-infected persons. In addition, rates of cutaneous reaction are unusually high among patients with AIDS. Physicians advising these travelers need to consider the problems that may arise from the use of agents such as antimalarial drugs, medications for altitude acclimatization, or antidiarrheal compounds; one example is increased cutaneous sensitivity to sulfonamides. Since zidovudine (AZT) is metabolized by hepatic glucuronidation, inhibitors of this process may elevate serum levels of the drug. Though quinine does not affect levels of zidovudine, there are no relevant data on chloroquine, primaquine, or mefloquine. Furthermore, it is not known whether the antagonistic effect of zidovudine on pyrimethamine has clinical relevance in the treatment or prevention of plasmodial infections.

CHRONIC ILLNESS, DISABILITY, AND TRAVEL
Chronic health problems should not prevent travel, but special attention can make it safer and more comfortable.

Heart Disease   Cardiovascular events are the main cause of deaths among travelers and of in-flight emergencies on commercial aircraft. Persons with underlying heart disease should review their itineraries with a physician prior to departure; travel in harsh environments or to remote destinations is not wise. Extra supplies of all medications should be kept in carry-on luggage, along with a recent copy of an electrocardiogram and the name and telephone number of the traveler's physician at home. Pacemakers are not affected by airport security devices, but electronic telephone checks of pacemaker function cannot be transmitted by international satellites. The traveler may benefit from supplemental oxygen, which should be ordered by a physician (since oxygen delivery systems are not standardized) 48 to 72 h before flight time. Personal oxygen tanks are not permitted on aircraft. Travelers should request aisle seating and should walk, perform stretching and flexing exercises, and remain hydrated during the flight to prevent venous thrombosis and pulmonary embolism.

Chronic Lung Disease Chronic obstructive pulmonary disease (COPD) is one of the most common diagnoses in patients who require emergency-room evaluation for symptoms occurring during airline flights. Patients with COPD experience dyspnea, edema, wheezing, cyanosis, and chest pain. The best predictor of the development of these symptoms is the sea level Pa_{O_2}. A Pa_{O_2} of at least 72 mmHg corresponds to an in-flight arterial Pa_{O_2} of 55 mmHg when the cabin is pressurized to 8000 ft. Therefore, if the traveler's baseline Pa_{O_2} is <72 mmHg, the provision of supplemental oxygen during the flight should be considered. Pulmonary function is also maximized by continuing bronchodilator treatment and the use of steroids as prescribed. Contraindications to flight include active bronchospasm, lower respiratory infection, phlebitis, pulmonary hypertension, and recent thoracic surgery (within the preceding 3 weeks) or pneumothorax. Consideration should be given to decreasing the amount of outdoor activity at the destination if there is excessive air pollution.

Diabetes Mellitus Alterations in glucose control and changes in insulin requirements are common problems when diabetics travel. Changes in time zone, in the amount and timing of food intake, and in physical activity demand more vigilant assessment of metabolic control. The diabetic traveler should pack medication (including a bottle of regular insulin for emergencies), insulin syringes and needles, equipment and supplies for glucose monitoring, and snacks in carry-on luggage. Insulin is stable for about 3 months at room temperature but should be kept as cool as possible. The name and telephone number of the home physician and a card and necklace listing the medical problems and the type and dose of insulin used should accompany the traveler. When six or more time zones are crossed, insulin requirements may be temporarily altered, depending on food intake and physical activity. In traveling eastward (e.g., from the United States to Europe), the morning insulin dose on arrival may need to be decreased. The blood glucose can then be checked during the day to determine whether additional insulin is required. For flights westward, with lengthening of the day, an additional dose of regular insulin may be required. Comfortable footwear is essential for the diabetic traveler.

Other Special Groups Other groups for whom special travel measures are now being encouraged include patients undergoing dialysis, those with transplants, and those with other disabilities. Up to 13 percent of travelers have some disability, but few advocacy groups and tour companies dedicate themselves to this growing population. The key to safe travel in each case is adequate research ahead of time. Patients undergoing chronic ambulatory peritoneal dialysis may ship their dialysis solutions to their destinations before traveling. They should carry essential medical records as well as antibiotics for self-treatment of presumed peritonitis. Hemodialysis patients need to reserve appointments at dialysis centers prior to their departure from home. Travel by transplant recipients to distant destinations should ideally be scheduled at least 1 year after surgery, as most rejection episodes occur early. Medication interactions are a source of serious concern for these travelers, and appropriate medical information should be carried, along with the home physician's name and telephone number. Some travelers taking steroids carry stress doses in case they become ill. Immunization of these immunocompromised travelers may result in less than adequate protection against certain diseases. Thus, the traveler and physician must carefully consider which destinations are appropriate.

PROBLEMS AFTER RETURN The most frequent medical problems encountered by travelers after their return home are diarrhea, fever, respiratory illnesses, and skin diseases. Frequently ignored problems are fatigue and emotional stress, especially in long-stay travelers. The approach to diagnosis requires some knowledge of geographic medicine, in particular the epidemiology and clinical presentation of infectious disorders. A geographic history should focus on the traveler's exact itinerary, including dates of arrival and departure, exposure history (food indiscretions, drinking-water sources, freshwater contact, sexual activity, animal contact, insect bites), location and style of travel (urban vs. rural, first-class hotel accommodation vs. camping), immunization history, and use of antimalarial chemosuppression.

Fever Because death from *P. falciparum* malaria can occur after an illness of only several days, fever in a traveler who has returned from a malarious area should be considered a medical emergency. Although "fever from the tropics" does not always have a tropical cause, malaria should be the first diagnosis considered. The risk of *P. falciparum* malaria is highest among travelers returning from Africa or Oceania and among those who become symptomatic within the first 2 months after return. Other important causes of fever after travel include viral hepatitis (hepatitis A and E), typhoid fever, bacterial enteritis, arbovirus infections (e.g., dengue fever), rickettsial infections (including tick and scrub typhus or Q fever) and—in rare instances—leptospirosis, acute HIV infection, and amebic liver abscess. In at least 25 percent of cases, no etiology can be found, and the illness resolves spontaneously. Clinicians should keep in mind that no present-day antimalarial agent guarantees protection from malaria and that some immunizations—notably, those against typhoid and cholera—are only partially protective.

Skin Diseases Pyodermas, sunburn, insect bites, skin ulcers, and cutaneous larva migrans are the most frequent skin conditions encountered in travelers after their return home. In those with persistent skin ulcers, the diagnoses of cutaneous leishmaniasis, mycobacterial infection, or fungal infection should be considered. Careful, complete inspection of the skin is important in detecting the rickettsial eschar in a febrile patient or the central breathing hole in a "boil" due to myiasis.

Emerging Infectious Diseases In recent years, travel and commerce have fostered the worldwide spread of HIV infection, led to the reemergence of cholera as a global health threat, and created considerable fear about the possible spread of Ebola virus infection and plague. For travelers, there are more realistic concerns. One of the largest outbreaks of dengue fever ever documented is now raging in Latin America; schistosomiasis is being described in previously unaffected lakes in Africa; and antibiotic-resistant strains of sexually transmitted and enteric pathogens are emerging at an alarming rate in the developing world. As Nobel Laureate Dr. Joshua Lederberg pointed out, "The microbe that felled one child in a distant continent yesterday can reach yours today and seed a global pandemic tomorrow." The vigilant clinician understands that the importance of a thorough travel history cannot be overemphasized.

BIBLIOGRAPHY

Barry M, Bia F: Pregnancy and travel. JAMA 261:728, 1989

Bia FS, Barry M: Special health considerations for travelers. Med Clin North Am 76:1295, 1992

Caumes E et al: Dermatoses associated with travel to tropical countries: A prospective study of the diagnosis and management of 269 patients presenting to a tropical disease unit. Clin Infect Dis 20:542, 1995

DuPont HL, Capsuto EG: Persistent diarrhea in travelers. Clin Infect Dis 22:124, 1996

Kelsall BL, Guerrant RL: Evaluation of diarrhea in the returning traveler. Infect Dis Clin North Am 6:413, 1992

Laguna F et al: Gastrointestinal leishmaniasis in human immunodeficiency virus–infected patients: Report of five cases and review. Clin Infect Dis 19:48, 1994

Phillips–Howard PA, Wood D: The safety of antimalarial drugs in pregnancy. Drug Safety 14:131, 1996

Rhoads JL et al: Safety and immunogenicity of multiple conventional immunizations administered during early HIV infection. J Acquir Immune Defic Syndr 4:724, 1991

Schwartz JS et al: Air travel and hypoxemia with chronic obstructive lung disease. Ann Intern Med 100:473, 1984

Steffen R, Lobel HO: Epidemiologic basis for the practice of travel medicine. J Wilderness Med 5:56, 1994

Strickland GT: Fever in the returned traveler. Med Clin North Am 76:1375, 1992

Svenson JE et al: Imported malaria. Clinical presentation and examination of symptomatic travelers. Arch Intern Med 155:861, 1995

Wilson ME et al: Infections in HIV-infected travelers: Risks and prevention. Ann Intern Med 114:582, 1991

124 *Robert S. Munford*

SEPSIS AND SEPTIC SHOCK

DEFINITIONS (See Table 124-1) The host's reaction to invading microbes involves a rapidly amplifying polyphony of signals and responses that may spread beyond the invaded tissue. Fever or hypothermia, tachypnea, and tachycardia often herald the onset of *sepsis*, the systemic inflammatory response to microbial invasion. When counterregulatory control mechanisms are overwhelmed, often as the microbe moves from a local site to invade the bloodstream, homeostasis may fail, and dysfunction of major organs may supervene (*severe sepsis*). Further failure of counterregulatory control leads to *septic shock*, which is characterized by hypotension as well as organ dysfunction. As sepsis progresses to septic shock, the risk of dying increases substantially. Early sepsis is usually reversible, whereas patients with septic shock often succumb despite aggressive therapy.

The *systemic inflammatory response syndrome* (SIRS), as defined recently by critical-care specialists, may have an infectious or a noninfectious etiology. If infection is suspected or proven, a patient with SIRS is said to have sepsis.

ETIOLOGY Sepsis can be a response to any class of microorganism. Microbial invasion of the bloodstream is not essential for the development of sepsis; local or systemic spread of microbial signal molecules or toxins can also elicit the response. Blood cultures yield bacteria or fungi in approximately 20 to 40 percent of cases of severe sepsis and 40 to 70 percent of cases of septic shock. Individual gram-negative or gram-positive bacteria account for approximately 75 to 85 percent of these isolates; the remainder are fungi or a mixture of microorganisms. In patients whose blood cultures are negative, the etiologic agent is often established by culture or microscopic examination of infected material from a local site. In some case series, a majority of patients with a clinical picture of severe sepsis or septic shock have had negative microbiological results.

EPIDEMIOLOGY Sepsis is now a contributing factor in more than 100,000 deaths per year in the United States. The annual incidence is probably between 300,000 and 500,000 cases. Approximately two-thirds of cases occur in patients hospitalized for other illnesses. Factors that predispose to gram-negative bacillary bacteremia include diabetes mellitus, lymphoproliferative diseases, cirrhosis of the liver, burns, invasive procedures or devices, and treatment with drugs that cause neutropenia. Major risk factors for gram-positive bacteremia include vascular catheterization, the presence of indwelling mechanical devices, burns, and intravenous drug use. Fungemia occurs most often in immunosuppressed patients with neutropenia, often after broad-spectrum antimicrobial therapy. The increasing incidence of sepsis in the United States is attributable to the aging of the population, the increasing longevity of patients with chronic diseases, and the relatively high frequency of this condition among patients with AIDS. The widespread use of antimicrobial agents, glucocorticoids, indwelling catheters, mechanical devices, and mechanical ventilation also plays a role.

PATHOPHYSIOLOGY The septic response is usually triggered when microorganisms spread from the gastrointestinal tract or skin into contiguous tissues. Localized tissue infection may then lead to bacteremia or fungemia. Alternatively, microorganisms may be introduced directly into the bloodstream (for example, via intravenous catheters). In a minority of cases, no primary site of infection is apparent. In general, the septic response occurs when an invading microbe has circumvented the host's innate and acquired immune defenses. Host factors that allow microbial growth (such as deficiencies of antibody, complement factors, or cell-mediated immunity) are therefore critical.

Microbial Signals Animals recognize certain microbial molecules as signals that microorganisms have invaded. Lipopolysaccharide (LPS, also called endotoxin) is the most potent and best-studied gram-negative bacterial signal molecule. A plasma protein (LPS-binding protein, or LBP) transfers LPS to CD14 on the surfaces of monocytes, macrophages, and neutrophils. This interaction rapidly triggers the production and release of mediators, such as tumor necrosis factor (TNF) α (see below), that amplify the LPS signal and transmit it to other cells and tissues. Soluble CD14 may also bind LPS in plasma and transfer it to vascular endothelial cells, which lack cell-surface CD14. The peptidoglycan and lipoteichoic acids of gram-positive bacteria, certain polysaccharides, extracellular enzymes, and toxins elicit responses in animals that are similar to those induced by LPS. The molecular basis for the stimulatory potency of these molecules is poorly understood, although some of them may also bind cell-surface or soluble CD14 before activating cells. CD14 may therefore be a receptor that facilitates responses to many microbial signals. Other innate immune mechanisms that recognize microbial molecules include complement (principally the alternative pathway; see Chap. 305), mannose-binding protein, and C-reactive protein.

Host Responses The septic response involves complex interactions among microbial signal molecules, leukocytes, humoral mediators, and the vascular endothelium.

Cytokines Inflammatory cytokines amplify and diversify the response. These proteins can exert endocrine, paracrine, and autocrine effects (Chap. 305). TNFα stimulates leukocytes and vascular endothelial cells to release other cytokines (as well as additional TNFα), to express cell-surface adhesion molecules, and to increase arachidonic acid turnover. Blood levels of TNFα are high in most patients with severe sepsis. Moreover, intravenous infusion of TNFα can elicit

Table 124-1

Definitions Often Used to Describe the Condition of Septic Patients

Bacteremia (fungemia)	Presence of viable bacteria (fungi) in the blood, as evidenced by positive blood cultures
Septicemia	Systemic illness caused by the spread of microbes or their toxins via the bloodstream
Systemic inflammatory response syndrome (SIRS)*	At least 2 of the following 4 conditions: (1) oral temperature of >38°C or <36°C; (2) respiratory rate of >20 breaths/min or Pa_{CO_2} of <32 mmHg; (3) heart rate of >90 beats/min; (4) leukocyte count of >12,000/μL or <4,000/μL or >10% bands
Sepsis*	SIRS that has a proven or suspected microbial etiology
Severe sepsis* (similar to "sepsis syndrome")	Sepsis with one or more signs of organ dysfunction, hypoperfusion, or hypotension, such as metabolic acidosis, acute alteration in mental status, oliguria, or adult respiratory distress syndrome
Hypotension*	Systolic blood pressure <90 mmHg—or 40 mmHg less than patient's baseline blood pressure—in the absence of other reasons for hypotension
Septic shock*	Sepsis with hypotension that is unresponsive to fluid resuscitation plus organ dysfunction or perfusion abnormalities as listed above for severe sepsis
Refractory septic shock	Septic shock that lasts for >1 h and does not respond to fluid and pressor administration
Multiple-organ dysfunction syndrome (MODS)*	Dysfunction of more than one organ, requiring intervention to maintain homeostasis

* Term preferred by the American College of Chest Physicians/Society of Critical Care Medicine Consensus Conference, 1992.

many of the characteristic abnormalities of sepsis, including fever, tachycardia, tachypnea, leukocytosis, myalgias, and somnolence. In animals, large doses of TNFα induce shock, disseminated intravascular coagulation (DIC), and death. Specific TNFα antagonists can abrogate the septic response and prevent the deaths of experimental animals challenged with endotoxin.

Although TNFα is a central mediator, it is only one of many cytokines that contribute to the septic process. Interleukin (IL)-1β, for example, which exhibits many of the same activities as TNFα, seems to play an increasingly significant role as the septic process intensifies. TNFα, IL-1β, interferon γ, IL-8, and other cytokines probably interact synergistically with one another and with additional mediators. Moreover, some mediators (such as IL-1β and TNFα) may enhance their own rates of synthesis by positive feedback. As sepsis progresses, the mixture of cytokines and other mediators becomes very complex: elevated blood levels of more than 30 pro- and anti-inflammatory molecules have been found in patients with septic shock. In animal models, the septic response can be interrupted by early interventions that neutralize one or another of its many components; this observation testifies to the importance of mediator interactions in the overall outcome. Unfortunately, it has been much more difficult to rescue animals from severe sepsis and septic shock.

Phospholipid-derived mediators Arachidonic acid, released from membrane phospholipids by phospholipase A₂, is converted by the cyclooxygenase pathway into prostaglandins and thromboxanes. Prostaglandin E₂ and prostacyclin cause peripheral vasodilation, whereas thromboxane is a vasoconstrictor and promotes platelet aggregation. Leukotrienes are also potent mediators of ischemia and shock; the fact that the reaction to endotoxin challenge is normal in mice that lack the 5-lipoxygenase gene, however, casts doubt on the role of leukotrienes in the septic response.

Another important phospholipid-derived mediator is platelet-activating factor (PAF, or 1-*O*-alkyl-2-acetyl-*sn*-glycerol-3-phosphocholine). PAF potently stimulates neutrophil aggregation and degranulation, promotes platelet aggregation, and may contribute to tissue injury.

Coagulation factors Intravascular fibrin deposition, thrombosis, and DIC are important features of the septic response. TNFα promotes intravascular coagulation initially by inducing blood monocytes to express tissue factor (see Chap. 60). When tissue factor is expressed on monocytes, it binds to factor VIIa to form an active complex that can convert factors X and IX to enzymatically active forms. The result is activation of both extrinsic and intrinsic clotting pathways, culminating in the generation of fibrin. Clotting is also favored by impaired function of the protein C–protein S inhibitory pathway, while fibrinolysis is prevented by increased plasma levels of plasminogen activator inhibitor 1. Thus, there may be a striking propensity for intravascular fibrin deposition, thrombosis, and bleeding. Contact-system activation occurs during sepsis but contributes more to the development of hypotension than to DIC.

Complement C5a and other products of complement activation may promote neutrophil reactions such as chemotaxis, aggregation, degranulation, and oxygen-radical production. When administered to animals, C5a induces hypotension, pulmonary vasoconstriction, neutropenia, and vascular leakiness due in part to endothelial damage.

Activation of the vascular endothelium Many tissues may be damaged by sepsis. The probable underlying mechanism is widespread vascular endothelial injury, with fluid extravasation and microthrombosis that decrease oxygen and substrate utilization by the affected tissues. Leukocyte-derived mediators and platelet-leukocyte-fibrin thrombi contribute to this injury, but the vascular endothelium itself seems to play an active role. Stimuli such as TNFα induce vascular endothelial cells to produce and release cytokines, procoagulant molecules, PAF, endothelium-derived relaxing factor (nitric oxide), and other mediators. In addition, regulated cell-adhesion molecules promote the adherence of leukocytes to endothelial cells. While these responses may attract phagocytes to infected sites and activate their antimicrobial arsenals, endothelial cell activation can also promote increased vascular permeability, microvascular thrombosis, DIC, and hypotension. Moreover, vascular integrity may be damaged by neutro-

phil enzymes (such as elastase) and toxic oxygen metabolites so that local hemorrhage ensues. Blocking the adhesion of leukocytes to endothelial cell surfaces, as with monoclonal antibodies to intercellular adhesion molecule 1, can prevent tissue necrosis in response to endotoxin administration in animals.

Septic shock Much evidence now implicates nitric oxide, produced by inducible nitric oxide synthase (*iNOS*), as a mediator of septic shock in experimental animals and probably in humans. Mice that lack the *iNOS* gene may not be resistant to endotoxic shock, however. Other prominent hypotensive molecules are β-endorphin, bradykinin, PAF, and prostacyclin. Agents that inhibit the synthesis or action of each of these mediators can prevent or reverse endotoxic shock in animals.

Control mechanisms Elaborate host mechanisms regulate both microbial signals and the inflammatory response. While plasma LBP promotes the inflammatory response by facilitating the interaction of LPS with monocyte cell-surface CD14, LBP and soluble CD14 can also prevent LPS signaling by transferring LPS molecules into plasma lipoprotein particles. The relative plasma concentrations of LPS, LBP, CD14, and lipoprotein therefore may determine LPS signal intensity. The mechanisms that control the inflammatory response are complex, overlapping, and poorly understood. Glucocorticoids inhibit cytokine synthesis by monocytes in vitro and, when administered with or shortly after an inflammatory stimulus, may protect animals from septic shock. The increase in blood cortisol levels early in the septic response presumably plays a similar inhibitory role. Certain cytokine antagonists also may contribute. Blood levels of IL-1 receptor antagonist often greatly exceed those of circulating IL-1β, and this excess may result in inhibition of the binding of IL-1β to its receptors. Transforming growth factor β (TGFβ) and IL-10 also can inhibit LPS-induced responses of human monocytes in vitro and prevent endotoxic death in animals. Blood and tissue levels of prostaglandin E₂, TGFβ, α-melanocyte-stimulating hormone, cortisol, IL-1 receptor antagonist, soluble TNF receptors, and IL-10 increase during the septic response, and these molecules probably act in concert to diminish its intensity. Indeed, blood leukocytes from patients with severe sepsis may be hyporesponsive to agonists such as LPS. The fact that plasma concentrations of many of these anti-inflammatory molecules may be very high in the patient with septic shock, however, indicates that they are unable to control the inflammatory response when it is most severe.

CLINICAL MANIFESTATIONS The systemic inflammatory response often intensifies over time from mild (sepsis) to extremely severe (septic shock). The rate at which the response increases may differ from patient to patient, and there are striking individual variations in its manifestations. For example, some septic patients have a normal temperature or are hypothermic; the absence of fever is most common among neonates, elderly patients, and persons with uremia or alcoholism.

Hyperventilation is often an early sign. Disorientation, confusion, and other manifestations of encephalopathy may also develop early in the septic response, particularly in the elderly and in individuals with preexisting neurologic impairment. Focal neurologic signs are uncommon, although preexisting focal deficits may become more prominent.

Hypotension and DIC predispose to acrocyanosis and ischemic necrosis of peripheral tissues, most commonly the digits. Cellulitis, pustules, bullae, or hemorrhagic lesions may develop when hematogenous bacteria or fungi seed the skin or underlying soft tissue. Bacterial toxins may also be distributed hematogenously, eliciting diffuse cutaneous reactions. On occasion, skin lesions may be suggestive of specific pathogens. When sepsis is accompanied by cutaneous petechiae or purpura, infection with *Neisseria meningitidis* (or, less commonly, *Haemophilus influenzae*) should be suspected; in a patient who has been bitten by a tick while in an endemic area, petechial lesions also suggest Rocky Mountain spotted fever. A cutaneous lesion seen almost exclusively in neutropenic patients is ecthyma gangrenosum, usually caused by *Pseudomonas aeruginosa* or *Aeromonas hydrophila*. It is a bullous lesion, surrounded by edema, that undergoes central hemorrhage and necrosis. Histopathologic examination shows bacteria in and around the wall of a small vessel, with little or no neutrophilic response. Hemorrhagic or bullous lesions in a septic patient who has recently eaten raw oysters suggest *Vibrio vulnificus* bacteremia, while such lesions in a patient who has recently suffered a dog bite may indicate bloodstream infection due to *Capnocytophaga canimorsus* or *Capnocytophaga cynodegmi*. Generalized erythroderma in a septic patient suggests the toxic shock syndrome due to *Staphylococcus aureus* or *Streptococcus pyogenes*.

Gastrointestinal manifestations such as nausea, vomiting, diarrhea, and ileus may be indicative of acute gastroenteritis. Stress ulceration can lead to upper gastrointestinal bleeding. Cholestatic jaundice, with elevated levels of serum bilirubin (mostly conjugated) and alkaline phosphatase, may precede other signs of sepsis. Hepatocellular or canalicular dysfunction appears to underlie most cases, and the results of hepatic function tests return to normal with resolution of the infection. Prolonged or severe hypotension may induce acute hepatic injury or ischemic bowel necrosis.

Blood lactate levels rise early, in part because of increased glycolysis with impaired clearance of the resulting lactate and pyruvate by the liver and kidneys. As hypoperfusion develops, tissue hypoxia generates more lactic acid, contributing to metabolic acidosis. The blood glucose concentration often increases, particularly in diabetics, although impaired gluconeogenesis and excessive insulin release on occasion produce hypoglycemia. The cytokine-driven acute-phase response inhibits the synthesis of albumin and transthyretin while enhancing the production of C-reactive protein, LBP, fibrinogen, and complement components. Protein catabolism is often markedly accelerated.

MAJOR COMPLICATIONS   Cardiopulmonary Complications   Ventilation-perfusion mismatching produces a fall in arterial P_{O_2} early in the course. Increasing alveolar capillary permeability results in an increased pulmonary water content, which decreases pulmonary compliance and interferes with oxygen exchange. Progressive diffuse pulmonary infiltrates, decreasing compliance, and arterial hypoxemia (whose frequent refractoriness to supplemental oxygen therapy indicates right-to-left shunting) signal the development of the adult respiratory distress syndrome (ARDS, or "shock lung"). ARDS develops in 20 to 50 percent of patients with sepsis, and sepsis is the leading cause of this syndrome. The failure of the respiratory muscles can exacerbate hypoxemia and hypercapnia. An elevated pulmonary capillary wedge pressure (>18 mmHG) suggests fluid volume overload or cardiac failure rather than ARDS. Pneumonia caused by viruses or *Pneumocystis carinii* infection may be clinically indistinguishable from ARDS.

Septic shock usually results from a severe decrease in systemic vascular resistance, a generalized maldistribution of blood flow, and functional hypovolemia that is due, at least in part, to diffuse capillary leakage of intravascular constituents. Other factors that may decrease effective intravascular volume include dehydration from antecedent disease or insensible fluid losses, vomiting or diarrhea, and polyuria. Cardiac output is initially normal or elevated. Indeed, normal or increased cardiac output and decreased systemic vascular resistance distinguish septic shock from cardiogenic, extracardiac obstructive, and hypovolemic shock; other processes that can produce this combination include anaphylaxis, beriberi, cirrhosis of the liver, and overdoses of nitroprusside or narcotics.

Depression of myocardial function, manifested as increased end-diastolic and systolic ventricular volumes with a decreased ejection fraction, develops within 24 h in most patients with advanced sepsis. Cardiac output is maintained despite the low ejection fraction because ventricular dilation permits a normal stroke volume. In survivors, myocardial function returns to normal over several days. While myocardial dysfunction may contribute to hypotension, refractory hypoten-

sion is usually due to a low systemic vascular resistance, and death results from refractory shock or the failure of multiple organs rather than from cardiac dysfunction per se.

Renal Complications   Oliguria, azotemia, proteinuria, and nonspecific urinary casts are frequently found. Many patients are inappropriately polyuric; hyperglycemia may exacerbate this tendency. Most renal failure is due to acute tubular necrosis induced by hypotension or capillary injury, although some patients also have glomerulonephritis, renal cortical necrosis, or interstitial nephritis. Drug-induced renal damage may complicate therapy, particularly when hypotensive patients are given aminoglycoside antibiotics.

Coagulation   Although thrombocytopenia occurs in 10 to 30 percent of patients, the underlying mechanism(s) are not understood. Platelet counts are usually very low (i.e., below $50,000/\mu L$) in patients with DIC; these low counts typically reflect diffuse endothelial injury (see Chap. 315).

Neurologic Complications   When the septic illness lasts for weeks to months, "critical-illness" polyneuropathy may prevent weaning from ventilatory support and produce distal motor weakness. Electrophysiologic studies are diagnostic. Guillain-Barré syndrome, metabolic disturbances, and toxin activity must be ruled out.

LABORATORY FINDINGS   In early sepsis, abnormalities may include leukocytosis with a left shift, thrombocytopenia, hyperbilirubinemia, and proteinuria. Leukopenia may develop. The neutrophils may contain toxic granulations, Döhle bodies, or cytoplasmic vacuoles. As the septic response becomes more severe, thrombocytopenia worsens (often with prolongation of the thrombin time, a decrease in fibrinogen, and the presence of D-dimers, suggesting DIC), azotemia and hyperbilirubinemia become more prominent, and levels of aminotransferases rise. Active hemolysis suggests clostridial bacteremia, malaria, a drug reaction, or DIC; in the case of DIC, microangiopathic changes may be seen on a blood smear.

During early sepsis, hyperventilation induces respiratory alkalosis. With respiratory-muscle fatigue and the accumulation of lactate, metabolic acidosis (with an increased anion gap) typically supervenes. Evaluation of arterial blood gases reveals hypoxemia, which is initially correctable with supplemental oxygen but whose later refractoriness to 100% oxygen inhalation indicates right-to-left shunting. The chest radiograph may be normal or may show evidence of underlying pneumonia, volume overload, or diffuse infiltrates of ARDS. The electrocardiogram may show only sinus tachycardia or nonspecific ST-T wave abnormalities.

Most diabetics with sepsis develop hyperglycemia. Severe infection may precipitate diabetic ketoacidosis, which may exacerbate hypotension (see Chap. 334). Hypoglycemia occurs rarely. The serum albumin level, initially within the normal range, declines as sepsis continues. Serum lipid concentrations are often elevated. Hypocalcemia is rare.

DIAGNOSIS   There is no specific test. Diagnostically sensitive findings in a patient with suspected or proven infection include fever or hypothermia, tachypnea, tachycardia, and leukocytosis or leukopenia (see Table 124-1); acutely altered mental status, thrombocytopenia, or hypotension also suggest the diagnosis. The septic response can be quite variable, however. In one study, 36 percent of patients with sepsis had a normal temperature, 40 percent had a normal respiratory rate, 10 percent had a normal pulse rate, and 33 percent had normal white blood cell counts. Moreover, the systemic responses of uninfected patients with other conditions may be similar to those characteristic of sepsis. Noninfectious etiologies of SIRS (see Table 124-1) include pancreatitis, burns, trauma, adrenal insufficiency, pulmonary enbolism, dissecting or ruptured aortic aneurysm, myocardial infarction, occult hemorrhage, cardiac tamponade, post-cardiopulmonary bypass syndrome, anaphylaxis, and drug overdose.

Definitive etiologic diagnosis requires the isolation of the microorganism from the blood or a local site of infection. At least two blood samples (10 mL each) should be obtained (from different venipuncture sites) for culture. Because gram-negative bacteremia is typically low-grade (fewer than 10 organisms per milliliter of blood), multiple blood cultures or prolonged incubation of cultures may be necessary;

S. aureus grows more readily and is detectable in blood cultures within 48 h in most instances. In many cases, blood cultures are negative; this result can reflect prior antibiotic administration, the presence of slow-growing or fastidious organisms, or the absence of microbial invasion of the bloodstream. In these cases, Gram's staining and culture of material from the primary site of infection or from infected cutaneous lesions may help establish the microbial etiology. The skin and mucosae should be examined carefully and repeatedly for lesions that might yield diagnostic information. With overwhelming bacteremia (e.g., pneumococcal sepsis in splenectomized individuals or fulminant meningococcemia), microorganisms are sometimes visible on buffy-coat smears of peripheral blood.

Detection of endotoxin in blood by the limulus lysate test may portend a poor outcome, but this assay is not useful for diagnosing gram-negative bacterial infections, including gram-negative bacteremia. Although blood levels of IL-6 also may correlate with prognosis, cytokine assays are poorly standardized and currently have limited clinical value.

℞ TREATMENT

Sepsis can kill quickly. Successful management requires urgent measures to treat local infection, to provide hemodynamic and respiratory support, and to eliminate the offending microorganism. The outcome is also influenced by the patient's underlying disease, which should be managed aggressively.

Antimicrobial agents Antimicrobial chemotherapy should be initiated as soon as samples of blood and other relevant sites have been cultured. The choice of initial therapy is based on knowledge of the likely pathogens at specific sites of local infection. Available information about patterns of antimicrobial susceptibility among bacterial isolates from the community, the hospital, and the patient also should be taken into account. It is important, pending culture results, to initiate empirical antimicrobial therapy that is effective against both gram-positive and gram-negative bacteria (see Table 124-2). Maximal recommended doses of antimicrobial drugs should be given intravenously, with adjustment for impaired renal function when necessary. When culture results become available, the regimen can often be simplified, as a single antimicrobial agent is frequently adequate for the treatment of a known pathogen. Most patients require antimicrobial therapy for at least 1 week; the duration of treatment is typically influenced by factors such as the site of tissue infection, the adequacy of surgical drainage, the patient's underlying disease (see Chap. 136), and the antimicrobial susceptibility of the bacterial isolate(s).

Removal of the source of infection Removal or drainage of a focal source of infection is essential. Sites of occult infection should be sought carefully. Indwelling intravenous catheters should be removed, the tip rolled over a blood agar plate for quantitative culture, and a new catheter inserted at a different site. Foley and drainage catheters should be replaced. The possibility of paranasal sinusitis (often caused by hospital-acquired gram-negative bacteria) should be considered if the patient has undergone nasal intubation. In the neutropenic patient, cutaneous sites of tenderness and erythema, particularly in the perianal region, must be carefully sought. In patients with sacral or ischial decubitus ulcers, it is important to exclude pelvic or other soft-tissue pus collections (by computed tomography or magnetic resonance imaging, if necessary). In patients with severe sepsis arising from the urinary tract, sonography or computed tomography should be used to rule out ureteral obstruction, perinephric abscess, and renal abscess. These studies are not so urgent in patients with less severe urosepsis, provided that a clinical response is evident within 48 to 72 h.

Hemodynamic, respiratory, and metabolic support (See also Chap. 38) Here the primary goal is to restore adequate oxygen and substrate delivery to the tissues. Adequate organ perfusion is essential. Effective intravascular volume depletion is common in septic patients, and the initial management of hypotension should include the administration of intravenous fluids—typically 1 to 2 L of normal saline over 1 to 2 h. The pulmonary capillary wedge

Table 124-2

Initial Antimicrobial Therapy for Severe Sepsis with No Obvious Source in Adults with Normal Renal Function

Type of Patient	Antimicrobial Regimens*
Immunocompetent adult	The many acceptable regimens include (1) ticarcillin-clavulanate *or* piperacillin-tazobactam (6.2 and 7.5 g q6h, respectively) *plus* gentamicin or tobramycin (1.5 mg/kg q8h); (2) ampicillin (30 mg/kg q4h) *plus* gentamicin (1.5 mg/kg q8h) *plus* clindamycin (900 mg q8h); and (3) imipenem-cilastatin (0.5 g q6h). If the patient is allergic to β-lactam agents, ciprofloxacin (400 mg q12h) *or* aztreonam (2 g q8h) should be substituted for ampicillin in regimen 2.
Neutropenic patient (<500 neutrophils/μL)	Regimens include (1) ticarcillin, mezlocillin, or piperacillin (3 g q4h) *or* ceftazidime (2 g q8h) *plus* tobramycin (1.5 mg/kg q8h) and (2) imipenem-cilastatin (0.5 g q6h) *or* ceftazidime. If the patient is allergic to β-lactam agents, aztreonam or ciprofloxacin should be used with tobramycin. If the patient has an infected vascular catheter or if the involvement of staphylococci is suspected, vancomycin (15 mg/kg q12h) should be added.
Splenectomized patient	Cefotaxime (2 g q4h) *or* ceftriaxone (2 g q12h) should be used. If the local prevalence of cephalosporin-resistant pneumococci is high, add vancomycin. If the patient is allergic to β-lactam drugs, vancomycin (15 mg/kg q12h) *plus* ciprofloxacin (400 mg q12h) *or* aztreonam (2 g q8h) should be used.
Intravenous drug user	Nafcillin *or* oxacillin (2 g q4h) *plus* gentamicin (1.5 mg/kg q8h) should be used. If the local prevalence of methicillin-resistant *Staphylococcus aureus* is high or if the patient is allergic to β-lactam drugs, vancomycin (15 mg/kg q12h) with gentamicin should be used.
AIDS patient	Ticarcillin-clavulanate (3 g q4h) *plus* tobramycin (1.5 mg/kg q8h) should be used. If the patient is allergic to β-lactam drugs, ciprofloxacin (400 mg q12h) *plus* vancomycin (15 mg/kg q12h) *plus* tobramycin should be used.

* All administered intravenously.

pressure or the central venous pressure must be monitored in patients with refractory shock or underlying cardiac or renal disease. To avoid pulmonary edema, the pulmonary capillary wedge pressure should be maintained at 14 to 18 mmHg or the central venous pressure at 10 to 12 cmH$_2$O. The urine output should be kept above 30 mL/h by continuing fluid administration; a diuretic such as furosemide may be used if needed. In about one-third of patients, hypotension and organ hypoperfusion respond to fluid resuscitation; a reasonable goal is to maintain a mean arterial blood pressure of >60 mmHg (systolic pressure, >90 mmHg) and a cardiac index of ≥4 (L/min)/m^2. If these guidelines cannot be met by volume infusion, inotropic and vasopressor therapy is indicated (see Chap. 38).

Adrenal insufficiency should be considered in septic patients with refractory hypotension, fulminant *N. meningitidis* bacteremia, prior glucocorticoid use, disseminated tuberculosis, or AIDS. The cosyntropin (α^{1-24}-ACTH) stimulation test (see Chap. 332) may suggest absolute or partial adrenal insufficiency. Supplemental hydrocortisone (50 mg intravenously every 6 h) may be given while the results of the cosyntropin test are awaited.

Ventilator therapy is indicated for progressive hypoxemia, hypercapnia, neurologic deterioration, or respiratory muscle failure.

Intubation is often undertaken to ensure adequate oxygenation, divert blood from the muscles of respiration, and reduce the cardiac afterload. Blood or erythrocyte transfusion is indicated if oxygen delivery is compromised by a low hemoglobin concentration (<8 to 10 g/dL).

Bicarbonate is sometimes administered for severe metabolic acidosis (arterial pH $<$ 7.2). DIC, if complicated by major bleeding, should be treated with transfusion of fresh frozen plasma and platelets. Successful treatment of the underlying infection is essential for the reversal of both acidosis and DIC. In patients with prolonged sepsis, nutritional supplementation may reduce the impact of protein hypercatabolism.

These are consensus recommendations; none of these generally accepted components of resuscitative care has been validated in randomized clinical trials.

Other measures Despite aggressive management, many patients with severe sepsis or septic shock die. Two kinds of agents that may help prevent these deaths are being investigated: (1) drugs that neutralize bacterial endotoxin and that thereby may benefit the fraction (approximately half) of septic patients who have gram-negative bacterial infections and (2) drugs that interfere with one or more mediators of the inflammatory response and may benefit all patients with sepsis.

ANTIENDOTOXIN AGENTS Lipid A, the toxic moiety of endotoxin, is conserved in the LPS of gram-negative bacteria. Despite much effort to develop drugs that bind lipid A and neutralize endotoxin in vivo, the potential of endotoxin as a target for therapeutic intervention remains controversial. In placebo-controlled clinical trials, two monoclonal antibodies to endotoxin failed to prevent the death of patients with severe gram-negative bacterial sepsis. In retrospective studies, these antibodies did not bind to LPS with high affinity, and one was reported to be a polyreactive autoantibody. Antibodies with improved binding properties are being evaluated. A theoretically more promising agent is bactericidal permeability-increasing protein, a human neutrophil protein that neutralizes the toxicity of lipid A and may be bactericidal to many gram-negative microorganisms. Other investigational drugs include nontoxic lipid A analogs that reduce host responses to endotoxins, a polymyxin B–dextran conjugate that binds endotoxins, and lipoproteins (such as high-density lipoprotein) that bind and neutralize endotoxin in the circulation.

ANTIMEDIATOR AGENTS Other adjunctive therapies are intended to control the inflammatory response, regardless of the microbial stimulus. Unfortunately, numerous agents that interfere directly or indirectly with the actions of inflammatory mediators have not prevented the death of patients with severe sepsis or septic shock. Anticytokine drugs tested in unsuccessful clinical trials include methylprednisolone, recombinant IL-1 receptor antagonist, genetically engineered soluble receptors for TNFα, and monoclonal antibodies to TNFα. Because TNFα and IL-1β doubtless play key roles in antimicrobial host defense, antagonizing these cytokines could be detrimental in some cases. In fact, recent studies suggest that many anti-inflammatory molecules may already be present at high concentrations in the plasma of patients with septic shock. Identifying beneficial regimens of treatment with drugs that neutralize TNFα and IL-1β may therefore be very difficult. Other compounds tested in recent clinical trials include PAF antagonists, bradykinin antagonists, and ibuprofen. Additional investigational agents include pentoxifylline, α-melanocyte-stimulating hormone, ketoconazole, inhibitors of *iNOS*, and recombinant anticoagulant proteins.

All of the recent clinical trials have enrolled patients with severe sepsis or septic shock. Neither the ability of adjunctive agents to *prevent* severe sepsis or septic shock in high-risk patients nor the value of combination therapy with two or more adjunctive drugs has been tested.

PROGNOSIS Approximately 25 to 35 percent of patients with severe sepsis and 40 to 55 percent of patients with septic shock die within 30 days. Others die within the ensuing 5 months. Late deaths often result from poorly controlled infection, complications of intensive care, failure of multiple organs, or underlying disease.

Several prognostic stratification systems that factor in the patient's age, underlying condition, and various physiologic variables yield estimates of the risk of dying of severe sepsis. Of the individual covariates, underlying disease most strongly influences the risk of dying. Septic shock is also a strong predictor of short- and long-term mortality. Case-fatality rates are similar for culture-positive and culture-negative severe sepsis and septic shock.

PREVENTION Prevention offers the best opportunity to reduce morbidity and mortality from sepsis. Most episodes of severe sepsis and septic shock are nosocomial. These cases might be prevented by reducing the number of invasive procedures undertaken, by limiting the use (and duration) of indwelling vascular and bladder catheters, by reducing the incidence and duration of profound neutropenia (<500 neutrophils/μL), and by more aggressively treating localized nosocomial infections. Increasing evidence supports the administration of enteral feeding supplements to traumatized patients at risk for infection. Indiscriminate use of antimicrobial agents and glucocorticoids should be avoided, and optimal infection-control measures (see Chap. 138) should be used. In addition, prompt and aggressive management of patients with early sepsis is imperative. Research is needed to identify patients at high risk for severe sepsis and to develop adjunctive agents that can damp the septic response before organ dysfunction or hypotension develops.

BIBLIOGRAPHY

AMERICAN COLLEGE OF CHEST PHYSICIANS/SOCIETY OF CRITICAL CARE MEDICINE CONSENSUS CONFERENCE COMMITTEE: Definitions for sepsis and organ failure and guidelines for the use of innovative therapies in sepsis. Crit Care Med 20:864, 1992

ASTIZ ME et al: Intravascular volume and fluid therapy for severe sepsis. New Horizons 1:127, 1993

BERNARD GR: Sepsis trials. Intersection of investigation, regulation, funding, and practice. Am J Respir Crit Care Med 152:4, 1995

BOLTON CF et al: The neurological complications of sepsis. Ann Neurol 33:94, 1993

EIDELMAN LA et al: The spectrum of septic encephalopathy. Definitions, etiologies, and mortalities. JAMA 275:470, 1996

HARRIS RL et al: Manifestations of sepsis. Arch Intern Med 147:1895, 1987

LEVI M et al: Pathogenesis of disseminated intravascular coagulation in sepsis. JAMA 270:975, 1993

LYNN WA, COHEN J: Adjunctive therapy for septic shock: A review of experimental approaches. Clin Infect Dis 20:143, 1995

MARTIN MA et al: Gram-negative sepsis and the adult respiratory distress syndrome. Clin Infect Dis 14:1213, 1992

PERL TM et al: Long-term survival and function after suspected gram-negative sepsis. JAMA 274:338, 1995

PINNER RW et al: Trends in infectious disease mortality in the U.S. JAMA 275:189, 1996

RANGEL-FRAUSTO MS et al: The natural history of the systemic inflammatory response syndrome (SIRS). A prospective study. JAMA 273:117, 1995

125 *Jeffrey A. Gelfand, Charles A. Dinarello*

FEVER OF UNKNOWN ORIGIN*

DEFINITION AND CLASSIFICATION

Fever of unknown origin (FUO) was defined by Petersdorf and Beeson in 1961 as (1) temperatures higher than 38.3°C (101°F) on several occasions, (2) a duration of fever of more than 3 weeks, and (3) failure to reach a diagnosis despite 1 week of inpatient investigation. While this classification has stood for more than 30 years, Durack and Street have proposed a new system for classification of FUO: (1) classic FUO, (2) nosocomial FUO, (3) neutropenic FUO, and (4) FUO associated with human immunodeficiency virus (HIV) infection (Table 125-1).

---

* Sheldon M. Wolff, M.D., now deceased, was an author in the previous edition of this revised chapter, and it is to his memory that the chapter is dedicated.

Table 125-1

Categories of FUO*

Feature	Nosocomial	Neutropenic	HIV-Associated	Classic
			Category of FUO	
Patient's situation	Hospitalized, acute care, no infection when admitted	Neutrophil count either less than 500/μL or expected to reach that level in 1–2 days	Confirmed HIV-positive	All others with fevers for ≥3 weeks
Duration of illness while under investigation	3 days†	3 days†	3 days† (or 4 weeks as outpatient)	3 days† or three outpatient visits
Examples of cause	Septic thrombophlebitis, sinusitis, *Clostridium difficile* colitis, drug fever	Perianal infection, aspergillosis, candidemia	MAI‡ infection, tuberculosis, non-Hodgkin's lymphoma, drug fever	Infections, malignancy, inflammatory diseases, drug fever

* All require temperatures of ≥38.3°C (101°F) on several occasions.
† Includes at least 2 days' incubation of microbiology cultures.
‡ *M. avium/M. intracellulare.*
SOURCE: Modified from Durack and Street.

CLASSIC FUO This category corresponds closely to the earlier definition of FUO, differing only with regard to the prior requirement for 1 week's study in the hospital; the new definition is broader, stipulating three outpatient visits or 3 days in the hospital without elucidation of a cause or 1 week of "intelligent and invasive" ambulatory investigation. In our opinion, a 2-week period of fever is sufficient grounds for entertaining the diagnosis of FUO when other criteria have been met.

NOSOCOMIAL FUO In nosocomial FUO, a temperature of ≥38.3°C (101°F) develops on several occasions in a hospitalized patient who is receiving acute care and in whom infection was not manifest or incubating on admission. Three days of investigation, including at least 2 days' incubation of cultures, is the minimum requirement for this diagnosis. In hospitalized patients, occult nosocomial infections, infected intravascular lines, recurrent pulmonary embolism, transfusion-related viral infection, and drug-related fever are possible diagnoses. In this setting, the approach is to focus on sites where occult infections might be sequestered (such as the sinuses of intubated patients and prosthetic devices) or on nosocomial complications such as acalculous cholecystitis, *Clostridium difficile* toxin in the stool (in cases including diarrhea), and drug reactions. Blood cultures are mandatory. Appropriate diagnostic maneuvers include ultrasonography and computed tomography (CT) of the abdomen, indium 111–labeled white blood cell or immunoglobulin scans, sinus x-rays, and discontinuation of treatment with suspect drugs.

NEUTROPENIC FUO This condition is defined as a temperature of ≥38.3°C (101°F) on several occasions in a patient whose neutrophil count is <500/μL or is expected to fall to that level in 1 to 2 days. The diagnosis of neutropenic FUO is invoked if a specific cause is not identified after 3 days of investigation, including at least 2 days' incubation of cultures. Neutropenic patients are susceptible to focal bacterial and fungal infections, to bacteremic infections, to infections involving catheters (including septic thrombophlebitis), and to perianal infections. *Candida* and *Aspergillus* infections are common.

Infections due to herpes simplex virus or cytomegalovirus (CMV) are sometimes causes of FUO in this group. While the duration of illness is far shorter in these patients, the consequences of untreated infection may be catastrophic.

HIV-ASSOCIATED FUO This disorder is defined by a temperature of ≥38.3°C (101°F) on several occasions over a period of more than 4 weeks for outpatients or more than 3 days for hospitalized patients with HIV infection. This diagnosis is invoked if appropriate investigation over 3 days, including 2 days' incubation of cultures, reveals no source. In this group of patients, HIV infection alone may be a cause of fever. Infection due to *Mycobacterium avium* or *Mycobacterium intracellulare* (together known as MAI), toxoplasmosis, CMV infection, tuberculosis, *Pneumocystis carinii* infection, salmonellosis, cryptococcosis, histoplasmosis, non-Hodgkin's lymphoma, and (of particular importance) drug fever are all possible causes of FUO.

Adoption of these categories of FUO on a wide scale in the literature would allow a more rational compilation of data regarding these disparate groups. In the remainder of this chapter, the discussion will focus on classic FUO unless otherwise specified.

CAUSES OF CLASSIC FUO

Table 125-2 summarizes the findings of a number of large studies of FUO carried out since the advent of the antibiotic era. Coincident with the widespread use of antibiotics, increasingly useful diagnostic technologies—both noninvasive and invasive—have been developed. Newer studies reflect not only changing patterns of disease but also the impact of diagnostic techniques that make it possible to eliminate many patients with specific illness from the FUO category. The ubiquitous use of microbiologic cultures and the widespread use of potent broad-spectrum antibiotics may have decreased the number of infections causing FUO. The wide availability of ultrasonography, CT, and magnetic resonance imaging (MRI) has enhanced the detection of occult neoplasms and lymphomas in patients previously thought to

Table 125-2

Classic FUO in Adults

Authors	Years of Study	No. of Cases	Infections (%)	Neoplasms (%)	Collagen Vascular Diseases (%)	Causes (%)	
						Miscellaneous Causes	Undiagnosed Causes
Petersdorf and Beeson	1952–57	100	36	19	13	25	7
Jacoby and Swartz	1957–71	128	40	20	15	17	8
Howard et al.	1969–76	100	37	31	19	8	5
Larson and Featherstone	1970–80	105	30	31	16	10	12
Knockaert and Vanneste	1980–89	199	22.5	7	21.5*	26.5*	2.5*

* Authors' raw data retabulated to conform to prior diagnostic categories.

have FUO. Likewise, the widespread availability of highly specific and sensitive immunologic testing has reduced the number of undetected cases of systemic lupus erythematosus (SLE) and other autoimmune diseases.

Several generalizations can be made. Infections, especially extrapulmonary tuberculosis, remain the leading cause of FUO. Prolonged mononucleosis syndromes caused by Epstein-Barr virus, CMV, or HIV are conditions whose consideration as a cause of FUO is sometimes confounded by delayed antibody responses. Intraabdominal abscesses (sometimes poorly localized) and renal, retroperitoneal, and paraspinal abscesses continue to be difficult to diagnose. Renal malacoplakia, with submucosal plaques or nodules involving the urinary tract, may cause FUO and is often fatal if untreated. It is associated with coliform infection, is seen most often in patients with defects of intracellular bacterial killing, and is treated with fluoroquinolones or trimethoprim-sulfamethoxazole. Occasionally, other organs may be involved. Osteomyelitis, especially where prosthetic devices have been implanted, and infective endocarditis must be considered. Although true culture-negative infective endocarditis is rare, one may be misled by slow-growing organisms of the HACEK group (*Haemophilus aphrophilus*, *Actinobacillus actinomycetemcomitans*, *Cardiobacterium hominis*, *Eikenella corrodens*, and *Kingella kingae*; see Chap. 152), *Bartonella* species (previously *Rochalimaea*), *Legionella* species, *Coxiella burnetii*, *Chlamydia psittaci*, and fungi. Prostatitis, dental abscesses, sinusitis, and cholangitis continue to be sources of occult fever.

Fungal disease, most notably histoplasmosis involving the reticuloendothelial system, may cause FUO. FUO with headache should prompt examination of spinal fluid for *Cryptococcus neoformans*. Malaria (which may result from transfusion, the failure to take a prescribed prophylactic agent, or infection with a drug-resistant strain) continues to be a cause, particularly of nonsynchronized FUO.

In most early series, neoplasms were the next most common cause of FUO after infections (Table 125-3). In a series of 199 patients studied between 1980 and 1989, a decrease in the percentage of FUO cases due to malignancy was attributed to the improvement in diagnostic technologies. This observation does not diminish the importance of considering neoplasia in the initial diagnostic evaluation of a patient with fever. A large number of patients in this series had diseases such as temporal arteritis, adult Still's disease, drug-related fever, and factitious fever. In most series, approximately 10 percent of cases of FUO remained undiagnosed. The general term "collagen vascular diseases" is used somewhat loosely to apply not only to SLE and temporal arteritis but also to systemic rheumatologic or vasculitic diseases such as polymyalgia rheumatica and adult Still's disease.

In the elderly, multisystem disease is the most frequent cause of FUO, giant-cell arteritis being the leading etiologic entity in this category. Tuberculosis is the most common infection causing FUO in the elderly, and colon cancer is an important cause of FUO with malignancy.

Many diseases have been grouped in the various studies as "miscellaneous." At the top of this list are the granulomatous diseases, including sarcoidosis, Crohn's disease, and granulomatous hepatitis. Additional diagnoses include drug fever, erythema multiforme, pulmonary embolism, factitious fever, familial Mediterranean fever, Behçet's syndrome, Fabry's disease, and Whipple's disease (now attributed to the bacillus *Tropheryma whippelii*).

Table 125-3

Malignancies That Commonly Cause FUO

Hodgkin's disease
Non-Hodgkin's lymphoma
Leukemia (including preleukemic and aleukemic phases)
Renal cell carcinoma
Hepatoma

Table 125-4

Causes of FUO Lasting More than 6 Months

Cause	Percentage of Cases
None identified	19
Miscellaneous causes	13
Factitious causes	9
Granulomatous hepatitis	8
Neoplasm	7
Still's disease	6
Infection	6
Collagen vascular disease	4
Familial Mediterranean fever	3
No fever*	27

* No actual fever observed during 2 to 3 weeks of inpatient observation. Includes patients with exaggerated circadian rhythm.

SOURCE: From a study of 347 patients referred to the National Institutes of Health from 1961 to 1977 with a presumptive diagnosis of FUO of >6 months' duration (Aduan et al).

A drug-related etiology must be considered in any case of prolonged fever. Any febrile pattern may be elicited by a drug, and both relative bradycardia and hypotension are uncommon. Eosinophilia and/or rash is found in only one-fifth of patients with drug fever. Fever usually begins 1 to 3 weeks after the start of therapy and remits 2 to 3 days after therapy is stopped. Virtually all classes of drugs cause fever, but antimicrobials (especially β-lactam antibiotics), cardiovascular drugs (e.g., quinidine), antineoplastic drugs, and drugs acting on the central nervous system (e.g., phenytoin) are particularly common causes.

It is axiomatic that, as the duration of fever increases, the likelihood of an infectious cause decreases (Table 125-4). In a series of 347 patients referred to the National Institutes of Health from 1961 to 1977, only 6 percent had an infection. A significant number (9 percent) had *factitious fevers*—i.e., fevers due either to false elevations of temperature or to self-induced disease. A substantial number of these factitious cases were in young women in the health professions. It is worth noting that 8 percent of the patients with prolonged fevers (some of whom had completely normal liver function studies) had granulomatous hepatitis, and 6 percent had adult Still's disease. After prolonged investigation, 19 percent of cases still had no specific diagnosis. A total of 27 percent of patients either had no actual fever during the weeks of inpatient observation or had an exaggerated circadian temperature rhythm without chills, elevated pulse, or other abnormalities. The conditions that may be considered in a differential diagnosis of classic FUO in adults are listed in Table 125-5. While this list applies strictly to the United States, the frequency of global travel underscores the need for a detailed travel history.

SPECIALIZED DIAGNOSTIC STUDIES IN CLASSIC FUO

Certain specific diagnostic maneuvers become critical in dealing with prolonged fevers. If factitious fever is suspected, numbered thermometers should be used, temperature-taking should be supervised, and simultaneous urine and body temperatures should be measured. Any tissue removed during prior relevant surgery should be reexamined; slides should be requested and, if need be, paraffin blocks of fixed pathologic material should be reexamined and additional special studies performed. Relevant x-rays should be reexamined; reviewing of prior radiologic reports may be insufficient. Serum should be set aside in the laboratory as soon as possible and retained for future examination for rising antibody titers. *Febrile agglutinins* is a vague term that in most laboratories refers to serologic studies for salmonellosis, brucellosis, and rickettsial diseases. These studies are seldom useful, having low sensitivity and variable specificity. Rising titers of antibody to *Brucella* are usually diagnostic, but false-positive results may be obtained in typhoid fever, tularemia, and yersinial infections. Infection with *Brucella canis* may be missed with standard antibody tests for

Salmonella infection elevates antibody titers to the H and O antigens. High titers of antibody to the H antigen persist for years and may reflect previous infection or immunization. The measurement of specific antirickettsial titers should be requested for the diagnosis of Rocky Mountain spotted fever and Q fever. Multiple blood samples—no fewer than three, rarely more than six—should be cultured in the laboratory for at least 2 weeks to ensure that any HACEK-group organisms that may be present have ample time to grow (see Chap. 152). Lysis-centrifugation blood culture techniques should be employed in cases where prior antimicrobial therapy or fungal or atypical mycobacterial infection is suspected. Blood culture media

should be supplemented with L-cysteine or pyridoxal to assist in the isolation of nutritionally variant streptococci. It should be noted that sequential cultures positive for multiple organisms may reflect self-injection of contaminated substances. Urine cultures, including cultures for mycobacteria, fungi, and CMV, are indicated. Liver biopsy, even when the results of liver function studies are normal, should be considered and pursued if the diagnosis remains elusive. Specimens should be cultured for mycobacteria and fungi. Likewise, bone marrow

Table 125-5

Causes of FUO in Adults in the United States

Infections
Localized pyogenic infections
  Appendicitis
  Cat-scratch disease
  Cholangitis
  Cholecystitis
  Dental abscess
  Diverticulitis/abscess
  Lesser sac abscess
  Liver abscess
  Mesenteric lymphadenitis
  Osteomyelitis
  Pancreatic abscess
  Pelvic inflammatory disease
  Perinephric/intrarenal abscess
  Prostatic abscess
  Renal malacoplakia
  Sinusitis
  Subphrenic abscess
  Suppurative thrombophlebitis
  Tuboovarian abscess
Intravascular infections
  Bacterial aortitis
  Bacterial endocarditis
  Vascular catheter infection
Systemic bacterial infections
  Bartonellosis
  Brucellosis
  Campylobacter infection
  Cat-scratch disease/bacillary angiomatosis
    (*B. henselae*)
  Gonococcemia
  Legionnaires' disease
  Leptospirosis
  Listeriosis
  Lyme disease
  Melioidosis
  Meningococcemia
  Rat-bite fever
  Relapsing fever
  Salmonellosis
  Syphilis
  Tularemia
  Typhoid fever
  Vibriosis
  Yersinia infection
Mycobacterial infections
  M. avium/M. intracellulare infections
  Other atypical mycobacterial infections
  Tuberculosis
Fungal infections
  Aspergillosis
  Blastomycosis
  Candidiasis
  Coccidioidomycosis
  Cryptococcosis
  Histoplasmosis
  Mucormycosis
  Paracoccidioidomycosis
  Sporotrichosis

Other bacterial infections
  Actinomycosis
  Nocardiosis
  Whipple's disease
Rickettsial infections
  Ehrlichiosis
  Murine typhus
  Q fever
  Rickettsialpox
  Rocky Mountain spotted fever
Mycoplasmal infections
Chlamydial infections
  Lymphogranuloma venereum
  Psittacosis
  TWAR (*C. pneumoniae*) infection
Viral infections
  Colorado tick fever
  Coxsackievirus group B infection
  Cytomegalovirus infection
  Dengue
  Epstein-Barr virus infection
  Hepatitis A, B, C, D, and E
  Human immunodeficiency virus infection
  Lymphocytic choriomeningitis
  Parvovirus B19 infection
Parasitic infections
  Amebiasis
  Babesiasis
  Chagas' disease
  Leishmaniasis
  Malaria
  P. carinii infection
  Strongyloidiasis
  Toxocariasis
  Toxoplasmosis
  Trichinosis
Presumed infections, agent undetermined
  Kawasaki's disease (mucocutaneous lymph
    node syndrome)
  Kikuchi's disease (necrotizing
    lymphadenitis)
Neoplasms
Malignant
  Colon cancer
  Hepatoma
  Hodgkin's lymphoma
  Immunoblastic lymphadenopathy
  Leukemia
  Lymphomatoid granulomatosis
  Malignant histiocytosis
  Nephroma
  Non-Hodgkin's lymphoma
  Pancreatic cancer
  Sarcoma
Benign
  Atrial myxoma
  Renal angiomyolipoma

Collagen vascular/hypersensitivity diseases
  Adult Still's disease
  Behçet's disease
  Erythema multiforme
  Erythema nodosum
  Giant-cell arteritis/polymyalgia rheumatica
  Hypersensitivity pneumonitis (e.g., "metal
    fume fever," "farmer's lung," "air-
    conditioner lung")
  Hypersensitivity vasculitis
  Mixed connective-tissue disease
  Polyarteritis nodosa
  Relapsing polychondritis
  Rheumatic fever
  Rheumatoid arthritis
  Systemic lupus erythematosus
  Takayasu's aortitis
  Weber-Christian disease
  Wegener's granulomatosis
Granulomatous diseases
  Crohn's disease
  Idiopathic granulomatous hepatitis
  Midline granuloma
  Sarcoidosis
Miscellaneous conditions
  Aortic dissection
  Drug fever
  Gout
  Hematomas
  Hemolytic diseases/hemoglobinopathies
  Laennec's cirrhosis
  Postmyocardial infarction syndrome
  Recurrent pulmonary emboli
  Subacute thyroiditis (de Quervain's)
  Tissue infarction/necrosis
Inherited and metabolic diseases
  Adrenal insufficiency
  Cyclic neutropenia
  Deafness, urticaria, and amyloidosis
  Fabry's disease
  Familial Mediterranean fever
  Hyperimmunoglobulinemia D and periodic
    fever
  Type V hypertriglyceridemia
Thermoregulatory disorders
  Central
    Brain tumor
    Cerebrovascular accident
    Encephalitis
    Hypothalamic dysfunction
  Peripheral
    Hyperthyroidism
    Pheochromocytoma
Factitious fevers
"Afebrile" FUO (<38.3°C)
Habitual hyperthermia (exaggerated circadian
  rhythm)

SOURCE: Modified from RK Root, RG Petersdorf, in *Harrison's Principles of Internal Medicine*, 12th ed, JD Wilson et al (eds). New York, McGraw-Hill, 1991.

biopsy (not simple aspiration) should be used to obtain specimens for histology and culture. The blood smear should be examined for *Plasmodium, Babesia, Trypanosoma, Leishmania,* and *Borrelia.*

In an FUO workup, the erythrocyte sedimentation rate (ESR) should be determined. Striking elevation of the ESR and anemia of chronic disease are frequently seen in association with giant-cell arteritis or polymyalgia rheumatica, common causes of FUO in patients over 50 years of age. Still's disease is also suggested by elevations of ESR, leukocytosis, and anemia and is often accompanied by arthralgias, polyserositis (pleuritis, pericarditis), lymphadenopathy, splenomegaly, and rash. Antinuclear antibody should be measured to rule out other collagen vascular diseases. Another cause of an extremely high ESR may be a "false-positive" value attributable to a cold agglutinin with a broad thermal amplitude. The ESR test is nonspecific, yielding values that depend on certain serum proteins (most notably fibrinogen) known to interfere with the zeta-potential that keeps erythrocytes from clumping. When fibrinogen levels go up, the zeta-potential is inhibited, erythrocytes clump, and the ESR is high. A cold agglutinin, by binding to erythrocytes, can produce a "false-positive" agglutinin that mimics an acute-phase response; cold agglutinins may be seen in *Mycoplasma* and Epstein-Barr virus infections and in lymphomas.

With rare exceptions, the intermediate-strength purified protein derivative (PPD) skin test should be used to screen for tuberculosis in patients with classic FUO. Concurrent control tests, such as the CMI test (Connaught Labs, Swiftwater, PA), which is especially effective, should be employed. It should be kept in mind that a negative PPD skin test plus negative results of the control tests may be seen with miliary tuberculosis, sarcoidosis, Hodgkin's disease, malnutrition, or AIDS. Noninvasive procedures should include an upper gastrointestinal contrast study with small-bowel follow-through and barium enema to include the terminal ileum and cecum. Chest x-rays should be repeated if new symptoms arise. In some cases, pulmonary function studies may be necessary. A diminished carbon monoxide diffusing capacity ($D_{L_{CO}}$) may indicate a restrictive lung disease such as sarcoidosis, even with a normal chest x-ray. In such cases, transbronchial biopsy may prove diagnostic. Flexible colonoscopy may be advisable, since colon carcinoma is a cause of FUO and easily escapes detection by ultrasound and CT.

CT of the chest and abdomen should be performed. If a spinal or paraspinal lesion is suspected, however, MRI is preferred. MRI may be superior to CT in demonstrating intraabdominal abscesses and aortic dissection, but the relative utility of MRI and CT in the diagnosis of FUO is unknown. At present, it would appear that abdominal CT should be used unless MRI is specifically indicated. Ultrasonography of the abdomen is useful for the investigation of the hepatobiliary tract, kidneys, spleen, and pelvis. Echocardiography may be helpful in an evaluation for bacterial endocarditis, pericarditis, nonbacterial thrombotic endocarditis, and atrial myxomas. Transesophageal echocardiography is especially sensitive for these lesions.

Radionuclide scanning procedures using technetium (Tc)-99m sulfur colloid, gallium (Ga) citrate, or indium (In) 111–labeled leukocytes or immunoglobulin may be useful in identifying and/or localizing inflammatory processes. In a recent study, Ga scintigraphy yielded useful diagnostic information in almost one-third of cases, and it was suggested that this procedure might actually be used before other imaging techniques if no specific organ is suspected of being abnormal. Tc bone scan should be undertaken to look for osteomyelitis or bony metastases; Ga scan may be used to identify sarcoidosis or *P. carinii* in lungs or Crohn's disease in the abdomen. ^{111}In-labeled white blood cell scan may be used to locate abscesses; ^{111}In-labeled immunoglobulin scan also shows promise in this regard. With both Ga and In white blood cell scans, false-positive and false-negative findings are common.

Biopsy of the liver and bone marrow should be considered routine in the workup of FUO if the studies mentioned above are unrevealing or if fever is prolonged. It goes without saying that areas of suspected abnormality should be sampled for pathologic examination whenever

practical. When possible, a section of the tissue block should be retained for further sections or stains. Polymerase chain reaction technology makes it possible to identify and speciate mycobacterial DNA in paraffin-embedded, fixed tissues. Thus, in some cases, it is possible to make a retrospective diagnosis based on studies of long-fixed pathologic tissues. In a patient over age 50 (or occasionally in a younger patient) with the appropriate symptoms and laboratory findings, "blind biopsy" of one or both temporal arteries may yield a diagnosis of arteritis. If noted, tenderness or decreased pulsation should guide the selection of a site for biopsy. Lymph node biopsy may be helpful if nodes are enlarged, but inguinal nodes are often palpable and are seldom diagnostically useful.

Exploratory laparotomy has been performed when all other diagnostic procedures fail but has largely been replaced by modern imaging and guided-biopsy techniques.

℞ TREATMENT

Patients with neutropenic FUO may be treated by a variety of empirical protocols. The regimen usually combines an aminoglycoside with an antipseudomonal β-lactam antibiotic or consists of imipenem or ceftazidime alone. Vancomycin should be added to the regimen if intravenous catheter–associated infection is suspected. If vancomycin is administered and fever continues, the addition of amphotericin B should be considered.

Empirical therapy for nosocomial FUO must be guided by the clinical situation. While empirical antibiotic therapy may be indicated, it should be remembered that complications of drug therapy (including *C. difficile*–associated colitis and drug-related fever), rather than infection, may be the cause of the fever.

The treatment of HIV-associated FUO depends on many factors and is discussed in Chap. 308. MAI, CMV, drugs administered to the patient, and HIV itself are probably the most common causes of FUO in this group once *P. carinii* infection, cryptococcosis, toxoplasmosis, tuberculosis, and bacterial sinusitis have been ruled out. Discontinuing or changing drugs is often necessary, and empirical therapy for these infections may be indicated.

The emphasis in patients with classic FUO is on continued observation and examination, with the avoidance of "shotgun" empirical therapy. Empirical treatment for endocarditis, for example, should be avoided unless there are specific reasons beyond fever to invoke this diagnosis. Every patient with FUO should undergo an exhaustive examination for tuberculosis. If the PPD skin test is positive or if granulomatous hepatitis or other granulomatous disease is present with anergy (and sarcoid seems unlikely), then a therapeutic trial with isoniazid and rifampin (and possibly a third drug) should be undertaken, with treatment usually continued for up to 6 weeks. A failure of the fever to respond over this period suggests an alternative diagnosis.

Q fever may cause noncaseating granulomatous hepatitis. Doxycycline is the drug of choice for a therapeutic trial if this etiology is suspected.

The response of rheumatic fever and Still's disease to aspirin and nonsteroidal anti-inflammatory agents (NSAIDs) may be dramatic. The effects of glucocorticoids on temporal arteritis, polymyalgia rheumatica, and granulomatous hepatitis are equally dramatic. Colchicine is highly effective in preventing attacks of familial Mediterranean fever but is of little use once an attack is well under way. The ability of glucocorticoids and NSAIDs to mask fever while permitting the spread of infection dictates that their use be avoided unless infection has been largely ruled out and unless inflammatory disease is both probable and debilitating or threatening.

When no underlying source of FUO is identified after prolonged observation (>6 months), the prognosis is generally good, however vexing the fever may be to the patient. Under such circumstances, debilitating symptoms are treated with NSAIDs, and glucocorticoids are the last resort. The initiation of empirical therapy does not mark the end of the diagnostic workup; rather, it commits the physician to continued thoughtful reexamination and evaluation. Patience, compassion, equanimity, and intellectual flexibility are indispensable attributes for the clinician in dealing successfully with FUO.

ADUAN R et al: Prolonged fever of unknown origin. Clin Res 26:558A, 1978

———— et al: Factitious fever and self-induced infection. Ann Intern Med 90:230, 1979

CUNHA BA: Fever of unknown origin. Infect Dis Clin North Am 10:111, 1996

DATA FL, THORNE DA: Gastrointestinal tract radionuclide activity on In-111 labeled leukocyte imaging: Clinical significance in patients with fever of unknown origin. Radiology 160:635, 1986

DEKLEIJN EM et al: Utility of scintigraphic methods in patients with fever of unknown origin. Arch Intern Med 155:1989, 1995

DINARELLO CA, WOLFF SM: Fever of unknown origin, in *Principles and Practice of Infectious Diseases*, 3d ed, GL Mandell et al (eds). New York, Wiley, 1990, pp 468–479

DURACK DT, STREET AC: Fever of unknown origin—reexamined and redefined, in *Current Clinical Topics in Infectious Diseases,* JS Remington, MN Swartz (eds). Cambridge, MA, Blackwell, 1991

GRANOWITZ EV et al: Interleukin-1 receptor antagonist production during experimental endotoxaemia. Lancet 338:1423, 1991

HOLTZ T et al: Liver biopsy in fever of unknown origin. J Clin Gastroenterol 17:29, 1993

HOWARD P JR et al: Fever of unknown origin: A prospective study of 100 patients. Tex Med 73:56, 1977

HUGGINS JW et al: Prospective, double-blind, concurrent placebo-controlled clinical trial of intravenous ribavirin therapy of hemorrhagic fever with renal syndrome. J Infect Dis 164:1119, 1991

HUGHES WT et al: Guidelines for the use of antimicrobial agents in neutropenic patients with unexplained fever. J Infect Dis 161:381, 1990

ISAAC B et al (eds): *Unexplained Fever.* Boca Raton, CRC Press, 1991

JACOBY GA, SWARTZ MN: Fever of undetermined origin. N Engl J Med 289:1407, 1973

KNOCKAERT DC, VANNESTE LJ: Fever of unknown origin in the 1980s. Arch Intern Med 152:51, 1992

———— et al: Fever of unknown origin in elderly patients. J Am Geriatr Soc 41:1187, 1993

———— et al: Clinical value of gallium-67 scintigraphy in evaluation of fever of unknown origin. Clin Infect Dis 18:601, 1994

LARSON EB, FEATHERSTONE HJ: Fever of undetermined origin: Diagnosis and follow-up of 105 cases, 1970–80. Medicine 61:269, 1982

MEYERS SP, WIENER SN: Diagnosis of hematogenous pyogenic vertebral osteomyelitis by magnetic resonance imaging. Arch Intern Med 151:683, 1991

MITCHELL MA et al: Bilateral renal parenchymal malacoplakia presenting as fever of unknown origin: Case report and review. Clin Infect Dis 18:704, 1994

ORR PH et al: Febrile urinary infection in the institutionalized elderly. Am J Med 100:71, 1996

PETERSDORF RC: Fever of unknown origin. An old friend revisited [editorial]. Arch Intern Med 152:21, 1992

———— RG, BEESON PB: Fever of unexplained origin. Medicine 40:1, 1961

ROSENBERG MR, GREEN M: Neuroleptic malignant syndrome. Arch Intern Med 149:1927, 1989

ROWLAND MD, DEL BENE VE: Use of body computed tomography to evaluate fever of unknown origin. J Infect Dis 156:408, 1987

RUBIN RH et al: 111In-labeled nonspecific immunoglobulin scanning in the detection of focal infection. N Engl J Med 321:935, 1989

SABBOOR SA et al: Detection of mycobacterial DNA in sarcoidosis and tuberculosis with polymerase chain reaction. Lancet 339:1012, 1992

SCHMIDT KG et al: Indium-111 granulocyte scintigraphy in the evaluation of patients with fever of undetermined origin. Scand J Infect Dis 19:339, 1987

SIMON HB, WOLFF SM: Granulomatous hepatitis and prolonged fever of unknown origin: A study of 13 patients. Medicine 52:1, 1973

SMITH JW: Southwestern internal medicine conference: Fever of undetermined origin: Not what it used to be. Am J Med Sci 292:56, 1986

SPACH DH et al: *Bartonella (Rochalimaea) quintana* bacteremia in inner-city patients with chronic alcoholism. N Engl J Med 332:424, 1995

STEINMETZ HT et al: Increase in interleukin-6 serum level preceding fever in granulocytopenia and correlation with death from sepsis. J Infect Dis 171:225, 1995

WEINSTEIN L: Clinically benign fever of unknown origin: A personal retrospective. Rev Infect Dis 7:692, 1985

WILSON ME: *A World Guide to Infections: Diseases, Distribution, Diagnosis.* New York, Oxford University Press, 1991

WOLFF SM et al: A syndrome of periodic hypothalamic discharge. Am J Med 36:956, 1964

———— et al: Unusual etiologies of fever and their evaluation. Annu Rev Med 26:277, 1975

ZANGWILL KM et al: Cat scratch disease in Connecticut—epidemiology, risk factors, and evaluation of a new diagnostic test. N Engl J Med 329:8, 1993

126 *Donald Kaye*

INFECTIVE ENDOCARDITIS

Infective endocarditis is a disease that produces vegetations on the endocardium. It is virtually always fatal if untreated. A heart valve is usually involved, but the infection may develop on a septal defect or on the mural endocardium. Infection of an arteriovenous shunt or coarctation of the aorta is more properly called *endarteritis* but produces a similar clinical syndrome. The discussion of endocarditis in this chapter also applies to endarteritis.

CLASSIFICATION

Endocarditis can be classified in three categories: native valve endocarditis, endocarditis in intravenous drug abusers, and prosthetic valve endocarditis. These categories have different infecting microorganisms and run different courses. Endocarditis also can be classified as acute or subacute. Acute endocarditis most frequently is caused by *Staphylococcus aureus*, occurs on a normal heart valve, is rapidly destructive, produces metastatic foci, and, if untreated, is fatal in less than 6 weeks. Subacute endocarditis usually is caused by viridans streptococci, occurs on damaged valves, does not produce metastatic foci, and, if untreated, takes more than 6 weeks—perhaps as long as a year—to be fatal. Correlations between organism and course are not perfect; viridans streptococci can be associated with an acute course and *S. aureus* with a subacute course. The most important basis for classification is the infecting organism (e.g., *S. aureus* endocarditis), because the organism has implications for therapy as well as course.

NATIVE VALVE ENDOCARDITIS Etiology Although almost any bacteria can produce endocarditis, streptococci, enterococci, and staphylococci account for the vast majority of cases.

Streptococci Streptococci cause about 55 percent of cases of native valve endocarditis in patients who do not abuse intravenous drugs. Viridans streptococci [most commonly *Streptococcus sanguis*, *Streptococcus mutans*, *Streptococcus mitis* (formerly *S. mitior*), or *Streptococcus milleri*] account for about 75 percent of these cases; *Streptococcus bovis* and other streptococci cause 20 and 5 percent, respectively. Viridans streptococci are normal inhabitants of the oropharynx and generally are highly susceptible to penicillin. Two group D streptococci, *S. bovis* and *Streptococcus equinus*, are also highly susceptible to penicillin G. *S. bovis* endocarditis occurs in elderly individuals; 80 percent of cases are in persons over 60 years of age. More than a third of these individuals have a malignant or premalignant gastrointestinal lesion, most often colonic cancer or a villous adenoma or polyp of the colon.

Group A beta-hemolytic streptococci attack normal or damaged heart valves and may cause their rapid destruction. Group B streptococci, which have been reported more frequently as a cause of endocarditis in recent years, also attack normal valves and result in large, friable vegetations and large emboli. Other streptococci are much more likely to infect damaged valves and rarely cause rapid valve destruction. *S. milleri* can cause metastatic abscesses, which are uncommon with other streptococci.

Enterococci Enterococci cause about 6 percent of cases of native valve endocarditis. Enterococci are alpha-, beta-, or gamma-hemolytic and are normal inhabitants of the gastrointestinal tract, the anterior urethra, and occasionally the mouth. All enterococci are in Lancefield's group D and can be distinguished from streptococci by biochemical tests. They are relatively resistant to penicillin G; an aminoglycoside must be added to achieve a bactericidal effect. Enterococcal endocarditis is more common among males, who develop infection at an average age of 60 years. Many patients have a recent history of genitourinary tract manipulation, trauma, or disease (e.g., cystoscopy, urethral catheterization, prostatectomy, abortion, pregnancy, or cesarean section).

Staphylococci   Staphylococci cause about 30 percent of cases of native valve endocarditis (with *S. aureus* 5 to 10 times more frequent than *Staphylococcus epidermidis*). *S. aureus* attacks normal or damaged heart valves, often causing rapid destruction. The course is often fulminant, with death from bacteremia within days or from heart failure within weeks. Abscesses are common at multiple sites (e.g., kidneys, lungs, and brain). *S. epidermidis* usually infects prosthetic valves.

HACEK organisms   The HACEK group of bacteria (*Haemophilus, Actinobacillus, Cardiobacterium, Eikenella,* and *Kingella*) are part of the oropharyngeal flora. They produce endocarditis with a subacute presentation and large vegetations. HACEK organisms are difficult to isolate from blood (see Chap. 152).

Other bacteria   Almost all species of bacteria are occasional causes of acute or subacute endocarditis, including *Streptococcus pneumoniae, Neisseria gonorrhoeae,* enteric gram-negative bacilli, *Pseudomonas, Salmonella, Streptobacillus, Serratia marcescens, Bacteroides, Brucella, Mycobacterium, Neisseria meningitidis, Listeria, Legionella,* and *Corynebacterium*.

Fungi   Fungi rarely cause native valve endocarditis in persons who do not abuse intravenous drugs. However, *Candida* and *Aspergillus* endocarditis can occur in patients with intravascular catheters who frequently have received glucocorticoids, broad-spectrum antimicrobial drugs, or cytotoxic agents. The course is usually subacute. Large friable vegetations are common and give rise to large emboli, often to the lower extremities. The prognosis is grave, partly because of the relatively poor activity of available antifungal agents.

Other microorganisms   Spirochetes (e.g., *Spirillum minus*), cell wall–deficient bacteria, rickettsiae (*Coxiella burnetii*), and chlamydiae (*Chlamydia psittaci, Chlamydia pneumoniae,* and *Chlamydia trachomatis*) are rare causes of endocarditis.

Epidemiology   Of patients with native valve endocarditis, more are male than female, and most are over age 50. Endocarditis is uncommon in children.

Between 60 and 80 percent of patients have an identifiable predisposing cardiac lesion. *Rheumatic valvular disease* accounts for about 25 percent of cases. The mitral valve is most commonly involved and the aortic valve next most commonly. The tricuspid valve is involved in rare cases.

Congenital heart disease other than mitral valve prolapse is the underlying lesion in about 10 to 20 percent of patients with endocarditis. Predisposing lesions include patent ductus arteriosus, ventricular septal defect, tetralogy of Fallot, coarctation of the aorta, pulmonary stenosis, and bicuspid aortic valve but not uncomplicated atrial septal defect. *Mitral valve prolapse* is the underlying lesion in about 10 to 33 percent of cases.

Degenerative heart disease predisposes to endocarditis. *Calcific aortic stenosis* (from degenerative disease or bicuspid valve) is an important lesion in the elderly. Other predisposing but unusual lesions are *asymmetric septal hypertrophy, Marfan's syndrome,* and *syphilitic aortic valve. Arterioarterial* or *arteriovenous fistulas* are also reported as underlying lesions. In 20 to 40 percent of patients with infective endocarditis, *no underlying heart disease* can be recognized.

ENDOCARDITIS IN INTRAVENOUS DRUG ABUSERS   Drug abusers with endocarditis are frequently young males. The skin is most often the source of microorganisms responsible for endocarditis in these cases; contamination of drugs is less common. *S. aureus* causes more than 50 percent of cases, streptococci and enterococci about 20 percent, and fungi (mainly *Candida*) and gram-negative bacilli (usually *Pseudomonas* species) about 6 percent each. Infection with multiple organisms is common. The onset is usually acute. Only about 20 percent of addicts experiencing their first episode of endocarditis have previously damaged heart valves. The tricuspid valve is infected in about 50 percent of cases, the aortic valve in 25 percent, the mitral valve in about 20 percent, and multiple valves in the rest. More than 75 percent of patients with *S. aureus* infection and a much lower percentage of those infected with other organisms have tricuspid

valve endocarditis. Pulmonary emboli or pneumonia consequent to septic pulmonary emboli is common in tricuspid valve endocarditis, and murmurs are frequently absent.

PROSTHETIC VALVE ENDOCARDITIS   Any intravascular prosthesis predisposes to endocarditis and makes cure difficult. Infections of prosthetic valves now account for 10 to 20 percent of cases of endocarditis. Intravascular sutures, pacemaker wires, and Teflon-Silastic tubes also can be foci of infection. Most patients with prosthetic valve endocarditis are males over age 60. Endocarditis occurs in 1 to 2 percent of these patients during the first year after surgery and in about 0.5 percent per year thereafter. Aortic valve prostheses are much more likely to be involved than mitral valve prostheses. The infection is usually on the suture line.

Early-onset endocarditis (onset of symptoms within 60 days of surgery) is usually a consequence of valve contamination during the procedure or of perioperative bacteremia. *Late-onset endocarditis* (onset of symptoms after 60 days) may have the same pathogenesis as early endocarditis (especially during the first year) but with a long incubation period; it also may result from transient bacteremia.

About half of all episodes of early-onset endocarditis and one-third of all episodes of late-onset endocarditis are caused by staphylococci, and *S. epidermidis* is more frequently involved than *S. aureus*. Gram-negative bacilli cause up to 15 percent, and fungi (most commonly *Candida*) up to 10 percent, of early-onset cases; they are less common in late-onset endocarditis. A prosthetic valve may malfunction because of large vegetations (often fungal). Streptococci are the most frequent single cause of late-onset endocarditis (about 40 percent of cases) but are uncommon in early-onset endocarditis.

Early-onset prosthetic valve endocarditis is often associated with valvular dysfunction or dehiscence and a fulminant course. Although late-onset endocarditis may be similarly fulminant, the course is commonly indistinguishable from that of endocarditis in patients without prosthetic valves, especially when the infecting organism is a streptococcus.

PATHOGENESIS AND PATHOLOGY

The characteristic lesions of infective endocarditis are vegetations on valves or elsewhere on the endocardium. The disease usually is secondary to the colonization by microorganisms of sterile vegetations composed of platelets and fibrin. Sterile vegetations, which represent *nonbacterial thrombotic endocarditis,* form over areas of trauma to the endothelium (from intracardiac foreign bodies, for example), in areas of turbulence (as on deformed valves), over scars, or in the setting of wasting disease, particularly malignancy (marantic endocarditis).

Infection of a sterile vegetation is most likely when bacteremia involves bacteria that adhere well to platelets, fibrin, and fibronectin. The vegetation of infective endocarditis then results from deposition of platelets and fibrin over the bacteria, which forms a "protected site" into which phagocytic cells penetrate poorly.

Endocarditis tends to occur in high-pressure areas (i.e., on the left side of the heart) and downstream from sites where blood flows at high velocity through a narrow orifice from a high- to a low-pressure chamber (e.g., distal to the constriction in coarctation of the aorta). Endocarditis is unusual in sites with a small pressure gradient, as in atrial septal defects. The disease occurs more frequently in patients with valvular incompetence than in those with pure stenosis, and the lesion characteristically is located on the atrial side of a regurgitant mitral valve and on the ventricular surface of a regurgitant aortic valve. A high-velocity stream of blood can produce satellite infected lesions at distant points of impact.

Microorganisms that possess little pathogenicity in other situations (e.g., viridans streptococci) usually implant only on deformed heart valves exhibiting nonbacterial thrombotic endocarditis, but more virulent microorganisms (e.g., *S. aureus* and *S. pneumoniae*) can infect apparently normal valves.

Transient bacteremia is common in various infections and during traumatic procedures involving epithelial surfaces that are colonized by a bacterial flora (oropharynx, genitourinary and gastrointestinal tracts, and skin). For example, after trauma to tissues of the mouth, viridans streptococci are the most common bacteria isolated from blood, either alone or—more often—mixed with other bacteria. The frequency and magnitude of bacteremia are related to the severity of periodontal disease and the severity of trauma. The portal of entry for the infecting organism in the initiating episode of bacteremia is usually not apparent in viridans streptococcal endocarditis. Dental procedures, the most common cause of apparent portals of entry, precede viridans streptococcal endocarditis in only 15 to 20 percent of cases.

Bacteremia also is common with prostatic surgery, cystoscopy, urethral dilation or catheterization, and procedures involving the female reproductive tract. The infecting organisms are usually enterococci and gram-negative bacilli. About 50 percent of patients with enterococcal endocarditis have recently undergone surgery or instrumentation of the genitourinary or gastrointestinal tract. About 35 percent of patients with staphylococcal endocarditis have had a preceding staphylococcal infection at a remote site.

The clinical features of endocarditis result from the vegetations and from an immune reaction to the infection. Extensive vegetations, especially in fungal endocarditis, may occlude the valve orifice. Rapid valve destruction with consequent regurgitation may occur, especially with *S. aureus*. Healing may cause scar formation, with subsequent valvular stenosis or regurgitation. Infection may extend into the myocardium, producing burrowing abscesses. Conduction abnormalities, fistulas (between chambers of the heart and the pericardium or major vessels), or rupture of the chordae, of a papillary muscle, or of the ventricular septum may result.

Pieces of vegetation may break off and cause embolisms in the heart, brain, kidney, spleen, liver, extremities, and lung (in right-sided endocarditis). Infarcts and occasionally abscesses result. Septic embolization to the vasa vasorum or direct bacterial invasion of the arterial wall may lead to the formation of mycotic aneurysms, which may rupture. Mycotic aneurysms most often develop in the cerebral arteries, aorta, sinuses of Valsalva, ligated ductus arteriosus, and superior mesenteric, splenic, coronary, and pulmonary arteries.

Patients with endocarditis usually have high titers of antibody to the infecting microorganism. This factor contributes to formation of circulating immune complexes that may result in glomerulonephritis (focal, membranoproliferative, or diffuse), arthritis, or various mucocutaneous manifestations of vasculitis.

Myocarditis may be due to small coronary-artery emboli, myocardial abscesses, or immune-complex vasculitis.

CLINICAL MANIFESTATIONS

Symptoms of endocarditis generally start within 2 weeks of the precipitating event. The frequencies of occurrence of some prominent clinical manifestations are shown in Table 126-1. With organisms of low pathogenicity (e.g., viridans streptococci), the *onset* is usually gradual, with mild fever and malaise. With organisms of high pathogenicity (e.g., *S. aureus*), the onset is often acute, with high fever. *Fever* is present in almost all patients with endocarditis (except occasionally in the elderly or in patients with renal failure, congestive heart failure, or severe debility). The fever is usually low-grade (less than 39.4°C) except in acute disease. Arthralgias and myalgias, especially low-back pain, are common, and arthritis develops occasionally.

Cardiac murmurs are almost always present except in patients with early acute endocarditis and in intravenous drug abusers with tricuspid valve infection. True changes in murmurs or the appearance of a new murmur is uncommon except in acute endocarditis, where a new murmur (particularly aortic regurgitation) is frequent. Changes in intensities of murmurs are often due to changes in heart rate and/or cardiac output (e.g., from anemia) and not necessarily to progressive valvular damage.

Splenomegaly and *petechiae* tend to occur in disease of long duration. Petechiae are most frequently found on the conjunctivae, palate, buccal mucosa, and upper extremities. *Splinter hemorrhages* are sub-ungual, linear, dark-red streaks that may appear in endocarditis but also commonly result from trauma. *Roth's spots* are oval, retinal hem-

Table 126-1

Frequencies of Occurrence of Prominent Clinical and Laboratory Manifestations in Endocarditis

Manifestation	Percentage of Cases
CLINICAL MANIFESTATIONS	
Fever	>95
Arthralgias and/or myalgias	25–45
Murmur	>85
Splenomegaly	25–60
Petechiae	20–40
Splinter hemorrhages	10–30
Roth's spots	<5
Osler's nodes	10–25
Janeway lesions	<5
Clubbing	10–20
Clinically apparent emboli	25–45
Neurologic manifestations	20–40
LABORATORY MANIFESTATIONS	
Anemia	70–90
Leukocytosis	20–30
Proteinuria	50–65
Microscopic hematuria	30–50
Elevated serum creatinine level	10–20
Elevated erythrocyte sedimentation rate	>90
Rheumatoid factor	50
Circulating immune complexes	65–100
Decreased serum complement level	5–40

orrhages with a clear, pale center; they may also occur in connective tissue disease and severe anemia. Likewise, *Osler's nodes* (small, tender nodules, usually on the finger or toe pads, which persist for hours to days) may also develop in other diseases. *Janeway lesions* are small hemorrhages with a slightly nodular character on the palms and soles and are most commonly seen in acute endocarditis. *Clubbing* of the fingers is reported in some patients with long-standing disease. *Embolic episodes* may occur during or after therapy. Emboli to large arteries (e.g., femoral arteries) are often the result of fungal endocarditis, with its large, friable vegetations. Pulmonary emboli are common in drug abusers with right-sided endocarditis and may be seen in patients with left-sided endocarditis who have left-to-right cardiac shunts.

Mycotic aneurysms occur in about 10 percent of patients. Symptoms are usually lacking but may be those of an expanding mass. The aneurysms can rupture during or even years after therapy. *Neurologic manifestations* are more common with left-sided endocarditis than with right-sided disease and with *S. aureus* infection than with viridans streptococcal infection. Clinically apparent cerebral emboli occur in about 20 percent of patients; encephalopathy (from microemboli with or without microabscess formation) in 10 percent; leakage from a mycotic aneurysm in fewer than 5 percent; and meningitis or a macroscopic brain abscess in fewer than 5 percent. Major cerebral emboli as well as mycotic aneurysms usually involve the middle cerebral artery system. Most patients with brain abscess or purulent meningitis have *S. aureus* endocarditis.

Heart failure may occur during the course of endocarditis or long after its cure. Contributing factors are valve destruction, myocarditis, coronary artery emboli with infarction, and myocardial abscesses. *Myocardial abscess* is most common in acute endocarditis (particularly that caused by *S. aureus*) or with a prosthesis. Conduction defects may result from ventricular septal invasion secondary to extension from a valve (most frequently the aortic valve). A valve-ring abscess—or, less commonly, a myocardial abscess—may extend into the epicardium and cause pericarditis. Echocardiography may be helpful in the diagnosis of myocardial abscess, and surgery is often indicated, especially with a prosthesis. *Renal disease* exists in most patients with endocarditis and is due to renal emboli or immune-complex glomerulonephritis. Renal insufficiency may result.

LABORATORY FEATURES

The frequencies of occurrence of some laboratory manifestations are shown in Table 126-1. Normocytic normochromic anemia is usual in infective endocarditis. The white blood cell and differential counts are often normal. However, in acute disease, leukocytosis without anemia may be present. Proteinuria and/or microscopic hematuria is found in most patients, and the serum creatinine level may be elevated. The erythrocyte sedimentation rate is almost always elevated except in cases with heart failure.

About 50 percent of patients with endocarditis of at least 6 weeks' duration have a positive serum test for rheumatoid factor, and most have circulating immune complexes, which tend to disappear with cure. The serum complement level may be decreased, especially with diffuse glomerulonephritis. Bacteria can be seen inside leukocytes in buffy-coat preparations of blood in about 50 percent of cases of endocarditis.

The critical diagnostic finding in endocarditis is bacteremia or fungemia. Blood cultures are positive in more than 95 percent of patients. The bacteremia is continuous; if any cultures are positive, all are likely to be positive. There is no advantage to obtaining samples for cultures at any particular time or body temperature. Arterial blood or bone marrow offers no advantage over antecubital vein blood.

In suspected subacute disease and in the absence of previous therapy, three sets of blood samples for culturing should be obtained over 3 to 6 h and therapy initiated. With previous therapy, it is justifiable to delay treatment until an attempt has been made to obtain positive blood cultures. In general, in acute disease, therapy should not be delayed for more than 2 to 3 h while cultures are obtained. Only one culture should be performed for each venipuncture; anaerobic as well as aerobic techniques should be used. Samples should be collected at least 30 to 60 min apart to demonstrate continuous bacteremia. The rate of positive cultures is increased by observation of the cultures over 3 weeks, with periodic sampling for Gram's stain and subculture even in the absence of turbidity.

Blood cultures may be negative in infections with fastidious organisms, such as *Haemophilus parainfluenzae*. Fifty percent of patients with *Candida* endocarditis and almost all with *Aspergillus*, *Histoplasma*, or *C. burnetii* endocarditis have negative blood cultures. With fungi, large peripheral emboli are common, necessitating embolectomy. Histologic examination and culture of the embolus may be diagnostic. Serologic tests for *C. burnetii* and *C. psittaci* are positive in endocarditis caused by these organisms.

Echocardiography has added a great deal to the ability to confirm or reject a diagnosis of infective endocarditis. All patients in whom infective endocarditis is suspected should at least undergo baseline transthoracic echocardiography (TTE) to determine the size and location of the vegetation, to obtain a picture that can be used for comparative purposes should cardiac complications arise, and to define underlying cardiac abnormalities. Transesophageal echocardiography (TEE) can detect vegetations as small as 1 to 1.5 mm, whereas the smallest size detectable by TTE is 2 to 3 mm. It follows that TEE is much more sensitive than TTE in detecting vegetations (90 percent vs. about 65 percent). This difference is even greater for the detection of prosthetic valve vegetations (about 75 percent vs. about 25 percent) and myocardial abscesses (85 percent vs. 25 percent). TEE should be performed for any patient with suspected infective endocarditis who has a prosthetic valve, for any patient with suspected myocardial or valve-ring abscess, and for any patient in whom TTE is technically unsatisfactory. In addition, any candidate for cardiac surgery should undergo TEE to delineate the cardiac architecture. Finally, a negative result of TEE

Table 126-2

Clinical Diagnosis of Infective Endocarditis

I. *Definite infective endocarditis:* Two major criteria *or* one major and three minor criteria *or* five minor criteria
  A. Major criteria
    1. Isolation of viridans streptococci, *S. bovis*, HACEK-group organisms, or (in the absence of a primary focus) community-acquired *S. aureus* or *Enterococcus* from two separate blood cultures *or* isolation of a microorganism consistent with endocarditis in (1) blood cultures ≥12 h apart or (2) all of three or most of four or more blood cultures, with first and last at least 1 h apart
    2. Evidence of endocardial involvement on echocardiography: oscillating intracardiac mass or abscess or new partial dehiscence of prosthetic valve *or* new valvular regurgitation
  B. Minor criteria
    1. Predisposing lesion or intravenous drug use
    2. Fever of ≥38.0°C
    3. Major arterial emboli, septic pulmonary infarcts, mycotic aneurysm, intracranial hemorrhage, conjunctival hemorrhages, Janeway lesions
    4. Glomerulonephritis, Osler's nodes, Roth's spots, rheumatoid factor
    5. Positive blood cultures not meeting the major criterion (excluding single cultures positive for organisms that do not typically cause endocarditis) or serologic evidence of active infection with an organism that causes endocarditis
    6. Echocardiogram consistent with endocarditis but not meeting the major criterion
II. *Possible infective endocarditis:* Findings that fall short of "definite" but do not fall into the "rejected" category
III. *Rejected:* Alternative diagnosis or resolution of syndrome or no evidence of infective endocarditis at surgery or autopsy with ≤4 days of antibiotic therapy

SOURCE: After Durack et al.

is strong evidence against infective endocarditis in patients with an equivocal syndrome.

Serial phonocardiography and cineradiography may be useful in evaluating infection on prosthetic valves. Disappearance of an opening click or sound produced by a closing valve suggests the presence of a vegetation. With dehiscence, cineradiography of the valve will show abnormal motion.

DIAGNOSIS

Recently introduced clinical criteria for the definitive diagnosis of infective endocarditis are shown in Table 126-2. These criteria depend heavily on blood culture and cardiac echocardiography.

Endocarditis should be suspected in patients who have a heart murmur and unexplained fever lasting for at least 1 week and in febrile intravenous drug abusers, even in the absence of a murmur.

Atrial myxoma, nonbacterial thrombotic endocarditis, acute rheumatic fever, lupus erythematosus, and sickle cell disease can duplicate the syndrome of infective endocarditis. Any patient with an existing heart murmur can develop fever related to another occult illness or to drugs. Therefore, in the absence of positive blood cultures and/or echocardiographic evidence, a search must be made for other causes of fever.

Following cardiac surgery, fever may be related to infection at other sites, to the postcardiotomy syndrome, or to a "postpump syndrome."

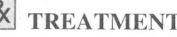 **TREATMENT**

Principles of Therapy   Cure of endocarditis requires eradication of all microorganisms from the vegetation. Therefore, microbicidal drug regimens must be used in high enough concentrations and for a long enough duration to sterilize the vegetation. Regimens including penicillins, cephalosporins, and vancomycin give far better results than are obtained when these agents cannot be used because of resistant organisms or drug reactions.

The minimal inhibitory concentration (MIC) and minimal bactericidal concentration (MBC) should be determined. In monitoring the therapeutic efficacy of a drug regimen, it may be useful to measure the bactericidal activity of the patient's serum against his or her isolate. A bactericidal titer of ≥1:8 in serum drawn 30 min after drug infusion probably indicates adequate therapy. While this determination is not necessary in most cases, it may be useful when infection is caused by organisms other than gram-positive cocci, when treatment has failed, or when the regimens being used do not include penicillins, cephalosporins, or vancomycin. Except in unusual circumstances, antibiotic administration should be parenteral to guarantee adequate absorption of drugs. The infecting microorganism should be saved for future testing (e.g., assessment of serum antibacterial activity, evaluation of different antibiotics, or comparison with a strain isolated during relapse).

Specific Antimicrobial Regimens THERAPY BEFORE CULTURE RESULTS ARE KNOWN The treatment of subacute infective endocarditis on a native valve while culture results are awaited should cover enterococci, which are more resistant to antibiotics than streptococci.

With an acute course, therapy should be directed against *S. aureus*. In intravenous drug abusers, initial therapy should be directed against *S. aureus*, and gentamicin (in a dose of 1.7 mg/kg every 8 h) should be included for the coverage of gram-negative bacilli. In many cities, most *S. aureus* isolates from drug abusers are methicillin-resistant, and vancomycin must be used. With prosthetic valves, vancomycin plus gentamicin should be used because of the high incidence of methicillin-resistant *S. epidermidis* and the need to cover enterococci.

Once the organism is isolated, the regimen should be altered appropriately. If cultures remain sterile and culture-negative endocarditis is likely, treatment is continued provided that the response is adequate.

STREPTOCOCCI WITH PENICILLIN G MICs OF ≤0.1 μg/mL Most streptococci are inhibited by concentrations of penicillin G of 0.1 μg/mL. Suggested regimens are listed in Table 126-3. Penicillin G or ceftriaxone alone for 4 weeks (regimens A and C in Table 126-3) gives cure rates of 98 percent. Addition of gentamicin to penicillin (regimen B) results in a more rapid bactericidal effect and gives equivalent cure rates in 2 weeks. Regimen B should be standard for uncomplicated infection treated in the hospital, but regimen A or C is preferred in patients likely to have side effects with aminoglycosides (i.e., those with renal insufficiency or eighth-nerve disease and those older than 65 years). Regimen B should not be used in patients with complications (e.g., metastatic abscesses). Regimen C is preferred for home treatment and can also be used in patients with a history of a delayed rash in response to penicillin. Regimen D should be used in patients with a history of anaphylaxis to penicillin.

STREPTOCOCCI WITH PENICILLIN G MICs OF >0.1 μg/mL BUT < 0.5 μg/mL Endocarditis caused by streptococci with MICs of penicillin G of >0.1 but <0.5 μg/mL is managed with regimen E.

ENTEROCOCCI OR STREPTOCOCCI WITH PENICILLIN G MICs OF ≥0.5 μg/mL OR NUTRITIONALLY VARIANT VIRIDANS STREPTOCOCCI Penicillin, ampicillin, and vancomycin are not bactericidal for most enterococci. However, the addition of an aminoglycoside results in a synergistic bactericidal effect. Enterococcal endocarditis requires penicillin, ampicillin, or vancomycin plus an aminoglycoside for cure in most cases (regimens F and G, with G used for patients hypersensitive to penicillin G). An alternative to regimen G consists of skin testing with major and minor determinants of penicillin, with subsequent attempts at desensitization to penicillin. This process involves a scratch test through a drop of penicillin G (100 units per

---

Table 126-3

Therapy for Infective Endocarditis

STREPTOCOCCI WITH PENICILLIN G MICs OF ≤0.1 μg/mL

Regimen A	Penicillin G, 12–18 million units per day IV in divided doses q4h × 4 weeks
Regimen B	Penicillin as in regimen A plus gentamicin, 1 mg/kg IV q8h, both × 2 weeks
Regimen C	Ceftriaxone, 2 g IV or IM once daily × 4 weeks
Regimen D	Vancomycin, 15 mg/kg IV q12h × 4 weeks

STREPTOCOCCI WITH PENICILLIN G MICs OF >0.1 BUT <0.5 μg/mL

Regimen E	Penicillin G, 18 million units per day IV in divided doses q4h × 4 weeks, plus gentamicin, 1 mg/kg IV q8h for the first 2 weeks; or regimen D if patient is allergic to penicillin

ENTEROCOCCI OR STREPTOCOCCI WITH PENICILLIN G MICs OF ≥0.5 μg/mL OR NUTRITIONALLY VARIANT VIRIDANS STREPTOCOCCI

Regimen F	Penicillin G, 18–30 million units per day IV, or ampicillin, 12 g/d IV, in divided doses q4h, plus gentamicin, 1 mg/kg IV q8h, both × 4–6 weeks
Regimen G	Vancomycin, 15 mg/kg IV q12h, plus gentamicin as in regimen F, both × 4–6 weeks

METHICILLIN-SUSCEPTIBLE STAPHYLOCOCCI ON A NATIVE VALVE

Regimen H	Nafcillin or oxacillin, 2 g IV q4h × 4–6 weeks, with or without gentamicin, 1 mg/kg IV q8h × the first 3–5 d
Regimen I	Cefazolin*, 2 g IV q8h × 4–6 weeks, with or without gentamicin as in regimen H
Regimen J	Vancomycin, 15 mg/kg IV q12h × 4–6 weeks, with or without gentamicin as in regimen H

METHICILLIN-RESISTANT STAPHYLOCOCCI OR *CORYNEBACTERIUM* SPP. ON A NATIVE VALVE

Regimen K	Vancomycin as in regimen J, with or without gentamicin as in regimen H, for staphylococci; continue gentamicin × 4–6 weeks for *Corynebacterium* spp.

THE ABOVE ORGANISMS ON A PROSTHETIC VALVE

Streptococci or enterococci: Regimen F or G. Streptococci: Penicillin or vancomycin × 6 weeks, with gentamicin × the first 2 weeks or longer. Enterococci: Penicillin or vancomycin plus an aminoglycoside × 6–8 weeks
Methicillin-susceptible staphylococci: Regimen H, I, or J × 6–8 weeks, with gentamicin × the first 2 weeks and rifampin (300 mg orally q8h) for the entire course
Methicillin-resistant staphylococci: Regimen J × 6–8 weeks, with gentamicin × the first 2 weeks and rifampin (300 mg orally q8h) for the entire course

HACEK BACTERIA

Regimen L	Use regimen C

---

* Another first-generation cephalosporin may be used instead of cefazolin.

NOTE: Serum concentrations of gentamicin should be about 3 μg/mL 1 h after a 20- to 30-min IV infusion or IM injection. Streptomycin may be substituted for gentamicin in regimens B, E, F, and G at 7.5 mg/kg IM every 12 h; serum concentrations should be about 20 μg/mL 1 h after injection. The maximal dose of vancomycin is 1 g every 12 h; serum concentrations of vancomycin 1 h after completion of the infusion should be 30–45 μg/mL.

milliliter), followed in 30 min by intradermal inoculation of graded amounts of penicillin, beginning at 0.01 unit in 0.1 mL of saline solution and continuing in tenfold increments every 30 min; with increasing amounts, administration is changed to the subcutaneous, the intramuscular, and finally the intravenous route. An oral desensitization regimen is also available, as described by Wendel et al. Epinephrine and diphenhydramine should be on hand for emergency use during the procedure in case of anaphylaxis, and, if possible, the procedure should be carried out in an intensive care unit. If a reaction occurs, alternative therapy should be initiated.

Therapy is usually given for 4 weeks but is prolonged to 6 weeks when symptoms have been present for longer than 3 months or the course is complicated. Cephalosporins cannot be used in enterococcal endocarditis because these organisms are highly resistant.

Penicillin and aminoglycosides exert a synergistic bactericidal effect against enterococci only when growth is inhibited by gentamicin at 500 μg/mL or streptomycin at 2000 μg/mL. Synergism is most likely with gentamicin. However, enterococci resistant to gentamicin at 500 μg/mL are now common. Some of these gentamicin-resistant strains are inhibited by streptomycin at 2000 μg/mL, but most are resistant to all aminoglycosides. With aminoglycoside-resistant strains, it is best to exclude aminoglycosides from the regimen and treat for 6 to 8 weeks. However, relapses may occur. Isolates of enterococci that are highly resistant to penicillin (owing to either production of penicillinase or other mechanisms) or to vancomycin have been observed with increasing frequency. A high percentage of strains of *Enterococcus faecium* and occasional strains of *Enterococcus faecalis* are highly resistant to penicillin and/or vancomycin. *E. faecium* accounts for about 15 percent of all enterococcal isolates from cases of endocarditis and *E. faecalis* for close to 85 percent. In vitro susceptibility testing of enterococci is required in the selection of appropriate therapy.

Endocarditis caused by streptococci with MICs of penicillin G of ≥0.5 μg/mL or by nutritionally variant viridans streptococci is managed in the same way as enterococcal endocarditis.

STAPHYLOCOCCI   Methicillin-susceptible *S. aureus* and *S. epidermidis* are treated with regimen H or I. Methicillin-resistant staphylococci are resistant to all penicillins and cephalosporins. In these instances and in those involving patients who cannot tolerate penicillins or cephalosporins, vancomycin must be used as in regimens J and K. Some experts advocate addition of gentamicin for the first 3 to 5 days because of an increase in the rate of bactericidal activity. However, clinical evidence of improved outcome is lacking, and routine use of this drug is not recommended. Four weeks' therapy is standard, but with metastatic or intracardiac abscess (or other complications), therapy should be extended to 6 weeks or even longer.

Evidence is mounting that vancomycin is inferior to β-lactam antibiotics in the treatment of staphylococcal endocarditis. Possible explanations include vancomycin's unpredictable pharmacokinetics, slower bactericidal activity, and poorer penetration into vegetations.

In intravenous drug users with *S. aureus* endocarditis localized to the tricuspid valve, excellent cure rates have been achieved with 2 weeks of treatment with nafcillin (but not vancomycin) plus an aminoglycoside.

STREPTOCOCCI, ENTEROCOCCI, AND STAPHYLOCOCCI IN PROSTHETIC VALVE ENDOCARDITIS   Prolonged therapy (Table 126-3) and combinations with an aminoglycoside for streptococci or enterococci and with an aminoglycoside plus rifampin for staphylococci are recommended for prosthetic valve infection.

OTHER ORGANISMS   Endocarditis due to HACEK organisms should be treated with regimen L and that due to *Corynebacterium* spp. with regimen K. In endocarditis caused by other organisms, bactericidal antibiotics—preferably a penicillin, a cephalosporin, or vancomycin with or without an aminoglycoside—should be given and therapy continued for 4 to 6 weeks. With gram-negative bacilli,

the penicillin or cephalosporin that displays the greatest potency against the infecting bacteria in vitro should be administered in large doses intravenously along with an aminoglycoside to which the bacterium is susceptible—e.g., ampicillin (2 g every 4 h), piperacillin (3 g every 4 h), cefotaxime (2 g every 4 to 6 h), or ceftazidime (2 g every 8 h) plus gentamicin (1.7 mg/kg every 8 h). A quinolone such as ciprofloxacin alone, which is bactericidal for gram-negative bacilli, also may be useful.

Therapy for fungal endocarditis with amphotericin B or an imidazole, such as fluconazole, usually has been unsuccessful. Such therapy plus cardiac surgery has generally been required for cure.

When the infecting organisms are resistant to penicillins, cephalosporins, quinolones, and vancomycin, therapy will probably be unsuccessful. Under these circumstances, treatment should consist of the bactericidal drug grouping with the best activity in vitro. If the response is poor or relapse occurs, antimicrobial therapy plus valve replacement will probably be necessary.

Home Therapy   Home Therapy is cost-effective and has been used successfully with stable individuals who are not intravenous drug users and are highly motivated, able to administer the therapy, and living with someone else. Regimen C or D has been used most frequently for streptococcal endocarditis and regimen J for staphylococcal endocarditis.

Surgery in the Management of Endocarditis   When curative microbicidal therapy is not available (as in most cases of fungal endocarditis), when positive blood cultures persist during therapy, or when relapse occurs after appropriate therapy, replacement of the valve should be considered. Ideally, surgery should be performed only after several days of the best available antimicrobial therapy. With organisms that tend to produce metastatic foci, therapy should then be continued long enough to eradicate these foci. Persistence of infection with the same organism following valve replacement has been uncommon. Immediate replacement (even after only hours of therapy) is essential in patients developing heart failure secondary to severe valvular regurgitation. Surgery is necessary to drain myocardial or valve-ring abscesses. Surgery should be considered when there are recurrent emboli despite adequate antimicrobial therapy. However, the frequency of emboli decreases dramatically with the initiation and continuation of antimicrobial therapy. Surgery also should be considered in patients with aortic valve endocarditis who develop first- and second-degree atrioventricular block. In some centers, the presence of a large vegetation on echocardiography has been considered an indication for surgery, but this point is controversial.

Replacement of a prosthesis is often necessary for infections with organisms other than streptococci. Some indications are valvular dysfunction or dehiscence and myocardial invasion. The latter is common with prosthetic valves and is suggested by continued fever after 10 days of therapy, a new regurgitant murmur, and/or atrioventricular conduction disturbance.

COURSE

Defervescence usually follows 3 to 7 days of antimicrobial therapy. Blood cultures should be obtained periodically during treatment; they generally become negative after several days of therapy. Both defervescence and the eradication of bacteremia have been slower when *S. aureus* endocarditis is treated with regimens containing vancomycin. Lack of response of fever and bacteremia may be associated with myocardial or metastatic abscess formation (especially associated with *S. aureus*).

The most common cause of persistent or recurrent fever during therapy is a drug reaction; less commonly, emboli are responsible. If a rash develops, therapy can be continued, and antihistamines or even glucocorticoids can be given to suppress the reaction. If the rash is severe, therapy should be altered.

Weight gain and a rise in hemoglobin may not be seen until weeks after therapy has been completed. Petechiae, Osler's nodes, and emboli may occur during and for weeks after successful antimicrobial therapy.

Mycotic aneurysms may regress during drug therapy or may rupture weeks to years later. Heart failure may occur during or after therapy and is the principal cause of death.

Anticoagulants should not be used in an attempt to prevent embolization from vegetations. Rather, they should be used only with a pressing indication (such as the presence of certain prosthetic valves) because of an increased risk of hemorrhage (especially intracranial). Warfarin is preferable to heparin. Blood cultures performed 2 and 4 weeks after discontinuation of therapy detect the vast majority of relapses. However, relapses are almost always clinically apparent.

PROGNOSIS

Factors that predispose to a poor prognosis are (1) nonstreptococcal disease, (2) development of heart failure, (3) aortic valve involvement, (4) infection on a prosthetic valve, (5) older age, and (6) valve-ring or myocardial abscess. The cure rate in streptococcal endocarditis is about 90 percent. Failures of therapy are due not to uncontrolled infection but to death from heart failure, embolus, rupture of a mycotic aneurysm, or renal failure. The mortality rate in nonaddicts with *S. aureus* endocarditis is at least 40 percent, and most deaths are due to overwhelming infection or heart failure. In drug addicts with *S. aureus* infection on the tricuspid valve, cure rates are over 90 percent. Results are poor in endocarditis caused by fungi and gram-negative bacilli resistant to penicillins and cephalosporins. Large vegetations (detected by echocardiography) may indicate a poorer prognosis than small or no vegetations. About 10 percent of patients will have additional episodes of endocarditis months or years later. The prognosis in early prosthetic valve endocarditis is much worse than that in late disease, with mortality rates of 40 to 80 percent versus 20 to 40 percent.

ANTIMICROBIAL PROPHYLAXIS OF ENDOCARDITIS

Although the risk of endocarditis is small and there is no proof of the efficacy of preventive therapy, prophylaxis is recommended for patients with predisposing cardiac lesions who are undergoing procedures known to cause bacteremia. The conditions in which prophylaxis is recommended are valvular or congenital heart disease (except uncomplicated atrial septal defect), intracardiac prostheses, asymmetric septal hypertrophy, and previous endocarditis. Mitral valve prolapse is associated with a low to moderate increase in the risk of endocarditis. However, this condition is so common that it is neither risk- nor cost-effective to give prophylaxis to all patients with prolapse for all procedures. It is, however, reasonable to use prophylaxis in individuals with mitral valve prolapse who have mitral regurgitation and who presumably are at greatest risk. Patients who have thickened, redundant mitral valve leaflets on echocardiography also appear to be at high risk.

Oral hygiene must be as good as possible in patients with cardiac lesions that predispose to endocarditis, especially those who are to have prosthetic cardiac valves implanted. For dental and other procedures in the mouth, nose, or throat that are likely to cause bleeding or significant trauma, prophylaxis is aimed at viridans streptococci. The regimen recommended by the American Heart Association is amoxicillin, 3 g orally 1 h before the procedure and 1.5 g 6 h after the initial dose. With penicillin allergy, the recommendation is 800 mg of oral erythromycin ethylsuccinate or 1.0 g of erythromycin stearate 2 h before the procedure or 300 mg of oral clindamycin 1 h before the procedure, in each case followed by half the dose 6 h after the initial dose. In high-risk patients (e.g., those with prosthetic valves), an alternative but optional and more stringent regimen is ampicillin (2 g intramuscularly or intravenously) plus gentamicin (1.5 mg/kg intramuscularly or intravenously)—both 30 min before the procedure—followed by amoxicillin (1.5 g orally) 6 h later or, with penicillin allergy, vancomycin (1 g intravenously) over 1 h starting 1 h before the procedure.

For genitourinary and gastrointestinal tract procedures likely to cause significant trauma (e.g., cystoscopy, prostatic surgery, and colonic or gallbladder surgery), prophylaxis is directed against enterococci. The recommended regimen is ampicillin plus gentamicin followed by amoxicillin, as delineated above. With penicillin allergy, the vancomycin regimen described above is given, but gentamicin at 1.5 mg/kg, given intravenously or intramuscularly, is added 1 h before the procedure. For low-risk patients, amoxicillin (3 g orally) may be used 1 h before the procedure, with 1.5 g administered 6 h later. Fiberoptic endoscopy, even with biopsy, carries such a low risk of endocarditis that prophylaxis is difficult to justify. Prophylaxis should be used only in high-risk patients, if at all.

Prophylaxis for cardiac surgery involving the placement of intracardiac prostheses, patches, or sutures is directed against staphylococci and has usually consisted of 2 g of cefazolin intravenously plus gentamicin at 1.5 mg/kg intravenously starting immediately preoperatively, with repeated doses 8 and 16 h later. However, since hospital strains of *S. epidermidis* and *S. aureus* may be methicillin-resistant, substitution of vancomycin for cefazolin (15 mg/kg intravenously over 1 h, starting 1 h before the procedure; 10 mg/kg after completion of bypass; and then 7.5 mg/kg every 6 h for 3 doses) is reasonable. Vancomycin also can be used when patients are hypersensitive to penicillins and cephalosporins.

Patients with coronary artery bypass grafts or transvenous pacemakers in place do not require prophylaxis for endocarditis, nor do patients undergoing cardiac catheterization.

BIBLIOGRAPHY

BAYER AS: Infective endocarditis. Clin Infect Dis 17:313, 1993

DAJANI AS et al: Prevention of bacterial endocarditis: Recommendations by the American Heart Association. JAMA 264:2919, 1990

DANIEL WG et al: Comparison of transthoracic and transesophageal echocardiography for detection of abnormalities of prosthetic and bioprosthetic valves in the mitral and aortic positions. Am J Cardiol 71:210, 1993

DINUBILE MJ: Short-course antibiotic therapy for right-sided endocarditis caused by *Staphylococcus aureus* in injection drug users. Ann Intern Med 121:873, 1994

DURACK D: Prophylaxis of infective endocarditis, in *Principles and Practice of Infectious Diseases*, 4th ed, GL Mandell et al (eds). New York, Churchill Livingstone, 1995

―――― et al: New criteria for diagnosis of infective endocarditis: Utilization of specific echocardiographic findings. Am J Med 96:200, 1994

FRANCIOLI PB: Ceftriaxone and outpatient treatment of infective endocarditis. Infect Dis Clin North Am 7:97, 1993

HEINLE S et al: Value of transthoracic echocardiography in predicting embolic events in active infective endocarditis. Am J Cardiol 74:799, 1994

KAYE D (ed): *Infective Endocarditis*, 2d ed. New York, Raven Press, 1992

―――― : Treatment of infective endocarditis. Ann Intern Med 124:606, 1996

MULLANY CJ et al: Early and late survival after surgical treatment of culture-positive active endocarditis. Mayo Clin Proc 70:517, 1995

SCHELD M, SANDE M: Endocarditis and intravascular infections, in *Principles and Practice of Infectious Diseases*, 4th ed, GL Mandell et al (eds). New York, Churchill Livingstone, 1995

STECKELBERG JM et al: Emboli in infective endocarditis. The prognostic value of echocardiography. Ann Intern Med 114:635, 1991

STEWART WJ, SHAN K: The diagnosis of prosthetic valve endocarditis by echocardiography. Semin Thorac Cardiovasc Surg 7:7, 1995

THRELKELD M, COBBS G: Infectious disorders of prosthetic valves and intravascular devices, in *Principles and Practice of Infectious Diseases*, 4th ed, GL Mandell et al (eds). New York, Churchill Livingstone, 1995

TUNKEL AR, KAYE D: Neurologic complications of infective endocarditis. Neurol Clin 11:419, 1993

WENDEL GD JR et al: Penicillin allergy and desensitization in serious infections during pregnancy. N Engl J Med 312:1229, 1985

WILSON WR et al: Antibiotic treatment of adults with infective endocarditis due to viridans streptococci, enterococci, staphylococci, and HACEK microorganisms. JAMA 274:1706, 1995

YU VL et al: Prosthetic valve endocarditis: Superiority of surgical valve replacement versus medical therapy only. Ann Thorac Surg 58:1073, 1994

127

Dori F. Zaleznik, Dennis L. Kasper

INTRAABDOMINAL INFECTIONS AND ABSCESSES

Intraperitoneal infections generally arise because a normal anatomic barrier is disrupted. This disruption may occur when the appendix, a diverticulum, or an ulcer ruptures; when the bowel wall is weakened by ischemia, tumor, or inflammation (e.g., in inflammatory bowel disease); or with adjacent inflammatory processes, such as pancreatitis or pelvic inflammatory disease, in which enzymes (in the former case) or organisms (in the latter) may leak into the peritoneal cavity. Whatever the inciting event, once inflammation develops and organisms usually contained within the bowel or another organ enter the normally sterile peritoneal space, a predictable series of events takes place. Intraabdominal infections occur in two stages: peritonitis and—if it goes untreated—abscess formation. The types of microorganisms predominating in each stage of infection are responsible for the pathogenesis of disease.

PERITONITIS

The peritoneal cavity is large but is divided into compartments. The upper and lower peritoneal cavities are divided by the transverse mesocolon; the greater omentum extends from the transverse mesocolon and from the lower pole of the stomach to line the lower peritoneal cavity. The pancreas, duodenum, and ascending and descending colon are located in the anterior retroperitoneal space; the kidneys, ureters, and adrenals are found in the posterior retroperitoneal space. The other organs, including liver, stomach, gallbladder, spleen, jejunum, ileum, transverse and sigmoid colon, cecum, and appendix, are found within the peritoneal cavity itself. Normally the cavity is lined with a serous membrane that can serve as a conduit for fluids—a property utilized in peritoneal dialysis. A small amount of fluid, sufficient to allow movement of organs, is normally present in the peritoneal space. This fluid is serous, with a protein content (consisting mainly of albumin) of <30 g/L and fewer than 300 white blood cells (WBCs, generally mononuclear cells) per microliter. In the presence of infection, some of these compartments collect fluid or pus more often than others. These compartments include the pelvis (the lowest portion), the subphrenic spaces on the right and left sides, and Morrison's pouch, which is a posterosuperior extension of the subhepatic spaces and is the lowest part of the paravertebral groove when a patient is recumbent. The falciform ligament separating the right and left subphrenic spaces appears to act as a barrier to the spread of infection; consequently, it is unusual to find bilateral subphrenic collections.

SPONTANEOUS BACTERIAL PERITONITIS   Peritonitis is either primary (without an apparent source of contamination) or secondary. The types of organisms found and the clinical presentation of these two processes are different. In adults, primary or spontaneous bacterial peritonitis (SBP) occurs most commonly in conjunction with cirrhosis of the liver (frequently the result of alcoholism). Patients with preexisting ascites are predisposed to infection at this site. Nevertheless, it is not a common event, occurring in no more than 10 percent of cirrhotic patients. The cause of SBP has not been established definitively but is believed to involve hematogenous spread of organisms in a patient in whom a diseased liver and altered portal circulation result in a defect in the usual filtration function. Organisms are able to multiply in ascites, a good medium for growth. The proteins of the complement cascade have been found in peritoneal fluid, with lower levels in cirrhotic patients than in patients with ascites of other etiologies. The opsonic and phagocytic properties of neutrophils are decreased in patients with advanced liver disease.

The presentation of SBP differs from that of secondary peritonitis. The most common manifestation is fever, which is reported in as many as 80 percent of patients. Ascites is found but virtually always predates infection. Abdominal pain, an acute onset of symptoms, and peritoneal irritation detected during physical examination can be helpful diagnostically, but the absence of any of these findings does not exclude this often-subtle diagnosis. It is vital to sample the peritoneal fluid of any cirrhotic patient with ascites and fever. The finding of more than 300 polymorphonuclear leukocytes (PMNs) per microliter is diagnostic for SBP, according to Conn. The microbiology of SBP also is distinctive. While enteric gram-negative bacilli such as *Escherichia coli* are the organisms most commonly encountered, gram-positive organisms such as streptococci, enterococci, or even pneumococci are sometimes found. The characteristic microbiologic features of SBP are that generally only a single bacterial species is recovered and anaerobes are found infrequently. This microbiologic picture contrasts with that of secondary peritonitis, in which a mixed flora including anaerobes is the rule. In fact, if SBP is suspected and multiple organisms including anaerobes are recovered from the peritoneal fluid, the diagnosis must be reconsidered and a source of secondary peritonitis sought.

The diagnosis of SBP is not easy. The level of suspicion needs to be high. It may be difficult to recover organisms from cultures of peritoneal fluid, presumably because the burden of organisms is low. The yield can be improved if 10 mL of peritoneal fluid is placed directly into a blood culture bottle. Bacteremia may accompany SBP; therefore, blood should be cultured simultaneously. No specific radiographic studies are helpful in the diagnosis of SBP. A plain film of the abdomen would be expected to show ascites. Chest and abdominal radiography should be performed in patients with abdominal pain to exclude free air, which signals a perforation.

Treatment for SBP is directed at the isolate from blood or peritoneal fluid. Gram's staining of peritoneal fluid often gives negative results in primary peritonitis; therefore, until culture results become available, empirical therapy should cover gram-negative aerobic bacilli and gram-positive cocci. Ampicillin plus gentamicin is a reasonable initial regimen. Third-generation cephalosporins, carbapenems, or broad-spectrum penicillin/β-lactamase inhibitor combinations also are options. Empirical coverage for anaerobes is not necessary. After the infecting organism is identified, therapy should be narrowed to treat that specific pathogen.

SECONDARY PERITONITIS   Secondary peritonitis develops when bacteria contaminate the peritoneum as a result of spillage from a ruptured intraabdominal viscus. The organisms found almost always constitute a mixed flora in which facultative gram-negative bacilli and anaerobes predominate, especially when the contaminating source is colonic. Early in the course of infection, when the host response is directed toward containment of the infection, exudate containing fibrin and PMNs is found. Early death in this setting is attributable to gram-negative bacillary sepsis and to potent endotoxins circulating in the bloodstream (see Chap. 124). Gram-negative bacilli, particularly *E. coli*, are common bloodstream isolates, but *Bacteroides fragilis* bacteremia occurs as well. The severity of abdominal pain and the clinical course depend on the inciting process. The species of organisms isolated from the peritoneum also vary with the source of the initial process and the normal flora present at that site. Peritonitis can result primarily from chemical irritation or bacterial contamination. For example, as long as the patient is not achlorhydric, a ruptured gastric ulcer will release low-pH gastric contents that will serve as a chemical irritant. The normal flora of the stomach comprises the same organisms found in the oropharynx (see Chap. 169) but in lower numbers. The surfaces of teeth contain approximately 10^7 aerobic and 10^7 anaerobic organisms per milliliter of saliva; the normally acidic stomach contains an equal ratio of aerobic and anaerobic species, but in concentrations more in the range of 10^5 per milliliter. After meals, when gastric acidity is highest, this number may fall to 10^3. Thus, the bacterial burden in a ruptured gastric ulcer—or even a duodenal ulcer—is negligible compared with that in a ruptured appendix. The normal flora of the colon below the ligament of Treitz contains about 10^{11} anaerobic organisms per gram of feces but only 10^8 aerobes per gram; therefore, anaerobic species account for 99 percent of the bacteria.

Leakage of colonic contents (pH 7 to 8) does not cause significant chemical peritonitis, but infection is intense because of the heavy bacterial load.

Depending on the inciting event, local symptoms may initially be found in secondary peritonitis—for example, epigastric pain from a ruptured gastric ulcer. In appendicitis (see Chap. 290), the initial presenting symptoms often are vague, with periumbilical discomfort and nausea followed in a number of hours by pain more localized to the right lower quadrant. Unusual locations of the appendix (including a retrocecal position) can complicate this presentation further. Once infection has spread to the peritoneal cavity, however, pain increases, particularly with infection involving the parietal peritoneum, which is innervated extensively. Patients usually lie motionless, often with knees drawn up to avoid stretching the nerve fibers of the peritoneal cavity. Coughing and sneezing, which increase pressure within the peritoneal cavity, are associated with sharp pain. There may or may not be pain localized to the infected or diseased organ from which secondary peritonitis has arisen. Patients with secondary peritonitis generally have abnormal findings on abdominal examination, with marked voluntary and involuntary guarding of the anterior abdominal musculature. Later findings include tenderness, especially rebound tenderness. In addition, there may be localized findings in the area of the inciting event. In general, patients are febrile, with marked leukocytosis and a left shift of the WBCs to earlier granulocyte forms.

While recovery of organisms from peritoneal fluid is easier in secondary than in primary peritonitis, a tap of the abdomen is rarely the procedure of choice in secondary peritonitis. An exception is in cases involving trauma, where the possibility of a hemoperitoneum may need to be excluded early. Treatment for secondary peritonitis includes early administration of antibiotics aimed particularly at aerobic gram-negative bacilli and anaerobes (see below) as well as etiologic studies. Secondary peritonitis usually requires both surgical intervention to address the inciting process and antibiotic administration to treat early bacteremia, to decrease the incidence of abscess formation and wound infection, and to prevent more distant spread of infection. In SBP in adults, surgery is rarely indicated. In secondary peritonitis, surgery may be life-saving.

PERITONITIS IN PATIENTS UNDERGOING CAPD A third type of peritonitis arises in patients who are undergoing continuous ambulatory peritoneal dialysis (CAPD). Unlike primary and secondary peritonitis, which are caused by endogenous bacteria, peritonitis in CAPD patients usually involves skin organisms. The pathogenesis of infection is similar to that of intravascular-device infection, in which skin organisms migrate along the catheter, which both serves as an entry point and exerts the effects of a foreign body. Exit-site or tunnel infection may or may not accompany CAPD peritonitis. Like primary peritonitis, CAPD peritonitis is usually caused by a single organism. Peritonitis is, in fact, the most common reason for discontinuation of CAPD. Improvements in equipment design, especially that of the Y-set connector, have resulted in a decrease from one case of peritonitis per 9 months of CAPD to one case per 15 months.

The clinical presentation of CAPD peritonitis resembles that of secondary peritonitis in that diffuse pain and peritoneal signs are common. The dialysate is usually cloudy and contains more than 100 WBCs per microliter, more than 50 percent of which are neutrophils. The most common etiologic organism is coagulase-negative *Staphylococcus*, which accounts for approximately 30 percent of cases. *Staphylococcus aureus* causes about 10 percent of cases and is more commonly identified among patients who are nasal carriers of the organism. Gram-negative bacilli and fungi such as *Candida* species are also found. The finding of more than one organism in dialysate culture should prompt a search for a cause of secondary peritonitis. As with primary peritonitis, culture of dialysate fluid in blood culture bottles improves the yield.

Empirical treatment is directed at coagulase-negative *Staphylococcus*, *S. aureus*, and gram-negative bacilli; intraperitoneal vancomycin plus gentamicin is a commonly used regimen. Vancomycin, when administered at a dose of 2 g and allowed to remain in the peritoneal cavity for 6 h, produces a reasonable level for 7 days. A loading dose of 70 to 140 mg of gentamicin is followed by maintenance therapy with 20 mg/L for a single daily exchange or with 4 to 8 mg/L per exchange for multiple daily exchanges. The clinical response is rapid; if the patient has not responded after 48 h of treatment, catheter removal should be considered.

INTRAPERITONEAL ABSCESSES

Abscess formation is common in untreated peritonitis if overt gram-negative sepsis either does not develop or develops but is not fatal. In experimental models of abscess formation, mixed aerobic and anaerobic organisms have been implanted intraperitoneally. Without therapy directed at anaerobes, animals develop intraabdominal abscesses. As in humans, these experimental abscesses may stud the peritoneal cavity, lie within the omentum or mesentery, or even develop on the surface of or within viscera such as the liver.

PATHOGENESIS AND IMMUNITY There is often disagreement about whether an abscess represents a disease state or a host response. In a sense, it represents both: While an abscess is an infection in which viable infecting organisms and PMNs are contained in a fibrous capsule, it is also a process by which the host confines microbes to a limited space, thereby preventing further spread of infection. Experimental work has helped to define both the host cells and the bacterial virulence factors responsible—most notably, in the case of *B. fragilis*. This organism, although accounting for only 0.5 percent of the normal colonic flora, is the anaerobe most frequently isolated from intraabdominal infections and is the most common anaerobic bloodstream isolate. On clinical grounds, therefore, *B. fragilis* appears to be uniquely virulent. Moreover, *B. fragilis* causes abscesses in animal models of intraabdominal infection, whereas most other *Bacteroides* species must act synergistically with a facultative organism to induce abscess formation.

Of the several virulence factors identified in *B. fragilis*, one is critical—the capsular polysaccharide complex (CPC) found on the bacterial surface. The CPC comprises two distinct surface polysaccharides, PS A and PS B. Structural analysis of each polysaccharide in the CPC has shown an unusual motif of oppositely charged sugars. Polysaccharides having these zwitterionic characteristics evoke a host response in the peritoneal cavity that localizes bacteria into abscesses. Although abscesses characteristically contain PMNs, the process of abscess induction depends on the stimulation of T lymphocytes by these unique polysaccharides. Animals depleted of CD4+/CD8+ T cells cannot form abscesses. The other host factors that have been found to participate in abscess formation include the alternative pathway of complement and fibrinogen.

While antibodies to the CPC are not critical in immunity to abscesses, they enhance bloodstream clearance of *B. fragilis*. When administered subcutaneously, *B. fragilis* PS A has immunomodulatory characteristics and stimulates T cells to inhibit the host response of abscess formation to intraperitoneal challenge with *B. fragilis*. Treatment of experimental animals with PS A can actually prevent the formation of abscesses, even in the face of provocation by the complete contents of the cecum, with its hundreds of bacterial species.

CLINICAL PRESENTATION Most intraperitoneal abscesses result from SBP due to fecal spillage from a colonic source, such as an inflamed appendix. Of all intraabdominal abscesses, 74 percent are intraperitoneal or retroperitoneal and are not associated with a specific organ. Abscesses also can arise from a number of other processes. They usually form within weeks of the development of peritonitis and may be found in a variety of locations, from omentum to mesentery, pelvis to psoas muscles, and subphrenic space to a visceral organ such as the liver, where they may develop either on the surface of the organ or within it. Infections of the female genital tract and pancreatitis are among the more common causative events. When abscesses occur in the female genital tract—either as a primary infection (e.g., tuboovarian abscess) or as an infection extending into the pelvic cavity or peritoneum—*B. fragilis* figures prominently among the organisms isolated. *B. fragilis* is not found in large numbers in the normal vaginal flora. It is encountered less commonly in pelvic inflammatory disease and endometritis, for example, without an associated abscess. In pancreatitis with leakage of damaging pancreatic enzymes, inflammation is prominent. Therefore, clinical findings such as fever, leukocytosis, and even abdominal pain do not distinguish pancreatitis itself from complications such as pancreatic pseudocyst, pancreatic abscess, or intraabdominal collections of pus. Some authors have advocated early needle aspiration of pancreatic collections under computed tomographic (CT) guidance as a means of distinguishing pseudocysts from abscesses, but this procedure is somewhat hazardous, and the recovery of organisms is not of clear significance.

The psoas muscle of the anterior back is another location in which abscesses are encountered. These abscesses may arise from a presumed hematogenous source, by contiguous spread from an intraabdominal or pelvic process, or by contiguous spread from nearby bony structures such as vertebral bodies. Associated osteomyelitis due to spread from bone to muscle or from muscle to bone is common in psoas abscesses. When Pott's disease was common, *Mycobacterium tuberculosis* was a frequent cause of psoas abscess. Currently in the United States, the usual isolates from psoas abscesses are either *S. aureus* or a mixture of enteric organisms including aerobic gram-negative bacilli. *S. aureus* is most likely to be isolated when a psoas abscess arises from hematogenous spread or a contiguous focus of osteomyelitis; a mixed enteric flora is most likely when the abscess has an intraabdominal or pelvic source.

DIAGNOSIS A variety of scanning procedures have considerably facilitated the diagnosis of intraabdominal abscesses. Abdominal CT scans probably have the highest yield, although ultrasonography is particularly useful for the right upper quadrant, kidneys, and pelvis. Both indium-labeled WBCs and gallium tend to localize in abscesses and may be useful in finding a collection. Since gallium is taken up in the bowel, indium-labeled WBCs may have a slightly greater yield for abscesses near the bowel. Neither indium-labeled WBC nor gallium scans serve as a basis for a definitive diagnosis, however; both need to be followed by other, more specific studies, such as CT, if an area of possible abnormality is identified. Abscesses contiguous with or contained within outpouchings of bowel are particularly difficult to diagnose with scanning procedures. Occasionally, a barium enema may detect a diverticular abscess not diagnosed by other procedures, although barium should not be injected if a free perforation is suspected. If one study is negative, a second study sometimes reveals a collection. On occasion, exploratory laparotomy still must be undertaken if an abscess is strongly suspected on clinical grounds, although this procedure has been less commonly used since the advent of CT.

℞ **TREATMENT**

The treatment of intraabdominal infections involves the determination of the initial focus of infection, the administration of broad-spectrum antibiotics targeted at organisms involved in the associated infection, and the performance of a drainage procedure if one or more definitive abscesses have formed already. It cannot be overemphasized that antimicrobial therapy, in general, is adjunctive to drainage and/or surgical correction of an underlying lesion or process in intraabdominal abscesses. Unlike the intraabdominal abscesses precipitated by most infections, for which drainage of some kind generally is required, abscesses associated with diverticulitis usually wall off locally after rupture of a diverticulum, so that surgical intervention is not routinely required.

A number of antimicrobial agents exhibit excellent activity against aerobic gram-negative bacilli. Since mortality in intraabdominal sepsis is linked to gram-negative bacteremia, empirical therapy for intraabdominal infection always needs to include adequate coverage of gram-negative aerobic and facultative organisms. Aminoglycosides and second- and third-generation cephalosporins are the agents most widely tested and used in intraabdominal processes. Newer antibiotics, such as aztreonam, imipenem, ticarcillin/clavulanic acid, piperacillin/tazobactam, and quinolones (e.g., ciprofloxacin), cover these organisms as well, although at a higher cost. Second-generation cephalosporins, such as cefoxitin or cefotetan, are not as uniformly active as the other agents against all of the aerobic gram-negative species. Aztreonam, ciprofloxacin, aminoglycosides, and most of the third-generation cephalosporins are not active against anaerobes; for the treatment of intraabdominal infections, these drugs need to be used in combination with another antibiotic. Since a number of antibiotics highly effective against anaerobes are available, third-generation cephalosporins generally should not be considered for use against the anaerobic bacteria involved in intraabdominal sepsis.

The most active and cost-effective antibiotic for anaerobic coverage currently is metronidazole (see Chap. 169). Only rare isolates of *B. fragilis* have been reported to be resistant to this drug. In a recent study from 10 geographic locations in the United States over a 5-year period, rates of resistance and susceptibility among *B. fragilis* isolates were analyzed for a number of antibiotics. The three that were most consistently active in vitro were metronidazole, imipenem, and piperacillin/tazobactam, with resistance rates of 0, 0.1, and 0.2 percent, respectively. In contrast, cefoxitin resistance was found in 6 percent of the 2800 isolates tested, and clindamycin resistance in 14 percent. Of the cephamycins, cefoxitin was more active than cefotetan or cefmetazole, with resistance observed in 27 and 20 percent of isolates, respectively. *Bacteroides* species other than *B. fragilis* often are highly resistant to the latter two drugs. Despite increasing reports of in vitro resistance of *B. fragilis* to a number of agents, clinical failures are still limited to case reports; therefore, the clinical significance of antimicrobial resistance in anaerobes is uncertain. One report describes a bloodstream isolate of *B. fragilis* with resistance to metronidazole and with reduced susceptibility to imipenem and amoxicillin/clavulanic acid that became resistant to both of the latter two drugs after treatment of the patient with imipenem. Among newer agents, imipenem, ticarcillin/clavulanic acid, piperacillin/tazobactam, meropenem, and ampicillin/sulbactam are highly active against anaerobes. Chloramphenicol, which exhibits strong activity against *B. fragilis* in vitro, nevertheless should probably not be considered a first-line drug for use against anaerobes, since failures of treatment have been documented in both experimental and clinical intraabdominal infections. Neither metronidazole nor clindamycin covers aerobic gram-negative bacilli; thus, these drugs must be combined with other agents for use in this setting.

VISCERAL ABSCESSES Liver Abscesses The liver is the organ most subject to the development of abscesses. Altemeier and associates studied 540 intraabdominal abscesses over a 12-year period. Of these abscesses 26 percent were visceral. Liver abscesses made up 13 percent of the total number of abscesses, or 48 percent of all visceral abscesses. Liver abscesses may be solitary or multiple; they may arise from hematogenous spread of bacteria or from local spread from contiguous sites of infection within the peritoneal cavity. In the past, appendicitis with rupture and subsequent spread of infection was the most common route for the development of a liver abscess. Currently, associated disease of the biliary tract is most often the etiology. Suppurative pylephlebitis, arising usually from infection in the pelvis but sometimes from infection elsewhere in the peritoneal cavity, is another common source for bacterial seeding of the liver.

Fever is the most common presenting sign of liver abscess. Some patients, particularly those with active associated disease of the biliary tract, have symptoms and signs localized to the right upper quadrant, including pain, guarding, punch tenderness, and even rebound tenderness. Nonspecific symptoms, such as chills, anorexia, weight loss, nausea, and vomiting, also may develop. Only 50 percent of patients with liver abscesses, however, have hepatomegaly, right-upper-quadrant tenderness, or jaundice; thus, half of patients have no symptoms or signs that would direct attention to the liver. Fever of unknown origin (FUO) may be the only presenting manifestation of liver abscess, especially in the elderly. Diagnostic studies of the abdomen, especially the right upper quadrant, should be a part of any FUO workup. The single most reliable laboratory finding is an elevated serum concentration of alkaline phosphatase, which is documented in 90 percent of patients with liver abscesses. Other tests of liver function may yield normal results, but 50 percent of patients have elevated serum levels of bilirubin, and 48 percent have elevated concentrations of aspartate aminotransferase. Other associated laboratory findings include leukocytosis in 77 percent of patients, anemia (usually normochromic, normocytic) in 50 percent, and hypoalbuminemia in 33 percent. Concomitant bacteremia is found in one-third of patients. A liver abscess is sometimes suggested by chest radiography, especially if a new elevation of the right hemidiaphragm is seen; other suggestive findings include a right basilar infiltrate and a right pleural effusion.

Imaging studies are the most reliable methods for diagnosing liver abscesses. These studies include ultrasonography, CT scan, indium-labeled WBC or gallium scans, and even magnetic resonance imaging. In an occasional case, more than one such study may be required. Organisms recovered from liver abscesses vary with the etiology. In liver infection arising from the biliary tree, enteric gram-negative aerobic bacilli and enterococci are common isolates. Unless previous surgery has been performed, anaerobes are not generally involved in liver abscesses arising from biliary infections. In contrast, in liver abscesses arising from pelvic and other intraperitoneal sources, a mixed flora including aerobic and anaerobic species (especially *B. fragilis*) is common. With hematogenous spread of infection, usually only a single organism is encountered; this species may be *S. aureus* or a streptococcal species such as *Streptococcus milleri.*

Liver abscesses also may be caused by *Candida* species; such abscesses usually follow fungemia in patients receiving chemotherapy for cancer and often present as a return of neutrophils after a period of neutropenia. Treatment of candidal liver abscesses usually entails lengthy administration of amphotericin B, although recent reports have described successful maintenance therapy with fluconazole after an initial course of amphotericin (see Chap. 207).

Amebic liver abscesses are not an uncommon problem (see Chap. 215). Amebic serologic testing gives positive results in more than 95 percent of cases; thus, a negative result helps to exclude this diagnosis.

While drainage—either percutaneous (with a pigtail catheter kept in place) or surgical—remains the mainstay of therapy for intraabdominal abscesses (including liver abscesses), there is growing interest in medical management alone for pyogenic liver abscesses. The drugs used in empirical broad-spectrum antibiotic therapy include the same ones used in intraabdominal sepsis. Usually, a diagnostic aspirate of abscess contents should be obtained before the initiation of empirical therapy, and antibiotic choices adjusted when the results of Gram's staining and culture become available. Cases treated without definitive drainage generally require longer courses of antibiotic therapy. When percutaneous drainage was compared with open surgical drainage, the average length of hospital stay for the former was almost twice that for the latter, although both the time required for fever to resolve and mortality were the same for the two procedures. Mortality was appreciable despite treatment, averaging 15 percent. Several factors may predict the failure of percutaneous drainage and therefore may favor primary surgical intervention. These factors include the presence of multiple, sizable abscesses; viscous abscess contents that tend to plug the catheter; associated disease (e.g., disease of the biliary tract) that requires surgery; or the lack of a clinical response to percutaneous drainage in 4 to 7 days.

Splenic Abscesses Splenic abscesses are much less common than liver abscesses. In fact, no splenic abscesses were observed in Altemeier's series of 540 intraabdominal abscesses. The incidence of splenic abscesses has ranged from 0.14 to 0.7 percent in various autopsy series. The clinical setting and the organisms isolated usually differ from those for liver abscesses. The degree of clinical suspicion for splenic abscess needs to be high, as this condition frequently is fatal if left untreated. Even in the most recently published series, diagnosis was made only at autopsy in 37 percent of cases. While splenic abscesses may arise occasionally from contiguous spread of infection or from direct trauma to the spleen, hematogenous spread of infection is the usual mode of development. Bacterial endocarditis is the most common associated infection. Splenic abscesses can develop in patients who have received extensive immunosuppressive therapy (particularly those with malignancy involving the spleen) and in patients with hemoglobinopathies or other hematologic disorders (especially sickle cell anemia).

While approximately 50 percent of patients with splenic abscesses have abdominal pain, the pain is localized to the left upper quadrant in only half of these cases. Splenomegaly is found in approximately 50 percent of patients. Fever and leukocytosis generally are present; the development of fever preceded diagnosis by an average of 20 days in one series. Left-sided chest findings may include abnormalities to auscultation, and chest radiographic findings may include an infiltrate or a left-sided pleural effusion. When splenic abscesses are being considered in a differential diagnosis, CT scan of the abdomen has been the most sensitive diagnostic tool. Ultrasonography can yield the diagnosis, but cases have been missed with this modality. Liver-spleen scan or gallium scan also may be useful. Streptococcal species are the most common bacterial isolates from splenic abscesses, and *S. aureus* is the next most common; presumably these prevalences reflect the bacterial cause of the associated endocarditis. An increase in the frequency of isolation of gram-negative aerobic organisms from splenic abscesses has been reported; these organisms often derive from a urinary tract focus, with associated bacteremia, or from another intraabdominal source. *Salmonella* species are seen fairly commonly, especially in patients with sickle cell hemoglobinopathy. Anaerobic species accounted for only 5 percent of isolates in the largest collected series, but the reporting of a number of "sterile abscesses" may indicate that optimal techniques for the isolation of anaerobes were not employed. Because of the high mortality figures reported for splenic abscesses, the treatment of choice is splenectomy with adjunctive antibiotics. However, percutaneous drainage has been successful. The most important factor in successful treatment of splenic abscesses is early consideration of the diagnosis.

Perinephric and Renal Abscesses Perinephric and renal abscesses are not common: The former accounted for only about 0.02 percent of hospital admissions and the latter for about 0.2 percent in Altemeier's series of 540 intraabdominal abscesses. While liver abscesses generally arise from contiguous foci of infection or track from other intraabdominal sources and splenic abscesses usually arise from hematogenous spread (e.g., spread from bacterial endocarditis), perinephric and renal abscesses have a different pathogenesis. Before antibiotics became available, most renal and perinephric abscesses were hematogenous in origin, with *S. aureus* most commonly recovered. Now, in contrast, more than 75 percent of perinephric and renal abscesses arise from an initial urinary tract infection. Infection ascends from the bladder to the kidney, with pyelonephritis occurring first. Bacteria may directly invade the renal parenchyma from medulla to cortex. Local vascular channels within the kidney may also facilitate the transport of organisms. Areas of abscess developing within the parenchyma may rupture into the perinephric space. The kidneys and adrenal glands are surrounded by a layer of perirenal fat that, in turn, is surrounded by Gerota's fascia, which extends superiorly to the diaphragm and inferiorly to the pelvic fat. When abscesses extend into the perinephric space, tracking may occur through Gerota's fascia into the psoas or transversalis muscles, into the anterior peritoneal cavity, superiorly to the subdiaphragmatic space, or inferiorly to the pelvis. Of the several risk factors that have been associated with the development of perinephric abscesses, the most important is the presence of concomitant nephrolithiasis producing local obstruction to urinary flow. Of patients with perinephric abscess, 20 to 60 percent have renal stones. In addition, other structural abnormalities of the urinary tract, a history of urologic surgery, trauma, and diabetes mellitus all have been identified as risk factors.

The organisms most frequently encountered in perinephric and renal abscesses are *E. coli*, *Proteus* species, and *Klebsiella* species. *E. coli*, the aerobic species most commonly found in colonic flora, seems to have unique virulence properties in the urinary tract, including factors promoting adherence to uroepithelial cells. The urease of *Proteus* species splits urea, thereby creating a more alkaline and hospitable environment for bacterial proliferation. *Proteus* species frequently are found in association with large struvite stones caused by the precipitation of magnesium ammonium sulfate in an alkaline environment. These stones serve as a nidus for recurrent urinary tract infection. While a single bacterial species usually is recovered from a perinephric or renal abscess, multiple species also may be found. If a urine culture is not contaminated with periurethral flora and is found to contain more than one organism, a perinephric abscess or renal abscess should be considered in the differential diagnosis. Urine cultures also may be polymicrobial in cases of bladder diverticulum.

Candida species should be considered in the etiology of renal abscesses. This fungus may spread to the kidney via the hematogenous route or by ascension from the bladder. The hallmark of the latter route of infection is ureteral obstruction with large fungal balls.

The presentation of perinephric and renal abscesses is quite nonspecific. Flank pain and abdominal pain are common. At least 50 percent of patients are febrile. Pain may be referred to the groin or leg, particularly with extension of infection. The diagnosis of perinephric abscess, like that of splenic abscess, is frequently delayed, and mortality in some series is appreciable, although lower than in the past. Perinephric or renal abscess should be most seriously considered when a patient presents with symptoms and signs of pyelonephritis and remains febrile after 4 or 5 days, by which time the fever should have resolved. Moreover, when a urine culture yields a polymicrobial flora, when a patient is known to have renal stone disease, or when fever and pyuria coexist with a sterile urine culture, the diagnosis of perinephric or renal abscess should be entertained.

Renal ultrasonography and abdominal CT scan are the most useful diagnostic modalities. If a renal abscess or perinephric abscess is diagnosed, nephrolithiasis should be excluded, especially when a high urinary pH suggests the presence of a urea-splitting organism. Treatment for perinephric or renal abscesses, like that for other intraabdominal abscesses, includes drainage of pus and antibiotic therapy directed at the organism(s) recovered. For perinephric abscesses, percutaneous drainage usually is successful.

BIBLIOGRAPHY

ALDRIDGE KE et al: A five-year multicenter study of the susceptibility of the *Bacteroides fragilis* group isolates to cephalosporins, cephamycins, penicillins, clindamycin, and metronidazole in the United States. Diagn Microbiol Infect Dis 18:235, 1994

ALTEMEIER WA et al: Intra-abdominal abscesses. Am J Surg 125:70, 1973

CHUN CH et al: Splenic abscess. Medicine 59:50, 1980

FINEGOLD SM: Anaerobic bacteria: General concepts, in *Mandell, Douglas and Bennett's Principles and Practice of Infectious Diseases*, 4th ed, GL Mandell et al (eds). New York, Churchill Livingstone, 1995

HUTCHISON FN, KAYSEN GA: Perinephric abscess: The missed diagnosis. Med Clin North Am 72:993, 1988

LEVISON ME, BUSH LM: Peritonitis and other intra-abdominal infections, in *Mandell, Douglas and Bennett's Principles and Practice of Infectious Diseases*, 4th ed, GL Mandell et al (eds). New York, Churchill Livingstone, 1995

MAHER JA et al: Successful medical treatment of pyogenic liver abscess. Gastroenterology 77:681, 1979

McDOWELL RK, DAWSON SL: Evaluation of the abdomen in sepsis of unknown origin. Radiol Clin North Am 34:177, 1996

SHULER FW et al: Nonoperative management for intra-abdominal abscesses. Am Surg 62:218, 1996

SOLOMKIN JS et al: Results of a randomized trial comparing sequential intravenous/oral treatment with ciprofloxacin plus metronidazole to imipenem/cilastatin for intra-abdominal infections. Ann Surg 223:303, 1996

TURNER et al: Simultaneous resistance to metronidazole, co-amoxiclav, and imipenem in clinical isolates of *Bacteroides fragilis*. Lancet 345:1275, 1995

TZIANABOS AO et al: Structural features of polysaccharides that induce intraabdominal abscesses. Science 262:416, 1993

——— et al: Polysaccharide-mediated protection against abscess formation in experimental intra-abdominal sepsis. J Clin Invest 96:2727, 1995

128

Joan R. Butterton, Stephen B. Calderwood

ACUTE INFECTIOUS DIARRHEAL DISEASES AND BACTERIAL FOOD POISONING

Ranging from mild annoyances during vacations to devastating dehydrating illnesses that can kill within hours, acute gastrointestinal illnesses rank second only to acute upper respiratory illnesses as the most common diseases worldwide. In children less than 5 years old, attack rates range from 2 to 3 illnesses per child per year in developed countries to as high as 10 to 18 illnesses per child per year in developing countries. In Asia, Africa, and Latin America, acute diarrheal illnesses are not only a leading cause of morbidity in children—with an estimated 1 billion cases per year—but also the major cause of mortality, being responsible for 4 to 6 million deaths per year, or a sobering total of 12,600 deaths per day. In some areas, more than 50 percent of deaths of children are directly attributable to acute diarrheal illnesses. In addition, by contributing to malnutrition and thereby reducing resistance to other infectious agents, gastrointestinal illnesses may be indirect factors in a far greater burden of disease.

The wide range of clinical manifestations of acute gastrointestinal illnesses is matched by the wide variety of infectious agents involved, including viruses, bacteria, and parasitic pathogens (Table 128-1). This chapter will discuss factors that enable gastrointestinal pathogens to cause disease, will review host defense mechanisms, and will delineate an approach to the evaluation and treatment of patients presenting with acute diarrhea. Individual organisms causing acute gastrointestinal illnesses are discussed in detail in subsequent chapters.

PATHOGENIC MECHANISMS Enteric pathogens have developed a variety of tactics to overcome host defenses. Understanding the virulence factors employed by these organisms is important in the diagnosis and treatment of clinical disease.

Inoculum Size The number of microorganisms that must be ingested to cause disease varies considerably from species to species. In the case of *Salmonella* or *Vibrio cholerae*, for example, 10^5 to 10^8 organisms must be ingested orally to cause disease, whereas for *Shigella*, *Giardia lamblia*, or *Entamoeba*, as few as 10 to 100 bacteria or cysts can produce infection. The ability of organisms to overcome host defenses has important implications for transmission; *Shigella*, *Entamoeba*, and *Giardia* can spread by person-to-person contact, whereas bacteria such as *Salmonella* may have to grow in food for several hours before reaching an effective infectious dose.

Adherence Many organisms must adhere to the gastrointestinal mucosa as an initial step in the pathogenic process; thus, organisms that can compete with the normal bowel flora and colonize the mucosa have an important advantage in causing disease. Specific cell-surface proteins involved in attachment of bacteria to intestinal cells are important virulence determinants. *V. cholerae*, for example, adheres to the brush border of small-intestinal enterocytes via specific surface adhesins, including the toxin-coregulated pilus and other accessory colonization factors. Enterotoxigenic *Escherichia coli* produces an adherence protein called *colonization factor antigen* that is necessary for colonization of the upper small intestine by the organism prior to the production of enterotoxin. Enteropathogenic and enterohemorrhagic strains of *E. coli* produce virulence determinants that allow these organisms to attach to and efface the brush border of the intestinal epithelium.

Toxin Production The production of one or more exotoxins is important in the pathogenesis of numerous enteric organisms. Such toxins include *enterotoxins*, which cause watery diarrhea by acting directly on secretory mechanisms in the intestinal mucosa; *cytotoxins*, which cause destruction of mucosal cells and associated inflammatory diarrhea; and *neurotoxins*, which act directly on the central or peripheral nervous system. Some exotoxins act by more than one mechanism; *Shigella dysenteriae* type 1, for example, produces an exotoxin that has both enterotoxic and cytotoxic activities.

The prototypical enterotoxin is cholera toxin, a heterodimeric protein composed of one A and five B subunits. The A subunit contains the enzymatic activity of the toxin, while the B subunit pentamer binds holotoxin to the enterocyte surface receptor, the ganglioside G_{M1}. After the binding of holotoxin, a fragment of the A subunit is translocated across the eukaryotic cell membrane into the cytoplasm, where it catalyzes the ADP-ribosylation of a GTP-binding protein and causes persistent activation of adenylate cyclase. The end result is an increase of cyclic AMP in the intestinal mucosa, which increases Cl^- secretion and decreases Na^+ absorption, leading to loss of fluid and the production of diarrhea.

Enterotoxigenic strains of *E. coli* may produce a protein called *heat-labile enterotoxin* (LT) that is similar to cholera toxin and causes secretory diarrhea by the same mechanism. Alternatively, enterotoxigenic strains of *E. coli* may produce *heat-stable enterotoxin* (ST), one form of which causes diarrhea by activation of guanylate cyclase and elevation of intracellular cyclic GMP. Some enterotoxigenic strains produce both LT and ST.

Bacterial cytotoxins, in contrast, destroy intestinal mucosal cells and produce the syndrome of dysentery, with bloody stools containing inflammatory cells. Enteric pathogens that produce such cytotoxins include *S. dysenteriae*, *Vibrio parahaemolyticus*, and *Clostridium difficile*. Enterohemorrhagic strains of *E. coli*, most commonly serotype O157:H7 in the United States, also produce potent cytotoxins that are highly related to Shiga toxin from *S. dysenteriae* and have been termed *Shiga-like toxins*. Such strains of *E. coli* have been associated with outbreaks of hemorrhagic colitis and hemolytic-uremic syndrome.

Neurotoxins usually are produced by the responsible organism outside the host and therefore cause symptoms soon after ingestion. Included are the staphylococcal and *Bacillus cereus* toxins, which act on the central nervous system to produce vomiting.

Invasion   Dysentery may result not only from the production of cytotoxins but also from bacterial invasion and destruction of intestinal mucosal cells. Infections due to *Shigella* and enteroinvasive *E. coli*, for example, are characterized by the organisms' invasion of mucosal epithelial cells, intraepithelial multiplication, and subsequent spread to adjacent cells. *Salmonella*, on the other hand, causes inflammatory diarrhea by invasion of the bowel mucosa but generally is not associated with the destruction of enterocytes or the full clinical syndrome of dysentery. *Salmonella typhi* and *Yersinia enterocolitica* can penetrate intact intestinal mucosa, multiply intracellularly in Peyer's patches and intestinal lymph nodes, and then disseminate through the bloodstream to cause enteric fever, a syndrome characterized by fever, headache, relative bradycardia, abdominal pain, splenomegaly, and leukopenia.

HOST DEFENSES   Given the enormous number of microorganisms ingested with every meal, it is evident that the normal host must possess effective defense mechanisms to combat a constant influx of potential enteric pathogens. Studies of infections in patients with alterations in these defenses have led to a greater understanding of the variety of ways in which the normal host can protect itself against disease.

Normal Flora   The large numbers of bacteria that normally inhabit the intestine act as an important host defense by preventing colonization by potential enteric pathogens. Persons with fewer intestinal bacteria, such as infants who have not yet developed normal enteric colonization or patients receiving antibiotics, are at significantly greater risk of developing infections with enteric pathogens. The composition of the intestinal flora is as important as the number of organisms present. More than 99 percent of the normal colonic flora is made up of anaerobic bacteria, and the acidic pH and volatile fatty acids produced by these organisms appear to be critical elements in the resistance to colonization conferred by the normal enteric flora.

Gastric Acid   The acidic pH of the stomach is an important barrier to enteric pathogens, and an increased frequency of infections

Table 128-1

Gastrointestinal Pathogens Causing Acute Diarrhea

Mechanism	Location	Illness	Stool Findings	Examples of Pathogens Involved
Noninflammatory (enterotoxin)	Proximal small bowel	Watery diarrhea	No fecal leukocytes	*Vibrio cholerae* Enterotoxigenic *Escherichia coli* (LT and/or ST) *Clostridium perfringens* *Bacillus cereus* *Staphylococcus aureus* *Aeromonas hydrophila* *Plesiomonas shigelloides* Rotavirus Norwalk-like viruses Enteric adenoviruses *Giardia lamblia* *Cryptosporidium*
Inflammatory (invasion or cytotoxin)	Colon or distal small bowel	Dysentery or inflammatory diarrhea	Fecal polymorphonuclear leukocytes	*Shigella* spp. *Salmonella* spp. *Campylobacter jejuni* Enterohemorrhagic *E. coli* Enteroinvasive *E. coli* *Yersinia enterocolitica* *Vibrio parahaemolyticus* *Clostridium difficile* ?*Aeromonas hydrophila* ?*Plesiomonas shigelloides* *Entamoeba histolytica*
Penetrating	Distal small bowel	Enteric fever	Fecal mononuclear leukocytes	*Salmonella typhi* *Yersinia enterocolitica*

SOURCE: After Guerrant.

due to *Salmonella, Shigella, G. lamblia,* and a variety of helminths has been reported among patients who have undergone gastric surgery or are achlorhydric for some other reason. Neutralization of gastric acid with antacids or with H$_2$ blockers—common among hospitalized patients—similarly increases the risk of enteric colonization. Some microorganisms, however, can survive the extreme acidity of the gastric environment; rotavirus, for example, is highly stable to acidity.

Intestinal Motility Normal peristalsis is the major mechanism for clearance of bacteria from the proximal small intestine, although gastric acidity and secreted immunoglobulins also play a role in limiting the number of organisms present. When intestinal motility is impaired—for example, by treatment with opiates or other antimotility drugs, anatomic abnormalities (diverticula, fistulas, or afferent-loop stasis following surgery), or hypomotility states (as in diabetes mellitus or scleroderma)—the frequency of bacterial overgrowth and infection of the small bowel with enteric pathogens is much increased. Some patients in whom *Shigella* infection is treated with diphenoxylate hydrochloride with atropine (Lomotil) experience prolonged fever and shedding of organisms, while patients treated with opiates for mild *Salmonella* gastroenteritis have a higher frequency of bacteremia than those not treated with opiates.

Immunity Both cellular immune responses and antibody production play important roles in protecting susceptible hosts from enteric infections. The wide spectrum of viral, bacterial, parasitic, and fungal gastrointestinal infections in patients with AIDS highlights the significance of cell-mediated immunity in protecting the normal host from these pathogens. Humoral immunity is also important and consists of systemic IgG and IgM as well as secretory IgA. Growing evidence supports the concept of a mucosal immune system for secretory IgA in which binding of bacterial antigens to the luminal surface of M cells in the distal small bowel and subsequent presentation of the antigens to subepithelial lymphoid tissue lead to the proliferation of sensitized lymphocytes. These lymphocytes circulate and populate all of the mucosal tissues of the body as IgA-secreting plasma cells.

—————————— *Approach to the Patient* ——————————

The approach to the patient with possible infectious diarrhea or bacterial food poisoning is shown in Fig. 128-1.

History The answers to questions with high discriminating value can quickly narrow the range of potential causes of diarrhea and help determine whether treatment is needed. Important elements of the narrative history are detailed in Fig. 128-1.

Physical Examination The examination of patients for signs of dehydration provides essential information about the severity of the diarrheal illness and the need for rapid therapy. Mild dehydration is indicated by thirst, dry mouth, decreased axillary sweat, decreased urine output, and slight weight loss. Signs of moderate dehydration include an orthostatic fall in blood pressure, skin tenting, and sunken eyes (or, in infants, a sunken fontanelle). Signs of severe dehydration range from hypotension and tachycardia to confusion and frank shock.

Diagnostic Approach After the severity of illness is assessed, the most important distinction that the clinician must make is between *inflammatory* and *noninflammatory* disease. Using the history and epidemiologic features of the case as guides in making this distinction, the clinician can rapidly evaluate the need for further efforts to define a specific etiology and for therapeutic intervention. Examination of a stool sample is an important supplement to the narrative history. Grossly bloody or mucoid stool suggests an inflammatory process, but all stools should be examined for fecal leukocytes; the latter task is accomplished by the preparation of a thin smear of the stool on a glass slide, the addition of a drop of methylene blue, and examination of the wet mount. Causes of acute infectious diarrhea, categorized as inflammatory and noninflammatory, are listed in Table 128-1.

EPIDEMIOLOGY **Travel History** Of the 12 to 20 million people who travel from temperate industrialized countries to tropical regions of Asia, Africa, and Central and South America each year, 20 to 50 percent will experience a sudden onset of abdominal cramps, anorexia, and watery diarrhea; thus *traveler's diarrhea* is the most common travel-related illness (see Chap. 123). The time of onset is usually 3 days to 2 weeks after the traveler's arrival in a tropical area; most cases begin within the first 3 to 5 days. The illness is generally self-limited, lasting 1 to 5 days. The high rate of diarrhea among travelers to underdeveloped areas is related to the ingestion of contaminated food or water.

The organisms that cause traveler's diarrhea vary considerably with location. In all areas, enterotoxigenic *E. coli* is the most common isolate from persons with the classic secretory traveler's diarrhea syndrome; the proportion of cases accounted for by this organism ranges from a high of approximately 50 percent in Latin America to a low of 15 percent in Asia. *Shigella, Salmonella,* and *Campylobacter* spp. are classically considered to cause more invasive dysenteric disease than enterotoxigenic *E. coli,* but clinical differentiation of infections attributable to these organisms can be difficult. *Shigella, Salmonella,* and *Campylobacter* are isolated in 1 to 15 percent of cases, with different organisms being more common in different locations. *Vibrio* species are most common in Asia, although *V. cholerae* disease reached epidemic proportions in parts of Central and South America in 1991 and has become a significant concern to travelers to these regions. Less common bacteria are *Aeromonas hydrophila* and *Plesiomonas shigelloides,* which have been isolated from travelers to Thailand. Parasitic causes of traveler's diarrhea include *Entamoeba histolytica,* which is responsible for up to 5 percent of cases in Mexico and Thailand, and *G. lamblia,* which has been associated with contaminated freshwater supplies in many areas of the world. *Giardia* is found in association with zoonotic reservoirs in the northern United States and poses a risk to hikers and campers who drink from freshwater streams. A striking association of *Giardia* with contaminated water supplies has likewise been noted in St. Petersburg in the former Soviet Union. *Cryptosporidium* has been recognized as a problem in travelers to the Commonwealth of Independent States, Mexico, and Africa and has caused large-scale urban outbreaks of infection in the United States. Viruses such as rotavirus and Norwalk-like viruses have been isolated from up to 12 percent of visitors to Latin America, Asia, and Africa.

Location Day-care centers are sites of particularly high attack rates of enteric infections. Rotavirus is most common among children less than 2 years old, with attack rates of 75 to 100 percent among those exposed. *G. lamblia* is more common among older children, with somewhat lower attack rates. Other common organisms, often spread by fecal-oral contact, are *Shigella, Campylobacter jejuni,* and *Cryptosporidium.* A characteristic feature of infection in day-care centers is the high rate of secondary cases among family members.

Similarly, hospitals are sites for concentrations of enteric infections. In medical intensive-care units and pediatric wards, diarrhea is among the most common nosocomial infections. *C. difficile* and *Salmonella* species are predominant causes of nosocomial diarrhea in the United States; viral pathogens, especially rotavirus, can spread rapidly in pediatric wards. Enteropathogenic *E. coli* has been associated with outbreaks of diarrhea in newborn nurseries. One-third of elderly patients in chronic-care institutions develop a significant diarrheal illness each year. Surveillance stool cultures suggest that 25 percent of the residents of these institutions harbor cytotoxin-producing *C. difficile,* which causes more than half of all cases of diarrhea in this population. Antimicrobial therapy can predispose to pseudomembranous colitis by altering the normal colonic flora and allowing the multiplication of *C. difficile.*

Age Most of the morbidity and mortality from enteric pathogens involves children less than 5 years of age. Breast-fed infants are protected from contaminated food and water and derive some protection from maternal antibodies, but their risk of infection rises dramatically when they begin to eat solid foods. Infants and younger children are more likely than adults to develop rotaviral disease, while older children and adults are more commonly infected with Norwalk-like viruses. Other organisms with higher attack rates among children than among adults include enterotoxigenic and enteropathogenic *E. coli,*

C. jejuni, and *G. lamblia*. In children, the incidence of *Salmonella* infections is highest among infants under 1 year of age, while the attack rate for *Shigella* infections is greatest among children aged 6 months to 4 years.

Bacterial Food Poisoning If the history and the stool examination indicate a noninflammatory etiology of diarrhea and there is evidence of a common-source outbreak, questions concerning the ingestion of specific foods and the time of onset of the diarrhea after a meal can provide clues to the bacterial cause of the illness. Potential causes of bacterial food poisoning are shown in Table 128-2.

Bacterial disease caused by an enterotoxin elaborated outside the host, such as that due to *Staphylococcus aureus* or *B. cereus*, has the shortest incubation period (1 to 6 h) and generally lasts less than 12 h. Most cases of staphylococcal food poisoning are caused by contamination from infected human carriers. Staphylococci can multiply at a wide range of temperatures; thus, if food is left to cool slowly and remains at room temperature after cooking, the organisms will have the opportunity to form enterotoxin. Outbreaks following picnics where potato salad, mayonnaise, and cream pastries have been served offer classic examples of staphylococcal food poisoning. Diarrhea, nausea, vomiting, and abdominal cramping are common, while fever is less so.

B. cereus can produce either a syndrome with a short incubation period—the *emetic* form, mediated by a staphylococcal type of enterotoxin—or one with a longer incubation period (8 to 16 h)—the *diarrheal* form, caused by an *E. coli* LT type of enterotoxin, in which diarrhea and abdominal cramps are characteristic but vomiting is uncommon. The emetic form of *B. cereus* food poisoning is associated with contaminated fried rice; the organism is common in uncooked rice, and its heat-resistant spores survive boiling. If cooked rice is not refrigerated, the spores can germinate and produce toxin. Frying before serving may not destroy the preformed, heat-stable toxin.

Food poisoning due to *Clostridium perfringens* also has a slightly longer incubation period (8 to 14 h) and results from the survival of heat-resistant spores in inadequately cooked meat, poultry, or legumes. After ingestion, toxin is produced in the intestinal tract, causing moderately severe abdominal cramps and diarrhea; vomiting is rare, as is fever. The illness is self-limited, rarely lasting for more than 24 h.

Not all food poisoning has a bacterial cause. Diagnostic confusion can result from diarrhea caused by nonbacterial agents of short-incubation food poisoning, including capsaicin, which is found in hot peppers, and a variety of toxins found in fish and shellfish (Table 128-3).

LABORATORY EVALUATION Many cases of noninflammatory diarrhea are self-limited or can be treated empirically, and in these instances the clinician may not need to determine a specific etiology. Potentially pathogenic *E. coli* cannot be distinguished from normal fecal flora by routine culture. Special tests to detect LT and

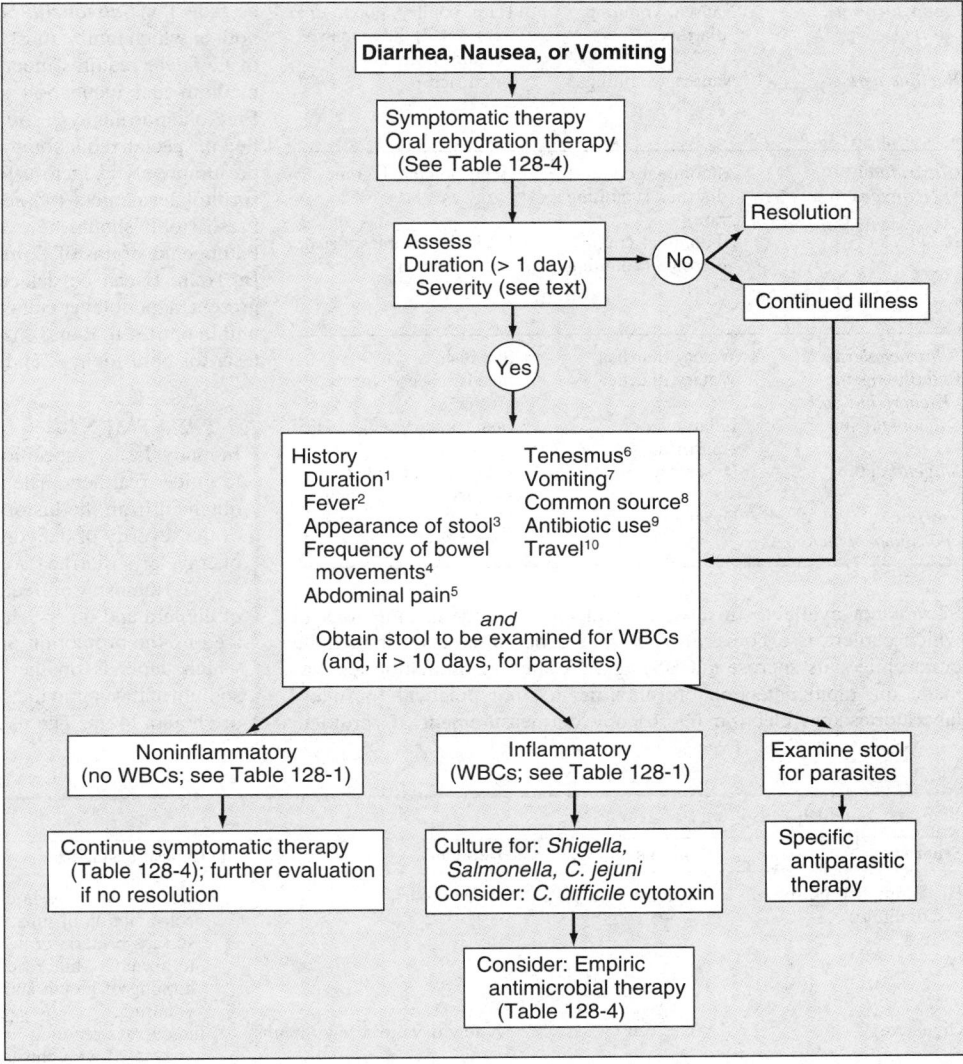

FIGURE 128-1 Clinical algorithm for the approach to patients with possible infectious diarrhea or food poisoning. Key to superscripts: 1. Diarrhea lasting more than 2 weeks generally is defined as chronic; in such cases, many of the causes of acute diarrhea are much less likely, and a new spectrum of causes needs to be considered. 2. Fever often implies invasive disease, although fever and diarrhea also may result from infection outside the gastrointestinal tract, as in malaria. 3. Stools that contain blood or mucus indicate ulceration of the large bowel. Bloody stools without fecal leukocytes should alert the laboratory to the possibility of infection with Shiga-like toxin–producing enterohemorrhagic *Escherichia coli*. Bulky white stools suggest a small intestinal process that is causing malabsorption. Profuse "rice-water" stools suggest cholera or a similar toxigenic process. 4. The number of stools over a given period can be the first warning of impending dehydration. 5. Abdominal pain may be most severe in inflammatory processes like those due to *Shigella, Campylobacter,* and necrotizing toxins. Painful abdominal muscle cramps, caused by electrolyte loss, can develop in severe cases of cholera. Bloating is common in giardiasis. An appendicitis-like syndrome should prompt a culture for *Yersinia enterocolitica* with cold enrichment. 6. Tenesmus (cramps in the rectum felt after a bowel movement) may be a feature of cases with inflammation of the rectum, as in shigellosis. 7. Vomiting implies an acute infection (e.g., a toxin-mediated illness or food poisoning) but can also be prominent in a variety of systemic illnesses (e.g., malaria) and in intestinal obstruction. 8. Asking patients whether anyone else they know is sick is a more efficient means of identifying a common source than is constructing a list of recently eaten foods. If a common source seems likely, specific foods can be investigated. See text for a discussion of bacterial food poisoning. 9. Stop antibiotic treatment if possible and consider culture for cytotoxigenic *Clostridium difficile*. Antibiotic use may increase the risk of other infections, such as salmonellosis. 10. See text for a discussion of traveler's diarrhea. (*After Guerrant and Guerrant and Bobak.*)

Table 128-2

Bacterial Food Poisoning

Organisms	Symptoms	Common Food Sources
1 TO 6 h INCUBATION		
Staphylococcus aureus	Nausea, vomiting, diarrhea	Ham, poultry, potato or egg salad, mayonnaise, cream pastries
Bacillus cereus	Nausea, vomiting, diarrhea	Fried rice
8 TO 16 h INCUBATION		
Clostridium perfringens	Abdominal cramps, diarrhea (vomiting rare)	Beef, poultry, legumes, gravies
B. cereus	Abdominal cramps, diarrhea (vomiting rare)	Meats, vegetables, dried beans, cereals
>16 h INCUBATION		
Vibrio cholerae	Watery diarrhea	Shellfish
Enterotoxigenic Escherichia coli	Watery diarrhea	Salads, cheese, meats, water
Salmonella spp.	Inflammatory diarrhea	Beef, poultry, eggs, dairy products
Shigella spp.	Dysentery	Potato or egg salad, lettuce, raw vegetables
Vibrio parahaemolyticus	Dysentery	Mollusks, crustaceans

ST are not available in most clinical laboratories. In situations in which cholera is a concern, stool should be cultured on thiosulfate citrate bile salts sucrose (TCBS) agar. A latex agglutination test has made the rapid detection of rotavirus in stool practical for many laboratories, but electron microscopy or measurement of serologic response with a radioimmunoassay is still necessary for the identification of Norwalk-like viruses. At least three stool specimens should be examined for *Giardia* cysts or stained for *Cryptosporidium* if the level of clinical suspicion regarding the involvement of these organisms is high.

All patients with fever and evidence of inflammatory disease should have stool cultured for *Salmonella*, *Shigella*, and *Campylobacter*. *Salmonella* and *Shigella* can be selected on MacConkey's agar as non-lactose-fermenting (colorless) colonies or can be grown on *Salmonella-Shigella* agar or in selenite enrichment broth, both of which inhibit most organisms except these pathogens. Isolation of *C. jejuni* requires inoculation of fresh stool onto selective growth medium and incubation at 42°C in a microaerophilic atmosphere. Enterohemorrhagic *E. coli* strains of serotype O157:H7 can be identified in specialized laboratories by serotyping but also can be identified presumptively as lactose-fermenting, indole-positive colonies of non-sorbitol fermenters (white colonies) on sorbitol MacConkey plates. Fresh stools should be examined for amebic cysts and trophozoites. Pathogenic strains of *C. difficile* generally produce two toxins, A and B. Toxin B can be detected with a cytotoxin assay; if the toxin is present, a monolayer culture of fibroblasts will show cytopathic effects within 6 to 24 h. Rapid enzyme immunoassays and latex agglutination tests for both toxin A and toxin B have recently been developed.

℞ TREATMENT

In many cases, a specific diagnosis is not necessary or not available to guide treatment. The clinician can proceed with the information obtained from the history, by stool examination, and by evaluation of the severity of dehydration. Empirical regimens for the treatment of traveler's diarrhea are listed in Table 128-4.

The mainstay of treatment is adequate rehydration. The treatment of cholera and other dehydrating diarrheal diseases was revolutionized by the promotion of oral rehydration solutions, the efficacy of which depends on the fact that glucose-facilitated absorption of sodium and water in the small intestine remains intact in the presence of cholera toxin. The use of oral rehydration solutions has reduced

Table 128-3

Fish and Shellfish Poisoning Syndromes

Syndrome	Incubation Period	Duration	Clinical Features
Histamine fish poisoning (scombroid)	5 min to 1 h	A few hours	Infection develops in coastal states and Hawaii and is associated with consumption of tuna, mackerel, and dolphin. Toxin is formed when surface bacteria grow on flesh, releasing free histidine, which leads to histamine-like reactions, with flushing, headache, dizziness, burning of mouth and throat, palpitations, nausea, diarrhea, and vomiting.
Ciguatera	1 to 6 h	A few days to a few months	Infection is reported in Hawaii, Florida, and the Caribbean and is associated with consumption of carnivorous reef fish such as barracuda and grouper. Toxin is produced by dinoflagellates and acquired by fish through the food chain. Vomiting, watery diarrhea, and cramps develop. Other symptoms include numbness and tingling of the lips and extremities, a reversal of hot and cold sensation, tooth pain, blurred vision, tremor, ataxia, hypotension, and bradycardia.
Paralytic shellfish poisoning	5 min to 4 h	A few hours to a few days	Infection is acquired in temperate coastal areas. Toxin is produced by dinoflagellates and concentrated in bivalve mollusks, often in association with "red tides." Symptoms include paresthesias of the mouth and extremities, headache, ataxia, vertigo, cranial-nerve dysfunction, and muscle paralysis. The case-fatality rate due to respiratory failure is 8 to 9 percent.
Neurotoxic shellfish poisoning	5 min to 4 h	A few hours to a few days	Infection is found in coastal Florida. Toxin is produced by dinoflagellates and concentrated in mollusks. Illness is milder than in paralytic shellfish poisoning, with paresthesias, ataxia, vomiting, and diarrhea but no paralysis.
Tetrodotoxin poisoning	10 min to 3 h	A few days	Infection is acquired in Japan and is caused by a neurotoxin concentrated in the skin and viscera of puffer fish (*Fugu*). Symptoms include lethargy, paresthesias, hyperemesis, salivation, weakness, ataxia, and dysphagia; severe cases may include ascending paralysis, respiratory failure, hypotension, and bradycardia. Mortality is 59 percent.

SOURCE: After Tauxe and Hughes.

Table 128-4

Treatment of Traveler's Diarrhea on the Basis of Clinical Features

Clinical Syndrome	Suggested Therapy
Watery diarrhea (no blood in stool or fever), 1–2 unformed stools per day without distressing enteric symptoms	Oral fluids (Pedialyte, Lytren, or flavored mineral wateR) and saltine crackers
Watery diarrhea (no blood in stool or fever), 1–2 unformed stools per day with distressing enteric symptoms	Bismuth subsalicylate (for adults): 30 mL or 2 tablets (262 mg/tablet) every 30 min for 8 doses; or loperamide*: 4 mg initially followed by 2 mg after passage of each unformed stool, not to exceed 8 tablets (16 mg) per day (prescription dose) or 4 caplets (8 mg) per day (over-the-counter dose); drugs can be taken for 2 days
Watery diarrhea (no blood in stool, distressing abdominal pain, or fever), >2 unformed stools per day	Antibacterial drug† plus (for adults) loperamide* (see dose above)
Dysentery (passage of bloody stools) or fever (>37.8°C)	Antibacterial drug†
Vomiting, minimal dirrhea	Bismuth subsalicylate (for adults; see dose above)
Diarrhea in infants (<2 y old)	Fluids and electrolytes (Pedialyte, Lytren); continue feeding, especially with breast milk; seek medical attention for moderate dehydration, fever lasting >24 h, bloody stools, or diarrhea lasting more than several days
Diarrhea in pregnant women	Fluids and electrolytes; can consider attapulgite, 3 g initially, with dose repeated after passage of each unformed stool or every 2 h (whichever is earlier), for a total dosage of 9 g/d
Diarrhea despite trimethoprim-sulfamethoxazole prophylaxis	Fluoroquinolone—with loperamide (see dose above) if no fever or blood in stool, alone in cases of fever/dysentery
Diarrhea despite fluoroquinolone prophylaxis	Bismuth subsalicylate (see dose above) for mild to moderate disease; consult physician for moderate to severe disease or if disease persists

* Loperamide should not be used by patients with fever or dysentery; its use may prolong diarrhea in patients with infection due to *Shigella* or other invasive organisms.
† The recommended antibacterial drugs are as follows:

Travel to Mexican interior, summer   *Adults:* Trimethoprim-sulfamethoxazole (TMP-SMZ), 160 mg/800 mg bid for 3 days
Children: TMP-SMZ, 4/20 mg/kg/d, given bid for 3 days

Travel to other areas in other seasons   *Adults:* Norfloxacin, 400 mg bid; ciprofloxacin, 500 mg bid; ofloxacin, 300 mg bid; or fleroxacin, 400 mg/d, for 3 days
Children: TMP-SMZ (above dose) plus erythromycin at dose based on weight (<11 kg, 250 mg/d; 11–18 kg, 375 mg/d; 18.5–25 kg, 500 mg/d; 25.5–36 kg, 750 mg/d; and >36 kg, 1000 mg/d) in four divided doses for 5 days; alternative single agent: furazolidone, 7.5 mg/kg/d in four divided doses for 5 days

All patients should take oral fluids (Pedialyte, Lytren, or flavored mineral water) plus saltine crackers. If moderate to severe diarrhea develops, if fever persists, or if bloody stools or dehydration develops, the patient should seek medical attention.

SOURCE: After Dupont.

mortality due to cholera from greater than 50 percent (in untreated cases) to less than 1 percent. The World Health Organization recommends a solution containing 3.5 g of sodium chloride, 2.5 g of sodium bicarbonate, 1.5 g of potassium chloride, and 20 g of glucose (or 40 g of sucrose) per liter of water. Patients who are severely dehydrated or in whom vomiting precludes the use of oral therapy should receive intravenous solutions such as Ringer's lactate.

Although most secretory forms of traveler's diarrhea—usually due to enterotoxigenic *E. coli*—can be treated effectively with rehydration, bismuth subsalicylate, or antiperistaltic agents, antimicrobial agents can shorten the duration of illness from 3 to 4 days to 24 to 36 h.

PROPHYLAXIS Improvements in hygiene to limit fecal-oral spread of enteric pathogens will be necessary if the prevalence of diarrheal diseases is to be significantly reduced in developing countries. Travelers can reduce their risk of diarrhea by eating only hot, freshly cooked food; by avoiding raw vegetables, salads, and unpeeled fruit; and by drinking only boiled or treated water and avoiding ice.

Bismuth subsalicylate is an inexpensive agent for the prophylaxis of traveler's diarrhea; it is taken at a dosage of 2 tablets (525 mg) four times a day. Treatment appears to be effective and safe for up to 3 weeks. Prophylactic antimicrobial agents, although effective, are not generally recommended for the prevention of traveler's diarrhea. The risk of side effects and the possibility of developing an infection with a drug-resistant organism or with more harmful, invasive bacteria make it more reasonable to institute a short course of treatment once symptoms have developed.

The possibility of exerting a major impact on the worldwide morbidity and mortality associated with diarrheal diseases has led to intense efforts to develop effective vaccines against the common bacterial and viral enteric pathogens. Recent research has shown promising advances in the development of vaccines against rotavirus, *Shigella*, *V. cholerae*, *S. typhi*, and enterotoxigenic *E. coli*.

BIBLIOGRAPHY

Advice for travelers. Med Lett Drugs Ther 38:17, 1996
ALTEKRUSE SF, SWERDLOW DL: The changing epidemiology of foodborne diseases. Am J Med Sci 311:23, 1996
DUPONT HL: Travelers' diarrhea, in *Infections of the Gastrointestinal Tract*, MJ Blaser et al (eds). New York, Raven Press, 1995, chap 22
———, ERICSSON CD: Prevention and treatment of traveler's diarrhea. N Engl J Med 328:1821, 1993
EASTAUGH J, SHEPHERD S: Infectious and toxic syndromes from fish and shellfish consumption. Arch Intern Med 149:1735, 1989
GUERRANT RL: Principles and syndromes of enteric infection, in *Mandell, Douglas and Bennett's Principles and Practice of Infectious Diseases*, 4th ed, GL Mandell et al (eds). New York, Churchill Livingstone, 1995, chap 75
———, BOBAK DA: Bacterial and protozoal gastroenteritis. N Engl J Med 325:327, 1991
TAUXE RV, HUGHES JM: Food-borne disease, in *Mandell, Douglas and Bennett's Principles and Practice of Infectious Diseases*, 4th ed, GL Mandell et al (eds). New York, Churchill Livingstone, 1995, chap 81

129   *King K. Holmes, H. Hunter Handsfield*

SEXUALLY TRANSMITTED DISEASES: OVERVIEW AND CLINICAL APPROACH

In all societies, sexually transmitted diseases (STDs) are among the most common of all infections. Moreover, STDs figure prominently among the world's major emerging/reemerging infections. Many new sexually transmitted pathogens have been recognized and characterized since 1980, including human immunodeficiency virus (HIV) types 1 and 2, human T cell lymphotropic virus (HTLV) types I and II, many genotypes of human papillomavirus (HPV), *Mycoplasma genitalium*, two species of *Mobiluncus*, and the Kaposi's sarcoma–associated herpesvirus. Certain well-known STD pathogens, including *Neisseria gonorrhoeae* and *Haemophilus ducreyi*, often lead the way in acquiring resistance to new antimicrobials. In developing countries, such factors as the population explosion (especially in the adolescent and young-adult age groups), rural-to-urban migration, wars, and poverty create steady pressure that favors the emergence of new STDs. In addition, in the developing countries, HIV infection and three bacterial STDs—gonorrhea, chlamydial infection, and syphilis—rank among the top 10 to 20 diseases causing the loss of years of healthy, productive life. Among the viral STDs, infection with HIV has become the leading cause of death in persons 25 to 44 years of age in the United States and in developing countries. Two of the most common sexually transmitted viruses—HPV and hepatitis B virus (HBV)—are important causes of cervical, vaginal, vulvar, and penile carcinomas and of hepatocellular carcinoma, respectively. In industrialized nations, sexually transmitted herpes simplex virus (HSV) infections are the most common cause of genital ulceration that may facilitate HIV transmission, and perinatally transmitted HSV frequently causes serious morbidity among infants. There is also growing evidence of the sexual transmission of HTLV-I in many developing countries of Latin America, Africa, and the Caribbean. Although the bacterial STDs remain extremely common in developing countries, their incidence is now rapidly declining in most industrialized countries. However, rates of gonorrhea, chancroid, and syphilis remain higher in the United States than in any other industrialized country except for Russia and several other eastern European nations that are now experiencing major epidemics of STDs. The Centers for Disease Control and Prevention (CDC) in Atlanta estimates that at least 12 million U.S. residents acquire an STD each year, and some authorities estimate that at least half of all Americans acquire a sexually transmitted infection by age 35. The total annual costs attributable to STDs other than HIV infection for the United States in 1994 have been estimated at $10 billion. In industrialized countries, certain incurable viral STDs [e.g., HPV infection, genital herpes, and cytomegalovirus (CMV) infection] remain very common in all segments of the adult population. The marked enhancement of the efficiency of transmission of HIV by both the genital ulcerative and the genital mucosal STDs adds to the urgency of STD prevention and control.

CLASSIFICATION AND GENERAL APPROACH

STDs can be classified on the basis of either cause or clinical manifestations. Table 129-1 summarizes the etiologic classification of STDs. Several of the pathogens listed are also transmitted nonsexually, but in each instance sexual transmission is clinically and epidemiologically important.

No single STD can be regarded as an isolated problem because multiple infections are common and because the presence of one STD denotes high-risk sexual behavior that is often associated with other, more serious infections. Most STDs are rarely if ever transmitted by fomites, food, flies, or casual contact. *At least one sexual partner is always infected*; the apparent exceptions usually can be attributed to prolonged subclinical infection in one or both partners. Therefore, risk assessment (including elicitation of a sexual history) and management of sexual partners are of paramount importance.

Persons with overt genital discharge, lesions, or pain usually cease sexual activity and seek medical care. Accordingly, those who transmit infection usually are asymptomatic or have mild symptoms and do not seek medical attention spontaneously. Physicians must examine and treat or refer such partners. In the United States, local health departments will usually help to identify and treat or counsel contacts of patients with syphilis, gonorrhea, and (in some jurisdictions) chlamydial or HIV infection; for most STDs, however, this responsibility is shared by the patient and the clinician.

In general, persons with a new-onset STD have a *source contact* from whom it was acquired; in addition, they may have a *secondary contact* (also known as a *spread contact* or *exposed contact*). The identification and treatment of both types of contacts are important but generally for different reasons. Treatment of the source contact (often a casual contact who, by definition, is transmitting infection) benefits the community by preventing further transmission. Treatment of the recently exposed secondary contact (more often a spouse or another steady sexual partner) prevents both the development of serious complications, such as pelvic inflammatory disease (PID), in the partner and reinfection of the index patient.

The increasing importance of the viral STDs, most of which are incurable and lifelong, underscores the central role of preventing infection. Whereas early detection and curative treatment can help curtail the spread of the bacterial STDs, control of the viral STDs depends entirely on the avoidance of unprotected exposure to infected persons the sole exception is vaccination against HBV infection.

STDs disproportionately affect women and newborn children. Many STDs (e.g., genital herpes, gonorrhea, and HIV infection) are transmitted more efficiently from men to women than from women to men. Once infection occurs, many STDs produce complications more often in women than in men, for several reasons. For anatomic or physiologic reasons, for example, women appear to be intrinsically more susceptible to genital cancers complicating HPV infection, to upper genital tract infections, and to puerperal complications. Furthermore, early in the course, women are more likely than men to have subclinical infections or minor, nonspecific symptoms—a situation that can result in delayed diagnosis. The lesser specificity of clinical findings and the lesser sensitivity of several microbiologic tests in women than in men make the diagnosis of STDs more difficult in women. Thus prevention of STDs is a women's health issue. CDC epidemiologists identified 150,737 deaths attributable to STDs in

Table 129-1

Sexually Transmitted Pathogens

Bacteria	Viruses	Other*
TRANSMITTED IN ADULTS PREDOMINANTLY BY SEXUAL INTERCOURSE		
Neisseria gonorrhoeae	Human immunodeficiency virus (types 1 and 2)	*Trichomonas vaginalis*
Chlamydia trachomatis		*Phthirus pubis*
Treponema pallidum	Human T cell lymphotropic virus type I	
Haemophilus ducreyi	Herpes simplex virus type 2	
Calymmatobacterium granulomatis	Human papillomavirus (multiple genotypes)	
Ureaplasma urealyticum	Hepatitis B virus†	
	Cytomegalovirus	
	Molluscum contagiosum virus	
SEXUAL TRANSMISSION REPEATEDLY DESCRIBED BUT NOT WELL DEFINED OR NOT THE PREDOMINANT MODE		
Mycoplasma hominis	Human T cell lymphotropic virus type II	*Candida albicans*
Mycoplasma genitalium	(?) Hepatitis C, D viruses	*Sarcoptes scabiei*
Gardnerella vaginalis and other vaginal bacteria	Herpes simplex virus type 1	
Group B *Streptococcus*	(?) Epstein-Barr virus	
	Kaposi's sarcoma–associated herpesvirus	
TRANSMITTED BY SEXUAL CONTACT INVOLVING ORAL-FECAL EXPOSURE; OF DECLINING IMPORTANCE IN HOMOSEXUAL MEN		
Shigella spp.	Hepatitis A virus	*Giardia lamblia*
Campylobacter spp.		*Entamoeba histolytica*

* Includes protozoa, ectoparasites, and fungi.
† Among U.S. patients for whom a risk factor can be ascertained, most hepatitis B virus infections are sexually transmitted.

U.S. women from 1973 to 1992; 29 percent of these deaths were attributable to HIV, 59 percent to cervical cancer, 11 percent to hepatitis, and the remainder to other STDs. STDs are propagated most efficiently in populations with frequent changes of sexual partners and with poor access to or low motivation in obtaining early treatment. In most of the United States, these groups consist predominantly of young unmarried individuals of low socioeconomic status. These individuals often reside within circumscribed, deteriorating, crowded urban neighborhoods, although rates of STDs are also high in some rural areas (in the southeastern United States, for example). The treatable bacterial STDs, such as syphilis, gonorrhea, and chancroid, are increasingly concentrated in "core populations" and increasingly affect prostitutes and their sexual partners as well as persons involved in the use of illicit drugs, particularly crack cocaine in the United States. Members of these core populations have been difficult to reach for the purposes of education and contact tracing and may continue to be sexually active despite STD symptoms. Other STDs are more evenly distributed in society. For example, in the absence of diagnostic testing and partner treatment, chlamydial infections can persist for many months (often asymptomatically) and can be propagated widely in populations that do not share all of the characteristics of core groups associated with gonorrhea, syphilis, chancroid, or HIV infection. Similarly, genital HPV infection is incurable and therefore persists and spreads efficiently in relatively low-risk populations.

Various STDs differ in the extent to which their spread and persistence in the population depend on high rates of sexual partner change. In general, the initial rate of spread of any STD pathogen within a population depends on the product of three factors: rate of exposure, efficiency of transmission per exposure, and duration of infectivity of those infected. For any given sexually transmitted infection, Anderson and May express this idea as $R_0 = c \times \beta \times D$, where R_0 represents the "reproductive rate" of a pathogen (i.e., the average number of new secondary cases arising from an infected person); c reflects the average rate and variance in the rate of partner change in the population and patterns of partner mixing; β represents the average efficiency of transmission per exposure of a susceptible person to an infected person; and D is the mean duration of infectivity for infected persons. For diseases with a high efficiency of transmission and/or a long duration of infectiousness, rates of partner change need not be very high to sustain an epidemic. For STDs with a low efficiency of transmission (e.g., HIV infection) or a short duration of infectiousness (e.g., chancroid), high rates of partner change may be necessary to sustain an epidemic. Efforts to prevent and control STDs involve attempts to decrease the duration of infectiousness (through early diagnosis and treatment), to decrease the efficiency of transmission (e.g., through promotion of condom use), and to decrease the rate of partner change (e.g., through provision of information, health education, and counseling and efforts to change the norms of sexual behavior).

MANAGEMENT OF COMMON STD SYNDROMES

Table 129-2 lists some of the most common clinical STD syndromes and their associated complications. Strategies for the management of some of the common STD syndromes are outlined below. Infections with human retroviruses are discussed in Chaps. 192 and 308.

An overall approach to the management of a patient with an STD begins with risk assessment (of sexual orientation, number of recent and current sexual partners, sexual practices, recent STD history of the partner, STD history of the patient, and sociodemographic and other markers for high risk) and clinical assessment (elicitation of information on specific current symptoms and signs of STDs). Confirmatory diagnostic tests or screening tests (e.g., culture, antigen detection tests, genetic probe or amplification tests, serologic tests) may then be ordered. In developing countries and in office practices in most industrialized countries, initial treatment is usually syndrome-based and is selected to cover the most likely causes. For certain syndromes in industrialized countries, rapid tests may be used to narrow the spectrum of this initial therapy (e.g., wet mount of vaginal

Table 129-2

Common STD Syndromes and Sexually Transmitted (ST) Etiologic Agents

Syndrome	Primary ST Agents
AIDS	HIV types 1 and 2
Urethritis: males	*Neisseria gonorrhoeae, Chlamydia trachomatis, Ureaplasma urealyticum, Trichomonas vaginalis,* HSV
Epididymitis	*C. trachomatis, N. gonorrhoeae*
Lower genital tract infections: females	
Cystitis/urethritis	*C. trachomatis, N. gonorrhoeae,* HSV
Mucopurulent cervicitis	*C. trachomatis, N. gonorrhoeae*
Vulvovaginitis	*Candida albicans, T. vaginalis*
Bacterial vaginosis (BV)	BV-associated bacteria (see text)
Acute pelvic inflammatory disease	*N. gonorrhoeae, C. trachomatis,* BV-associated bacteria
Infertility	*N. gonorrhoeae, C. trachomatis,* BV-associated bacteria
Ulcerative lesions of the genitalia	HSV-1, HSV-2, *Treponema pallidum, Haemophilus ducreyi, C. trachomatis* (LGV strains), *Calymmatobacterium granulomatis*
Intestinal infections	
Proctitis	*C. trachomatis, N. gonorrhoeae,* HSV, *T. pallidum*
Proctocolitis or enterocolitis	*Campylobacter* spp., *Shigella* spp., *Entamoeba histolytica,* other enteric pathogens
Enteritis	*Giardia lamblia, Cryptosporidium,* Microsporidia
Acute arthritis with urogenital infection or viremia	*N. gonorrhoeae* (e.g., DGI), *C. trachomatis* (e.g., Reiter's syndrome), HBV
Genital and anal warts	HPV (genital types)
Mononucleosis syndrome	CMV, HIV, EBV
Viral hepatitis	HBV, *T. pallidum,* CMV, EBV
Neoplasias	
Squamous cell dysplasias and cancers of the cervix, anus, vulva, vagina, or penis	HPV (especially types 16, 18, 31, 45)
Kaposi's sarcoma (KS), body-cavity lymphomas	KS-associated herpesvirus
T cell leukemia	HTLV-I
Hepatocellular carcinoma	HBV
Tropical spastic paraparesis	HTLV-I
Scabies	*Sarcoptes scabiei*
Pubic lice	*Phthirus pubis*

NOTE: HIV, human immunodeficiency virus; HSV, herpes simplex virus; LGV, lymphogranuloma venereum; DGI, disseminated gonococcal infection; HPV, human papillomavirus; CMV, cytomegalovirus; EBV, Epstein-Barr virus; HBV, hepatitis B virus; HTLV, human T cell lymphotropic virus.

fluid for women with vaginal discharge, Gram's stain of urethral discharge for men with such a discharge). After the institution of syndrome-based treatment or (when rapid tests have been diagnostic) of specific treatment, it is essential to complete the first phase of STD management with proper measures for prevention and control (see below). The following approach to the management of common STD syndromes is geared toward clinicians in industrialized countries, where rapid tests and confirmatory tests are widely available but less widely used than they should be.

URETHRITIS IN MEN   Urethritis is the most commonly recognized STD syndrome in men. During the past decade, the incidence of gonococcal urethritis has fallen precipitously in nearly all industrialized countries, while that of nongonococcal urethritis (NGU) remains high—a pattern suggesting that measures for control of NGU have so far been relatively ineffective. Gonorrhea and NGU occur with similar frequencies among men seen in STD clinics in the United

States, whereas NGU is much more common than gonorrhea among men seen by physicians in most other clinical settings.

About 30 to 40 percent of NGU cases are caused by *Chlamydia trachomatis*, although the proportion of cases due to this organism may have declined in populations where chlamydial control programs have been implemented. HSV and *Trichomonas vaginalis* each cause a small proportion of NGU cases in the United States, but most cases cannot be attributed to any of these three pathogens. *Ureaplasma urealyticum* has been implicated in case-control studies as a probable cause of many *Chlamydia*-negative cases, and *M. genitalium* was found by polymerase chain reaction (PCR) tests of urethral specimens to be associated with NGU in two recent case-control studies. A few cases are caused by coliform bacteria in men who are the insertive partners in unprotected anal intercourse. The initial diagnosis of urethritis in men usually does not include specific tests for pathogens aside from *N. gonorrhoeae* and *C. trachomatis*. The following steps should be taken in evaluating sexually active men with symptoms of urethral discharge and/or dysuria.

1. *Establish the presence of urethritis.* The first step is examination for purulent or mucopurulent urethral discharge. Sometimes the urethra must be milked after the patient has not voided for several hours, preferably overnight. Whether or not an abnormal discharge is evident, inflammation should be evaluated by examination of a Gram-stained smear after passage of a small swab 2 to 3 cm into the urethra; the presence of 5 or more neutrophils per 1000× field in areas containing cells suggests urethritis. Alternatively, the centrifuged sediment of the first 20 to 30 mL of voided urine can be examined for inflammatory cells, either by microscopy or by the leukocyte esterase test. Patients with symptoms who lack objective evidence of urethritis may have functional rather than organic problems and generally do not benefit from repeated courses of antibiotics.

2. *Evaluate for complications or alternative diagnoses.* Epididymitis and systemic complications, such as disseminated gonococcal infection and Reiter's syndrome, should be excluded by a brief history and examination. Bacterial prostatitis and cystitis should be excluded by appropriate testing of men with dysuria who lack evidence of urethritis and of sexually inactive men with urethritis. Digital examination of the prostate gland is seldom informative in the evaluation of sexually active young men with urethritis.

3. *Evaluate for gonococcal and chlamydial infection.* Gonorrhea is diagnosed by the demonstration of typical gram-negative diplococci within neutrophils, and a preliminary diagnosis of NGU is warranted if gram-negative diplococci are not found. However, as the incidence of gonorrhea declines and the infection becomes uncommon in many clinical settings, fewer clinicians and laboratories may have sufficient expertise to rely solely on stained smears for diagnosis or exclusion of gonococcal infection. Therefore, culture or genomic detection tests for *N. gonorrhoeae* and culture, antigen, or genomic detection tests for *C. trachomatis* should be routinely used in most clinical settings. Genetic amplification using ligase chain reaction or PCR appears to be sensitive and highly specific for either organism; such tests are likely to become widely used for screening and perhaps in diagnostic testing for chlamydial infection and gonorrhea. Diagnostic testing for *C. trachomatis* is recommended, even if empirical treatment for chlamydial infection is planned, because the results predict the patient's prognosis and guide the counseling given to the patient and the management of the patient's sexual partner(s).

4. *Treat the urethritis.* In practice, if gonorrhea is excluded by Gram's stain, urethritis is treated with a regimen effective for NGU—e.g., doxycycline (100 mg orally twice daily for 7 days) or azithromycin (1.0 g orally in a single dose). If gonococci are demonstrated by Gram's stain or if no diagnostic tests are performed, treatment should also include one of the single-dose regimens for gonorrhea

(see Chap. 150) plus azithromycin or a 7-day course of doxycycline for possible chlamydial infection. Sexual partners should be tested for gonorrhea and chlamydial infection and should receive the regimen given to the male index case.

EPIDIDYMITIS Acute epididymitis is almost always unilateral and must be differentiated from testicular torsion, tumor, and trauma. Torsion, a surgical emergency, usually occurs in the second or third decade of life and is suggested by a sudden onset of pain, elevation of the testicle within the scrotal sac, rotation of the epididymis from a posterior to an anterior position, and absence of blood flow on Doppler examination or ^{99m}Tc scan. Testicular tumor is suggested by the persistence of symptoms after a course of therapy. In sexually active men under age 35, acute epididymitis is caused most frequently by *C. trachomatis* and less commonly by *N. gonorrhoeae* and is usually associated with overt or subclinical urethritis. Acute epididymitis in older men or following urinary tract instrumentation is usually caused by gram-negative bacilli or other urinary pathogens. Similarly, epididymitis in men who have been the insertive partners in rectal intercourse is often caused by Enterobacteriaceae. Urethritis is usually absent in these cases, but bacteriuria is detected.

Antimicrobial agents are the mainstays of therapy; an optimal agent for syndrome-based treatment of epididymitis is ofloxacin (300 mg orally, twice daily for 10 days), which is effective against both *N. gonorrhoeae* and *C. trachomatis* as well as against Enterobacteriaceae. Alternatively, ceftriaxone (250 mg intramuscularly) followed by doxycycline (100 mg orally, twice daily for 10 days) is effective for epididymitis caused by *N. gonorrhoeae* or *C. trachomatis*.

LOWER GENITOURINARY TRACT INFECTION IN WOMEN Infections of the female lower urinary tract, cervix, vulva, and vagina produce various combinations of dysuria, vulvar irritation, dyspareunia, and increased or altered vaginal discharge. Two steps are required in the evaluation of symptoms of the lower genitourinary tract in women: (1) differentiation among cystitis, urethritis, vulvovaginitis, and cervicitis and (2) exclusion of associated upper tract disease (e.g., pyelonephritis, salpingitis).

Urethritis and the Urethral Syndrome *C. trachomatis*, *N. gonorrhoeae*, and occasionally HSV cause symptomatic urethritis—known as the *urethral syndrome*—characterized by "internal" dysuria (usually without urinary urgency or frequency) and pyuria, with *Escherichia coli* or other uropathogens not present at counts of ≥10^2 per milliliter of urine. In contrast, the dysuria associated with vulvar herpes or vulvovaginal candidiasis (and perhaps with trichomoniasis) is often described as "external," being caused by painful contact of urine with the inflamed labia or introitus.

Among women with acute dysuria and frequency, costovertebral pain and tenderness or fever suggest acute pyelonephritis. The management of bacterial urinary tract infection (UTI) is discussed in Chap. 131. Signs of vulvovaginitis, coupled with symptoms of external dysuria, suggest vulvar or vaginal infection. Among women without signs of vulvovaginitis, bacterial UTI must be differentiated from the urethral syndrome by assessment of risks, evaluation of the pattern of symptoms and signs, and specific microbiologic testing. An STD etiology is suggested by young age, more than one current sexual partner or a new partner within the past month, or coexisting mucopurulent cervicitis (see below). Bacterial cystitis is suggested by acute onset, association with urinary urgency or frequency, hematuria, or suprapubic bladder tenderness. The finding of a single conventional urinary pathogen, such as *E. coli* or *Staphylococcus saprophyticus*, in a concentration of ≥10^2/mL in a properly collected specimen of midstream urine from a symptomatic woman with pyuria indicates probable bacterial UTI, whereas pyuria with <10^2 conventional uropathogens per milliliter of urine ("sterile" pyuria) suggests acute urethral syndrome due to *C. trachomatis* or *N. gonorrhoeae*. Gonorrhea and chlamydial infection should be evaluated by cervical culture or other specific tests. Among women with "sterile" pyuria caused by chlamydial infection, treatment with doxycycline (100 mg twice daily for 7 days) alleviates dysuria.

Vulvovaginal Infections Vulvovaginal symptoms rank among the most common reasons for visits to physicians by young women.

Further, certain vulvovaginal infections may have serious sequelae, and trichomoniasis and vulvovaginal candidiasis may increase the rate of sexual transmission of HIV. Vaginal trichomoniasis and bacterial vaginosis early in pregnancy are independent predictors of premature onset of labor. Bacterial vaginosis also appears to be a risk factor for anaerobic bacterial infection of the upper genital tract. Vaginitis may be an early and prominent feature of toxic shock syndrome, and recurrent or chronic vulvovaginal candidiasis develops with increased frequency among women with systemic illnesses, such as diabetes mellitus or HIV infection with impaired immunity (although only a very small proportion of women with recurrent vulvovaginal candidiasis in the United States actually have a serious predisposing illness). Vaginal discharge may be the presenting manifestation of genital herpes and occasionally reflects mucopurulent cervicitis or PID caused by gonorrhea or chlamydial infection.

Thus vulvovaginal symptoms or signs warrant careful evaluation and appropriate therapy that is specific for the anatomic site and type of infection. A careful pelvic examination should usually precede more invasive or expensive tests in the evaluation of women with vulvovaginal, pelvic, or abdominal symptoms.

Bacterial vaginosis is the most common cause of vulvovaginal symptoms in most clinical settings; it is closely followed in frequency by vulvovaginal candidiasis. Trichomoniasis is much less common in most settings in developed countries. Vaginal infection may be characterized by one or more of the following: increased volume of discharge; abnormal yellow color of discharge caused by increased concentration of polymorphonuclear leukocytes; vulvar pruritus, irritation, or burning, often with external dysuria; vulvar dyspareunia; and vaginal malodor. An important component of the clinical evaluation of vaginal discharge is ascertaining by speculum examination whether this discharge emanates from the vagina or the cervix and whether it is objectively abnormal. The diagnosis and treatment of the three common types of vaginal infection are summarized in Table 129-3. A DNA probe test for the detection of *T. vaginalis*, *Candida albicans*, and the increased vaginal concentrations of *Gardnerella vaginalis* found in bacterial vaginosis is now commercially available but has not been extensively evaluated. The general approach to the management of these conditions is outlined below.

Vaginal trichomoniasis (See also Chap. 220) *T. vaginalis* is sexually transmitted. Although many infected women and most infected men are asymptomatic, treatment of asymptomatic as well as symptomatic cases reduces rates of transmission and prevents later development of symptoms.

Table 129-3

Diagnostic Features and Management of Vaginal Infection

Feature	Normal Vaginal Examination	Vulvovaginal Candidiasis	Trichomonal Vaginitis	Bacterial Vaginosis
Etiology	Uninfected; lactobacilli predominant	*Candida albicans*	*Trichomonas vaginalis*	Associated with *Gardnerella vaginalis*, various anaerobic bacteria, and mycoplasmas
Typical symptoms	None	Vulvar itching and/or irritation	Profuse purulent discharge; vulvar itching	Malodorous, slightly increased discharge
Discharge				
Amount	Variable; usually scant	Scant	Profuse	Moderate
Color*	Clear or white	White	Yellow	White or gray
Consistency	Nonhomogeneous, floccular	Clumped; adherent plaques	Homogeneous	Homogeneous, low viscosity; uniformly coats vaginal walls
Inflammation of vulvar or vaginal epithelium	None	Erythema of vaginal epithelium, introitus; vulvar dermatitis common	Erythema of vaginal and vulvar epithelium; colpitis macularis	None
pH of vaginal fluid†	Usually ≤4.5	Usually ≤4.5	Usually ≥5.0	Usually >4.5
Amine ("fishy") odor with 10% KOH	None	None	May be present	Present
Microscopy‡	Normal epithelial cells; lactobacilli predominant	Leukocytes, epithelial cells; mycelia or pseudomycelia in up to 80% of *C. albicans* culture-positive persons with typical symptoms	Leukocytes; motile trichomonads seen in 80% to 90% of symptomatic patients, less often in the absence of symptoms	Clue cells; few leukocytes; lactobacilli outnumbered by profuse mixed flora, nearly always including *G. vaginalis* plus anaerobic species on Gram's stain
Usual treatment	None	Miconazole or clotrimazole intravaginally, 100 mg nightly for 3 to 7 nights Fluconazole, 150 mg orally (single dose)	Metronidazole, 2 g orally (single dose) Metronidazole, 500 mg orally, twice daily for 7 days	Metronidazole, 500 mg orally, twice daily for 7 days Clindamycin, 2% vaginal cream, each night for 7 days Metronidazole, 0.75% vaginal gel, twice daily for 5 days Metronidazole, 2 g orally (single dose)§
Usual management of sexual partner	None	None; topical treatment if candidal dermatitis of penis is detected	Examination for STD; treatment with metronidazole, 2 g orally (single dose)	Examination for STD; no treatment if normal

* Color of discharge is best determined by examination against the white background of a swab.
† pH determination is not useful if blood is present.
‡ To detect fungal elements, vaginal fluid is digested with 10% KOH prior to microscopic examination; to examine for other features, fluid is mixed (1:1) with physiologic saline. Gram's stain is also excellent for detecting yeasts and pseudomycelia and for distinguishing normal flora from the mixed flora seen in bacterial vaginosis, but it is less sensitive than the saline preparation for detection of *T. vaginalis*.
§ Single-dose regimen is less effective than 7-day metronidazole regimen.

Symptomatic trichomoniasis characteristically produces a profuse, yellow, purulent, homogeneous vaginal discharge and vulvar irritation. The vaginal and vulvar epithelium may be visibly inflamed, and colposcopy reveals petechial lesions on the cervix ("strawberry cervix") in about 50 percent of cases. The pH of vaginal fluid is usually 5.0 or greater. In women with typical symptoms and signs of trichomoniasis, microscopic examination of vaginal discharge mixed with saline usually reveals motile trichomonads and polymorphonuclear leukocytes. In such cases, wet-mount examination is at least 80 percent as sensitive as culture. However, in women without symptoms or signs, culture is often required for detection of the organism. In men, the diagnosis of *T. vaginalis* infection requires culture of early-morning first-voided urine sediment or of a urethral swab specimen obtained before voiding. Methods of identifying *T. vaginalis* by immunofluorescence or by use of oligonucleotide probes are under investigation and may prove diagnostically helpful for cases in both men and women.

Only nitroimidazoles consistently cure trichomoniasis. A single 2.0-g oral dose of metronidazole is the treatment of choice and is as effective as more prolonged regimens. Other nitroimidazoles such as tinidazole and ornidazole have longer half-lives than metronidazole but do not clearly give better results in trichomoniasis. Routine treatment of sexual partners reduces both the risk of reinfection and the reservoir of infection. Vaginal treatment with 0.75% metronidazole gel, although effective for bacterial vaginosis (see below), is not highly effective for vaginal trichomoniasis. Metronidazole is not recommended during the first trimester of pregnancy but is considered safe thereafter. Alcohol must be avoided for 24 h after its use because of occasional disulfiram-like effects. When practical, the partners of patients with trichomoniasis (or with any sexually transmitted infection, for that matter) should be seen in person, examined, and counseled, but it is common practice to dispense metronidazole to the male partner via the infected female patient.

Bacterial vaginosis Vaginal discharge not associated with *T. vaginalis*, yeast, or cervical infection is usually due to bacterial vaginosis. This syndrome (formerly termed *nonspecific vaginitis*, *anaerobic vaginitis*, or *Gardnerella-associated vaginal discharge*) is characterized by vaginal malodor and a slightly to moderately increased white discharge that is homogeneous, is low in viscosity, and smoothly coats the vaginal mucosa. The syndrome is associated with STD risk factors, such as multiple sexual partners and recent intercourse with a new partner, but no single sexually transmitted pathogen has been clearly implicated as the cause, and antibiotic treatment of male partners so far has not reduced the rate of recurrence among affected women. Formerly considered a benign condition, bacterial vaginosis has been implicated as a risk factor for acute salpingitis, premature labor, and related neonatal and perinatal complications.

The prevalence and concentrations of *G. vaginalis*, *Mycoplasma hominis*, and several anaerobic bacteria [e.g., *Mobiluncus* spp., *Prevotella* spp. (formerly *Bacteroides* spp.), and some *Peptostreptococcus* spp.] are markedly greater in vaginal fluid of women with bacterial vaginosis than in that of women without this syndrome. However, none of these organisms is found only among women with bacterial vaginosis, and *G. vaginalis* has been isolated in low concentrations from the vagina of up to 50 percent of healthy women. Hydrogen peroxide–producing *Lactobacillus* spp., which constitute most of the normal vaginal flora, are usually absent from the vagina in bacterial vaginosis. This situation may permit overgrowth of the vagina by anaerobic bacteria, *M. hominis*, and *G. vaginalis*. Vaginal douching, use of intravaginal nonoxynol-9 spermicide, and new sexual partners are associated with loss of vaginal colonization by hydrogen peroxide–producing lactobacilli.

Bacterial vaginosis is conventionally diagnosed by demonstration of any three of the following four abnormalities:

1. *Objective signs of increased white homogeneous vaginal discharge and exclusion of candidal and trichomonal vaginitis and*

mucopurulent cervicitis. This process must include the collection of endocervical specimens to be tested for *C. trachomatis* and *N. gonorrhoeae.*

2. *Liberation of a distinct fishy odor immediately after mixing of vaginal secretions with a 10% solution of KOH.* This odor is attributable to volatile amines (e.g., trimethylamine, putrescine, and cadaverine) resulting from anaerobic bacterial metabolism in the vaginal fluid.

3. *A vaginal discharge pH of >4.5.* The elevated pH may be partly due to the presence of amines as well as to the decreased production of lactate. (Testing of cervical secretions, which typically have a pH of about 7.0, should be avoided.)

4. *Microscopic demonstration of "clue cells."* Clue cells are vaginal epithelial cells coated with coccobacillary organisms. On a wet mount prepared by mixing of vaginal secretions with normal saline in a ratio of approximately 1:1, clue cells have a granular appearance and indistinct borders (Fig. 129-1). Alternatively, the laboratory diagnosis of bacterial vaginosis can be based upon the detection of clue cells in a Gram-stained smear of vaginal discharge. The normally predominant lactobacilli (large, gram-positive rods) are mostly or completely replaced by a profusion of bacterial morphotypes consistent with *G. vaginalis* and anaerobic organisms. The demonstration of many clue cells by wet-mount microscopy and the documentation of a characteristically altered vaginal flora by Gram's stain are the most sensitive, specific, and objective criteria for the diagnosis of bacterial vaginosis in women with symptoms and/or signs of this condition.

Attempts to isolate *G. vaginalis*, genital mycoplasmas, or anaerobic bacteria are of little use in the diagnosis of bacterial vaginosis because these organisms are components of the vaginal flora in many women without the syndrome.

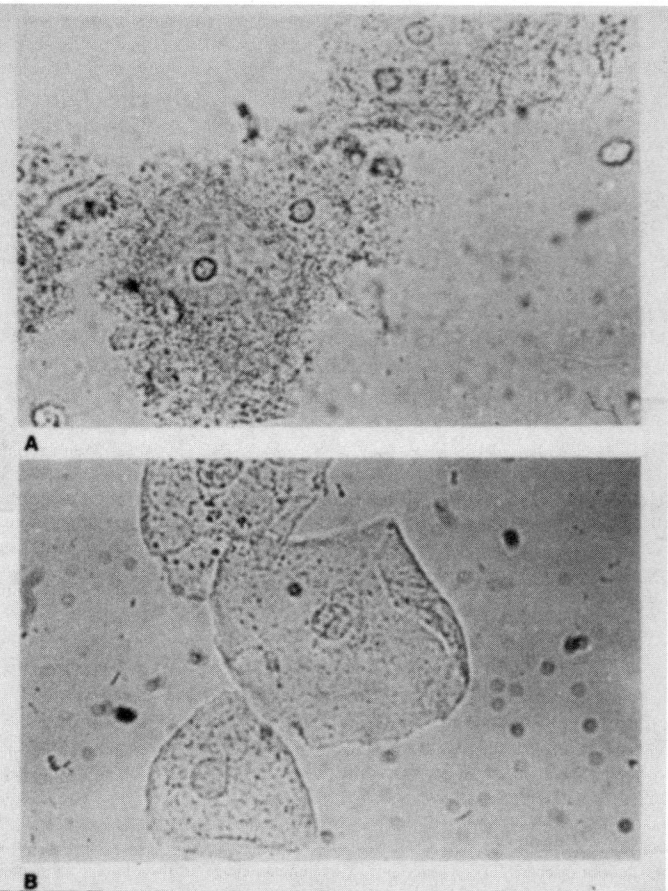

FIGURE 129-1 *A.* Vaginal epithelial "clue cells." Note granular appearance due to adherent *G. vaginalis* and indistinct cell margins (400×). *B.* Normal vaginal epithelial cells. The cell margins are distinct and lack granularity.

The standard regimen for the treatment of bacterial vaginosis has been metronidazole (500 mg orally, twice daily for 7 days). Clindamycin (300 mg orally, twice daily for 7 days) is also effective but not preferred. Intravaginal treatment with 2% clindamycin cream [one applicator full (5 g containing 100 mg of clindamycin phosphate) each night for 7 nights] or 0.75% metronidazole gel [one applicator full (5 g containing 37.5 mg of metronidazole) twice daily for 5 days] is also effective and does not elicit systemic adverse reactions. A single 2-g oral dose of metronidazole can also be used but produces short-term recurrence rates somewhat higher than those obtained with the 7-day metronidazole regimen. Long-term recurrence (i.e., after several months) is distressingly common, and its frequency is not reduced by treatment of male partners with metronidazole. Nonetheless, a new sexual partner has been implicated as a risk factor for recurrence.

No controlled data support the use of vaginal or oral preparations of *Lactobacillus* spp. in the treatment or prevention of recurrence of bacterial vaginosis. However, few if any of the available commercial preparations of lactobacilli contain hydrogen peroxide–producing vaginal strains that adhere to vaginal epithelium. Since adherence may be required for successful colonization, studies with such isolates will be of interest.

Vulvovaginal candidiasis The predominant symptom in vulvovaginal candidiasis is vulvar pruritus or irritation. There is usually no distinct odor, and symptoms of vaginal discharge are not characteristic. Signs of vulvar erythema, edema, and fissures are common. The vaginal discharge typically is white and scant and sometimes takes the form of white thrushlike plaques or cottage cheese–like curds adhering loosely to the vaginal mucosa. *C. albicans* accounts for at least 80 percent of yeasts isolated from the vagina, while *Torulopsis glabrata* and less commonly encountered *Candida* spp. are found in the remainder. Most cases of vulvovaginal candidiasis probably arise from endogenous strains of *C. albicans* that have colonized the vagina or the intestinal tract. Some men whose partners have vulvovaginal candidiasis develop symptomatic candidal dermatitis of the penis.

The diagnosis of vulvovaginal candidiasis involves the demonstration of fungi by microscopic examination of vaginal fluid in saline or 10% KOH or by Gram's stain. Demonstration of pseudohyphae or hyphae strengthens the diagnosis of vaginitis due to *C. albicans*. Polymorphonuclear leukocytes usually are present. Microscopic examination is less sensitive than culture but correlates better with symptoms. Culture does identify *C. albicans* in some women with symptoms and signs of vulvovaginal candidiasis in conjunction with negative results upon microscopic examination but also commonly detects coincidental colonization in women without such symptoms or signs. The pH of vaginal secretions is usually ≤4.5, and no amine odor is produced when vaginal secretions are mixed with 10% KOH. The superficial vulvar erosions or fissures of vulvovaginal candidiasis must be differentiated from the manifestations of genital herpes and other causes of genital ulcer.

In most circumstances, therapy for candidal vaginal infection is indicated only if the patient is symptomatic or has signs of vulvovaginitis. The usual treatment is intravaginal administration of any of several imidazole antibiotics (e.g., miconazole or clotrimazole) for 3 to 7 days. Over-the-counter marketing of such preparations has reduced the cost of care and made treatment more convenient for many women with recurrent yeast vulvovaginitis. However, the symptoms of this condition are nonspecific, and self-treatment of presumed vulvovaginal candidiasis may delay detection and treatment of more serious infections. Therefore, self-treatment should be strictly limited to women with classic symptoms of vulvar pruritus in whom previous episodes of yeast vulvovaginitis have been documented by an experienced clinician. Single-dose oral treatment with fluconazole (150 mg) is also effective and is preferred by many patients. Prolonged or periodic oral therapy with fluconazole or ketoconazole may be indicated for especially severe or frequently recurrent cases or for those that do not respond to intravaginal or single-dose oral therapy. Such patients probably should be evaluated for diabetes or HIV infection, although such systemic illnesses are uncommon explanations for recurrent vulvovaginal candidiasis. Treatment of sexual partners is not routinely indicated.

Mucopurulent Cervicitis *Mucopurulent cervicitis* refers to inflammation of the columnar epithelium and subepithelium of the endocervix and of any contiguous columnar epithelium that lies exposed in an ectopic position on the exocervix. Mucopurulent cervicitis in women is the "silent partner" of urethritis in men, being equally common and caused by the same agents but more difficult to recognize. It is the most common major STD syndrome in women, can be a harbinger or sign of PID, and—in pregnant women—can lead to obstetric complications. Mucopurulent cervicitis is caused most commonly by *C. trachomatis* and sometimes by *N. gonorrhoeae*; the relative proportions of cases due to these two organisms depend on their prevalence in the community. In the United States, however, at least half of all cases are associated with neither of these organisms and currently remain idiopathic. The syndrome usually can be differentiated clinically from cervicitis caused by HSV, which produces ulcerative lesions on the stratified squamous epithelium of the exocervix as well as on the columnar epithelium.

The diagnosis is based on the detection of yellow mucopurulent discharge from the cervical os or of increased numbers of polymorphonuclear leukocytes in Gram-stained or Papanicolaou smears of endocervical mucus. Edematous cervical ectopy (see below) and endocervical bleeding induced by gentle swabbing are also common signs of mucopurulent cervicitis due to *C. trachomatis*. The color of cervical mucus on a white swab removed from the endocervix should be noted; a yellow color indicates the presence of polymorphonuclear leukocytes. The mucus should be rolled *thinly* on a slide for Gram's staining. The presence of 20 to 30 or more polymorphonuclear cells per $1000\times$ microscopic field within strands of cervical mucus not contaminated by vaginal squamous epithelial cells or vaginal bacteria suggests cervicitis. When carefully collected endocervical specimens are examined by experienced personnel, Gram's staining of endocervical mucus is also an insensitive but fairly specific test for gonorrhea; intracellular gram-negative diplococci indicate gonococcal infection. Culture or other specific and sensitive tests for *N. gonorrhoeae* and *C. trachomatis* are also indicated.

Treatment usually should be administered when the clinical diagnosis is made—i.e., before the etiology is known. In settings where both gonorrhea and chlamydial infection are common, therapy should include a single-dose regimen effective for gonorrhea, such as cefixime (400 mg orally), followed by doxycycline (100 mg orally, twice daily for 1 week) or by azithromycin (1.0 g orally in a single dose). In settings where gonorrhea is much less common than chlamydial infection, initial therapy for mucopurulent cervicitis may cover chlamydial infection only (e.g., a regimen of azithromycin or doxycycline). The sexual partner(s) of a woman with mucopurulent cervicitis should be examined and given a regimen similar to that chosen for the woman unless results of tests for gonorrhea or chlamydial infection in either partner warrant a change in therapy.

Cervical Ectopy Cervicitis must be differentiated from *cervical ectopy*, which is often mislabeled "cervical erosion." Ectopy represents the presence of the one-cell-thick columnar epithelium extending from the endocervix out onto the visible ectocervix. In ectopy, the cervical os may contain clear or slightly cloudy mucus but usually does not contain yellow mucopus. Colposcopy shows that the epithelium is intact and not ulcerated. Ectopy is normally found during early adolescence and gradually recedes as squamous metaplasia replaces the ectopic columnar epithelium. Oral contraceptive use favors the persistence or reappearance of ectopy. Cauterization for the elimination of ectopy is not warranted. Ectopy may make the cervix more susceptible to infection with *N. gonorrhoeae* or *C. trachomatis* by exposing a larger area of susceptible columnar epithelium. Moreover, ectopy appears to enhance susceptibility to HIV infection. If mucopurulent cervicitis supervenes, the area of ectopy becomes edematous and fragile. Edema may result in eversion of the os, with enlargement of the apparent area of ectopy.

PELVIC INFLAMMATORY DISEASE The term *PID* refers to various combinations of endometritis, salpingitis, and pelvic peritonitis resulting from ascending genital infection, which usually arises from gonococcal or chlamydial mucopurulent cervicitis and/or from bacterial vaginosis. PID predominantly affects sexually active adolescents and young women, in whom at least 90 percent of cases are sexually acquired. Although sometimes clinically severe, with overt pelvic peritonitis or tuboovarian abscess (especially, it now appears, among women with HIV infection), most cases of acute PID are relatively mild or even subclinical. However, even subclinical PID can result in significant tubal damage, as evidenced by the frequent lack of history of clinically diagnosed PID in *Chlamydia*-seropositive women with tubal infertility or ectopic pregnancy. Accordingly, the clinician must not be slow to consider PID in the differential diagnosis of mild or even trivial abdominal pain in young women. This approach represents a shift in thinking from the days when PID was considered likely only in women with severe adnexal tenderness plus an elevation in temperature, white blood cell count, or erythrocyte sedimentation rate.

The proportion of cases of PID caused by *N. gonorrhoeae* recently has declined in most industrialized countries, a trend reflecting the declining incidence of gonococcal infections in general. *C. trachomatis* remains a common cause of PID in many settings. However, in geographic areas and health maintenance organizations that have implemented widespread screening of sexually active young women for chlamydial infection, the incidence of chlamydial PID has declined. Numerous other pathogens contribute to PID, including *M. hominis* and various anaerobic members of the vaginal flora found in bacterial vaginosis. PID occurs with increased frequency for a short period after insertion of an intrauterine contraceptive device, and endometritis can result from induced abortion or from childbirth (especially after cesarean section). Vaginal douching has been found to be an important risk factor for ascending pelvic infection, perhaps because the practice depletes hydrogen peroxide–producing *Lactobacillus* spp. Clinicians should not prescribe douching (which has not been demonstrated to be effective for treatment or prevention of any condition) and should strongly discourage douching for genital hygiene. PID is discussed in detail in Chap. 130.

ULCERATIVE LESIONS OF THE GENITALIA The etiology of genital ulcer disease has not been systematically studied in industrialized countries for more than 20 years except in recent outbreaks involving syphilis and chancroid in New Orleans, Louisiana, and Jackson, Mississippi. Table 129-4 approximates the differential diagnosis in patients attending STD clinics and, by extension, in young, sexually active persons in other clinical settings.

The incidence and etiology of ulcerative lesions of the genitalia vary greatly in different areas of the world. In Asia and Africa, genital

Table 129-4

Etiologies of Genital Ulcer Disease in Industrialized and Tropical Developing Countries

| | Percent of Cases | |
Diagnosis	Industrialized Countries	Tropical Developing Countries
Genital herpes	50–70	10–30*
Syphilis	10–20	10–30
Chancroid	0–10†	50–60
Lymphogranuloma venereum	<1	0–5
Donovanosis	<1	<1‡
Other/unknown	5–20	5–30

* The proportion of genital ulcers caused by HSV appears to be increasing as the prevalence of HIV infection increases in developing countries.
† The proportion is highly variable, depending on time, place, and population group. Chancroid may account for more than 25% of cases in STD clinic populations in selected U.S. cities during chancroid outbreaks.
‡ Donovanosis accounts for higher proportions of cases in some geographic areas (e.g., southern Africa, western Australia, Papua New Guinea, and the Indian subcontinent) than in others.

ulcers are seen as frequently as gonorrhea in some STD clinics; chancroid is the most common cause. Genital herpes was considered relatively uncommon until serologic studies and PCR testing of genital ulcers showed it to be common, especially among persons infected with HIV. In industrialized western countries, genital ulcers are considerably less common than urethritis, mucopurulent cervicitis, and vaginitis; genital herpes is the most common cause, and chancroid is relatively uncommon. Syphilis is the second most common form of genital ulcer in most areas of the world, and the possibility of syphilis must always be excluded. Lymphogranuloma venereum (LGV) and donovanosis (granuloma inguinale) are very rare in North America and Europe, although an unusual outbreak of LGV occurred in the Bahamas during the 1980s in association with crack cocaine use and epidemic HIV infection. Other causes of genital ulcer include candidiasis and traumatized genital warts, both of which usually are readily recognized. Trauma per se is an uncommon cause of genital ulcer unless there is a clear history of definite injury accompanied by bleeding. The differential diagnosis of genital ulceration is broad, and other conditions are more common in older patients, those at low risk for STDs, and those who present with lesions due to genital involvement of more widespread dermatoses, such as genital mucosal ulceration in Stevens-Johnson syndrome.

Chancroid, syphilis, genital herpes, and probably all causes of genital ulcer enhance the efficiency of sexual transmission and acquisition of HIV. Moreover, genital ulcers, especially those of chancroid and syphilis, are most common in sexually active inner-city populations with low socioeconomic status and high rates of prostitution and illicit drug use—independent risk factors for HIV infection. In the late 1980s in the United States, chancroid and syphilis spread at epidemic rates in such populations, although these rates declined rapidly from 1990 through 1995.

In industrialized countries, the differential diagnosis of genital ulceration in young, sexually active patients usually includes genital herpes, syphilis, and chancroid; together, these infections probably account for more than 90 percent of cases in which discrete genital ulcers are present in patients without generalized dermatoses. The clinical findings are occasionally definitive (e.g., the presence of herpetic vesicles), and clinical findings plus epidemiologic considerations can usually guide initial therapy pending the results of further studies. Nevertheless, most genital ulcerations cannot be diagnosed confidently on clinical grounds. It is axiomatic to exclude syphilis in all cases. Although syphilis serology should be routine, about one-quarter of patients with primary syphilis have not yet seroconverted when they first present for medical attention. All lesions except those highly characteristic of infection with HSV should therefore be subjected to dark-field examination or a direct immunofluorescence test for *Treponema pallidum*. Selective enrichment media are available for isolation of *H. ducreyi*. Use of simultaneous multiple PCR tests (e.g., for HSV, *T. pallidum*, and *H. ducreyi*) has proven valuable in recent studies of genital ulcer, identifying an etiologic agent in up to 95 percent of cases. Such tests are not yet commercially available.

The following general guidelines are recommended for management of ulcerative genital lesions.

Lesions Typical of Genital Herpes A clinical diagnosis of genital herpes is warranted if typical vesicles or pustules are evident or if there is a cluster of painful ulcers that was preceded by vesiculopustular lesions. These clinical presentations are sufficiently typical that confirmation of the diagnosis by isolation of HSV or immunochemical detection of the virus is optional. A serologic test for syphilis should be performed not only for diagnostic purposes but also because screening is indicated in all patients with a newly diagnosed STD.

All Other Acute Genital Ulcers The appearance of genital herpetic lesions is highly variable, and—except in the relatively clear-cut cases described above—a specific test for HSV is required to establish a diagnosis. "Nonspecific" or clinically trivial ulcers may be more common manifestations of genital herpes than classic vesiculopustular lesions. Isolation of HSV by culture, immunochemical identification of antigens, or detection of genetic material should be attempted. Culture or direct immunofluorescence tests allow typing of

HSV if it is detected, while enzyme-linked immunosorbent assays currently do not. Type-specific serologic tests are available for research and are now being developed to aid in the identification of HSV-2-seronegative persons who might benefit from future vaccines. However, commercially available serologic tests do not distinguish between antibodies to the two types of HSV and are of little use (see Chap. 184). Cytologic methods (Tzanck preparation with Wright-Giemsa or Papanicolaou staining) for the detection of HSV-infected multinucleated cells are insensitive except in the presence of intact vesicles and are seldom useful in diagnosing genital ulcer disease.

An attempt should be made to isolate *H. ducreyi* if the genital ulcer is painful and is not typical of herpes, especially when inguinal lymphadenopathy with fluctuance or overlying erythema is noted; if chancroid is prevalent in the community; if the patient is at high risk for chancroid (e.g., through the use of injection drugs or crack cocaine or through prostitution); or if the patient has recently had a sexual exposure in a chancroid-endemic area (e.g., a developing country or certain North American cities). Enlarged, fluctuant lymph nodes should be aspirated for culture and Gram's staining to detect *H. ducreyi* and pyogenic bacteria. A diagnosis of syphilis should be excluded by dark-field examination and serologic testing, and the latter should be repeated 1 to 2 weeks later if the results are initially negative and if another diagnosis cannot be established.

Lesions Typical of Syphilis   If lesions are at all suggestive of syphilis (e.g., painless, nontender, indurated); if there is firm, nontender inguinal adenopathy; or if there are epidemiologic reasons to suspect syphilis (e.g., recent exposure), dark-field examination and a rapid serologic test for syphilis should be performed. If the results are negative and the patient is reliable in terms of follow-up and sexual abstinence, two more dark-field examinations should be conducted on successive days before treatment is attempted, and the serologic test should be repeated 1, 2, and 6 weeks later. Direct immunofluorescence staining of *T. pallidum* is quite reliable and should be used if dark-field examination by experienced examiners is impossible.

Chronic Genital Ulceration   When genital ulcers persist beyond the usual course of herpes (2 to 3 weeks) or chancroid or syphilis (up to 6 weeks) and do not resolve with syndrome-based antimicrobial therapy, then—in addition to the usual tests for herpes, syphilis, and chancroid—biopsy is indicated to exclude donovanosis, carcinoma, and other nonvenereal dermatoses. A test for HIV infection should be done, since chronic, persistent genital herpes is common in HIV infection with immunosuppression.

Treatment of Genital Ulcers   Ideally, treatment for genital ulceration should be withheld until the diagnosis is secure. However, immediate syndrome-based treatment for acute genital ulcerations (after collection of all necessary diagnostic specimens) is sometimes necessary—e.g., when it is believed that a patient may not return for follow-up or may continue to be sexually active. Initial treatment in such cases should generally include 2.4 million units of benzathine penicillin G for possible primary syphilis. Immediate empirical therapy for chancroid also is indicated if the patient has been exposed in an area where chancroid is endemic and especially if regional lymph node suppuration is evident or appears imminent. Prompt systemic therapy with acyclovir is indicated for patients with initial episodes of genital or anorectal herpes (see Chap. 184). Finally, empirical antimicrobial therapy may be indicated if ulcers persist and the diagnosis remains unclear after 1 to 2 weeks of observation and repeated attempts to diagnose herpes, syphilis, and chancroid.

Candidate vaccines against HSV-2 are undergoing clinical trials; one candidate subunit vaccine recently appeared to be ineffective in preventing HSV-2 infection. If any vaccine proves effective in preventing genital herpes, potential target populations for HSV-2 immunization include the uninfected partners of persons with genital herpes and perhaps all young persons before the onset of sexual activity. Candidate vaccines are also being investigated for their efficacy in moderating the course of recurrent genital herpes.

PROCTITIS, PROCTOCOLITIS, ENTEROCOLITIS, AND ENTERITIS   Sexually acquired proctitis, or inflammation limited to the rectal mucosa, results from direct rectal inoculation of typical STD pathogens. In contrast, inflammation extending from the rectum to the colon (proctocolitis), involving both the small and the large bowel (enterocolitis), or involving the small bowel alone (enteritis) can result from ingestion of typical intestinal pathogens through oral-fecal exposure during sexual contact. Anorectal pain and mucopurulent, bloody rectal discharge suggest proctitis or proctocolitis. Proctitis is commonly associated with tenesmus (causing frequent attempts to defecate, but not true diarrhea) and constipation, whereas proctocolitis and enterocolitis are more often associated with true diarrhea. In all three conditions, anoscopy usually shows mucosal exudate and easily induced mucosal bleeding (i.e., a positive "wipe test"), sometimes with petechiae or mucosal ulcers. Exudate should be sampled for microbiologic studies and Gram's staining. Sigmoidoscopy or colonoscopy shows inflammation limited to the rectum (in proctitis) or disease extending at least into the sigmoid colon (in proctocolitis).

Most cases of sexually transmitted intestinal infection in the past have involved homosexual men. During the AIDS era, however, there has been an extraordinary shift in the clinical and etiologic spectrum of intestinal infections among homosexual men. The number of AIDS-related opportunistic intestinal infections has risen rapidly; most such infections are associated with chronic rather than acute intestinal symptoms. At the same time, the number of cases of the usually more acute sexually transmitted intestinal infections described below has fallen rapidly as high-risk sexual behaviors have become less common in this group.

Most infectious proctitis is due to the acquisition of *N. gonorrhoeae*, HSV, or *C. trachomatis* during receptive anorectal intercourse. Primary and secondary syphilis also can produce anal or anorectal lesions, with or without symptoms. Proctitis due to *N. gonorrhoeae* or to common strains of *C. trachomatis* typically involves the most distal rectal mucosa and the anal crypts and is clinically mild, without systemic manifestations. In contrast, primary proctitis due to HSV and proctocolitis due to the strains of *C. trachomatis* that cause LGV usually produce severe anorectal pain and often cause fever. Perianal ulcers and inguinal lymphadenopathy, most commonly due to HSV, also can occur in LGV or syphilis. Sacral nerve root radiculopathies, usually presenting as urinary retention, laxity of the anal sphincter, or constipation, are common in primary herpetic proctitis. In LGV, biopsy typically shows crypt abscesses, granulomas, and giant cells—findings resembling those in Crohn's disease. Syphilis also can produce rectal granulomas, usually in association with infiltration by plasma cells or other mononuclear cells.

Diarrhea and abdominal bloating or cramping pain without anorectal symptoms and with normal findings on anoscopy and sigmoidoscopy occurs with inflammation of the small intestine (enteritis) or with proximal colitis. In homosexual men without HIV infection, enteritis is often attributable to *Giardia lamblia*. Sexually acquired proctocolitis is most often due to *Campylobacter* spp., *Shigella* spp., or *Entamoeba histolytica*.

ACUTE ARTHRITIS   The gonococcal arthritis-dermatitis syndrome and Reiter's syndrome are among the most common forms of acute arthritis in sexually active young adults. These two syndromes must be differentiated from each other, from other forms of infective arthritis, from various diseases associated with immune-complex deposition, from crystal-induced arthritis, from acute rheumatoid arthritis, and from other, less common rheumatic disorders, such as systemic lupus erythematosus. Meningococcemia, infection with *Yersinia*, sarcoidosis, and syphilis are other occasional causes of acute arthritis in young adults.

Demonstration of *N. gonorrhoeae* by culture or by a specific immunochemical method in synovial fluid, blood, skin lesions, or cerebrospinal fluid is diagnostic of disseminated gonococcal infection (DGI). Even when such tests fail to detect the organism, gonococcal arthritis is highly probable if *N. gonorrhoeae* is recovered from a mucosal site of infection or from the patient's sexual partner in the presence of typical pustular or hemorrhagic skin lesions distributed primarily on the extremities. Suspected and confirmed cases of DGI should be treated promptly with an antibiotic effective against antibiotic-sensitive and antibiotic-resistant gonococci, such as ceftriaxone (see Chap. 150).

Reiter's syndrome occurs in a sporadic (apparently sexually transmitted) form that usually follows chlamydial infection and in a postdysenteric form that usually follows infection with *Yersinia*, *Campylobacter*, or *Shigella* spp. Discrete epidemics of the latter form are sometimes documented (see Chap. 317).

HUMAN PAPILLOMAVIRUS INFECTION AND GENITAL WARTS Genital warts and infection with HPV were long considered inconvenient but benign conditions. Most genital warts are caused by HPV types 6 and 11, which are rarely if ever associated with invasive cancers. However, evolving evidence implicates some strains of HPV—e.g., types 16, 18, 31, 33, 35, 39, 45, 52, 55, 56, and 58—in the development of moderate to severe squamous dysplasia and of overt cancer of the cervix, anus, vulva, vagina, and penis. Accordingly, HPV infection is now recognized as one of the most important STDs. The number of visits to clinicians because of genital warts has been estimated at more than 1.2 million each year in the United States. However, most HPV infections are subclinical, and increasingly sensitive tools for the detection of HPV (e.g., PCR) show that most sexually active young men and women seen at STD clinics have genital HPV infection, usually without visible clinical abnormalities. A recent study of university women followed from their initial sexual intercourse through their first two or three sexual partners suggested that about half became infected with HPV, many with oncogenic HPV types. Genital HPV infection was five times as common as all other sexually transmitted infections combined in this population.

Treatment of symptomatic external genital warts usually consists of provider-administered cryotherapy or podophyllin resin (10 to 25 percent resin in tincture of benzoin) or of patient-administered podophyllotoxin (podophylox), which is available as a 0.5 percent solution or gel. In special circumstances, surgery is used (e.g., scissor excision, electrodesiccation, laser vaporization). However, surgery does not cure subclinical infection of adjacent tissues. Thus the primary goal of treatment of genital warts is cosmetic, and therapy should be conservative. Although genital warts are no more predictive than other STDs of severe cervical dysplasia (since the types of HPV that commonly cause genital warts are not the types that cause severe dysplasia or invasive cancer), women with any STD should undergo routine cervical cytologic screening. These conditions are addressed further in Chap. 190.

HEPATITIS B VIRUS INFECTION Sexually transmitted HBV infection (Chap. 295) was an extremely common problem among homosexual and bisexual men until the mid-1980s, and sexual contact among men continues to account for 5 to 10 percent of adult HBV infections in the United States. About 25 percent of cases of hepatitis B in U.S. adults currently are attributed to heterosexual transmission and 30 percent to sharing of injection equipment by illicit drug users. The route of acquisition is unknown in 35 to 40 percent of cases, but the age distribution and other behavioral characteristics are consistent with sexual acquisition. Hepatitis B is the only STD for which an effective vaccine is available, and current recommendations in the United States include not only universal vaccination of infants but also targeted vaccination of adolescents in high-risk communities, people with multiple sexual partners or other STDs, sexual partners of individuals with acute hepatitis B, and seronegative sexual partners of chronic carriers of the hepatitis B surface antigen.

CYTOMEGALOVIRUS CMV is carried in blood and shed in semen and cervical secretions; it can be transmitted through sexual and perinatal exposure. Sexual contact is the most important mode of transmission of CMV between adults in many settings in industrialized countries. Among initially seronegative women attending STD clinics, the annual incidence of seroconversion is 8 to 30 percent. CMV (Chap. 187) is among the most common causes of congenital neurodevelop-mental abnormalities and of life-threatening morbidity in patients with advanced cellular immunodeficiency due to HIV, malignancy, or chemotherapy. Until an effective vaccine is developed, the prevention of sexually transmitted CMV infection will be problematic.

HUMAN T-CELL LYMPHOTROPIC VIRUS HTLV-I is transmitted perinatally, especially through breast feeding, and parenterally, especially through blood transfusions; it is also endemic as a sexually transmitted virus in parts of the Caribbean, Latin America, Asia, and Africa. HTLV-I (Chap. 192) is associated with T cell leukemia and tropical spastic paresis (HTLV-I–associated myelopathy), although only the latter has been seen after adult acquisition. HTLV-II is found in up to 15 to 20 percent of injection drug users in the United States, in whom it appears to be parenterally transmitted, and is also found in some Native American tribes. The clinical consequences of infection with HTLV-II have yet to be defined. Small case-control studies have implicated other sexually transmitted infections as possible risk factors for sexual acquisition of HTLV-I and HTLV-II.

KAPOSI'S SARCOMA–ASSOCIATED HERPESVIRUS (See Chap. 187) Early in the AIDS era, epidemiologic studies suggested that Kaposi's sarcoma in HIV-infected persons was due to a separate sexually transmissible agent. More recently, DNA sequences consistent with a previously unrecognized gamma herpes-group virus were identified in Kaposi's sarcoma lesions of homosexually active men with AIDS. This Kaposi's sarcoma–associated herpesvirus has since been associated with body-cavity lymphomas and Castleman's disease in preliminary studies. Rapid progress in cultivation and characterization of this virus and future development of specific serologic tests will eventually elucidate the epidemiologic features of the agent and will help to define whether and how it is involved in the pathogenesis of Kaposi's sarcoma and other conditions.

PREVENTION AND CONTROL OF STDs

Although rates of all curable STDs have been falling in the United States during the 1990s, all other industrialized countries of comparable economic development have made greater progress. For example, Sweden has virtually eliminated the transmission of gonorrhea, syphilis, and chancroid and has achieved very low rates of HIV transmission. Elimination of syphilis as an endemic disease might also be a plausible intermediate-term objective in the United States, but much stronger efforts toward prevention and control of all STDs are necessary.

Prevention and control of STDs rest on the reduction of the average risk of sexual exposure through (1) reduction of the average rate of partner change in all population groups; (2) reduction of the efficiency of transmission by promoting safer sexual practices, use of condoms during casual or commercial sex, hepatitis B immunization, and many other approaches; and (3) shortening of the duration of infectivity of STDs through early detection and curative or suppressive treatment.

Many barriers stand in the way of each of these three approaches. For example, sex education of children and young adults is hindered by the taboo surrounding the discussion of sexuality in the United States. Opposition to use of schools and the media as vehicles for sex education contrasts with frequent use of the media for the promulgation of explicit sexual messages in programs and advertising.

Clinicians have traditionally focused on early detection and treatment of curable STDs to reduce the duration of infectivity. They generally have relatively little training or experience in or time for counseling on risk reduction, treatment of sexual contacts, or condom promotion. Certain constraints imposed on time and finances by managed-care practice patterns may further curtail prevention efforts. Even the efforts of clinicians simply to detect and treat STDs are severely limited at several steps, as outlined in Fig. 129-2. As implied by this figure, improved detection and treatment of STDs depend in part on societal efforts to teach young people how to recognize symptoms of STDs; to motivate those with symptoms to seek care promptly; and to make such care accessible, affordable, and acceptable, especially to the young indigent patients most likely to acquire an STD. Clinicians must develop and maintain their skills in recognition of symptoms and signs of STDs and in treatment. The primary care clinician is

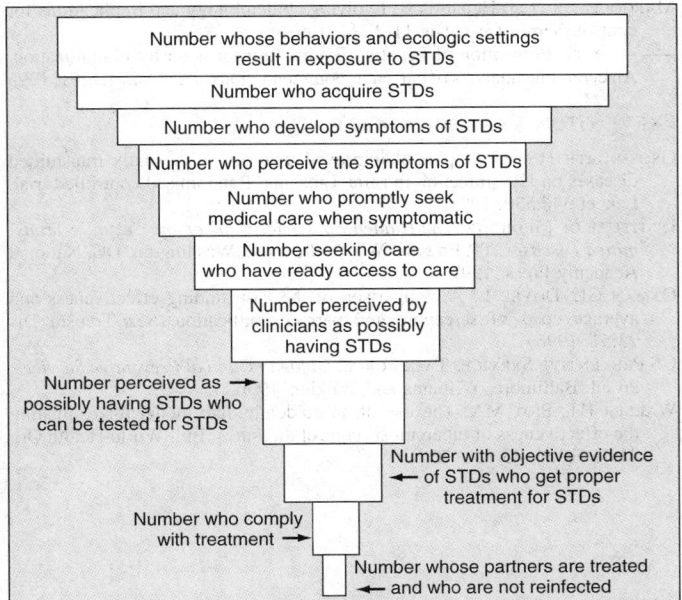

| Number whose behaviors and ecologic settings result in exposure to STDs |
| Number who acquire STDs |
| Number who develop symptoms of STDs |
| Number who perceive the symptoms of STDs |
| Number who promptly seek medical care when symptomatic |
| Number seeking care who have ready access to care |
| Number perceived by clinicians as possibly having STDs |

Number perceived as → possibly having STDs who can be tested for STDs

Number with objective evidence ← of STDs who get proper treatment for STDs

Number who comply with treatment →

Number whose partners are treated ← and who are not reinfected

FIGURE 129-2 Schematic representation of the levels of potential breakdown in the steps required for preventing and controlling STDs. Each level represents an important point for public health or clinical intervention. *(Adapted from Waller and Piot and from "Resource allocation model for public health planning—a case study of tuberculosis control," a supplement to volume 84 of the Bulletin of the World Health Organization, 1973.)*

also responsible for "the 4 Cs" of STD case management: ensuring *c*ompliance with therapy, arranging treatment of *c*ontacts, promoting the use of *c*ondoms, and *c*ounseling on risk reduction. Further, given that many infected individuals develop no symptoms or fail to recognize and report symptoms, clinicians should routinely perform an STD risk assessment for teenagers and young adults and should use the information obtained to selectively screen for STDs, to interpret symptoms and signs, and to identify individuals in need of counseling.

Screening tests for gonorrhea, chlamydial infection, and HIV as well as cervical cytology should be used in populations at risk in the United States according to the U.S. Preventive Services Task Force Guidelines. With few exceptions, sexually active females from 14 to 20 years of age should be tested for *C. trachomatis* whenever they present for health care (at least once a year), regardless of whether their sexual behavior appears to place them at risk; older women should be tested if they have more than one sexual partner, if they have begun a new sexual relationship since the previous test, or if they have another STD diagnosed. In other countries and in a few locations in the United States, widespread selective screening of young women for cervical *C. trachomatis* infection has been associated with a 50 to 60 percent drop in the prevalence of chlamydial infection; as noted above, such screening protects the individual woman from PID. Sexually active young men also can be screened for urethral *C. trachomatis* infection. Although definitive selective screening criteria have not yet been published, sensitive urine-based genetic amplification tests permit expansion of screening to men and teenage boys and to women in settings where a pelvic examination is not planned or is impractical.

Although gonorrhea is substantially less common than chlamydial infection, some persons should still be screened routinely, including women and teenage girls attending STD clinics and sexually active teens and women from impoverished environments, settings of substance abuse, or areas of high gonorrhea prevalence. Routine screening of asymptomatic men for urethral gonorrhea usually is unproductive in the primary care setting. However, if genetic amplification tests for *N. gonorrhoeae* become available at sufficiently low cost, combination with *C. trachomatis* testing in a single assay may facilitate the prevention and control of both infections in the populations at highest risk.

All patients with STDs or at high risk for STDs and all pregnant women should be routinely encouraged to undergo serologic testing for syphilis and HIV infection, with appropriate counseling before and after testing. In the primary care setting, such counseling is usually straightforward and can present opportunities for further risk-reduction counseling. Serologic tests for syphilis and HIV infection currently are not advocated for routine premarital use. Preimmunization serologic testing for antibody to HBV is indicated for unvaccinated persons who are known to be at high risk, such as homosexually active men and injection drug users. In most young persons, however, it is more cost-effective to vaccinate against HBV without serologic screening.

In summary, clinicians and public health agencies share responsibility for the prevention and control of STDs, including HIV infection, and it is likely in the managed-care era that the role of primary care clinicians will become increasingly important in prevention as well as in diagnosis and treatment.

BIBLIOGRAPHY

GENERAL

ANDERSON RM, MAY R: *Infectious Diseases of Humans: Dynamics and Control*. New York, Oxford Univ Press, 1991

BOEKELOO BO et al: Frequency and thoroughness of STD/HIV risk assessment by physicians in a high-risk metropolitan area. Am J Public Health 81:1645, 1991

BRANDT AM: *No Magic Bullet: A Social History of Venereal Disease in the United States Since 1890*, 2d ed. New York, Oxford Univ Press, 1989

CENTERS FOR DISEASE CONTROL AND PREVENTION: 1993 sexually transmitted disease treatment guidelines. Morb Mort Week Rep 42(RR-14):1, 1993

———: Update: Barrier protections against HIV infection and other sexually transmitted diseases. Morb Mort Week Rep 42:589, 1993

———: *Sexually Transmitted Disease Surveillance, 1994*. Atlanta, U.S. Public Health Service, 1995

Drugs for sexually transmitted diseases. Med Lett Drugs Ther 37:117, 1995

EBRAHIM SH et al: Mortality related to sexually transmitted diseases in women, US, 1973–1992. Am J Public Health, 1997

HANDSFIELD HH: *Color Atlas and Synopsis of Sexually Transmitted Diseases*. New York, McGraw-Hill, 1992

HOLMES KK: Human ecology and behavior and sexually transmitted bacterial infections. Proc Natl Acad Sci USA 91:2448, 1994

——— et al (eds): *Sexually Transmitted Diseases*, 3d ed. New York, McGraw-Hill, 1997

LAUMANN EO et al: *The Social Organization of Sexuality: Sexual Practices in the United States*. Chicago, Univ of Chicago Press, 1994

LEE HH et al: Diagnosis of *Chlamydia trachomatis* genitourinary infection in women by ligase chain reaction assay of urine. Lancet 345:213, 1995

MORSE SA et al: *Atlas of Sexually Transmitted Diseases*, 2d ed. Baltimore, Mosby-Wolfe, 1996

ORIEL JD: *The Scars of Venus: A History of Venereology*. London, Springer-Verlag, 1994

ROSS PE, LANDIS SE: Development and evaluation of a sexual history-taking curriculum for first- and second-year family practice residents. Fam Med 26:293, 1994

SMITH KR et al: Evaluation of ligase chain reaction for use with urine for identification of *Neisseria gonorrhoeae* in females attending a sexually transmitted disease clinic. J Clin Microbiol 33:455, 1995

WASSERHEIT JN: Effect of changes in human ecology and behavior on patterns of sexually transmitted diseases, including human immunodeficiency virus infection. Proc Natl Acad Sci USA 91:2430, 1994

URETHRITIS IN MALES

BOWIE WR et al: Etiology of nongonococcal urethritis. Evidence for *Chlamydia trachomatis* and *Ureaplasma urealyticum*. J Clin Invest 59:735, 1977

KRIEGER JN et al: Clinical manifestations of trichomoniasis in men. Ann Intern Med 118:844, 1993

MARTIN DH, BOWIE WR: Urethritis in males, in *Sexually Transmitted Diseases*, 3d ed, KK Holmes et al (eds). New York, McGraw-Hill, 1997, Chap 60

——— et al: A controlled trial of a single dose of azithromycin for the treatment of chlamydial urethritis and cervicitis. N Engl J Med 327:921, 1992

SHAFER MA et al: Urinary leukocyte esterase screening test for asymptomatic chlamydial and gonococcal infection in males. JAMA 262:2562, 1989

STAMM WE et al: Azithromycin for empirical treatment of the nongonococcal urethritis syndrome in men: A randomized double-blind study. JAMA 274:545, 1995

TAYLOR-ROBINSON D: The history and role of *Mycoplasma genitalium* in sexually transmitted diseases. The Harrison Lecture, Genitourin Med 71:1, 1995

EPIDIDYMITIS

BERGER RE: Epididymitis, in *Sexually Transmitted Diseases*, 3d ed, KK Holmes et al (eds). New York, McGraw-Hill, 1997, Chap 61

URETHRAL SYNDROME

STAMM WE, HOOTON TM: Management of urinary tract infections in adults. N Engl J Med 329:1328, 1993

VAGINAL INFECTIONS

ESCHENBACH DA et al: Diagnosis and clinical manifestations of bacterial vaginosis. Am J Obstet Gynecol 158:819, 1988
HAUTH JC et al: Reduced incidence of preterm delivery with metronidazole and erythromycin in women with bacterial vaginosis. N Engl J Med 333:1732, 1995
HAWES SE et al: Hydrogen peroxide–producing lactobacilli and acquisition of vaginal infections. J Infect Dis 174:1058, 1996
HILLIER SL et al: The relationship of hydrogen peroxide–producing lactobacilli to bacterial vaginosis and genital microflora in pregnant women. Obstet Gynecol 79:369, 1992
———— et al: Association between bacterial vaginosis and preterm delivery of a low-birth-weight infant. N Engl J Med 333:1737, 1995
WØLNER-HANSSEN P et al: Clinical manifestations of vaginal trichomoniasis. JAMA 261:571, 1989

MUCOPURULENT CERVICITIS

BRUNHAM RC et al: Mucopurulent cervicitis—the ignored counterpart in women of urethritis in men. N Engl J Med 311:1, 1984

GENITAL ULCERS

COREY L: The current trends in genital herpes: Progress in prevention. Sex Transm Dis 21(Suppl 2):S38, 1994
KOUTSKY LA et al: Underdiagnosis of genital herpes by current clinical and viral isolation procedures. N Engl J Med 326:1533, 1992
ORLE KA et al: Simultaneous PCR detection of *Haemophilus ducreyi, Treponema pallidum,* and herpes simplex virus types 1 and 2 from genital ulcers. J Clin Microbiol 34:49, 1996
WALD A et al: Virologic characteristics of subclinical and symptomatic genital herpes infections. N Engl J Med 333:770, 1995

PROCTITIS, PROCTOCOLITIS, ENTEROCOLITIS, AND ENTERITIS

QUINN TC et al: The polymicrobial etiology of intestinal infections in homosexual men. N Engl J Med 309:576, 1983

ARTHRITIS

RICE P, HANDSFIELD HH: Arthropathies, in *Sexually Transmitted Diseases*, 3d ed, KK Holmes et al (eds). New York, McGraw-Hill, 1997, Chap 68

PELVIC INFLAMMATORY DISEASE

HILLIER SL et al: Role of bacterial vaginosis–associated microorganisms in endometritis. Am J Obstet Gynecol 175:435, 1996
SCHOLES D et al: Prevention of pelvic inflammatory disease by screening for cervical chlamydial infection. N Engl J Med 334:1362, 1996
SOPER DE: Diagnosis and laparoscopic grading of acute salpingitis. Am J Obstet Gynecol 164:1370, 1991

HPV/WARTS

BAKEN LA et al: Genital human papillomavirus infection among male and female sex partners: Prevalence and type-specific concordance. J Infect Dis 171:429, 1995
KOUTSKY LA et al: A cohort study of the risk of cervical intraepithelial neoplasia grade 2 or 3 in relation to papillomavirus infection. N Engl J Med 327:1272, 1992

HBV, CMV, HTLV-I, AND HTLV-II

COLLIER AC et al: Cytomegalovirus infection in women attending a sexually transmitted disease clinic. J Infect Dis 162:46, 1990
GOTUZZO E et al: HTLV-I infection among female sex workers in Peru. J Infect Dis 169:754, 1994

MARGOLIS HS et al: Hepatitis B: Evolving epidemiology and implications for control. Semin Liver Dis 11(2):84, 1991
———— et al: Prevention of hepatitis B virus transmission by immunization. An economic analysis of current recommendations. JAMA 274:1201, 1995

PREVENTION AND CONTROL OF STDs

GROSSKURTH H et al: Impact of improved treatment of sexually transmitted diseases on HIV infection in rural Tanzania: Randomised controlled trial. Lancet 346:530, 1995
INSTITUTE OF MEDICINE: *The Hidden Epidemic: Confronting Sexually Transmitted Diseases*, TR Eng and WT Butler (eds). Washington, DC, National Academy Press, 1997
OXMAN GL, DOYLE L: A comparison of the case finding effectiveness and average costs of screening and partner notification. Sex Transm Dis 23:51, 1996
US PREVENTIVE SERVICES TASK FORCE: *Guide to Clinical Preventive Services*, 2d ed. Baltimore, Williams and Wilkins, 1996
WALLER HT, PIOT MA: The use of an epidemiologic model for estimating the effectiveness of tuberculosis control measures. Bull World Health Org 41:75, 1969; 43:1, 1970

130 *King K. Holmes*

PELVIC INFLAMMATORY DISEASE

DEFINITION The term *pelvic inflammatory disease* (PID) usually refers to ascending infection of the endometrium and/or fallopian tubes. Intrauterine infection can be primary (spontaneously occurring and usually sexually transmitted) or secondary to invasive intrauterine surgical procedures (e.g., dilatation and curettage, termination of pregnancy, insertion of an intrauterine device, or hysterosalpingography) or to parturition. Endometritis or endomyometritis is particularly common following delivery by cesarean section.

PID is uncommon during pregnancy itself. The uterotubal junction is closed as early as the seventh week of pregnancy, and the chorioamnion becomes approximated to the endocervical os, sealing off the intrauterine cavity, at the twelfth to fifteenth week of gestation. As a consequence, ascending intrauterine infection prior to the twelfth week of gestation may be associated (as either cause or effect) with endometritis and spontaneous abortion, while ascending infection after the twelfth week may be associated with chorioamnionitis. In rare instances, infection extends secondarily to the pelvic organs from adjacent foci of inflammation (e.g., sites of appendicitis, regional ileitis, or diverticulitis), as a result of hematogenous dissemination (e.g., of tuberculosis), or as a rare complication of certain tropical diseases (e.g., schistosomiasis).

Spontaneously occurring PID can be of the chronic or the acute type. Chronic PID due to *Mycobacterium tuberculosis* has become uncommon in industrialized countries. However, subacute or chronic PID caused by chronic infection with *Chlamydia trachomatis* is thought to be common.

The term *PID* is most often used today to refer to cases of acute, spontaneously occurring infection ascending from the cervix or vagina. The clinical diagnosis of PID is imprecise. Use of endometrial biopsy together with laparoscopy provides evidence of a continuum progressing from cervicitis alone to endometritis, to salpingitis, to pelvic peritonitis, and finally to generalized peritonitis, perihepatitis, or pelvic abscess. In this chapter, *PID* is used to refer to the clinical syndrome that includes each of these conditions, and the term *salpingitis* is restricted to cases of visually or histopathologically confirmed inflammation of the fallopian tubes. The distinction between endometritis and salpingitis and the distribution of cases of each infection may be important, because long-term sequelae are common after salpingitis. These sequelae include infertility due to bilateral tubal occlusion, peritubal adhesions, ectopic pregnancy due to tubal damage without occlusion, chronic pelvic pain, and recurrent PID.

ETIOLOGY The etiology of PID has seemed to vary greatly in several studies for reasons related to the selection of patients, the prevalence of sexually transmitted disease (STD) pathogens at the time and place of the study, and methodology. As is summarized in Table 130-1, the agents most often implicated in acute PID include those that are primary causes of cervicitis (*Neisseria gonorrhoeae* and *C. trachomatis*) and those that can be regarded as normal components of the vaginal flora.

During the 1980s, *N. gonorrhoeae* and/or *C. trachomatis* were found in 65 percent of women with a clinical diagnosis of PID at San Francisco General Hospital and in 85 percent of patients with proven salpingitis and endometritis in Seattle; in both studies, gonorrhea was nearly twice as common as chlamydial infection and dual infection was common. However, in Scandinavian countries, where gonococcal infection is under much better control, endocervical gonococcal infection has been found in a declining proportion of women with PID during the past decade, while chlamydial infection remains more common in this group. In general, PID is most often associated with gonorrhea where there is a high incidence of gonorrhea—e.g., in developing countries and in indigent, inner-city populations in developed countries. In several studies of women with PID, up to two-thirds of women with endocervical cultures positive for *N. gonorrhoeae* have also had endometrial, peritoneal, or tubal cultures positive for this organism. Similarly, studies of women with proven PID have shown that *C. trachomatis* can be demonstrated by culture or immunofluorescent staining in the endometrium or tubes of the majority of those who have endocervical chlamydial infection.

Anaerobic and facultative anaerobic organisms (especially *Prevotella* species, peptostreptococci, *Escherichia coli*, and group B streptococci) and genital mycoplasmas have been isolated from specimens obtained at laparoscopy from the peritoneal fluid or fallopian tubes in a varying proportion—typically one-fourth to one-third—of women with PID studied in the United States. These vaginal organisms can be found in association with chlamydial or gonococcal infection as well as in the absence of such infection. The importance of vaginal organisms in salpingitis has probably been overestimated in studies based on culture of specimens obtained by culdocentesis or endometrial aspiration, procedures in which contamination of the aspirated specimen by vaginal flora is possible. However, specimens obtained by laparoscopy from some patients with PID also have contained anaerobic and facultative species. It is extremely difficult to determine the exact microbial etiology of an individual case of PID because of the frequency of mixed infection, the difficulty in sampling the fallopian tube itself, and the complexity of the microbiologic techniques required to detect the various fastidious pathogens involved.

In general, first episodes of acute PID are particularly likely to be caused by *N. gonorrhoeae* and/or *C. trachomatis*. These sexually transmitted pathogens are implicated somewhat less often in recurrent bouts of acute PID, in episodes occurring in women with intrauterine devices (IUD), and in episodes precipitated by invasive intrauterine diagnostic or therapeutic procedures, which are often associated with ascending infection caused by certain components of the endogenous vaginal flora.

EPIDEMIOLOGY It has been estimated that about 850,000 cases of PID occurred in the United States each year during the mid-1970s. PID is not a reportable disease in the United States; surveillance

of physicians in private practice and of hospital discharges suggests that the incidence of PID increased from the mid-1960s through the mid-1970s and may then have decreased. Hospitalization for acute PID declined steadily from 1982 through 1993, but visits to physicians' offices remained constant during that period.

Acute PID is almost exclusively a disease of sexually active women. Important risk factors include a history of salpingitis, a recent history of vaginal douching, and the use of an IUD, particularly the Dalkon shield. In most studies, the relative risk of PID among IUD users is higher in nulliparous than in parous women and is greatest during the first few months after IUD insertion. The increased risk of PID among IUD users is evident mainly among those with multiple sex partners. In contrast, women using oral contraceptives appear to be at decreased risk of PID. Barrier methods of contraception also make PID less likely by reducing the risk of chlamydial and gonococcal infection. Tubal sterilization reduces (but does not completely eliminate) the risk of salpingitis by preventing intraluminal spread of infection into the tubes.

PATHOGENESIS Factors cited as possibly contributing to intracanalicular upward spread of gonococci and chlamydiae from the endocervix to the endometrium and endosalpinx include estrogen-dominated (thin) cervical mucus, attachment to sperm that migrate upward into the tubes, use of an IUD, vaginal douching, and menstruation. The onset of symptoms of *N. gonorrhoeae*–associated and *C. trachomatis*–associated PID often occurs during or soon after the menstrual period. In fallopian tube organ cultures in vitro, gonococci attach to the surface of the secretory columnar cells (but not the ciliated cells) of the endosalpinx. Gonococcal pili and perhaps other surface proteins are important in this attachment. Gonococci then are taken into the secretory cells by endocytosis. They pass through the cells—and perhaps between cells—and are extruded through the base of the cell into the submucosal connective tissue. Ciliary motion ceases, and then ciliated cells, although not directly invaded by gonococci, are sloughed from the mucosa—a factor that may render the tubes more susceptible to superinfection by other organisms. It is uncertain whether this loss of ciliated cells is irreversible in vivo. Gonococcal endotoxin and peptidoglycan as well as certain cytokines appear to be responsible for these cytotoxic effects. Gonococci associated with PID are significantly less susceptible to penicillin and less likely to belong to the Arg-Hyx-Ura auxotype than are strains causing uncomplicated gonorrhea.

C. trachomatis also infects the columnar cells of the fallopian tube but produces little damage in tubal organ cultures, perhaps because the host response is more important than directly toxic effects of bacterial products in the pathogenesis of chlamydial salpingitis. In chlamydial mucopurulent cervicitis (MPC), cervical biopsies show inclusions containing chlamydiae within columnar cells; columnar epithelial infiltration by neutrophils; submucosal and stromal infiltration by plasma cells, lymphocytes, histiocytes, and neutrophils; and lymphoid aggregates containing transformed lymphocytes. Routine endometrial biopsies from consecutive women with chlamydial MPC show endometritis in approximately one-half of cases. Although endometritis detected in this way is sometimes associated with uterine tenderness, abnormal menstrual bleeding, and leukocytosis, symptoms of abdominal pain and fever as well as signs of adnexal tenderness are usually lacking; this point underscores the subclinical nature or minimal clinical manifestations of many cases of upper genital tract chlamydial infection. It is not known what proportion of women with endometritis also have salpingitis, since laparoscopy has not been performed in the absence of more suggestive symptoms and signs of salpingitis. However, among women with chlamydial MPC who do have such symptoms and signs, the great majority of those who undergo endometrial biopsy and laparoscopy have both endometritis and salpingitis. Chlamydial inclusions are demonstrable by direct immunofluorescence in columnar epithelial cells of the endometrium and endosalpinx. The endometrial biopsies usually show neutrophils infiltrating

Table 130-1

Cervical and Vaginal Organisms Most Often Implicated in Acute PID

Cervical Pathogens	Vaginal Flora Components
Neisseria gonorrhoeae *Chlamydia trachomatis*	Anaerobic bacteria *Prevotella*, *Peptostreptococcus*, *Mobiluncus*, and *Actinomyces* species Facultative bacteria Enterobacteriaceae, *Haemophilus influenzae*, *Gardnerella vaginalis*, group B *Streptococcus* Mycoplasmas *Mycoplasma hominis*, *Ureaplasma urealyticum*

the epithelium and plasma cells infiltrating the stroma, findings also seen in gonococcal endometritis but not in the uninfected endometrium. Other inflammatory changes analogous to those seen in the cervix are also found in the endometrium with chlamydial infection. Experimental inoculation of the fallopian tubes of lower primates produces mild acute salpingitis and ciliary sloughing that is transient and reversible. However, if experimental tubal inoculation is preceded by repeated inoculation of the fallopian tubes or cervix, a more intense salpingitis results and progresses to peritubular scarring. The implication is that in the female genital tract, as in the eye, repeated exposure to *C. trachomatis* leads to the greatest degree of tissue inflammation and damage.

The pathogenesis of PID attributable to mycoplasmas or other vaginal anaerobic or facultative organisms is less well studied. It is possible that other vaginal organisms implicated in PID often cause tubal infection in women whose tubes have already been damaged by a primary sexually transmitted pathogen (i.e., *N. gonorrhoeae* or *C. trachomatis*). The vaginal organisms implicated in PID are found in the vagina most often and in greatest concentration in bacterial vaginosis, and there is epidemiologic evidence that bacterial vaginosis itself is a predisposing factor for PID (just as poor oral hygiene is a risk factor for aspiration pneumonia).

Certain other iatrogenic factors, such as dilatation and curettage or cesarean section, are known to increase the risk of PID in women with endocervical gonococcal or chlamydial infection. Recent evidence indicates that among women undergoing cesarean section, the presence of bacterial vaginosis increases the risk of postpartum endometritis.

CLINICAL MANIFESTATIONS **Tuberculous Salpingitis**
Unlike nontuberculous salpingitis, genital tuberculosis often occurs in older women, about half of whom are postmenopausal. In a large review in Sweden, 38 percent of women with tuberculous salpingitis had had tuberculosis diagnosed previously. The most common presenting symptoms were abnormal vaginal bleeding, pain (including dysmenorrhea), and infertility. Most of these women had normal findings on bimanual pelvic examination, though about one-quarter had adnexal masses. The most common basis for diagnosis was endometrial biopsy showing tuberculous granulomas, often in association with a positive culture.

Nontuberculous Salpingitis The evolution of symptoms of nontuberculous salpingitis classically proceeds from a mucopurulent vaginal discharge caused by cervicitis to midline abdominal pain and abnormal vaginal bleeding caused by endometritis and then to bilateral lower abdominal and pelvic pain caused by salpingitis, with nausea and vomiting and increased abdominal tenderness caused by peritonitis. Some patients have diffuse abdominal pain caused by generalized peritonitis or pleuritic right upper quadrant pain caused by perihepatitis. The pattern in which symptoms evolve varies from patient to patient and is also related to the etiology of the PID.

The onset of IUD-associated PID is typically gradual and may be preceded by the malodorous vaginal discharge characteristic of bacterial vaginosis. The onset of gonococcal PID has been more acute than that of chlamydial PID in some but not all studies, and PID of either etiology usually presents during the first half of the menstrual cycle.

The abdominal pain in nontuberculous salpingitis is usually described as dull or aching. In some cases, pain is lacking or is atypical, and active inflammatory changes are found in the course of an unrelated evaluation or procedure, such as a tubal ligation or a laparoscopic evaluation for infertility. Abnormal uterine bleeding precedes or coincides with the onset of pain in about 40 percent of women with PID, symptoms of urethritis (dysuria) occur in 20 percent, and symptoms of proctitis (anorectal pain, tenesmus, and rectal discharge or bleeding) occasionally are seen in women with gonococcal or chlamydial infection.

Speculum examination shows evidence of MPC in the majority of women with gonococcal or chlamydial PID. Cervical motion tenderness is produced by stretching of the adnexal attachments on the side toward which the cervix is pushed. Bimanual examination reveals uterine fundal tenderness due to endometritis and abnormal adnexal

tenderness due to salpingitis that is usually, but not necessarily, bilateral. Adnexal swelling is palpable in about one-half of women with acute salpingitis, but evaluation of the adnexae in a patient with marked tenderness—even by an experienced examiner—is not reliable. The initial temperature is >38°C in only about one-third of patients with acute salpingitis; thus fever is not required for the diagnosis.

Laboratory findings include elevation of the erythrocyte sedimentation rate (ESR) in 75 percent of patients with acute salpingitis and elevation of the peripheral white blood cell count in up to 60 percent. Microscopic examination of a saline wet-mount preparation of vaginal fluid has revealed either more than one polymorphonuclear leukocyte per vaginal epithelial cell or findings consistent with bacterial vaginosis in nearly all patients with laparoscopically confirmed salpingitis in Swedish studies. However, exceptions have not been uncommon in U.S. studies.

Certain clinical manifestations of acute PID have been correlated with etiologic findings. For example, the onset of salpingitis is related to menses in women with gonococcal or chlamydial infection. Women with *N. gonorrhoeae*– or *C. trachomatis*–associated salpingitis are significantly younger than women with salpingitis of other etiologies. In a Swedish study, women with *Chlamydia*-associated salpingitis had more indolent disease, with mild symptoms of significantly longer duration and less fever, than women with gonorrhea-associated salpingitis. It is suspected that, for all recognized cases of symptomatic acute chlamydial salpingitis, there is a comparable number of unrecognized cases of indolent or mildly symptomatic chlamydial salpingitis. Furthermore, it is thought that subclinical chronic or recurrent chlamydial salpingitis may be a major cause of female infertility.

IUD-associated PID has been much less common since withdrawal of the Dalkon shield from the market. This infection tends to be indolent and is associated less often with fever, but more often with adnexal masses, than is PID not associated with IUD use.

Perihepatitis and Periappendicitis Symptoms of perihepatitis, including pleuritic upper abdominal pain and tenderness (usually localized to the right upper quadrant), develop in 3 to 10 percent of women with acute PID. The onset of symptoms of perihepatitis takes place during or after the onset of symptoms of PID and may overshadow lower abdominal symptoms, thereby leading to a mistaken diagnosis of cholecystitis. In perhaps 5 percent of cases of acute salpingitis, early laparoscopy reveals inflammation ranging from edema and erythema of the liver capsule to exudate with fibrinous adhesions between the visceral and parietal peritoneum. When treatment is delayed and laparoscopy is performed late, dense "violin-string" adhesions are seen over the liver; chronic exertional or positional right upper quadrant pain ensues when traction is placed on the adhesions. Although perihepatitis, also known as the *Fitz-Hugh–Curtis syndrome*, was for many years attributed to gonococcal PID, most cases are now associated with chlamydial salpingitis. In patients with chlamydial salpingitis, serum titers of microimmunofluorescent antibody to *C. trachomatis* are typically much higher when perihepatitis is present than when it is absent, and it has been suggested that repeated chlamydial infections are responsible for perihepatitis.

Physical findings include right upper quadrant tenderness and usually include adnexal tenderness and cervicitis, even in patients whose symptoms are not suggestive of salpingitis. Liver function tests are nearly always normal, since inflammation is largely limited to the liver capsule and usually spares the parenchyma. Oral cholecystography may show nonfunction of the gallbladder, but ultrasonography of the right upper quadrant is normal. The presence of MPC and pelvic tenderness in a young woman with subacute pleuritic right upper quadrant pain and normal ultrasonography of the gallbladder points to a diagnosis of perihepatitis.

Periappendicitis (appendiceal serositis without involvement of the intestinal mucosa) has been found in approximately 5 percent of patients undergoing appendectomy for suspected appendicitis and can occur as a complication of gonococcal or chlamydial salpingitis.

Influence of Human Immunodeficiency Virus Infection Several studies have yielded inconsistent results with regard to the influence of infection with human immunodeficiency virus (HIV) on certain clinical manifestations of PID, such as fever, clinical severity, and etiology. However, HIV-infected women with PID do appear to be more likely than women without HIV infection to present with tubo-ovarian abscess, to require hospitalization, and to require surgery for PID.

DIAGNOSIS   Early diagnosis and initiation of therapy are essential to minimize tubal scarring. Recent reanalysis of Weström's cohort of Swedish women with proven salpingitis showed that those who delayed seeking care were three times more likely than those who sought care promptly to experience subsequent infertility or ectopic pregnancy. Appropriate treatment must not be withheld from patients who have an equivocal diagnosis. Since delay in therapy may lead to progression of tubal scarring, it is better to err on the side of overdiagnosis and overtreatment. On the other hand, it is essential to differentiate between salpingitis and other pelvic pathology, particularly surgical emergencies such as appendicitis and ectopic pregnancy.

No clinical finding or laboratory test short of laparoscopy definitively identifies salpingitis, and routine laparoscopy to confirm suspected salpingitis is generally impractical. Most patients with acute PID have lower abdominal pain of less than 3 weeks' duration, pelvic tenderness on bimanual pelvic examination, and evidence of lower genital tract infection (e.g., white blood cells outnumbering all other cells in the vaginal fluid). Approximately 60 percent of such patients have salpingitis at laparoscopy. Among the patients with these findings, a rectal temperature above 38°C, a palpable adnexal mass, and elevation of the ESR over 15 mm/h also raise the probability of salpingitis, which has been found at laparoscopy in 68 percent of patients with one of these additional findings, 90 percent of patients with two or fewer, and 96 percent of patients with three or fewer. However, only 17 percent of all patients with laparoscopy-confirmed salpingitis have had all three additional findings.

MPC is probably responsible for the presence of neutrophils in vaginal fluid in PID. In a woman with pelvic pain and tenderness, demonstration of an increased number of neutrophils ($\geq$30 per 1000$\times$ microscopic field in strands of cervical mucus) increases the predictive value of a clinical diagnosis of acute PID.

Several clinical features other than the presence of cervicitis also favor the diagnosis of acute PID. These include onset with menses, history of recent menstrual bleeding, presence of an IUD, history of salpingitis, and sexual exposure to a male with urethritis. Detection of polymorphonuclear leukocytes in fluid aspirated by culdocentesis supports a diagnosis of suspected salpingitis. Urethritis or proctitis may occur in chlamydial or gonococcal infection but also may represent a urinary tract source or an intestinal source, respectively, for the patient's symptoms. Appendicitis or another disorder of the gut is favored by the early onset of anorexia, nausea, or vomiting; the onset of pain later than day 14 of the menstrual cycle; or unilateral pain limited to the right or left lower quadrant. A missed menstrual period dictates an evaluation for ectopic pregnancy. The more sensitive assays for human beta-chorionic gonadotropin are usually positive. Ultrasonography is sometimes useful for the identification of tuboovarian or pelvic abscess, and intravaginal ultrasound assessment of the tubes has recently been reported to show increased tubal diameter, intratubal fluid, or tubal wall thickening in some cases of salpingitis.

Laparoscopy is the most specific method for diagnosis of acute salpingitis. Although laparoscopic findings may be normal if inflammation is limited to the endosalpinx or the endometrium, patients with suspected PID who have a normal laparoscopy have a better prognosis (with no sequelae at all or fewer sequelae) than patients who have abnormal laparoscopic findings. The primary and uncontested value of laparoscopy in women with lower abdominal pain is for the exclusion of other surgical problems. Table 130-2 clearly shows that the most common and serious problems that may be confused with salpingitis are usually unilateral. Unilateral pain or pelvic mass, though not incompatible with PID, is a strong indication for laparoscopy unless the clinical picture warrants laparotomy instead. Atypical clinical findings, such as the absence of lower genital tract infection, a missed menstrual period, or failure to respond to appropriate therapy, are other frequent indications for laparoscopy.

Table 130-2

Laparoscopic Findings in Patients with False-Positive or False-Negative Clinical Diagnoses of Acute PID

False-Positive Clinical Diagnosis		False-Negative Clinical Diagnosis, Unexpected PID at Laparoscopy	
Laparoscopic Diagnosis	Percent	Clinical Diagnosis	Percent
Acute appendicitis	24	Ovarian tumor	20
Endometriosis	16	Acute appendicitis	18
Corpus luteum bleeding	12	Ectopic pregnancy	16
Ectopic pregnancy	11	Chronic salpingitis	6
Pelvic adhesions only	7	Acute peritonitis	6
Benign ovarian tumor	7	Endometriosis	5
Chronic salpingitis	6	Uterine myoma	5
Miscellaneous	15	Atypical pelvic pain	6
		Miscellaneous	6

Laparoscopic criteria used for the diagnosis of salpingitis include (1) erythema of the fallopian tube, (2) edema of the fallopian tube, and (3) seropurulent exudate or fresh, easily lysed adhesions at the fimbriated end or on the serosal surface of a fallopian tube.

Endometrial biopsy is relatively sensitive and specific for the diagnosis of endometritis when the endometrial changes described above are found, and the presence of endometritis correlates well with the presence of salpingitis. Endometritis is found in at least three-fourths of women with laparoscopically confirmed salpingitis and is not found in women without PID.

The etiologic diagnosis of PID can be further studied by culture or other testing of specimens obtained by endocervical swab, endometrial aspiration, or culdocentesis or by laparoscopy or laparotomy. Endocervical swab specimens should be examined by Gram's staining for neutrophils and gram-negative diplococci and by culture or DNA amplification test for *N. gonorrhoeae*. Compared with culture, the sensitivity of Gram's staining is about 60 percent, and the specificity is more than 95 percent. The endocervical swab specimen also should be tested for *C. trachomatis* by culture, antigen detection, or assays for chlamydial DNA or RNA. Although detection of either *N. gonorrhoeae* or *C. trachomatis* in the endocervix does not prove that either agent is also present in the upper genital tract, this finding strongly supports the diagnosis of PID. The clinical diagnosis of PID made by expert gynecologists is confirmed by laparoscopy or endometrial biopsy in only about 60 percent of all consecutive patients but in about 90 percent of those who also have cultures positive for *N. gonorrhoeae* or *C. trachomatis*. There is no evidence that the isolation of anaerobes or facultative aerobes from the cervix or vagina correlates with the presence of these organisms in the upper genital tract in acute PID, but this point has not been well studied. The value of culture of culdocentesis and endometrial aspirate specimens is disputed because of the risk of contamination of the specimen with components of the vaginal flora. When laparoscopy is performed, material can be obtained directly from the cul-de-sac or the fimbriated opening of the tube or by tubal aspiration if pyosalpinx is present. Such specimens should be cultured for anaerobic and facultative pathogens as well as for *N. gonorrhoeae* and *C. trachomatis*.

℞ TREATMENT

Hospitalization should be considered in all cases of PID and is strongly recommended when (1) the diagnosis is uncertain and surgical emergencies such as appendicitis and ectopic pregnancy cannot be excluded, (2) pelvic abscess is suspected, (3) severe illness or nausea and vomiting preclude outpatient management, (4) the patient is pregnant, (5) the patient is an adolescent (since the compliance of adolescents is less predictable than that of adults), (6) the patient has HIV infection, (7) the patient is assessed as unable to follow or tolerate an outpatient regimen, (8) the patient has failed to respond to outpatient therapy, or (9) clinical follow-up after 48 to 72 h of antibiotic treatment cannot be arranged. Treatment should cover *N. gonorrhoeae*, *C. trachomatis*, gram-negative facultative bacteria (especially *E. coli*), vaginal anaerobes, and group B streptococci. No single agent is active against the entire spectrum of pathogens (Table 130-3). Several antimicrobial combinations do provide a broad spectrum of activity against the major pathogens in vitro, but many have not been adequately evaluated for clinical efficacy in PID.

Examples of Combination Regimens with Broad Activity Against Major Pathogens in PID Clinicians have had extensive experience with the following two inpatient regimens, which have given nearly identical results in a multicenter randomized trial:

1. Doxycycline [100 mg twice a day, given intravenously (IV) or orally] plus cefoxitin (2.0 g IV every 6 h) or cefotetan (2.0 g IV every 12 h). Administration of these drugs by the IV route should be continued for at least 48 h after the patient's condition improves, then followed with doxycycline (100 mg by mouth, twice a day) to complete 14 days of therapy. This regimen provides excellent coverage for *N. gonorrhoeae*, including penicillinase-producing strains, and for *C. trachomatis*.

2. Clindamycin (900 mg IV every 8 h) plus gentamicin (2.0 mg/ kg IV followed by 1.5 mg/kg IV every 8 h) in patients with normal renal function. Treatment with these drugs should be continued for at least 48 h after the patient's condition improves, then followed with doxycycline (100 mg orally twice a day) or with clindamycin (450 mg orally four times a day) to complete 14 days of therapy. This regimen is active against anaerobes and facultative gram-negative rods as well as against *C. trachomatis* and *N. gonorrhoeae*. In cases with tuboovarian abscess, many experts use clindamycin rather than doxycycline for continued therapy in order to provide better coverage for anaerobic infection.

Patients who are not hospitalized also should receive a combined regimen with broad activity, such as ceftriaxone [250 mg intramuscularly (IM)] followed by doxycycline (100 mg by mouth, twice a day for 14 days). Cefoxitin (2.0 g IM) given concurrently with probenecid (1.0 g orally) or another parenteral third-generation cephalosporin (e.g., ceftizoxime or cefotaxime) can be used in place of ceftriaxone. An alternative outpatient regimen that provides good coverage of the major pathogens is ofloxacin (400 mg twice daily) plus either metronidazole (500 mg twice daily) or clindamycin (450 mg four times daily) for 14 days.

Management of Sexual Partners Sexual partners of patients with acute PID—particularly those who have been partners within the 1 or 2 months before the onset of symptoms of PID—should be examined for STDs and promptly treated with a regimen effective against uncomplicated gonococcal and chlamydial infection. Treatment of PID should be considered inadequate until sexual partners have been properly evaluated and treated.

Follow-Up Hospitalized patients should show substantial clinical improvement within 3 to 5 days. Women treated as outpatients should be clinically reevaluated within 72 h. A follow-up telephone survey of women seen in an emergency room and given a prescription for 10 days of oral doxycycline for PID found that 28 percent never filled the prescription and 41 percent stopped taking medication early (after an average of 4.1 days), often because of persistent symptoms, lack of symptoms, or side effects. Women not responding favorably to ambulatory therapy should be hospitalized. After completion of treatment, tests for persistent or recurrent infection with *N. gonorrhoeae* or *C. trachomatis* should be performed if symptoms persist or recur or if the patient has not complied with therapy or has been reexposed to an untreated sex partner.

Removal of an IUD Although a beneficial impact of IUD removal on the response of acute salpingitis to antimicrobial therapy and on the risk of recurrent salpingitis has not been proven, removal of the IUD 2 or 3 days after antimicrobial therapy has been initiated seems reasonable. When an IUD is removed, contraceptive counseling is essential.

Surgery Surgery is necessary for the treatment of salpingitis only in the face of life-threatening infection (such as rupture or threatened rupture of a tuboovarian abscess) or for drainage of an abscess. Ultrasonography is useful for diagnosing and monitoring pelvic abscesses. When surgery is performed, conservative procedures are usually sufficient. Pelvic abscesses often can be drained by posterior colpotomy, and peritoneal lavage can be used if there is generalized peritonitis.

PROGNOSIS Among 900 women who underwent long-term follow-up for a mean period of 8 years after successful treatment of an acute episode of PID with various regimens in Sweden, late sequelae included infertility due to bilateral tubal occlusion, ectopic pregnancy due to tubal scarring without occlusion, chronic pelvic pain, and recurrent salpingitis. Chronic pain lasting longer than 6 months was seen in 18 percent of patients and infertility due to tubal occlusion in 17 percent; 4 percent of the pregnancies that did occur were ectopic, representing approximately a sixfold increase over the expected rate of ectopic pregnancies. The rate of infertility after salpingitis was found to be related to the age of the patient, the duration of symptoms when treatment was started, the severity of salpingitis (as determined by laparoscopy) at the time of diagnosis, and the number of episodes of salpingitis. The postsalpingitis risk of infertility due to tubal occlusion among sexually active women not using contraceptives was 14 percent at 15 to 24 years of age and 26 percent at 25 to 34 years of age; the risk for women of all ages combined was 11 percent after one episode of salpingitis, 23 percent after two episodes, and 54 percent after three or more episodes. The risk of infertility after gonococcal salpingitis was comparable to the risk after chlamydial salpingitis in one small prospective study. A study of outcomes of PID at the University of Washington found a sevenfold increase in the risk of ectopic pregnancy and an eightfold increase in the rate of hysterectomy after PID.

In several countries, a striking relationship has also been found between

Table 130-3

Relative Activities of the Antimicrobial Agents Most Commonly Used to Treat PID

Agent	Relative Activity Against Indicated Pathogen*					
			Vaginal Anaerobes		PID-Associated Facultative	
	N. gonorrhoeae	C. trachomatis	GPC†	GNR‡	GNR	M. hominis
Ampicillin/amoxicillin	2+	2+	4+	2+	2+	0
Doxycycline	2+	4+	2+	1+	1+	2+
Cefoxitin, cefotetan	3+	0	4+	3+	3+	0
Ceftriaxone§	4+	0	3+	2+	4+	0
Gentamicin/tobramycin	2+	0	1+	0	4+	2+ ?
Ofloxacin	4+	3+	1+	1+	4+	1+
Azithromycin	2+	4+	2+	?+	2+	?
Clindamycin	1+	3+	4+	4+	0	3+
Metronidazole	0	0	4+	4+	0	0

* No single antimicrobial agent offers optimal activity against all of these pathogens, but certain combinations (e.g., cefoxitin plus doxycycline, gentamicin plus clindamycin, and ofloxacin plus metronidazole) have complementary activity. Relative activity is indicated on a scale of 0 to 4+.
† GPC, gram-positive cocci (peptostreptococci).
‡ GNR, gram-negative rods (anaerobic GNR include *Prevotella*; facultative GNR include Enterobacteriaceae and *Haemophilus influenzae*).

infertility due to tubal occlusion and the prevalence and titer of anti-body to *C. trachomatis*. Recurrent salpingitis has been seen in approximately 15 to 25 percent of women treated for salpingitis in various studies.

PREVENTION   Prevention of PID depends first on the effective control of gonococcal and chlamydial infection in the general population. Effective methods include the promotion of changes in sexual behavior and the use of barrier contraceptives in the context of ready access to modern methods of diagnosis and effective treatment of sex partners to control further spread. The decline in popularity of the IUD, particularly among nulliparous women, has undoubtedly helped to reduce the incidence of PID. It is also possible, but not proven, that the use of oral contraceptives and the avoidance of vaginal douching may reduce the risk of PID.

A 1996 report presented the results of a randomized controlled trial designed to determine whether selective screening for chlamydial infection reduced the risk of subsequent PID. Women at high risk for chlamydial infection were identified by means of a questionnaire mailed to all women 18 to 34 years of age who were enrolled in the Group Health Cooperative of Puget Sound in Washington. Women randomized to undergo chlamydial screening had a 56 percent lower rate of PID over the following year than did women receiving the usual care without screening. This report strongly supports risk-based screening for *Chlamydia* among young women receiving health care in managed-care organizations or other settings.

The complications of salpingitis can be minimized by early diagnosis and prompt treatment. It seems logical, but is unproven, that broad-spectrum therapy effective against all of the common causes of PID offers the best outcome. Although few methodologically sound clinical trials (especially with prolonged follow-up) have been conducted, one meta-analysis by Dodson showed a benefit of providing good coverage against anaerobes. Similarly, hospitalization to ensure rest and adequate compliance may improve the rather dismal long-term prognosis for tubal function. One placebo-controlled study showed that concurrent anti-inflammatory therapy with prednisolone hastened the reduction of acute inflammatory changes but did not improve the end results, as measured by fertility, hysterosalpingographic findings, or chronic pain. The potential value of anti-inflammatory therapy remains to be evaluated adequately.

BIBLIOGRAPHY

CATES WJ et al: Worldwide patterns of infertility: Is Africa different? Lancet 2:596, 1985

CENTERS FOR DISEASE CONTROL AND PREVENTION: Policy guidelines for the prevention and management of pelvic inflammatory disease. Morb Mort Week Rep 40(RR-5):1, 1992

————: 1993 Sexually transmitted disease treatment guidelines. Morb Mort Week Rep 42(RR-14):T-102, 1993

DODSON MG: Antibiotic regimens for treating acute pelvic inflammatory disease. An evaluation. J Reprod Med 39:285, 1994

ESCHENBACH DA et al: Polymicrobial etiology of acute pelvic inflammatory disease. N Engl J Med 293:166, 1975

FALK V et al: Genital tuberculosis in women. Am J Obstet Gynecol 138:974, 1980

FERRIS DG et al: Women's use of over-the-counter antifungal medications for gynecologic symptoms. J Fam Pract 42:595, 1996

GERMAINE A et al: *Reproductive Tract Infections: Global Impact and Priorities for Women's Reproductive Health.* New York, Plenum, 1992

HASSELQUIST MB, HILLIER S: Susceptibility of upper-genital tract isolates from women with pelvic inflammatory disease to ampicillin, cefpodoxime, metronidazole, and doxycycline. Sex Transm Dis 18:146, 1991

HEMSELL DL et al: Comparison of three regimens recommended by the Centers for Disease Control and Prevention for the treatment of women hospitalized with acute pelvic inflammatory disease. Clin Infect Dis 19:729, 1994

HILLIER SL et al: Role of bacterial vaginosis–associated microorganisms in endometritis. Am J Obstet Gynecol 175:435, 1996

HILLIS SD et al: Delayed care of pelvic inflammatory disease as a risk factor for impaired fertility. Am J Obstet Gynecol 168:1503, 1993

KAMENGA MC et al: The impact of human immunodeficiency virus infection on pelvic inflammatory disease: A case-control study in Abidjan, Ivory Coast. Am J Obstet Gynecol 172:919, 1995

KIMANI J et al: Risk factors for *Chlamydia trachomatis* pelvic inflammatory disease among sex workers in Nairobi, Kenya. J Infect Dis 173:1437, 1996

KIVIAT N et al: Endometrial histopathology in patients with culture-proven upper genital tract infection and laparoscopically diagnosed acute salpingitis. Am J Surg Pathol 14:167, 1990

LANDERS DV et al: Combination antimicrobial therapy in the treatment of acute pelvic inflammatory disease. Am J Obstet Gynecol 164:849, 1991

PEIPERT JF et al: Laboratory evaluation of acute upper genital tract infection. Obstet Gynecol 87(pt 1):730, 1996

PLUMMER FA et al: Postpartum upper genital tract infections in Nairobi, Kenya: Epidemiology, etiology, and risk factors. J Infect Dis 156:92, 1987

REED SD et al: Antibiotic treatment of tuboovarian abscess: Comparison of broad-spectrum beta-lactam agents versus clindamycin-containing regimens. Am J Obstet Gynecol 164:1556, 1991

SCHOLES D et al: Prevention of pelvic inflammatory disease by screening for cervical chlamydial infection. N Engl J Med 334:1362, 1996

ST JOHN RK, BROWN ST (eds): International symposium on pelvic inflammatory disease. Am J Obstet Gynecol 138:845, 1980

SVENSSON L et al: Infertility after acute salpingitis—with special reference to *Chlamydia trachomatis*–associated infections. Fertil Steril 40:322, 1983

WALKER CK et al: Pelvic inflammatory disease: Meta-analysis of antimicrobial regimen efficacy. J Infect Dis 168:969, 1993

WASHINGTON AE, KATZ P: Cost of and payment source for pelvic inflammatory disease: Trends and projections, 1983 through 2000. JAMA 266:2565, 1991

WASSERHEIT JN et al: Microbial causes of proven pelvic inflammatory disease and efficacy of clindamycin with tobramycin. Ann Intern Med 104:187, 1986

WØLNER-HANSSEN P: Silent pelvic inflammatory disease: Is it overstated? Obstet Gynecol 86:321, 1995

131   *Walter E. Stamm*

URINARY TRACT INFECTIONS AND PYELONEPHRITIS

DEFINITIONS   Acute infections of the urinary tract can be subdivided into two general anatomic categories: lower tract infection (urethritis, cystitis, and prostatitis) and upper tract infection (acute pyelonephritis and intrarenal and perinephric abscesses). Infections at these various sites may occur together or independently and may either be asymptomatic or present as one of the clinical syndromes outlined below. Infections of the urethra and bladder are often considered superficial (or mucosal) infections, while prostatitis, pyelonephritis, and renal suppuration signify tissue invasion.

From a microbiologic perspective, urinary tract infection exists when pathogenic microorganisms are detected in the urine, urethra, bladder, kidney, or prostate. In most instances, growth of more than 10^5 organisms per milliliter from a properly collected midstream "clean-catch" urine sample indicates infection. However, significant bacteriuria is lacking in some cases of true urinary infection. Especially in symptomatic patients, a smaller number of bacteria (10^2 to 10^4 per milliliter of midstream urine) may signify infection. In urine specimens obtained by suprapubic aspiration or "in-and-out" catheterization and in samples from a patient with an indwelling catheter, colony counts of 10^2 to 10^4 per milliliter generally indicate infection. Conversely, colony counts in excess of 10^5 per milliliter of midstream urine are occasionally due to specimen contamination. That is especially likely to be the explanation when multiple species are found.

Infections that recur after antibiotic therapy can be due to the persistence of the originally infecting strain (as judged by species, antibiogram, serotype, and molecular type) or to reinfection with a new strain. "Same-strain" recurrent infections that become evident within 2 weeks of cessation of therapy can be the result of unresolved renal or prostatic infection (termed *relapse*) or of persistent vaginal or intestinal colonization leading to rapid reinfection of the bladder.

Symptoms of dysuria, urgency, and frequency that are unaccompanied by significant bacteriuria have been termed the *acute urethral syndrome*. Although widely used, this term lacks anatomic precision because many cases so designated are actually bladder infections. Moreover, since the causative agent can usually be identified in these patients, the term *syndrome*—implying unknown causation—is inappropriate.

Chronic pyelonephritis refers to chronic interstitial nephritis believed to result from bacterial infection of the kidney (see Chap. 276). Many noninfectious diseases also cause an interstitial nephritis that is indistinguishable pathologically from chronic pyelonephritis.

ACUTE INFECTIONS OF THE URINARY TRACT: URETHRITIS, CYSTITIS, AND PYELONEPHRITIS

EPIDEMIOLOGY Epidemiologically, urinary tract infections should be subdivided into catheter-associated (or nosocomial) infections and non-catheter-associated (or community-acquired) infections. Infections in either category may be symptomatic or asymptomatic. Acute infections are very common in noncatheterized patients (more so among women than among men) and account for more than 6 million office visits annually in the United States. These infections occur in 1 to 3 percent of schoolgirls and then increase markedly in incidence with the onset of sexual activity in adolescence. The vast majority of acute symptomatic infections involve young women. Acute symptomatic urinary infections are unusual in men under the age of 50. The development of asymptomatic bacteriuria parallels that of symptomatic infection and is rare among men under 50 but common among women between 20 and 50. Asymptomatic bacteriuria is quite common among elderly men and women, with rates as high as 40 to 50 percent in some studies.

ETIOLOGY Many different microorganisms can infect the urinary tract, but by far the most common agents are the gram-negative bacilli. *Escherichia coli* causes approximately 80 percent of acute infections in patients without catheters, urologic abnormalities, or calculi. Other gram-negative rods, especially *Proteus* and *Klebsiella* and occasionally *Enterobacter*, account for a smaller proportion of uncomplicated infections. These organisms, plus *Serratia* and *Pseudomonas*, assume increasing importance in recurrent infections and in infections associated with urologic manipulation, calculi, or obstruction. They play a major role in nosocomial, catheter-associated infections (see below). *Proteus* species, by virtue of urease production, and *Klebsiella* species, through the production of extracellular slime and polysaccharides, predispose to stone formation and are isolated more frequently from patients with calculi.

Gram-positive cocci play a lesser role in urinary tract infections. However, *Staphylococcus saprophyticus*, a novobiocin-resistant, coagulase-negative staphylococcus, accounts for 10 to 15 percent of acute symptomatic urinary tract infections in young females. Enterococci occasionally cause acute uncomplicated cystitis in women. More commonly, enterococci and *Staphylococcus aureus* cause infections in patients with renal stones or previous instrumentation. Isolation of *S. aureus* from the urine should arouse suspicion of bacteremic infection of the kidney.

About one-third of women with dysuria and frequency have either an insignificant number of bacteria in midstream urine cultures or completely sterile cultures and have been previously defined as having the urethral syndrome. About three-quarters of these women have pyuria, while one-quarter have no pyuria and little objective evidence of infection. In the women with pyuria, two groups of pathogens account for most infections. Low quantities (10^2 to 10^4 bacteria per milliliter) of typical bacterial uropathogens such as *E. coli*, *S. saprophyticus*, *Klebsiella*, or *Proteus* are found in midstream urine specimens from most of these women. These bacteria are probably the causative agents in these infections because they can usually be isolated from a suprapubic aspirate, are associated with pyuria, and respond to appropriate antimicrobial therapy. In other women with acute urinary symptoms, pyuria, and urine that is sterile (even when obtained by suprapubic aspiration), sexually transmitted urethritis-producing agents such as *Chlamydia trachomatis*, *Neisseria gonorrhoeae*, and herpes simplex virus are etiologically important. These agents are found most frequently in young, sexually active women with new sexual partners.

The causative role of nonbacterial pathogens in urinary tract infections remains poorly defined. *Ureaplasma urealyticum* has frequently been isolated from the urethra and urine of patients with acute dysuria and frequency but is also found in specimens from many patients without urinary symptoms. Ureaplasmas probably account for some cases of urethritis and cystitis. *U. urealyticum* and *Mycoplasma hominis* have been isolated from prostatic and renal tissues of patients with acute prostatitis and pyelonephritis and are probably responsible for some of these infections as well. Adenoviruses cause acute hemorrhagic cystitis in children and in some young adults, often in epidemics. Although many other viruses can be isolated from urine (cytomegalovirus, for example), they are thought not to cause urinary infection. Colonization of the urine of catheterized patients or diabetics by *Candida* and other fungal species is common and sometimes progresses to symptomatic invasive infection (see Chap. 207). → *Mycobacterial infection of the genitourinary tract is discussed in Chap. 171.*

PATHOGENESIS AND SOURCES OF INFECTION The urinary tract should be viewed as a single anatomic unit that is united by a continuous column of urine extending from the urethra to the kidney. In the vast majority of urinary tract infections, bacteria gain access to the bladder via the urethra. Ascent of bacteria from the bladder may follow and is probably the pathway for most renal parenchymal infections.

The vaginal introitus and distal urethra are normally colonized by diphtheroids, streptococcal species, lactobacilli, and staphylococcal species but not by the enteric gram-negative bacilli that commonly cause urinary tract infections. In females prone to the development of cystitis, however, enteric gram-negative organisms residing in the bowel colonize the introitus, the periurethral skin, and the distal urethra before and during episodes of bacteriuria. The factors that predispose to periurethral colonization with gram-negative bacilli remain poorly understood but probably include alteration of the normal perineal flora by antibiotics, other genital infections, or contraceptives, especially diaphragms and spermicide. Small numbers of periurethral bacteria probably gain entry to the bladder frequently, a process that is facilitated in some cases by urethral massage during intercourse. Whether bladder infection ensues depends on interacting effects of the pathogenicity of the strain, the inoculum size, and the local and systemic mechanisms of host defense.

Under normal circumstances, bacteria placed in the bladder are rapidly cleared, partly through the flushing and dilutional effects of voiding but also as a result of the antibacterial properties of urine and the bladder mucosa. Owing mostly to a high urea concentration and high osmolarity, the bladder urine of many normal persons inhibits or kills bacteria. Prostatic secretions possess antibacterial properties as well. Polymorphonuclear leukocytes in the bladder wall also appear to play a role in clearing bacteriuria. The role of locally produced antibody remains unclear.

Hematogenous pyelonephritis occurs most often in debilitated patients who either are chronically ill or are receiving immunosuppressive therapy. Metastatic staphylococcal or candidal infections of the kidney may follow bacteremia or fungemia, spreading from distant foci of infection in the bone, skin, endothelium, or elsewhere.

CONDITIONS AFFECTING PATHOGENESIS *Gender and Sexual Activity* The female urethra appears to be particularly prone to colonization with colonic gram-negative bacilli because of its proximity to the anus, its short length (about 4 cm), and its termination beneath the labia. Sexual intercourse causes the introduction of bacteria into the bladder and is temporally associated with the onset of cystitis; it thus appears to be important in the pathogenesis of urinary infections in younger women. (Voiding after intercourse has been shown to reduce the risk of cystitis, probably because it promotes the clearance of bacteria introduced during intercourse.) In addition, use of a diaphragm and/or a spermicide dramatically alters the normal introital bacterial flora and has been associated with marked increases in vaginal colonization with *E. coli* and in the risk of urinary infection. In males, prostatitis and urethral obstruction due to prostatic hypertrophy are important factors predisposing to bacteriuria. Homosexuality also is associated with an increased risk of cystitis, which probably is related to rectal intercourse. Men infected with human immunodeficiency virus (HIV) who have CD4 + T cell counts of <200/μL have recently been shown to be at increased risk of both bacteriuria and symptomatic urinary tract infection. Finally, lack of circumcision has been identified as a risk factor for urinary tract infection in both neonates and young men.

Pregnancy Urinary infections are detected in 2 to 8 percent of pregnant women, the exact figure depending on socioeconomic status. Symptomatic upper tract infections, in particular, are unusually common during pregnancy; fully 20 to 30 percent of pregnant women with asymptomatic bacteriuria subsequently develop pyelonephritis. This predisposition to upper tract infection during pregnancy results from decreased ureteral tone, decreased ureteral peristalsis, and temporary incompetence of the vesicoureteral valves. Bladder catheterization during or after delivery causes additional infections. Cystitis and pyelonephritis are no more common among women with toxemia of pregnancy than among other pregnant women. Increased prevalences of premature delivery and newborn mortality may result from urinary infections during pregnancy, particularly those involving the upper urinary tract.

Obstruction Any impediment to the free flow of urine—tumor, stricture, stone, or prostatic hypertrophy—results in hydronephrosis and a greatly increased frequency of urinary tract infection. Infection superimposed on urinary tract obstruction may lead to rapid destruction of renal tissue. It is of utmost importance, therefore, when infection is present, to repair obstructive lesions. On the other hand, when an obstruction is minor and is not progressive or associated with infection, great caution should be exercised in attempting surgical correction. The introduction of infection in such cases may be more damaging than an uncorrected minor obstruction that does not significantly impair renal function.

Neurogenic Bladder Dysfunction Interference with the nerve supply to the bladder, as in spinal cord injury, tabes dorsalis, multiple sclerosis, diabetes, and other diseases, may be associated with urinary tract infection. The infection may be initiated by the use of catheters for bladder drainage and is favored by the prolonged stasis of urine in the bladder. An additional factor often operative in these cases is bone demineralization due to immobilization, which causes hypercalciuria, calculus formation, and obstructive uropathy.

Vesicoureteral Reflux Defined as reflux of urine from the bladder cavity up into the ureters and sometimes into the renal pelvis, vesicoureteral reflux occurs during voiding or with elevation of pressure in the bladder. In practice, this condition is demonstrated by the finding of retrograde movement of radiopaque or radioactive material during a voiding cystourethrogram. An anatomically impaired vesicoureteral junction facilitates reflux of bacteria and thus upper tract infection. However, since a fluid connection between the bladder and the kidney always exists, even in the normal urinary system, some retrograde movement of bacteria probably takes place during infection but is not detected by radiologic techniques.

Vesicoureteral reflux is common among children with anatomic abnormalities of the urinary tract as well as among children with anatomically normal but infected urinary tracts. In the latter group, reflux disappears with advancing age and probably is attributable to factors other than urinary infection. Long-term follow-up of children with urinary tract infection who have reflux has established that renal damage correlates with marked reflux, not with infection.

The routine search for reflux would be aided by the development of noninvasive tests applicable to young children, in whom the need for an effective technique is greatest. In the meantime, it appears reasonable to search for reflux in anyone with unexplained failure of renal growth or with renal scarring, because urinary tract infection per se is an insufficient explanation for these abnormalities. On the other hand, it is doubtful that all children who have recurrent urinary tract infections but whose urinary tract appears normal on pyelography

should be subjected to voiding cystoureterography merely for the detection of the rare patient with marked reflux not revealed by the intravenous pyelogram.

Bacterial Virulence Factors Bacterial virulence factors markedly influence the likelihood that a given strain, once introduced into the bladder, will cause urinary tract infection. Not all strains of *E. coli*, for example, are equally able to infect the intact urinary tract. Most strains that cause symptomatic urinary tract infections in noncatheterized patients belong to a small number of specific O, K, and H serogroups, produce hemolysin, and share certain other "uropathogenic" properties. Adherence of bacteria to uroepithelial cells is a critical first step in the initiation of infection. For both *E. coli* and *Proteus*, fimbriae (hairlike proteinaceous surface appendages) mediate the attachment of bacteria to specific receptors on epithelial cells. Nearly all strains of *E. coli* that cause pyelonephritis in patients with anatomically normal urinary tracts possess a particular pilus (the P pilus or gal-gal pilus) that mediates attachment to the digalactoside portion of glycosphingolipids present on uroepithelium. In addition, strains that cause pyelonephritis usually produce hemolysin, have aerobactin (a siderophore for scavenging iron), and are resistant to the bactericidal action of human serum. Since most strains that produce acute pyelonephritis in the intact host possess all or nearly all of these virulence factors, the concept has arisen that only a few uropathogenic clones cause most such cases of infection. In contrast, infections in patients with structural or functional abnormalities of the urinary tract are generally caused by bacterial strains that lack these uropathogenic properties; the implication is that these properties are not needed for infection of the compromised urinary tract.

Genetic Factors Increasing evidence suggests that host genetic factors influence susceptibility to urinary infection. The number and type of receptors on uroepithelial cells to which bacteria may attach are at least in part genetically determined. Many of these structures are components of blood group antigens and are present on both erythrocytes and uroepithelial cells. For example, P fimbriae mediate attachment of *E. coli* to P-positive erythrocytes and are found on nearly all strains causing acute uncomplicated pyelonephritis. Conversely, P blood group–negative individuals, who lack these receptors, have a decreased likelihood of pyelonephritis. It has also been demonstrated that nonsecretors of blood group antigens are at increased risk of recurrent urinary infection; this predisposition may relate to a different profile of genetically determined glycolipids on uroepithelial cells.

LOCALIZATION OF INFECTION Infections involving the upper urinary tract usually cause a significant rise in serum antibodies to the O antigen of the infecting strain. They also produce a temporary defect in renal concentrating ability in many patients and may be associated with the formation of leukocyte casts. Lower tract infections rarely result in increased antibody titers, concentrating defects, or white cell casts. Unfortunately, these methods of distinguishing renal parenchymal infection from cystitis are neither reliable nor convenient enough for routine clinical use. More sensitive tests for distinguishing pyelonephritis from cystitis (bilateral ureteral catheterization and the bladder washout technique originated by Fairley) are inherently invasive and are too complex for routine clinical practice. A simpler, noninvasive test by which to distinguish upper from lower tract infections on the basis of antibody coating of bacteria in the urine is not sufficiently sensitive or specific to be of value in the routine clinical management of patients. An elevated level of C-reactive protein often accompanies acute pyelonephritis and is rare in cystitis, but this acute-phase reactant is nonspecific since it is also detectable in infections other than pyelonephritis.

CLINICAL PRESENTATION Clinical signs and symptoms cannot be relied on as an accurate basis for the diagnosis or localization of urinary tract infection. Many patients with significant bacteriuria (including some with upper tract infection) have no symptoms at all. Of those with significant bacteriuria and symptoms of cystitis, about two-thirds have lower tract infection and about one-third have clinically silent upper tract infection that becomes evident only on the performance of localization studies. Clinical symptoms and signs of pyelonephritis, though usually suggestive, do not always indicate upper tract infection. Finally, among women presenting with acute dysuria and frequency, only 60 to 70 percent have significant bacteriuria, but most of those without significant bacteriuria also have infections of the kidneys, bladder, or urethra.

Enumeration of the number and type of bacteria in the urine is an extremely important diagnostic procedure. In symptomatic infections of the urinary tract, uropathogenic bacteria are usually demonstrable in the urine in large numbers. As a rule, quantitative estimation of the number of bacteria in voided urine specimens makes it possible to distinguish contamination from true bacteriuria, and a bacterial colony count of $\geq 10^5$/mL has been the criterion traditionally used for this purpose. However, in symptomatic women with pyuria, colony counts of 10^2 to 10^4 *E. coli, Klebsiella, Proteus,* or *S. saprophyticus* per milliliter of midstream urine usually indicate infection, not contamination, and should not be disregarded. In asymptomatic patients, two consecutive urine specimens should be examined bacteriologically before therapy is instituted, and 10^5 or more bacteria of a single species per milliliter should be demonstrable in both specimens. Since the large number of bacteria in the bladder urine is due in part to bacterial multiplication during residence in the bladder cavity, samples of urine from the ureters or renal pelvis may contain fewer than 10^5 bacteria per milliliter and yet indicate infection. Similarly, the presence of bacteriuria of any degree in suprapubic aspirates or of 10^2 or more bacteria per milliliter of urine obtained by catheterization usually indicates infection. In some circumstances (antibiotic treatment, high urea concentration, high osmolarity, low pH), urine inhibits bacterial multiplication, resulting in relatively low bacterial colony counts despite infection. For this reason, antiseptic solutions should not be used in washing the periurethral area before collection of the urine specimen. Water diuresis or recent voiding also reduces bacterial counts in urine.

Rapid methods of detection of bacteriuria have been developed as alternatives to standard culture methods. These methods detect bacterial growth by photometry, bioluminescence, or other means and provide results rapidly, usually in 1 to 2 h. Compared with urine cultures, these techniques generally exhibit a sensitivity of 95 to 98 percent and a negative predictive value of >99 percent when bacteriuria is defined as 10^5 colony forming units per milliliter. However, the sensitivity of these tests falls to 60 to 80 percent when 10^2 to 10^4 colony forming units per milliliter is the standard of comparison.

Microscopy of urine from symptomatic patients can be of great diagnostic value. Microscopic bacteriuria, which is best assessed with Gram-stained uncentrifuged urine, is found in more than 90 percent of specimens from patients whose infections are associated with colony counts of at least 10^5/mL, and this finding is very specific. However, bacteria cannot usually be detected microscopically in infections with lower colony counts (10^2 to 10^4/mL). The detection of bacteria by urinary microscopy constitutes firm evidence of infection, but the absence of microscopically detectable bacteria does not exclude the diagnosis. When carefully sought by means of chamber-count microscopy, pyuria is a highly sensitive indicator of urinary tract infection in symptomatic patients. Pyuria is demonstrated in nearly all acute bacterial urinary tract infections, and its absence calls the diagnosis into question. The leukocyte esterase "dipstick" method is less sensitive than microscopy in identifying pyuria but is a useful alternative where microscopy is not feasible. Pyuria in the absence of bacteriuria (sterile pyuria) may indicate infection with unusual bacterial agents such as *C. trachomatis, U. urealyticum,* and *Mycobacterium tuberculosis* or with fungi. Alternatively, sterile pyuria may be demonstrated in noninfectious urologic conditions such as calculi, anatomic abnormality, nephrocalcinosis, vesicoureteral reflux, interstitial nephritis, or polycystic disease.

Cystitis Patients with dysuria, frequency, urgency, and suprapubic pain usually have cystitis. The urine often becomes grossly cloudy and malodorous, and it is bloody in about 30 percent of cases. White cells and bacteria can be detected by examination of unspun urine in most cases. However, some women with cystitis have only 10^2 to 10^4 bacteria per milliliter of urine, and in these instances bacteria cannot be seen in a Gram-stained preparation of unspun urine. Physical examination generally reveals only tenderness of the urethra or the suprapubic area. If a genital lesion or a vaginal discharge is evident, especially in conjunction with fewer than 10^5 bacteria per milliliter on urine culture, then pathogens that may cause urethritis, vaginitis, or cervicitis, such as *C. trachomatis, N. gonorrhoeae, Trichomonas, Candida,* and herpes simplex virus, should be considered. Prominent systemic manifestations such as a temperature of >38.3°C (>101°F), nausea, and vomiting usually indicate concomitant renal infection, as does costovertebral angle tenderness. However, the absence of these findings does not ensure that infection is limited to the bladder and urethra.

Acute Pyelonephritis Symptoms of acute pyelonephritis generally develop rapidly over a few hours or a day and include a temperature of ≥ 39.4°C (≥ 103°F), shaking chills, nausea, vomiting, and diarrhea. Symptoms of cystitis may or may not develop. Besides fever, tachycardia, and generalized muscle tenderness, physical examination reveals marked tenderness on deep pressure in one or both costovertebral angles or on deep abdominal palpation. In some patients, signs and symptoms of gram-negative sepsis predominate. Most patients have significant leukocytosis, pyuria with leukocyte casts in the urine, and bacteria detectable in Gram-stained unspun urine. Hematuria may be demonstrated during the acute phase of the disease; if it persists after acute manifestations of infection have subsided, a stone, a tumor, or tuberculosis should be considered.

Except in individuals with papillary necrosis or urinary obstruction, the manifestations of acute pyelonephritis usually respond to therapy within 48 to 72 h. However, despite the absence of symptoms, bacteriuria or pyuria may persist. In severe pyelonephritis, fever subsides more slowly and may not disappear for several days, even after appropriate antibiotic treatment has been instituted.

Urethritis Approximately 30 percent of women with acute dysuria, frequency, and pyuria have midstream urine cultures that show either no growth or insignificant bacterial growth. Clinically, these women cannot readily be distinguished from those with cystitis. In this situation, a distinction should be made between women infected with sexually transmitted pathogens, such as *C. trachomatis, N. gonorrhoeae,* or herpes simplex virus, and those with low-count *E. coli* or staphylococcal infection of the urethra and bladder. Chlamydial or gonococcal infection should be suspected in women with a gradual onset of illness, no hematuria, no suprapubic pain, and more than 7 days of symptoms. The additional history of a recent sex-partner change, especially if the patient's partner has recently had chlamydial or gonococcal urethritis, should heighten the suspicion of a sexually transmitted infection, as should the finding of mucopurulent cervicitis. Gross hematuria, suprapubic pain, an abrupt onset of illness, a duration of illness of less than 3 days, and a history of previous urinary tract infections favor the diagnosis of *E. coli* urinary tract infection.

Catheter-Associated Urinary Tract Infections Bacteriuria develops in at least 10 to 15 percent of hospitalized patients with indwelling urethral catheters. The risk of infection is about 3 to 5 percent per day of catheterization. *Proteus, Pseudomonas, Klebsiella,* and *Serratia,* in addition to *E. coli,* usually cause these infections. Many infecting strains display markedly greater antimicrobial resistance than organisms that cause community-acquired urinary infections. Factors associated with an increased risk of infection include female sex, prolonged catheterization, severe underlying illness, disconnection of the catheter and drainage tube, other types of faulty catheter care, and lack of systemic antimicrobial therapy.

Infection occurs when bacteria reach the bladder by one of two routes: by migrating through the column of urine in the catheter lumen (intraluminal route) or by moving up the mucous sheath outside the catheter (periurethral route). Hospital-acquired pathogens reach the patient's catheter or urine-collecting system on the hands of hospital personnel, in contaminated solutions or irrigants, and via contaminated instruments or disinfectants. Bacteria usually enter the catheter system at the catheter–collecting tube junction or at the drainage bag portal. The organisms then ascend intraluminally into the bladder within 24 to 72 h. Alternatively, the patient's own bowel flora may colonize the perineal skin and periurethral area and reach the bladder via the external surface of the catheter. This route is particularly common in women. Recent studies have demonstrated the importance of the attachment and growth of bacteria on the inner surface of the catheter in the pathogenesis of catheter-associated urinary tract infection. Such bacteria growing in biofilms on the inner surface of the catheter eventually produce encrustations consisting of bacteria, bacterial glycocalyces, host urinary proteins, and urinary salts. These encrustations provide a refuge for bacteria and may protect them from antimicrobials and phagocytes.

Clinically, most catheter-associated infections cause minimal symptoms and no fever and often resolve after withdrawal of the catheter. The frequency of upper tract infection associated with catheter-induced bacteriuria is unknown. Gram-negative bacteremia, which follows catheter-associated bacteriuria in 1 to 2 percent of cases, is the most significant recognized complication of catheter-induced urinary infections. The catheterized urinary tract has repeatedly been demonstrated to be the most common source of gram-negative bacteremia in hospitalized patients, generally accounting for about 30 percent of cases.

Catheter-associated urinary tract infections can sometimes be prevented in patients catheterized for less than 2 weeks by use of a sterile closed collecting system, by attention to aseptic technique during insertion and care of the catheter, and by measures to minimize cross-infection. Other preventive approaches, including short courses of systemic antimicrobial therapy, topical application of periurethral antimicrobial ointments, use of preconnected catheter–drainage tube units, and addition of antimicrobials to the drainage bag, have all been protective in one or more controlled trials but are not recommended for general use. Despite precautions, the majority of patients catheterized for longer than 2 weeks eventually develop bacteriuria. The need for treatment as well as the optimal type and duration of treatment for such patients with asymptomatic bacteriuria have not been established. Removal of the catheter in conjunction with a short course of antibiotics to which the organism is susceptible probably constitutes the best course of action and nearly always eradicates bacteriuria. Treatment of asymptomatic catheter-associated bacteriuria may be of greatest benefit to elderly women, who most often develop symptoms if left untreated. If the catheter cannot be removed, antibiotic therapy usually proves to be unsuccessful and may in fact result in infection with a more resistant strain. In this situation, the bacteriuria should be ignored unless the patient develops symptoms or is at high risk of developing bacteremia. In these cases, use of systemic antibiotics or urinary bladder antiseptics may reduce the degree of bacteriuria and the likelihood of bacteremia. Because of spinal cord injury, incontinence, or other factors, some patients in hospitals or nursing homes require long-term or semipermanent bladder catheterization. Measures intended to prevent infection have been largely unsuccessful, and essentially all such chronically catheterized patients develop bacteriuria. If feasible, intermittent catheterization by a nurse or by the patient appears to reduce the incidence of bacteriuria and associated complications in such patients. Treatment should be provided when symptomatic infections arise, but treatment of asymptomatic bacteriuria in such patients has no apparent benefit.

DIAGNOSTIC TESTING Although many authorities have recommended that urine culture and antimicrobial susceptibility testing be performed for any patient with a suspected urinary tract infection, it may be more practical and cost-effective to manage women who have symptoms characteristic of acute uncomplicated cystitis without an initial urine culture. Two approaches to presumptive therapy have generally been used. In the first, treatment is initiated solely on the basis of a typical history and/or typical findings on physical examination. In the second, women with symptoms and signs of acute cystitis and without complicating factors are managed with urinary microscopy (or, alternatively, with a leukocyte esterase test). A positive result for pyuria and/or bacteriuria provides enough evidence of infection to indicate that urine culture and susceptibility testing can be omitted

and the patient treated empirically. Urine should be cultured, however, when a woman's symptoms and urine-examination findings leave the diagnosis of cystitis in question. Pretherapy cultures and susceptibility testing also are essential in the management of all patients with suspected upper tract infections and of those with complicating factors, as in these situations any of a variety of pathogens may be involved and antibiotic therapy is best tailored to the individual organism.

℞ TREATMENT

The following principles underlie the treatment of urinary tract infections:

1. In most circumstances, a quantitative urine culture, a Gram stain, or an alternative rapid diagnostic test should be performed to confirm infection before treatment is begun. When culture results become available, antimicrobial sensitivity testing should be used to direct therapy.
2. Factors predisposing to infection, such as obstruction and calculi, should be identified and corrected if possible.
3. Relief of clinical symptoms does not always indicate bacteriologic cure.
4. Each course of treatment should be classified after its completion as a failure (symptoms and/or bacteriuria not eradicated during therapy or in the immediate posttreatment culture) or a cure (resolution of symptoms and elimination of bacteriuria). Recurrent infections should be classified as same-strain or different-strain and as early (occurring within 2 weeks of the end of therapy) or late.
5. In general, uncomplicated infections confined to the lower urinary tract respond to short courses of therapy, while upper tract infections require longer treatment. After therapy, early recurrences due to the same strain may result from an unresolved upper tract focus of infection but often (especially after short-course therapy for cystitis) result from persistent vaginal colonization rather than from recurrent bladder infection. Recurrences more than 2 weeks after the cessation of therapy nearly always represent reinfection with a new strain.
6. Community-acquired infections, especially initial infections, are usually due to antibiotic-sensitive strains.
7. In patients with repeated infections, instrumentation, or recent hospitalization, the presence of antibiotic-resistant strains should be suspected.

The anatomic location of a urinary tract infection greatly influences the success or failure of a therapeutic regimen. Bladder bacteriuria (cystitis) can usually be eliminated with nearly any antimicrobial to which the infecting strain is sensitive; in the past, it was demonstrated that as little as a single dose of 500 mg of intramuscular kanamycin eliminated bladder bacteriuria in most cases. With upper tract infections, however, single-dose therapy fails in the majority of cases, and even a 7-day course is unsuccessful in many instances. Longer periods of treatment (2 to 6 weeks) aimed at eradicating a persistent focus of infection may be necessary in some cases.

In *acute uncomplicated cystitis*, more than 80 percent of infections are due to *E. coli*, and, although resistance patterns vary geographically, most strains are sensitive to many antibiotics. Single doses of trimethoprim-sulfamethoxazole (four single-strength tablets), trimethoprim alone (400 mg), sulfa alone (2.0 g), and most fluoroquinolones (norfloxacin, ciprofloxacin, ofloxacin) have been used successfully to treat acute uncomplicated episodes of cystitis. A single 3-g dose of amoxicillin appears to result in lower cure rates than these other agents, especially when infection is due to amoxicillin-resistant strains. In most areas, about one-third of *E. coli* strains causing acute cystitis are amoxicillin-resistant.

The advantages of single-dose therapy include less expense, ensured compliance, fewer side effects, and perhaps less intense pressure favoring the selection of resistant organisms in the intestinal, vaginal, or perineal flora. However, several studies have suggested that more recurrences develop shortly after single-dose therapy than after 3 to 7 days of treatment and that single-dose therapy does not eradicate vaginal colonization with *E. coli*. Nevertheless, single-dose therapy does appear to be safe and efficacious for women presenting with acute uncomplicated cystitis. Single-dose therapy should be used only for reliable patients whose posttreatment follow-up can be ensured and for patients who have had symptoms for less than 7 days. A 3-day course of therapy with trimethoprim-sulfamethoxazole, trimethoprim, norfloxacin, ciprofloxacin, or ofloxacin appears to preserve the low rate of side effects of single-dose therapy while improving efficacy. Neither single-dose nor 3-day therapy should be used for women with symptoms or signs of pyelonephritis, urologic abnormalities or stones, or previous infections due to antibiotic-resistant organisms. Males with urinary tract infection often have urologic abnormalities or prostatic involvement and hence are not candidates for single-dose or 3-day therapy. They should generally receive a 7- to 14-day course.

The choice of treatment for women with acute urethritis depends on the etiologic agent involved. In chlamydial infection, doxycycline (100 mg orally bid for 7 days) should be used. Women with acute dysuria and frequency, negative urine cultures, and no pyuria usually do not respond to antimicrobial agents.

In women, *acute uncomplicated pyelonephritis* without accompanying clinical evidence of calculi or urologic disease is due to *E. coli* in most cases. Although the optimal route and duration of therapy have not been established, a 14-day course of trimethoprim-sulfamethoxazole, a fluoroquinolone, an aminoglycoside, or a third-generation cephalosporin is usually adequate. Ampicillin or amoxicillin should not be used as initial therapy because 20 to 30 percent of strains of *E. coli* are now resistant to these drugs in vitro. In some areas, more than 20 percent of *E. coli* strains causing acute pyelonephritis are resistant to trimethoprim-sulfamethoxazole; alternative therapies should be used in such areas. For at least the first few days of treatment, antibiotics should probably be given intravenously to most patients, but patients with mild symptoms can be treated with 2 weeks of an oral antibiotic (usually trimethoprim-sulfamethoxazole, ciprofloxacin, or ofloxacin). Patients who fail to respond to treatment within 72 h or who relapse after therapy should be evaluated for unrecognized suppurative foci, calculi, or urologic disease. If the results are negative, re-treatment for 2 to 6 weeks to eliminate a presumed upper tract focus causing recurrent bacteriuria should be given.

Complicated urinary tract infections (those arising in a setting of catheterization, instrumentation, urologic anatomic or functional abnormalities, stones, obstruction, immunosuppression, renal disease, or diabetes) are typically due to hospital-acquired bacteria, including *E. coli*, *Klebsiella*, *Proteus*, *Serratia*, *Pseudomonas*, enterococci, and staphylococci. Many of the infecting strains are antibiotic-resistant. Empirical antibiotic therapy ideally provides broad-spectrum coverage against these pathogens. In patients with minimal symptoms, oral therapy with a fluoroquinolone, such as ciprofloxacin or ofloxacin, can be administered until culture results and antibiotic sensitivities are known. In patients with more severe illness, including acute pyelonephritis or suspected urosepsis, hospitalization and parenteral therapy should be undertaken. Commonly used empirical regimens include imipenem alone, a penicillin or cephalosporin plus an aminoglycoside, and (when the involvement of enterococci is unlikely) ceftriaxone or ceftazidime. When information on the antimicrobial sensitivity pattern of the infecting strain becomes available, a more specific antimicrobial regimen can be selected. Therapy should generally be administered for 7 to 21 days, with the exact duration depending on the severity of the infection and the susceptibility of the infecting strain. Follow-up cultures 2 to 4 weeks after cessation of therapy should be performed to demonstrate cure.

In *pregnancy*, acute cystitis can be managed with 3 to 7 days of treatment with amoxicillin, nitrofurantoin, or a cephalosporin. All pregnant women should be screened for asymptomatic bacteriuria during the first trimester and, if bacteriuric, should be treated with one of the regimens just outlined. After treatment, a culture should be performed to ensure cure, and cultures should be repeated monthly thereafter until delivery. Acute pyelonephritis in pregnancy should be managed with hospitalization and parenteral antibiotic therapy, generally with a cephalosporin or an extended-spectrum penicillin. Continuous low-dose prophylaxis with nitrofurantoin should be given to women who have recurrent infections during pregnancy.

Asymptomatic bacteriuria should be documented by at least two positive cultures before treatment is given. Seven days of therapy with an oral agent to which the organism is sensitive should be given initially. If bacteriuria persists, it can be monitored without further treatment in most patients. High-risk patients with neutropenia, renal transplants, or other complicating conditions may require longer treatment.

UROLOGIC EVALUATION   Very few women with recurrent urinary tract infections have correctable lesions discovered at cystoscopy or upon intravenous pyelography, and these procedures should not be undertaken routinely in such cases. Urologic evaluation should be performed in selected instances—namely, in women with relapsing infection, a history of childhood infections, stones or painless hematuria, or recurrent pyelonephritis. Most males with urinary infection should be considered to have complicated infection and thus should be evaluated urologically. Possible exceptions include young men who have cystitis associated with sexual activity, who are uncircumcised, or who have AIDS. Men or women presenting with acute infection and signs or symptoms suggestive of an obstruction or stones should undergo urologic evaluation, generally by means of ultrasound.

PROGNOSIS   In patients with uncomplicated cystitis or pyelonephritis, treatment ordinarily results in complete resolution of symptoms. Lower tract infections in women are of concern mainly because they cause discomfort, morbidity, loss of time from work, and substantial health-care costs. Cystitis also may result in upper tract infection or in bacteremia (especially during instrumentation), but little evidence suggests that renal impairment follows. When repeated episodes of cystitis occur, they are nearly always reinfections, not relapses.

Acute uncomplicated pyelonephritis in adults rarely progresses to renal functional impairment and chronic renal disease. Repeated upper tract infections often represent relapse rather than reinfection, and a vigorous search for renal calculi or an underlying urologic abnormality should be undertaken. If neither is found, 6 weeks of chemotherapy may be useful in eradicating an unresolved focus of infection.

Repeated symptomatic urinary tract infections in children and in adults with obstructive uropathy, neurogenic bladder, structural renal disease, or diabetes progress to chronic renal disease with unusual frequency. Asymptomatic bacteriuria in these groups as well as in adults without urologic disease or obstruction predisposes to increased numbers of episodes of symptomatic infection but does not result in renal impairment in most instances.

PREVENTION   Patients with frequent symptomatic infections may benefit from long-term administration of low-dose antibiotics directed at preventing recurrences. Daily or thrice-weekly administration of a single dose of trimethoprim/sulfamethoxazole (80/400 mg), trimethoprim alone (100 mg), or nitrofurantoin (50 mg) has been particularly effective. Prophylaxis should be initiated only after bacteriuria has been eradicated with a full-dose treatment regimen. Women who have more than two infections every 6 months are candidates for such prophylaxis. The same regimens can be used after sexual intercourse to prevent episodes of symptomatic infection in women in whom these episodes are temporally related to intercourse. Other patients for whom prophylaxis appears to have some merit include men with chronic prostatitis; patients undergoing prostatectomy, both during the operation and in the postoperative period; and pregnant women with asymptomatic bacteriuria. All pregnant women should be screened for bacteriuria in the first trimester and should be treated if bacteriuria is demonstrated.

When infection of the renal pyramids develops in association with vascular diseases of the kidney or with urinary tract obstruction, renal papillary necrosis is likely to result. Patients with diabetes, sickle cell disease, chronic alcoholism, and vascular disease seem peculiarly susceptible to this complication. Hematuria, pain in the flank or abdomen, and chills and fever are the most common presenting symptoms. Acute renal failure with oliguria or anuria sometimes develops. Rarely, sloughing of a pyramid may take place without symptoms in a patient with chronic urinary infection, and the diagnosis is made when the necrotic tissue is passed in the urine or identified as a "ring shadow" on pyelography. If renal function deteriorates suddenly in a diabetic individual or a patient with chronic obstruction, the diagnosis of renal papillary necrosis should be entertained, even in the absence of fever or pain. Renal papillary necrosis is often bilateral; when it is unilateral, however, nephrectomy may be a life-saving approach to the management of overwhelming infection.

RENAL AND PERINEPHRIC ABSCESS

See Chap. 127

PROSTATITIS

The term *prostatitis* has been used for various inflammatory conditions affecting the prostate, including acute and chronic infections with specific bacteria and, more commonly, instances in which signs and symptoms of prostatic inflammation are present but no specific organisms can be detected. Patients with acute bacterial prostatitis can usually be identified on the basis of typical symptoms and signs, pyuria, and bacteriuria. To classify a patient with suspected chronic prostatitis correctly, first-void and midstream urine specimens, a prostatic expressate, and a postmassage urine specimen should be quantitatively cultured and evaluated for numbers of leukocytes. On the basis of the results of these studies, patients can be classified as having chronic bacterial prostatitis, chronic nonbacterial prostatitis, or prostatodynia. Patients with suspected chronic prostatitis usually have low back pain, perineal or testicular discomfort, mild dysuria, and lower urinary obstructive symptoms. Microscopic pyuria may be the only objective manifestation of prostatic disease.

ACUTE BACTERIAL PROSTATITIS When it occurs spontaneously, this disease generally affects young men; however, it may also be associated with an indwelling urethral catheter. It is characterized by fever, chills, dysuria, and a tense or boggy, extremely tender prostate. Although prostatic massage usually produces purulent secretions with a large number of bacteria on culture, bacteremia may result from manipulation of the inflamed gland. For this reason and because the etiologic agent can usually be identified by Gram's staining and culture of urine, vigorous prostatic massage should be avoided. In non-catheter-associated cases, the infection is generally due to common gram-negative urinary tract pathogens (*E. coli* or *Klebsiella*). Initially, intravenous trimethoprim-sulfamethoxazole, a cephalosporin, a fluoroquinolone, or an aminoglycoside can be administered if gram-negative rods are visible in urine, and a cephalosporin or nafcillin can be given if gram-positive cocci are detected. Although many of these drugs do not readily diffuse into the noninflamed prostate gland, the response to antibiotics in acute bacterial prostatitis is usually prompt, perhaps because drugs penetrate more readily into the acutely inflamed prostate. In catheter-associated cases, the spectrum of etiologic agents is broader, including hospital-acquired gram-negative rods and enterococci. The urinary Gram stain may be particularly helpful in such cases. Imipenem, an aminoglycoside, a fluoroquinolone, or a third-generation cephalosporin should be used for initial therapy until the organism has been isolated and its susceptibilities have been determined. The long-term prognosis is good, although in some instances acute infection may result in abscess formation, epididymoorchitis, seminal vesiculitis, septicemia, and residual chronic bacterial prostatitis. Since the advent of antibiotics, the frequency of acute bacterial

prostatitis has diminished markedly. In many instances, infections diagnosed as acute prostatitis are probably cases of posterior urethritis.

CHRONIC BACTERIAL PROSTATITIS This entity is now infrequent but should be considered in men with a history of recurrent bacteriuria. Symptoms are usually lacking, and the prostate usually feels normal on palpation. Obstructive symptoms or perineal pain develops in some patients. Intermittently, infection spreads to the bladder, producing frequency, urgency, and dysuria. A pattern of relapsing infection in a middle-aged man strongly suggests chronic bacterial prostatitis. Classically, the diagnosis is established by culture of *E. coli*, *Klebsiella*, *Proteus*, or other uropathogenic bacteria from the expressed prostatic secretion or postmassage urine in higher quantities than are found in first-void or midstream urine. Antibiotics promptly relieve the symptoms associated with acute exacerbations but have been less effective in eradicating the focus of chronic infection in the prostate. The relative ineffectiveness of antimicrobials for long-term cure results in part from the poor penetration of the prostate by most of these drugs; the low pH that prevails in this organ precludes the passage of most agents. Fluoroquinolones, including ciprofloxacin and ofloxacin, have been more successful than other antimicrobials, but they must be given for at least 12 weeks to be effective. Patients with frequent episodes of acute cystitis can be managed with prolonged courses of antimicrobials (usually a sulfonamide, trimethoprim, or nitrofurantoin), with a view toward suppressing symptoms and keeping the bladder urine sterile. Total prostatectomy obviously results in the cure of chronic prostatitis but is associated with considerable morbidity. Transurethral prostatectomy is safer but cures only one-third of patients.

NONBACTERIAL PROSTATITIS Patients who present with symptoms and signs of prostatitis, increased leukocytes in expressed prostatic secretion and postmassage urine, no bacterial growth in cultures, and no history of recurrent episodes of bacterial prostatitis are classified as having nonbacterial prostatitis. Prostatic inflammation can be considered present when the expressed prostatic secretion and postmassage urine contain at least 10-fold more leukocytes than the first-void and midstream urine specimens or when the expressed prostatic secretion contains ≥1000 leukocytes per microliter.

The presumably infectious etiology of this condition remains unidentified. Evidence for a causative role of both *U. urealyticum* and *C. trachomatis* has been presented but is not conclusive. Since most cases of nonbacterial prostatitis occur in young, sexually active men and since many cases follow an episode of nonspecific urethritis, the causative agent may well be sexually transmitted. The effectiveness of antimicrobial agents in this condition remains uncertain. Some patients benefit from a 4- to 6-week course of treatment with erythromycin, doxycycline, trimethoprim-sulfamethoxazole, or a fluoroquinolone, but controlled trials are lacking.

PROSTATODYNIA Patients who have symptoms and signs of prostatitis but no evidence of prostatic inflammation (normal leukocyte counts) and negative urine cultures are classified as having prostatodynia. Despite their symptoms, these patients most likely do not have prostatic infection and should not be given antimicrobial agents.

BIBLIOGRAPHY

AGACE W et al: Host resistance to urinary tract infection, in *Molecular Pathogenesis and Clinical Management*, HLT Mobley, JW Warren (eds). Washington, DC, ASM Press, 1996, pp 221–245

BAILEY RR: Management of lower urinary tract infections. Drugs 45(Suppl 3):139, 1993

BERGERON MG: Treatment of pyelonephritis in adults. Med Clin North Am 79:619, 1995

EISENSTADT J, WASHINGTON JA: Diagnostic microbiology for bacteria and yeasts causing urinary tract infections, in *Molecular Pathogenesis and Clinical Management*, HLT Mobley, JW Warren (eds). Washington, DC, ASM Press, 1996, pp 29–67

GRATACOS E et al: Screening and treatment of asymptomatic bacteriuria in pregnancy prevent pyelonephritis. J Infect Dis 169:1390, 1994

HOOTON TM et al: A prospective study of risk factors for symptomatic urinary tract infection in young women. N Engl J Med 335:468, 1996

JOHNSON JR: Virulence factors in *E. coli* urinary tract infections. Clin Microbiol Rev 4:80, 1991

————: Treatment and prevention of urinary tract infections, in *Molecular Pathogenesis and Clinical Management,* HLT Mobley, JW Warren (eds). Washington, DC, ASM Press, 1996, pp 95–118

KUNIN CM: Urinary tract infection in females. Clin Infect Dis 18:1, 1994

LIPSKY BA: Urinary tract infections in men. Ann Intern Med 110:138, 1989

SCHAEFFER AJ: Urinary tract infection in men—state of the art. Infection (Suppl 1):S19, 1994

STAMM WE, HOOTON TM: Management of urinary tract infections in adults. N Engl J Med 329:1328, 1993

————: Catheter-associated urinary tract infections: Epidemiology, pathogenesis, prevention. Am J Med 91(Suppl 3B):655, 1991

132	*James H. Maguire*

OSTEOMYELITIS

Osteomyelitis, an infection of bone, is caused most commonly by pyogenic bacteria and mycobacteria. Classification of cases on the basis of the causative agent and the route, duration, and anatomic location of infection provides a useful framework for evaluating the patient and planning treatment.

PATHOGENESIS AND PATHOLOGY Microorganisms enter bone by the hematogenous route, by direct introduction from a contiguous focus of infection, or by a penetrating wound. Trauma, ischemia, and foreign bodies enhance the susceptibility of bone to microbial invasion by exposing sites to which bacteria can bind. Phagocytes attempt to contain the infections and, in the process, release enzymes that lyse bone. Pus spreads into vascular channels, raising intraosseous pressure and impairing the flow of blood; as the untreated infection becomes chronic, ischemic necrosis of bone results in the separation of large devascularized fragments (*sequestra*). When pus breaks through the cortex, subperiosteal or soft tissue abscesses form, and the elevated periosteum deposits new bone (the *involucrum*) around the sequestrum. Bacteria escape host defenses by adhering tightly to damaged bone and by coating themselves and underlying surfaces with a protective polysaccharide-rich biofilm.

Microorganisms, infiltrates of neutrophils, and congested or thrombosed blood vessels are the principal histologic findings of acute osteomyelitis. The distinguishing feature of chronic osteomyelitis is necrotic bone, which is characterized by the absence of living osteocytes. Mononuclear cells predominate in chronic infections, and granulation and fibrous tissues replace bone that has been resorbed by osteoclasts. In the chronic stage, organisms may be too few to be seen.

HEMATOGENOUS OSTEOMYELITIS Hematogenous infection accounts for approximately 20 percent of cases of osteomyelitis and primarily affects children, in whom the long bones are infected, and older adults and intravenous drug users, in whom the spine is the usual site of infection.

Acute Hematogenous Osteomyelitis Infection usually involves a single bone, most commonly the tibia, femur, or humerus. Bacteria settle in the well-perfused metaphysis, where functioning phagocytes are scarce, a network of venous sinusoids slows the flow of blood, and fenestrations in capillaries allow organisms to escape into the extravascular space. Because vascular anatomy changes with age, hematogenous infection of long bones is uncommon during adulthood and, when it occurs, usually involves the diaphysis.

In children, the source of bacteremia is often inapparent, although there may have been recent blunt trauma to the extremity leading to a small intraosseous hematoma or vascular obstruction. On presentation, the child usually appears acutely ill, with high fever, chills, localized pain and tenderness, and leukocytosis. Cutaneous erythema

and swelling indicate extension of pus through the cortex. During infancy and after puberty, infection may spread through the epiphysis into the joint space. In children of other ages (i.e., between infancy and puberty), extension of infection through the cortex results in involvement of joints if the metaphysis is intracapsular. Thus, septic arthritis of the elbow, shoulder, and hip may complicate osteomyelitis of the proximal radius, humerus, and femur, respectively.

Plain radiographs initially show soft tissue swelling, but the first change in bone—a periosteal reaction—is not evident until at least 10 days after the onset of infection. Lytic changes can be detected after 2 to 6 weeks, when 50 to 75 percent of bone density has been lost. Rarely, a well-circumscribed lytic lesion, or *Brodie's abscess*, is seen in a child who has been in pain for several months but has had no fever.

Chronic Hematogenous Osteomyelitis With prompt treatment, fewer than 5 percent of cases of acute hematogenous osteomyelitis progress to chronic osteomyelitis. On average, 10 days are required for the formation of necrotic bone, but plain radiographs are unable to detect sequestra or sclerotic new bone for many weeks.

A protracted clinical course, long periods of quiescence, and recurrent exacerbations are characteristic of chronic osteomyelitis. Sinus tracts between bone and skin may drain purulent material and occasionally pieces of necrotic bone. An increase in drainage, pain, or the erythrocyte sedimentation rate (ESR) signals an exacerbation. Fever is unusual except when obstruction of a sinus tract leads to soft tissue infection. Rare late complications include pathologic fractures, squamous cell carcinoma of the sinus tract, and amyloidosis.

Vertebral Osteomyelitis Organisms reach the well-perfused vertebral body of adults via spinal arteries and quickly spread from the end plate into the disk space and then to the adjacent vertebral body. The infection may originate in the urinary tract and reach the spine via the prostatic venous (Batson's) plexus; such cases develop particularly often among elderly men. Other sources of bacteremia include endocarditis, soft tissue infection, and a contaminated intravenous line; these sources usually are obvious. Diabetes mellitus, hemodialysis, and intravenous drug use carry an increased risk of spinal infection. Penetrating injuries and surgical procedures to the spine may cause nonhematogenous vertebral osteomyelitis or infection localized to the disk.

Most patients with vertebral osteomyelitis report neck or back pain; 15 percent describe atypical pain in the chest, the abdomen, or an extremity that is due to irritation of nerve roots. Symptoms are localized to the lumbar spine more often than to the thoracic spine (more than 50 percent vs. 35 percent of cases) or the cervical spine in pyogenic infections, but the thoracic spine is involved most commonly in tuberculous spondylitis (Pott's disease). Percussion over the involved vertebra elicits tenderness, and physical examination may reveal spasm of the paraspinal muscles and a limitation of motion. More than 50 percent of patients experience a subacute illness in which a vague, dull pain gradually intensifies over the course of 2 to 3 months; fever is low grade or absent, and the white blood cell count is normal. An acute presentation with high fever and toxicity is less common and suggests ongoing bacteremia.

Usually, by the time the patient seeks medical attention, the ESR is elevated, and plain radiographs show irregular erosions in the end plates of adjacent vertebral bodies and narrowing of the intervening disk space. This radiographic pattern is virtually diagnostic of bacterial infection because tumors and other diseases of the spine rarely cross the disk space. Computed tomography (CT) or magnetic resonance imaging (MRI) may demonstrate epidural, paraspinal, retropharyngeal, mediastinal, retroperitoneal, or psoas abscesses that originate in the spine. An epidural abscess may evolve suddenly or over the course of several weeks; irreversible paralysis may be the consequence of failure to recognize the classic clinical presentation of a spinal epidural abscess, consisting of spinal pain progressing to radicular pain and weakness.

Microbiology More than 95 percent of cases of hematogenous osteomyelitis are caused by a single organism. *Staphylococcus aureus* accounts for 50 percent of isolates. Other common pathogens include group B streptococci and *Escherichia coli* during the newborn period and group A streptococci and *Haemophilus influenzae* in early childhood. Vertebral osteomyelitis is due to *E. coli* and other enteric bacilli in approximately 25 percent of cases. *S. aureus, Pseudomonas aeruginosa,* and *Serratia* infections are associated with intravenous drug use in some parts of the United States and may involve the sacroiliac, sternoclavicular, or pubic joints as well as the spine. *Salmonella* spp. and *S. aureus* are the major causes of long-bone osteomyelitis complicating sickle cell anemia and other hemoglobinopathies. Tuberculosis and brucellosis affect the spine more often than other bones. Other common sites of tuberculous osteomyelitis include the small bones of the hands and feet, the metaphyses of long bones, the ribs, and the sternum.

Unusual causes of hematogenous osteomyelitis include disseminated histoplasmosis, coccidioidomycosis, and blastomycosis in endemic areas. Immunocompromised persons on rare occasions develop osteomyelitis due to atypical mycobacteria or to species of *Candida, Cryptococcus, Aspergillus,* or *Pneumocystis.* Syphilis, yaws, varicella, and vaccinia may involve bone. The etiology of chronic relapsing multifocal osteomyelitis, an inflammatory condition of children that is characterized by recurrent episodes of painful lytic lesions in multiple bones, has not yet been identified.

OSTEOMYELITIS SECONDARY TO A CONTIGUOUS FOCUS OF INFECTION   Clinical Features   This broad category of osteomyelitis includes infections introduced by penetrating injuries and surgical procedures and by direct extension of infection from adjacent soft tissues. It accounts for the greatest number of cases of osteomyelitis and occurs most commonly in adults.

Frequently, the diagnosis is not made until the infection has already become chronic. The pain, fever, and inflammatory signs due to acute osteomyelitis may be attributed to the original injury or soft tissue infection. An indolent infection may become apparent only weeks or months later, when a sinus tract develops, a surgical wound breaks down, or a fracture fails to heal. It may be impossible to distinguish radiographic abnormalities due to osteomyelitis from those due to the precipitating condition.

A special type of contiguous-focus osteomyelitis occurs in the setting of peripheral vascular disease and nearly always involves the small bones of the feet of adult diabetic patients. Diabetic neuropathy exposes the foot to frequent trauma and pressure sores, and the patient may be unaware of infection as it spreads into bone. Poor tissue perfusion impairs normal inflammatory responses and wound healing and creates a milieu that is conducive to anaerobic infections. It is often during the evaluation of a nonhealing ulcer, a swollen toe, or acute cellulitis that a radiograph provides the first evidence of osteomyelitis. If bone is palpable during examination of the base of an ulcer with a blunt surgical probe, osteomyelitis is likely.

Microbiology   *S. aureus* is a pathogen in more than half of cases of contiguous-focus osteomyelitis. However, in contrast to hematogenous osteomyelitis, these infections often are polymicrobial and are more likely to involve gram-negative and anaerobic bacteria. Hence a mixture of staphylococci, streptococci, enteric organisms, and anaerobic bacteria may be isolated from a diabetic foot infection or pelvic osteomyelitis underlying a decubitus ulcer. Aerobic and anaerobic bacteria cause osteomyelitis following surgery or soft tissue infection of the oropharynx, paranasal sinuses, gastrointestinal tract, or female genital tract. *S. aureus* is the principal cause of postoperative infections; coagulase-negative staphylococci are common pathogens after implantation of orthopedic appliances; and these organisms as well as gram-negative enteric bacilli, atypical mycobacteria, and *Mycoplasma* may cause sternal osteomyelitis after cardiac surgery. Infection with *P. aeruginosa* is frequently associated with puncture wounds of the foot or with thermal burns, and *Pasteurella multocida* infection commonly follows cat bites (see Chap. 135).

DIAGNOSIS   Early diagnosis of acute osteomyelitis is critical because prompt antibiotic therapy may prevent the necrosis of bone. The evaluation usually begins with plain radiographs because of their ready availability, although they frequently show no abnormalities during early infection. The ESR and C-reactive protein levels are

elevated in most cases of active osteomyelitis, including those in which constitutional symptoms and leukocytosis are lacking. These findings are not specific to osteomyelitis, however, and the ESR is occasionally normal in early infections. In 95 percent of cases, the technetium radionuclide scan using ^{99m}Tc diphosphonate is positive within 24 h of the onset of symptoms. Falsely negative scans usually indicate obstruction of blood flow to the bone. Because the uptake of technetium reflects osteoblastic activity and skeletal vascularity, the bone scan cannot differentiate osteomyelitis from fractures, tumors, infarction, or neuropathic osteopathy. ^{67}Ga citrate– and ^{111}In-labeled leukocyte or immunoglobulin scans, which have greater specificity for inflammation, may help distinguish infectious from noninfectious processes and indicate inflammatory changes within bones that for other reasons are already abnormal on radiography and technetium scanning. Ultrasound can be used to diagnose osteomyelitis by the detection of subperiosteal fluid collections, soft tissue abscesses adjacent to bone, and periosteal thickening and elevation.

MRI is as sensitive as the bone scan for the diagnosis of acute osteomyelitis because it is able to detect changes in the water content of marrow. MRI yields better anatomic resolution of epidural abscesses and other soft tissue processes than CT and is currently the imaging technique of choice for vertebral osteomyelitis (see Fig. 132-1).

The role of diagnostic imaging in chronic osteomyelitis is to determine the presence of active infection and delineate the extent of debridement necessary to remove necrotic bone and abnormal soft tissues. Although plain films accurately reflect chronic changes, the CT scan is more sensitive for the detection of sequestra, sinus tracts, and soft tissue abscesses. Both CT and ultrasound are useful for

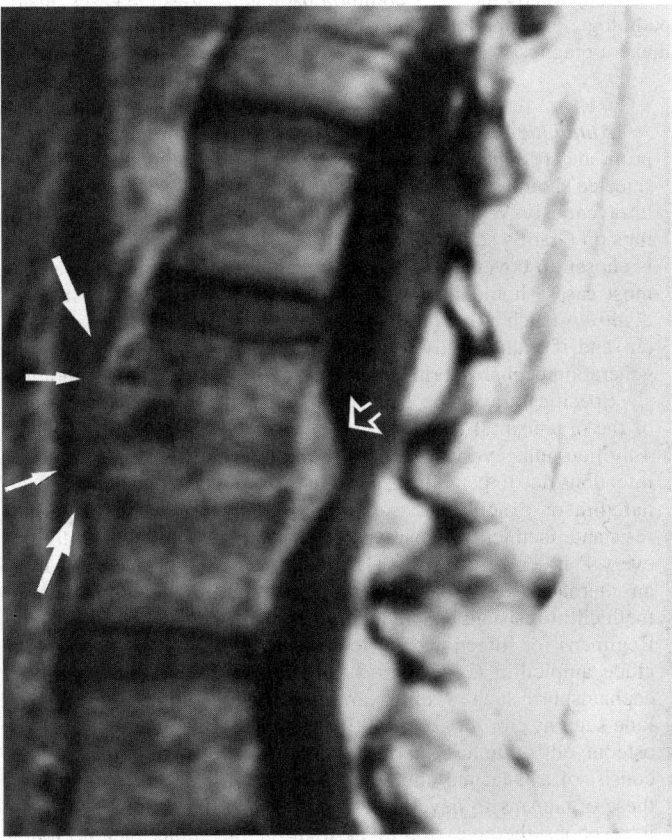

FIGURE 132-1   Osteomyelitis of the lumbar spine demonstrated on a sagittal T1-weighted magnetic resonance image after the administration of intravenous gadolinium. At L2–L3 there is involvement of the adjacent vertebral bodies and intervening disk. An epidural abscess compresses the thecal sac (open arrow), and the inflammatory process extends into the anterior prevertebral space (closed arrows).

guiding percutaneous aspiration of subperiosteal and soft tissue fluid collections. Sequential technetium and gallium or indium scans may help determine whether infection is active and may distinguish infection from noninflammatory bone changes; these methods do not, however, provide good anatomic detail. MRI provides detailed information about the activity and the anatomic extent of infection but does not always distinguish osteomyelitis from healing fractures and tumors. MRI is particularly useful in distinguishing cellulitis from osteomyelitis in the diabetic foot; however, no imaging modality consistently distinguishes infection from neuropathic osteopathy.

Appropriate samples for microbiologic studies should be obtained in all cases of suspected osteomyelitis before the initiation of antimicrobial therapy. Blood cultures are indicated in acute cases and are positive in more than one-third of cases of hematogenous osteomyelitis in children and in 25 percent of cases of vertebral osteomyelitis in adults. If the clinical picture demands immediate antibiotic therapy or if blood cultures are negative, samples from needle aspiration of pus in bone or soft tissues or from a bone biopsy should be obtained for culture.

The results of culture of specimens obtained by swabbing of a sinus tract or the base of an ulcer correlate poorly with the organisms infecting the bone. For this reason, in cases of chronic osteomyelitis and contiguous-focus osteomyelitis, samples for aerobic and anaerobic culture should be obtained from several sites by percutaneous needle aspiration, percutaneous biopsy, or intraoperative biopsy at the time of debridement. Isolates of coagulase-negative staphylococci and other organisms of low virulence should not automatically be disregarded as contaminants, especially in the presence of prosthetic materials. Special culture media may be necessary for the isolation of mycobacteria, fungi, and other, less common pathogens. In some cases, histopathologic examination of biopsy specimens may be the only way to make a diagnosis.

℞ **TREATMENT**

Antibiotic Therapy Antibiotics are administered only after appropriate specimens have been obtained for culture. The antibiotics selected should be bactericidal and, at least initially, should be given intravenously. When necessary, empirical therapy is guided by findings on Gram's staining of a specimen from the bone or abscess or is chosen to cover the most likely pathogens. Empirical therapy in most cases should include high doses of an agent active against *S. aureus* (such as oxacillin, nafcillin, a cephalosporin, or vancomycin) and, if gram-negative organisms are likely to be involved, a third-generation cephalosporin, an aminoglycoside, or a fluoroquinolone.

Specific intravenous therapy is based on the in vitro susceptibility of the organism(s) isolated from bone or blood. Penicillin G (3 to 4 million units every 4 h) is the drug of choice for the treatment of infections due to penicillin-sensitive staphylococci and streptococci; nafcillin or oxacillin (2 g every 4 h) is preferred for penicillin-resistant, methicillin-sensitive staphylococci. Cefazolin (1 to 2 g every 8 h) or vancomycin [15 mg/kg (up to 1 g) every 12 h] is an alternative for persons allergic to penicillins. Infections due to methicillin-resistant staphylococci are treated with vancomycin. Regimens for infections due to susceptible gram-negative rods include ampicillin (2 g every 4 h), cefazolin, a second-generation cephalosporin such as cefuroxime (1.5 g every 8 h), or a fluoroquinolone such as ciprofloxacin (400 mg every 12 h). Initial therapy for osteomyelitis due to *P. aeruginosa* or *Enterobacter* spp. should not consist of a β-lactam antibiotic alone because of the potential for these organisms to develop resistance during therapy. Appropriate intravenous therapies for *P. aeruginosa* infections include tobramycin (1.7 mg/kg every 8 h, or 5 to 7 mg/kg every 24 h) and a broad-spectrum β-lactam compound such as ticarcillin (3 g every 4 h), ceftazidime (1 to 2 g every 8 h), or aztreonam (1 to 2 g every 8 h); a fluoroquinolone may be substituted for one of the latter. *Enterobacter* infections can be treated with a fluoroquinolone alone or with combinations of a broad-spectrum β-lactam antibiotic and

gentamicin in the same doses as tobramycin. Serum levels of aminoglycosides should be monitored closely to avoid toxicity.

The duration of therapy is typically 4 to 6 weeks; at-home intravenous administration of antibiotics or oral therapy is appropriate for motivated and medically stable patients. Antibiotics that require infrequent dosing, such as ceftriaxone and vancomycin, facilitate home therapy. Children with acute hematogenous osteomyelitis routinely receive oral antibiotics after 5 to 10 days of parenteral therapy if signs of active infection have resolved; such treatment has been as successful as standard parenteral therapy. The doses of oral penicillins or cephalosporins required for the treatment of osteomyelitis are several times higher than the doses of these drugs given for common infections. Adults may not tolerate these high doses as well as children, and, except in the case of the fluoroquinolones, few data support the use of oral antibiotics by adults. Oral administration of an agent such as ciprofloxacin (750 mg every 12 h) or ofloxacin (400 mg every 12 h) has been as successful as intravenous administration of β-lactam antibiotics. Caution should be exercised in the use of fluoroquinolones as the sole agents for treatment of infection due to *S. aureus* or *P. aeruginosa* because resistance may develop during therapy. Oral administration of clindamycin (300 to 450 mg every 6 h) or metronidazole (500 mg every 8 h) results in high drug levels in serum and can take the place of intravenous regimens for the treatment of *Bacteroides* infections. Oral clindamycin has produced good results in therapy for osteomyelitis due to *S. aureus*, especially in children.

Serum minimal bactericidal concentrations (MBCs) against isolates of the responsible pathogen can be measured to document compliance and adequate serum levels in patients who receive an oral antibiotic. Otherwise, few data support the routine use of the MBC to monitor therapy for osteomyelitis.

Acute Osteomyelitis Early treatment of acute hematogenous osteomyelitis of childhood with 4 to 6 weeks of an appropriate antibiotic is usually successful; treatment for less than 3 weeks has resulted in a 10-fold greater rate of failure. Surgical intervention in childhood cases is indicated for intraosseous or subperiosteal abscesses, concomitant septic arthritis, and failure of the acute signs of infection to improve in 24 to 48 h. Acute hematogenous osteomyelitis of bones other than the spine in adults often requires surgical debridement.

Vertebral Osteomyelitis A 4- to 6-week course of treatment with an appropriate antibiotic is usually sufficient to cure vertebral osteomyelitis. Failure of the ESR to drop to no more than two-thirds of pretreatment levels is an indication for longer treatment. Surgery is seldom necessary, even in cases of many months' duration, except in instances of spinal instability, new or progressive neurologic deficits, large soft tissue abscesses that cannot be drained percutaneously, or a failure of medical treatment. Patients should maintain bed rest until back pain has declined to the point at which ambulation is possible. Body casts are no longer used. Spontaneous fusion of involved vertebrae occurs in the majority of cases after successful treatment.

Contiguous-Focus Osteomyelitis Even when diagnosed early, contiguous-focus osteomyelitis usually requires surgery in addition to 4 to 6 weeks of appropriate antibiotic therapy because of underlying soft tissue infection or damage to bone from an injury or surgery.

Chronic Osteomyelitis The risks and benefits of aggressive therapy for chronic osteomyelitis should be weighed before any attempt is made to eradicate the infection. Some patients with extensive disease prefer to live with their infections rather than undergo multiple surgical procedures, take prolonged courses of antimicrobial therapy, and face the risk of loss of an extremity. Such persons often benefit from intermittent courses of oral antibiotics to suppress acute exacerbations.

Once the decision has been made to treat chronic osteomyelitis aggressively, the patient's nutritional and metabolic status should be optimized to expedite healing of soft tissues and bone. Antibiotic administration should be started several days before surgery to reduce inflammation if the etiology of the infection is known preoperatively.

If not, antibiotic therapy should be withheld until surgical debridement. An empirical antibiotic regimen is started intraoperatively after culture specimens are obtained. A 4- to 6-week course of appropriate antibiotic therapy is given postoperatively on the basis of the susceptibility pattern of organisms isolated from the bone. The benefit of prolonged oral antibiotic therapy after 4 to 6 weeks of parenteral therapy remains unproven. There is insufficient information to recommend the routine use of hyperbaric oxygen to enhance the killing of microorganisms by phagocytes or of instillation pumps and antibiotic-impregnated methacrylate beads to deliver high levels of antibiotics to the bone.

The success of therapy for chronic osteomyelitis rests largely on the complete surgical removal of necrotic bone and abnormal soft tissues. Modern imaging techniques allow accurate preoperative delineation of tissues to be debrided, but it remains difficult for the surgeon to determine intraoperatively whether all necrotic and infected tissue has been removed. In the past, the inability to repair large defects in bone and soft tissue limited the extent of debridement. Muscle flaps and skin grafts are now used routinely to cover large soft tissue defects and fill dead space, and bone grafts and vascularized bone transfer may restore a seriously compromised bone to a functional state.

In infections of recent fractures, internal fixators are often left in place, and the infection is controlled by limited debridement and suppressive antibiotic therapy. Definitive surgical/antimicrobial therapy is delayed until after bony union of the fracture is achieved. If there is nonunion of the fracture or loosening of the fixator, the appliance should be removed, the bone debrided, and an external fixator or a new internal fixator applied.

Osteomyelitis of the small bones of the feet in persons with vascular disease also requires surgical treatment. The effectiveness of the surgery is limited by the blood supply to the site and the body's ability to heal the wound. Revascularization of the extremity is indicated if the vascular disease involves large arteries. In cases of decreased perfusion due to small-vessel disease, foot-sparing surgery may fail, and the best option is suppressive therapy or amputation. The duration of antibiotic therapy depends on the surgical procedure performed. When the infected bone is removed entirely but residual infection of soft tissues remains, antibiotic therapy should be given for 2 weeks; if amputation eliminates infected bone and soft tissue, standard surgical prophylaxis is given; otherwise, postoperative antibiotics must be given for 4 to 6 weeks.

BIBLIOGRAPHY

BRYSON YJ et al: High dose oral dicloxacillin treatment of acute staphylococcal osteomyelitis in children. J Pediatr 94:673, 1979

CAPUTO GM et al: Assessment and management of foot disease in patients with diabetes. N Engl J Med 331:854, 1994

CUNNINGHAM R et al: Clinical and molecular aspects of the pathogenesis of *Staphylococcus aureus* bone and joint infections. J Med Microbiol 44:157, 1996

DAROUICHE RO et al: Osteomyelitis associated with pressure sores. Arch Intern Med 154:753, 1994

ECKARDT JJ et al: An aggressive surgical approach to the management of chronic osteomyelitis. Clin Orthop 298:229, 1994

ESOLEN LM et al: *Pneumocystis carinii* osteomyelitis in a patient with common variable immunodeficiency. N Engl J Med 326:999, 1992

HENRY SL, GALLOWAY KP: Local antibacterial therapy for the management of orthopaedic infections. Pharmacokinetic considerations. Clin Pharmacokinet 29:36, 1995

HOPKINS KL et al: Gadolinium-DPTA-enhanced magnetic resonance imaging of musculoskeletal infectious processes. Skeletal Radiol 24:325, 1995

JAUREGUI LE: *Diagnosis and Management of Bone Infections.* New York, Marcel Dekker, 1995

LEW DP, WALDVOGEL FA: Quinolones and osteomyelitis: State-of-the-art. Drugs 49(Suppl 2):100, 1995

MAUCERI AA: Treatment of bone and joint infections utilizing a third-generation cephalosporin with an outpatient drug delivery device. HIAT Study Group. Am J Med 97(2a):14, 1995

MAY JW JR et al: Treatment of chronic traumatic bone wounds. Microvascular free tissue transfer: A 13-year experience in 96 patients. Ann Surg 214:241, 1991

MEIER JL, BEEKMANN SE: Mycobacterial and fungal infections of bones and joints. Curr Opin Rheumatol 7:329, 1995

NORDEN C et al: *Infections in Bones and Joints.* Boston, Blackwell Scientific, 1994

OSTERMANN PA et al: Local antibiotic therapy for severe open fractures. J Bone Joint Surg [Br] 77:93, 1995

SAPICO FL et al: Bone and joint infections in patients with infective endocarditis: Review of a 4-year experience. Clin Infect Dis 22:783, 1996

TORDA AJ et al: Pyogenic vertebral osteomyelitis: Analysis of 20 cases and review. Clin Infect Dis 20:320, 1995

WALDVOGEL FA et al: Osteomyelitis: A review of clinical features, therapeutic considerations, and unusual aspects. N Engl J Med 282:198, 1970

———, VASEY H: Osteomyelitis: The past decade. N Engl J Med 303:360, 1980

133

Dennis L. Stevens

INFECTIONS OF THE SKIN, MUSCLE, AND SOFT TISSUES

ANATOMIC RELATIONSHIPS: CLUES TO THE DIAGNOSIS OF SOFT TISSUE INFECTIONS Protection against infection of the epidermis is dependent on the mechanical barrier afforded by the stratum corneum, since the epidermis itself is devoid of blood vessels (Fig. 133-1). Disruption of this layer by burns, bites, abrasions, or foreign bodies allows penetration of bacteria to the deeper structures. Similarly, the hair follicle can serve as a portal either for components of the normal flora (e.g., *Staphylococcus*) or for extrinsic bacteria (e.g., *Pseudomonas* in hot-tub folliculitis). Intracellular infection of the squamous epithelium with vesicle formation may arise from cutaneous inoculation [as in infection with herpes simplex virus (HSV) type 1], from the dermal capillary plexus (as in varicella and infections due to other viruses associated with viremia), or from cutaneous nerve roots (as in herpes zoster). Bacteria infecting the epidermis, such as *Streptococcus pyogenes*, may be translocated laterally to deeper structures via lymphatics, an event that results in the rapid superficial spread of erysipelas. Later, engorgement or obstruction of lymphatics causes flaccid edema of the epidermis, another characteristic of erysipelas.

The rich plexus of capillaries beneath the dermal papillae provides nutrition to the stratum germinativum, and physiologic responses of this plexus produce important clinical signs and symptoms. For exam-

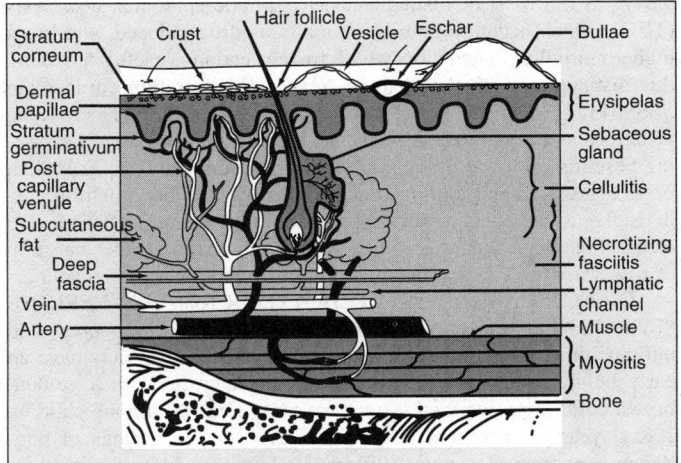

FIGURE 133-1 Structural components of the skin and soft tissue are identified at the left. Superficial infections are depicted along the top of the figure, and infections of the deeper structures of the soft tissue at the right. The rich capillary network beneath the dermal papillae plays a key role in the localization of infection and in the development of the acute inflammatory reaction.

ple, infective vasculitis of the plexus results in petechiae, Osler's nodes, Janeway lesions, and palpable purpura, which are important clues to the existence of endocarditis (Chap. 126). In addition, metastatic infection within this plexus can result in cutaneous manifestations of disseminated fungal infection (Chap. 207), gonococcal infection (Chap. 150), *Salmonella* infection (Chap. 158), *Pseudomonas* infection (i.e., ecthyma gangrenosum) (Chap. 157), meningococcemia (Chap. 149), and staphylococcal infection (Chap. 142). The plexus also provides access for bacteria to the circulation, thereby facilitating local spread or bacteremia. The postcapillary venules of this plexus are a major site of polymorphonuclear leukocyte sequestration, diapedesis, and chemotaxis to the site of cutaneous infection.

Exaggeration of these physiologic mechanisms by excessive levels of cytokines or bacterial toxins causes leukostasis, venous occlusion, and pitting edema. Edema with purple bullae and ecchymosis suggests loss of vascular integrity and necessitates exploration of the deeper structures for evidence of necrotizing fasciitis or myonecrosis. To make an early diagnosis, one must exercise a high level of suspicion in instances of unexplained fever and of pain and tenderness in the soft tissue, even in the absence of acute cutaneous inflammation.

INFECTIONS ASSOCIATED WITH VESICLES (Table 133-1) Vesicle formation due to infection is caused by viral proliferation within the epidermis. In varicella and variola, viremia precedes the onset of a diffuse centrifugal rash that progresses from macules to vesicles, then to pustules, and finally to scabs over the course of 1 to 2 weeks. Vesicles of varicella have a "dewdrop" appearance and develop in crops randomly about the trunk, extremities, and face over 3 to 4 days. Herpes zoster occurs in a single dermatome; the appearance of vesicles is preceded by pain for several days. Zoster may occur in persons of any age but is most common among immunosuppressed individuals and elderly patients, whereas most cases of varicella occur in young children. Vesicles due to HSV are found on or around the lips (HSV-1) or genitals (HSV-2) but may appear on the head and neck of young wrestlers (herpes gladiatorum) or on the digits of health care workers (herpetic whitlow). Coxsackievirus A16 characteristically causes vesicles on the hands, feet, and mouth of children. Orf is caused by a DNA virus related to smallpox virus and infects the fingers of individuals who work around goats and sheep. Molluscum contagiosum virus induces flaccid vesicles on the skin of healthy and immunocompromised individuals.

INFECTIONS ASSOCIATED WITH BULLAE (Table 133-1) Staphylococcal scalded-skin syndrome (SSSS) in neonates is caused by a toxin (exfoliatin) from phage group II *Staphylococcus aureus*. SSSS must be distinguished from toxic epidermal necrolysis (TEN), which occurs primarily in adults, is drug-induced, and has a higher mortality. Punch biopsy with frozen section is useful in making this distinction since the cleavage plane is the stratum corneum in SSSS (Fig. 133-1) and the stratum germinativum in TEN. Necrotizing fasciitis and gas gangrene also induce bulla formation (see "Necrotizing Fasciitis" below). Halophilic vibrio infection (see Chap. 161) can be as aggressive and fulminant as necrotizing fasciitis; a helpful clue in its diagnosis is a history of exposure to waters of the Gulf of Mexico or the Atlantic seaboard or (in a patient with cirrhosis) the ingestion of raw seafood. This organism is highly susceptible to tetracycline.

INFECTIONS ASSOCIATED WITH CRUSTED LESIONS (Table 133-1) Impetigo contagiosa is caused by *S. pyogenes*, and bullous impetigo is due to *S. aureus*. Both skin lesions may have an early bullous stage but then appear as thick crusts with a golden-brown color. Streptococcal lesions are most common among children 2 to 5 years of age, and epidemics may occur in settings of poor hygiene, particularly among children of lower socioeconomic status in tropical climates. It is important to recognize impetigo contagiosa because of its relationship to poststreptococcal glomerulonephritis. Superficial dermatophyte infection (ringworm) can occur on any skin surface, and skin scrapings with KOH staining are diagnostic. Primary infections with dimorphic fungi such as *Blastomyces* (Chap. 205) and

Table 133-1

Skin and Soft Tissue Infections

Lesion, Clinical Syndrome	Infectious Agent	Chapter
Vesicles		
Smallpox	Variola virus	188
Chickenpox	Varicella-zoster virus	185
Shingles (herpes zoster)	Varicella-zoster virus	185
Cold sores, herpetic whitlow, herpes gladiatorum	Herpes simplex virus	184
Hand-foot-and-mouth disease	Coxsackievirus A16	195
Orf	Parapoxvirus	188
Molluscum contagiosum	Pox-like virus	188
Bullae		
Staphylococcal scalded-skin syndrome	*Staphylococcus aureus*	142
Necrotizing fasciitis	*Streptococcus pyogenes, Clostridium* spp., mixed aerobes and anaerobes	169
Gas gangrene	*Clostridium* spp.	148
Halophilic vibrio	*Vibrio vulnificus*	161
Crusted lesions		
Bullous impetigo	*S. aureus*	142
Impetigo contagiosa	*S. pyogenes*	143
Ringworm	Superficial dermatophyte fungi	210
Sporotrichosis	*Sporothrix schenckii*	210
Histoplasmosis	*Histoplasma capsulatum*	203
Coccidioidomycosis	*Coccidioides immitis*	204
Blastomycosis	*Blastomyces dermatitidis*	205
Cutaneous leishmaniasis	*Leishmania* spp.	216
Cutaneous tuberculosis	*Mycobacterium tuberculosis*	171
Nocardiosis	*Nocardia asteroides*	167
Folliculitis		
Furunculosis	*S. aureus*	142
Hot-tub folliculitis	*Pseudomonas aeruginosa*	157
Swimmer's itch	*Schistosoma* spp.	224
Acne vulgaris	*Propionibacterium acnes*	55
Ulcers with or without eschars		
Anthrax	*Bacillus anthracis*	144
Ulceroglandular tularemia	*Francisella tularensis*	163
Bubonic plague	*Yersinia pestis*	164
Buruli ulcer	*Mycobacterium ulcerans*	173
Leprosy	*Mycobacterium leprae*	172
Cutaneous tuberculosis	*M. tuberculosis*	171
Erysipelas	*S. pyogenes*	143
Necrotizing fasciitis		
Streptococcal gangrene	*S. pyogenes*	143
Fournier's gangrene	Mixed aerobic and anaerobic bacteria	169
Myositis and myonecrosis		
Pyomyositis	*S. aureus*	142
Streptococcal necrotizing myositis	*S. pyogenes*	143
Gas gangrene	*Clostridium* spp.	148
Nonclostridial (crepitant) myositis	Mixed aerobic and anaerobic bacteria	169
Synergistic nonclostridial anaerobic myonecrosis	Mixed aerobic and anaerobic bacteria	169

Sporothrix schenckii (Chap. 210) can initially present as crusted skin lesions resembling ringworm. Disseminated infection with *Coccidioides immitis* (Chap. 204) also can involve the skin, and biopsy and culture should be performed on crusted lesions in patients from endemic areas. Crusted nodular lesions caused by *Mycobacterium chelonae* have recently been described in patients positive for human immunodeficiency virus. Treatment with clarithromycin looks promising.

FOLLICULITIS (Table 133-1) Hair follicles serve as a portal of entry for a number of bacteria, though *S. aureus* is the most common cause of localized folliculitis. Sebaceous glands empty into hair follicles and ducts and if blocked form sebaceous cysts, which may resemble staphylococcal abscesses or may become secondarily infected. Infection of sweat glands (hidradenitis suppurativa) can also mimic infection of hair follicles, particularly in the axillae. Chronic folliculitis is uncommon except in acne vulgaris, where constituents of the normal flora (e.g., *Propionibacterium acnes*) may play a role.

Diffuse folliculitis occurs in two settings. "Hot-tub folliculitis" is caused by *Pseudomonas aeruginosa* in waters that are insufficiently chlorinated and maintained at temperatures between 37 and 40°C. Infection is usually self-limited, though bacteremia and shock have been reported. Swimmer's itch occurs when a skin surface is exposed to water infested with freshwater avian schistosomes. Warm water temperatures and alkaline pH are suitable for molluscs that serve as intermediate hosts between bird and human. Free-swimming schistosomal cercariae (see Chap. 224) readily penetrate human hair follicles or pores but quickly die and elicit a brisk allergic reaction causing intense itching and erythema.

ULCERS WITH OR WITHOUT ESCHARS (Table 133-1) Cutaneous anthrax begins as a pruritic papule, which develops within days into an ulcer with surrounding vesicles and edema and then into an enlarging ulcer with black eschar. Cutaneous diphtheria may cause chronic nonhealing ulcers with an overlying dirty-gray membrane, though lesions may also mimic psoriasis, eczema, or impetigo. Ulceroglandular tularemia may have associated ulcerated skin lesions with painful regional adenopathy. Although buboes are the major cutaneous manifestation of plague (see Chap. 164), in 25 percent of cases ulcers with eschars, papules, or pustules are also present.

Mycobacterium ulcerans typically causes chronic skin ulcers on the extremities of individuals living in the tropics. *Mycobacterium leprae* may be associated with cutaneous ulcerations in patients with lepromatous leprosy related to Lucio's phenomenon or during reversal reactions. *Mycobacterium tuberculosis* may also cause ulcerations, papules, or erythematous macular lesions of the skin in both normal and immunocompromised patients.

Decubitus ulcers are due to tissue hypoxia secondary to pressure-induced vascular insufficiency and may become secondarily infected with components of the skin and gastrointestinal flora, including anaerobes. Ulcerative lesions on the anterior shins may be due to pyoderma gangrenosum, which must be distinguished from similar lesions of infectious etiology by histologic evaluation of biopsy sites.

ERYSIPELAS (Table 133-1) Erysipelas is due to *S. pyogenes* (see Chap. 143) and is characterized by an abrupt onset of fiery-red swelling of the face or extremities. The distinctive features of erysipelas are well-defined indurated margins, particularly along the nasolabial fold; rapid progression; and intense pain. Flaccid bullae may develop during the second or third day of illness, but extension to deeper soft tissues is rare. Treatment with penicillin is effective; swelling may progress despite appropriate treatment, though fever, pain, and the intense red color diminish. Desquamation of the involved skin occurs 5 to 10 days into the illness. Infants and elderly adults are most commonly afflicted, and the severity of systemic toxicity varies.

CELLULITIS Cellulitis is an acute inflammatory condition of the skin that is characterized by localized pain, erythema, swelling, and heat. Cellulitis may be caused by indigenous flora colonizing the skin and appendages (e.g., *S. aureus* and *S. pyogenes*) or by a wide variety of exogenous bacteria. Because the exogenous bacteria involved in cellulitis occupy unique niches in nature, a thorough history provides important clues to etiology (see Table 133-1 and text below).

Bacteria may gain access to the epidermis through cracks in the skin, abrasions, cuts, burns, insect bites, surgical incisions, and intravenous catheters. Cellulitis caused by *S. aureus* spreads from a central localized infection, such as an abscess, folliculitis, or an infected foreign body (e.g., a splinter, a prosthetic device, or an intravenous catheter). In contrast, cellulitis due to *S. pyogenes* is a more rapidly spreading, diffuse process frequently associated with lymphangitis and fever. Recurrent streptococcal cellulitis of the lower extremities may be caused by organisms of group A, C, or G in association with chronic venous stasis or with saphenous venectomy for coronary artery bypass surgery. Streptococci also cause recurrent cellulitis among patients with chronic lymphedema resulting from elephantiasis, lymph node dissection, or Milroy's disease. Recurrent staphylococcal cutaneous infections are more common among individuals who have eosinophilia and elevated serum levels of IgE (Job's syndrome) and among nasal

carriers of staphylococci. Cellulitis caused by *Streptococcus agalactiae* (group B streptococci) occurs primarily in patients with diabetes mellitus or peripheral vascular disease. *Haemophilus influenzae* typically causes periorbital cellulitis in children in association with sinusitis, otitis media, or epiglottitis. It is unclear whether this form of cellulitis will (like meningitis) become less common as a result of the impressive efficacy of the *H. influenzae* type b vaccine.

Many other bacteria also cause cellulitis. Fortunately, these organisms occur in such characteristic settings that a good history provides useful clues to the diagnosis. Cellulitis associated with cat bites and, to a lesser degree, with dog bites is commonly caused by *Pasteurella multocida*, though in the latter case *Staphylococcus intermedius* and *Capnocytophaga canimorsus* (DF-2) must also be considered. Sites of cellulitis and abscesses associated with dog bites and human bites also contain a variety of anaerobic organisms. *Pasteurella* is notoriously resistant to dicloxacillin and nafcillin but is sensitive to all other β-lactam antimicrobials as well as to quinolones, tetracycline, and erythromycin. Ampicillin/clavulanate, ampicillin/sulbactam, and cefoxitin are good choices for the treatment of animal or human bite infections. *Aeromonas hydrophila* causes aggressive cellulitis in tissues surrounding lacerations sustained in fresh water (lakes, rivers, and streams). This organism remains sensitive to aminoglycosides, fluoroquinolones, chloramphenicol, trimethoprim-sulfamethoxazole, and third-generation cephalosporins; it is resistant to ampicillin, however.

P. aeruginosa causes three types of soft tissue infection: ecthyma gangrenosum in neutropenic patients, hot-tub folliculitis, and cellulitis following penetrating injury. Most commonly, *P. aeruginosa* is introduced into the deep tissues when a person steps on a nail; this scenario is referred to as the "sweaty tennis shoe syndrome." Treatment includes surgical inspection and drainage, particularly if the injury also involves bone or joint capsule. Choices for empirical treatment while antimicrobial susceptibility data are awaited include an aminoglycoside, a third-generation cephalosporin (ceftazidime, cefoperazone, or cefotaxime), a semisynthetic penicillin (ticarcillin, mezlocillin, or piperacillin), or a fluoroquinolone (though drugs of the last class are not indicated for the treatment of children less than 13 years old).

Gram-negative bacillary cellulitis, including that due to *P. aeruginosa*, is most common among hospitalized, immunocompromised hosts. Cultures and sensitivity tests are critically important in this setting because of multidrug resistance (see Chap. 157).

The gram-positive aerobic rod *Erysipelothrix rhusiopathiae*, which causes cellulitis in bone renderers and fishmongers, remains susceptible to penicillin, erythromycin, clindamycin, tetracycline, and cephalosporins but is resistant to sulfonamides and chloramphenicol. Fish food containing the water flea *Daphnia* is sometimes contaminated with *Mycobacterium marinum*, which can cause cellulitis or granulomas on skin surfaces exposed to the water in aquariums or injured in swimming pools. Rifampin plus ethambutol has been an effective combination in some cases, though no comprehensive studies have been undertaken. In addition, some strains of *M. marinum* are susceptible to tetracycline or to trimethoprim-sulfamethoxazole.

The etiology of cellulitis can be suggested by epidemiologic data (see above). When there is drainage, an open wound, or an obvious portal of entry, Gram's stain and culture provide a definitive diagnosis. In the absence of these findings, the bacterial etiology of cellulitis is difficult to establish. Even with needle aspiration of the leading edge or a punch biopsy of the cellulitis tissue itself, cultures are positive in only 20 percent of cases. This observation suggests that relatively low numbers of bacteria may cause cellulitis and that the expanding area of erythema within the skin may be a direct effect of extracellular toxins or of the soluble mediators of inflammation elicited by the host.

NECROTIZING FASCIITIS (Table 133-1) Necrotizing fasciitis, formerly called streptococcal gangrene, may be associated with group A *Streptococcus* or mixed aerobic-anaerobic bacteria or may occur as part of gas gangrene caused by *Clostridium perfringens*. Early diagnosis may be difficult when pain or unexplained fever is the only presenting manifestation. Swelling then develops and is followed by brawny edema and tenderness. With progression, dark red induration of the epidermis appears along with bullae filled with blue or purple fluid. Later the skin becomes friable and takes on a bluish, maroon, or black color. By this stage, thrombosis of blood vessels in the dermal papillae is extensive (see Fig. 133-1). Extension of infection to the level of the deep fascia causes it to take on a brownish-gray appearance. Rapid spread occurs along fascial planes, through venous channels and lymphatics. Patients in the later stages are toxic and frequently manifest shock and multiorgan failure.

Necrotizing fasciitis caused by mixed aerobic-anaerobic bacteria begins with a breach in the integrity of a mucous membrane barrier, such as the mucosa of the gastrointestinal or genitourinary tract. The portal can be a malignancy, diverticulum, hemorrhoid, anal fissure, or urethral tear. Other predisposing factors include peripheral vascular disease, diabetes mellitus, surgery, and penetrating injury to the abdomen. Leakage into the perineal area results in a syndrome called *Fournier's gangrene*, characterized by massive swelling of the scrotum and penis with extension into the perineum or the abdominal wall and legs.

Necrotizing fasciitis caused by *S. pyogenes* has increased in frequency and severity since 1985. It frequently begins deep at the site of a nonpenetrating minor trauma such as a bruise or a muscle strain. Seeding of the site via transient bacteremia is likely, though most patients deny antecedent streptococcal infection. Alternatively, *S. pyogenes* may reach the deep fascia from a site of cutaneous infection or penetrating trauma. Toxicity is severe, and renal impairment may precede the development of shock. In 20 to 40 percent of cases, myositis occurs concomitantly, and, as in gas gangrene (see below), serum creatinine phosphokinase values may be markedly elevated. Necrotizing fasciitis due to mixed aerobic-anaerobic bacteria may be associated with gas in the deep tissue, but gas is not usually present when the cause is *S. pyogenes*. Prompt surgical exploration down to the deep fascia and muscle is essential. Necrotic tissue must be surgically removed, and Gram's staining and culture of excised tissue are useful in establishing whether group A streptococci, mixed aerobic-anaerobic bacteria, or *Clostridium* spp. are present (see "Treatment" below).

MYOSITIS (Table 133-1)   Muscle involvement can occur with virus infection [influenza, dengue, coxsackievirus B (pleurodynia)]; or parasitic invasion [*Trichinella spiralis* (trichinosis), *Taenia solium* (cysticercosis), *Toxoplasma gondii* (toxoplasmosis)]. Although myalgia can occur in most of these infections, severe muscle pain is the hallmark of pleurodynia, trichinosis, and bacterial infection. Acute rhabdomyolysis predictably occurs with clostridial and streptococcal myositis but may also be associated with influenza virus, echovirus, coxsackievirus, Epstein-Barr virus, and *Legionella* infection.

Pyomyositis is usually due to *S. aureus*, is common in tropical areas, and generally has no known portal of entry. Infection remains localized, and, unless organisms produce toxic shock syndrome toxin 1 or certain enterotoxins, shock does not develop. In contrast, *S. pyogenes* may induce primary myositis referred to as *streptococcal necrotizing myositis*, which is associated with severe systemic toxicity. Myonecrosis occurs concomitantly with necrotizing fasciitis in about 50 percent of cases. Both are part of the streptococcal toxic shock syndrome.

Gas gangrene usually follows severe penetrating injuries that result in interruption of the blood supply and introduction of soil into wounds. Such cases of traumatic gangrene are usually caused by *C. perfringens*, *Clostridium septicum*, or *Clostridium histolyticum*. Rarely, latent or recurrent gangrene can occur years after penetrating trauma, most

likely owing to dormant spores that reside at the site of previous injury. Spontaneous nontraumatic gangrene among patients with neutropenia, gastrointestinal malignancy, diverticulosis, or recent radiation therapy to the abdomen is caused by *C. septicum*. The tolerance of this anaerobe to oxygen probably explains why it can initiate infection spontaneously in normal tissue anywhere in the body.

Synergistic nonclostridial anaerobic myonecrosis, also known as necrotizing cutaneous myositis and synergistic necrotizing cellulitis, is a variant of necrotizing fasciitis caused by mixed aerobic and anaerobic bacteria with the exclusion of clostridial organisms (see "Necrotizing Fasciitis" above).

℞ TREATMENT

Early and aggressive surgical exploration is essential in patients with suspected necrotizing fasciitis, myositis, or gangrene in order to (1) visualize the deep structures, (2) remove necrotic tissue, (3) reduce compartment pressure, and (4) obtain suitable material for Gram's staining and for aerobic and anaerobic cultures. Appropriate empirical antibiotic treatment for mixed aerobic-anaerobic infections could consist of ampicillin/sulbactam, cefoxitin, or the following combination: (1) clindamycin (600 to 800 mg intravenously every 8 h) or metronidazole (750 mg every 6 h) plus (2) ampicillin or ampicillin/sulbactam (2 to 3 g intravenously every 6 h) plus (3) gentamicin (1.0 to 1.5 mg/kg every 8 h). Group A streptococcal and clostridial infection of the fascia and/or muscle carries a mortality rate of 20 to 50 percent with penicillin treatment. In experimental models of streptococcal and clostridial necrotizing fasciitis/myositis, clindamycin has exhibited markedly superior efficacy, but no comparative trials have been performed in humans. Hyperbaric oxygen treatment may also be useful in gas gangrene due to clostridial species. Antibiotic treatment should be continued until all signs of systemic toxicity have resolved, all devitalized tissue has been removed, and granulation tissue has developed (Chaps. 143, 148, and 169).

In summary, infections of the skin and soft tissues are diverse in presentation and severity and offer a great challenge to the clinician. This chapter provides an approach to diagnosis and understanding of the pathophysiologic mechanisms involved in these infections. More in-depth information is found in chapters on specific infections.

BIBLIOGRAPHY

BISNO AI, STEVENS DL: Streptococcal infections in skin and soft tissues. N Engl J Med 334:240, 1996

FRANCIS JS, NEFF J: Viral infections of the skin and soft tissues, in *Atlas of Infectious Diseases*, DL Stevens (ed). Philadelphia, Churchill Livingstone, 1994

GOLDSTEIN EJC: Bite wounds and infection. Clin Infect Dis 14:633, 1992

HOOK EW et al: Microbiologic evaluation of cutaneous cellulitis in adults. Arch Intern Med 146:295, 1986

SIMMONS RL, AHRENHOLZ DH: Infections of the skin and soft tissue, in *Surgical Infectious Diseases*, 2d ed, RJ Howard, RL Simmons (eds). Norwalk, CT, Appleton & Lange, 1988, p 377

STEVENS DL et al: Effect of antibiotics on toxin production and viability of *Clostridium perfringens*. Antimicrob Agents Chemother 31:213, 1987

——— et al: Spontaneous, nontraumatic gangrene due to *Clostridium septicum*. Rev Infect Dis 12:286, 1990

———: Invasive group A streptococcus infections. Clin Infect Dis 14:2, 1992

——— et al: Evaluation of hyperbaric oxygen therapy for treatment of experimental *Clostridium perfringens* infection. Clin Infect Dis 17:231, 1993

——— et al: Penicillin binding protein expression at different growth stages determines penicillin efficacy in vitro and in vivo: An explanation for the inoculum effect. J Infect Dis 167:1401, 1993

———: Necrotizing infections of the skin and soft tissues, in *Atlas of Infectious Diseases*, DL Stevens (ed). Philadelphia, Churchill Livingstone, 1994

———: Streptococcal toxic shock syndrome: Spectrum of disease, pathogenesis and new concepts in treatment. Emerging Infect Dis 1:69, 1995

WALLACE RJ et al: Clinical trial of clarithromycin for cutaneous (disseminated) infection due to *Mycobacterium chelonae*. Ann Intern Med 119:482, 1993

INFECTIONS (EXCLUDING AIDS) IN INJECTION DRUG USERS

The injection of illicit drugs is a widespread practice whose prevalence has increased dramatically since the 1950s in association with successive epidemics of heroin and cocaine use. Injection drug users are a hidden population, engaging in an illegal activity of which society disapproves. It is impossible to determine their precise number or, consequently, the true incidence of infectious complications in this population.

A markedly higher age-specific mortality rate among injection drug users than in the general population was documented even before the epidemic of infection with human immunodeficiency virus (HIV) and AIDS (see Chap. 308). For example, in New York City between 1965 and 1972, the death rate among relatively young (20- to 54-year-old) adult heroin addicts not involved in drug-treatment programs was estimated to be five times greater than that among age-matched, non-heroin-addicted adults (28.2 per 1000 versus 5.6 per 1000). A substantial portion of this excess mortality was the result of infectious complications of injection drug use. Data from the New York City Medical Examiner during the 1960s indicated that 27 percent of narcotic-related deaths were associated with infections. During this period, a wide array of infectious complications of injection drug use were described. More recently, as a consequence of the HIV epidemic, overall mortality and cause-specific mortality secondary to both AIDS and bacterial infections have dramatically increased in this population. Mortality rates of 3.41 per 100 person-years from AIDS and 1.08 per 100 person-years from bacterial infection preceding AIDS have been reported in HIV-infected injection drug users.

Most infectious complications in injection drug users reflect the events surrounding drug injection and associated life-style issues rather than the direct effects of the illicit drugs themselves. Drugs are purchased in powdered form and often contain adulterants such as quinine, talc, and dextrose. The drugs are dissolved in water (obtained from any available source) or occasionally in saliva in bottle caps or "cookers," filtered through cotton wool or gauze, aspirated into tuberculin or diabetic syringes, and injected intravenously or subcutaneously. Skin preparation is usually minimal and may consist of rubbing saliva on the injection site. A small amount of blood may remain in the needle and syringe after use and may merely be diluted by rinsing in tap water or bleach. Needles and syringes are often shared among injection drug users, either by a few friends or relatives or by larger numbers of users sequentially and anonymously in "shooting galleries." These clandestine locations, where injection drug users gather to rent injection equipment and administer drugs, are ideal sites for the transmission of bloodborne infectious agents.

In this setting, the characteristics of injection drug users that increase the risk of infection are (1) increased rates of skin, mucous membrane, and nasopharyngeal carriage of pathogenic organisms, particularly staphylococci; (2) unsterile injection technique resulting in the introduction of components of the dermal or nasopharyngeal flora into soft tissues or the bloodstream; (3) contamination of injection equipment or drugs with viral, bacterial, and parasitic microorganisms, which may be present in residual blood in shared injection equipment or in contaminated water used to dissolve drugs before injection or to rinse equipment afterward; (4) humoral, cell-mediated, and phagocytic defects induced by HIV infection and/or drug use (even before the HIV/AIDS epidemic, injection drug users were known to have abnormal immunologic parameters, including high levels of globulins, false-positive serologic reactions to multiple antigens, and abnormalities in phagocytosis, and these defects have been markedly exacerbated by HIV-induced B- and T-cell dysfunction); (5) poor dental hygiene and drug-induced impairment of gag and cough reflexes; (6) alteration of the normal microbial flora owing to intermittent antibiotic use; (7) low socioeconomic status, with increased prevalence of exposure to certain pathogens (notably *Mycobacterium tuberculosis*); (8) behaviors associ-

ated with injection drug use, such as cigarette smoking, alcohol use, or exchange of sex for drugs or money; and (9) decreased access to and/or lack of appropriate use of preventive and primary health care services, resulting in low levels of immunization and prophylaxis and delay in the diagnosis and treatment of minor infectious complications.

SPECIFIC INFECTIONS AMONG INJECTION DRUG USERS

SKIN AND SOFT TISSUE INFECTIONS (See also Chap. 133) Infections of the skin and soft tissues are the most common bacterial infectious complication of injection drug use and, before the AIDS epidemic, were the most common cause of hospital admissions of injection drug users. The clinical spectrum of infection is broad, ranging from simple cellulitis and abscess to life-threatening necrotizing fasciitis and septic thrombophlebitis. The high frequency of skin and soft tissue infections is attributable to several factors: the practice of injecting drugs subcutaneously ("skin popping"), the extravasation of drugs into soft tissue during intravenous injection, the presence in injected material of adulterants that may cause tissue necrosis, and the increased skin carriage of pathogenic organisms.

Most skin and soft tissue infections occur on the upper and lower extremities, but occasionally atypical sites (e.g., the abdomen or back, groin, scrotum, and neck) may be involved as a result of injection into the jugular or femoral veins. Cellulitis may extend from a fresh injection site or may result from superinfection of an open wound sustained earlier. The clinical appearance is often atypical because of chronic damage to the skin and to venous and lymphatic systems in both the upper and the lower extremities, with resultant underlying lymphedema, hyperpigmentation, scarring, and regional lymphadenopathy. Nevertheless, careful examination often reveals characteristic redness, warmth, and tenderness, with tender inguinal or axillary lymph nodes. Fever is variable and bacteremia infrequent.

Uncomplicated cellulitis is most often due to group A streptococci, other streptococci, or *Staphylococcus aureus*. Unless an associated open draining wound is present or bacteremia develops, the precise microbial etiology is difficult to determine. For localized abscesses presenting either as draining lesions or as fluctuant subcutaneous masses, Gram's staining and culture of pus or aspirated material are required. Although these abscesses are usually staphylococcal in etiology, they are sometimes due to a complex mixture of anaerobic and aerobic bacteria. A foul odor and characteristic findings on Gram's staining of pus suggest a polymicrobial etiology.

Treatment of skin infections consists of hospitalization in most cases, incision and drainage in instances of abscess formation, and administration of intravenous antistaphylococcal β-lactam antibiotics such as oxacillin or nafcillin. Cefazolin (4 to 6 g/d) may be an alternative choice. In areas where methicillin-resistant *S. aureus* is highly prevalent, vancomycin should be used empirically, pending the results of susceptibility tests. The total duration of therapy should be 10 to 14 days; for the latter part of this course, oral agents may or may not be used, depending on the individual's clinical response. For injection drug users who have an established relationship with a health care provider, mild infections may be treated with oral agents on an outpatient basis; therapy should be followed by frequent visits at which the response is assessed.

Indolent skin ulcers are common. These lesions are shallow and indurated and may become superinfected. Their etiology is unclear, but they are likely the result of foreign-body inflammatory changes, necrosis, and low-grade infection. They usually respond to local wound care and oral or topical antibiotic treatment. Occasionally, these ulcers are extensive enough to require skin grafting. When the lesions heal, they leave depressed, hyperpigmented scars.

Necrotizing fasciitis and myositis and septic thrombophlebitis are life-threatening local complications of injection drug use. Although infrequent, they should always be considered when skin or soft tissue infection develops in injection drug users. The presence of fasciitis and myositis is associated with exquisite pain and tenderness at the injection site and with toxicity and hemodynamic instability out of proportion to the local lesion. Crepitus may be noted, and soft tissue radiographs may reveal gas in tissues. Immediate surgical exploration, with extensive drainage and debridement of infected and nonviable tissue, is required. These infections often have a polymicrobial etiology that includes *S. aureus*, aerobic and anaerobic streptococci, enteric gram-negative bacilli, and other anaerobes. Parenteral antibiotic therapy aimed at gram-positive and gram-negative organisms, with anaerobic coverage, is essential. Several regimens—including vancomycin or nafcillin plus metronidazole or clindamycin plus an aminoglycoside, a third-generation cephalosporin, or a broad-spectrum penicillin—are indicated.

Septic thrombophlebitis of extremity, jugular, or femoral veins often appears as septic pulmonary emboli. Bacteremia is invariably found, and pus may be expressed from injection sites of infected vessels. Parenteral antibiotic therapy as well as ligation and excision of infected thrombosed veins (if technically feasible) are advocated. The value of heparin remains unproved, and its use is generally not recommended.

Other, infrequent complications of injection drug use under unsterile circumstances include wound botulism, tetanus, malaria, and disseminated candidiasis. The first two have been sporadically reported, usually in long-term users and often in "skin poppers," whereas outbreaks of malaria have resulted from the sharing of needles contaminated with infected blood. Botulism should be considered in patients with unusual, progressive cranial nerve palsies; wounds should be cultured for *Clostridium botulinum*. Tetanus should be suspected in drug users with seizures, muscle rigidity, and autonomic hyperactivity.

ENDOCARDITIS (See Chap. 126)   The potential for life-threatening complications and the usual need for prolonged intravenous antibiotic therapy in the hospital make bacterial endocarditis a disease of great consequence in injection drug users. In several studies of consecutive hospital admissions of injection drug users before the AIDS epidemic, endocarditis accounted for 5 to 16 percent of admissions and for 2 to 8 percent of all deaths.

Microbiology   The predominant organism causing endocarditis in injection drug users is *S. aureus*. In various published series, this organism has caused from 60 to more than 90 percent of cases. In many geographic locations, a substantial and increasing proportion of *S. aureus* isolates are resistant to methicillin. Although the organism was originally believed to be a contaminant of drugs and injection paraphernalia, it is now clear that *S. aureus* is part of the patient's own flora, carried in the nares and oropharynx and on the skin and subsequently introduced into the bloodstream by unsterile injection.

Right-sided endocarditis is caused by *S. aureus* in more than 80 percent of cases in injection drug users, whereas the organisms isolated in aortic or mitral valve endocarditis are more similar to those found in other patients. Streptococci and enterococci, including alpha-hemolytic viridans streptococci and *Enterococcus faecalis*, are the second most common organisms but account for only 5 to 10 percent of cases of endocarditis in various series. Geographic and temporal clustering of more unusual infecting organisms has occasionally been reported. These organisms include *Pseudomonas aeruginosa*, *Pseudomonas cepacia*, *Serratia marcescens*, enterococci, and, recently, methicillin-resistant *S. aureus*. Infrequent cases of endocarditis due to *Candida* spp., *Bacillus* spp., diphtheroids, and fastidious gram-negative or anaerobic components of the oral flora have been described as well. Polymicrobial endocarditis due to both gram-positive and gram-negative organisms has been documented.

Pathogenesis and Clinical Presentation   Longer duration and higher frequency of drug injection are associated with increased risk of endocarditis. The site most frequently involved is the tricuspid valve, possibly because of its proximity to the injection site. Injection of particulate matter, including talc and cotton, may cause pitting

and disruption of the smooth endothelial lining—changes that may facilitate the attachment of pathogenic organisms. Left-sided endocarditis may occur with or without right-sided involvement and usually develops in the setting of underlying valvular heart disease.

The various characteristic clinical presentations depend on the site of valvular involvement. In tricuspid valve endocarditis, the predominant picture is one of an abrupt illness with persistent high fever, pulmonary involvement, and an absence of systemic embolic or microvascular phenomena. Approximately 50 percent of patients present with cough and pleuritic chest pain, and some exhibit hemoptysis—all the result of multiple septic pulmonary emboli and infarctions. The characteristic murmur of tricuspid regurgitation may be heard in 50 percent of patients. This is a medium-pitched, midsystolic murmur at the lower left sternal border that increases in intensity with inspiration. Characteristically, chest radiography shows multiple patchy or nodular infiltrates that progress to cavitation during therapy and eventually resolve.

Endocarditis involving the mitral and aortic valves also has an acute onset, with high fever, toxicity, and signs and symptoms resulting from multiple systemic emboli (including arterial emboli and septic infarcts of the skin, liver, spleen, kidneys, and central nervous system). Toxic encephalopathy, focal neurologic abnormalities (the result of mycotic aneurysm or brain abscess), and bacterial meningitis may ensue. Petechiae and splenomegaly occur in approximately 50 percent of patients, and aortic and mitral regurgitant murmurs are reported in almost all cases.

Diagnosis   The diagnosis of endocarditis in injection drug users can be problematic, even in the emergency room setting, where most febrile drug users are evaluated and this diagnosis is often suspected. Right-sided endocarditis may be particularly difficult to diagnose because systemic emboli and a regurgitant murmur are usually absent. The diagnosis rests on a composite of clinical, microbiologic, radiologic, and imaging data.

The clinical criteria used include sustained bacteremia involving an organism likely to cause endocarditis and the presence of compatible pulmonary, systemic, or cardiac findings. The diagnostic accuracy of emergency room evaluation in predicting endocarditis in febrile injection drug users is quite low. Of 87 consecutive febrile injection drug users in one study, 13 percent ultimately met the case definition for definite or probable endocarditis. Only 4 of the 12 injection drug users suspected of having endocarditis in the emergency room proved to have this diagnosis, while 8 of 30 admitted with other diagnoses ultimately proved to have endocarditis. Bacterial pneumonia and minor illnesses were more frequent than endocarditis. The authors concluded that the accuracy of emergency room diagnosis is insufficient to distinguish between endocarditis and other conditions and that febrile injection drug users seen in emergency rooms should therefore be admitted for observation and/or therapy.

Injection drug users may self-medicate with oral antibiotics. This behavior, which is not always disclosed when the patient's medical history is taken, may be critically important in the evaluation of patients with suspected endocarditis because blood cultures may be falsely negative. The use of nonprescribed antibiotics before admission to the hospital is an important factor predicting endocarditis due to methicillin-resistant *S. aureus* among drug injectors.

All febrile injection drug users should have a careful history taken, with an emphasis on the frequency and type of drug injection and on antibiotic use. The physical examination should focus attention on the presence of septic emboli in the skin and on mucosal surfaces and the existence of regurgitant murmurs. Chest radiography should be used to detect the characteristic septic emboli or focal infections that may result in bacteremia. Ideally, three sets of blood samples—collected over several hours, as clinical exigency permits—should be cultured. Cardiac imaging studies are a valuable adjunct to diagnosis, although they cannot usually be undertaken at the time of initial presentation and are of variable sensitivity and specificity; false-negative results are frequent in right-sided involvement, and false-positive results also have been documented. Echocardiography may be invaluable in following patients with potentially unstable lesions (i.e., valvular incompetence or intramyocardial abscess).

After blood has been obtained for cultures, empirical antibiotic therapy should be instituted if patients are acutely ill, if left-sided endocarditis is strongly suspected, and/or if septic pulmonary emboli are seen on radiographs. However, it is not necessary to institute therapy for endocarditis in all injection drug users with fever. In fact, it is often reasonable to withhold antibiotics and to observe the patient carefully until the results of blood cultures are known. Some patients will be found to have a minor transient illness or a pyrogenic or hypersensitivity reaction to injected drugs and will defervesce within 24 h. In others, an alternative diagnosis will become apparent.

Appropriate empirical antibiotic therapy should be given parenterally and should always include an antistaphylococcal agent. Depending on local susceptibility patterns and the severity of the patient's illness, the agent selected is usually either a β-lactam antibiotic, such as oxacillin or nafcillin, or—if infection with methicillin-resistant *S. aureus* is suspected—vancomycin. If local patterns warrant, gram-negative coverage with an added aminoglycoside may be appropriate. For endocarditis due to methicillin-susceptible staphylococci, conventional therapy consists of 4 weeks of oxacillin or nafcillin at a dose of 1.5 to 2 g every 4 hours. In severe endocarditis, some clinicians add an aminoglycoside, usually gentamicin (1.5 mg/kg every 8 h) for the first 2 weeks of therapy; this addition may result in more rapid resolution of bacteremia, although an improved outcome has never been shown. In cases of allergy to penicillin or infection with methicillin-resistant *S. aureus*, vancomycin (1 g every 12 h) is given. Therapy targeting other organisms should be selected on the basis of antimicrobial susceptibility patterns. Treatment is usually given for 4 weeks. Successful treatment of uncomplicated right-sided endocarditis with a 2-week course of a β-lactam antibiotic plus an aminoglycoside has been reported. Given the difficulty of obtaining long-term secure intravenous access, this alternative regimen may prove valuable in selected cases. Most experts advocate parenteral therapy for the duration of the course, although this decision often necessitates the placement of an indwelling central line.

The prognosis of right-sided staphylococcal endocarditis in this population is excellent, with only rare deaths and an infrequent lack of response to medical therapy. Endocarditis caused by other organisms and left-sided involvement carry a more serious prognosis, with higher complication and fatality rates. The role of surgery remains controversial in this as in other populations with endocarditis (see Chap. 126). The criteria for surgical intervention should be the same as in other populations: intractable heart failure, undrained myocardial abscess, and failure of medical therapy, particularly in candidal or fungal endocarditis. The surgical approach varies with the cardiac valve(s) involved. Valve excision alone appears to be sufficient for severe tricuspid endocarditis. In mitral and aortic valve endocarditis, valve replacement is required and usually can be accomplished safely. Concerns about subsequent reinfection in the setting of continued injection drug use engender heated debates and require joint decisions by medical and surgical personnel and the patient.

PNEUMONIA (See also Chap. 255)   Community-acquired bacterial pneumonia, most often caused by *Streptococcus pneumoniae* and *Haemophilus influenzae*, was commonly described among drug injectors in the 1960s and 1970s. These infections were thought to be more frequent among drug users than among the general population. The putative risk factors in drug users included pulmonary aspiration resulting from intermittent overdose, deleterious effects of opiates on lung defenses and cough reflex, hypoventilation due to respiratory depression, and smoking.

These factors have all been outweighed by HIV infection, which has dramatically increased the risk of bacterial pneumonia in drug injectors. Beginning in the mid-1980s, epidemiologic surveillance data from New York City showed rising mortality from bacterial pneumonia and other bacterial infections among drug injectors—a phenomenon linked to HIV infection. In some cases, HIV-infected drug users died

from pyogenic bacterial infections even before the diagnosis of AIDS. Prospective studies demonstrated that even when they were not actively injecting drugs, HIV-infected drug users had a four- to fivefold greater risk of bacterial pneumonia and sepsis (up to 10 cases per 100 person-years) than their HIV-seronegative counterparts. Among febrile drug users presenting to an emergency room, pneumonia was the single largest diagnostic category, accounting for 38 percent of admissions.

The 1993 Revised AIDS Case Definition of the Centers for Disease Control and Prevention includes recurrent bacterial pneumonia in persons with HIV infection as an AIDS-defining condition. The organisms involved in HIV-related pneumonia among drug injectors are predominantly those reported in the earlier literature on community-acquired pneumonia in this group—*S. pneumoniae* and *H. influenzae*.

The clinical presentation of bacterial pneumonia and the strategies for its diagnosis and therapy are similar in injection drug users and in other populations, despite a wider array of differential diagnostic possibilities in the former group. The typical presentation includes fever, productive cough, pleuritic chest pain, and findings of consolidation and segmental or lobar infiltrates on chest radiography. Specific etiologic diagnosis requires cultures of sputum and/or blood. For uncomplicated community-acquired bacterial pneumonia, therapy aimed at *S. pneumoniae* and/or *H. influenzae*, given for 10 days to 2 weeks, is recommended. Many clinicians begin therapy with cefuroxime (1.5 g every 8 h). Therapeutic modifications are based on Gram's stain and culture results and on the clinical presentation and course. For uncomplicated pneumococcal pneumonia caused by a susceptible organism, penicillin G in a dose of 2 to 3 million units daily remains the drug of choice.

Among the infectious entities to be considered in the differential diagnosis of pulmonary infiltrates in this population of patients are septic pulmonary emboli, tuberculosis, and *Pneumocystis carinii* pneumonia (in patients infected with HIV). Noninfectious pulmonary complications of injection drug use also should be considered. Heroin-induced pulmonary edema, the most common of these complications, occurs most often in drug-use neophytes but also develops in experienced users exposed to particularly potent opiates and in persons who have resumed drug injection after a period of abstinence; this complication rapidly causes death by asphyxiation unless treated promptly with a narcotic antagonist (e.g., naloxone) and respiratory support.

The virtual universality of heavy cigarette smoking among drug injectors may not only predispose them to the usual sequelae of this behavior but also complicate the differential diagnosis of pulmonary symptoms (e.g., cough, shortness of breath, sputum production).

TUBERCULOSIS (See also Chap. 171)   The other important pulmonary infection described in drug injectors is tuberculosis. Infections due to *M. tuberculosis* were well documented in drug users before the AIDS epidemic, accounting for greater morbidity and mortality in this population than in the non-drug-using population. Although some authors attributed this greater impact to poverty, poor housing, and the social and demographic factors associated with both drug use and tuberculosis, others found an elevated risk of tuberculosis among drug users even after attempting to control for these other factors. AIDS has now overwhelmed all other potential risk factors and has resulted in a new epidemic of resurgent tuberculosis among HIV-infected drug users and their contacts (see Chaps. 171 and 308). Among persons with HIV infection, tuberculosis has disproportionately affected injection drug users. This observation may reflect higher levels of latent infection with *M. tuberculosis* in drug-using populations and associated environmental factors. In parts of the urban northeastern United States, where 20 percent of drug injectors have evidence of latent *M. tuberculosis* infection and 50 percent are infected with HIV, the overlap of these two endemic infections has resulted in an unprecedented increase in the incidence of tuberculosis since 1985. Both high rates of reactivation of latent infection (8 percent per 100 person-years) and increased transmission to susceptibles in community and hospital settings are responsible. Aggressive chemoprophylaxis with isoniazid, active case finding, and therapy are all essential.

Pulmonary tuberculosis should always be suspected and included in the differential diagnosis of pneumonia in injection drug users. Particularly among those with HIV infection, extrapulmonary tuberculosis has increased greatly in frequency. The unusually high incidence of both single-drug-resistant and multidrug-resistant (MDR) tuberculosis among injection drug users further complicates diagnosis and treatment in this population. MDR tuberculosis should be suspected in individuals with a history of treatment for tuberculosis, recent hospitalization or incarceration, or contact with a known case. The therapy administered to injection drug users is similar to that given to other populations. For nonresistant tuberculosis, a 2-month course of treatment with four drugs—isoniazid (5 mg/kg daily; maximum, 300 mg/d), rifampin (10 mg/kg daily; maximum, 600 mg/d), ethambutol (15 mg/kg daily; maximum, 1200 mg/d), and pyrazinamide (25 mg/kg daily; maximum, 2 g/d)—is followed by a 4-month course of isoniazid and rifampin alone. In patients with HIV infection, the duration of treatment is usually extended to 9 to 12 months. The treatment of MDR tuberculosis requires multiple additional drugs, usually including a quinolone and ethionamide. Special efforts must be made to ensure long-term adherence to the regimen, including direct observation of compliance with therapy.

SKELETAL INFECTIONS (See Chap. 132) Skeletal infections in injection drug users result both from hematogenous dissemination and, less commonly, from contiguous spread from chronically infected skin and soft tissue sites to underlying bone. In one series, skeletal infections represented 9 percent of admissions of injection drug users to a large urban hospital. Septic arthritis of large synovial joints may be seen during the course of staphylococcal endocarditis or of bacteremia arising from other infected sites and may appear as a complication of disseminated gonococcal disease. The joints most frequently involved are the knees, hips, shoulders, and elbows, but there is a predilection for the involvement of unusual joints as well—e.g., the vertebral column; the symphysis pubis; and the sternoclavicular, sternochondral, and sacroiliac joints. These infections are usually unilateral and subacute, with an indolent, progressive course characterized by pain, limitation of motion, and absence of fever. The diagnosis may be easily overlooked. Point tenderness over the affected joint is usually elicited. Sternoarticular infections are often associated with soft tissue swelling of the chest wall and bacteremia. Vertebral osteomyelitis may be associated with paraspinal soft tissue masses and (in cases of posterior extension) with the formation of spinal epidural abscesses. Radiologic and imaging studies may suggest the diagnosis by findings that are most characteristic of vertebral osteomyelitis, where the disk space is lost, contiguous bone erosion and new bone formation are evident, and several vertebrae are involved. Infection of the sacroiliac joints and symphysis pubis results in joint-space separation and erosion of the articular surfaces.

S. aureus is the pathogen most commonly isolated from sites of skeletal infection, but gram-negative organisms—notably *P. aeruginosa*, *S. marcescens*, and fungi—also have been well documented. *M. tuberculosis* should be included in the differential diagnosis, particularly in cases of vertebral osteomyelitis. Because etiologic agents and their antimicrobial susceptibilities vary, efforts should be made to obtain a specific microbiologic diagnosis. This process may involve diagnostic aspiration or closed or open biopsy, with fluid or material sent for staining and culture for bacterial, mycobacterial, and fungal pathogens.

Treatment consists of a combination of drainage of the synovial joints and the contiguous soft tissue collections and prolonged administration of appropriate high-dose antimicrobial therapy. For *S. aureus*, oxacillin—or, in cases of intolerance or resistance, vancomycin—is given for 4 to 6 weeks. *Pseudomonas* infections require an active third-generation cephalosporin and an aminoglycoside.

CENTRAL NERVOUS SYSTEM COMPLICATIONS The nervous system—in particular, the central nervous system—is an important site for adverse sequelae of drug injection. Drug injectors are at increased risk for certain noninfectious complications, including intracerebral hemorrhage and other stroke syndromes (especially with cocaine and amphetamine use), particulate emboli to the brain and spinal cord, vasculitis, and the consequences of head trauma. Among the infectious complications, the most common is systemic embolization to the brain as a result of bacterial endocarditis or bacteremia, which frequently involves multiple small septic emboli from either aortic or mitral valve vegetations. Patients may present with focal neurologic deficits, seizures, altered mental status, and/or meningismus. *S. aureus* and other bacteria that cause endocarditis in drug injectors are most commonly involved in these manifestations. Cerebral mycotic aneurysms and spinal and epidural abscesses also have been described as complications of endocarditis in this population. Less commonly, drug users have been reported to be at risk for focal brain abscesses that are unrelated to endocarditis and are caused by organisms such as *Aspergillus*, *Mucor*, other fungi, and *Nocardia*. There is also evidence that tuberculous meningitis and focal tuberculomas of the brain may be more common among drug users than among other patients with tuberculosis, with or without HIV infection. Finally, ocular infections, including episcleritis, chorioretinitis, and endophthalmitis, have been well described in drug injectors, involving such organisms as *Bacillus cereus*, *Aspergillus*, and *Candida albicans*.

HEPATITIS (See also Chaps. 295 and 297) Injection drug users have long been known to be at high risk for hepatitis, primarily through parenteral transmission. The acquisition of hepatitis B is a relatively early event for most drug injectors, occurring within the first several years of illicit drug use. Since the 1970s, seroprevalence studies in a wide range of drug-using populations have indicated that 75 to 90 percent of long-term drug injectors have serologic evidence of past exposure to hepatitis B. Approximately 5 to 10 percent of these individuals will remain chronic carriers of hepatitis B surface antigen; the remainder will develop immunity to hepatitis, producing antibody to hepatitis B core antigen and/or to hepatitis B surface antigen.

Another infectious agent commonly found in drug injectors is hepatitis D virus, previously referred to as the *delta agent*. This defective hepatotropic RNA virus depends on coexisting infection with hepatitis B virus for expression and replication. Antibody to hepatitis D virus has been found in 10 to 15 percent of patients with antibody to hepatitis B surface or core antigen and in as many as 50 to 70 percent of patients with chronic carriage of hepatitis B surface antigen. Fulminant hepatitis B may show a characteristic biphasic pattern in the setting of hepatitis D coinfection. Moreover, hepatitis D has been associated among drug users with chronic active hepatitis and persistent abnormalities of liver function.

The third significant bloodborne agent of hepatitis in injection drug users is hepatitis C virus. In seroprevalence studies in the United States and Europe, antibody to hepatitis C virus has been detected at levels of 70 percent or higher among drug injectors—a rate reflecting a level of infection comparable to that for hepatitis B. Like hepatitis B, hepatitis C appears to be acquired relatively soon after the start of illicit drug injection. Hepatitis C has been associated with chronic active hepatitis, persistent abnormalities of liver function, and cirrhosis. Interferon α may be of benefit in patients with progressive hepatitis B or hepatitis C. Treatment with interferon α has not yet been widely administered to drug users, however, and its requisite duration is unknown.

Although not considered to be a bloodborne infection, hepatitis A has been associated with injection drug use. Several surveillance-based investigations have indicated that injection drug users may have up to a 50-fold higher risk of acquiring hepatitis A than non-injection drug users. In addition, recent outbreaks of hepatitis A have been linked to groups of injection drug users in both the United States and Europe. Investigation of these outbreaks has suggested that fecal-oral contamination, close personal contact, and poor hygiene were more likely than viral contamination of drugs or injection equipment to be responsible for spread of the disease.

These observations suggest that in long-term drug injectors with known past exposure to hepatitis B and/or hepatitis C, hepatitis A (and—for chronic carriers of hepatitis B—hepatitis D) should be strongly considered in the differential diagnosis of new-onset acute hepatitis syndromes. The acquisition of bloodborne hepatitis soon after the start of illicit injection drug use suggests the importance of developing public health strategies that will reach adolescent and young-adult drug users with information about preventive interventions (such as hepatitis B vaccine) and risk-reducing behaviors.

While most hepatitis infections in drug users do not progress to chronic forms of clinically significant hepatitis or cirrhosis, at least 40 percent of most series of entrants into drug-treatment programs exhibit abnormalities of liver function. In addition to infectious causes, the toxic effects of adulterants used in the production of illicit drugs and the hepatotoxic effects of alcohol are responsible in part for these abnormalities. Hepatic cirrhosis in drug users is most often associated with coexisting alcohol abuse.

HTLV-I/II Injection drug users are at relatively high risk not only for infection with HIV but also for that with human T-cell lymphotropic virus (HTLV) types I and II (see Chap. 192). In the United States, injection drug use has been the most important behavioral factor associated with the presence of antibody to HTLV-I/II in blood donors screened for retroviral infection. Seroprevalence studies in the United States have documented HTLV-I/II infection in more than 10 percent of certain populations of drug users. HTLV infection has often been associated with black race, older age, and a history of heroin injection. Rates of infection have shown wide geographic variation. More than three-fourths of the HTLV infections in drug injectors are due to HTLV-II; this observation may account for the relatively low rate of clinical disease reported to date in patients with such infections. Two studies have suggested, however, that coinfection with HTLV-I/II and HIV may be associated with more rapid progression of HIV infection and earlier mortality.

HARM REDUCTION FOR INJECTION DRUG USERS

The myriad infectious consequences of injection drug use mandate the development of preventive harm-reduction strategies based on the principle that, since many drug users will continue to inject drugs, they should do so in a way that minimizes harm to themselves and others. Prevention of the infectious complications of injection and education about more hygienic injection practices are primary goals. Legalization of the purchase and possession of needles and syringes and institution of needle- and syringe-exchange programs are the most obvious examples of the harm-reduction approach. In addition to the distribution or exchange of injection equipment, needle-exchange programs typically include AIDS education, condom distribution, and enrollment in a variety of medical and social services.

Provision of primary medical care services linked to drug-abuse treatment is a way to promote preventive regimens to enhance harm reduction. In this and all other clinical settings, injection drug users should be routinely screened for hepatitis B, latent *M. tuberculosis* infection, and syphilis and other sexually transmitted diseases. They should be offered pneumococcal, influenza, tetanus, and hepatitis B immunization and (when appropriate) prophylaxis for tuberculosis and complications of HIV disease.

Clearly, the ultimate goal of harm-reduction strategies should be the reduction or prevention of illicit drug use itself, with the elimination of its root causes. Nonetheless, a high priority must also be assigned to the development of strategies that will minimize the serious medical consequences of drug abuse.

BIBLIOGRAPHY

ALCABES P, FRIEDLAND G: Injection drug use and human immunodeficiency virus infection. Clin Infect Dis 20:1467, 1995

ALLAND D et al: Transmission of tuberculosis in New York City: An analysis by DNA fingerprinting and conventional epidemiologic methods. N Engl J Med 330:1710, 1994

CENTERS FOR DISEASE CONTROL AND PREVENTION: Initial therapy for tuberculosis in the era of multi-drug resistance. Morb Mort Week Rep 42(RR-7):1, 1993

————: National action plan to combat multi-drug-resistant tuberculosis; meeting the challenge of multi-drug-resistant tuberculosis; management of persons exposed to multi-drug-resistant tuberculosis. Morb Mort Week Rep 41(RR-11):1, 1992

CHAMBERS HF et al: *Staphylococcus aureus* endocarditis: Clinical manifestations in addicts and non-addicts. Medicine 62:170, 1983

———— et al: Right-sided *Staphylococcus aureus* endocarditis in intravenous drug users: Two-week combination therapy. Ann Intern Med 109:619, 1988

CHANDRASEKAR PH, NARULA AP: Bone and joint infections in intravenous drug abusers. Rev Infect Dis 8:904, 1986

CHERUBIN CE, SAPIRA JD: The medical complications of drug addiction and the medical assessment of the intravenous drug user: 25 years later. Ann Intern Med 119:1017, 1993

FELTON CP: Pulmonary infections in the addict, in *Medical Aspects of Drug Abuse*, RW Richter (ed). Hagerstown, MD, Harper & Row, 1975

FRIEDEN TR et al: The emergence of drug-resistant tuberculosis in New York City. N Engl J Med 328:521, 1993

HAVERKOS HW, LANGE WR: Serious infections other than human immunodeficiency virus among intravenous drug users. J Infect Dis 161:894, 1990

HIRSCHTICH RE et al: Bacterial pneumonia in persons infected with the human immunodeficiency virus. N Engl J Med 333:845, 1995

ISEMAN MD et al: Directly observed treatment of tuberculosis. N Engl J Med 328:576, 1993

KHABBAZ RA et al: Seroprevalence of HTLV-I and HTLV-II among intravenous drug users and persons in clinics for sexually transmitted diseases. N Engl J Med 326:375, 1992

LETTAU LA et al: Outbreak of severe hepatitis due to delta and hepatitis B viruses in parenteral drug abusers and their contacts. N Engl J Med 317:1256, 1987

LEVINE DP, SOBEL JD (eds): *Infections in Intravenous Drug Abusers.* New York, Oxford University Press, 1991

LURIE P et al: *The Public Health Impact of Needle-Exchange Programs in the United States and Abroad.* San Francisco, University of California, 1993

MARANTZ PR et al: Inability to predict diagnosis in febrile intravenous drug abusers. Ann Intern Med 106:823, 1978

SANDE MA et al: Endocarditis in intravenous drug users, in *Infective Endocarditis*, 2d ed, D Kaye (ed). New York, Raven Press, 1992, pp 345–359

SELWYN PA et al: Clinical manifestations and predictors of disease progression in drug users with human immunodeficiency virus infection. N Engl J Med 327:1697, 1992

STONEBURNER RL et al: A larger spectrum of severe HIV-1 related disease in intravenous drug users in New York City. Science 242:916, 1988

135 *Lawrence C. Madoff*

INFECTIONS FROM BITES, SCRATCHES, AND BURNS

The skin is an essential component of the nonspecific immune system, protecting the host from potential pathogens in the environment. Breaches in this protective barrier thus represent a form of immunocompromise that predisposes the patient to infection. Bites and scratches from animals and humans allow the inoculation of microorganisms past the skin's protective barrier into deeper, susceptible host tissues. Thermal burns may cause massive destruction of the integument as well as derangements in humoral and cellular immunity, enabling environmental opportunists and components of the host's own skin flora to cause infection.

ANIMAL BITES AND SCRATCHES   Each year in the United States, between 1 and 2 million animal-bite wounds are sustained; the vast majority are inflicted by pet dogs and cats, which number more than 100 million. Other bite wounds are a consequence of encounters with animals in the wild or in occupational settings. While many of these wounds require minimal or no therapy, a significant number result in infection, which may be life-threatening. The microbiology of bite-wound infections in general reflects the oropharyngeal flora of the biting animal, although organisms from the soil, the skin of the animal and victim, and the animal's feces may also be involved.

Dog Bites Dogs are responsible for approximately 80 percent of bite wounds, an estimated 15 to 20 percent of which become infected. Most dog bites are provoked and inflicted by the victim's pet or by a dog known to the victim. These bites frequently occur during efforts to break up a dogfight. Victims tend to be male, and bites most often involve a lower extremity. Infection typically manifests 8 to 24 h after the bite as pain at the site of injury with cellulitis accompanied by purulent, sometimes foul-smelling discharge. Septic arthritis and osteomyelitis may develop if the canine tooth penetrates synovium or bone. Systemic manifestations such as fever, lymphadenopathy, and lymphangitis also may occur. The microbiology of dog-bite wound infections is usually mixed and includes alpha-hemolytic streptococci, *Staphylococcus* species, *Pasteurella multocida*, *Eikenella corrodens*, and *Capnocytophaga canimorsus* (formerly designated DF-2). Many wounds also include anaerobic bacteria such as *Actinomyces*, *Fusobacterium*, *Prevotella*, and *Porphyromonas* species.

While most infections resulting from dog-bite injuries are localized to the area of injury, many of the microorganisms involved are capable of causing systemic infection, including bacteremia, meningitis, brain abscess, endocarditis, and chorioamnionitis. These infections are particularly likely in hosts with edema or compromised lymphatic drainage in the involved extremity (e.g., after radical or modified radical mastectomy) and in patients who are immunocompromised by medication or disease (e.g., glucocorticoid use, systemic lupus erythematosus, acute leukemia, or hepatic cirrhosis). In addition, dog bites and scratches may result in systemic illnesses such as rabies (Chap. 199) and tetanus (Chap. 146).

Infection with *C. canimorsus* following dog-bite wounds may result in fulminant sepsis, disseminated intravascular coagulation, and renal failure, particularly in hosts who have impaired hepatic function, who have undergone splenectomy, or who are immunosuppressed. This organism is a thin gram-negative rod that is difficult to culture on most solid media but grows in a variety of liquid media. The bacteria are occasionally seen within polymorphonuclear leukocytes on Wright-stained smears of peripheral blood from septic patients.

Cat Bites Although less common than dog bites, more than half of all cat bites and scratches result in infection. Because the narrow, sharp feline incisors penetrate deeply into tissue, cat bites are more likely than dog bites to cause septic arthritis and osteomyelitis; the development of these conditions is particularly likely when punctures are located over or near a joint, especially in the hand. Women sustain cat bites more frequently than do men. These bites most often involve the hands and arms. Both bites and scratches from cats are prone to infection from organisms in the cat's oropharynx. *P. multocida*, a normal component of the feline oral flora, is a small gram-negative coccobacillus implicated in the majority of cat-bite wound infections. Like that of dog-bite wound infections, however, the microflora of cat-bite wound infections is usually mixed. Other microorganisms causing infection after cat bites are similar to those causing dog-bite wound infections.

The same risk factors for systemic infection following dog-bite wounds apply to cat-bite wounds. *Pasteurella* infections tend to advance rapidly, often within hours, causing severe inflammation accompanied by purulent drainage; *Pasteurella* may also be spread by respiratory droplets from animals, resulting in pneumonia or bacteremia. Like dog-bite wounds, cat-bite wounds may result in the transmission of rabies or in the development of tetanus. Infection with *Bartonella henselae* causes cat-scratch disease (Chap. 165) and is an important late consequence of cat bites and scratches. Tularemia (Chap. 163) has also been reported to follow cat bites.

Other Animal Bites Infections have been attributed to bites from many animal species, often as a consequence of occupational exposure (farmers, laboratory workers, veterinarians) or recreational exposure (hunters and trappers, wilderness campers, owners of exotic pets). Generally, the microflora of bite wounds reflects the oral flora of the biting animal. Most members of the cat family, including feral cats, harbor *P. multocida*. Bite wounds from aquatic animals such as alligators or piranhas may contain *Aeromonas hydrophila*. Venomous snakebites (Chap. 392) result in severe inflammatory responses and tissue necrosis, which renders these injuries prone to infection. The snake's oral flora includes many species of aerobes and anaerobes, such as *Pseudomonas aeruginosa*, *Proteus* species, *Staphylococcus epidermidis*, *Bacteroides fragilis*, and *Clostridium* species. Bites from nonhuman primates are highly susceptible to infection with pathogens similar to those isolated from human bites (which are discussed later in this chapter). Bites from Old World monkeys (*Macaca*) may also result in the transmission of B virus (*Herpesvirus simiae*, cercopithecine herpesvirus), a cause of serious infection of the human central nervous system. Bites of seals, walruses, and polar bears may cause a chronic suppurative infection known as seal finger, which is probably due to one or more species of *Mycoplasma* colonizing these animals.

Rat-bite fever Small rodents, including rats, mice, and gerbils, as well as animals that prey on rodents may transmit *Streptobacillus moniliformis* (a microaerophilic, pleomorphic gram-negative rod) or *Spirillum minor* (a spirochete), which cause a clinical illness known as rat-bite fever. The vast majority of cases in the United States are streptobacillary, whereas *Spirillum* infection occurs mainly in Asia.

In the United States, the risk of rodent bite mainly affects laboratory workers or inhabitants of rodent-infested dwellings (particularly children). Rat-bite fever is distinguished from acute bite-wound infection by its typical manifestation after the initial wound has healed. Streptobacillary disease follows an incubation period of 3 to 10 days. Fever, chills, myalgias, headache, and severe migratory arthralgias are usually followed by a maculopapular rash, which characteristically involves the palms and soles and may become confluent or purpuric. Complications include endocarditis, myocarditis, meningitis, pneumonia, and abscesses in many organs. *Haverhill fever* is an *S. moniliformis* infection acquired from contaminated milk or drinking water and has similar manifestations. Streptobacillary rat-bite fever was frequently fatal in the preantibiotic era. The differential diagnosis includes Rocky Mountain spotted fever, Lyme disease, leptospirosis, and secondary syphilis. The diagnosis is made by direct observation of the causative organisms in tissue or blood, by culture on enriched media, or by serologic testing with specific agglutinins.

Spirillum infection (referred to in Japan as *sodoku*) causes pain and purple swelling at the site of the initial bite, with associated lymphangitis and regional lymphadenopathy, after an incubation period of 1 to 4 weeks. The systemic illness includes fever, chills, and headache. The original lesion may eventually progress to an eschar. The infection is diagnosed by direct visualization of the spirochetes in blood or tissue or by animal inoculation.

Erysipeloid This distinctive skin infection is caused by direct cutaneous inoculation with *Erysipelothrix rhusiopathiae*. Because this organism is most often associated with fish and domestic swine, erysipeloid most commonly results from an occupational injury related to fishing ("fish-handler's disease") or slaughterhouse work; it may also follow contact with other animals or contact with fish or meat in a household setting. After an incubation period of several days, pain (often severe), edema, and a well-demarcated, purplish-red lesion develop. Systemic manifestations are unusual, but bacteremia and endocarditis have occasionally been reported. Definitive diagnosis requires isolation of the bacteria from a biopsy specimen, a tissue aspirate, or blood.

Human bite infections Human bites may be self-inflicted, may be sustained by medical personnel caring for patients, or may take place during fights or domestic abuse or during sexual activity. Human bites more frequently become infected than do bites inflicted by other animals. These infections reflect the diverse oral microflora of humans, which includes multiple species of aerobic and anaerobic bacteria. Common aerobic isolates include viridans streptococci, *Staphylococcus aureus*, *E. corrodens* (which is particularly common in clenched-fist injury; see below), and *Haemophilus influenzae*. Anaerobic species, including *Fusobacterium nucleatum* and *Prevotella*, *Porphyromonas*, *Peptococcus*, and *Peptostreptococcus* species, are isolated from 50 percent of human-bite wound infections; many of these isolates produce β-lactamases. The oral flora of hospitalized and debilitated patients often includes Enterobacteriaceae in addition to the usual organisms. Human immunodeficiency virus and hepatitis B virus have both been reported to be transmitted by human bite, but these instances appear to be quite rare.

Human bites are categorized as *occlusional* injuries, which are inflicted by actual biting, and *clenched-fist* injuries, which are sustained when the fist of one individual strikes the teeth of another, causing traumatic laceration of the hand. For several reasons, clenched-fist injuries result in particularly serious infections. The deep spaces of the hand, including the bone, joint, and tendons, are frequently inoculated with organisms in the course of such injuries. The clenched position of the fist during injury, followed by extension of the hand, may further promote the introduction of bacteria as contaminated tendons retract beneath the skin's surface. Moreover, medical attention often is sought only after frank infection develops.

℞ TREATMENT

Initial Assessment A careful history should be elicited, including the type of biting animal, the type of attack (provoked or unprovoked), and the amount of time elapsed since injury. Local and regional authorities should be contacted to determine whether an individual species could be rabid and/or to locate and observe the biting animal when rabies prophylaxis may be indicated. Suspicious human-bite wounds should provoke careful questioning regarding domestic or child abuse. Details on antibiotic allergies, immunosuppression, splenectomy, liver disease, mastectomy, and immunization history should be obtained. The wound should be inspected carefully for evidence of infection, including redness, exudate, and foul odor. The type of wound (puncture, laceration, or scratch), the depth of penetration, and the possible involvement of joints, tendons, nerves, and bone should be assessed. It is often useful to include a diagram or photograph of the wound in the medical record. In addition, a general physical examination should be conducted and should include an assessment of vital signs as well as an evaluation for evidence of lymphangitis, lymphadenopathy, dermatologic lesions, and functional limitations. Injuries to the hand warrant consultation with a hand surgeon for the assessment of tendon, nerve, and muscular damage. Radiographs should be obtained when the bone may have been penetrated or a tooth fragment may be present. Culture and Gram's staining of all infected wounds are essential; anaerobic cultures should be undertaken if abscesses, devitalized tissue, or foul-smelling exudate is present. A small-tipped swab may be used to culture deep punctures or small lacerations. It is also reasonable to culture samples from uninfected wounds due to bites inflicted by animals other than dogs and cats, since the microorganisms causing disease are less predictable in these cases. A white blood cell count should be determined and blood cultured if systemic infection is suspected.

Wound Management Wound closure is controversial in bite injuries. Many authorities prefer not to attempt primary closure of wounds that are or may become infected, preferring to irrigate these wounds copiously, debride devitalized tissue, remove foreign bodies, and approximate the wound edges. Delayed primary closure may be undertaken after the risk of infection is over. Small uninfected wounds may be allowed to close by secondary intention. Puncture wounds due to cat bites should be left unsutured because of the high rate at which they become infected. Facial wounds are usually sutured after thorough cleaning and irrigation because of the importance of a good cosmetic result in this area and because anatomic factors such as an excellent blood supply and the absence of dependent edema lessen the risk of infection.

Antibiotic Therapy Antibiotics should be administered in all established bite-wound infections and should be chosen in light of the most likely potential pathogens, as indicated by the biting species and by Gram's stain and culture results (Table 135-1). For dog and cat bites, antibiotics should be effective against *S. aureus*, *P. multocida*, *C. canimorsus*, streptococci, and oral anaerobes. For human bites, agents with activity against *S. aureus*, *H. influenzae*, and β-lactamase-positive oral anaerobes should be used. The combination of an extended-spectrum penicillin with a β-lactamase inhibitor (amoxicillin/clavulanic acid, ticarcillin/clavulanic acid, ampicillin/sulbactam) appears

to offer the most reliable coverage for these pathogens. Second-generation cephalosporins (cefuroxime, cefoxitin) also offer substantial coverage. The choice of antibiotics in penicillin-allergic patients (particularly those in whom immediate-type hypersensitivity makes the use of cephalosporins hazardous) is more difficult and is based primarily on in vitro sensitivity since data on clinical efficacy are inadequate. The combination of an antibiotic active against gram-positive cocci and anaerobes (such as clindamycin) with trimethoprim-sulfamethoxazole or a fluoroquinolone, which has activity against many of the other potential pathogens, would appear reasonable.

Antibiotics are normally given for 10 to 14 days, but the response to therapy must be carefully monitored. Failure to respond should prompt a consideration of diagnostic alternatives and surgical evaluation for possible drainage or debridement. Complications such as osteomyelitis or septic arthritis mandate a longer duration of therapy.

Management of *C. canimorsus* sepsis requires a 2-week course of intravenous penicillin G (2 million units intravenously every 4 h) and supportive measures. Alternative agents for the treatment of *C. canimorsus* infection include cephalosporins and fluoroquinolones. Serious infection with *P. multocida* (e.g., pneumonia, sepsis, or meningitis) should also be treated with intravenous penicillin G. Alternative agents include second- or third-generation cephalosporins or ciprofloxacin.

Bites by venomous snakes may not require antibiotic treatment, but it is often difficult to distinguish signs of infection from tissue damage caused by the envenomation. Thus many authorities continue to recommend treatment directed against the snake's oral flora—i.e., the administration of broadly active agents such as ceftriaxone (1 to 2 g intravenously every 12 to 24 h) or ampicillin/sulbactam (1.5 to 3.0 g intravenously every 6 h).

Seal finger appears to respond to doxycycline (100 mg twice daily). *E. rhusiopathiae* is sensitive to most β-lactam antibiotics, including penicillin, as well as to ciprofloxacin. Its resistance to vancomycin, which is unusual among gram-positive bacteria, is of potential clinical significance since this agent is sometimes used in empirical therapy for skin infection.

The use of antibiotics in patients presenting early after bite injury (within 8 h) is controversial. Although symptomatic infection will not yet be manifest in many of these wounds at this point, many early wounds will harbor pathogens, and many will become infected. Studies of the use of prophylactic antibiotics in wound infections are limited and have often included small numbers of cases in which various types of wounds have been managed according to various protocols. A recent meta-analysis of eight randomized trials of prophylactic antibiotics in patients with dog-bite wounds demonstrated a reduction of the rate of infection by approximately 50 percent with prophylaxis. However, in the absence of sound clinical trials, many clinicians base the decision to treat bite wounds presumptively with empirical antibiotics on the species of the biting animal; the location, severity, and extent of the bite wound; and the existence of comorbid conditions in the host (Table 135-1). All human- and monkey-bite wounds should be treated presumptively because of the high rate of infection. Most cat-bite wounds, particularly those involving the hand, should be treated. Other factors favoring treatment for bite wounds include severe injury, as in crush wounds; potential bone or joint involvement; involvement of the hands or genital region; host immunocompromise, including that due to liver disease or splenectomy; and prior mastectomy on the side of an involved upper extremity. When prophylactic antibiotics are administered, they are usually given for 3 to 5 days.

Rabies prophylaxis, consisting of both passive administration of rabies immune globulin and active immunization with the human diploid vaccine, should be given in consultation with local and regional public health authorities for many wild-animal (and some domestic-animal) bites and scratches as well as for certain nonbite exposures (see Chap. 199). Rabies is endemic in a variety of animals, including dogs and cats in many areas of the world. Many local

Table 135-1

Management of Wound Infections Following Animal Bites

Biting Species	Commonly Isolated Pathogens	Preferred Antibiotic(s)*	Alternative Agent for Penicillin-Allergic Patient	Recommendation for Prophylaxis in Patients with Recent Uninfected Wounds	Other Considerations
Dog	*Staphylococcus aureus, Pasteurella multocida,* anaerobes, *Capnocytophaga canimorsus*	Amoxicillin/clavulanic acid (250–500 mg PO tid); or ampicillin/sulbactam (1.5–3.0 g IV q6h)	Clindamycin (150–300 mg PO qid) plus either TMP-SMZ (1 double-strength tablet bid) or ciprofloxacin (500 mg PO bid)	Sometimes†	Consider rabies prophylaxis.
Cat	*P. multocida, S. aureus,* anaerobes	Amoxicillin/clavulanic acid or ampicillin/sulbactam, as for dog bite	Clindamycin plus either TMP-SMZ or a fluoroquinolone	Usually	Consider rabies prophylaxis; carefully evaluate for joint/bone penetration.
Human; occlusional bite	Viridans streptococci, *S. aureus, Haemophilus influenzae,* anaerobes	Amoxicillin/clavulanic acid or ampicillin/sulbactam, as for dog bite	Erythromycin, fluoroquinolone	Always	—
Human; clenched-fist injury	As for occlusional bite plus *Eikenella corrodens*	Ampicillin/sulbactam as for dog bite or imipenem	Cefoxitin‡ (1.5 g IV q6h)	Always	Examine for tendon/nerve/joint involvement.
Monkey	As for human bite	As for human bite	As for human bite	Always	For macaque monkeys, consider B virus prophylaxis with acyclovir.
Snake	*Pseudomonas aeruginosa, Proteus* species, *Bacteroides fragilis, Clostridium* species	Ampicillin/sulbactam as for dog bite	Clindamycin plus either TMP-SMZ or a fluoroquinolone	Sometimes, especially for venomous snakebite	Use antivenin for venomous snakebite.
Rodent	*Streptobacillus moniliformis, Leptospira* species, *P. multocida*	Penicillin VK (500 mg PO bid)	Doxycycline (100 mg PO qd)	Sometimes†	—

* Antibiotic choices should be based on culture data, when available. These suggestions for empirical therapy need to be tailored to individual circumstances and local conditions. Intravenous regimens should be used for hospitalized patients. When the patient is to be discharged after initial management, a single intravenous dose of antibiotic may be given and followed by oral therapy. TMP-SMZ, trimethoprim-sulfamethoxazole.
† Prophylactic antibiotics are suggested for severe or extensive wounds, facial wounds, or crush injuries; when bone or joint may be involved; or when comorbidity exists (see text).
‡ Cefoxitin may be hazardous to patients with immediate-type hypersensitivity to penicillin.

health authorities require the reporting of all animal bites. A tetanus booster immunization should be given if the patient has undergone primary immunization but has not received a booster dose in the past 5 years. Patients who have not previously undergone primary immunization should be immunized and should also receive tetanus immune globulin. Elevation of the site of injury is an important adjunct to antimicrobial therapy. Immobilization of the infected area, especially the hand, is also beneficial.

INFECTIONS CAUSED BY *AEROMONAS* AND *PLESIO-MONAS* Two species of gram-negative bacilli, members of the family Pseudomonadaceae, are found in fresh and brackish coastal waters and are occasional causes of human disease. *Aeromonas* species may be inoculated into wounds exposed to salt water or freshwater or into injuries caused by fish or shellfish implicated in skin and soft tissue infection. Bacteremic illness may occur in immunocompromised patients and in those with hepatobiliary disease. *Aeromonas* has also been associated with diarrhea, particularly among travelers. *Plesiomonas shigelloides* has also been implicated in diarrhea, usually that developing in association with exposure to contaminated food or water. This organism can cause bacteremia and meningitis; most cases involve immunocompromised patients. Both *Aeromonas* and *Plesiomonas* exhibit variable antibiotic sensitivities but are most often susceptible to chloramphenicol, trimethoprim-sulfamethoxazole, quinolones, imipenem, and third-generation cephalosporins.

BURNS **Epidemiology** More than 2 million burn injuries are brought to medical attention in the United States each year. While many burn injuries are minor and require little or no intervention,

approximately 70,000 persons are hospitalized for these injuries, and 20,000 of this number are burned severely enough to require admission to a specialized burn unit. Scalds, structural fires, and flammable liquids and gases are the major causes of burns, but electrical, chemical, and smoking-related sources are also important. Burns predispose to infection by damaging the protective barrier function of the skin, thus facilitating the entry of pathogenic microorganisms, and by inducing systemic immunosuppression. It is therefore not surprising that infectious complications are the major cause of morbidity and mortality in serious burn injury and that as many as 10,000 patients in the United States die of burn-related infections each year.

Pathophysiology Loss of the cutaneous barrier facilitates entry of the patient's own flora and of organisms from the hospital environment into the burn wound. The wound often contains devitalized or frankly necrotic tissue that quickly becomes contaminated with bacteria. Invasive infection—localized and/or systemic—occurs when bacteria penetrate viable tissue, usually below the eschar. Streptococci and staphylococci were the predominant causes of burn-wound infection in the preantibiotic era and remain important pathogens at present. With the advent of antimicrobial agents, *P. aeruginosa* became a major problem in burn-wound management. As antibiotics more effective against *Pseudomonas* have become available, fungal infections (particularly those due to *Candida albicans, Aspergillus* species, and the agents of mucormycosis) have emerged as increasingly important pathogens in burn-wound patients. Herpes simplex virus infection has also been found in burn wounds, especially on the face.

The frequency of infection parallels the extent and severity of burn injury. Severe burns cause defects in both cellular and humoral immunity that have a major impact on infection. For example, decreases in the number and activity of circulating helper T cells, increases in suppressor T cells, and diminution in levels of immunoglobulin follow major burns. Neutrophil function has also been shown to be impaired after burns. The increased levels of multiple cytokines detected in burn patients are compatible with the widely held belief that the inflammatory response becomes dysregulated in these individuals. Increased permeability of the gut wall to bacteria and their components, such as endotoxin, also contributes to immune dysregulation and sepsis. Thus, the burn patient is predisposed to infection at remote sites (see below) as well as at the sites of burn injury.

Clinical Manifestations Since clinical indications of wound infection are difficult to interpret, wounds must be monitored carefully for changes that may reflect infection. A margin of erythema frequently surrounds the sites of burns and by itself is not usually indicative of infection. Signs of infection include the conversion of a partial-thickness to a full-thickness burn, color changes (e.g., the appearance of a dark brown or black discoloration of the wound), the new appearance of erythema or violaceous edema in normal tissue at the wound margins, the sudden separation of the eschar from subcutaneous tissues, and the degeneration of the wound with the appearance of a new eschar. The appearance of a green discoloration of the wound or subcutaneous fat or the development of ecthyma gangrenosum at a remote site points to a diagnosis of invasive *P. aeruginosa* infection. Changes in body temperature, hypotension, tachycardia, altered mentation, neutropenia or neutrophilia, thrombocytopenia, and renal failure may result from invasive burn wounds and sepsis. However, because profound alterations in homeostasis occur as a consequence of burns per se and because inflammation without infection is a normal component of these injuries, the assessment of these changes is complicated. Alterations in body temperature, for example, are attributable to thermoregulatory dysfunction; tachycardia and hyperventilation accompany the metabolic changes induced by extensive burn injury and are not necessarily indicative of bacterial sepsis.

Given the difficulty of evaluating burn wounds solely on the basis of clinical observation and laboratory data, wound biopsies are necessary for definitive diagnosis of infection. The timing of these biopsies can be guided by clinical changes, but in some centers burn wounds are routinely biopsied at 48-h intervals. The biopsy specimen is examined for histologic evidence of bacterial invasion, and quantitative microbiologic cultures are performed. The presence of $>10^5$ viable bacteria per gram of tissue is highly suggestive of invasive infection and of a dramatically increased risk of sepsis. Histopathologic evidence of invasion of viable tissue by microorganisms is a more definitive indicator of infection. A blood culture positive for the same organism seen in high quantities in biopsied tissue is a reliable indicator of burn sepsis. Surface cultures may provide some indication of the microorganisms present in the hospital environment but are not indicative of the etiology of infection.

In addition to infection of the burn wound itself, a number of other infections due to the immunosuppression caused by extensive burns and the manipulations necessary for clinical care put burn patients at risk. Pneumonia, now the most common infectious complication among hospitalized burn patients, most often is nosocomially acquired via the respiratory route; septic pulmonary emboli may also occur. Suppurative thrombophlebitis may complicate the vascular catheterization necessary for fluid and nutritional support in burns. Endocarditis, urinary tract infection, bacterial chondritis (particularly in patients with burned ears), and intraabdominal infection also complicate serious burn injury.

℞ TREATMENT

The ultimate goal of burn-wound management is closure and healing of the wound. Early surgical excision of burned tissue, with extensive debridement of necrotic tissue and grafting of skin or skin substitutes, greatly decreases the mortality associated with severe burns. In addition, the three widely used topical antimicrobial agents—silver sulfadiazine cream, mafenide acetate cream, and silver nitrate—dramatically decrease the bacterial burden of burn wounds and reduce the incidence of burn-wound infection; they are routinely applied to partial- and full-thickness burns. All three agents are broadly active against many bacteria and against some fungi and are useful before bacterial colonization is established. Silver sulfadiazine is often used initially, but its value can be limited by bacterial resistance. Mafenide acetate has broader activity; the cream penetrates eschars and thus can prevent or treat infection beneath the eschars. The foremost disadvantages of this agent are that it can inhibit carbonic anhydrase, resulting in metabolic acidosis, and that it elicits hypersensitivity reactions in up to 7 percent of patients. This agent is most often used when gram-negative bacteria invade the burn wound and when treatment with silver sulfadiazene fails.

When invasive wound infection is diagnosed, topical therapy should be changed to mafenide acetate. Subeschar clysis (the direct instillation of an antibiotic, often piperacillin, under the eschar into wound tissues) is a useful adjunct to surgical and systemic antimicrobial therapy. Systemic treatment with antibiotics active against the pathogens present in the wound should be instituted. In the absence of culture data, treatment with an antibiotic active against gram-positive pathogens, such as oxacillin (2 g intravenously every 4 h), and with antibiotics active against *P. aeruginosa*, such as mezlocillin (3 g intravenously every 4 h) and gentamicin (5 mg/kg intravenously per day), should be started. In the penicillin-allergic patient, vancomycin (1 g intravenously every 12 h) may be substituted for oxacillin (and is efficacious when methicillin-resistant *S. aureus* is present), and ciprofloxacin (400 mg intravenously every 12 h) may be substituted for mezlocillin. It has frequently been noted that patients with burn wounds have alterations in metabolism and renal clearance mechanisms that mandate the monitoring of serum antibiotic levels; the levels achieved with standard doses are often subtherapeutic.

In general, prophylactic systemic antibiotics have no role in the management of burn wounds (except for minor burns in outpatients) and can in fact lead to colonization with resistant microorganisms. An exception involves cases requiring burn-wound manipulation. Since procedures such as debridement, excision, or grafting frequently result in bacteremia, prophylactic systemic antibiotics are administered at the time of burn-wound manipulation; the particular agents used should be chosen on the basis of data obtained by wound culture or data on the hospital's resident flora. All burn-injury patients should undergo tetanus booster immunization if they have completed primary immunization but have not received a booster dose in the past 5 years. Patients without prior immunization should receive tetanus immune globulin and undergo primary immunization. Infection control measures play a major role in preventing burn-wound infection and limiting the spread of antibiotic-resistant nosocomial pathogens.

BIBLIOGRAPHY

CUMMINGS P: Antibiotics to prevent infection in patients with dog bite wounds: A meta-analysis of randomized trials. Ann Emerg Med 23:535, 1994

FALLOUJI MA: Traumatic love bites. Br J Surg 77:100, 1990

GOLDSTEIN EJ: Bite wounds and infection. Clin Infect Dis 14:633, 1992

HOLMES GP et al: Guidelines for the prevention and treatment of B-virus infections in exposed persons. The B Virus Working Group. Clin Infect Dis 20:421, 1995

KULLBERG BJ et al: Purpura fulminans and symmetrical peripheral gangrene caused by *Capnocytophaga canimorsus* (formerly DF-2) septicemia—a complication of dog bite. Medicine (Baltimore) 70:287, 1991

MCMANUS WF et al: Subeschar antibiotic infusion in the treatment of burn wound infection. J Trauma 20:1021, 1980

PRUITT BJ et al: The changing epidemiology of infection in burn patients. World J Surg 16:57, 1992

WEBER DJ et al: Infections resulting from animal bites. Infect Dis Clin North Am 5:663, 1991

YOUN YK et al: The role of mediators in the response to thermal injury. World J Surg 16:30, 1992

YURT R: Burns, in *Mandell, Douglas and Bennett's Principles and Practice of Infectious Diseases*, 4th ed, G. Mandell et al (eds). New York, Churchill Livingstone, 1995, pp 2761–2765

136 | *Robert Finberg, Joyce Fingeroth*

INFECTIONS IN TRANSPLANT RECIPIENTS

The evaluation of infections in transplant recipients involves consideration of both the donor and the recipient of the transplanted organ. Infections following transplantation are complicated by the use of drugs that are necessary to enhance the likelihood of survival of the transplanted organ but that also cause the host to be immunocompromised. Thus what might have been a latent or asymptomatic infection in an immunocompetent donor becomes a life-threatening problem for the immunocompromised recipient.

A variety of organisms have been transmitted by organ transplantation (Table 136-1). Careful attention to the sterility of the medium used to handle the organ combined with meticulous culturing to detect contamination may reduce rates of transmission of infectious material. From 2 percent to more than 20 percent of donor kidneys are estimated to be contaminated with bacteria—in most cases, the organisms that colonize the skin or grow in the tissue culture medium used to bathe the donor kidney while it awaits transplantation. The reported rate of bacterial contamination of transplanted bone marrow is as high as 17 percent but is most commonly around 1 percent. It is not surprising that the use of enrichment columns and monoclonal-antibody depletion procedures results in a higher incidence of contamination. Approximately 2 percent of cryopreserved marrow and peripheral blood stem cells transfused as part of treatment for cancer are contaminated. In one series of patients receiving contaminated products, 14 percent had fever or positive blood cultures, but none died. Results of cultures performed at the time of cryopreservation and at the time of thawing were helpful in guiding therapy for the recipient.

In many organ transplantation centers, transmission of diseases that may be latent or clinically inapparent in the donor has resulted in the development of specific protocols for the screening of transplanted organs. In addition to ordering serologic studies focusing on viruses such as herpes simplex virus (HSV), varicella-zoster virus (VZV), cytomegalovirus (CMV), Epstein-Barr virus (EBV), hepatitis B and C viruses, and human immunodeficiency virus (HIV) and on parasites such as *Toxoplasma gondii*, clinicians caring for organ donors should also consider assessing stool (for parasites) and testing for tuberculosis. In this chapter, we will consider aspects unique to various transplant settings.

INFECTIONS IN BONE MARROW TRANSPLANT RECIPIENTS

Bone marrow transplantation for either immune deficiency or cancer results in a transient state of complete immune incompetence. Immediately after transplantation, both phagocytes and immune cells (T cells and B cells) are absent, and the host is extremely susceptible

Table 136-1

Organisms Transmitted by Organ Transplantation

Viruses	Parasites
Cytomegalovirus	*Plasmodium falciparum*
Epstein-Barr virus	*Toxoplasma gondii*
Herpes simplex virus	*Strongyloides stercoralis*
Hepatitis B and C viruses	*Trypanosoma cruzi*
Human immunodeficiency virus	
Fungi	
Candida albicans	
Histoplasma capsulatum	
Cryptococcus	

to infection. The reconstitution that follows transplantation has been likened to maturation of the immune system in neonates. The analogy does not entirely predict infections seen in bone marrow transplant (BMT) recipients, however, because the new marrow is usually expressed in an old host who has several latent infections already.

TIMING OF INFECTIONS In the first month after bone marrow transplantation, infectious complications are similar to those in granulocytopenic patients receiving chemotherapy for acute myelocytic or acute lymphocytic leukemia (see Chap. 87 and Fig. 136-1). Because of the anticipated 2- to 4-week duration of neutropenia in this population, many centers give prophylactic antibiotics to patients with the initiation of chemotherapy. Prophylactic trimethoprim-sulfamethoxazole or ciprofloxacin decreases the incidence of gram-negative bacteremia among these patients.

In the second month after transplantation, a major concern (particularly in allogeneic BMT recipients) is CMV disease (see Chap. 187), which rarely has its onset earlier than 14 days after transplantation and may become evident up to 4 months after the procedure. In cases in which the donor marrow is depleted of T cells [to prevent graft-versus-host disease (GVHD) or to eliminate a T cell tumor], the disease may be manifested earlier. Patients who are treated with ganciclovir (either prophylactically or because of positive antigen tests or cultures) may develop CMV infection even later than 4 months after transplantation; treatment appears to delay the development of the normal immune response to CMV infection. Although CMV infection may present as isolated fever or gastrointestinal disease, the cause of death from CMV infection in this setting is pneumonia.

The diagnosis of pneumonia in BMT recipients poses some special problems (see Table 87-5). Because they have undergone treatment with multiple chemotherapeutic agents as well as irradiation, their differential diagnosis should include CMV pneumonitis, diffuse alveolar hemorrhage, pneumonia of viral or fungal etiology, and parasitic infection. Since fungal disease and viruses such as adenovirus are also causes of pneumonia in this setting, it is important to diagnose CMV specifically (see below).

The late posttransplantation period (6 months after bone marrow reconstitution) is marked by episodes of bacteremia due to encapsulated organisms and reactivation of VZV. Because of the high risk of *Pneumocystis carinii* pneumonia (especially among patients being treated for hematologic malignancies), most patients should be maintained on prophylactic doses of trimethoprim-sulfamethoxazole. Such prophylaxis may also protect patients seropositive for *T. gondii*, which may cause pneumonia in the early weeks after transplantation or central nervous system (CNS) lesions later on. The advantages of maintaining patients on daily trimethoprim-sulfamethoxazole for 1 year after transplantation include protection against late bacterial infections with pneumococci and *Haemophilus influenzae*, which are a consequence of the inability of the immature bone marrow to respond to polysaccharide antigens (Fig. 136-1).

VIRAL INFECTIONS FOLLOWING BONE MARROW TRANSPLANTATION BMT recipients are susceptible to infection with a variety of viruses, including reactivation syndromes caused by most human herpesviruses (Table 136-2) and infections caused by viruses that circulate in the community.

Herpes Simplex Virus Within the first 6 weeks after transplantation, most patients who are seropositive for HSV type 1 excrete the virus in the oropharynx. The ability to isolate HSV declines with time. Because of the association between cultivability of virus and severity of mucositis, many clinicians administer prophylactic acyclovir to seropositive BMT recipients in order to reduce mucositis and prevent HSV pneumonia (a rare condition reported almost exclusively in BMT recipients). Both esophagitis (usually due to HSV-1) and anogenital disease (induced by HSV-2) may be prevented by acyclovir prophylaxis. → *For further discussion, see Chap. 184.*

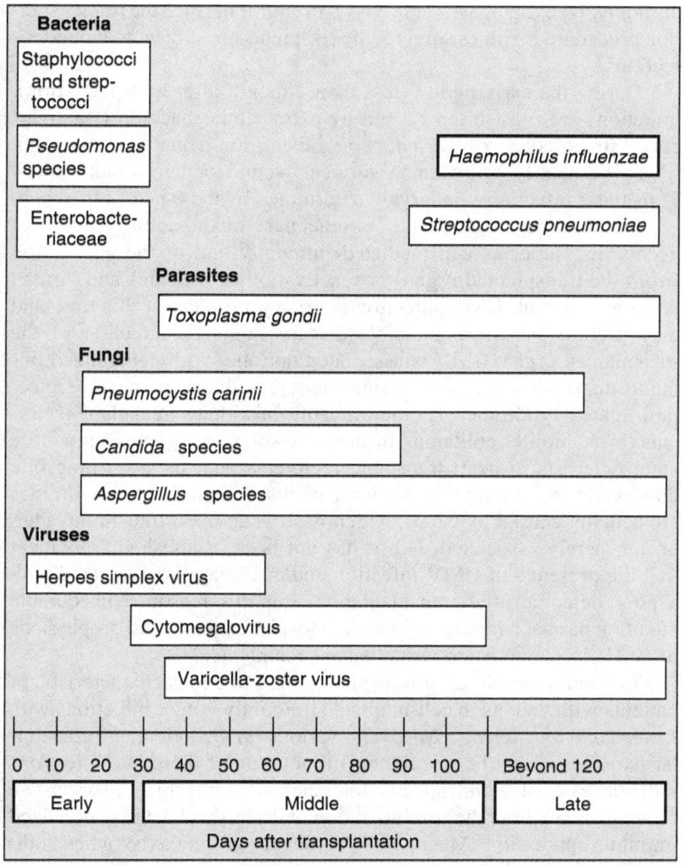

FIGURE 136-1   Infections after bone marrow transplantation.

Cytomegalovirus   The onset of CMV infection usually comes between 30 and 90 days after transplantation, when the granulocyte count is adequate but immunologic reconstitution has not occurred. CMV infection may cause interstitial pneumonia, bone marrow suppression, or graft failure. With the standard use of CMV-negative or filtered blood products, primary CMV infection should be a risk in allogeneic transplantation only when the donor is CMV-seropositive and the recipient is CMV-seronegative. Reactivation disease or superinfection with another strain from the donor is also common in CMV-positive recipients, and most seropositive patients who undergo bone marrow transplantation excrete CMV, with or without clinical findings.

Table 136-2

Herpes-Group Virus Syndromes in Transplant Recipients

Virus	Reactivation Disease
Herpes simplex virus type 1	Oral lesions, sometimes with spread (pneumonia described in bone marrow transplant recipients)
Herpes simplex virus type 2	Severe and/or persistent anogenital lesions
Varicella-zoster virus	Zoster (with possible dissemination)
Cytomegalovirus	Associated with graft rejection, fever, esophagitis, colitis, pneumonitis, hepatitis, neuropathy, glomerulopathy, and bone marrow failure
Epstein-Barr virus	Runaway infectious mononucleosis and B cell lymphoproliferative disease
Human herpesvirus 6	Fever, rash,* pneumonitis, bone marrow suppression
Human herpesvirus 7	Undefined
Kaposi's sarcoma–associated virus (human herpesvirus 8)	Kaposi's sarcoma

* A characteristic rash (seen in primary infection) has not been well defined.

Serious CMV disease is much more common among allogeneic BMT recipients and is often associated with GVHD. In addition to pneumonia and graft failure (or marrow suppression), manifestations of CMV disease in BMT recipients include fever with or without arthralgias, myalgias, hepatitis, and esophagitis. CMV ulcerations occur in both the lower and the upper gastrointestinal tract, and it is often difficult to distinguish diarrhea due to GVHD from that due to CMV infection. The finding of CMV in the liver of a patient with GVHD does not necessarily mean that CMV is responsible for hepatic enzyme abnormalities.

Because of the high fatality rate associated with CMV pneumonia in bone marrow transplantation and the difficulty of early diagnosis of CMV infection, prophylactic ganciclovir is given in some centers during the period of maximal vulnerability (from engraftment to day 120 after transplantation). The foremost problem with the administration of this drug relates to its adverse effects, which include dose-related neutrophil and platelet suppression. Because the frequency of CMV pneumonia is lower among autologous BMT recipients (2 to 7 percent) than among allogeneic BMT recipients (10 to 40 percent), prophylaxis in the former group will not become the rule until a less toxic antiviral agent becomes available. A common practice at many centers treating allogeneic BMT patients is to culture blood and urine (and bronchial secretions in some cases) and to give ganciclovir as prophylaxis for CMV pneumonia to those patients who have cultures positive for CMV. The use of the leukocyte antigen test for CMV disease (fluorescent staining of leukocytes for CMV antigens) permits earlier diagnosis but leads to the treatment of more patients, which is associated with an increase in very late disease (>120 days after transplantation). Treatment of CMV pneumonia in BMT recipients requires both intravenous immunoglobulin and ganciclovir, although ganciclovir alone is effective prophylactically. Transfusion of CMV-specific T cells from the donor decreased viral replication in one small series of patients. This result suggests that, in the future, immunotherapy may play a role in the treatment of this disease. → *For further discussion, see Chap. 187.*

Varicella-Zoster Virus   Reactivation of herpes zoster may occur as early as 1 month but more commonly occurs several months after transplantation (see Plate ID-38). Reactivation rates are approximately 40 percent for allogeneic BMT recipients and 25 percent for autologous BMT recipients. Localized zoster can spread in an immunosuppressed patient. Fortunately, disseminated disease can usually be controlled with high doses of acyclovir. Because of the high incidence of dissemination of herpes zoster among patients with skin lesions, acyclovir is given prophylactically in some centers to prevent severe disease. Low doses of acyclovir (400 mg orally, three times daily) appear to be effective in preventing reactivation of VZV. However, acyclovir also inhibits the development of VZV-specific immunity. Thus, its administration for only 6 months after transplantation does not prevent zoster from occurring when treatment is stopped. Some data suggest that administration of low doses of acyclovir for an entire year after transplantation is effective and may eliminate most cases of posttransplantation zoster. → *For further discussion, see Chap. 185.*

Epstein-Barr Virus   Primary EBV infection can be fatal to transplant recipients; EBV reactivation can cause B cell lymphoproliferative disease (EBV lymphoproliferative syndrome), which may also be fatal to patients taking immunosuppressive drugs. The localization of EBV to B cells leads to several interesting phenomena in marrow transplants. The marrow ablation that occurs as part of the bone marrow transplantation procedure may eliminate latent EBV from the host. The disease can then be reacquired after transplantation when a susceptible pool of B cells is regenerated.

The EBV lymphoproliferative syndrome can develop in the recipient's B cells (if any should survive marrow ablation) but is more likely to be a consequence of reactivation in donor cells. Reactivation of EBV is more likely during immunosuppression (e.g., it is associated with GVHD and the use of antibodies to T cells). Although less likely in autologous transplantation, reactivation can occur in T cell–depleted autologous BMT recipients (e.g., patients being treated for a T cell lymphoma with marrow depletion using antibodies to T cells). The EBV lymphoproliferative syndrome, which usually becomes apparent 1 to 3 months after engraftment, can cause high fevers and cervical adenopathy resembling the symptoms of infectious mononucleosis but more commonly resembles disseminated lymphoma. The incidence of 0.6 percent among allogeneic BMT recipients contrasts with figures of approximately 5 percent for renal transplant recipients and up to 20 percent for cardiac transplant patients. In all cases, EBV lymphoproliferative syndrome is more likely to occur with continued immunosuppression (especially that caused by the use of antibodies to T cells and cyclosporine). EBV-specific T cells generated from the donor have been used to treat EBV lymphoproliferative syndrome in the recipient. → *For further discussion, see Chap. 186.*

Other (Nonherpes) Viruses Both respiratory syncytial virus (RSV) and parainfluenza virus type 3 can cause severe or even fatal pneumonia in BMT recipients. Infections with both of these agents sometimes occur as disastrous nosocomial epidemics. Therapy with ribavirin reportedly lessens the severity of disease. Influenza is also seen in BMT recipients and generally mirrors the presence of infection in the community. In addition, adenovirus can be isolated from BMT recipients at rates varying from 5 to 18 percent. Although hemorrhagic cystitis, pneumonia, and fatal disseminated infection have been reported, adenovirus infection, which (like CMV infection) usually occurs in the first or second month after transplantation, is often asymptomatic. Infections with parvovirus B19 (presenting as anemia) and enteroviruses (sometimes fatal) can occur, rotaviruses are a common cause of gastroenteritis, and BK and JC viruses (polyomavirus hominis 1 and 2, respectively) are sometimes found in urine.

INFECTIONS IN SOLID ORGAN TRANSPLANT RECIPIENTS

Morbidity and mortality among solid organ transplant recipients have been reduced by the use of more effective antibiotics. The most important cause of early death among kidney transplant recipients, for example, was infection with organisms not susceptible to conventional antibiotic therapy. These infections developed in patients requiring prolonged courses of glucocorticoids and other immunosuppressive drugs.

The organisms that cause infections in recipients of solid organ transplants are different from those that infect BMT recipients because solid organ recipients do not go through a period of neutropenia. On the other hand, since organ transplant patients are immunosuppressed for more prolonged periods (usually permanently), they are susceptible to the same organisms as cancer patients with impaired T cell immunity (see Chap. 87, Table 87-1). In addition, since the transplantation procedure involves surgery, the recipients are subject to wound infections.

During the early period (less than 1 month after transplantation), infections are most often caused by extracellular bacteria (staphylococci, streptococci, *Escherichia coli*, other gram-negative organisms), which frequently originate in surgical wound or anastomotic sites. Thus these infections are largely determined by the type of transplant.

In subsequent weeks, the consequences of the administration of agents that suppress cell-mediated immunity and of the acquisition (from the transplanted organ) or reactivation of parasites and viruses become apparent. CMV infection is often a problem at this time and may present as severe systemic disease or as an infection of the transplanted organ. CMV is associated not only with generalized immunosuppression but also (in some series) with organ-specific, rejection-related syndromes: glomerulopathy in kidney transplant recipients, bronchiolitis obliterans in lung transplant recipients, premature atherosclerosis in heart transplant recipients, and the vanishing bile duct syndrome in liver transplant recipients. Whether these syndromes are actually caused by CMV, which itself is an opportunistic invader, or are merely associated with it has not been established. It is clear that the presence of CMV infection and/or disease is associated with a poor outcome after transplantation. For this reason, considerable attention has been focused on the diagnosis, treatment, and prophylaxis of CMV infection in organ transplant recipients.

Beyond 6 months after transplantation, infections characteristic of patients with defects in cell-mediated immunity—e.g., infections with *Listeria monocytogenes*, *Nocardia*, various fungi, and other intracellular parasites—may be a problem. Elimination of these late infections will not be possible until specific tolerance to the transplanted organ can be achieved without the administration of drugs that lead to generalized immunosuppression. Meanwhile, vigilance, prophylaxis (when indicated), and rapid diagnosis and treatment of infections can be lifesaving in solid organ transplant recipients, who, unlike most BMT recipients, continue to be immunosuppressed.

Solid organ transplant recipients are susceptible to EBV lymphoproliferative disease from as early as 2 months to many years after transplantation. The prevalence of this complication is increased by potent immunosuppressive drugs; the condition may be reversed (in some cases) by decreasing the degree of immunosuppression. Among organ transplant patients, those with lung and heart transplants are most likely to develop EBV-induced B cell proliferation, particularly in the lungs. Whether the tendency of EBV lymphoproliferation to take place in the transplanted organ relates to local factors (e.g., lack of access of host T cells to the transplanted organ because of disturbed lymphatics) or to the differences in major histocompatibility loci between the host T cells and the organ (which may lead to lack of cell migration or lack of effective T cell/macrophage cooperation) has not been established.

KIDNEY TRANSPLANTATION

(Table 136-3) **Early Infections** Infections developing soon after kidney transplantation are often caused by bacteria associated with skin or wound infections. Some data indicate a role for perioperative antibiotic prophylaxis, and many centers give cephalosporins or a penicillin with an aminoglycoside to decrease the risk of postoperative complications. Urinary tract infections manifesting immediately after transplantation are usually related to anatomic alterations resulting from surgery. Such early infections may require prolonged treatment (e.g., 6 weeks of antibiotic administration for pyelonephritis). Urinary tract infections that occur more than 6 months after transplantation do not seem to be associated with the high rate of

Table 136-3

Infections After Kidney Transplantation

	Infections in Indicated Period after Transplantation		
Site	Early, <1 Month	Middle, 1–6 Months	Late, >6 Months
Urinary tract	Bacteria (*Escherichia coli*, *Klebsiella*, Enterobacteriaceae, *Pseudomonas*, *Enterococcus*), associated with bacteremia and pyelonephritis, *Candida*	CMV (fever alone is common)	Bacteria; late UTIs usually not associated with bacteremia
Lungs	Bacteria (including *Legionella* in endemic settings)	CMV diffuse interstitial pneumonitis, *Pneumocystis carinii*, *Aspergillus*, *Legionella*	*Nocardia*, *Aspergillus*, *Mucor*
Central nervous system	—	*Listeria monocytogenes*, bacteremia and meningitis, CMV encephalitis, toxoplasmosis	CMV retinitis, listerial meningitis, cryptococcal meningitis, *Aspergillus*, *Nocardia*

NOTE: CMV, cytomegalovirus; UTIs, urinary tract infections.

pyelonephritis or relapse seen with infections that occur in the first 3 months and therefore may be treated for shorter periods.

Prophylaxis with trimethoprim-sulfamethoxazole [1 double-strength tablet (160 mg of trimethoprim and 800 mg of sulfamethoxazole) per day] for the first 4 months after transplantation decreases the incidence of early and middle-period infections (see below, Table 136-4).

Middle-Period Infections Because of continuing immunosuppression, kidney transplant recipients are predisposed to lung infections characteristic of those in patients with T cell deficiencies (i.e., infections with *Listeria*, *Mycobacterium*, *Nocardia*, fungi, viruses, and parasites). The high mortality associated with *Legionella pneumophila* infection (Chap. 153) led to the closing of renal transplant units in hospitals with endemic *Legionella*. Fifty percent of all renal transplant recipients presenting with fever 1 to 4 months after transplantation have evidence of CMV disease; CMV itself accounts for the fever in more than two-thirds of cases and thus is the predominant pathogen during this period. CMV infection (Chap. 187) may also present as arthralgias or myalgias. This infection can result in primary disease (in the case of a seronegative recipient who receives a kidney from a seropositive donor) or can present as either reactivation disease or superinfection during this interval. Patients may have atypical lymphocytosis. Unlike immunocompetent patients, however, they often do not have lymphadenopathy or splenomegaly. Therefore, clinical suspicion (and laboratory confirmation) are necessary for diagnosis. The clinical syndrome may be accompanied by bone marrow suppression (particularly leukopenia). CMV also causes glomerulopathy and is associated with an increased incidence of other opportunistic infections (e.g., fungal infections). Because of the frequency and severity of CMV disease, a considerable effort has been made to prevent and treat it in renal transplant recipients. Administration of an immune globulin preparation enriched with antibodies to CMV (CMV-Ig) decreases the incidence in the group at highest risk for severe infections (seronegative recipients of seropositive kidneys). Ganciclovir is useful for the treatment of serious CMV disease.

Infection with the other herpes-group viruses may become evident within 6 months after transplantation or later. Early after transplantation, HSV may cause either oral or anogenital lesions that are usually responsive to acyclovir. Large ulcerating lesions in the anogenital area may lead to bladder and rectal dysfunction as well as predisposing to bacterial infection. VZV may cause fatal disseminated infection in nonimmune kidney transplant recipients, but in immune patients reactivation zoster usually does not disseminate outside the dermatome; thus disseminated VZV infection is a less fearsome complication in kidney transplantation than in bone marrow transplantation.

EBV reactivation disease is more serious; it often presents as a polyclonal proliferation of B cells that invade the CNS, nasopharynx, liver, small bowel, heart, and transplanted kidney. The disease is diagnosed by the finding of a proliferation of EBV-positive B cells. The incidence of the syndrome is higher among patients given high doses of cyclosporine. Fortunately, the B cells usually regress, with or without antiviral therapy (acyclovir), when immunocompetence is restored. Human herpesvirus 6 infection and reactivation also follow renal transplantation.

The papovaviruses BK (polyomavirus hominis 1) and JC (polyomavirus hominis 2) have been cultured from the urine of kidney transplant recipients (as they have from that of BMT recipients). The excretion of BK virus is associated with ureteral strictures and that of JC virus with progressive multifocal leukoencephalopathy. Adenoviruses may persist with continued immunosuppression in these patients.

Kidney transplant recipients are also subject to infections with other intracellular organisms. These patients are likely to have pulmonary infections with *Nocardia*, *Aspergillus*, and *Mucor* as well as infections with other pathogens in which the T cell/macrophage axis plays an important role. In patients without intravenous catheters, *L. monocytogenes* is the most common cause of bacteremia 1 month or more after transplantation. Kidney transplant recipients may have *Salmonella* bacteremia, which can lead to endovascular infections and require prolonged therapy. Pulmonary infections with *P. carinii* are common unless the patient is maintained on trimethoprim-sulfamethoxazole prophylaxis. The addition of cyclosporine to azathioprine and prednisone is probably associated with an increased risk of *P. carinii* pneumonia. *Nocardia* infection (Chap. 167) may present in the skin, bones, lungs, or CNS (where it usually takes the form of single or multiple brain abscesses). *Nocardia* infection generally occurs 1 month or more after transplantation and may follow immunosuppressive treatment for an episode of rejection. Pulmonary findings are nonspecific: localized disease with or without cavities is most common, but the disease may disseminate. The diagnosis is made by culture of the organism from sputum or from the involved nodule. Most of these infections are now cured with prolonged sulfonamide therapy. Prophylaxis with trimethoprim-sulfamethoxazole also appears to be efficacious in the prevention of disease. The occurrence of *Nocardia* infections more than 2 years after transplantation suggests that a long-term prophylaxis regimen is justified.

Toxoplasmosis develops in seropositive patients, usually in the first few months after kidney transplantation. In endemic areas, histoplasmosis, coccidioidomycosis, and blastomycosis may cause pulmonary infiltrates or disseminated disease.

Late Infections Late infections (more than 6 months after transplantation) include CMV retinitis and a variety of CNS complications. Patients (particularly those whose degree of immunosuppression has been increased) are at risk for subacute meningitis due to *Cryptococcus*. Cryptococcal disease may present in an insidious manner (sometimes as a skin infection before the development of clear CNS findings). *Listeria* meningitis may have an acute presentation and requires prompt therapy to avoid a fatal outcome.

Patients who continue to take glucocorticoids are predisposed to infection. "Transplant elbow" is a recurrent bacterial infection in and around the elbow that is thought to result from a combination of poor tensile strength of the skin of steroid-treated patients and steroid-induced proximal myopathy that requires patients to push themselves up with their elbows to get out of chairs. Bouts of cellulitis (usually caused by *Staphylococcus aureus*) recur until patients are provided with elbow protection.

Table 136-4

Prophylaxis of Infections in Transplant Recipients

Risk Factor	Infection or Organism	Prophylactic Antibiotics	Examinations
Travel or residence in area with known risk of fungal infection	Coccidioidomycosis, histoplasmosis, blastomycosis	Imidazoles or amphotericin B	Chest radiography
Latent viruses	HSV, VZV, EBV, CMV	Acyclovir after BMT for HSV and VZV; ganciclovir in some settings	Serologic testing for HSV, VZV, CMV, EBV
Latent fungi/parasites	*Pneumocystis carinii*, *Toxoplasma gondii*	Trimethoprim-sulfamethoxazole or dapsone plus pyrimethamine	Serologic testing for *Toxoplasma*
History of exposure to tuberculosis	*Mycobacterium tuberculosis*	Isoniazid in cases with recent conversion of chest x-ray to positive and no previous treatment	PPD skin testing and chest radiography

NOTE: HSV, herpes simplex virus; VZV, varicella-zoster virus; EBV, Epstein-Barr virus; CMV, cytomegalovirus; BMT, bone marrow transplantation; PPD, purified protein derivative.

Kidney transplant recipients are susceptible to other fungal infections—with *Aspergillus* and *Rhizopus*, for example, which may present as superficial lesions before dissemination. Mycobacterial infection (particularly that with *Mycobacterium marinum*) can be diagnosed by skin examination. Infection with *Prototheca wickerhamii* (an achlorophyllic alga) has been diagnosed by skin biopsy. Warts caused by human papillomaviruses are a late consequence of persistent immunosuppression; local therapy is usually satisfactory.

HEART TRANSPLANTATION Early Infections Mediastinitis is an early complication of heart transplantation. An indolent course is common, with fever or a mildly elevated white blood cell count preceding the development of site tenderness or drainage. Clinical suspicion based on evidence of sternal instability and failure to heal may lead to the diagnosis. Although common residents of the skin, such as *S. aureus* and *Staphylococcus epidermidis*, are often involved, mediastinitis in these patients can also be due to *Mycoplasma hominis* (Chap. 180). Since this organism requires an anaerobic environment for growth and may be difficult to see on conventional medium, the laboratory should be alerted that *M. hominis* infection is suspected. *M. hominis* mediastinitis has been cured with a combination of surgical debridement (sometimes requiring muscle-flap placement) plus clindamycin and tetracycline. Other organisms, including *Pseudomonas aeruginosa* and *Candida*, can cause mediastinitis. The organisms may be cultured from accompanying pericardial fluid.

Middle-Period Infections *T. gondii* (Chap. 219) may be transmitted to a seronegative recipient in the heart of a seropositive donor. Thus serologic screening for *T. gondii* infection is important in the months after transplantation. The incidence of disease is so high in this setting that some centers have advocated prophylaxis with pyrimethamine. CMV and HIV have also been transmitted by heart transplantation. CNS infections can be caused by *Toxoplasma*, *Nocardia*, and *Aspergillus*. *L. monocytogenes* meningitis should be considered in heart transplant recipients with fever and headache.

CMV infection is associated with poor outcomes after heart transplantation. The virus is usually cultivable 1 to 2 months after transplantation, causes manifestations (usually fever and atypical lymphocytosis, often associated with leukopenia and thrombocytopenia) at 2 to 3 months, and produces severe disease (e.g., pneumonia) at 3 to 4 months. Seropositive recipients usually develop cultivable virus faster than patients whose primary CMV infection is a consequence of transplantation. Between 40 and 70 percent of patients develop symptomatic CMV disease: (1) CMV pneumonia, the most likely form of CMV disease to be fatal; (2) CMV esophagitis and gastritis, sometimes accompanied by abdominal pain with or without ulcerations and bleeding; and (3) the CMV syndrome consisting of CMV in the blood, fever, leukopenia, thrombocytopenia, and hepatic enzyme abnormalities. Ganciclovir is efficacious in the treatment of CMV infection; prophylaxis with ganciclovir may reduce the incidence of CMV-related disease.

Late Infections EBV infection usually presents as a lymphoma-like proliferation of B cells late after heart transplantation, particularly with increased immunosuppression. A subset of heart-lung transplant recipients may develop early (within 2 months) fulminant EBV lymphoproliferative disease, often in the transplanted lung. Prophylaxis for *P. carinii* infection is required for these patients (see below).

LUNG TRANSPLANTATION Early Infections It is not surprising that lung transplants are predisposed to the development of pneumonia. The combination of ischemia and the resulting mucosal damage together with accompanying denervation and lack of lymph drainage probably contributes to the high rate of pneumonia (66 percent in one series). The prophylactic use of high doses of broad-spectrum antibiotics for the first 3 or 4 days after surgery decreases the incidence of pneumonia. Gram-negative pathogens (Enterobacteriaceae and *Pseudomonas* species) are troublesome in the first 2 weeks after surgery (the period of maximal vulnerability). Pneumonia can also be caused by *Candida* (possibly as a result of colonization of the donor lung), *Aspergillus*, and *Cryptococcus*.

Mediastinitis may occur at an even higher rate among lung transplant recipients than among heart transplant recipients. *Staphylococcus*, *M. hominis*, and *Candida albicans* are common causes of mediastinitis that develops within 2 weeks of surgery. Mediastinitis due to CMV (which may be transmitted as a consequence of transplantation) usually presents between 2 weeks and 3 months after surgery, with primary disease occurring later than reactivation disease. The incidence of CMV infection, either reactivated or primary, is between 75 and 100 percent if either the donor or the recipient is seropositive for CMV. CMV-induced disease appears to be most severe in recipients of lung and heart-lung transplants. Whether this severity relates to the mismatch in lung antigen-presenting and host immune cells or is attributable to other (nonimmune) factors is not known. More than half of lung transplant recipients with symptomatic CMV disease have pneumonia, and difficulty in distinguishing the radiographic picture of CMV infection from organ rejection further complicates therapy. CMV can also cause bronchiolitis obliterans in lung transplants. The development of pneumonitis related to HSV has led to the prophylactic use of acyclovir. Such prophylaxis may also decrease rates of CMV disease and isolation. Ganciclovir is routinely used in therapy for CMV disease in lung transplant recipients.

Late Infections The incidence of *P. carinii* infection (which may present with a paucity of findings) is high among lung and heart-lung transplant recipients. Some form of prophylaxis for *P. carinii* pneumonia is indicated in all organ transplant situations (Table 136-4). Trimethoprim-sulfamethoxazole prophylaxis for 12 months after transplantation may be sufficient to prevent *P. carinii* disease in patients whose degree of immunosuppression is not increased.

As in other transplant recipients, infection with EBV may cause either a mononucleosis-like syndrome or lymphoproliferative disease in recipients of lung transplants. The tendency of the B cell blasts to present in the lung appears to be greater after lung transplantation than after the transplantation of other organs. Allograft disease may be of donor origin. Reduction of the cyclosporine dosage causes remission in some cases, but lymph node compression can be fatal. Prophylactic use of acyclovir or ganciclovir may prevent the spread of EBV to naive recipients and decrease the rate of development of runaway mononucleosis as well as other manifestations of lymphoproliferative disease.

LIVER TRANSPLANTATION Early Infections As in other types of transplantation, early bacterial infections are a major problem after liver transplantation. Many centers administer systemic broad-spectrum antibiotics for the first 5 days after surgery, even in the absence of documented infection. However, despite prophylaxis, infectious complications are common and are correlated with the duration of the surgical procedure and the type of biliary drainage. An operation lasting longer than 12 h is associated with an increased likelihood of infection. Patients who have a choledochojejunostomy with drainage of the biliary duct to a Roux-en-Y jejunal bowel loop have more fungal infections than those whose bile is drained via a choledochocholedochostomy (with anastomosis of the donor common bile duct to the recipient common bile duct).

Peritonitis and intraabdominal abscesses are common complications of liver transplantation. Bacterial peritonitis may result from biliary leaks and primary or secondary infection after leakage of bile. Peritonitis in liver transplant recipients is often polymicrobial, commonly involving enterococci, aerobic gram-negative bacteria, staphylococci, anaerobes, or *Candida*. Only one-third of patients with intraabdominal abscesses have bacteremia. Abscesses within the first month after surgery may occur not only over the liver but also in the spleen, pericolic area, and pelvis. Treatment includes antibiotic administration and drainage as necessary.

Like other transplant recipients, liver transplant patients have a high incidence of fungal infections, and the occurrence of fungal infection (often candidiasis) correlates with the preoperative use of glucocorticoids, a long duration of treatment with antibacterial agents, and posttransplantation use of immunosuppressive agents.

Middle-Period Infections The development of postsurgical biliary stricture predisposes patients to cholangitis. These patients may lack the characteristic signs and symptoms of cholangitis: fever, abdominal pain, and jaundice. Alternatively, these findings may be present but may suggest graft rejection. The diagnosis of cholangitis in liver transplant recipients therefore requires documentation of bacteremia or demonstration of aggregated neutrophils in bile duct biopsy specimens. Unfortunately, invasive studies of the biliary tract (either T-tube cholangiography or endoscopic retrograde cholangiopancreatography) may lead to cholangitis. For this reason, many clinicians recommend prophylaxis with antibiotics covering gram-negative organisms and anaerobes when these procedures are performed in liver transplant recipients.

Viral Infections Viral hepatitis is a common complication of liver transplantation (see Chap. 295). As in other transplant settings, reactivation disease with herpes-group viruses is common (Table 136-2). HSV, human herpesvirus 6, and CMV can be transmitted in donor organs. Although CMV hepatitis occurs in about 4 percent of liver transplant recipients, it is usually not so severe as to require retransplantation. CMV disease develops in the majority of seronegative recipients of organs from CMV-positive donors, but fatality rates are lower in liver transplant recipients than in lung or heart-lung transplant recipients. Disease due to CMV is associated with the vanishing bile duct syndrome after liver transplantation. Patients respond to treatment with ganciclovir; prophylaxis with CMV-Ig and acyclovir may modify disease. EBV lymphoproliferative disease after liver transplantation shows a propensity for involvement of the liver, and such disease may be of donor origin.

PANCREAS TRANSPLANTATION Transplantation of the pancreas is complicated by early abdominal infection in approximately 20 percent of cases. To prevent contamination of the allograft with enteric bacteria and yeasts, some surgeons, instead of draining the pancreas through the bowel, drain secretions into the urinary tract or bladder. A cuff of duodenum is often used in the anastomosis between the pancreatic graft and the bladder. In addition to bicarbonate loss, this technique causes a high rate of urinary tract infection (30 to 40 percent) that may be related to the retention of the duodenum. An alternative method—the transplantation of islet cells only—may eliminate the problems characteristically posed by wound and urinary tract sepsis in pancreas transplant recipients.

Issues related to the development of CMV infection, EBV lymphoproliferative disease, and infection with opportunistic pathogens in patients receiving a pancreas are similar to those discussed for other solid organ transplant recipients.

VACCINATION OF TRANSPLANT RECIPIENTS

In addition to receiving antibiotic prophylaxis, transplant recipients should be vaccinated against likely pathogens (Table 136-5). In the case of BMT recipients, optimal responses cannot be achieved until after reconstitution; despite previous immunization of both donor and recipient, recipients of allogeneic BMTs must be reimmunized if they are to be protected against pathogens. The situation is complex in the case of autologous transplantation. T and B cells in the peripheral blood may reconstitute the response if they are transferred in adequate numbers. However, cancer patients (particularly those with Hodgkin's disease, in whom vaccination has been extensively studied) who are undergoing chemotherapy do not respond normally to immunization, and titers of antibodies to infectious agents fall more rapidly than in healthy individuals. Therefore, even immunosuppressed patients who have not had marrow transplants may need booster vaccine injections. If memory cells are specifically eliminated as part of a marrow "cleanup" procedure, it will be necessary to reimmunize the recipient with a new primary series. Optimal times for immunizations of different transplant populations are being evaluated.

In the absence of compelling data as to optimal timing, it is reasonable to administer the pneumococcal and *H. influenzae* conjugate vaccines to both autologous and allogeneic BMT recipients 12 months after transplantation and again 12 months later (since the response to the initial vaccine dose is weak in the early posttransplantation period). These two vaccines are particularly important for patients who have undergone splenectomy. In addition, *Neisseria meningitidis* polysaccharide vaccine, diphtheria vaccine, tetanus vaccine, and inactivated polio vaccine can all be given at these same intervals (12 and 24 months after transplantation). Some authorities recommend instead a new primary series for tetanus-diphtheria and inactivated polio vaccine (vaccination 12, 14, and 16 months after transplantation). Because of the risk of spread, household contacts of BMT recipients (or of patients immunosuppressed as a result of chemotherapy) should also receive inactivated polio vaccine. Live virus measles/mumps/rubella vaccine (MMR) can be given to autologous BMT recipients 24 months after transplantation and to most allogeneic BMT recipients at the same point if they are not receiving maintenance therapy with immunosuppressive drugs and do not have ongoing GVHD. The risk of spread from a household contact is lower for MMR than for polio vaccine. In patients who have active GVHD and/or are taking high maintenance doses of glucocorticoids, it may be prudent to avoid all live virus vaccines.

In the case of solid organ transplant recipients, administration of all the usual vaccines and of the indicated booster doses should be completed before immunosuppression, if possible, to maximize responses. For patients taking immunosuppressive agents, the administration of pneumococcal vaccine should be repeated every 6 years. No data are available for meningococcal polysaccharide vaccine, but it is probably reasonable to administer it along with the pneumococcal vaccine. *H. influenzae* conjugate vaccine is safe and should be efficacious in this population; therefore, its administration before transplantation is recommended. Booster doses of this vaccine are not recommended for adults. Solid organ transplant recipients who continue to receive immunosuppressive drugs (glucocorticoids, cyclosporine) should not receive live virus vaccines. Thus a person in this group exposed to measles should be given immune globulin. Similarly, an immunocompromised patient who is seronegative for varicella and who comes into contact with a person who has chickenpox should be given varicella-zoster immune globulin as soon as possible (certainly within 96 h).

Table 136-5

Vaccination for Bone Marrow or Solid Organ Transplant Recipients

Vaccine	Use with Indicated Type of Transplantation	
	Bone Marrow	**Solid Organ**
Streptococcus pneumoniae, Haemophilus influenzae, Neisseria meningitidis infections	Immunize after transplantation (optimal timing not established); preimmunize*	Immunize before transplantation and every 6 years for Pneumovax (others not established)
Seasonal influenza	Vaccinate in the fall	Vaccinate before transplantation if possible
Poliomyelitis	Administer inactivated vaccine	Administer inactivated vaccine; live vaccine may be given before immunosuppression
Measles/mumps/rubella	Immunize 24 months after transplantation if graft-versus-host disease does not develop	Immunize before transplantation
Tetanus, diphtheria	Reimmunize after transplantation	Immunize before transplantation; give boosters at 10 years or as required; a new primary series is not required

* Studies indicate that it is possible to "immunize the graft" before transplantation.

Immunocompromised patients who travel benefit from some but not all vaccines. In general, they should receive any killed or inactivated vaccine preparation appropriate to the area they are visiting; this recommendation includes the vaccines for Japanese encephalitis, hepatitis A and B, poliomyelitis, meningococcal infection, and typhoid. The live typhoid vaccines are not recommended for use in most immunocompromised patients, but inactivated typhoid or the purified polysaccharide vaccine can be used. Live yellow fever vaccine should not be administered. Phenol-inactivated cholera vaccine is probably of little use in this setting. On the other hand, immunization with the purified protein hepatitis B vaccine is reasonable if patients are likely to be exposed. Inactivated hepatitis A vaccine should be used in the appropriate setting (see Chap. 122). If hepatitis A vaccine is not administered, travelers should consider receiving passive protection with immune globulin (the dose depending on the duration of travel in the high-risk area). Patients who will remain for longer than 6 months in areas where hepatitis B is common (Africa, Southeast Asia, the Middle East, eastern Europe, parts of South America, and the Caribbean) should receive hepatitis B vaccine.

BIBLIOGRAPHY

BRAYMAN KL: Analysis of infectious complications occurring after solid-organ transplantation. Arch Surg 127:38, 1992

FOX BC et al: A prospective, randomized, double-blind study of trimethoprim-sulfamethoxazole for prophylaxis of infection in renal transplantation: Clinical efficacy, absorption of trimethoprim-sulfamethoxazole, effects on the microflora, and the cost-benefit of prophylaxis. Am J Med 89:255, 1990

GOTTESDIENER KM: Transplanted infections: Donor-to-host transmission with the allograft. Ann Intern Med 110:1001, 1989

HOYLE C et al: Life-threatening infections occurring more than 3 months after BMT. Bone Marrow Transplant 14:247, 1994

KEATING MR et al: Strategies for prevention of infection after cardiac transplantation. May Clin Proc 67:676, 1992

LJUNGMAN P et al: Immunisations after bone marrow transplantation: Results of a European survey and recommendations from the Infectious Diseases Working Party of the European Group for Blood and Marrow Transplantation. Bone Marrow Transplant 15:455, 1995

MARTINEZ-MARCOS F et al: Prospective study of renal transplant infections in 50 consecutive patients. Eur J Clin Microbiol Infect Dis 13:1023, 1994

MOLRINE DC et al: Donor immunization with *Haemophilus influenzae* type b (HIB) conjugate vaccine in allogeneic bone marrow transplantation. Blood 87:3012, 1996

ROONEY CM et al: Use of gene-modified virus-specific T lymphocytes to control Epstein-Barr virus–related lymphoproliferation. Lancet 345:9, 1995

WEBB IJ et al: Sources and sequelae of bacterial contamination of hematopoietic stem cell products: Implications for safety and hematotherapy and graft engineering. Transfusion 36:782, 1996

137 *Dori F. Zaleznik*

HOSPITAL-ACQUIRED AND INTRAVASCULAR DEVICE–RELATED INFECTIONS

Nosocomial infections are defined as infections acquired during or as a result of hospitalization. Generally, a patient who has been in the hospital for less than 48 h and develops an infection is considered to have been incubating the infection before hospital admission. Most infections that become manifest after 48 h are considered to be nosocomial. A patient may develop a nosocomial infection after being discharged from the hospital if the organism apparently was acquired in the hospital. Surgical wound infection developing in the weeks after hospital discharge is an example of such nosocomial infection.

INCIDENCE AND COSTS Nosocomial infections contribute significantly to morbidity and mortality as well as to excess costs for hospitalized patients. It is estimated that 5 percent of patients admitted to an acute care hospital in the United States acquire a new infection, with more than 2 million nosocomial infections per year and an annual cost in excess of $2 billion. Some authorities estimate that the odds of death are doubled for patients who develop a nosocomial infection, although clearly such factors as underlying disease and severity of illness also play an important role in outcome.

Although immunosuppressed hosts are especially vulnerable to infections acquired in a hospital, common nosocomial infections occur even in immunocompetent hosts. The National Nosocomial Infections Surveillance (NNIS) Registry has been monitoring nosocomial infection rates since 1970. Its most recent report covers the period from January 1993 to April 1995 and includes both teaching and nonteaching hospitals and both small and large facilities. While the most common nosocomial infections have remained the same, the frequency distribution has altered in recent years. Urinary tract infection remains the most common type but now accounts for only 28 percent of hospital-acquired infections (as opposed to 40 percent in the past). Surgical wound infection and pneumonia—at 19 and 17 percent, respectively—are the next most common nosocomial infections. The frequency of primary bloodstream infection, often associated with intravascular devices, has risen from 7 to 16 percent.

The potential impact of nosocomial infections is considerable when assessed in terms of incidence, morbidity, mortality, and financial burden. Analyses of these factors examine nosocomial infections as both medical and economic issues. The clinical problem facing the physician is the development of a new fever in a patient in the hospital. In the evaluation of such a patient, information about the most common categories of infection may not be sufficient. Rather, the clinician must also use clinical clues from the patient's presentation and hospitalization to diagnose a nosocomial infection.

The evaluation of a hospitalized patient with new fever should include a careful history. Particular attention should be paid to symptoms of headache, cough, abdominal pain, diarrhea, flank pain, dysuria, urinary frequency, and leg pain. Other features related to the patient's hospitalization also are important, such as the presence and type of intravenous devices, the past or current use of a urinary catheter, the surgical procedure conducted (if any), and the new medications administered, including those for surgical prophylaxis. The physical examination should be directed at possible sources of infection and should focus particularly on the skin (with a search for rash or embolic lesions); the lungs; the abdomen (especially the right upper quadrant); the costovertebral angles; surgical wounds; the calves; and current and old intravenous access sites (for signs of phlebitis). The laboratory evaluation of all hospitalized patients with new fever should include a complete blood count with differential, a chest radiograph, and blood and urine cultures. Other diagnostic tests to consider include liver function tests; plain-film or other studies of the abdomen; routine aerobic cultures of sputum, stool, or other relevant body fluids; and (in cases of diarrhea) testing of stool for *Clostridium difficile* toxin.

CATEGORIES OF INFECTION **Pneumonia** Certainly the astute clinician will question the patient thoroughly and perform a rapid comprehensive physical examination. One way to continue the approach to the development of fever in a hospitalized patient is to consider potential infections that may be life-threatening, such as pneumonia. Most at risk for developing nosocomial pneumonia are patients in an intensive care unit (ICU), especially those who are intubated; patients with an altered level of consciousness, especially those with nasogastric tubes; elderly patients; patients with chronic lung disease; postoperative patients; and any of the above patients taking H_2 blockers or antacids. Nosocomial pneumonia in the NNIS Registry is diagnosed 4 to 7 times per 1000 hospitalizations. Among patients on ventilators, the occurrence of pneumonia is estimated at 15 cases per 1000 ventilator days in medical and surgical ICUs. Mortality figures for nosocomial pneumonia are as high as 50 percent.

Oropharyngeal and gastric colonization plays a critical role in the pathogenesis of pneumonia in hospitalized patients. The oropharynx can become colonized by many species of aerobic gram-negative organisms within 48 h of the patient's hospitalization; aspiration occurs commonly during sleep and is increased by such factors as a nasogastric tube, altered consciousness, decreased gag reflex, or delayed gastric emptying. As for gastric colonization, bacterial counts in the stomach rise in the presence of medications that raise gastric pH, such as H_2 blockers and antacids, as well as in malnourished, achlorhydric, and some elderly patients. The prevalence of pneumonia is reportedly two to three times higher among intubated patients receiving H_2 blockers or antacids for stress-ulcer prophylaxis than among intubated patients receiving sucralfate, a medication that heals ulcers without altering gastric pH. Gastric colonization is believed to influence the development of pneumonia by retrograde colonization of the oropharynx. Ventilated patients are also at risk of developing pneumonia by exposure to bacteria leaking around the cuff of the endotracheal tube or to bacteria from nebulizers, condensate within ventilator circuits, or humidifiers.

Outside the ICU, pneumonia should be suspected when a patient develops a new cough, fever, leukocytosis, sputum production, and a new infiltrate on chest x-ray. Diagnosis can be complicated in patients with congestive heart failure who have concomitant chest x-ray abnormalities or in patients with chronic sputum production. Some organisms, such as *Legionella* spp., may not be associated with peripheral leukocytosis.

In ICU patients, especially those who are intubated, the signs of pneumonia are relatively subtle, and thus the diagnosis often is relatively complex. In particular, the chest x-ray films are difficult to interpret, because fluid overload, congestive heart failure, and adult respiratory distress syndrome (ARDS) are all common findings in intubated patients. Polymorphonuclear leukocytes (PMNs) often are present on Gram-stained preparations of the purulent secretions commonly obtained from these patients. An important clue to pneumonia is a change in the output or character of these secretions. If their volume or thickness increases or their color changes, a sputum Gram's stain should be performed and pneumonia seriously considered in the differential diagnosis. Serial Gram's stains are useful, as the number of PMNs may increase substantially and the type(s) of organisms may shift with the development of pneumonia. For example, the baseline sputum sample from an intubated patient may contain about 25 PMNs per high-power field and have mixed gram-positive and gram-negative organisms of several morphologic types in moderate numbers. On the day of a new fever, the same patient may have copious amounts of more tenacious sputum with more PMNs and a predominance of enteric-appearing gram-negative rods. Even without distinct changes in the chest x-ray, this patient would be considered to have developed pneumonia. Another subtle sign of pneumonia in the intubated patient is a requirement for change in ventilator settings in the absence of fluid overload, a mechanical alteration (e.g., a shift in endotracheal tube placement), or a pneumothorax.

The major organisms of concern in nosocomial pneumonia are gram-negative aerobic bacteria. *Pseudomonas aeruginosa*, *Staphylococcus aureus*, and *Klebsiella pneumoniae* are frequent pathogens in nosocomial pneumonia. While surveys of organisms are useful, it is essential to know which pathogens are common in a given institution, as hospitals and especially ICUs differ in their resident flora. In some institutions, methicillin-resistant *S. aureus*, *Stenotrophomonas* (formerly *Xanthomonas*) *maltophilia*, *Flavobacterium* spp., and even *Legionella* spp. may be of particular concern. Viruses such as respiratory syncytial virus and adenovirus are receiving increased attention as etiologic agents of nosocomial pneumonia in both adults and children. In the past, viruses have been underrepresented in statistics on the agents of nosocomial pneumonia because the diagnosis of viral infection is more difficult and because many microbiology laboratories do not have the capability to isolate viruses.

Antibiotic resistance is another important issue to address in the management of a hospitalized patient. In addition to knowing the sensitivity patterns of the hospital flora, one must consider whether a patient has received continuous or multiple courses of antibiotic therapy. To reduce the likelihood of altering the sensitivity patterns of the patient's flora, antibiotic courses for pneumonia should be kept as short as possible, with coverage as narrow as is possible for the organism(s) involved.

Bacteremia Another potentially life-threatening nosocomial infection to consider in the evaluation of the patient with a new fever is bacteremia, which usually is related to the presence of an intravascular device (see also Chap. 138). While many common nosocomial infections such as pneumonia or urinary tract infection can be accompanied by bacteremia, primary bacteremia is defined by isolation of a recognized pathogen from the blood without an infection at another site. One carefully controlled study reported bloodstream infection in 2.7 percent of admissions to a surgical ICU, with 50 percent mortality and a prolongation of hospitalization by 24 days in survivors.

One difficulty in assessing the significance of bacteremia is to distinguish true pathogens from contaminating skin flora. This distinction is especially important in establishing an infection of an indwelling intravascular catheter because organisms that inhabit the skin, such as coagulase-negative staphylococci, also frequently cause infection. The most common point of entry for infection related to intravascular devices is the insertion site, with spread of the infection along the outside of the device initially. Other means of entry for infecting organisms include introduction via contaminated infusates or tubing, ports, or leaking connections and hematogenous seeding of a catheter during bacteremia. While gram-negative aerobic bacilli are probably the most feared nosocomial bloodstream pathogens, the NNIS data for 1980 through 1989 showed that the isolation of these organisms had not increased in frequency over the decade. The frequency of bloodstream isolation increased the most for coagulase-negative staphylococci, with the next highest increase for *Candida* spp. Other leading causes of line-related bacteremia were *S. aureus* and enterococci. Recent studies have confirmed these findings.

Establishing an infection of an intravascular device or primary bacteremia as the cause of fever in a hospitalized patient is a diagnosis of exclusion. If a patient has a fever and signs of cutaneous involvement (erythema, induration, tenderness, or purulent drainage) at the insertion site of a catheter, full cultures should be performed, the vascular-access line removed, and the catheter tip sent for quantitative culture. Studies have correlated the growth of 15 colonies or more from a catheter tip with infection of the line. More commonly, the exit site does not show signs of infection, and there is considerable debate about the necessity of removing a line from a febrile patient at that point. Unless another site of infection is obvious, it is generally advisable to remove the line when a patient develops a new fever. While central-line changes over a guidewire have been shown to be safe, it is not clear that maintaining the same insertion site is wise in cases of possible line infection. In general, when a line is removed because of possible infection, the site should be changed. If vascular access is a problem and one wishes to continue intravascular therapy despite the intravascular-device infection, it is probably not necessary to change the line over a guidewire. The traditional teaching is that an infected intravenous device should be removed. In current practice, however, especially with surgically implanted intravenous catheters, a decision may be made to attempt treatment with antibiotics while leaving the catheter in place. This practice is often successful when the infecting organism is a coagulase-negative *Staphylococcus* but is less often effective with other organisms, particularly *Candida* spp.

Another controversial management issue is whether to draw blood for culture through a line. While some studies report a correlation in the 90 percent range between culture results for blood drawn through vascular-access lines and those for peripheral blood, the former cultures can be either false-positive or false-negative. If the line culture is positive and no peripheral blood has been drawn, it is impossible to determine whether the patient has true bacteremia or the culture merely reflects bacteria associated with the line. Conversely, if multiple peripheral blood cultures are positive, it is reasonable to assume that the line is at least infected secondarily. Whether bacteremia is high- or low-grade and whether it is sustained or transient may influence the duration of antibiotic therapy and cannot be determined from cultures of specimens obtained through a line.

Surgical Wound Infection Evaluation of fever in the postoperative patient must include careful evaluation of the surgical wound. Although surgical wound infection reportedly accounts for 19 percent of nosocomial infections, the true incidence of postoperative wound infection is difficult to assess, particularly at a time when many patients are hospitalized for relatively short periods. In a number of studies, careful follow-up for the development of wound infections after discharge—especially observation of the wound by a trained observer, such as a nurse—has shown the actual rates of wound infections in all categories of surgery to be greater than the reported rates. Surgical procedures have long been classified as clean, clean-contaminated, contaminated, and dirty-infected. A more sophisticated risk index is based on the American Society of Anesthesiologists preoperative assessment score, the surgery classification (as either contaminated or dirty-infected), and the duration of surgery. With this index, rates of surgical wound infection have varied from 1.5 to 13 per 100 operations.

Other risk factors for the development of postoperative wound infection include the presence of a drain; a long preoperative length of stay, with the rates doubling for each week of preoperative hospitalization; preoperative shaving of the field, especially if performed 24 h or more beforehand; a long duration of surgery; the presence of an untreated remote infection; and the surgeon. Perioperative antibiotic prophylaxis has been shown to decrease rates of wound infection in a number of careful studies, including those of clean surgical procedures. Antibiotic coverage after the surgical wound is closed has not been shown to provide additional benefit.

A surgical wound should be examined for erythema extending more than 2 cm beyond the margin of the wound, localized tenderness and induration, fluctuance, drainage of purulent material, and dehiscence of sutures. Mechanical factors, as well as infection, can cause wound dehiscence. Sternal wounds following cardiac surgery are of special concern because the consequences of infection can be severe. The surface of the wound may not present an obvious cause for concern, but, in some patients, ongoing fevers and especially the development of rocking or instability of the sternum may be sufficient cause for surgical exploration of the wound. Mediastinitis or sternal osteomyelitis is a severe complication of cardiac surgery. Wounds associated with the placement of prosthetic devices such as mechanical joints also are of special concern. Infection of these wounds can lead to infection of the prosthesis, and clearance of prosthetic joint infections generally requires surgical removal of the device.

Urinary Tract Infection Urinary tract infection (UTI), the most common type of nosocomial infection, generally is the easiest to treat and has the least severe sequelae. Four principal risk factors have been associated repeatedly with the development of UTI in hospitalized patients: female sex, prolonged urinary catheterization, lack of systemic antibiotic therapy, and breach of appropriate catheter care. The administration of systemic antibiotics to patients with urinary catheters in place for 1 to 5 days has been associated with a decrease in rates of bacteriuria. For patients with catheters in place for 6 or more days, however, this benefit is not observed.

The pathogenesis of catheter-associated UTI appears to differ in men and women. In women, the typical mechanism involves periurethral colonization with fecal flora and tracking of organisms up the catheter to the bladder and thus resembles the pathogenesis of UTI in noncatheterized female patients, in whom bacteria track up the short female urethra. In contrast, periurethral colonization often cannot be demonstrated in men; most infections seem to arise from intraluminal spread of organisms to the bladder. Some organisms, such as *Proteus* and *Pseudomonas* spp., appear to facilitate the growth along the inside of the urinary catheter of a biofilm that encrusts and obstructs the flow of urine.

UTI is certainly an extremely common nosocomial infection; however, it is important to define this type of infection precisely. Especially in the evaluation of a febrile hospitalized patient, it is crucial to think carefully about all possible sources of infection and not to assume that UTI is the probable cause. In patients who have had urinary catheters in place for a number of days, fever, dysuria, frequency, leukocytosis, and especially flank pain or costovertebral angle tenderness are highly suggestive of bladder infection or pyelonephritis. In patients with fever but no other symptoms or signs referable to the urinary tract, one should look for ancillary findings suggestive of urinary tract involvement, such as white blood cells without epithelial cells in the urine sediment or leukocyte esterase or nitrite on urinalysis. A urine culture positive for a single organism should not be accepted as definitive evidence of UTI in an asymptomatic patient. While one might treat the febrile patient who has a positive urine culture with antibiotics, it is prudent to repeat the culture before the institution of therapy. Inability to recover any organism or the same organism on repeat culture, particularly if the patient does not respond to antibiotics, should raise questions about the validity of the diagnosis of UTI. In addition, isolation of two or more bacteria from a single specimen is most likely due to contamination unless there is reason to suspect a bladder diverticulum or a perinephric abscess.

Other Infectious Sources of Fever Several other types of infection may cause fever in the hospitalized patient and should be considered in the differential diagnosis of new fever. In patients who have received antibiotics (even a single dose as surgical prophylaxis), antibiotic-associated diarrhea may develop. This condition is usually caused by the spore-forming organism *C. difficile*, which produces toxins that cause diarrhea. Some patients may appear quite toxic with this infection, with high fevers, leukocytosis, and profuse diarrhea. The organism is quite hardy and is difficult to eradicate from the hospital environment. The hands of hospital personnel have been implicated as a mode of transmission of this organism, as have electronic rectal thermometers (despite the use of individual covering sheaths for each patient). The colon may become colonized with *C. difficile* while the patient is in the hospital, but—particularly if the patient is still taking antibiotics when sent home—diarrhea may not develop until after discharge.

Other infections to consider in the hospitalized patient include decubitus ulcers, particularly in patients in chronic-care wards or confined to bed rest for prolonged periods, and sinusitis, especially in intubated patients.

NONINFECTIOUS SOURCES OF FEVER A consideration of several common noninfectious causes of fever in hospitalized patients is part of a thorough evaluation of new fever. Drug treatment is the foremost noninfectious cause of fever. Drug fever may occur with or without an accompanying rash or eosinophilia and can be caused by a new medication or by medications the patient has been receiving for some time. Particular agents associated with drug fever include phenytoin, H_2 blockers, procainamide, and antibiotics, most notably sulfonamides. Even drug-associated fevers can be quite high in some patients and may take up to 5 days to resolve after discontinuation of treatment with the offending agent. Other noninfectious causes of fever include phlebitis, often at the site of an old intravenous line and sometimes followed by suppurative thrombophlebitis with clots or septic emboli, and pulmonary emboli, especially in patients undergoing prolonged bed rest; prophylactic heparin or mechanical boots often are used to reduce the risk of pulmonary embolism in the latter patients.

CONCLUSION The range of possibilities for the etiology of a new fever in a hospitalized patient is quite broad. An attention to detail, a careful history and physical examination, and a knowledge of the infections and organisms likely to cause nosocomial problems usually lead to an accurate diagnosis.

BIBLIOGRAPHY

BRONSEMA DA et al: Secular trends in rates and etiology of nosocomial urinary tract infections at a university hospital. J Urol 150:414, 1993

CRAVEN DE, STEGER KA: Epidemiology of nosocomial pneumonia: New perspectives on an old disease. Chest 108:1S, 1995

CULVER DH et al: Surgical wound infection rates by wound class, operative procedure, and patient risk index. Am J Med 91(S3B):152S, 1991

FAGON J-Y et al: Mortality attributable to nosocomial infections in the ICU. Infect Control Hosp Epidemiol 15:428, 1994

GEORGE DL: Nosocomial pneumonia, in *Hospital Epidemiology and Infection Control*, CG Mayhall (ed). Baltimore, Williams & Wilkins, 1996, p 175

JARVIS WR: Epidemiology of nosocomial fungal infections, with emphasis on *Candida* species. Clin Infect Dis 20:1526, 1995

National Nosocomial Infections Surveillance (NNIS) Semiannual Report, May 1995. Am J Infect Control 23:377, 1995

PITTET D et al: Nosocomial bloodstream infection in critically ill patients. JAMA 271:1598, 1994

| 138 | *Robert A. Weinstein* |

INFECTION CONTROL IN THE HOSPITAL

The costs of nosocomial (hospital-acquired) infections are great, whether measured in dollars or in morbidity and mortality (see Chap. 137). Although infection-control and hospital epidemiology activities have been the subjects of increasing scientific study over the past 25 years, efforts to lower infection risks have been continually challenged by the growing numbers of immunocompromised patients, of antibiotic-resistant bacteria, of fungal and viral superinfections, and of invasive devices and procedures. Three international decennial conferences on infection control, organized by the Centers for Disease Control and Prevention (CDC), have clearly documented these formidable trends. This chapter reviews the basic surveillance and prevention activities that have been developed to deal with these problems and that form the foundation for current hospital epidemiology programs.

ORGANIZATION AND RESPONSIBILITIES OF INFECTION-CONTROL PROGRAMS   The standards of the Joint Commission on Accreditation of Healthcare Organizations require all accredited hospitals to have an active program for surveillance, prevention, and control of nosocomial infections; a multidisciplinary infection-control committee usually oversees the program. The agents of the committee are the chairperson, who is preferably an infectious disease physician, and the infection-control practitioners, who are usually trained in nursing or medical technology and in epidemiology and public health. Education of physicians in infection control and hospital epidemiology is offered in some infectious disease fellowship programs and is available in courses provided by professional societies, primarily the Society for Healthcare Epidemiology of America.

In the 1970s, the CDC's extensive Study on the Efficacy of Nosocomial Infection Control found that nosocomial infection rates fell by 32 percent in hospitals that established programs with organized surveillance and control activities; a trained, effectual infection-control physician; and one infection-control practitioner per 250 beds. In contrast, rates in hospitals without effective programs increased by 18 percent. Since that study, however, the responsibilities and roles of hospital epidemiology programs have expanded in several directions. Diagnosis-related reimbursement has led hospital administrators to place increased emphasis on cost containment and on documentation of the cost-effectiveness of infection control. The quality-improvement movements and the Joint Commission's Agenda for Change have redirected infection-control attention, in part, beyond the mere writing of policies and procedures to improvement of the actual processes and optimization of outcomes. In a few hospitals, epidemiology programs have even taken on additional pharmacoepidemiologic and antibiotic-use review responsibilities. Finally, all programs must now respond to increasing governmental regulation of hospital waste and to Occupational Safety and Health Administration (OSHA)–mandated standards for protecting health care workers from occupational exposure to bloodborne pathogens and tuberculosis.

SURVEILLANCE   Traditionally, infection-control practitioners survey inpatients for nosocomial infections (defined as those neither present nor incubating at the time of admission). Surveillance involves a review of microbiology laboratory results, "shoe-leather" epidemiology on the nursing wards, application of standardized definitions of infection, ongoing dialogue with hospital workers, and com-

mon sense. Some innovative infection-control programs have taken advantage of the increased use of computerized pharmacy, microbiology, and other databases in hospitals to create algorithm-driven surveillance activities.

Because total hospital surveillance leaves little time for data analysis and education, most hospitals now aim surveillance at infections that are associated with a high level of morbidity [e.g., intensive care unit (ICU)–related infections and nosocomial pneumonia], are costly (e.g., cardiac surgery wound infections) or difficult to treat (e.g., infections due to antibiotic-resistant bacteria), pose recurring epidemic problems (e.g., *Clostridium difficile*–related diarrhea), and are potentially preventable (e.g., vascular access–related infections). Quality-assurance activities in infection control have led to increased surveillance of the compliance of personnel with policies (e.g., monitoring of the actual adherence to isolation precautions).

The results of surveillance are expressed as rates; for example, 5 to 10 percent of patients develop nosocomial infections. Although such overall statistics are often requested of hospitals by administrators or surveyors, they have little value unless qualified by site of infection, by patient population, and by exposure to risk factors. Meaningful denominators for infection rates include the number of patients exposed to a specific risk (e.g., rates of pneumonia among patients using mechanical ventilators) and the number of intervention days (e.g., rates of pneumonia per 1000 patient-days on a ventilator).

Temporal trends in rates should be reviewed, and rates ideally should be compared with regional and national norms. However, even comparison rates generated by the CDC's ongoing National Nosocomial Infection Surveillance System, which collects data from more than 200 hospitals that use standardized definitions of nosocomial infections, have not been validated independently and represent a nonrandom sample of hospitals. Interhospital comparisons are easily confounded by the wide range in risk factors and in severity of underlying illnesses; unless rates are adjusted for these factors, comparisons may be misleading. Unfortunately, systems for making such adjustments either are rudimentary or have not been well validated.

The ongoing analysis of an individual hospital's infection rates helps to determine whether control efforts are succeeding and where increased education and control measures should be focused. Knowledge of infection rates is also useful in discussions with the hospital administration regarding areas to which additional resources should be directed.

PREVENTION AND CONTROL MEASURES   Epidemiologic Basis and General Measures   Nosocomial infections follow basic epidemiologic patterns that can help to direct prevention and control measures. Nosocomial pathogens have reservoirs, follow predictable routes of transmission, and require susceptible hosts. Reservoirs and sources exist in the inanimate environment (e.g., tap water contaminated with *Legionella*) and in the animate environment (e.g., infected or colonized health care workers, patients, and hospital visitors). The mode of transmission most often is either cross-infection (e.g., indirect spread of pathogens from one patient to another on the inadequately washed hands of hospital personnel) or autoinoculation (e.g., aspiration of oropharyngeal flora into the lung along an endotracheal tube). Occasionally, pathogens (e.g., group A streptococci and many respiratory viruses) are spread indirectly from person to person via infectious droplets released by coughing or sneezing. Much less common—but often devastating in terms of epidemic risk—is true airborne spread of droplet nuclei (as in nosocomial chickenpox) or common-source spread by contaminated materials (e.g., iodophors contaminated with *Pseudomonas*). Factors that increase host susceptibility include underlying conditions (discussed elsewhere in this text) and the many medical-surgical interventions and procedures that bypass or compromise normal host defenses.

The hospital's infection-control committee, through its infection-control program, must determine the general and specific measures used to control infections and must review and recommend specific antiseptics and disinfectants for hospital use. Given the prominence of cross-infection, hand washing is the single most important preventive measure in hospitals. Many studies have examined the antimicrobial activity of a wide variety of antiseptic-containing hand-washing agents. The use of such agents is important before invasive procedures and possibly in ICU settings. Given the poor general compliance with hand-washing recommendations, the importance of using any hand cleanser between patient contacts cannot be overemphasized (Table 138-1).

The fact that 25 to 50 percent of nosocomial infections are due to the combined effect of the patient's own flora and invasive devices highlights the importance of improvements in the use and design of such devices. Intensive educational programs can be associated with at least a temporary reduction in infection rates through improved asepsis in handling and earlier removal of invasive devices, but the maintenance of such gains is often difficult. It is encouraging that epidemiologic studies have been used increasingly to assess the value of newer devices and site-specific control measures (discussed below) and to debunk some traditional yet ineffective and costly measures, such as routine culturing of the environment and personnel for "pathogens."

Urinary Tract Infections   Approaches to the prevention of urinary tract infections (UTIs) have included the use of topical meatal antimicrobials, drainage bag disinfectants, antimicrobial-coated catheters, and sealed catheter–drainage tube junctions to eliminate inadvertent breaks in the system. Because of conflicting study results, none of these measures is considered routine. Systemic antimicrobials given for other purposes decrease the risk of UTI during the first 4 days of catheterization, after which resistant bacteria or yeasts emerge as pathogens. Selective decontamination of the gut also is associated with a reduced risk. Again, however, neither approach is routine. Moreover, irrigation of catheters, with or without antimicrobials, may actually increase the risk of infection.

Pneumonia   Control measures for pneumonia are aimed at the remediation of risk factors in general patient care (e.g., minimizing aspiration-prone supine positioning and possibly avoiding prophylactic gastric alkalization because of the increased risk of colonization with gram-negative rods when the gastric pH is >4) and at meticulous aseptic care of respirator equipment (e.g., disinfecting or sterilizing all in-line reusable components such as nebulizers, replacing tubing circuits at intervals of more than 48 h—rather than more frequently—to lessen the number of breaks in the system, and teaching aseptic technique for suctioning). More controversial is the infection-control benefit of sucralfate, which provides stress-ulcer prophylaxis without

Table 138-1

Examples of Ways in Which Physicians Can Contribute to
Infection-Control Efforts

- Act as role models for other personnel by paying careful attention to hand-washing recommendations and barrier precautions during contact with patients and by observing posted isolation precautions.
- Give corrective feedback to caregivers who do not adhere to hand-washing recommendations or isolation precautions.
- Place invasive devices based on clinical need (not just on convenience).
- Remove invasive devices promptly when they are no longer needed clinically.
- Limit surgical antimicrobial prophylaxis to the perioperative period.
- Exercise care in initial empirical antibiotic selection (avoid "shotgun" approaches).
- Narrow the spectrum of antibiotic therapy once a pathogen is recovered.
- Discontinue antibiotic therapy in a timely fashion.
- Become familiar with the hospital's bloodborne pathogen and tuberculosis control plans.
- Order appropriate isolation precautions promptly for infected patients.
- During patient rounds, alert nursing staff to lapses in asepsis (e.g., soiled dressings at sites of intravascular catheters) and to infection-predisposing situations (e.g., aspiration-prone positioning of patients).
- Notify infection-control practitioners of potential infection-control problems (e.g., surgical wound infections that manifest after a patient's discharge).

altering gastric pH, and of selective decontamination of the oropharynx and gut with nonabsorbable antimicrobials. Each approach merits further investigation.

Surgical Wound Infections   The most important control measures for surgical wound infections include the use of antimicrobial prophylaxis at the start of high-risk procedures, attention to technical surgical issues and operating-room asepsis (e.g., not shaving the operative site until surgery and avoiding open or prophylactic drains), and preoperative therapy for any active infection. Reporting of surveillance results to surgeons has been associated with reductions in infection rates. This association, in conjunction with the increasingly extensive review of infection rates by regulatory agencies and third-party payers, emphasizes the importance of stratifying rates by patient-related risk factors and of developing meaningful systems for interhospital comparisons and for wound surveillance after the patient's discharge from the hospital or clinic (when more than 50 percent of infections first become apparent).

Infections Related to Vascular Access and Monitoring (See also Chap. 137)   Control measures for infections associated with vascular access and monitoring include the moving of peripheral or arterial catheters to a new site at specified intervals (e.g., every 72 h for peripheral intravenous catheters), which may be facilitated by use of an intravenous team; the application of disposable transducers and aseptic technique for the accessing of transducers or other vascular ports; and the removal of "idle" catheters. Unresolved issues include the best frequency for the rotation of central venous catheter sites (guidewire-assisted catheter changes at the same site do not lessen infection risk); the best antiseptics for site preparation and for catheter dressing; the appropriate role for mupirocin ointment, a topical antibiotic with excellent antistaphylococcal activity, in site care; the relative degrees of risk posed by percutaneous central catheters and by newer designs—tunneled, totally implanted, or peripherally inserted central catheters (PICC lines); and the role of other costly catheter innovations, such as the impregnation of the catheter with antimicrobials or the attachment of subcutaneous cuffs that contain bactericidal silver. In several studies, the use of semitransparent polyurethane dressings has increased infection rates, although these dressings can offer nursing benefits (ease of bathing and site inspection and protection of the site from secretions).

Isolation Techniques   Written policies for the isolation of infectious patients are a standard component of infection-control programs. The CDC is in the process of revising its isolation guidelines; their current system recommends that hospitals use either category-specific isolation (based on suspected infection) or disease-specific isolation (based on likely mode of transmission). The category-specific system includes *strict isolation* (e.g., for chickenpox), *contact isolation* (e.g., for staphylococcal wound infections), *respiratory isolation* (e.g., for untreated bacterial meningitis), and *acid-fast bacillus isolation* (for *Mycobacterium tuberculosis* infection, which has specific ventilation requirements, as described below), as well as *enteric precautions* (e.g., for *C. difficile*–associated bacterial diarrhea) and *drainage/secretion precautions* (e.g., for minor wound infections). Some hospitals also use blood and body-fluid precautions, although universal precautions have largely supplanted these measures. For each of the six category-specific modes, a door sign lists the necessary protective measures (e.g., gown, gloves, and mask for strict isolation). In the disease-specific system, the caregiver checks off the appropriate measures on a generic isolation sign on the basis of an understanding of the patient's infection and its specific mode(s) of transmission. The pending revision of the CDC's recommendations will offer greater guidance in the isolation of patients on the basis of presenting syndromes (before the recovery of specific infectious agents); will emphasize more standard, routine use of barrier precautions; and will simplify the categories of isolation.

In body-substance isolation, the preceding systems are abandoned in favor of instructing personnel to wear gloves for contact with any body substance or mucous membrane. Other barriers, such as gowns, are required if soiling or splashing is anticipated. For patients with airborne pathogens such as *M. tuberculosis*, additional isolation precautions are required (see below).

In addition to these three alternative systems, all hospitals are required by OSHA to provide annual in-service training in, and to monitor compliance with, universal precautions to protect health care workers from bloodborne pathogens, including human immunodeficiency virus (HIV) and hepatitis B and C viruses. In essence, these precautions require gloves, gown, mask, and/or eye protection, varying with the likelihood of contact or splashing with blood or *any* other potentially contaminated body fluid. Some hospitals use additional guidelines for infected mothers and their newborns and antibiotic-resistance precautions for patients colonized or infected with problematic strains.

EPIDEMIC PROBLEMS Outbreaks are always big news but probably account for fewer than 5 percent of nosocomial infections. The investigation and control of epidemics in hospitals require that infection-control personnel develop a case definition, confirm that an outbreak really exists (since many apparent epidemics are actually pseudo-outbreaks due to surveillance or laboratory artifacts), review aseptic practices and disinfectant use, determine the extent of the outbreak, perform an epidemiologic investigation to determine modes of transmission, work closely with microbiology personnel to culture for common sources or personnel carriers as appropriate and to type epidemiologically important isolates, and heighten surveillance to judge the effect of control measures. Control measures generally include the early reinforcement of routine aseptic practices during a search for compliance problems that may have fostered the outbreak, the ensuring of the appropriate isolation of cases (and the institution of cohort isolation and nursing if needed), and the implementation of further controls on the basis of the findings of the investigation. Examples of some potential epidemic problems follow.

Chickenpox When health care workers are exposed to chickenpox in the community or through patients with initially unrecognized infections, or when these employees work during the 24 h before developing chickenpox, infection-control practitioners institute a varicella exposure investigation and control plan. In this plan, the names of exposed workers and patients are obtained; medical histories are reviewed, and (if necessary) serologic tests for immunity are conducted; physicians are notified of susceptible exposed patients; prophylactic varicella-zoster immune globulin and/or early acyclovir treatment (where appropriate) is administered; and susceptible exposed employees are furloughed during the at-risk period for disease. The recently approved varicella vaccine should markedly decrease risk for susceptible employees.

Tuberculosis The resurgence of pulmonary tuberculosis in the United States since 1987 and a series of nosocomial outbreaks of infection with multidrug-resistant strains—primarily involving patients with AIDS and their caregivers—have led to a reevaluation of tuberculosis control. Important control measures include prompt recognition, isolation, and treatment of cases; recognition of atypical presentations (e.g., lower-lobe infiltrates without cavitation); use of negative pressure, 100 percent exhaust, private isolation rooms with closed doors, and six air changes per hour; use of face masks (approved by the National Institute for Occupational Safety and Health) by caregivers entering isolation rooms; possible use of HEPA (high-efficiency particulate air) filter units and/or ultraviolet lights for disinfecting air when other engineering controls are not feasible or reliable; and follow-up skin-testing of susceptible personnel who have been exposed to infectious patients before isolation.

Group A Streptococci The potential for a group A streptococcal outbreak should be considered when even a single nosocomial case occurs. Most outbreaks involve surgical wounds and are due to the presence of an asymptomatic carrier in the operating room. Investigation can be confounded by carriage at extrapharyngeal sites such as the rectum and vagina. Health care workers in whom carriage has been linked to nosocomial transmission of group A streptococci are removed from the patient-care setting and are not permitted to return until carriage has been eliminated by antimicrobial therapy.

Aspergillus *Aspergillus* spores are common in the environment, particularly on dusty surfaces. When hospital ceiling tiles are removed to provide access for electrical wiring or plumbing or when dusty areas are disturbed during hospital renovation, the spores become airborne. Inhalation of spores by immunosuppressed (particularly neutropenic) patients creates a risk of pulmonary and/or paranasal sinus infection and disseminated aspergillosis. Routine surveillance among neutropenic patients for infections with filamentous fungi, such as *Aspergillus* and *Fusarium*, helps hospitals to determine whether they have unduly large environmental loads of these organisms. To lower the risk, hospitals should inspect and clean air-handling equipment on a routine schedule, review all planned hospital renovations with infection-control personnel and subsequently construct appropriate barriers, remove immunosuppressed patients from renovation sites, and consider the use of HEPA filters for air supplied to rooms housing immunosuppressed patients.

Legionella Sporadic and epidemic cases of nosocomial *Legionella* pneumonia are most often due to the contamination of potable water or air-handling systems and predominantly affect immunosuppressed patients, particularly those receiving glucocorticoid medication. The risk varies greatly among geographic regions and within a given region, depending on the extent of hospital hot-water contamination, on the presence or absence of high-risk patient populations, and on specific hospital practices (e.g., inappropriate use of nonsterile water in respiratory therapy equipment). Laboratory-based surveillance for nosocomial *Legionella* should be performed, and a diagnosis of legionellosis should probably be considered more often than it is. If cases are detected, environmental samples (e.g., hot-water tank sediment, faucets, and showerheads) should be cultured. If cultures yield *Legionella* and if typing of clinical and environmental isolates reveals a correlation, eradication measures should be pursued (see Chap. 153). An alternative approach is to periodically culture water tanks and water on wards housing high-risk patients. If *Legionella* is found, a concerted effort should be made to culture samples from all patients with nosocomial pneumonia for *Legionella*.

Antibiotic-Resistant Bacteria Outbreaks of antibiotic resistance begin with Darwinian selection of bacterial chromosomal mutations, spread of plasmid- and/or transposon-borne resistance among bacterial species, and/or (re)admission to the hospital of patients chronically infected with resistant bacteria. After the introduction of resistant strains, dissemination occurs by cross-infection on unwashed hands of caregivers or, occasionally, via personnel carriage and/or environmental contamination. Outbreak control depends on close laboratory surveillance, with early detection of problems; on the reinforcement of routine asepsis (e.g., hand washing); on the implementation of barrier precautions for all colonized and/or infected patients; on the use of patient-surveillance cultures to more fully ascertain the extent of patient colonization; and on the timely initiation of an epidemiologic investigation when rates increase. Colonized personnel who are implicated in nosocomial transmission and patients who pose a threat may be decontaminated; for example, colonization with methicillin-resistant *Staphylococcus aureus* may be controlled with oral antibiotics, including trimethoprim-sulfamethoxazole and rifampin, and with topical agents, including hexachlorophene or chlorhexidine and mupirocin. In a few ICUs, selective decontamination has been used successfully as a temporary emergency control measure for outbreaks of infection due to gram-negative bacilli.

The most recent bacterial-resistance problem to plague hospitals is the emergence of vancomycin-resistant enterococci (VRE). Initially an ICU problem, VRE have now spread onto general wards in many hospitals. VRE are particularly problematic because of a substantial "iceberg" effect (i.e., the fact that, for each individual with a clinical infection, many other patients are colonized); the occurrence of both gastrointestinal and skin colonization (reflecting fecal contamination on the skin of ill, hospitalized patients); and the propensity for these organisms to contaminate the patient's environment, which may increase the risk of cross-infection. Control of VRE requires strict attention to hand washing by personnel, concerted use of barrier precautions for patients known to be colonized or infected, and emphasis on thorough cleaning of the rooms of these patients.

Because the excessive use of broad-spectrum antibiotics underlies many resistance problems, antibiotic-control policies (Table 138-2) must be considered a cornerstone of resistance-control efforts. Although the efficacy of antibiotic-control measures in reducing rates of antimicrobial resistance has not been proved in prospective controlled trials, it seems worthwhile to restrict the use of particular agents to narrowly defined indications or to cycle the use of antibiotic classes to limit the selective pressure on the nosocomial flora. Timely examples include the replacement of oral vancomycin with metronidazole for the treatment of *C. difficile* diarrhea, the elimination of oral vancomycin from prophylactic regimens administered to neutropenic patients, and the limitation of the empirical use of parenteral vancomycin for the treatment of fever in neutropenic patients.

EMPLOYEE HEALTH SERVICE ISSUES An institution's employee health service (EHS) is a critical component of its infection-control efforts. New employees should be processed through the EHS, where a contagious-disease history can be taken; evidence of immunity to a variety of diseases, such as hepatitis B, chickenpox, measles, and rubella, can be sought; immunizations for hepatitis B, measles, rubella, and varicella can be given as needed, and a reminder about the need for yearly influenza immunization can be imparted; a baseline PPD (purified protein derivative of tuberculin) skin test can be performed; and education about personal responsibility for infection control can be initiated. Evaluations of employees should be codified to meet the requirements of accrediting and regulatory agencies; for example, the CDC recommends at least annual PPD skin testing of susceptible caregivers, and OSHA requires that employees who may be exposed to blood or blood-containing fluids either receive hepatitis B vaccine at no cost or sign a specific refusal form.

The EHS must have protocols for dealing with employees who have been exposed to contagious diseases. A new problem is the counseling, treatment, and monitoring of personnel after percutaneous or mucosal exposure to the blood of patients infected with HIV or hepatitis C virus. The available data indicate that postexposure HIV prophylaxis with zidovudine is beneficial. Protocols are also needed for dealing with caregivers who have common contagious diseases, such as chickenpox, group A streptococcal infections, respiratory infections, and infectious

diarrhea, and for those who have less common but high-visibility public health problems, such as chronic hepatitis B or C or HIV infection, for which exposure-control guidelines have been published by the CDC and by the Society for Healthcare Epidemiology of America.

BIBLIOGRAPHY

BENNETT JV, BRACHMAN PS (eds): *Hospital Infections*, 4th ed. Boston, Little, Brown, 1996

CENTERS FOR DISEASE CONTROL: Report of the National Nosocomial Infections Surveillance (NNIS) System: Nosocomial infection rates for interhospital comparison: Limitations and possible solutions. Infect Control Hosp Epidemiol 12:609, 1991

CENTERS FOR DISEASE CONTROL AND PREVENTION: Draft guideline for isolation precautions in hospitals. Part I. Evolution of isolation precautions. Part II. Recommendations for isolation precautions in hospitals. Fed Regist 59:55552, 1994

GOLDMANN DA et al: Strategies to prevent and control the emergence and spread of antimicrobial-resistant microorganisms in hospitals—A challenge to hospital leadership. JAMA 275:234, 1996

MARTONE WJ, GARNER JS (eds): Proceedings of the Third Decennial International Conference on Nosocomial Infections. Am J Med 91(Suppl 3B):1S, 1991

MAYHALL CG (ed): *Hospital Epidemiology and Infection Control*. Baltimore, Williams & Wilkins, 1995

Table 138-2

Elements of an Antibiotic-Control Program

- Review antimicrobial agents and select a basic formulary.
- Establish prophylactic, empirical, and therapeutic guidelines.
- Restrict the use of agents that have special limited indications, cause excessive toxicity, or are costly.
- Release restricted agents for use in predetermined circumstances or after prospective approval.
- Ensure that the antibiotics on the formulary are the same as those being used for susceptibility testing by the microbiology laboratory.
- Monitor patterns of antibiotic susceptibility and trends in antibiotic use, providing regular feedback to the medical staff.
- Audit the use of specific antibiotics.
- Conduct ongoing educational programs.
- Regulate in-hospital promotional efforts of pharmaceutical companies.

SOURCE: After JP Flaherty, RA Weinstein, Infect Control Hosp Epidemiol 17:236, 1996.

SECTION 4

BACTERIAL DISEASES: GENERAL CONSIDERATIONS

139   *Gerald B. Pier*

MOLECULAR MECHANISMS OF BACTERIAL PATHOGENESIS

The past decade has seen an explosion of information about the bacterial and host molecules that contribute to the processes of infection and disease. These processes are thought by many to occur in three stages: (1) bacterial entry and colonization of the host; (2) bacterial invasion and growth in host tissues, along with elaboration of toxic substances; and (3) the host response. These three stages reflect the more traditional concepts of *infection* (presence of bacteria in a host) and *disease* (reaction to the infection)—terms that are often used interchangeably. Bacterial pathogenesis is the measure of an organism's capacity to cause disease and is a function of the myriad pathogenic or virulence factors elaborated by bacteria. These virulence factors may be classified in two groups: those that promote bacterial colonization and infection (usually surface molecules) and those that cause disease (often, but not exclusively, secreted toxins or toxic

metabolites). In addition, the host's inflammatory response to infection can contribute greatly to the observed disease and its attendant clinical signs and symptoms. Knowledge of the molecular architecture of the bacterial surface (Fig. 139-1), its interaction with the host, and the host response is critical to an understanding of the basic processes of infection and disease.

CELL WALL STRUCTURE OF GRAM-POSITIVE AND GRAM-NEGATIVE BACTERIA

GRAM-POSITIVE BACTERIA Gram-positive bacteria have a typical lipid bilayer cytoplasmic membrane surrounded by a rigid cell wall, which gives the organisms their characteristic shape, differentiates them from eukaryotic cells, and allows them to survive in osmotically unfavorable environments. The cell wall is composed mainly of peptidoglycan, a polymer of *N*-acetylglucosamine and its lactyl ether, *N*-acetylmuramic acid, with peptide side chains covalently bound to the lactyl group. The peptide chains consist of alternating D and L amino acids and are usually linked to each other by a pentaglycine bridge that binds a terminal D-alanine on one peptide substituent to the penultimate L-lysine on a neighboring peptide. Variations in this basic structure have been described for a number of bacterial genera.

In addition, the cell walls of gram-positive bacteria contain teichoic acids, phosphate-linked polymers of ribitol or glycerol that can have additional compounds linked to available side groups. Lipid tails anchor these acids to the cytoplasmic membrane, giving rise to lipoteichoic acids. Various substituents on teichoic acids are often responsible for the biologic and immunologic properties associated with disease due to pathogenic gram-positive bacteria.

Most pathogenic gram-positive bacteria have additional extracellular structures. These include surface polysaccharides (such as the group antigens of streptococci), capsular polysaccharides, and surface proteins and polypeptide capsules, which are needed for survival in blood and are useful for epidemiologic classification.

GRAM-NEGATIVE BACTERIA   In addition to having a cytoplasmic membrane and a peptidoglycan layer similar to but thinner than the one found in gram-positive organisms, gram-negative bacteria are characterized by an outer membrane that is covalently linked to the tetrapeptides of the peptidoglycan layer by a lipoprotein; this protein also contains a special lipid substituent on the terminal cysteine that embeds the lipoprotein in the outer membrane. The external surface of the outer membrane contains the lipopolysaccharide (LPS) constituent, and embedded in this membrane are special proteins that have important functions, including maintaining the outer membrane's integrity, acting as a selective barrier for diffusion of molecules into the cell, serving as receptors for bacteriophages, and binding siderophores that scavenge iron for transport into the bacterial cell.

Lipopolysaccharide   The LPS comprises lipid A and a polysaccharide. Lipid A is made up of a relatively conserved di-N-acetylglucosamine backbone that is linked $\beta 1 \rightarrow 6$ and has phosphate groups on the reducing 1 and nonreducing 4′ carbons. Hydroxyl and amino groups on various carbons are esterified with fatty acids of varying length. Lipid A likely possesses most of the important biologic properties associated with LPS or endotoxin. Attached to carbon 6′ is the inner polysaccharide core, which is usually, but not always, composed of a di- or trisaccharide of 2-keto-3-deoxyoctonate (KDO). Additional sugar substituents are linked to the inner core, forming a complete core that is somewhat conserved among related gram-negative pathogens. Attached to the complete core of LPS-smooth strains are the O-polysaccharide side chains, which, when present, confer serologic variability on different strains within a species and protect the cell from host proteins such as lytic complement components. O polysaccharides can be composed of a variety of monosaccharides, ranging from the common pentoses and hexoses to more complex and often unique sugars. These sugars can be substituted by a variety of components, such as formyl, acetyl, and hydroxybutyryl side chains; amino acids or peptides; and phosphate groups. This high level of chemical variability is thought to be central to bacterial pathogenesis, in that it allows various strains of pathogenic organisms to avoid host defenses.

Pili   Pili or fimbriae extend through the outer membrane into the external environment. They are seen in electron micrographs as hair-

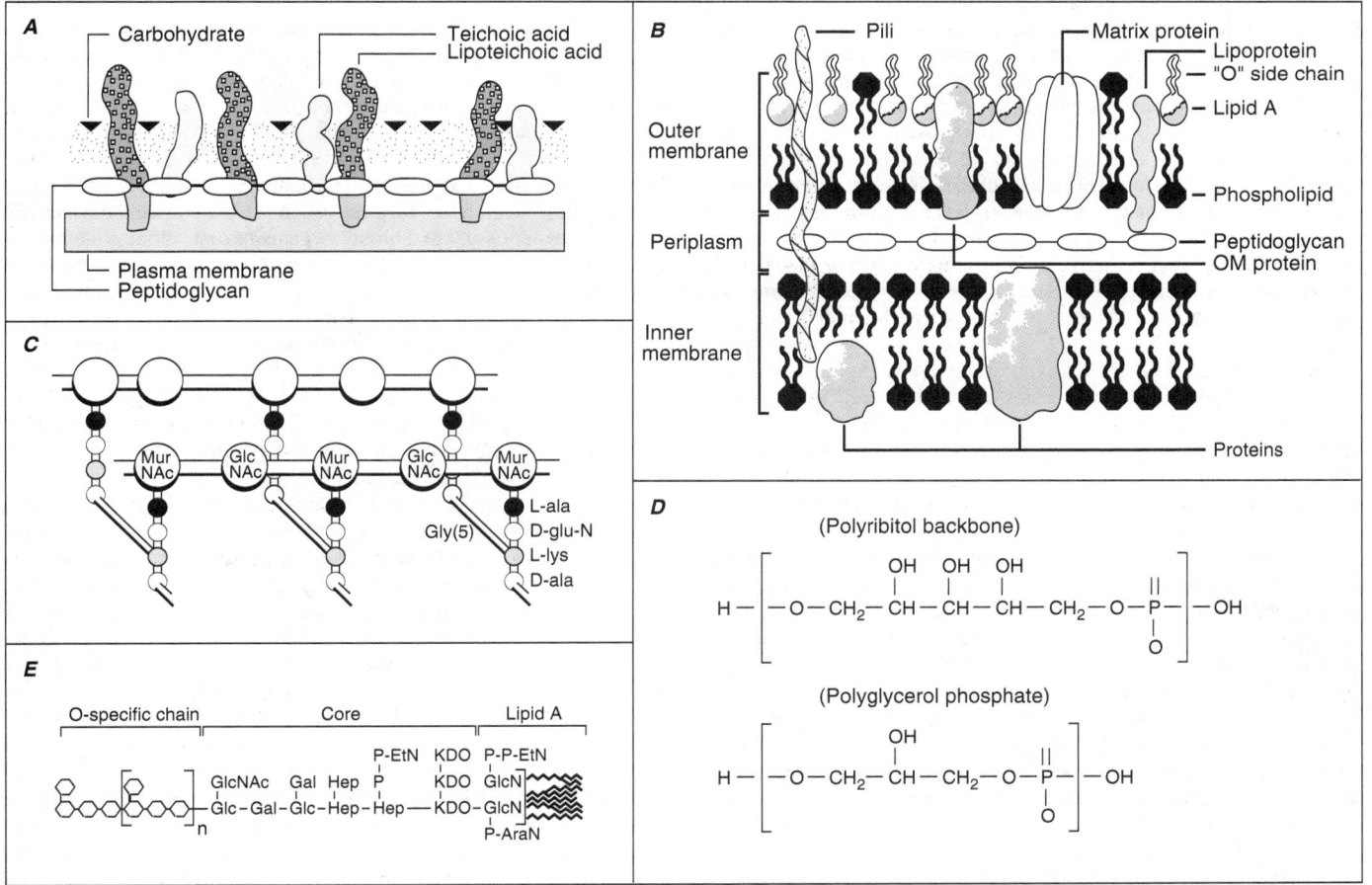

FIGURE 139-1   Schematic representations of bacterial surface structures. *A.* Cytoplasmic membrane and cell wall typical of gram-positive bacteria. *B.* Outer structure of a gram-negative organism (OM = outer membrane). *C.* Detailed structure of peptidoglycan showing backbone of *N*-acetylmuramic acid (MurNac) and *N*-acetylglucosamine (GlcNac); tetrapeptide bridges composed of L-alanine (L-ala), D-glutamate (D-glu-N), L-lysine (L-lys), and D-alanine (D-ala); and pentaglycine [Gly(5)] cross-bridges. *D.* Teichoic acid backbone.

E. Detailed structure of lipopolysaccharide typical of *Salmonella* spp., including the lipid A sugars glucosamine (GlcN) and 4-amino arabinose (AraN) and the core sugars 2-keto-3-deoxyoctonate (KDO), heptose (Hep), glucose (Glc), galactose (Gal), and *N*-acetylglucosamine (GlcNAc). Hexagons depicting the O-specific chain represent variable monosaccharide residues that comprise this structure. *(Drawing courtesy of T. J. DiCesare.)*

like projections, which may be confined to one end of the organism (polar pili) or distributed more evenly over the surface, with up to several hundred per cell. An individual cell may make multiple pili with different functions. Most pili consist of a major pilin protein subunit with a molecular weight of 17,000 to 30,000 that polymerizes to form the pilus. Some pili, such as the gal-gal–binding pili of *Escherichia coli*, have additional proteins located at their tips that are functionally critical. The major function attributed to pili to date is mediation of the binding of bacteria to host tissues.

Flagella Flagella are long appendages attached to either one or both ends of the bacterial cell (polar flagella) or distributed over the entire cell surface (peritrichous flagella). Flagella, like pili, are composed of a polymerized or aggregated basic protein. In flagella, the protein subunits form a tight helical structure and show serologic variability among different species. Spirochetes such as *Treponema pallidum* and *Borrelia burgdorferi* have axial filaments similar to flagella running down the long axis of the center of the cell and swim by rotation around these filaments. Some bacteria can glide over a surface in the absence of obvious motility structures.

INITIAL STAGE OF BACTERIAL INFECTION: COLONIZATION OF HOST SURFACES

Most bacterial pathogens initially enter the host through a mucosal surface of the respiratory, ocular, gastrointestinal, or genitourinary tract. The skin can be an important site of bacterial colonization (particularly for staphylococci), and direct inoculation of pathogens into the host is always a risk factor for subsequent disease. Successful colonization usually requires bacterial adherence to the mucosal surface. The ability to adhere is most often attributed to the pili, capsular polysaccharides, and lipoteichoic acids exposed on the cell surface, although any surface structure is capable of mediating adherence to host tissues. Host targets for bacterial adherence are either the epithelial cells lining mucosal tracts or the mucous layer itself. In the latter case, the bacteria must circumvent the host's normal ability to clear mucus-embedded cells. Such circumvention is thought to occur in states like ciliary dyskinesis in the respiratory tract or chronic *Pseudomonas aeruginosa* colonization of the respiratory tract of individuals with cystic fibrosis.

It now appears that an individual bacterial cell expresses multiple, often serologically variable adhesins and that the cell uses different adhesins during different stages of colonization. For example, most strains of *E. coli* express type 1 pili, whose binding to host tissues is inhibited by D-mannose. These pili appear to help these organisms bind to mucus. Strains of *E. coli* causing pyelonephritis express a different adhesin, the Pap or P pilus, that mediates binding to digalactose residues on globosides of the human P blood groups. Adherence here is due to minor components of the pilus proteins that are found only on the tip. In a recent study, a mutant strain of *E. coli* that (owing to a single base-pair mutation in the gene *papG*) lacked the pilus tip protein mediating bacterial binding to renal tissues failed to cause pyelonephritis in cynomolgus monkeys but did cause bladder infections. *E. coli* cells causing diarrheal disease express receptors for enterocytes on the small bowel, along with other receptors termed *colonization factors*. These receptors include the S and G fimbriae and a family of adhesins that bind to the complement regulatory factor designated *decay-accelerating factor*, a protein that also expresses the human Dr blood-group antigen.

A common type of pilus found in *Neisseria* spp., *Moraxella* spp., *Vibrio cholerae*, and *P. aeruginosa* appears to be involved in adherence of these organisms to target surfaces. These pili tend to have a relatively conserved amino-terminal region and a more variable carboxy-terminal region. For some species, such as *Neisseria gonorrhoeae* and *Neisseria meningitidis*, the pili are critical for attachment to mucosal epithelial cells; recent work shows that the principal pilus subunit of *Neisseria* also contains a minor component, the PilC protein, that is crucial for

bacterial binding to host tissue. For other species, such as *P. aeruginosa*, the pili mediate only some of the epithelial cell adherence. *V. cholerae* cells appear to use two different types of pili for intestinal colonization. While interference with this stage of colonization would appear to be an effective antibacterial strategy, attempts to develop pilus-based vaccines for human diseases have not been highly successful to date. Although there are claims that pilus vaccines prevent diarrhea due to *E. coli* in pigs, calves, and lambs, this ability has not been validated in a clinical trial, and a trial of a gonococcal pilus vaccine in humans failed to demonstrate efficacy. The serologic variability among pili is one barrier to this approach.

Other bacterial structures involved in adherence to host tissues include specific proteins found among staphylococci that bind to human proteins such as fibrin, fibronectin, laminin, and collagen and that have been called MSCRAMMs (microbial surface components recognizing adhesive matrix molecules). These bacterial structures probably promote the normal colonization of the nares and skin. Fibronectin appears to be a commonly used receptor for various pathogens; a particular sequence—Arg-Gly-Asp, or RGD—is critical to binding. Surface lipoteichoic acids promote adherence of streptococci to mucosal surfaces. The mucoid exopolysaccharide or alginate capsule of *P. aeruginosa* promotes binding of mucoid strains to respiratory mucins. Coagulase-negative staphylococci have emerged as important pathogens through their ability to colonize prosthetic devices and catheters commonly used in medical care; the surface capsular polysaccharide of these organisms promotes binding to the prosthetic material.

TISSUE INVASION AND TISSUE TROPISM

TISSUE INVASION Bacteria may invade deeper layers of mucosal tissue via intracellular uptake by epithelial cells or via traversal of epithelial cell junctions. Among virulent *Shigella* strains and invasive *E. coli*, outer-membrane proteins are critical to epithelial cell invasion and bacterial multiplication. Staphylococci and streptococci elaborate a variety of extracellular enzymes, such as hyaluronidase, lipases, nucleases, and hemolysins, that are probably important in breaking down cellular and matrix structures and allowing the bacteria access to deeper tissues and blood. Organisms that colonize the gastrointestinal tract can often translocate through the mucosa into the blood and, under circumstances in which host defenses are inadequate, cause bacteremia. *Yersinia enterocolitica* can invade the mucosa through the activity of the invasin protein. Some bacteria (e.g., *Brucella*) can be carried from a mucosal site to a distant site by phagocytic cells (e.g., polymorphonuclear leukocytes, or PMNs) that ingest but fail to kill the organisms. However, it has been shown that shedding of viable epithelial cells with bound and ingested bacteria can protect tissues such as the bladder from bacterial infection.

A number of major pathogens cause disease without further invasion of host tissues; these include *Bordetella pertussis*, *V. cholerae*, *Clostridium tetani*,*Clostridium botulinum*, *Corynebacterium diphtheriae*, *Mycobacterium tuberculosis*, and *Mycobacterium leprae*. Other pathogens can cause both local disease (such as pharyngitis and epiglottitis, skin ulcerations, or diarrhea) and disease due to tissue invasion. Some pathogens require a breach in host tissues to cause deeper infections; an example of this situation is peritonitis due to *Bacteroides fragilis* or other intestinal organisms after bursting of the appendix or intestinal trauma. In such cases, bacterial factors are not critical for invasion.

TISSUE TROPISM The propensity of certain bacteria to cause disease by infecting specific tissues has been known since the early days of bacteriology, yet the molecular basis for this propensity is much less well understood than is viral tissue tropism. By analogy, receptor-ligand interactions may be expected to underlie bacterial tissue tropism, and some good evidence from studies of gastrointestinal infection supports this possibility. However, there is no well-accepted explanation of why *N. gonorrhoeae* colonizes and infects the human genital tract, while the closely related species *N. meningitidis* principally colonizes the human oropharynx. *N. gonorrhoeae* can use the enzyme sialyltransferase from host tissues to add *N*-acetylneuraminic acid (sialic acid) to its LPS O side chain, and this alteration appears to make the organism resistant to host defenses. Whether this enzyme is present in a special form or amount in the genital tract of humans is not known. Bacteria with sialic acid sugars in their capsules, such as *N. meningitidis*, *E. coli* K1, and group B streptococci, have a propensity to cause meningitis, but this generalization has many exceptions. For example, all six recognized serotypes of group B streptococci contain sialic acid in their capsules, but only one of these serotypes (type III) is responsible for most cases of meningitis due to infection by these organisms. In addition, both *Haemophilus influenzae* and pneumococci can readily cause meningitis, and these organisms do not have sialic acid in their capsules.

COMPONENTS OF THE DISEASE PROCESS

Disease is a complex phenomenon resulting from bacterial colonization, invasion, and toxin elaboration and the host's response to these events. Toxin elaboration is one of the best-characterized molecular mechanisms of bacterial pathogenesis, while host factors such as interleukin (IL) 1 and IL-6, tumor necrosis factor (TNF) α, kinins, inflammatory proteins and products of complement activation, and mediators derived from arachidonic acid metabolites (leukotrienes) and cellular degranulation (histamines) readily contribute to the severity of disease.

TOXINS Among the first diseases caused by bacterial infection to be understood were those due to toxin-elaborating organisms. Diphtheria, botulism, and tetanus toxins are responsible for the disease associated with local infections due to *C. diphtheriae*, *C. botulinum*, and *C. tetani*, respectively. Enterotoxins produced by *E. coli*, *Salmonella*, *Shigella*, *Staphylococcus*, and *V. cholerae* contribute to diarrheal disease caused by these organisms. Staphylococci, streptococci, *P. aeruginosa*, and *Bordetella* elaborate a variety of toxins that cause or contribute to disease, including toxic shock syndrome toxin 1 (TSST-1), erythrogenic toxin, exotoxin A, and pertussis toxin. A number of toxins (e.g., cholera toxin, diphtheria toxin, pertussis toxin, *E. coli* heat-labile toxin, and *P. aeruginosa* exotoxin) have adenosine diphosphate (ADP)–ribosyltransferase activity, wherein the toxins enzymatically catalyze the transfer of the ADP-ribosyl portion of nicotinamide adenine diphosphate to target proteins and inactivate them. The staphylococcal enterotoxins, TSST-1, and streptococcal pyogenic exotoxins are known as "superantigens," stimulating certain T cells to proliferate without processing of the protein toxin by antigen-presenting cells. Part of this process involves stimulation of the antigen-presenting cells to produce IL-1 and TNFα, which have been implicated in many of the clinical features of diseases such as staphylococcal toxic shock syndrome, scarlet fever, and the increasingly recognized streptococcal toxic shock syndrome.

ENDOTOXIN The lipid A portion of gram-negative LPS has potent biologic activities that are thought to cause many of the clinical features seen in gram-negative bacterial sepsis. These include fever, muscle proteolysis, uncontrolled intravascular coagulation, and shock. This effect appears to be mediated by production from mononuclear cells of IL-1, TNFα, and perhaps IL-6. These molecules exhibit potent hyperthermic activity via effects in the hypothalamus, increase vascular permeability, alter the activity of endothelial cells, and induce these cells to show procoagulant activity. Unfortunately, to date, most therapeutic strategies aimed at neutralizing the effects of endotoxin—including the use of antibodies to lipid A and to TNF and the administration of the IL-1 receptor antagonist, which blocks the binding of IL-1 to its cellular receptor—have not proved clinically useful.

BACTERIAL INVASION Some diseases are likely caused primarily by the presence of bacteria in tissue sites that are normally sterile. Invasion of the bloodstream by gram-negative rods gives rise to sepsis and bacteremia without obvious exotoxin involvement, although endotoxin is very important in this situation. Pneumococcal pneumonia is mostly attributed to the growth of *Streptococcus pneumoniae* in the lung and the attendant host inflammatory response. Disease following bacteremia and invasion of the meninges by meningitis-producing bacteria such as *N. meningitidis*, *H. influenzae*, *E. coli* K1, and group B streptococci appears to be due solely to the ability of these organisms to get into these tissues and multiply. Most of the tissue destruction here results from bacterial growth and host inflammation.

If organisms are to effectively invade host tissues (particularly the blood), they must avoid the major host defenses of complement and phagocytic cells. This avoidance is most often accomplished through the presence of cell-surface polysaccharides—either capsular polysaccharides or long O-side-chain antigens characteristic of the smooth LPS of gram-negative bacteria. These polysaccharides appear to function by preventing activation and/or deposition of complement opsonins or by limiting access of phagocytic cells with receptors for complement opsonins to these molecules when they are deposited on the bacterial surface below the capsular layer. Another potential mechanism of microbial virulence is the ability of some organisms to present the capsule as an apparent self-antigen via molecular mimicry. For example, the polysialic acid capsule of group B *N. meningitidis* is chemically identical to an oligosaccharide found on human brain cells. The M proteins of group A streptococci appear to convey resistance to phagocytic activity in blood. Some bacteria, such as *Brucella*, *Yersinia*, *Listeria*, *Francisella*, and *Mycobacterium*, resist destruction inside phagocytic cells. Even when an obvious bacteremic phase is lacking (as, for example, in shigellosis), production of a smooth LPS is critical for bacterial pathogenesis and disease.

Immunochemical studies of capsular polysaccharides have led to an appreciation of the tremendous chemical diversity that can result from the linking of a few monosaccharides. For example, three different hexoses can link up in more than 300 different and potentially serologically distinct ways, while three different amino acids have only six possible peptide combinations. This immunochemical diversity may be the reason why many pathogenic bacteria use capsular polysaccharides to avoid host defenses. Capsular polysaccharides have been employed as effective vaccines against meningococcal meningitis as well as pneumococcal and *H. influenzae* infections and are currently under development as vaccines against infections due to group B streptococci, *P. aeruginosa*, *Klebsiella*, *Staphylococcus aureus*, and *Staphylococcus epidermidis*. In fact, capsular polysaccharides can function as a vaccine against any organism expressing a nontoxic, immunogenic capsular polysaccharide. In addition, most encapsulated pathogens become virtually avirulent when capsule production is interrupted via genetic manipulation; this observation emphasizes the importance of this structure in bacterial pathogenesis. Some encapsulated bacteria may alter their expression of capsular antigens during pathogenesis, producing a capsule when avoiding host defenses (such as during bloodstream dissemination) but not when adhering to and invading an epithelial cell during mucosal colonization.

HOST RESPONSE The inflammatory response of the host is critical for interruption and resolution of the infectious process but also is often responsible for the signs and symptoms of disease. Bacterial infection promotes a complex series of host responses involving the complement, kinin, and coagulation pathways. Most likely, the initial recognition of a foreign pathogen involves the activation of complement, and the generation of molecules such as C3a and C5a initiates inflammation. Consequently, changes take place in endothelial membranes; receptors for inflammatory cells are produced on the luminal side of the blood vessel, causing these cells to adhere to the endothelium and migrate through the vessel wall to the site of infection. The subsequent production of factors such as IL-1, IL-6, and TNF leads to fever, muscle proteolysis, and other effects noted above. An inability to kill or contain the microbe usually results in further damage due to the progression of inflammation and infection. For example, in many chronic infections, degranulation of host inflammatory cells can lead to release of host proteases, elastases, histamines, and other toxic substances that can degrade host tissues. Chronic inflammation in any tissue will eventually lead to the destruction of that tissue and to clinical disease associated with loss of organ function, such as sterility from pelvic inflammatory disease caused by chronic infection with *N. gonorrhoeae*.

The nature of the host response is often a critical factor in the type of pathology associated with a particular infection. Most bacterial pathogens provoke either local or systemic inflammation or the formation of a granuloma or an abscess. Local inflammation, as noted above, produces local tissue damage, while systemic inflammation, such as that seen during sepsis, can result in the signs and symptoms of septic shock. The latter can occur with either gram-negative or gram-positive infections, and its severity is associated with the degree of production of host effectors such as IL-1 and TNFα. Disease due to intracellular parasitism arising from infection with bacteria that cause tuberculosis, leprosy, or brucellosis results from the formation of granulomas, wherein the host attempts to wall off the parasite inside a fibrotic lesion surrounded by fused epithelial cells that make up so-called multinucleated giant cells. Levels of the cytokine IL-1α produced by macrophages can markedly affect the fate of intracellular microbes. A number of pathogens, particularly anaerobic bacteria, staphylococci, and streptococci, provoke the formation of an abscess. It has been shown that bacterial polysaccharides that contain both a positive and a negative charge (i.e., a free amino acid and a free carboxylate group) can induce abscesses following inoculation into the peritoneum of experimental animals. *B. fragilis*, a frequent cause of peritoneal abscesses, actually produces two surface polysaccharides capable of inducing these abscesses. IL-8 plays a role in recruiting and activating PMNs during abscess formation. The outcome of a bacterial infection will depend on the balance between an effective host response that eliminates a pathogen and an excessive inflammatory response that is associated with an inability to eliminate a pathogen and with the resultant tissue damage that leads to disease.

BIBLIOGRAPHY

BITTERSUERMANN D: Influence of bacterial polysialic capsules on host defense: Masquerade and mimicry, in *Polysialic Acid*, J Roth et al (eds). Basel, Birkhauser-Verlag, 1993, p 11

BOSLEGO JW et al: Efficacy trial of a parenteral gonococcal pilus vaccine in men. Vaccine 9:154, 1991

DAVIS BD: Bacterial architecture, in *Microbiology*, 4th ed, BD Davis et al (eds). Philadelphia, Lippincott, 1990, p 21

GLAUSER MP et al: Pathogenesis and potential strategies for prevention and treatment of septic shock: An update. Clin Infect Dis 18(Suppl 2):S205, 1994

MEKALANOS JJ: Environmental signals controlling expression of virulence determinants in bacteria. J Bacteriol 174:1, 1992

MELULENI GJ et al: Mucoid *Pseudomonas aeruginosa* growing in a biofilm in vitro are killed by opsonic antibodies to the mucoid exopolysaccharide capsule but not by antibodies produced during chronic lung infection in cystic fibrosis patients. J Immunol 155:2029, 1995

PATTI JM et al: MSCRAMM-mediated adherence of microorganisms to host tissues. Annu Rev Microbiol 48:585, 1994

ROBERTS JA et al: The Gal(alpha 1-4)Gal-specific tip adhesin of *Escherichia coli* P-fimbriae is needed for pyelonephritis to occur in the normal urinary tract. Proc Natl Acad Sci USA 91:11889, 1994

RUDEL T et al: Neisseria PilC protein identified as type-4 pilus tip-located adhesin. Nature 373:357, 1995

SCHAFER R et al: Superantigens and their role in infectious disease. Adv Pediatr Infect Dis 10:369, 1995

SCHLIEVERT PM et al: Severe invasive group A streptococcal disease: Clinical description and mechanisms of pathogenesis. J Lab Clin Med 127:13, 1996

SOUTHWICK FS, PURICH DL: Intracellular pathogenesis of listeriosis. N Engl J Med 334:770, 1996

STEVENS DL: Streptococcal toxic-shock syndrome. Emerging Infect Dis 1:69, 1995

TZIANABOS AO et al: Structural features of polysaccharides that induce intraabdominal abscesses. Science 262:416, 1993

140   *Gordon L. Archer, Ronald E. Polk*

TREATMENT AND PROPHYLAXIS OF BACTERIAL INFECTIONS

The development of drugs able to prevent and cure bacterial infections is one of the twentieth century's major contributions to human longevity and quality of life. Antibacterial agents are among the most commonly prescribed drugs of any kind worldwide. Used appropriately, these drugs are lifesaving. However, their indiscriminate use drives up the cost of health care, leads to a plethora of side effects and drug interactions, and fosters the emergence of bacterial resistance, rendering previously valuable drugs useless. The rational use of antibacterial agents is dependent on an understanding of their mechanisms of action, pharmacokinetics, toxicities, and interactions; bacterial strategies for resistance; and bacterial susceptibility in vitro. In addition, patient-associated parameters, such as the site of infection and the immune and the excretory status of the host, are critically important to appropriate therapeutic decisions.

This chapter provides specific data required for making an informed choice of antibacterial agent. Throughout the chapter the term *antibacterial agent* is used to refer to all natural, synthetic, and semisynthetic compounds that kill bacteria or inhibit their growth. The term *antibiotic* is reserved for those compounds produced by living organisms.

MECHANISMS OF ACTION

Antibacterial agents, like all antimicrobial drugs, are directed against unique targets not present in mammalian cells. The goal is to limit toxicity to the host and maximize chemotherapeutic activity affecting invading microbes only. The mechanisms of action of the antibacterial agents to be discussed in this section are summarized in Table 140-1.

INHIBITION OF CELL-WALL SYNTHESIS One major difference between bacterial and mammalian cells is the presence in bacteria of a rigid wall external to the cell membrane. The wall protects bacterial cells from osmotic rupture, which would result from the fact that the cell is usually markedly hyperosmolar (by up to 20 atm) to the host environment. The structure conferring cell-wall rigidity and resistance to osmotic lysis in both gram-positive and gram-negative bacteria is peptidoglycan, a large, covalently linked sacculus that surrounds the bacterium. In gram-positive bacteria, peptidoglycan is the only layered structure external to the cell membrane and is thick (20 to 80 nm); in gram-negative bacteria, there is an outer membrane external to a very thin (1-nm) peptidoglycan layer.

Chemotherapeutic agents directed at any stage of the synthesis, export, assembly, or cross-linking of peptidoglycan lead to inhibition of bacterial cell growth and, in most cases, to cell death. Peptidoglycan is composed of (1) a backbone of two alternating sugars, *N*-acetylglucosamine and *N*-acetylmuramic acid; (2) a chain of four amino acids that extends down from the backbone (stem peptides); and (3) a peptide bridge that cross-links the peptide chains. Peptidoglycan is formed by the addition of subunits (a sugar with its five attached amino acids) that are assembled in the cytoplasm and transported through the cytoplasmic membrane to the cell surface. Subsequent cross-linking is driven by cleavage of the terminal stem-peptide amino acid. Antibacterial agents act to inhibit cell-wall synthesis in several ways, as described below.

Bacitracin, a cyclic peptide antibiotic, inhibits the conversion to its active form of the lipid carrier that moves the water-soluble cytoplasmic peptidoglycan subunits through the cell membrane to the cell exterior. Cell-wall subunits accumulate in the cytoplasm and cannot be added to the growing peptidoglycan chain.

Glycopeptides (vancomycin and teicoplanin) are high-molecular-weight antibiotics that bind to the terminal D-alanine–D-alanine component of the stem peptide while the subunits are external to the cell membrane but still linked to the lipid carrier. This binding sterically inhibits the addition of subunits to the peptidoglycan backbone.

β-*Lactam antibiotics* (penicillins, cephalosporins, carbapenems, and monobactams; see Table 140-2), characterized by a four-membered β-lactam ring, prevent the cross-linking reaction called *transpeptidation*. The energy for attaching a peptide cross-bridge from the stem peptide of one peptidoglycan subunit to another is derived from the cleavage of a terminal D-alanine residue from the subunit stem peptide. The cross-bridge amino acid is then attached to the penultimate D-alanine by transpeptidase enzymes. The β-lactam ring of the antibiotic forms an irreversible covalent acyl bond with the transpeptidase enzyme (probably because of the antibiotic's steric similarity to the enzyme's D-alanine–D-alanine target), preventing the cross-linking reaction. Transpeptidases and similar enzymes involved in cross-linking are called *penicillin-binding proteins (PBPs)* because they all have active sites that bind β-lactam antibiotics.

Virtually all the antibiotics that inhibit bacterial cell-wall synthesis are bactericidal. That is, they eventually result in the cell's death due to osmotic lysis. However, much of the loss of cell-wall integrity following treatment with cell wall–active agents is due to the bacteria's own cell-wall remodeling enzymes (autolysins) that cleave peptidoglycan bonds in the normal course of cell growth. In the presence of antibacterial agents that inhibit cell-wall growth, autolysis proceeds without normal cell-wall repair; weakness and eventual cellular lysis occur.

INHIBITION OF PROTEIN SYNTHESIS Most of the antibacterial agents that inhibit protein synthesis interact with the bacterial ribosome. The difference between the composition of bacterial and mammalian ribosomes gives these compounds their selectivity.

Aminoglycosides (gentamicin, kanamycin, tobramycin, streptomycin, netilmicin, neomycin, and amikacin) are a group of structurally related compounds containing three linked hexose sugars. They exert a bactericidal effect by binding irreversibly to the 30S subunit of the bacterial ribosome and blocking initiation of protein synthesis. The reason for the lethal effect of aminoglycosides (as opposed to the largely bacteriostatic effect of other protein synthesis–inhibiting antibacterial drugs, including the macrolides, the lincosamides, chloramphenicol, and tetracycline) is not completely understood. Uptake of aminoglycosides and their penetration through the cell membrane constitute an aerobic, energy-dependent process. Thus, aminoglycoside activity is markedly reduced in an anaerobic environment. *Spectinomycin*, an aminocyclitol antibiotic, also acts on the 30S ribosomal subunit but has a different mechanism of action from the aminoglycosides and is bacteriostatic rather than bactericidal.

Macrolides (erythromycin, clarithromycin, and azithromycin) are antibiotics that consist of a large lactone ring to which sugars are attached. They bind specifically to the 50S portion of the bacterial ribosome. After attachment of mRNA to the initiation site of the 30S ribosomal subunit (the process blocked by aminoglycosides), the 50S subunit becomes bound to the 30S component to form the 70S ribosomal complex, and protein chain elongation proceeds. Binding of macrolides to the 50S ribosomal subunit inhibits protein chain elongation.

Table 140-1

Mechanisms of Action of and Resistance to Major Classes of Antibacterial Agents

Antibacterial Agent*	Major Cellular Target	Mechanism of Action	Major Mechanisms of Resistance
β-Lactams (penicillins and cephalosporins)	Cell wall	Inhibit cell-wall cross-linking	1. Drug inactivation (β-lactamase) 2. Insensitivity of target (altered penicillin-binding proteins) 3. Decreased permeability (altered gram-negative outer-membrane porins)
Vancomycin	Cell wall	Interferes with the addition of new cell-wall subunits (muramyl pentapeptides)	Alteration of target (substitution of terminal amino acid of peptidoglycan subunit)
Bacitracin	Cell wall	Prevents addition of cell-wall subunits by inhibiting recycling of membrane lipid carrier	Not defined
Macrolides (erythromycin)	Protein synthesis	Bind to 50S ribosomal subunit	1. Alteration of target (ribosomal methylation) 2. Drug interaction 3. Decreased intracellular drug accumulation (active efflux)
Lincosamides (clindamycin)	Protein synthesis	Bind to 50S ribosomal subunit	Alteration of target (ribosomal methylation)
Chloramphenicol	Protein synthesis	Binds to 50S ribosomal subunit	Drug inactivation (chloramphenicol acetyltransferase)
Tetracyclines	Protein synthesis	Bind to 30S ribosomal subunit	1. Decreased intracellular drug accumulation (active efflux) 2. Insensitivity of target
Aminoglycosides (gentamicin)	Protein synthesis	Bind to 30S ribosomal subunit	Drug inactivation (aminoglycoside-modifying enzyme)
Mupirocin	Protein synthesis	Inhibits isoleucine tRNA synthetase	Insensitivity of target (mutation of target gene or acquisition of gene for new, insensitive enzyme)
Sulfonamides and trimethoprim	Cell metabolism	Competitively inhibit enzymes involved in two steps of folic acid biosynthesis	Production of insensitive targets (dihydropteroic acid [sulfonamides] and dihydrofolic acid [trimethoprim]) that bypass metabolic block
Rifampin	DNA synthesis	Inhibits DNA-dependent RNA polymerase	Insensitivity of target (mutation of polymerase gene)
Metronidazole	DNA synthesis	Intracellularly generates short-lived reactive intermediates by electron transfer system	Not defined
Quinolones (ciprofloxacin)	DNA synthesis	Inhibit DNA gyrase (A subunit)	1. Insensitivity of target (mutation of gyrase genes) 2. Decreased intracellular drug accumulation (active efflux)
Novobiocin	DNA synthesis	Inhibits DNA gyrase (B subunit)	Not defined
Polymyxins (polymyxin B)	Cell membrane	Disrupt membrane permeability by charge alteration	Not defined
Gramicidin	Cell membrane	Forms pores	Not defined

* Compounds in parentheses are major representatives for the class.

Lincosamides (clindamycin and lincomycin), although structurally unrelated to macrolides, bind to a site on the 50S ribosome nearly identical to the binding site for macrolides. Although the mechanism and site of action of macrolides and lincosamides are similar, the number and types of bacteria against which these two groups of agents are active differ.

Chloramphenicol, a small antibiotic with a single aromatic ring and short side chain, binds reversibly to the 50S portion of the bacterial ribosome at a site close to but not identical with the binding sites of the macrolides and lincosamides. The ribosomal binding of chloramphenicol inhibits peptide bond formation.

Tetracyclines (tetracycline, doxycycline, and minocycline) consist of four aromatic rings with various substituent groups. They interact reversibly with the bacterial 30S ribosomal subunit, blocking the binding of aminoacyl tRNA to the mRNA-ribosome complex. This mechanism is markedly different from that of the aminoglycosides, which also bind to the 30S subunit. The specificity of tetracyclines for bacteria depends both on their selectivity for bacterial ribosomes and on their requirement for active, energy-dependent transport into the bacterial cell by a system not found in mammalian cell membranes.

Mupirocin (pseudomonic acid) is produced by the bacterium *Pseudomonas fluorescens*. Its mechanism of action is unique in that it inhibits the enzyme isoleucine tRNA synthetase by competing with bacterial isoleucine for its binding site on the enzyme. Inhibition of this enzyme depletes cellular stores of isoleucine-charged tRNA and therefore leads to a cessation of protein synthesis. The antibiotic is selective for bacteria because mammalian isoleucine tRNA synthetase lacks affinity for the compound.

INHIBITION OF BACTERIAL METABOLISM The *antimetabolites* are all synthetic compounds that interfere with bacterial synthesis of folic acid. Products of the folic acid synthesis pathway function as coenzymes for the one-carbon transfer reactions that are essential for the synthesis of thymidine, all purines, and several amino acids. Inhibition of folate synthesis leads to cessation of cell growth and, in some cases, to bacterial cell death. The principal antibacterial antimetabolites are sulfonamides (sulfisoxazole, sulfadiazine, and sulfamethoxazole) and trimethoprim.

Sulfonamides are structural analogues of *p*-aminobenzoic acid (PABA), one of the three structural components of folic acid (the other two being pteridine and glutamate). The first step in the synthesis of folic acid is the addition of PABA to pteridine by the enzyme dihydropteroic acid synthetase. Sulfonamides compete with PABA as substrates for the enzyme. The selective effect of sulfonamides is due to the fact that bacteria synthesize folic acid, while mammalian cells cannot synthesize the cofactor and must have exogenous supplies. However, the activity of sulfonamides can be greatly reduced in the presence of excess PABA or by the exogenous addition of end products of one-carbon transfer reactions (e.g., thymidine and purines). High concentrations of the latter substances may be present in some infections as a result of tissue and white cell breakdown, compromising sulfonamide activity.

Trimethoprim is a diaminopyrimidine, a structural analogue of the pteridine moiety of folic acid. It is a competitive inhibitor of dihydrofolate reductase, the enzyme responsible for reduction of dihydrofolic acid to tetrahydrofolic acid, the essential final component in the folic acid synthesis pathway that is necessary for all one-carbon transfer reactions. Like the sulfonamides, trimethoprim is bactericidal in the absence of thymine but is only bacteriostatic when this pyrimidine is present in high concentration. The selective antibacterial activity of trimethoprim is based on the extreme sensitivity of bacterial dihydrofolate reductase to inhibition by this drug in comparison with the mammalian enzyme. The bacterial enzyme is approximately 50,000 times more sensitive to such inhibition.

INHIBITION OF NUCLEIC ACID SYNTHESIS OR ACTIVITY Numerous antibacterial compounds have disparate effects on nucleic acids. The *quinolones*, including nalidixic acid and its fluorinated derivatives (norfloxacin, ciprofloxacin, ofloxacin, and lomefloxacin), are synthetic compounds that inhibit the activity of one of the subunits (the A subunit) of the bacterial enzyme DNA gyrase. DNA gyrase is responsible for negative supercoiling of DNA, an essential conformation for DNA replication in the intact cell. Inhibition of the activity of DNA gyrase is lethal to bacterial cells. The antibiotic *novobiocin* also interferes with the activity of DNA gyrase, but it interferes with the B subunit.

Rifampin, used primarily as an antituberculous agent, is an antibiotic that is also active against a variety of bacteria other than *Mycobacterium tuberculosis*. Rifampin binds tightly to bacterial DNA-dependent RNA polymerase, thus inhibiting transcription of DNA into RNA. Mammalian-cell RNA polymerase is not sensitive to the compound.

Nitrofurantoin, a synthetic compound, causes DNA damage. The nitrofurans, compounds containing a single five-membered ring, are reduced by a bacterial enzyme to highly reactive, short-lived intermediates that are thought to cause DNA strand breakage, either directly or indirectly.

Metronidazole, a synthetic compound, is an imidazole that has activity against a wide range of anaerobic bacteria and protozoa. This activity is totally dependent on the organism's system for anaerobic energy production. In the presence of the anaerobic electron-transport system, the nitro group of metronidazole is reduced to a series of transiently produced, reactive intermediates that are thought to cause DNA damage. Although the unique redox system of anaerobes accounts for the selective antibacterial activity of metronidazole, this

Table 140-2

Classification of β-Lactam Antibiotics

Class	Route of Administration	
	Parenteral	**Oral**
Penicillins		
β-Lactamase–susceptible		
Narrow-spectrum	Penicillin G	Penicillin V
Enteric-active	Ampicillin	Amoxicillin, ampicillin
Enteric-active and antipseudomonal	Carbenicillin, ticarcillin, mezlocillin, azlocillin, piperacillin	Indanyl carbenicillin
β-Lactamase–resistant		
Antistaphylococcal	Methicillin, oxacillin, nafcillin	Cloxacillin, dicloxacillin
Combined with β-lactamase inhibitors	Ticarcillin plus clavulanic acid, ampicillin plus sulbactam, piperacillin plus tazobactam	Amoxicillin plus clavulanic acid
Cephalosporins		
First-generation	Cefazolin, cephalothin, cephapirin	Cephalexin, cephradine, cefadroxil
Second-generation		
Haemophilus-active	Cefamandole, cefuroxime, cefonicid, ceforanide	Cefaclor, cefuroxime axetil, cefixime,* cefprozil, cefpodoxime,* loracarbef
Bacteroides-active	Cefoxitin, cefotetan, cefmetazole	None
Third-generation		
Extended-spectrum	Ceftriaxone, cefotaxime, ceftizoxime	None
Extended-spectrum and antipseudomonal	Ceftazidime, cefoperazone	None
Carbapenems	Imipenem-cilastatin	None
Monobactams	Aztreonam	None

* Some sources classify cefixime and cefpodoxime as third-generation oral agents because of a marginally broader spectrum.

compound is also a mutagen and a radiosensitizer of hypoxic mammalian cells.

ALTERATION OF CELL-MEMBRANE PERMEABILITY

The *polymyxins* (polymyxin B and colistin, or polymyxin E) are cyclic, basic polypeptides. They behave as cationic, surface-active compounds that disrupt the permeability of both the outer and the cytoplasmic membranes of gram-negative bacteria.

Gramicidin A is a polypeptide of 15 amino acids that acts as an ionophore, forming pores or channels in lipid bilayers.

MECHANISMS OF RESISTANCE

Some bacteria are *intrinsically resistant* to certain classes of antibacterial agents (e.g., obligate anaerobic bacteria to aminoglycosides and gram-negative bacteria to vancomycin). Clearly these agents can never be used alone in the treatment of infections caused by resistant bacteria. In addition, bacteria that are ordinarily susceptible to antibacterial agents can acquire resistance. *Acquired resistance* is one of the major limitations to effective antibacterial chemotherapy. Resistance can develop by mutation of resident genes or by acquisition of new genes. New genes mediating resistance are usually spread from cell to cell by way of mobile genetic elements such as plasmids, transposons, and bacteriophages. The resistant bacterial populations flourish in areas of high antimicrobial use, where they enjoy a selective advantage over susceptible populations.

The major mechanisms used by bacteria to resist the action of antimicrobial agents are inactivation of the compound, alteration or overproduction of the antibacterial target, decreased permeability of the cell envelope to the agent, and active elimination of the compound from the interior of the cell. Specific mechanisms of bacterial resistance to the major antibacterial agents are outlined below and are summarized in Table 140-1.

β-LACTAMS Bacteria develop resistance to β-lactam antibiotics by a variety of mechanisms. Most common is the destruction of the drug by β-lactamases. These enzymes have a higher affinity for the antibiotic than the antibiotic has for its target. Binding results in hydrolysis of the β-lactam ring. Genes encoding β-lactamases have been found in both chromosomal and extrachromosomal locations and in both gram-positive and gram-negative bacteria; these genes are often on mobile genetic elements. One strategy that has been devised for circumventing resistance mediated by β-lactamases is to combine the susceptible β-lactam with an inhibitor that avidly binds the inactivating enzyme, preventing its attack on the antibiotic. Unfortunately, the inhibitors (e.g., clavulanic acid and sulbactam) do not bind all classes of β-lactamase and thus cannot be depended on to prevent the inactivation of β-lactam antibiotics by all β-lactamases. No β-lactam antibiotic or inhibitor has been produced that can resist all of the many β-lactamases that have been identified.

A second mechanism of bacterial resistance to β-lactam antibiotics is an alteration in PBP targets so that the PBPs have a markedly reduced affinity for the drug. While this alteration may occur by mutation of existing genes, the acquisition of new PBP genes (as in staphylococcal resistance to methicillin) or of new pieces of PBP genes (as in pneumococcal, gonococcal, and meningococcal resistance to penicillin) is more important.

A final resistance mechanism is the alteration by gram-negative bacteria of their outer membrane so that it is no longer permeable to the antibiotic. Mutations of genes encoding the outer-membrane proteins called *porins* mediate this alteration in permeability. The resistance of Enterobacteriaceae to some cephalosporins and that of *Pseudomonas* spp. to ureidopenicillins are the best examples of this mechanism. Two or more resistance mechanisms commonly coexist in the same bacterial cell.

VANCOMYCIN Clinically important resistance to vancomycin was first described among enterococci in France in 1988. Vancomycin-resistant enterococci have subsequently become disseminated worldwide. The genes encoding resistance are carried on plasmids that can transfer themselves from cell to cell. Resistance is mediated by enzymes that substitute a different molecule for the terminal amino acid on the peptidoglycan stem peptide so that there is no longer an appropriate target for vancomycin binding. This alteration does not appear to affect cell-wall integrity, however. Acquired vancomycin resistance is so far confined to enterococci. Most clinically important staphylococci (i.e., *S. aureus* and *S. epidermidis*) remain susceptible.

AMINOGLYCOSIDES The most common resistance mechanism is inactivation of the antibiotic. Aminoglycoside-modifying enzymes, usually encoded on plasmids, transfer phosphate, adenyl, or acetyl residues from intracellular molecules to hydroxyl or amino side groups on the antibiotic. The modified antibiotic is less active because of decreased transport across the cytoplasmic membrane and diminished binding to its ribosomal target. Modifying enzymes that can inactivate any of the available aminoglycosides have been found in both gram-positive and gram-negative bacteria.

A second resistance mechanism that is uncommon but has been identified in clinical isolates of *Pseudomonas aeruginosa* is decreased antibiotic uptake, presumably due to alterations in the outer membrane.

MACROLIDES AND LINCOSAMIDES Resistance in gram-positive bacteria, the usual target organisms for macrolides and lincosamides, is due to the production of an enzyme—most commonly plasmid-encoded—that methylates ribosomal RNA, interfering with binding of the antibiotics to their target. Methylation mediates resistance to erythromycin, newer macrolides, and clindamycin.

CHLORAMPHENICOL Most bacteria resistant to this antibiotic produce a plasmid-encoded enzyme, chloramphenicol acetyltransferase, that inactivates the compound by acetylation.

TETRACYCLINES The most common mechanism of resistance in gram-negative bacteria is a plasmid-encoded active-efflux pump that is inserted into the cytoplasmic membrane and extrudes antibiotic from the cell. Resistance in gram-positive bacteria is due either to active efflux or to ribosomal alterations that diminish binding of the antibiotic to its target. Genes involved in ribosomal protection are found on mobile genetic elements.

MUPIROCIN Although this topical compound was only recently introduced into clinical use, resistance is already becoming widespread in some areas. The mechanisms appear to be mutation of the target isoleucine tRNA synthetase so that it is no longer inhibited by the antibiotic and plasmid-encoded production of a form of the target enzyme that binds mupirocin poorly.

TRIMETHOPRIM AND SULFONAMIDES The most prevalent resistance mechanism in both gram-positive and gram-negative bacteria is the acquisition of plasmid-encoded genes that produce a new, drug-insensitive target. Bacteria produce an insensitive dihydrofolate reductase for trimethoprim and an altered dihydropteroate synthetase for sulfonamides.

QUINOLONES Resistance to the newer fluoroquinolones emerged rapidly among *Staphylococcus* and *Pseudomonas* species after the introduction of these agents. The most common mechanism is the development of one or more mutations in target DNA gyrases so that the antibacterial agent no longer interferes with the activity of the enzyme. Some gram-negative bacteria also acquire mutations in their outer-membrane porins so that cells are no longer permeable to the drugs; some gram-positive bacteria develop a mutation that allows them to actively pump the antibacterial agents from the cell.

RIFAMPIN Bacteria rapidly become resistant to rifampin by developing mutations in RNA polymerase that render the enzyme unable to bind the antibiotic. The rapid selection of resistant mutants is the major limitation to the use of this antibiotic against otherwise susceptible staphylococci and requires that it be used in combination with another antistaphylococcal agent.

MULTIPLE ANTIBIOTIC RESISTANCE The acquisition by one bacterium of resistance to multiple antibacterial agents is becoming increasingly common. The two major mechanisms are the acquisition of multiple unrelated resistance genes and the development of mutations in a single gene or gene complex that mediate resistance to a series of unrelated compounds. The construction of multiresistant strains by acquisition of multiple genes occurs by sequential steps of gene transfer and environmental selection in areas of high antimicrobial use. In contrast, mutations in a single gene can conceivably be selected in a single step. Bacteria that are multiresistant by virtue of the acquisition of new genes include hospital-associated gram-negative bacteria, enterococci, and staphylococci and community-acquired strains of salmonellae, gonococci, and pneumococci. Most of the latter bacterial isolates originated in other countries but have become established in some areas of the United States. Mutations that confer resistance to multiple unrelated antimicrobial agents occur in the outer-membrane proteins (porins) of gram-negative bacteria. These mutations affect the permeability of these bacteria to β-lactams, quinolones, tetracycline, chloramphenicol, and trimethoprim. Multiresistant bacterial isolates pose increasing problems in U.S. hospitals; strains resistant to all available antibacterial chemotherapy have already been identified.

PHARMACOKINETICS

The *pharmacokinetic profile* of an antibacterial agent refers to concentrations in serum and tissue versus time after administration and reflects the processes of absorption, distribution, metabolism, and excretion. Important characteristics include peak and trough serum concentrations and mathematically derived parameters such as half-life, clearance, and distribution volume. Pharmacokinetic information is useful for estimating the appropriate antibacterial dose and frequency of administration, for adjusting dosages in patients with impaired excretory capacity, and for comparing one drug with another.

ABSORPTION Data on absorption can refer to oral, intramuscular, or intravenous administration.

Oral Administration Most patients with infection are treated with oral antibacterial agents in the outpatient setting. Advantages of oral therapy over parenteral therapy include lower cost, generally fewer adverse effects (including complications of indwelling lines), and greater acceptance by patients. The percentage of an orally administered antibacterial agent that is absorbed (i.e., the agent's *bioavailability*) ranges from as little as 10 to 20 percent (erythromycin and penicillin G) to nearly 100 percent (clindamycin, metronidazole, doxycycline, and trimethoprim-sulfamethoxazole). These differences in bioavailability are not clinically important as long as concentrations at the site of infection are sufficient to inhibit or kill the pathogen. However, therapeutic efficacy may be compromised when absorption is reduced as a result of physiologic or pathologic conditions (such as the presence of food for some drugs or the shunting of blood away from the gastrointestinal tract in patients with hypotension), drug interactions (such as that of quinolones and metal cations), or noncompliance. The oral route is usually used for patients with relatively mild infections in whom absorption is not thought to be compromised by the preceding conditions.

Intramuscular Administration Although the intramuscular route of administration usually results in 100 percent bioavailability, it is not as widely used in the United States as the oral and intravenous routes, in part because of the pain often associated with intramuscular injections and the relative ease of intravenous access in the hospitalized patient. Intramuscular injection may be suitable for specific indications requiring an "immediate" and reliable effect (e.g., with long-acting forms of penicillin, including benzathine and procaine, and with single doses of ceftriaxone for uncomplicated gonococcal infection).

Intravenous Administration The intravenous route is appropriate when oral antibacterial agents are not effective against a particular pathogen, when bioavailability is uncertain, or when larger doses are required than are feasible with the oral route. After intravenous administration, bioavailability is 100 percent, and serum concentrations peak at the end of the infusion. For many patients requiring long-term therapy, outpatient intravenous administration with the use of convenient portable pumps may be cost-effective and safe when oral therapy is not feasible. Alternatively, some newer oral antibacterial

drugs are sufficiently active against some organisms to rival parenteral therapy; their use may allow the patient to return home earlier or to avoid hospitalization entirely.

DISTRIBUTION After absorption, the serum concentrations of most antibacterial agents must exceed the minimum concentration required to inhibit bacterial growth (MIC; see Chap. 121) to be effective. Since most infections are extravascular, an antibiotic also must *distribute* to the site of infection. Concentrations of most antibacterials in interstitial fluid are similar to free drug concentrations in serum. However, when the infection is located in a "protected" site where penetration is poor, such as cerebrospinal fluid (CSF), the eye, the prostate, or infected cardiac vegetations, high parenteral doses or local administration for prolonged periods may be required for cure. In addition, even though an antibacterial agent may penetrate to the site of infection, its activity may be antagonized by local factors, such as an unfavorable pH or inactivation by cellular degradation products. For example, since the activity of aminoglycosides is reduced at acidic pH, the acidic environment in many infected tissues may be partly responsible for the relatively poor efficacy of aminoglycoside monotherapy. In addition, the abscess milieu reduces the activity of many antibacterial compounds, so that surgical drainage is required for cure.

Most bacteria that cause human infections are located extracellularly. Intracellular pathogens such as *Legionella*, *Chlamydia*, *Brucella*, and *Salmonella* may persist or cause relapse if the antibacterial agent does not enter the cell. In general, β-lactams, vancomycin, and aminoglycosides penetrate cells poorly, whereas macrolides, tetracyclines, metronidazole, chloramphenicol, rifampin, trimethoprim-sulfamethoxazole, and quinolones penetrate cells well.

METABOLISM AND ELIMINATION Like other drugs, antibacterial agents are disposed of by hepatic elimination (metabolism or biliary elimination), by renal excretion in unchanged or metabolized form, or by a combination of the two processes. For most antibacterial drugs, metabolism leads to loss of in vitro activity, although some agents, such as cefotaxime, rifampin, and clarithromycin, have bioactive metabolites that may contribute to their overall efficacy.

The most practical consequence of the mode of excretion of an antibacterial agent is the need to adjust the dosage when elimination capability is impaired. Direct, nonidiosyncratic toxicity from antibacterial drugs most often results from failure to reduce the dosage appropriately in a patient with impaired elimination. For agents that are primarily cleared intact by glomerular filtration, drug clearance is linearly correlated with creatinine clearance. Commonly used antibacterial drugs that require dosage adjustment in patients with renal impairment are listed in Table 140-3. Unfortunately, for drugs whose elimination is primarily hepatic, no simple marker (such as serum creatinine) is useful for dosage adjustment in subjects with liver disease. Even in patients with severe hepatic disease, residual metabolic capability is usually sufficient for the avoidance of accumulation and toxic effects. However, for drugs that undergo hepatic metabolism and have a narrow therapeutic index (such as chloramphenicol), alternative therapy may be warranted in patients with liver disease, since the technology for the monitoring of serum levels is not widely available.

PRINCIPLES OF ANTIBACTERIAL CHEMOTHERAPY

The choice of an antibacterial compound for a particular patient and a specific infection involves more than just a knowledge of the agent's mechanism of action and pharmacokinetic profile. The basic tenets of chemotherapy, to be elaborated below, include the following: First, whenever possible, material containing the infecting organism(s) should be obtained so that presumptive identification can be made by microscopic examination of stained specimens and the organism can be grown for definitive identification and susceptibility testing. Second, once the organism is identified and its susceptibility to antibacterial agents is determined, the regimen with the narrowest effective spectrum should be chosen. Third, the choice of antibacterial agent is guided by the pharmacokinetic and adverse-reaction profile of active compounds, the site of infection, the immune status of the host, and evidence of efficacy from well-performed clinical trials. Finally, if all other factors are equal, the antibacterial regimen that is the least expensive should be chosen.

SUSCEPTIBILITY OF BACTERIA TO ANTIBACTERIAL DRUGS IN VITRO The determination of the susceptibility of the patient's infecting organism to a panel of appropriate antibacterial agents is an essential first step in devising a chemotherapeutic regimen. The details of susceptibility testing are discussed elsewhere (Chap. 121). Such testing is designed to estimate the susceptibility of a bacterial isolate to an antibacterial drug under standardized conditions that favor rapidly growing aerobic or facultative organisms and to assess bacteriostasis only. Specialized testing is required for the assessment of bactericidal antimicrobial activity; for the detection of resistance among such fastidious organisms as obligate anaerobes, *Haemophilus* spp., and pneumococci; and for the determination of resistance phenotypes with variable expression, such as resistance to methicillin or oxacillin among staphylococci.

RELATIONSHIP OF PHARMACOKINETICS AND IN VITRO SUSCEPTIBILITY TO CLINICAL RESPONSE The relationship between the report of susceptibility in vitro and the clinical pharmacokinetics of the antibacterial agent helps predict clinical response. Bacteria are usually considered to be *susceptible* to a drug if the achievable peak serum concentration exceeds the MIC by at least fourfold. The *breakpoint* is the concentration of the antibiotic that separates susceptible from resistant bacteria. When a majority of the isolates of a given bacterial species are inhibited at concentrations below the breakpoint, the species is within the spectrum of the drug (see "Choice of Antibacterial Therapy" below). Antibacterial agents are frequently administered every three to four half-lives, since serum concentrations will by then be below the breakpoint and may be below the MIC for the organism. These relationships are illustrated in Fig. 140-1. *Pharmacodynamics* refers to the quantitative relationship among drug concentrations in serum and tissues, in vitro susceptibility, and microbial response at the site of infection. Pharmacodynamic parameters that appear to correlate with reduction in the number of bacteria at the site of infection include the ratio of the area under the serum concentration curve to the MIC (especially for aminoglycosides and quinolones), the length of time that concentrations exceed the MIC (especially for β-lactams), and the postantibiotic effect (PAE, or length of time that bacterial growth is inhibited after concentrations fall below the MIC). For some drugs with a PAE, such as the aminoglycosides, it may not be necessary to maintain serum concentrations above the MIC for the entire dose interval. Newer dosage regimens, such as the administration of the entire daily dosage of an aminoglycoside in a single dose, are designed to take advantage of this property. Many microbiology laboratories report quantitative susceptibilities (MICs); Table 140-3 lists peak serum concentrations and breakpoints for some common antibacterial agents.

STATUS OF THE HOST Various host factors must be considered when devising antibacterial chemotherapy. The host's antibacterial *immune function* is of importance, particularly as it relates to opsonophagocytic function. Since the major host defense against acute, overwhelming bacterial infection is the polymorphonuclear leukocyte, patients with neutropenia must be treated aggressively and empirically with bactericidal drugs for suspected infection (see Chap. 87). Likewise, patients who have deficient humoral immunity (e.g., those with chronic lymphocytic leukemia and multiple myeloma) and individuals with surgical or functional asplenia (e.g., those with sickle cell disease) should be treated empirically for infections with encapsulated organisms, especially the pneumococcus.

Pregnancy increases the risk of toxicity of certain antibacterial drugs for the mother (e.g., the hepatic toxicity of tetracycline), affects drug disposition and pharmacokinetics, and—because of the risk of fetal toxicity—severely limits the choice of agents for treating infections. Certain antibacterials are contraindicated in pregnancy either because their safety has not been established or because they are known to be toxic. These agents include all fluoroquinolones, clarithromycin, erythromycin estolate (but not erythromycin base), and tetracyclines. Data on the safety of many other antibacterial drugs are limited, but these drugs may be used cautiously when there is no suitable alternative and the perceived benefit outweighs the risk. These agents include the

Table 140-3

Pharmacokinetics of Selected Antibacterial Agents

Drug	Dose, Route	Peak Serum Concentration, μg/mL	Breakpoint,* μg/mL	Half-life, h	Dose Alteration in Renal Disease
Penicillin G	2×10^6 units, IV	60	0.1†	0.5	Yes
Ampicillin	1000 mg, IV	40	8‡	1	Yes
Dicloxacillin	500 mg, PO	15	2	1	No
Nafcillin	1000 mg, IV	40	2	1	No
Ticarcillin	3000 mg, IV	160	16‡	1	Yes
Cefazolin	1000 mg, IV	188	8	2	Yes
Cefaclor	500 mg, PO	15	8	1	Yes
Cephalexin	500 mg, PO	15	8	1	Yes
Cefoxitin	1000 mg, IV	110	8	1	Yes
Cefuroxime	1000 mg, IV	100	8	1.5	Yes
Ceftriaxone	1000 mg, IV	150	8	8	Slight
Ceftazidime	2000 mg, IV	170	8	2	Yes
Aztreonam	2000 mg, IV	200	8	2	Yes
Imipenem	500 mg, IV	43	4	1	Yes
Gentamicin	1.5 mg/kg, IV	8	4	2	Yes
Amikacin	7.5 mg/kg, IV	35	16	2	Yes
Doxycycline	100 mg, PO	2.5	4	18	Yes
Tetracycline	500 mg, PO	4	4	8	§
Erythromycin	500 mg, PO	1	0.5	0.5–2.0	No
Clindamycin	600 mg, IV	10	0.5	2.4	No
Metronidazole	500 mg, PO	10	NA¶	6	No
Vancomycin	1000 mg, IV	30	4	6	Yes
Trimethoprim-sulfamethoxazole	160/800 mg, PO	2/40	2/38	11/9	Yes
Ciprofloxacin	500 mg, PO	3	1	4	Yes
Ofloxacin	400 mg, PO	6	2	6	Yes

* For fully susceptible organisms.
† For most gram-positive organisms.
‡ For Enterobacteriaceae.
§f Contraindicated in renal impairment.
¶ NA = not applicable.

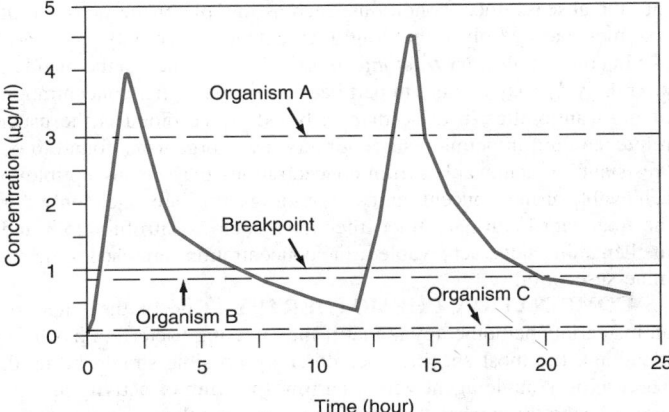

FIGURE 140-1 Relationship between pharmacokinetics of an antibiotic and susceptibility. Organism A is resistant, organism B is moderately susceptible, and organism C is very susceptible.

aminoglycosides, azithromycin, clindamycin, imipenem, metronidazole, trimethoprim, and vancomycin. The following drugs are contraindicated in the third trimester but can be used cautiously in the first two trimesters: chloramphenicol, nitrofurantoin, and the sulfonamides.

In patients with *concomitant viral infections*, the incidence of adverse reactions to antibacterial drugs may be unusually high. For example, persons with infectious mononucleosis and those infected with human immunodeficiency virus (HIV) may react more often to ampicillin and folic acid synthesis inhibitors, respectively.

In addition, the patient's age, sex, racial heritage, and excretory status all determine the incidence and type of side effects that can be expected with certain antibacterial agents.

SITE OF INFECTION The location of the infected site may play a major role in the choice and dose of antimicrobial drug. Patients with suspected *meningitis* should receive drugs that can cross the blood-CSF barrier; in addition, because of the relative paucity of phagocytes and opsonins at the site of infection, the agents should be bactericidal. Chloramphenicol, one of the standard drugs used in the treatment of meningitis, is bactericidal for common organisms causing meningitis (i.e., meningococci, pneumococci, and *Haemophilus influenzae*, but *not* enteric gram-negative bacilli), is highly lipid-soluble, and enters the CSF well. However, β-lactams, the mainstay of therapy for most of these infections, do not normally reach high levels in CSF. Their efficacy is based on the increased permeability of the blood-brain and blood-CSF barriers to hydrophilic molecules during inflammation and the extreme susceptibility of most infectious organisms to even small amounts of β-lactam drug.

The vegetation that is the major site of infection in *bacterial endocarditis* is also a focus that is protected from normal host-defense mechanisms. Antibacterial therapy needs to be bactericidal, with the selected agent administered parenterally over a long period and at a dose that produces serum levels at least eight times higher than the minimum bactericidal concentration (MBC) for the infecting organism. Likewise, *osteomyelitis* involves a site that is somewhat resistant to opsonophagocytic removal of infecting bacteria; furthermore, avascular bone (sequestrum) represents a foreign body that thwarts normal host-defense mechanisms. *Chronic prostatitis* is exceedingly difficult to cure because most antibiotics do not penetrate the nonfenestrated capillaries serving the prostate, especially when acute inflammation is absent. Drugs that are "ion trapped" after entering prostatic tissue, such as trimethoprim and fluoroquinolones, may be uniquely effective because of this mechanism. *Intraocular infections*, especially endophthalmitis, are difficult to treat because drug penetration into the vitreous from blood is hindered by retinal capillaries lacking fenestration. Inflammation does little to disrupt this barrier. Thus, direct injection into the vitreous is necessary in many cases. Antibiotic penetration into *abscesses* is usually poor. Even when an antibiotic does penetrate into the abscess, local conditions, such as low pH or the presence of enzymes that hydrolyze the drug, may antagonize activity.

In contrast, *urinary tract infections*, when confined to the bladder, are relatively easy to cure, in part because of the higher concentration of most antibiotics in urine than in blood. Since blood is the usual reference fluid in defining susceptibility, even organisms found to be "resistant" to achievable serum concentrations may be susceptible to achievable urine concentrations. For drugs that are used only for the treatment of urinary tract infections, such as nitrofurantoin and methenamine salts, achievable urine concentrations are used to determine susceptibility.

COMBINATION CHEMOTHERAPY One of the tenets of antibacterial chemotherapy is that if the infecting bacterium has been identified, the most specific chemotherapy possible should be used. The use of a single agent with a narrow spectrum of activity against the pathogen diminishes the alteration of normal flora and thus limits the overgrowth of resistant nosocomial organisms (e.g., *Candida albicans*, enterococci, *Clostridium difficile*, or methicillin-resistant staphylococci), avoids the potential toxicity of multiple-drug regimens, and

reduces cost. However, certain circumstances call for the use of more than one antibacterial agent. These are summarized below.

1. *Prevention of the emergence of resistant mutants.* Spontaneous mutations occur at a detectable frequency in certain genes encoding the target proteins for some antibacterial agents. The use of these agents can eliminate the susceptible population, select out resistant mutants at the site of infection, and result in the failure of chemotherapy. Resistant mutants are usually selected when the MIC of the antibacterial agent for the infecting bacterium is close to achievable levels in serum or tissues and/or when the site of infection limits the access or activity of the agent. The most common examples are rifampin for staphylococci, imipenem for *Pseudomonas*, and ciprofloxacin for staphylococci and *Pseudomonas*. Small-colony variants of staphylococci resistant to aminoglycosides also emerge during monotherapy with these antibiotics. A second antibacterial agent with a mechanism of action different from that of the first is added to prevent the emergence of these resistant mutants (e.g., imipenem plus an aminoglycoside for systemic *Pseudomonas* infections). However, since resistant mutants have emerged following combination chemotherapy, this approach is not uniformly successful.

2. *Synergistic or additive activity.* Against some bacteria, two antibacterial agents are clearly more active than one; whether or not this is the case is usually judged on the basis of testing in vitro. *Synergistic* or *additive activity* is defined as a lowering of the MIC or MBC of *each* of two drugs tested in combination against a specific bacterium. Thus *each* agent is more active when combined with a second drug than it would be alone. The best examples of a synergistic or additive effect, confirmed both in vitro and by animal studies, are the enhanced bactericidal activities of certain β-lactam–aminoglycoside combinations against enterococci, viridans streptococci, and *P. aeruginosa*. The synergistic or additive activity of these combinations also has been demonstrated for selected isolates of enteric gram-negative bacteria and staphylococci. The combination of trimethoprim and sulfamethoxazole also has synergistic or additive activity against many enteric gram-negative bacteria. Most other antimicrobial combinations show indifferent activity (i.e., the combination is *no better* than the more active of the two agents alone), and some combinations (e.g., penicillin plus tetracycline against pneumococci) may be antagonistic (i.e., the combination is *worse* than either drug alone).

3. *Therapy directed against multiple potential pathogens.* For certain infections, either a mixture of pathogens is suspected or the patient is desperately ill with an as-yet-unidentified infection. In these situations, the most important of the likely infecting bacteria need to be covered by therapy until culture and susceptibility results become available. Examples of the former infections are intraabdominal or brain abscesses and infections of limbs in diabetic patients with microvascular disease. The latter situations include fevers in neutropenic patients, acute pneumonia from aspiration of oral flora by hospitalized patients, and septic shock or sepsis syndrome. However, in circumstances where empirical therapy with more than one agent is begun, monotherapy should always be given subsequently if a single infecting bacterium that can be treated effectively with one agent is identified.

CHOICE OF ANTIBACTERIAL THERAPY

The antibacterial spectrum of specific agents and the infections for which they represent the treatment of choice are detailed below. No attempt has been made to include all the potential situations in which antibacterial agents may be used. A more detailed discussion of specific bacteria and infections that they cause can be found elsewhere in this volume.

β-LACTAMS (Table 140-2) All *penicillins* (except for the semisynthetic, penicillinase-resistant antistaphylococcal agents) are hydrolyzed by β-lactamases and are ineffective against isolates that produce these enzymes. Penicillin G has a spectrum that includes spirochetes (*Treponema pallidum*, *Borrelia*, and *Leptospira*), strepto-cocci (groups A and B, viridans, and *Streptococcus pneumoniae*), enterococci, most *Neisseria* species, a few staphylococci, many fastidi-ous oral bacteria [*Bacteroides* (*Porphyromonas* and *Prevotella*), strep-tococci, *Actinomyces*, and *Fusobacterium*], *Clostridium* species (ex-cept *C. difficile*), *Pasteurella multocida*, *Erysipelothrix rhusiopathiae*, and *Streptobacillus moniliformis*. However, resistance is widespread among staphylococci; is increasing rapidly among gonococci, entero-cocci, and pneumococci; and is emerging among meningococci and oral anaerobes such as *Porphyromonas* and *Prevotella*. Penicillin G is the drug of choice for syphilis, yaws, leptospirosis, group A and B streptococcal infections, actinomycosis, oral and periodontal infec-tions, meningococcal meningitis and meningococcemia, viridans strep-tococcal endocarditis, clostridial myonecrosis, tetanus, anthrax, rat-bite fever, *P. multocida* infections, and erysipeloid (*E. rhusiopathiae*).

Ampicillin extends the spectrum of penicillin G to some gram-negative rods. It is active against some isolates of *Escherichia coli*, *Proteus mirabilis*, *Salmonella*, *Shigella*, and *H. influenzae* and is one of the drugs of choice for susceptible organisms causing urinary tract infections, salmonellosis, *H. influenzae* meningitis and epiglottitis, and *Listeria monocytogenes* meningitis. High rates of resistance have lessened its value as empirical therapy in some situations. For example, more than 80 percent of isolates of *E. coli* and *P. mirabilis* are resistant in some hospitals, as are 10 to 30 percent of isolates of *H. influenzae*; moreover, in some outbreaks of infection due to salmonellae, all iso-lates are ampicillin-resistant.

The *penicillinase-resistant penicillins* are used solely for the treat-ment of staphylococcal infections and are the drugs of choice for systemic or deep staphylococcal infections caused by susceptible or-ganisms. Unfortunately, on average, approximately 20 percent of *S. aureus* isolates and more than 60 percent of coagulase-negative staphy-lococcal isolates acquired in U.S. hospitals are resistant to these agents (i.e., methicillin-resistant). The spectrum of these agents also includes most of the same gram-positive bacteria that are susceptible to penicil-lin G.

The spectrum of the *antipseudomonal penicillins* includes the bac-teria covered by ampicillin as well as some additional nonpseudomonal enteric gram-negative bacilli. For example, piperacillin is active against many indole-positive *Proteus*, *Enterobacter*, *Klebsiella*, *Pro-videncia*, and *Serratia* species. However, the susceptibility of these penicillins to β-lactamase markedly limits their utility as empirical therapy when infections caused by gram-negative enteric organisms are suspected. The major use of these compounds is in the treatment of proven or suspected infections with *P. aeruginosa* and *Acineto-bacter*, for which they are among the drugs of choice. Their relative antipseudomonal activities can be ranked as follows: piperacillin > mezlocillin/ticarcillin > carbenicillin.

The addition of β-*lactamase inhibitors* (clavulanic acid, sulbactam, or tazobactam) to ampicillin, amoxicillin, ticarcillin, or piperacillin extends the spectrum of these agents to include many organisms that are resistant by virtue of β-lactamase production. These organisms include *E. coli*, *Klebsiella*, all *Proteus* species, *H. influenzae*, *Mora-xella* (formerly *Branhamella*) *catarrhalis*, *Providencia*, and *Bacteroi-des fragilis*. Such combinations are also active against staphylococci that produce β-lactamase but are not methicillin-resistant. However, the efficacy of these combinations in serious staphylococcal infections has not been adequately proven. Furthermore, *Enterobacter*, *Pseudomonas*, *Acinetobacter*, and various enteric gram-negative isolates either pro-duce β-lactamases not inhibited by these compounds or develop resis-tance attributable to non-β-lactamase-mediated mechanisms.

The *first-generation cephalosporins* have a spectrum that includes penicillinase-producing, methicillin-susceptible staphylococci and streptococci. While these drugs may be used when infections with gram-positive bacteria are suspected, they are *not* the drugs of choice for such infections. They have excellent activity against many isolates of *E. coli*, *Klebsiella pneumoniae*, and *P. mirabilis* and are among the drugs of choice in presumptive therapy for non-hospital-acquired urinary tract infections. They have no activity against *B. fragilis*, enterococci, methicillin-resistant staphylococci, *Pseudomonas*, *Aci-netobacter*, *Enterobacter*, indole-positive *Proteus*, and *Serratia* and poor activity against *H. influenzae*.

The *parenteral second-generation cephalosporins* extend the gram-negative spectrum of first-generation compounds. The various second-generation agents have differing activities. Cefuroxime and cef-amandole retain activity against gram-positive cocci and are also active against *H. influenzae*, *Neisseria*, some *Enterobacter* isolates, and in-dole-positive *Proteus* but exhibit poor activity against *B. fragilis*. Cefox-itin and cefotetan have reasonably good activity against *B. fragilis*, but cefotetan is less effective against some other *Bacteroides* species (see Chaps. 127 and 169). Both of the latter drugs display poor activity against gram-positive cocci and *Enterobacter*. No second-generation cephalosporin is active against *Pseudomonas* or *Acinetobacter*.

Oral second-generation cephalosporins have fair activity against gram-positive cocci and *H. influenzae* and are widely used in outpatient therapy for otitis media, sinusitis, and lower respiratory tract infections, although cheaper agents that are equally effective are preferable. Cefixime, cefuroxime axetil, and cefpodoxime are among the drugs of choice for single-dose treatment of gonococcal urethritis.

Third-generation cephalosporins all have a broad spectrum of activity against enteric gram-negative rods and are especially useful for treating hospital-acquired infections caused by multiresistant or-ganisms. In addition, ceftazidime has excellent antipseudomonal activ-ity. Cefoperazone has modest antipseudomonal activity, and the other third-generation cephalosporins have poor antipseudomonal activity. Since resistance to third-generation cephalosporins is increasing among all nosocomial gram-negative rods, the use of these agents should be guided by susceptibility testing. The gram-positive spectrum of the third-generation cephalosporins is variable, the relative rank being cefotaxime/ceftizoxime/ceftriaxone > cefoperazone > ceftazi-dime. Because of its excellent gram-negative spectrum, its activity against *Haemophilus*, *S. pneumoniae*, and penicillin-resistant *Neisse-ria*, its long serum half-life, and its high serum and CSF levels, ceftriax-one has become one of the drugs of choice for empirical therapy for bacterial meningitis (except that caused by *Listeria*), all gonococcal infections, salmonellosis, and typhoid fever. It is also a drug of choice for nonpseudomonal hospital-acquired pneumonia. Third-generation cephalosporins have poor activity against *B. fragilis* and no activity against methicillin-resistant staphylococci, *Enterococcus*, *Acineto-bacter*, or *Xanthomonas*.

The only *carbapenem* currently available in the United States is imipenem. This drug is marketed in combination with the renal dipeptidase inhibitor cilastatin, which enables imipenem to escape renal inactivation and thus to reach higher urinary levels. Imipenem has excellent activity in vitro against virtually all bacterial pathogens except *Xanthomonas*, methicillin-resistant staphylococci, and *Entero-coccus faecium*. Limitations to its use are its relatively low blood levels, short serum half-life, central nervous system side effects, and high cost. Resistance to imipenem is a problem only among nosocomial isolates of *P. aeruginosa*, approximately 20 percent of which are resistant. Imipenem is *not* the drug of choice for any bacterial infection, but, because of its broad spectrum, it can be used as empirical therapy for serious nosocomial infections thought to be caused by multiple bacterial species or multiresistant organisms. This antibiotic often is held in reserve as therapy for nosocomial infections due to gram-negative pathogens resistant to third-generation cephalosporins.

The only *monobactam* currently available is aztreonam. This antibi-otic has a spectrum limited to facultative gram-negative enteric bacilli. It has no activity against any gram-positive or anaerobic bacterium. Its gram-negative spectrum is similar to that of ceftazidime, with equally good activity against *Pseudomonas*. Its primary advantages are its theo-retical ability to preserve the normal gram-positive and anaerobic flora and the lack of cross-reactive immediate hypersensitivity in patients who have had this type of reaction to other β-lactam antibiotics.

VANCOMYCIN The spectrum of vancomycin is limited to gram-positive cocci, especially enterococci, streptococci, and staphylococci. Vancomycin serves as second-line therapy for most gram-positive bacterial infections but is the drug of choice for infections caused by methicillin-resistant staphylococci or *Corynebacterium jeikeium* and for serious infections in penicillin-allergic patients. Given orally (a route by which it is not absorbed), vancomycin can be used to treat antibiotic-associated pseudomembranous colitis caused by *C. difficile* in patients who have failed to respond to metronidazole, the drug of choice. Resistance to vancomycin is increasing rapidly among isolates of *E. faecium* in large hospitals, particularly in areas of high-level vancomycin use. Because of the growing threat of vancomycin-resistant enterococci and the potential for staphylococci to acquire resistance genes, a national advisory committee has established guidelines for appropriate and limited use of this antibiotic.

AMINOGLYCOSIDES The aminoglycosides are rapidly bactericidal in vitro at low concentrations, with activity limited to facultative gram-negative bacteria and staphylococci. They have no activity against anaerobic bacteria and are not effective in environments that are acidic or have a low oxygen tension. However, their spectrum includes virtually all gram-negative bacteria that are not strict anaerobes, and they are among the drugs of choice for any suspected gram-negative bacteremic infection, particularly in neutropenic patients. Aminoglycosides are synergistically bactericidal in combination with a penicillin for the treatment of staphylococcal, enterococcal, or viridans streptococcal endocarditis and are usually combined with a β-lactam antibiotic for the treatment of gram-negative bacteremia. Aminoglycosides are also among the drugs of choice for severe infections of the upper urinary tract. The major limitations to use of aminoglycosides are their renal and otic toxicity, their diminished activity at certain sites of infection (e.g., abscesses and the central nervous system), the resistance of target bacteria, and the need to monitor serum levels. Among the available agents, gentamicin is generally preferred because of its low cost; however, tobramycin has slightly greater activity against *P. aeruginosa*, and amikacin retains activity against many tobramycin- and gentamicin-resistant gram-negative bacteria because it is inactivated by fewer aminoglycoside-modifying enzymes. Streptomycin is still one of the drugs of choice in initial therapy for tularemia, plague, glanders, and brucellosis and is a second-line agent for the treatment of tuberculosis.

MACROLIDES Erythromycin has broad-spectrum activity against gram-positive bacteria, with additional activity against *Legionella*, *Mycoplasma*, *Campylobacter*, and some *Chlamydia* isolates. It is the drug of choice for infections due to *Legionella*, *Campylobacter*, and *Mycoplasma* and is among the drugs of choice for pneumococcal pneumonia and pharyngitis and for skin and soft-tissue infections due to group A streptococci in penicillin-allergic patients. However, resistance to erythromycin among group A streptococci and pneumococci is increasing in some countries. Erythromycin also appears to be one of the drugs of choice for infections caused in immunocompromised patients by the newly identified agent of bacillary angiomatosis (*Bartonella henselae*). The newer macrolides clarithromycin and azithromycin have an antibacterial spectrum similar to that of erythromycin in vitro. However, azithromycin has greater activity against *Chlamydia*. Clarithromycin, in combination with a proton pump inhibitor, has been designated a drug of choice for the treatment of gastric infections due to *Helicobacter pylori* (gastritis, gastric and duodenal ulcers). Both are active against nontuberculous mycobacteria, and both appear to have fewer gastrointestinal side effects than does erythromycin.

LINCOSAMIDES The only lincosamide used in the United States is clindamycin. It shares the gram-positive coccal spectrum of erythromycin but is more active, in some cases showing bactericidal activity, against susceptible staphylococci. However, resistance among staphylococci and many streptococci, mediated by the same genes responsible for macrolide resistance, limits clindamycin's usefulness against gram-positive cocci. In general, all gram-positive cocci resistant to erythromycin should be considered resistant to clindamycin regardless of the results of in vitro susceptibility testing. Clindamycin is one of the drugs of choice for anaerobic infections because of its broad spectrum of activity against both gram-positive and gram-negative strict anaerobes. In contrast, clindamycin, like erythromycin, has no clinically significant activity against facultative gram-negative enteric bacilli. Appropriate use is limited only by resistance or the development of pseudomembranous colitis, the major serious side effect of this drug.

CHLORAMPHENICOL Chloramphenicol has a broad spectrum of activity against gram-positive and gram-negative bacteria, although plasmid-mediated resistance has diminished its effective spectrum. This antibiotic is rarely used in adult infections because of the rare idiosyncratic side effect of irreversible bone-marrow aplasia and the availability of other agents with similar activity. It remains one of the drugs of choice for the treatment of typhoid fever and plague and is still useful for the treatment of brucellosis and both pneumococcal and meningococcal meningitis in penicillin-allergic patients.

TETRACYCLINES Tetracyclines have a broad spectrum of bacteriostatic activity against gram-positive and gram-negative bacteria and are widely used in a variety of non-hospital-acquired infections. These agents are among the drugs of choice for chronic bronchitis, granuloma inguinale, brucellosis (with streptomycin), tularemia, glanders, melioidosis, spirochetal infections caused by *Borrelia* (Lyme disease and relapsing fever; doxycycline), infections caused by *Vibrio vulnificus*, some *Aeromonas* infections, infections caused by *Xanthomonas* (minocycline), plague, and ehrlichiosis (doxycycline). The tetracyclines are also used in penicillin-allergic patients for the treatment of leptospirosis, syphilis, actinomycosis, and skin and soft-tissue infections caused by gram-positive cocci. They are among the drugs of choice for infections due to chlamydiae (doxycycline), rickettsiae, and ehrlichiae and for granulomatous skin infection due to *Mycobacterium marinum* (minocycline).

SULFONAMIDES AND TRIMETHOPRIM The folic acid synthesis inhibitors have a broad spectrum of bacteriostatic activity individually; in combination, they can be bactericidal against facultative gram-negative bacteria and staphylococci. The fixed combination of sulfamethoxazole and trimethoprim, the major folic acid synthesis inhibitors used in therapy for bacterial infections, has only modest activity against some streptococci and no activity against strict anaerobes. The individual sulfonamides are rarely used in the treatment of bacterial infections but are among the drugs of choice for the treatment of nocardial infections, leprosy (dapsone, a sulfone), and toxoplasmosis (sulfadiazine). Trimethoprim-sulfamethoxazole is the drug of choice for the treatment of uncomplicated urinary tract infections (except for those caused by enterococci) and is widely used in the treatment of otitis media. It can be used in therapy for upper respiratory tract infections in which *H. influenzae* and *M. catarrhalis* are suspected, gonococcal and meningococcal infections, chancroid, and infections thought to be caused by *Aeromonas*, *Xanthomonas*, *Pseudomonas cepacia*, *Acinetobacter*, and *Yersinia enterocolitica*. For nosocomial infections due to *Xanthomonas*, trimethoprim-sulfamethoxazole is the drug of choice.

FLUOROQUINOLONES The fluoroquinolones have excellent activity against most facultative gram-negative rods, fair activity against staphylococci, variable to poor activity against streptococci, and no activity against obligate anaerobes. They are the oral agents with greatest activity against *P. aeruginosa*; ciprofloxacin is the most active against this species. The oral absorption of all the quinolones is good to excellent; ciprofloxacin and ofloxacin are also administered as intravenous formulations. Treatment with norfloxacin can be used for urinary tract infections and has been recommended for infectious diarrhea. However, quinolones other than norfloxacin should be used for systemic gram-negative infections. The quinolones are among the drugs of choice for complicated urinary tract infections, bacterial gastroenteritis, and enteric fever and may be useful in therapy for chronic infections caused by gram-negative organisms, such as osteomyelitis and chronic otitis externa in adults. The use of quinolones is limited by the development of resistance among staphylococci and *P. aeruginosa* and by interactions with other drugs.

RIFAMPIN Rifampin has been used in combinations for the treatment of serious infections due to methicillin-resistant staphylococci (e.g., coagulase-negative staphylococcal foreign-body infections). Because the spontaneous selection of rifampin-resistant mutants occurs rapidly, rifampin should never be used alone in the treatment of staphylococcal infections. Rifampin is also used for chemoprophylaxis in persons at risk of meningococcal meningitis and for the treatment of *Legionella* pneumonia.

METRONIDAZOLE Metronidazole has a spectrum limited to anaerobic bacteria. It is one of the drugs of choice for the treatment of any abscess in which the involvement of obligate anaerobes is suspected (e.g., lung, brain, or intraabdominal abscesses) because of its spectrum and its ability to penetrate into the area of infection. Other antibacterial agents should be used in combination with metronidazole if additional facultative and aerobic pathogens are thought to be involved. Metronidazole is the drug of choice for the treatment of bacterial vaginosis and antibiotic-associated pseudomembranous colitis.

URINARY TRACT ANTISEPTICS Urinary tract antiseptics are active only in the lower urinary tract and cannot be used for the treatment of upper urinary tract or systemic infections. Their activity is limited to susceptible gram-negative enteric bacteria. The available agents in this category include nitrofurantoin and methenamine salts.

TOPICAL ANTIBACTERIAL AGENTS Mupirocin is available only as a topical preparation for use against staphylococci and streptococci. Its major applications are for impetigo and eradication of the staphylococcal carrier state. It is the drug of choice for the elimination of nasal carriage of both methicillin-susceptible and methicillin-resistant staphylococci. Unfortunately, the emergence of resistance is limiting its usefulness in some hospitals.

Although their efficacy has never been well documented, topical preparations that include sulfonamides, polymyxin B, neomycin, bacitracin, gramicidin, and novobiocin in a variety of combinations are widely used as eye drops, irrigation solutions, and ointments for superficial skin infections.

ADVERSE REACTIONS

Adverse drug reactions are frequently classified by mechanism as either dose-related ("toxic") effects or unpredictable reactions. Unpredictable reactions are further categorized as either idiosyncratic or allergic. Dose-related reactions include aminoglycoside-induced nephrotoxicity, penicillin-induced seizures, and vancomycin-induced anaphylactoid reactions. Many of these reactions can be avoided by reducing dosage, limiting the duration of therapy, or reducing the frequency or rate of administration. Adverse reactions to antibacterial agents are a common cause of morbidity, requiring alteration in therapy and additional expense, and they occasionally result in death. The elderly, often those with the more severe infections, may be especially prone to certain adverse reactions. These reactions to antibacterial agents are summarized below.

β-LACTAMS The therapeutic index for β-lactam antibiotics is broad, and dose-related adverse reactions are uncommon and largely preventable. The greatest concern is allergic reactions. All types can occur, including anaphylaxis (type 1, hypersensitivity reactions), nephritis and Coombs-positive hemolytic anemia (type 2, cytotoxic reactions), drug fever and serum sickness (type 3, immune-complex formation), contact dermatitis (type 4, cell-mediated effects), and maculopapular eruption (type 5, idiopathic reactions). Approximately 1 to 4 percent of treatment courses result in an allergic reaction, and approximately 0.004 to 0.015 percent of treatment courses result in anaphylaxis. Fewer than half the patients who claim an allergy to penicillin react to skin testing with the major and minor determinants (penicilloyl-polylysine and benzylpenicillin degradation products, respectively); those with negative skin tests only rarely react adversely to subsequent therapeutic doses. Generally, a suitable alternative to β-lactams is available for patients who have a severe allergy, and penicillin desensitization can be carefully undertaken if there is no suitable alternative. A small proportion (fewer than 2 percent) of persons who are allergic to penicillin react similarly when a cephalosporin is administered; thus, cephalosporins are contraindicated in patients with a history of an immediate reaction to penicillin, although

they are often used in patients with a history of mild reactions. The same precaution applies to imipenem, but aztreonam is antigenically distinct and can be administered safely to the penicillin-allergic patient.

Other reactions thought to have an allergic basis include nephritis (associated with methicillin), hepatitis (related to oxacillin), leukopenia (following high doses of most β-lactams administered for prolonged periods), and severe skin rashes (toxic epidermal necrolysis and Stevens-Johnson syndrome). These reactions are not IgE-mediated, and skin testing is not predictive of their occurrence. For unclear reasons, most patients who have infectious mononucleosis develop a rash when given ampicillin.

Miscellaneous reactions to β-lactams include gastrointestinal side effects ranging in severity from mild diarrhea (5 to 10 percent) to pseudomembranous colitis (<1 percent). Drugs excreted to a large extent through the bile, such as ampicillin, ceftriaxone, and cefoperazone, may be especially prone to cause diarrhea. The addition of clavulanic acid to amoxicillin further increases the frequency of diarrhea. Ceftriaxone, because of extremely high concentrations in bile, can cause "sludging" in the gallbladder and occasionally produces symptoms compatible with acute cholecystitis.

In high doses—and most often in patients with renal impairment who receive an excessive dose—penicillins (especially ticarcillin and penicillin G) can cause bleeding from impaired platelet aggregation. Bleeding also is associated occasionally with the use of cephalosporins containing a methylthiotetrazole group at the 3' position (most commonly, cefamandole and cefoperazone); this reaction may result from impairment of prothrombin formation. These same cephalosporins can cause a disulfiram-like reaction if ethanol is ingested concurrently. Carbenicillin and ticarcillin are disodium salts and in high doses can cause hypokalemia and fluid overload.

Seizures are occasionally observed with β-lactams, especially penicillin G and imipenem. This reaction is most common when excessive doses relative to renal function are administered or in patients with a history of seizures.

VANCOMYCIN When vancomycin was first used clinically in 1956, local intolerance at the infusion site was common, as were systemic reactions, including ototoxicity and nephrotoxicity. Current formulations are of higher purity and, when proper dosage guidelines are followed, are very safe, although phlebitis can still be troublesome. The most common adverse reaction is called *red man syndrome* and is characterized by pruritus, flushing, and erythema of the head and upper torso. This anaphylactoid reaction usually follows the first dose, is dependent on dose and infusion time, and results from vancomycin-induced release of histamine. The reaction is usually mild in adult patients who receive 1 g over 60 min and diminishes with repeated doses. If vancomycin is mistakenly given as a bolus, severe hypotension may result. In unusually sensitive patients, extending the infusion time or administering H_1 receptor antagonists is usually effective in preventing this reaction or reducing its severity. Patients with this reaction must not be mislabeled as having an allergy to vancomycin, since vancomycin may be the only effective treatment for certain infections, such as those due to methicillin-resistant staphylococci.

Nephrotoxicity from vancomycin is mild and occurs in fewer than 5 percent of patients. Although some data suggest that aminoglycosides and vancomycin are synergistically nephrotoxic, this point is difficult to prove, and the simultaneous use of these agents should not be avoided if clinically indicated, as in the treatment of enterococcal endocarditis in penicillin-allergic patients.

Ototoxicity from vancomycin is rare as long as doses are appropriately reduced in patients with renal insufficiency. Other uncommon adverse reactions include leukopenia, skin rashes, and true allergy.

AMINOGLYCOSIDES Aminoglycoside antibiotics have a narrow therapeutic index. The two most common adverse reactions are nephrotoxicity and ototoxicity. Rarely, respiratory depression is observed. Nephrotoxicity results from accumulation of the aminoglycoside in the peritubular space, with damage to the proximal tubule and a corresponding reduction in the glomerular filtration rate. The incidence of nephrotoxicity, defined as a greater than 0.5 percent increase over baseline in the serum creatinine level, is approximately 5 to 10 percent among adult patients who receive a therapeutic course for 10 to 14 days. However, many cofactors also influence the frequency of toxicity, such as extremes of age (toxicity is uncommon among children, more common among the elderly), concomitant drug therapy, and hydration status. Nephrotoxicity is manifested clinically by a gradual rise in serum creatinine levels after a few days of therapy and is reversible if the dosage is reduced or treatment is discontinued. Serum creatinine levels should be monitored every 3 to 5 days or more often if changes are seen. There is not an important difference among the most useful agents (gentamicin, tobramycin, and amikacin) in terms of the frequency of nephrotoxicity; streptomycin is a rare cause of nephrotoxicity.

Ototoxicity from aminoglycoside therapy presents as either auditory or vestibular damage. Since the aminoglycosides can destroy hair cells in the inner ear, ototoxicity may be permanent. The risk of ototoxicity increases with prolonged therapy, higher serum concentrations (especially in patients with renal impairment), hypovolemia, and concurrent treatment with other ototoxins, especially ethacrynic acid. Clinically apparent ototoxicity, manifested by diminished acuity or vestibular imbalance, is uncommon (probably occurring in fewer than 1 percent of cases) when serum concentrations are monitored and the duration of therapy is kept to a minimum. With more sensitive monitoring (e.g., audiograms), asymptomatic high-tone hearing loss is more commonly noted. There are no clinically important differences among the aminoglycosides in the overall frequency of ototoxicity.

Neuromuscular depression from aminoglycosides is caused by reduced acetylcholine activity at postsynaptic membranes and can result in rare but severe respiratory depression. Risk factors include hypocalcemia, peritoneal administration, use of neuromuscular blockers, and preexisting respiratory depression. This complication can be largely avoided if the aminoglycoside is administered intravenously over 30 min or by intramuscular injection; if respiratory depression occurs, it is reversed by the administration of calcium.

Fear of toxicity should not prevent the use of aminoglycosides for a legitimate indication, since toxicity is usually mild and reversible. Serum concentrations are monitored both to minimize the risk of toxicity and to ensure that sufficient drug is administered to treat targeted infections.

MACROLIDES   Serious adverse reactions to the macrolide antibiotics are very rare. Gastrointestinal effects, such as burning, nausea, and vomiting, are the most common adverse reactions to the macrolides; depending on dosage, these reactions may occur in up to 50 percent of patients, occasionally requiring early discontinuation of therapy. The mechanism is thought to be the binding of erythromycin to motilin receptors, with a consequent increase in gastrointestinal motility. Gastrointestinal side effects appear equally common for all the oral formulations and also occur with intravenous administration. Clarithromycin and azithromycin are better tolerated than erythromycin, although gastrointestinal distress is still their most common adverse effect.

Less common reactions include hepatotoxicity and ototoxicity. Hepatotoxicity is a rare, nonfatal complication that is usually associated with erythromycin estolate and presents as an allergic cholestatic jaundice. Ototoxicity is rare after oral administration but may occur in a dose-dependent pattern in up to 20 percent of adults who receive intravenous erythromycin (4 g/d) and have audiograms performed. Ototoxicity is usually reversible and mild. Allergic cutaneous reactions are observed in rare cases.

LINCOSAMIDES   The most common adverse effect of clindamycin is gastrointestinal distress. Diarrhea has been reported in up to 20 percent of patients, and pseudomembranous colitis in 0.01 to 10 percent. The mechanism of pseudomembranous colitis is production of a toxin by *C. difficile* (see Chap. 148). *C. difficile* colonizes the gastrointestinal tract and may produce a toxin when the normal flora

is suppressed by clindamycin. This toxin causes mucosal damage that results in cramps, pain, and diarrhea that may be bloody. Pseudomembranous colitis may follow both intravenous and oral administration and may not become manifest until after completion of therapy. Oral metronidazole or oral vancomycin is effective in treating symptomatic patients with toxin-positive stools, but some spores may survive, and relapse is frequent. Although diarrhea and pseudomembranous colitis can be caused by most antibacterial agents, the incidence in relation to the amount used appears to be highest for clindamycin. Allergic reactions (such as rashes and fever), hepatotoxicity, and neutropenia are observed only rarely.

CHLORAMPHENICOL   Chloramphenicol causes two types of bone marrow suppression; a dose-related, reversible suppression of all elements, which occurs commonly during therapy at the maximal recommended doses (4 g/d in adults), and an idiosyncratic, irreversible aplastic anemia, which occurs in approximately 1 in every 25,000 to 40,000 exposures. The irreversible form has been reported to follow all types of chloramphenicol treatment, including ocular administration, and often develops months after therapy is discontinued.

In premature neonates and infants, chloramphenicol can cause a dose-related "gray syndrome" that is characterized by cyanosis, hypotension, and death and that results from an inability of the newborn to metabolize the drug. These potentially serious toxicities and the availability of newer drugs have substantially reduced the indications for chloramphenicol.

TETRACYCLINES   Gastrointestinal effects are the most common adverse reactions to the tetracyclines. These problems may be related to a direct irritant effect, since tetracyclines also can cause esophageal ulceration when they dissolve before reaching the stomach. Concurrent food intake may improve tolerance, but absorption of tetracycline HCl is impaired when it is taken with food.

Hepatotoxicity has been reported after administration of more than 2 g of tetracycline intravenously and at lower doses during pregnancy. There are currently no indications for intravenous tetracycline treatment in pregnancy. All tetracyclines can cause phototoxic skin reactions; these reactions are most common with doxycycline. Other dermal reactions, including rash, are uncommon. Tetracyclines are contraindicated in children less than 8 years of age because of mottling of the permanent teeth; doxycycline may be less likely than the other tetracyclines to cause this problem. Worsening of renal function in patients with preexisting renal dysfunction has been reported with use of tetracycline, although some of the increased azotemia may be due to amino acid catabolism. Doxycycline and perhaps minocycline appear to be free from these renal side effects. Alternative effective agents are nearly always available for use in patients with renal dysfunction. Minocycline can cause vertigo in up to 70 percent of women receiving therapeutic doses and in a lower percentage of men.

SULFONAMIDES AND TRIMETHOPRIM   The sulfonamides are generally safe, but the list of possible adverse reactions is very long. These compounds occasionally cause a number of allergic reactions, from relatively minor skin rashes (including maculopapular rashes and urticarial reactions typically appearing after a week of therapy) to severe or even life-threatening reactions such as erythema multiforme, Stevens-Johnson syndrome, and toxic epidermal necrolysis. The severe hypersensitivity reactions have occurred most commonly after treatment with the long-acting sulfonamides, such as sulfamethoxypyridazine, which are no longer used. Pyrimethamine plus sulfadoxine (Fansidar), used for malaria prophylaxis, may cause severe allergic reactions, including hepatic and hematologic toxicities, in addition to dermatologic toxicity. Photosensitivity reactions are also relatively common with sulfonamides.

Many patients infected with HIV who receive trimethoprim-sulfamethoxazole have adverse dermatologic reactions. These reactions are usually not life-threatening and appear to regress in many cases despite continuation of therapy. In high doses, trimethoprim interferes with the renal secretion of potassium. Hyperkalemia is relatively common among HIV-positive patients and is most often found after 7 days of trimethoprim-sulfamethoxazole therapy for pneumonia caused by *Pneumocystis carinii*.

Sulfonamides and trimethoprim also may cause severe hematologic complications, including agranulocytosis, hemolytic and megaloblastic anemia, and thrombocytopenia. These dose-related side effects may be greater in patients with renal insufficiency. Hemolytic anemia is most common in patients with glucose-6-phosphate dehydrogenase deficiency who take long-acting compounds; trimethoprim-sulfamethoxazole rarely causes hemolysis in such subjects. Granulocytopenia from trimethoprim-sulfamethoxazole is especially common in HIV-infected patients, occurring in 10 to 50 percent of subjects.

Renal insufficiency, caused by crystals of the relatively insoluble acetyl metabolite, is observed primarily with the long-acting sulfonamides. Many cases of crystalluria in HIV-infected patients taking sulfadiazine for toxoplasmosis have been reported. A high level of fluid intake may prevent this complication.

It is recommended that sulfonamides not be administered to the newborn because of concerns that bilirubin may be displaced from protein-binding sites, with subsequent jaundice and kernicterus.

In addition to the preceding problems, sulfonamides may occasionally cause drug fever with serum sickness, hepatic toxicity (including necrosis), and systemic lupus erythematosus.

FLUOROQUINOLONES   Fluoroquinolones are relatively safe; adverse reactions rarely require discontinuation of therapy. The most common reactions include gastrointestinal distress, such as nausea or diarrhea (<5 percent), and central nervous system effects, including insomnia and dizziness (<5 percent). Phototoxicity can be severe, especially with lomefloxacin. Rarely, hepatic and renal dysfunction and anaphylactoid and allergic reactions are observed. The use of these drugs is contraindicated in children less than 18 years of age because of evidence in animals of cartilage damage in developing joints. In carefully selected situations in which the perceived benefits outweigh the risks, such as in adolescent patients with cystic fibrosis who have pulmonary exacerbations, fluoroquinolones may be useful for short-term therapy. They are contraindicated in pregnancy because of concern for the developing fetus.

RIFAMPIN   Rifampin is generally well tolerated but has several important side effects. Some patients have transient rises in hepatic aminotransferases, but these levels usually return to normal without discontinuation of the drug. Although hepatitis from rifampin itself develops only rarely, the drug is thought by some investigators to potentiate the hepatic toxicity of concomitantly administered isoniazid. Intermittent administration of rifampin, usually less than three times per week, has been associated with symptoms that seem to have an immunologic basis. These include flulike symptoms and (rarely) hemolysis, thrombocytopenia, shock, and renal failure. Minor gastrointestinal side effects, skin rashes, and interstitial nephritis also have been reported. Patients should be warned that rifampin and its metabolites cause secretions such as urine, tears, sweat, and saliva to turn orange and that contact lenses may be stained.

METRONIDAZOLE   Serious adverse reactions to metronidazole are uncommon. Gastrointestinal side effects such as nausea are most frequent but rarely necessitate discontinuation of therapy. Pseudomembranous colitis in association with metronidazole has been reported but is very rare. A metallic taste is relatively common, and stomatitis and glossitis are occasionally reported. Disulfiram-like reactions can occur if ethanol is ingested concurrently. Peripheral neuropathy develops in some patients, and seizures and encephalopathy have been reported after high doses and in patients with hepatic failure.

Concerns about mutagenicity and carcinogenicity from metronidazole have led to recommendations that it not be used in pregnancy (especially during the first trimester) when alternative agents are available. Although retrospective studies have found no association between metronidazole and carcinogenesis, long-term administration of high doses should be avoided when therapeutic alternatives exist.

DRUG INTERACTIONS

Historically, clinically important interactions involving antibacterial drugs were generally of little concern, since β-lactams were the most widely used agents and rarely interacted with other drugs in a manner that affected the patient adversely. However, fluoroquinolones, macrolides, and rifampin are now more widely used, and interactions are of increasing concern. Table 140-4 lists the most common and best-documented interactions of antibacterial agents with other drugs and characterizes the clinical relevance of these interactions. Coadministration of drugs paired in Table 140-4 does not necessarily have clinically important adverse consequences. The result depends on the timing of administration, the dose and duration of therapy, the baseline serum concentration of the non-antibacterial drug administered, the patient's susceptibility to the pharmacologic effect of the non-antibacterial drug, and other, less well described cofactors. Recognition of the potential for an interaction before the administration of an antibacterial agent is crucial to the rational use of these drugs, since adverse consequences often can be prevented if the interaction is anticipated. Table 140-4 is intended only to heighten awareness of the potential for an interaction. Additional sources should be consulted to identify appropriate options.

MACROLIDES   Erythromycin can inhibit the hepatic metabolism of many concurrently administered drugs, such as theophylline, carbamazepine, terfenadine, warfarin, and ergot alkaloids—an effect leading to increased serum concentrations and toxicity. The magnitude of the theophylline interaction is highly variable and is proportional to the dose and duration of erythromycin treatment. In contrast, cyclosporine levels predictably increase when erythromycin is admin-

Table 140-4

Interactions of Antibacterial Agents with Other Drugs

Antibacterial Agent (A), Drug (B)	Effect	Clinical Relevance*
Erythromycin		
Theophylline	Increased levels of B	1
Carbamazepine	Increased levels of B	1
Digoxin	Increased levels of B	3
Triazolam	Increased levels of B	2
Ergotamine	Increased levels of B	1
Warfarin	Increased levels of B	2
Cyclosporine	Increased levels of B	1
Terfenadine/astemizole	Increased levels of B	1
Valproate	Increased levels of B	2
Fluoroquinolones		
Theophylline	Increased levels of B†	2
Divalent/trivalent cations (Al, Fe, Mg, etc.)	Decreased levels of A	1
Tetracyclines		
Divalent/trivalent cations	Decreased levels of A	1
Digoxin	Increased levels of B	3
Sulfonamides		
Oral hypoglycemic agents	Increased levels of B	2
Phenytoin	Increased levels of B	2
Warfarin	Increased levels of B	2
Metronidazole		
Ethanol	Disulfiram-like reaction	2
Warfarin	Increased levels of B	2
Rifampin		
Warfarin	Decreased levels of B	1
Oral contraceptives	Decreased levels of B	1
Cyclosporine	Decreased levels of B	1
Oral hypoglycemic agents	Decreased levels of B	1
Glucocorticoids	Decreased levels of B	1
Methadone	Decreased levels of B	1
Digoxin/digitoxin	Decreased levels of B	1
Quinidine	Decreased levels of B	1
Azole antifungal agents	Decreased levels of B	2
Phenytoin	Decreased levels of B	2
Zidovudine	Decreased levels of B	1
Diltiazem	Decreased levels of B	1
Verapamil	Decreased levels of B	1

* 1 = a well-documented interaction with clinically important consequences; 2 = an interaction of uncertain frequency but possible clinical importance; 3 = an unusual interaction of possible clinical importance in some patients.
† Enoxacin > ciprofloxacin > norfloxacin/ofloxacin > lomefloxacin.

istered, since erythromycin inhibits the specific enzyme responsible for cyclosporine metabolism. Decreased metabolism of terfenadine and probably of astemizole has been reported to cause severe cardiac dysfunction. Clarithromycin appears to be similar to erythromycin in its inhibitory potential, although azithromycin may have little effect on the metabolism of other drugs. In approximately 10 percent of patients receiving digoxin, concentrations increase when erythromycin is also given; the mechanism is increased absorption of digoxin because of the killing of digoxin-metabolizing bacteria by erythromycin.

TETRACYCLINES The most important interaction involving tetracyclines is the reduction in absorption when these drugs are coadministered with di- and trivalent cations, such as antacids, iron compounds, or dairy products. A similar interaction is seen with quinolones (see below). Food also adversely affects absorption of most tetracyclines. Inducers of hepatic isoenzymes, such as phenytoin and barbiturates, increase the clearance of doxycycline; although the clinical significance of this effect is unknown, use of an alternative antibiotic may be appropriate.

SULFONAMIDES Sulfonamides may increase the hypoprothrombinemic effect of warfarin by inhibition of metabolism of the more potent isomer of this agent and possibly by protein-binding displacement. Sulfonamides also may potentiate the effects of oral hypoglycemic agents and phenytoin through reduction in metabolism or displacement from serum protein.

FLUOROQUINOLONES There are two clinically important drug interactions involving fluoroquinolones. First, like tetracyclines, all fluoroquinolones are chelated by divalent and trivalent cations, which prevent most of the dose from being absorbed. Second, certain fluoroquinolones (enoxacin, ciprofloxacin, and to a lesser extent norfloxacin and ofloxacin, but not lomefloxacin) can inhibit hepatic enzymes that metabolize theophylline, with resultant theophylline toxicity. The same mechanism accounts for increases in serum caffeine concentrations, but the clinical significance of this interaction is unknown. Scattered reports indicate that quinolones also can potentiate the nephrotoxicity of cyclosporine, exaggerate the effects of warfarin, and increase neurotoxicity when coadministered with nonsteroidal anti-inflammatory agents. However, these interactions have not been confirmed by controlled trials.

RIFAMPIN Rifampin is an excellent inducer of many cytochrome P450 enzymes and increases the hepatic clearance of a number of drugs, including the following (with the indicated predictable outcomes): oral contraceptives (pregnancy), warfarin (decreased prothrombin times), cyclosporine and prednisone (organ rejection or exacerbations of any underlying inflammatory condition), and verapamil and diltiazem (increased dosage requirements).

METRONIDAZOLE Metronidazole can cause a disulfiram-like syndrome when alcohol is ingested; thus, patients taking metronidazole should be instructed to avoid alcohol. Inhibition of the metabolism of warfarin by metronidazole leads to significant rises in prothrombin times.

PROPHYLAXIS OF BACTERIAL INFECTIONS

Antibacterial agents are occasionally indicated for use in patients who have no evidence of infection but who have been or are expected to be exposed to bacterial pathogens under circumstances that constitute a major risk of infection. The basic tenets of antimicrobial prophylaxis are as follows: First, the risk or potential severity of infection should be greater than the risk of side effects from the antibacterial agent. Second, the antibacterial agent should be given for the shortest period necessary to prevent target infections. Third, the antibacterial agent should be given before the expected period of risk (e.g., surgical prophylaxis) or as soon as possible after contact with an infected individual (e.g., prophylaxis for meningococcal meningitis).

Table 140-5 lists the major indications for antibacterial prophylaxis in adults. (The use of antibacterial agents in children to prevent rheumatic fever and otitis media under certain circumstances is also common practice.) The table includes only those indications that are widely accepted, supported by well-designed studies, or recommended by expert panels. Prophylaxis is also used but is less widely accepted for recurrent cellulitis in conjunction with lymphedema, recurrent pneumococcal meningitis in conjunction with deficiencies in humoral immunity or CSF leaks, traveler's diarrhea, gram-negative sepsis in conjunction with neutropenia, and spontaneous bacterial peritonitis in conjunction with ascites.

The major use of antibacterial prophylaxis in the United States is for infections following surgical procedures. Antibacterial agents are administered just before the surgical procedure—and, for long operations, during the procedure as well—to ensure high levels in serum and tissues during surgery. The objective is to eradicate bacteria originating from the air of the operating suite, the skin of the surgical team, or the patient's own flora that may contaminate the wound. In all but colorectal surgical procedures, prophylaxis is predominantly directed against staphylococci. Prophylaxis is in-

Table 140-5

Prophylaxis of Bacterial Infections in Adults

Condition	Antibacterial Agent	Timing or Duration of Prophylaxis
Nonsurgical		
Cardiac lesions susceptible to bacterial endocarditis	Amoxicillin*	Before and after procedures causing bacteremia
Recurrent *S. aureus* infections	Mupirocin	5 days (intranasal)
Contact with patient with meningococcal meningitis	Rifampin Ciprofloxacin or ofloxacin	2 days Single dose
Bite wounds†	Penicillin V or amoxicillin–clavulanic acid	3–5 days
Recurrent cystitis	Trimethoprim-sulfamethoxazole	3 times per week for up to 1 year or after sexual intercourse
Surgical		
Clean (cardiac, vascular, neurologic, or orthopedic surgery)	Cefazolin (vancomycin)‡	Before and during procedure
Ocular	Topical combinations and subconjunctival cefazolin	During and at end of procedure
Clean-contaminated (head and neck, high-risk gastroduodenal or biliary tract surgery; cesarean section; hysterectomy)	Cefazolin (or clindamycin for head and neck)	Before and during procedure
Clean-contaminated (colorectal surgery or appendectomy)	Cefoxitin or cefotetan (add oral neomycin + erythromycin for colorectal)	Before and during procedure
Dirty† (ruptured viscus)	Cefoxitin or cefotetan ± gentamicin (clindamycin + gentamicin) or another appropriate regimen directed at anaerobes and gram-negative aerobes	Before and for 3–5 days after procedure
Dirty† (traumatic wound)	Cefazolin	Before and for 3–5 days after trauma

* Gentamicin should be added to the amoxicillin regimen for high-risk gastrointestinal and genitourinary procedures.
† In these cases, use of antibacterial agents actually constitutes treatment of infection rather than prophylaxis.
‡ Vancomycin is recommended only in institutions that have a high incidence of infection with methicillin-resistant staphylococci.

tended to prevent wound infection or infection of implanted devices, not all infections that may occur during the postoperative period (e.g., urinary tract infections or pneumonia). Prolonged prophylaxis merely alters the normal flora and favors infections with organisms resistant to the antibacterial agents used.

ANTIBACTERIAL COSTS AND INAPPROPRIATE USE

Use of antibacterial agents in hospitals in the United States accounts for 20 to 50 percent of all drug costs and represents the largest expenditure for any pharmacologic class. In the outpatient setting, the costs of antibacterial drugs are second only to those of cardiovascular agents. A survey of office-based physicians found that between 1980 and 1992 there was a marked increase in the use of expensive broad-spectrum antimicrobials. It is not unusual for the purchase cost (in 1995 dollars) of a newer parenteral antibiotic to be $1000 to $2000 for a 10- to 14-day course of treatment. Therapy with a new oral antibiotic can easily cost $50 to $60. Administration costs, monitoring costs, and pharmacy charges must be added to these figures. While some newer antibacterial agents undeniably represent important advances in therapy, many newer drugs offer no advantage over older, less expensive agents.

Clinicians are understandably confused by the bewildering array of available drugs. Numerous surveys have reported that approximately 50 percent of antibiotic use is in some way "inappropriate." Aside from the monetary cost of unnecessary antibiotics, there are the costs of excess morbidity from adverse effects and drug interactions and the eventual costs of treating more resistant organisms. The following suggestions are intended to provide guidance through the antibiotic maze.

First, objective evidence regarding the merits of newer drugs is available through publications such as *The Medical Letter*, including the annual update of *Drugs of Choice*. Second, clinicians should become comfortable using a few drugs recommended by independent experts and should resist the temptation to use a new drug unless the merits are clear. A new antibacterial agent with a "broader spectrum and greater potency" or a "longer half-life and higher tissue levels" does not necessarily mean greater clinical efficacy. Third, the clinician must become familiar with local bacterial susceptibility profiles. It may not be necessary to use a new drug with "improved activity against *P. aeruginosa*" if that pathogen is rarely encountered or if it retains full susceptibility to older drugs. Finally, with regard to inpatient use of antibacterial drugs, appropriate empirical treatment with one or more broad-spectrum agents may often be simplified, with use of a narrower-spectrum agent or even an oral drug, once the results of cultures and susceptibility tests become available. While there is an understandable temptation not to alter effective therapy, switching to a more specific agent, once the patient has improved clinically, does not compromise eventual outcome. If these guidelines are followed, the care of patients will not be undermined, many unnecessary complications and expenses will be avoided, and the useful life of valuable drugs will be extended.

BIBLIOGRAPHY

Anné S, Reisman RE: Risk of administering cephalosporin antibiotics to patients with histories of penicillin allergy. Ann Allergy Asthma Immunol 74:167, 1995

Antimicrobial prophylaxis in surgery. Med Lett Drugs Ther 37:79, 1995

Gillum JG et al: Pharmacokinetic drug interactions with antimicrobial agents. Clin Pharmacokinet 25:450, 1993

Hooper DC, Wolfson JS: Fluoroquinolone antimicrobial agents. N Engl J Med 324:384, 1991

Hospital Infection Control Practices Advisory Committee: Recommendations for preventing the spread of vancomycin resistance. Infect Control Hosp Epidemiol 16:105, 1995

McCaig LF, Hughes JM: Trends in antimicrobial drug prescribing among office-based physicians in the United States. JAMA 273:214, 1995

Neu HC: The crisis in antibiotic resistance. Science 257:1064, 1992

Nicolau DP et al: Antibiotic kinetics and dynamics for the clinician. Med Clin North Am 79:477, 1995

The choice of antibacterial drugs. Med Lett Drugs Ther 38:25, 1996

SECTION 5

DISEASES CAUSED BY GRAM-POSITIVE BACTERIA

---

141 *Daniel M. Musher*

PNEUMOCOCCAL INFECTIONS

HISTORY AND DEFINITION *Streptococcus pneumoniae* (the pneumococcus) was recognized as a major cause of pneumonia in the 1880s and has been a central focus of study leading to a modern understanding of humoral immunity. Before the start of the twentieth century, immunization with killed pneumococci was shown to protect rabbits against subsequent challenge with viable pneumococci. Serum from immunized rabbits or from humans who had recovered from pneumococcal pneumonia conferred protection. Early in the twentieth century, field trials of vaccination of South African miners with killed pneumococci demonstrated protection. Shortly thereafter, evidence implicated the capsule as the basis for resistance to phagocytosis; in the 1920s, antibody specific for capsular polysaccharide was determined to facilitate the ingestion and killing of *S. pneumoniae*. In 1936, pneumococcal capsular polysaccharide vaccine was used to abort an epidemic of pneumococcal pneumonia. In the 1940s, experiments involving capsular transformation among pneumococci first identified DNA as the material that carries genetic information.

The name *Diplococcus pneumoniae* was assigned to the organism in 1926 on the basis of its appearance in Gram-stained sputum. In 1974, the organism was renamed *Streptococcus pneumoniae* because of its growth in chains in liquid medium. Around 1900, pneumococcal serotypes were recognized after it was observed that the injection of killed organisms into a rabbit stimulated the production of serum antibody that agglutinated and caused increased capsular density of the immunizing strain as well as of some but not all other pneumococcal isolates. Ninety serotypes are now known to exist, each possessing a unique polysaccharide capsule.

MICROBIOLOGY Pneumococci are identified in the clinical laboratory as gram-positive cocci that grow in chains and are catalase-negative. They produce alpha hemolysin, a toxin that breaks down hemoglobin into a greenish degeneration product and causes alpha hemolysis on blood agar. More than 98 percent of pneumococcal isolates are susceptible to ethylhydrocupreine (optochin), and virtually all pneumococcal colonies are dissolved by bile salts.

Peptidoglycan and teichoic acid are the principal constituents of the pneumococcal cell wall. The cell wall's integrity depends on the presence of numerous peptide side chains cross-linked by the activity of enzymes such as trans- and carboxypeptidases. β-Lactam antibiotics inactivate these enzymes by covalent binding at their active site. Unique to *S. pneumoniae* and uniformly present in all strains is C-substance, a polysaccharide that is a teichoic acid containing a phosphorylcholine residue. An antigenically variable protein, PspA, is partially exposed on the cell surface. Nearly every clinical isolate of *S. pneumoniae* has a polysaccharide capsule. There are two systems for numbering the 90 known distinct capsules of *S. pneumoniae*. In the American system, serotypes are numbered in the order in which they were identified. The strains that most frequently cause human disease were generally the earliest to be identified and thus tend to have lower numbers. The more widely accepted Danish system places serotypes into groups based on antigenic similarities; for example, Danish group 19 includes types 19F, 19A, 19B, and 19C, which in the American system would be types 19, 57, 58, and 59, respectively. Serotyping was clinically relevant in the 1930s, when type-specific antisera were administered as therapy, and (although genetic typing is more specific) it has again become important for epidemiologic studies of the spread of antibiotic-resistant isolates in communities and among countries.

EPIDEMIOLOGY *S. pneumoniae* colonizes the nasopharynx and can be isolated from 5 to 10 percent of healthy adults and from 20 to 40 percent of healthy children. Once the organisms have colonized an adult, they are likely to persist for 2 to 6 months. Pneumococci spread from one individual to another as a result of extensive close contact; transmission may be enhanced by poor ventilation. Day-care centers have been a site of spread of penicillin-resistant strains, especially those of serotypes 6B, 14, 19F, and 23F. Epidemics among adults are associated with crowded living conditions—e.g., in military barracks, prisons, and shelters for the homeless. The risk of pneumococcal pneumonia is not increased by contact in schools or workplaces (including hospitals).

The incidence of pneumococcal bacteremia is relatively high among infants up to 2 years of age and low among teenagers and young adults; rates increase steadily beginning at around age 55. A recent surveillance study in South Carolina showed the incidences of pneumococcal bacteremia among infants, young adults, and persons ≥70 years of age to be 160, 5, and 70 cases per 100,000 population, respectively. Most cases of pneumococcal bacteremia in adults are due to pneumonia, and there are three to four cases of nonbacteremic pneumonia for every bacteremic case. Thus, it is estimated that there are 20 cases of pneumonia annually per 100,000 young adults and 280 cases annually per 100,000 persons over the age of 70. The incidence of pneumococcal bacteremia among adults exhibits a distinct midwinter peak and a striking dip in summer. In children, the incidence of otitis media increases in midwinter, but bacteremia is relatively constant throughout the year except for a marked dip in midsummer.

PATHOGENETIC MECHANISMS *S. pneumoniae* attaches to human nasopharyngeal cells through the specific interaction of bacterial surface adhesins with epithelial cell receptors that contain the disaccharide GlcNAcβ1–4Gal. Once the nasopharynx has been colonized, infection results if the organisms are carried into anatomically contiguous areas such as the eustachian tubes or the nasal sinuses and if their clearance is hindered by mucosal edema (for example, due to allergy or viral infection). Similarly, pneumonia ensues if organisms are inhaled or aspirated into the bronchioles or alveoli and then are not cleared—in many cases, because viral infection or cigarette smoke or other toxic substances have damaged ciliary action and other mechanisms of clearance. A mechanism by which pneumococci may bind to pneumocytes after viral infection has been suggested. Pneumocytes activated by cytokines have been shown to express the receptor for platelet-activating factor. This receptor binds the phosphorylcholine residue on pneumococcal C-substance, facilitating the adherence of pneumococci, which is coupled to invasion. Studies suggest that pneumococci may invade tissues by penetrating mucosal layers; the clinical significance of this finding remains to be determined.

Once pneumococci reach an area where they do not naturally belong, they activate complement by classic and alternative pathways and stimulate cytokine production, which leads to the attraction of polymorphonuclear neutrophils (PMNs). The polysaccharide capsule, however, renders the organisms resistant to phagocytosis. In the absence of anticapsular antibody, alveolar macrophages have a limited capacity to ingest and kill pneumococci; a large bacterial inoculum and/or the compromise of phagocytic function allows the initiation of lung infection. Infection of the meninges, joint spaces, bones, and peritoneal cavity results from the spread of pneumococci through the bloodstream, usually but not always from a recognized focus of infection in the respiratory tract.

The capacity to cause disease reflects the ability of pneumococci to escape ingestion and killing by host phagocytic cells, on the one hand, and to stimulate an inflammatory response, on the other. Some pneumococcal constituents may directly damage mammalian tissues. Encapsulated pneumococci are poorly ingested and killed in vivo in the immunologically naive host or in vitro by mammalian phagocytic cells in the absence of anticapsular antibody and complement. Unencapsulated pneumococci virtually never cause invasive disease (although they can cause conjunctivitis), and mutants lacking a capsule are essentially avirulent in experimental animals. Symptoms of disease are largely attributable to the generation of an inflammatory response that may cause pain by increasing pressure (as in otitis media) or may interfere with vital bodily functions, such as oxygenation of blood (as in pneumonia) or cerebral function (as in meningitis). Cell-wall constituents of *S. pneumoniae*, probably including both teichoic acid and peptidoglycan, activate complement by the alternative pathway; the reaction between cell-wall structures and antibody also activates the classic complement pathway. The result is the release of C5a, a potent attractant for PMNs, into the surrounding medium. Inflammation is also facilitated by the ability of peptidoglycan to stimulate cytokine production, which activates endothelial cells to express selectin and integrin receptors for inflammatory cells. Inflammation in the central nervous system (CNS) during meningitis is a major contributor to neuronal cell injury. Pneumolysin, a thiol-activated toxin, exerts a variety of effects on ciliary cells and PMNs and also activates the classic complement pathway by direct binding of Clq. Injection of pneumolysin into the lungs of experimental animals produces the histologic features of pneumonia; in mice, immunization with this substance or challenge with genetically engineered mutants that do not produce pneumolysin is associated with a significant reduction in virulence. Autolysin may contribute to the pathogenesis of pneumococcal disease by lysing the bacteria, thereby releasing bacterial constituents and heightening the reaction with human tissues. The release of excitatory amino acids in neuronal tissue may contribute to damage caused by meningitis.

HOST DEFENSE MECHANISMS Mechanisms of host defense may be immunologically nonspecific or specific. Nonspecific mechanisms include laminar airflow across mucous layers that filter inspired air, the glottal reflex, laryngeal closure, the cough reflex, the clearance of organisms from the lower airways by ciliated cells, and the ingestion by pulmonary macrophages and PMNs of small bacterial inocula that manage to reach alveolar spaces. Respiratory virus infection, chronic pulmonary disease, or heart failure compromises these mechanisms, predisposing to the development of pneumococcal pneumonia. Antibody to PspA and other pneumococcal constituents such as pneumolysin may be prevalent in the population and may contribute to nonspecific immunity to infection.

Anticapsular antibody provides serotype-specific protection against pneumococcal infection. However, most healthy adults lack IgG antibody to most pneumococcal capsular polysaccharides. Antibody appears after colonization, infection, or vaccination. In the first few weeks after colonization, nonspecific mechanisms probably protect the host from infection. Thereafter, newly developed anticapsular antibody provides a high degree of specific protection. In contrast to this normal situation, adults who are at risk of aspirating pharyngeal contents and/or who have diminished mechanisms of lower airway clearance are at risk of developing pneumonia before antibody is produced, and children whose nasal mucosal membranes become acutely congested around the time of colonization are at risk of developing otitis media. Persons with a diminished capacity to form antibody remain susceptible for as long as they are colonized.

The risk of serious pneumococcal infection is greatly increased in persons with conditions that compromise IgG synthesis and/or phagocytic function of PMNs and macrophages (Table 141-1). The susceptibility of elderly individuals to pneumococcal pneumonia may reflect senescence of the immune system, especially that due to diminished production of immunoglobulin, but debilitation, malnutrition, and comorbid diseases undoubtedly contribute to this susceptibility as well. Prior hospitalization either predisposes to or serves as a strong

Table 141-1

CHAPTER 141
Pneumococcal Infections   **871**

Common Conditions Predisposing to Pneumococcal Infection

Defective antibody formation
   Common variable hypogammaglobulinemia
   Selective IgG-subclass deficiency
   Multiple myeloma
   Chronic lymphocytic leukemia
   Lymphoma
Defective complement function
Defective clearance of pneumococcal bacteremia*
   Congenital asplenia, hyposplenia
   Splenectomy
   Sickle cell disease
Multifactorial conditions
   Infancy and aging
   Chronic disease, hospitalization
   Glucocorticoid treatment
   Malnutrition
   Infection with human immunodeficiency virus
   Alcoholism
   Cirrhosis of the liver
   Renal insufficiency
   Diabetes mellitus
   Fatigue, stress, and/or exposure to cold
Increased risk of exposure
   Day-care centers
   Military training camps
   Prisons
   Shelters for the homeless
Respiratory infection, inflammation†
   Influenza, other viral respiratory infections
   Air pollution
   Allergies
   Cigarette smoking
   Chronic obstructive pulmonary disease
   Other causes of chronic pulmonary inflammation or obstruction
Anatomic disruption of meninges (dural tear)‡

---

* The absence of a spleen predisposes to more fulminant infection (see text).
† Predisposes specifically to infections of the upper or lower respiratory tract.
‡ Predisposes to recurrent bacterial meningitis.

marker for pneumococcal infection. Once a pneumococcal infection has been initiated, the absence of a spleen predisposes to fulminant disease. The liver is able to remove opsonized (antibody-coated) pneumococci from the circulation; in the absence of antibody, however, only the slow passage of blood through the splenic sinuses and prolonged contact with reticuloendothelial cells in the cords of Billroth allow time for bacterial clearance. Patients without spleens may die of pneumococcal pneumonia and sepsis at such an early stage of the illness that pulmonary consolidation is not evident on x-ray but rather is found only at autopsy.

SPECIFIC INFECTIONS CAUSED BY *S. PNEUMONIAE*

S. pneumoniae causes infections of the middle ear, sinuses, trachea, bronchi, and lungs (Table 141-2) by spreading directly from the nasopharyngeal site of colonization. Infections of the CNS, heart valves, bones, joints, and peritoneal cavity usually arise by hematogenous spread; in rare cases peritoneal infection develops via ascent through the fallopian tubes. The CNS may also be infected by contiguous spread of organisms, as in patients who have a tear in the dura. Primary bacteremia—i.e., the presence of pneumococci in the blood with no

Table 141-2

Most Common Infections Caused by *Streptococcus pneumoniae*

Acute sinusitis	Osteomyelitis
Pneumonia	Septic arthritis
Acute purulent	Peritonitis
tracheobronchitis	Endocarditis
Otitis media	Pericarditis
Empyema	Endometritis
Meningitis	Cellulitis
Primary bacteremia	Brain abscess

NOTE: The order of the list very roughly approximates the order of frequency among adults, from most to least common.

apparent source—occurs commonly in children under 2 years of age and infrequently in adults; if no therapy is given, a source may become apparent. Pleural infection results either from direct extension of pneumonia to the visceral pleura or from hematogenous spread of bacteria from a pulmonary or extrapulmonary focus; the route cannot be determined in any individual case.

Otitis Media and Sinusitis When fluid from the middle ear is cultured during acute otitis media or fluid from a paranasal sinus is cultured during acute sinusitis, *S. pneumoniae* is the most common isolate or is second only to nontypable *Haemophilus influenzae*. Whether in adults or in children, pneumococci are identified in about 40 to 50 percent of cases of otitis in which an etiologic agent is isolated. Prior infection by a respiratory virus or allergy is thought to contribute significantly to these pneumococcal infections by causing congestion of the openings to the eustachian tubes or the paranasal sinuses. Prospective studies of young children have shown that colonization precedes infection in most cases. For reasons that are unclear, serotypes 6, 14, 19F, and 23F predominate both as colonizing and as infecting organisms of children; therefore, these serotypes are currently being studied most intensively for use in vaccines to be administered to young children.

Meningitis Except during outbreaks of meningococcal infection, *S. pneumoniae* is the most common etiologic agent of bacterial meningitis in adults. Because of the remarkable success of *H. influenzae* type b vaccine, *S. pneumoniae* now predominates among cases in infants and toddlers as well (but not among those in newborns). Meningitis develops either by the direct extension of infection from the sinuses or the middle ear or as a result of bacteremia with seeding of the choroid plexus. Favoring the former possibility are the association between acute otitis media and meningitis as well as the well-documented role of *S. pneumoniae* as the most common cause of recurrent bacterial meningitis associated with head trauma, cerebrospinal fluid (CSF) leak, and/or dural tear. Favoring the latter are the association between pneumococcal bacteremia from any source and meningitis as well as an autopsy study of temporal bone from children who died of bacterial meningitis, which yielded no evidence of extension from the middle ear. In the meninges and subarachnoid space, pneumococcal cell-wall antigens like peptidoglycan stimulate an intense inflammatory response mediated by the release of C5a, tumor necrosis factor, interleukins, and other proinflammatory cytokines. This inflammatory response and the local effect of pneumococci result in raised intracranial pressure, brain edema, and decreased blood flow leading to meningismus, drowsiness, or coma. Focal neurologic signs may result from suppurative vasculitis with venous or arterial thrombosis, from cranial neuropathy due to entrapment or infarction, from local cerebritis, from subdural effusion, or from brain herniation (see Chap. 377).

No distinctive clinical or laboratory feature differentiates meningitis due to *S. pneumoniae* from that due to other bacteria. Patients note the sudden onset of fever, headache, and stiffness or pain in the neck. Without treatment, there is a progression, over 24 to 48 h, to confusion and then obtundation. On physical examination, the patient looks acutely ill and has a rigid neck. In these cases lumbar puncture should not be delayed for computed tomography (CT) of the head unless papilledema or focal neurologic signs are evident. Typical CSF findings consist of pleocytosis (500 to 10,000 cells/μL) with a predominance of PMNs, an elevated protein level (100 to 500 mg/dL), and a decrease in glucose content. If antibiotics have not been given, large numbers of pneumococci can be seen in a Gram-stained specimen of CSF in nearly all cases. If an effective antibiotic has already been administered, the number of bacteria may be greatly decreased; in this situation, immunologic methods for the detection of pneumococcal capsule in the CSF may identify an etiologic agent in up to two-thirds of cases. However, these methods have fallen out of favor. Cultures will eventually turn positive in the great majority of cases, and most physicians prefer to continue empirical broad-spectrum antibiotic therapy until the etiologic agent has been definitively identified.

Pneumonia The distinctive symptoms and signs of pneumococcal pneumonia are (1) cough and sputum production, which reflect the proliferation of bacteria and the resulting inflammatory response in the alveoli; (2) fever; and (3) radiographic detection of an infiltrate.

Predisposing conditions Pneumococcal pneumonia is most common at the extremes of age. Despite the undisputed role of *S. pneumoniae* as a major pathogenic bacterium for humans, the great majority of adults with pneumococcal pneumonia have underlying diseases that predispose to infection. Otherwise healthy military recruits involved in outbreaks of infection may be an exception to this rule; however, many of those affected have an antecedent viral-type illness that may reduce normal host resistance. In addition to prior viral respiratory illness, the most common predisposing conditions are alcoholism, malnutrition, chronic pulmonary disease of any kind, infection with human immunodeficiency virus (HIV), diabetes mellitus, cirrhosis of the liver, renal insufficiency, and congestive heart failure. HIV infection is such an important predisposing factor that some authorities recommend that any young adult with pneumococcal pneumonia be tested for antibody to HIV.

Presenting symptoms Patients often present with a preexisting respiratory condition that has distinctly deteriorated. If a viral upper respiratory illness is the predisposing factor, the patient may have felt unwell for several days, with coryza or a nonproductive cough and low-grade fever; at the time of onset of pneumonia, the temperature rises to 38.9 to 39.4°C (102 to 103°F), and sputum production becomes prominent. In a patient who has chronic bronchitis, the sputum may increase in volume, become yellow or green and thicker than usual, and be associated with a fever that becomes progressively higher over 48 to 72 h. In a small proportion of cases, the onset of disease follows a hyperacute pattern in which the patient—often a healthy young individual—suddenly has a single episode of shaking chills followed by sustained fever and a cough productive of blood-tinged sputum. This clinical picture is unfortunately called "classic," a vague term that is best avoided because many physicians believe that it means "most common," which is clearly not the case. In elderly subjects, the onset of disease may be especially insidious and may not suggest pneumonia at all. Persons in their 80s may have minimal cough, no sputum production, and even no fever, instead appearing tired or confused or simply becoming hypothermic and going into shock. For the reasons noted above, the most abrupt progression of pneumococcal disease is that in patients who have previously undergone splenectomy; these individuals may go from apparent good health to death in as little as 24 h. In pneumonia, pleuritic chest pain may result from extension of the inflammatory process to the visceral pleura; persistence of this pain, especially after the first day or two of treatment, raises concern about empyema (see "Complications," below). Nausea and vomiting or diarrhea, sometimes quite prominent, occur in up to 20 percent of cases. Clearly, the range of symptoms is sufficiently broad that there is no characteristic presentation to distinguish pneumococcal from other types of bacterial pneumonia (and from some types of nonbacterial pneumonia).

Physical findings Patients with pneumococcal pneumonia usually appear ill and have a grayish, anxious appearance that differs from that of persons with viral or mycoplasmal pneumonia. Typically, the temperature is 38.9 to 39.4°C (102 to 103°F), the pulse 90 to 110 beats per minute, and the respiratory rate >20 breaths per minute. Elderly patients may have only a slight temperature elevation or be afebrile. A lack of fever in young or middle-aged adults is associated with increased morbidity and mortality, as is hypothermia. Herpes labialis appears in a small percentage of cases. Pain may cause diminished respiratory excursion (splinting) on the affected side. Dullness to percussion is noted in about half of cases, and vocal fremitus is increased. Breath sounds may be bronchial or tubular, and crackles are heard regularly on careful auscultation. Flatness to percussion at the lung base and inability to detect the expected degree of diaphragmatic motion suggest the presence of pleural fluid, which raises the possibility of empyema; the failure to assess fremitus, to distinguish dullness

from flatness by percussion, or to examine for diaphragmatic excursion may leave the physician at the mercy of often ambiguous radiologic interpretations. The finding of a heart murmur raises concern about endocarditis, a rare but serious complication. Confusion may result from hypoxia or the generalized response to pneumonia; obtundation or neck stiffness should lead to an immediate consideration of meningitis.

Radiographic findings In most cases of pneumococcal pneumonia, the chest x-ray reveals an area of infiltration involving less than a full segment. Whereas true consolidation with an air bronchogram is common among relatively healthy young adults, pneumonia superimposed on severe chronic lung disease causes a more moth-eaten, less homogeneous appearance. Segmental or lobar consolidation is apparent in fewer than half of cases, although most bacteremic patients exhibit such a radiologic pattern. Multilobar involvement is not uncommon. In rare instances, pneumococcal pneumonia leads to a lung abscess. Although some pleural fluid may actually be present in half of cases, no more than 20 percent of patients have a sufficient volume of fluid to allow aspiration, and in only a minority of these patients is empyema documented.

General laboratory findings The peripheral-blood white blood cell (WBC) count is >12,000/μL in the great majority of patients with pneumococcal pneumonia. However, the count is <6000/μL in 5 to 10 percent of persons hospitalized for pneumococcal pneumonia. Such a low count is often but not always associated with bone marrow suppression due to alcohol ingestion; this finding connotes a high risk of death. The serum bilirubin level may be increased to 4 mg/dL (68 μmol/L); hypoxia, inflammatory changes in the liver, and breakdown of red blood cells in the lung are all thought to contribute to this increase. Levels of lactate dehydrogenase may be elevated. A variety of other abnormalities may be present, reflecting the contributory role of underlying diseases. → *Abnormalities of pleural fluid in empyema are reviewed in Chap. 255.*

Diagnostic microbiology An etiologic role for the pneumococcus in pneumonia is strongly suggested by the demonstration of large numbers of PMNs and slightly elongated gram-positive cocci in pairs and chains in the sputum (Fig. 141-1). Examined areas of the slide must be free of epithelial cells, because organisms found in these locations may represent contamination by the oral bacterial flora. Capsules may be seen surrounding the bacterial forms. In this setting, the diagnosis can be confirmed by the identification of *S. pneumoniae* in sputum culture. However, culture is less sensitive than Gram's staining for identifying pneumococci. Since most pneumococci do not produce distinctively mucoid colonies, their identification in the laboratory depends on the ability to select putative pneumococcal colonies for further study from among alpha-hemolytic streptococci of the mouth. In short, laboratory diagnosis by sputum culture relies on the quality of the specimen provided, the care with which the relevant purulent component is separated for culture, and the assiduity with which alpha-hemolytic colonies are studied. These factors need

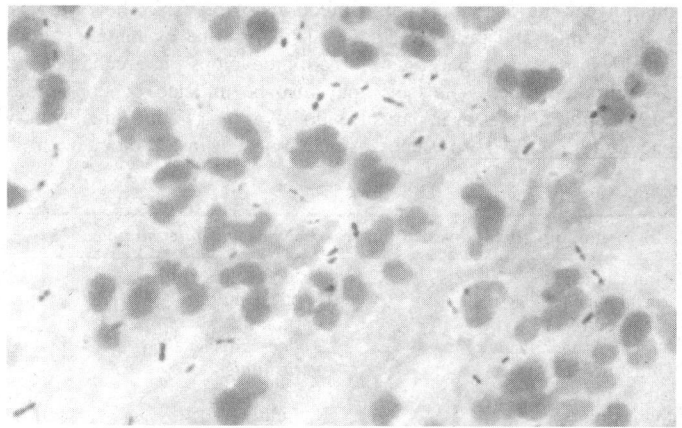

FIGURE 141-1 The microbiologist can easily identify *Streptococcus pneumoniae* as the etiologic agent of pneumonia when microscopic examination of a Gram-stained sputum specimen reveals this kind of picture.

to be considered when sputum cultures from patients who appear to have pneumococcal pneumonia are said to yield only "normal mouth flora" and when the medical literature describes what appear to be poor results of sputum culture. Because of the central role of Gram's stain in diagnosis, physicians should review the slides with the microbiologist. Blood cultures yield *S. pneumoniae* in about 20 percent of cases of pneumococcal pneumonia. Modern, automated systems often yield positive blood cultures within 12 h after the sample is obtained.

Complications Empyema is the most common complication of pneumococcal pneumonia, occurring in about 2 percent of cases. As noted above, some fluid appears in the pleural space in a substantial proportion of cases of pneumococcal pneumonia, but this parapneumonic effusion usually reflects an inflammatory response to infection that has been contained within the lung, and its presence is self-limited. When bacteria reach the pleural space—either hematogenously or as a result of contiguous spread, possibly across lymphatics of the visceral pleura—empyema results. The finding of frank pus, a positive result on Gram's staining, or the presence of fluid with a pH of ≤7.1 indicates the need for aggressive and complete drainage, preferably by prompt insertion of a chest tube, with verification by CT that fluid has been removed. If there is no response, thoracotomy is indicated. Persistence of fever (even if low-grade) and leukocytosis after 4 or 5 days of appropriate antibiotic treatment for pneumococcal pneumonia suggests empyema; in this setting, the diagnosis is exceedingly likely if the x-ray shows the persistence of pleural fluid; at this stage, thoracotomy is often needed for cure. Aggressive drainage is likely to reduce morbidity and mortality from empyema.

Other Syndromes The appearance of pneumococcal infection at other, usually sterile body sites indicates hematogenous spread, either during frank pneumonia or, in a smaller proportion of cases, from an inapparent focus of infection. A case of pneumococcal endocarditis is seen every few years at large tertiary-care hospitals. Purulent pericarditis due to this organism, occurring as a separate entity or together with endocarditis, is even rarer. Most cases of spontaneous bacterial peritonitis in children and some cases in adults are caused by *S. pneumoniae*. Peritonitis in women may be related to the use of an intrauterine contraceptive device, and pneumococcal infections of the female reproductive organs continue to be described. Septic arthritis can arise spontaneously in a natural or prosthetic joint or as a complication of rheumatoid arthritis. Osteomyelitis in adults tends to involve vertebral bones. Epidural and brain abscesses are rarely described. Cellulitis can develop and does so most often in persons who have connective tissue diseases or HIV infection. The appearance of any of these unusual pneumococcal infections in a young adult may suggest that tests for HIV infection should be undertaken.

R̽ TREATMENT

Antibiotic Susceptibility β-Lactam antibiotics, the cornerstone of therapy for serious pneumococcal infection, act by binding covalently to and thereby blocking the action of the cell-membrane enzymes (endo-, trans-, and carboxypeptidases) that are responsible for cell-wall synthesis. These enzymes were identified by their reaction with radiolabeled penicillin and thus are called penicillin-binding proteins. In the 1960s, virtually all clinical isolates of *S. pneumoniae* were susceptible to penicillin (i.e., were inhibited in vitro by concentrations of <0.06 μg/mL). During the past 15 years in Europe and the past 5 years or so in the United States, a steadily increasing number of pneumococcal isolates have shown some degree of resistance to penicillin, often together with resistance to other antibiotics (Table 141-3). Resistance results from spontaneous mutation or acquisition of new genetic material leading to the alteration of penicillin-binding proteins in a manner that necessitates a

higher concentration of penicillin for their saturation. The genetic information acquired also conveys resistance to other antibiotics. Mutation and selection of strains in communities in the United States—especially in areas of high antibiotic use, such as day-care centers—and spread of identifiable strains from other countries where antibiotics are available without prescription have both contributed to the prevalence of resistance.

For most of the antibiotic era, pneumococcal susceptibility was not studied in vitro because of the organism's high degree of susceptibility to virtually all antibiotics. Clearly, the situation has changed, and it seems reasonable to expect routine study of pneumococcal isolates, as of other organisms, for antibiotic susceptibility. In 1995, about 15 to 20 percent of strains isolated in the United States showed intermediate resistance to penicillin [minimum inhibitory concentration (MIC), 0.1 to 1.0 μg/mL], and 2 to 5 percent exhibited high-level resistance (MIC ≥2 μg/mL). A varying proportion of intermediately resistant isolates are also resistant to erythromycin and the newer macrolides, tetracyclines, trimethoprim-sulfamethoxazole, and clindamycin (Table 141-3), as are a greater proportion of highly resistant strains; certain of the latter isolates are also resistant to second-generation and some third-generation cephalosporins. So far, the majority of strains have retained susceptibility to cefotaxime, ceftriaxone, and imipenem. Given the relatively poor activity of ciprofloxacin against *S. pneumoniae*, most experts do not consider ciprofloxacin or ofloxacin reliable for the treatment of pneumococcal infection. Better alternative agents are almost always available, even for use against resistant strains. Some of the newer quinolones appear to be more effective in vitro against penicillin-resistant pneumococcal strains. Nearly all pneumococcal isolates remain susceptible to vancomycin, although the acquisition of resistance to this antibiotic is feared because of the increasing prevalence of vancomycin resistance among enterococci and among other gram-positive bacteria that may eventually transfer genetic material to pneumococci. The reader must be warned that this situation is fluid and that susceptibility patterns may vary greatly between and even within individual communities.

General Therapy Despite increased emphasis on outpatient therapy in the past decade, the author prefers to hospitalize all patients with pneumococcal pneumonia when it is feasible to do so. Patients who are elderly, have undergone splenectomy, appear sick, have oxygen desaturation, are confused, or have underlying lung disease, heart failure, cirrhosis, or renal insufficiency should certainly be hospitalized. Direct admission to an intensive care unit should be considered for all persons thought to have pneumococcal pneumonia who have hypotension, substantial oxygen desaturation or an increase in P_{CO_2} relative to their own baseline, radiographic involvement of more than one lobe, or a low peripheral WBC count (<6000/μL), even though it has been difficult to prove that such care enhances outcome.

Specific Antibiotic Therapy PNEUMONIA Pneumonia caused by penicillin-susceptible or intermediately penicillin-resistant pneu-

Table 141-3

Penicillin Susceptibility Status of Pneumococci Resistant to Other Antimicrobial Agents

Status of Strain	Percentage of Isolates Resistant to Indicated Agent											
	Amox	Amox/ Clav	Tet	Em	TMP-SMZ	Cfur	Ctax or Ctri	Cm	Newer Mac	Quin	Imi	Vm
Pen-S	0	0	20	2	10	0	0	0	0	?0	0	0
Pen-I	?	?	40	10	25	0	0	<10	10	?0	0	0
Pen-R	100	100	50	50	50	25	10	50	50	?0	10	0

Abbreviations: Pen-S, sensitivity to penicillin; Pen-I, intermediate resistance to penicillin; Pen-R, resistance to penicillin; Amox, amoxicillin; Clav, clavulanate; Tet, tetracycline; Em, erythromycin; TMP-SMZ, trimethoprim-sulfamethoxazole; Cfur, cefuroxime; Ctax, cefotaxime; Ctri, ceftriaxone; Cm, clindamycin; Mac, macrolides; Quin, quinolones; Imi, imipenem; Vm, vancomycin.

NOTE: These percentages reflect a composite of the data available in October 1995; actual results vary with the time and locale studied. A question mark indicates that the clinical significance of in vitro susceptibility results is uncertain, as discussed in the text.

mococcal isolates appears to be readily treatable with penicillin. The dosages that follow are acceptable for use against intermediately resistant strains and are somewhat excessive for susceptible isolates; it is a problem that pneumococcal susceptibility-test results do not become available until 24 to 72 h after treatment has begun (see below). Most patients hospitalized for pneumococcal pneumonia are treated with intravenous medications; 1 million units of penicillin every 4 h is excellent for this purpose. A first-generation cephalosporin given intravenously (for example, 1 g of cefazolin every 8 h) or procaine penicillin G given intramuscularly (2.4 million units to start, followed by 1.2 million units every 12 h) should be adequate. Amoxicillin has a substantially broader spectrum than is necessary for the treatment of pneumococcal infection. Nevertheless, its reliable and complete absorption after oral administration, substantially longer half-life, and antibacterial effect exceeding that of penicillin make this drug a good choice for the oral treatment of pneumococcal pneumonia in a dosage of 500 mg to start and then 250 mg every 8 h. Clindamycin is also highly effective against susceptible and intermediately resistant strains. Many isolates are resistant to tetracycline, and increasing numbers are resistant to erythromycin, newer macrolides, and trimethoprim-sulfamethoxazole; thus, the emphasis on "empirical" treatment of pneumonia is likely to become increasingly problematic. For highly penicillin-resistant isolates, intravenous treatment with cefotaxime (1 g every 6 h), ceftriaxone (1 g every 12 h), or imipenem (500 mg every 6 h) will be effective in about 90 percent of cases, and the course of therapy can be concluded with oral cefpodoxime. Vancomycin must be administered when the isolate is resistant to these drugs. Newer quinolones, streptogramins, oxazolidinones, and advanced tetracyclines are currently being studied in vivo, having shown in vitro activity against antibiotic-resistant *S. pneumoniae.*

Because the degree of susceptibility of a pneumococcal strain is not known when therapy is begun, it seems reasonable to treat a patient who has any of the markers that specifically suggest life-threatening pneumococcal pneumonia with cefotaxime or ceftriaxone. If resistance to ceftriaxone becomes prevalent, it may be necessary to administer vancomycin as well. Since bacteremic pneumococcal pneumonia is a life-threatening disease, this initial approach might be considered in all patients hospitalized for presumed pneumococcal pneumonia. Subsequent therapy should be based on the results of susceptibility testing. Patients with severe allergic reactions to β-lactam antibiotics should receive an advanced macrolide, clindamycin, or vancomycin until the results of susceptibility testing become available. The lack of a prompt response to therapy should raise the possibility of resistance, even if the laboratory has reported susceptibility, and treatment with vancomycin should be begun. In such instances, susceptibility testing should be repeated, and evidence of loculated infections (such as empyema) and/or other causes of fever should be sought.

The optimal duration of treatment for pneumococcal pneumonia is still uncertain. Pneumococci disappear from sputum within several hours of the first dose of penicillin, and a single dose of procaine penicillin, which produces an effective antimicrobial level persisting for 24 h, has been said to be curative in otherwise healthy young adults. Most older physicians treated pneumococcal pneumonia for 5 to 7 days. Although the failure of such therapy has not been reported, younger physicians seem to be treating this infection for 10 to 14 days. Prolongation of therapy is a two-edged sword, especially in debilitated patients, because the risk of complications increases with each day of antibiotic treatment, particularly in the hospital. Three to five days of close observation with parenteral therapy and a final few days of oral treatment—in all, not exceeding 5 days after the patient has become afebrile [temperature <37.2°C (<99°F)]—may be the best approach.

OTITIS MEDIA Treatment of acute otitis media may be more difficult than that of pneumonia. In the absence of diagnostic tympanocentesis, the etiologic diagnosis is nearly always presumptive

rather than proven. Many authorities continue to recommend amoxicillin. However, because penetration into a closed space is required for therapeutic efficacy, infection caused by intermediately resistant strains may not respond to penicillin or amoxicillin, and cefuroxime or cefpodoxime may be preferable. Once therapy has been initiated, patients must be monitored closely to be certain that they are responding. Although pneumococcal DNA has been detected by molecular analysis in middle-ear fluid, chronic serous otitis ("glue ear") is probably not due to active infection and does not require antibiotic therapy.

MENINGITIS Meningitis is the most life-threatening of pneumococcal infections. The author recommends that pneumococcal meningitis be treated initially with cefotaxime (2 g every 6 h) or ceftriaxone (1 g every 12 h) plus vancomycin (500 mg every 6 h or 1 g every 12 h) unless resistance to third-generation cephalosporins has not been reported in the community. Two drugs are given because the cephalosporin is likely to be effective against most isolates and readily penetrates the blood-brain barrier, whereas vancomycin is uniformly effective but has a somewhat unpredictable capacity to enter the CSF. Once an isolate is shown to be penicillin-susceptible, treatment can be continued with 24 million units of penicillin every 24 h, given every 4 h in divided doses or continuously. If the isolate exhibits intermediate resistance to penicillin but is susceptible to cefotaxime or ceftriaxone, the administration of vancomycin may be discontinued. Rifampin inhibits the bactericidal activity of β-lactam antibiotics and probably should not be added to the regimen. The total duration of therapy for pneumococcal meningitis is 10 to 14 days. Despite the central pathogenic role of inflammation in meningitis, the use of glucocorticoids or other anti-inflammatory agents is controversial, even in children, in whom most of the relevant studies have been done. Data simply do not exist on which to base an informed decision regarding the administration of glucocorticoids or cyclooxygenase inhibitors to adults with pneumococcal meningitis (see Chap. 377).

ENDOCARDITIS Pneumococcal endocarditis is associated with rapid destruction of heart valves. Vancomycin should be given pending assays for the minimal bactericidal concentrations of β-lactam antibiotics. There is no clear evidence that the addition of another antibiotic to the regimen is beneficial; aminoglycosides are somewhat synergistic and rifampin or quinolones are antagonistic with β-lactams. Endocarditis and meningitis should be treated initially in an intensive care unit, with the participation of appropriate consultants. Patients with meningitis should probably be seen by a neurologist as well as by a specialist in infectious diseases; those with endocarditis should be observed by an infectious disease consultant and a cardiologist, with a cardiovascular surgeon notified.

Other Therapeutic Modalities A variety of agents that block the action of tumor necrosis factor α, interleukin 1, or platelet-activating factor have conferred no benefit in and may have had a detrimental effect on pneumococcal sepsis. Similar results have been obtained with glucocorticoids.

PREVENTION Pneumococcal vaccine contains 25 μg of capsular polysaccharide from the 23 most prevalent serotypes; vaccination stimulates antibody to most serotypes in most recipients. In adults under 55 years old, protection rates are at least 85 percent, even 5 years or longer after vaccination. The level and duration of protection decrease with advancing age, such that persons in their eighties have 50 percent protection for 3 years and very little or no protection thereafter. In subgroups of the population who are most at risk (e.g., debilitated elderly persons and individuals with severe chronic lung disease), vaccine has not been shown conclusively to be effective. Persons who most need the vaccine because of compromised immunity are not likely to respond to immunization with significant increases in antibody level. Nevertheless, the poor average rate of response should not deter the physician from administering vaccine to a person at increased risk of pneumococcal infection. In light of the data demonstrating the safety, low cost, and efficacy of vaccine and the emergence of antibiotic-resistant strains, the failure to vaccinate elderly persons and individuals who have conditions predisposing to pneumococcal disease can be viewed as a missed opportunity in public health policy.

The Immunization Practices Advisory Committee of the Centers for Disease Control and Prevention recommends that pneumococcal vaccine be administered to adults who are generally regarded as immunocompetent but who are unusually likely to develop pneumococcal infection and/or a serious complication of such infection; this category includes (but is not limited to) persons with chronic pulmonary disease, advanced cardiovascular disease, diabetes mellitus, alcoholism, cirrhosis, chronic renal insufficiency, or CSF leak as well as all persons older than 65 years. A second category includes (but is not limited to) persons in whom immunosuppression is associated with an increased risk of pneumococcal disease or its complications, such as those with splenic dysfunction or asplenia, multiple myeloma, lymphoma, Hodgkin's disease, HIV infection, or organ transplantation.

There are, at the time of this writing, no official recommendations regarding revaccination. Nevertheless, in light of available data on the decline of antibody levels, the author believes that persons in these categories, especially those who have undergone splenectomy, should be revaccinated every 5 to 7 years.

With the increasing prevalence of penicillin-resistant pneumococci, the conditions under which the vaccine is administered may be liberalized. For example, pneumococcal vaccine could be given routinely to members of ethnic or racial groups that appear to have a particularly high incidence of pneumococcal infection (e.g., certain Native American populations) or to persons living in crowded settings, such as military camps or prisons. Adults over the age of 60 could be vaccinated and then revaccinated every 7 to 10 years or (after the age of 75) every 3 to 5 years. If penicillin-resistant pneumococci continue to increase in prevalence, routine immunization of children over the age of 2 should also be considered. Pneumococcal vaccine is not useful in children younger than 2 years because they do not respond well to polysaccharide antigens. Protein conjugate vaccines, currently under investigation, may eventually provide protection for infants and children.

BIBLIOGRAPHY

AFESSA B et al: Pneumococcal bacteremia in adults: A 14-year experience in an inner-city university hospital. Clin Infect Dis 21:345, 1995

AVERY OT et al: Studies on the chemical nature of the substance inducing transformation of pneumococcal types: Induction of transformation by a desoxyribonucleic acid fraction isolated from pneumococcus type III. J Exp Med 79:137, 1944

BOULNOIS GJ: Pneumococcal proteins and the pathogenesis of disease caused by Streptococcus pneumoniae. J Gen Microbiol 138:249, 1992

BREIMAN RF et al: Pneumococcal bacteremia in Charleston County, South Carolina: A decade later. Arch Intern Med 150:1401, 1990

———— et al: Emergence of drug-resistant pneumococcal infections in the United States. JAMA 271:1831, 1994

BURMAN LA et al: Invasive pneumococcal infections: Incidence, predisposing factors, and prognosis. Rev Infect Dis 7:133, 1985

DINUBILE MJ et al: Pneumococcal soft-tissue infections: Possible association with connective tissue diseases. J Infect Dis 63:897, 1991

FEDSON DS, MUSHER DM: Pneumococcal vaccine, in Vaccines, 2d ed, SA Plotkin, EA Mortimer Jr (eds). Philadelphia, Saunders, 1994, p 517

FRANKLIN C et al: Reduced mortality of pneumococcal bacteremia after early intensive care. J Intensive Care Med 6:302, 1991

FRIEDLAND IR, MCCRACKEN GH JR: Management of infections caused by antibiotic-resistant Streptococcus pneumoniae. N Engl J Med 331:377, 1994

GRAY BM, DILLON HC JR: Epidemiological studies of Streptococcus pneumoniae in infants: Antibody to types 3, 6, 14, and 23 in the first two years of life. J Infect Dis 158:948, 1988

HEFFRON R: Pneumonia: With special reference to pneumococcus lobar pneumonia. A Commonwealth Fund Book, © 1939. Reprinted by Harvard University Press, Cambridge, MA, 1979

JANOFF EN et al: Streptococcus pneumoniae colonization, bacteremia, and immune response among persons with human immunodeficiency virus infection. J Infect Dis 167:49, 1993

KIM PE et al: Invasive pneumococcal disease and the association with season, atmospheric temperature and isolation of respiratory viruses. Clin Infect Dis 20:100, 1996

MARKIEWICZ A, TOMASZ A: Variation in penicillin-binding protein patterns of penicillin-resistant clinical isolates of pneumococci. J Clin Microbiol 27:405, 1989

MURPHY TF, SETHI S: Bacterial infection in chronic obstructive pulmonary disease. Am Rev Respir Dis 146:1067, 1992

MUSHER DM: Streptococcus pneumoniae, in Mandell, Douglas and Bennett's Principles and Practice of Infectious Diseases, 4th ed, GL Mandell et al (eds). New York, Churchill Livingstone, 1994, p 1811

———— et al: Antibody to capsular polysaccharides of Streptococcus pneumoniae in adults: Prevalence, persistence, relation to carriage, and resistance to infection. Clin Infect Dis 17:66, 1993

ORT S et al: Pneumococcal pneumonia in hospitalized patients. JAMA 249:214, 1983

ORTQVIST A: Prognosis in community-acquired pneumonia requiring treatment in hospital. Importance of predisposing and complicating factors, and of diagnostic procedures. Scand J Infect Dis (Suppl) 65:1, 1990

POWDERLY WG et al: Pneumococcal endocarditis: Report of a series and review of the literature. Rev Infect Dis 8:786, 1986

RODRIGUEZ MC et al: Unusual manifestations of pneumococcal infection in HIV-infected individuals: The past revisited. Clin Infect Dis 14:192, 1992

SHAPIRO ED et al: The protective efficacy of polyvalent pneumococcal polysaccharide vaccine. N Engl J Med 325:1453, 1991

SIMBERKOFF MS et al: Efficacy of pneumococcal vaccine in high risk patients: Results of a Veterans Administration cooperative study. N Engl J Med 315:1318, 1986

SPANGLER SK et al: Activities of RPR 106972 (a new oral streptogramin), cefditoren (a new oral cephalosporin), two new oxazolidinones (U-100592 and U-100766), and other oral and parenteral agents against 203 penicillin-susceptible and -resistant pneumococci. Antimicrob Agents Chemother 40:481, 1996

TUOMANEN EI et al: Pathogenesis of pneumococcal infection. N Engl J Med 332:1280, 1995

VERSALOVIC J et al: Penicillin-resistant Streptococcus pneumoniae strains recovered in Houston: Identification and molecular characterization of multiple clones. J Infect Dis 167:850, 1993

VIÐARSSON G et al: Opsonization and antibodies to capsular and cell wall polysaccharides of Streptococcus pneumoniae. J Infect Dis 170:592, 1994

---

142 *Robert L. Deresiewicz, Jeffrey Parsonnet*

STAPHYLOCOCCAL INFECTIONS

The staphylococci are hardy and ubiquitous colonizers of human skin and mucous membranes and were among the first human pathogens identified. They cause a variety of syndromes, including superficial and deep pyogenic infections, systemic intoxications, and urinary tract infections. Staphylococci are the leading cause of bacteremia, surgical wound infections, and infections of bioprosthetic materials in the United States; in addition, they are the second leading cause of nosocomial infections overall. Organisms of this genus are also a significant cause of bacterial food poisoning.

Staphylococcus aureus is the most important human pathogen in the genus. It remains a major public health concern due to its tenacity, potential destructiveness, and increasing resistance to antimicrobial agents. Although less virulent, the coagulase-negative staphylococci (CNS), especially *Staphylococcus epidermidis*, adhere avidly to prosthetic materials and are increasingly important nosocomial pathogens, especially of compromised hosts. Another CNS species, *Staphylococcus saprophyticus*, is a common cause of urinary tract infections.

TAXONOMY AND MICROBIOLOGY Members of the genus *Staphylococcus* are nonmotile, nonsporulating gram-positive cocci, 0.5 to 1.5 μm in diameter, that occur singly and in pairs, short chains, and the irregular three-dimensional clusters from which their name is derived (Greek *staphulé*, "grape-like"). Staphylococci can grow over a wide range of environmental conditions, but they grow best at temperatures between 30°C and 37°C and at a pH around neutrality. They are resistant to desiccation and to chemical disinfectants, and they tolerate NaCl concentrations up to 12%. With rare exceptions, the staphylococci are facultatively anaerobic and catalase-positive. The more virulent staphylococci can clot plasma (coagulase-positive), while the less virulent cannot (coagulase-negative). Of the five recognized coagulase-positive staphylococcal species, the only important human pathogen is *S. aureus*, whose colonies are larger than those of *S. epidermidis*, are often pigmented (golden yellow), and are usually β-hemolytic on sheep blood agar. Twenty-seven species of CNS are recognized. Of these, *S. epidermidis* is by far the most common nonurinary human isolate. Strains of *S. epidermidis* are typically white and nonhemolytic and may be tenaciously adherent as a result of their production of polysaccharide adhesin. *S. epidermidis* is followed in frequency by *Staphylococcus haemolyticus* and *Staphylococcus warneri*. *S. saprophyticus* is the most common staphylococcal urinary isolate.

STAPHYLOCOCCUS AUREUS

EPIDEMIOLOGY Humans constitute the major reservoir of *S. aureus* in nature; the cross-sectional carriage rate in adults is 15 to 40 percent. The mucous membranes of the anterior nasopharynx are the principal site of carriage; other sites include the axillae, the vagina, and the perineum and occasionally the gastrointestinal tract. Among postmenarcheal U.S. women, the rate of vaginal colonization by *S. aureus* ranges from 5 to 15 percent but rises to 30 percent during menses—a change that is relevant to the pathogenesis of the toxic shock syndrome (TSS). Colonization by *S. aureus* may be intermittent or persistent and is probably influenced by both microbial and host factors as well as by the nature of the competing nonstaphylococcal flora. Carriage is more common among persons with frequent staphylococcal exposure and those with habitual or chronic disruption of cutaneous epithelial integrity. Thus, health care workers, dialysis patients, diabetic patients, injection drug users, and persons with chronic dermatologic conditions are often colonized. Colonization of mucocutaneous sites is an important risk factor for staphylococcal infection; for example, wound infection following cardiothoracic surgery is more frequent among patients who harbor *S. aureus* in the nares preoperatively than among those who do not.

In reference laboratories, a number of techniques are available to assess strain relatedness in potential epidemic situations. These include phage typing, determination of plasmid profile or antibiotic resistance pattern, DNA fingerprinting, ribotyping, and polymerase chain reaction–based genetic polymorphism analysis. At present, no one technique is clearly superior to the others.

PATHOGENESIS AND HOST DEFENSE *S. aureus* causes two types of syndrome: *intoxications* and *infections*. The clinical manifestations of intoxications are attributable solely to the action of one or a few secreted products of the microorganism (toxins), and these clinical features can be reproduced by administration of the toxin(s) in the absence of the microorganism. The toxin can be produced either in vivo (as in TSS or staphylococcal scalded skin syndrome) or in a suitable vector that subsequently delivers it to the host (as in staphylococcal food poisoning). Infections, on the other hand, involve bacterial proliferation, invasion or destruction of host tissues, and—in most cases—local and systemic responses by the host to these events. Although the ability of a microorganism to infect is predicated on its capacity to produce certain products that enable it to survive and prosper in the host (*virulence factors*), no single product is responsible for all manifestations of the infection. *S. aureus* is a particularly well-armed bacterium and produces an array of putative virulence factors.

Steps in Pathogenesis The pathogenesis of staphylococcal intoxications is straightforward and involves four steps: colonization by a toxigenic strain of the bacterium, toxin production, toxin absorption, and intoxication. The pathogenesis of staphylococcal infections is more complex and the steps less discrete. They include colonization, invasion of the bacterium across epithelial barriers, adherence to materials in the extracellular matrix, evasion or neutralization of host defenses, and destruction of host tissues. For both intoxications and infections, the entire process is carefully orchestrated by the bacterium in response to specific environmental conditions.

Physical preservation of cellular integrity Staphylococci are robust and adaptable organisms that can survive under relatively harsh environmental conditions. A rigid cell wall confers shape and strength to the organisms. The major component of the cell wall, *peptidoglycan*, is responsible for its physical properties. Disruption of peptidoglycan cross-linking by cell wall–active antibiotics (β-lactams or glycopeptides) renders the staphylococci susceptible to lysis mediated by endogenous peptidoglycan hydrolases (*autolysins*). Other important components of the staphylococcal cell wall include ribitol teichoic acid and protein A.

The osmotolerance exhibited by *S. aureus* enables the organism to grow without microbial competition in foods of low water activity and so sets the stage for contamination of food by staphylococcal enterotoxins. If ingested, these toxins can cause staphylococcal food poisoning.

Colonization Staphylococcal adherence to the nasal mucosa is mediated by cell wall and cell membrane teichoic acid. Whether teichoic acid also mediates adherence to other mucosal surfaces (e.g., the vaginal mucosa) is unknown. After colonization, the production of certain staphylococcal toxins [toxic shock syndrome toxin 1 (TSST-1), exfoliative toxins, or enterotoxins] can ensue if the appropriate environmental signals are present. Other circumstances (e.g., toxin absorption, a nonimmune host) can lead to systemic intoxication. Alternatively, colonization may persist for a while before the organism is cleared. If in the meantime the organism gains access to deeper tissues, the process of infection may begin.

Invasion and adherence to the extracellular matrix Staphylococci generally cannot invade through intact epithelial surfaces, which represent the primary line of antistaphylococcal defense. Invasion is facilitated by a mechanical break in the epithelium or by plugging of a gland or hair follicle. Once the epithelial barrier is breached, *S. aureus* can adhere to any of several molecules present either on cell surfaces or in the extracellular matrix. These molecules include fibrinogen, fibronectin, laminin, thrombospondin, collagen, elastin, vitronectin, and bone sialoprotein.

Destruction of host cells and alteration of the host microenvironment A number of products of *S. aureus* alter the host environment in a way that benefits the bacterium. *Coagulase* is a secreted enzyme that binds prothrombin and thereby causes the conversion of fibrinogen to fibrin; it may aid in the establishment of an environment within host tissues that is protected from cells of the immune system or from antibiotics. *S. aureus* also produces a number of *lipases*, which may enhance the organism's survival in sebaceous areas of the human body. *Hyaluronidase* hydrolyzes hyaluronic acid, a mucopolysaccharide present in extracellular ground substance; its action may ease the spread of the organism through the extracellular matrix. *Fatty acid-modifying enzyme* inactivates mammalian staphylocidal lipids, which accumulate during development of the staphylococcal abscess and which are thought to be a component of the body's nonspecific antistaphylococcal defense. *Staphylokinase, thermonuclease,* and *serine protease* are other extracellular enzymatic products that may play roles in pathogenesis.

S. aureus also produces a number of membrane-active toxins that probably contribute to pathogenesis by damaging host cells. These toxins include α-, β-, and δ-hemolysins and the synergohymenotropic toxins (γ-hemolysin and Panton-Valentine leukocidin). α-*Hemolysin* (α-toxin) is the prototypic pore-forming toxin; it inserts into the cell membrane, creating ion-conductive channels that destroy membrane integrity. The toxin is dermonecrotic on subcutaneous injection. It is responsible for the β-hemolytic phenotype exhibited by many *S. aureus* strains when they are grown on sheep erythrocytes. β-*Hemolysin* is a sphyngomyelinase that exhibits species-specific hemolytic activity dependent on the sphyngomyelin content of the target cell membrane. Little is known about δ-*hemolysin*, although it appears to exert a detergent-like effect on cell membranes. The *synergohymenotropic toxins* are a newly described family of bicomponent toxins. Their name derives from the fact that their two components, which are secreted separately, are tropic for cell membranes and are synergistically active against them. Like α-toxin, the synergohymenotropic toxins are pore-forming toxins. *Panton-Valentine leukocidin* is most active against polymorphonuclear cells, monocytes, and macrophages. It is dermonecrotic to rabbit skin, and strains producing it are strongly associated with human furunculosis. γ-*Hemolysin* is active against a wide range of mammalian erythrocytes.

Evasion of host defense   Once staphylococci have breached mucosal or epithelial barriers, the host's immune response is directed at containing and eliminating them, principally by polymorphonuclear recruitment and phagocytic killing. The bacteria fight back by cloaking antigenic determinants on their surface, by interfering with the function of opsonins, by directly killing the phagocytes, and by developing strategies to survive within them. The pyogenic abscess, the histologic hallmark of staphylococcal infection, represents the battlefield for this encounter and in some sense benefits both the microorganism and the host—the microorganism by providing an environment in which leukocyte function is impaired and into which antibiotics penetrate poorly, and the host by containing the spread of the bacteria.

Certain staphylococcal components and products are direct chemoattractants for polymorphonuclear leukocytes; others provoke the release of chemoattractant cytokines that recruit phagocytic cells to the infected area. Histologic sections of early lesions typically reveal a central focus of organisms surrounded by a zone of necrotic debris, which in turn is surrounded by a zone of viable inflammatory cells. The toxic action of staphylococcal leukocidin may in part explain the zone of necrosis. After several days, fibroblasts populate the margin of the abscess and there elaborate collagen, which creates a true capsule around the abscess.

Staphylococcal cell wall peptidoglycan activates complement, which is an important opsonin in persons lacking antibody to staphylococcal surface components. Peptidoglycan also acts as a general stimulator of inflammatory cytokine release but is much weaker in this regard than gram-negative lipopolysaccharide.

Opsonic antibodies specific for peptidoglycan or capsule also mediate phagocytosis. There is considerable interstrain variation in susceptibility to opsonization, and acquired protective immunity to staphylococcal infection is generally thought not to develop. At least two staphylococcal products mitigate against opsonization. *Polysaccharide capsule* is produced by about 80 percent of clinical isolates and lies external to the cell wall; it physically interferes with opsonization by complement. *Protein A*, an important cell surface component, binds the Fc portion of IgG subclasses 1, 2, and 4 and thereby interferes with antibody-mediated opsonization. Acquired antibody-mediated immunity to systemic staphylococcal intoxications (as opposed to infections) does occur.

Opsonized organisms are efficiently ingested by polymorphonuclear leukocytes and macrophages. Most are then killed rapidly by the oxidative burst within the phagosome. Staphylococcal catalase, which converts hydrogen peroxide to oxygen and water, detoxifies oxygen radicals and potentiates intracellular bacterial survival. Staphylococci are also taken up by nondedicated phagocytes, such as endothelial cells and osteoblasts, and may survive within them. Yet another staphylococcal strategy for intracellular survival is the genesis of so-called small-colony variants. These slow-growing cells exhibit alterations in electron transport and generally produce reduced amounts of virulence determinants such as α-toxin. They are relatively resistant to antibiotics and appear capable of persisting intracellularly for extended periods. Their existence may in part explain the startling capacity of certain *S. aureus* infections (e.g., chronic osteomyelitis) to recrudesce after years of dormancy.

Hosts at particular risk for staphylococcal infection include those with frequent or chronic disruptions in epithelial integrity, such as injection drug users or persons with chronic onychomycoses of the fingers or toes; those with disordered leukocyte chemotaxis, such as patients with the Chédiak-Higashi or Wiskott-Aldrich syndrome; those whose phagocytes are defective in oxidative killing, as in chronic granulomatous disease; and those with indwelling foreign bodies, which provide a matrix for staphylococcal adherence and biofilm formation. Patients with disorders of immunoglobulin or complement are also at increased risk for *S. aureus* infection, as are patients infected with human immunodeficiency virus.

Superantigens   The superantigens are V$_\beta$-restricted T cell mitogens: they bind directly and without prior processing to major histocompatibility class II molecules on the surface of antigen-presenting cells, thereby stimulating T cells on the basis of the sequence of the variable region of the β chain of the T cell receptor rather than on the basis of the epitope specified by this receptor. Accordingly, a superantigen may be able to stimulate up to about 10 percent of the T cells in a given individual—a percentage much higher than the approximately 1 in 10^6 cells stimulated by conventional antigens. This massive T cell stimulation provokes an exuberant and dysregulated immune response characterized by the release of the cytokines interleukins 1 and 2, tumor necrosis factor, and interferon γ. *S. aureus* produces a number of superantigens, including the staphylococcal enterotoxins (SEs), TSST-1, and possibly the exfoliative toxins (ETs). Eight SEs are currently known (enterotoxins A, B, C$_{1-3}$, D, E, and H) and are the causative agents of staphylococcal food poisoning. The mechanism by which the SEs cause vomiting is uncertain but may involve direct neural stimulation of the autonomic nervous system rather than a local effect on the gastrointestinal mucosa. The superantigenic properties of TSST-1 are thought to explain its ability to cause TSS, although the exact mechanism by which it crafts the various clinical manifestations of TSS is uncertain. There is conflicting evidence as to whether the ETs, which cause scalded skin syndrome, are superantigens; structural data suggest that they may instead be related to the serine proteases.

Genetic Regulation of Virulence Genes   The production of virulence factors by bacteria is typically tightly and coordinately regulated by genetic apparatuses that sense and respond to environmental cues. Such coordinate regulation enables an organism to rapidly tailor its repertoire of proteins to suit its changing needs, either as it passes between microenvironments or as the environment evolves around it. Many of the staphylococcal exoproteins are typical virulence factors in this regard. For example, α-, β-, and δ-hemolysins, TSST-1, staphylococcal enterotoxin B, serine protease, and thermonuclease are all produced during the late logarithmic phase of growth in batch culture, at a time when nutrients become scarce and cell density reaches saturation. Their production is coordinately regulated and occurs reciprocally to that of the cell wall–associated staphylococcal proteins protein A and coagulase. Several genetic regulatory loci modulate these events, as do specific environmental conditions that presumably operate through those genetic loci. Foreign materials that increase the risk of TSS and conditions in food that predispose to staphylococcal food poisoning probably do so by presenting microenvironments that stimulate production of the relevant toxins. Similar events are undoubtedly operative within the environment of host tissues during infection, even in the absence of a foreign body.

At least three separate genetic loci regulate exoprotein production in *S. aureus*: *agr* (accessory gene regulator), *xpr* (extracellular protein regulator), and *sar* (staphylococcal accessory regulator). All three loci affect gene expression primarily at the level of transcription, and all three activate the expression of secreted proteins and diminish the expression of cell wall–associated proteins during the late logarithmic phase of bacterial growth. Recent data suggest that *agr* may function primarily as a "quorum sensor," an apparatus that informs the bacterium of the density of staphylococci in its environment. Exoprotein regulation in *S. aureus* apparently results from a complex interplay of environmental factors and gene products.

STAPHYLOCOCCAL   INTOXICATIONS   Toxic   Shock Syndrome   TSS is an acute, life-threatening intoxication characterized by fever, hypotension, rash, multiorgan dysfunction, and desquamation during the early convalescent period (Fig. 142-1). The disease was first characterized in 1978 but gained notoriety in 1980 upon the recognition of a large outbreak in menstruating women. It is a relatively uncommon illness, with a reported incidence (among menstruating

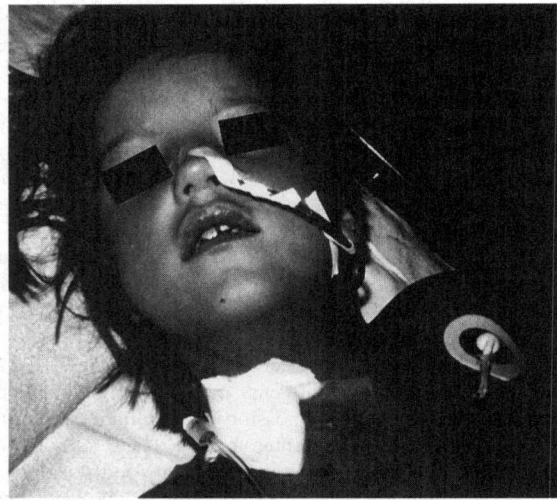

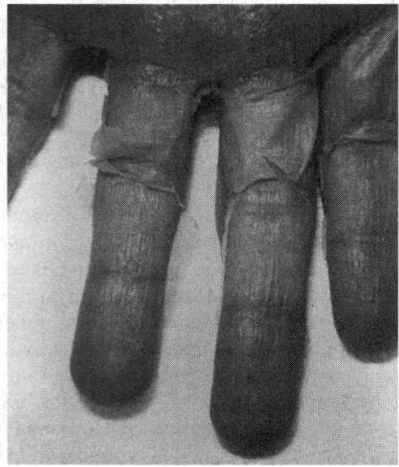

FIGURE 142-1 Cutaneous manifestations of toxic shock syndrome. The patient was a 7-year-old child with osteomyelitis and nonmenstrual TSS. *Top:* Diffuse erythroderma. The rubor was intense on the chest wall of this patient and is accurately represented in this black-and-white photograph. Circumoral pallor is evident. *Bottom:* Desquamation of the fingers during convalescence. *(From Deresiewicz, with permission.)*

women) of 1 case per 100,000; it is likely, however, that the disease is substantially underreported. About half of all cases occur in settings other than menstruation and are distributed among individuals of both sexes and all ages. Menstrual and nonmenstrual cases are clinically indistinguishable. Among cases reported to the Centers for Disease Control and Prevention between 1985 and 1994, the minimum case-fatality rate was 2.5 percent for menstrual cases and 6.4 percent for nonmenstrual cases.

TSS is caused by any of several related toxic exoproteins produced by *S. aureus.* TSST-1 is the toxin most frequently implicated and staphylococcal enterotoxin B the second most frequent. For illness to develop, an individual must be colonized or infected with a toxigenic strain of *S. aureus* and must lack a protective level of antibody to the toxin made by that strain. That TSS is primarily a disease of the young reflects the fact that more than 90 percent of individuals have antibodies to TSS toxins by adulthood.

Menstruation remains the most common setting for TSS, but the disease can also complicate the use of barrier contraceptives, the puerperium, septic abortion, and nonobstetric gynecologic surgery. Moreover, nonmenstrual TSS can complicate skin lesions of many types, including chemical or thermal burns, insect bites, varicella lesions, and surgical wounds. Postoperative disease can develop from

hours to weeks after a surgical procedure. Overt infection with *S. aureus* is not required for the development of TSS; mere colonization with a toxigenic strain may suffice. Accordingly, the primary site of toxin production in TSS may appear entirely benign. TSS has also been associated with musculoskeletal infections and respiratory infections caused by *S. aureus* and occasionally with staphylococcal bacteremia.

TSS remains a clinically defined syndrome (Table 142-1); patients meeting the case definition are severely ill. The illness begins precipitously, with high fever and a complex of symptoms that may include nausea, vomiting, abdominal pain, diarrhea, muscular pain, sore throat, and headache. Dizziness is a common manifestation of orthostatic or frank hypotension. The characteristic macular erythroderma develops over the first 2 days of illness. It is usually generalized but is sometimes locally confined; it can be evanescent or persistent. The patient's mental status is often abnormal to a degree that is out of proportion to the degree of hypotension. Conjunctival suffusion, pharyngeal injection, and peripheral edema are evident in many cases; a so-called strawberry tongue develops in up to half of patients. In menstrual disease, the vaginal mucosa may be erythematous and a purulent vaginal discharge may be present, but these findings are not universal. Common laboratory abnormalities include azotemia, hypoalbuminemia, hypocalcemia, hypophosphatemia, creatine phosphokinase elevation, leukocytosis or leukopenia with a left shift, thrombocytopenia, and pyuria.

The early signs and symptoms of TSS resolve within the first few days of illness, after which complications of organ hypoperfusion, such as renal and myocardial dysfunction, massive edema, and adult respiratory distress syndrome, dominate the picture. After about a week of illness, desquamation begins with superficial flaking of the skin of the torso, face, and extremities, which is followed by full-thickness desquamation of the palms, soles, and digits. Common late sequelae include peripheral gangrene, reversible nail and hair loss, muscle weakness, and neuropsychiatric dysfunction.

The differential diagnosis of TSS is that of a severe febrile exanthem with hypotension. In the setting of menstruation accompanied by purulent vaginal discharge, the diagnosis may be obvious. The challenge is to recognize the less obvious cases, in which the exanthem may be fleeting, multiorgan dysfunction may be subtle, or (in nonmenstrual cases) a primary site of infection may be inapparent. Other

Table 142-1

Staphylococcal Toxic Shock Syndrome: Case Definition

1. Fever: temperature of ≥38.9°C (102°F)
2. Rash: diffuse macular erythroderma ("sunburn" rash)
3. Hypotension: systolic blood pressure of ≤90 mmHg (adults) or <5th percentile for age (children under 16 years of age); or orthostatic hypotension (orthostatic drop in diastolic blood pressure by ≥15 mmHg, orthostatic dizziness, or orthostatic syncope)
4. Involvement of at least three of the following organ systems
   a. Gastrointestinal: vomiting or diarrhea at onset of illness
   b. Muscular: severe myalgias or serum creatine phosphokinase level at least twice the upper limit of normal
   c. Mucous membranes: vaginal, oropharyngeal, or conjunctival hyperemia
   d. Renal: blood urea nitrogen or creatinine level at least twice the upper limit of normal; or pyuria (≥5 leukocytes per high-power field) in the absence of urinary tract infection
   e. Hepatic: total serum bilirubin or aminotransferase (alanine or aspartate) level at least twice the upper limit of normal
   f. Hematologic: thrombocytopenia (platelet count, ≤100,000/μL)
   g. Central nervous: disorientation or alteration in consciousness but no focal neurologic signs at a time when fever and hypotension are absent
5. Desquamation: 1 to 2 weeks after the onset of illness (typically palms and soles)
6. Evidence against an alternative diagnosis: negative results of cultures of blood, throat, or CSF (if performed);* no rise in titers of antibody to the agents of Rocky Mountain spotted fever, leptospirosis, and rubeola (if obtained)

---

* Blood culture may be positive for *S. aureus.*

SOURCE: AL Reingold et al, Ann Intern Med 96(part 2):875, 1982.

diagnoses to consider include streptococcal TSS (toxic shock-like syndrome), staphylococcal scalded skin syndrome, Kawasaki syndrome, Rocky Mountain spotted fever, leptospirosis, meningococcemia, gram-negative sepsis, exanthematous viral syndromes, and severe drug reactions. Staphylococcal TSS and streptococcal TSS (see Chap. 143) can be clinically indistinguishable.

Treatment of TSS involves decontamination of the site of toxin production, aggressive fluid resuscitation, and administration of antistaphylococcal drugs. Recent surgical wounds should be explored and irrigated, even when signs of inflammation are lacking. Pressors should be used for sustained hypotension that is unresponsive to fluids. Electrolyte abnormalities, particularly hypocalcemia and hypomagnesemia, must be corrected. Semisynthetic penicillins (nafcillin, oxacillin) have been widely used in TSS; however, a growing body of clinical and laboratory evidence indicates that a protein synthesis inhibitor, such as clindamycin, might be superior. The authors recommend therapy with clindamycin (900 mg intravenously every 8 h), either alone or in combination with a β-lactam antibiotic or vancomycin. For a seriously ill patient in whom the diagnosis is uncertain, broad-spectrum antibiotics are appropriate until the diagnosis is confirmed. A 14-day course of therapy—some of which may be administered perorally—is reasonable. Patients whose illness is severe enough to warrant vasopressors, who require mechanical ventilation, who have worsening renal function, or who have an undrainable focus of infection should be treated with intravenous immunoglobulin, which contains high levels of neutralizing antibody to TSS toxins. A single infusion of 400 mg/kg generates a protective level of antibody to TSST-1 that persists for weeks. Steroids should not be administered routinely.

Because vaginal staphylococcal carriage can be sustained or recurrent and because in more than half of all cases TSS does not elicit immunity, recurrent menstrual TSS is a concern; recurrent nonmenstrual TSS has also been reported. The risk of recurrent illness can be assessed by tests for seroconversion to TSST-1. Women who do not seroconvert after acute illness (or who are not tested for antibody) should refrain indefinitely from using tampons or barrier contraceptives.

Staphylococcal Scalded Skin Syndrome This syndrome encompasses a range of cutaneous diseases of varying severity caused by ET-producing strains of *S. aureus*. The most severe form of staphylococcal scalded skin syndrome is termed *Ritter's disease* in newborns and *toxic epidermal necrolysis* (TEN) in older individuals. Milder and more common forms include *pemphigus neonatorum* and (in children and adults) *bullous impetigo* (see "Skin and Soft Tissue Infections" below). A portion of cases of so-called *staphylococcal scarlet fever* are also due to intoxication with ETs, although others are probably mild cases of TSS.

Persons over the age of 5 years rarely develop staphylococcal TEN; those who do almost invariably have underlying disease (renal insufficiency, systemic immunosuppression). The rarity of the syndrome in adults has been ascribed to acquired immunity to the inciting toxins, to enhanced renal clearance of the toxins, and perhaps to diminished sensitivity to the action of the toxins. Most adults have antibodies to the ETs as they do to other staphylococcal exotoxins. The syndrome has followed infections in a variety of sites, the most common being purulent rhinitis. Staphylococcal bacteremia is detected in only about 3 percent of children with this syndrome but in up to half of adults.

Staphylococcal TEN or Ritter's disease often begins with a nonspecific prodrome. The acute phase starts with the onset of an erythematous rash. The erythema begins in the periorbital and perioral areas and spreads to the trunk and centrifugally to the limbs. Pastia's lines may be apparent. The skin has a sandpaper texture and is often tender to the touch. Periorbital edema is common. In infants and children, fever and irritability or lethargy are common, but systemic toxicity is not. Within hours or days, wrinkling and sloughing of the epidermis begins; sloughing can be provoked by gentle stroking of the skin (Nikolsky's sign), even in areas that appear uninvolved. The denuded areas are red and glistening but not purulent, and staphylococci are not present. Exfoliation may continue in large sheets or in ragged snippets of tissue. Large, flaccid bullae may develop. As in thermal

burns, significant fluid and electrolyte loss can occur at this stage, as can secondary infection. Within about 48 h, the exfoliated areas dry and secondary desquamation begins. The entire illness resolves within about 10 days. Mortality (from hypovolemia or sepsis) is about 3 percent among children but approaches 50 percent among adults. Treatment includes the administration of antistaphylococcal agents, fluid and electrolyte management, and local care to the denuded skin.

Staphylococcal Food Poisoning Between 2 and 6 h after ingestion of contaminated food, staphylococcal food poisoning begins abruptly with nausea, vomiting, crampy abdominal pain, and diarrhea. The diarrhea is usually noninflammatory and is of lower volume than that in cholera or toxigenic *Escherichia coli* infection. Fever and rash are absent, and the patient is neurologically normal. The majority of cases are self-limited and resolve between 8 and 24 h after onset. In severe cases, hypovolemia and hypotension can develop. Although most cases probably do not come to medical attention or are not diagnosed, staphylococcal intoxication is the second or third leading cause of diagnosed food poisoning in the United States.

Food poisoning is caused by the ingestion of any of the SEs, which are produced by *S. aureus* in contaminated food before it is eaten. The presence of SEs in the food vector before its consumption accounts for the short incubation period of this illness. The SEs are heat stable, thus tolerating cooking conditions that kill the organisms that produced them. The disease has a high attack rate and is somewhat more common during the summer than at other times of the year. Processed meats and custard-filled baked goods are common food vectors, perhaps because staphylococci can tolerate conditions of high protein, salt, or sugar and so grow without competition in these environments. The most important epidemiologic risk factor in outbreaks of this disease is the ingestion of food that has been left at room temperature for prolonged periods, thereby allowing toxin production to occur before consumption. Contaminated preparation equipment and poor personal hygiene of food handlers are frequently implicated as well.

When a common-source food-borne outbreak of staphylococcal food poisoning is suspected, health authorities should be promptly consulted so that they can determine the etiology, isolate the source, and correct the conditions that led to the outbreak. A variety of immunologic techniques are available for the detection of SEs in foodstuffs.

STAPHYLOCOCCAL INFECTIONS *S. aureus* causes invasive disease by breaching host defense barriers, often after disruption or dysfunction of such barriers. The most common portals of entry leading to staphylococcal invasion are the skin and associated structures. A nidus for staphylococcal colonization and subsequent invasion is provided by chronic skin conditions, such as eczema and psoriasis; acute breaks in the skin, such as puncture wounds, abrasions, and lacerations; and abnormalities of skin appendages, such as hair follicles and nails. Colonization of the nasopharynx predisposes to respiratory tract infection after aspiration, obstruction (e.g., of a bronchus by carcinoma or of sinus ostia by trauma, edema, or polyps), or impaired ciliary function (e.g., in chronic bronchitis or acute viral infection). Intubation of the trachea provides a conduit by which upper respiratory flora, including pathogens such as *S. aureus*, can reach the lower respiratory tract. Less common portals of entry for *S. aureus* are the urinary and gastrointestinal tracts.

Skin and Soft Tissue Infections *S. aureus* is the most common etiologic agent of skin and soft tissue infections. Such infections are usually caused by endogenous flora—i.e., strains of *S. aureus* that are harbored in the nares or other sites of colonization. Infection may represent a primary pathologic process, with direct invasion of skin and adjacent tissues, or a secondary process complicating preexisting lesions.

Staphylococcal infections originating in hair follicles range in severity from trivial to life-threatening. *Folliculitis* is an infection of follicular ostia; the appearance is that of domed, yellow pustules with a narrow red margin. Infection is often self-limited, although healing may be hastened by topical antiseptics and more severe cases may benefit from topical or systemic antibiotics. A *furuncle* (often called a *boil*) is a deep-seated necrotic infection of a hair follicle, most often located on the buttocks, face, or neck. Furuncles are painful and tender, and their appearance is often accompanied by fever and constitutional symptoms. Surgical drainage and systemic antibiotic treatment are often required to hasten recovery and limit scar formation. Furunculosis may recur if there is continued colonization with a pathogenic strain of *S. aureus*. Deep infection of a group of contiguous follicles is called a *carbuncle*. This type of painful necrotic lesion, which is often accompanied by high fever and malaise, occurs most commonly on the back of the neck, shoulders, hips, and thighs, typically in middle-aged or elderly men. There is intense inflammation of surrounding and underlying connective tissue, and illness may be complicated by bacteremia. Surgical drainage and systemic antibiotic administration are indicated. *S. aureus* is also the most common cause of acute *paronychia*, infection of the lateral nail folds.

S. aureus causes *bullous impetigo*, a superficial cutaneous disorder occurring predominantly in children. An epidermal split caused by ET results in the formation of 1- to 2-cm bullae containing neutrophils and organisms. *Nonbullous impetigo* is most frequently caused by β-hemolytic streptococci, but *S. aureus* can secondarily infect impetiginous lesions. Treatment of impetigo with a topical antibiotic, such as mupirocin, may suffice for mild and localized infection, whereas systemic therapy is indicated for widespread or severe disease or for infection accompanied by lymphadenopathy.

Cellulitis, a spreading infection of subcutaneous tissue, is occasionally caused by *S. aureus*, but β-hemolytic streptococci are much more common agents of this disease (see Chap. 143). Secondary infection of surgical and traumatic wounds is more likely to be staphylococcal in etiology than is cellulitis arising from minor or inapparent breaks in the skin, and empiric treatment directed against both *S. aureus* and streptococci is reasonable in these settings. *Erysipelas*, the hallmark of which is a well-demarcated raised border, is a more superficial infection of the dermis and subcutaneous tissue; it is usually caused by group A streptococci and only rarely, if ever, by *S. aureus*.

Respiratory Tract Infections   *S. aureus* can gain access to the lung parenchyma by two routes: aspiration of upper respiratory flora and hematogenous spread. Staphylococcal pneumonia is a relatively uncommon but severe infection, characterized clinically by chest pain, systemic toxicity, and dyspnea and pathologically by intense neutrophilic infiltration, necrosis, and abscess formation. Only rarely does *S. aureus* cause pneumonia without predisposing epidemiologic or host factors that favor colonization of the respiratory tract and/or that impair defense mechanisms. Residence in a chronic care facility, recent use of antibiotics, and hospitalization favor colonization—and hence respiratory tract infection—with *S. aureus*. Staphylococcal pneumonia most commonly follows tracheal intubation of a hospitalized patient or viral infection of the respiratory tract. Influenza virus is known both to increase respiratory colonization by *S. aureus* and to impair ciliary function (and therefore clearance of staphylococci). In a classic scenario, a patient (often elderly and/or institutionalized) develops a flulike respiratory illness and then, after several days, deteriorates rapidly, with high fever, dyspnea, productive cough, and obtundation. The diagnosis is readily established by Gram's staining of expectorated sputum, which reveals abundant clusters of gram-positive cocci.

Hematogenous seeding of the lungs with *S. aureus* follows embolization from an intravascular nidus of infection. Common settings for septic pulmonary embolization are right-sided endocarditis (especially common among injection drug users) and septic thrombophlebitis, which is most often a complication of an indwelling venous catheter. Pneumonia is heralded by the acute onset of pleuritic chest pain and dyspnea; although diagnostic sputum may be lacking, a chest radiograph typically shows multiple nodular infiltrates and thus provides an important clue to both the diagnosis and the pathogenesis of disease. *Empyema* is a common sequela of staphylococcal pneumonia and increases the already-considerable morbidity associated with this infection.

Although not typically considered in the differential diagnosis of sore throat, *S. aureus* is occasionally isolated as the dominant organism from patients (especially children) with exudative *pharyngitis*. The illness may be accompanied by a scarlatiniform rash and may result in severe toxicity (like that seen in TSS). Staphylococcal *tracheitis* may be diagnosed in patients who have systemic toxicity and positive respiratory cultures but who lack pulmonary infiltrates. *S. aureus* is a prominent cause of *chronic sinusitis*, typically following the selection pressure of antimicrobial regimens that lack activity against this organism. Finally, *S. aureus* is a major etiologic agent of *sphenoid sinusitis*.

Infections of the Central Nervous System   *S. aureus* gains access to structures of the central nervous system by hematogenous spread or by direct extension from contiguous structures. This organism is a prominent cause of *brain abscess*, especially as a result of embolization during mitral or aortic valve endocarditis. Such abscesses are often multiple, small, and scattered diffusely throughout the brain. Brain abscess can also develop by direct extension from frontoethmoid or sphenoid sinuses or from infected soft tissue after surgery or penetrating trauma. Patients with staphylococcal brain abscesses are more likely to have fever, meningismus, and other signs of infection than are patients with anaerobic bacterial or mixed-etiology brain abscesses. Purulent *meningitis* may accompany staphylococcal brain abscess or may develop during bacteremia in the absence of demonstrable abscesses.

S. aureus is the organism most likely to cause a variety of other space-occupying, suppurative intracranial infections. *Subdural empyema* usually develops by direct extension of osteomyelitis of the skull, after surgery or trauma, or in the setting of sinusitis. This condition may be accompanied by meningitis, epidural abscess, or intracranial phlebitis. The cardinal features of subdural empyema are fever, headache, vomiting, and signs of meningeal irritation. As the infection progresses, cerebral edema, often with infarction, may ensue and may be accompanied by alteration in mental status, seizures, and focal neurologic signs, which sometimes progress rapidly. The diagnosis should be suspected in any patient with meningeal signs and focal neurologic findings. Magnetic resonance imaging (MRI) is the diagnostic procedure of choice; lumbar puncture is contraindicated because of the danger of brainstem herniation. Early surgical drainage and treatment with an antibiotic that penetrates well into the central nervous system may be curative, although neurologic sequelae are not uncommon.

S. aureus is the most common cause of *spinal epidural abscess*, which develops most often in association with vertebral osteomyelitis or diskitis. The diagnosis is suggested by fever, back pain, radicular pain, lower-extremity weakness, bowel or bladder dysfunction, and leukocytosis, but the presentation is often subtle. Patients may report only difficulty in walking or weakness, and objective findings may initially be lacking. The principal danger is the potential for necrosis of the spinal cord by compression and/or venous involvement. Early recognition of this condition is critical if long-term sequelae, such as paraplegia, are to be averted. An MR scan of the spine establishes whether or not an epidural collection is present; if it is, needle aspiration or open drainage confirms the infectious etiology. Prompt surgical decompression by laminectomy is often required for preservation of neurologic function, although a trial of antibiotic therapy alone may be considered if no focal neurologic deficits are detected. The pathogenesis of *intracerebral epidural abscess* is similar to that of subdural empyema, with staphylococcal infection usually following sinusitis, craniotomy, or trauma. Clinical manifestations reflect the anatomy of the underlying osteomyelitis plus the mass effect of the abscess, cerebral edema, and (often) secondary involvement of the subdural space. Emergent surgical drainage is usually required for cure.

Finally, *S. aureus* is the most common cause of *septic intracranial thrombophlebitis*, typically following sinusitis, mastoiditis, or soft tissue infection of the face. Clinical manifestations reflect the underlying condition and the anatomic structures in contiguity with the infected vein or sinus. Focal neurologic deficits, particularly of cranial nerve function, are characteristic of cavernous sinus thrombosis. Sagittal sinus thrombosis may be manifested by leg and arm weakness and by altered mental status; infections of the lateral and petrosal sinuses also produce characteristic clinical syndromes. Intracranial phlebitis may accompany epidural abscess, subdural empyema, and meningitis and is sometimes clinically indistinguishable from other types of intracranial infection. MRI is the diagnostic procedure of choice.

Urinary Tract Infections S. aureus is an uncommon cause of urinary tract infection. Ascending infection almost exclusively follows instrumentation of the bladder (e.g., cystoscopy or placement of an indwelling catheter). Under other circumstances, the presence of S. aureus in the urine, even in low numbers, suggests staphylococcal bacteremia and hematogenous seeding of the kidneys, with or without abscess formation; staphylococcal endocarditis should be considered in this setting.

Endovascular Infections S. aureus is the most common cause of acute bacterial *endocarditis* of both native and prosthetic valves. Staphylococcal endocarditis presents as an acute febrile illness, rarely of more than a few weeks' duration; complications such as meningitis, brain or visceral abscess, peripheral vascular embolization, valvular incompetence with heart failure, myocardial abscess, and purulent pericarditis have often developed by the time a patient seeks medical attention. The valves most commonly involved are the mitral and/or the aortic except among injection-drug users, in whom infection of the tricuspid valve is most common. The diagnosis is suggested by a heart murmur and the presence of conjunctival hemorrhages, subungual petechiae, or purpuric lesions on the distal extremities; it is readily confirmed by multiple positive blood cultures and echocardiography showing valvular vegetations. Echocardiography also helps establish which valve(s) are infected, the degree of valvular dysfunction or destruction, the quality of left ventricular function, and the presence or absence of annular or myocardial abscess.

Staphylococcal endocarditis carries a high mortality rate (on the order of 40 to 60 percent) and mandates prompt initiation of antimicrobial therapy. In addition to blood cultures and echocardiography, evaluation may include computed tomography (CT) of the head and lumbar puncture if brain abscess or meningitis is suspected; a radionucleotide study if osteomyelitis is suspected; and abdominal CT if visceral abscesses are suggested by abdominal pain or persistent fever or bacteremia. Indications for valve replacement are the same as those in endocarditis caused by other organisms: persistent bacteremia (beyond 5 to 7 days of therapy), valvular dysfunction resulting in heart failure, perivalvular or myocardial abscess, or recurrent embolization. Early consultation with a cardiothoracic surgeon is advisable because of the high percentage of patients with S. aureus endocarditis (around half) who develop one of these complications and therefore require valve replacement, often urgently. Once there is an indication for removal of an infected valve, nothing is gained and much can be lost by delaying surgery.

Right-sided endocarditis, which most often develops in association with injection drug use or venous catheterization, is frequently complicated by septic pulmonary emboli but otherwise carries a lower rate of serious complications than left-sided disease. Surgery is rarely required for right-sided disease. A relatively short course of parenteral therapy (2 weeks) may be curative, and the prognosis is relatively good. In contrast, S. aureus infection of a prosthetic valve (as an early or a late complication of valve replacement) almost always requires surgery for one of the above indications.

The propensity of S. aureus to adhere to and infect damaged tissues makes it the foremost cause of endovascular infections other than endocarditis. Vascular infection may be a consequence of hematogenous seeding of damaged vessels, especially large arteries with atheromatous plaques, resulting in the development of a mycotic aneurysm. It may also develop by spread from a contiguous focus of infection (e.g., after vascular surgery), often resulting in an infected pseudoaneurism, or by contamination of an intravascular device, resulting in septic phlebitis. Staphylococcal infection of an atherosclerotic artery (most commonly the abdominal aorta or iliac arteries), which may be aneurysmal to begin with, is a potentially catastrophic event. Such infections are associated with high-grade bacteremia, may result in rupture and massive hemorrhage, and are almost never curable without surgical

resection and bypass of the infected vessel. Septic phlebitis is also associated with high-grade bacteremia and systemic toxicity but is less likely than arteritis to result in rupture. Persistent bacteremia suggests the need for surgical removal of infected thrombus or vein, but the technical difficulty of such surgery may warrant an attempt at cure with antibiotics and anticoagulants alone.

A classic clinical scenario is that of a patient presenting with S. aureus bacteremia but without a demonstrable primary site of infection. Even in the absence of a changing murmur, peripheral embolic lesions, or a diagnostic echocardiogram, the possibility of endocarditis must be considered carefully in this situation. It is often hard to differentiate between endocarditis and bacteremia arising from another primary site; in addition, S. aureus may secondarily seed endovascular sites, such as heart valves or atheromatous plaques. Several criteria increase the probability that a patient has endocarditis as opposed to simple bacteremia: community (vs. nosocomial) acquisition of infection, absence of a primary site of infection, and evidence of metastatic infection. The evaluation of a bacteremic patient should be tailored to the individual but may include (in addition to an echocardiogram) an abdominal CT scan and a bone scan or gallium scan to detect an occult visceral abscess or osteomyelitis. Persistent bacteremia in conjunction with negative results in these studies may warrant a transesophageal echocardiogram, which is more sensitive than a transthoracic echo in detecting valvular vegetations.

Complications of S. aureus bacteremia include abscesses of abdominal viscera, brain abscess, meningitis, septic arthritis, osteomyelitis, endocarditis (if not already present), and mycotic aneurysm. High-grade or persistent bacteremia mandates a thorough evaluation for these complications, even if a primary site of infection has been identified.

Musculoskeletal Infections S. aureus is the most common cause of *acute osteomyelitis* in adults and one of the leading causes in children. Acute osteomyelitis develops as a result of either hematogenous seeding of bone (especially damaged bone) or direct extension from a contiguous focus of infection. The most common sites of hematogenous staphylococcal osteomyelitis in adults are the vertebral bodies; in children, the highly vascular metaphyses of long bones are most often affected. Acute osteomyelitis in adults usually presents as constitutional symptoms and pain over the affected area, often developing over several weeks or months; the diagnosis may be subtle, however, in the absence of localizing symptoms. Leukocytosis and an elevated erythrocyte sedimentation rate are laboratory clues to the diagnosis. Bacteremia may or may not be demonstrable. Four to six weeks of parenteral antibiotic therapy is usually curative.

S. aureus is also a prominent cause of *chronic osteomyelitis*, which develops at sites of previous surgery, trauma, or devascularization. In light of the hectic pace of many infections caused by S. aureus, chronic staphylococcal osteomyelitis can be impressively indolent; the infection may be asymptomatic for years or even decades, only to reawaken spontaneously and cause pain, sinus tract formation, and purulent drainage. A plain film of the affected area usually reveals bony destruction. The staphylococcal etiology of infection is best established by biopsy and culture of bone, as cultures of superficial or sinus tract drainage may yield misleading results. Cure requires surgical debridement of necrotic bone followed by a prolonged course of antibiotics.

A special form of osteomyelitis is that associated with prosthetic joints or with internal or external fixation devices. Pain, fever, swelling, and decreased range of motion are cardinal features of an infected prosthesis. A plain film may suggest loosening of the prosthesis, often as radiolucency at the interface between bone and cement. S. aureus osteomyelitis associated with a prosthesis can rarely be cured by antibiotics alone. Clinical sepsis, persistent bacteremia, or clinical or radiologic evidence of loosening is an absolute indication for removal of the prosthesis. S. aureus infection of fixation devices requires their removal, although this procedure is frequently delayed long enough to allow healing of the underlying fracture. Late relapses after apparent medical cure are not uncommon. A strategy of microbial suppression with oral antibiotics after a course of high-dose parenteral therapy is occasionally employed when removal of hardware is deemed too aggressive a measure for a particular patient.

S. aureus is a major cause of *septic arthritis* in adults. Predisposing factors include injection drug use, rheumatoid arthritis, use of systemic or intraarticular steroids, penetrating trauma, and joints previously damaged by trauma or disease. Knees, hips, and sacroiliac joints are most frequently infected. In addition to parenteral antibiotics, cure requires either repeated joint aspirations—the end points being sterilization of the joint space, a decrease in the number of leukocytes in the joint aspirate, and no reaccumulation of fluid—or open or arthroscopic debridement and drainage. Failure to adequately drain joints infected with *S. aureus* poses a risk of permanent loss of function. *S. aureus* is also the most common cause of *septic bursitis*.

S. aureus infection of muscle (*pyomyositis*) is relatively uncommon in temperate climates. *Psoas abscess* is the main exception. The psoas muscle is seeded either hematogenously or by direct extension from the site of vertebral osteomyelitis; the results are pain upon extension of the hip and fever. Although formerly an occasional cause of fever of unknown origin, psoas abscess is now relatively easy to diagnose by abdominal CT or MRI. Psoas abscesses are occasionally amenable to drainage via a percutaneous catheter; if not, then surgical drainage is indicated. For reasons that are not well understood, most other cases of staphylococcal pyomyositis occur in the tropics (tropical pyomyositis); in the United States, pyomyositis is seen most often in patients with underlying conditions such as diabetes mellitus, alcoholism, immunosuppressive therapy, or hematologic malignancy.

DIAGNOSIS The diagnosis of *S. aureus* infection is generally straightforward and is based on the isolation of the organism either from purulent material or from a normally sterile body fluid. Rarely if ever should *S. aureus* growing from even a single blood culture be considered a contaminant. Clinical samples require no special transport media to preserve the viability of the organisms. Gram's staining of purulent material from a staphylococcal abscess invariably reveals abundant neutrophils and intra- and extracellular cocci, which may be found singly or in pairs, short chains, tetrads, or clusters. *S. aureus* grows readily on standard laboratory media such as blood and chocolate agar. Colonies that are catalase positive and coagulase or thermonuclease positive may be identified presumptively as *S. aureus*. Many commercial kits are now available for the identification of grampositive cocci and are generally reliable for the identification of *S. aureus*.

The diagnosis of staphylococcal intoxications may be more difficult and may in fact rely entirely on clinical data (e.g., the diagnosis of TSS). The contribution of the laboratory may be confirmatory—for example, the demonstration of seroconversion to TSST-1 following a compatible illness, the demonstration of toxin production in vitro by a strain isolated from a patient, or the detection of SE in a food sample.

℞ **TREATMENT**

The essential elements of therapy for staphylococcal infections are drainage of purulent collections of pus, debridement of necrotic tissue, removal of foreign bodies, and administration of antimicrobial agents. The importance of adequate drainage cannot be overemphasized; all but the smallest of staphylococcal abscesses require drainage for cure. In skin and soft tissue infections, surgical drainage is occasionally all that is required for cure. It is almost impossible to eradicate *S. aureus* infection in the presence of a foreign body, such as a piece of orthopedic hardware, an intravascular catheter or other device, or a pacemaker. Only under extraordinary circumstances should an attempt be made to cure such infections without removal or debridement of foreign material.

Antimicrobial Resistance The relentless spread of antibiotic resistance among strains of *S. aureus* is one of the great challenges facing clinicians today. Within 4 years of the introduction of penicil-

lin G into clinical practice in 1941, β-lactamase-mediated resistance to penicillin was reported. As additional antibiotics (chloramphenicol, tetracyclines, macrolides, aminoglycosides) became available in the 1950s, resistance rapidly emerged to them as well. Penicillin resistance in *S. aureus* is due to the production of β-lactamase, a serine peptidase that enzymatically degrades penicillin's β-lactam ring, thereby inactivating the drug. β-Lactamase is related to the penicillin-binding proteins (PBPs), a group of transpeptidases that catalyze the terminal steps in peptidoglycan assembly. Methicillin-sensitive *S. aureus* (MSSA) produces four PBPs, all of which are inhibited by β-lactam antibiotics and three of which are essential for bacterial multiplication. Unlike β-lactamases from gram-negative organisms, some of which are more active against cephalosporins than against penicillins, the staphylococcal β-lactamases are principally penicillinases. Their transcription is induced by the presence of β-lactam molecules in the medium. Today, all but a very small percentage of *S. aureus* strains produce β-lactamase.

Methicillin, the first β-lactamase-stable semisynthetic penicillin, was introduced in 1960; the very next year, a methicillin-resistant strain of *S. aureus* (MRSA) was isolated. In recent years, the percentage of staphylococcal isolates from U.S. hospitals that are methicillin resistant has risen substantially, a trend that has been driven by indiscriminate antibiotic use. In some tertiary care institutions, more than 40 percent of *S. aureus* isolates are now resistant to methicillin, although rates of 5 to 10 percent are more typical. Community-acquired MRSA carriage remains rare except in certain high-risk groups, such as injection drug users.

Methicillin resistance is most accurately determined by the standard agar screen for MRSA. Classic methicillin resistance is encoded by the methicillin resistance determinant (*mec*), a 30- to 50-kb transposon-like segment of DNA that is present in MRSA strains and absent in MSSA strains. The *mecA* gene, which resides on *mec*, encodes a variant PBP called *PBP2'* or *PBP2a*. PBP2' has reduced affinity for β-lactam antibiotics and is able to substitute for the essential PBPs if they have been inactivated by β-lactams. MRSA strains are resistant to the action of all β-lactam antibiotics, including penicillins, cephalosporins, and carbapenems. These strains tend to be resistant to most other antibiotics as well, most often because they carry large conjugative plasmids bearing multiple resistance determinants. They remain uniformly sensitive to vancomycin, although the days of glycopeptide resistance may soon be upon us: transfer of such resistance from *Enterococcus faecalis* to *S. aureus* has been demonstrated in the laboratory.

An additional mechanism is responsible for a borderline methicillin-resistant phenotype (the so-called borderline-resistant, or BORSA, phenotype): hyperproduction of β-lactamase. These strains lack the *mecA* gene and are killed by oxacillin at the level used in the standard agar screen for methicillin resistance. BORSA infections can probably be treated successfully with high doses of semisynthetic penicillins.

Selection of Antibiotics Although most pathogenic strains of *S. aureus* are resistant to penicillin, the development of penicillins and cephalosporins that are resistant to β-lactamase has allowed these classes of antibiotics to remain useful for treatment of *S. aureus* infections. Nafcillin and oxacillin, both of which are β-lactamase-resistant penicillins, are the drugs of choice for parenteral treatment of serious staphylococcal infections. Penicillin remains the drug of choice for infections caused by susceptible organisms. Drug combinations consisting of a penicillin plus a β-lactamase inhibitor are also effective but are best reserved for treatment of mixed infections. Penicillin-allergic patients can usually be given a cephalosporin, although caution should be exercised if the adverse reaction to penicillin was anaphylaxis. Of the cephalosporins, the first-generation agents (e.g., cefazolin) are preferred for reasons related to cost, potency, and breadth of spectrum. The best alternative for parenteral administration is vancomycin. Dicloxacillin and cephalexin are recommended for oral treatment of minor infections or for continuation therapy. Several other agents are also available for use against susceptible strains.

In most clinical settings, no significant benefit is attained by treating *S. aureus* infections with more than one drug to which the organism is known to be susceptible. Synergy has been demonstrated in vitro for aminoglycoside/β-lactam combinations, which hasten sterilization of the blood in endocarditis. Accordingly, therapy for *S. aureus* bacteremia is often initiated with such a combination for a brief period (e.g., 5 to 7 days)—a strategy to which the authors are sympathetic. Thereafter, the toxicity of an aminoglycoside cannot be justified on the basis of available data. Use of rifampin in conjunction with a β-lactam antibiotic (or vancomycin) occasionally results in sterilization of sites of otherwise refractory infections, particularly those involving foreign bodies or avascular tissue; the results can be dramatic. Nevertheless, routine use of rifampin for serious *S. aureus* infections is not recommended because of potential added toxicity and theoretical antimicrobial antagonism. Rifampin should be reserved for refractory, usually inoperable infections and should never be administered as monotherapy, which rapidly leads to resistance.

Route and Duration of Therapy Because of poor bioavailability or tolerability of most oral antistaphylococcal agents, parenteral therapy should be used for infections that require high concentrations of antibiotic, such as endovascular infections, infections of poorly vascularized tissue, and infections of the central nervous system. Given the propensity of *S. aureus* to adhere to endovascular and devitalized or damaged tissues, high doses of antibiotics (e.g., 12 g of nafcillin per day) should be used for bacteremic infections. When high serum levels of antibiotic are required to produce adequate tissue levels (e.g., in endocarditis or osteomyelitis), the parenteral route should be used for the duration of therapy. Oral agents may suffice for the treatment of nonbacteremic infections in which high serum levels of antibiotic are not requisite (e.g., skin, soft tissue, and upper respiratory tract infections).

With the notable exceptions of bacteremia and osteomyelitis, the duration of therapy for *S. aureus* infections can be tailored to the severity of illness, the immunologic status of the host, and the response to treatment. Because antibiotics penetrate bone poorly, treatment of acute osteomyelitis in adults requires 4 to 6 weeks of parenteral therapy, with the actual duration depending on the vascular supply at the site of infection and the response to treatment. Chronic osteomyelitis is occasionally treated with 6 to 8 weeks of parenterally administered antibiotics followed by several months of oral therapy, especially if the adequacy of debridement is uncertain.

Acute endocarditis and other endovascular infections caused by *S. aureus* should be treated with parenteral antibiotics for 4 weeks (6 weeks in the case of prosthetic valves). Simple bacteremia, as might occur with a removable or drainable focus of infection, requires a shorter duration of therapy, but a 2-week course of *parenteral* therapy is recommended *for all patients* with *S. aureus* bacteremia, even under these circumstances. The cost and effort implicit in this recommendation are apparent, but shorter courses of therapy are associated with an unacceptable rate of secondary complications. One of the more challenging aspects of treating staphylococcal bacteremia is deciding whether to administer parenteral therapy for 2 or 4 weeks. A conservative approach (one that is supported by numerous studies) dictates that *4 weeks* should be standard unless specific criteria are met (Table 142-2).

PREVENTION AND CONTROL Nosocomial staphylococcal outbreaks and the spread of resistant strains of *S. aureus* are serious global problems. Within an institution, the most important vector of transmission of *S. aureus* is the hands of health care workers. Patients with exposed wounds or with nasal colonization are important reservoirs of the organisms. Transmission of *S. aureus*—and hence the incidence of staphylococcal infection within an institution—can be reduced most effectively by meticulous hand washing before and after contact with patients.

More stringent infection-control measures must be taken to prevent the nosocomial spread of MRSA. Such measures include assigning patients colonized or infected with MRSA to private rooms, wearing gloves for contact with contaminated wounds and mucous membranes

Table 142-2

Criteria for the Selection of Short-Course (2-Week) Parenteral Antibiotic Therapy for Patients with *S. aureus* Bacteremia

Subjects with *S. aureus* bacteremia who meet *all* criteria may be treated with parenteral antibiotics for 2 rather than 4 weeks.
1. No serious underlying condition, such as hematologic malignancy, poorly controlled diabetes, cirrhosis, severe malnutrition, rheumatoid arthritis, or AIDS
2. No hemodynamically significant valvular dysfunction
3. No "seedable sites," such as prosthetic heart valve, aortic aneurysm, necrotic bone, transvenous pacemaker, or prosthetic joint
4. A primary focus of infection that is readily apparent and amenable to removal (e.g., intravenous catheter) or surgical drainage
5. A short interval between the presumed onset of bacteremia and initiation of therapy (e.g., removal of catheter and start of antibiotics)
6. A staphylococcal isolate that proves to be susceptible to antibiotic(s) chosen initially
7. A prompt response to removal of the catheter and initiation of antibiotic treatment: defervescence within 72 h, negative blood cultures after catheter removal
8. No suppurative phlebitis at the catheter entry site
9. No evidence of metastatic foci of infection during the first 2 weeks of therapy

as well as a gown if contamination of clothing is likely, and hand washing with an antiseptic after patient contact. Patients who are colonized but not infected with MRSA should not be treated with vancomycin merely for the sake of eliminating carriage of this organism. *S. aureus* is the most common cause of postoperative wound infection. The incidence of staphylococcal infection in this situation can be reduced by perioperative administration of any of a number of antibiotics with favorable pharmacokinetic properties, including cefazolin, cefuroxime, and vancomycin.

Staphylococcal skin and soft tissue infections may recur once a person has been colonized with a virulent strain. In this context, therapy directed at the elimination of staphylococcal colonization may be warranted, especially for patients at particular risk for complications of infection. Use of an oral β-lactam antibiotic alone is ineffective, but combination therapy for 10 days with dicloxacillin or cephalexin (500 mg four times a day) plus rifampin (300 mg twice a day) plus mupirocin (2% ointment applied topically to both nares) is usually effective at clearing the carrier state.

COAGULASE-NEGATIVE STAPHYLOCOCCI

CNS are a major cause of nosocomial infection and are the organisms most frequently isolated from the blood of hospitalized patients. The frequency with which they cause opportunistic infection in immunocompromised hosts attests more to the increased vulnerability of such hosts in modern medical practice than to the intrinsic virulence of the organisms. Despite the weak pathogenicity of these bacteria, the global impact of CNS infection is considerable, including increased length and cost of hospital stay; increased use of antibiotics in general; and increased use of vancomycin in particular, which has contributed to the recent emergence of vancomycin-resistant enterococci.

Although the variety of clinical syndromes caused by CNS is impressive, several characteristics apply to most such infections (with notable exceptions). First, they tend to be *indolent*. There is often a long latent period between the time of contamination (e.g., of a medical device) and the onset of clinical illness; bacteremia in neutropenic patients can be an exception to this rule. Second, most CNS infections are nosocomial in origin; important exceptions are native valve endocarditis and *S. saprophyticus* infections of the urinary tract. Third, most clinically significant infections are caused by strains of CNS that are resistant to multiple antibiotics, including penicillins and cephalosporins. Finally, most CNS infections are associated with a medical device of some kind, and removal of such devices is usually required for cure.

EPIDEMIOLOGY AND PATHOGENESIS CNS, particularly *S. epidermidis*, are invariable and prominent constituents of the normal human skin flora. Infection most often results from direct inoculation of a foreign body at the time it is inserted, although hematogenous seeding can also occur. Patients and hospital personnel are the principal reservoirs for strains in the nosocomial environment.

CNS are the quintessential pathogens of medical devices. The array of virulence factors produced by CNS is meager compared with that of the virulence factors produced by *S. aureus*, but among these few factors are substances that promote bacterial adherence to and persistence on foreign bodies. A variety of surface antigens that promote colonization of medical devices by CNS (particularly *S. epidermidis*) have been identified; the best-studied of these is polysaccharide adhesin, which promotes the initial interaction of the bacteria and a foreign body. *S. epidermidis* also produces an exopolysaccharide known as *slime*, which is important in the persistence of infection; slime thwarts host defenses by coating foreign materials and impairing phagocytic killing. CNS appear not to make important exoproteins or toxins; rather, they cause disease by tenaciously persisting on foreign materials, resulting in a local and occasionally a systemic inflammatory response.

The most important risk factor for infection with CNS is the presence of a foreign body, especially an indwelling catheter. The likelihood of catheter-related infection depends upon a number of variables, including the experience and skill of the person who inserts the catheter, the length of time that a catheter is left in place, the adequacy of host immunity (especially granulocyte number and function), and the quality of postinsertion care of the catheter site. A second major risk factor for infection is deficient phagocyte function—especially neutropenia, which is most often an iatrogenic complication of chemotherapy for cancer but may also reflect an underlying disease process (such as leukemia). CNS only rarely cause infections in immunologically normal hosts and typically do so only under extenuating circumstances—e.g., subacute endocarditis involving an abnormal native valve or sternal osteomyelitis following cardiac surgery.

CLINICAL SYNDROMES Because CNS can adhere to a variety of materials, virtually all *foreign bodies* are susceptible to colonization by these organisms. CNS are the most common pathogens complicating the use of intravenous catheters, hemodialysis shunts and grafts, cerebrospinal fluid (CSF) shunts, peritoneal dialysis catheters, pacemaker wires and electrodes, prosthetic joints, vascular grafts, and prosthetic valves. CNS infection of intravenous catheters may or may not be accompanied by signs of inflammation at the site of catheter insertion, and the degree of systemic toxicity (including fever) ranges from minimal to considerable. The diagnosis can be established by the performance of multiple cultures of blood drawn from the catheter and by venipuncture. Infection of CSF shunts is usually evident within several weeks of implantation. Signs of meningitis are sometimes readily apparent but more often are subtle or absent. Malfunction of the shunt may be the only manifestation of shunt infection. CNS infection of a prosthetic joint often does not become evident until long after implantation, although the inciting contamination usually occurs at the time of implantation. Infection of vascular grafts may result in the development of an aneurysm or a pseudoaneurysm, with catastrophic consequences.

CNS are a prominent cause of *bacteremia* in immunosuppressed patients. While such infections in immunocompetent hosts are relatively benign, patients with neutropenia may have high-grade bacteremia that results in significant systemic toxicity and even death. A serious consequence of bacteremia is the seeding of a secondary foreign body, such as a prosthetic heart valve or joint or a pacemaker.

CNS are the organisms most commonly responsible for *prosthetic valve endocarditis*, causing the majority of infections that develop within several months of implantation as well as a substantial percentage of late infections. CNS are a less frequent but important cause of *native valve endocarditis*, accounting for fewer than 5 percent of

such infections and usually affecting abnormal valves. The syndrome generally consists of subacute endocarditis (thus contrasting with the syndrome produced by *S. aureus*), with an illness that is clinically indistinguishable from that caused by viridans streptococci. Infection of prosthetic valves is often complicated by valvular dysfunction secondary either to dehiscence of the sewing ring or obstruction of the valve's orifice by bulky vegetations.

S. saprophyticus is a prime cause of *urinary tract infection*, especially among sexually active young women, in whom it is second only to *E. coli* in frequency. *S. saprophyticus* produces a syndrome indistinguishable from that caused by other etiologic agents, with pyuria and symptoms of dysuria, frequency, and abdominal pain. Infection with *S. saprophyticus* is readily amenable to therapy with most agents commonly used to treat urinary tract infections. CNS can also cause urinary tract infection in hospitalized patients who have undergone invasive procedures; such infections are especially likely to be asymptomatic and may be difficult to treat because of antimicrobial resistance.

DIAGNOSIS Although CNS are the most common cause of nosocomial bacteremia, they are also the most common contaminant of blood cultures; differentiation between infection and contamination often poses a challenge with major therapeutic implications. Positive blood cultures are more likely to be "true positives" when there is a clinical illness suggestive of infection, when there is an indwelling catheter or some other risk factor for CNS infection, and when cultures of blood drawn from multiple sites are positive for phenotypically similar organisms with the same antimicrobial susceptibility patterns. Except in the setting of neutropenia, physicians often have the luxury of awaiting the results of repeat cultures when the significance of CNS growing from a blood culture is questionable.

℞ **TREATMENT**

Removal of the foreign body (especially when it is an intravenous catheter) often constitutes adequate therapy for CNS infection related to that device. Most infections of a foreign body require the removal of the device—whether a prosthetic valve, prosthetic joint, CSF shunt, vascular graft, pacemaker and associated hardware, or hemodialysis shunt. Cures of all such infections with antibiotics alone have been reported, however, and a patient's poor medical condition or the hazards of surgery occasionally warrant an attempt at medical cure without extirpation of the device (see below). Infections of peritoneal dialysis catheters can be cured with antibiotics alone often enough that an attempt should be made to do so. CNS infections of central venous catheters are also amenable to medical therapy, although relapses are common. Persistent bacteremia during therapy is an absolute indication for removal of a catheter, and bacteremia after a catheter's removal suggests seeding of a secondary site.

It is difficult to make generalizations about the optimal duration of therapy for CNS infections. In general, the duration of treatment is the same as for infection syndromes caused by other bacteria. For example, native valve endocarditis should be treated for 4 weeks, prosthetic valve endocarditis for 6. Transient bacteremia in an immunocompetent host may require no antimicrobial therapy after removal of an offending catheter. The efficacy of therapy can occasionally be enhanced by the delivery of antibiotics directly to the site of infection—e.g., by intraventricular administration of vancomycin and gentamicin for central nervous system infections or by intraperitoneal administration of these drugs for infections of peritoneal dialysis catheters.

Despite the low degree of pathogenicity of CNS, treatment of serious infections due to these organisms is usually problematic because of the high percentage of strains that are resistant to commonly used antibiotics, including most oral agents. Most strains of CNS isolated from patients in U.S. hospitals are resistant not only to penicillin but also to the penicillinase-resistant penicillins and cephalosporins. Nosocomial isolates are usually resistant to other classes of antibiotics as well. Vancomycin, to which CNS remain uniformly susceptible, is of necessity the drug of choice for *empiric* therapy for serious CNS infections. Strains proven to be susceptible to nafcillin (oxacillin) or penicillin should be treated with one of these agents or with a first-generation cephalosporin.

Synergistic combinations of antibiotics are often useful in the treatment of CNS infections. Rifampin plays a unique role in this endeavor by virtue of its potency against most staphylococci, its excellent penetration into tissues (including those that are poorly vascularized), and the high levels it reaches within human cells. Unfortunately, rifampin must be used in combination with other antibiotics because of the frequent and rapid emergence of microbial resistance to the drug when it is used alone. If an effort must be made to eradicate infection of a medical device without its removal, the concomitant use of a β-lactam antibiotic to which the organism is susceptible plus rifampin (300 mg twice daily by mouth) plus an aminoglycoside (usually gentamicin) affords the best chance for success. Vancomycin can be substituted for the β-lactam agent if so dictated by an organism's susceptibility pattern or by a patient's drug allergy.

BIBLIOGRAPHY

BAILEY CJ et al: The epidermolytic (exfoliative) toxins of *Staphylococcus aureus*. Med Microbiol Immunol 184:53, 1995

DERESIEWICZ RL: Staphylococcal toxic shock syndrome, in *Superantigens: Molecular Biology, Immunology, and Relevance to Human Disease*, DYM Leung et al (eds). New York, Marcel Dekker, 1997, pp 435–479

GUANGYONG J et al: Cell density control of staphylococcal virulence mediated by an octapeptide pheromone. Proc Natl Acad Sci USA 92:12055, 1995

JERNIGAN JA, FARR BM: Short-course therapy of catheter-related *Staphylococcus aureus* bacteremia: A meta-analysis. Ann Intern Med 119:304, 1993

MARRACK P, KAPPLER J: The staphylococcal enterotoxins and their relatives. Science 248:705, 1990

MULLIGAN ME et al: Methicillin-resistant *Staphylococcus aureus*: A consensus review of the microbiology, pathogenesis, and epidemiology with implications for prevention and management. Am J Med 94:313, 1993

MUSHER DM et al: The current spectrum of *Staphylococcus aureus* infection in a tertiary care hospital. Medicine 73:186, 1994

NEU HC: The crisis of antibiotic resistance. Science 257:1064, 1992

PRASAD GS et al: Structure of toxic shock syndrome toxin 1. Biochemistry 32:13761, 1993

RUPP ME, ARCHER GL: Coagulase-negative staphylococci: Pathogens associated with medical progress. Clin Infect Dis 19:231, 1994

SHEAGREN JN: *Staphylococcus aureus*: The persistent pathogen. N Engl J Med 310:1368, 1437, 1984

143 *Michael R. Wessels*

STREPTOCOCCAL AND ENTEROCOCCAL INFECTIONS

Many varieties of streptococci are found as part of the normal human flora colonizing the respiratory, gastrointestinal, and genitourinary tracts. Several species are important causes of human disease. Group A *Streptococcus*, or *Streptococcus pyogenes*, is the organism responsible for streptococcal pharyngitis, one of the most common bacterial infections of school-age children, and for the postinfectious syndromes of acute rheumatic fever and poststreptococcal glomerulonephritis. Group B *Streptococcus*, or *Streptococcus agalactiae*, is the leading cause of bacterial sepsis and meningitis in newborn infants and a major cause of endometritis and fever in parturient women. Enterococci are significant causes of urinary tract infection, intraabdominal infection, and endocarditis. Viridans streptococci are the most common cause of bacterial endocarditis.

Streptococci are gram-positive bacteria of spherical to ovoid shape that characteristically form chains when grown in liquid media. Most streptococci that cause human infections are facultative anaerobes, although some are strict anaerobes. Streptococci are relatively fastidious organisms, requiring enriched media for growth in the laboratory. No single scheme for classification of streptococci is entirely satisfactory. Consequently, clinicians and clinical microbiologists often identify streptococci by any of several classification systems, including

hemolytic pattern, Lancefield group, species name, and common or trivial name. Many of the streptococci associated with human infection produce a zone of complete hemolysis around the bacterial colony when cultured on blood agar, a pattern known as beta hemolysis. The beta-hemolytic streptococci can be classified by the Lancefield system, a serologic grouping based on the reaction of specific antisera with cell-wall carbohydrate antigens of the bacteria. With rare exceptions, organisms belonging to Lancefield groups A, B, C, and G are all beta-hemolytic streptococci, and each is associated with characteristic patterns of human infection. Other streptococci produce a zone of partial, or alpha, hemolysis, often imparting a greenish appearance to the agar. These alpha-hemolytic streptococci are identified more specifically by biochemical testing and include *Streptococcus pneumoniae*, an important cause of pneumonia, meningitis, and other infections (discussed in Chap. 141), and several species of streptococci referred to collectively as the viridans streptococci, which are part of the normal oral flora and are prominent as agents of subacute bacterial endocarditis. Finally, some streptococci are nonhemolytic, a pattern sometimes called gamma hemolysis. The classification of the major groups of streptococci responsible for human infections is outlined in Table 143-1. Among the organisms classified serologically as group D streptococci, the enterococci are now considered to constitute a separate genus on the basis of DNA homology studies. Thus, species previously designated as *Streptococcus faecalis* and *Streptococcus faecium* have been renamed *Enterococcus faecalis* and *Enterococcus faecium*, respectively.

GROUP A STREPTOCOCCI

Lancefield group A consists of a single species, *S. pyogenes*. As its species name implies, this organism is associated with a variety of suppurative infections. In addition, group A streptococci have the

Table 143-1

Classification of Streptococci Responsible for Human Infections

Lancefield Group	Representative Species	Hemolytic Pattern	Typical Infections
A	*S. pyogenes*	Beta	Pharyngitis, impetigo, cellulitis, scarlet fever
B	*S. agalactiae*	Beta	Neonatal sepsis and meningitis, puerperal infection, urinary tract infection, diabetic ulcer infection, endocarditis
C	*S. equi*	Beta	Cellulitis, bacteremia, endocarditis
D	Enterococci: *E. faecalis* *E. faecium*	Usually nonhemolytic	Urinary tract infection, wound infection, endocarditis
	Nonenterococci: *S. bovis*	Usually nonhemolytic	Bacteremia, endocarditis
G	*S. canis*	Beta	Cellulitis, bacteremia, endocarditis
Variable or nongroupable	Viridans streptococci: *S. mutans* *S. sanguis*	Alpha	Endocarditis, dental abscess, brain abscess
	Intermedius or *milleri* group: *S. intermedius*	Variable	Brain abscess, visceral abscess
	Anaerobic streptococci: *Peptostreptococcus magnus*	Usually nonhemolytic	Sinusitis, pneumonia, empyema, brain abscess, liver abscess

capacity to trigger the postinfectious syndromes of acute rheumatic fever and poststreptococcal glomerulonephritis, which are uniquely associated with these organisms. → *Acute rheumatic fever and glomerulonephritis are discussed in Chap. 236 and Chap. 274, respectively.*

PATHOGENESIS Group A streptococci elaborate a number of cell-surface components and extracellular products important both in the pathogenesis of infection and in the immune response of the human host. The cell wall contains a carbohydrate antigen that may be released by treatment with acid. The reaction of such acid extracts with group A–specific antiserum is the basis for the definitive identification of a streptococcal strain as *S. pyogenes*. The major surface protein of group A streptococci is M protein, which occurs in more than 80 antigenically distinct types and is the basis for the serotyping of strains with specific antisera. The M protein molecules are fibrillar structures anchored in the cell wall of the organism and extending as hairlike projections away from the cell surface. The amino acid sequence of the distal or amino-terminal portion of the M protein molecule is quite variable, accounting for the antigenic variation of the different M types, while more proximal regions of the protein are relatively conserved. The presence of M protein correlates with the capacity of a strain to resist phagocytic killing in fresh human blood; this phenomenon appears to be due, at least in part, to the binding of plasma fibrinogen to M protein molecules on the streptococcal surface, which interferes with complement activation and deposition of opsonic complement fragments on the bacterial cell. This resistance to phagocytosis may be overcome by M protein–specific antibodies, and thus individuals with antibodies to a given M type acquired as a result of prior infection are protected against subsequent infection with organisms of the same M type but not against that with different M types. Group A streptococci also elaborate (to varying degrees) a polysaccharide capsule composed of hyaluronic acid. The production of large amounts of hyaluronic acid capsule by certain strains results in a characteristic mucoid appearance of the bacterial colonies. The capsular polysaccharide also plays an important role in protecting the organisms from ingestion and killing by phagocytes. In contrast to M protein, the hyaluronic acid capsule is a weak immunogen, presumably because of the apparent structural identity between streptococcal hyaluronic acid and the hyaluronic acid of mammalian connective tissues. Antibodies to hyaluronate have not been shown to be important in protective immunity.

Group A streptococci produce a large number of extracellular products that may be important in local and systemic toxicity and in the spread of infection through tissues. These products include streptolysins S and O, toxins that damage cell membranes and account for the hemolysis produced by the organisms; streptokinase; DNases; protease; and pyrogenic exotoxins A, B, and C. The pyrogenic exotoxins, previously known as erythrogenic toxins, cause the rash of scarlet fever. Relatively recently, pyrogenic exotoxin-producing strains of group A *Streptococcus* have been linked to unusually severe invasive infections, including necrotizing fasciitis, and a systemic syndrome termed the *streptococcal toxic shock-like syndrome*. Several extracellular products stimulate specific antibody responses useful in the serodiagnosis of recent streptococcal infection. Tests for these antibodies are used primarily for the detection of preceding streptococcal infection in cases of suspected acute rheumatic fever or poststreptococcal glomerulonephritis.

PHARYNGITIS Although seen in patients of all ages, group A streptococcal pharyngitis is one of the most common bacterial infections of childhood, accounting for 20 to 40 percent of all cases of exudative pharyngitis in children. It is rare among those under the age of 3, who may manifest streptococcal infection with a syndrome of fever, malaise, and lymphadenopathy without exudative pharyngitis. Infection is acquired through contact with another individual carrying the organism. Respiratory droplets are the usual mechanism of spread, although other routes, including food-borne outbreaks, have been well described.

The incubation period of streptococcal pharyngitis is 1 to 4 days. Symptoms include sore throat, fever and chills, malaise, and sometimes abdominal complaints and vomiting, particularly in children. Both symptoms and signs are quite variable, ranging from mild throat discomfort with minimal physical findings to high fever and severe sore throat associated with intense erythema and swelling of the pharyngeal mucosa and the presence of purulent exudate over the posterior pharyngeal wall and tonsillar pillars. Enlarged, tender anterior cervical lymph nodes commonly accompany exudative pharyngitis.

The differential diagnosis of streptococcal pharyngitis encompasses the many other bacterial and viral causes of pharyngitis. Other infections that frequently produce exudative pharyngitis include infectious mononucleosis and adenovirus infection. Now rare in the United States, the pseudomembrane of diphtheria may give a similar appearance. *Corynebacterium (Arcanobacterium) haemolyticum* may cause pharyngitis, often in association with a scarlet fever-like rash. Other causes of pharyngitis, usually without a purulent exudate, include infections with coxsackievirus, influenza virus, mycoplasmas, or *Neisseria gonorrhoeae* and acute infection with human immunodeficiency virus. Because of the range of clinical presentations of streptococcal pharyngitis and the large number of other agents that can produce the same clinical picture, the diagnosis of streptococcal pharyngitis on clinical grounds alone is not reliable.

The throat culture remains the gold standard for diagnosis. Culture of a throat specimen that is properly collected (i.e., by vigorous rubbing of a sterile swab over both tonsillar pillars) and properly processed is the most sensitive and specific means available by which to make a definitive diagnosis. Rapid diagnostic kits using latex agglutination or enzyme immunoassay of swab specimens are now widely available and can serve as a useful adjunct to the throat culture. While precise figures on sensitivity and specificity vary among studies, the rapid diagnostic kits generally are highly (more than 95 percent) specific. Thus a positive result can be relied on for definitive diagnosis and eliminates the need for a throat culture. However, because the rapid diagnostic tests are less sensitive than throat culture (with a relative sensitivity ranging from 55 to 90 percent in comparative studies), a negative result should be confirmed with a throat culture.

In the usual course of uncomplicated streptococcal pharyngitis, symptoms resolve after 3 to 5 days. The course is shortened little by treatment, which is given primarily to prevent suppurative complications and rheumatic fever. Prevention of rheumatic fever depends on eradication of the organism from the pharynx, not simply on resolution of symptoms, and requires penicillin treatment—either a single intramuscular dose of benzathine penicillin G or a 10-day course of oral penicillin (Table 143-2). Erythromycin may be substituted for penicillin in the treatment of individuals allergic to penicillin. Follow-up culture after treatment is no longer routinely recommended but may

Table 143-2

Treatment of Group A Streptococcal Infections

Infection	Treatment*
Pharyngitis	Benzathine penicillin G, 1.2 million units IM; or penicillin V, 250 mg PO qid × 10 days (Children <27 kg: Benzathine penicillin G, 600,000 units IM; or penicillin V, 125 mg PO qid × 10 days)
Impetigo	Same as pharyngitis
Erysipelas/cellulitis	Severe: Penicillin G, 1–2 million units IV q4h Mild to moderate: Procaine penicillin, 1.2 million units IM bid
Necrotizing fasciitis/ myositis	Surgical debridement plus penicillin G, 2–4 million units IV q4h
Pneumonia/empyema	Penicillin G, 2–4 million units IV q4h plus drainage of empyema

* Penicillin allergy: Erythromycin (10 mg/kg PO qid up to a maximum of 250 mg per dose) may be substituted for oral penicillin. Alternative agents for parenteral therapy include first-generation cephalosporins—if the penicillin allergy does not manifest as immediate hypersensitivity (anaphylaxis or urticaria) or as another potentially life-threatening reaction (e.g., severe rash and fever)—and vancomycin.

be warranted in selected cases, such as those involving patients or families with frequent streptococcal infections or those occurring in situations in which the risk of rheumatic fever is thought to be high (for example, when cases of rheumatic fever have recently been reported in the community).

Suppurative complications of streptococcal pharyngitis have become uncommon with the widespread use of antibiotics for most cases of symptomatic streptococcal infection. These complications result from the spread of infection from the pharyngeal mucosa to deeper tissues, either by direct extension or by the hematogenous or lymphatic route, and may include cervical lymphadenitis, peritonsillar or retropharyngeal abscess, sinusitis, otitis media, meningitis, bacteremia, endocarditis, and pneumonia. Local complications, such as abscess formation in the peritonsillar or parapharyngeal space, should be considered in a patient with unusually severe or prolonged symptoms or localized pain associated with high fever and a toxic appearance.

ASYMPTOMATIC CARRIER STATE Surveillance cultures have shown that up to 20 percent of individuals in certain populations may have asymptomatic pharyngeal colonization with group A streptococci. There are no definitive guidelines for management of these asymptomatic carriers or of asymptomatic individuals who still have a positive throat culture after a full course of treatment for symptomatic pharyngitis. A reasonable course of action is to give a single 10-day course of penicillin for symptomatic pharyngitis and, if positive cultures persist, not to re-treat unless symptoms recur. Studies of the natural history of streptococcal carriage and infection have shown that the risk both of developing rheumatic fever and of transmitting infection to others is substantially lower among asymptomatic carriers than among individuals with symptomatic pharyngitis. Therefore, aggressive attempts to eradicate carriage probably are not justified under most circumstances. An exception to this general statement is the situation in which an asymptomatic carrier is a potential source of infection to others. Outbreaks of food-borne infection and nosocomial puerperal infection have been traced to asymptomatic carriers who may harbor the organisms in the throat, on the skin, or in the vagina or anus. In cases in which a carrier is transmitting infection, attempts to eradicate carriage are warranted, although data are limited on the best regimen to use to clear the organism after penicillin alone has failed. The combination of penicillin and rifampin has been used to eliminate pharyngeal carriage, and the addition of oral vancomycin has led to success in eradicating rectal colonization; however, experience is not extensive with any regimen for this indication.

SCARLET FEVER Scarlet fever consists of streptococcal infection, usually pharyngitis, accompanied by a characteristic rash. The rash arises from the effects of one of three toxins, which are currently designated streptococcal pyrogenic exotoxins A, B, and C and previously were known as erythrogenic or scarlet fever toxins. In the past, scarlet fever was thought to reflect infection of an individual lacking toxin-specific immunity with a toxin-producing strain of group A *Streptococcus*. Susceptibility to scarlet fever was correlated with results of the Dick test. A small amount of erythrogenic toxin injected intradermally produced local erythema in susceptible individuals but elicited no reaction in those with specific immunity. Subsequent studies have suggested that development of the scarlet fever rash may reflect a hypersensitivity reaction requiring prior exposure to the toxin. For reasons that are not clear, scarlet fever has become less common in recent years, although strains of group A streptococci that produce pyrogenic exotoxins continue to be prevalent in the population.

The symptoms of scarlet fever are the same as those of pharyngitis alone. The rash typically begins on the first or second day of illness over the upper trunk, spreading to involve the extremities but sparing the palms and soles. The rash is made up of minute papules, giving a characteristic "sandpaper" texture to the skin. Associated findings include circumoral pallor, "strawberry tongue" (enlarged papillae on a coated tongue, which later may become denuded), and accentuation of the rash in the skin folds (Pastia's lines). Subsidence of the rash after 6 to 9 days is followed after several days by desquamation of the palms and soles. The differential diagnosis of scarlet fever includes other causes of fever and generalized rash, such as measles and other viral exanthems, Kawasaki disease, toxic shock syndrome, and systemic allergic reactions (e.g., drug eruptions).

SKIN AND SOFT TISSUE INFECTIONS Group A streptococci—and occasionally other streptococcal species—cause a variety of infections involving the skin, subcutaneous tissues, muscles, and fascia. While several clinical syndromes, recognized according to the tissues involved, offer a useful means for classification of skin and soft tissue infections, not all cases fit exactly into a single category. The classic syndromes should be considered as general guides to predicting the level of tissue involvement in a particular patient, the probable clinical course, and the likelihood that surgical intervention or aggressive life-support measures will be required.

Impetigo (Pyoderma) Impetigo is a superficial infection of the skin caused primarily by group A streptococci and occasionally by other streptococci or by *Staphylococcus aureus*. This condition is seen most often in young children, tends to occur during the warmer months, and is more common in semitropical or tropical climates than in cooler regions. The infection occurs especially often among children living under conditions of poor hygiene. Prospective studies have shown that colonization of unbroken skin with group A streptococci precedes the development of clinical infection. Minor trauma, such as a scratch or an insect bite, may then serve to inoculate organisms into the skin. Impetigo is best prevented, therefore, by attention to adequate hygiene. The usual sites of involvement are the face (particularly around the nose and mouth) and the legs, although lesions may occur at other locations. Individual lesions begin as red papules, which evolve quickly into vesicular and then pustular lesions that break down and coalesce to form characteristic honeycomb-like crusts. Lesions generally are not painful, and patients do not appear ill. Fever is not a feature of impetigo and, if present, suggests either infection extending to deeper tissues or another diagnosis.

The classic presentation of impetigo usually poses little diagnostic difficulty. Cultures of impetiginous lesions often yield *S. aureus* as well as group A streptococci, but longitudinal studies have shown that, in almost all cases, streptococci can be isolated initially, with staphylococci appearing later, presumably as secondary colonizing flora. Previously, the nearly universal effectiveness of penicillin in these infections, despite the resistance of most staphylococcal strains, supported the primary role of streptococci. More recent studies, however, have reported treatment failures with penicillin and have suggested that *S. aureus* has become a significant cause of impetigo. *Bullous impetigo* is a distinctive form of *S. aureus* infection characterized by the presence of more extensive, bullous lesions that break down and leave thin paperlike crusts instead of the thick amber crusts of streptococcal impetigo. Other skin lesions that may be confused with impetigo include herpetic lesions—either those of orolabial herpes simplex or those of chickenpox or zoster. Herpetic lesions can generally be distinguished by their appearance as more discrete, grouped vesicles and by a positive Tzanck test (see Chap. 184). In diagnostically difficult cases, cultures of vesicle fluid should yield group A streptococci in impetigo and the responsible virus in herpes virus infection.

Agents active against *S. aureus* and streptococci (such as dicloxacillin, cephalexin, or topical mupirocin ointment) provide the most reliable treatment for impetigo, although penicillin or erythromycin is cheaper and equally effective in cases due to group A streptococci. Rheumatic fever is not a sequel to streptococcal skin infections (as opposed to pharyngitis), although poststreptococcal glomerulonephritis may follow either skin or throat infection. The reason for this difference is not known. One hypothesis is that the immune response necessary for the development of rheumatic fever occurs only after infection of the pharyngeal mucosa. In addition, the strains of group A streptococci that cause pharyngitis generally have a different type of M protein than those associated with skin infections; thus, the strains that cause pharyngitis may have rheumatogenic potential, while the skin-infecting strains may not.

Cellulitis Inoculation of organisms into the skin may lead to infection involving the skin and subcutaneous tissues, or cellulitis. The portal of entry may be a traumatic or surgical wound, an insect bite, or any other break in the skin's integrity. Often, no entry site is apparent.

One form of streptococcal cellulitis, known as *erysipelas*, is characterized by a bright red appearance of the involved skin, which forms a plateau sharply demarcated from the surrounding normal skin. The lesion is warm to the touch, may be tender, and appears shiny and swollen. The skin often has a *peau d'orange* texture, which is thought to reflect involvement of superficial lymphatics; superficial blebs or bullae may form, usually 2 or 3 days after onset. The lesion typically develops over a few hours and is associated with fever and chills. Erysipelas tends to occur in certain characteristic locations: the malar area of the face (often with extension over the bridge of the nose to the contralateral malar region) and the lower extremities. After one episode, recurrence at the same site—sometimes years later—is not uncommon.

Classic cases of erysipelas, with the typical features described above, are almost always due to group A streptococci. Often, however, the appearance of streptococcal cellulitis is not sufficiently distinctive to permit a specific diagnosis on clinical grounds. The area of involvement may not be one of the typical sites for erysipelas; the lesion may be less intensely red than usual and may fade into surrounding skin; and/or the patient may appear only mildly ill. In such cases, it is prudent to broaden the spectrum of empirical antimicrobial therapy to include other pathogens, particularly *S. aureus*, that can produce cellulitis with the same appearance.

Streptococcal cellulitis tends to develop at anatomic sites in which normal lymphatic drainage has been disrupted, such as sites of prior episodes of cellulitis, the arm ipsilateral to a mastectomy and axillary lymph-node dissection, a lower extremity previously involved in deep venous thrombosis or chronic lymphedema, and the leg from which a saphenous vein has been harvested for coronary artery bypass grafting. The organism may enter via a breach in the dermal barrier at a location some distance from the eventual site of clinical cellulitis. For example, some patients with recurrent episodes of leg cellulitis following saphenous vein removal have stopped having recurrent episodes only after treatment of tinea pedis on the foot of the affected extremity, fissures in the skin presumably having served as a portal of entry for streptococci, which then produced infection more proximally in the leg at the site of previous injury. Streptococcal cellulitis may also involve recent surgical wounds. Group A streptococci are among the few bacterial pathogens that typically produce signs of wound infection and surrounding cellulitis within the first 24 h after surgery. These wound infections are usually associated with a thin exudate and may spread rapidly, either as cellulitis in the skin and subcutaneous tissue or as a deeper tissue infection (see below). Streptococcal wound infection or localized cellulitis may also be associated with *lymphangitis*, manifested by red streaks extending proximally along superficial lymphatics from the site of infection.

Deep Soft Tissue Infections *Necrotizing fasciitis*, also referred to as *hemolytic streptococcal gangrene*, is an infection involving the superficial and/or deep fascia investing the muscles of an extremity or the trunk. The source of the infection is either the skin, with organisms introduced into the tissue as a result of trauma (which may be trivial), or the bowel flora, with organisms released during abdominal surgery or from an occult enteric source, such as a diverticular or appendiceal abscess. The site of inoculation in both forms of necrotizing fasciitis may be inapparent and often is some distance from the site of clinical involvement; for example, the introduction of organisms via minor trauma to the hand may be associated with clinical infection of the tissues overlying the shoulder or chest. In cases associated with the bowel flora, the infection is usually polymicrobial, involving a mixture of anaerobic bacteria (such as *Bacteroides fragilis* or anaerobic streptococci) and facultative organisms (usually gram-negative bacilli). Cases unrelated to contamination from bowel or-

ganisms are most commonly caused by group A streptococci, either alone or in combination with other organisms (most often *S. aureus*). Overall, group A streptococci are implicated in about 60 percent of cases of necrotizing fasciitis.

The onset of symptoms is usually quite acute and is marked by severe pain at the site of involvement, malaise, fever, chills, and a toxic appearance. The physical findings, particularly early in the illness, may not be striking, with only minimal erythema of the overlying skin. Pain and tenderness are usually severe; in contrast, in more superficial cellulitis, the appearance of the skin is more abnormal, but pain and tenderness are only mild or moderate. As the infection progresses (often in a matter of several hours), the severity and extent of symptoms worsen, and skin changes become more evident, with the appearance of dusky or mottled erythema and edema. The marked tenderness of the involved area may evolve into anesthesia as the spreading inflammatory process produces infarction of cutaneous nerves. Once the diagnosis is suspected, early surgical exploration is both diagnostically and therapeutically indicated. Surgery reveals necrosis and inflammatory fluid tracking along the fascial planes above and between muscle groups, without involvement of the muscles themselves. The process usually is found to extend beyond the area of clinical involvement, and extensive debridement is required. Drainage and debridement are central to the management of necrotizing fasciitis; antibiotic treatment is a useful adjunct (Table 143-2), but surgery is life-saving.

Although this syndrome is due more commonly to *S. aureus* infection, group A streptococci occasionally produce abscesses in skeletal muscles (*streptococcal myositis*), with little or no involvement of the surrounding fascia or overlying skin. The presentation is usually subacute, but a fulminant form has been described in association with severe systemic toxicity, bacteremia, and a high mortality rate. The fulminant form may reflect the same basic disease process as that seen in necrotizing fasciitis, but with the necrotizing inflammatory process extending into the muscles themselves rather than remaining limited to the fascial layers. Treatment for streptococcal myositis consists of surgical drainage—usually by an open procedure that permits evaluation of the extent of the infection and ensures adequate debridement of involved tissues—and high-dose penicillin (Table 143-2).

PNEUMONIA AND EMPYEMA Group A streptococci are an occasional cause of pneumonia, generally in previously healthy individuals. The onset of symptoms may be abrupt or gradual. Pleuritic chest pain, fever, chills, and dyspnea are the characteristic symptoms. Cough is usually present but may not be prominent. Approximately one-half of patients with group A streptococcal pneumonia have an accompanying pleural effusion. In contrast to the sterile parapneumonic effusions typically seen with pneumococcal pneumonia, the effusions that complicate streptococcal pneumonia are almost always infected. The empyema fluid is usually visible by chest radiography on initial presentation and may increase rapidly in volume. These pleural collections should be drained early, as they tend to become loculated quickly, resulting in a chronic fibrotic reaction that may necessitate thoracotomy for removal.

BACTEREMIA, PUERPERAL SEPSIS, AND STREPTO-COCCAL TOXIC SHOCK-LIKE SYNDROME Group A streptococcal bacteremia is usually associated with an identifiable local infection. Bacteremia occurs rarely with otherwise uncomplicated pharyngitis, occasionally with cellulitis or pneumonia, and relatively frequently with necrotizing fasciitis. Bacteremia without an identified source raises the possibility of endocarditis, an occult abscess, or osteomyelitis. A variety of focal infections may arise secondarily from streptococcal bacteremia, including endocarditis, meningitis, septic arthritis, osteomyelitis, peritonitis, and visceral abscesses.

Group A streptococci are occasionally implicated in infectious complications of childbirth, usually endometritis and associated bacteremia. In the preantibiotic era, puerperal sepsis was commonly caused by group A streptococci, but currently it is more often caused by group B streptococci. Several nosocomial outbreaks of puerperal infection due to group A streptococci have been traced to an asymptomatic carrier, usually an individual present at the time of delivery of the infant. The site of carriage may be the skin, throat, anus, or vagina.

Beginning in the late 1980s, several reports described patients who had group A streptococcal infections associated with shock and multisystem organ failure. This syndrome has been called the *streptococcal toxic shock-like syndrome* because it shares certain features with staphylococcal toxic shock syndrome. In 1993, a case definition for streptococcal toxic shock syndrome was formulated by a working group of clinicians, microbiologists, and epidemiologists in conjunction with the Centers for Disease Control and Prevention (Table 143-3). The general features of the illness include fever, hypotension, renal impairment, and respiratory distress syndrome. Various types of rash have been described, but rash usually does not develop. Laboratory abnormalities include a marked shift to the left in the white blood cell differential, with many immature granulocytes; hypocalcemia; hypoalbuminemia; and thrombocytopenia, which usually becomes more pronounced on the second or third day of illness. In contrast to those with staphylococcal toxic shock, most patients with the streptococcal syndrome are bacteremic. The most common associated infection is a soft tissue infection—necrotizing fasciitis, myositis, or cellulitis—although a variety of other local infections have been described in association with the syndrome, including pneumonia, peritonitis, osteomyelitis, and myometritis. Streptococcal toxic shock syndrome is associated with a mortality rate of 30 percent, with most deaths secondary to shock and respiratory failure. Because of its rapidly progressive and lethal course, early recognition of the syndrome is essential. Patients should be given aggressive supportive care in the form of fluid resuscitation, pressors, and mechanical ventilation in addition to antimicrobial therapy and, in cases associated with necrotizing fasciitis, surgical debridement. Exactly why certain patients develop this fulminant syndrome is not known; however, early studies of the streptococcal strains isolated from these patients demonstrated a strong association with the production of pyrogenic exotoxin A. In more recent case series, particularly from Europe, the syndrome has also been associated with strains producing either exotoxin B or exotoxin C.

Table 143-3

Proposed Case Definition for the Streptococcal Toxic Shock Syndrome*

I. Isolation of group A streptococci (*Streptococcus pyogenes*)
  A. From a normally sterile site (e.g., blood, cerebrospinal fluid, pleural or peritoneal fluid, tissue biopsy, surgical wound)
  B. From a nonsterile site (e.g., throat, sputum, vagina, superficial skin lesion)
II. Clinical signs of severity
  A. Hypotension: Systolic blood pressure of ≤90 mmHg in adults or in the 5th percentile for age in children

and

  B. Two or more of the following signs:
    1. Renal impairment: Serum creatinine level of ≥177 μmol/L (≥2 mg/dL) for adults or at least twice the upper limit of normal for age; in patients with preexisting renal disease, an elevation over the baseline level by a factor of 2 or more
    2. Coagulopathy: Platelet count of ≤100 × 10⁹ per liter (100,000/μL) or disseminated intravascular coagulation defined by prolonged clotting times, low fibrinogen level, and the presence of fibrin degradation products
    3. Liver involvement: Alanine aminotransferase (SGOT), aspartate aminotransferase (SGPT), or total bilirubin level at least twice the upper limit of normal for age; in patients with preexisting liver disease, an elevation over the baseline level by a factor of 2 or more
    4. Adult respiratory distress syndrome, defined by acute onset of diffuse pulmonary infiltrates and hypoxemia in the absence of cardiac failure; or evidence of diffuse capillary leakage manifested by acute onset of generalized edema; or pleural or peritoneal effusions with hypoalbuminemia
    5. Generalized erythematous macular rash that may desquamate
    6. Soft-tissue necrosis, including necrotizing fasciitis or myositis, or gangrene

---

* An illness fulfilling criteria IA, IIA, and IIB is defined as a *definite* case. An illness fulfilling criteria IB, IIA, and IIB is defined as a *probable* case if no other etiology is identified.

SOURCE: Working Group on Severe Streptococcal Infections, 1993.

In light of the possible role of these or other streptococcal toxins in streptococcal toxic shock syndrome, treatment of the affected patients with clindamycin has been advocated by some authorities, who argue that, through its direct action on protein synthesis, clindamycin is more effective in rapidly terminating toxin production than penicillin—a cell-wall agent. Support for this view comes from studies of an experimental model of streptococcal myositis, in which mice treated with clindamycin had a higher rate of survival than those given penicillin. Comparable data on the treatment of human infections are not available.

Intravenous immunoglobulin has been suggested as adjunctive therapy for streptococcal toxic shock; pooled immunoglobulin preparations are likely to contain antibodies capable of neutralizing the effects of streptococcal toxins. Anecdotal reports have suggested favorable clinical responses to intravenous immunoglobulin, but no controlled trials of this modality of therapy have yet been reported.

STREPTOCOCCI OF GROUPS C AND G

Group C and group G streptococci are beta-hemolytic bacteria that occasionally cause human infections similar to those caused by group A streptococci, including pharyngitis, pneumonia, cellulitis and soft-tissue infection, bacteremia, septic arthritis, and endocarditis. Group C or G streptococcal bacteremia occurs most often in patients who are elderly or chronically ill and, in the absence of an obvious local infection, is likely to reflect endocarditis. Septic arthritis due to these organisms, sometimes involving multiple joints, may complicate endocarditis or may develop in the absence of endocarditis. The response to treatment is slow, and patients with joint infections often require repeated aspiration or open drainage and debridement for cure. Penicillin is the drug of choice for therapy of infections due to group C or G streptococci. Because of the poor clinical response of some patients treated with penicillin alone, the addition of gentamicin (1 mg/kg every 8 h for patients with normal renal function) is recommended for the treatment of endocarditis or septic arthritis.

GROUP B STREPTOCOCCI

Identified first as a cause of mastitis in cows, streptococci belonging to Lancefield group B have since been recognized as a major cause of sepsis and meningitis in human neonates. Group B streptococci also are a frequent cause of peripartum fever in women and an occasional cause of serious infection in nonpregnant adults. Lancefield group B consists of a single species, *S. agalactiae*. This organism is definitively identified by means of serologic studies with antiserum specific for the group B cell wall–associated carbohydrate antigen. A streptococcal isolate can be classified presumptively as belonging to group B on the basis of biochemical tests, including hydrolysis of sodium hippurate (in which 99 percent of isolates are positive), hydrolysis of bile esculin agar (in which 99 to 100 percent are negative), bacitracin susceptibility (in which 92 percent are resistant), and production of CAMP factor (in which 98 to 100 percent are positive). CAMP factor is a phospholipase produced by group B streptococci that results in synergistic hemolysis with beta lysin produced by certain strains of *S. aureus*. Its presence can be demonstrated by cross-streaking of the test isolate and an appropriate staphylococcal strain on a blood agar plate. Group B streptococci causing human infections are encapsulated by one of nine antigenically distinct polysaccharides. The capsular polysaccharide has been shown experimentally to be important in the virulence of the organism. Antibodies to the capsular polysaccharide afford protection against group B streptococci of the same (but not of a different) capsular type.

INFECTION IN NEONATES Two general types of group B streptococcal infection in infants are defined by the age of the patient at presentation. Early-onset infections occur within the first week of life, with a median age of 20 h at the onset of illness. Approximately half of these infants have signs of group B streptococcal disease at birth. The infection is acquired during or shortly before birth from organisms colonizing the maternal genital tract. Surveillance studies have shown that 5 to 40 percent of women are vaginal or rectal carriers of group B streptococci. Approximately 50 percent of infants delivered vaginally by carrier mothers become colonized, although only 1 to 2 percent of those colonized develop clinically evident infection. Prematurity and maternal risk factors (prolonged labor, obstetric complications, and maternal fever) are often involved. The presentation of early-onset infection is the same as that of other forms of neonatal sepsis. Typical findings include respiratory distress, lethargy, and hypotension. Essentially all infants with early-onset disease are bacteremic, one-third to one-half have pneumonia and/or respiratory distress syndrome, and one-third have meningitis.

Late-onset infections occur in infants between 1 week and 3 months of age, with a mean age at onset of 3 to 4 weeks. The infecting organism may be acquired during birth (as in early-onset cases) or during later contact with a colonized mother, nursery personnel, or another source. Meningitis is the most common manifestation of late-onset infection and in most cases is associated with a strain of capsular type III. Infants present with fever, lethargy or irritability, poor feeding, and seizures. Poor prognostic signs include presentation with hypotension, coma, status epilepticus, or neutropenia. Up to 50 percent of survivors have some degree of long-term neurologic impairment, ranging from mild language delay or hearing loss to profound mental retardation, blindness, and uncontrolled seizures. A variety of other types of late-onset infection occur, including bacteremia without an identified source, osteomyelitis, septic arthritis, and facial cellulitis associated with submandibular or preauricular adenitis.

Penicillin is the treatment of choice for all group B streptococcal infections. Empirical broad-spectrum therapy for suspected neonatal bacterial sepsis, consisting of ampicillin and gentamicin, is generally administered until culture results become available. If cultures yield group B streptococci, many pediatricians continue to administer gentamicin, along with ampicillin or penicillin, for a few days until clinical improvement becomes evident. This practice is based on in vitro studies showing synergistic killing of group B streptococci by gentamicin and either of the latter two agents in combination. For infants with group B streptococcal meningitis, combined therapy for the first few days certainly is recommended, although rigorous clinical data to support this view are lacking. Therapy with penicillin alone should be continued for 10 days for bacteremia and local infections and for a minimum of 14 days for meningitis because of the risk of relapse in patients treated with shorter courses.

The incidence of group B streptococcal infection is unusually high among infants of women with risk factors: preterm delivery, early rupture of membranes (>24 h before delivery), prolonged labor, fever, or chorioamnionitis. Because the usual source of the organisms infecting a neonate is the mother's birth canal, efforts have been made to prevent group B streptococcal infections by the identification of high-risk carrier mothers and the administration of various forms of antibiotic or immunoprophylaxis. Prophylactic administration of ampicillin or penicillin to such patients during delivery has been shown to reduce the risk of infection in the newborn. This approach has been hampered by the logistical difficulties of identifying colonized women before delivery, since the results of vaginal cultures early in pregnancy are poor predictors of carrier status at the time of delivery. The Centers for Disease Control and Prevention have suggested the following approach to the prevention of neonatal group B streptococcal infection: Women should be screened for anogenital colonization at 35 to 37 weeks of pregnancy by means of a swab culture of the lower vagina and anorectum, and intrapartum chemoprophylaxis should be offered to all carriers and *recommended* to those carriers with any of the risk factors noted above, those anticipating multiple births, and those who have previously given birth to an infant with group B streptococcal infection. The recommended regimen is 5 million units of penicillin

G followed by 2.5 million units every 4 h until delivery. Clindamycin or erythromycin may be substituted in women allergic to penicillin.

There is controversy about whether to recommend chemoprophylaxis to carriers without risk factors: Although 25 percent of neonatal infections occur in infants born to women without risk factors, the risk of infection in such neonates is much lower than that in infants delivered to women with risk factors. Treatment of all carriers will result in the exposure of 15 to 25 percent of pregnant women and newborns to antibiotics, with the attendant risks of allergic reactions and selection for resistant organisms. A group B streptococcal vaccine—still in the developmental stages—ultimately may offer a better method of prevention. Because transplacental passage of maternal antibodies produces protective antibody levels in the newborn, efforts are under way to develop a vaccine against group B streptococci that can be given to women of childbearing age before or during pregnancy.

INFECTION IN ADULTS   The majority of group B streptococcal infections in adults are related to pregnancy and parturition. Peripartum fever, the most common manifestation, is sometimes accompanied by symptoms and signs of endometritis or chorioamnionitis (abdominal distention and uterine or adnexal tenderness). Blood cultures often are positive, as are cultures of vaginal swabs. Bacteremia is usually transitory but occasionally results in meningitis or endocarditis. Infections in adults that are not associated with the peripartum period generally involve individuals who are elderly or have some underlying chronic illness, such as diabetes mellitus or a malignancy. Infections that develop with some frequency in adults include cellulitis and soft-tissue infection (including infected diabetic skin ulcers), urinary tract infection, pneumonia, endocarditis, and septic arthritis. Less commonly reported infections include meningitis, osteomyelitis, and intraabdominal or pelvic abscesses.

Group B streptococci are less sensitive to penicillin than group A organisms, requiring drug concentrations 10 to 100 times higher for inhibition of growth in vitro. Therefore, somewhat higher doses of penicillin are needed for the treatment of group B infections. Adults with serious localized infections (pneumonia, pyelonephritis, abscess) should receive doses in the range of 12 million units of penicillin G daily, while patients with endocarditis or meningitis should receive 18 to 24 million units per day in divided doses. Vancomycin is an acceptable alternative for patients allergic to penicillin.

ENTEROCOCCI AND GROUP D STREPTOCOCCI

Lancefield group D includes the enterococci, organisms now classified in a separate genus from other streptococci, and nonenterococcal group D streptococci. Enterococci are distinguished from nonenterococcal group D streptococci by their ability to grow in the presence of 6.5 percent sodium chloride and by the results of other biochemical tests. The enterococcal species that are significant pathogens for humans are *E. faecalis* and *E. faecium*. These organisms tend to produce infection in patients who are elderly or debilitated or in whom mucosal or epithelial barriers have been disrupted or the balance of the normal flora altered by antibiotic treatment. Urinary tract infections due to enterococci are quite common, particularly among patients who have received antibiotic treatment or undergone instrumentation of the urinary tract. Enterococci account for 10 to 20 percent of cases of bacterial endocarditis on both native and prosthetic valves. The presentation of enterococcal endocarditis is usually subacute but may also be acute, with rapidly progressive valve destruction. Enterococci frequently are cultured from bile and are involved in infectious complications of biliary surgery and in liver abscesses. Moreover, enterococci often are isolated from polymicrobial infections arising from the bowel flora (e.g., intraabdominal abscesses), from abdominal surgical wounds, and from diabetic foot ulcers. While such mixed infections frequently are cured by antimicrobials not active against enterococci, specific therapy directed against enterococci is warranted when these organisms are the predominant species or are isolated from blood cultures.

Unlike other streptococci, enterococci are not reliably killed by penicillin or ampicillin alone at concentrations achieved clinically in the blood or tissues. Because in vitro testing has shown evidence of synergistic killing of most enterococcal strains by the combination of penicillin or ampicillin with an aminoglycoside, combined therapy is recommended for serious enterococcal infections. Ampicillin reaches sufficiently high urinary concentrations to constitute adequate single-drug therapy for uncomplicated urinary tract infections. For other types of enterococcal infection, however, the addition of gentamicin at moderate doses (e.g., 1 mg/kg every 8 h for patients with normal renal function) is recommended. Vancomycin, in combination with gentamicin, may be substituted for penicillin in the treatment of allergic patients. Enterococci are resistant to all cephalosporins; therefore, this class of antibiotics should not be used for the treatment of enterococcal infections.

The antimicrobial susceptibility of enterococcal isolates from patients with serious infections should be evaluated routinely and therapy adjusted according to the results (Table 143-4). Most enterococci are resistant to streptomycin, and this drug should not be used for the treatment of enterococcal infection unless in vitro testing of the strain indicates susceptibility. Though less widespread than streptomycin resistance, high-level resistance to gentamicin [minimum inhibitory concentration (MIC), greater than 2000 μg/mL] has become common. Gentamicin-resistant enterococci should be tested for susceptibility to other aminoglycosides; occasional gentamicin-resistant enterococci are sensitive to streptomycin. If the isolate is resistant to all aminoglycosides, treatment with penicillin or ampicillin alone may be successful. The prolonged administration (i.e., for at least 6 weeks) of high-dose ampicillin (e.g., 12 g/day) is recommended for endocarditis due to these highly resistant enterococci.

Enterococci may be resistant to penicillins by two distinct mechanisms. The first is the production of β-lactamase (mediating resistance to penicillin and ampicillin), which has been reported for *E. faecalis* isolates from several locations in the United States and other countries. Because the amount of β-lactamase produced by enterococci may be insufficient for detection by routine antibiotic susceptibility testing, isolates from serious infections should be screened specifically for β-lactamase production with use of a chromogenic cephalosporin or by another method. For the treatment of infections caused by β-lactamase–producing strains, vancomycin, ampicillin/sulbactam, amoxicillin/clavulanate, or imipenem may be used in combination with gentamicin.

The second mechanism of penicillin resistance is not mediated by β-lactamase and may be due to altered penicillin-binding proteins. This intrinsic penicillin resistance is common among isolates of *E. faecium*, which routinely are more resistant to β-lactam antibiotics than are isolates of *E. faecalis*. Moderately resistant enterococci (MICs of penicillin and ampicillin, 16 to 64 μg/mL) may be susceptible to high-dose penicillin or ampicillin in combination with gentamicin, but strains with MICs of ≥200 μg/mL must be considered resistant to clinically achievable levels of β-lactam antibiotics, including imipenem. Vancomycin plus gentamicin is the recommended regimen for infections due to enterococci with high-level intrinsic resistance to β-lactams.

Vancomycin-resistant enterococci, first reported from clinical sources in the late 1980s, have become relatively common in many hospitals. Three major vancomycin resistance phenotypes have been described: VanA, VanB, and VanC. The VanA phenotype is associated with high-level resistance to vancomycin and to teicoplanin, a related glycopeptide antibiotic not currently available in the United States. VanB and VanC strains are resistant to vancomycin but susceptible to teicoplanin, although teicoplanin resistance may develop during treatment in VanB strains. For enterococci resistant to both vancomycin and β-lactams, there are no established therapies. Regimens that have been tried with some success in individual cases or experimentally include ciprofloxacin plus rifampin plus gentamicin; ampicillin plus vancomycin (particularly if in vitro testing shows synergistic bacteriostatic activity); and chloramphenicol or tetracycline (if the strain is susceptible in vitro).

The main nonenterococcal group D streptococcal species that causes human infections is *Streptococcus bovis*. *S. bovis* endocarditis is often associated with neoplasms of the gastrointestinal tract—most frequently a colon carcinoma or polyp. When occult gastrointestinal lesions are carefully sought, abnormalities are found in at least 60 percent of patients with *S. bovis* endocarditis. In contrast to the enterococci, nonenterococcal group D streptococci like *S. bovis* are reliably killed by penicillin as a single agent, and penicillin is the treatment of choice for *S. bovis* infections.

VIRIDANS AND OTHER STREPTOCOCCI

Consisting of multiple species of alpha-hemolytic streptococci, the viridans streptococci are a heterogeneous group of organisms that are important as agents of bacterial endocarditis. Several species of viridans streptococci, including *Streptococcus salivarius*, *Streptococcus mutans*, *Streptococcus sanguis*, and *Streptococcus mitis*, are part of the normal flora of the mouth, where they live in close association with the teeth and gingiva. Some species contribute to the development of dental caries. The transient viridans streptococcal bacteremia induced by eating, tooth-brushing, flossing, and other sources of minor trauma, together with adherence to biologic surfaces, is thought to account for the tendency of these organisms to cause endocarditis. Viridans streptococci are also isolated, often as part of a mixed flora, from sites of sinusitis, brain abscess, and liver abscess.

Viridans streptococcal bacteremia occurs relatively frequently in neutropenic patients, particularly after bone marrow transplantation or high-dose chemotherapy for cancer. Some of these patients develop a sepsis syndrome with high fever and shock. Risk factors for viridans streptococcal bacteremia include antibiotic prophylaxis with trimethoprim-sulfamethoxazole or a fluoroquinolone, mucositis, treatment with antacids or histamine antagonists, and profound neutropenia. Because many of the viridans streptococci isolated from the blood in the setting of neutropenia are resistant to penicillin, neutropenic patients with bacteremia should be treated presumptively with vancomycin until the results of susceptibility testing become available.

The organisms referred to as the *Streptococcus intermedius* or *Streptococcus milleri* group (*Streptococcus intermedius*, *Streptococcus anginosus*, and *Streptococcus constellatus*) often are considered to be viridans streptococci, although they differ somewhat from other viridans streptococci in both their hemolytic pattern (they are often beta-hemolytic) and the disease syndromes they cause. These organisms commonly produce suppurative infections, particularly abscesses of brain and abdominal viscera.

As noted above, isolates from neutropenic patients with bacteremia frequently are resistant to penicillin; viridans streptococci isolated in other clinical settings usually are sensitive to penicillin. Occasional isolates cultured from the blood of patients with endocarditis fail to grow when subcultured on solid media. These *nutritionally variant*

Table 143-4

Treatment Options for Antibiotic-Resistant Enterococcal Infections

Resistance Pattern	Recommended Therapy
β-Lactamase production	Gentamicin plus ampicillin/sulbactam, amoxicillin/clavulanate, imipenem, or vancomycin
β-Lactam resistance, but no β-lactamase production	Gentamicin plus vancomycin
High-level gentamicin resistance	Streptomycin-sensitive isolate: Streptomycin plus ampicillin or vancomycin
	Streptomycin-resistant isolate: No proven therapy (continuous-infusion ampicillin, prolonged treatment)
Vancomycin resistance	Ampicillin plus gentamicin
Vancomycin and β-lactam resistance	Unknown; teicoplanin active against strains with low-level vancomycin resistance (VanB or VanC phenotype, but not VanA)

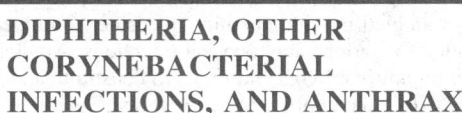

DIPHTHERIA, OTHER CORYNEBACTERIAL INFECTIONS, AND ANTHRAX

streptococci require supplemental thiol compounds or active forms of vitamin B_6 (pyridoxal or pyridoxamine) for growth in the laboratory. Because treatment failure and relapse appear to be more common for cases of endocarditis due to nutritionally variant streptococci than for those due to nutritionally standard viridans streptococci, the addition of gentamicin (1 mg/kg every 8 h for patients with normal renal function) to the penicillin regimen is recommended for therapy of endocarditis due to these organisms.

Streptococcus suis is an important pathogen in swine and has been reported to cause meningitis in humans, usually in individuals with occupational exposure to pigs. Strains of *S. suis* associated with human infections have generally reacted with Lancefield group R typing serum and sometimes with group D typing serum as well. Isolates may be alpha- or beta-hemolytic and have been shown to be sensitive to penicillin.

Anaerobic streptococci, or peptostreptococci, are part of the normal flora of the oral cavity, bowel, and vagina. They are involved, usually along with other organisms, in brain abscess, sinusitis, dental abscess, and other odontogenic infections (Ludwig's angina, abscesses of the retropharyngeal or lateral pharyngeal space); in aspiration pneumonia, lung abscess, and empyema; and in intraabdominal and pelvic abscesses. Anaerobic and microaerophilic streptococci, together with facultative bacteria, may also play a role in invasive soft-tissue infections—generally those related to trauma or surgical wounds. Management of these infections involves debridement of infected tissues and treatment with high-dose penicillin (12 to 18 million units per day for serious infections).

BIBLIOGRAPHY

BASILIERE JL et al: Streptococcal pneumonia. Am J Med 44:580, 1968

BISNO AL: Group A streptococcal infections and acute rheumatic fever. N Engl J Med 325:783, 1991

————, STEVENS DL: Streptococcal infections of skin and soft tissues. N Engl J Med 334:240, 1996

CENTERS FOR DISEASE CONTROL AND PREVENTION: Prevention of perinatal group B streptococcal disease: A public health perspective. Morb Mort Week Rep 45(RR-7):1, 1996

EDWARDS MS, BAKER CJ: *Streptococcus agalactiae* (group B *Streptococcus*), in *Principles and Practice of Infectious Diseases*, 4th ed, GL Mandell et al (eds). New York, Churchill Livingstone, 1995, p 1835

ELIOPOULOS GM: Increasing problems in the therapy of enterococcal infections. Eur J Clin Microbiol Infect Dis 12:409, 1993

ELTING LS et al: Septicemia and shock syndrome due to viridans streptococci: A case-control study of predisposing factors. Clin Infect Dis 14:1201, 1992

KLEIN RS et al: Association of *Streptococcus bovis* with carcinoma of the colon. N Engl J Med 297:800, 1977

LANCEFIELD RC: A serological differentiation of human and other groups of hemolytic streptococci. J Exp Med 57:571, 1933

MOELLERING RC JR: Emergence of *Enterococcus* as a significant pathogen. Clin Infect Dis 14:1173, 1992

STEVENS DL et al: Severe group A streptococcal infections associated with a toxic shock-like syndrome and scarlet fever toxin A. N Engl J Med 321:1, 1989

VARTIAN C et al: Infections due to Lancefield group G streptococci. Medicine 6:75, 1985

VIGLIONESE A et al: Recurrent group A streptococcal carriage in a health care worker associated with widely separated nosocomial outbreaks. Am J Med 91(Suppl 3B):329S, 1991

WANNAMAKER LW: Differences between streptococcal infections of the throat and of the skin. N Engl J Med 282:23, 78, 1970

WELLS VD et al: Infections due to beta-lactamase-producing, high-level gentamicin-resistant *Enterococcus faecalis*. Ann Intern Med 116:285, 1992

WORKING GROUP ON SEVERE STREPTOCOCCAL INFECTIONS: Defining the group A streptococcal toxic shock syndrome. JAMA 269:390, 1993

YODER EL et al: Spontaneous gangrenous myositis induced by *Streptococcus pyogenes*: Case report and review of the literature. Rev Infect Dis 9:382, 1987

DIPHTHERIA

DEFINITION   Diphtheria is a localized infection of mucous membranes or skin caused by *Corynebacterium diphtheriae*. A characteristic pseudomembrane may be present at the site of infection. Some strains of *C. diphtheriae* produce diphtheria toxin, a protein that can cause myocarditis, polyneuritis, and other systemic toxic effects. Respiratory diphtheria is usually caused by toxinogenic (tox[+]) *C. diphtheriae*, but cutaneous diphtheria is frequently caused by nontoxinogenic (tox[−]) strains.

ETIOLOGIC AGENT   *C. diphtheriae* is an aerobic, nonmotile, nonsporulating, irregularly staining, gram-positive rod. The bacteria are 2 to 6 μm long, 0.5 to 1 μm wide, club-shaped, and often arranged in clusters (*Chinese letters*) or parallel arrays (*palisades*). *C. diphtheriae* forms gray to black colonies on selective media containing tellurite. Three biotypes, designated *gravis*, *mitis*, and *intermedius*, are distinguished on the basis of colonial morphology and laboratory tests. Both tox[+] and tox[−] strains cause infections, and tox[+] strains of all three biotypes can cause severe disease.

The gene for diphtheria toxin is present in specific corynephages. Nontoxinogenic *C. diphtheriae* acquires the ability to produce diphtheria toxin by infection with tox[+] phages, a process termed *phage conversion*. Growth of *C. diphtheriae* under low-iron conditions mimicking the environment of host tissues induces the synthesis of diphtheria toxin and the expression of a siderophore-dependent, high-affinity iron uptake system.

IMMUNOLOGY   Treatment of diphtheria toxin with formaldehyde converts it to a nontoxic product called *diphtheria toxoid*. Immunization with toxoid elicits antibody (*antitoxin*) that neutralizes the toxin and prevents diphtheria. No specific amount of antitoxin provides absolute protection against diphtheria, but the attack rate and the mortality rate for diphtheria are much lower in individuals with >0.01 unit of antitoxin per milliliter. This antitoxin level is often used, therefore, as an index of immunity in epidemiologic studies. Antitoxin neither prevents colonization by *C. diphtheriae* nor eradicates the carrier state. If most individuals in a population have antitoxic immunity, however, the carriage of tox[+] strains of *C. diphtheriae* decreases to a low level. Thus, herd immunity reduces the risk that nonimmune individuals in the population will be exposed to tox[+] *C. diphtheriae*. Nonimmune individuals may contract diphtheria if they travel to regions where the disease is present or if tox[+] strains of *C. diphtheriae* are introduced into their community.

EPIDEMIOLOGY AND IMMUNITY   Humans are the reservoir for *C. diphtheriae*. The organism is transmitted primarily by close contact of diphtheria patients or carriers with susceptible individuals, but the risk of transmission from patients appears to be substantially greater than that of transmission from asymptomatic carriers. Transmission involving fomites and indirect routes is less common, although *C. diphtheriae* can survive for weeks to months in the environment. The incubation period for respiratory diphtheria is typically 2 to 5 days and rarely up to 8 days. Cutaneous diphtheria is usually a secondary infection whose signs develop an average of 7 days (range, 1 to >21 days) after the appearance of primary skin lesions.

In populations in temperate climates, diphtheria primarily involves the respiratory tract; occurs throughout the year, with a peak incidence in colder months; and is usually caused by tox[+] strains. Before the introduction of active immunization, diphtheria was generally a disease of children; it affected up to 10 percent of individuals in this group and sometimes occurred in devastating epidemics. Most infants were immune because of transplacental transfer of maternal IgG antitoxin, but children became susceptible by 6 to 12 months of age. Approximately 75 percent of individuals became immune by age 10 as a result of clinical or subclinical infection with *C. diphtheriae*. Mortality rates of 30 to 40 percent were common in untreated disease and sometimes exceeded 50 percent in epidemics. Treatment with antitoxin reduced the case-fatality rate to 5 to 10 percent.

Routine immunization of children in the United States resulted in a progressively decreasing incidence of diphtheria (from more than 206,000 cases in 1921 to few or no cases per year recently) that was accompanied by a shift of cases to older age groups; however, the case-fatality rate remained at 5 to 10 percent. High rates of immunization (96 percent) are now achieved by the time of school entry, but rates for younger children are substantially lower. Among adults over 20 years of age, 20 to 60 percent are susceptible to diphtheria. Large local outbreaks of diphtheria occurred in San Antonio, TX, in 1969 to 1970 (201 cases) and in Seattle, WA, in 1972 to 1982 (1100 cases). Alcoholism, low socioeconomic status, crowded living conditions, and Native American ethnic background were significant risk factors in these and other recent outbreaks. A report from England in 1992 described pharyngeal infections with tox⁻ *C. diphtheriae* developing predominantly among homosexual men; they often caused symptomatic pharyngitis and sometimes resulted in a tonsillar exudate.

A massive and expanding epidemic of diphtheria has been under way since 1990 in 14 of the 15 new independent states of the former Soviet Union, with 47,802 cases and 1746 deaths reported for 1994. Approximately 70 percent of cases have occurred in persons ≥15 years of age. Case-fatality rates have varied from 2.8 percent in the Russian Federation to 23 percent in Lithuania and Turkmenistan. Twenty imported cases related to this epidemic have already been reported in European countries, and two cases have been acquired by U.S. citizens in Russia and Ukraine.

In the tropics, cutaneous diphtheria is more common than respiratory diphtheria, occurs throughout the year, and often develops as a secondary infection complicating other dermatoses. Isolates of *C. diphtheriae* from skin lesions are more often tox⁻ than tox⁺. A study in Rangoon, Burma, demonstrated *C. diphtheriae* (18.5 percent tox⁺ strains) in more than 60 percent of bacterially infected skin lesions in patients under 12 years of age. Eighty percent of isolates were from impetiginous scabies, and most other isolates were from impetiginous eczema or impetigo. Cutaneous diphtheria has also been recognized increasingly in temperate climates during the past two decades; it accounted for 86 percent of the 1100 cases in the Seattle outbreak of 1972 to 1982.

PATHOLOGY AND PATHOGENESIS   *C. diphtheriae* infects mucous membranes, most commonly in the respiratory tract, and also invades open skin lesions resulting from insect bites or trauma. In infections caused by tox⁺ *C. diphtheriae*, initial edema and hyperemia are often followed by epithelial necrosis and acute inflammation. Coagulation of the dense fibrinopurulent exudate produces a pseudomembrane, and the inflammatory reaction accompanied by vascular congestion extends into the underlying tissues. The pseudomembrane contains large numbers of *C. diphtheriae*, but the bacterium is rarely isolated from the blood or internal organs.

Diphtheria toxin acts both locally and systemically. Very small amounts cause dermonecrosis, and toxin presumably contributes to pseudomembrane formation. The lethal dose of diphtheria toxin for nonimmune humans and highly susceptible animals is about 0.1 μg/kg of body weight. Absorbed toxin can cause myocarditis, neuritis, and focal necrosis in various organs, including the kidneys, liver, and adrenal glands. Early changes in diphtheritic myocarditis include cloudy swelling of muscle fibers and interstitial edema. These changes are followed within weeks by hyaline and granular degeneration of muscle fibers (sometimes with fatty degeneration of the myocardium) progressing to myolysis and finally to the replacement of lost muscle by fibrosis. Thus, diphtheria can cause permanent cardiac damage. In diphtheritic polyneuritis, pathologic changes include patchy breakdown of myelin sheaths in peripheral and autonomic nerves, but recovery of nerve damage is the rule if the patient survives.

Diphtheria toxin is produced by *C. diphtheriae* as an extracellular polypeptide. It is cleaved by proteases to form nicked toxin consisting of fragments A and B. Fragment B binds to a plasma-membrane receptor (a precursor of a heparin-binding growth factor resembling epidermal growth factor) on cells from humans or susceptible animals, and the bound toxin is internalized by receptor-mediated endocytosis. Fragment A is translocated across the endosomal membrane and released into the cytoplasm, where it catalyzes the transfer of the adenosine diphosphate ribose moiety from nicotinamide adenine dinucleotide (NAD) to a modified histidine residue (diphthamide) on elongation factor 2 (EF-2), thereby inactivating EF-2 and inhibiting protein synthesis. One molecule of fragment A in the cytoplasm can kill a cell. Other metabolic alterations in intoxicated cells are secondary to inhibition of protein synthesis.

CLINICAL MANIFESTATIONS   Patients with *C. diphtheriae* in the respiratory tract are classified as diphtheria cases if they have symptoms consistent with local infection and as diphtheria carriers if they are asymptomatic. Signs and symptoms vary with the site and severity of the local infection, the patient's age, and the patient's status with regard to preexisting nasopharyngeal disease and concomitant systemic disease. The onset is often gradual, but most patients seek medical care within a few days of becoming ill. Sore throat is the most common symptom, but children are less likely than adults to complain of sore throat and are more likely to have nausea and vomiting. Fever of 37.8 to 38.9°C (100 to 102°F) and dysphagia are documented in about half of patients; cough, hoarseness, chills, and rhinorrhea are less common. Systemic manifestations are due primarily to the effects of diphtheria toxin. Patients without toxicity exhibit discomfort and malaise associated with local infection, whereas severely toxic patients may develop listlessness, pallor, and tachycardia that can progress rapidly to vascular collapse.

Primary infection in the respiratory tract is most often tonsillopharyngeal (one-half to two-thirds of cases) but also may be (in decreasing order of frequency) laryngeal, nasal, and tracheobronchial. Multiple sites are frequently involved, and secondary spread of pharyngeal infection upward to the nasal mucosa or downward to the larynx and tracheobronchial tree is much more common than primary infection at those sites. Systemic toxicity is usually less severe in nasal diphtheria than in tonsillopharyngeal diphtheria and is most severe when pseudomembrane extends from the tonsils and pharynx into contiguous regions. A small percentage of patients present with malignant, or "bull-neck," diphtheria, with abrupt onset, extensive pseudomembrane formation, foul breath, massive swelling of the tonsils and uvula, thick speech, cervical lymphadenopathy, striking edematous swelling of the submandibular region and anterior neck, and severe toxicity.

In tonsillopharyngeal diphtheria, only erythema may be noted initially, but isolated spots of gray or white exudate are common. These spots often extend and coalesce within a day to form a confluent, sharply demarcated pseudomembrane that becomes progressively thicker, more tightly adherent to the underlying tissue, and darker gray. Unlike the exudate in streptococcal pharyngitis, the diphtheritic pseudomembrane often extends beyond the margin of the tonsils onto the tonsillar pillars, palate, or uvula. Dislodgement of the membrane is likely to cause bleeding. Estimates of the proportion of patients with pharyngeal diphtheria who develop typical pseudomembranes vary widely, from as few as one-third to almost all. Patients with nasal diphtheria often present with serosanguineous nasal discharge, which may be unilateral or bilateral and may cause irritation of the nares or the lip. Laryngeal diphtheria often presents as hoarseness and cough. Demonstration of laryngeal pseudomembrane by laryngoscopy is helpful for distinguishing diphtheria from other infectious forms of laryngitis. Primary or secondary diphtheritic infection occasionally involves other mucous membranes, including the conjunctiva and the membranes of the genitourinary and gastrointestinal tracts.

Cutaneous diphtheria usually presents as an infection by *C. diphtheriae* of preexisting dermatoses involving, in decreasing order of frequency, the lower extremities, upper extremities, head, or trunk. The clinical features are similar to those of other secondary cutaneous bacterial infections. In the tropics, the presentation of cutaneous diphtheria occasionally includes morphologically distinct "punched-out" ulcers that are covered by necrotic slough or membrane and have well-demarcated edges.

C. diphtheriae is an occasional cause of invasive infections, including endocarditis and septic arthritis. Risk factors for such infections include preexisting cardiac abnormalities, abuse of intravenous drugs, and alcoholic cirrhosis.

COMPLICATIONS Obstruction of the respiratory tract, presenting as tachypnea, dyspnea, stridor, cyanosis, and use of accessory muscles of respiration, can be caused by extensive pseudomembrane formation and swelling during the first few days of the disease or by sloughed pseudomembrane that becomes lodged in the airways at a later stage in the disease. The risk of respiratory obstruction is greater when infection involves the larynx or the tracheobronchial tree and is higher in children because of the small size of the airways.

Myocarditis and polyneuritis are the most prominent toxic manifestations of diphtheria. The risk of developing these manifestations is proportional to the severity of local disease, and the two can occur together in the same patient. Myocarditis may present during the acute phase of illness, develop as local disease is resolving, or begin insidiously after several weeks. One-half to two-thirds of patients with typical diphtheria have subtle evidence of cardiac dysfunction, including electrocardiographic abnormalities, but clinically apparent myocarditis develops in 10 to 25 percent of patients and is usually more severe when the onset is early. Electrocardiographic abnormalities include ST-T-wave changes, varying degrees of heart block, and arrhythmias, including atrial fibrillation, ventricular premature beats, ventricular tachycardia, and ventricular fibrillation. Clinical signs include diminished heart sounds, gallop rhythm, systolic murmurs, and (less commonly) acute or insidiously progressive congestive heart failure. Serum levels of aspartate aminotransferase reflect the intensity of myocardial damage and can be used to monitor its course.

Polyneuritis is uncommon in mild diphtheria but occurs in approximately 10 percent of cases of average severity and in up to 75 percent of severe cases. Bulbar dysfunction typically develops during the first 2 weeks. Palatal and pharyngeal paralysis usually develop first. Swallowing is difficult, the voice sounds nasal, and ingested fluids may be regurgitated through the nose. With unilateral pharyngeal infection, ipsilateral palatal paralysis is more common than contralateral or bilateral paralysis. Additional bulbar signs may develop over several weeks, with oculomotor and ciliary paralysis occurring more often than facial or laryngeal paralysis. Peripheral polyneuritis typically begins from 1 to 3 months after the onset of diphtheria with proximal weakness of the extremities that spreads distally. The severity of this condition varies from mild weakness of the pelvic muscles with unsteady gait to total paralysis, including failure of respiration. Paresthesias may develop and most often have a glove-and-stocking distribution. Approximately half of patients with diphtheritic neuropathy have evidence of cardiac vagal denervation, and fewer have abnormal baroreceptor function. Polyneuritis usually resolves completely, with the time needed for improvement approximately equal to that elapsing from exposure to the development of symptoms. Since severe muscular weakness may develop 1 to 2 weeks before maximal abnormalities in peripheral-nerve conduction velocity are demonstrated, there may be a striking dissociation between clinical and electrophysiologic findings. Cerebrospinal fluid (CSF) most often contains moderately increased levels of albumin, occasionally with pleocytosis, but the abnormalities in CSF do not determine prognosis.

Pneumonia occurs in more than half of fatal cases of diphtheria. Less common complications include renal failure, encephalitis, cerebral infarction, pulmonary embolism, and bacteremia or endocarditis due to invasive infection by *C. diphtheriae*. Serum sickness may result from antitoxin therapy.

COURSE AND PROGNOSIS Most cases of diphtheria develop in nonimmunized patients. The attack rate, severity of disease, and risk of complications are much lower in immunized patients. The

pseudomembrane may continue to increase in size during the first day after administration of antitoxin. During the next several days to a week, it becomes softer, less adherent, and nonconfluent and eventually disappears. In the preantibiotic era, *C. diphtheriae* persisted in the throat for about 2 weeks in one-half of patients and for 1 month or more in about one-fifth. Mortality increases with the severity of local disease, the extent of pseudomembrane formation, and the interval between onset of local disease and administration of antitoxin. The death rate is highest during the first week of illness; among patients with bull-neck diphtheria; among patients with myocarditis who develop ventricular tachycardia, atrial fibrillation, or complete heart block; among patients with laryngeal or tracheobronchial involvement; among infants and patients over 60 years of age; and among alcoholics. Both mortality and the risk of myocarditis or peripheral neuropathy are significantly lower in cutaneous diphtheria than in respiratory diphtheria.

DIAGNOSIS A characteristic pseudomembrane on the mucosa of the oropharynx, palate, nasopharynx, nose, or larynx suggests diphtheria but is not uniformly present. Diphtheritic pseudomembrane must be distinguished from other pharyngeal exudates, including those of group A beta-hemolytic streptococcal infections, infectious mononucleosis, viral pharyngitides, fusospirochetal infection, and candidiasis. A diagnosis of diphtheria should be considered in patients with sore throat, cervical adenopathy or swelling, and low-grade fever, especially when these manifestations are accompanied by systemic toxicity, hoarseness, stridor, palatal paralysis, or serosanguineous nasal discharge with or without demonstrable pseudomembrane. Treatment with diphtheria antitoxin should be begun as soon as the clinical diagnosis of diphtheria is made.

The definitive diagnosis of diphtheria depends on the isolation of *C. diphtheriae* from local lesions. The laboratory should be notified that diphtheria is suspected to ensure the use of selective tellurite medium appropriate for the isolation of *C. diphtheriae*. All isolates of *C. diphtheriae* should be subjected to toxicity testing. Primary isolates can be screened rapidly for toxinogenicity by the polymerase chain reaction, although occasional strains of *C. diphtheriae* that carry an inactive toxin gene give false-positive results. The biochemical tests needed to differentiate *C. diphtheriae* from corynebacteria of the normal flora (diphtheroids) require several days. Group A beta-hemolytic streptococci and *Staphylococcus aureus* are also isolated frequently from patients with diphtheria.

Cutaneous diphtheria may present as a characteristic punched-out ulcer with a membrane, but it is more often indistinguishable from other inflammatory dermatoses. Its diagnosis depends on a high degree of suspicion and on culture of cutaneous lesions on laboratory media appropriate for the isolation of *C. diphtheriae*. Throat samples from all patients with cutaneous diphtheria should be cultured for *C. diphtheriae*.

℞ **TREATMENT**

The decision to administer diphtheria antitoxin must be based on the clinical diagnosis of diphtheria without definitive laboratory confirmation, since each day of delay in treatment is associated with increased mortality. Because diphtheria antitoxin is produced in horses, it is necessary to inquire about possible allergy to horse serum and to perform a conjunctival or intracutaneous test with diluted antitoxin for immediate hypersensitivity. Epinephrine must be available for immediate administration to patients with severe allergic reactions. Patients with immediate hypersensitivity should be desensitized before a full therapeutic dose of antitoxin is given. The dose of diphtheria antitoxin currently recommended by the Committee on Infectious Diseases of the American Academy of Pediatrics is based on the site of the primary infection and the duration and severity of disease: 20,000 to 40,000 units for disease that has been present for 48 h or less and involves the pharynx or larynx; 40,000 to 60,000 units for nasopharyngeal infections; and 80,000 to 100,000 units for disease that is extensive, has been present for 3 days or longer, or is accompanied by diffuse swelling of the neck. Antitoxin is administered intravenously by infusion in saline over 60 min to neutralize unbound toxin rapidly. The approximately 10 percent risk of serum sickness is acceptable because of the established therapeutic value of antitoxin in decreasing mortality from respiratory diphtheria. During the early phase of the Seattle epidemic, all patients with cutaneous diphtheria received 20,000 units of antitoxin. Later, when most isolates were tox⁻, antitoxin was withheld initially and administered only to patients from whom tox⁺ strains were isolated. The potential systemic complications of cutaneous diphtheria must be weighed against the potential adverse effects of antitoxin treatment; authorities are not unanimous in recommending antitoxin therapy for cutaneous diphtheria.

Antibiotics have little demonstrated effect on the healing of local infection in diphtheria patients treated with antitoxin. The primary goal of antibiotic therapy for patients or carriers is therefore to eradicate *C. diphtheriae* and prevent its transmission from the patient to susceptible contacts. Erythromycin, penicillin G, rifampin, or clindamycin is recommended by most authorities. The commonly recommended regimen for the treatment of adults with respiratory diphtheria is erythromycin (500 mg four times daily, given parenterally or orally) or intramuscular procaine penicillin G (600,000 units at 12-h intervals) for 14 days. Patients with cutaneous diphtheria and carriers can be treated orally with erythromycin (500 mg four times daily) or rifampin (600 mg once daily) for 7 days. If compliance is in question, a single dose of benzathine penicillin G (1.2 to 2.4 million units intramuscularly) can be substituted. Eradication of *C. diphtheriae* should be documented by negative cultures of samples taken on two or three successive days, beginning at least 24 h after the completion of antibiotic therapy. Some authorities also recommend a repeat throat culture 2 weeks later. The small percentage of patients who continue to be infected with *C. diphtheriae* after treatment should receive an additional 10-day course of oral erythromycin or rifampin. Plasmid-mediated erythromycin resistance of the MLS type emerged transiently in *C. diphtheriae* during the Seattle epidemic, but its frequency declined dramatically after the routine use of erythromycin was discontinued.

Patients with respiratory or cutaneous diphtheria caused by tox⁺ strains or by strains of unknown toxinogenicity should be hospitalized, kept in bed initially, handled with isolation procedures appropriate for the site of infection, and given supportive care as needed. Respiratory and cardiac function must be monitored closely. Early intubation or tracheostomy is recommended when the larynx is involved or signs of impending airway obstruction are detected. Tracheobronchial membrane can sometimes be removed mechanically via the endotracheal tube or tracheostomy. Primary or secondary pneumonia should be diagnosed and treated promptly. Sedative or hypnotic drugs that may mask respiratory symptoms are contraindicated. Close electrocardiographic monitoring, treatment of arrhythmias, and electrical pacing for heart block are essential. Congestive heart failure should be treated as described in Chap. 233. Glucocorticoids do not reduce the risk of diphtheritic myocarditis or polyneuritis. Oral therapy with DL-carnitine (100 mg/kg per day, given in twice-daily doses for 4 days) may have a beneficial effect in diphtheritic myocarditis, but such therapy should be considered experimental until additional data become available. Ulcerative or ecthymatous cutaneous lesions should be treated with Burow's solution applied on wet compresses after debridement of necrotic areas, and treatment for associated conditions such as pediculosis, scabies, or underlying dermatoses should be instituted.

PREVENTION Vaccines available in the United States for immunization against diphtheria include diphtheria and tetanus toxoids and pertussis vaccine adsorbed (DTP), diphtheria and tetanus toxoids and acellular pertussis vaccine adsorbed (DTaP), diphtheria and tetanus toxoids adsorbed (DT; for pediatric use), and tetanus and diphtheria toxoids adsorbed (Td; for adult use). The adsorbent is alum, which functions as an adjuvant and enhances the immunogenicity of the vaccines. Td contains less diphtheria toxoid than DTP, DTaP, or DT and causes fewer adverse reactions in adults.

The recommended schedule for primary immunization against diphtheria for children from 2 months of age up to the seventh birthday consists of five doses of vaccine administered intramuscularly: three doses of DTP at 2-month intervals beginning at age 2 months, a fourth dose 6 to 12 months after the third dose, and a fifth dose at the age of 4 to 6 years—before entry into kindergarten or elementary school. DTaP can be substituted for DTP for doses 4 and 5 in children aged 15 months or older. Some preparations of DTP and *Haemophilus influenzae* type b conjugate vaccine are approved for administration as a single injection to children scheduled to receive the two vaccines separately. DT is substituted for DTP if pertussis vaccine is contraindicated. The fifth (preschool) dose of DTP, DTaP, or DT is omitted if the fourth dose is administered after the fourth birthday.

If immunization is delayed until after the seventh birthday, the recommended primary series consists of two doses of Td given 1 to 2 months apart and followed by a third dose 6 to 12 months after the second dose. If primary immunization is interrupted, the series should simply be completed; there is no need to start a new series. Adults with an uncertain history of immunization against diphtheria should receive a primary series.

Periodic booster doses of diphtheria toxoid are required to maintain immunity. The Task Force on Adult Immunization currently supports two regimens. Either doses of Td should be given at 10-year intervals after the completion of primary immunization and throughout adult life, or a single dose of Td should be given at age 50 to individuals who have completed a full primary series and have received a teenage/young adult booster dose. Among patients who require tetanus toxoid for wound management, use of DTP, DTaP, DT, or Td as appropriate, given the individual's age and specific contraindications, is recommended for the maintenance of immunity to diphtheria as well as tetanus. All patients should undergo active immunization after treatment for diphtheria, since infection does not necessarily confer immunity.

Close contacts of patients with diphtheria should be cultured for *C. diphtheriae*, kept under surveillance for 1 week, and treated with appropriate antibiotics if cultures are positive. Previously immunized close contacts should receive an appropriate booster injection including diphtheria toxoid if their last booster dose was given more than 5 years previously. If their immunization status is uncertain, close contacts should receive an antibiotic regimen appropriate for carriers and a primary immunization series appropriate for their age.

OTHER CORYNEBACTERIAL INFECTIONS

DEFINITION Medically important *coryneform bacteria* (formerly called *diphtheroids*) include members of the normal flora that cause opportunistic infections, human pathogens of relatively low virulence, and animal pathogens that cause occasional zoonotic infections. Reported infections caused by coryneform bacteria have increased substantially in number over the past two decades. Isolates of *Corynebacterium jeikeium* and group D-2 coryneform bacteria are often resistant to multiple antibiotics.

ETIOLOGIC AGENTS AND LABORATORY DIAGNOSIS Because coryneform bacteria are potential pathogens, it is important not to dismiss them as constituents of the normal flora or as contaminants when they are found in clinical specimens. Laboratory differentiation of coryneform bacteria is important when they are isolated repeatedly, when they are recovered in pure culture or in large numbers, or when they form pigmented or hemolytic colonies.

The coryneform bacteria are a large, taxonomically heterogeneous, poorly classified group of gram-positive, pleomorphic, irregularly staining bacilli or coccobacilli that superficially resemble *C. diphtheriae*. The scheme recommended by the Centers for Disease Control and Prevention (CDC) for the classification of coryneform bacteria assigns them to several genera, including *Actinomyces*, *Arcanobacterium*, *Corynebacterium*, *Oerskovia*, and *Rhodococcus*, as well as to several groups that have not yet been categorized at the genus and species level.

ECOLOGY AND EPIDEMIOLOGY Humans are the probable natural reservoir for *Corynebacterium xerosis*, *Corynebacterium* *pseudodiphtheriticum* (formerly *Corynebacterium hofmannii*), *Corynebacterium striatum*, *Corynebacterium minutissimum*, *Corynebacterium jeikeium* (fomerly CDC group JK), *Arcanobacterium haemolyticum* (formerly *Corynebacterium haemolyticum*), and members of CDC coryneform groups A-4, D-2, G, I, 1, and 2. Animals are the probable natural reservoir for *Actinomyces pyogenes* (formerly *Corynebacterium pyogenes*; cows, sheep, pigs), *Corynebacterium ulcerans* (cows, horses), and *Corynebacterium pseudotuberculosis* (sheep, goats, horses). The natural habitat for *Rhodococcus equi* (formerly *Corynebacterium equi*) is soil. The ecologic niches for most other coryneform bacteria of medical importance are not well defined.

The coryneform bacteria found most frequently as components of the normal flora include *C. pseudodiphtheriticum* (pharynx, skin), *C. xerosis* (conjunctival sac, nasopharynx, skin), and *C. striatum* (anterior nares, skin). Coryneform bacteria that frequently colonize the skin of hospitalized patients include *C. jeikeium* (axilla, groin, perineum) and CDC group D-2. *C. jeikeium* most frequently colonizes patients with malignancies or severe immunodeficiency; it is also isolated from environmental sources (surfaces, air) in hospitals and from the hands of ward staff. *C. ulcerans* infections are acquired by consumption of raw milk. *C. pseudotuberculosis* infections are acquired by contact with animals or animal products or by consumption of raw milk.

PATHOGENESIS AND CLINICAL MANIFESTATIONS

C. jeikeium was recognized in 1976 as a cause of infections in immunocompromised hosts. It also causes infections in immunocompetent hosts, but severe infections continue to be most frequent in patients with hematologic malignancies and neutropenia. Colonization of the skin precedes clinical infection. Additional risk factors for nosocomial *C. jeikeium* sepsis include prolonged hospitalization, breaks in the integument, chronic intravascular catheterization, and prior treatment with broad-spectrum antibiotics. Other presentations of *C. jeikeium* infection include endocarditis, device-related infections, pulmonary infiltrates, cutaneous septic emboli, soft tissue infections, and rashes. Endocarditis due to *C. jeikeium* occurs primarily in patients with prosthetic heart valves. *C. jeikeium* is a rare cause of central nervous system infections in patients with ventricular shunts.

Group D-2 coryneform bacteria were identified in 1985 as a significant cause of nosocomial urinary tract infections, including acute and chronic cystitis and pyelonephritis. These organisms closely resemble *C. jeikeium* but differ from the latter in that they produce urease and fail to convert glucose to acidic metabolites. Hydrolysis of urea by urease causes alkalinization of the urine and formation of ammonium magnesium phosphate (struvite) stones. Group D-2 bacteria cause alkaline-encrusted cystitis in patients with preexisting bladder lesions, which serve as foci for precipitation of struvite crystals. Risk factors associated with symptomatic urinary tract infections include preexisting immunosuppression, recent urologic procedures (including renal transplantation), underlying disorders of the genitourinary tract, and a history of urinary tract infections.

A. haemolyticum causes pharyngitis, with 90 percent of cases occurring in patients between 10 and 30 years old. In this age group, *A. haemolyticum* pharyngitis is 5 to 13 percent as frequent as *Streptococcus pyogenes* pharyngitis. An erythematous rash is present in 30 to 67 percent of cases. The rash is usually scarlatiniform and most pronounced on the extremities, but it sometimes resembles urticaria or erythema multiforme. Because rash is more frequent in *A. haemolyticum* infections than in *S. pyogenes* infections, older children and adults presenting with the scarlet fever syndrome are as likely to have *A. haemolyticum* as *S. pyogenes* infection. Infection due to *A. haemolyticum* can also present as extensive pharyngeal exudate and can mimic diphtheria. *A. haemolyticum* occasionally causes peritonsillar abscess, sepsis, endocarditis, or meningitis.

C. minutissimum is frequently isolated from the lesions of erythrasma, a common superficial skin infection characterized by the presence in intertriginous areas of reddish-brown, scaly, pruritic, macular patches that exhibit coral-red fluorescence under a Wood's light.

The etiology of erythrasma has not been definitively established; infection of the skin by *C. minutissimum* has been shown to follow the onset of maceration and scaling. Deep infections caused by *C. minutissimum* are rare and include abscesses, bacteremia, and endocarditis.

Among coryneform bacteria that cause disease in animals and occasionally in humans, *R. equi* is emerging as a potentially important, intracellular, opportunistic pathogen in immunocompromised patients. Most reported cases are pulmonary infections that resemble tuberculosis in patients with severely defective cell-mediated immunity. Several cases of *R. equi* infection have recently been documented in patients with AIDS. *A. pyogenes* causes bovine mastitis, a disease transmitted by flies. Yearly epidemics of leg ulcers infected with *A. pyogenes* occurred among schoolchildren in Thailand between 1979 and 1984 and were postulated to have resulted from introduction of the organism into traumatic skin lesions by flies. Reported *A. pyogenes* infections among adults in Denmark have included abscesses, cystitis, intraabdominal infections, and mastoiditis with bacteremia. *C. ulcerans* infections in humans usually present as pharyngitis and can mimic respiratory diphtheria, whereas infections caused by *C. pseudotuberculosis* typically present as suppurative granulomatous lymphadenitis. Some strains of *C. ulcerans* and *C. pseudotuberculosis* can produce diphtheria toxin. Human infections caused by tox[+] strains of *C. ulcerans*—but not by tox[+] strains of *C. pseudotuberculosis*—have been reported.

C. pseudodiphtheriticum, a commensal of low virulence, is an uncommon cause of pneumonia in men with AIDS and of endocarditis, necrotizing tracheitis, tracheobronchitis, and urinary tract infection in patients without known immune deficiencies. Likewise, *C. xerosis* and *C. striatum* only occasionally cause human infections.

DIAGNOSIS   The clinical features of *C. jeikeium* infections are not pathognomonic. The diagnosis of these infections is based on a high index of suspicion, identification of the organism by culture from appropriate clinical specimens, and exclusion of other likely causes of infection.

Group D-2 coryneform bacteria often are not detected by routine urine cultures; rather, it is necessary to incubate the cultures for 24 to 48 h on blood agar or on special media. Cultivation should be prolonged in selected cases—i.e., those involving patients (especially elderly men with preexisting genitourinary abnormalities) who have alkaline urine, ammonium magnesium phosphate stones, gram-positive bacilli in the urine, or negative standard urine cultures despite clinical evidence of bacteriuria. Other microbes that can cause urinary tract infections with alkaline urine include *Proteus*, *Ureaplasma*, and some staphylococci and streptococci. Alkaline-encrusted cystitis is an anatomic diagnosis made by cystoscopy.

The differential diagnosis of *A. haemolyticum* pharyngitis with rash includes scarlet fever; rubella; staphylococcal and streptococcal toxic shock syndromes; infections caused by Epstein-Barr virus, cytomegalovirus, and enteroviruses (especially coxsackieviruses); disseminated gonococcal infection; secondary syphilis; and drug allergy. Routine diagnostic methods for throat cultures are not ideal for the detection of *A. haemolyticum*, nor is this organism detected by the rapid tests for *S. pyogenes* that are sometimes substituted for throat cultures. Pharyngitis caused by *A. haemolyticum* in adolescents and adults is likely to be underdiagnosed until improved tests for the organism are used by diagnostic laboratories.

Erythrasma is diagnosed clinically. Because of uncertainty about the etiologic role of *C. minutissimum*, culture of erythrasma lesions is not currently recommended. Pharyngitis caused by tox[+] strains of *C. ulcerans* may be clinically indistinguishable from diphtheria. The presentations of infections caused by other coryneform bacteria are not usually diagnostic; cultures are required for identification of the causal organisms.

℞ TREATMENT

Strains of *C. jeikeium* are typically resistant to most antibiotics except vancomycin, which is the drug of choice for the treatment of infections caused by this organism. Some recent isolates of *C. jeikeium* are susceptible or only moderately resistant to β-lactam antibiotics; infections due to fully susceptible strains can be treated with β-lactam antibiotics alone, and those due to moderately resistant strains can be treated with β-lactam antibiotics plus an aminoglycoside. Quinolones, especially ciprofloxacin, have excellent in vitro activity against *C. jeikeium*. For device-related *C. jeikeium* infections, removal of the infected device is usually required in addition to appropriate antibiotic therapy.

Group D-2 coryneform bacteria are often resistant to the antibiotics used commonly for the treatment of urinary tract infections. Early isolates were uniformly susceptible to vancomycin and quinolones, but recent isolates have exhibited increasing resistance to norfloxacin and ciprofloxacin. Isolates are often susceptible to erythromycin, rifampin, novobiocin, and tetracyclines. Treatment of urinary tract infections due to group D-2 strains is often difficult; several courses of antibiotic therapy may be necessary for bacteriologic cure. Patients with alkaline-encrusted cystitis require resection of the encrusted lesions in addition to antibiotic therapy.

Controlled trials of treatment for infections caused by *A. haemolyticum* have not been performed. In vitro tests have demonstrated susceptibility to erythromycin but tolerance or relative resistance to penicillin. Limited data suggest that the clinical course of *A. haemolyticum* pharyngitis may be shortened by treatment with erythromycin.

Infections with *C. ulcerans* that present like diphtheria or that are known to be caused by tox⁺ strains of *C. ulcerans* should be treated like diphtheria. Oral erythromycin is usually effective for the treatment of erythrasma. Initial treatment of infections caused by other coryneform bacteria should be based on the identity of the organism and on published data regarding antibiotic susceptibility. Therapy should be modified, when necessary, in light of the results of antibiotic susceptibility tests. All isolates of *Corynebacterium* and of coryneform bacteria reported to date have been susceptible to vancomycin.

ANTHRAX

DEFINITION Anthrax is an acute bacterial infection caused by *Bacillus anthracis*. It occurs most frequently in herbivorous animals. Humans become infected when spores of *B. anthracis* are introduced into the body by contact with infected animals or contaminated animal products, insect bites, inhalation, or ingestion. In humans, the most common form is cutaneous anthrax, which is characterized by the development of a localized skin lesion with a central eschar surrounded by marked nonpitting edema. Inhalation anthrax (woolsorters' disease) typically involves hemorrhagic mediastinitis, rapidly progressive systemic infection, and a very high mortality rate. Gastrointestinal anthrax is rare and is associated with a high mortality rate.

ETIOLOGIC AGENT *B. anthracis* is a large (1 to 1.5 μm by 4 to 10 μm), nonmotile, encapsulated, chain-forming, aerobic, gram-positive rod that forms oval spores. Oxygen is required for sporulation but not for germination of spores, and sporulation does not take place in living animals. The rectangular shape of the individual bacteria gives chains of *B. anthracis* a boxcar-like appearance. On blood agar, virulent *B. anthracis* usually forms nonhemolytic or weakly hemolytic, grayish-white, rough colonies; however, if the medium contains bicarbonate and incubation takes place in the presence of excess CO_2, the colonies are smooth and mucoid. Virulent strains of *B. anthracis* are pathogenic for animals, including mice and guinea pigs. Known virulence factors include three proteins collectively called *anthrax toxin* (see below) and an antiphagocytic capsular polypeptide composed of D-glutamic acid residues linked by peptide bonds involving the gamma carboxyl group. The genes that determine the production of anthrax toxin and that of capsular polypeptide are located on separate plasmids of *B. anthracis*. Determination of susceptibility to bacillus phage gamma and demonstration of species-specific antigens are helpful in laboratory identification of *B. anthracis*. Spores of *B. anthracis* can survive for years in dry earth but are destroyed by boiling for about 10 min, by treatment with oxidizing agents such as potassium permanganate or hydrogen peroxide, or by dilute formaldehyde. Most strains of *B. anthracis* are susceptible to penicillin.

EPIDEMIOLOGY The distribution of anthrax is worldwide. All animals are susceptible to varying degrees, but the disease is most prevalent among domestic herbivores (including cattle, sheep, horses, and goats) and wild herbivores.

Grazing animals become infected when they are foraging for food in areas contaminated with spores of *B. anthracis* under appropriate climatic conditions. Anthrax in herbivores tends to be severe, with a high mortality rate. Terminally ill animals have overwhelming bacteremic infections and often bleed from the nose, mouth, and bowel, thereby contaminating soil or watering places with vegetative *B. anthracis* that can subsequently sporulate and persist in the environment. The carcasses of infected animals provide additional potential foci of contamination. Epidemics among animals may spread from an initial focus to contiguous geographic areas in a pattern consistent with the movement of infected animals. Biting flies have also been implicated as vectors for the spread of anthrax, and vultures that feed on infected carcasses occasionally spread spores from a contaminated area to noncontiguous areas, probably by the contamination of surface water pools.

The natural resistance of humans to anthrax is greater than that of herbivorous animals. It is difficult to determine the annual worldwide incidence of human anthrax, because many cases do not receive medical attention and are not reported; estimates of 20,000 to 100,000 cases per year have been made. Human cases are classified as agricultural or industrial on the basis of the epidemiologic setting in which they occur. Agricultural cases result most often from contact with animals that have anthrax (for example, during skinning, butchering, or dissecting), from bites of contaminated or infected flies, and (in rare instances) from consumption of contaminated meat. Industrial cases are associated with exposure to contaminated hides, goat's hair, wool, or bones. Anthrax in animals has been a long-standing problem in Iran, Turkey, Pakistan, and Sudan, and the probability is high that animal products (especially goat's hair) originating from these areas will be contaminated with anthrax spores.

Only three cases of cutaneous anthrax were reported to the CDC in the United States from 1984 through 1993, and gastrointestinal anthrax has never been documented in this country. Large epidemics of anthrax occurred in the former Soviet Union at Sverdlovsk in 1979 and in Zimbabwe between 1978 and the early 1980s. Initially, the cases in Sverdlovsk were reported to be cutaneous and gastrointestinal anthrax and were attributed to exposure to meat from infected animals. Intense international interest was stimulated by the suspicion that the release of *B. anthracis* from a nearby military facility was responsible for the outbreak. Recent analyses of epidemiologic data from the Sverdlovsk outbreak and autopsy findings on most of the fatal cases determined that the disease was, in fact, inhalation anthrax. The outbreak in Zimbabwe involved more than 9700 cases of agricultural anthrax in humans. This massive outbreak occurred during wartime and was associated with disruption of the veterinary and medical infrastructure and the cessation of veterinary anthrax vaccination programs (see below).

PATHOGENESIS *B. anthracis* is an extracellular pathogen that can evade phagocytosis, invade the bloodstream, multiply rapidly to a high population density in vivo, and kill quickly. Capsular polypeptide and anthrax toxin are the principal virulence factors of *B. anthracis*. The capsule of *B. anthracis* consists of poly-D-glutamic acid and confers resistance to phagocytosis. Anthrax toxin consists of three proteins called *protective antigen* (PA), *edema factor* (EF), and *lethal factor* (LF). The toxin was discovered in studies demonstrating that the transfer of sterile blood from guinea pigs dying of anthrax to uninfected guinea pigs killed the recipients.

PA binds to plasma membranes of target cells and is cleaved by a cellular protease into two fragments. The larger fragment remains on the cell surface, displays a single binding site for a domain that is present in both EF and LF, and serves as a specific receptor that mediates endocytic entry of EF or LF into the target cells. The activity of EF, a calmodulin-dependent adenylate cyclase, is expressed within human or animal cells that provide both the calmodulin activator and the ATP substrate for EF. The biologic effects of EF, which include formation of edema in anthrax lesions and the inhibition of polymorphonuclear leukocyte functions, are mediated by the cyclic AMP that is formed intracellularly by the enzymatic action of EF. PA-mediated entry of LF into susceptible cells leads to cell death by an unknown mechanism.

Cutaneous anthrax is initiated when spores of *B. anthracis* are introduced into the skin through cuts or abrasions or by biting flies. The spores germinate within hours, and the vegetative cells multiply and produce anthrax toxin. Histologically, the lesion in cutaneous anthrax is characterized by necrosis, vascular congestion, hemorrhage, and gelatinous edema. The number of leukocytes is disproportionately small in comparison with the amount of tissue damage. The clinical description of this lesion as a "malignant pustule" is not in concordance with the pathologic findings.

In inhalation anthrax, *B. anthracis* spores in airborne particles <5 μm in diameter are deposited directly into the alveoli or alveolar ducts. The spores are phagocytized by alveolar macrophages, and some are carried to and germinate in mediastinal nodes. Hemorrhagic necrosis of the nodes, in association with hemorrhagic mediastinitis and overwhelming *B. anthracis* bacteremia, may develop rapidly. Secondary pneumonia sometimes occurs.

Gastrointestinal anthrax usually results from ingestion of inadequately cooked meat from animals with anthrax. Primary infection can be initiated in the intestine by organisms that survive passage through the stomach, but an oropharyngeal form of the disease also has been described. Lesions in the throat or intestine are usually accompanied by hemorrhagic lymphadenitis.

B. anthracis bacteremia can develop in any form of anthrax and occurs in almost all fatal cases. Autopsies reveal large numbers of bacteria in blood vessels, lymph nodes, and many organs.

CLINICAL MANIFESTATIONS Approximately 95 percent of human cases of anthrax are the cutaneous form and about 5 percent the inhalation form. Gastrointestinal anthrax is rare. Anthrax meningitis occurs in a small percentage of all cases and is a frequent complication of overwhelming *B. anthracis* bacteremia.

Cutaneous Anthrax The cutaneous lesion in anthrax is most often found on exposed areas of skin. In Zimbabwe, lesions in children under 5 years old were significantly more likely to be on the head, neck, or face and less likely to be on the upper limbs than lesions in adults. This distribution correlates with the fact that children have less contact with carcasses of infected animals and are more likely to acquire infection through fly bites.

Within days after inoculation of *B. anthracis* spores into the skin, a small red macule appears. During the next week, the lesion typically progresses through papular and vesicular or pustular stages to the formation of an ulcer with a blackened necrotic eschar surrounded by a highly characteristic, expanding zone of brawny edema. The early lesion may be pruritic, and the fully developed lesion is painless. Small satellite vesicles may surround the original lesion, and painful nonspecific regional lymphadenitis is common. Most patients are afebrile, with mild or no constitutional symptoms; in severe cases, however, edema may be extensive and associated with shock. Spontaneous healing occurs in 80 to 90 percent of untreated cases, but edema may persist for weeks. In the 10 to 20 percent of untreated patients who have progressive infection, bacteremia develops and is often associated with high fever and rapid death. The differential diagnosis includes staphylococcal skin infections, tularemia, plague, and orf. Cutaneous anthrax should be considered when patients have painless ulcers associated with vesicles and edema and have had contact with animals or animal products.

Inhalation Anthrax The frequent similarity of the presenting symptoms of inhalation anthrax (woolsorters' disease) to those of severe viral respiratory diseases makes early diagnosis difficult. After 1 to 3 days, an acute phase supervenes, with increasing fever, dyspnea, stridor, hypoxia, and hypotension usually leading to death within 24 h. Occasionally, patients present with fulminant disease. A characteristic radiologic finding associated with hemorrhagic mediastinitis is symmetric mediastinal widening.

Gastrointestinal Anthrax Symptoms of gastrointestinal anthrax are variable and include fever, nausea and vomiting, abdominal pain, bloody diarrhea, and sometimes rapidly developing ascites. Diarrhea is occasionally massive in volume, causing hemoconcentration and severe contraction of intravascular volume. The major features of oropharyngeal anthrax are fever, sore throat, dysphagia, painful regional lymphadenopathy, and toxemia; respiratory distress may be evident. The primary lesion is most often on the tonsils.

LABORATORY DIAGNOSIS *B. anthracis* is present in large numbers in cutaneous lesions of anthrax and can be demonstrated by Gram's staining, direct fluorescent antibody staining, or culture unless the patient has been treated with antibiotics. A small proportion of patients with anthrax have bacteremia, but the disease may progress to death before blood cultures become positive. Patients with anthrax meningitis have bloody spinal fluid containing large numbers of *B. anthracis* organisms demonstrable by staining or culture. The virulence of suspected isolates of *B. anthracis* can be demonstrated by inoculation of guinea pigs; death occurs within 24 h with positive cultures of heart blood. Patients with mild disease usually have normal leukocyte counts, but patients with disseminated disease typically have polymorphonuclear leukocytosis. Tests for antibody to *B. anthracis* are useful in confirming the diagnosis of anthrax. A sensitive and specific polymerase chain reaction method developed for the detection of spores of *B. anthracis* may be useful for rapid testing of potentially contaminated animal or agricultural products.

℞ **TREATMENT**

Viable *B. anthracis* organisms disappear from the lesions of cutaneous anthrax within 5 h of the initiation of treatment with parenteral penicillin G. The recommended therapeutic regimen for adults is 2 million units of penicillin G at intervals of 6 h until edema subsides, with the subsequent administration of oral penicillin to complete a 7- to 10-day course. For penicillin-sensitive adults, treatment with ciprofloxacin, erythromycin, tetracycline, or chloramphenicol can be substituted. Antibiotics decrease local edema and systemic toxicity in cutaneous anthrax but do not prevent eschar formation. Cutaneous lesions should be cleaned and covered, and used dressings should be decontaminated. For inhalation anthrax, high-dose penicillin therapy (2 million units at 2-h intervals) is recommended; for gastrointestinal anthrax or anthrax meningitis, the recommended regimen is the same. A rational case can be made for passive immunization with anthrax antitoxin in addition to antibiotic therapy in severely ill patients with anthrax, but no appropriate antitoxin is commercially available.

PREVENTION Inhalation anthrax was essentially eliminated in England before 1940 through the development of methods to decontaminate wool and goat's hair and the improvement of working conditions for handlers of animal products.

Nonliving vaccines consisting of alum-precipitated or aluminum hydroxide–adsorbed extracellular components of unencapsulated *B. anthracis* are used in the United Kingdom and the United States for the immunization of agricultural workers, veterinary personnel, and others at risk of exposure to anthrax. The major active component of these vaccines is PA. Live attenuated vaccines containing spores of *B. anthracis* are used in both developed and developing countries to immunize domestic herbivores; these preparations are also used to immunize humans in Russia but not in the United States. The probable basis for attenuation of the original Pasteur spore vaccine is partial loss of the plasmid that encodes anthrax toxin during prolonged incubation of *B. anthracis* cultures at 42°C. The basis for attenuation of the current Sterne spore vaccine is loss of the plasmid that encodes capsular polypeptide.

Improved anthrax vaccines for humans are needed, because the current vaccines are impure and chemically complex, elicit only slow-onset protective immunity, provide incomplete protection, and cause significant adverse reactions. In addition to agricultural and industrial anthrax, the possible use of *B. anthracis* as an agent of biological warfare is a stimulus for the development of an improved vaccine. Current strategies for vaccine development include purification of candidate protective antigens, expression of protective antigens in recombinant microbial vaccines, and construction of improved live attenuated strains of *B. anthracis*.

Carcasses of animals that succumb to anthrax should be buried intact or cremated. Necropsy or butchering of infected animals should be avoided, because sporulation of *B. anthracis* occurs only in the presence of oxygen.

PROGNOSIS   The mortality rate for cutaneous anthrax is 10 to 20 percent in the absence of treatment but is very low with appropriate antibiotic therapy. In contrast, the mortality rate for inhalation anthrax approaches 100 percent, and therapy is usually unsuccessful. The mortality rate for treated gastrointestinal anthrax is approximately 50 percent. Anthrax meningitis is usually fatal.

BIBLIOGRAPHY

ACP Task Force on Adult Immunization and Infectious Diseases Society of America: *Guide for Adult Immunization*, 3d ed. Philadelphia, American College of Physicians, 1994, p 19

Aksaray N et al: Cutaneous anthrax. Trop Geogr Med 42:168, 1990

Centers for Disease Control and Prevention: Diphtheria epidemic—new independent states of the former Soviet Union, 1990–1994. Morb Mort Week Rep 44(10):177, 1995

————: Diphtheria acquired by U.S. citizens in the Russian Federation and Ukraine—1994. Morb Mort Week Rep 44(12):237, 1995

Cohen Y et al: *Corynebacterium pseudodiphtheriticum* pulmonary infection in AIDS patients. Lancet 340:114, 1992

Committee on Infectious Diseases: Diphtheria, in *Report of the Committee on Infectious Diseases*, 23d ed. Elk Grove Village, IL, American Academy of Pediatrics, 1994, p 177

Coyle MB, Lipsky BA: Coryneform bacteria in infectious diseases: Clinical and laboratory aspects. Clin Microbiol Rev 3:227, 1990

Creange A et al: Diphtheritic neuropathy. Muscle Nerve 18:1460, 1995

Damade R et al: Septic arthritis due to *Corynebacterium diphtheriae*. Clin Infect Dis 16:446, 1993

Farizo KM et al: Fatal respiratory disease due to *Corynebacterium diphtheriae*: Case report and review of guidelines for management, investigation, and control. Clin Infect Dis 16:59, 1993

George S et al: An outbreak of anthrax meningoencephalitis. Trans R Soc Trop Med Hyg 88:206, 1994

Hardy IRB et al: Current situation and control strategies for resurgence of diphtheria in newly independent states of the former Soviet Union. Lancet 347:1739, 1996

Hedlund KW: Anthrax toxin: History and recent advances and perspectives. J Toxicol Toxin Rev 11:41, 1992

Höfler W: Cutaneous diphtheria. Int J Dermatol 30:845, 1991

Kain KC et al: *Arcanobacterium haemolyticum* infection: Confused with scarlet fever and diphtheria. J Emerg Med 9:33, 1991

Laforce FM: Anthrax. Clin Infect Dis 19:1009, 1994

Meselson M et al: The Sverdlovsk anthrax outbreak of 1979. Science 266:1202, 1994

Popovic T et al: Molecular epidemiology of diphtheria in Russia, 1985–1994. J Infect Dis 174:1064, 1996

Rakhmanova AG et al: Diphtheria outbreak in St. Petersburg: Clinical characteristics of 1,860 adult patients. Scand J Infect Dis 28:37, 1996

Rozdzinski E et al: *Corynebacterium jeikeium* bacteremia at a tertiary care center. Infection 19:201, 1991

Soriano F et al: Urinary tract infection caused by *Corynebacterium* group D2: Report of 82 cases and review. Rev Infect Dis 12:1019, 1990

Tiley SM et al: Infective endocarditis due to nontoxigenic *Corynebacterium diphtheriae*: Report of seven cases and review. Clin Infect Dis 16:271, 1993

Turnbull PCB: Anthrax vaccines: Past, present and future. Vaccine 9:533, 1991

Wilson APR et al: Unusual non-toxigenic *Corynebacterium diphtheriae* in homosexual men. Lancet 339:998, 1992

145   *Anne Schuchat, Claire V. Broome*

INFECTIONS CAUSED BY *LISTERIA MONOCYTOGENES*

Listeria monocytogenes is a gram-positive rod that can be isolated from soil, vegetation, and many animal reservoirs. Human disease due to *L. monocytogenes* generally occurs in the setting of pregnancy or immunosuppression caused by illness or medication. Increasing evidence suggests that a substantial portion of cases of human listeriosis are attributable to the food-borne transmission of *L. monocytogenes*. Unlike most food-borne pathogens, which cause primarily gastrointestinal illness, *L. monocytogenes* causes invasive syndromes, such as meningitis, sepsis, chorioamnionitis, and stillbirth.

ETIOLOGY   Listeriae are aerobic or facultatively anaerobic nonsporulating bacilli that grow at 1 to 45°C and typically have tumbling motility when cultured at 20 to 25°C. Characteristics that help distinguish *L. monocytogenes* from other *Listeria* species include the formation of a narrow zone of beta hemolysis on sheep blood agar and the production of acid from glucose, maltose, L-rhamnose, and α-methyl-D-mannoside but not from D-xylose. Determination of the serotype of *L. monocytogenes* is based on somatic (O) and flagellar (H) antigens. Most cases of human disease are caused by serotypes 1/2a, 1/2b, and 4b. Molecular subtyping techniques, including multilocus enzyme electrophoresis, phage typing, and DNA fingerprinting methods, have made it easier to discriminate among strains of *Listeria* and thus to link environmental or food isolates with clinical infections.

PATHOGENESIS   *L. monocytogenes* is an intracellular pathogen, a characteristic consistent with its predilection for causing illness in persons with deficient cell-mediated immunity. The organism can be found as part of the gastrointestinal flora in healthy individuals. Lack of gastric acidity and abnormal gastrointestinal functioning may increase the risk of invasive disease following exposure to the organism in the gastrointestinal tract. Invasion, intracellular multiplication, and cell-to-cell spread of the organism appear to be mediated through proteins such as internalin, the hemolysin listeriolysin O, and phospholipase C. The increased risk of *L. monocytogenes* infection in pregnant women may be due to both systemic and local immunologic changes associated with pregnancy. For example, local immunosuppression at the maternal-fetal interface of the placenta may facilitate intrauterine infection following transient maternal bacteremia.

EPIDEMIOLOGY   Long recognized as a veterinary pathogen, *L. monocytogenes* causes basilar meningitis ("circling disease") and stillbirth in sheep and cattle. The occurrence of listeriosis among humans has received increasing attention as the role of contaminated foods in the pathogenesis of epidemic listeriosis has been recognized and reports of disease associated with the expanding immunosuppressed population have accumulated.

Invasive listeriosis—confirmed by culture of blood or cerebrospinal fluid—occurs in approximately 4.4 individuals per million population annually in the United States, for an estimated 1092 cases per year. Perinatal listeriosis complicates 9 births per 100,000. A 40 percent decline in incidence since the period from 1986 through 1990 may be attributable to aggressive food regulation and industrial cleanup efforts. Multistate surveillance for sporadic listeriosis suggests that 23 percent of infections are fatal or result in stillbirth, although higher case-fatality rates have been reported during listeriosis epidemics and were described in early series. Most cases of disease due to *L. monocytogenes* are sporadic; however, investigation of several outbreaks of listeriosis during the 1980s and 1990s demonstrated common-source food-borne transmission as a cause of human illness and showed that the incubation period for disease following consumption of contaminated food can be 2 to 6 weeks. The largest North American outbreak, which took place in Los Angeles in 1985, involved more than 100 cases and 48 deaths or stillbirths. A nationwide outbreak in France in

1992 involved 279 cases and 63 deaths. Foods implicated in outbreaks of listeriosis include contaminated coleslaw, pasteurized milk, soft cheeses, pâté, and ready-to-eat pork products, while epidemiologic studies have implicated undercooked chicken, uncooked hot dogs, soft cheeses, and food from store delicatessen counters in sporadic disease. Listerial contamination of foods is relatively common. Among foods contaminated with the organism, those that are purchased ready to eat, are contaminated with serotype 4b, and are contaminated at a relatively high level may be the most likely to cause illness. The long incubation period associated with listeriosis contributes to the difficulty of implicating specific foods as the cause of either common-source outbreaks or sporadic cases.

Although food-borne transmission appears to be the foremost cause of epidemic and sporadic disease, several clusters of late-onset neonatal infection suggest nosocomial transmission of *L. monocytogenes*. Contaminated multiuse materials and equipment have been suggested as causes of some nosocomial clusters. Listeriosis has been reported in veterinarians and other persons in close contact with infected animals.

CLINICAL PRESENTATION *Pregnancy-associated listeriosis* may occur during any stage of pregnancy, although most infections are detected during the third trimester, possibly because of failure to obtain specimens for bacterial culture earlier during gestation in instances of abortion and stillbirth. One-half to two-thirds of pregnant women with perinatal listeriosis experience a mild illness that is characterized by fever, myalgias, malaise, and backache, which sometimes are accompanied by diarrhea, abdominal pain, nausea, and/or vomiting during the bacteremic phase. Blood cultures should be used for diagnosis, since isolation of the organism from rectal or vaginal culture is not diagnostic. Transplacental spread of the organism results in intrauterine infection, which can lead to chorioamnionitis, premature labor, intrauterine fetal demise, or early-onset disease of the newborn. Women with listeriosis diagnosed during pregnancy have a favorable clinical outcome after antibiotic therapy or delivery. Although often included in the differential diagnosis of recurrent spontaneous abortion, infection with *L. monocytogenes* appears to cause fewer than 2 percent of stillbirths.

Neonatal listeriosis can be classified under the same categories used for group B streptococcal infection, with early-onset disease evident during the first week of life and late-onset disease developing thereafter. Infants may be symptomatic at birth; most infants with early-onset disease are symptomatic by the second day of life. Aspiration of infected amniotic fluid contributes to the pathogenesis. Early-onset disease may include sepsis, respiratory distress, skin lesions, and the syndrome called *granulomatosis infantisepticum*, which is characterized by disseminated abscesses involving the liver, spleen, adrenal glands, lungs, and other sites. Infants with late-onset neonatal disease are more likely than those with early-onset disease to develop meningitis. While early-onset disease is often associated with obstetrical complications such as premature delivery and chorioamnionitis, late-onset disease typically affects infants born at term by uncomplicated deliveries. Infants may acquire *L. monocytogenes* during passage through the birth canal; except in several clusters of late-onset neonatal infections linked to nosocomial transmission, the pathogenesis of late-onset disease is not well understood.

Listeriosis not associated with pregnancy usually affects persons with immunosuppressive conditions, although invasive disease can also affect immunocompetent adults, particularly elderly persons. The most common underlying conditions in nonpregnant adults with listeriosis are chronic glucocorticoid therapy, solid or hematologic malignancies, diabetes mellitus, renal disease, liver disease, and AIDS. Although the prevalence of listeriosis among persons infected with human immunodeficiency virus (HIV) is much higher than that in the general population, listeriosis is a relatively uncommon opportunistic infection in AIDS.

Sepsis Recent studies of clinical series have shown that bacteremic infection without an evident focus is the most common clinical manifestation of listeriosis among immunocompromised hosts, while infection of the central nervous system (CNS) ranks second in frequency. Listerial sepsis cannot be distinguished clinically from bacteremia involving other organisms. Patients are usually febrile, often appear extremely ill, and may have prodromal symptoms including myalgia, nausea, vomiting, and diarrhea. Immunocompromised patients with listeriosis are less likely than other adults to present with CNS infection. Immunocompromised patients may be especially likely to have blood cultured during febrile episodes, whereas in other adults transient bacteremia due to *L. monocytogenes* may go unrecognized.

CNS Infection The most common presentation of CNS infection due to *L. monocytogenes* is meningitis. Meningitis due to *L. monocytogenes* is not distinguishable clinically from other types of bacterial meningitis; presenting symptoms include fever, headache, and an altered level of consciousness. Examination of cerebrospinal fluid (CSF) usually reveals pleocytosis, increased protein concentrations, and normal glucose levels, although other patterns are sometimes found. As in other forms of bacterial meningitis, Gram's stain may not be revealing. The diagnosis is made when *L. monocytogenes* is identified on culture. Despite its name, *L. monocytogenes* is rarely associated with monocytosis of either CSF or blood. Other syndromes seen in CNS infection include meningoencephalitis; cerebritis; and brainstem, spinal cord, or intracranial abscesses. The unusual syndrome of rhombencephalitis includes asymmetrical cranial nerve palsies, altered consciousness, cerebellar signs, and motor or sensory loss. Symptoms of other nonmeningitic CNS infections include fever, ataxia, seizures, personality changes, and coma. Nuchal rigidity is rare in nonmeningitic infections. CSF cultures may be sterile; blood cultures are usually diagnostic.

Endocarditis Like most forms of bacterial endocarditis, endocarditis due to *L. monocytogenes* typically occurs in patients with prosthetic or previously damaged valves. The organism has a predilection for the left side of the heart. Endocarditis due to *L. monocytogenes* is often associated with systemic embolization.

Focal Infections Other focal infections that can follow unrecognized bacteremia include endophthalmitis, peritonitis, osteomyelitis, visceral abscess, pleuropulmonary infection, and cholecystitis. Cutaneous lesions may develop without systemic involvement and have been reported in veterinarians and poultry workers.

Recurrences Recurrent infection with *L. monocytogenes* has been reported but is rare. Many recurrences are due to the subtype responsible for the initial infection, which suggests that recurrence results either from insufficient treatment of a focus of primary infection or from repeated exposure to a persistently contaminated source.

Gastrointestinal Illness Recent investigations of common-source outbreaks of acute gastroenteritis suggest that *L. monocytogenes* can cause an acute diarrheal syndrome in persons without immunocompromising conditions. The importance of *L. monocytogenes* in sporadic diarrheal illness is unclear. Although the organism is not identified by the culture methods routinely used for stool specimens, studies using selective enrichment media for evaluation of consecutive specimens from patients hospitalized with acute diarrhea have suggested that *L. monocytogenes* is not a major cause of sporadic diarrhea.

DIAGNOSIS Invasive listeriosis is diagnosed when the organism is cultured from a site that is usually sterile, such as blood, CSF, or amniotic fluid. The organism will grow readily within 36 h on routine culture media, but morphologic similarities between *Listeria* and both diphtheroids and streptococci make it necessary to use biochemical tests to identify the species. Serologic assays with whole-cell antigens have not been useful for the diagnosis of listeriosis, both because exposure to the organism (and thus the presence of antibody) may be common and because infected individuals may not produce antibody after infection. Assays for antibody to listeriolysin O have been applied in epidemiologic investigations and, retrospectively, in the diagnosis of culture-negative CNS infection. Culture of the organism from nonsterile sites such as the vagina and rectum is not useful for clinical diagnosis, as the organism may be carried at these sites by approximately 5 percent of healthy individuals.

Differential diagnosis of prematurity, spontaneous abortion, or stillbirth includes infectious diseases such as group B streptococcal infection, congenital syphilis, and toxoplasmosis; pathogens such as group B streptococci and *Escherichia coli* are more common than *L. monocytogenes* as causes of meningitis and sepsis in the newborn period. Because *L. monocytogenes* is not sensitive to cephalosporins, these agents should not be used for single-agent empirical treatment of neonatal sepsis and meningitis. Listerial infection should always be considered in the differential diagnosis of meningitis in immunosuppressed persons, particularly transplant recipients and others receiving glucocorticoid treatment, patients with hematologic malignancy, and HIV-infected patients. Among healthy adults, meningitis is much more likely to be caused by *Neisseria meningitidis, Streptococcus pneumoniae*, or viral pathogens than by *L. monocytogenes*.

℞ TREATMENT

The treatment of choice for listeriosis is intravenous administration of either ampicillin or penicillin, often in combination with an aminoglycoside for synergy. Trimethoprim-sulfamethoxazole is bactericidal against *L. monocytogenes* and has been used successfully in the treatment of patients with penicillin allergy. *L. monocytogenes* is susceptible in vitro to penicillin G, ampicillin, erythromycin, trimethoprim-sulfamethoxazole, chloramphenicol, rifampin, tetracyclines, aminoglycosides, and imipenem. However, chloramphenicol and rifampin may antagonize the bactericidal effect of penicillins. Cephalosporins are not recommended.

Dosages and durations of therapy have not been subjected to controlled trials. For nonpregnant adults with listeriosis, the therapy of choice is either ampicillin (12 g intravenously per day in six divided doses) or penicillin G (15 to 20 million units intravenously per day in six divided doses); for immunosuppressed patients with meningitis, some experts add gentamicin (1.3 mg/kg intravenously every 8 h) for synergy. Penicillin-allergic patients may be treated with trimethoprim-sulfamethoxazole (15/75 mg/kg intravenously per day in three equal portions every 8 h). Meningitis in an immunocompetent patient may require 2 to 3 weeks of antibiotic therapy after defervescence. Meningitis, bacteremia, endocarditis, and nonmeningitic listeriosis in immunosuppressed patients should be treated longer, probably for 4 to 6 weeks. Neonatal listeriosis can be treated with a 2-week course of ampicillin. Infants weighing less than 2000 g should receive 100 mg/kg per day in two equal doses during the first week of life and 150 mg/kg per day during the second week. Infants weighing 2000 g or more should receive 150 mg/kg per day in three equal doses during the first week of life and 200 mg/kg per day during the second week. The addition of an aminoglycoside should be considered for neonatal infection (gentamicin, 5 mg/kg per day in two divided doses during the first week of life; 7.5 mg/kg per day in three equal doses during the second week). For listeriosis in pregnant women, a 2-week course of ampicillin (4 to 6 g per day in four equal doses) is recommended. During the last month of pregnancy, infected women with serious penicillin allergies may be treated with erythromycin.

PROGNOSIS Treatment of maternal bacteremia during pregnancy can prevent neonatal infection. Antibiotic therapy for the newborn can limit sequelae, although the widely disseminated disease characteristic of granulomatosis infantisepticum is frequently fatal regardless of treatment. Early-onset disease carries a higher mortality risk than late-onset infection, and immunocompromised hosts have a worse prognosis than do otherwise healthy adults with listeriosis.

PREVENTION *L. monocytogenes* is frequently isolated from food; the Food and Drug Administration, the U.S. Department of Agriculture, and manufacturers are pursuing further measures to reduce *L. monocytogenes* contamination of foods that have been subjected to listericidal processing. Prevention of listeriosis requires dietary counseling of persons at increased risk of disease (Table 145-1). There is no role for the administration of prophylaxis to contacts of patients with listeriosis. Clinicians are encouraged to report cases of listeriosis to local or state health departments and thus to facilitate early recognition of outbreaks and prevention of subsequent cases.

Table 145-1

Dietary Recommendations for the Prevention of Food-Borne Listeriosis

Recommendations to all individuals:
1. Thoroughly cook raw food from animal sources, such as beef, pork, and poultry.
2. Wash raw vegetables thoroughly before eating them.
3. Keep uncooked meats separate from vegetables and from cooked and ready-to-eat foods.
4. Avoid raw (unpasteurized) milk or foods made from raw milk.
5. Wash hands, knives, and cutting boards after handling uncooked foods.

Additional recommendations to high-risk individuals*:
- Avoid soft cheeses such as Mexican-style, feta, Brie, Camembert, and blue-veined cheese. There is no need to avoid hard cheeses, cream cheese, cottage cheese, or yogurt.
- Leftover foods or ready-to-eat foods, such as hot dogs, should be reheated until steaming hot before being eaten.
- Although the risk of listeriosis associated with foods from delicatessen counters is relatively low and poorly characterized, pregnant women and immunosuppressed persons may choose to avoid these foods or to thoroughly reheat cold cuts before eating them.

* Persons immunocompromised by illness or medications; pregnant women.

BIBLIOGRAPHY

BERCHE P et al: Detection of anti-listeriolysin O for serodiagnosis of human listeriosis. Lancet 335:624, 1990

CHERUBIN CE et al: Epidemiologic spectrum and current treatment of listeriosis. Rev Infect Dis 13:1108, 1991

NIEMAN RE, LORBER B: Listeriosis in adults: A changing pattern. Report of eight cases and review of the literature, 1968–1978. Rev Infect Dis 2:207, 1980

PINNER RW et al: Role of foods in sporadic listeriosis: II. Microbiologic and epidemiologic investigation. JAMA 267:2046, 1992

PORTNOY DA et al: Molecular determinants of *Listeria monocytogenes* pathogenesis. Infect Immun 60:1263, 1992

RIEDO FX et al: A point-source foodborne listeriosis outbreak: Documented incubation period and possible mild illness. J Infect Dis 170:693, 1994

SCHLECH WF et al: Epidemic listeriosis—evidence for transmission by food. N Engl J Med 308:203, 1983

SCHUCHAT A et al: Role of foods in sporadic listeriosis: I. Case-control study of dietary risk factors. JAMA 267:2041, 1992

——— et al: Epidemiology of human listeriosis. Clin Microbiol Rev 4:169, 1991

SEELIGER HPR: *Listeriosis.* Basel, Karger, 1961

SKOGBERG K et al: Clinical presentation and outcome of listeriosis in patients with and without immunosuppressive therapy. Clin Infect Dis 14:815, 1992

SOUTHWICK FS, PURICH DL: Intracellular pathogenesis of listeriosis. N Engl J Med 334:770, 1996

SWAMINATHAN B et al: *Listeria,* in *Manual of Clinical Microbiology,* PR Murray et al (eds). Washington, DC, ASM Press, 1995, p 341

TAPPERO JW et al: Reduction in the incidence of human listeriosis in the United States—effectiveness of prevention efforts? JAMA 273:1118, 1995

146 *Elias Abrutyn*

TETANUS

DEFINITION Tetanus is a neurologic disorder, characterized by increased muscle tone and spasms, that is caused by tetanospasmin, a powerful protein toxin elaborated by *Clostridium tetani.* Tetanus occurs in several clinical forms, including generalized, neonatal, and localized disease.

ETIOLOGIC AGENT *C. tetani* is an anaerobic, motile gram-positive rod that forms an oval, colorless, terminal spore and thus assumes a shape resembling a tennis racket or drumstick. The organism is found worldwide in soil, in the inanimate environment, in animal feces, and occasionally in human feces. Spores may survive for years in some environments and are resistant to various disinfectants and to boiling for 20 min. Vegetative cells, however, are easily inactivated and are susceptible to several antibiotics (metronidazole, penicillin, and others).

Tetanospasmin is formed in vegetative cells under plasmid control. It is a single-polypeptide chain. With autolysis, the single-chain toxin is released and cleaved to form a heterodimer consisting of a heavy chain (100 kDa), which mediates binding to nerve-cell receptors and entry into these cells, and a light chain (50 kDa), which acts to block neurotransmitter release. The amino acid structures of the two most powerful toxins known, botulinum toxin and tetanus toxin, are partially homologous.

EPIDEMIOLOGY Tetanus occurs sporadically and almost always affects nonimmunized persons, partially immunized persons, or fully immunized individuals who fail to maintain adequate immunity with booster doses of vaccine. Although tetanus is entirely preventable by immunization, the burden of disease is large worldwide. The disease is common in areas where soil is cultivated, in rural areas, in warm climates, during summer months, and among males. In countries without a comprehensive immunization program, tetanus occurs predominantly in neonates and other young children; an estimated 515,000 neonates died of tetanus worldwide in 1993. In the United States and other nations with successful immunization programs, neonatal tetanus is rare and the disease affects other age groups and groups inadequately covered by immunization (such as nonwhites). The elderly in particular are prominently involved. Only 27 percent of persons aged 70 years or older have a protective level of antibody to *C. tetani*, whereas 88 percent of children 6 to 11 years of age are protected. Overall, fewer than 60 cases of tetanus were reported to the Centers for Disease Control and Prevention each year during the period 1991 through 1994; 95 percent of all cases involved persons 20 years of age or older, and 53 percent involved persons 70 years of age or older. The burden of illness, however, is greater than the statistics indicate because reporting is incomplete.

In the United States, most cases of tetanus follow an acute injury, such as a puncture wound, laceration, or abrasion. Tetanus is often acquired indoors or during farming, gardening, and other outdoor activities. The injury may be major but often is trivial, so that medical attention is not sought; in some instances no injury can be identified. The disease may complicate chronic conditions such as skin ulcers, abscesses, and gangrene. Tetanus is also associated with burns, frostbite, middle-ear infection, surgery, abortion, childbirth, and drug abuse, notably "skin popping." In some patients no portal of entry for the organism can be identified.

PATHOGENESIS Contamination of wounds with spores of *C. tetani* is probably frequent. Germination and toxin production, however, take place only in wounds with low oxidation-reduction potential, such as those with devitalized tissue, foreign bodies, or active infection. *C. tetani* does not itself evoke inflammation, and the portal of entry retains a benign appearance unless infection with other organisms is present.

Toxin released in the wound binds to peripheral motor neuron terminals, enters the axon, and is transported to the nerve-cell body in the brainstem and spinal cord by retrograde intraneuronal transport. The toxin then migrates across the synapse to presynaptic terminals, where it blocks release of the inhibitory neurotransmitters glycine and gamma-aminobutyric acid (GABA). The blocking of neurotransmitter release by tetanospasmin, a zinc metalloprotease, involves the cleavage of protein(s) critical to proper function of the synaptic vesicle release apparatus. With diminished inhibition, the resting firing rate of the alpha motor neuron increases, producing rigidity. With lessened activity of reflexes, which limits polysynaptic spread of impulses (a glycinergic activity), agonists and antagonists may be recruited rather than inhibited, with the consequent production of spasms. Loss of inhibition also may affect preganglionic sympathetic neurons in the lateral gray matter of the spinal cord and produce sympathetic hyperactivity and high circulating catecholamine levels. Tetanospasmin, like botulinum toxin, may block neurotransmitter release at the neuromuscular junction and produce weakness or paralysis; recovery requires sprouting of new nerve terminals.

In local tetanus, only the nerves supplying the affected muscles are involved. Generalized tetanus occurs when toxin released in the wound enters the lymphatics and bloodstream and is spread widely to distant nerve terminals; the blood-brain barrier blocks direct entry into the central nervous system. If it is assumed that intraneuronal transport times are equal for all nerves, short nerves are affected before long nerves: this fact explains the sequential involvement of nerves of the head, trunk, and extremities in generalized tetanus.

CLINICAL MANIFESTATIONS Generalized tetanus, the most common form of the disease, is characterized by increased muscle tone and generalized spasms. The median time of onset after injury is 7 days; 15 percent of cases occur within 3 days and 10 percent after 14 days.

Typically, the patient first notices increased tone in the masseter muscles (trismus, or lockjaw). Dysphagia or stiffness or pain in the neck, shoulder, and back muscles appears concurrently or soon thereafter. The subsequent involvement of other muscles produces a rigid abdomen and stiff proximal limb muscles; the hands and feet are relatively spared. Sustained contraction of the facial muscles results in a grimace or sneer (risus sardonicus), and contraction of the back muscles produces an arched back (opisthotonos). Some patients develop paroxysmal, violent, painful, generalized muscle spasms that may cause cyanosis and threaten ventilation. These spasms occur repetitively and may be spontaneous or provoked by even the slightest stimulation. A constant threat during generalized spasms is reduced ventilation or apnea or laryngospasm. The severity of illness may be mild (muscle rigidity and few or no spasms), moderate (trismus, dysphagia, rigidity, and spasms), or severe (frequent explosive paroxysms). The patient may be febrile, although many have no fever; mentation is unimpaired. Deep tendon reflexes may be increased. Dysphagia or ileus may preclude oral feeding.

Autonomic dysfunction commonly complicates severe cases and is characterized by labile or sustained hypertension, tachycardia, arrhythmia, hyperpyrexia, profuse sweating, peripheral vasoconstriction, and increased plasma and urinary catecholamine levels. Periods of bradycardia and hypotension also may be documented. Sudden cardiac arrest sometimes occurs, but its basis is unknown. Other complications include pneumonia, fractures, muscle rupture, deep vein thrombophlebitis, pulmonary emboli, decubitus ulcer, and rhabdomyolysis.

Neonatal tetanus usually occurs as the generalized form and is usually fatal if left untreated. It develops in children born to inadequately immunized mothers, frequently after unsterile treatment of the umbilical cord stump. Its onset generally comes during the first 2 weeks of life. Poor feeding, rigidity, and spasms are typical features of neonatal tetanus.

Local tetanus is an uncommon form in which manifestations are restricted to muscles near the wound. The prognosis is excellent.

Cephalic tetanus, a rare form of local tetanus, follows head injury or ear infection. Trismus and dysfunction of one or more cranial nerves, often the seventh nerve, are found. The incubation period is a few days and the mortality is high.

DIAGNOSIS The diagnosis of tetanus is based entirely on clinical findings. Tetanus is unlikely if a reliable history indicates the completion of a primary vaccination series and the receipt of appropriate booster doses. Wounds should be cultured in suspected cases. However, *C. tetani* can be isolated from wounds of patients without tetanus and frequently cannot be recovered from wounds of those with tetanus. The leukocyte count may be elevated. Cerebrospinal fluid examination yields normal results. Electromyograms may show continuous discharge of motor units and shortening or absence of the silent interval normally seen after an action potential. Nonspecific changes may be evident on the electrocardiogram. Muscle enzyme levels may be raised. Serum antitoxin levels of 0.01 unit/mL or higher are considered protective and make tetanus unlikely, although cases developing despite protective antitoxin levels have been reported.

The differential diagnosis includes local conditions also producing trismus, such as alveolar abscess, strychnine poisoning, dystonic drug reactions (e.g., to phenothiazines and metoclopramide), and hypocalcemic tetany. Other conditions sometimes confused with tetanus include meningitis/encephalitis, rabies, and an acute intraabdominal process (because of the rigid abdomen). Markedly increased tone in central muscles (face, neck, chest, back, and abdomen) with superimposed generalized spasms and relative sparing of the hands and feet strongly suggests tetanus.

℞ TREATMENT

General Measures The goals of therapy are to eliminate the source of toxin, neutralize unbound toxin, prevent muscle spasms, and provide support—especially respiratory support—until recovery. Patients should be admitted to a quiet room in an intensive care unit, where observation and cardiopulmonary monitoring can be maintained continuously but stimulation can be minimized. Protection of the airway is vital. Wounds should be explored, carefully cleansed, and thoroughly debrided.

Antibiotic Therapy Although of unproven value, antibiotic therapy is administered to eradicate vegetative cells—the source of toxin. The use of penicillin (10 to 12 million units intravenously, given daily for 10 days) has been recommended, but metronidazole (500 mg every 6 h or 1 g every 12 h) is preferred by some experts on the basis of this drug's excellent antimicrobial activity, a survival rate higher than that obtained with penicillin in one nonrandomized trial, and the absence of the GABA antagonistic activity seen with penicillin. Clindamycin and erythromycin are also alternatives for the treatment of penicillin-allergic patients. Additional specific antimicrobial therapy should be given for active infection with other organisms.

Antitoxin Given to neutralize circulating toxin and unbound toxin in the wound, antitoxin effectively lowers mortality; toxin already bound to neural tissue is unaffected. Human tetanus immune globulin (TIG) is the preparation of choice and should be given promptly. The dose is 3000 to 6000 units intramuscularly, usually in divided doses because the volume is large. The optimal dose is not known, however, and results from one study indicated that a 500-unit dose was as effective as higher doses. Pooled intravenous immunoglobulin may be an alternative to TIG. It may be best to administer antitoxin before manipulating the wound; the value of injecting a dose proximal to the wound or infiltrating the wound is unclear. Additional doses are unnecessary because the half-life of antitoxin is long. Antibody does not penetrate the blood-brain barrier. Intrathecal administration should be considered experimental. Equine tetanus antitoxin (TAT) is also available. It is cheaper than human antitoxin, but its half-life is shorter and its administration commonly elicits hypersensitivity and serum sickness. Doses of up to 100,000 units are given, part intramuscularly and part intravenously, but 10,000 units may suffice.

Control of Muscle Spasms Many agents, alone and in combination, have been used to treat the muscle spasms, which are painful and can threaten ventilation by causing laryngospasm or sustained contraction of ventilatory muscles. The ideal therapeutic regimen would abolish spasmodic activity without causing oversedation and hypoventilation. Diazepam, a benzodiazepine and GABA agonist, is in wide use. The dose is titrated, and large doses (250 mg/d or more) may be required. Lorazepam, with a longer duration of action, and midazolam, whose short half-life necessitates administration by continuous intravenous infusion, are other options. Barbiturates and chlorpromazine are considered second-line agents. Mechanical ventilation and therapeutic paralysis with a nondepolarizing neuromuscular blocking agent may be required for the treatment of spasms unresponsive to medication or spasms that threaten ventilation. However, prolonged paralysis after the discontinuation of therapy with such agents has been described, and both the need for continued paralysis and the occurrence of complications should be assessed daily. Alternative agents include propofol, which is expensive, and dantrolene and baclofen, which are being investigated in the hope of shortening the period of therapeutic paralysis.

Respiratory Care Intubation or tracheostomy, with or without mechanical ventilation, may be required for hypoventilation due to oversedation or laryngospasm or for the avoidance of aspiration by patients with trismus, disordered swallowing, or dysphagia. The need for these procedures should be anticipated, and they should be undertaken electively and early.

Autonomic Dysfunction The optimal therapy for sympathetic overactivity has not been defined. Agents that have been considered include labetalol (an alpha- and beta-adrenergic blocking agent that is recommended by some experts but that reportedly has caused sudden death), esmolol administered by continuous infusion (a beta blocker whose short half-life may be advantageous in the event of severe hypertension from unopposed alpha-adrenergic activity), clonidine (a central-acting antiadrenergic drug), and morphine sulfate. Parenteral magnesium sulfate and continuous spinal or epidural anesthesia have been used but may be more difficult to administer and monitor. The relative efficacy of these modalities has yet to be determined. Hypotension or bradycardia may require volume expansion, use of vasopressors or chronotropic agents, or pacemaker insertion.

Vaccine Patients recovering from tetanus should be actively immunized (see below) because immunity is not induced by the small amount of toxin that produces disease.

Additional Measures Additional therapeutic measures include hydration to control insensible and other fluid losses, which may be significant; the meeting of the patient's increased nutritional requirements by enteral or parenteral means; physiotherapy to prevent contractures; and administration of heparin or another anticoagulant to prevent pulmonary emboli. Bowel, bladder, and renal function must be monitored. Gastrointestinal bleeding and decubitus ulcers must be prevented, and intercurrent infection should be treated.

PREVENTION **Active Immunization** All partially immunized and unimmunized adults should receive vaccine, as should those recovering from tetanus. The primary series for adults consists of three doses: the first and second doses are given 4 to 8 weeks apart, and the third dose is given 6 to 12 months after the second. A booster dose is required every 10 years and may be given at mid-decade ages—35, 45, and so on. Combined tetanus and diphtheria toxoid (Td) adsorbed (for adult use), rather than single-antigen tetanus toxoid, is preferred for persons over 7 years of age.

Wound Management Proper wound management requires consideration of the need for (1) passive immunization with TIG and (2) active immunization with vaccine, preferably Td in persons over age 7. For clean minor wounds, Td is administered to persons who have (1) unknown tetanus immunization histories; (2) received fewer than three doses of adsorbed tetanus toxoid; (3) received three or more doses of adsorbed vaccine, with the last dose given more than 10 years previously; and (4) received three doses of *fluid* (nonadsorbed) vaccine. The recommendations for contaminated or severe wounds are identical, except that vaccine should be given to those who have received three or more doses of adsorbed tetanus toxoid if more than 5 years have elapsed since the last dose. Passive immunization with TIG is not recommended for clean minor wounds but is given for all other wounds if the patient's vaccination history indicates unknown or partial immunization. The dose of TIG for passive immunization of persons with wounds of average severity is 250 units intramuscularly, which produces a protective antibody level in the serum for at least 4 to 6 weeks; the appropriate dose of TAT is 3000 to 6000 units. Vaccine and tetanus antitoxin should be administered at separate sites in separate syringes.

Neonatal Tetanus Measures aimed at preventing neonatal tetanus include maternal vaccination, even during pregnancy; efforts to increase the proportion of births that take place in the hospital; and the provision of training for nonmedical birth attendants.

PROGNOSIS The application of methods to support respiration has markedly improved the prognosis in tetanus; mortality rates as low as 10 percent have been reported from units accustomed to handling such cases. In the United States, 11 deaths from tetanus were reported in 1990, 11 in 1991, and 9 in 1992. The outcome is poor in neonates and the elderly and in patients with a short incubation period, a short interval from the onset of symptoms to admission, or a short period from onset of symptoms to the first spasm (period of onset).

The course of tetanus extends over 4 to 6 weeks, and patients may require ventilatory support for 3 weeks during this period. Increased tone and minor spasms can last for months, but recovery is usually complete.

BIBLIOGRAPHY

ABRUTYN E, BERLIN JA: Intrathecal therapy of tetanus: A meta-analysis. JAMA 266:2262, 1991

AHMADSYAH I, SALIM A: Treatment of tetanus: An open study to compare the efficacy of procaine penicillin and metronidazole. BMJ 291:648, 1985

BAGETTA G, NISTICO B: Tetanus toxin as a neurobiological tool to study mechanisms of neuronal cell death in the mammalian brain. Pharmacol Ther 62:29, 1994

BLECK TP: *Clostridium tetani*, in *Principles and Practice of Infectious Diseases*, vol 2, 4th ed, GL Mandell et al (eds). New York, Churchill Livingstone, 1995

CENTERS FOR DISEASE CONTROL: Diphtheria, tetanus, and pertussis: Recommendations for vaccine use and other preventive measures. Recommendations of the Immunization Practices Advisory Committee. Morb Mort Week Rep 40(RR-10):1, 1991

CRONE NE, REDER AT: Severe tetanus in immunized patients with high anti-tetanus titers. Neurology 42:761, 1992

GERGEN PJ et al: A population-based serologic survey of immunity to tetanus in the United States. N Engl J Med 332:761, 1995

LEE DC, LEDERMAN HM: Anti-tetanus toxoid antibodies in intravenous gamma globulin: An alternative to tetanus immune globulin. J Infect Dis 166:642, 1992

SANFORD JP: Tetanus—forgotten but not gone. N Engl J Med 332:812, 1995

SCHIAVO G et al: Intracellular targets and metalloprotease activity of tetanus and botulinum neurotoxins. Curr Top Microbiol Immunol 195:257, 1995

WASSILAK SGF et al: Tetanus toxoid, in *Vaccines*, 2d ed, SA Plotkin and EA Mortimer Jr (eds). Philadelphia, Saunders, 1994

WESLEY AG, PATHER M: Tetanus in children: An 11-year review. Ann Trop Paediatr 7:32, 1987

YEN JM et al: Role of quinine in the high mortality of intramuscular injection tetanus. Lancet 344:786, 1994

147	*Elias Abrutyn*

BOTULISM

DEFINITION Botulism is a paralytic disease that begins with cranial nerve involvement and progresses caudally to involve the extremities. It is caused by potent protein neurotoxins elaborated by *Clostridium botulinum*. Cases may be classified as (1) *food-borne botulism*, from ingestion of preformed toxin in food contaminated with *C. botulinum*; (2) *wound botulism*, from toxin produced in wounds contaminated with the organism; (3) *infant botulism*, from ingestion of spores and production of toxin in the intestine of infants; or (4) *undetermined classification*, a group that includes some cases in older children and adults in which disease is produced by a mechanism similar to that described for infant botulism.

ETIOLOGIC AGENT *C. botulinum*, a heterogeneous group of anaerobic gram-positive organisms that form subterminal spores, is found in soil and marine environments throughout the world and elaborates the most potent bacterial toxin known. Organisms of types A through G have been distinguished by the antigenic specificities of their toxins; a classification system based on physiologic characteristics has also been described. Rare strains of other clostridial species—*C. butyricum* and *C. baratii*—also have been found to produce toxin. *C. botulinum* strains with proteolytic activity can digest food and produce

a spoiled appearance; nonproteolytic types leave the appearance of food unchanged.

Of the eight distinct toxin types described (A, B, C_1, C_2, D, E, F, and G), all except for C_2 are neurotoxins; C_2 is a cytotoxin of unknown clinical significance. Botulinum neurotoxin, whether ingested or produced in the intestine or a wound, enters the vascular system and is transported to peripheral cholinergic nerve terminals, including neuromuscular junctions, postganglionic parasympathetic nerve endings, and peripheral ganglia. The central nervous system is not involved. Active neurotoxin (150 kDa) is composed of a heavy chain (100 kDa) and a light chain (50 kDa). The steps involved in neurotoxin activity include (1) specific binding to presynaptic nerve cells at the myoneural junction, (2) internalization of the toxin inside the nerve cell in vesicles of unknown nature, (3) translocation of the toxin into the cytosol, and (4) proteolysis by toxin (a zinc endopeptidase) of components of the neuroexocytosis apparatus that curtails the release of the neurotransmitter acetylcholine. Cure follows sprouting of new nerve terminals.

Toxin can be inactivated during home cooking by exposure to a temperature of 100°C for 10 min. In the gastrointestinal tract, toxin is complexed with nontoxin proteins and resists degradation. Spores are highly heat-resistant, and their inactivation requires exposure to a temperature of 120°C (e.g., in steam sterilizers or pressure cookers).

Toxin types A, B, E, and (in rare instances) F cause human disease; type G (now called *C. argentinense*) has been associated with sudden death, but not with neuroparalytic illness, in a few patients in Switzerland; and types C and D cause animal disease.

EPIDEMIOLOGY Human botulism occurs worldwide. In the United States, the geographic distribution of cases by toxin type parallels the distribution of organism types found in the environment. Type A predominates west of the Rocky Mountains; type B is generally distributed but is more common in the East; and type E is found in the Pacific Northwest, Alaska, and the Great Lakes area. In the United States, food-borne botulism has been associated primarily with home-canned food, particularly vegetables, fruit, and condiments, and less commonly with meat and fish. Type E outbreaks are frequently associated with fish products. Commercial products occasionally cause outbreaks, but some of these outbreaks have resulted from improper handling after purchase. Outbreaks in restaurants, schools, and private homes have been traced to uncommon sources (commercial potpies, beef stew, turkey loaf, sauteed onions, baked potatoes, and chopped garlic in oil). Food-borne botulism can occur when (1) a food to be preserved is contaminated with spores, (2) preservation does not inactivate the spores but kills other putrefactive bacteria that might inhibit the growth of *C. botulinum* and provides anaerobic conditions at a pH and temperature that allow germination and toxin production, and (3) food is not heated to a temperature that destroys toxin before being eaten.

CLINICAL MANIFESTATIONS **Food-Borne Botulism** Following ingestion of food containing toxin, illness varies from a mild condition for which no medical advice is sought to very severe disease that can result in death within 24 h. The incubation period is usually 18 to 36 h but, depending on toxin dose, can extend from a few hours to several days. Symmetric descending paralysis is characteristic and can lead to respiratory failure and death. Cranial nerve involvement, which almost always marks the onset of symptoms, usually produces diplopia, dysarthria, and/or dysphagia; weakness progresses, often rapidly, from the head to involve the neck, arms, thorax, and legs; the weakness is occasionally asymmetric. Nausea, vomiting, and abdominal pain may precede or follow the onset of paralysis. Dizziness, blurred vision, dry mouth, and very dry, occasionally sore throat are common. Patients are generally alert and oriented, but they may be drowsy, agitated, and anxious. Typically, they have no fever. Ptosis is frequent; the pupillary reflexes may be depressed, and fixed or dilated pupils are noted in half of patients. The gag reflex may be suppressed, and deep tendon reflexes may be normal or decreased. Paralytic ileus, severe constipation, and urinary retention are common.

Wound Botulism When wounds are contaminated with *C. botulinum* spores, the spores may germinate into vegetative organisms that produce toxin. This rare condition resembles food-borne illness except that the incubation period is longer, averaging about 10 days, and gastrointestinal symptoms are lacking. Wound botulism has been documented after traumatic injury involving contamination with soil, in chronic drug abusers, and after cesarean delivery. The illness has occurred even after antibiotics have been given to prevent wound infection. When present, fever is probably attributable to concurrent infection with other bacteria. The wound may appear benign.

Infant Botulism In infant botulism, the most common form of the disease, toxin is produced in and absorbed from the intestine after the germination of ingested spores. The severity ranges from mild illness with failure to thrive to fulminant severe paralysis with respiratory failure and may be one cause of sudden infant death. The identification of contaminated honey as one source of spores has led to the recommendation that honey not be fed to children less than 12 months of age. Most cases cannot be attributed to a particular food source. The factors permitting intestinal colonization with *C. botulinum* are not fully defined, but cases usually involve infants under 6 months of age; susceptibility may decrease as the normal intestinal flora develops.

Undetermined Classification This group of cases includes those in which a specific food cannot be implicated. In some cases, the disease resembles infant botulism in that toxin is produced in the intestine of persons colonized with the organism. Toxin and organisms may be found in the stool over prolonged periods, and spores—but not toxin—may be found in the suspect food. Gastrointestinal disease or surgery may predispose to illness. Descriptive names for this illness include *adult enteric infectious botulism*, *adult infectious botulism of unknown source*, and *adult infant botulism*.

DIAGNOSIS A diagnosis of botulism must be considered in afebrile, mentally intact patients who have symmetric descending paralysis without sensory findings. The diagnosis must be suspected on clinical grounds in the context of an appropriate history. Conditions often confused with botulism include myasthenia gravis, which may be ruled out by electromyography and antibody studies, and Guillain-Barré syndrome, which is characterized by ascending paralysis, sensory abnormalities, and elevation of the protein concentration in cerebrospinal fluid. The Fisher variant of Guillain-Barré—a descending paralysis—can indeed be difficult to differentiate from botulism. Other conditions that may resemble botulism include Lambert-Eaton syndrome, poliomyelitis, tick paralysis, diphtheria, and intoxications from mushrooms, medications, or chemicals. Hypermagnesemia should be considered.

The demonstration of toxin in serum by bioassay in mice is definitive, but this test may be negative, particularly in wound and infant botulism. It is performed only by specific laboratories, which can be identified through regional public health authorities. The demonstration of the organism or its toxin in vomitus, gastric fluid, or stool is strongly suggestive of the diagnosis, because intestinal carriage is rare. Isolation of the organism from food without toxin is insufficient grounds for the diagnosis. Wound cultures yielding the organism are suggestive of botulism. The edrophonium chloride (Tensilon) test for myasthenia gravis may be falsely positive in botulism but is usually less dramatically positive than in the former condition. Nerve conduction velocity is normal, but action potentials on routine electromyography are decreased with a supramaximal stimulus, and facilitation is evident after repetitive stimulation at high frequency. Single-fiber electromyography may be helpful. The white blood cell count and sedimentation rate are normal.

℞ **TREATMENT**
Patients should be hospitalized and monitored closely, both clinically and by spirometry, pulse oximetry, and measurement of arterial blood gases for incipient respiratory failure. Intubation and mechanical ventilation should be strongly considered when the vital capacity is less than 30 percent of predicted, especially when paralysis is progressing rapidly and hypoxemia with absolute or relative hypercarbia is documented (see Chap. 266). Serial measurements of the maximal static inspiratory pressure may be useful in predicting respiratory failure.

In food-borne illness, trivalent (types A, B, and E) equine antitoxin should be administered as soon as possible after specimens are obtained for laboratory analysis. The initiation of treatment should not await laboratory confirmation, which may take days. After testing for hypersensitivity to horse serum, two vials of antitoxin are given, one intravenously and one intramuscularly; repeated doses probably are not necessary but may be given 2 to 4 h later. Anaphylaxis and serum sickness are risks inherent in use of the equine product, and desensitization of allergic patients may be required. If there is no ileus, cathartics and enemas may be given to purge the gut of toxin; emetics or gastric lavage can also be used if the time since ingestion is brief (only a few hours). Use of antibiotics to eliminate an intestinal source for possible continued toxin production and of guanidine hydrochloride and other drugs to reverse paralysis is of unproven value. In the United States, antitoxin as well as help in clinical management and laboratory confirmation are available at *any* time from state health departments or the Centers for Disease Control and Prevention.

Treatment of infant botulism requires supportive care. Neither equine antitoxin nor antibiotics have been shown to be beneficial, and the value of human botulism immune globulin, an experimental preparation, is still being evaluated. In wound botulism, equine antitoxin is administered. The wound should be thoroughly explored and debrided, and an antibiotic such as penicillin should be given to eradicate *C. botulinum* from the site, even though the benefit of this therapy is unproven. Results of wound cultures should guide the use of other antibiotics.

PROGNOSIS Type A disease is generally more severe than type B, and mortality from botulism is higher among patients above age 60 than among younger patients. With improved respiratory and intensive care, the case-fatality rate in food-borne illness has been reduced to about 7.5 percent and is low in infant botulism as well. Artificial respiratory support may be required for months in severe cases. Some patients experience residual weakness and autonomic dysfunction for as long as a year after disease onset.

BOTULINUM TOXIN THERAPY Botulinum toxin is being used as therapy for strabismus, blepharospasm, and other dystonias and appears safe and effective.

BIBLIOGRAPHY

CARDOSO F, JANKOVIC J: Clinical use of botulinum neurotoxins. Curr Top Microbiol Immunol 195:123, 1995

DAVIS LE: Botulinum toxin: From poison to medicine. West J Med 158:25, 1993

FERRARI ND III, WEISSE ME: Botulism. Adv Pediatr Infect Dis 10:81, 1995

HATHEWAY CL: Botulism: The present status of disease. Curr Top Microbiol Immunol 195:55, 1995

JAHN R, NIEMANN H: Molecular mechanisms of clostridial neurotoxins. Ann NY Acad Sci 733:245, 1994

MCCROSKEY LM, HATHEWAY CL: The large intestine as the site of *Clostridium botulinum* colonization in human infant botulism. J Clin Microbiol 26:1052, 1988

MECHEM CC, WALTZER FG: Wound botulism. Vet Hum Toxicol 36:233, 1994

OGUMA K et al: Structure and function of *Clostridium botulinum* toxins. Microbiol Immunol 39:161, 1995

ROBLOT P et al: Retrospective study of 108 cases of botulism in Poitiers, France. J Med Microbiol 40:379, 1994

SCHIAVO G et al: Intracellular targets and metalloprotease activity of tetanus and botulism neurotoxins. Curr Top Microbiol Immunol 195:257, 1995

SCHWARZ PJ, ARNON SS: Botulism immune globulin for infant botulism arrives—one year and a Gulf War later. West J Med 156:197, 1991

SMITH LDS, SUGIYAMA H: *Botulism: The Organism, Its Toxins, the Disease*, 2d ed. Springfield, IL, Charles C Thomas, 1988

WEBER JT et al: Wound botulism in a patient with a tooth abscess: Case report and review. Clin Infect Dis 16:635, 1993

Wound botulism—California, 1995. Morb Mortal Wkly Rep 44:889, 1995

148 *Dennis L. Kasper, Dori F. Zaleznik*

GAS GANGRENE, ANTIBIOTIC-ASSOCIATED COLITIS, AND OTHER CLOSTRIDIAL INFECTIONS

DEFINITION Bacteria of the genus *Clostridium* are gram-positive, spore-forming, obligate anaerobes that are ubiquitous in nature. There are more than 60 recognized species of clostridia, many of which are generally considered saprophytic. Some of these species are pathogenic for humans and animals, particularly under conditions of lowered oxidation-reduction potential. Infections associated with these organisms range from localized wound contamination to overwhelming systemic disease. The four major disease categories for which clostridia are responsible are intestinal disorders, deep tissue suppurative infections, skin and soft tissue infections, and bacteremia (see Table 148-1). Toxins play a major role in some of these syndromes.

ETIOLOGY In humans, clostridia normally reside in the gastrointestinal tract and in the female genital tract, although they occasionally are isolated from the skin or the mouth. Of the known species of the genus *Clostridium*, at least 30 have been isolated from human infections. Like several other pathogenic anaerobic bacterial species, clostridia are quite aerotolerant, but they do not grow on artificial media in the presence of oxygen. Clostridia characteristically produce abundant gas in artificial media and form subterminal endospores. *Clostridium perfringens*, one of the most important species, is encapsulated and nonmotile and rarely sporulates in artificial media; the spores usually can be destroyed by boiling. *Clostridium tetani* and *Clostridium botulinum* are discussed in detail in Chaps. 146 and 147, respectively.

Clostridia are present in the normal colonic flora at concentrations of 10^9 to 10^{10} per gram. Of the 30 or more species that normally colonize humans, *Clostridium ramosum* is the most common and is followed in frequency by *C. perfringens*. These organisms are universally present in soil at concentrations of up to 10^4 per gram. Clostridia are gram-positive organisms; however, in clinical specimens or stationary-phase cultures, many species may appear to be gram-negative. Therefore, the results of Gram's staining of cultures or clinical material should be interpreted with great care.

C. perfringens is the most common of the clostridial species isolated from tissue infections and bacteremias; next in frequency are *Clostridium novyi* and *Clostridium septicum*. In the category of enteric infections, *Clostridium difficile* is an important cause of antibiotic-associated colitis, and *C. perfringens* is associated with food poisoning and enteritis necroticans.

PATHOGENESIS Despite the isolation of clostridial species from many serious traumatic wounds, the prevalence of severe infec-

Table 148-1

Classification of Diseases Caused by Clostridia

1. Intestinal syndromes
   a. Food poisoning
   b. Enteritis necroticans
   c. Antibiotic-associated colitis
2. Suppurative deep tissue infections
   a. Mixed bacterial infections
   b. Monobacterial infections
3. Skin and soft tissue infections
   a. Simple contamination
   b. Local infection without systemic signs
   c. Spreading cellulitis and fasciitis
   d. Myonecrosis (gas gangrene)
4. Bacteremia
   a. Transient bacteremia
   b. Sepsis

tions due to these organisms is low. Two factors that appear to be essential to the development of severe disease are tissue necrosis and a low oxidation-reduction potential. *C. perfringens* requires about 14 amino acids and at least six additional growth factors for optimal growth. These nutrients are not found in appreciable concentrations in normal body fluids but are present in necrotic tissue. When *C. perfringens* grows in necrotic tissue, a zone of tissue damage due to the toxins elaborated by the organism allows for progressive growth. In contrast, when only a few bacteria leak into the bloodstream from a small defect in the intestinal wall, the organisms do not have the opportunity to multiply rapidly because blood as a medium for growth is relatively deficient in certain amino acids and growth factors. Therefore, in a patient without tissue necrosis, bacteremia is usually benign.

C. perfringens possesses at least 17 possible virulence factors, including 12 active tissue toxins and enterotoxins. This species has been divided into five types (A through E) on the basis of four major toxins: alpha, beta, epsilon, and iota. The alpha toxin is a phospholipase C (lecithinase) that splits lecithin into phosphorylcholine and diglyceride. This alpha toxin has been associated with gas gangrene and is known to be hemolytic, to destroy platelets and polymorphonuclear leukocytes, and to cause widespread capillary damage. When injected intravenously, it causes massive intravascular hemolysis and damages liver mitochondria. Alpha toxin may be important in the initiation of muscle infections that may progress to gas gangrene. Experimentally, the higher the concentration of alpha toxin present in the culture fluid, the smaller the dose of *C. perfringens* required to produce infection. The protective effect of antiserum is directly proportional to its content of alpha antitoxin. Beta, epsilon, and iota toxins are also known to increase capillary permeability.

C. difficile produces two major toxins, designated A and B. In experimental models of intestinal inflammation, toxin A mediates alteration in fluid secretion, enhances inflammation, and induces postcapillary venules to leak albumin. Toxin B appears to be more active than toxin A in causing damage to and exfoliation of superficial epithelial cells. Toxin B inhibits ADP ribosylation of Rho proteins. Both toxins cause disruption and condensation of F actin, which result in electrophysiologic alterations of colonic tissue. Diarrheal disease due to *C. difficile* is toxin mediated. Earlier teaching about the pathogenesis of this disease centered on the overgrowth of *C. difficile* when antibiotics suppress the normal bowel flora. Actually, the mechanism is probably more complex, since many of the antibiotics that cause this disease are active against *C. difficile* as well as other members of the bowel flora and since many patients who become colonized with *C. difficile* do not develop diarrhea. Critical features in the pathogenesis of this disease include mechanisms of toxin production and the interaction of *C. difficile* with other components of the bowel flora. Some antibiotics may actually trigger toxin production by the organism. In turn, other constituents of the bowel flora may suppress or inhibit toxin production. *Clostridium sordellii*, for example, neutralizes cytotoxin B in vitro. In addition, when antibiotics eliminate more sensitive members of the bowel flora, more resistant organisms may produce enzymes such as β-lactamases that can inactivate antibiotics and thereby facilitate the growth of *C. difficile*.

CLINICAL MANIFESTATIONS **Intestinal Disorders** *Food poisoning* *C. perfringens* is the second or third most common cause of food poisoning in the United States (see Chap. 128). Outbreaks generally have resulted from problems in the cooling and storage of food cooked in bulk. The food sources primarily involved are meat, meat products, and poultry. Generally, the implicated meats have been cooked, allowed to cool, and then recooked the following day, often in a stew or hash. Strains of *C. perfringens* that contaminate meat manage to survive initial cooking. During reheating, the organisms sporulate and germinate. The disease is associated with an attack rate that is often as high as 70 percent. Symptoms of food poisoning from type A strains develop 8 to 24 h after ingestion of foods heavily contaminated with the organism. The primary symptoms include epigastric pain, nausea, and watery diarrhea usually lasting 12 to 24 h. Fever and vomiting are uncommon. Diarrhea appears to be caused by a heat-labile protein enterotoxin. The enterotoxin inhibits glucose transport, damages the intestinal epithelium, and causes protein loss into the intestinal lumen.

C. perfringens has also been implicated in a more severe form of diarrhea than that of classic food poisoning. This more severe disease tends to occur in the elderly and has been associated with antibiotic use in hospitalized populations. In this form of disease, diarrhea is generally more profuse, of longer duration, and accompanied by abdominal pain. Blood and mucus have been detected in the feces of the affected patients. In one hospital-based study of a cluster of cases, widespread environmental contamination with *C. perfringens* spores was documented.

Enteritis necroticans Necrotizing enteritis (enteritis necroticans, or *pigbel*) is caused by beta toxin produced by type C strains of *C. perfringens* following ingestion of a high-protein meal in conjunction with trypsin inhibitors (e.g., in sweet potatoes) by a susceptible host who has limited intestinal proteolytic activity. This disease has been reported among children and adults in New Guinea. A similar disease, *darmbrand*, was epidemic in Germany after World War II. Clinical features of pigbel include acute abdominal pain, bloody diarrhea, vomiting, shock, and peritonitis; 40 percent of patients die. Pathologic studies reveal an acute ulcerative process of the bowel restricted to the small intestine. The mucosa is lifted off the submucosa, with the formation of large denuded areas. Pseudomembranes composed of sloughed epithelium are common, and gas may dissect into the submucosa. The source of the organisms may be the patient's own intestinal flora; cultures of ingested pork have failed to yield the organism. Antibodies to the beta toxin of *C. perfringens* have been of considerable benefit in changing the course of established disease. In a large-scale trial, children immunized with *C. perfringens* beta toxoid were protected.

Antibiotic-associated colitis Currently, strains of *C. difficile* that produce toxins detectable in the stool are the only identified cause of colitis induced by antibiotic use. The diagnosis of this type of colitis requires that there be no other identifiable cause of diarrhea and that the onset of symptoms occur either during antimicrobial administration or within 4 weeks after treatment with the implicated agent has been discontinued. Essentially any antibiotic can cause this syndrome; even metronidazole and vancomycin, which are used to treat the disease, have been implicated as etiologic agents in some cases. On a per-use basis, clindamycin, which was the first antibiotic described to cause this entity, is the most commonly implicated antibiotic. However, since other antibiotics are prescribed more often than clindamycin in the United States, cephalosporins are currently the antibiotics that most commonly cause *C. difficile* enterocolitis, and penicillins rank next in frequency.

Antimicrobial-associated diarrhea can be divided into four categories based on the appearance of the colon: (1) normal colonic mucosa; (2) mild erythema with some edema; (3) granular, friable, or hemorrhagic mucosa; and (4) pseudomembrane formation. Most patients with antibiotic-associated diarrhea have a normal, minimally erythematous colonic mucosa with some edema. Occasionally, colitis is more severe and is characterized by a granular, friable, or hemorrhagic mucosa. Examination of stool from the affected patients may reveal large numbers of red blood cells and some leukocytes. Biopsy shows subepithelial edema with round cell infiltration of the lamina propria and focal extravasation of erythrocytes. *C. difficile* cytotoxin B has been found in 15 to 75 percent of stools from patients in the first three categories, which suggests that other factors are involved in the pathogenesis of antibiotic-associated diarrhea.

The most characteristic form of antibiotic-associated colitis caused by *C. difficile* is pseudomembranous colitis (PMC). More than 95 percent of patients with documented PMC have positive stool toxin assays. Close inspection of pseudomembranes reveals exudative, punctate, raised plaques with skip areas or edematous hyperemic mucosa. These plaques can enlarge and coalesce over large segments of intestine in the later stages of disease. The clinical spectrum of antibiotic-associated PMC is diverse. Diarrhea is the key feature and is usually watery, voluminous, and without gross blood or mucus. Most patients have abdominal cramps and tenderness, fever, and leukocytosis. However, the symptoms vary considerably. At one end of the spectrum are many patients with annoying diarrhea but no systemic signs or symptoms, while at the other end are those with severe systemic toxicity, fever (temperatures of 40 to 40.6°C, or 104 to 105°F), and peripheral white blood cell counts of up to 50,000/μL with a marked left shift. Fecal examination frequently reveals leukocytes. Without specific therapy, the course is highly variable. Some patients, particularly those with clinically mild disease, experience prompt resolution of symptoms with discontinuation of drug treatment, while others have protracted diarrhea with large stool volumes for up to 8 weeks, with resultant hypoalbuminemia and electrolyte imbalance. Severely ill patients with toxic megacolon and colonic perforation have been reported. Among patients who are severely ill mortality rates may be as high as 30 percent, while in most of those with minimal symptoms disease may resolve with the discontinuation of antibiotic treatment alone. In the majority of patients, symptoms begin 4 to 10 days after antibiotic therapy is initiated. However, about 25 percent of patients do not develop symptoms until use of the implicated antimicrobial has been discontinued, in some instances as long as 4 weeks afterward. Some cases have been reported within hours after initiation of antibiotic therapy or after a single dose of antibiotic administered for surgical prophylaxis.

Suppurative Deep Tissue Infections Clostridia are recovered frequently from various suppurative conditions in conjunction with other anaerobic and aerobic bacteria but also can be the only organisms isolated. These suppurative conditions, which exist with severe local inflammation but usually without the characteristic systemic signs induced by clostridial toxins, include intraabdominal sepsis, empyema, pelvic abscess, subcutaneous abscess, frostbite with gas gangrene, infection of a stump in an amputee, brain abscess, prostatic abscess, perianal abscess, conjunctivitis, infection of a renal cell carcinoma, and infection of an aortic graft.

Clostridia are isolated from approximately two-thirds of patients with intraabdominal infections resulting from intestinal perforation. *C. ramosum*, *C. perfringens*, and *Clostridium bifermentans* are the most commonly isolated species. The presence of clostridial species does not affect the clinical presentation or outcome of these infections (see Chap. 169).

An association has been made between malignancy and the isolation of *C. septicum* in the absence of grossly contaminated deep traumatic wounds. A major site for such a malignancy is the gastrointestinal tract, particularly the colon. An association with leukemia or with other solid tumors also has been noted. Some of these patients present with *C. septicum* bacteremia; these cases have a fulminant clinical course (discussed below). Others develop localized suppurative infection in the abdomen or the abdominal wall without bacteremia. Presumably, this infection arises from a silent perforation that leads to intraabdominal abscess formation.

Clostridia have been isolated from suppurative infections of the female genital tract, particularly tuboovarian and pelvic abscesses. The major species involved has been *C. perfringens*. Most of these are mild suppurative infections without evidence of uterine gangrene. *C. perfringens* has been isolated from as many as 20 percent of diseased gallbladders at surgery. One clinical syndrome, emphysematous cholecystitis, is caused by clostridial species at least 50 percent of the time. In this syndrome, gas forms in the biliary radicles and the wall of the gallbladder. It is seen most often in diabetic patients. Although the mortality rate in this entity is higher than in more common forms of cholecystitis, there is no evidence of myonecrosis.

Clostridia are among the many organisms found in empyema fluid or isolated by transtracheal aspiration from patients with lung abscesses. There is no unique clinical clue to the presence of clostridia (as opposed to other organisms) in these infections. *C. perfringens* has been reported as a cause of empyema arising from aspiration pneumonia, pulmonary emboli, and infarction. However, the majority of cases of clostridial empyema are secondary to trauma.

Skin and Soft Tissue Infections Various categories of traumatic wound infections due to clostridia have been described: simple contamination, anaerobic cellulitis, fasciitis with or without systemic manifestations, and anaerobic myonecrosis.

Simple contamination Clostridia are cultured most often from wounds in the absence of clinical signs of sepsis. As many as 30 percent of battle wounds are contaminated by clostridia without signs of suppuration, and 16 percent of penetrating abdominal wounds yield clostridia on culture despite treatment with cephalothin and kanamycin. In cases of trauma, clostridia are isolated with equal frequency from suppurative and well-healing wounds. Thus the diagnosis of clostridial infection should be based on clinical rather than bacteriologic criteria.

Localized infection of the skin and soft tissue without systemic signs This condition, originally referred to as *anaerobic cellulitis*, is a localized infection involving the skin and soft tissue and is due to clostridia alone or with other bacteria. There are no systemic signs of toxicity, although the infection may invade locally, producing necrosis. These infections tend to be relatively indolent, spreading slowly to contiguous areas. Localized infections are relatively free of pain and edema. Perhaps because of the lack of edema, gas that is limited to the wound and the immediately surrounding tissue may be more evident than in gas gangrene. In these localized infections, gas is never found intramuscularly. Cellulitis, perirectal abscesses, and diabetic foot ulcers are typical infections from which clostridial species can be isolated. If inadequately treated, these localized infections advance by extension through subcutaneous tissue and fascial planes into muscle and may produce severe systemic disease with signs of toxemia.

A localized form of suppurative myositis has been described in heroin addicts. These patients develop local pain and tenderness in discrete areas (particularly the thigh and forearm), with the subsequent appearance of fluctuance and crepitance that require surgical drainage. The unusual aspect of these infections is that they remain localized without systemic signs of toxicity. Moreover, the affected local areas are not necessarily sites of trauma or heroin injection. Pathologic examination reveals subcutaneous abscesses, purulent myositis, and fasciitis from which clostridia are recovered in pure culture; on occasion, mixed infections involving aerobes and anaerobes are found.

Spreading cellulitis and fasciitis with systemic toxicity This condition involves diffuse spreading cellulitis and fasciitis, without myonecrosis and with only mild inflammation in muscle. Patients present with the abrupt onset of a syndrome that progresses rapidly (within hours) through the fascial planes. In cases with suppuration and gas in soft tissues as well as overwhelming toxemia, the infection is rapidly fatal. On physical examination there is subcutaneous crepitance but little localized pain. Surgery is of no proven value because there are no discretely involved tissues amenable to resection, as may be the case in myonecrosis. However, in rapidly advancing fasciitis, incision of the affected area is still the cornerstone of therapy. The initial local lesion may be quite innocuous and arises from an area involved by tumor or other infection and not by injury. The systemic toxic effects include hemolysis and injury of capillary membranes. Usually, this infection is uniformly fatal within 48 h, despite intensive therapy involving antitoxin and exchange transfusion. This syndrome is seen most commonly in patients with carcinoma, especially of the sigmoid or the cecum. Presumably, the tumor invades the fascia, and colonic contents leak into the abdominal wall. Patients present with extreme toxicity and occasionally with total-body crepitance. The syndrome differs from necrotizing fasciitis caused by other organisms in three respects: (1) rapid mortality, (2) rapid tissue invasion, and (3) the systemic effects of the toxin, typified by massive hemolysis.

Clostridial myonecrosis (gas gangrene) Clostridial myonecrosis occurs when bacteria invade healthy muscle from adjacent traumatized muscle or soft tissue. The infection originates in a wound contaminated with clostridia. Although more than 30 percent of deep wounds are infected with clostridia, the incidence of clostridial myonecrosis is quite low. These infections occur in both military and civilian settings. An essential factor in the genesis of gas gangrene appears to be trauma, particularly involving deep muscle laceration. The entity of clostridial myonecrosis is relatively uncommon after simple, through-and-through bullet wounds without shattering of bone and is relatively common following shrapnel fragmentation wounds, particularly when deep muscle is involved. In civilian cases, gas gangrene can follow trauma, surgery, or intramuscular injection. The trauma need not be severe; however, the wound must be deep, necrotic, and without communication to the surface.

The incubation period of gas gangrene is usually short: almost always less than 3 days and frequently less than 24 h. Eighty percent of cases are caused by *C. perfringens*, while *C. novyi*, *C. septicum*, and *Clostridium histolyticum* cause most of the other cases. Typically, gas gangrene begins with the sudden onset of pain in the region of the wound, which helps to differentiate it from spreading cellulitis. Once established, the pain increases steadily in severity but remains localized to the infected area and spreads only if the infection spreads. Soon after pain develops, local swelling and edema—accompanied by a thin, often hemorrhagic exudate—appear. Patients frequently develop marked tachycardia, but elevation in temperature may be only minimal. Gas usually is not obvious at this early stage and may be completely absent. Frothiness of the wound exudate may be noted. The skin is tense, white, often marbled with blue, and cooler than normal. The symptoms progress rapidly; swelling, edema, and toxemia increase, and a profuse serous discharge, which may have a peculiar sweetish smell, appears. Gram's staining of the wound exudate shows many gram-positive rods with relatively few inflammatory cells.

At surgery, muscle may appear pale because of the intensity of edema, but it does not contract when probed with a scalpel. When dissected, the muscle is beefy red and nonviable and can progress to become black, friable, and gangrenous. It is important to establish a diagnosis early, preferably by frozen-section biopsy of muscle.

Despite hypotension, renal failure, and (often) body crepitance, patients with myonecrosis frequently have a heightened awareness of their surroundings until just before death, when they lapse into toxic delirium and coma. In untreated cases, as the local wounds progress, the skin becomes bronzed; bullae appear, become filled with dark red fluid, and are accompanied by dark patches of cutaneous gangrene. Gas appears in later phases but may not be as obvious as in anaerobic cellulitis. Jaundice is rare in wound gas gangrene (in contrast to uterine infections) and, when it does appear, is almost invariably associated with hemoglobinuria, hemoglobinemia, and septicemia. Cases of clostridial myonecrosis without a history of trauma have been reported. These patients have bullous lesions and crepitance of the skin; they present with a rapidly worsening course that includes myonecrosis, especially of the extremities.

Bacteremia and Clostridial Sepsis The relatively common entity of transient clostridial bacteremia can arise in any hospitalized patient but is most common with a predisposing focus in the gastrointestinal tract, biliary tract, or uterus. Fever frequently resolves within 24 to 48 h without therapy. Despite the finding of clostridial bacteremia following septic abortions and the frequent isolation of clostridia from the lochia, most of the patients involved do not have evidence of sepsis. In one series of 60 patients with clostridial bacteremia, half had an infected site that could be associated with the bacteremia, while the other half had a totally unrelated illness, such as tuberculous pneumonia, meningitis, or benign gastroenteritis. By the time blood culture reports are returned, patients frequently are completely well and sometimes have been discharged. Therefore, when a blood culture is positive for clostridia, the patient must be assessed clinically rather than simply treated on the basis of the culture result.

Clostridial sepsis is an uncommon but almost invariably fatal illness following clostridial infection—primarily that of the uterus, colon, or biliary tract. This entity must be differentiated from transient clostridial bacteremia, which is much more common. *C. perfringens* causes the majority of cases of sepsis as well as the majority of cases of transient bacteremia. *C. septicum*, *C. sordellii*, and *C. novyi* account for most of the remainder of cases. Clostridia account for 1 to 2.5 percent of all positive blood cultures in major hospital centers.

The majority of cases of clostridial sepsis originate from the female genital tract and follow septic abortion. Introduction of a foreign body is a common antecedent event. In the uterus, residual necrotic fetal and placental tissues and traumatized endometrium may allow the growth of clostridia. Only a small fraction of cases of septic abortion (1 percent) are followed by serious sepsis. In these patients, sepsis, fever, and chills begin from 1 to 3 days after the attempted abortion. The initial signs are malaise, headache, severe myalgias, abdominal pain, nausea, vomiting, and occasionally diarrhea. Frequently, a bloody or brown vaginal discharge is noted. Patients may rapidly develop oliguria, hypotension, jaundice, and hemoglobinuria. The hemolysis, which is secondary to *C. perfringens* alpha toxin, causes a characteristic bronzing of the skin. As in myonecrosis, the mental status of severely ill patients is characterized by increased alertness and apprehension. Local examination of the pelvis reveals foul cervical discharge, occasionally with gas. Frequently, laceration marks around the cervix or perforation of the cervical segment are evident. If the infection involves the myometrium or has spread to the adnexa, extreme tenderness, guarding, and an adnexal mass may be found.

Laboratory studies in patients with sepsis reveal an elevated white blood cell count and may show pink, hemoglobin-tinged plasma. Anemia is proportional to the degree of hemolysis, and the hematocrit may be extremely low. Platelet counts may be reduced, and there is often evidence of disseminated intravascular coagulation. Oliguria or anuria, increasingly refractory hypotension, and hemorrhage and bruising may develop.

Clostridia may enter the bloodstream from the gastrointestinal or biliary tract. This occurrence is associated with ulcerative lesions or obstruction of the small or large intestine, necrotic or infiltrating malignancy, bowel surgery, or various abdominal catastrophes. The patient may present with an acute febrile illness, with chills and fever but no other signs of localized infection. Intravascular hemolysis occurs in as many as half of such cases. Biliary or gastrointestinal symptoms, if present, may be the only clue to the etiology. Positive blood cultures provide the definitive clue to the diagnosis.

Patients with malignant disease also can develop rapidly fatal clostridial sepsis, particularly from a gastrointestinal focus. The most common species in this setting is *C. septicum*. Characteristic signs and symptoms include fever, tachycardia, hypotension, abdominal pain or tenderness, nausea, vomiting, and (preterminally) coma. The tachycardia may be out of proportion to the fever. Only about 20 to 30 percent of patients develop hemolysis. A striking feature of this syndrome is the rapidity of death, which frequently occurs in less than 12 h.

DIAGNOSIS The diagnosis of clostridial disease, in association with positive cultures, must be based primarily on clinical findings. Because of the presence of clostridia in many wounds, their mere isolation from any site, including the blood, does not necessarily indicate severe disease. Smears of wound exudates, uterine scrapings, or cervical discharge may show abundant large gram-positive rods as well as other organisms. Cultures should be placed in selective media and incubated anaerobically for identification of clostridia. The diagnosis of clostridial myonecrosis can be established by frozen-section biopsy of muscle.

The urine of patients with severe clostridial sepsis may contain protein and casts, and some patients may develop severe uremia. Profound alterations of circulating erythrocytes are seen in severely toxemic patients. Patients have hemolytic anemia, which develops extremely rapidly, along with hemoglobinemia, hemoglobinuria, and elevated levels of serum bilirubin. Spherocytosis, increased osmotic and mechanical red blood cell fragility, erythrophagocytosis, and methemoglobinemia have been described. Disseminated intravascular coagulation may develop in patients with severe infection. In patients with severe sepsis, Wright's or Gram's staining of a smear of peripheral blood or buffy coat may demonstrate clostridia.

X-ray examination sometimes provides an important clue to the diagnosis by revealing gas in muscles, subcutaneous tissue, or the uterus. However, the finding of gas is not pathognomonic for clostridial infection. Other anaerobic bacteria, frequently mixed with aerobic organisms, may produce gas.

The diagnosis of *C. difficile*–associated colitis is made by the identification of *C. difficile* toxin in stool. Diagnostic evaluation of patients with PMC should include examination of the stool for *C. difficile* cytotoxin. Although several assays are available, the tissue culture assay is the most practical and sensitive. The assay is performed by incubation of stool filtrates with tissue culture cells and monitoring for a cytopathic effect that can be neutralized by antitoxin to either *C. sordellii* (which is cross-reactive with *C. difficile* but does not cause PMC) or *C. difficile*. Identical cytopathic and actinomorphic changes in fibroblasts are induced by toxins A and B; however, the standard assay is about 1000-fold more sensitive for toxin B. Most strains produce both toxins when grown under similar conditions. Endoscopy, although useful in establishing the presence of PMC, does not establish the etiology and should be reserved for cases with more serious disease manifestations, in which it can be used to exclude alternative diagnoses. Isolation of *C. difficile* from stool cultures is difficult. Moreover, *C. difficile* may be part of the "normal" flora of asymptomatic patients, particularly infants.

℞ TREATMENT

Traditionally, the treatment of choice for severe clostridial infection has been penicillin G (20 million units a day in adults). Recently, penicillin G treatment of gas gangrene has become more controversial because of increasing resistance to this drug and data obtained from animal models of infection. In a mouse model of gas gangrene, Stevens et al. demonstrated that antibiotics that inhibit protein synthesis may be preferable to cell wall–active drugs. Clindamycin treatment enhanced survival more than therapy with penicillin. The combination of clindamycin and penicillin was superior to penicillin alone. For severe clostridial sepsis, clindamycin may be used at a dose of 600 mg every 6 h in combination with high-dose penicillin. Although no clinical trials validate this choice, it is gaining acceptance in the infectious disease community.

In cases of penicillin sensitivity or allergy, other antibiotics should be considered, but all should be tested for in vitro activity because of the occasional isolation of resistant strains. Clostridia are frequently, but not universally, susceptible in vitro to cefoxitin, carbenicillin, chloramphenicol, clindamycin, metronidazole, doxycycline, imipenem, minocycline, tetracycline, third-generation cephalosporins, and vancomycin. For severe clostridial infections, sensitivity testing should be done before an antimicrobial with unpredictable activity is used. Simple contamination of a wound with clostridia should not be treated with antibiotics. Localized skin and soft tissue infection can be managed by debridement rather than with systemic antibiotics. Drugs are required when the process extends into adjacent tissue or when fever and systemic signs of sepsis are present. Surgery is a mainstay of therapy for clostridial myonecrosis or gas gangrene. Amputation may be required for rapidly spreading infection involving a limb. Hysterectomy is required for uterine myonecrosis. Abdominal wall myonecrosis usually continues despite initial aggressive surgery and antibiotic therapy and requires repeated surgical debridement of all involved muscle.

Suppurative infections should be treated with antibiotics. Frequently, broad-spectrum antibiotics must be used because of the mixed flora involved in these infections. Aminoglycosides can be used for the aerobic gram-negative bacteria involved in mixed infections.

The use of a polyvalent gas gangrene antitoxin is still recommended by some authorities. At present, no such antitoxin is produced in the United States, and most centers have discontinued its use in the management of patients with suspected gas gangrene or clostridial postabortion sepsis because of questionable efficacy and the substantial risk of hypersensitivity to horse serum, from which the antitoxin is derived.

The use of hyperbaric oxygen in the treatment of gas gangrene is also controversial. Studies in humans are not well designed to answer questions on efficacy, but several knowledgeable authors believe that hyperbaric oxygen therapy has contributed to dramatic clinical improvement. Such therapy may, however, be associated with untoward effects due to oxygen toxicity and high atmospheric pressure. Some centers without hyperbaric chambers have reported acceptable mortality rates; thus expert surgical and medical management and control of complications are probably the most important factors in the treatment of gas gangrene.

The treatment of *C. difficile*–associated colitis requires discontinuation of therapy with the offending antimicrobial agent. In some patients, symptoms will resolve over a period of 2 weeks if the infection is left untreated. However, specific therapy shortens the duration of symptoms.

The most widely used agent in the treatment of antibiotic-associated diarrhea ascribed to *C. difficile* is oral vancomycin. Most strains of *C. difficile* are susceptible to achievable concentrations of this agent. Vancomycin is poorly absorbed after oral administration and reaches high levels in the stool. The usual initial schedule is 125 mg orally four times a day for 7 to 10 days, but in cases of extremely severe disease the dose may be increased to 500 mg orally four times a day. A randomized trial comparing vancomycin with metronidazole demonstrated equal efficacy and relapse rates of 8 to 9 percent for the two regimens. The dose of metronidazole used was 250 mg four times a day, although 500 mg three times a day should be equally effective. Both because metronidazole is considerably less costly than vancomycin and because oral vancomycin has been implicated in the emergence of vancomycin-resistant enterococci, treatment should begin with metronidazole. If diarrhea persists, therapy should be changed to vancomycin. In patients with refractory symptoms and fever unresponsive to either regimen, the combination of rifampin with vancomycin has sometimes been beneficial. Since resistance to rifampin can develop, this agent should not be used alone.

A number of patients who respond to initial therapy present with a relapse of symptoms and a repeat positive toxin assay. Relapses following therapy are much more frequent than failures to respond to initial therapy. Most relapses occur 3 to 10 days after discontinuation of treatment. Most relapsing patients respond to a second course of antibiotics, but some go on to suffer multiple relapses. A number of options are available in this situation. Some patients have been shown to acquire a different strain of *C. difficile* despite the appearance of relapsing disease. These patients respond to a second course of the same agent used to treat the first episode. Alternatively, patients who receive vancomycin and who then have a relapse can be treated with metronidazole, and vice versa. Some authors report success with tapering regimens of vancomycin given daily or every other day for 1 to 2 months to avoid relapse. The resin cholestyramine binds the cytotoxin of *C. difficile* and has been used with some success to treat severe cases. Since cholestyramine also binds vancomycin, the two agents should not be used in combination. Repopulation of the normal colonic flora has also been tried in relapsing disease. Ingestion of capsules of the yeast *Saccharomyces boulardii* showed some promise in one trial. It appears that all of these regimens are effective in some cases but that no regimen is universally efficacious in relapsing disease.

BIBLIOGRAPHY

Bartlett JG: *Clostridium difficile:* History of its role as an enteric pathogen and the current state of knowledge about the organism. Clin Infect Dis 18:S265, 1994

————: Antibiotic-associated diarrhea. Clin Infect Dis 15:573, 1992

————: Gas gangrene (other clostridium-associated diseases), in *Principles and Practice of Infectious Diseases,* 3d ed, GL Mandell et al (eds). New York, Churchill Livingstone, 1990

———— et al: Antibiotic-associated pseudomembranous colitis due to toxin-producing clostridia. N Engl J Med 298:531, 1978

Borriello SP: Clostridial disease of the gut. Clin Infect Dis 20:S242, 1995

Finegold SM: *Anaerobic Bacteria in Human Disease.* New York, Academic, 1977

————: Anaerobic infections and *Clostridium difficile* colitis emerging during antibacterial therapy. Scand J Infect Dis (Suppl) 49:160, 1986

Gorbach SL, Thadepalli H: Isolation of *Clostridium* in human infections: Evaluation of 114 cases. J Infect Dis 131:S81, 1975

Jendrzejewski JW et al: Nontraumatic clostridial myonecrosis. Am J Med 65:542, 1978

Johnson S et al: Enteritis necroticans among Khmer children at an evacuation site in Thailand. Lancet 2:496, 1987

Just I et al: Glucosylation of Rho proteins by *Clostridium difficile* toxin B. Nature 375:500, 1995

Koransky JR et al: *Clostridium septicum* bacteremia. Am J Med 66:63, 1979

Kurose I et al: *Clostridium difficile* toxin A–induced microvascular dysfunction: Role of histamine. J Clin Invest 94:1919, 1994

Pritchard JA, Whalley PJ: Abortion complicated by *Clostridium perfringens* infection. Am J Gynecol 111:484, 1971

Riegler M et al: *Clostridium difficile* toxin B is more potent than toxin A in damaging human colonic epithelium in vitro. J Clin Invest 95:2004, 1995

Smith LDS: Virulence factors of *Clostridium perfringens.* Rev Infect Dis 1:254, 1979

Stevens DL et al: Comparison of clindamycin, rifampin, tetracycline, metronidazole, and penicillin for efficacy in prevention of experimental gas gangrene due to *Clostridium perfringens.* J Infect Dis 155:220, 1987

————: Effect of antibiotics on toxin production and viability of *Clostridium perfringens.* Antimicrob Agents Chemother 31:213, 1987

————: Comparison of single and combination antimicrobial agents for prevention of experimental gas gangrene caused by *Clostridium perfringens.* Antimicrob Agents Chemother 31:312, 1987

Teasley DG et al: Prospective, randomized trial of metronidazole versus vancomycin for *Clostridium difficile*–associated diarrhea and colitis. Lancet 2:1043, 1983

Tibbles PM, Edelsberg JS: Medical progress: Hyperbaric-oxygen therapy. N Engl J Med 334:1642, 1996

SECTION 6

DISEASES CAUSED BY GRAM-NEGATIVE BACTERIA

---

149   *Claus O. Solberg*

MENINGOCOCCAL INFECTIONS

DEFINITION *Neisseria meningitidis* can cause a variety of infections; bacteremia and meningitis are by far the most common. Meningococcal disease remains a worldwide problem and occurs sporadically, as localized outbreaks, or as widespread epidemics. The clinical manifestations are varied and range from transient bacteremia to fulminant disease culminating in death within hours of the onset of symptoms. Few, if any, infectious diseases rival severe meningococcemia in fulminance.

ETIOLOGIC AGENT *N. meningitidis* is a gram-negative diplococcus whose adjacent sides are flattened to produce its characteristic biscuit shape. The microorganism grows best on enriched media such as Mueller-Hinton or chocolate agar and at 37°C in an atmosphere of 5 to 10% CO_2. Because meningococci are highly susceptible to drying or chilling, cultures should be promptly inoculated and incubated. *Neisseria* spp. are differentiated by their ability to use sugars as sources of energy. Typically, meningococci use glucose and maltose and not sucrose or lactose.

In contrast to other neisseriae, meningococci are surrounded by a polysaccharide capsule. On the basis of antigenic differences among their capsular polysaccharides, the microorganisms are divided into at least 13 serogroups. Although encapsulated meningococci from all serogroups frequently colonize the nasopharynx and have the potential to cause systemic disease, more than 99 percent of meningococcal infections are caused by strains of serogroups A, B, C, 29E, W-135, and Y. The serogroups are further divided into serotypes, subtypes, and immunotypes according to differences in outer-membrane proteins and lipopolysaccharides (LPSs). In addition to being classified serologically, the meningococci are divided into clonal types based on characterization of the bacterial genome. These classification systems have been of great value for epidemiologic surveillance.

EPIDEMIOLOGY Meningococci are confined entirely to humans; the natural habitat of these bacteria is the nasopharynx. The organisms are presumably transmitted from person to person through the inhalation of droplets of infected nasopharyngeal secretions and by direct or indirect oral contact. In nonepidemic periods, the overall rate of nasopharyngeal carriage is about 10 percent but may approach 60 to 80 percent in closed populations, such as those at military recruit camps or schools. Rates of carriage are also high among family members and other close contacts of patients with meningococcal disease. Carriage usually persists for a few months; chronic carriage is not uncommon. Nasopharyngeal acquisition is followed by a rise in titers of specific serum antibodies to the colonizing strain, and colonization only rarely proceeds to disease. Observations during epidemics suggest that invasive meningococcal disease is most likely to occur within a few days of acquisition of a new strain, i.e., before the development of specific serum antibodies.

In temperate climates, the annual incidence of meningococcal infection is generally 1 to 2 cases per 100,000 population; the attack rate is highest in the first quarter of the year. Most infections occur among children 6 months to 3 years of age. The annual attack rate in this group is usually 10 to 15 cases per 100,000 population, with the peak incidence at 6 to 12 months of age. A second group at risk is the adolescent population between 14 and 20 years of age. As in infectious mononucleosis, the girls in this risk group who develop meningococcal infection are on average 2 years younger than the boys. In epidemics, the age distribution of the patients is shifted to older individuals, and more cases develop among individuals 3 to 20 years of age. When sporadic cases occur in families, the attack rate among household contacts may increase dramatically to 1 in 1000.

Major outbreaks of meningococcal disease are regularly reported from Africa, China, and South America. These epidemics may involve thousands of individuals and cause many deaths. Serogroup A meningococci are the primary cause of the epidemics. In the "meningitis belt" of sub-Saharan Africa, the incidence of meningococcal disease rises sharply towards the end of the dry and dusty season and falls with the onset of rains. It has been postulated that the presence of dust interferes with local IgA secretion in the nasopharynx, reducing host defenses against meningococci.

Serogroup A strains caused most outbreaks of meningococcal disease in Europe and the United States in the first half of the twentieth century. Since World War II, meningococci of serogroups B and C have become predominant. Currently, group B strains account for 50 percent of sporadic cases. Serogroup C strains have caused more infections in older age groups, and serogroup B strains have been especially common in very young children. Outbreaks occur more frequently among the poorest segments of the population, where overcrowding and poor sanitation are common.

PATHOGENESIS Meningococcal infection begins in the nasopharynx. Shortly after adherence to the nasopharyngeal mucosa, encapsulated meningococci are transported through nonciliated epithelial cells in large, membrane-bound phagocytic vacuoles. Within 24 h the microorganisms are observed in the submucosa in close proximity to local immune cells and blood vessels. In most instances, this nasopharyngeal infection is subclinical, but mild symptoms occasionally develop. After mucosal penetration and presumably a phase of adaptation, the bacteria may gain access to the circulation. In the vascular compartment, the invading meningococci either may be killed by the combined actions of serum bactericidal antibodies, complement, and phagocytic cells or may multiply, initiating the bacteremic stage. The symptoms and signs of systemic disease appear concurrently with meningococ-

cemia and usually precede symptoms of meningitis by 24 to 48 h. Meningococci are capable of replicating at an astonishing rate; within hours, a patient may deteriorate from good health to irreversible shock, marked hemorrhagic diathesis, and death.

Role of LPS Endotoxin (LPS) of the meningococcal outer membrane seems to play a central role in the development of severe disease. LPS is released into the circulation during multiplication and autolysis of meningococci, and a fair correlation has been established between LPS levels in plasma and disease severity: patients with minor symptoms have low or undetectable levels of LPS, while patients with fulminant meningococcemia have among the highest LPS levels detected in human plasma. In fulminant disease, major cascade systems associated with inflammation (including the coagulation, complement, fibrinolysis, and kallikrein-kinin systems) as well as the production of cytokines [tumor necrosis factor α (TNFα), interleukin (IL) 1, IL-6, IL-8, and IL-10] and nitric oxide are all triggered and upregulated simultaneously by native LPS. This dose-dependent inflammatory response results in marked vasodilation, reduced cardiac performance, platelet aggregation, disseminated intravascular coagulation (DIC), and capillary leak. The end results of these complicated processes are septic shock, adult respiratory distress syndrome, and multiple-organ failure (Chap. 124).

Although systemic meningococcal infection is primarily a bacteremic disease, *N. meningitidis* exhibits marked tropism for the meninges and skin and to a lesser degree for synovia, serosal surfaces, and adrenal glands. The most common clinical presentation is a composite of bacteremia and meningitis. Infection of the central nervous system may begin in the vicinity of the ependyma that lines the cerebral ventricles, subsequently spreading to the subarachnoid space. Meningococci appear to adhere readily to the cerebrovascular endothelium and (by yet poorly defined mechanisms) to penetrate the vessel walls. Later, the permeability of the blood-brain barrier may be further increased by locally produced inflammatory mediators such as TNFα, IL-1, and IL-6 induced by increasing levels of LPS in the cerebrospinal fluid (CSF). In patients with meningococcal meningitis, LPS levels in CSF are 100 to 1000 times higher than those in simultaneously collected plasma. This compartmentalized bacterial growth is also reflected in the higher CSF levels of bioactive TNFα, IL-1, IL-6, and IL-10 in patients with meningitis than in patients with septic shock or mild bacteremia.

Host Immunity The development of invasive disease is most dependent on host factors. Invasive meningococcal disease occurs almost exclusively in individuals who lack protective bactericidal antibodies to the infecting strain. Infants are protected from meningococcal disease for the first few months of life by passively transferred maternal antibodies and by a very low rate of meningococcal acquisition. As maternal antibodies are lost, susceptibility rises, peaking at 6 to 12 months; it then falls progressively as antibodies are acquired through colonization with closely related but nonpathogenic bacteria such as *N. lactamica*, avirulent *N. meningitidis*, or other bacteria expressing surface antigens in common with virulent meningococcal strains. *N. lactamica* colonizes the nasopharynx earlier during life than *N. meningitidis*, and colonized infants develop antibodies that prompt complement-mediated lysis and opsonophagocytosis of a broad spectrum of potentially pathogenic meningococci.

As children grow older, colonization with *N. meningitidis* gradually replaces that with *N. lactamica*, whose carriage is rare among teenagers. Colonization with *N. meningitidis* induces antibodies to the infecting strain and to other strains; thus naturally acquired immunity is reinforced and broadened. Many enteric bacteria have capsules or other antigens that are chemically similar to those of meningococci. Colonization with these unrelated yet immunologically similar bacteria may be important in the development of natural immunity to meningococci.

Immunologic Deficiencies The complement system plays a critical role in host defenses against invasive meningococcal disease, and activated complement brings about bacterial cell death by direct lysis or opsonophagocytosis. Occasional individuals who experience recurrent attacks of meningococcal disease have a high prevalence of a familial deficiency in a terminal complement component. This deficiency results in an inability to assemble the membrane attack complex (C5 to C9). The population prevalence of terminal complement-component deficiency is very low (about 0.03 percent), but approximately 50 percent of affected individuals experience an attack of meningococcal disease at some time. In these individuals the infection is usually mild and the mortality low. This milder illness may be due to intact opsonophagocytic mechanisms that do not require the terminal cascade and to diminished release of LPS from invading bacteria as a consequence of the host's inability to directly lyse bacteria in the serum. Patients with complement deficiency tend to be infected with strains of the less common W-135, X, Y, Z, and 29E serogroups. Several systemic diseases (e.g., systemic lupus erythematosus and membranoproliferative glomerulonephritis) can lead to secondary complement-component deficiencies and sporadic meningococcal disease.

Individuals with properdin deficiency, a sex-linked inherited disorder, have an intact classic complement pathway but impaired alternative pathway activation. More than half of the males in this group develop meningococcal disease, the course of which is frequently fulminant, with a case-fatality rate approaching 75 percent. Vaccination of properdin-deficient individuals is likely to reduce the risk of meningococcal disease as the generation of complement-fixing antibodies leads to the activation of complement via the classic pathway and to the consequent lysis and opsonophagocytosis of bacteria. Individuals with hypogammaglobulinemia, primary isolated IgM deficiency, and functional asplenia are also at increased risk of sporadic meningococcal disease, although pneumococcal infection is a more common complication in this group.

Other Risk Factors An association between respiratory virus infections and meningococcal infection has been postulated. While infection with influenza A virus seems to predispose to meningococcal disease, this association appears to be less likely for other viral infections.

Reasons for epidemics of meningococcal disease are poorly understood. Overcrowding is clearly a prominent risk factor. Moreover, it has been suggested that epidemic meningococcal strains are clonal and that important surface structures vary cyclically, providing a new bacterial surface that allows evasion of host defense systems.

CLINICAL MANIFESTATIONS *N. meningitidis* typically causes an acute infective illness, and more than 90 percent of the patients who become ill have meningococcemia and/or meningitis. A sequential development of clinical manifestations can be discerned, the usual sequence consisting of initial infection of the upper respiratory tract followed by meningococcemia, meningitis, and less common focal manifestations.

Upper Respiratory Tract Infection The portal of entry of meningococci is the nasopharynx. Most patients are asymptomatic or report fever alone before the onset of systemic manifestations. Some patients with invasive meningococcal disease describe mild prodromal symptoms of sore throat, rhinorrhea, cough, headache, and conjunctivitis in the week before hospital admission. Whether these manifestations are due to infection with the meningococcus or with other microorganisms that may facilitate meningococcal invasion is not known.

Meningococcemia Between 30 and 40 percent of patients with meningococcal disease have meningococcemia without clinical signs of meningitis. The clinical manifestations vary from minor symptoms of transient bacteremia to fulminating disease of a few hours' duration. The onset is usually sudden, with fever, chills, nausea, vomiting, rash, myalgia, and arthralgia. Fever, usually between 39 and 41°C, is almost universal, although occasional patients with fulminant disease may be afebrile or even hypothermic. Most patients suffer from nausea and vomiting and are distressed. One-third of patients have myalgias and/or arthralgias. The most striking feature is rash, which develops in

three-fourths of patients and may be maculopapular, petechial, or ecchymotic. The maculopapular rash appears soon after the onset of disease; the lesions are pink, 2 to 10 mm in diameter, and sparsely distributed on the trunk and extremities. Often petechiae appear in the center of the macules. The rash may progress within hours to become hemorrhagic as the general condition of the patient deteriorates. The petechial lesions are 1 to 2 mm in diameter and are distributed mainly on the trunk and lower extremities but also on the face, palate, and conjunctivae. In relatively severe cases, petechiae may become confluent and develop into hemorrhagic bullae, with extensive ulcerations. Widespread petechial eruption, hypotension, reduced peripheral circulation, and lack of meningism are all indicators of poor prognosis. Ecchymoses and fulminant purpuric rash are common among patients with fulminant meningococcemia.

Fulminant meningococcemia, previously called Waterhouse-Friderichsen syndrome, differs from the milder form in its rapid progression and overwhelming character. It occurs in 10 to 20 percent of patients with meningococcal disease and is characterized by the development of shock, DIC, and multiple-organ failure. The onset is abrupt; purpuric lesions, hypotension, and peripheral vasoconstriction with cold cyanotic extremities frequently develop within hours. The state of consciousness is variable, but many patients remain alert despite hypotension. The purpuric lesions enlarge rapidly and involve skin, mucous membranes, and internal organs such as skeletal muscle, adrenal glands, and occasionally the pituitary gland. Myocardial depression contributing to shock is evidenced by impaired myocardial contractility, lowered cardiac index, increased wedge pressure, and elevated serum levels of creatinine phosphokinase. Metabolic acidosis, serum electrolyte derangement, oliguria, leukopenia, and low levels of coagulation factors are common. Despite advanced intensive care management, 50 to 60 percent of patients die, usually from cardiac and/or respiratory failure. Patients who recover may have severe skin lesions necessitating plastic surgery or loss of parts of limbs due to gangrene.

Chronic meningococcemia makes up only 1 to 2 percent of all cases of meningococcal disease. This syndrome of recurrent fever, maculopapular rash, and arthralgia may last for weeks to months. The rash may also be petechial. During afebrile periods, patients appear remarkably well. Failure to diagnose and treat chronic meningococcemia may result in the development of systemic disease.

Meningitis Meningitis is frequently associated with meningococcemia; in patients with systemic disease, the onset of meningitis may be inapparent. However, most patients with meningitis soon develop symptoms of meningeal inflammation, including severe headache, confusion, lethargy, and vomiting. Signs of meningeal irritation are present in most but not all cases. The symptoms and signs associated with meningococcal meningitis cannot be differentiated from those associated with meningitis due to other organisms (see Chap. 377). Infants present particularly often with nonspecific symptoms and without localizing signs, although they may have a tense, bulging fontanelle. Meningitis may also occur without specific signs in elderly patients or in those with fulminant meningococcemia. As the infection advances, lethargy may progress to coma, and seizures, cranial nerve palsies, and hemiparesis or other focal neurologic signs may appear.

Less Common Manifestations A number of less common manifestations of meningococcal infections have been reported. These include arthritis, pneumonia, sinusitis, otitis media, conjunctivitis, endophthalmitis, endocarditis, pericarditis, urethritis, and endometritis. Arthritis occurs in 5 to 10 percent of patients and may develop at any stage of the acute illness. Large joints are most commonly affected, particularly the knee. Meningococci are infrequently isolated from the synovial fluid, and the majority of cases, especially when arthritis develops after the initiation of therapy, are immunologically mediated. Sequelae are rare. Primary meningococcal pneumonia is well recognized, particularly in association with serogroup Y strains. The clinical syndrome is similar to that of other bacterial pneumonias. Since the introduction of antibiotics, endocarditis and pericarditis have become very unusual features of acute meningococcal disease.

Complications The complications of meningococcal infections include intercurrent infections and damage to the central nervous system. Most pyogenic complications have become uncommon. However, superinfection of the respiratory tract with microorganisms other than meningococci may develop, particularly during assisted ventilation of seriously ill patients. Neurologic complications may result from direct infection of brain parenchyma (cerebritis or brain abscess), injury to cranial nerves as they pass through the inflamed meninges, venous or arterial infarction (seizures, focal deficits), cerebral edema (raised intracranial pressure), interruption of CSF pathways (hydrocephalus), or effusions into the subdural space producing mass effects. Nonetheless, permanent neurologic sequelae are infrequent, occurring in fewer than 5 percent of survivors of acute meningococcal meningitis. As in other severe infections, herpes labialis is prevalent in the acute stage of meningococcal disease.

LABORATORY FINDINGS Meningococci usually can be isolated from blood and CSF of patients with meningococcal disease and occasionally are found in petechial aspirate and synovial, pleural, or pericardial fluid. The growth of meningococci in blood culture bottles can be inhibited by sodium polyanetholesulfonate, a frequent additive to media. Gram-negative diplococci may be demonstrated in CSF, petechiae, or buffy coat smears from at least half of patients. Group-specific capsular polysaccharides can be detected in CSF, synovial fluid, serum, or urine by counterimmunoelectrophoresis or latex agglutination assays. However, these tests give false-negative results in 50 percent of culture-proven cases. The combined use of cultures, gram-stained smears, and immunoassays will provide a diagnosis in more than 95 percent of cases. The immunoassays may be particularly useful in situations where cultures are of limited value because of prior antibiotic administration. The polymerase chain reaction (PCR) may also be a valuable tool in these situations. CSF examinations indicate that the specificity and sensitivity of PCR for the diagnosis of meningococcal meningitis are at least 90 percent. A specific antibody response during convalescence may also be diagnostic.

Other laboratory data offer limited support in the diagnosis of meningococcal disease. Elevated counts of polymorphonuclear leukocytes with a left shift are common, but normal counts are not unusual. Patients with fulminant meningococcemia usually have neutropenia and markedly reduced platelet counts; prothrombin and partial thromboplastin times are prolonged, plasma fibrinogen levels are diminished, and fibrinogen degradation product titers are elevated as a result of DIC (see Chap. 124). Decreased P_{CO_2} and metabolic acidosis secondary to tissue hypoperfusion are frequent. CSF findings in meningitis include increased pressure, increased protein content, low glucose concentrations, and (in most cases) 100 to 20,000 polymorphonuclear leukocytes per microliter (see Chap. 377).

DIAGNOSIS Meningococcal infections in their early stages may resemble any acute systemic infection, including influenza or another common viral infection, and the distinction between the latter infections and early meningococcemia may be most difficult. In contrast to the prevalence of neurologic symptoms in meningococcal meningitis, the lack of such symptoms in meningococcemia may prevent early recognition of this severe form of meningococcal disease. However, early in meningococcal disease there is often a generalized, mottled erythema or a light pink maculopapular rash resembling the rose spots of typhoid fever. By careful examination of the patient, the physician can detect these lesions and establish a presumptive diagnosis. As the disease progresses, a petechial or purpuric rash usually develops, and the diagnosis becomes more obvious. The rash seen in some common viral exanthems, *Mycoplasma* infection, Rocky Mountain spotted fever, endemic typhus, and vascular purpura may be confused with that of meningococcemia. In the absence of rash or other manifestations of bacteremia, meningococcal meningitis is indistinguishable from meningitis caused by other pathogens (see Chap. 377). The ultimate diagnosis of meningococcal disease depends on the recovery of *N. meningitidis* or the detection of its antigens in various body fluids or petechial aspirates. Isolation of meningococci from the nasopharynx only confirms the carrier state and cannot be used alone to establish the diagnosis of systemic infection.

℞ **TREATMENT**

Despite the availability of potent antibiotics and advances in intensive care management, overall mortality from meningococcal disease is about 10 percent, rising to as high as 50 to 60 percent among patients with meningococcemia and shock. To improve the prognosis, early diagnosis and treatment are of utmost importance, particularly in patients with meningococcemia. Any febrile patient with a petechial rash should be considered to have meningococcal infection. Blood for cultures should be taken immediately and treatment begun without awaiting confirmation. If the patient is not initially seen in the hospital, intravenous penicillin G (60,000 to 100,000 units per kilogram) should be given and the patient immediately admitted. In the outpatient setting, if vascular access is problematic, antibiotics can be given intramuscularly (at several injection sites in light of the large volume). If the patient is first seen in the hospital, intravenous access should be established immediately, blood obtained for cultures, and antibiotics administered as soon as possible. Initiation of therapy in patients with signs of circulatory insufficiency or rapid deterioration in cerebral condition should not await lumbar puncture.

Antibiotics Penicillin G remains the drug of choice for meningococcal disease. Prior to the identification of the etiologic agent, the choice of antibiotics depends upon the age of the patient, the status of the patient's underlying host-defense system, and the prevalence of antimicrobial resistance in the community. *Streptococcus pneumoniae* as well as *Haemophilus influenzae* and other gram-negative bacteria may cause a clinical picture similar to that of meningococcal infection. The third-generation cephalosporins cefotaxime and ceftriaxone are recommended as empiric therapy. Although mortality and long-term morbidity among patients given cephalosporins for the treatment of meningococcal disease are similar to those among patients treated with penicillin, the cephalosporins are preferred because of their high level of activity against other common meningeal pathogens, including most penicillin-resistant pneumococci; their excellent penetration into the CSF; their lack of toxicity; and the convenience of using a single agent that can be administered three times daily (cefotaxime) or once or twice daily (ceftriaxone).

As part of their empiric regimen, patients undergoing immunosuppressive therapy, newborns, and the elderly should receive high-dose penicillin to cover *Listeria monocytogenes*. The cephalosporins are also highly active against *N. meningitidis* strains with reduced sensitivity to penicillin. Such strains have been reported from several countries and have been described especially often in reports from South Africa and Spain. The usual daily dosage of cefotaxime is 150 to 200 mg/kg intravenously up to a maximum daily dosage of 12 g; that of ceftriaxone is 75 to 100 mg/kg intravenously up to a maximum daily dosage of 5 g. Once meningococci have been isolated and shown to be sensitive to penicillin G, the therapeutic regimen can be changed to penicillin G. Chloramphenicol is as effective as penicillin G for the treatment of meningococcal disease and can be used in patients allergic to penicillins or cephalosporins. The usual daily dosage of penicillin G is 200,000 to 300,000 units per kilogram intravenously in divided doses every 6 h up to a maximum daily dosage of 24 million units; that of chloramphenicol is 75 to 100 mg/kg intravenously in divided doses every 6 h up to a maximum daily dosage of 4 g. A 7-day course of high-dose parenteral therapy is adequate for both meningococcal meningitis and meningococcemia. The dose should not be tapered over the course of therapy.

Supportive Care The course of meningococcal disease is highly unpredictable. All patients with invasive meningococcal infection, whatever their clinical condition on admission, should be considered to have potentially life-threatening infection and should be carefully observed during the first 48 h in the hospital, with monitoring of arterial blood pressure, pulse, perfusion, urine output, and core and peripheral temperature. Many patients who do not appear acutely ill on admission may deteriorate suddenly in the following hours, with the development of severe shock and profound DIC. Patients with a rapidly progressive purpuric rash, a low peripheral white cell count, and no evidence of meningeal involvement are likely to deteriorate very soon after admission.

The most important manifestation requiring urgent intervention is severe meningococcemia with shock. Patients with this form of meningococcal disease have a severe capillary leak syndrome and myocardial dysfunction. Strategies to reverse circulatory failure include optimizing preload, decreasing afterload, and improving myocardial contractility. Intravenous fluid administration together with ionotropic support with dobutamine (1 to 10 µg/kg per minute) or dopamine (2 to 10 µg/kg per minute) should be started immediately and tailored to the needs of each patient on the basis of clinical assessment and of monitoring of systemic arterial pressure and central venous or pulmonary wedge pressure (see Chap. 38). Vasodilators should be administered with extreme caution to patients with severe shock. In marked tissue edema in adults, the administration of as much as 8 to 10 L of intravenous fluid may be necessary during the first 24 h. Because the risk of pulmonary edema is considerable, patients in severe shock should be electively ventilated, even if they are ventilating adequately. Several controlled studies of patients with septic shock have demonstrated no beneficial effect of high-dose glucocorticoid treatment. Although these studies have included only small numbers of patients with meningococcemia, a beneficial effect of glucocorticoids in fulminant meningococcemia seems unlikely.

Some patients present in profound respiratory failure, even if they have not received intravenous fluid. Such patients should be ventilated immediately to prevent acute respiratory collapse. Adult respiratory distress syndrome is heralded by an increase in oxygen requirement and a reduction of pulmonary compliance and tends to follow initial resuscitation and correction of hypovolemia. Management in this situation depends on measures to improve myocardial function, assisted ventilation, and removal of extravascular fluid (if necessary, by dialysis).

Patients with severe meningococcemia usually have a complex derangement of serum electrolytes, acid-base balance, and metabolism. Metabolic acidosis is a result of poor tissue perfusion in shock. Serum electrolytes and acid-base balance should be measured frequently and abnormalities corrected immediately. Correction is often hampered by oliguria or anuria, and dialysis is often required. Because dialysis is a highly effective means of reducing extravascular fluid accumulation and correcting electrolytic and metabolic derangements, it should be instituted early in patients with severe meningococcemia. Continuous plasma filtration or dialysis may also be necessary in proximal tubular necrosis due to meningococcal disease.

Virtually all patients with severe meningococcemia have marked DIC. Routine heparinization for patients with DIC has failed to improve prognosis and is not recommended. However, in patients with impending peripheral gangrene and severe coagulopathy, the administration of low-dose heparin (10 units/kg per hour) together with fresh frozen plasma may be tried. The administration of large quantities of fresh frozen plasma may also restore depleted levels of antithrombin III, protein C, and protein S.

Brain damage in bacterial meningitis may result in part from cytokines produced in the inflammatory response to bacterial products, and the reduction of brain injury by anti-inflammatory agents has been demonstrated in animals. In studies of children with *H. influenzae* meningitis, dexamethasone has significantly reduced the severity of neurologic sequelae, particularly deafness. Firm conclusions on the efficacy of dexamethasone in reducing neurologic sequelae in meningococcal meningitis cannot be derived from these studies, and the use of this agent in meningococcal meningitis remains controversial (see Chap. 377).

Symptom-based treatment of raised intracranial pressure is best administered in an intensive care setting. Elevation of the head to 30°, modest hyperventilation, and fluid restriction may be useful. Infusion of mannitol (0.25 to 1 g/kg) results in a rapid shift of fluid from the extravascular to the intravascular space and may be associated with a prompt reduction of intracranial pressure. In patients whose condition is unstable, insertion of an intracranial pressure monitor may aid in the management of this complication of meningitis. Airway obstruction, cardiac insufficiency, and convulsions may lead to hypoxia, impaired brain perfusion, and enhanced cerebral edema. Measures to optimize respiration and cardiac output and to control convulsions also are important in reducing intracranial pressure.

A number of experimental forms of therapy, including the use of monoclonal antibodies to endotoxin, TNFα, IL-1, and leukocyte adhesion molecules, have shown promise in animal models of meningitis or septic shock. The results of clinical trials have been less promising, but several trials are still in progress.

PROGNOSIS Meningococcal disease was usually fatal before the antibiotic era. After the introduction of antibiotics, overall mortality declined to 10 to 15 percent and has remained at about 10 percent despite early appropriate chemotherapy and advances in intensive care management. The mortality rate is less than 5 percent among patients with meningococal meningitis but can be as high as 50 to 60 percent among patients with fulminant meningococcemia, primarily because these patients are often in severe shock when admitted to the hospital. Most deaths from fulminant meningococcemia occur within 24 to 48 h of admission. Permanent sequelae of meningococcal meningitis, including deafness, cranial nerve paralysis, and mental deficiency, are uncommon.

PREVENTION Attack rates are approximately 100-fold higher among household contacts of patients with meningococcal disease than in the general population. The risk is highest in the first week after the index case has presented with infection. Chemoprophylaxis helps avert secondary cases of infection and should be administered to intimate contacts in the household, day-care center, and nursery school and also to anyone who has had oral contact with the index case (kissing, mouth-to-mouth resuscitation). The recommended regimen for prophylaxis consists of rifampin at a dosage of 10 mg/kg (up to 600 mg) every 12 h for 2 days for adults and children over 1 year of age and 5 mg/kg every 12 h for 2 days for children less than 1 year old. Ciprofloxacin or ofloxacin (a single oral dose of 500 or 400 mg, respectively) is a suitable alternative for adults but is not recommended for children or pregnant women. A single 250-mg intramuscular dose of ceftriaxone is recommended for pregnant contacts; for children less than 12 years of age, 125 mg of ceftriaxone can be given.

Vaccines are available against four serogroups of meningococci: A, C, W-135, and Y. No effective serogroup B vaccine is presently available. The efficacy rate of a single dose of serogroup A or serogroup C vaccine is at least 90 percent in adults and children over 2 years of age, and routine immunization of recruits has eliminated nearly all disease among military personnel. To prevent late secondary cases, close contacts of patients with sporadic disease caused by strains of serogroup A or C should receive a single dose of polysaccharide vaccine. Travelers to areas where disease is epidemic as well as individuals with splenic dysfunction or deficiencies in complement or properdin should be immunized. Conjugate serogroup A and serogroup C vaccines have been developed and are now undergoing clinical trials. If these vaccines provide young infants with long-lasting protection, they may be used in outbreak management as well as in routine infant-immunization programs. Serogroup B vaccines are also being developed.

BIBLIOGRAPHY

BRANDTZAEG P: Pathogenesis of meningococcal infections, in *Meningococcal Disease*, K Cartwright (ed). Chichester, John Wiley, 1995, pp 71–114

CARTWRIGHT K: Meningococcal carriage and disease, in *Meningococcal Disease*, K Cartwright (ed). Chichester, John Wiley, 1995, pp 115–146

DENSEN P et al: Familial properdin deficiency and fatal meningococcemia: Correction of the bactericidal defect by vaccination. N Engl J Med 316:922, 1987

FRASCH CE: Meningococcal vaccines: Past, present and future, in *Meningococcal Disease*, K Cartwright (ed). Chichester, John Wiley, 1995, pp 245–283

GRIFFISS JM: Mechanisms of host immunity, in *Meningococcal Disease*, K Cartwright (ed). Chichester, John Wiley, 1995, pp 35–70

GUTTORMSEN H-K et al: Cross-reacting serum opsonins in patients with meningococcal disease. Infect Immun 60:2777, 1992

HALSTENSEN A et al: Case fatality of meningococcal disease in western Norway. Scand J Infect Dis 19:35, 1987

LYNN WA, COHEN J: Adjunctive therapy of septic shock: A review of experimental approaches. Clin Infect Dis 20:143, 1995

NAESS A et al: Sequelae one year after meningococcal disease. Acta Neurol Scand 89:139, 1994

PARILLO JE: Pathogenetic mechanisms of septic shock. N Engl J Med 328:1471, 1993

ROSS SC et al: Killing of *Neisseria meningitidis* by human neutrophils: Implications for normal and complement-deficient individuals. J Infect Dis 155:1266, 1987

SCHILDKAMP RL et al: Clinical manifestations and course of meningococcal disease in 562 patients. Scand J Infect Dis 28:47, 1996

| 150 | *King K. Holmes, Stephen A. Morse* |

GONOCOCCAL INFECTIONS

DEFINITION Gonorrhea, an infection of columnar and transitional epithelium caused by *Neisseria gonorrhoeae*, is the most common reportable communicable disease in the United States. Anatomic sites that can be infected directly by the gonococcus include the urethra, rectum, conjunctiva, pharynx, and endocervix. Local complications include endometritis, salpingitis, peritonitis, perihepatitis, and bartholinitis in the female and periurethral abscess and epididymitis in the male. Systemic manifestations of gonococcemia include arthritis, dermatitis, endocarditis, and meningitis as well as myopericarditis and hepatitis.

ETIOLOGIC AGENT *N. gonorrhoeae* is a gram-negative coccus usually found in pairs with flattened adjacent sides. It forms oxidase-positive colonies and is differentiated from other *Neisseria* species by its ability to utilize glucose but not maltose, sucrose, or lactose; by nucleic acid probes; and by specific immunologic reactions.

Organisms present in colonies examined within 20 h of inoculation from clinical specimens are covered by fimbriae (*pili*). Pili mediate attachment to various epithelial cells and interfere with neutrophil phagocytosis. Each pilus is composed of repeating peptide (*pilin*) subunits, which have a molecular weight of about 20,000. The pilin subunits consist of conserved and variable regions. Pili undergo both antigenic and phase variation. Chromosomal rearrangements, leading to expression of any one of a large number of incomplete (silent) pilin genes, lead to *antigenic variation* in pili. If the rearrangement involves a defective pilin gene, piliated gonococci (pil⁺) produce nonpiliated variants (pil⁻), a process known as *phase variation*. Piliated organisms cause infection and urethritis after inoculation into the urethras of male volunteers, whereas nonpiliated organisms do not. Binding to epithelial cells requires the presence of another phase-variable protein, PilC, which is located at the tip of the pili. Antigenic variation of pilin subunits may allow gonococci to attach to different types of epithelial surfaces and to evade the host's antibody response to pilin. Phase variation from pil⁺ to pil⁻ may permit gonococcal detachment and facilitate spread. The synthesis of pilin is essential for competence in transformation of *N. gonorrhoeae*. Genetic transformation presumably is responsible for recombination between chromosomal genes of different gonococcal lineages.

The trilaminar outer-membrane of the gonococcus contains several classes of proteins, including proteins I, II, and III, and lipopolysaccharide (LPS) (Fig. 150-1). Like pili, protein II [now referred to as *opacity-associated outer-membrane proteins* (OPAs)] is thought to function as a ligand, mediating the attachment of gonococci to various types of human cells. An individual gonococcus can possess about a dozen OPA genes and can express zero to three or more OPAs at a time. Gonococci possessing certain OPAs adhere to and are phagocytosed by human neutrophils in the absence of serum. Certain OPAs may be responsible for the clumping of gonococci that is so evident on Gram-stained smears of urethral exudate.

Opaque colonies contain organisms that express OPAs and predominate in isolates from the male urethra and in cervical isolates obtained from women in midcycle. Transparent colonies often lack OPAs and predominate in cervical isolates obtained from women during menses and in isolates from blood, synovial fluid, or fallopian tubes.

From a quantitative point of view, protein I is the major outer-membrane protein; it exhibits intrastrain differences in molecular mass, with variation between 34.6 and 37.7 kDa. Protein I molecules associate in a trimeric structure, forming anion-selective transmembrane channels (*porins*) that permit the exchange of hydrophilic molecules through the outer membrane. Protein I also interacts with other outer-membrane components, such as protein III and LPS, to form complex outer-membrane structures. Protein I molecules have been shown to move rapidly from gonococcal outer membranes to the more fluid cytoplasmic membrane of human cells, where they form pores. This process may initiate endocytosis of the gonococcus, the first step in gonococcal invasion of the epithelium.

The LPS of the gonococcus contains lipid A and an oligosaccharide. Features that distinguish gonococcal LPS from enteric LPS are the highly branched oligosaccharide structure and the absence of repeating O-antigen subunits; thus gonococcal LPS is often referred to as *lipooligosaccharide* (LOS). Gonococcal LOS exhibits antigenic variation, which may be a mechanism for evading host defenses. The type of LOS produced can be altered by a mechanism that is not well understood but is thought to have to do with transcriptional regulation

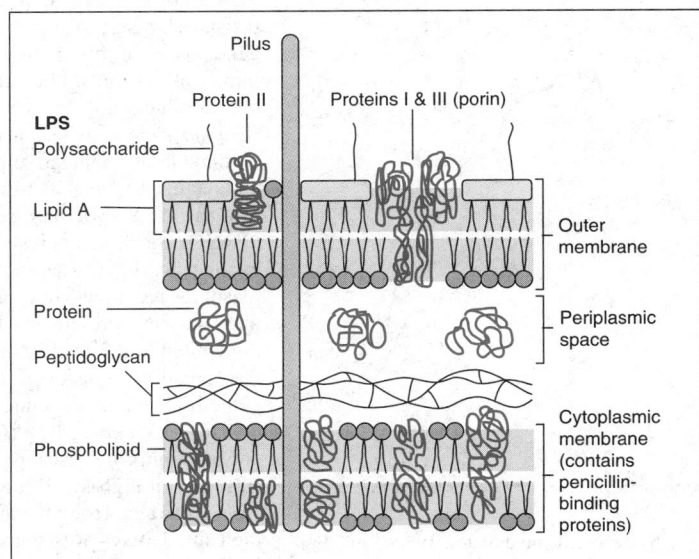

FIGURE 150-1 Diagram of the envelope of *N. gonorrhoeae*, showing structures thought to influence pathogenesis, antimicrobial susceptibility, and antigenicity.

of glycosyltransferases involved in LOS biosynthesis. Host-derived cytidine monophospho-*N*-acetylneuraminic acid can be used by gonococci to sialylate the oligosaccharide component of a LOS. This sialylation results in the conversion of a serum-sensitive organism into one that is serum-resistant and markedly reduces nonopsonic interactions of OPA-expressing gonococci with human neutrophils. The fact that gonococci observed in urethral exudate are sialylated indicates that sialylation occurs in vivo. Recent structural and immunochemical analyses of gonococcal LOS have revealed that the antigenicity and immunogenicity of the LOS is complex, in part because of the structural similarity of the oligosaccharide to host glycosphingolipids. No capsular polysaccharide has been isolated, but high-molecular-weight surface polyphosphates that may have functions similar to those of capsular polysaccharides in other organisms have been demonstrated.

For the past decade, gonococcal strains have been typed for epidemiologic studies on the basis of nutritional requirements (*auxotyping*) or antigenic differences of protein I (*serotyping*). Unlike pili and protein II, the protein I expressed by any single strain of gonococcus is antigenically stable, although there is considerable antigenic heterogeneity of protein I between strains. There are two structurally related forms of protein I, known as IA and IB; individual strains contain either but not both. Protein IA and IB genes are alleles of the same gene. Monoclonal antibodies to different epitopes of protein IA and protein IB can be used to classify gonococci into a large number of serovariants, known as serovars IA1 to IA24 and IB1 to IB32. In most populations, only a limited number of auxotype/serovar classes account for the majority of isolates. New techniques based on DNA polymorphism [e.g., restriction fragment length polymorphism (RFLP)] or OPA typing permit enhanced discrimination.

EPIDEMIOLOGY The only natural hosts for *N. gonorrhoeae* are humans. In the United States, the annual age-specific incidence rates tripled from 1963 to 1975, when more than 1 million cases were reported and an equal number probably went unreported. During this period of epidemic gonorrhea, the incidence increased fastest among young white females. As shown in Fig. 150-2, the reported incidence of gonorrhea has decreased from a peak of 473 cases per 100,000 in 1975 to about 150 per 100,000 in 1995—approximately the same incidence as when the epidemic began 30 years ago. Nonetheless, this incidence is unsurpassed by that of any other industrialized country. For example, it is 50 times higher than the incidence of 3 per 100,000 in 1995 in Sweden, which has essentially eliminated endemic transmission of gonorrhea.

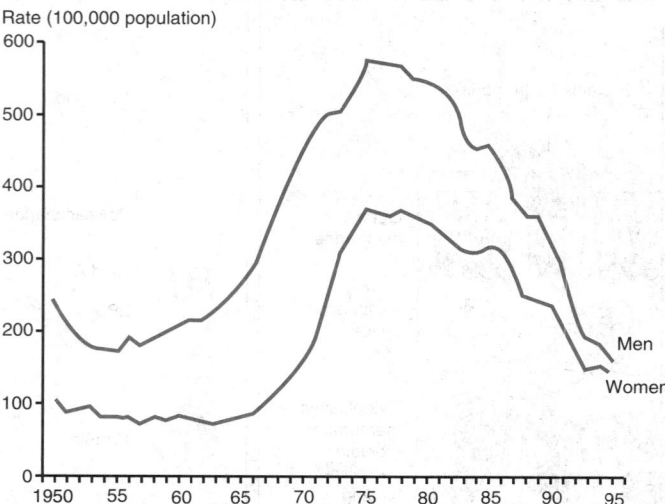

Rate (100,000 population)

FIGURE 150-2 Gonorrhea rates by gender: United States, 1950–1995. Figures for 1950–1955 are based on fiscal-year reporting; those for 1956–1995 are based on calendar-year reporting. (*Unpublished data courtesy of Russell Roegner, Centers for Disease Control and Prevention, Atlanta.*)

Gonorrhea incidence and prevalence rates are known to be related to age, sex, sexual preference, race, socioeconomic status, marital status, residential setting (urban, suburban, rural), and level of education—risk factors that influence sexual behavior, illness-related behavior, and accessibility of health care. Among sexually active individuals, the rates are highest in teenagers, in nonwhites, in the poor and poorly educated, in residents of large cities, and in unmarried persons—particularly those who live alone. Many such individuals make up a core group of "efficient transmitters" who play a disproportionate role in the spread of gonorrhea. The incidence of gonorrhea has continued to fall among white and Hispanic men and women since 1985 and has declined among black men and women since 1990. Beginning in the mid-1980s and continuing through the mid-1990s, gonorrhea, like syphilis and chancroid, has been associated with the "crack" cocaine epidemic and with the exchange of sex by women for illegal drugs such as cocaine. The incidence of gonorrhea is higher among men than among women, while the prevalence is higher among women. Routine testing by endocervical culture or newer methods is still advocated for gonorrhea case detection in asymptomatic young women who are considered to be at high risk because of their sexual behavior or the demographic factors cited above. Outreach to such women in selected settings, such as teen clinics, juvenile detention centers, jails, and drug treatment centers, remains most productive and often involves combined testing for gonorrhea and chlamydial infection. However, as the incidence and prevalence of gonorrhea continue to fall, greater reliance should be placed on partner notification (contact tracing) than on routine endocervical tests, which are expensive and often do not focus on the individuals most likely to transmit the infection. The single most important axiom about the epidemiology of this disease is that *gonorrhea is usually spread by carriers who have developed no symptoms or have ignored symptoms*. Symptomatic patients, male or female, have usually been recently infected by such carriers, who must in turn be traced and treated to prevent further transmission. *Men and women with symptomatic gonorrhea should always be interviewed to identify their recent sexual contacts, who should be examined and treated if infected.*

There are interesting regional differences in the antibiotic resistance of *N. gonorrhoeae*. In 1976, penicillinase-producing strains of *N. gonorrhoeae* (PPNG) that were completely resistant to penicillin and ampicillin appeared almost simultaneously in West Africa and Asia. PPNG first became established and then spread in areas of the world where prostitution is exceptionally common and where access to subcurative antimicrobial therapy is unrestricted. PPNG now account for 50 percent or more of all gonococci in many areas of Africa, Asia, and Latin America and have become well established in many regions of the United States and Europe. Plasmid-borne penicillin resistance results from the presence of a TEM-1-type β-lactamase gene on one of five small R factors that make up a very closely related family of plasmids. Plasmid-borne tetracycline resistance results from the introduction of the streptococcal resistance determinant *tetM* into *N. gonorrhoeae*, where it resides on a plasmid derived in part from a gonococcal conjugative plasmid. This plasmid is self-transmissible and retains the capacity to mobilize some of the β-lactamase plasmids. Strains of *N. gonorrhoeae* with tetracycline resistance plasmids (TRNG) are clinically resistant to tetracycline, minocycline, and doxycycline. Strains possessing both penicillin and tetracycline resistance plasmids are now widespread; one or both of these two types of plasmid were present in about 14 percent of gonococcal isolates in the United States by 1994 (Fig. 150-3). Of equal importance has been the spread of gonococci with chromosomally mediated resistance to penicillin and tetracycline, referred to as chromosomally mediated resistant *N. gonorrhoeae* (CMRNG). Overall, one-third of U.S. gonococcal strains are resistant to penicillin and/or tetracycline. Recently, strains with high-level fluoroquinolone resistance have been reported from Australia, Hong Kong, the Philippines, the United Kingdom, and the United States. Resistance to fluoroquinolones is not yet widespread in the United States. Auxotyping, monoclonal antibody serotyping, and RFLP analysis have shown that in a midsized metropolitan city, as many as 60 to 100 different gonococcal strains are circulating, and

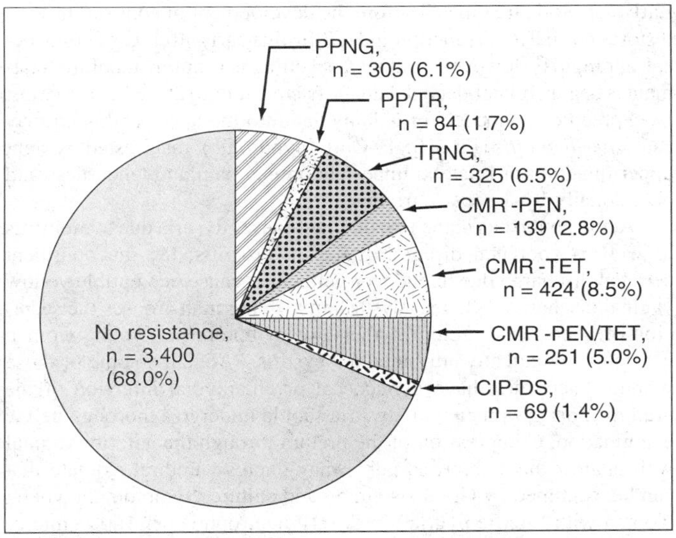

FIGURE 150-3 Antimicrobial resistance in *N. gonorrhoeae*. PPNG, penicillinase-producing *N. gonorrhoeae* (plasmid-mediated); TRNG, tetracycline-resistant *N. gonorrhoeae* [minimal inhibitory concentration (MIC), $\geq$16 μg/mL; presumably plasmid-mediated]; PP/TR, penicillinase-producing and tetracycline-resistant *N. gonorrhoeae*; CMR-PEN, chromosomal resistance to penicillin (MIC, $\geq$2 μg/mL); CMR-TET, chromosomal resistance to tetracycline (MIC, 2.0–8.0 μg/mL); CMR-PEN/TET, chromosomal resistance to penicillin and tetracycline; CIP-DS, decreased susceptibility to ciprofloxacin (MIC, $\geq$0.125–0.5 μg/mL; two isolates with MICs of 4.0 and 8.0 μg/mL, respectively). [*U.S. CDC Gonococcal Isolate Surveillance Project 1994 (5000 isolates). Courtesy of Kimberly Fox and W. L. Whittington.*]

new strains are being continuously introduced. Against this background, local outbreaks of infection due to PPNG, TRNG, CMRNG, or strains with high-level fluoroquinolone resistance belonging to a single auxotype-serovar class have been identified. Public health efforts have at times been successfully focused on the control of such strains.

Recent epidemiologic studies have shown interesting relationships between gonorrhea and human immunodeficiency virus (HIV) infection. Gonorrhea in female prostitutes has been associated with increased susceptibility to HIV infection; gonococcal urethritis has been related to increased shedding of cell-free HIV in the seminal plasma and of cell-associated HIV in the urethral exudate of HIV-seropositive men; in both instances, shedding is eliminated or decreased by treatment and cure of the urethritis. HIV infection in prostitutes has been associated with both increased risk of gonococcal reinfection and increased risk of clinical signs of salpingitis when gonococcal infection occurs.

IMMUNOLOGY AND PATHOGENESIS Epidemiologic data suggest that only about one-third of men become infected after a single exposure to *N. gonorrhoeae*; under experimental conditions an inoculum of about 10^3 organisms appears necessary to establish urethral infection in 50 percent of male volunteers. Various gonococcal virulence factors influence the size of the inoculum required. Factors that may confer resistance to infection remain undefined. However, components of the urethral or vaginal flora, such as *Candida albicans*, *Staphylococcus epidermidis*, and certain types of lactobacilli, can inhibit *N. gonorrhoeae* in vitro and may provide some natural resistance in vivo.

In humans, most extracellular iron is bound by the major iron-binding proteins transferrin and lactoferrin. The resulting concentration of free iron ($10^{-18} M$) is far too low to support gonococcal growth. Under these iron-limiting conditions, gonococci produce iron-repressible proteins that help remove iron from transferrin and lactoferrin. Gonococci bind only human transferrin and lactoferrin. This specificity may explain why gonococci in nature infect only humans. *N. gonorrhoeae* presumably competes with the lactoferrin present at mucosal surfaces for the iron required for growth of the organism. Gonococcal strains requiring arginine, hypoxanthine, and uracil for growth (AHU auxotype) are generally unable to remove iron from lactoferrin;

this inability may in part explain the tendency of such strains to cause asymptomatic mucosal infections.

Gonococci infect mucus-secreting epithelial surfaces, and mucus may be a physical barrier or a competitive inhibitor. Pili and protein II partially mediate the attachment of gonococci to mucosal cells. Local antibody to pili or protein II can partially block attachment. Pili also impede phagocytosis of gonococci by neutrophils, and antibody to pili (as well as antibody to protein II) is opsonic. An enzyme produced by the pathogenic neisseriae—IgA1 protease, which inactivates sIgA1—may interfere with IgA-mediated antiadherence activity, resulting in increased attachment.

After attachment to columnar or transitional epithelium, gonococci penetrate through or between cells to reach the subepithelial connective tissue. Transfer of gonococcal protein I into the host cell may initiate endocytosis into the epithelial cell. Gonococcal LOS produces mucosal damage in fallopian tube organ cultures. Recent evidence suggests that gonococcal LOS stimulates the production of tumor necrosis factor in fallopian tube organ cultures; inhibition of tumor necrosis factor with specific antiserum prevents tissue damage. Peptidoglycan fragments also damage the fallopian tube mucosa and may contribute to the intense inflammatory reactions characteristic of gonococcal disease. Gonococci produce several proteases, peptidases, and phospholipases that may play a role in pathogenesis. In subepithelial tissue as well as in blood, gonococci presumably interact with serum antibody, including natural IgM antibody to LOS antigens. These immune complexes activate complement, with generation of the chemotactic factor C5a and formation of the bactericidal C5b-C9 attack complex. Insertion of the attack complex into the outer membrane of serum-sensitive gonococci results in gonococcal cell lysis, making antibody to LOS (like antibody to protein I) bactericidal. Certain gonococci that tend to be associated with gonococcal bacteremia resist killing by normal human serum. The attack complex formed when serum interacts with such gonococci has an abnormal configuration, and its insertion into the outer membrane of the organism does not result in the usual rapid cell lysis. Furthermore, some human sera contain complement-fixing IgG antibody to epitopes on protein III, which blocks bactericidal antibodies to other gonococcal antigens. Protein III has extensive homology to the enterobacterial OmpA protein and the meningococcal class 4 protein. Since Enterobacteriaceae and *Neisseria meningitidis* are common commensal microorganisms, it is possible that the protein III–blocking antibodies result from prior exposure to cross-reacting proteins from other microbial species.

Oxygen-independent antimicrobial mechanisms contribute significantly to intraleukocytic killing of gonococci following their phagocytosis by neutrophils. Despite effective intraleukocytic killing of gonococci in vitro, a small but reproducible number of organisms survive. Whether gonococci survive within neutrophils in vivo remains a subject of controversy.

Spread of gonococci from the cervix to the endometrium and salpinges may be enhanced in women using an intrauterine device. Menstruation further increases the risk of intraluminal ascent from the cervix and also predisposes to gonococcal bacteremia.

CLINICAL MANIFESTATIONS The clinical spectrum of gonococcal infection depends on the site of inoculation, the duration of infection, the virulence of the infecting strain, and whether or not the organism spreads locally or systemically. The influence of inoculum size, variations in host susceptibility, and coinfection with *Chlamydia trachomatis* or other genital pathogens on clinical manifestations has not been well defined.

Gonorrhea in the Male The usual incubation period of gonococcal urethritis ("clap") in the male is 2 to 5 days, although the interval can be longer and some men never develop symptoms. In one study, one auxotype—the AHU auxotype—was associated with 96 percent of asymptomatic infections and with only 40 percent of symptomatic infections. Symptoms of urethritis include a purulent urethral discharge, which develops in 90 to 95 percent of men with urethral gonococcal infection and is usually associated with dysuria, and meatal erythema. Most symptomatic men seek treatment and are removed from the infectious pool. The remaining men—who never develop symptoms or who ignore their symptoms—accumulate in number over time and constitute about two-thirds of all infected men at any point in time. Together with those who have just become infected, have begun to shed organisms, but have not yet developed symptoms, they serve as the source of spread of infection to women. Before antibiotic treatment became available, symptoms of urethritis persisted for an average of 8 weeks, and unilateral epididymitis occurred in 5 to 10 percent of untreated men. Epididymitis is now an uncommon complication (see below), and gonococcal prostatitis occurs rarely if at all. Other local complications of gonococcal urethritis that are now unusual include inguinal lymphadenitis, edema of the penis due to dorsal lymphangitis or thrombophlebitis, submucous inflammatory "soft" infiltration of the urethral wall, periurethral abscess or fistula, unilateral inflammation or abscess of Cowper's gland (which lies between the thumb and forefinger when the forefinger is in the anal canal and the thumb is positioned anteriorly on the perineum), and (in rare cases) seminal vesiculitis. Urethral stricture presumably results from poorly managed urethritis due to gonococci, chlamydiae, or less common causes.

Among homosexual men, the frequency of gonococcal infection fell by 90 percent or more throughout the United States during the early AIDS era of the 1980s, but a disturbing resurgence of gonorrhea in young homosexual men has been seen in several cities during the 1990s. Gonococcal isolates from homosexual men tend to be more resistant to antimicrobials than are isolates from heterosexuals. The reason may be that certain highly susceptible strains are rapidly killed by bile salts and fatty acids in feces and thus are rarely found in homosexual men, while gonococci with a mutation resulting in multidrug resistance (*mtr*) are more resistant to bile salts and fatty acids and thus are found with increased frequency in homosexual men. The *mtr* mutation involves a DNA-binding protein and results in the derepression of genes encoding an efflux mechanism of resistance. Rectal infection may be asymptomatic from the outset or may produce anorectal pain, pruritus, tenesmus, and a bloody, mucopurulent rectal discharge. Proctoscopy and appropriate laboratory studies are essential to exclude several other conditions that cause similar symptoms (see Chap. 129). These symptoms may subside without treatment, leaving a chronic asymptomatic carrier state. Pharyngeal gonococcal infection occurs in approximately 20 percent of homosexual men or heterosexual women exposed via fellatio and in a smaller proportion of heterosexual men exposed via cunnilingus. Pharyngeal infection may produce exudative tonsillitis but frequently is asymptomatic; asymptomatic pharyngeal gonococcal infection usually clears spontaneously over several weeks, even without therapy.

Gonorrhea in the Female   Gonococcal infection in the female involves the endocervix, urethra, rectum, and pharynx, in decreasing order of frequency. Endocervical inflammation produces mucopurulent (yellow) endocervical discharge, which may result in a yellow vaginal discharge, and causes easily induced cervical bleeding. Upward extension of infection from the endocervix to the fallopian tubes occurs in at least 15 percent of women with gonorrhea. This extension tends to come soon after the acquisition of infection or during menstruation and results in *acute endometritis*—with abnormal menstrual bleeding, midline low-abdominal pain and tenderness, and dyspareunia—followed by *acute salpingitis*, the major complication of gonorrhea. Salpingitis can be subclinical but typically produces symptoms of bilateral lower-quadrant pain and tenderness and signs of cervical motion and abnormal adnexal mass. Endometritis and salpingitis may cause fever, leukocytosis, and abnormalities in serum acute-phase reactants (e.g., elevation of the erythrocyte sedimentation rate or of levels of C-reactive protein). Coexisting *C. trachomatis* infection may increase the rate of pelvic inflammatory disease (PID). Extension of infection to the pelvis may produce symptoms and signs of pelvic peritonitis accompanied by nausea and vomiting and may lead to pelvic abscess.

Early antibiotic treatment (before the development of adnexal masses) restores normal tubal function and fertility in nearly all cases of gonococcal salpingitis. However, if adnexal swelling is prominent before treatment is begun, bilateral tubal damage occurs in 15 to 25 percent of cases.

Spread of gonococci or chlamydiae into the upper abdomen may cause *perihepatitis* (Fitz-Hugh–Curtis syndrome), manifested by right upper quadrant or bilateral upper-abdominal pain and tenderness and occasionally by a hepatic friction rub.

Acute gonorrhea in the female often causes dysuria due to urethritis as well as anorectal discomfort due to proctitis; the mucopurulent cervical discharge due to endocervicitis may cause perceptible yellow vaginal discharge. Whereas dysuria in a young man arouses the suspicion of gonococcal urethritis, the same symptom in a young woman is often automatically attributed to "cystitis." Actually, some of those without bacteriuria have gonococcal or chlamydial infection of the urethra. Young women with dysuria should undergo a thorough pelvic examination. Compression of the urethra through the anterior vaginal wall against the symphysis pubis may express urethral exudate that can be examined by Gram's staining and culture. Symptomatic young women with "sterile pyuria" (i.e., ≥ 10 neutrophils per $100\times$ microscopic field in the centrifuged sediment of clean-catch midstream urine or a positive urine leukocyte esterase test, with no uropathogens isolated from the urine) should be evaluated for gonococcal and chlamydial infection. Acute symptoms of gonococcal urethritis in the female may subside spontaneously or after subcurative therapy with sulfonamides or urinary antiseptics. The proportion of women with gonorrhea who never develop symptoms is undefined but may be one-half or more.

Acute inflammation of Bartholin's gland is usually unilateral and frequently is due to gonococcal infection. The acutely infected duct is surrounded by a red halo and exudes pus at the posterior third of the labium majus. Occlusion of the duct results in formation of a Bartholin abscess. Chronic Bartholin cysts are rarely caused by active gonococcal infection.

There is evidence that peripartum endocervical gonococcal infection is associated with premature rupture of membranes, preterm delivery, and postpartum endometritis. In a recent randomized trial comparing a single dose of ceftriaxone with a single dose of placebo given at 28 to 34 weeks of gestation to women in Nairobi, the ceftriaxone regimen resulted in a significant increase in birth weight and a significant reduction in rates of postpartum endometritis and postpartum gonorrhea.

Gonorrhea in the Child   During childbirth, the gonococcus may infect the conjunctiva, pharynx, respiratory tract, or anal canal of the newborn. The risk of infection increases with prolonged rupture of membranes. Prevention of gonococcal ophthalmia by prophylactic use of 1% silver nitrate eyedrops or ophthalmic preparations containing erythromycin or tetracycline is a cost-effective measure in most areas of the world, including the United States. However, it is not certain whether ophthalmic tetracycline prophylaxis is effective in preventing neonatal conjunctivitis caused by TRNG. Since neonates and young infants lack bactericidal IgM antibody to *N. gonorrhoeae*, they may be at increased risk for gonococcal bacteremia. During the first year of life, infection of the infant usually results from accidental contamination of the eye or vagina by organisms from an adult under very poor hygienic conditions. In the United States, many cases of gonorrhea in children between 1 year of age and puberty involve vulvovaginitis in females who have been molested, and medicolegal considerations necessitate a complete bacteriologic diagnosis and a child welfare consultation. Auxotyping and serotyping of isolates from the sexual assault victim and the accused assailant have been used as evidence in court.

Disseminated Gonococcal Infection   The incidence of disseminated gonococcal infection (DGI) varies with time and place in relation to the local incidence of infection with strains of gonococci that have a propensity to produce bacteremia and to produce few or no symptoms or signs of inflammation at the local mucosal site of infection. Approximately two-thirds of patients with DGI are women, and symptoms of bacteremia often begin during menses.

Patients typically present either with manifestations of gonococcemia or with purulent arthritis affecting one or two joints. The onset of gonococcemia is characterized by fever, polyarthralgias, and the appearance (usually on the distal extremities) of 3 to 20 papular, petechial, pustular, hemorrhagic, or necrotic skin lesions. Initial joint manifestations are characteristically limited to tenosynovitis involving several joints asymmetrically. The wrists, fingers, knees, and ankles are most often involved. Circulating immune complexes have been demonstrated at this stage of infection, but serum complement levels are normal (except in individuals with complement deficiency), and the role of immune complexes, if any, is uncertain. Without treatment, the duration of gonococcemia is variable; the systemic manifestations of bacteremia can subside spontaneously within a week. Alternatively, septic arthritis can ensue, often without prior symptoms of fever, polyarthralgias, or skin lesions. Pain and swelling then increase in one or (very occasionally) more joints, with accumulation of purulent synovial fluid leading to progressive destruction of the joint if treatment is delayed.

IgM antibody to gonococcal LOS, present in normal human serum, is bactericidal for most strains of gonococci in the presence of complement. Gonococci isolated from patients with DGI exhibit stable resistance to normal human serum. Isolates from patients with tenosynovitis and skin lesions are even more serum-resistant than are isolates from patients with purulent arthritis; this difference suggests that the two DGI syndromes may be determined by characteristics of the causative organism. Gonococci associated with DGI usually contain outer-membrane protein IA and are highly susceptible to penicillin unless they produce β-lactamase. They often belong to the AHU auxotype. The decline in the incidence of such strains in the United States during the past two decades has been associated with a sharp decline in the incidence of DGI as well. Patients deficient in complement components C5, C6, C7, and C8 are uniquely susceptible to gonococcemia and meningococcemia because they cannot mount a serum bactericidal response to gonococci or meningococci. Although only perhaps 5 percent of patients with a first episode of gonococcemia or meningococcemia are complement-deficient, the proportion is higher among those with recurrent gonococcemia or meningococcemia. Strains isolated from complement-deficient patients may not be resistant to normal human serum.

The probability of positive blood cultures decreases after 48 h of illness, and the probability of recovery of gonococci from synovial fluid increases with the duration of illness. Gonococci are infrequently recovered from early effusions containing fewer than 20,000 leukocytes/μL but are usually recovered from effusions containing more than 80,000 leukocytes/μL. The organisms are seldom recovered simultaneously from blood and synovial fluid of the same patient.

Other common manifestations of DGI include mild myopericarditis and "toxic" hepatitis. Endocarditis and meningitis are infrequent but severe complications. Endocarditis is suggested by pathologic or changing heart murmurs, major embolic phenomena, severe myocarditis, deterioration of renal function, or an unusually large number of skin lesions.

DIFFERENTIAL DIAGNOSIS Gonococcal infection produces several common clinical syndromes that have multiple possible etiologies or that mimic other conditions. In particular, the epidemiologic and clinical features of *C. trachomatis* infections closely resemble those of gonococcal infections. The differential diagnosis of urethritis, epididymitis, and proctitis in men; cervicitis in women; vaginitis in prepubertal girls; and acute arthritis in young adults is discussed in Chap. 129. The differential diagnosis of PID is discussed in Chap. 130.

LABORATORY DIAGNOSIS The presence of intracellular gram-negative diplococci within leukocytes on Gram-stained smears of urethral or endocervical exudate warrants a presumptive diagnosis of gonorrhea. The diagnosis is equivocal if only extracellular or atypical gram-negative diplococci are seen and is ruled out if no gram-negative diplococci are seen. When experienced microbiologists employ these criteria, the sensitivity and specificity of Gram's staining of the urethral exudate approach 100 percent. The specificity of Gram's staining of purulent cervical exudate also is high, but the sensitivity is only about 50 percent. A presumptive diagnosis of gonorrhea cannot be made on the basis of gram-negative diplococci in smears from the pharynx, where other *Neisseria* species are components of the normal flora.

The "gold standard" for diagnosis of gonorrhea is the isolation of the organism by culture, which allows testing of isolates for antimicrobial resistance. Selective media (i.e., regular or modified Thayer-Martin medium), which contain antibiotics that selectively inhibit most other organisms, are most useful for recovering the gonococcus from the urethra, endocervix, pharynx, and rectum. After inoculation, the medium should be placed in a chamber with 70 percent humidity and an atmosphere containing 3 to 10% CO_2 to permit growth of the gonococcus. Inoculated media should be incubated at 35 to 37°C for 24 to 48 h, and putative gonococcal colonies should be confirmed by oxidase reaction; Gram's staining; and sugar utilization tests, rapid enzyme tests, nucleic acid probes, or agglutination reactions with antibodies specific for *N. gonorrhoeae*. The last four tests are especially important for isolates from the pharynx and rectum; for isolates obtained from populations with a low prevalence of gonorrhea, such as prenatal patients; and for isolates from victims of rape or sexual child abuse.

For diagnosis in men with incubating or chronic asymptomatic urethral infection without exudate or as a test of cure following treatment, a very thin urogenital swab should be inserted 2 cm into the anterior urethra and used to inoculate Thayer-Martin or another selective medium. Samples from the pharynx and rectum of homosexual men with suspected gonorrhea should be obtained for culture.

The endocervical culture is positive on a single examination in approximately 80 to 90 percent of women with gonorrhea. This diagnostic yield can be increased by the performance of a second endocervical culture and cultures of the rectum, urethra, and pharynx.

Another diagnostic approach has been the detection of gonococcal antigen in urethral or cervical secretions by enzyme-linked immunosorbent assay. In men with urethritis, Gram's staining is just as accurate, quicker, and cheaper; in women, the positive predictive value of antigen detection tests has been poor in populations with a low prevalence of gonorrhea. A nucleic acid probe test appears to be quite sensitive and specific in the detection of urethral and endocervical infections in populations with a relatively high prevalence of gonorrhea. Experience with pharyngeal and rectal specimens suggests that the probe test may be less sensitive than culture. The results of the probe test should be considered presumptive, particularly in low-prevalence populations. Promising DNA amplification tests, which make use of polymerase chain reaction or ligase chain reaction technology, have been developed for the diagnosis of gonococcal and chlamydial infections. The eventual utility of these tests may be greater for the diagnosis of chlamydial infection than for the diagnosis of gonorrhea, but the possibility of a single technology that could be used to detect either infection is attractive.

Standard blood-culture broth medium should be used for the culture of blood and is also recommended for the culture of synovial fluid. The broth should be vented and incubated under increased CO_2 tension. Synovial fluid also can be plated onto chocolate agar rather than a selective medium because it is not likely to be contaminated with commensal bacteria. In pus from skin lesions, *N. gonorrhoeae* is often demonstrable by immunofluorescent staining, but this test is seldom performed.

Techniques designed to detect gonococcal infection by testing of a single serum sample for antibody to *N. gonorrhoeae* have been limited by an inability to differentiate antibody due to past gonorrhea from antibody due to current infection and by false-positive results caused by cross-reactive antibody to *N. meningitidis*. For these reasons, serologic tests for gonorrhea have had a very low predictive value and are not used in clinical practice.

A false-positive diagnosis of gonorrhea can have medicolegal and psychosocial implications for both the physician and the patient.

℞ TREATMENT

Although long-acting forms of penicillin (such as benzathine penicillin G) are effective in therapy for syphilis, they have *no place* in the treatment of gonorrhea. Penicillin V and the isoxazolyl penicillins are not recommended for the treatment of gonococcal infection.

Similarly, first-generation cephalosporins are not used for gonorrhea. In 1993, the Centers for Disease Control and Prevention (CDC) published new guidelines for the treatment of gonorrhea. These 1993 guidelines are based on several observations: the importance of single-dose efficacy; the substantial proportion (over 30 percent in the United States and over 50 percent in many developing countries) of infections due to gonococci that are resistant to the penicillins (including ampicillin and amoxicillin) and/or the tetracyclines; the high frequency of coexisting chlamydial infections in persons with gonorrhea; and the severity of complications of gonococcal and chlamydial infections. The guidelines do not represent a comprehensive list of all possible treatment regimens.

As is shown in Table 150-1, for uncomplicated urethral, endocervical, rectal, or pharyngeal gonococcal infections in adults, the 1993 CDC guidelines recommend a regimen combining a single dose of any of the four most effective drugs for gonorrhea (ceftriaxone, cefixime, ciprofloxacin, or ofloxacin) with a 7-day course of doxycycline (for potential coinfection with chlamydiae). A single 1-g oral dose of azithromycin is a highly effective and convenient—but more expensive—alternative to doxycycline for chlamydial infections; potential drug interactions and adverse reactions resulting from the use of azithromycin in combination with gonorrhea therapy have not yet been well studied. These combination regimens can be expected to provide adequate therapy for gonorrhea at any site and will eliminate coexisting infections due to *C. trachomatis*. Although gonococci with high-level resistance to the fluoroquinolones remain uncommon in the United States as of 1997, an increasing incidence of such strains in the future could limit the usefulness of ciprofloxacin or ofloxacin, which can no longer be considered highly reliable for

gonorrhea in parts of Southeast Asia (e.g., the Philippines, Malaysia, Hong Kong, and Cambodia). A 2-g dose of azithromycin appears to be effective so far for gonorrhea but causes unacceptable gastrointestinal side effects.

Pregnant women who cannot tolerate a cephalosporin can receive a single dose of spectinomycin (2 g intramuscularly) for gonorrhea. Pregnant women should not receive doxycycline for chlamydial coverage but can instead take erythromycin base or stearate (500 mg by mouth four times daily for 7 days) or equivalent doses of erythromycin ethylsuccinate. If these doses of erythromycin are not well tolerated, 250 mg four times daily can be given for 14 days. Amoxicillin (500 mg orally three times daily for 7 to 10 days) can also be used for coexisting chlamydial infection in pregnancy.

All patients with gonorrhea should have a serologic test for syphilis at the time of diagnosis and should be offered confidential testing for HIV infection. Patients who have incubating seronegative syphilis without clinical signs of syphilis are likely to be cured of syphilis by the recommended ceftriaxone/doxycycline regimen. The quinolones are not effective for the treatment of syphilis, and the efficacy of cefixime for incubating syphilis has not been established, but the administration of doxycycline for 1 week to cure coexisting chlamydial infection also undoubtedly cures many cases of incubating syphilis. Nonetheless, patients with gonorrhea who also have syphilis or who are established contacts of someone with syphilis should be given additional treatment appropriate to the stage of syphilis (see Chap. 174).

Follow-Up and Treatment Failure Failure of combined therapy with ceftriaxone or cefixime and doxycycline is exceedingly rare. In the United States, the same is still true for therapy with ciprofloxacin or ofloxacin plus doxycycline. Therefore, at present, a follow-up culture is not essential after treatment with any of the recommended regimens for uncomplicated gonococcal infection. Patients should be advised to return for reexamination if any symptoms persist or recur after completion of treatment. Persistent or recurrent symptoms or signs after treatment for gonorrhea should be evaluated by culture for *N. gonorrhoeae* and by a specific test for chlamydial infection. Any posttreatment gonococcal isolate should be tested for antibiotic susceptibility. Recurrent gonococcal infections after treatment with the recommended schedule are almost always due to reinfection and indicate a need for improved referral of patients' sexual partners and education of patients themselves.

Postgonococcal urethritis (PGU) usually becomes apparent about 2 to 3 weeks after treatment of gonorrhea with a penicillin or a cephalosporin. PGU often is caused by *C. trachomatis*, which sometimes is acquired at the same time as *N. gonorrhoeae* but does not produce clinical symptoms until later because of a longer incubation period. When PGU occurs, it can be managed, like nongonococcal urethritis, with doxycycline (100 mg orally twice daily) or tetracycline (0.5 g four times a day) for 7 days. Similarly, mucopurulent cervicitis in women often persists or appears after treatment of gonorrhea with a single dose of a cephalosporin, a fluoroquinolone, or spectinomycin. This condition is frequently caused by *C. trachomatis* and can be treated like PGU. Men and women exposed to gonorrhea should be examined, have specimens obtained for culture, and be treated according to one of the recommended schedules.

Gonococcal arthritis can be treated satisfactorily with several regimens. Gonococci recovered from patients with gonococcal arthritis are generally less resistant to penicillin or tetracycline than isolates from patients with uncomplicated gonorrhea. However, several cases of DGI caused by PPNG have been reported. Because of the threat of endocarditis, meningitis, and joint sepsis, patients with DGI should be hospitalized and treated with ceftriaxone intravenously (1 g once a day) or with an alternative listed in Table 150-1. Patients without endocarditis or meningitis whose compliance is reliable can be discharged 24 to 48 h after symptoms resolve and can then complete a 7- to 10-day course of therapy with oral cefixime (400 mg twice a day) or ciprofloxacin (500 mg twice a day). A patient's failure to improve despite the administration of appropriate antimicrobial regimens strongly suggests a diagnosis other than DGI.

Table 150-1

Recommended Treatment for Gonococcal Infection: 1993 Guidelines of the Centers for Disease Control and Prevention

Diagnosis	Treatment of Choice
Uncomplicated infection of urethra, cervix, rectum, or pharynx	Ceftriaxone, 125-mg single IM dose *or* Cefixime, 400-mg single PO dose *or* Ciprofloxacin, 500-mg single PO dose *or* Ofloxacin, 400-mg single PO dose *plus* A regimen effective against possible coinfection with chlamydiae, such as: Doxycycline, 100 mg PO bid for 7 days *or* Azithromycin, 1-g single PO dose
Treatment failure	True treatment failure with ceftriaxone or cefixime is rare so far. Evaluate for reinfection or alternative diagnosis. In cases of ciprofloxacin or ofloxacin failure, also evaluate for gonococcal resistance to quinolones.
Alternative regimens	Spectinomycin, 2-g single IM dose Ceftizoxime, 500-mg single IM dose Cefotaxime, 500-mg single IM dose
Disseminated gonococcal infection, initial therapy*	Ceftriaxone, 1 g IV or IM q 24 h *or* Cefotaxime or ceftizoxime, 1 g IV q 8 h *or†* Spectinomycin, 2 g IM q 12 h
Pelvic inflammatory disease	See Chap. 130.
Epididymitis	See Chap. 129.
Pediatric gonococcal infection	See text.

* Hospitalization is recommended to exclude endocarditis, meningitis, and other diagnoses. See text for information on duration of inpatient and subsequent outpatient therapy.
† Spectinomycin is given if the patient is allergic to β-lactam agents.

Repeated joint aspiration or closed irrigation of the joint with sterile saline may be required to reduce inflammation in patients with high synovial-fluid leukocyte counts. Open drainage is seldom if ever required for gonococcal arthritis except in infants with hip infection. Temporary immobilization of the joint may reduce discomfort and may facilitate walking by patients with persistent effusions of the knee or ankle. Antibiotics should not be injected directly into the joint. Once the diagnosis of gonococcal arthritis is proven, occasional patients benefit from treatment with anti-inflammatory agents along with antimicrobial drugs. However, if the diagnosis is suspected but not proven, the early use of anti-inflammatory drugs will make it impossible to monitor the response to antimicrobial therapy, which is usually rapid and often of diagnostic importance in gonococcal arthritis.

Meningitis and endocarditis caused by the gonococcus require high-dose intravenous therapy with an agent effective against the strain causing the disease. Ceftriaxone (1 to 2 g intravenously every 12 h) is given for 10 to 14 days for meningitis and for at least 1 month for endocarditis. Patients with gonococcal endocarditis or meningitis—and perhaps all patients with DGI—should be evaluated for complement deficiency.

Gonococcal conjunctivitis in adults or in children weighing more than 20 kg should be managed by prompt irrigation of the conjunctiva with saline and administration of a single 1-g intramuscular dose of ceftriaxone, which was found to be effective in all of 12 adults with gonococcal conjunctivitis in a recent North American study. All patients must undergo careful ophthalmologic evaluation, including slit-lamp examination.

Treatment of Pediatric Gonococcal Infection The infant born to a mother with gonorrhea is at high risk of infection and requires prophylaxis with a single dose of ceftriaxone (25 to 50 mg/kg intravenously or intramuscularly, not to exceed 125 mg). Ceftriaxone should be given with caution to hyperbilirubinemic infants, especially premature babies. Topical prophylaxis for neonatal ophthalmia does not provide adequate protection against infections at other sites. Infants with gonococcal infection at any site (e.g., the eye) should be hospitalized and evaluated for signs of DGI (e.g., sepsis, arthritis, meningitis). Those with DGI should be treated for 7 days with ceftriaxone (25 to 50 mg/kg in a single daily intravenous or intramuscular dose); a treatment duration of 10 to 14 days is recommended if meningitis is documented. Alternatively, cefotaxime can be administered intravenously or intramuscularly in a dose of 25 mg/kg twice daily. Limited data suggest that uncomplicated gonococcal ophthalmia in the infant can be cured with a single injection of ceftriaxone (25 to 50 mg/kg, with a maximum dose of 125 mg). Irrigation of the eyes with saline or buffered ophthalmic solutions should be performed immediately and then repeated as often as necessary to eliminate discharge. Topical antibiotic preparations alone are neither sufficient nor required when appropriate systemic antibiotic therapy is given. Both parents of a newborn with gonococcal ophthalmia should be evaluated and treated for gonorrhea. The parents and infant also should be tested for chlamydial infection.

Children who weigh 45 kg or more should be treated with adult regimens. Children who weigh less than 45 kg should be treated as follows: For uncomplicated vulvovaginitis, cervicitis, urethritis, proctitis, and pharyngitis, the recommended regimen is a single intramuscular dose of ceftriaxone (125 mg), and the alternative regimen is a single intramuscular dose of spectinomycin (40 mg/kg, with a maximum dose of 2 g). In addition, children 8 years of age or older can be given doxycycline (100 mg twice a day for 7 days). Children with suspected gonorrhea should be evaluated by standard culture systems for isolation and identification of *N. gonorrhoeae* and should be tested for coexisting syphilis and chlamydial infection. Sexual abuse is the most common cause of gonococcal infection in prepubescent children after the age of 1 year; anorectal and pharyngeal sites are most often infected and are frequently asymptomatic.

Topical and/or systemic estrogen therapy is of no benefit in gonococcal vulvovaginitis. All children should have follow-up cultures, and the source of infection should be identified, examined, and treated. The possibility of sexual abuse should be carefully considered and evaluated. For the treatment of complicated disease, the alternative regimens recommended for adults may be used in appropriate pediatric dosages.

Treatment of Gonorrhea in Developing Countries The proportion of gonococcal infections caused by PPNG, TRNG, CMRNG, or strains resistant to ciprofloxacin is highest in developing countries, which can least afford ceftriaxone, cefixime, spectinomycin, or other new antimicrobials effective against these strains and where the newer cephalosporins are not widely available in any case. Inexpensive alternatives to penicillin G and tetracycline, the traditional mainstays of gonorrhea therapy, have been disappointing. For example, a sulfonamide-trimethoprim combination that initially cured more than 95 percent of cases of gonorrhea in African countries was found to be effective in fewer than 75 percent of cases within 2 years after it became a popular regimen in Kenya. Norfloxacin, ciprofloxacin, and ofloxacin are increasingly prescribed or dispensed without prescription for urethritis and other conditions in developing countries. Ciprofloxacin has been on the UNICEF essential-drug list and is widely available. However, none of these drugs is effective as a single-dose regimen for chlamydial urethritis. Furthermore, the emergence of high-level fluoroquinolone resistance in Asia means that one of the few relatively inexpensive, widely available, oral antimicrobials is no longer reliable for the treatment of gonorrhea in Asia. Another approach has been the administration of 4.8 million units of procaine penicillin G intramuscularly plus 1.0 g of probenecid orally together with 125 mg of clavulanic acid (in the form of one capsule of amoxicillin/clavulanate) to inhibit gonococcal β-lactamase. This inexpensive regimen was effective in small-scale trials in Kenya, even against PPNG infections, but would not be highly effective again CMRNG. Gentamicin, in a single 280-mg intramuscular dose, also has been used in this setting. Use of newer cephalosporins in lower-than-recommended doses to reduce cost should be discouraged. There is a growing need for less expensive regimens and for ongoing surveillance of in vitro sensitivity of *N. gonorrhoeae*.

PREVENTION AND CONTROL Gonorrhea probably provides the most striking illustration of the failure of a specific treatment alone to eradicate a communicable disease. No vaccine is available. A field trial of a purified gonococcal pilus vaccine in U.S. soldiers in Korea showed that the vaccine was not effective. Use of a condom can prevent transmission. The extensive use of condoms for contraception may be responsible for the low rates of gonorrhea in some countries (e.g., Japan). Spermicidal preparations used with a diaphragm or cervical sponges impregnated with nonoxynol-9 offer some protection against gonorrhea and chlamydial infection. Prophylactic antibiotics (e.g., 200 mg of minocycline or doxycycline taken soon after sexual exposure) have reduced the risk of infection but are not recommended for general use or for use by individuals with known exposure to gonorrhea, who should receive one of the regimens recommended for established gonorrhea.

To contain the increasing spread of antimicrobial-resistant gonococci, several measures are important: (1) routine use of highly effective antibiotics, such as ceftriaxone, to prevent gonorrhea treatment failures; (2) rapid identification and treatment of sexual partners of patients with gonorrhea, particularly partners of those with recurrent infection and those known to be infected with resistant strains; (3) in patients in whom treatment appears to have failed, routine diagnosis by cultures and testing of isolates for antimicrobial resistance or β-lactamase production; and (4) much greater emphasis on prevention by methods other than diagnosis and treatment—for example, by public health education and individual patient counseling to promote fewer sexual partners and condom use during casual and commercial sexual encounters.

BIBLIOGRAPHY

BRITIGAN BE, SPARLING PF: Gonococcal infection: A model of molecular pathogenesis. N Engl J Med 312:1683, 1985

CENTERS FOR DISEASE CONTROL AND PREVENTION: 1993 Sexually transmitted diseases treatment guidelines. Morb Mort Week Rep 42(RR-14):1, 1993

————: Fluoroquinolone resistance in *Neisseria gonorrhoeae*—Colorado and Washington, 1995. Morb Mort Week Rep 44:761, 1995

COHEN MS, SPARLING PF: Mucosal infection with *Neisseria gonorrhoeae.* Bacterial adaptation and mucosal defenses. J Clin Invest 89:1699, 1992

———— et al: Human experimentation with *Neisseria gonorrhoeae:* Rationale, methods, and implications for the biology of infection and vaccine development. J Infect Dis 169:532, 1994

HANDSFIELD HH et al: A comparison of single-dose cefixime with ceftriaxone as treatment for uncomplicated gonorrhea. N Engl J Med 325:1337, 1991

———— et al: Multicenter trial of single-dose azithromycin vs. ceftriaxone in the treatment of uncomplicated gonorrhea. Sex Transm Dis 21:107, 1994

HOLMES KK et al: Impact of a gonorrhea control program, including selective mass treatment, in female sex workers. J Infect Dis 174(Suppl 2):S230, 1996

KNAPP JS et al: Serologic classification of *Neisseria gonorrhoeae* using monoclonal antibodies directed against outer membrane protein I. J Infect Dis 150:44, 1985

MANALASTOS R et al: Fluoroquinolone resistance in *Neisseria gonorrhoeae* in the Republic of the Philippines. Antimicrob Agents Chemother 1997, in press

MORAN JS, LEVINE WC: Drugs of choice for the treatment of uncomplicated gonococcal infection. Clin Infect Dis 20(Suppl 1):S47, 1995

MORSE SA et al: High-level tetracycline resistance in *Neisseria gonorrhoeae* is result of acquisition of streptococcal *tet*M determinant. Antimicrob Agents Chemother 30:664, 1986

———— et al (eds): Perspectives on pathogenic *Neisseria* spp. Clin Microbiol Rev 2(Suppl 1S), 1989

MOSS G et al: Human immunodeficiency virus DNA in urethral secretions in men: Association with gonococcal urethritis and CD4 cell depletion. J Infect Dis 172:1469, 1995

O'ROURKE M et al: Opa-typing: A high-resolution tool for studying the epidemiology of gonorrhea. Mol Microbiol 17:865, 1995

PETERSEN BH et al: *Neisseria meningitidis* and *Neisseria gonorrhoeae* bacteremia associated with C6, C7, or C8 deficiency. Ann Intern Med 90:917, 1979

RICE PA et al: Immunoglobulin G antibodies directed against protein III block killing of serum-resistant *Neisseria gonorrhoeae* by immune serum. J Exp Med 164:1735, 1986

———— et al: Sociodemographic distribution of gonorrhea incidence: Implications for prevention and behavioral research. Am J Public Health 81:1252, 1991

SMITH KR et al: Evaluation of ligase chain reaction for use with urine for identification of *Neisseria gonorrhoeae* in females attending a sexually transmitted disease clinic. J Clin Microbiol 33:455, 1995

TEMMERMAN M et al: Mass antimicrobial treatment in pregnancy. A randomized placebo-controlled trial in a population with high rates of sexually transmitted diseases. J Reprod Med 40:176, 1995

VAN PUTTEN JPM: Iron acquisition and the pathogenesis of meningococcal and gonococcal disease. Med Microbiol Immunol 179:289, 1990

YORKE JA et al: Dynamics and control of the transmission of gonorrhea. Sex Transm Dis 5:51, 1978

---

151 *Daniel M. Musher*

MORAXELLA (BRANHAMELLA) CATARRHALIS, OTHER *MORAXELLA* SPECIES, AND *KINGELLA*

MORAXELLA (BRANHAMELLA) CATARRHALIS

The gram-negative coccus now known as *Moraxella catarrhalis* has undergone three changes of name in as many decades. Originally called *Micrococcus catarrhalis,* it was renamed *Neisseria catarrhalis* in the 1960s because of its morphologic similarity to *Neisseria* species. Then, in 1970, it was elevated to the status of a distinct genus, *Branhamella,* on the basis of DNA homology. In 1979 this organism was placed into the genus *Moraxella,* of which *Branhamella* may be a subgenus. Some authorities continue to call it *Moraxella (Branhamella) catarrhalis.* A component of the normal bacterial flora of the upper airways, *M. catarrhalis* has been increasingly recognized as a cause of otitis media, sinusitis, and bronchopulmonary infection.

BACTERIOLOGY AND IMMUNITY On Gram's staining, *M. catarrhalis* appears as gram-negative cocci, often occurring in pairs and retaining the side-by-side kidney-bean configuration of *Neisseria.* These cocci tend to retain crystal violet during the decolorizing step and may be confused with *Staphylococcus aureus.* Colonies grow well on blood or chocolate agar and are readily distinguishable from *Neisseria* species by biochemical tests.

M. catarrhalis shows a surprising degree of homogeneity of outer-membrane proteins. Antibody to certain of these proteins is generally present in serum of children over the age of 4 years; however, colonizing isolates or those that cause disease may survive in serum despite this naturally present antibody and complement. Bactericidal antibody emerges following natural infection and may be directed against one or more conserved outer-membrane proteins, a property of potential value in vaccine development. An 81-kDa outer-membrane protein is associated with virulence in mice; antibody to this protein is protective.

EPIDEMIOLOGY With the use of selective media, *M. catarrhalis* can be isolated from the upper respiratory tract or saliva of 50 percent of healthy schoolchildren and up to 7 percent of healthy adults. The rate of nasopharyngeal colonization is higher among children who have otitis media. Investigators in both the Northern and Southern Hemispheres have reported a striking seasonal variation in the isolation of this organism from clinical specimens, with a peak in late winter/early spring and a nadir in late summer/early fall. Direct contact has not been shown to contribute to community-acquired infection, but nosocomial spread of infection has been documented occasionally.

OTITIS MEDIA, SINUSITIS *M. catarrhalis* has repeatedly been shown to be the third most common bacterial isolate from middle-ear fluid of children who have otitis media, being surpassed only by *Streptococcus pneumoniae* and nontypable *Haemophilus influenzae.* Recent studies have shown this organism to be a prominent isolate from sinus cavities in acute and chronic sinusitis.

PURULENT TRACHEOBRONCHITIS, PNEUMONIA *M. catarrhalis* causes acute exacerbations of chronic bronchitis (increased production and/or purulence of sputum), purulent tracheobronchitis (the latter also involving fever and leukocytosis), and pneumonia. The great majority of infected persons are older than 50 years and have a long history of cigarette smoking and underlying chronic obstructive pulmonary disease (COPD); lung cancer is often present as well. In one recent study, 76 percent of affected persons had COPD (often severe), and one-third of those with COPD had lung cancer; most patients also had clinical evidence of malnutrition. In one extensive series of cases, *M. catarrhalis* pneumonia did not occur in otherwise healthy hosts.

Symptoms of patients with *M. catarrhalis* pneumonia have been regarded as modest in severity, perhaps more because of a diminished febrile response (due to the advanced age and underlying diseases of the affected individuals) than because of any lack of pathogenic capacity of this organism. Both cough and the amount and purulence of the sputum are usually increased above baseline. Chills are reported in one-quarter of patients, pleuritic pain in one-third, and malaise in 40 percent. Most patients have peak temperatures of $<101°F$ (38.3°C), and peripheral white blood cell counts are $<10,000/\mu L$ in nearly one-quarter of cases. Microscopic examination of a good sputum specimen following Gram's staining regularly reveals profuse organisms (approximately 2×10^8 colony forming units per milliliter). The radiologic appearance is variable; in one study, 43 percent of subjects had segmental or lobar infiltrates, and the remainder had a mixed pattern of subsegmental, segmental, interstitial, and diffuse involvement. These clinical, laboratory, and radiographic findings do not differ from those of pneumococcal pneumonia in an older patient population. However, a far lesser degree of bloodstream invasion occurs in *M. catarrhalis* infection; in one series, none of 25 patients with *M. catarrhalis* pneumonia had bacteremia. Nevertheless, pneumonia due to *M. catarrhalis* is a marker for severe underlying disease, in that nearly one-half of patients die within 3 months of onset.

OTHER SYNDROMES   Local extension causing empyema is very uncommon, and, as might be inferred from the low rate of bacteremia, metastatic complications of *M. catarrhalis* pneumonia, such as septic arthritis, are exceedingly rare. As of 1990, 27 cases of bacteremic infection due to *M. catarrhalis* had been reported, mainly in children less than 10 years old or adults more than 60 years old; most of these patients were immunocompromised. The syndromes reported have included bacteremia with no apparent focus, endocarditis, and meningitis. A petechial or purpuric rash, reminiscent of that observed in meningococcal sepsis and associated with disseminated intravascular coagulation, has been described in a few cases, nearly all in children.

℞ TREATMENT

Treatment of presumed *M. catarrhalis* infection with a penicillin/clavulanic acid combination seems highly appropriate. Penicillin resistance first appeared in *Branhamella* isolates in the mid-1970s and is now found in 85 percent of clinical isolates. Resistance is mediated by two closely related β-lactamases, BRO-1 and BRO-2 (acronyms derived from *Branhamella* and *Moraxella*), which are present in 90 and 10 percent, respectively, of resistant isolates. These enzymes are active against penicillin, ampicillin, and amoxicillin but less so against cephalosporins, especially third-generation cephalosporins, and they bind avidly to clavulanic acid and sulbactam.

Cephalosporins, especially those of the second and third generations, are effective alternatives. A 5-day course of therapy has been shown to cure respiratory infection, although a slightly longer course may be required in sinusitis. Isolates in the United States are nearly uniformly susceptible to tetracycline, erythromycin, trimethoprim-sulfamethoxazole, quinolones, and chloramphenicol, although tetracycline resistance, perhaps due to TetB determinants, is increasing in Europe and Asia and has been documented in two isolates in the United States.

During the period between the identification of gram-negative cocci in a Gram-stained specimen and the final identification of the organisms by culture, the severity of the condition and the potential presence of other infecting organisms should dictate antibiotic selection. For example, an exacerbation of bronchitis caused by *M. catarrhalis* might be treated with tetracycline or trimethoprim-sulfamethoxazole; however, in a patient with pneumonia, the possibility that pneumococci resistant to these agents also might be present dictates the choice of ampicillin/sulbactam or a third-generation cephalosporin, at least until results of culture are available.

OTHER *MORAXELLA* SPECIES AND *KINGELLA KINGAE*

Other *Moraxella* species cause a wide range of infections, including bronchitis, pneumonia, empyema, endocarditis, meningitis, conjunctivitis, urinary tract infection, septic arthritis, and wound infection. In a report of all *Moraxella* isolates submitted to the Centers for Disease Control and Prevention (CDC) between 1953 and 1980, certain clinical associations were apparent (Table 151-1). *M. osloensis* and *M. nonliquefaciens* were the most common species, having been cultured from a wide range of normally sterile body sites, including blood, cerebrospinal fluid, and joints. *M. osloensis* was the *Moraxella* species most commonly isolated from blood; *M. nonliquefaciens* tended to be isolated from the ears, nose, or throat (47 percent) or the sputum (8 percent). *M. canis* (formerly *Moraxella* M-5) had a striking association with infected wounds from dog bites (72 percent of all isolates), whereas *M. lacunata* was associated with conjunctivitis and keratitis (70 percent of isolates). *M. urethralis* was isolated most often from urine and the genital tract and probably represents the *Moraxella* species implicated previously in urethritis. More than one-half of isolates of *M. phenylpyruvica* and *M. atlantae* were obtained from normally sterile sites. The clinical features of infections due to *Moraxella* species other than *M. catarrhalis* and the nature of the hosts in which they occur have not been fully characterized.

Table 151-1

Moraxella Species and *Kingella kingae*

Species	Number of Isolates	Common Sites/Clinical Association	Number (Percent) for Each Site
*M. osloensis**	199	Blood	44 (22)
		CSF	18 (9)
		Urine	17 (9)
		Respiratory tract	24 (12)
M. nonliquefaciens	356	Blood	27 (8)
		CSF	6 (2)
		Respiratory tract	196 (55)
M. canis	74	Dog-bite wound	53 (72)
M-6	47	Blood, bone	15 (32)
M. lacunata	33	Conjunctivitis, keratitis	23 (70)
M. urethralis	28	Urine	16 (57)
		Genital tract	3 (11)
M. phenylpyruvica	73	Blood	19 (26)
		CSF	8 (11)
		Urine	12 (16)
M. atlantae	44	Blood	20 (45)
		CSF	5 (11)
Kingella kingae	79	Blood	38 (48)
		Joint	10 (13)
		Bone	11 (14)

* Some of these isolates would now be distinguished as a new species, *M. lincolnii*.
SOURCE: Adapted from a summary of CDC experience (Graham et al).

Kingella kingae was originally designated *Moraxella* new species 1 (M-1) and was subsequently named in honor of Dr. Elizabeth King of the CDC, who first described it. A fastidious organism, *K. kingae* has been found to cause endocarditis, arthritis, and osteomyelitis (see Table 151-1); isolated instances of other infections have been recorded. Most bone and joint infections occur in young children. One-half of all cases of septic arthritis in one recently reported series of children younger than 24 months were due to *K. kingae*. The fact that this organism is not implicated more frequently as a cause of pneumonia may indicate a true tissue tropism for heart valve, bones, and joints, or it may reflect the difficulty of separating *Kingella* from the normal respiratory flora on sputum culture.

Most moraxellae and kingellae remain susceptible to penicillins, cephalosporins, tetracyclines, and chloramphenicol, but some strains of *Moraxella* produce BRO β-lactamases, and clinical specimens must be tested for lactamase production and antibiotic susceptibility. Initial therapy with a penicillin or cephalosporin is reasonable pending susceptibility testing.

BIBLIOGRAPHY

CATLIN BW: *Branhamella catarrhalis:* An organism gaining respect as a pathogen. Clin Microbiol Rev 3:293, 1990
DEGROOT R et al: Bone and joint infections caused by *Kingella kingae:* Six cases and review of the literature. Rev Infect Dis 10:998, 1988
GRAHAM D et al: Infections caused by *Moraxella, Moraxella urethralis, Moraxella*-like groups M-5 and M-6, and *Kingella kingae* in the United States, 1953–1980. Rev Infect Dis 12:423, 1990
HAGER H et al: *Branhamella catarrhalis* respiratory infections. Rev Infect Dis 9:1140, 1987
HELMINEN ME et al: A large, antigenically conserved protein on the surface of *Moraxella catarrhalis* is a target for protective antibodies. J Infect Dis 170:867, 1994
IOANNIDIS JPA et al: Spectrum and significance of bacteremia due to *Moraxella catarrhalis.* Clin Infect Dis 21:390, 1995
KIBSEY PC et al: Disk diffusion versus broth microdilution susceptibility testing of *Haemophilus* species and *Moraxella catarrhalis* using seven oral antimicrobial agents: Application of updated susceptibility guidelines of the National Committee for Clinical Laboratory Standards. J Clin Microbiol 32:2786, 1994
MORRISON VA, WAGNER KF: Clinical manifestations of *Kingella kingae* infections: Case report and review. Rev Infect Dis 11:776, 1989
VERGHESE A, BERK SL: *Moraxella (Branhamella) catarrhalis.* Infect Dis Clin North Am 5:523, 1991

WALLACE RJ JR et al: Antibiotic susceptibilities and drug resistance in *Moraxella (Branhamella) catarrhalis*. Am J Med 88(Suppl 5A):46S, 1990

WRIGHT PW et al: A descriptive study of 42 cases of *Branhamella catarrhalis* pneumonia. Am J Med 88(Suppl 5A):2S, 1990

YAGUPSKY P et al: Epidemiology, etiology, and clinical features of septic arthritis in patients younger than 24 months. Arch Pediatr Adolesc Med 149:537, 1994

---

152   *Timothy F. Murphy, Dennis L. Kasper*

INFECTIONS DUE TO *HAEMOPHILUS INFLUENZAE*, OTHER *HAEMOPHILUS* SPECIES, THE HACEK GROUP, AND OTHER GRAM-NEGATIVE BACILLI

HAEMOPHILUS INFLUENZAE

MICROBIOLOGY   *Haemophilus influenzae* was first recognized in 1892 by Pfeiffer, who erroneously concluded that the bacterium was the cause of influenza. The bacterium is a small (~1- by 0.3-μm) gram-negative organism of variable shape; hence, it is often described as a pleomorphic coccobacillus. In clinical specimens such as cerebrospinal fluid (CSF) and sputum, it frequently stains only faintly with phenosafranin and therefore can easily be overlooked.

H. influenzae grows both aerobically and anaerobically. Its aerobic growth requires two factors: hemin (X factor) and nicotinamide adenine dinucleotide (V factor). These requirements are used in the clinical laboratory to identify the bacterium. Six major serotypes of *H. influenzae* have been identified; designated *a* through *f*, they are based on antigenically distinct polysaccharide capsules. In addition, some strains lack a polysaccharide capsule and are referred to as *nontypable* strains. Type b and nontypable strains are the most relevant strains clinically, although encapsulated strains other than type b can cause disease. *H. influenzae* is the first free-living organism whose entire genome has been sequenced.

The antigenically distinct type b capsule is a linear polymer composed of ribosyl-ribitol phosphate. Strains of *H. influenzae* type b (Hib) cause disease primarily in infants and children under the age of 6 years. Nontypable strains are primarily mucosal pathogens, although the incidence of invasive disease caused by these strains is increasing.

EPIDEMIOLOGY AND TRANSMISSION   *H. influenzae* is an exclusively human pathogen. Nontypable strains colonize the upper respiratory tract of up to three-fourths of healthy adults. Colonization with nontypable *H. influenzae* is a dynamic process; new strains are acquired and other strains are replaced periodically.

Hib strains colonize the nasopharynx of children at a rate of 3 to 5 percent; before the introduction of type b vaccine, higher rates were seen in day-care centers. The rate of nasopharyngeal colonization by Hib strains is decreasing with the widespread use of conjugate vaccines to prevent invasive infections caused by Hib. The organism is spread by airborne droplets or by direct contact with secretions or fomites.

Certain population groups have a higher incidence of invasive Hib disease than the general population. The incidence of meningitis due to Hib has been three to four times higher among black children than among white children in several studies. In some Native American groups, the incidence of invasive Hib disease is 10 times higher than that in the general population. Although this increased incidence has not yet been accounted for, several factors may be relevant, including age at exposure to the bacterium, socioeconomic conditions, and genetic differences in the ability to mount an immune response.

PATHOGENESIS   Hib strains cause systemic disease by invasion and hematogenous spread to distant sites such as the meninges, bones, and joints. The type b polysaccharide capsule is an important virulence factor affecting the bacterium's ability to avoid opsonization and cause systemic disease.

Nontypable strains cause disease by local invasion of mucosal surfaces. Otitis media results when bacteria reach the middle ear by way of the eustachian tube. Lower respiratory infection develops in adults with chronic bronchitis when nontypable strains gain access to and colonize the lower respiratory tract. The incidence of invasive disease caused by nontypable strains is low but increasing.

IMMUNE RESPONSE   Antibody to capsule is important in protection from infection by Hib strains. The level of (maternally acquired) serum antibody to the capsular polysaccharide, which is a polymer of polyribitol ribose phosphate and thus is sometimes designated PRP, declines from birth to 6 months of age and, in the absence of vaccination, remains low until around 2 or 3 years of age. The age at the antibody nadir correlates with that of the peak incidence of type b disease. Antibody to PRP then appears partly as a result of exposure to Hib or cross-reacting antigens. Systemic Hib disease is unusual after the age of 6 years because of the presence of protective antibody. Vaccines in which PRP is conjugated to protein carrier molecules have been developed and are now used widely. These vaccines generate an antibody response to PRP in infants and are effective in preventing invasive infections in infants and children.

Since nontypable strains lack a capsule, the immune response to infection is directed at noncapsular antigens. These noncapsular antigens of *H. influenzae* have generated considerable interest as targets of the human immune response and as potential vaccine components.

CLINICAL MANIFESTATIONS   *H. influenzae* **Type b**   The most serious manifestation of infection with Hib is meningitis. The age of peak incidence varies somewhat among populations, depending in part on the use of vaccine, but this infection primarily affects infants under 2 years of age. The clinical manifestations of meningitis caused by Hib are similar to those of meningitis caused by other bacterial pathogens. Fever and altered central nervous system function are the most common features at presentation. Nuchal rigidity may or may not be evident. Subdural effusion, the most common complication, is suspected when, despite 2 or 3 days of appropriate antibiotic therapy, the infant has seizures, hemiparesis, or continued obtundation. The overall mortality from meningitis caused by Hib is approximately 5 percent, and the rate of morbidity is high. Six percent of survivors have permanent sensorineural hearing loss, and about one-fourth have a significant handicap of some type. If more subtle handicaps are sought, up to half of survivors are found to have some neurologic sequelae, such as partial hearing loss and delay in language development.

Epiglottitis is a life-threatening infection involving cellulitis of the epiglottis and supraglottic tissues. It can lead to acute upper airway obstruction. Its unique epidemiologic features are its occurrence in an older age group (2 to 7 years old) than other Hib infections and its absence among Navajo Indians and Alaskan Eskimos. Sore throat and fever rapidly progress to dysphagia, drooling, and airway obstruction.

Cellulitis due to Hib occurs in young children. The most common location is on the head or neck, and the involved area sometimes takes on a characteristic bluish-red color. Most patients have bacteremia, and 10 percent have an additional focus of infection.

Hib causes pneumonia in infants. The infection is clinically indistinguishable from other types of bacterial pneumonia (e.g., pneumococcal pneumonia) except that it is more likely to involve the pleura.

Several less common invasive conditions can be important clinical manifestations of Hib infection in children. These include osteomyelitis, septic arthritis, pericarditis, orbital cellulitis, endophthalmitis, urinary tract infection, abscesses, and bacteremia without an identifiable focus. As has already been mentioned, infections due to Hib are unusual among patients older than 6 years.

Nontypable *H. influenzae*   Nontypable *H. influenzae* is the second most common cause (after *Streptococcus pneumoniae*) of community-acquired bacterial pneumonia in adults. Nontypable *H. influenzae* pneumonia is especially common among patients with chronic obstructive pulmonary disease (COPD) or AIDS. The clinical features of pneumonia due to *H. influenzae* are similar to those of other types of bacterial pneumonia (including pneumococcal pneumonia). Patients present with fever, cough, and purulent sputum, usually of several days' duration. Chest radiography reveals alveolar infiltrates in a patchy or lobar distribution. Gram-stained sputum contains a predominance of small, pleomorphic, coccobacillary gram-negative bacteria.

Exacerbations of COPD caused by nontypable *H. influenzae* are characterized by increased cough, sputum production, and shortness of breath. Fever is low-grade, and no infiltrates are evident on chest x-ray.

Nontypable *H. influenzae* is one of the three most common causes of childhood otitis media (the other two being *S. pneumoniae* and *Moraxella catarrhalis*). Infants are febrile and irritable, while older children report ear pain. Symptoms of viral upper respiratory infection often precede otitis media. The diagnosis is made by pneumatic otoscopy. An etiologic diagnosis, although not routinely sought, can be established by tympanocentesis and culture of middle-ear fluid. Nontypable *H. influenzae* also causes puerperal sepsis and is an important cause of neonatal bacteremia. Nontypable strains tend to be of biotype IV and cause invasive disease after colonizing the female genital tract.

Nontypable *H. influenzae* causes sinusitis in adults and children. In addition, the bacterium is a less common cause of various invasive infections that are reported primarily as small series descriptions and case reports. These infections include empyema, adult epiglottitis, pericarditis, cellulitis, septic arthritis, osteomyelitis, endocarditis, cholecystitis, intraabdominal infections, urinary tract infections, mastoiditis, aortic graft infection, and bacteremia without a detectable focus. Before the early 1980s, nontypable strains were frequently misidentified as Hib because of their autoagglutination when serotypes were determined in agglutination assays.

DIAGNOSIS The most reliable method for establishing a diagnosis of Hib infection is recovery of the organism in culture. The CSF of a patient in whom meningitis is suspected should be subjected to Gram's staining and culture. The presence of gram-negative coccobacilli in Gram-stained CSF is strong evidence for Hib meningitis. Recovery of the organism from CSF confirms the diagnosis. Cultures of other normally sterile body fluids, such as blood, joint fluid, pleural fluid, pericardial fluid, and subdural effusion, are confirmatory in other infections.

Detection of PRP is an important adjunct to culture in rapid diagnosis. Immunoelectrophoresis, latex agglutination, coagglutination, and enzyme-linked immunosorbent assay are effective in detecting PRP. These assays are particularly helpful when patients have received prior antimicrobial therapy and thus are especially likely to have negative cultures.

Since nontypable *H. influenzae* is primarily a mucosal pathogen, it is a component of a mixed flora; this situation makes etiologic diagnosis challenging. Nontypable *H. influenzae* infection is strongly suggested by the predominance of gram-negative coccobacilli among abundant polymorphonuclear leukocytes in a Gram-stained sputum specimen from a patient in whom pneumonia or tracheobronchitis is suspected. A sputum culture is helpful when interpreted along with the results of Gram's staining. Although bacteremia is detectable in a small proportion of patients with pneumonia due to nontypable *H. influenzae*, most such patients have negative blood cultures.

A diagnosis of otitis media is based on the detection by pneumatic otoscopy of fluid in the middle ear. An etiologic diagnosis requires tympanocentesis but is not routinely sought. An invasive procedure is also required to determine the etiology of sinusitis; thus, treatment is often empirical once the diagnosis is suspected in light of clinical symptoms and sinus radiographs.

℞ **TREATMENT**

Initial therapy for meningitis due to Hib should consist of a cephalosporin such as ceftriaxone or cefotaxime. An alternative regimen for initial therapy is ampicillin plus chloramphenicol. Therapy should continue for a total of 1 to 2 weeks.

Administration of glucocorticoids to patients infected with *H. influenzae* reduces the incidence of neurologic sequelae. The pre-

sumed mechanism is reduction of the inflammation induced by bacterial cell-wall mediators of inflammation when cells are killed by antimicrobial agents. Dexamethasone (0.6 mg/kg per day intravenously in four divided doses for 4 days) is recommended for the treatment of Hib meningitis in children over 2 months of age.

Invasive infections other than meningitis are treated with the same antimicrobial agents. Epiglottitis constitutes a medical emergency, and maintenance of an airway is critical. The duration of therapy is determined by the clinical response. A course of 1 to 2 weeks is usually appropriate.

Many infections caused by nontypable strains of *H. influenzae*, such as otitis media, sinusitis, and exacerbations of COPD, can be treated with oral antimicrobial agents. Approximately 25 percent of nontypable strains produce β-lactamase and are resistant to ampicillin. Infections caused by ampicillin-resistant strains can be treated with a variety of agents, including trimethoprim-sulfamethoxazole, erythromycin/sulfisoxazole, amoxicillin/clavulanic acid, various extended-spectrum cephalosporins, fluoroquinolones, and clarithromycin.

PREVENTION **Vaccination** The development of conjugate vaccines that prevent invasive infections by Hib in infants and children has been a dramatic success. Four such vaccines are licensed in the United States. In addition to eliciting protective antibody, these vaccines prevent disease by reducing pharyngeal colonization with Hib.

All children should be immunized with an Hib conjugate vaccine, receiving the first dose at approximately 2 months of age, the rest of the primary series between 2 and 6 months of age, and a booster dose at 12 to 15 months of age. Specific recommendations vary for the different conjugate vaccines. The reader is referred to the recommendations of the American Academy of Pediatrics.

Currently no vaccines are available for the prevention of disease caused by nontypable *H. influenzae*.

Chemoprophylaxis The risk of secondary disease is greater than normal among household contacts of patients with Hib disease. The attack rate is as high as 4 percent among susceptible infants. Therefore, all members (children and adults) of households where there are contacts less than 4 years old should receive prophylaxis with oral rifampin. (This rule does not apply when all household contacts under the age of 4 years have been completely immunized with conjugate vaccine.) Children under 12 years old should receive rifampin at a dose of 20 mg/kg once daily for 4 days, and adults should receive 600 mg daily for 4 days. The index case should receive rifampin before or at the time of discharge from the hospital because antimicrobial agents used for the treatment of meningitis do not reliably eradicate Hib from the nasopharynx.

The data on secondary cases among contacts outside the household (e.g., in day-care settings) are conflicting. The administration of rifampin prophylaxis to contacts in day-care centers should be considered, but each decision should be individualized and in part based on the contacts' immunization history, the size of the center, the extent of contact, and whether the exposure is to a single case or to multiple cases.

HAEMOPHILUS INFLUENZAE BIOGROUP AEGYPTIUS

H. influenzae biogroup aegyptius was formerly called *Haemophilus aegyptius* because of phenotypic characteristics distinct from those of *H. influenzae*. However, more recent studies involving DNA hybridization and DNA transformation have demonstrated that *H. aegyptius* and *H. influenzae* are members of the same species.

H. influenzae biogroup aegyptius has long been associated with conjunctivitis. Moreover, this strain is now known to be the cause of Brazilian purpuric fever (BPF), which was first recognized in 1984 in the rural Brazilian town of Promissao. The sharing of many phenotypic and genotypic characteristics by the various strains of *H. influen-*

zae biogroup aegyptius that cause BPF indicates that these strains represent a clone of *H. influenzae*. The age of peak incidence of BPF is 1 to 4 years, with a range of 3 months to 8 years. The illness can occur sporadically or in outbreaks. Typically, after an episode of purulent conjunctivitis, high fever occurs in association with vomiting and abdominal pain. Within 12 to 48 h after onset, the patient develops petechiae, purpura, and peripheral necrosis and experiences vascular collapse. The characteristic laboratory features are thrombocytopenia, prolonged prothrombin time, uniformly unrevealing CSF findings, and blood cultures positive for *H. influenzae* biogroup aegyptius. Initial reports cited high mortality (~70 percent), but subsequent studies have indicated that milder forms of the illness exist. Most patients have resolved or resolving purulent conjunctivitis, and culture of the conjunctiva is positive in approximately one-third of cases. BPF has been seen in several towns in Brazil and on two occasions in Australia.

HAEMOPHILUS DUCREYI

Haemophilus ducreyi is the etiologic agent of chancroid, a sexually transmitted disease characterized by genital ulceration and inguinal adenitis. *H. ducreyi* poses a significant health problem in developing countries. Although this infection is less common in the United States, its incidence has increased dramatically in the past several years. In addition to being a cause of morbidity in itself, chancroid is associated with infection with human immunodeficiency virus (HIV) because of the role of genital ulceration in the transmission of HIV.

MICROBIOLOGY *H. ducreyi* is a highly fastidious coccobacillary gram-negative bacterium whose growth requires X factor (hemin). Although, in light of this requirement, the bacterium has been classified in the genus *Haemophilus*, DNA homology and chemotaxonomic studies have established substantial differences between *H. ducreyi* and other *Haemophilus* species. Taxonomic reclassification of the organism is likely in the future but awaits further study.

EPIDEMIOLOGY AND PREVALENCE Chancroid is a common cause of genital ulcers in developing countries. Several large outbreaks of chancroid have occurred in the United States since 1981. Recurring epidemiologic themes have been apparent in these outbreaks: (1) transmission has been predominantly heterosexual, (2) males have outnumbered females by ratios of 3:1 to 25:1, and (3) prostitutes have been important in transmission of the infection. The incidence of chancroid in the United States will undoubtedly increase in the coming years, and the genital ulcers associated with this infection will continue to play a role in the transmission of HIV.

CLINICAL MANIFESTATIONS Infection is acquired as the result of a break in the epithelium during sexual contact with an infected individual. After an incubation period of 4 to 7 days, the initial lesion—a papule with surrounding erythema—appears. In 2 to 3 days, the papule evolves into a pustule, which spontaneously ruptures and forms a sharply circumscribed ulcer that is generally not indurated. The ulcers are painful and bleed easily; little or no inflammation of the surrounding skin is evident. Approximately half of patients develop enlarged, tender inguinal lymph nodes, which frequently become fluctuant and spontaneously rupture.

The presentation of chancroid does not usually include all of the typical clinical features and is sometimes atypical. Multiple ulcers can coalesce to form giant ulcers. Ulcers can appear and then resolve, with inguinal adenitis and suppuration following 1 to 3 weeks later; this clinical picture can be confused with that of lymphogranuloma venereum. Multiple small ulcers can resemble folliculitis. Other differential diagnostic considerations include the various infections causing genital ulceration, such as primary syphilis, condyloma latum of secondary syphilis, genital herpes, and donovanosis. In rare cases chancroid lesions become secondarily infected with bacteria; the result is extensive inflammation.

DIAGNOSIS Clinical diagnosis of chancroid is often inaccurate, and laboratory confirmation should be attempted in suspected cases. Gram's staining of a swab of the lesion may reveal a predominance of characteristic gram-negative coccobacilli, but the presence of other bacteria often makes it difficult to interpret this result. An accurate diagnosis of chancroid relies on cultures of *H. ducreyi* from the lesion. Since the organism can be difficult to grow, the use of selective and supplemented media is necessary.

℞ TREATMENT

Clinical isolates of *H. ducreyi* often exhibit plasmid-mediated resistance to ampicillin, chloramphenicol, tetracyclines, and sulfonamides. Nevertheless, chancroid can be treated effectively with several regimens, including (1) ceftriaxone, 250 mg intramuscularly as a single dose; (2) erythromycin, 500 mg orally four times daily for 7 days; (3) trimethoprim-sulfamethoxazole, one double-strength tablet twice daily for 7 days (in regions where resistant strains are not prevalent); and (4) ciprofloxacin, 500 mg orally twice daily for 3 days. Isolates from patients who do not respond promptly to treatment should be tested for antimicrobial susceptibility.

OTHER HAEMOPHILUS SPECIES

Haemophilus species are often recovered as components of the flora of the normal human upper respiratory tract. However, these bacteria are infrequent causes of infection because of their low pathogenic potential. *Haemophilus* species have fastidious growth requirements and are generally rather slow-growing. The species implicated in human infections include *Haemophilus parainfluenzae*, *Haemophilus aphrophilus*, and *Haemophilus paraphrophilus* (see "HACEK Group Organisms" below); *Haemophilus parahaemolyticus*; *Haemophilus haemolyticus*; and *Haemophilus segnis*. *Haemophilus* species are differentiated from one another by several characteristics, primarily their requirements for X and V factors. Species designated *para-* require V factor but not X factor for growth, whereas the others require either X and V or X only.

A variety of infections involving almost all organ systems can be caused by *Haemophilus* species. Most of these unusual manifestations have been reported as single cases and small series.

The antimicrobial susceptibility characteristics of other *Haemophilus* species are similar to those of *H. influenzae*. Some strains produce β-lactamase and are thereby resistant to ampicillin. Other strains are sensitive to ampicillin, and this agent has been used successfully to treat many infections. Alternative agents with good activity against most *Haemophilus* species include trimethoprim-sulfamethoxazole, third-generation cephalosporins, tetracycline, chloramphenicol, and aminoglycosides. Endocarditis caused by ampicillin-sensitive strains should be treated with ampicillin plus an aminoglycoside.

HACEK GROUP ORGANISMS

HACEK organisms are a group of fastidious, slow-growing, gram-negative organisms whose growth requires an atmosphere of carbon dioxide. Species belonging to this group include several *Haemophilus* species (the most important of which are *H. aphrophilus*, *H. parainfluenzae*, and *H. paraphrophilus*), *Actinobacillus actinomycetemcomitans*, *Cardiobacterium hominis*, *Eikenella corrodens*, and *Kingella kingae*. These organisms frequently require prolonged incubation for isolation from blood cultures (at least 7 days). Cultures of blood from patients with suspected endocarditis due to HACEK organisms may require up to 30 days to become positive. These organisms are found less commonly in clinical specimens than *H. influenzae*, perhaps because they are less virulent. HACEK bacteria normally reside in the oral cavity and have been associated with local infections in the mouth. They are also known to cause severe systemic infections—most often bacterial endocarditis.

Of the HACEK group, the *Haemophilus* species, *A. actinomycetemcomitans*, and *C. hominis* are most frequently associated with endocarditis, which can develop on either native or prosthetic valves. In large series of cases of infective endocarditis, about 1 percent of cases are attributable to HACEK organisms, with the *Haemophilus* species most commonly isolated. The clinical course of HACEK endocarditis tends to be subacute; however, embolization is common. The overall prevalence of major emboli associated with endocarditis due to these organisms is 28 percent; rates have been as high as 60 percent in some series.

Thirty-three percent of patients with HACEK native-valve endocarditis due to *Haemophilus* species have a history of cardiac valvular disease, 60 percent have been ill for less than 2 months before presentation, and 50 percent are anemic at presentation. Nineteen percent of patients develop congestive heart failure. Mortality rates as high as 30 percent (with most deaths attributed to cerebral embolism) have been reported. Despite these grim statistics for endocarditis on native valves, the cure rate for HACEK prosthetic-valve endocarditis appears to be high. Frequently (in more than 80 percent of cases), cure is achieved with antibiotic treatment alone and without surgical intervention. The better success in prosthetic-valve than in native-valve endocarditis is most likely due to earlier detection of infection.

Therapy for HACEK endocarditis due to *Haemophilus* species should be based on antibiotic sensitivity testing. Empirical combination therapy with ampicillin and gentamicin, which tend to be synergistic against some isolates, is a reasonable initial approach. Ceftriaxone (2 g/d) has also been used successfully.

A. actinomycetemcomitans, another slow-growing inhabitant of the oral cavity, can be isolated from soft tissue infections and abscesses in association with *Actinomyces israelii*. About 30 percent of actinomycotic lesions also yield *A. actinomycetemcomitans* on culture. *A. actinomycetemcomitans* has been associated with severe destructive periodontal disease, characterized by loss of alveolar bone of the molars and incisors, in both children and adults. This organism has also been associated with endocarditis, especially in patients with severe periodontal disease and underlying cardiac valvular damage; high rates of embolic phenomena are associated with endocarditis. *A. actinomycetemcomitans* has been isolated from patients with brain abscesses, meningitis, parotitis, osteomyelitis, urinary tract infection, pneumonia, and empyema, among other infections. Most isolates are susceptible to third-generation cephalosporins, semisynthetic penicillins like mezlocillin, trimethoprim-sulfamethoxazole, quinolones, and azithromycin. However, because of variability among strains, susceptibility testing should be undertaken. Endocarditis should be treated for 4 weeks, whereas prosthetic-valve infections or infections in patients with complications such as embolization justify 6 weeks of therapy.

C. hominis primarily causes endocarditis in patients with underlying valvular heart disease or with prosthetic valves. Many patients have signs and symptoms of long-standing infection before diagnosis. As in endocarditis due to other HACEK organisms, embolization, mycotic aneurysms, and congestive heart failure are frequent. Antibiotic sensitivity testing of *C. hominis* is difficult. Most cases of infection due to *C. hominis* are treated with penicillin, either alone or in combination with an aminoglycoside. The value of the aminoglycoside in this situation has not been established.

E. corrodens, a fastidious facultative gram-negative organism, is part of the endogenous flora of the mouth and nasopharynx. It is most frequently recovered from sites of infection in conjunction with other bacterial species. Clinical sources of *E. corrodens* include sites of human bite wounds (clenched-fist injuries), endocarditis, soft tissue infections of the head and neck, soft tissue infections in drug abusers, osteomyelitis, respiratory infections, chorioamnionitis, gynecologic infections associated with intrauterine devices, meningitis and brain abscesses, and visceral abscesses. *E. corrodens*–associated infections can be treated with ampicillin or with second- or third-generation cephalosporins. The organism is susceptible to the fluoroquinolones in vitro but is resistant to metronidazole and clindamycin. → *Kingella kingae* is discussed in Chap. 151.

OTHER GRAM-NEGATIVE BACILLI

ALCALIGENES XYLOSOXIDANS This gram-negative bacillus is probably part of the endogenous intestinal flora and has been isolated from water sources. Immunocompromised hosts appear to be at increased risk for infection with this organism. Nosocomial sources to which outbreaks of infection with *A. xylosoxidans* have been attributed include contaminated intravenous fluids, pressure transducers, and disinfectants. Clinical illness has been associated with isolates from many sites, including blood, urine, respiratory secretions, peritoneal and pleural fluids, and endocarditic prosthetic valves. In vitro susceptibility testing of all clinically relevant isolates is essential to the selection of appropriate therapy.

AGROBACTERIUM TUMEFACIENS This organism has been associated with intravascular catheter–related infections in immunocompromised hosts, especially individuals infected with HIV. Clinically important infections associated with *A. tumefaciens* include prosthetic-joint and prosthetic-valve infections, bacteremia, peritonitis, and urinary tract infections. Antibiotic sensitivity testing is essential in the choice of therapy.

***CAPNOCYTOPHAGA* SPECIES** This genus of fusiform, long, thin gram-negative rods is facultatively anaerobic and requires an atmosphere enriched in carbon dioxide for optimal growth. *Capnocytophaga ochracea*, *Capnocytophaga gingivalis*, and *Capnocytophaga sputigena* are normal inhabitants of the human oral cavity and have been isolated from the female genital tract. Their isolation has also been reported from blood, CSF, and respiratory fluids (including pleural collections). These organisms have been associated with sepsis in immunocompromised hosts; particularly at risk are patients with acute myelogenous leukemia or acute lymphocytic leukemia. In the immunocompetent host, these three species probably play a role in localized juvenile periodontitis; however, they have been isolated from many other sites as well, usually as part of a polymicrobial infection. In vitro sensitivity testing of these organisms is difficult because they are slow-growing and fastidious. Although penicillin has been considered first-line therapy, an increasing number of isolates reportedly produce β-lactamase. Clindamycin or drug combinations including a penicillin derivative plus a β-lactamase inhibitor—such as ampicillin/sulbactam or amoxicillin/clavulanate—are currently recommended for empiric therapy.

Capnocytophaga canimorsus and *Capnocytophaga cynodegmi* are endogenous to the canine mouth. Patients infected with these species frequently have a history of dog bites or of exposure to dogs without scratches or bites. Asplenia, glucocorticoid therapy, and alcohol abuse are predisposing conditions and are associated with relatively fulminant infections. The interval from dog bite to presentation averages 5 days but ranges from 1 day to 1 month. *C. canimorsus* causes a wide range of infections, including severe sepsis with shock and disseminated intravascular coagulation, meningitis, endocarditis, cellulitis, and septic arthritis. In the asplenic individual who has recently sustained a dog bite, infection with this organism must be considered early because of a potentially rapid progression to death. Penicillin is the drug of choice for infections with *C. canimorsus*. This agent should also be given prophylactically to asplenic patients sustaining dog-bite injuries. Patients with suspected *C. canimorsus* infection should be treated empirically, because identification of this organism and determination of its antibiotic sensitivity can take many days. Other drugs to which *C. canimorsus* is reportedly susceptible include clindamycin, imipenem, quinolones, and third-generation cephalosporins.

CHROMOBACTERIUM VIOLACEUM This organism is rarely a human pathogen but reportedly has been responsible for life-threatening infections with severe sepsis and metastatic abscesses. A slender, slightly curved, gram-negative rod that is facultatively anaerobic, *C. violaceum* inhabits tropical water and soil and causes infection after contamination of skin wounds. Patients with defective neutrophil function (e.g., those with chronic granulomatous disease) are infected by this organism with unusual frequency. The mortality rate in the United States from infection with *C. violaceum* has been reported at >60 percent. The organism is generally susceptible to ciprofloxacin, trimethoprim-sulfamethoxazole, gentamicin, and chloramphenicol.

FLAVOBACTERIUM MENINGOSEPTICUM The most important of the *Flavobacterium* species isolated from humans, *F. menin-*

gosepticum is associated with nosocomial infections transmitted by fluids such as disinfectants and arterial catheter flush solutions. This organism has also been associated with neonatal sepsis and meningitis. Adults have sometimes developed infection after receiving aerosolized antibiotics or while immunocompromised. *F. meningosepticum* has been reported to cause meningitis, endocarditis, bacteremia, and respiratory infections. Antibiotic treatment should be based on susceptibility results because of the high likelihood that *F. meningosepticum* will produce β-lactamase.

PLESIOMONAS SHIGELLOIDES This freshwater organism is a cause of acute diarrhea (see Chap. 128) and occasionally of serious extraintestinal disease. *P. shigelloides* is transmitted to humans via contaminated water or food. This motile, facultatively anaerobic gram-negative rod most often produces mild diarrhea with mucoid, bloody feces containing leukocytes. Severe extraintestinal infections have been reported most commonly in immunocompromised hosts and include bacteremia, cellulitis, neonatal sepsis and meningitis, and septic arthritis. There is great variability among strains in terms of antibiotic sensitivity patterns, and isolates must be tested before appropriate therapy can be selected.

MISCELLANEOUS ORGANISMS Many other gram-negative rods have been reported to cause occasional infections in hosts who are immunologically unprepared to deal with relatively avirulent organisms or who are unfortunate enough to encounter an exceptionally large inoculum. Such organisms include *Weeksella* species; various CDC groups, such as EF-4, Ve-2 (*Flavimonas* species), IVc-2, NO-1, WO-1, and Gilardi Group WO-1; *Sphingobacterium* species; *Protomonas* species; *Ochrobactrum anthropi*; *Oligella urethralis*; and *Achromobacter* species. The reader is advised to consult subspecialty texts and references for further guidance on these organisms.

BIBLIOGRAPHY

BARBOUR ML et al: The impact of conjugate vaccine on carriage of *Haemophilus influenzae* type b. J Infect Dis 171:93, 1995

BILGRAMI S et al: *Capnocytophaga* bacteremia in a patient with Hodgkin's disease following bone marrow transplantation: Case report and review. Clin Infect Dis 14:1045, 1992

BRUCKNER DA, COLONNA P: Nomenclature for aerobic and facultative bacteria. Clin Infect Dis 16:598, 1993

CAMPBELL JR, EDWARDS MS: *Capnocytophaga* species infections in children. Pediatr Infect Dis J 10:944, 1991

CIESLAK TJ, RASZKA WV: Catheter-associated sepsis due to *Alcaligenes xylosoxidans* in a child with AIDS. Clin Infect Dis 16:592, 1993

CLARK RB et al: Fatal *Plesiomonas shigelloides* septicaemia in a splenectomized patient. J Infect 23:89, 1991

COLDING H et al: Ribotyping for differentiating *Flavobacterium meningosepticum* isolates from clinical and environmental sources. J Clin Microbiol 32:501, 1994

COMMITTEE ON INFECTIOUS DISEASES: *Haemophilus influenzae* infections, in *1994 Red Book, Report of the Committee on Infectious Diseases,* G Peter et al (eds). Elk Grove Village, IL, American Academy of Pediatrics, 1994

DECRE D et al: A beta-lactamase-overproducing strain of *Alcaligenes denitrificans* subsp. *xylosoxidans* isolated from a case of meningitis. J Antimicrob Chemother 30:769, 1992

FARLEY MM et al: Invasive *Haemophilus influenzae* disease in adults. Ann Intern Med 116:806, 1992

FLEISCHMANN RD et al: Whole-genome random sequencing and assembly of *Haemophilus influenzae* Rd. Science 269:496, 1995

FLOOD JM et al: Multistrain outbreak of chancroid in San Francisco, 1989–91. J Infect Dis 167:1106, 1993

FUJII T et al: Purification and properties of inducible penicillin beta-lactamase isolated from *Alcaligenes faecalis*. Antimicrob Agents Chemother 27:608, 1985

HARABUCHI Y et al: Nasopharyngeal colonization with nontypeable *Haemophilus influenzae* and recurrent otitis media. J Infect Dis 170:862, 1994

HOLMBERG SD et al: *Plesiomonas* enteric infections in the United States. Ann Intern Med 105:690, 1986

HULSE M et al: *Agrobacterium* infection in humans: Experience at one hospital and review. Clin Infect Dis 16:112, 1993

JANDA JM, ABBOTT SL: Expression of hemolytic activity by *Plesiomonas shigelloides*. J Clin Microbiol 31:1206, 1993

KULLBERG JB et al: Purpura fulminans and symmetrical peripheral gangrene caused by *Capnocytophaga canimorsus* (formerly DF-2) septicemia—a complication of dog bite. Medicine 70:287, 1991

KURIKKA S et al: Comparison of five different vaccination schedules with *Haemophilus influenzae* type b–tetanus toxoid conjugated vaccine. J Pediatr 128:524, 1996

MURPHY TF, SETHI S: Bacterial infection in chronic obstructive pulmonary disease. Am Rev Respir Dis 146:1067, 1992

——— et al: Declining incidence of *Haemophilus influenzae* type b disease since introduction of vaccination. JAMA 269:246, 1993

PATRICK WD et al: Infective endocarditis due to *Eikenella corrodens:* Case report and review of the literature. Can J Infect Dis 1:139, 1990

PICKETT MJ et al: Miscellaneous gram-negative bacteria, in *Manual of Clinical Microbiology,* 5th ed, A Balows et al (eds). Washington, DC, American Society for Microbiology, 1991, pp 410–428

POKRUKA M et al: A *Flavobacterium meningosepticum* outbreak among intensive care patients. Am J Infect Control 21:139, 1993

POLLNER JH et al: Severe soft-tissue infection caused by *Eikenella corrodens.* Clin Infect Dis 15:740, 1992

RAMIREZ FC et al: *Agrobacterium tumefaciens* peritonitis mimicking tuberculosis. Clin Infect Dis 15:938, 1992

ROBISON WJ, VITELLI AS: Infectious endocarditis caused by *Cardiobacterium hominis.* South Med J 78:1020, 1985

ROSCOE DL et al: Antimicrobial susceptibilities and β-lactamase characterization of *Capnocytophaga* species. Antimicrob Agents Chemother 36:2197, 1992

SCHEIFELE DW: Recent trends in pediatric *Haemophilus influenzae* type b infections in Canada. Immunization Monitoring Program, Active (IMPACT) of the Canadian Paediatric Society and the Laboratory Centre for Disease Control. Can Med Assoc J 154:1041, 1996

SORENSON RU et al: *Chromobacterium violaceum* adenitis acquired in the northern United States as a complication of chronic granulomatous disease. Pediatr Infect Dis 4:701, 1985

STEINHART R et al: Invasive *Haemophilus influenzae* infections in men with HIV infection. JAMA 268:3350, 1992

TAVERAS JM III et al: Apparent culture-negative endocarditis of the prosthetic valve caused by *Cardiobacterium hominis.* South Med J 86:1439, 1993

TI T-Y et al: Nonfatal and fatal infections caused by *Chromobacterium violaceum.* Clin Infect Dis 17:505, 1993

VADHEIM CM et al: Eradication of *Haemophilus influenzae* type b disease in southern California. Arch Pediatr Adolesc Med 148:51, 1994

WALSH RD et al: *Achromobacter xylosoxidans* osteomyelitis. Clin Infect Dis 16:176, 1993

WILSON ME: Prosthetic valve endocarditis and paravalvular abscess caused by *Actinobacillus actinomycetemcomitans.* Rev Infect Dis 11:665, 1989

153

Lutfiye Mulazimoglu, Victor L. Yu

LEGIONELLA INFECTION

DEFINITION *Legionellosis* refers to the two clinical syndromes caused by bacteria of the genus *Legionella*. *Pontiac fever* is an acute, febrile, self-limited illness that has been serologically linked to *Legionella* species, whereas *Legionnaires' disease* is the designation for pneumonia caused by these species.

HISTORY Legionnaires' disease was first recognized in 1976, when an outbreak of pneumonia took place at a hotel in Philadelphia during the American Legion Convention. Investigators from the Centers for Disease Control and Prevention (CDC) identified the causative aerobic gram-negative bacterium in lung specimens obtained from the victims at autopsy and named this organism *Legionella pneumophila*. Retrospective studies of stored serum samples revealed that an epidemic of Legionnaires' disease had occurred in 1957 in Austin, Minnesota. In this epidemic (the earliest documented so far), 78 persons were hospitalized with acute respiratory infection. Antibody determinations showed seroconversion to *L. pneumophila* in most cases.

MICROBIOLOGY At present, the family Legionellaceae comprises 41 species with 63 serogroups. The species *L. pneumophila* causes 80 to 90 percent of human infections and includes at least 14 serogroups; serogroups 1, 4, and 6 are most commonly implicated in human infections. To date, 17 species other than *L. pneumophila* have been associated with human infections, among which *L. micdadei* (Pittsburgh pneumonia agent), *L. bozemanii*, *L. dumoffii*, and *L. longbeachae* are the most common.

Members of the Legionellaceae are aerobic, thin, gram-negative bacilli that do not grow on routine microbiologic media. Buffered charcoal yeast extract (BCYE) agar is the medium used to grow *Legionella*. This highly enhanced medium contains the amino acid L-cysteine, which is an absolute growth requirement for *Legionella*. Growth of the organism on BCYE medium is usually visible in 3 to 5 days at 35 to 37°C. *L. micdadei* and *L. maceachernii* produce blue colonies on BCYE medium containing bromocresol purple and bromothymol blue dyes, while the other species produce green colonies.

Antimicrobial agents, including polymyxin B, cefamandole, and vancomycin, are used in *Legionella*-selective media to suppress competing components of the microflora. Although *L. pneumophila* is relatively tolerant to these antibiotics, the drugs may inhibit the growth of other legionellae; for example, cefamandole-containing media suppress the growth of *L. micdadei*.

Traditional biochemical tests are not particularly helpful in distinguishing one *Legionella* species from another. Fatty-acid profile determination by gas-liquid chromatography and ubiquinone analysis allow identification to the genus level. The direct fluorescent antibody (DFA) test can definitively identify a number of individual species. In *L. pneumophila*, lipopolysaccharide is a prominent constituent of the outer membrane, and the serogroup-specific antigen and antibodies detected by immunofluorescence are directed primarily at the lipopolysaccharide. Both polyclonal and monoclonal DFA reagents are commercially available. The monoclonal antibody reagent (Genetic Systems, Seattle, WA) is less cross-reactive but is specific for *L. pneumophila*. Genetic analysis has been considered the definitive arbiter for the identification of individual species, with the degree of DNA sequence homology the most common criterion employed. A nucleic-acid hybridization probe reactive to *Legionella* ribosomal RNA, used with a single reagent, can identify a member of the genus within hours.

ECOLOGY AND TRANSMISSION The natural habitats for *L. pneumophila* are aquatic bodies, including lakes and streams; *L. longbeachae* has been isolated from soil. Legionellae can survive under a wide range of environmental conditions; for example, the organisms can live for years in refrigerated water samples. Natural bodies of water contain only small numbers of legionellae. However, once the organisms enter human-constructed aquatic reservoirs (such as cooling towers or water-distribution systems), they can grow and proliferate. Factors known to enhance colonization by and amplification of legionellae include warm temperatures (25 to 42°C), stagnation, and scale and sediment. The presence of symbiotic microorganisms, including algae, amebas, ciliated protozoa, and other water-dwelling bacteria, likewise promotes growth of *L. pneumophila*.

Hot-water tanks colonized with *L. pneumophila* are significantly more likely than uncolonized tanks to be cooler (<60°C), to have a vertical configuration, to be older, and to have higher concentrations of calcium and magnesium. Vertical tanks, especially those that are electric coil-heated rather than gas-heated, have a pronounced temperature stratification and thick sediment accumulation at the bottom. Studies have shown that neither a high degree of outward cleanliness nor routine application of maintenance measures decreases the frequency or intensity of *Legionella* colonization. Thus, engineering guidelines and building codes, although often advocated as preventive measures, have relatively little impact on *Legionella* colonization.

The source of *Legionella* is water, but the mode of transmission from the environmental reservoir to the patient remains controversial. Early investigations that implicated cooling towers antedated the discovery that the organism could also exist in potable water distribution systems. It is now known that, in many outbreaks, cases of Legionnaires' disease continued to occur despite disinfection of cooling towers and the potable water supply was the actual source. Koch's postulates have been fulfilled in epidemiologic studies using molecular fingerprinting methods to link potable water sources (unlike cooling towers) to *Legionella* infection in humans. Community-acquired Legionnaires' disease has been linked to colonization of residential and industrial water supplies.

The modes of transmission of *Legionella* to humans are probably multiple: evidence exists for transmission due to aerosolization, aspiration, and direct instillation into the lung during respiratory tract manipulations. Aspiration may be the predominant mode of transmission, but it is unclear whether *Legionella* enters the lung via oropharyngeal colonization or directly via the drinking of contaminated water. Nasogastric tubes have been linked to nosocomial Legionnaires' disease in several reports; microaspiration of contaminated water was the hypothesized mode of transmission. Surgery with general anesthesia is a known risk factor that is consistent with aspiration. Especially compelling is the reported 30 percent incidence of postoperative *Legionella* pneumonia among patients undergoing head and neck surgery in a hospital with a contaminated water supply; aspiration is a recognized sequela in such cases. Studies of patients with hospital-acquired Legionnaires' disease showed that these individuals underwent endotracheal intubation significantly more often and for a significantly longer duration than patients with nosocomial pneumonia of other etiologies.

Aerosolization of legionellae by devices filled with tap water, including nebulizers and humidifiers, has caused cases of Legionnaires' disease. An ultrasonic mist machine in the produce section of a grocery store was implicated in a community outbreak. Pontiac fever has been linked to *Legionella*-containing aerosols from water-using machinery, a cooling tower, air-conditioners, and whirlpools.

EPIDEMIOLOGY The incidence of Legionnaires' disease depends on the degree of contamination of the aquatic reservoir, the susceptibility and immune status of the persons exposed to the water from that reservoir, the intensity of exposure, and the availability of specialized laboratory tests on which the correct diagnosis can be based.

Numerous prospective studies have found *Legionella* to rank among the top three microbial causes of community-acquired pneumonia (*Streptococcus pneumoniae* and *Haemophilus influenzae* usually ranking first and second), accounting for 3 to 15 percent of cases. On the basis of a multihospital study of community-acquired pneumonia in Ohio, the CDC has estimated that only 3 percent of sporadic cases of Legionnaires' disease are correctly diagnosed. Legionellae are responsible for 10 to 50 percent of nosocomial pneumonias when a hospital's water system is colonized with the organisms. One situation in which the diagnosis of Legionnaires' disease should be considered is that in which the presenting patient has been hospitalized within 10 days before the onset of symptoms. In one study, a number of patients had been discharged from the hospital and readmitted with Legionnaires' disease; molecular fingerprinting showed that the isolates obtained from patients and the isolate from the hospital's water supply were similar.

The most common risk factors for Legionnaires' disease are cigarette smoking, chronic lung disease, advanced age, and immunosuppression. The disease most often develops in elderly men; this predilection is probably related to cigarette smoking. Surgery is a prominent predisposing factor in nosocomial infection, with transplant recipients at highest risk. Nosocomial cases are now being recognized among neonates and among children with immunosuppression or underlying pulmonary disease.

Pontiac fever occurs in epidemics. The high attack rate (above 90 percent) reflects airborne transmission.

PATHOGENESIS Legionellae enter the lungs via aspiration or direct inhalation. The organisms possess pili that may mediate adherence to respiratory tract epithelial cells. Thus, conditions that impair mucociliary clearance, including cigarette smoking, lung disease, or alcoholism, predispose to Legionnaires' disease.

Cell-mediated immunity is the primary mechanism of host defense against *Legionella*, as it is against other intracellular pathogens, including *Mycobacterium tuberculosis*, *Listeria*, and *Toxoplasma*. Alveolar macrophages readily phagocytose legionellae. However, the organisms are not killed and proliferate intracellularly until the cells rupture; the bacteria are then phagocytosed again by newly recruited phagocytes, and the cycle begins anew. Legionnaires' disease is more common and the disease manifestations are more severe in patients with depressed cell-mediated immunity, including transplant recipients, patients infected with human immunodeficiency virus, and patients receiving glucocorticoids. The disease also occurs with unusual frequency among patients with hairy cell leukemia (which is characterized by monocyte deficiency and dysfunction) but not among patients with other types of leukemia.

The role of neutrophils in immunity appears to be minimal: neutropenic patients are not predisposed to Legionnaires' disease. Although *L. pneumophila* is susceptible to oxygen-dependent microbiologic systems in vitro, it resists killing by neutrophils.

The humoral immune system is active against *Legionella*. Type-specific IgM and IgG antibodies are measurable within weeks of infection. In vitro, antibodies promote killing of legionellae by phagocytes (neutrophils, monocytes, and alveolar macrophages). However, antibodies neither enhance lysis by complement nor inhibit intracellular multiplication within phagocytes. Immunized animals develop a specific antibody response, with subsequent resistance to *Legionella* challenge.

Some *L. pneumophila* strains are clearly more virulent than others, although the precise factors mediating virulence remain uncertain. For example, although multiple strains may colonize water-distribution systems, only a few cause disease in patients exposed to that water. At least one surface epitope of *L. pneumophila* serogroup 1 is associated with virulence. *L. pneumophila* serogroup 6 is more commonly involved in nosocomial Legionnaires' disease and is more likely to be associated with a poor outcome.

PATHOLOGY The consistent pathologic features of Legionnaires' disease are confined to the lungs. Findings in infected lung tissue range from multifocal pneumonia with patchy lobular inflammation to extensive multilobar consolidation. Visible abscesses with central necrosis were seen in 20 percent of autopsied cases in one study. On histologic examination, fibrinopurulent pneumonia with intensive alveolitis and bronchiolitis is evident. Lesions of longer standing can have a nodular appearance with a central area of necrosis surrounded by macrophages and other cells. The alveoli are filled with fibrin, neutrophils, and alveolar macrophages.

Usual tissue stains, including Gram's, hematoxylin and eosin, Brown-Brenn, and methenamine silver, do not reveal the organism. Giminez stain can be used for imprints on fresh or fixed tissue. Dieterle's silver stain or modified Giminez stain, although nonspecific and relatively insensitive, can be used for paraffin-fixed specimens. The DFA stain is not only specific but also the most sensitive option for visualization of the organism in tissues. Polyvalent DFA stains but not monoclonal DFA stain can be used for formalinized specimens. Because the DFA stains are species and serogroup specific, false-negative results can be obtained if the incorrect reagent is used. Thus culture is the preferred method for diagnosis based on clinical specimens.

CLINICAL AND LABORATORY FEATURES **Pontiac Fever** Pontiac fever is an acute, self-limiting, flulike illness with a 24- to 48-h incubation period. Pneumonia does not develop in Pontiac fever. Malaise, fatigue, and myalgias are the most frequent symptoms, occurring in 97 percent of cases. Fever (usually with chills) develops in 80 to 90 percent of cases and headache in 80 percent. Other symptoms (seen in fewer than 50 percent of cases) include arthralgias, nausea, cough, abdominal pain, and diarrhea. Modest leukocytosis with a neutrophilic predominance is sometimes detected. Complete recovery takes place within only a few days without antibiotic therapy; a few patients may experience lassitude for many weeks thereafter. The diagnosis is established by antibody seroconversion.

Table 153-1

Clinical Clues Suggestive of Legionnaires' Disease

Diarrhea
High fever (>40°C)
Numerous neutrophils but no organisms revealed by Gram's staining of respiratory secretions
Hyponatremia (serum sodium level of <131 meq/L)
Failure to respond to β-lactam drugs (penicillins or cephalosporins) and aminoglycoside antibiotics
Occurrence of illness in an environment in which the potable water supply is known to be contaminated with *Legionella*
Onset of symptoms within 10 days after discharge from the hospital

Legionnaires' Disease (Pneumonia) Clinical findings that raise the possibility of Legionnaires' disease are summarized in Table 153-1. Although these manifestations may provide clues to the diagnosis, prospective comparative studies have shown that they are generally nonspecific and do not serve to distinguish Legionnaires' disease from pneumonia of other etiologies. Legionnaires' disease is often included in the differential diagnosis of "atypical pneumonia," along with infection due to *Chlamydia pneumoniae*, *Chlamydia psittaci*, *Mycoplasma pneumoniae*, *Coxiella burnetii*, and some viruses. The clinical similarities among these types of pneumonia include a relatively nonproductive cough and a low incidence of grossly purulent sputum. However, the clinical manifestations of Legionnaires' disease are usually more severe than those of most "atypical" pneumonias, and the course and prognosis of *Legionella* pneumonia more resemble those of bacteremic pneumococcal pneumonia than those of pneumonia due to other "atypical" pathogens. Patients with community-acquired Legionnaires' disease are significantly more likely than patients with pneumonia of other etiologies to be admitted to an intensive care unit upon presentation.

The incubation period for Legionnaires' disease is 2 to 10 days. The symptoms and signs may range from a mild cough and a slight fever to stupor with widespread pulmonary infiltrates and multisystem failure. Nonspecific symptoms—malaise, fatigue, anorexia, and headache—are seen early in the illness. Myalgias and arthralgias are uncommon but are unusually marked in a few patients. Upper respiratory symptoms, including coryza, are rare.

The mild cough of Legionnaires' disease is only slightly productive. Sometimes the sputum is streaked with blood. Chest pain—either pleuritic or nonpleuritic—can be a prominent feature and, when coupled with hemoptysis, can lead to an incorrect diagnosis of pulmonary embolism. Shortness of breath is reported by one-third to one-half of patients.

Gastrointestinal difficulties are often pronounced; abdominal pain, nausea, and vomiting affect 10 to 20 percent of patients. Diarrhea (watery rather than bloody) is reported in 25 to 50 percent of cases. The most common neurologic abnormalities are confusion or changes in mental status; however, the multitudinous neurologic symptoms reported range from headache and lethargy to encephalopathy.

Patients with Legionnaires' disease virtually always have fever. Temperatures in excess of 40.5°C were recorded in 20 percent of the cases in one series. Relative bradycardia has been overemphasized as a useful diagnostic finding; it occurs infrequently, primarily affecting older patients with severe pneumonia. Chest examination reveals rales early in the course and evidence of consolidations as the disease progresses. Abdominal examination may reveal generalized or local tenderness.

Diarrhea and hyponatremia occur significantly more often in Legionnaires' disease than in other forms of pneumonia. Hyponatremia is most common in severe cases. The mechanism of hyponatremia does not appear to be related to inappropriate secretion of antidiuretic hormone but instead to salt and water loss. Besides hyponatremia, other laboratory abnormalities include abnormal liver function tests, hypophosphatemia, hematuria, hematologic abnormalities, and thrombocytopenia; although common, these abnormalities are not found significantly more frequently in Legionnaires' disease than in pneumonias of other etiologies.

Extrapulmonary Legionellosis Since the portal of entry for legionellae is the lung in virtually all cases, extrapulmonary manifestations usually result from bloodborne dissemination from the lung. In a prospective survey of patients with Legionnaires' disease diagnosed by isolation of the organism from sputum, legionellae were isolated from the blood by a special culture method in 38 percent of cases.

Legionella has been identified in the spleen, liver, or kidneys in 50 percent of autopsied cases of Legionnaires' disease. The organism has also been isolated from intrathoracic and inguinal lymph nodes— a finding suggesting dissemination by lymphatic pathways. Extrapulmonary involvement, including sinusitis, peritonitis, pyelonephritis, cellulitis, and pancreatitis, has been documented predominantly in immunosuppressed patients.

The most common extrapulmonary site of legionellosis is the heart; numerous reports have described myocarditis, pericarditis, postcardiotomy syndrome, and prosthetic-valve endocarditis. Most cases have been hospital-acquired. Since many of the patients involved have not had overt pneumonia, the lung may not have been the portal of entry. Rather, in these cardiac infections, the organisms may have gained entry via a postoperative sternal wound exposed to contaminated tap water or via a mediastinal-tube insertion site.

Various other sources of or factors promoting *Legionella* infection at various extrapulmonary sites have been postulated, including the presence of foreign bodies, such as sutures and draining tubes (wound infection following cardiothoracic surgery); immersion in a Hubbard tank (superinfection of a hip wound); bloodborne dissemination from a pulmonary infection site (perirectal abscess); and ingestion of contaminated water (peritonitis).

Chest Radiographic Abnormalities Virtually all patients with Legionnaires' disease have abnormal chest radiographs showing pulmonary infiltrates at the time of clinical presentation. In a few cases of nosocomial disease, fever and respiratory tract symptoms have preceded the appearance of the infiltrate on chest radiography. Findings on chest radiography are nonspecific and do not serve to distinguish Legionnaires' disease from pneumonias of other etiologies. Pleural effusion is evident in one-third of cases, and the diagnosis is often based on culture and antigen testing (by the method designed for use with urine) of pleural fluid obtained by thoracentesis.

In immunosuppressed patients, especially those receiving glucocorticoids, distinctive rounded nodular opacities may be seen; these lesions may expand and cavitate (Fig. 153-1). Likewise, pulmonary abscesses can occur in immunosuppressed hosts. The progression of infiltrates on chest radiography despite appropriate antibiotic therapy is common, and radiographic improvement lags behind clinical improvement by several days. Complete clearing of infiltrates requires 1 to 4 months.

DIAGNOSIS The diagnosis of Legionnaires' disease requires special microbiologic tests (Table 153-2). The sensitivity of bronchoscopy specimens is approximately the same as that of sputum samples; if sputum is not available, bronchoscopy specimens may yield the

Table 153-2

Utility of Special Laboratory Tests for the Diagnosis of Legionnaires' Disease

Test	Sensitivity, %	Specificity, %
Culture		
Sputum*	80	100
Transtracheal aspirate	90	100
DFA staining of sputum	50–70	96–99
Urinary antigen testing†	70	100
Antibody serology‡	40–60	96–99

* Use of multiple selective media with dyes.
† Serogroup 1 only.
‡ IgG and IgM testing of both acute- and convalescent-phase sera. A single titer of ≥1:128 is considered presumptive, while a single titer of ≥1:256 or fourfold seroconversion is considered definitive.

organism. Bronchoalveolar lavage fluid gives higher yields than bronchial wash specimens. Thoracentesis should be performed if pleural effusion is found, and the fluid should be evaluated by DFA staining, culture, and the antigen test designed for use with urine.

Staining Gram's staining of material from normally sterile sites, such as pleural fluid or lung tissue, occasionally suggests the diagnosis; efforts to detect legionellae in sputum by Gram's staining typically reveal numerous leukocytes, but no organisms. When they are visualized, the organisms appear as small, pleomorphic, faint, gram-negative bacilli. *L. micdadei* organisms can be detected as weakly or partially acid-fast bacilli in clinical specimens. Modified acid-fast staining substitutes 1% sulfuric acid for the traditional 3% hydrochloric acid; the less aggressive decolorizer increases the yield of *L. micdadei*. *Legionella*-infected patients have often been treated empirically with antituberculosis medications because of false-positive acid-fast smears.

Culture The definitive method for diagnosis of *Legionella* infection is isolation of the organism from respiratory secretions or other specimens. As has been mentioned, BCYE agar supplemented with antibiotics and dyes is the most sensitive medium, and colonies grow slowly, requiring 3 to 5 days to become grossly visible. When culture plates are overgrown with other microflora, pretreatment of the specimen with acid or heat can markedly improve the yield. *L. pneumophila* is often isolated from sputum that is not grossly or microscopically purulent; sputum containing more than 25 epithelial cells per high-power field (a finding that classically suggests contamination) may still yield *L. pneumophila*.

DFA The DFA test is rapid and highly specific but is less sensitive than culture because large numbers of organisms are required for microscopic visualization. This test is more likely to be positive in advanced than in early disease.

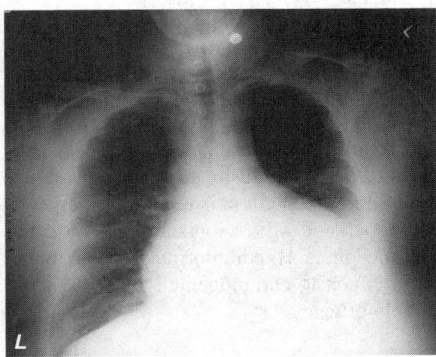
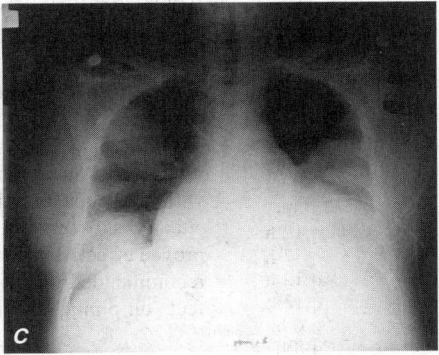
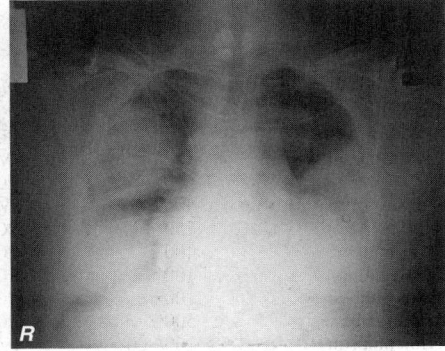

FIGURE 153-1 Chest radiographic findings in a 52-year-old man who presented with pneumonia subsequently diagnosed as Legionnaires' disease. The patient was a cigarette smoker with chronic obstructive pulmonary disease and alcoholic cardiomyopathy; he had received glucocorticoids. *L. pneumophila* was identified by DFA staining and culture of sputum. *Left:* Baseline chest radiograph showing long-standing cardiomegaly. *Center:* Admission chest radiograph showing new rounded opacities. *Right:* Chest radiograph taken 3 days after admission, during treatment with erythromycin. (*Courtesy of Dr. Feng-Yee Chang.*)

Antibody Detection   Antibody testing of both acute- and convalescent-phase sera may be necessary. A fourfold rise in titer is diagnostic; 4 to 12 weeks are often required for the detection of an antibody response, and some patients never seroconvert. A single titer of 1:128 in a patient with pneumonia constitutes presumptive (but not definitive) evidence for Legionnaires' disease. Serology is of use primarily in epidemiologic studies. The specificity of serology for the non–*L. pneumophila* species is uncertain; there is cross-reactivity with *L. pneumophila* and some gram-negative bacilli.

Urinary Antigen   The assay for *Legionella* soluble antigen in urine (Binax, South Portland, ME) is rapid, relative inexpensive, easy to perform, second only to culture in terms of sensitivity, and highly specific (Table 153-2). Its use in every clinical laboratory is recommended. The test is available only for *L. pneumophila* serogroup 1, which, as has been mentioned, causes about 80 percent of *Legionella* infections. Antigen in urine is detectable 3 days after the onset of clinical disease, even if specific therapy has been started; furthermore, urinary antigen persists for several weeks.

Molecular Methods   Polymerase chain reaction (PCR) with DNA probes may prove more sensitive and specific than other methods. PCR has proved useful in the identification of legionellae from environmental water specimens. Evaluation of the sensitivity of this technique for the testing of clinical specimens is under way.

℞ TREATMENT

Regimens of value in the treatment of *Legionella* infections are listed in Table 153-3. Prospective, controlled evaluations of therapy for Legionnaires' disease have not been conducted. In the 1976 American Legion outbreak, cases treated with erythromycin and tetracycline appeared to have a better outcome than those treated with other agents. These two antibiotics also exhibit intracellular activity against legionellae and, unlike other antimicrobials, are effective in animal models.

The preference for erythromycin in the treatment of *Legionella* infections has evolved over time, although use of the intravenous dosage recommended specifically for Legionnaires' disease (4 g/d) has unmasked adverse effects that have led to management problems. These problems include the necessity for a large fluid volume, which is challenging because so many patients with Legionnaires' disease have underlying cardiac disease and prolongation of the QT interval. Symptomatic ototoxicity was confirmed by audiography in 21 percent of patients receiving the 4-g dose as empirical therapy for community-acquired pneumonia; ototoxicity was reversible when the administration of erythromycin was discontinued. Gastrointestinal side effects are especially troublesome, given the promi-

nent gastrointestinal symptoms in some cases of Legionnaires' disease.

Compared with erythromycin, the new macrolides (azithromycin, clarithromycin, roxithromycin, josamycin) display superior in vitro activity against legionellae and greater intracellular and lung tissue penetration. Clinical experience is most extensive with azithromycin, but anecdotal reports have indicated that all of the newer macrolides are effective in the treatment of Legionnaires' disease. Given that adverse effects are notably less pronounced with the newer macrolides than with erythromycin and that the improved pharmacokinetics of the newer agents allows once- or twice-daily administration, it is anticipated that—once intravenous formulations become available—these drugs will supplant erythromycin as the antibiotics of choice for Legionnaires' disease.

Moreover, the newer macrolides (especially azithromycin) may be preferred for the treatment of immunocompetent patients with community-acquired pneumonia in whom Gram's staining of sputum shows many neutrophils but a paucity or absence of organisms. Such a result is compatible not only with infection due to *Legionella* but also with that due to *M. pneumoniae* or *C. pneumoniae*, which can also be treated with these new macrolides. Finally, the newer macrolides are active against *S. pneumoniae*, *H. influenzae*, *Moraxella catarrhalis*, and *Staphylococcus aureus*—common pathogens in community-acquired pneumonia. (Clarithromycin is the least active of these drugs against *H. influenzae*.)

The quinolones (ciprofloxacin, ofloxacin, pefloxacin) are highly active against *Legionella* in vitro, in dilution susceptibility tests and intracellular models, and in animal models. Furthermore, in open noncomparative studies of pneumonia, numerous cases of Legionnaires' disease have been successfully treated with quinolones. Ciprofloxacin is the preferred antibiotic for *Legionella*-infected transplant recipients because both macrolides and rifampin interact pharmacologically with transplant-immunosuppressive medications, including cyclosporine and tacrolimus.

For severely ill patients with Legionnaires' disease, the combination of rifampin plus a macrolide or a quinolone is recommended as initial treatment. Alternative agents include tetracycline and its analogues (doxycycline, minocycline) and trimethoprim-sulfamethoxazole. Anecdotal reports have described success with imipenem and clindamycin, but these agents probably should not be used until more experience in the treatment of humans has accumulated.

The clinical response to intravenous treatment usually occurs within 3 to 5 days, after which the switch to oral therapy can be made. The recommended total duration of therapy is 10 to 14 days; a longer course (3 weeks) may be appropriate for immunosuppressed patients with advanced disease. With appropriate and timely antibiotic therapy, mortality is low among immunocompetent patients (although in nosocomial infection the figure has sometimes approached 40 to 50 percent).

Pontiac fever requires only symptom-based treatment, not antimicrobial therapy.

PREVENTION   Disinfection of the water supply is the ultimate preventive measure. Although many disinfection modalities have been tried, only two methods have proved reliable and cost-effective. The superheat and flush method requires heating of the water so that the distal-outlet temperature is 70 to 80°C and flushing of the distal outlets with hot water for at least 30 min. This method is ideal for emergency situations. A commercial copper and silver ionization method has proved effective in numerous hospitals. Hyperchlorination is no longer recommended because of its expense, carcinogenicity, corrosive effects on piping, and unreliable efficacy.

Table 153-3

Antibiotic Therapy for *Legionella* Infection

Antimicrobial Agent	Dose, mg*	Route	Frequency
Azithromycin	500†	PO, IV‡	q 24 h
Clarithromycin	500	PO, IV‡	q 12 h
Roxithromycin	300‡	PO	q 12 h
Erythromycin	1000 (1 g)	IV	q 6 h
	500	PO	q 6 h
Ciprofloxacin	400	IV	q 8 h
	750	PO	q 12 h
Ofloxacin	400	PO, IV	q 12 h
Doxycycline	100†	PO, IV	q 12 h
Minocycline	100†	PO, IV	q 12 h
Tetracycline	500	PO, IV	q 6 h
Trimethoprim-sulfamethoxazole	160/800	IV	q 8 h
	160/800	PO	q 12 h
Rifampin	600	PO, IV	q 12 h

* Except as indicated.
† Doubling first dose should be considered.
‡ Investigational in the United States.

BIBLIOGRAPHY

BARBAREE JM et al: *Legionella: Current status and emerging perspectives.* Washington, DC, American Society for Microbiology, 1993
CARRATALA J et al: Risk factors for nosocomial *Legionella pneumophila* pneumonia. Am J Respir Crit Care Med 149:625, 1994

EDELSTEIN PH: Antimicrobial chemotherapy for Legionnaires' disease: A review. Clin Infect Dis 21:5265, 1995

FALCO V et al: *L. pneumophila*—a cause of severe community acquired pneumonias. Chest 100:1007, 1991

FANG GD: Disease due to *Legionella* (other than *Legionella pneumophila*): Historical, microbiological, clinical and epidemiologic review. Medicine 68:116, 1989

——— et al: New and emerging etiologies for community-acquired pneumonia with implications for therapy: A prospective multicenter study of 359 cases. Medicine 69:37, 1990

HEATH CH et al: Delay in appropriate therapy of *Legionella* pneumonia associated with increasing mortality. Eur J Clin Microbiol Infect Dis 15:286, 1996

LOWRY PW, TOMPKINS LS: Nosocomial legionellosis: A review of pulmonary and extrapulmonary syndromes. Am J Infect Control 21:21, 1993

ROIG J et al: Legionnaires' disease. Chest 105:1827, 1994

STRAUSS WL et al: Risk factors for domestic acquisition of Legionnaires' disease. Arch Intern Med 156:1685, 1996

YU VL: Could aspiration be the major mode of transmission for *Legionella*? Am J Med 95:13, 1993

154 *George R. Siber, Matthew H. Samore*

PERTUSSIS

DEFINITION Pertussis, or whooping cough, is an acute infection of the respiratory tract caused by *Bordetella pertussis*. The name *pertussis*, coined by Sydenham in 1679, means "violent cough" and describes the most characteristic feature of this disease. The Chinese call this illness "the cough of 100 days" because of the chronic nature of the cough. A dramatic inspiratory whoop following a paroxysmal cough is a hallmark of severe pertussis in children but is frequently lacking, particularly in infants and adults. Thus the term *whooping cough* may mislead clinicians by implying that whoops are an essential feature of the disease.

The clinical features that should suggest pertussis are a chronic cough lasting 2 weeks or longer and coughing spells that are typically sudden in onset and paroxysmal in nature. The episodes may, in severe cases, be followed by a whoop or by vomiting. Fever is absent or low except in cases of superinfection. An absolute lymphocytosis may provide an additional clue to the diagnosis, particularly in unimmunized children.

MICROBIOLOGY *B. pertussis* was first isolated by Bordet and Gengou in 1900 from the medium that bears their names. Humans are the only known host of *B. pertussis*. Other species in the genus *Bordetella* include *B. parapertussis*, which is associated with a milder respiratory illness in humans, and *B. bronchiseptica*, an animal pathogen that on rare occasions causes respiratory or opportunistic infections in humans.

B. pertussis is a small, nonmotile, gram-negative coccobacillus that is slow growing and fastidious in its growth requirements. After 3 to 16 days of growth at 36°C on special medium such as Bordet-Gengou agar, glistening pinpoint colonies with surrounding zones of hemolysis appear. Preliminary identification is accomplished by direct fluorescent antibody staining or by agglutination with antiserum to *B. pertussis*. This species is distinguished from *B. bronchiseptica* and *B. parapertussis* by further tests, such as motility and nitrate reduction. *B. pertussis*, *B. parapertussis*, and *B. bronchiseptica* show extensive DNA homology and share many enzymes not related to virulence as well as some virulence factors. However, only *B. pertussis* expresses pertussis toxin.

Like many other bacterial pathogens, *B. pertussis* possesses a precise mechanism for coordinated regulation of its virulence factors. Antigenic modulation involves reversible downregulation of virulence factors (i.e., pertussis toxin, filamentous hemagglutinin, pertactin, fimbriae, adenyl cyclase, dermonecrotic toxin) and upregulation of other proteins in response to a variety of environmental stimuli. Phase variation, which abolishes the expression of virulence factors, involves mutations of a regulatory locus at a frequency of 10^{-3} to 10^{-6} organisms. Both antigenic modulation and phase variation occur in vitro and in vivo, but their role in the ecology of *B. pertussis* is unknown. It has been suggested that phase variation or antigenic modulation may facilitate expulsion of the organism from the respiratory tract by lowering its adherence, may enable it to survive hostile environmental conditions during transmission, or may allow it to survive intracellularly in a quiescent state, protected from attack by immune mechanisms directed toward its virulence factors.

PATHOGENESIS *B. pertussis* initiates colonization of the respiratory tract by adhering to ciliated epithelial cells; grows to high numbers, causing local mucosal damage; and induces the paroxysmal cough that enhances its expulsion and transmission to contacts. A number of virulence factors responsible for this cycle of events have been described. Fimbriae, hairlike appendages on the surface of the organism, may play a role in the initial stages of adherence to ciliated cells. The fimbriae induce serotype-specific agglutinating antibodies (agglutinins) and are therefore called *agglutinogens*. Filamentous hemagglutinin (a large, 220-kDa, rodlike surface protein) and pertactin (a 69-kDa protein residing in the outer membrane) enable the organism to adhere closely to ciliated and other mammalian cells. Both of these adherence factors have arginine-glycine-aspartic acid repeat sequences (RGD) typical of eukaryotic adhesins that stick to the integrin family of mammalian cell-surface proteins.

A variety of toxins then impair local defenses (tracheal cytotoxin by inducing ciliostasis and adenyl cyclase by inhibiting phagocytes) and cause local tissue damage (tracheal cytotoxin and dermonecrotic toxin), thereby enhancing the supply of nutrients and perhaps facilitating systemic absorption of pertussis toxin. Pertussis toxin conforms to the general A/B model of enzymatic bacterial exotoxins. It contains an enzymatic moiety, the A subunit, which consists of a single peptide (S1), and a binding moiety, the B oligomer, which consists of four peptides (S2, S3, S4, and S5) in a molar ratio of 1:1:2:1. The B oligomer adheres to mammalian cells and delivers the A subunit to its targets; it exerts some biologic functions directly (e.g., mitogenesis of T cells) and may contribute to adherence of the whole organism to mammalian cells. The A subunit transfers ADP-ribose from NAD to certain members of a family of guanine nucleotide–binding regulatory membrane proteins (G proteins) in target cells. By this mechanism, pertussis toxin produces a variety of biologic effects, including lymphocytosis (lymphocytosis-promoting factor); the sensitization of mice to histamine and serotonin (histamine-sensitizing factor); the enhancement of insulin secretion in response to regulatory signals, such as beta-adrenergic stimulation (islet-activating protein); and the enhancement of certain immune functions, such as the production of IgG and IgE antibodies.

The mechanisms whereby *B. pertussis* produces the paroxysmal cough typical of pertussis have not been elucidated. The best evidence that pertussis toxin plays a critical role in producing the pertussis syndrome was provided by studies in which infants immunized only with pertussis toxoid had an 80 to 90 percent lower rate of severe pertussis than did controls.

EPIDEMIOLOGY Pertussis is a highly communicable disease, with attack rates of 90 to 100 percent among nonimmune household contacts. Transmission of the organism is mediated by exposure to respiratory droplets expelled in large numbers by symptomatic individuals.

Before the introduction of pertussis vaccine in the late 1940s, 115,000 to 270,000 cases of pertussis were reported annually in the United States (average incidence, 150 cases/100,000 population per year). Epidemics of pertussis recurred at intervals of 3 to 4 years without significant seasonality. During the years 1940 to 1948, pertussis caused more deaths among infants than did diphtheria, polio, measles, meningitis, and scarlet fever combined.

The incidence of pertussis declined 100- to 150-fold after the adoption of universal whole-cell pertussis vaccination, and mortality rates decreased even more dramatically, primarily as a result of improvements in health care. Discontinuation or reduction of pertussis vaccination was associated with a rapid resurgence of pertussis in Great Britain, Sweden, and Japan. In the United States, the incidence of pertussis fell to a nadir in the mid-1970s, with 1010 cases reported in 1976, and subsequently increased, with peaks in 1983, 1986, 1990, and 1993. In 1992 to 1994, a total of 15,286 cases of pertussis were reported to the Centers for Disease Control and Prevention (CDC). Infants <1 year of age accounted for 41 percent of these reported pertussis cases and for 78 percent of pertussis deaths. The case-fatality rate was 0.2 percent overall but was 0.6 percent among infants <6 months of age. Of children between 7 months and 4 years of age who developed pertussis, approximately half had not received the appropriate number of doses of vaccine for their age group.

Persons aged 20 years or older accounted for 11 percent of pertussis cases reported during 1992 to 1994. However, epidemiologic studies suggest that the actual incidence of pertussis in this age group is much higher than is indicated by estimates based on passive reporting to the CDC. Serologic studies show that 12 to 30 percent of episodes of persistent paroxysmal cough (i.e., episodes lasting longer than 2 weeks) in healthy adults are due to pertussis. In a recent seroprevalence study, the incidence of pertussis among U.S. adults was estimated to be 176 cases/100,000 person-years—a figure 500- to 1000-fold higher than that based on reported cases.

The high degree of transmissibility of *B. pertussis* in susceptible adolescent and adult populations is demonstrated by the large outbreaks of pertussis that have occurred in schools, nursing homes, hospitals, and residential facilities. Furthermore, careful studies of household contacts of pertussis cases show that 40 to 80 percent of family members have serologic evidence of infection and that only one-third to one-half of these infections are clinically symptomatic. It is now widely recognized that symptomatic undiagnosed pertussis in adults is an important source of transmission to infants and children and a mechanism for perpetuation of the disease in the population.

Studies of pertussis outbreaks suggest that protective immunity induced by whole-cell vaccine wanes rapidly. Child contacts appear to resist transient colonization and seroconversion for 2 years after their last vaccination, transiently develop asymptomatic or minimally symptomatic colonization and seroconvert at 3 to 5 years, and develop prolonged cough—frequently along with other symptoms of pertussis—at 6 to 12 years. The whole-cell vaccine does not offer protection beyond 12 years after immunization. Although it was once thought that natural pertussis offered lifelong protection, recent studies show that adults who have had pertussis again become susceptible to the disease after 20 years. Indeed, the rate of adult pertussis in Germany, where most adults are immune as a result of natural infection, resembles that in the United States (133 cases/100,000 population per year).

CLINICAL MANIFESTATIONS Pertussis is typically a prolonged illness, with an average duration of 6 to 8 weeks. The incubation period ranges from 5 to 14 days but is usually 7 to 10 days. The symptoms of pertussis generally evolve through three stages: the catarrhal, the paroxysmal, and the convalescent. The *catarrhal stage* lasts 1 and 2 weeks and is characterized by nonspecific symptoms of coryza, mild cough, lacrimation, malaise, and low-grade fever. The *paroxysmal stage*, which usually lasts 2 to 4 weeks, is characterized by paroxysmal cough, defined as sudden, forceful, repetitive coughing. The number of coughs per spasm is variable, ranging from 10 to 30; the paroxysms of pertussis characteristically occur during a single exhalation, a feature useful in distinguishing this illness from the repetitive cough caused by other pathogens, in which there are inspirations between coughs. In severe cases, the physical effort associated with each spasm may be extreme, with neck-vein distention, bulging of the eyes, and cyanosis. The distinctive whoop is heard in half of pediatric cases and is due to sudden inspiration against a closed glottis at the end of the paroxysm. Often resulting in the expectoration of viscous respiratory secretions, the paroxysm may be triggered by external stimuli, such as loud noises or physical contact. Typically, 10 to 25 paroxysms occur per 24-h period, with disruption of nocturnal

sleep. Posttussive vomiting is common and should be considered suggestive of pertussis. Fever is generally absent during the paroxysmal stage except in cases of bacterial superinfection. Most complications of pertussis develop during the paroxysmal stage. The *convalescent stage* is defined by the gradual waning in intensity of the cough. Complete resolution of the cough may require several months. Superimposed viral or bacterial respiratory infections may lead to severe clinical exacerbations, with the recurrence of paroxysmal coughing.

An absolute lymphocytosis is a characteristic but not universal laboratory finding in children with pertussis. Typically, the total white blood cell count ranges from 10,000 to 30,000 cells/μL, with 50 to 75 percent lymphocytes. Lymphocytosis is much less common among teenagers and adults, presumably because of antitoxin immunity.

The most common presentation of pertussis in adolescents and adults is cough, with or without paroxysms, persisting for 2 weeks or more (Table 154-1). Whooping is less common than it is among children, and lymphocytosis is rare. Useful clinical clues include shortness of breath during coughing spells, nocturnal cough, a tingling sensation in the back of the throat, posttussive vomiting, and a history of exposure to other patients with prolonged coughing illness.

B. pertussis has been isolated from human immunodeficiency virus–infected patients with chronic respiratory symptoms and may persist in these patients for many months. It is not known whether the incidence of pertussis is unusually high in this group.

COMPLICATIONS Minor complications of pertussis secondary to increased intrathoracic pressure include subconjunctival hemorrhage and upper torso petechiae. Episodes of cyanosis and apnea are common among infants and small children (prevalence, 20 to 50 percent). Malnutrition and weight loss may result from inadequate caloric intake. The major respiratory complication of pertussis is pneumonia, usually due to superinfection by encapsulated bacterial pathogens such as *Streptococcus pneumoniae* and *Haemophilus influenzae*. Pneumonia is more common among infants (incidence, 21 percent) than among children between 1 and 2 years of age (12 percent) or among adults (3 percent). Nonimmune infants may develop severe primary pneumonia due to *B. pertussis*. Neurologic complications, which are infrequent, include encephalopathy (0.7 percent) and seizures (2 percent). The potential mechanisms of pertussis-associated encephalopathy, though unknown, are postulated to include hypoxia and/or hypoglycemia due to pertussis toxin, hemorrhages secondary to increased venous pressure, direct neurotoxic effects, and coinfection by neurotoxic viruses.

DIAGNOSIS Laboratory confirmation should be attempted in all cases of suspected pertussis. The standard diagnostic test is the isolation of *B. pertussis* from nasopharyngeal swab culture. A calcium alginate swab is inserted into the nares and maintained in contact with the nasopharynx for 10 s to permit moistening. The swab should be placed immediately into transport medium (such as Regan-Lowe charcoal medium) or plated directly onto fresh Bordet-Gengou agar or another suitable agar. A nasopharyngeal aspirate collected with a syringe attached to a fine plastic catheter is a suitable alternative specimen. Growth typically requires 3 to 5 days of incubation at

Table 154-1

Clinical Features of Pertussis in Adolescents and Adults

Feature	Percentage of Patients
Cough	100
Prolonged (>14–21 days)	60–90
Paroxysmal	60–90
Worse at night	50–80
Whooping	5–20
Posttussive vomiting	15–60
Cold symptoms	60–75
Lymphocytosis	<5
Laboratory evidence of *B. pertussis*	
Culture	50–80 early, <5 late
Polymerase chain reaction	50–80 early, <5 late
Serology	20–50 early, 50–80 late

36°C. Suspicious colonies may be presumptively identified by direct fluorescent antibody staining or agglutination. Nasopharyngeal cultures are positive in 70 to 80 percent of children and in 30 to 60 percent of adults when specimens are obtained within 2 weeks of the onset of symptoms (during the catarrhal or early paroxysmal stage). The diagnostic yield declines rapidly thereafter. By 4 weeks, cultures are rarely positive. Detection of *B. pertussis* DNA in nasopharyngeal specimens by the polymerase chain reaction (PCR) may increase the diagnostic yield over that obtained by culture, particularly when the patient has received antibiotics. Again, however, the rate of positive results in PCR declines rapidly with the increasing duration of symptoms.

Thus, serologic assays are the only method currently available for the diagnosis of pertussis in patients with cough persisting for longer than 2 to 3 weeks. Enzyme-linked immunosorbent assays (ELISAs) for IgG or IgA antibodies to pertussis toxin and filamentous hemagglutinin are most frequently used. Seroconversion (a two- to fourfold rise in titer) is useful in previously nonimmune individuals, but previously immune individuals typically have already mounted an anamnestic response by the time the diagnosis is considered. Therefore, a single high titer (≥ 2 standard deviations above the mean for appropriately matched controls) is the most useful diagnostic test in such patients and has a sensitivity of 50 to 80 percent. Unfortunately, adequately standardized serologic assays for pertussis are not yet available in most areas of the United States.

DIFFERENTIAL DIAGNOSIS   The classical presentation of pertussis—the constellation of prolonged paroxysmal cough accompanied by whoops and lymphocytosis—is highly specific. *B. parapertussis* typically causes a milder respiratory illness and is not associated with lymphocytosis. Although the organisms are distinct species, *B. parapertussis* and *B. pertussis* are occasionally associated epidemiologically. They have been isolated from the same patients simultaneously or sequentially. Although viruses such as respiratory syncytial virus and adenovirus have been isolated from patients with clinical pertussis (with or without the isolation of *B. pertussis*), it is unlikely that these viruses alone can cause the full pertussis syndrome with whooping and lymphocytosis.

The infectious and noninfectious differential diagnosis of prolonged cough without whooping and lymphocytosis, a typical presentation of pertussis in adolescents and adults, is much broader. Influenza virus, adenovirus, *Mycoplasma pneumoniae*, *Chlamydia pneumoniae*, and pyogenic bacteria such as *S. pneumoniae* are common causes of acute respiratory infection. In general, the diagnosis of pertussis should be considered when an individual has an unexplained cough lasting for more than 2 weeks, has severe paroxysmal coughing of any duration, or has cough or upper respiratory symptoms of any duration after contact with a patient with pertussis.

℞ **TREATMENT**

Antibiotics   The major aim of antibiotic therapy for pertussis is to eradicate *B. pertussis* from the respiratory tract. Erythromycin (preferably in the estolate form), at a dose of 50 mg/kg per day (maximum, 2 g/d) in two to four divided doses, reliably eradicates the organism from the nasopharynx within 5 days. Treatment should be continued for a full 14 days to prevent bacteriologic relapse. Therapy with erythromycin ameliorates clinical illness when begun during the catarrhal phase and may also reduce the severity of the disease when begun within 2 weeks of the onset of paroxysmal cough.

Other macrolide antibiotics, such as azithromycin and clarithromycin, have exhibited excellent in vitro activity against *B. pertussis*, but clinical data on their effectiveness are currently lacking. Another alternative of unproven efficacy for patients unable to tolerate erythromycin is trimethoprim-sulfamethoxazole (8/40 mg/kg per day in two divided doses). Resistance to erythromycin has been described in only a single instance; in this case a *B. pertussis* strain recovered from an infant who deteriorated clinically during erythromycin treatment proved to be fully resistant to the drug.

Supportive Care   Infants have the highest rates of complications and death due to pertussis. Accordingly, most infants and those older patients with severe pertussis should be hospitalized. Supportive care includes monitoring for apnea and cyanosis, gentle nasotracheal suctioning, oxygen supplementation, hydration, and nutritional support. Glucocorticoids and the beta-adrenergic stimulant albuterol (salbutamol) have been advocated but have not been proved to be effective. Cough suppressants are ineffective.

Isolation of Hospitalized Patients   Persons caring for hospitalized patients with pertussis should use precautions appropriate for infectious agents transmitted by large respiratory droplets. Wearing of a surgical-type mask within 3 ft of the infected patient is considered to provide adequate protection. Isolation should be continued for 5 days after initiation of erythromycin treatment or for 3 weeks if the patient is unable to tolerate antimicrobial therapy.

PREVENTION   Management of Contacts   All household and other close contacts, irrespective of age or immunization status, should receive chemoprophylaxis with erythromycin (preferably the estolate) at 40 to 50 mg/kg per day in four divided doses (maximum, 2 g/d) for 14 days. Erythromycin is effective in limiting secondary transmission if administered within 2 weeks of the onset of symptoms in the index case. For children younger than 7 years, pertussis immunization should be initiated or continued according to the recommended schedule.

Vaccines   Diphtheria-tetanus-pertussis (DTP) vaccine, which is currently used for primary immunization of infants, consists of killed whole-cell *B. pertussis* organisms combined with diphtheria and tetanus toxoids adsorbed to aluminum phosphate adjuvant. The standard schedule involves three primary doses at 2-month intervals (with the first dose given at 6 to 8 weeks of age) and booster doses given at 15 to 18 months and 4 to 6 years of age. Vaccination above the age of 6 years is not recommended but has been used in special circumstances for the control of nosocomial outbreaks.

The best whole-cell vaccines are 80 to 95 percent efficacious in protecting individuals from pertussis for 2 to 3 years. Thereafter, protective immunity wanes, with attack rates reaching 90 percent among household contacts exposed more than 12 years after immunization. Some whole-cell vaccines are less efficacious, perhaps because of their low content of protective antigens. Widespread administration of whole-cell vaccines to children reduces the incidence of clinical pertussis in the population by >90 percent.

Injection of DTP vaccine containing the whole-cell pertussis component is associated with high rates of local reactions and fever (30 to 50 percent). In rare instances, reactions are more severe; these reactions include a temperature of >40.5°C, persistent crying, unusual high-pitched crying, seizures, hypotonic hyporesponsive episodes, and anaphylaxis. The occurrence of the more severe of these adverse events constitutes a contraindication to further use of DTP vaccine. The physician should refer to package inserts for details.

The risk of acute encephalopathy appears to be unusually high during the 7 days after DTP immunization (1 in 140,000 doses; excess risk, 0 to 10.5 per 1 million doses). Children with DTP-related acute encephalopathy are at excess risk of subsequent chronic neurologic disease and death; their risk is similar to that of children with DTP-unrelated acute encephalopathy. It remains uncertain whether DTP causes encephalopathy or triggers the disease in children with underlying brain or metabolic abnormalities.

In recently completed trials, a variety of acellular pertussis vaccines have exhibited a degree of efficacy similar to that of whole-cell vaccines in infants, with significantly fewer side effects. Pertussis vaccines containing only pertussis toxoid appear to be about as efficacious as multicomponent vaccines in preventing severe pertussis (i.e., >3 weeks of paroxysmal cough). However, the inclusion of the adherence factors pertactin, fimbriae, and filamentous hemagglutinin appears to contribute additional protection against milder illness, particularly in the setting of household exposure or epidemic disease.

Two acellular pertussis (aP) vaccines formulated with diphtheria and tetanus toxoids (DTaP) are licensed in the United States for use as booster doses at 15 to 18 months and 4 to 6 years of age in children previously immunized with three primary doses of whole-cell DTP vaccine. A variety of DTaP vaccines are expected to be licensed for the primary immunization of infants.

Neither DTaP vaccine nor whole-cell DTP vaccine is currently approved for use in adults. Whole-cell vaccine has been used rarely in the control of hospital outbreaks of pertussis but is associated with high rates of adverse reactions in adults. Both DTaP and aP vaccines are associated with much lower rates of adverse reactions and induce strong antibody responses in adults.

The Future of Immunoprophylaxis   Key issues that will need to be evaluated include (1) whether the various acellular vaccines differ in terms of the rates at which they elicit severe adverse reactions; (2) whether these vaccines differ detectably in efficacy or effectiveness in the United States, where pertussis is endemic rather than epidemic; (3) whether aP vaccine, perhaps formulated with adult doses of tetanus and diphtheria toxoids (TdaP), should be introduced into the routine immunization schedules for adolescents and adults to reduce the high rates of disease in these age groups and to reduce transmission of infection to young infants; and (4) whether immunization of mothers reduces the frequency or severity of pertussis in young infants.

B. pertussis is known to be a pathogen only in humans and is believed to be spread primarily by symptomatic individuals. Thus routine immunization of the entire population with aP vaccine has the potential to eradicate this pathogen.

BIBLIOGRAPHY

AOYAMA T et al: Pertussis in adults. Am J Dis Child 146:163, 1992

CATTANEO LA et al: The seroepidemiology of *Bordetella pertussis* infections: A study of persons ages 1–65 years. J Infect Dis 173:1256, 1996

CENTERS FOR DISEASE CONTROL AND PREVENTION: Pertussis—United States, January 1992–1995. Morb Mort Week Rep 44:28, 1995

DEEN JL et al: Household contact study of *Bordetella pertussis* infections. Clin Infect Dis 21:1211, 1995

DEVILLE JG et al: Frequency of unrecognized *Bordetella pertussis* infections in adults. Clin Infect Dis 21:639, 1995

GRECO D et al: A controlled trial of two acellular vaccines and one whole-cell vaccine against pertussis. N Engl J Med 334:341, 1996

GUSTAFSSON L et al: A controlled trial of a two-component acellular, a five-component acellular, and a whole-cell pertussis vaccine. N Engl J Med 334:349, 1996

HE Q et al: Outcomes of *Bordetella pertussis* infection in different age groups of an immunized population. J Infect Dis 170:873, 1994

MARCHANT CD et al: Pertussis in Massachusetts, 1981–1991: Incidence, serologic diagnosis, and vaccine effectiveness. J Infect Dis 169:1297, 1994

MINK CAM et al: A search for *Bordetella pertussis* infection in university students. Clin Infect Dis 14:464, 1992

NENNIG ME et al: Prevalence and incidence of adult pertussis in an urban population. JAMA 275:1672, 1996

OLSON LC: Pertussis. Medicine 54:427, 1975

PITTMAN M: The concept of pertussis as a toxin-mediated disease. Pediatr Infect Dis J 3:467, 1984

SCHMITT-GROHE S et al: Pertussis in German adults. Clin Infect Dis 21:860, 1995

SHEFER A et al: Use and safety of acellular pertussis vaccine among adult hospital staff during an outbreak of pertussis. J Infect Dis 171:1053, 1995

TROLLFORS B et al: A placebo-controlled trial of a pertussis-toxoid vaccine. N Engl J Med 333:1045, 1995

WEBER DJ, RUTALA WA: Management of healthcare workers exposed to pertussis. Top Occup Med 15:411, 1994

WIRSING VON KÖNIG CH et al: Pertussis in adults: Frequency of transmission after household exposure. Lancet 346:1326, 1995

WRIGHT SW et al: Pertussis infection in adults with persistent cough. JAMA 273:1044, 1995

155   *Barry I. Eisenstein, Vish Watkins*

DISEASES CAUSED BY GRAM-NEGATIVE ENTERIC BACILLI

The gram-negative enteric bacilli are a diverse group of bacteria that reside in the human colon. They also colonize a number of other habitats with which many hospitalized patients come into contact. Because of their ubiquity, they often cause opportunistic infections such as pneumonia in debilitated patients. As a group, the enteric bacteria account for about one-third of all septicemia isolates, two-thirds of bacterial gastroenteritis isolates, and three-quarters of urinary tract infection isolates. One of these organisms, *Escherichia coli*, is the most frequent cause of urinary tract infection and one of the most important causes of bacterial diarrhea.

GENERAL PROPERTIES

CLASSIFICATION AND PHYSIOLOGY   On a genetic basis, the gram-negative enteric bacilli belong to the family Enterobacteriaceae, which includes other pathogens (*Shigella, Edwardsiella, Salmonella, Citrobacter, Yersinia*) discussed elsewhere in this volume. Members of this family lack the ability to form spores, can grow both aerobically and anaerobically (i.e., are facultative anaerobes), can ferment glucose to acid, are oxidase negative, and have variable motility (depending on the presence or absence of flagella).

STRUCTURE   Like all typical bacteria, Enterobacteriaceae have a peptidoglycan-containing cell wall, a single circular chromosome consisting of double-stranded DNA that is located throughout the cytoplasm, and prokaryote-type ribosomes. What distinguishes gram-negative bacteria from other bacteria is the unique multilayered nature of the cell envelope, which, in addition to the inner (or cytoplasmic) membrane and the surrounding polymeric peptidoglycan, also has a complex outer membrane. The medically important elements of the outer layer include lipopolysaccharide (LPS, or endotoxin), which is toxic to humans, and porins, multimeric proteins that form channels for the passage of antimicrobial agents and nutrients. The LPS of all gram-negative bacteria has a core that contains the moiety lipid A, which triggers endotoxic septic shock (see Chap. 124). Most pathogenic strains (at least those of *E. coli*) also have repeating polysaccharide side chains (O antigens) attached to the core LPS (see Chap. 139).

Three classes of surface antigens have been used in serologic tests for the clonal identification of *E. coli* and *Salmonella* strains: (1) the O (somatic) antigens of LPS, (2) the H (flagellar) antigens, and (3) the K (capsular) antigens. Clonal identification is of taxonomic and epidemiologic importance. In *E. coli*, a number of the O, H, and K serogroupings act as markers for clones capable of causing particular infectious diseases; these clones possess other virulence factors required for pathogenesis of those diseases. The O serogroups may be markers for a specific clustering of virulence properties. Thus, some O serogroups possess adhesive factors and toxins needed to cause urinary tract infections, while other O serogroups have adhesins and toxins needed to produce gastroenteritis. The O157:H7 serogroup is associated with hemorrhagic colitis and the hemolytic-uremic syndrome. The K, or capsular, antigen of the K1 type is an epidemiologic marker (and virulence factor) for neonatal meningitis, bacteremia, and urinary tract infection. Today, genetics-based tests are supplanting analysis of surface antigens as the preferred method of differentiating bacterial clones.

THE HOST-PARASITE INTERACTION   Many enteric bacteria colonize the gastrointestinal tract without causing symptoms. Significant disease requires an exceptionally virulent organism, a defect in host defenses, or a combination of the two. Thus, a virulent bacterium like *Shigella dysenteriae* can produce dysentery even in normal hosts. A commensal strain of *E. coli* can produce peritonitis in a healthy individual with a ruptured appendix (a breach in physical defenses) or bacteremia in a person who is granulocytopenic from treatment with an antineoplastic drug (a defect in host immunity).

Regardless of the initial state of the host defenses, disease due to enteric bacterial infection consists of several sequential stages, beginning with entry into and colonization of the gastrointestinal tract, nasopharynx, oropharynx, or urinary tract. Those bacteria that are successful at colonizing the gastrointestinal tract, whether they are pathogenic or commensal, must survive the harsh environmental excesses of high acidity in the stomach and then the alkalinity and high concentrations of detergent (bile salts) and digestive enzymes in the small intestine, not to mention the immune system's IgA and phagocytic and lymphocytic cells. The compact texture of the cell wall of gram-negative bacteria enables them to cope with these challenges. To avoid being dislodged by the passing intestinal contents, these bacteria attach to specific receptors on the epithelial cell or in the cell-associated mucus by hairlike, proteinaceous organelles known as fimbriae or pili, which cover the entire surface of each bacterium. Strains of *E. coli* that cause gastroenteritis have fimbriae that bind specifically to receptors in the gastrointestinal tract. Other strains of *E. coli* that are associated with urinary tract infections contain P fimbriae (so called because of affinity for the P blood-group antigen found on uroepithelial cells) that bind specifically to receptors in the urinary tract. P fimbriae are also called PAP, for *p*yelonephritis-*a*ssociated *p*ili.

The normal host defenses limit most bacterial interactions to benign commensalism. To produce disease in healthy hosts, these organisms need special attributes, known as virulence factors. For localized diseases (e.g., diarrhea, dysentery), the bacteria use secretory and cytologic toxins and, occasionally, cellular invasive factors. For survival in the bloodstream, the organisms have capsules (e.g., K1) that enable them to resist opsonization. In addition, the polysaccharide chains of O antigens, along with particular outer-membrane proteins, enable the bacteria to resist the bactericidal activity of serum by preventing the cylindrical membrane-attack complex of the terminal components of complement from inserting efficiently into the bacterial membrane and thus causing bacterial lysis.

In contrast to infections in normal hosts, those in debilitated individuals are often caused by relatively avirulent organisms. Such organisms are robust enough to survive in various hospital environments, including water supplies and the hands of caregivers, and are sufficiently drug resistant to be part of the flora of an antibiotic-treated host. A debilitated host recovering from surgery or trauma can become ill merely from the inadvertent relocation of a commensal strain to a site either normally sterile or normally not colonized with enteric bacteria. For example, aspiration of gram-negative bacteria colonizing the upper airways can lead to pneumonia, and contamination of surgical wounds or previously sterile intravascular or urinary catheters can cause wound infection, bacteremia, and urinary tract infection, respectively. These "opportunistic" infections can be severe if the debilitated host cannot mount a normal immune response. Moreover, the bacteria in the antimicrobial-laden hospital environment are preselected for drug resistance and may be particularly difficult to treat.

Whether the pathogen is a virulent invader or an opportunistic commensal, the host response, together with appropriate antimicrobial therapy, mediates recovery. Paradoxically, the normal immune response can also potentiate the disease by mediating inflammatory responses beyond those needed for bacterial containment. Complement activation, the liberation of cytokines (e.g., tumor necrosis factor and the numerous interleukins), leukocyte mobilization and degranulation, and platelet and coagulation-pathway activation can mediate the lethal manifestations of endotoxemia, including excessive fluid extravasation and circulatory collapse, renal tubular necrosis, adult respiratory distress syndrome, and (when the organism has entered the cerebrospinal fluid) meningitis. Recent efforts to treat severe gram-negative infection have been directed not only at eliminating the invading microbe but also at attenuating the immune response.

DRUG RESISTANCE AND VIRULENCE FACTORS The success of therapy for bacterial infection depends on the use of antimicrobial agents to which the infecting microbe is susceptible. Unfortunately, bacteria have an evolutionary ability to avoid the effects of these drugs (see Chap. 140) by mechanisms that include alteration of the antibacterial target site, decreased permeability to influx of drug,

active export of drug to the outside, and enzymatic destruction of drug. Mutation of preexisting DNA can result in drug resistance, particularly through target-site alteration but also through alteration of the amount or affinity of drug-destroying enzymes. Most drug resistance results from the acquisition of new genes, usually in the form of transposons. Transposons are usually found on R-plasmids, which are self-replicating, nonchromosomal units of DNA that can be transferred by conjugation from one bacterial cell to another (even to a cell of a different species).

The genetic organization of these genes promotes their spread throughout the Enterobacteriaceae. Since R-plasmids move across bacterial populations readily, the presence of several antimicrobials in the environment selects those bacteria that contain multiple drug-resistance elements. With time and the continued use of different drugs in hospitals and in agriculture, R-plasmids have become larger; each now consists of many different transposons strung together like pearls on a necklace. The genes encoding many virulence factors, including colonization factors, enterotoxins, and hemolysin, are found on plasmids (occasionally on R-plasmids), and this situation promotes their spread.

ESCHERICHIA COLI INFECTIONS

ETIOLOGY, EPIDEMIOLOGY, AND MANIFESTATIONS
Enteric Infections *E. coli* is a major cause of bacterial gastroenteritis in U.S. residents traveling abroad. This organism comes in many pathogenic varieties, each with a different mechanism of disease production. The most important are enterotoxigenic *E. coli* (ETEC), an important cause of traveler's diarrhea; enteropathogenic or enteroadherent *E. coli* (EPEC), an important cause of childhood diarrhea; enteroinvasive *E. coli* (EIEC), which causes a dysentery-like disease; and enterohemorrhagic *E. coli* (EHEC), which causes hemorrhagic colitis and has been associated with the hemolytic-uremic syndrome (HUS) in children.

Traveler's diarrhea occurs in individuals from industrialized countries who visit tropical or subtropical regions that lack advanced hygienic conditions. The organism, commonly ETEC, is acquired through the fecal-oral route, usually through consumption of unbottled water or uncooked vegetables. The inoculum of organisms must be high enough to resist destruction by acid in the stomach. (Individuals with achlorhydria are especially susceptible.) The major manifestations are a consequence of the copious outpouring of fluid from the gastrointestinal tract due to the action of one of two types of enterotoxin on the gastrointestinal mucosa. The heat-labile toxin activates intracellular adenylate cyclase, with a subsequent increase in intracellular levels of cyclic adenosine monophosphate. The heat-stable toxin activates guanylate cyclase, with the subsequent elevation of intracellular levels of cyclic guanosine monophosphate. The elevated cyclic monophosphate levels stimulate chloride secretion and inhibit sodium chloride absorption—effects that result in net intestinal secretion. Within 1 or 2 days of exposure in most cases, the patient develops abdominal cramps and frequent explosive bowel movements; these symptoms last 3 to 4 days. Traveler's diarrhea is treated with oral trimethoprim-sulfamethoxazole or a fluoroquinolone. For social convenience or for medical reasons (e.g., for diabetics prone to dehydration with serious consequences or for persons with underlying inflammatory bowel disease), chemoprophylaxis with bismuth subsalicylate, trimethoprim-sulfamethoxazole, or fluoroquinolones may be reasonable.

EPEC strains cause childhood diarrhea, especially in underdeveloped countries and in nursery outbreaks. These bacteria bind to the membranous cells of Peyer's patches and disrupt the overlying mucous gel of the host cell. In contrast to ETEC and EPEC, EIEC strains (rare in the United States) invade the host cell and provoke a significant inflammatory response. The manifestations are those of bacterial dysentery, with fever and bloody diarrheal stool containing polymorphonuclear leukocytes. Treatment consists of fluid replacement. Because these organisms are often resistant to antibiotics, the role of specific treatment is limited. Antibiotics usually are not needed. In severe cases, trimethoprim-sulfamethoxazole, fluoroquinolones, and sometimes intravenous third-generation cephalosporins may be indicated.

Every year, EHEC strains, typically of serotype O157:H7, cause about 20,000 cases of colitis (often hemorrhagic) in the United States. Young children and the elderly can develop HUS characterized by microangiopathic hemolytic anemia, thrombocytopenia, and acute renal failure; central nervous system manifestations, including seizures, hemiparesis, and coma, may develop. Hemorrhage and edema in the lamina propria, accompanied by focal necrosis, hemorrhage, and inflammation of the superficial mucosa, are found in the colon. Injury to the glomerular capillary endothelial cell and microvascular angiopathy elsewhere, especially in the central nervous system, are the predominant pathologic features of HUS. Shiga-like cytotoxins produced by the organisms are thought to participate in the pathogenesis of this disease by their lethality to human colonic cells and their ability to damage endothelial cells. The diagnosis is confirmed by culture from stool of *E. coli* strains that, unlike most commensal strains, fail to ferment sorbitol. These strains also agglutinate with antiserum to O157. Treatment consists of supportive measures. Patients are monitored for signs of HUS for 1 week after the onset of diarrhea. In young children and the elderly, blood counts, peripheral-blood smears, serum creatinine levels, and the urinary sediment are monitored. Antimotility agents should be avoided, as they exacerbate illness and facilitate the development of HUS. Patients with renal failure may need dialysis.

Urinary Tract Infection (See Chap. 131) Unlike the gastrointestinal tract, the urinary tract is normally sterile. Most uncomplicated infections are due to *E. coli*. The typical acute infection occurs in a sexually active female following bacterial colonization of the periurethral region and ascension up the urethra; disease includes asymptomatic bacteriuria, urethritis, cystitis, pyelitis, and pyelonephritis. Complications, including obstruction of the urinary tract, the presence of foreign bodies or anatomic defects, prior surgery, pregnancy, or stones, increase a patient's chance of infection with other Enterobacteriaceae and strains of *Pseudomonas* and of chronic or relapsing infection, loss of renal tissue, and bacteremia.

Intraabdominal Infections (See Chap. 127) *E. coli* represents a small part of the normal bowel flora—more than 99 percent of the bacteria in this population are strict anaerobes—yet it is a significant pathogen in infections resulting from spillage of normal bowel contents into previously sterile environments. Studies of experimental infections in animals suggest that the aerobic bowel flora (including *E. coli*) is responsible for the often lethal early septicemia associated with bowel spillage, whereas anaerobic species cause late-onset abscesses (with aerobic bacteria acting as potentiators). Thus, in cases of peritonitis resulting from a perforated viscus, *E. coli* is usually cultured from the local site and, in severe cases, from the blood. It can also be associated with intraabdominal abscesses in any location as well as with cholecystitis and ascending cholangitis. Intraabdominal infections can be particularly severe in patients with ischemia of the bowel or other organs—e.g., many patients with diabetes and atherosclerotic vascular disease. Such individuals are at unusually high risk of developing acute emphysematous cholecystitis, which is characterized by gangrene and perforation, and septic thrombophlebitis of the portal vein (pylephlebitis), which leads to liver abscesses. *E. coli* is a prominent pathogen in each of these processes.

Bacteremia Because of its association with septic shock (Chap. 124), bloodstream invasion by *E. coli* is the most serious event associated with this pathogen and the one most likely to lead to multiorgan failure and death. In these cases, the sequential biologic responses of the host to the invading pathogen or to its circulating constituents (e.g., LPS) result in the clinical progression of disease from a systemic inflammatory response syndrome (SIRS) through syndromes of sepsis and severe sepsis to septic shock. *SIRS* is defined as the combination of any two of the following: fever or hypothermia; tachycardia (>90 beats per minute); tachypnea (>20 breaths per minute); and leukocyto-

sis, leukopenia, or >10 percent immature leukocytes in a differential white blood cell count. *Septic shock* is sepsis-induced hypotension that persists in spite of fluid resuscitation and involves hypoperfusion abnormalities, including lactic acidosis, oliguria, and an acute change in mental status, accompanied by organ dysfunction. In a significant proportion of patients, combinations of uremia, hepatic failure, respiratory failure (adult respiratory distress syndrome), and stupor and coma develop. Antecedent diseases include urinary tract infection, biliary or intraperitoneal sepsis, and nosocomial infections such as pneumonia and intravascular catheter–related infections. Patients in whom bacteremia persists despite adequate therapy often have an undrained abscess, most typically intraabdominal. Some patients, especially those with poor filtering capacity in the liver (i.e., those with cirrhosis or portosystemic shunts), diminished reticuloendothelial function, or diminished numbers of circulating phagocytic cells, have no obvious portal of bacterial entry. In most of these cases, the gastrointestinal tract is the source.

Other Manifestations As a consequence of bacteremia or contiguous spread, *E. coli* can be found in abscesses anywhere in the body. Individuals with vascular disease (which is especially common in conjunction with diabetes mellitus) are prone to infections of the distal extremities and surgical wounds, whereas those with diminished numbers of circulating phagocytes are prone to perianal abscesses. Many of these subcutaneous infections are polymicrobial, involving anaerobic as well as aerobic organisms. *E. coli* may cause septic arthritis, perinephric abscess, endophthalmitis, suppurative thyroiditis, brain abscess, endocarditis, osteomyelitis, sinusitis, pneumonia, and other infections. Neonates, particularly premature infants, are especially susceptible to bacteremia and meningitis with K1 encapsulated *E. coli*.

DIAGNOSIS The diagnosis of *E. coli* infection depends on the combination of suspicious clinical findings (e.g., signs and symptoms of urinary tract infection) and isolation of *E. coli* by the clinical microbiology laboratory. Infection with *E. coli* can be a monomicrobial condition developing either at a previously sterile site (e.g., urinary tract infection, meningitis) or in a nonsterile setting (e.g., gastroenteritis); alternatively, it can be part of a polymicrobial process (e.g., a ruptured appendix, or an infected foot in a diabetic). These distinctions are important in the interpretation of laboratory results. Because *E. coli* is present normally in stool, the diagnosis of *E. coli* gastroenteritis is problematic, but it can be made with techniques that exploit unique properties of specific strains that cause these infections (e.g., sorbitol negativity in EHEC). Whether the recovery of *E. coli* from tracheal aspirates in intubated patients indicates colonization or infection (i.e., tracheitis from local inflammation induced by the endotracheal tube or bacterial pneumonia) must be decided in the context of the patient's clinical state. In contrast, any growth of *E. coli* in a normally sterile locale—the bloodstream, cerebrospinal fluid, biliary tract, pleural fluid, or peritoneal cavity—should be assumed to be diagnostic of *E. coli* infection at that site.

Gram's staining can rapidly identify gram-negative bacilli at the site of infection. Unfortunately, this technique cannot differentiate *E. coli* from other gram-negative bacteria that cause similar infectious diseases. Newer techniques, particularly those incorporating amplification of nucleic acid, show promise in identifying virulence genes associated with specific microbes or drug-resistance genes. Although the culture method is slow, isolation of the microbe can be followed by antimicrobial susceptibility testing, which is particularly important with the emergence of drug-resistant pathogens.

℞ **TREATMENT**

As for any infectious disease, the mainstay of treatment for *E. coli* infections is twofold: antimicrobial therapy and elimination of pus, necrotic tissue, and foreign bodies. General principles of treatment will be discussed here. For treatment of specific infections and for information about specific antibiotics, the reader is referred to the chapters on particular infectious syndromes and to the chapter on antimicrobial chemotherapy (Chap. 140).

Several classes of antibiotics and various antibiotics within those classes have recently become available for the treatment of infections caused by members of the Enterobacteriaceae, including *E. coli*

(Table 155-1). The antibiotic selected, its dose, and the duration of treatment depend on (1) the site of infection, (2) the presence or absence of complicating illnesses, (3) the susceptibility or resistance of the isolated strain, (4) the severity of illness, (5) a history—or lack thereof—of allergy to a potentially useful antibiotic, (6) the cost of the regimen, and (7) other factors (such as whether or not the patient is pregnant and how old the patient is). Urinary tract infections serve as an example to show how these factors influence therapy. Uncomplicated cystitis in a healthy woman is treated for 3 days with oral trimethoprim-sulfamethoxazole. A patient allergic to sulfonamides may be treated with a fluoroquinolone for 3 days. A diabetic or pregnant patient with this infection requires 7 days of treatment. For the pregnant patient, the choice of agents is limited to amoxicillin, macrocrystalline nitrofurantoin, or cefpodoxime proxetil. The patient with mild uncomplicated pyelonephritis can be treated with oral trimethoprim-sulfamethoxazole or a fluoroquinolone for 10 to 14 days. The pregnant patient with pyelonephritis and any patient with severe pyelonephritis should be given intravenous antibiotics in the hospital; the choices are ceftriaxone, ciprofloxacin, gentamicin with or without ampicillin, aztreonam, imipenem/cilastatin, or an extended-spectrum penicillin. After acute symptoms resolve, an oral antibiotic should replace the intravenous antibiotic for a total duration of 14 to 21 days. Again, the choice is dictated by the factors mentioned above—e.g., avoidance of aminoglycosides if the patient has diabetes mellitus; avoidance of imipenem if the patient has renal failure; and, if the patient is pregnant, avoidance of fluoroquinolones and caution with gentamicin (which may cause eighth-cranial-nerve toxicity in the fetus).

KLEBSIELLA, ENTEROBACTER, AND SERRATIA INFECTIONS

Klebsiella, *Enterobacter*, and *Serratia* belong to the tribe Klebsielleae. These genera are typically differentiated only by certain amino acid decarboxylase tests and the facts that strains of *Klebsiella* are usually nonmotile and form large mucoid colonies when grown on solid media. Like *E. coli*, all of these organisms colonize the human gastrointestinal tract, yet they rarely cause disease in the normal host; rather, they are a major cause of nosocomial and opportunistic infection. In many hospitals, strains of *Klebsiella* are among the most antimicrobial-resistant microbes isolated; they readily acquire R-plasmids carrying aminoglycoside-inactivating enzymes, a wide variety of β-lactamases, and other drug-resistance genes.

Klebsiella pneumoniae (Friedlander's bacillus) is a well-recognized cause of community-acquired lobar pneumonia found typically in alcoholic men over 40 years of age with such underlying conditions as diabetes mellitus and chronic obstructive pulmonary disease. Pneumonia due to *K. pneumoniae* mimics pneumococcal pneumonia except for the greater tendency of *Klebsiella* pneumonia to progress to lung abscess and empyema. Occasionally, this necrotic process causes the radiographic features of bulging fissures and loss of lung volume, which are sometimes seen in severe bacterial pneumonia of any etiology. Gram's staining of the sputum can help in the diagnosis; it shows a predominance of short, plump, gram-negative bacilli, often surrounded by a capsule that appears as a clear space.

In the hospital, *K. pneumoniae* and its tribal relatives are major causes of infections of the urinary tract, lower respiratory tract, biliary tract, and surgical wounds. Many of these infections are associated with bacteremia and life-threatening septic shock. *K. pneumoniae* infections are usually treated with a cephalosporin. In severe infections, some specialists add an aminoglycoside for synergy, usually for a short duration (e.g., 3 or 4 days). The antibiotic selected, its dosage, and the duration of therapy depend on the factors discussed above in the section on treatment of *E. coli* infections. Treatment of infections due to resistant organisms depends on the results of susceptibility tests. Less common conditions caused by strains closely related to *K. pneumoniae* include rhinoscleroma, a chronic granulomatous disease that involves the mucosa of the upper respiratory system, occasionally leads to bony invasion and airway obstruction, and is associated with *Klebsiella rhinoscleromatis*; and ozena, a chronic severe rhinitis involving turbinate atrophy and progressive anosmia that is associated with *Klebsiella ozaenae*. DNA-relatedness studies have shown that these strains, which are indole negative, actually belong to the species *K. pneumoniae* and that indole-positive strains of *K. pneumoniae* belong to a new species, *Klebsiella oxytoca*.

The genus *Enterobacter* consists of *Enterobacter aerogenes*, *Enterobacter cloacae*, *Enterobacter agglomerans* (formerly called *Erwinia*), and several other species. *E. cloacae* accounts for most hospital-acquired infections with this genus. Like *Enterobacter*, *Serratia* is

Table 155-1

Antibiotics Used in the Treatment of Infections with Enterobacteriaceae

Antibiotic Class	Representative Antibiotics	Properties to Consider
Early penicillins	Ampicillin (parenteral), amoxicillin (oral)	Resistance (30%) among bacteria causing urinary infections in the U.S.; inexpensive; bactericidal
Extended-spectrum penicillins	Ticarcillin, piperacillin	Useful in some infections with resistant *Enterobacter* spp. when combined with an aminoglycoside; useful in some polymicrobial infections (e.g., diabetic foot infections) when combined with a β-lactamase inhibitor
First-generation cephalosporins	Cephalothin, cefazolin	Inexpensive; bactericidal; useful in many infections with *Escherichia coli* and in some infections with *Klebsiella* spp. and *Proteus mirabilis*
Third-generation cephalosporins	Ceftriaxone, cefotaxime, ceftizoxime, cefpodoxime (oral)	Broad-spectrum; bactericidal; intravenous forms excellent for treating meningitis; resistance in many *Enterobacter* spp.; oral agents useful in uncomplicated urinary infections caused by susceptible bacteria (most *E. coli*, *Klebsiella pneumoniae*)
Carbacephems	Loracarbef (oral)	Similar to oral third-generation cephalosporins, with activity against common urinary tract pathogens but not *Enterobacter* spp.
Carbapenems	Imipenem/cilastatin	Broad-spectrum; may cause seizures in patients with renal failure or central nervous system lesions; useful in infections with resistant *Enterobacter* spp.
Sulfonamides	Trimethoprim-sulfamethoxazole	Inexpensive; useful in urinary infections; intravenous form useful in serious infections (meningitis) caused by *Enterobacter* spp.
Monobactams	Aztreonam	Useful in patients allergic to penicillin; may be used in pregnant patients
Quinolones	Ciprofloxacin, ofloxacin, norfloxacin, lomefloxacin, enoxacin	Useful in traveler's diarrhea, urinary infections, osteomyelitis, and infections with resistant *Enterobacter* spp.; should not be used by pregnant patients
Aminoglycosides	Gentamicin, tobramycin, amikacin	Once-daily dosing may reduce toxicity; should not be used by patients with renal dysfunction and diabetes mellitus unless absolutely necessary; prolonged therapy to be avoided; useful in infections with resistant *Enterobacter* spp.

an opportunist that has been recognized as a human pathogen only since the 1960s. *Serratia marcescens* and *Serratia liquefaciens* have been predominantly associated with human disease. The epidemiology of *S. marcescens* differs from that of other Enterobacteriaceae in that *S. marcescens* appears less likely to colonize the gastrointestinal tract but more likely to colonize the respiratory and urinary tracts of hospitalized adults.

Numerous strains of *Enterobacter*, *Serratia*, and *Klebsiella* have become resistant to many of the β-lactam antibiotics by three different mechanisms. The use of newer cephalosporins has led to a higher frequency of *Enterobacter* strains that are resistant to β-lactam antibiotics, a higher frequency of infections caused by these strains, and a higher rate of mortality from infections caused by the resistant strains than by the sensitive strains. The basis of this resistance is an enzyme that inactivates all clinically available cephalosporins. Unless there is prior exposure to cephalosporins, the gene encoding this cephalosporinase lies dormant in the bacterial chromosome; the fact that the enzyme is not expressed gives the erroneous impression on susceptibility testing that the organism is sensitive to the newer cephalosporins. This *inducible* gene is also present in *Citrobacter freundii*, *Serratia* spp., and indole-positive *Proteus*. Mutations in this gene have enabled many *Enterobacter* strains to produce large amounts of the cephalosporinase constitutively (i.e., continuously, without the need for induction). A second form of resistance is the production of plasmid-encoded enzymes, the extended-spectrum β-lactamases, which cause resistance to all available β-lactam antibiotics except the carbapenems. A third form of resistance has recently been identified in which some strains, by exposure to the carbapenems, acquire mutant porins that no longer allow these antibiotics to enter the bacterial cells. Thus, the carbapenems can no longer reach their normal target sites and kill the bacteria. Table 155-1 provides suggestions for treating *Enterobacter* infections.

PROTEUS, MORGANELLA, AND *PROVIDENCIA* INFECTIONS

Proteeae are actively motile bacteria that do not ferment lactose. DNA studies show this tribe to consist of at least three genera—*Proteus*, *Morganella*, and *Providencia*—and seven species: *Proteus vulgaris*, *Proteus mirabilis*, *Proteus myxofaciens*, *Morganella morganii* (previously *Proteus morganii*), *Providencia alcalifaciens*, *Providencia stuartii*, and *Providencia rettgeri* (previously *Proteus rettgeri*). Virtually all strains of *P. mirabilis*, which causes most *Proteus* infections, are indole negative, whereas virtually all other strains in the tribe are indole positive. *Proteus* strains are unique in their ability to swarm on moist agar media, which is due to the presence of hundreds of flagella per cell. These organisms are part of the normal fecal flora and are found in soil, water, and sewage. Except for urinary tract infections, *Proteus* rarely causes primary disease in otherwise healthy individuals. *Proteus* is an important cause of chronic urinary tract infection, in part because it possesses the enzyme urease, which splits urea into ammonium hydroxide and raises urinary pH to levels that promote the formation of struvite stones. These stones act as foreign bodies that obstruct urinary flow, serve as a nidus for persistent infection, and exacerbate destruction of the renal parenchyma. *Proteus* species are common opportunistic invaders in debilitated individuals undergoing broad-spectrum antimicrobial therapy. Like other gram-negative bacteria, they can contaminate burns, decubitus ulcers, and surgical wounds. Similarly, they have been associated with destructive chronic infections of the middle ear and mastoid, occasionally leading to deafness or malignant extension to the central nervous system with lateral sinus thrombosis, meningitis, brain abscess, and death. Following trauma to the eye, these organisms can cause corneal ulcers, leading to panophthalmitis. Like other gram-negative bacteria, *Proteus* can cause bacteremia and septic shock. The urinary tract serves as the portal of entry in most cases; next in frequency are the biliary tree, the gastrointestinal tract, and other foci. A surgical procedure often

precedes bloodstream invasion. Like *Proteus*, *P. rettgeri* and *P. stuartii* are important nosocomial urinary tract pathogens. The latter organisms are often resistant to many antibiotics.

Treatment of these infections is similar to that of infections due to other gram-negative bacteria, with two differences. Most strains of *P. mirabilis* are sensitive to most β-lactam antibiotics and aminoglycosides and are less difficult to treat. Nevertheless, the association of struvite stones with urinary tract infections due to these urea-splitting organisms poses compensatory challenges. Because contaminated stones provide a nidus of bacterial persistence, surgical intervention is often required for the eradication of infection. Untreated obstruction leads to rapid renal destruction and sepsis.

ACINETOBACTER INFECTIONS

Acinetobacter organisms are saprophytes ubiquitous in water and soil that, along with the genera *Moraxella*, *Neisseria*, and *Kingella*, make up the family Neisseriaceae. The two well-characterized variants are *Acinetobacter calcoaceticus* var. *lwoffii*, formerly called *Mima polymorpha*, and *Acinetobacter calcoaceticus* var. *anitratus*, formerly called *Herellea vaginicola*. Like other family members, these organisms have the appearance of gram-negative diplococci when grown on agar but differ from the latter by their typically negative oxidase reaction, their simple growth requirements, and their bacillary appearance when grown in broth. Unlike Enterobacteriaceae, they give a negative nitrate reaction.

The infections caused by *Acinetobacter* are similar to those caused by the Enterobacteriaceae, particularly nosocomial and community-acquired infections of the urinary tract, meninges, and lower respiratory tract and bacteremia. *Acinetobacter* strains also cause both subacute and acute bacterial endocarditis. With their low innate virulence but high prevalence on the skin of normal individuals, these bacteria are opportunistic and tend to invade the bloodstream of patients with intravenous catheters, surgical wounds, or burns. Occasionally, a bacteremic episode may be fulminant and suggestive of meningococcemia, with high fever, shock, and petechiae. Many cases of bacteremia are polymicrobial.

Given the ubiquity of *Acinetobacter*, disease due to this organism must be distinguished from mere colonization. True infection may be difficult to treat because it occurs in debilitated patients and because these bacteria have grown increasingly resistant to standard antimicrobials. While the results of sensitivity testing are awaited, treatment with an extended-spectrum β-lactam plus an aminoglycoside should be provided in conjunction with the removal of foreign bodies and the debridement of necrotic tissue.

BIBLIOGRAPHY

ENTEROBACTERIACEAE: GENERAL

BONE RC: The pathogenesis of sepsis. Ann Intern Med 115:457, 1991

MURRAY BE: New aspects of antimicrobial resistance and the resulting therapeutic dilemmas. J Infect Dis 163:1184, 1991

NICOLLE LE et al: Infections and antibiotic resistance in nursing homes. Clin Microbiol Rev 9:1, 1996

RANGEL-FRAUSTO MS et al: The natural history of the systemic inflammatory response syndrome (SIRS). JAMA 273:117, 1995

SANDERS CS, SANDERS WE: Resistance in gram-negative bacteria: Global trends and clinical impact. Clin Infect Dis 15:824, 1992

SCHABERG DR et al: Major trends in the microbial etiology of nosocomial infection. Am J Med 91(Suppl 3B):72S, 1991

ESCHERICHIA COLI INFECTIONS

GRANSDEN WR et al: Bacteremia due to *Escherichia coli:* A study of 861 episodes. Rev Infect Dis 12:1008, 1990

RUBINOFF MJ, FIELD M: Infectious diarrhea. Annu Rev Med 42:403, 1991

KLEBSIELLA-ENTEROBACTER-SERRATIA INFECTIONS

BODEY GP et al: Bacteremia caused by *Enterobacter*: 15 years of experience in a cancer hospital. Rev Infect Dis 13:550, 1991

CARPENTER JL: *Klebsiella* pulmonary infections: Occurrence at one medical center and review. Rev Infect Dis 12:672, 1990

CHOW JW et al: *Enterobacter* bacteremia: Clinical features and emergence of antibiotic resistance during therapy. Ann Intern Med 115:585, 1991

JOHNSON MP, RAMPHAL R: β-Lactam-resistant *Enterobacter* bacteremia in febrile neutropenic patients receiving monotherapy. J Infect Dis 162:981, 1990

SCHWIMMBECK PL, OLDSTONE MB: Molecular mimicry between human leukocyte antigen B27 and *Klebsiella*. Consequences for spondyloarthropathies. Am J Med 85:51, 1988

WOLFF MA et al: Antibiotic therapy for enterobacter meningitis: A retrospective review of 13 episodes and review of the literature. Clin Infect Dis 16:772, 1993

PROTEUS INFECTIONS

RAIMONDI A et al: Imipenem- and meropenem-resistant mutants of *Enterobacter cloacae* and *Proteus rettgeri* lack porins. Antimicrob Agents Chemother 35:1174, 1991

ACINETOBACTER INFECTIONS

BERGOGNE-BÉRÉZIN E, TOWNER KJ: *Acinetobacter* spp. as nosocomial pathogens: Microbiological, clinical, and epidemiological features. Clin Microbiol Rev 9:148, 1996

156 *John C. Atherton, Martin J. Blaser*

HELICOBACTER INFECTIONS

DEFINITION   Most human *Helicobacter* infections are caused by *Helicobacter pylori* and a few by *Helicobacter heilmanii* (formerly *Gastrospirillum hominis*) and other *Helicobacter* species (for example, *Gastrospirillum suis*). The current level of interest in *H. pylori* infection is high because of its etiologic importance in peptic ulcer disease and in gastric malignancy.

ETIOLOGIC AGENTS   Helicobacters are gram-negative, spiral, flagellate bacilli. Many species exist, most of which colonize specific animal hosts. *H. pylori* naturally infects humans and monkeys and has recently been described in domestic cats. It is noninvasive, living in the mucus that overlies gastric-type mucosae; a small proportion of the bacterial cells are adherent to the mucosa. Its spiral shape and flagellae render *H. pylori* motile in the mucous environment, and its efficient urease protects it against acid by catalyzing urea hydrolysis to produce ammonia. Urease plays a role in colonization and may be important in the maintenance of infection, although the deep gastric mucus is far less acidic than the gastric lumen. In vitro, *H. pylori* is microaerophilic and requires complex growth media; its major metabolic pathways are still poorly understood. It grows slowly, and old cultures contain slowly metabolizing coccoid forms that may or may not be important in the natural history of the infection. *H. heilmanii* is a longer, more tightly coiled spiral and also produces urease. It cannot be cultured in vitro by current techniques. Unlike *H. pylori* and most other helicobacters, *H. heilmanii* readily colonizes a range of animal species.

EPIDEMIOLOGY   The prevalence of *H. pylori* infection is about 30 percent in the United States and other developed countries as opposed to 80 percent in most developing countries. In the United States, prevalence varies with age: the figure is around 50 percent among 60-year-old persons and 25 percent among those 30 years old. Most studies show that spontaneous acquisition or loss of infection in adulthood is uncommon; thus most infections are thought to be acquired in childhood. The age association is largely but not exclusively due to a cohort effect. In other words, persons who are now 60 years old more commonly acquired the infection as children than did those who are now 30 years old. Other than age, the main risk factor for infection is low income. Humans are the major—if not the only—reservoir of *H. pylori*, but the exact route and source of infection are unknown. The fact that members of a family often carry the same strain of *H. pylori* implies that they acquire the infection from one another or from a common source; children may be the usual source of infection. Given that the bacteria can be cultured from feces, fecal-oral spread is likely, but oral-oral spread also is possible, and the relative contribution of each route to overall transmission is not known. *H. pylori* DNA has been identified in water sources, and cats may harbor the infection; however, whether either water sources or cats are important reservoirs of infection is unknown.

The prevalence of *H. heilmanii* infection is less than 1 percent. This *Helicobacter* species colonizes a number of animals, including domestic pets, and infection in humans is thought to be a zoonosis. Concurrent infection of the same human host with *H. pylori* and *H. heilmanii* has been described.

CLINICAL MANIFESTATIONS   Although *H. pylori* infection is usually asymptomatic, essentially all *H. pylori*–infected persons have gastric inflammation (Fig. 156-1). *H. pylori* infection is the foremost cause of peptic ulcer disease, which occurs at some point in the lifetime of about 15 percent of infected persons in developed countries. The main lines of evidence for a causal role of *H. pylori* are (1) that the presence of infection is a risk factor for the development of ulcers, (2) that ulcers do not develop in the absence of infection (except in cases with other known etiologic factors, such as treatment with nonsteroidal anti-inflammatory drugs), (3) that cure of the infection results in a dramatic drop in the rate of ulcer relapse (from about 80 percent to 15 percent in the first year, with even lower rates thereafter), and (4) that experimental infection of gerbils and mice causes gastroduodenal injury.

Prospective case-control studies have shown that *H. pylori* also is a risk factor for adenocarcinomas of the stomach other than those arising in the gastric cardia. The relative risk of these adenocarcinomas associated with *H. pylori* infection is about ninefold after adjustment for the inaccuracy of serologic testing in the elderly. The attributable risk of noncardia gastric adenocarcinoma to *H. pylori* has been estimated to be 75 percent in the United States and 85 percent in some developing countries. Infection due to *H. pylori* appears to be a major risk factor for primary gastric non-Hodgkin's lymphoma. It is strongly associated with low-grade B cell mucosa-associated lymphoid tissue (MALT) lymphoma, which is antigen driven and regresses in about half of cases when *H. pylori* infection is eradicated with antimicrobial agents. *H. pylori* infection may also increase the risk of aggressive diffuse large cell lymphoma of the stomach; patients with this tumor are 7.4 times more likely than controls to have been infected.

Whether *H. pylori* infection causes symptoms in the absence of ulcers or malignancy is unknown. The prevalence of *H. pylori* is

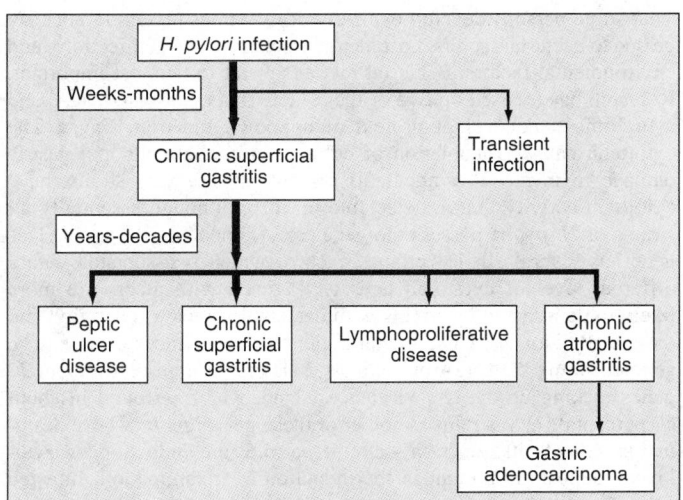

FIGURE 156-1   Natural history of infection with *Helicobacter pylori*. Some infected persons develop transient infection after exposure to *H. pylori*, while others develop chronic superficial gastritis within months after acquisition of the organism. In the absence of antimicrobial treatment, this process persists in most hosts for life. A minority of hosts develop clinically relevant conditions such as peptic ulceration, lymphoproliferative disease, or severe chronic atrophic gastritis leading to adenocarcinoma of the distal stomach. (*After Blaser and Parsonnet, with permission.*)

approximately 20 percent higher among patients with so-called non-ulcer dyspepsia than among matched controls; some but not all trials of *H. pylori* eradication in nonulcer dyspepsia have documented the alleviation of symptoms in some proportion of patients. Thus, some patients with nonulcer dyspepsia may benefit from treatment targeting *H. pylori,* but at present there is no prospective method for identifying this group. Peptic ulcers and nonulcer dyspepsia have been described in association with *H. heilmanii* infection, but it is unclear whether this association is causal.

PATHOLOGY AND PATHOGENESIS   Infection with *H. pylori* induces chronic superficial gastritis, which includes both mononuclear and polymorphonuclear cell infiltration of the mucosa and injury to epithelial cells. (The term *gastritis* should be used specifically to describe histologic features; it has also been used to describe endoscopic appearances and even symptoms, neither of which have been linked to microscopic findings or to *H. pylori* infection.) The immune response to *H. pylori* infection includes both the production of antibody (local and systemic) and a cell-mediated response but is ineffective in clearing the infection. *H. pylori* and associated inflammation are most evident in the stomach but are also found elsewhere in areas of gastric metaplasia and heterotopia (e.g., the duodenal bulb). In the United States, the most common pattern of gastric inflammation is antral-predominant, and this is the pattern most closely linked with duodenal ulceration. In developing countries, the predominant form is pangastritis, which is epidemiologically linked with gastric ulceration and gastric carcinoma. Longitudinal analyses of gastric biopsy specimens taken from the same patient on occasions many years apart show that inflammation may progress to atrophy, intestinal metaplasia, and dysplasia and then, by implication, to carcinoma. Patients with atrophic gastritis are at risk of developing vitamin B_{12} deficiency with the associated hematologic and neurologic sequelae. The individual's age at acquisition of the infection may influence the pattern of infection in the stomach and the pattern of disease. Thus, infection during early childhood may lead to gastric ulcers and gastric carcinoma, whereas infection later in childhood may lead to antral-predominant gastritis and duodenal ulceration.

Like *H. pylori*, *H. heilmanii* is associated with chronic gastritis. However, infection due to *H. heilmanii* is patchier and may clear spontaneously.

Most *H. pylori*–infected persons do not develop clinical sequelae. That some persons develop overt disease whereas others do not may be due to bacterial factors, host factors (including age at infection), and environmental factors. Bacterial factors appear to be most important. Research has focused on two of these factors: a cytotoxin, VacA, and a high-molecular-weight protein of unknown function, CagA. The cytotoxin causes vacuolation of cultured epithelial cells and gastric damage in mice. Only about 50 percent of *H. pylori* strains have cytotoxin activity that is detectable in vitro, although essentially all strains of *H. pylori* possess the gene (*vacA*) encoding the toxin. This gene has several allelic variants, each of which is associated with a different level of cytotoxin activity. Patients with ulcers are more likely to be infected by strains with detectable cytotoxin activity, and the sla allele of *vacA* is an even better marker of ulcer disease. The gene encoding the CagA protein, *cagA,* is one of a group of about 20 genes making up the *cag* virulence island, which is found in about 60 percent of U.S. strains. Another of these genes, *picB* (whose designation reflects its function—i.e., it *p*ermits the *i*nduction of *c*ytokines), appears important in the induction of inflammation. Infected patients with ulcers or gastric adenocarcinoma are more likely to have CagA-positive strains than persons without these conditions.

One puzzling question regarding *H. pylori* has been how a gastric infection causes duodenal ulceration. Colonization of areas of gastric heterotopia or metaplasia in the duodenum appears important, as does an *H. pylori*–induced increase in acid secretion. The latter phenomenon is due both to hypergastrinemia and to increased responsivity of the parietal cell mass to gastrin. The number of antral G cells (which produce gastrin) is unchanged, but the number of D cells (which

produce somatostatin) is decreased. Somatostatin has a negative feedback on gastrin release and on stimulated acid production, and the reduction of this negative feedback may account for the observed changes. Whether the resulting hyperacidity causes duodenal ulceration per se or induces gastric metaplasia in the duodenum—which subsequently becomes infected and inflamed, then ulcerates—is still unclear. After the eradication of *H. pylori* in patients with duodenal ulcer disease, the level of acid secretion falls.

DIAGNOSIS   Tests for *H. pylori* infection can be divided into two groups: invasive tests, which require upper gastrointestinal endoscopy and are based on the analysis of gastric biopsy specimens, and noninvasive tests (Table 156-1). At present, invasive tests are preferred in the initial management of dyspeptic patients because the decision about whether to treat the infection depends on ulcer disease status. The most convenient endoscopy-based test is the biopsy urease test. In this procedure, two antral biopsy specimens are put into a gel containing urea and an indicator. The presence of *H. pylori* urease elicits a color change, which often takes place within minutes but can require up to 24 h; a complicating issue is that at 24 h the result of the test is sometimes falsely positive. Histologic examination of biopsy specimens is accurate. Special stains (e.g., a modified Giemsa or silver stain) permit optimal visualization of *H. pylori*. Histologic study also yields additional information, including the degree and pattern of inflammation, atrophy, metaplasia, and dysplasia. However, these details are rarely of clinical use. Microbiologic culture is most specific, although failure of this test is common except in expert hands. The identity of *H. pylori* can be confirmed by its typical appearance on Gram's staining and its positive reactions in oxidase, catalase, and urease tests. Once bacteria have been cultured, antibiotic sensitivities can be determined, but this information is not used routinely at present in the selection of treatment regimens. Biopsy specimens containing *H. heilmanii* are only weakly positive in the urease test. The diagnosis of *H. heilmanii* infection is based on the characteristic histologic appearance of the organism since it cannot be cultivated in vitro.

The simplest tests for *H. pylori* infection are serologic, involving the assessment of specific IgG levels in serum. Both standard and rapid office tests are available. When these tests are properly done, their diagnostic accuracy parallels that of invasive tests, although not all tests are equally accurate. A drop in antibody titer between matched serum samples taken before and 6 months after treatment (no sooner because of a lag in antibody decline) accurately indicates that *H. pylori* infection has been eradicated. The other major noninvasive tests are the ^{13}C and ^{14}C urea breath tests. In these simple tests, the patient drinks a labeled urea solution and then blows into a tube. The urea is labeled with either the nonradioactive isotope ^{13}C or a minute dose of the radioactive isotope ^{14}C (which exposes the patient to less radiation than a standard chest x-ray). If *H. pylori* urease is present, the

Table 156-1

Tests Commonly Used in the Diagnosis of *Helicobacter pylori* Infection

Test	Advantages	Disadvantages
INVASIVE (ENDOSCOPY- AND BIOPSY-BASED)		
Biopsy urease	Quick, simple	Rapid test not fully sensitive, 24-h test not fully specific
Histology	Widely available; may give additional histologic information	Sensitivity dependent on experience
Culture	Permits determination of antibiotic susceptibilities	Sensitivity dependent on experience
NONINVASIVE		
Serology	Cheap and convenient	Cannot be used for early follow-up
Urea breath	Safer and cheaper than endoscopy	Low-dose irradiation required for ^{14}C test

urea is hydrolyzed and labeled carbon dioxide is detected in breath samples. Both urea breath tests and serology may be more accurate than biopsy-based tests, as they are not subject to the sampling error involved in the collection of biopsy specimens. Unlike serologic tests, urea breath tests can be used to assess the outcome of treatment 1 month after its completion and thus may replace endoscopy for this purpose. Neither urea breath tests nor endoscopy-based tests can be used to assess treatment outcome earlier since, even when treatment is unsuccessful, the load of organisms may be too small to render the test positive.

℞ TREATMENT

At present, the only clear indications for treatment are *H. pylori*–related duodenal and gastric ulceration and the rare low-grade B cell MALT lymphoma. *H. pylori* infection should be treated in patients with ulcer disease, whether or not the ulcers are currently active, to reduce the likelihood of relapse. In the future, the indications for therapy may be broader, but at present treatment is not recommended for nonulcer dyspepsia. Neither is routine prophylaxis against ulcers or gastric adenocarcinoma recommended, although it may be reasonable to treat the infection in persons with a strong family history of gastric cancer. Reasons for avoiding treatment for "soft" indications include the expense, the induction of morbidity in otherwise healthy people, and the risk of widespread antibiotic resistance.

Treatment of *H. pylori* infection is becoming increasingly simple and effective, although multidrug regimens are required. *H. pylori* is susceptible to many antibiotics in vitro, but these drugs often fail in vivo, perhaps because they are not delivered to the site of infection in effective concentrations and in a fully active form. Initial failure of monotherapy has led to the use of multidrug regimens (still not approved by the Food and Drug Administration), the most widely tested of which is "standard triple therapy" with bismuth subsalicylate, tetracycline, and metronidazole, which is given for 2 weeks and eradicates *H. pylori* in about 90 percent of cases (Table 156-2). However, good compliance is crucial to the success of this complex regimen and is difficult to ensure. Thus, there is much interest in simpler 1-week triple-therapy regimens involving agents that inhibit gastric acidity (Table 156-2). These regimens have yielded promising early results, and the newly approved ranitidine bismuth citrate may be a reasonable substitute for proton pump inhibitors. Problems remain, for example, with regimens containing metronidazole or clarithromycin: resistance to these agents often arises in *H. pylori* after treatment failure, and the previous use of metronidazole for the treatment of an intercurrent infection, even many years earlier, commonly leads to metronidazole resistance. Paradoxically, metronidazole-containing regimens are still effective against around 60 percent of resistant infections. Resistance to amoxicillin, tetracycline, bismuth compounds, and proton pump inhibitors has not been described for *H. pylori*.

Successful treatment of *H. heilmanii* infections with bismuth compounds alone has been reported. However, it is unclear whether this treatment has been truly successful or whether the good outcome has merely reflected the natural history of the infection.

Because of the uncertainties surrounding the efficacy of treatment for *H. pylori* infection, it is reasonable to retest for the infection; to this end, the urea breath test or endoscopy should be undertaken no sooner than 1 month after treatment. The knowledge gained will elucidate prognosis and facilitate management. Once treatment regimens with confirmed efficacy are available, such a strategy may be unnecessary except when there is good reason to suspect that treatment has failed. Matched pretreatment and late posttreatment serology may then become the norm.

PREVENTION *H. pylori* infection is a major public health problem in developing countries, and gastric adenocarcinoma is the second leading cause of cancer death worldwide. The most immediate solution is vaccination, and experimental immunization of animals has given promising results. In the United States and other developed countries, the incidences of *H. pylori* infection and its clinical sequelae are dropping, possibly because of improvements in living standards. Thus the prevention of infection in these countries may be necessary for populations at high risk of gastric cancer. In the United States, these groups include African, Asian, Hispanic, and Native Americans.

BIBLIOGRAPHY

ATHERTON JC, SPILLER RC: The urea breath test for *Helicobacter pylori*. Gut 35:723, 1994

BLASER MJ, PARSONNET J: Parasitism by the "slow" bacterium *Helicobacter pylori* leads to altered gastric homeostasis and neoplasia. J Clin Invest 94:4, 1994

———: The bacteria behind ulcers. Sci Am 274:104, 1996

DOOLEY CP et al: Prevalence of *Helicobacter pylori* infection and histologic gastritis in asymptomatic persons. N Engl J Med 321:1562, 1989

HANSSON L-E et al: The risk of stomach cancer in patients with gastric or duodenal ulcer disease. N Engl J Med 335:242, 1996

KUIPERS E et al: Atrophic gastritis and *Helicobacter pylori* infection in patients with reflux esophagitis treated with omeprazole or fundoplication. N Engl J Med 334:1018, 1996

MARSHALL BJ, WARREN JR: Unidentified curved bacilli in the stomach of patients with gastritis and peptic ulceration. Lancet 1:1311, 1984

NIH CONSENSUS DEVELOPMENT PANEL: *Helicobacter pylori* and peptic ulcer disease. JAMA 272:65, 1994

NOMURA A et al: *Helicobacter pylori* infection and gastric carcinoma in a population of Japanese-Americans in Hawaii. N Engl J Med 325:1132, 1991

PARSONNET J et al: *Helicobacter pylori* infection and gastric lymphoma. N Engl J Med 330:1267, 1994

——— et al: Modelling cost-effectiveness of *Helicobacter pylori* screening to prevent gastric cancer: A mandate for clinical trials. Lancet 348:150, 1996

WOTHERSPOON AC et al: *Helicobacter pylori*–associated gastritis and primary B cell gastric lymphoma. Lancet 338:1175, 1991

Table 156-2

Recommended Regimens for the Eradication of *Helicobacter pylori* Infection

Drug 1	Drug 2	Drug 3	Duration
STANDARD TRIPLE-THERAPY REGIMEN			
Bismuth subsalicylate (2 tabs qid)	Tetracycline HCl (500 mg qid*)	Metronidazole (250 mg tid)	2 weeks
TRIPLE-THERAPY REGIMENS WITH ACID REDUCTION			
Omeprazole (20 mg bid)	Clarithromycin (250 mg bid)	Metronidazole (500 mg bid)	1 week
Omeprazole (20 mg bid)	Clarithromycin (500 mg bid)	Amoxicillin (1 g bid)	1 week

* Amoxicillin (500 mg qid) may be substituted for tetracycline, although meta-analysis suggests that this substitution results in a small drop in efficacy.

NOTE: These regimens have not yet been approved for this indication by the Food and Drug Administration.

157 *Matthew Pollack*

INFECTIONS DUE TO *PSEUDOMONAS* SPECIES AND RELATED ORGANISMS

Pseudomonas species and phylogenetically related bacteria are ubiquitous, free-living, opportunistic gram-negative pathogens. *Pseudomonas aeruginosa*, the most common human pathogen in this group, is the primary subject of this chapter. Also discussed are *Burkholderia cepacia* (formerly *Pseudomonas cepacia*), primarily an opportunistic pathogen; *Stenotrophomonas maltophilia* (formerly *Xanthomonas maltophilia*), which primarily infects hospitalized patients; *Burkholderia pseudomallei* (formerly *Pseudomonas pseudomallei*), an organism that inhabits soil and water (primarily in the tropics) and that causes melioidosis—a systemic disease with acute or chronic manifestations—in nonimmunocompromised patients; and *Burkholderia mallei* (formerly *Pseudomonas mallei*), a pathogen of animal origin that occasionally produces glanders in humans.

INFECTIONS DUE TO *P. AERUGINOSA*

P. aeruginosa is a small, aerobic gram-negative rod belonging to the family Pseudomonadaceae. It is motile by virtue of its single polar flagellum. More than half of all clinical isolates produce the blue-green pigment pyocyanin; this pigment is helpful in the identification of the organism and accounts for the species name *aeruginosa*, which refers to the distinctive color of copper oxide. *P. aeruginosa* is readily identified in the clinical laboratory. It is a straight or slightly curved, nonsporulating, motile gram-negative rod that grows aerobically on most common media.

EPIDEMIOLOGY *P. aeruginosa* is widespread in nature, inhabiting soil, water, plants, and animals (including humans). It has a predilection for moist environments. This organism occasionally colonizes the skin, external ear, upper respiratory tract, or large bowel of healthy humans. Rates of carriage are relatively low, however, except among patients who have serious underlying disease, whose host defenses have been naturally or iatrogenically compromised, who have previously received antibiotic therapy, and/or who have been exposed to the hospital environment. Under these circumstances, colonization with *P. aeruginosa* frequently precedes infection, and factors that predispose to the former also increase the likelihood of the latter.

Most *P. aeruginosa* infections are hospital acquired. Many potential reservoirs of infection have been identified, including respiratory equipment, cleaning solutions, disinfectants, sinks, vegetables, flowers, endoscopes, and physiotherapy pools. Most reservoirs are associated with moisture. It is assumed that the organism is transmitted to patients via the hands of hospital personnel or via fomites.

While some infecting strains of *P. aeruginosa* appear to be endemic within the hospital environment, others are traced to a common source associated with a specific outbreak or epidemic. Epidemiologic investigation is facilitated by serotyping (immunotyping) of strains on the basis of differences in lipopolysaccharide structure and by the use of DNA or RNA probes.

PATHOGENESIS That the pathogenesis of infections due to *P. aeruginosa* is complex is evidenced by the clinical diversity of the diseases related to this organism and by the multiplicity of virulence factors it produces. *P. aeruginosa* rarely causes disease in the healthy host. It may undergo a "malignant" transformation, however, when normal cutaneous or mucosal barriers have been breached or bypassed (e.g., as a result of burn injury, penetrating trauma, surgery, endotracheal intubation, urinary bladder catheterization, or intravenous drug abuse); when immunologic defense mechanisms have been compromised (e.g., by chemotherapy-induced neutropenia, hypogammaglobulinemia, extremes of age, diabetes mellitus, cystic fibrosis, cancer, or AIDS); when the protective function of the normal bacterial flora has been disrupted by broad-spectrum antibiotic therapy; and/or when the patient has been exposed to reservoirs associated with a hospital environment. The ubiquity of the organism, its flexible nutritional and metabolic requirements, its environmental resiliency, and its relative resistance to antibiotics help account for the frequency and success with which it acts as an opportunistic pathogen.

Infections caused by *P. aeruginosa* usually begin with bacterial attachment and superficial colonization of cutaneous or mucosal surfaces and progress to localized bacterial invasion and damage to underlying tissues. This process may continue with bloodstream invasion, dissemination, systemic inflammatory-response syndrome (SIRS), multiple-organ dysfunction, and ultimately death. Alternatively, the infection may remain anatomically localized or may spread by direct extension to contiguous structures. The organism and its products may cause tissue injury at primary and secondary sites of infection, while the release of systemically acting toxins or inflammatory mediators

of the infected host may contribute directly or indirectly to the sepsis syndrome.

The initial attachment of *P. aeruginosa* to the respiratory epithelium and other epithelial surfaces appears to be mediated by bacterial organelles called *pili* or *fimbriae* and by the mucoid exopolysaccharide *alginate*, which is produced by mucoid strains. Receptors for these adhesins are found, for example, on tracheal epithelial cells and tracheobronchial mucin and are composed, at least in part, of *N*-acetylneuraminic acid (sialic acid) and *N*-acetylglucosamine, respectively.

Surface moieties of *P. aeruginosa*, including exopolysaccharide and lipopolysaccharide, may protect the organism from direct antibody- and complement-mediated bactericidal mechanisms and from opsonophagocytosis. Meanwhile, the organism produces a number of extracellular enzymes, including alkaline protease, elastase, phospholipase, cytotoxin, and exoenzymes (or exotoxins) A and S. The breakdown of host tissues by these extracellular bacterial products creates conditions conducive to enhanced bacterial proliferation, invasion, and tissue injury.

The preceding process is particularly likely to culminate in bloodstream invasion and dissemination in the face of immune compromise such as that resulting from profound neutropenia. The sepsis syndrome, or SIRS, due to *P. aeruginosa* shares many of the features of gram-negative sepsis caused by other bacteria, and the lipopolysaccharide or endotoxin produced by this organism, like that produced by other bacterial species, is thought to play a pivotal role in the pathogenesis of this syndrome.

In addition to lipopolysaccharide, which is a structural component of the bacterial outer membrane, the extracellular enzyme exotoxin A—a diphtheria-like toxin—is produced by most clinical isolates of *P. aeruginosa*. Exotoxin A inhibits mammalian protein synthesis by transferring the adenosine diphosphate (ADP) ribose moiety of the nicotinamide adenine dinucleotide into covalent linkage with elongation factor 2, an enzyme that catalyzes the elongation step in polypeptide assembly but is inactivated by exotoxin-mediated ADP ribosylation. Exotoxin A appears to cause both local and systemic disease. It is cytotoxic in vitro and necrotizing in vivo and produces fatal shock in experimental animals, including nonhuman primates. Toxigenic clinical isolates are more virulent than nontoxigenic strains. Moreover, the rate of survival is higher among patients with *P. aeruginosa* bacteremia in the presence than in the absence of adequate preexisting levels of exotoxin A–specific serum antibodies.

CLINICAL MANIFESTATIONS AND DIAGNOSIS **Respiratory Tract Infections** Lower respiratory tract infections due to *P. aeruginosa* occur mainly in immunocompromised patients. *Primary* or *nonbacteremic pneumonia* results from aspiration of upper respiratory tract secretions; often develops in patients with chronic lung disease, congestive heart failure, or AIDS; and is most common in an intensive care setting in association with mechanical ventilator use. *Bacteremic pneumonia*, in contrast, complicates hematopoietic malignancies, especially after chemotherapy that induces severe neutropenia. Chronic infection of the lower respiratory tract with *P. aeruginosa* is prevalent among patients with cystic fibrosis. It occurs typically in older children or young adults and is caused almost exclusively by mucoid strains.

Primary or nonbacteremic pneumonia caused by *P. aeruginosa* may present as an acute, life-threatening infection characterized by fever, chills, severe dyspnea, cyanosis, productive cough, apprehension, confusion, and other signs of severe systemic toxicity. Chest roentgenograms typically show bilateral bronchopneumonia with nodular infiltrates and small areas of radiolucency; pleural effusions are common; empyema is relatively uncommon; and lobar consolidation is occasionally seen. Pathologic lesions include alveolar necrosis, focal hemorrhages, and microabscesses. Cavitary lesions are particularly common in AIDS patients with *P. aeruginosa* pneumonia.

Bacteremic pneumonia due to *P. aeruginosa*, typically associated with neutropenia, begins as a respiratory infection, but subsequent bloodstream invasion and resulting metastatic spread produce characteristic lesions in the lung and other viscera. Alveolar hemorrhage and necrosis are common. The signs and symptoms of this fulminant disease include those described for nonbacteremic pneumonia caused by this organism as well as those associated with gram-negative sepsis.

Chest roentgenograms characteristically demonstrate a rapid progression from pulmonary vascular congestion to interstitial edema, then to pulmonary edema, and finally to diffuse necrotizing bronchopneumonia with cavity formation. The patient typically dies 3 or 4 days after initial presentation.

Mucoid strains of *P. aeruginosa* infect the lower respiratory tract of patients with cystic fibrosis, contributing to the acute exacerbations and chronic progression that characterize pulmonary disease in these individuals. Colonization with *P. aeruginosa* correlates with bronchial airway disease in cystic fibrosis patients. It is unclear whether mucus plugging precedes infection or vice versa. The uncertainty notwithstanding, airway obstruction appears to begin with bronchiolitis, which causes mucus plugging and predisposes to *P. aeruginosa* infection. The latter produces more mucus plugging, chronic suppuration, bronchiectasis, atelectasis, and ultimately fibrosis. This process progresses to pulmonary insufficiency, hypoxemia, and alterations in cardiopulmonary dynamics resulting in pulmonary hypertension and cor pulmonale.

Clinical manifestations of lower respiratory tract infections due to *P. aeruginosa* in cystic fibrosis vary with the severity and duration of underlying lung disease and with the frequency and intensity of acute episodes. Early in the disease, patients may experience recurrent upper respiratory symptoms followed by a lingering cough. Episodes of pneumonia develop later, with persistent cough between acute episodes. Eventually, patients exhibit a chronic productive cough, diminished appetite, weight loss, growth retardation, and decreased activity. Other symptoms may include wheezing, tachypnea, and irritability. Acute exacerbations are typically accompanied by low-grade fever and heightened respiratory symptoms. Physical signs include evidence of malnutrition, an increase in anteroposterior diameter, intercostal retractions, cyanosis, inspiratory and expiratory wheezing, rhonchi, moist rales, abdominal distention, and clubbing of the fingers and toes. Laboratory abnormalities include leukocytosis with a left shift and hypoxemia with or without hypercarbia. Tests of pulmonary function demonstrate obstructive and restrictive defects. Chest roentgenograms reveal overaeration, patchy atelectasis, peribronchial fibrosis, and patchy infiltrates associated with pneumonia. In more advanced disease, there may be evidence of severe overaeration, depressed diaphragm, increased anteroposterior diameter, extensive peribronchial infiltration, generalized bronchiectasis, and cyst formation.

Bacteremia   *P. aeruginosa* causes one of the most common and life-threatening gram-negative bloodstream infections in immunocompromised patients. *P. aeruginosa* bacteremia is usually associated with nosocomial infections and is frequently iatrogenic. It is either primary (with no identifiable source) or secondary to a discrete extravascular focus. *P. aeruginosa* bacteremia is associated with underlying conditions such as hematologic malignancies, neutropenia, immunoglobulin deficiencies, severe burns, dermatitis, diabetes mellitus, AIDS, and prematurity. Predisposing iatrogenic factors include cancer chemotherapy resulting in neutropenia or mucosal ulceration, genitourinary instrumentation or catheterization, placement of intravascular hardware, recent surgery, steroid therapy, and antibiotic administration.

The clinical features of *P. aeruginosa* bacteremia are similar to those of other forms of bacteremia. Common primary sites of infection include the urinary tract, gastrointestinal tract, lungs, intravascular foci, skin, and soft tissues. Fever, tachypnea, tachycardia, and prostration are common. Disorientation, confusion, or obtundation may be evident. Hypotension can progress to refractory shock. Renal failure, adult respiratory distress syndrome, or disseminated intravascular coagulation sometimes occurs as a complication. Jaundice is seen more commonly in *P. aeruginosa* bacteremia than in other forms of gram-negative sepsis.

Pathognomonic skin lesions termed *ecthyma gangrenosum* develop in a relatively small minority of patients with *P. aeruginosa* bacteremia. The lesions begin as small hemorrhagic vesicles surrounded by a rim of erythema and undergo central necrosis with subsequent ulceration. They occur singly or in small numbers on the perineum, buttocks, and extremities; in the axillae; or elsewhere. Ecthyma-like lesions are occasionally noted on the mucous membranes of the mouth or gingiva. Histologic study shows that these lesions contain numerous bacteria invading blood vessels but few inflammatory cells. Bacteria are readily visible on Gram's staining and may be cultured from aspirated material.

Endocarditis   *P. aeruginosa* infects native heart valves in intravenous drug users as well as prosthetic heart valves. The source of *P. aeruginosa* strains infecting drug users appears to be standing water contaminating drug paraphernalia. Moreover, foreign materials that are mixed with heroin may cause injury to valve leaflets or mural endocardium, with consequent fibrosis. These factors, combined with the apparent high affinity of the organism for human endocardium, may explain the association between *P. aeruginosa* endocarditis and intravenous drug use. The particularly frequent exposure of the tricuspid valve to both trauma and bacteria apparently accounts for the high incidence of tricuspid involvement in association with intravenous drug use.

The pulmonic, mitral, or aortic valve or the mural endocardium of either atrium also may be affected in *P. aeruginosa* endocarditis. Multiple-valve infections are common. Tricupsid or right-sided involvement is often associated with septic pulmonary emboli. Right-sided *P. aeruginosa* endocarditis usually presents subacutely, while the appearance of left-sided disease is likely to be more acute or even fulminant. Fever is a virtually invariable feature, and murmurs are usually detectable at initial presentation or shortly thereafter. Septic pulmonary emboli associated with right-sided disease result in cough, pleuritic chest pain, sputum production, pulmonary infiltration (with or without abscess formation), and pleural effusion. Left-sided infections may present as intractable heart failure or large systemic emboli. Mycotic aneurysms, cerebritis, or brain abscess may occur; septic infarcts are occasionally found in the spleen; but skin and soft tissue manifestations, including Janeway lesions, Osler's nodes, and ecthyma gangrenosum, are relatively uncommon.

The diagnosis of *P. aeruginosa* endocarditis is based on a positive blood culture in the absence of an extracardiac source; an indication of valvular dysfunction or vegetation on an echocardiogram; evidence of septic pulmonary lesions on a chest roentgenogram (in right-sided disease); and the actual demonstration of infected heart valves at the time of surgery.

Central Nervous System Infections   *P. aeruginosa* infections of the central nervous system include meningitis and brain abscess. These infections follow extension from a contiguous parameningeal structure such as the ear, mastoid, or paranasal sinus; direct inoculation into the subarachnoid space or brain through head trauma, surgery, or diagnostic procedures; or bacteremic spread from a distant site such as the urinary tract, lung, or heart valve. Like *P. aeruginosa* infections at other anatomic sites, central nervous system infections are documented almost exclusively in patients with compromised local or systemic immune-defense mechanisms. Predisposing factors include recent neurosurgical procedures, penetrating head trauma, lumbar puncture or spinal anesthesia, cancer of the head and neck, parameningeal infection, and *P. aeruginosa* infections at distant sites in association with bloodstream invasion.

The clinical signs of *P. aeruginosa* meningitis, like those of other forms of acute bacterial meningitis, include fever, headache, stiff neck, confusion, and obtundation. The onset of illness may be acute or even fulminant, particularly in bacteremic patients, with a precipitous downhill course, shock, coma, and early death. In nonbacteremic patients, *P. aeruginosa* meningitis or brain abscess may present more insidiously, with a paucity of systemic symptoms. This presentation is especially common in infections resulting from recent neurosurgery, cancer of the head and neck, or direct extension from a parameningeal focus of chronic infection. Occasionally, *P. aeruginosa* meningitis runs a subacute or relapsing course that is thought to be related to the intermittent release of bacteria from a loculated site of infection. Chronic or recurrent meningitis may result from altered cranial anatomy associated with central nervous system tumors, traumatic injury, neurosurgical procedures, indwelling hardware, or cerebrospinal fluid leaks.

Ear Infections   *P. aeruginosa* is often found in the external auditory canal, particularly under moist conditions and in the presence of inflammation or maceration (as in "swimmer's ear"). Moreover, this organism is the predominant pathogen associated with external otitis, a usually benign inflammatory process affecting the external auditory canal. This self-limited condition provides a local environment conducive to the growth of *P. aeruginosa*, which, in turn, appears to contribute to the inflammatory process. The ear is painful or merely itchy, there is a purulent discharge, and pain is elicited by pulling on the pinna. The external canal appears edematous and is filled with detritus that often prevents visualization of the tympanic membrane.

P. aeruginosa occasionally penetrates the epithelium overlying the floor of the external auditory canal at the junction between bone and cartilage and invades underlying soft tissue. The ensuing invasive process, which involves soft tissue, cartilage, and cortical bone, is typically slow but destructive. Termed *malignant external otitis*, this condition occurs predominantly in elderly diabetic patients but is reported occasionally in infants with other underlying diseases and rarely in elderly nondiabetic patients. Virtually all cases of malignant external otitis are caused by *P. aeruginosa*. From the external ear, the infection advances to the retromandibular area or parotid space and enters the mastoid air cells and temporal bone. Advancing osteomyelitis at the base of the skull often involves the seventh, ninth, tenth, and eleventh cranial nerves. The cavernous sinus can become involved, as can the contralateral petrous apex. The middle ear is commonly spared; meningitis and brain abscess are relatively rare complications.

Otalgia and otorrhea are common presenting symptoms of malignant external otitis. Facial-nerve paralysis tends to occur early, while other cranial-nerve palsies appear later. There may be a loss of hearing, the pinna of the ear is typically tender, and trismus indicates temporomandibular involvement. Constitutional symptoms such as fever and weight loss are relatively uncommon. Physical examination almost always reveals abnormalities of the external auditory canal, including swelling, erythema, purulent discharge, debris, and granulation tissue in the canal wall. The tympanic membrane is often hidden from view and is sometimes perforated. Inflammation may involve the pinna as well as the periauricular, retromandibular, and mastoid areas. Bilateral disease is unusual but does occur.

Peripheral leukocytosis is relatively infrequent in malignant external otitis, while the erythrocyte sedimentation rate usually is markedly elevated. Cerebrospinal fluid occasionally exhibits pleocytosis and an elevation in the protein level. Computed tomography (CT) or polytomography of the mastoid or temporal bone typically reveals bony erosions and new bone formation, while the floor of the skull may have soft tissue densities associated with areas of cellulitis. Magnetic resonance imaging (MRI) may delineate soft tissue involvement with greater sensitivity and accuracy than CT. In addition, technetium 99m bone scans and gallium 67 scans frequently give positive results. Cultures of samples from the external auditory canal and of surgical specimens are almost always positive for *P. aeruginosa*.

P. aeruginosa is commonly implicated in chronic suppurative otitis media in children and adults. It either is the sole bacterial isolate or is among the organisms isolated from the middle or external ear in a majority of cases, and it is thought to play a central pathogenic role.

Eye Infections (See also Chap. 28) *P. aeruginosa* causes bacterial keratitis or corneal ulcer and endophthalmitis in the human eye. Keratitis due to *P. aeruginosa* may result from even minor corneal injury, which interrupts the integrity of the superficial epithelial surface and permits bacterial access to the underlying stroma. Corneal ulcer may complicate contact lens use, particularly when extended-wear soft contact lenses are involved. Contact lens solutions or the lenses themselves may be the source of the organism, which is probably inoculated into the eye at sites of minor lens-induced corneal damage. Patients who have sustained serious burns, have undergone ocular irradiation or tracheostomy, have been exposed to the intensive care environment, and/or are in a coma are also susceptible to *P. aeruginosa*–associated corneal ulcers. *P. aeruginosa* keratitis usually starts as a small central ulcer; spreads concentrically to involve a large portion of the cornea, sclera, and underlying stroma; and in some cases progresses to posterior corneal perforation.

The clinical manifestations of *P. aeruginosa* keratitis include a rapidly expanding, necrotic stromal infiltrate in the bed of an epithelial injury; surrounding epithelial edema; an anterior chamber reaction; and mucopurulent discharge adherent to the ulcer's surface. Corneal ulcer due to *P. aeruginosa* may advance rapidly to involve the entire cornea in 2 days or less or may evolve subacutely over several days. Systemic symptoms are uncommon. Complications include corneal perforation, anterior chamber involvement, and endophthalmitis.

P. aeruginosa endophthalmitis may complicate penetrating injuries of the eye, intraocular surgery, hematogenous spread from other sites of *Pseudomonas* infection, or posterior perforation of corneal ulcers. It is typically a rapidly progressive, sight-threatening condition that demands immediate therapeutic intervention. Clinical manifestations may include eye pain, conjunctival hyperemia, chemosis, lid edema, decreased visual acuity, hypopyon, severe anterior uveitis, and signs of possible vitreous involvement. Panophthalmitis may result from this intraocular infection.

Bone and Joint Infections Vertebral osteomyelitis due to *P. aeruginosa* is associated with complicated urinary tract infection, genitourinary instrumentation or surgery, and intravenous drug abuse. Vertebral infections associated with a urinary tract source most often develop in the elderly and usually affect the lumbosacral spine. Drug use–related infections typically occur in younger patients and may affect the cervical or lumbosacral spine. *P. aeruginosa* vertebral osteomyelitis is usually an indolent disease. Accordingly, symptoms may develop weeks or even months before diagnosis. Back or neck pain is generally reported, while fever and systemic symptoms are relatively uncommon. Local tenderness and decreased range of motion of the affected spine are typical. Neurologic deficits are documented in a minority of patients. Leukocytosis may be noted, the erythrocyte sedimentation rate is almost always markedly elevated, and blood cultures are sometimes positive. Roentgenograms reveal loss of bone density, narrowed intervertebral space, destruction of vertebral end plates, lytic lesions of vertebral bodies, sclerosis, and possible osteophyte formation. CT or MRI may be the most sensitive means of defining lesions. Technetium bone scans and gallium scans usually yield positive results, while myelograms are revealing only if granulation tissue impinges on the epidural space. An etiologic diagnosis requires the culture of material obtained by needle aspiration or biopsy of the affected spine under fluoroscopic guidance; open biopsy is occasionally needed.

Sternoclavicular pyarthrosis caused by *P. aeruginosa* is another complication of intravenous drug abuse; in some cases it is associated with *P. aeruginosa* endocarditis, but more often it is not. Joint involvement is usually monoarticular, with the sternoclavicular joint more often affected than sternochondral joints. Localized pain in the anterior chest wall is the usual presenting complaint, movement of the homolateral shoulder may be restricted by discomfort, associated fever is common, and symptoms typically last for months (although some cases do have more acute presentations). Physical examination reveals tenderness, erythema, and swelling over the affected joint. Leukocytosis is common, and the erythrocyte sedimentation rate is almost invariably elevated. Roentgenograms show soft tissue edema, bone demineralization, lytic lesions, and periosteal elevation of the clavicular head, rib, or sternum. Material obtained by arthrocentesis or synovial biopsy yields *P. aeruginosa* in culture.

P. aeruginosa infections of the symphysis pubis are associated with pelvic surgery and intravenous drug use. The symphysis pubis, like other fibrocartilaginous joints, exhibits a peculiar susceptibility to bloodborne infection with *P. aeruginosa*. Affected patients report pain in the groin, hip, thigh, and/or lower abdomen that is made worse by walking. Fever is variable, and the duration of symptoms before diagnosis ranges from days to months. As in other bone and joint infections caused by *P. aeruginosa*, leukocytosis is variable, while the erythrocyte sedimentation rate is markedly elevated. Roentgenograms show irregularities of the pubic margins, separation of the symphysis pubis, and osteomyelitic abnormalities of the pubic rami that may be extensive. Bone scans are usually positive. Needle aspiration or biopsy is necessary to obtain material for culture. A positive culture is particularly important for the discrimination of *P. aeruginosa* infections and other pyogenic infections from osteitis pubis, which is thought to be a noninfectious condition complicating pelvic surgery, childbirth, or trauma.

P. aeruginosa osteochondritis of the foot follows puncture wounds of the foot, primarily in children. The organism infects the small joints and bones of the foot, including the proximal phalanges, metatarsals, metatarsophalangeal joints, tarsal bones, and calcaneus. *P. aeruginosa* shows a particular predilection for cartilage. Systemic symptoms are usually lacking. On average, symptoms last for several weeks. There may be plantar cellulitis over the involved area or tenderness upon deep palpation. Results of roentgenograms and bone scans are generally positive. Aspiration of the affected joint usually yields purulent material in which *P. aeruginosa* can be demonstrated by Gram's staining and by culture.

P. aeruginosa is one of the most common causative agents in a variety of other, less specific syndromes involving nonhematogenous infections of bones and joints and collectively referred to as *chronic contiguous osteomyelitis*. These infections may result, for example, from compound fractures, contamination associated with open reduction and fixation of closed fractures, sternotomy performed in conjunction with cardiac surgery, contiguous spread from infected ischemic ulcers related to peripheral vascular disease or diabetes mellitus, and cellulitis in general. The chronicity, indolence, and heterogeneity of these infections explain their varied clinical manifestations and the frequent need for complicated long-term management.

Gastrointestinal Infections *P. aeruginosa* infections involving virtually every portion of the human gastrointestinal tract—from oropharynx to rectum—have been documented. *P. aeruginosa*–associated gastrointestinal disease is most common among infants and among adults with hematologic malignancies and neutropenia. Moreover, asymptomatic large-bowel colonization resulting from prolonged exposure to the hospital environment and the selective pressure of antibiotics may be a silent source of organisms that subsequently invade the bloodstream during severe chemotherapy-induced neutropenia or other forms of immunosuppression.

P. aeruginosa causes necrotizing enterocolitis in infants and a similar disease in neutropenic patients with cancer. The most common sites of involvement are the distal ileum, cecum, and colon. The pathologic lesions are hemorrhagic and necrotic ulcers that begin in the bowel mucosa and extend into the submucosa. Vascular invasion by bacteria may be documented in the submucosa in association with bacteremia, local spread to the muscularis and serosa, and subsequent perforation leading to peritonitis. Necrotic ulcers are also documented occasionally in the oropharynx, esophagus, stomach, or proximal small bowel. Typhlitis, a disease developing most frequently in patients with leukemia, involves localized lesions of the cecum that are associated with necrosis and gangrene and that sometimes result in perforation, bacterial peritonitis, and early death; *P. aeruginosa* is the agent most commonly identified in this condition. This organism is also among the pathogens most frequently isolated from rectal abscesses in neutropenic patients with cancer. These lesions, which may be associated with few signs and symptoms, must be carefully sought in susceptible patients because they may give rise to life-threatening sepsis if not surgically drained.

P. aeruginosa has been implicated in epidemics of moderate to severe diarrhea in children, in a form of enteric fever sometimes referred to as *Shanghai fever*, and in a cholera-like illness attributed to a putative but still-unidentified *Pseudomonas* enterotoxin.

Urinary Tract Infections *P. aeruginosa* is one of the most common causes of complicated and nosocomial infections of the urinary tract. These infections may result from urinary tract catheterization, instrumentation, surgery, or obstruction; they may arise from persistent foci (e.g., the prostate or stones) and may be chronic or recurrent. The urinary tract may be a target for bloodborne infection in patients with *P. aeruginosa* bacteremia but more often is the source of bacteremia. Chronic *P. aeruginosa* infections of the urinary tract are relatively common among patients with indwelling Foley catheters, altered urinary tract anatomy secondary to diversionary procedures, and paraplegia.

The clinical features of urinary tract infections due to *P. aeruginosa* are usually indistinguishable from those of other bacterial infections. However, *P. aeruginosa* infections exhibit a propensity for persistence, chronicity, resistance to antibiotic therapy, and recurrence. More unusual forms of urinary tract involvement peculiar to *P. aeruginosa* include ulcerative lesions of the renal pelvis, ureters, and bladder that cause sloughing of vesical membrane in the urine and bacterial invasion of renal blood vessels that produces ecthyma-like lesions in association with *Pseudomonas* sepsis.

Skin and Soft Tissue Infections As indicated above, *P. aeruginosa* bacteremia may be associated with ecthyma gangrenosum. These disseminated skin lesions, which frequently begin as small vesicles, are characterized by hemorrhage, necrosis, surrounding erythema, and histologic evidence of blood vessel invasion by bacteria. *P. aeruginosa* can almost always be cultured from the lesions. Less common skin manifestations of *P. aeruginosa* sepsis include vesicular or pustular lesions, bullae, subcutaneous nodules, deep abscesses, and cellulitis. Metastatic lesions of the skin or mucous membranes complicate *Pseudomonas* sepsis and occasionally produce massive necrosis or gangrene of the extremities, perineum, face, or oropharynx.

Primary *P. aeruginosa* pyoderma occurs when the skin breaks down secondary to trauma, burn injury, dermatitis, or ulcers related to peripheral vascular disease or pressure sores. Moist conditions, such as those in the perineum or diaper area of infants, contribute to the development of *P. aeruginosa* pyoderma. Neutropenia also may predispose to this condition. The clinical appearance of primary *P. aeruginosa* pyoderma, which frequently includes hemorrhage and necrosis, resembles that of metastatic *P. aeruginosa* skin lesions. Histologic studies document vascular invasion by bacteria in both diseases. A rare distinguishing feature of *P. aeruginosa* pyoderma is its association with a blue-green exudate and a characteristic fruity odor.

P. aeruginosa wound sepsis complicating extensive third-degree burn injuries results from colonization of the burn site or burn eschar, invasion of the subeschar space and underlying dermis, vascular invasion, and systemic spread. The development and progression of *P. aeruginosa* burn wound sepsis are facilitated by the injury-associated breakdown of normal skin, antibiotic selection, and burn-related immune defects. Local manifestations include black, dark brown, or violaceous discoloration of the burn eschar; degeneration of underlying granulation tissue, hemorrhage, and premature eschar separation; edema, hemorrhage, and necrosis of skin adjacent to the burn site; erythematous nodular lesions in unburned skin; and formation of brown or black neoeschars. Systemic manifestations include fever or hypothermia, confusion or obtundation, oliguria, hypotension, ileus, and sometimes respiratory failure or pneumonia. The diagnosis of *P. aeruginosa* burn sepsis is based on these local and systemic clinical manifestations and on a burn wound biopsy that reveals both $>10^5$ colony-forming units of *P. aeruginosa* per gram of tissue and histologic evidence of bacterial invasion of unburned tissue, vasculitis, or intense inflammation at the burn margin.

P. aeruginosa causes diffuse pruritic maculopapular and vesiculopustular rashes associated with exposure to contaminated hot tubs, spas, whirlpools, and swimming pools. Most cases of *P. aeruginosa* dermatitis have occurred as part of a common-source outbreak. At least two nosocomial common-source outbreaks—one related to a physiotherapy pool—have been reported. Skin rashes may be limited to areas covered by swimsuits or may be more diffuse, sparing only the head and neck. Associated symptoms may include dizziness, headache, earache, sore eyes, sore nose, sore throat, swollen breasts, or abdominal cramps. Low-grade fever is uncommon. The illness is usually self-limited, and the rash resolves without specific therapy after cessation of exposure. One nosocomial outbreak involving immunocompromised patients, however, resulted in *P. aeruginosa* folliculitis evolving into full-blown ecthyma gangrenosum.

℞ TREATMENT

Most types of *P. aeruginosa* disease are treated with one or more antibiotics to which the infecting organism is sensitive. Exceptions are external otitis (nonmalignant) and dermatitis associated with exposure to contaminated water. Both of these infections are self-limited and usually require no specific antimicrobial therapy.

In general, the choice of antibiotics with antipseudomonal activity includes the aminoglycosides (e.g., gentamicin, tobramycin, netilmicin, amikacin), selected third-generation cephalosporins (e.g., ceftazidime, cefoperazone), selected extended-spectrum penicillins (e.g., ticarcillin, ticarcillin/clavulanate, piperacillin, piperacillin/tazobactam, mezlocillin, azlocillin), carbapenems (e.g., imipenem, meropenem), monobactams (e.g., aztreonam), and fluoroquinolones (e.g., ciprofloxacin, ofloxacin, enoxacin, lomefloxacin, norfloxacin). (For information on dosages and schedules, see Chap. 140.) All these agents except enoxacin, lomefloxacin, and norfloxacin are available in parenteral form; ciprofloxacin and ofloxacin are available in both oral and intravenous forms. It is noteworthy that because of sometimes variable antimicrobial activity against *P. aeruginosa* or distinctive pharmacokinetic properties, different members of a particular antibiotic class are not always interchangeable in the treatment of all *P. aeruginosa* infections. Ciprofloxacin, for example, demonstrates somewhat higher in vitro activity against many clinical isolates of *P. aeruginosa* than do other fluoroquinolones. Conversely, certain multiresistant strains of *P. aeruginosa* exhibit cross-resistance to antibiotics of different classes. Thus, local patterns of antimicrobial susceptibility should influence the initial choice of antibiotic agents, while the susceptibility profile of the isolate from a particular case should dictate definitive antibiotic therapy.

In most severe or life-threatening infections due to *P. aeruginosa*, two antibiotics to which the infecting strain is (or is likely to be) sensitive should be administered together. The combination of an aminoglycoside and a β-lactam antibiotic is usually appropriate. The goals of combined therapy are to achieve additive or synergistic killing, to exploit the pharmacologic strengths and offset the pharmacologic limitations of each agent, and to prevent the emergence of antibiotic resistance. Particularly in acute or fulminant infections, antibiotics should be employed at the maximal doses consistent with safety. Likewise, when sites of infection are relatively inaccessible (e.g., the central nervous system or the heart), maximal or even supramaximal antibiotic doses may be required for the attainment of therapeutic concentrations in infected tissues. In relatively indolent, self-limited, and often chronic infections due to *P. aeruginosa* (e.g., certain cases of chronic contiguous osteomyelitis or malignant external otitis), a single antimicrobial agent may be employed; an oral fluoroquinolone such as ciprofloxacin or ofloxacin may be appropriate under these circumstances, although such oral therapy must often be protracted if infection is to be eradicated. In addition, certain urinary tract infections due to *P. aeruginosa*, which are limited to the lower urinary tract, may be amenable to short-term treatment with a single antibiotic active against *P. aeruginosa*.

The appropriate duration of antibiotic therapy for disease caused by *P. aeruginosa* depends on the type, location, and severity of infection. Precise, prospectively defined treatment guidelines are sometimes problematic; it may be more appropriate to tailor the duration of therapy to the specific circumstances of a case, including the initial response to treatment. In general, chronic infections associated with extensive tissue injury, disruption of normal anatomy, foreign or prosthetic material, or suboptimal antibiotic accessibility require therapy for weeks or even months rather than days. More acute infections may be treated aggressively but for shorter periods.

P. aeruginosa infections of the lower respiratory tract in patients with cystic fibrosis pose a special challenge because these infections represent long-standing, chronic conditions complicated by acute exacerbations and a downhill course. Antibiotic therapy for acute exacerbations clearly results in clinical improvement. A more aggressive approach featuring periodic expectant courses of antimicrobial therapy may limit disease progression. Frequent pulmonary toileting is important in the management of this disease, while periodic bronchial lavage has been employed to good effect to relieve symptoms associated with mucus plugging. Aerosolized antibiotics also have been used successfully in some instances. Finally, lung transplantation has been employed with good results in selected cystic fibrosis patients with severe progressive lower respiratory tract infections due to *P. aeruginosa*.

Optimal management of infections due to *P. aeruginosa* often requires surgical intervention as well as antimicrobial therapy. The presence of necrotic tissue or of prosthetic or foreign material necessitates surgical debridement (e.g., in malignant external otitis and in some cases of chronic osteomyelitis or osteochondritis); loculated pus demands drainage (e.g., in sternoclavicular pyarthrosis, brain abscess, and endophthalmitis); left-sided endocarditis is an indication for early valve replacement; perforated bowel requires laparotomy and bowel resection (e.g., in necrotizing enterocolitis); and urinary tract obstruction may necessitate appropriate surgery.

PROGNOSIS All infections caused by *P. aeruginosa* are treatable and—with the possible exception of lung infections in patients with cystic fibrosis—are potentially curable. The heterogeneity of these infections, however, accounts for substantial differences in short- and long-term prognosis. At one end of the spectrum are acute fulminant infections such as bacteremic pneumonia, septicemia, burn wound sepsis, and meningitis, which are associated with extremely high mortality despite appropriate therapy. At the other end of the spectrum are more chronic, indolent infections, including certain cases of chronic contiguous osteomyelitis, malignant external otitis, and lower respiratory tract infections in patients with cystic fibrosis. Although the latter infections may not be imminently life-threatening, they are often difficult to eradicate and (as in the case of cystic fibrosis lung disease) may end fatally in the longer term.

INFECTIONS CAUSED BY OTHER *PSEUDOMONAS* SPECIES OR RELATED BACTERIA

Burkholderia cepacia (formerly *P. cepacia*), like *P. aeruginosa*, is primarily an opportunistic pathogen that is implicated in both endemic infections and occasional nosocomial outbreaks. Hospital epidemics are most frequently associated with a liquid reservoir or a moist environmental surface. Under these circumstances, the organism may colonize various body sites, with the subsequent development of invasive disease. The distinction between colonization and true infection is often difficult and may hinge on the presence of clinical signs of infection as well as a positive culture. *B. cepacia* has been reported to cause pneumonia, urinary tract infections, meningitis, peritonitis, surgical and burn wound infections, bacteremia, and endocarditis related to injection drug use. In addition, *B. cepacia* has been implicated, either alone or together with *P. aeruginosa*, in chronic infections of the lower respiratory tract in patients with cystic fibrosis. In some of these patients, the appearance of *B. cepacia* has been associated with fulminant necrotizing pneumonia, bacteremia, and a rapid downhill course.

The treatment of *B. cepacia* infections is complicated by the resistance of the organism to aminoglycosides and to many β-lactam agents. Although trimethoprim-sulfamethoxazole and chloramphenicol have been used successfully in the treatment of *B. cepacia* infections, resistance to these two antimicrobial agents has been reported. Third-generation cephalosporins and fluoroquinolones have variable activity against *B. cepacia*. However, ciprofloxacin and ampicillin/sulbactam may be considered as alternative agents for use against sensitive strains. While in vitro synergy has been demonstrated for certain antibiotic combinations, such as ciprofloxacin, imipenem, and rifampin, the clinical efficacy of such combinations has not been fully documented.

Stenotrophomonas maltophilia (formerly *X. maltophilia*) is a ubiquitous, free-living opportunistic pathogen that colonizes and occasionally infects hospitalized patients, particularly in an intensive care setting. This organism has been associated with pneumonia, urinary tract infection, wound infection, peritonitis, cholangitis, meningitis, bacteremia, and endocarditis. *S. maltophilia*, like *Pseudomonas* species, has been implicated in pseudoinfections, particularly pseudobacteremia related to contaminated blood-drawing materials. It is thus essential to consider clinical signs and symptoms in distinguishing exogenous contamination or simple colonization from genuine infection. Urinary tract infection is usually associated with a chronic indwelling urinary catheter or with urinary tract instrumentation; line-related sepsis complicates intravenous therapy; peritonitis has occurred in patients undergoing chronic ambulatory peritoneal dialysis; native valve endocarditis has been described in intravenous drug users; and prosthetic valve endocarditis also has been reported. Acute *S. maltophilia* pneumonia, an often devastating disease associated with bacteremia, is being seen with increasing frequency in debilitated patients on intensive care units.

Antibiotic resistance in *S. maltophilia*, based on both low outer-membrane permeability and inducible β-lactamases, is at least partly responsible for the emergence of this organism as a nosocomial pathogen under the selective pressure of antibiotic treatment. Trimethoprim-sulfamethoxazole is often useful for the treatment of infections due to drug-resistant strains. Alternative agents include ticarcillin/clavulanate, ciprofloxacin, and minocycline or doxycycline. The third-generation cephalosporins cefoperazone and ceftazidime may be active against *S. maltophilia* in some instances, but in vitro susceptibilities should be tested in each case. The aminoglycosides and imipenem are usually inactive.

Pseudomonas fluorescens occasionally causes human disease; it is implicated particularly often in infections related to the administration of contaminated (stored) blood products and in pseudoinfections. Additional bacterial species that are associated only rarely with human infections include *Pseudomonas putida*, *Pseudomonas stutzeri*, *Pseudomonas pseudoalcaligenes*, and (all formerly *Pseudomonas* species) *Burkholderia pickettii*, *Comamonas acidovorans*, *Comamonas testosteroni*, *Brevundimonas diminuta*, and *Brevundimonas vesicularis*.

MELIOIDOSIS Infections caused by *B. pseudomallei* constitute a broad spectrum of acute and chronic, local and systemic, clinical and subclinical disease processes collectively called *melioidosis*. *B. pseudomallei* and the infections it causes are found mainly in the tropics and are endemic in Southeast Asia and surrounding areas. *B. pseudomallei* is a free-living, small, motile, aerobic gram-negative rod previously classified in the rRNA homology group II of *Pseudomonas* and related species. The organism is a saprophyte that is normally found in soil, ponds, and rice paddies and on produce from endemic areas. It is occasionally a pathogen for animals. Humans contract the disease through soil contamination of abrasions, ingestion, nasal instillation, or inhalation. Person-to-person transmission is apparently rare.

Acute infections most often involve the lungs, although lesions sometimes develop in other organs. Pulmonary lesions tend to be more extensive and dissemination to other organs tends to be more widespread in subacute melioidosis. Acute abscesses exhibit necrosis, polymorphonuclear leukocyte infiltration, and surrounding hemorrhage; multinucleated histiocytes are observed in areas of necrosis. Subacute lesions, in contrast, are characterized by caseation necrosis, with mononuclear and plasma cell infiltration.

Melioidosis presents in different forms. High rates of seropositivity in endemic areas such as Vietnam, Thailand, and Malaysia suggest that many infections are clinically inapparent. The occasional diagnosis based solely on abnormal routine chest roentgenograms represents asymptomatic pulmonary infection. Acute, localized, suppurative skin infections associated with nodular lymphangitis and regional lymphadenitis result from direct inoculation at sites of minor skin trauma. Acute pulmonary infections may originate in the respiratory tract or result from hematogenous spread, their severity varying from mild bronchitis to extensive necrotizing pneumonia. Onset may be sudden or gradual. Fever, productive cough, and marked tachypnea are frequent. Chest roentgenograms typically reveal upper lobe consolidation or thin-walled cavities. Progressive upper lobe disease mimics tuberculosis.

Acute suppurative infections or pulmonary disease may give rise to hematogenous dissemination and the acute septicemic form of melioidosis. This progression is more likely in chronically debilitated patients, such as those with diabetes mellitus or alcoholism. Patients with pulmonary infections in particular may present with severe tachypnea, confusion, headache, pharyngitis, diarrhea, and pustular lesions of the head, trunk, and extremities. The skin may be flushed or cyanotic; signs of meningitis or arthritis may be apparent; the liver and spleen may be enlarged; and muscle tenderness may be striking. Chest roentgenograms show diffuse nodular densities that may expand, coalesce, and finally cavitate. The acute septicemic form of melioidosis usually follows a rapid downhill course, ending in early death unless arrested by early and aggressive therapy.

Chronic suppurative melioidosis is characterized by acute or chronic abscesses of the skin and various organs. Recrudescent disease arising from inactive sites of infection and perhaps triggered by intercurrent illness or other events may present in any acute or chronic form.

The diagnosis of melioidosis should be entertained when a febrile patient who has been in an endemic area presents with an acute lower respiratory tract illness associated with tachypnea, exhibits unusual skin or subcutaneous lesions, or has a chest roentgenogram suggesting tuberculosis in the absence of sputum-associated tubercle bacilli. An etiologic diagnosis may be made by microscopic demonstration of small, irregularly staining, gram-negative rods in exudate material; by characteristic bipolar ("safety-pin") staining of organisms with methylene blue; and by a culture positive for *B. pseudomallei* and/or a fourfold or greater rise in the titer of serum antibody to the organism.

℞ TREATMENT

The mainstay of treatment for melioidosis is antibiotic administration combined with appropriate surgical drainage of abscesses and aggressive support for patients with septicemic forms of the disease. The guidelines for antibiotic therapy are somewhat imprecise. Subclinical infection or mere seropositivity does not usually require specific therapy. Ceftazidime appears to be the agent of choice for clinical disease, while trimethoprim-sulfamethoxazole, cefotaxime, imipenem, and amoxicillin/clavulanate are possible alternatives. Therapy with a combination such as ceftazidime plus trimethoprim-sulfamethoxazole is indicated in severe forms of melioidosis. However, the resistance of many strains of *B. pseudomallei* to trimethoprim-sulfamethoxazole, particularly in Southeast Asia, necessitates other antibiotic choices. Acute septicemic infections probably should be treated with combinations of multiple agents administered parenterally. Patients with acute pulmonary infections should receive antibiotics for 60 to 150 days, while chronic disease associated with persistently positive sputum cultures may require longer treatment. Extrapulmonary suppurative disease is appropriately treated for 6 months to 1 year. When initial therapy for acute infections involves a third-generation cephalosporin such as ceftazidime, a switch can often be made after 30 days to an oral agent such as trimethoprim-sulfamethoxazole or amoxicillin/clavulanate.

Most cases of melioidosis are curable if appropriately treated. However, septicemic infections are still associated with very high mortality despite optimal therapy, while all forms of melioidosis are subject to possible early or very late recrudescence.

GLANDERS Glanders is primarily a systemic equine disease that is caused by *B. mallei* and is associated with pulmonary involvement, subcutaneous ulcerative lesions, and lymphangitis. Once widespread, glanders still occurs in Africa, Asia, and South America but not in the United States or western Europe. The infection may be communicated to humans during close contact with horses, mules, or donkeys, probably by cutaneous inoculation or nasal exposure to contaminated discharges. Glanders assumes the following forms in humans: acute localized suppurative infection, acute pulmonary infection, acute septicemic infection, and chronic suppurative infection. Inoculation of *B. mallei* into the skin usually produces a nodule with an area of lymphangitis. Fever, malaise, and prostration are common. Mucous membrane infection results in the production of a mucopurulent discharge from the eye, nose, or lips, with the subsequent development of granulomatous ulcers. Pulmonary infection secondary to inhalation of the organism is accompanied by typical local and systemic signs and symptoms of pneumonia. Lymphadenopathy and splenomegaly may be documented. Chest roentgenograms reveal circumscribed densities suggesting early lung abscesses; bronchopneumonia or lobar consolidation also may be evident. Chronic suppurative infection presents as multiple subcutaneous and intramuscular abscesses, particularly often involving the extremities; visceral lesions are documented in some patients. The acute septicemic form of glanders may be associated with a diffuse papular or pustular eruption, severe systemic symptoms, and early death.

The diagnosis of glanders may be suggested by the clinical setting (including a history of close contact with equines) and confirmed by culture of the causative agent from clinical material and by demonstration of *B. mallei*–specific seroconversion.

℞ TREATMENT

Optimal antimicrobial therapy for glanders has not been adequately defined. Sulfadiazine has proven effective historically both in animals and in humans. It has been suggested, however, that rational therapy consists of the same antibiotics recommended for the treatment of melioidosis, with the specific agent chosen on the basis of in vitro susceptibility testing. Antibiotics are administered for at least 30 days in uncomplicated infections and longer in complicated cases. Abscesses may require surgical drainage, and appropriate supportive measures are necessary in acute septicemic forms of the disease.

BIBLIOGRAPHY

P. AERUGINOSA INFECTIONS

Baltch AL, Smith RP (eds): *Pseudomonas aeruginosa Infections and Treatment.* New York, Marcel Dekker, 1994

Barker LF: The clinical symptoms, bacteriologic findings and postmortem appearances in cases of infection of human beings with the *Bacillus pyocyaneus.* JAMA 29:213, 1897

Bodey GP et al: *Pseudomonas* bacteremia: Retrospective analysis of 410 episodes. Arch Intern Med 145:1621, 1985

Fick RB (ed): *Pseudomonas aeruginosa: The Opportunist, Pathogenesis and Disease.* Boca Raton, CRC, 1992

Korvick JA, Yu VL: Antimicrobial agent therapy for *Pseudomonas aeruginosa.* Antimicrob Agents Chemother 35:2167, 1991

Morrison AF, Wenzel RP: Epidemiology of infections due to *Pseudomonas aeruginosa.* Rev Infect Dis 6(Suppl):S267, 1984

Pollack M: The virulence of *Pseudomonas aeruginosa.* Rev Infect Dis 6(Suppl):S617, 1984

———: *Pseudomonas aeruginosa,* in *Principles and Practice of Infectious Diseases,* 4th ed, GL Mandell et al (eds). New York, Churchill Livingstone, 1995, pp 1980–2003

INFECTIONS DUE TO RELATED ORGANISMS

Elting LS, Bodey GP: Septicemia due to *Xanthomonas* species and non-*aeruginosa Pseudomonas* species: Increasing incidence of catheter-related infections. Medicine 69:296, 1990

Goldmann DA, Klinger JD: *Pseudomonas cepacia:* Biology, mechanisms of virulence, epidemiology. J Pediatr 108:806, 1986

Murray AR et al: Blood transfusion–associated *Pseudomonas fluorescens* septicemia: Is this an increasing problem? J Hosp Infect 9:243, 1987

Pollack M: *Pseudomonas,* in *Infectious Diseases,* SL Gorbach et al (eds). Philadelphia, Saunders, 1992, pp 1502–1513

Tomashefski JF et al: *Pseudomonas cepacia*–associated pneumonia in cystic fibrosis. Arch Pathol Lab Med 112:166, 1988

MELIOIDOSIS

Leelarasamee A, Bovornkitti S: Melioidosis: Review and update. Rev Infect Dis 11:413, 1989

Sanford JP: *Pseudomonas* species (including melioidosis and glanders), in *Principles and Practice of Infectious Diseases,* 4th ed, GL Mandell et al (eds). New York, Churchill Livingstone, 1995, pp 2003–2009

---

158 Gerald T. Keusch

SALMONELLOSIS

The prototypic *Salmonella, S. choleraesuis,* mistakenly described by Theobald Smith in 1894 as the cause of the viral disease hog cholera, was named in honor of Smith's supervisor, Dr. Daniel Salmon. The genus is both vast and diverse. Of its more than 2300 distinguishable organisms, some can cause infections in humans, including typhoid fever (also known as enteric fever); focal systemic infections; septicemia; and (most commonly) diarrhea, varying from acute watery diarrhea to bloody diarrhea or dysentery. Salmonellae are ecologically entrepreneurial and exist in a multiplicity of habitats; this characteristic adaptability, which accounts for the ubiquity of the organisms in nature and for the many ways in which they encounter potential new human hosts, is related to their genetic plasticity.

ETIOLOGY Salmonellae are gram-negative bacillary members of the family Enterobacteriaceae that are almost always motile by means of multiple peritrichous flagella and with two exceptions are nonencapsulated. (*S. typhi* and *S. paratyphi* C express the Vi capsular polysaccharide.) The salmonellae are facultatively anaerobic and typically do not ferment lactose; these properties form the basis for their identification during initial screening in the microbiology laboratory. Taxonomy, typically the staid and stable domain of a few cognoscenti, has been in a state of flux for *Salmonella* in recent years, as the number of recognized species classified within the genus has varied from one to a few thousand. The current classification, based on DNA relatedness, recognizes only two species, *S. enterica* and *S. bongori,* the latter of which is not a human pathogen (Table 158-1). The choice of the designation *S. enterica* reflects a desire to avoid confusion with the prototypic organism described by Smith, *S. choleraesuis,* and the fact that none of the named isolates has previously been called *enterica. S. enterica* encompasses six subspecies, each of which includes multiple members (serovars). Most human pathogenic salmonellae fall within subspecies *enterica.*

The huge number of salmonellae distinguishable by serologic methods reflects the ability of the organisms to create mosaic flagellin genes through multiple recombinational events and horizontal transfer, point mutations, and gene duplications and alterations in length, all of which together may constitute an adaptive response to host immune defense systems. Since subspecies members are distinguished by serologic markers on polysaccharide somatic O antigens and protein flagellar H antigens, individual salmonellae are properly considered *serovars.* Thus, *S. typhi* should be called *S. enterica* subspecies *enterica* serovar typhi, while *S. typhimurium* would properly be designated *S. enterica* subspecies *enterica* serovar typhimurium. Because the majority of serovars have been named after the place in which they were first detected (for example, Heidelberg or Newport), *Salmonella* nomenclature seems more geographic than microbiologic. Nevertheless,

Table 158-1

Taxonomy of the Genus *Salmonella*, with Serogroups and Representative Serovars

Species	Subspecies	Serogroup	Common Serovars
S. enterica	(I) *enterica*	A	paratyphi A
		B	typhimurium, agona, derby, heidelberg, paratyphi B
		C	choleraesuis, infantis, virchow
		D	dublin, enteritidis, typhi
		E	anatum
	(II) *salamae*		
	(IIIa) *arizonae*		
	(IIIb) *diarizonae*		
	(IV) *houtenae*		
	(VI) *indica*		
*S. bongori**	—		

* Formerly subspecies V of *S. enterica.*

clinicians continue to use convenient abbreviated names such as *S. heidelberg* or *S. newport* to refer to these organisms. Therefore, this chapter also makes use of this shorthand system.

Another commonly used historic classification system for salmonellae groups isolates on the basis of the major representatives of the 60 phase-1 somatic antigens they express. These *serogroups* are designated by letters (A, B, C, etc.). Most human pathogenic salmonellae are members of groups A through D (Table 158-1); indeed, the serogroup designation is typically the first piece of specific data about an isolate to emerge from the clinical microbiology laboratory. Because just a few serovars cause most cases of human disease (see below), serogrouping offers a useful initial clue to the exact identity of the organism involved and also provides clinically useful diagnostic, prognostic, and therapeutic information.

Some salmonellae are highly adapted to human or other animal hosts. Animal-adapted strains generally do not cause human disease, while human-adapted strains often cause typhoid fever. The rest of the salmonellae are non-host-adapted organisms that may infect both humans and other animals. These organisms are the most common causes of *Salmonella* diarrhea.

TYPHOID FEVER

Typhoid fever is a distinctive acute systemic febrile infection of the mononuclear phagocytes and deserves separate consideration. Since it may be caused by several serovars (*S. typhi*, *S. paratyphi* A, *S. paratyphi* B, and occasionally *S. typhimurium*), many clinicians prefer the term *enteric fever*. However, because typhoid is fundamentally not an enteric disease, this term is also inappropriate. On balance, *typhoid fever* is still the best term, for it is understood by nearly all clinicians to describe a particular syndrome that is, in fact, due primarily to *S. typhi*.

EPIDEMIOLOGY Because the cause of clinical typhoid fever is almost always a human-adapted *Salmonella*, most cases can be traced to a human carrier. The proximate cause is most often water but may also be food contaminated by a human carrier. Chronic carriers are generally over 50 years old, are more commonly women than men, and often have gallstones. *S. typhi* resides in the bile (even inside stones), intermittently reaches the lumen of the bowel, and is excreted in the stool, thereby contaminating water or food.

With improvements in environmental sanitation in the United States, the incidence of *S. typhi* infection has dropped to a low level. From 1930 to 1950, the typhoid incidence—initially around 22 per 100,000—diminished by 90 percent (Fig. 158-1). From 1985 to 1994, an average of only 508 cases per year were identified in the United States, accounting for just over 1 percent of all *Salmonella* isolates.

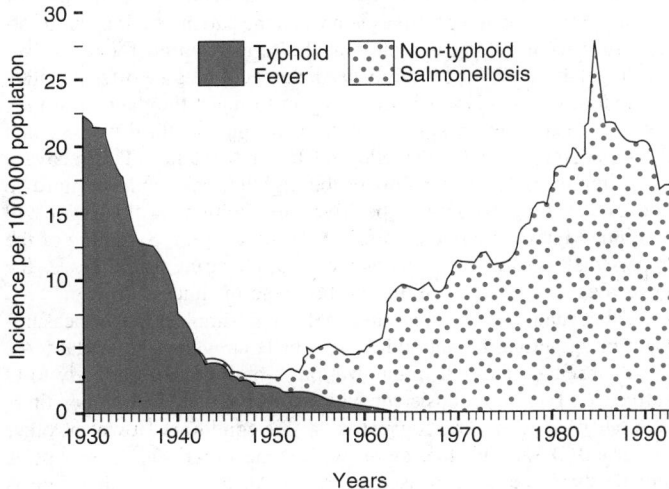

FIGURE 158-1 Incidence of typhoid fever and nontyphoidal salmonellosis in the United States, 1930–1994. (*Courtesy of Robert V. Tauxe, M.D., Centers for Disease Control and Prevention, Atlanta.*)

Even this small number greatly exceeds the figures for the isolation of paratyphoid organisms in the United States, of which two-thirds are *S. paratyphi* B. The majority of *S. typhi* infections take the form of active disease or convalescent carriage rather than chronic asymptomatic carriage. This pattern is consistent with the decline of domestically acquired infections in the United States. Most active cases are now acquired during travel abroad and involve children, adolescents, and young adults, whereas chronic carriers are most often in the seventh decade of life. In New York City, the proportion of typhoid cases that were related to travel increased from two-thirds to four-fifths from 1980 to 1990, and most of these cases followed travel to southern and Southeast Asia. Mexico remains the leading source of typhoid among residents of the United States, especially those in border states and traveling students; because there are so many travelers to Mexico, this problem is seen frequently even though the rate of acquisition of typhoid in Mexico is relatively low. Known global hotspots for typhoid fever include Peru, Alexandria (Egypt), Jakarta (Indonesia), India, Pakistan, and Nepal. In Santiago, Chile, the previously high endemic rate of typhoid has recently been reduced markedly by improvements in water quality and in the sanitation infrastructure.

Typhoid contracted in the United States is usually due either to contact with carriers or to large (common-source) or small (family-related) food-borne outbreaks, which are often associated with food handlers or domestic workers who are immigrants from endemic countries. Also at continuing risk of typhoid are bacteriology laboratory workers. The number of patients in the United States is clearly underestimated, and an unknown proportion of cases escape detection because appropriate cultures are not done or antibiotic treatment is administered before samples for culture can be obtained.

In *S. typhi*–endemic regions, the rate of clinical typhoid among persons positive for human immunodeficiency virus (HIV) is approximately 25-fold higher than that among HIV-negative individuals in the 15- to 35-year-old age group and is as much as 60-fold higher than that in the general population. Asymptomatic HIV-positive patients have a typical clinical presentation and response to therapy; AIDS patients can present with fulminant diarrhea and/or colitis and are far more likely to relapse. While this enhanced sensitivity has little practical significance for AIDS patients in countries with a low typhoid incidence, it may become a problem for those who travel to highly endemic countries.

PATHOGENESIS Infection is initiated by oral ingestion of organisms, which must pass the gastric acid barrier to establish infection. While experiments with volunteers have suggested that 10^5 organisms are required for the initiation of infection, buffering of acid by food lowers the necessary inoculum in natural exposures, and the actual infectious dose is probably considerably less than 10^5. Analysis of multiple studies of experimental *S. typhi* infection in healthy young adults, which generally have used a single laboratory strain (Quailes), has suggested no significant association between dose and severity of illness, although both a direct relation between dose and attack rate and an indirect relation between dose and incubation period exist (Table 158-2). Severity is determined by both host and microbial properties (as discussed below).

Salmonella exhibits a genetic adaptive acid-tolerance response: exposure to acid leads to synthesis of at least 40 proteins, some of which may play a role in pathogenesis. Bacteria successfully evading

Table 158-2

Response of Volunteers to Experimental Infection with *S. typhi*

Inoculum	Attack Rate	Mean Incubation Period, days
10^3	0/13 (0)	—
10^5	77/200 (38.5)	9.3
10^7	13/27 (48.1)	7.4
10^8–10^9	24/25 (96.0)	4.7

"acid death" in the stomach pass on to the distal ileum and colon, where they penetrate the mucosal barrier. Most new information about *Salmonella* pathogenesis has been derived from a combination of studies in cell culture and experimental infection with *S. typhimurium* in mice (which results in a typhoid-like illness in this species). It is curious that the infection of mice with *S. typhi* produces no clinical illness. The mechanism of penetration of mammalian cells by *S. typhi* appears to be similar to that for nontyphoidal salmonellae and is discussed below in relation to the latter organisms.

Initial bacterial invasion results in transient asymptomatic bacteremia, as organisms are rapidly ingested by mononuclear phagocytes within which they survive and multiply. This process is favored by a lack of bactericidal antibodies in the susceptible host; in contrast, opsonized salmonellae are taken up by neutrophils and killed. Opsonophagocytosis is limited by the capsular Vi polysaccharide of *S. typhi* (also expressed by *S. paratyphi* C and *Citrobacter freundii*), which enhances resistance to complement activation and bacterial lysis by the alternative pathway as well as to peroxide-mediated killing. Another apparent microbial determinant of the host-pathogen interaction is flagellar type. Flagellar type H1-j bacteria, which have been associated with infection only in Indonesia, affect older individuals and cause milder illness than flagellar type H1-d bacteria. The fate of organisms within macrophages depends both on microbial factors that promote resistance to killing and on specific host T lymphocyte–activated, cell-mediated immune mechanisms that are under the genetic control of the *ity* locus in mice. This locus, which was identified in studies of the resistance of inbred mouse strains to infection with *S. typhimurium*, turned out to be of more general relevance and identical to the *lsh* and *bcg* loci mediating resistance to other intracellular pathogens such as *Leishmania* species and *Mycobacterium bovis* strain BCG. The human variant of the *ity/lsh/bcg* locus, *Nramp* (natural resistance-associated macrophage protein), is present on chromosome 2q35. *Nramp*, which is actually a family of at least three genes linked to the genes for the interleukin (IL) 1 receptor and the IL-8 receptor gene cluster, encodes a macrophage-specific membrane transport protein needed for the early killing of intracellular pathogens by a mechanism that remains uncertain but is distinct from those of activated macrophages.

When intracellular multiplication has proceeded enough to permit the initiation of persistent bacteremia, the clinical phase of typhoid fever begins with invasion of the gallbladder and Peyer's patches of the intestine. The sustained bacteremia is responsible for the persistent fever of clinical typhoid, while inflammatory responses to tissue invasion determine the pattern of clinical expression (cholecystitis, intestinal hemorrhage, or perforation). With invasion of the gallbladder and Peyer's patches, bacteria regain entry to the bowel lumen and may be recovered in stool cultures beginning in the second week of clinical disease. Seeding of the kidney leads to positive urine cultures, albeit in a much lower percentage of patients than have positive blood cultures. The lipopolysaccharide (endotoxin) of *S. typhi* may contribute to fever, leukopenia, and other systemic symptoms, but the occurrence of such symptoms in individuals rendered tolerant to endotoxin supports a role for other factors, such as cytokines released from infected mononuclear phagocytes, that can mediate inflammation (see Chap. 17).

CLINICAL MANIFESTATIONS The incubation period of typhoid fever is variable and depends on both the inoculum size and the state of the host's defenses. A range of 3 to 60 days has been reported. The disease classically presents with a steplike daily increase in temperature (up to 40 to 41°C) associated with headache, malaise, and chills. The hallmark of typhoid fever is prolonged, persistent fever (4 to 8 weeks in untreated patients). The illness may be mild and brief; however, in some cases, acute, severe infection with disseminated intravascular coagulation and central nervous system involvement rapidly results in death. In other instances, necrotizing cholecystitis or intestinal bleeding and perforation can occur in the third or fourth week of illness, when the patient is otherwise improving. In most cases, the onset of these complications is dramatic and clinically

obvious. Intestinal perforation appears to be less common among children under 5 years of age.

Early intestinal manifestations include constipation (especially in adults) or mild diarrhea (in children) associated with abdominal tenderness. Mild hepatosplenomegaly is detectable in the majority of patients. Bradycardia relative to the height of the fever may be a clinical clue to typhoid but is present in only a minority of patients. Epistaxis may be noted in the early stages of illness. "Rose spots," appearing as small, pale red, blanching, slightly raised macules, are occasionally seen on the chest and abdomen during the first week. They can evolve into nonblanching small hemorrhages that are difficult to see in dark-skinned patients. The major characteristics of untreated typhoid are persistent high fever, severe anorexia, weight loss, and changes in sensorium, but a variety of other complications also may develop, including hepatitis, meningitis, nephritis, myocarditis, bronchitis, pneumonia, arthritis, osteomyelitis, parotitis, and orchitis. Except for that of relapse, the frequency of all these complications, including hemorrhage and perforation, is reduced by prompt use of appropriate antibiotics. Typhoid, long considered to be uncommon and typically mild in young children, may in reality be frequent and severe in this group. Neonatal typhoid, which can be acquired vertically from infected mothers or from exogenous sources, is often a severe, life-threatening septicemic illness with a high case-fatality rate.

Multidrug-resistant *S. typhi* is becoming more prevalent in many endemic countries. Patients infected with resistant strains present with more severe illness, look "toxic," and have a higher incidence of disseminated intravascular coagulation and hepatomegaly and a three-fold higher mortality rate that is thought to be related to the longer duration of disease and to prior ineffective oral antibiotic therapy.

Around 3 to 5 percent of patients become long-term asymptomatic carriers, some for life unless treated. Many carriers give no history of typhoid fever and probably have had an undiagnosed mild infection.

LABORATORY FINDINGS AND DIAGNOSIS In around 25 percent of patients, leukopenia and neutropenia are evident. In most patients, the white blood cell count is normal, albeit low in relation to the degree of fever; this pattern may be a clue to the diagnosis. Severe leukopenia (<2000 cells/µL) is found in rare instances. In the event of intestinal perforation or pyogenic complications, secondary leukocytosis develops. The anemia of blood loss may be superimposed on the anemia of chronic infection.

Whereas definitive diagnosis still depends on isolation of the organism, the overall yield of culture is disappointingly low. The yield is affected by several variables: when the cultures are performed, what is cultured, and whether the patient has taken antibiotics. The rate of recovery of organisms from blood is highest in the first week of illness, approaching 90 percent among untreated patients; the figure falls to less than 50 percent by the third week. Yields can approach 100 percent when blood and bone marrow both are cultured; bone marrow cultures are frequently positive even when the patient is taking antibiotics. Buffy-coat culture can shorten the time required for a positive result, but this technique is rarely used. Stool cultures are often negative in the first week, when it is most urgent to make the diagnosis; they become positive in 75 percent of cases during the third week, when the organism reinvades the bile and Peyer's patches. The recovery rate diminishes to 10 percent by the eighth week, and one-third to one-half of the patients with positive stool cultures at this point will continue to have positive cultures for at least 1 year. Sampling of the upper-small-bowel secretions by means of the string test increases the yield over that of stool culture at this stage of illness.

Other diagnostic tests are available. The simplest is the measurement of agglutinating antibodies to O or H antigens (the Widal test). In the absence of recent immunization, a high titer of antibody to O antigen (>1:160) is consistent with acute typhoid, and higher titers (>1:640) are even more suggestive of this condition. However, other serogroup D salmonellae, along with some organisms in groups A and B, share the antigen used in the Widal test, which therefore is not specific. Antibodies to H antigens may be found in even higher titer but, because of their broad cross-reactivity, are difficult to interpret. A fourfold rise in antibody titer between paired serum samples is strong evidence for infection; however, such a rise is of little use in the management of the acutely ill patient, and the antibody response may be blunted by early, effective antibiotic therapy. Recently developed latex agglutination or coagglutination tests for antibody to the Vi antigen appear to be much more specific and sensitive than classic Widal tests. Sensitivities are 95 percent or higher, with very low rates of false negativity; however, these new tests either are not commercially available or are not in common use. In some studies in developing countries with high incidences of typhoid fever, coagglutination is much more reliable than culture because so many patients have already taken antibiotics before being seen by a physician. Promising new enzyme immunoassays that detect *S. typhi* outer-membrane proteins are being evaluated. A sensitive and specific multiplex polymerase chain reaction for Vi antigen promises to be highly sensitive and specific, but its value has not been proved in clinical studies, nor is it available yet.

DIFFERENTIAL DIAGNOSIS When all the classic clinical manifestations are present, including rose spots, prolonged fever, relative bradycardia, and leukopenia, the diagnosis of typhoid will be strongly suggested. However, most cases do not fit this "typical" profile. Differential diagnosis includes infections associated with prolonged fever, such as the rickettsioses, brucellosis, tularemia, leptospirosis, miliary tuberculosis, viral hepatitis, infectious mononucleosis, cytomegalovirus infections, and malaria, as well as noninfectious causes of fever, such as lymphoma (see Chap. 17). In the United States, typhoid should be considered in any patient with prolonged, unexplained fever, especially after recent travel to places with endemic typhoid fever.

℞ TREATMENT

Since its introduction, chloramphenicol has been the antimicrobial "gold standard" for treatment. No drug has been better in promoting a favorable clinical response, which usually becomes apparent within 24 to 48 h of the start of treatment in the appropriate dosages (3 to 4 g/d in adults or 50 to 75 mg/kg of body weight per day in young children). The drug is given orally for 2 weeks; the dose may be reduced to 2 g/d or 30 mg/kg per day when the patient becomes afebrile—usually by day 5 of treatment. However, because of the specter of aplastic anemia associated with chloramphenicol, the drug is little used in the United States. Other effective oral regimens include amoxicillin (4 to 6 g/d in four divided doses in adults or 100 mg/kg per day in children), trimethoprim-sulfamethoxazole (640 and 3200 mg, respectively, in two divided doses daily in adults or 185 mg of the trimethoprim component per square meter of body surface area per day in children), or—for patients over 17 years of age—a 4-fluoroquinolone such as ciprofloxacin or ofloxacin.

A variety of intravenous drugs are also effective. Both chloramphenicol and trimethoprim-sulfamethoxazole can be given intravenously to patients who cannot take oral medications. Other effective parenteral antimicrobials include high-dose ampicillin, cefotaxime, cefoperazone, and the 4-fluoroquinolones. However, none has been as rapidly acting or as effective as ceftriaxone, which rivals or betters chloramphenicol in rapidity of defervescence. Initial recommendations for a 7-day course of ceftriaxone have been pared down (to 3 days of 2 to 4 g once daily in adults or 5 days of 50 to 80 mg/kg once daily in children) without apparent loss of efficacy. In addition, compared with that for other drugs, the relapse rate for ceftriaxone appears lower.

The prevalence of resistance to multiple first-line oral drugs has been rising among strains of *S. typhi* in developing countries, especially in the Indian subcontinent and Southeast Asia, due to the acquisition of plasmids encoding inactivating β-lactamases and chloramphenicol acetyl transferases. Where multidrug resistance is a problem, ceftriaxone or a 4-fluoroquinolone should be administered initially to adults over 17 years of age, and ceftriaxone is the best choice for children because of concerns about quinolone-induced arthropathy and cartilage damage in this age group. Recent safety studies employed magnetic resonance imaging in the evaluation of children 8 months to 13 years of age who had received ciprofloxacin

at a daily dosage of 15 to 25 mg/kg for 9 to 16 days; these studies found no bone or cartilage damage, and follow-up measurements 2 years later detected no abnormality in height. Short-course (3-day) quinolone therapy has been shown to be effective against multidrug-resistant typhoid in children, and its use further reduces the likelihood of drug toxicity. Alternative oral agents that reportedly are effective for this indication include furazolidone (7.5 mg/kg per day) and cefixime (5 mg/kg every 12 h). The high cost of ceftriaxone is somewhat offset by the efficacy of a short course and the economy of once-daily dosing.

Studies in Indonesia of patients with severe typhoid who presented with central nervous system manifestations and/or evidence of disseminated intravascular coagulation suggested that intravenous dexamethasone (3 mg/kg as a loading dose over 30 min, followed by 1 mg/kg every 6 h for 24 to 48 h), used along with parenteral antimicrobials, reduces mortality. Salicylates should be avoided to diminish the danger of intestinal hemorrhage. Prompt surgical management of bleeding and bowel perforation reduces mortality, since a fatal outcome is associated primarily with peritonitis. Bowel perforations should be closed in two layers for best results. The antibiotics selected should cover not only *S. typhi* but also the facultative and anaerobic bowel flora. Selective angiography, radioisotopic scanning methods, and sometimes endoscopy (see Chap. 282) to localize the bleeding site can facilitate operative repair. In developing countries, however, patients often present late after perforation, are poor surgical candidates, and may be severely malnourished, and only limited surgical and postoperative care may be available. Supportive medical care and antibiotics alone have been recommended in this setting, although limited surgery to close the perforation site without bowel resection is increasingly favored. With double-layer closure of the lesion, aggressive fluid replacement, and administration of an inexpensive broad-spectrum antibiotic regimen including chloramphenicol, gentamicin, and metronidazole, mortality rates have been reduced from 25 to 30 percent to well under 10 percent.

The early use of effective antimicrobials is associated with a relatively high rate of relapse; relapse rates of 20 percent can be expected, whereas the figure is only 5 to 10 percent in untreated patients. Presumably, prompt therapy inhibits the development of an adequate immune response. Relapses are usually milder than the initial attack and respond to the same antimicrobial used initially.

Eradication of the chronic carrier state, especially in the presence of gallstones, is notoriously difficult. Traditional regimens have used ampicillin or amoxicillin (100 mg/kg per day) plus probenecid (30 mg/kg per day) or trimethoprim-sulfamethoxazole (160/800 mg twice daily) plus rifampin (600 mg once daily) for at least 6 weeks. Recent studies suggest that a 4-week course of a 4-fluoroquinolone is at least as good and probably much better because the organism is exquisitely sensitive in vitro and the drugs reach the gut lumen, liver, gallbladder, and bile in active form. The new quinolones provide the best chance of eradicating *S. typhi* in the presence of gallstones; for reasons of simplicity and safety, they should be the first-choice agents for the treatment of patients without stones as well. The optimal dose and duration of quinolone treatment have yet to be defined. These drugs are the best choice for chronic suppression of typhoid relapse in AIDS patients.

PREVENTION AND CONTROL Worldwide experience has shown that improvement of environmental sanitation, including sewage disposal and water supplies, will sharply reduce the incidence of typhoid fever. Where this approach is not yet possible and for travelers, immunization has been used. Traditional heat-killed, phenol-extracted whole typhoid vaccine is no longer recommended because of its limited efficacy and duration of protection and the high frequency of local reactions and fever. One option for children over 6 years of age and adults consists of three doses of a first-generation live oral vaccine (Ty21a), which is invasive but metabolically defective and dies after a few cycles of replication. This vaccine is safe, provides as much protection as the killed vaccine, and continues to be protective for at least several years. One dose of purified Vi polysaccharide vaccine has proved as effective and long-lasting as multiple doses of Ty21a and may be used in children over 2 years of age and in at-risk HIV-infected patients. New genetically engineered live typhoid vaccine strains are being developed, not only for immunization against typhoid but also for use as live vectors into which extraneous genes can be cloned for oral delivery of protective antigens from unrelated species. In addition, Vi-protein conjugates are being evaluated as immunogens suitable for infants, especially in endemic regions where infantile typhoid is prevalent and remains a dangerous disease.

Typhoid is a reportable disease in the United States. Patients should be monitored for prolonged carriage and treated if necessary. Precautions in food handling by carriers and in disposal of their stools are obviously important (see Chap. 138).

PROGNOSIS Appropriate therapy for typhoid fever, especially if patients present for medical care in the early stage of disease, is highly successful. The mortality rate should be under 1 percent, and few complications other than relapse should occur.

NONTYPHOIDAL SALMONELLOSIS

An infection caused by any *Salmonella* organism other than *S. typhi* is termed *nontyphoidal salmonellosis*. Such an infection can present as acute diarrhea, a septicemic syndrome, focal abscesses, meningitis, osteomyelitis, endocarditis, or mycotic aneurysm or can be asymptomatic.

EPIDEMIOLOGY The species *S. enterica* includes a diverse group of host-adapted and non-host-adapted serovars. Two human-adapted serovars, *S. paratyphi* A and *S. schottmuelleri* (more often called *S. paratyphi* B), mimic *S. typhi* and cause a mild form of typhoid fever. Of the more than 2300 known serovars, just 10 account for two-thirds of all human-disease isolates in the United States, and four serovars (*S. typhimurium*, *S. enteritidis*, *S. heidelberg*, and *S. newport*) cause about three-fifths of all disease cases (Table 158-3). Periodic increases in the recovery of certain serovars represent either the introduction of a new transmission source or the occurrence of a large outbreak. A fivefold increase in the recovery of *S. enteritidis* isolates between 1976 and 1986 was due to ingestion of contaminated intact grade-A eggs, primarily in the northeastern United States. The number of infections from this source continued to increase, and by 1992 *S. enteritidis* overtook *S. typhimurium* as the most frequently isolated *Salmonella* serovar in the United States and in all countries of Europe. These changes suggested a new global pandemic related primarily to infected poultry eggs.

Surveillance data in the United States indicate that not only the number but also the incidence of nontyphoidal *Salmonella* isolates is increasing (Fig. 158-1). The incidence of disease is five times higher among young children than among older subjects and increases again in adults over 70 years of age. Between 1970 and 1986, the median age of infected individuals rose from 6 years to 20 years and has since remained the same. The greatest increase has been in the 20- to 39-year-old population; this observation suggests that foods consumed by young adults are important vehicles or that persons in this age group are traveling more to endemic areas. For example, the emergence of serious systemic infections in southern California due to *S. dublin* carrying a high-virulence plasmid has been associated with the ingestion of unpasteurized dairy products or nontraditional nutritional treatments containing raw calf-liver extracts contaminated with this serotype. A reasonable estimate of the total incidence of symptomatic nontyphoidal *Salmonella* infection in the United States is around 2 million cases per year. The degree of morbidity represented by this figure implies a significant economic impact in terms of lost productivity and medical costs and, by extension, a serious and underestimated cause of mortality.

Because nontyphoidal salmonellae are so often non-host-adapted, many kinds of domestic animals can harbor the organisms and serve as a source for human infection. From 50 to 75 percent of broiler and layer chicken flocks in Canada are infected with a wide variety of *Salmonella* serovars, many of which are virulent for humans. At laying, intact eggs of naturally infected layer flocks may be positive for low numbers of organisms belonging to serovars virulent for humans; however, growth to large numbers quickly takes place if the eggs are not kept at 4°C. At such levels of contamination, viable organisms will survive cooking by any method. If an egg rests for a short time on infected hen feces or even on the dry bedding of an infected hen, *Salmonella* can penetrate the surface of the shell through microscopic pores normally present in the shell. Because the epidemic due to *S. enteritidis* is so extensive and thus so unlike salmonellosis associated with cracked eggs, and because it has involved free-range as well as commercial henhouse eggs, a transovarian route is most likely and poses a problem for infection control. The conditions in which raising, shipping, slaughtering, and marketing take place contribute to the spread of *Salmonella* in the food supply. Introduction of the organism into processed foods, including commercial milk-chocolate products, can result in widespread dissemination, and contamination of such common foods as eggs or milk leads to large-scale outbreaks, including nosocomial epidemics. Dried or frozen foods preserve viable salmonellae. For these reasons, salmonellosis is more a disease of the industrialized world than of the developing world. Additional sources of human infection are animals sold as pets, including baby chicks, ducks, and turtles, and medical products of animal origin, such as carmine dye (from insects), pancreatin, bile salts, or tissue extracts from thyroids, adrenals, stomachs, or rattlesnakes.

A potentially serious problem is the selection of antibiotic-resistant salmonellae by unregulated drug use in animal husbandry. Persistent and severe salmonellosis also has been recognized as a problem among patients with AIDS (see Chap. 308).

PATHOGENESIS As with *S. typhi*, the events following ingestion of other salmonellae are determined by environmental factors (dose), microbial factors (the ability to invade epithelial cells, to multiply within mononuclear phagocytes, and to resist intestinal peptide antibiotic defensins), and host resistance factors (the effects of gastric acid, the rapid mobilization of phagocytic cells, and the activation and expansion of clones of T cells involved in protection, such as V gamma 9–bearing γ/δ T cells). As few as 10^3 virulent organisms may cause disease, especially in persons who have achlorhydria or who have recently received antimicrobial therapy. Systemic invasion is more likely in patients with "reticuloendothelial blockade" due to hemolysis (e.g., in malaria, barto-

Table 158-3

The Ten Most Common *S. enterica* Isolates in the United States in 1994

Rank	Serovar	Serogroup	No. of Isolations	Percentage (Cumulative Percentage) of All *Salmonella* Isolations
1	enteritidis	D	10,009	26.1 (26.1)
2	typhimurium	B	8479	22.1 (48.2)
3	heidelberg	B	1855	4.8 (53.0)
4	newport	C_2	1698	4.4 (57.4)
5	hadar	C_2	1033	2.7 (60.1)
6	agona	B	766	2.0 (62.1)
7	montevideo	C_1	639	1.7 (63.8)
8	oranienburg	C_1	616	1.6 (65.4)
9	muenchen	C_2	562	1.5 (66.9)
10	thompson	C_1	560	1.5 (68.4)

SOURCE: Centers for Disease Control and Prevention, Annual Surveillance Report, 1994.

nellosis, leptospirosis, or sickle cell anemia) or intracellular infections (e.g., histoplasmosis) and may be facilitated by the expression of bacterial plasminogen receptors, the conversion of bound plasminogen to enzymatically active plasmin, and subsequent degradation of the extracellular matrix. Documented bacteremia varies in incidence from 5 to 45 percent but is assumed to occur early in the course of many, and possibly all, *Salmonella* infections. Bacteremia is quickly cleared by patients infected with most *S. enteritidis* serovars. *S. dublin*, *S. infantis*, *S. virchow*, *S. panama*, and *S. newport* may be especially invasive; virulence is associated with an 80-kb plasmid in *S. dublin*. *S. typhimurium* isolates from the bloodstream are significantly more likely to hybridize with a probe from the highly conserved *Eco*RI fragment of the *S. dublin* plasmid than are fecal isolates (rate of hybridization, 76 vs. 42 percent). Bacteremia may lead to focal tissue infections. *S. choleraesuis*, a highly invasive serotype, usually causes a septicemia syndrome and is commonly isolated from blood but not from stool. Microbial factors that determine the invasiveness of salmonellae include motility and the presence of chromosomal and plasmid genes needed for invasion and replication within mononuclear phagocytes. Many of these genes are turned on by contact of the organism with host cells and are regulated by a two-component sensing/signaling system, *PhoP/PhoQ*.

Invasion occurs across the small-intestinal mucosa. In *Shigella* infection, the organism multiplies within epithelial cells; in contrast, in *Salmonella* infection, epithelial cells represent a barrier to be crossed by the organism, not an ecologic niche for its survival. Invading salmonellae induce a dramatic ruffling of the plasma membrane of the mammalian cell that is regulated by *PhoP/PhoQ* and reflects cytoskeletal rearrangements leading to uptake of the organism within phagosome-like vesicles, its transit across the cell, and its release into the lamina propria. A multigene chromosomal locus, *inv*, encodes the invasive phenotype and shares homology with genes of other invasive bacteria. *PhoP/PhoQ* also regulates the resistance of salmonellae to host intestinal antibacterial defensins. Invasion activates cell signaling pathways, including mitogen-activated protein kinase; phospholipase A_2; release of arachidonic acid; production of prostaglandins and leukotrienes (especially leukotriene D_4); and a sharp increase in intracellular calcium level. Many of these changes are known to alter electrolyte transport and may cause diarrhea. Invasion and inflammation are necessary but not sufficient to cause *Salmonella* diarrhea in experimental animal models, and transepithelial signals that recruit neutrophils are also involved via induced local chemokine (IL-8) production. Some salmonellae appear to produce a molecule similar to cholera toxin that increases electrolyte and fluid secretion. However, the importance of this molecule in causing diarrhea remains uncertain.

CLINICAL MANIFESTATIONS Gastroenteritis The incubation period of *Salmonella* gastroenteritis is generally short (24 to 48 h). Sporadic illness is likely to go undiagnosed because specimens are not taken for culture. Large outbreaks, often considered "food poisoning" and characterized by self-limited fever and diarrhea, are more likely to be investigated and diagnosed. Diarrhea may be associated with nausea, vomiting, and abdominal cramps and occasionally is bloody or even dysenteric when the colon becomes involved. Direct microscopic examination of stool shows many leukocytes, which offer a clue to the invasive nature of the infection. The illness is generally mild and resolves without specific therapy, but it may cause severe dehydration or disseminate and lead to death in debilitated elderly patients or neonates. Blood cultures obtained initially often become positive as the patient's condition is improving. Treatment may be discontinued after identification of the organism unless there is an underlying immunosuppressive disease (e.g., sickle cell disease, AIDS, or a malignancy such as a lymphoma) or the patient is receiving glucocorticoid or immunosuppressive drug therapy. In these conditions, an appropriate antibiotic should be administered for 7 to 10 days. Carriage of salmonellae in the stool continues for several weeks after the resolution of symptomatic disease but rarely persists for longer than 2 months.

Localization of Systemic Infections Bloodborne salmonellae can invade any tissue or organ. The most common isolates are *S.*

typhimurium, *S. enteritidis*, *S. virchow*, *S. dublin*, and *S. choleraesuis*. Localized infections usually follow intestinal infection, although there may be no prior diarrhea. Endocarditis is rare but, when it occurs, may include destructive cardiac lesions such as valve perforations or ring or septal abscesses. Therapy may require both the administration of appropriate antimicrobials and surgery (see Chap. 126).

Arterial infection generally occurs in persons with preexisting arteriosclerotic infrarenal aortic aneurysms and is especially likely in men over the age of 50 years. *S. choleraesuis* accounts for about 20 percent of arterial infections but is isolated from fewer than 1 percent of patients with *Salmonella* diarrhea; this distribution reflects the capacity of this organism to cause systemic invasive disease. *S. typhimurium* accounts for approximately 25 percent of isolates in arterial infections—a finding consistent with its high prevalence in gastrointestinal salmonellosis. In addition to treatment with antimicrobials, eradication usually requires prompt excision and drainage with bypass through uninvolved tissue. The disease should be suspected when elderly men develop prolonged fever accompanied by back, abdomen, or chest pain following gastroenteritis; when bacteremia occurs or recurs after therapy for the initial illness; or when bacteremia develops in patients with vertebral osteomyelitis or prosthetic valves.

Cholecystitis, other *hepatobiliary infection*, and *splenic abscess* are the most common intraabdominal localized infections due to *Salmonella*. In addition to *S. typhimurium* and *S. enteritidis*, *S. typhi* is an important cause.

Urinary tract infections due to *Salmonella* sometimes develop. These illnesses are especially likely in patients who have urolithiasis, structural abnormalities, or immunosuppressive diseases or who are receiving immunosuppressive therapy. *Salmonella* urinary tract infections can coexist with renal tuberculosis or with *Schistosoma haematobium* infection.

Pneumonia or *empyema* caused by *Salmonella* is rare. These conditions usually involve patients with preexisting abnormalities of the lungs or pleura or with conditions that predispose to infection, including malignancy, diabetes, glucocorticoid use, sickle cell disease, or alcohol abuse.

Meningitis caused by *Salmonella* is also rare and is most prevalent among infants and young children. Gram's stains of cerebrospinal fluid are usually positive. Mortality rates of 40 and 60 percent are reported for children and adults, respectively. In survivors, residua include seizures, hydrocephalus, subdural empyemas, and permanent disabilities such as retardation, paresis, athetosis, and visual disturbances.

Septic arthritis due to *Salmonella* is associated with positive joint-fluid cultures and should not be confused with reactive arthritis (a culture-negative inflammatory joint disease following invasive diarrheas, especially in HLA-B27–positive patients). Common underlying conditions include glucocorticoid or immunosuppressive drug therapy, sickle cell disease, prosthetic joints, or aseptic necrosis. Drainage may be needed in addition to appropriate antibiotic therapy.

Salmonella osteomyelitis is predictably associated with sickle cell disease. It generally affects the long bones and occurs primarily in young patients. Blood cultures are often positive; the most common isolate is *S. typhimurium*.

Bacteremia Sepsis, with prolonged fever and positive blood cultures but generally without prior diarrhea, occurs most commonly with *S. choleraesuis* or *S. dublin* infection. While this presentation is "typhoidal," typical manifestations of typhoid (rose spots, relative bradycardia, leukopenia) are lacking, and the illness is more acute in onset than typhoid. *S. choleraesuis* or *S. dublin* sepsis is a severe disease that is associated with high mortality.

Intermittent symptomatic *Salmonella* bacteremia is seen in patients with hepatosplenic or urinary schistosomiasis. Clinically severe *Salmonella* sepsis due to *S. typhimurium* also occurs in AIDS patients (see Chap. 308), is often recurrent, and is an AIDS-defining event. The infection may be refractory to treatment or recurrent despite appropriate therapy. The incidence of salmonellosis among AIDS patients in the United States is estimated at 46 to 384 per 100,000, which is 100- to 1000-fold greater than the incidence in the general population (0.3 per 100,000).

DIAGNOSIS Specific diagnosis depends on the isolation of salmonellae from stool, blood, or tissue fluids. All clinical laboratories should be able to make the initial isolation and identify common serovars. Uncommon serovars usually must be sent to reference laboratories for identification.

℞ TREATMENT

Choice of antibiotic is complicated by the increasing prevalence of antimicrobial resistance (including multiple-drug resistance) among nontyphoidal salmonellae as well as in *S. typhi*. The use of antibiotics in commercial animal rearing, the prevalence of *Salmonella* in the global food chain, and the growing international commerce in meat, poultry, and processed food products are contributing to the wider distribution of resistant clones.

In the face of these complications, treatment for focal systemic infections requires the selection of the most appropriate antibiotic and, at times, drainage or resection of infected tissue. Bactericidal antibiotics, administered by the parenteral route, are usually chosen. The regimen may include ampicillin (6 to 12 g/d for adults or 100 mg/kg for young children, in divided doses) or appropriate doses of third-generation cephalosporins such as ceftriaxone. Unless resistance is prevalent, chloramphenicol (2 to 4 g/d for adults or 50 mg/kg for children, in divided doses) remains a good choice in developing countries because it can be given orally and is inexpensive. The new quinolones are highly effective, in part because they act on the intracellular compartment and thus affect bacteria within host mononuclear cells; while concerns remain about their safety in infants and children, increasing evidence suggests that the risk of cartilage damage is small.

The proper treatment of *Salmonella* gastroenteritis is not clear; the traditional dogma has been that antibiotics do not shorten the illness but do increase the duration of convalescent carriage. For this reason, it has generally been recommended that antimicrobial agents not be used in this illness. Initial highly favorable results with the new quinolones are now balanced by a number of contradictory studies. The best recommendation at present is that antimicrobial therapy be reserved for patients with severe disease and for patients at high risk of invasive disease.

Positive blood cultures in the setting of otherwise uncomplicated gastroenteritis do not warrant antibiotic therapy. When an infant under 3 months of age has diarrhea and signs of systemic invasion, a workup to localize the septic process should be initiated and presumptive treatment with a third-generation cephalosporin administered until culture results are available. Fever is often absent in very young infants and is not a reliable indicator of systemic infection. Asymptomatic patients with salmonellae other than *S. typhi* in the stool should *not* receive antimicrobial treatment, since active disease may be provoked and the carriage state is generally self-limiting. A quinolone would be a good choice for the treatment of long-term carriers.

PREVENTION AND CONTROL It is not possible to eradicate nontyphoidal salmonellosis because the organisms are so widespread in nature. Reduced animal-feed use of antimicrobials employed for the treatment of human infection and improved animal-rearing and animal-marketing practices would be useful. Vigilance in food preparation and in quality testing of the known and commonly contaminated foods should help as well. It is recommended that eggs not be eaten raw or partially cooked, especially by persons at high risk of infection; however, even fully cooked eggs can harbor viable *Salmonella*. If universal body-substance precautions are not routinely utilized, hospital staff caring for patients with salmonellosis should observe "enteric precautions," wearing gowns and gloves when handling stool and urine and carefully washing their hands after patient contact (see Chap. 138).

During outbreaks, food handlers may be responsible for transmission. Much effort is given to the identification (by stool culture) of asymptomatic food handlers who are carriers during food-borne outbreaks; these individuals are usually kept away from work until they become culture-negative. (The predictive value of three consecutive stool cultures negative for *Salmonella* is 95 percent.) However, it is more important that standards are maintained to ensure the environmental and personal hygiene of food handlers and thus to prevent the problem in the first place, since carriage may be intermittent and is often not uniform within a single stool sample and since foods contaminated with the organism require improper handling to permit the growth of a sufficient inoculum to cause disease. It may be justifiable to restrict carriers from the workplace only in the course of a hospital outbreak or when workers refuse to improve their personal hygiene.

The development of effective vaccines for nontyphoidal salmonellosis may be difficult because of the great number of serovars involved in infection. Some progress has been made with galactose epimerase and aroA vaccine mutants of *S. typhimurium* for use in animals, and these vaccines may ultimately be tested in humans. It would be most useful to have vaccines for *S. choleraesuis*, *S. typhimurium*, and *S. enteritidis*. *S. dublin* and *S. virchow*, while quite virulent, are still uncommon causes of human disease.

BIBLIOGRAPHY

ACHARYA G et al: Treatment of typhoid fever: Randomized trial of a three-day course of ceftriaxone versus a fourteen-day course of chloramphenicol. Am J Trop Med Hyg 52:162, 1995

CELLIER M et al: Human natural resistance–associated macrophage protein: cDNA cloning, chromosomal mapping, genomic organization, and tissue-specific expression. J Exp Med 180:1741, 1994

DUPONT HL: Quinolones in *Salmonella typhi* infection. Drugs 45(Suppl 3):119, 1993

GLYNN JR et al: Infecting dose and severity of typhoid: Analysis of volunteer data and examination of the influence of the definition of illness used. Epidemiol Infect 115:23, 1995

GRUNEWALD R et al: Relationship between human immunodeficiency virus infection and salmonellosis in 20- to 59-year-old residents of New York City. Clin Infect Dis 18:358, 1994

GUINEY DG et al: Plasmid-mediated virulence genes in non-typhoid *Salmonella* serovars. FEMS Microbiol Lett 124:1, 1994

HENNESSY TW et al: A national outbreak of *Salmonella enteritidis* infections from ice cream. N Engl J Med 334:1281, 1996

IVANOFF B et al: Vaccination against typhoid fever: Present status. Bull World Health Organ 72:957, 1994

LAHTEENMAKI K et al: Bacterial plasminogen receptors: In vitro evidence for a role in degradation of the mammalian extracellular matrix. Infect Immun 63:3659, 1995

LEE LA et al: Increase in antimicrobial-resistant *Salmonella* infections in the United States, 1989–1990. J Infect Dis 170:128, 1994

McCORMICK BA et al: Transepithelial signaling to neutrophils by salmonellae: A novel virulence mechanism for gastroenteritis. Infect Immun 63:2302, 1995

MILLS SD, FINLAY BB: Comparison of *Salmonella typhi* and *Salmonella typhimurium* invasion, intracellular growth and localization in cultured human epithelial cells. Microb Pathog 17:409, 1994

PAVIA AT et al: Epidemiologic evidence that prior antimicrobial exposure decreases resistance to infection by antimicrobial-sensitive *Salmonella*. J Infect Dis 161:255, 1990

PRADHAN KM et al: Safety of ciprofloxacin therapy in children: Magnetic resonance images, body fluid levels of fluoride and linear growth. Acta Paediatr 84:555, 1995

RIESENBERG-WILMES MR et al: Role of the acid tolerance response in virulence of *Salmonella typhimurium*. Infect Immun 64:1085, 1996

SCHAAD UB: Use of the quinolones in paediatrics. Drugs 45(Suppl 3):37, 1993

TRAN TH et al: Short-course ofloxacin for treatment of multidrug-resistant typhoid. Clin Infect Dis 20:917, 1995

TUMBARELLO M et al: The impact of bacteraemia on HIV infection. Nine years experience in a large Italian university hospital. J Infect 31:123, 1996

WILCOX MH, SPENCER RC: Quinolones and *Salmonella* gastroenteritis. J Antimicrob Chemother 30:221, 1992

WORKMAN MR et al: *Salmonella* bacteraemia in sickle cell disease at King's College Hospital: 1976–1991. J Hosp Infect 27:195, 1994

SHIGELLOSIS

DEFINITION *Shigellosis* is an acute infectious inflammatory colitis due to one of the members of the genus *Shigella*. Although the disease is often referred to as "bacillary dysentery," many patients have only mild watery diarrhea and never develop dysenteric symptoms. Less severe illness predominates in industrialized countries such as the United States, whereas more severe, often fatal dysentery occurs in patients in developing countries.

ETIOLOGIC AGENT Shigellae are slender, gram-negative, nonmotile bacilli and are members of the family Enterobacteriaceae and the tribe Escherichieae. They are so closely related to *Escherichia coli* that the two genera cannot be distinguished by DNA hybridization methods. In fact, *Shigella* can be thought of as a differentiated pathogenic *E. coli*. The four *Shigella* species (*S. dysenteriae*, *S. flexneri*, *S. boydii*, and *S. sonnei*) are defined on the basis of surface somatic O antigens and carbohydrate fermentation patterns. Most are lactose-negative (*S. sonnei* is a late lactose fermenter) and produce acid but not gas from glucose, resulting in a typical acid butt and alkaline slant in triple sugar iron agar without H_2S production. The genus is characterized by its ability to invade intestinal epithelial cells and to cause infection and illness in humans, even when the inoculum is small (a few hundred to a few thousand organisms).

EPIDEMIOLOGY Worldwide, it is estimated that at least 140 million cases of shigellosis and almost 600,000 deaths due to shigellosis occur annually among children under the age of 5 years, primarily in developing countries. The organism is found everywhere in the world but is most common where poor environmental sanitation and crowding facilitate transmission from person to person. A major outbreak took place in the makeshift camps for refugees fleeing the Rwandan civil war in 1994, with thousands of cases and high mortality.

Data collected by the Centers for Disease Control and Prevention in the United States from 1967 through 1988 suggest an average annual incidence of 6 *Shigella* infections per 100,000 population, with periodic hyperendemic increases (primarily due to large outbreaks of *S. sonnei* infection) raising the rate to between 9 and 10 per 100,000. On the basis of these data, the annual number of episodes of shigellosis in the United States is estimated at 25,000 to 30,000. Incidence rates approximate 27 per 100,000 among children 1 to 4 years of age but are only 2.6 per 100,000 among persons 20 years of age or older. Cases are detected most commonly in counties with a relatively high proportion of low-income minority-group residents, including African Americans, Hispanics, and Native Americans; rates are especially high in poor urban communities, in day-care centers, and among retarded children in custodial care.

A comparison with rates among rural Guatemalan Indian children during the same period puts this disease burden into perspective. A prospective surveillance study among 321 such children revealed an annual incidence of nearly 10,000 per 100,000.

Since the description of the genus *Shigella*, major global shifts in the prevalence of its four species have been noted. Until World War I, *S. dysenteriae* type 1 was the predominant isolate, frequently causing devastating epidemics with high mortality until it was replaced by *S. flexneri*. Since World War II, however, *S. flexneri* has been steadily replaced by *S. sonnei* in the industrialized countries. The reasons for these shifts are not clear. *S. boydii*, the fourth species, has remained largely confined to the Indian subcontinent.

Shigella is highly host-adapted and is a natural pathogen only of humans and a few other primates. Transmission from person to person takes place by the fecal-oral route, generally via direct contact but sometimes through contaminated vectors such as food, water, flies, and fomites. The organism can even be transmitted during participation in recreational water sports in fecally contaminated pools or lakes and can spread rapidly among confined populations in close contact—for example, in day-care centers, in institutions for the mentally retarded, on cruise ships, or among military personnel. *Shigella* is one of several pathogens associated with *gay bowel syndrome*. These cases are commonly transmitted by anal-oral sexual practices and are almost always due to *S. flexneri*; homosexual young men may be a major reservoir for these organisms in the United States (see Chap. 308).

Shigellosis is associated with a high rate of secondary household transmission. As many as 40 percent of children and 20 percent of adults who are household contacts of a case (generally a preschool child) will develop *Shigella* infection; the infection is often symptomatic in children but asymptomatic in adults, who seem to have an acquired immunity. In contrast, epidemic disease affects all ages, with clusters of severe and fatal cases in the very young and the very old. Since 1969, epidemic *S. dysenteriae* type 1 has reappeared in Latin America, in the Indian subcontinent and elsewhere in Asia, and in central and southern Africa and has been associated with relatively high mortality rates due to antimicrobial resistance and inadequate diagnosis and case management. Prolonged asymptomatic carriage is uncommon; unless there is underlying malnutrition, the organisms are generally cleared in a few weeks.

PATHOGENESIS AND PATHOLOGY Shigellae are orally ingested and, because they survive low pH more easily than other enteric pathogens (a genetically regulated property), seem to have little difficulty in passing the gastric acid barrier. An essential step in pathogenesis is invasion of colonic epithelial cells and cell-to-cell spread of infection. This step involves initial attachment of the organism to colonic cells, entry by an endocytic mechanism in which organisms are initially encased in and then escape from plasma membrane–enclosed vesicles, and a jet propulsion–like movement to the epithelial cell surface that is powered by bacterium-induced actin polymerization at the trailing end of the organism. This sequence of events not only provides the organism with a means to evade host defenses but also allows its effective local spread. Although invasion is initially innocuous, subsequent intracellular multiplication causes cell damage and death, ultimately resulting in characteristic mucosal ulcerations.

These events are extremely complicated and require the functions of multiple genes and regulatory elements encoded on both the chromosome and a large 120- to 140-MDa plasmid present in all virulent shigellae as well as on enteroinvasive *E. coli* (EIEC), which cause a *Shigella*-like disease. The number of structural and regulatory genes known to be involved in pathogenesis continues to increase as the process continues to be dissected. Some of these gene products induce the phagocytosis-like uptake of the organism by causing rearrangements of the host cell's cytoskeleton. Once a single *Shigella* organism has invaded a single host cell, the entire process of bacterial escape from the phagocytic vesicle into the host cell's cytoplasm, multiplication, and cell-to-cell spread can take place without exposure of the bacterium to the extracellular milieu and to the host's defenses.

It was originally thought that shigellae invade the host across the intestinal epithelial cells; however, recent studies using cell culture or a rabbit-ileum in vivo model suggest that the initial invasion may occur via the antigen-sampling M cell. The resulting limited penetration by organisms initiates an inflammatory response and alters the functional integrity of tight junctions between epithelial cells. These changes allow more organisms to breach the mucosal barrier at intercellular junctions. Subsequent neutrophil infiltration of the lamina propria appears to be essential to the development of illness and is associated with dramatically increased invasion. If neutrophil migration is directly inhibited by the treatment of animals with antibody to CD18, the escalating invasion by microorganisms does not take place.

Escape from the phagocytic vesicle is necessary for the virulence of shigellae and permits multiplication of the organisms in the cytoplasm. The multiplying organisms spread within the cytoplasm to the plasma membrane of the host cell and then from cell to cell. This spread is achieved by the polymerization of actin at the back end of the dividing bacteria (defined relative to the subsequent direction of motion). Binding and cross-linking by the host protein plastin result in a sphincter-like contraction that provides a forward propulsive force. This so-called actin motor is energized by ATP generated by a microbial-encoded ATPase called *IcsA*, which is, at the same time, phosphorylated and regulated by cyclic nucleotide-dependent protein kinases of the host. Phosphorylation may serve as a molecular host-defense mechanism to modulate virulence, limiting microbial spread.

Another important host protein involved in pathogenesis of shigellosis is the cadherin L-CAM, which is essential in the cell-to-cell spread of infection. Mutations in L-CAM alter the long finger-like protrusions induced by shigellae when they reach the plasma membrane and impair their subsequent fusion with the plasma membrane of the adjacent cell, thus inhibiting the transfer of the bacterium from one cell to another. Ultimately, the invaded host cell dies, possibly as a result of apoptosis induced by or during the process of microbial invasion.

Another property of apparent importance in virulence for *S. dysenteriae* type 1 is the ability to produce Shiga toxin, which is encoded by the iron-regulated chromosomal gene *stx*. Shiga toxin is composed of two distinct peptide subunits, each with highly conserved active regions. The first, located on the larger A subunit, is an *N*-glycosidase that hydrolyzes adenine from specific sites of ribosomal RNA of the mammalian 60S ribosomal subunit, irreversibly inhibiting protein synthesis. The second common region is a binding site on the B subunit that recognizes glycolipids of target cell membranes that terminate in a galactose $\alpha1\rightarrow4$-galactose disaccharide. The glycolipid Gb3, containing a gal-gal-glu trisaccharide, is a specific receptor present on toxin-sensitive rabbit intestinal villus cells but not crypt cells, and toxin action is specific for the former.

Wild-type toxigenic *S. dysenteriae* causes more severe illness in primates than does an isogenic toxin-negative mutant. The toxin of this organism, the prototype of a family of related toxin proteins produced by enterohemorrhagic *E. coli* (EHEC), appears to play a role in the pathogenesis of microangiopathic complications, hemolytic-uremic syndrome (HUS), and thrombotic thrombocytopenic purpura: only toxin-producing shigellae and *E. coli* are associated with these systemic illnesses. Two new *Shigella* enterotoxins, ShET-1 and -2, have been described; the former is restricted almost exclusively to *S. flexneri* 2a, whereas the latter is distributed more widely (e.g., on the physiologically similar EIEC). The two enterotoxins are encoded by chromosomal and plasmid genes, respectively. Both toxins alter electrolyte transport by segments of gut in vitro and cause net fluid secretion in vivo in ligated rabbit ileal loops. Moreover, both toxins induce antibody in infected humans. However, their role (if any) in the pathogenesis of the watery diarrhea phase of shigellosis remains uncertain.

In shigellosis, the epithelial surface of the human colon shows extensive ulcerations, with an exudate consisting of desquamated colonic cells, polymorphonuclear leukocytes, and erythrocytes; the ulcerations may resemble a pseudomembrane in severely affected areas. Marked mucus depletion and increased mitotic activity are evident in the crypt regions and presumably reflect a response to the loss of surface colonic cells. The lamina propria is edematous and hemorrhagic and is infiltrated by neutrophils and plasma cells. There is also swelling of capillary and venular endothelial cells, with margination of neutrophils. At the ultrastructural level, bacteria can be seen within vesicles as well as free in the cytoplasm. Histologic examination of colon from dysenteric humans shows an alteration of mucosal endothelial cells similar to that induced by endotoxin (lipopolysaccharide, or LPS). Shiga toxin (protein) targets endothelial cells as well, especially when toxin receptor expression is upregulated by exposure to LPS or proinflammatory cytokines. Levels of circulating LPS are high in *S. dysenteriae* type 1 infection and somewhat lower in *S. flexneri* infection, even without bacteremia. The frequency of endotoxemia in shigellosis suggests a broader role for LPS in the pathogenesis of the disease. One likely mechanism is related to the ability of LPS to induce cytokine gene transcription and the strong association of cyto-

kine secretion and inflammation. However, bacterial invasion of the mucosa itself activates the transcription factor NF-kappa B, which is involved in regulation of cytokine synthesis. Cytokine-producing cells are present in the mucosa of patients infected with *S. dysenteriae* or *S. flexneri* and in their stools as well. In fact, the number of cells producing interleukin 1, interleukin 6, interferon α, and tumor growth factor β is directly related to the severity of the inflammation. Inflammatory changes in *Shigella* infection thus appear to be components of the pathogenesis of dysentery as much as they are a consequence of the bacterial invasive process.

Epidemiologic evidence indicates that immunity develops and is serotype specific. The precise nature of this immunity is not known. Common surface outer-membrane proteins involved in invasion elicit serum antibodies; however, these are cross-reactive among *Shigella* species and serotypes and do not seem to be protective. The serotype-specific determinants are likely to be somatic antigens, as serum antibody to LPS predicts resistance to infection, and there is evidence of IgA-mediated mucosal responses to LPS during convalescence from shigellosis.

CLINICAL MANIFESTATIONS The spectrum of clinical shigellosis was shown in a study in which volunteers ingested 10,000 organisms of *S. flexneri* type 2a. While approximately one-quarter of the volunteers never became ill, over the first 24 to 48 h approximately 25 percent developed transient fever, another 25 percent had fever and self-limited watery diarrhea, and the remaining 25 percent had fever and watery diarrhea that progressed to bloody diarrhea and dysentery. In young children in particular, the temperature can rise rapidly to 40° to 41°C, and fever sometimes results in generalized seizures. These seizures rarely recur or result in serious sequelae. Dysentery is characterized by frequent passage (usually 10 to 30 times per day) of small-volume stools consisting of blood, mucus, and pus; this diarrhea is accompanied by abdominal cramps and tenesmus—the painful straining with stooling that may lead to rectal prolapse, especially in young children. Severe dysentery is most likely in infection due to *S. dysenteriae* type 1 or *S. flexneri* and least likely in *S. sonnei* infection. Patients with mild disease generally recover without specific therapy in a few days to a week. Severe shigellosis can progress to toxic dilatation and colonic perforation, which may be fatal.

Endoscopy shows the mucosa to be hemorrhagic, with mucous discharge and focal ulcerations and sometimes with overlying exudate. The majority of lesions are in the distal colon and progressively diminish in the more proximal segments of large bowel. Mild dehydration is common among patients with watery diarrhea; severe dehydration is very rare. With extensive colonic involvement, protein-losing enteropathy can occur and can have important adverse nutritional consequences, especially for already poorly nourished children.

A variety of *extraintestinal complications* of shigellosis have been described. The majority arise in patients in developing countries and are related both to the prevalence of infections due to *S. dysenteriae* type 1 and *S. flexneri* and to the poor nutritional state of the host. For example, bacteremia, thought to be relatively infrequent in the United States, develops in up to 8 percent of patients hospitalized for shigellosis in Dacca, Bangladesh. The causative *Shigella* species is isolated from half the patients; other Enterobacteriaceae are found in the remainder. Bacteremia is associated with higher-than-usual mortality and is more common among infants under 1 year of age and among persons with protein-energy malnutrition. Persistent and clinically severe *Shigella* bacteremia has been encountered in the United States in patients with AIDS (see Chap. 308).

HUS may occur with *S. dysenteriae* type 1 infection. In the United States, the more likely cause of HUS is one of the hemorrhagic colitis–causing strains of *E. coli* (such as *E. coli* O157:H7) that produce high levels of Shiga-family toxins. HUS usually develops toward the end of the first week of shigellosis, when dysentery is already resolving. Oliguria and a marked drop in hematocrit (by as much as 10 percent within 24 h) are the first signs and may progress to anuria with renal failure and to severe anemia with congestive heart failure, respectively. Even with advanced therapy, 5 to 10 percent of patients with HUS die of the acute illness. In addition, renal damage progresses slowly over several decades in survivors, an estimated 50 percent of whom develop significant renal failure and most of whom require long-term dialysis or renal transplantation. Leukemoid reactions, with leukocyte counts of more than 50,000/μL, may occur along with HUS; thrombocytopenia (with 30,000 to 100,000 platelets/μL) is common. Profound hyponatremia and severe hypoglycemia may be documented. Central nervous system abnormalities include encephalopathic symptoms, seizures, altered consciousness, and bizarre posturing.

Less common extraintestinal manifestations include seizures in some patients and reactive arthritis in others; both of these manifestations are usually due to infection with *S. flexneri* strains. In patients expressing histocompatibility antigen HLA-B27, the full triad of Reiter's syndrome sometimes develops (see Chap. 317). Pneumonia, meningitis, vaginitis (in prepubertal girls), keratoconjunctivitis, and "rose spot" rashes are rare events.

DIAGNOSIS AND LABORATORY FINDINGS Shigellosis is the principal bacterial cause of dysentery and should be considered whenever a patient presents with bloody diarrhea. However, in the United States, because *S. sonnei* is the most common species, most patients present with fever and nonbloody watery diarrhea indistinguishable from signs caused by other bacterial or viral agents of mild to moderate diarrhea, while many patients with bloody diarrhea have EHEC as the cause. The specific diagnosis is based on culture of *Shigella* from the stool; however, diagnosis by the polymerase chain reaction is possible, and a commercial enzyme immunoassay to detect Shiga-family toxins in stool can identify most patients infected with *S. dysenteriae* type 1 or EHEC within 3 h. The yield of *Shigella* is increased if the organism is sought by stool culture when the patient has fecal leukocytes or bloody diarrhea. The organism is very labile and must be transferred quickly to plates or holding media (such as buffered glycerol saline) if it is to survive. Stool samples are preferable to swabs; when the latter are used, a rectal sample should be obtained. More than one selective medium should be used for culture—i.e., MacConkey and one other, such as Hektoen enteric or xylose-lysine-deoxycholate.

Serologic tests can be performed, since antibodies to somatic antigens develop early in the acute phase of disease. However, the resources for such tests are not generally available, and serologic assessments usually are used only for epidemiologic studies.

The differential diagnosis includes inflammatory colitis due to other microbial agents: EHEC, EIEC, *Campylobacter jejuni*, *Salmonella enteritidis*, *Yersinia enterocolitica*, *Clostridium difficile*, and the protozoan *Entamoeba histolytica*. Ulcerative colitis and Crohn's colitis are among the conditions with "noninfectious" causes that should be considered (see Chap. 286). All these infections except that due to *E. histolytica* are associated with the presence of large numbers of fecal leukocytes. Amebiasis can be diagnosed by the detection of erythrophagocytic trophozoites in the stool (see Chap. 215).

Other laboratory studies are nonspecific and may disclose neutrophilic leukocytosis, anemia due to blood loss with hemorrhagic diarrhea, prerenal azotemia, or (if watery diarrhea has been pronounced) hyperchloremic acidosis. Laboratory findings in shigellosis complicated by HUS are discussed above.

℞ **TREATMENT**

The mild to moderate dehydration in shigellosis is readily corrected with oral rehydration solutions (see Chap. 161). The role of antibiotic therapy is variable and depends on the organism and the severity of disease. Since *S. sonnei* infection is usually self-limited, culture results generally do not become available until the patient is better and there is little clinical need for further therapy. The use of antibiotics in severe cases with bloody diarrhea or dysentery reduces the duration of illness and can shorten the carriage state. Resistance to sulfonamides, streptomycin, chloramphenicol, and tetracyclines is almost universal, and many shigellae are now resistant to ampicillin and trimethoprim-sulfamethoxazole as well. Knowledge of the pattern of resistance in a given population, which can change with time, is useful. In the United States, multiresistant strains are most likely to be acquired during travel abroad, and either ampicillin (50 to 100 mg/kg per day in children or 2 g/d in adults, in divided doses) or trimethoprim-sulfamethoxazole (8/40 mg/kg per day in children or 2 regular-strength tablets twice a day in adults, given for 5 days) is generally recommended. Short courses of treatment (1 or 3 days) or even single doses of drugs like tetracycline and ciprofloxacin have been employed with success and may soon become the standard. Amoxicillin should *not* be substituted for ampicillin because it is not effective against shigellosis. In developing countries, where resistance to both of these drugs is commonplace, the drug of choice for the treatment of multiresistant *S. dysenteriae* type 1 infections has been nalidixic acid (55 mg/kg per day for 5 days); however, resistance to the latter agent is increasing in prevalence. The 4-fluoroquinolones (e.g., ciprofloxacin) are highly effective against all strains (see Chap. 140) but are currently too costly in the Third World and are not yet approved for use in children under 17 in the United States; these drugs have caused cartilage damage in young rodents during toxicity tests, although there is no evidence for a similar effect of therapeutic doses in humans. Alternative drugs shown to be effective include oral pivamdinocillin (amdinocillin, pivoxil, pivmecillinam; still not available in the United States) and intravenous ceftriaxone (50 mg/kg per day for 5 days). In small-scale clinical trials, cephalexin has had no effect in limiting symptoms; single doses of ceftriaxone may be effective, but more information is needed. No antibiotic treatment is recommended for the convalescent carrier state, which usually lasts no more than several weeks. Patients with AIDS may develop chronic carriage of *Shigella* and may be subject to relapsing infection with bacteremia (see Chap. 308). This cycle may be interrupted by prolonged (several weeks') treatment with a quinolone.

The role of antimotility agents such as atropine sulfate and diphenoxylate (Lomotil) and loperamide (Imodium) in the early phases of shigellosis is controversial. Loperamide, in particular, may reduce diarrhea and in one study was highly effective in combination with antimicrobials. However, these antimotility drugs are suspected of enhancing the severity of disease by delaying excretion of organisms and thus facilitating further invasion of the mucosa. Therefore, they are contraindicated for the treatment of infants and young children. In adults, these agents are contraindicated for use in the dysenteric phase of disease.

Treatment of complications of shigellosis often differs in developed and developing countries. For example, antibiotic-unresponsive toxic megacolon, with or without perforation, is often managed by colectomy in the United States. Surgery is less often employed in developing countries because of a lack of availability or difficulties in ileostomy management. HUS often requires dialysis. In developing countries, dialysis may be needed relatively infrequently because azotemia is slow to develop and the risk of significant hyperkalemia is often diminished by a preexisting deficiency in total-body potassium, with malnutrition and wasting of lean body mass. The management of hyponatremia, usually caused by inappropriate secretion of antidiuretic hormone (vasopressin), is governed by the severity of the condition and the symptomatic state of the patient, as outlined in Chap. 49. Infusion of glucose can reverse clinical manifestations caused by hypoglycemia, and responses can be monitored by fingerstick blood glucose tests if no biochemistry laboratory is available. Optimal nutritional management is needed to correct deficiencies due to underlying malnutrition as well as the superimposed catabolic stress and protein-losing enteropathy of shigellosis. Nutritional support should begin during the acute illness and may be required for months thereafter (see Chap. 78).

PREVENTION Direct-contact transmission of shigellosis can be prevented by appropriate environmental and personal hygiene. Hand washing with soap and water, decontamination of water supplies, use of sanitary latrines or toilets, and precautions in the preparation and storage of food can all reduce the primary and secondary transmission of *Shigella* infection. In highly endemic developing countries, infants are protected during the period of exclusive breast feeding, which should be encouraged. Any measures that reduce the burden of malnutrition will also reduce the burden of shigellosis in the population. Stool precautions should be instituted for hospitalized infected patients to ensure safe disposal of infected excreta and linens, and hospital personnel must wash their hands and medical instruments (such as stethoscopes) after each contact with an infected patient. Cohorting of asymptomatic infected children, use of antibiotics to reduce infectiousness, and scrupulous attention to hygiene are usually successful in nosocomial outbreaks. Children in day care must be kept at home while clinically ill and ideally should have a negative stool culture before returning to the day-care facility. Likewise, food handlers who develop shigellosis should be culture-negative before returning to work. Antibiotic treatment is not indicated for the asymptomatic carrier state. No effective vaccine is available.

BIBLIOGRAPHY

ACHESON DWK et al: The family of Shiga and Shiga-like toxins, in *Sourcebook of Bacterial Protein Toxins*, JE Alouf, JH Freer (eds). London, Academic Press, 1991, pp 415–433

BENNISH ML, SALAM MA: Rethinking options for the treatment of shigellosis. J Antimicrob Chemother 30:243, 1992

BRIAN MJ et al: Evaluation of the molecular epidemiology of an outbreak of multiply resistant *Shigella sonnei* in a day-care center by using pulsed-field gel electrophoresis and plasmid DNA analysis. J Clin Microbiol 31:2152, 1993

COLES FB et al: Shigellosis outbreaks at summer camps for the mentally retarded in New York State. Am J Epidemiol 130:966, 1989

CRUZ JR et al: Infection, diarrhea and dysentery caused by *Shigella* species and *Campylobacter jejuni* among Guatemalan rural children. Pediatr Infect Dis J 13:216, 1994

FASANO A et al: Shigella enterotoxin 1: An enterotoxin of *Shigella flexneri* 2a active in rabbit small intestine in vivo and in vitro. J Clin Invest 95:2853, 1995

GOLDBERG MB, SANSONETTI PJ: *Shigella* subversion of the cellular cytoskeleton: A strategy for epithelial colonization. Infect Immun 61:4941, 1993

GOMA EPIDEMIOLOGY GROUP: Public health impact of Rwandan refugee crisis: What happened in Goma, Zaire, in July 1994? Lancet 345:339, 1995

HOFFMAN RE, SHILLAM PJ: The use of hygiene, cohorting, and antimicrobial therapy to control an outbreak of shigellosis. Am J Dis Child 144:219, 1990

KRISTJANSSON M et al: Polymicrobial and recurrent bacteremia with *Shigella* in a patient with AIDS. Scand J Infect Dis 26:411, 1994

LEE LA et al: Hyperendemic shigellosis in the United States: A review of surveillance data for 1967–1988. J Infect Dis 164:894, 1991

LEVINE OS, LEVINE MM: Houseflies (*Musca domestica*) as mechanical vectors of shigellosis. Rev Infect Dis 13:688, 1991

LINDBERG AA, PAL T: Strategies for development of potential candidate *Shigella* vaccines. Vaccine 11:168, 1993

MATHAN MM, MATHAN VI: Morphology of rectal mucosa of patients with shigellosis. Rev Infect Dis 13(Suppl 4):S314, 1991

PERDOMO OJ et al: Acute inflammation causes epithelial invasion and mucosal destruction in experimental shigellosis. J Exp Med 180:1307, 1994

RAQUIB R et al: Persistence of local cytokine production in shigellosis in acute and convalescent stages. Infect Immun 63:289, 1995

SANSONETTI PJ et al: Role of interleukin-1 in the pathogenesis of experimental shigellosis. J Clin Invest 96:884, 1995

SCHAAD UB et al: Use of fluoroquinolones in pediatrics: Consensus report of an International Society of Chemotherapy commission. Pediatr Infect Dis J 14:1, 1995

TAUXE RV et al: The persistence of *Shigella flexneri* in the United States: The increased role of the adult male. Am J Public Health 78:1432, 1988

ZYCHLINSKY A et al: Molecular and cellular mechanisms of tissue invasion by *Shigella flexneri*. Ann NY Acad Sci 730:197, 1994

160

Martin J. Blaser

INFECTIONS DUE TO *CAMPYLOBACTER* AND RELATED SPECIES

DEFINITION Bacteria of the genus *Campylobacter* and of the related genera *Arcobacter* and *Helicobacter* cause a variety of pyogenic infections. Although acute diarrheal illnesses are most common, these organisms may cause infections in virtually all parts of the body, especially in compromised hosts, and these infections may have late nonsuppurative sequelae. The designation *Campylobacter* comes from the Greek for "curved rod" and refers to the organism's vibrio-like morphology.

ETIOLOGY Campylobacters are motile, non-spore-forming, curved gram-negative rods. Originally known as *Vibrio fetus*, these bacilli were reclassified as a new genus in 1973 after it was recognized that they were quite dissimilar from other vibrios. Since then, more than 15 species have been identified. These species are currently divided into three genera: *Campylobacter*, *Arcobacter*, and *Helicobacter*. Not all of the species are pathogens of humans. The human pathogens can be divided into two major groups: those that primarily cause diarrheal disease and those that cause extraintestinal infection. The principal diarrheal pathogen is *Campylobacter jejuni*, which accounts for 80 to 90 percent of all cases of recognized illness due to campylobacters. Other organisms that cause diarrheal disease include *Campylobacter coli*, *Campylobacter upsaliensis*, *Campylobacter lari*, and *Campylobacter fetus*. The major species causing extraintestinal illnesses is *C. fetus*; however, any of the diarrheal agents may cause systemic or localized infection as well. Neither aerobes nor strict anaerobes, these microaerophilic organisms are adapted for survival in the gastrointestinal mucous layer. This chapter will focus on *C. jejuni* and *C. fetus* as the major pathogens and prototypes for their groups; the key features of infection are listed by species (excluding *C. jejuni*, described in detail in the text below) in Table 160-1.

EPIDEMIOLOGY Campylobacters are found in the gastrointestinal tract of many animals used for food (including poultry, cattle, sheep, and swine) and of many household pets (including birds, dogs, and cats). These microorganisms usually do not cause illness in their animal hosts. In most cases, campylobacters are transmitted to humans in raw or undercooked food products or through direct contact with infected animals. In the United States and other developed countries, ingestion of contaminated poultry that has not been sufficiently cooked is the most common means of acquiring infection (50 to 70 percent of cases). Other modes of transmission include ingestion of raw (unpasteurized) milk or untreated water, contact with infected household pets, travel to developing countries (campylobacters being among the causes of traveler's diarrhea), and (occasionally) contact with an index case who is incontinent of stool.

Campylobacter infections are not rare. Several studies indicate that, in the United States, diarrheal disease due to campylobacters is more common than that due to *Salmonella* and *Shigella* combined. Infections occur throughout the year, but their incidence peaks during summer and early autumn. Persons of all ages are affected; however, attack rates for *C. jejuni* are highest among young children and young adults, while those for *C. fetus* are highest at the extremes of age. Systemic infections due to *C. fetus* (and to other *Campylobacter* and related species) are most common in compromised hosts. Persons at increased risk include those with AIDS, hypogammaglobulinemia, neoplasia, liver disease, diabetes mellitus, and generalized atherosclerosis as well as pregnant women. However, apparently healthy nonpregnant persons occasionally develop transient *Campylobacter* bacteremia.

In developing countries, *C. jejuni* infections are hyperendemic, with the highest rates among children <2 years old. Infection rates fall with age, as does the illness-to-infection ratio; these observations suggest that frequent exposure to *C. jejuni* leads to the acquisition of immunity.

PATHOLOGY AND PATHOGENESIS   Many *C. jejuni* infections are subclinical, especially in partially immune hosts. Most illnesses occur within 2 to 4 days (range, 1 to 7 days) of exposure to the organism in food or water. The sites of tissue injury include the jejunum, ileum, and colon. Biopsies show an acute nonspecific inflammatory reaction, with neutrophils, monocytes, and eosinophils in the lamina propria, as well as damage to the epithelium, including loss of mucus, glandular degeneration, and crypt abscesses. Biopsy findings may be consistent with Crohn's disease or ulcerative colitis, but these "idiopathic" chronic inflammatory diseases should not be diagnosed unless infectious colitis, *specifically including* that due to infection with *Campylobacter*, has been ruled out.

The high frequency of *C. jejuni* infections and their severity and recurrence among hypogammaglobulinemic patients suggest that antibodies are important in protective immunity. The pathogenesis of infection is uncertain. Both the motility of the strain and its capacity to adhere to host tissues appear to favor disease, but classic enterotoxins and cytotoxins (although described) do not appear to play any substantial role in tissue injury or disease production. In contrast, the organisms have been visualized in the epithelium, albeit in low numbers. The documentation of a significant tissue response and occasionally of *C. jejuni* bacteremia further suggests that tissue invasion is clinically significant.

The pathogenesis of *C. fetus* infections is better defined. Virtually all clinical isolates of *C. fetus* possess a proteinaceous capsule-like structure (an S layer) that renders the organism resistant to complement-mediated killing and opsonization. As a result, *C. fetus* can cause bacteremia and can seed sites beyond the intestinal tract. The ability of the organism to switch the S-layer proteins expressed, a phenomenon that results in antigenic variability, may contribute to the chronicity and high rate of recurrence of these infections in compromised hosts.

CLINICAL MANIFESTATIONS OF *C. JEJUNI* AND *C. FETUS* INFECTIONS   The clinical features of infections due to all of the *Campylobacter* and related species causing enteric disease appear to be highly similar. There is often a prodrome, with fever, headache, myalgia, and/or malaise, 12 to 48 h before the onset of diarrheal symptoms. The most common symptoms of the intestinal phase are diarrhea, abdominal pain, and fever. The degree of diarrhea varies from several loose stools to grossly bloody stools; most patients presenting for medical attention have 10 or more bowel movements on the worst day of illness. Abdominal pain usually consists of cramping and may be the most prominent symptom. Pain usually is generalized but may become localized; *C. jejuni* infection may cause pseudoappendicitis. Fever may be the only initial manifestation of *C. jejuni* infection, a situation mimicking the early stages of typhoid fever. Febrile young children may develop convulsions. *Campylobacter* enteritis generally is self-limited; however, symptoms persist for longer than 1 week in 10 to 20 percent of patients seeking medical attention, and relapses occur in 5 to 10 percent of untreated patients.

C. fetus may cause a diarrheal illness similar to that due to *C. jejuni*, especially in normal hosts, or may cause either intermittent diarrhea or nonspecific abdominal pain without localizing signs. Sequelae are uncommon, and outcome is benign. *C. fetus* also may cause a prolonged relapsing systemic illness (with fever, chills, and myalgias) that has no obvious primary source; this manifestation is especially common in compromised hosts. Secondary seeding of an organ (e.g., meninges, brain, bone, urinary tract, or soft tissue) complicates the course, which may be fulminant. *C. fetus* infections have a tropism for vascular sites: endocarditis, mycotic aneurysm, and septic thrombophlebitis all may occur. Infection during pregnancy often leads to fetal death. *Helicobacter cinaedi* causes recurrent cellulitis with fever and bacteremia in immunocompromised hosts.

COMPLICATIONS   Except in the case of infection with *C. fetus* or *H. cinaedi*, bacteremia is uncommon, developing most often in immunocompromised hosts and at the extremes of age. Three patterns of extraintestinal infection have been noted: (1) transient bacteremia in a normal host with enteritis (benign course, no specific treatment needed); (2) sustained bacteremia or focal infection in a normal host (bacteremia originating from enteritis, with patients responding well to antimicrobial therapy); and (3) sustained bacteremia or focal infection in a compromised host. Enteritis may not be demonstrated. Antimicrobial therapy, possibly prolonged, is necessary for suppression or cure of the infection.

Campylobacter infections in patients with AIDS or hypogammaglobulinemia may be severe, persistent, and extraintestinal; relapse after cessation of therapy is common. Hypogammaglobulinemic patients also may develop osteomyelitis and an erysipelas-like rash.

Table 160-1

Clinical Features Associated with Infection due to "Atypical" *Campylobacter* and Related Species Implicated as Causes of Human Illness

Species	Common Clinical Features	Less Common Clinical Features	Additional Information
Campylobacter coli	Fever, diarrhea, abdominal pain	Bacteremia	Clinically indistinguishable from *C. jejuni*
Campylobacter fetus	Bacteremia, sepsis, meningitis, vascular infections	Diarrhea, relapsing fevers	Not usually isolated from media containing cephalothin
Campylobacter upsaliensis	Watery diarrhea, low-grade fever, abdominal pain	Bacteremia, abscesses	Difficult to isolate because of cephalothin susceptibility
Campylobacter lari	Abdominal pain, diarrhea	Colitis, appendicitis	Seagulls frequently colonized; organism often transmitted to humans via contaminated water
Campylobacter hyointestinalis	Watery or bloody diarrhea, vomiting, abdominal pain	Bacteremia	Causes proliferative enteritis in swine
Helicobacter fennelliae	Chronic mild diarrhea, abdominal cramps, proctitis	Bacteremia*	Best treated with fluoroquinolones
Helicobacter cinaedi	Chronic mild diarrhea, abdominal cramps, proctitis	Bacteremia*	Best treated with fluoroquinolones; identified in healthy hamsters
Campylobacter jejuni subspecies *doylei*	Diarrhea	Chronic gastritis, bacteremia†	Uncertain role as human pathogen
Arcobacter cryaerophila	Diarrhea	Bacteremia	Cultured under aerobic conditions
Arcobacter butzleri	Fever, diarrhea, abdominal pain, nausea	Bacteremia, appendicitis	Cultured under aerobic conditions; enzootic in nonhuman primates
Campylobacter sputorum	Pulmonary, perianal, groin, and axillary abscesses	None described	Three clinically relevant biovars: *C. sputorum* subspecies *sputorum*, *C. sputorum* subspecies *bubulus*, and *Campylobacter mucosalis*

* In children and HIV-infected persons.
† In children.

SOURCE: Allos and Blaser.

Local suppurative complications of infection include cholecystitis, pancreatitis, and cystitis; distant complications include meningitis, endocarditis, arthritis, peritonitis, cellulitis, and septic abortion. All are rare. Hepatitis, interstitial nephritis, and the hemolytic-uremic syndrome occasionally complicate acute infection. Reactive arthritis and other rheumatologic complaints may develop several weeks after infection, especially in persons with the HLA-B27 phenotype. Guillain-Barré syndrome follows *Campylobacter* infections uncommonly (i.e., in 1 of every 1000 to 2000 cases). However, because of their high incidence, it is now estimated that *Campylobacter* infections may trigger 20 to 40 percent of all cases of Guillain-Barré syndrome.

LABORATORY FINDINGS In patients with *Campylobacter* enteritis, peripheral leukocyte counts reflect the severity of the inflammatory process. However, stools from nearly all patients presenting for medical attention in the United States contain leukocytes or erythrocytes. Fecal smears should be treated with Gram's or Wright's stain and examined in all suspected cases. When the diagnosis of *Campylobacter* enteritis is suspected on the basis of findings of inflammatory diarrhea (fever, fecal leukocytes), clinicians can ask the laboratory to attempt the visualization of organisms with characteristic vibrioid morphology by direct microscopic examination of stools with Gram's staining or to use phase-contrast or dark-field microscopy to identify the organisms' characteristic "darting" motility. Confirmation of the diagnosis of *Campylobacter* infection is based on identification of an isolate from cultures of stool, blood, or another site. *Campylobacter*-specific media should be used to culture stools from all patients with inflammatory or bloody diarrhea. Since all *Campylobacter* species are fastidious, they will not be isolated unless selective media or other selective techniques are used. Not all media are equally useful for isolation of the broad array of campylobacters; therefore, failure to isolate campylobacters from stool does not entirely rule out their presence. The detection of the organisms in stool almost always implies infection; there is a brief period of postconvalescent fecal carriage and no commensalism. In contrast, *Campylobacter sputorum* and related organisms found in the oral cavity are commensals without known pathogenic significance.

DIFFERENTIAL DIAGNOSIS The symptoms of *Campylobacter* enteritis are not sufficiently unusual to distinguish this illness from that due to *Salmonella*, *Shigella*, or *Yersinia*, among other pathogens. The combination of fever and fecal leukocytes or erythrocytes is indicative of inflammatory diarrhea, and definitive diagnosis is based on culture. Similarly, extraintestinal *Campylobacter* illness is diagnosed by culture. Infection due to *Campylobacter* should be suspected in the setting of septic abortion and that due to *C. fetus* specifically in the setting of septic thrombophlebitis. It is important to reiterate that the presentation of *Campylobacter* enteritis may mimic that of ulcerative colitis or Crohn's disease, that *Campylobacter* enteritis is much more common than either of the latter (especially among young adults), and that biopsy may not distinguish among these entities. Thus a diagnosis of inflammatory bowel disease should not be made until *Campylobacter* infection has been ruled out, especially in persons with a history of foreign travel, significant animal contact, immunodeficiency, or practices incurring a high risk of transmission.

℞ **TREATMENT**

Fluid and electrolyte replacement is central to the treatment of diarrheal illnesses (see Chap. 128). Even among patients presenting for medical attention with *Campylobacter* enteritis, fewer than half will clearly benefit from specific antimicrobial therapy. Indications for such therapy include high fever, bloody diarrhea, severe diarrhea, persistence for more than 1 week, and worsening of symptoms. A 5- to 7-day course of erythromycin (250 mg orally four times daily or—for children—30 to 50 mg/kg per day, in divided doses) is the regimen of choice. Although no relevant clinical trials have been conducted, the in vitro susceptibility of *Campylobacter* species to macrolides such as clarithromycin and azithromycin suggests that these organisms also would be useful therapeutic agents. An alternative regimen for adults is ciprofloxacin (500 mg orally twice daily) for 5 to 7 days, but resistance to this agent is increasing. Other alternatives include tetracycline, norfloxacin, and furazolidone. Use of antimotility agents, which may prolong the duration of symptoms and has been associated with deaths, is not recommended.

For systemic infections, treatment with gentamicin, imipenem, or chloramphenicol should be started empirically, but susceptibility testing should then be performed. Ciprofloxacin and amoxicillin/clavulanate are alternative agents. For immunocompromised patients with systemic infections due to *C. fetus*, prolonged therapy is usually necessary.

PROGNOSIS Nearly all patients recover fully from *Campylobacter* enteritis, either spontaneously or after antimicrobial therapy. Volume depletion likely contributes to the few deaths that are reported. As stated above, occasional patients develop reactive arthritis or Guillain-Barré syndrome. Systemic infection with *C. fetus* is much more often fatal than that due to related species; this higher mortality reflects in part the population affected. Prognosis is dependent on the rapidity with which appropriate therapy is begun. Otherwise healthy hosts usually survive *C. fetus* infections without sequelae. Compromised hosts often have recurrent infections.

BIBLIOGRAPHY

ALLOS BM, BLASER MJ: *Campylobacter jejuni* and the expanding spectrum of related infections. Clin Infect Dis 20:1092, 1995

BLASER MJ et al: *Campylobacter* enteritis in the United States: A multicenter study. Ann Intern Med 98:360, 1983

NACHAMKIN I et al (eds): *Campylobacter jejuni: Current Strategy and Future Trends.* Washington, American Society for Microbiology, 1992, pp 1–300

161 *Gerald T. Keusch, Robert L. Deresiewicz*

CHOLERA AND OTHER VIBRIOSES

Members of the genus *Vibrio* cause a number of important infectious syndromes. Classic among them is cholera, a devastating diarrheal disease caused by *Vibrio cholerae* group O1 that has been responsible for seven global pandemics and much suffering over the past two centuries. Epidemic cholera remains a major public health concern and is dealt with at length in this chapter. Recently, other vibrioses have been described, including syndromes of diarrhea, soft tissue infection, or primary sepsis caused by additional named species in the genus *Vibrio*. These, too, are considered below.

All members of the genus are actively motile, facultatively anaerobic, curved gram-negative rods with one or more polar flagella. Except for *V. cholerae* and *Vibrio mimicus*, all require salt for growth ("halophilic vibrios"). In nature, vibrios most commonly reside in tidal rivers and bays under conditions of moderate salinity. They proliferate in the summer months when water temperatures exceed about 20°C. As might be expected, the illnesses they cause also increase in frequency during the warm months.

CHOLERA

DEFINITION Cholera is an acute diarrheal disease that can, in a matter of hours, result in profound, rapidly progressive dehydration and death. Accordingly, cholera gravis (the severe form of cholera) is a much-feared disease, particularly in its epidemic presentation. Fortunately, prompt, aggressive fluid repletion and supportive care can obviate the high mortality that it has historically wrought. While the term *cholera* occasionally has been applied to any severely dehydrating secretory diarrheal illness, whether infectious in etiology or not, it generally refers to disease caused by *V. cholerae* serogroup O1. Epidemic and endemic O1 cholera has raged in Africa since the early 1970s and appeared in Latin America for the first time in this century in 1991. In 1992, a new epidemic serotype emerged on the Indian subcontinent and has since killed thousands of people.

ETIOLOGY AND EPIDEMIOLOGY   The species *V. cholerae* comprises a host of organisms classified on the basis of the carbohydrate determinants of their somatic O antigens. Some 140 serogroups have been recognized. They are divided into those that agglutinate in antisera to the O1 group antigen (*V. cholerae* O1) and those that do not (non-O1 *V. cholerae*). Although some strains of non-O1 *V. cholerae* occasionally cause sporadic outbreaks of diarrhea, serogroup O1 was, until recently, the exclusive cause of epidemic cholera. That paradigm changed in late 1992 with the identification of serogroup O139 Bengal as the cause of a large epidemic of cholera in southern India and Bangladesh along the Bay of Bengal. *V. cholerae* O139 Bengal is discussed in greater detail below.

V. cholerae O1 exists in two biotypes, *classic* and *El Tor*, that are distinguished on the basis of a number of characteristics, including phage susceptibility and hemolysin production. Each biotype is further subdivided into two serotypes, termed *Inaba* and *Ogawa*. Serotyping is a useful tool in field epidemiologic studies. Newer molecular epidemiologic techniques, such as ribotyping and other gene-based methods, now make it possible to trace the source and origin of cholera strains from around the world.

The natural habitat of *V. cholerae* is coastal salt water and brackish estuaries, where the organism lives in close relation to plankton and where it may survive in a viable but noncultivable form. Humans become infected incidentally but, once infected, can act as vehicles for spread. Ingestion of water contaminated by human feces is the most common means of acquisition of *V. cholerae*. Consumption of contaminated food in the home, in restaurants, or from street vendors can also contribute to spread. There is no known animal reservoir. While the infectious dose is relatively high, it is markedly reduced in hypochlorhydric persons, in those using antacids, and when gastric acidity is buffered by a meal. Cholera is predominantly a pediatric disease in endemic areas, but it affects adults and children equally when newly introduced into a population. In endemic areas, the disease is more common in the summer and fall months. While this seasonality has not been explained fully, it may be due to environmental conditions that affect the multiplication of vibrios or to seasonal alterations in human behavior that affect contact with water. Asymptomatic infections are frequent and more common with the El Tor than the classic biotype. In endemic areas, children under 2 years of age are less likely to develop severe cholera than are older children, perhaps because of passive immunity acquired from breast milk. For unexplained reasons, susceptibility to cholera is significantly influenced by ABO blood group status; those with type O blood are at greatest risk, while those with type AB are at least risk.

Cholera is native to the Ganges delta in the Indian subcontinent. Since 1817, seven global pandemics have occurred. The current (seventh) pandemic, the first due to the El Tor biotype, began in Indonesia in 1961 and spread throughout Asia, with *V. cholerae* El Tor displacing the endemic classic strain in many areas. It briefly invaded Europe, but effective public health measures and the high level of sanitation combined to limit its impact. In the early 1970s, El Tor cholera struck in Africa, causing major epidemics before becoming a persistent endemic problem. Its recent history in Africa has been punctuated by severe outbreaks, often fed by the chaos of war and genocide. Such was the case in the camps for Rwandan refugees set up in 1994 around Goma, Zaire. Tens of thousands of cases occurred and mortality was high. In 1995, the occurrence of hundreds of cases in Romania and the Black Sea states of the former Soviet Union demonstrated the epidemic potential of this organism whenever public health measures break down.

Since 1973, sporadic endemic infections due to vibrios related to the seventh-pandemic strain have been recognized along the U.S. Gulf Coast of Louisiana and Texas. These infections are typically associated with the consumption of contaminated, locally harvested shellfish. Occasionally, cases in U.S. locations remote from the Gulf Coast have been linked to shipped-in Gulf Coast seafood.

Although the event was long expected, it was not until 1991 that the current cholera pandemic reached Latin America. Beginning along the Peruvian coast in January 1991, the disease was carried by fishermen to Ecuador and Colombia. It then spread in an explosive epidemic to virtually all of South and Central America and to Mexico (Fig. 161-1). About 400,000 cases were reported in the first year of the outbreak, and more than 1 million had been reported by the end of 1994. While the cumulative mortality rate has been under 1 percent, the mortality rate approached 30 percent in the communities first affected, where a lack of familiarity with the disease led initially to the deployment of wholly ineffective treatment. Intensive education of health care providers and of the community at large has enhanced awareness of the disease and its appropriate management and has greatly diminished mortality. As it did in Africa two decades earlier, the epidemic El Tor strain proved capable of establishing itself in inland waters rather than in its classic niche of coastal salt waters; the organism has already become endemic in many of the Latin American countries into which it was recently introduced.

Cases linked to the Latin American epidemic have occurred in the United States. For example, 11 people in New York and New Jersey were infected in two separate outbreaks in 1991 after eating boiled crabmeat illegally transported by travelers from Ecuador. Although secondary spread of this strain has not taken place in the United States, these events underscore the need for vigilance among health care professionals, even in locations remote from an epidemic.

In October 1992, a large-scale outbreak of clinical cholera occurred in the port city of Madras and surrounding towns in southern India. The etiologic agent proved to be a novel strain of *V. cholerae* belonging neither to the O1 serogroup that typically causes epidemic cholera nor to any of the 137 other serogroups known at the time. This strain spread rapidly up and down the coast of the Bay of Bengal, reaching Bangladesh in December 1992. There alone, it caused more than 100,000 cases of cholera in the first 3 months of 1993. It subsequently

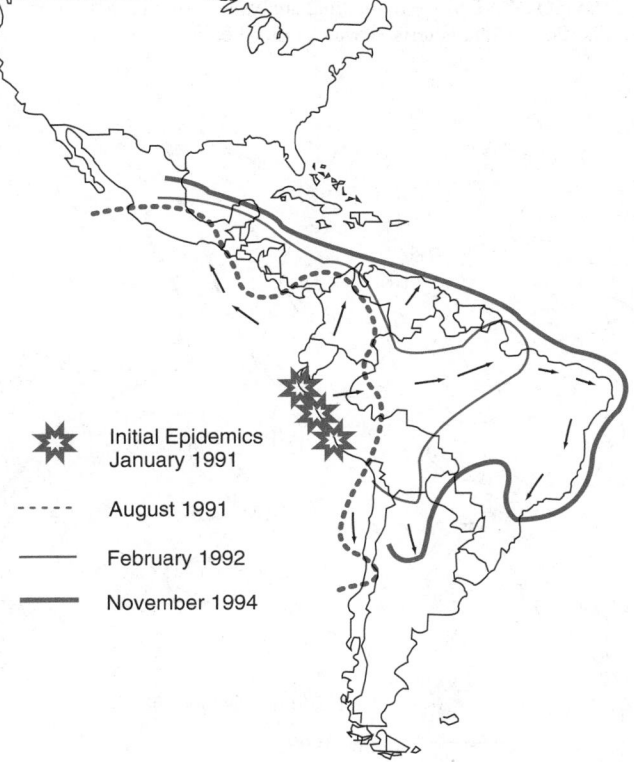

Initial Epidemics January 1991
- - - - - August 1991
——— February 1992
━━━━ November 1994

FIGURE 161-1   Spread of *Vibrio cholerae* O1 in the Americas, 1991–1994. (Courtesy of Dr. Robert V. Tauxe, Centers for Disease Control and Prevention, Atlanta.)

spread across the Indian subcontinent and to neighboring countries, affecting Pakistan, Nepal, western China, Thailand, and Malaysia by the end of 1994 (Fig. 161-2). The organism has since been designated *V. cholerae* O139 Bengal, in recognition of its novel somatic O antigen and its geographic origin.

The clinical manifestations and epidemiologic features of the disease caused by strain O139 Bengal are indistinguishable from those of O1 cholera. Immunity to the latter, however, is not protective against the former. Thus, although O139 Bengal cholera has been restricted almost exclusively to O1-endemic areas, it has affected patients of all ages, with most cases in adults. Moreover, populations into which strain O139 Bengal has been introduced have responded as virgin populations with respect to severe, lethal cholera. Because naturally acquired immunity to *V. cholerae* O1 does not cross-protect against the O139 Bengal strain, vaccines being developed against the former are unlikely to be effective against the latter.

Like the O1 epidemics in cholera-naive areas before it, the O139 epidemic was initially devastating. Some authorities believed that the emergence of *V. cholerae* O139 signaled the beginning of the eighth global cholera pandemic. Indeed, just as O1 El Tor replaced the classic biotype that preceded it, O139 Bengal in 1993 rapidly replaced O1 El Tor as the most common environmental isolate and the predominant cause of clinical cholera in the areas in which it had appeared (Fig. 161-3). Surprisingly and unexpectedly, however, by the beginning of 1994, O1 El Tor had resumed its dominance in Bangladesh, relegating O139 Bengal cholera to the status of a background endemic infection. This trend continued in 1995. That notwithstanding, the potential for global spread of O139 Bengal was underscored by an intercontinental food-borne outbreak that occurred in early 1994 among passengers on a cruise ship in Southeast Asia. Six of the 630 travelers (five from the United States and one from Great Britain) became ill, their symptoms beginning only after they returned home. They likely acquired the organism during a stopover in Thailand. A specific rice dish eaten during a specific meal at a specific restaurant was the probable source.

PATHOGENESIS In the final analysis, cholera is a toxin-mediated disease. Its characteristic watery diarrhea is due to the action of

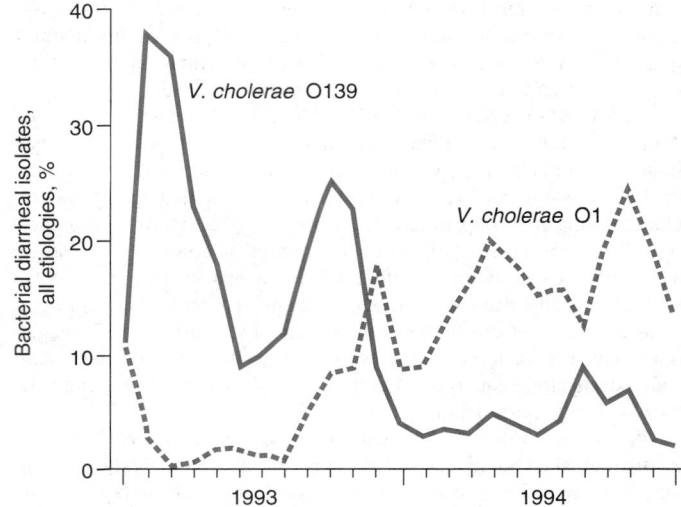

FIGURE 161-3 Isolations of *Vibrio cholerae* O1 and *V. cholerae* O139 in Bangladesh, 1993–1994, by month. (Courtesy of Dr. John Albert and Dr. A S G Faruque, International Centre for Diarrhoeal Disease Research, Bangladesh.)

cholera toxin (CTX), a potent protein enterotoxin elaborated by the organism in the small intestine. However, for *V. cholerae* to colonize the small intestine and produce CTX, it must first recognize, contend with, and traverse several hostile environments. The first of these is the acidic milieu of the stomach. *V. cholerae* lacks genetically controlled mechanisms of acid resistance (such as those that exist in *Shigella*). Rather, it relies on a large inoculum size to allow some organisms to elude the bactericidal effects of gastric acidity.

If successful, it must next traverse the mucous layer of the upper small bowel. Several properties of the organism enhance its ability to accomplish this feat, including its motility, its chemotaxis, and its production of hemagglutinin/protease. This last substance, originally named cholera lectin, is closely related to the *Pseudomonas aeruginosa* elastase and is both an agglutinin and a zinc-dependent protease. It is able to cleave mucin and fibronectin as well as the A subunit of CTX. Hemagglutinin/protease may also serve to detach vibrios bound to the small-bowel surface, thus facilitating their spread within the intestine and excretion in the stool.

Having successfully negotiated the barriers of gastric acidity and small-intestinal mucus, the vibrios must finally adhere to the bowel wall. Their attachment is mediated by the toxin-coregulated pilus (TCP), so named because its synthesis is regulated in parallel with that of CTX.

CTX, TCP, and several other virulence factors, including an accessory colonization factor and various hemagglutinins, are coordinately regulated by the *toxR* gene product. ToxR protein is a "master switch" that modulates the expression of virulence genes in response to signals that it senses in the environment, the most important of which, at least in vitro, are changes in osmolarity and pH and the presence of certain free amino acids. Coordinate regulation presumably enables the organism to tailor its repertoire of proteins to suit its needs as it passes from one microenvironment to another. Regulation of the *toxR* type has become a paradigm for similar systems that have been discovered in a wide range of pathogenic bacteria.

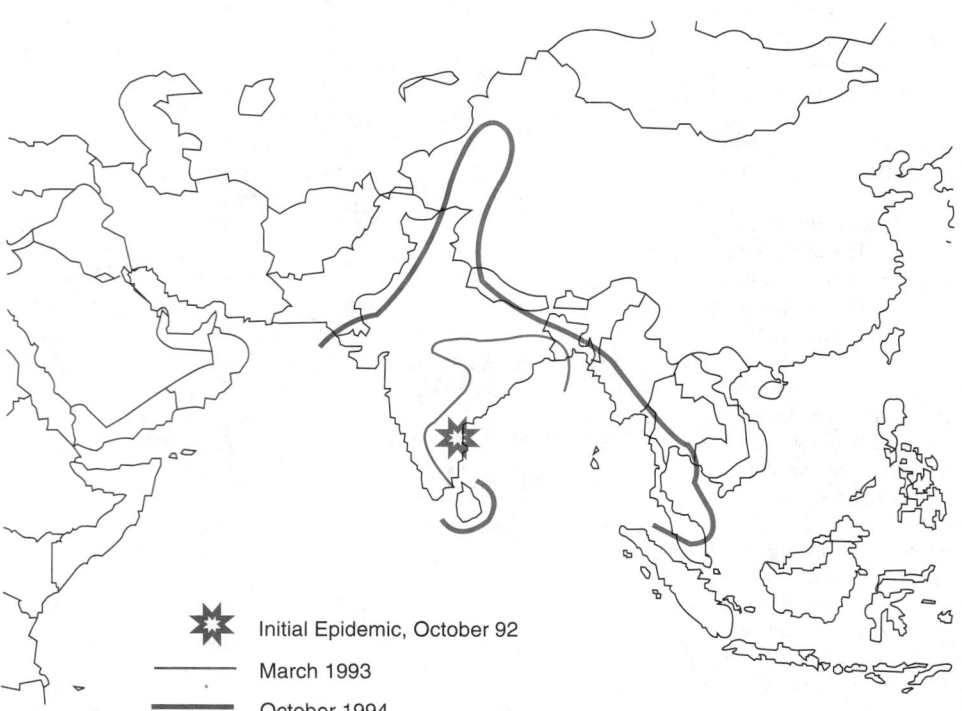

Initial Epidemic, October 92

——— March 1993

——— October 1994

FIGURE 161-2 Spread of *Vibrio cholerae* O139 in the Indian subcontinent and elsewhere in Asia, 1992–1994. (Courtesy of Dr. Robert V. Tauxe, Centers for Disease Control and Prevention, Atlanta.)

Once established, the organism produces CTX, which consists of a monomeric enzymatic moiety (the A subunit) and a pentameric binding moiety (the B subunit). The B pentamer binds to G_{M1} ganglioside, a glycolipid receptor on the surface of jejunal epithelial cells, and this binding makes possible the delivery of the A subunit to its cytosolic target. The activated A subunit (A_1) irreversibly transfers ADP-ribose from nicotinamide adenine dinucleotide to its specific target protein, the GTP-binding regulatory component of adenylate cyclase in intestinal epithelial cells. When ADP-ribosylated, this G protein up-regulates the cyclase catalytic subunit; the result is the intracellular accumulation of high levels of cyclic AMP. In turn, cyclic AMP inhibits the absorptive sodium transport system in villus cells and activates the excretory chloride transport system in crypt cells, and these events lead to the accumulation of sodium chloride in the intestinal lumen. Since water moves passively to maintain osmolality, isotonic fluid accumulates in the lumen. When the volume of that fluid exceeds the capacity of the rest of the gut to resorb it, watery diarrhea results. Unless the wasted fluid and electrolytes are adequately replaced, shock (due to profound dehydration) and acidosis (due to loss of bicarbonate) follow.

Although perturbation of the adenylate cyclase pathway is the primary mechanism by which CTX causes excess fluid secretion, it is not the only one. Increasing evidence indicates that CTX also enhances intestinal secretion via prostaglandins and/or neural histamine receptors. It is possible that the redundancy of secretory mechanisms activated by CTX accounts for the profound diarrhea and dehydration characteristic of severe cholera.

The genes encoding CTX (*ctxAB*) have for some time been known to reside on the so-called CTX *genetic element*, a 7- to 9.7-kb segment of DNA occupying a particular position on the chromosomes of toxigenic strains and absent in nontoxigenic strains. The element carries at least four open reading frames in addition to *ctxAB*: *cep* (encoding core-encoded pilin), *orfU* (encoding a product for which no function has been assigned), *ace* (encoding accessory cholera enterotoxin), and *zot* (encoding zonula occludens toxin). On the basis of the element's structural organization and its failure readily to self-transmit in vitro, it had been assumed to represent a transposon. Recent work has demonstrated conclusively that the element is not a transposon but a lysogenic filamentous bacteriophage (CTXΦ). Cep, the *orfU* gene product, Ace, and Zot, which were originally thought to be accessory virulence factors, may actually function in phage morphogenesis.

The surface receptor for CTXΦ on *V. cholerae* is TCP. Accordingly, the phage is transferred far more efficiently under conditions of high rather than low TCP expression. Moreover, enhanced transmission of CTXΦ has been detected in vivo in a murine intestinal colonization model. This finding provides strong genetic evidence for expression of TCP in vivo and demonstrates the critical role of environmental signaling in shaping the behaviors of these microorganisms. The discovery of CTXΦ establishes that horizontal transfer of virulence genes takes place in *V. cholerae* and may be one mechanism by which novel virulent serogroups emerge. Whether transfer to attenuated vaccine strains of *V. cholerae* can also occur remains to be determined. The attenuated strain currently in use, which is discussed in more detail below, has been carefully studied in field trials and appears to have an excellent safety profile.

Molecular analysis of *V. cholerae* O139 Bengal has suggested the basis of its origin and the reasons it was able to cause an explosive epidemic of cholera. Both phenotypically and genotypically, strain O139 Bengal is closely related to the O1 El Tor strains of the seventh pandemic, and it seems to have arisen from them by horizontal gene transfer. It shares the virulence attributes and general pathogenic mechanisms of O1 vibrios, including possession of the same CTX genetic element, the same TCP, and the *toxR* regulon. In all ways but two, strain O139 Bengal is virtually identical to the seventh-pandemic strain of *V. cholerae* O1 El Tor. Those differences are its production of the novel O139 lipopolysaccharide (LPS) and of an immunologically related O-antigen polysaccharide capsule. Both are putative virulence factors, independently enhancing colonization in a murine infection model. The ability to produce the O139 LPS is due to a replacement of the DNA in the central region of the O1 antigen biosynthetic complex with an 11-kb segment containing the genes encoding O139

LPS. At least one of those genes is involved in the production of both the O139 LPS and the capsule. Encapsulation is not a feature of O1 strains and may explain the resistance of O139 strains to human serum in vitro as well as the occasional development of O139 bacteremia.

CLINICAL MANIFESTATIONS After a 24- to 48-h incubation period, cholera begins with the sudden onset of painless watery diarrhea that may quickly become voluminous and often is followed shortly by vomiting. In severe cases, stool volume can exceed 250 mL/kg in the first 24 h. If fluids and electrolytes are not replaced, hypovolemic shock and death ensue. Fever is usually absent. Muscle cramps due to electrolyte disturbances are common. The stool has a characteristic appearance: a nonbilious, gray, slightly cloudy fluid with flecks of mucus, no blood, and a somewhat sweet, inoffensive odor. It has been called "rice-water" stool because of its resemblance to the water in which rice has been washed. Clinical symptoms parallel volume contraction: At losses of 3 to 5 percent of normal body weight, thirst develops; at 5 to 8 percent, postural hypotension, weakness, tachycardia, and decreased skin turgor; and above 10 percent, oliguria, weak or absent pulses, sunken eyes (and, in infants, sunken fontanelles), wrinkled ("washerwoman") skin, somnolence, and coma. Complications derive exclusively from the effects of volume and electrolyte depletion and include renal failure due to acute tubular necrosis. Thus, if the patient is adequately treated with fluid and salt, complications are averted and the process is self-limited, resolving in a few days.

Laboratory data usually reveal an elevated hematocrit (due to hemoconcentration) in nonanemic patients; mild neutrophilic leukocytosis; elevated levels of blood urea nitrogen and creatinine consistent with prerenal azotemia; normal sodium, potassium, and chloride levels; a markedly reduced bicarbonate level (<15 mmol/L); and an elevated anion gap (due to increases in serum lactate, protein, and phosphate). Arterial pH is usually low (about 7.2).

DIAGNOSIS The clinical suspicion of cholera can be confirmed by the identification of *V. cholerae* in stool; however, the organism must be specifically sought. In experienced hands, it can be detected directly by dark-field microscopy on a wet mount of fresh stool, and its serotype can be discerned by immobilization with Inaba- or Ogawa-specific antiserum. Laboratory isolation of the organism requires the use of a selective medium. The best of these is thiosulfate–citrate–bile salts–sucrose (TCBS) agar, on which the organism grows as a flat yellow colony. If a delay in sample processing is expected, Carey-Blair transport medium and/or alkaline-peptone water-enrichment medium should be inoculated as well. In endemic areas there is little need for biochemical confirmation and characterization, although these tasks may be worthwhile in places where *V. cholerae* is an uncommon isolate. Standard microbiologic biochemical testing for Enterobacteriaceae will suffice for identification of *V. cholerae*. All vibrios are oxidase-positive. *V. cholerae* can be distinguished from the otherwise similar *V. mimicus* by its ability to ferment sucrose.

The yield of stool cultures for the diagnosis of *V. cholerae* infection declines late in the course of the illness or when effective antibacterial therapy is initiated. Although not generally evaluable in clinical laboratories, serum vibriocidal antibody titers can be used to confirm the diagnosis in non-cholera-endemic regions of the world. Monoclonal antibody–based diagnostic kits and methods based on the polymerase chain reaction and on DNA probes have been developed for *V. cholerae* O1 and O139 but are unlikely to become available in U.S. clinical laboratories.

℞ **TREATMENT**

Cholera is simple to treat; only the rapid and adequate replacement of fluids, electrolytes, and base is required. The mortality rate for appropriately treated disease is usually less than 1 percent. However, analysis of a large outbreak of cholera among airline travelers from an endemic country to the United States revealed frequent misdiagnoses by U.S. health professionals and poor appreciation on their part of the principles of management. Compounding these problems was the general unavailability of appropriate oral fluids. Even intravenous fluid therapy typically was not optimal.

It has been proved conclusively that fluid may be given orally. This approach takes advantage of the hexose-Na$^+$ cotransport mechanism to move Na$^+$ across the gut mucosa together with an actively transported molecule such as glucose. Since Na$^+$ losses in the stool are high, a fluid containing Na$^+$ at 90 mmol/L has been recommended by the World Health Organization (WHO) (Table 161-1). This amount of Na$^+$ is higher than that needed to treat diarrhea due to most other causes. The solution is safe, even for infants, if its intake is alternated with the consumption of sodium-free fluids such as breast milk or water. For the sake of simplicity, WHO advises routine use of this single solution for diarrheal disease rather than attempts to choose among multiple formulations according to etiology.

Cereal-based formulations are receiving increased attention as alternative oral rehydration solutions. Because of their lower osmolarity, they may reduce stool output. A mixture with a lower sugar and salt content has also been evaluated in cholera patients, with favorable results. However, concerns have been raised over the safety of its use—in particular, whether it could cause significant hyponatremia in patients with moderate or severe diarrhea. Because commercial oral rehydration solutions also contain concentrations of glucose and sodium lower than those of the WHO formulation, they should not yet be used routinely to treat cholera.

For initial management of severely dehydrated patients, intravenous fluid replacement is preferable, if available. Because profound acidosis (pH < 7.2) is common in this group, Ringer's lactate is the best choice among commercial products (Table 161-2). It must be used with additional potassium supplements, preferably given by mouth. The total fluid deficit in severely dehydrated patients (10 percent or more of body weight) can be replaced safely within the first 4 h of therapy, half within the first hour. Thereafter, oral therapy usually can be initiated, with the goal of maintaining fluid intake equal to fluid output. However, patients with continued large-volume diarrhea may require prolonged intravenous treatment to keep up with gastrointestinal fluid losses. Severe hypokalemia can develop but will respond to potassium given either intravenously or orally. In the absence of adequate staff to monitor the patient's progress, the oral route of rehydration and potassium replacement is safer than the intravenous route and is physiologically regulated by thirst and urine output.

Although not necessary for cure, the use of an antibiotic to which the organism is susceptible will diminish the duration and volume of fluid loss and will hasten clearance of the organism from the stool. Single-dose tetracycline (2 g) or doxycycline (300 mg) is effective in adults but is not recommended for children under 8 years of age because of possible deposition in bone and developing teeth. Emerging drug resistance is an ever-present concern. For adults with cholera in areas where tetracycline resistance is prevalent,

Table 161-1

Composition of World Health Organization Oral Rehydration Solution (ORS)*·†

Constituent	Concentration, mmol/L
Na$^+$	90
K$^+$	20
Cl$^-$	80
Citrate‡	10
Glucose	110

* Contains (per package, to be added to 1 L of drinking water): NaCl, 3.5 g; Na$_3$C$_6$H$_5$O$_7$·2H$_2$O, 2.9 g; KCl, 1.5 g; and glucose, 20 g.

† If prepackaged ORS is unavailable, a simple homemade alternative can be prepared by combining 5 g NaCl (about 1 level teaspoon) with either 50 g precooked rice cereal or 40 g sucrose in 1 L of drinking water. In that case, potassium must be supplied separately (e.g., in orange juice or coconut water).

‡ 10 mmol citrate per liter, which supplies 30 mmol HCO$_3$/L.

Table 161-2

Electrolyte Composition of Cholera Stool and of Intravenous Rehydration Solution

Substance	Concentration, mmol/L			
	Na$^+$	K$^+$	Cl$^-$	Base
Stool				
Adult	135	15	90	30
Child	100	25	90	30
Ringer's lactate	130	4*	109	28

* Potassium supplements, preferably administered by mouth, are required to replace the usual potassium losses from stool.

ciprofloxacin—either in a single dose (30 mg/kg, not to exceed a total dose of 1 g) or in a short course (15 mg/kg bid for 3 days, not to exceed a total daily dose of 1 g)—or erythromycin (a total of 40 mg/kg daily in three divided doses for 3 days) is a clinically effective substitute. Both drugs are highly effective in reducing total stool output, and each is significantly better than trimethoprim-sulfamethoxazole. Because of the high cost of quinolones, WHO recommends erythromycin as the first alternative to tetracycline. For children, furazolidone has been the recommended agent and trimethoprim-sulfamethoxazole the second choice. It is of note that *V. cholerae* O139 is resistant to both of these drugs but is susceptible to quinolones, erythromycin, tetracycline, and ampicillin (among others). Because of cost and/or toxicity issues related to the other drugs, erythromycin is a good choice for pediatric cholera, especially where O139 Bengal is present. The efficacy of single-dose erythromycin therapy for cholera has not been demonstrated.

CONTROL In outbreaks, efforts should first be made to identify case contacts and to treat incubating carriers. Next, epidemiologic studies should be undertaken to establish the modes of transmission to define the best strategy to interrupt them. Both the establishment of rehydration centers and instruction in rehydration techniques are essential to the reduction of mortality.

PREVENTION Provision of safe water and facilities for sanitary disposal of feces, improved nutrition, and attention to food preparation and storage in the household could significantly reduce the incidence of cholera. Much effort has been devoted to the development of a cholera vaccine over the past two decades, with a particular focus on the use of live oral vaccine strains. Traditional killed cholera vaccine given intramuscularly provides little protection to nonimmune subjects and predictably causes adverse effects, including pain at the injection site, malaise, and fever. The vaccine's limited efficacy is at least partially due to its failure to induce a local immune response at the intestinal mucosal surface.

Two types of oral cholera vaccines are under development. The first is the killed whole-cell vaccine, which has been prepared both with and without the inclusion of the nontoxic B subunit of CTX (WC/BS and WC vaccine, respectively). The second is the live attenuated vaccine. In trials in Bangladesh, both of the killed vaccines were compared with placebo and conferred about 50 percent protection over a 3-year evaluation period. The protective efficacy of WC/BS was superior to that of WC during the initial 8 months of follow-up (69 versus 41 percent) but equivalent or inferior thereafter. Immunity was relatively sustained in persons vaccinated at an age of >5 years but not well sustained in younger vaccinees.

Live attenuated vaccine strains are being developed in several laboratories, with the use of various starting strains and attenuation strategies. A strain can be attenuated by the isolation or creation of mutants lacking certain virulence factors. Three criteria must be met in live vaccine design: The vaccine strain must induce protective immunity, it must be safe to administer, and it must be minimally reactogenic. *Safety* refers to the vaccine strain's potential to regain virulence, either spontaneously or via horizontal gene transfer from environmental strains. *Reactogenicity* refers to its potential to cause symptoms such as fever or diarrhea in vaccinees.

Strain CVD 103-HgR, an oral live cholera vaccine licensed in Europe, was created from a classic strain of *V. cholerae* by the deletion of the CTX A subunit gene and the insertion in the hemolysin gene of a mercury resistance marker. Although poorly excreted in the stool of human vaccinees, CVD 103-HgR produces a significant increase in the titer of vibriocidal antibody in about 75 percent of recipients, including children between the ages of 2 and 4 years, when given in single dose. This vaccine is more effective against classic than against El Tor cholera. It is marketed in Europe by the Swiss Serum and Vaccine Institute but is unavailable in the United States. This vaccine has an acceptable safety record. Nevertheless, the recent discoveries of CTXΦ and of its capacity for horizontal transfer in vivo mandate reconsideration of vaccine strategies that utilize live cholera strains attenuated only by deletion of toxin genes. Such strains are presumably still capable of infection by wild-type CTXΦ and therefore have at least the theoretical potential for reversion to virulence.

Other vaccine candidate strains have been prepared from El Tor and from O139 vibrios. These strains have been attenuated by the removal of the entire CTX genetic element and its flanking site-specific RS1 insertion sequences, as well as attRS1, the chromosomal target for insertion of the CTX operon. The *recA* gene, which mediates homologous recombination, has also been deleted. These modifications make it virtually impossible for the organisms to regain virulence. To enhance the protective immune response elicited by these strains, the gene encoding the CTX B subunit has been restored to their chromosomes under the control of a strong promoter. In some formulations, spontaneously arising motility-deficient strains have been used to further reduce the potential for reactogenicity. These vaccines are all still years away from licensing. At present, because of the minimal efficacy of existing parenteral vaccines, cholera immunization is recommended for U.S. travelers only if it is mandated by the countries they plan to visit.

OTHER *VIBRIO* SPECIES

In recent years, the taxonomic, epidemiologic, pathophysiologic, and clinical features of the non-O1 vibrios have become increasingly well understood. Ten human pathogens are currently recognized in the genus *Vibrio*. Included are species associated primarily with gastrointestinal illness (*V. parahaemolyticus*, non-O1 *V. cholerae*, *V. mimicus*, *V. fluvialis*, *V. hollisae*, and *V. furnissii*) and species associated primarily with soft tissue infections (*V. vulnificus*, *V. alginolyticus*, and *V. damsela*). In addition, *V. vulnificus* has emerged as a cause of primary sepsis in certain compromised hosts. Vibrios are abundant in coastal waters the world over and tend to concentrate in the tissues of filter-feeding mollusks. Under optimal conditions, some can double in number in as little as 9 min. Consequently, seawater and raw or undercooked shellfish are important sources of human infection (Table 161-3). Vibrios grow best at temperatures between about 28°C and 44°C but not at all below 4°C or above 60°C. Most can be cultured on blood or MacConkey agar, each of which contains enough salt to support the growth of the halophilic organisms (≥0.5 percent). As with *V. cholerae*, TCBS is the best selective medium. The species can be differentiated in the laboratory by standard biochemical tests. The most important members of the group are *V. parahaemolyticus*, a major cause of gastroenteritis in the Far East, and *V. vulnificus*, a notable cause of sepsis in certain immunosuppressed patients in the United States. These and selected other species are considered below in greater detail.

SPECIES ASSOCIATED PRIMARILY WITH GASTROINTESTINAL ILLNESS *V. parahaemolyticus* First implicated as a cause of enteritis by Japanese workers in 1953, *V. parahaemolyticus* is now recognized as an important intestinal pathogen in

many parts of the world. In one study from Japan, 24 percent of reported cases of food poisoning were attributed to this organism, presumably owing to the widespread consumption of raw seafood there. In the United States, *V. parahaemolyticus* has been responsible for several well-documented common-source outbreaks of diarrhea, typically linked to ingestion of undercooked or improperly handled seafood or of other foods that have been contaminated by seawater. Most reports have come from the Atlantic Coast, the Gulf of Mexico, and Hawaii. The organism is ubiquitous in marine environments and is able to grow in saline concentrations up to about 8 to 10 percent. The ability to cause hemolysis on Wagatsuma agar (the so-called Kanagawa phenomenon) is closely linked to enteropathogenicity. In one study, 96.5 percent of isolates from patients with diarrhea were hemolytic versus only about 1 percent of isolates from seawater. Hemolysis is attributed to a 42-kDa heat-stable protein, the exact pathophysiologic role of which is uncertain. The mechanism by which *V. parahaemolyticus* causes diarrhea is not clear.

V. parahaemolyticus has been associated with two distinct gastrointestinal presentations. The more common is a syndrome of watery diarrhea, accompanied in most cases by abdominal cramps, nausea, and vomiting and in about one-quarter of cases by fever and chills. The incubation period ranges from 4 h to 4 days, and the symptomatic period lasts for a median of 3 days. The vast majority of North American cases have been of this type. The less common syndrome is one of dysentery, described in India and Bangladesh and characterized by severe abdominal cramps, nausea, vomiting, and bloody or mucoid stools. Most cases of either type are self-limited and require neither antimicrobial treatment nor hospitalization. The occasional severe case should be treated with fluid replacement and antibiotics, as described above for cholera. Death is very rare. There are no reliable differential diagnostic features. *V. parahaemolyticus* should be considered as a possible cause in all cases of diarrhea that can be epidemiologically linked to seafood consumption or to the sea itself.

In addition to gastrointestinal disease, *V. parahaemolyticus* is a rare cause of extraintestinal infections, including wound infections, otitis, and—very rarely—sepsis.

Non-O1 *V. cholerae* The heterogeneous non-O1 *V. cholerae* organisms are biochemically indistinguishable from *V. cholerae* O1 on routine testing but fail to agglutinate in O1 antiserum. While technically a non-O1 vibrio, *V. cholerae* O139 Bengal is not grouped with these pathogens because of its epidemic potential, as detailed above. Non-O1 *V. cholerae* strains have been responsible for several well-described food-borne outbreaks of gastroenteritis as well as for sporadic cases of otitis media, wound infection, and bacteremia. About half of all U.S. isolates are obtained from stool specimens. Like other vibrios, non-O1 *V. cholerae* organisms are widely distributed in marine environments; unlike most other vibrios, however, they require only trace amounts of NaCl to survive (i.e., they are nonhalophilic). Recognized U.S. cases invariably have been associated either with the consumption of raw oysters or with recent travel, typically to Mexico. The clinical spectrum of diarrheal disease caused by non-O1 *V. cholerae* is

Table 161-3

Features of Selected Noncholera Vibrioses

Organism	Vehicle or Activity	Host at Risk	Syndrome
V. parahaemolyticus	Shellfish, seawater	Normal	Gastroenteritis
	Seawater	Normal	Wound infection
Non-O1 *V. cholerae*	Shellfish, travel	Normal	Gastroenteritis
	Seawater	Normal	Wound infection, otitis media
V. vulnificus	Shellfish	Immunosuppressed*	Sepsis, secondary cellulitis
	Seawater	Normal	Wound infection, cellulitis
V. alginolyticus	Seawater	Normal	Wound infection, cellulitis, otitis
	Seawater	Burned, other immunosuppressed	Sepsis

* Especially with liver disease or hemochromatosis.

broad and likely reflects the heterogeneous virulence attributes of the group. Occasional isolates make a protein enterotoxin very similar to CTX. Others produce cytotoxins, hemolysins, or invasins.

Gastroenteritis due to non-O1 *V. cholerae* typically has an incubation period of less than 2 days. Stools may be copious and watery, and their passage may leave the patient severely dehydrated, as in cholera; alternatively, the stools may be partly formed, less voluminous, and bloody or mucoid. Abdominal cramps, nausea, vomiting, and fever are often reported. In one series, 11 percent of patients were hospitalized; in another, the figure was 50 percent. The duration of illness ranges from about 2 to 7 days. As in cholera, patients with significant dehydration should be treated with oral or intravenous fluids. The role of antibiotics is uncertain.

Wound infection and otitis media each account for about 10 percent of non-O1 *V. cholerae* isolates. Bacteremia accounts for another 20 percent. Patients with extraintestinal infection often have a history of occupational or recreational exposure to seawater. Bacteremia is more likely to develop in the presence of liver disease. Extraintestinal infections should be treated with antibiotics. There is a paucity of information to guide the choice of a specific agent and schedule. Most strains are sensitive in vitro to tetracycline, chloramphenicol, and other agents.

SPECIES ASSOCIATED PRIMARILY WITH SOFT TISSUE INFECTION OR BACTEREMIA   *V. vulnificus*   Though it represents only a small minority of the *Vibrio* species found in nature (4 percent of Atlantic Coast isolates in one study), *V. vulnificus* is perhaps the most important cause of severe *Vibrio* infections in the United States (0.8 cases per 100,000 population in one study from Louisiana). Formerly included in the species *V. parahaemolyticus*, *V. vulnificus* was distinguished in the 1970s by its ability to ferment lactose and to cause distinct clinical syndromes. Like most vibrios, it proliferates in the warm summer months. It requires a saline environment for growth but prefers concentrations lower than those preferred by *V. parahaemolyticus* and *V. alginolyticus* (range, up to about 8 percent; optimal, about 1 percent). Infections in humans typically occur in coastal states between May and October and most often involve men over age 40. *V. vulnificus* has been linked unequivocally to two distinct syndromes: primary sepsis, typically in patients with antecedent liver disease, and primary wound infections, usually in people without underlying disease. Some authors have suggested that this organism causes gastroenteritis, but the evidence for this association is tenuous.

V. vulnificus is remarkably invasive in animal models. It is endowed with a number of virulence attributes, including an antiphagocytic capsule, serum resistance, a cytotoxin/hemolysin (the organism is Kanagawa-positive), collagenase, elastolytic protease, phospholipase, and siderophores. Its virulence, as measured by the 50 percent lethal dose in mice, is markedly enhanced under conditions of iron overload, a fact consonant with its propensity to infect patients with hemochromatosis.

Primary sepsis occurs most commonly in patients with cirrhosis or hemochromatosis but also has developed in patients with hematopoietic disorders or chronic renal insufficiency, in persons using immunosuppressive medications or alcohol, and (rarely) in individuals without apparent underlying disease. Most of those affected have ingested raw oysters within 2 days of onset (median incubation period, 16 h). The process begins precipitously with malaise, chills, fever (mean temperature, 39.8°C), and prostration. Hypotension develops in one-third of cases, often by the time of admission. Cutaneous manifestations, which develop in three-quarters of cases (usually by 36 h after onset), typically involve the extremities—lower more often than upper. A common sequence is the evolution of erythematous patches followed by ecchymoses, vesicles, and bullae. (Indeed, the presence of sepsis and bullous skin lesions suggests the diagnosis in an appropriate setting.) Necrosis and sloughing may occur. Laboratory study reveals leukopenia more often than leukocytosis, thrombocytopenia, and (occasionally) elevated levels of fibrin split products. *V. vulnificus* can be cultured from blood or cutaneous lesions.

Mortality approaches 50 percent, with most deaths due to uncontrolled sepsis. Accordingly, prompt treatment is critical and should include empirical antibiotic administration, aggressive debridement, and general supportive care. *V. vulnificus* is sensitive to a number of antimicrobials in vitro, including tetracycline, gentamicin, and third-generation cephalosporins. No compelling clinical data from studies of humans support the preferential use of any one of these agents. Tetracycline is demonstrably superior in a murine model and on that basis is considered the drug of choice (0.5 to 1 g intravenously every 12 h), either alone or in combination with gentamicin. The duration of therapy is guided by the clinical response.

Wound infections with *V. vulnificus* can develop in patients with or without underlying disease and invariably follow contact of seawater with either a prior or a fresh wound. The incubation period is brief (4 h to 4 days; mean, 12 h). The disease begins with swelling, erythema, and—in many cases—intense pain around the wound. Rapidly spreading cellulitis follows, with vesicular, bullous, or necrotic lesions developing in some instances. Metastatic events do not generally occur. Fever (median temperature, 38.9°C) and leukocytosis are demonstrable in most cases. The organism can be cultured from skin lesions and occasionally from blood. Prompt antibiotic therapy and debridement are usually curative.

V. alginolyticus   This species was first recognized as a human pathogen in 1973 and is now known to cause occasional wound, ear, and eye infections. It is the most salt-tolerant of the vibrios, able to grow in concentrations exceeding 10 percent. Most clinical isolates come from superinfected wounds, which presumably became contaminated at the beach. Infection varies in severity but is generally not serious and responds well to antibiotic therapy and drainage. A few reports have described otitis externa, otitis media, or conjunctivitis. Therapy with tetracycline is usually curative. *V. alginolyticus* is a rare cause of bacteremia in immunocompromised hosts.

BIBLIOGRAPHY

ALI A et al: *Vibrio vulnificus* sepsis in solid organ transplantation: A medical nemesis. J Heart Lung Transplant 14:598, 1995

BEGUE RE et al: Community-based assessment of safety and immunogenicity of the whole cell plus recombinant B subunit (WC/rBS) oral cholera vaccine in Peru. Vaccine 13:691, 1995

BESSER RE et al: Diagnosis and treatment of cholera in the United States. Are we prepared? JAMA 272:1203, 1994

BHAN MK et al: Clinical trials of improved oral rehydration salt formulations: A review. Bull WHO 72:945, 1994

COLWELL RR, HUQ A: Environmental reservoir of *Vibrio cholerae*, the causative agent of cholera. Ann NY Acad Sci 740:44, 1994

COSTER TS et al: Safety immunogenicity, and efficacy of live attenuated *Vibrio cholerae* O139 vaccine prototype. Lancet 345:949, 1995

HOGE CW et al: Epidemiological study of *Vibrio cholerae* O1 and O139 in Thailand: At the advancing edge of the eighth pandemic. Am J Epidemiol 143:263, 1996

KAPER JB et al: Cholera. Clin Microbiol Rev 8:48, 1995

KHAN WA et al: Comparative trial of five antimicrobial compounds in the treatment of cholera in adults. Trans R Soc Trop Med Hyg 89:103, 1995

LACEY SW: Cholera: Calamitous past, ominous future. Clin Infect Dis 20:1409, 1995

LEVINE WC, GRIFFIN PM: Vibrio infections on the Gulf Coast: Result of first year of regional surveillance. J Infect Dis 167:479, 1993

MEKALANOS JJ, SADOFF JC: Cholera vaccines: Fighting an ancient scourge. Science 265:1387, 1994

MORRIS JG JR: Non-O1 *V. cholerae*: A look at the epidemiology of an occasional pathogen. Epidemiol Rev 12:179, 1990

TAYLOR DN et al: Cholera among Americans living in Peru. Clin Infect Dis 22:1108, 1996

WALDOR MK et al: Emergence of a new cholera pandemic: Molecular analysis of virulence determinants in *Vibrio cholerae* O139 and development of a live vaccine prototype. J Infect Dis 170:278, 1994

——— et al: The *Vibrio cholerae* O139 serogroup antigen includes an O-antigen capsule and lipopolysaccharide virulence determinants. Proc Natl Acad Sci USA 91:11388, 1994

———, MEKALANOS JJ: Lysogenic conversion by a filamentous phage encoding cholera toxin. Science 272:1910, 1996

WEBER JT et al: Cholera in the United States, 1965–1991. Risks at home and abroad. Arch Intern Med 154:551, 1994

BRUCELLOSIS

DEFINITION   Brucellosis is a zoonosis transmitted to humans from infected animals. Its clinical features are not disease specific. Brucellosis and its etiologic agents are named after David Bruce, a Scottish physician who discovered the latter in 1887 while stationed in Malta. *Brucellosis* has many synonyms derived from the geographical regions in which the disease occurs (e.g., Mediterranean fever, Malta fever, Gibraltar fever, Cyprus fever); from the remittent character of its fever (e.g., undulant fever); or from its resemblance to malaria and typhoid (e.g., typhomalarial fever, intermittent typhoid).

ETIOLOGIC AGENTS   Human brucellosis can be caused by any of four species: *Brucella melitensis* (the most common cause worldwide) is acquired primarily from goats, sheep, and camels; *Brucella abortus* from cattle; *Brucella suis* from hogs; and *Brucella canis* from dogs. These small aerobic gram-negative bacilli are unencapsulated, nonmotile, non-spore-forming, facultative intracellular parasites. Brucellae are killed by boiling or pasteurization of milk and milk products. They survive for up to 8 weeks in unpasteurized, white, soft cheese made from goat's milk and are not killed by freezing. The organisms remain viable for up to 40 days in dried soil contaminated with infected-animal urine, stool, vaginal discharge, and products of conception and for longer periods in damp soil.

EPIDEMIOLOGY   The global incidence of human brucellosis is not known because of the variable quality of disease reporting and notification systems in many countries. Worldwide, the only countries believed to be free of brucellosis are Norway, Sweden, Finland, Denmark, Iceland, Switzerland, the Czech and Slovak republics, Romania, the United Kingdom (including the Channel Islands), the Netherlands, Japan, Luxembourg, Cyprus, and Bulgaria; the U.S. Virgin Islands are also free of the disease. Reports indicate that, even in developed nations, the true incidence of brucellosis may be up to 26 times higher than official figures suggest. In the United States, about 200 new cases are reported every year; however, it is estimated that only 4 to 10 percent of cases are recognized and reported. Consumption of imported cheese, travel abroad, and occupation-related exposures are the most frequently identified sources of infection. In communities where brucellosis occurs in children, the disease may be endemic and family members of infected persons are at risk. Even in countries where animal brucellosis is controlled, the disease occasionally develops among farmers, meat-processing workers, veterinarians, and laboratory workers.

Brucella is transmitted most commonly through the ingestion of untreated milk or milk products, raw meat, or bone marrow. However, the organism can be contracted via inhalation during contact with animals, especially by children and by slaughterhouse, farm, and laboratory workers. Other routes of infection for at-risk workers include skin abrasion, autoinoculation, and conjunctival splashing. The organism has been transmitted from person to person through the placenta, during breast feeding, and (in rare instances) during sexual activity.

IMMUNITY AND PATHOGENESIS   Immunity to *Brucella* is determined by phagocytosis mediated by specific antibodies and by cell-mediated mechanisms. *Brucella* organisms are phagocytosed by polymorphonuclear leukocytes and by activated macrophages. *Brucella* antigens are capable of inducing the production of specific antibodies. Serum IgM antibodies appear early after infection and are followed later by IgG and IgA. Inflammatory responses or granulomas may develop, and caseation, necrosis, and abscess formation have been described. Endogenous interleukin (IL)-12 has a strong inducing effect on interferon γ–producing T cells (see Chap. 305), which also play a key role in the host's defense against *Brucella* infection; in contrast, IL-10 downregulates protective immunity to *Brucella*. Intracellular multiplication of the organism takes place in lymph nodes and reticuloendothelial tissues. Other organs may also be affected through hematogenous spread.

CLINICAL FEATURES   The protean manifestations of brucellosis may mimic the features of other febrile illnesses. The incubation period lasts for about 1 to 3 weeks but may be as long as several months. The onset of symptoms may be either abrupt (over 1 to 2 days) or gradual (over 1 week or more). The most common symptoms are fever, chills, diaphoresis, headaches, myalgia, fatigue, anorexia, joint and low-back pain, weight loss, constipation, sore throat, and dry cough. Physical examination often reveals no abnormalities, and patients can look deceptively well. Some patients, in contrast, are acutely ill, with pallor, lymphadenopathy, hepatosplenomegaly, arthritis, spinal tenderness, epididymoorchitis, skin rash, meningitis, cardiac murmurs, or pneumonia. The fever of brucellosis has no distinctive pattern but may exhibit diurnal variation, with normal temperatures in the morning and high temperatures in the afternoon and evening. Table 162-1 lists the frequencies of key historical features, symptoms, and signs among 500 patients with brucellosis due to *B. melitensis*.

Bones and Joints   Although monarticular septic arthritis occurs, 30 to 40 percent of patients have reactive asymmetric polyarthritis involving the knees, hips, shoulders, and sacroiliac and sternoclavicular joints. The total white cell count in synovial fluid ranges from 4000 to 40,000/μL, with 60 percent polymorphonuclear leukocytes. The synovial fluid glucose concentration may be reduced and the protein concentration elevated; cultures of synovial fluid are positive in about 50 percent of cases.

Brucella osteomyelitis commonly affects the lumbar vertebrae, starting at the superior end plate (an area with a rich blood supply) and occasionally progressing to involve the entire vertebra, disk space, and adjacent vertebrae. Extraspinal *Brucella* osteomyelitis is rare. In *Brucella* septic arthritis and osteomyelitis, the peripheral white cell

Table 162-1

Relevant Historical Features and Symptoms and Signs in 500 Patients with Brucellosis due to *Brucella melitensis*

Feature	No. (%) of Patients
HISTORY	
Animal contact	368 (74)
Raw milk/cheese ingestion	350 (70)
Raw liver ingestion	147 (29)
Family history of brucellosis	188 (38)
SYMPTOM/SIGN	
Fever	464 (93)
Chills	410 (82)
Sweats	437 (87)
Aches	457 (91)
Lack of energy	473 (95)
Joint and back pain	431 (86)
Arthritis	202 (40)
Spinal tenderness	241 (48)
Headache	403 (81)
Loss of appetite	388 (78)
Weight loss	326 (65)
Constipation	234 (47)
Abdominal pain	225 (45)
Diarrhea	34 (7)
Cough	122 (24)
Testicular pain/epididymoorchitis	62 (21*)
Rash	72 (14)
Sleep disturbances	185 (37)
Ill appearance	127 (25)
Pallor	110 (22)
Lymphadenopathy	160 (32)
Splenomegaly	125 (25)
Hepatomegaly	97 (19)
Jaundice	6 (1)
Central nervous system abnormalities	20 (4)
Cardiac murmur	17 (3)
Pneumonia	7 (1)

* Among 290 males.

count is normal, while the erythrocyte sedimentation rate may be either normal or elevated.

Heart   Cardiovascular complications of brucellosis include endocarditis, myocarditis, pericarditis, aortic root abscess, mycotic aneurysms, thrombophlebitis with pulmonary aneurysm, and pulmonary embolism. *Brucella* endocarditis may develop on valves previously damaged by rheumatic fever or congenital malformation but also occurs on previously normal valves. The clinical features are indistinguishable from those of endocarditis caused by other organisms (see Chap. 126). In the past, endocarditis was the leading cause of death in brucellosis. In recent years, the outcome of *Brucella* endocarditis has been more favorable because of advances in early diagnosis, antibiotic treatment, and cardiac surgery. Physicians of patients with culture-negative endocarditis who, because of environmental exposure, may be at risk for *Brucella* infection should notify the bacteriology laboratory performing the blood culture so that extended incubation, specific media, and biohazard precautions can be employed.

Respiratory Tract   *Brucella* can produce respiratory symptoms. A flulike illness with sore throat, tonsillitis, and dry cough is common and usually mild. Hilar and paratracheal lymphadenopathy, pneumonia, solitary or multiple pulmonary nodules, lung abscesses, and empyema have been reported.

Gastrointestinal Tract   Gastrointestinal manifestations of *Brucella* infection are generally mild and may include nausea, vomiting, constipation, acute abdominal pain, and/or diarrhea. Pathologic examination of the liver may reveal any of several changes, including noncaseating granuloma, suppurative abscesses, or mononuclear cell infiltration. Hepatic and splenic enlargement may be documented in 15 to 20 percent of cases, and abscesses may develop in the liver and spleen. Mild jaundice may be evident, with elevated levels of bilirubin and hepatic enzymes.

Genitourinary Tract   Various genitourinary infections have been attributed to *Brucella*, including unilateral or bilateral epididymoorchitis, which is a self-limiting manifestation. Prostatitis, seminal vesiculitis, dysmenorrhea, tuboovarian abscess, salpingitis, cervicitis, and acute pyelonephritis have also been documented. *Brucella* has been cultured from the urine in up to 50 percent of cases of genitourinary tract infection.

Central Nervous System   Neurobrucellosis is uncommon but serious and includes meningoencephalitis, multiple cerebral or cerebellar abscesses, ruptured mycotic aneurysms, myelitis, Guillain-Barré syndrome, cranial nerve lesions, hemiplegia, sciatica, myositis, and rhabdomyolysis. Papillitis, papilledema, retrobulbar neuritis, optic atrophy, and ophthalmoplegia due to lesions in cranial nerves III, IV, and VI may occur in *Brucella* meningoencephalitis. Cerebrospinal fluid (CSF) pressure is usually elevated; the fluid may appear clear, turbid, or hemorrhagic; the protein concentration and cell count (predominantly lymphocytes) are elevated; and the glucose concentration may be either reduced or normal. In *Brucella* meningitis, the organism may be cultured from the CSF.

Other Manifestations   Splashing of the eyes with virulent brucellae or with organisms in veterinary vaccines may result in keratitis, corneal ulcers, uveitis, retinal detachment, and endophthalmitis.

Skin manifestations of brucellosis are uncommon. They include maculopapular eruptions, purpura and petechiae, chronic ulcerations, multiple cutaneous and subcutaneous abscesses, discharging sinuses, superficial thrombophlebitis, erythema nodosum, and pemphigus.

Brucellosis during human pregnancy can cause fetal death. *Brucella* has been isolated from the human placenta and fetus.

Endocrinologic findings in brucellosis include thyroiditis, adrenal insufficiency, and the syndrome of inappropriate secretion of antidiuretic hormone.

DIAGNOSIS   The combination of potential exposure, consistent clinical features, and raised levels of *Brucella* agglutinin (with or without positive cultures of blood or tissues) confirms the diagnosis of brucellosis. Serum antibodies to *Brucella* can be detected by several methods, including standard tube agglutinins (STA), the 2-mercaptoethanol agglutination test, Coombs' test, and an enzyme-linked immunosorbent assay. *B. abortus* antigens, which are commonly used for serologic tests, cross-react with *B. melitensis* and *B. suis* but not with *B. canis*. Specific antigen is required for the diagnosis of *B. canis* infection; although the materials required for testing are not commercially available, *B. canis* antibody titers can be determined in the United States at the Centers for Disease Control and Prevention in Atlanta. A false-negative result in the STA may be obtained because of the presence of IgA and IgG blocking antibodies. This so-called prozone phenomenon can be avoided by testing of sera at both low and high dilutions. In endemic areas a *Brucella* antibody titer of 1:320 or 1:640 is significant, while in nonendemic areas an antibody titer of 1:160 is considered significant. Detection of elevated levels of antibody to *Brucella* in the absence of symptoms during the screening of potential blood donors is common in endemic areas. To establish a diagnosis in these regions, clinical and serologic evaluation should be repeated after 2 to 4 weeks and a further rise in titer sought. A high titer of specific IgM suggests recent exposure, while a high titer of specific IgG suggests active disease. Lower titers of IgG may indicate past exposure or treated infection. Several studies have demonstrated that the polymerase chain reaction is specific and highly sensitive for the detection of *Brucella*.

Cooperation and consultation with a microbiologist are important when brucellosis is suspected. It may be necessary to hold culture bottles for up to 6 weeks. Subcultures should be prepared on duplicate blood agar plates (with and without an atmosphere of 10% CO_2) and special media. Cultures of blood or bone marrow are positive in 50 to 70 percent of cases. The peripheral white cell count is usually normal but may be low, with relative lymphocytosis. Thrombocytopenia and disseminated intravascular coagulation may be documented. Levels of hepatic enzymes and serum bilirubin may be raised.

Radiologic investigations aimed at detecting skeletal involvement include plain radiography, bone scintigraphy, computed tomography (CT), and magnetic resonance imaging (MRI). Bone scintigraphy is more sensitive than conventional radiography in detecting areas of spinal and extraspinal involvement, particularly in the early stage of infection. CT is useful for further evaluation of spinal lesions and of the extension of infection into the spinal canal. MRI is the modality of choice for the assessment of *Brucella* spondylitis and is more sensitive than scintigraphy or CT for demonstration of the extent of disease.

Plain lateral radiography of the spine may reveal bone sclerosis, with destruction and erosion of the superior end plate anteriorly. As the disease progresses, healing with osteophyte formation and reduction of disk space may take place. In *Brucella* septic monarthritis, plain radiography may show effusion and soft tissue swelling without bone or joint destruction. Scintigraphy may document increased uptake in sacroiliac joints or lumbar vertebrae even when plain radiography gives normal results. MRI shows diffuse, high signal intensity of the affected vertebrae and may reveal narrowing of the spinal canal as well as loss of definition of the posterior aspect of the vertebrae.

R𝗑 TREATMENT
Single-agent therapy for brucellosis has now been abandoned because of the high incidence of failure and relapse and the potential development of resistance. Relatively short courses (less than 8 weeks) of treatment with antibiotic combinations have similarly been associated with high rates of relapse. The combination of doxycycline and an aminoglycoside (streptomycin, gentamicin, or netilmicin) for 4 weeks followed by the combination of doxycycline and rifampin for 4 to 8 weeks is the most effective regimen. Doxycycline (which is preferred over tetracycline) is given orally in a dose of 100 mg twice daily. Netilmicin (which is preferred to streptomycin) is given (intramuscularly to outpatients, intravenously to inpatients) in a dose of 2 mg/kg every 12 h; trough levels in plasma should be monitored regularly and maintained at ≤2 μg/mL. Streptomycin is given intramuscularly in a dose of 1 g once daily to patients

under 45 years of age and in a dose of 0.5 to 0.75 g/d to older patients. Gentamicin is given intramuscularly or as a slow intravenous infusion (3 to 5 mg/kg per day in divided doses every 8 h). Tetracycline is given orally in a dose of 250 mg every 6 h and rifampin as a single daily dose of 600 to 900 mg. An alternative regimen consists of the doxycycline/rifampin combination given for 8 to 12 weeks. The doxycycline/netilmicin (or doxycycline/ streptomycin) combination is more effective than the doxycycline/ rifampin combination in that rifampin reduces levels of doxycycline in plasma.

When used alone, fluoroquinolones—antibiotics with good intracellular penetration and efficacy against *Brucella* in vitro—have been associated with the development of quinolone resistance and with high rates of failure and relapse. At present, clinical data are inadequate for the formulation of recommendations regarding the combination of fluoroquinolones with doxycycline, rifampin, or streptomycin.

Third-generation cephalosporins (e.g., ceftriaxone), although active in vitro against *Brucella* when used alone, have also been associated with a high incidence of clinical failure and relapse. These agents may be useful in combination with other drugs for the treatment of *Brucella* meningitis.

In pregnancy, trimethoprim-sulfamethoxazole (TMP-SMZ) can be given in combination with rifampin for 8 to 12 weeks. Children below the age of 7 years can also be treated with rifampin and TMP-SMZ for 8 to 12 weeks, while older children should receive the same antibiotics as adults in the following doses: doxycycline, 100 mg/d orally; an aminoglycoside; and rifampin, 15 mg/kg per day orally or by slow intravenous infusion. TMP-SMZ is given orally every 12 h in a dose that depends on the patient's age (birth to 6 months, 120 mg; 6 months to 6 years, 240 mg).

In cases of neurobrucellosis, aortic root abscess, and endocarditis, rifampin should be added to the doxycycline/aminoglycoside combination. Cardiac surgery may be needed along with antibiotic therapy in the acute stage, particularly in cases of *Brucella* endocarditis and aortic root abscess. In instances of renal failure, doxycycline can be used safely. In contrast, the use of aminoglycosides requires facilities for the monitoring of plasma levels; if such facilities are not available, then the doxycycline/rifampin combination should be administered for 8 to 12 weeks.

Within 4 to 14 days after the initiation of therapy, patients become afebrile and constitutional symptoms disappear. The enlarged liver and spleen return to their normal size within 2 to 4 weeks. An acute, intense flare-up of symptoms may follow the start of treatment, especially that with tetracyclines. This reaction is transient and does not necessitate the discontinuation of therapy. In endemic areas the coexistence of brucellosis and tuberculous spondylitis may result in a failure to respond to appropriate treatment. Treated patients whose infections are apparently cured should be followed up clinically and serologically, with repeat blood cultures, every 3 to 6 months for 2 years.

PREVENTION Efforts at prevention should be aimed at the source of infection. Immunization of animals and boiling or pasteurization of milk and milk products are important. Workers in the meat and dairy industries in the former Soviet Union, China, and France have been vaccinated; the vaccine (two injections given 2 weeks apart, each containing 1 mg of an insoluble fraction of phenol-extracted bacteria) has markedly reduced the rate of infection. However, immunity is short-lived, and vaccination should be repeated every 2 years. This vaccine is not used in the United States.

PROGNOSIS Deaths attributable to brucellosis should be avoidable. Even before the discovery of antibiotics, mortality was less than 2 percent and endocarditis was most frequently the cause of death. Morbidity due to brucellosis remains significant; its severity depends on the infecting *Brucella* species and is greatest with *B. melitensis*. Spinal damage, paraplegia, and other neurologic deficits may occur. Nerve deafness due to meningitis or secondary to treatment with streptomycin has been documented.

BIBLIOGRAPHY

AL-KASAB S et al: Management of *Brucella* endocarditis with aortic root abscess. Chest 98:1532, 1990

AL MAJED SA et al: Use of antibiotics in the treatment of human brucellosis. Curr Ther Res Clin Exp 57:175, 1996

ARIZA J et al: Treatment of human brucellosis with doxycycline plus rifampin or doxycycline plus streptomycin: A randomized double-blind study. Ann Intern Med 117:25, 1992

CENTERS FOR DISEASE CONTROL AND PREVENTION: Brucellosis outbreak at a pork processing plant—North Carolina, 1992. JAMA 271:1734, 1994

CHEVALIER P et al: Fatal *Brucella* pancarditis. Presse Med 25:628, 1996

CHOMEL BB et al: Changing trends in the epidemiology of human brucellosis in California from 1973 to 1992: A shift toward foodborne transmission. J Infect Dis 170:1216, 1994

COMENERO JD et al: Possible implications of doxycycline-rifampin interaction for treatment of brucellosis. Antimicrob Agents Chemother 38:2798, 1994

GARCIA-RODRIGUEZ JA et al: Susceptibilities of *Brucella melitensis* to clinafloxacin and four other new fluoroquinolones. Antimicrob Agents Chemother 39:1194, 1995

HADJICHRISTODOVLOV C et al: Tolerance of the human brucellosis vaccine and the intradermal reaction test for brucellosis. Eur J Clin Microbiol Infect Dis 13:129, 1994

MADKOUR MM: *Brucellosis*. London, Butterworths, 1989

———— et al: Osteoarticular brucellosis; results of bone scintigraphy in 140 patients. Am J Roentgenol 150:1101, 1988

———— et al: Occupational related infectious arthritis, in *Baillier's Clinical Rheumatology: Occupational Rheumatic Diseases*, GP Balint (ed). London, Saunders, 1989, pp 157–192

ROMERO C et al: Specific detection of *Brucella* DNA by PCR. J Clin Microbiol 33:615, 1995

ZHAN Y, CHEERS C: Endogenous interleukin-12 is involved in resistance to *Brucella abortus* infection. Infect Immun 63:1387, 1995

163 *Richard F. Jacobs*

TULAREMIA

DEFINITION Tularemia is a zoonosis caused by *Francisella tularensis*, so named in 1974 in recognition of the contributions of Edward Francis. Humans of any age, sex, or race are universally susceptible to this systemic infection. Tularemia is primarily a disease of wild animals and persists in contaminated environments, ectoparasites, and animal carriers. Human infection is incidental and usually results from interaction with biting or blood-sucking insects, wild or domestic animals, or the environment. Tularemia is common in Arkansas, Oklahoma, and Missouri, where more than 50 percent of the cases in the United States occur. An increasing number of cases of tularemia have been reported from the Scandinavian countries, eastern Europe, and Siberia. The illness is characterized by various clinical syndromes, the most common of which consists of an ulcerative lesion at the site of inoculation, with regional lymphadenopathy and lymphadenitis. Systemic manifestations, including pneumonia, typhoidal tularemia, and fever without localizing findings, pose a greater diagnostic challenge.

ETIOLOGY AND EPIDEMIOLOGY *F. tularensis* is the etiologic agent of tularemia, which, with rare exceptions, is the only disease produced by this genus. The organism is a small, gram-negative, pleomorphic, nonmotile, non-spore-forming bacillus measuring 0.2×0.2 to 0.7 μm. Bipolar staining results in a coccoid appearance. The organism is a thinly encapsulated, nonpiliated strict aerobe that invades host cells.

In nature, *F. tularensis* is a hardy organism that persists for weeks or months in mud, water, and decaying animal carcasses. Dozens of biting and blood-sucking insects, especially ticks and tabanid flies, serve as vectors. Ticks and wild rabbits are the source for most of the human cases in the endemic areas of the southeastern United States and the Rocky Mountain states. In Utah, Nevada, and California, tabanid flies are the most common vectors. Animal reservoirs include wild rabbits, squirrels, birds, sheep, beavers, muskrats, and domestic dogs and cats.

The two main biovars of *F. tularensis*—*tularensis* (type A) and *palearctica* (type B)—are both found in the United States. Type A produces more serious disease in humans; without treatment, the associated fatality rate is approximately 5 percent. Type B produces a milder, often subclinical infection that is usually contracted from water or marine mammals.

Ticks pass the organism to their offspring via a transovarian route. The organism is found in tick feces but not in large quantities in tick salivary glands. In the United States, the disease can be carried by *Dermacentor andersoni* (Rocky Mountain wood tick), *Dermacentor variabilis* (American dog tick), *Dermacentor occidentalis* (Pacific coast dog tick), and *Amblyomma americanum* (Lone Star tick). *F. tularensis* is transmitted frequently during blood meals taken by embedded ticks following hours of attachment. It is the taking of a blood meal through a fecally contaminated field that transmits the organism. Tularemia is more common among men. Person-to-person transmission is rare or nonexistent. Transmission of the organism by ticks and tabanid flies takes place mainly in the spring and summer. However, continued transmission in the winter months by trapped or hunted animals has been documented. The organism is extremely infectious. Biosafety level 2 is recommended for clinical laboratory work with material whose contamination is suspected, and biosafety level 3 is required for culture of the organism in large quantities.

PATHOGENESIS AND PATHOLOGY   The most common portal of entry for human infection is through skin or mucous membranes, either directly—through the bite of a tick, other arthropods, or other animals—or via inapparent abrasions. Inhalation or ingestion of *F. tularensis* can also result in infection. Although more than 10^8 organisms are usually required to produce infection via the oral route (oropharyngeal or gastrointestinal tularemia), fewer than 50 organisms will result in infection when injected into the skin (ulceroglandular/glandular tularemia) or inhaled (pneumonia). After inoculation into the skin, the organism multiplies locally; within 2 to 5 days (range, 1 to 10 days), it produces an erythematous, tender, or pruritic papule. The papule rapidly enlarges and forms an ulcer with a black base (chancriform lesion). The bacteria spread to regional lymph nodes, producing lymphadenopathy (buboes), and, with bacteremia, may spread to distant organs.

Tularemia is characterized by mononuclear cell infiltration with pyogranulomatous pathology. The histopathologic findings can be quite similar to those in tuberculosis, although tularemia develops more rapidly. As a facultatively intracellular bacterium, *F. tularensis* is capable of parasitizing both phagocytic and nonphagocytic host cells and of surviving intracellularly for prolonged periods. In the acute phase of infection, the primary organs affected (skin, lymph nodes, liver, and spleen) include areas of focal necrosis, initially surrounded by polymorphonuclear leukocytes. Subsequently, granulomas form, with epithelioid cells, lymphocytes, and multinucleated giant cells surrounded by areas of necrosis. These areas may resemble caseation necrosis but later coalesce to form abscesses.

Conjunctival inoculation can result in infection of the eye, with regional lymph node enlargement (preauricular lymphadenopathy, Parinaud's complex). Aerosolization and inhalation or hematogenous spread of organisms can result in pneumonia. In the lung, an inflammatory reaction—with foci of alveolar necrosis and cell infiltration (initially polymorphonuclear and later mononuclear) with granulomas—develops. Chest roentgenograms usually reveal bilateral patchy infiltrates rather than large areas of consolidation. Pleural effusions are common and may contain blood. Lymphadenopathy occurs in regions draining infected organs. Therefore, in pulmonary infection, mediastinal adenopathy may be evident, while patients with oropharyngeal tularemia develop cervical lymphadenopathy. In gastrointestinal or typhoidal tularemia, mesenteric lymphadenopathy may follow the in-

gestion of large numbers of organisms. The term *typhoidal tularemia* may be used to describe severe bacteremic disease, irrespective of the mode of transmission or portal of entry. Meningitis has been reported as a primary or secondary manifestation of bacteremia. Patients may also present with fever and no localizing signs.

IMMUNOLOGY   Infection with *F. tularensis* stimulates the host to produce antibodies. However, this antibody response probably plays only a minor role in the containment of infection. In contrast, cell-mediated immunity, which develops over 2 to 4 weeks, plays a major role in containment and eradication of the infection. Macrophages, once activated, are capable of killing *F. tularensis*.

Immunospecific protection against tularemia can be afforded either by natural infection or by vaccination with live attenuated strains of *F. tularensis*. Killed vaccines, on the other hand, induce no protection against virulent *F. tularensis*. After natural infection or vaccination, serum antibodies to surface-exposed carbohydrate antigens predominate, whereas T cell determinants are located on membrane proteins beneath the bacterial capsule. T cell responses are thought to be due to priming by the organism. The anamnestic T cell response to *F. tularensis* seems to involve a multitude of microbial proteins, each with a distinct set of T cell determinants. A predominant role for CD4+ T cells is supported by the results of experiments in mice, which indicated that resistance to infection was restricted at the level of the MHC class II determinants. Humans primed to *F. tularensis* (like those primed to *Mycobacterium tuberculosis*) show a T_H1-like response. T cell proliferation is associated with the production of interleukin (IL) 2 and interferon γ but with little or no production of IL-4.

Recent investigations of neutrophils in cases of tularemia have suggested that polymorphonuclear neutrophils (PMNs) are needed for defense against primary infection. PMNs may restrict the growth of *F. tularensis* before the organism becomes intracellular.

CLINICAL MANIFESTATIONS   Tularemia often starts with a sudden onset of fever, chills, headache, and generalized myalgias and arthralgias (Table 163-1). This onset takes place when the organism penetrates the skin, is ingested, or is inhaled. An incubation period of 2 to 10 days is followed by the formation of an ulcer at the site of penetration, with local inflammation. The ulcer may persist for several months as organisms are transported via the lymphatics to the regional lymph nodes. These nodes enlarge and may become necrotic and suppurating. If the organism enters the bloodstream, widespread dissemination as well as signs and symptoms of endotoxemia may result.

In the United States, most patients with tularemia (75 to 85 percent) acquire the infection by inoculation of the skin. In adults, the most common localized form is inguinal/femoral lymphadenopathy; in children, it is cervical lymphadenopathy. About 20 percent of patients develop a generalized maculopapular rash, which occasionally becomes pustular. Erythema nodosum occurs infrequently. The clinical manifestations of tularemia have been divided into various syndromes, which are listed in Table 163-2.

Ulceroglandular/Glandular Tularemia   These two forms of tularemia account for approximately 75 to 85 percent of cases. The predominant form in children involves cervical or posterior auricular lymphadenopathy and is usually related to tick bites on the head and neck area. In adults, the most common form is inguinal/femoral

Table 163-1

Clinical Presentation of Tularemia

Sign or Symptom	Rate of Occurrence, %	
	Children	Adults
Lymphadenopathy	96	65
Fever (≥38.3°C)	87	21
Ulcer/eschar/papule	45	51
Myalgias/arthralgias	39	2
Headache	9	5
Cough	9	5
Pharyngitis	43	—
Diarrhea	43	—

SOURCE: Adapted from Jacobs et al.

Table 163-2

CHAPTER 163
Tularemia
973

Clinical Syndromes of Tularemia

Syndrome	Rate of Occurrence, %	
	Children	Adults
Ulceroglandular	45	51
Glandular	25	12
Pulmonary (pneumonia)	14	18
Oropharyngeal	4	—
Oculoglandular	2	—
Typhoidal	2	12
Unclassified	6	11

SOURCE: Adapted from Jacobs et al.

lymphadenopathy resulting from insect and tick exposures on the lower limbs. In cases related to wild game, the usual portal of entry for *F. tularensis* is either an injury sustained while skinning or cleaning an animal carcass or a bite (usually on the hand). Epitrochlear lymphadenopathy/lymphadenitis is common in patients with bite-related injuries.

In ulceroglandular tularemia, the ulcer is erythematous, indurated, and nonhealing, with a punched-out appearance that lasts from 1 to 3 weeks. The papule may begin as an erythematous lesion that is tender or pruritic; it evolves over several days into an ulcer with sharply demarcated edges and a yellow exudate. The ulcer gradually develops a black base, and simultaneously the regional lymph nodes become tender and severely enlarged. The affected lymph nodes may become fluctuant and drain spontaneously, but usually the condition resolves with effective treatment. Late suppuration of lymph nodes has been described in up to 25 percent of patients with ulceroglandular/glandular tularemia. Examination of material taken from these late fluctuant nodes after successful antimicrobial treatment has revealed sterile necrotic tissue. In 5 to 10 percent of patients, the skin lesion may be inapparent, with lymphadenopathy plus systemic signs and symptoms the only physical findings. This clinical syndrome is designated *glandular tularemia*. Conversely, a tick or deerfly bite on the trunk may result in an ulcer without evident lymphadenopathy.

Oculoglandular Tularemia In about 1 percent of patients, the portal of entry for *F. tularensis* is the conjunctiva. Usually, the organism reaches the conjunctiva through contact with contaminated fingers. The inflamed conjunctiva is painful, with numerous yellowish nodules and pinpoint ulcers. Purulent conjunctivitis with regional lymphadenopathy (preauricular, submandibular, or cervical) is evident. Because of debilitating pain, the patient may seek medical attention before regional lymphadenopathy develops. Painful preauricular lymphadenopathy is unique to tularemia and distinguishes it from cat-scratch disease, tuberculosis, sporotrichosis, and syphilis. Corneal perforation may occur.

Oropharyngeal and Gastrointestinal Tularemia Rarely, tularemia follows the ingestion of contaminated undercooked meat, the oral inoculation of *F. tularensis* from the hands in association with the skinning and cleaning of animal carcasses, or the consumption of contaminated food or water. Oral inoculation may result in acute, exudative, or membranous pharyngitis associated with cervical lymphadenopathy or in ulcerative intestinal lesions associated with mesenteric lymphadenopathy, diarrhea, abdominal pain, nausea, vomiting, and gastrointestinal bleeding. Infected tonsils become enlarged and develop a yellowish-white pseudomembrane, which can be confused with that of diphtheria. The clinical severity of gastrointestinal tularemia varies from mild, unexplained, persistent diarrhea with no other symptoms to a rapidly fulminant, fatal disease. In fatal cases, the extensive intestinal ulceration found at autopsy suggests an enormous inoculum.

Pulmonary Tularemia Tularemia pneumonia presents as variable parenchymal infiltrates that are unresponsive to treatment with β-lactam antibiotics. Tularemia must be considered in the differential diagnosis of atypical pneumonia in a patient with a history of travel to an endemic area. The disease can result from either inhalation of an infectious aerosol or spread to the lungs and pleura after bloodstream dissemination. Inhalation-related pneumonia has been described in laboratory workers after exposure to contaminated materials and is associated with a relatively high mortality rate. Exposure to *F. tularensis* in aerosols from live domestic animals or dead wildlife (including birds) has been reported to cause pneumonia. Hematogenous dissemination to the lungs occurs in 10 to 15 percent of cases of ulceroglandular tularemia and in about half of cases of typhoidal tularemia. Previously, tularemia pneumonia was thought to be a disease of older patients, but as many as 10 to 15 percent of children with clinical manifestations of tularemia have parenchymal infiltrates detected by chest roentgenography. Patients with pneumonia usually have a nonproductive cough and may have dyspnea or pleuritic chest pain. Roentgenograms of the chest usually reveal bilateral patchy infiltrates (described as ovoid or lobar densities), lobar parenchymal infiltrates, and cavitary lesions. Pleural effusions may have a predominance of mononuclear leukocytes or PMNs and sometimes red blood cells. Empyema may develop. Patients with tularemia pneumonia can have blood cultures positive for *F. tularensis*.

Typhoidal Tularemia Once thought to represent up to 10 percent of all cases of tularemia, the typhoidal presentation is now considered to be rare in the United States. In this presentation, fever develops without apparent skin lesions or lymphadenopathy. In the absence of a history of possible contact with a vector, diagnosis can be extremely difficult. Blood cultures may be positive and patients may present with classic sepsis or septic shock in this acute systemic form of the infection. Typhoidal tularemia is usually associated with a huge inoculum or with a preexisting compromising condition. High continuous fevers, signs of endotoxemia, and severe headache are common findings. The patient may be delirious and may develop prostration and shock. If presumptive antibiotic therapy in culture-negative cases does not include an aminoglycoside, the mortality rate can approach 30 percent.

Other Manifestations *F. tularensis* infection has been associated with meningitis, pericarditis, hepatitis, peritonitis, endocarditis, osteomyelitis, and sepsis and septic shock with rhabdomyolysis and acute renal failure. In the rare cases of tularemia meningitis, a predominantly lymphocytic response can be demonstrated in cerebrospinal fluid.

DIFFERENTIAL DIAGNOSIS When patients in endemic areas present with fever, chronic ulcerative skin lesions, and large tender lymph nodes, a diagnosis of tularemia should be made presumptively, and confirmatory diagnostic testing and appropriate therapy should be undertaken. When the possibility of tularemia is considered in a patient with this presentation in a nonendemic area, an attempt should be made to determine whether the individual has come into contact with a potential animal vector. The level of suspicion of tularemia should be especially high in hunters, trappers, game wardens, veterinarians, laboratory workers, and individuals with a history of exposure to an insect or other animal vector. However, up to 40 percent of patients with tularemia have no known history of epidemiologic contact with an arthropod or other animal vector.

The characteristic presentation of ulceroglandular tularemia does not pose a diagnostic problem, but a less classic progression of regional lymphadenopathy or glandular tularemia must be differentiated from other diseases. The skin lesion may resemble those seen in sporotrichosis; skin infection with *Staphylococcus aureus*, *Streptococcus pyogenes*, or *Mycobacterium marinum*; syphilis; anthrax; rat-bite fever (due to *Spirillum minus*); or rickettsiosis (scrub typhus). In the latter infections, regional lymphadenopathy is usually not as impressive as in tularemia. The lymphadenopathy of tularemia (especially glandular tularemia) must be differentiated from that of plague, lymphogranuloma venereum, and cat-scratch disease. In children, the differentiation from cat-scratch disease is made more difficult by the chronic papulovesicular lesion associated with *Bartonella henselae* infection (see Chap. 165).

Oropharyngeal tularemia can resemble and must be differentiated from pharyngitis due to group A beta-hemolytic streptococci, *Arcano-*

bacterium haemolyticum, or *Corynebacterium diphtheriae* as well as from infectious mononucleosis. Tularemia pneumonia may resemble any of the atypical pneumonias, including those due to various viruses, *Mycoplasma pneumoniae*, *Chlamydia pneumoniae*, *Chlamydia psittaci*, *Legionella pneumophila*, *Coxiella burnetii*, and (occasionally) *Histoplasma capsulatum*. Typhoidal tularemia may resemble typhoid fever, other *Salmonella* bacteremias, rickettsial infections (Rocky Mountain spotted fever, ehrlichiosis), brucellosis, infectious mononucleosis, acquired toxoplasmosis, miliary tuberculosis, sarcoidosis, and hematologic or reticuloendothelial malignancies.

LABORATORY DIAGNOSIS Direct microscopic examination of polychromatically stained tissue smears or clinical specimens reveals *F. tularensis* organisms, singly and in groups, both intra- and extracellularly. Gram's staining of clinical or biopsy material is of little value, as the small, weakly staining organisms cannot be readily distinguished from the background. An indirect fluorescent antibody test with commercially available antisera can be useful, although false-positive results due to *Legionella* species have been reported.

The diagnosis of tularemia is most frequently confirmed by serologic testing. In the standard tube agglutination test, a single titer of ≥1:160 is interpreted as a presumptive positive result. A fourfold increase in titer between paired serum samples collected 2 to 3 weeks apart is considered diagnostic. False-negative serologic responses are obtained early in infection; up to 30 percent of patients infected for 3 weeks have sera that test negative. Late in infection, titers into the thousands are common, and titers of 1:20 to 1:80 may persist for years. A microagglutination test that may be as much as 100-fold more sensitive than the standard tube agglutination test has been described and is currently being used in many clinical microbiology laboratories. Enzyme-linked immunosorbent assays have proven useful for the detection of both antibodies and antigens. Analysis of urine for *F. tularensis* antigen has yielded promising results in clinical trials, but facilities for this type of analysis are not widely available. A skin test for delayed hypersensitivity to *F. tularensis* turns positive during the first week of illness and remains positive for years. The skin-test antigen, which is not commercially available, can boost titers of agglutinating antibody.

Culture and isolation of *F. tularensis* are difficult. In one study the organism was isolated in only 10 percent of more than 1000 human cases, 84 percent of which were confirmed by serology. The medium of choice is cysteine-glucose-blood agar. *F. tularensis* can be isolated directly from infected ulcer scrapings, lymph-node biopsy specimens, gastric washings, sputum, and blood cultures. Colonies are blue-gray, round, smooth, and slightly mucoid. On media containing blood, a small zone of alpha hemolysis usually surrounds the colony. Slide agglutination tests or direct fluorescent antibody tests with commercially available antisera can be applied directly to culture suspensions for identification.

The polymerase chain reaction has been used to detect *F. tularensis* DNA, primarily in blood. However, this test has not been shown to be more sensitive than direct culture and at present remains a research tool.

℞ **TREATMENT**

F. tularensis cannot be subjected to standardized antimicrobial susceptibility testing because the organism will not grow on the media used. A wide variety of antibiotics, including all β-lactam antibiotics and the newer cephalosporins, are ineffective for the treatment of this infection. Recent studies indicated that third-generation cephalosporins were active against *F. tularensis* in vitro, but clinical case reports suggested a nearly universal failure rate of ceftriaxone in pediatric patients with tularemia. Although in vitro data indicate that imipenem may be active, therapy with imipenem, sulfanilamides, and macrolides is not presently recommended because of the lack of clinical data. Fluoroquinolones have shown promise in terms of their relatively low toxicity and their potential for oral administration. Chloramphenicol

and tetracycline have been used successfully for treatment of the acute stages of tularemia but have been associated with higher relapse rates (up to 20 percent) than conventionally used agents.

Streptomycin, given intramuscularly at a dose of 7.5 to 10 mg/kg every 12 h, is considered the drug of choice for adults. In severe cases, 15 mg/kg every 12 h may be used for the first 48 to 72 h. Streptomycin is also considered the drug of choice for children; the appropriate dose is 30 to 40 mg/kg daily in two divided doses administered intramuscularly. In children, after a clinical response is demonstrated at 3 to 5 days, the dose can be reduced to 10 to 15 mg/kg daily in two divided doses. Therapy is typically continued for 7 to 10 days; however, in mild to moderate cases of tularemia in which the patient becomes afebrile within the first 48 to 72 h of streptomycin treatment, a 5- to 7-day course has been successful.

Gentamicin, at a dose of 1.7 mg/kg given intravenously or intramuscularly every 8 h, is also effective. The published experience in adults consists of two reports describing, respectively, nine and eight patients who were treated effectively with gentamicin. The eight patients in one of the reports all had fever before treatment, and all eight became afebrile within 24 to 72 h. In a recent pediatric study, other symptoms, such as tender lymphadenitis and pharyngitis, also responded within 24 to 72 h of the start of gentamicin therapy.

Virtually all strains of *F. tularensis* are susceptible to streptomycin and gentamicin. In successfully treated patients, defervescence usually occurs within 2 days, but skin lesions and lymph nodes may take 1 to 2 weeks to heal. When therapy is not initiated within the first several days of illness, defervescence may be delayed. Relapses are uncommon with streptomycin or gentamicin therapy. Late lymph-node suppuration, however, occurs in approximately 40 percent of children, regardless of the treatment received. These nodes have typically been found to contain sterile necrotic tissue without evidence of active infection. Patients with fluctuant nodes should receive several days of antibiotic therapy before drainage to minimize the risk to hospital personnel. Unlike streptomycin and gentamicin, tobramycin is ineffective in the treatment of tularemia and should not be used.

PROGNOSIS If tularemia goes untreated, symptoms usually last 1 to 4 weeks but may continue for months. The mortality rate from severe untreated infection (including all cases of untreated tularemia pneumonia and typhoidal tularemia) can be as high as 30 percent. However, the overall mortality rate for untreated tularemia is less than 8 percent. Mortality is less than 1 percent with appropriate treatment. Poor outcomes are often associated with long delays in diagnosis and treatment. Lifelong immunity usually follows tularemia.

PREVENTION The prevention of tularemia is based on avoidance of exposure to biting and blood-sucking insects, especially ticks and deerflies. An intradermal vaccine made from live attenuated *F. tularensis* is available from the Centers for Disease Control and Prevention. This vaccine is effective in reducing the frequency and severity of infection. Vaccination of high-risk individuals working with large quantities of cultured organisms is recommended. Others who come into contact with the organisms, such as veterinarians, hunters, or game wardens, should consider vaccination, particularly if they live in endemic areas. The avoidance of skinning wild animals, especially rabbits, and the wearing of gloves while handling animal carcasses decrease the risk of transmission. Use of insect repellents and preparations that prevent tick attachment as well as prompt removal of ticks can be helpful. Prophylaxis of tularemia has not proved effective in patients with embedded ticks or insect bites. However, in patients who are known to have been exposed to large quantities of organisms (e.g., in the laboratory) and who have incubating infection with *F. tularensis*, early treatment can prevent the development of significant clinical disease.

BIBLIOGRAPHY

BAKER CN et al: Antimicrobial susceptibility testing of *Francisella tularensis* with a modified Mueller-Hinton broth. J Clin Microbiol 22:212, 1985

BERNARD K et al: Early recognition of atypical *Francisella tularensis* strains lacking a cysteine requirement. J Clin Microbiol 32:551, 1994

CROSS JT, JACOBS RF: Tularemia: Treatment failures with outpatient use of ceftriaxone. Clin Infect Dis 17:976, 1993

ENDERLIN G et al: Streptomycin and alternative agents for the treatment of tularemia: Review of the literature. Clin Infect Dis 19:42, 1994

JACOBS RF, NARAIN JP: Tularemia in children. Pediatr Infect Dis J 2:487, 1983

——— et al: Tularemia in adults and children: A changing presentation. Pediatrics 76:818, 1985

LONG GW et al: Detection of *Francisella tularensis* in blood by polymerase chain reaction. J Clin Microbiol 31:152, 1993

MASON WL et al: Treatment of tularemia, including pulmonary tularemia, with gentamicin. Am Rev Respir Dis 121:39, 1980

PENN RL, KINASEWITZ GT: Factors associated with a poor outcome in tularemia. Arch Intern Med 147:265, 1987

RUBIN SA: Radiographic spectrum of pleuropulmonary tularemia. Am J Roentgenol 131:277, 1978

SCHMID GP et al: Granulomatous pleuritis caused by *Francisella tularensis*: Possible confusion with tuberculous pleuritis. Am Rev Respir Dis 128:314, 1983

SJOSTEDT A et al: Neutrophils are critical for host defense against primary infection with the facultative intracellular bacterium *Francisella tularensis* in mice and participate in defense against reinfection. Infect Immun 62:2779, 1994

TARNVIK A: Nature of protective immunity to *Francisella tularensis*. Rev Infect Dis 11:440, 1989

——— et al: *Francisella tularensis*—a model for studies of the immune response to intracellular bacteria in man. Immunology 76:349, 1992

TAYLOR JP et al: Epidemiologic characteristics of human tularemia in the southwest-central states, 1981–1987. Am J Epidemiol 133:1032, 1991

| 164 | *Grant L. Campbell, David T. Dennis* |

PLAGUE AND OTHER *YERSINIA* INFECTIONS

PLAGUE

DEFINITION Plague is an acute, febrile, zoonotic disease caused by infection with *Yersinia pestis*. Although human cases are infrequent and are curable with antibiotics, plague is one of the most virulent and potentially lethal infectious diseases known. The plague bacterium occurs in widely scattered foci in Asia, Africa, and the Americas, where its usual hosts are wild and peridomestic rodents. It is transmitted to humans typically by flea bite and less commonly by direct contact with infected animal tissues or by airborne droplet. The principal clinical forms of plague are bubonic, septicemic, and pneumonic. Most cases are sporadic, occurring singly or in small clusters, although the potential for epidemic spread still exists in some countries.

ETIOLOGIC AGENT *Y. pestis* is a gram-negative coccobacillus in the family Enterobacteriaceae. It is microaerophilic, nonmotile, nonsporulating, oxidase and urease negative, and biochemically unreactive. The organism is nonfastidious and infective for laboratory rodents. It grows well, if slowly, on routinely used microbiologic media (e.g., sheep blood agar, brain-heart infusion broth, and MacConkey agar). *Y. pestis* can multiply within a wide range of temperatures ($-2°C$ to $45°C$) and pH values (5.0 to 9.6), but optimal growth occurs at $28°C$ and at pH ~7.4. When incubated on agar plates, colonies are pinpoint in size at 24 h and 1 to 2 mm in diameter at 48 h. Colonies are gray-white with irregular surfaces that are often described as having a "hammered-metal" appearance when viewed microscopically. In broth culture, *Y. pestis* grows without turbidity in clumps clinging to the sides of tubes. When stained with a polychromatic stain (e.g., Wayson or Giemsa), *Y. pestis* isolated from clinical specimens exhibits a characteristic bipolar appearance, often resembling closed safety pins. The bacterium is nonencapsulated but when grown at $\geq 30°C$ produces an immunogenic cell-surface envelope glycoprotein, fraction 1 (F1).

HISTORIC BACKGROUND Plague's deadly epidemic potential is notorious and well documented. The Justinian pandemic (542 to 767 A.D.) spread from central Africa to the Mediterranean littoral and thence to Asia Minor, causing an estimated 40 million deaths. The second pandemic began in central Asia, was carried to Sicily by ship from Constantinople in 1347, and swept through Europe and the British Isles in successive waves over the next four centuries. At its height, it killed as many as a quarter of the affected population and became known as the Black Death. In the third (modern) pandemic, plague appeared in Yunnan, China, in the latter half of the nineteenth century; established itself in Hong Kong in 1894; and spread by ship to Bombay in 1896 and subsequently to major port cities throughout the world, including San Francisco and several other West Coast and Gulf Coast ports in the United States. The plague bacillus was first cultured by Alexandre Yersin in Hong Kong in 1894. In 1898, Paul-Louis Simond, a French scientist sent to investigate epidemic bubonic plague in Bombay, identified the bacillus in the tissues of dead rats and proposed transmission by rat fleas. Waldemar Haffkine, also in Bombay at that time, developed a crude vaccine.

By 1910, plague had circled the globe and established itself in rodent populations on all inhabited continents other than Australia. After 1920, however, the spread of plague was largely halted by international regulations that mandated control of rats in harbors and inspection and rat-proofing of ships. Before the third pandemic subsided, it resulted in an estimated 26 million plague cases and more than 12 million deaths, the vast majority in India. By 1950, plague outbreaks around the world had become isolated, sporadic, and manageable with modern techniques of surveillance, flea and rat control, and antimicrobial treatment of patients. From 1969 through 1993, a median of 1356 human plague cases were reported annually to the World Health Organization, with around 10 to 15 countries reporting cases each year. Plague has practically disappeared from cities and now occurs mostly in rural and semirural areas, where it is maintained in wild rodents. In the United States, the last outbreak of urban plague occurred in Los Angeles in 1924 and 1925, and human cases since then have resulted from zoonotic exposures in rural areas of western states.

Plague, because of its pandemic history, remains one of three quarantinable diseases subject to international health regulations (the other two being cholera and yellow fever). The alarm that plague is still able to evoke was highlighted by the public panic over and exaggerated international response to reports of outbreaks of bubonic and pneumonic plague in India in 1994.

EPIDEMIOLOGY *Y. pestis* is maintained in enzootic cycles involving relatively resistant wild rodents and their fleas in mostly remote, lightly populated areas of Asia, Africa, and the Americas and in limited rural foci in extreme southeastern Europe near the Caspian Sea. Humans and other nonrodent mammals are incidental hosts. Enzootic transmission places humans at low risk, and cases are typically infrequent and sporadic. Epizootic transmission involving susceptible rodents and efficient flea vectors (both are amplifying hosts) results in local or even widespread depopulation of susceptible rodents and poses a more serious threat to humans than does enzootic transmission. In the United States, the principal epizootic hosts are various ground squirrels, prairie dogs, and chipmunks; a variety of burrowing rodents act as epizootic hosts in rural areas elsewhere in the world. *Y. pestis* occasionally spills over from wild rodents to commensal rat species that inhabit cultivated fields and adjacent homes, villages, and towns. The organism can then be transported from towns to cities by these relatively cosmopolitan rats and their fleas. Urban plague is reported from a few countries in southern Asia, such as Vietnam and Myanmar, and occurs only sporadically elsewhere.

Plague in populated areas is most likely to develop when sanitation is poor and rats are numerous—especially the common black or roof rat (*Rattus rattus*) and the larger brown sewer or Norway rat (*R. norvegicus*). A high mortality rate from plague in these susceptible rat populations forces their fleas to seek alternative hosts, including humans. The virtually ubiquitous oriental rat flea *Xenopsylla cheopis* and (in southern Africa and Brazil) the related species *X. brasiliensis* are efficient vectors of the plague bacillus among rats and are also efficient vectors to humans. *Y. pestis* can multiply to enormous numbers in the foregut (proventriculus) of these fleas, resulting in a bolus of organisms and clotted blood that blocks the passage of subsequent blood meals. Regurgitation by a "blocked" flea while it feeds facilitates transmission of the plague bacillus to the new host.

Except for large outbreaks of pneumonic plague in Manchuria in the early part of the twentieth century, person-to-person respiratory transmission of plague during and since the third pandemic has occurred only sporadically and has been limited to clusters of close contacts of pneumonic plague patients, such as household members and caregivers. The 1994 outbreak of pneumonic plague in the city of Surat, India, although reported to be extensive, most likely involved fewer than 100 cases and 50 deaths.

International health regulations require immediate reporting of plague cases. From 1979 through 1993, 16,312 human plague cases and 1668 deaths (mortality, 10 percent) were reported by 20 countries to the World Health Organization. In the same 15-year period, the United States reported 227 plague cases (mean, 15 cases per year) and 32 deaths (mortality, 14 percent). Cases reported by the United States are confirmed by the plague laboratory at the Centers for Disease Control and Prevention (CDC). Enzootic and epizootic plague occurs in 17 contiguous western states, extending from the Great Plains states and eastern Texas to the Pacific Coast; around 80 percent of human cases in this country occur in New Mexico, Arizona, and Colorado and around 10 percent in California. Although plague in the United States is a rural disease, more than 50 percent of cases are thought to be caused by peridomestic exposures, especially in the southwestern states, where homes are often situated in natural surroundings that provide a favorable habitat for plague-susceptible animals (such as rock squirrels and wood rats) and their fleas. In the Sierra Nevadas of California and Nevada, epizootic plague in chipmunks and ground squirrels poses a risk to visitors in public parks. Hikers, campers, and hunters in natural areas throughout the western states are at a small but finite risk of exposure to plague, especially in the summer months.

Plague can be transmitted during the skinning and handling of carcasses of wild animals such as rabbits and hares, prairie dogs, wildcats, and coyotes. Such direct inoculation of mammal-adapted organisms is associated with primary septicemia and high mortality. Oropharyngeal plague can result from the ingestion of undercooked contaminated meat and perhaps from the manual transfer of infected fluids to the mouth during the handling of infected animal tissues.

Carnivores, including dogs and cats, can become infected with *Y. pestis* by eating infected rodents and perhaps by being bitten by fleas from infected rodents. Although clinical plague commonly develops in infected cats, it rarely does so in infected dogs, which thus do not directly expose humans to infection. However, both dogs and cats may transport infected fleas from rodent-infested areas to the home environment.

From 1950 through 1994, 373 plague cases were reported in the United States. Of the 364 evaluable cases, 313 cases (86 percent) presented as primary lymphadenitic (bubonic) plague, almost all of them thought to be associated with flea bites; 44 cases (12 percent) presented as primary septicemic plague, many of them following direct animal exposures; and 7 cases (2 percent) presented as primary pneumonic plague, 6 resulting from the inhalation of respiratory droplets released by infected cats. The last case of human-to-human plague transmission in the United States occurred in the Los Angeles outbreak of 1924/1925.

PATHOGENESIS AND PATHOLOGY *Y. pestis* is among the most invasive bacteria known. The mechanisms by which the organism causes disease are incompletely understood, but both chromosome- and plasmid-encoded gene products are probably involved. Three plasmids encode for a variety of known or presumed virulence factors, including the F1 envelope antigen, which confers bacterial resistance to phagocytosis by polymorphonuclear leukocytes (PMNs) in vitro; a murine exotoxin; the V antigen, which is essential for virulence, may immunocompromise the host by suppressing the synthesis of interferon γ and tumor necrosis factor α, and stimulates

protective immunity in laboratory animals; pesticin, a bactericidal protein of unknown function and importance; a protease that can activate plasminogen and degrade serum complement and that is thought to play a role in the dissemination of *Y. pestis* from peripheral sites of infection; a coagulase; and a fibrinolysin. A lipopolysaccharide endotoxin, believed to be chromosomally encoded, is probably important in the pathogenesis of septicemic plague and disseminated intravascular coagulation (DIC).

Y. pestis organisms inoculated through the skin or mucous membranes usually invade cutaneous lymphatic vessels and reach regional lymph nodes, although direct bloodstream inoculation may take place. Mononuclear phagocytes, which can phagocytize *Y. pestis* organisms without destroying them, may play a role in dissemination of the infection to distant sites. Plague can involve almost any organ, and untreated plague generally results in widespread and massive tissue destruction. In the early stages, infected lymph nodes (buboes, Fig. 164-1) are characterized by edema and congestion without inflammatory infiltrates or apparent vascular injury. Fully developed buboes contain huge numbers of infectious plague organisms and show distorted or obliterated lymph node architecture with vascular destruction and hemorrhage, serosanguineous effusion, necrosis, and a mild neutrophilic infiltration. At this stage, the effusion often involves perinodal tissues. If several adjacent lymph nodes are involved, a boggy edematous mass can result.

Primary septicemic plague results from the direct inoculation of infected fluids or tissues or from an infective flea bite in the apparent absence of a bubo; secondary septicemic plague occurs when lymphatic and other host defenses are breached and the plague bacillus multiplies within the bloodstream. In either primary or secondary septicemic plague, renal glomeruli often contain fibrin thrombi. Diffuse interstitial myocarditis with cardiac dilatation may develop. Multifocal necrosis of the liver is common, as is diffuse hemorrhagic splenic necrosis. If DIC ensues, vascular necrosis may lead to widespread cutaneous, mucosal, and serosal ecchymoses and petechiae.

Pneumonic plague arises from primary exposure to infective respiratory droplets from a person or cat with respiratory plague or secondary to hematogenous spread in a patient with bubonic or septicemic plague. Pneumonic plague can also result from accidental inhalation of *Y. pestis* in the laboratory. Primary plague pneumonia generally begins as a lobular process and then extends by confluence, becoming lobar and then multilobar (Fig. 164-2). Plague organisms typically are most numerous in the alveoli. Secondary plague pneumonia begins more diffusely, with organisms usually most numerous in the interstitium. In untreated cases of both primary and secondary plague pneumo-

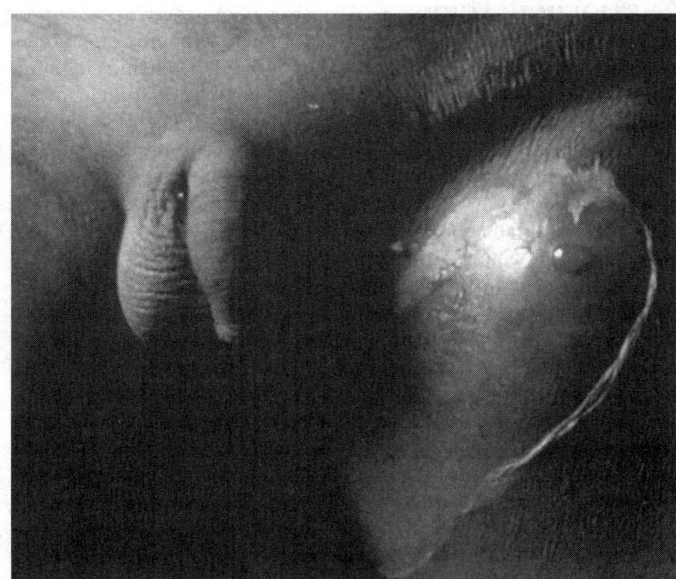

FIGURE 164-1 Left inguinal and femoral buboes, with surrounding edema and overlying desquamation.

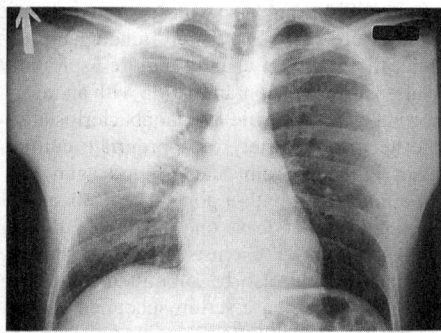 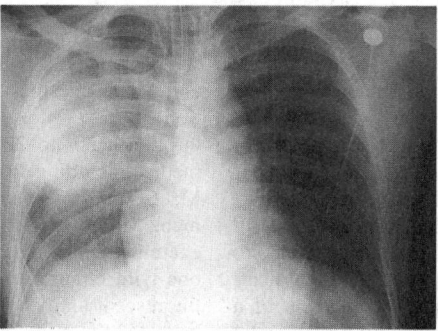 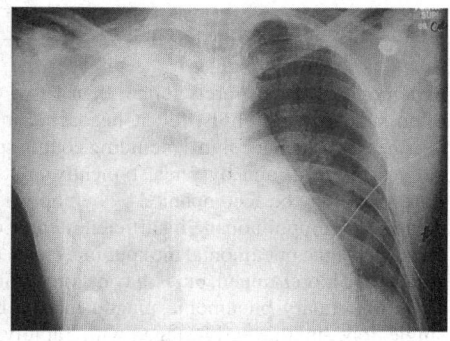

FIGURE 164-2 Sequential chest radiographs of a patient with fatal primary plague pneumonia. *Left:* Upright posteroanterior film taken at admission to hospital emergency department on third day of illness, showing segmental consolidation of right upper lobe. *Center:* Portable anteroposterior film taken 8 h after admission, showing extension of pneumonia to right middle and right lower lobes. *Right:* Portable anteroposterior film taken 13 h after admission (when patient had clinical ARDS), showing diffuse infiltration throughout right lung and patchy infiltration of left lower lung. A cavity later developed at the site of initial right upper lobe consolidation.

nia, diffuse hemorrhage, necrosis, and scant neutrophilic infiltration develop.

MANIFESTATIONS Plague is characterized by a rapid onset of fever and other systemic manifestations of gram-negative bacterial infection. If it is not quickly and correctly treated, plague can follow a toxic course, resulting in shock, multiple-organ failure, and death. In humans, the three principal forms of plague are bubonic, septicemic, and pneumonic. Bubonic plague, the most common form, is almost always caused by the bite of an infected flea but occasionally results from direct inoculation of infectious tissues or fluids. Septicemic and pneumonic plague can be either primary or secondary to metastatic spread. Unusual secondary forms include plague meningitis, endophthalmitis, and lymphadenitis at multiple sites. Primary plague pharyngitis has been documented by culture of organisms from throat swabs, but its clinical and epidemiologic features have not been completely described.

Bubonic plague usually has an incubation period of 2 to 6 days, occasionally longer. Typically, the patient experiences chills; fever, with temperatures that rise within hours to 38°C or higher; myalgias; arthralgias; headache; and a feeling of weakness. Soon—usually within 24 h—the patient notices tenderness and pain in one or more regional lymph nodes proximal to the site of inoculation of the plague bacillus (Fig. 164-1). Because fleas often bite the legs, femoral and inguinal nodes are most commonly involved; axillary and cervical nodes are next most commonly affected. The enlarging bubo becomes progressively painful and tender, sometimes exquisitely so. The patient usually guards against palpation and limits movement, pressure, and stretch around the bubo. The surrounding tissue often becomes edematous, sometimes markedly so, and the overlying skin may be erythematous, warm, and tense. Inspection of the skin surrounding or distal to the bubo sometimes reveals the site of a flea bite marked by a small papule, pustule, scab, or ulcer. Large eschars develop rarely (Fig. 164-3). A list of lymphadenitic conditions that could be confused with a plague bubo would include *Staphylococcus aureus* and group A beta-hemolytic streptococcal infections, cat-scratch disease, and tularemia. The bubo of plague is distinguishable from lymphadenitis of most other causes, however, by its rapid onset, its extreme tenderness, the accompanying signs of toxemia, and the absence of cellulitis or obvious ascending lymphangitis.

Treated in the uncomplicated state with an appropriate antibiotic, bubonic plague usually responds quickly, with defervescence and alleviation of other systemic manifestations over 2 to 5 days. Buboes often remain enlarged and tender for a week or more after the initiation of antimicrobial treatment and can become fluctuant. Without effective antimicrobial treatment, patients with typical bubonic plague manifest an increasingly toxic state of fever, tachycardia, lethargy leading to prostration, agitation and confusion, and (occasionally) convulsions and delirium. Secondary plague sepsis may result in an alarmingly rapid and refractory cascade of DIC, bleeding, shock, and organ failure. Mild forms of bubonic plague, called *pestis minor*, have been described in South

America and elsewhere; in these cases, the patients are ambulatory, are only mildly febrile, and have subacute buboes.

Septicemic plague is a progressive, overwhelming bacterial infection. Primary septicemia develops in the absence of apparent regional lymphadenitis, and the diagnosis of plague often is not suspected until preliminary blood culture results are reported to be positive by the laboratory. *Y. pestis*, however, can also be cultured from the blood of most bubonic plague patients, and bacteremia should be distinguished from septicemia, in which the patient is desperately ill and requires aggressive care. Patients with septicemic plague often present with gastrointestinal symptoms of nausea, vomiting, diarrhea, and abdominal pain, which may further confound the correct diagnosis. If not treated early with appropriate antibiotics, septicemic plague can be fulminant and fatal. In the United States in 1950 through 1994, 64 cases of septicemic plague and 18 deaths were reported, for a case-fatality rate of 28 percent. Petechiae, ecchymoses, bleeding from puncture wounds and orifices, and gangrene of acral parts are manifestations of DIC; refractory hypotension, renal shutdown, obtundation, and other signs of shock are preterminal events. Adult respiratory distress syndrome (ARDS), which can occur at any stage of septicemic plague, is sometimes confused with other conditions such as Hantavirus pulmonary syndrome.

Of all forms of the disease, pneumonic plague develops most rapidly and is most frequently fatal. The incubation period for primary

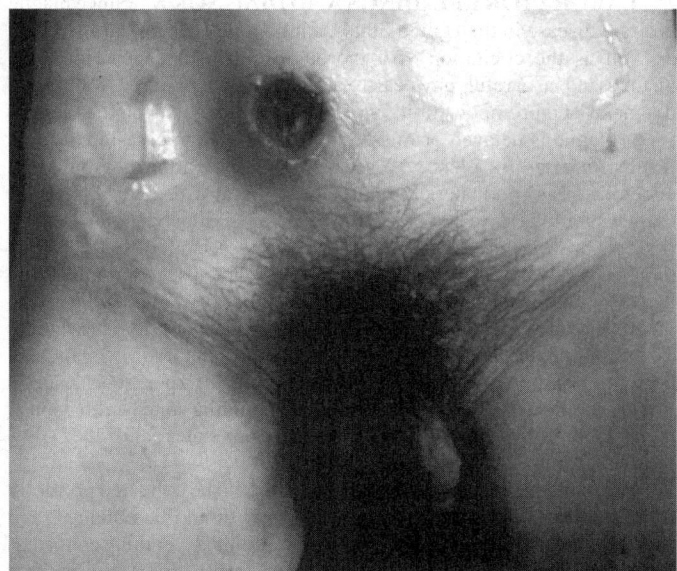

FIGURE 164-3 Large abdominal ulceration with eschar at presumed site of inoculation of *Y. pestis* by flea bite, accompanied by right inguinal bubo and erythema of overlying skin.

pneumonic plague is rarely longer than 1 to 4 days. The onset is most often sudden, with chills, fever, headache, myalgias, weakness, and dizziness. Pulmonary signs, including cough, sputum production, chest pain, tachypnea, and dyspnea, typically arise on the second day of illness and may be accompanied by hemoptysis, increasing respiratory distress, cardiopulmonary insufficiency, and circulatory collapse. In primary plague pneumonia, the sputum is most often watery or mucoid, frothy, and blood-tinged, but it may become frankly bloody. Pulmonary signs in primary pneumonic plague may indicate involvement of a single lobe in the early stage, with rapidly developing segmental consolidation before bronchopneumonic spread to other lobes of the same and opposite lungs. Liquefaction necrosis and cavitation may occur early in areas of consolidation and may or may not leave significant residual scarring.

Secondary plague pneumonia manifests first as diffuse interstitial pneumonitis in which sputum production is scant; since the sputum is more likely to be inspissated and tenacious in character than the sputum found in primary pneumonia, it may be less infectious. In the United States in 1950 through 1994, 39 cases of secondary pneumonic plague and 7 cases of primary pneumonic plague were reported, with no known transmission to contacts and an overall case-fatality rate of 41 percent. Observers in the early twentieth century remarked on the relative lack of auscultatory findings, the usual presence of toxemia, and the frequency of sudden death in patients with pneumonic plague as compared to patients with other bacterial pneumonias.

Meningitis is an unusual manifestation of plague. In the United States, there were 12 meningitis cases among the 373 plague cases reported in 1950 through 1994. All cases of meningitis were complications of bubonic plague, and all patients survived. Although meningitis may be a part of the initial presentation of plague, its onset is often delayed and is a manifestation of insufficient treatment. Recent cases in the United States have occurred during the first and second weeks of antibiotic treatment for bubonic plague. Chronic relapsing meningeal plague over periods of weeks or even months was described in the preantibiotic era. The affected patients typically presented with fever, headache, meningismus, and pleocytosis.

Plague pharyngitis presents as fever, sore throat, cervical lymphadenitis, and headache and is often indistinguishable clinically from pharyngitis of other infectious etiologies. Caregivers working in plague-endemic areas must be alert to the possibility of plague to avoid misdiagnosis leading to delayed and/or inappropriate treatment.

LABORATORY FINDINGS AND DIAGNOSIS Since plague is a rare disease in the United States, a high index of clinical suspicion as well as the elicitation of a thorough clinical and epidemiologic history and a careful physical examination are required for timely diagnosis and prompt institution of specific therapy. When the diagnosis of plague is delayed or missed altogether, a high case-fatality rate results; infected travelers who seek medical care after they have left endemic areas (peripatetic plague cases) are at especially high risk. Plague should always be considered when a previously healthy person presents with septic shock in the southwestern United States. When the diagnosis of plague is being considered, close communication between clinicians and the diagnostic laboratory and between the diagnostic laboratory and a qualified reference laboratory is essential. Tests for plague are highly reliable when conducted by laboratory personnel experienced with *Y. pestis*, but such expertise is usually limited to selected reference laboratories, including state health department laboratories in some plague-endemic states and the CDC plague laboratory.

When plague is suspected, specimens should be collected promptly for laboratory studies, chest roentgenograms should be obtained, and specific antimicrobial therapy should be initiated pending confirmation. Appropriate diagnostic specimens for smear and culture include citrated or heparinized whole blood from all patients with suspected plague, bubo aspirates from those with suspected buboes, sputum samples or tracheal aspirates from those with suspected pneumonic plague, and cerebrospinal fluid (CSF) from those with suspected plague meningitis. Since early buboes are often exquisitely tender and are seldom fluctuant or necrotic, these lesions usually require aspiration under local anesthesia and after surface decontamination with an injection of 1 to 2 mL of normal saline (sterile but nonbacteriostatic) through a 20- to 22-gauge needle. A variety of appropriate culture media (including brain-heart infusion broth, sheep blood agar, and MacConkey agar) should be inoculated with a portion of each specimen. Moreover, for each specimen, at least one smear should be examined immediately with Wayson or Giemsa stain and at least one with Gram's stain; a smear should also be submitted for direct fluorescent antibody testing. An acute-phase serum specimen should be tested for antibody to *Y. pestis*; whenever possible, a convalescent-phase serum specimen collected 3 to 4 weeks later should also be tested. When a patient dies and plague is suspected, appropriate autopsy tissues for culture and fluorescent antibody testing include buboes, all solid organs (especially liver, spleen, and lung), and bone marrow. If culture of such specimens is to be attempted, they should be sent to the laboratory either fresh or frozen on dry ice, not in preservatives or fixatives. If necessary, Cary-Blair or a similar medium can be used to transport *Y. pestis*–infected tissues.

Laboratory confirmation of plague depends on the isolation of *Y. pestis* from cultures of body fluids or tissues. Cultures of three blood samples taken over a 45-minute period before treatment will usually result in isolation of the bacterium. *Y. pestis* strains are readily distinguished from those of the closely related species *Yersinia pseudotuberculosis* by differences in biochemical profile, temperature-dependent susceptibility to lysis by a *Y. pestis*–specific bacteriophage, and motility. Automated bacteriologic test systems can be used to assist in the identification of isolates as *Y. pestis*, but such strains can be misidentified (e.g., as *Y. pseudotuberculosis*) or overlooked if these systems are improperly programmed.

In the absence of isolation of *Y. pestis*, plague cases can be confirmed by the demonstration of seroconversion (a fourfold or greater titer rise) to *Y. pestis* F1 antigen by passive hemagglutination testing of acute- and convalescent-phase serum specimens or by detection of an antibody titer of >128 in a single serum sample from a patient with a plague-compatible illness who has not received plague vaccine. The specificity of a positive passive-hemagglutination test requires confirmation with the F1 antigen hemagglutination-inhibition test. A few plague patients seroconvert to F1 antigen as early as 5 days after the onset of illness. Most seroconvert between 1 and 2 weeks after onset; a few seroconvert 3 weeks or more after onset; and a few (fewer than 5 percent) fail to seroconvert at all. Early, specific antibiotic treatment may delay seroconversion by several weeks. After seroconversion, positive serologic titers diminish gradually over months to years. Enzyme-linked immunosorbent assays (ELISAs) for IgM and IgG antibodies to *Y. pestis* have only recently been developed.

Detection of F1 antigen in tissues or fluids by direct fluorescent antibody testing is presumptive evidence of plague, as is an F1 antibody titer of >10 in a single serum sample from a patient with a plague-compatible illness who has not received plague vaccine. Visualization of characteristic bipolar bacilli in a Giemsa- or Wayson-stained smear constitutes supportive evidence of plague. Tularemia, especially the glandular, typhoidal, and pneumonic forms, can sometimes be confused clinically and epidemiologically with plague, but the results of microbiologic and serologic tests should readily distinguish these two diseases.

Patients with plague typically have white blood cell (WBC) counts of 15,000 to 25,000/μL, with a predominance of PMNs and a left shift. Leukemoid reactions with WBC counts as high as 100,000/μL can occur. Modest thrombocytopenia is usually documented, and fibrin-fibrinogen split products are often detected even in patients without frank DIC. Serum levels of aminotransferases and bilirubin may be elevated. Chest roentgenograms of patients with pneumonic plague usually show patchy bronchopneumonic infiltrates as well as lobar or segmental consolidation with or without confluence (Fig. 164-2); they occasionally show cavitation. Stained sputum samples usually contain PMNs and characteristic bipolar-staining bacilli. In

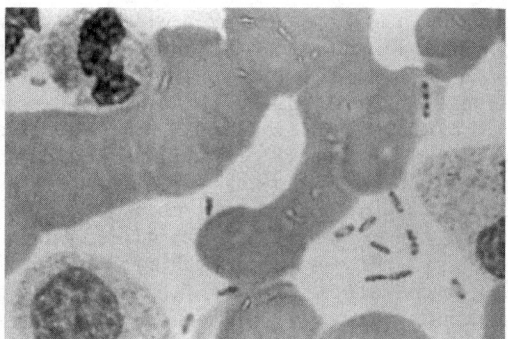

FIGURE 164-4 Peripheral blood smear from a patient with fatal plague septicemia and shock, showing characteristic bipolar-staining *Y. pestis* bacilli (Wright's stain, oil immersion).

Y. pestis septicemia, visualization of the characteristic bacilli in a routine blood smear or a buffy-coat smear is an uncommon but grave prognostic sign (Fig. 164-4). In patients with plague meningitis, pleocytosis with a predominance of PMNs is the rule, and the characteristic bacilli are usually visible in stained CSF smears.

℞ TREATMENT

Left untreated, plague is fatal in more than 50 percent of cases of bubonic disease and in nearly all cases of septicemic, pneumonic, and meningeal disease. The overall mortality rate for plague cases in the United States in the past 25 years has been ~15 percent; deaths are almost always due to delays in seeking treatment, misdiagnosis, delays in the institution of treatment, or incorrect treatment. Rapid diagnosis and appropriate antimicrobial therapy are essential.

Guidelines for the treatment of plague are given in Table 164-1. Streptomycin is the drug of choice. Alternative antibiotics include the tetracyclines and chloramphenicol; these agents are usually given orally with initial loading doses but may be given intravenously to critically ill patients and to patients unable to tolerate oral medication. Gentamicin is increasingly used for the treatment of plague in the United States because of its ready availability; it is probably as effective as streptomycin, although results of controlled studies have not yet been published. Penicillins, cephalosporins, and macrolides are suboptimal and should not be used. Doxycycline may be as effective as other tetracyclines or even more so, but comparative evaluations have not been made. Trimethoprim-sulfamethoxazole

has been used successfully to treat bubonic plague but is not considered a first-line choice. Chloramphenicol is indicated for the treatment of plague meningitis, pleuritis, endophthalmitis, and myocarditis because of its superior tissue penetration; it is used alone or in combination with streptomycin. In general, antimicrobial treatment should be continued for 10 days or for at least 3 days after the patient has become afebrile and has made a clinical recovery. Patients initially given intravenous antibiotics may be switched to oral regimens upon clinical improvement. Such improvement is usually evident 2 or 3 days after the start of treatment, even though fever may continue for several more days; as noted earlier, buboes can persist for days or even weeks.

Consequences of delayed treatment of plague include DIC, ARDS, and other complications of gram-negative sepsis. Patients with these disorders require intensive monitoring and close physiologic support, as outlined elsewhere (see Chaps. 118 and 265). Buboes may require surgical drainage. Abscessed nodes can cause recurrent fever in patients who have apparently recovered; this relation may be occult if intrathoracic or intraabdominal nodes are involved. Viable *Y. pestis* organisms have been isolated from affected nodes 1 to 2 weeks after clinical recovery from acute disease. Antibiotic-resistant strains of *Y. pestis* have rarely been identified, and the plague bacillus is considered to be genetically stable.

PREVENTION AND CONTROL Persons at greatest risk for plague in the United States are those who live, work, and participate in outdoor recreational activities in areas of those western states in which plague is enzootic. Surveillance, education, and environmental management are the cornerstones of prevention and control. A network of biologists and public health specialists coordinates these activities through local and state health departments and the CDC. Personal protective measures include the avoidance of areas with known epizootic plague (which may be posted) and of sick or dead animals; the use of repellents, insecticides, and protective clothing when at risk of exposure to rodents' fleas; and the wearing of gloves when handling animal carcasses. Short-term antibiotic prophylaxis (Table 164-2) is recommended for persons known to have had face-to-face or other direct contact with a patient with suspected or confirmed pneumonic plague; it may also be advisable occasionally for persons who are unable to avoid an area where a plague outbreak is in progress or who are caring for patients with plague. To decrease the risk of pneumonic transmission, all patients in whom plague is suspected should be placed in respiratory isolation (to prevent droplet spread) until pneumonia has been ruled out or until 48 h of specific antimicrobial therapy has been administered, after which only standard precautions are generally necessary.

Rodent food (garbage, pet food) and habitats (brush piles, junk heaps, woodpiles) should be eliminated in domestic, peridomestic,

Table 164-1

Guidelines for the Treatment of Plague

Drug	Daily Dosage	Interval, h	Route(s) of Administration
Streptomycin			
Adults	2 g	12	IM
Children	30 mg/kg	12	IM
Gentamicin			
Adults	4.5 mg/kg	8	IM or IV
Children	6.0–7.5 mg/kg	8	IM or IV
Infants/neonates	7.5 mg/kg	8	IM or IV
Tetracycline			
Adults	2 g	6	PO or IV
Children ≥9 y	25–50 mg/kg	6	PO or IV
Doxycycline			
Adults	200 mg	12 or 24	PO or IV
Children ≥9 y	4 mg/kg	12 or 24	PO or IV
Oxytetracycline			
Adults	250–300 mg	8, 12, or 24	PO or IM
Children ≥9 y	15–25 mg/kg	8, 12, or 24	PO or IM
Chloramphenicol			
Adults	75–100 mg/kg	6	PO or IV
Children ≥1 y	75–100 mg/kg	6	PO or IV

* Maximum, 250 mg/d.

SOURCE: Adapted with permission from DT Dennis, in *Conn's Current Therapy 1996*, RE Rakel (ed). Philadelphia, Saunders, 1996.

Table 164-2

Guidelines for Plague Prophylaxis

Drug	Daily Dosage	Interval, h	Route of Administration
Tetracycline			
Adults	1–2 g	6 or 12	PO
Children ≥9 y	25–50 mg/kg	6 or 12	PO
Doxycycline			
Adults	100–200 mg	12 or 24	PO
Children ≥9 y	2–4 mg/kg	12 or 24	PO
Trimethoprim-sulfamethoxazole			
Adults	1.6–3.2 g*	12	PO
Children ≥2 mo	40 mg/kg*	12	PO

* Sulfamethoxazole component.

SOURCE: Adapted with permission from DT Dennis, in *Conn's Current Therapy 1996*, RE Rakel (ed). Philadelphia, Saunders, 1996.

and working environments; buildings and food stores should be rodent-proofed. The control of fleas with insecticides is a key public health measure in situations where epizootic plague activity places humans at high risk; this effort includes dusting and spraying of rodent burrows, rodent runs, and other sites where rodents and their fleas are found. In plague-endemic areas of the western United States, persons should keep their dogs and cats free of fleas and restrained. The decision to control plague by killing rodents should be left to public health authorities, and such a program should be carried out only in conjunction with effective flea control. Killing of rodents has no lasting benefit without environmental sanitation.

A killed, whole-cell plague vaccine is available in the United States. The efficacy of this vaccine in humans has not been evaluated in controlled studies, although reviews of vaccine use during the Vietnam War provide indirect evidence that it is at least partially protective against plague transmitted by fleas. The vaccine does not appear to offer protection against primary pneumonic plague. As recommended by the manufacturer, primary immunization consists of a series of three injections followed by booster doses as warranted (at intervals of 6 months or more). The degree and duration of the immune response vary, and persons at continuing risk may need to have their antibody levels monitored. Adverse reactions are usually mild after injection of the first dose but may increase with repeated doses. Vaccination is recommended for laboratory personnel who routinely work with *Y. pestis* and should also be considered for persons whose vocation brings them into regular contact with wild rodents and their fleas in areas experiencing enzootic or epizootic plague. Military personnel in some situations are vaccinated, but vaccination is not routinely indicated for civilians living in areas with enzootic plague (such as the western United States), for medical personnel, for travelers to countries that have reported plague cases, or for the control of plague epidemics.

OTHER *YERSINIA* INFECTIONS

DEFINITION Yersiniosis is an uncommon bacterial zoonosis caused by infection with either of the two enteropathogenic *Yersinia* species: *Yersinia enterocolitica* or *Yersinia pseudotuberculosis*. Reservoir hosts of these bacteria include swine and other wild and domestic animals. These yersiniae are transmitted to humans predominantly via the oral route. Both sporadic cases and common-source outbreaks occur. The most frequent acute clinical manifestations are (1) enteritis or enterocolitis with self-limited diarrhea (especially with *Y. enterocolitica*), and (2) mesenteric adenitis and terminal ileitis (especially with *Y. pseudotuberculosis*), which can be difficult to distinguish from acute appendicitis. Septicemia and metastatic focal infections are less common. Some cases of yersiniosis are complicated by nonsuppurative, extraintestinal, inflammatory sequelae (e.g., reactive arthritis and erythema nodosum).

ETIOLOGIC AGENTS *Y. enterocolitica* and *Y. pseudotuberculosis* are pleomorphic gram-negative bacilli in the family Enterobacteriaceae. They are aerobic or facultatively anaerobic, motile at 25°C, nonmotile at 37°C, oxidase negative, urease positive, able to ferment glucose, unable to ferment lactose, and usually able to reduce nitrates. They grow well, if slowly, on nonselective media (e.g., blood agar) and on most of the routine media used to select for enteric bacteria (e.g., MacConkey agar). They can multiply within a wide temperature range ($-1°C$ to $45°C$). The most clinically and epidemiologically useful methods for identifying pathogenic *Y. enterocolitica* isolates are biotyping based on biochemical profiles and serotyping according to somatic O and H antigens. Six biotypes and more than 60 serotypes of *Y. enterocolitica* are recognized. A separate serotyping system for *Y. pseudotuberculosis* (also based on somatic antigens) has distinguished six major serotypes (I through VI) and their subtypes.

EPIDEMIOLOGY *Y. enterocolitica* is distributed worldwide and has been isolated from soil, fresh water, contaminated foodstuffs

(e.g., meat, milk, and vegetables), and a wide variety of wild and domestic animals, including mammals, birds, amphibians, fish, and shellfish. Many serotypes isolated from environmental sources, however, evidently are not human pathogens. Most human infections have been caused by *Y. enterocolitica* serotypes O:3, O:5, O:8, and O:9, which are primarily associated with wild and domestic mammals. The incidence of these infections and their sequelae is highest in Scandinavia and some other northern European countries, but this observation may be in part an artifact of underrecognition in other countries. Because many individuals with enteric *Y. enterocolitica* infection are asymptomatic or minimally symptomatic and do not seek medical attention, reliable population-based estimates of incidence are unavailable. However, in many clinical microbiology laboratories in recent decades, *Y. enterocolitica* has been the fourth most common bacterial pathogen isolated from patients' fecal specimens, trailing *Salmonella* (the most frequently isolated), *Campylobacter*, and *Shigella* species. In one multistate pediatric study in the United States, *Y. enterocolitica* strains were isolated from 1 percent of submitted fecal specimens and accounted for 16 percent of all bacterial pathogens isolated from fecal samples. This yield was comparable to that of *Shigella* or *Campylobacter* and about 40 percent as great as that of *Salmonella*.

All age groups are susceptible to *Y. enterocolitica* infections, but the majority of cases of enterocolitis are in children aged 1 to 4. Moreover, these infections show a modest predilection for males. Mesenteric adenitis and terminal ileitis are most common among older children and young adults. Risk factors for *Y. enterocolitica* septicemia and metastatic focal infections include chronic liver disease, malignancy, diabetes mellitus, immunosuppressive therapy, alcoholism, malnutrition, advanced age, iron overload (see below), and hemolytic anemias (including the thalassemias). The nonsuppurative sequelae of yersiniosis are most common among adults. HLA-B27 is expressed in 70 to 80 percent of patients who develop reactive arthritis associated with yersiniosis. HLA-B27 is not a risk factor for *Yersinia*-induced erythema nodosum; females with this condition outnumber males by 2 to 1. In Europe, *Y. enterocolitica* infections are more common in the cooler months than in warmer weather. In North America, no consistent seasonal pattern has been documented.

For several decades, serotypes O:3 and O:9 have predominated among *Y. enterocolitica* isolates from patients in Europe. Serotype O:3 has also predominated in Canada and Japan. In the United States, serotype O:3 emerged in the 1980s to surpass serotype O:8 in frequency of isolation from patients. The incidence of *Yersinia*-induced nonsuppurative sequelae reportedly is 10 to 30 percent in Scandinavia and much lower in most other countries, including the United States. No convincing explanation for this observation has been confirmed, but reasonable possibilities include population genetic factors and geographic strain variation.

Common-source outbreaks of *Y. enterocolitica* enteritis have been traced to such vehicles as raw milk, contaminated pasteurized milk, and foods prepared with contaminated fresh water. In Belgium, the ingestion of ground raw pork (a regional custom) is a significant risk factor for sporadic infection with *Y. enterocolitica* serotypes O:3 and O:9. These serotypes commonly colonize the oral cavity and intestines of European swine, and *Y. enterocolitica* infection is an occupational risk of swine butchers in Europe. In the United States, sporadic cases and one outbreak of *Y. enterocolitica* O:3 infection have been associated with the preparation or ingestion of raw pork intestines (chitterlings). In some cases of yersiniosis, circumstantial evidence suggests transmission via contact with dogs and cats or their feces. Several nosocomial outbreaks of *Y. enterocolitica* infection have been described; fecal-oral transmission from person to person was suspected. Fecal-oral transmission among family members may also explain occasional secondary cases in households. In a prospective study of 50 children with *Y. enterocolitica* enteritis, fecal excretion of the organism persisted for an average of 27 days (range, 4 to 79 days) after the cessation of symptoms. A chronic carrier state, however, has not been demonstrated. *Y. enterocolitica* is a rare but often lethal cause of transfusion-associated septicemia. The explanation is that blood donors occasionally have transient, occult *Y. enterocolitica* bacteremia and that this organism can slowly multiply to high concentrations in blood refrigerated for at least 10 to 20 days.

The ecology of *Y. pseudotuberculosis* seems to parallel that of *Y. enterocolitica* closely. *Y. pseudotuberculosis* is also widespread in wild and domestic animals and is isolated from many environmental sources. Human infections with *Y. pseudotuberculosis*, however, appear to be rare. In North America and Europe, most such infections have been with serotype I, but outbreaks involving other serotypes have occurred in Japan and Scandinavia. Swine appear to be an important reservoir for pathogenic strains of *Y. pseudotuberculosis*.

PATHOGENESIS AND PATHOLOGY Except in rare instances of transmission via contaminated blood products or direct cutaneous inoculation, the enteropathogenic yersiniae are thought to enter the host via the oral route. The 50 percent infectious dose in humans is uncertain but may be $\geq 10^9$. The incubation period averages 5 days (range, 1 to 11 days). Studies of animals have shown that the organisms initially invade the ileal epithelium, then are translocated via M cells into the lamina propria, and finally enter Peyer's patches, where they are able to replicate. They subsequently drain into the mesenteric lymph nodes, which undergo hyperplasia and from which the bacteria can be distributed systemically. The mesenteric lymph nodes can become intensely swollen and matted and are occasionally detected on physical examination as a tender right lower quadrant mass. Intestinal inflammation (most commonly of the distal ileum and less commonly of the ascending colon) develops and may be accompanied by mucosal ulcerations and by the shedding of PMNs and red blood cells into the intestinal lumen. In relatively severe cases, thrombosis of mesenteric blood vessels, intestinal hemorrhage, and necrosis can occur. In patients with enteropathogenic yersinial infections who undergo exploratory laparotomy, the appendix usually is histologically normal or shows only lymphoid hyperplasia, but frank suppuration is sometimes evident.

A plasmid of ~70 kb is essential for virulence of the enteropathogenic yersiniae because it encodes at least six *Yersinia* outer-membrane proteins, some of which confer to bacterial strains such properties as cytotoxicity; resistance to phagocytosis by PMNs; and the ability to suppress the host's expression of tumor necrosis factor α, to interfere with platelet aggregation and host complement activation, and to dephosphorylate host proteins. A chromosomal gene (*inv*) encodes for the surface protein invasin, which is necessary for yersinial invasion of nonphagocytic host cells (e.g., epithelial cells) in vitro and which facilitates the translocation of bacteria across the intestinal epithelium. Both *Y. enterocolitica* and *Y. pseudotuberculosis* can express at least one protein superantigen that selectively stimulates the proliferation of T cells. Many strains of *Y. enterocolitica* produce a heat-stable enterotoxin that is similar to *Escherichia coli* enterotoxin. The cell walls of *Y. enterocolitica* and *Y. pseudotuberculosis* contain a lipopolysaccharide (endotoxin). The roles of superantigens, enterotoxin, and endotoxin in the pathogenesis of yersiniosis are unclear. Some *Yersinia* strains are unable to synthesize bacterial iron chelators called *siderophores*. However, they can exploit host-chelated iron stores and the drug deferoxamine (a siderophore produced by *Streptomyces pilosus*). Therefore, iron overload (e.g., caused by hemodialysis or multiple transfusions) and deferoxamine therapy appear to be independent risk factors for *Y. enterocolitica* bacteremia (especially that involving serotypes O:3 and O:9) and to a lesser degree for *Y. pseudotuberculosis* bacteremia.

Immunogenetic factors are clearly involved in the pathogenesis of reactive arthritis following infection with the enteropathogenic yersiniae. As noted above, most patients with *Yersinia*-induced reactive arthritis express HLA-B27. In addition, *Y. pseudotuberculosis* shares at least one cross-reactive epitope with HLA-B27. In patients with reactive arthritis following *Y. enterocolitica* infection, yersinial antigens are commonly detectable in synovial fluid cells in the apparent absence of whole organisms. Thus, it is unknown whether the arthritis results from occult bacterial persistence through self-tolerance of HLA-B27 with a failure of cross-reactive immune responses to yersiniae, from an immune response to common antigenic determinants shared by the bacteria and host HLA-B27 (i.e., molecular mimicry), or from other mechanisms. Local T cell immune responses appear to be particularly important in the pathogenesis of reactive arthritis. The pathogenesis of *Yersinia*-induced erythema nodosum is obscure.

In some assays, patients with Graves' disease have an increased prevalence of serum antibodies to *Y. enterocolitica*, and the immunoglobulins of patients recovering from *Y. enterocolitica* infections react with the human thyroid-stimulating hormone receptor. However, a link between *Y. enterocolitica* infection and the subsequent development of autoimmune thyroiditis has not been convincingly demonstrated.

MANIFESTATIONS The principal clinical manifestations of *Y. enterocolitica* infection are enteritis, enterocolitis, mesenteric adenitis, and terminal ileitis. Less common manifestations include exudative pharyngitis, septicemia, metastatic focal infections, reactive polyarthritis, and erythema nodosum. When age groups are combined, the most common presentation of *Y. enterocolitica* infection is acute diarrhea from enteritis or enterocolitis. Low-grade fever and cramping abdominal pain occur in most cases, nausea and vomiting in 15 to 40 percent, hematochezia in up to 30 percent, and a generalized maculopapular skin rash in a few cases. Diarrhea persists for an average of 2 weeks (range, 1 day to many months), during which the frequency of bowel movements diminishes. Uncommonly, enteritis or enterocolitis can be complicated by severe abdominal pain and high fever. Rare (and sometimes fatal) complications include diffuse inflammation, ulceration, hemorrhage, and necrosis of the small bowel and colon; intestinal perforation; peritonitis; ascending cholangitis; mesenteric vein thrombosis; diverticulitis; toxic megacolon; and ileocecal intussusception.

The syndrome of mesenteric adenitis and terminal ileitis without diarrhea is easily confused with appendicitis. Low-grade fever and right lower quadrant pain, tenderness, guarding, and rebound tenderness are common. During six recognized common-source outbreaks in the United States, 10 percent of 444 patients with symptomatic undiagnosed *Y. enterocolitica* infections underwent laparotomy for suspected appendicitis; surgical incisions became infected with *Y. enterocolitica* in a few of these cases.

Acute pharyngitis and pharyngotonsillitis, with or without cervical adenitis or intestinal illness, are less common but potentially lethal manifestations of *Y. enterocolitica* infection, particularly in adults. *Y. enterocolitica* septicemia generally presents as a severe illness with fever and leukocytosis, often with abdominal pain and jaundice and without localized signs of infection. Metastatic focal *Y. enterocolitica* infections can occur with or without clinically apparent bacteremia and can affect almost any organ system. Examples include abscess formation (e.g., in liver, spleen, kidney, lung, skeletal muscle, lymph node, or cutaneous tissue), osteomyelitis, meningitis, peritonitis, urinary tract infection, pneumonia, empyema, endocarditis, pericarditis, mycotic aneurysm, septic arthritis, suppurative conjunctivitis, panophthalmitis, Parinaud's oculoglandular syndrome, and cutaneous pustules or bullae.

In Scandinavia, the incidence of reactive arthritis following *Y. enterocolitica* infection among adults is estimated to be at least 10 percent. About 80 percent of these patients have preceding symptoms such as fever, diarrhea, or abdominal pain. Typically, these symptoms precede the arthritis by 1 week and are of short duration. The most commonly affected joints are the knees and ankles, but other joints can be involved. Typically, multiple (two to eight) joints become involved sequentially and asymmetrically over a period of a few days to 2 weeks, after which no additional joints are affected. Monoarticular arthritis occurs less commonly. In two-thirds of cases, the acute arthritis remits spontaneously within 1 to 3 months. Chronic joint disease is documented in a minority of cases. A few HLA-B27-positive patients with *Y. enterocolitica*–induced arthritis have subsequent ankylosing spondylitis, but this development is best explained by the fact that HLA-B27 is a major risk factor for each of these diseases. Mild, self-limited myocarditis accompanies about 10 percent of cases of *Yersinia*-induced arthritis and can occur independently. Typical manifestations include cardiac murmurs and transient electrocardiographic abnormalities, including prolongation of the PR interval and nonspecific ST-segment and T-wave changes. The syndrome of *Yersinia*-induced arthritis and carditis can be confused with acute rheumatic fever. In Scandinavia, erythema nodosum occurs in 15 to 20 percent of patients with yersiniosis, usually within a few days to 3 weeks after the onset of intestinal illness. Lesions typically are located on the lower extremities and resolve within 1 month. Less commonly reported nonsuppurative sequelae of *Y. enterocolitica* infections include reactive uveitis, iritis, conjunctivitis, urethritis, and glomerulonephritis. The complete triad of Reiter's syndrome (arthritis, conjunctivitis, and urethritis) is seen in 5 to 10 percent of patients with *Yersinia*-induced arthritis.

The most common clinical presentation of *Y. pseudotuberculosis* infection is fever and abdominal pain caused by mesenteric adenitis; diarrheal illness is less common than in *Y. enterocolitica* infection. Systemic manifestations, including septicemia, focal infections, reactive arthritis, and erythema nodosum, generally are similar to those associated with *Y. enterocolitica* infection. In addition, *Y. pseudotuberculosis* has been associated with a scarlet fever–like syndrome, acute interstitial nephritis, and hemolytic-uremic syndrome.

LABORATORY FINDINGS AND DIAGNOSIS Results of routine laboratory tests in most patients with yersiniosis are nonspecific. Leukocyte counts are usually normal or slightly elevated, often with a modest left shift. Standard microbiologic methods are sufficient to isolate *Y. enterocolitica* and *Y. pseudotuberculosis* from otherwise-sterile sites, such as blood, CSF, lymph node tissue, and peritoneal fluid, and from abscesses. Isolation of these organisms from feces is impeded by their slow growth and the overgrowth of normal fecal flora on culture media routinely used to select for enteric bacteria. When routine enteric media are used, the yield of yersinial isolates from feces is increased by incubation at 22 to 25°C for 48 h. The yield from feces and other grossly contaminated specimens can be further increased by the use of *Yersinia*-selective cefsulodin-Irgasan-novobiocin (CIN) agar and by cold enrichment (i.e., inoculation of feces into buffered saline and incubation at 4°C for 2 to 4 weeks, with periodic plating onto enteric media). Because bacteriologic procedures designed to isolate yersiniae from feces are not considered cost-effective, many laboratories undertake them by special request only.

The results of serologic tests can be used to support a diagnosis of yersiniosis. Agglutination tests or ELISAs are used most commonly. The existence of multiple serotypes makes routine serologic tests laborious; thus these tests are generally conducted only in research laboratories or large commercial laboratories. Since these tests are experimental and are neither standardized nor well validated, and since some strains of *Yersinia* cross-react with other bacteria (e.g., *Brucella*, *Salmonella*, and *Vibrio*) and with serum from some patients with thyroiditis, results should be interpreted with caution. In typical uncomplicated cases of yersiniosis, agglutinin titers begin to rise within the first week of illness, peak in the second week, and then gradually diminish and return to normal within 3 to 6 months, although agglutinating antibody may remain detectable for several years in some cases. Because an initial serum specimen is often collected a week or more after the onset of illness, when agglutinin titers are already high, it is usually impossible to document a fourfold or greater rise in titer between paired specimens (although a fourfold or greater fall in titer may be found).

In patients with *Yersinia*-induced reactive arthritis, synovial fluid is sterile and the leukocyte count ranges from a few hundred to 60,000/μL, with a majority of PMNs. The erythrocyte sedimentation rate is often >100 mm/h. Rheumatoid factor and antinuclear antibodies are usually absent. The diagnosis of *Yersinia*-induced reactive arthritis or other nonsuppurative inflammatory sequelae can be difficult, especially when triggering infections are asymptomatic or clinically mild or occur several weeks before the diagnosis is attempted. Because the isolation of a pathogenic *Yersinia* strain from feces is the most specific diagnostic test in such cases, it should be attempted. Since culture is of limited sensitivity in this clinical setting, a high index of suspicion and positive results of serologic tests for *Y. enterocolitica* or *Y. pseudotuberculosis* usually are required for diagnosis.

℞ **TREATMENT**

The effectiveness of antimicrobial agents in the treatment of yersinial enteritis, enterocolitis, mesenteric adenitis, or terminal ileitis has not been established. These conditions are usually self-limited, and their treatment is symptom-based and supportive. In uncomplicated cases, diarrhea should be treated with fluid and electrolyte replacement, with the route of delivery dependent on clinical severity. Enteric precautions are advisable for patients hospitalized with yersinial diarrhea. In general, antimicrobial treatment should be reserved for patients with septicemia, metastatic focal infections, or immunosuppression and enterocolitis. Controlled clinical comparisons of antimicrobial agents in the treatment of severe cases of yersiniosis have not yet been conducted. In such cases, drug selection should ultimately be guided by clinical response and bacterial sensitivity patterns. Clinical isolates of *Y. enterocolitica* and *Y. pseudotuberculosis* are usually susceptible in vitro to aminoglycosides, third-generation cephalosporins, chloramphenicol, quinolones, tetracyclines, and trimethoprim-sulfamethoxazole. In laboratory animals infected with enteropathogenic yersiniae, the fluoroquinolones have exerted the strongest bactericidal effects in vivo; clinical experience with these drugs against these pathogens in humans is promising but limited. Because they produce β-lactamases, isolates typically are resistant to penicillin, ampicillin, carbenicillin, and first-generation and most second-generation cephalosporins. Optimal dosages and durations of therapy have not been established. Mortality from *Y. enterocolitica* septicemia has been estimated at 25 to 50 percent despite treatment. However, in a recent retrospective, population-based study of 53 cases in France, mortality was 7.5 percent. Focal extraintestinal infections may require at least 3 weeks of therapy. No role for antimicrobial agents in the management of the nonsuppurative inflammatory manifestations of yersiniosis has been established. Patients with reactive arthritis may benefit from treatment with nonsteroidal anti-inflammatory drugs, intraarticular steroid injections, and physical therapy.

PREVENTION AND CONTROL The importance of safe food-handling and food-preparation practices in the prevention of yersiniosis cannot be overemphasized. Caution is particularly warranted in the case of pork and other animal products. The consumption of raw or undercooked meats, especially pork, should be avoided. Increased efforts to prevent the spread of enteric pathogens in household, pet-care, day-care, and hospital settings and in the food industry would be likely to decrease the incidence of yersiniosis. Current regulations of the Food and Drug Administration require visual inspection of packed red cell units before transfusion, with the discarding of units in which bacterial contamination is suspected on the basis of darkening (reflecting decreased oxygen saturation and hemolysis). Since the risk is minimal, more specific measures to further decrease the likelihood of transfusion of *Y. enterocolitica*–contaminated blood products (e.g., limiting the period for which red cells can be stored before transfusion) are not considered cost-effective.

Yersiniosis is not routinely reportable to public health authorities in most jurisdictions. However, clinicians who suspect a common-source outbreak (e.g., because they have documented a familial case cluster or have diagnosed the disease in several apparently unrelated patients over a short period) or some other public health threat (e.g., because they have found occult *Y. enterocolitica* bacteremia in a recent blood donor) should consult promptly with local public health officials.

BIBLIOGRAPHY

PLAGUE

BARNES AM: Surveillance and control of bubonic plague in the United States, in *Animal Disease in Relation to Animal Conservation*, MA Edwards, U McDonnell (eds). New York, Academic Press, 1982, p 237

BRUBAKER RR: Factors promoting acute and chronic diseases caused by yersiniae. Clin Microbiol Rev 4:309, 1991

BUTLER T: *Yersinia* infections: Centennial of the discovery of the plague bacillus. Clin Infect Dis 19:655, 1994

CAMPBELL GL, HUGHES JM: Plague in India: A new warning from an old nemesis; editorial. Ann Intern Med 122:151, 1995

CENTERS FOR DISEASE CONTROL AND PREVENTION: Prevention of plague: Recommendations of the Advisory Committee on Immunization Practices (ACIP). Morb Mort Week Rep 45(RR-14):1, 1996

CRAVEN RB et al: Reported cases of human plague infections in the United States, 1970–1991. J Med Entomol 30:758, 1993

LEARY SE et al: Active immunization with recombinant V antigen from *Yersinia pestis* protects mice against plague. Infect Immun 63:2854, 1995

NAKAJIMA R et al: Suppression of cytokines in mice by protein A-V antigen fusion peptide and restoration of synthesis by active immunization. Infect Immun 63:3021, 1995

POLITZER R: *Plague.* WHO monograph series 22:1. Geneva, World Health Organization, 1954

RUSSELL P et al: Doxycycline or ciprofloxacin prophylaxis and therapy against experimental *Yersinia pestis* infection in mice. J Antimicrob Chemother 37:769, 1996

OTHER YERSINIA INFECTIONS

BEUSCHER HU et al: Bacterial evasion of host immune defense: *Yersinia enterocolitica* encodes a suppressor for tumor necrosis factor alpha expression. Infect Immun 63:1270, 1995

BOTTONE EJ: *Yersinia enterocolitica.* A panoramic view of a charismatic microorganism. CRC Crit Rev Microbiol 5:211, 1977

——— (ed): *Yersinia enterocolitica.* Boca Raton, FL, CRC Press, 1981

BRUBAKER RR: Factors promoting acute and chronic diseases caused by yersiniae. Clin Microbiol Rev 4:309, 1991

COVER TL, ABER RC: *Yersinia enterocolitica.* N Engl J Med 321:16, 1989

GAYRAUD M et al: Antibiotic treatment of *Yersinia enterocolitica* septicemia: A retrospective review of 43 cases. Clin Infect Dis 17:405, 1993

HERMANN E et al: HLA-B27-restricted CD8 T cells derived from synovial fluids of patients with reactive arthritis and ankylosing spondylitis. Lancet 342:646, 1993

KIHLSTROM E et al: Intestinal symptoms and serological response in patients with complicated and uncomplicated *Yersinia enterocolitica* infections. Scand J Infect Dis 24:57, 1992

LEE LA et al: *Yersinia enterocolitica* O:3: An emerging cause of pediatric gastroenteritis in the United States. J Infect Dis 163:660, 1991

LEINO R et al: Yersiniosis as a gastrointestinal disease. Scand J Infect Dis 19:63, 1987

OSTROFF SM et al: Clinical features of sporadic *Yersinia enterocolitica* infections in Norway. J Infect Dis 166:812, 1992

PEPE JC, MILLER VL: *Yersinia enterocolitica* invasin: A primary role in the initiation of infection. Proc Natl Acad Sci USA 90:6473, 1993

PRESTON MA et al: Antimicrobial susceptibility of pathogenic *Yersinia enterocolitica* isolated in Canada from 1972 to 1990. Antimicrob Agents Chemother 38:2121, 1994

RESETKOVA E et al: Seroreactivity to bacterial antigens is not a unique phenomenon in patients with autoimmune thyroid diseases in Canada. Thyroid 4:269, 1994

TAUXE RV et al: *Yersinia enterocolitica* infections and pork: The missing link. Lancet 1:1129, 1987

ZHANG Y et al: Antibiotic prophylaxis and treatment of reactive arthritis. Lessons from an animal model. Arthritis Rheum 39:1238, 1996

---

165   *Lucy Stuart Tompkins*

BARTONELLA INFECTIONS, INCLUDING CAT-SCRATCH DISEASE

Bartonella species, including *B. bacilliformis*, *B. henselae*, and *B. quintana*, are tiny gram-negative bacilli that can invade mammalian cells, including endothelial cells and erythrocytes. Previously classified as *Rochalimaea* species within the rickettsia group, *Bartonella* species have now been removed from the order Rickettsiales on the grounds that they are not obligate intracellular parasites. These agents cause a wide spectrum of clinical illnesses, including trench fever, cat-scratch disease (CSD), bacillary angiomatosis, endocarditis, Oroya fever, and verruga peruana. The pathologic manifestations of *Bartonella* disease vary with the immune status of the host.

OROYA FEVER AND VERRUGA PERUANA

DEFINITION   Oroya fever and verruga peruana are caused by *B. bacilliformis*. Oroya fever is characterized by fever, profound anemia, and—unless antibiotic treatment is given—high mortality. The lesions referred to as verruga peruana may develop during the convalescent phase of Oroya fever or during chronic infection with *B. bacilliformis*. In 1885 Daniel Carrión, a Peruvian medical student, inoculated himself with blood from a patient with verruga peruana and subsequently died of Oroya fever, thus proving that both diseases are caused by a single agent.

EPIDEMIOLOGY   Infection with *B. bacilliformis* follows the bite of the sandfly vector *Phlebotomus*, an insect found in the river valleys of the Andes Mountains at altitudes of 600 to 2500 m. Oroya fever develops in nonimmune individuals who are not residents of the endemic region, whereas verruga peruana occurs in persons who apparently have been exposed in the past, including those who have recently had Oroya fever. The disease has rarely been described in the United States.

PATHOLOGY   During initial infection in the nonimmune host, *B. bacilliformis* cells adhere to erythrocytes and produce indentations in the cell membrane; the bacteria subsequently enter the erythrocytes and cause persistent deformation of the cytoskeleton. The parasitized erythrocytes are ultimately phagocytosed and destroyed. Although the life span of infected erythrocytes is markedly shortened, not all of this change can be attributed to the mechanical fragility induced by the internalization of bacteria. Decreased bone marrow erythropoiesis also contributes to anemia.

CLINICAL MANIFESTATIONS   The onset of symptoms in Oroya fever may be either insidious or abrupt, after an incubation period of approximately 3 weeks. The subacute presentation may include low-grade fever, malaise, headache, and anorexia. Sudden-onset disease commences with high fever, chills, diaphoresis, headaches, and changes in mental status. These manifestations are followed by the sudden development of profound anemia, which is due to a marked decrease in erythrocyte numbers and is associated with macrocytic changes, poikilocytosis, Howell-Jolly bodies, nucleated erythrocytes, and immature myeloid cells. The leukocyte differential usually shifts to the left, although the total leukocyte count may be normal. The erythrocyte count may fall to extremely low levels. In eosin/thiazine-stained peripheral-blood smears, numerous microorganisms can be seen adhering to most erythrocytes.

During the acute phase, muscle and joint pain and headache may be severe; central nervous system changes include insomnia, delirium, and decreased level of consciousness. Thrombocytopenic purpura may develop. If the patient survives, a convalescent phase ensues, characterized by the sudden disappearance of bacteria from blood smears, declining fever, and an increase in the erythrocyte count. While much of the mortality associated with Oroya fever is due to profound anemia and toxicity, secondary bacterial infections (including salmonellosis and other enteric infections, malaria, and tuberculosis) are often an important contributing factor.

After convalescence from acute Oroya fever, verrugas may develop. These red or purple cutaneous lesions may be either tiny and sessile or large, pedunculated, and nodular. They bear a marked resemblance to the lesions of bacillary angiomatosis and to Kaposi's sarcoma.

DIAGNOSIS   During acute infection, bacteria can be cultured from the blood on agar containing rabbit blood, with incubation at 28°C. The hallmark of verruga peruana is the formation of new blood vessels (angiogenesis) at the sites of bacterial replication.

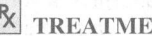 **TREATMENT**

Oroya fever responds to a variety of antimicrobial agents, including chloramphenicol, tetracyclines, penicillin, and streptomycin. Chloramphenicol is used most often because of its efficacy against most

Salmonella infections (as salmonellosis may develop intercurrently). Verruga peruana may respond similarly; however, failure to respond to therapy and relapse are common and require the reinstitution of prolonged therapy.

BACILLARY ANGIOMATOSIS

DEFINITION AND ETIOLOGY Bacillary angiomatosis was initially described as a condition occurring primarily in patients with AIDS and characterized by vascular cutaneous lesions resembling Kaposi's sarcoma. The disease can disseminate to involve virtually any organ system. Immunocompromised individuals, especially those infected with human immunodeficiency virus (HIV), are at particularly high risk for bacillary angiomatosis, although in rare instances the patient is not obviously immunosuppressed. Both *B. henselae* and *B. quintana* (the infectious agent initially associated with trench fever) produce bacillary angiomatosis in persons with immunodeficiency.

EPIDEMIOLOGY Acquisition of *B. henselae* has been significantly associated with exposure to young cats infested with fleas (*Ctenocephalides felis*). Since a high percentage of cats are seropositive, it has been suggested that patients with HIV infection avoid exposure to these animals. The recent finding that a large proportion of cats with fleas have persistent asymptomatic *B. henselae* bacteremia suggests that the domestic cat is the animal reservoir of this microorganism. The flea may serve as a transmitting vector in the cross-infection of cats, but its role in human infection is not clear. Tick-associated cases of *B. henselae* bacteremia have been reported in healthy immunocompetent individuals.

Person-to-person transmission of *B. quintana* by the human body louse (*Pediculus humanis corporis*) was documented during World War I under conditions of poor personal hygiene and sanitation. Recent cases of infection have most often involved homeless people; the implication is that ectoparasites, including mites and lice, may transmit infection from person to person. However, this point has not been proven, and the reservoir of *B. quintana* has not been identified.

MICROBIOLOGY *B. henselae* can be demonstrated in tissue by Warthin-Starry staining. Clumps and clusters of pleomorphic bacilli appear as purple deposits in tissue stained with hematoxylin and eosin. Although the bacteria may be difficult to cultivate in the laboratory, they can eventually be isolated from cultures of blood and of material from other sites. Colonies develop after prolonged incubation (1 to 4 weeks) on blood-containing media; bacterial cells are gram-negative.

Classification of *B. henselae* was first accomplished when molecular techniques were used to analyze bacterial ribosomal genes extracted from tissue samples. Definitive identification of *Bartonella* species is based on sequence analysis of 16S ribosomal DNA.

PATHOGENESIS AND PATHOLOGY Bacillary angiomatosis is characterized by a lobular proliferation of new blood vessels (angiogenesis) and a neutrophilic inflammatory response to myriad bacilli located within collagen-rich microscopic and macroscopic nodules. The endothelial cells lining the vascular spaces have a typical epithelioid appearance, and the lesions may resemble Kaposi's sarcoma histopathologically, although the characteristic spindle cell of the latter disease is usually absent. The bacterial and eukaryotic host factors that elicit the pathologic response are unknown.

CLINICAL MANIFESTATIONS The skin lesions of bacillary angiomatosis (also called *epithelioid angiomatosis*) are vascular nodules, papules, or tumors that range from tiny lesions resembling cherry angiomas or pyogenic granulomas to large, pedunculated, exophytic masses (Fig. 165-1). Characteristically, the lesions are red or purple, resembling Kaposi's sarcoma; they may be surrounded by an epithelial collarette, may be located anywhere on the skin, and may involve mucous membranes. The overlying epidermis may be focally ulcerated, and the underlying bone may be invaded and destroyed.

Dissemination of *B. henselae* infection occurs primarily in patients with cellular immune defects. Clinical manifestations accompanying

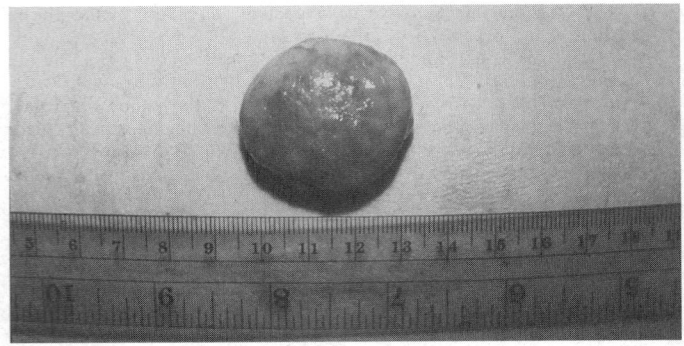

FIGURE 165-1 Characteristic skin lesion of bacillary angiomatosis in an HIV-positive young woman. This large, pedunculated tumor exhibits the typical angiomatous appearance. The patient was treated with oral erythromycin, with nearly complete resolution of the lesion; however, upon discontinuation of antibiotic therapy after a 4-week course, the lesion recurred.

dissemination are often nonspecific and include persistent fever, abdominal pain, weight loss, and malaise. Although the liver, spleen, bone marrow, and lymph nodes are primarily affected, HIV-infected patients may also develop central nervous system abnormalities (including psychiatric disorders and brain lesions), which are responsive to antibiotic therapy. Skin lesions usually are not evident in disseminated infection. Involvement of the liver or spleen may produce bacillary peliosis hepatis. Patients with the latter condition may report localized pain on palpation of the abdomen. Nodular lesions of variable size can be demonstrated by computed tomography or magnetic resonance imaging, with or without contrast agents.

DIAGNOSIS The diagnosis of bacillary angiomatosis is based primarily on the typical histopathologic findings of angiomas in association with clumps of tiny bacilli revealed by Warthin-Starry silver stain. Infection due to *B. henselae* can also be established by culture or by identification of specific DNA sequences. *B. henselae* is most easily isolated from blood through a lysis-centrifugation system. Colonies may be detected on blood-containing agar (rabbit blood is preferred) incubated with 5 to 10% CO_2 at 37°C for 2 to 4 weeks. *B. quintana* may be isolated from BACTEC (Becton Dickinson, Sparks, MD) aerobic bottles containing resin. Isolation from skin lesions and other tissues is more difficult but should be attempted when feasible. Initial reports suggested that cocultivation with endothelial cell monolayers was necessary; however, isolation by direct plating onto freshly prepared agar media has also been successful. Bacilli picked from new colonies but not subcultured may not stain, even with acridine orange; they stain weakly with safranin. Identification of *B. henselae* and *B. quintana* is based primarily on cellular fatty-acid analysis and on polymerase chain reaction (PCR)-based restriction fragment length polymorphism analysis. Definitive identification of *Bartonella* species depends on DNA sequence analysis of 16S ribosomal RNA genes. The diagnosis of CSD (see next section) can be made by specific serologic testing that detects *B. henselae*–specific antibodies, but the sensitivity and specificity of this method in patients with cutaneous and disseminated bacillary angiomatosis have not been determined.

DIFFERENTIAL DIAGNOSIS The differential diagnosis of cutaneous bacillary angiomatosis includes Kaposi's sarcoma, angiomas, and pyogenic granulomas. These conditions can be distinguished by histopathologic examination of biopsied material.

Cutaneous bacillary angiomatosis caused by *B. henselae* or *B. quintana* resembles verruga peruana, which is not seen outside of South America. In patients with AIDS, Kaposi's sarcoma lesions and bacillary angiomatosis may coexist.

℞ **TREATMENT**

Cutaneous lesions have been treated with a wide variety of antimicrobial drugs, including macrolides, tetracyclines, and antituberculous agents; *B. henselae* is susceptible to most antibiotics in vitro. Erythromycin (2 g/d), given orally for 3 weeks, is usually effective; however, relapse may require prolonged therapy with antibiotics that reach an intracellular compartment, such as erythromycin (2 g/d), ciprofloxacin (1 to 1.5 g/d), or doxycycline (200 mg/d). Patients with peliosis hepatis should be treated with intravenous antibiotics, and those with disseminated disease or bacteremia should be treated with a prolonged course (3 weeks to 2 months) of systemic antibiotics, such as macrolides (erythromycin, 2 g/d) or quinolones (ciprofloxacin, 800 mg/d). Cutaneous lesions may or may not regress spontaneously, perhaps depending on the status of the host's immunity. The safety of ciprofloxacin in pregnant or lactating women has not been established. Moreover, no antimicrobial has been studied prospectively, and information on efficacy comes from only a few case reports.

CAT-SCRATCH DISEASE

DEFINITION AND ETIOLOGY   Typical CSD is manifested by painful regional lymphadenopathy persisting for several weeks or months after a cat scratch. Occasionally, infection may disseminate and produce more generalized lymphadenopathy and systemic manifestations, which may be confused with the manifestations of lymphoma. *B. henselae* is the causative agent of CSD. There is no evidence that *B. quintana* or *Afipia felis* (originally proposed as the agent of CSD) can cause this disease, nor are those two species carried by cats.

EPIDEMIOLOGY   Approximately 60 percent of cases of CSD in the United States occur in children. Exposure to bacteremic young cats that either are flea-infested or have been in contact with another cat carrying fleas poses a significant risk of infection. Most infections are caused by a scratch and only rare cases by a bite or by licking. Most cases occur in the warmer months, when fleas are active. Regions of the United States where fleas are endemic have higher rates of infection. The flea may serve to transmit infection between cats; it is not known whether humans can be infected through the bite of an infected flea.

CLINICAL MANIFESTATIONS   A localized papule, progressing to a pustule that often crusts over, develops 3 to 5 days after a cat scratch. Tender regional lymphadenopathy develops within 1 to 2 weeks after inoculation; by this time, the papule may have healed spontaneously. Scratches are most often sustained on the hands or face, producing epitrochlear, axillary, pectoral, and cervical lymph node involvement. The involved nodes occasionally become suppurative; bacterial superinfection with staphylococci or other cutaneous pathogens may develop. Although most patients do not have fever, systemic symptoms are frequent and include malaise, anorexia, and weight loss. Without treatment, lymphadenopathy persists for weeks or even months and may be confused with lymphatic malignancy. Other manifestations in apparently immunocompetent patients include encephalitis, seizures and coma (especially in children), meningitis, transverse myelitis, granulomatous hepatitis and splenitis, osteomyelitis, and disseminated infection. Conjunctival inoculation may cause Parinaud's oculoglandular syndrome, with conjunctivitis and preauricular lymphadenopathy.

PATHOLOGY   The histopathologic hallmark of CSD is granulomatous inflammation with stellate necrosis but no evidence of angiogenesis. Thus, infection by *B. henselae* can produce two entirely different pathologic reactions, depending on the immune status of the host: CSD or bacillary angiomatosis.

DIAGNOSIS   CSD should be suspected if the patient has a history of exposure to cats and develops lymphadenopathy and a skin lesion. The diagnosis can be confirmed by pathologic examination of the involved nodes. Tiny bacilli in clusters can sometimes be seen in biopsy samples stained with Warthin-Starry silver. The CSD skin test, in which lymph node material obtained from patients with CSD serves as an antigen, is no longer used for diagnosis because of concerns about the transmission of viral agents. A specific serologic test has been developed recently and may produce a positive result in 70 to 90 percent of patients with intact immunity. The identification of *B. henselae* 16S ribosomal RNA genes in biopsy material by PCR amplification with specific oligonucleotide primers can also be diag-

nostically useful; however, these methods are not yet commercially available. Cultures of lymph nodes, cerebrospinal fluid, or other tissues are rarely positive.

 TREATMENT
Although CSD is generally self-limited, tender regional lymphadenopathy and systemic symptoms may be debilitating. Patients with encephalitis or other serious manifestations should be treated with antibiotics, even though the efficacy of such therapy is unclear. No comparative trials of antibiotic treatment have been performed, and no anecdotal reports of treatment failures have appeared. Several reports suggest that aminoglycoside treatment (e.g., intravenous gentamicin at standard doses calculated to result in therapeutic levels) is effective in patients with encephalitis and other systemic infections. The oral agents that appear to be useful are those that also are most effective for the treatment of bacillary angiomatosis; they include ciprofloxacin, doxycycline, and possibly erythromycin (at the dosages recommended for bacillary angiomatosis). Many patients with established CSD have no apparent response to antibiotics; the necessary duration of therapy is variable.

TRENCH FEVER

Trench fever was first described as a debilitating febrile illness associated with prolonged *B. quintana* bacteremia in soldiers fighting in Europe during World War I. Although not usually fatal, the illness accounted for substantial morbidity. In recent years, trench fever has reemerged in the United States and has been caused by either *B. henselae*—the agent of CSD and bacillary angiomatosis—or *B. quintana*.

EPIDEMIOLOGY   Although trench fever was thought to have disappeared from the United States, recent cases have been diagnosed in homeless persons (*B. quintana*) and in persons bitten by ticks (*B. henselae*). During World War I, trench fever was transmitted from person to person by the human body louse. Transmission by ectoparasites is suspected in the recent cases of *B. quintana* infection but has not been firmly documented. Patients with trench fever have apparently normal immune defenses.

CLINICAL MANIFESTATIONS   Trench fever is characterized by the sudden onset of headache, aseptic meningitis, persistent fever (which can be high-grade and is commonly paroxysmal), malaise, weight loss, and other nonspecific symptoms. Severe musculoskeletal pain is more common among immunocompetent than among immunocompromised patients. Bacteremia can persist for days or weeks, and relapses have followed short courses of antibiotic therapy. Localized findings are uncommon.

DIAGNOSIS   Trench fever is diagnosed by the finding of sustained bacteremia. *B. henselae* and *B. quintana* grow slowly. Colonies develop on rabbit blood agar after 1 to 4 weeks of incubation under conditions of increased CO_2. Serologic tests for this disease have not yet been standardized.

 TREATMENT
A prolonged course (4 weeks) of antimicrobial therapy may be required. Agents that can cross the mammalian cell membrane are most effective, including erythromycin (2 g/d) or azithromycin (500 mg/d). Data on the efficacy of these agents come from a limited number of case reports.

OTHER *BARTONELLA* INFECTIONS

The application of molecular methods to the detection of microorganisms that are difficult to cultivate in the laboratory has revealed new *Bartonella* species and has established *Bartonella* species as a cause of endocarditis cases previously classified as being of unknown etiology. One new species, *Bartonella elizabethae*, has been identified as an agent of endocarditis, and cases of endocarditis associated with *B. quintana* and *B. henselae* have been reported recently. Therefore, the possibility of *Bartonella* infection should be considered and appropriate laboratory methods employed in an effort to isolate and identify *Bartonella* species in cases of "culture-negative" endocarditis or bacteremia.

BIBLIOGRAPHY

ARIAS-STELLA J et al: Histology, immunohistochemistry, and ultrastructure of the verruga in Carrion's disease. Am J Surg Pathol 10:595, 1986

BOGUE CW et al: Antibiotic therapy for cat-scratch disease? JAMA 262:813, 1989

CARITHERS HA: Cat scratch disease: An overview based on a study of 1,200 patients. Am J Dis Child 139:1124, 1985

COCKERELL DJ, LeBOIT PE: Bacillary angiomatosis: A newly characterized, pseudoneoplastic, infectious, cutaneous vascular disorder. J Am Acad Dermatol 22:501, 1990

DOLAN MJ et al: Syndrome of *Rochalimaea henselae* adenitis suggesting cat scratch disease. Ann Intern Med 118:331, 1993

HOLLEY HP JR: Successful treatment of cat-scratch disease with ciprofloxacin. JAMA 265:1563, 1991

KOEHLER JE et al: Isolation of *Rochalimaea* species from cutaneous and osseous lesions of bacillary angiomatosis. N Engl J Med 23:1625, 1992

———, TAPPERO JW: AIDS commentary: Bacillary angiomatosis and bacillary peliosis in patients infected with human immunodeficiency virus. Clin Infect Dis 17:612, 1993

——— et al: *Rochalimaea henselae* infection: A new zoonosis with the domestic cat as reservoir. JAMA 271:531, 1994

LUCEY D et al: Relapsing illness due to *Rochalimaea henselae* in immunocompetent hosts: Implication for therapy and new epidemiological associations. Clin Infect Dis 14:683, 1992

PERKOCHA LA et al: Clinical and pathological features of bacillary peliosis hepatis in association with human immunodeficiency virus infection. N Engl J Med 323:148, 1990

REGNERY RL et al: Characterization of a novel *Rochalimaea* species, *R. henselae*, sp.nov., isolated from blood of a febrile, human immunodeficiency virus–positive patient. J Clin Microbiol 30:265, 1992

RELMAN DA et al: The agent of bacillary angiomatosis: An approach to the identification of uncultured pathogens. N Engl J Med 323:1573, 1990

RICKETTS WE: Clinical manifestations of Carrion's disease. Arch Intern Med 84:751, 1949

SHINALL EA: Cat-scratch disease: A review of the literature. Pediatr Dermatol 7:11, 1990

SLATER LN et al: A newly recognized fastidious gram-negative pathogen as a cause of fever and bacteremia. N Engl J Med 323:1587, 1990

SPACH DH et al: *Bartonella (Rochalimaea) quintana* bacteremia in inner-city patients with chronic alcoholism. N Engl J Med 332:425, 1995

STRONG RO (ed): *Trench Fever: Report of Commission, Medical Research Committee, American Red Cross.* Oxford, Oxford University Press, 1918, p 40

TAPPERO JW et al: The epidemiology of bacillary angiomatosis and bacillary peliosis. JAMA 269:770, 1993

ZANGWILL KM et al: Cat scratch disease in Connecticut: Epidemiology, risk factors, and evaluation of a new diagnostic test. N Engl J Med 329:8, 1993

166 *King K. Holmes*

DONOVANOSIS (GRANULOMA INGUINALE)

DEFINITION Donovanosis (granuloma inguinale) is a mildly contagious, chronic, indolent, progressive, autoinoculable, ulcerative disease involving the skin and lymphatics of the genital or perianal areas. The disease appears to be sexually transmitted and is associated with the presence in affected tissues of an intracellular microorganism, identified morphologically as the Donovan body.

ETIOLOGY Donovanosis was described by McLeod in India in 1882. In 1905 Donovan described the intracellular bodies that are thought to cause the disease. During the 1940s, encapsulated bacteria resembling Donovan bodies were recovered from pseudobuboes of granuloma inguinale by inoculation of chick embryo yolk sacs or yolk-agar medium. These bacteria, which are known as *Calymmatobacterium granulomatis*, measure 1.5 by 0.7 μm. Since such isolates are no longer available and *C. granulomatis* has not been reproducibly cultivable, the organism has not been characterized. However, investigators in South Africa have recently reported cultivation and propagation of a *C. granulomatis*–like organism in mononuclear cells, and other researchers have used polymerase chain reaction amplification of the *phoE* or ribosomal genes of material obtained directly from donovanosis ulcers in attempts to identify the causative organism. Definitive characterization of *C. granulomatis* awaits further research. Electron-microscopic studies of Donovan bodies show their morphologic resemblance to gram-negative bacteria.

EPIDEMIOLOGY Donovanosis is endemic in the tropics, particularly in Papua New Guinea, southern India, southern Africa, and parts of Australia, Brazil, and the Caribbean. In the United States, the disease is rare. In reported cases, the sex ratio of males to females is nearly 10:1. The disease is uncommon in Caucasians. The frequency of donovanosis in sexual partners of chronically infected patients is highly variable, ranging from 1 percent to over 50 percent. Evidence for sexual transmission includes the age-specific incidence, which corresponds to that of other sexually transmitted diseases; the frequent concomitant presence of syphilis; the predilection for genital involvement in heterosexuals and for anorectal infection in homosexually active men; and the fact that outbreaks of clusters of cases of donovanosis have been traced to sexual exposure to a single-source contact. A significant association of human immunodeficiency virus (HIV) infection with donovanosis has been found among men in Durban, South Africa.

CLINICAL MANIFESTATIONS The incubation period for donovanosis ranges from 8 days to 12 weeks, but most lesions appear within 30 days after sexual exposure. The disease begins as a papule that ulcerates and develops into a painless elevated zone of clean, beefy-red, friable granulation tissue. The edges are irregular and spread by continuity or by autoinoculation of approximated skin surfaces. Secondary anaerobic infection may produce pain and a foul-smelling exudate. Less common complications of the disease include deep ulcerations, chronic cicatricial lesions, phimosis, lymphedema, and exuberant epithelial proliferation that grossly resembles carcinoma. In men, the lesions are usually located on the glans, prepuce, or shaft of the penis or in the perianal area, while infection of the labia is most common in women. Lesions in women often arise at the fourchette and progress anteriorly in a V pattern along the vulva. Extragenital lesions may develop, involving the face, neck, mouth, and/or other sites. The chronicity of the disease is of diagnostic importance, since several months often elapse before patients seek treatment. Extension to the inguinal region by autoinoculation, by continuity, or via the lymphatics results in a diffuse intradermal and subcutaneous swelling or suppuration known as a *pseudobubo* because involvement of the underlying lymph nodes is minimal. Locally destructive lesions and secondary infection may cause severe morbidity or death. Fatal disseminated disease involving the bones, joints, or liver has been reported. Rates of disseminated infection are apparently elevated during pregnancy. The relationship of donovanosis to subsequent carcinoma of the genitalia is uncertain.

DIAGNOSIS Early donovanosis may be mistaken for the primary chancre or condyloma latum of syphilis. Epithelial proliferation resembling carcinoma in the genital or perianal region in a young individual should always raise the suspicion of donovanosis if unnecessary destructive surgery is to be avoided. Chronic ulcerative or cicatricial changes may resemble those of lymphogranuloma venereum.

Amebiasis can produce penile lesions resembling the lesions of donovanosis. In the United States, *Haemophilus ducreyi* frequently has been isolated from lesions resembling those of donovanosis; these *H. ducreyi*–associated lesions have been termed *pseudo–granuloma inguinale chancroid*. Histologic studies in donovanosis reveal marked acanthosis and pseudoepitheliomatous hyperplasia. The dermis contains an inflammatory infiltrate consisting mainly of plasma cells and histiocytes. Because Donovan bodies are seldom detectable in sections stained with hematoxylin and eosin, these changes may lead to an erroneous diagnosis of carcinoma and to unnecessary and destructive surgery. Although silver impregnation techniques are useful for the demonstration of Donovan bodies in sections, the diagnosis is best made by examination of impression smears prepared from specimens obtained by punch biopsy of granulation tissue from the periphery of a lesion; the deep portion of the specimen is removed and crushed between two slides, which are air-dried, fixed in methanol, and stained with Wright-Giemsa. In these stained smears, Donovan bodies appear as rounded coccobacilli of 1 by 2 μm lying within cystic spaces in the cytoplasm of large mononuclear cells. The capsule stains as a dense acidophilic zone surrounding the bacterium, which resembles a closed safety pin because of bipolar condensation of chromatin. The pathognomonic mononuclear cell is 25 to 90 μm in diameter and has many cystic areas containing Donovan bodies. Donovan bodies also have been identified within histiocytes in cervical Papanicolaou smears.

Perianal donovanosis may resemble condylomata lata of secondary syphilis. Other venereal diseases, particularly syphilis, frequently co-exist with donovanosis. Repeated negative dark-field examinations of lesions and negative serologic tests exclude syphilis but should not be rigidly required while treatment is withheld from potentially non-compliant patients. In countries where donovanosis is endemic, the persistence of suspected condylomata lata after appropriate penicillin therapy for syphilis is highly suggestive of donovanosis.

℞ TREATMENT

The antimicrobials currently effective in the treatment of dono-vanosis in various parts of the world include trimethoprim-sulfameth-oxazole, tetracycline, erythromycin, newer quinolones, gentamicin, and chloramphenicol or the related drug thiamphenicol (not available in the United States). Recent studies have found azithromycin or ceftriaxone to be effective. Streptomycin, once commonly used for this condition, is not widely used today. Ampicillin is not recommended for the treatment of donovanosis. Unfortunately, no comparative trials have been conducted with the currently used antimicrobi-

als, and in vitro susceptibility testing is not possible. The minimum duration of treatment is not well established; it is customary, though perhaps not essential, to continue therapy until lesions have completely healed over. Thus treatment for large lesions is generally more prolonged than that for small lesions, whose healing is usually apparent within 3 weeks. As the lesions heal, they become pale and flatter and peripheral reepithelialization begins. Lack of an objective clinical response within 7 days should lead to reassessment of the diagnosis and therapy. Donovan bodies disappear from lesions within a few days after the initiation of therapy. Typical dosages of the commonly used drugs include 500 mg four times daily for tetracy-cline or erythromycin and 160/800 mg twice daily for trimethoprim-sulfamethoxazole.

BIBLIOGRAPHY

BASSA AG et al: Granuloma inguinale (donovanosis) in women. An analysis of 61 cases from Durban, South Africa. Sex Transm Dis 20:164, 1993

BOWDEN FJ et al: Pilot study of azithromycin in the treatment of genital donovanosis. Genitourin Med 72:17, 1996

KUBERSKI T: Granuloma inguinale (donovanosis). Sex Transm Dis 7:29, 1980

MEIN J et al: Donovanosis: Sequelae of severe disease and successful azithro-mycin treatment. Int J STD AIDS 7:448, 1996

MERIANOS A et al: Ceftriaxone in the treatment of chronic donovanosis in central Australia. Genitourin Med 70:84, 1994

O'FARRELL N: Clinico-epidemiological study of donovanosis in Durban, South Africa. Genitourin Med 69:108, 1993

——— et al: A rapid stain for the diagnosis of granuloma inguinale. Genitourin Med 66:200, 1990

——— et al: HIV-1 infection among heterosexual attendees of a sexually transmitted disease clinic in Durban. S Afr Med J 80:17, 1991

RAMANAN C et al: Treatment of donovanosis with norfloxacin. Int J Dermatol 29:298, 1990

RICHENS J: The diagnosis and treatment of donovanosis (granuloma inguinale). Genitourin Med 67:441, 1991

ROSEN T et al: Granuloma inguinale. J Am Acad Dermatol 11:433, 1984

SECTION 7

MISCELLANEOUS BACTERIAL INFECTIONS

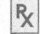

167 *Gregory A. Filice*

NOCARDIOSIS

DEFINITION The term *nocardiosis* refers to invasive disease associated with *Nocardia* species, aerobic actinomycetes that cause several characteristic syndromes. Pneumonia and disseminated disease, both thought to follow inhalation of fragmented bacterial mycelia, are most common. Three syndromes follow transcutaneous inoculation: cellulitis, a lymphocutaneous syndrome, and actinomycetoma. Keratitis follows inoculation into the eye at the time of corneal trauma.

ETIOLOGIC AGENTS Nocardiae are common bacterial inhabitants of soil, where they contribute to the decay of organic matter. Seven *Nocardia* species have been associated with human disease: *N. asteroides*, *N. brasiliensis*, *N. otitidiscaviarum* (formerly *N. caviae*), *N. farcinica*, *N. nova*, *N. transvalensis*, and *N. pseudobrasiliensis*.

EPIDEMIOLOGY Nocardiosis occurs throughout the world. Approximately 1000 cases are diagnosed annually in the United States, 85 percent of them pulmonary and/or systemic. The disease is more common among adults than among children and among males than among females. Outbreaks are rare, and person-to-person spread has not been well documented.

The risk of pulmonary or disseminated disease is greater than usual among people with deficient cell-mediated immunity, especially

deficiency associated with lymphoma, transplantation, or AIDS. Nocardiosis has also been associated with pulmonary alveolar proteinosis, tuberculosis, and chronic granulomatous disease.

Nocardia is one of the several actinomycete genera associated with antinomycetoma, which occurs mainly in tropical and subtropical regions, especially those of Mexico, Central and South America, Africa, and India. The most important risk factor for actinomycetoma is frequent contact with soil or vegetable matter.

PATHOLOGY AND PATHOGENESIS The characteristic histologic feature of pulmonary or systemic nocardial infection is an abscess extensively infiltrated with neutrophils. Granulation tissue usually surrounds the lesions, but extensive fibrosis or encapsulation is uncommon. Actinomycetoma is characterized by suppurative inflammation with sinus tract formation. The lesions of actinomycetoma and their drainage contain granules composed of dense masses of bacterial filaments.

Nocardiae have evolved a number of properties that enable them to survive within phagocytes, including neutralization of oxidants, prevention of phagosome-lysosome fusion, and prevention of phagosome acidification. Neutrophils phagocytose the organisms and limit their growth but do not kill them efficiently. Cell-mediated immunity is important for definitive control and elimination of the organisms.

CLINICAL MANIFESTATIONS **Pulmonary Disease** Nocardial pneumonia is typically subacute; persons generally seek medical care several days or weeks after the development of symptoms.

The onset may be more acute in immunosuppressed patients. Cough is prominent and productive of small amounts of thick, purulent sputum that is not malodorous. Fever, anorexia, weight loss, and malaise are common; dyspnea, pleuritic pain, and hemoptysis are less common. Tracheitis and bronchitis are uncommon. Obstructive bronchial masses have been reported. Remissions and exacerbations over periods of several weeks are frequent.

Roentgenologic patterns are variable. Infiltrates vary in size and are usually of moderate or greater density. Nodules and cavitation are common. Empyema is evident in one-third of cases.

Pulmonary nocardiosis may spread directly from the lungs to involve adjacent tissues. Pericarditis, mediastinitis, and the superior vena cava syndrome have all been reported. Spread through the chest wall is rare.

Nocardia species are sometimes isolated from respiratory secretions of patients without apparent nocardial disease. Most of these patients have chronic pulmonary disease with abnormal airways or parenchyma.

Extrapulmonary Dissemination   In half of all cases of pulmonary nocardiosis, disease appears outside the lungs. One-fifth of patients with disseminated disease present only with extrapulmonary disease, which has probably spread hematogenously from an inapparent or healed pulmonary focus. The most common sites are the brain, skin and supporting structures, kidneys, bone, and muscle, but dissemination to nearly every organ has been reported. Peritonitis and endocarditis have been described. The typical manifestation of extrapulmonary dissemination is a subacute or chronic abscess. A minority of abscesses outside the lungs or central nervous system (CNS) form fistulas and discharge small amounts of pus. All *Nocardia* species are associated with disseminated disease, but most invasive strains previously classified as *N. brasiliensis* have been grouped in the new species *N. pseudobrasiliensis*.

The CNS is the most common location for disseminated disease. Usually there are one or more supratentorial brain abscesses, often multiloculated. Brain abscesses tend to burrow into the ventricles or out into the subarachnoid space. The symptoms and signs are somewhat more indolent than those of brain abscess due to other bacteria. Meningitis without apparent brain abscess is rare. The organism is not easily recovered from cerebrospinal fluid.

Disease Following Transcutaneous Inoculation   As has already been mentioned, infection following transcutaneous inoculation usually takes one of three forms: cellulitis, lymphocutaneous syndrome, or actinomycetoma. Cellulitis generally begins 1 to 3 weeks after a recognized breach of the skin. Often the wound has been contaminated with soil. Subacute cellulitis, with pain, swelling, erythema, and warmth, develops over days or weeks. The lesions are usually firm and nonfluctuant. The process may progress to involve underlying muscles, tendons, bones, and joints. Dissemination is rare. *N. asteroides* is common in colder climates, while *N. brasiliensis* predominates in warmer climates.

In the lymphocutaneous syndrome, there is typically a pyodermatous lesion at the site of inoculation, with central ulceration and purulent or honey-colored drainage. Subcutaneous nodules often appear along lymphatics that drain the primary lesion. The lymphangitic form closely resembles lymphocutaneous sporotrichosis (see Chap. 210). Most cases of the lymphocutaneous syndrome are associated with *N. brasiliensis*.

Actinomycetoma usually begins with a nodular swelling, sometimes in conjunction with local trauma. Lesions typically develop on the feet or the hands but may involve the posterior part of the neck, the upper back, the head, and other sites. The nodule eventually breaks down and a fistula appears. This fistula is soon accompanied by others. The fistulas tend to come and go, with new ones forming as old ones disappear. The discharge is serous or purulent, may be bloody, and often contains 0.1- to 2-mm white granules consisting of masses of mycelia. The lesions spread slowly along fascial planes to involve adjacent areas of skin, subcutaneous tissue, and bone. Over a period

of months to years, there may be extensive deformation of the affected part. Lesions involving soft tissues are only mildly painful, whereas those affecting bones or joints are more so. Systemic symptoms are minimal or lacking altogether. Infection rarely disseminates from actinomycetoma, and lesions on the hands and feet usually cause only local disability. Lesions on the head, neck, and trunk can invade locally to involve deep organs and result in severe disability or death.

Keratitis   *Nocardia* species (most often *N. asteroides*) are uncommon causes of subacute keratitis. The infection usually follows eye trauma. Nocardial infection of lacrimal glands has been reported. Disease involving deeper eye structures is usually a manifestation of dissemination.

DIAGNOSIS   The first step in the diagnosis of nocardiosis is the examination of sputum or pus for crooked, branching, beaded, gram-positive filaments 1 μm in width and up to 50 μm long. Most nocardiae are acid-fast in direct smears if a weak acid is used for decolorization (e.g., in the modified Kinyoun, Ziehl-Neelsen, and Fite-Faraco methods). The organisms often take up silver stains. Nocardiae grow relatively slowly; colonies may take up to 2 weeks to appear and may not develop their characteristic appearance for up to 4 weeks. Their pattern of growth is quite different from those of more common pathogens; thus, the laboratory should always be alerted when nocardial infection is suspected so that the likelihood of its recovery is maximized. In difficult cases, paraffin baiting can be employed, as nocardiae are among the few aerobic microorganisms that can use paraffin as a carbon source.

Smears are often negative. In such cases, invasive procedures are necessary for diagnosis. Transtracheal aspiration should be avoided, as it frequently leads to nocardial cellulitis in tissues around the puncture wound.

Growth of nocardiae from sputum may represent colonization and not disease. Findings that make disease more likely are the detection of nocardiae on Gram-stained preparations and the isolation of the organisms from multiple cultures. A positive culture of sputum from an immunosuppressed patient usually reflects disease.

A careful history should be obtained and a thorough physical examination performed to evaluate the possibility of dissemination in patients with nocardial pneumonia. Suggestive symptoms or signs should be pursued with further diagnostic tests. Computed tomography or magnetic resonance imaging of the head, with and without contrast material, should be undertaken if there are signs or symptoms suggesting brain involvement.

Biphasic culture bottles incubated aerobically for up to 30 days often yield nocardiae, but routine blood cultures are usually negative. If clinically indicated, specimens of cerebrospinal fluid or urine should be concentrated and then cultured. In cases of actinomycetoma, an effort should be made to find granules in the discharge. Suspect particles should be washed in saline, examined microscopically, and cultured.

Several presumptive diagnostic tests have been studied, including tests for antibodies and nocardial metabolites in serum or cerebrospinal fluid. None of these tests is ready for clinical use at this time.

℞ TREATMENT

Sulfonamides are the drugs of choice for nocardiosis. Initially, 6 to 8 g of sulfadiazine or sulfisoxazole per day in four divided doses should be used. After the disease is under control, 4 g per day can be used to complete the course of therapy. (For durations, see below.) In difficult cases, sulfonamide levels in serum should be measured and dosages adjusted to keep serum concentrations between 100 and 150 μg/mL. The combination of sulfamethoxazole and trimethoprim is equivalent or possibly slightly more effective but poses a modestly greater risk of hematologic toxicity. Initially, 10 to 20 mg of trimethoprim per kilogram and 50 to 100 mg of sulfamethoxazole per kilogram should be given each day in two divided doses. Later, the daily dose can be dropped to as little as 5 mg of trimethoprim and 25 mg of sulfamethoxazole per kilogram. Sulfonamides given for prophylaxis of other infectious diseases appear to reduce the risk of nocardiosis.

Antimicrobial susceptibility testing has not been developed to the point where its clinical relevance is certain, and initial choices of antimicrobials should be based on published clinical experience. However, isolates should be sent to a reference laboratory for definitive identification and susceptibility testing with methods developed specifically for *Nocardia*. The results may help guide therapy if initial choices do not work or if toxicity develops. Nocardiae are generally susceptible to sulfonamides, minocycline, amikacin, cefotaxime, ceftizoxime, ceftriaxone, and imipenem and resistant to ampicillin and erythromycin. *N. farcinica* strains differ in that most are resistant to cephalosporins and one-fifth are resistant to imipenem. Strains of *N. pseudobrasiliensis* often show resistance to minocycline or amoxicillin/clavulanic acid and exhibit susceptibility to ciprofloxacin or clarithromycin.

Minocycline is the best-established alternative oral drug for use against all species and should be given in doses of 100 to 200 mg twice a day. Other tetracyclines are usually ineffective. Infections due to *N. nova* can be treated with erythromycin (500 to 750 mg four times a day) and/or ampicillin (1 g four times a day), but other *Nocardia* species are usually resistant to both of these drugs. Amoxicillin combined with clavulanate (500 and 125 mg, respectively, given three times a day) can be used except against *N. nova*, in which clavulanate induces β-lactamase production. Ofloxacin (400 mg twice a day) and clarithromycin (500 mg twice a day) have each been used successfully in a few cases.

Amikacin, the best-established drug for parenteral use, is given in doses of 5 to 7.5 mg/kg every 12 h. Serum levels should be monitored if therapy is prolonged, if renal function is diminished, or if the patient is elderly. Newer β-lactam antibiotics, including cefotaxime, ceftizoxime, ceftriaxone, and imipenem, are usually effective except against *N. farcinica*.

The administration of immunosuppressive agents should be continued if necessary for the treatment of underlying disease or the prevention of organ-transplant rejection. In many cases, two or more antimicrobials have been used to treat nocardiosis, often in combinations including a sulfonamide or minocycline. Whether therapy with two or more agents is better than therapy with a single agent is not known, however, and therapy with multiple drugs increases the risk of toxicity.

A brain abscess should be aspirated, drained, or excised if the diagnosis is unclear, if the abscess is large and accessible, or if it fails to respond to chemotherapy. Small abscesses and those in inaccessible or critical locations should be treated medically. In cases managed medically, clinical improvement should be noticeable within 1 to 2 weeks. Anatomic resolution often lags behind clinical improvement and should be monitored with repeated imaging.

Antimicrobial therapy usually suffices for nocardial actinomycetoma. In cases of deep or extensive disease, drainage or excision of heavily involved tissue may facilitate healing, but structure and function should be preserved whenever possible.

Because nocardial infections tend to relapse, long courses of antimicrobial therapy are necessary. Nocardiosis is particularly tenacious and likely to relapse in people with chronic granulomatous disease. When the patient is immunocompetent, the treatment of pulmonary or systemic nocardiosis outside the CNS should be continued for 6 to 12 months. Ordinarily, treatment of CNS nocardiosis should be continued for 1 year. If all apparent sites of CNS disease have been excised, it may be possible to reduce the duration of therapy to 6 months. When the patient is immunosuppressed, the treatment of pulmonary or systemic nocardiosis should be continued for 1 year. In some patients with AIDS, it has been necessary to continue therapy indefinitely. If nocardial disease is unusually extensive or if the response to therapy is slow, these recommendations should be exceeded.

Patients with cellulitis or the lymphocutaneous syndrome should be treated for 2 months if the infection is limited to soft tissues and for 4 months if bone is involved. Unusually extensive cases or cases in immunosuppressed people should be treated longer. Therapy for actinomycetoma should be continued for 6 to 12 months after clinical cure. Keratitis should be treated with oral and topical sulfonamides until the infection appears to be cured and then with oral sulfonamides alone for an additional 2 to 4 months.

PROGNOSIS The mortality for pulmonary or disseminated nocardiosis outside the CNS should be less than 5 percent. CNS disease poses a greater risk of death. Patients should be followed carefully for at least 6 months after therapy has ended. Any child with nocardiosis and no known cause of immunosuppression should undergo tests to determine the adequacy of the phagocytic respiratory burst.

BIBLIOGRAPHY

ARDUINO RC et al: Nocardiosis in renal transplant recipients undergoing immunosuppression with cyclosporine. Clin Infect Dis 16:505, 1993

BERKEY P, BODEY GP: Nocardial infection in patients with neoplastic disease. Rev Infect Dis 11:407, 1989

FILICE GA, SIMPSON GS: Management of *Nocardia* infections, in *Current Clinical Topics in Infectious Diseases*, JS Remington, MN Swartz (eds). New York, McGraw-Hill, 1984, vol 5, pp 49–64

KING CT et al: Recurrent nocardiosis in a renal transplant recipient. South Med J 86:225, 1993

LEBLANG SD et al: CNS *Nocardia* in AIDS patients: CT and MRI with pathologic correlation. J Comput Assist Tomogr 19:15, 1995

MCNEIL MM et al: Infections due to *Nocardia transvalensis*: Clinical spectrum and antimicrobial therapy. Clin Infect Dis 15:453, 1992

PALMER DL et al: Diagnostic and therapeutic considerations in *Nocardia asteroides* infection. Medicine 53:391, 1974

PETERSON EA et al: Minocycline treatment of pulmonary nocardiosis. JAMA 250:930, 1983

RUIMY R et al: *Nocardia pseudobrasiliensis* sp. nov., a new species of *Nocardia* which groups bacterial strains previously identified as *Nocardia brasiliensis* and associated with invasive diseases. Int J Syst Bacteriol 46:259, 1996

SATTERWHITE TK, WALLACE RJ JR: Primary cutaneous nocardiosis. JAMA 242:333, 1979

TIGHT RR, BARTLETT MS: Actinomycetoma in the United States. Rev Infect Dis 3:1139, 1981

UTTAMCHANDANI RB et al: Nocardiosis in 30 patients with advanced human immunodeficiency virus infection: Clinical features and outcome. Clin Infect Dis 18:348, 1994

WALLACE RJ JR et al: Antimicrobial susceptibility patterns of *Nocardia asteroides*. Antimicrob Agents Chemother 32:1776, 1988

——— et al: Cefotaxime-resistant *Nocardia asteroides* strains are isolates of the controversial species *Nocardia farcinica*. J Clin Microbiol 28:2726, 1990

——— et al: Clinical and laboratory features of *Nocardia nova*. J Clin Microbiol 29:2407, 1991

——— et al: New *Nocardia* taxon among isolates of *Nocardia brasiliensis* associated with invasive disease. J Clin Microbiol 33:1528, 1995

168 *Thomas A. Russo*

ACTINOMYCOSIS

Actinomycosis is an indolent, slowly progressive bacterial infection caused by a variety of gram-positive, non-spore-forming anaerobic or microaerophilic rods, most of which are of the genus *Actinomyces*. Actinomycosis was common in the preantibiotic era but is less frequent now, and consequently so is its timely recognition. The clinical presentations of this disease, which can affect nearly every organ and body site, are myriad, but most characteristic are the formation of "sulfur granules" and the violation of normal tissue plane barriers as infection spreads and creates draining sinuses. Actinomycosis has been called "the most misdiagnosed disease," and it has been said that "no disease is so often missed by experienced clinicians." An awareness of the full spectrum of the disease is needed to expedite its diagnosis and treatment and to minimize the unnecessary morbidity and mortality that are reported all too often.

ETIOLOGIC AGENTS Actinomycosis is most commonly caused by *Actinomyces israelii*. *Actinomyces naeslundii*, *Actinomyces odontolyticus*, *Actinomyces viscosus*, *Actinomyces meyeri*, *Actinomyces gerencseriae*, and *Propionibacterium propionicum* (formerly *Arachnia propionica*) are established but less common causes of disease.

Most if not all actinomycotic infections are polymicrobial. *Actinobacillus actinomycetemcomitans*, *Eikenella corrodens*, Enterobacteriaceae, and species of *Fusobacterium*, *Bacteroides*, *Capnocytophaga*, *Staphylococcus*, and *Streptococcus* are commonly isolated with actinomycetes in various combinations, depending on the site of infection. The contribution of these other species to pathogenesis in actinomycosis is uncertain.

EPIDEMIOLOGY   The agents of actinomycosis are members of the normal oral flora and are often cultured from the bronchi, the gastrointestinal tract, and the female genital tract. Infection occurs throughout life, with a peak incidence in the middle decades. Males have a threefold higher incidence of infection, possibly because of poorer dental hygiene and/or more frequent trauma. Likely contributing factors to the decrease in the incidence of actinomycosis since the start of the antibiotic era include improved dental hygiene and the initiation of antimicrobial treatment early on—before the full development of the disease. Individuals who do not have access to health care may well be at higher risk.

PATHOGENESIS AND PATHOLOGY   A vital step in the development of actinomycosis is disruption of the mucosal barrier, which allows the actinomycetes to invade beyond their endogenous habitat in the mouth, lower gastrointestinal tract, and female genitourinary tract. Local infection, subsequent extension, and (in rare instances) distant hematogenous seeding may ensue. Initial acute inflammation is followed by the characteristic chronic, indolent phase. Lesions usually appear as single or multiple indurations. Cental fluctuance, with pus containing neutrophils and sulfur granules, may develop. Granules are gritty in vivo conglomerations of organisms that are virtually diagnostic of actinomycosis (Fig. 168-1). The fibrous walls of the mass are typically described as woody and, in the absence of suppuration, are sometimes confused with neoplasms. Once established, actinomycosis spreads contiguously in a slow, progressive manner. Tissue planes are ignored; with time, sinus tracts that can spontaneously close and reopen will form and extend to skin, adjacent organs, or bone.

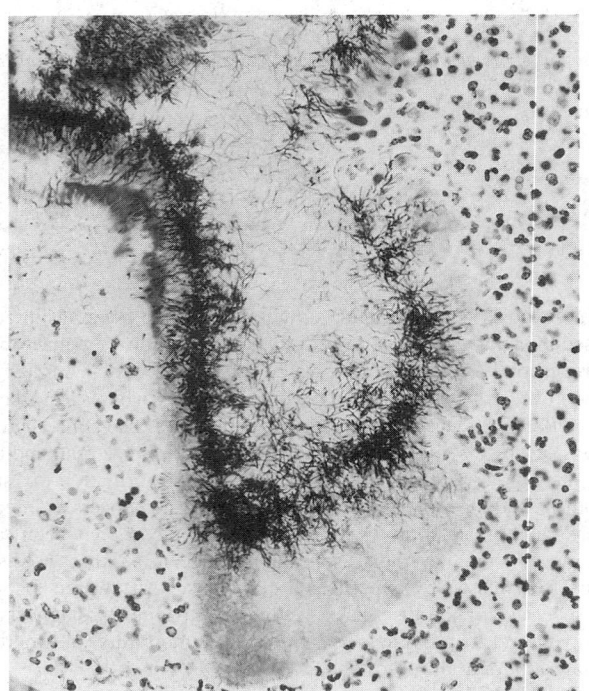

FIGURE 168-1   Actinomycotic sulfur granule surrounded by inflammatory cells. The delicate branched filaments of *Actinomyces* are surrounded by the proteinaceous eosinophilic coating of the granule (Slendore-Hoeppli phenomenon).

An association of pelvic actinomycosis with use of an intrauterine contraceptive device (IUD) suggests that this foreign body contributes to pathogenesis. In addition, an increasing number of reports have described an association of actinomycosis with infection due to human immunodeficiency virus (HIV). Ulcerative mucosal infections (caused, for example, by herpes simplex virus or cytomegalovirus) and abnormalities in host defenses may facilitate the development of actinomycosis in the latter setting.

CLINICAL MANIFESTATIONS   Oral-Cervicofacial Disease   Actinomycosis occurs most frequently at an oral, cervical, or facial site, usually as a soft tissue swelling, abscess, or mass lesion that is often mistaken for a neoplasm. The angle of the jaw is generally involved, but a diagnosis of actinomycosis should be considered with any mass lesion or relapsing infection in the head and neck. Otitis, sinusitis, and canaliculitis can also develop. Pain, fever, and leukocytosis are variably reported. Contiguous extension to the cranium, cervical spine, or thorax is a potential sequela.

Thoracic Disease   Thoracic actinomycosis usually follows an indolent, progressive course, with involvement of the pulmonary parenchyma and/or the pleural space. Chest pain, fever, and weight loss are common. A cough, when present, is variably productive. The usual radiographic appearance is either a mass lesion or pneumonitis. Cavitary disease or hilar adenopathy may develop. More than 50 percent of cases include pleural thickening, effusion, or empyema. Rarely, pulmonary nodules or endobronchial lesions occur. Pulmonary lesions suggestive of actinomycosis may cross fissures or pleura; may involve the mediastinum, contiguous bone, or chest wall; or may be associated with a sinus tract. In the absence of these findings, thoracic actinomycosis is usually mistaken for a neoplasm or for pneumonitis due to more usual causes (see Chap. 255).

Mediastinal infection is uncommon, usually arising from thoracic extension but rarely resulting from perforation of the esophagus, from trauma, or from head-and-neck or abdominal disease. The structures in the mediastinum and the heart can be involved in various combinations; consequently, the possible presentations are diverse. Isolated disease of the breast has been described.

Abdominal Disease   Abdominal actinomycosis poses a great diagnostic challenge. Months or years usually pass from the inciting event (e.g., appendicitis, diverticulitis, peptic ulcer disease, foreign-body perforation, or bowel surgery) to the clinical recognition of disease. Because of the flow of peritoneal fluid and/or the direct extension of primary disease, virtually any abdominal organ, region, or space can be involved. The disease usually presents as an abscess or a mass lesion that is often fixed to underlying tissue and mistaken for a tumor. Infiltrative disease with irregular contrast enhancement may be seen on computed tomography. Sinus tracts to the abdominal wall or perianal region may develop. Recurrent disease or a wound or fistula that fails to heal (in the absence of inflammatory bowel disease) suggests actinomycosis.

Hepatic infection usually presents as single or multiple abscesses or masses. Isolated disease presumably develops via hematogenous seeding from cryptic foci. The imaging and percutaneous techniques that now are available have resulted in improved diagnosis and treatment.

All levels of the urogenital tract can be infected. Renal disease usually presents as pyelonephritis and/or renal and perinephric abscess. Bladder involvement, usually due to extension of pelvic disease, may result in ureteral obstruction or fistulas to bowel, skin, or uterus.

Pelvic Disease   Actinomycotic involvement of the pelvis occurs most commonly in association with an IUD. Although the risk has not yet been quantified, it appears to be small. The disease rarely develops unless the IUD has been in place for at least 2 years, but it can present months after the removal of the device. Symptoms are typically indolent, with fever, weight loss, abdominal pain, and abnormal vaginal bleeding or discharge being the most common. The earliest stage of disease—often endometritis—commonly progresses to limited pelvic masses or a tubo-ovarian abscess. Unfortunately, because diagnosis is often delayed, a "frozen pelvis" mimicking malignancy or endometriosis can develop by the time of recognition.

An unresolved issue is whether the isolation of *Actinomyces*-like organisms (ALOs) from cultures of screening cervical or endometrial specimens or the detection of ALOs by immunofluorescence is correlated with IUD-associated disease. Until more quantitative data become available, detection of ALOs or immunofluorescence-positive organisms in conjunction with symptoms that cannot be accounted for appears to warrant removal of the IUD and initiation of a 14-day course of empirical treatment for possible early pelvic actinomycosis. If such organisms are detected in the absence of symptoms, education of the patient and close follow-up are warranted, but removal of the IUD is not required.

Central Nervous System Disease   Actinomycosis of the central nervous system is rare. Single or multiple brain abscesses are most common, usually appearing on computed tomography as a ring-enhancing lesion with a thick wall that may be irregular or nodular.

Musculoskeletal Infection   Actinomycotic infection of the bone is usually due to adjacent soft-tissue infection but may be associated with trauma (e.g., fracture of the mandible) or hematogenous spread. Because of slow disease progression, new-bone formation and bone destruction are seen concomitantly. Infection of an extremity is uncommon and is usually a result of trauma. Skin, subcutaneous tissue, muscle, and bone (with periostitis or acute or chronic osteomyelitis) are involved alone or in various combinations.

Disseminated Disease   Hematogenous dissemination of disease from any location rarely results in multiple-organ involvement. The lungs and the liver are most commonly affected, with the presentation of multiple nodules mimicking disseminated malignancy. The clinical presentation may be surprisingly indolent given the extent of disease.

DIAGNOSIS   Actinomycotic sulfur granules consist of aggregated microorganisms; are usually yellow; can be oval, round, or U-shaped; and, if sought, can be identified macroscopically and/or microscopically in drainage from sinus tracts or other purulent material. Their detection makes the diagnosis of actinomycosis likely. Botryomycosis, mycetoma, and pseudoactinomycotic radiate granules need to be excluded. The isolation of an agent of actinomycosis from granules or from a sterile site confirms the diagnosis. Microbiologic identification is possible in only a minority of cases, often being precluded by prior antimicrobial therapy. Therefore, for optimal yield, the avoidance of even a single dose of antibiotics is mandatory. The microbiology laboratory should be alerted so that cultures are processed appropriately. Primary isolation usually requires 5 to 7 days but may take as long as 2 to 4 weeks. Immunofluorescence testing for *A. israelii*, *A. naeslundii*, and *P. propionicum* (available through the Centers for Disease Control and Prevention in Atlanta) has become a useful diagnostic alternative. Because these organisms are components of the normal oral and genital-tract flora, their identification in sputum, bronchial washings, and cervicovaginal secretions is of little significance in the absence of sulfur granules. *Actinomyces* can be detected in urine by means of appropriate staining and culture.

℞ **TREATMENT**

Actinomycosis must be treated with high doses of antimicrobials for a prolonged period. Although therapy needs to be individualized, the intravenous administration of 18 to 24 million units of penicillin for 2 to 6 weeks, followed by oral therapy with penicillin or amoxicillin for 6 to 12 months, is a reasonable guideline for serious infections. Less extensive disease, particularly that involving the oral-cervicofacial region, may require less intensive therapy. If therapy is extended beyond the point of resolution of measurable disease, the risk of relapse—one of the clinical hallmarks of this infection—will be minimized. For the treatment of penicillin-allergic patients, tetracycline has been used most extensively; erythromycin, minocycline, and clindamycin are other suitable alternatives. First-generation cephalosporins may be an option, depending on the nature of the penicillin allergy and the degree of infection. Of the newer antimicrobial agents, imipenem and ceftriaxone have been described as successful in anecdotal reports. Metronidazole and the aminoglycosides are unreliable. Although the role of "companion" microbes in actinomycosis is unclear, many of these isolates are pathogens in their

own right; therefore, an initial therapeutic regimen that covers these organisms is reasonable.

Combined medical-surgical therapy is still advocated by some authorities. Since antimicrobial therapy alone can cure extensive disease, it is unclear how often surgical intervention is actually necessary. Moreover, percutaneous drainage has become an additional option. If the patient's condition is stable and the response to therapy can be monitored, an attempt to cure the infection with medical therapy alone seems justified. However, when the patient is critically ill or disease is documented at a critical site (e.g., the central nervous system), a combined approach seems prudent.

BIBLIOGRAPHY

BENNHOFF D: Actinomycosis: Diagnostic and therapeutic considerations and a review of 32 cases. Laryngoscope 94:1198, 1984

CINTRON JR et al: Abdominal actinomycosis. Dis Colon Rectum 39:105, 1996

FIORINO AS: Intrauterine contraceptive device–associated actinomycotic abscess and *Actinomyces* detection on cervical smear. Obstet Gynecol 87:142, 1996

GOODMAN HM, CENTENO BA: Case records of the Massachusetts General Hospital, Case 10-1992. N Engl J Med 326:692, 1992

RUSSO TA: Actinomycosis, in *Principles and Practice of Infectious Diseases*, 4th ed, GL Mandell et al (eds). New York, Churchill Livingstone, 1995, p 2280

169   *Dennis L. Kasper*

INFECTIONS DUE TO MIXED ANAEROBIC ORGANISMS

DEFINITIONS   *Anaerobic* bacteria are organisms that require reduced oxygen tension for growth, failing to grow on the surface of solid media in 10% CO_2 in air. *Microaerophilic* bacteria can grow in 10% CO_2 in air or under anaerobic or aerobic conditions; however, these organisms grow best in the presence of only a small amount of atmospheric oxygen. *Facultative* bacteria can grow in the presence or absence of air. This chapter describes infections caused by nonsporulating anaerobic bacteria. In general, anaerobes associated with human infections are relatively aerotolerant. They can survive for as long as 72 h in the presence of oxygen, although generally they will not multiply in this environment. A far smaller number of pathogenic anaerobic bacteria (which are also part of the normal flora) die after brief contact with oxygen, even in low concentrations.

The nonsporulating anaerobic bacteria exist as components of the normal flora on the mucosal surfaces of humans and animals. The major reservoirs of these bacteria are the mouth, gastrointestinal tract, skin, and female genital tract. Among the constituents of the oral flora, anaerobes are the predominant commensal organisms, ranging in concentration from 10^9/mL in saliva to 10^{12}/mL in gingival scrapings. In the oral cavity, the ratio of anaerobic to aerobic bacteria ranges from 1:1 on the surface of a tooth to 1000:1 in the gingival crevice. Anaerobic bacteria are not found in appreciable numbers in the normal intestine until the distal ileum. In the colon, the proportion of anaerobes increases significantly, as does the overall bacterial count. For example, in the colon there are 10^{11} to 10^{12} organisms per gram of stool, with a ratio of anaerobes to aerobes of approximately 1000:1. In the female genital tract, there are approximately 10^9 organisms per milliliter of secretions, with a ratio of anaerobes to aerobes of approximately 10:1.

Hundreds of species of anaerobic bacteria have been identified as part of the normal flora of humans. Identification of as many as 500 different anaerobic species in fecal specimens reflects the diversity of the anaerobic flora. Despite the complex array of bacteria in the normal flora, relatively few species are isolated commonly from human infection.

Anaerobic infections occur when the harmonious relationship between the host and the bacteria is disrupted. Any site in the body is susceptible to infection with these indigenous organisms when a mucosal barrier or the skin is compromised by surgery, trauma, tumor, or ischemia or necrosis, which reduce local tissue redox potentials. Because the sites that are colonized by anaerobic bacteria contain many species of bacteria, disruption of anatomic barriers allows penetration of many organisms, resulting in mixed infections involving multiple species of anaerobes combined with facultative or microaerophilic organisms. Such mixed infections are seen in the head and neck (chronic sinusitis, chronic otitis media, Ludwig's angina, and periodontal abscesses). Brain abscesses and subdural empyema are the most frequent anaerobic infections of the central nervous system. Anaerobes are responsible for pleuropulmonary diseases such as aspiration pneumonia, necrotizing pneumonia, lung abscess, and empyema. These organisms also play an important role in various intraabdominal infections, such as peritonitis and intraabdominal and liver abscesses (see Chap. 127). They are isolated frequently in female genital tract infections, such as salpingitis, pelvic peritonitis, tuboovarian abscess, vulvovaginal abscess, septic abortion, and endometritis (see Chaps. 129 and 130). Anaerobic bacteria also are frequently found in infections of the skin, soft tissues, and bones and in bacteremia.

ETIOLOGY The major anaerobic gram-positive cocci that produce disease are *Peptostreptococcus* species. The major species involved in infections are *P. magnus*, *P. asaccharolyticus*, *P. anaerobius*, and *P. prevotii*. Clostridia are gram-positive rods that are isolated from wounds, abscesses, sites of abdominal infection, and blood; they are discussed in Chap. 148. The principal anaerobic gram-negative bacilli are the members of the *Bacteroides* "family," which includes the *Bacteroides fragilis* group, fusobacteria, *Prevotella*, and *Porphyromonas*.

The *B. fragilis* group contains the anaerobic pathogens most frequently isolated from clinical infections. Members of this group are part of the normal bowel flora; they include several distinct species, such as *B. fragilis*, *B. thetaiotaomicron*, *B. distasonis*, *B. vulgatus*, *B. uniformis*, and *B. ovatus*. Of this group, *B. fragilis* is the most important clinical isolate. However, *B. fragilis* is isolated from the normal fecal flora at a lower frequency than other *Bacteroides* species.

A second major group of phenotypically similar organisms is part of the indigenous oral flora. These are primarily pigment-producing bacteria that were previously classified under the species *Bacteroides melaninogenicus*, now known as *Prevotella melaninogenica*. The nomenclature of this group has changed so that several distinct species are recognized, including *Porphyromonas gingivalis*, *Porphyromonas asaccharolytica*, and *P. melaninogenica*. The asaccharolytic pigmented *Porphyromonas* species seldom cause systemic infections in humans.

In female genital tract infections, *Prevotella bivia* and *Prevotella disiens* are the most frequent isolates, although *B. fragilis* is not uncommon. Fusobacteria are also isolated from clinical infections, including necrotizing pneumonia and abscesses. *Bilophila wadsworthia* is an anaerobic, gram-negative organism that is frequently resistant to several antimicrobials, including imipenem, cefoxitin, and other beta-lactam agents. This organism has been reported to cause serious infections, including bacteremia, necrotizing fasciitis, and abscesses.

Infections caused by anaerobic bacteria most frequently are due to more than one organism. These infections may be due to one or several anaerobic species or to a combination of anaerobic organisms and aerobic bacteria acting synergistically.

Approach to the Patient

The physician must consider several points when approaching the patient with presumptive infection due to anaerobic bacteria. (1) Most of these organisms are harmless commensals; very few cause disease. (2) For these organisms to cause infection, they must spread beyond the normal mucosal barriers. (3) Conditions favoring the propagation of these bacteria, particularly a lowered oxidation-reduction potential, are necessary. These conditions exist at sites of trauma, tissue destruction, compromised vascular supply, and complication of preexisting infection that produces necrosis. (4) There is a complex array of infecting flora. For example, as many as 12 different types of organisms can be isolated from a suppurative site. (5) Anaerobic organisms tend to be found in abscess cavities or in necrotic tissue. The failure of an abscess to yield organisms on routine culture is a clue that the abscess is likely to contain anaerobic bacteria. Often smears of this "sterile pus" are found to be teeming with bacteria when Gram's stain is applied. Malodorous pus suggests anaerobic infection. Although some facultative organisms, such as *Staphylococcus aureus*, also are capable of causing abscesses, abscesses in organs or deeper body tissues should call to mind anaerobic infection. (6) Treatment need not be directed at all the organisms in the infectious site. However, some species (the best example being the *B. fragilis* group) require specific therapy. Many of these synergistic infections can be cured with antibiotics directed at some but not all of the organisms involved. Antibiotic therapy, combined with debridement and drainage, disrupts the interdependent relationship among the bacteria, and some species that are resistant to the antibiotic do not survive without the coinfecting organisms. (7) Manifestations of disseminated intravascular coagulation are unusual in patients with anaerobic infection.

EPIDEMIOLOGY Difficulties in the performance of appropriate cultures, contamination of cultures by aerobic bacteria or components of the normal flora, and the lack of readily available, reliable culture techniques have made it impossible to obtain accurate incidence or prevalence data. However, these infections are encountered frequently in hospitals with active surgical, trauma, and obstetric and gynecologic services. In some centers, anaerobic bacteria, particularly *B. fragilis*, account for approximately 8 to 10 percent of positive blood cultures.

PATHOGENESIS Anaerobic bacterial infections usually occur when an anatomic barrier becomes disrupted and constituents of the local flora enter a site that was previously sterile. The bacteria isolated from infected sites have survived changes in oxidation-reduction potential and exposure to host defenses. Because of the specific growth requirements of anaerobic organisms and their presence as commensals on mucosal surfaces, conditions must arise that allow these organisms to penetrate mucosal barriers and enter tissue with a lowered oxidation-reduction potential. Therefore, tissue ischemia, trauma, surgery, perforated viscus, shock, and aspiration provide environments conducive to the proliferation of anaerobes. Some highly fastidious anaerobes lack the enzyme superoxide dismutase, which in other organisms reduces toxic superoxide radicals and thereby lessens the potentially lethal effects of superoxide. In the case of a perforated viscus, hundreds of species of anaerobic bacteria are spilled into the peritoneal cavity, but many of these organisms are unable to survive because the highly vascularized tissue provides an adequate oxygen supply. The entry of oxygen into the environment results in the selection of aerotolerant organisms.

The ability of an organism to adhere to host tissues is important to the establishment of infection. Some oral species adhere to crevicular epithelium in the oral cavity. *P. melaninogenica* actually attaches to other microorganisms; *P. gingivalis* is a common isolate in periodontal disease. These organisms have fimbriae that facilitate attachment. Some unencapsulated *Bacteroides* strains appear to be piliated, a characteristic that may account for their ability to adhere.

The most extensively studied virulence factor of the nonsporulating anaerobes is the polysaccharide capsule of *B. fragilis*. This polysaccharide possesses distinct biologic properties, such as the ability (owing to a unique motif of charged sugars) to promote abscess formation in a rodent model of intraabdominal sepsis. Abscess induction is a T cell–dependent phenomenon. Immunization with the capsule confers protection against abscess induction following challenge with *B. fragilis* or other intestinal microorganisms capable of inducing abscesses. This protection is mediated by a T cell circuit that blocks the tissue response of abscess formation. Although some clinicians have viewed abscess formation as a protective host response that localizes and contains infecting bacteria, abscess formation in patients with sepsis often results in severe and chronic illness that requires surgical drainage in combination with antimicrobial therapy.

Anaerobic bacteria produce a number of exoproteins that are capable of enhancing the organisms' virulence. These enzymes include a heparinase elaborated by *B. fragilis* that may contribute to intravascular clotting and necessitate increased doses of heparin for patients receiving heparin therapy. Collagenase, produced by *P. gingivalis*, may enhance tissue destruction. Alteration of the secretory cytoskeleton of intestinal epithelial cells by an enterotoxin from *B. fragilis* has been described. Both *B. fragilis* and *P. melaninogenica* possess lipopolysaccharides (endotoxins) that lack the biologic potency characteristic of endotoxins associated with aerobic gram-negative bacteria. The biologic inactivity of the endotoxin may account for the lower frequency of disseminated intravascular coagulation and purpura in *Bacteroides* bacteremia than in facultative and aerobic gram-negative bacillary bacteremia.

CLINICAL MANIFESTATIONS   Anaerobic Infections of the Mouth, Head, and Neck (See Chap. 30)   Infections of the mouth can arise from either the supragingival or the subgingival dental plaque. Supragingival plaque formation begins with the adherence of gram-positive bacteria to the tooth surface. This form of plaque is influenced by salivary and dietary components, oral hygiene, and local host factors. Once the supragingival plaque is established, the acquisition of pathogenic bacteria and an increase in the amount of plaque are responsible for the ultimate development of gingivitis. Early bacteriologic changes in the supragingival plaque initiate an inflammatory response in the gingiva, including edema, swelling, and increase in gingival fluid, and cause the development of caries and endodontic (pulp) infections. In addition, these changes contribute to the subsequent pathogenic alteration in the subgingival plaque that arises from poor or inadequate oral hygiene.

Subgingival plaque is associated with periodontal disease and disseminated infection arising from the oral cavity. Bacteria that colonize the subgingival area are primarily anaerobic. The black-pigmented gram-negative anaerobic bacilli, principally *P. gingivalis* and *P. melaninogenica*, are the most important. Infections in this area are frequently mixed and involve both anaerobic and aerobic bacteria. After establishment of local infection either in root canals or in the periodontal area, infection may extend into the mandible, causing osteomyelitis; to the maxillary sinuses; or to local tissues in the submandibular or submental spaces, depending on which teeth are involved. Periodontitis also may result in spreading infection that can involve adjacent bone or soft tissues.

Gingivitis   Gingivitis may become a necrotizing infection (trench mouth, Vincent's stomatitis). The onset of disease is usually sudden and is associated with tender bleeding gums, foul breath, and a bad taste. The gingival mucosa, especially the papillae between the teeth, becomes ulcerated and may be covered by a gray exudate, which is removable with gentle pressure. Patients may become systemically ill, developing fever, cervical lymphadenopathy, and leukocytosis. Occasionally, ulcerative gingivitis can spread to the buccal mucosa, the teeth, and the mandible or maxilla, resulting in widespread destruction of bone and soft tissue. This infection is termed *acute necrotizing ulcerative mucositis* (cancrum oris, noma). It destroys tissue rapidly, causing the teeth to fall out and large areas of bone—or even the whole mandible—to be sloughed. A strong putrid odor is frequently detected, although the lesions are not painful. The gangrenous lesions eventually heal, leaving large disfiguring defects. This infection is seen most commonly following a debilitating illness or in severely malnourished children. It has been known to complicate leukemia or to develop in individuals with a genetic deficiency of catalase.

Acute necrotizing infections of the pharynx   These infections usually occur in association with ulcerative gingivitis. Symptoms include an extremely sore throat, foul breath, and a bad taste accompanied by fever and a sensation of choking. Examination of the pharynx demonstrates that the tonsillar pillars are swollen, red, ulcerated, and covered with a grayish membrane that peels easily. Lymphadenopathy and leukocytosis are common. The disease may last for only a few days or, if not treated, may persist for weeks. Lesions begin unilaterally but may spread to the other side of the pharynx or the larynx. Aspiration of the infected material by the patient can result in lung abscesses. Soft tissue infection of the oral-facial area may or may not be odontogenic. *Ludwig's angina*, a periodontal infection usually arising from the tissues surrounding the third molar, may produce submandibular cellulitis that results in marked local swelling of tissues, with pain, trismus, and superior and posterior displacement of the tongue. Submandibular swelling of the neck can impair swallowing and cause respiratory obstruction. In some cases, tracheotomy may be life-saving.

Fascial infections   These infections arise from the spread of organisms originating in the upper airways to potential spaces formed by the fascial planes of the head and neck. Perimandibular space infection most commonly involves the submandibular, peritonsillar, and parapharyngeal spaces. Peritonsillar abscesses occur in association with pharyngitis. Complicated dental infections spread to the submandibular and buccal spaces. Entry of organisms by either portal can result in parapharyngeal space infections. Although there are few well-documented reports on the microbiology of these syndromes, anaerobes from the oral flora have been implicated in many cases. *S. aureus* and *Streptococcus pyogenes* infections may arise from boils or impetigo, whereas anaerobes are associated with space infections either occurring spontaneously or arising from diseases of the mucous membranes or from dental manipulations.

Sinusitis and otitis   The role of anaerobic bacteria in acute sinusitis may be underestimated because of improper collection of specimens. In a study of chronic sinusitis, anaerobic bacteria were found in 52 percent of specimens collected during external frontoethmoidotomy or radical antrotomy. Anaerobic bacteria are much more easily implicated in chronic suppurative otitis media than in acute otitis media. Purulent exudate from chronically draining ears has been found to contain anaerobes, particularly *Bacteroides* species, in up to 50 percent of cases. *B. fragilis* has been isolated from up to 28 percent of patients with chronic otitis media.

Complications of anaerobic head and neck infections   Contiguous craniad spread of these infections may result in osteomyelitis of the skull or mandible or in intracranial infections such as brain abscess and subdural empyema. Caudad spread can produce mediastinitis or pleuropulmonary infection. Hematogenous complications also may result from anaerobic infections of the head and neck. Bacteremia, which occasionally is polymicrobial, can lead to endocarditis or other distant infections. When infections spread to produce suppurative thrombophlebitis of the internal jugular vein, a destructive syndrome—with prolonged fever, bacteremia, septic emboli to both the lung and the brain, and multiple metastatic foci of suppurative infection—may develop. This syndrome has been reported with fusobacterial septicemia following exudative pharyngitis but is uncommon in this era of antimicrobial agents.

Central Nervous System Infections   Brain abscesses are frequently associated with anaerobic bacteria (see Chap. 377). If optimal bacteriologic techniques are employed, as many as 85 percent of brain abscesses yield anaerobic bacteria—most often anaerobic gram-positive cocci, which are followed in frequency by fusobacteria and *Bacteroides* species. Facultative or microaerophilic streptococci and coliforms often are part of a mixed infecting flora in brain abscesses.

Pleuropulmonary Infections   Anaerobic pleuropulmonary infections result from the aspiration of oropharyngeal contents, often in the context of an altered state of consciousness or an absent gag reflex. Four clinical syndromes are associated with anaerobic pleuropulmonary infection produced by aspiration: simple aspiration pneumonia, necrotizing pneumonia, lung abscess, and empyema.

Aspiration pneumonitis   Aspiration pneumonitis must be distinguished from two other clinical syndromes associated with aspiration that are not of bacterial etiology. One syndrome results from aspiration of solids, usually food. Obstruction of major airways typically results in atelectasis and moderate nonspecific inflammation. Therapy consists of removal of the foreign body.

The second aspiration syndrome is more easily confused with bacterial aspiration. This is the so-called Mendelson's syndrome, resulting from regurgitation of stomach contents and aspiration of chemical material, usually gastric juices. Pulmonary inflammation—including the destruction of the alveolar lining, with transudation of fluid into the alveolar space—occurs with remarkable rapidity. Typically this syndrome develops within hours, often following anesthesia when the gag reflex is depressed. The patient becomes tachypneic, hypoxic, and febrile. The leukocyte count may rise, and the chest x-ray may evolve suddenly from normal to a complete "whiteout" bilaterally within 8 to 24 h. Sputum production is minimal. The pulmonary signs and symptoms can resolve quickly with symptom-based therapy or can culminate in respiratory failure with the subsequent development of bacterial superinfection over a period of days. Antibiotic therapy is not indicated unless bacterial infection supervenes. The signs of bacterial infection include sputum production, persistent fever, leukocytosis, and clinical evidence of sepsis.

In contrast to these syndromes, bacterial aspiration pneumonia develops more slowly. It is seen in patients who are hospitalized and have a depressed gag reflex, impaired swallowing, or a tracheal or nasogastric tube; elderly patients; or those with transient impaired consciousness in the wake of seizures, cerebrovascular accidents, or alcoholic blackouts. Patients who enter the hospital with this syndrome typically have been ill for several days and generally complain of low-grade fever, malaise, and sputum production. Usually the history reveals a predisposition for aspiration, such as alcohol overdose or residence in a nursing home. Sputum characteristically is not malodorous unless the process has been going on for at least a week. A mixed bacterial flora with many polymorphonuclear leukocytes is evident on Gram's staining; cultures are reliable only if contamination with the normal oral flora is avoided—that is, by transtracheal aspiration. In general, this procedure is not indicated in the evaluation of these patients. The most commonly encountered anaerobes in these infections are pigmented and nonpigmented *Prevotella* spp., *Fusobacterium nucleatum*, *Peptostreptococcus* spp., and *Bacteroides* spp. Chest x-rays show consolidation in dependent pulmonary segments: in the basilar segments of the lower lobes if the patient has aspirated while upright or sitting and in either the posterior segment of the upper lobe (usually on the right side) or the superior segment of the lower lobe if the patient has aspirated while supine. The organisms isolated reflect the pharyngeal flora; *P. melaninogenica*, *Fusobacterium* species, and anaerobic cocci are the most frequent isolates. The patient who aspirates in the hospital also may have a mixed infection involving enteric gram-negative rods.

Necrotizing pneumonitis This form of anaerobic pneumonitis is characterized by numerous small abscesses that spread to involve several pulmonary segments. The process can be indolent or fulminating. This syndrome is less common than either aspiration pneumonia or lung abscess and includes features of both types of infection.

Anaerobic lung abscesses These abscesses result from subacute anaerobic pulmonary infection. The clinical syndrome typically involves a history of constitutional symptoms, including malaise, weight loss, fever, chills, and foul-smelling sputum, perhaps over a period of weeks (see Chap. 255). Patients who develop lung abscesses characteristically have dental infection and periodontitis, but lung abscesses in edentulous patients have been reported. Abscess cavities may be single or multiple and generally occur in dependent pulmonary segments. Anaerobic abscesses must be distinguished from those associated with tuberculosis, neoplasia, and other conditions. Oral anaerobes predominate, although *B. fragilis* is isolated in up to 10 percent of cases. *S. aureus* may be found as well.

For many years penicillin was considered the gold standard of therapy for lung abscesses. Recent clinical trials have shown that clindamycin therapy results in a better clinical outcome than penicillin,

presumably because clindamycin has a better spectrum of activity against oral anaerobes. Thus, a combination of penicillin and metronidazole or another antibiotic combination that treats both oral anaerobes and aerobes is likely to be as effective as clindamycin. Bronchoscopy is indicated only to rule out the presence of airway obstruction, but it should be delayed until the antimicrobial has begun to affect the disease process so that it does not spread the infection. Bronchoscopy has no role in enhancing drainage. Surgery is almost never indicated because of the danger of spilling the abscess contents into the lungs.

Empyema Empyema is a manifestation of long-standing anaerobic pulmonary infection. The clinical presentation, which includes the presence of foul-smelling sputum, resembles that of other anaerobic pulmonary infections. Patients may complain of pleuritic chest pain and marked chest-wall tenderness.

Empyema may be masked by overlying pneumonitis and should be considered especially in cases of persistent fever in a patient receiving antibiotic therapy. Diligent physical examination and the use of ultrasound to localize a loculated empyema are important diagnostic tools. The collection of a foul-smelling exudate by thoracentesis is typical. Cultures of infected pleural fluid yield an average of 3.5 anaerobes and 0.6 facultative or aerobic bacterial species. Drainage is required. Defervescence, a return to a feeling of well-being, and resolution of the process may require several months.

Extension from a subdiaphragmatic infection also may result in anaerobic empyema. Septic pulmonary emboli may originate from intraabdominal or female genital tract infections and can produce anaerobic pneumonia.

Intraabdominal Infections (See Chap. 127) Enterotoxigenic *B. fragilis* has been associated with watery diarrhea in a small number of young children and adults. In case-control studies of children with undiagnosed diarrheal disease, enterotoxigenic *B. fragilis* was isolated from as many as 20 percent of the children with diarrhea but from fewer than 5 percent of the control children. The role of this enterotoxin and of enterotoxigenic *B. fragilis* in diarrheal disease remains unclear.

Pelvic Infections The vagina of a healthy woman is one of the major reservoirs of anaerobic and aerobic bacteria. In the normal flora of the female genital tract, anaerobes outnumber aerobes by a ratio of approximately 10:1 and include anaerobic gram-positive cocci and *Bacteroides* species. Anaerobes are isolated from most patients with infections of the genital tract not caused by a sexually transmitted pathogen. The major anaerobic pathogens are *B. fragilis*, *P. bivia*, *P. disiens*, *P. melaninogenica*, anaerobic cocci, and clostridial species. Anaerobes frequently are encountered in tuboovarian abscess, septic abortion, pelvic abscess, endometritis, and postoperative wound infection, particularly following hysterectomy. Although these infections are frequently mixed, involving both anaerobes and coliforms, pure anaerobic infections without coliform or other facultative bacterial species occur more often in pelvic than in intraabdominal sites and are characterized by drainage of foul-smelling pus or blood from the uterus, generalized uterine or local pelvic tenderness, and continued fever and chills. Suppurative thrombophlebitis of the pelvic veins may complicate the infections and lead to repeated episodes of septic pulmonary emboli. Anaerobic bacteria have been thought to be contributing factors in the etiology of bacterial vaginosis. This syndrome is characterized by a profuse malodorous discharge and an increase in the number of bacteria in the vagina, including *Gardnerella vaginalis*, *Prevotella* spp., *Mobiluncus* spp., peptostreptococci, and genital mycoplasmas. Anaerobic bacteria are thought to play a role in the etiology of pelvic inflammatory disease (see Chap. 130), and several investigations have shown an association between bacterial vaginosis and the development of pelvic inflammatory disease.

Skin and Soft Tissue Infections Injury to skin, bone, or soft tissue by trauma, ischemia, or surgery creates a suitable environment for anaerobic infections. These infections are most frequently found in sites prone to contamination with feces or with upper airway secretions—for example, wounds associated with intestinal surgery, decubitus ulcers, or human bites. Anaerobic bacteria can be isolated in cases of crepitant cellulitis, synergistic cellulitis, or gangrene and necrotizing fasciitis. Moreover, these organisms have been isolated from cutaneous abscesses, rectal abscesses, and axillary sweat gland infections (hydradenitis suppurativa). Anaerobes frequently have been cultured from foot ulcers in diabetic patients.

These soft tissue or skin infections are usually polymicrobial. A mean of 4.8 bacterial species are isolated, with a roughly 3:2 ratio of anaerobes to aerobes. The most frequently isolated organisms include *Bacteroides* species, anaerobic streptococci, enterococci, clostridial species, and *Proteus* species. The presence of anaerobes in these types of infections is associated with a higher frequency of fever, foul-smelling lesions, or visible foot ulcer.

Anaerobic bacterial *synergistic gangrene* (Meleney's gangrene) is characterized by exquisite pain, redness, and swelling followed by induration. Erythema surrounds a central zone of necrosis. A granulating ulcer, which may heal, forms at the original center as necrosis and erythema extend outward. Symptoms are limited to pain; fever is not typical. These infections usually involve a combination of anaerobic cocci and *S. aureus;* the usual site of infection is an abdominal surgical wound or the area surrounding an ulcer on an extremity. Treatment includes surgical removal of necrotic tissue and antimicrobial therapy.

Necrotizing fasciitis This rapidly spreading destructive disease of the fascia is usually attributed to group A streptococci but can also be caused by anaerobic bacteria, including *Peptostreptococcus* and *Bacteroides* species. Similarly, myonecrosis can be associated with mixed anaerobic infection. Fournier's gangrene consists of cellulitis involving the scrotum, perineum, and anterior abdominal wall, with mixed anaerobic organisms spreading along deep external fascial planes and causing extensive loss of skin.

Bone and Joint Infections Although *actinomycosis* (see Chap. 168) accounts on a worldwide basis for most anaerobic infections in bone, organisms including anaerobic or microaerophilic cocci, *Bacteroides* species, *Fusobacterium* species, and *Clostridium* species can also be found. These infections frequently arise adjacent to soft tissue infections. Hematogenous seeding of bone is uncommon. Oral *Bacteroides* species are seen in infections involving the maxilla and mandible, whereas *Clostridium* species have been reported as anaerobic pathogens in cases of osteomyelitis of the long bones following fracture or trauma. Fusobacteria have been isolated in pure culture from sites of osteomyelitis adjacent to the perinasal sinuses. Anaerobic and microaerophilic cocci have been reported as significant pathogens in infections involving the skull or mastoid.

In cases of anaerobic septic arthritis, the most common isolates are *Fusobacterium* species. Most of the patients involved have uncontrolled peritonsillar infections progressing to septic cervical venous thrombophlebitis and resulting in hematogenous dissemination with a predilection for the joints. Antibiotic treatment of peritonsillar abscess has decreased the prevalence of dissemination to the joints; thus, since the beginning of the antibiotic era, the isolation of *Fusobacterium* species from joints has been less common. Unlike anaerobic osteomyelitis, anaerobic pyoarthritis in most cases is not polymicrobial and may be acquired hematogenously. Anaerobes are important pathogens in infections involving prosthetic joints; in these infections, the causative organisms (such as anaerobic gram-positive cocci and *Propionibacterium acnes*) are part of the normal skin flora.

In patients with osteomyelitis (see Chap. 132), the most reliable source of culture is a bone biopsy sample free of normal uninfected skin and subcutaneous tissue. If a mixed flora is isolated from a bone biopsy specimen, all isolates should be covered by the regimen selected for treatment. When an anaerobic isolate is recognized as a major or sole pathogen infecting a joint, the duration of treatment should be similar to that used for arthritis caused by aerobic bacteria. Therapy includes the management of underlying disease states, appropriate antimicrobial therapy, temporary joint immobilization, percutaneous drainage of effusions, and usually the removal of infected prostheses or internal fixation devices. Surgical drainage and debridement procedures such as sequestrectomy are essential for the removal of necrotic tissue that would sustain anaerobic infections.

Bacteremia Transient bacteremia is a well-known event in healthy people whose anatomic mucosal barriers have been injured (e.g., during dental extractions or dental scaling). These bacteremic episodes, which are often due to anaerobes, have no pathologic consequences. However, anaerobic bacteria are found in cultures of blood from clinically ill patients when proper culture techniques are used. *B. fragilis* is the single most common anaerobic isolate. In recent years, the rate of isolation of anaerobic bacteria from blood cultures has been decreasing. Studies from the 1970s and early 1980s found that 10 to 15 percent of positive blood cultures yielded anaerobes. More recently, similar surveys have found lower rates. The cause of this change is unknown but may be related to the administration of antibiotic prophylaxis before intestinal surgery, the earlier recognition of localized infections, and the empirical use of broad-spectrum antibiotics for presumed infection.

Once the organism has been identified, both the portal of bloodstream entry and the underlying problem that probably led to seeding of the bloodstream can often be deduced from an understanding of the organism's normal place of residence. For example, mixed anaerobic bacteremia including *B. fragilis* usually implies colonic pathology with mucosal disruption from neoplasia, diverticulitis, or some other inflammatory lesion. The initial manifestations are determined by the portal of entry and reflect the localized condition. When bloodstream invasion occurs, patients can become extremely ill, with rigors and hectic fevers ranging up to 40.6°C (105°F). The clinical picture may be quite similar to that seen in sepsis involving aerobic gram-negative bacilli. Although other complications of anaerobic bacteremia, such as septic thrombophlebitis and septic shock, have been reported, the incidence of these complications in association with anaerobic bacteremia is low. Anaerobic bacteremia is potentially fatal and requires rapid diagnosis and appropriate therapy. Mortality appears to increase with the age of the patient (with reported rates of more than 66 percent among patients over 60 years old), with the isolation of multiple species from the bloodstream, and with the failure to surgically remove a focus of infection.

Endocarditis (See Chap. 126) Endocarditis due to anaerobes is uncommon. However, anaerobic streptococci, which are often classified incorrectly, are responsible for this disease more frequently than is generally appreciated. Gram-negative anaerobes are unusual causes of endocarditis.

DIAGNOSIS Because of the time and difficulty involved in the isolation of anaerobic bacteria, diagnosis of these infections must frequently be based on presumptive evidence. Certain sites (such as avascular necrotic tissues) with lowered oxidation-reduction potential favor the diagnosis of an anaerobic infection. When infections occur in proximity to mucosal surfaces normally harboring an anaerobic flora, such as the gastrointestinal tract, female genital tract, or oropharynx, anaerobes should be considered as potential etiologic agents. A foul odor is often indicative of anaerobes, which produce certain organic acids as they proliferate in necrotic tissue. Although the presence of these odors is nearly pathognomonic for anaerobic infection, the absence of odor does not exclude these organisms as etiologic agents. Because anaerobes often coexist with other bacteria to cause mixed or synergistic infection, Gram's staining of exudate frequently reveals numerous pleomorphic cocci and bacilli suggestive of anaerobes. Sometimes these organisms will have morphologic characteristics associated with specific species.

The presence of gas in tissues is highly suggestive, but not diagnostic, of anaerobic infection. When cultures of obviously infected sites yield no growth, streptococci only, or a single aerobic species such as *Escherichia coli*, and Gram's staining reveals a mixed flora, the implication is that the anaerobic microorganisms failed to grow because of inadequate transport and/or culture techniques. Failure of a patient to respond to antibiotics that are not active against anaerobes—for example, aminoglycosides and in some circumstances penicillin, cephalosporins, or tetracyclines— suggests the possibility of anaerobic infection.

There are three critical steps in the diagnosis of anaerobic infection: (1) proper specimen collection; (2) rapid transport of the specimens to the microbiology laboratory, preferably in anaerobic transport media; and (3) proper handling of the specimens by the laboratory.

Specimens must be collected by meticulous sampling of infected sites and avoidance of contamination with the normal flora. When contamination of a specimen with the normal flora is likely, the specimen is unacceptable for processing by the bacteriology laboratory. Examples of specimens unacceptable for anaerobic culture include (1) sputum collected by expectoration or nasal tracheal suction, (2) bronchoscopy specimens, (3) samples collected directly through the vaginal vault, (4) urine collected by voiding, and (5) feces. Specimens that can be cultured for anaerobes include blood, pleural fluid, transtracheal aspirates, pus obtained by direct aspiration from an abscess cavity, fluid obtained by culdocentesis, suprapubic bladder aspirates, cerebrospinal fluid, and lung puncture specimens.

Because even brief exposure to oxygen may kill some anaerobic organisms and result in a failure to isolate them in the laboratory, air must be expelled from the syringe used to aspirate the abscess cavity, and the needle must be capped with a sterile rubber stopper. Proper precautions should be used in the handling of contaminated needles. Specimens can be injected into transport bottles containing a reduced medium or taken immediately in syringes to the laboratory for direct culture on anaerobic media. In general, swabs should not be used. If a swab must be used, it should be placed in a reduced semisolid carrying medium before transport to the laboratory. Delays in transport may lead to a failure to isolate anaerobes due to exposure to oxygen or overgrowth of facultative organisms, which may eliminate or obscure the anaerobes that are present. All clinical specimens from suspected anaerobic infections should be Gram-stained and examined for organisms with characteristic morphology. It is not unusual for organisms to be observed on Gram's staining but not isolated in culture. If purulent materials are found to be sterile or organisms are seen on Gram's staining but do not grow in the culture, the involvement of anaerobes should be suspected.

℞ TREATMENT

Successful therapy for anaerobic infections involves a combination of appropriate antibiotics, surgical resection, debridement of devitalized tissues, and drainage. Perforations must be closed promptly, closed spaces drained, tissue compartments decompressed, and an adequate blood supply established. Abscess cavities should be drained as soon as fluctuation or localization occurs. While surgery was formerly required to establish drainage, with the advent of computed tomography, magnetic resonance imaging, and ultrasound, diagnostic radiologists now are able to drain a number of abscess sites percutaneously.

Patients with infections due to anaerobic bacteria require treatment with appropriate antibiotics. Antibiotic susceptibility testing of anaerobic bacteria has been difficult and controversial. Owing to the slow growth rate of many anaerobes, the lack of standardized methodology, the lack of clinically related standards for resistance, and the generally good results obtained with empirical therapy, susceptibility testing has been recommended only for the study of resistance patterns in regional centers or local hospitals, for the prediction of the efficacy of new antibiotics, and for the management of selected patients. The selection of initial antibiotic therapy should be based on knowledge of the pathogens likely to be present in a specific clinical condition in combination with the Gram's stain findings, which should suggest the likelihood of certain species of organisms. In many infections, anaerobes tend to be mixed with coliforms and other facultative organisms. The best therapeutic regimens, therefore, are usually those with activity against both aerobic and anaerobic bacteria. The choice of empirical antibiotics for the anaerobes can nearly always be made reliably, since patterns of antimicrobial susceptibility are usually predictable (see Chap. 140 and Table 169-1).

Anaerobic gram-negative rods that are frequently resistant to penicillin are listed in Table 169-2. Organisms belonging to the *B. fragilis* group are essentially all resistant to penicillin. This clinically significant resistance mandates that anaerobic infections arising be-

Table 169-1

Antimicrobial Therapy for Infections Involving Commonly Encountered Anaerobic Gram-Negative Rods

Group 1 (<1% Resistance)	Group 2 (<15% Resistance)	Group 3 (Variable Resistance)	Group 4 (Resistance)
Metronidazole*	Clindamycin	Penicillin	Aminoglycosides
Ampicillin/sulbactam	Cefoxitin	Cephalosporins	Quinolones
Ticarcillin/clavulanic acid	High-dose	Tetracycline	Monobactams
Piperacillin/tazobactam	antipseudo-	Vancomycin	
Imipenem	monal peni-	Erythromycin	
Meropenem	cillins		
Chloramphenicol†			

* Usually needs to be given in combination with aerobic bacterial coverage. For infections originating below the diaphragm, aerobic gram-negative coverage is essential. For infections from an oral source, aerobic gram-positive coverage is added. Metronidazole also is not active against *Actinomyces* or *Propionibacterium* and is unreliable against peptostreptococci.
† Chloramphenicol is probably not as effective as other group 1 antimicrobials in treating anaerobic infections.

low the diaphragm be treated with specific therapy directed at *B. fragilis* (see Table 169-1). Recently, β-lactamase production has been reported in strains that are usually isolated from infections originating above the diaphragm. Forty to sixty percent of the clinical isolates classified as *Prevotella* or *Porphyromonas*, non–*B. fragilis* species of *Bacteroides*, or *Fusobacterium* species have been reported as producing β-lactamase. The clinical implications of this resistance have not been completely clarified. However, clindamycin does appear to be superior to penicillin for the treatment of lung abscesses. Although most oral anaerobic infections and cases of anaerobic pneumonia still respond to penicillin therapy, some infections due to oral organisms fail to respond, and in these cases the use of a drug that is effective against penicillin-resistant anaerobes is recommended (see Table 169-1). Life-threatening infections involving the anaerobic flora of the mouth, such as space infections of the head and neck, should be treated empirically as if penicillin-resistant anaerobes are involved. Less serious infections involving the oral microflora can be treated with penicillin alone; metronidazole can be added (or clindamycin can be substituted) if the patient responds poorly to therapy. If metronidazole is used in the treatment of mixed anaerobic and aerobic infections, it is imperative that other appropriate antibiotics be used in conjunction. Metronidazole is inactive against aerobic bacteria, *Actinomyces*, and *Propionibacterium*. The sensitivity of peptostreptococci to metronidazole is unpredictable. Therapy for intraabdominal sepsis (see Chap. 127) must include drugs active against the aerobic flora of the bowel. Combinations of antibiotics used in the treatment of mixed infections of oral origin must include antibiotics active against the aerobic flora of the mouth.

Table 169-2

Frequency of Penicillin Resistance among Commonly Encountered Anaerobic Gram-Negative Rods

Organism	Frequency of Penicillin Resistance*
Bacteroides fragilis	High
Bacteroides thetaiotaomicron	High
Bacteroides ovatus	High
Bacteroides distasonis	High
Bacteroides vulgatus	High
Bacteroides gracilis	High
Bilophila wadsworthia	High
Fusobacterium nucleatum	Low
Fusobacterium necrophorum	Low
Fusobacterium mortiferum	Low
Fusobacterium varium	Low
Prevotella species	Moderate
Porphyromonas species	Low

* High: >90 percent of strains; moderate: 5 to 90 percent of strains; low: <5 percent of strains.

Infections arising from a colonic source are likely to involve *B. fragilis*. Many therapeutic failures have been noted in patients with documented *B. fragilis* infection who are treated with penicillin or first-generation cephalosporins. In intraabdominal sepsis, the use of antibiotics effective against penicillin-resistant anaerobes has clearly reduced the incidence of postoperative infection and serious infectious complications. The number of antimicrobial agents effective against *B. fragilis* has expanded, and there are currently several useful choices (see Table 169-1). In general, cure rates of greater than 80 percent can be achieved in patients with *B. fragilis* infection by means of appropriate antimicrobial therapy and drainage.

Recommendations for the treatment of anaerobic infections with antibiotics are usually based on known resistance patterns in certain species and the likelihood of encountering a given species in the case at hand. Antibiotics active against the *B. fragilis* group, penicillin-resistant *Prevotella* and *Porphyromonas*, non–*B. fragilis* species of *Bacteroides*, and *Fusobacterium* species can be grouped into four categories on the basis of their predicted activity against anaerobes (see Table 169-1).

Resistance of *B. fragilis* to metronidazole has been reported rarely. This well-tolerated drug reaches significant levels in serum and also can be found at high levels in abscess cavities. It should be considered first-line therapy against *B. fragilis* infection. If a patient fails to respond to one of the group 1 or 2 drugs (Table 169-1), consideration should be given to alternative therapy and to determination of the resistance patterns among *B. fragilis* group isolates. Although in vitro resistance to chloramphenicol has not been reported, this drug may not be as effective as other group 1 drugs. Ampicillin/sulbactam, ticarcillin/clavulanic acid, piperacillin/tazobactam, imipenem, and meropenem have been effective in the treatment of *B. fragilis* infection. Ciprofloxacin and other currently available quinolones should not be used as primary agents against *B. fragilis*. Penicillin remains the drug of choice for use against peptostreptococci.

Specific regimens must be tailored to the initial infecting site in clinical situations. In the treatment of intraabdominal sepsis, a group 1 drug must be included for broad-spectrum coverage (see Chap. 127). If the involvement of gram-positive bacteria is suspected, an appropriate penicillin should be added. Chloramphenicol has been used successfully in patients with anaerobic central nervous system infections at a dose of 30 to 60 mg/kg per day, depending on the severity of illness. However, penicillin G and metronidazole also cross the blood-brain barrier and are bactericidal for many anaerobic organisms (see Chap. 377).

Nearly all the drugs mentioned have toxic side effects, which are described in detail in Chap. 140.

Anaerobic infections that have failed to respond to treatment or that have relapsed should be reassessed. Consideration should be given to additional surgical drainage or debridement. Superinfections with resistant gram-negative facultative or aerobic bacteria should be ruled out. The possibility of drug resistance also must be entertained; repeated cultures should yield the pathogenic organism.

Other supportive measures in the management of anaerobic infections include careful attention to fluid and electrolyte balance (since extensive local edema may lead to hypoalbuminemia); hemo-dynamic support for septic shock; immobilization of infected extremities; maintenance of adequate nutrition during chronic infections by parenteral hyperalimentation; relief of pain; and anticoagulation with heparin for thrombophlebitis. Hyperbaric oxygen therapy is advocated by some experts but is of no proven value.

BIBLIOGRAPHY

APPELBAUM PC et al: β-Lactamase production and susceptibilities to amoxicillin, amoxicillin-clavulanate, ticarcillin, ticarcillin-clavulanate, cefoxitin, imipenem, and metronidazole of 320 non–*Bacteroides fragilis Bacteroides* isolates and 129 fusobacteria from 28 U.S. centers. Antimicrob Agents Chemother 34:1546, 1990

BARTLETT JG: Infections caused by anaerobic bacteria, in *Infectious Diseases*, SL Gorbach et al (eds). Philadelphia, Saunders, 1992

————, FINEGOLD SM: Anaerobic infections of the lung and pleural space. Am Rev Respir Dis 110:56, 1974

CRABB JH et al: T-cell regulation of *Bacteroides fragilis*–induced intraabdominal abscesses. Rev Infect Dis 12:S178, 1990

DORSHER CW et al: Anaerobic bacteremia: Decreasing rate over a 15-year period. Rev Infect Dis 13:633, 1991

FINEGOLD SM: Anaerobic bacteria: General concepts, in *Principles and Practice of Infectious Diseases*, 4th ed, GL Mandell et al (eds). New York, Churchill Livingstone, 1995

————: Overview of clinically important anaerobes. Clin Infect Dis 20:S205, 1995

————, GEORGE WL: *Anaerobic Infections in Humans*. San Diego, Academic, 1989

GIBBS RS: Microbiology of the female genital tract. Am J Obstet Gynecol 156:491, 1987

HORN J et al: Role of anaerobic bacteria in perimandibular space infections. Ann Otol Rhinol Laryngol (Suppl) 154:34, 1991

LEVIN S, GOODMAN LJ: Selected overview of nongynecologic surgical intraabdominal infections: Prophylaxis and therapy. Am J Med 79:146, 1985

MATHISEN GE et al: Brain abscess and cerebritis. Rev Infect Dis 6:S101, 1984

NAKATA MN, LEWIS RP: Anaerobic bacteria in bone and joint infections. Rev Infect Dis 6:S165, 1984

NEWMAN MG: Anaerobic oral and dental infections. Rev Infect Dis 6:S107, 1984

NICHOLS RL: Surgical infections: Prevention and treatment—1965 to 1995. Am J Surg 172:68, 1996

ONDERDONK AB et al: Animal model system for studying virulence of and host response to *Bacteroides fragilis*. Rev Infect Dis 12:S169, 1990

PANTOSTI A et al: Immunochemical characterization of two surface polysaccharides of *Bacteroides fragilis*. Infect Immun 59(5):1690, 1991

SEARS CL et al: Enterotoxigenic *Bacteroides fragilis*. Clin Infect Dis 20:S142, 1995

SUMMANEN PH et al: *Bilophila wadsworthia* isolates from clinical specimens. Clin Infect Dis 20:S210, 1995

SWEET RL: Role of bacterial vaginosis in pelvic inflammatory disease. Clin Infect Dis 20:S271, 1995

THORNSBERRY C: Antimicrobial susceptibility testing of anaerobic bacteria: Review and update on the role of the National Committee for Clinical Laboratory Standards. Rev Infect Dis 12:S218, 1990

TZIANABOS AO et al: Structural features of polysaccharides that induce intraabdominal abscesses. Science 262:416, 1993

ZALEZNIK DF: Role of bacterial virulence factors in pathogenesis of anaerobic infections, in *Anaerobic Infections in Humans*, S Finegold (ed). Orlando, Academic, 1989

SECTION 8
MYCOBACTERIAL DISEASES

170 *Paul W. Wright, Richard J. Wallace, Jr.*

ANTIMYCOBACTERIAL AGENTS

The physician is greatly challenged to provide optimal therapy for mycobacterial illnesses because of the advent of AIDS, the increase in both drug-susceptible and multidrug-resistant tuberculosis, and the plethora of new antibiotics with antimycobacterial potential. This chapter reviews the agents used for the treatment of tuberculosis, leprosy (Hansen's disease), and diseases caused by pathogenic nontuberculous mycobacteria including *Mycobacterium avium-intracellulare* (MAI), *Mycobacterium kansasii*, the rapidly growing mycobacteria, and *Mycobacterium marinum*. The use of antimycobacterial agents in patients with renal or hepatic disease and in pregnant women is summarized in Table 170-1. The effects of major antimycobacterial agents on the levels, activity, and toxicity of other commonly used drugs are summarized in Table 170-2.

Table 170-1

Use of Antimycobacterial Agents in Patients with Renal or Hepatic Disease and in Pregnant Women

Agent	Severe Hepatic Disease	Renal Disease: Creatinine Clearance Rate		Pregnancy*
		>30 mL/min	≤30 mL/min	
Azithromycin	No change	No change	?Decrease dose	No evidence of risk (B)
Clarithromycin	No change	No change	Decrease dose	Risk cannot be ruled out (C)
Ethambutol	No change	No change	Decrease dose	Risk cannot be ruled out (?C)
Isoniazid	Avoid use or decrease dose	No change	Decrease dose	Risk cannot be ruled out (?C)
Pyrazinamide	Avoid use or decrease dose	No change	Decrease dose†	Risk cannot be ruled out (C)
Rifabutin	No change	No change	No change	No evidence of risk (B)
Rifampin	Avoid use or decrease dose	No change	No change	Risk cannot be ruled out (C)
Streptomycin	No change	Decrease dose	Decrease dose and frequency	Definite evidence of risk (D)

* Based on Food and Drug Administration pregnancy categories of A–D, X.
† Prudent but not absolutely necessary.

TUBERCULOSIS

Drugs used to treat tuberculosis are classified as first-line and second-line agents. *First-line essential* antituberculous agents are the most effective and are a necessary component of any short-course therapeutic regimen. The two drugs in this category are isoniazid and rifampin. *First-line supplemental* agents either can shorten chemotherapy (e.g., pyrazinamide) or are highly effective and infrequently toxic (ethambutol and streptomycin). *Second-line* antituberculous drugs are clinically much less effective than first-line agents and much more frequently elicit severe reactions. These drugs are rarely used in therapy and then only by caregivers experienced with their use. They include

para-aminosalicylic acid (PAS), ethionamide, cycloserine, kanamycin, amikacin, capreomycin, viomycin, and thiacetazone. *Newer* antitubercular drugs, which have not yet been placed in the above categories, include rifabutin and the quinolones, especially ciprofloxacin, ofloxacin, and sparfloxacin.

FIRST-LINE ESSENTIAL DRUGS Isoniazid

Perhaps the best antituberculous drug available, isoniazid should be included in all tuberculosis treatment regimens unless the organism is resistant. It is inexpensive, readily synthesized, available worldwide, very selective for mycobacteria, and well tolerated, with only 5 percent of patients exhibiting adverse effects.

Mechanism of action Isoniazid is the hydrazide of isonicotinic acid, a small water-soluble molecule that easily penetrates the cell. Its mechanism of action involves inhibition of mycolic acid cell-wall synthesis via oxygen-dependent pathways such as the catalase-peroxidase reaction. Isoniazid is bacteriostatic against resting bacilli and bactericidal against rapidly multiplying organisms, both extracellularly and intracellularly. The minimal inhibitory concentrations (MICs) of isoniazid for wild-type (untreated) strains of *Mycobacterium tuberculosis* are <0.1 μg/mL, while those for *M. kansasii* usually are 0.5 to 2.0 μg/mL. The MICs of this drug for other mycobacteria are much higher.

Pharmacology Both oral and intramuscular preparations of isoniazid are readily absorbed. A 300-mg oral dose generally produces peak serum levels of 3 to 5 μg/mL. Isoniazid diffuses well throughout the body and reaches therapeutic concentrations in serum, cerebrospinal fluid (CSF), and infected tissue, including caseous granulomas. Isoniazid is metabolized in the liver via acetylation and hydrolysis; its metabolites are excreted into the urine. The rate of acetylation is genetically controlled. The usual daily dose for the treatment of tuberculosis is 5 mg/kg for adults and 10 to 20 mg/kg for children, with a maximal daily dose of 300 mg for both groups. For intermittent therapy (usually directly observed), a maximal dose of 900 mg twice or three times weekly is used. Even in moderate or severe renal failure, the adult dose rarely needs to be reduced below 200 mg/d.

Adverse effects (Table 170-3) The two most important adverse effects of isoniazid therapy are hepatotoxicity and peripheral neuropathy. Other adverse reactions are either rare or less significant and include rash (2 percent), fever (1.2 percent), anemia, acne, arthritic symptoms, a systemic lupus erythematosus–like syndrome, optic atrophy, seizures, and psychiatric symptoms. Isoniazid-associated hepatitis is idiosyncratic and increases in incidence with age. It occurs in 0.3 percent of treated persons under 35 years of age, 1.2 percent of those under 49 years of age, and 2.3 percent of those over 50 years of age. The risk of isoniazid-associated hepatitis is increased by daily alcohol consumption,

Table 170-2

Effect of Major Antimycobacterial Agents on Levels/Activity/Toxicity of Other Commonly Used Drugs

Rifampin	Isoniazid	Clarithromycin	Rifabutin*	Agents with No/Minimal Drug Effects
Analgesics (↓)	Alcohol (↑ risk of hepatitis)	Astemizole (↑)	(↓ In same drugs as rifampin but to a lesser degree)	Amikacin
Anticonvulsants (↓)		Carbamazepine (↑)		Azithromycin
Barbiturates (↓)	Carbamazepine (↑)	Digoxin (↑)		Capreomycin
β blockers (↓)		Rifabutin (↑)		Ethambutol
Chloramphenicol (↓)	Diphenylhydantoin (↑)	Ritonavir (↑)		Streptomycin
Clarithromycin (↓)		Terfenadine (↑)		Pyrazinamide
Clofibrate (↓)	Enflurane (↑ risk of renal failure)	Zidovudine (↓)		
Cyclosporine (↓)	Warfarin (↑)			
Dapsone (↓)				
Diazepam (↓)				
Digoxin (↓)				
Disopyramide (↓)				
Glucocorticoids (↓)				
Halothane (↓)				
Indinavir (↓)				
Ketoconazole (↓)				
Mexiletine (↓)				
Narcotics (↓)				
Oral contraceptives (↓)				
Oral hypoglycemic agents (↓)				
Probenecid (↓)				
Progestins (↓)				
Quinidine (↓)				
Ritonavir (↓)				
Saquinavir (↓)				
Theophylline (↓)				
Verapamil (↓)				
Warfarin (↓)				
Zidovudine (↓)				

* Rifabutin induces the cytochrome P450 system but to a lesser degree than rifampin. All drugs whose half-life is decreased by rifampin induction of hepatic microsomal enzymes may be subject to the same effect when coadministered with rifabutin; however, this point has not yet been studied.

concomitant rifampin administration, and slow acetylation of isoniazid. Mortality from isoniazid-induced hepatitis has been reported to be 6 to 12 percent, but the real risk is certainly much lower: the reported rates were documented in high-risk patients who continued to take the drug despite progressive symptoms of hepatitis and without monitoring of liver enzyme levels. Liver enzymes are monitored in most settings among high-risk patients, and administration of the drug is discontinued at the onset of hepatitis. The American Thoracic Society recommends that serum concentrations of aspartate or alanine aminotransferase (AST or ALT) be determined at baseline in patients over 35 years of age who are receiving isoniazid for chemoprophylaxis, with monthly determinations thereafter. The benefit of such routine monitoring remains controversial, however. Measurement of the ALT or AST level is certainly mandatory whenever a patient notices the onset of symptoms suggestive of isoniazid-associated hepatitis (e.g., fever, anorexia, nausea, vomiting, and/or a flulike syndrome including fever and myalgias), and treatment should immediately be discontinued until the relationship between therapy and symptoms is ascertained. The American Thoracic Society also recommends that, even in the absence of these symptoms, discontinuation of isoniazid be strongly considered whenever an AST or ALT level exceeds 150 to 200 IU (three to five times the upper limit of normal) in a high-risk patient. When these guidelines are followed, death from isoniazid-associated hepatitis has occurred at a rate of only 14 per 100,000 treated patients. Twelve percent of patients who have initially normal liver function and take isoniazid may experience transient elevations of AST. If AST elevation persists, if AST is elevated to more than five times the normal level, or if symptoms of hepatitis develop, therapy must be discontinued. Several recent studies have demonstrated that many patients with isoniazid intolerance can be desensitized.

Peripheral neuritis associated with isoniazid develops at a dose-dependent rate of 2 to 20 percent and probably relates to interference with pyridoxine metabolism. This rate can be reduced to 0.2 percent with the prophylactic administration of 10 to 50 mg of pyridoxine (vitamin B$_6$) daily.

Resistance Isoniazid-resistant mutants of *M. tuberculosis* occur spontaneously at a rate of 1 in 10^5 to 10^6 organisms. The molecular sites of isoniazid resistance have recently been detailed. Almost all isoniazid-resistant strains have amino acid changes in the catalase-peroxidase gene (*katG*) or a two-gene locus known as *inhA*. Missense mutations or deletion of *katG* are also associated with reduced catalase and peroxidase activity. Primary isoniazid resistance is detected in 7 percent of untreated patients in native U.S. populations, but the percentage is much higher in many immigrant populations.

Rifampin Rifampin, a semisynthetic derivative of *Streptomyces mediterranei*, is the second most important antituberculous agent, exhibiting efficacy against *M. tuberculosis* comparable to that of isoniazid. It is also active against a wide spectrum of other organisms, including some gram-positive and gram-negative bacteria, *Legionella* species, *M. kansasii*, *M. marinum*, and some strains of MAI.

Pharmacology Rifampin is a fat-soluble complex macrocyclic antibiotic that is absorbed readily either orally or intravenously. Serum levels of 10 to 20 μg/mL follow a standard oral dose of 600 mg. Rifampin distributes well throughout most body tissues, including inflamed meninges. The fact that rifampin turns body fluids (urine, saliva, sputum, tears) to a red-orange color makes it simple and inexpensive to check on a patient's compliance with therapy. Rifampin is excreted primarily through the bile and the enterohepatic circulation, while 30 to 40 percent of a dose is excreted via the kidneys. The drug is administered either twice weekly or daily at a dose of 600 mg for adults (10 mg/kg) and 10 to 20 mg/kg for children.

Mechanism of action Rifampin has both intracellular and extracellular bactericidal activity. It blocks RNA synthesis by specifically binding and inhibiting DNA-dependent RNA polymerase. Susceptible strains of *M. tuberculosis* as well as *M. kansasii* and *M. marinum* are inhibited by ≤1 μg/mL.

Adverse effects (Table 170-3) Rifampin is generally well tolerated; the most common adverse event is gastrointestinal upset. Patients with chronic liver disease, especially those with alcoholism and those who are elderly, appear to be at unusually high risk for the most serious adverse reaction: hepatitis. Concomitant administration of rifampin increases the risk of isoniazid-associated hepatitis. Other adverse effects of rifampin include rash (0.8 percent), hemolytic anemia (<1 percent), thrombocytopenia, and immunosuppression of unknown clinical importance. Rifampin is a potent inducer of the hepatic microsomal enzymes and thereby decreases the half-life of a number of drugs, including digoxin, warfarin, prednisone, cyclosporine, methadone, oral contraceptives, clarithromycin, zidovudine, and quinidine (Table 170-2).

Resistance Resistance to rifampin results from spontaneous point mutations that alter the β subunit of the RNA polymerase (*rpoB*) gene. Recent studies have shown that 96 percent of rifampin-resistant strains have a missense mutation within a 91-bp central core region of the gene. Rifampin-resistant strains of *Mycobacterium leprae* have similar mutations that alter a single serine residue (Ser-425) in the same core region of the *rpoB* gene.

Rifabutin Rifabutin, a semisynthetic rifamycin spiropiperidyl derivative, shares many characteristics with rifampin, including activity against *M. tuberculosis*. Rifabutin is active against some strains of rifampin-resistant *M. tuberculosis* and is more active than rifampin against MAI and other nontuberculous mycobacteria. To date, rifabutin has been most useful in the prophylaxis of disseminated MAI infection and in the treatment of drug-resistant tuberculosis. Because it seems

Table 170-3

Monitoring Side Effects of Common Antituberculous Drugs

Drug	Side Effect	Management
Isoniazid	Hepatitis	Monitor AST/limit alcohol consumption/monitor for hepatitis symptoms/educate patient/stop drug at first symptoms of hepatitis (nausea, vomiting, anorexia, flulike syndrome)
	Peripheral neuritis	Administer vitamin B$_6$
	Optic neuritis	Administer vitamin B$_6$
	Seizures	Administer vitamin B$_6$
Rifampin	Rash	Observe patient
	Liver dysfunction	Monitor AST/limit alcohol consumption/monitor for hepatitis symptoms
	Flulike syndrome	Administer at least twice weekly/limit dose to 10 mg/kg (adults)
	Red-orange urine	Reassure patient
	Drug interactions	Consider monitoring drug levels when possible, especially with contraceptives, anticoagulants, and digoxin/avoid use with protease inhibitors
Pyrazinamide	Hepatitis	Monitor AST/limit dosage to 15–30 mg/kg/d
	Hyperuricemia	Monitor uric acid level only in cases of gout or renal failure
Ethambutol	Optic neuritis	Use lower dose (15 mg/kg/d) when possible/monitor visual acuity (eye chart) and red-green color vision (Ishihara Color Book) monthly and with any visual complaint/educate patient/stop drug at first change in vision
Streptomycin, amikacin, capreomycin	Ototoxicity, renal toxicity	Limit dose and duration of therapy as much as possible/avoid daily therapy in patients >50 years old/monitor BUN and serum creatinine levels and possibly conduct audiometry before and as needed during therapy/question patient regularly about tinnitus, dizziness, vertigo, and decreased hearing/measure serum drug levels if possible/educate patient/stop drug at first development of adverse effect

NOTE: AST, aspartate aminotransferase; BUN, blood urea nitrogen.

to show more antituberculous activity than rifampin in vitro and in animals, its possible advantages over rifampin are being evaluated. In a multinational trial with either rifampin (600 mg/d) or rifabutin (150 mg/d) in combination with isoniazid plus 2 months of pyrazinamide and ethambutol, rifampin and rifabutin were equally effective and well tolerated in the treatment of newly diagnosed pulmonary tuberculosis. Rifabutin may be preferable to rifampin in the treatment of individuals positive for human immunodeficiency virus (HIV) who are also taking a protease inhibitor.

Pharmacology The pharmacology of rifabutin is dramatically different from that of rifampin. Rifabutin is readily absorbed after a single oral dose of 300 mg and reaches peak serum levels (0.35 μg/mL) in 2 to 4 h. This lipophilic drug distributes best to tissue: tissue levels are 5 to 10 times higher than plasma levels. CSF concentrations are 30 to 70 percent of plasma levels in HIV-infected patients who have meningitis. The drug's slow clearance via hepatic metabolism and renal excretion results in a mean serum half-life of 45 h, which is much longer than the 3- to 5-h half-life of rifampin. Clarithromycin (but not azithromycin) and fluconazole appear to block the hepatic metabolism of rifabutin, with consequent increases in serum levels. When rifabutin is administered orally with food, its rate of absorption is slowed, but the extent of absorption is unchanged. Adjustment of dosage is usually unnecessary in elderly patients and in patients with reduced hepatic or renal function.

Mechanism of action In *Escherichia coli* and *Bacillus subtilis*, rifabutin inhibits DNA-dependent RNA polymerase in the same manner as rifampin. Its mode of action against mycobacteria is believed to be the same.

Adverse effects Most adverse effects of rifabutin are dose related and occur most frequently in patients receiving >300 mg/d. Discontinuation of therapy because of adverse reactions is reported in 16 percent of patients receiving rifabutin as opposed to 8 percent of those receiving a placebo. The most common symptoms are gastrointestinal; other reactions include rash, fever, headache, asthenia, chest pain, myalgia, and insomnia. Like those taking rifampin, most patients taking rifabutin have discolored (orange to tan) urine and other body fluids. Less common adverse reactions include a flulike syndrome, hepatitis, *Clostridium difficile*–associated diarrhea, and skin discoloration. After a rifabutin dose of 450 or 600 mg in combination with clarithromycin, anterior uveitis is reported in up to 40 percent of patients; also reported are hyperpigmentation and a polymyalgia/arthralgia syndrome, both of which are reversible when treatment is discontinued. Laboratory abnormalities include neutropenia, leukopenia, thrombocytopenia, and increased levels of liver enzymes.

Rifabutin induces the hepatic cytochrome P450 enzymes but does so much less strongly than rifampin. Drugs whose metabolism is enhanced by rifabutin include anticoagulants, quinidine, oral contraceptives, sulfonylureas, analgesics, dapsone, narcotics, glucocorticoids, clarithromycin, zidovudine, and cardiac glycosides.

Resistance Resistance to rifabutin occurs by the same mechanism as that to rifampin—i.e., spontaneous point mutations involving the *rpoB* gene. However, of the 14 mutant *rpoB* alleles that confer resistance to rifampin, only nine confer high-level resistance to rifabutin, while the remaining five result in only small changes in rifabutin MICs (all remain at ≤0.5 μg/mL). The MIC of rifabutin for susceptible strains of *M. tuberculosis* is low (<0.06 μg/mL), and the drug is considered clinically active against partially resistant strains that are inhibited by plasma levels of ≤0.5 μg/mL. Thus rifabutin inhibits about one-quarter of rifampin-resistant strains of *M. tuberculosis*.

FIRST-LINE SUPPLEMENTAL DRUGS Pyrazinamide
A derivative of nicotinic acid, pyrazinamide is an important bactericidal drug used in short-course therapy for tuberculosis.

Pharmacology Pyrazinamide is well absorbed after oral administration, with a plasma concentration of 45 μg/mL in 2 h and excellent distribution throughout the body. The drug is hydrolyzed in the liver into several metabolites, one of which, pyrazinoic acid, is considered

the active form. Pyrazinoic acid is then hydroxylated to 5-hydroxypyrazinoic acid, which is subsequently excreted by renal glomerular filtration.

Mechanism of action Pyrazinamide is similar to isoniazid in its narrow spectrum of antibacterial activity, which essentially includes only *M. tuberculosis*. At plasma levels of 12.5 μg/mL, the drug is bactericidal to slowly metabolizing organisms located within the acidic environment of the phagocyte or caseous granuloma (being active only at a pH of <6.0). The mode of action of pyrazinamide and the mechanism of resistance to pyrazinamide are unknown.

Adverse effects (Table 170-3) At the high dosages used in the past, hepatotoxicity was a prominent complication of pyrazinamide therapy. However, at the currently recommended daily dosage of 15 to 30 mg/kg, with a maximum of 2 g (which can be given in one dose), the frequency of hepatotoxicity is not higher than that for concomitant isoniazid and rifampin therapy. Hyperuricemia is a common adverse effect of pyrazinamide therapy that is probably reduced by concurrent rifampin therapy. Clinical gout is seen only rarely in patients receiving pyrazinamide. Polyarthralgias are encountered fairly commonly but are not related to hyperuricemia.

Ethambutol A derivative of ethylenediamine, ethambutol is a water-soluble compound that is active only against mycobacteria. Susceptible species include *M. tuberculosis*, *M. marinum*, *M. kansasii*, and MAI. Among first-line drugs, it is the least potent against *M. tuberculosis*. It is used most often with rifampin in the treatment of tuberculosis in patients who are unable to tolerate isoniazid or who are thought or known to be infected with isoniazid-resistant organisms.

Mechanism of action Ethambutol is bacteriostatic against rapidly growing mycobacteria. Neither the mechanism of action nor the mechanism of resistance has been elucidated for this drug.

Pharmacology After oral administration, 75 to 80 percent of a dose of ethambutol is absorbed from the gastrointestinal tract. Serum levels peak at 2 to 4 μg/mL 2 to 4 h after a dose of 15 mg/kg. The drug's distribution throughout the body is adequate except in the CSF, where it reaches only low levels. However, ethambutol can reach CSF levels up to 50 percent as high as peak plasma levels when administered at a dose of 25 mg/kg to a patient with inflamed meninges. Almost all of the dose is excreted by the kidneys within 24 h of ingestion, either unchanged or as metabolites. The usual daily adult dosage of ethambutol is 25 mg/kg (which may be given in one dose) for the first 2 months, with a subsequent reduction to 15 mg/kg. In cases where retreatment is necessary, the higher dose may be given for the duration. For intermittent therapy, the dosage is 50 mg/kg twice weekly or 30 mg/kg three times weekly. The dosage must be lowered for patients with renal insufficiency (a creatinine clearance rate of <25 mL/min) to prevent drug accumulation and toxicity.

Adverse effects (Table 170-3) Ethambutol is usually well tolerated. Retrobulbar optic neuritis is the most serious adverse effect; axial or central neuritis—the only form reported in patients taking daily doses of <30 mg/kg—involves the papillomacular bundle of fibers and results in reduced visual acuity, central scotoma, and loss of the ability to see green. Symptoms of ocular toxicity typically develop several months after the initiation of therapy, but rapid-onset optic neuritis has been reported. The risk of optic neuritis depends on the dose and duration of therapy: this reaction develops in 5 percent of patients receiving a daily dose of 25 mg/kg but in fewer than 1 percent of patients given a daily dose of 15 mg/kg. Patients should be tested monthly (and whenever there is a subjective visual change) for visual acuity and red-green color discrimination. Optic neuritis with associated visual loss is usually reversible, but recovery may take 6 months or longer.

Other adverse effects of ethambutol are infrequent. Hyperuricemia occurs but is usually asymptomatic. The drug is not recommended for young children, in whom visual complications are difficult to monitor.

Streptomycin An aminoglycoside isolated from *Streptomyces griseus*, streptomycin is available for intramuscular and intravenous administration only. In the United States, it is the least used first-line supplemental drug for tuberculosis because of its toxicity, the difficulty in obtaining adequate CSF levels, and the inconvenience of its parenteral administration. In developing countries, however, streptomycin is frequently used because of its low cost. The drug is active against untreated strains of *M. tuberculosis*, *M. kansasii*, and *M. marinum* and against some strains of MAI at readily achievable serum levels.

Pharmacology Serum levels of streptomycin peak at 25 to 40 μg/mL after a 1.0-g dose. Streptomycin is bactericidal for rapidly dividing extracellular mycobacteria but is ineffective in the acidic environment within the macrophage. It diffuses poorly into the meninges and reaches CSF levels in patients with meningitis that are only 20 percent of serum levels.

The usual adult dose of streptomycin is 0.5 to 1.0 g (10 to 15 mg/kg) daily or five times per week; the pediatric dose is 20 to 40 mg/kg per day, with a maximum of 1 g/d. Because streptomycin is eliminated almost exclusively by the kidneys, the dosage must be lowered and the frequency of administration reduced (to only two or three times per week) in most patients over 50 years of age and in any patient with renal impairment.

Mechanism of action Streptomycin inhibits protein synthesis by disruption of ribosomal function.

Adverse effects (Table 170-3) Adverse reactions to streptomycin therapy occur in 10 to 20 percent of patients. Ototoxicity and renal toxicity are the most common and the most serious. Renal toxicity, usually manifested as nonoliguric renal failure, is less common with streptomycin than with other commonly used aminoglycosides, such as gentamicin. Ototoxicity involves both hearing loss and vestibular dysfunction. The latter is more common and includes loss of balance, vertigo, and tinnitus. Patients receiving streptomycin must be monitored carefully for these adverse effects. Less serious effects include perioral paresthesias, eosinophilia, rash, and drug fever.

Resistance Spontaneous resistance to streptomycin occurs in 1 in 10^5 to 10^7 organisms. In two-thirds of streptomycin-resistant strains of *M. tuberculosis*, mutations have been identified in one of two targets: a 16S rRNA gene (*rrs*) and the gene encoding ribosomal protein S12 (*rpsL*). Both targets are believed to be involved in streptomycin ribosomal binding. No mutational change has been identified in the other one-third of resistant isolates. Strains of *M. tuberculosis* that are resistant to streptomycin are not cross-resistant to capreomycin or amikacin.

SECOND-LINE DRUGS Second-line antituberculous agents are used either for drug-resistant tuberculosis or when first-line supplemental drugs are not available. The more important second-line drugs are discussed below in the general (descending) order of usefulness.

Quinolones A surprisingly large number of fluorinated quinolones are being developed and studied as inhibitors of mycobacteria. Their mode of action presumably is the prevention of DNA synthesis through the inhibition of DNA gyrase. Ofloxacin and ciprofloxacin, the best-studied quinolones, are active against many mycobacteria, including *M. tuberculosis*, *M. marinum*, *M. kansasii*, and *Mycobacterium fortuitum*. These two drugs are well absorbed orally, reach high serum levels, and distribute well to body tissues and fluids. While not approved for antituberculous therapy in the United States, ofloxacin—used in combination with isoniazid and rifampin for the treatment of pulmonary tuberculosis—was shown to be as active and safe as ethambutol in initial trials. Adverse effects are relatively uncommon, occurring in 0.5 to 10 percent of cases, and consist mostly of benign reactions such as gastrointestinal intolerance, rashes, dizziness, and headache. However, more serious adverse effects are now being reported and include confusion, seizures, interstitial nephritis, skin vasculitis, and acute renal failure.

Mycobacterial resistance to the fluoroquinolones develops rapidly. Its molecular basis is complex; only some strains exhibit missense mutations in the A subunit (*gyrA* gene) of DNA gyrase. Fluoroquinolone-resistant tuberculosis is a source of growing concern: 22 such cases were reported recently from New York City. Antituberculous therapy with quinolones should be reserved for patients with multidrug resistance or those who are intolerant to first-line drugs.

Capreomycin Capreomycin, a complex cyclic polypeptide antibiotic derived from *Streptomyces capreolus*, is similar to streptomycin

in terms of dosing, mechanism of action, pharmacology, and toxicity. It is administered only by the intramuscular route in doses of 10 to 15 mg/kg daily or five times per week (maximum daily dose, 1 g), with peak blood levels of 20 to 40 μg/mL. After 2 to 4 months, the dosage should be reduced to 1 g two or three times a week. Cross-resistance to kanamycin and amikacin—but not to streptomycin—is common. After streptomycin, capreomycin is the injectable drug of choice for tuberculosis.

Amikacin and Kanamycin These well-known aminoglycosides are bactericidal to extracellular organisms. Kanamycin is rarely used because of its toxicity. Amikacin is active against *M. tuberculosis* and several of the nontuberculous species, including the rapidly growing mycobacteria, *Mycobacterium scrofulaceum*, *M. leprae*, and MAI. The usual adult dosage is 10 to 15 mg/kg intramuscularly or intravenously three to five times a week.

Para-Aminosalicylic Acid PAS, a calcium or sodium salt that inhibits the growth of *M. tuberculosis* by impairing folate synthesis, is rarely indicated for the treatment of tuberculosis because of its low level of antituberculous activity and its high gastrointestinal toxicity (manifesting as nausea, vomiting, and diarrhea). A recently approved PAS formulation, enteric-coated PAS granules (4 g every 8 h), may be better tolerated and results in higher therapeutic blood levels. PAS is well absorbed after oral administration but reaches only low concentrations in the CSF. The drug has a short half-life (1 h), and 80 percent of the dose is excreted in the urine.

Thiacetazone Also called amithiozone, thiacetazone is not available in the United States but—because it is inexpensive and readily available—is widely used in the developing world as a single-tablet combination with isoniazid to treat tuberculosis. The usual daily dosage is 150 mg. Thiacetazone is structurally related to isoniazid but is bacteriostatic and more toxic. The World Health Organization advises against the use of thiacetazone by HIV-infected patients because of an unacceptably high rate of severe adverse (gastrointestinal) and fatal (skin) reactions.

Viomycin A complex basic polypeptide antibiotic, viomycin has properties similar to those of capreomycin, amikacin, and kanamycin and must be administered by intramuscular injection. Ninety percent of strains of multidrug-resistant *M. tuberculosis* are inhibited by viomycin levels of 1 to 10 μg/mL. Toxic effects are more common and severe than with other polypeptide antibiotics. This drug is not available in the United States.

Ethionamide Like isoniazid and pyrazinamide, ethionamide is a derivative of isonicotinic acid. This agent is bacteriostatic against metabolizing *M. tuberculosis* and some nontuberculous mycobacteria. It is most useful in therapy for multidrug-resistant tuberculosis. However, its use is severely limited by its toxicity and frequent side effects, which include intense gastrointestinal intolerance (anorexia, vomiting, and dysgeusia), serious neurologic reactions, reversible hepatitis (5 percent of cases), hypersensitivity reactions, and hypothyroidism. Ethionamide is well absorbed orally and is widely distributed throughout the body at sites including the CSF.

Cycloserine Cycloserine (D-4-amino-3-isoxazolidinone) is produced by *Streptomyces orchidaceus* and is active against a broad spectrum of bacteria, including *M. tuberculosis*. Cycloserine is well absorbed after oral administration and is widely distributed throughout the body fluids, including the CSF. Serious side effects limit the use of this drug and include psychosis (with suicide in some cases), seizures, peripheral neuropathy, headaches, somnolence, and allergic reactions. Cycloserine should not be given to patients with epilepsy, active alcohol abuse, severe renal insufficiency, or a history of depression or psychosis.

Miscellaneous Drugs A number of other drugs are being evaluated for their antituberculous activity. This group includes amoxicillin/clavulanic acid, clofazimine, clarithromycin, and new rifamycins such as rifapentine and KRM-1648 (a newly synthesized benzoxazinorifamycin).

LEPROSY (HANSEN'S DISEASE)

Therapy for leprosy remains difficult, especially in developing countries, because of the long duration of therapy required, the high cost and low availability of most drugs, the frequency of adverse reactions to drugs, the acquisition of drug resistance, the difficulty of determining a disease end point or cure, and (given that *M. leprae* still cannot be grown in vitro) the difficulty of conducting susceptibility testing. While many drugs are active against *M. leprae*, efficacy in the treatment of leprosy has been established only for dapsone, rifampin, clofazimine, and ethionamide.

Dapsone Dapsone (4,4′-diaminodiphenylsulfone) inhibits bacterial folic acid synthesis. It is considered the drug of choice in most cases of Hansen's disease because of its ready availability, low cost, and low toxicity and the susceptibility of untreated strains of *M. leprae* to very low concentrations.

Pharmacology Dapsone is well absorbed orally and distributes well throughout the body. The usual daily dosage is 100 mg for adults and 0.9 to 1.4 mg/kg for children. Plasma concentrations peak within 1 to 3 h. The median half-life of elimination is 22 h. Dapsone is cleared by acetylation in the liver, with genetic variation similar to that documented for the acetylation of isoniazid. The drug is 70 percent bound to plasma protein. Usual daily doses produce serum concentrations of 10 to 15 μg/mL, which far exceed the MIC for *M. leprae* (0.01 to 0.001 μg/mL).

Adverse effects Hemolysis and methemoglobinemia are common untoward reactions to dapsone. Patients should be screened for glucose-6-phosphate dehydrogenase deficiency to prevent drug-induced hemolysis. However, most patients tolerate dapsone therapy well with adequate clinical and laboratory supervision. Other side effects include gastrointestinal intolerance, headache, pruritus, peripheral neuropathies, nephrotic syndrome, fever, and rash. In lepromatous and borderline lepromatous leprosy, erythema nodosum leprosum (ENL) may occur. This reaction may be difficult to distinguish from reactions of leprosy, including drug reactions and the infectious mononucleosis–like dapsone syndrome.

Rifampin The use of rifampin, the second most useful drug in leprosy therapy, is limited by its cost. This drug is markedly bactericidal against *M. leprae* and rapidly reduces the number of viable bacilli in the patient's tissues. It must be combined with other antileprosy drugs to prevent the development of resistance. For reasons of cost, the drug is given at a dose of 600 mg once a month (supervised) outside the United States, but it is given daily in the United States.

Clofazimine A phenazine iminoquinone dye, clofazimine is weakly bactericidal against *M. leprae*. It is useful in treating dapsone-resistant leprosy and may lessen the severity of ENL. Clofazimine's mode of action is not well understood, but the drug may inhibit DNA binding. It is absorbed orally and is distributed to the fatty tissues and the reticuloendothelial system. Its serum half-life is about 60 to 70 days; only a small proportion of the dose is excreted daily into the urine or bile. Bactericidal activity is very slow and is evident for about 50 days after administration. The usual adult dosage is 50 to 100 mg daily, 100 mg three times a week, or 300 mg/d for treatment of ENL. Untoward effects include skin discoloration and, less commonly, gastrointestinal intolerance. Recently, clofazimine was reported to be responsible for a case of cardiotoxicity induced via ventricular arrhythmia. Even though clofazimine-resistant disease has been reported only rarely when this agent is used alone, it should be used with other effective antibiotics. Clofazimine is active in vitro against some of the nontuberculous mycobacterial species, including MAI, *M. kansasii*, *Mycobacterium simiae*, and *Mycobacterium abscessus*.

Ethionamide While ethionamide (250 mg/d) has not been approved by the Food and Drug Administration for the treatment of leprosy, it is sometimes used in the United States in combination with rifampin (600 mg/d) to treat dapsone-resistant leprosy in patients who cannot accept the skin-depigmentation effect of clofazimine. Because

resistance to ethionamide develops quickly when the drug is used alone, it must be used with other effective agents. Patients should be monitored closely for hepatotoxicity when taking ethionamide (especially in combination with rifampin), and treatment should be discontinued if the patient's ALT levels exceed 2.5 times the normal value.

Prothionamide, a congener of ethionamide that is not available in the United States, has pharmacologic properties similar to those of ethionamide and is widely used throughout the world.

Other Agents A number of other drugs exhibit significant activity against *M. leprae*, but clinical experience with these agents is lacking. Thalidomide may be useful in suppressing ENL but acts as a tranquilizer and also is extremely teratogenic; it is available as an investigational drug in the United States (Gillis W. Long Hansen's Disease Center, Carville, LA). The newer macrolide antibiotics (particularly clarithromycin), minocycline (a long-acting tetracycline), and a number of the fluoroquinolones (including ofloxacin, sparfloxacin, and pefloxacin) have shown promising bactericidal activity against *M. leprae* in studies of mice and in early clinical trials. All of these newer leprosy drugs have low toxicity profiles, modes of action different from those of the established agents, and powerful bactericidal activity against *M. leprae*. However, their levels of bactericidal activity are still lower than that of rifampin.

NONTUBERCULOUS MYCOBACTERIA

Although less pathogenic than *M. tuberculosis*, the nontuberculous mycobacteria can cause pulmonary, skin, bone and joint, lymph node, and soft tissue infection as well as disseminated disease in immunocompromised hosts, including patients with AIDS. MAI and *M. kansasii* are the two most common causes of nontuberculous mycobacterial pulmonary infection. Up to 40 percent of AIDS patients develop disseminated disease with MAI.

Clarithromycin Clarithromycin (6-*O*-methylerythromycin) is a new macrolide that is similar to erythromycin in its mechanism of action. However, unlike erythromycin, it is well absorbed with or without meals and elicits little gastrointestinal intolerance at low doses. Clarithromycin distributes well into body tissues and fluids and is highly concentrated in macrophages. The drug is metabolized in the liver, and approximately 30 percent of a given dose is excreted in the urine. The dosage should be reduced if the creatinine clearance rate is ≤30 mL/min. Like erythromycin, clarithromycin binds with plasma proteins (65 to 70 percent) and can raise the levels of drugs such as theophylline and carbamazepine. As noted earlier, serum levels of clarithromycin are reduced by the concomitant administration of rifampin and to a lesser degree by that of rifabutin; clarithromycin treatment increases serum levels of rifabutin and some antihistamines (e.g., terfenadine), thus increasing their toxicity. Clarithromycin and (probably) azithromycin are the most active agents for the treatment of MAI infections; one of these drugs is considered an essential component of any regimens used for this purpose. However, because of mutational drug resistance, clarithromycin should be given in combination with other agents, such as ethambutol and rifampin or rifabutin. The drug is also highly active against almost all other nontuberculous mycobacteria, including *M. marinum*, *M. kansasii*, *M. haemophilum*, *M. genavense*, *M. xenopi*, *M. abscessus*, *M. chelonae*, and most isolates of *M. fortuitum*. Standard antimycobacterial doses have been 500 mg twice daily; doses of 1000 mg twice daily have been associated with increased mortality in patients with AIDS and disseminated MAI disease. The more common side effects of high doses include nausea, vomiting, a bitter taste, and (occasionally) abnormal liver-function tests. Most side effects can be minimized by reducing the dose, usually by 50 percent. Clarithromycin is teratogenic in laboratory animals and is in category C for use in pregnancy (Table 170-1). Mutational resistance occurs in one in 10^8 to 10^9 organisms and develops rapidly with monotherapy, especially that for disseminated MAI disease. Resistance results from point mutations involving A2058 or A2059 in the 23*S* ribosomal binding site.

Azithromycin Azithromycin is a macrolide that belongs to the family of azalides. It reaches much lower serum levels than clarithromycin (usually ≤0.5 μg/mL) but attains high tissue and macrophage concentrations and has a longer half-life that suggests the feasibility of intermittent therapy. Azithromycin appears to be as active as clarithromycin against MAI. It is involved in few drug interactions since it does not affect the cytochrome P450 system. No alteration in dose is required in renal failure. The usual dose is 250 to 500 mg/d. The most common side effects are gastrointestinal symptoms and reversible hearing loss. Resistance to azithromycin develops by the same mechanism as that to clarithromycin, with cross-resistance between the two macrolides.

THERAPY FOR SPECIFIC NONTUBERCULOUS MYCO-BACTERIA MAI First-line antituberculous drugs are much less active against MAI than against *M. tuberculosis.* Therapy for MAI is controversial because of the lack of controlled clinical trials. In 1990 the American Thoracic Society recommended the following four-drug regimen for MAI lung disease in HIV-negative patients: 18 to 24 months of isoniazid (300 mg), rifampin (600 mg), and ethambutol (25 mg/kg, then 15 mg/kg beginning in the third month), with intermittent streptomycin. However, two subsequent events—the demonstration of the dramatic activity of clarithromycin against both pulmonary and disseminated MAI infection and the introduction of rifabutin—have altered the therapeutic approach to MAI infection. Clarithromycin (500 mg twice daily) now replaces isoniazid, and rifabutin (300 mg/d) is often used in place of rifampin. Therapy for pulmonary disease is generally continued until cultures have been negative for 12 months.

For disseminated disease in AIDS, one of the newer macrolides (clarithromycin or azithromycin) plus ethambutol (15 mg/kg) are considered essential components of any treatment regimen, with rifabutin (300 mg) a commonly used third drug in patients not taking a protease inhibitor for their HIV infection. Other alternative drugs include ciprofloxacin, streptomycin, and amikacin. Clofazimine appears to increase mortality and should be avoided. For the prophylaxis of disseminated MAI disease, rifabutin (300 mg/d), clarithromycin (500 mg twice daily), and azithromycin (1200 mg once weekly) have all been demonstrated to be effective in controlled or comparative clinical trials.

Mycobacterium kansasii M. kansasii is usually sensitive to most antituberculous drugs except for pyrazinamide. Current recommendations for the treatment of *M. kansasii* pulmonary disease are 18 to 24 months of daily isoniazid (300 mg), rifampin (600 mg), and ethambutol (15 mg/kg). The potential advantages of the highly active rifabutin and the newer macrolides have not been studied.

Rapidly Growing Mycobacteria *M. fortuitum, M. abscessus,* and *M. chelonae* account for more than 80 percent of cases of clinical disease due to rapidly growing mycobacteria. These organisms are resistant to antituberculous agents other than amikacin but are variably susceptible to several other antibiotics. Clarithromycin has dramatically changed the approach to therapy for infection with these organisms, as it inhibits all rapidly growing mycobacteria—except for 20 percent of *M. fortuitum* strains and most *Mycobacterium smegmatis* strains—at concentrations of ≤4 μg/mL. Other drugs with good activity include amikacin (which inhibits 80 to 100 percent of strains), cefoxitin (80 percent of *M. abscessus* and *M. fortuitum* strains), doxycycline (50 percent of *M. fortuitum* strains), imipenem (100 percent of *M. fortuitum* strains, 70 percent of *M. chelonae* strains, and 70 percent of *M. abscessus* strains), the fluorinated quinolones ciprofloxacin and ofloxacin (100 percent of *M. fortuitum* strains), and sulfonamides (90 percent of *M. fortuitum* strains).

Mycobacterium marinum M. marinum, a photochromogen, is typically susceptible to minocycline, rifampin, ethambutol, clarithromycin, and trimethoprim-sulfamethoxazole and is resistant to isoniazid.

Mycobacterium haemophilum Infection due to *M. haemophilum* occurs most commonly as disseminated disease in immunocompromised patients with and without AIDS. This organism can cause bone and joint infection and skin infection. Isolates typically show in vitro resistance to most drugs but may be susceptible to rifampin, rifabutin, quinolones, and clarithromycin.

Mycobacterium xenopi In the United States, *M. xenopi* most often causes nosocomial infections; these infections most commonly occur in the environment of the hospital's hot-water system. In one study from Brooklyn, New York, *M. xenopi* was the second most common pathogenic nontuberculous mycobacterial species; of the 86 hospitalized patients from whom it was isolated, 41 percent were HIV-positive. Drug therapy for *M. xenopi* infection is difficult because in vitro sensitivity tests do not reliably predict clinical results. *M. xenopi* is often resistant to first-line antituberculous agents but susceptible to the newer macrolides, quinolones, streptomycin, and ethionamide.

Mycobacterium genavense M. genavense is a newly recognized organism that grows only in liquid media, such as Bactec 12B or 13A. This organism almost exclusively infects AIDS patients, causing disseminated disease and being isolated from blood, bone marrow, liver, lymph node, spleen, and intestinal cultures. The in vitro susceptibility profile of *M. genavense* has not been well established. Some isolates are susceptible to amikacin, clarithromycin, ofloxacin, rifampin, and rifabutin.

BIBLIOGRAPHY

AD HOC COMMITTEE OF THE SCIENTIFIC ASSEMBLY ON MICROBIOLOGY, TUBERCULOSIS, AND PULMONARY INFECTIONS: Treatment of tuberculosis and tuberculosis infection in adults and children. Am J Respir Crit Care Med 149:1359, 1994

Antimycobacterial drugs, in *Drug Evaluations Annual 1995.* Chicago, American Medical Association, pp 1685–1725

BOBROWITZ D: Ethambutol in tuberculous meningitis. Chest 61:629, 1972

BROGDEN RN, FITTON A: Rifabutin: A review of its antimicrobial activity, pharmacokinetic properties and therapeutic efficacy. Drugs 47:983, 1994

Clinical update: Impact of HIV protease inhibitors on the treatment of HIV-infected tuberculosis patients with rifampin. Morb Mort Week Rep 45:921, 1996

GELBER RH: Chemotherapy of lepromatous leprosy: Recent developments and prospects for the future. Eur J Clin Microbiol Infect Dis 13:942, 1994

GOBLE M et al: Treatment of 171 patients with pulmonary tuberculosis resistant to isoniazid and rifampin. N Engl J Med 328:527, 1993

GONZALES-MONTANER LJ: Rifabutin for the treatment of newly diagnosed pulmonary tuberculosis: A multinational, randomized, comparative study versus rifampicin. Tubercle Lung Dis 75:341, 1994

GRANGE JM et al: Clinically significant drug interactions with antituberculosis agents. Drug Saf 11:242, 1994

HAVLIR DV et al: Prophylaxis against disseminated *Mycobacterium avium* complex with weekly azithromycin, daily rifabutin, or both. N Engl J Med 335:392, 1996

KOPANOFF DE et al: Isoniazid-related hepatitis. Am Rev Respir Dis 117:991, 1978

LEIBOLD JE: The ocular toxicity of ethambutol and its relation to dose. Ann NY Acad Sci 135:904, 1966

MUSSER JM: Antimicrobial agent resistance in mycobacteria: Molecular genetic insights. Clin Microbiol Rev 8:496, 1995

NIGHTINGALE SD et al: Two controlled trials of rifabutin prophylaxis against *Mycobacterium avium* complex infection in AIDS. N Engl J Med 329:828, 1993

PIERCE M et al: A randomized trial of clarithromycin as prophylaxis against disseminated *Mycobacterium avium* complex infection in patients with advanced acquired immunodeficiency syndrome. N Engl J Med 335:384, 1996

REYNOLDS JEF (ed): *Martindale, the Extra Pharmacopoeia,* 30th ed. London, The Pharmaceutical Press, 1993

SHAFRAN SD et al: A comparison of two regimens for the treatment of *Mycobacterium avium* complex bacteremia in AIDS: Rifabutin, ethambutol, and clarithromycin versus rifampin, ethambutol, clofazimine, and ciprofloxacin. N Engl J Med 335:377, 1996

STARKE JR et al: Medical progress: Resurgence of tuberculosis in children. J Pediatr 120:839, 1992

UNDERLIED CB: Antimycobacterial agents: In vitro susceptibility testing, spectrums of activity, mechanism of action and resistance, and assays for activity in biological fluid, in *Antibiotics in Laboratory Medicine,* 3d ed, V Lorian (ed). Baltimore, Williams & Wilkins, 1991, pp 134–197

WOLINSKY E: Nontuberculous mycobacteria and associated diseases. Am Rev Respir Dis 119:107, 1979

171 *Mario C. Raviglione, Richard J. O'Brien*

TUBERCULOSIS

DEFINITION Tuberculosis is caused by bacteria belonging to the *Mycobacterium tuberculosis* complex. The disease usually affects the lungs, although in up to one-third of cases other organs are involved. If properly treated, tuberculosis caused by drug-susceptible strains is curable in virtually all cases. If untreated, the disease may be fatal within 5 years in more than half of cases. Transmission usually takes place through the airborne spread of droplet nuclei produced by patients with infectious pulmonary tuberculosis.

HISTORY That tuberculosis is one of the oldest diseases known to affect humanity has been proved by the finding of tuberculous spinal disease in Egyptian mummies. The Greeks called the disease *phthisis* ("consumption"), emphasizing the dramatic aspect of general wasting associated with chronic untreated cases. During the industrial revolution and the period of related urbanization in the seventeenth and eighteenth centuries, tuberculosis became a problem of epidemic proportions in Europe, causing at least 20 percent of all deaths in England and Wales in 1650. In the eastern part of the United States, the annual mortality rate from tuberculosis in the early nineteenth century was approximately 400 per 100,000 population.

The infectious etiology of tuberculosis was debated until Robert Koch's discovery of the tubercle bacillus in 1882. Improvement of socioeconomic conditions and isolation of infectious patients in sanatoria had a favorable impact on the epidemiology of tuberculosis in the first half of the twentieth century. In Europe and the United States, mortality rates began to decrease decades before the introduction of antimycobacterial drugs in the middle of the century.

ETIOLOGIC AGENT Mycobacteria belong to the family Mycobacteriaceae and the order Actinomycetales. Of the pathogenic species belonging to the *M. tuberculosis* complex, the most frequent and important agent of human disease is *M. tuberculosis* itself. Closely related organisms that also infect humans include *Mycobacterium bovis* (the bovine tubercle bacillus, once an important cause of tuberculosis transmitted by unpasteurized milk and currently the cause of a small percentage of cases in developing countries) and *Mycobacterium africanum* (isolated in a small proportion of cases in West and Central Africa). In addition, *M. tuberculosis* is related to various other human pathogens belonging to the genus *Mycobacterium*, such as the agent of leprosy (*Mycobacterium leprae*; see Chap. 172) and mycobacteria other than tuberculosis or nontuberculous mycobacteria (see Chap. 173); some of the latter organisms are becoming increasingly important opportunistic pathogens.

M. tuberculosis is a rod-shaped, non-spore-forming, thin aerobic bacterium measuring about 0.5 μm by 3 μm. Mycobacteria, including *M. tuberculosis*, do not stain readily and are often neutral on Gram's staining. However, once stained, the bacilli cannot be decolorized by acid alcohol, a characteristic justifying their classification as acid-fast bacilli (AFB). Acid fastness is due mainly to the organisms' high content of mycolic acids, long-chain cross-linked fatty acids, and other cell-wall lipids. Microorganisms other than mycobacteria that display some acid fastness include species of *Nocardia* and *Rhodococcus*, *Legionella micdadei*, and the protozoa *Isospora* and *Cryptosporidium*. In the mycobacterial cell wall, lipids (e.g., mycolic acids) are linked to underlying arabinogalactan and peptidoglycan. This structure is responsible for the very low permeability of the cell wall and thus for the ineffectiveness of most antibiotics against the organism. In addition, lipids such as acylated trehaloses, or "cord factors," may play a role in the virulence of *M. tuberculosis* by inducing cytokine-mediated events. Another molecule in the mycobacterial cell wall, lipoarabinomannan, is involved in the pathogen-host interaction and facilitates the survival of *M. tuberculosis* within macrophages. The several proteins characteristic of *M. tuberculosis* include those in purified protein derivative (PPD) tuberculin, a mixture of non-species-specific molecules in an extract from a culture filtrate.

EPIDEMIOLOGY Approximately 3.8 million new cases of tuberculosis (all forms, pulmonary and extrapulmonary), 90 percent of them from developing countries, were reported annually to the World Health Organization in the early 1990s. However, because of a low level of case detection and poor reporting in many national programs, reported cases represent only a fraction of the total. It is estimated that 8.8 million cases of tuberculosis occurred worldwide in 1995, 95 percent of them in developing countries of Asia (5.5 million), Africa (1.5 million), the Middle East (745,000), and Latin America (600,000). It is also estimated that nearly 3 million deaths from tuberculosis occurred in 1995, 98 percent of them in developing countries.

Beginning in the mid-1980s in many industrialized countries, the number of tuberculosis case notifications, which had been falling steadily, stabilized or even began to increase. This phenomenon was first noted in the United States but was soon observed in many European countries as well. In the United States in 1995, 22,813 cases of tuberculosis (8.7 cases per 100,000 population) were reported to the Centers for Disease Control and Prevention; this figure represented an increase of 2.8 percent over the lowest-ever number of cases reported (22,201 in 1985). A number of factors—most notably infection due to human immunodeficiency virus (HIV); immigration from countries with high prevalences of tuberculosis; and social problems such as poverty, homelessness, and drug abuse—have been implicated in the increasing rates of tuberculosis in this country. In some areas (e.g., New York City), deterioration in the public health system and dismantling of tuberculosis management services have also contributed to the worsening situation. In the United States, tuberculosis is uncommon among young adults of European descent, who have only rarely been exposed to *M. tuberculosis* infection during recent decades. In contrast, because of a high risk in the past, the prevalence of *M. tuberculosis* infection is relatively high among the elderly Caucasian population, who remain at increased risk of developing active tuberculosis. Tuberculosis in this nation is a disease of young adult members of the HIV-infected, immigrant, and disadvantaged/marginalized populations. Similarly, in Europe, tuberculosis has reemerged as an important public health problem, mainly as a result of cases among immigrants from high-prevalence countries.

In developing countries of Africa and Asia, tuberculosis trends over the past several decades are not entirely clear. However, in sub-Saharan African countries with reliable reporting systems, the recent spread of the HIV epidemic has been accompanied by doubling or tripling of the number of reported cases of tuberculosis during a period as short as 10 years. At the same time, the growing number of young adults with *M. tuberculosis* infection has fueled the rates of active tuberculosis in many developing countries. If the tuberculosis-control situation worldwide remains as it is now, 90 million new cases and 30 million deaths due to tuberculosis are expected during the 1990s.

From Exposure to Infection *M. tuberculosis* is most commonly transmitted from a patient with infectious pulmonary tuberculosis to other persons by droplet nuclei, which are aerosolized by coughing, sneezing, or speaking. The tiny droplets dry rapidly; the smallest (<5 to 10 μm in diameter) may remain suspended in the air for several hours and may gain direct access to the terminal air passages. There may be as many as 3000 infectious nuclei per cough. In the past, a frequent source of infection was raw milk containing *M. bovis* from tuberculous cows. Other routes of transmission of tubercle bacilli, such as through the skin or the placenta, are uncommon and of no epidemiologic significance.

The probability of contact with a source case of *M. tuberculosis* infection, the intimacy and duration of that contact, the degree of infectiousness of the case, and the environment of the contact are all important determinants of transmission. Several studies of close contacts have clearly demonstrated that tuberculosis patients whose sputum contains AFB visible by microscopy play the greatest role in the spread of infection. These patients have cavitary pulmonary disease or tuberculosis of the respiratory tract (endobronchial or laryngeal tuberculosis) and produce sputa containing as many as 10^5 AFB/mL. Patients with sputum smear–negative/culture-positive tuberculosis are much less infectious, and those with culture-negative pulmonary disease and extrapulmonary tuberculosis are essentially noninfectious. Crowding in poorly ventilated rooms is one of the most important factors in the transmission of tubercle bacilli, since it increases the intensity of contact with a case.

In short, the risk of acquiring *M. tuberculosis* infection is determined mainly by exogenous factors. Because of delays in seeking care and in diagnosis, an estimated two or three contacts will usually be infected by each AFB-positive case before detection.

From Infection to Disease Unlike the risk of acquiring infection with *M. tuberculosis*, the risk of developing disease after being infected depends largely on endogenous factors, such as the individual's innate susceptibility to disease and level of function of cell-mediated immunity. Clinical illness directly following infection is classified as *primary tuberculosis* and is common among children up to 4 years of age. Although this form is often severe and disseminated, it is usually not transmissible. When infection is acquired later in life, the chance is greater that the immune system will contain it, at least temporarily. The majority of infected individuals who will ultimately develop tuberculosis do so within the first year or two after infection. Dormant bacilli, however, may persist for years before being reactivated to produce *secondary tuberculosis*, which is often infectious. Overall, it is estimated that about 10 percent of infected persons will eventually develop active tuberculosis. *Reinfection* of a previously infected individual, which is probably common in areas with high rates of tuberculosis transmission, may also favor the development of disease. Restriction fragment length polymorphism (RFLP) is an analytical tool by which the results of standard epidemiologic investigations can be confirmed. RFLP yields a unique and stable strain-specific pattern of nucleic acid bands of variable sizes after digestion with restriction enzymes (a "fingerprint"). Analysis and comparison of fingerprints from various strains of *M. tuberculosis* have suggested that up to one-third of cases of active tuberculosis in U.S. inner-city communities are due to recent transmission rather than to reactivation of latent infection.

As implied above, age is an important determinant of the risk of disease after infection. Among infected persons, the incidence of tuberculosis is highest during late adolescence and early adulthood; the reasons are unclear. The incidence among women peaks at 25 to 34 years of age. In this age group rates among women are usually higher than those among men, while at older ages the opposite is true. The risk may increase in the elderly, possibly because of waning immunity.

A variety of diseases favor the development of active tuberculosis. The most potent risk factor for tuberculosis among infected individuals is clearly HIV coinfection, which suppresses cellular immunity. The risk that latent *M. tuberculosis* infection will proceed to active disease is directly related to the patient's degree of immunosuppression. In a recent study of HIV-infected, PPD-positive persons, this risk varied from 2.6 to 13.3 cases per 100 person-years and depended upon the CD4+ cell count. The risk of developing tuberculosis is several times higher among HIV-infected than among HIV-uninfected hosts. Other conditions known to increase the risk of active tuberculosis among persons infected with tubercle bacilli include silicosis; lymphoma, leukemia, and other malignant neoplasms; hemophilia; chronic renal failure and hemodialysis; insulin-dependent diabetes mellitus; immunosuppressive treatment; and conditions associated with malnutrition, such as gastrectomy and jejunoileal bypass surgery. Moreover, the presence of old, self-healed, fibrotic tuberculous lesions constitutes a serious risk of active disease.

NATURAL HISTORY OF DISEASE Studies conducted in various countries before the advent of chemotherapy clearly showed that untreated tuberculosis is often fatal. About one-third of patients died within 1 year after diagnosis and one-half within 5 years. Five-year mortality among sputum smear–positive cases was 65 percent. Of the survivors at 5 years, about 60 percent had undergone spontaneous remission, while the remainder were still excreting tubercle bacilli.

The introduction of effective chemotherapy has markedly affected the natural history of tuberculosis. With proper treatment, patients have a good chance of being cured. However, improper use of antituberculosis drugs, while reducing mortality, may also result in large numbers of chronic infectious cases, often with drug-resistant bacilli.

PATHOGENESIS AND IMMUNITY The interaction of *M. tuberculosis* with the human host begins when droplet nuclei containing microorganisms from infectious patients are inhaled. While the majority of inhaled bacilli are trapped in the upper airways and expelled by ciliated mucosal cells, a fraction (usually fewer than 10 percent) reach the alveoli. There, nonspecifically activated alveolar macrophages ingest the bacilli. The balance between the bactericidal activity of the macrophage and the virulence of the bacillus is probably linked to the bacterium's lipid-rich cell wall and to its glycolipid capsule, which confers resistance to complement and free radicals of the phagocyte. The number of invading bacilli is also important.

Several observations suggest that genetic factors also play a key role in innate nonimmune resistance to infection with *M. tuberculosis*. The existence of this resistance is suggested by the differing degrees of susceptibility to tuberculosis in different populations. In mice, an allele called *bcg* appears to be responsible for resistance to bacille Calmette-Guérin (BCG). The protein product of the *bcg* gene, designated Nramp (natural resistance–associated macrophage protein), seems to regulate resistance and susceptibility to *M. tuberculosis* infection through macrophages. The existence of a human homologue of Nramp remains to be investigated.

In the initial stage of host-bacterium interaction, either the hosts macrophages contain bacillary multiplication by producing proteolytic enzymes and cytokines or the bacilli begin to multiply. If the bacilli multiply, their growth quickly kills the macrophage, which lyses. Nonactivated monocytes attracted from the bloodstream to the site by various chemotactic factors ingest the bacilli released from the lysed macrophages. These initial stages of infection are usually asymptomatic.

Two to four weeks after infection, two additional host responses to *M. tuberculosis* develop: a tissue-damaging response and a macrophage-activating response. The *tissue-damaging response* is the result of a delayed-type hypersensitivity (DTH) reaction to various bacillary antigens; it destroys nonactivated macrophages that contain multiplying bacilli. The *macrophage-activating response* is a cell-mediated phenomenon resulting in the activation of macrophages that are capable of killing and digesting tubercle bacilli. Although both of these responses can inhibit mycobacterial growth, it is the balance between the two that determines the form of tuberculosis that will develop subsequently.

With the development of specific immunity and the accumulation of large numbers of activated macrophages at the site of the primary lesion, granulomatous lesions (*tubercles*) are formed. These lesions consist of lymphocytes and activated macrophages, such as epithelioid cells and giant cells. Initially, the newly developed tissue-damaging response is the only event capable of limiting mycobacterial growth within macrophages. This response, mediated by various bacterial products, not only destroys macrophages but also produces early solid necrosis in the center of the tubercle. Although *M. tuberculosis* can survive, its growth is inhibited within this necrotic environment by low oxygen tension, low pH, and other factors. At this point, some lesions may heal by fibrosis and calcification, while others undergo further evolution.

Cell-mediated immunity is critical at this early stage. In the majority of infected individuals, local macrophages are activated when bacillary antigens processed by macrophages stimulate T lymphocytes to release interferon γ (IFNγ) and other lymphokines. These activated cells aggregate around the lesion's center and effectively neutralize tubercle bacilli without causing further tissue destruction. In the central part of the lesion, the necrotic material assumes the aspect of soft cheese (caseous necrosis). Even when healing takes place, viable bacilli may remain dormant within macrophages or in the necrotic material for years or even throughout the patient's lifetime. These "healed" lesions in the lung parenchyma and hilar lymph nodes may later undergo calcification (*Ranke complex*).

In a minority of cases, the macrophage-activating response is weak, and mycobacterial growth can be inhibited only by intensified DTH reactions, which lead to tissue destruction. The lesion tends to enlarge further, and the surrounding tissue is progressively damaged. At the center of the lesion, the caseous material liquefies. Bronchial walls as well as blood vessels are invaded and destroyed, and cavities are formed. The liquefied caseous material, containing large numbers of bacilli, is drained through bronchi. Within the cavity walls, tubercle bacilli can now multiply well and can spread into the airways and the environment through expectorated sputum.

In the early stages of infection, bacilli are usually transported by macrophages to regional lymph nodes, from which they disseminate widely to many organs and tissues. The resulting lesions may undergo the same evolution as those in the lungs, although most tend to heal. In young children with poor natural immunity, hematogenous dissemination may result in fatal miliary tuberculosis or tuberculous meningitis.

Cell-mediated immunity confers partial protection against *M. tuberculosis*, while humoral immunity has no defined role in protection. Two types of cells are essential: macrophages, which directly phagocytize tubercle bacilli, and T lymphocytes, which induce protection through the production of lymphokines.

After infection with *M. tuberculosis*, alveolar macrophages secrete a number of cytokines: interleukin (IL) 1 contributes to fever; IL-6 contributes to hyperglobulinemia; and tumor necrosis factor α (TNFα) contributes to the killing of mycobacteria, the formation of granulomas, and a number of systemic effects, such as fever and weight loss. Macrophages are also critical in processing and presenting antigens to T lymphocytes; the result is a proliferation of CD4+ lymphocytes, which are crucial to the host's defense against *M. tuberculosis*. Qualitative and quantitative defects of CD4+ T cells explain the inability of HIV-infected individuals to contain mycobacterial proliferation. CD4+ lymphocytes are important producers of IFNγ, whose role in tuberculosis is probably to stimulate macrophages to produce TNFα and 1,25-dihydroxyvitamin D—both effective mycobacterial inhibitors. After stimulation with IFNγ and TNFα, macrophages may release nitric oxide, which is essential for their bactericidal activity. Among CD4+ cells, two subpopulations, Th1 and Th2 cells, produce different cytokines whose interplay may determine the host's response to mycobacteria. Gamma-delta cells also appear to participate in the host's response to infection.

M. tuberculosis possesses various protein antigens. Some are present in the cytoplasm and cell wall; others are secreted. That the latter are more important in eliciting a T lymphocyte response is suggested by experiments documenting the appearance of protective immunity in animals only after immunization with live, protein-secreting mycobacteria. Among the antigens with a potential protective role are the 30- and 32-kDa molecules of the BCG85 complex, which may mediate the adhesion and invasion of bacilli, and the 10-kDa antigen (BCG-a), which stimulates the proliferation of lymphocytes. The 65-kDa heat-shock protein, previously believed to be of importance in immunity, is now recognized as a weak antigen.

Coincident with the appearance of immunity, DTH to *M. tuberculosis* develops. This abnormal host reactivity is revealed by the PPD skin test, currently the only test that reliably detects *M. tuberculosis* infection in persons without symptoms. The cellular mechanisms responsible for PPD reactivity are related mainly to previously sensitized CD4+ lymphocytes, which are attracted to the skin-test site. There, they proliferate and produce cytokines.

In 1891, Robert Koch discovered components of *M. tuberculosis* in a concentrated liquid culture medium. Subsequently named "old tuberculin" (OT), this material was initially believed to be useful in the treatment of tuberculosis (although this idea was later disproved). It soon became clear that OT was capable of eliciting a skin reaction when injected subcutaneously into patients with tuberculosis. In 1932, Seibert and Munday purified this product by ammonium sulfate precipitation. The result was an active protein fraction known as tuberculin

purified protein derivative. However, the complexity and diversity of the constituents of PPD rendered its standardization difficult. PPD-S, developed by Seibert and Glenn in 1941, was chosen as the international standard. Later, the World Health Organization and UNICEF sponsored large-scale production of a master batch of PPD, termed *RT23*, and made it available for general use. The greatest limitation of PPD is its lack of mycobacterial species specificity, a property that is due to the large number of proteins in this product that are highly conserved in the various species of mycobacteria.

While DTH is associated with protective immunity (PPD-positive persons being less susceptible to a new *M. tuberculosis* infection than PPD-negative persons), it by no means guarantees protection against reactivation. In fact, severe cases of active tuberculosis are often accompanied by strongly positive skin-test reactions.

CLINICAL MANIFESTATIONS   Tuberculosis is usually classified as pulmonary or extrapulmonary. Before the recognition of HIV infection, more than 80 percent of all cases of tuberculosis were limited to the lungs. However, up to two-thirds of HIV-infected patients with tuberculosis may have both pulmonary and extrapulmonary disease or extrapulmonary disease alone.

Pulmonary Tuberculosis   Pulmonary tuberculosis can be categorized as primary or postprimary (secondary).

Primary disease   Primary pulmonary tuberculosis results from an initial infection with tubercle bacilli. In areas of high tuberculosis prevalence, this form of disease is often seen in children and is frequently localized to the middle and lower lung zones. The lesion forming after infection is usually peripheral and accompanied by hilar or paratracheal lymphadenopathy, which may not be detectable on chest radiography. In the majority of cases, the lesion heals spontaneously and may later be evident as a small calcified nodule (*Ghon lesion*).

In children with impaired immunity, such as those with malnutrition or HIV infection, primary pulmonary tuberculosis may progress rapidly to clinical illness. The initial lesion increases in size and can evolve in different ways. Pleural effusion, a frequent finding, results from the penetration of bacilli into the pleural space from an adjacent subpleural focus. In the majority of cases, the effusion resolves spontaneously, although tuberculous empyema may ensue in the presence of severe multibacillary pulmonary disease. In severe cases, the primary site rapidly enlarges, its central portion undergoes necrosis, and acute cavitation develops (progressive primary tuberculosis). Tuberculosis in young children is almost invariably accompanied by hilar or mediastinal lymphadenopathy due to the spread of bacilli from the lung parenchyma through lymphatic vessels. Enlarged lymph nodes may compress bronchi, causing obstruction and subsequent segmental or lobar collapse. Partial obstruction may cause obstructive emphysema, and bronchiectasis may also develop. Hematogenous dissemination, which is common and is often asymptomatic, may result in the most severe manifestations of primary *M. tuberculosis* infection. Bacilli reach the bloodstream from the pulmonary lesion or the lymph nodes and disseminate into various organs, where they may produce granulomatous lesions. Although healing frequently takes place, immunocompromised subjects (e.g., persons with HIV infection and those recovering from measles) may develop miliary tuberculosis and/or tuberculous meningitis.

Postprimary disease   Also called adult-type, reactivation, or secondary tuberculosis, postprimary disease results from endogenous reactivation of latent infection and is usually localized to the apical and posterior segments of the upper lobes, where the high oxygen concentration favors mycobacterial growth. In addition, the superior segments of the lower lobes are frequently involved. The extent of lung parenchymal involvement varies greatly, from small infiltrates to extensive cavitary disease. With cavity formation, liquefied necrotic contents ultimately are discharged into the airways, resulting in satellite lesions within the lungs that may in turn undergo cavitation. Massive involvement of pulmonary segments or lobes, with coalescence of lesions, produces tuberculous pneumonia. While up to one-third of untreated patients reportedly succumb to severe pulmonary tuberculosis within a few weeks or months after onset, others undergo a process of spontaneous remission or proceed along a chronic, progressively debilitating course ("consumption"). Under these circumstances, some pulmonary lesions become fibrotic and may later calcify, but cavities persist in other parts of the lungs. Individuals with such chronic disease continue to discharge tubercle bacilli into the environment. Most patients have a definite clinical response to treatment, with defervescence, decreasing cough, weight gain, and a general improvement in well-being within several weeks.

Early in the course of disease, symptoms and signs are often nonspecific and insidious, consisting mainly of fever and night sweats, weight loss, anorexia, general malaise, and weakness. However, in the majority of cases, cough eventually develops—perhaps initially non-productive and subsequently accompanied by the production of purulent sputum. Blood streaking of the sputum is frequently documented. Massive hemoptysis may ensue as a consequence of the erosion of a fully patent vessel located in the wall of a cavity. Hemoptysis, however, may also result from rupture of a dilated vessel in a cavity (Rasmussen's aneurysm) or from aspergilloma formation in an old cavity. Pleuritic chest pain sometimes develops in patients with subpleural parenchymal lesions but can also be the consequence of muscle strain due to persistent coughing. Extensive disease may produce dyspnea and (occasionally) adult respiratory distress syndrome (ARDS).

Physical findings are of limited use in pulmonary tuberculosis. Many patients have no abnormalities detectable by chest examination, while others have detectable rales in the involved areas during inspiration, especially after coughing. Occasionally, rhonchi due to partial bronchial obstruction and classical amphoric breath sounds in areas with large cavities may be heard. Systemic features include fever (often low-grade and intermittent) and wasting. In some cases, pallor and finger clubbing develop. The most common hematologic findings are mild anemia and leukocytosis. Hyponatremia due to the syndrome of inappropriate secretion of antidiuretic hormone (SIADH) has also been found.

Extrapulmonary Tuberculosis   In order of frequency, the extra-pulmonary sites most commonly involved in tuberculosis are the lymph nodes, pleura, genitourinary tract, bones and joints, meninges, and peritoneum. However, virtually all organ systems may be affected. As a result of hematogenous dissemination in HIV-infected individuals, extrapulmonary tuberculosis is seen more commonly today than in the past.

Pleural tuberculosis   Involvement of the pleura is common in primary tuberculosis and results from penetration by a few tubercle bacilli into the pleural space. Depending on the extent of reactivity, the effusion may be small, remain unnoticed, and resolve spontaneously or may be sufficiently large to cause symptoms such as fever, pleuritic chest pain, and dyspnea. Physical findings are those of pleural effusion: dullness to percussion and absence of breath sounds. A chest radiograph reveals the effusion and, in no more than one-third of cases, also shows a parenchymal lesion. Thoracentesis is required to ascertain the nature of the effusion. The fluid is straw colored and at times hemorrhagic; it is an exudate with a protein concentration more than 50 percent of that in serum, a normal to low glucose concentration, a pH that is generally <7.2, and detectable white blood cells (usually 500 to 2500/μL). Neutrophils may predominate in the early stage, while mononuclear cells are the typical finding later. Mesothelial cells are generally rare or absent. AFB are very rarely seen on direct smear, but cultures may be positive for *M. tuberculosis* in up to one-third of cases. Needle biopsy of the pleura is often required for diagnosis and reveals granulomas and/or yields a positive culture in up to 70 percent of cases. This form of pleural tuberculosis responds well to chemotherapy and may resolve spontaneously.

Tuberculous empyema is a less common complication of pulmonary tuberculosis. It is usually the result of the rupture of a cavity, with delivery of a large number of organisms into the pleural space, or of a bronchopleural fistula from a pulmonary lesion. A chest radiograph may show pyopneumothorax with an air-fluid level. The effusion is purulent and thick and contains large numbers of lymphocytes. An acid-fast smear of pleural fluid is often found to be positive when examined by microscopy, as is culture of the pleural fluid. Surgical drainage is usually required as an adjunct to chemotherapy. Tuberculous empyema may result in severe pleural fibrosis and restrictive lung disease.

Tuberculosis of the upper airways   Nearly always a complication of advanced cavitary pulmonary tuberculosis, tuberculosis of the upper airways may involve the larynx, pharynx, and epiglottis. Symptoms include hoarseness and dysphagia in addition to chronic productive cough. Findings depend on the site of involvement, and ulcerations may be seen on laryngoscopy. Acid-fast smear of the sputum is often positive, but biopsy may be necessary in some cases to establish the diagnosis. Cancer may have similar features but is usually painless.

Lymph-node tuberculosis (tuberculous lymphadenitis)   One of the commonest presentations of extrapulmonary tuberculosis (being documented in more than 25 percent of cases), lymph-node disease is particularly frequent among HIV-infected patients. In the United States, children and women (particularly non-Caucasians) also seem to be especially susceptible. Lymph-node tuberculosis presents as painless swelling of the lymph nodes, most commonly at cervical and supraclavicular sites. Lymph nodes are usually discrete in early disease but may be inflamed and have a fistulous tract draining caseous material. Systemic symptoms are usually limited to HIV-infected patients, and concomitant lung disease may or may not be present. The diagnosis is established by fine-needle aspiration or surgical biopsy. AFB are seen in up to 50 percent of cases, cultures are positive in 70 to 80 percent, and histologic examination shows granulomatous lesions. Among HIV-infected patients, granulomas usually are not seen. Differential diagnosis includes a variety of infectious conditions as well as neoplastic diseases such as lymphomas or metastatic carcinomas (see Chap. 61).

Pericardial tuberculosis (tuberculous pericarditis)   Due to direct progression of a primary focus within the pericardium, to reactivation of a latent focus, or to rupture of an adjacent lymph node, pericardial tuberculosis has often been a disease of the elderly in countries with low tuberculosis prevalence but develops frequently in HIV-infected patients. The onset may be subacute, although an acute presentation, with fever, dull retrosternal pain, and a friction rub, is possible. An effusion eventually develops in many cases; cardiovascular symptoms and signs of cardiac tamponade may ultimately appear (see Chap. 240). The effusion, detectable on chest radiography, is exudative in nature, with a high count of leukocytes (predominantly mononuclear cells). Hemorrhagic effusion is frequent. Culture of the fluid reveals *M. tuberculosis* in about 30 percent of cases, while biopsy has a higher yield. Without treatment, pericardial tuberculosis is usually fatal. Even with treatment, complications may develop, including chronic constrictive pericarditis with thickening of the pericardium, fibrosis, and sometimes calcification, which may be visible on a chest radiograph. A short course of glucocorticoids may prevent constriction.

Genitourinary tuberculosis   Genitourinary tuberculosis accounts for about 15 percent of all extrapulmonary cases, may involve any portion of the genitourinary tract, and is usually due to hematogenous seeding following primary infection. Local symptoms predominate. Urinary frequency, dysuria, hematuria, and flank pain are common presentations. However, patients may be asymptomatic and the disease discovered only after severe destructive lesions of the kidneys have developed. Urinalysis gives abnormal results in 90 percent of cases, revealing pyuria and hematuria. The documentation of culture-negative pyuria in acidic urine raises the suspicion of tuberculosis. An intravenous pyelogram helps in diagnosis. Culture of three morning urine specimens yields a definitive diagnosis in nearly 90 percent of cases.

Genital tuberculosis is diagnosed more commonly in females than in males. In females, it affects the fallopian tubes and the endometrium and may cause infertility, pelvic pain, and menstrual abnormalities. Diagnosis requires biopsy or culture of specimens obtained by dilatation and curettage. In males, tuberculosis preferentially affects the epididymis, producing a slightly tender mass that may drain externally through a fistulous tract; orchitis and prostatitis may also develop. In almost half of cases of genitourinary tuberculosis, urinary tract disease is also present. Genitourinary tuberculosis responds well to chemotherapy.

Skeletal tuberculosis   In early series of cases of extrapulmonary tuberculosis, disease of the bones and joints was responsible for 8 to

9 percent of cases. Today, rates are lower since skeletal tuberculosis is only infrequently described among HIV-infected patients. In bone and joint disease, pathogenesis is related to reactivation of hematogenous foci or to spread from adjacent paravertebral lymph nodes. Weight-bearing joints (spine, hips, and knees—in that order) are affected most commonly. Spinal tuberculosis (Pott's disease or tuberculous spondylitis) often involves two or more adjacent vertebral bodies. While the upper thoracic spine is the most common site of spinal tuberculosis in children, the lower thoracic and upper lumbar vertebrae are usually affected in adults. From the anterior superior or inferior angle of the vertebral body, the lesion reaches the adjacent body, also destroying the intervertebral disk. With advanced disease, collapse of vertebral bodies results in kyphosis (*gibbus*). A paravertebral "cold" abscess may also form. In the upper spine, this abscess may track to the chest wall as a mass; in the lower spine, it may reach the inguinal ligaments or present as a psoas abscess. Computed tomography (CT) or magnetic resonance imaging (MRI) reveals the characteristic lesion and suggests its etiology, although the differential diagnosis includes other infections and tumors. Aspiration of the abscess or bone biopsy confirms the tuberculous etiology, as cultures are usually positive and histologic findings highly typical. A catastrophic complication of Pott's disease is paraplegia, which is usually due to an abscess or a lesion compressing the spinal cord. Paraparesis due to a large abscess is a medical emergency and requires abscess drainage. Tuberculosis of the hip joints causes pain and limping; tuberculosis of the knee produces pain and swelling and sometimes follows trauma. If the disease goes unrecognized, the joints may be destroyed. Skeletal tuberculosis responds to chemotherapy, but severe cases may require surgery.

Gastrointestinal tuberculosis Any portion of the gastrointestinal tract may be affected by tuberculosis. Various pathogenetic mechanisms are involved: swallowing of sputum with direct seeding, hematogenous spread, or (rarely) ingestion of milk from cows affected by bovine tuberculosis. The terminal ileum and the cecum are the sites most commonly involved. Abdominal pain, at times similar to that associated with appendicitis, diarrhea, obstruction, hematochezia, and a palpable mass in the abdomen, are common findings at presentation. Fever, weight loss, and night sweats are also frequent. With intestinal-wall involvement, ulcerations and fistulae may simulate Crohn's disease. Anal fistulae should prompt an evaluation for rectal tuberculosis. As surgery is required in most cases, the diagnosis can be established by histologic examination and culture of specimens obtained intraoperatively.

Tuberculous peritonitis follows either the direct spread of tubercle bacilli from ruptured lymph nodes and intraabdominal organs or hematogenous seeding. Nonspecific abdominal pain, fever, and ascites should raise the suspicion of tuberculous peritonitis. The coexistence of cirrhosis (see Chap. 298) in patients with tuberculous peritonitis complicates the diagnosis. In tuberculous peritonitis, paracentesis reveals an exudative fluid with a high protein content and leukocytosis that is usually lymphocytic (although neutrophils occasionally predominate). The yield of direct smear and culture is relatively low; culture of a large volume of ascitic fluid can increase the yield, but peritoneal biopsy is often needed to establish the diagnosis.

Miliary or disseminated tuberculosis Miliary tuberculosis is due to hematogenous spread of tubercle bacilli. While in children it is often the consequence of a recent primary infection, in adults it may be due to either recent infection or reactivation of old disseminated foci. Lesions are usually yellowish granulomas 1 to 2 mm in diameter that resemble millet seeds (thus the term *miliary*, coined by nineteenth-century pathologists).

Clinical manifestations are nonspecific and protean, depending on the predominant site of involvement. Fever, night sweats, anorexia, weakness, and weight loss are presenting symptoms in the majority of cases. At times, patients have a cough and other respiratory symptoms due to pulmonary involvement as well as abdominal symptoms. Physical findings include hepatomegaly, splenomegaly, and lymphadenopathy. Eye examination may reveal choroidal tubercles, which are pathognomonic of miliary tuberculosis, in up to 30 percent of cases. Meningismus occurs in fewer than 10 percent of cases.

A high index of suspicion is required for the diagnosis of miliary tuberculosis. Frequently, chest radiography reveals a miliary reticulonodular pattern (more easily seen on underpenetrated film), although no radiographic abnormality may be evident early in the course and among HIV-infected patients. Other radiologic findings include large infiltrates, interstitial infiltrates (especially in HIV-infected patients), and pleural effusion. A sputum smear is negative in 80 percent of cases. Anemia with leukopenia or leukocytosis with neutrophilia may be documented, and disseminated intravascular coagulation has been reported. Elevation of alkaline phosphatase levels and other abnormal values in liver function tests are detected in patients with severe hepatic involvement. The PPD test may be negative in up to half of cases, but reactivity may be restored during chemotherapy. Bronchoalveolar lavage and transbronchial biopsy are more likely to permit bacteriologic confirmation, and granulomas are evident in liver or bone-marrow biopsy specimens from many patients. If it goes unrecognized, miliary tuberculosis is lethal; with proper treatment, however, it is amenable to cure.

A rare presentation seen in the elderly is *cryptic miliary tuberculosis*, which has a chronic course characterized by mild intermittent fever, anemia, and—ultimately—meningeal involvement preceding death. An acute septicemic form, *nonreactive miliary tuberculosis*, occurs very rarely and is due to massive hematogenous dissemination of tubercle bacilli. Pancytopenia is common in this form of disease, which is rapidly fatal. At postmortem examination, multiple necrotic but nongranulomatous ("nonreactive") lesions are detected.

Tuberculous meningitis and tuberculoma Tuberculosis of the central nervous system accounts for about 5 percent of extrapulmonary cases. It is seen most often in young children but also develops in adults, especially those who are infected with HIV. Tuberculous meningitis results from the hematogenous spread of primary or postprimary pulmonary disease or from the rupture of a subependymal tubercle into the subarachnoid space. In more than half of cases, evidence of old pulmonary lesions or a miliary pattern is found on chest radiography. The disease may present subtly as headache and mental changes or acutely as confusion, lethargy, altered sensorium, and neck rigidity. Typically, the disease evolves over 1 or 2 weeks—a course longer than that of bacterial meningitis. Paresis of cranial nerves (ocular nerves in particular) is a frequent finding, and the involvement of cerebral arteries may produce focal ischemia. Hydrocephalus is common. Lumbar puncture is the cornerstone of diagnosis. In general, examination of the cerebrospinal fluid (CSF) reveals a high leukocyte count (usually with a predominance of lymphocytes but often with a predominance of neutrophils in the early stage), a protein content of 1 to 8 g/L (100 to 800 mg/dL), and a low glucose concentration; however, any of these three parameters can be within the normal range. AFB are seen on direct smear of CSF sediment in only 20 percent of cases, but repeated lumbar punctures increase the yield. Culture of CSF is diagnostic in up to 80 percent of cases. Imaging studies (CT and MRI) may show hydrocephalus and abnormal enhancement of basal cisterns or ependyma. If unrecognized, tuberculous meningitis is uniformly fatal. This disease responds to chemotherapy; however, neurologic sequelae are documented in 25 percent of treated cases, in most of which the diagnosis has been delayed. Glucocorticoids are a useful adjunct to chemotherapy, especially in cases with cerebral edema or high CSF protein levels.

Tuberculoma, an uncommon manifestation of tuberculosis, presents as one or more space-occupying lesions and usually causes seizures and focal signs. CT or MRI reveals contrast-enhanced ring lesions, but biopsy is necessary to establish the diagnosis.

Less common extrapulmonary forms Tuberculosis may cause chorioretinitis, uveitis, panophthalmitis, and painful hypersensitivity-related phlyctenular conjunctivitis. Tuberculous otitis is rare and presents as hearing loss, otorrhea, and tympanic membrane perforation. In the nasopharynx, tuberculosis may simulate Wegener's granulomatosis. Cutaneous manifestations of tuberculosis include primary infection due to direct inoculation, abscesses and chronic ulcers, scrofuloderma, lupus vulgaris, miliary lesions, and erythema nodosum. Adrenal tuberculosis is a manifestation of advanced disease presenting as signs of adrenal insufficiency. Finally, congenital tuberculosis results from transplacental spread of tubercle bacilli to the fetus or from ingestion of contaminated amniotic fluid. This rare disease affects the liver, spleen, lymph nodes, and various other organs.

HIV-Associated Tuberculosis Tuberculosis is an important opportunistic disease among HIV-infected persons worldwide. In developing countries of Africa, Southeast Asia, and Latin America, an estimated 8.5 million persons were coinfected as of the middle of 1996. In the United States, coinfection with HIV and *M. tuberculosis* is common in certain segments of the population, including drug users and some minorities. A person with skin test–documented *M. tuberculosis* infection who acquires HIV infection has a 3 to 15 percent annual risk of developing active tuberculosis.

The association between tuberculosis and HIV is supported by other epidemiologic observations. First, HIV seropositivity is several times higher among patients with tuberculosis than among the general population: in New York City the rate is nearly 50 percent, and in African countries it reaches 60 to 70 percent. Second, marked increases in numbers of tuberculosis cases have been reported at locations hard hit by the HIV epidemic, such as Zambia, Tanzania, Malawi, northern Thailand, and New York City. Globally, the proportion of tuberculosis cases associated with HIV infection is growing rapidly and may reach 14 percent by the year 2000.

HIV directly attacks the critical immune mechanisms involved in protection against tuberculosis. Tuberculosis can appear at any stage of HIV infection, but its presentation varies with the stage. When cell-mediated immunity is only partially compromised, pulmonary tuberculosis presents as a typical pattern of upper lobe infiltrates and cavitation, without significant lymphadenopathy or pleural effusion. In late stages of HIV infection, a primary tuberculosis–like pattern, with diffuse interstitial or miliary infiltrates, little or no cavitation, and intrathoracic lymphadenopathy, is more common. Overall, sputum smears may be positive less frequently among tuberculosis patients with HIV infection than among those without; thus the diagnosis of tuberculosis may be unusually difficult, especially in view of the variety of HIV-related pulmonary conditions mimicking tuberculosis.

As has been mentioned, extrapulmonary tuberculosis is common among HIV-infected patients. In various series studied in the United States and many developing countries, extrapulmonary tuberculosis—alone or in association with pulmonary disease—has been documented in 40 to 60 percent of all cases. The most common forms are lymph nodal, disseminated, pleural, and pericardial. Mycobacteremia and meningitis are also frequent, particularly in advanced HIV disease.

The diagnosis of tuberculosis in HIV-infected patients may be difficult not only because of the increased frequency of sputum-smear negativity (up to 40 percent in culture-proven pulmonary cases) but also because of atypical radiographic findings, a lack of classic granuloma formation in the late stages, and negative results in PPD skin tests. Delays in treatment may prove fatal. The response to short-course chemotherapy is similar to that in HIV-seronegative patients. However, adverse effects may be more pronounced, including severe or even fatal skin reactions to amithiozone (thiacetazone).

DIAGNOSIS The key to the diagnosis of tuberculosis is a high index of suspicion. Diagnosis is not difficult with a high-risk patient—e.g., a homeless alcoholic who presents with typical symptoms and a classic chest radiograph showing upper lobe infiltrates with cavities. On the other hand, the diagnosis can easily be missed in an elderly nursing-home resident or a teenager with a focal infiltrate.

Often, the diagnosis is first entertained when the chest radiograph of a patient being evaluated for respiratory symptoms is abnormal. If the patient has no complicating medical conditions that favor immunosuppression, the chest radiograph may show the typical picture of upper lobe infiltrates with cavitation. The longer the delay between the onset of symptoms and the diagnosis, the more likely is the finding of cavitary disease. On the other hand, immunosuppressed patients, including those with HIV infection, may have "atypical" findings on chest radiography—e.g., lower zone infiltrates without cavity formation.

AFB Microscopy A presumptive diagnosis is commonly based on the finding of AFB upon microscopic examination of a diagnostic specimen such as a smear of expectorated sputum or of tissue (for example, a lymph node biopsy). Most modern laboratories processing large numbers of diagnostic specimens use auramine-rhodamine staining and fluorescence microscopy. The more traditional method—light microscopy of specimens stained with Kinyoun or Ziehl-Neelsen basic fuchsin dyes—is satisfactory, although more time-consuming. For patients with suspected pulmonary tuberculosis, three sputum specimens, preferably collected early in the morning, should be submitted to the laboratory for AFB smear and mycobacteriology culture. If tissue is obtained, it is critical that the portion of the specimen intended for culture not be put in formaldehyde.

Mycobacterial Culture Definitive diagnosis is dependent on the isolation and identification of *M. tuberculosis* from a diagnostic specimen—in most cases, a sputum specimen obtained from a patient with a productive cough. Specimens may be inoculated onto egg- or agar-based medium (e.g., Löwenstein-Jensen or Middlebrook 7H10) and incubated at 37°C under 5% CO_2. Because most species of mycobacteria, including *M. tuberculosis*, are slow growing, 4 to 8 weeks may be required before growth is detected. Although *M. tuberculosis* may be presumptively identified on the basis of growth time and colony pigmentation and morphology, a variety of biochemical tests have traditionally been used to speciate mycobacterial isolates. In today's laboratories, the use of liquid media with radiometric growth detection (e.g., BACTEC-460) and the identification of isolates by nucleic acid probes have replaced the traditional methods of isolation on solid media and identification by biochemical tests. These new methods have decreased the time required for isolation and speciation to 2 to 3 weeks.

Radiographic Procedures As noted above, the initial suspicion of pulmonary tuberculosis is often based on abnormal chest radiograph findings in a patient with respiratory symptoms. Although the "classic" picture is that of upper lobe disease with infiltrates and cavities, virtually any radiographic pattern—from a normal film or a solitary pulmonary nodule to diffuse alveolar infiltrates in a patient with ARDS—may be seen. In the era of AIDS, no radiographic pattern can be considered pathognomonic.

PPD Skin Testing Skin testing with PPD is most widely used in screening for *M. tuberculosis* infection (see below). The test is of limited value in the diagnosis of active tuberculosis because of its low sensitivity and specificity. False-negative reactions are common in immunosuppressed patients and in those with overwhelming tuberculosis. Positive reactions are sometimes obtained when patients have been infected with *M. tuberculosis* but do not have active disease and when persons have been sensitized by nontuberculous mycobacteria (see Chap. 173) or BCG vaccination. Although BCG vaccine is not commonly used in the United States, many immigrants will have received it. In the absence of a history of BCG vaccination, a positive skin test may provide additional support for the diagnosis of tuberculosis in culture-negative cases.

Drug Susceptibility Testing In general, the initial isolate of *M. tuberculosis* should be tested for susceptibility to the primary drugs used for treatment: isoniazid, rifampin, ethambutol, pyrazinamide, and streptomycin. In addition, drug susceptibility tests are mandatory when patients fail to respond to initial therapy or experience a relapse after the completion of treatment (see below). Susceptibility testing may be conducted directly (with the clinical specimen) or indirectly (with mycobacterial cultures) on solid or liquid medium. Results are obtained most rapidly by direct susceptibility testing on liquid medium, with an average reporting time of 3 weeks. With indirect testing on solid media, results may not be available for 8 weeks or longer.

Additional Diagnostic Procedures Other diagnostic tests may be used when pulmonary tuberculosis is suspected. Sputum induction by ultrasonic nebulization of hypertonic saline may be useful for patients unable to produce a sputum specimen spontaneously. Frequently, patients with radiographic abnormalities that are consistent with other diagnoses (e.g., bronchogenic carcinoma) undergo fiberoptic bronchoscopy with bronchial brushings or transbronchial biopsy of the lesion. Bronchoalveolar lavage of a lung segment containing an abnormality may also be performed. In all cases, it is essential that specimens be submitted for AFB smear and mycobacterial culture. For the diagnosis of primary pulmonary tuberculosis in children, who often do not expectorate sputum, specimens from early-morning gastric lavage may yield positive cultures.

Invasive diagnostic procedures are also indicated for patients with suspected extrapulmonary tuberculosis. In addition to specimens of involved sites (e.g., CSF for tuberculous meningitis, pleural fluid and biopsy samples for pleural disease), bone marrow and liver biopsy and culture have a good diagnostic yield in disseminated (miliary) tuberculosis. Blood from HIV-infected patients with suspected tuberculosis should be cultured.

In some cases, cultures will be negative, and a clinical diagnosis of tuberculosis will be supported by consistent epidemiologic evidence (e.g., a history of close contact with an infectious patient), a positive PPD skin test, and a compatible clinical and radiographic response to treatment. In the United States and other industrialized countries with low rates of tuberculosis, a significant percentage of patients with abnormal chest radiographs and sputum positive for AFB may have pulmonary disease due to organisms of the *Mycobacterium avium* complex (MAC) or *Mycobacterium kansasii* (see Chap. 173). Factors favoring the diagnosis of nontuberculous mycobacterial disease over tuberculosis include an absence of risk factors for tuberculosis, a negative PPD skin test, and underlying chronic obstructive pulmonary disease.

Patients with HIV-associated tuberculosis pose several diagnostic problems, as noted above in the description of clinical manifestations. Moreover, HIV-infected patients with sputum culture–positive and AFB-positive tuberculosis may present with a normal chest radiograph. Thus, in a patient with HIV infection, the finding of a normal chest radiograph does not rule out the diagnosis of pulmonary tuberculosis. An additional consideration is that, among relatively severely immunosuppressed AIDS patients in Europe and North America, MAC disease is more common than tuberculosis, usually presenting as a disseminated condition without pulmonary parenchymal involvement.

Adjunctive Diagnostic Tests A number of methods have been proposed as adjuncts to standard laboratory diagnosis. The most thoroughly investigated is serologic diagnosis based on detection of antibody to a variety of mycobacterial antigens. However, tests with most of the target antigens have a low predictive value when used in a population with a presumably low probability of disease. Tests aimed at detection of mycobacterial antigen by serologic methods have generally not been sufficiently sensitive to be useful. More promising are tests using biochemical and other methods to detect molecules that may be present in small amounts in diagnostic specimens. One example of a test that may be of some use, though its performance is presently limited to research laboratories, is the detection of tuberculostearic acid by gas-liquid chromatography in CSF from patients with tuberculous meningitis.

One of the most promising diagnostic techniques involves the amplification and detection of specific segments of DNA by polymerase chain reaction (PCR). The early problem with false-positive reactions due to amplicon contamination appears to have been solved. However, lingering problems with the preparation of specimens, particularly sputum specimens, have limited the sensitivity of the method. PCR may be most useful for the diagnosis of paucibacillary forms of pulmonary tuberculosis or extrapulmonary disease. Because of significant commercial interest, it is expected that the use of PCR in the diagnosis of tuberculosis will ultimately become established as technical problems are solved.

℞ **TREATMENT**

Chemotherapy for tuberculosis became possible with the discovery of streptomycin in the mid-1940s. Randomized clinical trials clearly indicated that the administration of streptomycin to patients with chronic tuberculosis reduced mortality and led to cure in a number of cases. However, monotherapy with streptomycin was frequently associated with the development of resistance to streptomycin and the attendant failure of treatment. With the discovery of para-aminosalicylic acid (PAS) and isoniazid, it became axiomatic that cure of tuberculosis required the concomitant administration of at least two agents to which the organism was susceptible. Furthermore, early clinical trials demonstrated that a long period of treatment—i.e., 12 to 24 months—was required to prevent the recurrence of tuberculosis.

The introduction of rifampin in the early 1970s heralded the era of effective short-course chemotherapy, with a treatment duration of less than 12 months. The discovery that pyrazinamide, which was first used in the 1950s, augmented the potency of isoniazid/rifampin regimens led to the use of a 6-month course of this triple-drug regimen as standard therapy.

Drugs Five major drugs are considered the first-line agents for the treatment of tuberculosis (see Chap. 170 for a detailed discussion): isoniazid, rifampin, pyrazinamide, ethambutol, and streptomycin (Table 171-1). The first four, which are usually given orally, are well absorbed, with peak serum levels at 2 to 4 h and nearly complete elimination within 24 h. These agents are recommended on the basis of their bactericidal activity (ability to rapidly reduce the number of viable organisms), their sterilizing activity (ability to kill all bacilli and thus sterilize the affected organ, measured in terms of the ability to prevent relapses), and their low rate of induction of drug resistance.

Because of a lower degree of efficacy and a higher degree of intolerability and toxicity, a number of second-line drugs are used only for the treatment of patients with tuberculosis resistant to first-line drugs. Included in this group are the injectable drugs kanamycin, amikacin, and capreomycin and the oral agents ethionamide, cycloserine, and PAS. Recently, quinolone antibiotics have been added to the list; although ofloxacin is generally recommended, sparfloxacin and levofloxacin have been more active in experimental studies. Other second-line drugs include clofazimine, amithiozone (thiacetazone, widely used with isoniazid in less wealthy countries but not marketed in North America or Europe), and amoxicillin/clavulanic acid. Long-acting rifamycin derivatives are also being evaluated for the treatment of tuberculosis, including rifabutin, which is used for prophylaxis against MAC disease in AIDS patients and is probably active against some tubercle bacilli with low-level resistance to rifampin, and rifapentine, which may be effective when given only once weekly.

Regimens Short-course regimens are divided into an initial or bactericidal phase and a continuation or sterilizing phase. During the initial phase, the majority of the tubercle bacilli are killed, symptoms

Table 171-1

Recommended Drugs and Dosages for the Initial Treatment of Tuberculosis in Adults*

Drug	Dosage	
	Daily	Thrice Weekly†
Isoniazid	5 mg/kg, max. 300 mg	15 mg/kg, max. 900 mg
Rifampin	10 mg/kg, max. 600 mg	10 mg/kg, max. 600 mg
Pyrazinamide	15–30 mg/kg, max. 2 g	50–70 mg/kg, max. 3 g
Ethambutol	15–25 mg/kg	25–30 mg/kg
Streptomycin	15 mg/kg, max. 1 g	25–30 mg/kg, max. 1.5 g

* Dosages for children are similar, except that some authorities recommend higher doses of isoniazid (10–20 mg/kg daily; 20–40 mg/kg intermittent) and rifampin (10–20 mg/kg).

† Dosages for twice-weekly administration are the same except for pyrazinamide (maximum, 4 g/d) and ethambutol (50 mg/kg).

SOURCE: Based on recommendations of the American Thoracic Society and the Centers for Disease Control and Prevention, 1994.

resolve, and the patient becomes noninfectious. The continuation phase is required to eliminate semidormant "persisters."

The treatment regimen of choice for virtually all forms of tuberculosis in both adults and children consists of a 2-month initial phase of isoniazid, rifampin, and pyrazinamide followed by a 4-month continuation phase of isoniazid and rifampin (Table 171-2). Except for patients who seem unlikely on epidemiologic grounds to be initially infected with a drug-resistant strain, ethambutol (or streptomycin) should be included in the regimen for the first 2 months or until the results of drug susceptibility testing become available. Treatment is most commonly given daily throughout the course, although intermittent regimens (either three times weekly throughout the course or a daily initial phase followed by twice-weekly treatment during the continuation phase) produce equivalent results. For patients with sputum culture–negative pulmonary tuberculosis, the duration of treatment may be reduced to a total of 4 months. Pyridoxine (10 to 25 mg/d) should be added to the regimen given to persons at high risk of vitamin deficiency (e.g., alcoholics; malnourished persons; pregnant and lactating women; and patients with conditions such as chronic renal failure, diabetes, and HIV infection or AIDS, which are also associated with neuropathy).

Patients' lack of adherence to treatment regimens is recognized worldwide as the most important impediment to cure. Moreover, the mycobacterial strains infecting patients who do not adhere to the prescribed regimen are especially likely to develop acquired drug resistance. Both patient- and provider-related factors may affect compliance. Patient-related factors include a lack of belief that the illness is significant and/or that treatment will have a beneficial effect; the existence of concomitant medical conditions (notably substance abuse); lack of social support; and poverty, with attendant joblessness and homelessness. Provider-related factors that may promote compliance include the education and encouragement of patients, the offering of convenient clinic hours, and the provision of incentives such as bus tokens.

In addition to specific measures addressing noncompliance, two other strategic approaches are used: direct observation of treatment and provision of drugs in combined formulations. Because it is difficult to predict which patients will adhere to the recommended treatment, all patients should have their therapy directly supervised, especially during the intensive phase. In the United States, personnel to supervise therapy are usually available through tuberculosis control programs of local public health departments. Supervision increases the proportion of patients completing treatment and greatly lessens the chances of relapse and acquired drug resistance. Combination products (isoniazid/rifampin and isoniazid/rifampin/pyrazinamide) are available and are strongly recommended as a means of minimizing the likelihood of prescription error and of the development of drug resistance (as the result of treatment with only one agent). In some formulations of these combination products, the bioavailability of rifampin has been found to be substandard. In North America and Europe, regulatory authorities ensure that combination products are of good quality; however, this type of monitoring cannot be assumed to take place in less affluent countries. Alternative regimens for patients who exhibit drug intolerance or adverse reactions are listed in Table 171-2.

Monitoring of the Response to Treatment Bacteriologic evaluation is the preferred method of monitoring the response to treatment for tuberculosis. Patients with pulmonary disease should have their sputum examined monthly until cultures become negative. With the recommended 6-month regimen, more than 80 percent of patients will have negative sputum cultures at the end of the second month of treatment. By the end of the third month, virtually all patients should be culture-negative. In some patients, especially those with extensive cavitary disease and large numbers of organisms, AFB smear conversion may follow culture conversion. This phenomenon is presumably due to the expectoration and microscopic visualization of dead bacilli. When a patient's sputum cultures remain positive at or beyond 3 months, treatment failure and drug resistance should be suspected (see below). A sputum specimen should be collected at the end of treatment to document cure. If mycobacterial cultures are not practical, then monitoring by AFB smear examination should be undertaken at 2, 5, and 6 months. Smears positive after 5 months should be considered indicative of treatment failure.

Bacteriologic monitoring of patients with extrapulmonary tuberculosis is more difficult and often is not feasible. In these cases, the response to treatment must be assessed clinically.

Monitoring of the response to treatment by serial chest radiographs is not recommended. Radiographic changes may lag behind bacteriologic response and are not highly sensitive. However, a chest radiograph at the end of treatment may be useful for comparative purposes should the patient develop symptoms of recurrent tuberculosis. After the completion of treatment, neither follow-up sputum examination nor chest radiography is recommended. However, patients should be instructed to report promptly for medical assessment should they develop any symptoms consistent with recurrent tuberculosis.

During treatment, patients should be monitored for drug toxicity. The most common adverse reaction of significance is hepatitis. Pa-

Table 171-2

Recommended Regimens for the Treatment of Tuberculosis

	Initial Phase		Continuation Phase	
Indication	**Duration, Months**	**Drugs**	**Duration, Months**	**Drugs**
New smear- or culture-positive case	2	HRZE*	4	HR*
New culture-negative case	2	HRZE*	2	HR*
Intolerance to H	2	RZE	7	RE
Intolerance to R	2	HES (±Z)	16	HE
Intolerance to Z	2	HRE	7	HR
Pregnancy	2	HRE	7	HR
Failure and relapse†	—	—	—	—
Standard retreatment (susceptibility testing unavailable)	3	HRZES‡	5	HRE
Resistance to H + R	Throughout (12–18)	ZE + O + S (or another injectable agent§)	—	—
Resistance to all first-line drugs	Throughout (24)	1 injectable agent§ + 3 of these 4: ethionamide, cycloserine, PAS, O	—	—

* All drugs can be given daily or intermittently (three times weekly throughout or twice weekly after the initial phase of daily therapy).
† Regimen is tailored according to the results of drug susceptibility tests.
‡ Streptomycin treatment should be discontinued after 2 months.
§ Amikacin, kanamycin, or capreomycin. Treatment with all of these agents should be discontinued after 2 to 6 months, depending upon the patient's tolerance and response.

NOTE: H, isoniazid; R, rifampin; Z, pyrazinamide; E, ethambutol; S, streptomycin; O, ofloxacin; PAS, para-aminosalicylic acid.

tients should be carefully educated about the signs and symptoms of drug-induced hepatitis (e.g., dark urine, loss of appetite) and should be instructed to discontinue treatment promptly and see their health care provider should these symptoms occur. Although biochemical monitoring is not routinely recommended, all adult patients should undergo baseline assessment of liver function (e.g., measurement of levels of hepatic aminotransferases and serum bilirubin). Older patients, those with histories of hepatic disease, and those using alcohol daily should be monitored especially closely, with repeated measurements of aminotransferases, during the initial phase of treatment. Up to 20 percent of patients have small increases in aspartate aminotransferase (up to three times the upper limit of normal) that are accompanied by no symptoms and are of no consequence. For patients with symptomatic hepatitis and those with marked elevations in aspartate aminotransferase, treatment should be stopped and drugs reintroduced one at a time after liver function has returned to normal.

Hypersensitivity reactions usually require the discontinuation of administration of all drugs and rechallenge to determine which agent is the culprit. Because of the variety of regimens available, it is usually not necessary—although it is possible—to desensitize patients. Hyperuricemia and arthralgia caused by pyrazinamide can usually be managed by the administration of acetylsalicylic acid; however, pyrazinamide treatment should be stopped if the patient develops gouty arthritis. Individuals who develop autoimmune thrombocytopenia secondary to rifampin therapy should not receive the drug thereafter. Similarly, the occurrence of optic neuritis with ethambutol and the development of eighth-nerve damage with streptomycin are indications for permanent discontinuation of these respective drugs. Other common manifestations of drug intolerance, such as pruritus and gastrointestinal upset, can generally be managed without the interruption of therapy.

Treatment Failure and Relapse   As stated above, treatment failure should be suspected when a patient's sputum cultures remain positive after 3 months or when AFB smears remain positive after 5 months. In the management of such patients, it is imperative that the current isolate be tested for susceptibility to first- and second-line agents. When the results of susceptibility testing are expected to become available within several weeks, changes in the regimen can be postponed until that time. However, if the patient's clinical condition is deteriorating, an earlier change in regimen may be indicated. A cardinal rule in the latter situation is always to add more than one drug at a time to a failing regimen: at least two and preferably three drugs that have never been used should be added. The patient may continue to take isoniazid and rifampin along with these new agents pending the results of susceptibility tests.

The mycobacterial strains infecting patients who experience a relapse after apparently successful treatment are less likely to have acquired drug resistance (see below) than are strains from patients in whom treatment has failed. However, if the regimen administered initially does not contain rifampin (and thus is not a short-course regimen), the probability of isoniazid resistance is high. Acquired resistance is uncommon among strains from patients who relapse after completing a short course of therapy. However, it is prudent to begin the treatment of all relapses with all five first-line drugs pending the results of susceptibility testing. In less affluent countries and other settings where facilities for culture and drug susceptibility testing are not available, a standard regimen should be used in all instances of relapse and treatment failure (Table 171-2).

Drug-Resistant Tuberculosis   Strains of *M. tuberculosis* resistant to individual drugs arise by spontaneous point mutations in the mycobacterial genome, which occur at low but predictable rates. Because there is no cross-resistance among the commonly used drugs, the probability that a strain will be resistant to two drugs is the product of the probabilities of resistance to each drug and thus is low. The development of drug-resistant tuberculosis is invariably

the result of monotherapy—i.e., the failure of the health care provider to prescribe at least two drugs to which tubercle bacilli are susceptible or of the patient to take properly prescribed therapy.

Drug-resistant tuberculosis may be either primary or acquired. *Primary* drug resistance is that in a strain infecting a patient who has not previously been treated. *Acquired* resistance develops during the course of treatment with an inappropriate regimen. In North America and Europe, rates of primary resistance are generally low, and isoniazid resistance is most common. Much attention has been focused on disease due to isoniazid/rifampin-resistant or multidrug-resistant (MDR) tuberculosis. As noted above, drug-resistant tuberculosis can be prevented by adherence to the principles of sound therapy: the inclusion of at least two bactericidal drugs to which the organism is susceptible (in practice, four drugs are commonly given in the initial phase) and the verification that patients complete the prescribed course.

Although the 6-month regimen described in Table 171-2 is highly effective for patients with initial isoniazid-resistant disease, it is prudent to extend treatment to 9 months and to include ethambutol throughout. For disease with high-level isoniazid resistance, isoniazid probably does not contribute to a successful outcome and can be dropped from the regimen. MDR tuberculosis is more difficult to manage than is disease caused by a drug-susceptible organism, especially because resistance to other first-line drugs as well as to isoniazid and rifampin is common. For strains resistant to isoniazid and rifampin, combinations of ethambutol, pyrazinamide, and streptomycin (or, for those with streptomycin resistance as well, another injectable agent such as amikacin), given for 12 to 18 months and for at least 9 months after sputum culture conversion, may be effective. Many authorities would add ofloxacin to this regimen. For patients with bacilli resistant to all of the first-line agents, cure may be attained with a combination of three drugs chosen from ethionamide, cycloserine, PAS, and ofloxacin plus one drug chosen from amikacin, kanamycin, and capreomyin (Table 171-2). The optimal duration of therapy for MDR tuberculosis is not known; however, patients are commonly treated for up to 24 months. Because the management of patients with MDR tuberculosis is complicated by both social and medical factors, care of these patients should be restricted to specialists and tuberculosis control programs. For patients with localized disease and sufficient pulmonary reserve, lobectomy or pneumonectomy can lead to cure.

Special Clinical Situations   Although comparative clinical trials of treatment for extrapulmonary tuberculosis are limited, the available evidence indicates that all forms of disease can be treated with the 6-month regimen recommended for patients with pulmonary disease. However, the American Academy of Pediatrics recommends that children with bone and joint tuberculosis, tuberculous meningitis, or miliary tuberculosis receive a minimum of 12 months of treatment.

Treatment for tuberculosis may be complicated by underlying medical problems that require special consideration. As a rule, patients with chronic renal failure should not receive aminoglycosides and should receive ethambutol only if serum levels can be monitored. Isoniazid, rifampin, and pyrazinamide may be given in the usual doses in cases of mild to moderate renal failure, but the dosages of isoniazid and pyrazinamide should be reduced for all patients with severe renal failure except those undergoing hemodialysis. Patients with hepatic disease pose a special problem because of the hepatotoxicity of isoniazid, rifampin, and pyrazinamide. Patients with severe hepatic disease may be treated with ethambutol and streptomycin and, if required, with isoniazid and rifampin under close supervision. The use of pyrazinamide by patients with liver failure should be avoided. Silicotuberculosis necessitates the extension of therapy by at least 2 months. Finally, patients with HIV infection or AIDS appear to respond well to standard 6-month therapy, although treatment may need to be prolonged if the response is suboptimal.

The regimen of choice for pregnant women is 9 months of treatment with isoniazid and rifampin supplemented by ethambutol for the first 2 months. When required, pyrazinamide may be given, although there are no data concerning its safety in pregnancy. Streptomycin is contraindicated because it is known to cause eighth-cranial-nerve damage in the fetus. Treatment for tuberculosis is not a contraindication to breast feeding; most of the drugs administered will be present in small quantities in breast milk, albeit at concentrations far too low to provide any therapeutic or prophylactic benefit to the child.

PREVENTION   By far the best way to prevent tuberculosis is the rapid diagnosis of infectious cases with appropriate treatment until cure. Additional strategies include BCG vaccination and preventive chemotherapy.

BCG Vaccination   BCG was derived from an attenuated strain of *M. bovis* and was first administered to humans in 1921. Many BCG vaccines are available worldwide; all are derived from the original strain, but the vaccines vary in efficacy. In fact, estimates of efficacy from randomized, placebo-controlled trials have ranged from 80 percent to nil. A similar range of efficacy was found in recent observational studies (case-control, historical cohort, and cross-sectional studies) in areas where infants are vaccinated at birth. These studies also found higher rates of efficacy in the protection of infants and young children from relatively serious forms of tuberculosis, such as tuberculous meningitis and miliary tuberculosis.

BCG vaccine is safe and rarely causes serious complications. The local tissue response begins 2 to 3 weeks after vaccination, with scar formation and healing within 3 months. Side effects—most commonly, ulceration at the vaccination site and regional lymphadenitis—occur in 1 to 10 percent of vaccinated persons. Some vaccine strains have caused osteomyelitis in approximately one case per million doses administered. Disseminated BCG infection and death have occurred in 1 to 10 cases per 10 million doses administered, although this problem is restricted almost exclusively to persons with impaired immunity, such as those with HIV infection. BCG vaccination induces PPD reactivity. The presence or size of PPD skin-test reactions after vaccination does not predict the degree of protection afforded.

BCG vaccine is recommended for routine use at birth in countries with high tuberculosis prevalences. However, because of the low risk of transmission of tuberculosis in the United States and the unreliable protection afforded by BCG, the vaccine has never been recommended for general use in the United States. Currently, vaccination is recommended only for PPD-negative infants and children who are at high risk of intimate and prolonged exposure to patients with MDR tuberculosis and who cannot take prophylactic isoniazid and for infants and children in groups in which the rate of new *M. tuberculosis* infections exceeds 1 percent per year.

Preventive Chemotherapy   A major component of tuberculosis control in the United States involves the administration of isoniazid to persons with latent tuberculosis and a high risk of active disease. This intervention is based on the results of a large number of randomized, placebo-controlled clinical trials demonstrating that a 6- to 12-month course of isoniazid reduces the risk of active tuberculosis in infected people by 90 percent or more. In the absence of reinfection, the protective effect is believed to be lifelong. More recently, limited clinical trials have also shown that isoniazid prophylaxis reduces rates of tuberculosis among persons with HIV infection.

In most cases, candidates for prophylaxis (Table 171-3) are identified by PPD skin testing of high-risk groups of individuals. For skin testing, 5 tuberculin units of polysorbate-stabilized PPD should be injected intradermally into the volar surface of the forearm (Mantoux method). Multipuncture tests, which may be useful for screening large populations, are not recommended for this purpose; any positive reaction to a multipuncture test must be confirmed by Mantoux testing. Reactions are read at 48 to 72 h as the transverse diameter in millimeters of induration; the diameter of erythema is not considered. In some persons, PPD reactivity wanes with time but can be recalled by a second skin test administered 1 week or more after the first (i.e., two-step testing). For persons undergoing periodic PPD skin testing, such as health care workers and individuals admitted to long-term-care institutions, a repeat test in instances of an initially negative result

Table 171-3

Recommendations for Isoniazid Prophylaxis

Risk Group	Tuberculin Reaction, mm	Duration of Treatment, months
HIV-infected persons	≥5*	12
Close contacts of tuberculosis patients	≥5†	6 (9 for children)
Persons with fibrotic lesions on chest radiography	≥5	12
Recently infected persons	≥10	6
Persons with high-risk medical conditions‡	≥10	6–12
High-risk group, <35 years of age§	≥10	6
Low-risk group, <35 years of age	≥15	6

* Anergic HIV-infected persons with an estimated risk of *M. tuberculosis* infection of 10 percent may also be considered candidates.

† Tuberculin-negative contacts, especially children, should receive prophylaxis for 2 or 3 months after contact ends and should then be retested with PPD. Those whose results remain negative should discontinue prophylaxis.

‡ Includes diabetes mellitus, prolonged therapy with systemic glucocorticoids, other immunosuppressive therapy, some hematologic and reticuloendothelial diseases, injection drug use (with HIV seronegativity), end-stage renal disease, and clinical situations associated with rapid weight loss.

§ Includes persons born in high-prevalence countries, members of medically underserved low-income populations, and residents of long-term-care facilities.

SOURCE: Based on recommendations of the American Thoracic Society and the Centers for Disease Control and Prevention, 1994.

may preclude the misclassification of persons with boosted reactions as PPD converters.

The cutoff for a positive skin test (and thus for prophylaxis) is related both to the probability that the reaction represents true infection and to the likelihood that the individual, if truly infected, will develop tuberculosis. Thus positive reactions for close contacts of infectious cases, persons with HIV infection, and previously untreated persons whose chest radiograph is consistent with healed tuberculosis are defined as an area of induration ≥5 mm in diameter. A 10-mm cutoff is used to define positive reactions in most other at-risk persons. For persons with a very low risk of developing tuberculosis if infected, a cutoff of 15 mm is used.

Some PPD-negative individuals are also candidates for prophylaxis. Infants and children who have come into contact with infectious cases should be given prophylactic isoniazid and should have a repeat skin test 2 or 3 months after contact ends. Those whose test results remain negative should discontinue prophylaxis. HIV-infected persons who have a negative skin test and are at increased risk of tuberculosis may receive prophylaxis if they are found to be anergic on testing with other DTH antigens, such as *Candida* and mumps. Finally, some authorities recommend that all HIV-infected contacts of infectious cases be considered candidates for prophylaxis.

Isoniazid is administered in a dose of 5 mg/kg per day (up to 300 mg) for 6 to 12 months; the longer course is recommended for persons with HIV infection and for those with abnormal chest radiographs. On the basis of cost-benefit analyses, the shorter period is recommended for individuals in other categories. However, the American Academy of Pediatrics recommends that children receive a 9-month course of therapy. When supervised prophylaxis is desirable and feasible, isoniazid may be given at a dose of 15 mg/kg (up to 900 mg) twice weekly.

Contraindications to isoniazid prophylaxis include the presence of active liver disease. Since the major adverse reaction to this drug is hepatitis, persons at increased risk of toxicity (e.g., those aged 35 years or older, those consuming alcohol daily, and those with a history of liver disease) should undergo baseline and then monthly assessment of liver function during treatment. All patients should be carefully educated about hepatitis and instructed to discontinue use of the drug immediately should any symptoms develop. Moreover, patients should be seen and questioned about adverse reactions monthly during therapy and should be given no more than 1 month's supply of drug at each visit.

It may be more difficult to ensure compliance with a prophylactic regimen than with a therapeutic regimen for active tuberculosis. If family members of active cases are being treated, compliance and monitoring may be easier. For high-risk patients (such as HIV-infected injection-drug users) and persons who are institutionalized, twice-weekly supervised therapy may be useful. As in active cases, the provision of incentives may also be helpful.

BASICS OF CONTROL   The highest priority in any tuberculosis control program is the prompt detection of cases and the provision of directly observed short-course chemotherapy to all tuberculosis patients, with emphasis on the cure of sputum smear–positive cases. In addition, in low-prevalence countries with adequate resources, screening of high-risk groups (such as immigrants from high-prevalence countries and HIV-seropositive persons) is recommended. Identification of active cases of tuberculosis should be followed by treatment and that of PPD positivity in high-risk persons by prophylaxis. Contact investigation is also an important component of efficient tuberculosis control. In the United States, a great deal of attention has been given to the transmission of tuberculosis (particularly in association with HIV infection) in institutional settings such as hospitals, homeless shelters, and prisons. Measures to limit such transmission include respiratory isolation of persons with suspected tuberculosis until they are proven to be noninfectious (i.e., by sputum AFB smear negativity), proper ventilation in rooms of patients with infectious tuberculosis, use of ultraviolet lights in areas of increased risk of tuberculosis transmission, and periodic screening of personnel who may come into contact with known or unsuspected cases of tuberculosis. In the past, radiographic surveys, especially those conducted with portable equipment and miniature films, were advocated for case-finding. Today, however, the prevalence of tuberculosis in industrialized countries is sufficiently low that "mass miniature radiography" is not cost-effective.

In high-prevalence countries, tuberculosis control programs should be based on the following key elements: (1) case detection, predominantly through passive case-finding (e.g., microscopic examination of sputum from patients who present spontaneously to health care facilities with cough of more than 3 weeks' duration); (2) administration of standard short-course chemotherapy to all sputum smear–positive patients under proper case-management conditions—namely, supervised administration of drugs; (3) establishment and maintenance of a system of regular drug supply; and (4) establishment and maintenance of an effective system for patient evaluation and program management. This system should allow an analysis of treatment outcomes (e.g., cure, completion of treatment without proof of cure, death, treatment failure, and default) in all cases registered.

BIBLIOGRAPHY

AMERICAN THORACIC SOCIETY AND CENTERS FOR DISEASE CONTROL: Control of tuberculosis in the United States. Am Rev Respir Dis 146:1623, 1992
————: Treatment of tuberculosis and tuberculosis infection in adults and children. Am J Respir Crit Care Med 149:1359, 1994
ANTONUCCI G et al: Risk factors for tuberculosis in HIV-infected persons. A prospective cohort study. JAMA 274:143, 1995
BLOOM BR (ed): *Tuberculosis. Pathogenesis, Protection, and Control.* Washington, DC, American Society for Microbiology, 1994
CANTWELL MF et al: Epidemiology of tuberculosis in the United States, 1985 through 1992. JAMA 272:535, 1994
CENTERS FOR DISEASE CONTROL: Guidelines for preventing the transmission of tuberculosis in health-care settings, with special focus on HIV-related issues. Morb Mortal Week Rep 39(RR-17):1, 1990

CROFTON J et al: *Clinical Tuberculosis.* London, Macmillan Education, 1992
FINE PEM: Bacille Calmette-Guérin vaccines: A rough guide. Clin Infect Dis 20:11, 1995
HOPEWELL PC: Impact of human immunodeficiency virus infection on the epidemiology, clinical features, management, and control of tuberculosis. Clin Infect Dis 15:540, 1992
ISEMAN MD: Treatment of multidrug-resistant tuberculosis. N Engl J Med 329:784, 1993
MITCHISON DA: The action of antituberculosis drugs in short-course chemotherapy. Tubercle 66:219, 1985
O'BRIEN RJ: Preventive therapy for tuberculosis, in *Clinical Tuberculosis,* PDO Davies (ed). London, Chapman & Hall, 1994, pp 279–295
RAVIGLIONE MC et al: Global epidemiology of tuberculosis. Morbidity and mortality of a worldwide epidemic. JAMA 273:220, 1995
REICHMAN LB, HERSHFIELD ES (eds): *Tuberculosis. A Comprehensive International Approach.* New York, Mercel Dekker, 1993
SMALL PM et al: The epidemiology of tuberculosis in San Francisco: A population-based study using conventional and molecular methods. N Engl J Med 330:1703, 1994
SUMARTOJO E: When tuberculosis treatment fails. A social behavioral account of patient adherence. Am Rev Respir Dis 147:1311, 1993
STYBLO K: Epidemiology of tuberculosis, in *Selected Papers,* vol 24. The Hague, Royal Netherlands Tuberculosis Association, 1993
WORLD HEALTH ORGANIZATION: *Treatment of Tuberculosis. Guidelines for National Programmes.* Geneva, WHO, 1993

| 172 | *Richard A. Miller* |

LEPROSY (HANSEN'S DISEASE)

DEFINITION AND ETIOLOGY   Leprosy (Hansen's disease) is a chronic granulomatous infection of humans that attacks superficial tissues, especially the skin and peripheral nerves. *Mycobacterium leprae,* the causal agent, is an acid-fast rod assigned to the family Mycobacteriaceae on the basis of morphologic, biochemical, antigenic, and genetic similarities to other mycobacteria. Although it has not been cultivated in artificial media or tissue culture, *M. leprae* can be propagated in armadillos and in the footpads of mice. The bacillus multiplies exceedingly slowly, with an estimated optimal doubling time of 11 to 13 days during logarithmic growth in mouse footpads. The mouse model has been used extensively for the study of antileprosy drugs, and the high bacterial yield from armadillos has been crucial for immunologic and genetic studies. The genome of *M. leprae* has been completely mapped, and the genes for the major protein antigens have been cloned and sequenced.

The cellular components of *M. leprae* that are responsible for its pathogenicity and ability to survive within the host are poorly understood. The best-characterized virulence factor is phenolic glycolipid I, a prominent surface lipid specific to *M. leprae.* Phenolic glycolipid I can bind to complement component C3, which in turn mediates phagocytosis of the bacterium by mononuclear phagocytes via CR1, CR3, and CR4 receptors on their cell surfaces. Once the bacterium is inside the phagocyte, phenolic glycolipid I helps to protect it from oxidative killing by chemically scavenging hydroxyl radicals and superoxide anions.

EPIDEMIOLOGY   The number of leprosy cases worldwide has dropped dramatically in the past decade, from an estimated 10 to 12 million cases to 1.8 million cases. The explanation for this decline is controversial and undoubtedly multifactorial. Possible contributing factors include improved case detection, use of short-course multidrug therapeutic regimens, expanded bacillus Calmette-Guérin (BCG) vaccination programs, and increasing global urbanization. Leprosy remains largely a disease of the rural poor. In 1995, five countries—India, Brazil, Bangladesh, Indonesia, and Myanmar—accounted for 76 percent of the estimated number of cases in the world.

The distribution of infected individuals within countries is very nonhomogeneous. In some locales, 20 percent of the population is affected. The distribution of cases across the spectrum of leprosy also varies among countries, with lepromatous disease predominating in some countries, such as Mexico, and tuberculoid disease in others, such as India. Ninety percent of the cases diagnosed in the United States in the past two decades have occurred in immigrants from leprosy-endemic countries. Indigenous transmission takes place primarily in Hawaii, the Pacific Island territories, and (sporadically) along the Gulf Coast. The incidence of leprosy in the United States has fallen from a peak of 360 cases in 1985 (associated with an influx of immigrants from Southeast Asia) to an average of 150 cases per year.

Leprosy can present in persons of any age, although cases in infants less than 1 year of age are extremely rare. The age-specific incidence peaks during childhood in most developing countries; up to 20 percent of cases occur in children under 10. The sex ratio of leprosy presenting during childhood is 1:1, but males predominate by a 2:1 ratio among adult patients.

It is humbling to realize how little is known about the modes of transmission and acquisition of leprosy, given that the communicable nature of the infection has been recognized for millennia and that the etiologic agent was identified over 100 years ago. Direct human-to-human transmission is believed to be responsible for most cases of leprosy, although a history of exposure can be elicited from fewer than half of all patients. Animal reservoirs exist among feral armadillos and possibly among nonhuman primates, but in only a few human cases has zoonotic transmission been implicated. Detection of *M. leprae* in hematophagous insects and of phenolic glycolipid I in soil has led to speculation about environmental acquisition of infection. Among close family contacts of untreated lepromatous patients, the risk of disease is increased by approximately eightfold, and the attack rate can be as high as 10 percent. Development of clinical disease in contacts of tuberculoid patients is less common, although immunologic tests suggest that most of these contacts have been sensitized to *M. leprae*. The site of entry remains a matter of conjecture but is probably either the skin or the mucosa of the upper respiratory tract. The chief portal of exit is thought to be the nasal mucosa of untreated lepromatous patients.

The incubation period is frequently 3 to 5 years but has been reported to range from 6 months to several decades.

PATHOGENESIS The early events following the entry of *M. leprae* into the body have not been described in humans. The bacilli are surrounded by a dense, nearly inert lipid capsule; produce no exotoxins; and engender little inflammatory response. Immunologic and epidemiologic studies suggest that only a small fraction (possibly 10 to 20 percent) of the persons infected develop signs of indeterminate leprosy and that only about 50 percent of those with indeterminate disease experience a progression to full-blown clinical leprosy.

The intensity of the specific cell-mediated immune response to *M. leprae* correlates with the clinical and histologic disease class. Individuals with polar tuberculoid disease have an intense cellular response to *M. leprae* and a low bacillary load, whereas patients with lepromatous leprosy have no detectable cellular immunity to the leprosy bacillus. There is evidence from family studies that specific HLA-associated genes may be linked to different classes of disease. HLA-DR2 is inherited preferentially by children with polar tuberculoid disease, whereas HLA-MT1 and HLA-DQ1 are associated with polar lepromatous disease. The antigenic epitopes recognized by some of these major histocompatibility complex (MHC) molecules have been identified. The effect of the HLA-associated genes is limited to an influence on the type of leprosy that develops; there is no association between HLA haplotypes and overall susceptibility to leprosy.

The defect in cell-mediated immunity in lepromatous patients is extremely specific. These individuals do not suffer increased morbidity following infection by pathogens such as viruses, protozoa, or fungi, for which cellular immunity is important, and they are not at increased risk of neoplasia. In lepromatous leprosy, cells of the monocyte-macrophage family become engorged with *M. leprae* and are unable to kill or digest the organisms. However, when studied in vitro, monocytes from these patients respond normally to cytokines and display normal phagocytic and microbicidal activity. Patients with lepromatous leprosy have been shown to have an increased number of circulating CD8 + ("suppressor") lymphocytes that can be specifically activated by *M. leprae* antigens, and the lymphocytes present in their cutaneous

granulomas are almost exclusively CD8 + . In contrast, CD4 + 4B4 + ("helper") cells predominate among the T cells in the cutaneous lesions of tuberculoid patients. In addition to these differences in lesional T cell populations, local cytokine production in lepromatous lesions is distinctly different from that in tuberculoid lesions. Lesions of tuberculoid leprosy characteristically have a predominant Th1 cytokine response, with high levels of production of interleukin (IL) 2, interferon γ (IFNγ), and IL-12. In contrast, IL-4 and IL-10 are dominant in lepromatous lesions, consistent with a Th2-like response. These observations have led to renewed interest in adjunctive therapy with immunomodulatory agents and may be crucial for vaccine development.

Intense bacillemia is very common in lepromatous leprosy, and organisms can often be seen in stained smears of peripheral blood or buffy coats; however, high fever and signs of systemic toxicity are absent. Even in the most advanced cases, destructive lesions are limited to the skin, peripheral nerves, anterior portions of the eyes, upper respiratory passages above the larynx, testes, and structures of the hands and feet. One feature common to these sites is that they are all usually several degrees cooler than 37°C. Two sites of preferential involvement are the ulnar nerves near the elbow and the peroneal nerves where they pass around the head of the fibula; above and below these areas, where these nerves take deeper courses, they are less severely involved. In patients with lepromatous leprosy, collections of bacilli are also found in the liver, spleen, and bone marrow, but no visceral organ system dysfunction has been associated with the presence of these bacilli.

CLINICAL AND HISTOPATHOLOGIC MANIFESTATIONS The variable immune response to infection with *M. leprae* results in a wide spectrum of histologic and clinical manifestations. Since there is a strong concordance between clinical findings and dermal histopathology, they will be discussed together.

Early or Indeterminate Leprosy The first signs of leprosy are usually cutaneous. The lesions of indeterminate leprosy are very subtle and are most commonly diagnosed during the examination of contacts of known leprosy patients. One or more hypopigmented or hyperpigmented macules or plaques may be seen. Often an anesthetic or paresthetic patch is the first symptom noted by the patient, but skin involvement can be found on careful examination. Sensation is often relatively preserved in these early lesions, particularly those on the face. The lesions may clear spontaneously in a year or two, but specific treatment is recommended.

Tuberculoid Leprosy The initial lesion of tuberculoid leprosy, one of the "poles" of the clinical and immunologic spectrum, is often a hypopigmented macule that is sharply demarcated and hypesthetic. Later the lesions enlarge by peripheral spread, and the margins become elevated and circinate or gyrate (Fig. 172-1). The central area in turn becomes atrophic and depressed. Fully developed lesions are densely anesthetic and have lost the normal skin organs (sweat glands and hair follicles). The lesions are single or few in number. Nerve involvement occurs early, and the superficial nerves leading from the lesions may

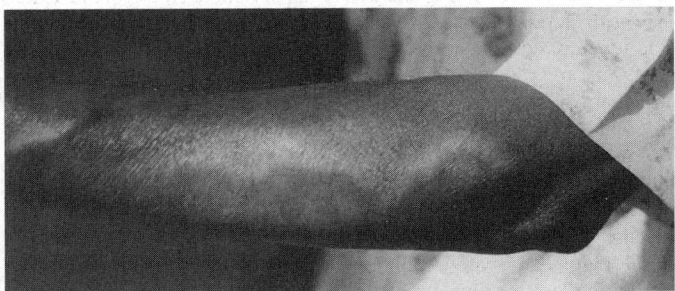

FIGURE 172-1 Tuberculoid leprosy. The large, solitary lesion has a raised, indurated border. The central clear area of the lesion is hypesthetic, with thinning of the dermis and loss of dermal structures such as sweat glands and hair follicles.

be enlarged. The larger peripheral nerves (especially the ulnar, peroneal, and greater auricular nerves and those closest to the skin lesion) may be palpably and visibly enlarged. The patient may experience severe neuritic pain. Neural involvement leads to muscle atrophy, especially of the small muscles of the hand. Contractures of the hand and foot are frequent. Trauma, especially from burns and splinters and from excessive pressure, leads to secondary infection of the hands and to plantar ulcers. Later, resorption and loss of phalanges may supervene. When the facial nerves are involved, there may be lagophthalmos, exposure keratitis, and corneal ulceration leading to blindness.

The histologic picture consists of noncaseating granulomas comprising lymphocytes, epithelioid cells, and perhaps giant cells; bacilli are frequently absent or difficult to demonstrate.

Lepromatous Leprosy   Lepromatous leprosy is the other polar form. Cutaneous involvement is extensive and roughly bilaterally symmetric across the midline of the host. Individual skin lesions are highly variable and can include macules, nodules, plaques, or papules. The borders of the lesions are ill defined, and the centers of raised lesions are indurated and convex (rather than concave, as in tuberculoid disease). There is diffuse infiltration of the dermis between discrete lesions, and apparently normal skin usually contains bacilli demonstrable by staining. The sites of predilection are the face (cheeks, nose, brows), ears, wrists, elbows, buttocks, and knees. At times, involvement with infiltration and little or no nodulation may progress so subtly that the disease goes unnoticed. Loss of the lateral portions of the eyebrows is common. Much later the skin of the face and forehead becomes thickened and corrugated (leonine facies), and the earlobes become pendulous.

Nasal "stuffiness," epistaxis, and obstructed breathing are common early symptoms. Complete nasal obstruction, laryngitis, and hoarseness also develop. Septal perforation and nasal collapse lead to saddlenose. Invasion of the anterior portion of the eye can result in keratitis and iridocyclitis. Painless inguinal and axillary lymphadenopathy occurs. In men, infiltration and scarring of the testes lead to sterility. Gynecomastia is common.

Involvement of the major nerve trunks is less prominent in the lepromatous than in the tuberculoid form, but diffuse hypesthesia involving the peripheral portions of the extremities is common in advanced disease. Pathologic studies reveal that the peripheral nerves are heavily infected but often better preserved than in the tuberculoid form.

Histologic examination detects a diffuse granulomatous reaction with macrophages, large foam (Virchow or lepra) cells, and many intracellular bacilli, frequently in spheroidal masses (globi). Epithelioid cells and giant cells are not found.

Borderline Leprosy   The borderline portion of the leprosy spectrum lies between the tuberculoid and lepromatous poles and is usually subdivided into borderline tuberculoid, borderline (or dimorphous), and borderline lepromatous classes. Classification within the borderline region of the spectrum is less precise than at the poles. Lesions tend to increase in number and heterogeneity but decrease in individual size as the lepromatous pole is approached. The skin lesions of borderline tuberculoid leprosy generally resemble those of tuberculoid disease but are more numerous and have less well-defined borders. Involvement of multiple peripheral nerve trunks is more common than in polar tuberculoid disease.

Increasing variability in the appearance of the skin lesions is characteristic of borderline leprosy. Papules and plaques may coexist with macular lesions. Anesthesia is less prominent than in tuberculoid disease. The earlobes may be slightly thickened, but the eyebrows and nasal regions are spared. Skin lesions become even more numerous in borderline lepromatous disease, but the distribution lacks the bilateral symmetry typical of polar lepromatous disease (Fig. 172-2).

The histopathology of the granulomas in borderline leprosy changes from an epithelioid cell predominance in borderline tuberculoid disease to a macrophage predominance as the lepromatous pole

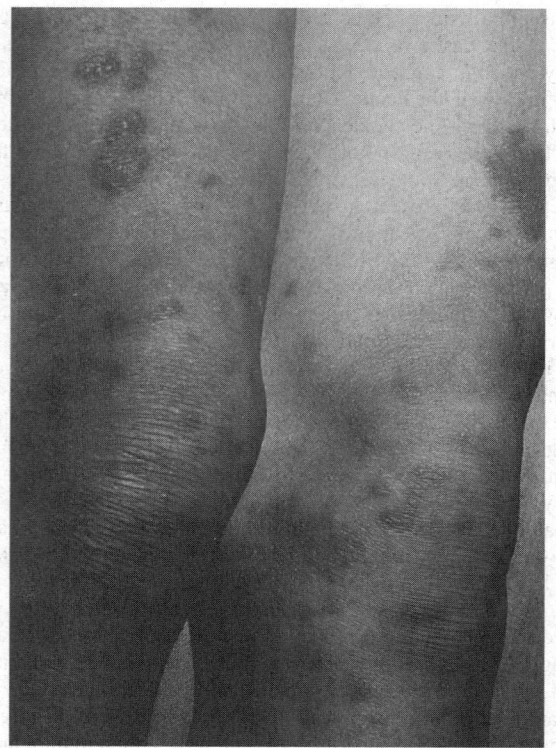

FIGURE 172-2   Borderline lepromatous leprosy. Multiple macules, papules, and nodules have an asymmetric distribution. Individual lesions are small but may become confluent.

is approached. The presence and number of lymphocytes are variable and correlate poorly with disease class. Bacilli are present in large numbers in the skin granulomas of borderline and borderline lepromatous patients. For this reason, these categories of disease, together with polar lepromatous leprosy, are referred to as *multibacillary leprosy*. The borderline tuberculoid, polar tuberculoid, and indeterminate classes are grouped together as *paucibacillary leprosy*.

The borderline disease states are unstable and may shift toward the lepromatous form in the untreated patient or toward the tuberculoid pole during treatment. Change of either polar type to the other is exceedingly rare.

In all forms of leprosy, peripheral nerve involvement is a constant feature. In any histologic section, involvement of nerves tends to be more severe than involvement of other tissues. Much of the neural destruction appears to result from the granulomatous reaction of the host rather than from an innate neurotoxic property of the bacillus. Albeit uncommonly, neural involvement can occur in the absence of cutaneous lesions (pure neural leprosy).

REACTIONAL STATES   The general course of leprosy is indolent but may be interrupted by two types of reaction. Both reactions can occur in untreated patients but more often emerge as complications of chemotherapy.

Erythema Nodosum Leprosum   Erythema nodosum leprosum (ENL), or type 2 lepra reaction, develops in lepromatous and borderline lepromatous patients, most frequently in the latter half of the initial year of treatment. Tender, inflamed subcutaneous nodules develop, usually in crops. Each nodule lasts a week or two, but new crops may continue to appear. Thus ENL may last only a week or two or may persist for long periods. Fever, lymphadenopathy, and arthralgias can accompany severe ENL. Histologically, ENL is characterized by polymorphonuclear leukocyte infiltration and deposits of IgG and complement, resembling an Arthus reaction. The precise factors responsible for initiating attacks of ENL are unclear, but in vitro and in vivo data have established the central roles of IFNγ and tumor necrosis factor α (TNFα) in producing the observed clinical and immunologic abnormalities. In one study, exogenous IFNγ induced ENL in 6 of 10 lepromatous patients, probably through increased secretion of TNFα by activated monocytes. Patients with ENL often have elevated serum levels of TNFα, and the alleviation of ENL by thalidomide is mediated through specific inhibition of TNFα production.

Reversal Reaction The reversal reaction, or type 1 lepra reaction, can complicate all three borderline categories. Existing skin lesions develop erythema and swelling, and new lesions may appear. An early influx of lymphocytes into existing lesions is followed by edema and a shift toward tuberculoid histology. Cellular immunity increases. Reversal reactions can be differentiated from disease progression or relapse by mouse inoculations to test bacillary viability and by histologic studies. *Downgrading reactions*, which clinically mimic reversal reactions, are most common in untreated patients and in women during the third trimester of pregnancy. Skin biopsies reveal a shift toward lepromatous histology and reflect a decrease in cellular immunity.

COMPLICATIONS Leprosy is probably the most frequent cause of crippling of the hand in the world (Fig. 172-3). Trauma and secondary chronic infections can lead to loss of digits or distal extremities. Blindness is also common.

The *Lucio phenomenon*, characterized by arteritis, is limited to patients with diffuse, infiltrative, nonnodular lepromatous disease. Severe cases clinically resemble other forms of necrotizing vasculitis and are associated with a high mortality rate.

Secondary amyloidosis is a complication of severe lepromatous disease, especially that complicated by chronic ENL.

Leprosy and Human Immunodeficiency Virus (HIV) Infection Surprisingly, given the experience with other mycobacterial diseases and the intricate immune response to *M. leprae*, concurrent infection with HIV appears to have little effect on the clinical manifestations or natural history of leprosy. Anecdotal reports suggest that the relapse rate after completion of therapy for paucibacillary disease may be slightly higher than usual among HIV-infected patients. In addition, HIV-positive patients with early or subclinical leprosy may be more likely to develop overt disease. Concurrent leprosy also may accelerate the course of HIV disease.

DIAGNOSIS The demonstration of acid-fast bacilli in skin smears made by the scraped-incision method is strong evidence for leprosy, but in tuberculoid disease bacilli may not be demonstrable. Wherever possible, a skin biopsy specimen from the affected area should be sent to a pathologist knowledgeable in leprosy. The histologic involvement of peripheral nerves is pathognomonic, even in the absence of bacilli. Work is underway on the development of tests using genetic probes for the rapid identification and speciation of mycobacteria in clinical specimens, but current polymerase chain reaction (PCR) technology offers little improvement in sensitivity over conventional microscopy.

Hematologic and blood chemistry tests are of little help in establishing the diagnosis. Lepromatous patients frequently have mild ane-

mia, an elevated erythrocyte sedimentation rate, and hyperglobulinemia. Between 10 and 20 percent of lepromatous patients have low-titer false-positive serologic tests for syphilis or autoantibodies directed against nuclear or cellular antigens.

Lepromin is a suspension of killed *M. leprae* prepared from heavily infected human or armadillo tissue. Intradermal injection elicits, somewhat variably, a tuberculin-like reaction at 48 h (the Fernandez reaction) and, more consistently, a papular reaction at 3 to 4 weeks (the Mitsuda reaction). The Mitsuda reaction is usually positive in tuberculoid patients and is always negative in lepromatous patients. However, because it is also positive in nearly all healthy adults, even those residing in areas free of endemic leprosy, it has no diagnostic value. Lepromin is not commercially available.

A specific serodiagnostic test for leprosy has been developed. Based on the detection of antibody to phenolic glycolipid I, this assay has a sensitivity of over 95 percent in polar lepromatous disease and about 30 percent in tuberculoid disease. The apparent correlation of the level of antibody with the bacillary load explains the high false-negative rate in polar tuberculoid disease. Despite this limitation, the near 100 percent specificity of this assay makes it potentially useful as a means of confirming the diagnosis of leprosy and as an epidemiologic tool for studying disease incubation and transmission.

The differential diagnosis includes lupus erythematosus, lupus vulgaris, sarcoidosis, yaws, dermal leishmaniasis, and a host of more mundane skin diseases. The skin lesions of leprosy, especially of tuberculoid disease, are characterized by hypesthesia, and peripheral nerve involvement can always be demonstrated. Peripheral neuropathy from other causes and syringomyelia may be confused with leprosy, although skin involvement is not a feature of these other diseases. The combination of a chronic skin disease and peripheral nerve involvement should always lead to the consideration of leprosy.

℞ TREATMENT

The management of leprosy involves a broad multidisciplinary approach, including consultative services such as orthopedic surgery, ophthalmology, and physical therapy in addition to antimicrobial chemotherapy.

Specific Chemotherapy Dapsone (4,4′-diaminodiphenylsulfone, DDS, diphenylsulfone), a folate antagonist, is the mainstay of therapy. The daily dosage is 50 to 100 mg in adults. Dapsone is very inexpensive, is safe in pregnancy, and has a long serum half-life of about 24 h that allows once-daily administration. Major side effects, which are relatively uncommon, include hemolysis, agranulocytosis, hepatitis, and potentially fatal exfoliative dermatitis. In lepromatous disease, enough bacilli are killed during the first 10 to 12 weeks of dapsone monotherapy to render mouse footpad inoculations negative. However, in this form of the disease, nonviable bacilli disappear slowly and may be found in the tissues for 5 to 10 years. Moreover, a few viable bacilli (persisters) may survive in the tissues for many years and cause a relapse if treatment is discontinued.

Years of dapsone monotherapy have led to the emergence of dapsone-resistant strains of *M. leprae*. Secondary resistance, which develops in 2 to 30 percent of lepromatous patients receiving dapsone monotherapy, presents as a clinical and bacteriologic relapse after several years of apparently successful regular therapy. Primary dapsone resistance in previously untreated patients has complicated empiric therapy in many parts of the world but remains uncommon (present in fewer than 3 percent of cases) in the United States. To counteract this problem, the World Health Organization (WHO) recommended in 1982 that defined-duration, multiple-drug therapy be administered to all leprosy patients. The results of multiple-drug therapy have exceeded expectations. The epidemic of dapsone resistance has been aborted, and active-case loads have fallen as patients have been declared cured.

Rifampin is the most rapidly mycobactericidal drug known for use against *M. leprae*. The viability of skin bacilli falls to undetect-

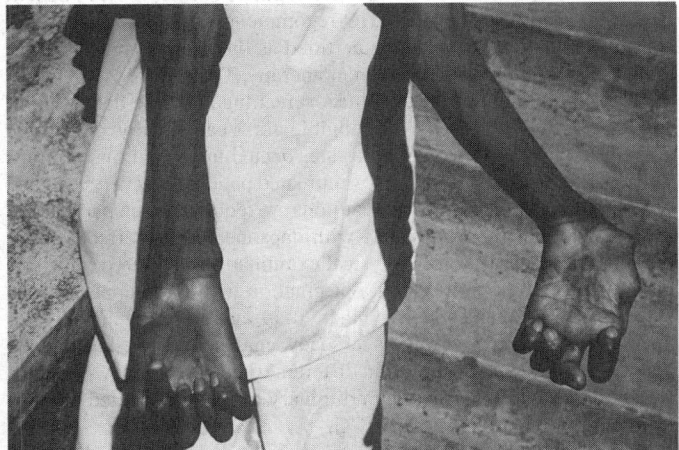

FIGURE 172-3 Borderline tuberculoid leprosy. Bilateral claw hand deformities result from ulnar and median nerve damage. Note the severe loss of muscle tissue in the forearms secondary to neuropathic and disuse atrophy.

able levels within 5 days after a single 1500-mg dose of oral rifampin. The usual dosage is 600 mg/d. The high cost of rifampin has limited its use in the developing world and has led to regimens in which it is given at a dosage of 600 or 900 mg once per month. Many leprologists prefer to treat with daily or twice-weekly rifampin if cost is not a crucial issue. Rare cases of rifampin-resistant *M. leprae* have been reported. Rifampin has not been approved for the intermittent treatment of leprosy by the Food and Drug Administration.

Clofazimine, a compound derived from a phenazine dye, is highly lipophilic and accumulates in the skin, the gastrointestinal tract, and macrophages and monocytes. It is usually given in a dosage of 50 to 200 mg/d and has an apparent half-life of over 70 days. Its major toxicity is restricted to the skin and the intestinal tract. The reddish skin pigmentation (often accompanied by ichthyosis) that is associated with clofazimine use is unacceptable to many light-skinned patients and can lead to poor compliance. The agent's intestinal toxicity is dose-related and is reflected in diarrhea and cramping abdominal pain. Clofazimine is not safe for use during pregnancy.

The several older agents with limited activity against *M. leprae* include ethionamide, prothionamide, thiambutosine, and amithiozone. All these drugs have significant toxicities, and none has yet been approved for the treatment of leprosy by the Food and Drug Administration. An extremely important and exciting development in the past few years has been the identification of several new antimicrobials with impressive activity against *M. leprae*. The most promising agents are minocycline, ofloxacin, and clarithromycin. These agents exhibit less bactericidal activity against *M. leprae* than does rifampin but are more active than dapsone or clofazimine. Combinations of these newer drugs will be important for the treatment of the rare cases of disease caused by rifampin-resistant *M. leprae*. Again, none of these drugs has yet been approved for the treatment of leprosy by the Food and Drug Administration.

Therapy for multibacillary disease should consist of three drugs, usually dapsone, rifampin, and clofazimine. If the organism is known to be dapsone-sensitive, the combination of dapsone and rifampin may be adequate for borderline and borderline lepromatous cases, but the likelihood of secondary dapsone resistance makes the addition of a third drug advisable in lepromatous disease. Objective measures of the response to therapy, including skin scrapings and biopsies, should be monitored and therapy continued at least until morphologically intact bacilli are consistently absent and the inflammatory cell infiltrate has resolved. The optimal duration of therapy is unknown, but a minimum of 2 years is recommended by WHO. An approach commonly used in the United States is to administer two or three drugs for the first 3 to 5 years and then to institute lifelong dapsone therapy.

Therapeutic regimens containing two drugs, usually dapsone and rifampin, are adequate for paucibacillary leprosy. WHO recommends a 6-month course and reports an annual failure rate after completion of only 0.1 percent. Standard practice in the United States is to use dapsone and rifampin for the first 6 to 12 months (depending on the clinical response) and then to use dapsone alone to complete a total of 24 months of therapy.

Evidence of clinical improvement should be visible by the second or third month of treatment. The clinical response to therapy may be obscured by intercurrent reactional states, but the disease stops progressing and the skin lesions gradually improve. Recovery from neurologic impairment is limited.

On the basis of promising results from preliminary studies, WHO is currently planning a large-scale trial comparing the combination of rifampin and ofloxacin with the conventional regimen of dapsone, rifampin, and clofazimine for the treatment of multibacillary disease. It is hoped that the duration of treatment can be shortened from the current minimum of 24 months to less than 6 months. Long-term follow-up is essential for the evaluation of all new regimens, as relapses continue to occur for more than 8 years after the completion of therapy with the dapsone/rifampin/clofazimine regimen.

Treatment of Reactional States Mild ENL is managed with antipyretics and anti-inflammatory agents. Severe cases can be rapidly controlled with high dosages of prednisone (60 to 120 mg/d). Antimicrobial therapy should be continued, since glucocorticoid therapy promotes the viability of *M. leprae* in mice not given antileprosy drugs. Rifampin enhances the metabolism of glucocorticoids by the liver, necessitating the administration of larger doses to achieve a given therapeutic effect. Thalidomide is the most effective drug for ENL. The usual initial dosage of 200 mg twice a day can be gradually tapered to a maintenance dosage of 50 to 100 mg/d for patients with chronic ENL. Thalidomide is absolutely contraindicated in women of childbearing age because of its teratogenicity but has proved relatively free of major side effects in other leprosy patients. This drug has not been approved by the Food and Drug Administration but is available through the Hansen's Disease Center, Carville, Louisiana, as an investigational agent. Clofazimine has anti-inflammatory properties as well as antimycobacterial activity and can be valuable in the treatment of chronic ENL; however, because it takes at least 3 to 4 weeks for clofazimine to reach effective levels, this drug is of little use in acute attacks. Other anti-inflammatory agents, including chloroquine, cyclosporine, and cytotoxic drugs, have been used in difficult cases; in general, these unusual situations should be managed in consultation with a leprosy specialist.

Reversal reactions are often acute and can lead to rapid and irreversible neurologic damage. Mild episodes may be managed with nonsteroidal anti-inflammatory agents, but glucocorticoids are essential in severe reversal reactions. Prolonged maintenance therapy is often necessary. Reversal reactions do not respond to thalidomide.

Other Measures Many of the deformities and disabilities of leprosy are preventable. Plantar ulcers, which are very common, may be prevented by rigid-soled footwear or walking plaster casts, and contractures of the hand may be prevented by physical therapy and application of casts. Reconstructive surgery is sometimes helpful. Nerve and tendon transplants and release of contractures can give patients more functional ability. All patients should undergo a thorough ophthalmologic examination, as up to 48 percent may have evidence of sight-threatening ocular complications. Vocational retraining is often necessary for those with permanent disability. Plastic surgery for facial deformities facilitates the acceptance of patients in society. The psychological trauma that historically resulted from prolonged segregation is now minimized by home therapy in virtually all cases.

CONTROL Case finding and chemotherapy form the present basis for the control of leprosy. Because infectiousness can be quickly suppressed with chemotherapy, early detection of cases is important. In endemic countries, early detection requires the establishment of local clinics or traveling teams. Family members and other close contacts of cases need to be examined regularly for leprosy. A benefit of the short (6- to 24-month) WHO-recommended multidrug treatment regimens is that patients can be certified as disease-free much sooner than was possible with dapsone monotherapy. Thus leprosy case workers can devote more effort to contact screening and case detection. In the United States, patients are eligible for treatment by the Public Health Service, and special clinics are located in several major cities. The risk of transmission—even by untreated patients—is very low, and no unusual infection-control precautions are required when patients are hospitalized. Chemoprophylaxis with dapsone may be effective, but contact screening by yearly physical examinations is preferred to empiric therapy in most situations. Vaccination with BCG appears to be more effective against leprosy than it is against tuberculosis. For unclear reasons, the vaccine's efficacy against leprosy has ranged widely (from 20 to 80 percent) in different trials. Several new vaccines are undergoing field trials, but preliminary results have failed to show significant improvement over BCG.

BIBLIOGRAPHY

BLAKE LA et al: Environmental nonhuman sources of leprosy. Rev Infect Dis 9:562, 1987

Cambau E et al: Multidrug-resistance to dapsone, rifampicin, and ofloxacin in *Mycobacterium leprae*. Lancet 349:103, 1997

Dana M et al: Ocular manifestations of leprosy in a noninstitutionalized community in the United States. Arch Ophthalmol 112:626, 1994

Editorial: Serological tests for leprosy. Lancet 1:533, 1986

Goodless DR et al: Reactional states in Hansen's disease: Practical aspects of emergency management. South Med J 84:237, 1991

Grosset J: Progress in the chemotherapy of leprosy. Int J Lepr Other Mycobact Dis 62:268, 1994

Hastings RC (ed): *Leprosy*. New York, Churchill Livingstone, 1985

Jacobson R: The face of leprosy in the United States today. Arch Dermatol 126:1627, 1990

Karonga Prevention Trial Group: Randomized controlled trial of single BCG, repeated BCG, or combined BCG and killed *Mycobacterium leprae* vaccine for prevention of leprosy and tuberculosis in Malawi. Lancet 348:17, 1996

Miko TL et al: Damage and regeneration of peripheral nerves in advanced treated leprosy. Lancet 342:521, 1993

Miller RA: Leprosy and AIDS. Int J Lepr Other Mycobact Dis 59:639, 1991

Noorden SK: Eliminating leprosy as a public health problem; why the optimism is justified. Int J Lepr Other Mycobact Dis 63:559, 1995

Ponnighaus JM et al: Efficacy of BCG vaccine against leprosy and tuberculosis in northern Malawi. Lancet 339:636, 1992

Sampaio EP et al: Influence of thalidomide on the clinical and immunologic manifestations of erythema nodosum leprosum. J Infec Dis 168:408, 1993

Yamamura M et al: Defining protective responses to pathogens: Cytokine profiles in leprosy lesions. Science 254:277, 1991

173 | *Bernard Hirschel*

INFECTIONS DUE TO NONTUBERCULOUS MYCOBACTERIA

Mycobacteria are slightly curved or straight, rod-shaped or coccoid bacilli traditionally identified by the property of acid-fastness: once stained, the organisms are not easily decolorized, even with acid-alcohol, because of the composition of their cell walls. The genetic relation of mycobacteria with one another is evidenced by their ribosomal RNA sequence homology, which can be used for diagnostic purposes.

Because of the overwhelming clinical importance of tuberculosis, mycobacteriologists have distinguished the *Mycobacterium tuberculosis* complex (consisting of *M. tuberculosis*, *M. bovis*, and *M. africanum*) from all other mycobacteria. Except for *Mycobacterium leprae* (see Chap. 172), the other mycobacteria are referred to as atypical mycobacteria, mycobacteria other than tuberculosis (MOTT), or nontuberculous mycobacteria (NTM). The isolation of NTM—or the lack thereof—from an individual patient or laboratory specimen must be interpreted with the following facts in mind:

1. Some NTM require special media and/or growth conditions. The laboratory must be alerted and cultures for acid-fast bacilli requested if the diagnosis of these infections is not to be missed.
2. NTM grow slowly. Even the so-called rapid growers take 3 to 7 days to form visible colonies on solid media, whereas slow-growing mycobacteria take weeks or do not grow at all on artificial media.
3. The slow growth of mycobacteria complicates antibiotic susceptibility testing. During prolonged incubation, antibiotics may be degraded and disappear from the culture medium. Long delays reduce the clinical usefulness of whatever results are eventually obtained.
4. Data on in vitro susceptibility correlate poorly with clinical results. For example, clarithromycin, azithromycin, and clofazimine are highly and variably concentrated in tissues; consequently, the concentrations necessary for determining resistance are difficult to establish in vitro. Sensitivity testing, based on achievable serum levels, would have predicted that these drugs would have little efficacy in vivo; in fact, the opposite is true, both in animal models and in humans.

5. In contrast to *M. tuberculosis*, NTM are ubiquitous in the environment. Therefore, isolation of NTM from a site that is not normally sterile (such as sputum, urine, skin, or feces) does not constitute proof of disease. In Switzerland between 1983 and 1988, for example, only 23 of 513 human immunodeficiency virus (HIV)–negative patients with NTM isolates had clinically significant disease. Clusters of unusual isolates are more likely to suggest contamination—e.g., from tap water or bronchoscopy equipment—than to represent an epidemic of disease.

The original method for the classification of NTM, developed between 1950 and 1980, depends on speed of growth, morphology, and pigmentation of colonies on solid media as well as biochemical reactions. Although reliable and inexpensive, these procedures take a long time; a period of 12 weeks is often required for definitive identification. Of course, such delayed results are of little use in the care of patients.

The isolation of NTM from blood cultures requires the use of a special medium for lysis-centrifugation or radiometric broth culture. The lysis-centrifugation method (lysis of blood cells followed by centrifugation and plating of the pellet with the bacteria on solid medium) permits quantification of bacteremia; however, some mycobacteria (e.g., *M. genavense*) do not grow well on solid medium and will not be detected by this method. Culture in liquid broth, such as that used in the radiometric Bactec system, shortens the time needed to identify a positive culture but also precludes the study of colonial morphology and pigmentation. Molecular probes are now used for rapid identification of the most important species (*M. avium*, *M. intracellulare*, *M. gordonae*, *M. kansasii*, and the *M. tuberculosis* complex) in a positive culture; a color is produced upon hybridization of the probe to specific sequences of the mycobacterial ribosome.

Twenty years ago, the field of mycobacteriology was something of a backwater. Tuberculosis was incorrectly perceived as a disappearing problem, and NTM were causing only rare and chronic diseases. AIDS, however, has brought mycobacterial infections to the forefront of clinical medicine once more. HIV and *M. tuberculosis* make a volatile mixture, and disseminated infections with NTM are extremely frequent in the advanced stages of AIDS (see Chap. 308). In this setting, it is fortunate that new molecular techniques based on DNA amplification promise to accelerate diagnosis, identify common sources of infection, and reveal new types of NTM, while new antibiotics, such as the macrolides, the rifamycins, and the fluoroquinolones, offer improved options for treatment and prevention.

DISSEMINATED NTM INFECTIONS IN AIDS AND OTHER IMMUNODEFICIENCIES

ETIOLOGY   The majority of mycobacterial infections in immunocompromised hosts are caused by organisms belonging to the group referred to as the *M. avium* complex (MAC). This group has always been considered to include *M. avium* and *M. intracellulare* (designated by the abbreviation *MAI*) and in the past encompassed *M. scrofulaceum* as well (hence the abbreviation *MAIS*). With the development and marketing of diagnostic probes that distinguish *M. avium* from *M. intracellulare*, it has become clear that the vast majority of disseminated "MAC" infections in AIDS are actually caused by *M. avium*. Thus, from a microbiologic standpoint, this designation is now obsolete. However, it is still used in clinical practice and will be employed in that context herein.

M. genavense causes systemic infections similar to those caused by MAC organisms. It is difficult to estimate the relative frequencies of *M. genavense* and MAC infections because *M. genavense* does not grow well in culture and may therefore be missed in some instances. However, in a series of nearly 200 disseminated NTM infections from Switzerland, 13 percent of cases were due to *M. genavense*. Other NTM, including *M. xenopi*, *M. simiae*, *M. scrofulaceum*, *M. malmoense*, and *M. celatum*, may also be involved in such cases. In addition, AIDS patients with localized NTM diseases often have positive blood cultures (e.g., patients with skin disease due to *M. haemophilum* or with lung disease due to *M. kansasii*).

EPIDEMIOLOGY AND HOST FACTORS Because gastrointestinal symptoms often predominate in NTM infection and because the intestinal submucosa is intensely involved, ingestion seems logical as a primary route of infection. Many environments and animals teem with NTM (especially MAC organisms), including swamps in the southeastern United States, swine almost everywhere, piped water in New England and in Finland, and soil from potted plants in San Francisco. Birds are frequently infected with *M. genavense*. Skin-test data and humoral antibody patterns point to widespread exposure to NTM. However, a direct connection of the environment to the patient is often lacking, and it is not always clear whether strains found in the environment are pathogenic in humans. In an exhaustive study of dietary factors, patients with NTM were found to have consumed more hard cheese than controls without NTM, but no NTM could be found in samples of cheese. At present, the epidemiologic evidence is not strong enough to serve as a basis for dietary recommendations in persons at high risk of NTM infection. There is no evidence for nosocomial spread of NTM from patient to patient; however, hospital hot-water systems have been suspected as the source of isolated clusters of cases. Whereas regional variations in the environmental frequency of NTM are striking, it is difficult to correlate these variations with the frequency of NTM infection among HIV-infected patients.

Disseminated infections with NTM occur almost exclusively in severely immunosuppressed patients, usually those with AIDS. Rarely, such infections are found in patients immunosuppressed for other reasons, including transplant recipients and patients with any of several ill-defined congenital immunodeficiencies, leukemia (in particular, hairy-cell leukemia), or lymphoma. Finally, rare cases of dissemination occur in immunocompetent patients who have extensive pulmonary disease.

In patients with AIDS, the risk of NTM infection correlates well with the degree of depletion of CD4 lymphocytes. For example, among patients with fewer than 10 CD4 lymphocytes per microliter, the actuarial probability of having a blood culture positive for NTM reaches 40 percent after 1 year. NTM may ultimately infect most such patients unless they first die for another reason. In the early 1990s, because prophylaxis of *Pneumocystis carinii* pneumonia was so successful, more patients survived to develop NTM infection. It remains to be proven whether prophylaxis of NTM infection with rifabutin or clarithromycin will alleviate this problem, although studies have found these drugs to be effective in reducing the risk of disseminated MAC infection.

DIAGNOSIS Blood cultures on special media are the cornerstone of the diagnosis of NTM infection, both in patients with organ involvement and in those without. In most symptomatic patients, the intensity of mycobacteremia is such that most or all blood cultures are positive. Therefore, the performance of multiple, repetitive cultures at short intervals is not worthwhile. Rather, in clinical practice, two or three blood cultures are sufficient. In one study, the results of prospective cultures varied, and these variations (positive followed by negative or vice versa) were unrelated to symptom status. As mentioned above, liquid cultures (e.g., the Bactec system) are likely to become positive earlier (within 7 to 14 days) and are therefore preferred to cultures on solid medium. In patients infected with *M. genavense* or *M. xenopi* and in patients being treated for MAC infection, the interval to culture positivity may be much longer. In rare cases, organ involvement in NTM infection may be found to be widespread at autopsy despite multiple negative blood cultures during life.

Because the liver and bone marrow are often involved in disseminated NTM infection, the bacteria may be visible in acid-fast–stained biopsy samples from these sites. Presumptive diagnosis by examination of a biopsied liver specimen saves time. The yield has been as high as 50 percent in patients with clearly abnormal values in liver function tests. However, the yield of this method has been disappointing in patients with suspected NTM infection, negative blood cultures, and normal or nearly normal results in liver function tests.

CLINICAL MANIFESTATIONS Disseminated infection with NTM is essentially a disease of advanced immunodeficiency. In HIV-infected patients, the median CD4 lymphocyte count at the time of diagnosis is around 10/μL. Certainly, other diagnoses should be considered first when a patient with symptoms suggestive of NTM infection has more than 100 CD4 cells per microliter. Prospective monthly blood cultures have shown that NTM bacteremia often causes few or no symptoms. In clinical practice, however, cultures are not performed if the patient is asymptomatic.

Disseminated NTM infection should be suspected on the basis of prolonged fever (sometimes of varying intensity—particularly at first—and accompanied by night sweats) and weight loss. Signs of abdominal involvement that may be evident on computed tomography or ultrasonography include enlargement of the liver and spleen and swelling of abdominal lymph nodes, which may result in diarrhea and/or abdominal pain. Anemia and leukopenia are frequently documented; although it is tempting to relate these abnormalities to infection of bone marrow by NTM, multiple factors are usually involved.

In short, the clinical picture of infection with NTM is not distinctive. Many other conditions, including abdominal lymphoma, the HIV wasting syndrome, *Salmonella* or *Campylobacter* infection, cryptosporidiosis, or microsporidiosis, may mimic (and coexist with) disseminated NTM infection. As stated earlier, suspicion of such infection should prompt a request for blood cultures.

℞ TREATMENT

Compared with *M. tuberculosis*, NTM are of low virulence. NTM tend to affect severely immunosuppressed patients, who usually have many other medical problems. Treatment is complex and frequently needs to be continued indefinitely since the eradication of NTM is difficult and relies on the use of multiple drugs with numerous adverse effects. At the beginning of the AIDS era, many physicians and activists took a dim view of drug therapy for NTM infection. The pendulum has now swung the other way, for the following reasons:

1. Patients with AIDS and disseminated NTM infection do not survive as long as comparable patients without NTM infection. Moreover, among those AIDS patients with disseminated NTM infection, treatment is associated with longer survival. Although not proof of a cause-and-effect relation (without randomization, it is always possible that untreated patients are sicker than treated patients at the time of diagnosis), such indirect evidence can guide clinical practice until data from prospective studies become available.
2. In many cases, symptoms are dramatically alleviated after the initiation of treatment. Some of this improvement (e.g., a decrease in fatigue and an increase in energy) may be difficult to quantify but is nonetheless of great importance to the patient.
3. Newer drugs exhibit increased activity against NTM both in vitro and in vivo.

The drugs used for the treatment of disseminated NTM infection are different from those used against tuberculosis (see Chap. 170). In particular, isoniazid has little effect on MAC organisms. The best method for antibiotic sensitivity testing of NTM is controversial, and the question of what relation—if any—exists between in vitro resistance and treatment failure remains unanswered. From the clinician's viewpoint, growth inhibition in liquid (Bactec) cultures is preferred to other methods of sensitivity testing because the results become available within 7 days.

The agents most active against MAC organisms are the macrolides clarithromycin and azithromycin. Both of these drugs are well absorbed from the gastrointestinal tract and well concentrated in macrophages and tissues, where their levels exceed those in plasma by more than 10-fold. Given alone, either drug can render blood cultures negative in a substantial proportion of cases. However, resistance (due to a single point mutation in the gene coding for the large ribosomal subunit) invariably develops, and NTM reappears in the bloodstream.

A majority of MAC strains are sensitive to ethambutol, ciprofloxacin, clofazimine, amikacin, rifampin, and rifabutin; that is, the concentrations of these drugs attainable in serum are inhibitory in vitro. However, none of these drugs consistently reduces the intensity of mycobacteremia when used alone. Trials to identify the best drug combination are ongoing. In the meantime, the following suggestions for therapy are made:

1. Include either clarithromycin (500 mg bid) or azithromycin (500 mg/d) in all regimens unless the mycobacterial strain is known to be resistant to these drugs in broth culture.
2. Include ethambutol (15 to 25 mg/kg per day) in treatment regimens. Most MAC strains are sensitive to this drug, and studies of immunosuppressed mice with disseminated MAC infection have documented excellent activity in vivo.
3. Add a third oral drug to the regimen: rifabutin (300 mg/d; higher doses—600 mg/d—have caused uveitis in up to 40 percent of patients when the drug is used together with clarithromycin), clofazimine (100 mg/d), rifampin (600 mg/d), or ciprofloxacin (500 mg bid). On the basis of in vitro data, results in experimental animals, and findings in one clinical trial, rifabutin is preferred. The rifamycins stimulate cytochrome P450 enzymes in the liver; drug interactions occur frequently (see Chap. 170). Compliance is an important issue in the treatment of patients with advanced immunodeficiency, who must ingest many drugs.
4. The inclusion of intravenous amikacin in multidrug regimens has not conferred additional benefit. Nonetheless, this drug may be useful in certain cases—for example, when resistance to clarithromycin develops or when severe gastrointestinal symptoms interfere with oral therapy. In addition, amikacin may prevent the emergence of resistance to clarithromycin when the two drugs are used concurrently.

It is not clear how long therapy needs to be administered. Older regimens did not eradicate MAC, and many experts recommended lifelong treatment. Unfortunately, multidrug regimens are often poorly tolerated. In patients whose symptoms have lessened, whose blood cultures have become negative, and who desire to simplify their regimen, it is currently considered reasonable to cut back to two drugs (usually clarithromycin and ethambutol) after 3 months.

In vitro and in experimental animals, cytokines such as interleukin 12, granulocyte-macrophage colony-stimulating factor, and interferon γ act synergistically with antibiotics against MAC. In a small-scale pilot trial including seven HIV-negative patients, interferon γ was beneficial.

Encapsulation of many drugs into liposomes enhances their effect in animal models because both liposomes and MAC are ingested by macrophages. Relevant data from studies of humans are still scarce, however. Disseminated infections caused by NTM other than MAC have been too rare for therapy to be evaluated in controlled trials. The presently recommended treatment for these infections is the same as that for disseminated MAC infections (Table 173-1). In particular, *M. genavense* seems to be sensitive to clarithromycin and rifabutin.

Table 173-1

The Most Important Nontuberculous Mycobacteria

Mycobacterial Species	Disseminated Infections	Localized Infections			Contaminant/ Commensal	Recommended Therapy	Percentage of Strains
		Lung	Lymphadenitis	Skin and Soft Tissue			
M. abscessus	—	—	—	Typical, linked to surgery	Typical	Debridement; clarithromycin, clofazimine, amikacin	<1
M. avium	Typical in AIDS with CD4 count of <50/μL; rare in other immunodeficiencies	See *M. intracellulare*	In children (rare)	In disseminated infection (rare)	Typical in sputum and feces	Clarithromycin,* ethambutol, rifabutin	30–50
M. celatum	AIDS (rare)	Rare	—	—	—	See *M. avium*	<1
M. chelonae	Rare	—	—	Typical, linked to surgery	Typical	See *M. abscessus*	<1
M. fortuitum	Rare	Rare	—	Typical	Typical	Amikacin, ciprofloxacin, sulfonamides, clofazimine, clarithromycin	1
M. genavense	Typical in AIDS	—	Rare	—	—	See *M. avium*	5
M. gordonae	Rare	—	—	Rare	Typical	—	10–30
M. haemophilum	Typical in AIDS and other immunodeficiencies	—	—	Typical, in AIDS		See *M. avium*	<1
M. intracellulare	See *M. avium*	Cavities in CF or COPD† Lingular infection in normal hosts	In children (rare)	See *M. avium*	Possible in sputum	See *M. avium*	4–8
M. kansasii	In AIDS (rare)	Typical, resembling tuberculosis	Rare	Rare	Possible in sputum	Rifampin, isoniazid, ethambutol, clarithromycin, sulfonamides	2–4
M. malmoense	Rare	Rare	—	—	—	See *M. avium*	1–4
M. marinum	Rare	—	—	Typical		Trimethoprim-sulfamethoxazole‡	1
M. scrofulaceum	Rare	Rare	Typical	—	—	See *M. avium*	1
M. simiae	In AIDS (rare)	Rare	—	—	Possible	See *M. avium*	1
M. szulgai	—	Rare	—	Typical	—	Rifampin, isoniazid, ethambutol	<1
M. xenopi	Rare	Rare	—	—	Typical	See *M. avium*	10–20

* Or azithromycin.
† CF, cystic fibrosis; COPD, chronic obstructive pulmonary disease.
‡ Or minocycline.

SOURCE: Data are from J Clin Microbiol 31:1882, 1993 (335 strains) and the Mycobacteriology Laboratory of the University Hospital in Geneva (1993–1994, 313 strains, Dr. P. Rohner).

PREVENTION As has been discussed, disseminated infection with MAC occurs almost exclusively in persons severely immunocompromised by HIV infection. Prophylaxis with rifabutin (300 mg/d), clarithromycin (500 mg once or twice daily), or azithromycin (1200 mg weekly) decreases the incidence of positive blood cultures by about 60 percent in patients with fewer than 200 CD4 lymphocytes per microliter. Patients receiving prophylaxis have also had less fever, experienced less fatigue, and survived longer than patients not receiving prophylaxis. Although breakthrough bacteremia involving resistant organisms is a concern, this condition has not developed with rifabutin prophylaxis and is rare with clarithromycin. Prophylaxis should therefore be considered for patients with fewer than 100 CD4 cells/μL. Some physicians are more restrictive in their indications and treat only those patients with fewer than 75 or 50 CD4 cells/μL; their rationale is that most disseminated MAC infections occur at very low CD4 counts, that prophylaxis is expensive (e.g., the cost of drugs to prevent one case of MAC infection is 50- to 100-fold greater than the cost of drugs to prevent a single case of *P. carinii* pneumonia), and that MAC prophylaxis heightens the potential for adverse reactions and drug interactions.

LOCALIZED INFECTIONS DUE TO NTM

PULMONARY DISEASE Etiology The NTM most frequently causing pulmonary infections are *M. intracellulare, M. avium,* and *M. kansasii.* Many other species, such as *M. xenopi* and *M. malmoense,* can also be involved in these infections. Identification of the specific pathogen is important in the choice among the various therapeutic strategies. For example, *M. kansasii* responds to antituberculosis drugs, including isoniazid.

Epidemiology and Host Factors As has already been noted, NTM are ubiquitous in the environment, but their pathogenicity is low. Preexisting lung disease (e.g., chronic obstructive airway disease, cancer, previous tuberculosis, bronchiectasis, cystic fibrosis, and silicosis, with cavities and bronchiectases) is the main predisposing factor for pulmonary disease due to NTM.

Anecdotal evidence suggests that the proportion of patients without underlying lung pathology who are developing pulmonary disease due to NTM is increasing. These patients are usually elderly; many are women with pectus excavatum or scoliosis. In the latter elderly women, the lingula and the right middle lobes are particularly involved. Somewhat whimsically, the disease in these patients has been called "Lady Windermere syndrome" after the main character in Oscar Wilde's play *Lady Windermere's Fan,* who went to extremes to refrain from coughing.

The significance of isolation of NTM from the airways of AIDS patients merits special discussion. *M. avium* only rarely causes significant pulmonary disease in AIDS; its isolation from sputum in the absence of radiographic changes is usually without clinical significance (except that in patients with fewer than 50 CD4 lymphocytes per microliter it may signal an increased likelihood of positive blood cultures in the future). In contrast, the isolation of *M. kansasii* from the lung is clinically significant: this organism causes a disease—often predominant in the upper lobes—that resembles pulmonary tuberculosis, with fever, cough, infiltrates, and cavities.

Clinical Manifestations Most patients with pulmonary NTM infection present with chronic cough, low-grade fever, and malaise; some present with hemoptysis. These symptoms may be masked by those of the underlying disease process. AIDS patients with pulmonary *M. kansasii* infection may develop severe symptoms mimicking pulmonary tuberculosis.

Diagnosis In contrast to the isolation of *M. tuberculosis,* of which even a single colony—whatever its origin—is clinically significant, the isolation of NTM from the sputum never in itself proves the existence of disease. NTM are frequently commensals and colonize both diseased and normal airways. Because treatment of NTM infection is compli-

cated, it is important that the diagnosis be certain. The American Thoracic Society has formulated the following minimal guidelines for the diagnosis of pulmonary NTM disease: "evidence, such as an infiltrate visible on a chest roentgenogram, of disease, the cause of which has not been determined by careful clinical and laboratory studies, and . . . isolation of multiple colonies of the same strain of mycobacteria repeatedly, usually in the absence of other pathogens." For patients who have pulmonary infiltrates but not cavities, these criteria may not be specific enough; some patients are found to have cleared NTM after a 1-month trial of bronchial hygiene alone (inhalation of saline and bronchodilators to induce cough and sputum production). The detection by computed tomography of bronchiectases and nodular infiltrates in the same lobe may be particularly suggestive of NTM infection.

℞ TREATMENT

Lung disease due to NTM may be managed by follow-up without treatment, by resection, or by drug therapy. No randomized trial has determined which is the best option. In retrospectively analyzed case series, patients undergoing surgery have had a better outcome than those treated only with drugs. However, selection bias has probably influenced these results since patients with extensive lung disease are poor candidates for surgery.

Patients with minimal disease (in particular, HIV-infected patients with NTM in sputum or bronchoalveolar lavage fluid but little evidence of lung damage) do not need treatment at all. Likewise, NTM disease may present as a solitary pulmonary nodule that, once resected (to confirm or exclude a diagnosis of cancer), requires no further drug treatment.

Most other patients with pulmonary NTM disease are treated with antimicrobials; in addition, they may or may not undergo surgery. The drugs available for the treatment of infection with *M. avium* or *M. intracellulare* have already been discussed. The regimens recommended for disseminated MAC infection are preferred, although large doses of clarithromycin are often poorly tolerated by elderly patients. *M. intracellulare* may be easier to treat and eradicate than *M. avium.* In two small open studies, single-agent treatment with clarithromycin (500 mg bid) led to improvements detected by chest radiography and sputum culture.

Indications for surgery are difficult to establish but include a disappointing response to antibiotics, the presence of localized disease, and the absence of contraindications (especially impaired respiratory functions). Ideally, drug treatment should begin before surgery and should render the sputum negative by the time of the operation.

In contrast to MAC organisms, *M. kansasii* is predictably sensitive to antituberculosis agents. Treatment should consist of isoniazid (300 mg/d), rifampin (600 mg/d), and ethambutol (15 to 25 mg/kg per day), whether or not the patient is infected with HIV; the optimal duration of therapy is unknown, but most patients have been treated for 18 to 24 months. Recent data suggest that 12 months may suffice. Sulfamethoxazole is recommended for the occasional patient whose infection relapses after *M. kansasii* becomes resistant to rifampin.

LYMPHADENITIS NTM are among the causes of localized lymphadenitis. This disease occurs mostly in children between the ages of 1 and 5 years. Painless swelling of one node or a group of nodes usually affects the anterior cervical chain. Nodes may rapidly increase in size, with the formation of fistulas to the skin. *M. scrofulaceum* or MAC organisms most commonly cause NTM lymphadenitis, although many other species may be involved. Once tuberculosis has been excluded, the treatment of choice is excision without chemotherapy. When excision is dangerous because of proximity to the facial nerve, aspiration combined with chemotherapy may be effective.

SKIN DISEASE DUE TO NTM Swimming-Pool and Fish-Tank Granuloma Between 1 week and 2 months (usually 2 to 3 weeks) after contact with contaminated tropical fish tanks, swimming pools, or saltwater fish, a small violet nodule or pustule may appear at a site of minor trauma. This lesion may evolve to form a crusted ulcer or small abscess or may remain warty. Lesions are multiple and disseminated on occasion—particularly, but not exclusively, in immunosuppressed patients. The causative organism is *M. marinum*. The patient's clinical history, combined with the isolation of *M. marinum* after biopsy and culture, establishes the diagnosis. Lesions often heal spontaneously. In cases of persistence or dissemination, rifampin (300 to 600 mg/d) in combination with ethambutol (15 to 25 mg/kg per day), trimethoprim-sulfamethoxazole (160/800 mg/bid), or minocycline (100 mg/d) may be tried for a period of at least 3 months. Very rarely, a similar clinical picture is produced by *M. gordonae*, a frequently isolated but usually nonpathogenic species.

Buruli Ulcer In many tropical areas throughout the world, *M. ulcerans* may cause an itching nodule on the arms or legs, which then breaks down to form a shallow ulcer of variable size. The course of this condition is usually prolonged. *M. ulcerans* is difficult to culture; plates need to be incubated at low temperature. Excision constitutes the usual therapy. Treatment with rifampin, clofazimine, or trimethoprim-sulfamethoxazole has met with variable success.

NTM Skin Disease in Patients with AIDS and Other Deficits of Cell-Mediated Immunity MAC organisms, which frequently cause disseminated disease with positive blood cultures in AIDS, also are rarely associated with heterogeneous skin manifestations, such as nodules, ulcers, areas of erythema, pustules, abscesses, or panniculitis. Skin biopsies and blood cultures establish the diagnosis.

In contrast to MAC organisms, *M. haemophilum* has a tendency to involve the skin, bones, joints, and lungs, although most patients also have positive blood cultures. Skin lesions are nodular, may ulcerate, and are disseminated. In the absence of specific data, treatment should follow the guidelines for MAC infection.

NTM INFECTIONS OF SOFT TISSUE, TENDONS, BONES, AND JOINTS Infections Linked to Injections and Surgery Occasionally, mycobacteria are isolated from nodular skin lesions of hospitalized patients, particularly those who are immunosuppressed; in some instances there is associated lymphatic spread. Many cases are linked to injection; diabetic patients are at especially high risk. In ophthalmology, mycobacteria may cause keratitis and corneal ulceration after surgery or injury. Epidemics of mycobacterial infection following cardiac surgery have been linked to contaminated ice packs and contaminated porcine heart valves. These infections are usually due to *M. fortuitum*, *M. chelonae*, or *M. abscessus*, which are referred to collectively as the *M. fortuitum* complex. These are the so-called rapidly growing mycobacteria: colonies on solid medium appear 3 to 7 days after inoculation. As organisms may fail to grow at 37°C, incubation at 30 to 33°C is recommended. These mycobacteria are notoriously resistant to most antituberculosis drugs. Debridement is best combined with administration of two or three of the antibiotics mentioned in Table 173-1.

Infections of Tendons, Joints, and Bones In rare cases, mycobacteria invade deep tissues after direct inoculation, via contiguous spread from superficial sites of infection, or through the bloodstream. MAC organisms and *M. ulcerans* are most often cited in these instances. *M. szulgai* seems to be involved particularly frequently in olecranon bursitis.

BIBLIOGRAPHY

Diagnosis and treatment of disease caused by nontuberculous mycobacteria. Am Rev Respir Dis 142:940, 1990

HOOVER DR et al: Clinical manifestations of AIDS in the era of *Pneumocystis* prophylaxis. Multicenter AIDS Cohort Study. N Engl J Med 329:1922, 1993

HORSBURGH CR: *Mycobacterium avium* complex infection in the acquired immunodeficiency syndrome. N Engl J Med 324:1332, 1991

ISEMAN MD: *Mycobacterium avium* complex and the normal host: The other side of the coin. N Engl J Med 321:896, 1989

NOLTE FS, METCHOCK B: Mycobacteria, in *Manual of Clinical Microbiology*, 7th ed, PR Murray et al (eds). Washington, ASM Press, 1995, pp 400–437

WOLINSKY E: Mycobacterial lymphadenitis in children: A prospective study of 105 nontuberculous cases with long-term follow-up. Clin Infect Dis 20:954, 1995

SECTION 9

SPIROCHETAL DISEASES

---

174 *Sheila A. Lukehart, King K. Holmes*

SYPHILIS

DEFINITION Syphilis, a chronic systemic infection caused by *Treponema pallidum* subspecies *pallidum*, is usually sexually transmitted and is characterized by episodes of active disease interrupted by periods of latency. After an incubation period averaging 3 weeks, a primary lesion appears, often associated with regional lymphadenopathy. A secondary bacteremic stage, associated with generalized mucocutaneous lesions and generalized lymphadenopathy, is followed by a latent period of subclinical infection lasting many years. In about one-third of untreated cases, the tertiary stage is characterized by progressive destructive mucocutaneous, musculoskeletal, or parenchymal lesions; aortitis; or symptomatic central nervous system (CNS) disease.

ETIOLOGY Schaudinn and Hoffman discovered *T. pallidum* in syphilitic material in 1905. *T. pallidum* is one of the many spiral-shaped microorganisms that propel themselves by spinning around their longitudinal axis. The Spirochaetales include three genera that are pathogenic for humans and for a variety of other animals: *Leptospira*, whose species cause human leptospirosis; *Borrelia*, including *Borrelia recurrentis* and *Borrelia vincentii*, which cause relapsing fever and Vincent's angina, respectively, as well as *Borrelia burgdorferi*, the causative agent of Lyme disease; and *Treponema*, whose members are responsible for the diseases known as treponematoses. The genus *Treponema* includes *T. pallidum* subspecies *pallidum* (hereafter called *T. pallidum*), which causes venereal syphilis; *T. pallidum* subspecies *pertenue*, which causes yaws; *T. pallidum* subspecies *endemicum*, which causes endemic syphilis or bejel; and *Treponema carateum*, which causes pinta (see Chap. 175). Other *Treponema* species found in the human mouth, genital mucosa, and gastrointestinal tract have no proven pathogenic role. These spirochetes can be confused with *T. pallidum* on dark-field examination. Riviere and co-workers have described a new oral treponeme that is very closely related to *T. pallidum* antigenically and is significantly associated with periodontitis and acute necrotizing ulcerative gingivitis. Its etiologic role in these gum diseases is unknown.

T. pallidum, a thin, delicate organism with 6 to 14 spirals and tapered ends, measures 6 to 15 μm in total length and 0.2 μm in width. The cytoplasm is surrounded by a trilaminar cytoplasmic membrane, which in turn is surrounded by a delicate peptidoglycan layer providing some structural rigidity. This layer is surrounded by a lipid-rich outer membrane that contains relatively few integral membrane proteins, although a putative surface-exposed porin molecule was recently described. Six endoflagella wind around the cell body in a space between the inner cell wall and the outer membrane and may be the elements responsible for motility. None of the four pathogenic treponemes has yet been cultured in vitro in quantity, and no convincing genetic, morphologic, serologic, or metabolic differences among them has been discerned. They are distinguished primarily according

134,255 in 1990. The number of new cases of infectious syphilis reached a peak in 1947 and then fell to approximately 6000 in 1956; since then, a rather steady increase in infectious syphilis has been punctuated by four cycles of 7 to 10 years, each with a rapid rise and fall in incidence (with peaks in 1965, 1975, 1982, and 1990). Since 1990, the number of reported cases of infectious syphilis has again declined by more than 50 percent. In 1994, there were 20,627 reported cases of primary and secondary syphilis and 32,012 cases of early latent syphilis.

The populations at highest risk for acquiring syphilis have changed. Between 1977 and 1982, approximately half of all patients with early syphilis in the United States were homosexual or bisexual men. Largely because of changing sexual practices in this population due to the AIDS epidemic, this proportion has decreased. The most recent epidemic of syphilis predominantly involved black heterosexual men and women (Fig. 174-2) and occurred largely in urban areas, where infectious syphilis has been significantly correlated with the exchange of sex for "crack" cocaine. The incidence of syphilis peaks at 15 to 34 years of age. The reported incidence of syphilis is much higher among blacks than in other ethnic groups and is higher in urban than in rural areas. In addition, there is a striking concentration of cases in the southeastern United States.

The incidence of congenital syphilis roughly parallels that of infectious syphilis in females. The number of reported cases of congenital syphilis in infants ≤1 year of age was lowest (107 cases) in 1978, when infectious syphilis was most prevalent among homosexual and bisexual men. The dramatic increase in the incidence of primary and secondary syphilis among women from 1986 to 1990 resulted in a proportionate increase in the number of infants born with congenital syphilis—to 3275 infants in 1991. It is important to note, however, that the case definition for congenital syphilis was broadened in 1989 and now includes all live or stillborn infants delivered to women with untreated or inadequately treated syphilis at delivery.

Approximately one of every two individuals named as sexual contacts of persons with infectious syphilis becomes infected. Many sexual contacts will already have developed manifestations of syphilis when they are first seen, and about 30 percent of apparently uninfected contacts who are examined within 30 days of exposure actually have incubating infection and will later develop infectious syphilis if not treated. Thus, the identification and "epidemiologic" treatment of all recently exposed sexual contacts constitute an important aspect of syphilis control. Also important is the identification of infected persons by serologic testing of pregnant women, persons admitted to hospitals, military inductees, and persons undergoing examination in physicians' offices. Still controversial are laws and regulations requiring routine premarital serologic testing for syphilis, where—though national data are not available—the yield is undoubtedly lower.

NATURAL COURSE AND PATHOGENESIS OF UNTREATED SYPHILIS

T. pallidum rapidly penetrates intact mucous membranes or microscopic abrasions in skin and within a few hours enters the lymphatics and blood to produce systemic infection and metastatic foci long before the appearance of a primary lesion. Blood from a patient with incubating or early syphilis is infectious. The generation time of *T. pallidum* during early active disease in vivo is estimated to be 30 to 33 h, and the incubation period of syphilis is inversely proportional to the number of organisms inoculated. The concentration of treponemes generally reaches at least 10^7 per gram of tissue before the appearance of a clinical lesion. Experimental infection

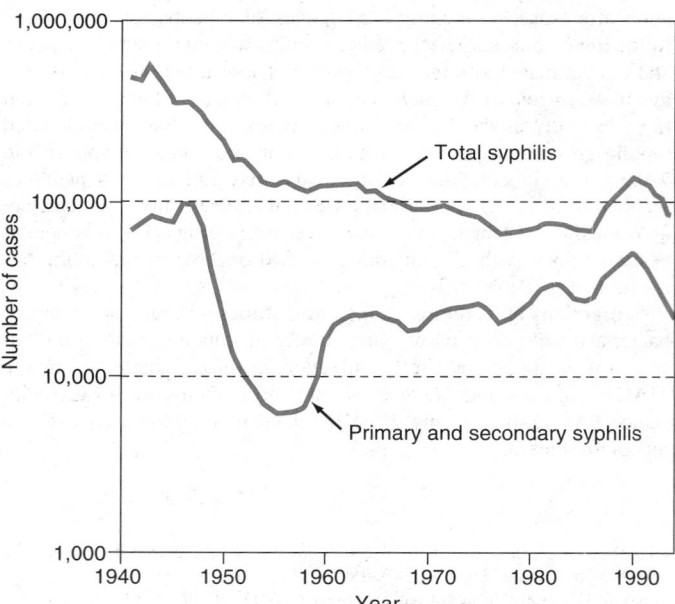

FIGURE 174-1 Number of cases of total syphilis and primary and secondary syphilis reported annually in the United States, 1940–1994. (*Data from the Centers for Disease Control and Prevention.*)

to the clinical syndrome they produce. The only known natural host for *T. pallidum* is the human. *T. pallidum* can infect many mammals, but only humans, higher apes, and a few laboratory animals regularly develop syphilitic lesions. Virulent strains of *T. pallidum* are grown and maintained in rabbits.

EPIDEMIOLOGY Nearly all cases of syphilis are acquired by sexual contact with infectious lesions (i.e., the chancre, mucous patch, skin rash, or condyloma latum). Less common modes of transmission include nonsexual personal contact and infection in utero or following blood transfusions.

The total number of cases of syphilis reported annually in the United States (Fig. 174-1) fell steadily from 575,593 in 1943 to a low of 64,621 in 1987—an 88 percent decrease—but then increased to

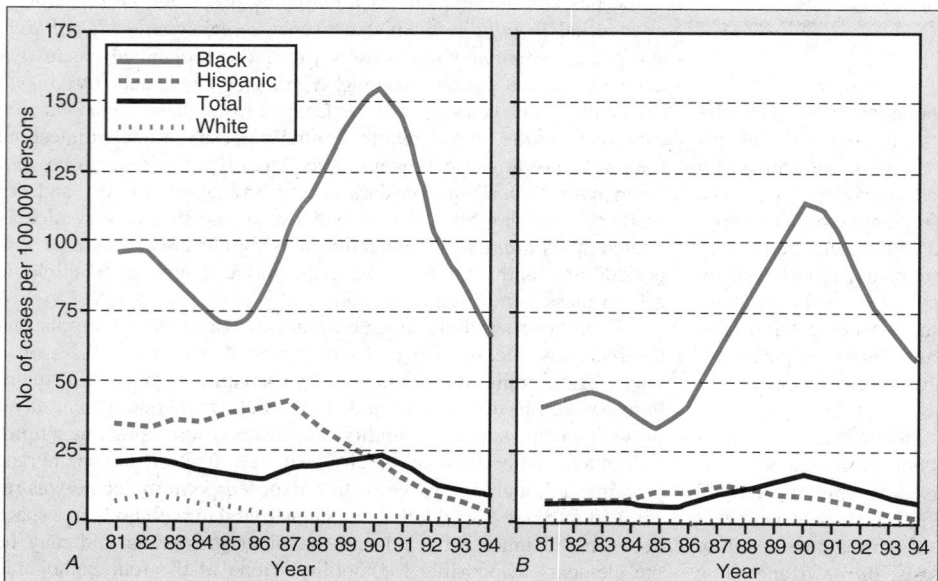

FIGURE 174-2 Rates of primary and secondary syphilis among (*A*) men and (*B*) women in the United States, by ethnic origin, 1981–1994. (*Data from the Centers for Disease Control and Prevention.*)

of rabbits or humans with very few treponemes leads to a discernible lesion only after several weeks, although histopathologic changes are evident earlier. In contrast, intradermal injection of 10^6 organisms usually produces a lesion within 72 h. On the basis of intradermal injection of graded doses of *T. pallidum* into eight volunteers, the 50 percent infectious dose was calculated to be 57 organisms. The median incubation period in humans (about 21 days) suggests an average inoculum of 500 to 1000 infectious organisms for naturally acquired disease. The incubation period (from inoculation until the primary lesion becomes discernible) rarely exceeds 6 weeks. Subcurative therapy during the incubation period may delay the onset of the primary lesion, but it is not certain that such treatment reduces the probability that symptomatic disease will ultimately develop.

The primary lesion appears at the site of inoculation, usually persists for 2 to 6 weeks, and then heals spontaneously. Histopathologic examination of primary lesions shows perivascular infiltration, chiefly by lymphocytes (including CD8 + and CD4 + cells), plasma cells, and macrophages, with capillary endothelial proliferation and subsequent obliteration of small blood vessels. The CD4 + infiltration displays a T_H1-type cytokine profile consistent with the activation of macrophages. At this time *T. pallidum* is demonstrable in the chancre in spaces between epithelial cells; within invaginations or phagosomes of epithelial cells, fibroblasts, plasma cells, and the endothelial cells of small capillaries; within lymphatic channels; and in the regional lymph nodes. Phagocytosis of organisms by activated macrophages ultimately causes their destruction, which results in spontaneous resolution of the chancre.

The generalized parenchymal, constitutional, and mucocutaneous manifestations of secondary syphilis usually appear about 6 to 8 weeks after healing of the chancre, although 15 percent of patients with secondary syphilis still have persisting or healing chancres. In other patients, secondary lesions may appear several months after the chancre has healed, and some patients may enter the latent stage without ever recognizing secondary lesions. The histopathologic features of secondary maculopapular skin lesions are hyperkeratosis of the epidermis, capillary proliferation with endothelial swelling in the superficial corium, and dermal papillae with transmigration of polymorphonuclear leukocytes and, in the deeper corium, perivascular infiltration by monocytes, plasma cells, and lymphocytes. Treponemes are found in many tissues, including the aqueous humor of the eye and the cerebrospinal fluid (CSF). Invasion of the CNS by *T. pallidum* occurs during the first weeks or months of infection, and CSF abnormalities are detected in as many as 40 percent of patients during the secondary stage. Clinical hepatitis and immune complex–induced membranous glomerulonephritis are relatively rare but recognized manifestations of secondary syphilis; liver function tests may yield abnormal results in up to a quarter of patients with early syphilis. Generalized nontender lymphadenopathy is noted in 85 percent of patients with secondary syphilis. The paradoxical appearance of secondary manifestations despite high titers of antibody (including immobilizing antibody) to *T. pallidum* is unexplained. Secondary lesions subside within 2 to 6 weeks, and the infection enters the latent stage, which is detectable only by serologic testing. In the preantibiotic era, up to 25 percent of untreated patients experienced one or more subsequent generalized or localized mucocutaneous relapses during the first 2 to 4 years after infection. Since 50 percent of such infectious relapses occur during the first year, identification and examination of sexual contacts are most important for patients with syphilis of less than 1 year's duration. Recurrent generalized rash is now rare.

In the preantibiotic era, about one-third of patients with untreated latent syphilis developed clinically apparent tertiary disease; today, in industrialized countries, specific treatment and coincidental therapy of early and latent syphilis have all but eliminated tertiary disease except for sporadic cases of neurosyphilis in persons infected with human immunodeficiency virus (HIV). In the past, the most common type of tertiary disease was the gumma, a usually benign granulomatous lesion. Today, gummas are very uncommon. Tertiary lesions are caused by obliterative small-vessel endarteritis, usually involving the vasa vasorum of the ascending aorta and less often involving the CNS.

Asymptomatic CNS involvement is demonstrable in up to 25 percent of patients with late latent syphilis. The factors that contribute to the development and progression of tertiary disease are unknown.

The course of untreated syphilis was studied retrospectively in a group of nearly 2000 patients with primary or secondary syphilis diagnosed clinically (the Oslo Study, 1891–1951); prospectively in 431 black men with seropositive latent syphilis of 3 or more years' duration (the notorious Tuskegee Study, 1932–1972); and retrospectively in a review of 198 autopsies of patients with untreated syphilis (the Rosahn Study, 1917–1942).

In the Oslo Study, 24 percent of patients developed relapsing secondary lesions within 4 years, and 28 percent eventually developed one or more manifestations of tertiary syphilis. Cardiovascular syphilis, including aortitis, was detected in 10 percent of patients, none of whom had been infected before age 15; 7 percent of patients developed symptomatic neurosyphilis, and 16 percent developed benign tertiary syphilis (gummas of the skin, mucous membranes, and skeleton). Syphilis was the primary cause of death in 15 percent of men and 8 percent of women. Cardiovascular syphilis was documented in 35 percent of men and 22 percent of women who eventually came to autopsy. In general, serious late complications were nearly twice as common among men as among women.

The Tuskegee Study showed that the death rate among untreated black men with syphilis (25 to 50 years old) was 17 percent higher than that among uninfected subjects and that 30 percent of all deaths were attributable to cardiovascular or CNS syphilis. The ethical issues eventually raised by this study, begun in the preantibiotic era but continuing into the early 1970s, had a major influence on the development of current guidelines for human medical experimentation, and the history of the study may still contribute to a reluctance of some African-Americans to participate as subjects in clinical research. By far the most important factor in increased mortality was cardiovascular syphilis. Anatomic evidence of aortitis was found in 40 to 60 percent of autopsied subjects with syphilis (versus 15 percent of control subjects), while CNS syphilis was found in only 4 percent. Rates of hypertension were also higher among the infected subjects.

These studies each showed that about one-third of patients with untreated syphilis develop clinical or pathologic evidence of tertiary syphilis, that about one-fourth die as a direct result of tertiary syphilis, and that there is additional excess mortality not directly attributable to tertiary syphilis.

MANIFESTATIONS **Primary Syphilis** The typical primary chancre usually begins as a single painless papule that rapidly becomes eroded and usually becomes indurated, with a characteristic cartilaginous consistency on palpation of the edge and base of the ulcer (Fig. 174-3). In heterosexual men the chancre is usually located on the

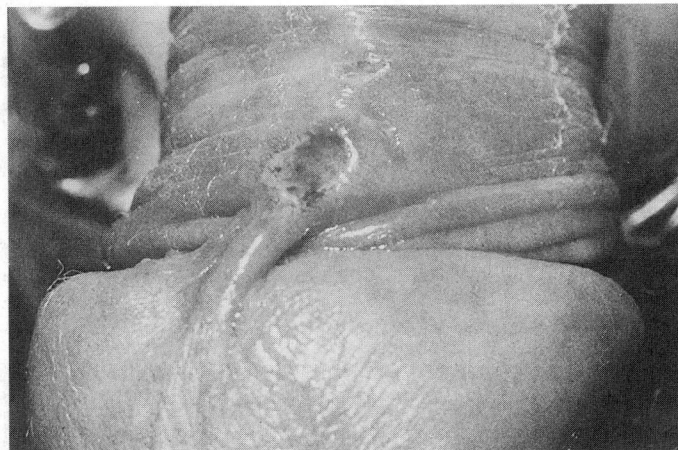

FIGURE 174-3 Primary syphilitic chancre on the penis. (*From E Stoltz: Sexually Transmitted Diseases. Rotterdam, Boehringer Ingelheim, 1977.*)

penis, whereas in homosexual men it is often found in the anal canal or rectum, in the mouth, or on the external genitalia. In women, common primary sites are the cervix and labia. Consequently, primary syphilis goes unrecognized in women and homosexual men more often than in heterosexual men.

Atypical primary lesions are common. The clinical appearance depends on the number of treponemes inoculated and on the immunologic status of the patient. A large inoculum produces a dark-field–positive ulcerative lesion in nonimmune volunteers but may produce a small dark-field–negative papule, an asymptomatic but seropositive latent infection, or no response at all in individuals with a history of syphilis. A small inoculum may produce only a papular lesion, even in nonimmune individuals. Therefore, syphilis should be considered even in the evaluation of trivial or atypical dark-field–negative genital lesions. The genital lesions that most commonly must be differentiated from those of primary syphilis include traumatic superinfected lesions, lesions of herpes simplex virus infection (see Chap. 184), and lesions of chancroid (see Chap. 152). *Primary genital herpes* may produce inguinal adenopathy, but the nodes are tender and the lesions consist of multiple painful vesicles, which later ulcerate and often are accompanied by systemic symptoms, including fever. *Recurrent genital herpes* typically begins with a unilateral cluster of painful vesicles, usually without associated adenopathy. *Chancroid* produces painful, superficial, exudative, nonindurated ulcers, more often multiple than in syphilis; adenopathy is common, can be either unilateral or bilateral, is tender, and may be suppurative.

Regional lymphadenopathy usually accompanies the primary syphilitic lesion, appearing within 1 week of the onset of the lesion. The nodes are firm, nonsuppurative, and painless. Inguinal lymphadenopathy is bilateral and may occur with anal as well as with external genital chancres, since lymphatic drainage of the anus involves inguinal nodes. Rectal chancres result in perirectal lymphadenopathy, while chancres of the cervix and vagina result in iliac or perirectal adenopathy. The chancre generally heals within 4 to 6 weeks (range, 2 to 12 weeks), but lymphadenopathy may persist for months.

Secondary Syphilis   The protean manifestations of the secondary stage usually include localized or diffuse symmetric mucocutaneous lesions and generalized nontender lymphadenopathy. The healing primary chancre is still present in 15 percent of cases. The skin rash consists of macular, papular, papulosquamous, and occasionally pustular syphilides; often more than one form is present simultaneously. The eruption may be very subtle. Approximately 25 percent of patients with a discernible rash of secondary syphilis may be unaware that they have dermatologic manifestations. Initial lesions are bilaterally symmetric, pale red or pink, nonpruritic, discrete, round macules that measure 5 to 10 mm in diameter and are distributed on the trunk and

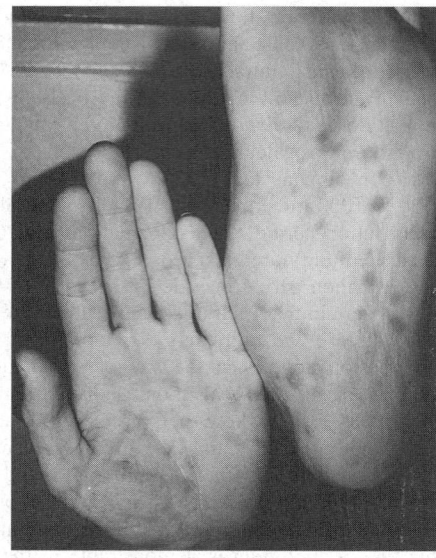

FIGURE 174-5   Secondary syphilitic rash on the palm and sole. [*From R Roddy, in Gynecology and Obstetrics, JW Sciarra (ed). New York, Harper & Row, 1985.*]

proximal extremities (Fig. 174-4). After several days or weeks, red papular lesions 3 to 10 mm in diameter also appear. These lesions, which may progress to necrotic lesions (resembling pustules) in association with increasing endarteritis and perivascular mononuclear infiltration, are distributed widely, frequently involve the palms and soles (Fig. 174-5), and may occur on the face and scalp. Tiny papular *follicular syphilides* involving hair follicles may result in patchy alopecia (alopecia areata), with loss of scalp hair, eyebrows, or beard in up to 5 percent of cases. Progressive endarteritis obliterans and ischemia result in superficial scaling of papules (*papulosquamous syphilides*) and eventually may lead to central necrosis (*pustular syphilides*).

In warm, moist, intertriginous areas, including the perianal area, vulva, scrotum, inner thighs, axillae, and skin under pendulous breasts, papules can enlarge and become eroded to produce broad, moist, pink or gray-white, highly infectious lesions called *condylomata lata*; these lesions develop in 10 percent of patients with secondary syphilis. Superficial mucosal erosions, called *mucous patches*, occur in 10 to 15 percent of patients and may involve the lips, oral mucosa, tongue (Fig. 174-6), palate, pharynx, vulva and vagina, glans penis, or inner prepuce. The typical mucous patch is a painless silver-gray erosion surrounded by a red periphery. During relapses of secondary syphilis, condylomata lata are particularly common, and skin lesions tend to be asymmetrically distributed and more infiltrated, resembling skin

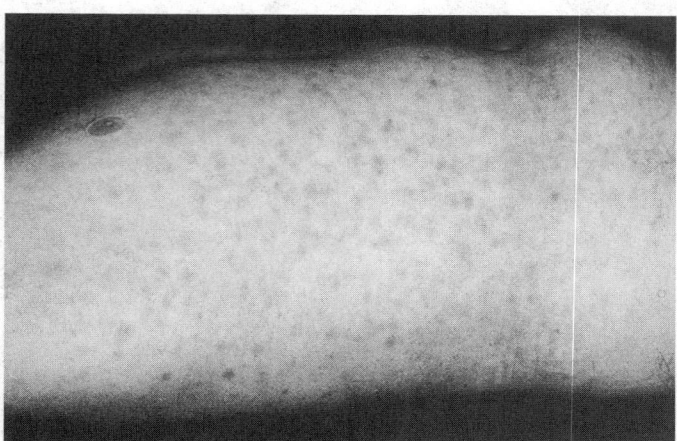

FIGURE 174-4   Maculopapular rash of secondary syphilis. (*From E Stoltz: Sexually Transmitted Diseases. Rotterdam, Boehringer Ingelheim, 1977.*)

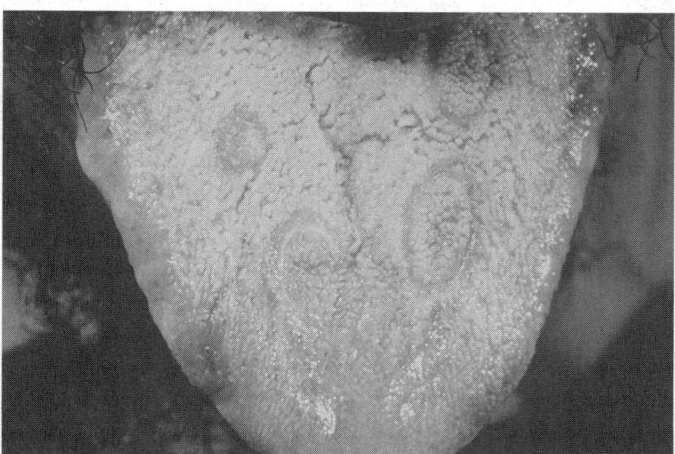

FIGURE 174-6   Mucous patches on the tongue of a patient with secondary syphilis. [*From R Roddy, in Sexually Transmitted Diseases, 2d ed. KK Holmes et al (eds). New York, McGraw-Hill, 1990.*]

lesions of late syphilis. These characteristics may reflect increasing cellular immunity.

Constitutional symptoms that may accompany or precede secondary syphilis include sore throat (15 to 30 percent), fever (5 to 8 percent), weight loss (2 to 20 percent), malaise (25 percent), anorexia (2 to 10 percent), headache (10 percent), and meningismus (5 percent). *Acute meningitis* occurs in only 1 to 2 percent of cases, but numbers of cells and levels of protein in CSF are increased in 30 percent of cases or more. *T. pallidum* has been recovered from CSF during primary and secondary syphilis in 30 percent of cases; this finding is often but not always associated with other CSF abnormalities.

Less common complications of secondary syphilis include hepatitis, nephropathy, gastrointestinal involvement (hypertrophic gastritis, patchy proctitis, ulcerative colitis, or a rectosigmoid mass), arthritis, and periostitis. Ocular findings that suggest secondary syphilis include otherwise unexplained pupillary abnormalities, optic neuritis, and a retinitis pigmentosa syndrome as well as the classic iritis (especially granulomatous iritis) or uveitis. The diagnosis of secondary syphilis is often considered only after the patient fails to respond to steroid therapy. Anterior uveitis has been reported in 5 to 10 percent of patients with secondary syphilis, and *T. pallidum* has been demonstrated in the aqueous humor from these patients. *Syphilitic hepatitis* is distinguished by an unusually high serum level of alkaline phosphatase and by a nonspecific histologic appearance that is unlike that of viral hepatitis and includes moderate inflammation with polymorphonuclear leukocytes and lymphocytes, some hepatocellular damage, and no cholestasis. *Renal involvement* produces proteinuria associated with an acute nephrotic syndrome (or rarely with hemorrhagic glomerulonephritis) and is characterized by subepithelial electron-dense deposits and glomerular immune complexes—findings suggesting immune-complex glomerulonephritis.

Latent Syphilis Positive reaginic and specific treponemal antibody tests for syphilis, together with a normal CSF examination and the absence of clinical manifestations of syphilis, indicate a diagnosis of latent syphilis. The diagnosis is often suspected on the basis of a history of primary or secondary lesions, a history of exposure to syphilis, or the delivery of an infant with congenital syphilis. A previous negative serologic test or a history of lesions or exposure may help establish the duration of latent infection. *Early latent* syphilis encompasses the first year after infection, while *late latent* syphilis (beginning 1 year or longer after infection in the untreated patient) is associated with relative immunity to infectious relapse and with increasing resistance to reinfection. *T. pallidum* may still seed the bloodstream intermittently during this stage. Pregnant women with latent syphilis may infect the fetus in utero. Moreover, syphilis has been transmitted through the transfusion of blood from patients with latent syphilis of many years' duration. It was previously thought that untreated late latent syphilis had three possible outcomes: (1) it could persist throughout the lifetime of the infected individual, (2) it could end in the development of late syphilis, or (3) it could end with the spontaneous cure of infection, with reversion of serologic tests to negative. It is now apparent, however, that the more sensitive treponemal antibody tests rarely, if ever, become negative without treatment. About 70 percent of untreated patients with latent syphilis never develop clinically evident late syphilis, but the occurrence of spontaneous cure is in doubt.

Late Syphilis The slowly progressive inflammatory disease leading to tertiary manifestations begins early during the pathogenesis of syphilis, although these manifestations may not become clinically apparent for years. Early syphilitic aortitis becomes evident soon after secondary lesions subside, and patients who develop CSF abnormalities during the early stages of syphilis appear to be at highest risk of late neurologic complications.

Asymptomatic neurosyphilis CNS syphilis represents a continuum comprising early invasion, usually within the first weeks or months of infection, and asymptomatic involvement, which may or may not lead to neurologic manifestations. Traditionally, the diagnosis of asymptomatic neurosyphilis has been made in patients who no longer have manifestations of primary or secondary syphilis, who lack

neurologic symptoms and signs, and who have certain CSF abnormalities. Such abnormalities are found in up to one-quarter of patients with untreated late latent syphilis, and it is these patients who are known to be at risk for neurologic complications. However, in early syphilis, *T. pallidum* can be isolated from CSF even in the absence of other CSF abnormalities. In approximately 40 percent of patients with primary or secondary syphilis, *T. pallidum* can be isolated from the CSF and/or abnormalities of the CSF consistent with asymptomatic neurosyphilis can develop. Although the therapeutic implications of these findings in early syphilis are uncertain, it seems appropriate to conclude that even patients with early syphilis who have such findings do indeed have asymptomatic neurosyphilis. In patients with untreated asymptomatic neurosyphilis, the overall cumulative probability of progression to clinical neurosyphilis is about 20 percent in the first 10 years but increases with time; the likelihood is highest among patients with the greatest degree of pleocytosis or protein elevation. Patients with untreated latent syphilis and normal CSF probably run no risk of subsequently developing neurosyphilis.

Symptomatic neurosyphilis Although mixed features are common, the major clinical categories of symptomatic neurosyphilis include meningeal, meningovascular, and parenchymatous syphilis. The last category includes general paresis and tabes dorsalis. The interval from infection to onset of symptoms is a few months to 20 years for meningeal syphilis (usually less than a year) and for meningovascular syphilis (average, 7 years), 20 years for general paresis, and 25 to 30 years for tabes dorsalis. However, symptomatic neurosyphilis, particularly in the antibiotic era, often presents not as a classic picture but rather as mixed and subtle or incomplete syndromes.

Meningeal syphilis may involve either the brain or the spinal cord, and patients may present with headache, nausea, vomiting, neck stiffness, cranial nerve palsies, seizures, and changes in mental status. *Meningovascular syphilis* reflects diffuse inflammation of the pia and arachnoid together with evidence of focal or widespread arterial involvement of small, medium, or large vessels. The most common presentation is a stroke syndrome involving the middle cerebral artery of a relatively young adult; however, unlike the usual thrombotic or embolic stroke syndrome of sudden onset, meningovascular syphilis often becomes manifest after a subacute encephalitic prodrome, with headaches, vertigo, insomnia, and psychological abnormalities, which is followed by a gradually progressive vascular syndrome.

The manifestations of *general paresis* reflect widespread parenchymal damage and include abnormalities corresponding to the mnemonic *paresis*: *p*ersonality, *a*ffect, *r*eflexes (hyperactive), *e*ye (e.g., Argyll Robertson pupils), *s*ensorium (illusions, delusions, hallucinations), *i*ntellect (a decrease in recent memory and in the capacity for orientation, calculations, judgment, and insight), and *s*peech. *Tabes dorsalis* presents as symptoms and signs of demyelination of the posterior columns, dorsal roots, and dorsal root ganglia. Symptoms include ataxic wide-based gait and footslap; paresthesias; bladder disturbances; impotence; areflexia; and loss of position, deep pain, and temperature sensations. Trophic joint degeneration (Charcot's joints) and perforating ulceration of the feet can result from loss of pain sensation. The small, irregular Argyll Robertson pupil, a feature of both tabes dorsalis and paresis, reacts to accommodation but not to light. *Optic atrophy* also occurs frequently in association with tabes.

Cardiovascular syphilis Cardiovascular manifestations are attributable to endarteritis obliterans of the vasa vasorum, which provide the blood supply to large vessels. This condition produces medial necrosis with destruction of elastic tissue, particularly in the ascending and transverse segments of the aortic arch, resulting in uncomplicated aortitis, aortic regurgitation, saccular aneurysm, or coronary ostial stenosis. Symptoms appear from 10 to 40 years after infection. Cardiovascular complications occur more often and at an earlier age among men than among women and may be more common among blacks than among whites. In the preantibiotic era, symptomatic cardiovascular complications developed in about 10 percent of persons with late untreated syphilis, and aortic regurgitation was two to four times as common as aneurysm. However, syphilitic aortitis was demonstrated at autopsy in about one-half of black men with untreated syphilis.

Linear calcification of the ascending aorta on chest x-ray films suggests asymptomatic syphilitic aortitis, as arteriosclerosis seldom produces this sign. Aortic dilation and a tambour quality to the sound of aortic closure are unreliable signs of aortitis. Syphilitic aneurysms—usually saccular, occasionally fusiform—do not lead to dissection. Approximately 1 in 10 aortic aneurysms of syphilitic origin involve the abdominal aorta, but these aneurysms tend to occur above the renal arteries, whereas arteriosclerotic abdominal aneurysms usually are found below the renal arteries. With increasing age, the nervous system is also affected in up to 40 percent of patients with cardiovascular syphilis.

Late lesions of the eyes   Iritis associated with pain, photophobia, and dimness of vision or chorioretinitis occurs not only during secondary syphilis but also as a relatively common manifestation of late syphilis. Adhesions of the iris to the anterior lens may produce a fixed pupil, not to be confused with Argyll Robertson pupil.

Late benign syphilis (gumma)   Gummas may be multiple or diffuse but are usually solitary lesions that range from microscopic size to several centimeters in diameter. From a histologic perspective, gummas consist of a granulomatous inflammation with a central area of necrosis surrounded by mononuclear, epithelioid, and fibroblastic cells, occasional giant cells, and perivasculitis. Although rarely demonstrated microscopically, *T. pallidum* has reportedly been recovered from these lesions. The most commonly involved sites include the skin and skeletal system, the mouth and upper respiratory tract, the larynx, the liver, and the stomach; however, any organ may be involved. Gummas of the skin produce painless and indurated nodular, papulosquamous, or ulcerative lesions that form characteristic circles or arcs, with peripheral hyperpigmentation. Gummas are usually indolent and may heal spontaneously with scarring, but they may also be explosive in onset and are often destructive. These lesions may resemble those of many other chronic granulomatous conditions, including tuberculosis and sarcoidosis, leprosy, and deep fungal infections. Skeletal gummas most frequently involve the long bones of the legs, although any bone may be affected. Trauma may predispose a specific site to involvement. Presenting symptoms usually include focal pain and tenderness. Radiographic abnormalities with advanced gummas of bone include periostitis or destructive or sclerosing osteitis. Upper respiratory gummas can lead to perforation of the nasal septum or palate. Gummatous hepatitis may produce epigastric pain and tenderness as well as low-grade fever and may be associated with splenomegaly and anemia.

The histopathology and extensive tissue necrosis associated with gummas suggest delayed hypersensitivity to *T. pallidum*. Certain individuals appear to develop an exaggerated delayed-hypersensitivity response to *T. pallidum*, which presumably is mediated by sensitized T lymphocytes and macrophages. Since the histologic changes may be suggestive but are nonspecific, the diagnosis of late benign syphilis is confirmed by serologic testing and by therapeutic trial. Treatment with penicillin results in rapid healing of active gummatous lesions.

Congenital Syphilis   Transmission of *T. pallidum* from a syphilitic woman to her fetus across the placenta may occur at any stage of pregnancy, but the lesions of congenital syphilis generally develop after the fourth month of gestation, when fetal immunologic competence begins to develop. This timing suggests that the pathogenesis of congenital syphilis depends on the immune response of the host rather than on a direct toxic effect of *T. pallidum*. The risk of infection of the fetus during untreated early maternal syphilis is estimated to be 75 to 95 percent, decreasing to about 35 percent for maternal syphilis of longer than 2 years' duration; some risk of fetal infection apparently continues throughout late latent maternal syphilis. Adequate treatment of the mother before the 16th week of pregnancy should prevent fetal damage. Untreated maternal infection may result in a rate of fetal loss of up to 40 percent (with stillbirth more common than abortion because of the late onset of fetal pathology), prematurity, neonatal death, or nonfatal congenital syphilis. In one series of mothers with untreated syphilis of less than 2 years' duration, 21 percent aborted or had a stillbirth, 13 percent gave birth to infants who died within 2 months, 43 percent had infants with syphilis who were still alive at 2 months, and 23 percent had nonsyphilitic infants. Among infants born alive, only fulminant congenital syphilis is clinically apparent at birth, and these babies have a very poor prognosis. The most common clinical problem is the healthy-appearing baby born to a mother with a positive serologic test. Routine serologic testing in early pregnancy is considered cost-effective in virtually all populations, even in areas with a low prenatal prevalence of syphilis. To ensure prompt treatment, rapid plasma reagin (RPR) screening should be performed on site when pregnancy is detected in a woman who may prove noncompliant. Where the prevalence of syphilis is high and when the patient is at high risk, syphilis serology should be repeated in the third trimester and at delivery.

The manifestations of congenital syphilis can be divided into three types according to their timing: (1) early manifestations, which appear within the first 2 years of life (often between 2 and 10 weeks of age), are infectious, and resemble the manifestations of severe secondary syphilis in the adult; (2) late manifestations, which appear after 2 years and are noninfectious; and (3) residual stigmata. The earliest sign of congenital syphilis is usually rhinitis ("snuffles"), which is soon followed by other mucocutaneous lesions. These may include bullae (syphilitic pemphigus), vesicles, superficial desquamation, petechiae, and (later) papulosquamous lesions, mucous patches, and condylomata lata. The most common early manifestations are osteochondritis and osteitis (particularly involving the metaphyses of long bones), which progress in severity during the first 6 months of life and then spontaneously subside, and periostitis, which continues to progress after the first 6 months. Hepatosplenomegaly, lymphadenopathy, anemia, jaundice, thrombocytopenia, and leukocytosis are common. The anemia is usually hypoproliferative but may be hemolytic. The nephrotic syndrome in early congenital syphilis, as in adult secondary syphilis, represents immune complex–induced glomerulonephritis. A compilation of clinical presentations of congenital syphilis in nine studies involving a total of 212 infants included abnormal bone radiographs (61 percent), hepatomegaly (51 percent), splenomegaly (49 percent), petechiae (41 percent), other skin rashes (35 percent), anemia (34 percent), lymphadenopathy (32 percent), jaundice (30 percent), pseudoparalysis (28 percent), and snuffles (23 percent).

Neonatal congenital syphilis must be differentiated from other generalized congenital infections, including rubella, cytomegalovirus or herpes simplex virus infection, and toxoplasmosis, as well as from erythroblastosis fetalis. Neonatal death is usually due to pulmonary hemorrhage, secondary bacterial infection, or severe hepatitis. Pathologic findings include interstitial and perivascular inflammation followed by variable fibroblastic proliferation (with involvement of the skin, bones, liver, kidneys, pancreas, spleen, lungs, and intestines) and by extramedullary hematopoiesis.

Late congenital syphilis is defined as congenital syphilis that remains untreated after 2 years of age. In perhaps 60 percent of cases, the infection remains subclinical; the clinical spectrum in the remainder of cases differs in certain respects from that of acquired late syphilis in the adult. For example, cardiovascular syphilis rarely develops in late congenital syphilis, whereas interstitial keratitis is much more common and occurs between the ages of 5 and 25. Other manifestations associated with interstitial keratitis are eighth-nerve deafness and recurrent arthropathy. Bilateral knee effusions are known as *Clutton's joints*. Examination of CSF discloses asymptomatic neurosyphilis in about one-third of untreated patients without other late clinical manifestations; moreover, clinical neurosyphilis occurs in one-quarter of individuals over 6 years of age who have untreated congenital syphilis. The clinical manifestations of congenital neurosyphilis correspond to those of adult neurosyphilis. Gummatous periostitis occurs between the ages of 5 and 20 and, as in nonvenereal endemic childhood syphilis, tends to cause destructive lesions of the palate and nasal septum.

Characteristic stigmata include *Hutchinson's teeth*—centrally notched, widely spaced, peg-shaped upper central incisors—and "mulberry" molars—sixth-year molars with multiple, poorly developed cusps. The abnormal facies of congenital syphilis includes frontal bossing, saddle nose, and poorly developed maxillae. Saber shins, characterized by anterior tibial bowing, are rare. *Rhagades* are linear scars at the angles of the mouth and nose that are caused by secondary bacterial infection of the early facial eruption. Other stigmata include unexplained nerve deafness, old chorioretinitis, optic atrophy, and corneal opacities due to past interstitial keratitis.

LABORATORY EXAMINATIONS **Dark-Field Examination Technique** Dark-field examination is essential in evaluating moist cutaneous lesions, such as the chancre of primary syphilis or the condylomata lata of secondary syphilis. The surface of the suspected ulcerated lesion should be cleaned with saline and gauze and then gently abraded further with dry gauze, taking care not to induce bleeding. The lesion is then squeezed to express a serous transudate, a drop of which is picked up on the surface of a glass slide. A drop of saline (without bacteriostatic additives) may be mixed with the transudate if necessary, and this preparation is then covered with a coverslip and examined immediately for *T. pallidum* with a dark-field or phase-contrast microscope by an experienced individual. The identification of a single characteristic motile organism by a trained observer is sufficient for diagnosis. Examination of oral lesions and anal ulcers by this method is not recommended, as it is difficult to differentiate *T. pallidum* from other spirochetes that may be present. A single negative examination does not exclude the possibility of syphilis, since at least 10^4 treponemes per microliter of transudate must be present to be seen; furthermore, prior use of topical antiseptic or cleansing by the patient may confuse the results and therefore should be avoided. Ideally, the dark-field examination should be repeated on three successive days before being considered negative.

Direct Immunofluorescence Most syphilis is diagnosed in the offices of private physicians, where dark-field microscopy is not available; alternative methods for the identification of *T. pallidum* in exudate are needed. The direct fluorescent antibody *T. pallidum* (DFA-TP) test, available at central laboratories, uses fluorescein-conjugated polyclonal antitreponemal antibody for the detection of *T. pallidum* in fixed smears prepared from suspect lesions. A refinement of this technique uses a monoclonal antibody specific to the pathogenic treponemes but is not yet commercially available. The polymerase chain reaction is currently being evaluated for the detection of *T. pallidum* and other genital ulcer pathogens.

Demonstration of *T. pallidum* in Tissue It is often necessary to demonstrate *T. pallidum* in tissue when clinical or histopathologic features suggest the diagnosis of syphilis. Although the organism can be found in tissue with appropriate silver stains, these results should be interpreted with caution because artifacts resembling *T. pallidum* are often seen. Treponemes can be demonstrated more reliably in tissue by immunofluorescent or immunohistochemical methods using specific monoclonal or polyclonal antibodies to *T. pallidum*.

Serologic Tests for Syphilis The profusion of serologic tests for syphilis causes much unnecessary confusion. Syphilitic infection produces two types of antibodies—antilipid "reaginic" antibody and specific antitreponemal antibody—that are measured by the nontreponemal and treponemal tests, respectively (Table 174-1). Both types of tests are reactive in persons with any treponemal infection, including yaws, pinta, and endemic syphilis.

The nontreponemal antibodies produced in syphilis contain both IgG and IgM directed against a cardiolipin-lecithin-cholesterol antigen complex. The term *reagin* is unfortunate, since the unrelated IgE antibody involved in certain allergic phenomena is also known as reagin. The most widely used nontreponemal or reagin antibody tests for syphilis are the RPR test, which can be automated (ART); the Venereal Disease Research Laboratory (VDRL) slide test; and the toluidine red unheated serum test (TRUST). Less frequently used nontreponemal tests include the unheated serum reagin (USR) test and the reagin screen test (RST). In these tests, antibody is detected by the microscopic (VDRL and USR tests) or macroscopic (RPR test,

Table 174-1

Common Serologic Tests for Syphilis

Nontreponemal (reagin) tests	
Microscopic flocculation	Venereal Disease Research Laboratory (VDRL) test
Macroscopic flocculation	Rapid plasma reagin (RPR) test
	Toluidine red unheated serum test (TRUST)
Treponemal tests	
Immunofluorescence	Fluorescent treponemal antibody–absorbed (FTA-ABS) test; 19S IgM FTA-ABS test
Hemagglutination	*T. pallidum* hemagglutination assay (MHA-TP, TPHA)

TRUST, and RST) flocculation of the antigen suspension (see Table 174-1). New ELISA-based methods are being evaluated.

The RPR test is often more expensive than the VDRL test, but it is easier to perform and uses unheated serum; it is the test of choice for rapid serologic diagnosis in a clinic or office setting. The VDRL test, however, remains the standard for use with CSF.

The RPR and VDRL tests are equally sensitive and may be used for initial screening or for quantitation of serum antibody. The titer reflects the activity of the disease. A fourfold or greater rise in titer may be seen during the evolution of early syphilis. VDRL titers usually reach 1:32 or higher in secondary syphilis. A persistent fall of two dilutions (fourfold) or greater following treatment of early syphilis provides essential evidence of an adequate response to therapy. VDRL titers do not correspond directly to RPR titers, and sequential quantitative testing (as for response to therapy) must employ a single test.

There are two standard treponemal tests: the fluorescent treponemal antibody–absorbed (FTA-ABS) test and the microhemagglutination assay for antibodies to *T. pallidum* (MHA-TP). Another hemagglutination test, the *T. pallidum* hemagglutination (TPHA) test, is widely used in Europe but is not available in the United States. Both the hemagglutination and the FTA-ABS tests are very specific and, when used for confirmation of positive reaginic antibody tests, have a very high positive predictive value for the diagnosis of syphilis. However, even these tests give false-positive results at rates as high as 1 to 2 percent when used for the screening of normal populations. The *T. pallidum* immobilization (TPI) test, in which live *T. pallidum* organisms are immobilized by immune serum plus complement, is the most specific treponemal test but is more laborious than other methods and, in the United States, is available only in research laboratories.

The relative sensitivities of the VDRL test, the FTA-ABS test, and MHA-TP in the various stages of syphilis are shown in Table 174-2. The nontreponemal tests are nonreactive in about one-quarter of patients presenting with primary or late syphilis. In early primary syphilis, the detection of antibody can be maximized either by the performance of an FTA-ABS test or simply by repetition of a VDRL test after 1 to 2 weeks if the initial VDRL result is negative. However, a reagin antibody test alone is not sufficient for the detection of late

Table 174-2

Sensitivity of Serodiagnostic Tests in Untreated Syphilis

Test*	Mean Percentage Positive (Range) at Indicated Stage of Disease†			
	Primary	**Secondary**	**Latent**	**Tertiary**
VDRL	78 (74–87)	100	95 (88–100)	71 (37–94)
FTA-ABS	84 (70–100)	100	100	96
MHA-TP	76 (69–90)	100	100	94

* The specificity for each of these tests is 97 to 99 percent.
† In CDC studies.

SOURCE: Modified from Larsen et al.

symptomatic syphilis; the more sensitive FTA-ABS test should be performed routinely in suspected late syphilis. The hemagglutination tests may be less sensitive than the reagin tests in primary syphilis but are as sensitive as the FTA-ABS test in other stages. All treponemal and nontreponemal tests are reactive during secondary syphilis, and a nonreactive result virtually excludes syphilis in a patient with otherwise compatible mucocutaneous lesions. (Fewer than 1 percent of patients with secondary syphilis have a VDRL test that is nonreactive or weakly reactive with undiluted serum but is positive at higher serum dilutions—the *prozone* phenomenon.) While the nontreponemal tests will become nonreactive or will be reactive in lower titers following therapy for early syphilis, the treponemal tests often remain reactive after therapy and therefore are not helpful in determining the infection status of persons with past syphilis.

The presence of specific IgM antibody has been proposed as a marker for active syphilis, with the claim that IgM disappears following adequate therapy. However, because the rate at which IgM declines after therapy is quite variable from patient to patient, the use of this criterion for cure is not recommended. A new 19S IgM FTA-ABS test for syphilis has been approved by the Centers for Disease Control and Prevention (CDC) for the evaluation of infants with suspected congenital syphilis.

False-Positive Serologic Tests for Syphilis   Because the antigen used in nontreponemal tests is found in other tissues, the tests may be reactive in persons without treponemal infection, although rarely do titers exceed 1:8 in such patients. In a population selected for screening because of clinical suspicion, history of exposure, or increased risk for sexually transmitted infections, fewer than 1 percent of reactive tests are falsely positive. False-positive reagin tests are classified as acute if they become negative within 6 months and as chronic if they persist for 6 months or longer. Pregnancy is often mentioned as a cause of false-positive reactivity. However, a number of studies have shown a very low rate of false-positive results among pregnant women, and a reactive VDRL or RPR test in such patients should be pursued aggressively. The high rates of false-positive reactivity reported several decades ago among patients with leprosy, infectious mononucleosis, and miscellaneous other infections were obtained mostly in studies with early lipoidal tests. The modern VDRL and RPR tests are 97 to 99 percent specific, and false-positive reactions are now limited largely to those conditions listed in Table 174-3. Reagin tests yield false-positive results in up to 25 percent of intravenous narcotic addicts. False positivity is also common among persons with autoimmune disorders. The prevalence of false-positive reagin tests increases with advancing age; 10 percent of people over 70 years

of age have false-positive reactions. In the patient with a false-positive reagin test, syphilis is excluded by a nonreactive treponemal test.

For practical purposes, most clinicians need to be familiar with the three uses of serologic tests for syphilis: (1) testing of large numbers of sera for screening or diagnostic purposes (e.g., the RPR or VDRL test), (2) quantitative measurement of the reagin antibody titer to assess the clinical activity of syphilis or to monitor the response to therapy (e.g., the VDRL or RPR test), and (3) confirmation of the diagnosis of syphilis in a patient with a positive reagin antibody test or with a suspected clinical diagnosis of syphilis (e.g., the FTA-ABS test or MHA-TP).

Evaluation for Asymptomatic Neurosyphilis   Asymptomatic involvement of the CNS is detected by examination of CSF for pleocytosis, increased protein concentration, and VDRL activity. CSF abnormalities can be demonstrated in up to 40 percent of cases of primary or secondary syphilis and in 25 percent of cases of latent syphilis. *T. pallidum* has been recovered by rabbit inoculation from up to 30 percent of patients with primary or secondary syphilis but rarely from those with latent syphilis. The demonstration of *T. pallidum* in CSF is often associated with other CSF abnormalities; however, organisms can be recovered from patients with otherwise normal CSF. Before the advent of penicillin, the risk of developing clinical neurosyphilis was roughly proportional to the intensity of CSF changes in early syphilis. CSF examination is essential in the evaluation of any seropositive patient with neurologic signs and symptoms and is recommended for all patients with untreated syphilis of unknown duration or of greater than 1 year's duration. The possibility of asymptomatic neurosyphilis in some patients with early disease is not addressed by these recommendations. Because standard therapy with penicillin G benzathine (benzathine benzylpenicillin) for early syphilis fails to result in treponemicidal levels in the CSF, some experts advise lumbar puncture in secondary and early latent syphilis, with follow-up examinations for patients with abnormalities.

The CSF VDRL test is highly specific if the fluid is not contaminated with blood. This test is relatively insensitive, however, and may be nonreactive even in cases of progressive symptomatic neurosyphilis. The degree of sensitivity is highest in meningovascular syphilis and paresis and is lower in asymptomatic neurosyphilis and tabes dorsalis. Measures of intrathecal antitreponemal IgM or IgG have proved to be insensitive. The unabsorbed FTA test on CSF is reactive far more often than the CSF VDRL test in all stages of syphilis, but FTA reactivity may reflect passive transfer of serum antibody into the CSF. A nonreactive CSF FTA test, however, may be used to rule out neurosyphilis. Even in the absence of confirmatory CSF examination, a therapeutic trial of penicillin in doses adequate for neurosyphilis is warranted in any patient with a positive serum treponemal antibody test who also has neurologic findings consistent with neurosyphilis.

Evaluation for Syphilis in Patients Infected with HIV   Because persons at highest risk for syphilis (inner-city populations, homosexually active men, and people in many developing countries) are also at increased risk for HIV infection, these two infections are frequently found in the same patient. There is evidence that syphilis and other genital-ulcer diseases may be important risk factors for the acquisition and transmission of HIV infection.

The manifestations of syphilis may be altered in patients with concurrent HIV infection, and multiple cases of neurologic relapse following standard therapy have been reported in HIV-infected patients. *T. pallidum* has been isolated from the CSF of several patients after therapy for early syphilis with penicillin G benzathine. A recent multicenter U.S. study of early syphilis found similar therapeutic responses in persons with and without concurrent HIV infection, although the study lacked sufficient statistical power to exclude an effect of HIV and 41 percent of subjects were lost to follow-up. This investigation confirmed the high rate of CNS invasion in early syphilis and the persistence of *T. pallidum* after standard therapy: 11 of 43 HIV-infected patients and 21 of 88 HIV-uninfected patients had *T. pallidum* detectable in CSF before therapy; 7 of the 35 patients who underwent lumbar puncture after therapy (some HIV-infected and others uninfected) still had *T. pallidum* detectable in CSF.

Table 174-3

Causes of False-Positive Reactions in Nontreponemal Serologic Tests for Syphilis

Cause	Rate of False-Positive Reactions, %*
ACUTE FALSE-POSITIVE REACTION (<6 MONTHS)	
Recent viral illness or immunization	1–2
Genital herpes	4.4
Human immunodeficiency virus infection	1–4
Mycoplasma pneumoniae infection	1–2
Malaria	11
Parenteral drug use	20–25
CHRONIC FALSE-POSITIVE REACTION (≥6 MONTHS)	
Aging	9–11
Autoimmune disorders	1–20
Systemic lupus erythematosus	11–20
Rheumatoid arthritis	5
Parenteral drug use	20–25

* Data were collected from a variety of published reports.

The frequency of unusual clinical and laboratory manifestations of syphilis among patients coinfected with HIV is unknown. Such changes may be dependent on the stage of HIV infection and the degree of immunosuppression. There is no clear evidence that the sensitivity of serologic tests for syphilis or the serologic response to therapy in the vast majority of HIV-infected patients with early syphilis differs from the corresponding findings in patients not infected with HIV. Interpretation of serologic results should be the same for the two groups.

The evaluation of all syphilis patients should include serologic testing for HIV, with the patient's consent. Conversely, persons with newly diagnosed HIV infection should be tested for syphilis. Currently, some authorities, persuaded by reports of the persistence of *T. pallidum* in the CSF of HIV-infected persons after standard penicillin benzathine therapy for early syphilis, recommend examination of CSF for evidence of neurosyphilis for all coinfected patients, regardless of the clinical stage of syphilis, with treatment for neurosyphilis if CSF abnormalities are found or if CSF examination is not performed. Others do not recommend routine CSF examination for HIV-coinfected patients with early syphilis and believe that standard therapy is sufficient. Serologic testing after treatment is important for all patients with syphilis, particularly those also infected with HIV.

℞ TREATMENT

Treatment of Acquired Syphilis Penicillin G is the drug of choice for all stages of syphilis. *T. pallidum* is killed by very low concentrations of penicillin G, although a long period of exposure to penicillin is required because of the unusually slow rate of multiplication of the organism. The efficacy of penicillin for syphilis remains undiminished after 50 years of use. Other antibiotics effective in syphilis include the tetracyclines, erythromycin, and the cephalosporins. Aminoglycosides and spectinomycin inhibit *T. pallidum* only in very large doses, and the sulfonamides and the quinolones are inactive.

Serum levels of penicillin G of 0.03 μg/mL or more for at least 7 days are considered necessary for the cure of early syphilis. Recurrence rates for a given regimen increase as infection progresses from incubating to seronegative primary to seropositive primary to secondary to late syphilis. Therefore, it is probable but unproven that a longer duration of therapy is required to effect cure as the infection progresses. For these reasons, some authorities use more prolonged penicillin therapy than that recommended by the U.S. Public Health Service when treating secondary, latent, or late syphilis.

The treatment regimens recommended for syphilis are summarized in Table 174-4 and are described in more detail below.

EARLY SYPHILIS Preventive (abortive, "epidemiologic") treatment is recommended for seronegative individuals without signs of syphilis who have been exposed to infectious syphilis within the previous 3 months. Before treatment is given, every effort should be made to establish a diagnosis by examination and serologic testing. *The regimens recommended for prevention are the same as those recommended for early syphilis.*

Penicillin G benzathine is the most widely used agent for the treatment of early syphilis (including primary, secondary, and early latent syphilis),

although it is more painful on injection than penicillin G procaine. A single dose of 2.4 million units cures more than 95 percent of cases of primary syphilis. Because the drug's efficacy in secondary syphilis may be slightly lower, some physicians administer a second dose of 2.4 million units 1 week after the initial dose at this stage of disease. Clinical relapse can follow treatment with penicillin G benzathine in patients with both HIV infection and early syphilis. Examination of CSF from HIV-seropositive individuals with syphilis of any stage is recommended by some experts. Furthermore, treatment with regimens effective against neurosyphilis has been proposed by some authorities for all HIV-seropositive individuals with syphilis of any stage.

For penicillin-allergic patients with early syphilis, a 2-week course of therapy with doxycycline or tetracycline is recommended. These regimens appear to be effective, although no well-controlled studies have been performed, and poor compliance may be problematic. Although ceftriaxone and azithromycin have shown activity against *T. pallidum* in animals, human trials have not been of sufficient scope to permit the recommendation of either drug for any stage of syphilis.

LATE LATENT AND LATE SYPHILIS Lumbar puncture should be performed in the evaluation of latent syphilis of more than 1 year's duration, in suspected neurosyphilis, and in late complications other than symptomatic neurosyphilis (since asymptomatic neurosyphilis may coexist with other late complications). In older asymptomatic seropositive individuals, the yield of lumbar puncture is relatively low. CSF examination is most clearly indicated in the following situations: neurologic signs or symptoms, treatment failure, a serum reagin titer of ≥1:32, HIV antibody positivity, other evidence of active syphilis (e.g., aortitis, gumma, visual or hearing changes), or plans to administer nonpenicillin therapy. The recommended treatment for late latent syphilis with normal CSF, for cardiovascular syphilis, and for late benign syphilis (gumma) is penicillin G benza-

Table 174-4

Recommendations for the Treatment of Syphilis*

Stage of Syphilis	Patients without Penicillin Allergy	Patients with Confirmed Penicillin Allergy
Primary, secondary, or early latent	Penicillin G benzathine (single dose of 2.4 million units IM, 1.2 million units in each buttock)	Tetracycline hydrochloride (500 mg PO qid) or doxycycline (100 mg PO bid) for 2 weeks
Late latent (or latent of uncertain duration), cardiovascular, or benign tertiary	Lumbar puncture CSF normal: Penicillin G benzathine (2.4 million units IM weekly for 3 weeks) CSF abnormal: treat as neurosyphilis	Lumbar puncture CSF normal: tetracycline hydrochloride (500 mg PO qid) or doxycycline (100 mg PO bid) for 4 weeks CSF abnormal: treat as neurosyphilis
Neurosyphilis† (asymptomatic or symptomatic)	Aqueous penicillin G (12–24 million units/d IV, given in divided doses every 4 h) for 10–14 days *or* Aqueous penicillin G procaine (2.4 million units/d IM) plus oral probenecid (500 mg qid), both for 10–14 days	Desensitization and treatment with penicillin if allergy is confirmed by skin testing
Syphilis in pregnancy	According to stage	Desensitization and treatment with penicillin if allergy is confirmed by skin testing

* See text for discussion of syphilis therapy in HIV-infected individuals.
† Some authorities recommend following these regimens with three doses of 2.4 million units of penicillin G benzathine, given IM 1 week apart. Penicillin G benzathine alone has given inferior results when used for the treatment of neurosyphilis. Drugs other than penicillin are not recommended. Many patients who give a history of penicillin allergy prove negative when skin-tested for immediate hypersensitivity to penicillin and can be given aqueous crystalline penicillin G for CNS syphilis under close supervision in the hospital.
SOURCE: These recommendations are modified from those issued by the Centers for Disease Control and Prevention in 1993.

thine, 2.4 million units intramuscularly once a week for 3 successive weeks (7.2 million units total). Doxycycline or tetracycline (given for 1 month) offers an untested alternative for penicillin-allergic patients with latent or late syphilis and normal CSF. If CSF abnormalities are found, the patient should be treated for neurosyphilis.

No studies of penicillin G benzathine for cardiovascular syphilis have been reported, and the efficacy of penicillin therapy in any form for this condition has not been proven. The response of cardiovascular syphilis to penicillin is seldom dramatic because aortic aneurysm and aortic regurgitation cannot be reversed by antibiotic treatment, although further progression of these lesions may be arrested. In contrast, the response of benign tertiary syphilis and of meningovascular syphilis to penicillin G is usually impressive. The response of parenchymal neurosyphilis has been variable. In Hahn's 1959 cooperative study of the treatment of 1086 general paretics with penicillin, the frequency of clinical improvement or termination of progression ranged from 38 percent among persons with severe involvement to 81 percent among those with mild involvement. Tabes dorsalis or optic atrophy responds less often. In general, treatment of inactive neurosyphilis in which neurologic damage has already been done may produce no clinical change, and retreatment of such cases is not warranted. However, the persistence of CSF pleocytosis or its recurrence after an initial response to treatment indicates continuing active infection, which should respond to additional treatment. The CDC's 1993 treatment guidelines for neurosyphilis are presented in Table 174-4. Penicillin G benzathine, given in total doses of up to 7.2 million units to adults or 50,000 units per kilogram to infants, does not produce detectable concentrations of penicillin G in CSF, and asymptomatic neurosyphilis may relapse in up to one-quarter of adults treated with 2.4 million units. Therefore, the use of penicillin G benzathine alone for the treatment of neurosyphilis is not recommended. On the other hand, administration of intravenous penicillin G in doses of 12 million units or more per day for 10 days or longer is thought to ensure treponemicidal concentrations of penicillin G in CSF and occasionally cures infection in patients who fail to respond to other therapy.

Several recent publications have reported neurologic relapse after high-dose intravenous penicillin therapy for neurosyphilis in HIV-infected patients. No alternative therapies have been explored, but careful follow-up is essential, and retreatment is warranted in such patients.

No data support the use of antibiotics other than penicillin G for the treatment of neurosyphilis; however, some of the third-generation cephalosporins may deserve further evaluation. In patients with penicillin allergy demonstrated by skin testing, desensitization may be the best course (see Chap. 126).

MANAGEMENT OF SYPHILIS IN PREGNANCY Every pregnant woman should undergo a nontreponemal test at her first prenatal visit, and women at high risk of exposure should have a repeat test in the third trimester and at delivery. In the pregnant patient with presumed syphilis (evidenced by a reactive serology, with or without clinical manifestations) and with no history of treatment for syphilis, expeditious evaluation and initiation of treatment are essential. Therapy should be administered according to the stage of the disease, as for nonpregnant patients. Patients should be warned of the risk of a Jarisch-Herxheimer reaction, which may be associated with mild premature contractions but rarely results in premature delivery.

Penicillin is the only recommended therapy for syphilis in pregnancy. If the patient has a well-documented penicillin allergy that is confirmed by the demonstration of an immediate wheal-and-flare response to skin testing with penicilloyl polylysine or penicillin G minor-determinant mixture, desensitization and penicillin treatment should be undertaken in a hospital according to the 1993 sexually transmitted diseases treatment guidelines issued by the CDC. After treatment, a quantitative reagin test should be repeated monthly throughout pregnancy. Treated women whose titers rise fourfold or

who do not show a fourfold decrease in titer in a 3-month period should be retreated.

Evaluation and Management of Congenital Syphilis Newborn infants of mothers with reactive VDRL or FTA-ABS tests may themselves have reactive tests, whether or not they have become infected, because of transplacental transfer of maternal IgG antibody. Rising or persistent titers indicate infection, and the infant should be treated. Neonatal IgM antibody can be detected in cord or neonatal serum with the 19S IgM FTA-ABS test, in which IgM is enriched by column chromatography (which removes IgG) and is detected by fluorescein-labeled anti-human IgM. This test avoids the specificity and sensitivity problems associated with earlier versions of the IgM FTA-ABS test. Alternatively, monthly quantitative reagin tests may be performed on asymptomatic infants born to women treated adequately with penicillin during pregnancy.

If the seropositive mother has received inadequate penicillin treatment or therapy with a drug other than penicillin, if her treatment status is unknown, or if the infant may be difficult to follow, the infant should be treated at birth. It is unwise to require proof of diagnosis before treatment in such cases. The CSF should be examined to obtain baseline values before treatment. Penicillin is the only recommended drug for syphilis in infants. The penicillin dosage used for the treatment of the patient with late congenital syphilis is calculated in the same way as that used in the infant, until dosage based on weight reaches that used for adult neurosyphilis. Specific recommendations for the treatment of infants are included in the CDC's 1993 guidelines.

Jarisch-Herxheimer Reaction A dramatic though usually mild reaction consisting of fever (average temperature elevation, 1.5°C), chills, myalgias, headache, tachycardia, increased respiratory rate, increased circulating neutrophil count (average total white blood cell count, 12,500/μL), and vasodilation with mild hypotension may follow the initiation of treatment for syphilis. This reaction occurs in approximately 50 percent of patients with primary syphilis, 90 percent of those with secondary syphilis, and 25 percent of those with early latent syphilis. The onset comes within 2 h of treatment, the temperature peaks at about 7 h, and defervescence takes place within 12 to 24 h. The reaction is more delayed in neurosyphilis, with fever peaking after 12 to 14 h. In patients with secondary syphilis, erythema and edema of the mucocutaneous lesions increase; occasionally, subclinical or early mucocutaneous lesions may first become apparent during the reaction. The pathogenesis of this reaction is undefined, although recent studies have demonstrated the induction of inflammatory mediators such as tumor necrosis factors by treponemal lipoproteins. Patients should be warned to expect such symptoms, which can be managed by bed rest and aspirin. Adjunctive steroid therapy has not been shown to prevent the Jarisch-Herxheimer reaction in syphilis and is not recommended.

Follow-Up Evaluation of Responses to Therapy The response of early syphilis to treatment should be determined by monitoring of the quantitative VDRL or RPR titer 1, 3, 6, and 12 months after treatment. More frequent serologic examination (1, 2, 3, 6, 9, and 12 months) is recommended for patients concurrently infected with HIV. Because the FTA-ABS and hemagglutination tests remain positive in most patients treated for seropositive early syphilis, these tests are not useful in following the response to therapy. After successful treatment of seropositive first-episode primary or secondary syphilis, the VDRL titer progressively declines, becoming negative by 12 months in 40 to 75 percent of seropositive primary cases and in 20 to 40 percent of secondary cases. Two years after treatment for first-episode primary syphilis, at least 60 percent of patients have a negative VDRL test, although 25 to 58 percent of patients with secondary disease and a higher proportion of those treated for early latent syphilis maintain low reagin titers. Patients with a history of syphilis have less rapid declines in titer and are less likely to become VDRL- or RPR-negative. If the VDRL test becomes negative or if VDRL titers drop to a fixed low value within 1 or 2 years, lumbar puncture is unnecessary since the CSF examination is almost invariably normal and there is little risk of subsequent neurosyphilis.

However, if a VDRL titer of 1:8 or more fails to fall at least fourfold within 12 months, if the VDRL titer rises fourfold, or if clinical symptoms persist or recur, retreatment is indicated. Every effort should be made to differentiate treatment failure from reinfection, and the CSF should be examined. Patients in whom treatment failure is suspected, especially those with abnormal CSF, should be treated as described for neurosyphilis. If the patient remains seropositive but asymptomatic after such retreatment, no further therapy is necessary. Patients treated for late latent syphilis frequently have low VDRL titers before therapy and may not have a fourfold drop after therapy with penicillin; about half of these patients remain seropositive (with low titers) for years after therapy. Retreatment is not warranted unless the titer rises or signs and symptoms of syphilis appear.

The activity of neurosyphilis correlates best with the degree of CSF pleocytosis. Changes in the CSF cell count and, to a lesser extent, in the CSF protein concentration provide the most sensitive index of response to treatment. CSF should be examined every 3 to 6 months for 3 years after the treatment of asymptomatic or symptomatic neurosyphilis or until CSF findings return to normal. An elevated CSF cell count falls to $\leq 10/\mu L$ in 3 to 12 months in 95 percent of adequately treated cases and becomes normal in all cases within 2 to 4 years. Elevated levels of CSF protein fall more slowly, and the CSF reagin titer declines gradually over a period of several years. Some evidence suggests that serum and CSF parameters may normalize more slowly in HIV-infected patients with neurosyphilis than in persons not infected with HIV.

Persistence of Treponemal Forms The persistence of *T. pallidum* in the aqueous humor, CSF, lymph nodes, brain, inflamed temporal arteries, and other tissues after "adequate" penicillin treatment has been suggested by dark-field microscopy, immunofluorescent antibody and silver staining techniques, rabbit inoculation, and polymerase chain reaction. Because the data on persisting treponemes are scanty, no modification of the treatment recommendations seems warranted for HIV-uninfected persons. Adherence to recommendations regarding CSF examination before the selection of therapy should minimize the possibility that *T. pallidum* will persist in the CSF.

IMMUNITY TO AND PREVENTION OF SYPHILIS About 30 to 50 percent of contacts of patients with primary and secondary syphilis become infected, but the actual risk of infection from a single exposure is probably much lower. The rate of development of acquired resistance to *T. pallidum* after natural or experimental infection is related to the amount of the antigenic stimulus, which depends on both the size of the infecting inoculum and the duration of infection before treatment. The role of serum antibody in conferring immunity to syphilis remains controversial. Reagin (VDRL) antibody is not protective, although it is opsonic for *T. pallidum*. Passively administered antibody prevents or delays the appearance of clinical manifestations of syphilis in the rabbit model; it does not prevent infection. Cellular immunity is considered to be of major importance in the healing of early lesions and the control of syphilitic infection. The cellular infiltration of early lesions predominantly involves T lymphocytes and macrophages; specifically sensitized T lymphocytes develop early in the course of infection in humans and experimentally infected rabbits. The cytokine milieu of primary and secondary lesions is of the T_H1 type, consistent with the clearance of organisms by activated macrophages. Specific antibody enhances phagocytosis and is required for macrophage-mediated killing of *T. pallidum*.

Inability to cultivate pathogenic treponemes in vitro has hindered the analysis of treponemal antigens. Attempts to induce immunity to syphilis by vaccination have shown limited promise, although repeated injection of rabbits with gamma-irradiated motile strains has conferred immunity to rechallenge. The outer membrane of *T. pallidum* contains few integral membrane proteins, although the first surface-exposed antigen, a porin molecule, has recently been identified. Many of the major antigens are lipoproteins, which are probably associated via their lipid tail with the inner membrane, projecting into the periplasmic space. None of these identified antigens has been shown to induce protective immunity. Until a practical and effective vaccine is developed, the prevention of syphilis will depend on the use of condoms and on the detection and treatment of infectious cases.

BIBLIOGRAPHY

BERRY CD et al: Neurologic relapse after benzathine penicillin therapy for secondary syphilis in a patient with HIV infection. N Engl J Med 316:1587, 1987

BLANCO DR et al: Porin activity and sequence analysis of a 31-kilodalton *Treponema pallidum* subsp. *pallidum* rare outer membrane protein (Tromp 1). J Bacteriol 177:3556, 1995

CENTERS FOR DISEASE CONTROL: Guidelines for the prevention and control of congenital syphilis. Morb Mort Week Rep 37(S-1):1, 1988

CENTERS FOR DISEASE CONTROL AND PREVENTION: Summary of notifiable disease 1993. Morb Mort Week Rep 42(53):1, 1993

———: 1993 sexually transmitted diseases treatment guidelines. Morb Mort Week Rep 42(RR-14):1, 1993

DOWELL ME et al: Response of latent syphilis or neurosyphilis to ceftriaxone therapy in persons infected with human immunodeficiency virus. Am J Med 93:481, 1992

GORDON SM et al: The response of symptomatic neurosyphilis to high-dose intravenous pencillin G in patients with human immunodeficiency virus infection. N Engl J Med 331:1469, 1994

KATZ DA et al: Neurosyphilis in acquired immunodeficiency syndrome. Arch Neurol 46:895, 1989

LARSEN SA et al: Laboratory diagnosis and interpretation of tests for syphilis. Clin Microbiol Rev 8:1, 1995

LUKEHART SA et al: Invasion of the central nervous system by *Treponema pallidum*: Implications for diagnosis and treatment. Ann Intern Med 109:855, 1988

MARRA CM et al: Resolution of serum and cerebrospinal fluid abnormalities after treatment of neurosyphilis: Influence of concomitant human immunodeficiency virus infection. Sex Transm Dis 23:184, 1996

MCLEISH WM et al: The ocular manifestations of syphilis in the human immunodeficiency virus type 1–infected host. Ophthalmology 97:196, 1990

MOHR JA et al: Neurosyphilis and penicillin in cerebrospinal fluid. JAMA 236:2208, 1976

MUSHER DM et al: Effect of human immunodeficiency virus infection on the course of syphilis and on the response to treatment. Ann Intern Med 113:872, 1990

RADOLF JD et al: Outer membrane ultrastructure explains the limited antigenicity of virulent *Treponema pallidum*. Proc Natl Acad Sci USA 86:2051, 1989

ROMANOWSKI B et al: Serologic response to treatment of infectious syphilis. Ann Intern Med 114:1005, 1991

SIMON RP: Neurosyphilis. Arch Neurol 42:606, 1985

THOMAS JC et al: Syphilis in the South: Rural rates surpass urban rates in North Carolina. Am J Public Health 85:1119, 1995

THOMAS SB: The Tuskegee syphilis study, 1932 to 1972: Implications for HIV education and AIDS risk education programs in the black community. Am J Public Health 81:1498, 1991

VAN VOORHIS WC et al: Primary and secondary syphilis lesions contain mRNA for T_H1 cytokines. J Infect Dis 173:491, 1996

WENDEL GD et al: Penicillin allergy and desensitization in serious infections during pregnancy. N Engl J Med 312:1229, 1985

175 *Peter L. Perine*

ENDEMIC TREPONEMATOSES

GENERAL CONSIDERATIONS Nonvenereal treponematoses occur in less developed areas of the world. Yaws, pinta, and endemic syphilis are distinguished from venereal syphilis solely by clinical and epidemiologic features since they are caused by treponemes with no demonstrated significant morphologic or genetic differences from *Treponema pallidum*. The etiologic agents of endemic syphilis and yaws are generally held to be identical to *T. pallidum* and have been designated as *T. pallidum* ssp. *endemicum* and ssp. *pertenue*, respectively. Pinta is caused by *Treponema carateum* and involves the skin alone; yaws affects skin and bones; and endemic syphilis involves the skin, bones, and mucous membranes. Each disease tends to progress by stages, but these are neither as distinct nor as predictable as in venereal syphilis. Congenital infections and cardiovascular and central nervous system involvement occur rarely, if ever, in the nonvenereal treponematoses but are common in venereal syphilis. It is unclear whether the clinical and epidemiologic differences among yaws, pinta, endemic syphilis, and venereal syphilis are determined by environmental and host factors alone or are also attributable in part to undefined biologic differences among the causal treponemes. The relationships among the treponematoses are summarized in Table 175-1.

EPIDEMIOLOGY Treponemal antibodies are demonstrable in some proportion of nonhuman primates in regions of Africa where human yaws and endemic syphilis are common. Pathogenic treponemes have been found in skin lesions and lymph nodes of seropositive animals; these treponemes have produced yawslike lesions in susceptible monkeys and hamsters. No epidemiologic evidence indicates that these treponemes play a significant role in the epidemiology of yaws in humans.

Yaws and endemic syphilis are diseases of young children. Yaws occurs throughout the world between the tropics of Cancer and Capricorn in humid, warm environments. Transmission of yaws among children is favored by scanty clothing, poor hygiene, and frequent skin trauma. Spread occurs by direct contact with infected lesions and perhaps by passive transfer of treponemes by insects. Endemic syphilis occurs in arid subtropical or temperate climates in Africa, the eastern Mediterranean, the Arabian peninsula, and central Asia. It is not found in the western hemisphere. Skin-to-skin transmission is less important than in yaws; instead, infection of mucous membranes results from direct mouth-to-mouth contact or from contaminated fomites, such as shared drinking or eating utensils.

Although cutaneous pigmentary changes resembling late stages of pinta occur in yaws and endemic syphilis, pinta is a separate, more benign disease that occurs only in the western hemisphere. The onset is typically later than in yaws or endemic syphilis, usually between 10 and 20 years of age. Pinta is not highly contagious, and its mode of transmission is not well defined.

The WHO/UNICEF-assisted mass campaigns for eradication of endemic nonvenereal treponematoses from 1948 to 1969 were unusually successful. More than 160 million people were examined in 46 countries, and approximately 50 million cases, contacts, and latent infections were treated. The impact of this program was remarkable. The prevalence of active yaws lesions was reduced from over 20 percent to less than 1 percent in many rural areas. In Bosnia, endemic syphilis was eradicated—the only example of eradication of an endemic treponematosis.

Relaxation of active surveillance efforts since the mass campaigns has led to a resurgence of yaws, particularly in Africa. Yaws has not been eradicated in any large area. A large reservoir of yaws remains in West Africa and encompasses the Ivory Coast, Ghana, Togo, Benin, and the pygmies of Zaire and the Central African Republic. Yaws is also prevalent in Indonesia; Papua, New Guinea; and the Solomon Islands of the western Pacific. The Sahelian African nations of Mali, Niger, Burkina Faso, and Senegal have endemic syphilis prevalence rates of 10 to 15 percent in some areas. These rates exceed those reported before the mass treatment campaigns. Seroreactivity and late manifestations of endemic syphilis persist among nomads in Saudi Arabia. The resurgence of yaws and endemic syphilis led to a new yaws campaign in Ghana in 1980, and other national campaigns are planned to control resurgent yaws and endemic syphilis in Africa.

Antitreponemal and reaginic seroreactivity has been detected in a small percentage of children without clinical disease born after the mass campaigns in some areas (e.g., Nigeria, New Guinea, and Bosnia). This reactivity may represent attenuated or asymptomatic infection or may simply reflect the decrease in the predictive value of serologic tests (i.e., in the probability that disease is present if the test is positive) when the prevalence of disease is sharply reduced.

In the Americas, foci of yaws persist in Haiti; Dominica, St. Lucia, and St. Vincent; Peru, Colombia, and Ecuador; a few areas of Brazil; and Guyana and Surinam. Pinta is confined to Central America and northern South America, where it appears to have receded to remote Indian villages. Its prevalence today is probably less than 1 percent of that 20 years ago.

BIOLOGIC RELATIONSHIPS Specific humoral antibodies to *T. pallidum* are produced in individuals with yaws, pinta, or endemic syphilis, but the time of appearance of antibodies after the onset of infections is variable. The fluorescent treponemal antibody absorption (FTA-ABS) test, the *T. pallidum* hemagglutination (TPHA) test, and the *T. pallidum* immobilization (TPI) test cannot differentiate among the treponematoses.

In addition to the clinical and epidemiologic differences among the treponematoses in humans, the range of susceptible animal hosts and some manifestations of experimental infection are different. In particular, *T. carateum* has produced an infection in chimpanzees that resembles pinta, but attempts to infect other experimental animals have been unsuccessful. Individuals who have had yaws or pinta are considered relatively immune to syphilis, and persons with active pinta or syphilis cannot be superinfected with *T. pallidum* ssp. *pertenue* by experimental inoculation.

CLINICAL MANIFESTATIONS Yaws Also known as *pian*, *framboesia*, or *bouba*, yaws is a chronic infectious disease of childhood caused by *T. pallidum* ssp. *pertenue*. The disease is characterized by the development of one or more initial skin lesions and then of relapsing, nondestructive secondary lesions of

Table 175-1

Etiology, Epidemiology, and Clinical Manifestations of the Treponematoses

	Finding in Indicated Disease			
Feature	Venereal Syphilis	Endemic Syphilis	Yaws	Pinta
Organism	*T. pallidum* ssp. *pallidum*	*T. pallidum* ssp. *endemicum*	*T. pallidum* ssp. *pertenue*	*T. carateum*
Transmission	Sexual, transplacental*	Household contacts: mouth-to-mouth or via shared drinking/eating utensils	Skin-to-skin; insect vector?	Skin-to-skin; insect vector?
Usual age	Adulthood	Early childhood	Early childhood	Adolescence
Primary lesion	Cutaneous ulcer (chancre)	Rarely seen	Framboesioma (raspberry), or "mother yaw"	Nonulcerating papule with satellites
Secondary lesion	Mucocutaneous lesions; occasional periostitis	Florid mucocutaneous lesions (mucous patch, split papule, condyloma latum); osteoperiostitis	Cutaneous papulosquamous lesions; osteoperiostitis	Pintides
Tertiary	Gummas, cardiovascular and CNS lues	Destructive cutaneous osteoarticular gummas	Destructive cutaneous osteoarticular gummas	Dyschromic, achromic macules

* Since the nonvenereal treponematoses are usually acquired in childhood and treponemal bacteremia ceases with time, only in adult-onset venereal syphilis is there any likelihood that a mother will give birth to an infected child.

skin and bones. In the late stages, destructive lesions of skin, bones, and joints occur.

The incubation period following experimental inoculation of the causative organism into susceptible human beings is 3 to 4 weeks. Disruption of the skin by insect bites, abrasions, or injuries promotes the acquisition of natural infection from infected contacts, most likely by fingers contaminated directly or indirectly with material from early yaws lesions. The initial early lesion is a single papule, which is usually located on a leg. The lesion enlarges and becomes papillomatous (Fig. 175-1). This lesion, known as a *framboesioma* (raspberry) or "mother yaw," becomes superficially eroded and covered by a thin yellow crust of serous exudate containing *T. pallidum* ssp. *pertenue*. Erythema and induration do not occur. The lesion is mildly pruritic, and regional lymphadenopathy develops. The initial lesion usually heals in 6 months. As a result of treponemal bacteremia and autoinoculation, a generalized secondary eruption of similar lesions appears either before or after the initial lesion has healed and is most extensive on the exposed surfaces of the body. These early cutaneous lesions of yaws have a variety of forms, including desquamative macular and papular as well as papillomatous types. Painful papillomata on the soles of the feet result in a crablike gait referred to as "crab yaws." Early lesions are infectious and heal slowly. They may result in scarring, hyperpigmentation, or depigmentation; the pigmentary changes resemble those seen in pinta. Histologic findings include mononuclear cell infiltration, acanthosis, hyperkeratosis, and many treponemes.

Other manifestations of early yaws include lymphadenopathy and nocturnal bone pain and polydactylitis due to periostitis. Fever and other constitutional symptoms are rare unless lesions become secondarily infected. Infectious cutaneous relapses are characteristic during the first 5 years after infection. Late yaws lesions occur in about 10 percent of cases, starting 5 years or more after infection, and differ histologically from early lesions in that they exhibit endarteritis. Late lesions include gummas of the skin and long bones, particularly of the legs; hyperkeratoses of the soles and palms; osteitis; periostitis; juxtaarticular fibromatous nodes; and hydrarthrosis.

Late lesions of yaws are characteristically extensive and usually destructive. Destruction of the nose, maxilla, palate, and pharynx, termed *gangosa* or *rhinopharyngitis mutilans*, occurs in late yaws as well as in leprosy and leishmaniasis. Hypertrophic paranasal maxillary osteitis produces distinctive facies known as *goundou*.

The clinical features of yaws have become less reliable for diagnosis as the prevalence of yaws has decreased. Thus the use of easily performed serologic tests, such as the rapid plasma reagin (RPR) card test, has become necessary. *T. pallidum* ssp. *pertenue* can be demonstrated by dark-field examination in early cutaneous lesions but should not be confused with other spirochetes found in tropical ulcers. The serum reagin antibody tests become positive after 1 month, and the FTA-ABS test is also positive.

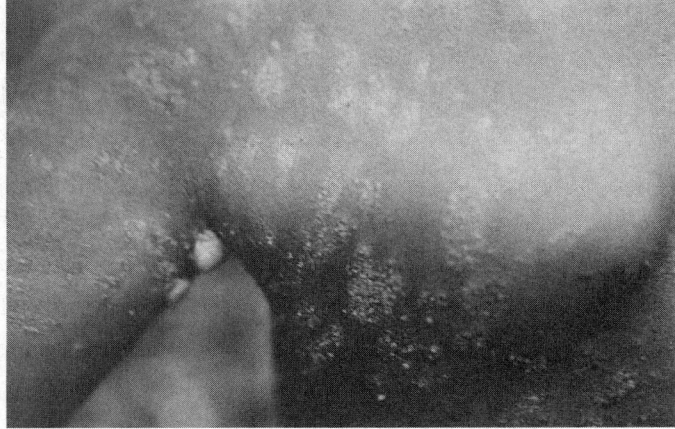

FIGURE 175-1 Squamous micropapules of early yaws with papillomas in the axilla and scapular area.

Endemic Syphilis Endemic syphilis (also called *bejel, siti, dichuchwa, njovera,* and *skerljevo*) is a chronic nonvenereal treponemal infection of childhood characterized by early mucous membrane or mucocutaneous lesions, a latent period of indeterminate duration, and late complications including gummas of bone and skin. The causative organism, *T. pallidum* ssp. *endemicum,* is indistinguishable from *T. pallidum* ssp. *pallidum.* Endemic syphilis differs from congenital syphilis in that dental changes, interstitial keratitis, and neurosyphilis rarely, if ever, occur. Cardiovascular complications are considered rare in both endemic and congenital syphilis.

Primary cutaneous lesions are infrequent and, when present, are extragenital. The earliest manifestation of endemic syphilis is usually an intraoral mucous patch or mucocutaneous lesion resembling the split papules or condylomata of secondary syphilis. Periostitis is common. Regional lymphadenopathy occurs, but generalized lymphadenopathy is unusual. Treponemes are abundant in the moist early lesions and in aspirates from regional lymph nodes. After a variable latent period, late lesions may develop. These lesions, which are the most frequent clinical manifestations, resemble the lesions of late benign syphilis and include osseous or cutaneous gummas. Destructive gummas, osteitis, and gangosa are more common than in late yaws. Gummas develop on the nipples of mothers who have previously had endemic syphilis and who breast-feed infants with oral lesions. Both early and late forms of endemic syphilis thus may coexist in the same family. The tertiary lesions of endemic syphilis sometimes result from repeated exposure of a previously sensitized host to reinfection.

Pinta Also known as *mal del pinto, carate, azul,* or *purupuru,* pinta is an infectious disease of the skin caused by *T. carateum.* This disease has three cutaneous stages characterized by marked changes in the skin color, does not involve osseous tissue or viscera, and causes no disability other than that associated with cosmetic disfigurement.

The initial lesion is a small papule that appears 7 to 30 days after exposure and is located most often on the extremities, face, neck, or buttocks. It slowly increases in size by peripheral extension and by coalescence with smaller satellite papules. Regional lymphadenopathy occurs. A secondary eruption not associated with generalized lymphadenopathy appears 1 month to 1 year after the appearance of the initial lesion. The secondary lesions are termed *pintides,* may be numerous, and evolve into a psoriatic or circinate configuration. Pintides are initially red but become deeply pigmented, turning a slate-blue color after an interval whose length is related to exposure to sun. Pigmentation changes occur most rapidly on the exposed parts of the body. Tertiary pigmented lesions are known as *dyschromic macules* and contain treponemes that are located principally in the epidermis in older lesions. Histologic study reveals deposition of pigment in the dermis, with decreased melanin in the basal cell layer. Within 3 months to a year, most of the pintides show varying degrees of depigmentation, becoming brown and finally white and giving the skin a mottled appearance. The porcelain-white achromic lesions represent the "late" stage of the disease, in which the epidermis is atrophic and melanocytes and melanin are absent. *T. carateum* can be demonstrated in transudates from initial, early secondary, or dyschromic lesions. Reaginic and antitreponemal antibody tests are positive but may take four times longer to become positive in pinta than in venereal syphilis.

℞ TREATMENT

Treatment is similar for all the endemic treponematoses. Intramuscular administration of 2.4 million units of benzathine penicillin G to adults and of half this dose to children results in rapid resolution of lesions and prevents recurrence. A regimen of procaine penicillin G in oil and 2% aluminum monostearate (PAM) has been used extensively. When patients are allergic to penicillin, tetracycline hydrochloride in a dose similar to that used for infectious syphilis (see Chap. 174) is effective. In areas where fewer than 5 percent of the population have active disease, cases are managed on an individual basis, and all contacts of infected persons are treated with antibiotics.

PREVENTION Although the nonvenereal treponematoses are less amenable to eradication than smallpox, the resurgence of yaws has led some authorities to suggest that selective epidemiologic control, like that used in smallpox eradication, be applied to yaws control. This strategy emphasizes ongoing active surveillance, investigation of outbreaks, and treatment of active cases and their contacts rather than mass treatment. There is concern that the epidemiology and course of yaws and endemic syphilis will be adversely affected by the human immunodeficiency virus (HIV) pandemic in Africa and Asia. It is feared that, in HIV-infected individuals, cutaneous lesions may last longer, may more easily become secondarily infected, and may serve as a portal for nonvenereal transmission of HIV.

BIBLIOGRAPHY

BURKE JP et al (eds): International symposium on yaws and other endemic treponematoses. Rev Infect Dis 7:S217, 1985

ENGELKENS HJH et al: Endemic treponematosis. Int J Dermatol 30:77, 1991

GUTHE T: Clinical, serological and epidemiological features of framboesia tropica (yaws) and its control in rural communities. Acta Dermatol Venereol 49:343, 1969

KOFF AB, ROSEN T: Nonvenereal treponematoses: Yaws, endemic syphilis, and pinta. J Am Acad Dermatol 29:519, 1993

NOORDHOEK GT, VAN EMBDEN JDA: Yaws, an endemic treponematosis reconsidered in the HIV era. Eur J Clin Microbiol Infect Dis 10:4, 1991

MEHEUS A, ANTAL GM: Endemic treponematoses: Not yet eradicated. World Health Stat Q 45:228, 1992

PERINE PL et al: *Handbook of Endemic Treponematoses*. Geneva, World Health Organization, 1984

Treponematoses Research: Report of a WHO Scientific Group, WHO Technical Report Series 674, 1982

176 *Peter Speelman*

LEPTOSPIROSIS

Leptospirosis is an infectious disease caused by pathogenic leptospires and is characterized by a broad spectrum of clinical manifestations, varying from inapparent infection to fulminant, fatal disease. In its mild form, leptospirosis may present as an influenza-like illness with headache and myalgias. Severe leptospirosis, characterized by jaundice, renal dysfunction, and hemorrhagic diathesis, is referred to as *Weil's syndrome.*

ETIOLOGIC AGENTS Leptospires are spirochetes belonging to the order Spirochaetales and the family Leptospiraceae. Traditionally, the genus *Leptospira* comprised two species: the pathogenic *L. interrogans* and the free-living *L. biflexa.* Although seven species of pathogenic leptospires are now recognized on the basis of their DNA relatedness, it is more practical clinically and epidemiologically to use a classification based on serologic differences. The pathogenic leptospires are divided into serovars according to their antigenic composition. More than 200 serovars make up the 23 serogroups.

Leptospires are coiled, thin, highly motile organisms with hooked ends and two periplasmic flagella, which enable the organisms to burrow into tissue. These organisms are 6 to 20 μm long and about 0.1 μm wide; they stain poorly but can be seen microscopically by dark-field examination and after silver impregnation staining. Leptospires require special media and conditions for growth; it may take weeks for cultures to become positive.

EPIDEMIOLOGY Leptospirosis is a zoonosis with a worldwide distribution that affects at least 160 mammalian species. Rodents, especially rats, are the most important reservoir, although dogs, other wild mammals, fish, and birds may also harbor these microorganisms. Leptospires establish a symbiotic relationship with their host and can persist in the renal tubules for years. Some serovars are associated with particular animals—e.g., icterohaemorrhagiae/copenhageni with

rats, grippotyphosa with voles, hardjo with cattle, canicola with dogs, and pomona with pigs.

Transmission of leptospires may follow direct contact with urine, blood, or tissue from an infected animal or exposure to a contaminated environment; human-to-human transmission is rare. Since leptospires are excreted in the urine and can survive in water for many months, water is an important vehicle in their transmission. Leptospirosis occurs most commonly in the tropics because the climate as well as the sometimes poor working and hygienic conditions favor the pathogen's survival.

Humans are not commonly infected with leptospires. However, in the United States, the 40 to 120 cases reported annually to the Centers for Disease Control and Prevention certainly represent a significant underestimation of the total number. Certain occupational groups are at especially high risk; included are veterinarians, agricultural workers, sewage workers, slaughterhouse employees, and workers in the fishing industry. Such individuals may acquire leptospirosis through direct exposure to or contact with contaminated water and soil.

In western countries, recreational exposure and domestic-animal contact are also prominent sources of leptospirosis. Recreational water use, such as canoeing, windsurfing, swimming, and waterskiing, place persons at risk for leptospirosis. Sometimes the infection is acquired during travel abroad. In a recent study in the Netherlands, 14 percent of patients with confirmed leptospirosis had acquired the infection while traveling in tropical countries, mostly in Southeast Asia. Transmission via laboratory accidents has been reported but is rare. Occasionally, leptospirosis develops after unanticipated immersion in contaminated water (e.g., in an automobile accident). Most cases occur in men, with a peak incidence during the summer and fall in western countries and during the rainy season in the tropics.

PATHOGENESIS The pathogenesis of leptospirosis is incompletely understood. Leptospires may enter the host through abrasions in the skin or through intact mucous membranes, especially the conjunctiva and the lining of the oro- and nasopharynx. Drinking of contaminated water may introduce leptospires through the mouth, throat, or esophagus. After entry of the organisms, leptospiremia develops, with subsequent spread to all organs. Multiplication takes place in blood and in tissues, and leptospires can be isolated from blood and cerebrospinal fluid (CSF) during the first 4 to 10 days of illness. It is not clear why the presence of leptospires in the CSF does not cause damage. An important role for a toxin in the pathogenesis of the disease has been suggested but not proved.

Leptospire-inflicted damage to the capillary endothelium results in vasculitis, which is responsible for the most important manifestations of the disease. Although leptospires mainly infect the kidneys and liver, any organ may be affected. In the kidney, leptospires migrate to the interstitium, renal tubules, and tubular lumen, causing interstitial nephritis and tubular necrosis. Hypovolemia due to dehydration or altered capillary permeability may contribute to the development of renal failure. In the liver, centrilobular necrosis with proliferation of Kupffer cells may be found. However, severe hepatocellular necrosis is not a feature of leptospirosis. Pulmonary involvement is the result of hemorrhage and not of inflammation. Invasion of skeletal muscle by leptospires results in swelling, vacuolation of the myofibrils, and focal necrosis. In severe leptospirosis, vasculitis may ultimately impair the microcirculation and increase capillary permeability, resulting in fluid leakage and hypovolemia.

When antibodies are formed, leptospires are eliminated from all sites in the host except the eye, the proximal renal tubules, and perhaps the brain, where they may persist for weeks or months. The persistence of leptospires in the aqueous humor occasionally causes chronic or recurrent uveitis. The systemic immune response is effective in eliminating the organism but may also produce symptomatic inflammatory reactions. A rise in antibody titer coincides with the development of meningitis; this association suggests that an immunologic mechanism is responsible.

After the start of antimicrobial treatment for leptospirosis, a Jarisch-Herxheimer reaction similar to that seen in other spirochetal diseases may develop. Although frequently described in older publications, this reaction seems to be a rare event in leptospirosis and is certainly less frequent in this infection than in other spirochetal diseases.

CHAPTER 176
Leptospirosis

1037

CLINICAL MANIFESTATIONS Serologic evidence of past inapparent infection is found in 15 to 40 percent of persons who have been exposed but have not become ill. In symptomatic cases of leptospirosis, clinical manifestations vary from mild to serious or even fatal. More than 90 percent of symptomatic persons have the relatively mild and usually anicteric form of leptospirosis, with or without meningitis. Severe leptospirosis with profound jaundice (Weil's syndrome) develops in 5 to 10 percent of infected individuals.

The incubation period is usually 1 to 2 weeks but ranges from 2 to 26 days. Typically, an acute leptospiremic phase is followed by an immune leptospiruric phase. The distinction between the first and second phases is not always clear, and milder cases do not always include the second phase.

Anicteric Leptospirosis Leptospirosis may present as an acute influenza-like illness, with fever, chills, severe headache, nausea, vomiting, and myalgias. Muscle pain, which especially affects the calves, back, and abdomen, is an important feature of leptospiral infection. Less common features include sore throat and rash. The patient usually has an intense headache (frontal or retroorbital) and sometimes develops photophobia. Mental confusion may be evident. Pulmonary involvement, manifested in most cases by cough and chest pain and in a few cases by hemoptysis, is not uncommon.

The most common finding on physical examination is fever with conjunctival suffusion. Less common findings include muscle tenderness, lymphadenopathy, pharyngeal injection, rash, hepatomegaly, and splenomegaly. The rash may be macular, maculopapular, erythematous, urticarial, or hemorrhagic. Mild jaundice may be present.

Most patients become asymptomatic within 1 week. After an interval of 1 to 3 days, the illness recurs in a number of cases. The start of this second (immune) phase coincides with the development of antibodies. Symptoms are more variable than during the first (leptospiremic) phase. Usually the symptoms last for only a few days, but occasionally they persist for weeks. Often the fever is less pronounced and the myalgias are less severe than in the leptospiremic phase. An important event during the immune phase is the development of aseptic meningitis. Although no more than 15 percent of all patients have symptoms and signs of meningitis, many patients may have CSF pleocytosis. Meningeal symptoms usually disappear within a few days but may persist for weeks. Similarly, pleocytosis generally disappears within 2 weeks but occasionally persists for months. Iritis, iridocyclitis, and chorioretinitis—late complications that may persist for years—can become apparent as early as the third week but often present several months after the initial illness.

Severe Leptospirosis (Weil's Syndrome) Weil's syndrome, the most severe form of leptospirosis, is characterized by jaundice, renal dysfunction, hemorrhagic diathesis, and high mortality. This syndrome is frequently but not exclusively associated with infection due to serovar icterohaemorrhagiae/copenhageni. The onset of illness is no different from that of less severe leptospirosis; however, after 4 to 9 days, jaundice as well as renal and vascular dysfunction generally develop. Although some degree of defervescence may be noted after the first week of illness, a biphasic disease pattern like that seen in anicteric leptospirosis is lacking. The jaundice of Weil's syndrome, which can be profound and give an orange cast to the skin, is usually not associated with severe hepatic necrosis. Death is rarely due to liver failure. Hepatomegaly and tenderness in the right upper quadrant are usually detected. Splenomegaly is found in 20 percent of cases.

Renal failure may develop, often during the second week of illness. Hypovolemia and decreased renal perfusion contribute to the development of acute tubular necrosis with oliguria or anuria. Dialysis is sometimes required, although a fair number of cases can be managed without dialysis. Renal function may be completely regained.

Pulmonary involvement occurs frequently, resulting in cough, dyspnea, chest pain, and blood-stained sputum and sometimes in hemoptysis or even respiratory failure. Hemorrhagic manifestations are seen in Weil's syndrome: epistaxis, petechiae, purpura, and ecchymo-

ses are found commonly, while severe gastrointestinal bleeding and adrenal or subarachnoid hemorrhage are detected rarely.

Rhabdomyolysis, hemolysis, myocarditis, pericarditis, congestive heart failure, cardiogenic shock, adult respiratory distress syndrome, and multiorgan failure have all been described during severe leptospirosis.

LABORATORY AND RADIOLOGIC FINDINGS The kidneys are invariably involved in leptospirosis. Related findings range from urinary sediment changes (leukocytes, erythrocytes, and hyaline or granular casts) and mild proteinuria in anicteric leptospirosis to renal failure and azotemia in severe disease.

The erythrocyte sedimentation rate is usually elevated. In anicteric leptospirosis, peripheral leukocyte counts range from 3000 to 26,000/ μL, with a left shift; in Weil's syndrome, leukocytosis is often marked. Mild thrombocytopenia occurs in up to 50 percent of patients and is associated with renal failure.

In contrast to patients with acute viral hepatitis, those with leptospirosis typically have elevated serum levels of bilirubin and alkaline phosphatase as well as mild increases (up to 200 U/L) in serum levels of aminotransferases. In Weil's syndrome, the prothrombin time may be prolonged but can be corrected with vitamin K. Levels of creatine phosphokinase, which are elevated in up to 50 percent of patients with leptospirosis during the first week of illness, may help to differentiate this infection from viral hepatitis.

When a meningeal reaction develops, polymorphonuclear leukocytes predominate initially and the number of mononuclear cells increases later. The protein concentration in the CSF may be elevated; CSF glucose levels are normal.

In severe leptospirosis, pulmonary radiographic abnormalities are more common than would be expected on the basis of physical examination. These abnormalities most frequently develop 3 to 9 days after the onset of illness. The most common radiographic finding is a patchy alveolar pattern that corresponds to scattered alveolar hemorrhage. Radiographic abnormalities most often affect the lower lobes in the periphery of the lung fields.

DIAGNOSIS A definite diagnosis of leptospirosis is based either on isolation of the organism from the patient or on seroconversion or a rise in antibody titer in the microscopic agglutination test (MAT). For a presumptive diagnosis of leptospirosis, an antibody titer of $\geq$1:100 in the MAT or a positive macroscopic slide agglutination test in the presence of a compatible clinical illness is required. Antibodies generally do not reach detectable levels until the second week of illness. The antibody response can be affected by early treatment.

The macroscopic slide agglutination test with killed antigen is useful for screening but is not specific. The MAT, which uses a battery of live leptospiral strains, and the enzyme-linked immunosorbent assay (ELISA), which uses a broadly reacting antigen, are the standard serologic procedures. These tests usually are available only in specialized laboratories and are used for the determination of the antibody titer and for the tentative identification of the serovar involved (thus the importance of using antigens representative of the serovars prevalent in the particular geographic area). Since cross-reactions occur frequently, however, it is often impossible to identify the infecting serovar. Serologic testing cannot be used as the basis for a decision about whether to start treatment.

In addition to the MAT and the ELISA, various other tests with diagnostic value have been developed. Some tests, such as an indirect hemagglutination test, a microcapsule agglutination test, and an IgM ELISA, are commercially available. Recently, dot-ELISA, gold immunoblot, and polymerase chain reaction techniques have been developed, but these techniques are not yet used for routine diagnosis.

Leptospires can be isolated from blood and/or CSF during the first 10 days of illness and from urine for several weeks beginning at around 1 week. Sometimes urine cultures remain positive for months or years after the start of illness. For isolation of leptospires from body fluids or tissues, Ellinghausen-McCullough-Johnson-Harris (EMJH) medium is useful; other possibilities are Fletcher medium and Korthoff medium. Specimens can be mailed to a reference laboratory for culture since leptospires remain viable in anticoagulated blood for up to 11 days. Isolation of leptospires is important since it is the only way the infecting serovar can be correctly identified. Dark-field examination of blood or urine frequently results in misdiagnosis and should not be used.

DIFFERENTIAL DIAGNOSIS Leptospirosis should be differentiated from other febrile illnesses associated with headache and muscle pain, such as malaria, enteric fever, viral hepatitis, dengue, Hantavirus infections, and rickettsial diseases. In light of the strong similarity in epidemiology and clinical presentation between leptospirosis and Hantavirus infections and given the reported occurrence of dual infections, it is advisable to conduct serologic testing for Hantavirus in cases of suspected leptospirosis. When patients have a flulike disease with disproportionately severe myalgia or aseptic meningitis, a diagnosis of leptospirosis should be considered.

 TREATMENT

The effect of antimicrobial therapy for the mild febrile form of leptospirosis is controversial, but such treatment is indicated for more severe forms. Treatment should be initiated as early as possible; nevertheless, contrary to previous reports, treatment started after the first 4 days of illness is effective.

For severe cases of leptospirosis, intravenous administration of penicillin G, amoxicillin, ampicillin, or erythromycin is recommended (Table 176-1). In milder cases, oral treatment with tetracycline, doxycycline, ampicillin, or amoxicillin should be considered. Although several other antibiotics, including newer cephalosporins, are highly active against leptospires in vitro, no clinical experience has yet been gained with these drugs.

In rare cases, a Jarisch-Herxheimer reaction develops within hours after the start of antimicrobial therapy (see "Pathogenesis" above). The only effective mode of management of this reaction is supportive. Patients with severe leptospirosis and renal failure may require dialysis. Those with Weil's syndrome may need transfusions of whole blood and/or platelets. Intensive care may be necessary.

Most patients with leptospirosis recover. Mortality is highest among patients who are elderly and those who have Weil's syndrome. Leptospirosis during pregnancy is associated with high fetal mortality. Long-term follow-up of patients with renal failure and hepatic dysfunction has documented good recovery of renal and hepatic function.

PREVENTION Individuals who may be exposed to leptospires through their occupations or their involvement in recreational water activities should be informed about the risks. Measures for controlling leptospirosis include avoidance of exposure to urine and tissues from infected animals, vaccination of animals, and rodent control. The animal vaccine used in a given area should contain the serovars known to be present in that area. Unfortunately, some vaccinated animals still excrete leptospires in their urine. Vaccination of humans against a specific serovar prevalent in an area has been undertaken in some European and Asian countries and has proved effective. Chemoprophylaxis with doxycycline (200 mg once a week) has appeared to be efficacious in military personnel but is indicated only in rare instances of sustained short-term exposure.

BIBLIOGRAPHY

FARR RW: Leptospirosis. Clin Infect Dis 21:1, 1995
FEIGIN RD, ANDERSON DC: Human leptospirosis. Crit Rev Clin Lab Sci 5:413, 1975
MCCLAIN JBL et al: Doxycycline therapy for leptospirosis. Ann Intern Med 100:696, 1984
O'NEILL KM et al: Pulmonary manifestations of leptospirosis. Rev Infect Dis 13:705, 1991
SHAKED Y et al: Leptospirosis in pregnancy and its effect on the fetus: Case report and review. J Infect Dis 17:241, 1993
VAN CREVEL R et al: Leptospirosis in travelers. Clin Infect Dis 19:132, 1994
WATT G et al: Placebo-controlled trial of intravenous penicillin for severe and late leptospirosis. Lancet 1:433, 1988
——— et al: Skeletal and cardiac muscle involvement in severe, late leptospirosis. J Infect Dis 162:266, 1990

David T. Dennis, Grant L. Campbell

177 RELAPSING FEVER

DEFINITION The term *relapsing fever* describes two distinct borrelial disease entities: louse-borne relapsing fever (LBRF) and tick-borne relapsing fever (TBRF). Both are characterized by recurrent acute episodes of spirochetemia and fever alternating with spirochetal clearance and apyrexia.

ETIOLOGY A clinical and epidemiologic distinction between LBRF and similar fevers of different etiology, such as typhus fever, was made in Scotland in the mid-nineteenth century. Spirochetes were first seen in the blood of patients with relapsing fever by Obermeier in Germany in 1868, and spirochete-infected blood was shown to be infectious shortly thereafter. The worldwide distribution of relapsing spirochetal fevers was recognized in the early part of the twentieth century, and the causative agents were shown to be transmitted by lice and ticks. Relapsing-fever spirochetes were described as borreliae belonging to the family Spirochaetaceae. *Borrelia recurrentis* was identified as the cause of LBRF, and strains of borreliae causing TBRF were identified and named, often according to the species of *Ornithodoros* tick responsible for their transmission (Table 177-1).

Relapsing-fever borreliae are gram-negative helical bacteria that average 0.2 to 0.5 μm in width and 5 to 20 μm in length. They comprise an outer membrane, an intermediate peptidoglycan layer, and an inner cytoplasmic membrane, which encloses the protoplasmic cylinder. Periplasmic flagella (15 to 20 at each end of the bacterium) are situated beneath the outer membrane. Relapsing-fever borreliae are slow-growing and microaerophilic; they grow best at 30 to 35°C. TBRF spirochetes grow well in a modification of Kelly's medium, Barbour-Stoenner-Kelly (BSK) medium; LBRF spirochetes are more fastidious in the laboratory and grow poorly on artificial medium.

Relapsing-fever borreliae are distinguished by remarkable antigenic variability and strain heterogeneity. New *Borrelia* serotypes spontaneously emerge at a high rate, resulting from a unique process of DNA rearrangement within genes located on linear plasmids. These genes code for variable major proteins (VMPs) located on the spirochete's outer-membrane surface. This antigenic variation, generated by sequential expression of previously silent *vmp* genes for serotype-specific VMPs, allows the borreliae to escape the immune response

Table 176-1

Treatment and Chemoprophylaxis of Leptospirosis

Purpose of Drug Administration	Regimen
Treatment	
Mild leptospirosis	Doxycycline, 100 mg orally bid
	or
	Ampicillin, 500–750 mg orally qid
	or
	Amoxicillin, 500 mg orally qid
Moderate/severe leptospirosis	Penicillin G, 1.5 million units IV qid
	or
	Ampicillin, 1 g IV qid
	or
	Amoxicillin, 1 g IV qid
	or
	Erythromycin, 500 mg IV qid
Chemoprophylaxis	Doxycycline, 200 mg orally once a week

NOTE: All regimens used for treatment are administered for 7 days.

of the host and results in the relapse phenomenon characteristic of infection with these organisms.

EPIDEMIOLOGY **Louse-Borne Relapsing Fever** Body lice (*Pediculus humanus* var. *corporis*) become infected with *B. recurrentis* by feeding on spirochetemic humans, the only reservoirs of infection. In lice, *B. recurrentis* spirochetes are found almost exclusively in the hemolymph; humans acquire infection when infected body lice are crushed and their fluids contaminate mucous membranes or bite wounds or other breaks in the skin (such as abrasions caused by scratching of pruritic louse bites). Louse-borne spirochetes are transmitted neither by the bite of a louse (anterior station transmission) nor by inoculation of louse feces (posterior station transmission). Lice have a short life span, feed at frequent intervals, and survive only a few days off the human host. Louse infestation of patients and the environmental circumstances of exposure are easily identified. Persons of all ages and both sexes are equally susceptible to infection.

LBRF has severely affected military and civilian populations disrupted by war and other disasters. During the Industrial Revolution, the disease was common among slum dwellers, prisoners, and other impoverished and overcrowded groups in Great Britain and Europe. Outbreaks occurred in the mid-nineteenth century in Philadelphia and other east coast cities and in the mining camps of the western United States. LBRF and louse-borne typhus were epidemic in eastern Europe and in Russia in the early part of the twentieth century. During the Second World War, LBRF spilled out of Ethiopia and spread across the Sudan to West Africa, causing many thousands of cases and deaths. Most recently, outbreaks of LBRF have occurred in northeastern Africa among refugees fleeing war and famine. LBRF has disappeared over large regions of the world as improvements have been made in standards of living, sanitation, and hygiene; it is now an important endemic disease only in northeastern Africa, especially the highlands of Ethiopia, where an estimated 10,000 cases occur annually. In Ethiopia, the disease affects mostly homeless men crowded together in unhygienic circumstances, especially during the cool rainy season, when it is more difficult for them to change and wash their clothing. LBRF does not pose a significant risk to tourists or other casual visitors but can be acquired from lice by persons (such as relief workers) in intimate contact with those affected as well as through accidental needle stick or mucocutaneous contact with infected blood.

Tick-Borne Relapsing Fever Soft ticks (Argasidae, *Ornithodoros* spp.) transmit TBRF. The ticks become infected by feeding on spirochetemic mammalian hosts. Except for *Borrelia duttoni* (a prominent cause of TBRF in sub-Saharan Africa), TBRF borreliae are zoonotic disease agents found naturally in rodents (rats, mice, chipmunks, and squirrels) and in lagomorphs (rabbits and hares). In ticks, TBRF borreliae invade all tissues, including the salivary glands and the ovaries. The spirochetes are transmitted to humans and animals via saliva and coxal fluid when the tick feeds. Infection in ticks is transmitted vertically from one stage to the next; in some tick species, infection is transmitted transovarially over several generations. Soft ticks are hardy and can survive for 10 years or more with only an occasional blood meal. These ticks feed painlessly, relatively quickly (for 20 to 45 minutes), and usually at night while

hosts are sleeping; thus patients with TBRF are often unaware of tick exposures.

TBRF borreliae are widely distributed throughout the world. TBRF is most highly endemic in sub-Saharan Africa but is also found in countries of the Mediterranean littoral, Middle Eastern states, southern Russia, the Indian subcontinent, and China. In the United States, this disease occurs west of the Mississippi River, especially in mountainous areas, where *B. hermsii* is the causative agent. TBRF is reported at low frequency throughout Latin America. The disease typically occurs sporadically or in small—often familial—clusters. Infected soft ticks may cause repeated infections among persons living or sleeping in the same dwelling. In sub-Saharan Africa, *O. moubata*, the vector of *B. duttoni*, infests native huts and rest houses, hiding in crevices of floors and walls during the day and emerging at night to feed on sleeping inhabitants. In the United States, *B. hermsii* infections most often occur during spring and summer months in mountain cabins. Infections of humans are sometimes precipitated by the disappearance of rodents (e.g., as a result of epizootic plague) that nest in foundations, wall spaces, and attics and that serve as the usual maintenance hosts for *O. hermsi* ticks. Outbreaks caused by *B. hermsii* have recently taken place among persons staying in rustic cabins along the north rim of the Grand Canyon and in the mountains of California, Idaho, and Colorado. Rodent-infested caves in southwestern states are associated with occasional cases of human infection with *B. turicatae*.

PATHOGENESIS AND PATHOLOGY In humans, relapsing-fever borreliae penetrate the skin or mucous membranes, multiply in the blood, and circulate in great numbers during febrile periods. The organisms also may be found in the liver, spleen, central nervous

Table 177-1

Characteristics and Distribution of Louse-Borne and Tick-Borne Borreliae

Borrelia Species	Arthropod Vector	Animal Reservoir	Distribution	Type(s) of Relapsing Fever
*B. recurrentis**	*Pediculus humanus* var. *corporis*	Humans	Worldwide	Louse-borne, epidemic
B. duttoni	*Ornithodoros moubata*	Humans	Central, eastern, southern Africa	East African tick-borne, endemic
B. hispanica	*O. erraticus* (large variety)	Rodents	Spain, Portugal, Morocco, Algeria, Tunisia	Hispano-African tick-borne
B. crocidurae, *B. merionesi,* *B. microti,* *B. dipodilli*	*O. erraticus* (small variety)	Rodents	Morocco, Libya, Egypt, Iran, Turkey, Senegal, Kenya	North African tick-borne
B. persica	*O. tholozani*†	Rodents	From western China and Kashmir to Iraq and Egypt, former USSR, India	Asiatic-African tick-borne
B. caucasica	*O. verrucosus*	Rodents	Caucasus to Iraq	Caucasian tick-borne
B. latyschewii	*O. tartakovskyi*	Rodents	Iran, Central Asia	Caucasian tick-borne
B. hermsii	*O. hermsi*	Rodents	Western United States	American tick-borne
B. turicatae	*O. turicata*	Rodents	Southwestern United States	American tick-borne
B. parkeri	*O. parkeri*	Rodents	Western United States	American tick-borne
B. mazzotti	*O. talaje*‡	Rodents	Southern United States, Mexico, Central and South America	American tick-borne
B. venezuelensis	*O. rudis*§	Rodents	Central and South America	American tick-borne

* Synonyms: *B. obermeyeri, B. novyi.*
† Synonyms: *O. papillipes, O. crossi?*
‡ Synonym: *O. dugesi?*
§ Synonym: *O. venezuelensis.*
SOURCE: From Burgdorfer and Schwan.

system, bone marrow, and other tissues and may be sequestered at these sites during periods of remission. The severity of disease is positively related to spirochete density in the blood; however, the role of borreliae in causing the systemic manifestations of relapsing fever is incompletely understood. Even though the pathophysiologic manifestations of the disease resemble responses to endotoxin, and although plasma from some patients with relapsing fever coagulates *Limulus* amebocyte lysates, borreliae and other spirochetes have not been shown to contain endotoxin. Infection with *B. recurrentis* does, however, activate protein mediators of inflammation, such as Hageman factor, prekallikrein, and proteins of the complement system; further, a spirochetal heat-stable pyrogenic factor stimulates mononuclear phagocytes to express increased amounts of leukocyte pyrogen and thromboplastin.

The Jarisch-Herxheimer reaction in LBRF patients is associated with a release of various cytokines into the plasma, including tumor necrosis factor, interleukin 6, interleukin 8, and C-reactive protein. These mediators of inflammation and fever most likely underlie many manifestations of relapsing fever, especially the complex series of pathophysiologic events that occur while spirochetes are being cleared rapidly from the blood, either during a spontaneous crisis or in response to antibiotic treatment. Meptazinol, a partial opioid agonist, diminishes the Jarisch-Herxheimer reaction in LBRF; this effect may indicate an exhaustion of endogenous opioids.

Findings at autopsy of relapsing-fever patients most often include enlargement of the liver and spleen and variable edema and swelling of other organs, such as the brain, lungs, and kidneys. On microscopic examination, the spleen is congested and contains multiple microabscesses of mononuclear cells that replace the white pulp, the myocardium displays diffuse histiocytic inflammation and interstitial edema, and the liver has areas of midzonal necrosis. Petechial hemorrhages are commonly evident over the surfaces of the meninges, pleura, heart, spleen, liver, kidneys, and mesentery. Subcapsular and parenchymal hemorrhagic infarcts of the spleen, heart, liver, and brain are sometimes grossly visible. Icterus is a common finding in severe and fatal cases of relapsing fever.

CLINICAL MANIFESTATIONS The clinical manifestations of LBRF and TBRF are similar. The mean incubation period is 7 days (range, 2 to 18 days), and the onset of illness is sudden, with fever, headache, shaking chills, sweats, myalgias, and arthralgias. The arthralgia of relapsing fever can be severe, involving small and large joints, but there is no evidence of arthritis. Dizziness, nausea, and vomiting are common. Sleep may be difficult and is sometimes accompanied by disturbing dreams. The patient is coherent but withdrawn, thirsty, and disinterested in food and other outside stimuli. The fever is high from the first (with a usual temperature of ≥40°C), is most often irregular in pattern, and is sometimes accompanied by delirium. Patients become progressively prostrate as the disease advances. The pulse is rapid and the patient is mildly tachypneic. Meningism may be found. The conjunctivae are often injected, and the patient usually exhibits photophobia. The sclerae are sometimes icteric, most commonly in the later stages of illness. The mucous membranes are often dry, and the patient is mildly dehydrated. Scattered petechiae develop on the trunk, extremities, and mucous membranes in one-third or more of LBRF patients and in fewer TBRF patients. A nonproductive cough is common, but chest sounds are usually normal; pleuritic pain and an accompanying pleuritic rub are sometimes noted. Cardiac findings are compatible with a high-output state; tachycardia and summation gallop are common. Upper quadrant abdominal tenderness and slight or moderate enlargement of the spleen and liver frequently characterize the acute phase of illness.

Epistaxis and blood-tinged sputum are common complications; clinically apparent gastrointestinal and central nervous system hemorrhage occur infrequently. Other complications of variable incidence include iridocyclitis, meningitis, coma, isolated cranial-nerve palsy, pneumonitis, myocarditis, and rupture of the spleen. Infection during

pregnancy can result in spontaneous abortion, stillbirth, or neonatal infection. Life-threatening complications are unusual in otherwise healthy persons, especially if the illness is diagnosed and treated early.

Without treatment, symptoms intensify over a 2- to 7-day period (average, 5 days in LBRF and 3 days in TBRF), ending in a spontaneous crisis during which spirochetes disappear from the circulation. Treatment with one of the rapidly acting antibiotics, such as erythromycin, a tetracycline, or chloramphenicol, regularly precipitates a Jarisch-Herxheimer reaction within 1 to 4 h. This reaction is indistinguishable from the spontaneous crisis; its severity is positively correlated with the density of spirochetes in the blood at the time of treatment. In the first phase of the crisis or reaction (the *chill phase*), rigors and rising fever are accompanied by an increasing metabolic rate, alveolar hyperventilation, high cardiac output, increasing peripheral vascular resistance, and decreased pulmonary arterial pressure. The body temperature commonly rises to 41.5°C or higher. This high fever is accompanied often by agitation and confusion and sometimes by delirium. Fever can be partially controlled by the use of a cooling blanket and ice packs and by sponging of the patient with tepid water and alcohol. The chill phase terminates after 10 to 30 min, giving way to a *flush phase* characterized by a fall in body temperature, drenching sweats, and sometimes (more commonly in LBRF) a potentially dangerous fall in systemic arterial pressure and rise in pulmonary arterial pressure. Although cardiac output is maintained at high levels, the effective circulating blood volume decreases as peripheral vascular resistance falls. Vital signs must be monitored carefully during this period of the reaction, which usually lasts 8 h or less. Clinical and electrocardiographic evidence of myocarditis and myocardial dysfunction includes a prolonged QT_c interval, a third heart sound (S_3), elevated central venous pressure, arterial hypotension, and pulmonary edema.

The crisis is followed by a period of exhaustion, sleep, and a rapid and uneventful recovery. Not uncommonly, in the first week of convalescence, patients experience 1 or 2 days of mild fever unassociated with detectable spirochetemia. In untreated cases, spirochetemia and symptoms may recur after a period of several days or weeks (average interval to first relapse, 9 days in LBRF and 7 days in TBRF). Only one or two relapses characteristically occur in untreated LBRF, while as many as 10 (average, three) can occur in untreated TBRF. In most cases, the illness becomes shorter and milder and the afebrile intervals longer with each relapse. Because of the great antigenic variation among *Borrelia* strains, infection does not confer protective immunity, and repeated infections of the same individual have been recorded.

Diseases that should be considered in the differential diagnosis of relapsing fever or that may complicate relapsing fever include typhus fever, typhoid, nontyphoid salmonellosis, malaria, dengue and other arboviral illnesses, tuberculosis, and leptospirosis. In the United States, the geographic distribution of Colorado tick fever overlaps that of TBRF, and the two diseases have similar manifestations early in their courses.

LABORATORY FINDINGS AND DIAGNOSIS The diagnosis of relapsing fever is confirmed most easily by the detection of spirochetes in blood, bone marrow aspirates, or cerebrospinal fluid. Motile spirochetes can be seen when fresh blood is examined by darkfield microscopy, and fixed organisms are clearly visible in Wright-, Giemsa-, or acridine orange-stained preparations of thin or dehemoglobinized thick smears of peripheral blood or buffy-coat preparations (Fig. 177-1). Organisms are found in blood taken during periods of fever preceding the crisis; smears from 70 percent or more of LBRF patients and from fewer TBRF patients are positive. In reference laboratories, relapsing-fever spirochetes are cultured from blood by the inoculation of BSK medium or by the intraperitoneal inoculation of immature laboratory mice. The detection of agglutinins against *Proteus* OX-K (Weil-Felix reaction) in convalescent-phase serum supports the diagnosis. Serum antibodies to *Borrelia* can be detected by enzyme immunoassays, but these tests are unstandardized and subject to insensitivity due to antigenic variations among strains. Serologic cross-reactions occur with other spirochetes, including *Borrelia burgdorferi*, the agent of Lyme disease, and *Treponema pallidum*.

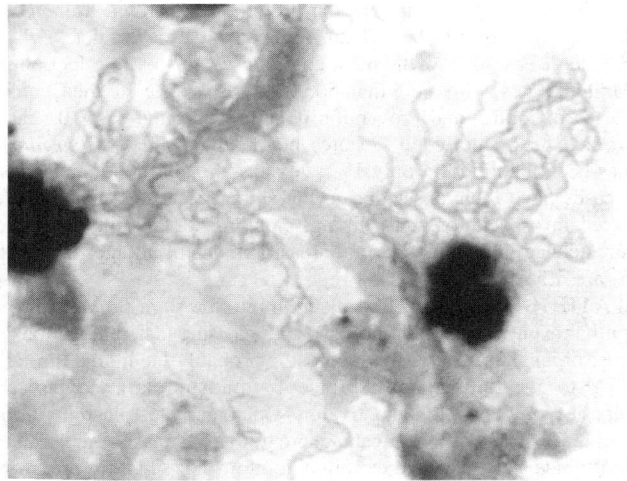

FIGURE 177-1 Blood smear (dehemoglobinized thick film) from a patient with louse-borne relapsing fever, showing multiple spirochetes (Wright's stain, × 600).

Other laboratory findings in relapsing fever are generally nonspecific. The leukocyte count is normal or moderately elevated, with an unremarkable cell differential. Serum bilirubin levels are generally only slightly elevated. Thrombocytopenia (mean platelet count about 50,000/μL) is evident in LBRF patients at admission and rebounds during early convalescence. Prothrombin and partial thromboplastin times are moderately prolonged during acute illness, as are standardized bleeding times. Fibrinogen concentrations in the blood are normal, and fibrinolysis is mild or absent. Results of the Rumpel-Leede tourniquet test are negative, despite the presence of petechiae.

℞ TREATMENT

Relapsing-fever borreliae are exquisitely sensitive to antibiotics. Treatment with erythromycin, a tetracycline, chloramphenicol, or penicillin produces rapid clearance of spirochetes and a remission of symptoms (Table 177-2). For children less than 9 years of age and for pregnant women, erythromycin and penicillin are the preferred drugs. The use of delayed-release intramuscular penicillin may prolong or delay the clearance of spirochetes and attenuate the accompanying Jarisch-Herxheimer reaction, but this response is not predictable; furthermore, single-dose penicillin treatment sometimes results in relapse of spirochetemia and symptoms. Although a single dose of erythromycin, a tetracycline, or chloramphenicol is highly effective in the treatment of LBRF, less is known about the efficacy of single-dose treatment of TBRF. Empirical treatment of TBRF for 7 days is therefore recommended to reduce the risk of persisting or

Table 177-2

Antibiotic Treatment of Louse-Borne and Tick-Borne Relapsing Fever in Adults

Medication	Louse-Borne Relapsing Fever (Single Dose)	Tick-Borne Relapsing Fever (7-Day Schedule)
Oral		
Erythromycin	500 mg	500 mg q 6 h
Tetracycline	500 mg	500 mg q 6 h
Doxycycline	100 mg	100 mg q12 h
Chloramphenicol	500 mg	500 mg q 6 h
Parenteral*		
Erythromycin	500 mg	500 mg q 6 h
Tetracycline	250 mg	250 mg q 6 h
Doxycycline	100 mg	100 mg q 12 h
Chloramphenicol	500 mg	500 mg q 6 h
Penicillin G (procaine)	600,000 IU	600,000 IU daily

* For tick-borne relapsing fever, parenteral therapy is used only until oral treatment is tolerated.

relapsing borreliosis. Glucocorticoids and nonsteroidal anti-inflammatory agents do not prevent or significantly modify the cardio-pulmonary disturbances of the Jarisch-Herxheimer reaction, although hydrocortisone and acetaminophen given at the same time as antibiotics reduce peak body temperature. Close monitoring of fluid balance, arterial and venous pressures, and myocardial function is advised in supportive management of the Jarisch-Herxheimer reaction in LBRF patients. The management of patients with myocardial dysfunction requires caution in the administration of intravenous fluids and, in some cases, rapid digitalization. Bleeding is not controlled by heparin, and clinical studies do not suggest that disseminated intravascular coagulopathy is important. Vitamin K and other soluble vitamins are sometimes given to counter dietary deficiencies in LBRF patients. Because postural hypotension is often pronounced during the acute phase of relapsing fever and in the early stage of recovery, patients should be assisted when arising from bed.

Untreated LBRF has a high case-fatality rate, especially in persons in otherwise poor health, such as those in famine-affected populations. The fatality rate among treated persons is usually less than 5 percent. In general, TBRF is a milder disease than LBRF: the spontaneous crisis and the Jarisch-Herxheimer reactions are less pronounced and the case-fatality rates are lower for TBRF than for LBRF.

PREVENTION AND CONTROL LBRF can be prevented by elimination of circumstances that promote louse infestation (crowding, poverty, homelessness), by use of personal hygienic practices that eliminate or reduce numbers of body lice (bathing, washing clothes, changing clothes at frequent intervals), and by application of acaricides to clothing. Secondary complications and the spread of infection can be prevented by early case detection and treatment. Historically, outbreaks of LBRF have been controlled by mass delousing. In situations like those in refugee camps, individuals, their clothes, and their bedding should be deloused with appropriate acaricides, such as lindane (1% dust), malathion (1% dust), or pyrethrins; in addition, provisions should be made for washing and changing of clothing. Impregnation of clothing with permethrin, a residual acaricide, can provide long-term protection against infestation. In outbreaks of fever that involve louse-infested populations, empirical single-dose treatment with doxycycline will be effective against typhus as well as LBRF. *B. recurrentis* has a fragile life cycle and is eradicable.

TBRF can be prevented by the avoidance of rodent- and tick-infested dwellings and infested natural sites in areas endemic for relapsing fever. Limiting rodent access to the foundations and attics of homes and vacation cabins and eliminating harborage for rodents in and around these dwellings reduce the potential for tick exposure. Rodents and rodent nests should be removed from infested buildings and their surroundings. Tick harborages of infested buildings or other circumscribed sites, such as rodent burrows and nests in hollow logs surrounding dwellings and in rodent-infested caves, can be chemically treated by pest-control specialists using various acaricides, such as carbaryl, diazinon, chlorpyrifos, pyrethrins, and malathion. Persons who enter tick-infested sites can protect themselves by wearing clothing that denies ticks access to the skin, by applying repellents to exposed skin and to clothing, and by applying an acaricide containing permethrin to clothing. Reporting of suspected cases of relapsing fever to public health authorities is important so that an epidemiologic investigation and control measures can be initiated promptly.

BIBLIOGRAPHY

BARBOUR AG: Antigenic variation of relapsing fever *Borrelia* species. Annu Rev Microbiol 44:155, 1990

BURGDORFER W, SCHWAN TG: *Borrelia*, in *Manual of Clinical Microbiology 6*, PR Murray et al (eds). Washington, DC, American Society for Microbiology, 1995, pp 626–635

FEKADE D et al: Prevention of Jarisch-Herxheimer reactions by treatment with antibodies against tumor necrosis factor α. N Engl J Med 335:311, 1996

HORTON JM, BLASER MJ: The spectrum of relapsing fever in the Rocky Mountains. Arch Intern Med 145:871, 1985

PERINE PL, TEKLU B: Antibiotic treatment of louse-borne relapsing fever in Ethiopia: A report of 377 cases. Am J Trop Med Hyg 32:1096, 1983

SPACH DH et al: Tick-borne diseases in the United States. N Engl J Med 329:936, 1993

178   Allen C. Steere

LYME BORRELIOSIS

DEFINITION Lyme borreliosis, a tick-transmitted spirochetal illness, usually begins with a characteristic expanding skin lesion, erythema migrans (EM; stage 1, localized infection). After several days or weeks, the spirochete may spread hematogenously to many different sites (stage 2, disseminated infection). Possible manifestations of disseminated infection include secondary annular skin lesions, meningitis, cranial or peripheral neuritis, carditis, atrioventricular nodal block, or migratory musculoskeletal pain. Months to years later (usually after periods of latent infection), intermittent or chronic arthritis, chronic encephalopathy or polyneuropathy, or acrodermatitis may develop (stage 3, persistent infection). Most patients experience early symptoms of the illness during the summer, but the infection may not become symptomatic until it progresses to stage 2 or 3. Despite regional variations, the basic stages of the illness are similar worldwide.

ETIOLOGIC AGENT *Borrelia burgdorferi*, the causative agent of the disease, is a fastidious, microaerophilic bacterium that grows best at 33°C in a complex liquid medium called Barbour, Stoenner, Kelly (BSK) medium. Culture of the spirochete from clinical specimens (except for biopsy samples of skin at sites of EM or acrodermatitis) has been difficult. Three groups of *B. burgdorferi* organisms, together referred to as *B. burgdorferi sensu lato*, have been identified, and more groups surely exist. To date, most North American strains have belonged to the first group, *B. burgdorferi sensu stricto*. Although all three of the identified groups have been found in Europe and Asia, most isolates there have been strains of group 2 (*B. garinii*) or group 3 (*B. afzelii*). These differences may well account for the clinical variations in the disease in different geographic regions.

EPIDEMIOLOGY The distribution of Lyme borreliosis correlates closely with the geographic ranges of certain ixodid ticks—*Ixodes dammini* (also called *I. scapularis*), *I. pacificus*, *I. ricinus*, and *I. persulcatus*. *I. dammini* is the principal vector in the northeastern United States from Massachusetts to Maryland and in the midwestern states of Wisconsin and Minnesota. Surveys in these regions have documented infection in at least 20 percent of *I. dammini* ticks; most cases of Lyme disease in the United States have occurred in these areas. *I. pacificus* is the vector in the western states of California and Oregon. The disease is acquired throughout Europe (from Great Britain to Scandinavia to European Russia), where *I. ricinus* is the vector, and in Asian Russia, China, and Japan, where *I. persulcatus* is the vector. These ticks transmit other diseases that may have similar symptoms. In the United States, *I. dammini* also transmits babesiosis and ehrlichiosis; in Europe and Asia, *I. ricinus* and *I. persulcatus* also transmit tick-borne encephalitis.

The *Ixodes* ticks have different animal hosts. For *I. dammini*, the white-footed mouse is the preferred host of the immature larval and nymphal ticks. It is critical that both of the tick's immature stages feed on the same host, because the life cycle of the spirochete depends on horizontal transmission: in early summer from infected nymphs to mice and in late summer from infected mice to larvae, which then molt to become the infected nymphs that will begin the cycle again the following year. White-tailed deer, which are not involved in the life cycle of the spirochete, are the preferred host for *I. dammini*'s adult stage and seem to be critical to the survival of the tick.

Lyme disease is now the most common vector-borne infection in the United States, with more than 50,000 cases reported to the Centers for Disease Control and Prevention (CDC) during the past 10 years. Cases have been reported in 47 states, but the life cycle of *B. burgdorferi* has been identified in only 19 states. As already mentioned, most new cases have their onset during the summer months. Cases have occurred in association with hiking, camping, or hunting trips and with residence in wooded or rural areas. Persons of all ages and both sexes are affected.

PATHOGENESIS After injection into the skin, *B. burgdorferi* may migrate outward, producing EM, and may spread hematogenously to other organs. Spread within the host is probably facilitated through binding to the spirochete's surface by human plasminogen and urokinase-type plasminogen activator, which activates plasmin, a potent protease. The spirochete can adhere to many types of mammalian cells; it binds specifically to certain ubiquitous host integrin receptors in the extracellular matrix, to vitronectin and fibronectin, and to matrix glycosaminoglycans. *B. burgdorferi* seems to have a particular tropism for tissues of the skin, nervous system, and joints, from all of which it has been cultured, seen in histologic sections, or (more commonly) detected (via its DNA) by the polymerase chain reaction (PCR). These findings and the response of all stages of the disease to antibiotic therapy suggest that the organism persists in affected tissues throughout the illness, but the mechanisms of persistent infection are not yet clear.

The immune response in Lyme disease develops gradually. After the first several weeks of infection, mononuclear cells generally exhibit heightened responsiveness to *B. burgdorferi* antigens, and evidence of B-cell hyperactivity is found, including elevated total serum IgM levels, cryoprecipitates, and circulating immune complexes. Titers of specific IgM antibody to *B. burgdorferi* peak between the third and sixth week after disease onset. The specific IgG response develops gradually over months, with response to an increasing array of 12 or more spirochetal polypeptides and maximal expansion during the period of arthritis. The spirochete is a potent inducer of proinflammatory cytokines, including tumor necrosis factor α and interleukin 1β. Histologic examination of all affected tissues reveals an infiltration of lymphocytes and plasma cells with some degree of vascular damage (including mild vasculitis or hypervascular occlusion), suggesting that the spirochete may have been present in or around blood vessels.

CLINICAL MANIFESTATIONS **Early Infection: Stage 1 (Localized Infection)** After an incubation period of 3 to 32 days, EM, which occurs at the site of the tick bite, usually begins as a red macule or papule that expands slowly to form a large annular lesion, most often with a bright red outer border and partial central clearing. Because of the small size of ixodid ticks, most patients do not remember the preceding tick bite. The center of the lesion sometimes becomes intensely erythematous and indurated, vesicular, or necrotic. In other instances, the expanding lesion remains an even, intense red; several red rings are found within an outside ring; or the central area turns blue before the lesion clears. Although EM can be located anywhere, the thigh, groin, and axilla are particularly common sites. The lesion is warm but not often painful. Perhaps as many as 25 percent of patients do not exhibit this characteristic skin manifestation.

Early Infection: Stage 2 (Disseminated Infection) Within days or weeks after the onset of EM, the organism often spreads hematogenously to many sites. In these cases patients frequently develop secondary annular skin lesions similar in appearance to the initial lesion. Skin involvement is frequently accompanied by severe headache, mild stiffness of the neck, fever, chills, migratory musculoskeletal pain, arthralgias, and profound malaise and fatigue. Less common manifestations include generalized lymphadenopathy or splenomegaly, hepatitis, sore throat, nonproductive cough, conjunctivitis, iritis, or testicular swelling. Except for fatigue and lethargy, which are often constant, the early signs and symptoms of Lyme disease are typically intermittent and changing. Even in untreated patients, the early symptoms usually become less severe or disappear within several weeks.

Symptoms suggestive of meningeal irritation may develop early in Lyme disease when EM is present but usually are not associated with cerebrospinal fluid (CSF) pleocytosis or an objective neurologic deficit. After several weeks or months, about 15 percent of untreated patients develop frank neurologic abnormalities, including meningitis, subtle encephalitic signs, cranial neuritis (including bilateral facial palsy), motor or sensory radiculoneuropathy, mononeuritis multiplex, or myelitis—alone or in various combinations. In the United States, the usual pattern consists of fluctuating symptoms of meningitis accompanied by facial palsy and peripheral radiculoneuropathy. Lymphocytic pleocytosis (about 100 cells per microliter) is found in CSF, often along with elevated protein levels and normal or slightly low glucose concentrations. In Europe and Asia, the first neurologic sign is characteristically radicular pain, which is followed by the development of CSF pleocytosis (called Bannwarth's syndrome), but meningeal or encephalitic signs are frequently absent. These early neurologic abnormalities usually resolve completely within months, but chronic neurologic disease may occur later.

Within several weeks after the onset of illness, about 8 percent of patients develop cardiac involvement. The most common abnormality is a fluctuating degree of atrioventricular block (first-degree, Wenckebach, or complete heart block). Some patients have more diffuse cardiac involvement, including electrocardiographic changes indicative of acute myopericarditis, left ventricular dysfunction evident on radionuclide scans, or (in rare cases) cardiomegaly or pancarditis. Cardiac involvement usually lasts for only a few weeks but may recur. One case of chronic cardiomyopathy caused by *B. burgdorferi* has been reported.

During this stage, musculoskeletal pain is common. The typical pattern consists of migratory pain in joints, tendons, bursae, muscles, or bones (usually without joint swelling) lasting for hours or days and affecting one or two locations at a time.

Late Infection: Stage 3 (Persistent Infection) Months after the onset of infection, about 60 percent of patients in the United States who have received no antibiotic treatment develop frank arthritis. The typical pattern comprises intermittent attacks of oligoarticular arthritis in large joints (especially the knees), lasting for weeks to months in a given joint. Small joints and periarticular sites also may be affected, primarily during early attacks. The number of patients who continue to have recurrent attacks decreases each year. However, in a small percentage of cases, involvement of large joints—usually one or both knees—becomes chronic and may lead to erosion of cartilage and bone. These patients have a higher frequency of the class II major histocompatibility complex allele HLA-DR4 than patients with brief Lyme arthritis or normal control subjects.

White cell counts in joint fluid range from 500 to 110,000/μL (average, 25,000/μL); most of these cells are polymorphonuclear leukocytes. Tests for rheumatoid factor or antinuclear antibodies usually give negative results. Examination of synovial biopsy samples reveals fibrin deposits, villous hypertrophy, vascular proliferation, microangiopathic lesions, and a heavy infiltration of lymphocytes and plasma cells.

Although less common, chronic neurologic involvement may also become apparent months or years after the onset of infection, sometimes following long periods of latent infection. The most common form of chronic central nervous system involvement is subtle encephalopathy affecting memory, mood, or sleep and often accompanied by axonal polyneuropathy manifested as either distal paresthesias or spinal radicular pain. Patients with encephalopathy frequently have evidence of memory impairment in neuropsychological tests and abnormal results in CSF analyses. In cases with polyneuropathy, electromyography generally shows extensive abnormalities of proximal and distal nerve segments. Encephalomyelitis or leukoencephalitis, a rare manifestation of Lyme borreliosis, is a severe neurologic disorder that may include spastic parapareses, upper motor-neuron bladder dysfunction, and lesions in the periventricular white matter. The prolonged course of chronic neuroborreliosis following periods of latent infection is reminiscent of tertiary neurosyphilis.

Acrodermatitis chronica atrophicans, the late skin manifestation of the disorder, has been associated primarily with *B. afzelii* infection in Europe and Asia. It has been observed primarily in elderly women. The skin lesions, which are usually found on the acral surface of an arm or leg, begin insidiously with reddish-violaceous discoloration; they become sclerotic or atrophic over a period of years.

DIAGNOSIS Lyme disease is usually diagnosed by the recognition of a characteristic clinical picture with serologic confirmation. Although serologic testing may yield negative results during the first several weeks of infection, most patients have a positive antibody response to *B. burgdorferi* after that time. The limitation of serologic tests is that they do not clearly distinguish between active and inactive infection. Patients with previous Lyme disease—particularly in cases progressing to late stages—often remain seropositive for years, even after adequate antibiotic treatment. In addition, some patients are seropositive because of asymptomatic infection. If these individuals subsequently develop another illness, the positive serologic test for Lyme disease may cause diagnostic confusion. On the other hand, a few patients who receive inadequate antibiotic therapy during the first several weeks of infection develop subtle joint or neurologic symptoms but are seronegative. The important point is that seronegative Lyme disease is usually a mild, attenuated illness.

For serologic analysis in Lyme disease, the CDC recommends a two-step approach in which samples are first tested by ELISA and equivocal or positive results are then tested by western blotting. During the first month of infection, both IgM and IgG responses to the spirochete should be determined, preferably in both acute- and convalescent-phase serum samples. Approximately 20 to 30 percent of patients have a positive response detectable in acute-phase samples, whereas about 70 to 80 percent have a positive response during convalescence (2 to 4 weeks later). After that time, the great majority of patients continue to have a positive IgG antibody response, and a single test (that for IgG) is usually sufficient. In persons with illness of longer than 1 month's duration, a positive IgM test result alone is likely to be false-positive. According to current criteria adopted by the CDC, an IgM western blot is considered positive if two of the following three bands are present: 23, 39, and 41 kDa. However, the combination of the 23- and 41-kDa bands may still represent a false-positive result. An IgG blot is considered positive if 5 of the following 10 bands are present: 18, 23, 28, 30, 39, 41, 45, 58, 66, and 93 kDa.

Because serologic tests do not distinguish between active and inactive infection, tests that detect the spirochete directly are being researched. *B. burgdorferi* may be cultured from skin lesions of patients with the disorder, but its culture from other sites has been a low-yield proposition. Detection of spirochetal DNA by PCR may serve as a substitute for culture in cases of Lyme arthritis. In a recent study, *B. burgdorferi* DNA was detected in synovial fluid samples from 75 (85 percent) of 88 patients and in none of 64 control samples. However, the sensitivity of PCR determinations in CSF from patients with neuroborreliosis has not been as high. The role of PCR in the detection of *B. burgdorferi* DNA from blood or urine samples is not yet clear.

DIFFERENTIAL DIAGNOSIS The most common problem in diagnosis is to distinguish late Lyme disease from chronic fatigue syndrome or fibromyalgia. This difficulty is compounded by the fact that a small percentage of patients develop these chronic pain or fatigue syndromes in association with or soon after Lyme disease. Compared with Lyme disease, chronic fatigue syndrome (see Chap. 384) or fibromyalgia tends to produce more generalized and disabling symptoms, including marked fatigue, severe headache, diffuse musculoskeletal pain, multiple symmetric tender points in characteristic locations, pain and stiffness in many joints, diffuse dysesthesias, difficulty with concentration, and sleep disturbances. Patients with chronic fatigue syndrome or fibromyalgia lack evidence of joint inflammation; they have normal results in neurologic tests; and they usually have a greater degree of anxiety and depression than patients with chronic neuroborreliosis.

℞ **TREATMENT**

As outlined in the algorithm in Fig. 178-1, the various manifestations of Lyme disease can usually be treated successfully with orally administered antibiotics; the exceptions are objective neurologic abnormalities, which seem to require intravenous therapy. For early Lyme disease, doxycycline (100 mg twice a day) is effective in men and in nonpregnant women. An advantage of this regimen is that it is also effective against the agent of human granulocytic ehrlichiosis, which is transmitted by the same tick that transmits the Lyme disease agent. Amoxicillin (500 mg three times a day), cefuroxime axetil (500 mg twice a day), and erythromycin (250 mg four times a day) or its congeners are second-, third-, and fourth-choice alternatives, respectively. In children, amoxicillin is effective (50 mg/kg per day, but not more than 2 g/d) in divided doses; in cases of penicillin allergy, cefuroxime axetil or erythromycin may be used. For patients with infection localized to the skin, a 10-day course of therapy is generally sufficient; in contrast, for patients with disseminated infection, a 20- to 30-day course is recommended. Approximately 15 percent of patients experience a Jarisch-Herxheimer-like reaction during the first 24 h of therapy.

These oral antibiotic regimens, when given for 30 to 60 days, are effective for the treatment of Lyme arthritis. However, the response to therapy may be slow. A small percentage of patients with arthritis, particularly those with the HLA-DR4 allele and an immune response to the OspA or OspB protein of the spirochete, do not respond to antimicrobial therapy. Treatment with anti-inflammatory agents or synovectomy may be successful in such cases.

For objective neurologic abnormalities (with the possible exception of facial palsy alone), parenteral antibiotic therapy seems to be necessary. Intravenous ceftriaxone (2 g/d for 4 weeks) is most commonly used for this purpose, but intravenous cefotaxime (2 g three times a day) or intravenous penicillin G (20 million units per day in divided doses) for the same duration may also be effective. In patients with high-degree atrioventricular block or a PR interval of greater than 0.3 s, intravenous therapy for at least part of the course and cardiac monitoring are recommended. In patients with complete heart block or congestive heart failure, glucocorticoids may be of benefit if antimicrobial therapy alone does not result in improvement within 24 h.

It is unclear how and whether asymptomatic infection should be treated, but patients with such infection are often given a course of oral antibiotics. The appropriate treatment for Lyme disease during pregnancy is also unclear. Because the risk of maternal-fetal transmission seems to be very low, standard therapy for the documented stage and manifestation of the illness may be sufficient. Relapse may follow the use of any of the antibiotic regimens for Lyme disease, and a second course of therapy may be necessary. On the other hand, in patients who develop chronic fatigue syndrome or fibromyalgia after Lyme disease, further antibiotic therapy does not seem to be of benefit.

The risk of infection with *B. burgdorferi* after a recognized tick bite is so low that antibiotic prophylaxis is not routinely indicated. However, if the tick is engorged, if follow-up is difficult, or if the patient is quite anxious, therapy with amoxicillin or doxycycline for 10 days is likely to prevent Lyme disease. A vaccine for Lyme disease is currently being tested but is not yet available.

PROGNOSIS   The response to treatment is best early in the disease. Later treatment of Lyme borreliosis is still effective, but convalescence may be longer. Eventually, most patients recover with minimal or no residual deficit.

BIBLIOGRAPHY

Barbour AG, Hayes SF: Biology of *Borrelia* species. Microbiol Rev 50:381, 1986

Dressler F et al: Western blotting in the serodiagnosis of Lyme disease. J Infect Dis 167:392, 1993

Logigian EL et al: Chronic neurologic manifestations of Lyme disease. N Engl J Med 323:1438, 1990

Luft BJ et al: Azithromycin compared with amoxicillin in the treatment of erythema migrans. Ann Intern Med 124:785, 1996

McAlister HF et al: Lyme carditis: An important cause of reversible heart block. Ann Intern Med 110:339, 1989

Nocton JJ et al: Detection of *Borrelia burgdorferi* DNA by polymerase chain reaction in synovial fluid in Lyme arthritis. N Engl J Med 330:229, 1994

Pachner AR, Steere AC: The triad of neurologic manifestations of Lyme disease: Meningitis, cranial neuritis, and radiculoneuritis. Neurology 35:47, 1985

Rahn DW, Malawista SE: Lyme disease: Recommendations for diagnosis and treatment. Ann Intern Med 114:472, 1991

Saint Girons I et al: Molecular biology of *Borrelia*, bacteria with linear replicons. Microbiology 140:1803, 1994

——: Lyme disease. N Engl J Med 321:586, 1989

—— et al: The early clinical manifestations of Lyme disease. Ann Intern Med 99:76, 1983

—— et al: The clinical evolution of Lyme arthritis. Ann Intern Med 107:725, 1987

—— et al: Treatment of Lyme arthritis. Arthritis Rheum 37:878, 1994

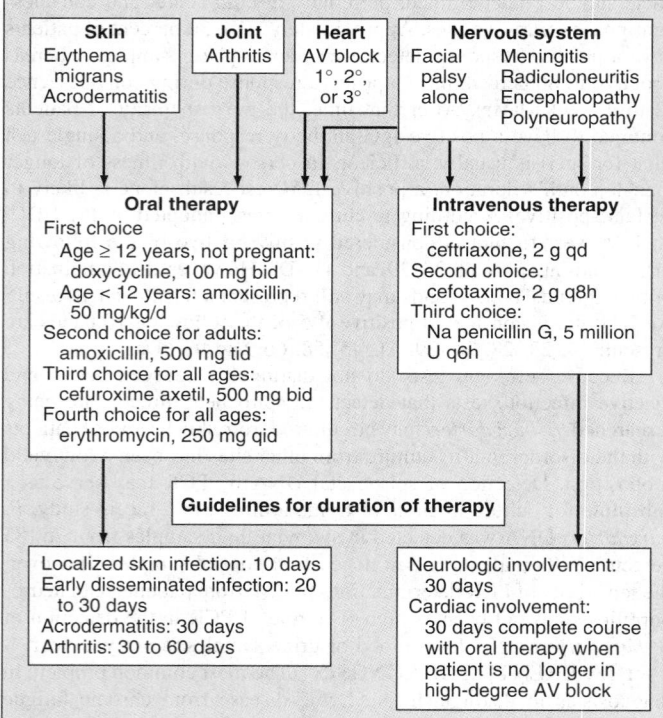

FIGURE 178-1   Algorithm for the treatment of the various acute or chronic manifestations of Lyme borreliosis. Relapse may occur with any of these regimens, and a second course of treatment may be necessary. AV, atrioventricular.

179 *David Walker, Didier Raoult, Philippe Brouqui, Thomas Marrie*

RICKETTSIAL DISEASES

The rickettsiae make up a family of gram-negative coccobacilli and short bacilli that grow strictly in eukaryotic cells. Characteristics of these organisms include their intracellular localization and persistence. The rickettsiae move through mammalian reservoirs; they are transmitted by insect vectors. Except for louse-borne typhus, humans are incidental hosts. Only *Coxiella burnetii* (the agent of Q fever) is able to survive for an extended period outside of the reservoir or vector. Clinical infections with rickettsiae can be classified into five general groups: (1) tick- and gamasid mite-borne spotted fever group (SFG) rickettsial diseases; (2) flea- and louse-borne typhus group rickettsial diseases; (3) chigger-borne scrub typhus; (4) ehrlichioses; and (5) Q fever.

TICK- AND MITE-BORNE SPOTTED FEVERS

ROCKY MOUNTAIN SPOTTED FEVER Rocky Mountain spotted fever (RMSF), a severe rickettsial disease, is caused by *Rickettsia rickettsii*, the prototype SFG organism. *R. rickettsii* has two major immunodominant surface-exposed proteins, OmpA and OmpB, which have species-specific conformational epitopes. OmpA functions as an adhesin for the host cell; OmpB, the most abundant outer-membrane protein, shares genetic sequences and limited antigens with typhus group rickettsiae. This small (0.3 μm by 1.0 μm) bacillus has a typical gram-negative cell wall structure (see Chap. 139); its lipopolysaccharide shares antigens mainly within the SFG and, in the quantities found in human infections, is not a potent endotoxin.

RMSF has been documented in 48 states and in Canada, Mexico, Costa Rica, Panama, Colombia, and Brazil. It is transmitted by *Dermacentor variabilis*, the American dog tick, in the eastern two-thirds of the United States and California; by *Dermacentor andersoni*, the Rocky Mountain wood tick, in the western United States; by *Rhipicephalus sanguineus* in Mexico; and by *Amblyomma cajennense* in Mexico and Central and South America. Although it is maintained principally by transovarian transmission from one generation of ticks to the next, *R. rickettsii* can be acquired by uninfected ticks through the ingestion of a blood meal from rickettsemic small mammals.

Humans become infected during the active season of the vector tick species. In northern areas, cases occur mainly in the spring; in warmer southern states, most cases occur from May to September, although some cases are reported in the winter. Four percent of *D. variabilis* ticks carry rickettsiae, the vast majority of which are nonpathogenic species such as *Rickettsia montana* and *Rickettsia bellii*. The likelihood of an individual tick's containing *R. rickettsii* is slight. From 1986 to 1992, approximately 600 cases of RMSF were reported annually. This number is probably an underestimate, since the diagnosis is difficult and reporting is incomplete. The incidence of infection is highest among 5- to 9-year-old children. In the preantibiotic era, the mortality rate was 20 to 25 percent; it still runs around 5 percent, primarily because of delayed diagnosis and delayed treatment. The case-fatality ratio is higher for males than for females and increases with each decade of life above age 20.

Pathogenesis *R. rickettsii* organisms are inoculated into the dermis along with secretions of the tick's salivary glands after ≥6 h of feeding. Rickettsiae spread throughout the body by the lymphatics and the bloodstream, attach via OmpA to the endothelial cell membrane, and induce their own engulfment. Once intracellularly located, they escape rapidly from the phagosome, replicate in the cytosol by binary fission, and spread from cell to cell, propelled by polar polymerization of the host cell's actin (Fig. 179-1). After an incubation period of approximately 1 week (range, 3 to 12 days; the length is

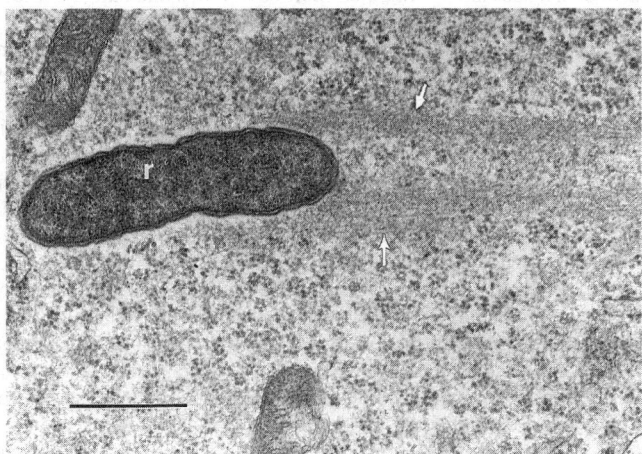

FIGURE 179-1 A spotted fever group rickettsia (r) in the cytosol of a cultured endothelial cell demonstrates a prominent actin tail (arrows), the source of the propulsive force that permits intracellular motion and intercellular spread. Bar = 0.5 μm. *(Courtesy of Dr. Vsevolod L. Popov.)*

dependent on the size of the rickettsial inoculum), numerous foci of contiguous, heavily infected endothelial cells that are extensive enough to manifest as injury develop. *R. rickettsii* is more invasive than other rickettsiae, routinely spreading to infect vascular smooth-muscle cells. Damage to these cells results in increased vascular permeability, edema, the development of a host mononuclear-cell tissue response, and hemorrhage.

Although occlusive thrombosis and ischemic necrosis are often cited as the pathologic basis for tissue and organ injury in RMSF, it is in fact increased vascular permeability, with resulting edema, hypovolemia, and ischemia, that is responsible. Indeed, immunohistologic studies of severely infected humans and animals have demonstrated numerous zones of infected endothelium, only a small proportion of which contain thrombi. The thrombi are usually located to one side of the lumen, which is not occluded. These hemostatic plugs appear to be an appropriate host response rather than a pathogenic process. Consumption of platelets may result in thrombocytopenia in up to half of infected patients, but disseminated intravascular coagulation with hypofibrinogenemia is rare in RMSF. Activation of platelets, generation of thrombin, and activation of the fibrinolytic system all appear to be homeostatic physiologic responses to endothelial injury.

Clinical Manifestations Early in the illness, when medical attention usually is first sought, RMSF is difficult to distinguish from many self-limiting viral illnesses. During the first 3 days, fever, headache, malaise, myalgia, nausea, vomiting, and anorexia are the most frequent symptoms. The untreated illness progresses insidiously as vascular infection and injury advance. In one large series, only one-third of patients were diagnosed with presumptive RMSF early in the clinical course and were treated appropriately as outpatients. All too often, RMSF is recognized only when its late severe manifestations, developing at the end of the first week or in the second week of illness in patients without appropriate treatment, prompt admission to the intensive care unit.

The progressive nature of the infection is clearly manifested in the skin. Rash is evident in 14 percent of patients on the first day of illness and in 49 percent during the first 3 days. Despite widespread hematogenous dissemination of rickettsiae to the skin during the incubation period, vascular injury usually makes its appearance between the third and the fifth febrile day as macules up to 5 mm in diameter on the wrists and ankles. Subsequently, similar lesions develop on the remainder of the extremities and the trunk. The pink foci of vasodilation become leaky, with local edema and conversion to maculopapules that blanch on compression. Later, more severe vascular damage results in frank hemorrhage at the center of the maculopapule, creating a petechia that does not disappear upon compression. Effective treatment may delay or abort this sequence of events. In fact, rash does not appear until day 6 or afterward in 20 percent of cases and does not develop at all in around 10 percent of cases, including some patients with severe visceral lesions that result in death. Overall, petechiae occur in about half of cases, developing on or after day 6 in most. Involvement of the palms and soles, often considered diagnostically important, usually occurs relatively late in the course (after day 5 in 43 percent of cases) and does not occur at all in many cases.

The systemic and pulmonary microcirculations are the target of the vascular changes induced by intracellular rickettsial infection, and clinical manifestations reflect the ensuing damage. Widespread increases in vascular permeability result in edema, decreased plasma volume, hypoalbuminemia, reduced serum oncotic pressure, and prerenal azotemia. Hypotension is reported in 17 percent of cases. Extensive infection of the pulmonary microcirculation is associated with noncardiogenic pulmonary edema in the face of normal or near-normal left ventricular function. True cardiac involvement is most frequently manifested as dysrhythmia, which is detected in up to 16 percent of cases. Pulmonary involvement with severe respiratory distress, often requiring mechanical ventilation, is frequently a prominent factor in fatal cases. In one series, 9 of 10 RMSF patients who required mechanical ventilation died.

Central nervous system involvement is the other important clinical feature of RMSF. Encephalitis due to vascular injury, presenting as confusion or lethargy, is apparent in 25 percent of cases. Progressively more severe encephalitis manifests as stupor or delirium, ataxia, coma, and seizures. Numerous other neurologic abnormalities have been seen, including cranial nerve palsies, hearing loss, severe vertigo, nystagmus, dysarthria, aphasia, unilateral corticospinal signs, ankle clonus, extensor toe signs, hyperreflexia, spasticity, fasciculations, athetosis, neurogenic bladder, hemiplegia, paraplegia, and complete paralysis. Meningoencephalitis results in cerebrospinal fluid (CSF) pleocytosis in about one-third of cases; usually there are 10 to 100 cells per microliter with a mononuclear predominance, but occasionally there are more than 100 cells per microliter with a polymorphonuclear predominance. The protein concentration in CSF may be increased, but the glucose concentration is usually normal.

Renal failure, a result of hypoperfusion of the kidneys, occurs in the more severely ill patients with RMSF. Hypovolemia and hypotension cause a reduction in the glomerular filtration rate and prerenal azotemia; these abnormalities are often reversible with rehydration. In the most severe cases, shock results in acute tubular necrosis–induced renal failure, which may require hemodialysis.

Hepatic injury is manifested in 38 percent of cases as mildly or moderately increased serum aminotransferase concentrations owing to focal necrosis of hepatocytes, but hepatic failure does not occur. An elevated serum bilirubin concentration and frank jaundice are sometimes found and are probably consequences of both hemolysis and hepatocyte injury. Many patients develop gastrointestinal symptoms, including abdominal pain, nausea, vomiting, and diarrhea.

Bleeding is a potentially life-threatening effect of severe vascular damage. Anemia develops in 30 percent of cases and may be severe enough to require transfusions of red blood cells. Blood is detected in the stools or vomitus of 10 percent of patients, and death has followed massive upper gastrointestinal hemorrhage.

Other characteristic findings include a normal white blood cell count with increased numbers of immature myeloid cells and increased plasma concentrations of proteins of the acute-phase response (C-reactive protein, fibrinogen, ferritin, and others). Hyponatremia is reported in 56 percent of cases and is due to the inappropriate secretion of antidiuretic hormone in response to the hypovolemic state. Skeletal muscle injury, clinically manifested as myositis, has been documented in several individual cases by the detection of marked elevations in serum creatine kinase levels or of histopathologic evidence of vascular injury in skeletal muscle and multifocal rhabdomyonecrosis. Ocular involvement includes conjunctivitis in 30 percent of cases and retinal vein engorgement, flame hemorrhages, arterial occlusion, and papilledema with normal CSF pressure in some instances.

In untreated cases, death usually occurs within 2 weeks after the onset of illness. A rare presentation, fulminant RMSF, is fatal within 5 days after onset. This fulminant presentation has been associated with RMSF in black males with a glucose-6-phosphate dehydrogenase deficiency and is believed to be related to an undefined effect of hemolysis on the rickettsial infection. Although survivors of RMSF usually appear to return to their previous state of health, patients who have been severely ill may sustain permanent sequelae, including neurologic deficits, and may need to have gangrenous extremities amputated.

Diagnosis The diagnosis of RMSF during the acute stage is more difficult than is generally appreciated. Clinical and epidemiologic considerations are more important than a laboratory diagnosis early in the illness. The most important epidemiologic factor is a history of exposure within 12 days before onset to a potentially tick-infested environment during a season of possible tick activity. However, only 60 percent of patients actually recall being bitten by a tick during the incubation period.

The differential diagnosis for early clinical manifestations of RMSF (fever, headache, and myalgia without a rash) includes influenza, enterovirus infection, infectious mononucleosis, viral hepatitis, leptospirosis, typhoid fever, gram-negative or gram-positive bacterial sepsis, and other rickettsial diseases. Enterocolitis may be suggested by nausea, vomiting, and abdominal pain; a prominence of abdominal tenderness has resulted in exploratory laparotomy. Central nervous system infection, including bacterial and viral meningoencephalitis, should be considered in the presence of seizures, coma, neurologic signs, and CSF abnormalities. Cough, pulmonary signs, and chest roentgenographic opacities may lead to the diagnostic consideration of bronchitis or pneumonia.

During the first 3 days of illness, only 3 percent of patients exhibit the classic triad of fever, rash, and history of tick exposure. When a rash appears, a diagnosis of RMSF should certainly be considered. However, many other illnesses considered in the differential diagnosis may also be associated with a rash, including rubeola, rubella, meningococcemia, disseminated gonococcal infection, secondary syphilis, toxic shock syndrome, drug hypersensitivity, idiopathic thrombocytopenic purpura, thrombotic thrombocytopenic purpura, Kawasaki syndrome, and immune complex vasculitis. The converse is also true: Any person in an endemic area with a provisional diagnosis of one of the above illnesses may have RMSF.

Serologic tests for RMSF are usually negative at the time of presentation for medical care, and treatment should not be delayed while a positive serologic result is awaited. The most common laboratory test for confirmation of the diagnosis is the indirect immunofluorescence assay. Between 7 and 10 days after the onset of illness, a diagnostic titer of ≥64 is usually detectable. Latex agglutination and a solid-state enzyme immunoassay are also available commercially. Latex agglutination usually yields a diagnostic titer of ≥128 at 1 week after onset.

The sensitivity and specificity of the indirect immunofluorescence assay are 94 to 100 percent and 100 percent, respectively; the latex agglutination test has a sensitivity of 71 to 94 percent and a specificity of 96 to 99 percent. The performance of the solid-state immunoassay has not been reported. The historically significant, but insensitive and nonspecific, Weil-Felix *Proteus vulgaris* OX-19 and OX-2 agglutination tests are unreliable and should not be used. Weil and Felix found that serum from a patient convalescing from typhus agglutinated a *Proteus* isolate (which they designated X-2) from the patient's urine. These researchers also found that another strain of *Proteus*, X-19, was similarly agglutinated but to a much higher titer. Because the X-2 and X-19 antigens were determined to be part of the heat-stable somatic or O antigen, these strains have commonly been referred to as OX strains. In 1934, Castaneda showed that *Proteus vulgaris* OX-19 and

Rickettsia prowazekii shared antigens. By studies with *Proteus* strains OX-19 and OX-2 as well as a third *Proteus* strain (OX-K, which was agglutinated by serum from patients with tsutsugamushi fever, or scrub typhus), it was possible to diagnose spotted fever, in which all three strains were agglutinated; scrub typhus, in which only strain OX-K was agglutinated; and epidemic (murine) typhus, in which only strain OX-19 was agglutinated. With the development of more specific tests, however, the Weil-Felix test has been abandoned. The test's rate of false positivity is about 20 percent, and it is insensitive.

The only diagnostic test that is useful during the acute illness is immunohistologic examination (immunofluorescence or immunoenzyme staining) of a cutaneous biopsy of a rash lesion for *R. rickettsii*. Examination of a 3-mm punch biopsy of such a lesion is 70 percent sensitive and 100 percent specific. Except in the preterminal stage, polymerase chain reaction (PCR) amplification and detection of *R. rickettsii* DNA in peripheral blood is an insensitive approach, since rickettsiae are present in large quantities in heavily infected foci of endothelial cells but in relatively low quantities in the circulation. Cultivation of rickettsiae in cell culture is technically feasible but is seldom undertaken because of biohazard and technologic concerns.

℞ TREATMENT

The drug of choice for the treatment of adults with RMSF is doxycycline, except for patients who are pregnant or are allergic to the drug. Because tetracyclines are known to stain the teeth of young children (<9 years old), their use by these children and by pregnant women may raise concern. Although perhaps not as effective, chloramphenicol has been used successfully for the treatment of RMSF and is recommended for use by pregnant women and perhaps by young children. Doxycycline is administered orally (or, in the presence of coma or vomiting, intravenously) at a dosage of 200 mg/d in two divided doses. Other regimens include oral tetracycline (25 to 50 mg/kg per day) in four divided doses or chloramphenicol (50 to 75 mg/kg per day) in four divided doses. The most seriously ill patients are managed in intensive care units, with careful administration of fluids to achieve optimal tissue perfusion without precipitating noncardiogenic pulmonary edema. In some severely ill patients, hypoxemia requires intubation and mechanical ventilation; oliguric or anuric acute renal failure requires hemodialysis; seizures necessitate the use of antiseizure medication; anemia or severe hemorrhage necessitates transfusions of packed red blood cells; and bleeding with severe thrombocytopenia necessitates platelet transfusions. Heparin is not a useful component of treatment, and there is no evidence that glucocorticoids, although frequently administered, affect the outcome of RMSF.

Prevention Avoidance of tick bites is the only available preventive approach. Protective clothing and tick repellents, which could reduce the risk, are seldom actually used. After possible exposure to ticks, it is wise to inspect the body once or twice a day and remove ticks before they inoculate rickettsiae.

MEDITERRANEAN SPOTTED FEVER (BOUTONNEUSE FEVER) AND OTHER SPOTTED FEVERS The etiologic agent of *Mediterranean spotted fever*, *Rickettsia conorii*, is prevalent in southern Europe (below the 45th parallel), all of Africa, and southwestern and south-central Asia. *Rhipicephalus sanguineus*, the brown dog tick, is the vector and reservoir. The names for this disease vary with the region in which it occurs; examples include *Mediterranean spotted fever* (also known as *boutonneuse fever*), *Kenya tick typhus*, *Indian tick typhus*, *Israeli spotted fever*, and *Astrakhan spotted fever*. Whatever the designation, the clinical manifestations are similar, characteristically including high fever, rash, and—in most geographic locales—an inoculation eschar (tâche noire) at the site of the tick bite. A clinically severe form of the disease, associated with a 50 percent mortality rate, has been observed in patients with diabetes, alcoholism, or heart failure.

A strain that has been referred to as *Rickettsia africae* is prevalent among *Amblyomma* ticks in central, eastern, and southern Africa. *R. africae* causes *African tick-bite fever*, which appears to be milder than

classic Mediterranean spotted fever, with 2 to 5 days of fever and a tâche noire. *Rickettsia japonica* causes *Japanese* or *Oriental spotted fever*. Patients present with fever, a cutaneous eruption, and an inoculation eschar.

In Australia, two spotted fevers have been described. *Queensland tick typhus* is due to *Rickettsia australis* and is transmitted by *Ixodes holocyclus*. The skin rash in this disease is usually maculopapular but is sometimes vesicular, and there is an inoculation eschar. The spotted fever observed on *Flinders Island* (near Tasmania) is due to *Rickettsia honei*.

The diagnosis of these other tick-borne spotted fevers is based on clinical and epidemiologic findings and is confirmed by isolation of rickettsiae (by techniques not available in most laboratories) or by serology (Table 179-1). In an endemic area, patients presenting with fever, rash, and/or a skin lesion consisting of a black necrotic area or a crust surrounded by erythema should be considered to have one of these rickettsial spotted fevers. Treatment is outlined in Table 179-1.

RICKETTSIALPOX Rickettsialpox was first described in 1946 by a general practitioner in New York City and soon afterwards was shown to be caused by a distinct rickettsial species, *Rickettsia akari*. This species is isolated from mice and their mites (*Liponyssoides sanguineus*), which maintain the organisms by transovarian transmission. *R. akari* shares lipopolysaccharide antigens with other members of the SFG.

More than 100 cases of rickettsialpox were diagnosed annually in the northeastern United States in the late 1940s and 1950s, and outbreaks occurred in the Ukraine in the 1950s. However, few cases are diagnosed currently. Recently, a culture-confirmed case of rickettsialpox was documented in southern Europe. This case was initially misdiagnosed as Mediterranean spotted fever on the basis of the development of serum antibodies cross-reactive with *R. conorii*. Recent cases of rickettsialpox have also been reported in Arizona, Utah, and Ohio.

In rickettsialpox, a papule forms at the site of the mite-bite inoculation of rickettsiae. The lesion develops a central vesicle that becomes a 1- to 2.5-cm painless black crusted eschar surrounded by an erythematous halo. Enlargement of the lymph nodes draining the region of the eschar is typical. After a 10-day incubation period, during which the eschar and regional lymphadenopathy frequently go unnoticed, the onset of illness is marked by malaise, chills, fever, headache, and myalgia. A macular rash appears 2 to 6 days later and evolves sequentially into papules, vesicles, and crusts that heal without scarring. In some cases the rash remains macular or maculopapular. Some patients suffer nausea, vomiting, abdominal pain, cough, conjunctivitis, or photophobia.

The diagnosis and treatment of rickettsialpox are summarized in Table 179-1. Untreated rickettsialpox is not fatal, with fever lasting 6 to 10 days.

FLEA- AND LOUSE-BORNE RICKETTSIAL DISEASES

ENDEMIC (MURINE) TYPHUS (FLEA-BORNE) Murine typhus was postulated to be a distinct disease, with rats as the reservoir and fleas as the vector, by Maxcy in 1926. Dyer isolated *Rickettsia typhi* from rats and fleas in 1931. By the end of World War II, murine typhus was known to be a global disease. Recently, a novel typhus-group *Rickettsia* has been shown by Azad and coworkers to be maintained transovarially in cat fleas and to cause human infection. This flea-transmitted typhus-group species shares epitopes of the surface protein homologous to SFG rickettsial OmpB and of lipopolysaccharide, but it totally lacks OmpA. Clear differences between the genes for the 17-kDa lipoprotein citrate synthase and 16S rRNA indicate that *R. typhi* and the novel cat-flea rickettsia are separate species. This novel organism, designated *Rickettsia felis* (previously called the ELB agent), has been found in 4 percent of cat fleas and in 33 percent of opossums collected in the vicinity of human murine typhus cases in southern Texas.

Epidemiology *R. typhi* is maintained in mammalian host/flea cycles, with rats (*Rattus rattus* and *Rattus norvegicus*) and the Oriental rat flea (*Xenopsylla cheopis*) as the classic zoonotic niche. Fleas acquire *R. typhi* from rickettsemic rats and carry the organisms for the rest of their lives. Nonimmune rats and humans are infected when rickettsia-laden flea feces are "scratched" into pruritic bite lesions; less frequently, the flea bite itself transmits the organisms. Yet another possible route of transmission is the inhalation of aerosols of flea feces. Infected rats appear healthy, although they are rickettsemic for approximately 2 weeks.

Currently, fewer than 100 cases of endemic typhus are reported annually in the United States. These cases occur mainly in southern Texas and in southern California—locations where the classic rat/flea cycle is absent and a cycle involving the opossum and the cat flea (*Ctenocephalides felis*) is prominent. Although *X. cheopis* fleas are inefficient at the transovarian maintenance of *R. felis*, cat fleas are highly effective at the transovarian transmission of this organism, whose natural occurrence has been detected in fleas in California, Texas, and Oklahoma. *R. felis*–infected opossums and cat fleas as well as a case of human infection were reported from Corpus Christi, Texas, in the same environment where humans, opossums, and cat fleas are infected with *R. typhi*. Cases of endemic typhus occur year-round, mainly in warm (often coastal) areas. The peak prevalence in southern Texas is from April through June and elsewhere is during the warm months of summer and early fall. Although patients seldom recall a fleabite or exposure to fleas, exposure to animals such as cats, opossums, raccoons, skunks, and rats is reported by nearly 40 percent of those who are questioned.

Clinical Manifestations The incubation period of experimental murine typhus in volunteers averages 11 days, with a range of 8 to 16 days. Close observation during this period reveals prodromal symptoms of headache, myalgia, arthralgia, nausea, and malaise devel-oping 1 to 3 days before the abrupt onset of chills and fever. Nearly all patients experience nausea and vomiting early in the illness.

The duration of untreated illness averages 12 days (range, 9 to 18 days). Rash is present in only 13 percent of patients at the time of presentation for medical care (about 4 days after the onset of symptoms), appearing an average of 2 days later in half of the remaining patients and never appearing in the other half. The initial macular rash is often detected by careful inspection of the axilla or the inner surface of the arm. Subsequently, the rash becomes maculopapular, involving the trunk more often than the extremities; it is seldom petechial and rarely involves the face, palms, or soles. A rash is detected in only 20 percent of patients with dark brown or black skin.

Pulmonary involvement is frequently prominent in murine typhus. Thirty-five percent of patients have a hacking, nonproductive cough, and 23 percent of those who undergo chest radiography are found to have pulmonary densities due to interstitial pneumonia, pulmonary edema, and pleural effusions. Bibasilar rales are the most common pulmonary sign. Less commonly observed symptoms and signs include abdominal pain, confusion, stupor, seizures, ataxia, coma, and jaundice. Laboratory studies frequently reveal anemia and leukopenia early in the course and leukocytosis late in the course, thrombocytopenia, hyponatremia, hypoalbuminemia, mildly increased serum levels of hepatic aminotransferases, and prerenal azotemia. Complications may include respiratory failure requiring intubation and mechanical ventilation, hematemesis, cerebral hemorrhage, and hemolysis (in patients with glucose-6-phosphate dehydrogenase deficiency and in those with some hemoglobinopathies). The illness is severe enough to necessitate the admission of 10 percent of hospitalized patients to an intensive care unit. A greater degree of severity is generally associated with old age, underlying disease, and treatment with a sulfa drug; the case-fatality rate in these situations is 1 percent. In a study of children with murine typhus, 50 percent suffered only nocturnal fevers, feeling well enough for active daytime play.

Diagnosis and Treatment See Table 179-1.

EPIDEMIC TYPHUS (LOUSE-BORNE) Epidemic typhus due to infection with *R. prowazekii* is transmitted by the human body louse (*Pediculus humanus corporis*), which lives in clothes and is

Table 179-1

Laboratory Diagnosis and Treatment of Selected Rickettsial Diseases

Disease(s)	Laboratory Diagnosis	Treatment
Mediterranean spotted fever Japanese or Oriental spotted fever Queensland tick typhus Flinders Island spotted fever	Isolation of rickettsiae, shell-vial culture; serology, IFA* (IgM, ≥1:64; or IgG, ≥1:128); PCR amplification of DNA from tissue specimens (especially for *R. japonica*)	Doxycycline (100 mg bid PO for 1–5 days) *or* Ciprofloxacin (750 mg bid PO for 5 days) *or* Chloramphenicol (500 mg qid PO for 7–10 days) *or* (in pregnancy) Josamycin† (3 g/d PO for 5 days)
Rickettsialpox	IFA: seroconversion to a titer of ≥1:64 or a single titer of ≥1:128; cross-absorption to eliminate antibodies to shared antigens necessary for a specific diagnosis of the spotted fever rickettsial species	Doxycycline (100 mg bid PO for 1–5 days) *or* Ciprofloxacin (750 mg bid PO for 5 days) *or* Chloramphenicol (500 mg qid PO for 7–10 days) *or* (in pregnancy) Josamycin† (3 g/d PO for 5 days)
Endemic (murine) typhus	IFA: fourfold rise to a titer of ≥1:64 or a single titer of ≥1:128; immunohistology: skin biopsy; PCR amplification of *R. typhi* or *R. felis* DNA from blood; dot ELISA* and immunoperoxidase methods also available	Doxycycline (100 mg bid PO for 7–15 days) *or* Chloramphenicol (500 mg qid for 7–15 days)
Epidemic typhus	IFA: titer of ≥1:128; necessary to use clinical and epidemiologic data to distinguish among louse-borne epidemic typhus, flying-squirrel typhus, and Brill-Zinsser disease	Doxycycline (200 mg PO as a single dose or until patient is afebrile for 24 h)
Scrub typhus	IFA: titer of ≥1:200; PCR amplification of *Orientia tsutsugamushi* DNA from blood of febrile patients	Doxycycline (100 mg bid PO for 7–15 days) or chloramphenicol (500 mg qid PO for 7–15 days; for children, 150 mg/kg per day for 5 days); azithromycin more effective than doxycycline in vitro against both doxycycline-susceptible and -resistant strains of *O. tsutsugamushi*

* IFA, indirect immunofluorescence assay; ELISA, enzyme-linked immunosorbent assay.
† Not approved by the Food and Drug Administration.

found in conditions of poor hygiene. The infected louse defecates during its blood meal, and the patient autoinoculates the organisms by scratching. Since the louse does not pass the organism to its offspring, the disease usually is spread from person to person by the louse-borne route. This epidemic form of typhus is associated with poverty, cold weather, war, and disasters and is currently prevalent in mountainous areas of Africa, South America, and Asia. In the United States, sporadic cases are transmitted by flying-squirrel fleas.

Brill-Zinsser disease is a recrudescent, mild form of epidemic typhus occurring years after the acute disease, probably as a result of immunosuppression or old age. Nathan Brill first identified recrudescent typhus in New York in 1898. In 1923, Hans Zinsser noted that more than 90 percent of patients with recrudescent typhus had emigrated from typhus-endemic areas of Europe. Strains of *R. prowazekii* indistinguishable from classic strains were isolated from patients with recrudescent typhus. Furthermore, *R. prowazekii* was isolated from the lymph nodes of patients undergoing elective surgery who had had typhus years earlier. Thus, the typhus rickettsiae can remain dormant for years and can reactivate with waning immunity.

Clinical Manifestations After an incubation period of 1 week, the onset of illness is abrupt, with prostration, severe headache, and rapidly rising temperatures of 38.8 to 40.0°C (102 to 104°F). A rash begins on the upper trunk by the fifth day of fever and later becomes generalized, involving all of the body except the face, palms, and soles. Initially, this rash is macular; without treatment, it becomes maculopapular, petechial, and confluent. Photophobia, with considerable conjunctival injection and eye pain, is frequent. The tongue may be dry, brown, and furred. Skin necrosis and gangrene of the digits have been noted in severe cases. Untreated disease is fatal in up to 40 percent of cases, with outcome depending primarily on the condition of the host. Patients with untreated infections develop renal insufficiency and multivisceral involvement, with prominent neurologic manifestations in 12 percent of cases. North American *R. prowazekii* infection transmitted by flying-squirrel ectoparasites is a much milder illness than epidemic louse-borne typhus—whether because of host-related factors (e.g., health status) or organism-related factors (e.g., virulence). Brill-Zinsser disease is similar to epidemic typhus in terms of symptoms but is usually a milder illness.

Diagnosis and Treatment See Table 179-1.

CHIGGER-BORNE SCRUB TYPHUS

The etiologic agent of scrub typhus is a small, obligately intracellular bacterium of the family Rickettsiaceae that differs substantially from other family members in its genetic and cell-wall composition; for example, this organism lacks lipopolysaccharide and peptidoglycan. Consequently, it has been classified as a species in a separate genus, *Orientia tsutsugamushi*.

O. tsutsugamushi is maintained in nature by transovarian transmission in trombiculid mites, mainly of the genus *Leptotrombidium*. After hatching, infected mite larvae (the only stage that feeds on an animal host) inoculate organisms into the skin while feeding. Scrub typhus is found in environments that harbor the infected chiggers, particularly areas of heavy scrub vegetation—e.g., where forest is regrowing after being cleared and along riverbanks. Human infections occur during the wet season, when the mites lay their eggs. The disease is endemic in eastern and southern Asia, northern Australia, and islands of the western Pacific Ocean. Scrub typhus is also found in tropical areas of India, Sri Lanka, and Bangladesh; in temperate areas of Japan, Korea, far-eastern Russia, Tadzhikistan, and the Himalayan Mountains; and in nontropical areas of China. Those infected include indigenous rural workers, residents of suburban areas, and Westerners visiting endemic areas for military, business, or recreational purposes. Infections are more prevalent than the number of clinical diagnoses would suggest: in some areas more than 3 percent of the population is infected or reinfected each month. (Immunity wanes over 1 to 3 years.)

Clinical Manifestations The illness resulting from scrub typhus varies in severity from mild and self-limiting to fatal. After an incuba-

tion period of 6 to 21 days (usually 8 to 10 days), the onset of disease is characterized by fever, headache, myalgia, cough, and gastrointestinal symptoms. Some patients develop no further signs or symptoms and recover spontaneously after a few days. The classic case description includes an eschar at the site of chigger feeding, regional lymphadenopathy, and a maculopapular rash—signs that are seldom observed in indigenous patients. Fewer than 50 percent of western patients develop eschars; fewer than 40 percent develop a rash on day 4 to 6 of illness. Severe cases typically include prominent encephalitis and interstitial pneumonia as key features of vascular injury. Severe illness in persons deficient in glucose-6-phosphate dehydrogenase has been accompanied by hemolysis. The case-fatality rate for untreated classic cases is 7 percent; however, the figure would probably be lower if all relatively mild cases (which are underdiagnosed) were included.

Diagnosis and Treatment See Table 179-1.

EHRLICHIOSES

Two members of the genus *Ehrlichia* have emerged as etiologic agents of life-threatening human disease in the United States. *Ehrlichia chaffeensis*, which targets mainly macrophages and monocytes, causes human monocytic ehrlichiosis; an *Ehrlichia equi*–like organism causes human granulocytic ehrlichiosis (Table 179-2). Ehrlichiae are small, gram-negative, obligately intracellular bacteria that grow as microcolonies in phagosomes (Fig. 179-2). The appearance of the cytoplasmic inclusion, a vacuolar cluster of Giemsa-stained ehrlichiae in phagocytes, accounts for its name, *morula*, the Latin word for mulberry.

Ehrlichiae were discovered by veterinary scientists: *Anaplasma marginale* in 1910, *Cowdria ruminantium* in 1925, *Ehrlichia canis* in 1935, and *Ehrlichia phagocytophila* in 1940. The veterinary investigation of ehrlichiae was further stimulated by an outbreak of fatal canine ehrlichiosis among military dogs during the Vietnam War and by the recognition of equine monocytic ehrlichiosis along the Potomac River in 1979. The agent of a human disease resembling infectious mononucleosis was isolated in Japan in 1953 and was subsequently designated as *Ehrlichia sennetsu*.

The taxonomy of *Ehrlichia* is being resolved by the tools of molecular phylogeny. Present knowledge suggests that three separate genetic clusters may represent three different genera. *E. chaffeensis* belongs among other tick-borne organisms, such as *E. canis* and *C. ruminantium*. The human granulocytic ehrlichiae fit into another genogroup of tick-borne bacteria that includes *E. equi*, *E. phagocytophila*, and *A. marginale*. *E. sennetsu* belongs to the group of organisms that parasitize fish-infesting flukes. This fish helminth occupies an interesting evolutionary niche as far from those of the human ehrlichial pathogens found in the United States as their substantial genetic divergence would suggest. The

Table 179-2

Comparison of Two Human Ehrlichioses: Human Monocytic Ehrlichiosis (HME) and Human Granulocytic Ehrlichiosis (HGE)

Feature	HME	HGE
Etiologic agent	*E. chaffeensis*	*E. equi*–like organism
Tick vector(s)	*Amblyomma americanum, Dermacentor variabilis* (dog tick)	*Ixodes scapularis* (deer tick), *I. ricinus*
Seasonality	April through September	Year-round; peak May through July
Major target cell	Monocyte	Granulocyte
Morulae seen	Rarely	Frequently
Antigen used in IFA*	*E. chaffeensis*	*E. equi*
Diagnostic titer	Fourfold rise or single titer of ≥1:128; cutoff for negative titer, 1:64	Fourfold rise; cutoff for negative titer, 1:80
Treatment of choice	Doxycycline	Doxycycline
Mortality	2–3%	5%

* IFA, indirect immunofluorescence assay.

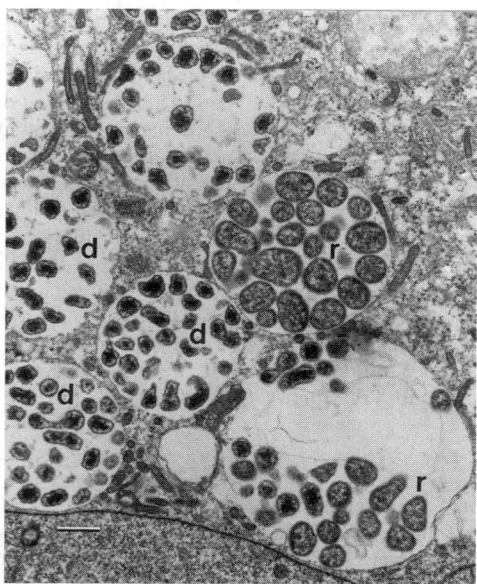

FIGURE 179-2 *Ehrlichia chaffeensis* microcolonies (morulae) within cytoplasmic vacuoles manifest as two morphologic forms: reticulate cells (r) and dense-core cells (d). Bar = 1 μm. (*Courtesy of Dr. Vsevolod L. Popov.*)

ecologic niche of the tick-borne *Ehrlichia* species involves a persistently infected mammalian reservoir from which immature ticks acquire organisms that are maintained during stage-to-stage molting (but not transovarially) and are transmitted by tick bite.

HUMAN MONOCYTIC EHRLICHIOSIS **Epidemiology** Hundreds of cases of *E. chaffeensis* infection have been documented serologically in 30 states, mostly in the south-central, southeastern, and mid-Atlantic regions, as well as in Europe and Africa. The Lone Star tick (*Amblyomma americanum*) is the major vector, and the white-tailed deer is an important reservoir host. Most patients recall tick bites or exposures during the 3 weeks before the onset of illness; usually these events take place during the season of greatest tick activity—i.e., from April to September, with a peak from May through July. Human monocytic ehrlichiosis (HME) is most common in rural areas. The median age of patients is 44 years (older than for RMSF), and 75 percent of patients are male.

Clinical Manifestations After the tick-bite inoculation of *E. chaffeensis* and a median incubation period of 9 days, only one-third of persons who seroconvert actually become ill. However, in documented cases, the illness lasts for a median of 23 days; 62 percent of patients are hospitalized, and 2 to 3 percent die. The clinical signs and symptoms, which do not point to a specific diagnosis, include fever (97 percent), headache (81 percent), myalgia (68 percent), anorexia (66 percent), nausea (48 percent), vomiting (37 percent), rash (6 percent at onset, 25 percent during the first week, and 36 percent overall), cough (26 percent), pharyngitis (26 percent), diarrhea (25 percent), lymphadenopathy (25 percent), abdominal pain (22 percent), and confusion (20 percent). Severe illness may be manifested as respiratory insufficiency (in some cases with pulmonary infiltrates); neurologic involvement, with seizures, coma, CSF pleocytosis (including the presence of ehrlichiae); acute renal failure; gastrointestinal hemorrhage; and opportunistic fungal or viral infection. Laboratory abnormalities that are indicative of multisystem illness and are often diagnostically useful include thrombocytopenia, leukopenia (absolute lymphopenia and/or neutropenia), and elevated levels of serum aspartate and alanine aminotransferases. The bone marrow is usually hyperplastic and contains noncaseating granulomas. *Ehrlichia*-containing monocytes are seldom seen in the peripheral blood, but macrophages with ehrlichial morular inclusions have been demonstrated in bone marrow, spleen, liver, lymph node, lung, kidney, and CSF.

Diagnosis Clinical suspicion, based on fever and exposure to ticks in an endemic area during the prior 3 weeks, is essential to the diagnosis of HME. The finding of leukopenia and thrombocytopenia supports a presumptive diagnosis and the institution of empirical treatment with doxycycline. Serologic confirmation of the diagnosis is generally possible during convalescence, when antibodies to *E. chaffeensis* antigens are detected by indirect immunofluorescence assay at a titer of ≥64. Laboratory diagnosis during the acute stage of illness can be established by PCR amplification of *E. chaffeensis* DNA from blood.

℞ TREATMENT

Tetracycline drugs such as doxycycline (100 mg twice daily) have been shown to shorten the course of HME. However, no controlled trials of antimicrobial therapy have been conducted. Moreover, the required duration of administration of doxycycline is not known. Retrospective analysis has revealed that the administration of doxycycline markedly reduces the likelihood that an outpatient will require hospitalization and significantly shortens the duration of illness in a hospitalized patient. Although chloramphenicol also appears to shorten the course of illness, some patients do not respond to treatment with this agent, and *E. chaffeensis* is resistant to chloramphenicol in cell culture. Persistent ehrlichial infection has been documented after treatment with tetracycline and chloramphenicol.

HME is prevented by the avoidance of tick bite in endemic areas. Valuable precautions include the wearing of protective clothing; the use of tick repellent; and careful, frequent checking of the body, with prompt removal of ticks.

Ehrlichial infection is most likely controlled by a combination of cell-mediated and humoral immune mechanisms. Successful treatment is followed by an unusual rebound lymphocytosis of predominantly γ/δ T lymphocytes.

HUMAN GRANULOCYTIC EHRLICHIOSIS **Epidemiology** As of 1995, approximately 150 cases of human granulocytic ehrlichiosis (HGE) had been documented in 11 states, mostly in the upper midwestern and northeastern regions, with a distribution similar to that of Lyme disease. Since the first report of a series of cases of HGE by Bakken and colleagues in 1994, the frequency of its recognition has increased rapidly, but its geographic limits still are not known precisely. Most cases have been diagnosed within the range of various *Ixodes ricinus*–complex ticks, particularly *Ixodes scapularis (dammini)*, but some cases have been found in the range of southern-type *I. scapularis*, *Ixodes pacificus* (in the far-western states), and *I. ricinus* (in Europe). Agents of HGE have been detected in *I. scapularis (dammini)* in the upper Midwest and the Northeast as well as in the blood of deer in the upper Midwest and California and of horses and dogs in the upper Midwest, the Northeast, and Sweden. A role for rodents and deer in maintaining HGE in nature is suspected but not yet defined.

The agent of HGE is virtually indistinguishable from *E. equi*, which is transmitted to horses by *I. pacificus* in California, or from *E. phagocytophila*, which is transmitted to deer, cattle, and sheep by *I. ricinus* in Europe. Indeed, transfusion of human blood containing the agent of HGE into horses causes typical equine granulocytic ehrlichiosis and confers protective immunity against subsequent challenge with *E. equi*. The HGE agent, *E. equi*, and *E. phagocytophila* may in fact be different strains of a single species.

The incidence of HGE peaks in June and July, but the disease occurs throughout the year in conjunction with human exposure to *Ixodes* ticks. HGE predominantly affects males (79 percent of cases) and older persons (median age, 58 years).

Clinical Manifestations After a median incubation period of 8 days, patients with HGE usually suffer a flulike illness with fever (100 percent), chills (98 percent), malaise (98 percent), headache (85 percent), nausea (39 percent), and vomiting (34 percent). Some patients develop a cough (29 percent) or confusion (17 percent)—generally later in the course. Rash and seizures are rare. Patients frequently develop thrombocytopenia, leukopenia, anemia, and elevated serum aminotransferase concentrations. Bone marrow examination has demonstrated hypercellularity or normal marrow. Severe disease affects elderly patients in particular; however, children are also susceptible to the infection. The illness as presently recognized has a moderate to severe course unless treated early. The natural history of untreated HGE in adults is a 3- to 11-week illness with a possibly fatal outcome. One child who was not treated with an antiehrlichial drug was febrile for a shorter period (10 days). Overall, 56 percent of cases have required hospitalization, 7 percent have resulted in admission to an intensive care unit, and 5 percent have ended in death. Autopsies in fatal cases of HGE have revealed opportunistic fungal pneumonia due to *Aspergillus fumigatus*, *Cryptococcus neoformans*, or *Candida albicans*. This finding suggests compromised host defenses, similar to the defective function of neutrophils and of T and B lymphocytes documented in sheep infected with *E. phagocytophila*. Coinfection with the agent of HGE and *Borrelia burgdorferi* or *Babesia microti*—which are transmitted by the same vector, *I. scapularis (dammini)*—probably occurs on occasion. Serologic studies have demonstrated antibodies to the agent of HGE in substantial portions of patients with Lyme disease, and both this agent and *B. burgdorferi* have been found in individual ticks. It is possible that microbial interactions in this situation lead to more severe disease than infection with a single agent.

Diagnosis   HGE should be suspected clinically when patients from an endemic area have a flulike febrile illness and have been exposed to an environment infested with *I. scapularis*, *I. pacificus*, or *I. ricinus* ticks. The detection of thrombocytopenia should increase the level of suspicion. Thorough examination of a peripheral-blood smear reveals neutrophils containing *Ehrlichia*-filled vacuoles in many but by no means all cases. PCR based upon primers specific for 16S rDNA sequences of the *E. phagocytophila* genogroup is diagnostically sensitive when performed under optimal laboratory conditions. Serodiagnosis by indirect immunofluorescence assay, with *E. equi*–infected equine neutrophils as antigen, is highly sensitive but is useful mainly for retrospective documentation of seroconversion to a titer of 80 or greater during convalescence.

 TREATMENT
Doxycycline is an effective therapeutic drug. Of 35 HGE patients treated with doxycycline, 94 percent defervesced within 24 to 48 h. One patient who did not receive doxycycline had the agent of HGE detected by PCR in the blood on day 28 of illness.

Like HME, HGE is prevented by avoidance of tick bite and prompt removal of attached ticks.

Q FEVER

Q fever results from infection with *Coxiella burnetii*. This small gram-negative microorganism (0.2 μm × 0.7 μm) exists in two antigenic forms: phase I and phase II. When *C. burnetii* is passaged in cell cultures or embryonated eggs, its lipopolysaccharide undergoes changes that result in an antigenic shift called *phase variation*. In humans and other animals, the organism exists in the phase I form, which is extremely infectious. Passage in cell culture or embryonated eggs results in a shift to the phase II form, which is avirulent. The ability of *C. burnetii* to form spores allows it to survive in harsh environments. Indeed, it can survive for more than 40 months in skim milk at room temperature and is readily recovered from soil up to 1 month after contamination. Three different plasmids have been described in various isolates of *C. burnetii*.

Q fever encompasses two broad clinical syndromes: acute and chronic infection. It is likely that the host's immune response (rather than characteristics of the infecting strain) determines whether or not chronic Q fever develops.

Epidemiology   Q fever is a zoonosis. The primary sources of human infection are infected cattle, sheep, and goats. However, infected cats, rabbits, and dogs have also been shown to transmit *C. burnetii* to humans. The extensive wildlife reservoir for *C. burnetii* includes mammals, birds, and ticks. In the infected female mammal, *C. burnetii* localizes to the uterus and the mammary glands; infection is reactivated during pregnancy, and high concentrations of *C. burnetii* are found in the placenta. At parturition, *C. burnetii* is dispersed as

an aerosol, and infection follows inhalation of these organisms by a susceptible host. Infected female animals shed the organism in milk for weeks or months after parturition. In rare instances, human-to-human transmission has followed childbirth by an infected woman or autopsy on an infected patient. *C. burnetii* has been transmitted via blood transfusion. It is evident that the persons at risk for Q fever include abattoir workers, veterinarians, and others who vocationally or avocationally come into contact with infected animals. Exposure to infected newborn animals or to infected products of conception poses the highest risk. Sexual transmission has been demonstrated experimentally in mice, as has transmission during artificial insemination in cattle. Whether *C. burnetii* is sexually transmitted in humans is not yet known. While the experimental evidence on this point is contradictory, the ingestion of contaminated milk in some areas is probably a major route of infection.

Infections due to *C. burnetii* occur in most countries. Indeed, the only areas known to be free of *C. burnetii* are New Zealand and Antarctica. The primary manifestation of acute Q fever differs from place to place. In Nova Scotia (Canada) it is pneumonia, while in Marseille (France) it is granulomatous hepatitis. In the Basque country of Spain, both pneumonia and granulomatous hepatitis occur. It has been suggested that these differences may reflect the route of infection—i.e., that the ingestion of contaminated milk results in hepatitis while the inhalation of contaminated aerosols results in pneumonia.

Clinical Manifestations   The incubation period for *acute Q fever* ranges from 3 to 30 days. The clinical presentations include flu-like syndromes, prolonged fever, pneumonia, hepatitis, pericarditis, myocarditis, meningoencephalitis, and infection during pregnancy. The symptoms of acute Q fever are nonspecific; common among them are fever, extreme fatigue, and severe headache. Other symptoms include chills, sweats, nausea, vomiting, and diarrhea, which occur in 5 to 20 percent of patients. Cough develops in about half of all patients with Q fever pneumonia. Neurologic manifestations of acute Q fever are uncommon. However, in one outbreak in the West Midlands of the United Kingdom, 23 percent of 102 patients had neurologic signs and symptoms as the major manifestation of acute Q fever. A nonspecific skin rash may be evident in some patients. The white blood cell count is usually normal. Thrombocytopenia is present in about 25 percent of patients, and reactive thrombocytosis (with platelet counts of up to 1 million/μL [1×10^{12}/L]) frequently develops during recovery. This thrombocytosis may account for cases of deep-vein thrombophlebitis complicating acute Q fever in some series. Uncommon manifestations of acute Q fever include optic neuritis, extrapyramidal neurologic disease, Guillain-Barré syndrome, inappropriate secretion of antidiuretic hormone, epididymitis, orchitis, priapism, hemolytic anemia, mediastinal lymphadenopathy mimicking lymphoma, pancreatitis, erythema nodosum, and mesenteric panniculitis. Chest radiography may show an opacity that is indistinguishable from those seen in pneumonia of other causes. Multiple rounded opacities are common. In the appropriate epidemiologic setting, these opacities are highly suggestive of Q fever pneumonia; however, right-sided endocarditis resulting in septic pulmonary emboli can produce the same radiographic appearance.

Chronic Q fever almost always implies endocarditis. This infection usually occurs in patients with previous valvular heart disease, immunosuppression, or chronic renal insufficiency. Fever is usually absent or, if present, is low grade. Patients may have nonspecific symptoms for up to 1 year before diagnosis. Valvular vegetations have been seen in only 12 percent of patients with transthoracic echocardiograms, but the rate of detection may be higher with the use of transesophageal echocardiography. A high index of suspicion is necessary for a correct diagnosis. All patients with valvular heart disease and an unexplained purpuric eruption, renal insufficiency, stroke, and/or progressive heart failure should be tested for *C. burnetii* infection. Patients with chronic Q fever have hepatomegaly and/or splenomegaly. These two findings, especially in combination with positive rheumatoid factor, high erythrocyte sedimentation rate, high C-reactive protein level, and/or increased gamma globulin concentrations, suggest this diagnosis. Other manifestations of chronic Q fever include infection of vascular prostheses, aneurysms, and bone.

Diagnosis *C. burnetii* can be isolated from buffy-coat blood samples or tissue specimens by a shell-vial technique; however, most laboratories are not currently permitted to attempt the isolation of *C. burnetii*, since it is considered highly infectious. PCR can be used to amplify *C. burnetii* DNA from tissue or biopsy specimens. This technique can also be used on paraffin-embedded tissues. Serology, however, is the most commonly used diagnostic tool. Three techniques are available: complement fixation, indirect immunofluorescence, and enzyme-linked immunosorbent assay. Indirect immunofluorescence is sensitive and specific and is the method of choice. Rheumatoid factor should be absorbed from the specimen before testing. An IgG titer of ≥1:800 to phase I antigen is suggestive of chronic Q fever. In almost all instances of chronic Q fever, the phase I antibody titer is much higher than the phase II antibody titer. The reverse is true in acute Q fever. In addition, in acute Q fever, it is usually possible to demonstrate a fourfold rise in titer between acute- and convalescent-phase samples.

℞ TREATMENT

Treatment of acute Q fever with doxycycline (100 mg twice daily for 14 days) is usually successful. Quinolones are also effective. Treatment of chronic Q fever should include at least two antibiotics active against *C. burnetii*. The combination of rifampin and doxycycline has been used with success. Doxycycline should be given as 100 mg twice daily and rifampin as 300 mg once daily. The optimal duration of antibiotic therapy for chronic Q fever remains undetermined. We recommend a minimum of 3 years of treatment. Therapy should be discontinued only if the phase I IgA antibody titer is ≤1:50 and the phase I IgG titer is ≤1:200. Another therapeutic option under investigation is the combination of doxycycline (100 mg twice daily) with hydroxychloroquine (600 mg once daily). In vitro, the addition of hydroxychloroquine at a concentration of 1 mg/mL renders doxycycline bactericidal for *C. burnetii*. A vaccine has been shown to be effective in preventing Q fever in abattoir workers in Australia.

BIBLIOGRAPHY

ARCHIBALD LK, SEXTON DJ: Long-term sequelae of Rocky Mountain spotted fever. Clin Infect Dis 20:1122, 1995

AZAD AF: Epidemiology of murine typhus. Annu Rev Entomol 35:553, 1990
——— et al: Genetic characterization and transovarial transmission of a typhus-like rickettsia found in cat fleas. Proc Natl Acad Sci USA 89:43, 1992

BAKKEN JS et al: Human granulocytic ehrlichiosis in the upper midwest United States. A new species emerging? JAMA 272:212, 1994

BROUQUI P, RAOULT D: In vitro antibiotic susceptibility of the newly recognized agent of ehrlichiosis in humans, *Ehrlichia chaffeensis*. Antimicrob Agents Chemother 36:2799, 1992

DALTON MJ et al: National surveillance for Rocky Mountain spotted fever, 1981–1982: Epidemiologic summary and evaluation of risk factors for fatal outcome. Am J Trop Med Hyg 52:405, 1995

DAWSON JE et al: Isolation and characterization of an *Ehrlichia* sp. from a patient diagnosed with human ehrlichiosis. J Clin Microbiol 29:2741, 1991

DUMLER JS et al: Clinical and laboratory features of murine typhus in south Texas, 1980 through 1987. JAMA 266:1365, 1991

FICHTENBAUM CJ et al: Ehrlichiosis presenting as a life-threatening illness with features of the toxic shock syndrome. Am J Med 95:351, 1993

FISHBEIN DB et al: Human ehrlichiosis in the United States, 1985 to 1990. Ann Intern Med 120:736, 1994

HELMICK CG et al: Rocky Mountain spotted fever: Clinical, laboratory, and epidemiological features of 262 cases. J Infect Dis 150:480, 1984

HIGGINS JA et al: *Rickettsia felis*: A new species of pathogenic rickettsia isolated from cat fleas. J Clin Microbiol 34:671, 1996

KASS EM et al: Rickettsial pox in a New York City hospital, 1980–1989. N Engl J Med 331:1612, 1994

MARRIE TJ: Q fever, in *Q Fever*, vol 1, TJ Marrie (ed). Boca Raton, FL, CRC Press, 1990

O'CONNOR LF et al: A cluster of murine typhus cases in Western Australia. Med J Aust 165:24, 1996

RAOULT D, DRANCOURT M: Antimicrobial therapy of rickettsial diseases. Antimicrob Agents Chemother 35:2457, 1991

RATNASAMY N et al: Central nervous system manifestations of human ehrlichiosis. Clin Infect Dis 23:314, 1996

RIKIHISA Y: The tribe *Ehrlichieae* and ehrlichial diseases. Clin Microbiol Rev 4:286, 1991

SCHRIEFER ME et al: Identification of a novel rickettsial infection in a patient diagnosed with murine typhus. J Clin Microbiol 32:949, 1994

SILPAPOJAKUL K et al: Murine typhus in Thailand: Clinical features, diagnosis and treatment. Q J Med 86:43, 1993

STRICKMAN D et al: *In vitro* effectiveness of azithromycin against doxycycline-resistant and -susceptible strains of *Rickettsia tsutsugamushi*, etiologic agent of scrub typhus. Antimicrob Agents Chemother 39:2406, 1995

WALKER DH et al: Fulminant Rocky Mountain spotted fever. Its pathologic characteristics associated with glucose-6-phosphate dehydrogenase deficiency. Arch Pathol Lab Med 107:121, 1983

YEVICH SJ et al: Seroepidemiology of infections due to spotted fever group *Rickettsia* and *Ehrlichia* species in military personnel exposed in areas of the United States where such infections are endemic. J Infect Dis 171:1266, 1995

---

180 *Gail H. Cassell, Gregory C. Gray, K. B. Waites*

MYCOPLASMA INFECTIONS

Mycoplasmas are the smallest free-living microorganisms and are commonly found in plants, animals, and humans. Individual cells range in diameter from 100 to 300 nm. Many of the biologic properties of mycoplasmas, including resistance to β-lactam antibiotics and marked cellular pleomorphism, stem from the lack of a cell wall. The extremely small size of the mycoplasmal genome severely limits the organism's biosynthetic capabilities, helps explain the complex nutritional requirements for its cultivation, and necessitates a parasitic or saprophytic existence. Mycoplasmas most commonly colonize mucosal surfaces and typically cause chronic inflammatory diseases of the respiratory tract, urogenital tract, and joints of a wide variety of animal species. Fourteen mycoplasmal species are known to occur in humans, some only rarely. *Mycoplasma orale* and *Mycoplasma salivarium* are common oral commensals. *Mycoplasma pneumoniae* is a common cause of pneumonia in all age groups. Both *Ureaplasma urealyticum* and *Mycoplasma hominis* often colonize the genitourinary tract of normal asymptomatic individuals but are important opportunistic pathogens in adults and newborn infants. *Mycoplasma genitalium*, *Mycoplasma fermentans*, and *Mycoplasma penetrans* have been detected in the respiratory and genitourinary tracts and warrant further attention as potential causes of human disease. However, these species have been described relatively recently, and detailed information concerning their true ecologic niche is lacking. They appear to be even more fastidious than other *Mycoplasma* species found in humans.

MECHANISMS OF PATHOGENICITY

Adhesion to host cells is a prerequisite for mycoplasmal colonization and for infection. *M. pneumoniae* adheres and attaches by a complex and multifactorial process requiring a number of accessory proteins; adhesion is followed by induction of ciliostasis. Factors involved in the adherence of *U. urealyticum* and *M. hominis* have not been characterized. While most mycoplasmas reside attached to the cell surface, intracellular localization of *M. fermentans*, *M. penetrans*, and (to a limited extent) *M. pneumoniae* has now been documented. This intracellular localization can protect mycoplasmas from antibodies and antibiotics, contributing to the chronicity of disease and to the difficulties encountered in cultivation of the organisms on artificial media.

The pathogenic properties of *U. urealyticum* and *M. hominis* have not been elucidated. However, surface antigens of both organisms undergo variation at a high rate that may be related to mycoplasmal persistence at invasive sites. One important property of *M. hominis* is its ability to metabolize arginine and thus to release large, potentially cytotoxic amounts of ammonia. *M. pneumoniae* and *M. hominis* produce hydrogen peroxide, which is also thought to play a role in cell injury.

Ureaplasmas differ from all other genera within the class Mollicutes in that they possess urease activity. Like other prokaryotes that have urease activity, *U. urealyticum* can induce urinary calculi. Ureaplasmas—but not *M. hominis* or *M. pneumoniae*—exhibit specific protease activity through which they can degrade human IgA1 but not IgA2; this activity is believed to be a virulence factor.

M. pneumoniae, like many other species of mycoplasmas, can nonspecifically stimulate B lymphocytes and—to a lesser extent—T lymphocytes. Certain individuals infected with *M. pneumoniae* develop autoantibodies, including those reactive with brain, heart, and muscle; erythrocyte I antigen; intermediate filaments; and mitotic spindles of dividing cells. Infection with *M. pneumoniae* may evoke IgM autoantibodies that agglutinate human erythrocytes at 4°C (cold agglutinins). This effect sometimes causes complications. *M. pneumoniae* uses specific long-chain sialooligosaccharides at the host-cell surface as receptors. These sialooligosaccharides contain I antigen in their backbones and are richly expressed at the primary site of infection—the ciliated bronchial epithelium—and on erythrocytes. The autoantibodies to I antigen are directed to cell membrane receptors and may be triggered by an autoimmunogenic mycoplasma-receptor complex in which the lipid-rich microorganism serves as an adjuvant. Cold agglutinins are thought to contribute to the anemia often seen in *M. pneumoniae*–infected patients. With the exception of cold agglutinins, the role of immunologic factors in *M. pneumoniae*–induced disease is unknown.

MYCOPLASMA PNEUMONIAE

EPIDEMIOLOGY Approximately 10 to 20 percent of all pneumonias are due to *M. pneumoniae*. This organism is a common cause of tracheobronchitis and other respiratory syndromes such as bronchiolitis and pharyngitis. Symptoms can persist for weeks or months. *M. pneumoniae* is spread by aerosol from person to person. However, in contrast to that of other respiratory infections, person-to-person spread of mycoplasmal infections by aerosols is slow, even among family members. The incubation period is 1 to 3 weeks long. In large urban areas, *M. pneumoniae* infection appears to be endemic and occurs throughout the year. Epidemics can occur every 3 to 7 years.

M. pneumoniae was previously thought to be rare among children under 5 years of age and to cause only acute, self-limited respiratory disease. However, recent studies indicate that the incidence may actually be highest among 3 and 4 year olds and that the rate of hospitalization for *M. pneumoniae* pneumonia among children under 5 is high. Recent studies of adults (mean age, 62 years) have indicated that *M. pneumoniae* accounts for as many as 15 percent of cases of community-acquired pneumonia in this age group. Prospective studies of adults (mean age, 56 years) requiring hospitalization for community-acquired pneumonia have confirmed that up to 18 percent of these cases are caused by *M. pneumoniae*. The common misconception that *M. pneumoniae* disease is rare among the very young and among older adults has led to a failure of physicians even to consider this condition in the differential diagnosis.

CLINICAL MANIFESTATIONS Although *M. pneumoniae* is best known as the primary cause of "walking" or "atypical" pneumonia, the clinical syndrome for which it is most frequently responsible is tracheobronchitis, often accompanied by upper respiratory tract symptoms. Typical complaints include sore throat, headache, chills, coryza, and general malaise. The throat may be erythematous, but cervical adenopathy is uncommon. Myringitis and otitis sometimes develop. Severe mycoplasmal respiratory disease has been thought to be uncommon, yet recent reports suggest that the disease spectrum is wider than was previously thought and that severe pulmonary involvement is possible in otherwise healthy children and adults of all ages. Lung abscesses, pneumatoceles, extensive lobar consolidation, respira-

tory distress, and pleural effusion may develop. Small effusions are found in 20 percent of cases. *M. pneumoniae* is sometimes isolated from the pleural fluid in relatively severe cases.

EXTRAPULMONARY COMPLICATIONS Meningoencephalitis, aseptic meningitis, encephalitis, ascending paralysis, and transverse myelitis have been reported. Some cases with neurologic complications are fatal. Recovery from neurologic dysfunction is often slow, and some patients are left with a permanent neurologic deficit. The initial failure of investigators to demonstrate direct invasion of the central nervous system (CNS) by mycoplasmas and the fact that many reported cases were diagnosed solely on the basis of serologic testing led many investigators to regard the association of *M. pneumoniae* infection with CNS disease as rather tenuous. However, CNS infection has now been documented by polymerase chain reaction and cultural isolation of *M. pneumoniae* from cerebrospinal fluid and from brain tissue obtained at autopsy in the absence of other infectious agents and other identifiable causes of clinical manifestations. As already mentioned, *M. pneumoniae* frequently evokes cold agglutinins. A positive Coombs test and detection of reticulocytosis suggest that subclinical anemia may be common. Other complications include hemolytic anemia, paroxysmal cold hemoglobinuria, Raynaud's phenomenon, disseminated intravascular coagulation, thrombocytopenia, and renal failure.

Cardiac involvement is generally thought to be rare, but the true incidence is unknown. Myocardial dysfunction is often associated with hemolytic anemia and may mimic infarction. Myopericarditis, hemopericardium, congestive heart failure, and complete heart block have been reported, and marked electrocardiographic changes may be evident without cardiac symptoms. *M. pneumoniae* has been isolated in pure culture from pericardial fluid and cardiac tissue.

Mucocutaneous lesions are found in approximately 25 percent of *M. pneumoniae* infections. Erythematous maculopapular and vesicular exanthems are most common. Half of patients with mucocutaneous lesions also have ulcerative stomatitis and conjunctivitis. In many cases, throat and bulla-fluid cultures are positive for *M. pneumoniae*.

M. pneumoniae infection occasionally is associated with joint manifestations, including arthritis. Illnesses suggestive of rheumatic fever have been described. About 25 percent of cases of *M. pneumoniae* infection include nausea, vomiting, and/or diarrhea.

DIAGNOSIS The possibility of *M. pneumoniae* infection should be considered in patients of any age who have respiratory manifestations. Although complications appear to be uncommon, their true incidence may have been underestimated. Because of the mistaken impression that severe pneumonia and extrapulmonary complications are inconsistent with *M. pneumoniae* disease, this etiology often is not included in the differential diagnosis. Extrapulmonary manifestations usually begin 1 to 21 days after respiratory symptoms. However, some patients have no history of respiratory symptoms, and others report only upper respiratory illness. Extrapulmonary manifestations have been reported in all age groups.

Routine laboratory tests usually yield normal results. About one-fourth of all patients with mycoplasmal pneumonia develop leukocytosis, and one-third have an elevated erythrocyte sedimentation rate. Chest radiographs of patients with mycoplasmal pneumonia may reveal diffuse reticulonodular or interstitial infiltrates, usually located in the lower lobes and often appearing as streaks radiating from the hilus to the base. Lung involvement tends to be unilateral but can be bilateral. Clinical, radiologic, and laboratory findings in *M. pneumoniae* infections are sufficiently indistinct to serve as a basis for an accurate diagnosis. *Chlamydia pneumoniae*, *Chlamydia psittaci*, *Streptococcus pneumoniae*, *Haemophilus influenzae*, *Moraxella catarrhalis*, *Francisella tularensis*, *Bordetella pertussis*, *Coxiella burnetii*, *Legionella* species, and several viruses (including adenoviruses) can produce infections that are clinically indistinguishable from *M. pneumoniae* infection and may in fact occur simultaneously with mycoplasmal infections. Although a cold agglutinin response is not specific for *M. pneumoniae* and is detected in ≤50 percent of cases, it suggests the diagnosis, is easy to document, and may be evident within the first week of infection. To detect this response, the patient's serum is mixed with type O erythrocytes, the mixture is incubated at 0°C for several minutes, and the presence or absence of hemagglutination is noted. A titer of 1:32 is suggestive of infection with *M. pneumoniae*. A rapid bedside test can also be performed: A 1-mL volume of the patient's blood is drawn into a tube containing anticoagulant. The tube is cooled in wet ice or in a standard refrigerator for 3 to 4 min, and the contents are examined for hemagglutination.

At present, no rapid diagnostic methods for the detection of *M. pneumoniae* in clinical specimens are commercially available. In addition, culture services often are not readily available, a positive result takes time to obtain, and the collection of proper diagnostic specimens in some types of respiratory infections is impractical. Therefore, serologic tests are most commonly used to confirm *M. pneumoniae* infection. The enzyme-linked immunosorbent assay is the preferred serologic method. Definitive diagnosis requires seroconversion documented by paired specimens obtained 2 to 4 weeks apart. Although single-titer IgM assays purported to detect current infection have recently become commercially available, it is not clear how long IgM persists after acute infection, and as many as 50 percent of adults may not mount a detectable IgM response. Conversely, some children may not mount an IgG response. Therefore, reliance on a single serologic test could be clinically misleading, and paired assays for both IgM and IgG are recommended. While complement fixation is acceptable, this technique is not satisfactory for the detection of IgG and is also rather insensitive.

℞ **TREATMENT**

Orally administered erythromycin (250 to 500 mg every 6 h for adults, 20 to 50 mg/kg daily in three or four doses for children) is the drug of choice for mycoplasmal respiratory infections, although tetracycline (250 to 500 mg every 6 h) or doxycycline (100 mg every 12 h) are suitable alternatives for older children and adults. Clindamycin is active in vitro but may not be active in vivo and should not be considered a first-line agent. Fluoroquinolones such as ciprofloxacin (500 mg every 12 h) exhibit some antimycoplasmal activity in vitro but not nearly as much as the macrolides and tetracyclines; therefore, fluoroquinolones should not be used when alternatives are available. Newer agents such as clarithromycin (500 mg every 12 h for adults, 15 mg/kg daily in two doses for children) and azithromycin[1] (500 mg on day 1, then 250 mg daily) are highly effective in vitro against *M. pneumoniae* at concentrations equivalent to or lower than those of erythromycin, demonstrate similar clinical efficacy, and are available as pediatric suspensions. Moreover, they are better tolerated, cause fewer gastrointestinal side effects, and have a longer half-life that allows less frequent administration. Like that of erythromycin, the administration of clarithromycin may cause an increase in serum theophylline concentrations. Because mycoplasmas are slow-growing organisms, it is logical to expect infections to respond better to longer courses of treatment than might be offered for other types of infections. Therefore, a 14- to 21-day course of oral therapy with most agents is appropriate.

In addition to antimicrobials, preparations such as cough suppressants, antipyretics, and analgesics should be given as needed to relieve headache and other systemic symptoms caused by *M. pneumoniae* infection. Since most extrapulmonary manifestations are diagnosed late in the course of disease, the benefit of early or prolonged treatment in preventing them or diminishing their severity is unknown.

---

[1] This drug has not been approved by the Food and Drug Administration for use against *M. pneumoniae*.

UREAPLASMA UREALYTICUM AND MYCOPLASMA HOMINIS

EPIDEMIOLOGY Genital mycoplasmas may be found throughout the lower urogenital tract of asymptomatic women. In addition, mycoplasmas have been isolated from the urine, the semen, and the distal urethra of asymptomatic men. *U. urealyticum* is detected in the vagina of 40 to 80 percent of sexually mature, asymptomatic women and *M. hominis* in 21 to 53 percent; the incidence of each is somewhat lower in males.

Both ureaplasmas and *M. hominis* can be isolated from amniotic fluid in the presence of intact membranes as early as 12 to 20 weeks of gestation. Up to 14 percent of the isolates of *U. urealyticum* and up to 30 percent of the isolates of *M. hominis* from endotracheal aspirates collected at birth from infants whose birth weight is <2500 g are from infants born by cesarean section to women with intact membranes. These figures indicate that in utero acquisition is rather common, at least among preterm infants. *U. urealyticum* and *M. hominis* can be acquired in utero either by an ascending route secondary to colonization of the mother's genital tract or transplacentally from the mother's blood. Both organisms have been isolated from maternal and umbilical-cord blood. The rate of vertical transmission of *U. urealyticum* and *M. hominis* among infants ranges from 18 to 55 percent. Rates of colonization among healthy full-term infants decline after 3 months of age. Fewer than 10 percent of older children and sexually inexperienced adults are colonized with either ureaplasmas or *M. hominis*.

DISEASES OF THE GENITOURINARY TRACT OF ADULTS Three conditions of the urinary tract definitively shown to be caused by mycoplasmas are urethritis due to *U. urealyticum* in males, urinary calculi due to *U. urealyticum*, and pyelonephritis due to *M. hominis*. Although the exact proportion of cases for which it is responsible is unknown, *M. hominis* is considered to be a cause of pelvic inflammatory disease (PID). Inoculation of *M. hominis* into fallopian tubes of monkeys induces parametritis and salpingitis within 3 days, and inoculation of human fallopian tube explants produces ciliostasis; the organism has been isolated in pure cultures from the fallopian tubes of approximately 8 percent of women with salpingitis diagnosed by laparoscopy; the figure for women without lesions is zero. *M. hominis* is sometimes isolated from the endometrium. In addition, a role for this organism in cases of PID associated with neither *Neisseria gonorrhoeae* nor *Chlamydia trachomatis* is supported by significant increases in specific antibody. While *U. urealyticum* can be isolated directly from affected fallopian tubes, it is usually found in the presence of other known pathogens.

Given that *M. hominis* is a cause of salpingitis, it is reasonable to assume that severe tubal infections with this organism can lead to occlusion and infertility. However, prospective studies are needed to prove this point. Although the possibility that *U. urealyticum* plays a role in involuntary infertility in humans was first raised more than 20 years ago, the association remains speculative.

PERINATAL MORBIDITY AND MORTALITY *U. urealyticum* is a common cause of histologic chorioamnionitis. Individual case reports provide compelling evidence that, in at least some individuals, *U. urealyticum* alone causes spontaneous abortion and premature birth. Rates of placental isolation of ureaplasmas are inversely related to infants' gestational age and birth weight. *M. hominis* also commonly invades the chorioamnion and amniotic fluid but is rarely found in the absence of other organisms, particularly ureaplasmas. Therefore, it is unclear whether *M. hominis* alone causes histologic chorioamnionitis or clinical amnionitis.

U. urealyticum is the single most common organism isolated from the CNS and lower respiratory tract of newborn infants, particularly those delivered prematurely and weighing <1000 g. The isolation of the organism in pure culture from pleural fluid, lung biopsy, and lung tissue obtained at autopsy from infants with pneumonia, along with the production of similar histologic lesions in lungs of newborn mice and prematurely born nonhuman primates with these isolates, proves that this organism can cause pneumonia in newborn infants. Ureaplasmal pneumonia may play a role in the development of chronic lung disease. While the occurrence of clinically significant hydrocephalus and meningitis is variable in CNS infections with *U. urealyticum* and *M. hominis*, it is clear that in some cases the organisms cause these conditions. *M. hominis* is also a cause of septicemia, pneumonia, pericarditis, adenitis, and abscesses of the subcutaneous tissue in newborn infants.

EXTRAGENITAL INFECTIONS IN CHILDREN AND ADULTS While *U. urealyticum* and *M. hominis* typically remain localized in the lower genital tract, both organisms can cause extragenital infections. Infections at extragenital sites have been reported in patients of both sexes and a broad range of ages (14 to 76 years). Disseminated infection has been reported in otherwise healthy hosts, but most infections follow genitourinary manipulation or trauma of the genitourinary tract or develop in individuals with underlying immunosuppression.

The ability of *M. hominis* to infect surgical wounds or sites of trauma is well documented. Heart-lung transplant recipients commonly develop sternal wound infections due to *M. hominis*, with associated mediastinitis and empyema. *M. hominis* has been identified in cases of meningitis following trauma and in brain abscesses of immunocompromised patients. In addition, *M. hominis* has been reported as a cause of lower respiratory tract infection and pneumonia in immunosuppressed and other compromised patients. *U. urealyticum* is the predominant cause of sinopulmonary disease and progressive lung failure in agammaglobulinemic patients. Both *U. urealyticum* and *M. hominis* have been isolated from pericardial fluid and/or pericardial tissue of patients with large pericardial effusions requiring surgical drainage. Prosthetic valve endocarditis and persistent and fatal bloodstream infection due to *M. hominis* have been reported. Peritonitis following organ transplantation and renal dialysis can also result from *M. hominis* infection. Both *M. hominis* and *U. urealyticum* are common causes of postpartum bacteremia, endometritis, and cesarean wound infection. *M. hominis* has also been associated with postpartum pneumonia and arthritis.

Approximately 20 percent of individuals with agammaglobulinemia develop joint inflammation; evidence suggests that mycoplasmas may be responsible for the majority of cases. Furthermore, both *U. urealyticum* and *M. hominis* can cause arthritis in other types of immunosuppressed or otherwise compromised patients (i.e., those with prosthetic joints). In most reported cases, the arthritis has been persistent, lasting from several months to more than 1 year. Aggressive, erosive arthritis can progress despite anti-inflammatory therapy and gamma globulin replacement. Osteomyelitis has been reported in association with invasive infection with both *U. urealyticum* and *M. hominis*.

DIAGNOSIS *M. hominis* and *U. urealyticum* grow more rapidly than *M. pneumoniae* in culture and can be detected in 2 to 5 days. While commercial media are available for the culture of genital mycoplasmas, no commercial serologic assays or rapid detection tests are available for routine diagnosis.

℞ TREATMENT

Oral tetracyclines, given for at least 7 days in the same doses used for mycoplasmal respiratory infections, have historically been the drugs of choice for the treatment of urogenital infections due to *M. hominis*; however, 20 to 40 percent of clinical isolates are now resistant to these agents. Clindamycin (150 to 450 mg every 6 h for adults, 10 to 40 mg/kg daily in three or four doses for children) is an alternative agent for the treatment of tetracycline-resistant *M. hominis* infection. Either erythromycin or tetracyclines can be used in therapy for *U. urealyticum* infections, but tetracycline resistance occurs in 10 to 15 percent of clinical isolates. The activity of quinolones is not affected by tetracycline resistance caused by the tetM transposon. Ciprofloxacin is generally less active than ofloxacin in vitro against either species. A 7-day course of oral ofloxacin (200 to 400 mg every 12 h for adults) appears to be adequate for urethritis, but studies of this regimen have focused on *C. trachomatis* rather than on *U. urealyticum*. A single (1-g) dose of azithromycin is

approved for treatment of urethritis due to *C. trachomatis* and has been shown to work as well clinically as 7 days of doxycycline therapy in persons with infection due to *U. urealyticum*. *M. hominis* is resistant to macrolides.

Infections in immunocompromised hosts may be caused by resistant organisms refractory to antimicrobial therapy and may require prolonged administration of a combination of intravenous antimicrobials, intravenous immunoglobulin, and/or antisera prepared specifically against the infecting species. Despite aggressive therapy, relapses are likely. No specific treatment guidelines for neonates with systemic mycoplasmal or ureaplasmal infections have been established, and no controlled trials of clinical efficacy have been conducted. However, appropriately modified dosages of the same drugs used for older children have been used successfully in numerous reported cases in neonates.

BIBLIOGRAPHY

CASSELL GH et al: *Ureaplasma urealyticum* intrauterine infection: Role in prematurity and disease in the newborn. Clin Microbiol Rev 6:69, 1993
———: The changing role of mycoplasmas in respiratory disease and AIDS. Clin Infect Dis 17(Suppl):S1, 1993
——— et al: Genital mycoplasmal infections, in *Current Pediatric Therapy*, FD Burg et al (eds). Orlando, Saunders, 1995, p 673
CHAN ED, WELSH CH: Fulminant *Mycoplasma pneumoniae* pneumonia. West J Med 162:133, 1995

---

181 *Walter E. Stamm*

CHLAMYDIAL INFECTIONS

The genus *Chlamydia* contains three species that infect humans: *Chlamydia psittaci*, *Chlamydia trachomatis*, and *Chlamydia pneumoniae* (formerly the TWAR agent). *C. psittaci* is widely distributed in nature, producing genital, conjunctival, intestinal, or respiratory infections in many mammalian and avian species. Genital infections with *C. psittaci* have been well characterized in several species and cause complications such as abortion and infertility. Although mammalian strains of *C. psittaci* are not known to infect humans, avian strains occasionally do so, causing pneumonia and the systemic illness known as psittacosis.

C. pneumoniae is a fastidious chlamydial species that appears to be a frequent cause of upper respiratory tract infection and pneumonia, primarily in children and young adults, and is a cause of recurrent respiratory infections in older adults. No animal reservoir has been identified for *C. pneumoniae*; it appears to be a human pathogen spread via the respiratory route through close personal contact. To date, all strains of *C. pneumoniae* studied have been serologically homologous.

C. trachomatis is exclusively a human pathogen and was identified as the cause of trachoma in the 1940s. Since then, *C. trachomatis* has been recognized as a major cause of sexually transmitted and perinatal infection.

Chlamydiae are obligate intracellular parasites. They possess both DNA and RNA, have a cell wall and ribosomes similar to those of gram-negative bacteria, and are inhibited by antibiotics such as tetracycline. Chlamydiae are classified as bacteria belonging to their own order (Chlamydiales).

A unique feature of all chlamydiae is their complex reproductive cycle. Two forms of the microorganism—the extracellular elementary body and the intracellular reticulate body—participate in this cycle. The elementary body is adapted for extracellular survival and is the infective form transmitted from one person to another. Elementary bodies attach to susceptible target cells (usually columnar or transitional epithelial cells) and enter the cells within a phagosome. Within 8 h, the elementary bodies reorganize into reticulate bodies. These forms are adapted to intracellular survival and multiplication. They undergo binary fission, eventually producing numerous replicates contained within the membrane-bound "inclusion body," which occupies much of the infected host cell. Chlamydial inclusions resist lysosomal fusion until late in the developmental cycle. After 24 h, the reticulate bodies condense and form elementary bodies still contained within the inclusion. The inclusion then ruptures, releasing elementary bodies from the cell to initiate infection of adjacent cells.

Recent studies using monoclonal antibodies to and nucleotide sequencing of the major outer-membrane protein have delineated at least 20 serotypes of *C. trachomatis*. According to the serovar classification system of Wang and Grayston, strains associated with trachoma have generally been those of the A, B, Ba, and C serovars, while serovars D through K have largely been associated with sexually transmitted and perinatally acquired infections. Serovars L_1, L_2, and L_3 produce lymphogranuloma venereum (LGV) and hemorrhagic proctocolitis. The LGV strains demonstrate unique biologic behavior in that they are more invasive than the other serovars, produce disease in lymphatic tissue, grow readily in cell culture systems and macrophages, and are fatal when inoculated intracerebrally into mice and monkeys. Non-LGV strains of *C. trachomatis* characteristically produce superficial infections involving the columnar epithelium of the eye, genitalia, and respiratory tract.

C. trachomatis has been reported as an infrequent cause of endocarditis, peritonitis, pleuritis, and possibly periappendicitis and may occasionally cause respiratory infections in older children and adults. Immunosuppressed patients with pneumonia have had, in some cases, either serologic or cultural evidence of *C. trachomatis* infection, but more data are necessary to define the role of *Chlamydia* in these patients.

SEXUALLY TRANSMITTED AND PERINATAL INFECTIONS DUE TO *C. TRACHOMATIS*

SPECTRUM OF *C. TRACHOMATIS* GENITAL INFECTIONS Genital infections caused by *C. trachomatis* represent the most common bacterial sexually transmitted diseases (STDs) in the United States. An estimated 4 million cases occur each year. In adults the clinical spectrum of sexually transmitted *C. trachomatis* infections parallels the spectrum of gonococcal infections (Table 181-1). Chlamydial and gonococcal infections have been associated with urethritis, proctitis, and conjunctivitis in both sexes; with epididymitis in men; and with mucopurulent cervicitis (MPC), acute salpingitis, bartholinitis, and the Fitz-Hugh–Curtis syndrome (perihepatitis) in women. Moreover, both types of infection can be associated with systemic complications, particularly arthritis. In general, however, chlamydial infections produce fewer symptoms and signs than corresponding gonococcal infections at the same anatomic site; in fact, the former are often totally asymptomatic. Increasing evidence suggests that many chlamydial infections of the genital tract, especially in women, persist for months without producing symptoms. Simultaneous infection with *C. trachomatis* often occurs in women with cervical gonococcal infection and in heterosexual men with gonococcal urethritis.

EPIDEMIOLOGY Infections due to *C. trachomatis* have now been made reportable in many states, and national incidence data show steadily rising numbers of reported infections, undoubtedly reflecting both increased testing and increased reporting. The annual occurrence of nongonococcal urethritis (NGU) has been measured through surveys of diagnoses made by physicians in private practice and has been used as a surrogate measure of trends in chlamydial infection. The incidence of NGU increased dramatically during the 1960s and 1970s, a period when chlamydiae caused 30 to 50 percent of such cases. Even as the incidence of gonococcal urethritis fell during the 1980s, the incidence of NGU stabilized in the United States, probably reflecting the relative lack of implementation of programs to control chlamydial infections. More recently, the implementation of such programs in some regions has been associated with a decline in the proportion of NGU cases

Table 181-1

Clinical Parallels Between Sexually Transmitted Infections due to *Neisseria gonorrhoeae* and *Chlamydia trachomatis*

	Clinical Syndrome Caused by	
Site of Infection	*N. gonorrhoeae*	*C. trachomatis*
MEN		
Urethra	Urethritis	Nongonococcal or post-gonococcal urethritis
Epididymis	Epididymitis	Epididymitis
Rectum	Proctitis	Proctitis
Conjunctiva	Conjunctivitis	Conjunctivitis
Systemic	Disseminated gonococcal infection	Reiter's syndrome
WOMEN		
Urethra	Acute urethral syndrome	Acute urethral syndrome
Bartholin's gland	Bartholinitis	Bartholinitis
Cervix	Cervicitis	Cervicitis
Rectum	Proctitis	Proctitis
Endometrium	Endometritis	Endometritis
Fallopian tube	Salpingitis	Salpingitis
Conjunctiva	Conjunctivitis	Conjunctivitis
Liver capsule	Perihepatitis	Perihepatitis
Systemic	Disseminated gonococcal infection	Reiter's syndrome

caused by chlamydiae; thus trends in NGU may now be less reliable as a surrogate for trends in the incidence of chlamydial infection.

The age of peak incidence of genital *C. trachomatis* infections, as of other sexually transmitted infections, is the late teens and early twenties. The prevalence of chlamydial urethral infection among young men is 3 to 5 percent for those seen in general medical settings, over 10 percent for asymptomatic soldiers undergoing routine physical examination, and 15 to 20 percent for heterosexual men seen in STD clinics. In areas where chlamydial control programs have been implemented, prevalence may be markedly reduced. In short, prevalence varies widely with the population group studied and with the geographic locale. Urethral chlamydial infection is less common among homosexual than among heterosexual men, but rectal infections occur in homosexual men who practice receptive anorectal intercourse without condoms. The ratio of chlamydial to gonococcal urethritis is highest for heterosexual men and for those with high socioeconomic status and is lowest for homosexual men and indigent populations.

The prevalence of cervical infection among women is approximately 5 percent for asymptomatic college students and prenatal patients in the United States, over 10 percent for women seen in family planning clinics, and over 20 percent for women seen in STD clinics. As in men, prevalence varies substantially by geographic locale. In the United States, the prevalence of *C. trachomatis* in the cervix of pregnant women is 5 to 10 times higher than that of *Neisseria gonorrhoeae*. The prevalence of genital infection with either agent is highest among individuals who are single, non-Caucasian, and between ages 18 and 24. Oral contraceptive use and the presence of cervical ectopy also confer an increased risk of chlamydial infection. The proportion of infections that are asymptomatic appears to be higher for *C. trachomatis* than for *N. gonorrhoeae*, and symptomatic *C. trachomatis* infections are clinically less severe. It is suspected that mild or asymptomatic chlamydial infections of the fallopian tubes may nonetheless cause ongoing tubal damage and infertility. Furthermore, because the total number of *C. trachomatis* infections exceeds the total number of *N. gonorrhoeae* infections in industrialized countries, the total morbidity caused by *C. trachomatis* genital infections in these countries equals or exceeds that caused by *N. gonorrhoeae*. The prevalence of *C. trachomatis* is higher than that of *N. gonorrhoeae* in industrialized countries, in part because measures such as treatment of sex partners and routine cultures for case detection in asymptomatic individuals have been applied much more effectively to the control of gonorrhea than to the control of *C. trachomatis* infection.

CLINICAL MANIFESTATIONS   Nongonococcal and Postgonococcal Urethritis

NGU is a diagnosis of exclusion that is applied to men with symptoms and/or signs of urethritis who do not have gonorrhea. Postgonococcal urethritis (PGU) refers to nongonococcal urethritis developing in men 2 to 3 weeks after treatment of gonococcal urethritis with single doses of agents such as amoxicillin or cephalosporins that lack sufficient activity against chlamydiae. Since current treatment for gonorrhea also includes tetracycline, doxycycline, or azithromycin for concomitant chlamydial infection, both the incidence of PGU and the causative role of chlamydiae in this syndrome have declined. *C. trachomatis* causes 20 to 40 percent of the cases of NGU and PGU in heterosexual men but is less commonly isolated from homosexual men with these syndromes. The cause of most of the remaining cases is uncertain, although considerable evidence suggests that *Ureaplasma urealyticum* causes many of these infections, while *Trichomonas vaginalis* and herpes simplex virus (HSV) cause some cases of NGU.

NGU is diagnosed by documentation of a leukocytic urethral exudate and by exclusion of gonorrhea by Gram's staining or culture. *C. trachomatis* urethritis is generally less severe than gonococcal urethritis, although in an individual patient these two forms of urethritis cannot be reliably differentiated solely on clinical grounds. Symptoms include urethral discharge, dysuria (often whitish and mucoid rather than frankly purulent), and urethral itching. Physical examination may reveal meatal erythema and tenderness and a urethral exudate that is often demonstrable only by stripping of the urethra. At least one-third of males with *C. trachomatis* urethral infection have no demonstrable signs or symptoms of urethritis. Asymptomatic chlamydial urethritis has been demonstrated in 5 to 10 percent of sexually active adolescent males screened in teen clinics. Such patients frequently have first-glass pyuria ($\geq$15 leukocytes per 400$\times$ microscopic field in the sediment of first-voided urine), a positive leukocyte esterase test, or an increased number of leukocytes on Gram-stained smear prepared from a urogenital swab inserted 1 to 2 cm into the anterior urethra. For the enumeration of leukocytes, the smear is first scanned at low power to identify areas of the slide containing the highest concentration of leukocytes. These areas are then examined under oil immersion (1000$\times$). An average of four or more leukocytes in at least three of five 1000$\times$ (oil-immersion) fields is indicative of urethritis and correlates with the recovery of *C. trachomatis*. To differentiate between true urethritis and functional symptoms among symptomatic patients or to make a presumptive diagnosis of *C. trachomatis* infection in asymptomatic men (e.g., male patients in STD clinics, sex partners of women with nongonococcal salpingitis or MPC, fathers of children with inclusion conjunctivitis), the examination of an endourethral specimen for increased leukocytes is useful if specific diagnostic tests for chlamydiae are not available. Alternatively, noninvasive screening for urethritis can be accomplished by testing of a first-void urine sample for pyuria, either by microscopy or by the leukocyte esterase test. Urine can also be directly tested for chlamydiae or gonococci by DNA amplification methods, as described below.

Epididymitis   *C. trachomatis* is the major cause of epididymitis in sexually active heterosexual men under 35 years of age, accounting for about 70 percent of cases. *N. gonorrhoeae* causes most of the remaining cases, and some men have simultaneous infections with both pathogens, usually accompanied by asymptomatic urethritis as defined above. In homosexual men, sexually transmitted coliform infection acquired via rectal intercourse may cause epididymitis. Coliform bacteria and *Pseudomonas aeruginosa*, usually in association with preceding urologic instrumentation or surgery, are the most common causes of epididymitis in men over 35. Men with epididymitis typically present with unilateral scrotal pain, fever, and epididymal tenderness or swelling on examination. The illness may be mild enough to treat on an outpatient basis or severe enough to require hospitalization. Testicular torsion should be excluded promptly by radionuclide scan, Doppler flow study, or surgical exploration in a teenager or young adult who presents with acute unilateral testicular pain without urethritis. The possibility of testicular tumor or chronic infection (e.g.,

tuberculosis) should be excluded when a patient with unilateral intrascrotal pain and swelling does not respond to appropriate antimicrobial therapy.

Reiter's Syndrome   Reiter's syndrome consists of conjunctivitis, urethritis (or cervicitis in females), arthritis, and characteristic mucocutaneous lesions (see Chap. 317). *C. trachomatis* has been recovered from the urethra of up to 70 percent of men with untreated nondiarrheal Reiter's syndrome and associated urethritis. In the absence of overt urethritis, it is important to exclude subclinical urethritis in the men in whom this diagnosis is suspected.

The pathogenesis of Reiter's syndrome remains obscure. However, since more than 80 percent of affected patients have the HLA-B27 phenotype and since other mucosal infections (with *Salmonella*, *Shigella*, or *Campylobacter*, for example) produce an identical syndrome, chlamydial infection is thought to initiate an aberrant and hyperactive immune response that produces inflammation at the involved target organs in these genetically predisposed individuals. Evidence of exaggerated cell-mediated and humoral immune responses to chlamydial antigens in Reiter's syndrome supports this hypothesis. The presumptive demonstration of chlamydial elementary bodies and chlamydial DNA in the joint fluid and synovial tissue of patients with Reiter's syndrome suggests that chlamydiae may actually spread from genital to joint tissues in these patients, perhaps in macrophages.

Proctitis   *C. trachomatis* strains of either the genital immunotypes D through K or the LGV immunotypes cause proctitis in homosexual men who practice receptive anorectal intercourse. In the United States, the vast majority of cases are due to immunotypes D through K and present either as asymptomatic infection or as mild proctitis not unlike gonococcal proctitis. These infections may develop in heterosexual women as well. Patients present with mild rectal pain, mucous discharge, tenesmus, and (occasionally) bleeding. Nearly all have neutrophils in their rectal Gram's stain. Anoscopy in these non-LGV cases of chlamydial proctitis reveals mild, patchy mucosal friability and mucopurulent discharge, and the disease process is limited to the distal rectum. LGV strains produce more severe ulcerative proctitis or proctocolitis that can be confused clinically with HSV proctitis (severe rectal pain, bleeding, discharge, and tenesmus) and that histologically resembles Crohn's disease in that giant cell formation and granulomas can be seen (see Chap. 286). In the United States, these cases occur almost exclusively in homosexual men.

Mucopurulent Cervicitis   Although many women with *C. trachomatis* infection of the cervix have no symptoms or signs, a careful speculum examination reveals evidence of MPC in 30 to 50 percent of cases. As is discussed more fully in Chap. 130, MPC is associated with yellow mucopurulent discharge from the endocervical columnar epithelium and with $\geq$20 neutrophils per 1000$\times$ microscopic field within strands of cervical mucus on a thinly smeared, Gram-stained preparation of endocervical exudate. Other characteristic findings include edema of the zone of cervical ectopy and a propensity of the mucosa to bleed on minor trauma—e.g., when specimens are collected with a swab. A pap smear shows increased numbers of neutrophils as well as a characteristic pattern of mononuclear inflammatory cells, including plasma cells, transformed lymphocytes, and histiocytes. Cervical biopsy shows a predominantly mononuclear cell infiltrate of the subepithelial stroma, often with follicular cervicitis.

Pelvic Inflammatory Disease (PID)   *C. trachomatis* plays an important causative role in salpingitis. Infection with *C. trachomatis* has been demonstrated in laparoscopically verified salpingitis, the organism has been recovered from the fallopian tubes in the absence of other pathogens, and serologic evidence of recent *C. trachomatis* infection has been found in women with PID. In the United States, *C. trachomatis* has been identified in the fallopian tubes or endometrium of up to 50 percent of women with PID, and its role as an important etiologic agent in this syndrome is well accepted.

PID occurs via ascending intraluminal spread of *C. trachomatis* from the lower genital tract. MPC is thus followed by endometritis, endosalpingitis, and finally pelvic peritonitis. Evidence of MPC is usually found in women with laparoscopically verified salpingitis. Similarly, endometritis, demonstrated by endometrial biopsy showing plasma cell infiltration of the endometrial epithelium, is documented in most women with laparoscopically verified chlamydial (or gonococcal) salpingitis. Chlamydial endometritis also can occur in the absence of clinical evidence of salpingitis: approximately 40 to 50 percent of women with MPC have plasma cell endometritis. Histologic evidence of endometritis has been correlated with an "endometritis syndrome" consisting of vaginal bleeding, lower abdominal pain, and uterine tenderness in the absence of adnexal tenderness. It is not known what proportion of women who have chlamydial endometritis without adnexal tenderness also have salpingitis. However, chlamydial salpingitis may produce milder symptoms than does gonococcal salpingitis and may be associated with less marked adnexal tenderness. Mild adnexal or uterine tenderness in sexually active women with cervicitis suggests PID.

Infertility associated with fallopian-tube scarring has been strongly linked to antecedent *C. trachomatis* infection in serologic studies. Since many infertile women with tubal scarring and antichlamydial antibody have no history of PID, it appears that subclinical tubal infection ("silent salpingitis") may produce scarring. Ectopic pregnancy, which occurs in more than 70,000 women in the United States annually, is also thought to be related to *Chlamydia*-induced tubal scarring in many cases. While the pathogenesis of *Chlamydia*-induced tubal scarring remains poorly understood, antibodies to the chlamydial 60-kDa heat-shock protein have been correlated with tubal infertility, ectopic pregnancy, and Fitz-Hugh–Curtis syndrome (see below). Thus this antigen may initiate an immune-mediated process that ultimately damages the fallopian tube. Host genetic susceptibility, as defined by HLA type, may also play an important role.

Perihepatitis, or the Fitz-Hugh–Curtis syndrome, was originally described as a complication of gonococcal PID. However, cultural and/or serologic evidence of *C. trachomatis* infection is found in three-quarters of women with this syndrome. *C. trachomatis* has also been cultured from exudate on the hepatic capsule in laparoscopically verified cases. This syndrome should be suspected whenever a young, sexually active woman presents with an illness resembling cholecystitis (fever and right upper quadrant pain of subacute or acute onset). Symptoms and signs of salpingitis may be minimal. High titers of antibodies to *C. trachomatis* are generally present.

Urethral Syndrome in Women In the absence of infection with uropathogens such as coliforms or *Staphylococcus saprophyticus*, *C. trachomatis* is the pathogen most commonly isolated from college women with dysuria, frequency, and pyuria (see Chap. 131). *Chlamydia* also can be isolated from the urethra of women without symptoms of urethritis, and up to 25 percent of female STD clinic patients with chlamydial urogenital infection have cultures positive for *C. trachomatis* from the urethra only.

C. trachomatis Infection in Pregnancy *C. trachomatis* in pregnancy has been associated in some studies (but not in others) with premature delivery and with postpartum endometritis. Whether these complications are in part attributable to *C. trachomatis* is not clear.

PERINATAL INFECTIONS: INCLUSION CONJUNCTIVITIS AND PNEUMONIA **Epidemiology** Studies in the United States have demonstrated that 5 to 25 percent of pregnant women have *C. trachomatis* infections of the cervix. In these studies, approximately one-half to two-thirds of children exposed during birth have acquired *C. trachomatis* infection. Roughly half of the infected infants (or 25 percent of the group exposed) have developed clinical evidence of inclusion conjunctivitis. In addition to infecting the eye, *C. trachomatis* has been isolated frequently and persistently from the nasopharynx, rectum, and vagina of infants, occasionally for periods exceeding 1 year in the absence of treatment. Pneumonia develops in about 10 percent of children infected perinatally, and otitis media may in some cases result from perinatally acquired chlamydial infection.

Inclusion Conjunctivitis of the Newborn (Neonatal Chlamydial Conjunctivitis) Neonatal chlamydial conjunctivitis has an acute onset and often produces a profuse mucopurulent discharge. In the newborn, chlamydial conjunctivitis generally has a longer incubation period than gonococcal conjunctivitis (usually 5 to 14 days vs. 1 to 3 days); however, this guideline is not reliable for the diagnosis of individual cases, and in any event it is impossible to differentiate chlamydial conjunctivitis from other forms of neonatal bacterial conjunctivitis on clinical grounds; instead, laboratory diagnosis is required. Besides *C. trachomatis* and *N. gonorrhoeae*, the other important infectious causes of conjunctivitis in newborns include *Haemophilus influenzae*, *Streptococcus pneumoniae*, and HSV. Inclusions within epithelial cells are often detected in Giemsa-stained conjunctival smears, but these smears are less sensitive than cultures or antigen detection tests. Gram-stained smears may show gonococci or occasional small gram-negative coccobacilli in *Haemophilus* conjunctivitis, but smears should be accompanied by cultures for these agents. Very rarely, a trachoma-like eye disease occurs in children who have chlamydial infection and who live in areas that do not have endemic trachoma. Since concomitant pharyngeal infection is often present, neonatal chlamydial conjunctivitis should be treated with oral antimicrobials in order to prevent chlamydial pneumonia.

Infant Pneumonia *C. trachomatis* causes a distinctive pneumonia syndrome in infants. Recent epidemiologic studies have linked chlamydial pulmonary infection in infants with increased occurrence of subacute lung disease (bronchitis, asthma, wheezing) in later childhood.

LYMPHOGRANULOMA VENEREUM **Definition** LGV is a sexually transmitted infection caused by *C. trachomatis* strains of the L_1, L_2, and L_3 serovars. In the United States, most cases are caused by L_2 organisms. Acute LGV in heterosexual men is characterized by a transient primary genital lesion followed by multilocular suppurative regional lymphadenopathy. Women, homosexual men, and—in occasional instances—heterosexual men may develop hemorrhagic proctitis with regional lymphadenitis. Acute LGV is almost always associated with systemic symptoms such as fever and leukocytosis but is rarely associated with systemic complications such as meningoencephalitis. After a latent period of years, late complications include genital elephantiasis due to lymphatic involvement; strictures; and fistulas of the penis, urethra, and rectum.

Epidemiology LGV is usually sexually transmitted, but occasional transmission by nonsexual personal contact, fomites, or laboratory accidents has been documented. Laboratory work involving the creation of aerosols of LGV organisms (e.g., sonication, homogenization) must be conducted only with appropriate measures for biologic containment.

The peak incidence of LGV corresponds to the age of greatest sexual activity: the second and third decades of life. The worldwide incidence of LGV is falling, but the disease is still endemic and a major cause of morbidity in Asia, Africa, South America, and parts of the Caribbean. In the Bahamas, an apparent outbreak of LGV has been described in association with a concurrent increase in heterosexual infection with human immunodeficiency virus. However, only 235 cases were reported in the United States in 1994.

The frequency of infection following exposure is believed to be much lower than that for gonorrhea and syphilis. Early manifestations are recognized far more often in men than in women, who usually present with late complications. In the United States, where the reported male-to-female ratio of cases is 3.4 : 1, most cases have involved homosexually active men and persons returning from abroad (travelers, sailors, and military personnel). The main reservoir of infection, although it has not been directly demonstrated, is presumed to be asymptomatically infected individuals.

Clinical Manifestations In heterosexuals, a *primary genital lesion* develops from 3 days to 3 weeks after exposure. It is a small, painless vesicle or nonindurated ulcer or papule located on the penis in men and on the labia, posterior vagina, or fourchette in women. The primary lesion is noticed by fewer than one-third of men with LGV and only rarely by women. It heals in a few days without scarring and, even when noticed, usually is recognized as LGV only in retrospect. LGV strains of *C. trachomatis* have occasionally been recovered from genital ulcers and from the urethra of men and the endocervix of women who present with inguinal adenopathy; these areas may be the primary site of infection in some cases.

In women and homosexual men, *primary anal* or *rectal infection* develops after receptive anorectal intercourse. In women, rectal infection with LGV (or non-LGV) strains of *C. trachomatis* presumably can also arise by the contiguous spread of infected secretions along the perineum (as in rectal gonococcal infections in women) or perhaps by spread to the rectum via the pelvic lymphatics.

From the site of the primary urethral, genital, anal, or rectal infection, the organism spreads via the regional lymphatics. Penile, vulvar, or anal infection can lead to inguinal and femoral lymphadenitis. Rectal infection produces hypogastric and deep iliac lymphadenitis. Upper vaginal or cervical infection results in enlargement of the obturator and iliac nodes.

The most common presenting picture in heterosexual men is the *inguinal syndrome*, which is characterized by painful inguinal lymphadenopathy beginning 2 to 6 weeks after presumed exposure; in rare instances, the onset comes after a few months. The inguinal adenopathy is unilateral in two-thirds of cases, and palpable enlargement of the iliac and femoral nodes is often evident on the same side as the enlarged inguinal nodes. The nodes are initially discrete, but progressive periadenitis results in a matted mass of nodes that becomes fluctuant and suppurative. The overlying skin becomes fixed, inflamed, and thin and finally develops multiple draining fistulas. Extensive enlargement of chains of inguinal nodes above and below the inguinal ligament ("the sign of the groove") is not specific and, although not uncommon, is documented in only a minority of cases. On histologic examination, infected nodes are initially found to have characteristic small stellate abscesses surrounded by histiocytes. These abscesses coalesce to form large, necrotic, suppurative foci. Spontaneous healing usually takes place after several months; inguinal scars or granulomatous masses of various sizes persist for life. Massive pelvic lymphadenopathy in women or homosexual men may lead to exploratory laparotomy.

As cultures and serologic tests for *C. trachomatis* are being used more often, increasing numbers of cases of LGV proctitis are being recognized in homosexual men. Such patients present with anorectal pain and mucopurulent, bloody rectal discharge. Although these patients may complain of diarrhea, they are often referring not to diarrhea but rather to frequent, painful, unsuccessful attempts at defecation (tenesmus). Sigmoidoscopy reveals ulcerative proctitis or proctocolitis, with purulent exudate and mucosal bleeding. The histopathologic findings in the rectal mucosa include granulomas with giant cells, along with crypt abscesses and extensive inflammation. These clinical, sigmoidoscopic, and histopathologic findings may closely resemble those of Crohn's disease of the rectum.

Constitutional symptoms are common during the stage of regional lymphadenopathy and, in cases of proctitis, may include fever, chills, headache, meningismus, anorexia, myalgias, and arthralgias. These findings in the presence of lymphadenopathy sometimes are mistakenly interpreted as representing malignant lymphoma. Other systemic complications are infrequent but include arthritis with sterile effusion, aseptic meningitis, meningoencephalitis, conjunctivitis, hepatitis, and erythema nodosum. Chlamydiae have been recovered from the cerebrospinal fluid and in one case were isolated from the blood of a patient with severe constitutional symptoms—a result indicating the dissemination of infection. Laboratory-acquired infections suspected of being due to the inhalation of aerosols have been associated with mediastinal lymphadenopathy, pneumonitis, and pleural effusion.

Complications of untreated anorectal infection include perirectal abscess; fistula in ano; and rectovaginal, rectovesical, and ischiorectal fistulas. Secondary bacterial infection probably contributes to these complications. Rectal stricture is a late complication of anorectal infection and usually develops 2 to 6 cm from the anal orifice—i.e., at a site within reach on digital rectal examination. Proximal extension of the stricture for several centimeters may lead to a mistaken clinical and radiographic diagnosis of carcinoma.

A small percentage of cases of LGV in men present as chronic progressive infiltrative, ulcerative, or fistular lesions of the penis, urethra, or scrotum. Associated lymphatic obstruction may produce elephantiasis. When urethral stricture occurs, it usually involves the posterior urethra and causes incontinence or difficulty with urination.

APPROACH TO THE DIAGNOSIS AND TREATMENT OF *C. TRACHOMATIS* GENITAL INFECTIONS

Four types of laboratory procedure are available to confirm *C. trachomatis* infection: direct microscopic examination of tissue scrapings for typical intracytoplasmic inclusions or elementary bodies; isolation of the organism in cell culture; detection of chlamydial antigens or nucleic acid by immunologic or hybridization methods; and detection of antibody in serum or in local secretions.

Except in conjunctivitis, direct microscopic examination of Giemsa-stained cell scrapings for typical inclusions has an unacceptably low degree of sensitivity, and false-positive interpretations by inexperienced observers are common. Even for conjunctivitis, this approach has been replaced by direct fluorescent antibody staining of conjunctival smears to identify chlamydial elementary bodies (see below).

Cell culture techniques for isolation of *C. trachomatis* are available in most large medical centers but not in other clinical settings. In addition to limited availability, other disadvantages of cell culture include its low and variable level of sensitivity (60 to 80 percent), its requirement for rigorous transport conditions, and its high cost and technically demanding nature. Therefore, nonculture alternatives utilizing antigen detection or nucleic acid hybridization have been developed. In the immunofluorescent slide test, potentially infected genital or ocular secretions are smeared onto a slide, fixed, and stained with fluorescein-conjugated monoclonal antibody specific for chlamydial antigens. The observation of fluorescing elementary bodies confirms the diagnosis. Compared with culture, this test is 70 to 85 percent sensitive, and it is quite specific when used for confirmation of urethral, cervical, or ocular infection in high-risk patients with suspected *C. trachomatis* infection. The sensitivity and specificity of the test depend directly upon the skill of the microscopist. The apparently lower sensitivity of the test in low-risk populations, along with its relatively labor-intensive nature, limits its value as a screening tool.

Enzyme-linked immunosorbent assay (ELISA) techniques for the detection of chlamydial antigens provide another alternative to culture. The reported sensitivity and specificity of these tests for genital infections (as compared with culture) have been 60 to 80 percent and 97 to 99 percent, respectively, in high-risk populations. Sensitivities have generally been higher in cervical infection and lower in urethritis among males. Like the direct fluorescent antibody slide test, the ELISA is less accurate in low-prevalence populations. ELISAs are better suited to screening than is direct immunofluorescence because large numbers of specimens can easily be processed.

Assays using nucleic acid probes have also been developed for chlamydial diagnosis. One such test uses DNA-RNA hybridization and appears to be approximately equal to the best ELISAs in terms of sensitivity and specificity. Recently, nucleic acid probes have been developed for use in amplification assays such as ligase chain reaction and polymerase chain reaction (PCR). These tests are now the most sensitive chlamydial diagnostic methods available, being the first nonculture assays actually to surpass culture itself in sensitivity. The ability of these tests to detect chlamydial genes in urine with a high degree of sensitivity and specificity allows their use with urine specimens rather than with conventional urethral and cervical swabs. The use of urine specimens is particularly appealing for public-health chlamydial screening programs.

Serologic tests are of limited usefulness in the diagnosis of chlamydial oculogenital infections. The complement fixation (CF) test with heat-stable, genus-specific antigen has been used with some success to diagnose LGV but is insensitive in infections due to non-LGV strains of *C. trachomatis*. The microimmunofluorescence (micro-IF) test with *C. trachomatis* antigens is more sensitive but is generally available only in research laboratories. The test measures antibodies by serovar specificity and by immunoglobulin class (IgM, IgG, IgA, secretory IgA) in both serum and local secretions. Serologic diagnosis by the micro-IF test may be useful in infant pneumonia (in which high-titer IgM antibody and/or fourfold rises in titer are often demonstrated), in chlamydial salpingitis (especially Fitz-Hugh–Curtis syndrome), and in LGV.

Table 181-2 summarizes the diagnostic tests of choice for patients with suspected chlamydial infection. With few exceptions, the most suitable method for diagnosis is demonstration of the agent by either cell culture or one of the newer nonculture techniques. Selection of the most appropriate of these tests often depends upon local availability and expertise. However, it is clear that, in most settings and for most purposes, sensitivity and specificity will be greatest with nucleic acid amplification techniques. For patients to whom medicolegal considera-

tions may apply (victims of sexual or child abuse), cultures or nucleic acid amplification methods should always be used. Since *C. trachomatis* is an intracellular pathogen, adequate specimens for chlamydial diagnostic testing must include epithelial cells. Cultures or nonculture tests of pus are less often positive. In urethritis, a thin-shafted urogenital swab should be inserted at least 2 cm into the urethra to obtain an appropriate specimen. Although cultures of urine for chlamydiae are less sensitive than urethral cultures, recent studies suggest that nucleic acid amplification testing of a first-void urine specimen from men is a more sensitive and less painful diagnostic alternative to the more invasive urethral swab–based tests. The first 30 mL of voided urine should be collected for testing. When a cervical sample is collected, the external os should first be cleaned of debris and purulent material; a plastic-shafted swab should then be inserted into the cervix, rotated slowly several times, and withdrawn. For the diagnosis of infections in women, testing of a first-void urine specimen by nucleic acid amplification methods is at least as sensitive as testing of a cervical swab. When conjunctival specimens are sought, the epithelium should be swabbed to remove cells rather than just purulent material. All specimens for chlamydial culture should be placed immediately into transport medium and then either refrigerated (if they will reach the labora-

Table 181-2

Diagnostic Tests for *Chlamydia trachomatis* Infection

Infection	Suggestive Signs/Symptoms	Presumptive Diagnosis*	Confirmatory Test of Choice
MEN			
NGU, PGU	Discharge, dysuria	Gram's stain with >4 neutrophils per oil-immersion field; no gonococci	Urethral culture or nonculture test for *C. trachomatis*; urine PCR or LCR for *C. trachomatis*
Epididymitis	Unilateral intrascrotal swelling, pain, tenderness; fever; NGU	Gram's stain with >4 neutrophils per oil-immersion field; no gonococci; urinalysis with pyuria	Urethral culture or nonculture test for *C. trachomatis*; urine PCR or LCR for *C. trachomatis*
WOMEN			
Cervicitis	Mucopurulent cervical discharge, bleeding and edema of the zone of cervical ectopy	Cervical Gram's stain with ≥20 neutrophils per oil-immersion field in cervical mucus	Cervical culture or nonculture test for *C. trachomatis*; urine PCR or LCR for *C. trachomatis*
Salpingitis	Lower abdominal pain, cervical motion tenderness, adnexal tenderness or masses	*C. trachomatis* always potentially present in salpingitis	Cervical culture or nonculture test for *C. trachomatis*; urine PCR or LCR for *C. trachomatis*
Urethritis	Dysuria and frequency without urgency or hematuria	MPC; sterile pyuria; negative routine urine culture	Urethral and cervical cultures or nonculture test for *C. trachomatis*; urine PCR or LCR for *C. trachomatis*
ADULTS OF EITHER SEX			
Proctitis	Rectal pain, discharge, tenesmus, bleeding; history of receptive anorectal intercourse	Negative gonococcal culture and Gram's stain; at least 1 neutrophil per oil-immersion field in rectal Gram's stain	Rectal culture or direct immunofluorescence test for *C. trachomatis*
Reiter's syndrome	NGU, arthritis, conjunctivitis, typical skin lesions	Gram's stain with >4 neutrophils per oil-immersion field; lack of gonococci indicative of NGU	Urethral culture or nonculture test for *C. trachomatis*
LGV	Regional adenopathy, primary lesion, proctitis, systemic symptoms	None	Isolation of LGV strain from node or rectum, occasionally from urethra or cervix; LGV CF titer, ≥1:64; micro-IF titer, ≥1:512
NEONATES			
Conjunctivitis	Purulent conjunctival discharge 6 to 18 days postdelivery	Negative culture and Gram's stain for gonococci, *Haemophilus* species, pneumococci, staphylococci	Conjunctival culture or nonculture test for *C. trachomatis*; Giemsa-stained scraping of conjunctival material capable of providing more rapid diagnosis but less sensitive
Infant pneumonia	Afebrile, staccato cough, diffuse rales, bilateral hyperinflation, interstitial infiltrates	None	Chlamydial culture of sputum, pharynx, eye, rectum; micro-IF antibody to *C. trachomatis*— fourfold change in IgG or IgM antibody titer

* A presumptive diagnosis of chlamydial infection is often made in the syndromes listed when gonococci are not found. A positive test for *Neisseria gonorrhoeae* does not exclude the involvement of *C. trachomatis*, which often is present in patients with gonorrhea.

NOTE: CF, complement-fixing; LCR, ligase chain reaction; LGV, lymphogranuloma venereum; micro-IF, microimmunofluorescence; MPC, mucopurulent cervicitis; NGU, nongonococcal urethritis; PCR, polymerase chain reaction; PGU, postgonococcal urethritis.

tory within 12 to 18 h) or frozen at −70°C (if longer storage is anticipated). A major advantage of the nonculture diagnostic techniques is their less rigid transport requirements; neither refrigeration nor rapid transport is needed.

From a public health viewpoint, the most effective use of chlamydial diagnostic testing has not been established and varies with the clinical population, local resources, and laboratory expertise. The Centers for Disease Control and Prevention have recommended empiric treatment (without diagnostic testing if resources are not available for testing) of selected high-risk groups. These include men with NGU or sexually transmitted epididymitis; women with MPC or PID; asymptomatic sex partners of patients with these syndromes; women and heterosexual men with gonorrhea (because of the high proportion of these patients who also have *C. trachomatis* infection); and sexual contacts of men or women with gonorrhea. However, diagnostic testing (in addition to empiric therapy) offers several potential benefits in the management of these patients, including confirmation of infection and support of the clinical diagnosis (especially in women with MPC or PID), enhancement of sex-partner referral and compliance with drug therapy, determination of prognosis, and education of physicians regarding the correlation of signs and symptoms with culture results. Since chlamydial diagnostic testing has become more widely available, its use for specific diagnosis in such patients should be promoted. From a public health perspective, high priority should be given to the screening of asymptomatic high-risk women who would not otherwise receive treatment for presumptive chlamydial infection, especially those seen in high-risk settings (e.g., STD clinics or abortion clinics) and those with a high-risk profile (e.g., sexually active and ≤21 years of age, new sex partner within the preceding 2 months, or more than one current sex partner). Similar screening programs should be used to detect and treat asymptomatic urethritis in high-risk adolescent males. Screening programs of this type have been associated with reductions in the prevalence of chlamydial infection and of the complications of chlamydial infection, such as PID.

ANTIMICROBIAL SUSCEPTIBILITY In laboratory tests that evaluate the growth of chlamydiae in cell cultures, the tetracyclines, erythromycin, rifampin, certain fluoroquinolones (especially ofloxacin), and the new macrolide azithromycin are all highly active against these organisms. Sulfonamides and clindamycin are also active against *C. trachomatis,* but to a lesser degree. Penicillin and ampicillin suppress chlamydial multiplication but do not eradicate the organism in vitro. The cephalosporins appear to be relatively ineffective against *C. trachomatis.* Streptomycin, gentamicin, neomycin, kanamycin, vancomycin, ristocetin, spectinomycin, and nystatin are not effective at concentrations inhibitory for most bacteria and fungi. There does not appear to be much strain-to-strain variation in susceptibility to antibiotics, and no clinically significant antimicrobial resistance in chlamydiae has been described. Thus antimicrobial susceptibility testing is not needed in the routine management of patients with chlamydial infection.

℞ TREATMENT

Until the introduction of azithromycin, chlamydial infections could not be eradicated by single-dose or short-term antimicrobial regimens. In most situations in adults, 7 days of treatment with doxycycline or tetracycline should be given for uncomplicated genital infections, but a 2-week course of therapy is recommended for complicated chlamydial infections (e.g., PID, epididymitis) and at least a 3-week course for LGV. Failure of treatment of genital infections with a tetracycline usually indicates poor compliance or reinfection rather than the involvement of a drug-resistant strain.

Therapy for *C. trachomatis* urethritis is more effective than therapy for nonchlamydial NGU. *C. trachomatis* is eradicated from the urethra by treatment with tetracycline hydrochloride (500 mg qid for 7 days) or doxycycline (100 mg by mouth bid for 7 days). An effective alternative regimen is erythromycin at a dose of 500 mg qid for 7 days.

Eradication of *C. trachomatis* from the cervix by tetracycline, doxycycline, and erythromycin, given at similar doses and for similar durations, has been demonstrated. Erythromycin base (500 mg qid for 10 to 14 days) is the regimen of choice for pregnant women with *C. trachomatis* infection. Amoxicillin (500 mg tid for 10 days) has also been used successfully in pregnant women. Tetracycline hydrochloride (500 mg qid) or doxycycline (100 mg bid) for 14 days produces clinical and microbiologic cure of epididymitis and PID associated with *C. trachomatis* infection, but in this situation tetracycline should always be used together with a drug that is highly effective against gonorrhea.

Two other antimicrobial agents can be used for the treatment of uncomplicated chlamydial genital infections in men and women. Ofloxacin (300 mg orally bid for 7 days) is as effective as doxycycline for the treatment of chlamydial infection and appears to be safe and well tolerated. It cannot be used in pregnancy. Azithromycin, a macrolide, is highly active against *C. trachomatis*, exhibits prolonged bioavailability, and is concentrated intracellularly. In comparative trials, a 1-g single dose of azithromycin has been as effective as 7 days of doxycycline for uncomplicated chlamydial infection. Azithromycin causes fewer adverse gastrointestinal reactions than do older macrolides like erythromycin. Both ofloxacin and azithromycin offer alternatives for treatment that may be of value in selected patients who are allergic to or intolerant of tetracyclines and erythromycin, but they are considerably more expensive than these standard regimens. The single-dose regimen of azithromycin has great appeal for the treatment of patients with uncomplicated chlamydial infection (especially those without symptoms and those with a likelihood of poor compliance) and of sexual partners of infected patients. Although not approved by the U.S. Food and Drug Administration, the 1-g single-dose regimen of azithromycin has been safe and effective in the treatment of pregnant women.

Treatment of Sex Partners The continued high prevalence of chlamydial infections in most parts of the United States is due primarily to the failure to diagnose—and therefore treat—patients with symptomatic or asymptomatic infection and their sex partners. Patients with NGU, epididymitis, Reiter's syndrome, or MPC sometimes are not treated with antimicrobials, and their sex partners are treated even less often. *C. trachomatis* urethral or cervical infection has been well documented in a high proportion of the sex partners of patients with NGU, epididymitis, Reiter's syndrome, salpingitis, or endocervicitis. If possible, confirmatory laboratory tests for *Chlamydia* should be undertaken in these individuals, but even those without evidence of clinical disease who have recently been exposed to proven or possible chlamydial infection (for example, NGU) should be offered therapy.

Treatment of Neonates and Infants In neonates with conjunctivitis or infants with pneumonia, erythromycin ethylsuccinate or estolate can be given orally in a dose of 50 mg/kg per day, preferably as 12.25 mg/kg qid, for 2 weeks. Careful attention must be given to compliance with therapy—a frequent problem. Relapses of eye infection are common following treatment with topical erythromycin or tetracycline ophthalmic ointment and may also occur after oral erythromycin therapy. Thus follow-up cultures should be performed after treatment. Both parents should be examined for *C. trachomatis* infection and, if diagnostic testing is not readily available, should be treated with doxycycline or azithromycin.

PREVENTION Efforts to develop a vaccine for chlamydial infection have not yet been successful. Early diagnosis and treatment shorten the duration of infectiousness of the carrier and therefore constitute primary prevention of chlamydial infection. By the early 1990s, one of the 10 regions of the United States (Region X, the Pacific Northwest) had formally undertaken a chlamydial control program involving widespread testing. Approximately 500,000 tests per year were conducted in 150 family planning clinics throughout the region in women meeting the criteria for high risk. Within 5 years, the prevalence of chlamydial infection had fallen from 10 percent to 5 percent. While other regions of the United States have now initiated similar programs, many family planning and STD clinics still do not offer chlamydial testing. The availability of highly sensitive and specific diagnostic tests that can be done with urine specimens and of single-dose therapy makes it feasible to mount an effective chlamydial control program nationwide.

TRACHOMA AND ADULT INCLUSION CONJUNCTIVITIS

DEFINITION Trachoma is a chronic conjunctivitis associated with infection by *C. trachomatis* serovar A, B, Ba, or C. It has been responsible for an estimated 20 million cases of blindness throughout the world and remains an important cause of preventable blindness. Inclusion conjunctivitis is an acute ocular infection caused by sexually transmitted *C. trachomatis* strains (usually serovars D through K) in adults exposed to infected genital secretions and in their newborn offspring.

EPIDEMIOLOGY Epidemiologically, two types of eye disease are caused by *C. trachomatis*. In trachoma-endemic areas where the classic eye disease is seen, transmission is from eye to eye via hands, flies, towels, and other fomites and usually involves serovar A, B, Ba, or C. In nonendemic areas, organisms of serovars D through K can be transmitted from the genital tract to the eye, usually causing only the inclusion conjunctivitis syndrome, occasionally with keratitis. Rarely, the eye disease acquired in this way progresses, with the development of pannus and scars similar to those seen in endemic trachoma. These cases may be referred to as paratrachoma to differentiate them epidemiologically from eye-to-eye-transmitted endemic trachoma.

The worldwide incidence and severity of trachoma have decreased dramatically during the past 35 years, mainly as a result of improving hygienic and economic conditions. Endemic trachoma is still the major cause of preventable blindness in northern Africa, sub-Saharan Africa, the Middle East, and parts of Asia. The endemic disease is transmitted primarily through close personal contact, particularly among young children in rural communities with limited water supplies. In endemic areas, trachoma is associated with repeated exposure and reinfection, but the infection can also be latent. In the United States a mild form of endemic trachoma still occurs in Mexican Americans as well as in immigrants from areas where trachoma is endemic. Acute relapse of old trachoma occasionally follows treatment with cortisone eye ointment or develops in very old persons who were exposed in their youth.

CLINICAL MANIFESTATIONS Both endemic trachoma and adult inclusion conjunctivitis present initially as a conjunctivitis characterized by small lymphoid follicles in the conjunctiva. In regions with hyperendemic classic blinding trachoma, the disease usually starts insidiously before the age of 2 years. Reinfection is common and probably contributes to the pathogenesis of trachoma. Studies using PCR techniques indicate that chlamydial DNA is often present in the ocular secretions of patients with trachoma, even in the absence of positive cultures. Thus persistent infection may be more common than was previously thought.

The cornea becomes involved, with inflammatory leukocytic infiltrations and superficial vascularization (pannus formation). As the inflammation continues, conjunctival scarring eventually distorts the eyelids, causing them to turn inward so that the inturned lashes constantly abrade the eyeball (trichiasis and entropion); eventually the corneal epithelium is abraded and may ulcerate, with subsequent corneal scarring and blindness. Destruction of the conjunctival goblet cells, lacrimal ducts, and lacrimal gland may produce a "dry-eye" syndrome, with resultant corneal opacity due to drying (xerosis) or secondary bacterial corneal ulcers.

Communities with blinding trachoma often experience seasonal epidemics of conjunctivitis due to *H. influenzae* that contribute to the intensity of the inflammatory process. In such areas the active infectious process usually resolves spontaneously in affected persons between 10 and 15 years of age, but the conjunctival scars continue to shrink, producing trichiasis and entropion and subsequent corneal scarring in adults. In areas with milder and less prevalent disease, the process may be much slower, with active disease continuing into adulthood; blindness is rare in these cases.

Eye infection with genital *C. trachomatis* strains in sexually active young adults presents as the acute onset of unilateral follicular conjunctivitis and preauricular lymphadenopathy similar to that seen in acute adenovirus or herpesvirus conjunctivitis. If untreated, the disease may persist for 6 weeks to 2 years. It is frequently associated with corneal inflammation in the form of discrete opacities ("infiltrates"), punctate epithelial erosions, and minor degrees of superficial corneal vascularization. Very rarely, conjunctival scarring and eyelid distortion occur, particularly in patients treated for many months with topical glucocorticoids. Recurrent eye infections develop most often in patients whose sexual consorts are not treated with antimicrobials.

DIAGNOSIS The clinical diagnosis of classic trachoma can be made if two of the following signs are present:

1. Lymphoid follicles on the upper tarsal conjunctiva
2. Typical conjunctival scarring
3. Vascular pannus
4. Limbal follicles or their sequelae, Herbert's pits

The clinical diagnosis of endemic trachoma should be confirmed by laboratory tests in children with more marked degrees of inflammation. Intracytoplasmic chlamydial inclusions are found in 10 to 60 percent of Giemsa-stained conjunctival smears in such populations, but isolation in cell cultures, newer antigen detection testing, or chlamydial PCR is more sensitive. Follicular conjunctivitis in adult Europeans or Americans living in trachomatous regions is rarely due to trachoma.

Sporadic cases of adult inclusion conjunctivitis must be differentiated from keratoconjunctivitis due to adenovirus or HSV and from bacterial conjunctivitis during the first 15 days after onset; later, they must be distinguished from other forms of chronic follicular conjunctivitis. Demonstration of chlamydiae by Giemsa- or immunofluorescent-stained smears, by isolation in cell cultures, or by newer nonculture tests constitutes definitive evidence of infection. Genital examination and tests for genital chlamydial infection are indicated. Serum antibody does not constitute evidence of chlamydial eye infection since many sexually active adults have acquired serum antibody from genital infection.

DIFFERENTIAL DIAGNOSIS OF CONJUNCTIVITIS AND KERATOCONJUNCTIVITIS The eye and its adnexa may be infected during the course of many cutaneous and systemic viral diseases. Sometimes these ocular infections produce minor manifestations, such as the transient loss of accommodation in dengue and the milder forms of conjunctivitis in systemic adenovirus infections. Other virus infections, however, such as herpes simplex (see Chap. 184), herpes zoster (see Chap. 185), measles (see Chap. 196), and vaccinia (see Chap. 188), occasionally produce serious and permanent visual loss. In addition, congenital infections are an important cause of blindness, particularly rubella, which leads to cataracts and microphthalmos; cytomegalic inclusion disease with retinal involvement; and syphilis with interstitial keratitis or optic neuritis. Among the viral infections limited to the outer eye and manifested as follicular conjunctivitis are epidemic keratoconjunctivitis, herpes simplex keratoconjunctivitis, Newcastle disease virus conjunctivitis, and acute hemorrhagic conjunctivitis.

℞ **TREATMENT**

Public health control programs for endemic trachoma have consisted of the mass application of tetracycline or erythromycin ointment to the eyes of all children in affected communities for 21 to 60 days or on an intermittent schedule. These programs also include surgical correction of inturned eyelids by a mobile surgical team that visits each locale. Single-dose azithromycin therapy offers an alternative method of mass antibiotic treatment for trachoma of young children and pregnant women that is now being evaluated.

Adult inclusion conjunctivitis responds well to treatment with full doses of systemic tetracycline or erythromycin for 3 weeks. Treatment of all sexual consorts of the patient simultaneously is also necessary to prevent ocular reinfection and to avoid genital disease due to chlamydial infection. Topical antibiotic treatment is not required for patients who receive systemic antibiotics.

PREVENTION Efforts to develop a trachoma vaccine have not yet been successful. General hygienic measures associated with improved living standards are effective in the elimination of endemic trachoma. An adequate water supply for personal cleanliness may be a key factor. In some areas the reduction of numbers of flies in the household is important.

PSITTACOSIS

DEFINITION Psittacosis is primarily an infectious disease of birds that is caused by *C. psittaci*. Transmission of infection from birds to humans results in a febrile illness characterized by pneumonitis and systemic manifestations. Inapparent infections or mild influenza-like illnesses may also occur. The term *ornithosis* is sometimes applied to infections contracted from birds other than parrots or parakeets, but *psittacosis* is the preferred generic term for all forms of the disease.

EPIDEMIOLOGY Almost any avian species can harbor *C. psittaci*. Psittacine birds (parrots, parakeets, budgerigars) are most commonly infected, but human cases have been traced to contact with pigeons, ducks, turkeys, chickens, and many other birds. Psittacosis may be considered an occupational disease of pet-shop owners, poultry workers, pigeon fanciers, taxidermists, veterinarians, and zoo attendants. During the past 20 years, there has been an increase in incidence, with cases and outbreaks occurring primarily among employees of poultry-processing plants. It is suspected that many cases go undiagnosed and unreported. The disease appears to be especially common in England, where budgerigars are popular household pets and where restrictions on the importation of these birds have been eased.

The agent is present in nasal secretions, excreta, tissues, and feathers of infected birds. Although the disease can be fatal, infected birds frequently show only minor evidence of illness, such as ruffled feathers, lethargy, and anorexia. Asymptomatic avian carriers are common, and complete recovery may be followed by continued shedding of the organism for many months.

Psittacosis is almost always transmitted to humans by the respiratory route. On rare occasions the disease may be acquired from the bite of a pet bird. Prolonged contact is not essential for transmission of the disease; a few minutes spent in an environment previously occupied by an infected bird has resulted in human infection. The severity of the disease in humans bears no apparent relationship to closeness or duration of contact, although sick birds are more likely to transmit infection than healthy ones. A psittacosis-like agent has been transmitted among hospital personnel, with severe and sometimes fatal infections. There is evidence that these "human" strains are more virulent than avian organisms. There is no record of infection acquired by the ingestion of poultry products.

PATHOGENESIS The psittacosis agent gains entrance to the body through the upper part of the respiratory tract, spreads via the bloodstream, and eventually localizes in the pulmonary alveoli and in the reticuloendothelial cells of the spleen and liver. Invasion of the lung probably takes place by way of the bloodstream rather than by direct extension from the upper air passages. A lymphocytic inflammatory response occurs on both the interstitial and the respiratory surfaces of the alveoli as well as in the perivascular spaces. The alveolar walls and interstitial tissues of the lung are thickened, edematous, necrotic, and occasionally hemorrhagic. Histologic examination of the affected areas reveals alveolar spaces filled with fluid, erythrocytes, and lymphocytes. The picture is not pathognomonic of psittacosis unless macrophages containing characteristic cytoplasmic inclusion bodies [Levinthal-Coles-Lillie (LCL) bodies] can be identified. The respiratory epithelium of the bronchi and bronchioles usually remains intact.

CLINICAL MANIFESTATIONS The clinical manifestations and course of psittacosis are extremely variable. After an incubation period of 7 to 14 days or longer, the disease may start abruptly with shaking chills and fever, with temperatures ranging as high as 40.5°C (105°F); however, the onset is often gradual, with fever increasing over a 3- to 4-day period. Headache is almost always a prominent symptom; it is usually diffuse and excruciating and is often the patient's chief complaint.

Many patients present with a dry hacking cough that is usually nonproductive, but small amounts of mucoid or bloody sputum may be raised as the disease progresses. Cough may begin early in the course of the disease or as late as 5 days after the onset of fever. Chest pain, pleurisy with effusion, or a friction rub may all occur but are rare. Pericarditis and myocarditis have been reported. Most patients have a normal or slightly increased respiratory rate; marked dyspnea with cyanosis occurs only in severe psittacosis with extensive pulmonary involvement. In psittacosis, as in most nonbacterial pneumonias, the physical signs of pneumonitis tend to be less prominent than symptoms and x-ray findings would suggest. The initial examination may reveal fine sibilant rales, or clinical evidence of pneumonia may be completely lacking. Rales usually become audible and more numerous as the illness progresses. Signs of frank pulmonary consolidation are usually absent. Symptoms of upper respiratory tract infection are not prominent, although mild sore throat, pharyngitis, and cervical adenopathy are often documented; on occasion, the last may be the only manifestation of illness. Epistaxis is encountered early in the course of nearly one-fourth of cases. Photophobia is also a common complaint.

Patients often report generalized myalgia, and spasm and stiffness of the muscles of the back and neck may lead to an erroneous diagnosis of meningitis. Lethargy, mental depression, agitation, insomnia, and disorientation have been prominent features of the illness in some epidemics but not in others; delirium and stupor develop near the end of the first week in severe cases. Occasional patients are comatose when first seen, and the diagnosis of psittacosis may be elusive in these cases. Gastrointestinal problems such as abdominal pain, nausea, vomiting, or diarrhea are noted in some cases; constipation and abdominal distention sometimes occur as late complications. Icterus, the result of severe hepatic involvement, is a rare and ominous finding. A faint macular rash (Horder's spots) simulating the rose spots of typhoid fever has been described.

Patients without cough or other clinical evidence of respiratory involvement present with fever of unknown origin (see Chap. 125). The pulse rate is slow in relation to the fever. When splenomegaly is noted in a patient with acute pneumonitis, psittacosis should be considered; the reported incidence of splenomegaly in this disease ranges from 10 to 70 percent. Nontender hepatic enlargement also occurs, but jaundice is rare. Thrombophlebitis is not unusual during convalescence; indeed, pulmonary infarction is sometimes a late complication and may be fatal.

In untreated cases of psittacosis, sustained or mildly remittent fever persists for 10 days to 3 weeks or occasionally for as long as 3 months. Over this period, the respiratory manifestations gradually abate. Psittacosis contracted from parrots or parakeets is more likely to be a severe, prolonged illness than infection acquired from pigeons or barnyard fowl. Relapses occur but are rare. Occasional patients develop endocarditis, and *C. psittaci* infection should be considered in cases of culture-negative endocarditis. Secondary bacterial infections are uncommon. Immunity to reinfection is probably permanent.

LABORATORY FINDINGS The chest x-ray in psittacosis is nonspecific and may show pneumonic lesions that are usually patchy in appearance but can be hazy, diffuse, homogeneous, lobar, atelectatic, wedge-shaped, nodular, or miliary. The white blood cell count is normal or moderately decreased in the acute phase of the disease but may rise in convalescence. The erythrocyte sedimentation rate frequently is not elevated. Transient proteinuria is common. The cerebrospinal fluid sometimes contains a few mononuclear cells but is otherwise normal. Despite hepatomegaly, the results of liver function tests are generally normal or mildly elevated.

The diagnosis can be confirmed only by isolation of the causative microorganism or by serologic studies. The agent is present in the blood during the acute phase of the disease and in the bronchial secretions for weeks or sometimes years after infection, but it is difficult to isolate. Further, the organism is hazardous to work with in the laboratory, and most clinical laboratories do not offer culture for *C. psittaci*. Thus psittacosis is most readily diagnosed by the demonstration of a rising titer of CF antibody in the serum of a patient with a compatible clinical syndrome. Both an acute-phase and a convalescent-phase specimen should always be tested. *C. trachomatis*, *C. psittaci*, and *C. pneumoniae* all share a genus-specific "group" antigen, which is the basis of the CF test. Thus acute infections with *C. trachomatis* or *C. pneumoniae* can also produce titer rises in the CF test. However, these three species have different major outer-membrane proteins that are the principal antigens in the micro-IF test. If there is doubt as to the interpretation of the CF test, the micro-IF test can be used to differentiate among them. The prompt initiation of treatment with tetracycline has been shown to delay an antibody rise in convalescence for several weeks or months.

DIFFERENTIAL DIAGNOSIS A history of exposure to birds may be the only clinical basis for differentiating psittacosis from a variety of infectious and noninfectious febrile disorders. The list of pulmonary diseases that may be confused with psittacosis includes *Mycoplasma* pneumonia, *C. pneumoniae* pneumonia, legionellosis, viral pneumonia, Q fever, coccidioidomycosis, tuberculosis, enterovirus infection, carcinoma of the lung with bronchial obstruction, and common bacterial pneumonias. In the early stages, before pneumonitis appears, psittacosis may be mistaken for influenza, typhoid fever, miliary tuberculosis, or infectious mononucleosis.

℞ TREATMENT

The tetracyclines are consistently effective in the treatment of psittacosis. Defervescence and alleviation of symptoms usually take place within 24 to 48 h after the institution of therapy with 2 g daily in four divided doses. To avoid relapse, treatment should probably be continued for at least 7 to 14 days after defervescence. In severe cases, hospitalization and pulmonary intensive care may be indicated. Sulfonamides are not active against *C. psittaci*. Erythromycin can be used in patients allergic to or intolerant of tetracyclines.

C. PNEUMONIAE INFECTIONS

A third chlamydial species, *C. pneumoniae*, has been described in the past decade. *C. pneumoniae* can be distinguished from the other two species on the basis of DNA hybridization and restriction endonuclease analyses. Although *C. pneumoniae* can be grown in a variety of cell cultures, it is considerably more difficult to culture than other chlamydiae, especially from clinical specimens. HL cells appear to be the most effective cell line for isolation of *C. pneumoniae*.

Knowledge of the epidemiology of *C. pneumoniae* infections has been derived primarily from serologic studies. Infections begin to occur in late childhood, achieve peak incidence in young adults, but continue throughout adult life. Seroprevalence in the many adult populations that have been tested throughout the world exceeds 40 percent—a figure suggesting that *C. pneumoniae* infections are ubiquitous. Secondary episodes (reinfections) appear to occur in older adults throughout life. In Scandinavia, *C. pneumoniae* produces epidemics of pneumonia and respiratory illness followed by periods of infrequent infection. The incidence of infections outside of epidemics remains poorly defined. Transmission appears to be from person to person, probably primarily in schools and family units.

The clinical spectrum of *C. pneumoniae* infection includes acute pharyngitis, sinusitis, bronchitis, and pneumonitis, primarily in young adults. The clinical manifestations of primary infection appear to be more severe and prolonged than those of reinfection. The pneumonitis resembles that of *Mycoplasma pneumoniae* pneumonia in that leukocytosis is frequently lacking and patients often have prominent antecedent upper respiratory tract symptoms, fever, nonproductive cough, a mild to moderate degree of illness, minimal findings on chest auscultation, and small segmental infiltrates on chest x-ray. In elderly patients, pneumonia due to *C. pneumoniae* can be especially severe and may necessitate hospitalization and respiratory support.

Epidemiologic studies have demonstrated an association between serologic evidence of *C. pneumoniae* infection and atherosclerotic disease of the coronary and other arteries. In addition, *C. pneumoniae* has been identified in atherosclerotic plaques by electron microscopy, DNA hybridization, and immunocytochemistry. The clinical significance of these findings is not yet clear.

Diagnosis of *C. pneumoniae* infection is currently difficult because cell culture techniques are not available for routine clinical use and nonculture tests using antigen detection methods or DNA probes have not been developed. Acute- and convalescent-phase sera can be tested for chlamydial CF antibody to make a retrospective diagnosis. However, this test does not distinguish *C. pneumoniae* infection from infection due to *C. trachomatis* or *C. psittaci*. Although controlled treatment trials have not been conducted, *C. pneumoniae* is inhibited in vitro by erythromycin and tetracycline. Recommended therapy consists of 2 g per day of either agent for 10 to 14 days.

BIBLIOGRAPHY

BAUWENS JE et al: Diagnosis of *Chlamydia trachomatis* urethritis in men by polymerase chain reaction assay of first catch urine. J Clin Microbiol 31:3013, 1993

CATES W JR, WASSERHEIT JN: Genital chlamydial infections: Epidemiology and reproductive sequelae. Am J Obstet Gynecol 164:1771, 1991

CENTERS FOR DISEASE CONTROL AND PREVENTION: Recommendations for the prevention and management of *Chlamydia trachomatis* infections, 1993. Morb Mortal Week Rep 42(RR-12):1, 1993

COULTS II et al: Clinical and radiographic features of psittacosis infection. Thorax 40:530, 1985

GRAYSTON JT: Infections caused by *Chlamydia pneumoniae*, strain TWAR. Clin Infect Dis 15:757, 1992

——— et al: A new *Chlamydia psittaci* strain, TWAR, isolated in acute respiratory tract infections. N Engl J Med 315:161, 1986

HOLMES KK: Lower genital tract infections in women: Cystitis, urethritis, vulvovaginitis, and cervicitis, in *Sexually Transmitted Diseases*, 2d ed, KK Holmes et al (eds). New York, McGraw-Hill, 1990

LEE HH et al: Diagnosis of *Chlamydia trachomatis* genitourinary infection in women by ligase chain reaction assay of urine. Lancet 345:213, 1995

MARTIN DH et al: A controlled trial of a single dose of azithromycin for the treatment of chlamydial urethritis and cervicitis. N Engl J Med 327:921, 1992

RETTIG PJ: Perinatal infections with *Chlamydia trachomatis*. Clin Perinatol 15:321, 1988

SCHACHTER J, STAMM WE: Chlamydia, in *Manual of Clinical Microbiology*, PR Murray et al (eds). Washington, DC, ASM Press, 1995

——— et al: Experience with the routine use of erythromycin for chlamydial infections in pregnancy. N Engl J Med 314:276, 1986

SCHOLES D et al: Prevention of pelvic inflammatory disease by screening for cervical chlamydial infection. N Engl J Med 334:1362, 1996

SOPER D: Pelvic inflammatory disease. Infect Dis Clin North Am 8:821, 1994

STAMM WE: Towards control of sexually transmitted chlamydial infections. Ann Intern Med 119:432, 1993

———, HOLMES KK: *Chlamydia trachomatis* infections in adults, in *Sexually Transmitted Diseases*, 2d ed, KK Holmes et al (eds). New York, McGraw-Hill, 1990

——— et al: Azithromycin for empirical treatment of the nongonococcal urethritis syndrome in men. A randomized double-blind study. JAMA 274:545, 1995

——— et al: *Chlamydia trachomatis* urethral infections in men. Prevalence, risk factors, and clinical manifestations. Ann Intern Med 100:47, 1984

STERGACHIS A et al: Selective screening for *Chlamydia trachomatis* infections in a primary care population of women. Am J Epidemiol 138:143, 1993

WEINSTOCK H et al: *Chlamydia trachomatis* infections. Infect Dis Clin North Am 8:797, 1994

182 Fred Wang, Elliott Kieff

MEDICAL VIROLOGY

HISTORICAL PERSPECTIVE

Although descriptions of poxvirus and herpesvirus infections extend back to antiquity, the field of virology is barely 100 years old. In contrast, bacteriology was developing rapidly through much of the second half of the nineteenth century. By the end of the nineteenth century, many types of bacteria could be grown on media and could be identified in cultures and in tissues by light microscopy; growth media could be sterilized by passage through porcelain filters; and Henle and Koch had written postulates for establishing the bacterial etiology of disease. In 1892, Ivanofsky in Russia showed that the infectious agent of mosaic tobacco-leaf disease was not a bacterium because it passed through a porcelain filter. Over the next 20 years, several animal infections were shown to be caused by filterable agents, and the term *virus* began to be applied to these agents. From the 1920s through the 1950s, research on bacterial, plant, and animal (including human) viral infections of cells, tissues, organs, and organisms led to improved techniques for the culture of cells and viruses in vitro. Improved culture techniques made it feasible to study the biochemical and genetic properties of viruses. Viruses came to be recognized as genetically simple tools for learning about fundamental biologic and biochemical processes in cells, tissues, organs, and animals, including humans.

DEFINING A VIRUS

Viruses consist of a nucleic acid surrounded by one or more proteins. Some viruses also have an outer-membrane envelope. Viruses differ from other replicating organisms in that they do not have ribosomes or enzymes for high-energy phosphate generation or for protein, carbohydrate, or lipid metabolism. Viruses are obligate intracellular parasites—that is, they require cells in order to replicate. Typically, viral nucleic acids encode proteins necessary for replicating and packaging the nucleic acids into new viral particles.

Viruses differ from viroids, prions, and virusoids. *Virusoids* are nucleic acids that depend on helper viruses to package the nucleic acids into virus-like particles. *Viroids* are simply molecules of naked, cyclical, mostly double-stranded, small RNAs and are restricted to plants. *Prions* are abnormal cellular proteins that can spread from cell to cell and effect changes in normal cellular proteins, thereby disrupting cellular function and propagating themselves. Prions have been implicated in neurodegenerative conditions such as Creutzfeldt-Jakob disease, kuru, and Gerstmann-Sträussler syndrome. Recently, prions have also been implicated in the putative human transmission of bovine spongiform encephalopathy.

VIRAL STRUCTURE

Viruses have from a few to 200 genes. These genes may be embodied in a single-strand or double-strand DNA genome or in a single-strand sense, a single-strand or segmented antisense, or a double-strand segmented RNA genome. Sense-strand RNA genomes can be translated directly into protein. Sense and antisense genomes are also referred to as positive-strand and negative-strand genomes, respectively. The viral nucleic acid is usually associated with one or more virus-encoded nucleoproteins in the core of the viral particle. The viral nucleic acid is almost always enclosed in a protein shell called a capsid. Because of the limited genetic complexity of viruses, their capsids are usually composed of multimers of identical capsomers. Capsomers are in turn composed of one or a few proteins. The capsomers assemble into capsids with icosahedral or helical symmetry. Icosahedral structures

approximate spheres but have two-, three-, and fivefold axes of symmetry, while helical structures have only a twofold axis of symmetry. Capsids filled with nucleic acid are called nucleocapsids. Many human viruses have a simple nucleocapsid structure; others are more complex and have an outer envelope that is derived from membranes of the infected cell. The membrane that composes the viral envelope has been modified by the insertion of virus-encoded glycoproteins. Enveloped viruses frequently have matrix or tegument proteins that fill the space between the nucleocapsid and the envelope. In general, enveloped viruses are sensitive to solvents and nonionic detergents that can disrupt the envelope, while viruses that consist only of nucleocapsids are usually more resistant. The schematic diagram of a herpesvirus shown in Fig. 182-1 illustrates the components of a complicated DNA virus. Prototypical pathogenic human viruses are listed in Table 182-1. The relative sizes and structures of typical pathogenic human viruses are shown in Fig. 182-2.

TAXONOMY OF PATHOGENIC HUMAN VIRUSES

As is apparent from Table 182-1 and Fig. 182-2, the classification of viruses into orders and families is based on nucleic acid composition, nucleocapsid size and symmetry, and envelopment status. Viruses of a single family have similar types of genomes and are morphologically similar in electron micrographs. Further subclassification into genus is dependent on similarities in epidemiology and biologic effects and on the degree of colinear nucleic acid sequence homology. In general, each human virus has a common name related to its pathologic effects or the circumstances of its discovery and a formal species name assigned by the International Committee on Taxonomy of Viruses (http://www.ncbi.nlm.nih.gov/ICTV). The latter designation consists of the name of the host followed by the family or genus of the virus and a number. This dual terminology has created a confusing situation in which viruses are referred to and referenced by either name—e.g., varicella-zoster virus (VZV) or human herpesvirus type 3.

VIRAL INFECTION IN VITRO

STAGES OF INFECTION At the cellular level, viral infection proceeds in stages: (1) viral interactions at the cell surface, (2) viral gene expression and replication, and (3) viral assembly and egress.

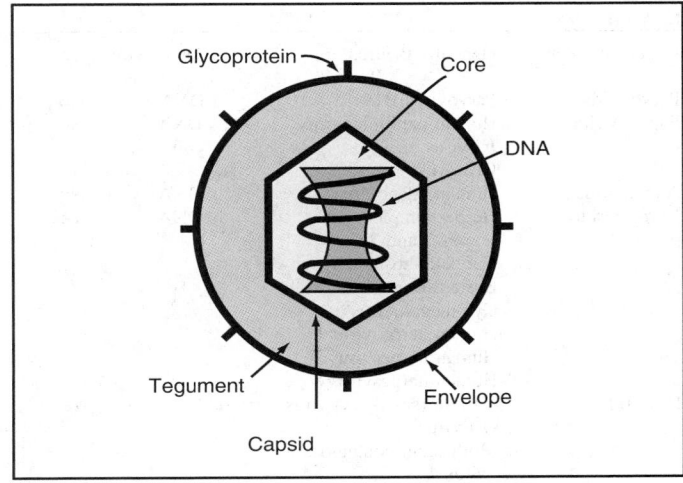

FIGURE 182-1 Schematic diagram of an enveloped herpesvirus with an icosahedral nucleocapsid. The approximate respective dimensions of the nucleocapsid and the enveloped particles are 100 μm and 180 μm. The capsid is composed of 162 capsomeres: 150 with sixfold and 12 with fivefold axes of symmetry.

Table 182-1

Virus Families Pathogenic for Humans

Family	Representative Viruses	Type of RNA/DNA	Lipid Envelope
RNA VIRUSES			
Picornaviridae	Poliovirus Coxsackievirus Echovirus Enterovirus Rhinovirus Hepatitis A virus	(+) RNA	No
Caliciviridae	Norwalk agent Hepatitis E virus	(+) RNA	No
Togaviridae	Rubella virus Eastern equine encephalitis virus Western equine encephalitis virus	(+) RNA	Yes
Flaviviridae	Yellow fever virus Dengue virus St. Louis encephalitis virus Hepatitis C virus Hepatitis G virus	(+) RNA	Yes
Coronaviridae	Coronavirus	(+) RNA	Yes
Rhabdoviridae	Rabies virus Vesicular stomatitis virus	(−) RNA	Yes
Filoviridae	Marburg virus Ebola virus	(−) RNA	Yes
Paramyxoviridae	Parainfluenza virus Respiratory syncytial virus Newcastle disease virus Mumps virus Rubeola (measles) virus	(−) RNA	Yes
Orthomyxoviridae	Influenza A, B, and C viruses	(−) RNA, 8 segments	Yes
Bunyaviridae	Hantavirus California encephalitis virus Sandfly fever virus	(−) RNA, 3 circular segments	Yes
Arenaviridae	Lymphocytic choriomeningitis virus Lassa fever virus South American hemorrhagic fever virus	(−) RNA, 2 circular segments	Yes
Reoviridae	Rotavirus Reovirus Colorado tick fever virus	ds RNA, 10–12 segments	No
DNA VIRUSES			
Hepadnaviridae	Hepatitis B virus	ds DNA with ss portions	Yes
Parvoviridae	Parvovirus B19	ss DNA	No
Papovaviridae	Human papillomavirus JC virus BK virus	ds DNA	No
Adenoviridae	Human adenovirus	ds DNA	No
Herpesviridae	Herpes simplex virus types 1 and 2* Varicella-zoster virus† Epstein-Barr virus‡ Cytomegalovirus§ Human herpesvirus 6 Human herpesvirus 7 Human herpesvirus 8	ds DNA	Yes
Poxviridae	Variola (smallpox) virus Orf virus Molluscum contagiosum virus	ds DNA	Yes

* Also called human herpesvirus (HHV) 1 and 2, respectively.
† Also called HHV-3.
‡ Also called HHV-4.
§ Also called HHV-5.
ABBREVIATIONS: ds, double-strand; ss, single-strand.

Viral Interactions at the Cell Surface First, virus adsorbs to a receptor on the cell surface. Adsorption is the consequence of a molecular interaction of a viral surface protein with a molecule on the cell's plasma membrane. For example, a poliovirus capsid protein binds to a cell plasma-membrane protein of the immunoglobulin superfamily type; a rhinovirus capsid protein binds to intracellular adhesion molecule 1; an echovirus capsid protein binds to an integrin; the influenza virus envelope hemagglutinin protein binds to sialic acid; the envelope glycoprotein of human immunodeficiency virus (HIV) binds to CD4 and to chemokine receptors; the herpes simplex virus (HSV) envelope glycoproteins bind to heparan sulfate and to a tumor necrosis factor receptor; and an Epstein-Barr virus (EBV) glycoprotein binds to the B lymphocyte complement receptor CD21. Adsorption characteristically proceeds almost as well at 4°C as at 37°C, and adsorbed virus can still be neutralized by antibody.

After adsorption, viruses penetrate through or fuse with the cell membrane and are uncoated as they enter the cytoplasm. Penetration and uncoating as well as subsequent steps in viral replication depend on the cell's energy metabolism and on biochemical changes in the cell's plasma membrane and cytoskeleton. Therefore, penetration proceeds slowly at temperatures below 37°C. The process of penetration is frequently initiated by the interaction of viral surface proteins with cellular receptors during adsorption. The viral protein that engages the receptor is displayed on the surace of the virus in at least several copies. Similarly, the cell's plasma membrane has at least several and usually hundreds of receptor molecules. The interaction of virus with its receptors usually induces receptor aggregation at the site of viral adsorption. Receptor aggregation triggers signaling events in the cytoplasm and active changes in the plasma membrane. The cell usually perceives that the receptor has encountered its "normal ligand." Frequently, the aggregated receptor is internalized through an endocytic process that involves clathrin-coated pits. The virus is thereby brought into endosomes in the cytoplasm. Endocytosis is important in the entry of viruses as diverse as picornaviruses, influenza viruses, adenoviruses, and herpesviruses. In many instances, further fusion of the virus with the endosomal membrane is dependent on lowering of the endosomal pH. The effect of pH on viral penetration has been well studied in the case of influenza virus. Influenza hemagglutinin mediates adsorption, receptor aggregation, and endocytosis. In low-pH endosomes, changes in the conformation of the hemagglutinin expose amphipathic domains that interact chemically with the cell membrane and initiate the fusion of the viral and cellular membranes. Little is known about the biochemical details of the fusion and uncoating processes for most viral capsids or envelopes. The end result of fusion is the mixture of viral envelope lipids and proteins with the lipids and proteins of cell membranes. In the case of complex viruses, viral surface proteins other than the protein that mediates adsorption may mediate fusion with the cell membrane. For some viruses, there is evidence of different receptors or membrane-fusion partners on different tissues or on different surfaces of polarized epithelial cells.

Viral Gene Expression and Replication As a result of the interaction of viruses with their receptors and subsequent steps in uncoating, viral nucleic acids and associated viral proteins are released into the cell's cytoplasm. Viral nucleic acid and virion structural proteins must be synthesized, and the nucleic acid and proteins must be assembled into progeny virions. Most viruses differentially regulate the transcription of their messenger RNAs (mRNAs), which are then translated into proteins. Most RNA viruses replicate their nucleic acid and assemble entirely in the cytoplasm, while most DNA viruses replicate their nucleic acid and assemble into nucleocapsid complexes in the nucleus.

Positive-strand RNA viruses Genomic RNA from positive-strand RNA viruses is released into the cytoplasm without associated enzymes. The recognition and association of cell ribosomes with an internal ribosome entry sequence in the viral genomic RNA permit the translation of a polyprotein that is a fusion of many or all of the viral proteins. The viral RNA polymerase and other viral proteins are cleaved from the polyprotein by protease components of the polyprotein. Antigenomic RNA is then transcribed from the genomic RNA

Positive-strand RNA viruses

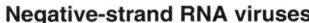
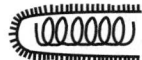
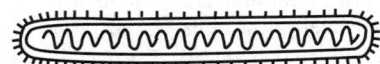
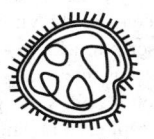

	Picornaviridae	Caliciviridae	Togaviridae	Flaviviridae	Coronaviridae
Genome size (kb)	7.2–8.4	8	12	10	16–21
Envelope	No	No	Yes	Yes	Yes
Capsid symmetry	Icosahedral	Icosahedral	Icosahedral	Icosahedral?	Helical

Negative-strand RNA viruses

	Rhabdoviridae	Filoviridae	Paramyxoviridae
Genome size (kb)	13–16	13	16–20
Envelope	Yes	Yes	Yes
Capsid symmetry	Helical	Helical	Helical

Segmented negative-strand RNA viruses

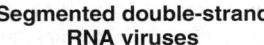

Segmented double-strand RNA viruses

	Orthomyxoviridae	Bunyaviridae	Arenaviridae	Reoviridae
Genome size (kb)	14	13–21	10–14	16–27
Envelope	Yes	Yes	Yes	No
Capsid symmetry	Helical	Helical	Helical	Icosahedral

Retroviruses

	Retroviridae
Genome size (kb)	3–9
Envelope	Yes
Capsid symmetry	Icosahedral

DNA viruses

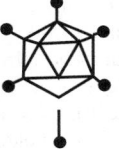
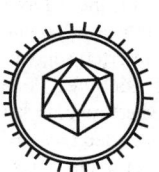
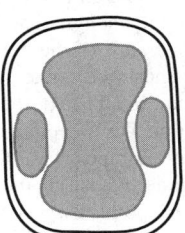

	Parvoviridae	Papovaviridae	Adenoviridae	Herpesviridae	Poxviridae
Genome size (kb)	5	5–9	36–38	100–250	240
Envelope	No	No	No	Yes	Yes
Capsid symmetry	Icosahedral	Icosahedral	Icosahedral	Icosahedral	Complex

100 nm

FIGURE 182-2 Schematic diagrams of the major virus families including species that infect humans. The viruses are grouped by genome type and are drawn approximately to scale. Key: |———|, 100 nm.

template. Positive-strand genomes and mRNAs are next transcribed from the antigenomic RNA by the viral RNA polymerase. Positive-strand genomic RNA is encapsidated in the cytoplasm.

Negative-strand RNA viruses Negative-strand RNA virus genomes are released into the cytoplasm with an associated RNA polymerase. Most negative-strand RNA viruses replicate entirely in the cytoplasm. The RNA polymerase transcribes mRNAs as well as full-length antigenomic RNA, which is the template for replication of genomic RNA. The mRNAs encode for RNA polymerase and accessory factors as well as for viral structural proteins. Influenza virus is an unusual segmented negative-strand RNA virus that transcribes its mRNAs and antigenomic RNA in the cell's nucleus. The infecting RNA segments must make their way to the nucleus with their associ-

ated RNA polymerase and accessory proteins. The nuclear localization of influenza RNA permits the use of two cell-nuclear processes: (1) the incorporation of cell mRNA cap sequences to enhance ribosomal recognition and translational initiation of viral mRNAs, and (2) the splicing of some influenza virus mRNAs. Negative-strand RNA viruses, including influenza virus, assemble in the cytoplasm.

DNA viruses Most DNA viruses except for poxviruses must get to the cell's nucleus for their DNA to be transcribed by cellular RNA polymerase II. Except for a few viral proteins that contribute to transcriptional regulation, DNA viruses depend on the cell for mRNA synthesis and processing. Herpesvirus nucleocapsids are released into the cytoplasm along with tegument proteins. The complex is then transported along microtubules to nuclear pores, and the DNA is released into the nucleus along with a viral tegument protein that can activate transcription of viral immediate-early genes. Immediate-early genes require only a component of the viral tegument and preexisting cellular transcription factors to be actively transcribed. In herpesvirus infections, immediate-early proteins are stringently required to turn on viral early-gene transcription. Other DNA viruses do not depend absolutely on the immediate-early transactivators encoded from the viral genome for early-gene transcription. Most early genes encode proteins that are necessary for viral DNA synthesis and for the turn-on of late-gene transcription. Late genes encode mostly viral structural proteins or viral proteins necessary for the assembly and egress of the virus from the infected cell. Late-gene transcription is continuously dependent on DNA replication. Therefore, inhibitors of DNA replication also stop late-gene transcription.

Each DNA virus family uses unique mechanisms for replicating its DNA. Herpesvirus DNAs are linear in the virion but circularize in the infected cell. The circular viral genome is replicated into linear concatemers through a "rolling-circle" mechanism. Herpesviruses encode their own polymerase and several enzymes that increase the pool of nucleotide precursors. Adenovirus genomes are linear in the virion and are replicated into complementary linear copies by a virus-encoded DNA polymerase and an initiator protein complex. The double-strand circular papovavirus genomes are replicated into progeny circular DNA molecules by cellular DNA replication enzymes. A single viral early protein contributes to the initiation of viral DNA replication. The early papovavirus proteins stimulate cellular DNA synthesis, thus facilitating viral DNA replication. Occasionally, papovaviruses (e.g., papillomaviruses) integrate into the host chromosome; overexpression of viral proteins and excessive stimulation of cellular growth result. Sometimes the consequence is the development of malignancies such as cervical cancer (see "Role of Persistent Viral Infections in Human Cancers" below).

Poxviruses are unique among the DNA viruses in replicating entirely in the cytoplasm. Pox virions have virus-encoded transcription factors and an RNA polymerase as well as enzymes for RNA capping and polyadenylation. Poxvirus DNA also has a unique structure. The two strands of the double-strand linear DNA are covalently linked at the ends so that the genome is also a covalently closed single-strand circle. In addition, there are inverted repeats at the ends of the DNA. During DNA replication, the genome is cleaved within the terminal inverted repeat, and the inverted repeats self-prime complementary-strand synthesis by the virus-encoded DNA polymerase. Like herpesviruses, poxviruses encode several enzymes that increase nucleotide levels and thus facilitate viral DNA synthesis.

Viruses with both RNA and DNA genomes   Retroviruses, lentiviruses, and hepatitis B virus are not purely RNA or DNA viruses.

Retroviruses and lentiviruses are enveloped RNA viruses with diploid sense-strand genomes and associated reverse transcriptase and integrase enzymes. Retroviruses and lentiviruses differ from all other viruses in that they reverse-transcribe themselves into partially duplicated double-strand DNA copies and then routinely integrate into the host genome as part of their replication strategy. Viral mRNAs and genomic RNAs are then transcribed from a single integrated proviral promoter. Remnants of simple retroviral DNA in the human genome suggest the possibility of replication-competent simple human retroviruses, but little other evidence supports their existence. Human T cell leukemia virus (HTLV) types I and II are more complicated retroviruses that are endemic in specific human populations, where they cause tropical spastic paraparesis and adult T cell leukemia. HTLV transcripts include both the full-length genomic transcripts characteristic of all retroviruses (encoding Gag, polymerase/integrase, and envelope glycoprotein) and spliced transcripts (encoding Tax and Rex, which are regulators of transcription and RNA processing). HIV types 1 and 2 are full-fledged lentiviruses that cause AIDS and a milder immunodeficiency syndrome; these viruses have a larger number of spliced viral transcripts that encode the regulatory proteins Tat, Rev, Nef, Vpr, Vpu, and Vif. All of the viral transcripts and proteins are

usually expressed in HTLV- or HIV-infected cells. Retroviruses and lentiviruses assemble near the plasma membrane. The nucleocapsid is composed of two copies of a full genomic transcript, cellular transfer RNA, and proteins cleaved from the viral Gag protein. The nucleocapsid is enveloped at sites in the plasma membrane that have been modified by viral glycoprotein insertion.

Hepatitis B virus is an enveloped virus with an incomplete double-strand circular DNA genome. On entry into the cytoplasm, virion polymerase completes DNA synthesis; the covalently closed circular genome resides in the nucleus. Viral mRNAs are transcribed from the closed circular viral episome by cellular RNA polymerase II. A capped and polyadenylated, full-genome-length, terminally redundant transcript is packaged into viral core particles in the cytoplasm of infected cells. This RNA is associated with the viral polymerase, which has reverse transcriptase activity and converts the full-length, terminally redundant, core-particle, encapsidated RNA genome into partially double-strand DNA.

Viral Assembly and Egress   As viral nucleic acid and structural proteins are synthesized, nucleic acid and proteins begin to assemble. The assembly and egress of mature infectious virus mark the end of the eclipse phase of infection, during which infectious virus cannot be recovered from the infected cell. Nucleic acids from RNA viruses and poxviruses assemble into nucleocapsids in the cytoplasm. For all DNA viruses except poxviruses, viral DNA assembles into nucleocapsids in the nucleus. In general, the capsid proteins of viruses with icosahedral nucleocapsids can self-assemble into densely packed and highly ordered capsid structures. Viral nucleic acid or nucleoprotein complex then enters or spools into the assembled capsid. In contrast, helical nucleocapsids frequently appear to assemble around the nucleic acid, which contributes to capsid organization.

Viruses must egress from the infected cell and not bind back to its plasma membrane. In many cases, enveloped viruses simply egress and acquire their envelope by budding through the cell's plasma membrane. Excess viral membrane protein is synthesized to saturate cell receptors and facilitate viral envelopment. Other viruses encode membrane proteins with enzymatic activity for receptor destruction. Influenza virus, for example, encodes a glycoprotein with neuraminidase activity, which destroys sialic acid on the infected cell's plasma membrane. Herpesvirus nucleocapsids acquire their initial envelope by budding through the nuclear membrane. Enveloped herpesviruses are released from the cell either by maturation in cytoplasmic vesicles, which fuse with the plasma membrane and release the virus by exocytosis, or by "de-envelopment" and release of the nucleocapsid into the cytoplasm and "re-envelopment" at the plasma membrane. In most instances, nonenveloped nucleocapsid viruses appear to depend on the death and dissolution of the infected cell for their release.

FIDELITY OF VIRAL REPLICATION   While cells grow by doubling their genome and dividing, viral replication typically results in the release of 10 to 1000 infectious progeny and of many more partially assembled genomes and structures. Replication can alter the viral genomic sequence by various mechanisms. In general, viral nucleic acid replication is more error-prone than cellular nucleic acid replication. For RNA viruses and retroviruses, RNA polymerase and reverse transcriptase are intrinsically more error-prone than DNA polymerases. These errors can lead to the emergence of mutant viral strains capable of evading immune-system recognition or resisting the action of antiviral drugs. For DNA viruses, errors are probably due to less adequate postreplication repair (proofreading) in the virus-infected cell. Other mechanisms for introducing change into viral nucleic acid sequences include reassortment of segmented RNA genomes, as in influenza viruses, and recombination of homologous nucleic acid sequences between related viral strains. Defective viruses, consisting of empty nucleocapsids or viruses with deletions or rearrangements of the viral genome, are produced frequently by many viruses but are of uncertain pathophysiologic significance. For most viruses, there are 5 to 10 times more mature-appearing viral particles than fully infectious virions.

OTHER VIRAL GENES   Many RNA and DNA viruses also have genes encoding proteins that are not directly involved in replication or packaging of the viral nucleic acid, in virion assembly, or in regulation of the transcription of viral genes involved in those processes. Many of these genes have provided important insights into normal cell biology and may play a role during viral infection of humans. Most of these proteins fall into four classes: (1) proteins that directly or indirectly alter cell growth; (2) proteins that inhibit cellular DNA, RNA, or protein synthesis so that viral mRNA can be efficiently transcribed or translated; (3) proteins that promote the cell's survival or inhibit apoptosis so that progeny virus can mature and escape from the infected cell; and (4) proteins that downregulate host inflammatory or immune responses so that viral infection can proceed in the infected patient. As the basic processes of viral replication have become better understood, contemporary virology has focused increasingly on these more sophisticated issues of cellular and organismal biology.

HOST RANGE The cell types in which a virus can replicate define the host range for that virus. For the most part, the host-range limitations of a virus are defined by specific cell-surface proteins required for its adsorption or penetration. Another common basis for host-range limitation involves transcription. DNA viruses depend not only on cellular RNA polymerase II and the basal components of the cellular transcription complex but also on activated components and transcriptional accessory factors, both of which differ among differentiated tissues; among cells at various phases of the cell cycle; and among resting, G_0, and cycling cells.

The concept of host range needs to be modified in the cases of papovaviruses and herpesviruses. Some cell types may be permissive for infection with these viruses and nonpermissive or partially permissive for their replication. A papovavirus or herpesvirus may persist in a latent state in a cell that is nonpermissive for its replication. Human papillomaviruses infect cells of the basal layer of the skin but replicate only when the cells further differentiate into keratinocytes. HSV infects cells of the dorsal root ganglia but cannot replicate in these cells until they are stimulated by fever, skin injury, or psychic trauma, all of which somehow turn on transcription of the viral immediate-early genes in previously latently infected neurons. EBV, another herpesvirus, establishes latency in B lymphocytes, in which it initially expresses proteins that cause the proliferation of the latently infected cells. This virus also expresses a protein that prevents lymphocytes from becoming activated and turning on viral replication in response to src-family kinase-mediated signal transduction events. This blockade must be bypassed when the lymphocytes traffic near the oropharyngeal epithelium so that these cells can become permissive for viral replication and the virus can be released into saliva to complete its life cycle in humans.

VIRAL CYTOPATHIC EFFECTS AND INHIBITION OF APOPTOSIS The replication of almost all viruses has adverse effects on the infected cell, inhibiting cellular synthesis of DNA, RNA, or proteins. This inhibitory effect probably stems from the viruses' need to prevent or limit the induction of interferon and to replicate rapidly and efficiently, thereby gaining a foothold before an effective host immune response is mounted. Most commonly, viruses specifically inhibit host protein synthesis by attacking a component of the translational initiation complex—frequently, a component that is not required for efficient translation of viral RNAs. Poliovirus protease 2A, for example, cleaves a cellular component of the complex that ordinarily facilitates translation of cellular mRNAs by interacting with their 5′ cap structure. Poliovirus RNA is efficiently translated without a 5′ cap since it has an internal ribosome entry sequence. Influenza virus inhibits the processing of mRNA by snatching 5′ cap structures from nascent cellular RNAs and using them as primers in the synthesis of viral mRNA. HSV has a virion tegument protein that inhibits cellular mRNA translation.

A frequent corollary of the inhibition of cellular macromolecular synthesis is the induction of apoptosis. While this event may be important for the release of virions (particularly in the case of nonenveloped viruses), viruses have also acquired genes or parts of genes that enable them to forestall infected-cell apoptosis. Some adenoviruses and some herpesviruses encode analogues of the cellular protein Bc12, which inhibits apoptosis in lymphocytes. In addition, some papillo-

maviruses and adenoviruses have proteins that counteract the action of p53 in inducing cell-cycle arrest and apoptosis in virus-infected cells.

VIRAL INFECTION IN VIVO

The capsid and envelope of a virus enable the genome to escape degradation, to spread from cell to cell, and to spread among humans or to humans from other animals, including insects. Most common viral infections are spread by inhalation of aerosolized particles, by ingestion of contaminated water or food, or by direct contact. In all of these situations, infection begins on an epithelial or mucosal surface and spreads along it or from it to deeper tissues. Infection may then spread through the body via the bloodstream, lymphatics, or neural circuits. Parenteral inoculation also serves to transmit some viral infections among humans or from animals (including insects) to humans.

PRIMARY INFECTION The duration of primary (first-episode) viral infection usually varies from several days to several weeks. During this period, the concentration of virus at sites of infection rises and then falls, usually to unmeasurable levels. The rate at which the intensity of viral infection rises and falls at a given site depends on the accessibility of that organ or tissue to both the virus and systemic immune effectors, the intrinsic ability of the virus to replicate at that site, and endogenous nonspecific and specific resistance. Typically, infections with enterovirus, mumps virus, measles virus, rubella virus, rotavirus, influenza virus, adenovirus, HSV, and VZV are cleared from almost all sites within 3 to 4 weeks. Some of these viruses can alter or evade the immune response; primary infection then lasts for several months. Characteristically extending beyond several weeks are primary infections due to hepatitis virus (B, C, or D), EBV, cytomegalovirus (CMV), HIV, papillomavirus, and molluscum contagiosum virus. Primary infection with CMV may last for several months, and that with HIV, papillomavirus, or molluscum contagiosum virus may last even longer.

Disease manifestations usually arise as a consequence of viral replication at a specific site but do not necessarily correlate with levels of replication at that site. For example, the clinical manifestations of limited infection with poliovirus, enterovirus, rabies virus, measles virus, mumps virus, or HSV in neural cells are severe relative to the level of viral replication at mucosal surfaces. Similarly, severe morbidity may be associated with fetal infections with rubella virus or CMV.

Primary infections are cleared by specific and nonspecific immune responses. Thereafter, an immunocompetent person is usually immune to the disease manifestations of reinfection by the same virus. Immunity does not prevent transient surface colonization on reexposure to virus.

PERSISTENT AND LATENT INFECTIONS Relatively few viruses cause persistent or latent infections. Hepatitis B and C viruses, rabies virus, measles virus, HIV, HTLV, papovaviruses, herpesviruses, and some poxviruses are notable exceptions. In part, RNA viruses can escape immune destruction because their genomes can change over time during the infection of an individual. Hepatitis C virus and HIV undergo significant evolution during the course of primary and persistent infection in individual patients. Double-strand DNA replication is less error-prone, and DNA viruses appear not to change significantly during their persistence in humans. Papovaviruses and herpesviruses persist by establishing long-term latency in some cells. In the latent state, the viruses are mostly hidden from the normal immune response. When reactivated at epithelial surfaces, papovaviruses and herpesviruses are shed intermittently or continuously at a low level by healthy humans. The continued production of these viruses by humans despite an immune response that is adequate to suppress most or all manifestations of disease creates a continuous supply of these viruses and permits viral spread to children and to susceptible adults, ensuring viral perpetuation in human populations.

Molluscum contagiosum virus is a poxvirus causing a proliferative and hypertrophic wart-like disease that can persist for several months or years. The hypertrophic nature of other poxvirus infections has been attributed to viral homologues of cellular growth factors, including an epidermal growth factor homologue. However, the DNA sequence of molluscum contagiosum virus shows no homology to known epidermal or fibroblast growth factors. The DNA sequence does reveal a chemokine homologue that is likely to block inflammatory responses and a class I major histocompatibility analogue that may block cytotoxic T lymphocyte attack.

ROLE OF PERSISTENT VIRAL INFECTIONS IN HUMAN CANCERS Estimates of the fraction of human malignancies that result directly from viral infection range from 10 to 20 percent. Most hepatocellular carcinomas are presumed to be caused by infection with hepatitis B or C virus, almost all cervical carcinomas by infection with "high-risk" strains of genital papillomavirus, all anaplastic nasopharyngeal carcinomas by infection with EBV, and most adult cutaneous T cell lymphomas/leukemias by infection with HTLV-I. The presumption of a causal relationship between the hepatitis viruses and hepatocellular carcinoma is based on epidemiologic data and on studies with experimental models, which indicate that chronic liver injury attributable to these viruses can cause hepatocellular cancer in rodents. Hepatitis B viral DNA can integrate into cellular DNA, and this integration can contribute to oncogenicity. For cervical cancer, nasopharyngeal carcinoma, and adult T cell leukemia, the corresponding presumptions are based on epidemiologic data, the universal presence of viral DNA in tumor cells, the ability of the viruses to transform human cells in culture, and the pathophysiologic links between specific viral genes expressed in premalignant or malignant cells and cell-transforming effects in various assays in vitro. EBV has been implicated in lymphoproliferative diseases in immunosuppressed patients, in some B and T lymphocyte malignancies, in some gastric cancers, in muscle tumors in AIDS patients, and in a significant fraction of cases of Hodgkin's disease. Specific EBV genes and gene products have been genetically and pathophysiologically linked to effects on cell growth. Recent evidence suggests that a newly identified herpesvirus may cause Kaposi's sarcoma. Formal proof of the viral etiology of these malignancies will most likely come from efforts to prevent or intervene in infections with the putative oncogenic human viruses.

RESISTANCE TO VIRAL INFECTIONS Resistance to viral infection is initially provided by factors that are not specific for individual viruses. Physical protection is afforded by the cornified layers of the skin and by mucous secretions that continuously sweep over mucosal surfaces. Once the first cell is infected, interferons become important as local resistance factors. Viral infection may also cause the release of other cytokines from infected cells. Viral protein epitopes expressed on the cell surface in the context of histocompatibility proteins can attract T cells with appropriate receptors. Cytokines, inflammatory agents, and antigens released by virus-induced cell death attract inflammatory cells, granulocytes, natural killer cells, and lymphocytes to the site of initial infection. Interferons and natural killer cells are particularly important in containing viral infection for the first several days. Granulocytes and macrophages also are important in the phagocytosis and degradation of viruses, particularly after the onset of an antibody response.

Near the end of the first week or the beginning of the second week after infection, several responses can be detected: a virus-specific antibody response; a virus-specific, histocompatibility leukocyte antigen (HLA) class II–restricted, CD4 + helper T lymphocyte response; and a virus-specific, HLA class I–restricted, CD8 + cytotoxic T lymphocyte response. The magnitude of these responses, which are important in rapid recovery, typically increases over the second and third weeks of infection. Also between the second and third weeks, the antibody isotype usually changes from IgM to IgG, and virus-specific IgA antibody may be detected at mucosal surfaces. Antibody may neutralize virus directly by binding to its surface and preventing

its adsorption or penetration. Complement usually enhances virus neutralization. Antibody and complement can also lyse virus-infected cells that express viral proteins on their surface. A cell infected with an enveloped virus usually expresses viral glycoprotein components of the envelope on its surface. Thus, the infected cell is rendered subject to destruction by antibodies to the glycoprotein and complement.

The antibody response and the CD4 + and CD8 + T lymphocyte responses tend to persist for several months after primary infection. Antibody-producing lymphocytes persist in small numbers as memory cells and begin to proliferate rapidly in response to reexposure, providing an early barrier to reinfection with the same virus. Immunologic memory for T cell responses appears to be less long lived, and redevelopment of T cell immunity may take longer than secondary antibody responses, particularly when many years have elapsed between primary infection and reexposure. Some viruses have genes that alter the normal host response. Examples of viral genes that hinder host resistance include adenoviral VA RNAs, which prevent interferon from shutting off protein synthesis in adenovirus-infected cells; adenoviral E1A protein, which inhibits interferon responsiveness at specific promoters; adenoviral E3 proteins, which prevent cytolysis induced by tumor necrosis factor and block class I antigen synthesis by the infected cell; and herpes simplex viral ICP47 and cytomegaloviral US11, which block class I antigen presentation. Clearly, many viruses have evolved to include genes that inhibit interferon, natural killer, and CD8 + cytotoxic cell effects. The adoption of these strategies by viruses highlights the importance of these host resistance factors in containing viral infection and also highlights the redundancy in host resistance. Even when viruses block one or several effectors of host resistance, infection can still be contained in the vast majority of immunocompetent hosts.

Much has been written about the role of specific aspects of the host immune response in containment of specific viral infections. Certainly, T lymphocyte disorders are particularly associated with relatively severe primary and reactivated herpesvirus infections, and antibody responses are important in resistance to many RNA virus infections. However, that antibody responses are also important in resistance to herpesvirus infections is evidenced by the utility of immunoglobulin therapy in herpesvirus infections. In addition, T lymphocyte responses are important in resistance to RNA virus infections; this importance is exemplified by the presence of cytotoxic T cells specific for influenza virus nucleoprotein. Redundancy in host resistance allows interferon, natural killer cell, B lymphocyte, or T lymphocyte responses to compensate in most instances for a deficiency in one of these host resistance factors.

Redundancy in host resistance has its price. Clearly, aspects of the host response contribute to the pathophysiologic manifestations of viral infection. Inflammation at sites of infection is essential to an effective local response but also contributes to local and systemic symptoms and local cell death. The systemic immune balance can be altered by viral infection, and the change can result in an immune attack on neural or other cells. The notion has been put forward that some of these aberrant responses may be due in part to cross-reactivity between viral and cellular antigens. While such effects can be demonstrated in experimental models, their role in the autoimmune manifestations of primary or recurrent human viral infections is uncertain.

INTERFERONS All human cells can synthesize interferon α or β in response to viral infection. The induction of an interferon response is usually due to the presence of double-strand viral RNA, which can be made by both RNA and DNA viruses. Interferon γ is not directly related to interferons α and β and is produced mainly by natural killer cells and by immune T lymphocytes responding to interleukin 12. Interferons α and β bind to the interferon α receptor, while interferon γ binds to a different but related receptor. Both receptors signal through receptor-associated JAK kinases and other cytoplasmic proteins, including STAT proteins. These proteins are tyrosine phosphorylated by JAK kinases, translocate to the nucleus, and transactivate promoters for specific cellular genes. Three types of antiviral effect are induced by interferon at the transcriptional level. The first involves the induction of $2'$-$5'$ oligo(A) synthetases, which require double-strand RNA for activation. Activated synthetase polymerizes oligo(A) and thereby activates RNAse L, which in turn degrades single-strand RNA. The second effect involves the induction of PKR, a serine and threonine kinase that is also activated by double-strand RNA. PKR phosphorylates and negatively regulates the translational initiation factor eIF2 α, shutting down protein synthesis in the infected cell. The third effect entails the induction of Mx proteins, a family of GTPases that are particularly important in inhibiting the replication of influenza virus and vesicular stomatitis virus. None of these effects of interferons are specifically directed against the virus; infected-cell synthesis of RNA and proteins is inhibited globally. Interferon probably results in the death of the infected cell.

ANTIVIRAL AGENTS Twenty-five years ago, the field of clinically useful antiviral agents was limited to amantadine prophylaxis of influenza A virus infection. The synthesis of acycloguanosine and the discovery of its utility for the treatment of severe herpesvirus infections led to antiviral drug discovery programs at every major pharmaceutical company. Recent areas of focus include viral kinases, proteases, RNA polymerases, and polymerase accessory factors. The identification of HIV as the causative agent of AIDS led to worldwide efforts to develop antiretroviral drugs and renewed efforts to develop agents that would be effective against other viral infections in AIDS patients. The current status of clinically useful antivirals is summarized in Chap. 183.

Augmentation of the normal immune response by passive transfer of immunoglobulins or virus-specific T cells can be an effective mode of antiviral therapy. Human immunoglobulin enriched with antibodies to VZV is used to prevent disease in exposed susceptible individuals and to ameliorate disease in immunodeficient patients. Moreover, immunoglobulins are useful for prophylaxis of hepatitis and rabies virus infection and of CMV disease in transplant recipients; immunoglobulin administration appears to have a role in the treatment of parvovirus-induced aplastic anemia. Cellular immunotherapy effectively prevents and treats diseases induced by CMV and EBV in transplant recipients. In this instance, the number of virus-specific T cells is expanded in vitro, and the cells are readministered later, when the patient is at high risk for untoward consequences of viral infection.

DIAGNOSTIC VIROLOGY A wide variety of methods are now used to diagnose viral infection, but serology and viral isolation in tissue culture continue to form the backbone of diagnostic virology. Acute- and convalescent-phase sera with rising titers of antibody to virus-specific antigens and a shift from IgM to IgG antibodies are generally accepted as findings diagnostic of acute viral infection. Traditionally, virus-specific antibodies have been detected by hemadsorption, hemagglutination, or indirect immunofluorescence. Immunofluorescence assays use fixed virus-infected cells as a target for serum antibodies. Hemadsorption and hemagglutination assays measure the ability of serum antibodies to the hemagglutinin proteins of RNA viruses to inhibit virus-induced adsorption or agglutination of red cells. Serologic diagnosis is based on a greater than fourfold rise in IgG antibody concentration when acute- and convalescent-phase sera are analyzed at the same time. A simultaneous fall in IgM antibody confirms recent primary viral infection.

Immunofluorescence, hemadsorption, and hemagglutination assays are labor intensive and are being replaced by enzyme-linked immunoassays (ELISAs). ELISAs generally use specific viral proteins purified from virus-infected cells or produced by recombinant DNA technology. These viral antigens are attached to a solid phase, where they can be incubated with serum; washed to eliminate nonspecific antibodies; and allowed to react with an enzyme-linked reagent to detect either human IgG or IgM antibody specifically adhering to the viral antigen on the solid phase. The amount of antibody is then quantitated by the intensity of a color reaction mediated by the linked enzyme. ELISAs can be automated and can be more sensitive than immunofluorescence, hemagglutination, or hemadsorption assays.

Western blots measure antibody to multiple viral proteins simultaneously. The proteins are separated by size and transferred to an inert membrane, where they are incubated with serum antibodies. Western blots have an internal specificity control in that the level of reactivity for viral proteins can be compared with that for cellular proteins in

the same sample. Although western blots are useful for confirmatory testing, they require individual evaluation and are inherently difficult to quantitate.

The isolation of virus in tissue culture depends on the infection of susceptible cells and amplification through viral replication in infected cells. Viruses growing in tissue culture are frequently identified by their effect on the tissue culture, as detected under light microscopy. For example, HSV produces a typical cytopathic effect in rabbit kidney cells within 3 days. Other viral cytopathic effects may not be as definitively diagnostic and may require confirmation by staining with virus-specific monoclonal antibodies. Viruses growing in tissue culture can also be identified by hemadsorption, by interference (e.g., rubella virus–infected cells resist lysis induced by echoviral infection), or by electron microscopy (assuming that the specimen has altered cellular morphology detectable by ordinary light microscopy).

The efficiency and speed with which viruses are identified can be enhanced if short-term culture is combined with immune detection. With shell vials of tissue-culture cells growing on a coverslip, viral infection can be detected by staining with a monoclonal antibody to a specific viral protein expressed early in viral replication. Thus, virus-infected cells can be detected within hours or days of inoculation—i.e., before the several rounds of replication that would be required to produce a visible cytopathic effect.

The sensitivity of viral isolation is highly dependent on the collection of specimens from the appropriate site and their rapid transport in the appropriate medium to the virology laboratory. Rapid transport ensures viral viability and limits bacterial and fungal overgrowth. Lipid-enveloped viruses are generally much more sensitive than nonenveloped viruses to the effects of freezing and thawing. The most appropriate site for culture depends on the pathogenesis of the virus in question. Nasopharyngeal, tracheal, or endobronchial aspirates are most appropriate for the identification of respiratory viruses; sputum cultures generally are not appropriate because bacterial contamination and viscosity threaten tissue-culture cell viability. Aspirates of vesicular fluid are useful for the isolation of HSV and VZV. Nasopharyngeal aspirates and stool specimens may be useful in instances of fever and rash in which enteroviral infection is suspected. Adenoviruses can be cultured from the urine of patients with hemorrhagic cystitis. CMV can frequently be isolated from cultures of urine or the buffy-coat portion of peripheral blood. Material obtained by biopsy can be cultured effectively when viruses infect major organs—e.g., in herpesviral encephalitis or adenoviral pneumonia. Unlike serologic testing, the isolation of a virus does not establish the time of primary infection. Many viruses persistently or intermittently colonize normal human mucosal surfaces. Saliva is not infrequently positive for herpesviruses, and 1 percent of normal urine samples are positive for CMV. Isolations from blood, cerebrospinal fluid, or biopsy specimens are more likely to be diagnostic of significant viral infection.

Another method aimed at increasing the speed of viral diagnosis is direct antigen testing. Virus-infected cells obtained directly from the patient are detected by staining with virus-specific monoclonal antibodies; for example, epithelial cells obtained by nasopharyngeal aspiration can be stained with a variety of monoclonal antibodies to respiratory viruses. The Tzanck preparation used to detect multinucleated giant cells in lesions induced by HSV or VZV was the predecessor for these direct antigen tests, which can be enhanced by the use of monoclonal antibodies specific for HSV or VZV. Similarly, monoclonal antibodies can be applied to histopathology specimens to identify virus-infected cells.

Advances in nucleic acid technology may revolutionize diagnostic virology. Because of the speed and sensitivity of tests that directly amplify minute amounts of viral nucleic acids present in clinical specimens, detection no longer depends on viable virus and viral replication. For example, amplification and detection of nucleic acids of HSV leaking into the cerebrospinal fluid of patients with HSV encephalitis can be more sensitive than culture of HSV from cerebrospinal fluid.

The extreme sensitivity of these tests can also be problematic: trivial amounts of contamination can lead to false-positive results. Before their application in clinical diagnostic practice, these methods must be standardized and their clinical utility systematically evaluated.

Recent studies suggest that the progression of AIDS and the clinically significant emergence of drug-resistant variants can be detected by quantitative viral-load measurements based on the polymerase chain reaction. Thus, the Food and Drug Administration has approved nucleic acid tests to quantify HIV load. The usefulness of these tests in the cost-effective management of patients remains to be maximized.

IMMUNIZATION (See also Chap. 122)   The development of viral vaccines is among the outstanding accomplishments of twentieth-century science. The scourge of smallpox has been eradicated, and the eradication of poliovirus infection may soon follow. Rabies and measles can be contained or eradicated. The excess mortality due to influenza epidemics can be eliminated, and the threat of influenza pandemics is now minimal. Widespread use of hepatitis B virus vaccination has dramatically lessened the frequency of acute and chronic hepatitis and is expected to lead to a dramatic decrease in the incidence of hepatocellular carcinoma. The ease with which some viruses are attenuated in tissue culture has facilitated widespread immunization against rubella, measles, mumps, and chickenpox and reduction of their attendant morbidity. Recombinant DNA–based strategies will make it possible to prevent severe infections with many other viruses through the use of purified proteins or genetically engineered live-virus vaccines. Unfortunately, there are limits to these prospects. The evolutionary divergence of HIV and hepatitis C virus appears to preclude the development of highy effective immunogens for the prevention of infection with these agents. However, modestly effective immunogens may prove useful against exposure to very low doses of even these pathogens.

BIBLIOGRAPHY

ALKHATIB G et al: CC CKR5: A Rantes, MIP-1α, MIP-1β receptor as a fusion cofactor for macrophage-tropic HIV-1. Science 272:1955, 1996

FIELDS BN et al (eds): *Virology*, 3d ed. New York, Raven Press, 1996

LAKEMAN FD, WHITLEY RJ: Diagnosis of herpes simplex encephalitis: Application of polymerase chain reaction to cerebrospinal fluid from brain-biopsied patients and correlation with disease. National Institute of Allergy and Infectious Diseases Collaborative Antiviral Study Group. J Infect Dis 172:1641, 1995

MCFADDEN G (ed): *Viroreceptors, Virokines, and Related Immune Modulators Encoded by DNA Viruses.* Austin, TX, Landes, 1995

MONTGOMERY R et al: Herpes simplex virus-1 entry into cells mediated by a novel member of the TNF/NGF receptor family. Cell 87:427, 1996

SAAG MS et al: HIV viral load markers in clinical practice. Nat Med 2:625, 1996

SENKEVICH T et al: Genome sequence of a human tumorigenic poxvirus: Prediction of specific host response-evasion genes. Science 273:813, 1996

TELLING G et al: Evidence for the conformation of the pathologic isoform of the prion protein enciphering and propagating prion diversity. Science 274:2079, 1996

WIEDBRAUK DL, JOHNSTON SLG: *Manual of Clinical Virology.* New York, Raven, 1993

183   *Raphael Dolin*

ANTIVIRAL CHEMOTHERAPY

The use of antiviral compounds for chemotherapy and chemoprophylaxis of viral diseases is a new development in the field of infectious diseases, particularly relative to the more than 50 years of experience with antibacterial agents. The principles that underlie the use of antiviral compounds have been modeled after those successfully employed in the treatment of bacterial infections, as outlined in Chap. 140. However, application of these principles to antiviral chemotherapy and chemoprophylaxis presents a number of unique problems.

First, antiviral compounds must possess a high degree of selectivity because of the biologic properties of viruses. Bacteria can replicate extracellularly and have evolved metabolic and structural features that differ considerably from those of mammalian cells. In contrast, viruses must replicate intracellularly and often employ host cell enzymes, macromolecules, and organelles for the synthesis of virus particles. Therefore, safe and effective antiviral compounds must be able to discriminate with a high degree of efficiency between cellular and virus-specific functions. Inhibitors of virus replication that lack this selectivity are likely to be too toxic for clinical use.

Second, because of the nature of virus replication, the in vitro sensitivity of virus isolates to antiviral compounds must be evaluated in a complex culture system consisting of living cells (e.g., tissue culture). The results from such assay systems vary widely according to the type of tissue culture cells employed and the conditions of assay. Furthermore, the precise relationship between the in vitro sensitivity of an isolate and the outcome of antiviral therapy has not been well worked out for many viral infections.

Third, information regarding the pharmacokinetics of some antiviral compounds, particularly in diverse clinical settings, is limited, particularly when compared with that available for antibacterial agents. Assays to determine concentrations of antivirals, particularly of active moieties within cells, are not widely available. There are few guidelines with which to adjust dosage levels in order to maximize antiviral activity and minimize toxicity. Therefore, clinical use of antiviral compounds must be accompanied by particular vigilance for unanticipated adverse effects or toxicity.

Fourth, it is clear that highly complex host defense systems play critical roles in the course of viral infections. The presence or absence of preexisting immunity and the ability to mount humoral and/or cell-mediated immune responses are especially important determinants in the outcome of viral infections. The state of host defenses and their interactions with antiviral compounds need to be considered when antivirals are utilized or evaluated.

Finally, as with antibacterial agents, the optimal use of antiviral compounds requires that a specific and timely diagnosis be made. For some viral infections, such as herpes zoster, the clinical manifestations are so characteristic that a diagnosis can be made on clinical grounds alone. For other viral infections, such as influenza A, epidemiologic information (e.g., the documentation of a community-wide outbreak) can be used to make a presumptive diagnosis with a high degree of accuracy. However, for most other viral infections, including herpes simplex encephalitis, cytomegalovirus infections other than retinitis, and acute viral gastroenteritis, diagnosis on clinical grounds alone cannot be accomplished with certainty. For such infections, rapid noninvasive viral diagnostic techniques are sorely needed. Considerable progress has been made in recent years in the development of such tests for a number of viral infections.

Despite these complexities, the efficacy of a number of antiviral compounds has been clearly established in rigorously conducted and controlled studies. The compounds that are currently licensed or are likely to be licensed in the immediate future for clinical use are discussed below and summarized in Table 183-1.

ANTIVIRAL DRUGS

AMANTADINE AND RIMANTADINE   Amantadine (1-adamantanamine hydrochloride) and the closely related compound rimantadine (α-methyl-1-adamantanemethylamine hydrochloride) are primary symmetric amines with antiviral activity limited to influenza A viruses, whose replication they inhibit by interfering with the uncoating of virus after infection of the cell. This interference is attributable to the agents' interaction with the influenza A M2 matrix protein, during which the ion channel function of M2 is inhibited. A substitution of a single amino acid in the M2 protein can result in a virus that is resistant to amantadine and rimantadine.

Amantadine and rimantadine have been demonstrated to be effective in the prophylaxis of influenza A in large-scale studies of young adults and in less extensive studies of children and elderly subjects.

Table 183-1

Antiviral Chemotherapy and Chemoprophylaxis

Infection	Drug	Route	Dosage	Comment
Influenza A Prophylaxis	Amantadine or rimantadine	Oral	Adults: 200 mg/d for period at risk Children ≤9 yrs: 5 mg/kg per day (maximum, 150 mg/d)	Therapy must continue for duration of outbreak. Dosage should be reduced (more for amantadine) in patients with renal failure and the elderly. Drugs can be administered along with vaccine.
Treatment	Amantadine or rimantadine	Oral	As above for 5–7 days	Both drugs are effective in uncomplicated influenza. Neither has been thoroughly studied in complicated cases (e.g., pneumonia). Rimantadine is not approved for the treatment of children.
RSV infection	Ribavirin	Small-particle aerosol	Administered continuously from reservoir containing 20 mg/mL for 3–6 days	Ribavirin is used for treatment of infants and young children hospitalized with RSV pneumonia and bronchiolitis.
CMV retinitis in immunocompromised host	Ganciclovir Foscarnet	IV Oral IV	5 mg/kg bid for 14–21 days; then 5 mg/kg per day as maintenance dose 1 g tid as maintenance dose 60 mg/kg q 8 h for 14–21 days; then 90–120 mg/kg per day as maintenance dose	Both drugs are licensed for treatment of CMV retinitis in immunosuppressed patients, including those with AIDS. They are also used for colitis, pneumonia, or "wasting" syndromes associated with CMV and for prevention of CMV disease in transplant recipients. Foscarnet is not myelosuppressive and is active against acyclovir- and ganciclovir-resistant herpesviruses.
HIV infection	Zidovudine (ZDV)	Oral IV	200 mg q 8 h 1–2 mg/kg q 4 h	ZDV is licensed for treatment of patients with HIV infection and CD4 counts of $<500/\mu L$. The optimal time to initiate therapy is controversial. Administration during pregnancy, during delivery, and to newborns reduces rates of perinatal HIV transmission. Higher doses are preferred for AIDS-related dementia.
	Didanosine (ddI)	Oral	125–200 mg (tablets) bid	ddI is licensed for treatment of HIV-infected patients who are intolerant of or failing to respond to ZDV. Clinical benefit is evident when patients are switched from ZDV to ddI, even if they have been stable on the former.
	Zalcitabine (ddC)	Oral	0.75 mg q 8 h	ddC is licensed for use in combination with ZDV in patients with advanced HIV infection who are not responding to ZDV alone. ddC appears inferior to ZDV as monotherapy in patients with advanced disease (median CD4 count, $89/\mu L$). Combination of ZDV and ddC is superior to ZDV alone in patients with less advanced disease (median CD4 count, $354/\mu L$).
	Stavudine (d4T)	Oral	30–40 mg bid	Stavudine is licensed for treatment of patients with advanced HIV infection who are intolerant of or failing to respond to approved therapy. Patients with CD4 counts of $50–500/\mu L$ with ≥6 mo of ZDV therapy benefit from a switch to stavudine.
	Lamivudine (3TC)	Oral	150 mg bid	3TC is used in combination with ZDV or d4T in patients with HIV infection and clinical or immunologic disease progression. 3TC retards the emergence of phenotypic resistance to ZDV.
	Saquinavir	Oral	600 mg tid	This protease inhibitor is approved for combination therapy with nucleoside analogues in advanced HIV infection, is well tolerated, has a low level of oral bioavailability, and should be taken within 2 h of a meal; it is subject to important drug interactions via the P450 system.

(continued)

Table 183-1—(*Continued*)

Antiviral Chemotherapy and Chemoprophylaxis

Infection	Drug	Route	Dosage	Comment
HIV infection (continued)	Indinavir	Oral	800 mg q 8 h	This protease inhibitor is approved for antiretroviral therapy in HIV infection. The drug is associated with hyperbilirubinemia and nephrolithiasis. It should be taken on an empty stomach. Indinavir is subject to important interactions via the P450 system.
	Ritonavir	Oral	600 mg bid	This protease inhibitor is approved for antiretroviral therapy in HIV infection. In advanced disease, ritonavir is associated with improved survival and delayed disease progression. Because of frequent gastrointestinal intolerance, the drug should be taken with meals. It is subject to important drug interactions via the P450 system.
Varicella				
Immunocompetent host	Acyclovir	Oral	20 mg/kg (maximum, 800 mg) 4 or 5 times daily for 5 days	Treatment confers modest clinical benefit when administered within 24 h of onset of rash.
Immunocompromised host	Acyclovir	IV	500 mg/m^2 q 8 h for 7 days	No studies have compared IV acyclovir with vidarabine for varicella.
	Vidarabine	IV	10 mg/kg per day as 12-h infusion for 5 days	Limited data from placebo-controlled studies suggest similar effects for the two drugs.
Herpes simplex encephalitis	Acyclovir	IV	10 mg/kg q 8 h for 10 days	Acyclovir is the drug of choice on the basis of comparative trials with vidarabine. Results are optimal when therapy is initiated early.
	Vidarabine	IV	15 mg/kg per day as continuous infusion over 12 h for 10 days	Drug must be given as dilute solution. Therapy can result in substantial fluid load.
Neonatal herpes simplex	Vidarabine	IV	30 mg/kg per day as continuous infusion over 12 h for 14–21 days	Vidarabine and acyclovir are equivalent in clinical efficacy. Serious morbidity is frequent despite therapy.
	Acyclovir	IV	10 mg/kg q 8 h for 14–21 days	
Genital herpes simplex				
Primary (treatment)	Acyclovir	IV	5 mg/kg q 8 h for 5–10 days	The IV route is preferred for infections severe enough to warrant hospitalization or with neurologic complications.
		Oral	200 mg 5 times daily for 10 days	This is the preferred route for patients whose condition does not warrant hospitalization. Adequate hydration must be maintained.
		Topical	5% ointment; 4–6 applications daily for 7–10 days	Topical use—largely supplanted by oral therapy—may obviate systemic administration to pregnant women. Systemic symptoms and untreated areas are not affected.
Recurrent				
Treatment	Acyclovir	Oral	200 mg 5 times daily for 5 days	Clinical effect is modest and is enhanced if therapy is initiated early. Treatment does not affect recurrence rates.
	Famciclovir	Oral	125 mg bid for 5 days	
	Valacyclovir	Oral	500 mg bid for 5 days	
Suppression	Acyclovir	Oral	400 mg bid for ≥12 mo	Suppressive therapy is recommended only for patients with at least 6–10 recurrences per year. "Breakthrough" occasionally takes place, and asymptomatic shedding of virus occurs. Need for suppressive therapy should be reevaluated after 1 year
Mucocutaneous herpes simplex in immunocompromised host				
Treatment	Acyclovir	IV	250 mg/m^2 q 8 h for 7 days	Choice of intravenous or oral route depends on severity of infection and patient's ability to take oral medication. Oral or IV treatment has supplanted topical therapy except for small, easily accessible lesions.
		Oral	400 mg 5 times daily for 10 days	
		Topical	5% ointment; 4–6 applications daily for 7 days or until healed	

(continued)

Table 183-1—*(Continued)*

Antiviral Chemotherapy and Chemoprophylaxis

Infection	Drug	Route	Dosage	Comment
	Vidarabine	IV	10 mg/kg per day for 7 days as 12-h infusion	Efficacy has been demonstrated in HSV-1 infections and in patients older than 40. Vidarabine appears to be less useful than acyclovir in this setting.
Prevention of recurrences during intense immunosuppression	Acyclovir	Oral IV	200 mg qid 5 mg/kg q 12 h	Acyclovir is administered during periods when intense immunosuppression is expected—e.g., during antitumor chemotherapy or after transplantation. After therapy is discontinued, lesions recur.
Herpes simplex keratitis	Trifluridine	Topical	1 drop of 1% ophthalmic solution q 2 h while awake (maximum, 9 drops daily)	Therapy should be undertaken in consultation with an ophthalmologist.
	Vidarabine	Topical	0.5-in ribbon of 3% ophthalmic ointment 5 times daily	
Herpes zoster Immunocompromised host	Acyclovir Vidarabine	IV IV	500 mg/m^2 q 8 h for 7 days 10 mg/kg per day as 12-h infusion for 5 days	Both drugs are effective in localized zoster, particularly when given early; acyclovir appears to be more effective. Studies of treatment of disseminated zoster are under way. High-dose oral acyclovir (4 g/d) is also used for herpes zoster in these patients.
Immunocompetent host	Valacyclovir	Oral	1 g tid for 7 days	Valacyclovir may be more effective than acyclovir for relief of pain; otherwise, it has a similar effect on cutaneous lesions and should be given within 72 h of onset of rash.
	Famciclovir	Oral	500 mg q 8 h for 7 days	Duration of postherpetic neuralgia is shorter than with placebo. Famciclovir showed overall efficacy similar to that of acyclovir in a comparative trial. It should be given ≤72 h after onset of rash.
	Acyclovir	Oral	800 mg 5 times daily for 7–10 days	Acyclovir causes faster resolution of skin lesions than placebo and provides some relief of acute symptoms if given within 72 h of onset of rash.
Herpes zoster ophthalmicus	Acyclovir	Oral	600 mg 5 times daily for 10 days	Treatment reduces ocular complications, including ocular keratitis and uveitis.
Condyloma acuminatum	Interferon α2b	Intralesional	1 million units per wart (maximum of 5) thrice weekly for 3 weeks	Intralesional treatment frequently results in regression of warts, but lesions often recur. Parenteral administration may be useful if lesions are numerous.
	Interferon αn3	Intralesional	250,000 units per wart (maximum of 10) twice weekly for up to 8 weeks	
Chronic hepatitis, non-A, non-B/C	Interferon α2b	SC or IM	3 million units thrice weekly for 24 weeks	Serum alanine aminotransferase values return to normal in 40–50% of cases but relapse in half when treatment is stopped. Optimal duration and regimens are being studied.
Chronic hepatitis B	Interferon α2b	SC or IM	5 million units daily for 16 weeks	Hepatitis B **e** antigen and DNA are eliminated in 33–37% of cases. Histopathologic improvement is also evident.

NOTE: CMV, cytomegalovirus; HIV, human immunodeficiency virus; HSV, herpes simplex virus; RSV, respiratory syncytial virus.

In such studies, efficacy rates of 55 to 80 percent in the prevention of influenza-like illness were noted, and even higher rates were reported when virus-specific attack rates were calculated. Amantadine and rimantadine also have been demonstrated to be effective in the treatment of influenza A infection in studies involving predominantly young adults and, to a lesser extent, children. Administration of these compounds within 24 to 72 h after the onset of illness has resulted in a reduction of the duration of signs and symptoms by approximately 50 percent from that in a placebo-treated group. The effect on signs and symptoms of illness has been demonstrated to be superior to that of commonly used antipyretic-analgesics. Only anecdotal reports are available concerning the efficacy of amantadine or rimantadine in the prevention or treatment of complications of influenza (e.g., pneumonia).

Amantadine and rimantadine are available only in oral formulations and are ordinarily administered to adults once or twice daily in a dose of 100 to 200 mg/d. Despite their structural similarities, the pharmacokinetics of the two compounds are different. Amantadine is not metabolized and is excreted almost entirely by the kidney, with a half-life of 12 to 17 h and peak plasma concentrations of 0.4 μg/mL. Rimantadine is extensively metabolized to hydroxylated derivatives and has a half-life of 30 h. Only 30 to 40 percent of an orally administered dose is recovered in the urine. The peak plasma levels of rimantadine are approximately half those of amantadine, but rimantadine is concentrated in respiratory secretions to a greater extent than amantadine. For prophylaxis, the compounds must be administered daily for the period at risk (i.e., the peak duration of the outbreak).

For therapy, amantadine or rimantadine is generally administered for 5 to 7 days.

Although these compounds are generally well tolerated, 5 to 10 percent of amantadine recipients experience mild central nervous system side effects consisting primarily of dizziness, anxiety, insomnia, and difficulty in concentrating. These effects are rapidly reversible upon cessation of the drug's administration. At a dose of 200 mg/d, rimantadine is better tolerated than amantadine; in a large-scale study of young adults, adverse effects were no more frequent among rimantadine recipients than among placebo recipients. Seizures and worsening of congestive heart failure also have been reported in patients treated with amantadine, although a causal relationship has not been established. The dosage of amantadine should be reduced to 100 mg/d or less in patients with renal insufficiency [i.e., a creatinine clearance (CrCl) rate of <50 mL/min] and in the elderly. A rimantadine dose of 100 mg/d should be used for patients with a CrCl of <10 mL/min and in the elderly. Resistance to amantadine and rimantadine can be induced readily in vitro. The emergence and probable transmission of virus resistant to these drugs also have been noted in vivo after their use for the treatment of children or adults. In the United States, both amantadine and rimantadine are approved for the prophylaxis and treatment of influenza A in adults and for prophylaxis in children. Amantadine is also approved for the treatment of influenza A in children.

RIBAVIRIN   Ribavirin is a synthetic nucleoside analogue that inhibits a wide range of RNA and DNA viruses. The mechanism of action of ribavirin is not completely defined and may be different for different groups of viruses. Ribavirin-5′-monophosphate blocks the conversion of inosine-5′-monophosphate to xanthosine-5′-monophosphate and interferes with the synthesis of guanine nucleotides as well as that of both RNA and DNA. Ribavirin-5′-monophosphate also inhibits capping of virus-specific messenger RNA in certain viral systems. In studies demonstrating the effectiveness of ribavirin, the compound has been administered as a small-particle aerosol. It has been used to treat respiratory syncytial virus (RSV) infections in infants and—less extensively—to treat parainfluenza virus infections in children and influenza A and B virus infections in young adults. In infants with RSV infection who were given ribavirin by continuous aerosol for 3 to 6 days, illness and lower respiratory tract signs resolved more rapidly and arterial oxygen desaturation was less pronounced than in placebo-treated groups. Ribavirin has also had a beneficial clinical effect in infants with RSV infection who require mechanical ventilation. Aerosolized ribavirin has been administered to older children and adults with severe RSV and parainfluenza virus infections (including immunosuppressed patients), but the benefit of this treatment, if any, is unclear. Orally administered ribavirin has not been effective in the treatment of influenza A virus infections. Intravenous or oral ribavirin has reduced mortality among patients with Lassa fever; it has been particularly effective in this regard when given within the first 6 days of illness. Intravenous ribavirin has been reported to be of clinical benefit in the treatment of hemorrhagic fever with renal syndrome caused by Hantaan virus and as therapy for Argentinian hemorrhagic fever. Moreover, oral ribavirin has been recommended for the treatment and prophylaxis of Congo-Crimean hemorrhagic fever. Intravenous ribavirin is being evaluated as therapy for the hemorrhagic fever with pulmonary syndrome caused by newly described hantaviruses in the United States.

Large doses of ribavirin administered orally (800 to 1000 mg/d) have been associated with reversible hematopoietic toxicity, but this effect has not been observed with aerosolized ribavirin, apparently because little drug is absorbed systemically. Aerosolized administration of ribavirin is generally well tolerated but occasionally is associated with bronchospasm, rash, or conjunctival irritation. Aerosolized ribavirin has been licensed for treatment of RSV infection in infants and should be administered under close supervision—particularly in the setting of mechanical ventilation, where precipitation of the drug

is possible. Health care workers exposed to the drug have experienced minor toxicity, including eye and respiratory tract irritation. Because ribavirin is mutagenic, teratogenic, and embryotoxic, its use is generally contraindicated in pregnancy. Its administration as an aerosol poses a risk to pregnant health care workers.

ACYCLOVIR AND VALACYCLOVIR   Acyclovir, or 9-[(2-hydroxyethoxy)methyl]guanine, is a highly potent and selective inhibitor of the replication of certain herpesviruses, including herpes simplex virus (HSV) types 1 and 2 (HSV-1 and HSV-2), varicella-zoster virus (VZV), and Epstein-Barr virus (EBV). It is relatively ineffective in the treatment of human cytomegalovirus (CMV) infections. Valacyclovir, the L-valyl ester of acyclovir, is almost entirely converted to acyclovir after oral administration.

The high degree of selectivity of acyclovir is related to its mechanism of action, which requires that the compound first be phosphorylated to acyclovir monophosphate. This phosphorylation occurs efficiently in herpesvirus-infected cells by means of a virus-coded thymidine kinase. In uninfected mammalian cells, little phosphorylation of acyclovir occurs, and the drug is therefore concentrated in herpesvirus-infected cells. Acyclovir monophosphate is subsequently converted by host cell kinases to a triphosphate that is a potent inhibitor of virus-induced DNA polymerase but has relatively little effect on host cell DNA polymerase. Acyclovir triphosphate also can be incorporated into viral DNA, with early chain termination.

Acyclovir is available in intravenous, oral, and topical forms. Intravenous acyclovir is markedly effective in the treatment of mucocutaneous HSV infections in immunocompromised hosts, reducing time to healing, duration of pain, and virus shedding. When administered prophylactically during periods of intense immunosuppression (e.g., related to chemotherapy for leukemia or transplantation) and before the development of lesions, intravenous acyclovir reduces the frequency of HSV-associated disease. After prophylaxis is discontinued, HSV lesions recur. Intravenous acyclovir is also effective in the treatment of HSV encephalitis; two comparative trials have indicated that acyclovir is more effective than vidarabine for this indication (see below). Because VZV is generally less sensitive to acyclovir than is HSV, higher doses of acyclovir must be used to treat VZV infections. In immunocompromised patients with herpes zoster, intravenous acyclovir reduces the frequency of cutaneous dissemination and visceral complications and—in one comparative trial—was more effective than vidarabine. Acyclovir, administered orally at doses of 800 mg five times a day, had a modest beneficial effect on localized herpes zoster lesions in both immunocompromised and immunocompetent patients. The overall effect of acyclovir on postherpetic neuralgia is unclear and is being evaluated further in large-scale collaborative trials. A comparative study of acyclovir (800 mg orally five times daily) and valacyclovir (1 g orally three times daily) in immunocompetent patients with herpes zoster indicated that the latter drug may be more effective in eliciting the resolution of zoster-associated pain. Orally administered acyclovir (600 mg five times a day) reduced complications of herpes zoster ophthalmicus in a placebo-controlled trial.

In normal children with chickenpox, acyclovir—administered at 20 mg/kg four times a day, up to a maximum of 800 mg four times a day, within 24 h of the onset of rash—resulted in a modest overall clinical benefit. Intravenous acyclovir also has been reported to be effective in the treatment of immunocompromised children with chickenpox.

The most widespread use of acyclovir is in the treatment of genital HSV infections. Both intravenous and oral formulations have shortened the duration of symptoms, reduced virus shedding, and accelerated healing when employed for the treatment of primary genital HSV infections. Oral acyclovir has also had a modest effect on recurrent genital HSV infections. However, the failure of treatment of either primary or recurrent disease to reduce the frequency of subsequent recurrences has indicated that acyclovir is ineffective in eliminating latent infection. Chronic administration of oral acyclovir for periods of 1 to 6 years has been shown to reduce the frequency of recurrences markedly during therapy; once the drug is discontinued, lesions recur. In AIDS patients, chronic or intermittent administration of acyclovir has been associated with the development of HSV and VZV strains resistant to the action of the drug and with clinical failures. The most common mechanism of resistance is a deficiency of the virus-induced thymidine kinase. Patients with HSV or VZV infections resistant to acyclovir have frequently responded to foscarnet.

With the availability of the oral and intravenous forms, there are few indications for topical acyclovir, although treatment with this formulation has been modestly beneficial in primary genital HSV infections and in mucocutaneous HSV infections in immunocompromised hosts.

Overall, acyclovir is remarkably well tolerated and is generally free of toxicity. The most frequently encountered form of toxicity is renal dysfunction, particularly after rapid intravenous administration or with inadequate hydration. Central nervous system changes, including lethargy and tremors, are occasionally reported, primarily in immunosuppressed patients. However, whether these changes are related to acyclovir, to concurrent administration of other therapy, or to underlying infection remains unclear. Acyclovir is excreted primarily unmetabolized by the kidney, via both glomerular filtration and tubular secretion. Approximately 15 percent of a dose of acyclovir is metabolized to 9-[(carboxymethoxy)methyl]guanine or other minor metabolites. Reduction in dosage is indicated in patients with a CrCl of less than 50 mL/min per 1.73 m^2. The half-life of acyclovir is approximately 3 h in normal adults, and the peak plasma concentration after a 1-h infusion of a dose of 5 mg/kg is 9.8 μg/mL. Approximately 22 percent of an orally administered acyclovir dose is absorbed, and peak plasma concentrations of 0.3 to 0.9 μg/mL are attained after administration of a 200-mg dose. Acyclovir penetrates relatively well into the cerebrospinal fluid (CSF), with concentrations approaching half of those found in plasma.

Acyclovir causes chromosomal breakage at high doses, but its administration to pregnant women has not been associated with fetal abnormalities. Nonetheless, the potential risks and benefits of acyclovir should be carefully assessed before the drug is used in pregnancy.

Valacyclovir exhibits three to five times greater bioavailability than acyclovir. The concentration-time curve for valacyclovir, given as 1 g orally three times daily, is similar to that for acyclovir, given as 5 mg/kg intravenously every 8 h. The safety profiles of valacyclovir and acyclovir are similar, although thrombotic thrombocytopenic purpura/hemolytic-uremic syndrome has been reported in immunocompromised patients who have received high doses of valacyclovir. Valacyclovir is approved for the treatment of herpes zoster and recurrent genital HSV infections in immunocompetent adults. It is being studied for use against other herpesvirus infections in various clinical settings.

GANCICLOVIR An analogue of acyclovir, ganciclovir, or 9-[(1,3-dihydroxy-2-propoxy)methyl]guanine, is active against HSV and VZV and is markedly more active than acyclovir against CMV. Ganciclovir triphosphate inhibits CMV DNA polymerase and can be incorporated into CMV DNA, whose elongation it eventually terminates. In HSV- and VZV-infected cells, ganciclovir is phosphorylated by virus-encoded thymidine kinases; in CMV-infected cells, it is phosphorylated by a viral kinase encoded by the UL97 gene. Ganciclovir triphosphate is present in 10-fold higher concentrations in CMV-infected cells than in uninfected cells. Ganciclovir is approved for the treatment of CMV retinitis in immunosuppressed patients and for the prevention of CMV disease in transplant recipients. It is widely used for the treatment of other CMV-associated syndromes, including pneumonia, esophagogastrointestinal infections, hepatitis, and "wasting" illness.

Ganciclovir is available for intravenous or oral administration. Because its oral bioavailability is low (5 to 9 percent), relatively large doses (1 g orally three times daily) need to be administered by this route. Oral bioavailability is enhanced if the drug is administered with food, as recommended. The serum half-life of ganciclovir is 3.5 h after intravenous administration and 4.8 h after oral administration. The drug is excreted primarily by the kidney in unmetabolized form, and its dosage should be reduced in cases of renal failure. The most commonly employed dosage for initial therapy—5 mg/kg intravenously every 12 h for 14 to 21 days—is followed by a maintenance dose of 5 mg/kg intravenously per day or 5 times per week, possibly for as long as immunosuppression persists. Oral ganciclovir is approved as an alternative to the intravenous preparation in maintenance therapy for CMV retinitis, where it appears to be somewhat less effective although more convenient than intravenous therapy. Intraocular ganciclovir, given by either intravitreal injection or intraocular implantation, has also been used to treat CMV retinitis. The use of oral ganciclovir as prophylaxis against CMV disease in AIDS patients is currently being evaluated.

The administration of ganciclovir has been associated with profound bone marrow suppression, particularly neutropenia, which significantly limits the drug's use in many patients. Bone marrow toxicity is potentiated when other bone marrow suppressants, such as zidovudine, are used concomitantly.

Resistance has been noted in CMV isolates obtained after therapy with ganciclovir, especially in patients with AIDS. Such resistance may develop through a mutation in either the viral UL97 gene or the viral DNA polymerase. Ganciclovir-resistant isolates are usually sensitive to foscarnet (see below).

FAMCICLOVIR AND PENCICLOVIR Famciclovir is the diacetyl, 6-deoxyester of the guanosine analogue penciclovir (9-[4-hydroxy-3-hydroxymethylbut-1-yl]guanine). Famciclovir is well absorbed orally, with a bioavailability of 77 percent, and is rapidly converted by deacetylation and oxidation to penciclovir. Penciclovir's spectrum of activity and mechanism of action are similar to those of acyclovir. Penciclovir is phosphorylated initially by a virus-encoded thymidine kinase and subsequently by cellular kinases to penciclovir triphosphate, which inhibits HSV-1, HSV-2, and VZV DNA polymerases as well as hepatitis B virus. The serum half-life of penciclovir is 2 h, but the intracellular half-life of penciclovir triphosphate is 7 to 20 h—markedly longer than that of acyclovir triphosphate. Penciclovir is eliminated primarily in the urine by both glomerular filtration and tubular secretion. The recommended dosage interval (every 8 h) should be adjusted for renal insufficiency.

Two trials involving immunocompetent adults with herpes zoster showed that famciclovir was superior to placebo in eliciting the resolution of skin lesions and virus shedding and in shortening the duration of postherpetic neuralgia; moreover, it was least as effective as acyclovir administered orally at a dose of 800 mg five times daily. Famciclovir was well tolerated, with occasional headache, nausea, and diarrhea reported in frequencies similar to those among placebo recipients. The administration of high doses of famciclovir for 2 years was associated with an increased incidence of mammary adenocarcinomas in female rats, but the clinical significance of this effect is unknown.

Famciclovir is approved for the treatment of herpes zoster and recurrent genital HSV infections in immunocompetent adults. It is being studied for the treatment of herpes zoster in immunocompromised patients and of other HSV infections in various clinical settings.

FOSCARNET Foscarnet (phosphonoformic acid) is a pyrophosphate-containing compound that potently inhibits herpesviruses, including CMV. This drug inhibits DNA polymerases at the pyrophosphate binding site at concentrations that have relatively little effect on cellular polymerases. Foscarnet does not require phosphorylation to exert its antiviral activity and is therefore active against HSV and VZV isolates that are resistant to acyclovir because of deficiencies in thymidine kinase as well as against most ganciclovir-resistant strains of CMV. Foscarnet also inhibits the reverse transcriptase of human immunodeficiency virus (HIV) and is active against HIV in vivo.

Foscarnet is poorly soluble and must be administered intravenously via an infusion pump in a dilute solution over 1 to 2 h. The plasma half-life of foscarnet is 3 to 5 h and increases with decreasing renal function, since the drug is eliminated primarily by the kidneys. It has been estimated that 10 to 28 percent of a dose may be deposited in bone, where it can persist for months. The most common initial dosage of foscarnet—60 mg/kg every 8 h for 14 to 21 days—is followed by a maintenance dose of 90 to 120 mg/kg once a day.

Foscarnet is licensed for the treatment of CMV retinitis in patients with AIDS. In a comparative clinical trial, the drug appeared to be about as efficacious as ganciclovir against CMV retinitis but was associated with a longer survival period, possibly because of its anti-HIV activity. Intraocular foscarnet has been used to treat CMV retinitis. Foscarnet also has been employed to treat acyclovir-resistant HSV and VZV infections as well as ganciclovir-resistant CMV infections, although resistance to foscarnet has been reported in CMV isolated during therapy.

The major form of toxicity associated with foscarnet is renal impairment. Thus renal function should be monitored closely, particularly during the initial phase of therapy. Since foscarnet binds divalent metal ions, hypocalcemia, hypomagnesemia, hypokalemia, and hypo- or hyperphosphatemia can develop. Saline hydration and slow infusion appear to protect the patient against nephrotoxicity and electrolyte disturbances. Although hematologic abnormalities have been documented (most commonly anemia), foscarnet is not generally myelosuppressive and may be administered concomitantly with myelosuppressive medications such as zidovudine.

IDOXURIDINE   Idoxuridine (IUdR) inhibits the replication of herpesviruses and poxviruses. It was formerly used systemically to treat herpesvirus infections, but, because of associated toxicity and lack of proven efficacy, its systemic use has largely been abandoned. Topical IUdR is effective in the treatment of HSV keratitis, particularly in superficial infections, but has been supplanted by topically applied trifluridine and vidarabine (see below).

TRIFLURIDINE   Trifluridine (5-trifluoromethyl-2′-deoxyuridine) is a pyrimidine nucleoside active against HSV-1, HSV-2, and CMV. Trifluridine monophosphate irreversibly inhibits thymidilate synthetase, and trifluridine triphosphate inhibits viral and, to a lesser extent, cellular DNA polymerases. Because of systemic toxicity, its use is limited to topical therapy. Trifluridine is approved for treatment of HSV keratitis, for which trials have shown that it is more effective than topical IUdR but similarly effective to topical vidarabine. The drug has benefited some patients with HSV keratitis who have failed to respond to IUdR or vidarabine. Topical application of trifluridine to acyclovir-resistant HSV mucocutaneous infections has also been beneficial in some cases.

VIDARABINE   Vidarabine (9-β-D-arabinofuranosyladenine) is a purine nucleoside analogue with activity against HSV-1, HSV-2, VZV, and EBV. Vidarabine inhibits viral DNA synthesis through its 5′-triphosphorylated metabolite, although the precise molecular mechanisms of action are not completely understood. For systemic administration, vidarabine is available only as an intravenous preparation with poor solubility and is administered as a constant 12-h infusion; thus a substantial fluid load can result. At doses of 10 to 15 mg/kg per day vidarabine is generally well tolerated, but at somewhat higher doses (20 mg/kg per day) the drug has been associated with hematopoietic side effects, including anemia, leukopenia, and thrombocytopenia. Neurotoxicity has also been reported, particularly at high dosages and in patients with hepatic or renal insufficiency.

Vidarabine is clinically effective against varicella and mucocutaneous HSV infections in immunocompromised patients but has been supplanted by acyclovir because of the latter drug's ease of administration. Vidarabine has been ineffective in the treatment of acyclovir-resistant HSV infections in AIDS patients. In comparative trials, vidarabine was as effective as acyclovir in the treatment of neonatal HSV infections but was less effective than acyclovir in the treatment of herpes simplex encephalitis. A 3% vidarabine ophthalmic ointment is effective in the treatment of HSV keratitis.

OTHER ANTIVIRAL DRUGS   Sorivudine (BV-ARA-U) is a nucleoside analogue that potently inhibits VZV. It is also active against HSV-1 and EBV but not against HSV-2 or CMV. Sorivudine triphosphate inhibits viral DNA synthesis and is concentrated in virus-infected cells. It is well absorbed when given orally and is generally well tolerated. Administration of high doses (75 to 750 times the weight-adjusted human dose) has been associated with hepatic and testicular neoplasms in rodents. Sorivudine appears to be promising as therapy for VZV infections and is currently undergoing clinical trials for the treatment of herpes zoster in immunosuppressed patients and of varicella in immunocompromised adults.

Cidofovir is a phosphonomethylether derivative of cytosine that is highly active against CMV, including some ganciclovir- and foscarnet-resistant strains. This agent is administered intravenously and is cleared largely by the kidney, with a serum half-life of 2.6 h. Concomitant administration with probenecid markedly prolongs the half-life of cidofovir and protects recipients against the major form of toxicity elicited by the drug (nephrotoxicity). The intracellular half-life of cidofovir diphosphate—17 to 30 h—is the basis for its infrequent administration (once a week or once every other week). Cidofovir is currently being evaluated for the treatment of CMV retinitis in patients with AIDS.

ANTIRETROVIRAL DRUGS

ZIDOVUDINE   Zidovudine (ZDV), also known as azidothymidine (AZT), inhibits the replication of HIV-1 and HIV-2 through competitive inhibition of HIV reverse transcriptase (by ZDV triphosphate) and through chain termination of viral DNA synthesis. ZDV is usually administered orally, although an intravenous formulation is available as well. The plasma half-life of ZDV is approximately 1 h, and 90 percent of a dose is recovered in the urine, mostly as the glucuronide metabolite.

In 1987 a large-scale placebo-controlled trial involving patients with AIDS or advanced symptomatic HIV-associated disease demonstrated that administration of ZDV was associated with prolonged survival and with decreases in the frequency and severity of opportunistic infections. Subsequently, ZDV was shown to be beneficial in placebo-controlled trials involving patients with less advanced HIV disease, including persons with early symptomatic disease and asymptomatic patients with CD4 counts of ≤500/mL. However, the optimal point for initiation of ZDV therapy (i.e., during symptomatic or asymptomatic infection) remains controversial, and the use of this agent alone is inferior to its use in combination with various other antiretrovirals, according to recent trials. A recent study showed that the rate of perinatal transmission of HIV-1 was reduced by two-thirds when ZDV was administered at 14 to 34 weeks of pregnancy to women who had CD4 counts of >200/μL and who had received less than 6 months of previous antiretroviral therapy. In that study, ZDV was also administered intrapartum and subsequently was given to the newborn for 6 weeks.

The clinical benefits of ZDV monotherapy appear to wane after a variable period and often last for no more than 12 to 18 months in patients with advanced disease. The full explanation for this diminishing effect is unclear but may be related to the high frequency of resistance to ZDV among HIV-1 isolates from patients with advanced disease who have received the drug for 6 months or more. The development of resistance appears to be less frequent in asymptomatic patients and in patients with less advanced disease. ZDV resistance is associated with specific amino acid substitutions in the HIV reverse transcriptase through mutations at codons 41, 67, 70, 215, and 219. Strategies for the use of ZDV in combination with other agents are designed in part to decrease or otherwise modify the emergence of such resistant viruses.

The most frequently employed dosage of ZDV is 200 mg by mouth every 8 h, and comparative dosage studies indicate that total daily doses of 500 to 600 mg are as effective as and less toxic than the higher doses previously recommended. The major toxicities of ZDV are hematopoietic—most often anemia and granulocytopenia, which occur more frequently in patients with more advanced HIV disease. Nausea, headache, and malaise are also encountered frequently, and ZDV-related skeletal and cardiac myopathies can occur. Severe steatosis and lactic acidosis have been described with ZDV as well as with other nucleoside analogues.

DIDANOSINE   Didanosine (ddI) is a nucleoside analogue with activity against HIV-1 and HIV-2. It is an inhibitor of the HIV reverse transcriptase and also can act as a chain terminator for viral DNA elongation. ddI is phosphorylated and converted to ddATP, which is the active antiviral moiety. ddI is active in vitro against most HIV isolates that are resistant to ZDV. Resistance to ddI has been described and is associated with mutations at position 74 (and, to a lesser extent, at positions 135 and 184) in the reverse transcriptase.

Because ddI is given orally and is highly acid labile, it must be administered with buffers against stomach acidity. These buffers are incorporated into the powder or tablet preparations. ddI is 20 to 25 percent more bioavailable in tablets than in powder. The plasma half-life of ddI is 1.5 h, and approximately 50 percent of a dose is cleared by renal mechanisms. The intracellular half-life of ddATP is considerably longer (8 to 24 h) and provides the rationale for the recommended dosing schedule of every 12 h.

ddI was licensed originally on the basis of its favorable effects on "surrogate markers" of HIV disease (CD4 cell counts and p24 antigen concentrations) for use in patients who were intolerant of or failing to respond clinically or immunologically to treatment with ZDV. Subsequently, controlled studies have shown that switching such patients from ZDV to ddI monotherapy confers a clear clinical benefit, as does switching some patients to ddI who otherwise appear to be clinically stable on ZDV. Comparisons of ddI and ZDV as initial monotherapy in HIV disease have yielded conflicting results: ddI was superior to ZDV in a population with somewhat less advanced disease (median CD4 cell count, 354/μL), while ZDV appeared to be more effective in a population with more advanced disease (median CD4 count, 130/μL). ddI is also being evaluated as part of various two- and three-drug combinations.

The major toxicities encountered in the use of ddI have been pancreatitis and peripheral neuropathy. Overall rates of pancreatitis among recipients of ddI have been estimated at 5 to 9 percent, with rates at the upper end of this range among patients with advanced HIV disease. Most cases are mild to moderate in severity, but fatal cases have occurred rarely. Painful peripheral neuropathy, primarily involving the lower extremities, may develop and is generally reversible if it is recognized early and if drug administration is stopped. Medications or other factors that can cause pancreatitis or peripheral neuropathy should be avoided by patients who are taking ddI. ddI has not been associated with consistent hematopoietic toxicity; in fact, hemoglobin levels and white blood cell and platelet counts frequently improve during ddI therapy. Thus ddI may be particularly useful when hematopoietic suppression—either from drugs or from underlying diseases—is present or anticipated.

ZALCITABINE   Zalcitabine (ddC) is a nucleoside analogue that potently inhibits HIV-1 and HIV-2. The triphosphate of ddC (ddCTP) inhibits HIV reverse transcriptase activity and also acts as a chain terminator. ddC is administered orally, has a plasma half-life of 1.2 h, and is excreted primarily by the kidney. A study comparing ddC with ZDV in patients who had received ZDV for less than 3 months showed that ddC was less effective. Most of the interest in ddC has centered on its use for combination therapy. Because combinations of ZDV and ddC had beneficial effects on CD4 cell counts and p24 antigen concentrations, ddC was licensed for use with ZDV in patients failing to respond clinically or immunologically to ZDV alone. Recently, large-scale trials have indicated a greater clinical benefit of combinations of ZDV plus ddC than of ZDV alone, particularly in patients with less advanced HIV disease. Evaluations of other two- and three-drug combinations including ddC are under way.

The major toxicities of ddC are dose-related peripheral neuropathy and aphthous stomatitis. Hematologic toxicity, as manifested by anemia and neutropenia, has not been a particular problem. Resistance to ddC has been reported and involves substitutions in the reverse transcriptase at positions 65 and 69.

STAVUDINE   Stavudine (d4T) is a thymidine nucleoside analogue active against HIV-1 and HIV-2. It is phosphorylated by cellular kinases to stavudine triphosphate, which inhibits HIV reverse transcriptase and also causes DNA chain termination. Stavudine's relatively limited ability to inhibit cellular thymidine metabolism may account for its relative lack of toxicity in certain cell systems, such

as human bone marrow progenitor cells. Stavudine is well absorbed orally, with a plasma half-life of approximately 1 h; stavudine triphosphate has an intracellular half-life of 3.5 h. Forty percent of a dose is eliminated by renal mechanisms, and dose reductions are recommended for patients with a CrCl of ≤50 mL/min.

Stavudine has been licensed for use in patients with advanced HIV infection who are intolerant of or are failing to respond to approved therapies. This licensure was based on studies in which the drug's administration was associated with improvement in CD4 cell counts and p24 antigen concentrations. Recently, other studies have indicated that patients who are clinically stable after 6 months or more of therapy with ZDV, with CD4 counts between 50 and 500 cells/μL, benefit clinically from being changed to stavudine rather than continuing on ZDV. Stavudine is also being studied as part of various combination regimens. The recommended dose of stavudine (given orally) is 40 mg twice daily for patients weighing ≥60 kg and 30 mg twice daily for patients weighing <60 kg.

Stavudine is generally well tolerated. The major form of toxicity associated with its use is painful peripheral neuropathy. The development of resistance to this agent in vivo has been difficult to characterize, although resistance after serial passage in vitro has been associated with mutations at positions 50 and 75 in the reverse transcriptase.

OTHER ANTIRETROVIRAL AGENTS   Lamivudine (3TC) is another nucleoside analogue inhibitor of reverse transcriptase that is active against HIV-1 and HIV-2. Although well tolerated, it has been relatively unimpressive as monotherapy; moreover, resistance has emerged rapidly in association with mutation at position 184. However, when lamivudine is administered in combination with ZDV, the development of this mutation suppresses phenotypic resistance to ZDV. Clinical trials of ZDV/lamivudine combinations have revealed sustained beneficial effects on CD4 counts and virus loads. The clinical effects of these combinations are being studied.

Nonnucleoside reverse transcriptase inhibitors (nevirapine, delavirdine) are also being evaluated in clinical trials. These drugs are active against HIV-1 but not HIV-2. They are generally well tolerated, with rash as the most troublesome side effect. The rapid development of resistance has been noted during monotherapy; thus the role of these agents is likely to be in combination therapy with other antiretrovirals.

Among the most promising antiretrovirals are the protease inhibitors, including saquinavir, indinavir, and ritonavir. These potent inhibitors of HIV-1 and HIV-2, which have recently been approved by the FDA, interfere with the cleavage of the polyprotein product of viral mRNA. The development of these drugs has been hampered by problems with bioavailability and their other pharmacokinetic properties. Clinical trials of protease inhibitors have shown impressive improvement in CD4 counts and decreases in viral load markers, but viral resistance has emerged after variable periods. Large-scale trials with clinical endpoints are under way to evaluate therapy with these drugs, either singly or in combination with other antiretroviral drugs.

INTERFERONS

From the earliest descriptions of interferon, considerable interest has existed in its application to the prophylaxis and/or treatment of viral infections. Interferons are cytokines that exhibit a broad spectrum of antiviral activities as well as immunomodulating and antiproliferative properties. Early studies with human leukocyte interferon demonstrated an effect in the prophylaxis of experimentally induced rhinovirus infections in humans and in the treatment of VZV infections in immunosuppressed patients. DNA recombinant technology has made available highly purified α, β, and γ interferons that have been evaluated in a variety of viral infections. Results of such trials have confirmed the effectiveness of intranasally administered interferon in the prophylaxis of rhinovirus infections, although its use has been associated with nasal mucosal irritation. Studies have also demonstrated a beneficial effect of intralesionally or systemically administered interferons on genital warts. The effect of systemic administration consists primarily of a reduction in the size of lesions, and this mode of therapy may be useful in individuals who have numerous warts that cannot easily be treated by individual intralesional injection. However, lesions frequently recur after intralesional or systemic interferon therapy is discontinued.

Interferons have undergone extensive study in the treatment of chronic hepatitis B virus (HBV) infection. The administration of interferon α2b (5 million units daily for 16 weeks) to patients with stable chronic HBV infection resulted in loss of markers of HBV replication, such as hepatitis B **e** antigen (HBeAg) and HBV DNA, in 33 to 37 percent of cases; 10 to 20 percent of patients also became negative for hepatitis B surface antigen. In more than 80 percent of patients who lose HBeAg and HBV DNA markers, serum aminotransferases return to normal levels, and both short- and long-term improvements in liver histopathology have been described. Predictors of a favorable response to therapy include low pretherapy levels of HBV DNA, high pretherapy serum levels of alanine aminotransferase (ALT), a short duration of chronic HBV infection, and active liver histopathology. Adverse effects of the above dose of interferon are common and include fever, chills, myalgia, fatigue, neurotoxicity (primarily manifested as somnolence and confusion), and leukopenia. Approximately 25 percent of patients receiving a daily dose of 5 million units will require dose reduction, but fewer than 5 percent will require discontinuation of therapy.

Several interferon preparations, including α2a, α2b, and αL (lymphoblastoid), have been studied as therapy for chronic non-A, non-B/C hepatitis infections. A variety of regimens have been employed, of which the most common are 1 million and 3 million units three times per week for 6 months. A complete response, defined as a return to normal serum ALT values at the end of treatment, has been documented in approximately 40 percent of patients. In addition, liver biopsies have shown decreases in lobular and periportal inflammation. However, relapse has occurred in at least half of all cases upon discontinuation of therapy. Relapses have generally responded quickly to retreatment. Additional clinical studies aimed at developing more

effective regimens and defining prognostic variables in this patient population are under way. A recent study of patients with chronic hepatitis D showed that interferon α2a (9 million units three times per week for 48 weeks) resulted in reversion of ALT values to normal, loss of hepatitis D viral RNA, and histologic improvement in approximately 50 percent of cases. However, relapse was common after treatment was discontinued.

Interferon is licensed in the United States for the treatment of chronic HBV infection (α2b), chronic hepatitis non-A, non-B/C infection (α2b), condyloma acuminatum (α2b, αn3), hairy-cell leukemia (α2a, α2b), and Kaposi's sarcoma (α2a, α2b). Interferon γ (γ1b) is licensed for the treatment of chronic granulomatous disease.

BIBLIOGRAPHY

BEUTNER KR et al: Valacyclovir compared with acyclovir for improved therapy for herpes zoster in immunocompetent adults. Antimicrob Agents Chemother 39:1546, 1995

CONNOR EM et al: Reduction of maternal-infant transmission of human immunodeficiency virus type 1 with zidovudine treatment. N Engl J Med 331:1173, 1994

DOLIN R et al: A controlled trial of amantadine and rimantadine in the prophylaxis of influenza A infection. N Engl J Med 307:580, 1982

FISCHL M et al: The efficacy of azidothymidine (AZT) in the treatment of patients with AIDS and AIDS-related complex; a double-blind placebo-controlled trial. N Engl J Med 317:185, 1987

HALL CB et al: Aerosolized ribavirin treatment of infants with respiratory syncytial viral infection: A randomized double-blind study. N Engl J Med 308:1443, 1983

KAHN JO et al: A controlled trial comparing continued zidovudine with didanosine in human immunodeficiency virus infection. N Engl J Med 327:581, 1992

PERILLO RP et al: A randomized, controlled trial of interferon alfa-2b, alone and after prednisone withdrawal, in the treatment of chronic hepatitis B infection. N Engl J Med 323:295, 1990

REICHMAN RC et al: Treatment of condyloma acuminatum with three different interferons administered intralesionally: A double-blind, placebo-controlled trial. Ann Intern Med 108:675, 1988

STUDIES OF THE OCULAR COMPLICATIONS OF AIDS RESEARCH GROUP: Mortality in patients with the acquired immunodeficiency syndrome treated with either foscarnet or ganciclovir for cytomegalovirus retinitis. N Engl J Med 326:213, 1992

WHITLEY RJ et al: Herpes simplex encephalitis: Adenine arabinoside versus acyclovir therapies. N Engl J Med 314:144, 1986

SECTION 12
DNA VIRUSES

184

Lawrence Corey

HERPES SIMPLEX VIRUSES

DEFINITION Herpes simplex viruses (HSV-1, HSV-2; *Herpesvirus hominis*) produce a variety of infections involving mucocutaneous surfaces, the central nervous system (CNS), and—on occasion—visceral organs. The advent of effective chemotherapy for HSV infections has made prompt recognition of these syndromes even more clinically important than in the past. A related virus, herpes B, is enzootic in some monkey species but has caused rare cases of fatal infection in humans following contact with infected animals.

ETIOLOGIC AGENT The genome of HSV is a linear, double-stranded DNA molecule (molecular weight about 100×10^6) that encodes more than 70 gene products. The genomic structures of the two HSV subtypes are similar, and the overall sequence homology between HSV-1 and HSV-2 is about 50 percent. The homologous sequences are distributed over the entire genome map, and most of the polypeptides specified by one viral type are antigenically related to polypeptides of the other viral type. Many type-specific regions unique to HSV-1 and HSV-2 proteins do exist, however, and many of these regions appear to be important in host immunity. Restriction

endonuclease analysis of viral DNA can be used to distinguish between the two subtypes and among strains of each subtype. The variability of nucleotide sequences from clinical strains of HSV-1 and HSV-2 is such that HSV isolates obtained from two individuals can be differentiated by restriction enzyme patterns unless the isolates are from epidemiologically related sources, such as sexual partners, mother-infant pairs, or victims of a common-source outbreak.

The viral genome is packaged in a regular icosahedral protein shell (capsid) composed of 162 capsomers. The outer covering of the virus is a lipid-containing membrane (envelope) derived from modified cell membrane and acquired as the DNA-containing capsid buds through the inner nuclear membrane of the host cell. Between the capsid and lipid bilayer of the envelope is the tegument. Viral replication has both nuclear and cytoplasmic phases. The initial steps of replication include attachment, fusion between the viral envelope and the cell membrane to liberate the nucleocapsid into the cytoplasm of the cell, and disassembly of the nucleocapsid to release the viral DNA. Replication of HSV is highly regulated. Following fusion of the virion envelope with the host cell membrane, several viral proteins are released from the HSV virion. Some shut off host protein synthesis (by increasing cellular RNA degradation), while others "turn on" transcription of early genes of HSV replication. These early gene products, designated α *genes,* are required for synthesis of the subsequent polypeptide group, the β polypeptides, many of which are regulatory proteins and enzymes required for DNA replication. Most current antiviral drugs interfere with β proteins, such as the viral DNA polymerase enzyme. The third (γ) class of HSV genes requires viral DNA replication for expression and constitutes most of the structural proteins specified by the virus.

Following replication of the viral genome and synthesis of structural proteins, nucleocapsids are assembled in the nucleus of the cell. Envelopment occurs as the nucleocapsids bud through the inner nuclear membrane into the perinuclear space. In some cells, viral replication in the nucleus forms two types of inclusion bodies: type A basophilic Feulgen-positive bodies that contain viral DNA and an eosinophilic inclusion body that is devoid of viral nucleic acid or protein and represents a "scar" of viral infection. Virions are then transported via the endoplasmic reticulum and the Golgi apparatus to the cell surface.

HSV infection of some neuronal cells does not result in cell death. Instead, viral genomes are maintained by the cell in a repressed state compatible with survival and normal activities of the cell, a condition called *latency*. Latency is associated with transcription of only a limited number of virus-encoded proteins. Subsequently, activation of the viral genome may occur, resulting in the normal pattern of regulated viral gene expression, replication, and release of HSV. The release of virus from the neuron and its subsequent entry into epithelial cells result in viral replication. This process is termed *reactivation*. Whereas infectious virus rarely can be recovered from sensory or autonomic nervous system ganglia dissected from cadavers, maintenance and growth of the neural cells in tissue culture result in production of infectious virions (*explantation*) and in subsequent permissive infection of susceptible cells (*cocultivation*). The fact that HSV replication was first detected in neurons during reactivation in vitro suggested that the neuron harbors the latent virus in vivo. Viral DNA and RNA have since been found in neural tissue at times when infectious virus cannot be isolated. Two RNA "latency-associated" transcripts that overlap the immediate early (α) gene products, called ICP-O, are found in abundance in the nuclei of latently infected neurons. These latency-associated transcripts code proteins in an antisense direction. Deletion mutants of this region that can become latent have been made. However, the efficiency of their later reactivation is reduced; thus, the antisense transcripts may play a role in maintaining rather than in establishing latency. At present, the molecular mechanisms of the latency of HSV-1 and HSV-2 are not well understood, and strategies to interrupt latency or to maintain molecular latency in neurons are not available.

PATHOGENESIS Exposure to HSV at mucosal surfaces or abraded skin sites permits entry of the virus and initiation of its replication in cells of the epidermis and dermis. Initial HSV infection is often subclinical—i.e., without clinically apparent lesions. Both clinical acquisition and subclinical acquisition are associated with sufficient viral replication to permit infection of either sensory or autonomic nerve endings. Upon entry into the neuronal cell, the virus— or, more likely, the nucleocapsid—is transported intraaxonally to the nerve cell bodies in ganglia. In humans, the interval from inoculation of virus in peripheral tissue to spread to the ganglia is unknown. During the initial phase of infection, viral replication occurs in ganglia and contiguous neural tissue. Virus then spreads to other mucosal skin surfaces through centrifugal migration of infectious virions via peripheral sensory nerves. This mode of spread helps explain the large surface area involved, the high frequency of new lesions distant from the initial crop of vesicles that is characteristic in patients with primary genital or oral-labial HSV infection, and the recovery of virus from neural tissue distant from neurons innervating the inoculation site. Contiguous spread of locally inoculated virus also may take place and allow further mucosal extension of disease.

After the resolution of primary disease, infectious HSV can no longer be recovered in the ganglia. However, viral DNA can be found in 10 to 50 percent of ganglion cells in the anatomic region of the initial infection. Only about 1 percent of such cells express latency-associated transcripts of RNA detectable by current techniques. The mechanisms by which various stimuli cause the reactivation of HSV infection are unknown. Ultraviolet light, immunosuppression, and trauma to the skin or ganglia are associated with reactivation.

Analysis of the DNA from sequentially isolated strains of HSV or from isolates from multiple infected ganglia in any one individual has revealed identical restriction endonuclease patterns in most persons. Occasionally (most frequently in immunocompromised persons), multiple strains of the same viral subtype are detected in one individual. This finding suggests that exogenous infection with different strains of the same subtype is possible although very uncommon.

IMMUNITY Host responses to infection with HSV influence the acquisition of disease, the severity of infection, resistance to the development of latency, the maintenance of latency, and the frequency of recurrences. Both antibody-mediated and cell-mediated reactions are clinically important. Immunocompromised patients with defects in cell-mediated immunity experience more severe and more extensive HSV infections than those with deficits in humoral immunity, such as agammaglobulinemia. Experimental ablation of lymphocytes indicates that T cells play a major role in preventing lethal disseminated disease, although antibodies help reduce virus titers in neural tissue. Some aspects of the pathogenesis of HSV disease also may be related to the host immune response (e.g., stromal opacities associated with recurrent herpetic keratitis). The surface viral glycoproteins have been shown to be antigens recognized by antibodies mediating neutralization and immune-mediated cytolysis (antibody-dependent cell-mediated cytotoxicity). Monoclonal antibodies specific for each of the known viral glycoproteins have, in experimental infections, conferred protection against subsequent neurologic disease or ganglionic latency. Multiple cell populations, including natural killer cells, macrophages, a variety of T lymphocytes, and lymphokines generated by these cells, play a role in host defenses against HSV infections. In animals, passive transfer of primed lymphocytes confers protection from subsequent challenge. Maximum protection usually requires the activation of multiple T cell subpopulations, including cytotoxic T cells and T cells responsible for delayed hypersensitivity. The latter cells may confer protection by the antigen-stimulated release of lymphokines (e.g., interferons), which may have a direct antiviral effect or may activate other nonspecific effector cells. The HSV virion contains a gene called unique long gene no. 12 (UL-12) that can bind to the cellular transporter-activating protein TAP-1 and reduce the ability of this protein to bind HSV peptides to HLA class I. Thus, the virus may reduce the classic MHC class I expression of the cytotoxic T cell response to itself. This may be an important mechanism for the frequent reactivation of HSV.

EPIDEMIOLOGY Seroepidemiologic studies have documented HSV infections worldwide. Much of the humoral immune response to HSV is to type-common antigenic determinants. Serologic assays with whole-virus antigen preparations, such as complement fixation, neutralization, indirect immunofluorescence, passive hemagglutination, radioimmunoassay, and enzyme-linked immunosorbent assay, do not reliably distinguish between the two viral subtypes. Serologic assays that identify antibodies to type-specific surface proteins of the two subtypes have been developed. These assays, which are based on the demonstration of antibodies to type-specific epitopes of the virus, can reliably distinguish between the human antibody responses to HSV-1 and HSV-2. The most commonly used assays are those which measure antibodies to glycoprotein G of HSV-1 (gG1) and HSV-2 (gG2). A western blot assay that can detect several HSV type-specific proteins can also be used.

Infection with HSV-1 is acquired more frequently and earlier than infection with HSV-2. More than 90 percent of adults have antibodies to HSV-1 by the fifth decade of life. In populations of low socioeconomic status, most persons acquire HSV-1 infection before the third decade of life.

Antibodies to HSV-2 are not detected routinely until puberty. Antibody prevalence rates correlate with past sexual activity and vary greatly among different population groups. Recent serosurveys indicate that nearly 22 percent of the U.S. population has antibodies to

HSV-2—a 30 percent increase in the past 12 years. In most routine obstetric and family planning clinics, 25 percent of women have HSV-2 antibodies, although only 10 percent report a history of genital lesions. As many as 50 percent of heterosexual adults attending sexually transmitted disease clinics have antibodies to HSV-2. Antibody prevalence rates average about 5 percent higher among women than among men. The large reservoir of unidentified carriers of HSV-2 and the frequent asymptomatic reactivation of virus from the genital tract have fostered the continued spread of genital herpes throughout the world. HSV-2 infection has been shown to be an independent risk factor for the acquisition and transmission of infection with human immunodeficiency virus (HIV) type 1. Among coinfected persons, HIV-1 virions can be shed from herpetic lesions of the genital region. This shedding may facilitate the spread of HIV via sexual contact.

HSV infections occur throughout the year. The incubation period ranges from 1 to 26 days (median, 6 to 8 days). Transmission can result from contact with persons with active ulcerative lesions or with persons without clinical manifestations of infection who are shedding HSV or on whose mucosal surfaces the virus is replicating. Asymptomatic salivary excretion of HSV-1 by 2 to 9 percent of adults and 5 to 8 percent of children has been reported. Subclinical shedding of HSV-2 by both men and women infected with this virus has been detected on an average of 2 to 3 percent of days.

The frequency of subclinical reactivation varies greatly among individuals. Twenty percent of women seropositive for HSV-2 may subclinically shed culture-detected virus on >8 percent of days. Recently, polymerase chain reaction (PCR)–based systems have detected HSV-2 shedding on mucosal surfaces of immunocompetent young adults on 15 to 40 percent of days. These data indicate that subclinical reactivation of HSV on mucosal surfaces is more common than has been appreciated. The implication is that most seropositive persons are potential transmitters of the infection. Such data are supported by the continued rise in the seroprevalence of HSV infection worldwide.

CLINICAL SPECTRUM HSV has been isolated from nearly all visceral or mucocutaneous sites. The clinical manifestations and course of HSV infection depend on the anatomic site involved, the age and immune status of the host, and the antigenic type of the virus. First episodes of HSV disease, especially primary infections (i.e., first infections with either HSV-1 or HSV-2 in which the host lacks HSV antibodies in acute-phase serum), are frequently accompanied by systemic signs and symptoms, involve both mucosal and extramucosal sites, and have a longer duration of symptoms, a longer duration of virus isolation from lesions, and a higher rate of complications than recurrent episodes of disease. Both viral subtypes can cause genital and oral-facial infections, and the infections caused by the two subtypes are clinically indistinguishable. However, the frequency of reactivation of infection is influenced by anatomic site and virus type. Genital HSV-2 infection is twice as likely to reactivate and recurs 8 to 10 times more frequently than genital HSV-1 infection. Conversely, oral-labial HSV-1 infection recurs more frequently than oral-labial HSV-2 infection.

Oral-Facial Infections Gingivostomatitis and pharyngitis are the most frequent clinical manifestations of first-episode HSV-1 infection, while recurrent herpes labialis is the most frequent clinical manifestation of reactivation HSV infection. HSV pharyngitis and gingivostomatitis usually result from primary infection and are most commonly seen in children and young adults. Clinical symptoms and signs, which include fever, malaise, myalgias, inability to eat, irritability, and cervical adenopathy, may last from 3 to 14 days. Lesions may involve the hard and soft palate, gingiva, tongue, lip, and facial area. HSV-1 or HSV-2 infection of the pharynx usually results in exudative or ulcerative lesions of the posterior pharynx and/or tonsillar pillars. Lesions of the tongue, buccal mucosa, or gingiva may occur later in the course in one-third of cases. Fever lasting from 2 to 7 days and cervical adenopathy are common. It can be difficult to differentiate HSV pharyngitis clinically from bacterial pharyngitis, *Mycoplasma*

pneumoniae infections, and pharyngeal ulcerations of noninfectious etiologies (e.g., Stevens-Johnson syndrome). No substantial evidence suggests that reactivation oral-labial HSV infection is associated with symptomatic recurrent pharyngitis.

Reactivation of HSV from the trigeminal ganglia may be associated with asymptomatic virus excretion in the saliva, development of intraoral mucosal ulcerations, or herpetic ulcerations on the vermilion border of the lip or external facial skin. About 50 to 70 percent of seropositive patients undergoing trigeminal nerve root decompression and 10 to 15 percent of those undergoing dental extraction develop oral-labial HSV infection a median of 3 days after these procedures.

In immunosuppressed patients, infection may extend into mucosal and deep cutaneous layers. Friability, necrosis, bleeding, severe pain, and inability to eat or drink may result. The lesions of HSV mucositis are clinically similar to mucosal lesions caused by cytotoxic drug therapy, trauma, or fungal or bacterial infections. Persistent ulcerative HSV infections are among the most common infections in patients with AIDS. HSV and *Candida* infections often occur concurrently. Systemic acyclovir therapy speeds the rate of healing and relieves the pain of mucosal HSV infections in immunosuppressed patients. Patients with atopic eczema also may develop severe oral-facial HSV infections (eczema herpeticum), which may rapidly come to involve extensive areas of skin and occasionally disseminate to visceral organs. Extensive eczema herpeticum has resolved promptly with the administration of intravenous acyclovir. Erythema multiforme (EM) also may be associated with HSV infections; some evidence suggests that HSV infection is the precipitating event in about 75 percent of cases of cutaneous EM. HSV antigen has been demonstrated both in circulatory immune complexes and in skin lesion biopsy samples from these patients. Patients with severe HSV-associated EM are candidates for chronic suppressive oral antiviral therapy.

HSV-1 has recently been implicated in the etiology of Bell's palsy (flaccid paralysis of the mandibular portion of the facial nerve). Whether antiviral chemotherapy can alter the course of this infection is unclear.

Genital Infections First-episode primary genital herpes is characterized by fever, headache, malaise, and myalgias. Pain, itching, dysuria, vaginal and urethral discharge, and tender inguinal lymphadenopathy are the predominant local symptoms. Widely spaced bilateral lesions of the external genitalia are characteristic. Lesions may be present in varying stages, including vesicles, pustules, or painful erythematous ulcers. The cervix and urethra are involved in more than 80 percent of women with first-episode infections. First episodes of genital herpes in patients who have had prior HSV-1 infection are associated with less frequent systemic symptoms and faster healing than primary genital herpes. The clinical courses of acute first-episode genital herpes among patients with HSV-1 and HSV-2 infections are similar. However, the recurrence rates of genital disease differ with the viral subtype: the 12-month recurrence rates among patients with first-episode HSV-2 and HSV-1 infections are ~90 percent and 55 percent, respectively (median number of recurrences, 4 and <1, respectively). Recurrence rates for genital HSV-2 infections vary greatly among individuals and over time within the same individual. HSV has been isolated from the urethra and urine of men and women without external genital lesions. A clear mucoid discharge and dysuria are characteristics of symptomatic HSV urethritis. HSV has been isolated from the urethra of 5 percent of women with the dysuria-frequency syndrome. Occasionally, HSV genital tract disease is manifested by endometritis and salpingitis in women and by prostatitis in men.

Both HSV-1 and HSV-2 can cause symptomatic or asymptomatic rectal and perianal infections. HSV proctitis is usually associated with rectal intercourse. However, subclinical perianal shedding of HSV is detected both in heterosexual men and in women who report no rectal intercourse. This phenomenon is due to the establishment of latency in the sacral dermatome from prior genital tract infection, with subsequent reactivation in epithelial cells in the perianal region. Such reactivations are often subclinical. Symptoms of HSV proctitis include anorectal pain, anorectal discharge, tenesmus, and constipation. Sigmoidoscopy reveals ulcerative lesions of the distal 10 cm of the rectal mucosa. Rectal biopsies show mucosal ulceration, necrosis, polymorphonuclear and lymphocytic infiltration of the lamina propria, and (in occasional cases) multinucleated intranuclear inclusion–bearing cells. Perianal herpetic lesions are also found in immunosuppressed patients receiving cytotoxic therapy. Extensive perianal herpetic lesions and/or HSV proctitis is common among patients with HIV infection.

Herpetic Whitlow Herpetic whitlow—HSV infection of the finger—may occur as a complication of primary oral or genital herpes by inoculation of virus via a break in the epidermal surface or by direct introduction of virus into the hand through occupational or some other type of exposure. Clinical signs and symptoms include the abrupt onset of edema, erythema, and localized tenderness of the infected finger. Vesicular or pustular lesions of the fingertip that are indistinguishable from lesions of pyogenic bacterial infection are seen. Fever, lymphadenitis, and epitrochlear and axillary lymphadenopathy are common. The infection may recur. Prompt diagnosis (to avoid unnecessary and potentially exacerbating surgical therapy and/or transmission) is essential. Antiviral chemotherapy (to speed the healing of the process) is usually recommended (see below).

Herpes Gladiatorum HSV may infect almost any area of skin. Mucocutaneous HSV infections of the thorax, ears, face, and hands have been described among wrestlers. Transmission of these infections is facilitated by trauma to the skin sustained during wrestling. Prompt diagnosis and therapy are required to contain the spread of this infection.

Eye Infections HSV infection of the eye is the most frequent cause of corneal blindness in the United States. HSV keratitis presents with an acute onset of pain, blurring of vision, chemosis, conjunctivitis, and characteristic dendritic lesions of the cornea. Use of topical glucocorticoids may exacerbate symptoms and lead to involvement of deep structures of the eye. Debridement, topical antiviral treatment, and/or interferon therapy hastens healing. However, recurrences are common, and the deeper structures of the eye may sustain immunopathologic injury. Chorioretinitis, usually a manifestation of disseminated HSV infection, may occur in neonates or in patients with HIV infection. HSV and varicella-zoster virus can cause acute necrotizing retinitis as an uncommon but severe manifestation.

Central and Peripheral Nervous System Infections HSV is the most commonly identified cause of acute, sporadic viral encephalitis in the United States, accounting for 10 to 20 percent of all cases. The estimated incidence is about 2.3 cases per million persons per year. Cases are distributed throughout the year, and the age distribution appears to be biphasic, with peaks at 5 to 30 and >50 years of age. Subtype 1 virus causes more than 95 percent of cases of HSV encephalitis.

The pathogenesis of HSV encephalitis varies. In children and young adults, primary HSV infection may result in encephalitis; presumably, exogenously acquired virus enters the CNS by neurotropic spread from the periphery via the olfactory bulb. However, most adults with HSV encephalitis have clinical or serologic evidence of mucocutaneous HSV-1 infection prior to the onset of the CNS symptoms. In about 25 percent of the cases examined, the HSV-1 strains from the oropharynx and brain tissue of the same patient differ; thus some cases may result from reinfection with another strain of HSV-1 that reaches the CNS. Two theories have been proposed to explain the development of actively replicating HSV in localized areas of the CNS in persons whose ganglionic and CNS isolates are similar. Reactivation of latent HSV-1 infection in trigeminal or autonomic nerve roots may be associated with extension of virus into the CNS via nerves innervating the middle cranial fossa. HSV DNA has been demonstrated by DNA hybridization in brain tissue obtained at autopsy—even from healthy adults. Thus, reactivation of long-standing latent CNS infection may be another mechanism for the development of HSV encephalitis.

The clinical hallmark of HSV encephalitis has been the acute onset of fever and focal neurologic (especially temporal-lobe) symptoms. Differentiation of HSV encephalitis from other viral encephalitides, as well as from other focal infections and noninfectious processes, is difficult. The most sensitive noninvasive method for early diagnosis

of HSV encephalitis is the demonstration of HSV DNA in cerebrospinal fluid (CSF) by PCR. Although titers of CSF and serum antibodies to HSV increase in most cases of HSV encephalitis, they rarely do so earlier than 10 days into the illness and therefore, while useful retrospectively, are generally not helpful in establishing an early clinical diagnosis. Demonstration of HSV antigen, HSV DNA, or HSV replication in brain tissue obtained by biopsy is highly sensitive and has a low complication rate; examination of such tissue also provides the best opportunity to identify alternative, potentially treatable causes of encephalitis. Antiviral chemotherapy reduces the rate of death from HSV encephalitis. Intravenous acyclovir is more effective than vidarabine. Even with therapy, however, neurologic sequelae are frequent, especially in persons over 35 years of age. Most authorities recommend the administration of intravenous acyclovir to patients with presumed HSV encephalitis until the diagnosis is confirmed or an alternative diagnosis is made.

HSV has been isolated from the CSF of 0.5 to 3 percent of patients presenting to the hospital with aseptic meningitis. HSV meningitis, which is usually seen in association with primary genital HSV infection, is an acute, self-limited disease manifested by headache, fever, and mild photophobia and lasting from 2 to 7 days. Lymphocytic pleocytosis in the CSF is characteristic. Neurologic sequelae of HSV meningitis are rare. HSV is the most commonly identified cause of recurrent lymphocytic meningitis (Mollaret's meningitis). Demonstration of HSV antibodies in CSF or persistence of HSV DNA in CSF can establish the diagnosis. Daily administration of antiviral therapy aimed at reducing the likelihood of clinical HSV reactivation has been successful in such cases.

Autonomic nervous system dysfunction, especially of the sacral region, has been reported in association with both HSV and varicella-zoster virus infections. Numbness, tingling of the buttocks or perineal areas, urinary retention, constipation, CSF pleocytosis, and (in males) impotence may occur. Symptoms appear to resolve slowly over days to weeks. Occasionally, hypesthesia and/or weakness of the lower extremities may persist for many months. Rarely, transverse myelitis manifested by a rapidly progressive symmetric paralysis of the lower extremities or a Guillain-Barré syndrome may follow HSV infection. Similarly, peripheral nervous system involvement (Bell's palsy) or cranial polyneuritis also may be related to reactivation of HSV-1 infection. Transitory hypesthesia of the area of skin innervated by the trigeminal nerve and vestibular system dysfunction as measured by electronystagmography are the predominant signs of disease. Studies to determine whether antiviral chemotherapy may abort these signs or reduce their frequency and severity are unavailable.

Visceral Infections HSV infection of visceral organs usually results from viremia, and multiple-organ involvement is common. Occasionally, however, the clinical manifestations of HSV infection involve only the esophagus, lung, or liver. HSV esophagitis may result from direct extension of oral-pharyngeal HSV infection into the esophagus or may occur de novo by reactivation and spread of HSV to the esophageal mucosa via the vagus nerve. The predominant symptoms of HSV esophagitis are odynophagia, dysphagia, substernal pain, and weight loss. There are multiple oval ulcerations on an erythematous base with or without a patchy white pseudomembrane. The distal esophagus is most commonly involved. With extensive disease, diffuse friability may spread to the entire esophagus. Neither endoscopic nor barium examination can differentiate HSV esophagitis from *Candida* esophagitis or from esophageal ulcerations due to thermal injury, radiation, or corrosives. Endoscopically obtained secretions for cytologic examination and culture provide the most useful material for diagnosis. Systemic antiviral chemotherapy usually reduces symptoms and heals esophageal ulcerations.

HSV pneumonitis is uncommon except in severely immunosuppressed patients and may result from extension of herpetic tracheobronchitis into lung parenchyma. Focal necrotizing pneumonitis usually ensues. Hematogenous dissemination of virus from sites of oral or genital mucocutaneous disease also may occur and produce bilateral interstitial pneumonitis. Bacterial, fungal, and parasitic pathogens are commonly present in HSV pneumonitis. The mortality rate from untreated HSV pneumonia in immunosuppressed patients is high (>80 percent). HSV also has been isolated from the lower respiratory tract of persons with adult respiratory distress syndrome (ARDS). However, the relationship between the isolation of HSV and the pathogenesis of ARDS is unclear.

HSV is an uncommon cause of hepatitis in immunocompetent patients. HSV infection of the liver is associated with fever, abrupt elevations of bilirubin and the serum aminotransferases, and leukopenia (<4000 white blood cells per microliter). Disseminated intravascular coagulation also may develop.

Other reported complications of HSV infection include monarticular arthritis, adrenal necrosis, idiopathic thrombocytopenia, and glomerulonephritis. Disseminated HSV infection in immunocompetent patients is rare. In immunocompromised, burned, or malnourished patients, HSV occasionally disseminates to other visceral organs, such as the adrenal glands, pancreas, small and large intestines, and bone marrow. Rarely, primary HSV infection in pregnancy disseminates and may be associated with the death of both mother and fetus. This uncommon event is usually associated with the acquisition of primary infection in the third trimester.

Neonatal HSV Infection Neonates (infants <6 weeks of age) have the highest frequency of visceral and/or CNS infection of any HSV-infected patient population. If not treated, neonatal herpes undergoes dissemination or develops into CNS infection in >70 percent of cases. Without therapy, the overall rate of death from neonatal herpes is 65 percent; fewer than 10 percent of neonates with CNS infection develop normally. While skin lesions are the most commonly recognized features of disease, many infants do not develop lesions until well into the course of disease. Of the 70 percent of neonatal HSV infections caused by HSV-2, almost all result from contact with infected genital secretions at the time of delivery. However, congenitally infected infants have been reported. Usually these infants are born to mothers who have acquired primary HSV infection during pregnancy. In most series, 30 percent of neonatal HSV infections are due to HSV-1. Most of these cases are associated with the maternal acquisition of primary genital HSV-1 late in pregnancy and the consequent contact of the infant with infectious genital secretions at birth. Neonatal HSV-1 infections may also be acquired through postnatal contact with immediate family members who have symptomatic or asymptomatic oral-labial HSV-1 infection or through nosocomial transmission within the hospital. Antiviral chemotherapy has reduced the rate of death from neonatal herpes to 25 percent. However, the rate of morbidity, especially in infants with HSV-2 infection involving the CNS, is still very high.

DIAGNOSIS Both clinical and laboratory criteria are useful for establishing the diagnosis of HSV infections. A clinical diagnosis can be made accurately when characteristic multiple vesicular lesions on an erythematous base are present. However, it is increasingly being recognized that herpetic ulcerations may clinically resemble skin ulcerations of other etiologies. Mucosal HSV infections may also present as urethritis or pharyngitis without cutaneous lesions. Thus, laboratory studies to confirm the diagnosis and to guide therapy are recommended. Staining of scrapings from the base of the lesions with Wright's, Giemsa's (Tzanck preparation), or Papanicolaou's stain demonstrates characteristic giant cells or intranuclear inclusions of herpesvirus infection. These cytologic techniques are often useful as quick office procedures to confirm the diagnosis. Limitations of the cytologic method are that it does not differentiate between HSV and varicella-zoster virus infections, that it is relatively insensitive, and that the correct identification of giant cells requires experience.

HSV infection is best confirmed in the laboratory by isolation of virus in tissue culture or by demonstration of HSV antigens or DNA in scrapings from lesions. HSV causes a discernible cytopathic effect in a variety of cell culture systems, and most specimens can be identi-

fied within 48 to 96 h after inoculation. Spin-amplified culture with subsequent staining for HSV antigen has shortened the time needed to identify HSV to less than 24 h. The sensitivity of viral isolation depends on the stage of lesions (with higher sensitivity in vesicular than in ulcerative lesions), on whether the patient has a first or a recurrent episode of the disease (with higher sensitivity in first than in recurrent episodes), and on whether the sample is from an immunosuppressed or an immunocompetent patient (with more antigen in immunosuppressed patients). Antigen detection procedures have approached viral isolation in terms of sensitivity in detecting HSV in genital or oral-labial lesions; however, antigen detection appears to be only about 50 percent as sensitive as viral isolation for the identification of HSV in cervical or salivary secretions of asymptomatic patients. PCR techniques appear to be more sensitive for HSV than viral isolation, especially for the diagnosis of CNS infections and for the detection of HSV as a cause of late-stage ulcerative lesions. Laboratory confirmation permits subtyping of the virus; information on subtype may be useful epidemiologically and may help to predict the frequency of reactivation after first-episode oral-labial or genital HSV infection.

Acute- and convalescent-phase serum can be useful in demonstrating seroconversion during primary HSV-1 or HSV-2 infection. However, only 5 percent of patients with recurrent mucocutaneous HSV infections have a fourfold or greater rise in titer of antibody to HSV in the interval between the collection of the first and second samples. Serologic assays, especially type-specific assays, should be used to identify asymptomatic carriers of HSV-1 or HSV-2 infection.

Several studies have shown that persons seropositive for HSV-2 to whom the clinical manifestations of HSV have been explained are able to identify symptomatic reactivations. Individuals seropositive for HSV-2 should be told about the high frequency of subclinical reactivation in mucosal surfaces not visible to the eye (e.g., cervix, urethra, perianal skin) or in microscopic ulcerations that may not be clinically symptomatic. Transmission of infection during such episodes is well established.

℞ **TREATMENT**

Many aspects of mucocutaneous and visceral HSV infections are amenable to antiviral chemotherapy. For mucocutaneous infections, acyclovir and its congeners famciclovir and valacyclovir have been the mainstay of therapy. Several antiviral agents are available for topical use in HSV eye infections: idoxuridine, trifluorothymidine, topical vidarabine, and (recently) cidofovir. For HSV encephalitis and neonatal herpes, intravenous acyclovir is the treatment of choice.

Several compounds have been developed that are effective in the treatment of HSV infections. To date, all work by inhibiting HSV DNA polymerase. One class of drugs, typified by the drug acyclovir, is made up of substrates for the HSV enzyme thymidine kinase. Acyclovir, ganciclovir, famciclovir, and valacyclovir are all selectively phosphorylated to the monophosphate form in virus-infected cells. Cellular enzymes convert the monophosphate form of the drug to the triphosphate, which is then incorporated into the viral DNA chain.

Acyclovir is the best-studied and most frequently used agent for the treatment of HSV infections. Famciclovir, the oral formulation of penciclovir, is also clinically effective in the treatment of a variety of HSV-1 and HSV-2 infections. Currently, no intravenous preparation of penciclovir is available. Thus, for serious HSV infections, acyclovir is the current standard of treatment. Valacyclovir is a valyl ester of acyclovir that has greater bioavailability than acyclovir. Ganciclovir has activity against both HSV-1 and HSV-2; however, as it is more toxic than acyclovir, valacyclovir, and famciclovir, it is generally not recommended for the treatment of HSV infections.

Acyclovir has been shown to be effective in shortening the duration of symptoms and lesions of mucocutaneous HSV infections in immunocompromised patients (Table 184-1). Intravenous and oral acyclovir also prevents reactivation of HSV in seropositive immunocompromised patients during induction chemotherapy for acute leukemia or in the period immediately following bone marrow

Table 184-1

CHAPTER 184
Herpes Simplex Viruses

1085

Antiviral Chemotherapy for HSV Infection

Mucocutaneous HSV infections

Infections in immunosuppressed patients

Acute symptomatic first or recurrent episodes: IV acyclovir (5 mg/kg q 8 h) or oral acyclovir (400 mg qid for 7–10 days) relieves pain and speeds healing. With localized external lesions, 5% topical acyclovir ointment applied 4–6 times daily may be beneficial.

Suppression of reactivation disease: IV acyclovir (5 mg/kg q 8 h) or oral acyclovir (400 mg 3–5 times per day) prevents recurrences during high-risk periods, e.g., the immediate posttransplantation period. In HIV-infected persons, oral famciclovir (500 mg bid) reduces rates of HSV-1 and HSV-2 reactivation.

Genital herpes

First episodes: Oral acyclovir (200 mg 5 times per day or 400 mg tid) is given. Oral valacyclovir (1000 mg bid) or famciclovir (250 mg bid) for 10–14 days is effective. IV acyclovir (5 mg/kg q 8 h for 5 days) is given for severe disease or neurologic complications such as aseptic meningitis.

Symptomatic recurrent genital herpes: Oral acyclovir (200 mg 5 times per day for 5 days), valacyclovir (500 mg bid), or famciclovir (125 mg bid) is effective in shortening lesion duration and viral excretion time.

Suppression of recurrent genital herpes: Oral acyclovir (200-mg capsules bid or tid, 400 mg bid, or 800 mg qd), famciclovir (250 mg bid), or valacyclovir (500 mg bid, or 1000 mg qd) prevents symptomatic reactivation.

Oral-labial HSV infections

First episode: Oral acyclovir (200 mg) is given 4 or 5 times per day.

Recurrent episodes: Topical penciclovir cream is effective in speeding the healing of oral-labial HSV. Topical acyclovir cream is licensed in Europe. The ointment formulation of acyclovir available in the U.S. has no clinical benefit. Oral acyclovir has minimal benefit.

Suppression of reactivation of oral-labial HSV: Oral acyclovir (400 mg bid), if started before exposure and continued for the duration of exposure (usually 5–10 days), will prevent reactivation of recurrent oral-labial HSV infection associated with severe sun exposure.

Herpetic whitlow: Oral acyclovir (200 mg) is given 5 times daily for 7–10 days.

HSV proctitis: Oral acyclovir (400 mg 5 times per day) is useful in shortening the course of infection. In immunosuppressed patients or in patients with severe infection, IV acyclovir (5 mg/kg q 8 h) may be useful.

Herpetic eye infections: In acute keratitis, topical trifluorothymidine, vidarabine, idoxuridine, acyclovir, and interferon are all beneficial. Debridement may be required; topical steroids may worsen disease.

CNS HSV infections

HSV encephalitis: Intravenous acyclovir (10 mg/kg q 8 h; 30 mg/kg per day) for 10 days is preferred.

HSV aseptic meningitis: No studies of systemic antiviral chemotherapy exist. If therapy is to be given IV, acyclovir (15–30 mg/kg per day) should be used.

Autonomic radiculopathy: No studies are available.

Neonatal HSV infections: Acyclovir (45–60 mg/kg per day) is given. Neonates appear to tolerate this high dose of acyclovir. The recommended duration of treatment is 21 days.

Visceral HSV infections

HSV esophagitis: Systemic acyclovir (15 mg/kg per day) should be considered. In some patients with milder forms of immunosuppression, oral therapy with valacyclovir or famciclovir is effective.

HSV pneumonitis: No controlled studies exist. Systemic acyclovir (15 mg/kg per day) should be considered.

Disseminated HSV infections: No controlled studies exist. Intravenous acyclovir nevertheless should be tried. No definite evidence indicates that therapy will decrease the risk of death.

Erythema multiforme associated with HSV: Anecdotal observations suggest that oral acyclovir (400 mg bid or tid) will suppress erythema multiforme.

Infections due to acyclovir-resistant HSV: Foscarnet (40 mg/kg IV q 8 h) should be given until lesions heal. The optimal duration of therapy and the usefulness of its continuation to suppress lesions are unclear. Some patients may benefit from cutaneous application of trifluorothymidine or 5% cidofovir gel. Trials of systemic cidofovir are under way.

transplantation. Famciclovir is currently under study and is also likely to be effective.

Oral acyclovir, famciclovir, and valacyclovir have been shown to speed the healing and resolution of symptoms in first and recurrent episodes of genital HSV-1 and HSV-2 infections. Chronic daily suppressive therapy reduces the frequency of reactivation disease among patients with frequent genital herpes.

Intravenous acyclovir (30 mg/kg per day, given as a 10 mg/kg infusion over 1 h at 8-h intervals) is effective in reducing the rates of death and morbidity from HSV encephalitis. Early initiation of therapy is a critical factor in outcome. The major side effect associated with intravenous acyclovir is transient renal insufficiency, usually due to crystallization of the compound in the renal parenchyma. This adverse reaction can be avoided if the medication is given slowly over 1 h and the patient is well hydrated. Because CSF levels of acyclovir average only 30 to 50 percent of plasma levels, the dosage of acyclovir used for treatment of CNS infection (30 mg/kg per day) is double that used for treatment of mucocutaneous or visceral disease (15 mg/kg per day).

Acyclovir-resistant strains of HSV are being identified with increasing frequency, especially in HIV-infected persons. Almost all clinically significant acyclovir resistance has been seen in immunocompromised patients. Most acyclovir-resistant strains of HSV have an altered substrate specificity for phosphorylating acyclovir. Thus, cross-resistance to famciclovir is usually found. Occasionally, an isolate with altered thymidine kinase (TK) specificity will arise and will be sensitive to famciclovir but not to acyclovir. In some patients infected with TK-deficient virus, higher doses of acyclovir are associated with clearing of lesions. In others, clinical disease progresses despite high-dose therapy. Isolation of HSV from persisting lesions despite adequate dosages and blood levels of acyclovir should raise the suspicion of acyclovir resistance. Therapy with the antiviral drug foscarnet is useful (see Chap. 183). Because of its toxicity and cost, this drug is usually reserved for patients with extensive mucocutaneous infections. Cidofovir is a nucleotide analogue and exists as a phosphonate or monophosphate form. Most TK-deficient strains of HSV are sensitive to cidofovir. Cidofovir ointment has been shown to speed healing of acyclovir-resistant lesions. Clinical trials of systemic cidofovir are under way.

PREVENTION The large reservoir of persons with asymptomatic HSV-1 and HSV-2 infections indicates that the success of efforts to control HSV disease through suppressive antiviral chemotherapy and/or educational programs will be limited. Rather, control of HSV infection will require the prevention of infection—a goal most likely to be attained by vaccination. Several candidate vaccines are under investigation, and the prevention of HSV infection has been assigned a high public health priority.

Barrier forms of contraception, especially condoms, decrease the likelihood of transmission of HSV infection, especially during periods of asymptomatic viral excretion. However, when lesions are present, HSV infection may be transmitted by skin-to-skin contact despite the use of a condom. Nevertheless, the available data suggest that consistent condom use is an effective means of reducing the risk of genital HSV-2 transmission. Prevention of neonatal HSV requires the prevention of acquisition of HSV in the third trimester of pregnancy.

BIBLIOGRAPHY

ASHLEY R et al: Inability of enzyme immunoassays to accurately discriminate between infections with herpes simplex virus types 1 and 2. Ann Intern Med 115:520, 1991

BENEDETTI J et al: Recurrence rates in genital herpes after symptomatic first episode infection. Ann Intern Med 121:847, 1994

BROWN ZA et al: Neonatal herpes simplex virus infection in relation to asymptomatic maternal infection at the time of labor. N Engl J Med 324:1247, 1991

COREY L, SPEAR P: Infections with herpes simplex viruses. N Engl J Med 314:686, 1986

ERLICH KS et al: Acyclovir-resistant herpes simplex virus infections in patients with the acquired immunodeficiency syndrome. N Engl J Med 320:293, 1989

Hook EW et al: Herpes simplex virus infection as a risk factor for human immunodeficiency virus infection in heterosexuals. J Infect Dis 165:251, 1992

Lalezari JP et al: Treatment with intravenous (S)-1-[3-hydroxy-2-(phosphonylmethoxy)propyl]-cytosine of acyclovir-resistant mucocutaneous infection with herpes simplex virus in a patient with AIDS. J Infect Dis 170:570, 1994

Mertz GJ et al: Risk factors for the sexual transmission of genital herpes. Ann Intern Med 116:197, 1992

Oliver L et al: Seroprevalence of herpes simplex virus infections in a family medicine clinic. Arch Fam Med 4:228, 1995

Perry CM, Wagstaff AJ: Famciclovir. A review of its pharmacological properties and therapeutic efficacy in herpesvirus infections. Drugs 50:396, 1995

Safrin S et al: A controlled trial comparing foscarnet with vidarabine for acyclovir-resistant mucocutaneous herpes simplex in the acquired immunodeficiency syndrome. N Engl J Med 325:551, 1991

Stewart JA et al: Herpesvirus infections in persons infected with human immunodeficiency virus. Clin Infect Dis 21(Suppl 1):S114, 1995

Stone KM, Whittington WL: Treatment of genital herpes. Rev Infect Dis 12:S610, 1990

Tedder DG et al: Herpes simplex virus infection as a cause of benign recurrent lymphocytic meningitis. Ann Intern Med 121:334, 1994

Wald A et al: Suppression of subclinical shedding of herpes simplex virus type 2 with acyclovir. Ann Intern Med 124:8, 1996

Whitley RJ, Gnann JW Jr: Acyclovir: A decade later. N Engl J Med 327:782, 1992; 328:671, 1993

———, Lakeman F: Herpes simplex virus infections of the central nervous system: Therapeutic and diagnostic considerations. Clin Infect Dis 20:414, 1995

185 Richard J. Whitley

VARICELLA-ZOSTER VIRUS INFECTIONS

DEFINITION Varicella-zoster virus (VZV) causes two distinct clinical entities: varicella, or chickenpox, and herpes zoster, or shingles. Chickenpox, a ubiquitous and extremely contagious infection, is usually a benign illness of childhood characterized by an exanthematous vesicular rash. With reactivation of latent VZV (which is most common after the sixth decade of life), herpes zoster presents as a dermatomal vesicular rash, usually associated with severe pain.

ETIOLOGY A clinical association between varicella and herpes zoster has been recognized for nearly 100 years. Early in the twentieth century, similarities in the histopathologic features of skin lesions resulting from varicella and herpes zoster were demonstrated. Viral isolates from patients with chickenpox and herpes zoster produced similar alterations in tissue culture—specifically, the appearance of eosinophilic intranuclear inclusions and multinucleated giant cells; these results suggested that the viruses were biologically similar. Restriction endonuclease analyses of viral DNA from a patient with chickenpox who subsequently developed herpes zoster verified the molecular identity of the two viruses responsible for these different clinical presentations.

VZV is a member of the herpesvirus family, sharing with other members such structural characteristics as a lipid envelope surrounding a nucleocapsid with icosahedral symmetry, a total diameter of approximately 150 to 200 nm, and centrally located double-stranded DNA with a molecular weight of approximately 80 million.

PATHOGENESIS AND PATHOLOGY **Primary Infection** Transmission is most likely to take place by the respiratory route; the subsequent localized replication of the virus at an undefined site (presumably the nasopharynx) leads to seeding of the reticuloendothelial system and ultimately to the development of viremia. Viremia in patients with chickenpox is reflected in the diffuse and scattered nature of the skin lesions and can be verified in selected cases by the recovery of VZV from the blood. Vesicles involve the corium and dermis, with degenerative changes characterized by ballooning, the presence of multinucleated giant cells, and eosinophilic intranuclear inclusions. Infection may involve localized blood vessels of the skin, resulting in necrosis and epidermal hemorrhage. With the evolution of disease, the vesicular fluid becomes cloudy because of the recruitment of polymorphonuclear leukocytes and the presence of degenerated cells and fibrin. Ultimately, the vesicles either rupture and release their fluid (which includes infectious virus) or are gradually reabsorbed.

Recurrent Infection The mechanism of reactivation of VZV that results in herpes zoster is unknown. It is presumed that the virus infects the dorsal root ganglia during chickenpox, where it remains latent until reactivated. Histopathologic examination of representative dorsal root ganglia during active herpes zoster demonstrates hemorrhage, edema, and lymphocytic infiltration.

Active replication of VZV in other organs, such as the lung or the brain, can occur during either chickenpox or herpes zoster but is uncommon in the immunocompetent host. Pulmonary involvement is characterized by interstitial pneumonitis, multinucleated giant cell formation, intranuclear inclusions, and pulmonary hemorrhage. Central nervous system (CNS) infection leads to histopathologic evidence of perivascular cuffing similar to that encountered in measles and other viral encephalitides. Focal hemorrhagic necrosis of the brain, characteristic of herpes simplex virus encephalitis, is uncommon in VZV infection.

EPIDEMIOLOGY AND CLINICAL MANIFESTATIONS **Chickenpox** Humans are the only known reservoir for VZV. Chickenpox is highly contagious, with an attack rate of at least 90 percent among susceptible (seronegative) individuals. Individuals of both sexes and all races are infected equally often. The virus is endemic in the population at large; however, it becomes epidemic among susceptible individuals during seasonal peaks—namely, late winter and early spring in the temperate zone. Children between the ages of 5 and 9 are most commonly affected and account for 50 percent of all cases. Most other cases involve children aged 1 to 4 and those aged 10 to 14. Approximately 10 percent of the population of the United States over the age of 15 is susceptible to infection.

The incubation period of chickenpox ranges between 10 and 21 days but is usually between 14 and 17 days. Secondary attack rates in susceptible siblings within a household are between 70 and 90 percent. Patients are infectious approximately 48 h prior to the onset of the vesicular rash, during the period of vesicle formation (which generally lasts 4 to 5 days), and until all vesicles are crusted.

Clinically, chickenpox presents as a rash, low-grade fever, and malaise, although a few patients develop a prodrome 1 to 2 days before onset of the exanthem. In the immunocompetent patient, this is usually a benign illness that is associated with lassitude and with body temperatures of 37.8 to 39.4°C (100 to 103°F) of 3 to 5 days' duration. The skin lesions—the hallmark of the infection—include maculopapules, vesicles, and scabs in various stages of evolution. These lesions, which evolve from maculopapules to vesicles over hours to days, appear on the trunk and face and rapidly spread to involve other areas of the body. Most are small and have an erythematous base with a diameter of 5 to 10 mm. Successive crops appear over a 2- to 4-day period. Lesions also can be found on the mucosa of the pharynx and/or the vagina. Their severity varies from one individual to another. Some individuals have very few lesions, while others have as many as 2000. Younger children tend to have fewer vesicles than older individuals. Secondary and tertiary cases within families are associated with a relatively large number of vesicles. Immunocompromised individuals—both children and adults, particularly those with leukemia—have lesions (often with a hemorrhagic base) that are more numerous and take longer to heal than those of immunocompetent patients. Immunocompromised individuals are also at greater risk for visceral complications, which occur in 30 to 50 percent of cases and are fatal 15 percent of the time.

The most common infectious complication of varicella is secondary bacterial superinfection of the skin, which is usually caused by *Streptococcus pyogenes* or *Staphylococcus aureus*. This complication may result from excoriation of skin lesions after scratching. Gram's staining of skin lesions should help clarify the etiology of unusually erythematous and pustulated lesions.

CHAPTER 185
Varicella-Zoster Virus Infections **1087**

The most common extracutaneous site of involvement in children is the CNS. The syndrome of acute cerebellar ataxia and meningeal irritation generally appears around 21 days after the onset of the rash and rarely develops in the preeruptive phase. The cerebrospinal fluid (CSF) contains lymphocytes and elevated levels of protein. CNS involvement is a benign complication of VZV infection in children and generally does not require hospitalization. Aseptic meningitis, encephalitis, transverse myelitis, Guillain-Barré syndrome, and Reye's syndrome also can occur. Encephalitis is reported in 0.1 to 0.2 percent of children with chickenpox. Other than supportive care, no specific therapy is available for patients with CNS involvement.

Varicella pneumonia is the most serious complication following chickenpox, developing more commonly in adults (up to 20 percent of cases) than in children. It usually has its onset 3 to 5 days into the illness and is associated with tachypnea, cough, dyspnea, and fever. Cyanosis, pleuritic chest pain, and hemoptysis are frequent. Roentgenographic evidence of disease consists of nodular infiltrates and interstitial pneumonitis. Resolution of pneumonitis parallels improvement of the skin rash; however, patients may have persistent fever and compromised pulmonary function for weeks.

Other complications of chickenpox include myocarditis, corneal lesions, nephritis, arthritis, bleeding diatheses, acute glomerulonephritis, and hepatitis. Hepatic involvement, distinct from Reye's syndrome and usually asymptomatic, is common in chickenpox and is usually characterized by elevated levels of liver enzymes, particularly aspartate and alanine aminotransferases.

Perinatal varicella is associated with a high mortality rate when maternal disease develops within 5 days before delivery or within 48 h thereafter. Because the newborn does not receive protective transplacental antibodies and has an immature immune system, the illness may be unusually severe. The reported mortality rate has been as high as 30 percent in this group. Congenital varicella, with clinical manifestations of limb hypoplasia, cicatricial skin lesions, and microcephaly at birth, is extremely uncommon.

Herpes Zoster Herpes zoster, a sporadic disease, is the consequence of reactivation of latent VZV from the dorsal root ganglia. Most patients have no history of recent exposure to other individuals with VZV infection. Herpes zoster occurs at all ages, but its incidence is highest (5 to 10 cases per 1000 persons) among individuals in the sixth through the eighth decades of life. It has been suggested that approximately 2 percent of patients with herpes zoster will develop a second episode of infection.

Herpes zoster, also called shingles, is characterized by a unilateral vesicular eruption within a dermatome, often associated with severe pain. The dermatomes from T3 to L3 are most frequently involved. If the ophthalmic branch of the trigeminal nerve is involved, zoster ophthalmicus results. The factors responsible for the reactivation of VZV are not known. In children reactivation is usually benign, whereas in adults it can be debilitating. The continuum of pain from onset to resolution is known as *zoster-associated pain*. The onset of disease is heralded by pain within the dermatome that may precede lesions by 48 to 72 h; an erythematous maculopapular rash evolves rapidly into vesicular lesions. In the normal host, these lesions may remain few in number and continue to form only for a period of 3 to 5 days. The total duration of disease is generally between 7 and 10 days; however, it may take as long as 2 to 4 weeks for the skin to return to normal. In a few patients, characteristic localization of pain to a dermatome with serologic evidence of herpes zoster has been reported in the absence of skin lesions. When branches of the trigeminal nerve are involved, lesions may appear on the face, in the mouth, in the eye, or on the tongue. In Ramsay Hunt syndrome, pain and vesicles appear in the external auditory canal, and patients lose their sense of taste in the anterior two-thirds of the tongue while developing ipsilateral facial palsy. The geniculate ganglion of the sensory branch of the facial nerve is involved.

The most debilitating complication of herpes zoster, in both the normal and the immunocompromised host, is pain associated with acute neuritis and postherpetic neuralgia. Postherpetic neuralgia is uncommon in young individuals; however, at least 50 percent of patients over age 50 with zoster report some degree of pain in the involved dermatome months after the resolution of cutaneous disease. Changes in sensation in the dermatome, resulting in either hypo- or hyperesthesia, are common.

CNS involvement may follow localized herpes zoster. Many patients without signs of meningeal irritation have CSF pleocytosis and moderately elevated levels of CSF protein. Symptomatic meningoencephalitis is characterized by headache, fever, photophobia, meningitis, and vomiting. A rare manifestation of CNS involvement is granulomatous angiitis with contralateral hemiplegia, which can be diagnosed by cerebral arteriography. Other neurologic manifestations include transverse myelitis with or without motor paralysis.

Like chickenpox, herpes zoster is more severe in the immunocompromised host than in the normal individual. Lesions continue to form for over a week, and scabbing is not complete in most cases until 3 weeks into the illness. Patients with Hodgkin's disease and non-Hodgkin's lymphoma are at greatest risk for progressive herpes zoster. Cutaneous dissemination develops in about 40 percent of these patients. Among patients with cutaneous dissemination, the risk of pneumonitis, meningoencephalitis, hepatitis, and other serious complications is increased by 5 to 10 percent. However, even in immunocompromised patients, disseminated zoster is rarely fatal.

Patients who have received a bone marrow transplant are at particularly high risk of VZV infection. Thirty percent of cases of posttransplantation VZV infection occur within 1 year (50 percent of these within 9 months); 45 percent of the patients involved have cutaneous or visceral dissemination. The mortality rate in this situation is 10 percent. Postherpetic neuralgia, scarring, and bacterial superinfection are especially frequent in VZV infections occurring within 9 months of transplantation. Among infected patients, concomitant graft-versus-host disease increases the chance of dissemination and/or death.

DIFFERENTIAL DIAGNOSIS The diagnosis of chickenpox is not difficult. The characteristic rash and a history of recent exposure should lead to a prompt diagnosis. Other viral infections that can mimic chickenpox include disseminated herpes simplex virus infection in patients with atopic dermatitis and the disseminated vesiculopapular lesions sometimes associated with coxsackievirus infection, echovirus infection, or atypical measles. However, these rashes are more commonly morbilliform with a hemorrhagic component rather than vesicular or vesiculopustular. Rickettsialpox can be confused with chickenpox; however, it can be distinguished easily by detection of the "herald spot" at the site of the mite bite and the development of a more pronounced headache. Serologic testing is useful in differentiating rickettsialpox from varicella.

Unilateral vesicular lesions in a dermatomal pattern should lead rapidly to the diagnosis of herpes zoster, although the occurrence of shingles without a rash has been reported. Both herpes simplex virus infections and coxsackievirus infections can cause dermatomal vesicular lesions. Supportive diagnostic virology and fluorescent staining of skin scrapings with monoclonal antibodies are helpful in ensuring the proper diagnosis. In the prodromal stage of herpes zoster, the diagnosis can be exceedingly difficult and may be made only after lesions have appeared or by retrospective serologic assessment.

LABORATORY FINDINGS Unequivocal confirmation of the diagnosis is possible only through the isolation of VZV in susceptible tissue-culture cell lines, by the demonstration of seroconversion, or by the demonstration of a fourfold or greater rise in antibody titer between convalescent- and acute-phase serum specimens. A rapid impression can be obtained by a Tzanck smear, with scraping of the base of the lesions in an attempt to demonstrate multinucleated giant cells, although the sensitivity of this method is low. Polymerase chain reaction technology for the detection of viral DNA in vesicular fluid is available in some diagnostic laboratories. Direct immunofluorescent staining of cells from the lesion base or detection of viral antigens by other assays (such as the immunoperoxidase assay) is also useful, although these tests are not commercially available. The most frequently employed serologic tools for assessing host response are the immunofluorescent detection of antibodies to VZV membrane antigens, the fluorescent antibody to membrane antigen (FAMA) test, immune adherence hemagglutination, and enzyme-linked immunosorbent assay (ELISA). The FAMA test and the ELISA appear to be the most sensitive.

PROPHYLAXIS While chickenpox in the otherwise healthy host is relatively benign, it can cause morbidity and death. Furthermore, the parents of a child with chickenpox often lose a significant amount of time from work. Recently, a live attenuated varicella vaccine was licensed for administration to all immunocompetent children.

The immunocompromised individual is at significant risk for developing progressive varicella; modalities of prevention include passive immunization or experimental administration of the same live attenuated vaccine used in the immunocompetent child. Immune prophylaxis can consist of the administration of specific zoster immune globulin (ZIG) derived from patients with herpes zoster, varicella-zoster immune globulin (VZIG), or the intravenous formulation of zoster immune plasma (ZIP). Both ZIG and VZIG should be given within 96 h (preferably within 72 h) of exposure to ensure efficacy. It is likely that ZIP can be given somewhat later. Indications for the administration of VZIG are summarized in Table 185-1.

Clinical trials in Japan and the United States have demonstrated the efficacy of live attenuated VZV vaccine (OKA) in both immunocompetent and immunocompromised hosts. This live attenuated vaccine has now been licensed in the United States and is recommended for routine pediatric immunization and for immunization of susceptible adults.

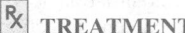 **TREATMENT**
Medical management of chickenpox in the immunologically normal host is directed toward the prevention of avoidable complications. Obviously, good hygiene includes daily bathing and soaks. Secondary bacterial infection of the skin can be avoided by meticulous skin care, particularly with close cropping of fingernails. Pruritus can be decreased with topical dressings or the administration of antipruritic drugs. Tepid water baths and wet compresses are better than drying lotions for the relief of itching. Aluminum acetate soaks for the management of herpes zoster can be both soothing and cleansing. Administration of aspirin to children with chickenpox should be avoided because of the association of aspirin derivatives with the development of Reye's syndrome. Acyclovir therapy (800 mg by mouth five times daily for 5 to 7 days) is recommended for adoles-

cents and adults with chickenpox of ≤24 h duration. Acyclovir therapy for children <12 years of age may likewise be of benefit if initiated early in the disease (<24 h) at a dose of 20 mg/kg every 6 h.

Patients with herpes zoster benefit from oral acyclovir therapy, as evidenced by accelerated healing of lesions and resolution of zoster-associated pain. The dosage is 800 mg 5 times daily for 7 to 10 days. Recently, two new drugs have been licensed for the treatment of herpes zoster (see Chap. 183). Famciclovir, the prodrug of penciclovir, is at least as effective as acyclovir and perhaps more so. One recent study showed twofold faster resolution of postherpetic neuralgia in famciclovir-treated patients with zoster than in recipients of placebo. The dose is 500 mg by mouth three times daily for 7 to 10 days. Valacyclovir, the prodrug of acyclovir, accelerates healing and resolution of zoster-associated pain more promptly than acyclovir. The dose is 1 g by mouth three times daily for 7 to 10 days. Both of these new drugs offer the advantage of a lower dosing frequency.

Both chickenpox and herpes zoster in the immunocompromised host should be treated with intravenous acyclovir, which reduces the occurrence of visceral complications but has no effect on healing of skin lesions or pain. The dose is 10 to 12.5 mg/kg every 8 h for 7 days. These treatment recommendations apply to immunocompromised patients with disseminated herpes zoster as well. Oral acyclovir therapy is not recommended for the treatment of VZV infections in immunocompromised patients. Concomitant with the administration of intravenous acyclovir, it is desirable to attempt to wean these patients from immunosuppressive treatment.

Patients with varicella pneumonia may require removal of bronchial secretions and ventilatory support. Persons with zoster ophthalmicus should be referred immediately to an ophthalmologist. Therapy for this condition consists of the administration of analgesics for severe pain and the use of atropine. Acyclovir will accelerate healing.

The management of acute neuritis and/or postherpetic neuralgia can be particularly difficult. In addition to the judicious use of analgesics, ranging from nonnarcotics to narcotic derivatives, drugs such as amitriptyline hydrochloride and fluphenazine hydrochloride have been reported to be beneficial for pain relief. In one study, glucocorticoid therapy administered early in the course of localized herpes zoster significantly accelerated such quality-of-life improvements as a return to usual activity and termination of analgesia. The dose of prednisone administered orally was 60 mg/d on days 1 through 7, 30 mg/d on days 8 through 14, and 15 mg/d on days 15 through 21. This regimen is appropriate only for relatively healthy elderly persons who have moderate or severe pain. Patients with osteoporosis, diabetes mellitus, glycosuria, or hypertension may not be appropriate candidates. Glucocorticoids should not be used without concomitant antiviral therapy.

Table 185-1

Recommendations for VZIG Administration

Exposure criteria
A. Both exposure to person with chickenpox or zoster as:
  1. Continuous household contact
  2. Playmate for >1 h indoors
  3. Hospital contact (same room or prolonged face-to-face)
  4. Mother (see C below)
B. And time elapsed ≤96 h (preferably ≤72 h)

Candidates (provided they have significant exposure) include
A. Immunocompromised susceptible children
B. Immunocompetent susceptible adolescents (≥15 years old) and adults, especially pregnant women
C. Newborn infants of mothers with onset of chickenpox <5 days before or <2 days after delivery
D. Hospitalized premature infants
  1. ≥28 weeks of gestation when mother has no history of chickenpox
  2. <28 weeks of gestation and/or birth weight of ≤1000 g, regardless of maternal history

SOURCE: Adapted from American Academy of Pediatrics, in Red Book, Report of the Committee on Infectious Diseases, G Peter (ed), Elk Grove Village, IL, American Academy of Pediatrics, 1994.

BIBLIOGRAPHY

BALFOUR HH JR et al: Acyclovir treatment of varicella in otherwise healthy adolescents. J Pediatr 120:627, 1992

BEUTNER KR et al: Valacyclovir compared with acyclovir for improved therapy for herpes zoster in immunocompetent adults. Antimicrob Agents Chemother 39:1547, 1995

BRUNELL PA et al: Prevention of varicella by zoster immune globulin. N Engl J Med 280:1191, 1969

DUNKLE LM et al: A controlled trial of acyclovir for chickenpox in normal children. N Engl J Med 325:1539, 1991

ESSMAN V et al: Prednisone does not prevent postherpetic neuralgia. Lancet 2:126, 1987

GERSHON AA et al: Live attenuated varicella vaccine. JAMA 252:355, 1984

HOPE-SIMPSON RE: The nature of herpes zoster: A long-term study and a new hypothesis. Proc R Soc Med 58:9, 1965

LOCKSLEY RM et al: Infection with varicella-zoster virus after marrow transplantation. J Infect Dis 152:1172, 1985

PROBER CG et al: Acyclovir therapy of chickenpox in immunosuppressed children—a collaborative study. J Pediatr 101:622, 1982

SHEPP D et al: Treatment of varicella-zoster virus in severely immunocompromised patients: A randomized comparison of acyclovir and vidarabine. N Engl J Med 314:208, 1987

TYRING S et al: Famciclovir for the treatment of acute herpes zoster. Effects on acute disease and postherpetic neuralgia: A randomized, double-blind, placebo-controlled trial. Ann Intern Med 123:89, 1995

WEIBEL RE et al: Live attenuated varicella virus vaccine: Efficacy trial in healthy children. N Engl J Med 310:1409, 1984

WELLER TH: Varicella and herpes zoster: Changing concepts of the natural history, control, and importance of a not-so-benign virus. N Engl J Med 309:1362, 1983

WHITLEY RJ et al: Early vidarabine therapy to control the complications of herpes zoster in immunosuppressed patients. N Engl J Med 307:971, 1982

——— et al: Vidarabine therapy of varicella in immunosuppressed patients. J Pediatr 1:125, 1982

——— et al: Varicella-zoster virus infections, in *Antiviral Agents and Viral Diseases of Man*, GJ Galasso et al (eds). New York, Raven, 1984, vol 2, pp 517–542

——— et al: Disseminated herpes zoster in the immunocompromised host: A comparative trial of acyclovir and vidarabine. J Infect Dis 165:450, 1992

——— et al: Acyclovir with and without prednisone for the treatment of herpes zoster: A randomized, placebo-controlled trial. Ann Intern Med 125:376, 1996

WOOD MJ et al: A randomized trial of acyclovir for 7 days or 21 days with and without prednisolone for treatment of acute herpes zoster. N Engl J Med 330:896, 1994

ZAIA JA et al: Evaluation of varicella-zoster immune globulin: Protection of immunosuppressed children after household exposure to varicella. J Infect Dis 147:737, 1983

186   *Jeffrey I. Cohen*

EPSTEIN-BARR VIRUS INFECTIONS, INCLUDING INFECTIOUS MONONUCLEOSIS

DEFINITION   Epstein-Barr virus (EBV) is the cause of heterophile-positive infectious mononucleosis (IM), which is characterized by fever, sore throat, lymphadenopathy, and atypical lymphocytosis. EBV is also associated with several human tumors, including nasopharyngeal carcinoma, Burkitt's lymphoma, Hodgkin's disease, and—in patients with immunodeficiencies (including AIDS)—B-cell lymphoma. The virus, initially discovered in Burkitt's lymphoma cells, is a member of the family Herpesviridae. The viral genome consists of a linear, double-stranded DNA core surrounded by an icosahedral nucleocapsid and by the viral envelope, which contains glycoproteins. The two types of EBV that are widely prevalent in nature are not distinguished by conventional serologic tests.

EPIDEMIOLOGY   EBV infections occur worldwide. These infections are most common in early childhood, with a second peak during late adolescence. By adulthood, more than 90 percent of individuals have been infected and have antibodies to the virus. IM is usually a disease of young adults. In lower socioeconomic groups and in areas of the world with lower standards of hygiene (e.g., developing countries), EBV tends to infect children at an early age, and symptomatic IM is uncommon. In areas with higher standards of hygiene (e.g., the United States), infection with EBV is often delayed until adulthood, and IM is more prevalent.

EBV is spread by contact with oral secretions. The virus is frequently transmitted from adults to infants and among young adults by transfer of saliva during kissing. Transmission by less intimate contact is rare. EBV has been transmitted by blood transfusion and by bone marrow transplantation. While earlier studies suggested that 20 percent of asymptomatic seropositive individuals shed the virus in oropharyngeal secretions, more sensitive studies suggest a figure of more than 90 percent, with up to one-fourth of seropositive persons secreting virus on most days. Rates of virus shedding are especially high among patients with IM and among immunosuppressed patients.

PATHOGENESIS   EBV is transmitted by salivary secretions, usually from asymptomatic persons shedding the virus. The virus infects the epithelium of the oropharynx and the salivary glands and is shed from these cells. While B cells may become infected after contact with epithelial cells, recent studies suggest that lymphocytes in the tonsillar crypts can be infected directly. The virus then spreads through the bloodstream and disseminates throughout the body. The proliferation and expansion of EBV-infected B cells along with reactive T cells during IM result in enlargement of lymphoid tissue. During the acute phase of IM, about 1 in every 1000 B cells in the peripheral blood is infected by EBV, while after recovery, about 1 in every million B cells is infected. Recent data suggest that the B cell, not the epithelial cell, is the reservoir for EBV in the body: Shedding of EBV from the oropharynx stops but the virus persists in B cells when patients are treated with acyclovir.

The EBV receptor (CD21), present on the surface of B cells and epithelial cells, is also the receptor for the C3d component of complement. EBV infection of epithelial cells results in replication of the virus, with the production of virions. When B cells are infected by EBV in vitro, they become transformed and can proliferate indefinitely. During latent infection of B cells, only the EBV nuclear antigens (EBNAs), latent membrane proteins, and small EBV RNAs are expressed in vitro. EBV-transformed B cells secrete immunoglobulin; only a small fraction of cells produce virus.

Acute infection with EBV is accompanied by polyclonal activation of B cells, and antibodies are made to both host-cell and viral proteins. During the first week of infection, the number of T cells increases. Moreover, the percentage of CD4 + T cells decreases, while the percentage of CD8 + T cells increases; the result is an inverted CD4 +/CD8 + ratio. Cellular immunity is more important than humoral immunity in controlling EBV infection. In the initial phase of infection, suppressor T cells, natural killer cells, and nonspecific cytotoxic T cells are important in controlling the proliferation of EBV-infected B cells. Levels of markers of T-cell activation and serum interferon γ are elevated. Later in infection, HLA-restricted cytotoxic T cells that can recognize EBNAs and latent membrane proteins and can destroy EBV-infected cells are generated. Recent studies have shown that one of the late genes expressed during EBV replication, *BCRF1*, exhibits a high degree of amino acid homology with interleukin 10 and can inhibit the production of interferon γ by mononuclear cells in vitro.

If T-cell immunity is compromised, EBV-infected B cells may begin to proliferate. When EBV is associated with lymphoma, its mechanisms of B-cell stimulation are diverse and, in general, EBV-induced proliferation is one step in a multistep process of neoplastic transformation.

CLINICAL MANIFESTATIONS   Most EBV infections in infants and young children either are asymptomatic or present as mild pharyngitis with or without tonsillitis. In contrast, up to 75 percent of infections in adolescents present as IM.

Signs and Symptoms   The incubation period for IM in young adults is about 4 to 6 weeks. A prodrome of fatigue, malaise, and myalgia may last for 1 to 2 weeks before the onset of fever, sore throat, and lymphadenopathy. Fever is usually low-grade and is most common in the first 2 weeks of the illness; however, it may persist for over a month. Common signs and symptoms are listed along with their frequencies in Table 186-1. Lymphadenopathy and pharyngitis are most prominent during the first 2 weeks of the illness, while splenomegaly is more prominent during the second and third weeks. Lymphadenopathy most often affects the posterior cervical nodes but may be generalized. Enlarged lymph nodes are frequently tender and symmetrical but are not fixed in place. Pharyngitis, often the most prominent sign, can be accompanied by enlargement of the tonsils with an exudate resembling that of streptococcal pharyngitis. A morbilliform or papular rash, usually on the arms or trunk, develops in about 5 percent of cases. Most patients treated with ampicillin develop a macular rash; this rash is not predictive of future adverse reactions to penicillins. Erythema nodosum and erythema multiforme have also been described (see Chap. 57). Most patients have symptoms for 2 to 4 weeks, but malaise and difficulty concentrating can persist for months.

Symptomatic IM is uncommon in infants and young children. IM in the elderly presents relatively often as nonspecific symptoms, including prolonged fever, fatigue, myalgia, and malaise; in contrast,

Table 186-1

Signs and Symptoms of Infectious Mononucleosis

Manifestation	Median Percentage of Patients (Range)
SYMPTOMS	
Sore throat	75 (50–87)
Malaise	47 (42–76)
Headache	38 (22–67)
Abdominal pain, nausea, or vomiting	17 (5–25)
Chills	10 (9–11)
SIGNS	
Lymphadenopathy	95 (83–100)
Fever	93 (60–100)
Pharyngitis or tonsillitis	82 (68–90)
Splenomegaly	51 (43–64)
Hepatomegaly	11 (6–15)
Rash	10 (0–25)
Periorbital edema	13 (2–34)
Palatal enanthem	7 (3–13)
Jaundice	5 (2–10)

pharyngitis, lymphadenopathy, splenomegaly, and atypical lymphocytes are relatively rare in elderly patients.

Laboratory Findings The white blood cell count is usually elevated and peaks at 10,000 to 20,000/μL during the second or third week of illness. Lymphocytosis is usually demonstrable, with more than 10 percent atypical lymphocytes. The latter cells are enlarged lymphocytes that have abundant cytoplasm, vacuoles, and indentations of the cell membrane. CD8 + cells predominate among the atypical lymphocytes. Low-grade neutropenia and thrombocytopenia are common during the first month of illness. Liver function is abnormal in more than 90 percent of cases. Serum levels of aminotransferases and alkaline phosphatase are usually mildly elevated; the serum concentration of bilirubin is elevated in about 40 percent of cases.

Complications Most cases of IM are self-limited. Deaths are very rare and most often are due to central nervous system (CNS) complications, splenic rupture, upper airway obstruction, or bacterial superinfection.

CNS complications usually develop during the first 2 weeks of EBV infection; in some patients, especially children, they are the only clinical manifestations of IM. Heterophile antibodies and atypical lymphocytes may be absent. Meningitis and encephalitis are the most common neurologic abnormalities, and patients may present with headache, meningismus, or cerebellar ataxia; acute hemiplegia and psychosis have also been described. The cerebrospinal fluid (CSF) contains mainly lymphocytes, with occasional atypical lymphocytes. Most cases resolve without neurologic sequelae. Acute EBV infection has also been associated with cranial nerve palsies (especially ones involving cranial nerve VII), Guillain-Barré syndrome, acute transverse myelitis, and peripheral neuritis.

Autoimmune hemolytic anemia occurs in about 2 percent of cases during the first 2 weeks. In most cases the anemia is Coombs'-test positive, with cold agglutinins directed against the i red blood cell antigen. Most patients with hemolysis have mild anemia that lasts for 1 or 2 months, but some patients have severe disease with hemoglobinuria and jaundice. Nonspecific antibody responses may also include rheumatoid factor, antinuclear antibodies, anti-smooth muscle antibodies, antiplatelet antibodies, and cryoglobulins. IM has been associated with red-cell aplasia, severe granulocytopenia, pancytopenia, and hemophagocytic syndrome. The spleen ruptures in fewer than 0.5 percent of cases. Splenic rupture is more common among males than among females and may be manifest as abdominal pain, referred shoulder pain, or hemodynamic compromise.

Hypertrophy of lymphoid tissue in the tonsils or adenoids can result in upper airway obstruction, as can inflammation and edema of the epiglottis, pharynx, or uvula. About 10 percent of patients with IM develop streptococcal pharyngitis after their initial sore throat resolves.

Other rare complications associated with acute EBV infection include hepatitis (which can be fulminant), myocarditis or pericarditis with electrocardiographic changes, pneumonia with pleural effusion, interstitial nephritis, and vasculitis.

OTHER DISEASES ASSOCIATED WITH EBV INFECTION EBV-associated lymphoproliferative disease has been described in patients with congenital or acquired immunodeficiency, including those with ataxia-telangiectasia, severe combined immunodeficiency, or AIDS; recipients of bone marrow transplants; and recipients of organ transplants who are receiving immunosuppressive drugs (especially cyclosporine). Proliferating EBV-infected B cells infiltrate lymph nodes and multiple organs, and patients present with fever and lymphadenopathy or gastrointestinal symptoms. Pathologic studies show B-cell hyperplasia or poly- or monoclonal lymphoma. The X-linked lymphoproliferative syndrome (Duncan's disease) is a recessive disorder of young boys who have a normal response to childhood infections but develop fatal lymphoproliferative disorders after infection with EBV. Most patients with this syndrome die of acute IM; others develop hypogammaglobulinemia, malignant B-cell lymphomas, aplastic anemia, or agranulocytosis. IM has also proved fatal to some patients with no obvious preexisting immune abnormality.

Oral hairy leukoplakia is an early manifestation of infection with human immunodeficiency virus (HIV) in adults (see Chap. 308). Most patients present with raised, white corrugated lesions on the tongue (and occasionally on the buccal mucosa) that contain EBV DNA. Children infected with HIV can develop lymphoid interstitial pneumonitis; EBV DNA is often found in lung tissue from these patients.

Patients with the chronic fatigue syndrome may have titers of antibody to EBV that are elevated but are not significantly different from those in healthy EBV-seropositive adults. While some patients have malaise and fatigue that persists for weeks or months after IM, persistent EBV infection is not a cause of the chronic fatigue syndrome. Chronic active EBV infection is very rare and is distinct from the chronic fatigue syndrome. The affected patients have an illness lasting more than 6 months with markedly elevated titers of antibody to EBV and evidence of organ involvement, including hepatosplenomegaly, lymphadenopathy, and pneumonitis, uveitis, or neurologic disease.

EBV is associated with several malignancies. About 15 percent of cases of Burkitt's lymphoma in the United States and about 90 percent of those in Africa are associated with EBV (see Chap. 113). African patients with Burkitt's lymphoma have high levels of antibody to EBV, and their tumor tissue usually contains viral DNA. Anaplastic nasopharyngeal carcinoma is uniformly associated with EBV; the affected tissues contain viral DNA and antigens. Patients with nasopharyngeal carcinoma often have elevated titers of antibody to EBV (see Chap. 89).

EBV has been associated with Hodgkin's disease, especially the mixed-cellularity type (see Chap. 113). Patients with Hodgkin's disease often have elevated titers of antibody to EBV, and in about half of cases viral DNA and antigens are found in Reed-Sternberg cells. In some cases, EBV DNA has been detected in tonsillar carcinoma, angioimmunoblastic lymphadenopathy, angiocentric immunoproliferative lesions, T-cell lymphoma, thymoma, gastric carcinoma, and CNS lymphoma tissues from patients with no underlying immunodeficiency. Recent studies have demonstrated viral DNA in leiomyosarcomas from AIDS patients and in smooth muscle tumors from organ transplant recipients. Virtually all CNS lymphomas in AIDS patients are associated with EBV.

DIAGNOSIS Serologic Testing The heterophile test is used for the diagnosis of IM in children and adults (Table 186-2). Heterophile antibody is an IgM antibody that does not bind EBV proteins. In the test for this antibody, human serum is absorbed with guinea pig kidney, and the heterophile titer is defined as the greatest serum dilution that agglutinates sheep, horse, or cow erythrocytes. A titer of 40-fold or greater is diagnostic of acute EBV infection in a patient who has symptoms compatible with IM and atypical lymphocytes. Tests for heterophile antibodies are positive in 40 percent of patients with IM during the first week of illness and in 80 to 90 percent during the third week. Therefore, repeated testing may be necessary, especially if the initial test is performed early. Tests usually remain positive for 3 months after the onset of illness, but heterophile antibodies can persist for up to 1 year. These antibodies usually are not detectable in children less than 5 years of age, in the elderly, or in patients presenting with symptoms not typical of IM. The commercially available monospot test for heterophile antibodies is somewhat more sensitive than the classic heterophile test. False-positive results in the monospot test are more common in children and in patients with other viral infections.

EBV-specific antibody testing is used for patients with suspected acute EBV infection who lack heterophile antibodies and for patients with atypical infections. Serologic tests are particularly useful in young children, who often do not develop heterophile antibodies. Titers of IgM and IgG antibodies to viral capsid antigen (VCA) are elevated in the serum of more than 90 percent of patients at the onset of disease. IgM antibody to VCA is useful for the diagnosis of acute IM because it is present at elevated titers only during the first 2 months of the disease; in contrast, IgG antibody to VCA is often used to assess exposure to EBV in the past because it persists for life.

Antibodies to early antigens (EAs) are found either in a diffuse pattern in the nucleus and cytoplasm of infected cells (EA-D antibody) or restricted to the cytoplasm (EA-R antibody). These antibodies are detectable 3 to 4 weeks after the onset of symptoms in patients with IM. About 70 percent of individuals with IM, especially those with relatively severe disease, have EA-D antibodies during the course of their illness. These antibodies usually persist for only 3 to 6 months. Levels of EA-D antibodies are also elevated in patients with nasopharyngeal carcinoma or chronic active EBV infection. EA-R antibodies are only occasionally detected in patients with IM but are often found at elevated titers in patients with African Burkitt's lymphoma or chronic active EBV infection.

IgA antibodies to EBV antigens have proved useful for the identification of patients with nasopharyngeal carcinoma and of persons at high risk for the disease. Seroconversion to EBNA positivity is also useful for the diagnosis of acute infection with EBV. Antibodies to EBNA are detectable relatively late (3 to 6 weeks after the onset of symptoms) in nearly all cases of acute EBV infection and persist for the lifetime of the patient. These antibodies may be lacking in immunodeficient patients and in those with chronic active EBV infection.

Other Studies Detection of EBV DNA, RNA, or proteins has been valuable in demonstrating the association of the virus with various malignancies. The polymerase chain reaction has been used to detect EBV DNA in the CSF of some AIDS patients with lymphomas and to monitor the amount of EBV DNA in the blood of patients with lymphoproliferative disease. Culture of EBV from throat washings or blood is not helpful in the diagnosis of acute infection, since EBV commonly persists in the oropharynx and in B cells for the lifetime of the infected individual.

Differential Diagnosis The differential diagnosis of IM and atypical lymphocytosis includes acute infection with cytomegalovirus, *Toxoplasma*, HIV, human herpesvirus 6, and hepatitis virus as well as drug hypersensitivity reactions. Cytomegalovirus is the most common cause of heterophile-negative mononucleosis, usually involves older patients, and is associated with a lower frequency of sore throat, splenomegaly, and lymphadenopathy than IM due to EBV. Other diseases that share some of the features of IM include rubella, acute infectious lymphocytosis in children, and lymphoma or leukemia.

Table 186-2

Serologic Features of EBV-Associated Diseases

		Anti-VCA		Anti-EA		
Condition	Heterophile	IgM	IgG	EA-D	EA-R	Anti-EBNA
Acute infectious mononucleosis	+	+	+ +	+	−	−
Convalescence	±	−	+	−	±	+
Past infection	−	−	+	−	−	+
Reactivation with immunodeficiency	−	−	+ +	+	+	±
Burkitt's lymphoma	−	−	+ + +	±	+ +	+
Nasopharyngeal carcinoma	−	−	+ + +	+ +	±	+

* VCA, viral capsid antigen; EA, early antigen; EA-D antibody, antibody to early antigen, diffuse pattern in nucleus and cytoplasm of infected cells; EA-R antibody, antibody to early antigen, restricted to the cytoplasm; and EBNA, Epstein-Barr nuclear antigen.

SOURCE: Adapted from Okano.

℞ TREATMENT

Therapy for IM consists of supportive measures, with rest and analgesia. Excessive physical activity during the first month should be avoided to reduce the possibility of splenic rupture. If splenic rupture occurs, splenectomy is required. Glucocorticoid therapy is not indicated for uncomplicated IM and in fact may predispose to bacterial superinfection. Prednisone (40 to 60 mg/d for 2 to 3 days, with subsequent tapering of the dose over 1 to 2 weeks) have been used for the prevention of airway obstruction in patients with severe tonsillar hypertrophy, for autoimmune hemolytic anemia, and for severe thrombocytopenia. These agents have also been used in a few selected patients with severe malaise and fever and in patients with severe CNS or cardiac disease.

Acyclovir has had no significant clinical impact on IM in controlled trials. However, at a dosage of 400 to 800 mg five times daily, it has been effective for the treatment of oral hairy leukoplakia (despite common relapses) and some cases of chronic active EBV disease. Acyclovir generally has not been beneficial for patients with lymphoproliferative syndromes. When possible, therapy for EBV lymphoproliferative disease should be directed toward the reduction of immunosuppressive medication. New therapies, including the use of interferon α and the infusion of donor T cells or EBV-specific cytotoxic T cells, are being studied.

The isolation of patients with IM is unnecessary. Vaccines directed against the major EBV glycoprotein have been effective in animal studies and are currently undergoing small-scale clinical trials.

BIBLIOGRAPHY

COHEN JI: Epstein-Barr virus lymphoproliferative disease associated with acquired immunodeficiency. Medicine 70:137, 1991

HESLOP HE et al: Long-term restoration of immunity against Epstein-Barr virus infection by adoptive transfer of gene-modified virus-specific T lymphocytes. Nat Med 2:551, 1996

KHANNA R et al: Immune regulation in Epstein-Barr virus-associated diseases. Microbiol Rev 59:387, 1995

OKANO M et al: Epstein-Barr virus and human diseases: Recent advances in diagnosis. Clin Microbiol Rev 1:300, 1988

PAPADOPOULOS EB et al: Infusions of donor leukocytes to treat Epstein-Barr virus-associated lymphoproliferative disorders after allogeneic bone marrow transplantation. N Engl J Med 330:1185, 1994

PATHMANATHAN R et al: Clonal proliferations of cells infected with Epstein-Barr virus in preinvasive lesions related to nasopharyngeal carcinoma. N Engl J Med 333:693, 1995

RICKINSON AB, KIEFF E: Epstein-Barr virus, in Fields Virology, 3d ed, BN Fields et al (eds). Philadelphia, Lippincott-Raven, 1996

SCHLOSSBERG D (ed): Infectious Mononucleosis, 2d ed. New York, Springer-Verlag, 1989

STRAUS SE et al: Epstein-Barr virus infections: Biology, pathogenesis, and management. Ann Intern Med 118:45, 1993

VAN DER HORST C et al: Lack of effect of peroral acyclovir for the treatment of infectious mononucleosis. J Infect Dis 164:788, 1991

187 | *Martin S. Hirsch*

CYTOMEGALOVIRUS AND HUMAN HERPESVIRUS TYPES 6, 7, AND 8

CYTOMEGALOVIRUS

DEFINITION Cytomegalovirus (CMV), which was initially isolated from patients with congenital cytomegalic inclusion disease, is now recognized as an important pathogen in all age groups. In addition to inducing severe birth defects, CMV causes a wide spectrum of disorders in older children and adults, ranging from an asymptomatic, subclinical infection to a mononucleosis syndrome in healthy individuals to disseminated disease in immunocompromised patients. Human CMV is one of several related species-specific viruses that cause similar diseases in various animals. All are associated with the production of characteristic enlarged cells—hence the name *cytomegalovirus*.

CMV is a member of the beta herpesvirus group and has double-stranded DNA, a protein capsid, and a lipoprotein envelope. Like other members of the herpesvirus group, CMV demonstrates icosahedral symmetry, replicates in the cell nucleus, and can cause either a lytic and productive or a latent infection. CMV can be distinguished from other herpesviruses by certain biologic properties, such as host range and type of cytopathology induced. Viral replication is associated with the production of large intranuclear inclusions and smaller cytoplasmic inclusions. The virus appears to replicate in a variety of cell types in vivo; in tissue culture it grows preferentially in fibroblasts. Although there is little evidence that CMV is oncogenic in vivo, the virus does transform fibroblasts in rare instances, and genomic transforming fragments have been identified.

EPIDEMIOLOGY CMV has a worldwide distribution. Approximately 1 percent of newborns in the United States are infected with CMV, and the percentage is higher in many less developed countries. Communal living and poor personal hygiene facilitate early spread. Perinatal and early childhood infections are common. Virus may be present in milk, saliva, feces, and urine. Transmission of CMV has been identified among young children in day-care centers and has been traced from infected toddler to pregnant mother to developing fetus. When an infected child introduces CMV into a household, 50 percent of susceptible family members seroconvert within 6 months.

The virus is not readily spread by casual contact but requires repeated or prolonged intimate exposure for transmission. In late ado-

lescence and young adulthood, CMV is often transmitted sexually, and asymptomatic viral carriage in semen or cervical secretions is common. CMV antibody is present at detectable levels in nearly 100 percent of female prostitutes and sexually active homosexual men. Sexually active adults may harbor several strains of CMV simultaneously. Transfusion of whole blood or certain blood products containing viable leukocytes also may transmit CMV, with a frequency of 0.14 to 10 percent per unit transfused.

Once infected, an individual probably carries the virus for life. The infection usually remains latent. However, CMV reactivation syndromes develop frequently when T lymphocyte–mediated immunity is compromised—for example, after organ transplantation or in association with lymphoid neoplasms and certain acquired immunodeficiencies (in particular, infection with human immunodeficiency virus or HIV; see Chap. 308). Most primary CMV infections in organ transplant recipients result from transmission of the virus in the graft itself. In CMV-seropositive transplant recipients, infection results from reactivation of latent virus or, less commonly, from reinfection by a new strain of CMV.

PATHOGENESIS Congenital CMV infection can result from either primary or reactivation infection of the mother. However, clinical disease in the fetus or newborn is almost exclusively related to primary maternal infection (Table 187-1). The factors determining the severity of congenital infection are unknown; a deficient capacity to produce precipitating antibodies and to mount T cell responses to CMV is associated with relatively severe disease.

Primary infection in late childhood or adulthood is often associated with a vigorous T lymphocyte response that may contribute to the development of a mononucleosis syndrome similar to that observed following Epstein-Barr virus infection (see Chap. 186). The hallmark of such infection is the appearance of atypical lymphocytes in the peripheral blood; these cells are predominantly activated CD8+ T lymphocytes. Polyclonal activation of B cells by the virus contributes to the development of rheumatoid factors and other autoantibodies during CMV mononucleosis.

Once acquired by symptomatic or asymptomatic primary infection, CMV persists indefinitely in tissues of the host. The sites of persistent or latent infection are unclear but probably include multiple cell types and various organs. Transmission following blood transfusion or organ transplantation is due to silent infections in these tissues. Autopsy studies suggest that salivary glands and bowel also may be areas of latent infection.

If the host's T cell responses become compromised by disease or by iatrogenic immunosuppression, latent virus can be reactivated to cause a variety of syndromes. Chronic antigenic stimulation in the presence of immunosuppression (for example, following tissue transplantation) appears to be an ideal setting for CMV activation and CMV-induced disease. Certain particularly potent suppressants of T cell immunity, such as antithymocyte globulin, are associated with a high rate of clinical CMV syndromes, which may follow either primary or reactivation infection. CMV may itself contribute to further T lymphocyte hyporesponsiveness, which often precedes superinfection with other opportunistic pathogens, such as *Pneumocystis carinii*. CMV and *P. carinii* are frequently found together in immunosuppressed patients with severe interstitial pneumonia. CMV may function as a cofactor to activate latent HIV infection.

PATHOLOGY Cytomegalic cells in vivo (presumed to be infected epithelial cells) are two to four times larger than surrounding cells and often contain an 8- to 10-μm intranuclear inclusion that is eccentrically placed and is surrounded by a clear halo, producing an

Table 187-1

CMV in the Immunocompromised Host

Population	Risk Factors	Principal Syndromes	Treatment	Prevention
Fetus	Primary maternal infection/early pregnancy	Cytomegalic inclusion disease	None	Avoidance of exposure
Organ transplant recipient	Seropositive donor, seronegative recipient; intensive immunosuppression, particularly with antilymphocyte globulins, cyclosporine	Febrile leukopenia; pneumonia; gastrointestinal disease	Ganciclovir	Donor matching; CMV immunoglobulin; ganciclovir or high-dose acyclovir
Bone marrow transplant recipient	Graft-vs.-host disease; older age; seropositive recipient; viremia	Pneumonia; gastrointestinal disease	Ganciclovir plus CMV immunoglobulin	Ganciclovir or high-dose acyclovir
Person with AIDS	<100 CD4+ cells per microliter; CMV seropositivity	Retinitis; gastrointestinal disease; neurologic disease	Foscarnet or ganciclovir	Trials under way; oral ganciclovir?

"owl's eye" appearance. Smaller granular cytoplasmic inclusions are demonstrated occasionally. Cytomegalic cells are found in a wide variety of organs, including salivary gland, lung, liver, kidney, intestine, pancreas, adrenal gland, and the central nervous system.

The cellular inflammatory response to infection consists of plasma cells, lymphocytes, and monocyte-macrophages. Granulomatous reactions occasionally develop, particularly in the liver. Immunopathologic reactions may contribute to CMV disease. Immune complexes have been detected in infected infants, sometimes in association with CMV-related glomerulopathies. Immune-complex glomerulopathy has been observed in some CMV-infected patients after renal transplantation.

CLINICAL MANIFESTATIONS   Congenital CMV Infection   Fetal infections range from inapparent to severe and disseminated. Cytomegalic inclusion disease develops in approximately 5 percent of infected fetuses and is seen almost exclusively in infants born to mothers who develop primary infections during pregnancy. Petechiae, hepatosplenomegaly, and jaundice are the most common presenting features (60 to 80 percent of cases). Microcephaly with or without cerebral calcifications, intrauterine growth retardation, and prematurity are reported in 30 to 50 percent of cases. Inguinal hernias and chorioretinitis are less common. Laboratory abnormalities, in decreasing order of frequency, include a serum IgM level of >0.20 g/L (>20 mg/dL), atypical lymphocytosis, elevated concentrations of liver aminotransferases, thrombocytopenia, hyperbilirubinemia, and a cerebrospinal fluid protein level of >0.20 g/L (>20 mg/dL). The prognosis for severely infected infants is poor; the mortality rate is 20 to 30 percent, and few of the patients who survive escape intellectual or hearing difficulties in later years. The differential diagnosis of cytomegalic inclusion disease in infants includes syphilis, rubella, toxoplasmosis, infection with herpes simplex virus or enterovirus, and bacterial sepsis.

Most congenital CMV infections are clinically inapparent at birth. Between 5 and 25 percent of asymptomatically infected infants develop significant psychomotor, hearing, ocular, or dental abnormalities over the next several years.

Perinatal CMV Infection   The newborn may acquire CMV at the time of delivery by passage through an infected birth canal or by postnatal contact with maternal milk or other secretions. Approximately 40 to 60 percent of infants who are breast-fed for longer than 1 month by seropositive mothers become infected. Iatrogenic transmission also can result from neonatal blood transfusion. Screening of blood products before they are transfused into low-birth-weight seronegative infants or into seronegative pregnant women decreases the risk of infection.

The great majority of infants infected at or after delivery remain asymptomatic. However, protracted interstitial pneumonitis has been associated with perinatally acquired CMV infection, particularly in premature infants, and occasionally has been accompanied by infection with *Chlamydia trachomatis*, *P. carinii*, or *Ureaplasma urealyticum*. Poor weight gain, adenopathy, rash, hepatitis, anemia, and atypical lymphocytosis also may be found, and CMV excretion often persists for months or years.

CMV Mononucleosis   The most common clinical manifestation of CMV infection in normal hosts beyond the neonatal period is a heterophil antibody–negative mononucleosis syndrome. This manifestation may develop spontaneously or may follow the transfusion of leukocyte-containing blood products. Although the syndrome occurs at all ages, it most often involves sexually active young adults. Incubation periods range from 20 to 60 days, and the illness generally lasts for 2 to 6 weeks. Prolonged high fevers, sometimes accompanied by chills, profound fatigue, and malaise, characterize this disorder. Myalgias, headache, and splenomegaly are frequent, but in CMV mononucleosis (as opposed to infectious mononucleosis caused by Epstein-Barr virus), exudative pharyngitis and cervical lymphadenopathy are rare. Occasional patients develop rubelliform rashes, often after exposure to ampicillin. Less commonly observed are interstitial or segmental pneumonia, myocarditis, pleuritis, arthritis, and encephalitis. In rare cases, Guillain-Barré syndrome complicates CMV mononucleosis. The characteristic laboratory abnormality is relative lymphocytosis in periph-

eral blood, with more than 10 percent atypical lymphocytes. Total leukocyte counts may be low, normal, or markedly elevated. Although significant jaundice is uncommon, serum aminotransferase and alkaline phosphatase levels are often moderately elevated. Heterophil antibodies are absent; however, transient immunologic abnormalities are common and may include the presence of cryoglobulins, rheumatoid factors, cold agglutinins, and antinuclear antibodies. Hemolytic anemia, thrombocytopenia, and granulocytopenia complicate recovery in rare instances.

Most patients recover without sequelae, although postviral asthenia may persist for months. The excretion of CMV in urine, genital secretions, and/or saliva often continues for months or years. Rare patients have recurrent episodes of fever and malaise, sometimes associated with autonomic nervous system dysfunction (e.g., attacks of sweating or flushing).

CMV Infection in the Immunocompromised Host (See also Table 187-1)   CMV appears to be the most common and important viral pathogen complicating organ transplantation. In recipients of kidney, heart, lung, and liver transplants, CMV induces a variety of syndromes, including fever and leukopenia, hepatitis, pneumonitis, esophagitis, gastritis, colitis, and retinitis. The period of maximal risk is between 1 and 4 months after transplantation, although retinitis may be a later complication. The risk of disease appears to be greater after primary infection than after reactivation. In addition, molecular studies indicate that seropositive transplant recipients are susceptible to reinfection with donor-derived, genotypically variant CMV, and such infection often results in disease. Reactivation infection, although frequent, is less likely than primary infection to be important clinically. Clinical disease is related to various factors (see Table 187-1), such as the degree of immunosuppression; patients receiving certain immunosuppressive agents, such as antithymocyte globulin, appear to be more likely to have severe infections than those receiving other agents, such as cyclosporine. The transplanted organ is particularly vulnerable as a target for CMV infection; thus, there is a tendency for CMV hepatitis to follow liver transplantation and for CMV pneumonitis to follow lung transplantation.

CMV pneumonia occurs in nearly 15 to 20 percent of bone marrow transplant recipients, with a case-fatality rate of 84 to 88 percent. The risk is greatest between 5 and 13 weeks after transplantation, and the several risk factors identified include certain types of immunosuppressive therapy, acute graft-versus-host disease, older age, viremia, and seropositivity before transplantation.

CMV is recognized as an important pathogen in patients with AIDS (see Chap. 308). In fact, CMV infection is nearly universal in these patients and often causes retinitis or disseminated disease, contributing to death. CMV-associated clinical syndromes occur predominantly when peripheral-blood CD4+ cell counts fall below 50 to 100/μL. CMV-induced immunosuppression probably contributes to the T lymphocyte deficiency initiated by the etiologic retrovirus.

Syndromes produced by CMV in the immunocompromised host often begin with prolonged fever, malaise, anorexia, fatigue, night sweats, and arthralgias or myalgias. Liver function abnormalities, leukopenia, thrombocytopenia, and atypical lymphocytosis may be observed during these episodes. The development of tachypnea, hypoxia, and unproductive cough signals respiratory involvement. Radiologic examination of the lung often demonstrates bilateral interstitial or reticulonodular infiltrates, which begin in the periphery of the lower lobes and spread centrally and superiorly; localized segmental, nodular, or alveolar patterns are less common. The differential diagnosis includes infection with *P. carinii*; infections due to other viral, bacterial, or fungal pathogens; pulmonary hemorrhage; and injury secondary to irradiation or to treatment with cytotoxic drugs.

Gastrointestinal CMV involvement may be localized or extensive and almost exclusively affects compromised hosts. Ulcers of the esophagus, stomach, small intestine, or colon may result in bleeding or perforation. CMV infection may lead to exacerbations of underlying ulcerative colitis. Hepatitis occurs frequently, particularly following liver transplantation, and CMV-associated acalculous cholecystitis and adrenalitis have been described.

CMV rarely causes meningoencephalitis in otherwise healthy individuals. Two forms of CMV encephalitis are seen in patients with AIDS. One resembles HIV encephalitis and presents as progressive dementia; the other is a ventriculoencephalitis characterized by cranial-nerve deficits, nystagmus, disorientation, lethargy, and ventriculomegaly. In immunocompromised patients, CMV also can cause subacute progressive polyradiculopathy, which is often reversible if recognized and treated promptly.

CMV retinitis is an important cause of blindness in immunocompromised patients, particularly patients with AIDS. Early lesions consist of small, opaque, white areas of granular retinal necrosis that spread in a centrifugal manner and are later accompanied by hemorrhages, vessel sheathing, and retinal edema (see **Plate III-1**). CMV retinopathy must be distinguished from that due to other conditions, including toxoplasmosis, candidiasis, and herpes simplex virus infection.

Fatal CMV infections often are associated with persistent viremia and the involvement of multiple organ systems. Progressive pulmonary infiltrates, pancytopenia, hyperamylasemia, and hypotension are characteristic features that are frequently found in conjunction with a terminal bacterial, fungal, or protozoan superinfection. Extensive adrenal necrosis with CMV inclusions is often documented at autopsy, as is CMV involvement of many other organs.

DIAGNOSIS The diagnosis of CMV infection usually cannot be made reliably on clinical grounds alone. Isolation of the virus from appropriate clinical specimens, together with demonstration of a fourfold or greater rise in antibody titers or persistently elevated antibody titers, is the preferred diagnostic approach. Virus excretion or viremia is readily detected by culture of appropriate specimens on human fibroblast monolayers. If viral titers are high, as is frequently the case in congenital disseminated infection or in patients with AIDS, characteristic cytopathic effects may be detected within a few days. However, in some situations—such as CMV mononucleosis—viral titers are low, and cytopathic effects may take several weeks to appear. Many laboratories expedite diagnosis by using an overnight tissue-culture method (shell vial assay) involving centrifugation and an immunocytochemical detection technique employing monoclonal antibodies to an immediate-early CMV antigen. Isolation of virus from urine or saliva does not, by itself, constitute proof of acute infection, since excretion from these sites may continue for months or years after illness. Detection of CMV viremia is a better predictor of acute infection. Detection of CMV immediate-early antigens (pp65) or DNA in peripheral-blood leukocytes may hasten the diagnosis of CMV disease in certain populations, including organ transplant recipients and persons with AIDS. Such assays may yield a positive result several days earlier than culture methods. The detection of CMV DNA in cerebrospinal fluid by the polymerase chain reaction is useful in the diagnosis of CMV encephalitis or polyradiculopathy.

A variety of serologic assays [complement fixation, immunofluorescence, indirect hemagglutination, enzyme-linked immunosorbent assay (ELISA)] are available to detect increases in titers of antibody to CMV antigens. An increased antibody level may not be detectable for up to 4 weeks after primary infection, and titers often remain high for years after infection. For this reason, single-sample antibody determinations are of no value in assessing the acuteness of infection. Detection of CMV-specific IgM is sometimes useful in the diagnosis of recent or active infection; circulating rheumatoid factors may result in occasional false-positive IgM tests.

℞ **TREATMENT**

Several prophylactic measures are useful for the prevention of CMV infection in patients at high risk. The use of blood from seronegative donors or of blood that has been frozen, thawed, and deglycerolized greatly decreases the rate of transfusion-associated transmission of CMV. Similarly, matching of organ or bone marrow transplants by CMV serology, using only organs from seronegative donors for seronegative recipients, reduces rates of primary infection following transplantation. Both live attenuated (Towne strain) and CMV subunit vaccines have been evaluated, but neither is close to approval for general use.

CMV immune globulin has been reported to reduce rates of occurrence of CMV-associated syndromes and fungal or parasitic superinfections among seronegative renal transplant recipients. Similar studies in bone marrow transplant recipients have produced conflicting results. Prophylactic acyclovir has been demonstrated to reduce CMV infection and disease in certain seronegative renal transplant recipients; acyclovir is not effective in the treatment of active CMV disease, however.

Ganciclovir (dihydroxypropoxymethylguanine, DHPG) is a guanosine derivative that has considerably more activity against CMV than its congener acyclovir. After intracellular conversion by a viral phosphotransferase encoded by CMV gene region UL97, ganciclovir triphosphate is a selective inhibitor of CMV DNA polymerase. Several clinical studies have indicated response rates of 70 to 90 percent among patients with AIDS given ganciclovir for the treatment of CMV retinitis or colitis. In bone marrow transplant recipients with CMV pneumonia, ganciclovir is less effective when given alone, but it elicits a favorable clinical response 50 to 70 percent of the time when it is combined with CMV immune globulin. Prophylactic or suppressive ganciclovir may be useful in high-risk bone marrow or organ transplant recipients (e.g., those who are CMV-seropositive before transplantation or who are CMV culture–positive afterward). In many patients with AIDS and CMV disease, clinical and virologic relapses occur promptly if treatment with ganciclovir is discontinued. Therefore, prolonged maintenance regimens are recommended. Resistance to ganciclovir is common among patients treated for more than 3 months and is usually related to mutations in the CMV UL97 gene.

Ganciclovir therapy for CMV retinitis consists of a 14- to 21-day induction course (5 mg/kg intravenously twice a day) followed by a prolonged intravenous or oral maintenance regimen. For parenteral maintenance, the dose is 5 mg/kg daily or 6 mg/kg 5 days per week. Peripheral-blood neutropenia develops in 16 to 29 percent of treated patients but is often ameliorated by granulocyte or granulocyte-macrophage colony-stimulating factor. Oral ganciclovir at a high dose (3 g/d) can also be used for maintenance, although the blood levels achieved are insufficient for acute induction regimens. Although progression (as assessed by funduscopy) is more rapid with oral than with intravenous ganciclovir maintenance (mean time to progression, 68 vs. 96 days; $p = 0.03$), the ease of administration and reduced toxicity of the oral preparation may make it an acceptable alternative for some patients. The use of oral ganciclovir as prophylaxis in high-risk AIDS patients (i.e., those with CD4+ cell counts of $<100/\mu L$) has been studied in two placebo-controlled trials, with somewhat contradictory results.

Foscarnet (sodium phosphonoformate) also acts against CMV infection by inhibiting viral DNA polymerase. Because this agent does not require phosphorylation to be active, it is also effective against ganciclovir-resistant CMV isolates. A comparative trial of foscarnet and ganciclovir in 234 patients with AIDS and CMV retinitis demonstrated equivalent activity against retinitis but longer survival (12.6 vs. 8.5 months) in the foscarnet group. Although the reasons for the latter difference are unclear, the antiretroviral activity of foscarnet and the greater use of zidovudine by foscarnet recipients are strong possibilities. Foscarnet is less well tolerated than ganciclovir and causes considerable toxicity, including renal dysfunction, hypomagnesemia, hypokalemia, hypocalcemia, genital ulcers, dysuria, nausea, and paresthesia. Moreover, foscarnet administration requires the use of an infusion pump and close clinical monitoring. With aggressive hydration and dose adjustments for renal dysfunction, the toxicity of foscarnet can be reduced. The use of foscarnet should be avoided when a saline load cannot be tolerated (e.g., in cardiomyopathy). The approved induction regimen is 60 mg/kg every

8 h for 2 weeks, although 90 mg/kg every 12 h is equally effective and no more toxic. Maintenance infusions should deliver 90 to 120 mg/kg once daily; no oral preparation is available. Foscarnet-resistant viruses may emerge during extended therapy.

Ganciclovir has recently been administered via a slow-release pellet sutured into the eye. Although this intraocular device provides good local protection, contralateral eye disease and disseminated disease are not affected, and early retinal detachment is possible. A combination of intraocular and systemic therapy is being studied, as are combinations of ganciclovir and foscarnet. New drugs are being investigated, and one, cidofovir (also known as HPMPC), is available through expanded-access programs.

HUMAN HERPESVIRUS TYPES 6, 7, AND 8

Human herpesvirus (HHV) type 6 was first isolated in 1986 from peripheral-blood leukocytes of six persons with various lymphoproliferative disorders. Although initially thought to be B-lymphotropic and thus designated *human B-lymphotropic virus*, HHV-6 is clearly primarily T-lymphotropic. The virus has a worldwide distribution, and two genetically distinct variants (HHV-6A and HHV-6B) are now recognized.

Infection with HHV-6 frequently develops during infancy as maternal antibody wanes. Although HHV-6A has not yet been associated with disease, HHV-6B can cause exanthem subitum (roseola infantum), a common illness characterized by fever with subsequent rash. HHV-6B is also a major cause of febrile seizures without rash during infancy. In older age groups, HHV-6B has been associated with mononucleosis syndromes, focal encephalitis, and (in immunocompromised hosts) pneumonitis and disseminated disease. As many as 80 percent of adults are seropositive for HHV-6. The virus may be transmitted by saliva and possibly by genital secretions. There is no established treatment or vaccine.

HHV-7 was isolated in 1990 from T lymphocytes from the peripheral blood of a healthy 26-year-old man. Other isolates have since been obtained. It appears that the virus is frequently acquired during childhood and is frequently present in the saliva of healthy adults. No human disease has yet been definitively linked to HHV-7, although some cases of exanthem subitum have been associated with HHV-7 infection.

Unique herpesvirus-like DNA sequences were reported during 1994 and 1995 in tissues derived from Kaposi's sarcoma and body cavity–based lymphoma occurring in patients with AIDS. These sequences are partially homologous to the DNA of Epstein-Barr virus and herpesvirus saimiri of squirrel monkeys. When subjected to representational-difference analyses, more than 90 percent of Kaposi's sarcoma tissue samples were found to contain these sequences, whereas appropriate control tissues did not. The same herpesvirus-like DNA sequences have been reported in Kaposi's sarcoma tissue from non-AIDS patients, in a subgroup of AIDS-related B-cell body cavity–based lymphomas, in certain brain tumors, and in some proliferative skin lesions of organ transplant recipients. Approximately 15 percent of non-Kaposi's-sarcoma tissue specimens from patients with AIDS contain these sequences, which have also been found in semen from both AIDS and non-AIDS patients. Because of the uniqueness of these sequences, some authors have tentatively called the virus from which they come HHV-8. Its role in Kaposi's sarcoma and other diseases remains to be established. The recent isolation of HHV-8 in cell culture should help define its role in disease by making diagnostic techniques more reliable.

BIBLIOGRAPHY

AKASHI K et al: Severe infectious mononucleosis-like syndrome and primary human herpesvirus 6 infection in an adult. N Engl J Med 329:168, 1993

BALFOUR HH et al: A randomized, placebo-controlled trial of oral acyclovir for the prevention of cytomegalovirus disease in recipients of renal allografts. N Engl J Med 320:1381, 1989

BOWDEN RA et al: Cytomegalovirus (CMV)–specific intravenous immunoglobulin for the prevention of primary CMV infection and disease after marrow transplant. J Infect Dis 164:483, 1991

BUHLES WC et al: Ganciclovir treatment of life- or sight-threatening cytomegalovirus infection: Experience in 314 immunocompromised patients. Rev Infect Dis 10:S495, 1988

CESARMAN E et al: Kaposi's sarcoma–associated herpesvirus-like DNA sequences in AIDS-related body-cavity based lymphomas. N Engl J Med 332:1186, 1995

CHANG Y et al: Identification of herpesvirus-like DNA sequences in AIDS-associated Kaposi's sarcoma. Science 266:1865, 1994

DREW WL et al: Oral ganciclovir as maintenance treatment for cytomegalovirus retinitis in patients with AIDS. N Engl J Med 333:615, 1995

HIRSCH MS: The treatment of cytomegalovirus in AIDS: More than meets the eye. N Engl J Med 326:262, 1992

HO M: *Cytomegalovirus: Biology and Infection*, 2d ed. New York, Plenum Press, 1991

JABS DA: Controversies in the treatment of cytomegalovirus retinitis: Foscarnet versus ganciclovir. Infect Agents Dis 4:131, 1995

LEACH CT et al: Human herpesvirus 6 infection of the female genital tract. J Infect Dis 169:1281, 1994

MANEZ R et al: Time to detection of cytomegalovirus (CMV) DNA in blood leukocytes is a predictor for the development of CMV disease in CMV-seronegative recipients of allografts from CMV-seropositive donors following liver transplantation. J Infect Dis 173:1072, 1996

MCCUTCHAN JA: Cytomegalovirus infections of the nervous system in patients with AIDS. Clin Infect Dis 20:747, 1995

MERIGAN TC et al: A controlled trial of ganciclovir to prevent cytomegalovirus disease after heart transplantation. N Engl J Med 326:1182, 1992

MONINI P et al: Kaposi's sarcoma–associated herpesvirus DNA sequences in prostate tissue and human semen. N Engl J Med 334:1168, 1996

ONORATO IM et al: Epidemiology of cytomegaloviral infections: Recommendations for prevention and control. Rev Infect Dis 7:479, 1985

PASS RF et al: Young children as a probable source of maternal and congenital cytomegalovirus infection. N Engl J Med 316:1366, 1987

RENNE R et al: Lytic growth of Kaposi's sarcoma–associated herpesvirus (human herpesvirus 8) in culture. Nature Med 2:342, 1996

SMYTH RL et al: Cytomegalovirus infection in heart-lung transplant recipients: Risk factors, clinical associations, and response to treatment. J Infect Dis 164:1045, 1991

SNYDMAN DR et al: Use of cytomegalovirus immune globulin to prevent cytomegalovirus disease in renal transplant recipients. N Engl J Med 317:1049, 1987

STUDIES OF OCULAR COMPLICATIONS OF AIDS RESEARCH GROUP, AIDS CLINICAL TRIALS GROUP: Mortality in patients with the acquired immunodeficiency syndrome treated with either foscarnet or ganciclovir for cytomegalovirus retinitis. N Engl J Med 326:213, 1992

———: Combination foscarnet and ganciclovir therapy vs monotherapy for the treatment of relapsed cytomegalovirus retinitis in patients with AIDS. The cytomegalovirus retreatment trial. Arch Ophthalmol 114:23, 1996

WYATT LS et al: Human herpesvirus 7 is a constitutive inhabitant of adult human saliva. J Virol 66:3206, 1992

188 *Fred Wang*

SMALLPOX, VACCINIA, AND OTHER POXVIRUSES

Poxviruses are characterized by a brick-shaped morphology and a large double-stranded DNA genome. These are the only DNA viruses that replicate in cytoplasm, where accumulated viral particles form eosinophilic inclusions, or Guarnieri bodies, visible by light microscopy. Poxviruses associated with human disease include variola, vaccinia, and molluscum contagiosum viruses as well as other agents that cause zoonotic infections (the most important being monkeypox virus).

SMALLPOX

The last case of endemic smallpox was reported in 1977 from Somalia. In 1980 the World Health Organization officially declared that smallpox had been eliminated worldwide as a result of a global vaccination and eradication program. Several features contributed to this unique accomplishment, including (1) universal interest in eliminating this costly disease with high morbidity and mortality, (2) the infection's long incubation period and low level of communicability, (3) the ease of diagnosis of skin lesions by characteristic histology or antigen detection, (4) the fact that humans were the sole reservoir of the infection, (5) the absence of a carrier state, and (6) the availability of an effective live-virus vaccine that could readily be delivered to less developed countries because of its resistance to chemicals, temperature changes, and drying. The only known remaining repositories of smallpox virus are two research laboratories (located in the United States and Russia, respectively), and the issue of whether these last samples should be maintained or destroyed remains controversial. However, there is currently a moratorium on destroying the virus before 1999.

Before the eradication of smallpox, variola virus existed as two related strains: *variola major* (smallpox), with a case-mortality rate of 20 to 50 percent, and *variola minor* (alastrim), which caused a clinically milder form of smallpox with a mortality of less than 1 percent. Smallpox was a relatively noncontagious disease whose transmission required close contact. Fever and macular rash appeared after an average incubation period of 12 days, with a progression to typical vesicular and pustular lesions over 1 to 2 weeks.

VACCINIA

The origin of vaccinia virus—the virus used for vaccination against smallpox—is uncertain, but it was probably derived from cowpox virus, variola virus, or a hybrid of the two. It is now a laboratory virus with no natural host. Experience has proven the effectiveness of live vaccinia-virus vaccine, although its efficacy and safety have not been established in controlled studies. Percutaneous administration of vaccinia virus vaccine results in protective cellular and humoral immune responses in more than 95 percent of primary vaccinees. Formation of a pustule and scab at the site of inoculation is indicative of immunity; because immunity wanes after 10 to 20 years, revaccination every 10 years is recommended for continued protection. Routine smallpox vaccination was discontinued in 1971 and has not been required for international travel since 1982. However, the development of recombinant vaccinia viruses for potential use in vaccines against other infectious agents or as immunotherapy against malignant diseases has led to the recommendation that laboratory and health care employees working directly with vaccinia virus vectors be considered for vaccination. Selected groups that may be exposed to poxviruses (e.g., some military personnel and individuals who work with animals) are also vaccinated.

The most frequent adverse complication of vaccination is inadvertent inoculation (usually autoinoculation) at other sites. More serious complications, which are more common among primary vaccinees and infants than among revaccinees and adults, include (1) generalized vaccinia in otherwise healthy individuals, which is generally self-limited; (2) eczema vaccinatum, which consists of disseminated cutaneous lesions in highly susceptible patients with eczema or other chronic skin diseases and is occasionally severe or even fatal; (3) progressive vaccinia (vaccinia necrosum), which is a severe, potentially fatal illness occurring in patients with immunodeficiency, whether congenital, acquired (e.g., via leukemia or lymphoma), iatrogenic (e.g., via chemotherapy or glucocorticoid treatment), or human immunodeficiency virus (HIV)–induced; and (4) postinfectious encephalitis, which is rare (3 cases per million primary vaccinees) but can be fatal in 15 to 25 percent of cases and can leave 25 percent of patients with permanent neurologic sequelae. Since vaccinees can transmit vaccinia virus to susceptible individuals, vaccination is contraindicated if the proposed recipient or his/her household contacts have eczema, are immunocompromised, or are pregnant. Vaccinia immune globulin (0.6 mL/kg) derived from the plasma of vaccinated persons may be useful for the treatment of severe generalized vaccinia, eczema vaccinatum, progressive vaccinia,

and ocular vaccinia resulting from inadvertent inoculation but is of no value for the treatment of postinfectious encephalitis.

MOLLUSCUM CONTAGIOSUM

Molluscum contagiosum is generally a benign disease characterized by pearly, flesh-colored, umbilicated skin lesions 2 to 5 mm in diameter. The infection can be transmitted by close contact, including sexual intercourse. Lesions typically occur in the genital region but can be found anywhere on the body except the palms and the soles. In most cases the disease is self-limited and has no systemic complications. Molluscum contagiosum develops especially often in association with the advanced stages of HIV infection, with a prevalence of 5 to 18 percent among HIV-infected patients (see Chap. 308). The disease is often more generalized, severe, and persistent in AIDS patients than in other groups, frequently involving the face and upper body. Extensive molluscum contagiosum has also been reported in conjunction with other types of immunodeficiency.

The diagnosis of molluscum contagiosum can be made by histologic demonstration of cytoplasmic eosinophilic inclusions characteristic of poxvirus replication. This poorly characterized virus cannot be propagated in vitro, but electron microscopy and molecular studies can be used for its identification.

There is no specific systemic treatment for molluscum contagiosum, but a variety of techniques for physical ablation have been used.

MONKEYPOX VIRUS AND OTHER POXVIRUSES

Monkeypox virus naturally infects nonhuman primates in the tropical rain forests of western and central Africa and can infect humans who come into direct contact with infected animals. Human disease is rare and is characterized by a vesicular rash similar to that of variola. The disease is occasionally fatal, especially to young children and individuals who have not received smallpox vaccine.

Other poxviruses can cause localized vesicular lesions when humans come into direct contact with infected animals. These viruses include cowpox virus (cows, rodents); milkers' node virus (cows); buffalopox virus (buffaloes); bovine papular stomatitis virus (cows); and orf virus, which is also known as contagious pustular dermatitis virus (sheep, goats).

BIBLIOGRAPHY

BREMAN JG, ARITA I: The confirmation and maintenance of smallpox eradication. N Engl J Med 303:1263, 1980

JEZEK Z et al: Human monkeypox: Clinical features of 282 patients. J Infect Dis 156:293, 1987

JOKLIK WK et al: Why the smallpox virus stocks should not be destroyed. Science 262:1225, 1993

MAHY BW et al: The remaining stocks of smallpox virus should be destroyed. Science 262:1223, 1993

MOSS B: Vaccinia virus: A tool for research and vaccine development. Science 252:1662, 1991

SCHWARTZ JJ, MYSKOWSKI PL: Molluscum contagiosum in patients with human immunodeficiency virus infection. A review of twenty-seven patients. J Am Acad Dermatol 27:583, 1992

Vaccinia (smallpox) vaccine. Recommendations of the Immunization Practices Advisory Committee (ACIP). Morb Mortal Week Rep 40:1, 1991

189 *Neil R. Blacklow*

PARVOVIRUS

DEFINITION The parvovirus group includes several species-specific viruses of animals. One parvovirus, designated B19, is known to be a human pathogen. B19 is a small (diameter, 20 to 25 nm), icosahedral, nonenveloped, single-stranded DNA virus with an outer capsid formed by two structural proteins. Individual virus particles contain DNA strands of positive or negative polarity. The virus is stable and retains infectivity after incubation at 60°C for 16 h. It has failed to grow in conventional cell culture lines and animal model systems but does replicate in vitro in erythroid progenitor cells derived from human bone marrow, umbilical cord, peripheral blood, or fetal liver sources.

During the 1980s, it was discovered that B19 causes a variety of disorders ranging from erythema infectiosum and acute arthropathy in otherwise healthy hosts to transient aplastic crisis and chronic anemia in compromised patients to fetal infection manifested by death or hydrops fetalis. Many of the severe manifestations of B19 viremia relate to the propensity of the virus to infect and lyse erythroid precursor cells in the bone marrow. The name B19 is derived from the code number of the human serum in which the virus was discovered.

PATHOGENESIS Two studies of adult volunteers have provided a basis for understanding the pathogenesis of B19 infection, which has two phases. The first phase is characterized by viremia that develops approximately 6 days after intranasal inoculation of B19 into susceptible individuals who lack serum antibodies to the virus. The viremia lasts about 1 week; its clearance is correlated with the development of IgM antibodies to B19, which remain detectable for up to a few months. IgG antibodies develop several days later and persist indefinitely. Nonspecific systemic symptoms lasting 2 or 3 days occur early during the viremic phase; these symptoms include headache, malaise, myalgia, fever, chills, and pruritus and are accompanied by reticulocytopenia and excretion of the virus from the respiratory tract. Several days after the onset of symptoms, a clinically insignificant decline in hemoglobin concentration is noted; the decreased level is maintained for 7 to 10 days, during which time examination of bone marrow samples reveals a marked depletion of erythroid precursor cells. Transient mild lymphopenia, neutropenia, and a drop in platelet count also may be found. A second phase of illness begins around 17 or 18 days after virus inoculation (after the clearance of viremia, the cessation of viral shedding in throat secretions, and the resolution of reticulocytopenia). This illness mimics erythema infectiosum in adults, with 2 or 3 days of fine maculopapular rash accompanied by arthralgias and arthritis that last another 1 or 2 days. This phase occurs in the presence of rising serum titers of antibody to B19.

The studies just described indicate that B19 disease in the otherwise *healthy host*, manifested by self-limited erythema infectiosum and/or arthropathy, is almost certainly an immune-complex disorder. This concept is supported by the induction of erythema infectiosum through the infusion of immunoglobulins into chronically viremic patients. In contrast, B19 disease in the *compromised host* (chronic hemolytic disease or immunodeficiency syndromes) is often serious, resulting from the destruction by B19 of erythroid precursor cells. Normal hosts can tolerate 7 to 10 days of shutoff of erythropoiesis; however, patients with hemolytic disease who require increased production of erythrocytes do not tolerate erythroid cell destruction and thus usually develop severe transient aplastic crisis. Patients who are immunodeficient may fail to clear B19 viremia, the results being persistent infection of red blood cells and chronic severe anemia. The fetus requires a higher level of red cell production than do adults and has an immature immune system; both these factors could explain B19-induced hydrops fetalis.

B19 binds specifically to a cellular receptor, erythrocyte P antigen; this specific binding explains the tropism of B19 for erythroid progenitor cells, particularly pronormoblasts and normoblasts. The few persons who lack P antigen cannot be infected with B19.

EPIDEMIOLOGY Although B19 infections occur year-round, they appear most commonly as outbreaks of erythema infectiosum in schools during winter and spring months. Between 20 and 60 percent of children in outbreaks are symptomatic, and many are asymptomatically infected. Seroepidemiologic studies indicate that approximately half of adults possess serum antibodies to B19. Antibody prevalence (reflecting prior exposure and probable immunity to the virus) rises rapidly between the ages of 5 and 18 years and continues to increase with age—a pattern probably indicating ongoing exposure during adulthood. B19 can be detected in throat swabbings, respiratory tract secretions, and serum, and its detection at these sites probably corre-

lates with infectiousness. Thus, patients with transient aplastic crisis are highly infectious. Their infectivity has been firmly documented as the source of one well-defined nosocomial outbreak of erythema infectiosum among nurses. In contrast, individuals with erythema infectiosum are much less infectious. The usual route of viral transmission under natural conditions is unknown but may be respiratory or through direct contact. B19 can be transmitted during therapy with clotting factor concentrate, even after exposure to steam or dry heat.

CLINICAL MANIFESTATIONS **Erythema Infectiosum** Erythema infectiosum is the most common manifestation of B19 infection and occurs predominantly in children. This entity is also called *fifth disease* because it was classified in the late nineteenth century as the fifth in a series of six exanthems of childhood. Normally a mild illness, erythema infectiosum typically presents as a facial rash with a "slapped-cheek" appearance that is sometimes preceded by low-grade fever. The rash may develop quickly on the arms and legs and usually has a lacy, reticular, erythematous appearance. The trunk, palms, and soles are less commonly involved. Occasionally, the rash appears with maculopapular, morbilliform, vesicular, purpuric, or pruritic characteristics. The typical rash resolves in about a week but can recur intermittently for several weeks, particularly after stress, exercise, exposure to sunlight, bathing, or change in environmental temperature. Arthralgia and arthritis are uncommon among children but are frequent among adults, in whom the rash is often absent or nonspecific, with a lack of the characteristic facial erythema.

Arthropathy B19 infection in adults most commonly presents as acute arthralgias and arthritis, sometimes accompanied by rash. The arthritis is characteristically symmetric and peripheral, involving the wrists, hands, and knees most frequently. It normally resolves in about 3 weeks and is nondestructive. However, a small percentage of patients have arthritis persisting for months or even (in rare cases) for years. It is not known whether these individuals have persistent infection or an abnormal immune response to the virus. Several case reports have suggested a link—as yet unproven—between B19 and idiopathic thrombocytopenic purpura, virus-associated hemophagocytic syndrome with pancytopenia, Lyme-like arthritis, recurrent paresthesia, fibromyalgia, systemic lupus erythematosus, and vasculitis (including polyarteritis nodosa, Wegener's granulomatosis, and Kawasaki disease).

Transient Aplastic Crisis B19 infection is the cause in most instances of transient aplastic crisis developing suddenly in patients with chronic hemolytic disease. Nearly all hemolytic conditions can be affected by B19 infection, including sickle cell disease, erythrocyte enzyme deficiencies, hereditary spherocytosis, thalassemias, paroxysmal nocturnal hemoglobinuria, and autoimmune hemolysis. B19-induced aplastic crisis also can occur in the setting of acute blood loss. Patients present with weakness, lethargy, pallor, and severe anemia, a syndrome often preceded by a few days of nonspecific symptoms. These patients have intense reticulocytopenia lasting 7 to 10 days, and their bone marrow contains no erythroid precursor cells despite a normal myeloid series. Transient aplastic crisis can produce life-threatening anemia and may require urgent transfusion therapy. Unlike patients with erythema infectiosum or arthropathy, those with transient aplastic crisis are viremic and can readily transmit B19 infection to other people.

Chronic Anemia in Immunodeficient Patients Immunodeficient patients may be unable to eliminate B19 infection, probably because they cannot produce adequate levels of virus-specific IgG antibodies. The result is persistent infection with destruction of erythroid precursor cells in the bone marrow and chronic transfusion-dependent anemia. This condition has been described in patients with immunodeficiency related to infection with human immunodeficiency virus, congenital immunodeficiencies, and acute lymphocytic leukemia during maintenance chemotherapy as well as in recipients of bone marrow transplants. In addition, some cases of idiopathic pure red-cell aplasia probably are caused by persistent B19 infection. B19-induced chronic anemia may be the presenting finding of an otherwise unrecognized immunodeficiency. Chronic anemia may fluctuate in intensity over time and may be cured or controlled by immunoglobulin therapy. Both the spectrum of immunodeficiencies associated with B19-induced chronic anemia and the frequency of the association remain to be determined.

Fetal and Congenital Infection Maternal B19 infections usually do not adversely affect the fetus. More often than not, in fact, the fetus remains uninfected. Therefore, couples in which the pregnant woman is infected should be counseled as to the relatively low risk of fetal infection. It is estimated that fewer than 10 percent of maternal B19 infections lead to fetal death; when fetal death does occur, it is usually attributable to the development of nonimmune hydrops fetalis, wherein the fetus succumbs to severe anemia and congestive heart failure. B19 can be detected in fetal tissues, with predominant infection of erythroblasts. Pregnant women with known exposure to B19 should have their serum monitored for IgM antibodies to the virus and for elevated levels of alpha fetoprotein; ultrasonic examinations of the fetus for hydrops should also be conducted. Some hydropic fetuses survive B19 infection and appear normal at delivery. Rarely, fetal infection with hydrops results in congenital anemia and hypogammaglobulinemia that is unresponsive to immunoglobulin therapy.

DIAGNOSIS Diagnosis most commonly relies on measurements of B19-specific IgM and IgG antibodies, which can be detected with commercially available immunoassay kits. The virus, its DNA, or its antigens are also detected in the serum or infected tissues of some patients. Acute infection can be proven by B19-compatible symptoms and the presence of IgM antibodies or virus itself, whereas past infection is documented by IgG antibodies. Individuals with erythema infectiosum and acute arthropathy usually have IgM antibodies without detectable virus in serum. Those with transient aplastic crisis may have IgM antibodies but typically possess high titers of virus and its DNA in serum; the bone marrow of these patients shows characteristic giant pronormoblasts and hypoplasia. Immunodeficient patients with anemia often lack readily detectable antibodies but have viral particles and DNA in serum. Fetal infection may be recognized by hydrops fetalis and the presence of B19 DNA in amniotic fluid or fetal blood in association with maternal IgM antibodies to B19.

℞ **TREATMENT**

Erythema infectiosum usually requires no treatment; the same is true for many cases of arthropathy. More severe cases of arthritis, particularly those involving chronic symptoms, can be treated with nonsteroidal anti-inflammatory agents. Transient aplastic crisis is usually treated with erythrocyte transfusions. In immunodeficient anemic patients, B19 infection should be treated with commercial intravenous immunoglobulin, which is known to contain IgG antibodies to B19. This therapy controls and may cure B19 infection. Prophylaxis of B19 infection with immunoglobulin should be considered for patients with chronic hemolysis or immunodeficiency and for pregnant women. The risk of infection for these persons may be reduced by hand washing before eating or after contact with respiratory or other secretions when B19 is known to be present in a community. Patients with transient aplastic crisis or chronic B19 infection (but not those with erythema infectiosum or arthropathy) pose a serious risk for nosocomial transmission of infection. They should be hospitalized in a private room with contact and respiratory isolation precautions. It is not known whether pre- or postexposure administration of immunoglobulin prevents infection. No vaccine for B19 is currently available; however, a baculovirus-infected insect cell line that expresses noninfectious immunogenic B19 capsid proteins is being evaluated as a vaccine candidate.

BIBLIOGRAPHY

ANDERSON LJ: Human parvoviruses. J Infect Dis 161:603, 1990

ANDERSON MJ et al: Experimental parvoviral infection in humans. J Infect Dis 152:257, 1985

BANSAL GP et al: Candidate recombinant vaccine for human B19 parvovirus. J Infect Dis 167:1034, 1993

BELL LM et al: Human parvovirus B19 infection among hospital staff members after contact with infected patients. N Engl J Med 321:485, 1989

BROWN KE et al: Congenital anemia after transplacental B19 parvovirus infection. Lancet 343:895, 1994

———— et al: Resistance to parvovirus B19 infection due to lack of virus receptor (erythrocyte P antigen). N Engl J Med 330:1192, 1994

BRUU AL, NORDBO SA: Evaluation of five commercial tests for detection of immunoglobulin M antibodies to human parvovirus B19. J Clin Microbiol 33:1363, 1995

CENTERS FOR DISEASE CONTROL: Risks associated with human parvovirus B19 infection. Morb Mort Week Rep 38:81, 1989

FINKEL TH et al: Chronic parvovirus B19 infection and systemic necrotising vasculitis: Opportunistic infection or aetiological agent? Lancet 343:1255, 1994

FRICKHOFEN N et al: Persistent B19 parvovirus infection in patients infected with human immunodeficiency virus type 1 (HIV-1): A treatable cause of anemia in AIDS. Ann Intern Med 113:926, 1990

HARRIS JW: Parvovirus B19 for the hematologist. Am J Hematol 39:119, 1992

KURTZMAN G et al: Pure red-cell aplasia of 10 years' duration due to persistent parvovirus B19 infection and its cure with immunoglobulin therapy. N Engl J Med 321:519, 1989

MOREY AL et al: Clinical and histopathological features of parvovirus B19 infection in the human fetus. Br J Obstet Gynaecol 99:566, 1992

NAIDES SJ et al: Rheumatologic manifestations of human parvovirus B19 infection in adults: Initial two-year clinical experience. Arthritis Rheum 33:1297, 1990

PLUMMER FA et al: An erythema infectiosum–like illness caused by human parvovirus infection. N Engl J Med 313:74, 1985

RODIS JF et al: Management and outcomes of pregnancies complicated by human B19 parvovirus infections: A prospective study. Am J Obstet Gynecol 163:1168, 1990

190 *Richard C. Reichman*

HUMAN PAPILLOMAVIRUS INFECTIONS

DEFINITION Human papillomaviruses (HPVs) selectively infect the epithelium of the skin and mucous membranes. These infections may be asymptomatic, produce warts, or be associated with a variety of benign and malignant neoplasias.

ETIOLOGIC AGENT Papillomaviruses are members of the *Papillomavirus* genus of the family Papovaviridae. They are nonenveloped, measure 50 to 55 nm in diameter, have icosahedral capsids composed of 72 capsomeres, and contain a double-stranded circular DNA genome of about 7900 base pairs. The genomic organization of all papillomaviruses is similar and consists of an early (E) region, a late (L) region, and a long-control region (LCR). Oncogenic HPV types can immortalize human keratinocytes, and this activity has been mapped to products of early genes E6 and E7. E6 protein mediates the degradation of the p53 tumor suppressor protein, and E7 protein binds the retinoblastoma gene product. The E1 and E2 proteins modulate viral DNA replication and regulate gene expression. The L1 gene codes for the major capsid protein, which makes up 80 percent of the virion mass. L2 codes for a minor capsid protein. Type-specific conformational antigenic determinants are located on the virion surface. Papillomavirus types are distinguished from one another by the degree of nucleic acid sequence homology. Distinct types share fewer than 90 percent of their DNA sequences in L1. More than 70 types of HPV are recognized, and individual types are associated with specific clinical manifestations (Table 190-1). HPVs are species-specific and have not been propagated in tissue culture or in common experimental animals. However, HPV types 1, 6, 11, and 16 have been produced in human tissues implanted in immunodeficient mice.

EPIDEMIOLOGY There are few good studies of the incidence or prevalence of warts in well-defined human populations. Common warts (verruca vulgaris) are found in as many as 25 percent of some groups and are most prevalent among young children. Plantar warts

Table 190-1

CHAPTER 190
Human Papillomavirus Infections **1099**

Correlation of Human Papillomavirus Type with Disease

Disease	Associated HPV Types
Plantar warts	1,* 2,* 4, 63
Common warts	1,* 2,* 4, 26, 27, 29, 41,† 57, 65, 77
Common warts of meat handlers	1, 2,* 3, 4, 7,* 10, 28
Flat warts	3,* 10,* 27, 38, 41,† 49, 75, 76
Intermediate warts	10,* 26, 28
Epidermodysplasia verruciformis	2,* 3,* 5,*† 8,*† 9,* 10,* 12,* 14,*† 15,* 17,*† 19, 20,† 21, 22, 23, 24, 25, 36, 37, 38,† 47, 50
Condyloma acuminatum	6,* 11,* 30,† 42, 43, 44, 45,† 51,† 54, 55, 70
Intraepithelial neoplasias	
Unspecified	30,† 34, 39,† 40, 53, 57, 59, 61, 62, 64, 66,† 67, 68, 69, 70, 71, 74
Low-grade	6,* 11,* 16,† 18,† 31,† 33,† 35,† 42, 43, 44, 45,† 51,† 52†
High-grade	6, 11, 16,*† 18,*† 31,† 33,† 35,† 39,† 42, 44, 45,† 51,† 52,† 56,† 58,† 66†
Bowen's disease	16,*† 31,† 34
Bowenoid papulosis	16,*† 34, 39,† 42, 45,† 55
Cervical carcinoma	16,*† 18,*† 31,† 33,† 35,† 39,† 45,† 51, 52,† 56,† 58,† 66†
Laryngeal papillomas	6,* 11*
Focal epithelial hyperplasia of Heck	13,* 32*
Conjunctival papillomas	6,* 11,* 16*†
Others	6, 11, 16,† 30,† 33,† 36, 37 38,† 41,† 48,† 60, 72, 73

* Most common associations.
† High malignant potential.

(verruca plantaris) are also widely prevalent; they occur most often among adolescents and young adults. Condyloma acuminatum (which manifests as anogenital warts) is one of the most common sexually transmitted diseases in the United States. HPV infection of the uterine cervix produces the squamous-cell abnormalities most frequently detected on Papanicolaou smears.

Most genital HPV infections are transmitted through direct contact with infectious lesions. Both direct contact and fomites play a role in transmission of cutaneous nongenital warts. Minor trauma at the site of inoculation may facilitate transmission. Recurrent respiratory papillomatosis in young children is an uncommon disease that is acquired from maternal genital tract infection; in adults orogenital sexual contact may transmit the disease.

HPV infection has been strongly associated with the development of dysplasia and cancer of the uterine cervix. More than 90 percent of cervical cancers contain DNA of oncogenic (high-risk) HPV types, such as 16, 18, and 31. HPV DNA is also present in the precursor lesions of cervical cancer, known as cervical intraepithelial neoplasias. Such lesions containing DNA of oncogenic HPV types are more likely to progress than those associated with low-risk types, such as 6 and 11. HPV DNA is transcribed in tumor tissues, and many epidemiologic studies have confirmed a relation between HPV infection (with or without cofactors) and the development of cervical cancer. Infection with specific HPV types has also been associated with squamous cell carcinomas and dysplasias of the penis, anus, vagina, and vulva. In patients with epidermodysplasia verruciformis, squamous cell cancers develop frequently at sites infected with specific HPV types, including 5 and 8.

Recent serologic studies employing virus-like particles as antigens have demonstrated a modest prevalence of antibodies among patients with HPV genital tract infections.

CLINICAL MANIFESTATIONS The clinical manifestations of HPV infection depend on the location of the lesions and the type

of virus. Common warts usually occur on the hands as flesh-colored to brown, exophytic, hyperkeratotic papules. Plantar warts may be quite painful; they can be differentiated from calluses by paring of the surface to reveal thrombosed capillaries. Flat warts (verruca plana) are most common among children and occur on the face, neck, chest, and flexor surfaces of the forearms and legs.

Anogenital warts develop on the skin and mucosal surfaces of the external genitalia and perianal areas. In men, warts are found most frequently at the frenum or coronal sulcus but may affect any part of the penis. They occur commonly at the urethral meatus and may extend proximally. Perianal warts are common among homosexual men but develop in heterosexual men as well. In women, warts appear first at the posterior introitus and adjacent labia. They then spread to other parts of the vulva and commonly involve the vagina and cervix. These lesions may be present without external warts. The differential diagnosis of anogenital warts includes condylomata lata of secondary syphilis, molluscum contagiosum, hirsutoid papillomatosis (pearly penile papules), fibroepitheliomas, and a variety of benign and malignant mucocutaneous neoplasms. Respiratory papillomatosis in young children may be life-threatening and presents as hoarseness, stridor, or respiratory distress. The disease in adults is usually mild.

Immunosuppressed patients, particularly those undergoing organ transplantation, often develop pityriasis versicolor–like lesions, from which DNA of several HPV types has been extracted. Occasionally, such lesions appear to undergo malignant transformation. Patients infected with human immunodeficiency virus (HIV) frequently have severe clinical manifestations of HPV infection and appear to be at unusually high risk for cervical and anal malignancies. HPV disease in patients with HIV infection is difficult to treat and often recurs.

Epidermodysplasia verruciformis is a rare autosomal recessive disease characterized by the inability to control HPV infection. Patients are often infected with unusual HPV types and frequently develop cutaneous squamous cell malignancies, particularly in sun-exposed areas. The lesions resemble flat warts or macules similar to those of pityriasis versicolor.

The complications of warts include itching and occasionally bleeding. In rare cases warts become secondarily infected with bacteria or fungi. Large masses of warts may cause mechanical problems, such as obstruction of the birth canal. Dysplasias of the uterine cervix are generally asymptomatic until frank carcinoma develops.

PATHOGENESIS The incubation period of HPV disease is usually 3 to 4 months, with a range of 1 month to 2 years. All types of squamous epithelium can be infected by HPV, and the gross and histologic appearances of individual lesions vary with the site of infection and the type of virus. The replication of HPV begins with the infection of basal cells. As cellular differentiation proceeds, HPV DNA replicates and is transcribed. Ultimately, virions are assembled in the nucleus and released when keratinocytes are shed. This process is associated with proliferation of all epidermal layers except the basal layer and produces acanthosis, parakeratosis, and hyperkeratosis. Koilocytes, large round cells with pyknotic nuclei, appear in the granular layer. Histologically normal epithelium may contain HPV DNA, and residual DNA after treatment can be associated with recurrent disease.

Episomal HPV DNA is present in the nuclei of infected cells in benign lesions caused by the virus. However, in severe dysplasias and cancers, HPV DNA is generally integrated, with disruption of the E1/E2 open reading frames. This disruption leads to upregulation of E6 and E7 and subsequent interference with cellular tumor suppressor proteins.

Host defense responses to HPV infection are incompletely understood, and immune correlates of protection from infection and resolution of disease have not been established. Because patients with defects in cell-mediated immune responses, including transplant recipients and patients with HIV infection, frequently develop severe HPV disease, such responses are probably important for the control of virus replication. Histologic studies demonstrating an epidermal lymphomonocytic infiltrate in resolving warts suggest that local immunity may be of particular importance in the resolution of disease. HPV infection can also elicit a serologic response, and antibodies to the viral capsid have been found in sera from patients with anogenital warts, cutaneous warts, and respiratory papillomatosis. Antibodies to E-region proteins, most notably E7, have been detected among patients with cervical carcinoma. Vaccine studies in animals have shown that the production of neutralizing antibodies can be associated with protection from papillomavirus infection.

DIAGNOSIS Most warts that are visible to the naked eye can be diagnosed correctly by history and physical examination alone. The use of a colposcope is invaluable in assessing vaginal and cervical lesions and is helpful in the diagnosis of oral and cutaneous HPV disease as well. Papanicolaou smears prepared from cervical scrapings often show cytologic evidence of HPV infection. Persistent or atypical lesions should be biopsied and examined by routine histologic methods. The most sensitive and specific methods of virologic diagnosis entail the use of techniques such as the polymerase chain reaction or the hybrid capture assay to detect HPV nucleic acids and to identify specific virus types. Serologic techniques to diagnose HPV infection are in the early stages of development and are not yet widely available.

Rx **TREATMENT**

Decisions regarding the initiation of therapy should be made with the knowledge that currently available modes of treatment are not completely effective and some have significant side effects. In addition, treatment may be expensive, and many HPV lesions resolve spontaneously. Frequently used therapies include cryosurgery, application of caustic agents, electrodesiccation, surgical excision, and ablation with a laser. Topical antimetabolites such as 5-fluorouracil also have been used. Both failure and recurrence have been well documented with all of these methods of treatment. Cryosurgery is the initial treatment of choice for condyloma acuminatum. Topically applied podophyllum preparations as well as podofilox may also be used. Various interferon preparations have been employed with modest success in the treatment of respiratory papillomatosis and condyloma acuminatum. A topically applied interferon inducer, imiquimod, appears to be of benefit in the treatment of condyloma

acuminatum. The diagnosis and management of anogenital dysplasias and of internal anogenital warts require special skills and resources, and patients with such lesions should be referred to a qualified specialist.

No effective methods for the prevention of HPV infections are available at present other than the avoidance of contact with infectious lesions. Barrier methods of contraception may be helpful in preventing the transmission of condyloma acuminatum and other HPV-associated diseases of the genital tract. Vaccine preparations including virus-like particles have shown promise in the prevention of papillomavirus infection and disease in some animal models.

BIBLIOGRAPHY

BONNEZ W et al: A randomized, double-blind, placebo-controlled trial of systemically administered alpha-, beta-, or gamma-interferon in combination with cryotherapy for the treatment of condyloma acuminatum. J Infect Dis 171:1081, 1995

——— et al: Current and future approaches to the treatment of condylomata acuminata (anogenital warts), in *Principles and Practice of Infectious Diseases Updates,* GL Mandell et al (eds). New York, Churchill Livingstone, 1996, vol 4, no 2

BOSCH FX et al: Prevalence of human papillomavirus in cervical cancer: A worldwide perspective. J Natl Cancer Inst 87:796, 1995

CARTER JJ et al: Use of human papillomavirus type 6 capsids to detect antibodies in people with genital warts. J Infect Dis 172:11, 1995

HO GYF et al: Persistent genital human papillomavirus infection as a risk factor for persistent cervical dysplasia. J Natl Cancer Inst 87:1365, 1995

KJAER SK et al: Human papillomavirus—the most significant risk determinant of cervical intraepithelial neoplasia. Int J Cancer 65:601, 1996

ORTH G, ZUR HAUSEN H: General features: Infections of the anogenital tract, in *Encyclopedia of Virology.* 1994, pp 1013–1026

REICHMAN RC, BONNEZ W: Papillomaviruses, in *Mandell, Douglas and Bennett's Principles and Practice of Infectious Diseases,* 4th ed, GL Mandell et al (eds). New York, Churchill Livingstone, 1995

ROSE RC et al: Human papillomavirus type 11 (HPV-11) virus-like particles (VLPs) induce the formation of neutralizing antibodies and detect genital HPV-specific antibodies in human sera. J Gen Virol 75:2075, 1994

SCHIFFMAN MH: Epidemiology of cervical human papillomavirus infections. Curr Top Microbiol Immunol 186:55, 1994

———, BRINTON LA: The epidemiology of cervical carcinogenesis. Cancer 76:1888, 1995

SUZICH JA et al: Systemic immunization with papillomavirus L1 protein completely prevents the development of viral mucosal papillomas. Proc Natl Acad Sci USA 92:11553, 1995

Section 13

DNA AND RNA RESPIRATORY VIRUSES

---

191   *Raphael Dolin*

COMMON VIRAL RESPIRATORY INFECTIONS

GENERAL CONSIDERATIONS Acute viral respiratory illnesses are among the most common of human diseases, accounting for one-half or more of all acute illnesses. The incidence of acute respiratory disease in the United States is from 3 to 5.6 cases per person per year. The rates are highest among children under 1 year old (6.1 to 8.3 cases per year) and remain high until age 6, when a progressive decrease begins. Adults have 3 to 4 cases per person per year. Morbidity from acute respiratory illnesses accounts for 30 to 50 percent of time lost from work by adults and for 60 to 80 percent of time lost from school by children.

It has been estimated that two-thirds to three-fourths of cases of acute respiratory illnesses are caused by viruses. More than 200 antigenically distinct viruses from 8 different genera have been reported to cause acute respiratory illness, and it is likely that additional

agents will be described in the future. The vast majority of these viral infections involve the upper respiratory tract, but lower respiratory tract disease can also develop, particularly in younger age groups and in certain epidemiologic settings.

The illnesses caused by respiratory viruses traditionally have been divided into multiple distinct syndromes, such as the "common cold," pharyngitis, croup (laryngotracheobronchitis), tracheitis, bronchiolitis, bronchitis, and pneumonia. Each of these general categories of illnesses has a certain epidemiologic and clinical profile; for example, croup occurs exclusively in very young children and has a characteristic clinical course. Some types of respiratory illnesses are more likely to be associated with certain viruses (e.g., the common cold with rhinoviruses), while others occupy characteristic epidemiologic niches (e.g., adenovirus infections in military recruits). The syndromes most commonly associated with infections with the major respiratory virus groups are summarized in Table 191-1. Most respiratory viruses clearly have the potential to cause more than one type of respiratory illness, and frequently features of several types of illness are found in the same patient. Moreover, the clinical illnesses induced by these viruses are rarely sufficiently distinctive to permit an etiologic diagnosis on

Table 191-1

Illnesses Associated with Respiratory Viruses

Virus	Frequency of Respiratory Syndromes		
	Most Frequent	Occasional	Infrequent
Rhinoviruses	Common cold	Exacerbation of chronic bronchitis and asthma	Pneumonia in children
Coronaviruses	Common cold	Exacerbation of chronic bronchitis and asthma	Pneumonia and bronchiolitis
Respiratory syncytial virus	Pneumonia and bronchiolitis in young children	Common cold in adults	Pneumonia in elderly and immunosuppressed patients
Parainfluenza viruses	Croup and lower respiratory tract disease in young children	Pharyngitis and common cold	Tracheobronchitis in adults; lower respiratory tract disease in immunosuppressed patients
Adenoviruses	Common cold and pharyngitis in children	Outbreaks of acute respiratory disease in military recruits*	Pneumonia in children; lower respiratory tract and disseminated disease in immunosuppressed patients
Influenza A viruses	Influenza-like illness†	Pneumonia and excess mortality in high-risk patients	Pneumonia in healthy individuals
Influenza B viruses	Influenza-like illness†	Rhinitis and pharyngitis alone	Pneumonia
Enteroviruses	Acute undifferentiated febrile illnesses‡	Rhinitis and pharyngitis	Pneumonia
Herpes simplex viruses	Gingivostomatitis in children; pharyngotonsillitis in adults	Tracheitis and pneumonia in immunocompromised patients	Disseminated infection in immunocompromised patients

* Serotypes 4 and 7.
† Fever, cough, myalgia, malaise.
‡ May or may not have a respiratory component.

clinical grounds alone, although the epidemiologic setting increases the likelihood that one group of viruses rather than another is involved. In general, laboratory methods must be relied on to establish a specific viral diagnosis.

This chapter reviews viral infections caused by five of the major groups of respiratory viruses: rhinoviruses, coronaviruses, respiratory syncytial viruses, parainfluenza viruses, and adenoviruses. Influenza viruses, which are a major cause of mortality as well as morbidity, are reviewed in Chap. 193. Herpesviruses, which occasionally cause pharyngitis and which also cause lower respiratory tract disease in immunosuppressed patients, are reviewed in Chap. 184. Enteroviruses, which account for occasional respiratory illnesses during the summer months, are reviewed in Chap. 195.

RHINOVIRUS INFECTIONS

ETIOLOGIC AGENT Rhinoviruses are members of the Picornaviridae family, small (15 to 30 nm) nonenveloped viruses that contain a single-stranded RNA genome. In contrast to other members of

the picornavirus family, such as enteroviruses, rhinoviruses are acid-labile and are almost completely inactivated at pH 3 or lower. Rhinoviruses grow preferentially at 33 to 34°C—the temperature of the human nasal passages—rather than at the higher temperature (37°C) of the lower respiratory tract. One hundred distinct serotypes and one subtype of rhinovirus are recognized.

EPIDEMIOLOGY Rhinoviruses are a major cause of the common cold and have been isolated from 15 to 40 percent of adults with common cold–like illnesses. Overall rates of infection with rhinoviruses are higher among infants and young children and decrease with increasing age. Rhinovirus infections occur throughout the year, with seasonal peaks in early fall and spring in temperate climates. Rhinovirus infections are most often introduced into families by preschool or grade-school children younger than 6 years old. Between 25 and 70 percent of initial illnesses in family settings are followed by secondary cases, with the highest attack rates among the youngest siblings at home. Attack rates also increase with family size.

Rhinoviruses appear to spread via direct contact with infected secretions, usually respiratory droplets. In some studies of volunteers, transmission was most efficient by hand-to-hand contact, with subsequent self-inoculation of the conjunctival or nasal mucosa. In other studies, transmission by large- or small-particle aerosol was demonstrated. Virus also can be recovered from plastic surfaces inoculated 1 to 3 h previously; this observation suggests that environmental surfaces contribute to transmission. In studies of married couples in which neither partner had detectable serum antibody, transmission was associated with prolonged contact (122 h or more) during a 7-day period. Transmission was infrequent unless virus was recoverable from the donor's hands and nasal mucosa, at least 1000 TCID$_{50}$ of virus was present in nasal washes from the donor, and the donor was at least moderately symptomatic with the "cold." Despite anecdotal observations, exposure to cold temperatures, fatigue, or sleep deprivation has not been associated with increased rates of rhinovirus-induced illness in volunteers.

Infection with rhinoviruses is worldwide in distribution. By the time they reach adulthood, nearly all individuals have neutralizing antibodies to multiple serotypes, although the prevalence of antibody to any one serotype varies widely. Multiple serotypes circulate simultaneously, and generally no single serotype or group of serotypes has been more prevalent than the others.

PATHOGENESIS Rhinoviruses infect cells via attachment to specific cellular receptors; the major group of such receptors has been identified as intercellular adhesion molecule 1 (ICAM-1). Relatively limited information is available on the histopathology and pathogenesis of acute rhinovirus infections in humans. Examination of biopsy specimens obtained during experimentally induced and naturally occurring illness indicates that the nasal mucosa is edematous, is often hyperemic, and—during acute illness—is covered by a mucoid discharge. There is a mild infiltrate with inflammatory cells, including neutrophils, lymphocytes, plasma cells, and eosinophils. Mucus-secreting glands in the submucosa appear hyperactive; the nasal turbinates are engorged, a condition that may lead to obstruction of nearby openings of sinus cavities.

The incubation period for rhinovirus illness is short, generally 1 or 2 days. Virus shedding coincides with the onset of illness or may begin shortly before symptoms develop. The mechanisms of immunity to rhinovirus are not well worked out. In some studies, the presence of homotypic antibody has been associated with significantly reduced rates of subsequent infection and illness, but data conflict regarding the relative importance of serum and local antibody in protection from rhinovirus infection.

CLINICAL MANIFESTATIONS The most common clinical manifestations of rhinovirus infections are those of the common cold. Initially, illness begins with rhinorrhea and sneezing accompanied by nasal congestion. The throat is frequently sore, and in some cases sore throat is the initial complaint. Systemic signs and symptoms, such as malaise and headache, are mild or absent, and fever is unusual. Illness generally lasts for 4 to 9 days and resolves spontaneously without sequelae. In children, bronchitis, bronchiolitis, and bronchopneumonia have been reported; nevertheless, it appears that rhinoviruses are not major causes of lower respiratory tract disease in children. Rhinoviruses also may cause exacerbations of asthma and chronic pulmonary disease in adults. The vast majority of rhinovirus infections resolve without sequelae, but complications related to obstruction of the eustachian tubes or sinus ostia, including otitis media or acute sinusitis, can develop.

DIAGNOSIS Although rhinoviruses are the most frequently recognized cause of the common cold, similar illnesses are caused by a variety of other viruses, and the etiologic diagnosis cannot be made on clinical grounds alone. Rather, rhinovirus infection is diagnosed by isolation of the virus from nasal washes or nasal secretions in tissue culture. In practice, this procedure is rarely undertaken because of the benign, self-limited nature of the illness. Given the many serotypes of rhinovirus, diagnosis by serum antibody tests is currently impractical. Likewise, common laboratory tests, such as white cell count and sedimentation rate, are not helpful.

℞ TREATMENT

Rhinovirus infections are generally mild and self-limited, so treatment is not necessary. Some patients may benefit from the use of analgesics and nasal decongestants, and reduction of activity is prudent in instances of significant discomfort or fatigability. Antibacterial agents should be used only if bacterial complications such as otitis media or sinusitis develop. Specific antiviral therapy is not available. Application of interferon sprays intranasally has been effective in the prophylaxis of rhinovirus infections but is also associated with local irritation of the nasal mucosa. Prevention of rhinovirus infection by antibodies directed against rhinovirus receptors or by the soluble purified receptors themselves is under study. Experimental vaccines to certain rhinovirus serotypes have been prepared, but their utility is questionable because of the myriad serotypes and the uncertainty regarding mechanisms of immunity. Thorough hand washing, environmental decontamination, and protection against autoinoculation may help to reduce rates of transmission of infection.

CORONAVIRUS INFECTIONS

ETIOLOGIC AGENT Coronaviruses are pleomorphic, single-stranded RNA viruses that measure 80 to 160 nm in diameter. The name derives from the crownlike appearance produced by the club-shaped projections that stud the viral envelope. Three antigenically distinct coronavirus subgroups, designated B814, 229E, and OC43, have been isolated from humans. Coronaviruses are fastidious and are difficult to culture in vitro. Some strains will grow only in human tracheal organ cultures rather than in tissue culture.

EPIDEMIOLOGY Only limited seroepidemiologic studies of coronavirus infections have been conducted. Seroprevalence studies of two strains, 229E and OC43, have demonstrated the presence of serum antibodies at rates ranging from 12 percent to more than 80 percent in various populations. Overall, coronaviruses account for 10 to 20 percent of common colds. Coronavirus infections appear to be particularly prevalent in late fall, winter, and early spring—an interval when rhinovirus infections are less common. A cyclical pattern has been suggested for outbreaks of infection with strains OC43 and 229E, with outbreaks occurring every 2 to 4 years.

CLINICAL FEATURES The clinical features of illness caused by coronaviruses are similar to those of illness caused by rhinoviruses. In studies of volunteers, the mean incubation period of illness induced by coronaviruses (3 days) is somewhat longer than that of illness caused by rhinoviruses, and the duration of illness is somewhat shorter (mean, 6 to 7 days). In some studies, the amount of nasal discharge was somewhat greater in colds induced by coronaviruses than in those

induced by rhinoviruses. Coronaviruses have been recovered from infants with pneumonia and from military recruits with lower respiratory tract disease and have been associated with worsening of chronic bronchitis. However, the overall significance of coronaviruses in lower respiratory tract disease in humans remains unclear.

℞ TREATMENT

The approach to the treatment of common colds caused by coronaviruses is similar to that discussed above for rhinovirus-induced illnesses. Because of uncertainty regarding the number and relative importance of coronavirus subgroups and the mechanisms of immunity, vaccines against coronaviruses have not been developed.

RESPIRATORY SYNCYTIAL VIRUS INFECTIONS

ETIOLOGIC AGENT Respiratory syncytial virus (RSV) is a member of the Paramyxoviridae family and comprises the genus *Pneumovirus*. RSV, an enveloped virus approximately 150 to 300 nm in diameter, is so named because its replication leads to the fusion of neighboring cells into large multinucleated syncytia. The single-stranded RNA genome codes for 10 virus-specific proteins. Viral RNA is contained in a helical nucleocapsid surrounded by a lipid envelope bearing two glycoproteins: the G protein, by which the virus attaches to cells, and the F (fusion) protein, which facilitates entry of the virus into the cell by fusing host and viral membranes. RSV was once considered to be of a single antigenic type, but two distinct groups (A and B) and multiple subtypes within each group have now been described. The epidemiologic and clinical significance of subtype differences is being investigated.

EPIDEMIOLOGY RSV is the major respiratory pathogen of young children and the foremost cause of lower respiratory disease in infants. Infection with RSV is seen throughout the world in annual epidemics that occur in late fall, winter, or spring and that last up to 5 months. The virus is rarely encountered during the summer. Rates of illness are highest among infants between 1 and 6 months of age, peaking between 2 and 3 months of age. The attack rates among susceptible infants and children are extraordinarily high, approaching 100 percent in settings such as day-care centers where large numbers of susceptible infants are present. RSV accounts for 20 to 25 percent of hospital admissions of young infants and children for pneumonia and for up to 75 percent of cases of bronchiolitis in this age group. It has been estimated that more than half of infants who are at risk will become infected during an RSV epidemic.

In older children and adults, reinfection with RSV is frequent but disease is milder than in infancy. A common cold–like syndrome is the illness most commonly associated with RSV infection in adults. Severe lower respiratory tract disease with pneumonitis can occur in elderly (often institutionalized) adults and in patients with immunocompromising disorders or treatment, including recipients of bone-marrow and solid-organ transplants. RSV is also an important nosocomial pathogen; during an outbreak; it can infect pediatric patients and up to 25 to 50 percent of the staff on pediatric wards. The spread of virus among families is efficient: up to 40 percent of siblings may become infected when RSV is introduced into the family setting.

RSV is transmitted primarily by close contact with contaminated fingers or fomites and by self-inoculation of the conjunctiva or anterior nares. Virus also may be spread by coarse aerosols produced by coughing or sneezing, but it is inefficiently spread by fine-particle aerosols. The incubation period of illness is approximately 4 to 6 days, and virus shedding may last for 2 weeks or longer in children and for shorter periods of time in adults.

PATHOGENESIS Little is known about the histopathology of minor RSV infection. Severe bronchiolitis or pneumonia is characterized by necrosis of the bronchiolar epithelium and a peribronchiolar infiltrate of lymphocytes and mononuclear cells. Interalveolar thickening and filling of alveolar spaces with fluid can also be found. The characteristics of the immune response to RSV are not well elucidated. Because reinfection occurs frequently and is often associated with illness, the immunity that develops after single episodes of infection obviously is not complete or long-lasting. However, the cumulative effect of multiple reinfections is to temper subsequent disease and to provide some temporary measure of protection against infection. Studies of experimentally induced disease in healthy volunteers indicate that the presence of nasal IgA neutralizing antibody correlates more closely with protection than does the presence of serum antibody. Studies in infants, however, suggest that maternally acquired antibody provides some protection from lower respiratory tract disease, although illness can be severe even in infants who have moderate levels of maternally derived serum antibody. The relatively severe disease observed in immunosuppressed patients and experimental animal models indicates that cell-mediated immunity is an important mechanism of host defense against RSV.

CLINICAL MANIFESTATIONS RSV infection leads to a wide spectrum of respiratory illnesses. In infants, 25 to 40 percent of infections result in lower respiratory tract involvement, including pneumonia, bronchiolitis, and tracheobronchitis. In this age group, illness begins most frequently with rhinorrhea, low-grade fever, and mild systemic symptoms, often accompanied by cough and wheezing. Most patients recover gradually over 1 to 2 weeks. In more severe illness, tachypnea and dyspnea develop, and eventually frank hypoxia, cyanosis, and apnea can ensue. Physical examination may reveal diffuse wheezing, rhonchi, and rales. Chest radiography shows hyperexpansion, peribronchial thickening, and variable infiltrates ranging from diffuse interstitial infiltrates to segmental or lobar consolidation. Illness may be particularly severe in children born prematurely and in those with congenital cardiac disease, bronchopulmonary dysplasia, nephrotic syndrome, or immunosuppression. One study documented a 37 percent mortality rate for infants with RSV pneumonia and congenital cardiac disease.

In adults, the most common symptoms of RSV infection are those of the common cold, with rhinorrhea, sore throat, and cough. Illness is occasionally associated with moderate systemic symptoms such as malaise, headache, and fever. RSV also has been reported to cause lower respiratory tract disease with fever in adults, including severe pneumonia in the elderly. RSV pneumonia can be a significant cause of morbidity and mortality in patients (particularly children) undergoing bone-marrow and solid-organ transplantation.

LABORATORY FINDINGS AND DIAGNOSIS The diagnosis of RSV infection can be suspected on the basis of a suggestive epidemiologic setting—that is, severe illness among infants during an outbreak of RSV in the community. Infections in older children and adults cannot be differentiated with certainty from those caused by other respiratory viruses. The specific diagnosis is established by isolation of RSV from respiratory secretions, including sputum, throat swabs, or nasopharyngeal washes. Virus is detected in tissue culture and is identified specifically through immunologic reactions detected by immunofluorescence, enzyme-linked immunosorbent assay (ELISA), or other techniques. Immunofluorescence microscopy of nasal scrapings or washings provides a rapid diagnosis. Serologic tests that depend on fourfold or greater rises in complement-fixing or neutralizing antibody titers are useful for diagnosis in older children and adults but are less sensitive in children under 4 months of age. ELISA is more sensitive than complement-fixation or neutralization tests in the detection of serum antibody. Serologic diagnosis requires comparison of acute- and convalescent-phase serum specimens and is therefore not useful during acute illness.

℞ **TREATMENT**

Treatment of upper respiratory tract RSV infection is aimed primarily at the alleviation of symptoms and is similar to that for other viral infections of the upper respiratory tract. For lower respiratory tract infections, respiratory therapy, including hydration, suctioning of secretions, and administration of humidified oxygen and antibronchospastic agents, is given as needed. In severe hypoxia, intubation and ventilatory assistance may be required. Studies of infants with RSV infection who were given aerosolized ribavirin, a nucleoside analogue active in vitro against RSV, have demonstrated a beneficial

effect on the resolution of lower respiratory tract illness, including alleviation of blood-gas abnormalities. No similar studies have been performed in adults with RSV pneumonitis, and the benefit of ribavirin in these patients is unknown. Immunoglobulins with high titers of antibodies to RSV conferred protection against severe lower respiratory tract disease when administered to infants at high risk for complications of RSV infection in a multicenter trial. This approach is undergoing further study.

Considerable interest exists in the development of vaccines against RSV. Inactivated whole-virus vaccines have been ineffective; in one study, they actually potentiated the disease in infants. Other approaches include immunization with purified F and G surface glycoproteins of RSV or generation of stable, live attenuated virus vaccines. In settings such as pediatric wards where rates of transmission are high, barrier methods for the protection of hands and conjunctivae may be useful in reducing the spread of virus.

PARAINFLUENZA VIRUS INFECTIONS

ETIOLOGIC AGENT Parainfluenza viruses are members of the Paramyxoviridae family and comprise the genus *Paramyxovirus*. Parainfluenza viruses are 150 to 250 nm in diameter, are enveloped, and contain a single-stranded RNA genome. The envelope is studded with two glycoproteins: one possessing both hemagglutinin and neuraminidase activity and the other containing fusion activity. The viral RNA genome is enclosed in a helical nucleocapsid and codes for seven or eight virus-specific proteins. All four distinct serotypes of parainfluenza viruses share certain antigens with other members of the Paramyxoviridae family, including mumps and Newcastle disease viruses.

EPIDEMIOLOGY Parainfluenza viruses are distributed throughout the world, although infection with type 4 (subtypes 4A and 4B) has been reported less widely, probably because type 4 is more difficult to grow in tissue culture. Infection is acquired in early childhood, so that by 8 years of age most children have antibodies to serotypes 1, 2, and 3. Types 1 and 2 cause epidemics during the fall, primarily in odd-numbered years. Type 3 infection has been detected during all seasons of the year, but epidemics have occurred annually in the spring.

The contribution of parainfluenza infections to respiratory disease varies with both the location and the year. In studies conducted in the United States, parainfluenza virus infections accounted for 4.3 to 22 percent of respiratory illnesses in children. In adults, parainfluenza infections are generally mild and account for fewer than 5 percent of respiratory illnesses. The major importance of parainfluenza viruses is as a cause of respiratory illness in young children, in whom they rank second only to RSV as causes of lower respiratory tract illness. Parainfluenza virus type 1 is the most frequent cause of croup (laryngotracheobronchitis) in children, while serotype 2 causes similar, although generally less severe, disease. Type 3 is an important cause of bronchiolitis and pneumonia in infants, while illnesses associated with type 4 have generally been mild. Unlike types 1 and 2, type 3 frequently causes illness during the first month of life, while passively acquired maternal antibody is still present. Parainfluenza viruses are spread through infected respiratory secretions, primarily by person-to-person contact and/or by large droplets. The incubation period has varied from 3 to 6 days in experimental infections but may be somewhat shorter for naturally occurring disease in children.

PATHOGENESIS Immunity to parainfluenza viruses is incompletely understood, but evidence suggests that immunity to infections with serotypes 1 and 2 is mediated by local IgA antibodies in the respiratory tract. Passively acquired serum neutralizing antibodies also confer some protection against infection with types 1, 2, and—to a lesser degree—3. Studies in experimental animal models and in immunosuppressed patients suggest that cell-mediated immunity may also be important in parainfluenza virus infections.

CLINICAL MANIFESTATIONS Parainfluenza virus infections occur most frequently among children, in whom initial infection with serotype 1, 2, or 3 is associated with an acute febrile illness 50 to 80 percent of the time. Children may present with coryza, sore throat, hoarseness, and cough that may or may not be croupy. In severe croup, fever persists, with worsening coryza and sore throat. A brassy or barking cough may progress to frank stridor. Most children recover over the next 1 or 2 days, although progressive airway obstruction and hypoxia ensue occasionally. If bronchiolitis or pneumonia develops, progressive cough accompanied by wheezing, tachypnea, and intercostal retractions may occur. In this setting, sputum production increases modestly. Physical examination shows nasopharyngeal discharge and oropharyngeal injection, along with rhonchi, wheezes, or coarse breath sounds. Chest x-rays can show air trapping and occasionally interstitial infiltrates.

In older children and adults, parainfluenza infections tend to be milder, presenting most frequently as a common cold or as hoarseness, with or without cough. Lower respiratory tract involvement in older children and adults is uncommon, but tracheobronchitis in adults has been reported. Severe, prolonged, and even fatal parainfluenza infection has been reported in children and adults with severe immunosuppression, including bone-marrow and solid-organ transplant recipients.

LABORATORY FINDINGS AND DIAGNOSIS Like other respiratory viral diseases, the clinical syndromes caused by parainfluenza viruses (with the possible exception of croup in young children) are not sufficiently distinctive to be diagnosed on clinical grounds alone. A specific diagnosis is established by detection of virus in respiratory tract secretions, throat swabs, or nasopharyngeal washings. Virus is detected by growth in tissue culture, either by hemagglutination or by a cytopathic effect, or by immunofluorescence of viral antigens in exfoliated cells from the respiratory tract. Serologic diagnosis is based on a fourfold or greater rise in antibody titer, as detected by hemagglutination inhibition or by complement-fixation or neutralization tests in acute- and convalescent-phase specimens. However, as frequent heterotypic responses occur among the parainfluenza serotypes, the serotype causing illness often cannot be identified by serologic techniques alone.

Acute epiglottitis caused by *Haemophilus influenzae* type b must be differentiated from viral croup. Influenza A virus also is a common cause of croup during epidemic periods.

℞ **TREATMENT**

For upper respiratory tract illness, symptoms can be treated as discussed for other viral respiratory tract illnesses. If complications such as sinusitis, otitis, or superimposed bacterial bronchitis develop, appropriate antibiotics should be administered. Mild cases of croup should be treated with bed rest and moist air generated by vaporizers. More severe cases require hospitalization and close observation for the development of respiratory distress. If acute respiratory distress develops, humidified oxygen and intermittent racemic epinephrine are usually administered. High-dose systemic glucocorticoids also may be of benefit. No specific antiviral therapy is available, although ribavirin is active against parainfluenza viruses in vitro and is being evaluated clinically. Effective vaccines against parainfluenza viruses have not been developed.

ADENOVIRUS INFECTIONS

ETIOLOGIC AGENT Adenoviruses are complex DNA viruses that measure 70 to 80 nm in diameter. Human adenoviruses belong to the genus *Mastadenovirus*, which includes at least 47 serotypes. Adenoviruses have a characteristic morphology consisting of an icosahedral shell composed of 20 equilateral triangular faces and 12 vertices. The protein coat (capsid) consists of hexon subunits with group-specific and type-specific antigenic determinants and penton subunits at each vertex primarily containing group-specific antigens. A fiber with a knob at the end projects from each penton; this fiber contains type-specific and some group-specific antigens. Human adenoviruses have been divided into six subgenera (A through F) on the basis of the homology of DNA genomes and other properties. The adenovirus genome is a linear double-stranded DNA that codes for structural and nonstructural polypeptides. The replicative cycle of adenovirus may result either in lytic infection of cells or in the establishment of a latent infection (primarily involving lymphoid cells). Some adenovirus types can induce oncogenic transformation, and tumor formation has been observed in rodents; however, despite intensive investigation, adenoviruses have not been associated with tumors in humans.

EPIDEMIOLOGY Adenovirus infections most frequently affect infants and children. Infections occur throughout the year but are most common from fall to spring. Adenoviruses account for 3 to 5 percent of acute respiratory infections in children but for fewer than 2 percent of respiratory illnesses in civilian adults. Nearly 100 percent of adults have serum antibody to multiple serotypes—a finding indicating that infection is common in childhood. Types 1, 2, 3, and 5 are the most frequent isolates from children. Certain adenovirus serotypes—particularly 4 and 7 but also 3, 14, and 21—are associated with outbreaks of acute respiratory disease in military recruits in winter and spring. Adenovirus infection can be transmitted by inhalation of aerosolized virus, by inoculation of virus into conjunctival sacs, and probably by the fecal-oral route as well. Type-specific antibody generally develops after infection and is associated with protection against infection with the same serotype.

CLINICAL MANIFESTATIONS In children, adenoviruses cause a variety of clinical syndromes. The most common is an acute upper respiratory tract infection, with prominent rhinitis. On occasion, lower respiratory tract disease, including bronchiolitis and pneumonia, also develops. Adenoviruses, particularly types 3 and 7, cause pharyngoconjunctival fever, a characteristic acute febrile illness of children that occurs in outbreaks, most often in summer camps. The syndrome is marked by bilateral conjunctivitis in which the bulbar and palpebral conjunctivae have a granular appearance. Low-grade fever is frequently present for the first 3 to 5 days, and rhinitis, sore throat, and cervical adenopathy develop. The illness generally lasts for 1 to 2 weeks and resolves spontaneously. Febrile pharyngitis without conjunctivitis also has been associated with adenovirus infection. Adenoviruses have been isolated from cases of whooping cough with or without *Bordetella pertussis;* the significance of adenovirus in that disease is unknown.

In adults, the most frequently reported illness has been acute respiratory disease caused by adenovirus types 4 and 7 in military recruits. This illness is marked by a prominent sore throat and the gradual onset of fever, which often reaches 39°C on the second or third day of illness. Cough is almost always present, and coryza and regional lymphadenopathy are frequently seen. Physical examination may show pharyngeal edema, injection, and tonsillar enlargement with little or no exudate. If pneumonia has developed, auscultation and x-ray of the chest may indicate areas of patchy infiltration.

Adenoviruses have been associated with a number of non–respiratory tract diseases, including acute diarrheal illness caused by adenovirus types 40 and 41 in young children and hemorrhagic cystitis caused by adenoviruses 11 and 21. Epidemic keratoconjunctivitis, caused most frequently by adenovirus types 8, 19, and 37, has been associated with contaminated common sources such as ophthalmic solutions and roller towels. Adenoviruses also have been implicated in disseminated disease and pneumonia in immunosuppressed patients, including patients with AIDS and recipients of solid-organ or bone-marrow transplants.

LABORATORY FINDINGS AND DIAGNOSIS Adenovirus infection should be suspected in the epidemiologic setting of acute respiratory disease and in certain of the clinical syndromes (such as pharyngoconjunctival fever or epidemic keratoconjunctivitis) in which outbreaks of characteristic illnesses occur. In most cases, however, illnesses caused by adenovirus infection cannot be differentiated from those caused by a number of other viral respiratory agents and *Mycoplasma pneumoniae.* A definitive diagnosis of adenovirus infection is established by culture or detection of the virus from sites such as the conjunctiva and oropharynx or from sputum, urine, or stool. Virus may be detected in tissue culture by cytopathic changes and specifically identified by immunofluorescence or other immunologic techniques. Adenovirus types 40 and 41, which have been associated with diarrheal disease in children, require special tissue-culture cells for isolation, and these serotypes are most commonly detected by direct ELISA of stool. Serum antibody rises can be demonstrated by complement-fixation or neutralization tests, ELISA, or radioimmunoassay. Hemagglutination inhibition tests also may be done for those adenoviruses that hemagglutinate red cells.

 TREATMENT

Only symptom-based treatment and supportive therapy are available for adenovirus infections, and no clinically useful antiviral compounds have been identified. Live vaccines have been developed against adenovirus types 4 and 7 and are widely used to control illness in military recruits. These vaccines consist of live, unattenuated virus administered in enteric-coated capsules. Infection of the gastrointestinal tract with types 4 and 7 does not cause disease but stimulates local and systemic antibodies that are protective against subsequent acute respiratory disease due to those serotypes. Vaccines prepared from purified subunits of adenovirus are being investigated.

BIBLIOGRAPHY

RHINOVIRUSES

GWALTNEY JM: Rhinoviruses, in *Principles and Practice of Infectious Diseases*, 4th ed, GF Mandell et al (eds). New York, Churchill Livingstone, 1995, pp 1656–1663

McKINLAY MA et al: Treatment of the picornavirus common cold by inhibitors of viral uncoating and attachment. Annu Rev Microbiol 46:635, 1992

ROSSMAN MG et al: Structure of a human common cold virus and functional relationships to other picornaviruses. Nature 317:145, 1985

TYRRELL DAJ: Common colds. Intervirology 25:177, 1986

CORONAVIRUSES

LARSON HE et al: Isolation of rhinoviruses and coronaviruses from 38 colds in adults. J Med Virol 5:221, 1980

McINTOSH K: Coronaviruses, in *Virology*, 3d ed, BN Fields (ed). New York, Raven, 1995, pp 1095–1103

MONTO AS: Medical reviews, coronaviruses. Yale J Biol Med 47:234, 1974

RESPIRATORY SYNCYTIAL VIRUS

ANDERSON LJ et al: Multicenter study of strains of respiratory syncytial virus. J Infect Dis 163:687, 1991

CHANOCK RM et al: Serious respiratory tract disease caused by respiratory syncytial virus: Prospects for improved therapy and effective immunization. Pediatrics 90:137, 1992

ENGLUND JA et al: Respiratory syncytial virus infection in immunocompromised adults. Ann Intern Med 109:203, 1988

GLEZEN WP et al: Risk of primary infection and reinfection with respiratory syncytial virus. Am J Dis Child 140:543, 1986

HALL CB et al: Aerosolized ribavirin treatment of infants with respiratory syncytial viral infection. A randomized double blind study. N Engl J Med 308:1443, 1983

HENDERSON FW et al: Respiratory syncytial virus infections, reinfections and immunity. N Engl J Med 300:530, 1979

PARAINFLUENZA VIRUSES

DENNY FW et al: Croup: An 11 year study in a pediatric practice. Pediatrics 71:871, 1983

HEILMAN CA: Respiratory syncytial and parainfluenza viruses. J Infect Dis 161:402, 1990

WRIGHT PF: Parainfluenzaviruses, in *Textbook of Human Virology*, 2d ed, RB Belshe (ed). St. Louis, Mosby, 1991, pp 342–350

ADENOVIRUSES

BAUM SG: Adenoviruses, in *Principles and Practice of Infectious Diseases*, 4th ed, G Mandell et al (eds). New York, Churchill Livingstone, 1995, pp 1382–1387

FOX JP et al: The Seattle virus watch. VII. Observations of adenovirus infections. Am J Epidemiol 105:362, 1977

HIERHOLZER JC: Adenoviruses in the immunocompromised host. Clin Microbiol Rev 5:262, 1992

ROSE HM et al: Adenoviral infection in military recruits. Arch Environ Health 21:356, 1970

SECTION 14
RNA VIRUSES

 Anthony S. Fauci, Dan L. Longo

THE HUMAN RETROVIRUSES

The retroviruses, which make up a large family (Retroviridae), infect mainly vertebrates. They have a unique replication cycle whereby their genetic information is encoded by RNA rather than DNA. Retroviruses contain an RNA-dependent DNA polymerase (a reverse transcriptase) that directs the synthesis of a DNA form of the viral genome after infection of a host cell. The designation *retrovirus* denotes that information in the form of RNA is transcribed into DNA in the host cell—a sequence that overturned a central dogma of molecular biology: that information passes unidirectionally from DNA to RNA to protein. Interest in this class of viruses was stimulated by the pioneering studies of Peyton Rous, who in 1911 identified an agent that was transmissible and filterable (that is, smaller than a cell) and that produced sarcoma in chickens, and by those of Ludwig Gross, who in the 1950s demonstrated a viral etiology for murine leukemia. The observation that RNA was the source of genetic information in the causative agents of these and other animal tumors led to a number of paradigm-shifting biologic insights regarding not only the direction of genetic-information passage but also the viral etiology of certain cancers and the concept of oncogenes as normal host genes scavenged and altered by a viral vector.

The family Retroviridae includes three subfamilies (Table 192-1): Oncovirinae, of which human T-cell lymphotropic virus (HTLV) type I is the most important in humans; Lentivirinae, of which human immunodeficiency virus (HIV) is the most important in humans; and Spumavirinae, the "foamy" viruses, named for the pathologic appearance of infected cells. A number of spumaviruses have been isolated from humans; however, they are not associated with any known disease and therefore are not discussed further in this chapter.

The wide variety of interactions of a retrovirus with its host range from completely benign events (e.g., silent carriage of endogenous retroviral sequences in the germ-line genome of many animal species) to rapidly fatal infections (e.g., exogenous infection with an oncogenic virus such as Rous sarcoma virus in chickens). The ability of retroviruses to acquire and alter the structure and function of host cell sequences has revolutionized our understanding of molecular carcinogenesis. The viruses can insert into the germ-line genome of the host cell and behave as a transposable or movable genetic element. They can activate or inactivate genes near the site of integration into the genome. They can rapidly alter their own genome by recombination and mutation under selective environmental stimuli.

Most human viral diseases occur as a consequence of either tissue destruction by the virus itself or the host's response to the virus. Although these mechanisms are operative in retroviral infections, retroviruses have additional mechanisms of inducing disease, including the malignant transformation of an infected cell and the induction of an immunodeficiency state that leads to opportunistic diseases (infections and neoplasms).

STRUCTURE AND LIFE CYCLE Despite the wide range of biologic consequences of retroviral infection, all retroviruses are similar in structure, genome organization, and mode of replication. Retroviruses are 70 to 130 nm in diameter and have a lipid-containing envelope surrounding an icosahedral capsid with a dense inner core. The core contains two identical copies of the single-stranded RNA genome (rendering retroviruses diploid). The RNA molecules are 8 to 10 kb long and are complexed with reverse transcriptase and tRNA. Other viral proteins, such as integrase, are also components of the virion particle. The RNA has features usually found in mRNA: a cap site at the 5' end of the molecule, which is important in the initiation of mRNA translation, and a polyadenylation site at the 3' end, a feature that seems to influence mRNA turnover (i.e., messages with shorter polyA tails turn over faster than messages with longer polyA tails). However, the retroviral RNA is not translated; instead it is transcribed into DNA. The DNA form of the retroviral genome is called a *provirus*.

The replication cycle of retroviruses proceeds in two phases (Fig. 192-1). In the first phase, the virus enters the cytoplasm after binding to a specific cell-surface receptor; the viral RNA and reverse transcriptase synthesize a double-stranded DNA version of the RNA template; and the provirus moves into the nucleus and integrates into the host cell genome. This proviral integration is permanent. Although some animal retroviruses integrate into a single specific site of the host genome in every infected cell, the four known pathogenic human retroviruses (HLTV-I, HTLV-II, HIV-1, and HIV-2) integrate randomly. This first phase of replication depends entirely on gene products in the virus. The second phase includes the synthesis and processing of viral genomes, mRNAs, and proteins using host cell machinery, often under the influence of viral gene products. Virions are assembled and released from the cell by budding from the membrane; host cell membrane proteins are frequently incorporated into the envelope of the virus. Proviral integration occurs during the S phase of the cell cycle; thus, in general, nondividing cells are resistant to retroviral infection. Only the lentiviruses are able to infect nondividing cells. Once a host is infected, it is infected for life.

Retroviral genomes include both coding and noncoding sequences (Fig. 192-2). In general, noncoding sequences are important recognition signals for DNA or RNA synthesis or processing events and are located in the 5' and 3' terminal regions of the genome. All retroviral genomes are terminally redundant, containing identical sequences called long terminal repeats (LTRs). The ends of the retroviral RNA genome differ slightly in sequence from the integrated retroviral DNA. In the latter, the LTR sequences are repeated in both the 5' and the 3' terminus of the virus. The LTRs contain sequences involved in initiating the expression of the viral proteins, the integration of the provirus, and the polyadenylation of viral RNAs. The primer binding site, which is critical for the initiation of reverse transcription, and the viral packaging sequences are located outside the LTR sequences. The coding regions include the *gag* (group-specific antigen, core protein), *pol* (RNA-dependent DNA polymerase), and *env* (envelope) genes. The *gag* gene encodes a precursor polyprotein that is cleaved to form three to five capsid proteins; a fraction of the Gag precursor proteins also contain a protease responsible for cleaving the Gag and Pol polyproteins. A Gag-Pol polyprotein gives rise to the protease that is responsible for cleaving the Gag-Pol polyprotein. The *pol* gene encodes three proteins: the reverse transcriptase, the integrase, and the protease. The reverse transcriptase functions to copy the viral RNA into the double-stranded DNA provirus, which can attach to the host cell DNA via the action of integrase. The protease functions to cleave the Gag-Pol polyprotein into smaller protein products. The *env* gene encodes the envelope glycoproteins: one protein that binds to specific surface receptors and determines what cell types can be infected and a smaller transmembrane protein that anchors the complex to the envelope. The cartoon in Fig. 192-3 shows how the retroviral gene products make up the virus structure.

HTLVs have a region between *env* and the 3' LTR that encodes at least two proteins in overlapping reading frames; Tax, a 40-kD protein that does not bind to DNA but induces the expression of host cell transcription factors that alter host cell gene expression; and Rex, a 27-kD protein that regulates the expression of viral mRNAs. These two proteins are produced from messages that are similar but that are spliced differently from overlapping but distinct exons.

The lentiviruses in general, and HIV-1 and -2 in particular, contain a larger genome than other pathogenic retroviruses; the size of this genome is related to the presence of an untranslated region between *pol* and *env* that encodes portions of several proteins, varying with the reading frame into which the mRNA is spliced. Tat is a 14-kD protein that augments the expression of virus from the LTR. The Rev protein regulates RNA splicing and/or RNA transport in HIV-1 and may function in a manner similar to the Rex protein of HTLV. The Nef protein appears to down-regulate CD4, the cellular receptor for HIV; to alter host T-cell activation pathways; and to enhance viral infectivity. The Vif protein is necessary for the proper assembly of the HIV nucleoprotein core in many types of cells; without Vif, proviral DNA is not efficiently produced in these infected cells. Vpr, Vpu (HIV-1 only), and Vpx (HIV-2 only) are viral proteins encoded by translation of the same message in different reading frames. As noted above, oncogenic retroviruses depend on cell proliferation for their replication; lentiviruses can infect nondividing cells, largely owing to effects mediated by Vpr. Vpr appears to facilitate transport of the provirus into the nucleus and can induce other cellular changes, such as G2 growth arrest and differentiation of some target cells. Vpx is structurally related to Vpr, but its functions are not fully defined. Vpu promotes the degradation of CD4 in the endoplasmic reticulum and stimulates the release of virions from infected cells.

Retroviruses can be either exogenously acquired by infection with a virion capable of replication or transmitted in the germ line as endogenous virus. Endogenous retroviruses are often replication-defective. The human genome contains endogenous retroviral se-

Table 192-1

Classification of Retroviruses: the Family Retroviridae

Subfamily	Group*	Example	Feature
Oncovirinae (oncogenic viruses)	Avian leukosis	Rous sarcoma virus	Contains *src* oncogene
	Mammalian C-type	Abelson leukemia virus	Contains *abl* oncogene
	B-type	Murine mammary tumor virus	Can be endogenous or exogenous
	D-type	Mason-Pfizer monkey virus	—
	HTLV-BLV	HTLV-I	Causes T-cell lymphoma and neurologic disease
Lentivirinae (slow viruses)	—	HIV-1, HIV-2	Causes AIDS
		Visna virus	Causes lung and brain diseases in sheep
		Feline immunodeficiency virus	Causes immunodeficiency in cats
Spumavirinae (foamy viruses)	—	Simian foamy virus, human foamy virus	Causes no known disease

Abbreviations: HTLV, human T-lymphotropic virus; BLV, bovine leukemia virus; HIV, human immunodeficiency virus.
* The Oncovirinae were originally grouped into types A–D on the basis of morphologic features (size, core location, budding) under electron microscopy; however, this system has been replaced by groupings based on relationships of genome structure and sequence.

quences, but there are no known replication-competent endogenous retroviruses in humans.

In general, viruses that contain only the *gag*, *pol*, and *env* genes either are not pathogenic or take a long time to induce disease because the pathogenesis of neoplastic transformation relies on the chance integration of the provirus at a spot in the genome that will result in the expression of a cellular gene (proto-oncogene) that becomes transforming by virtue of its unregulated expression. For example, avian leukosis virus causes B-cell leukemia by inducing the expression of *myc*. Some retroviruses possess captured and altered cellular genes near their integration site, and these viral oncogenes are capable of transforming the infected host cell. Viruses that have oncogenes often have lost a portion of their genome that is required for replication. Such viruses need helper viruses to reproduce, a feature that may explain why these acute transforming retroviruses are rare in nature. All human retroviruses identified to date are exogenous and are not acutely transforming (that is, they lack a transforming oncogene).

These remarkable properties of retroviruses have led to experimental efforts to use them as vectors to insert specific genes into particular cell types, a process known as *gene therapy* or *gene transfer*. The process could be used to repair a genetic defect or to introduce a new property that could be used therapeutically; for example, it could be possible to insert a gene (e.g., thymidine kinase) that would make a tumor cell susceptible to killing by a drug (e.g., ganciclovir). One source of concern about the use of retroviral vectors in humans is that replication-competent viruses might rescue endogenous retroviral replication, with unpredictable results. This concern is not merely hypothetical: The detection of proteins encoded by endogenous retroviral sequences on the surface of cancer cells implies that the genetic events leading to the cancer were able to activate the synthesis of these usually silent genes.

HUMAN T-CELL LYMPHOTROPIC VIRUS

HTLV-I was isolated in 1980 from a T-cell lymphoma cell line from a patient originally thought to have cutaneous T-cell lymphoma. Later it became clear that the patient had a distinct form of lymphoma (originally reported in Japan) called adult T-cell leukemia/lymphoma (ATL). Serologic data have determined that HTLV-I is the cause of at least two important diseases: ATL and tropical spastic paraparesis, also called HTLV-I–associated myelopathy (HAM).

Two years after the isolation of HTLV-I, HTLV-II was isolated from a patient with an unusual form of hairy cell leukemia that affected T cells. Although early epidemiologic studies of HTLV-II failed to reveal a consistent disease association, more recent studies suggest an association of HTLV-II with human disease (see "Associated Diseases"

under "Features of HTLV-II Infection" below), particularly among injection drug users.

BIOLOGY AND MOLECULAR BIOLOGY Because the biology of HTLV-I and that of HTLV-II are similar and because these viruses are generally grouped together, the following discussion will focus on HTLV-I.

The cellular receptor for HTLV-I has not yet been identified, but it maps to chromosome 17. Generally, only T cells are productively infected, but infection of B cells and other cell types is occasionally detected. The most common outcome of HTLV-I infection is latent

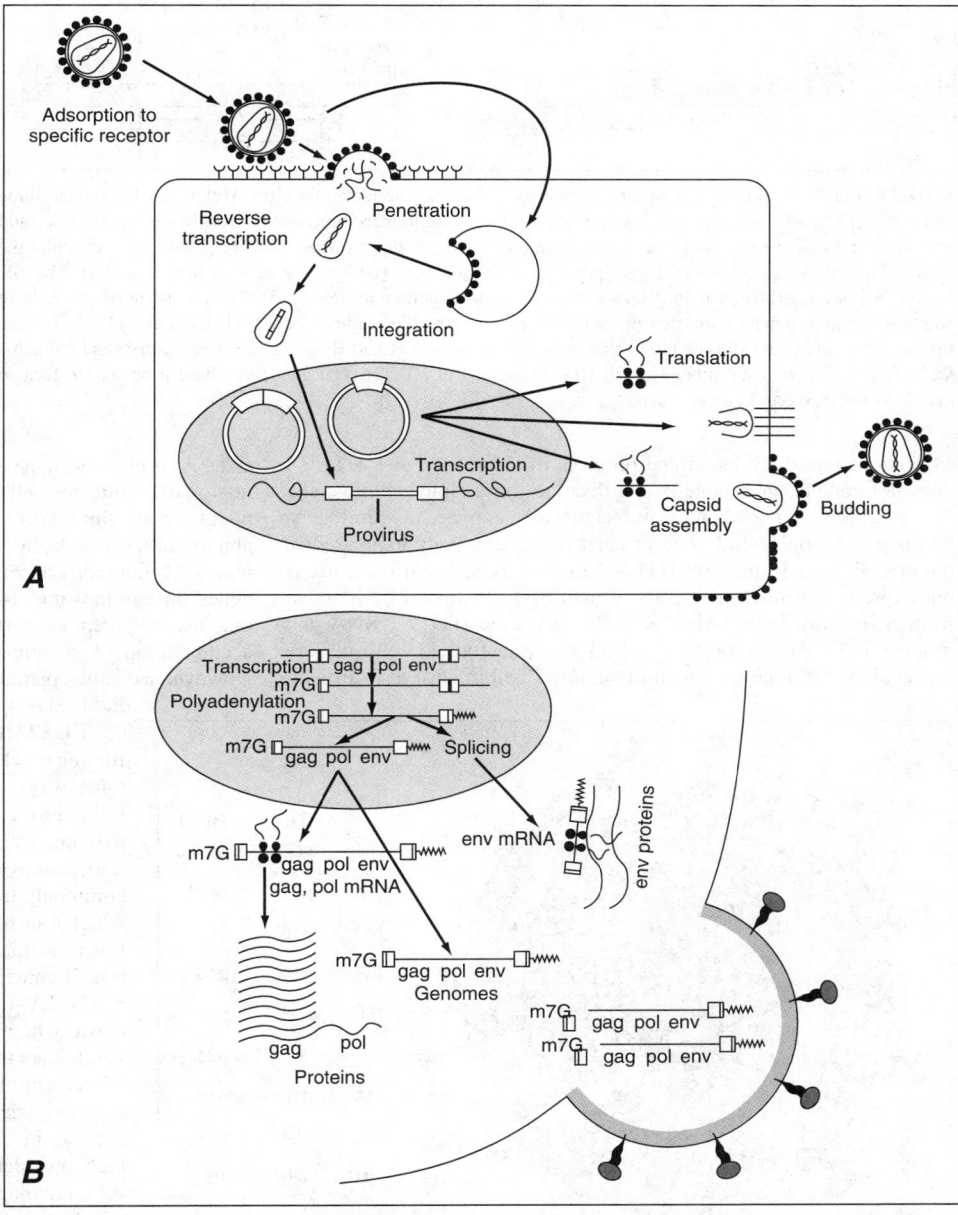

FIGURE 192-1 The life cycle of retroviruses. *A.* Overview of virus replication. The retrovirus enters a target cell by binding to a specific cell-surface receptor; once the virus is internalized, its RNA is released from the nucleocapsid and is reverse-transcribed into proviral DNA. The provirus is inserted into the genome and then transcribed into RNA; the RNA is translated; and virions assemble and are extruded from the cell membrane by budding. *B.* Overview of retroviral gene expression. The provirus is transcribed, capped, and polyadenylated. Viral RNA molecules then have one of three fates: They are exported to the cytoplasm, where they are packaged as the viral RNA in infectious viral particles; they are spliced to form the message for the envelope polyprotein; or they are translated into Gag and Pol proteins. Most of the messages for the Pol protein fail to initiate Pol translation because of a stop codon before its initiation; however, in a fraction of the messages, the stop codon is missed and the Pol proteins are translated. *(Modified from Coffin.)*

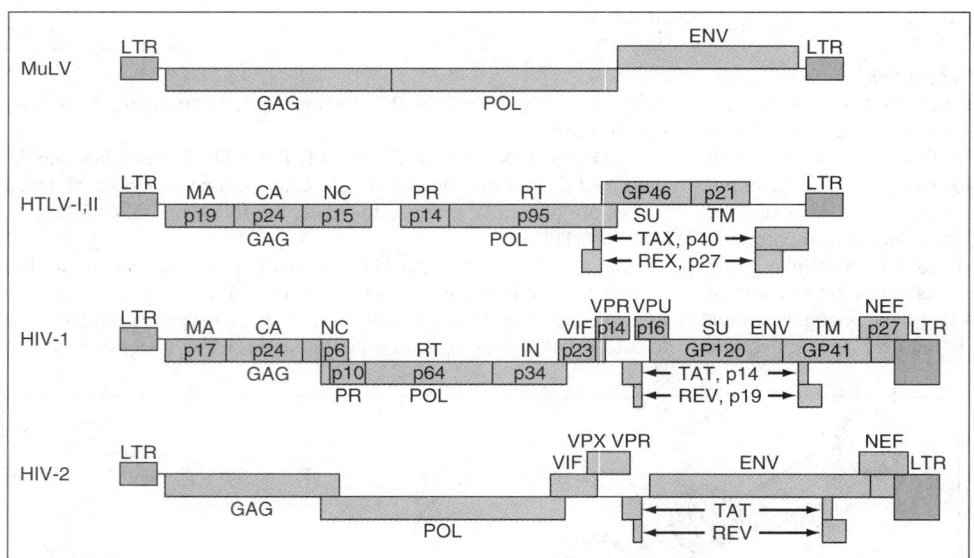

FIGURE 192-2 Genomic structure of retroviruses. The murine leukemia virus MuLV has the typical three structural genes: *gag*, *pol*, and *env*. The *gag* region gives rise to three proteins: matrix (MA), capsid (CA), and nucleic acid–binding (NC) proteins. The *pol* region encodes both a protease (PR) responsible for cleaving the viral polyproteins and a reverse transcriptase (RT). In addition, HIV *pol* encodes an integrase (IN). The *env* region encodes a surface protein (SU) and a small transmembrane protein (TM). The human retroviruses have additional gene products translated in each of the three possible reading frames. HTLV-I and HTLV-II have *tax* and *rex* genes with exons on either side of the *env* gene. HIV-1 and HIV-2 have six accessory gene products: *tat*, *rev*, *vif*, *nef*, *vpr*, and either *vpu* (in HIV-1) or *vpx* (in HIV-2). The genes for these proteins are located mainly between the *pol* and *env* genes.

carriage of randomly integrated provirus in CD4+ T cells. HTLV-I does not contain an oncogene and does not insert into a unique site in the genome. Indeed, most infected cells express no viral gene products. The only viral gene product that is routinely expressed in tumor cells transformed by HTLV-I in vivo is *tax*, and even *tax* is not expressed in the tumor cells of many ATL patients. Cells transformed in vitro, by contrast, actively transcribe HTLV-I RNA and produce infectious virions. Most HTLV-I–transformed cell lines are the result of the infection of a normal host T cell in vitro. It is difficult to establish cell lines derived from authentic ATL cells.

Although *tax* does not itself bind to DNA, it does induce the expression of a wide range of host-cell gene products, including transcription factors (especially *c-rel*, *ets*-1 and -2, and members of the *fos/jun* family), cytokines [e.g., interleukin (IL) 2, granulocyte-macrophage colony-stimulating factor, and tumor necrosis factor (TNF)], and membrane proteins and receptors [major histocompatibility (MHC) molecules and IL-2 receptor α]. The genes activated by *tax* are generally controlled by transcription factors of the *c-rel* and cyclic AMP response element binding (CREB) protein families. It is unclear how this induction of host gene expression leads to neoplastic transformation. Induction of a cytokine-autocrine loop has been proposed; however, IL-2 is not the crucial cytokine. The involvement of IL-4 and IL-7 has been proposed, and the newly identified cytokine IL-15 may play a role.

In light of the irregular expression of *tax* in ATL cells, it has been suggested that *tax* is important in the early phases of transformation but is not essential for the maintenance of the transformed state. As is clear from the epidemiology of HTLV-I infection, transformation of an infected cell is a rare event and may depend on heterogeneous second, third, or fourth genetic hits. No consistent chromosomal abnormalities have been described in ATL; however, individual cases with *p53* mutations and translocations involving the T-cell receptor genes on chromosome 14 have been reported. Recent data suggest that *tax* may repress certain DNA repair enzymes, permitting the accumulation of genetic damage that would normally be repaired. However, a detailed picture of the molecular pathogenesis of HTLV-I–induced neoplasia is not yet available.

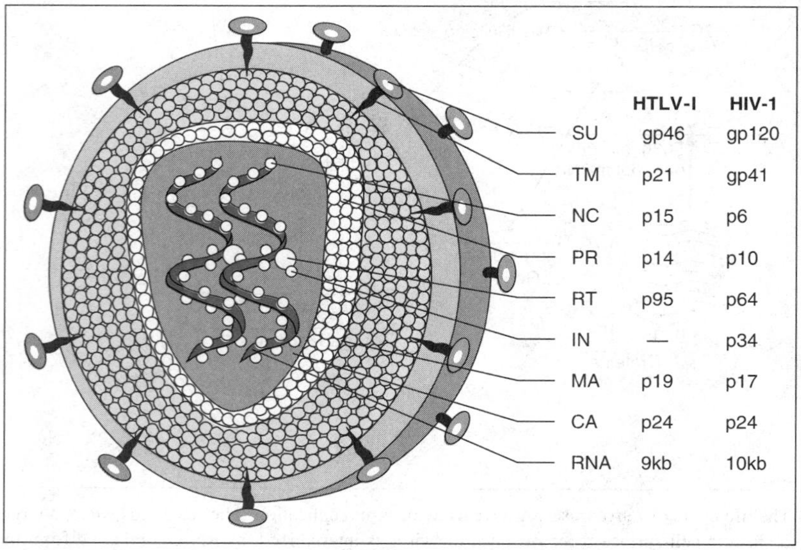

FEATURES OF HTLV-I INFECTION Epidemiology HTLV-I infection is transmitted in at least three ways: from mother to child, especially in breast milk; through sexual activity, more commonly from men to women; and through the blood—i.e., via contaminated transfusions or contaminated needles. The virus is most commonly transmitted perinatally. Compared with HIV, which can be transmitted in cell-free form, HTLV-I is less infectious, and its transmission usually requires cell-to-cell contact.

HTLV-I is endemic in southwestern Japan and Okinawa, where more than 1 million persons are infected. Antibodies to HTLV-I are present in the serum of up to 35 percent of Okinawans, 10 percent of residents of the Japanese island of Kyushu, and fewer than 1 percent of persons in nonendemic regions of Japan. Despite this high prevalence of infection, only about 500 cases of ATL are diagnosed in this area each year. Other clusters of infection have been noted in other areas of the Orient, such as Taiwan; in the Caribbean basin, including northeastern South America; in central Africa; in Italy; in Israel; in the Arctic; and in the southeastern part of the United States.

Although early epidemiologic studies indicated an increasing seroprevalence of HTLV-I among injection drug users, more recent investigations with the use of confirmatory serologic assays that reliably distinguish between HTLV-I and HTLV-II indicate that the vast

	HTLV-I	HIV-1
SU	gp46	gp120
TM	p21	gp41
NC	p15	p6
PR	p14	p10
RT	p95	p64
IN	—	p34
MA	p19	p17
CA	p24	p24
RNA	9kb	10kb

FIGURE 192-3 Schematic structure of human retroviruses. The surface glycoprotein (SU) is responsible for binding to receptors of host cells. The transmembrane protein (TM) anchors SU to the virus. NC is a nucleic acid–binding protein found in association with the viral RNA. A protease (PR) cleaves the polyproteins encoded by the *gag*, *pol*, and *env* genes into their functional components. RT is reverse transcriptase, and IN is an integrase present in some retroviruses (e.g., HIV-1) that facilitates insertion of the provirus into the host genome. MA is a Gag protein closely associated with the lipid of the envelope. The capsid protein (CA) forms the major internal structure of the virus, the core shell.

majority of HTLV infections among injection drug users are, in fact, due to HTLV-II (see below). The development of ATL is rare among persons infected by blood products; however, about 20 percent of patients with HAM acquire HTLV-I from contaminated blood.

A progressive spastic or ataxic myelopathy that develops in an individual who is HTLV-I positive (i.e., who has serum antibodies to HTLV-I) is likely to be due to direct nervous system infection with the virus; a similar disorder may result from infection with HIV or HTLV-II. In rare instances, patients with HAM are seronegative but have detectable antibody to HTLV-I in the cerebrospinal fluid (CSF).

The cumulative lifetime risk of developing ATL is 2 to 5 percent among HTLV-I–infected patients; a similar risk is projected for HAM. The distribution of the two diseases overlaps the distribution of HTLV-I, with more than 95 percent of affected patients showing serologic evidence of HTLV-I infection. The latent period between infection and the emergence of disease is 20 to 30 years for ATL. For HAM, the median latency period is about 3.3 years; the interval is usually shorter (one case occurred within 4 months of a contaminated transfusion) but can also be as long as 20 to 30 years.

Associated Diseases *Adult T-cell leukemia/lymphoma* Four clinical types of HTLV-I–induced neoplasia have been described: acute, lymphomatous, chronic, and smoldering. All of these tumors are monoclonal proliferations of CD4 + post-thymic T cells with clonal proviral integrations and clonal T-cell receptor gene rearrangements.

About 60 percent of patients who develop malignancy have classic *acute* ATL, which is characterized by a short clinical prodrome (~2 weeks between the first symptoms and the diagnosis) and an aggressive natural history (median survival period, 6 months). The clinical picture is dominated by rapidly progressive skin lesions, pulmonary involvement, hypercalcemia, and lymphocytosis with cells containing lobulated or "cloven-hoof" nuclei. The malignant cells have monoclonal proviral integrations and express CD4, CD3, and CD25 (low-affinity IL-2 receptors) on their surface. Serum levels of CD25 can be used as a tumor marker. Anemia and thrombocytopenia are rare. The skin lesions may be difficult to distinguish from those in mycosis fungoides. Lytic bone lesions, which are common, do not contain tumor cells but rather are composed of osteolytic cells, usually without osteoblastic activity. Despite the leukemic picture, bone marrow involvement is patchy in most cases.

The hypercalcemia of ATL is multifactorial; the tumor cells produce osteoclast-activating factors (TNFα, IL-1, lymphotoxin) and can also produce a parathyroid hormone–like molecule. The affected patients have an underlying immunodeficiency that makes them susceptible to opportunistic infections similar to those seen in patients with AIDS (see Chap. 308). The pathogenesis of the immunodeficiency is unclear. Pulmonary infiltrates in ATL patients reflect leukemic infiltration half the time and opportunistic infections with organisms such as *Pneumocystis carinii* and other fungi the other half. Gastrointestinal symptoms are nearly always related to opportunistic infection. Serum concentrations of lactate dehydrogenase (LDH) and alkaline phosphatase are often elevated. About 10 percent of patients have leptomeningeal involvement leading to weakness, altered mental status, paresthesias, and/or headache. Unlike other forms of central nervous system (CNS) lymphoma, ATL may be accompanied by normal CSF protein levels. The diagnosis depends on finding ATL cells in the CSF (see Chap. 113).

The *lymphomatous* type of ATL occurs in about 20 percent of patients and is similar to the acute form in its natural history and clinical course, except that circulating abnormal cells are rare and lymphadenopathy is evident. The histology of the lymphoma, which can fit any of five diagnostic types usually used for lymphoma classification, does not influence the natural history. In general, the diagnosis is suspected on the basis of the patient's birthplace and the presence of skin lesions and hypercalcemia. The diagnosis is confirmed by the detection of antibodies to HTLV-I in serum.

Patients with the *chronic* form of ATL generally have normal serum levels of calcium and LDH and no involvement of the CNS, bone, or gastrointestinal tract. The median duration of survival for

these patients is 2 years. In some cases, chronic ATL progresses to the acute form of the disease.

No more than 5 percent of patients have the *smoldering* form of ATL. In this form, the malignant cells have monoclonal proviral integration; fewer than 5 percent of peripheral-blood cells exhibit typical morphologic abnormalities; hypercalcemia, adenopathy, and hepatosplenomegaly do not develop; the CNS, the bones, and the gastrointestinal tract are not involved; and skin and pulmonary lesions may be present. The median survival period of this small subset of patients appears to be 5 years or longer.

HTLV-I–associated myelopathy (tropical spastic paraparesis)   In contrast to ATL, in which there is a slight predominance of male patients, HAM affects females disproportionately. HAM resembles multiple sclerosis in certain ways (see Chap. 379). The onset is insidious. Symptoms include weakness or stiffness in one or both legs, back pain, and urinary incontinence. Sensory changes are usually mild, but peripheral neuropathy may develop. The disease generally takes the form of slowly progressive and unremitting thoracic myelopathy; one-third of patients are bedridden within 10 years of diagnosis, and one-half are unable to walk unassisted by this point. Patients display spastic paraparesis or paraplegia with hyperreflexia, ankle clonus, and extensor plantar responses. Cognitive function is usually spared; cranial nerve abnormalities are unusual.

Magnetic resonance imaging (MRI) reveals lesions in both the white matter and the paraventricular regions of the brain as well as in the spinal cord. Pathologic examination of the spinal cord shows symmetrical degeneration of the lateral columns, including the corticospinal tracts; some cases involve the posterior columns as well. The spinal meninges and cord parenchyma contain an inflammatory infiltrate with myelin destruction.

HTLV-I usually is not found in cells of the CNS, but it may be detected in a small population of lymphocytes present in the CSF. In general, HTLV-I replication is greater in HAM than in ATL, and patients with HAM have a stronger immune response to the virus. Antibodies to HTLV-I are present in the serum and appear to be produced in the CSF of HAM patients, where titers are often higher than in the serum. It has been proposed that the pathophysiology of HAM involves the induction of autoimmune destruction of neural cells by T cells with specificity for viral components such as Tax or Env proteins. One theory is that susceptibility to HAM may be related to the presence of human leukocyte antigen (HLA) alleles capable of presenting viral antigens in a fashion that leads to autoimmunity. There are insufficient data at present to confirm such an HLA association.

Other putative HTLV-I–related diseases   In areas where HTLV-I is endemic, diverse inflammatory and autoimmune diseases have been attributed to the virus, including uveitis, dermatitis, pneumonitis, rheumatoid arthritis, and polymyositis. However, a causal relationship between HTLV-I and these illnesses has not been rigorously established.

Prevention of Disease   The principles of prevention of HTLV-I–induced disease are clear. Women in endemic areas should not breast-feed their children, and blood donors should be screened for serum antibodies to HTLV-I. As in the prevention of HIV infection, the practice of safe sex and the avoidance of needle sharing are important. Conscientious adherence to these principles should have an enormous impact on the prevalence of HTLV-I infection.

℞ TREATMENT
For the small number of patients who develop HTLV-I–related disease, therapies are not curative. In patients with the acute and lymphomatous types of ATL, the disease progresses rapidly. Hypercalcemia is generally controlled by glucocorticoid administration and cytotoxic therapy directed against the neoplasm. The tumor is highly responsive to combination chemotherapy that is employed against other forms of lymphoma; however, patients are susceptible to overwhelming bacterial and opportunistic infections, and ATL

relapses within 4 to 10 months after remission in most patients. The combination of interferon α and zidovudine reportedly elicits responses in a substantial fraction of patients with less toxicity than the usual lymphoma regimens. Survival may be extended by this treatment. Because viral replication is not clearly associated with ATL progression, zidovudine is probably effective through its cytotoxic effects (as a chain-terminating thymidine analogue) rather than its antiviral effects. An experimental approach using an yttrium 90–labeled antibody to the IL-2 receptor appears promising but is not widely available. Patients with the chronic or smoldering form of ATL may be managed with an expectant approach: Treat any infections, and watch and wait for signs of progression to acute disease.

Patients with HAM may obtain some benefit from the use of glucocorticoids to reduce inflammation. Antiretroviral regimens have not been effective. In one study, danazol (200 mg tid) produced significant neurologic improvement in five of six treated patients, with resolution of urinary incontinence in two cases, decreased spasticity in three, and the restoration of the ability to walk after confinement to a wheelchair in two. Physical therapy and rehabilitation are important components of management.

FEATURES OF HTLV-II INFECTION Epidemiology HTLV-II is endemic in certain Native American tribes. It is generally considered to be a New World virus that was brought from Asia to the Americas 10,000 to 40,000 years ago during the migration of infected populations across the Bering land bridge.

The mode of transmission of HTLV-II is probably the same as that of HTLV-I (see above). HTLV-II may be less readily transmitted sexually than HTLV-I.

Because of their biologic similarity and the previous lack of distinguishing serologic assays, HTLV-I and HTLV-II were often grouped together in seroepidemiologic studies. This practice led to the incorrect conclusion that HTLV-I was becoming quite prevalent among injection drug users in the United States. Studies of large cohorts of injection drug users with serologic assays that reliably distinguish HTLV-I from HTLV-II indicate that the vast majority of HTLV-positive subjects are infected with HTLV-II. The seroprevalence of HTLV in a cohort of 7841 injection drug users from drug treatment centers in Baltimore, Chicago, Los Angeles, New Jersey (Asbury Park and Trenton), New York City (Brooklyn and Harlem), Philadelphia, and San Antonio was 20.9 percent, with more than 97 percent of cases due to HTLV-II. The seroprevalence of HTLV-II was higher in the Southwest and the Midwest than in the Northeast. In contrast, the seroprevalence of HIV-1 was higher in the Northeast than in the Southwest or the Midwest. Approximately 3 percent of the cohort members were infected with both HTLV-II and HIV-1. The seroprevalence of HTLV-II increased linearly with age, as did that of HTLV-I in other studies. Women were significantly more likely to be infected with HTLV-II than were men; the virus is thought to be more efficiently transmitted from male to female than from female to male.

Associated Diseases Although HTLV-II was isolated from a patient with a T-cell variant of hairy cell leukemia, this virus has not been consistently associated with a particular disease and in fact has been thought of as "a virus searching for a disease." However, evidence is accumulating that HTLV-II may play a role in certain neurologic, hematologic, and dermatologic diseases. These data require confirmation, particularly in light of the previous confusion regarding the relative prevalences of HTLV-I and HTLV-II among injection drug users.

Prevention Given current information on the prevalence of HTLV-II among injection drug users in the United States, the impact of preventive measures could be substantial. Avoidance of needle sharing, safe-sex practices, screening of blood (by assays for HTLV-I, which also detect HTLV-II), and avoidance of breast-feeding by infected women are important principles in the prevention of spread of HTLV-II.

HUMAN IMMUNODEFICIENCY VIRUS (See Chap. 308)

HIV-1 and HIV-2 are members of the lentivirus subfamily of Retroviridae and are the only lentiviruses known to infect humans. The lentiviruses are slow-acting by comparison with viruses that cause acute infection (e.g., influenza virus) but not by comparison with other retroviruses. The features of acute primary infection with HIV resemble those of more classic acute infections. The characteristic chronicity of HIV disease is consistent with the designation *lentivirus*. HIV is discussed in considerable detail in Chap. 308. The following brief discussion focuses on those aspects of HIV that distinguish it from the other human retroviruses.

BIOLOGY AND MOLECULAR BIOLOGY Unlike HTLV-I and HTLV-II, which are oncogenic viruses that transform cells in culture, HIV-1 and HIV-2 are cytopathic in culture. The primary receptor for HIV is the CD4 molecule, which is present predominantly on the surface of a subset of T lymphocytes but also on monocytes. These two types of cell are thus the major targets of HIV infection. Other cell types express CD4 and are variably susceptible to HIV infection (see Chap. 308). In addition to CD4, other cell-surface molecules—referred to as *coreceptors*—function as accessory receptors in target cells that express CD4. In this regard, it has been demonstrated that certain cell-surface molecules that belong to the seven transmembrane G protein–coupled family of receptors serve as coreceptors for different strains of HIV-1. The molecule termed *fusin* is the coreceptor for T cell–tropic strains of HIV-1 (such as strain IIIB), while the β-chemokine receptor CCCKR5 is the coreceptor for macrophage-tropic strains of HIV-1 (such as strain Ba-L) (see Chap. 308). Certain cell-surface markers clearly enhance infection of CD4 + cells by HIV; these include Fc receptors (FcRs) or complement (C') receptors. The binding of virus by antibody may lead to increased efficiency of infection of FcR-positive cells, and the formation of immune complexes of HIV, antibody, and C' may lead to increased efficiency of infection of cells expressing C' receptors. It is still unclear whether FcRs and C' receptors can mediate infection independently of CD4. Finally, certain receptors may function as primary receptors in HIV infection of CD4− cells. For example, the glycolipid galactosyl ceramide (galactocerebroside, GalC) is one candidate cell-surface receptor for the infection of CD4− glial and neuroblastoma cells. Once the virus binds to the target cell, fusion with the cell membrane occurs via the gp41 molecule of the viral envelope, and the HIV genomic RNA is uncoated and internalized. HIV then proceeds with its life cycle as outlined in Fig. 192-1.

HIV has little sequence homology with the HTLVs; however, these viruses have some important similarities in genomic makeup. Both groups have flanking LTRs as well as the *gag*, *pol*, and *env* structural genes. The HIV equivalents of the HTLV *rex* and *tax* genes are *rev* and *tat*. However, HIV also possesses several auxiliary genes, including *nef*, *vpr*, *vpu* (HIV-1 only), and *vpx* (HIV-2 only) (see "Structure and Life Cycle" above). The LTRs of HIV include conventional regulatory sequences, such as the polyadenylation signal sequence and the TATA promoter sequence. The binding sites for both cellular and viral transcription factors have been mapped to the U3 and R regions of the LTR. Three functional domains in the U3 and R regions have been described: (1) a modulatory element that includes binding sites for activation protein 1 (AP-1), nuclear factor κB (NFκB), nuclear factor of activated T cells (NFAT), upstream stimulatory factor, and T-cell factor 1α; (2) a core promoter element that contains three binding sites for SP1 and the TATA sequence; and (3) a transactivator response (TAR) element that contains binding sites for both cellular and viral factors, including the viral Tat protein.

All of these factors may exert either positive or negative effects on viral RNA transcription. For example, the SP1, TATA, and TAR sequences as well as NFκB exert a positive effect on viral transcription. In contrast, some *upstream* sequences in the LTR exert negative effects on viral transcription and thus are designated the *negative regulatory element*. Stimulation of the initiation of transcription depends strictly on the presence of these factors in their active forms. Factors that exert a positive effect on viral transcription are abundant in activated cells; thus, the stimulation of viral RNA transcription depends on the state of activation of the target cells.

The mRNA species that are transcribed as a result of the binding of these factors to HIV LTR are multiply spliced (containing the viral LTR and the major viral regulatory genes *tat*, *rev*, and *nef*), singly spliced (containing the *env* coding sequences), or unspliced (containing the *gag-pol* sequences). Multiply spliced mRNA enters the cytoplasm, where it is translated. Tat is responsible for the upregulation of expression of all the other HIV genes, particularly *rev*. The principal function of the Rev protein is to allow for the cytoplasmic expression of the singly spliced and unspliced HIV mRNAs. In the absence of Rev, these mRNAs remain sequestered in the nucleus, where they ultimately are either degraded or multiply spliced. Accumulation of the Rev protein promotes the production of viral mRNAs that encode for structural proteins. The Rev protein interacts with the Rev responsive element (RRE); Rev-RRE binding is thought to mediate nuclear export and translation of unspliced or singly spliced mRNAs, resulting in the production of structural proteins such as Gag, Gag-Pol, and Env as well as of enzymatic proteins required for the creation of virus particles (Fig. 192-1). Virions are assembled at the inner surface of the plasma membrane of the infected cell; this process is regulated by the Gag polyprotein. The viral RNA contains a packaging sequence critical to the efficient incorporation of genomic RNA into virions. Assembly, budding, and maturation of virions take place in the absence of the envelope glycoprotein. Incorporation of the envelope protein occurs on the outer surface of the plasma membrane during the budding process. Once virus particles are released from the cell surface, Gag and Gag-Pol polyproteins are cleaved by viral protease.

MOLECULAR HETEROGENEITY Molecular analysis of various HIV isolates reveals variation over many parts of the viral genome. For example, the coding sequences of the viral envelope protein can differ by only a few percent or by as much as 50 percent. The percentage of actual envelope-protein sequence differences can be even greater. These changes tend to cluster in hypervariable regions. One such region, V3, is a target for neutralizing antibodies and contains recognition sites for T-cell responses. Variability in this region is probably due to selective pressure from the host's immune system. The extraordinary variability within HIV-1 contrasts markedly with the relative genetic stability of HTLV-I and HTLV-II. On the basis of this molecular heterogeneity, HIV-1 isolates have been categorized into two *groups*: group M, which is responsible for most of the infections in the world, and group O, which is a relatively rare outlier group currently found in Cameroon, Gabon, and France. The M group comprises eight sequence *subtypes* or *clades*, designed A through H. Subtype A viruses are most common worldwide, while subtype B viruses are found only in the United States. Phylogenetic-tree analysis and the distribution of various HIV-1 subtypes throughout the world are discussed in Chap. 308.

EPIDEMIOLOGY HIV is spread by sexual contact, contaminated blood or blood products, contaminated injection equipment, intrapartum and perinatal mother-child contact, and breast-feeding (see Chap. 308). HIV has caused a global pandemic, with the number of infected individuals worldwide estimated at approximately 20 million in 1996. The predominant mode of transmission around the world—particularly prominent in developing countries—is by heterosexual contact with an infected individual. Although heterosexual spread is increasing in frequency in developed countries, homosexual contact and injection drug use remain the predominant modes of transmission in the United States. Intrapartum/perinatal transmission from a mother to a fetus or an infant is a major source of infection in developing countries and is becoming more important in developed countries as rates of heterosexual spread rise.

HIV-1 is the predominant agent of HIV infection worldwide. HIV-2 is prominent in West Africa; moreover, it is now being documented in other regions of Africa as well as in Western Europe, in South America (particularly Brazil), and—to a much lesser extent—in Canada and the United States.

ASSOCIATED DISEASES HIV disease is characterized by progressive immunodeficiency associated with quantitative depletion and qualitative defects in CD4+ T cells. Advanced HIV disease is referred to as the acquired immunodeficiency syndrome, or AIDS. When the CD4+ T-cell count falls below a certain critical level, usually $200/\mu L$, the infected individual becomes highly susceptible to a number of opportunistic infections and neoplasms. These conditions are AIDS-defining illnesses; diminution of the CD4+ T-cell count to $<200/\mu L$, even if the individual is asymptomatic, still constitutes a diagnosis of AIDS. Compared with HIV-1, HIV-2 is believed to cause disease that is more indolent and that evolves to the advanced stages over a longer period. HIV-1 causes neurologic disease in a high proportion of patients. This form of disease may be manifested as AIDS dementia complex, aseptic meningitis, myelopathy, peripheral neuropathy, and/or myopathy. A number of organ-specific abnormalities are also associated with HIV infection.

PREVENTION Strategies for the prevention of HIV infection are similar to those for the prevention of HTLV infection (see above and Chap. 308). → *The treatment of HIV infection and its complications is discussed in detail in Chap. 308.*

BIBLIOGRAPHY

BARRE-SINOUSSI F et al: Isolation of a T-lymphotropic retrovirus from a patient at risk for acquired immune deficiency syndrome (AIDS). Science 220:868, 1983

BRIGGS NC et al: Seroprevalence of human T cell lymphotropic virus type II infection, with or without human immunodeficiency virus type I coinfection, among US intravenous drug users. J Infect Dis 172:51, 1995

COFFIN JM: Retroviridae and their replication, in *Fields Virology*, BN Fields, DM Knipe (eds). New York, Raven Press, 1990, p 1437

FAUCI AS: Multifactorial nature of human immunodeficiency virus disease: Implications for therapy. Science 262:1011, 1993

FRANCHINI G: Molecular mechanisms of human T-cell leukemia/lymphotropic virus type I infection. Blood 86:3619, 1995

GALLO RC: Human retroviruses in the second decade: A personal perspective. Nature Med 1:753, 1995

——— et al: Frequent detection and isolation of cytopathic retroviruses (HTLV-III) from patients with AIDS and at risk for AIDS. Science 224:500, 1984

GILL PS et al: Treatment of adult T-cell leukemia-lymphoma with a combination of interferon alpha and zidovudine. N Engl J Med 332:1744, 1995

HARRINGTON WJ JR et al: Tropical spastic paraparesis/HTLV-I-associated myelopathy (TSP/HAM): Treatment with an anabolic steroid danazol. AIDS Res Hum Retroviruses 7:1031, 1991

HOLLSBERG P, HAFLER DA: Pathogenesis of diseases induced by human lymphotropic virus type I infection. N Engl J Med 328:1173, 1993

KORBER BTM et al: Mutational trends in V3 loop protein sequences observed in different genetic lineages of human immunodeficiency virus type I. J Virol 68:6730, 1994

MYERS G: HIV: Between past and future. AIDS Res Hum Retroviruses 10:1317, 1994

PANTALEO G et al: The role of lymphoid organs in the pathogenesis of HIV infection. Semin Immunol 5:157, 1993

———, FAUCI AS: The acquired immunodeficiency syndrome (AIDS), in *Handbook of Experimental Immunology*, LA Herzenberg et al (eds). Oxford, Blackwell Scientific, 1996

POIESZ BJ et al: Detection and isolation of type C retrovirus particles from fresh and cultured lymphocytes of a patient with cutaneous T-cell lymphoma. Proc Natl Acad Sci USA 77:7415, 1980

TRONO D: HIV accessory proteins: Leading roles for the supporting cast. Cell 82:189, 1995

URBA WJ, LONGO DL: The clinical spectrum of human retroviral-induced diseases. Cancer Res 45:4637, 1985

——— et al: Adult T-cell leukemia/lymphoma, in *Clinical Oncology*, MD Abeloff et al (eds). New York, Churchill Livingstone, 1995, p 2173

WALDMANN TA: The multichain interleukin-2 receptor: A target for immunotherapy. Ann Intern Med 116:148, 1992

ZEHENDER G et al: High prevalence of human T-cell lymphotropic virus type II infection in patients affected by human immunodeficiency virus type I–associated predominantly sensory polyneuropathy. J Infect Dis 172:1595, 1995

193 *Raphael Dolin*

INFLUENZA

DEFINITION Influenza is an acute respiratory illness caused by infection with influenza viruses. The illness affects the upper and/or lower respiratory tract and is often accompanied by systemic signs and symptoms such as fever, headache, myalgia, and weakness. Outbreaks of illness of variable extent and severity occur nearly every winter. Such outbreaks result in significant morbidity in the general population and in increased mortality rates among certain high-risk patients, mainly as a result of pulmonary complications.

ETIOLOGIC AGENT Influenza viruses are members of the Orthomyxoviridae family. Influenza A and B viruses constitute one genus, and influenza C viruses make up the other. The designation of influenza viruses as type A, B, or C is based on antigenic characteristics of the nucleoprotein (NP) and matrix (M) protein antigens. Influenza A viruses are further subdivided (subtyped) on the basis of the surface hemagglutinin (H) and neuraminidase (N) antigens (see below); individual strains are designated according to the site of origin, isolate number, year of isolation, and subtype—for example, influenza A/Johannesburg/33/94 (H3N2). Influenza B and C viruses are similarly designated, but H and N antigens from these viruses do not receive subtype designations, since intratypic variations in these antigens are less extensive in these viruses.

Most of the information on the molecular biology of influenza viruses has come from studies of influenza A viruses, and less is known about the replicative cycle of influenza B and C viruses. Morphologically, influenza viruses A, B, and C are similar. The virions are irregularly shaped spherical particles, 80 to 120 nm in diameter, and have a lipid envelope from the surface of which the H and N glycoproteins project (Fig. 193-1). The hemagglutinin is the site by which virus binds to cell receptors, whereas the neuraminidase degrades the receptor and probably plays a role in the release of virus from infected cells after replication has taken place. Antibodies to the H antigen are the major determinants of immunity to influenza virus, while those to the N antigen limit viral spread and contribute to reduction of the infection. The inner surface of the lipid envelope contains the M proteins M1 and M2, the functions of which are incompletely understood but which may be involved in virus assembly and in stabilization of the lipid envelope. The virion also contains the NP antigen, which is associated with the viral genome, as well as three polymerase (P) proteins that are essential for transcription and synthesis of viral RNA. Two nonstructural (NS) proteins of unknown function are also present in infected cells.

The genome of influenza A virus consists of eight single-stranded RNA segments, which code for the structural and nonstructural proteins. Because the genome is segmented, the opportunity for reassortment of genes during infection is high, and reassortment occurs frequently during infection of cells with more than one influenza A virus.

EPIDEMIOLOGY Influenza outbreaks are recorded virtually every year, although their extent and severity vary widely. Localized outbreaks take place at variable intervals, usually every 1 to 3 years. Global epidemics or pandemics have occurred approximately every 10 to 15 years since the 1918–1919 pandemic (Table 193-1).

The most extensive and severe outbreaks are caused by influenza A viruses. In part, this predominance is a result of the remarkable propensity of the H and N antigens of influenza A virus to undergo periodic antigenic variation. Major antigenic variations are referred to as *antigenic shifts*, which may be associated with pandemics and are restricted to influenza A viruses. Minor variations are called *antigenic drifts*. These antigenic changes may involve the hemagglutinin alone or both the hemagglutinin and the neuraminidase. In human infections, three major antigenic subtypes of hemagglutinins (H1, H2, and H3) and two of neuraminidases (N1 and N2) have been recognized. The hemagglutinins formerly designated as H0 and Hsw1 are now classified as variants of H1. An example of an antigenic shift involving both the hemagglutinin and the neuraminidase is that of 1957, when the predominant influenza A virus subtype shifted from H1N1 to H2N2; this shift resulted in a severe pandemic, with an estimated 70,000 excess deaths (i.e., deaths in excess of the number expected without an influenza epidemic) in the United States alone. In 1968, an antigenic shift involving only the hemagglutinin occurred (H2N2 to H3N2); the subsequent pandemic was less severe than that of 1957. In 1977, an H1N1 virus emerged and caused a pandemic that primarily affected younger individuals (i.e., those born after 1957). As can be seen in Table 193-1, H1N1 viruses circulated from 1918 to 1956; thus, individuals born prior to 1957 would be expected to have some degree of immunity to H1N1 viruses. During most outbreaks of influenza A, a single subtype has circulated at a time. However, since 1977, H1N1 and H3N2 viruses have circulated simultaneously, resulting in outbreaks of varying severity. In some outbreaks, influenza B viruses have also circulated simultaneously with influenza A viruses.

The origin of pandemic strains is unknown. Given the marked differences between the primary structures of the hemagglutinins of different subtypes of influenza A viruses (H1, H2, and H3), it seems unlikely that antigenic shifts result from spontaneous mutations in the hemagglutinin gene. Because the segmented genome of influenza viruses may result in high rates of reassortment, it has been suggested that pandemic strains may emerge by reassortment of genes between human and animal viruses. Influenza B viruses do not have an animal reservoir and do not undergo antigenic shifts, although they do undergo antigenic drift.

Pandemics provide the most dramatic evidence of the impact of influenza. However, illnesses that occur between pandemics account for greater total mortality and morbidity, albeit over a longer period. From 1972 to 1991, interpandemic illness was associated with 20,000

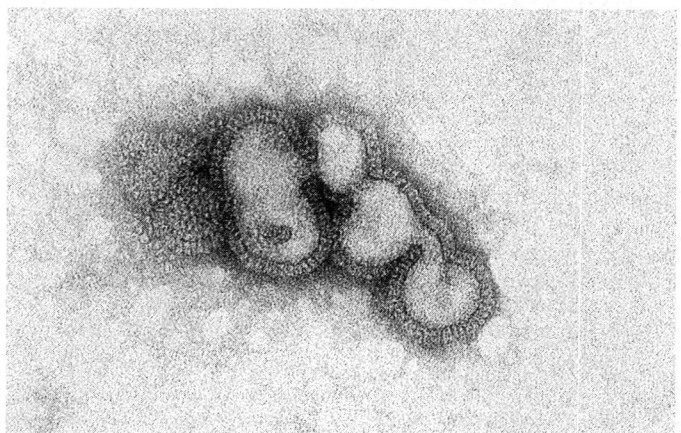

FIGURE 193-1 An electron micrograph of influenza virus (×143,000). (*From R Dolin, Am Fam Phys 14:74, 1976.*)

Table 193-1

Emergence of Antigenic Subtypes of Influenza A Virus Associated with Pandemic or Epidemic Disease

Year	Subtype	Extent of Outbreak
1889–90	H2N8*	Severe pandemic
1900–03	H3N8*	?Moderate epidemic
1918–19	H1N1† (formerly HswN1)	Severe pandemic
1933–35	H1N1† (formerly H0N1)	Mild epidemic
1946–47	H1N1	Mild epidemic
1957–58	H2N2	Severe pandemic
1968–69	H3N2	Moderate pandemic
1977–78‡	H1N1	Mild pandemic

* As determined by retrospective serologic survey of individuals alive during those years ("seroarcheology").

† Hemagglutinins formerly designated as Hsw and H0 are now classified as variants of H1.

‡ From this time until the present (1995–96), no new antigenic subtypes of influenza A virus have emerged. Rather, viruses of the H1N1 and H3N2 subtypes have circulated either in alternating years or concurrently.

or more excess deaths during each of 10 epidemics in the United States; more than 40,000 influenza-associated deaths occurred in each of three of these epidemics. Influenza A viruses that circulate between pandemics demonstrate antigenic drifts in the H antigen. These antigenic drifts apparently result from point mutations involving the RNA segment that codes for the hemagglutinin. Epidemiologically significant strains—that is, those with the potential to cause widespread outbreaks—exhibit changes in amino acids in at least two of the major antigenic sites in the hemagglutinin molecule. Since two point mutations are unlikely to occur simultaneously, it is believed that antigenic drifts result from point mutations occurring sequentially during the spread of virus from person to person. Antigenic drifts have been reported nearly annually since 1977 for H1N1 viruses and since 1968 for H3N2 viruses.

Influenza A epidemics begin abruptly, peak over a 2- to 3-week period, generally last for 2 to 3 months, and often subside almost as rapidly as they began. The first indication of influenza activity in a community is an increase in the number of children with febrile respiratory illnesses who present for medical attention. This increase is followed by increases in rates of influenza-like illnesses among adults and eventually by an increase in hospital admissions for patients with pneumonia, worsening of congestive heart failure, and exacerbations of chronic pulmonary disease. Rates of absence from work and school also rise at this time. An increase in the number of deaths caused by pneumonia and influenza is generally a late observation in an outbreak. Attack rates have been highly variable from outbreak to outbreak but most commonly are in the range of 10 to 20 percent of the general population. During the pandemic of 1957, it was estimated that the attack rate of clinical influenza exceeded 50 percent in urban populations and that an additional 25 percent or more of individuals in these populations may have been subclinically infected with influenza A virus. Among institutionalized populations and in semiclosed settings with a large number of susceptible individuals, even higher attack rates have been reported.

Epidemics of influenza occur almost exclusively during the winter months in the Northern and Southern Hemispheres. It is highly unusual to detect influenza A virus at other times, although serologic rises or even outbreaks have been noted rarely during warm-weather months. Where or how influenza A virus persists between outbreaks is unknown. It is possible that influenza A viruses are maintained in the human population on a worldwide basis by person-to-person transmission and that large population clusters support a low level of interepidemic transmission. Alternatively, human strains may persist in animal reservoirs. Convincing evidence to support either explanation is not available. In the modern era, rapid transportation may contribute to the transmission of viruses among widespread geographic locales.

The factors that result in the inception and termination of outbreaks of influenza are incompletely understood. A major determinant of the extent and severity of an outbreak is the level of immunity in the population at risk. With the emergence of an antigenically novel influenza virus to which little or no antibody is present in a community, extensive outbreaks may occur. When the absence of antibody is worldwide, epidemic disease may spread around the globe, resulting in a pandemic. Such pandemic waves can continue for several years, until immunity in the population reaches a high level. In the years following pandemic influenza, antigenic drifts among influenza viruses result in outbreaks of variable severity in populations with high levels of immunity to the pandemic strain that circulated earlier. This situation persists until another antigenically novel pandemic strain emerges. On the other hand, outbreaks sometimes end despite the persistence of a large pool of susceptible individuals in the population.

Occasionally, the emergence of a significantly different antigenic variant will result only in a localized outbreak. The swine influenza outbreak of 1976 in the United States, caused by an A/H1N1 virus antigenically similar to the virus that circulated in 1918–1919 (see Table 193-1), may be an example, although this outbreak may have represented simply the introduction of a swine influenza virus into a crowded human population without spread beyond that setting. It also has been suggested that certain viruses, such as recently circulating

A/H1N1 strains, may be intrinsically less virulent and cause less severe disease than other variants, even in immunologically virgin subjects. If so, then other undefined factors besides the level of preexisting immunity must play a role in the epidemiology of influenza.

Influenza B virus causes outbreaks that are generally less extensive and are associated with less severe disease than those caused by influenza A virus. The hemagglutinin and neuraminidase of influenza B virus undergo less frequent and less extensive variation than those of influenza A viruses; this characteristic may account, in part, for the lesser extent of disease. Influenza B outbreaks are seen most frequently in schools and military camps, although outbreaks in institutions in which elderly individuals reside also have been noted on occasion. The most serious complication of influenza B virus infection is Reye's syndrome (see Chap. 300). Influenza C virus has been only infrequently associated with human disease, although the wide prevalence of serum antibody to this virus indicates that asymptomatic infection may be common.

The morbidity and mortality caused by influenza outbreaks continue to be substantial. Most individuals who die in this setting have underlying diseases that place them at high risk for complications of influenza. Excess hospitalizations for adults with high-risk medical conditions have reached rates of 800 per 100,000 during recent outbreaks of influenza. The most prominent high-risk conditions are chronic cardiac and pulmonary diseases as well as old age. Mortality among individuals with chronic metabolic, renal, and certain immunosuppressive diseases has also been high, although lower than that among patients with chronic cardiopulmonary diseases. The morbidity attributable to influenza in the general population is considerable. For each of three outbreaks in the United States that were studied during the 1960s, it has been estimated that direct and indirect economic costs ranged from 1.5 to 3.5 billion dollars; today such costs would obviously be much greater.

PATHOGENESIS The initial event in influenza is infection of the respiratory epithelium with influenza virus acquired from respiratory secretions of acutely infected individuals. In all likelihood, transmission occurs via aerosols generated by coughs and sneezes, although hand-to-hand contact, other personal contact, and even fomite transmission may take place. Experimental evidence suggests that infection by a small-particle aerosol (particle diameter, less than 10 μm) is more efficient than that by larger droplets. Initially, viral infection involves the ciliated columnar epithelial cells, but it also may involve other respiratory tract cells, including alveolar cells, mucous gland cells, and macrophages. In infected cells, virus replicates within 4 to 6 h, after which infectious virus is released to infect adjacent or nearby cells. In this way, infection spreads from a few foci to a large number of respiratory cells over several hours. In experimentally induced infection, the incubation period of illness has ranged from 18 to 72 h, depending on the size of the virus inoculum. Histopathologic study reveals degenerative changes, including granulation, vacuolization, swelling, and pyknotic nuclei, in infected ciliated cells. The cells eventually become necrotic and desquamate; in some areas, previously columnar epithelium is replaced by flattened and metaplastic epithelial cells. The severity of illness is correlated with the quantity of virus shed in secretions; thus, the degree of viral replication itself may be an important mechanism in the pathogenesis of illness. Despite the frequent development of systemic signs and symptoms such as fever, headache, and myalgias, influenza virus has only rarely been detected in extrapulmonary sites (including the bloodstream), and the pathogenesis of systemic symptoms in influenza remains unknown.

The host response to influenza infections involves a complex interplay of humoral antibody, local antibody, cell-mediated immunity, interferon, and other host defenses. Serum antibody responses, which can be detected by the second week after primary infection, are measured by a variety of techniques: hemagglutination inhibition (HAI), complement fixation (CF), neutralization, enzyme-linked immunosorbent assay (ELISA), and antineuraminidase antibody assay. Antibodies directed against the hemagglutinin appear to be the most important mediators of immunity; in several studies, HAI titers of 40 or greater have been associated with protection from infection. Secretory antibodies produced in the respiratory tract are predominantly of the IgA class and also play a major role in protection against infection. Secretory antibody neutralization titers of 4 or higher also have been associated with protection. A variety of cell-mediated immune responses, both antigen-specific and non-antigen-specific, can be detected early after infection, depending on the prior immunity of the host. These responses include T-cell proliferative, T-cell cytotoxic, and natural killer cell activity. Interferons have been detected in respiratory secretions shortly after the shedding of virus has begun, and rises in interferon titers coincide with decreases in virus shedding.

The host defense factors responsible for cessation of virus shedding and resolution of illness have not been defined specifically. Virus shedding generally stops within 2 to 5 days after symptoms first appear, at a time when serum and local antibody responses often are not detectable by conventional techniques (although antibody rises may be detected earlier by use of highly sensitive techniques, particularly in individuals with previous immunity to the virus). It has been suggested that interferon, cell-mediated immune responses, and/or nonspecific inflammatory responses are important in the resolution of illness.

MANIFESTATIONS Influenza has been most frequently described as an illness characterized by the abrupt onset of systemic symptoms, such as headache, feverishness, chills, myalgia, or malaise, and accompanying respiratory tract signs, particularly cough and sore throat. In many cases, the onset is so abrupt that patients can recall the precise time they became ill. A typical case of naturally occurring influenza is depicted in Fig. 193-2. However, the spectrum of clinical presentations is wide, ranging from a mild, afebrile respiratory illness similar to the common cold (with either gradual or abrupt onset) to severe prostration with relatively few respiratory signs and symptoms. In most of the cases that come to a physician's attention, the patient has a fever, with temperatures of 38 to 41°C. A rapid temperature rise within the first 24 h of illness is generally followed by a gradual defervescence over a 2- to 3-day period, although, on occasion, fever may last for as long as a week. Patients report a feverish feeling and

chilliness, but true rigors are rare. Headache, either generalized or frontal, is often particularly troublesome. Myalgias may involve any part of the body but are most common in the legs and lumbosacral area. Arthralgias also may develop.

Respiratory complaints often become more prominent as systemic symptoms subside. Many patients have a sore throat or persistent cough, which may last for a week or more and which is often accompanied by substernal discomfort. Ocular signs and symptoms include pain on motion of the eyes, photophobia, and burning of the eyes.

Physical findings are usually minimal in cases of uncomplicated influenza. Early in the illness, the patient appears flushed and the skin is hot and dry, although diaphoresis and mottled extremities are sometimes evident, particularly in older patients. Examination of the pharynx may yield surprisingly unremarkable results despite a severe sore throat, but injection of the mucous membranes and postnasal discharge are apparent in some cases. Mild cervical lymphadenopathy may be noted, particularly in younger individuals. The results of chest examination are largely negative in uncomplicated influenza, although rhonchi, wheezes, and scattered rales have been reported with variable frequency in different outbreaks. Frank dyspnea, hyperpnea, cyanosis, diffuse rales, and signs of consolidation are indicative of pulmonary complications. Patients with apparently uncomplicated influenza have been reported to have a variety of mild ventilatory defects and increased alveolar-capillary diffusion gradients; thus, subclinical pulmonary involvement may be more frequent than is appreciated.

In uncomplicated influenza, the acute illness generally resolves over a 2- to 5-day period, and most patients have largely recovered in 1 week. In a significant minority (particularly the elderly), however, symptoms of weakness or lassitude (postinfluenzal asthenia) may persist for several weeks and may prove troublesome for persons who wish to resume their full level of activity promptly. The pathogenetic basis for this asthenia is unknown, although pulmonary function abnormalities may persist for several weeks after uncomplicated influenza.

COMPLICATIONS OF INFLUENZA The most common complication of influenza is pneumonia: "primary" influenza viral pneumonia, secondary bacterial pneumonia, or mixed viral and bacterial pneumonia. Primary influenza viral pneumonia is the least common but most severe of the pneumonic complications. It presents as acute influenza that does not resolve but instead progresses relentlessly, with persistent fever, dyspnea, and eventual cyanosis. Sputum production is generally scanty, but the sputum can contain blood. Few physical signs may be evident early in the illness. In more advanced cases, diffuse rales may be noted, and chest x-ray findings consistent with diffuse interstitial infiltrates and/or acute respiratory distress syndrome may be present. In such cases, arterial blood-gas determinations show marked hypoxia. Viral cultures of respiratory secretions and lung parenchyma, particularly if samples are taken early in illness, yield high titers of virus. In fatal cases of primary viral pneumonia, histopathologic examination reveals a marked inflammatory reaction in the alveolar septa, with edema and infiltration with lymphocytes, macrophages, occasional plasma cells, and variable numbers of neutrophils. Fibrin thrombi in alveolar capillaries, along with necrosis and hemorrhage, also have been noted. Eosinophilic hyaline membranes can be found lining alveoli and alveolar ducts.

Primary influenza viral pneumonia has a predilection for individuals with cardiac disease, particularly those with mitral stenosis, but also has been reported in otherwise healthy young adults as well as in older individuals with chronic pulmonary disorders. In some epidemics of influenza (notably those of 1918 and 1957), pregnancy increased the risk of primary influenza pneumonia.

Secondary bacterial pneumonia follows acute influenza. Improvement of the patient's condition over 2 to 3 days is followed by a reappearance of fever along with clinical signs and symptoms of bacterial pneumonia, including cough, production of purulent sputum, and physical and x-ray signs of consolidation. The most common bacterial pathogens in this setting are *Streptococcus pneumoniae*, *Staphylococcus aureus*, and *Haemophilus influenzae*—organisms that can colonize the nasopharynx and that cause infection in the wake of changes in bronchopulmonary defenses. The etiology can often be

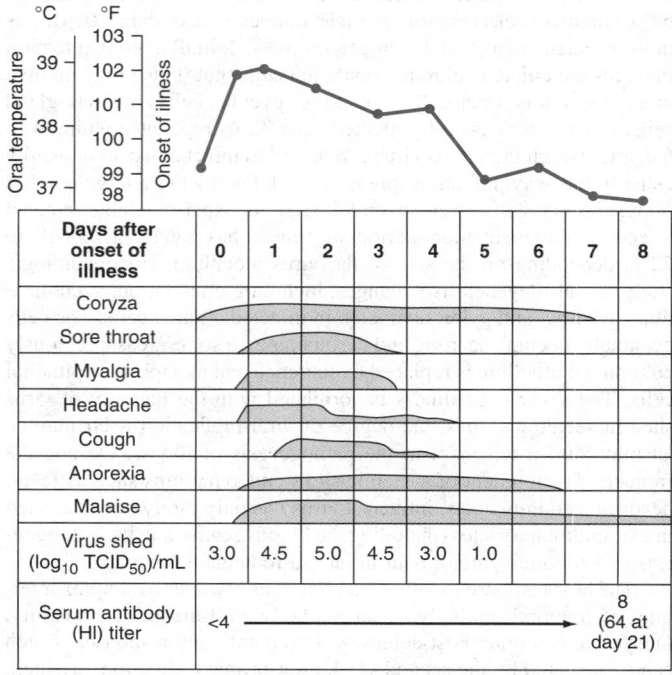

Days after onset of illness	0	1	2	3	4	5	6	7	8
Coryza									
Sore throat									
Myalgia									
Headache									
Cough									
Anorexia									
Malaise									
Virus shed (log$_{10}$ TCID$_{50}$)/mL	3.0	4.5	5.0	4.5	3.0	1.0			
Serum antibody (HI) titer	<4 ——————————————————————————→								8 (64 at day 21)

FIGURE 193-2 Clinical characteristics of a naturally occurring case of influenza A in an otherwise healthy 28-year-old man. (*From R Dolin, Am Fam Phys 14:74, 1976.*)

determined by Gram's staining and culture of an appropriately obtained sputum specimen. Secondary bacterial pneumonia occurs most frequently in high-risk individuals with chronic pulmonary and cardiac disease and in elderly individuals. Patients with secondary bacterial pneumonia often respond to antibiotic therapy when it is instituted promptly.

Perhaps the most common of the pneumonic complications during outbreaks of influenza is mixed viral and bacterial pneumonia. The clinical course of this complication includes features of both primary and secondary pneumonia. Patients may experience a gradual progression of their acute illness or may show transient improvement followed by clinical exacerbation, with eventual manifestation of the clinical features of bacterial pneumonia. Sputum cultures may contain both influenza A virus and one of the bacterial pathogens described above. Patchy infiltrates or areas of consolidation may be detected by physical examination and chest x-ray. Patients with mixed viral and bacterial pneumonia generally have less widespread involvement of the lung than those with primary viral pneumonia, and their bacterial infections may respond to appropriate antibiotics. Mixed viral and bacterial pneumonia occurs primarily in patients with chronic cardiovascular and pulmonary diseases.

Other pulmonary complications associated with influenza include worsening of chronic obstructive pulmonary disease and exacerbation of chronic bronchitis and asthma. In children, influenza infection may present as croup.

In addition to the pulmonary complications of influenza, a number of extrapulmonary complications may occur. These include *Reye's syndrome*, a serious complication in children that is associated with influenza B and to a lesser extent with influenza A virus infection as well as with varicella-zoster virus infection. An epidemiologic association between Reye's syndrome and aspirin therapy for the antecedent viral infection has been noted, and the incidence of Reye's syndrome has decreased markedly with widespread warnings regarding the use of aspirin by children with acute viral respiratory infections. → *A detailed description of Reye's syndrome is found in Chap. 300.*

Myositis, rhabdomyolysis, and myoglobinuria are occasional complications of influenza infection. Although myalgias are exceedingly common in influenza, true myositis is rare. Patients with acute myositis have exquisite tenderness of the affected muscles, most commonly in the legs, and may not be able to tolerate even the slightest pressure, such as the touch of bedsheets. In the most severe cases, there is frank swelling and bogginess of muscles. Serum levels of creatine phosphokinase and aldolase are markedly elevated, and an occasional patient has developed renal failure from myoglobinuria. The pathogenesis of influenza-associated myositis is also unclear, although the presence of influenza virus in affected muscles has been reported.

Myocarditis and pericarditis were reported in association with influenza virus infection during the 1918–1919 pandemic; these reports were based largely on histopathologic findings, and these complications have been reported only infrequently since that time. Electrocardiographic changes during acute influenza are common among patients who have cardiac disease but have been ascribed most often to exacerbations of the underlying cardiac disease rather than to direct involvement of the myocardium with influenza virus.

Central nervous system (CNS) diseases, including encephalitis, transverse myelitis, and Guillain-Barré syndrome, have been reported during influenza. The etiologic relationship of influenza virus to such CNS illnesses remains unestablished. Toxic shock syndrome caused by *S. aureus* infection following acute influenza infection has also been reported (see Chap. 142).

In addition to complications involving the specific organ systems described above, influenza outbreaks include a number of cases in which elderly and other high-risk individuals develop influenza and subsequently experience a gradual deterioration of underlying cardiovascular, pulmonary, or renal function—changes that occasionally are irreversible and lead to death. These fatalities contribute to the overall excess mortality associated with influenza A outbreaks.

LABORATORY FINDINGS AND DIAGNOSIS Laboratory diagnosis is accomplished during acute influenza by isolation of the virus from throat swabs, nasopharyngeal washes, or sputum. Virus usually is detected in tissue culture or less commonly is found in the amniotic cavity of chick embryos within 48 to 72 h after inoculation. Viral antigens may be detected somewhat earlier by immunodiagnostic techniques in tissue culture or directly in exfoliated nasopharyngeal cells obtained by washings, although currently the latter method is less sensitive than isolation of virus in tissue culture. The type of influenza virus (A or B) may be determined by either immunofluorescence or HAI techniques, and the hemagglutinin subtype of influenza A virus (H1, H2, or H3) may be identified by HAI with use of subtype-specific antisera. Serologic methods for diagnosis require comparison of antibody titers in sera obtained during the acute illness with those in sera obtained 10 to 14 days after the onset of illness and are useful primarily in retrospect. Fourfold or greater titer rises as detected by HAI or CF or significant rises as measured by ELISA are diagnostic of acute infection. CF tests are generally less sensitive than other serologic techniques, but, as they detect type-specific antigens, they may be particularly useful when subtype-specific reagents are not available.

Other laboratory tests are generally not helpful in making a specific diagnosis of influenza virus infection. Leukocyte counts are variable, frequently being low early in illness and normal or slightly elevated later. Severe leukopenia has been described in overwhelming viral or bacterial infection, while leukocytosis with more than 15,000 cells per microliter raises the suspicion of secondary bacterial infection.

DIFFERENTIAL DIAGNOSIS On clinical grounds alone, an individual case of influenza may be difficult to differentiate from an acute respiratory illness caused by any of a variety of respiratory viruses or by *Mycoplasma pneumoniae*. Severe streptococcal pharyngitis or early bacterial pneumonia may mimic acute influenza, although bacterial pneumonias generally do not run a self-limited course. Purulent sputum in which a bacterial pathogen can be detected by Gram's staining is an important diagnostic feature in bacterial pneumonia. The fact that influenza occurs in characteristic outbreaks during the winter months may facilitate a clinical diagnosis. When local health authorities indicate that influenza is present in the community, an acute febrile respiratory illness can be attributed to influenza with a high degree of certainty, particularly if the typical features of abrupt onset and systemic symptoms are present.

℞ **TREATMENT**

In uncomplicated cases of influenza, therapy with either acetaminophen or salicylates for the relief of headache, myalgia, and fever may be considered, but the use of salicylates should be avoided in children below 18 years of age because of the possible association of salicylates with Reye's syndrome. Since cough is ordinarily self-limited, treatment with cough suppressants generally is not indicated, although codeine-containing compounds may be employed if the cough is particularly troublesome. Patients should be advised to rest and maintain hydration during acute illness and should return to full activity only gradually after the illness has resolved, particularly if the illness has been severe.

Specific antiviral therapy in the form of amantadine and rimantadine is available for influenza A. These drugs are active only against influenza A viruses and have been licensed for the prophylaxis and therapy of influenza A virus infections in the United States. If begun within 48 h of the onset of illness, treatment with amantadine or rimantadine reduces the duration of systemic and respiratory symptoms of influenza by approximately 50 percent. In some studies, these drugs have been shown to be superior to antipyretic-analgesics in this regard. From 5 to 10 percent of individuals who receive amantadine will experience mild CNS side effects, primarily jitteriness, anxiety, insomnia, or difficulty in concentrating. These side effects disappear promptly upon cessation of the drug. Rimantadine appears to be equally efficacious and is associated with less frequent CNS side effects than is amantadine. In adults, the usual dose of amantadine or rimantadine is 200 mg/d for 3 to 7 days. Since both drugs are excreted via the kidney, the dose should be reduced to 100 mg/d or less in elderly patients and patients with renal insufficiency. Rimantadine has not been approved for the treatment of influenza A in children. Ribavirin, a nucleoside analogue with activity against a variety of viral agents, has been reported to be effective against both influenza A and influenza B virus infections when administered as an aerosol, although it is relatively ineffective when administered orally.

Studies demonstrating the therapeutic efficacy of antiviral compounds in influenza have almost exclusively included young adults with uncomplicated disease; it is not known whether such compounds are effective in the treatment of complications such as influenza pneumonia. Therapy for primary influenza pneumonia is directed at maintaining oxygenation and is most appropriately undertaken in an intensive care unit, with aggressive respiratory and hemodynamic support as needed. Bypass membrane oxygenators have been employed in this setting with variable results. When an acute respiratory distress syndrome develops, fluids must be administered cautiously, with close monitoring of blood gases and hemodynamic function.

Antibacterial drugs should be reserved for the therapy of bacterial complications of acute influenza, such as secondary bacterial pneumonia. The choice of antibiotics should be guided by Gram's staining and culture of appropriate specimens of respiratory secretions, such as sputum or transtracheal aspirates. If the etiology of a case of bacterial pneumonia is unclear from an examination of respiratory secretions, empirical antibiotics effective against the most common bacterial pathogens in this setting (*S. pneumoniae*, *S. aureus*, and *H. influenzae*) should be selected (see Chaps. 141, 142, and 152).

PROPHYLAXIS   The major public health measure for prevention of influenza has been the use of inactivated influenza vaccines derived from influenza A and B viruses that circulated during the previous influenza season. If the vaccine virus and the currently circulating viruses are closely related, 50 to 80 percent protection against influenza would be expected. Presently available vaccines have been highly purified and are associated with few reactions. Up to 5 percent of individuals experience low-grade fever and mild systemic symptoms 8 to 24 h after vaccination, and up to one-third develop mild redness or tenderness at the vaccination site. Since the vaccine is produced in eggs, individuals with true hypersensitivity to egg products either should be desensitized or should not be vaccinated. Although the 1976 swine influenza vaccine appears to have been associated with an increased frequency of Guillain-Barré syndrome, influenza vaccines administered since 1976 generally have not been. Possible exceptions were noted during 1990–1991 in 18- to 64-year-old vaccinees and during 1993–1994 among vaccine recipients. However, the risk of this syndrome following influenza outweighs the potential risk associated with vaccination. Live attenuated ("cold-adapted") influenza A vaccines also have been developed and appear to be promising in ongoing studies in adults and children. Such vaccines are administered intranasally and stimulate local antibody production more efficiently than conventional inactivated vaccines.

The U.S. Public Health Service recommends influenza vaccination for any individual older than 6 months of age who is at an increased risk for complications of influenza. Included are individuals with chronic cardiovascular or pulmonary disorders (including asthma) and residents of nursing homes and other chronic-care facilities. Other populations for whom the vaccine is recommended include healthy individuals over 65 years of age and individuals who have required regular medical attention for diabetes mellitus, renal disease, hemoglobinopathies, or immunosuppression. Individuals who provide care for high-risk patients or who come into frequent contact with such patients, including household members, also should receive vaccine to reduce the likelihood of transmission of infection. Since commercially available vaccines are inactivated ("killed"), they may be administered

safely to immunocompromised patients. Influenza vaccination is not associated with exacerbations of chronic nervous-system diseases such as multiple sclerosis. Vaccine should be administered early in the autumn before influenza outbreaks occur and should be repeated annually to maintain immunity against the most current influenza virus strains.

Studies have shown amantadine and rimantadine to be 70 to 100 percent effective in the prophylaxis of illness associated with influenza A virus infection. Such prophylaxis is most likely to be used for high-risk individuals who have not received influenza vaccine or in a situation where the vaccines previously administered are relatively ineffective because of antigenic changes in the circulating virus. During an outbreak, amantadine can be administered simultaneously with inactivated vaccine, since it will not interfere with an immune response to the vaccine. In fact, there is evidence that the protective effects of amantadine and vaccine may be additive. Amantadine has also been employed to control nosocomial outbreaks of influenza A. For prophylaxis, administration of amantadine or rimantadine should be instituted promptly when influenza A activity is detected and must be continued daily for the duration of the outbreak. The dosage most frequently employed has been 200 mg/d for adults, but the dose of amantadine should be reduced for patients with renal insufficiency and for the elderly. Viruses resistant to both amantadine and rimantadine can emerge quickly after therapy with these drugs, and the possible transmission of these resistant viruses has been reported.

BIBLIOGRAPHY

CENTERS FOR DISEASE CONTROL: Prevention and control of influenza. Morb Mort Week Rep 45(RR–5):1, 1996

DOLIN R et al: A controlled trial of amantadine and rimantadine in the prophylaxis of influenza A infection. N Engl J Med 307:580, 1982

GLEZEN WP: Serious morbidity and mortality associated with influenza epidemics. Epidemiol Rev 4:25, 1982

GROSS PA et al: Association of influenza immunization with reduction in mortality in an elderly population: A prospective study. Arch Intern Med 148:562, 1988

MURPHY BR, WEBSTER RG: Orthomyxoviruses, in *Virology*, 3d ed, BN Fields (ed). New York, Raven Press, 1995, pp 1091-1152

YINNON AM, DOLIN R: Using antivirals to fight influenza. J Respir Dis 12:1146, 1991

194   *Harry B. Greenberg*

VIRAL GASTROENTERITIS

In less developed countries, acute infectious diarrheal disease is a leading cause of morbidity in all age groups and of mortality in infants and young children. In developed countries, acute diarrheal illness remains an important cause of morbidity among both children and adults. Two distinct groups of viruses—the rotaviruses and the enteric caliciviruses, such as Norwalk virus—as well as a variety of bacterial pathogens (see Chap. 128) have emerged as important etiologic agents of gastroenteritis. The rotaviruses are primarily pathogens of young children. The Norwalk and related enteric caliciviruses affect adults as well as children.

ROTAVIRUS   Classification and Characterization   Rotaviruses are members of the Reoviridae family. The rotavirus virion consists of a 100-nm triple-shelled icosahedral capsid surrounding a genome composed of 11 segments of double-stranded RNA. The virus has two surface proteins, both of which are involved with viral neutralization. Because rotaviruses have a segmented genome, they are capable of undergoing gene reassortment at high frequency. The role of gene reassortment in generating rotavirus antigenic diversity is not known. In humans, rotavirus infection is characterized by replication that is localized almost exclusively in the small intestinal epithelial cells.

Epidemiology   Rotavirus infection occurs worldwide. By the age of 3 years, virtually every individual has been infected by rotaviruses at least once. In areas with a temperate climate, rotavirus infection is seasonal, occurring in the cooler winter months. In the United States, the annual seasonal rotavirus epidemic tends to spread from west to east, starting in California and ending in New England. In tropical areas, rotavirus infection tends to occur throughout the year, with some increase in incidence during the cooler rainy season.

Rotaviruses are the single most important cause of severe dehydrating diarrhea in infants and young children (under age 3) in both developed and less developed countries and account for 30 to 50 percent of all cases of diarrhea requiring hospitalization or intensive rehydration therapy. Although severe rotavirus infections are confined primarily to infants and small children, these agents are frequently associated with diarrhea in adults, particularly family members of affected infants, geriatric patients, and immunocompromised hosts. They account for up to 10 percent of cases of traveler's diarrhea (see Chap. 128). Rotaviruses also may be responsible for occasional cases of acute and chronic diarrhea in patients with AIDS.

The majority of rotavirus infections are subclinical or cause mild gastrointestinal illnesses that do not require hospitalization. Subclinical infections in neonates have been shown to protect these children against severe rotavirus gastroenteritis for up to 3 years.

At least nine distinct serotypes of human rotavirus have been described, but only four types are commonly encountered. The relationship of the frequency of infection with these serotypes to host immune status is unclear. A large variety of mammalian and avian species can be infected by rotavirus, but it appears that these animal rotavirus strains do not cause disease in humans very frequently. Rotaviruses are shed in very large numbers (up to 10^{10} particles per gram of feces) in the stool; it is presumed that transmission occurs via fecal-oral spread.

Pathophysiology Rotavirus infects and kills the mature villus tip cells of the small intestine. The mature epithelial cells are replaced by immature absorptive cells that cannot absorb carbohydrates or other nutrients efficiently. Rotavirus infection leads to osmotic diarrhea due to nutrient malabsorption. Changes in intracellular cyclic adenosine monophosphate or guanosine monophosphate are not involved in the etiology of rotavirus diarrhea.

Manifestations The manifestations of rotavirus infection range from subclinical infections through mild diarrhea to severe, occasionally fatal illness. Most information concerning the signs and symptoms of rotavirus infection has been derived from studies of hospitalized young children. The onset of illness is usually abrupt. More than 80 percent of affected children develop vomiting followed by diarrhea. About one-third of hospitalized children have a temperature of greater than 39°C (102.2°F). Gastrointestinal symptoms usually last between 2 and 6 days. Mucus is commonly found in the stool, but white and red blood cells are present in fewer than 15 percent of cases.

Rotavirus infection frequently occurs in conjunction with respiratory tract symptoms, but there is little evidence to indicate that rotavirus replicates in the respiratory tract. Rotavirus infection has been observed in association with a wide variety of other clinical syndromes, including sudden infant death syndrome, Reye's syndrome, encephalitis, aseptic meningitis, pneumonia, exanthema subitum, Kawasaki's syndrome, necrotizing enterocolitis, intussusception, Schönlein-Henoch purpura, hemolytic-uremic syndrome, disseminated intravascular coagulation, and Crohn's disease. The etiologic relationship between these clinical syndromes and rotavirus infection is probably coincidental rather than causal. Rotavirus infection may be especially severe, and even fatal, in immunocompromised children.

Clinical Immunity Relative immunity to rotavirus illness is acquired following infection early in childhood. Immunity is not complete, and adults with low levels of antibody can be symptomatically infected. Local humoral immunity appears to be the critical determinant in protection, and cellular immune mechanisms appear to be involved as well.

Diagnosis Because rotavirus is shed in large amounts in the stool, detection is relatively easy. A variety of specific commercial immunoassays are available to detect rotavirus antigen in fecal specimens. DNA probe diagnosis also appears to be sensitive and specific. There are no pathognomonic signs or symptoms of rotavirus infection,

but this infection is more frequently associated with severe dehydration than are infections caused by other enteric bacterial or viral pathogens.

 TREATMENT

Despite the fact that rotavirus diarrhea is caused by intestinal epithelial-cell lysis and death, it can be adequately treated by standard oral rehydration therapy. Only rarely is intravenous rehydration required. Since rotavirus infections have persisted in developed countries with advanced sanitation facilities and widely available clean water, it is unlikely that these infections will be preventable by hygienic measures alone. Progress with a number of candidate live attenuated vaccines suggests that prevention through vaccination may be feasible in the near future.

NORWALK AND RELATED ENTERIC CALICIVIRUSES

Classification and Characterization A variety of round 27- to 32-nm particles, some with clearly defined ultrastructure, have been identified in the stools of individuals with acute nonbacterial gastroenteritis. These agents have been difficult to classify because they are shed in the stool in small amounts for only a few days, and they have not been adapted to cell culture or to animal models. The Norwalk virus is the most extensively studied and best characterized member of this group of agents, which also includes such serologically distinct viruses as the Hawaii agent, the Snow Mountain agent, the W-Ditchling agent, and a number of agents described as calicivirus-like. The Norwalk virus and the Snow Mountain virus have a protein structure similar to that of typical caliciviruses. Recently, the genomes of Norwalk virus and several related viruses have been cloned and sequenced. The genomes are plus-stranded RNA molecules of approximately 7.5 kilobases. The genomic organization of Norwalk virus is similar to that of other members of the calicivirus family.

Epidemiology Norwalk infection occurs year-round and is common. More than 70 percent of adults in both developed and less developed countries have antibodies to this virus. Antibody acquisition occurs at a younger age among children in less developed countries than among those in developed areas; this observation is consistent with the presumption that Norwalk virus is spread by the fecal-oral route. In developed countries, the virus is responsible for approximately one-third of all epidemics of nonbacterial gastroenteritis. Norwalk virus has been incriminated in a variety of food-borne epidemics, and transmission vehicles have included oysters, green salad, and chocolate icing. The virus is a common cause of waterborne epidemics of gastroenteritis and has been shown to be the etiologic agent in nursing home, cruise ship, and institutional (summer camp and school) outbreaks. Norwalk virus is also responsible for a small proportion of cases of traveler's diarrhea. The role of Norwalk-like virus infection in childhood diarrhea is currently under investigation.

In less developed countries, the role of Norwalk-like virus infection in the etiology of diarrhea has not been thoroughly investigated. Preliminary studies indicate that Norwalk virus can cause mild diarrhea in young children, but it does not appear to cause severe illness in infants in either developed or less developed countries. The other serologically distinct calicivirus-like gastroenteritis agents must be studied in more detail before their epidemiology can be distinguished from that of Norwalk virus. It appears, however, that some human caliciviruses, especially those with well-defined ultrastructure, are primarily pathogens of young children rather than adults.

Pathophysiology Following infection with Norwalk or Hawaii virus, the proximal small intestinal architecture is altered, with villus shortening, crypt hyperplasia, and infiltration of the lamina propria by polymorphonuclear and mononuclear cells. No changes are observed in the stomach or colon. The cells in which viral replication occurs have not been identified. The histologic alterations are accompanied by mild steatorrhea, carbohydrate malabsorption, and decreased levels of some brush border enzymes. No changes in adenylate cyclase activity have been observed.

Manifestations   Norwalk illness has an incubation period of between 18 and 72 h. Disease is characterized by the abrupt onset of nausea and abdominal cramps followed by vomiting and/or diarrhea. Vomiting is reported more frequently for children than for adults. Low-grade fever [above 37.5°C (99.5°F)] develops in about half of affected individuals. Headache, myalgias, and abdominal pain are common. The white blood cell count is normal; rarely, there is leukocytosis with relative lymphopenia. Red and white cells are not found in the stool. The illness is usually mild and self-limited, lasting 24 to 48 h.

Clinical Immunity   Most people do not develop long-term resistance (i.e., resistance lasting 2 years or more) to Norwalk reinfection. In volunteers challenged with Norwalk agent, there is a paradoxical relationship between the level of antibody to Norwalk virus and susceptibility to illness: Low levels of Norwalk antibody in the serum and intestine are associated with clinical resistance to illness. It appears, therefore, that immune mechanisms are not the primary determinants of protection from Norwalk virus.

Diagnosis, Treatment, and Prevention   Enzyme-linked immunosorbent assays and polymerase chain reaction–based assays have recently been developed for Norwalk virus and several other 27- to 30-nm gastroenteritis agents. Because Norwalk illness is acute and self-limited, treatment is not usually required. In the rare case of severe vomiting or diarrhea, oral or intravenous rehydration is indicated. Because long-term immunity to Norwalk illness does not usually follow natural infection, the role of vaccination is unclear.

MISCELLANEOUS ENTERIC VIRAL PATHOGENS   Enteric adenoviruses are a minor cause of diarrheal illness in infants and children, accounting for 10 percent of cases. These viruses differ from other adenovirus strains in a variety of ways, including neutralization serotype, restriction endonuclease digestion pattern, and ability to grow in tissue culture. The role of enteric adenovirus illness in adults or in persons in less developed countries is not known.

Several strains of antigenically distinct rotaviruses, presently called atypical rotaviruses or groups B and C rotaviruses, have been identified as the cause of occasional episodes of diarrhea in humans and animals.

Preliminary epidemiologic studies have indicated that astroviruses are a relatively frequent cause of mild to moderate diarrhea in young children in developed and less developed countries, accounting for about half as much illness as group A rotaviruses. Astroviruses are 27 to 32 nm in diameter, have a characteristic icosahedral ultrastructure, and contain a plus-stranded RNA genome with a size of approximately 7.0 kilobases and a unique genomic organization. At least seven distinct serotypes have been identified. The recent availability of sensitive and specific diagnostic assays should facilitate more complete assessment of the importance of these agents. Preliminary studies indicate that astroviruses are a common cause of diarrhea in immunocompromised hosts, such as bone marrow transplant recipients and patients with AIDS.

Coronaviruses are frequent causes of diarrheal disease in a variety of animals. Several investigators, using electron microscopy, have identified putative coronavirus-like particles in the stools of patients with diarrhea. In most cases, however, these particles do not have the typical morphologic features of coronaviruses and may represent bacterial breakdown products or cellular fragments.

BIBLIOGRAPHY

BERNSTEIN DI: Evaluation of rhesus rotavirus monovalent and tetravalent reassortant vaccines in U.S. children. JAMA 273:1191, 1995

BLACKLOW NR, GREENBERG HB: Viral gastroenteritis. N Engl J Med 325:252, 1991

GLASS RI et al: Rotavirus vaccines: Success by reassortment. Science 265:1389, 1994

GROHMANN GS et al: Enteric viruses and diarrhea in HIV-infected patients. N Engl J Med 329:14, 1993

JIANG X et al: Sequence and genomic organization of Norwalk virus. Virology 195:51, 1993

LEWIS TL et al: Analysis of astrovirus serotype 1 RNA, identification of viral RNA-dependent RNA polymerase motif and expression of a viral structural protein. J Virol 68:77, 1994

OKHUYSEN PC: Viral shedding and fecal IgA after Norwalk virus infection. J Infect Dis 171:566, 1995

195   *Jeffrey I. Cohen*

ENTEROVIRUSES AND REOVIRUSES

ENTEROVIRUSES

CLASSIFICATION AND CHARACTERIZATION   Enteroviruses are so named because of their ability to multiply in the gastrointestinal tract. Despite their name, these viruses are not a prominent cause of gastroenteritis. Members of the picornavirus (Spanish *pico*, "a little bit" + RNA + virus) family, enteroviruses encompass 67 human serotypes: 3 serotypes of poliovirus, 23 serotypes of coxsackievirus A, 6 serotypes of coxsackievirus B, 31 serotypes of echovirus, and enteroviruses 68 through 71.

Human enteroviruses contain a single-stranded RNA genome that is translated to form a polyprotein; this polyprotein is cleaved into 11 different proteins. The RNA is surrounded by an icosahedral capsid comprising four viral proteins (VP1 through VP4). VP1 is the predominant target of neutralizing antibody. The three-dimensional structure of poliovirus has been determined by x-ray diffraction; a deep cleft on the surface is thought to contain the site of attachment to the cellular receptor. The receptor for poliovirus is a member of the immunoglobulin superfamily, the receptor for echovirus types 1 and 8 is VLA-2 integrin, and the receptor for enterovirus 7 is CD55, or decay-accelerating factor. Poliovirus infection is limited to primates, primarily because of the ability of these cells to express the poliovirus receptor. While cultured mouse cells cannot be infected with the virus, expression of the receptor in transgenic mice allows these animals to become infected with poliovirus and to develop central nervous system (CNS) disease. Several enterovirus genomes have been cloned, and cDNA copies of these genomes are infectious in cultured cells. Construction of recombinant viruses containing portions of virulent and attenuated genomes from these cDNAs has allowed mapping of viral sequences that are responsible for attenuation of the live oral poliovirus vaccines.

Enteroviruses have no lipid envelope and are stable in acidic environments, including the stomach. These viruses are resistant to inactivation by standard disinfectants (e.g., alcohol, detergents) and can persist for days at room temperature.

PATHOGENESIS AND IMMUNITY   Much of what is known about the pathogenesis of enteroviruses has been derived from studies of poliovirus infection. After ingestion, poliovirus is thought to infect epithelial cells in the mucosa of the gastrointestinal tract and then to spread to and replicate in the submucosal lymphoid tissue of the tonsils and Peyer's patches. The virus next spreads to the regional lymph nodes, enters the bloodstream during the first (minor) viremic phase, and replicates in organs of the reticuloendothelial system. In some cases poliovirus again infects the bloodstream (major viremia) and then replicates further in various tissues, sometimes causing symptomatic disease. It is uncertain whether poliovirus reaches the CNS during viremia or whether it also spreads via peripheral nerves. Since viremia precedes the onset of neurologic disease in humans and in experimentally infected chimpanzees, it has been assumed that the virus enters the CNS via the bloodstream. Recent studies demonstrating the poliovirus receptor in the end-plate region of muscle at the neuromuscular junction suggest that if the virus enters the muscle during viremia, it could travel across the neuromuscular junction up the axon to the anterior horn cells. Studies of monkeys or transgenic mice expressing the poliovirus receptor show that, after intramuscular injection, poliovirus does not reach the spinal cord if the sciatic nerve is cut. Taken together, these findings suggest that poliovirus can spread directly from muscle to the CNS by neural pathways.

Poliovirus can usually be cultured from the blood 3 to 5 days after infection, before the development of neutralizing antibodies. While viral replication at secondary sites begins to slow 1 week after infection, it continues in the gastrointestinal tract. Poliovirus is shed from the oropharynx for up to 3 weeks after infection and from the gastrointestinal tract for as long as 8 weeks; immunodeficient patients can shed poliovirus for very long periods. During replication in the gastrointestinal tract, attenuated oral poliovirus can mutate, reverting to a more neurovirulent phenotype within a few days. The clinical significance of this increased neurovirulence is unknown.

Humoral and secretory immunity in the gastrointestinal tract is important for the control of enterovirus infections. Enteroviruses induce specific IgM, which usually persists for less than 6 months, and specific IgG, which persists for life. Neutralizing antibody generally confers lifelong protection against subsequent disease caused by the same serotype but does not prevent infection or virus shedding. Enteroviruses also induce cellular immunity, but the importance of this mechanism in limiting infection is uncertain. Patients with impaired cellular immunity are not known to develop unusually severe disease when infected with enteroviruses. In contrast, the severe infections in patients with agammaglobulinemia emphasize the importance of humoral immunity in controlling enterovirus infections. IgA antibodies are important in reducing poliovirus replication in and shedding from the gastrointestinal tract. Breast milk contains IgA specific for enteroviruses and can protect humans from infection.

EPIDEMIOLOGY Enteroviruses have a worldwide distribution. More than 50 percent of nonpoliovirus enterovirus infections and more than 90 percent of poliovirus infections are subclinical. When symptoms do develop, they are usually nonspecific and occur in conjunction with fever and sometimes with upper respiratory tract manifestations; only a minority of infections are associated with specific clinical syndromes. The incubation period for most enterovirus infections ranges from 2 to 14 days but usually is less than a week.

Enterovirus infection is more common in socioeconomically disadvantaged areas, especially in those where conditions are crowded and in tropical areas where hygiene is poor. Infection is most common among infants and young children; serious illness develops most often during the first few days of life and in older children and adults. In developing countries, where children are infected at an early age, poliovirus infection has less often been associated with paralysis; in countries with better hygiene, older children and adults are more likely to be seronegative, become infected, and develop paralysis. The acquisition of maternal antibody reduces the risk of symptomatic infection in neonates. Young children are the most frequent shedders of enteroviruses and are usually the index cases in family outbreaks. In temperate climates enterovirus infections occur most often in the summer and fall; no seasonal pattern is apparent in the tropics.

Most enteroviruses are transmitted primarily by the fecal-oral route from fecally contaminated fingers or inanimate objects. Patients are most infectious shortly before and after the onset of symptomatic disease, when virus is present in the stool and throat. The ingestion of virus-contaminated food or water can also cause disease. Certain enteroviruses (such as enterovirus 70, which causes acute hemorrhagic conjunctivitis) can be transmitted by direct inoculation from the fingers to the eye. Airborne transmission is important for some viruses that cause respiratory tract disease, such as coxsackievirus A21. Enteroviruses can be transmitted across the placenta from mother to fetus, causing severe disease in the newborn. The transmission of enteroviruses through blood transfusions or insect bites has not been documented. Nosocomial spread of coxsackievirus and echovirus has taken place in hospital nurseries.

DIAGNOSIS Isolation of enterovirus in cell culture is the most common procedure for the diagnosis of infection. While cultures of stool, nasopharyngeal, or throat samples from patients with enterovirus diseases are often positive, isolation of the virus from these sites does not prove that it is directly associated with disease because these sites are frequently colonized for weeks in patients with subclinical infections. Isolation of virus from the throat is more likely to be associated with disease than isolation from the stool since virus is shed for shorter periods from the throat. Cultures of cerebrospinal fluid (CSF), serum, fluid from body cavities, or tissues are positive less frequently, but a positive result is indicative of disease caused by enterovirus. In some cases the virus can be isolated only from the blood or only from the CSF; therefore, it is important to culture multiple sites. Cultures are more likely to be positive early than later in the course of infection. Most human enteroviruses can be detected within a week after inoculation of cell cultures. Cultures may be negative because of the presence of neutralizing antibody, lack of susceptibility of the cells used, or inappropriate handling of the specimen. Coxsackievirus A may require inoculation into special cell-culture lines or into suckling mice.

Identification of the serotype of an enterovirus is useful primarily for epidemiologic studies and, with a few exceptions, has little clinical utility. It is important to identify serious infections with enterovirus during epidemics and to distinguish the vaccine strain of poliovirus from the other enteroviruses in the throat or in the feces. Stool and throat samples for culture as well as acute- and convalescent-phase serum specimens should be obtained from all patients with suspected poliomyelitis. In the absence of a positive CSF culture, a positive culture of stool obtained within the first 2 weeks after the onset of symptoms is most often used to confirm the diagnosis of poliomyelitis. If poliovirus is isolated, it should be sent to the Centers for Disease Control and Prevention (CDC) in Atlanta for identification as a wild-type or a vaccine virus.

The polymerase chain reaction (PCR) has been used to amplify viral nucleic acid from CSF, serum, and tissues. The high degree of homology among the different enterovirus serotypes at the 5′ end of the genome allows the detection of most (more than 92 percent) of the human serotypes with a single pair of PCR primers. With the proper controls, PCR of the CSF is highly sensitive ($\geq$95 percent) and specific (nearly 100 percent) and is more rapid and probably more sensitive than culture. PCR may be particularly helpful for the diagnosis and follow-up of enterovirus disease in immunodeficient patients receiving immunoglobulin therapy, whose viral cultures may be negative. Antigen detection and hybridization of enterovirus sequences in human tissues with a specific probe are additional options, but these techniques are generally less sensitive than PCR.

Serologic diagnosis of enterovirus infection is limited by the large number of serotypes and the lack of a common antigen. Demonstration of seroconversion may be useful in rare cases for confirmation of culture results, but serologic testing is usually limited to epidemiologic studies. Serum should be collected and frozen soon after the onset of disease and again about 4 weeks later. Measurement of neutralizing titers is the most accurate method for antibody determination; measurement of complement-fixation titers is usually less sensitive. Titers of virus-specific IgM are elevated in both acute and chronic infection.

℞ TREATMENT

Most enterovirus infections are mild and resolve spontaneously; however, intensive supportive care may be needed for cardiac, hepatic, or CNS disease. Intravenous, intrathecal, or intraventricular immunoglobulin has been used with apparent success for the treatment of chronic enterovirus meningoencephalitis and dermatomyositis in patients with hypo- or agammaglobulinemia. The disease may stabilize or resolve during therapy; however, some patients decline inexorably despite therapy. Intravenous administration of immunoglobulin with high titers of antibody to the infecting virus has been successful in the treatment of some cases of life-threatening neonatal infection; neonates with such infection may not have maternally acquired antibody. In a recent trial involving neonates with enterovirus infections, immunoglobulin containing very high titers of antibody to the infecting virus reduced rates of viremia; however, no substantial clinical benefit was apparent. The ability of the study to detect a difference in outcome was limited by the small number of patients included. While antiviral agents that inhibit the growth of enterovirus in vitro and in animal models have been developed, these drugs have not yet undergone clinical trials. Glucocorticoids are contraindicated.

Good hand-washing practices and the use of gowns and gloves are important in limiting nosocomial transmission of enteroviruses during epidemics. Enteric precautions are indicated for 7 days after the onset of enterovirus infections.

POLIOVIRUS

MANIFESTATIONS Most infections with poliovirus are asymptomatic. After an incubation period of 3 to 6 days, about 5 percent of patients present with a minor illness (abortive poliomyelitis) manifested by fever, malaise, sore throat, anorexia, myalgias, and headache. This condition usually resolves in 3 days. About 1 percent of patients present with aseptic meningitis (nonparalytic poliomyelitis). Examination of CSF reveals lymphocytic pleocytosis, a normal glucose level, and a normal or slightly elevated protein level; CSF polymorphonuclear leukocytes may be present early. In some patients, especially children, malaise and fever precede the onset of aseptic meningitis.

The least common presentation is that of paralytic disease. After one or several days, signs of aseptic meningitis are followed by severe back, neck, and muscle pain and by the rapid or gradual development of motor weakness. In some cases the disease appears to be biphasic, with aseptic meningitis followed first by apparent recovery but then (1 or 2 days later) by the return of fever and the development of paralysis; this form is more common among children than among adults. Weakness is generally asymmetric, is proximal more than distal, and may involve the legs (most commonly); the arms; or the abdominal, thoracic, or bulbar muscles. Paralysis develops during the febrile phase of the illness and usually does not progress after defervescence. Urinary retention may also occur. Examination reveals weakness, fasciculations, decreased muscle tone, and reduced or absent reflexes in affected areas. Transient hyperreflexia sometimes precedes the loss of reflexes. Patients frequently report sensory symptoms, but objective sensory testing usually yields normal results. Bulbar paralysis leads to dysphagia, difficulty in handling secretions, or dysphonia. Respiratory insufficiency due to aspiration, involvement of the respiratory center in the medulla, or paralysis of the phrenic or intercostal nerves may occur, and severe medullary involvement may lead to circulatory collapse. Most patients with paralysis recover some function weeks to months after infection. About two-thirds of patients have residual neurologic sequelae.

Paralytic disease is more common among older individuals, pregnant women, and persons exercising strenuously or undergoing trauma at the time of CNS symptoms. Tonsillectomy predisposes to bulbar poliomyelitis, and intramuscular injections increase the risk of paralysis in the involved limb(s).

At present, the only cases of poliomyelitis in the United States are due to live poliovirus vaccine; 5 to 10 such cases are reported each year. About half of these cases occur in vaccine recipients; vaccine-induced disease is most frequent among infants after the first dose. The median interval from vaccination to the onset of symptoms is 3 weeks. Most of the other cases develop in close contacts of these patients—usually persons over 20 years old who have not received a full course of vaccine. About 5 percent of the cases of poliomyelitis associated with vaccine occur in members of the community who have had no known direct contact with vaccinees. About 15 percent of all cases of vaccine-associated poliomyelitis involve immunodeficient children or adults, most of whom have hypo- or agammaglobulinemia. In these patients the median interval between vaccination and the onset of symptoms is 6 weeks, but disease can develop up to 6 months after vaccination. The risk of developing poliomyelitis after oral vaccination

is estimated at 1 case per 2.5 million doses administered. The risk of developing paralytic disease after oral vaccination is about 2000 times higher among immunodeficient patients than among immunocompetent children.

The postpolio syndrome presents as a new onset of weakness, fatigue, fasciculations, and pain with additional atrophy of the muscle group involved during the initial paralytic disease 20 to 30 years earlier. The onset is insidious, and weakness occasionally extends to muscles that were not involved during the initial illness. The prognosis is generally good; progression to further weakness is usually slow, with plateau periods that range from 1 to 10 years. The syndrome is thought to be due to progressive dysfunction and loss of motor neurons that compensated for the neurons lost during the original infection and not to persistent or reactivated poliovirus infection.

PREVENTION AND ERADICATION (See also Chap. 122) After a peak of 57,879 cases of poliomyelitis in the United States in 1952, the introduction of inactivated vaccine in 1955 and of oral vaccine in 1961 ultimately eradicated disease due to wild-type poliovirus in the western hemisphere. Such disease has not been documented in the United States since 1979, when cases occurred among religious groups who had declined immunization. In the western hemisphere, paralysis due to wild-type poliovirus was last documented in 1991.

In 1988 the World Health Organization adopted a resolution to eradicate poliomyelitis by the year 2000. From 1985 to 1994, the number of cases worldwide decreased by 84 percent, with 6241 cases reported from 51 countries in 1994. More than 70 percent of cases worldwide were from the Indian subcontinent; outbreaks of poliomyelitis in Europe and North America have been traced to cases imported from this region. Poliomyelitis still occurs in sub-Saharan Africa and in parts of Asia (including several republics of the former Soviet Union) and is a source of concern for unimmunized or partially immunized travelers to these regions. Clearly, global eradication of polio is necessary to eliminate the risk of importation of wild-type virus. Outbreaks are thought to have been facilitated by suboptimal rates of vaccination, isolated pockets of unvaccinated children, poor sanitation and crowding, improper vaccine-storage conditions, and a reduced level of response to one of the serotypes in the vaccine.

For the development of live oral poliovirus vaccine (OPV) containing all three serotypes, wild-type virus was attenuated by passage in monkey kidney cell cultures. OPV strains differ from the wild-type strain in a limited number of nucleotide changes (i.e., fewer than 60). Multiple doses are required to ensure infection and development of immunity to all three serotypes. OPV is given at 2, 4, and 6 to 18 months and at 4 to 6 years of age. While intramuscular injections of other vaccines (live or attenuated) can be given concurrently with OPV, unnecessary intramuscular injections should be avoided during the first month after vaccination because of the risk of vaccine-associated paralysis.

Inactivated poliovirus vaccine is generated by formalin inactivation of the three serotypes of live poliovirus. Since 1988 an enhanced–potency inactivated poliovirus vaccine (IPV-e) has been available in the United States. IPV-e is recommended for adults because of the slightly greater risk of paralysis with OPV in adults than in children. Either children or adults immunized with IPV-e should receive three doses; children should receive a fourth dose when entering school. Current indications and contraindications for OPV and IPV-e are listed in Table 195-1.

The efficacy of OPV after three doses is estimated to be nearly 100 percent. OPV and IPV-e induce antibodies that persist for at least 5 years. Both vaccines induce IgG and IgA antibodies. Compared with recipients of IPV-e, recipients of OPV shed less virus and less frequently develop reinfection with wild-type virus after exposure to poliovirus. Although IPV-e is safe and efficacious, OPV has been used for routine immunization in the United States because of its ease of administration, lower cost, and induction of intestinal immunity resulting in a reduction in the risk of community transmission of wild-type virus. While OPV has been the vaccine of choice for childhood immunization in the United States, the CDC recommended in late

1996 that children receive a sequential schedule of two doses of IPV-e followed by two doses of OPV. A four-dose schedule of either IPV-e or OPV is an acceptable option and may be preferred in certain circumstances. Vaccination with the sequential regimen is expected to reduce the number of cases of vaccine-associated poliomyelitis by 50 to 75 percent.

COXSACKIEVIRUS, ECHOVIRUS, AND OTHER ENTEROVIRUSES

An estimated 5 to 10 million cases of symptomatic enterovirus disease occur in the United States each year. Enteroviruses are the major cause of aseptic meningitis and nonspecific febrile illnesses of neonates. Certain clinical syndromes are more likely to be caused by certain serotypes (Table 195-2), but there is much overlap. From 1970 to 1983, 70 percent of enterovirus infections were caused by only 10 of the 67 human serotypes. Echoviruses 9 and 11 alone accounted for 24 percent of recognized enterovirus infections; echoviruses 4, 6, and 30 and coxsackieviruses A9 and B2 through B5 accounted for 46 percent.

Nonspecific Febrile Illness (Summer Grippe) The most common clinical manifestation of enterovirus infection is a nonspecific febrile illness. After an incubation period of 3 to 6 days, patients present with an acute onset of fever, malaise, and headache. Many cases include upper respiratory symptoms, and some cases include nausea and vomiting. Symptoms often last for 3 to 4 days, and most cases resolve in a week. While infections with other respiratory viruses occur more often from late fall to early spring, enterovirus febrile illness frequently occurs in the summer.

Generalized Disease of the Newborn Most serious enterovirus infections in infants develop during the first week of life, although severe disease can occur up to 3 months of age. Neonates often present with an illness resembling bacterial sepsis, with fever, irritability, and lethargy. Laboratory abnormalities include leukocytosis with a left shift, thrombocytopenia, elevated values in liver function tests, and CSF pleocytosis. The illness can be complicated by myocarditis and hypotension, fulminant hepatitis and disseminated intravascular coagulation, meningitis or meningoencephalitis, or pneumonia. It may be difficult to distinguish enterovirus infection from bacterial sepsis, although a history of a recent virus-like illness in the mother provides a clue.

Aseptic Meningitis and Encephalitis Enteroviruses are the cause of up to 90 percent of cases of aseptic meningitis in children and young adults in which an etiologic agent can be identified. Patients with aseptic meningitis typically present with an acute onset of fever, chills, headache, photophobia, and pain on eye movement. Nausea and vomiting are also common. Examination reveals meningismus without localizing neurologic signs; drowsiness or irritability may also be apparent. In some cases, a febrile illness may be reported that remits but returns several days later in conjunction with signs of meningitis. Other systemic manifestations may pro-

vide clues to an enteroviral cause, including pharyngitis and cough, diarrhea, myalgias, rash, pleurodynia, myocarditis, and herpangina. Examination of the CSF invariably reveals pleocytosis; early in the course, polymorphonuclear leukocytes may be present or even predominate, raising the possibility of bacterial or other nonviral causes of meningitis. Partially treated bacterial meningitis may be particularly difficult to exclude in some instances. A useful rule is that the CSF cell count in enteroviral meningitis shows a shift to lymphocytic predominance within 24 h of presentation, and the total count generally does not exceed 1000 cells/μL. Additional CSF findings consist of a normal glucose content and a normal or only slightly elevated (by $\leq$100 mg/mL) level of protein. Enteroviruses and mumps virus may produce a similar picture of meningitis with orchitis; a low CSF glucose level suggests mumps, whereas a normal CSF glucose level and transient CSF polymorphonuclear pleocytosis suggest enterovirus infection. Symptoms ordinarily resolve within a week, although CSF abnormalities can persist for several weeks. Neurologic sequelae are rare, and most patients have an excellent prognosis. Enteroviral encephalitis is much less common than enteroviral aseptic meningitis. Occasional highly inflammatory cases of enteroviral meningitis may be complicated by a mild form of encephalitis that is recognized on the basis of progressive lethargy, disorientation, and sometimes seizures. Less

Table 195-1

Indications for and Contraindications to Poliovirus Vaccination

INDICATIONS FOR IMMUNIZATION WITH ORAL POLIOVIRUS VACCINE (OPV)

1. Normal infants and children undergoing routine immunization*
2. Unimmunized or partially immunized children at imminent risk of exposure to poliovirus
3. Adults at future risk of exposure to poliomyelitis who have in the past received one or more doses of OPV or IPV(-e)

INDICATIONS FOR IMMUNIZATION WITH ENHANCED-POTENCY INACTIVATED POLIOVIRUS VACCINE (IPV-e)

1. Normal infants, children, or adults undergoing routine immunization*
2. Immunodeficient persons, including those infected with human immunodeficiency virus (HIV), who are unimmunized or partially immunized
3. Household contacts of an HIV-infected or otherwise immunodeficient person
4. Partially immunized or unimmunized adults in households (or other close contacts) of children receiving OPV, provided that timely immunization of the child can be ensured
5. Adults at future risk of exposure to poliomyelitis who have been partially immunized with IPV(-e) or OPV or have received a primary series of IPV(-e)†
6. Individuals refusing OPV vaccination

CONTRAINDICATIONS TO IMMUNIZATION

1. Pregnant women should not receive OPV or IPV-e unless immediate protection is needed.
2. Immunodeficient patients (e.g., those with AIDS, hypogammaglobulinemia, or generalized malignancy and recipients of immunosuppressive therapy) should not receive OPV.
3. Household contacts of immunodeficient persons should not receive OPV.
4. Families with a history of immunodeficient children should not receive OPV until the immune status of all family members is documented and immunodeficiency is excluded.

* A sequential schedule of two doses of IPV-e followed by two doses of OPV is now recommended by the CDC for infants and children (see text for details and options).
† OPV is also acceptable.
SOURCE: Modified from 1994 Redbook, Report of the Committee on Infectious Diseases.

Table 195-2

Manifestations Commonly Associated with Enterovirus Serotypes

Manifestation	Serotype(s) of Indicated Virus	
	Coxsackievirus	Echovirus (E) and Enterovirus (Ent)
Aseptic meningitis	A2, 4, 7, 9, 10; B1-5	E4, 6, 7, 9, 11, 16, 18, 30, 33; Ent70, 71
Exanthem	A4, 5, 9, 10, 16; B1, 3-5	E4-7, 9, 11, 16-19, 25, 30; Ent71
Generalized disease of the newborn	B2-5	E4-6, 9, 11, 14, 16, 19
Hand-foot-and-mouth disease	A5, 7, 9, 10, 16; B2, 5	Ent71
Herpangina	A1-10, 16, 22; B1-5	E6, 9, 11, 16, 17, 22, 25
Myocarditis, pericarditis	A4, 9, 16; B1-5	E6, 9, 11, 22
Paralysis	A4, 7, 9; B1-5	E2, 4, 6, 9, 11, 30; Ent70, 71
Pleurodynia	A1, 2, 4, 6, 9, 10, 16; B1-6	E1-3, 6–9, 11, 12, 14, 16, 19, 23–25, 30
Pneumonia	A9, 16; B1-5	E6, 7, 9, 11, 12, 19, 20, 30; Ent68, 71

commonly, severe primary encephalitis may develop. It is estimated that 10 to 20 percent of cases of viral encephalitis are due to enteroviruses. Immunocompetent patients generally have a good prognosis.

Patients with hypo- or agammaglobulinemia or severe combined immunodeficiency may develop chronic meningitis or encephalitis; about half of these patients have a dermatomyositis-like syndrome, with peripheral edema, rash, and myositis. They may also have chronic hepatitis. Patients may develop neurologic disease while receiving gamma globulin replacement therapy. Echoviruses (especially echovirus 11) are the most common pathogens in this situation.

Paralytic disease due to enteroviruses other than poliovirus occurs sporadically and is usually less severe than poliomyelitis. Most cases are due to enterovirus 70 or 71 or to coxsackievirus A7. Guillain-Barré syndrome is also associated with enterovirus infection. While some studies have suggested a link between enteroviruses and the chronic fatigue syndrome, most recent studies have not demonstrated such an association.

Pleurodynia (Bornholm Disease) Patients with pleurodynia present with an acute onset of fever and spasms of pleuritic chest or upper abdominal pain. Chest pain is more frequent in adults, and abdominal pain is more common in children. Paroxysms of severe, knifelike pain usually last 15 to 30 min and are associated with diaphoresis and tachypnea. Fever peaks within an hour after the onset of paroxysms and subsides when pain resolves. The involved muscles are tender to palpation, and a pleural rub may be detected. The white blood cell count and chest x-ray are usually normal. Most cases are due to coxsackievirus B and occur during epidemics. Symptoms resolve in a few days, and recurrences are rare. Treatment includes the administration of nonsteroidal anti-inflammatory agents or the application of heat to the affected muscles.

Myocarditis and Pericarditis Enteroviruses are estimated to cause up to one-third of cases of acute myocarditis. Coxsackievirus B and its RNA have been detected in pericardial fluid and myocardial tissue in some cases of acute myocarditis and pericarditis. Most cases of enteroviral myocarditis or pericarditis occur in newborns, adolescents, or young adults. More than two-thirds of patients are male. Patients often present with an upper respiratory tract infection that is followed by fever, chest pain, dyspnea, arrhythmias, and occasionally heart failure. A pericardial friction rub is documented in half of cases, and the electrocardiogram shows ST segment elevations or ST- and T-wave abnormalities. Serum levels of myocardial enzymes are often elevated. Neonates commonly have severe disease, while most older children and adults recover completely. Up to 10 percent of cases progress to chronic dilated cardiomyopathy. Chronic constrictive pericarditis may also be a sequela.

Exanthems Enterovirus infection is the leading cause of exanthems in children in the summer and fall. While exanthems are associated with many enteroviruses, certain types have been linked to specific syndromes. Echoviruses 9 and 16 have frequently been associated with exanthem and fever. Rashes may be discrete (rubelliform) or confluent (morbilliform), beginning on the face and spreading to the trunk and extremities. Echovirus 9 is the most common cause of rubelliform rash. Unlike the rash of rubella, the enteroviral rash occurs in the summer and is not associated with lymphadenopathy. Roseola-like rashes develop after defervescence, with macules and papules on the face and trunk. The Boston exanthem, caused by echovirus 16, is a roseola-like rash that often affects multiple members of a family. A variety of other rashes have been described, including erythema multiforme and vesicular, urticarial, petechial, or purpuric lesions. Enanthems also occur, including lesions that resemble the Koplik's spots seen with measles.

Hand-Foot-and-Mouth Disease After an incubation period of 4 to 6 days, patients with hand-foot-and-mouth disease present with fever, anorexia, and malaise; these manifestations are followed by the development of sore throat and vesicles on the buccal mucosa and often on the tongue and then by the appearance of tender vesicular lesions on the dorsum of the hands, sometimes with involvement of the palms. The vesicles may form bullae and quickly ulcerate. About one-third of patients also have lesions on the palate, uvula, or tonsillar pillars, and one-third have a rash on the feet (including the soles) or on the buttocks. The disease is highly infectious, with attack rates of close to 100 percent among young children. The lesions usually resolve in 1 week. Most cases are due to coxsackievirus A16.

Herpangina Herpangina is usually caused by coxsackievirus A and presents as acute-onset fever, sore throat, dysphagia, and grayish-white papulovesicular lesions on an erythematous base that ulcerate. The lesions can persist for weeks; are present on the soft palate, anterior pillars of the tonsils, and uvula; and are concentrated in the posterior portion of the mouth. In contrast to herpes stomatitis, enteroviral herpangina is not associated with gingivitis. Acute lympho-nodular pharyngitis associated with coxsackievirus A10 presents as white or yellow nodules surrounded by erythema in the posterior oropharynx. The lesions do not ulcerate.

Acute Hemorrhagic Conjunctivitis Patients with acute hemorrhagic conjunctivitis present with an acute onset of severe eye pain, blurred vision, photophobia, and watery discharge from the eye. Examination reveals edema, chemosis, and subconjunctival hemorrhage and often documents punctate keratitis and conjunctival follicles as well. Preauricular adenopathy is often found. Epidemics and nosocomial spread have been associated with enterovirus 70 and coxsackievirus A24. Systemic symptoms, including headache and fever, develop in 20 percent of cases, and recovery is usually complete in 10 days. The sudden onset and short duration of the illness help to distinguish acute hemorrhagic conjunctivitis from other ocular infections such as those due to adenovirus and *Chlamydia*. Paralysis has been associated with some cases of acute hemorrhagic conjunctivitis due to enterovirus 70 during epidemics.

Other Manifestations Enteroviruses are an infrequent cause of childhood pneumonia and the common cold. Coxsackievirus B has been isolated at autopsy from the pancreas of a few children presenting with insulin-dependent diabetes mellitus; however, most attempts to isolate the virus have been unsuccessful. Other diseases that have been associated with enterovirus infection include bronchitis, bronchiolitis, croup, infectious lymphocytosis, polymyositis, acute arthritis, and acute nephritis.

REOVIRUSES

Reoviruses are double-stranded RNA viruses encompassing three serotypes. Serologic studies indicate that most humans are infected with reoviruses during childhood; however, it has been difficult to establish a definite link of reovirus infection with a particular disease. It is likely that most infections either are asymptomatic or cause very mild disease. One outbreak of reovirus infection in children resulted in minor upper respiratory tract symptoms. Reovirus is considered a rare cause of mild gastroenteritis in infants and children. Speculation regarding an association of reovirus type 3 with idiopathic neonatal hepatitis and extrahepatic biliary atresia is based on a higher prevalence of antibody to reovirus in some of these patients and detection of virus in the porta hepatis in one case.

BIBLIOGRAPHY

ABZUG MJ et al: Neonatal enterovirus infection: Virology, serology, and effects of intravenous immune globulin. Clin Infect Dis 20:1201, 1995

CHEN RT et al: Seroprevalence of antibody against poliovirus in inner-city preschool children: Implications for vaccination policy in the United States. JAMA 275:1639, 1996

COCHI SL et al (eds): Global poliomyelitis eradication initiative; status report. J Infect Dis 175(Suppl 1):S1–S292, 1997

DALAKAS MC et al (eds): The postpolio syndrome: Advances in the pathogenesis and treatment. Ann NY Acad Sci 753:1, 1995

FADEN H: Long-term immunity to poliovirus in children immunized with live attenuated and enhanced-potency inactivated trivalent poliovirus vaccines. J Infect Dis 168:452, 1993

———— et al: Comparative evaluation of immunization with live attenuated and enhanced-potency inactivated trivalent poliovirus vaccines in childhood: Systemic and local immune responses. J Infect Dis 162:1291, 1990

IKEDA RM et al: Pleurodynia among football players at a high school. JAMA 270:2205, 1993

McKINNEY R et al: Chronic enteroviral meningoencephalitis in agammaglobulinemic patients. Rev Infect Dis 9:334, 1987

ROTBART HA (ed): *Human Enterovirus Infections.* Washington, DC, ASM Press, 1995

STREBEL PM et al: Epidemiology of poliomyelitis in the United States one decade after the last reported case of indigenous wild virus–associated disease. Clin Infect Dis 14:568, 1992

————— et al: Intramuscular injections within 30 days of immunization with oral poliovirus vaccine—a risk factor for vaccine-associated paralytic poliomyelitis. N Engl J Med 332:500, 1995

196 | *Anne Gershon*

MEASLES (RUBEOLA)

DEFINITION   Measles (rubeola) is a highly contagious, acute, exanthematous respiratory disease with a characteristic clinical picture and pathognomonic enanthem. A successful live attenuated measles vaccine became available in 1963 in the United States and elsewhere, and measles is now an unusual disease in most developed countries where this vaccine is widely used. However, measles continues to occur sporadically in mini-epidemics in the United States, and major epidemics in developing nations make this disease a persistent cause of childhood morbidity and mortality.

ETIOLOGIC AGENT   Measles virus is a member of the genus *Morbillivirus* and the family Paramyxoviridae. It is closely related to the viruses causing canine and porcine distemper, rinderpest of cattle, and *peste des petits ruminants* of goats and sheep. There is only one antigenic type, and the genome has been sequenced. Measles virions are pleomorphic spherical structures having a diameter of 100 to 250 nm and consisting of six proteins. The inner capsid is composed of a coiled helix of RNA and three proteins, and the outer envelope consists of a matrix protein bearing two types of short surface-glycoprotein projections or peplomers. One peplomer is a conical hemagglutinin (H) and the other a dumbbell-shaped fusion (F) protein.

EPIDEMIOLOGY   Measles has a worldwide distribution; humans are the only natural hosts although other primates can be experimentally infected. During the prevaccination era in the United States, measles epidemics occurred every 2 to 5 years in the winter and spring. In an epidemic year, roughly half a million measles cases were reported; 99 percent of adults had serologic evidence of previous measles infection. After the live attenuated vaccine became available, the number of cases reported to the Centers for Disease Control and Prevention (CDC) fell, with a nadir of 1497 cases in 1983. More recently, after an upsurge to more than 27,000 cases (with 89 deaths) in 1990, the disease was once more brought under control (with only 312 cases reported to the CDC in 1993), in part through the routine administration of two doses of vaccine. The foremost reason for the resurgence of measles was failure to immunize infants and young children, especially in inner-city areas. Primary vaccine failure (documented in about 5 percent of individuals) and secondary vaccine failure or waning immunity accounted for some cases. In recent years the majority of cases of measles have involved preschool children. Mortality is highest among children under 2 years of age and among adults. Patients with impaired cell-mediated immunity are at especially high risk for severe or even fatal measles. The measles-associated mortality rate in the United States is about 0.3 percent; in developing countries, mortality frequently exceeds 1 percent and sometimes approaches 10 percent.

Measles virus is transmitted by respiratory secretions, predominantly through exposure to aerosols but also through direct contact with larger droplets. Patients are contagious from 1 or 2 days before the onset of symptoms until 4 days after the appearance of the rash. Infectivity peaks during the prodromal phase. The mean intervals from infection to onset of symptoms and to appearance of rash are 10 and 14 days, respectively.

PATHOGENESIS AND PATHOLOGY   Measles virus invades the respiratory epithelium and spreads via the bloodstream to the reticuloendothelial system, from which it infects all types of white blood cells, thereby establishing infection of the skin, respiratory tract, and other organs. Both viremia and viruria develop. Multinucleated giant cells with inclusion bodies in the nucleus and cytoplasm (Warthin-Finkeldey cells) are found in respiratory and lymphoid tissues and are pathognomonic for measles. Direct invasion of T lymphocytes may play a role in the temporary depression of cellular immunity that accompanies and transiently follows measles. Infection of the entire respiratory tract accounts for the characteristic cough and coryza of measles and for the less frequent manifestations of croup, bronchiolitis, and pneumonia. Generalized damage to the respiratory tract, with resultant loss of cilia, predisposes to secondary bacterial infections such as pneumonia and otitis media.

Specific antibodies are not detectable before the onset of rash. Cellular immunity (consisting of cytotoxic T cells and possibly natural killer cells) plays a prominent role in host defense, and patients who are deficient in cellular immunity are at high risk for severe measles. Children with isolated agammaglobulinemia are not at increased risk. Immune reactions to the virus in the endothelial cells of dermal capillaries play a substantial role in the development of Koplik's spots (the pathognomonic enanthem) as well as in that of rash; in immunodeficient hosts, measles may be severe despite the absence of these manifestations. Measles antigens have been demonstrated in involved skin during early stages of the illness.

Pathologic changes in measles encephalitis include focal hemorrhage, congestion, and perivascular demyelination. Measles virus is rarely isolated from cerebrospinal fluid (CSF) in cases of encephalitis, which are thought to be due to the interaction of virus-infected cells with local cellular immune factors.

CLINICAL MANIFESTATIONS   Measles begins with a 2- to 4-day respiratory prodrome of malaise, cough, coryza, conjunctivitis with lacrimation, nasal discharge, and increasing fever [with temperatures as high as 40.6°C (105°F), probably reflecting secondary viremia]. At this stage of the illness, in which the rash has not yet developed, influenza may be suspected. Just before the onset of the rash, Koplik's spots appear as 1- to 2-mm blue-white spots on a bright red background. Without adequate illumination for examination, they may be overlooked. Koplik's spots are typically located on the buccal mucosa alongside the second molars and may be extensive; they are not associated with any other infectious disease. The spots wane after the onset of rash and soon disappear. The entire buccal and inner labial mucosa may be inflamed, and the lips may be reddened.

The characteristic erythematous, nonpruritic, maculopapular rash of measles begins at the hairline and behind the ears, spreads down the trunk and limbs to include the palms and soles, and often becomes confluent. At this time, the patient is at the most severe point of the illness. By the fourth day, the rash begins to fade in the order in which it appeared. Brownish discoloration of the skin and desquamation may occur later. Fever usually resolves by the fourth or fifth day after the onset of rash; prolonged fever suggests a complication of measles. Lymphadenopathy, diarrhea, vomiting, and splenomegaly are common features. The chest x-ray may be abnormal, even in uncomplicated measles, because of the propensity of this virus to invade the respiratory tract. The entire illness usually lasts about 10 days. The disease tends to be more severe in adults than in children, with higher fever, more prominent rash, and a higher incidence of complications.

Milder forms of the illness with less intense symptoms and a milder rash, termed *modified measles*, may occur in individuals with preexisting partial immunity induced by active or passive vaccination. These patients include infants under 1 year of age who retain some proportion of passively acquired maternal antibodies. On occasion, individuals with a history of immunization may develop modified measles.

COMPLICATIONS   The complications of measles can conveniently be divided into three groups, according to the site involved:

the respiratory tract, the central nervous system (CNS), and the gastrointestinal tract. Respiratory tract involvement, manifested as laryngitis, croup, or bronchitis, occurs in the majority of cases of uncomplicated measles. In young children, otitis media is the most common complication. Pneumonia is a frequent reason for hospitalization, especially of adults. The pneumonia is of viral origin in the majority of cases, but secondary bacterial infection (most commonly caused by streptococci, pneumococci, or staphylococci) also takes place with some frequency. Primary giant cell (Hecht's) pneumonia is most often documented in immunocompromised and/or malnourished patients.

Encephalographic abnormalities in the absence of symptoms of CNS disease are extremely frequent in measles. Symptomatic CNS disease, with fever, headache, drowsiness, coma, and/or seizures, occurs in about 1 case in 1000. Symptoms usually begin within days after the onset of rash but occasionally appear for the first time several weeks later. About 10 percent of patients do not survive acute measles encephalitis; a significant percentage of surviving patients develop permanent sequelae, such as mental retardation or epilepsy. Most cases appear to result from an immune-mediated response to myelin proteins (postinfectious encephalomyelitis) and not directly from viral infection of the CNS (see Chap. 376). Rarely, transverse myelitis follows measles. Immunocompromised patients are at risk for progressive fatal encephalitis 1 to 6 months after measles; in some cases, even though prior measles has not been recognized, the virus is identified at autopsy. Subacute sclerosing panencephalitis (SSPE)—a protracted, chronic, extremely rare form of measles encephalitis—sometimes follows measles and is particularly common among children who have measles before the age of 2 years (see Chap. 379). SSPE has virtually disappeared in the United States as a result of widespread vaccination. Typically, progressive dementia evolves over several months. SSPE is thought to be due to a complex interaction of the host with defective measles virus. It is associated with extremely high levels of antibodies to measles virus in the blood and CSF.

Gastrointestinal complications of measles include gastroenteritis, hepatitis, appendicitis, ileocolitis, and mesenteric adenitis. It is not uncommon to detect high levels of alanine and aspartate aminotransferases in the absence of gastrointestinal signs such as jaundice.

Other, rare complications include myocarditis, glomerulonephritis, and postinfectious thrombocytopenic purpura. Measles can exacerbate preexisting tuberculosis, presumably through depression of cellular immunity induced by the virus. Natural measles and immunization against measles can result in tuberculin skin-test anergy lasting for about 1 month.

ATYPICAL MEASLES   An atypical form of measles has been reported in individuals who received formalin-inactivated measles vaccine (used in the United States from 1963 through 1967 and in Canada until 1970) and subsequently were exposed to measles virus. After a several-day prodrome of fever, myalgia, and headache, the rash appears. Unlike the rash of typical measles, that of atypical measles begins peripherally and moves centrally; it can be urticarial, maculopapular, hemorrhagic, and/or vesicular. Fever is usually high and is accompanied by edema of the extremities, interstitial pulmonary infiltrates, hepatitis, and (on occasion) pleural effusion. The differential diagnosis often includes Rocky Mountain spotted fever, Henoch-Schönlein purpura, meningococcemia, drug allergy, toxic shock syndrome, and varicella. Despite the severity of atypical measles, patients invariably recover after a convalescence that may be prolonged. Measles virus is not isolated from these patients, and they do not spread the virus to others. This disease is believed to be due to hypersensitivity to measles virus induced by the inactivated vaccine. Formalin inactivation destroys the antigenicity of the F protein, antibodies to which are important in preventing spread of the virus from one cell to another. The role of cellular immunity in this process is unknown. Extremely high convalescent titers of antibody to measles virus (e.g., 1:1,000,000) are diagnostic of atypical measles. To prevent this syndrome, adults who received formalin-inactivated measles vaccine should be reimmunized with at least one dose of live attenuated measles vaccine. Since inactivated measles vaccine has not been available for more than 25 years, atypical measles has now virtually disappeared.

MEASLES IN THE IMMUNOCOMPROMISED HOST   Patients with defects in cell-mediated immunity are at risk for severe protracted and fatal measles. Included in this category are patients with congenital cellular immune defects or malignancy, recipients of immunosuppressive therapy, or persons infected with human immunodeficiency virus (HIV). In these patients, measles may not be accompanied by a rash. Complications are primary measles (giant cell) pneumonia, progressive encephalitis beginning weeks to months after initial infection, and (in HIV-infected patients) progression to AIDS.

MEASLES IN ADULTS   Measles is naturally a disease of childhood and, like many other viral infections, is more severe in adults than in children. About 3 percent of young adults with measles develop primary viral pneumonia and require hospitalization. Hepatitis and bronchospasm are more common among adults with measles than among children, and the rash is more severe and more confluent in adults. Bacterial superinfection is more common among adults, more than one-third of whom develop respiratory complications such as otitis media, sinusitis, and pneumonia. Adults may develop measles because they were never immunized or (more rarely) because their vaccine-induced immunity has waned. Very low titers of antibody to measles virus have been associated with lack of protection.

LABORATORY FINDINGS   Lymphopenia and neutropenia are common in measles and may be due to invasion of leukocytes by the virus, with subsequent cell death. Leukocytosis may herald a bacterial superinfection. Patients with measles encephalitis usually have an elevated protein concentration in CSF as well as lymphocytosis. A specific diagnosis of measles can be made quickly by immunofluorescent staining of a smear of respiratory secretions for measles antigen; monoclonal antibodies conjugated to fluorescein are commercially available for this purpose. Secretions can also be examined microscopically for multinucleated giant cells. Measles virus can be isolated from respiratory secretions or urine and rapidly identified in tissue culture with fluorescein-labeled monoclonal antibodies. A number of serologic tests are available for the diagnosis of measles; however, a serologic diagnosis cannot necessarily be made quickly since both acute- and convalescent-phase sera are usually tested, ideally at the same time. The older hemagglutination inhibition test has been replaced by enzyme immunoassay (EIA), which is more sensitive and simpler to perform. EIA can be used to measure specific IgM and thus to diagnose measles on the basis of an acute-phase serum sample alone. Specific IgM antibodies are detectable within 1 to 2 days after the appearance of rash, and the IgG titer rises significantly after 10 days. As already mentioned, atypical measles and SSPE are associated with extremely high titers of antibody.

DIFFERENTIAL DIAGNOSIS   Classic measles—with Koplik's spots, cough, coryza, conjunctivitis, and a rash beginning on the head—is easily diagnosed on clinical grounds. Modified measles is more difficult to diagnose clinically since one or more characteristic signs may be lacking. The differential diagnosis of measles includes Kawasaki's syndrome, scarlet fever, infectious mononucleosis, toxoplasmosis, drug eruption, and *Mycoplasma pneumoniae* infection. Most of these conditions can be identified by either culture or serologic assay. In the differential diagnosis of measles, attention should be paid to the current epidemiology of the disease in the community and to the patient's history of measles vaccination and foreign travel.

PREVENTION   The development of live attenuated measles vaccine by Enders and his colleagues was a milestone in American medicine. This vaccine, used in the United States for the routine immunization of children since 1963, induces seroconversion in about 95 percent of recipients and probably confers lifelong protection. Waning immunity to measles after immunization has been documented only on rare occasions. For the past 25 years, measles vaccine has been available as the combination vaccine of measles-mumps-rubella (MMR); this combination MMR vaccine should be administered to children between the ages of 12 and 15 months. (Vaccination at 12 months is preferred for infants whose mothers were immunized against measles in childhood. These mothers have lower antibody titers than women who have had natural measles, and their infants correspondingly have transplacental antibodies of lower titer and shorter duration.) A second dose of MMR vaccine is recommended at 4 to 5 years of age (CDC) or at 12 years of age (American Academy of Pediatrics). This policy was developed in the late 1980s in response to measles outbreaks in the United States. Since the institution of the two-dose regimen and the increased effort to immunize all children, measles has again become an unusual disease in the United States. Regional guidelines that reflect the current local epidemiology of measles should be followed.

Older susceptible persons should also be immunized. Individuals should be considered susceptible to measles unless they have documentation of physician-diagnosed measles or of the receipt of two doses of vaccine, have laboratory evidence of measles immunity, or were born before 1957. Rarely, individuals born before 1957 develop measles, and those who are at risk of exposure to measles (e.g., health workers, teachers, and international travelers) should be tested for measles antibody and immunized if necessary. Approximately 10 percent of healthy vaccinees develop a fever, with temperatures up to 39.4°C (103°F), 5 to 7 days after vaccination; this fever lasts 1 to 5 days and is accompanied by a transient rash. Individuals previously immunized only with killed vaccine are considered susceptible and should receive at least one dose—and preferably two doses—of MMR vaccine. Transient adverse reactions in these individuals include fever, malaise, and redness and swelling at the injection site.

Children with asymptomatic HIV infection should receive MMR vaccine. Strong consideration should also be given to the vaccination of symptomatic HIV-infected children because of the severity of measles in this group and the lack of reported problems following vaccination. Measles vaccine is contraindicated for persons with impaired cell-mediated immunity, for pregnant women, and for persons with a history of anaphylaxis due to egg protein or neomycin. Minor illnesses, with or without fever and a history of convulsions, are not contraindications to vaccination. Vaccination should be deferred for 6 to 11 months after the receipt of immune globulin or of blood products containing antibodies and for at least 3 months after the discontinuation of immunosuppressive treatment. Vaccine failures have been ascribed to faulty storage of the preparation used, immunization of infants with preexisting (maternally derived) antibodies, and simultaneous administration of measles vaccine and immune globulin.

Children and adults who are susceptible to measles and are exposed to the disease should receive postexposure prophylaxis. Standard immune globulin, given intramuscularly within 6 days of exposure, can exert a protective or modifying effect; the earlier it is given, the better the outcome. The dose is 0.25 mL/kg for healthy persons and 0.5 mL/kg for immunocompromised persons, with a maximum dose of 15 mL. Immune globulin is particularly strongly indicated for susceptible household contacts, especially those less than 1 year of age, and for immunocompromised persons. HIV-infected persons should be given immune globulin after exposure, regardless of immune status and whether or not they are receiving intravenous immunoglobulin. Vaccination within 72 h of exposure may also provide protection against clinical measles, but this strategy is contraindicated as postexposure prophylaxis for immunocompromised individuals. Vaccine and immune globulin should not be given concurrently.

TREATMENT

Therapy for measles is largely supportive and symptom-based. Patients with otitis media and pneumonia should be given standard antibiotics. Patients with encephalitis need supportive care, including observation for increased intracranial pressure. Controlled trials suggest clinical benefit from high doses of vitamin A in severe or potentially severe measles, especially in children under the age of 2 years. A dose of 50,000 IU is used for infants aged 1 to 6 months, 100,000 IU for infants aged 7 to 12 months, and 200,000 IU for children over 1 year. A single dose is administered on two consecutive days. Transient vomiting and headache may be associated with the administration of vitamin A. Ribavirin is effective against measles virus in vitro and may be considered for use in immunocompromised individuals.

BIBLIOGRAPHY

EBERHART-PHILLIPS JE et al: Measles in pregnancy: A descriptive study of 58 cases. Obstet Gynecol 82:797, 1993

FORNI AL et al: Severe measles pneumonitis in adults: Evaluation of clinical characteristics and therapy with intravenous ribavirin. Clin Infect Dis 19:454, 1994

GREMILLION DH et al: Measles pneumonia in young adults. An analysis of 106 cases. Am J Med 71:539, 1981

HUSSEY GD et al: A randomized, controlled trial of vitamin A in children with severe measles. N Engl J Med 323:160, 1990

KAPLAN LJ et al: Severe measles in immunocompromised patients. JAMA 267:1237, 1992

LA BOCCETTA AC et al: Measles encephalitis. Report of 61 cases. Am J Dis Child 107:247, 1964

MARKOWITZ LE et al: Duration of live measles vaccine–induced immunity. Pediatr Infect Dis J 9:101, 1990

PELTOLA H et al: The elimination of indigenous measles, mumps, and rubella from Finland by a 12-year, two-dose vaccination program. N Engl J Med 331:1397, 1994

SMARON MF et al: Diagnosis of measles by fluorescent antibody and culture of nasopharyngeal secretions. J Virol Methods 33:223, 1991

TAKAHASHI H et al: Detection and comparison of viral antigens in measles and rubella rashes. Clin Infect Dis 22:36, 1996

WATSON BM et al: Safety and immunogenicity of a combined live attenuated measles, mumps, rubella, and varicella vaccine (MMR(II)V) in children. J Infect Dis 173:731, 1996

197 *Anne Gershon*

RUBELLA (GERMAN MEASLES)

DEFINITION Rubella is an acute viral infection of children and adults that characteristically includes rash, fever, and lymphadenopathy and has a broad spectrum of other possible manifestations. However, a high percentage of rubella infections in both children and adults are subclinical. In addition, the illness can resemble a mild attack of measles (rubeola) and can cause arthritis, especially in adults. Rubella during pregnancy can lead to fetal infection, with the production of a significant constellation of malformations (*congenital rubella syndrome*) in a high proportion of infected fetuses.

ETIOLOGIC AGENT Rubella virus, a togavirus, is closely related to the alphaviruses. Unlike these agents, however, it does not require a vector for transmission. Moreover, there is no RNA sequence homology between rubella virus and the alphaviruses.

The rubella virion is composed of an inner helical capsid of RNA and protein that is surrounded by a lipid-containing envelope with a diameter of about 60 nm. The structural proteins associated with rubella virus are E1 and E2 (transmembrane envelope glycoproteins) and C (the capsid protein that surrounds the viral RNA).

EPIDEMIOLOGY In the United States during the prevaccine era, rubella was most common in the spring and most often affected school-age children; only 80 to 90 percent of adults were immune; and major epidemics occurred every 6 to 9 years. In 1968, 18,269 cases of rubella were reported in the United States, with 30 cases of congenital rubella syndrome. Since the introduction of live attenuated rubella vaccine in 1969, there have been no epidemics; limited outbreaks have been reported in settings where susceptible individuals come into close contact with one another (e.g., schools and workplaces). In 1994, only 227 cases of postnatally acquired rubella—most of them in young adults—and 7 cases of congenital rubella syndrome were reported to the Centers for Disease Control and Prevention (CDC).

Whether symptomatic or subclinical, rubella is contagious, albeit less so than measles. Its incubation period is 18 days on average, with a range of 12 to 23 days. The virus, which is spread in droplets shed in respiratory secretions, infects the respiratory tract and then the bloodstream. In postnatally acquired infections, rubella virus is shed during the prodromal phase of the illness, and shedding from the pharynx can continue for about a week after onset. Despite high titers of specific neutralizing antibodies, infants with congenital rubella may excrete rubella virus from the respiratory tract and in the urine until the age of 2 years. This excretion raises important issues related to infection control in hospital and day-care settings. Persons recently immunized with live attenuated rubella vaccine do not transmit the vaccine virus to others, although low titers of rubella virus may be detected transiently in the pharynx.

After an attack of rubella, specific antibodies and cell-mediated immunity develop and probably play a significant role in protection against future disease. Although asymptomatic reinfection is rarely if ever associated with viremia, it is common upon reexposure to the virus. Rubella virus has been cultured from respiratory secretions during reinfection. Fetal infection may occur during maternal reinfection but is acknowledged to be extremely rare because of the absence of maternal viremia under these circumstances. Viremia following reinfection of individuals immunized against rubella is also rare. Thus the current level of congenital rubella in the United States is exceedingly low.

PATHOGENESIS AND PATHOLOGY Little is known about the microscopic pathology of postnatally acquired rubella since the disease is invariably self-limited. Like that of measles, the rash of rubella is immunologically mediated; its onset coincides with the development of specific antibodies. Viremia can be demonstrated for about a week before and ends within a few days after the onset of rash.

The cause of the damage to cells and organs in congenital rubella is not well understood. Proposed mechanisms of fetal damage include mitotic arrest of cells, tissue necrosis without inflammation, and chromosomal damage. The growth of the fetus may be retarded. Other findings may include decreased numbers of megakaryocytes in the bone marrow, extramedullary hematopoiesis, and interstitial pneumonia.

CLINICAL MANIFESTATIONS **Postnatally Acquired Rubella** Infection acquired after birth usually results in an extremely mild or subclinical illness. A prodromal phase is uncommon in children; adults may have more severe disease, with a brief prodrome of malaise, fever, and anorexia. The foremost symptoms of postnatally acquired rubella include posterior auricular, cervical, and suboccipital lymphadenopathy; fever; and rash. The rash often begins on the face and spreads down the body. It is maculopapular but not confluent, is sometimes accompanied by mild coryza and conjunctivitis, and generally lasts for 3 to 5 days. A petechial enanthem on the soft palate, designated *Forschheimer spots*, may occur but is not specific for rubella. Fever may be absent entirely or may be present for only several days in the early phase of the illness.

Complications of postnatally acquired rubella are uncommon; bacterial superinfection is rare. One particularly troublesome complication is seen almost exclusively in women: arthritis, most frequently involving the fingers, wrists, and/or knees, develops as the rash is appearing and may take several weeks to resolve. Chronic arthritis resulting from rubella is extremely rare. Rubella virus has been isolated from joint fluid during acute rubella arthritis and from peripheral blood in chronic rubella arthritis.

Another complication of postnatally acquired rubella is hemorrhage due to both thrombocytopenia and vascular damage, which occurs in 1 of every 3000 patients. Thrombocytopenia may last for weeks or months; it can have long-term consequences if there is bleeding into organs such as the eye or the brain.

Both children and adults may develop encephalitis after rubella; the incidence is about five times lower than that of encephalitis following measles. Adults are more likely than children to develop encephalitis; the mortality rate from this complication is 20 to 50 percent. Mild hepatitis is an unusual complication. Immunosuppressed patients are not at increased risk for rubella as they are for measles.

Congenital Rubella Maternal infection in early pregnancy can lead to fetal infection, with resultant congenital rubella. The classic signs of congenital rubella are cataract, heart disease, and deafness, but a myriad of other defects have been reported. These abnormalities include signs and symptoms that are transient, such as low birth weight, thrombocytopenia, hepatosplenomegaly, jaundice, and pneumonia; those that are permanent, such as deafness, pulmonic stenosis, patent ductus arteriosus, glaucoma, and cataract; and those that are developmental, such as mental retardation, diabetes mellitus, and behavioral disorders.

The most important factor in the pathogenicity of rubella virus for the fetus is gestational age at the time of infection. Maternal infection during the first trimester leads to fetal infection in about 50 percent of cases; maternal infection early in the second trimester leads to fetal infection in about one-third of cases. Fetal malformations not only are more common after maternal infection in the first trimester but also tend to be more severe and to involve more organ systems. While a fetus infected in the fourth week of gestation may develop many problems, one infected later (e.g., in the 20th week) may have isolated deafness as the only symptom.

DIAGNOSIS Since postnatally acquired rubella is such a mild disease and since many cases are subclinical, diagnosis on clinical grounds can be difficult. Other diseases that may mimic rubella include toxoplasmosis, scarlet fever, modified measles, roseola, fifth disease (erythema infectiosum due to parvovirus B19), and enteroviral infection. Routine laboratory tests usually reveal leukopenia and atypical lymphocytes.

The isolation of rubella virus in cell cultures of throat samples, urine, or other secretions is difficult and expensive but is sometimes undertaken. This technique is most useful when congenital rubella is suspected. A laboratory diagnosis is more often made serologically. The most commonly used test is an enzyme-linked immunosorbent assay (ELISA) for IgG and IgM antibodies. Acute rubella is diagnosed by the documentation of a fourfold or greater rise in the titer of IgG antibodies in paired acute- and convalescent-phase serum specimens or by the detection of rubella-specific IgM antibodies in one serum specimen. However, false-negative and -positive IgM reactions are sometimes obtained. Moreover, true-positive IgM reactions can be obtained in both primary infection and reinfection. Congenital rubella is diagnosed by the isolation of rubella virus, the detection of IgM antibodies in a single serum sample, and/or the documentation of either the persistence of rubella antibodies in serum beyond 1 year of age or a rising antibody titer anytime during infancy in an unvaccinated child. Biopsied tissues and/or blood and cerebrospinal fluid have also been used for the demonstration of rubella antigens with monoclonal antibodies and for the detection of rubella RNA by in situ hybridization and polymerase chain reaction.

PREVENTION Live attenuated rubella vaccine was licensed in 1969, 7 years after the virus was first isolated in culture. This vaccine was developed as a strategy to prevent congenital rubella by ensuring that very few pregnant women would be susceptible and that there would be little circulating wild-type virus. Rubella vaccine induces seroconversion in more than 95 percent of recipients. Since its licensure, there have been no major epidemics in the United States, and the number of cases has declined by 98 percent. The last large-scale epidemic of rubella in the United States took place in 1964 to 1965; this epidemic resulted in the birth of tens of thousands of infants with the congenital rubella syndrome. The vaccine currently licensed in the United States, RA 27/3, is propagated in human diploid cells and is more immunogenic (particularly with regard to the stimulation of secretory immunity) than previously licensed vaccines. The present vaccination strategy, developed in part when measles was not being adequately controlled, is to immunize all infants at 12 to 15 months of age with measles-mumps-rubella (MMR) vaccine and to administer a second dose during childhood. Rubella vaccine may also be administered to anyone who is thought to be susceptible to the infection and is not pregnant; it is particularly important that hospital workers of either sex be immune to rubella so that nosocomial transmission is avoided. While there has been little change in the prevalence of immunity to rubella among women of childbearing age (about 80 percent), the incidence of congenital rubella is extremely low—about 10 cases annually. It is likely that, although antibody may be undetectable years after immunization, protection against infection—possibly due to cell-mediated immunity—is the rule. At present, there is little if any evidence of significant waning of clinically important immunity to rubella with time.

On occasion, rubella vaccine may cause arthralgia or arthritis, especially in young women. Very rarely, rubella vaccination results in chronic arthritis; however, even cases of frank arthritis in vaccinees are self-limited, lasting only about 1 week.

After investigation of a series of more than 400 women who were inadvertently immunized during pregnancy and who carried their infants to term, the CDC has concluded that vaccine-type rubella virus either does not cause the congenital rubella syndrome at all or does so at an incidence too low to be detected. Nonetheless, rubella vaccine is contraindicated for use in pregnant women, and it is recommended that pregnancy be avoided for at least 3 months after rubella vaccination. It is acceptable for rubella-susceptible children whose mothers are also susceptible to be immunized, since vaccinated individuals do not shed rubella virus or transmit it to susceptible individuals. Although it is recommended that rubella vaccine not be given to immunosuppressed persons, the vaccine is given to children infected with human immunodeficiency virus. No adverse effects of rubella vaccine have been reported in immunocompromised patients.

 TREATMENT

There is no specific therapy for rubella. At one time, immune globulin was used in an effort to prevent congenital rubella when pregnant women became infected. However, since administration of immune globulin did not prevent maternal viremia, this approach was discarded. Treatment is given for symptoms such as fever, arthralgia, and arthritis.

BIBLIOGRAPHY

BOSMA TJ et al: Use of PCR for prenatal and postnatal diagnosis of congenital rubella. J Clin Microbiol 33:2881, 1995

CHANTLER JK et al: Persistent rubella virus infection associated with chronic arthritis in children. N Engl J Med 313:1117, 1985

CUSI MG et al: Serological evidence of reinfection among vaccinees during rubella outbreak. Lancet 336:1071, 1991

GREGG NM: Congenital cataract following German measles in the mother. Trans Ophthalmol Soc Aust 3:35, 1941

HERRMANN KL: Available rubella serologic tests. Rev Infect Dis 7:S108, 1985

HORSTMANN D et al: Persistence of vaccine-induced immune responses to rubella. Rev Infect Dis 7:S80, 1985

MELLINGER AK et al: High incidence of congenital rubella syndrome after a rubella outbreak. Pediatr Infect Dis J 14:573, 1995

SKENDZEL LP: Rubella immunity: Defining the level of protective antibody. Am J Clin Pathol 106:170, 1996

SMITH CA et al: Rubella virus and arthritis. Rheum Dis Clin North Am 13:810, 1987

TOWNSEND JJ et al: Progressive rubella panencephalitis: Late onset after congenital rubella. N Engl J Med 292:990, 1975

WEIBEL RE, BENOR DE: Chronic arthropathy and musculoskeletal symptoms associated with rubella vaccines: A review of 124 claims submitted to the National Vaccine Injury Compensation Program. Arthritis Rheum 39:1529, 1996

 Anne Gershon

MUMPS

DEFINITION   Mumps is an acute, systemic, communicable viral infection whose most distinctive feature is swelling of one or both parotid glands. Involvement of other salivary glands, the meninges, the pancreas, and the gonads is also common.

ETIOLOGIC AGENT   Mumps virus, a paramyxovirus, is pleomorphic and has a diameter ranging from 100 to 600 nm. The virion is composed of RNA and five proteins. The RNA is surrounded by an envelope with glycoprotein projections. There are two envelope glycoproteins—a hemagglutinin-neuraminidase (HN) and a hemolysis cell fusion antigen (F)—as well as a matrix envelope protein (M). There are two internal components: a nucleocapsid protein (NP) and an RNA polymerase protein. There is only one antigenic type of mumps virus.

EPIDEMIOLOGY   After the introduction of mumps vaccine in 1967, the incidence of clinical mumps declined significantly in the United States. In 1968 (before widespread immunization), 152,209 cases of mumps were reported in this country. The 1537 cases reported in 1994 represent a reduction in the number of cases by >99 percent from prevaccine levels; this is the lowest number of cases ever reported in a year. Before widespread vaccination, the incidence of mumps was highest in the winter and spring, with epidemics every 2 to 5 years. At that time mumps was principally a disease of childhood, although today more than 50 percent of cases occur in young adults. Epidemics tended to occur in confined populations, such as those in schools and the military services.

The incubation period of mumps generally ranges from 14 to 18 days, with extremes of 7 and 23 days. However, because a contact may be shedding virus before the onset of clinical disease or (like one-third of patients) may have subclinical infection, the incubation period in individual cases is often uncertain. One attack of mumps usually confers lifelong immunity. Long-term immunity is also associated with immunization.

PATHOGENESIS   Mumps virus is transmitted by droplet nuclei, saliva, and fomites. Replication of the virus in the epithelium of the upper respiratory tract leads to viremia, which is followed by infection of glandular tissues and/or the central nervous system (CNS).

Little is known of the pathology of mumps since the disease is rarely fatal. The affected glands contain perivascular and interstitial mononuclear cell infiltrates with prominent edema. Necrosis of acinar and epithelial duct cells is evident in the salivary glands and in the germinal epithelium of the seminiferous tubules.

CLINICAL MANIFESTATIONS   The prodrome of mumps consists of fever, malaise, myalgia, and anorexia. Parotitis, if it develops, usually does so within the next 24 h but may be delayed for as long as a week; it is generally bilateral, although the onset on the two sides may not be synchronous and at times only one side is affected. The submaxillary and sublingual glands are involved less often than the parotid and are almost never involved alone. Swelling of the parotid is accompanied by tenderness and obliteration of the space between the ear lobe and the angle of the mandible. The patient frequently reports an earache and finds it difficult to eat, swallow, or talk. Glandular swelling increases for a few days and then gradually subsides, disappearing within a week. The orifice of Stensen's duct is commonly red and swollen. Presternal pitting edema has been described in about 5 percent of mumps cases, often in association with submandibular adenitis.

Other than parotitis, orchitis is the most common manifestation of mumps among postpubertal males, developing in about 20 percent of cases. The testis is painful and tender and is enlarged to several times its normal size; accompanying fever is common. Later, testicular atrophy develops in half of the affected men. Since orchitis is bilateral in fewer than 15 percent of cases, sterility after mumps is rare. Oophoritis in women—far less common than orchitis in men—may cause lower abdominal pain but does not lead to sterility.

Aseptic meningitis, which may develop before, during, after, or in the absence of parotitis, is a common manifestation of mumps in both children and adults. Symptoms include stiff neck, headache, and drowsiness. Pleocytosis of the cerebrospinal fluid (CSF), with up to 1000 cells/μL, may develop in up to 50 percent of cases of clinical mumps, but clinical signs of meningeal irritation are documented in only 5 to 25 percent of cases. Within the first 24 h, polymorphonuclear leukocytes may predominate in CSF, but by the second day nearly all the cells are lymphocytes. The glucose level in CSF may be abnormally low, and this finding may arouse suspicion of bacterial meningitis. Aseptic meningitis due to mumps without parotitis is indistinguishable clinically from that caused by other viruses. Mumps meningitis is almost invariably self-limited, although cranial nerve palsies have occasionally led to permanent sequelae, particularly deafness. More rarely, mumps virus may cause encephalitis, which presents as high fever with marked changes in the level of consciousness and frequently results in permanent sequelae in survivors. Other CNS problems occasionally associated with mumps include cerebellar ataxia, facial palsy, transverse myelitis, Guillain-Barré syndrome, and aqueductal stenosis leading to hydrocephalus.

Mumps pancreatitis, which may present as abdominal pain, is difficult to diagnose because an elevated serum amylase level can be associated with either parotitis or pancreatitis. Other unusual complications of mumps include myocarditis, mastitis, thyroiditis, nephritis, arthritis, and thrombocytopenic purpura. An excessive number of spontaneous abortions is associated with gestational mumps when the disease occurs during the first trimester. Mumps in pregnancy does not lead to premature birth or fetal malformations.

DIFFERENTIAL DIAGNOSIS   The diagnosis of mumps is made easily in patients with acute bilateral parotitis and a history of recent exposure. When parotitis is unilateral or absent or when sites other than the parotid gland are involved, laboratory diagnosis is required (see below).

The myriad causes of bilateral parotid swelling other than mumps virus include infection with other viruses, such as parainfluenza virus type 3, coxsackieviruses, and influenza A virus; metabolic diseases, such as diabetes mellitus and uremia; and drugs, such as phenylbutazone and thiouracil. Unilateral parotid swelling can result from a tumor, a cyst, or a ductal obstruction due to stones or strictures. Other conditions associated with chronic parotid swelling include sarcoidosis, Sjögren's syndrome, and infection with human immunodeficiency virus (HIV). Suppurative parotitis, usually caused by *Staphylococcus aureus*, is most often unilateral.

Other entities should be considered when manifestations consistent with mumps appear in organs other than the parotid. Testicular torsion may produce a painful scrotal mass resembling that seen in mumps orchitis. Other viruses (e.g., enteroviruses) may cause aseptic meningitis that is clinically indistinguishable from that due to mumps virus.

LABORATORY DIAGNOSIS   Mumps virus is readily isolated after inoculation of appropriate clinical specimens into a variety of host systems, such as rhesus monkey kidney cells and human embryonic lung fibroblasts. The virus can be rapidly identified by the use of cells grown in shell vials and of fluorescein-labeled monoclonal antibodies. Mumps virus may be recovered from saliva, throat, and urine during the first few days of illness and from the CSF of patients with mumps meningitis. Shedding of virus in the urine may persist for as long as 2 weeks. No particular peripheral blood cell count is characteristic of mumps.

Highly sensitive enzyme-linked immunosorbent assays (ELISA) are useful for diagnosis of mumps and for determination of susceptibility to the disease. Acute mumps can be diagnosed either by the examination of acute- and convalescent-phase sera for a significant increase in antibody titer or by the demonstration of specific IgM in one serum specimen. Use of a skin-test antigen to assess immunity to mumps has been replaced by serologic testing.

TREATMENT

Therapy for parotitis and other manifestations of mumps is symptom-based. The administration of analgesics and the application of warm or cold compresses to the parotid area may be helpful. Mumps immune globulin is of no value in the prophylaxis or treatment of established disease. Testicular pain may be minimized by the local application of cold compresses and gentle support for the scrotum. Anesthetic blocks may also be used. Neither the administration of

glucocorticoids nor incision of the tunica albuginea is of proven value for the treatment of severe orchitis. Anecdotal information on a small number of patients with orchitis suggests that administration of interferon α may be helpful.

PREVENTION   Live attenuated mumps vaccine (Jeryl Lynn strain) induces antibodies that protect against infection in more than 95 percent of cases. The subcutaneously administered vaccine may be given to children older than 1 year but is not recommended for younger infants because of the potential for interference by passive maternal antibodies. Mumps vaccine is usually administered as part of the measles-mumps-rubella (MMR) vaccine at the age of 15 months and again later in childhood. This MMR vaccine is also recommended for susceptible older children, adolescents, and adults, particularly adolescent males who have not had mumps. For these patients, either MMR or monovalent mumps vaccine may be given; two doses are preferred. Inadvertent immunization of individuals who are already immune is not associated with significant adverse reactions. Mumps vaccine is not recommended for pregnant women, for patients receiving glucocorticoids, or for other immunocompromised hosts. However, children with HIV infection can safely be immunized against mumps; MMR vaccine is usually used for this purpose.

BIBLIOGRAPHY

BROWN E et al: The Urabe AM9 mumps vaccine is a mixture of viruses differing at amino acid 335 of the hemagglutinin-neuraminidase gene with one form associated with disease. J Infect Dis 174:619, 1996
CENTERS FOR DISEASE CONTROL: Update on adult immunization: Recommendations of the Immunization Practices Advisory Committee (ACIP). Morb Mort Week Rep 40:22, 1991
————: Mumps surveillance—United States. Morb Mort Week Rep 44:1, 1995
CHAUDARY S et al: Fulminant mumps myocarditis. Ann Intern Med 110:569, 1989
GUT JP et al: Symptomatic mumps reinfections. J Med Virol 45:17, 1995
HAREL L et al: Mumps arthritis in children. Pediatr Infect Dis J 9:928, 1990
HERSH BS et al: Mumps outbreak in a highly vaccinated population. J Pediatr 119:187, 1991
LYON RP et al: Mumps epididymo-orchitis: Treatment by anesthetic block of the spermatic cord. JAMA 196:736, 1966
McDONALD JC et al: Clinical and epidemiologic features of mumps encephalitis and possible causes of vaccine-related disease. Pediatr Infect Dis J 8:751, 1989
RUTHER U et al: Successful interferon-alpha 2 therapy for a patient with acute mumps orchitis. Eur Urol 27:174, 1995

199   *Lawrence Corey*

RABIES VIRUS AND OTHER RHABDOVIRUSES

RABIES VIRUS

DEFINITION   Rabies is an acute viral disease of the central nervous system (CNS) that affects all mammals and that is transmitted by infected secretions, usually saliva. Most exposures to rabies are through the bite of an infected animal, but on occasion contact with a virus-containing aerosol or the ingestion or transplantation of infected tissues may initiate the disease process.

ETIOLOGY   The rabies virus is a bullet-shaped, enveloped, single-stranded RNA virus that is 75 to 80 nm in diameter and belongs to the rhabdovirus family. Within this family is the genus *Lyssavirus*, which includes the group of agents causing rabies in humans and other animals. Placement of a particular virus within the genus *Lyssavirus* is based on similarities in neutralization of prototype antisera, a feature related to the viruses' surface glycoprotein structure. The envelope glycoproteins are arranged in knoblike structures that cover the surface of the virion. The viral glycoproteins bind to acetylcholine receptors, contribute to the neurovirulence of rabies virus, elicit neutralizing and hemagglutination-inhibiting antibodies, and stimulate cytotoxic T cell immunity. The nucleocapsid antigen induces a complement-fixing antibody as well as T helper cell reactivity. Neutralizing antibodies to the surface glycoproteins appear to be protective. Most of the neutralizing antibodies appear to be directed at conformational epitopes of the viral envelope glycoprotein. The antibodies to rabies virus used in diagnostic immunofluorescence assays are generally directed against the nucleocapsid antigens. Isolates of rabies virus from different animal species and locales differ in their antigenic and biologic properties. These variations may account for differences in virulence between isolates. Interferon is induced by rabies virus, particularly in those tissues with high virus concentrations, and may play some role in retarding progressive infection.

EPIDEMIOLOGY Rabies is found in animals in all regions of the world except Australia and Antarctica. Rabies exists in two epidemiologic forms: *urban*, propagated chiefly by unimmunized domestic dogs and/or cats, and *sylvatic*, propagated by skunks, foxes, raccoons, mongooses, wolves, and bats. Infection in domestic animals usually represents a "spillover" from sylvatic reservoirs of infection, and human beings can be infected in either an urban or a sylvatic setting. Hence human infection tends to occur in locales where rabies is enzootic or epizootic, where there is a large population of unimmunized domestic animals, and where human contact with the outdoors is common. While only about 1000 rabies deaths are reported to the World Health Organization each year, the worldwide incidence of rabies is estimated at more than 30,000 cases per year. Southeast Asia, the Philippines, Africa, the Indian subcontinent, and tropical South America are areas where the disease is especially common. In some endemic areas, 1 to 2 percent of autopsies yield evidence of rabies. Increased spread of terrestrial rabies (i.e., rabies in animals that walk on the ground rather than rabies in animals that fly) and increased travel to countries where urban rabies exists have made the recognition of clinical rabies and its prevention of increasing importance. During the 1980s and 1990s, there has been continued spread of focal epidemics of terrestrial rabies within the United States and Europe. Antigenic analyses have shown that these epidemics arise from the introduction of particular viral strains within the wildlife population and the rapid dissemination of this variant within the animal populace. In the United States, human rabies is exceedingly rare, and most cases now originate either from animal bites in countries where canine rabies is endemic or from exposure to bats.

In most areas of the world, the dog is the most important vector of rabies virus for humans. However, the wolf (in eastern Europe and Arctic regions), the mongoose (in South Africa and the Caribbean), the fox (in western Europe), and the vampire bat (in Latin America) also may be prominent vectors. In the United States, feline rabies is now reported more frequently than canine rabies; thus the vaccination of domestic cats is extremely important. Rodents and lagomorphs are rarely infected with rabies virus. Although rabies in wildlife is common throughout both the developed and the undeveloped world, most cases of postexposure prophylaxis are associated with domesticated animals such as dogs and cats. Several cases of human-to-human transmission of rabies through corneal transplantation also have been documented.

PATHOGENESIS The first event in rabies is the introduction of live virus through the epidermis or onto a mucous membrane. Initial viral replication appears to occur within striated muscle cells at the site of inoculation. The peripheral nervous system is exposed at the neuro-muscular and/or neurotendinous spindles of unmyelinated sensory nerve cell endings. The virus then spreads centripetally up the nerve to the CNS, probably via peripheral nerve axoplasm, at a rate of approximately 3 mm/h. Viremia has been documented in experimental conditions but is thought not to play a role in naturally acquired disease. Once the virus reaches the CNS, it replicates almost exclusively within the gray matter and then passes centrifugally along autonomic nerves to other tissues—the salivary glands, adrenal medulla, kidneys, lungs, liver, skeletal muscles, skin, and heart. Passage of the virus into the salivary glands and viral replication in mucinogenic acinar cells facilitate further transmission via infected saliva. The incubation period of rabies is exceedingly variable, ranging from 7 days to over 1 year (mean,

1 to 2 months) and apparently depending on the amount of virus introduced, the amount of tissue involved, host defense mechanisms, and the actual distance that the virus has to travel from the site of inoculation to the CNS. Rates of infection and mortality are highest from bites on the face, intermediate from bites on the hands and arms, and lowest from bites on the legs. Cases of human rabies with an extended incubation period (2 to 7 years) have been reported, but they are rare. Host immune responses and viral strains also influence disease expression.

The neuropathology of rabies resembles that of other viral diseases of the CNS: hyperemia, varying degrees of chromatolysis, nuclear pyknosis, and neuronophagia of the nerve cells; infiltration by lymphocytes and plasma cells of the Virchow-Robin space; microglial infiltration; and parenchymal areas of nerve cell destruction. In experimental animal models, adenohypophyseal infection with rabies virus, with reduction in growth hormone and vasopressin release, is common. The most characteristic pathologic finding of rabies in the CNS is the formation of cytoplasmic inclusions called *Negri bodies* within neurons. Each eosinophilic mass measures approximately 10 nm and is made up of a finely fibrillar matrix and rabies virus particles. Negri bodies are distributed throughout the brain, particularly in Ammon's horn, the cerebral cortex, the brainstem, the hypothalamus, the Purkinje cells of the cerebellum, and the dorsal spinal ganglia. Negri bodies are not demonstrated in at least 20 percent of cases of rabies, and their absence from brain material does not rule out the diagnosis.

CLINICAL MANIFESTATIONS The clinical manifestations of rabies can be divided into four stages: (1) a nonspecific prodrome, (2) an acute encephalitis similar to other viral encephalitides, (3) a profound dysfunction of brainstem centers that produces the classic features of rabies encephalitis, and (4) death or—in rare cases—recovery.

The prodromal period usually lasts 1 to 4 days and is marked by fever, headache, malaise, myalgias, increased fatigability, anorexia, nausea and vomiting, sore throat, and a nonproductive cough. The prodromal symptom suggestive of rabies is the complaint of paresthesia and/or fasciculations at or around the site of inoculation of virus. These sensations, which may be related to the multiplication of virus in the dorsal root ganglion of the sensory nerve supplying the area of the bite, are reported by 50 to 80 percent of patients.

The encephalitic phase is usually ushered in by periods of excessive motor activity, excitation, and agitation. Confusion, hallucinations, combativeness, bizarre aberrations of thought, muscle spasms, meningismus, opisthotonic posturing, seizures, and focal paralysis soon appear. Characteristically, the periods of mental aberration are interspersed with completely lucid periods, but as the disease progresses the lucid periods get shorter until the patient lapses into coma. Hyperesthesia, with excessive sensitivity to bright light, loud noise, touch, and even gentle breezes, is very common. On physical examination, the temperature may be found to be as high as 40.6°C (105°F). Abnormalities of the autonomic nervous system include dilated irregular pupils, increased lacrimation, salivation, perspiration, and postural hypotension. Evidence of upper motor neuron paralysis, with weakness, increased deep tendon reflexes, and extensor plantar responses, is the rule. Paralysis of the vocal cords is common.

The manifestations of brainstem dysfunction begin shortly after the onset of the encephalitic phase. Cranial nerve involvement causes diplopia, facial palsies, optic neuritis, and the characteristic difficulty with deglutition. The combination of excessive salivation and difficulty in swallowing produces the traditional picture of "foaming at the mouth." Hydrophobia, the painful, violent, involuntary contraction of the diaphragmatic, accessory respiratory, pharyngeal, and laryngeal muscles initiated by swallowing liquids, is seen in about 50 percent of cases. Involvement of the amygdaloid nucleus may result in priapism and spontaneous ejaculation. The patient lapses into coma, and involvement of the respiratory center produces an apneic death. The prominence of early brainstem dysfunction distinguishes rabies from other viral encephalitides and accounts for the rapid downhill course. The median period of survival after the onset of symptoms is 4 days, with a maximum of 20 days, unless artificial supportive measures are instituted.

If intensive respiratory support is used, a number of late complications may appear. These include inappropriate secretion of antidiuretic hormone, diabetes insipidus, cardiac arrhythmias, vascular instability, adult respiratory distress syndrome, gastrointestinal bleeding, thrombocytopenia, and paralytic ileus. Recovery is very rare and, when it occurs, gradual.

Rabies may also present as an ascending paralysis resembling the Landry/Guillain-Barré syndrome (dumb rabies, *rage tranquille*). Initially, this clinical pattern was reported most frequently among persons bitten by vampire bats who were given postexposure rabies prophylaxis. Paralytic rabies also occurs in Southeast Asia among persons with canine exposures.

The difficulty of diagnosing rabies associated with ascending paralysis is illustrated by two cases of person-to-person transmission of the virus by tissue transplantation. Corneal transplants from two donors who died of presumed Landry/Guillain-Barré syndrome produced clinical rabies in and caused the deaths of the recipients. Retrospective pathologic examinations of the brains of both recipients demonstrated Negri bodies, and rabies virus was subsequently isolated from each donor's frozen eye.

LABORATORY FINDINGS Early in the disease, hemoglobin values and routine blood chemistry results are normal; abnormalities develop as hypothalamic dysfunction, gastrointestinal bleeding, and other complications ensue. The peripheral white blood cell count is usually slightly elevated (12,000 to 17,000/μL) but may be normal or as high as 30,000/μL.

As in any viral infection, the specific diagnosis of rabies depends on (1) the isolation of virus from infected secretions [saliva or—rarely—cerebrospinal fluid (CSF)] or tissue (brain), (2) the serologic demonstration of acute infection, (3) the detection of viral antigen in infected tissue (e.g., corneal impression smears, skin biopsies, or brain), or (4) the detection of viral nucleic acid (RNA) by polymerase chain reaction (PCR). Samples of brain obtained either on postmortem examination or at brain biopsy should be subjected to (1) mouse inoculation studies for virus isolation, (2) fluorescent antibody (FA) staining for viral antigen, and (3) histologic and/or electron-microscopic examination for Negri bodies or reverse transcription PCR for detection of rabies virus RNA. While mouse inoculation studies for virus isolation and direct FA staining for viral antigen are quite reliable and sensitive, "autosterilization" may occur and these tests may be negative if the patient's life has been prolonged and high levels of neutralizing antibody are present in serum and CSF. The use of FA staining of skin biopsies, corneal impression smears, and saliva to obtain evidence of rabies antigen has been helpful in diagnosing rabies during life. Confirmation of these findings, either serologically or by demonstration of virus or of viral antigen or RNA in the brain, should be sought.

If the patient has not been immunized against rabies, a fourfold rise in titer of neutralizing antibody to rabies virus in serial serum samples is diagnostic. If the patient has been vaccinated, a clue to the diagnosis may be obtained from the absolute titers of serum neutralizing antibody and the presence of neutralizing antibody in CSF. Postexposure rabies prophylaxis rarely produces CSF neutralizing antibody to rabies virus. If present after prophylaxis, it is usually found at a low titer (<1:64), whereas CSF titers in human rabies may vary from 1:200 to 1:160,000.

DIFFERENTIAL DIAGNOSIS There is little to distinguish rabies from other viral encephalitides. The most helpful clue to the diagnosis is a history of exposure. Other problems to be considered in the differential diagnosis include hysterical reactions to animal bites (pseudohydrophobia), Landry/Guillain-Barré syndrome, poliomyelitis, and allergic encephalomyelitis developing in response to rabies vaccine. The latter is most common after the use of nerve tissue–derived vaccine and usually begins 1 to 4 weeks after vaccination.

℞ **TREATMENT**

Each year more than 1 million Americans are bitten by animals. In each instance, a decision must be made whether to initiate postexposure rabies prophylaxis. In this decision, the following considerations apply: (1) whether the individual came into physical contact with saliva or another substance likely to contain rabies virus, (2) whether rabies is known or suspected in the species and area associated with the exposure (e.g., all persons within the continental United States bitten by a bat that escapes should receive postexposure prophylaxis), and (3) the circumstances surrounding the exposure (e.g., whether the bite was provoked or unprovoked). A guide for postexposure rabies prophylaxis is provided in Fig. 199-1.

If rabies is known or suspected to be present in the animal species involved in a human exposure, the implicated animal should be captured if possible. Any wild animal involved in a rabies exposure; any ill, unvaccinated, or stray domestic animal involved in a rabies exposure; and any animal inflicting an unprovoked bite, exhibiting abnormal behavior, or suspected of being rabid should be humanely killed. The animal's head should be sent immediately to an appropriate laboratory for rabies FA examination. If examination of the brain by the FA technique gives negative results, it can be assumed that the saliva contains no virus, and the exposed person need not be treated. Persons exposed to wild animals that subsequently escape, that are capable of carrying rabies (bats, skunks, coyotes, foxes, raccoons, etc.), and that inhabit an area where rabies is known or suspected to be present should undergo both passive and active immunization against rabies (see below).

In an area in which feline or canine rabies is not prevalent, a healthy biting dog or cat can be confined and observed for 10 days. If it becomes ill or behaves abnormally during the observation period,

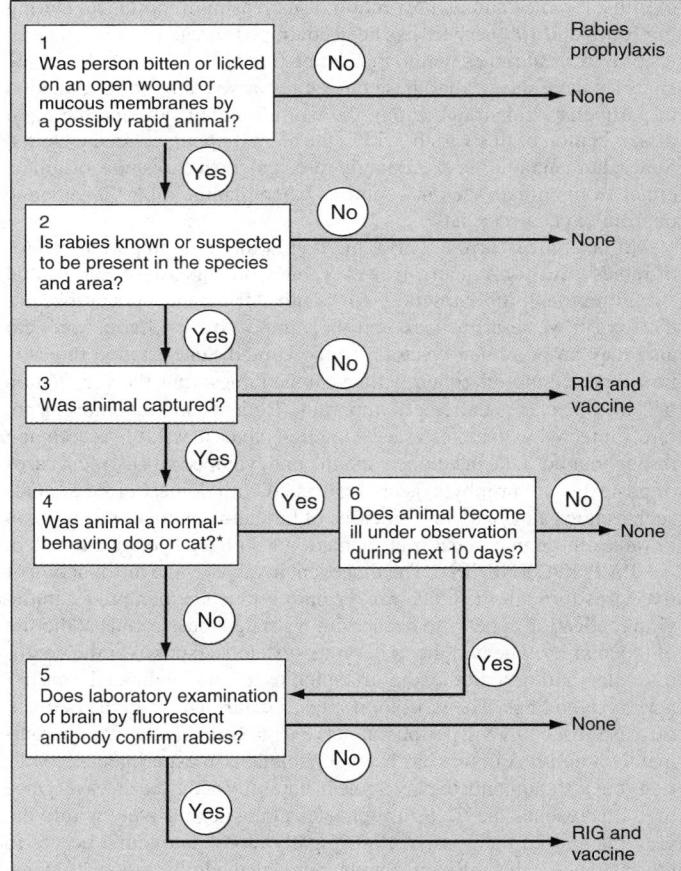

FIGURE 199-1 Postexposure rabies prophylaxis algorithm. *Instances of exposure to livestock or to normal-behaving, unvaccinated dogs or cats should be considered individually, and local and state public health officials should be consulted.

the animal should be killed for FA examination. Experimental and epidemiologic evidence suggests that animals that remain healthy for 10 days after a bite will not have transmitted rabies virus at the time of the bite. In areas of high endemicity for canine rabies, immediate examination of the animal's brain, especially in the case of a severe bite, may be warranted.

PREVENTION **Postexposure Prophylaxis** Postexposure prophylaxis of rabies includes local treatment of the wound and the administration of rabies vaccine together with antirabies immunoglobulin.

1. *Local wound therapy.* Local treatment of the bite wound is an important component of rabies prevention. The wound should be scrubbed with soap and then flushed with water. Both mechanical cleansing and chemical cleansing are important. Quaternary ammonium compounds such as 1 to 4% benzalkonium chloride or 1% cetrimonium bromide are useful because they inactivate the rabies virus. However, 0.1% benzalkonium solutions are less effective than 20% soap solutions. Usually tetanus toxoid and antibiotics should be administered.
2. *Passive immunization with antirabies antiserum of either equine or human origin.* Human rabies immune globulin (HRIG) is preferred because equine antiserum may cause serum sickness. Fifty percent of the total dose of 20 units per kilogram for HRIG and 40 units per kilogram for equine antiserum is given by local infiltration of the wound, and the rest is administered intramuscularly into the gluteal region.
3. *Active immunization with antirabies vaccine.* In the developed world, human diploid cell vaccine (HDCV) is the recommended rabies vaccine. In the United States, two products are licensed. One vaccine contains the Pitman-Moure strain of virus (Pasteur-Mérieux: Imovax), which is grown on human diploid cell cultures and inactivated with β-propiolactone. The other vaccine, rabies vaccine absorbed (RVA), is distributed by the Biologics Products Program of the Michigan Department of Public Health and is prepared from the Kissling strain of virus adapted to fetal rhesus lung diploid cells and adjuvanted with alum. The two vaccines are considered equally efficacious and safe but are expensive because the viral yield from diploid cells is limited. Severe reactions to HDCV are uncommon. Immediate hypersensitivity responses such as urticaria have been reported in approximately 1 of every 650 recipients. Systemic reactions such as fever, headache, and nausea are generally mild and are reported in 1 to 4 percent of recipients. Local reactions such as swelling, erythema, and induration at the injection site occur in 15 to 20 percent of vaccinees.

In the developing world, several other effective rabies vaccines have been licensed and used extensively. They include vaccines made in chick embryonic cells, primary hamster cells, Vero cells, and duck embryonic cells. These preparations appear to be safe, immunogenic, and effective for postexposure prophylaxis.

Five 1-mL doses of HDCV are given intramuscularly, preferably in the deltoid or anterolateral thigh area; the first dose is administered as soon as possible after exposure and should be accompanied by an injection of HRIG into the gluteal and local wound areas. The five doses of HDCV should be administered within 28 days on the following schedule: days 0, 3, 7, 14, and 28. The World Health Organization also recommends 21- and 90-day courses.

The combination of HRIG and HDCV elicits high titers of neutralizing antibodies in almost all recipients. Only rarely has this regimen proved unsuccessful in preventing the development of rabies. Administration of vaccine alone appears to be associated with a higher failure rate than use of the combination, especially in severe bite exposures. Because of cost, postexposure prophylaxis consisting of intradermal injections of rabies vaccine is being used increasingly in the developing world. The combination of HRIG plus 0.1-mL intradermal doses of HDCV at eight sites on day 0, four sites on day 7, and one site on days 28 and 91 produces good antibody responses and

has had excellent clinical results. Alternatively, the World Health Organization has approved a regimen of two 0.1-mL doses at two intradermal sites on days 0, 3, and 7 and a 0.1-mL intradermal injection at a single site on days 21 and 90.

Preexposure Prophylaxis Individuals at high risk of contact with rabies virus, including veterinarians, cave explorers, laboratory workers, and animal handlers, should receive preexposure prophylaxis with rabies vaccine. HDCV is the preferred preparation for preexposure prophylaxis; three 1-mL intramuscular or three 0.1-mL intradermal injections on days 0, 7, and 21 or 28 should be administered. RVA should not be used intradermally. The neutralizing antibody titer should be checked after vaccination. Concomitant chloroquine administration interferes with the antibody response to rabies vaccine. Depending on the level of risk, serologic testing should be done at 2- to 6-year intervals. When neutralizing titers fall below 1:5, booster doses should be given. Booster doses may be administered as a single 1-mL intramuscular or 0.1-mL intradermal injection. Postexposure prophylaxis in individuals previously given preexposure prophylaxis consists of two intramuscular doses of HDCV on days 0 and 3. HRIG is not given in these situations.

Booster doses of HDCV are associated with fever, headache, muscle aches, and joint pains in about 20 percent of recipients. Up to 6 percent of persons receiving intramuscular booster doses of HDCV develop an immune complex–like reaction characterized by urticaria, arthritis, nausea, vomiting, and occasionally angioedema. These reactions are self-limited and appear to be associated with the presence of β-propiolactone-altered human serum albumin in the vaccine and the development of IgE antibodies to this antigen. Persons who work in high-risk areas should undergo periodic measurement of antibodies, and booster doses are recommended for those with low antibody titers. Those at very low risk may elect not to receive routine booster doses but rather to undergo active immunization should any substantive exposure take place.

MOKOLA VIRUS

Mokola virus was first isolated from wild shrews captured in Nigeria and was subsequently shown to be related morphologically and serologically to rabies virus. However, neither of the two reported cases of human disease (both in children) had the classic clinical features of rabies. One patient had a nonfatal illness characterized by fever, pharyngitis, and convulsions; Mokola virus was recovered from CSF. In the second patient, fever with cough and vomiting was followed within several days by drowsiness, confusion, and generalized flaccid weakness. The CSF was normal. The patient progressed to deep coma and died within 10 days of onset. Mokola virus was isolated from the brain, and examination of histopathologic sections revealed finely granular cytoplasmic inclusions that were distinguishable from Negri bodies in many neurons.

VESICULAR STOMATITIS VIRUS

Vesicular stomatitis is a viral illness of animals that occasionally affects humans. It presents as an acute, self-limited, influenza-like disease. The disease in animals is found in the United States and South America and affects chiefly domestic cattle, horses, swine, wild deer, raccoons, skunks, and bobcats.

In animals, vesicular stomatitis is characterized by the development of vesicles on the oral mucosa, particularly the tongue; the udders; and the heels. The mode of spread is probably by direct contact; however, epidemics tend to occur in warm weather, and isolation of the virus from *Phlebotomus* sandflies in Panama and *Aedes* species in New Mexico suggests that these insects may be vectors. Two distinct serotypes, New Jersey and Indiana, have been recognized, and most outbreaks in North America have been attributed to the New Jersey strain. Vesicular stomatitis is most common among laboratory workers.

In one report, three-fourths of laboratory personnel handling experimentally infected animals or manipulating the virus developed neutralizing antibodies. The disease is also transmissible, however, under natural conditions among workers having direct contact with infected animals, especially cattle. An incubation period ranging from 1 to 6 days is followed by the sudden onset of fever [with temperatures of up to 40°C (104°F)], chills, profuse sweating, myalgias, malaise, headache, and pain on ocular movement. One-third to one-half of patients have a sore throat and cervical and/or submandibular adenopathy. Small raised vesicular lesions may appear on the buccal mucosa. Conjunctivitis and coryza are evident in about 20 percent of cases. Occasionally, small subcorneal, intraepithelial vesicles appear on the fingers, usually in association with direct inoculation of the virus. Symptoms generally last 3 to 4 days, but occasionally the course is diphasic. Inapparent infection is common: among laboratory workers with serologic evidence of infection, only about one-half reported symptoms. In some areas of Panama, 17 to 35 percent of the population have neutralizing antibodies to vesicular stomatitis virus.

The differential diagnosis includes hand-foot-and-mouth disease, herpangina, primary herpetic pharyngitis and other mucocutaneous syndromes, and influenza. The virus is not commonly isolated from patients. However, a rise in titer of complement-fixation and/or neutralizing antibody to vesicular stomatitis virus between acute- and convalescent-phase sera helps to confirm the diagnosis. Treatment is nonspecific.

BIBLIOGRAPHY

FISHBEIN DB, ROBINSON LE: Current concepts. Rabies. N Engl J Med 329:1632, 1993
IMMUNIZATION PRACTICES ADVISORY COMMITTEE (ACIP): Rabies prevention, United States, 1991. Morb Mort Week Rep 40(RR-3): 1, 1991
JAVADI MA et al: Transmission of rabies by corneal graft. Cornea 15:431, 1996
LOPEZ RA et al: Outbreak of human rabies in the Peruvian jungle. Lancet 339:408, 1992
SACRAMENTO D et al: PCR technique as an alternative method for diagnosis and molecular epidemiology of rabies virus. Mol Cell Probes 5:229, 1991
SMITH JS: New aspects of rabies with emphasis on epidemiology, diagnosis, and prevention of the disease in the United States. Clin Microbiol Rev 9:166, 1996
WARRELL MJ: Human deaths from cryptic bat rabies in the USA. Lancet 346:65, 1993
WHO EXPERT COMMITTEE: *Report on Rabies*, technical report series no. 824. Geneva, World Health Organization, 1992
WILDE H et al: Rabies in Thailand 1990. Rev Infect Dis 17:644, 1991
——— et al: Heterologous antisera and antivenins are essential biologicals: Perspectives on a worldwide crisis. Ann Intern Med 125:233, 1996

200 *C. J. Peters*

INFECTIONS CAUSED BY ARTHROPOD- AND RODENT-BORNE VIRUSES

Most viral infections that come to medical attention in office or hospital practice in the developed countries are caused by viruses that can be latent in the human host, such as the herpesviruses, or by viruses that are continuously transmitted among humans, such as measles virus, influenza virus, and human immunodeficiency virus. However, some other viruses are transmitted in nature without regard to humans and only incidentally infect and produce disease in humans; in addition, a few agents are regularly spread among humans by arthropods. Most of these viruses either are maintained by arthropods or chronically infect rodents. Obviously, the mode of transmission is not a rational basis for taxonomic classification. Indeed, zoonotic viruses from at least seven virus families act as significant human pathogens (Table

200-1). The virus families differ fundamentally from one another in terms of morphology, replication mechanisms, and genetics. Information on a virus's membership in a family or genus is enlightening with regard to maintenance strategies, sensitivity to antivirals, and some aspects of pathogenesis but does not necessarily predict which clinical syndromes—if any—the virus will cause in humans.

FAMILIES OF ARTHROPOD- AND RODENT-BORNE VIRUSES   The Arenaviridae   The Arenaviridae are spherical, 110- to 130-nm particles that bud from the cell's plasma membrane and utilize ambisense RNA genomes with two segments for replication. There are two main phylogenetic branches of Arenaviridae: the old world viruses, such as Lassa fever and lymphocytic choriomeningitis viruses, and the new world viruses, including those causing the South American hemorrhagic fevers (HFs). Arenaviruses persist in nature by chronically infecting rodents with a striking one-virus–one-rodent species relationship. These rodent infections result in long-term virus excretion and perhaps in lifelong viremia; vertical infection is common with some arenaviruses. Humans become infected through the inhalation of aerosols containing arenaviruses, which are then deposited in the terminal air passages, and probably also through close contact with rodents and their excreta, which results in the contamination of mucous membranes or breaks in the skin.

The Bunyaviridae   The family Bunyaviridae includes four medically significant genera. All of these spherical viruses have three negative-sense RNA segments maturing into 90- to 120-nm particles in the Golgi complex and exiting the cell by exocytosis. Viruses of the genus *Bunyavirus* are largely mosquito borne and have a viremic vertebrate intermediate host; many are also transovarially transmitted in their specific mosquito host. One serologic group also uses biting midges as vectors. Sandflies or mosquitoes are the vectors for the genus *Phlebovirus* (named after phlebotomus fever or sandfly fever, the best-known disease associated with the genus), while ticks serve as vectors for the genus *Nairovirus*. Viruses of both of these genera are also associated with vertical transmission in the arthropod host and with horizontal spread through viremic vertebrate hosts. The genus *Hantavirus* is unique among the Bunyaviridae in that it is not transmitted by arthropods but is maintained in nature by rodent hosts that chronically shed virus. Like the arenaviruses, the hantaviruses usually display striking virus-rodent species specificity. As far as is known, however, the hantaviruses do not cause chronic viremia in their rodent host and are transmitted only horizontally from rodent to rodent.

Other Families   The Flaviviridae are positive-sense, single-stranded RNA viruses that form particles of 40 to 50 nm in the endoplasmic reticulum. The flaviviruses discussed here are from the genus *Flavivirus* and make up two phylogenetically and antigenically distinct divisions transmitted among vertebrates by mosquitoes and ticks, respectively. The mosquito-borne viruses fall into phylogenetic groups that include yellow fever viruses, the four dengue viruses, and the encephalitis viruses, while the tick-borne group encompasses a geographically varied spectrum of species, some of which are responsible for encephalitis or for hemorrhagic disease with encephalitis. The Reoviridae are double-stranded RNA viruses with multisegmented genomes. These 80-nm particles are the only viruses discussed in this chapter that do not have a lipid envelope and thus are insensitive to detergents. The Togaviridae have a single positive strand RNA genome and bud particles of approximately 60 to 70 nm from the plasma membrane. The togaviruses discussed here are all members of the genus *Alphavirus* and are transmitted among vertebrates by mosquitoes in their natural cycle. Alphaviruses are divided phylogenetically into two groups: one seems to have developed in the new world, and the other is associated primarily with the old world. → *The Filoviridae and the Rhabdoviridae are discussed in Chaps. 201 and 199, respectively.*

PROMINENT FEATURES OF ARTHROPOD- AND RODENT-BORNE VIRUSES   Although this chapter discusses the major features of selected arthropod- and rodent-borne viruses, it does not deal with more than 500 other distinct recognized zoonotic viruses, about one-fourth of which infect humans. Zoonotic viruses are undergoing genetic evolution, "new" zoonotic viruses are being discovered, and the epidemiology of zoonotic viruses is continuing to evolve through environmental changes affecting vectors, reservoirs, and humans. These zoonotic viruses are most numerous in the tropics but are also found in temperate and frigid climates. Their distribution and seasonal activity may be variable and often depend largely on ecologic conditions such as rainfall and temperature, which in turn affect the density of vectors and reservoirs and the development of infection therein.

Maintenance and Transmission Arthropod-borne viruses infect their vectors after the ingestion of a blood meal from a viremic vertebrate. The vectors then develop chronic, systemic infection as the viruses penetrate the gut and spread throughout the body. The viruses eventually reach the salivary glands during a period that is referred to as *extrinsic incubation* and that typically lasts 1 to 3 weeks in mosquitoes. At this point an arthropod is competent to continue the chain of transmission by infecting another vertebrate when a subsequent blood meal is taken. The arthropod generally is unharmed by the infection, and the natural vertebrate partner usually has only transient viremia with no overt disease. An alternative mechanism for virus maintenance in its arthropod host is transovarial transmission, which is most common among members of the family Bunyaviridae.

Rodent-borne viruses such as the hantaviruses and arenaviruses are maintained in nature by chronic infection transmitted between rodents. As in arthropod-borne virus cycles, there is usually a high degree of rodent-virus specificity, and there is no overt disease in the reservoir/vector.

Epidemiology The distribution of arthropod- and rodent-borne viruses is restricted by the areas inhabited by their reservoir/vectors and provides an important clue in the differential diagnosis. Table 200-2 shows the approximate geographic distribution of the most important of these viruses. Members of each family, each genus, and even each serologically related group usually occur in each area but may not be pathogenic in all areas or may not be a commonly recognized cause of disease in all areas and so may not be included in the table. Although there is generally no overt disease in the vertebrate reservoirs, disease in nonhuman target species may be a useful diagnostic clue, and serologic testing of selected animals may be a useful way to monitor virus circulation.

Most of these diseases are acquired in a rural setting; a few have urban vectors. Seoul, sandfly fever, and Oropouche viruses are examples of urban viruses, but the most notable are yellow fever, dengue, and chikungunya viruses, which are transmitted between humans with the mosquito *Aedes aegypti* as a principal or alternate vector. A history of mosquito bite has little diagnostic significance in the individual; a

Table 200-1

Major Zoonotic Virus Families and Some Characteristics of Typical Members

Family	Genus or Group	Syndrome(s): Typical Viruses	Maintenance Strategy
Arenaviridae	Old world complex	FM, E: Lymphocytic choriomeningitis virus HF: Lassa fever virus	Chronic infection of rodents, often with persistent viremia; vertical transmission common
	New world or Tacaribe complex	HF: South American HF viruses (Machupo, Junin, Guanarito, Sabia)	Chronic infection of rodents, sometimes with persistent viremia; vertical infection may occur
Bunyaviridae	*Bunyavirus*	E: California serogroup viruses (La Crosse, Jamestown Canyon, California encephalitis)	Mosquito-vertebrate cycle; transovarial transmission in mosquito common
		FM: Bunyamwera, group C, Tahyna viruses	
		FM: Oropouche virus	Transmitted by *Culicoides*
	Phlebovirus	FM: Sandfly fever, Toscana viruses FM: Punta Toro virus	Sandfly transmission between vertebrates, with prominent transovarial component in sandfly
		HF, FM, E: Rift Valley fever virus	Mosquito-vertebrate transmission, with transovarial component in mosquito
	Nairovirus	HF: Crimean Congo HF virus	Tick-vertebrate, with transovarial transmission in tick
	Hantavirus	HF: Hantaan, Dobrava, Puumala viruses	Rodent reservoir; chronic virus shedding, but chronic viremia unknown
		HF: Sin Nombre and related hantaviruses	Sigmodontine rodent reservoir
Filoviridae*		HF: Marburg virus, Ebola viruses (4 subtypes)	Unknown
Flaviviridae	*Flavivirus* (mosquito-borne)	HF: Yellow fever virus	Mosquito-vertebrate
		FM, HF: Dengue viruses (4 subtypes)	
		E: St. Louis, Japanese, West Nile, and Murray Valley encephalitis viruses; Rocio viruses	
	Flavivirus (tick-borne)	E: Central European tick-borne encephalitis, Russian spring-summer encephalitis, Powassan viruses	Tick-vertebrate
		HF: Omsk HF, Kyasanur Forest disease viruses	
Reoviridae	*Coltivirus*	FM, E: Colorado tick fever virus	Tick-vertebrate
	Orbivirus	FM, E: Orungo, Kemerova viruses	Arthropod-vertebrate
Rhabdoviridae†	*Vesiculovirus*	FM: Vesicular stomatitis virus (Indiana, New Jersey); Chandipura, Piry viruses	Sandfly-vertebrate, with prominent transovarial component in sandfly
Togaviridae	*Alphavirus*	AR: Sindbis, chikungunya, Mayaro, Ross River, Barmah Forest viruses	Mosquito-vertebrate
		E: Eastern, western, and Venezuelan equine encephalitis viruses	

* The Filoviridae are discussed in Chap. 201.
† The Rhabdoviridae are discussed in Chap. 199.

NOTE: Abbreviations refer to the disease syndrome most commonly associated with the virus: FM, fever and myalgia; AR, arthritis and rash; E, encephalitis; HF, hemorrhagic fever.

history of tick-bite is more diagnostically specific. Rodent exposure is often reported by persons infected with an arenavirus or a hantavirus but again has little specificity. Indeed, aerosols may infect persons who have no recollection of having even seen rodents.

Syndromes Human disease caused by arthropod- and rodent-borne viruses is often subclinical. The spectrum of possible responses to infection is wide, and our knowledge of the outcome of most of these infections is limited. The usual disease syndromes associated with these viruses have been grouped into four categories: fever and myalgia, arthritis and rash, encephalitis, and hemorrhagic fever. Although for the purposes of this discussion most viruses have been placed in a single group, the categories often overlap. For example, West Nile and Venezuelan equine encephalitis viruses are discussed as encephalitis viruses, but during epidemics they may cause many cases of milder syndromes and relatively uncommon cases of encephalitis. Similarly, Rift Valley fever virus is best known as a cause of HF, but the attack rates for febrile disease are far higher, and encephalitis is occasionally seen as well. Lymphocytic choriomeningitis (LCM) virus is classified as a cause of fever and myalgia because this syndrome is its most common disease manifestation and, even when central nervous system (CNS) disease occurs, it is usually preceded by fever and myalgia. Dengue virus infection is considered as a cause of fever and myalgia (dengue fever) because this is by far the most common manifestation worldwide and is the syndrome most likely to be seen in the United States; however, dengue HF is also discussed in the HF section because of its complicated pathogenesis and importance in pediatric practice in certain areas of the world.

Diagnosis Laboratory diagnosis is required in any given case, although epidemics occasionally provide clinical and epidemiologic clues on which an educated guess as to etiology can be based. For most arthropod- and rodent-borne viruses, acute-phase serum samples (collected within 3 or 4 days of onset) have yielded isolates, and paired sera have been used to demonstrate rising antibody titers by a variety of tests. Intensive efforts to develop rapid tests for HF have resulted in an antigen-detection enzyme-linked immunosorbent assay (ELISA) and an IgM-capture ELISA that can provide a diagnosis based on a single serum sample within a few hours and are particularly useful in severe cases. More sensitive reverse transcription polymerase chain reaction (RT-PCR) tests may yield diagnoses based on samples without detectable antigen and may also provide useful genetic information about the virus. Preliminary data suggest that similar tests applied to some fever-myalgia syndromes would give positive results if developed further. Hantavirus infections differ from others discussed here in that severe acute disease is immunopathologic; patients present with serum IgM that serves as the basis for a sensitive and specific test. Every ELISA must include a control incorporating a negative antigen with each serum sample tested; the frequent failure to include such a control has resulted in numerous false-positive results in diagnostic tests.

At the time of diagnosis, patients with encephalitis generally are no longer viremic or antigenemic and usually do not have virus in cerebrospinal fluid (CSF). In this situation, the value of serologic methods is being validated. IgM capture is increasingly being used for the testing of serum and CSF. IgG ELISA or classic serology is useful in the evaluation of past exposure to the viruses, many of which circulate in areas with a minimal medical infrastructure and sometimes cause mild or subclinical infection.

The remainder of this chapter offers general descriptions of the broad syndromes caused by arthropod- and rodent-borne viruses and then addresses specific differences between diseases. It is important to remember that most of the diseases under consideration have not been studied in detail with modern medical approaches and thus available data may be incomplete or biased.

FEVER AND MYALGIA

Fever and myalgia constitute the syndrome most commonly associated with zoonotic virus infection. Many of the numerous viruses belonging to the families listed in Table 200-1 probably cause this syndrome, but several viruses have been selected for inclusion in the table because of their prominent associations with the syndrome and their biomedical importance.

The syndrome typically begins with the abrupt onset of fever, chills, intense myalgia, and malaise. Patients may also report joint

Table 200-2

Geographic Distribution of Some Important and Commonly Encountered Human Zoonotic Viral Diseases

Area	Arenaviridae	Bunyaviridae	Flaviviridae	Rhabdoviridae	Togaviridae
North America	Lymphocytic choriomeningitis	La Crosse, Jamestown Canyon, California encephalitis; hantavirus (pulmonary syndrome)	St. Louis, Powassan encephalitis; dengue	Vesicular stomatitis	Eastern, western equine encephalitis
South America	Bolivian, Argentine, Venezuelan, and Brazilian HF; lymphocytic choriomeningitis	Oropouche, group C, Punta Toro infection; hantavirus pulmonary syndrome	Yellow fever, dengue, Rocio virus infection	Vesicular stomatitis, Piry virus infection	Mayaro virus infection, Venezuelan equine encephalitis
Europe	Lymphocytic choriomeningitis	Tahyna, Toscana, sandfly fever, HF with renal syndrome	West Nile, Central European tick-borne, Russian spring-summer encephalitis	—	Sindbis virus infection
Middle East	—	Sandfly fever, Crimean Congo HF	West Nile encephalitis, dengue	—	—
Eastern Asia	—	Sandfly fever; Hantaan, Seoul virus infection	Dengue; Japanese, Russian spring-summer encephalitis; Omsk HF	Chandipura virus infection	—
Southwestern Asia	—	Sandfly fever, Crimean Congo HF	West Nile, Japanese encephalitis; dengue; Kyasanur Forest disease	—	Chikungunya
Southeast Asia	—	Seoul virus infection	Japanese encephalitis, dengue	—	Chikungunya
Africa	Lassa fever	Bunyamwera virus infection, Rift Valley fever	Yellow fever, dengue	—	Sindbis virus infection, chikungunya
Australia	—	—	Murray Valley encephalitis, dengue	—	Ross River, Barmah Forest virus infection

NOTE: HF, hemorrhagic fever.

pains, but no true arthritis is detectable. Anorexia is characteristic and may be accompanied by nausea or even vomiting. Headache is common and may be severe, with photophobia and retroorbital pain. Physical findings are minimal and usually are confined to conjunctival injection with pain on palpation of muscles or the epigastrium. The duration of symptoms is quite variable but generally is 2 to 5 days, with a biphasic course in some instances. The spectrum of disease varies from subclinical to temporarily incapacitating.

Less constant findings include a maculopapular rash. Epistaxis may occur but does not necessarily indicate a bleeding diathesis. A minority of the cases caused by some viruses are known or suspected to include aseptic meningitis, but this diagnosis is difficult in remote areas, given the patients' photophobia and myalgia as well as the lack of opportunity to examine the CSF. Although pharyngitis may be noted or radiographic evidence of pulmonary infiltrates found in some cases, these viruses are not primary respiratory pathogens. The differential diagnosis includes anicteric leptospirosis, rickettsial diseases, and the early stages of other syndromes discussed in this chapter. These diseases are often described as "flulike," but the usual absence of cough and coryza makes influenza an unlikely confounder except at the earliest stages.

Complete recovery is generally the outcome in this syndrome, although prolonged asthenia and nonspecific symptoms have been described in some cases, particularly after infection with LCM or dengue virus. Treatment is supportive, with aspirin avoided because of the potential for exacerbated bleeding and Reye's syndrome. Efforts at prevention are best based on vector control, which, however, may be expensive or impossible. For mosquito control, destruction of breeding sites is generally the most economically and environmentally sound approach; spraying to kill adult mosquitoes and thus to reduce their numbers transiently may have a preventive role in selected settings but has not been notably effective in the past. Measures taken by the individual to avoid the vector can be valuable. Avoiding the vector's habitat and times of peak activity, preventing the vector from entering dwellings by using screens or other barriers, judiciously applying arthropod repellents such as diethyltoluamide (DEET) to the skin, and wearing permethrin-impregnated clothing are all possible approaches, depending on the vector and its habits.

LYMPHOCYTIC CHORIOMENINGITIS LCM is transmitted from the common house mouse (*Mus musculus*) to humans by aerosols of excreta and secreta. LCM virus, an arenavirus, is maintained in the mouse mainly by vertical transmission from infected dams. The vertically infected mouse remains viremic for life, with high concentrations of virus in all tissues. Infected colonies of pet hamsters have also served as a link to humans. LCM virus is widely used in immunology laboratories as a model of T cell function and can silently infect cell cultures and passaged tumor lines, resulting in infections among scientists and animal caretakers. Patients with LCM may have a history of residence in rodent-infested housing or other exposure to rodents. An antibody prevalence of about 5 to 10 percent has been reported in the United States, Argentina, and endemic areas of Germany.

LCM differs from the general syndrome of fever and myalgia in that its onset is gradual. Among the conditions occasionally associated with LCM are orchitis, transient alopecia, arthritis, pharyngitis, cough, and maculopapular rash. An estimated one-fourth of patients or fewer suffer a febrile phase of 3 to 6 days and then, after a brief remission, develop renewed fever accompanied by severe headache, nausea and vomiting, and meningeal signs lasting for about a week. These patients virtually always recover fully, as do the uncommon patients with clear-cut signs of encephalitis. Recovery may be delayed by transient hydrocephalus.

During the initial febrile phase, leukopenia and thrombocytopenia are common and virus can usually be isolated from blood. During the CNS phase of the illness, virus may be found in the CSF, but antibodies are present in blood. The pathogenesis of LCM is thought to resemble that following direct intracranial inoculation of the virus into adult mice; the onset of the immune response leads to T cell–mediated immunopathologic meningitis. During the meningeal phase, CSF

mononuclear-cell counts range from the hundreds to the low thousands per microliter, and hypoglycorrhachia is found in one-third of cases. The IgM-capture ELISA of serum and CSF is usually positive; recently, RT-PCR assays have been developed for application to CSF.

Infection with LCM virus should be suspected in acutely ill febrile patients with marked leukopenia and thrombocytopenia. In cases of aseptic meningitis, the well-marked febrile prodrome, adult age, autumn seasonality, low CSF glucose levels, or mononuclear cell counts exceeding 1000/μL all should raise a suspicion of this viral infection.

In pregnant women, LCM virus infection may lead to fetal invasion with consequent congenital hydrocephalus and chorioretinitis. Since the maternal infection may be mild, consisting of only a short febrile illness, antibodies to the virus should be sought in both the mother and the fetus in suspicious circumstances.

BUNYAMWERA VIRUS INFECTION The mosquito-transmitted Bunyamwera serogroup viruses are found on every continent except Australia and Antarctica. Bunyamwera virus and its close relative Ilesha virus commonly cause febrile disease in Africa. Other related viruses are implicated in such disease in Southeast Asia (Batai virus), Europe (Calovo virus), and South America (Wyeomyia virus). In North America, Cache Valley virus has been implicated in febrile human disease and in rare instances of more serious systemic illness; the presence of serum antibodies to this virus may be associated with congenital malformations. In Central America, the closely related Fort Sherman virus causes the fever-myalgia syndrome.

GROUP C VIRUS INFECTION The group C viruses include at least 11 agents transmitted by mosquitoes in neotropical forests. These agents are among the most common causes of arboviral infection in humans entering American jungles and cause acute febrile disease.

TAHYNA VIRUS INFECTION This California-serogroup virus (see discussion of California encephalitis below) occurs in central and western Europe, and related viruses are emerging in Russia. The significance of Tahyna virus in human health has been well studied only in the Czech and Slovak Republics; there, the virus was found to be a prominent cause of febrile disease, in some cases causing pharyngitis, pulmonary syndromes, and aseptic meningitis. The potential for arboviruses to be unexpectedly involved in such cases in areas of high mosquito prevalence needs to be kept in mind.

OROPOUCHE FEVER Oropouche virus is transmitted in Central and South America by a biting midge, *Culicoides paraensis*, which often breeds to high density in cacao husks and other vegetable detritus found in towns and cities. Explosive epidemics involving thousands of cases have been reported from several towns in Brazil and Peru. Rash and aseptic meningitis have been detected in a number of cases.

SANDFLY FEVER The sandfly *Phlebotomus papatasi* transmits sandfly fever. Female sandflies may be infected by the oral route as they take a blood meal and may transmit the virus to offspring when they lay their eggs after a second blood meal. This prominent transovarial pattern was the first to be recognized among dipterans and complicates virus control. The former designation for sandfly fever, "3-day fever," instructively describes the brief, debilitating course associated with this essentially benign infection. There is neither a rash nor CNS involvement, and complete recovery is the rule.

Sandfly fever is found in the circum-Mediterranean area, extending to the east through the Balkans into China as well as into the Middle East and southwestern Asia. The vector is found in both rural and urban settings and is known for its small size, which enables it to penetrate standard mosquito screens and netting, and for its short flight range. Epidemics have been described in the wake of natural disasters and wars. In parts of Europe, sandfly populations and virus transmission were greatly reduced by the extensive residual spraying conducted after World War II to control malaria, and the prevalence continues to decline. A common pattern of disease in endemic areas consists of high attack rates among travelers and military personnel with little or no disease in the local population, who are protected after childhood infection. In addition to the two well-characterized, non-cross-protective Sicilian and Naples virus species, more than 30 related phleboviruses are transmitted by sandflies and mosquitoes, but most are of unknown significance in terms of human health.

TOSCANA VIRUS DISEASE Toscana virus is a *Phlebovirus* (family Bunyaviridae) transmitted primarily by the circum-Mediterranean sandfly *Phlebotomus perniciosus*. The vertebrate amplifying host, if one exists, is unknown. Toscana virus infection is common during the summer among rural residents and vacationers; a number of cases have been identified in travelers returning to Germany and Scandinavia. The disease may manifest as an uncomplicated febrile illness but is often associated with aseptic meningitis, with virus isolated from the CSF.

PUNTA TORO VIRUS DISEASE Of the several phleboviruses that are associated with new world sandflies and infect humans, Punta Toro virus is the best known. The disease caused by this virus is clinically similar to but epidemiologically different from that caused by the Naples or Sicilian sandfly fever viruses. Punta Toro virus infections are sporadic and are acquired in the tropical forest, where the vectors rest on tree buttresses. Epidemics have not been reported, but antibody prevalences among inhabitants of villages in the endemic areas indicate a cumulative lifetime exposure rate of more than 50 percent.

DENGUE FEVER All four distinct dengue viruses (dengue 1–4) have *A. aegypti* as their principal vector, and all cause a similar clinical syndrome. In rare cases, second infection with a serotype of dengue virus different from that involved in the primary infection leads to dengue HF with severe shock (see below). Sporadic cases are seen in the settings of endemic transmission and epidemic disease. Year-round transmission between latitudes 25°N and 25°S has been established, and seasonal forays of the viruses to points as far north as Philadelphia are thought to have taken place in the United States. With increasing spread of the vector mosquito throughout the tropics and subtropics, large areas of the world have become vulnerable to the introduction of dengue viruses, particularly through air travel by infected humans, and both dengue fever and the related dengue HF are becoming increasingly common. Conditions favorable to dengue transmission exist in the southern United States, and bursts of dengue fever activity are to be expected in this region, particularly along the Mexican border, where water may be stored in containers and *A. aegypti* numbers may therefore be greatest: this mosquito, which also is an efficient vector of the yellow fever and chikungunya viruses, typically breeds near human habitation, using relatively fresh water from sources such as water jars, vases, discarded containers, coconut husks, and old tires. *A. aegypti* usually inhabits dwellings and bites during the day.

After an incubation period of 2 to 7 days, the typical patient experiences the sudden onset of fever, headache, retroorbital pain, and back pain along with the severe myalgia that gave rise to the colloquial designation "break-bone fever." There is often a macular rash on the first day as well as adenopathy, palatal vesicles, and scleral injection. The illness may last a week, with additional symptoms usually including anorexia, nausea or vomiting, marked cutaneous hypersensitivity, and—near the time of defervescence—a maculopapular rash beginning on the trunk and spreading to the extremities and the face. Epistaxis and scattered petechiae are often noted in uncomplicated dengue, and preexisting gastrointestinal lesions may bleed during the acute illness.

Laboratory findings include leukopenia, thrombocytopenia, and, in many cases, serum aminotransferase elevations. The diagnosis is made by IgM ELISA or paired serology during recovery or by antigen-detection ELISA or RT-PCR during the acute phase. Virus is readily isolated from blood in the acute phase if mosquito inoculation or mosquito cell culture is used.

COLORADO TICK FEVER Several hundred cases of Colorado tick fever are reported annually in the United States. The infection is acquired between March and November through the bite of an infected *Dermacentor andersoni* tick in mountainous western regions at altitudes of 1200 to 3000 m (4000 to 10,000 ft). Small mammals serve as the amplifying host. The most common presentation consists of fever and myalgia; meningoencephalitis is not uncommon, and hemorrhagic disease, pericarditis, myocarditis, orchitis, and pulmonary presentations are also reported. Rash develops in a substantial minority of cases. The disease usually lasts 7 to 10 days and is often biphasic. The most important differential diagnostic considerations since the turn of the century have been Rocky Mountain spotted fever and tularemia.

Infection of erythroblasts and other marrow cells by Colorado tick fever virus results in the appearance and persistence (for several weeks) of erythrocytes containing the virus. This feature, detected in smears stained by immunofluorescence, can be diagnostically helpful. The clinical laboratory detects leukopenia and thrombocytopenia.

ORBIVIRUS INFECTION The orbiviruses encompass many human and veterinary pathogens. For example, Orungo virus is widely transmitted by mosquitoes in tropical Africa and causes febrile disease in humans. The Kemerova complex includes the Kemerova, Lipovnik, and Tribec viruses of Russia and central Europe; these viruses are transmitted by ticks and are associated with febrile and neurologic disease.

VESICULAR STOMATITIS See Chap. 199.

ENCEPHALITIS

Arboviral encephalitis is a seasonal disease, commonly occurring in the warmer months. Its incidence varies markedly with time and place, depending on ecologic factors. The causative viruses differ markedly in terms of case-infection ratio (i.e., the ratio of clinical to subclinical infection), mortality, and residua (Table 200-3). Humans are not an important amplifier of these viruses.

All the viral encephalitides discussed in this section have a similar pathogenesis as far as is known. An infected arthropod ingests a blood meal from a human and infects the host. The initial period of viremia is thought to originate most commonly from the lymphoid system. Viremia leads to CNS invasion, presumably through infection of olfactory neuroepithelium with passage through the cribriform plate or through infection of brain capillaries and multifocal entry into the CNS. During the viremic phase, there may be little or no recognized disease except in the case of tick-borne flaviviral encephalitis, in which there may be a clearly delineated phase of fever and systemic illness. The disease process in the CNS arises partly from direct neuronal infection and subsequent damage and partly from edema, inflammation, and other indirect effects. The usual pathologic picture is one of focal necrosis of neurons, inflammatory glial nodules, and perivascular lymphoid cuffing; the severity and distribution of these abnormalities vary with the infecting virus. Involved areas display the "luxury perfusion" phenomenon, with normal or increased total blood flow and low oxygen extraction.

The typical patient presents with a prodrome of nonspecific constitutional symptoms, including fever, abdominal pain, vertigo, sore throat, and respiratory symptoms. Headache, meningeal signs, photophobia, and vomiting follow quickly. Involvement of deeper structures may be signaled by lethargy, somnolence, and intellectual deficit (as disclosed by the mental status examination or failure at serial 7 subtraction); more severely affected patients will be obviously disoriented and may be comatose. Tremors, loss of abdominal reflexes, cranial nerve palsies, hemiparesis, monoparesis, difficulty in swallowing, and frontal lobe signs are all common. Convulsions and focal signs may be evident early or may appear during the course of the disease. Some patients present with an abrupt onset of fever, convulsions, and other signs of CNS involvement. The results of human infection range from no significant symptoms through febrile headache to aseptic meningitis and finally to full-blown encephalitis; the proportions and severity of these manifestations vary with the infecting virus.

The acute encephalitis usually lasts from a few days to as long as 2 to 3 weeks, but recovery may be slow, with weeks or months required for the return of maximal recoupable function. Common complaints during recovery include difficulty concentrating, fatigability, tremors, and personality changes. The acute illness requires management of a comatose patient who may have intracranial pressure elevations, inappropriate secretion of antidiuretic hormone, respiratory failure, and convulsions. There is no specific therapy for these viral encephalitides. The only practical preventive measures are vector management and personal protection against the arthropod transmitting the virus; for Japanese encephalitis or tick-borne encephalitis, vaccination should be considered in certain circumstances (see relevant sections below).

The diagnosis of arboviral encephalitis depends on the careful evaluation of a febrile patient with CNS disease, with rapid identification of treatable herpes simplex encephalitis, ruling out of brain abscess, exclusion of bacterial meningitis by serial CSF examination, and performance of laboratory studies to define the viral etiology. Leptospirosis and neurosyphilis should also be considered. The CSF examination usually shows a modest cell count—in the tens or hundreds or perhaps a few thousand. Early in the process, a significant proportion of these cells may be polymorphonuclear leukocytes, but usually there is a mononuclear cell predominance. CSF glucose levels are usually normal. There are exceptions to this pattern of findings. In eastern equine encephalitis, for example, polymorphonuclear leukocytes may predominate during the first 72 h of disease and hypoglycorrhachia may be detected. In LCM, lymphocyte counts may be in the thousands, and the glucose concentration may be diminished. Experience with imaging studies is still evolving; clearly, however,

both computed tomography (CT) and magnetic resonance imaging (MRI) may be normal except for evidence of preexisting conditions or sometimes may suggest diffuse edema. Several patients with eastern equine encephalitis have had focal abnormalities, and individuals with severe Japanese encephalitis have presented with bilateral thalamic lesions that have often been hemorrhagic. Electroencephalography usually shows diffuse abnormalities and is not directly helpful.

A humoral immune response is usually detectable at or near the onset of disease. Both serum and CSF should be examined for IgM antibodies. Virus generally cannot be isolated from blood or CSF, although Japanese encephalitis virus has been recovered from CSF in severe cases. Virus can be obtained from and viral antigen is present in brain tissue, although its distribution may be focal.

CALIFORNIA, LA CROSSE, AND JAMESTOWN CANYON VIRUS ENCEPHALITIS The isolation of California encephalitis virus established the California serogroup of viruses as a cause of encephalitis, and its use as a diagnostic antigen led to the description of many cases of "California encephalitis." In fact, however, this virus has been implicated in only a few cases of encephalitis, and the serologically related La Crosse virus is the major cause of encephalitis among viruses in the California serogroup. "California encephalitis"

Table 200-3

Prominent Features of Arboviral Encephalitis

Virus	Natural Cycle	Incubation Period, Days	Annual No. of Cases	Case-to-Infection Ratio	Age of Cases	Case-Mortality Rate, %	Residua
La Crosse	*Aedes triseriatus–*chipmunk (transovarial component in mosquito also important)	~3–7	70 (U.S.)	<1:1000	<15 years	<0.5	Recurrent seizures in ~10%; severe deficits in rare cases; decreased school performance and behavioral change suspected in small proportion
St. Louis	*Culex tarsalis, Culex pipiens, Culex quinquefasciatus–*birds	4–21	85 (hundreds to thousands in epidemic years) (U.S.)	<1:200	Milder cases in the young; more severe cases in adults >40 years old, particularly the elderly	7	Common in the elderly
Japanese	*Culex tritaeniorhyncus–*birds	5–15	>25,000	1:200–300	All ages; children in highly endemic areas	20–50	Common (approximately half of cases); may be severe
West Nile	*Culex* mosquitoes–birds	3–6	?	Very low	Mainly the elderly and children	—	Uncommon
Central European	*Ixodes ricinus–*rodents, insectivores	7–14	Thousands	1:12	All ages; milder in children	1–5	20%
Russian spring-summer	*Ixodes persulcatus–*rodents, insectivores	7–14	Hundreds	—	All ages; milder in children	20	Approximately half of cases; often severe; limb-girdle paralysis
Powassan	*Ixodes cookei–*wild mammals	~10	~1 (U.S.)	—	All ages; some predilection for children	~10	Common (approximately half of cases)
Eastern equine	*Culiseta melanura–*birds	~5–10	5 (U.S.)	1:40 adult 1:17 child	All ages; predilection for children	50–75	Common
Western equine	*Culex tarsalis–*birds	~5–10	~20 (U.S.)	1:1000 adult 1:50 child 1:1 infant	All ages; predilection for children <2 years old (increased mortality in elderly)	3–7	Common only among infants < 1 year old
Venezuelan equine (epidemic)	Unknown (multiple mosquito species and horses in epidemics)	1–5	?	1:250 adult 1:25 child (approximate)	All ages; predilection for children	~10	—

due to La Crosse virus infection is most commonly reported from the upper Midwest but is also found in other areas of the central and eastern United States, most often in West Virginia, North Carolina, and Georgia. The serogroup includes 13 other viruses, some of which may also be involved in human disease that is misattributed because of the complexity of the group's serology; these viruses include the Jamestown Canyon, snowshoe hare, Inkoo, and Trivittatus viruses, all of which have *Aedes* mosquitoes as their vector and all of which have a strong element of transovarial transmission in their natural cycles.

The mosquito vector of La Crosse virus is *Aedes triseriatus*. In addition to a prominent transovarial component of transmission, a mosquito can also become infected through feeding on viremic chipmunks and other mammals as well as through venereal transmission from another mosquito. The mosquito breeds in sites such as tree holes and abandoned tires and bites during daylight hours; these findings correlate with the risk factors for cases: recreation in forested areas, residence at the forest's edge, and the presence of abandoned tires around the home. Intensive environmental modification based on these findings has reduced the incidence of disease in a highly endemic area in the Midwest. Most cases occur from July through September. The recently introduced Asian tiger mosquito, *Aedes albopictus*, efficiently transmits the virus to mice and also transmits the agent transovarially in the laboratory; the possible impact of this aggressive anthropophilic mosquito, which has the capacity to urbanize, on transmission to humans is of concern.

An antibody prevalence of ≥20 percent in endemic areas indicates that infection is common, but CNS disease has been recognized primarily in children <15 years of age. The illness varies from a picture of aseptic meningitis accompanied by confusion to severe and occasionally fatal encephalitis. Although there may be prodromal symptoms, the onset of CNS disease is sudden, with fever, headache, and lethargy often joined by nausea and vomiting, convulsions (in one-half of patients), and coma (in one-third of patients). Focal seizures, hemiparesis, tremor, aphasia, chorea, Babinski's sign, and other evidence of significant neurologic dysfunction are common, but residua are not. Perhaps 10 percent of patients have recurrent seizures in the succeeding months. Other serious sequelae are rare, although a decrease in scholastic standing has been reported and mild personality change has occasionally been suggested. Treatment is supportive over a 1- to 2-week acute phase during which status epilepticus, cerebral edema, and inappropriate secretion of antidiuretic hormone are important concerns.

The blood leukocyte count is commonly elevated, sometimes reaching levels of >20,000/μL, and there is usually a left shift. CSF cell counts are typically 30 to 500/μL with a mononuclear cell predominance (although 25 to 90 percent of cells are polymorphonuclear in some cases). The protein level is normal or slightly increased, and the glucose level is normal. Specific virologic diagnosis based on IgM-capture assays of serum and CSF is efficient. The only human anatomic site from which virus has been isolated is the brain.

Jamestown Canyon virus has been implicated in several cases of encephalitis in adults; in these cases the disease was usually associated with a significant respiratory illness at onset. Human infection with this virus has been documented in New York, Wisconsin, Ohio, Michigan, Ontario, and other areas of North America where the vector mosquito, *Aedes stimulans*, feeds on its main host, the white-tailed deer.

ST. LOUIS ENCEPHALITIS   St. Louis encephalitis virus is transmitted between *Culex* mosquitoes and birds. This virus causes low-level endemic infection among rural residents of the western and central United States, where *Culex tarsalis* is the vector (see western equine encephalitis below), but the more urbanized mosquito species *Culex pipiens* and *Culex quinquefasciatus* have been responsible for epidemics resulting in hundreds or even thousands of cases in cities of the central and eastern United States. Most cases occur in June through October. The urban mosquitoes breed in accumulations of stagnant water and sewage with high organic content and readily bite humans in and around houses. The elimination of open sewers and

trash-filled drainage systems is expensive and may not be possible, but screening of houses and implementation of personal protective measures against the dusk-biting vectors may be an effective approach for individuals. The rural vector is most active at dusk and outdoors; its bites can be avoided by modification of activities and use of repellents.

Disease severity increases with age: infections that result in aseptic meningitis or mild encephalitis are concentrated in children and young adults, while severe and fatal cases primarily affect the elderly. Infection rates are similar in all age groups; thus the greater susceptibility of older persons to disease is a biologic consequence of aging. The disease has an abrupt onset, sometimes following a prodrome, and begins with fever, lethargy, confusion, and headache. In addition, nuchal rigidity, hypotonia, hyperreflexia, myoclonus, and tremor are common. Severe cases can include cranial nerve palsies, hemiparesis, and convulsions. Patients often complain of dysuria and may have viral antigen in urine as well as pyuria. The overall mortality is generally around 7 percent but may reach 20 percent among patients over the age of 60. Recovery is slow. Emotional lability, difficulties in concentration and memory, asthenia, and tremor are commonly prolonged in older patients.

The CSF of patients infected with St. Louis encephalitis virus usually contains tens to hundreds of cells, with a lymphocytic predominance and a normal glucose level. Leukocytosis with a left shift is often documented.

JAPANESE ENCEPHALITIS   Japanese encephalitis virus is found throughout Asia, including far eastern Russia, Japan, China, India, Pakistan, and Southeast Asia, and causes occasional epidemics on western Pacific islands. Recently, the virus has been detected in the Torres Strait islands near the Australian mainland. This flavivirus is particularly common in areas where irrigated rice fields attract the natural avian vertebrate hosts and provide abundant breeding sites for mosquitoes such as *Culex tritaeniorhyncus*, which transmit the virus to humans. Additional amplification by pigs, which suffer abortion, and horses, which develop encephalitis, may be significant as well. Vaccination of these additional amplifying hosts can reduce the transmission of the virus. An effective, formalin-inactivated vaccine purified from mouse brain is produced in Japan and licensed for human use in the United States. It is given on days 0, 7, and 30 or—with some sacrifice in serum neutralizing titer—on days 0, 7, and 14. Vaccination is indicated for summer travelers to rural Asia, where the risk of clinical disease may be 0.05 to 2.1/10,000 per week. The severe and often fatal disease reported in expatriates must be balanced against the 0.1 to 1 percent chance of a late systemic or cutaneous allergic reaction. These reactions are rarely fatal but may be severe and have been known to begin 1 to 9 days after vaccination, with associated pruritus, urticaria, and angioedema. Live attenuated vaccines are being used in China but are not recommended in the United States at this time.

WEST NILE VIRUS INFECTION   West Nile virus is transmitted among wild birds by *Culex* mosquitoes in Africa, the Middle East, southern Europe, and Asia. It is a frequent cause of febrile disease without CNS involvement, but it occasionally causes aseptic meningitis and severe encephalitis; these serious infections are particularly common among children and the elderly. In 1996, West Nile or a closely related virus caused more than 300 cases of CNS disease, with 10 percent mortality, in the Danube flood plains, including Bucharest. The febrile-myalgic syndrome caused by West Nile virus is distinguished from other such syndromes by the frequent appearance of a maculopapular rash concentrated on the trunk and lymphadenopathy. Headache, ocular pain, sore throat, nausea and vomiting, and arthralgia (but not arthritis) are common accompaniments. In addition, the virus has been implicated in severe and fatal hepatic necrosis in Central Africa.

West Nile virus falls into the same phylogenetic group of flaviviruses as St. Louis and Japanese encephalitis viruses, as do Murray Valley and Rocio viruses. The latter two viruses are both maintained in mosquitoes and birds and produce a clinical picture resembling that of Japanese encephalitis. Murray Valley virus has caused occasional epidemics and sporadic cases in Australia. Rocio virus caused recurrent epidemics in a focal area of Brazil in 1975 to 1977 and then virtually disappeared.

CENTRAL EUROPEAN TICK-BORNE ENCEPHALITIS AND RUSSIAN SPRING-SUMMER ENCEPHALITIS A spectrum of tick-borne flaviviruses has been identified across the Eurasian land mass. Many are known mainly as agricultural pathogens (e.g., louping ill virus in the United Kingdom). From Scandinavia to the Urals, central European tick-borne encephalitis is transmitted by *Ixodes ricinus*. Human cases occur between April and October, with a peak in June and July. A related and more virulent virus is that of Russian spring-summer encephalitis, which is associated with *Ixodes persulcatus* and is distributed from Europe across the Urals to the Pacific Ocean. The ticks transmit the disease primarily in the spring and early summer, with a lower rate of transmission later in summer. Small mammals are the vertebrate amplifiers for both viruses. The risk varies by geographic area and can be highly localized within a given area; human cases usually follow outdoor activities or consumption of raw milk from infected goats or other infected animals.

After an incubation period of 7 to 14 days or perhaps longer, the central European viruses classically result in a febrile-myalgic phase that lasts for 2 to 4 days and is thought to correlate with viremia. A subsequent remission for several days is followed by the recurrence of fever and the onset of meningeal signs. The CNS phase varies from mild aseptic meningitis, which is more common among younger patients, to severe encephalitis with coma, convulsions, tremors, and motor signs lasting for 7 to 10 days before improvement begins. Spinal and medullary involvement can lead to typical limb-girdle paralysis and to respiratory paralysis. Most patients recover, only a minority with significant deficits. Infections with the far eastern viruses generally run a more abrupt course. The encephalitic syndrome caused by these viruses sometimes begins without a remission and has more severe manifestations than the central European syndrome. Mortality is high, and major sequelae—most notably, lower motor neuron paralyses of the proximal muscles of the extremities, trunk, and neck—are common.

In the early stage of the illness, virus may be isolated from the blood. In the CNS phase, IgM antibodies are detectable in serum and/or CSF. Thrombocytopenia sometimes develops during the initial febrile illness, which resembles the early hemorrhagic phase of some other tick-borne flaviviral infections, such as Kyasanur Forest disease. Other tick-borne flaviviruses are less common causes of encephalitis, including louping ill virus in the United Kingdom and Powassan virus (see below).

There is no specific therapy for infection with these viruses. However, effective alum-adjuvanted, formalin-inactivated vaccines are produced in Austria, Germany, and Russia. Two doses of the Austrian vaccine separated by an interval of 1 to 3 months appear to be effective in the field, and antibody responses are similar when vaccine is given on days 0 and 14. Other vaccines have elicited similar neutralizing antibody titers. Since rare cases of postvaccination Guillain-Barré syndrome have been reported, vaccination should be reserved for persons likely to experience rural exposure in an endemic area during the season of transmission. Cross-neutralization for the central European and far eastern strains has been established, but there are no published field studies on cross-protection of formalin-inactivated vaccines. Because 0.2 to 4 percent of ticks in endemic areas may be infected, tick bites raise the issue of immunoglobulin prophylaxis. Prompt administration of high-titered specific preparations should probably be undertaken, although no controlled data are available to prove the efficacy of this measure. Immunoglobulin should not be administered late because of the risk of antibody-mediated enhancement.

POWASSAN ENCEPHALITIS Powassan virus is a member of the tick-borne encephalitis virus complex and is transmitted by *Ixodes cookei* among small mammals in eastern Canada and the United States, where it has been responsible for 20 recognized cases of human disease. Other ticks may transmit the virus in a wider geographic area, and there is some concern that *Ixodes dammini*, a competent vector in the laboratory, may become involved as it becomes more prominent in the United States. Patients with Powassan encephalitis—often children—present in May through December after outdoor exposure and an incubation period thought to be about 1 week. Powassan encephalitis is severe, and sequelae are common.

EASTERN EQUINE ENCEPHALITIS Eastern equine encephalitis is found primarily within endemic swampy foci along the eastern coast of the United States, with a few inland foci as far removed as Michigan. Human cases present from June through October, when the bird–*Culiseta* mosquito cycle spills over into other mosquito species such as *Aedes sollicitans*, or *Aedes vexans*, which are more likely to bite mammals. There is concern over the potential role of the introduced anthropophilic mosquito species *A. albopictus*, which has been found to be naturally infected and is an effective vector in the laboratory. Horses are a common target for the virus; if not vaccinated, they serve as a harbinger of human disease but probably do not play a significant role in amplification of the virus.

Eastern equine encephalitis is one of the most destructive of the arboviral conditions, with a brusque onset, rapid progression, high mortality, and frequent residua. This severity is reflected in the extensive necrotic lesions and polymorphonuclear infiltrates found at postmortem examination of the brain and the acute polymorphonuclear CSF pleocytosis often occurring during the first 1 to 3 days of disease. In addition, leukocytosis with a left shift is a common feature. A formalin-inactivated vaccine has been used to protect laboratory workers but is not generally available or applicable.

WESTERN EQUINE ENCEPHALITIS The primary maintenance cycle for western equine encephalitis virus in the United States is between *C. tarsalis* and birds, principally sparrows and finches. Equines and humans become infected, and both species suffer encephalitis without amplifying the virus in nature. St. Louis encephalitis is transmitted in a similar cycle in the same region but causes human disease about a month earlier than the period (July through October) in which western equine encephalitis virus is active. Large epidemics of western equine encephalitis took place in the western and central United States and Canada during the 1930s to 1950s, but in recent years the disease has been uncommon. There were 41 reported cases in the United States in 1987, but only 4 reported cases from 1988 to 1995. This decline in incidence may reflect in part the integrated approach to mosquito management that has been employed in irrigation projects and the increasing use of agricultural pesticides; it almost certainly reflects the increased tendency for humans to be indoors behind closed windows at dusk, the peak period of biting by the major vector.

Western equine encephalitis virus causes a typical diffuse viral encephalitis with an increased attack rate and increased morbidity in the young, particularly children under 2 years of age. In addition, mortality is high among the young and the very elderly. One-third of individuals who have convulsions during the acute illness have subsequent seizure activity. Infants under 1 year of age—particularly those in the first months of life—are at serious risk of motor and intellectual damage. Twice as many males as females develop clinical encephalitis after 5 to 9 years of age; this difference may be related to greater outdoor exposure of boys to the vector but is also likely to be due in part to biologic differences. A formalin-inactivated vaccine has been used to protect laboratory workers but is not generally available or applicable.

VENEZUELAN EQUINE ENCEPHALITIS There are six known types of virus in the Venezuelan equine encephalitis complex. An important distinction is between the "epizootic" viruses (subtypes IAB and IC) and the "enzootic" viruses (subtypes ID to IF and types II to VI). The epizootic viruses have an unknown natural cycle but periodically cause extensive epidemics in equines and humans in the Americas. These epidemics rely on the high-level viremia in horses and mules that results in the infection of several species of mosquitoes, which in turn infect humans and perpetuate virus transmission. Humans also have high-level viremia but probably are not important in virus transmission. Enzootic viruses are found primarily in humid tropical forest habitats and are maintained between *Culex* mosquitoes and rodents; these viruses cause human disease but are not pathogenic for horses and do not cause epizootics.

Epizootics of Venezuelan equine encephalitis occurred repeatedly in Venezuela, Colombia, Ecuador, Peru, and other South American countries at intervals of 10 years or less from the 1930s until 1969, when a massive epizootic spread throughout Central America and Mexico, reaching southern Texas in 1972. Genetic sequencing of the virus from the 1969 to 1972 outbreak suggested that it originated from residual "un-inactivated" virus in veterinary vaccines. The outbreak was terminated in Texas with the use of a live attenuated vaccine (TC-83) originally developed for human use by the U.S. Army; this virus was then used for further production of inactivated veterinary vaccines. No further epizootic disease was definitely identified until 1993 to 1995, when additional epizootics took place in Mexico, Colombia, and Venezuela. The viruses involved in these epizootics as well as previously epizootic subtype IC viruses have been shown to be close phylogenetic relatives of known enzootic subtype ID viruses. This finding suggests that active evolution and selection of epizootic viruses are under way in northern South America.

During epizootics, extensive human infection is the rule, with clinical disease in 10 to 60 percent of infected individuals. Most infections result in notable acute febrile disease, while relatively few result in encephalitis. A low rate of CNS invasion is supported by the absence of encephalitis among the many infections resulting from exposure to aerosols in the laboratory or from vaccine accidents. The most recent epizootic of Venezuelan equine encephalitis occurred in Colombia and Venezuela in 1995; of the more than 85,000 clinical cases, 4 percent (with a higher proportion among children than adults) included neurologic symptoms and 300 ended in death.

Enzootic strains of Venezuelan equine encephalitis virus are common causes of acute febrile disease, particularly in areas such as the Florida Everglades and the humid Atlantic coast of Central America. Encephalitis has been documented only in the Florida infections; the three cases were caused by type II enzootic virus, also called *Everglades virus*. All three patients had preexisting cerebral disease. Extrapolation from the rate of genetic change suggests that Everglades virus was introduced into Florida less than 200 years ago and that it is most closely related to the ID subtypes that appear to have given evolutionary rise to the epizootic strains active in South America.

The prevention of epizootic Venezuelan equine encephalitis depends on vaccination of horses with the attenuated TC-83 vaccine or with an inactivated vaccine prepared from that strain. Humans can be protected with similar vaccines, but the use of such products is restricted to laboratory personnel because of reactogenicity and limited availability. In addition, wild-type vaccine and perhaps TC-83 vaccine are thought to have some degree of fetal pathogenicity. Enzootic viruses are antigenically somewhat different from epizootic viruses, and protection against the former with vaccines prepared from the latter is relatively ineffective.

ARTHRITIS AND RASH

True arthritis is a common accompaniment of several viral diseases, such as rubella (caused by a non-alphavirus togavirus), parvovirus B19 infection, and hepatitis B; it is an occasional accompaniment of infection due to mumps virus, enteroviruses, herpesviruses, and adenoviruses. It is not generally appreciated that the alphaviruses are also common causes of arthritis. In fact, the alphaviruses discussed below all cause acute febrile diseases accompanied by the development of true arthritis and a maculopapular rash. Rheumatic involvement includes arthralgia alone, periarticular swelling, and (less commonly) joint effusions. Most of these diseases are less severe and have fewer articular manifestations in children than in adults. In temperate climates, these are summer diseases. No specific therapy or licensed vaccines for these viral diseases yet exist.

SINDBIS VIRUS INFECTION Sindbis virus is transmitted among birds by mosquitoes. Infections with the northern European strains of this virus (which cause, for example, Pogosta disease in Fin-

land, Karelian fever in the new independent states of the former Soviet Union, and Okelbo disease in Sweden) and with the genetically related southern African strains are particularly likely to result in the arthritis-rash syndrome. Exposure to a rural environment is commonly associated with this infection, which has an incubation period of less than 1 week.

The disease begins with rash and arthralgia. Constitutional symptoms are not marked, and fever is modest or lacking altogether. The rash, which lasts about a week, begins on the trunk, spreads to the extremities, and evolves from macules to papules that often vesiculate. The arthritis of this condition is multiarticular, migratory, and incapacitating, with resolution of the acute phase in a few days. Wrists, ankles, phalangeal joints, knees, elbows, and—to a much lesser extent—proximal and axial joints are involved. Persistence of joint pains and occasionally of arthritis is a major problem and may go on for months or even years despite a lack of deformity.

CHIKUNGUNYA VIRUS INFECTION It is likely that chikungunya virus ("that which bends up") is of African origin and is maintained among nonhuman primates on that continent by *Aedes* mosquitoes of the subgenus *Stegomyia* in a fashion similar to yellow fever virus. Like that flavivirus, chikungunya virus is readily transmitted among humans in urban areas by *A. aegypti*. The *A. aegypti*–chikungunya virus transmission cycle has also been introduced into Asia, where it poses a prominent health problem. The disease is endemic in rural areas of Africa, and intermittent epidemics take place in towns and cities of Africa and Asia. Chikungunya is one more reason (in addition to dengue and yellow fever) that *A. aegypti* must be controlled.

Full-blown disease is most common among adults, in whom the clinical picture may be dramatic. The brusque onset follows an incubation period of 2 to 3 days. Fever and severe arthralgia are accompanied by chills and constitutional symptoms such as headache, photophobia, conjunctival injection, anorexia, nausea, and abdominal pain. Migratory polyarthritis mainly affects the small joints of the hands, wrists, ankles, and feet, with lesser involvement of the larger joints. Rash may appear at the outset or several days into the illness; its development often coincides with defervescence, which takes place around day 2 or day 3 of disease. The rash is most intense on the trunk and limbs and may desquamate. Petechiae are occasionally seen, and epistaxis is not uncommon, but this virus is not a regular cause of the HF syndrome, even in children. A few patients develop leukopenia. Elevated levels of aspartate aminotransferase (AST) and C-reactive protein have been described, as have mildly decreased platelet counts. Recovery may require weeks. Some older patients continue to suffer from stiffness, joint pain, and recurrent effusions for several years; this persistence may be especially common in HLA-B27 patients. A live attenuated investigational vaccine has been developed but requires further testing.

A related virus, O'nyong-nyong, caused a major epidemic of arthritis and rash involving at least 2 million people as it moved across eastern and central Africa in the 1960s. After its mysterious emergence, the virus virtually disappeared, leaving only occasional evidence of its persistence in Kenya until a resurgence of activity in 1997.

MAYARO FEVER Mayaro virus is maintained in the forests of the Americas by *Haemagogus* mosquitoes and nonhuman primates. It causes a frequent endemic and sometimes epidemic infection of humans and appears to cause a syndrome resembling chikungunya.

EPIDEMIC POLYARTHRITIS (ROSS RIVER VIRUS INFECTION) Ross River virus has caused epidemics of distinctive clinical disease in Australia since the turn of the century and continues to be responsible for thousands of cases in rural and suburban areas annually. The virus is transmitted by *Aedes vigilax* and other mosquitoes, and its persistence is thought to involve transovarial transmission. No definitive vertebrate host has been identified, but several mammalian species, including wallabies, have been suggested. Endemic transmission has also been documented in New Guinea, and in 1979 the virus swept through the eastern Pacific Islands, causing hundreds of thousands of illnesses. The virus was carried from island to island by infected humans and was believed to have been transmitted among humans by *Aedes polynesiensis* and *A. aegypti*.

The incubation period is 7 to 11 days long, and the onset of illness is sudden, with joint pain usually ushering in the disease. The rash generally develops coincidentally or follows shortly but in some cases precedes joint pains by several days. Constitutional symptoms such as low-grade fever, asthenia, myalgia, headache, and nausea are not prominent and indeed are absent in many cases. Most patients are incapacitated for considerable periods by joint involvement, which interferes with sleeping, walking, and grasping. Wrist, ankle, metacarpophalangeal, interphalangeal, and knee joints are the most commonly involved, although toes, shoulders, and elbows may be affected with some frequency. Periarticular swelling and tenosynovitis are common, and one-third of patients have true arthritis. Only half of all arthritis patients can resume normal activities within 4 weeks, and 10 percent still must limit their activity at 3 months. Occasional patients are symptomatic for 1 to 3 years but without progressive arthropathy. Aspirin and nonsteroidal anti-inflammatory drugs are effective for the treatment of symptoms.

Clinical laboratory values are normal or variable in Ross River virus infection. Tests for rheumatoid factor and antinuclear antibodies are negative, and the erythrocyte sedimentation rate is acutely elevated. Joint fluid contains 1000 to 60,000 mononuclear cells per microliter, and Ross River virus antigen is demonstrable in macrophages. IgM antibodies are particularly valuable in the diagnosis of this infection. The isolation of the virus from blood by mosquito inoculation or mosquito cell culture is possible early in the illness. Because of the great economic importance of annual epidemics in Australia, an inactivated vaccine is being developed and has been found to be protective in mice.

Perhaps because of the high level of current interest in arboviruses in general and in Ross River virus in particular, other arthritogenic arboviruses have been identified in Australia, including Gan Gan virus, a member of the family Bunyaviridae; Kokobera virus, a flavivirus; and Barmah Forest virus, an alphavirus. The last virus is a common cause of infection and must be differentiated from Ross River virus by specific testing.

HEMORRHAGIC FEVERS

The viral HF syndrome is a constellation of findings based on vascular instability and decreased vascular integrity. An assault, direct or indirect, on the microvasculature leads to increased permeability and (particularly when platelet function is decreased) to actual disruption and local hemorrhage. Blood pressure is decreased, and in severe cases shock supervenes. Cutaneous flushing and conjunctival suffusion are examples of common, observable abnormalities in the control of local circulation. The hemorrhage is inconstant and is thought in most cases to be an indication of widespread vascular damage rather than a life-threatening loss of blood volume. Disseminated intravascular coagulation is occasionally found in any severely ill patient with HF but is thought to occur regularly only in the early phases of HF with renal syndrome, Crimean Congo HF, and perhaps some cases of filovirus HF. In some viral HF syndromes, specific organs may be particularly impaired, such as the kidney in HF with renal syndrome, the lung in hantavirus pulmonary syndrome, or the liver in yellow fever, but in all these diseases the generalized circulatory disturbance is critically important.

The pathogenesis of HF is poorly understood and varies among the viruses regularly implicated in the syndrome, which number more than a dozen. In some cases direct damage to the vascular system or even to parenchymal cells of target organs is important, whereas in others soluble mediators are thought to play the major role. The acute phase in most cases of HF is associated with ongoing virus replication and viremia. Exceptions are the hantavirus diseases and dengue HF/dengue shock syndrome (DHF/DSS), in which the immune response plays a major pathogenic role.

The HF syndromes all begin with fever and myalgia, usually of abrupt onset. Within a few days the patient presents for medical attention because of increasing prostration that is often accompanied by severe headache, dizziness, photophobia, hyperesthesia, abdominal or chest pain, anorexia, nausea or vomiting, and other gastrointestinal disturbances. Initial examination often reveals only an acutely ill patient with conjunctival suffusion, tenderness to palpation of muscles or abdomen, and borderline hypotension or postural hypotension, perhaps with tachycardia. Petechiae (often best visualized in the axillae), flushing of the head and thorax, periorbital edema, and proteinuria are common. Levels of AST are usually elevated at presentation or within a day or two thereafter. Hemoconcentration from vascular leakage, which is usually evident, is most marked in hantavirus diseases and in DHF/DSS. The seriously ill patient progresses to more severe symptoms and develops shock and other findings typical of the causative virus. Shock, multifocal bleeding, and CNS involvement (encephalopathy, coma, convulsions) are all poor prognostic signs.

One of the major diagnostic clues is travel to an endemic area within the incubation period for a given syndrome (Table 200-4). Except for Seoul, dengue, and yellow fever virus infections, which have urban vectors, travel to a rural setting is especially suggestive of a diagnosis of HF.

Early recognition is important because of the need for virus-specific therapy and supportive measures, including prompt, atraumatic hospitalization; judicious fluid therapy that takes into account the patient's increased capillary permeability; use of pressors to maintain blood pressure at levels that will support renal perfusion; treatment of the relatively common secondary bacterial infections; replacement of clotting factors and platelets as indicated; and the usual precautionary measures used in the treatment of patients with hemorrhagic diatheses. Disseminated intravascular coagulation should be treated only if clear laboratory evidence of its existence is found and if laboratory monitoring of therapy is feasible; there is no proven benefit of such therapy. The available evidence suggests that HF patients have a decreased cardiac output and will respond poorly to fluid loading as it is often practiced in the treatment of shock associated with bacterial sepsis. Specific therapy is available for several of the HF syndromes. In addition, several diseases considered in the differential diagnosis—malaria, shigellosis, typhoid, leptospirosis, and rickettsial disease—are treatable and potentially lethal. Strict barrier nursing and other precautions against infection of medical staff and visitors are indicated in HF except that due to hantaviruses, yellow fever, Rift Valley fever, and dengue.

LASSA FEVER Lassa virus is known to cause disease in Nigeria, Sierra Leone, Guinea, and Liberia. This virus and its relatives exist elsewhere in Africa, but their health significance is unknown. Like other arenaviruses, Lassa virus is spread to humans by small-particle aerosols from chronically infected rodents and may be acquired during the capture or eating of these animals; it can also be transmitted by person-to-person contact. The virus is often present in urine during convalescence and is suspected to be present in seminal fluid early in recovery. Nosocomial spread has occurred but is uncommon if proper sterile parenteral techniques are used. People of all ages and both sexes are affected; the incidence of disease is highest in the dry season, but transmission takes place year-round. In countries where Lassa virus is endemic, Lassa fever can be a prominent cause of febrile disease. For example, in one hospital in Sierra Leone, laboratory-confirmed Lassa fever is consistently responsible for one-fifth of admissions to the medical wards. There are probably tens of thousands of Lassa fever cases annually in West Africa alone.

The average case has a gradual onset (among the HF agents, only the arenaviruses are typically associated with a gradual onset) that gives way to more severe constitutional symptoms and prostration. Bleeding is seen in only about 15 to 30 percent of cases. A maculopapular rash is often noted in light-skinned Lassa patients. Effusions are common, and male-dominant pericarditis may develop late. The fetal death rate is 92 percent in the last trimester, when maternal mortality is also increased from the usual 15 percent to 30 percent; these figures suggest that interruption of the pregnancy of infected women should be considered. White blood cell counts are normal or slightly elevated, and platelet counts are normal or somewhat low. Deafness coincides with clinical improvement in about 20 percent of cases and is permanent and bilateral in some. Reinfection may occur but has not been associated with severe disease.

High-level viremia or a high serum concentration of AST predicts a fatal outcome. Thus patients with an AST level of >150 IU/mL should be treated with intravenous ribavirin. This antiviral nucleoside analogue appears to be effective in reducing mortality from rates among retrospective controls, and its only major side effect is reversible anemia that usually does not require transfusion. The drug should be given by slow intravenous infusion in a dose of 32 mg/kg; this dose should be followed by 16 mg/kg q 6 h for 4 days and then by 8 mg/kg q 8 h for 6 days.

SOUTH AMERICAN HF SYNDROMES (ARGENTINE, BOLIVIAN, VENEZUELAN, AND BRAZILIAN) These diseases are similar to one another clinically, but their epidemiology differs with the habits of their rodent reservoirs and the interactions of these animals with humans (Table 200-4). Person-to-person or nosocomial transmission is rare but has occurred.

The basic disease resembles Lassa fever with two marked differences. First, thrombocytopenia—often marked—is the rule, and bleeding is quite common. Second, CNS dysfunction is much more common than in Lassa fever and is often manifest by marked confusion, tremors of the arms and tongue, and cerebellar signs. Some cases follow a predominantly neurologic course, with a poor prognosis. The clinical laboratory is helpful in diagnosis since thrombocytopenia, leukopenia, and proteinuria are typical findings.

Argentine HF is readily treated with convalescent-phase plasma given within the first 8 days of illness. In the absence of passive antibody therapy, intravenous ribavirin in the dose recommended for Lassa fever is likely to be effective in all the South American HF syndromes. The transmission of the disease from men convalescing from Argentine HF to their wives suggests the need for counseling of arenavirus HF patients concerning the avoidance of intimate contacts for several weeks after recovery. A safe, effective, live attenuated vaccine exists for Argentine HF. In experimental animals, this vaccine is cross-protective against the Bolivian HF virus.

RIFT VALLEY FEVER This mosquito-borne virus is also a pathogen of domestic animals such as sheep, cattle, and goats. It is maintained in nature by transovarial transmission in floodwater *Aedes* mosquitoes and presumably in a vertebrate amplifier. Epizootics and epidemics occur when sheep or cattle become infected during particularly heavy rains; developing high-level viremia, these animals infect many different species of mosquitoes. Remote sensing via satellite can detect the ecologic changes associated with high rainfall that predict the likelihood of Rift Valley fever transmission; it can also detect the special depressions from which the floodwater *Aedes* mosquito vectors emerge. In addition, the virus is infectious when transmitted by contact with blood or aerosols from domestic animals or their abortuses. The slaughtered meat is not infectious. The natural range of Rift Valley fever virus is confined to sub-Saharan Africa, but the virus has recently been found in Madagascar and has been introduced into Egypt twice, with extensive epidemics occurring on both occasions (1977 to 1979 and 1993 to 1995). Neither person-to-person nor nosocomial transmission has been documented.

Table 200-4

Viral Hemorrhagic Fever (HF) Syndromes and Their Distribution

Disease	Incubation Period, Days	Case-Infection Ratio	Case-Mortality Rate, %	Geographic Range	Target Population
Lassa fever	5–16	Mild infections probably common	15	West Africa	All ages, both sexes
South American HF	7–14	Most infections (more than half) result in disease	15–30	Selected rural areas of Bolivia, Argentina, Venezuela, and Brazil	Bolivia: Men in countryside; all ages, both sexes in villages Argentina: All ages, both sexes; excess exposure and disease in men Venezuela: All ages, both sexes
Rift Valley fever	2–5	~1:100 (most infections result in fever and myalgia)	~50	Sub-Saharan Africa, Madagascar, Egypt	All ages, both sexes; more often diagnosed in men; preexisting liver disease may predispose
Crimean Congo HF	3–12	1:5 or higher	15–30	Africa, Middle East, Balkans, southern region of former Soviet Union, western China	All ages, both sexes; men more exposed in some settings
HF with renal syndrome	9–35	>3:4, Hantaan; 1:20, Puumala	5–15, Hantaan; <1, Puumala	Worldwide, depending on rodent reservoir	Excess of male patients (partly due to greater exposure); mainly adults
Hantavirus pulmonary syndrome	~7–28	Very high	40–50	Americas	Excess of male patients due to some occupational exposure; mainly adults
Marburg or Ebola HF	3–16	High	25–90	Sub-Saharan Africa	All ages, both sexes; children less exposed
Yellow fever	3–6	1:2–1:20	20	Africa, South America	All ages, both sexes; adults more exposed in jungle setting; preexisting flavivirus immunity may cross-protect
Dengue HF/dengue shock syndrome	2–7	1:10,000, nonimmune; 1:100, heterologous immune	<1 with supportive treatment	Tropics and subtropics worldwide	Predominantly children; previous heterologous dengue infection predisposes to HF
Kyasanur Forest/Omsk HF	3–8	Variable	0.5–10	Mysore State, India/western Siberia	Variable

Rift Valley fever virus is unusual in that it causes at least four different clinical syndromes. Most infections are manifested as the febrile-myalgic syndrome. A small proportion result in HF with especially prominent liver involvement. Perhaps 10 percent of otherwise mild infections lead to retinal vasculitis; funduscopic examination reveals edema, hemorrhages, and infarction, and some patients permanently lose partial vision. A small proportion of cases (<1 in 200) are followed by typical viral encephalitis. One of the complicated syndromes does not appear to predispose to another.

There is no proven therapy for any of the syndromes described above. The sensitivity of animal models of Rift Valley fever to antibody or ribavirin therapy suggests that either could be given intravenously to persons with HF. Both retinal disease and encephalitis occur after the acute febrile syndrome has ended and serum neutralizing antibody has developed—events suggesting that only supportive care need be given. Epidemic disease is best prevented by vaccination of livestock. The established ability of this virus to propagate after an introduction into Egypt suggests that other potentially receptive areas, including the United States, should have a response ready to use in such an eventuality. It seems likely that this disease, like Venezuelan equine encephalitis, can be controlled only with adequate stocks of an effective live attenuated vaccine, and there are no such global stocks. A formalin-inactivated vaccine confers immunity on humans, but quantities are limited and three injections are required; this vaccine is recommended for exposed laboratory workers and for veterinarians working in sub-Saharan Africa.

CRIMEAN CONGO HF This severe HF syndrome has a wide geographic distribution, potentially being found wherever ticks of the genus *Hyalomma* occur (see Table 200-4). The propensity of these ticks to feed on domestic livestock and certain wild mammals means that veterinary serosurveys are the most effective mechanism for the surveillance of virus circulation in a region. Human infection is acquired via a tick bite or during the crushing of infected ticks. Domestic animals do not become ill but do develop viremia; thus there is danger of infection at the time of slaughter and for a brief interval thereafter (through contact with hides or carcasses). A recent epidemic was associated with slaughter of tick-infested ostriches in South Africa. Nosocomial epidemics are common and are usually related to extensive blood exposure or needle sticks.

Although generally similar to other HF syndromes, Crimean Congo HF causes extensive liver damage, resulting in jaundice in some cases. Clinical laboratory values indicate disseminated intravascular coagulation and show elevations in AST, creatine phosphokinase, and bilirubin. Patients with fatal cases generally have more marked changes even in the early days of illness and also develop leukocytosis rather than leukopenia. Thrombocytopenia is also more marked and develops earlier in cases with a fatal outcome.

No controlled trials have been performed with intravenous ribavirin, but clinical experience and retrospective comparison of patients with ominous clinical laboratory values suggest that ribavirin is efficacious and should be given. No human or veterinary vaccines are recommended.

HF WITH RENAL SYNDROME This disease, the first to be identified as an HF, is widely distributed over Europe and Asia; the major causative viruses and their rodent reservoirs on these two continents are Puumala virus (bank vole, *Clethrionomys glareolus*) and Hantaan virus (striped field mouse, *Apodemus agrarius*), respectively. Other potential causative viruses exist, including Dobrava virus (yellow-necked field mouse, *Apodemus flavicollus*), which causes severe HF with renal syndrome in the Balkans. Seoul virus is associated with the Norway or sewer rat, *Rattus norvegicus*, and has a worldwide distribution through the migration of the rodent; it is associated with mild or moderate HF with renal syndrome in Asia, but in many areas of the world the human disease has been difficult to identify. Most cases occur in rural residents or vacationers; the exception is Seoul virus disease, which may be acquired in an urban or rural setting or from contaminated laboratory rat colonies. Classic Hantaan disease in Korea (Korean HF) and in rural China (epidemic HF) is most common in spring and fall and is related to rodent density and agricul-

tural practices. Human infection is acquired primarily through aerosols of rodent urine, although virus is also present in saliva and feces. Patients with hantavirus diseases are not infectious. HF with renal syndrome is the most important form of HF today, with more than 100,000 cases of severe disease in Asia annually and milder Puumala infections numbering in the thousands as well.

Severe cases of HF with renal syndrome caused by Hantaan virus evolve in identifiable stages: the febrile stage with myalgia, lasting 3 to 4 days; the hypotensive stage, often associated with shock and lasting from a few hours to 48 h; the oliguric stage with renal failure, lasting 3 to 10 days; and the polyuric stage with diuresis and hyposthenuria.

The *febrile period* is initiated by the abrupt onset of fever, headache, severe myalgia, thirst, anorexia, and often nausea and vomiting. Photophobia, retroorbital pain, and pain on ocular movement are common, and the vision may become blurred with ciliary body inflammation. Flushing over the face, the V area of the neck, and the back are characteristic, as are pharyngeal injection, periorbital edema, and conjunctival suffusion. Petechiae often develop in areas of pressure, the conjunctivae, and the axillae. Back pain and tenderness to percussion at the costovertebral angle reflect massive retroperitoneal edema. Laboratory evidence of mild to moderate disseminated intravascular coagulation is present. Other laboratory findings include proteinuria and an active urinary sediment.

The *hypotensive phase* is ushered in by falling blood pressure and sometimes by shock. The relative bradycardia typical of the febrile phase is replaced by tachycardia. Kinin activation is marked. The rising hematocrit reflects increasing vascular leakage. Leukocytosis with a left shift develops, and thrombocytopenia continues. Atypical lymphocytes—which in fact are activated CD8 + and to a lesser extent CD4 + T cells—circulate. Proteinuria is marked, and the urine's specific gravity falls to 1.010. The renal circulation is congested and compromised from local and systemic circulatory changes resulting in necrosis of tubules, particularly at the corticomedullary junction, and oliguria.

During the *oliguric phase*, hemorrhagic tendencies continue, probably in large part because of uremic bleeding defects. The oliguria persists for 3 to 10 days before renal function returns and marks the onset of the *polyuric stage*, which carries the danger of dehydration and electrolyte abnormalities.

Mild cases of HF with renal syndrome may be much less stereotyped. The presentation may include only fever, gastrointestinal abnormalities, and transient oliguria followed by hyposthenuria.

HF with renal syndrome should be suspected in patients with rural exposure in an endemic area. Prompt recognition of the disease will permit rapid hospitalization and expectant management of shock and renal failure. Useful clinical laboratory parameters include leukocytosis, which may be leukemoid and is associated with a left shift; thrombocytopenia; and proteinuria. Mainstays of therapy are the management of shock, reliance on pressors, modest crystalloid infusion, intravenous use of human serum albumin, and treatment of renal failure with prompt dialysis for the usual indications. Hydration may result in pulmonary edema, and hypertension should be avoided because of the possibility of intracranial hemorrhage. Use of intravenous ribavirin has reduced mortality and morbidity in severe cases provided treatment is begun within the first 4 days of illness. The case-mortality rate may be as high as 15 percent among unrecognized cases but with proper therapy should be <5 percent. Sequelae have not been definitely established, but there is a correlation in the United States between chronic hypertensive renal failure and the presence of antibodies to Seoul virus.

Infections with Puumala virus, the most common cause of HF with renal syndrome in Europe, result in a much attenuated picture but the same general presentation. The syndrome may be referred to by its former name, *nephropathia epidemica*. Bleeding manifestations are found in only 10 percent of cases, hypotension rather than shock is usually seen, and oliguria is present in only about half of patients. The dominant features may be fever, abdominal pain, proteinuria, mild oliguria, and sometimes blurred vision or glaucoma followed by polyuria and hyposthenuria in recovery. Mortality is <1 percent.

The diagnosis is readily made by IgM-capture ELISA, which should be positive at admission or within 24 to 48 h thereafter. The isolation of virus is difficult, but RT-PCR of a blood clot collected early in the clinical course or of tissues obtained postmortem will give positive results. Such testing is undertaken only if definitive identification of the infecting viral species is required.

HANTAVIRUS PULMONARY SYNDROME Hantavirus pulmonary syndrome was discovered in 1993, but retrospective identification of cases by immunohistochemistry (1978) and serology (1959) support the idea that it is a recently discovered rather than a truly new disease. The causative viruses are hantaviruses of a distinct phylogenetic lineage that is associated with the rodent subfamily Sigmodontinae. Sin Nombre virus chronically infects the deer mouse (*Peromyscus maniculatus*) and is the most important virus causing hantavirus pulmonary syndrome in the United States. In the southern states, the disease is also caused by a Sin Nombre virus variant from the white-footed mouse (*Peromyscus leucopus*), by Black Creek Canal virus (*Sigmodon hispidus*, the cotton rat), and by Bayou virus (*Oryzomys palustris*, the rice rat). Viruses such as Andes virus are responsible for cases of hantavirus pulmonary syndrome in Argentina, Brazil, Chile, and Paraguay. The disease is linked to rodent exposure and particularly affects rural residents living in dwellings permeable to rodent entry or working at occupations that pose a risk of rodent exposure. Each rodent species has its own particular habits; in the case of the deer mouse, these behaviors include living in and around human habitation.

The disease begins with a prodrome of about 3 to 4 days (range, 1 to 11 days) comprising fever, myalgia, malaise, and often gastrointestinal disturbances such as nausea, vomiting, and abdominal pain. Dizziness is common and vertigo occasional. Severe prodromal symptoms sometimes bring some individuals to medical attention, but patients more commonly present as the pulmonary phase begins. Typically, there is slightly lowered blood pressure, tachycardia, tachypnea, mild hypoxemia, and early radiographic signs of pulmonary edema. Physical findings in the chest are often surprisingly scant. The conjunctival and cutaneous signs of vascular involvement seen in other types of HF are absent. During the next few hours, decompensation may progress rapidly to severe hypoxemia and respiratory failure. Most patients surviving the first 48 h of hospitalization are extubated and discharged within a few days, with no apparent residua.

Management during the first few hours after presentation is critical. The goal is to prevent severe hypoxemia by oxygen therapy and, if needed, intubation and intensive respiratory management. During this period, hypotension and shock with increasing hematocrit invite aggressive fluid administration, but this intervention should be undertaken with great caution. Because of low cardiac output and increased pulmonary vascular permeability, shock should be managed expectantly with pressors and modest infusion of fluid guided by the pulmonary capillary wedge pressure. Mild cases can be managed by frequent monitoring and oxygen administration without intubation. Many patients require intubation to manage hypoxemia and also develop shock. Mortality remains at about 40 percent with good management. The antiviral drug ribavirin inhibits the virus in vitro and is undergoing clinical trials for efficacy but did not have a marked effect on patients treated in an open-label study.

During the prodrome, the differential diagnosis of hantavirus pulmonary infection is difficult, but by the time of presentation or within 24 h thereafter, a number of helpful clinical features become apparent. Cough is not usually present at the outset but may develop later. Interstitial edema is evident on the chest x-ray. Later, bilateral alveolar edema with a central distribution develops in the setting of a normal-sized heart; occasionally, the edema is initially unilateral. Pleural effusions are often visualized. Thrombocytopenia, circulating atypical lymphocytes, and a left shift (often with leukocytosis) are almost always evident. Hemoconcentration, proteinuria, and hypoalbuminemia should also be sought. Although thrombocytopenia virtually always develops and prolongation of the partial thromboplastin time is the rule, clinical evidence for coagulopathy or laboratory indications of disseminated intravascular coagulation are found in only a minority of cases, usually in severely ill patients. These patients also have acidosis and elevated serum levels of lactate. Mildly increased values in renal function tests are common, but patients with severe cases often have markedly elevated concentrations of serum creatinine; some of the viruses other than Sin Nombre virus have been associated with more kidney involvement, but few such cases have been studied. The differential diagnosis includes abdominal surgical conditions and pyelonephritis as well as rickettsial disease, sepsis, meningococcemia, plague, tularemia, influenza, and relapsing fever.

A specific diagnosis is best made by IgM testing of acute-phase serum, which has yielded a positive result even in the prodrome. Tests using a Sin Nombre virus antigen detect the related hantaviruses causing the pulmonary syndrome in the Americas. Occasionally, heterologous viruses will react only in the IgG ELISA, but this finding is highly suspicious given the very low seroprevalence of these viruses in normal populations. RT-PCR is usually positive when used to test blood clots obtained in the first 7 to 9 days of illness as well as tissues; this test is useful in identifying the infecting virus in areas outside the home range of the deer mouse and in atypical cases.

YELLOW FEVER Yellow fever virus caused major epidemics in the Americas, Africa, and Europe before the discovery of mosquito transmission in 1900 led to its control through attacks on its urban vector, *A. aegypti*. Only then was it found that a jungle cycle also existed in Africa, involving other *Aedes* mosquitoes and monkeys, and that colonization of the new world with *A. aegypti*, originally an African species, had established urban yellow fever as well as an independent sylvatic yellow fever cycle in American jungles involving *Haemagogus* mosquitoes and new world monkeys. Today, urban yellow fever transmission occurs only in some African cities, but the threat exists in the great cities of South America, where reinfestation by *A. aegypti* has taken place and dengue transmission by the same mosquito is common. As late as 1905, New Orleans suffered more than 3000 cases with 452 deaths from "yellow jack." Despite the existence of a highly effective and safe vaccine, several hundred jungle yellow fever cases occur annually in South America, and thousands of jungle and urban cases occur each year in Africa.

Yellow fever is a typical HF accompanied by prominent hepatic necrosis. A period of viremia, typically lasting 3 or 4 days, is followed by a period of "intoxication." During the latter phase in severe cases, the characteristic jaundice, hemorrhages, black vomit, anuria, and terminal delirium occur, perhaps related in part to extensive hepatic involvement. Blood leukocyte counts may be normal or reduced and are often high in terminal stages. Albuminuria is usually noted and may be marked; as renal function fails in terminal or severe cases, the level of blood urea nitrogen rises proportionately. Abnormalities detected in liver function tests range from modest elevations of AST levels in mild cases to severe derangement.

Urban yellow fever can be prevented by the control of *A. aegypti*. The continuing sylvatic cycle requires vaccination of all visitors to areas of potential transmission. Reactions to vaccine are minimal; immunity is provided within 10 days and lasts for at least 10 years. An egg allergy dictates caution in vaccine administration. Although there are no documented harmful effects of the vaccine on the fetus, pregnant women should be immunized only if they are definitely at risk of yellow fever exposure. Since vaccination has been associated with several cases of encephalitis in children under 6 months of age, it should be delayed until after 12 months of age unless the risk of exposure is very high. Timely information on changes in yellow fever distribution and yellow fever vaccine requirements can be obtained from Health Information for Travelers, Centers for Disease Control and Prevention, Atlanta, GA 30333; by fax request (404-332-4565; document number 220022#); by phone (404-332-4559); or on the World-Wide Web at http://www.cdc.gov.

DENGUE HEMORRHAGIC FEVER/DENGUE SHOCK SYNDROME A syndrome of HF noted in the 1950s among children in the Philippines and Southeast Asia was soon associated with dengue virus infections, particularly those occurring against a background of previous exposure to another serotype. The transient heterotypic protection after dengue virus infection is replaced within several weeks by the potential for heterotypic infection resulting in typical dengue fever (see above) or—uncommonly—for enhanced disease (secondary DHF/DSS). In rare instances, primary dengue infections lead to an HF syndrome, but much less is known about pathogenesis in this situation. In the past 20 years, *A. aegypti* has progressively reinvaded Latin America and other areas, and frequent travel by infected individuals has introduced multiple strains of dengue virus from many geographic areas. Thus the pattern of hyperendemic transmission of multiple dengue serotypes has now been established in the Americas and the Caribbean and has led to the emergence of DHF/DSS as a major problem there as well. Millions of dengue infections, including many thousands of cases of DHF/DSS, occur annually. The severe syndrome is unlikely to be seen in U.S. citizens since few children have the dengue antibodies that can trigger the pathogenetic cascade when a second infection is acquired.

Macrophage/monocyte infection is central to the pathogenesis of dengue fever and to the origin of DHF/DSS. Previous infection with a heterologous dengue-virus serotype may result in the production of nonprotective antiviral antibodies that nevertheless bind to the virion's surface and through interaction with the Fc receptor focus secondary dengue viruses on the target cell, the result being enhanced infection. The host is also primed for a secondary antibody response when viral antigens are released and immune complexes lead to activation of the classic complement pathway, with consequent phlogistic effects. Cross-reactivity at the T cell level results in the release of physiologically active cytokines, including interferon γ and tumor necrosis factor alpha. The induction of vascular permeability and shock depends on multiple factors, including the following:

1. *Presence of enhancing and nonneutralizing antibodies*—Transplacental maternal antibody may be present in infants <9 months old, or antibody elicited by previous heterologous dengue infection may be present in older individuals.
2. *Age*—Susceptibility to DHF/DSS drops considerably after 12 years of age.
3. *Sex*—Females are more often affected than males.
4. *Race*—Caucasians are more often affected than blacks.
5. *Nutritional status*—Malnutrition is protective.
6. *Sequence of infection*—For example, serotype 1 followed by serotype 2 is more dangerous than serotype 4 followed by serotype 2.
7. *Infecting serotype*—Type 2 is apparently more dangerous than other serotypes.

In addition, there is considerable variation among strains of a given serotype, with Southeast Asian serotype 2 strains having more potential to cause DHF/DSS than others.

Dengue HF is identified by the detection of bleeding tendencies (tourniquet test, petechiae) or overt bleeding in the absence of underlying causes such as preexisting gastrointestinal lesions. Dengue shock syndrome, usually accompanied by hemorrhagic signs, is much more serious and results from increased vascular permeability leading to shock. In mild DHF/DSS, restlessness, lethargy, thrombocytopenia (<100,000/μL), and hemoconcentration are detected 2 to 5 days after the onset of typical dengue fever, often at the time of defervescence. The maculopapular rash that often develops in dengue fever may also appear in DHF/DSS. In more severe cases, frank shock is apparent, with low pulse pressure, cyanosis, hepatomegaly, pleural effusions, ascites, and in some cases severe ecchymoses and gastrointestinal bleeding. The period of shock lasts only 1 or 2 days, and most patients respond promptly to close monitoring, oxygen administration, and infusion of crystalloid or—in severe cases—colloid. The mortality rates reported vary greatly with case ascertainment and the quality of treatment; however, most DHF/DSS patients respond well to supportive therapy, and overall mortality in an experienced center in the tropics is probably as low as 1 percent.

A virologic diagnosis can be made by the usual means, although multiple flavivirus infections lead to a broad immune response to several members of the group, and this situation may result in a lack of virus specificity of the IgM and IgG immune responses. A secondary antibody response can be sought with tests against several flavivirus antigens to demonstrate the characteristic wide spectrum of reactivity.

The key to control of both dengue fever and DHF/DSS is the control of *A. aegypti*, which also reduces the risk of urban yellow fever and chikungunya virus circulation. Control efforts have been handicapped by the presence of nondegradable tires and long-lived plastic containers in trash repositories, insecticide resistance, urban poverty, and an inability of the public health community to mobilize the populace to respond to the need to eliminate mosquito breeding sites. Live attenuated dengue vaccines are in the late stages of development and have produced promising results in early tests. Whether vaccines can provide safe, durable immunity to an immunopathologic disease such as DHF/DSS in endemic areas is an issue that will have to be tested, but it is hoped that vaccination will reduce transmission to negligible levels.

KYASANUR FOREST DISEASE AND OMSK HEMORRHAGIC FEVER Kyasanur Forest virus and Omsk HF virus are geographically restricted, tick-borne flaviviruses that cause a syndrome of viral HF during a wave of viremia and that may also enter the CNS to cause subsequent viral encephalitis (see discussion of tick-borne encephalitis above). There is no therapy for these infections, but an inactivated vaccine has been used in India against Kyasanur Forest disease. A new and related virus isolate has been obtained from butchers with HF in the Middle East; the implication is that there are more agents in this group.

FILOVIRUS HEMORRHAGIC FEVER → *See Chap. 201.*

BIBLIOGRAPHY

ZOONOTIC VIRUSES

CALISHER CH: Medically important arboviruses of the United States and Canada. Clin Microbiol Rev 7:89, 1994

KARABATSOS N: *International Catalogue of Arboviruses, Including Certain Other Viruses of Vertebrates*, 3d ed. San Antonio, TX, American Society of Tropical Medicine and Hygiene, 1985

MONATH TP (ed): *The Arboviruses: Epidemiology and Ecology*, vols I–V. Boca Raton, FL, CRC Press, 1988

TSAI TF: Arboviral infections in the US. Infect Dis Clin North Am 5:73, 1991

VASCONCELOS PFC et al: Clinical and ecoepidemiological situation of human arboviruses in Brazilian Amazonia. Ciencia e Cultura 44:117, 1992

HEMORRHAGIC FEVERS

CENTERS FOR DISEASE CONTROL AND PREVENTION: Management of patients with suspected viral hemorrhagic fever. Morb Mort Week Rep 37(S-3):1, 1988

———: Update: Management of patients with suspected viral hemorrhagic fever—United States. Morb Mort Week Rep 44:475, 1995

PETERS CJ et al: Management of patients infected with high-hazard viruses. Arch Virol 11(Suppl):141, 1996

———: Pathogenesis of viral hemorrhagic fevers, in *Viral Pathogenesis*, N Nathanson et al (eds). Philadelphia, Lippincott-Raven, 1996

——— et al: Viral hemorrhagic fevers, in *Atlas of Infectious Diseases*, vol 8, R Fekety (ed). Philadelphia, Current Medicine, 1997, pp 10.1–10.26

SMORODINTSEV AA et al: *Virus Hemorrhagic Fevers*. Jerusalem, Israel Program for Scientific Translations, 1964, 245 pp

ZAKI SR, PETERS CJ: Viral hemorrhagic fevers, in *The Pathology of Infectious Diseases*, DH Connor et al (eds). Stamford, CT, Appleton & Lange, 1997 pp 347–346

ARENAVIRUSES

BARRY M et al: Treatment of a laboratory-acquired Sabiá virus infection. N Engl J Med 333:294, 1995

ENRIA D, MAIZTEGUI JI: Antiviral treatment of Argentine hemorrhagic fever. Antiviral Res 23:23, 1994

JOHNSON KM et al: Hemorrhagic fevers of Southeast Asia and South America: A comparative appraisal. Prog Med Virol 9:105, 1967

———— et al: Clinical virology of Lassa fever in hospitalized patients. J Infect Dis 155:456, 1987

LARSEN PD et al: Hydrocephalus complicating lymphocytic choriomeningitis infection. Pediatr Infect Dis J 12:628, 1993

McCORMICK JB et al: A case-control study of the clinical diagnosis and course of Lassa fever. J Infect Dis 155:445, 1987

MOLINAS FC et al: Hemostasis and the complement system in Argentine hemorrhagic fever. Rev Infect Dis 11(Suppl 4):762, 1989

PETERS CJ: Arenaviruses, in *Clinical Virology*, DD Richman et al (eds). New York, Churchill Livingstone, 1997, pp 973–996

———— et al: Hemorrhagic fever in Cochabamba, Bolivia, 1971. Am J Epidemiol 99:425, 1974

SALAS R et al: Venezuelan hemorrhagic fever. Lancet 338:1033, 1991

BUNYAVIRIDAE

ANTONIADIS A et al: Direct genetic detection of Dobrava virus in Greek and Albanian haemorrhagic fever with renal syndrome (HFRS) patients. J Infect Dis 174:407, 1996

BRUNO P et al: The protean manifestations of hemorrhagic fever with renal syndrome. A retrospective review of 26 cases from Korea. Ann Intern Med 113:385, 1990

DUCHIN JS et al: Hantavirus pulmonary syndrome: A clinical description of 17 patients with a newly recognized disease. N Engl J Med 330:949, 1994

HUGGINS JW et al: Prospective, double-blind, concurrent, placebo controlled clinical trial of intravenous ribavirin therapy of hemorrhagic fever with renal syndrome. J Infect Dis 164:1119, 1991

KETAI LH et al: Hantavirus pulmonary syndrome (HPS): Radiographic findings in 16 patients. Radiology 191:665, 1994

KHAN AS et al: Hantavirus pulmonary syndrome: The first 100 U.S. cases. J Infect Dis 173:1297, 1996

LAUGHLIN LW et al: Epidemic Rift Valley fever in Egypt: Observations of the spectrum of human illness. Trans R Soc Trop Med Hyg 73:630, 1979

PETERS CJ, LeDuc JW: Bunyaviridae: bunyaviruses, phleboviruses, and related viruses, in *Textbook of Human Virology*, 2d ed, R Belshe (ed). St Louis, Mosby Year Book, 1991, pp 571–614

————, LINTHICUM KJ: Rift Valley fever, in *Handbook Series of Zoonoses, Section B: Viral Zoonoses*, 2d ed, GW Beran (ed). Boca Raton, FL, CRC Press, 1994, pp 125–138

SEXTON DJ et al: Life-threatening Cache Valley virus infection. N Engl J Med 336:547, 1997

SWANEPOEL R et al: Epidemiologic and clinical features of Crimean-Congo hemorrhagic fever in South Africa. Am J Trop Med Hyg 6:120, 1987

———— et al: The clinical pathology of Crimean-Congo hemorrhagic fever. Rev Infect Dis 11(Suppl 4):S794, 1989

SYMPOSIUM ON EPIDEMIC HEMORRHAGIC FEVER(May, 1954). Am J Med 16:1–617, 1954

ZAKI SR: Hantavirus-associated diseases, in *The Pathology of Infectious Diseases*, DH Connor et al (eds). Stamford, CT, Appleton & Lange, 1997

———— et al: Hantavirus pulmonary syndrome: Pathogenesis of an emerging infectious disease. Am J Pathol 146:552, 1995

FILOVIRUSES

CENTERS FOR DISEASE CONTROL AND PREVENTION: Update: Outbreak of Ebola viral hemorrhagic fever—Zaire, 1995. Morb Mort Week Rep 44:468, 1995

MARTINI GA, SIEGERT R (eds): *Marburg Virus Disease*. Berlin, Springer-Verlag, 1971

PETERS CJ et al: Filoviruses, in *Fields Virology*, 3d ed, BN Fields et al (eds). Philadelphia, Lippincott-Raven, 1996

WHO/INTERNATIONAL STUDY TEAM: Ebola hemorrhagic fever in Sudan, 1976. Bull World Health Organ 56:247, 1978

WORLD HEALTH ORGANIZATION: Ebola haemorrhagic fever in Zaire, 1976. Report of an international commission. Bull World Health Organ 56:271, 1978

FLAVIVIRUSES

BARROS MLB, BOECKEN G: Jungle yellow fever in the central Amazon. Lancet 348:969, 1996

HALSTEAD SB: Dengue and dengue hemorrhagic fever, in *Textbook of Pediatric Infectious Disease*, R Feigin and JD Cherry (eds). Philadelphia, Saunders, 1987, pp 1510–1521

————: Antibody, macrophages, dengue virus infection, shock, and hemorrhage: A pathogenic cascade. Rev Infect Dis 11(Suppl 4):S830, 1989

————, O'ROURKE EJ: Dengue viruses and mononuclear phagocytes. I. Infection enhancement by non-neutralizing antibody. J Exp Med 146:201, 1977

KERR JA: The clinical aspects and diagnosis of yellow fever, in *Yellow Fever*, GR Strode (ed). New York, McGraw-Hill, 1951, pp 385–425

KURANE I et al: Immunopathologic mechanisms of dengue hemorrhagic fever and dengue shock syndrome. Arch Virol 9:59, 1994

LUBY JP: St. Louis encephalitis, Rocio encephalitis, and West Nile fever, in *Kass Handbook of Infectious Diseases. Exotic Viral Infections*, JS Porterfield (ed). New York, Chapman and Hall, 1995, pp 183–202

MONATH TP, HEINZ FX: Flaviviruses, in *Fields Virology*, 3d ed, BN Fields et al (eds). Philadelphia, Lippincott-Raven, 1996, pp 961–1034

SABIN AB: Research on dengue during World War II. Am J Trop Med Hyg 1:30, 1952

TSAI T, YU XX: Japanese encephalitis vaccines, in *Vaccines*, 2d ed, SW Plotkin and E Mortimer (eds). Philadelphia, WB Saunders, 1994, pp 671–713

WALDVOGEL K et al: Severe tick-borne encephalitis following passive immunization. Eur J Pediatr 155:775, 1996

REOVIRUSES

EMMONS RW: Colorado tick fever, in *Handbook Series of Zoonoses, Section B: Viral Zoonoses, vol 1*, GW Beran (ed). Boca Raton, FL, CRC Press, 1981, pp 113–124

MONATH TP, GUIRAKHOO F: Orbiviruses and coltiviruses, in *Fields Virology*, 3d ed, BN Fields et al (eds). Philadelphia, Lippincott-Raven, 1996, pp 1735–1766

RHABDOVIRUSES

REIF JS: Vesicular stomatitis, in *Handbook Series of Zoonoses, Section B: Viral Zoonoses*, vol 1, 2d ed, GW Beran (ed). Boca Raton, FL, CRC Press, 1995, pp 113–124

TOGAVIRUSES

FRASER JRE: Epidemic polyarthritis and Ross River virus disease. Clin Rheum Dis 12:369, 1986

JOHNSTON RE, PETERS CJ: Alphaviruses, in *Fields Virology*, 3d ed, BN Fields et al (eds). Philadelphia, Lippincott-Raven, 1996, pp 843–898

MACKENZIE JS: Mosquito-borne viruses and epidemic polyarthritis. Med J Aust 164:90, 1996

NIKLASSON B: Sindbis and Sindbis-like viruses, in *The Arboviruses: Epidemiology and Ecology*, vol IV, TP Monath (ed). Boca Raton, FL, CRC Press, 1988, pp 167–176

PHILLIPS DA et al: Clinical and subclinical Barmah Forest virus infection in Queensland. Med J Aust 152:463, 1990

PINHEIRO FP et al: An outbreak of Mayaro virus disease in Belterra, Brazil. I. Clinical and virological findings. Am J Trop Med Hyg 30:674, 1981

RIVAS F et al: Epidemic Venezuelan equine encephalitis in La Guajira, Colombia, 1995. J Infect Dis 1997

ROBINSON MC: An epidemic of virus disease in Southern Province Tanganyika Territory, in 1952–53. I. Clinical features. Trans R Soc Trop Med Hyg 49:28, 1955

201   *Lawrence Corey*

MARBURG AND EBOLA VIRUSES (FILOVIRIDAE)

DEFINITION Both Marburg virus and Ebola virus cause an acute systemic febrile illness associated with high mortality. This illness is characterized by the abrupt onset of headache, myalgias, pharyngitis, rash, and hemorrhagic manifestations. Person-to-person and nosocomial contact may lead to secondary cases and intermittent outbreaks of infection.

ETIOLOGY The family Filoviridae includes two former members of the family Rhabdoviridae: Marburg virus, a unique agent with only one known subtype, and Ebola virus, which is antigenically distinct from Marburg virus and has three known subtypes. The Ebola virus subtypes (Zaire, Sudan, and Reston) have common as well as unique epitopes. The Reston subtype appears to be attenuated in its pathogenicity for humans. Antigenic and genomic analyses of the surface glycoprotein of the Sudan strains isolated from 1976 to 1979 appear identical; this finding is indicative of stability in the antigenic structure of the subtypes of Ebola virus. Both Ebola virus and Marburg virus can be isolated in a variety of cell culture systems, including vervet monkey kidney (Vero) cells. The virion contains one copy of linear, negative-sense, single-stranded RNA with a helical nucleocapsid and a lipid envelope derived from the host cell plasma membrane. Structurally, the virus appears as an 80- to 100-nm elongated filamentous particle with surface projections or peplomers. The viral genome is approximately 19 kb and codes for seven gene products. The surface glycoprotein makes up the surface spikes, mediates viral entry, and is highly glycosylated—a characteristic that may contribute to the rather low levels of neutralizing antibodies detected in infected individuals. Two matrix proteins called VP40 and VP24 appear to be involved in viral budding and uncoating. The viral nucleocapsid is composed of a major nucleoprotein and a minor protein (VP30). As in other negative-stranded RNA viruses, the virion contains an RNA polymerase protein. In infected cells, both Ebola virus and Marburg virus produce a nonstructural secreted glycoprotein that may play a role in interference with the host's immune responses. The viruses are stable and remain infectious for prolonged periods at room temperature. They are destroyed by heat (60°C, 30 min) and lipid solvents. Both viruses are biosafety level 4 pathogens and require maximal biologic containment facilities.

EPIDEMIOLOGY Marburg virus was first identified in Germany in 1967. The virus was isolated from laboratory workers exposed to African Green monkeys (*Cercopithecus aethiops*) that had been imported from Uganda. Virus was isolated from the blood and tissue of these monkeys and of several laboratory workers. Of the 25 cases of primary Marburg infection, 7 ended in death. Most of 6 secondary cases appeared to be related to accidental needle sticks or abrasions. Secondary spread to the wife of one patient was documented. Marburg virus was demonstrated in semen of the source contact despite the presence of circulating antibody. This secondary case is believed to have been acquired through sexual intercourse. Since this outbreak, isolated cases of Marburg infection have been reported, usually involving persons on the African continent.

In 1976, epidemics of severe hemorrhagic fever occurred simultaneously in Zaire and Sudan. Among 550 cases, there were more than 470 deaths. Ebola virus was isolated in both locations. Epidemic spread took place through close person-to-person contact and injections from reused needles. Both epidemics ended with the institution of strict quarantine procedures.

In 1989, numerous deaths from hemorrhagic fever among quarantined primates were noted in a primate import quarantine facility in Reston, Virginia. Ebola virus (Reston strain) was isolated from cynomolgus macaques from the Philippines and Indonesia that were being kept at the facility. Four employees were infected; none died.

In May 1995, an epidemic of hemorrhagic fever occurred in Kikwit, Zaire, resulting in 250 clinically identified cases and 80 percent mortality. Again, person-to-person spread within households and in hospitals facilitated secondary spread. During the outbreak, Ebola virus was isolated from sweat glands of symptomatic patients; thus contact with patients' perspiration may have facilitated the spread of the agent. Strict quarantine measures arrested the epidemic.

Despite extensive investigations, the reservoirs for the filoviruses are unknown. The viruses appear to be zoonotic, but all attempts to define the natural reservoir of infection have yielded unconvincing results. These viruses' similarity to Lassa virus suggests their persistence in an unidentified mammalian host. Whether subclinical filovirus infections occur in humans is still controversial.

PATHOLOGY Both Marburg virus and Ebola virus appear to be "pantropic"; viral replication takes place in almost all organs, including lymphoid tissue, liver, spleen, pancreas, adrenals, thyroid, kidneys, testes, skin, and brain. Focal necrosis of liver, lymphatic organs, kidneys, testes, and ovaries is common. In the liver, eosinophilic cytoplasmic bodies resembling the Councilman bodies of yellow fever have been noted. The lungs may exhibit interstitial pneumonitis as well as vascular lesions indicative of endarteritis in small arterioles. Neuropathologic changes consist of multiple small hemorrhagic infarcts with glial proliferation. The pathophysiology of the hemorrhagic manifestations of infection is unclear. Viral infection of endothelial cells, with in situ fibrin depletion, may be a factor. Inflammatory mediators of the "sepsis syndrome" may also play a role.

CLINICAL MANIFESTATIONS After an incubation period of 3 to 9 days, patients develop frontal and temporal headache, malaise, myalgias (especially in the lumbar area), nausea, and vomiting. Fever—with temperatures of 39.4 to 40°C (103 to 104°F)—is characteristic, and about half of all patients have conjunctivitis. Between 1 and 3 days after onset, watery diarrhea (often severe), lethargy, and a change in mentation are noted. An enanthem of the palate and tonsils and cervical lymphadenopathy also may become apparent during the first week of illness. The most reliable clinical feature is the appearance of a nonpruritic maculopapular rash, which begins on the fifth to seventh day on the face and neck and spreads centrifugally to the extremities. A fine desquamation of the affected skin, especially on the palms and soles, appears 4 to 5 days later. Hemorrhagic manifestations, including gastrointestinal, renal, vaginal, and/or conjunctival hemorrhages, generally develop between days 5 and 7 of disease.

During the first week, the temperature remains around 40°C (104°F), falling by lysis during the second week only to increase again between days 12 and 14. Other clinical signs apparent in the second week of disease include splenomegaly, hepatomegaly, facial edema, and scrotal or labial reddening. Complications include orchitis, which may lead to testicular atrophy; myocarditis, with irregular pulse and electrocardiographic abnormalities; and pancreatitis. Patients who die usually do so on the eighth to sixteenth days of illness. Recovery is often protracted over a 3- to 4-week period, during which loss of hair, intermittent abdominal pain, poor appetite, and prolonged psychotic disturbances have been noted. Late sequelae, including transverse myelitis and uveitis, have been reported. Marburg virus has been isolated from the anterior eye chamber and semen nearly 3 months after onset of disease.

LABORATORY FINDINGS Abnormalities in granulocyte function are found in filovirus infection. Leukopenia is detected as early as the first day, with leukocyte counts as low as 1000/µL and neutrophilia by the fourth day. Subsequently, atypical lymphocytes as well as neutrophils exhibiting the Pelger-Huët anomaly may appear. Thrombocytopenia develops early and is most marked (often with fewer than 10,000 cells/µL) between days 6 and 12. Fatal cases may include evidence of disseminated intravascular coagulation. Hypoproteinemia, proteinuria, and azotemia may develop. Elevations in aspartate and alanine aminotransferases are usual. Lumbar puncture may yield normal findings or reveal minimal pleocytosis. The erythrocyte sedimentation rate is usually low.

DIAGNOSIS The characteristic clinical course and epidemiologic features of filovirus infections form the basis for the diagnosis. Specific diagnosis requires isolation of the virus or detection of serologic evidence of infection in paired serum samples. In fatal filovirus infections, there is high-titer viremia and little evidence of a host immune response. Viremia coincides with the febrile stage of disease; virus has been isolated from tissue as well as from urine, semen, and throat and rectal swabs. *Attempts to isolate virus must be made only in specialized high-security laboratories.* Gamma irradiation is the most common way to inactivate virus. Staining for viral antigens and assays based on the reverse transcription polymerase chain reaction have been useful when conducted in specialized laboratories. Specimens should be sent to the Centers for Disease Control and Prevention, Atlanta, Georgia; the Central Public Health Laboratory, Colindale, London, England; or the National Institute of Virology, Sandringham, Republic of South Africa. Since person-to-person transmission is the means by which outbreaks are propagated, all patients should be managed under conditions of strict barrier isolation, and all specimens should be handled and shipped with extreme care according to World Health Organization guidelines.

℞ TREATMENT

Other than supportive care, no definitive treatment for filovirus infection is available. The administration of convalescent-phase serum from recovered patients has been proposed but has not been systematically evaluated. In any event, such serum is rarely available.

In vitro, neither Marburg virus nor Ebola virus is inhibited by the antiviral drug ribavirin.

BIBLIOGRAPHY

CENTERS FOR DISEASE CONTROL: Management of patients with suspected viral hemorrhagic fever. Morb Mort Week Rep 37(Suppl 3):1, 1988

ELLIOT LH et al: Improved specificity of testing methods for filovirus antibody. J Virol Methods 43:85, 1993

FISHER HOCH SP et al: Pathogenic potential of filovirus. J Infect Dis 166:753, 1992

GEISBERT TW et al: Differentiation of filoviruses by electron microscopy. Virus Res 39:129, 1995

JAAX NK et al: Lethal experimental infection of rhesus monkey with Ebola-Zaire (Mayinga) virus by the oral and conjunctival route of exposure. Arch Pathol Lab Med 120:140, 1996

PETERS CJ et al: Filoviruses as emerging pathogens. Semin Virol 5:147, 1994

SECTION 15

FUNGAL INFECTIONS

202   *John E. Bennett*

DIAGNOSIS AND TREATMENT OF FUNGAL INFECTIONS

MYCOLOGY FUNDAMENTALS

Fungi can appear microscopically as either rounded, budding forms (yeastlike organisms) or hyphae (molds). Yeastlike colonies are smooth, while mold colonies are fuzzy; fungi that grow as yeasts include species of *Candida* and *Cryptococcus*, while fungi that grow as molds include species of *Aspergillus*, *Rhizopus*, and dermatophytes (ringworm fungi). The fungi that cause histoplasmosis, blastomycosis, sporotrichosis, coccidioidomycosis, and paracoccidioidomycosis are called *dimorphic* ("having two forms") because they are rounded in tissue but grow like molds when cultured at room temperature. *Candida* species other than *Candida glabrata* appear in tissue as both budding yeasts and tubular elements called *pseudohyphae*.

Some fungi described in this text are given two different names. For example, *Histoplasma capsulatum* is also called *Ajellomyces capsulatus*, the latter being the name for the "perfect state." The diagnostic laboratory rarely sees a fungus growing in the perfect state and therefore does not use this name. One of the exceptions is *Scedosporium apiospermum*, which may be seen in the perfect state and is then called *Pseudallescheria boydii*. The reader is referred to standard textbooks of medical mycology for an explanation of the perfect state.

Most fungi that are pathogenic for humans are saprophytes in nature; they cause infection when airborne spores reach the lung or paranasal sinus or when hyphae or spores are accidentally inoculated into the skin or cornea. Acquisition of infection from another person or an animal has been reported in the case of ringworm but is very rare in other mycoses. Thus, hospitalized patients with fungal infections do not require special isolation. Most fungi infect hosts preferentially by one route and only infrequently by other routes. For example, the agents of ringworm, pityriasis versicolor, and piedra infect the epidermis and its appendages. Sporotrichosis and mycetoma usually arise from subcutaneous inoculation. Inhalation is the route of inoculation for the agents of most deep mycoses. Ingestion of fungi rarely causes infection; *Candida albicans*, a normal commensal in the mouth and intestine, reaches deeper tissues only when mucosal or cutaneous barriers are breached by disease, surgery, trauma, or catheterization. Histoplasmosis, blastomycosis, coccidioidomycosis, and paracoccidioidomycosis have been called "endemic" mycoses to emphasize their restricted geographic distribution. Some fungi, such as *Aspergillus*, are said to be opportunists in that they usually infect hosts with compromised immunity. This distinction is relative, not absolute.

Immunity after exposure to fungi may confer partial protection against reinfection. Residents of areas in which mycoses are endemic are less subject to infection than are newcomers. Predisposing factors are helpful in defining host defense. Immunoglobulin deficiencies do not appear to predispose to any mycosis, whereas neutropenia is common among patients who develop invasive aspergillosis or deep candidiasis. Cell-mediated immunity appears to be of paramount importance in most other deep mycoses.

DIAGNOSIS

Many fungi can be identified to the genus or even the species level by microscopic examination of smears or biopsy specimens. Calcofluor white staining with fluorescence microscopy is a sensitive technique for smears of sputum, bronchoalveolar lavage fluid, or pus. India ink smear remains the method of choice for detecting cryptococci in cerebrospinal fluid (CSF). Smears of vaginal or oral lesions for *Candida* pseudohyphae can be prepared by wet mounting or Gram's staining. For histopathology slides, Gomori methenamine silver and a neutral counterstain are preferred.

The method used has a marked effect on the rapidity and sensitivity of blood cultures for fungi, except in the case of *Candida* species, which are relatively easy to grow. For most other fungi, concentration of the blood by lysis centrifugation and culture on solid medium constitute the optimal technique. Commercially available nucleic acid hybridization techniques can speed the identification of slow-growing molds, such as *H. capsulatum* and *Coccidioides immitis*. Serology has limited value, but testing of serum or CSF for cryptococcal antigen or antibody to *C. immitis* can be diagnostic. Skin testing with fungal antigens is not useful in detecting active infection.

ANTIFUNGAL THERAPY

TOPICAL AGENTS   Imidazoles and Triazoles   These synthetic compounds act by inhibiting ergosterol synthesis in the fungal cell wall and, when given topically, may cause direct damage to the fungal cytoplasmic membrane. The imidazoles available for cutaneous application include clotrimazole, econazole, ketoconazole, sulconazole, oxiconazole, and miconazole. Vaginal formulations include four imidazoles (miconazole, clotrimazole, tioconazole, and butoconazole) and one triazole (terconazole). Miconazole lotion and vaginal preparations of both miconazole and clotrimazole are available without prescription. As yet, no substantial differences in the efficacy of or local intolerance to the various topical azoles have become apparent. All are effective in the treatment of cutaneous candidiasis, tinea (pityriasis) versicolor, and mild to moderately severe ringworm of the glabrous skin. Vaginal formulations are effective for vulvovaginal candidiasis. Clotrimazole is poorly absorbed from the gastrointestinal tract, but the oral troche is useful as a topical treatment for oral and esophageal candidiasis.

Polyene Macrolide Antibiotics   These broad-spectrum antifungal agents combine with sterol in the fungal cytoplasmic membrane, increasing membrane permeability. Topically, they are not active against ringworm but are effective against candidiasis of the skin and mucous membranes. Nystatin suspension is effective in oral thrush, and vaginal troches are effective in vulvovaginal candidiasis. Both nystatin and amphotericin B are available in topical preparations for cutaneous candidiasis.

Other Topical Antifungals   Ciclopirox olamine, haloprogin, terbinafine, and naftifine have the same clinical spectrum among the cutaneous mycoses as the imidazoles. Tolnaftate and undecylenic acid are effective against ringworm but not candidiasis. Keratolytic agents, such as salicylic acid, are helpful as accessory drugs for some hyperkeratotic skin lesions.

SYSTEMIC ANTIFUNGALS **Griseofulvin** Griseofulvin is a useful drug in the treatment of certain kinds of ringworm; however, it is ineffective in the treatment of candidiasis. The microcrystalline and ultramicrocrystalline preparations differ in dose but not in efficacy. Absorption of both is enhanced when the drug is ingested with fat-containing foods. Griseofulvin interacts with phenobarbital and coumarin-type anticoagulants.

Terbinafine Oral terbinafine (250 mg once daily) is at least as effective as itraconazole and more effective than griseofulvin in onychomycosis and ringworm. Gastrointestinal distress is the most common side effect. Rash, hepatitis, and pancytopenia have occurred, but serious adverse effects have been uncommon. Terbinafine decreases cyclosporine levels. Cimetidine increases and rifampin decreases terbinafine levels in blood.

Imidazoles and Triazoles *Ketoconazole* Absorption of ketoconazole is variable among individuals, is not affected by food, and is poor in patients with AIDS and those taking cimetidine or other H_2 blocking agents. Simultaneous administration of antacids also can impair the absorption of ketoconazole. Its metabolism is chiefly hepatic, but substantial liver disease has only a minimal effect on its concentrations in plasma. Ketoconazole plasma levels are decreased in patients taking rifampin and also in some taking isoniazid. Ketoconazole administration can elevate cyclosporine and cisapride levels in blood, can increase the likelihood of terfenadine or astemizole cardiotoxicity, and occasionally can enhance the anticoagulant effect of warfarin. The drug is contraindicated during pregnancy and, because it appears in breast milk, during breast-feeding. Neither renal disease nor hemodialysis affects the metabolism of ketoconazole.

The most common toxicities of ketoconazole are dose-related nausea, anorexia, and occasionally vomiting. Hepatotoxicity is idiosyncratic and usually mild (manifesting as transiently elevated levels of aminotransferases) but, in rare instances, can be serious and fatal. Several dose-related, temporary endocrine effects have been observed: decreased adrenal cortical reserve; gynecomastia; a decrease in serum testosterone level, libido, and potency in males; and menstrual irregularity in females. Pruritus or rash also may occur.

Ketoconazole is effective in blastomycosis, histoplasmosis, paracoccidioidomycosis, chronic mucocutaneous candidiasis, esophageal candidiasis, and some forms of disseminated coccidioidomycosis and pseudallescheriasis. The usual adult dose is 400 mg once daily. Partial improvement may follow ketoconazole treatment of cutaneous sporotrichosis and chromoblastomycosis. Although vulvovaginal candidiasis, ringworm, and tinea versicolor are responsive to the drug, the toxicity of oral ketoconazole makes topical imidazoles or other drugs preferable for these indications.

Itraconazole This triazole analogue of ketoconazole is superior to the parent compound in safety and efficacy. Hormonal suppression and hepatotoxicity are less marked with itraconazole than with ketoconazole. Clinical indications for the use of itraconazole include all those cited for ketoconazole but also extend to selected cases of onychomycosis, sporotrichosis, cryptococcosis, and aspergillosis. The drug is marketed as 100-mg capsules. No parenteral formulation is available. The usual dose is 200 mg once or twice a day by mouth with food (to enhance absorption). Itraconazole is metabolized in the liver, and its hydroxy metabolite retains antifungal activity. Concurrent therapy with rifampin, carbamazepine, and H_2 receptor antagonists or phenytoin decreases itraconazole blood levels. Cardiotoxicity due to digoxin, terfenadine, or astemizole and nephrotoxicity due to cyclosporine may occur during concomitant itraconazole therapy. Itraconazole inhibits the metabolism of tacrolimus, midazolam, triazolam, oral hypoglycemic agents, and cisapride. Its use during pregnancy is contraindicated.

Fluconazole This triazole can be administered in tablet form, as a suspension, or as an intravenous infusion. With a half-life of about 31 h, fluconazole can be given once a day. Its bioavailability when given by the oral route is excellent and is unimpaired by lack of gastric acid or the presence of food. Fluconazole therapy can elevate blood levels of phenytoin, cyclosporine, warfarin, rifabutin, and sulfonylureas. Approximately 80 percent of the drug is excreted unchanged in the urine. Patients with creatinine clearance rates of 21 to 50 mL/min and 11 to 20 mL/min should have their fluconazole doses reduced by 50 and 75 percent, respectively. The drug penetrates the CSF and other body fluids very well.

Nausea and abdominal distress are the most common forms of dose-limiting fluconazole toxicity. An allergic rash may develop and is particularly common among patients infected with human immunodeficiency virus (HIV). Fatal cases of Stevens-Johnson syndrome have been described in the HIV-infected population. Alopecia commonly follows prolonged administration of $\geq$400 mg daily but resolves when therapy is discontinued. Rare cases of anaphylaxis, hepatic necrosis, and neutropenia have been described.

Fluconazole is a useful drug in the treatment of adults with oropharyngeal and esophageal candidiasis. A single 150-mg tablet is effective in vulvovaginal candidiasis. Catheter-acquired candidemia in the immunocompetent host responds to 400 mg of fluconazole daily in conjunction with the removal of the infected catheter. Fluconazole is also effective in initial and maintenance therapy for cryptococcal meningitis in patients with AIDS, although most of these patients should initially receive a 2-week course of intravenous amphotericin B. Patients with coccidioidal meningitis can often be given fluconazole rather than intrathecal amphotericin B as maintenance therapy.

The incidence of deep candidiasis among recipients of allogeneic bone marrow transplants can be reduced by the administration of fluconazole (400 mg daily) for 75 days after initiation of the transplantation-preparative regimen. Prophylaxis in other neutropenic patients has not appeared useful. Fluconazole (200 mg daily) reduced the incidence of cryptococcosis and mucosal candidiasis among AIDS patients whose CD4+ cell counts were <200/μL and was particularly effective among those with counts of <50/μL. However, this regimen is not recommended because it does not reduce mortality, is expensive, and can lead to drug resistance.

Fluconazole is less effective than itraconazole in blastomycosis, histoplasmosis, and sporotrichosis. The drug is not active in aspergillosis or mucormycosis.

Amphotericin B A colloidal preparation of the polyene drug amphotericin B is available for intravenous or intrathecal administration. In-line filters with a 0.22-μm pore diameter may trap some of the colloid. The catabolism of amphotericin B is extremely slow and is not influenced by renal failure, hepatic failure, or hemodialysis. The drug's penetration into CSF and vitreous humor is poor; however, the concentrations in pleural, peritoneal, and articular exudates are adequate for many mycoses. Histoplasmosis, blastomycosis, paracoccidioidomycosis, candidiasis, and cryptococcosis are the most responsive mycoses; coccidioidomycosis, extraarticular sporotrichosis, aspergillosis, and mucormycosis are less responsive; and chromoblastomycosis, mycetoma, and pseudallescheriasis respond little, if at all. The usual course is 0.5 to 0.7 mg/kg daily for 8 to 10 weeks. Infusions are generally given in 5% dextrose over 2 to 4 h.

Initial doses of amphotericin B occasionally cause marked febrile reactions that may be poorly tolerated by adult patients with limited cardiac or pulmonary function. It may be prudent to give such patients an initial 1-mg test dose followed by rapidly escalating doses, depending on tolerance. Premedication with aspirin or acetaminophen or the addition of hydrocortisone (25 mg) to the infusion decreases chills and fever. Azotemia during treatment is usual, the extent depending on the daily dose. Saline infusions have been advocated to reduce azotemia. Permanent loss of renal function is related to the total dose of amphotericin B; this condition is generally noted in adults who have received more than 3 g. Other side effects include anemia, hypokalemia, renal tubular acidosis, nausea, anorexia, weight loss, phlebitis, and occasionally hypomagnesemia. Intrathecal amphotericin B has been used in coccidioidal meningitis and refractory cryptococcal meningitis, although this therapy is associated with considerable toxicity.

Newer formulations of intravenous amphotericin B have been marketed overseas and are in the process of becoming commercially available in the United States: amphotericin B lipid complex (ABLC), amphotericin B colloidal dispersion (ABCD), and a liposomal formulation (AmBisome). At doses two to five times higher than those used with the deoxycholate preparation, the nephrotoxicity of all three newer formulations has been minimal. Chills and hypokalemia have been reported with the latter two. No comparative efficacy trials have been conducted, and the indications for these more expensive formulations remain unknown. On the basis of uncontrolled trials, ABLC is marketed in the United States for the narrow indication of refractory aspergillosis; the recommended dose is 5 mg/kg daily. The deoxycholate formulation of amphotericin B has also been mixed with the intravenous lipid used for parenteral nutrition; the nephrotoxicity of this combination appears to be less than that of the deoxycholate formulation alone, but the effect of this mixing on antifungal efficacy remains to be determined.

Flucytosine Flucytosine (5-fluorocytosine) is a synthetic oral drug useful in cryptococcosis, candidiasis, and chromoblastomycosis. Within the fungal cell, flucytosine is converted to the antimetabolite 5-fluorouracil. Drug resistance appears rather rapidly when flucytosine is used alone. For this reason, the drug is generally used in combination with amphotericin B. The usual dose of flucytosine is 25 to 37.5 mg/kg every 6 h. Flucytosine is well absorbed from the gastrointestinal tract. The drug penetrates well into the CSF and is excreted unchanged in the urine. Even modest reductions in renal function may elevate flucytosine blood levels into the toxic range ($\geq$100 to 125 μg/mL). Elevated levels are associated with a significant incidence of neutropenia and thrombocytopenia and also seem to predispose to colitis, the other major toxic effect of this drug. Hepatotoxicity is idiosyncratic and uncommon. An allergic rash may develop.

BIBLIOGRAPHY

GENERAL

Kwon-Chung KJ, Bennett JE: *Medical Mycology.* Philadelphia, Lea & Febiger, 1992

THERAPY

Bennett JE: Antifungal agents, in *Mandell, Douglas and Bennett's Principles and Practice of Infectious Diseases,* 4th ed, GL Mandell et al (eds). New York, Churchill Livingstone, 1995, pp 401–410
Bowden RA et al: Phase 1 study of amphotericin B colloidal dispersion for the treatment of invasive fungal infections after bone marrow transplant. J Infect Dis 173:1208, 1996
Lazar JD, Hilligoss DM: The clinical pharmacology of fluconazole. Semin Oncol 17:14, 1990
Powderly WG et al: A randomized trial comparing fluconazole with clotrimazole troches for the prevention of fungal infections in patients with advanced human immunodeficiency virus infection. N Engl J Med 332:700, 1995
Slavin MA et al: Efficacy and safety of fluconazole prophylaxis for fungal infections after marrow transplantation—a prospective, randomized, double-blind trial. J Infect Dis 171:1545, 1995
Tucker RM et al: Adverse events associated with itraconazole in 189 patients on chronic therapy. J Antimicrob Chemother 26:561, 1991

203   *John E. Bennett*

HISTOPLASMOSIS

ETIOLOGIC AGENT *Histoplasma capsulatum* is a dimorphic fungus that grows as a mold in nature or on Sabouraud's agar at room temperature. Hyphae bear both large and small spores, which are used for identification. Nucleic acid hybridization can also be used to identify the organism in culture. *H. capsulatum* grows as a small

budding yeast in host tissue and on enriched agar, such as blood cysteine glucose, at 37°C. Despite its name, the fungus is unencapsulated. Coculture of isolates with opposite mating types can produce the perfect state called *Ajellomyces capsulatus.* (The reader is referred to standard textbooks of medical mycology for an explanation of the perfect state.)

EPIDEMIOLOGY Infection with *H. capsulatum* has been encountered in many areas of the world but is much more frequent in certain areas. Within the United States, infection is most common in the southeastern, mid-Atlantic, and central states. Endemicity is probably contingent on the availability of proper conditions in nature for growth of the fungus. *H. capsulatum* prefers moist surface soil, particularly soil enriched by droppings of certain birds and bats. The fungus has been isolated repeatedly from such sites, and many case clusters have occurred 5 to 18 days after the exposure of groups of people to dust, while (for example) raking, cleaning dirt-floored chicken coops, bulldozing, or cave exploring. Skin-test reactivity in many endemic areas indicates that 80 percent or more of residents over age 16 have been exposed.

PATHOGENESIS AND PATHOLOGY Microconidia, or small spores, of *H. capsulatum* are small enough to reach the alveoli on inhalation and are transformed there to budding forms. With time, an intense granulomatous reaction occurs. Caseation necrosis or calcification may mimic tuberculosis. In children, the primary infection usually heals completely but may leave spotty calcification in the hilar nodes or lung. Transient dissemination may leave calcified granulomas in the spleen. In adults, a rounded mass of scar tissue, with or without central calcification, may remain in the lung. This mass has been called a *histoplasmoma.* Previous exposure is thought to confer some protection against reinfection, but infection in persons with prior positive skin tests clearly has occurred.

In a small proportion of patients, histoplasmosis becomes a progressive, potentially fatal infection. The disease occurs either as chronic fibrocavitary pneumonia or, less commonly, as disseminated infection. Patients with either form lack a history of acute primary pulmonary histoplasmosis. Chronic pulmonary infection favors otherwise healthy males over the age of 40. A history of cigarette use is elicited from nearly all patients with chronic progressive pulmonary histoplasmosis. An acute, rapidly fatal course is most likely to be encountered among young children and immunosuppressed patients, including those with AIDS. A more chronic but equally lethal disseminated infection is more common among previously healthy adults.

CLINICAL MANIFESTATIONS The vast majority of infections are either asymptomatic or mild, and the diagnosis is elusive. Cough, fever, malaise, and chest x-ray findings of hilar adenopathy with or without one or more areas of pneumonitis are typical features. Erythema nodosum and erythema multiforme have been reported in a few outbreaks. Hilar adenopathy may cause temporary compression of the right-middle-lobe bronchus in children and young adults. Subacute pericarditis may develop, probably by extension from contiguous lymph nodes. Rarely, hilar nodes undergo a caseous, granulomatous reaction with perinodal fibrosis. Mediastinal structures become encased by progressive fibrosis, and compression of the pulmonary veins, superior vena cava, pulmonary arteries, and esophagus may take place over many years. Late in mediastinal disease, only rare nonviable *Histoplasma* cells can be found in caseous residua of lymph nodes.

Chronic pulmonary histoplasmosis is characterized by a gradual onset (over weeks or months) of increasing productive cough, weight loss, and sometimes night sweats. Chest x-ray reveals uni- or bilateral fibronodular apical infiltrates. Approximately one-third of cases stabilize or improve spontaneously early in the course. The remainder progress insidiously. Retraction and cavitation of the upper lobes occur, with spread to the apex of the lower lobes and other areas of the lung. Emphysema and bulla formation further compromise pulmonary function. Death from cor pulmonale, bacterial pneumonia, or histoplasmosis occurs after months or years.

Acute disseminated histoplasmosis may be mistaken for miliary tuberculosis (see Chap. 171). Common findings include fever, emaciation, hepatosplenomegaly, lymphadenopathy, jaundice, anemia, leukopenia, and thrombocytopenia. All these features may be noted in chronic dissemination as well, but chronic disease tends to be more localized. Indurated ulcers of the mouth, tongue, nose, or larynx are reported in about one-fourth of cases. Other focal findings include granulomatous hepatitis, Addison's disease, gastrointestinal ulceration, endocarditis, and chronic meningitis. Chest x-ray abnormalities are evident in half of cases and characteristically consist of discrete nodules or a miliary pattern.

The presumed *ocular histoplasmosis* syndrome is a distinct clinical form of uveitis. Although a positive histoplasmin skin test is a requisite for diagnosis, none of the patients involved has had active histoplasmosis.

Infection with *H. capsulatum* var. *duboisii* is rare outside of Africa. The yeast form is larger in tissue than that of *H. capsulatum* var. *capsulatum*. Clinical manifestations resemble those of blastomycosis more than those of histoplasmosis in that skin and bone lesions are very common.

DIAGNOSIS Culture of the etiologic organism is the preferred method for diagnosis of histoplasmosis but is often difficult. Blood cultures are best done by the lysis-centrifugation technique, with plates held at 30°C for at least 2 weeks. Approximately 15 mL of blood should be cultured from adults. Routine blood cultures in broth are generally unsuitable. Cultures of bone marrow, mucosal lesions, liver, and bronchoalveolar lavage fluid are diagnostically useful in disseminated histoplasmosis. Sputum culture is the preferred method for the diagnosis of chronic pulmonary histoplasmosis. However, growth may require 2 to 4 weeks to become visible, and other organisms may overgrow the plate. Diagnosis based on Giemsa-stained smears of blood or bronchoalveolar lavage fluid or on methenamine silver staining of infected lung, bone marrow, lymph node, or mucosal lesions requires considerable expertise, though these techniques yield results rapidly and provide specimens that can easily be sent to a referral laboratory. Organisms may be very scanty in lesions with marked caseous necrosis. A radioactive assay for *Histoplasma* antigen in blood or urine is commercially available and is useful both for diagnosis and for monitoring of the response to therapy in AIDS patients with disseminated infection. Tests for antibody to *H. capsulatum* have been of limited value. Histoplasmin skin testing has proven useful in epidemiologic studies but not in clinical diagnosis.

℞ TREATMENT

Acute pulmonary histoplasmosis requires no therapy. Patients with mediastinal fibrosis may benefit from surgery, but their ultimate prognosis is poor. All patients with disseminated or chronic fibronodular pulmonary histoplasmosis should receive chemotherapy. Intravenous amphotericin B (0.6 mg/kg daily) is the drug of choice for the initial treatment of patients who are severely ill or immunosuppressed or whose infection involves the central nervous system; the regimen can be changed to itraconazole (200 mg twice daily) once clinical improvement is evident in these patients. For AIDS patients with disseminated histoplasmosis who are known to have blood levels of itraconazole (measured by bioassay) of at least 2 µg/mL, the dose can be decreased to 200 mg once daily after 10 weeks. Maintenance therapy with itraconazole is continued for life in AIDS patients.

Immunocompetent patients can initially be given itraconazole (200 mg twice daily) and are generally treated for 6 to 12 months. Ketoconazole (400 to 800 mg once daily) can be used instead of itraconazole for the treatment of immunocompetent patients without central nervous system disease when the lower cost is more important than the higher complication rate. Alternatively, immunocompetent patients can be given a 10-week course of amphotericin B (0.5 mg/kg daily).

Whatever drug is administered, relapse is not rare, particularly among patients who are immunocompromised or have endocarditis.

BIBLIOGRAPHY

GOODWIN RA et al: Histoplasmosis in normal hosts. Medicine 60:231, 1981
RAYMOND LW et al: Scars without wounds: Spectrum of delayed manifestations of histoplasmosis outside of the endemic area. Crit Rev Diagn Imaging 14:37, 1980

WHEAT JL et al: Disseminated histoplasmosis in the acquired immune deficiency syndrome: Clinical findings, diagnosis and treatment, and review of the literature. Medicine 69:361, 1990
————: Endemic mycoses in AIDS: A clinical review. Clin Microbiol Rev 8:146, 1995
———— et al: Itraconazole treatment of disseminated histoplasmosis in patients with the acquired immunodeficiency syndrome. Am J Med 98:336, 1995

204 *John E. Bennett*

COCCIDIOIDOMYCOSIS

ETIOLOGIC AGENT *Coccidioides immitis* has two forms, growing as a white fluffy mold on most culture media but as a nonbudding spherical form (a spherule) in host tissue or under specialized conditions. The organism reproduces in host tissue by forming small endospores within mature spherules. After rupture of the spherule, the released endospores enlarge, become spherules, and repeat the cycle. The fungus is identified by its appearance and by the formation of thick-walled, barrel-shaped spores, called *arthrospores*, in the hyphae of the mold form.

EPIDEMIOLOGY, PATHOGENESIS, AND PATHOLOGY *C. immitis* is a soil saprophyte found in certain arid regions of the United States, Mexico, Central America, and South America. Within the United States, most cases of infection with *C. immitis* are acquired in California, Arizona, and western Texas. A few cases are acquired by exposure to fomites from endemic areas (e.g., in cotton bales).

Infection in humans and animals results from inhalation of windborne arthrospores from soil sites. This primary pulmonary infection is symptomatic in only 40 percent of cases, with symptoms ranging from a mild influenza-like illness to severe pneumonia. Mild self-limited infections may come to medical attention because of case clusters or hypersensitivity reactions: erythema nodosum, erythema multiforme, toxic erythema, arthralgia, arthritis, conjunctivitis, or episcleritis. Case clusters occur 10 to 14 days after a group of susceptible individuals is exposed to dust in an endemic area through such activities as unearthing Indian relics, rock hunting, participating in military maneuvers, or doing construction work. Windstorms can carry spores to adjacent nonendemic areas and cause case clusters. The usual course of primary pneumonia is complete healing, although an area of pneumonitis (detected on radiographs) may heal by the formation of a coinlike lesion called a *coccidioidoma*. Less commonly, a single thin-walled cavity remains as a chronic sequela in the area of consolidation. The consolidation may persist as chronic pneumonia or progress to fibronodular cavitary disease.

Pleural effusion may be the only manifestation of primary infection. Spontaneous healing of this form is common.

An uncommon but dreaded complication of coccidioidomycosis is dissemination beyond the lung and hilar lymph nodes. Dissemination is especially frequent among blacks, Filipinos, Native Americans, Mexican-Americans, pregnant women, and immunosuppressed patients, including those with AIDS.

C. immitis incites a chronic granulomatous reaction in host tissue, often with caseation necrosis. Lung and hilar node lesions may show calcification. Both IgM and IgG antibodies to *C. immitis* are induced by infection, but neither type of antibody appears to be protective. The amount of specific IgG antibody is a rough measure of the antigenic mass (i.e., of the intensity of infection), and a high titer is a poor prognostic sign. Appearance of delayed hypersensitivity to antigens of *C. immitis* is most common in clinical forms of disease with a good prognosis, such as self-limited primary pulmonary disease. In skin tests for *Coccidioides* antigens about half of patients with disseminated disease have negative results that portend a poor outcome.

CLINICAL MANIFESTATIONS   Symptomatic primary pulmonary infection is manifested by fever, cough, chest pain, malaise, and sometimes the hypersensitivity reactions listed above. Chest radiographs may show an infiltrate, hilar adenopathy, or pleural effusion. Mild peripheral-blood eosinophilia may be found. Spontaneous improvement begins after several days to 2 weeks of illness and usually culminates in complete recovery.

The symptoms of a chronic thin-walled cavity include cough or hemoptysis in half of cases; the other half are asymptomatic. Chronic progressive pulmonary coccidioidomycosis causes cough, sputum production, variable degrees of fever, and weight loss. The first indications of dissemination usually appear during primary infection. Reactivation with dissemination in later years occurs occasionally, especially if Hodgkin's disease, non-Hodgkin's lymphoma, renal transplantation, AIDS, or immunosuppression of some other etiology has supervened. Dissemination should be suspected when fever, malaise, hilar or paratracheal lymphadenopathy, elevated sedimentation rate, and high complement fixation titers signal abnormal persistence in patients with primary pulmonary coccidioidomycosis. With time, lesions appear in the bone, skin, subcutaneous tissue, meninges, joints, and other sites. Chronic meningitis may be the only presenting manifestation of disseminated coccidioidomycosis. Cultures and smears of cerebrospinal fluid (CSF) are most often negative, but antibody is usually detectable in CSF by complement fixation. Skin lesions are indolent and maculopapular; soft tissue and bony lesions contain pus and may present as a draining sinus. Without treatment, disseminated coccidioidomycosis progresses to death over weeks to years.

DIAGNOSIS   When coccidioidomycosis is suspected, sputum, urine, and pus should be examined for *C. immitis* by wet smear and culture. *The laboratory request should indicate clearly that coccidioidomycosis is suspected, because the mold form must be handled with extreme care to prevent infection of laboratory personnel.* On biopsy, smaller spherules must be distinguished from nonbudding forms of *Blastomyces* and *Cryptococcus*, but the appearance of the mature spherule is diagnostic.

Serologic tests are very helpful in the diagnosis of coccidioidomycosis. Latex agglutination and agar gel diffusion tests are useful in screening sera for antibody to *Coccidioides*. The complement fixation test is used for CSF determinations and for the confirmation and quantitation of serum antibody detected by screening tests. The number of cases with a positive complement fixation test depends on the severity of disease and on the laboratory performing the test. Positive tests are least common among patients with solitary pulmonary cavities or primary pulmonary infection, while sera from patients with disseminated disease in multiple organs are nearly all positive. Seroconversion is helpful in primary pulmonary coccidioidomycosis but may not occur for up to 8 weeks after onset. A positive complement fixation test of unconcentrated CSF is diagnostic of meningitis. Rarely, a parameningeal focus causes a positive complement fixation test of CSF.

Conversion of the skin test from negative to positive (≥ 5 mm of induration at 24 or 48 h) with either coccidioidin or spherulin, the two commercially available antigens, may take place between days 3 and 21 of symptoms in primary pulmonary coccidioidomycosis. Skin testing can be helpful in epidemiologic studies, such as investigations of case clusters or the definition of endemic areas. The utility of skin testing as a diagnostic tool is limited by the persistence of positive tests resulting from remote exposures to *Coccidioides* and by the frequency of negative skin tests among patients with either thin-walled cavities or disseminated coccidioidomycosis.

℞ **TREATMENT**

Primary pulmonary coccidioidomycosis usually resolves spontaneously. Some physicians give a few weeks of treatment with intravenous amphotericin B or itraconazole to patients with unusually severe or protracted primary infection in the hope of aborting disseminated or chronic pulmonary disease.

Patients with severe or rapidly progressing disseminated coccidioidomycosis are first given intravenous amphotericin B at a dose of 0.5 to 0.7 mg/kg daily. Patients whose condition improves after 2 to 3 months of treatment with amphotericin B or who have more indolent disseminated infection are given ketoconazole (400 mg/d), itraconazole (200 mg twice daily), or fluconazole (400 to 600 mg/d). These oral agents are useful for long-term suppression of infection, and treatment should be continued for years. Patients with coccidioidal meningitis usually are initially given fluconazole (400 to 800 mg/d) but may require intrathecal amphotericin B. Hydrocephalus is a frequent complication of uncontrolled meningitis. Surgical debridement of bone lesions or drainage of abscesses can be helpful. The prognosis for ultimate cure of disseminated coccidioidomycosis is guarded.

Resection of chronic progressive pulmonary lesions is a helpful adjunct to chemotherapy when infection is confined to the lung and to one lobe. A single thin-walled cavity tends to close spontaneously and ordinarily is not resected. Such a cavity responds poorly to chemotherapy.

BIBLIOGRAPHY

FISH DG et al: Coccidioidomycosis during human immunodeficiency virus infection. A review of 77 patients. Medicine 69:384, 1990

GRAYBILL JR et al: Itraconazole treatment of coccidioidomycosis. Am J Med 89:282, 1990

PEREZ JA et al: Fluconazole therapy in coccidioidal meningitis maintained with intrathecal amphotericin B. Arch Intern Med 155:1665, 1995

STEVENS DA: Coccidioidomycosis. N Engl J Med 332:1077, 1995

VINCENT T et al: The natural history of coccidioidal meningitis: VA-Armed Forces Cooperative Studies, 1955–58. Clin Infect Dis 16:247, 1993

205   *John E. Bennett*

BLASTOMYCOSIS

ETIOLOGIC AGENT   *Blastomyces dermatitidis* is a dimorphic fungus that grows at room temperature as a white or tan mold but grows within the host or at 37°C as budding, round yeastlike cells. The fungus can be identified on the basis of its appearance, its dimorphism, the small spores borne on hyphae of the mold form, or the results of nucleic acid hybridization. When isolates of the two opposite mating types are grown close together on special culture medium, such as yeast extract or soil extract agar, sporulating structures that characterize the perfect state, called *Ajellomyces dermatitidis*, appear. (The reader is referred to standard textbooks of medical mycology for an explanation of the perfect state.)

EPIDEMIOLOGY   The infection is restricted by geography and age. Blastomycosis is uncommon in any locality, but most cases occur in the southeastern, central, and mid-Atlantic areas of the United States, with occasional cases in other localities in the United States and Canada. Cases have also been encountered in Africa, Mexico, Central America, and (rarely) South America. Most patients are between 20 and 69 years old. The male-to-female ratio is about 10:1. There is no occupational predisposition to the development of blastomycosis.

PATHOGENESIS AND PATHOLOGY   Infection with *B. dermatitidis* appears to be acquired by inhalation of the fungus from soil, decomposed vegetation, or rotting wood. Several case clusters have resulted from participation in recreational activities in wooded areas along waterways. Infection is not transmissible from person to person. The initial pulmonary infection may either heal spontaneously or become chronic. Spread to other portions of the lung, cavitation, or endobronchial lesions may be found in chronic cases. Whether or not the lung lesion resolves spontaneously, infection commonly spreads hematogenously to the skin, subcutaneous tissue, bone, prostate, epididymis, or mucosa of the nose, mouth, or larynx. Less commonly, infection spreads to the brain, meninges, liver, lymph nodes, or spleen. Dissemination may not be evident for weeks or years after the appearance of the lung lesion. Progressive infection is only rarely attributable to an underlying disease or to immunosuppressive treatment. The inflammatory response includes lymphocytes, giant cells, and neutrophils. Pseudoepitheliomatous hyperplasia may be striking and may lead to a mistaken diagnosis of squamous cell carcinoma.

CLINICAL MANIFESTATIONS A few patients have acute, self-limited pneumonia. Fever, productive cough, myalgia, and malaise usually resolve within a month. Pulmonary infiltrates clear slowly as *B. dermatitidis* disappears from the sputum.

In the vast majority of cases, blastomycosis has an indolent onset and a chronically progressive course. Fever, cough, weight loss, lassitude, skin lesions, and chest ache are common. Skin lesions favor exposed areas and enlarge over many weeks from pimples to well-circumscribed, verrucous, crusted, or ulcerated lesions. Pain and regional lymphadenopathy are minimal. Large chronic lesions may undergo central healing with scarring and contracture. Mucous membrane lesions resemble squamous cell carcinoma. Chest x-ray findings are abnormal in two-thirds of cases, with one or more pneumonic or nodular infiltrates. Calcification, hilar adenopathy, and large pleural effusions are rare. Osteolytic lesions may be found in nearly any bone and present as a cold abscess or a draining sinus. Extension to a contiguous joint may cause indolent swelling, pain, and restricted motion. Prostatic and epididymal lesions clinically resemble those of tuberculosis.

DIAGNOSIS The diagnosis of blastomycosis is made by demonstration of the fungus in a culture of sputum, pus, or urine. An expert can diagnose blastomycosis on the basis of the appearance of the organism in wet smear or histopathologic section. The fungus may be visible in a sputum cytology smear but is easily overlooked.

℞ **TREATMENT**

A few patients have developed only transitory lung lesions, but no guidelines are known to distinguish these patients from those whose disease will progress locally or disseminate. Therefore, every patient should receive treatment. Intravenous amphotericin B is the drug of choice for patients with rapidly progressive infections, severe illness, or meningitis. Skin and noncavitary lung lesions should be treated for about 8 to 10 weeks. The recommended total dose for an adult is about 2.0 g. Cavitary lung disease or infection extending beyond the lung and skin should be treated for about 10 to 12 weeks with 2.5 g or more.

Itraconazole (200 mg twice daily with food) is the drug of choice for the treatment of patients who have indolent nonmeningeal blastomycosis of mild to moderate severity and who take the drug reliably. Ketoconazole (400 to 800 mg daily) is an effective alternative agent. Therapy with either itraconazole or ketoconazole is continued for 6 to 12 months.

The mortality rate in appropriately treated cases is 15 percent or less.

BIBLIOGRAPHY

BAUMGARDNER DJ et al: Epidemiology of blastomycosis in a region of high endemicity in north-central Wisconsin. Clin Infect Dis 15:629, 1992

BRADSHER RW: Blastomycosis: Fungal infections of the lung. Update 1989. Semin Respir Infect 5:105, 1990

MANGINO JE, PAPPAS PG: Itraconazole for the treatment of histoplasmosis and blastomycosis. Int J Antimicrob Agents 5:219, 1995

PAPPAS PG et al: Blastomycosis in immunocompromised patients. Medicine 72:311, 1993

206 *John E. Bennett*

CRYPTOCOCCOSIS

ETIOLOGIC AGENT Cryptococcosis is an infection caused by the yeastlike fungus *Cryptococcus neoformans*. This fungus reproduces by budding and forms round, yeastlike cells. Within the host and on certain culture media, a large polysaccharide capsule surrounds each yeast cell. The fungus grows well in smooth, creamy-white colonies on Sabouraud's or other simple media at 20 to 37°C. Certain culture media for ringworm contain cycloheximide, which inhibits the growth of *C. neoformans*. Identification of the organism is based on gross and microscopic appearance, biochemical test results, and growth at 37°C. The results of nucleic acid hybridization or the formation of brown pigment on Niger seed agar can also be used for identification.

The fungus has four capsular serotypes, designated A, B, C, and D. There are also two mating types. Coculture of opposite mating types creates a transient diploid state called *Filobasidiella neoformans* var. *neoformans* for serotypes A and D and *Filobasidiella neoformans* var. *bacillispora* for serotypes B and C. Organisms not cultured under mating conditions are designated *C. neoformans* var. *neoformans* for serotypes A and D and *C. neoformans* var. *gattii* for serotypes B and C; a simple color medium distinguishes the two varieties.

EPIDEMIOLOGY Weathered pigeon droppings commonly contain serotype A or D (*C. neoformans* var. *neoformans*). *C. neoformans* var. *gattii* has been isolated from the litter around eucalyptus trees of the species *Eucalyptus camaldulensis* and *Eucalyptus tereticornis*. The latter isolates have so far typed as serotype B. The distribution of these eucalyptus species in Australia corresponds to the distribution of infections due to *C. neoformans* var. *gattii* in that country. The high prevalence of these trees in other subtropical climates has been postulated to explain the relative restriction of such infections to warm climates.

Cryptococcosis due to *C. neoformans* var. *neoformans* is a common complication of late infection with human immunodeficiency virus (HIV), having occurred in 6.2% of the 274,150 AIDS patients reported to the Centers for Disease Control and Prevention as of September 1993. Patients who have undergone solid-organ transplantation or glucocorticoid therapy and those with sarcoidosis are also at increased risk for infections with *C. neoformans* var. *neoformans*. Almost all such infections are caused by serotype A, although serotype D occurs in up to 20 percent of cases in Western Europe. Infections with var. *gattii* have been rare among AIDS patients and other immunocompromised patients, even in subtropical climates, where var. *gattii* infection occurs in previously healthy individuals.

Animals, particularly cats, can acquire cryptococcosis but have not transmitted the infection to other animals or to humans. The source from which humans acquire the infection is unknown, with the rare exception of cases acquired through a transplanted cornea, kidney, or other solid organ. Cryptococcosis is rare before puberty.

PATHOGENESIS AND PATHOLOGY Infection is thought to be acquired by inhalation of fungus into the lungs. Pulmonary infection has a tendency toward spontaneous resolution and is frequently asymptomatic. Silent hematogenous spread to the brain leads to clusters of cryptococci in the perivascular areas of cortical gray matter, in the basal ganglia, and, to a lesser extent, in other areas of the central nervous system. The inflammatory response around these foci is usually scant. In the more chronic cases, a dense basilar arachnoiditis is typical. Lung lesions are characterized by intense granulomatous inflammation. Cryptococci are best seen in tissue by staining with methenamine silver or periodic acid–Schiff. Although a strongly positive result upon mucicarmine staining of tissue is diagnostic, staining varies from intense to absent.

CLINICAL MANIFESTATIONS Most patients have *meningoencephalitis* at the time of diagnosis. This form of the infection is invariably fatal without appropriate therapy; death occurs any time from 2 weeks to several years after the onset of symptoms. Early manifestations include headache, nausea, staggering gait, dementia, irritability, confusion, and blurred vision. Both fever and nuchal rigidity are often mild or lacking. Papilledema is evident in one-third of cases at the time of diagnosis. Cranial nerve palsies, typically asymmetric, occur in about one-fourth of cases. Other lateralized signs are rare. With progression of the infection, deepening coma and signs of brainstem compression appear. Autopsy often reveals cerebral edema in more acute cases and hydrocephalus in more chronic cases.

Pulmonary cryptococcosis causes chest pain in about 40 percent of patients and cough in 20 percent. The chest x-ray shows one or more dense infiltrates, which are often well circumscribed. Cavitation, pleural effusions, and hilar adenopathy are infrequent. Calcification is not evident, and fibrotic stranding is rarely noticeable.

Ten percent of patients with cryptococcosis have skin lesions, and the vast majority of patients with skin lesions have disseminated infection. One or a few asymptomatic tiny papular lesions appear and slowly enlarge; and they display a tendency toward central softening leading to ulceration. Osteolytic lesions occur in 4 percent of cases and usually present as a cold abscess. Rare manifestations of cryptococcosis include prostatitis, endophthalmitis, hepatitis, pericarditis, endocarditis, and renal abscess.

DIAGNOSIS Fever and headache in a patient with AIDS or with risk factors for HIV infection suggest the possibility of cryptococcosis, toxoplasmosis, or central nervous system lymphoma. Evidence of a focal lesion on magnetic resonance imaging is unusual in cryptococcosis. Most cryptococcal cerebral mass lesions occur in patients infected with *C. neoformans* var. *gattii* who also have meningitis. In patients without AIDS, meningitis due to *C. neoformans* resembles that due to *Mycobacterium tuberculosis*, *Histoplasma capsulatum*, *Coccidioides immitis*, or metastatic cancer. Lumbar puncture is the single most useful diagnostic test. An india ink smear of centrifuged cerebrospinal fluid (CSF) sediment reveals encapsulated yeast in more than half of cases, although artifacts can cause confusion. In patients without AIDS, levels of glucose in CSF are reduced in half of all cases; protein levels are usually increased; and lymphocytic pleocytosis is usually found. CSF abnormalities are less pronounced in patients with AIDS, though india ink smear is more often positive.

Approximately 90 percent of patients with cryptococcal meningoencephalitis, including all those with a positive CSF smear, have capsular antigen detectable in CSF or serum by latex agglutination. An enzyme immunoassay for cryptococcal antigen is also available. Occasional false-positive results in the above tests make culture the definitive diagnostic test. *C. neoformans* is often present in urine from patients with meningoencephalitis. Fungemia occurs in 10 to 30 percent of patients and is particularly common among AIDS patients.

Pulmonary cryptococcosis mimics malignancy with regard to radiographic findings and symptoms. Sputum culture is positive in only 10 percent of cases, and serum antigen tests are positive in only one-third. Occasionally, *C. neoformans* appears in one or more sputum specimens as an endobronchial saprophyte. Biopsy is usually required for diagnosis.

Cutaneous cryptococcosis may be mistaken for a comedo, basal cell carcinoma, or sarcoidosis. In AIDS patients, skin lesions may be numerous and are sometimes mistaken for molluscum contagiosum. Biopsy reveals myriad cryptococci. Osseous cryptococcosis resembles tuberculosis.

℞ **TREATMENT**

Patients with AIDS and cryptococcosis are treated initially with intravenous amphotericin B (with or without flucytosine) and later with fluconazole. During active infection, fluconazole (400 mg) is given once daily. After infection is controlled, treatment with a smaller dose of fluconazole (200 mg daily) is continued indefinitely. Itraconazole is less effective than fluconazole for maintenance therapy.

In patients without AIDS, cryptococcosis may be treated with amphotericin B alone or in combination with flucytosine. Amphotericin B is given in a dose of 0.5 to 0.7 mg/kg per day when used alone and in a dose of 0.3 to 0.5 mg/kg per day when used in combination with flucytosine. Flucytosine is given initially in a dose of 25 to 37.5 mg/kg every 6 h to patients with normal renal function. Although nomograms are available for adjusting flucytosine dosage in the presence of reduced renal function, the best way to prevent toxicity is to measure serum levels frequently and to maintain them between 50 and 100 μg/mL.

The duration of therapy in patients without AIDS is based on the results of lumbar punctures, which are best done weekly until culture conversion is clearly demonstrated. Six weeks of therapy may be adequate for patients whose CSF (2 to 4 mL) is cultured weekly and remains sterile for at least 4 weeks, whose india ink smear has become negative, and whose CSF glucose level is normal. Declining titers of cryptococcal antigen in CSF offer some assurance of therapeutic success; in contrast, serum antigen titers, while useful in diagnosis, have not proven useful in evaluation of the response to therapy. Approximately 50 to 70 percent of cases of cryptococcosis in non-AIDS patients are cured.

Hydrocephalus may be the presenting manifestation or a later complication of cryptococcosis. Blindness, dementia, and personality change are among the other sequelae. Daily lumbar puncture or CSF shunting has been advocated—in the hope of averting permanent blindness—for patients with marked cerebral edema who have incipient blurred vision.

Patients with extraneural cryptococcosis most often require treatment with intravenous amphotericin B, with or without flucytosine. Observation or excision of lesions may suffice for some patients who have previously been healthy; who have a single focus in lung, skin, or bone; and who have no cryptococci in CSF, urine, or blood. No guidelines are yet available for the use of fluconazole in non-AIDS patients. For reasons presented elsewhere (see Chap. 202), fluconazole is not recommended for the prevention of cryptococcosis in AIDS patients.

BIBLIOGRAPHY

MEYOHAS M-C et al: Pulmonary cryptococcosis: Localized and disseminated infections in 27 patients with AIDS. Clin Infect Dis 21:628, 1995

MURAKAWA GJ et al: Cutaneous *Cryptococcus* infection and AIDS: Report of 12 cases and review of the literature. Arch Dermatol 132:545, 1996

PINNER RW et al: Prospects for preventing cryptococcosis in persons infected with human immunodeficiency virus. Clin Infect Dis 21:S103, 1995

POWDERLY WG et al: Measurement of cryptococcal antigen in serum and cerebrospinal fluid: Value in the management of AIDS-associated cryptococcal meningitis. Clin Infect Dis 18:789, 1994

REX JR et al: Catastrophic visual loss due to *Cryptococcus neoformans* meningitis. Medicine 72:207, 1993

SPEED B, DUNT D: Clinical and host differences between infections with the two varieties of *Cryptococcus neoformans*. Clin Infect Dis 21:28, 1995

WHITE M et al: Cryptococcal meningitis: Outcome in patients with AIDS and patients with neoplastic disease. J Infect Dis 165:690, 1992

207   *John E. Bennett*

CANDIDIASIS

ETIOLOGIC AGENTS *Candida albicans* is the most common cause of candidiasis, but *Candida tropicalis*, *Candida parapsilosis*, *Candida guilliermondii*, *Candida glabrata*, *Candida krusei*, and a few other species can cause deep candidiasis that is sometimes fatal. *C. parapsilosis* is particularly notable for its ability to cause endocarditis. *C. tropicalis* accounts for about one-third of the cases of deep candidiasis in neutropenic patients.

All *Candida* species pathogenic for humans are also encountered as commensals of humans, particularly in the mouth, stool, and vagina. These species grow rapidly at 25 to 37°C on simple media as oval, budding cells. In special culture media and in tissue, hyphae or elongated branching structures called *pseudohyphae* are formed. *C. glabrata*, formerly called *Torulopsis glabrata*, differs from other members of the genus in that it forms no true hyphae or pseudohyphae in vitro or in infected tissue. *C. albicans* can be identified presumptively by its ability to form germ tubes in serum or by the formation of thick-walled large spores called *chlamydospores*. Final identification of all species requires biochemical tests.

PATHOGENESIS Candidiasis is often preceded by increased colonization of the mouth, vagina, and stool with *Candida* due to broad-spectrum antibiotic therapy. Additional local and systemic factors favor infection. Oropharyngeal thrush is particularly likely to occur in neonates and in patients with diabetes mellitus, human immunodeficiency virus (HIV) infection, or dentures. Vulvovaginal candidiasis is especially common in the third trimester of pregnancy. *Candida* from the perineum can enter the urinary tract via an indwelling bladder catheter. Cutaneous candidiasis most often involves macerated skin, such as that in the diapered area of infants, under pendulous breasts, or on hands constantly in water or covered by occlusive gloves. *Candida* can pass from the colonized surface into deep tissue when the integrity of the mucosa or skin is violated, as, for example, by perforation of the gastrointestinal tract through trauma, surgery, or peptic ulceration or by mucosal damage due to cytotoxic agents used for cancer chemotherapy. Although *Candida* is not normally a resident of the skin, secretions from the mouth, rectum, or vagina as well as drainage from surgical wounds or tracheostomy sites can contaminate the hub or skin site of a catheter in an umbilical or central vein, and this contamination can lead to severe *Candida* sepsis. Intravenous drug abuse or third-degree burns can also provide a skin portal for *Candida* that can lead to deep candidiasis. Once *Candida* has passed the integumentary barrier, very low birth weight (in neonates) and neutropenia or glucocorticoid therapy (in any patient) markedly decrease host defense. Hematogenous seeding is particularly evident in the retina, kidney, spleen, and liver.

CLINICAL MANIFESTATIONS *Oral thrush* presents as discrete and confluent adherent white plaques on the oral and pharyngeal mucosa, particularly in the mouth and on the tongue. These lesions are usually painless, but fissuring at the corners of the mouth can be painful. Unexplained oropharyngeal thrush raises the possibility of HIV infection. Oral thrush is common in acute HIV infection and becomes increasingly common as the CD4+ cell count falls. At CD4+ counts below 50/μL, esophageal thrush also becomes common. HIV infection appears not to be an independent risk factor for vulvovaginal thrush.

Cutaneous candidiasis presents as red macerated intertriginous areas, paronychia, balanitis, or pruritus ani. Candidiasis of the perineal and scrotal skin may be accompanied by discrete pustular lesions on the inner aspects of the thighs. *Chronic mucocutaneous candidiasis* or *Candida granuloma* typically presents as circumscribed hyperkeratotic skin lesions, crumbling dystrophic nails, partial alopecia in areas of scalp lesions, and both oral and vaginal thrush. Systemic infection is very rare, but disfigurement of the face and hands can be severe. Other findings may include chronic epidermophytosis, dental dysplasia, and hypofunction of the parathyroid, adrenal, or thyroid gland. A variety of defects in T cell function have been described in these patients. Vulvovaginal thrush causes pruritus, discharge, and sometimes pain on intercourse or urination. Speculum examination reveals an inflamed mucosa and a thin exudate, often with white curds.

Esophageal candidiasis is often asymptomatic but can cause substernal pain or a sense of obstruction on swallowing. Most lesions are in the distal third of the esophagus and appear on endoscopy as areas of redness and edema, focal white patches, or ulcers. Biopsy or brushing is required for the diagnosis and detection of concomitant infections, particularly herpes simplex in patients with hematologic malignancies and cytomegalovirus infection in AIDS patients. Esophagraphy is diagnostically insensitive but may reveal spasm or mucosal irregularities. *Candida* esophagitis can cause bleeding and impaired alimentation. Hematogenous dissemination from the esophagus probably occurs in some neutropenic patients but is rarely reported in HIV-infected patients.

Candida can cause cystitis, pyelitis, or renal papillary necrosis in an obstructed urinary tract. When a colonized urinary tract is operated on or instrumented, candidemia may result. However, most patients with *Candida* cultured from the urine simply have bladder colonization from a Foley catheter or a sizable volume of residual urine. Contamination of a voided midstream specimen by vaginal *Candida* is also common.

Hematogenous seeding can cause a wide spectrum of illnesses, ranging from septic shock to fever alone; the etiology of these conditions becomes clear later, when focal abscesses develop in multiple organs. Retinal lesions are visible on funduscopy within 2 weeks and

should be sought in all patients with candidemia. Blurred vision, scotoma, or ocular pain may not be noted for weeks, especially by obtunded or sedated patients. The earliest lesions are retinal exudates, unilateral in half of cases. Extension of lesions leads to vitreitis, vitreal abscess, retinal detachment, and hypopyon. Most cases with ocular involvement have occurred in nonneutropenic patients. In contrast, so-called hepatosplenic candidiasis is usually recognized in patients with acute leukemia who are recovering from profound neutropenia. This entity, better called *chronic disseminated candidiasis*, originates from intestinal seeding of the portal and venous circulation. Fever, modestly elevated serum concentrations of alkaline phosphatase, and multiple small abscesses evident on ultrasonography, magnetic resonance imaging, or computed tomography of the liver, spleen, or kidney suggest the diagnosis. During acute candidemia in neutropenic patients, small erythematous papules may appear anywhere on the skin. If the patient does not expire promptly from disseminated candidiasis, the lesions will develop a necrotic center. Painful muscle lesions may also be found. Punch biopsy of a skin lesion helps distinguish this extremely grave condition from *Malassezia* furunculosis, a similar-appearing but benign condition that can involve the cape area of the chest or the extremities of a sweaty febrile patient.

Hematogenous seeding in the neutropenic patient is occasionally visible radiologically as tiny pulmonary nodules. *Candida* pneumonia, apart from hematogenous candidiasis, is very rare. Organisms seeding a native or prosthetic cardiac valve originate principally from central venous catheters; occasionally, valvular seeding is encountered in intravenous drug abusers. Emboli to large arteries, such as the iliac or femoral artery, are characteristic. Intravenous injection of impure brown heroin has caused a clinical syndrome consisting of *Candida* endophthalmitis and purulent folliculitis, sometimes accompanied by vertebral osteomyelitis. This diffuse folliculitis favors hairy areas, including the scalp and the area under the beard.

Candida can cause indolent arthritis, most commonly of the knee, in patients who have received glucocorticoid injections into the joint, in patients who are immunosuppressed, and in low-birth-weight neonates. Prosthetic joints may become infected during implantation. Scanty growth of *Candida* from joint fluid can cause the laboratory to incorrectly dismiss the organism as a contaminant.

Hematogenous dissemination can lead to brain abscess or chronic meningitis. Diagnosis of infections of ventriculoperitoneal shunts is difficult because symptoms are indolent and cultures of lumbar fluid are usually sterile.

DIAGNOSIS Demonstration of pseudohyphae on wet smear with confirmation by culture is the procedure of choice for diagnosing superficial candidiasis. Scrapings for the smear may be obtained from skin, nails, and oral and vaginal mucosa. Culture alone is not diagnostic; however, recovery of *Candida* species from multiple superficial sites in immunosuppressed patients may portend visceral invasion.

Deeper lesions due to *Candida* may be diagnosed by histologic section of biopsy specimens or by culture of cerebrospinal fluid, blood, joint fluid, or surgical specimens. Blood cultures are useful in the diagnosis of *Candida* endocarditis and intravenous catheter–induced sepsis but are positive less often in other forms of disseminated disease. Serologic tests for antibody or antigen are not useful.

℞ **TREATMENT**

Cutaneous candidiasis of macerated areas responds to measures that reduce moisture and chafing plus topical application of an antifungal agent in a nonocclusive base. Nystatin powder or a cream containing ciclopirox or an azole is useful. Clotrimazole, miconazole, econazole, ketoconazole, sulconazole, and oxiconazole are available as creams or lotions. *Candida* vulvovaginitis responds better to an azole than to nystatin suppositories. There is little difference in efficacy among miconazole, clotrimazole, tioconazole, butoconazole, and terconazole vaginal formulations. Systemic treatment of *Candida* vulvovaginitis with a single 150-mg capsule of fluconazole is more convenient than topical treatment but also poses a higher risk of adverse effects. Clotrimazole troches, used five times a day, are more effective in oral and esophageal candidiasis than nystatin suspension. Ketoconazole (200 to 400 mg daily) or itraconazole (200 mg daily) is also useful in *Candida* esophagitis, but many patients absorb the drugs poorly because they are receiving H_2 receptor antagonists or have AIDS. In AIDS patients, fluconazole (100 to 200 mg daily) is the most effective azole for oral and esophageal candidiasis.

Management of recurrent oropharyngeal candidiasis in the HIV-infected patient presents special problems. Patients with CD4+ cell counts below 100/μL who have received prolonged fluconazole therapy are at risk of developing azole resistance, requiring an increased dose to mount a response, relapsing early, and eventually failing to respond well to any dose of fluconazole. Therapy with itraconazole, ketoconazole, or clotrimazole at this point results in only transient or no improvement. The increasing azole resistance in this population suggests that HIV-infected patients with oropharyngeal candidiasis should be treated for each individual episode and that only when episodes become intolerably frequent should weekly or daily preventive therapy be given and even then at the lowest dose required to maintain remission. In contrast, AIDS patients with *Candida* esophagitis are so prone to relapse that preventive therapy with fluconazole is recommended for all proven cases. Most HIV-infected patients with azole-resistant oropharyngeal candidiasis also have esophagitis. Nearly all patients with azole-resistant oropharyngeal or esophageal candidiasis respond to intravenous amphotericin B (0.3 to 0.5 mg/kg daily) but relapse promptly after the completion of therapy.

Bladder thrush responds to bladder irrigations with amphotericin B (50 μg/mL for 5 days). If no bladder catheter is in place, oral fluconazole can be used to control candiduria. In all forms of superficial candidiasis, relapse after successful treatment is common unless the underlying factor can be eliminated.

Intravenous amphotericin B is the drug of choice in disseminated candidiasis. The drug is usually given at a dosage of 0.5 to 0.7 mg/kg daily. In patients with no contraindication to the use of flucytosine, administration of that drug at a dosage of 100 to 150 mg/kg per day along with amphotericin B (0.3 to 0.5 mg/kg per day) is an effective alternative. Fluconazole in an adult dose of 100 mg daily is probably the drug of choice for chronic mucocutaneous candidiasis.

Candida isolated from a culture of a properly obtained blood sample should be considered significant; true false-positives are rare. All patients with *Candida* cultured from peripheral blood should receive intravenous amphotericin B to treat acute infection and prevent late sequelae. In immunocompetent patients with intravenous catheter-acquired *C. albicans* fungemia, the catheter should be removed in conjunction with the administration of either fluconazole (400 mg daily) or amphotericin B (0.5 mg/kg daily). Patients with suppurative phlebitis of a peripheral vein should have the infected portion of the vein excised. Therapy for candidemia is continued for 2 weeks after the patient becomes afebrile. The *Candida* species involved should be considered in choosing between fluconazole and amphotericin B. *C. krusei* causes about 1 percent of all cases of candidemia but is resistant to fluconazole in vitro. *C. glabrata* exhibits an intermediate level of susceptibility to fluconazole, but too few cases have been studied to determine whether candidemia involving that species will respond as well to fluconazole as to amphotericin B. Strains of *Candida lusitaniae* resistant to amphotericin B but susceptible to azoles have been encountered. In every case of candidemia, a funduscopic examination for endophthalmitis should be undertaken, and therapy should be continued until retinal lesions have resolved. Intravenous amphotericin B, with or without flucytosine, is the preferred treatment for *Candida* endophthalmitis, although cures have been reported with fluconazole. Pars plana vitrectomy may facilitate diagnosis and cure when a *Candida* vitreous abscess is present. Leaving amphotericin B in the vitreous cavity at the end of the vitrectomy procedure should be considered.

Injection of amphotericin B into an infected joint, pleural cavity, or peritoneum is rarely indicated. Removal of prostheses, including prosthetic joints, cardiac valves, peritoneal dialysis catheters, and central venous catheters, is usually essential. Collections of pus, such as those in the postoperative abdomen, need to be drained surgically or by percutaneous, computed tomography–guided catheterization; an exception relates to the numerous small abscesses in liver, spleen, or kidney in chronic disseminated candidiasis, which cannot be drained effectively and require prolonged antifungal therapy. In general, treatment should continue until the patient with chronic disseminated candidiasis has been afebrile and nonneutropenic for at least 2 weeks. Defects may persist on imaging studies long after cure. Relapse during another episode of neutropenia is common unless the patient is receiving amphotericin B. Repeat cytotoxic therapy or even bone marrow transplantation can be undertaken in patients with prior chronic disseminated candidiasis, but amphotericin B should be given prophylactically during neutropenia.

Fluconazole can decrease the incidence of deep candidiasis in recipients of allogeneic bone marrow transplants when 400 mg is given daily until engraftment. Although the incidence of superficial candidiasis is also decreased by fluconazole prophylaxis, superficial infection can be readily detected and treated. Aspergillosis is not prevented by prophylactic fluconazole. Studies of leukemic and other neutropenic patients have found no beneficial effect of prophylactic fluconazole. Empirical administration of fluconazole to febrile neutropenic patients not responding to broad-spectrum antibacterial agents is not currently recommended.

The role of newer formulations of amphotericin B in the treatment of deep candidiasis or in empirical therapy is under study.

BIBLIOGRAPHY

AKLER MA et al: Use of fluconazole in the treatment of candidal endophthalmitis. Clin Infect Dis 20:657, 1995

ANAISSIE E et al: Fluconazole therapy for chronic disseminated candidiasis in patients with leukemia and prior amphotericin B therapy. Am J Med 91:142, 1991

LAINE L et al: Fluconazole compared with ketoconazole for the treatment of candida esophagitis in AIDS. Ann Intern Med 117:655, 1992

LECCIONES JA et al: Vascular catheter-associated fungemia in patients with cancer: Analysis of 155 episodes. Clin Infect Dis 14:875, 1992

ODDS FC: *Candida and Candidosis.* Philadelphia, Saunders, 1988

REX JR et al: A randomized trial comparing fluconazole with amphotericin B for the treatment of candidemia in patients without neutropenia. N Engl J Med 331:1324, 1994

SLAVIN MA et al: Efficacy and safety of fluconazole prophylaxis for fungal infections after marrow transplantation—a prospective, randomized, double-blind study. J Infect Dis 171:1545, 1995

THALER M et al: Hepatic candidiasis in cancer patients: The evolving picture of the syndrome. Ann Intern Med 198:88, 1988

TOSTI A et al: Treatment of dermatophyte nail infections: An open randomized study comparing intermittent terbinafine with continuous terbinafine treatment and intermittent itraconazole therapy. J Am Acad Dermatol 34:595, 1996

WHITE A, GOETZ MB: Azole-resistant *Candida albicans:* Report of two cases of resistance to fluconazole and review. Clin Infect Dis 19:687, 1994

WINGARD JR: Importance of *Candida* species other than *C. albicans* as pathogens in oncology patients. Clin Infect Dis 20:115, 1995

WINSTON DJ et al: Fluconazole prophylaxis of fungal infections in patients with acute leukemia. Ann Intern Med 118:495, 1993

208 *John E. Bennett*

ASPERGILLOSIS

ETIOLOGIC AGENTS *Aspergillus fumigatus* is the most common cause of aspergillosis, but *Aspergillus flavus, Aspergillus niger,* and several other species can also cause disease. *Aspergillus* is a mold with septate hyphae about 2 to 4 μm in diameter. The fungus is identified by its gross and microscopic appearance in culture.

PATHOGENESIS AND PATHOLOGY   All the common species of *Aspergillus* that cause disease in humans are ubiquitous in the environment, growing on dead leaves, stored grain, compost piles, hay, and other decaying vegetation. Inhalation of *Aspergillus* spores must be extremely common, but disease is rare. Invasion of lung tissue is confined almost entirely to immunosuppressed patients, in roughly 90 percent of whom two of the following three conditions will be operative: a granulocyte count in peripheral blood of $<500/\mu L$, treatment with supraphysiologic doses of adrenal glucocorticoids, and a history of treatment with cytotoxic drugs such as cyclosporine. Invasive aspergillosis is an occasional complication of AIDS. *Aspergillus* infection is characterized by hyphal invasion of blood vessels, thrombosis, necrosis, and hemorrhagic infarction. Chronic granulomatous disease of childhood also predisposes to invasive pulmonary aspergillosis, but in that situation the inflammatory response is granulomatous and blood vessel invasion is rare.

Massive inhalation of *Aspergillus* spores by healthy persons can lead to acute, diffuse, self-limited pneumonitis. Epithelioid granulomas with giant cells and central pyogenic areas containing hyphae are detected in these cases. Spontaneous recovery taking several weeks is the usual course.

Aspergillus can colonize the damaged bronchial tree, pulmonary cysts, or cavities of patients with underlying lung disease. Balls of hyphae within cysts or cavities (aspergillomas), usually in the upper lobe, may reach several centimeters in diameter and may be visible on chest x-ray. Tissue invasion does not occur. The term *allergic bronchopulmonary aspergillosis* denotes the condition of patients with preexisting asthma who have eosinophilia, IgE antibody to *Aspergillus*, and fleeting pulmonary infiltrates from bronchial plugging (see Chap. 253).

CLINICAL MANIFESTATIONS   *Endobronchial saprophytic pulmonary aspergillosis* presents as chronic productive cough, often with hemoptysis, in a patient with prior chronic lung disease, such as tuberculosis, sarcoidosis, bronchiectasis, or histoplasmosis. *Aspergillus* may be spread from its endocavitary or endobronchial site to the pleura during the course of bacterial lung abscess or surgery. Patients reported to have chronic necrotizing *Aspergillus* pneumonia appear in most instances to have had saprophytic endobronchial colonization and a pulmonary process attributable to another disease, with or without superimposed bacterial infections. Patients with chronic pneumonia and *Aspergillus* in the sputum should be assumed to have either pneumonia of a different etiology (e.g., histoplasmosis) or *Aspergillus* pneumonia with underlying immunosuppression [e.g., chronic granulomatous disease or infection with human immunodeficiency virus (HIV)].

Invasive aspergillosis in the immunocompromised host presents as an acute, rapidly progressive, densely consolidated pulmonary infiltrate and is most common among patients with acute leukemia and recipients of tissue transplants. Infection progresses by direct extension across tissue planes and by hematogenous dissemination to lung, brain, and other organs. Computed tomography (CT) has been helpful in identifying early lung infiltrates and, as neutrophil counts rise, in defining central areas of cavitation. *Aspergillus* may invade immunosuppressed patients through the skin at a site of minor trauma or through the upper airway mucosa. Early lesions in the nose should be sought in neutropenic patients with fever and minimal epistaxis. Scarlet-red patches of the mucosa rapidly become necrotic and white, then black. Rapid extension into the adjacent paranasal sinus, orbit, or face is usual, with or without the appearance of lung lesions.

Aspergillus sinusitis in immunocompetent patients may take two forms. A ball of hyphae may form in a chronically obstructed paranasal sinus, without tissue invasion. Much less commonly, a chronic, fibrosing granulomatous inflammation associated with *Aspergillus* hyphae within tissue may begin in the sinus and spread slowly to the orbit and the brain. *Aspergillus* is a cause of allergic fungal sinusitis, darkwalled fungi (e.g., *Cladosporium, Alternaria*) being more common in this setting. Patients usually have a history of chronic allergic rhinitis, sometimes with nasal polyps, but are otherwise healthy, presenting with painless proptosis, nasal obstruction, or dull aching pain. On CT or magnetic resonance imaging, a solid soft tissue mass pushing out

the lateral wall of the ethmoid sinus or the medial wall of the maxillary sinus may be detected. On sinus exploration, the mucosa is found to be thickened and inflamed but intact. Within the sinus cavity, sticky mucopus with strands of neutrophils, eosinophils, Charcot-Leyden crystals, and occasional hyphae can be found.

Aspergillosis in HIV-infected patients most commonly involves the lung, presenting as fever, cough, and dyspnea. Typically, the CD4 cell count is below $50/\mu L$. Roughly half of these patients have neutropenia or have recently been treated with glucocorticoids. Bilateral diffuse or focal pulmonary infiltrates with a tendency to cavitate constitute the most common radiologic manifestation. Well-localized, white, necrotic pseudomembranes full of hyphae or ulcers may develop in the trachea or the major bronchi. Progression of bronchitis to pneumonia is usual, but hematogenous dissemination is uncommon. Either allergic or invasive *Aspergillus* sinusitis can occur in HIV-infected patients; the allergic form can develop even at CD4 cell counts above $50/\mu L$.

The growth of *Aspergillus* on cerumen and detritus within the external auditory canal is termed *otomycosis*. Trauma to the cornea may cause *Aspergillus* keratitis. Endophthalmitis follows the introduction of *Aspergillus* into the globe by trauma or surgery. *Aspergillus* may infect intracardiac or intravascular prostheses.

DIAGNOSIS   The repeated isolation of *Aspergillus* from sputum or the demonstration of hyphae in sputum or bronchoalveolar lavage fluid suggests endobronchial colonization or infection. Even a single isolation of *Aspergillus* from the sputum of a neutropenic patient with pneumonia, particularly a child or a nonsmoker, suggests the diagnosis of invasive aspergillosis. In patients with advanced AIDS, fever, and cough, the isolation of *Aspergillus* from respiratory secretions raises the possibility of aspergillosis and thus should prompt bronchoscopy. Fungus ball of the lung is usually detectable by chest x-ray. IgG antibody to *Aspergillus* antigens is demonstrable in the serum of many colonized patients and of virtually all patients with fungus ball.

Biopsy is usually required for the diagnosis of invasive aspergillosis of the lung, nose, paranasal sinus, bronchi, or sites of dissemination. Blood cultures are rarely positive, even in patients with infected cardiac valves (native or prosthetic). *Aspergillus* hyphae can be identified presumptively by histology, but culture is required for confirmation and for determination of the species. Only culture can reliably distinguish aspergillosis from pseudallescheriasis; drug therapy for these two diseases differs.

℞ TREATMENT

Patients with severe hemoptysis due to fungus ball of the lung may benefit from lobectomy. Poor pulmonary function in residual lung and dense pleural adhesions around the lesion can complicate the resection. Systemic chemotherapy is of no value in endobronchial or endocavitary aspergillosis.

Treatment with intravenous amphotericin B (1.0 to 1.5 mg/kg daily) has resulted in the arrest or cure of invasive aspergillosis when immunosuppression is not severe. Itraconazole (200 mg bid) is useful in some less immunosuppressed patients with indolent or slowly progressive invasive aspergillosis. Surgery is the only treatment needed for fungus ball of the sinus and for allergic fungal sinusitis. Antifungal therapy has little effect on either entity if used alone, but chronic suppressive therapy has been begun postoperatively for relapse of allergic fungal sinusitis. The prognosis for cure of invasive aspergillosis in the paranasal sinus is very poor when the patient has profound and unremitting neutropenia. The prognosis is better in less immunosuppressed patients.

BIBLIOGRAPHY

DENNING DW, STEVENS DA: Antifungal and surgical treatment of invasive aspergillosis: Review of 2121 published cases. Rev Infect Dis 12:1147, 1990

LOGAN PM et al: Invasive aspergillosis of the airways: Radiographic, CT and pathologic findings. Radiology 193:383, 1994

LOTHLOLARY O et al: Invasive aspergillosis in patients with acquired immuno-deficiency syndrome: Report of 33 cases. Am J Med 95:177, 1993

SHIRAKUSA T et al: Surgical treatment of pulmonary aspergilloma and *Aspergillus* empyema. Ann Thorac Surg 48:779, 1989

TALBOT GH et al: Invasive *Aspergillus* rhinosinusitis in patients with acute leukemia. Rev Infect Dis 13:219, 1991

209   *John E. Bennett*

MUCORMYCOSIS

ETIOLOGIC AGENTS   Species of *Rhizopus*, *Rhizomucor*, and *Cunninghamella* are most the common causes of mucormycosis, but species of *Apophysomyces*, *Saksenaea*, *Mucor*, and *Absidia* also are occasionally responsible for this infection. The organism in tissue is composed of broad, rarely septate hyphae of uneven diameter (diameter ranging from 6 to 50 μm). The organisms are inexplicably difficult to grow from infected tissue. When growth does take place, it is rapid and profuse on most media at room temperature. Identification is based on the gross and microscopic appearance of the mold.

Zygomycosis is a term that includes mucormycosis and ento-mophthoramycosis. The latter is a tropical infection of the subcutaneous tissue or paranasal sinuses caused by species of *Basidiobolus* or *Conidiobolus*.

EPIDEMIOLOGY AND PATHOLOGY   *Rhizopus* and *Rhizomucor* species are ubiquitous, appearing on decaying vegetation, dung, and foods of high sugar content. Mucormycosis is uncommon and is largely confined to patients with serious preexisting diseases. Mucormycosis originating in the paranasal sinuses and nose predominantly affects patients with poorly controlled diabetes mellitus. Patients who have undergone organ transplantation, who have a hematologic malignancy, or who are receiving long-term deferoxamine therapy are predisposed to mucormycosis of either sinus or lung. Gastrointestinal mucormycosis occurs in a variety of conditions, including uremia, severe malnutrition, and diarrheal diseases. The infection is acquired from nature, with no person-to-person spread. In all forms of mucormycosis, vascular invasion by hyphae is a prominent feature. Ischemic or hemorrhagic necrosis is the foremost histologic finding.

CLINICAL MANIFESTATIONS   Mucormycosis originating in the nose and paranasal sinuses produces a characteristic clinical picture. Low-grade fever, dull sinus pain, and sometimes nasal congestion or a thin, bloody nasal discharge are followed in a few days by double vision, increasing fever, and obtundation. Examination reveals a unilateral generalized reduction of ocular motion, chemosis, and proptosis. The nasal turbinates on the involved side may be dusky red or necrotic. A sharply delineated area of necrosis, strictly respecting the midline, may appear in the hard palate. The skin of the cheek may become inflamed. Fungal invasion of the globe or ophthalmic artery leads to blindness. Opacification of one or more sinuses is detected by computed tomography (CT) or by magnetic resonance imaging (MRI). Carotid arteriography may show invasion or obstruction of the carotid siphon. Coma is due to direct invasion of the frontal lobe. Early symptoms mimic those of bacterial sinusitis. Clouding of the sensorium may be attributed to diabetic acidosis. Cavernous sinus thrombosis may be considered when orbital invasion occurs. Without treatment, the patient may die after an interval ranging from a few days to a few weeks.

Pulmonary mucormycosis manifests as progressive severe pneumonia accompanied by high fever and toxicity. The necrotic center of large infiltrates may cavitate. Hematogenous spread to other areas of the lung, as well as to the brain and other organs, is common. Survival beyond 2 weeks is unusual. Gastrointestinal invasion presents as one or more ulcers that tend to perforate. Hematogenous dissemina-

tion can originate from the gastrointestinal tract, lung, or paranasal sinuses. Sometimes no portal of entry can be found.

DIAGNOSIS   CT or MRI is very helpful in assessing the extent of sinusitis before surgery and in evaluating the patient afterward. CT is better for detecting bony erosion; MRI better visualizes extension into the frontal lobe or carotid artery in the siphon. Lesions of the lung and craniofacial structures are best diagnosed by biopsy and histologic section. Cultural confirmation should be attempted. Wet smear of crushed tissue can provide a rapid diagnosis. Cultures of blood and cerebrospinal fluid are negative. Smear and culture of sputum may be positive during cavitation of a lung lesion.

 TREATMENT

Regulation of diabetes mellitus and a decrease in the dose of immuno-suppressive drugs facilitate the treatment of mucormycosis. Extensive debridement of craniofacial lesions appears to be very important. Orbital exenteration may be required. Intravenous amphotericin B is clearly of value in craniofacial mucormycosis and should be employed in the other forms of mucormycosis as well. The maximal tolerated doses are given until progression is halted. With the deoxycholate formulation, 1 to 1.5 mg/kg daily is indicated. Therapy is continued for a total of 10 to 12 weeks. Azoles are of no value. Appropriate management results in cure of about half of craniofacial infections. The survival of patients with pulmonary, gastrointestinal, or disseminated mucormycosis is rare.

BIBLIOGRAPHY

BOELAERT JR: Mucormycosis (zygomycosis): Is there news for the clinician? J Infect 28:S1, 1994

GALETTA SL et al: Rhinocerebral mucormycosis: Management and survival after carotid occlusion. Ann Neurol 28:103, 1990

INGRAM CW et al: Disseminated zygomycosis: Report of four cases and review. Rev Infect Dis 11:741, 1989

SINGH N et al: Invasive gastrointestinal zygomycosis in a liver transplant recipient: Case report and review of zygomycosis in solid-organ transplant recipients. Clin Infect Dis 20:617, 1995

TEDDER M et al: Pulmonary mucormycosis: Results of medical and surgical therapy. Ann Thorac Surg 57:1044, 1994

210   *John E. Bennett*

MISCELLANEOUS MYCOSES AND *PROTOTHECA* INFECTIONS

CHROMOBLASTOMYCOSIS   This chronic subcutaneous mycosis, rarely seen in the United States, presents as a verrucoid, ulcerated, or crusted skin lesion. The disease follows the introduction of any of several fungi into subcutaneous tissue by thorns or bits of vegetation. The infection spreads over ensuing months and years to contiguous tissue, causing few symptoms. The appearance of thick-walled, dark-colored, rounded forms ("copper pennies") in tissue is diagnostic. No satisfactory treatment is available.

DERMATOPHYTOSIS   **Definition**   Dermatophytosis, also known as ringworm or tinea, is a chronic fungal infection of the skin, hair, or nails.

Etiology   Species of *Trichophyton*, *Microsporum*, and *Epidermophyton* are called *dermatophytes*. These organisms grow in and remain confined to the keratinous structures of the body. Other mycoses, such as candidiasis, pityriasis versicolor, and tinea nigra, sometimes include fungal invasion of keratinous structures but traditionally are not called dermatophytoses.

Pathology and Pathogenesis   Dermatophyte species are referred to as *anthropophilic*, *zoophilic*, or *geophilic*, depending on whether their usual reservoir in nature appears to be humans, animals, or soil, respectively. The infectivity of organisms from all these sources is low, and outbreaks are largely confined to occasional clusters of cases of scalp infection in children. Acquisition of a dermatophytosis appears to be favored by minor trauma, maceration, and poor hygiene of the skin. Infection does not seem to confer solid immunity: Repeated infection with the same species is common, particularly with anthropophilic species. The infrequency of scalp infection among adults has been attributed to local factors rather than immunity.

Invasion of the stratum corneum by dermatophytes may cause inflammation that is either mild or (particularly with zoophilic fungi) intense. Shedding of the stratum corneum is increased by inflammation. To the extent that fungal growth cannot keep up with shedding, inflammation may help terminate infection. Conversely, infection is probably favored when shedding is reduced by treatment with glucocorticoids and cytotoxic drugs. Antifungal drugs interfere with the ability of fungal growth to keep up with shedding.

Clinical Manifestations   The disease varies with the site of infection and the fungal species involved. Foot infection (athlete's foot, tinea pedis) may present as fissuring of the toe webs, scaling of the plantar surfaces, or vesicles around the toe webs and soles. Interdigital lesions may be pruritic or, when bacterial superinfection occurs, may be painful. Hand infection is less common but resembles foot infection.

Scalp dermatophytosis (tinea capitis) is characterized by areas of alopecia and scaling. In so-called endothrix infection, the hair shaft breaks off at the skin surface, leaving the hairs visible as black dots in the scalp. Some forms of scalp infection include an area of intense boggy suppuration called a *kerion*.

Dermatophytosis of the glabrous skin (tinea corporis) presents as circumscribed lesions with a wide variety of appearances, including scales, vesicles, and pustules. Inflammation may be minimal or intense. Central healing of less inflamed lesions may take place. The serpiginous border of inflammation is the source of the name *ringworm*.

Dermatophytosis of the bearded area (tinea barbae) appears as a pustular folliculitis. Onychomycosis (tinea unguium) presents as a white discoloration of the nails or as thickening, chalkiness, and crumbling of the nails. Peeling and fissuring of paronychial nail folds or keratotic debris under the nail edge also may be evident.

Diagnosis   Discolored hairs, scales, and keratotic debris under infected nails should be collected for KOH smear and culture. In the scraping of skin lesions, a drop of water on the skin site may keep the removed scales from flying off and thus may aid in their collection. Culture is important in distinguishing dermatophytes from *Candida* and fungal saprophytes growing in keratinaceous debris.

℞ **TREATMENT**

Noninflammatory lesions of the trunk, groin, hands, and feet usually respond to twice-daily applications of clotrimazole, miconazole, ketoconazole, econazole, naftifine, terbinafine, or ciclopirox olamine cream. Hyperkeratotic lesions of the palms and soles respond slowly to these agents and may benefit from Whitfield's ointment initially to thin the keratin. Ointment should not be used between the toes, in the groin, or in the gluteal crease because maceration promotes bacterial infection.

Ringworm that is moderately severe, that is unresponsive to topical therapy, or that involves the scalp, nails, or bearded area should be treated systemically. The drug of choice is griseofulvin. Either 500 mg of the microcrystalline form or 375 mg of the ultramicrocrystalline form is given once daily or divided into two doses and given with meals. Double this amount has been recommended for refractory infections. Treatment must be continued until all infected keratin is gone. Cutting of infected hair and cleansing of interdigital webs can expedite cure. Secondary bacterial infection of the foot may require soaks or antibacterial agents. The likelihood of relapse of dermatophyte foot infections may be decreased by keeping the feet clean and dry. Griseofulvin-resistant cases may respond to itraconazole (200 mg once daily). Onychomycosis responds poorly to griseofulvin but may respond to itraconazole. Terbinafine (250 mg orally) is at least as effective as itraconazole in onychomycosis and ringworm, but the comparative safety of the two drugs is unclear.

Onychomycosis, which most often is due to *Trichophyton rubrum*, must be treated systemically until all infected portions of the nails grow out and are trimmed off. Deformed nails may grow more slowly than usual. Treatment should continue for at least 3 months. Cultures and smears can be helpful in determining the appropriate time to end therapy. Relapse is common.

PROTOTHECOSIS   *Prototheca* species are ubiquitous achlorophyllic algae that enter the skin through trauma or surgery and cause localized infections in the olecranon bursa, skin, subcutaneous tissue, tendon sheaths, or deeper tissue. Diagnosis is based on culture or histopathologic demonstration of sporangia with endospores in tissue. Surgical debridement and treatment with intravenous amphotericin B are useful.

FUSARIOSIS   *Fusarium* species can cause localized or hematogenously disseminated infection. Almost all patients with the latter have had hematopoietic malignancy and neutropenia. Abrupt onset of fever, sometimes with myalgia, is followed by distinctive skin lesions in two-thirds of cases. The lesions resemble ecthyma gangrenosum, tend to be multiple, progressively expand in size, and favor the extremities. A portal of infection is not usually apparent. Blood cultures have been positive in 59 percent of cases. Amphotericin B is probably the drug of choice for the treatment of fusariosis, but recovery depends on the diminution of neutropenia.

***MALASSEZIA* INFECTION (PITYRIASIS)**   *Malassezia furfur* is part of the normal flora of the human skin but can cause tinea (pityriasis) versicolor or catheter-acquired sepsis. Tinea versicolor appears as asymptomatic, well-delineated, hyperpigmented or hypopigmented macules centered on the upper trunk and upper arms. Confluent lesions may cover large areas, making the border difficult to find. A fine "branny" scale or folliculitis is sometimes visible. When examined microscopically by KOH mount, skin sections are seen to contain characteristic round and elongated cells. On inspection with Wood's light, lesions either do not fluoresce or appear yellow-green. Erythrasma resembles tinea versicolor but is characterized by gram-positive bacilli on smear and coral-red fluorescence. Azole creams are effective for the treatment of small areas of tinea versicolor; however, the application of selenium sulfide shampoo (Selsun) for 10 min daily, followed by showering to remove the shampoo, is more practical for large areas. Oral ketoconazole or itraconazole is also effective. Catheter-acquired sepsis due to *M. furfur* develops in patients (particularly neonates) receiving intravenous lipid. The organism requires special culture conditions for growth, and the infection is cured by catheter removal.

MYCETOMA   **Etiology**   *Actinomycetoma* refers to infection by actinomycetes of the genera *Nocardia, Nocardiopsis, Streptomyces,* and *Actinomadura. Eumycetoma* is caused by true fungi of many different genera. The predominant agent varies with the locality.

Pathogenesis and Pathology   The pathogens live in the soil and enter the skin through minor trauma. The most common site of infection is the foot. The infection runs a relentless course over many years, with destruction of contiguous bone and fascia. Grains are found in purulent foci surrounded by fibrosis and a mononuclear cell inflammatory response.

Clinical Manifestations   *Mycetoma* is a chronic suppurative infection originating in subcutaneous tissue and characterized by the presence of grains, which are tightly clumped colonies of the causative agent. The infected site is characterized by painless swelling, woody induration, and sinus tracts that discharge pus intermittently. Systemic symptoms do not develop, and spread to distant sites in the body does not take place.

Diagnosis   Although the clinical picture is characteristic, mycetoma is sometimes confused with chronic osteomyelitis or botryomycosis. The diagnosis requires demonstration of grains in pus from the draining sinus or in biopsy sections. Many histologic sections may need to be examined to locate a grain.

℞ TREATMENT

Actinomycetoma may respond to prolonged combination chemotherapy—e.g., with streptomycin and either dapsone or trimethoprim-sulfamethoxazole. Eumycetoma rarely responds to chemotherapy; some cases caused by *Madurella mycetomatis* have appeared to respond to ketoconazole or itraconazole.

PARACOCCIDIOIDOMYCOSIS Etiology Formerly called *South American blastomycosis*, this mycosis is caused by *Paracoccidioides brasiliensis*. A dimorphic fungus, *P. brasiliensis* grows as a budding yeast in tissue but may be grown as either a yeast or a mold on culture medium. The organism is identified by its gross and microscopic appearance. A superficial resemblance to *Blastomyces dermatitidis* may cause misdiagnosis.

Pathogenesis and Pathology Infection is thought to be acquired by inhalation of spores from environmental sources, but the organism's reservoir in nature remains obscure. Pulmonary infection produces few symptoms initially. Hematogenous spread to the mucous membranes of the mouth and nose, the lymph nodes, and other sites causes patients to seek medical attention. In fatal cases, the infection spreads to the adrenals, the gastrointestinal tract, and many other viscera.

Clinical Manifestations Common signs include indurated ulcers of the mouth, oropharynx, larynx, and nose; enlarged and draining lymph nodes; lesions of the skin and genitalia; and productive cough, weight loss, dyspnea, and sometimes fever. Paracoccidioidomycosis is acquired only in South America, Central America, and Mexico, but its extreme indolence may delay its recognition until many years after the patient has left the endemic area. Chest radiography most often shows bilateral patchy pneumonia.

Diagnosis Cultures of sputum, pus, and mucosal lesions are often diagnostic. The diagnosis can be made by smear or histologic section, although confirmation by culture is preferable. Serologic tests are useful in suggesting the diagnosis and monitoring the response to therapy.

℞ TREATMENT

Relatively mild cases of paracoccidioidomycosis may be cured by 1 year of treatment with oral ketoconazole or itraconazole (200 to 400 mg daily). More advanced cases are treated with intravenous amphotericin B followed by itraconazole.

PHAEOHYPHOMYCOSIS This is the name given to infections caused by fungi with dark-walled hyphae, excluding those given conventional names like chromoblastomycosis. Although an extraordinary variety of fungi and clinical syndromes are encompassed by this definition, most patients have brain abscess, subcutaneous abscess, or allergic fungal sinusitis. Most of the brain abscesses are due to *Cladosporium trichoides* and occur in previously healthy persons. Subcutaneous abscesses are usually single, arise at the site of minor trauma, and occur in both immunosuppressed and immunocompetent individuals.

Allergic fungal sinusitis develops in patients with allergic rhinitis and presents as an expanding mucoid mass in one or more paranasal sinuses. The tenacious mucus contains eosinophils, Charcot-Leyden crystals, and occasional hyphae. Surgical excision of phaeohyphomycotic lesions is important; the response to antifungal therapy is often unsatisfactory.

PSEUDALLESCHERIASIS Etiology Also called *Petriellidium boydii*, *Pseudallescheria boydii* is a mold frequently found in soil. When the fungus is isolated in the imperfect state, it is called *Scedosporium apiospermum*. (The reader is referred to standard textbooks of medical mycology for an explanation of the perfect and imperfect states.)

Pathogenesis and Pathology Wind-borne spores of *P. boydii*, arising from the soil, are the presumed source of infection. The fungus grows as a mold within tissue, causing necrosis and abscess formation.

Clinical Manifestations *P. boydii* resembles *Aspergillus* in its ability to colonize the endobronchial tree, to form fungus balls in the lungs or paranasal sinuses, and to invade the cornea or globe of the eye, the soft tissues, the joints, or the bones following trauma or surgery and in its propensity to invade the lungs and paranasal sinuses of immunosuppressed hosts, including AIDS patients. Hyphae of *P. boydii* in tissue may be difficult to distinguish from those of *Aspergillus*. Infection with *P. boydii* is much less common than that with *Aspergillus*. Nevertheless *P. boydii* is the single most common cause of mycetoma in the United States. Intravascular hyphae, a hallmark of invasive aspergillosis, are also found in pseudallescheriasis. Near-drowning in polluted water has led to severe *P. boydii* pneumonia, often with dissemination and fatal brain abscesses.

Diagnosis Demonstration of hyphae in tissue and culture confirmation are required for diagnosis.

℞ TREATMENT

Therapy with intravenous miconazole, itraconazole, or ketoconazole is recommended, but the response to all drugs has been poor.

Scedosporium prolificans, a fungus closely related to *P. boydii*, has caused infections in bones, joints, or soft tissue, usually following trauma. These infections have responded to surgical debridement. Disseminated infection with *S. prolificans* in immunosuppressed patients has been fatal. The response to treatment with all antifungal agents has been poor.

SPOROTRICHOSIS Etiology *Sporothrix schenckii* lives as a saprophyte on plants in many areas of the world. In nature and on culture at room temperature the fungus grows as a mold, but within host tissue or at 37°C on enriched media it grows as a budding yeast. It is identified by its appearance in mold and yeast forms.

Pathogenesis and Pathology Infection results from the inoculation of *S. schenckii* into subcutaneous tissue via minor trauma. Nursery workers, florists, and gardeners acquire the illness from roses, sphagnum moss, and other plants. Infection may be limited to the site of inoculation (plaque sporotrichosis) or extend along proximal lymphatic channels (lymphangitic sporotrichosis). Spread beyond an extremity—the usual site of infection—is rare, and hematogenous dissemination from the skin remains unproven. The portal for osteoarticular, pulmonary, and other extracutaneous forms of sporotrichosis is unknown but is likely the lung.

Untreated sporotrichosis shows little evidence of self-healing and is capable of chronicity. The inflammatory response includes both the clustering of neutrophils and a marked granulomatous response with epithelioid cells and giant cells.

Clinical Manifestations In lymphangitic sporotrichosis, by far the most common manifestation, a nearly painless red papule forms at the site of inoculation. Over the next several weeks, similar nodules form along proximal lymphatic channels. The nodules intermittently discharge small amounts of pus. Ulceration may occur. The proximal extension of these lesions, often with skip areas, is quite distinctive but may be mimicked by lesions of *Nocardia brasiliensis*, *Mycobacterium marinum*, or (in rare cases) *Leishmania braziliensis* or *Mycobacterium kansasii*.

Plaque sporotrichosis manifests as a nontender red maculopapular granuloma confined to the site of inoculation. Osteoarticular sporotrichosis presents as mono- or polyarticular arthritis of indolent onset and progression over months or years, involving the elbows, knees, wrists, ankles, and (rarely) smaller joints of the extremities. Periarticular bone develops areas of demineralization detectable on x-ray, and draining sinuses may appear over joints and bursae. Hematogenous spread to the skin may take place during polyarticular disease, but none of the skin lesions shows lymphangitic spread. Immunosuppression, including advanced infection with human immunodeficiency virus, predisposes to hematogenous spread. Pulmonary sporotrichosis usually presents as a single chronic cavitary upper-lobe lung lesion. Chronic meningitis can develop in the absence of skin or lung lesions. *S. schenckii* is difficult to recover from cerebrospinal fluid.

Diagnosis Culture of pus, joint fluid, sputum, or skin biopsy specimen is the preferred method of diagnosis. The appearance of *S. schenckii* in tissue is quite variable. In skin lesions, the organisms are hard to find.

 TREATMENT

Cutaneous sporotrichosis can be cured with a saturated solution of potassium iodide given orally in increasing divided daily doses up to 4.5 to 9 mL/d for adults, as tolerated. Gastrointestinal disturbance or acneiform rash over the cape area and face is common, but therapy should be continued for 1 month after the resolution of all lesions. Itraconazole (100 to 200 mg daily) is an effective and better-tolerated alternative. Extracutaneous sporotrichosis rarely responds to iodides, but more than half of cases have been cured by prolonged courses of intravenous amphotericin B. Itraconazole (200 mg once or twice daily) is effective in some cases of extracutaneous sporotrichosis.

TRICHOSPOROSIS *Trichosporon beigelii* causes asymptomatic small white concretions on hair shafts, a condition called *white piedra*, but can also cause hematogenously disseminated infection in neutropenic patients (mostly those with leukemia). Multiple erythematous or purpuric papules accompany the fungemia. The lesions can evolve into large, tense hemorrhagic bullae. Blood cultures are usually positive. Prosthetic-valve endocarditis due to *T. beigelii* has been well described. Intravenous amphotericin B is the drug of choice for the treatment of *T. beigelii* infection.

BIBLIOGRAPHY

AMMARI LK et al: Catheter-related *Fusarium solani* fungemia and pulmonary infection in a patient with leukemia in remission. Clin Infect Dis 16:148, 1993

ARENAS R et al: Open randomized comparison of itraconazole versus terbinafine in onychomycosis. Int J Dermatol 34:138, 1995

BARBER GR et al: Catheter-related *Malassezia furfur* fungemia in immunocompromised patients. Am J Med 95:365, 1993

BOYD AS et al: Cutaneous manifestations of *Prototheca* infections. J Am Acad Dermatol 32:758, 1995

HAY RJ et al: Mycetoma. J Med Vet Mycol 30(Suppl 1):41, 1992

IACOVIELLO VR: Protothecosis complicating prolonged endotracheal intubation: Case report and literature review. Clin Infect Dis 15:959, 1992

MARCON MJ, POWELL DA: Human infections due to *Malassezia* spp. Clin Microbiol Rev 5:101, 1992

MARTINO P et al: Clinical patterns of *Fusarium* infections in immunocompromised patients. J Infect 28(Suppl 1):7, 1994

MEYER RD et al: Fungal sinusitis in patients with AIDS: Report of 4 cases and review of the literature. Medicine 73:69, 1994

NARANJO MS et al: Treatment of paracoccidioidomycosis with itraconazole. J Med Vet Mycol 28:67, 1990

NIELSEN K et al: Disseminated *Scedosporium prolificans* infection in an immunocompromised adolescent. Pediatr Infect Dis J 12:882, 1993

RABODONIRINA M et al: *Fusarium* infections in immunocompromised patients: Case reports and literature review. Eur J Clin Microbiol Infect Dis 13:153, 1994

RESTREPO A: Treatment of tropical mycoses. J Am Acad Dermatol 31:S91, 1994

RUXIN TA et al: *Pseudallescheria boydii* in an immunocompromised host: Successful treatment with debridement and itraconazole. Arch Dermatol 132:382, 1996

SUPPARATPINYO K et al: *Penicillium marneffei* infection in patients infected with human immunodeficiency virus. Clin Infect Dis 14:871, 1992

VARTIVARIAN SE et al: Emerging fungal pathogens in immunocompromised patients: Classification, diagnosis, and management. Clin Infect Dis 17:487, 1993

WINN RE et al: Systemic sporotrichosis treated with itraconazole. Clin Infect Dis 17:210, 1993

WOOLRICH A et al: Cutaneous protothecosis and AIDS. J Am Acad Dermatol 31:920, 1994

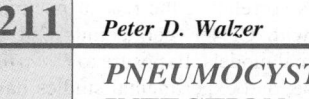

211 *Peter D. Walzer*

PNEUMOCYSTIS CARINII INFECTION

DEFINITION AND DESCRIPTION *Pneumocystis carinii* is an opportunistic pathogen whose natural habitat is the lung. The organism is an important cause of pneumonia in the compromised host.

The taxonomy of *P. carinii* has long been controversial; however, recent studies favor its placement in the fungal kingdom. Analysis of gene sequences of ribosomal RNA, mitochondrial proteins, and major enzymes (thymidylate synthase, dihydrofolate reductase) has demonstrated that *P. carinii* is more closely related to fungi than to protozoa. Moreover, biochemical studies have suggested that the cell wall of *P. carinii* contains glucans; drugs that inhibit 1,3-β-glucan synthesis in fungi are highly active against *P. carinii* in animal models. On the basis of this information, *P. carinii* is now considered a fungus in this textbook.

Study of the basic biology of *P. carinii* has been severely hampered by the lack of a reliable in vitro cultivation system. Major developmental stages of the organism include the small (1- to 4-μm) pleomorphic trophozoite or trophic form; the 5- to 8-μm cyst, which has a thick cell wall and contains up to eight intracystic bodies; and the precyst, an intermediate stage. The life cycle of *P. carinii* probably involves asexual replication by the trophic form and sexual reproduction by the cyst, which ends in release of the intracystic bodies; an intracellular stage has not been identified. Ultrastructurally, *P. carinii* has a primitive organelle system, but little is known about its metabolism.

P. carinii contains two prominent antigen groups. The 95- to 140-kDa major surface glycoprotein complex represents a family of proteins encoded by multiple genes. This complex plays a central role in the host-parasite relationship in *P. carinii* infection. The antigen facilitates the adherence of *P. carinii* to lung cells, contains protective epitopes, and is capable of antigenic variation. The other antigen, which migrates as a band of 35 to 55 kDa, is the most common antigen recognized by the host and thus may serve as a marker of infection.

EPIDEMIOLOGY *P. carinii* has a worldwide distribution among humans and has been found in a variety of animals. The organisms found in these hosts are morphologically identical, but molecular and antigenic data indicate that species and/or strain differences exist. Data about the fungal nature of *P. carinii* raise intriguing questions about previously undescribed developmental stages and environmental sources of the organism. Serologic surveys indicate that most healthy children have been exposed to the organism by 3 to 4 years of age. Animal model experiments have demonstrated that *P. carinii* is transmitted by the airborne route. Person-to-person transmission has been suggested by the occurrence of outbreaks of pneumocystosis among institutionalized debilitated infants and in hospitals caring for immunosuppressed patients. On the basis of animal studies, the incubation period is thought to be 4 to 8 weeks.

PATHOGENESIS AND PATHOLOGY *P. carinii* pneumonia occurs in the following hosts: premature, malnourished infants; children with primary immunodeficiency diseases; patients receiving immunosuppressive therapy (particularly glucocorticoids) for cancer, organ transplantation, and other disorders; and people with AIDS. The frequency of pneumocystosis among patients infected with human immunodeficiency virus (HIV) far exceeds that among other immunocompromised hosts. Despite the increased recognition of *P. carinii* and the wider use of chemoprophylaxis against it, the organism remains a leading cause of opportunistic infection and death among AIDS patients in industrialized countries.

Impaired cellular immunity is the major host factor that predisposes to pneumocystosis, although defects in B cell function also play a role. The importance of CD4+ cells in protection from *P. carinii* infection has been shown by studies correlating the risk of pneumocystosis in HIV-infected patients with CD4+ cell counts and by adoptive transfer experiments in animal models. Exposure to *P. carinii* stimulates a potent immune response, and experimental studies have shown that the cytokines tumor necrosis factor α and interleukin 1 play an important role in early host defenses against the organism. It has long been thought that *P. carinii* pneumonia develops by reactivation of latent infection, yet recent molecular evidence suggests that at least some episodes of the disease represent new bouts of infection.

Within the lung, *P. carinii* attaches firmly to the alveolar type I pneumocyte. This process is mediated by several factors, including extracellular proteins (fibronectin) and the mannose receptor. As the host's immune system becomes compromised, *P. carinii* organisms propagate slowly and gradually fill alveoli. These events are accompanied by an increase in alveolar-capillary permeability, a fall in surfactant phospholipids, a rise in surfactant proteins A and D, and damage to the type I cell.

On lung sections stained with hematoxylin and eosin, the alveoli are filled with a typical foamy, vacuolated exudate. Severe disease may include interstitial edema, fibrosis, and hyaline membrane formation. The host inflammatory changes usually consist of hypertrophy of alveolar type II cells, a typical reparative response, and a mild mononuclear cell interstitial infiltrate. Malnourished infants display an intense plasma cell infiltrate that gave the disease its early name: interstitial plasma cell pneumonia.

CLINICAL FEATURES   Patients with *P. carinii* pneumonia develop dyspnea, fever, and nonproductive cough. Symptoms in non-AIDS patients often begin after the glucocorticoid dose has been tapered and typically last 1 to 2 weeks. AIDS patients are usually ill for several weeks or longer and have relatively subtle manifestations. However, the clinical picture in individual patients is quite variable, and a high index of suspicion and elicitation of a careful history are key factors in early detection.

Physical findings include tachypnea, tachycardia, and cyanosis, but lung auscultation reveals few abnormalities. The white blood cell count is variable and is usually governed by the patient's underlying disease. Assessment of arterial blood gases demonstrates hypoxia, an increased alveolar-arterial oxygen gradient ($PA_{O_2} - Pa_{O_2}$), and respiratory alkalosis. There also may be changes in pulmonary function test values (diffusing capacity) and increased uptake with nuclear imaging techniques (gallium scan). Elevated serum concentrations of lactate dehydrogenase (LDH) have been reported; they probably reflect lung parenchymal damage but are not specific to *P. carinii* infection. In general, laboratory abnormalities are less severe in AIDS patients than in those without AIDS.

The classic findings on chest radiography consist of bilateral diffuse infiltrates beginning in the perihilar regions, but a variety of atypical manifestations (nodular densities, cavitary lesions) have also been reported. Patients who receive aerosolized pentamidine have an increased frequency of upper-lobe infiltrates and pneumothorax. Early in the course of pneumocystosis, the chest radiograph may be normal.

Although *P. carinii* usually remains confined to the lungs, cases of disseminated infection have occurred in both AIDS and non-AIDS patients. Estimates of the frequency of extrapulmonary pneumocystosis have ranged from <1 to 3 percent. One risk factor in HIV-infected patients appears to be the administration of aerosolized pentamidine. The most common sites of extrapulmonary involvement are the lymph nodes (40 to 50 percent of cases); next in frequency are the spleen, liver, and bone marrow (30 to 40 percent). Other common sites include the gastrointestinal and genitourinary tracts, adrenal and thyroid glands, heart, pancreas, eyes, ears, and skin. Clinical manifestations range from incidental findings at autopsy to specific organ involvement (low-density lesions in the spleen on computed tomography, cotton-wool spots on the retina). Histopathologic examination reveals the presence of *P. carinii* and the characteristic associated foamy material. Treatment for the extrapulmonary forms of pneumocystosis is the same as that for pneumonia.

DIAGNOSIS   Since the clinical picture of *P. carinii* infection can be produced by many other infectious and noninfectious agents, the diagnosis must be based on specific identification of the organism. A definitive diagnosis is made by histopathologic staining. Traditional stains have included reagents such as methenamine silver, toluidine blue, and cresyl echt violet, which selectively stain the wall of *P. carinii* cysts, and reagents such as Wright-Giemsa, which stain the nuclei of all developmental stages. Immunofluorescence with monoclonal antibodies is more sensitive than traditional staining but is also more expensive. Other reagents include nonspecific fluorochrome stains (calcofluor white) and Papanicolaou's stain. Selection of staining techniques is largely a matter of personal preference; frequently, more than one reagent is used to make the diagnosis. Molecular probes and the polymerase chain reaction offer promise in the diagnosis of *P. carinii* infection, but little progress has been made with culture or with antigen and antibody detection techniques.

Successful diagnosis of pneumocystosis requires an aggressive approach to the collection of proper specimens. In general, the yield from different diagnostic procedures is higher in AIDS patients than in non-AIDS patients, probably because of the higher organism burden in people with AIDS. In recent years, sputum induction has gained popularity as a simple, noninvasive technique; this procedure requires trained and dedicated personnel, and its success has varied at different institutions. Fiberoptic bronchoscopy with bronchoalveolar lavage (BAL), which is more sensitive and invasive than sputum induction, remains the mainstay of *P. carinii* diagnosis. This procedure provides information about the organism burden, the host inflammatory response, and the presence of other opportunistic infections. Transbronchial biopsy and open lung biopsy, which are the most invasive procedures, are reserved for situations in which a diagnosis cannot be made by lavage.

COURSE AND PROGNOSIS   In the typical case of untreated *P. carinii* pneumonia, progressive respiratory embarrassment leads to death. Therapy is most effective when instituted early in the course of the disease, before there is extensive alveolar damage. The most widely used prognostic indicators have been the arterial oxygen pressure and the alveolar-arterial oxygen gradient. Other factors that may influence survival include the organism burden, percentage of neutrophils in BAL fluid, chest radiographic abnormalities, serum LDH and albumin levels, and the expertise of the hospital in caring for AIDS patients. Concurrent pulmonary infections also complicate management, but the presence of cytomegalovirus does not usually affect the outcome of pneumocystosis.

℞ **TREATMENT**

Trimethoprim-sulfamethoxazole (TMP-SMZ), which acts by inhibiting folic acid synthesis, is considered the drug of choice for all forms of pneumocystosis. TMP-SMZ is administered orally or intravenously at a dosage of 15 to 20 mg of TMP/kg per day and 75 to 100 mg of SMZ/kg per day in three or four divided doses. This agent is well tolerated by non-AIDS patients, but more than half of AIDS patients experience serious adverse reactions, including fever, rash, neutropenia, thrombocytopenia, hepatitis, and hyperkalemia.

The other major drug used to treat *P. carinii* pneumonia is pentamidine isethionate. Although pentamidine has been available for many years, its mode of action against *P. carinii* is unclear. Pentamidine is given as a single dose of 4 mg/kg per day by slow intravenous infusion. Pentamidine is about as effective as TMP-SMZ but is toxic for almost all recipients. Its principal adverse effects are hypotension, cardiac arrhythmia, dysglycemia, azotemia, electrolyte changes, and neutropenia.

Several regimens have been developed for patients in whom therapy with TMP-SMZ or pentamidine is unsuccessful or intolerable. TMP plus dapsone, clindamycin plus primaquine, and atovaquone are less toxic oral regimens that are used in mild to moderate pneumocystosis. Parenteral trimetrexate has been used in severe disease.

Treatment of *P. carinii* pneumonia should be continued for 14 days in non-AIDS patients and for 21 days in persons with AIDS.

Since AIDS patients respond more slowly than non-AIDS patients, it is prudent to wait at least 7 days before concluding that therapy has failed. The addition of drugs to an existing regimen is no more effective than switching regimens and may increase the risk of toxicity.

There is increasing evidence that the host's inflammatory or immune response contributes to lung damage in *P. carinii* pneumonia, but the mechanisms involved are poorly understood. Several studies have shown that the administration of glucocorticoids to AIDS patients with moderate to severe pneumocystosis (a P_{O_2} of ≤ 70 mmHg or a $P_{A_{O_2}} - P_{a_{O_2}}$ of ≥ 35 mmHg) can prevent the early deterioration in respiratory function that frequently occurs after antimicrobial therapy and can improve the rate of survival. The administration of steroids should be started early in the course of the illness (usually when antimicrobial drugs are begun) for maximal benefit; the recommended regimen is 40 mg of prednisone orally twice daily, with tapering to a dose of 20 mg/d over a 3-week period. This regimen has generally proven to be safe despite concern about its effects on other opportunistic infections and Kaposi's sarcoma. The use of steroids as adjunctive therapy in non-AIDS patients remains to be evaluated.

Other important measures include the maintenance of oxygenation, nutrition, and electrolyte balance. Admission to the intensive care unit and mechanical ventilation (if instituted promptly) can improve the survival rate for patients who develop respiratory failure.

PREVENTION Primary prophylaxis is indicated for HIV-infected patients at high risk of developing pneumocystosis—that is, those who have CD4+ cell counts of $<200/\mu L$, unexplained fever [$>37.8°C$ ($>100°F$)] for ≥ 2 weeks, or a history of oropharyngeal candidiasis. Guidelines for the administration of primary prophylaxis to other immunocompromised hosts are less clear. Secondary prophylaxis is indicated for all patients who have recovered from *P. carinii* pneumonia. Among AIDS patients, the risk of recurrent episodes of pneumocystosis is high and lifelong; among non-AIDS patients, the risk is lower and exists for as long as the immunosuppressive condition persists.

One double-strength tablet of TMP-SMZ (160 mg of TMP, 800 mg of SMZ) per day is the prophylactic regimen of choice. The major limitation of TMP-SMZ is the high frequency of adverse reactions among HIV-infected patients. Recommended alternative regimens include TMP-SMZ at a reduced dose or frequency; dapsone alone; dapsone, pyrimethamine, and leucovorin; and aerosolized pentamidine (administered in a Respirgard II nebulizer).

Although there are no specific recommendations for preventing the spread of *P. carinii* in health care facilities, it seems prudent to prevent direct contact between patients with pneumocystosis and other susceptible hosts.

BIBLIOGRAPHY

BAUGHMAN RP: Current methods of diagnosis, in *Pneumocystis carinii Pneumonia*, P Walzer (ed). New York, Dekker, 1994, pp 381–401

BENNETT CL et al: The learning curve for AIDS-related *Pneumocystis carinii* pneumonia: Experience from 3981 cases in Veterans Affairs Hospitals 1987–1991. J Acquir Immun Defic Syndr Hum Retrovirol 8:373, 1995

CARTWRIGHT CP et al: Development and evaluation of a rapid and simple procedure for detection of *Pneumocystis carinii* by PCR. J Clin Microbiol 32:1634, 1994

HOFFMAN OA et al: *Pneumocystis carinii* stimulates tumor necrosis factor alpha release from alveolar macrophages through a beta-glucan-mediated mechanism. J Immunol 150:3932, 1993

HUGHES W et al: Comparison of atovaquone (566C80) with trimethoprim-sulfamethoxazole for the treatment of *Pneumocystis carinii* pneumonia in patients with AIDS. N Engl J Med 328:1521, 1993

KEELY SP et al: Genetic variation among *Pneumocystis carinii hominis* isolates in recurrent pneumocystosis. J Infect Dis 172:595, 1995

MASUR H: Drug therapy: Prevention and treatment of pneumocystis pneumonia. N Engl J Med 327:1853, 1992

NATIONAL INSTITUTES OF HEALTH—UNIVERSITY OF CALIFORNIA EXPERT PANEL FOR CORTICOSTEROIDS AS ADJUNCTIVE THERAPY FOR PNEUMOCYSTIS PNEUMONIA: Consensus statement on the use of corticosteroids as adjunctive therapy for pneumocystis pneumonia in the acquired immunodeficiency syndrome. N Engl J Med 323:1500, 1990

PEGLOW SL et al: Serologic responses to *Pneumocystis carinii* in health and disease. J Infect Dis 161:296, 1990

PHAIR J et al: The risk of *Pneumocystis carinii* pneumonia among men infected with human immunodeficiency virus type 1. N Engl J Med 322:161, 1990

SATTLER FR et al: Comparison of trimetrexate with leucovorin versus trimethoprim-sulfamethoxazole for moderate-to-severe episodes of *Pneumocystis carinii* pneumonia in patients with AIDS: A prospective, controlled multicenter investigation of the AIDS Clinical Trials Group protocol 029/031. J Infect Dis 170:165, 1994

SMULIAN AG et al: Analysis of *Pneumocystis carinii* organism burden, viability and antigens in bronchoalveolar lavage fluid in AIDS patients with pneumocystosis: Correlation with disease severity. AIDS 8:1555, 1994

STERNBERG RI et al: *Pneumocystis carinii* alters surfactant protein A concentrations in bronchoalveolar lavage fluid. J Lab Clin Med 125:462, 1995

TELZAK EE et al: Extrapulmonary *Pneumocystis carinii* infections. Rev Infect Dis 12:380, 1990

THEUS SA et al: Adoptive transfer of lymphocytes sensitized to the major surface glycoprotein of *Pneumocystis carinii* confers protection in the rat. J Clin Invest 95:2587, 1995

US PUBLIC HEALTH SERVICE/INFECTIOUS DISEASES SOCIETY OF AMERICA: Guidelines for the prevention of opportunistic infections in persons infected with human immunodeficiency virus: A summary. Morb Mort Week Rep 44(RR-8):1, 1995

WADA M et al: Antigenic variation by positional control of major surface glycoprotein gene expression in *Pneumocystis carinii*. J Infect Dis 171:1563, 1995

WALZER PD: *Pneumocystis carinii*: Recent advances in basic biology and their clinical application. AIDS 7:1293, 1993

SECTION 16

PROTOZOAL AND HELMINTHIC INFECTIONS: GENERAL CONSIDERATIONS

212 *Peter F. Weller*

APPROACH TO THE PATIENT WITH PARASITIC INFECTION

Because of the diversity of parasitic organisms that may infect humans, a range of factors are germane to an assessment of the possible parasitic etiology of a patient's disease. These factors include issues related to the patient's history, immune status, and presenting clinical and laboratory characteristics, especially eosinophilia. Complementing historical and immunologic information, a full clinical evaluation and laboratory testing provide additional data to direct the assessment for parasitic infection. The specific tests required, ranging from standard blood biochemical assays to imaging of selected organs, are dictated by the nature of the patient's illness. Additional diagnostic testing for parasitic infections (Chap. 213) completes the evaluation.

HISTORY Geographic History The history can provide valuable information about potential exposures to parasitic infections. A history of travel to, residence or work in, or immigration from areas of the world in which various parasites not endemic in the United States are encountered offers a clue to possible parasitic etiologies of a patient's disease. Some parasitic infections may become manifest early after a traveler's return home; paramount among these in terms of preventable mortality is malaria. If a patient has been in a region of the world where malaria is endemic (even only briefly, as in an airport layover), fever mandates a consideration of malaria, whether or not malaria chemoprophylaxis has been used. Falciparum malaria, which in a nonimmune patient may progress rapidly to serious and even life-threatening consequences (Chap. 216), is a potential medical emergency and must be considered at the initial evaluation, even if symptoms and fever patterns are suggestive of less specific flulike or gastrointestinal illness. Rarely, malaria transmission has been reported within the United States.

For patients with a history of recent travel, the onset of gastrointestinal symptoms only after return suggests protozoal diseases characterized by a 1- to 2-week delay between acquisition and appearance of symptoms—notably, giardiasis and cryptosporidiosis (Chap. 220). Gastrointestinal symptoms lasting longer than a week also suggest protozoan etiologies, including giardiasis, amebiasis, and cyclosporiasis. For patients who have traveled less recently, information on the specific countries and the types of regions (urban or rural) visited and on the nature and duration of the visit, whether for general tourism or for activities related to specific occupations, is helpful in concert with presenting clinical features and hematologic and other laboratory findings. Diseases that may become manifest only some years after an individual leaves an endemic region include schistosomiasis, some forms of filariasis, strongyloidiasis, echinococcosis, and cysticercosis.

For the illnesses of patients who have never left the United States, various parasitic etiologies should be considered, depending on the presenting disease. Trichomoniasis, trichinosis, strongyloidiasis, giardiasis, cryptosporidiosis, cyclosporiasis, echinococcosis, and pinworm are among the parasitic infections endemic in settings within the United States. Diseases that are more frequent where there is fecal contamination of soil or other environmental sites include hookworm, ascariasis, trichuriasis, amebiasis, and strongyloidiasis; dermal exposure, as by walking barefoot on soil contaminated with parasitic larvae, predisposes to the acquisition of cutaneous larva migrans, hookworm, and strongyloides by residents of such an area as well as by travelers.

Dietary History   If more than one patient develops similar symptoms in a given situation, common-source waterborne diseases (giardiasis, cryptosporidiosis, cyclosporiasis) should be considered. These infections are more likely to be acquired from surface water supplies, ranging from mountain streams to municipal reservoirs. Likewise, attention to dietary history may be helpful. Trichinosis should be considered when the patient may have consumed contaminated pork, bear, walrus, or other meat from carnivores. Ingestion of undercooked fish predisposes to anisakiasis and to infection with other fish-dwelling nematodes, tapeworms (*Diphyllobothrium latum*), or flukes (*Nanophyetus salmincola*). Ingestion of snails or of produce contaminated with land snails can lead to infection with *Angiostrongylus cantonensis* (eosinophilic meningitis; Chap. 221). Ingestion of more exotic animal foodstuffs, including snakes, can result in the transmission of gnathostomiasis (Chap. 221). For children with a propensity for pica, ingestion of soil containing *Toxocara* eggs may lead to visceral larva migrans. Rarely, eosinophilic meningitis due to *Baylisascaris procyonis* has also been described. Consumption of ground-grown vegetables, including those shipped in from distant fields contaminated with human feces, provides an opportunity for the ingestion of nematode eggs of *Ascaris lumbricoides* or *Trichuris trichiura*.

Other Exposure Histories   An antecedent blood transfusion raises the possibility of malaria (especially that due to *Plasmodium malariae* or *Plasmodium falciparum*), babesiosis, or Chagas' disease. A history of wading or swimming in fresh water is germane to the acquisition of schistosomiasis or avian schistosome dermatitis. Fresh water may be a source of infection with free-living amebae, and these

protozoa may cause ocular infections, especially in persons wearing contact lenses. Arthropod vector–borne parasitic infections include malaria and lymphatic filariasis (carried by mosquitoes) and babesiosis (carried by ticks); the latter is transmitted in some regions of the United States.

Residence in an institutional setting where fecal-oral hygiene may be imperfect raises the possibility of giardiasis, cryptosporidiosis, or strongyloidiasis. Child-care centers provide opportunities for young children and their family members to acquire giardiasis, cryptosporidiosis, and pinworm infections. Trichomoniasis is transmitted sexually; giardiasis, cryptosporidiosis, amebiasis, and strongyloidiasis can be transmitted during anal intercourse or oral-anal contact.

IMMUNE STATUS   The patient's immune status is relevant in determining which parasitic infections need to be considered. In patients infected with human immunodeficiency virus type 1, especially those with depressed CD4+ lymphocyte counts, specific protozoan diseases may develop opportunistically. These infections include toxoplasmosis, isosporiasis, cyclosporiasis, cryptosporidiosis, visceral leishmaniasis, American trypanosomiasis, microsporidiosis, and infections with free-living amebae (*Acanthamoeba* and related genera). In individuals infected with human T-lymphotropic virus type 1, strongyloidiasis is a prominent consideration. Patients who are asplenic are at risk not only for overwhelming infections due to encapsulated bacteria but also for fulminant infections caused by intraerythrocytic protozoa, including malaria and babesiosis. Patients with hypogammaglobulinemia or cystic fibrosis may develop refractory giardiasis. In patients developing symptoms of enterocolitis while receiving glucocorticoids, the possibility of an exacerbation of unsuspected strongyloidiasis or amebic colitis should be considered.

EOSINOPHILIA   The role of eosinophilia in the evaluation for parasitic infection is worth mentioning. Eosinophilia offers a hematologic clue to the presence of some parasites. Only two protozoan parasites have been associated with eosinophilia: *Isospora belli* and, on occasion, *Dientamoeba fragilis*. In the latter instance, eosinophilia may be due in part to concomitant infection with pinworms. Thus the detection of eosinophilia generally mandates a consideration of the multicellular helminthic parasites that characteristically elicit this abnormality. (Helminth-elicited eosinophilia, however, may be suppressed by glucocorticoid therapy or by intercurrent bacterial or viral infections.) The magnitude of eosinophilia tends to correlate with the extent of tissue invasion by helminths. Marked blood eosinophilia (more than 3000 eosinophils per microliter) develops during the early transpulmonary migration of intestinal nematodes, including *Ascaris* and hookworms, at a time when eggs (whose presence confirms the diagnosis) have not yet been produced in the intestinal tract. Eosinophilia is also marked in the early stages of fluke infections, including schistosomiasis (Katayama fever), paragonimiasis, clonorchiasis, and fascioliasis; during the stage of muscle invasion in trichinosis; during tissue migration of adult worms in loiasis and gnathostomiasis; and with heavy infections in visceral larva migrans. Eosinophilia persisting for more than a year may be indicative of hookworm infection, strongyloidiasis, visceral larva migrans (especially in children), filarial infection (including onchocerciasis, loiasis, and tropical pulmonary eosinophilia), fluke infections (including schistosomiasis, fascioliasis, clonorchiasis, and paragonimiasis), and cysticercosis. Leakage of fluids from echinococcal cysts can cause intermittent increases in eosinophilia. Eosinophilia sometimes provides the only clue to the presence of helminthic infection and should prompt an evaluation for such infection. Serologic testing for schistosomiasis, filariasis, visceral larva migrans, and strongyloidiasis will be helpful in an assessment for some of the diseases most likely to elicit eosinophilia. Serologic evaluation for strongyloidiasis is especially important since autoinfection may permit persistence of the organisms for decades and put the patient at risk for disseminated disease if immunosuppressive glucocorticoids are later administered for any reason.

BIBLIOGRAPHY

Gyorkos TW et al: Seroepidemiology of *Strongyloides* infection in the Southeast Asian refugee population in Canada. Am J Epidemiol 132:257, 1990

—— et al: Intestinal parasite infection in the Kampuchean refugee population 6 years after resettlement in Canada. J Infect Dis 166:413, 1992

KAPPUS KD et al: Intestinal parasitism in the United States: Update on a continuing problem. Am J Trop Med Hyg 50:705, 1994

LIBMAN MD et al: Screening for schistosomiasis, filariasis, and strongyloidiasis among expatriates returning from the tropics. Clin Infect Dis 17:353, 1993

MANNHEIMER SB, SOAVE R: Protozoal infections in patients with AIDS. Cryptosporidiosis, isosporiasis, cyclosporiasis, and microsporidiosis. Infect Dis Clin North Am 8:483, 1994

PRATLONG F et al: Leishmania–human immunodeficiency virus coinfection in the Mediterranean basin: Isoenzymatic characterization of 100 isolates of the Leishmania infantum complex. J Infect Dis 172:323, 1995

SELIK RM et al: Trends in infectious diseases and cancers among persons dying of HIV infection in the United States from 1987 to 1992. Ann Intern Med 123:933, 1995

SUN T: Current topics in protozoal diseases. Am J Clin Pathol 102:16, 1994

SVENSON JE et al: Imported malaria. Clinical presentation and examination of symptomatic travelers. Arch Intern Med 155:861, 1995

WELLER PF: Eosinophilia in travelers. Med Clin North Am 76:1413, 1992

213 *Charles E. Davis*

LABORATORY DIAGNOSIS OF PARASITIC INFECTIONS

The cornerstone for the diagnosis of parasitic infections is a thorough history of the patient's illness. Epidemiologic aspects of the illness are especially important because the risks of acquiring many parasites are closely related to occupation, recreation, or travel to areas of high endemicity. Without a basic knowledge of the epidemiology and life cycles of the major parasites, it is difficult to approach the diagnosis of parasitic infections systematically. Accordingly, the medical classi-

Table 213-1

Flatworm Infections

Parasite	Geographic Distribution	Intermediate (Transmission)	Definitive	Parasite Stage	Body Fluid or Tissue	Serologic Tests	Other
TAPEWORMS (CESTODES)							
Intestinal tapeworms							
Taenia saginata (beef tapeworm)	Worldwide	Beef	Humans	Ova, segments	Feces	—	Motile segments
Hymenolepis nana (dwarf tapeworm)	Worldwide	Grain beetles	Humans, mice*	Ova	Feces	—	—
Diphyllobothrium latum (fish tapeworm)	Worldwide	Copepods–fish‡	Humans, other mammals	Ova, segments	Feces	—	Megaloblastic anemia in 1%
Taenia solium† (pork tapeworm)	Worldwide	Swine	Humans	Ova, segments	Feces	WB	Especially Mexico, Central and South America, Africa
Somatic tapeworms							
Echinococcus granulosus (hydatid disease)	Sheep-raising and hunting areas	Sheep, camels, humans, others	Dogs	Hydatid	Lung, liver	WB	Chest radiography, CT, MRI
Echinococcus multilocularis (hydatid disease)	Subarctic areas	Rodents, humans	Foxes, dogs, cats	Hydatid	Liver	—	May resemble cholangiocellular carcinoma
Taenia solium† (pork tapeworm)	Worldwide	Swine, humans	Humans	Cysticercus	Muscles, CNS	WB	CT, MRI, radiography
FLUKES (TREMATODES)							
Intestinal flukes							
Fasciolopsis buski	China, India	Snails–water chestnuts	Humans	Ova	Feces	—	—
Heterophyes heterophyes	Far East, India	Snails–fish	Humans	Ova	Feces	—	—
Metagonimus yokogawai	Focal in Europe and North Africa	Snails–fish	Humans	Ova	Feces	—	—
Liver flukes							
Clonorchis sinensis	China, Southeast Asia	Snails–fish	Humans	Ova	Feces, bile	—	Recurrent bacterial cholangitis
Fasciola hepatica	Sheep-raising areas	Snails–watercress	Humans, sheep	Ova	Feces, bile	—	Cirrhosis, portal hypertension
Lung flukes							
Paragonimus spp.	Orient, Africa, South America	Snails–crabs/crayfish	Humans, other mammals	Adults, ova	Lung, sputum, CNS	WB	Chest radiography, CT, MRI
Blood flukes							
Schistosoma mansoni	Africa, Central and South America, West Indies	Snails	Humans	Ova, adults	Feces	EIA, WB	Rectal snips, liver biopsy
Schistosoma haematobium	Africa	Snails	Humans	Ova, adults	Urine	EIA, WB	Liver, urine, or bladder biopsy
Schistosoma japonicum	Far East	Snails	Humans	Ova, adults	Feces	EIA, WB	Liver biopsy

* Larvae also can mature in intestinal villi of humans and mice.
† *T. solium* can cause either intestinal infections or cysticercosis. Its ova are identical to those of *T. saginata*; scolices and segments of the two species differ.
‡ When there are two intermediate hosts, the first is separated from the second by a dash. Definitive hosts are infected by the second intermediate host.
NOTE: WB, western blot; CT, computed tomography; MRI, magnetic resonance imaging; CNS, central nervous system; EIA, enzyme immunoassay. Serologic tests listed in Tables 213-1, 213-2, and 213-3 are available from the Centers for Disease Control and Prevention, Atlanta, GA.

fication of important human parasites in this chapter emphasizes their geographic distribution, their transmission, and the anatomic location and stages of their life cycle in humans. The text and tables are intended to serve as a guide to the correct diagnostic procedures for the major parasitic infections and to direct the reader to other chapters that contain more comprehensive information about each infection. Tables 213-1, 213-2, and 213-3 summarize the geographic distributions, the anatomic locations, and the laboratory methods employed for the diagnosis of flatworm, roundworm, and protozoal infections, respectively.

In addition to selecting the correct diagnostic procedures, physicians must counsel their patients to ensure that specimens are collected properly and arrive at the laboratory promptly. For example, the diagnosis of bancroftian filariasis is unlikely to be confirmed by laboratory personnel unless blood is drawn near midnight, when the nocturnal microfilariae are active. Laboratory personnel and surgical pathologists should be notified in advance when a parasitic infection is suspected. Continuing interaction with the laboratory staff and the surgical pathologists increases the likelihood that parasites in body fluids or biopsy specimens will be examined carefully by the most capable individuals.

INTESTINAL PARASITES Most helminths and protozoa exit the body in the fecal stream. The patient or the patient's attendant should be instructed to collect feces in a clean cardboard container and to record the time of collection on the container. Contamination with water, which could contain free-living protozoa, or with urine should be avoided. Fecal samples should be collected before ingestion of barium or other contrast agents for radiologic procedures and before treatment with antidiarrheal agents and antacids, because these substances change the consistency of the feces and interfere with microscopic detection of parasites. Because of the cyclic shedding of most parasites in the feces, a minimum of three samples collected on alternate days should be examined. When delays in transport to the laboratory are unavoidable or specimens must be shipped by mail, fecal

Table 213-2

Roundworm Infections

| Parasite | Geographic Distribution | Life-Cycle Hosts | | Diagnosis | | | |
		Intermediate (Transmission)	Definitive	Parasite Stage	Body Fluid or Tissue	Serologic Tests	Other
INTESTINAL ROUNDWORMS							
Enterobius vermicularis (pinworm)	Temperate and tropical zones	Fecal-oral	Humans	Ova	Perianal skin	—	"Scotch tape" test
Trichuris trichiura (whipworm)	Temperate and tropical zones	Soil, fecal-oral	Humans	Ova	Feces	—	Rectal prolapse
Ascaris lumbricoides (roundworm of humans)	Temperate and tropical zones	Soil, fecal-oral	Humans	Ova	Feces	—	Sx of pulmonary migration
Ancylostoma duodenale (Old World hookworm)	Eurasia, Africa, Pacific	Soil→skin	Humans	Ova/larvae	Feces	—	Sx of pulmonary migration, anemia
Necator americanus (New World hookworm)	U.S., Africa, worldwide	Soil→skin	Humans	Ova/larvae	Feces	—	Sx of pulmonary migration, anemia
Strongyloides stercoralis (strongyloidiasis)	Moist tropics and subtropics	Soil→skin	Humans	Larvae	Feces, sputum, duodenal fluid	EIA	Dissemination in immunodeficiency
TISSUE ROUNDWORMS							
Trichinella spiralis (trichinosis)	Worldwide	Swine/humans	Swine/humans	Larvae	Muscle	BF, EIA	Muscle biopsy
Wuchereria bancrofti (filariasis)	Coastal areas in tropics and subtropics	Mosquitoes	Humans	Microfilariae	Blood, lymph nodes	—	Nocturnal periodicity*
Brugia malayi (filariasis)	Asia, Indian subcontinent	Mosquitoes	Humans	Microfilariae	Blood	—	Nocturnal
Loa loa (African eye worm)	West and Central Africa	Mango flies (*Chrysops*)	Humans	Microfilariae	Blood	—	May be visible in eye, diurnal
Onchocerca volvulus (river blindness)	Africa, Mexico, Central and South America	Blackflies	Humans	Adults/larvae	Skin/eye	—	Examine nodules or skin snips
Dracunculus medinensis (guinea worm)	Orient, Africa, West Indies, Brazil	*Cyclops*	Humans	Adults/larvae	Skin	—	May be visible in lesion
LARVA MIGRANS SYNDROMES							
Ancylostoma braziliense (creeping eruption)	Tropical and temperate zones	Soil→skin	Dogs/cats, humans	Larvae	Skin	—	Dog and cat hookworm
Toxocara canis and *cati* (visceral larva migrans)	Tropical and temperate zones	Soil, fecal-oral	Dogs/cats, humans	Larvae	Viscera, CNS, eye	EIA†	Also caused by roundworms of other species

* Blood should be drawn at midnight, except for infection acquired in the South Pacific.
† The presence of hemagglutinins is a useful clue.
NOTE: BF, bentonite flocculation; Sx, signs/symptoms; EIA, enzyme immunoassay; CNS, central nervous system.

samples should be kept in polyvinyl alcohol to preserve protozoal trophozoites. Refrigeration also will preserve trophozoites for a few hours and protozoal cysts and helminthic ova for several days.

Analysis of fecal samples consists of both a macroscopic and a microscopic examination. Watery or loose stools are more likely to contain protozoal trophozoites, but protozoal cysts and all stages of helminths may be found in formed feces. If adult worms or tapeworm segments are observed, they should be transported promptly to the laboratory or washed and preserved in fixative for later examination. The only tapeworm with motile segments is *Taenia saginata*, the beef tapeworm, which patients will sometimes bring to the physician.

Motility is an important distinguishing characteristic, because the ova of *T. saginata* and *Taenia solium*, the cause of cysticercosis, are morphologically indistinguishable.

Microscopic examination of feces (Table 213-4) is not complete until direct wet mounts have been evaluated and concentration techniques as well as permanent stains have been applied. Before accepting a report of negativity for ova and parasites as final, the physician should insist that the laboratory undertake each of these procedures.

Table 213-3

Protozoal Infections

Parasite	Geographic Distribution	Life-Cycle Hosts Intermediate (Transmission)	Definitive	Parasite Stage	Body Fluid or Tissue	Serologic Tests	Other
INTESTINAL PROTOZOANS							
Entamoeba histolytica (amebiasis)	Worldwide, especially tropics	Fecal-oral	Humans	Troph, cyst	Feces, liver	ID, EIA, IHA, antigen detection	Ultrasound, liver CT
Giardia lamblia (giardiasis)	Worldwide	Fecal-oral	Humans	Troph, cyst	Feces	Antigen detection	String test
Isospora belli	Worldwide	Fecal-oral	Humans	Oocyst	Feces	—	Acid-fast
Cryptosporidium	Worldwide	Fecal-oral	Humans, other animals	Oocyst	Feces	Antigen detection	Acid-fast, biopsy, PCR
Enterocytozoon bieneusi (microsporidiosis)	Worldwide?	?	Animals, humans	Spore	Feces	—	Modified trichrome, biopsy, PCR
FREE-LIVING AMEBAS							
Naegleria	Worldwide	Warm water	Humans	Troph, cyst	CNS, nares	—	Biopsy, nasal swab
Acanthamoeba	Worldwide	Soil, water	Humans	Troph, cyst	CNS, skin, cornea	—	Biopsy, scrapings
BLOOD AND TISSUE PROTOZOANS							
Plasmodium spp. (malaria)	Subtropics and tropics	Mosquitoes	Humans	Asexual	Blood	Little use	PCR
Babesia microti (babesiosis)	U.S., especially New England	Ticks	Rodents, humans	Asexual	Blood	IIF	Animal spp. in asplenia
Trypanosoma rhodesiense (African sleeping sickness)	Sub-Saharan East Africa	Tsetse flies	Humans, herbivores	Tryp	Blood, CSF	Card agglutination, IIF*	Also chancre, lymph nodes
Trypanosoma gambiense (African sleeping sickness)	Sub-Saharan West Africa	Tsetse flies	Humans, swine	Tryp	Blood, CSF	Card agglutination, IIF*	Also chancre, lymph nodes
Trypanosoma cruzi (Chagas' disease)	Mexico→ South America	Reduviid bugs (triatomes)	Humans, dogs, wild animals	Amastigote, tryp	Multiple organs/ blood	CF, IIF, EIA	Reactivation in immunosuppression
Leishmania tropica, etc.	Widespread in tropics and subtropics	Sandflies (*Phlebotomus*)	Humans, dogs, rodents	Amastigote	Skin	IFA†	Biopsy, scraping, culture
Leishmania braziliensis (mucocutaneous)	Mexico→ South America	Sandflies (*Lutzomyia*)	Humans, dogs, rodents	Amastigote	Skin, mucous membranes	IFA†	Biopsy, scraping, culture
Leishmania donovani (kala-azar)	Widespread in tropics and subtropics	Sandflies (*Phlebotomus*)	Humans, dogs, wild animals	Amastigote	RE system	IFA†	Biopsy, culture
Toxoplasma gondii (toxoplasmosis)	Worldwide	Humans, other mammals	Cats	Cyst, troph	CNS, eye, muscles, other	EIA, IIF	Reactivation in immunosuppression

* Card agglutination provided to endemic countries by the World Health Organization; IIF available intermittently—contact the WHO or the CDC.
† Limited specificity. Most sensitive for *L. donovani* (kala-azar).

NOTE: ID, immunodiffusion by commercial kit (not available from the CDC); IHA, indirect hemagglutination; CT, computed tomography; CF, complement fixation; troph, trophozoite; tryp, trypomastigote form; IIF, indirect immunofluorescence; RE, reticuloendothelial; PCR, polymerase chain reaction; EIA, enzyme immunoassay.

Table 213-4

Laboratory Diagnosis of Parasites Found in Feces*

Parasites and Fecal Stages	Alternative Diagnostic Procedures
TAPEWORMS (CESTODES)	
Taenia saginata ova and segments	Perianal "Scotch tape" test for ova
Hymenolepis nana ova	None
Diphyllobothrium ova and segments	None
Taenia solium ova and segments	Brain biopsy for neurocysticercosis; serology
FLUKES (TREMATODES)	
Fasciolopsis buski ova	None
Heterophyes heterophyes ova	None
Metagonimus yokogawai ova	None
Clonorchis (Opisthorchis) sinensis ova	Examination of bile for ova and adults in cholangitis
Fasciola hepatica ova	Examination of bile for ova and adults in cholangitis
Paragonimus spp. ova	Sputum; biopsy of lung or brain for ova; serology
Schistosoma ova	Rectal snips (especially for *S. mansoni*), urine (*S. haematobium*), liver biopsy and serology for all
ROUNDWORMS	
Enterobius vermicularis ova and adults	Perianal "Scotch tape" test for ova and adults
Trichuris trichiura ova	None
Ascaris lumbricoides ova and adults	Examination of sputum for larvae in lung disease
Hookworm ova and occasional larvae	Examination of sputum for larvae in lung disease
Strongyloides larvae	Duodenal aspirate or jejunal biopsy; sputum or lung biopsy for filariform larvae in disseminated disease; serology
Capillaria philippinensis ova†	None
PROTOZOANS	
Entamoeba histolytica trophozoites and cysts	Liver biopsy for trophozoites; serology
Giardia lamblia trophozoites and cysts	Duodenal aspirate or jejunal biopsy‡
Isospora belli oocysts	Duodenal aspirate or jejunal biopsy‡
Cryptosporidium oocysts	Duodenal aspirate or jejunal biopsy‡
Enterocytozoon bieneusi spores	Duodenal aspirate or jejunal biopsy‡

* Stains and concentration techniques are discussed in the text.
† Can be confused with *Trichuris trichiura*.
‡ Commercial string test or Crosby capsule are satisfactory; *Isospora* and *Cryptosporidium* are acid-fast.

Some intestinal parasites are more readily detected in material other than feces. For example, use of the string test (or one of its commercial substitutes) to sample duodenal contents is sometimes necessary to detect *Giardia lamblia*, *Cryptosporidium*, and *Strongyloides* larvae. Use of the "Scotch tape" technique to detect pinworm ova on the perianal skin sometimes also reveals ova of *T. saginata* deposited perianally when the motile segments disintegrate (see Table 213-4).

Two routine solutions are used to make wet mounts for the identification of the various life stages of helminths and protozoa: physiologic saline for trophozoites, cysts, ova, and larvae and dilute iodine solution for protozoal cysts and ova. Iodine solution must never be used to examine specimens for trophozoites because it kills the parasites and thus eliminates their characteristic motility.

The two most common concentration procedures for detecting small numbers of cysts and ova are formalin-ether sedimentation and zinc sulfate flotation. The formalin-ether technique is preferable, because all parasites sediment but not all float. Slides permanently stained for trophozoites should be prepared before concentration. Additional slides stained for cysts and ova may be made from the concentrate.

In many instances, especially in the differentiation of *Entamoeba histolytica* from other amebas, identification of parasites from wet mounts or concentrates must be considered tentative. Permanently stained smears allow study of the cellular detail necessary for definitive identification. The iron-hematoxylin stain is excellent for critical work, but the trichrome stain, which can be completed in 1 h, is a satisfactory alternative that also stains parasites in specimens preserved in polyvinyl alcohol fixative.

BLOOD AND TISSUE PARASITES Invasion of tissue by protozoa and helminths renders the choice of diagnostic techniques more difficult. For example, physicians must understand that aspiration of an amebic liver abscess rarely reveals *E. histolytica* because the trophozoites are located primarily in the abscess wall. They must remember that the urine sediment offers the best opportunity to detect *Schistosoma haematobium* in the Ethiopian youngster or the American traveler who returns from Africa with hematuria (Table 213-5). Tables 213-1, 213-2, and 213-3, which offer a quick guide to the geographic distribution and anatomic locations of the major tissue parasites, should help the physician to select the appropriate body fluid or biopsy site for microscopic examination. Tables 213-5, 213-6, and 213-7 provide additional information about the identification of parasites in samples from specific anatomic locations. The laboratory procedures for detection of parasites in other body fluids are similar to those used in the examination of feces. The physician should insist on wet mounts, concentration techniques, and permanent stains for all body fluids. The trichrome or iron-hematoxylin stains are satisfactory for all tissue helminths in body fluids other than blood, but microfilarial worms and blood protozoa are more easily visualized when stained with Giemsa or Wright's stain.

The most common parasites detected in Giemsa-stained blood smears are the plasmodia, microfilariae, and African trypanosomes

Table 213-5

Identification of Parasites in Blood and Other Body Fluids

Body Fluid, Parasite	Enrichment/Stain	Culture Technique
BLOOD		
Plasmodium spp.	Thick and thin smears/ Giemsa or Wright's	Not useful for diagnosis
Leishmania spp.	Buffy coat/Giemsa	Media available from CDC
African trypanosomes*	Buffy coat, anion column/wet mount and Giemsa	Mouse or rat inoculation†
Trypanosoma cruzi‡	As for African species	As above and xenodiagnosis
Toxoplasma gondii	Buffy coat/Giemsa	Fibroblast cell lines
Microfilariae§	Nuclepore filtration/ wet mount and Giemsa	None
URINE¶		
Schistosoma haematobium	Centrifugation/wet mount	None
Microfilariae (in chyluria)	As for blood	None
SPINAL FLUID		
African trypanosomes	Centrifugation, anion column/wet mount and Giemsa	As for blood
Naegleria fowleri	Centrifugation/wet mount and Giemsa or trichrome	Nonnutrient agar overlaid with *Escherichia coli*

* *Trypanosoma rhodesiense* and *T. gambiense.*
† Inject mice intraperitoneally with 0.2 mL of whole heparinized blood (0.5 mL for rats). After 5 days, tail blood should be checked daily for trypanosomes as described above.
‡ Detectable in blood by conventional techniques only during acute disease. Xenodiagnosis is successful in about 50 percent of patients with chronic Chagas' disease.
§ Day (1000–1400 h) and night (2200–0200 h) blood should be drawn to maximize the chance of detecting *Wuchereria* (nocturnal except for Pacific strains), *Brugia* (nocturnal), and *Loa loa* (diurnal).
¶ *Trichomonas vaginalis* is often detectable in urine, but examination of vaginal secretions is probably the preferable technique.

(see Table 213-5). Most patients with Chagas' disease present in the chronic phase, when *Trypanosoma cruzi* is no longer microscopically detectable in blood smears. Wet mounts are sometimes more sensitive than stained smears for the detection of microfilariae and African trypanosomes because these active parasites cause noticeable movement of the erythrocytes in the microscopic field. Nuclepore filtration of blood facilitates the detection of microfilariae. The intracellular amastigote forms of *Leishmania* spp. and *T. cruzi* can sometimes be visualized in stained smears of peripheral blood, but aspirates of the bone marrow, liver, and spleen are the best sources for microscopic detection and culture of *Leishmania* in kala-azar and of *T. cruzi* in chronic Chagas' disease.

The diagnosis of malaria and the critical distinction among the various *Plasmodium* species are made by microscopic examination of stained thick and thin blood films (see Table 213-6). Most malariologists prefer Giemsa stain because of its overall high quality, suitability for staining of both thick and thin smears, and stability in tropical climates. Wright's stain can produce high-quality thin smears and is widely used in the Americas, but it deteriorates rapidly in the tropics because its methanol base is highly hygroscopic. Specimens of capillary or venous blood should be obtained every 4 to 12 h until a diagnosis is established. The thin smear is made on clean slides exactly like a blood film for a white blood cell differential. The thick film is made by placing one drop of blood on the slide and stirring it in a circular motion to a diameter of about 2 cm. The erythrocytes in the

Table 213-6

Differential Diagnosis of *Plasmodium* Species in Blood Smears

Feature	*P. falciparum*	*P. vivax*	*P. malariae*	*P. ovale*
FEATURE OF RED CELLS				
Size	All sizes	Large (young)	Small (old)	Large (young)
Shape	Round; may be crenated	Round or oval	Round	Round or pear-shaped, fimbriated
Stippling	Maurer's clefts: large, red (up to 20)	Schüffner's dots: numerous, small, red	None	Schüffner's dots
FEATURE OF PARASITE				
Ring trophozoites	Thread-like, multiple infections, double chromatin dots, accolé forms*	Thicker	Compact	Compact
Mature trophozoites	Absent	Ameboid, may fill cell	More regular, smaller band forms†	Less ameboid and smaller than those of *P. vivax*
Schizonts	Absent	12 to 24 merozoites	8 to 12 merozoites, often rosetted around pigment	8 to 12 merozoites
Gametocytes	Banana-shaped, central chromatin (female) or diffuse (male)	Round, fills cell, pigment often central	Round, large, coarse pigment	Smaller and oval, but similar to those of *P. vivax*
DIAGNOSTIC KEYS				
	Gametocyte, multiple rings, double chromatin dots, accolé forms, heavy infections	Schizont, large RBCs, ameboid forms	Schizont, small RBCs, band forms	Schizont and large RBCs, pear-shaped, fimbriated RBCs

* At periphery of RBCs; may be flattened into rod shape.
† Stretch across RBCs, but not banana-shaped.
NOTE: RBCs, red blood cells.

Table 213-7

Minor Procedures for Diagnosis of Parasitic Infections

Procedure	Parasite(s) and Stage
Skin snips: Lift skin with a needle and excise about 1 mg to a depth of 0.5 mm from several sites. Weigh each sample, place it in 0.5 mL of saline for 4 h, and examine wet mounts and Giemsa stains of the saline either directly or after filtration. Count microfilariae.*	*Onchocerca volvulus* and *Mansonella streptocerca* microfilariae
Biopsies of subcutaneous nodules: Stain routine histopathologic sections and impression smears with Giemsa.	*Loa loa* adults and *O. volvulus* adults and microfilariae
Muscle biopsies: Excise about 1.0 g of deltoid or gastrocnemius muscle and squash between two glass slides for direct microscopic examination.	*Trichinella spiralis* larvae (and perhaps *Taenia solium* cysticerci)
Rectal snips: From four areas of mucosa take 2-mg snips, tease onto a glass slide, and flatten with a second slide before examining directly at 10×. Preparations may be fixed in alcohol or stained.	*Schistosoma* ova of all species, but especially *S. mansoni*
Aspirate of chancre or lymph node†: Aspirate center with 18-gauge needle, place a drop on a slide, and examine for motile forms. An otherwise insufficient volume of material may be stained with Giemsa.	*Trypanosoma gambiense* and *Trypanosoma rhodesiense* trypomastigotes
Corneal scrapings: Obtain sample from ophthalmologist for immediate Giemsa staining and culture on nutrient agar overlaid with *Escherichia coli.*	*Acanthamoeba* species trophozoites or cysts
Swabs, aspirates, or punch biopsies of skin lesions: Obtain specimen from margin of lesion for Giemsa staining of impression smears and section and culture on special media from CDC.	Cutaneous and mucocutaneous species of *Leishmania*

* Counts of >100/mg are associated with significant risk of complications.
† Lymph node aspiration is contraindicated in some infections and should be used judiciously.

thick film are lysed with water, but the thin film is fixed in methanol to preserve erythrocyte morphology.

Although most tissue parasites stain with the traditional hematoxylin and eosin, surgical biopsy specimens should also be stained with appropriate special stains. The surgical pathologist who is accustomed to applying silver stains for *Pneumocystis carinii* to induced sputum and transbronchial biopsies may have to be reminded to examine wet mounts and iron-hematoxylin–stained preparations of pulmonary specimens for helminthic ova and *E. histolytica*. The clinician also should be able to advise the surgeon and pathologist about optimal techniques for the identification of parasites in specimens obtained by certain specialized minor procedures (see Table 213-7). For example, the excision of skin snips for the diagnosis of onchocerciasis, the collection of rectal snips for the diagnosis of schistosomiasis, and punch biopsy of skin lesions for the identification and culture of cutaneous and mucocutaneous species of *Leishmania* are simple procedures, but the diagnosis can be missed if the specimens are improperly obtained or processed.

NONSPECIFIC TESTS Eosinophilia is a common accompaniment of infections with most of the tissue helminths; absolute numbers of eosinophils may be high in trichinosis and the migratory phases of filariasis (Table 213-8). Intestinal helminths provoke eosinophilia only during pulmonary migration of the larval stages. Eosinophilia is not a manifestation of protozoal infections, with the possible exceptions of those due to *Isospora* and *Dientamoeba fragilis*.

Like the hypochromic, microcytic anemia of heavy hookworm infections, other nonspecific laboratory abnormalities may suggest parasitic infection in patients with appropriate geographic and/or environmental exposures. Biochemical evidence of cirrhosis or an abnor-

mal urine sediment in an African immigrant certainly raises the possibility of schistosomiasis, and anemia and thrombocytopenia in a febrile traveler or immigrant are among the hallmarks of malaria. Computed tomography and magnetic resonance imaging also contribute to the diagnosis of infections with many tissue parasites and have become invaluable adjuncts in the diagnosis of neurocysticercosis and cerebral toxoplasmosis.

ANTIBODY AND ANTIGEN DETECTION As shown in Table 213-9, there are useful antibody assays for many of the important tissue parasites. The antibody assays listed in Table 213-9 are available from the Centers for Disease Control and Prevention (CDC) in Atlanta. The results of most serologic tests not listed in the tables and not offered by the CDC should be interpreted with caution.

The value of antibody assays is limited in the case of the filarial worms and plasmodia. The detection of antibody to plasmodia is primarily an epidemiologic tool and is of limited use for establishing the diagnosis of malaria in individual patients. Filarial antigens cross-react with those from other nematodes, and antibody assays do not distinguish between past and current infection. In contrast, a negative result in an American or European traveler virtually rules out the diagnosis of bancroftian or brugian filariasis. Promising assays for filarial antigens in lymphatic filariasis are not yet available in commercial kits or from the CDC.

Despite these specific limitations, the restricted geographic distribution of many of the tropical parasites increases the usefulness of antibody detection as a means of establishing diagnoses in travelers from industrialized countries. On the other hand, a large proportion of the world has been exposed to *Toxoplasma gondii*, and the presence of IgG antibody does not constitute proof of active disease.

Fewer antibody assays are available for the diagnosis of infection with intestinal parasites. Problems of cross-reactivity and lack of efficient cultivation techniques, along with the ability to establish diagnoses without invasive procedures, have discouraged intensive investigation of these methods. *E. histolytica* is the major exception. The availability of sensitive, specific serologic tests is an invaluable aid in the diagnosis of amebiasis. Commercial kits for the detection of

Table 213-8

Parasites Frequently Associated with Eosinophilia*

Parasite	Comment
TAPEWORMS (CESTODES)	
Echinococcus granulosus	When hydatid cyst leaks
Taenia solium	During muscle encystation and in CSF with neurocysticercosis
FLUKES (TREMATODES)	
Paragonimus spp.	Uniformly high in acute stage
Fasciola hepatica	May be high in acute stage
Clonorchis (Opisthorchis) sinensis	Variable
Schistosoma mansoni	50% of infected travelers
Schistosoma haematobium	25% of infected travelers
Schistosoma japonicum	Up to 6000/μL in acute infection
ROUNDWORMS	
Ascaris lumbricoides	During larval migration
Hookworm species	During larval migration
Strongyloides stercoralis	Profound during migration and early years of infection
Trichinella spiralis	Up to 7000/μL
Filarial species†	Varies but can reach 5000 to 8000/μL
Toxocara spp.	>3000/μL
Ancylostoma braziliense	With extensive cutaneous eruption
Gnathostoma spinigerum	In visceral larva migrans and eosinophilic meningitis
Angiostrongylus cantonensis	In eosinophilic meningitis
Angiostrongylus costaricensis	During larval migration in mesenteric vessels
POSSIBLE PROTOZOAL CAUSES	
Isospora belli	A few reports of profound eosinophilia
Dientamoeba fragilis	Possible pathogenicity and eosinophilia

* Virtually every helminth has been associated with eosinophilia. This table includes both common and uncommon parasites that frequently elicit eosinophilia during infection.
† *Wuchereria bancrofti*, *Brugia* spp., *Loa loa*, and *Onchocerca volvulus*.

Table 213-9

Serologic and Molecular Tests for Parasitic Infections

Parasite, Infection	Antibody	Antigen or DNA/RNA
TAPEWORMS		
Echinococcosis	WB, IHA	
Cysticercosis	WB	
FLUKES		
Paragonimiasis	WB	
Schistosomiasis	EIA, WB	
ROUNDWORMS		
Strongyloidiasis	EIA	
Trichinellosis	BF, EIA	
Toxocariasis	EIA	
PROTOZOANS		
Amebiasis	IHA, EIA	EIA
Giardiasis		EIA, IIF, DFA
Cryptosporidiosis		IIF, EIA, DFA, PCR
Malaria (all species)	IIF*	PCR
Babesiosis (*B. microti*)	IIF	
Chagas' disease	IIF, CF, EIA	
Leishmaniasis	IIF, CF	
Toxoplasmosis	IIF (IgM), EIA	
Microsporidiosis		PCR

* Of use primarily for screening blood donors.

NOTE: BF, bentonite flocculation; CF, complement fixation; EIA, enzyme immunoassay; WB, western blot; IHA, indirect hemagglutination; IIF, indirect immunofluorescence; DFA, direct fluorescent antibody; PCR, polymerase chain reaction. All antibody tests listed are available from the CDC. Antigen and parasite detection kits are available commercially. The PCRs listed are those currently available from the CDC.

antigen by enzyme-linked immunosorbent assay (ELISA) or of whole organisms by fluorescent antibody assay are now available for several protozoan parasites (Table 213-9).

MOLECULAR TECHNIQUES DNA hybridization with probes that are repeated many times in the genome of a specific parasite and amplification of a specific DNA fragment by the polymerase chain reaction (PCR) are promising techniques for the diagnosis of infections with parasites and other infectious agents. Although molecular techniques for the detection of many parasites are already being used in insect vectors, animal models, and human trials, few are available for routine use in patients at this time. The only available commercial kit is that for the identification of *Trichomonas vaginalis* by hybridization of secretions from vaginal swabs with synthetic oligonucleotide probes. Currently, the CDC will perform PCR for microsporidia and cryptosporidia on frozen stool, on stool fixed in potassium dichromate, and on biopsy specimens fixed in methanol or ethanol and for plasmodia (identification or speciation) on blood treated with EDTA or blotted on filter paper (Table 213-9).

BIBLIOGRAPHY

Despommier DD, Karapeleu JW: *Parasite Life Cycles.* New York, Springer-Verlag, 1987

Fleck SL, Moody AH: *Diagnostic Techniques in Medical Parasitology.* London, Wright, 1988

Garcia LS et al: Diagnosis of parasitic infections: Collection, processing, and examination of specimens, in *Manual of Clinical Microbiology*, 6th ed, PR Murray et al (eds). Washington, DC, ASM Press, 1995, pp 1145–1158

Gutierrez V, Little MD (eds): *Clinics in Laboratory Medicine: Diagnosis of Important Parasitic Diseases.* Philadelphia, Saunders, 1991, vol 11

Pearson RD, De Queiroz Sousa A: Clinical spectrum of leishmaniasis. Clin Infect Dis 22:1, 1996

Tomecki KJ (ed): *Dermatologic Clinics, Systemic Mycoses and Parasitic Diseases.* Philadelphia, Saunders, 1989, vol 7

Weber R et al: Improved light-microscopical detection of microsporidia spores in stool and duodenal aspirates. N Engl J Med 326:161, 1992

Weiss JB: DNA probes and PCR for diagnosis of parasitic infections. Clin Microbiol Rev 8:113, 1995

Weller PF: Eosinophilia in travelers. Med Clin North Am 76:1413, 1992

Wilson M et al: Diagnosis of parasitic infections: Immunologic and molecular methods, in *Manual of Clinical Microbiology*, 6th ed, PR Murray et al (eds). Washington, DC, ASM Press, 1995, pp 1159–1170

214 Leo X. Liu, Peter F. Weller

THERAPY FOR PARASITIC INFECTIONS

Chemotherapy for parasitic diseases is beset with potential problems. Knowledge of the fundamental biology and metabolism of eukaryotic parasites is still rudimentary. Many essential antiparasitic drugs, such as chloroquine and diethylcarbamazine, have been used for decades without a full understanding of their mechanisms of action. For a disease such as falciparum malaria, which causes tremendous suffering and mortality worldwide, the emergence of drug resistance poses an urgent problem. Because most parasitic infections primarily affect populations in poor developing countries, commercial incentives to develop and market antiparasitic drugs are limited.

Nevertheless, the introduction in recent years of several new agents, such as mefloquine, praziquantel, albendazole, and ivermectin, has led to improved therapy for several parasitic infections. Table 214-1 summarizes drug therapy for the more common parasitic diseases. Information regarding the indications, adverse effects, and contraindications for selected drugs is presented below. Drugs considered investigational by the Food and Drug Administration (FDA) for a given parasitic indication are marked with an asterisk (*). Other drugs, marked with a dagger (†), may not be generally available in the United States but can be obtained through the Centers for Disease Control and Prevention Drug Service, Atlanta, GA 30333 (telephone 404-639-3670). Antiparasitic drug treatment to be used for children and pregnant women or in certain unusual circumstances is detailed in the references.

Albendazole* This benzimidazole derivative is active against a variety of helminthic parasites but is still available only directly from the manufacturer (Smith Kline–Beecham). Albendazole is the drug of choice for the medical treatment of hydatid cysts and is also useful as an adjunct to surgical therapy. It is effective for cysticercosis, is promising for many intestinal and tissue nematode infections, and is less toxic than the older benzimidazoles. Adverse reactions to albendazole include occasional diarrhea and abdominal pain, and its use during pregnancy is contraindicated.

Benznidazole* This nitroimidazole derivative, not presently available in the United States, can ameliorate the course of acute Chagas' disease. Frequent side effects include rashes, nausea, and peripheral neuritis.

Bithionol† This drug is used for the treatment of fascioliasis and paragonimiasis. Adverse cutaneous and gastrointestinal reactions are common.

Chloroguanide* This pyrimidine derivative (also known as proguanil) is active against the preerythrocytic intrahepatic forms of *Plasmodium falciparum* and possibly *Plasmodium vivax*. Its use is largely limited to malaria prophylaxis (in combination with chloroquine) in parts of Africa where chloroquine-resistant *P. falciparum* is not yet widely prevalent. However, foci of resistance to chloroguanide exist in many regions, and clinical failures with this agent are common. Chloroguanide is not licensed in the United States but is sold in Canada, Europe, and Africa.

Chloroquine This mainstay of oral antimalarial therapy is a 4-aminoquinolone that rapidly kills schizonts and gametocytes of *P. vivax*, *Plasmodium ovale*, *Plasmodium malariae*, and susceptible strains of *P. falciparum*. Unfortunately, in many areas *P. falciparum* is resistant to chloroquine, and in Oceania resistance has emerged in *P. vivax*. Chloroquine is still effective for the treatment and prophylaxis of malaria in areas where resistance is not yet established. If chloroquine phosphate is not available, hydroxychloroquine sulfate (more commonly used as an antiarthritic agent) can be used effectively; 400 mg of the latter is equivalent to 500 mg of the former. Chloroquine is safe in children and pregnant women. Side effects may include abdominal discomfort, headache, and dizziness.

Diethylcarbamazine This piperazine derivative remains the drug of choice for lymphatic filariasis, despite adverse reactions. The mechanism of action of diethylcarbamazine is unclear, but the drug is microfilaricidal in vivo. Adverse reactions are generally proportional to the microfilarial burden and include fever, headache, dizziness, and transient exacerbation of lymphangitis. In patients with onchocerciasis, the drug elicits prominent pruritus and ocular and constitutional symptoms (the Mazzotti reaction) and thus has been supplanted by ivermectin. Diethylcarbamazine is effective for treatment and prophylaxis of *Loa loa* infection and has been used for visceral larva migrans. The drug is not commercially available in the United States; limited amounts may be obtained from the manufacturer (Wyeth-Ayerst).

Diloxanide Furoate† This amebicidal agent is poorly absorbed and is active only against luminal amebas. Its mode of action is unknown. Mild side effects include flatulence and gastrointestinal discomfort.

Eflornithine Commonly known as difluoromethylornithine or DFMO, this drug is effective in both hemolymphatic and central nervous system stages of *Trypanosoma brucei gambiense* infection (African trypanosomiasis). Eflornithine is available in the United States only from the manufacturer (Merrell Dow). It acts by irreversible inhibition of the trypanosomal ornithine decarboxylase, although *Trypanosoma brucei rhodesiense* is relatively insensitive to its effects. Adverse reactions—diarrhea, anemia, and leukopenia—are frequent but reversible.

Furazolidone This nitrofuran derivative is used as an alternative drug for the treatment of giardiasis. Unlike other drugs used for this

Table 214-1

Treatment of Parasitic Infections*

Infection (Etiologic Agent)	Treatment of Choice	Alternative Regimen
Amebiasis (*Entamoeba histolytica*)		
Asymptomatic infection	Diloxanide furoate 500 mg tid for 10 days	Iodoquinol 650 mg tid for 20 days, *or* paromomycin 25–30 mg/kg/d in 3 doses for 7 days
Mild to moderate disease	Metronidazole 750 mg tid for 10 days followed by iodoquinol 650 mg tid for 20 days	Tinidazole 2 g/d followed by iodoquinol as above
Severe intestinal disease	Metronidazole as above followed by iodoquinol as above	Tinidazole 600 mg bid or 800 mg tid for 5 days followed by iodoquinol as above
Hepatic abscess	Metronidazole as above for 5 days followed by iodoquinol as above	Tinidazole 600 mg bid or 800 mg tid for 5 days followed by iodoquinol as above
Amebic meningoencephalitis (*Naegleria*)	Amphotericin B 1 mg/kg/d IV for uncertain duration	—
Angiostrongyliasis		
Angiostrongylus cantonensis	Supportive therapy and glucocorticoids as needed	—
Angiostrongylus costaricensis	Thiabendazole 75 mg/kg/d in 3 doses for 3 days (max 3 g/d)	Mebendazole 200–400 mg tid for 10 days
Anisakiasis (*Anisakis*)	Surgical or endoscopic removal	—
Ascariasis (*Ascaris lumbricoides*)	Mebendazole 100 mg bid for 3 days, *or* piperazine 75 mg/kg (max 3.5 g) for 2 days	Pyrantel pamoate 11 mg/kg (max 1 g), *or* albendazole 400 mg once
Babesiosis (*Babesia*)	Clindamycin 1.2 g bid IV *or* 600 mg tid PO for 7 days plus quinine 650 mg tid PO for 7 days	—
Balantidiasis (*Balantidium coli*)	Tetracycline 500 mg qid for 10 days	Metronidazole 750 mg tid for 5 days
Capillariasis (*Capillaria philippinensis*)	Mebendazole 200 mg bid for 20 days	Albendazole 200 mg bid for 10 days, *or* thiabendazole 25 mg/kg/d in 2 doses for 30 days
Cryptosporidiosis (*Cryptosporidium*)	No effective specific therapy; self-limited in normal hosts; paromomycin 500–750 mg qid possibly effective in some HIV-infected patients	
Cutaneous larva migrans, or "creeping eruption" (hookworms, usually *Ancylostoma braziliense*)	Thiabendazole 10% suspension topically qid, *or* 25 mg/kg for 2–5 days	Ivermectin 150–200 μg/kg once, *or* albendazole 200 mg bid for 3 days
Cyclosporiasis (*Cyclospora cayetanensis*)	Trimethoprim-sulfamethoxazole 160/800 mg bid for 7 days	—
Cysticercosis (*Cysticercus cellulosae*)	Praziquantel 50 mg/kg/d in 3 doses for 15 days, *or* albendazole 15 mg/kg/d in 3 doses for 8–28 days, repeated as necessary, with concurrent glucocorticoids for CNS disease	Surgery
Dracunculiasis (*Dracunculus medinensis*)	Metronidazole 250 mg tid for 10 days plus worm removal	Thiabendazole 50–75 mg/kg/d in 2 doses for 3 days plus worm removal
Echinococcosis		
Echinococcus granulosus (hydatid cyst)	Surgical excision if possible and albendazole 400 mg bid for 20 days, repeated as necessary	—
Echinococcus multilocularis	Surgical excision	—
Enterobiasis (*Enterobius vermicularis*, pinworm)	Pyrantel pamoate 11 mg/kg once (max 1 g), *or* mebendazole 100 mg once, *or* albendazole 400 mg once; each repeated after 2 weeks	—
Filariasis		
Lymphatic filariasis (*Wuchereria bancrofti, Brugia malayi*)	Diethylcarbamazine Day 1: 50 mg PO Day 2: 50 mg tid Day 3: 100 mg tid Days 4–21: 6 mg/kg/d in 3 doses	—
Loiasis (*Loa loa*)	Diethylcarbamazine Day 1: 50 mg PO Day 2: 50 mg tid Day 3: 100 mg tid Days 4–21: 9 mg/kg/d in 3 doses	—
Mansonelliasis		
Mansonella ozzardi	Ivermectin 150 μg/kg single dose	—
M. perstans	Mebendazole 100 mg bid for 30 days	—
M. streptocerca	Diethylcarbamazine as for lymphatic filariasis	—
Tropical pulmonary eosinophilia	Diethylcarbamazine 6 mg/kg/d in 3 doses for 21 days	—
Onchocerciasis (*Onchocerca volvulus*)	Ivermectin 150 μg/kg once, repeated every 3–12 months	—

(continued)

Table 214-1 (*Continued*)

Treatment of Parasitic Infections*

Infection (Etiologic Agent)	Treatment of Choice	Alternative Regimen
Fluke infections		
Liver flukes (*Clonorchis sinensis*; *Opisthorchis viverrini*)	Praziquantel 75 mg/kg/d in 3 doses for 1 day	—
Sheep liver fluke (*Fasciola hepatica*)	Bithionol 30–50 mg/kg on alternate days for 10–15 doses	—
Intestinal flukes (*Fasciolopsis buski*, *Heterophyes heterophyes*, *Metagonimus yokogawai*)	Praziquantel 75 mg/kg/d in 3 doses for 1 day	—
Lung fluke (*Paragonimus westermani*)	Praziquantel 75 mg/kg/d in 3 doses for 2 days	Bithionol 30–50 mg/kg on alternate days for 10–15 doses
Giardiasis (*Giardia lamblia*)	Metronidazole 250 mg tid for 5 days	Tinidazole 2 g once, *or* paromomycin 25–30 mg/kg in 3 doses for 7 days, *or* furazolidone 100 mg qid for 7–10 days
Gnathostomiasis (*Gnathostoma spinigerum*)	Surgical removal plus albendazole 400–800 mg/d for 21 days	—
Hookworm (*Ancylostoma duodenale*, *Necator americanus*)	Mebendazole 100 mg bid for 3 days, *or* pyrantel pamoate 11 mg/kg (max 1 g) for 3 days	Albendazole 400 mg once
Isosporiasis (*Isospora belli*)	Trimethoprim-sulfamethoxazole 160/800 mg qid for 10 days, then bid for 3 weeks	Pyrimethamine 50–75 mg once daily for 3 weeks
Leishmaniasis: cutaneous, mucocutaneous, or visceral (*Leishmania braziliensis*, *L. mexicana*, *L. tropica*, *L. major*, *L. donovani*)	Stibogluconate sodium 20 mg/kg/d (max 800 mg/d) IV or IM for 20–28 days, *or* meglumine antimonate 20 mg/kg/d for 20–28 days; may be repeated or continued until response is demonstrated	Amphotericin B 0.25–1 mg/kg by slow infusion daily or every 2 days for up to 8 weeks, *or* pentamidine isethionate 2–4 mg/kg/d IM up to 15 doses
Malaria (*Plasmodium falciparum*, *P. ovale*, *P. vivax*, *P. malariae*)		
Treatment		
All except chloroquine-resistant *P. falciparum*		
Oral	Chloroquine phosphate 600 mg base (1 g), then 300 mg base (500 mg) at 6, 24, and 48 h	—
Parenteral	Quinidine gluconate 10 mg/kg loading dose (max 600 mg) over 1 h followed by continuous infusion of 0.02 mg/kg/min for 3 days maximum	—
Followed by (for *P. vivax* and *P. ovale* only)	Primaquine phosphate 15 mg base (26.3 mg)/d for 14 days or 45 mg base (79 mg)/wk for 8 weeks	—
Chloroquine-resistant *P. falciparum*		
Oral	Quinine sulfate 650 mg tid for 3 days plus pyrimethamine-sulfadoxine 3 tablets at once on last day of quinine, *or* plus tetracycline 250 mg qid for 7 days, *or* plus clindamycin 900 mg tid for 3 days	Mefloquine 750 mg followed by 500 mg 6–8 h later, *or* halofantrine 500 mg q6h for 3 doses, repeated in 1 week
Parenteral	Quinidine gluconate as above	—
Prophylaxis		
Chloroquine-sensitive areas	Chloroquine phosphate 300 mg base (500 mg salt) given PO once a week beginning 1 week before and continuing for 4 weeks after last exposure	—
Chloroquine-resistant areas	Mefloquine 250 mg given PO once a week and continuing for 4 weeks after last exposure, *or* doxycycline 100 mg/d during exposure and for 4 weeks afterward	Chloroquine phosphate as in chloroquine-sensitive areas plus pyrimethamine-sulfadoxine for presumptive treatment *or* plus proguanil† 200 mg/d in sub-Saharan Africa during exposure and for 4 weeks afterward
Schistosomiasis		
Schistosoma mansoni	Praziquantel 40 mg/kg/d in 2 doses for 1 day	Oxamniquine 15 mg/kg once; 30 mg/kg once in East Africa; 30 mg/kg once daily for 2 days in Egypt and South Africa
S. haematobium	Praziquantel 40 mg/kg/d in 2 doses for 1 day	—
S. japonicum, *S. mekongi*	Praziquantel 60 mg/kg/d in 3 doses for 1 day	—
Strongyloidiasis		
(*Strongyloides stercoralis*)	Thiabendazole 50 mg/kg/d in 2 doses (max 3 g/d) for 2 days; for disseminated disease, continue for 7 days (or longer if host is immunocompromised)	Ivermectin 200 μg/kg/d for 1–2 days, *or* albendazole 400 mg once daily for 3 days

(*continued*)

Table 214-1 (*Continued*)

Treatment of Parasitic Infections*

Infection (Etiologic Agent)	Treatment of Choice	Alternative Regimen
Tapeworm intestinal infections		
Diphyllobothrium latum—fish; *Taenia saginata*—beef; *T. solium*—pork; *Dipylidium caninum*—dog	Praziquantel 10–20 mg/kg once	—
Hymenolepis nana (dwarf tapeworm)	Praziquantel 25 mg/kg once	—
Toxoplasmosis		
(*Toxoplasma gondii*)	Pyrimethamine 25–100 mg/d plus sulfadiazine 1–1.5 g qid plus folinic acid 10 mg/d for 3–4 weeks	Clindamycin 1.8–2.4 g/d in divided doses plus pyrimethamine 25–100 mg/d plus folinic acid 10 mg/d for 3–4 weeks; *or* spiramycin 3–4 g/d in pregnancy continued until delivery
Trichinosis		
(*Trichinella spiralis*)	Glucocorticoids (for severe symptoms) plus mebendazole 200–400 mg tid for 3 days, then 400–500 mg tid for 10 days	—
Trichomoniasis		
(*Trichomonas vaginalis*)	Metronidazole 2 g once or 250 mg tid PO for 7 days, *or* tinidazole 2 g once	—
Trichostrongyliasis		
(*Trichostrongylus*)	Pyrantel pamoate 11 mg/kg once (max 1 g)	Mebendazole 100 mg bid for 3 days, *or* albendazole 400 mg once
Trichuriasis		
(*Trichuris trichiura*, whipworm)	Mebendazole 100 mg bid for 3 days, *or* albendazole 400 mg once	—
Trypanosomiasis		
Trypanosoma cruzi (Chagas' disease)	Nifurtimox 8–10 mg/kg/d PO in 4 doses for 120 days	Benznidazole 5–7 mg/kg/d for 30–120 days
T. brucei gambiense, T. brucei rhodesiense (sleeping sickness)		
Hemolymphatic stage	Suramin test dose of 100–200 mg IV, then 1 g IV on days 1, 3, 7, 14, 21; *or* eflornithine 100 mg/kg qid for 14 days, then 300 mg/kg/d PO for 3–4 weeks	Pentamidine isethionate 4 mg/kg/d IM for 10 days
Late stage with CNS involvement	Melarsoprol 2–3.6 mg/kg/d IV for 3 days, after 1 week 3.6 mg/kg/d IV for 3 days, repeated after 10–21 days; *or* eflornithine 100 mg/kg qid for 14 days, then 300 mg/kg/d PO for 3–4 weeks	Tryparsamide 30 mg/kg (max 2 g) IV q5d to total of 12 injections, sometimes repeated after 1 month; plus suramin 10 mg/kg IV q5d to total of 12 injections, sometimes repeated after 1 month
Visceral larva migrans		
(*Toxocara cani* or *T. cati*, toxocariasis)	Supportive therapy and glucocorticoids	Diethylcarbamazine 2 mg/kg tid for 7–10 days, *or* mebendazole 100–200 mg bid for 5 days, *or* albendazole 400 mg bid for 3–5 days

* For information on the treatment of infection due to *Pneumocystis carinii,* formerly considered a parasite but now classified as a fungus, see Chap. 211.
† Chloroguanide.

purpose, furazolidone is not bitter and is available in a liquid form useful for administration to young children. Nausea, vomiting, and allergic reactions occur. The drug is a monoamine oxidase (MAO) inhibitor and produces a disulfiram-like reaction when taken with alcohol.

Halofantrine This oral antimalarial drug has been used as an alternative for the treatment of malaria due to chloroquine-resistant *P. falciparum.* Adverse effects include abdominal pain, diarrhea, and pruritus. Halofantrine should not be used in pregnancy. Because this agent causes dose-related lengthening of the PR and QT$_c$ intervals and has caused first-degree atrioventricular block, it should not be given to patients with cardiac conduction defects. Cardiac monitoring during treatment is advisable.

Iodoquinol This halogenated oxyquinolone is used for the treatment of noninvasive amebiasis and *Dientamoeba fragilis* infection and as an alternative agent for *Balantidium coli* infection. Adverse effects are uncommon, but optic neuritis has developed with prolonged use of excessively high doses.

Ivermectin† This semisynthetic derivative of avermectin is now the drug of choice for *Onchocerca volvulus* infections. A single oral dose of ivermectin is active against microfilariae but has no effect on adult worms. The agent's mechanism of action has not been conclusively identified. Ivermectin also is active against a range of intestinal nematodes and is being investigated for the treatment of lymphatic filariasis. The drug is safe and well tolerated in children and adults, but its safety in pregnancy has not been specifically investigated.

Mebendazole This benzimidazole derivative is effective against a spectrum of intestinal and tissue nematodes, including *Ascaris, Ancylostoma, Necator, Enterobius,* and *Trichuris,* and is an investigational drug for use against *Capillaria.* Benzimidazoles may act by binding β-tubulin to disrupt microtubule formation and glucose uptake. Side effects include mild abdominal pain and diarrhea. Benzimidazoles can be teratogenic in experimental animals and so are avoided during pregnancy.

Mefloquine This antimalarial agent is active against the blood stages of all malarial species and the schizonts of *P. falciparum.* A 4-aminoquinolone derivative, mefloquine is the preferred agent for the prophylaxis and oral treatment of chloroquine-resistant malaria. Adverse effects are generally dose-related and include nausea and dizziness and (more rarely) vomiting, diarrhea, psychosis, and seizures. Because it has been associated with sinus bradycardia, mefloquine is contraindicated in persons taking beta-adrenoreceptor and calcium-channel blocking agents and should not be given concurrently with quinine or quinidine. Resistance to mefloquine has been documented in *P. falciparum* in parts of Southeast Asia and Africa and poses a growing problem. Since its safety in pregnancy has not been established, mefloquine should not be given to pregnant women.

Melarsoprol† This organic arsenical compound is used only to treat late-stage African trypanosomiasis involving the central nervous system. Only after intravenous administration does enough drug enter the cerebrospinal fluid to kill the trypanosomes. Severe adverse effects are common and include myocarditis, encephalopathy, and the Jarisch-Herxheimer reaction.

Metronidazole This 5-nitroimidazole exhibits potent activity against anaerobic bacteria and several protozoa, including *Entamoeba histolytica*, *Giardia lamblia*, *Trichomonas vaginalis*, and *B. coli*. Metronidazole is the drug of choice for the treatment of giardiasis (although it is not FDA approved for this indication) and for the initial treatment of invasive amebiasis. It is generally well tolerated, but mild abdominal pain, headache, nausea, and a persistent metallic taste are common. The drug is teratogenic in animals and should be avoided in early pregnancy. Because it produces a disulfiram-like reaction, abstinence from alcohol during treatment is advisable.

Nifurtimox† This synthetic nitrofuran compound is active in acute *Trypanosoma cruzi* infection. Response rates are variable, and the drug has little effect in chronic Chagas' disease. Adverse reactions, including nausea, vomiting, insomnia, headache, vertigo, tremor, paresthesias, and convulsions, are common and dose-dependent.

Oxamniquine This tetrahydroquinolone derivative is used as an alternative agent for the treatment of *Schistosoma mansoni* infection. Higher doses are needed in Egypt and South Africa than elsewhere, and resistant strains have been encountered. Oxamniquine is well tolerated, with occasional side effects including headache, dizziness, drowsiness, and gastrointestinal disturbances. It should not be used in pregnancy.

Paromomycin This orally administered, poorly absorbed aminoglycoside is used as an alternative agent for the treatment of noninvasive amebiasis. Paromomycin also has been used in lieu of metronidazole to treat amebiasis and giardiasis in pregnant women, although it has not been approved for this purpose.

Pentamidine Isethionate This stable aromatic diamine compound is active against several protozoal pathogens, including *Leishmania* spp. and *T. brucei gambiense*. Its mechanism of action remains uncertain. Adverse reactions to parenteral pentamidine are common and include reversible nephrotoxicity, acute hypotension, pancreatitis, hypoglycemia, cardiac arrhythmias, blood dyscrasias, and sterile abscesses at the injection site.

Piperazine This inexpensive drug, widely used in developing countries for the treatment of ascariasis and enterobiasis, is an anticholinergic agent that paralyzes worms, allowing them to be flushed out by peristalsis. Intestinal disturbances, hypersensitivity reactions, and dizziness are occasional adverse reactions. Piperazine and pyrantel pamoate have antagonistic modes of action and should not be administered together.

Praziquantel This agent is the drug of choice for most trematode (fluke) and many cestode infections. Its mechanism of action is unknown. In schistosomes, however, it causes paralysis and tegumental disruption, which may permit a synergistic host immune response. Praziquantel is highly active against all human schistosome parasites, intestinal tapeworms, cysticerci, and other flukes exclusive of *Fasciola hepatica*. Side effects include headache, dizziness, drowsiness, and abdominal discomfort. Use of higher doses and adjunctive treatment with anti-inflammatory glucocorticoids are recommended for neurocysticercosis.

Primaquine This 8-aminoquinolone derivative is the only standard drug active against the intrahepatic hypnozoite forms of malarial species and is used for the radical cure of *P. vivax* and *P. ovale* malaria following schizonticidal therapy. It is also an effective gametocidal agent. A potent oxidant, primaquine causes acute hemolysis in the presence of glucose-6-phosphate dehydrogenase deficiency, and at-risk patients should be screened before such therapy is instituted. Use of primaquine is contraindicated during pregnancy.

Pyrantel This well-tolerated pyrimidine derivative acts against intestinal nematodes by inducing neuromuscular paralysis in the worms, which allows them to be expelled. A single dose is usually curative for ascariasis, enterobiasis, and trichostrongyliasis, but several doses are recommended for hookworm infection. Pyrantel is safe for use in pregnancy.

Pyrimethamine-Sulfonamides Pyrimethamine combined with sulfadiazine is used in the treatment of toxoplasmosis. The high doses required for this indication often result in significant folate deficiency, necessitating folinic acid replacement. Abdominal symptoms and rashes are also common. Pyrimethamine combined with sulfadoxine is active against most strains of *P. falciparum*, although drug resistance has become increasingly widespread. As an adjunct to quinine, pyrimethamine-sulfadoxine is still useful in the oral treatment of chloroquine-resistant *P. falciparum* malaria but is no longer recommended for malaria prophylaxis because of occasional severe or even fatal skin hypersensitivity reactions and hepatitis.

Quinine and Quinidine These cinchona alkaloids have re-emerged as first-line drugs for the treatment of falciparum malaria because of widespread chloroquine resistance. Quinine in combination with a second active drug (to reduce the likelihood of recurrence) is recommended as oral therapy for *P. falciparum* malaria. For severe infections requiring intravenous therapy, only quinidine gluconate (which is at least as effective as parenteral quinine) is available in the United States. Cardiac monitoring during quinidine infusion is mandatory, and oral quinine should be substituted as soon as the patient is able to take it. Both quinine and quinidine can cause hypoglycemia. Symptoms of cinchonism, including tinnitus, headache, visual disturbances, nausea, and abdominal pain, often develop with treatment but are rarely grounds for discontinuing the drug. Oral quinine also is used with clindamycin to treat babesiosis.

Spiramycin This agent provides an alternative to antifolates in the treatment of toxoplasmosis, particularly for pregnant women, in whom it is safe.

Stibogluconate Sodium† (Sodium Antimony Gluconate)† This pentavalent antimonial parenteral solution is the drug of choice for all forms of leishmaniasis. Its mechanism of action is unknown. Adverse effects include muscle pain, joint stiffness, nausea, vomiting, and (less commonly) rash and cardiac or hepatic toxicity. Meglumine antimonate, another pentavalent antimonial drug, is used in many French- and Spanish-speaking countries.

Suramin† This complex derivative of urea is the drug of choice for the treatment of early African trypanosomiasis. It must be given intravenously and is excreted very slowly. Adverse effects are common, can be severe, and include vomiting, pruritus, urticaria, paresthesias, photophobia, peripheral neuropathy, anaphylaxis, and renal damage.

Tetracycline and Doxycycline Tetracycline is effective against *B. coli* and *D. fragilis* and is also used as an adjunct to quinine in the treatment of chloroquine-resistant falciparum malaria. Doxycycline (in once-daily form) may be used for chemoprophylaxis of chloroquine-resistant falciparum malaria. Tooth staining in children and photosensitivity are potential hazards.

Thiabendazole This older benzimidazole derivative is active against a variety of nematode parasites, but frequent and severe side effects limit its primary systemic use in the treatment of strongyloidiasis. These adverse reactions include dizziness, nausea, vomiting, drowsiness, pruritus, headache, neuropsychiatric disturbances, hepatitis, and hypersensitivity reactions (e.g., Stevens-Johnson syndrome). A topical suspension of thiabendazole is used for cutaneous larva migrans.

Tinidazole* This nitroimidazole is available only outside the United States for the treatment of amebiasis, giardiasis, and vaginal trichomoniasis. Tinidazole appears to be more effective and better tolerated than metronidazole.

Trimethoprim-Sulfamethoxazole This antifolate combination is active in *Cyclospora cayetanensis* and *Isospora belli* infections. Adverse effects are predominantly due to the sulfamethoxazole component and include skin, liver, and bone marrow toxicity.

BIBLIOGRAPHY

Abramowicz M (ed): Drugs for parasitic infections. Med Lett Drugs Ther 37:99, 1995

Liu LX, Weller PF: An update on antiparasitic drugs. N Engl J Med 334:1178, 1996

World Health Organization: *Model Prescribing Information: Drugs Used in Parasitic Diseases*, 2d ed. Geneva, WHO, 1995

215 | *Sharon L. Reed*

AMEBIASIS AND INFECTION WITH FREE-LIVING AMEBAS

AMEBIASIS

DEFINITION   Amebiasis is an infection with the intestinal protozoan *Entamoeba histolytica*. About 90 percent of infections are asymptomatic, and the remaining 10 percent produce a spectrum of clinical syndromes ranging from dysentery to abscesses of the liver or other organs.

LIFE CYCLE AND TRANSMISSION   *E. histolytica* is acquired by ingestion of viable cysts from fecally contaminated water, food, or hands. Food-borne exposure is most prevalent and is particularly likely when food handlers are shedding cysts or food is being grown with feces-contaminated soil, fertilizer, or water. Less common means of transmission include contaminated water, oral and anal sexual practices, and—in rare instances—direct rectal inoculation through colonic irrigation devices. Motile trophozoites are released from cysts in the small intestine and, in most patients, remain as harmless commensals in the large bowel. After encystation, infectious cysts are shed in the stool and can survive for several weeks in a moist environment. In some patients, the trophozoites invade either the bowel mucosa, causing symptomatic colitis, or the bloodstream, causing distant abscesses of the liver, lungs, or brain. The trophozoites may not encyst in patients with active dysentery, and motile hematophagous trophozoites are frequently present in fresh stools. Trophozoites are rapidly killed by exposure to air or stomach acid, however, and therefore cannot cause infection.

EPIDEMIOLOGY   About 10 percent of the world's population is infected with *E. histolytica*; amebiasis is the third most common cause of death from parasitic disease (after schistosomiasis and malaria). Areas of highest incidence (due to inadequate sanitation and crowding) include most developing countries in the tropics, particularly Mexico, India, and nations of Central and South America, tropical Asia, and Africa. The main groups at risk in developed countries are travelers, recent immigrants, homosexual men, and inmates of institutions.

All *E. histolytica* trophozoites and cysts are morphologically identical, but the wide spectrum of clinical disease is caused in part by infection with two different species of *Entamoeba*. Isolates of *E. histolytica* from patients with invasive amebiasis have unique isoenzymes, surface antigens, DNA markers, and virulence properties and now are classified as a separate species from the noninvasive species *Entamoeba dispar*.

Most asymptomatic carriers, including homosexual men and AIDS patients, harbor nonpathogenic strains and have self-limited infections. These findings suggest that nonpathogenic strains (i.e., *E. dispar*) are incapable of causing invasive disease, since *Cryptosporidium* and *Isospora belli*, which also cause only self-limited illnesses in immunocompetent people, cause devastating diarrhea in AIDS patients. However, host factors play a role as well: Some patients infected with strains shown (by isoenzyme patterns) to be pathogenic do not develop invasive amebiasis but rather remain asymptomatic. In one study, 10 percent of asymptomatic patients who were colonized with pathogenic strains went on to develop amebic colitis, while the rest remained asymptomatic and cleared the infection within 1 year.

PATHOGENESIS AND PATHOLOGY   Both trophozoites (Fig. 215-1) and cysts (Fig. 215-2) are found in the intestinal lumen, but only trophozoites invade tissue. The trophozoite is 20 to 60 µm in diameter and contains vacuoles and a nucleus with a characteristic central karyosome. In animals, depletion of intestinal mucus, diffuse inflammation, and disruption of the epithelial barrier occur before

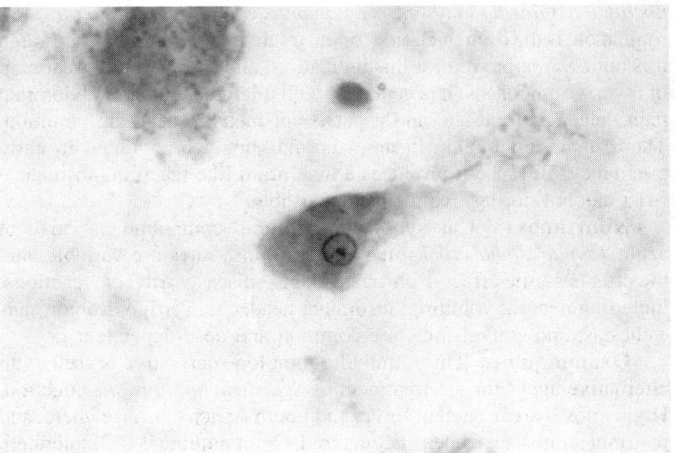

FIGURE 215-1   Trophozoite of *E. histolytica* demonstrating a single nucleus with a central, dotlike karyosome (trichrome stain).

trophozoites actually come into contact with the colonic mucosa. Trophozoites attach to colonic mucus and epithelial cells by a galactose-inhibitable lectin. The earliest intestinal lesions are microulcerations of the mucosa of the cecum, sigmoid colon, or rectum that release erythrocytes, inflammatory cells, and epithelial cells. Proctoscopy reveals small ulcers with heaped up margins and normal intervening mucosa. Submucosal extension of ulcerations under viable-appearing surface mucosa causes the classic "flask-shaped" ulcer containing trophozoites at the margins of dead and viable tissues. Although neutrophilic infiltrates may accompany the early lesions in animals, human intestinal infection is marked by a paucity of inflammatory cells, probably in part because of the killing of neutrophils by trophozoites. Treated ulcers characteristically heal with little or no scarring. Occasionally, however, full-thickness necrosis and perforation occur.

Rarely, intestinal infection results in the formation of a mass lesion, or ameboma, in the bowel lumen. The overlying mucosa is usually thin and ulcerated, while other layers of the wall are thickened, edematous, and hemorrhagic, resulting in exuberant formation of granulation tissue with little fibrous-tissue response.

A number of virulence factors have been linked to the ability of amebas to invade through the interglandular epithelium. One is an extracellular cysteine proteinase that degrades collagen, elastin, secre-

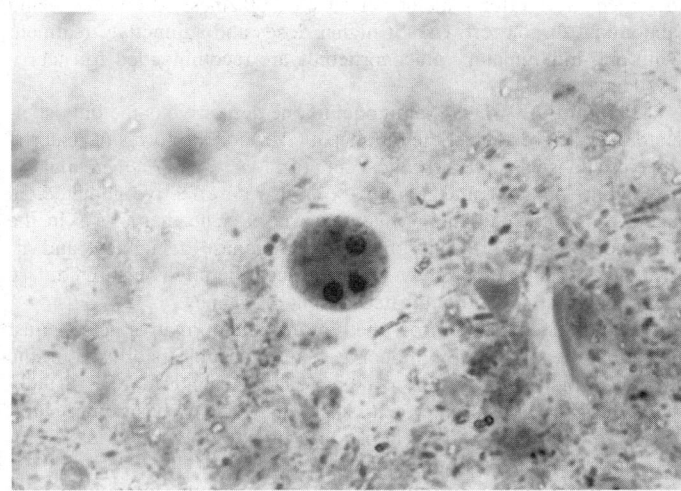

FIGURE 215-2   Cyst of *E. histolytica* showing three of the four nuclei (trichrome stain).

tory IgA, and the anaphylatoxins C3a and C5a. Other enzymes may disrupt glycoprotein bonds between mucosal epithelial cells in the gut. Amebas can lyse neutrophils, monocytes, lymphocytes, and cells of colonic and hepatic cell lines. The cytolytic effect of amebas appears to require direct contact with target cells and may be linked to the release of phospholipase A and pore-forming peptides.

Liver abscesses are always preceded by intestinal colonization, which may be asymptomatic. Blood vessels may be compromised early by lysis of the wall and thrombus formation. Trophozoites invade veins to reach the liver through the portal venous system. Pathogenic isolates are resistant to complement-mediated lysis, a property critical to survival in the bloodstream. In contrast, nonpathogenic strains are rapidly lysed by complement and are thus restricted to the bowel lumen. Inoculation of amebas into the portal system of hamsters results in an acute cellular infiltrate consisting predominantly of neutrophils. Later, the neutrophils are lysed by contact with amebas, and the release of neutrophil toxins may contribute to necrosis of hepatocytes. The liver parenchyma is replaced by necrotic material that is surrounded by a thin rim of congested liver tissue. The necrotic contents of a liver abscess are classically described as "anchovy paste," although the fluid is variable in color and is composed of bacteriologically sterile granular debris with few or no cells. Amebas, if seen, tend to be found only near the capsule of the abscess.

Clinical infection does not induce immunity to recurrent colonization with E. histolytica, but repeated episodes of colitis or liver abscess are unusual. Antibody is not protective; titers correlate with the length of illness rather than with the severity of disease. Studies of animals suggest that cell-mediated immunity may be important for protection, although patients with AIDS appear not to be predisposed to more severe disease.

CLINICAL SYNDROMES   Intestinal Amebiasis   The most common type of amebic infection is asymptomatic cyst passage. Even in highly endemic areas, most patients harbor nonpathogenic strains.

Symptomatic amebic colitis develops 2 to 6 weeks after the ingestion of infectious cysts. Lower abdominal pain and mild diarrhea develop gradually and are followed by malaise, weight loss, and diffuse lower abdominal or back pain. Cecal involvement may mimic acute appendicitis. Patients with full-blown dysentery may pass 10 to 12 stools per day. The stools contain little fecal material and consist mainly of blood and mucus. In contrast to those with bacterial diarrhea, fewer than 40 percent of patients with amebic dysentery are febrile. Virtually all patients have heme-positive stools.

More fulminant intestinal infection, with severe abdominal pain, high fever, and profuse diarrhea, is rare and occurs predominantly in children. Patients may develop toxic megacolon, in which there is severe bowel dilation with intramural air. Patients receiving glucocorticoids are at risk for severe amebiasis. Uncommonly, patients develop a chronic form of amebic colitis, which can be confused with inflammatory bowel disease. The positive association between severe amebiasis complications and steroid therapy emphasizes the importance of excluding amebiasis in any case in which inflammatory bowel disease is suspected. Amebomas are inflammatory mass lesions that develop owing to chronic intestinal forms of amebiasis. An occasional patient presents only with an asymptomatic or tender abdominal mass caused by an ameboma, which is easily confused with cancer on barium studies. A positive serologic test or biopsy can prevent unnecessary surgery in this setting. The syndrome of postamebic colitis—persistent diarrhea following documented cure of amebic colitis—is controversial; no evidence of recurrent amebic infection can be found, and re-treatment usually has no effect.

Amebic Liver Abscess   Extraintestinal infection by E. histolytica most often involves the liver. Of travelers who develop an amebic liver abscess after leaving an endemic area, 95 percent do so within 5 months. Young patients with an amebic liver abscess are more likely than older patients to present in the acute phase with prominent symptoms of less than 10 days' duration. Most patients are febrile and have right upper quadrant pain, which may be dull or pleuritic in nature and radiate to the shoulder. Point tenderness over the liver and right-sided pleural effusion are common. Jaundice is rare. Although

the initial site of infection is the colon, fewer than one-third of patients with an amebic abscess have active diarrhea. Older patients from endemic areas are more likely to have a subacute course lasting 6 months, with weight loss and hepatomegaly. About one-third of patients with chronic presentations are febrile. Thus, the clinical diagnosis of an amebic liver abscess may be difficult to establish because the symptoms and signs are often nonspecific. Since 10 to 15 percent of patients present only with fever, amebic liver abscess must be considered in the differential diagnosis of fever of unknown origin.

Complications of Amebic Liver Abscess   Pleuropulmonary involvement, which is reported in 20 to 30 percent of patients, is the most frequent complication of amebic liver abscess. Manifestations include sterile effusions, contiguous spread from the liver, and rupture into the pleural space. Sterile effusions and contiguous spread usually resolve with medical therapy, but frank rupture into the pleural space requires drainage. A hepatobronchial fistula may cause cough productive of large amounts of necrotic material that may contain amebas. This dramatic complication carries a good prognosis. Abscesses that rupture into the peritoneum may present as an indolent leak or an acute abdomen and require both percutaneous catheter drainage and medical therapy. Rupture into the pericardium, usually from abscesses of the left lobe of the liver, carries the gravest prognosis; it can occur during medical therapy and requires surgical drainage.

Other Extraintestinal Sites   The genitourinary tract may become involved by direct extension of amebiasis from the colon or by hematogenous spread of the infection. Painful genital ulcers, characterized by a punched-out appearance and profuse discharge, may develop secondary to extension from either the intestine or the liver. Both these conditions respond well to medical therapy. Cerebral involvement has been reported in fewer than 0.1 percent of patients in large clinical series. Symptoms and prognosis depend on the size and location of the lesion.

DIAGNOSTIC TESTS   Laboratory Diagnosis   Stool examinations, serologic tests, and noninvasive imaging of the liver are the most important procedures in the diagnosis of amebiasis. Fecal findings suggestive of amebic colitis include a positive test for heme, a paucity of neutrophils, and the presence of Charcot-Leyden crystal protein (double pyramid-shaped crystals normally found in the cytoplasm of eosinophils). The definitive diagnosis of amebic colitis is made by the demonstration of hematophagous trophozoites of E. histolytica (Fig. 215-1). Because trophozoites are killed rapidly by water, drying, or barium, it is important to examine at least three fresh stool specimens. Examination of a combination of wet mounts, iodine-stained concentrates, and trichrome-stained preparations of fresh stool and concentrates for cysts (Fig. 215-2) or trophozoites (Fig. 215-1) confirms the diagnosis in 75 to 95 percent of cases. Cultures of amebas are more sensitive but are not routinely available. If stool examinations are negative, sigmoidoscopy with biopsy of the edge of ulcers may increase the yield, but this procedure is dangerous during fulminant colitis because of the risk of perforation. Trophozoites in a biopsy specimen from a colonic mass confirm the diagnosis of ameboma, but trophozoites are rare in liver aspirates. Accurate diagnosis requires experience, since trophozoites may be confused with neutrophils and the cysts must be differentiated morphologically from Entamoeba hartmanni, Entamoeba coli, and Endolimax nana, which do not cause clinical disease and do not warrant therapy. Unfortunately, the cysts of pathogenic strains of E. histolytica cannot be distinguished microscopically from those of nonpathogenic strains. Future diagnostic tests will focus on the detection of antigens with monoclonal antibodies or DNA amplification as a means of differentiating E. histolytica from E. dispar.

Serology is an important addition to the methods used for the parasitologic diagnosis of invasive amebiasis. Kits for the performance of counterimmunodiffusion assays, agar gel diffusion assays, and ELISAs are commercially available, and the results of these tests are positive in more than 90 percent of patients with colitis, amebomas, or liver abscess. Positive results in conjunction with the appropriate clinical syndrome suggest active disease because serologic findings usually revert to negative within 6 to 12 months. Even in highly endemic areas such as South Africa, fewer than 10 percent of asymptomatic people have a positive amebic serology. The interpretation of the indirect hemagglutination test is more difficult because titers may remain positive for as long as 10 years. Up to 10 percent of patients with acute amebic liver abscess may have negative serologic findings; in suspected cases with an initially negative result, testing should be repeated in a week. In contrast to carriers of nonpathogenic strains, most asymptomatic carriers of pathogenic strains develop antibodies. Thus, serologic tests are helpful in assessing the risk of invasive amebiasis in asymptomatic, cyst-passing individuals in nonendemic areas. Serologic tests also should be performed in patients with ulcerative colitis before the institution of steroid therapy to prevent the development of severe colitis or toxic megacolon owing to unsuspected amebiasis.

Routine hematology and chemistry tests are usually not very helpful in the diagnosis of invasive amebiasis. About three-fourths of patients with an amebic liver abscess have leukocytosis (>10,000 cells per microliter); this condition is particularly likely if symptoms are acute or complications have developed. Invasive amebiasis does not elicit eosinophilia. Anemia, if present, is usually multifactorial. Even with large liver abscesses, liver enzyme levels are normal or minimally elevated. The alkaline phosphatase level is most often elevated and may remain so for months. Aminotransferase elevations suggest acute disease or a complication.

Radiographic Studies Radiographic barium studies are potentially dangerous in acute amebic colitis. Amebomas are usually identified first by a barium enema, but biopsy is necessary for differentiation from carcinoma.

Newer radiographic techniques have improved the detection of amebic liver abscesses. Liver scans, ultrasonography, computed tomography (Fig. 215-3), and magnetic resonance imaging are all useful for detection of the round or oval hypoechoic cyst. More than 80 percent of patients who have had symptoms for more than 10 days have a single abscess of the right lobe of the liver. Approximately 50 percent of patients who have had symptoms for less than 10 days have multiple abscesses. Findings associated with complications include large abscesses (>10 cm) in the superior part of the right lobe, which may rupture into the pleural space; multiple lesions, which must be differentiated from pyogenic abscesses; and lesions of the left lobe, which may rupture into the pericardium. Because abscesses resolve slowly and may increase in size in patients who are responding clinically to therapy, frequent follow-up ultrasonography may prove confusing. Complete resolution of a liver abscess within 6 months can be anticipated in two-thirds of patients, but 10 percent may have persistent abnormalities for a year.

DIFFERENTIAL DIAGNOSIS The differential diagnosis of intestinal amebiasis includes bacterial diarrheas caused by *Campylobacter*; enteroinvasive *Escherichia coli*; and *Shigella*, *Salmonella*, and *Vibrio* species. Although the typical patient with amebic colitis has less prominent fever than in these conditions and heme-positive stools with few neutrophils, correct diagnosis requires bacterial cultures, microscopic examination of stools, and amebic serologic testing. As has already been mentioned, amebiasis must be ruled out in any patient thought to have inflammatory bowel disease.

Because of the variety of presenting signs and symptoms, amebic liver abscess can easily be confused with pulmonary or gallbladder disease or with any febrile illness with few localizing signs, such as malaria or typhoid fever. The diagnosis should be considered in members of high-risk groups who have recently traveled outside the United States and in inmates of institutions. Once radiographic studies have identified an abscess in the liver, the most important differential diagnosis is between amebic and pyogenic abscess. Patients with pyogenic abscess typically are older and have a history of underlying bowel disease or recent surgery. Amebic serology is helpful, but aspiration of the abscess, with Gram staining and culture of the material, may be required for differentiation of the two diseases.

℞ **TREATMENT**

Intestinal Disease The drugs used to treat amebiasis can be classified according to their primary site of action. Luminal amebicides are poorly absorbed and reach high concentrations in the bowel, but their activity is limited to cysts and trophozoites close to the mucosa. Three luminal drugs are available in the United States: iodoquinol, paromomycin, and diloxanide furoate (Table 215-1). Indications for the use of luminal agents include eradication of cysts in patients with colitis or a liver abscess and treatment of asymptomatic carriers. Until probes are available for differentiating nonpathogenic from pathogenic cysts, it is prudent to treat asymptomatic individuals who pass cysts.

Tissue amebicides reach high concentrations in the blood and tissue after oral or parenteral administration. The development of nitroimidazole compounds, especially metronidazole, was a major advance in the treatment of invasive amebiasis. Patients with amebic colitis should be treated with intravenous or oral metronidazole (750 mg three times daily for 10 days). Side effects include nausea, vomiting, abdominal discomfort, and a disulfiram-like reaction.

Table 215-1

Drug Therapy for Amebiasis

Drug	Dosage
ASYMPTOMATIC CARRIER (LUMINAL AGENTS)	
Iodoquinol (650-mg tablets)	650 mg tid for 20 days
Diloxanide furoate* (500-mg tablets)	500 mg tid for 10 days
Paromomycin (250-mg tablets)	500 mg tid for 10 days
ACUTE COLITIS	
Metronidazole (250- or 500-mg tablets) plus	750 mg PO or IV tid for 5 to 10 days
Luminal agent as above	
AMEBIC LIVER ABSCESS	
Metronidazole	750 mg PO or IV tid for 5 to 10 days
Tinidazole†	2 g PO
Ornidazole† plus	2 g PO
Luminal agent as above	

* Available only through the Centers for Disease Control and Prevention at telephone number (404) 639-3356.
† Not available in the United States.

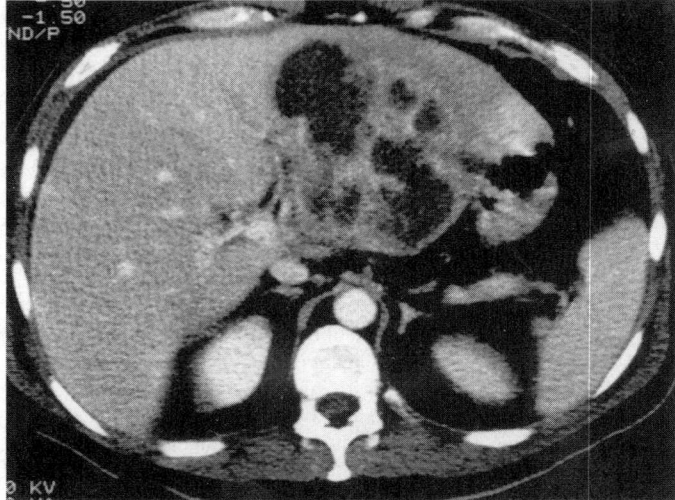

FIGURE 215-3 Abdominal computed tomography scan of a large amebic abscess of the left lobe of the liver. *(Courtesy of the Department of Radiology, UCSD Medical Center, San Diego.)*

Other imidazole compounds, such as tinidazole and ornidazole, are as effective but are not available in the United States. All patients should also receive a full course of therapy with a luminal agent, since metronidazole does not eradicate cysts. Resistance to metronidazole has not been identified. Relapses are not uncommon and probably represent reinfection or failure to eradicate amebas from the bowel because of an inadequate dosage or duration of therapy.

Amebic Liver Abscess Metronidazole is the drug of choice for amebic liver abscess. The usefulness of nitroimidazoles in single-dose or abbreviated regimens is important in endemic areas where access to hospitalization is limited. With early diagnosis and therapy, mortality from uncomplicated amebic liver abscess is less than 1 percent. The second-line therapeutic agents emetine and chloroquine should be avoided if possible because of the potential cardiovascular and gastrointestinal side effects of the former and the higher relapse rates with the latter. There is no evidence that combined therapy with two drugs is more effective than the single-drug regimen. Studies of South Africans with liver abscesses demonstrated that 72 percent of patients without intestinal symptoms were colonized asymptomatically with pathogenic strains; thus, all treatment regimens should include a luminal agent to eradicate cysts and prevent further transmission. Amebic liver abscess recurs rarely.

Aspiration of Liver Abscesses More than 90 percent of patients respond dramatically to metronidazole therapy with decreases in both pain and fever within 72 h. Indications for aspiration of liver abscesses are (1) the need to rule out a pyogenic abscess, particularly in patients with multiple lesions; (2) the failure to respond clinically in 3 to 5 days; (3) the threat of imminent rupture; and (4) the prevention of rupture of left-lobe abscesses into the pericardium. There is no evidence that aspiration, even of large abscesses (up to 10 cm), accelerates healing. Percutaneous drainage may be successful even if the liver abscess has already ruptured. Surgery should be reserved for instances of bowel perforation and rupture into the pericardium.

PREVENTION Amebic infection is spread by ingestion of food or water contaminated with cysts. Since an asymptomatic carrier may excrete up to 15 million cysts per day, prevention of infection requires adequate sanitation and eradication of cyst carriage. In high-risk areas, infection can be minimized by the avoidance of unpeeled fruits and vegetables and the use of bottled water. Because cysts are resistant to readily attainable levels of chlorine, disinfection by iodination (tetraglycine hydroperiodide) is recommended. There is no effective prophylaxis.

INFECTION WITH FREE-LIVING AMEBAS

EPIDEMIOLOGY Free-living amebas of the genera *Acanthamoeba* and *Naegleria* are distributed throughout the world and have been isolated from a wide variety of fresh and brackish water, including that from lakes, taps, hot springs, swimming pools, and heating and air-conditioning units, and even from the nasal passages of healthy children. Encystation may protect the protozoa from desiccation and food deprivation. The persistence of *Legionella pneumophila* in water supplies may be attributable in part to chronic infection of free-living amebas, particularly *Naegleria*.

NAEGLERIA **INFECTIONS** Altogether, more than 100 cases of primary amebic meningoencephalitis from *Naegleria fowleri* have been reported. Infection follows the aspiration of water contaminated with trophozoites or cysts or the inhalation of contaminated dust, leading to invasion of the olfactory neuroepithelium. After an incubation period of 2 to 15 days, severe headache, high fever, nausea, vomiting, and meningismus develop. Photophobia and palsies of the third, fourth, and sixth cranial nerves are common. Rapid progression to seizures and coma may follow, and most patients die within a week. Infection is most common in otherwise healthy children or young adults, who often report recent swimming in lakes or heated swimming pools.

Diagnosis depends on the detection of motile trophozoites in wet mounts of fresh spinal fluid. Other laboratory findings resemble those

for fulminant bacterial meningitis, with elevated intracranial pressure, high white blood cell counts (up to 20,000 cells per microliter), and elevated protein concentrations and low glucose levels in cerebrospinal fluid. The diagnosis should be considered in any patient who has purulent meningitis without evidence of bacteria on Gram staining, antigen detection assay, and culture. The prognosis is uniformly poor. Only four survivors, treated with high-dose amphotericin B and rifampin, have been reported. Antibodies to *Naegleria* spp. have been detected in normal adults; serologic testing is not useful in the diagnosis of acute infection.

ACANTHAMOEBA **INFECTIONS** **Granulomatous Amebic Encephalitis** Infection with *Acanthamoeba* species follows a more indolent course and occurs typically in chronically ill or debilitated patients. Risk factors include lymphoproliferative disorders, chemotherapy, glucocorticoid therapy, lupus erythematosus, and AIDS. Infection usually reaches the central nervous system hematogenously from a primary focus in the sinuses, skin, or lungs. In the central nervous system, the onset is insidious, and the syndrome often mimics a space-occupying lesion. Altered mental status, headache, and stiff neck may be accompanied by focal findings such as cranial nerve palsies, ataxia, and hemiparesis. Cutaneous ulcers or hard nodules containing amebas were detected in 8 of the 13 AIDS patients with disseminated *Acanthamoeba* infection described so far in the United States.

Examination of the cerebrospinal fluid for trophozoites may be diagnostically helpful, but lumbar puncture may be contraindicated because of increased intracerebral pressure. Computed tomography frequently reveals cortical and subcortical lesions of decreased density consistent with embolic infarcts. In other patients, multiple enhancing lesions with edema may mimic the computed tomographic appearance of toxoplasmosis. Demonstration of the trophozoites and cysts of *Acanthamoeba* on wet mounts or in biopsy specimens establishes the diagnosis. Culture on nonnutrient agar plates seeded with *Escherichia coli* may also be helpful. Fluorescein-labeled antiserum is available from the Centers for Disease Control and Prevention (CDC) for the detection of protozoa in biopsy specimens. At least nine cases of granulomatous amebic encephalitis have been reported in patients with AIDS, in whom the disease may have an accelerated course, with survival for only 3 to 40 days, because of their difficulty in forming granulomas. Although studies in animals suggest that rifampin may be useful, the infection is almost uniformly fatal. A similar syndrome may be caused by a leptomyxid ameba.

Keratitis The incidence of keratitis caused by *Acanthamoeba* has increased in the past 15 years; more than 250 infections have been reported to the CDC. The first of these infections to be recognized were associated with trauma to the eye and exposure to contaminated

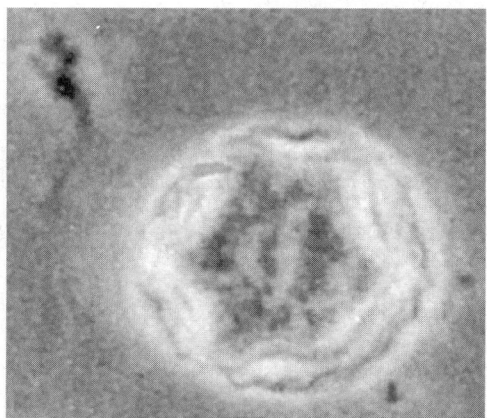

FIGURE 215-4 Double-walled cyst of *Acanthamoeba castellani*, as seen by phase-contrast microscopy. *[From DJ Krogstad et al, in Manual of Clinical Microbiology, 5th ed, A Balows et al (eds), Washington, DC, American Society for Microbiology, 1991.]*

water. At present, most infections are linked to extended-wear contact lenses. Risk factors include the use of homemade saline, the wearing of lenses while swimming, and inadequate disinfection. Since contact lenses presumably cause microscopic trauma, the early corneal findings may be nonspecific. The first symptoms usually include tearing and the painful sensation of a foreign body. Once infection is established, progression is rapid; the characteristic clinical sign is an annular, paracentral corneal ring representing a corneal abscess. Deeper corneal invasion and loss of vision may follow.

The differential diagnosis includes bacterial, mycobacterial, and herpetic infection. The irregular polygonal cysts of *Acanthamoeba* (Fig. 215-4) may be identified in corneal scrapings or biopsy material, and trophozoites can be grown on special media. Cysts are resistant to available drugs, and the results of medical therapy have been disappointing. Some reports have suggested partial responses to propamidine isethionate eyedrops. Severe infections usually require keratoplasty.

BIBLIOGRAPHY

AMEBIASIS

ALLASON-JONES E et al: *Entamoeba histolytica* as a commensal intestinal parasite in homosexual men. N Engl J Med 315:353, 1986

CLARK CG, DIAMOND LS: Ribosomal RNA genes of "pathogenic" and "nonpathogenic" *Entamoeba histolytica* are distinct. Mol Biochem Parasitol 49:297, 1991

IRUSEN EM et al: Asymptomatic intestinal colonization by pathogenic *Entamoeba histolytica* in amebic liver abscess: Prevalence, response to therapy, and pathogenic potential. Clin Infect Dis 14:889, 1992

KATZENSTEIN D et al: New concepts of amebic liver abscess derived from hepatic imaging, serodiagnosis, and hepatic enzymes in 67 consecutive cases in San Diego. Medicine 61:237, 1982

LIEPPE M et al: Cytolytic and antibacterial activity of synthetic peptides derived from amoebapore, the pore-forming peptide of *Entamoeba histolytica*. Proc Natl Acad Sci USA 91:1440, 1994

McCOY JJ et al: Adherence and cytotoxicity of *Entamoeba histolytica*, or how lectins let parasites stick around. Infect Immun 62:3045, 1994

McKERROW JH: Pathogenesis in amebiasis: Is it genetic or acquired? Infect Agents Dis 1:11, 1992

PETRI WA: Amebiasis and the *Entamoeba histolytica* Gal/GalNAc lectin: From bench to bedside. J Invest Med 44:24, 1996

————: Recent advances in amebiasis. CRC Crit Rev Clin Lab Sci 33:1, 1996

RAVDIN JI: Amebiasis. Clin Infect Dis 20:1453, 1995

REED SL et al: Cloning of a virulence factor of *Entamoeba histolytica*. Pathogenic strains possess a unique cysteine proteinase gene. J Clin Invest 91:1532, 1993

———— et al: *Entamoeba histolytica* infection and AIDS. Am J Med 90:269, 1991

STANLEY SL: Progress toward an amebiasis vaccine. Parasitol Today 12:7, 1996

THOMPSON JE et al: Amebic liver abscess: A therapeutic approach. Rev Infect Dis 7:171, 1985

ACANTHAMOEBA AND *NAEGLERIA*

LARKIN DFP: *Acanthamoeba* keratitis. Int Ophthalmol Clin 31:163, 1991

MA P et al: *Naegleria* and *Acanthamoeba* infections: Review. Rev Infect Dis 12:490, 1990

MARTINEZ AJ, VISVESVARA GS: Laboratory diagnosis of pathogenic freeliving amoebas: *Naegleria*, *Acanthamoeba*, and *Leptomyxid*. Clin Lab Med 11:861, 1991

SISON JP et al: Disseminated acanthamoeba infection in patients with AIDS: Case reports and review. Clin Infect Dis 20:1207, 1995

Nicholas J. White, Joel G. Breman

MALARIA AND OTHER DISEASES CAUSED BY RED BLOOD CELL PARASITES

MALARIA

Malaria is a protozoan disease transmitted by the bite of infected *Anopheles* mosquitoes. It is the most important of the parasitic diseases of humans, affecting more than 500 million people and causing between 1 and 3 million deaths each year. Malaria has now been eradicated from North America, Europe, and Russia but, despite enormous control efforts, has resurged in many parts of the tropics. Added to this resurgence are the increasing problems of drug resistance of the parasite and insecticide resistance of the vectors. Malaria remains today, as it has been for centuries, a heavy burden on tropical communities and a danger to travelers.

ETIOLOGY AND PATHOGENESIS Four species of the genus *Plasmodium* cause nearly all infections in humans (although rare infections involve species normally affecting other primates). These are *Plasmodium vivax*, *Plasmodium ovale*, *Plasmodium malariae*, and *Plasmodium falciparum* (Table 216-1). Almost all deaths are caused by falciparum malaria. Human infection begins when a female anopheline mosquito inoculates plasmodial sporozoites from its salivary gland during a blood meal (Fig. 216-1). These microscopic motile forms of the malarial parasite are carried rapidly via the bloodstream to the liver, where they invade hepatic parenchymal cells and begin a period of asexual reproduction. By this amplification process (known as intrahepatic or preerythrocytic schizogony or merogony), a single sporozoite eventually produces thousands of daughter merozoites. The swollen liver cell eventually bursts, discharging motile merozoites into the bloodstream; at this point the symptomatic stage of the infection begins. In *P. vivax* and *P. ovale* infections, a proportion of the intrahepatic forms do not divide immediately but remain dormant for months to years before reproduction begins. These dormant forms, or hypnozoites, are the cause of the relapses that characterize infection with these two species.

After entry into the bloodstream, merozoites rapidly invade erythrocytes and become trophozoites. Attachment is mediated via a specific erythrocyte surface receptor. In the case of *P. vivax*, this receptor is related to the Duffy blood-group antigen Fy^a or Fy^b. Most West Africans and people with origins in that region carry the Duffy-negative FyFy phenotype and are therefore resistant to *P. vivax* malaria. During the early stage of intraerythrocytic development, the small "ring forms" of the four parasitic species appear similar under light microscopy. As the trophozoites enlarge, species-specific characteristics become evident, pigment becomes visible, and the parasite assumes an irregular or ameboid shape. By the end of the 48-h intraerythrocytic life cycle (72 h for *P. malariae*), the parasite has consumed nearly all the hemoglobin and grown to occupy most of the red cell. Multiple nuclear divisions take place (schizogony or merogony), and the red cell ruptures to release 6 to 30 daughter merozoites, each capable of invading a new red cell and repeating the cycle. The disease in human beings is caused by the direct effects of red cell invasion and destruction by the asexual parasite and the host's reaction. During this process, some parasites develop into morphologically distinct sexual forms (gametocytes, still within the erythrocytes), which are long-lived.

After being ingested in the blood meal of a biting female anopheline mosquito, the male and female gametocytes form a zygote in the insect's midgut. This zygote matures into an ookinete, which penetrates and encysts in the mosquito's gut wall. The resulting oocyst expands by asexual division until it bursts to liberate myriad motile sporozoites, which then migrate in the hemolymph to the salivary gland of the mosquito to await inoculation into another human at the next feeding.

EPIDEMIOLOGY Malaria occurs throughout most of the tropical regions of the world. *P. falciparum* predominates in Africa, New Guinea, and Haiti; *P. vivax* is more common in Central America and the Indian subcontinent. The prevalence of these two species is approximately equal in South America, eastern Asia, and Oceania. *P.malariae* is found in most endemic areas, especially throughout sub-Saharan Africa, but is much less common. *P. ovale* is relatively unusual outside Africa.

The epidemiology of malaria is complex and may vary considerably even within relatively small geographic areas. Endemicity is traditionally defined in terms of palpable-spleen rates in children 2 to 9 years of age as hypoendemic (<10 percent), mesoendemic (11 to 50 percent), hyperendemic (51 to 75 percent), and holoendemic (>75 percent). In holo- and hyperendemic areas—e.g., certain regions of tropical Africa or coastal New Guinea, where there is intense *P. falciparum* transmission (up to one human bite per infected mosquito per day)—people are infected repeatedly throughout their lives. Here, morbidity and mortality during childhood are considerable. Immunity against disease is hard won, but by adulthood malarial infections are largely asymptomatic. This situation is termed *stable transmission*. In areas where transmission is low, erratic, or focal, full protective immunity is not acquired, and symptomatic disease may occur at all ages. This situation is termed *unstable transmission*. Even in areas with stable transmission, there is often an increased incidence coinciding with increased mosquito breeding during the rainy season. Malaria behaves like an epidemic disease in some areas, such as in northern India, Sri Lanka, Southeast Asia, Ethiopia, southern Africa, and Madagascar. An epidemic can develop when there are changes in environmental, economic, or social conditions, such as heavy rains following drought or migrations (usually of refugees or workers) from a nonmalarious region to an area of high transmission. This situation usually results in considerable mortality among all age groups.

The principal determinants of the epidemiology of malaria are the number (density), the human-biting habits, and the longevity of the anopheline mosquito vectors. More specifically, the transmission of malaria is directly proportional to the density of the vector, the square of the number of human bites per day per mosquito, and the tenth power of the probability of the mosquito's surviving for 1 day. In other words, the most effective mosquito vectors are those (such as *Anopheles gambiae* in western Africa) that occur in high densities, bite humans frequently, and are long-lived. Mosquito longevity is particularly important, because the portion of the parasite's life cycle that takes place within the mosquito—from gametocyte ingestion to subsequent inoculation—lasts for a minimum of 7 days (depending on ambient temperature); thus, to transmit malaria, the mosquito must survive for longer than 7 days. The entomologic inoculation rate—the number of sporozoite-positive mosquito bites per year—is the most common measure of malarial transmission and varies from <1 in some parts of Latin America and Southeast Asia to >300 in parts of tropical Africa.

ERYTHROCYTE CHANGES IN MALARIA After invading an erythrocyte, the growing parasite progressively consumes and degrades intracellular proteins, principally hemoglobin; the parasite also alters the red cell membrane by changing its transport properties, exposing cryptic surface antigens, and inserting new parasite-derived proteins. The red cell becomes more irregular in shape, more antigenic, and less deformable.

In *P. falciparum* infections, membrane protuberances appear on

Table 216-1

Characteristics of *Plasmodium* Species Infecting Humans

Characteristic	Finding for Indicated Species			
	P. falciparum	*P. vivax*	*P. ovale*	*P. malariae*
Duration of intra-hepatic phase (days)	5.5	8	9	15
Number of merozoites released per infected hepatocyte	30,000	10,000	15,000	15,000
Duration of erythrocytic cycle (hours)	48	48	50	72
Red cell preference	Younger cells (but can invade cells of all ages)	Reticulocytes	Reticulocytes	Older cells
Morphology	Usually only ring forms;* banana-shaped gametocytes	Irregularly shaped large rings and trophozoites; enlarged erythrocytes; Schüffner's dots	Infected erythrocytes, enlarged and oval; Schüffner's dots	Band or rectangular forms of trophozoites common
Pigment color	Black	Yellow-brown	Dark brown	Brown-black
Ability to cause relapses	No	Yes	Yes	No

* Parasitemia sometimes exceeds 2 percent with multiple infections of a single erythrocyte.

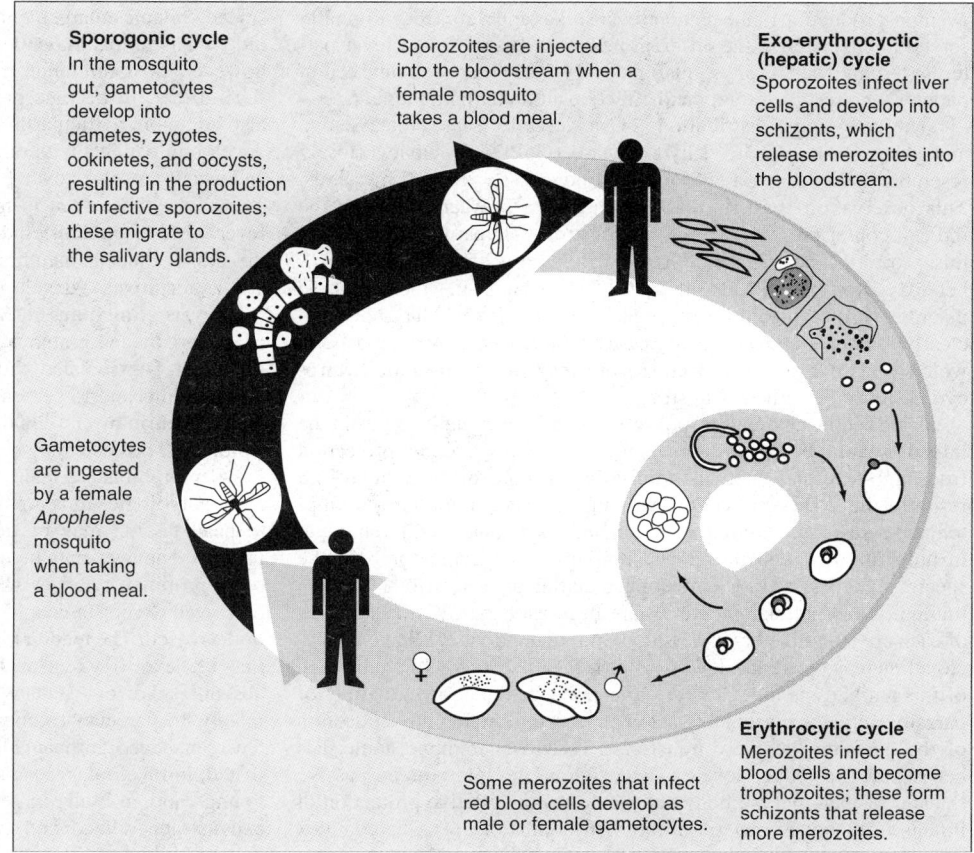

Sporogonic cycle
In the mosquito gut, gametocytes develop into gametes, zygotes, ookinetes, and oocysts, resulting in the production of infective sporozoites; these migrate to the salivary glands.

Sporozoites are injected into the bloodstream when a female mosquito takes a blood meal.

Exo-erythrocytic (hepatic) cycle
Sporozoites infect liver cells and develop into schizonts, which release merozoites into the bloodstream.

Gametocytes are ingested by a female *Anopheles* mosquito when taking a blood meal.

Some merozoites that infect red blood cells develop as male or female gametocytes.

Erythrocytic cycle
Merozoites infect red blood cells and become trophozoites; these form schizonts that release more merozoites.

FIGURE 216-1   The malaria transmission cycle.

the erythrocyte's surface in the second 24 h of the asexual cycle. These "knobs" extrude a high-molecular-weight, antigenically variant, strain-specific, adhesive protein that mediates attachment to receptors on venular and capillary endothelium—an event termed *cytoadherence*. Thus the infected erythrocytes sequester inside the small blood vessels. At the same stage, these *P. falciparum*–infected red cells may also adhere to uninfected red cells to form rosettes. The processes of cytoadherence and rosetting are central to the pathogenesis of falciparum malaria. They result in the sequestration of red cells containing mature forms of the parasite in vital organs (particularly the brain and heart), where they interfere with microcirculatory flow and metabolism. Sequestered parasites continue to develop out of reach of the principal host defense mechanism: splenic processing and filtration. As a consequence, only the younger ring forms of the asexual parasites are seen in the peripheral blood in falciparum malaria, and the level of peripheral parasitemia underestimates the true number of parasites within the body.

In the other three "benign" malarias, sequestration does not occur, and all stages of the parasite's development are evident on peripheral blood smears. Whereas *P. vivax*, *P. ovale*, and *P. malariae* show a marked predilection for either old red cells or reticulocytes and produce a level of parasitemia seldom exceeding 2 percent, *P. falciparum* can invade erythrocytes of all ages and may be associated with very high levels of parasitemia.

HOST RESPONSE   Initially, the host responds to plasmodial infection by activating nonspecific defense mechanisms. Splenic immunologic and filtrative clearance functions are augmented in malaria, and the removal of both parasitized and uninfected erythrocytes is accelerated. The parasitized cells escaping splenic removal are destroyed when the schizont ruptures. The material released induces the activation of macrophages and the release of proinflammatory mononuclear cell–derived cytokines, which cause fever and exert other pathologic effects. Temperatures of 40°C are schizonticidal; in untreated infections, the effect of such temperatures is to synchronize the parasitic cycle with eventual production of the regular fever spikes and rigors that originally served to characterize the different malarias. These regular fever patterns (tertian, every 2 days; quartan, every 3 days) are seldom seen in patients who receive prompt and effective antimalarial treatment.

The geographic distributions of sickle cell disease, thalassemia, and glucose-6-phosphate dehydrogenase (G6PD) deficiency closely resemble that of malaria before the introduction of control measures. This observation suggests that these genetic disorders affecting the red cell confer protection against death from falciparum malaria, and this protection has been confirmed in the case of hemoglobin A/S heterozygotes (the sickle cell trait). The mechanism whereby these disorders protect against severe plasmodial infection has not been clearly elucidated except in the case of Melanesian ovalocytosis, in which rigid erythrocytes resist merozoite invasion and the intraerythrocytic electrolyte milieu is hostile.

The specific immune response to malaria eventually controls the infection and, with exposure to sufficient strains, confers protection from high-level parasitemia and disease but not from infection. As a result of this state of infection without illness (premunition), asymptomatic parasitemia is common among adults and older children living in holo- or hyperendemic areas. Immunity is specific for both the species and the strain of infecting malarial parasite. Both humoral immunity and cellular immunity are necessary, but the mechanisms of each are incompletely understood. Immune individuals have a polyclonal increase in serum levels of IgM, IgG, and IgA, although much of this antibody is unrelated to protection. Antibodies to a variety of parasitic antigens presumably act in concert to limit in vivo replication of the parasite. Passively transferred IgG from immune adults has been shown to reduce levels of parasitemia in children, and passive transfer of maternal antibody contributes to the relative protection of infants from severe malaria in the first months of life. This complex immunity to disease is lost when a person lives outside an endemic area for several months or longer.

Several factors retard the development of cellular immunity. These factors include the absence of major histocompatibility antigens on the surface of infected red cells, which precludes direct T cell recognition; malaria antigen–specific immune unresponsiveness; and the enormous strain diversity of malarial parasites along with the ability of the parasites to express immunodominant variant antigens on the erythrocyte surface that change during the period of infection. Strain diversity also has an impact on the heterogeneity of the humoral antibody response. Immunity to all strains is never achieved. Parasites may persist in the blood for months (or, in the case of *P. malariae*, for many years) if treatment is not given. The complexity of the immune response in malaria, the sophistication of the parasites' evasion mechanisms, and the lack of a good in vitro correlate with clinical immunity have all slowed progress toward an effective vaccine.

CLINICAL FEATURES   The first symptoms of malaria are nonspecific; the lack of a sense of well-being, headache, fatigue, abdominal discomfort, and muscle aches followed by fever are all similar to the symptoms of a minor viral illness. In some instances, a prominence of headache, chest pain, abdominal pain, arthralgia, myalgia, or diarrhea may suggest another diagnosis. Although headache may be severe in malaria, there is no neck stiffness or photophobia resembling that in meningitis. While myalgia may be prominent, it is not usually as severe as in dengue fever, and the muscles are not tender as in leptospirosis or typhus. Nausea, vomiting, and orthostatic hypotension are common. The classic malarial paroxysms, in which fever spikes, chills, and rigors occur at regular intervals, suggest infection with *P. vivax* or *P. ovale*. The fever is irregular at first (that of falciparum malaria may never become regular); the temperature of nonimmune individuals and children often rises above 40°C in conjunction with tachycardia and sometimes delirium. Although childhood febrile convulsions may occur with any of the malarias, generalized seizures are specifically associated with falciparum malaria and may herald the development of cerebral disease. Many clinical abnormalities have been described in acute malaria, but most patients with uncomplicated infections have few abnormal physical findings other than fever, malaise, mild anemia, and (in some cases) a palpable spleen. Splenic enlargement is very common among otherwise-healthy individuals in malaria-endemic areas and reflects repeated infections; however, in nonimmune individuals with malaria, the spleen takes several days to become palpable. Slight enlargement of the liver is also common, particularly among young children. Mild jaundice may develop in patients with otherwise-uncomplicated falciparum malaria and usually resolves over 1 to 3 weeks. Malaria is not associated with a rash like those seen in meningococcal septicemia, typhus, enteric fever, viral exanthems, and drug reactions. Petechial hemorrhages in the skin or mucous membranes—features of viral hemorrhagic fevers and leptospirosis—develop only rarely in severe falciparum malaria.

Severe Falciparum Malaria   *Cerebral malaria*   Coma is a characteristic and ominous feature of falciparum malaria and, despite treatment, is associated with death rates of approximately 20 percent among adults and 15 percent among children. Lesser degrees of obtundation, delirium, and abnormal behavior should also be taken very seriously. The onset may be gradual or sudden following a convulsion.

Cerebral malaria manifests as diffuse symmetric encephalopathy; focal neurologic signs are unusual. Although some passive resistance to head flexion may be detected, signs of meningeal irritation are lacking. The eyes may be divergent and a pout reflex is common, but other primitive reflexes are usually absent. The corneal reflexes are preserved except in deep coma. Muscle tone may be either increased or decreased. The tendon reflexes are variable, and the plantar reflexes may be flexor or extensor; the abdominal and cremasteric reflexes are absent. Flexor or extensor posturing may be documented. Approximately 15 percent of patients have retinal hemorrhages. Fewer than 5 percent have significant bleeding or other clinical evidence of disseminated intravascular coagulation. Anemia is also common among young children living in areas with stable transmission. Convulsions, usually generalized and often repeated, are common, particularly among children with cerebral malaria. Whereas adults rarely suffer neurologic sequelae, approximately 10 percent of children surviving cerebral malaria—especially those with hypoglycemia, severe anemia, repeated seizures, and deep coma—have some residual neurologic deficit when they regain consciousness.

Hypoglycemia An important and common complication of severe malaria, hypoglycemia is associated with a poor prognosis and is particularly problematic in children and pregnant women. Hypoglycemia in malaria results from a failure of hepatic gluconeogenesis and an increase in the consumption of glucose by both host and parasite. To compound the situation, quinine and quinidine, the drugs of choice for the treatment of severe chloroquine-resistant malaria, are powerful stimulants of pancreatic insulin secretion. Hyperinsulinemic hypoglycemia is especially troublesome in pregnant women receiving quinine treatment. In severe disease, the clinical diagnosis of hypoglycemia is difficult as the usual physical signs (sweating, gooseflesh, tachycardia) are absent and the neurologic impairment caused by hypoglycemia cannot be distinguished from that caused by malaria.

Lactic acidosis Lactic acidosis commonly coexists with hypoglycemia in patients with malaria. Anaerobic glycolysis occurs in tissues where sequestered parasitized erythrocytes interfere with microcirculatory flow; lactate production by the parasites combines with a failure of hepatic lactate clearance to cause lactic acidosis. The prognosis of lactic acidosis is poor; acidotic breathing, a sign of poor prognosis in severe malaria, is usually followed by circulatory failure refractory to volume expansion or to treatment with inotropic drugs or by respiratory arrest.

Noncardiogenic pulmonary edema Adults with severe falciparum malaria may develop noncardiogenic pulmonary edema even after several days of antimalarial therapy. The pathogenesis of this variant of the adult respiratory distress syndrome is unclear. Mortality is over 80 percent. This condition can be aggravated by overly vigorous administration of intravenous fluid.

Renal impairment Renal impairment is common among adults with severe falciparum malaria but rare among children. The pathogenesis of renal failure is unclear but may be related to parasitized-erythrocyte sequestration interfering with renal microcirculatory flow and regional metabolism. Clinically and pathologically, this syndrome resembles acute tubular necrosis. Renal cortical necrosis never develops. Mortality in the initial phase of hypercatabolic acute renal failure is high; in survivors, urine flow resumes in a median of 4 days, and serum creatinine levels return to normal in a mean of 17 days (see Chap. 270). Dialysis considerably enhances the likelihood of a patient's survival.

Hematologic abnormalities Anemia results from accelerated red cell destruction and removal by the spleen in conjunction with ineffective erythropoiesis. In severe malaria in nonimmune individuals and in areas with unstable transmission, anemia can develop rapidly and transfusion is often required. In many areas of Africa, children may develop severe anemia due to repeated malarial infections. This is a common consequence of continued infection resulting from treatment with chloroquine (or other drugs) to which the parasites are resistant.

Slight coagulation abnormalities are common in falciparum malaria, and mild thrombocytopenia is usual. Fewer than 5 percent of patients with cerebral malaria have significant bleeding with evidence of disseminated intravascular coagulation. Hematemesis, presumably from stress ulceration or acute gastric erosions, may also occur.

Other complications Aspiration pneumonia following convulsions is an important cause of death in cerebral malaria. Malaria predisposes to bacterial superinfection, possibly through its effect on immune responsiveness. Chest infections and catheter-induced urinary tract infections are common among patients who are unconscious for more than 3 days. Spontaneous gram-negative septicemia develops occasionally in severe malaria, and *Salmonella* septicemia has been associated with *P. falciparum* infections in endemic areas.

Malaria in Pregnancy Falciparum malaria is an important cause of fetal death. In hyper- and holoendemic areas, malaria in primigravida and secundigravida is associated with low birth weight. In general, infected mothers remain asymptomatic despite intense parasitization of the placenta due to sequestration of parasitized erythrocytes in the placental microcirculation.

In areas with unstable transmission of malaria, pregnant women are prone to severe infections and are particularly vulnerable to high-level parasitemia with anemia, hypoglycemia, and acute pulmonary edema. Fetal distress, premature labor, and stillbirth or low birth weight are common results. Congenital malaria occurs in fewer than 5 percent of newborns whose mothers are infected and is related directly to the parasitic density in maternal blood and in the placenta.

Malaria in Children Most of the estimated 1 to 3 million persons who die of falciparum malaria each year are young African children. Convulsions, coma, hypoglycemia, metabolic acidosis, and severe anemia are relatively common among children with severe malaria, whereas deep jaundice, acute renal failure, and acute pulmonary edema are unusual. In general, children tolerate the antimalarial drugs well and respond rapidly to treatment.

Transfusion Malaria Malaria can be transmitted by blood transfusion, needle-stick injury, sharing of needles by infected drug addicts, or organ transplantation. The incubation period in these settings is often short because there is no preerythrocytic stage of development. The clinical features and management of these cases are the same as for naturally acquired infections, although falciparum malaria tends to be especially severe in drug addicts. Radical chemotherapy with primaquine is unnecessary for *P. vivax* and *P. ovale* infections.

CHRONIC COMPLICATIONS OF MALARIA **Tropical Splenomegaly (Hyperreactive Malarial Splenomegaly)** Chronic or repeated malarial infections produce hypergammaglobulinemia; normochromic, normocytic anemia; and—in certain situations—splenomegaly. Some residents of malaria-endemic areas in tropical Africa and Asia exhibit an abnormal immunologic response to repeated infections that is characterized by massive splenomegaly, hepatomegaly, marked elevations in serum titers of IgM and malarial antibody, hepatic sinusoidal lymphocytosis, and (in Africa) peripheral (B cell) lymphocytosis. This syndrome has been associated with the production of cytotoxic IgM antibodies to suppressor (CD8+) lymphocytes, which leads to uninhibited B cell production of IgM and the formation of cryoglobulins (IgM aggregates and immune complexes). This immunologic process stimulates reticuloendothelial hyperplasia and clearance activity and eventually produces splenomegaly. Patients with hyperreactive malarial splenomegaly (HMS) present with an abdominal mass or a dragging sensation in the abdomen and occasional sharp abdominal pains suggesting perisplenitis. Anemia and some degree of pancytopenia are usually evident, but in many cases malarial parasites cannot be found in peripheral blood smears. Vulnerability to respiratory and skin infections is increased; many patients die of overwhelming sepsis. Persons with HMS who are living in endemic areas should receive antimalarial chemoprophylaxis; the results are usually good. In nonendemic areas, treatment is advised. In some cases refractory to therapy, clonal lymphoproliferation may develop and then evolve into a malignant lymphoproliferative disorder.

Quartan Malarial Nephropathy Chronic or repeated infections with *P. malariae* may cause soluble immune-complex injury to the renal glomeruli, resulting in the nephrotic syndrome. Other, unidentified factors must contribute to this process since only a very small proportion of infected patients develop renal disease. The histologic appearance is that of focal or segmental glomerulonephritis with splitting of the capillary basement membrane. Subendothelial dense deposits are seen on electron microscopy, and immunofluorescence reveals deposits of complement and immunoglobulins; in samples of renal tissue from children, *P. malariae* antigens are often visible. A coarse-granular pattern of basement membrane immunofluorescent deposits (predominantly IgG3) with selective proteinuria carries a better prognosis than a fine-granular, predominantly IgG2 pattern with nonselective proteinuria. Quartan nephropathy usually responds poorly to treatment with either antimalarial agents or glucocorticoids and cytotoxic drugs.

Burkitt's Lymphoma and Epstein-Barr Virus Infection It is possible that malaria-related immunosuppression provokes infection with lymphoma viruses. Burkitt's lymphoma is strongly associated with Epstein-Barr virus. The prevalence of this childhood tumor is high in malarious areas of Africa.

DIAGNOSIS   Demonstration of the Parasite   The diagnosis of malaria rests on the demonstration of asexual forms of the parasite in peripheral blood smears subjected to Romanovsky staining. Giemsa at pH 7.2 is preferred; Wright's, Field's, or Leishman's stain can also be used. Both thin and thick blood smears should be examined.

The thin blood smear should be air-dried rapidly, fixed in anhydrous methanol, and stained, and the red cells in the tail of the film should then be examined under oil immersion. The level of parasitemia is expressed as the number of parasitized erythrocytes among 1000 cells, and this figure is then converted to the number of parasitized erythrocytes per microliter. A simple, sensitive, and specific diagnostic stick test that detects *P. falciparum* histidine-rich protein 2 in finger-prick blood samples has recently been introduced, and nucleic acid–based assays are being developed. The relation between parasitemia and prognosis is complex; in general, patients with more than 10^5 parasites per microliter are at increased risk of dying, but nonimmune patients may die with much lower counts. In severe malaria, a poor prognosis is indicated by a predominance of more mature *P. falciparum* parasites (i.e., more than 20 percent of parasites with visible pigment) or circulating schizonts in the peripheral blood film or by the presence of phagocytosed malarial pigment in more than 5 percent of neutrophils.

The thick blood film should be of uneven thickness. The smear should be dried thoroughly and stained without fixing. As many layers of erythrocytes overlie one another and are lysed during the staining procedure, the thick film has the advantage of concentrating the parasites (by 20- to 40-fold compared with a thin blood film) and thus increasing diagnostic sensitivity. Both parasites and white cells are counted, and the number of parasites per unit volume is calculated from the total leukocyte count. A minimum of 200 white cells should be counted. Interpretation of thick films requires some experience because artifacts are common. Before a thick smear is judged to be negative, 100 to 200 fields should be examined under oil immersion. Phagocytosed malarial pigment is sometimes seen inside peripheral blood monocytes or polymorphonuclear leukocytes and may provide a clue to recent infection if malarial parasites are not detectable. After the clearance of the parasites, malarial pigment is often evident for several days in peripheral blood phagocytes, bone marrow aspirates, or smears of fluid expressed after intradermal puncture. Staining of parasites with the fluorescent dye acridine orange allows more rapid diagnosis of cases in which the level of parasitemia is low.

Laboratory Findings   Normochromic, normocytic anemia is usually documented. The leukocyte count is generally low to normal, although it may be raised in very severe infections. The erythrocyte sedimentation rate, degree of plasma viscosity, and level of C-reactive protein are high. The platelet count is usually reduced to about 10^5 per microliter. Severe infections may be accompanied by prolonged prothrombin and partial thromboplastin times and by especially severe thrombocytopenia. Levels of antithrombin III are reduced even in mild infection. In uncomplicated malaria, plasma concentrations of electrolytes, blood urea nitrogen, and creatinine are usually normal. Findings in severe malaria may include metabolic acidosis, with low plasma concentrations of glucose, sodium, bicarbonate, calcium, phosphate, and albumin together with elevations in lactate, blood urea nitrogen, creatinine, urate, muscle and liver enzymes, and conjugated and unconjugated bilirubin. Hypergammaglobulinemia is usual in immune and semi-immune subjects, and urinalysis generally gives normal results. In adults and children with cerebral malaria, the mean opening pressure at lumbar puncture is about 160 mm of cerebrospinal fluid; the cerebrospinal fluid usually is normal or has a slightly elevated total protein level [<1.0 g/L (100 mg/dL)].

PREVENTION   In most of the tropics, the eradication of malaria is not feasible because of the widespread distribution of *Anopheles*

breeding sites, the great number of infected persons, and inadequacies in resources, infrastructure, and control programs. Where possible, the disease is contained by judicious use of insecticides to kill the mosquito vector, rapid diagnosis and appropriate patient management, and administration of chemoprophylaxis to high-risk groups. Despite massive investment in efforts to develop a malaria vaccine, no safe, effective, long-lasting vaccine is likely to be available for general use in the near future (see Chap. 122).

Personal Protection Against Malaria   Simple measures to reduce the frequency of mosquito bites in malarious areas are very important. These measures include the avoidance of exposure to mosquitoes at their peak feeding times (usually dusk and dawn) and the use of insect repellents, suitable clothing, and insecticide-impregnated bed nets. Widespread use of bed nets, particularly those treated with permethrin (a residual pyrethroid), often reduces the incidence of malaria and has recently been shown to reduce mortality in western and eastern Africa.

Chemoprophylaxis (See Table 216-2)   Few areas of therapeutics are as controversial as antimalarial drug prophylaxis. Recommendations for prophylaxis depend on a knowledge of local patterns of plasmodial drug sensitivity and the likelihood of acquiring malarial infection. Chemoprophylaxis is never entirely reliable, and malaria should always be considered in the differential diagnosis of fever in patients who have traveled to endemic areas, even if they are taking prophylactic antimalarial drugs.

All pregnant women at risk should receive prophylaxis. In addition, antimalarial prophylaxis should be considered for children between the ages of 3 months and 4 years in areas where malaria causes high childhood mortality. However, such prophylaxis may not be logistically feasible in many countries. Children born to nonimmune mothers in endemic areas (usually expatriates moving to these areas) should receive prophylaxis from birth.

Travelers should start taking antimalarial drugs at least 1 week before departure so that any untoward reactions can be detected and therapeutic antimalarial blood concentrations will be present when needed. Antimalarial prophylaxis should continue for 4 weeks after the traveler has left the endemic area.

Mefloquine has become the antimalarial prophylactic agent of choice for much of the tropics because it is usually effective against multidrug-resistant falciparum malaria and is reasonably well tolerated. Nausea, dizziness, muzziness, disturbed sleep patterns, and dysphoria are relatively common. Approximately 1 in every 10,000 recipients develops an acute reversible neuropsychiatric reaction manifest by confusion, psychosis, convulsions, or encephalopathy. In recent studies in Africa, mefloquine prophylaxis was found to be effective and safe during pregnancy.

Daily administration of doxycycline is an effective alternative to mefloquine that also exhibits some causal (preerythrocytic) prophylactic activity. It is generally well tolerated but may cause vulvovaginal thrush, diarrhea, and photosensitivity and cannot be used by children less than 8 years old or by pregnant women. Recent studies indicate that daily primaquine is effective for prophylaxis of *P. falciparum* and *P. vivax* malaria; further confirmatory studies are needed.

Chloroquine remains the drug of choice for the prevention of infection with drug-sensitive *P. falciparum* and with the other human malarial species (although chloroquine resistance in *P. vivax* has been reported recently from parts of eastern Asia and Oceania). This agent is generally well tolerated, although some patients are unable to take the drug because of dysphoria, headache, or—in dark-skinned patients—pruritus. (A concomitant filarial infection may provoke or aggravate chloroquine-induced pruritus.) Chloroquine is considered safe in pregnancy. With chronic administration over more than 5 years, a characteristic dose-related retinopathy may develop, but this condition is rare at the doses used for antimalarial prophylaxis. Idiosyncratic or allergic reactions are likewise rare. Skeletal and cardiac myopathy are rare and much more likely at the high doses used in the treatment of rheumatoid arthritis. Neuropsychiatric reactions and skin rashes are unusual. Amodiaquine, a related aminoquinoline, is associated with a high risk of agranulocytosis (approximately 1:2000) and is not recommended.

Table 216-2

Prophylaxis and Self-Treatment for Malaria

Drug	Usage	Adult Dosage	Child Dosage
Prophylaxis			
Mefloquine	Used in areas where chloroquine-resistant malaria has been reported	228 mg of base (250 mg of salt) orally, once/week*	<15 kg: 4.6 mg of base/kg (5 mg of salt/kg)
			15–19 kg: ¼ tablet/week
			20–30 kg: ½ tablet/week
			31–45 kg: ¾ tablet/week
			>45 kg: 1 tablet/week
Doxycycline	Used as alternative to mefloquine	100 mg orally, once/day	>8 years of age: 2 mg/kg per day orally; maximum dose, 100 mg/d
Chloroquine	Used in areas where chloroquine-resistant malaria has *not* been reported	300 mg of base (500 mg of salt) orally, once/week	5 mg of base/kg (8.3 mg of salt/kg) orally, once/week; maximum dose, 300 mg of base
Proguanil (not available in U.S.)	Used simultaneously *with* chloroquine as alternative to mefloquine or doxycycline	200 mg orally, once/day, in combination with weekly chloroquine	<2 years: 50 mg/d
			2–6 years: 100 mg/d
			7–10 years: 150 mg/d
			>10 years: 200 mg/d
Primaquine	Used for travelers only after testing for G6PD deficiency; postexposure prevention for relapsing malaria	15 mg of base (26.3 mg of salt) orally, once/day for 14 days	0.3 mg of base/kg (0.5 mg of salt/kg) orally, once/day for 14 days
Self-treatment			
Pyrimethamine-sulfadoxine†	In areas with chloroquine-resistant malaria, should be carried during travel by persons taking mefloquine or doxycycline	3 tablets (75 mg of pyrimethamine and 1500 mg of sulfadoxine) orally, as a single dose	5–10 kg: ½ tablet
			11–20 kg: 1 tablet
			21–30 kg: 1½ tablets
			31–45 kg: 2 tablets
			>45 kg: 3 tablets

* Tablets manufactured outside the United States may contain 250 mg of base.
† Regimen is used for treatment only.

In the past, the dihydrofolate reductase inhibitors pyrimethamine and proguanil (chloroguanide) have been administered widely, but resistant strains of both *P. falciparum* and *P. vivax* have limited their use. Whereas antimalarial quinolines such as chloroquine act on the erythrocyte stage of parasitic development, the dihydrofolate reductase inhibitors also inhibit preerythrocytic growth in the liver and development in the mosquito. Proguanil is safe and well tolerated, although mouth ulceration occurs in 8 percent of persons using this drug; it is considered the safest agent for antimalarial prophylaxis in pregnancy. The prophylactic use of the combination of pyrimethamine and sulfadoxine is not recommended because of an unacceptable incidence of severe toxicity, principally exfoliative dermatitis and other skin rashes, agranulocytosis, hepatitis, and pulmonary eosinophilia. The combination of pyrimethamine with dapsone (0.2/1.5 mg/kg weekly; 25/200 mg maximum) is a second-line drug available in some countries and can be used in areas with chloroquine-resistant *P. falciparum*. This combination is generally well tolerated; however, resistance is increasing, and dapsone may cause methemoglobinemia and allergic reactions and (at higher doses) may pose a significant risk of agranulocytosis.

Because of the increasing spread and intensity of plasmodial resistance to chloroquine in Africa and other areas of the world (Fig. 216-2), the Centers for Disease Control and Prevention, which recommends a weekly dose of mefloquine for all travelers, maintains an updated 24-h malaria information audiotape that can be accessed by touch-tone telephone (404-332-4555) and an interactive international travel information service that responds by fax (404-332-4565).

℞ TREATMENT

When a patient in or from a malarious area presents with fever, a blood smear should be prepared and examined to confirm the diagnosis and identify the species of infecting parasite. Patients with severe malaria or those unable to take oral drugs should receive parenteral antimalarial therapy. If there is any doubt about the resistance status of the infecting organism, then quinine or quinidine should be given. Several drugs are available for oral treatment, and the choice of drug depends on the likely sensitivity of the infecting parasites. Despite recent evidence of chloroquine resistance in *P. vivax* from Oceania, chloroquine remains the treatment of choice for the benign human malarias. Characteristics of various antimalarial agents are shown in Table 216-3, and regimens of drugs approved

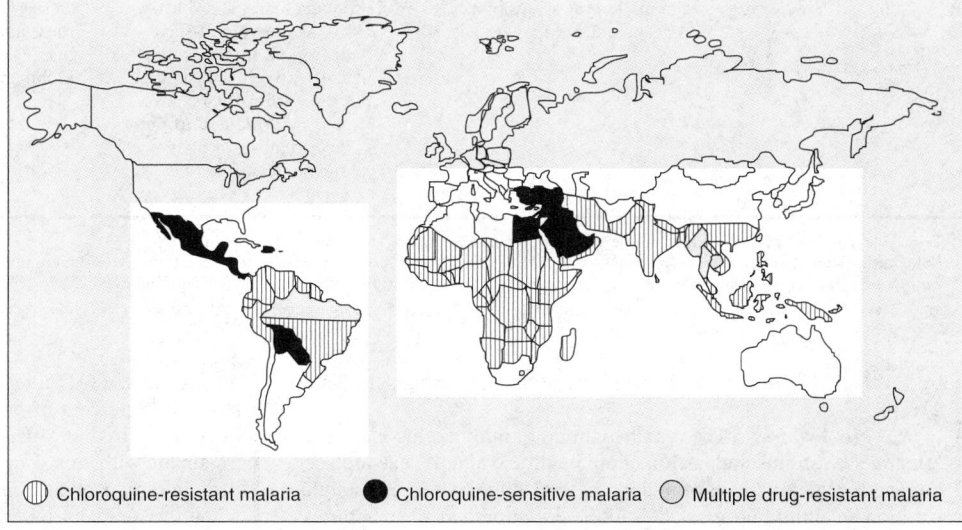

FIGURE 216-2 Worldwide distribution of malaria and drug-resistant *Plasmodium falciparum*, 1996.

⬛ Chloroquine-resistant malaria ● Chloroquine-sensitive malaria ○ Multiple drug-resistant malaria

Table 216-3

Properties of Antimalarial Drugs

Drug(s)	Pharmacokinetic Properties	Antimalarial Activity	Minor Toxicity	Major Toxicity
Quinine, quinidine	Good oral and IM absorption; Cl and V_d reduced, but plasma protein binding (principally to $\propto 1$ acid glycoprotein) increased (90%) in malaria; $t_{1/2}$: 16 h in malaria, 11 h in healthy persons	Acts mainly on trophozoite blood stage; kills gametocytes of *P. vivax*, *P. ovale*, and *P. malariae*; no action on liver stages	*Common:* Cinchonism: tinnitus, high-tone hearing loss, nausea, vomiting, dysphoria, postural hypotension; ECG QT_c interval prolongation *Rare:* Diarrhea, visual disturbance, rashes *Note:* Bitter taste	*Common:* Hypoglycemia *Rare:* Hypotension, blindness, deafness, cardiac arrhythmias, thrombocytopenia, hemolysis, hemolytic-uremic syndrome, cholestatic hepatitis, neuromuscular paralysis *Note:* Quinidine more cardiotoxic
Chloroquine	Good oral absorption, very rapid IM and SC absorption; complex pharmacokinetics; enormous Cl and V_d (unaffected by malaria); blood concentration profile determined by distribution processes in malaria; $t_{1/2}$: 1–2 months	As for quinine but more rapid	*Common:* Nausea, dysphoria, pruritus in dark-skinned patients, postural hypotension *Rare:* Accommodation difficulties, rash *Note:* Bitter taste, well tolerated	*Acute:* Hypotensive shock (parenteral), cardiac arrhythmias, neuropsychiatric reactions *Chronic:* Retinopathy (cumulative dose, >100 g), skeletal and cardiac myopathy
Mefloquine	Adequate oral absorption; no parenteral preparation; $t_{1/2}$: 14–20 days (shorter in malaria)	As for quinine	Nausea, giddiness, dysphoria, confusion, sleeplessness, nightmares	Neuropsychiatric reactions, convulsions, encephalopathy
Tetracycline, doxycycline*	Excellent absorption; $t_{1/2}$: 8 h for tetracycline, 18 h for doxycycline	Weak antimalarial activity; should not be used alone for treatment	Gastrointestinal intolerance, deposition in growing bones and teeth, photosensitivity, moniliasis, benign intracranial hypertension	Renal failure in patients with impaired renal function (tetracycline)
Halofantrine†	Highly variable absorption; $t_{1/2}$: 1–3 days (active desbutyl metabolite $t_{1/2}$: 2–7 days)	As for quinine but more rapid	Diarrhea	Prolonged ECG QT_c interval, AV conduction delay, cardiac arrhythmias
Artemisinin and derivatives (artemether, artesunate)	Good oral absorption, variable absorption of IM artemether; artesunate and artemether biotransformed to active metabolite dyhydroartemisinin; all drugs eliminated rapidly	Broader stage specificity and more rapid than other drugs; no action on liver stages	Reduction in reticulocyte count; fever	Neurotoxicity reported in animals, but no evidence in humans
Pyrimethamine	Good oral absorption, variable IM absorption; $t_{1/2}$: 4 days	For blood stages, acts mainly on mature forms; causal prophylactic	Well tolerated	Megaloblastic anemia, pancytopenia, pulmonary infiltration
Proguanil (chloroguanide)	Good oral absorption; biotransformed to active metabolite cycloguanil; $t_{1/2}$: 16 h	Causal prophylactic; not used for treatment	Well tolerated, with mouth ulcers and rare alopecia	Megaloblastic anemia in renal failure
Primaquine	Complete oral absorption; active compound not known; $t_{1/2}$: 7 h	Radical cure; some activity against blood-stage infection, used to eradicate exoerythrocytic (hepatic) forms of *P. vivax* and *P. ovale* and to prevent relapses; kills gametocytes of *P. falciparum*	Nausea, vomiting, diarrhea, abdominal pain, hemolysis, methemoglobinemia	Massive hemolysis in subjects with severe G6PD deficiency

* Tetracycline and doxycycline should not be given to pregnant women or to children <8 years of age.
† Halofantrine should not be used by patients with long ECG QT_c intervals or known conduction disturbances or by those taking drugs that may affect ventricular repolarization—e.g., quinidine, quinine, mefloquine, chloroquine, neuroleptics, tricyclic antidepressants, terfenadine, or astemizole.
NOTE: Cl, systemic clearance; V_d, total apparent volume of distribution; IM, intramuscular; SC, subcutaneous; ECG, electrocardiogram.

by the U.S. Food and Drug Administration are detailed in Table 216-4.

Severe Malaria The antiarrhythmic quinidine gluconate is as effective as quinine and, as it is more readily available, has replaced quinine for the treatment of malaria in the United States. The administration of quinidine must be closely monitored if dysrrhythmias and hypotension are to be avoided. Total plasma levels in excess of 8 μg/mL, a QT_c interval of greater than 0.6 s, or QRS widening beyond 25 percent of baseline are indications for slowing infusion rates. If arrhythmia or saline-unresponsive hypotension develops, treatment with this drug should be discontinued. Quinine is safer than quinidine, and cardiovascular monitoring is not required except when the recipient has cardiac disease. In some areas, the Chinese drugs derived from artemisinin (artemether and artesunate) have become first-line treatments for severe malaria. These agents are rapidly effective against multidrug-resistant falciparum malaria and appear to be safe. They are not available in the United States.

Severe falciparum malaria constitutes a medical emergency requiring intensive nursing care and careful management. The patient should be weighed and, if comatose, placed on his or her side and given a single parenteral dose of phenobarbital (5 to 20 mg/kg) to prevent convulsions. Frequent evaluation of the patient's condition is essential. Ancillary drugs such as high-dose glucocorticoids, urea, heparin, and dextran are of no value. The choice of antimalarial drug depends on a knowledge of the prevailing sensitivity of *P. falciparum* to antimalarials. If there is any doubt, quinine or quinidine should be given. Because the systemic clearance and apparent volume of distribution of these alkaloids are markedly reduced and plasma protein binding is increased in severe malaria, the blood concentrations attained with a given dose are higher. The optimal therapeutic range for quinine in severe malaria is not known with certainty, but total plasma concentrations between 8 and 20 μg/mL are effective and do not cause serious toxicity. An initial loading dose should be given so that therapeutic concentrations are reached as soon as possible. If the patient remains seriously ill or in acute renal failure for more than 2 days, the maintenance doses should be reduced by 30 to 50 percent to prevent toxic accumulation of the drugs. The initial doses should never be reduced. If chloroquine is given, dose reduction is unnecessary even in renal failure. Provided that it can be performed safely, exchange transfusion is indicated for patients with high-level parasitemia ($>$15 percent) and vital organ dysfunction. Exchange transfusion should be considered for severely ill patients with a level of parasitemia between 5 and 15 percent.

When the patient is unconscious, the blood glucose level should be measured every 4 to 6 h, and values below 2.2 mmol/L (40 mg/dL) should prompt treatment with intravenous dextrose. All patients treated with intravenous quinine or quinidine should receive a continuous infusion of 5 to 10% dextrose. The parasite count and hematocrit level should be measured every 6 to 12 h. Anemia develops rapidly; if the hematocrit level falls below 20 percent, then whole blood (preferably fresh) or packed cells should be transfused slowly, with careful attention to circulatory status and judicious use of small doses of a diuretic to prevent fluid overload. Exchange transfusion

should be strongly considered for patients with a high level of parasitemia ($>$10 percent) and altered mental status. Renal function should be checked daily. Management of fluid balance is difficult in severe malaria because of the thin dividing line between overhydration (leading to pulmonary edema) and underhydration (contributing to renal impairment). If necessary, pulmonary artery occlusion pressures should be measured and maintained in the low-normal range. As soon as the patient can take fluids, oral therapy should be substituted for parenteral treatment.

Uncomplicated Malaria Infections due to *P. vivax*, *P. malariae*, *P. ovale*, and known sensitive strains of *P. falciparum* should be treated with oral chloroquine (25 mg of base/kg). In Africa, chloroquine-resistant strains are usually sensitive to sulfadoxine-pyrimethamine. Where there is resistance to the latter combination as well, either quinine plus tetracycline/doxycycline or mefloquine should be used; tetracycline and doxycycline cannot be given to pregnant women or to children $<$8 years of age. Oral quinine is extremely bitter and regularly produces cinchonism, a complex of symptoms comprising tinnitus, high-tone deafness, nausea, vomiting, and dysphoria. Compliance is poor with the required 5- to 7-day regimens of this drug. Mefloquine can be given at a dosage of 25 mg/kg (15 mg/kg followed 8 to 12 h later by 10 mg/kg). Although significant resistance to mefloquine has been documented in Thailand, Burma, Vietnam, and Cambodia, this agent usually is effective against multidrug-resistant strains of *P. falciparum*.

Patients should be monitored for vomiting for 1 h after the administration of any oral antimalarial drug. Symptom-based treatment, with tepid sponging and acetaminophen administration, lowers fever and thereby reduces the patient's propensity to vomit these drugs. Minor central nervous system reactions (nausea, dizziness, sleep disturbances) are common. The incidence of serious adverse neuropsychiatric reactions to mefloquine treatment is approximately 1 in 1000. All the antimalarial quinolines (chloroquine, mefloquine, and quinine) exacerbate the orthostatic hypotension associated with malaria, and all are tolerated better by children than by adults. Pregnant women, young children, patients unable to tolerate oral

Table 216-4

Recommended Therapeutic Doses of Antimalarial Drugs

Drug	Uncomplicated Malaria (Oral)	Severe Malaria* (Parenteral)
Chloroquine	10 mg of base/kg followed by 10 mg/kg at 24 h and 5 mg/kg at 48 h *or* by 5 mg/kg at 12, 24, and 36 h (total dose, 25 mg/kg); for *P. vivax* or *P. ovale*, primaquine (0.25 mg of base/kg/d for 14 days†) added for radical cure	10 mg of base/kg by constant-rate infusion over 8 h followed by 15 mg/kg over 24 h *or* by 3.5 mg of base/kg by IM or SC injection every 6 h (total dose, 25 mg/kg)
Sulfadoxine/pyrimethamine	20/1 mg/kg, single oral dose (3 tablets for adults)	—
Mefloquine	For semi-immunes, 15 mg of base/kg as a single dose; in areas with mefloquine resistance or for nonimmunes, 15 mg/kg followed 8–12 h later by second dose of 10 mg/kg;	—
Quinine	10 mg of salt/kg q 8 h for 7 days combined with tetracycline‡ (4 mg/kg qid) or doxycycline (3 mg/kg once daily) for 7 days	20 mg of salt/kg by IV infusion over 4 h§ followed by 10 mg/kg over 2–8 h every 8 h
Quinidine gluconate	—	10 mg of base/kg by constant-rate infusion over 1–2 h followed by 0.02 mg/kg per min, with ECG monitoring¶
Artesunate	In combination with 25 mg of mefloquine/kg, 10–12 mg/kg given in divided doses over 3–5 days (e.g., 4 mg/kg for 3 days or 4 mg/kg followed by 1.5 mg/kg per day for 4 days); if used alone, same dose divided over 7 days (usually 4 mg/kg initially followed by 2 mg/kg on days 2 and 3 followed by 1 mg/kg on days 4–7)	2.4 mg/kg IV or IM stat followed by 1.2 mg/kg at 12 and 24 h and then daily
Artemether	Same regimen as for artesunate	3.2 mg/kg IM stat followed by 1.6 mg/kg/d

* Oral treatment should be substituted for parenteral therapy as soon as the patient can take tablets by mouth.

† In Oceania and Southeast Asia, the dose should be 0.33 to 0.5 mg of base/kg. This regimen should not be used in patients with severe variants of G6PD deficiency.

‡ Neither tetracycline nor doxycycline should be given to pregnant women or to children $<$8 years old.

§ Alternatively, infusion of 7 mg of salt/kg over 30 minutes can be followed by 10 mg of salt/kg over 4 h.

¶ Some authorities recommend a lower dose of intravenous quinidine: 6.2 mg of base/kg over 1–2 h followed by 0.0125 mg/kg per min.

NOTE: In severe malaria, quinine or quinidine should be used if there is any doubt about infecting strain's sensitivity to chloroquine. IM, intramuscular; SC, subcutaneous; IV, intravenous; ECG, electrocardiogram.

therapy, and nonimmune subjects (e.g., travelers) with suspected malaria should be hospitalized. If there is any doubt as to the identity of the infecting malarial species, treatment for falciparum malaria should be given. A negative blood smear does not rule out malaria; thick blood films should be checked 1 and 2 days later to exclude the diagnosis. Nonimmune subjects with malaria should have daily parasite counts performed until negative thick films indicate clearance of the parasite. If the level of parasitemia does not fall below 25 percent of the admission value in 48 h or if parasitemia has not cleared by 7 days (and compliance is assumed), drug resistance is likely and the regimen should be changed. Quinine (or quinidine) and tetracycline should be reserved for multidrug-resistant infections, but if falciparum malaria has been contracted in an area of known drug sensitivity, then treatment with chloroquine, sulfadoxine-pyrimethamine, or mefloquine is preferable because these agents are better tolerated and simpler to administer.

Primaquine (0.3 mg of base/kg; 15 mg of base, adult dose) should be given daily for 14 days to patients with *P. vivax* or *P. ovale* infections after laboratory tests for G6PD deficiency have proved negative. A dose of 22.5 to 30 mg is recommended for infections acquired in Southeast Asia and Oceania. If the patient has a mild variant of G6PD deficiency, primaquine can be given in a dose of 0.6 mg of base/kg (45 mg maximum) weekly for 8 weeks.

COMPLICATIONS Acute Renal Failure If the level of blood urea nitrogen or creatinine rises despite adequate rehydration, fluid administration should be restricted to prevent volume overload. The indications for dialysis are the same as those in other forms of hypercatabolic acute renal failure (see Chap. 270). Even with adequate peritoneal dialysis, secondary bacterial infections are common in the tropics, and hemodialysis or hemofiltration is preferable. Some patients will pass small volumes of urine sufficient to allow control of fluid balance; these cases can be managed conservatively if other indications for dialysis do not arise. Renal function usually improves within days, but full recovery may take weeks.

Other Complications Patients who develop spontaneous bleeding should be given fresh blood and intravenous vitamin K. Convulsions should be treated with intravenous or rectal benzodiazepines. Aspiration pneumonia should be suspected in any unconscious patient with convulsions, particularly with persistent hyperventilation. Intravenous antimicrobial agents and oxygen should be administered, and pulmonary toilet should be undertaken. Systemic *Salmonella* infections are common in African children with falciparum malaria. Hypoglycemia or gram-negative septicemia should be suspected when any patient suddenly deteriorates for no obvious reason while receiving antimalarial treatment.

BABESIOSIS

Babesiosis is a protozoan disease of animals that is transmitted by ticks; humans are infected incidentally and initially develop a nonspecific febrile illness. *Babesia* organisms enter red blood cells and resemble malarial parasites morphologically, thus posing a diagnostic problem.

ETIOLOGY AND NATURAL CYCLE Of the more than 100 species of *Babesia*, *Babesia microti* and *Babesia divergens* are the two that cause most human infections. Ixodid (or hard-bodied) ticks, in particular *Ixodes dammini* (*Ixodes scapularis*) and *Ixodes ricinus*, are the vectors of the parasite. Ticks ingest *Babesia* while feeding, and the parasite multiplies within the tick's gut wall. The organisms then spread to the salivary glands; their inoculation into a vertebrate host by a tick larva, nymph, or adult completes the cycle of transmission. Asexual reproduction of *Babesia* within red blood cells produces two or four parasites.

EPIDEMIOLOGY While *Babesia* infections in wild and domestic animals are distributed globally, almost all *B. microti* infections

in the United States occur along the northeastern coast, including Nantucket Island and Martha's Vineyard in Massachusetts, Long Island and Shelter Island in New York, and the nearby mainland, including Connecticut. Cases also have been reported from Wisconsin. *Babesia* isolates from patients in the states of Washington and California have been characterized recently as WA 1, a category that is genetically and antigenically distinct from *B. microti*. A strain isolated in Missouri differs from these isolates, suggesting that babesiosis may be an "emerging infection." The deer tick, *I. dammini*, is the vector associated with *B. microti*.

Transfusions are another source of babesiosis. In several transfusion-associated cases, no parasites were detected in blood donors, but serologic testing of their blood for *Babesia* gave positive results.

Infections with *B. divergens* have occurred sporadically in previously splenectomized patients in several countries in Europe. *I. ricinus* is probably the vector in these cases, as it is for the transmission of this organism among cattle. The infected persons were predisposed to illness by their asplenic status.

I. dammini feeds on rodents as a larva and a nymph and on deer as an adult; nymphs are abundant during the spring and summer and feed on humans readily. In some endemic areas, the seroprevalence in the human population may be greater than 2 percent. This figure indicates that asymptomatic infection is more frequent than is generally thought.

CLINICAL PRESENTATION The incubation period for *B. microti* infection is about 1 to 4 weeks. Immunosuppressed patients, splenectomized individuals, and the elderly have the most severe illness. The clinical presentation varies widely; symptoms and signs include a gradual onset of irregular fever, chills, sweating, muscle pain, and fatigue. Mild hepatosplenomegaly and mild hemolytic anemia may develop. The level of parasitemia may exceed 10 percent. The illness may continue for weeks or months.

Patients infected with *B. divergens* have a more severe illness, with a rapid onset of chills, fever, nausea, vomiting, and hemolytic anemia progressing to jaundice, hemoglobinemia, and renal failure. *B. divergens* infections are often fatal.

DIAGNOSIS Whether or not they have a history of exposure to ticks or tick bites, febrile persons living in endemic areas should have Giemsa-stained thick and thin blood films examined for small intraerythrocytic parasites. *B. microti* appears as a small ring form resembling *P. falciparum*. Unlike infection with *Plasmodium*, however, that with *Babesia* does not cause the production of pigment in parasites, nor are schizonts or gametocytes formed. Dividing within red blood cells, *B. microti* can form four daughter parasites attached by strands of cytoplasm; these "tetrad" forms are seen infrequently in human blood films but are a distinguishing feature. An indirect immunofluorescence antibody test is useful for the diagnosis of infection with *B. microti* but does not replace the blood smear. The serum antibody titer rises 2 to 4 weeks after the onset of illness and then wanes over 6 to 12 months; cross-reactions can occur with other species of *Babesia* and with *Plasmodium*. About half of patients infected with *B. microti* have antibody to *Borrelia burgdorferi*, the agent of Lyme disease (Chap. 178); this figure varies with the geographic area. The occurrence of mixed infections is not surprising since both organisms are transmitted by *I. dammini*. Intraperitoneal inoculation of blood from patients with babesiosis into hamsters or gerbils results in detectable parasitemia within 2 to 4 weeks.

℞ **TREATMENT**

B. microti infections in patients with intact spleens are generally self-limiting without treatment. Treatment with the combination of quinine sulfate (650 mg of salt orally, three times daily) and clindamycin (600 mg orally, three times daily; or 1.2 g parenterally, twice daily) for 7 to 10 days is effective in some cases but may not eliminate parasites. The pediatric dose is 20 to 40 mg/kg per day for quinine sulfate and 25 mg/kg per day for clindamycin, both in three doses given over 7 to 10 days. Atovaquone suspension (750 mg twice daily) plus azithromycin (500 to 1000 mg/d) may be effective when quinine and clindamycin fail. Symptoms may persist for months with or without treatment, although there are no permanent sequelae. More severe infections with high-level *B. microti* parasitemia in asplenic patients have been successfully treated with exchange transfusions in addition to quinine and clindamycin.

BIBLIOGRAPHY

BAIRD JK et al: Primaquine for prophylaxis against malaria among nonimmune transmigrants in Irian Jaya, Indonesia. Am J Trop Med Hyg 52:479, 1995

BOUSTANI MR, GELFAND JA: Babesiosis. Clin Infect Dis 22:611, 1996

BREMAN JG, STEKETEE RW: Malaria, in *Maxcy-Rosenau-Last Public Health and Preventive Medicine*, 13th ed, JM Last, RB Wallace (eds). Norwalk, CT, Appleton & Lange, 1992, pp 240–253

CENTERS FOR DISEASE CONTROL AND PREVENTION: *Health Information for International Travelers*. HHS publication no. (CDC) 96-8280. Washington, U.S. Department of Health and Human Services, 1996

GARNHAM PCC: Malaria parasites of man: Life cycles and morphology (excluding ultrastructure) in malaria, in *Principles and Practice of Malariology*, WH Wernsdorfer, I McGregor (eds). Edinburgh, Churchill Livingstone, 1988, pp 61–96

HERWALDT BL et al: Babesiosis in Wisconsin: A potentially fatal disease. Am J Trop Med Hyg 53:146, 1995

KITCHEN SF: Symptomatology: General considerations and falciparum malaria, in *Malariology*, vol 2, MF Boyd (ed). Philadelphia, Saunders, 1949, pp 996–1016

MOLINEAUX L, GRAMICCIA G: *The Garki Project. Research on the Epidemiology and Control of Malaria in the Sudan Savannah of West Africa*. Geneva, World Health Organization, 1980

PASLOSKE BL, HOWARD RJ: Malaria, the red cell and the endothelium. Annu Rev Med 45:283, 1994

PERSING DH et al: Infection with a *Babesia*-like organism in northern California. N Engl J Med 332:298, 1995

SHANKS GD: Malaria prevention and prophylaxis, in *Balliere's Clinical Infectious Diseases*, vol 2-2, G Pasvol (ed). London, Balliere Tindall, 1995, pp 331–349

SPITZ S: Pathology of acute falciparum malaria. Milit Med 99:555, 1946

STEKETEE RW et al: Malaria treatment and prevention in pregnancy: The indications for use and adverse events associated with use of chloroquine or mefloquine. Am J Trop Med Hyg 55(Suppl 1):50, 1996

WHITE NJ: The treatment of malaria. N Engl J Med 335:800, 1996

———, HO M: The pathophysiology of malaria. Adv Parasitol 31:84, 1992

WORLD HEALTH ORGANIZATION, DIVISION OF CONTROL OF TROPICAL DISEASES:Severe and complicated malaria. Trans R Soc Trop Med Hyg 84(Suppl 2):1, 1990

217   *Barbara L. Herwaldt*

LEISHMANIASIS

DEFINITION   The term *leishmaniases* refers collectively to various clinical syndromes that are caused by obligate intracellular protozoa of the genus *Leishmania* (order Kinetoplastida). Leishmaniasis is endemic in diverse ecologic settings in the tropics and subtropics, ranging from deserts to rain forests and from rural to periurban areas. It typically is a vector-borne zoonosis, with rodents, small mammals, and canines as common reservoir hosts and humans as incidental hosts. In humans, visceral, cutaneous, and mucosal leishmaniases result from infection of macrophages throughout the mononuclear-phagocyte system, in the skin, and in the naso-oropharyngeal mucosae, respectively. The age range of infected persons depends on such factors as the duration of leishmaniasis endemicity in the specific geographic area, sandfly behavior (e.g., whether the sandfly species typically is intra- or extradomiciliary), and host behavior and immunity. Current challenges in this field include the emergence of leishmaniasis in new geographic areas and host populations [e.g., visceral leishmaniasis in civil war–affected southern Sudan and in persons infected with human immunodeficiency virus (HIV)] and the need for field-applicable, rapid diagnostic tests; efficacious, safe, inexpensive, and short-course oral treatment regimens; and effective and affordable control measures and immunoprophylactic agents.

ETIOLOGY   Visceral leishmaniasis is typically but not exclusively caused by organisms of the *Leishmania donovani* complex (Table 217-1); Old World cutaneous leishmaniasis by *Leishmania tropica*, *Leishmania major*, and *Leishmania aethiopica*; New World (or American) cutaneous leishmaniasis by organisms of the *Leishmania mexicana* complex and the species now commonly placed in the subgenus *Viannia* (*Leishmania braziliensis*, *Leishmania guyanensis*, *Leishmania panamensis*, and *Leishmania peruviana*); and mucosal leishmaniasis by some organisms in the latter group.

Because all of the leishmanial parasites associated with human disease are morphologically similar, their identification and classification can be challenging. Information on factors such as setting of acquisition (epidemiologic and geographic) and clinical manifestations is valuable; however, this information does not serve to classify the organisms taxonomically since these factors are quite variable. Thus, data on the intrinsic characteristics of the parasites are needed. To this end, the biochemical characteristics of *Leishmania* have been studied by techniques such as isoenzyme analysis, the genetic characteristics by methods including kinetoplast-DNA hybridization, and the immunologic characteristics by approaches such as monoclonal antibody specificity determination and excreted-factor serotyping.

LIFE CYCLE   Leishmaniasis is transmitted by the bite of female phlebotomine sandflies [genus *Phlebotomus* (Old World) or *Lutzomyia* (New World)]. As the flies attempt to feed, they regurgitate the parasite's flagellated promastigote stage into the skin of mammalian hosts. The saliva of *Lutzomyia longipalpis* sandflies, which transmit *Leishmania chagasi* infection, contains an erythema-producing peptide (maxadilan) that may enhance the infectivity of promastigotes and influence the course of infection. Promastigotes attach to receptors on macrophages, are phagocytized, and transform within phagolysosomes into the nonflagellated amastigote stage, which multiplies by binary fission. After rupture of infected macrophages, amastigotes are phagocytized by other macrophages. If ingested by feeding sandflies, amastigotes transform back into promastigotes, which require at least 7 days to become infective.

IMMUNOLOGY   Advances in the understanding of the immunology of leishmaniasis have made this parasitic disease the paradigm for studies of the T cell subsets and cytokines that govern resistance and susceptibility to intracellular pathogens. The paradigm is best demonstrated in murine leishmaniasis. In inbred mice, the nature of the T cell response determines the outcome of *L. major* infection: T helper type 1 (Th1) cells, which produce interferon γ and interleukin (IL) 2, are involved in cell-mediated immunity and resistance (the healing phenotype), whereas T helper type 2 (Th2) cells, which produce IL-4, IL-5, and IL-10, confer susceptibility (the nonhealing phenotype).

Not all aspects of leishmaniasis in mice, whose susceptibility to leishmanial infection is genetically determined, apply to human infection, for which the genetic determinants have yet to be identified. However, a consistent principle is that healing and resistance to reinfection are associated with expanding numbers of *Leishmania*-specific Th1 cells, production of interferon γ, and activation of macrophages to kill intracellular amastigotes. Whereas IL-12 promotes the development of Th1 responses, factors such as IL-4 and transforming growth factor β (murine leishmaniasis) and IL-10 (human visceral leishmaniasis) suppress their development. In murine macrophages, nitrogen oxides mediate intracellular killing, which occurs by nonoxidative mechanisms.

DIAGNOSIS   Definitive diagnosis of leishmaniasis requires demonstration of the parasite. To identify amastigotes by light-microscopic examination, the specimen obtained from an infected site (e.g., thin smear, histologic section) should be stained with Giemsa or another Romanovsky stain and presumptive amastigotes (2 to 4 μm in diameter) examined under oil immersion for the presence of a nucleus and a rod-shaped kinetoplast; the latter is a specialized mitochondrial structure that contains extranuclear DNA. Other means of parasitologic confirmation include in vitro culture (e.g., on Novy-MacNeal-Nicolle medium), inoculation into animals (e.g., golden hamsters, BALB/c mice), and use of molecular techniques (e.g., polymerase chain reaction). The parasites can be identified to the species level by isoenzyme analysis of cultured promastigotes or by use of monoclonal antibodies or DNA probes.

Indirect immunologic methods for diagnosis include serologic assays (e.g., indirect immunofluorescence antibody testing) and tests for *Leishmania*-specific cell-mediated immunity (e.g., skin testing for delayed-type hypersensitivity reactions). The usefulness of such methods depends on the clinical syndrome (see, for example, the section on diagnosis of visceral leishmaniasis). However, traditional serologic assays do not reliably distinguish past from current infection, and no leishmanin skin-test preparation has yet been approved for use in the United States.

℞ TREATMENT

For decades, the pentavalent antimonial (Sb^v) compounds sodium stibogluconate (Pentostam; Wellcome Foundation, United Kingdom; 100 mg of Sb^v/mL) and meglumine antimonate (Glucantime; Rhône Poulenc, France; 85 mg of Sb^v/mL) have been the mainstay of therapy for leishmaniasis. The Centers for Disease Control and Prevention (CDC) in Atlanta makes sodium stibogluconate available to U.S.-licensed physicians through the CDC Drug Service (404-639-3670) under an investigational new-drug protocol. The CDC generally recommends a daily parenteral (either intravenous or intramuscular) dose of 20 mg of Sb^v/kg, with a duration of therapy of 20 consecutive days for cutaneous leishmaniasis and 28 consecutive days for visceral and mucosal leishmaniasis. Alternative Sb^v regimens (e.g., longer or shorter courses) may have merit in some circumstances. Toxicity

(manifested, for example, as myalgia, arthralgia, fatigue, hepatotoxicity, chemical pancreatitis, or electrocardiographic abnormalities) becomes increasingly common as the course of treatment progresses but usually does not limit therapy and is reversible.

Amphotericin B and pentamidine are the traditional parenteral alternatives to Sb^v but are generally considered more toxic. Amphotericin B elicits reactions such as fever, chills, hypotension, nephrotoxicity, hypokalemia, and anemia, while pentamidine can cause hypotension, hypoglycemia, diabetes, vomiting, and pain at the injection site. Many other agents have been advocated as alternatives or adjuncts to Sb^v, often on the basis of suboptimal data; even the results of well-conducted clinical trials may not be generalizable to the treatment of patients in other settings, particularly patients infected with other leishmanial species or strains. Even in the absence of a consensus about if, when, or how to use other agents, it is important to consider whether the patient's illness could result in substantial morbidity or in death and therefore requires expeditious treatment with a regimen that usually is highly effective.

PREVENTION AND CONTROL   The transmission of *Leishmania* species is typically focal, with local "hot spots." This pattern is due in part to the characteristics of sandflies, whose flight is noiseless and limited in range; because of their short, hopping flight style, they usually remain within a few hundred meters of their breeding site. They rest in dark, moist places and are found in habitats ranging from deserts to rain forests; peridomestic sandflies rest in debris or rubble near buildings.

Personal protective measures include the avoidance of outdoor activities when sandflies are most active (dusk to dawn); the use of mechanical barriers such as screens and bed-nets that keep out sandflies, which are about one-third the size of mosquitoes; the wearing of protective clothing; and the application of insect repellent to exposed skin. Impregnation of clothing, bed-nets, and screens with permethrin may also be useful, as may spraying of dwellings with residual-action insecticide. Vaccine strategies are being investigated. Treatment of human cases is an effective control measure only where humans are the primary reservoirs of infection. Vector control and elimination of reservoir hosts (e.g., domestic dogs) may be useful in some settings—for example, where transmission is intra- or peridomiciliary.

VISCERAL LEISHMANIASIS
Visceral leishmaniasis, which has been reported in 47 countries and continues to be epidemic in eastern India, has emerged in new geographic areas (e.g., southern Sudan, where persons of all ages have been affected), in new settings (e.g., suburban areas in northeastern Brazil, where most cases have occurred in children <10 years of age), and among new host populations (e.g., HIV-infected persons). The causative leishmanial species typically are species of the *L. donovani* complex (Table 217-1); *Leishmania amazonensis* in Latin America and *L. tropica* in the Old World also can cause visceral infection. The organisms can be transmitted not only by sandflies but also congenitally and parenterally (e.g., via blood transfusion or sharing of needles). Infection begins in macrophages at the inoculation site (e.g., in dermal macrophages at the site of a sandfly bite) and disseminates

Table 217-1

Major *Leishmania* Species That Cause Disease in Humans

Species*	Clinical Syndrome†	Geographic Distribution
SUBGENUS *LEISHMANIA*		
L. donovani complex		
L. donovani	VL (PKDL, OWCL)	China, Indian subcontinent, southwestern Asia, Ethiopia, Kenya, Sudan; possibly sporadic in sub-Saharan Africa
L. infantum	VL (OWCL)	China, central and southwestern Asia, Middle East, southern Europe, North Africa, Ethiopia, Sudan; sporadic in sub-Saharan Africa
L. chagasi	VL (NWCL)	Central and South America
L. mexicana complex		
L. mexicana	NWCL (DCL)	Texas, Mexico, Central and South America
L. amazonensis	NWCL (ML, DCL, VL)	Panama and South America
L. tropica	OWCL (VL)‡	Central Asia, India, southwestern Asia, Middle East, Turkey, Greece, North Africa, Ethiopia, Kenya, Namibia
L. major	OWCL§	Central Asia, India, southwestern Asia, Middle East, Turkey, North Africa, Sahel region of north-central Africa, Ethiopia, Sudan, Kenya
L. aethiopica	OWCL (DCL)	Ethiopia, Kenya
SUBGENUS *VIANNIA*		
L. (V.) braziliensis	NWCL (ML)	Central and South America
L. (V.) guyanensis	NWCL (ML)	South America
L. (V.) panamensis	NWCL (ML)	Central America, Venezuela, Colombia, Ecuador, Peru
L. (V.) peruviana	NWCL¶	Peru (western slopes of Andes)

* Other species besides those listed here have been reported to infect humans. The taxonomy of the *Leishmania* species has not been finalized.

† Abbreviations: VL, visceral leishmaniasis; PKDL, post–kala-azar dermal leishmaniasis; OWCL, Old World cutaneous leishmaniasis; NWCL, New World (American) cutaneous leishmaniasis; DCL, diffuse cutaneous leishmaniasis; ML, mucosal leishmaniasis. Clinical syndromes less frequently associated with the various species are shown in parentheses.

‡ *L. tropica* also causes leishmaniasis recidivans and viscerotropic leishmaniasis.

§ *L. major*–like organisms also cause New World cutaneous leishmaniasis.

¶ The cutaneous leishmaniasis syndrome caused by this species is called *uta*.

throughout the mononuclear-phagocyte system in the context of both specific (i.e., to leishmanial antigens) and nonspecific (e.g., to tuberculin) anergy.

Manifestations Visceral infection can remain subclinical or can become symptomatic, with an acute, subacute, or chronic course. In some settings, inapparent infections far outnumber clinically apparent ones; malnutrition is a risk factor for the development of disease. The incubation period usually ranges from weeks to months but can be as long as years. Whereas the general term *visceral leishmaniasis* covers a broad spectrum of severity and manifestations, the term *kala-azar* (Hindi for "black fever," indicating that the skin can turn gray) generally conjures up the classic image of profoundly cachectic, febrile patients who are heavily parasitized and have life-threatening disease. Splenomegaly (with the spleen most often soft and nontender) typically is more impressive than hepatomegaly, and the spleen can in fact be massive; both splenomegaly and hepatomegaly in visceral leishmaniasis result from reticuloendothelial cell hyperplasia. Peripheral lymphadenopathy is common in some geographic areas, including Sudan.

The abnormal laboratory findings associated with advanced disease include pancytopenia—anemia, leukopenia (neutropenia, marked eosinopenia, relative lymphocytosis and monocytosis), and thrombocytopenia—as well as hypergammaglobulinemia (chiefly involving IgG, from polyclonal B cell activation) and hypoalbuminemia. Causes of anemia can include bone-marrow infiltration, hypersplenism, autoimmune hemolysis, and bleeding.

Some patients develop post–kala-azar dermal leishmaniasis. This syndrome is manifested by skin lesions (including pigmented or depigmented macules, papules, nodules, and patches) that typically are most prominent on the face. These lesions can develop during or within a few months after therapy (e.g., in East Africa) or years after therapy (e.g., in India). Visceral infection can relapse. Persons with persistent skin lesions can serve as reservoirs of infection.

So-called *viscerotropic leishmaniasis* caused by *L. tropica*, which typically is dermotropic, has been recognized among U.S. soldiers who participated in Operation Desert Storm in the Persian Gulf. The affected persons have had light parasite burdens and either no symptoms or nonspecific symptoms such as fatigue, fever, and gastrointestinal problems.

Diagnosis Parasitologic diagnosis of visceral leishmaniasis is accomplished by demonstration of the parasite on stained slides or in cultures of a tissue aspirate or a biopsy specimen (e.g., of spleen, liver, bone marrow, or lymph node). The diagnostic yield is highest for splenic aspiration (specifically, as high as 98 percent for splenic aspirates vs. <90 percent for other specimens), but this procedure can cause hemorrhage. Patients who have kala-azar typically carry a relatively heavy parasite burden; develop high titers of antibody to *Leishmania* (diagnostically useful but not protective); and have undetectable *Leishmania*-specific cell-mediated immunity (with leishmanin skin-test reactivity as well as lymphocyte proliferation and interferon γ responses to leishmanial antigens noted only after recovery). In contrast, viscerotropic leishmaniasis can be difficult to diagnose because of a light parasite burden and a minimal antibody response.

The differential diagnosis of visceral leishmaniasis includes other tropical infectious diseases that cause fever or organomegaly (e.g., typhoid fever, miliary tuberculosis, brucellosis, malaria with tropical splenomegaly syndrome, and schistosomiasis) as well as diseases such as leukemia and lymphoma. Post–kala-azar dermal leishmaniasis should be differentiated from syphilis, yaws, and leprosy.

℞ TREATMENT

Because classic cases of kala-azar generally are fatal if not appropriately treated, highly effective therapy is essential, as is close monitoring for bleeding and intercurrent infectious conditions such as pneumonia and diarrhea. In general, use of a pentavalent antimonial agent (i.e., 20 mg of Sb^v/kg given intravenously or intramuscularly once daily for 28 consecutive days) still constitutes first-line therapy. However, parasite-related factors such as apparent primary drug resistance and host characteristics such as coinfection with HIV can complicate treatment so that prolonged Sb^v administration or use of an alternative or adjunctive agent may be indicated (see below).

Typically, patients feel better and become afebrile during the first week of treatment. Abnormal laboratory findings and splenomegaly improve during therapy but may take weeks or months to resolve; the reappearance of eosinophils in the leukocyte differential count is a good sign. The best indicator of permanent cure is freedom from clinical relapse during at least 6 months of follow-up. Repeat tissue sampling is indicated if the patient's status is in question. The results of repeat tissue sampling must be interpreted with caution: the persistence of some parasites is not necessarily a poor prognostic indicator, whereas the apparent absence of parasites does not ensure that the patient will not relapse. The possibility of HIV coinfection should be considered if the patient does not respond to therapy or repeatedly relapses.

In India, where unresponsiveness to Sb^v therapy is becoming increasingly problematic, amphotericin B (0.5 to 1.0 mg/kg daily or every other day, given intravenously for a total dose of 7 to 20 mg/kg) has been found to be a highly effective, though potentially toxic, alternative. Pentamidine (2 to 4 mg/kg daily or every other day, given intravenously or intramuscularly for at least 15 doses) is reasonably effective but may need to be administered in prolonged courses that are associated with toxicity. Formulations of liposomal amphotericin B may prove highly effective and less toxic: liposomes passively target amphotericin away from the kidneys to macrophage-rich organs.

Various parenteral agents have been advocated as adjuncts to accelerate or improve the response to Sb^v therapy. The aminoglycoside aminosidine (12 to 15 mg/kg per day, intravenously or intramuscularly), which is the chemical equivalent of paromomycin, is an effective adjunct but is not available in the United States. Cytokine immunotherapy with subcutaneous injections of recombinant interferon γ or granulocyte macrophage colony-stimulating factor, both of which activate macrophages, also shows promise as an adjunctive measure. The oral agents allopurinol and ketoconazole have been used as adjuncts, but, because of the highly variable results obtained, their use cannot be generally recommended.

Visceral Leishmaniasis in HIV-Infected Persons Visceral leishmaniasis is becoming an important opportunistic infection among persons infected with HIV-1 in geographic areas in which both infections are endemic. To date, most coinfections have been reported from southern Europe, where *Leishmania infantum* is endemic and visceral leishmaniasis is no longer primarily a disease of young children. In HIV-infected patients, even relatively avirulent leishmanial strains can disseminate to the viscera. Clinical leishmaniasis in patients with HIV infection can represent newly acquired or reactivated infection; most coinfected patients who have clinically evident leishmaniasis have fewer than 200 CD4 lymphocytes per microliter. A better understanding of the interaction of these two infections is needed.

A diagnosis of visceral leishmaniasis should be considered for HIV-infected patients who have ever been in leishmaniasis-endemic areas and who have such manifestations as unexplained fever, organomegaly, anemia, or pancytopenia. Coinfected patients can develop unusual manifestations of visceral leishmaniasis, in part because of atypical localization of the parasite (e.g., in the gastrointestinal tract).

The diagnostic sensitivity of classic serologic methods is lower in coinfected than in immunocompetent patients (about 50 percent vs. >90 percent). On the other hand, parasitologic diagnosis by noninvasive means is easier in the case of coinfected patients; parasites are more commonly found in the circulating blood monocytes of these patients, and sensitivities are about 50 percent for a Giemsa-stained peripheral-blood smear and 70 to 75 percent for a stained or cultured buffy-coat preparation. Invasive methods of parasitologic diagnosis (e.g., microscopic examination or culture of a bone-marrow aspirate) typically are highly sensitive, especially for previously untreated patients, who commonly have heavy parasite burdens.

Coinfected patients may initially respond well to antileishmanial therapy, albeit with more drug toxicity than is experienced by most immunocompetent persons. However, coinfected patients commonly have a chronic or relapsing course, seemingly irrespective of the drug regimens used for induction and suppression therapy. Comparative clinical trials of candidate drug regimens are urgently needed.

CUTANEOUS LEISHMANIASIS Cutaneous leishmaniasis, which has been reported from 61 countries, has traditionally been classified as New World (American) or Old World. Local names for New World disease include *chiclero ulcer, pian bois* (bush yaws), and *uta*; those for Old World disease include *oriental sore, bouton d'orient, Aleppo boil,* and *Baghdad sore*. In the Americas, the leishmaniasis-endemic area extends from southern Texas to northern Argentina; in many affected regions, most cases occur in men who have forest-related occupational exposures. The etiologic agents typically are those of the *L. mexicana* complex and the *Viannia* group (Table 217-1) but also include *L. major*–like organisms and *L. chagasi*. Old World cutaneous leishmaniasis is caused by *L. tropica, L. major,* and *L. aethiopica* as well as by *L. infantum* and *L. donovani*.

Clinical Manifestations Although the incubation period for clinically evident disease typically ranges from weeks to months, local trauma can activate latent infection. The first clinical manifestation is usually a papule at the site of the sandfly bite but is sometimes regional lymphadenopathy (sometimes bubonic) in *L. (V.) braziliensis* infection. Most skin lesions evolve from papular to nodular to ulcerative, with a central depression (which can be several centimeters in diameter) surrounded by a raised indurated border; some lesions persist as nodules or plaques. Multiple primary lesions, satellite lesions, regional adenopathy, sporotrichosis-like subcutaneous nodules, lesion pain or pruritus, and secondary bacterial infection are variably present. The infecting species, the location of the lesion, and the host's immune response are major determinants of the clinical manifestations and chronicity of untreated lesions. For example, in the New World, lesions caused by *L. mexicana* tend to be smaller and less chronic than those caused by *L. (V.) braziliensis*; in the Old World, *L. major* tends to cause "wet" exudative lesions that are less chronic than the "dry" lesions with central crusting that are caused by *L. tropica*. The spontaneous resolution of lesions, which may require weeks, months, or even years, does not preclude reactivation or reinfection.

The polyparasitic and oligoparasitic ends of the spectrum of cutaneous leishmaniasis are respectively represented by the rare syndromes of diffuse cutaneous leishmaniasis (DCL) and leishmaniasis recidivans, both of which are notoriously difficult to treat. DCL, caused by *L. aethiopica* (Old World) or by the *L. mexicana* complex (New World), develops in the context of *Leishmania*-specific anergy and is manifested by chronic, nonulcerative skin lesions; on histopathologic examination of samples of these lesions, abundant parasites but few lymphocytes are noted. Leishmaniasis recidivans, a hyperergic variant with scarce parasites, is usually caused by *L. tropica* and manifested by a chronic solitary lesion on the cheek that expands slowly despite central healing.

Diagnosis Dermal scrapings of debrided ulcerative lesions are useful for histologic examination, aspirates of skin lesions and lymph nodes for in vitro culture, and biopsy specimens for both examination and culture. Although examination of histologic sections of biopsy specimens can help exclude other diagnoses, amastigotes appear larger and are more easily recognizable on Giemsa-stained thin smears (e.g., smears of dermal scrapings, touch preparations of biopsy specimens). As lesions age, amastigotes become more scarce and parasitologic confirmation becomes more difficult.

Serologic testing is an insensitive means for diagnosing cutaneous leishmaniasis; antibody titers are at most minimally elevated except in patients who have DCL. In contrast, leishmanin skin-test reactivity usually is evident or develops in persons who have simple cutaneous or recidivans leishmaniasis but not in those who have DCL.

Cutaneous leishmaniasis is frequently confused with tropical, traumatic, and venous-stasis ulcers; foreign-body reactions; superinfected insect bites; impetigo; fungal infections (e.g., sporotrichosis); mycobacterial infections; and other diseases (e.g., sarcoidosis, neoplasms). DCL and leishmaniasis recidivans must be differentiated from lepromatous leprosy and lupus vulgaris, respectively.

℞ TREATMENT

In decisions about whether and how to treat cutaneous leishmaniasis, the possibility of mucosal dissemination should be considered, as should lesion location (the cosmetic implications), number, size, evolution, and chronicity. When optimal efficacy is important, Sb^v therapy is recommended. In general, a regimen of 20 mg of Sb^v/kg (intravenous or intramuscular) should be given once daily for 20 consecutive days; lower daily doses or shorter courses may have merit in some situations. The clinical response begins with lesion flattening and continues after the end of therapy, whereas relapse typically is manifested by clinical reactivation at the margin of the lesion.

A study in Colombia showed that pentamidine (3 mg/kg intramuscularly, every other day for four doses) is an effective parenteral alternative to Sb^v. The oral agents that are currently available—most notably, the imidazoles ketoconazole (adult dosage, 600 mg/d for 28 days) and itraconazole (adult dosage, 200 mg twice daily for 28 days); allopurinol; and dapsone—probably are modestly active at best and are effective only against some leishmanial species/strains. Adjunctive immunotherapy remains highly experimental but may be useful in DCL.

Unless used in an adjunctive role, local or topical therapy should be considered only for the treatment of infection that does not have the potential for dissemination (e.g., for relatively benign lesions caused by *L. mexicana* or *L. major*). Examples of local approaches include the application of an ointment containing paromomycin and methylbenzethonium chloride (not licensed in the United States), the intralesional administration of Sb^v (not an approved use of drug obtained through the CDC), heat therapy, and cryotherapy. Excisional biopsy poses a substantial risk for relapse and is not recommended.

MUCOSAL LEISHMANIASIS Leishmanial infection of the naso-oropharyngeal mucosae is a relatively rare but potentially disfiguring metastatic complication of cutaneous leishmaniasis. Mucosal disease develops despite antileishmanial cell-mediated immunity and most commonly is caused by organisms of the *Viannia* group [typically *L. (V.) braziliensis* but also *L. (V.) panamensis* and *L. (V.) guyanensis*]. Although mucosal disease usually becomes clinically evident within several years after the healing of the original cutaneous lesions, cutaneous and mucosal lesions can exist simultaneously or can appear decades apart. Typically, the original cutaneous lesions in these cases were not treated or were inadequately treated.

Mucosal involvement generally is manifested first by persistent unusual nasal symptoms (e.g., epistaxis), with erythema and edema of the nasal mucosae, and then by progressive, ulcerative, naso-oropharyngeal destruction. Supportive laboratory data (e.g., a positive serologic test) are useful, but the scarcity of amastigotes makes parasitologic confirmation difficult. The differential diagnosis includes sarcoidosis, neoplasms, midline granuloma, rhinoscleroma, paracoccidioidomycosis, histoplasmosis, syphilis, and tertiary yaws.

Pentavalent antimonial therapy (20 mg of Sb^v/kg per day, given intravenously or intramuscularly for 28 days) is moderately effective for mild mucosal disease, whereas advanced disease may not respond to such therapy or may relapse repeatedly. Therapy with amphotericin B is the best alternative currently available. Patients who develop signs of respiratory compromise during therapy may benefit from concomitant steroid treatment.

BIBLIOGRAPHY

BERMAN JD: Human leishmaniasis: Clinical, diagnostic, and chemotherapeutic developments in the last 10 years. Clin Infect Dis 24:684, 1997

DAVIDSON RN et al: Liposomal amphotericin B (AmBisome) in Mediterranean visceral leishmaniasis: A multi-centre trial. Q J Med 87:75, 1994

GRIMALDI G, TESH RB: Leishmaniases of the New World: Current concepts and implications for future research. Clin Microbiol Rev 6:230, 1993

HERWALDT BL, BERMAN JD: Recommendations for treating leishmaniasis with sodium stibogluconate (Pentostam) and review of pertinent clinical studies. Am J Trop Med Hyg 46:296, 1992

—— et al: The natural history of cutaneous leishmaniasis in Guatemala. J Infect Dis 165:518, 1992

—— et al: American cutaneous leishmaniasis in U.S. travelers. Ann Intern Med 118:779, 1993

HO JL et al: Cytokines in the treatment of leishmaniasis: From studies of immunopathology to patient therapy. Biotherapy 7:223, 1994

KALTER DC: Laboratory tests for the diagnosis and evaluation of leishmaniasis. Dermatol Clin 12:37, 1994

MAGILL AJ: Epidemiology of the leishmaniases. Dermatol Clin 13:505, 1995

—— et al: Visceral infection caused by *Leishmania tropica* in veterans of Operation Desert Storm. N Engl J Med 328:1383, 1993

PEARSON RD, DE QUEIROZ SOUSA A: Clinical spectrum of leishmaniasis. Clin Infect Dis 22:1, 1996

ROSENTHAL E et al: Visceral leishmaniasis and HIV-1 co-infection in southern France. Trans R Soc Trop Med Hyg 89:159, 1995

SEAMAN J et al: Epidemic visceral leishmaniasis in southern Sudan: Treatment of severely debilitated patients under wartime conditions and with limited resources. Ann Intern Med 124:664, 1996

WORLD HEALTH ORGANIZATION: Control of the leishmaniases. Technical Report Series 793. Geneva, World Health Organization, 1990

218

Louis V. Kirchhoff

TRYPANOSOMIASIS

CHAGAS' DISEASE

DEFINITION Chagas' disease, or American trypanosomiasis, is a zoonosis caused by the protozoan parasite *Trypanosoma cruzi*. Acute Chagas' disease is usually a mild febrile illness that results from initial infection with the organism. After spontaneous resolution of the acute illness, most infected persons remain for life in the indeterminate phase of chronic Chagas' disease, which is characterized by subpatent parasitemia, easily detectable antibodies to *T. cruzi*, and an absence of symptoms. In a minority of chronically infected patients, cardiac and gastrointestinal lesions develop that can result in serious morbidity and even death.

LIFE CYCLE AND TRANSMISSION *T. cruzi* is transmitted among its mammalian hosts by hematophagous triatomine insects, or reduviid bugs. The insects become infected by sucking blood from animals or humans who have circulating parasites. Ingested organisms multiply in the gut of the reduviids, and infective forms are discharged with the feces at the time of subsequent blood meals. Transmission to a second vertebrate host occurs when breaks in the skin, mucous membranes, or conjunctivae become contaminated with bug feces that contain infective parasites. *T. cruzi* also can be transmitted by the transfusion of blood donated by infected persons, from mother to fetus, and in laboratory accidents.

PATHOLOGY An indurated inflammatory lesion called a *chagoma* often appears at the site of the parasite's entry. Local histologic changes include the presence of parasites within leukocytes and cells of subcutaneous tissues and the development of interstitial edema, lymphocytic infiltration, and reactive hyperplasia of adjacent lymph nodes. After dissemination of the organisms through the lymphatics and the bloodstream, muscles (including the myocardium) may become heavily parasitized. The characteristic pseudocysts seen in sections of infected tissues are intracellular aggregates of multiplying parasites.

The pathogenesis of chronic Chagas' disease is poorly understood. The heart is the organ most commonly affected, and changes include biventricular enlargement, thinning of the ventricular walls, apical aneurysms, and mural thrombi. Widespread lymphocytic infiltration, diffuse interstitial fibrosis, and atrophy of myocardial cells are often demonstrated, but parasites are rarely seen in myocardial tissue. Conduction-system involvement often affects the right branch and the left anterior branch of the bundle of His. In chronic Chagas' disease of the gastrointestinal tract (megadisease), the esophagus and colon may ex-

hibit varying degrees of dilatation. On microscopic examination, focal inflammatory lesions with lymphocytic infiltration are seen, and the number of neurons in the myenteric plexus may be markedly reduced.

EPIDEMIOLOGY *T. cruzi* is found only in the Americas. Wild and domestic mammals harboring *T. cruzi* and infected reduviids are found in spotty distributions from the southern United States to southern Argentina. Humans become involved in the cycle of transmission when infected vectors take up residence in the primitive wood, adobe, and stone houses common in much of Latin America. Thus, human *T. cruzi* infection is a health problem primarily among the poor in rural areas of Central and South America. Most new *T. cruzi* infections in rural settings occur in children, but the incidence is unknown because most cases go undiagnosed. Thousands of individuals also become infected every year through blood transfusions in urban areas. Currently, it is estimated that 16 to 18 million people, more than a third of whom live in Brazil, are chronically infected with *T. cruzi*. Chronic Chagas' disease is a major cause of morbidity and mortality in many Latin American countries, including Mexico, since many chronically infected persons eventually develop symptomatic cardiac lesions or gastrointestinal disease.

Acute Chagas' disease is rare in the United States. Four cases of autochthonous transmission have been described, and three instances of transmission by blood transfusion have recently been reported. In addition, between 1971 and 1992, seven laboratory-acquired infections and nine imported cases of acute Chagas' disease were reported to the Centers for Disease Control and Prevention (CDC). In contrast, the prevalence of chronic *T. cruzi* infections in the United States has increased considerably in recent years. Since the mid-1970s, enormous numbers of Central Americans have emigrated to the United States. In one study conducted in Washington, D.C., 5 percent of Salvadoran and Nicaraguan immigrants were found to have chronic *T. cruzi* infections. Estimates based on the latter study and on a small number of studies done in U.S. blood banks put the total number of infected immigrants now living here at more than 50,000. The presence of these carriers of *T. cruzi* creates a substantial risk of transmission by blood transfusion, as is evidenced by the occurrence of the three transfusion-associated cases just cited.

CLINICAL COURSE The first signs of acute Chagas' disease develop at least 1 week after invasion by the parasites. When the organisms have entered through a break in the skin, an indurated area of erythema and swelling (the chagoma), accompanied by local lymphadenopathy, may appear. Romaña's sign—the classic finding in acute Chagas' disease, which consists of unilateral painless edema of the palpebrae and periocular tissues—can result when the conjunctiva is the portal of entry. These initial local signs are followed by malaise, fever, anorexia, and edema of the face and lower extremities. Generalized lymphadenopathy and mild hepatosplenomegaly may appear. Severe myocarditis develops rarely; most deaths in acute Chagas' disease are due to heart failure. Neurologic signs are not common, but meningoencephalitis has been reported. The acute symptoms resolve spontaneously in virtually all patients, who then enter the asymptomatic or indeterminate phase of chronic *T. cruzi* infection.

Symptomatic chronic Chagas' disease becomes apparent years or even decades after the initial infection. The heart is commonly involved, and symptoms are caused by rhythm disturbances, cardiomyopathy, and thromboembolism. Right bundle-branch block is the most common electrocardiographic abnormality, but other types of atrioventricular block, premature ventricular contractions, and tachy- and bradyarrhythmias are seen frequently. Cardiomyopathy often results in right-sided or biventricular heart failure. Embolization of mural thrombi to the brain or other areas may take place. Patients with megaesophagus suffer from dysphagia, odynophagia, chest pain, and regurgitation. Aspiration can occur, especially during sleep, and repeated episodes of aspiration pneumonitis are common. Weight loss, cachexia, and pulmonary infection can result in death. Patients with megacolon are plagued by abdominal pain and chronic constipation, and advanced megacolon can cause obstruction, volvulus, septicemia, and death.

DIAGNOSIS The diagnosis of acute Chagas' disease requires the detection of parasites. Microscopic examination of fresh anticoagulated blood or of the buffy coat is the simplest way to see the motile organisms. Parasites also can be seen in Giemsa-stained thin and thick blood smears. When repeated attempts to visualize the organisms are unsuccessful, mouse inoculation and culture of blood in specialized media should be performed. As a last resort, xenodiagnosis should be attempted. In this technique, uninfected reduviid bugs are allowed to feed on the patient's blood. Approximately 30 days after the blood meal, the intestinal contents of the bugs are examined for parasites. When done properly, this method is positive in virtually all cases of acute Chagas' disease and in approximately half of chronic infections. Since early treatment of acute Chagas' disease is extremely important, however, the decision to initiate therapy for *T. cruzi* infection despite negative wet preparations and smears must be made on clinical and epidemiologic grounds before the results of these indirect methods become available. Serologic testing is of limited usefulness in diagnosing acute Chagas' disease.

The diagnosis of chronic Chagas' disease is made by the detection of antibodies that bind to *T. cruzi* antigens. Demonstration of the parasite is not of primary importance. Several highly sensitive serologic tests for the detection of antibodies to *T. cruzi* are used widely in Latin America, including complement-fixation and immunofluorescence tests and enzyme-linked immunosorbent assay (ELISA). However, a persistent problem with these conventional assays is the occurrence of false-positive reactions, typically with sera from patients who have other parasitic infections or autoimmune diseases. For this reason, it is generally recommended that positivity in one assay be confirmed by two other tests and that well-characterized positive and negative comparison sera be included in each run. A highly sensitive and specific method for detecting antibodies to *T. cruzi* [approved by the Clinical Laboratory Improvement Amendment (CLIA) and available in the author's laboratory] employs immunoprecipitation of radiolabeled *T. cruzi* antigens and electrophoresis. Serodiagnostic assays that employ recombinant *T. cruzi* proteins as target antigens are being developed, as are tests based on the amplification of *T. cruzi* DNA sequences by polymerase chain reaction. However, these tests are not yet available for general use.

℞ TREATMENT

Therapy for Chagas' disease is unsatisfactory. Nifurtimox is the only drug active against *T. cruzi* that is available in the United States. In acute Chagas' disease, nifurtimox markedly reduces the duration of symptoms and parasitemia and decreases mortality. Nevertheless, its efficacy at eradicating parasites is low. Limited studies have shown that only approximately 50 percent of acute infections are cured parasitologically by a full course of treatment. Despite its limitations, nifurtimox treatment should be initiated as early as possible in acute Chagas' disease. Moreover, when laboratory accidents occur in which it appears likely that *T. cruzi* infection could become established, nifurtimox therapy should be initiated without waiting for clinical or parasitologic indications of infection.

The usefulness of nifurtimox in individuals with indeterminate-phase or symptomatic chronic Chagas' disease has not been established. No evidence suggests that patients in the indeterminate phase are less likely to develop symptomatic disease after treatment with nifurtimox, nor has this agent been shown to have any effect on symptomatic chronic disease. Moreover, posttreatment xenodiagnoses are positive in a large proportion of chronically infected patients given this drug. Hence there is no indication for nifurtimox treatment of chronic *T. cruzi* infections.

Common adverse effects of nifurtimox include abdominal pain, anorexia, nausea, vomiting, and weight loss. Neurologic reactions to the drug may include restlessness, disorientation, insomnia,

twitching, paresthesia, polyneuritis, and seizures. These symptoms usually disappear when the dosage is reduced or treatment is discontinued. The recommended daily dosage is 8 to 10 mg/kg for adults, 12.5 to 15 mg/kg for adolescents, and 15 to 20 mg/kg for children 1 to 10 years of age. The drug should be given orally in four divided doses each day, and therapy should be continued for 90 to 120 days. Nifurtimox is available from the Drug Service of the CDC in Atlanta, Georgia (telephone number, 770-639-3670).

Benznidazole is a second agent used to treat Chagas' disease. Its efficacy is similar to that of nifurtimox, and its adverse effects include peripheral neuropathy, rash, and granulocytopenia. The recommended oral dosage is 5 mg/kg per day for 60 days. Benznidazole is used widely in Latin America but is not available in the United States. In a recent poll, many Brazilian authorities on Chagas' disease indicated that they would treat patients in the indeterminate phase of the illness with benznidazole. It has not been shown, however, that such treatment reduces the likelihood of symptomatic disease. None of those polled favored using the drug for the treatment of symptomatic chronic Chagas' disease.

Recent studies have shown that allopurinol is not useful for the treatment of chronic *T. cruzi* infections. Studies in mice have shown that recombinant interferon γ decreases the duration and severity of acute *T. cruzi* infection; however, its usefulness in persons with acute Chagas' disease has not been evaluated systematically.

Patients who develop cardiac and/or gastrointestinal disease in association with *T. cruzi* infection should be referred to appropriate subspecialists for further evaluation and treatment.

PREVENTION Since drug therapy is unsatisfactory and vaccines are not available, the control of *T. cruzi* transmission in endemic countries must depend on reduction of domiciliary vector populations by spraying of insecticides and improvement of housing. In addition, in endemic areas, programs for the screening of donated blood for *T. cruzi* need to be expanded and improved to reduce rates of transmission by transfusion. Tourists traveling in endemic areas should avoid sleeping in dilapidated houses outside urban areas. Mosquito nets and insect repellent will provide additional protection.

In the United States, blood donations should not be accepted from immigrants from regions in which Chagas' disease is endemic, unless serologic assays indicate that the donor is not infected with *T. cruzi*. Moreover, all immigrants from endemic regions should be screened for serologic evidence of infection with the parasite. Identification of infected individuals in this group is important not only in preventing transmission by blood transfusion but also in prompting physicians who care for these patients to undertake appropriate diagnostic monitoring and supportive therapy when indicated. Laboratory personnel should wear gloves and eye protection when working with *T. cruzi* and infected vectors. Patients with end-stage chagasic cardiopathies should not undergo cardiac transplantation because the immunosuppression required after surgery often leads to reactivation of *T. cruzi* infection, with serious consequences and even death.

SLEEPING SICKNESS

DEFINITION Sleeping sickness, or African trypanosomiasis, is caused by flagellated protozoan parasites that belong to the *Trypanosoma brucei* complex and are transmitted to humans by tsetse flies. In untreated patients, the trypanosomes first cause a febrile illness that is followed months or years later by progressive neurologic impairment and death.

THE PARASITES AND THEIR TRANSMISSION The East African (*rhodesiense*) and the West African (*gambiense*) forms of sleeping sickness are caused, respectively, by two trypanosome subspecies: *T. brucei rhodesiense* and *T. brucei gambiense*. These subspecies are morphologically indistinguishable but cause illnesses that are epidemiologically and clinically distinct. The parasites are transmitted by blood-sucking tsetse flies of the genus *Glossina*. The insects acquire the infection when they ingest blood from infected mammalian hosts. After many cycles of multiplication in the midgut of the vector, the parasites migrate to the salivary glands. Their transmission takes place when they are inoculated during a subsequent blood meal. The injected trypanosomes multiply in the blood and other extracellular spaces and evade immune destruction in mammalian hosts for long periods by undergoing antigenic variation, a process by which the antigenic structure of their surface coat of glycoproteins changes periodically.

PATHOGENESIS AND PATHOLOGY A self-limited inflammatory lesion (trypanosomal chancre) may appear a week or so after the bite of an infected tsetse fly. A systemic febrile illness then evolves as the parasites are disseminated through the lymphatics and bloodstream. Systemic African trypanosomiasis without central nervous system (CNS) involvement is generally referred to as *stage I disease*. In this stage, widespread lymphadenopathy and splenomegaly reflect marked lymphocytic and histiocytic proliferation and invasion of morular cells, which are plasmacytes that may be involved in the production of IgM. Endarteritis, with perivascular infiltration of both parasites and lymphocytes, may develop in lymph nodes and spleen. Myocarditis develops frequently in patients with stage I disease and is especially common in *T. b. rhodesiense* infections.

Hematologic manifestations that accompany stage I trypanosomiasis include moderate leukocytosis, thrombocytopenia, and anemia. High levels of immunoglobulins, consisting primarily of polyclonal IgM, are a constant feature, and heterophile antibodies, antibodies to DNA, and rheumatoid factor are often detected. High levels of antigen-antibody complexes may play a role in the tissue damage and increased vascular permeability that facilitate dissemination of the parasites.

Stage II trypanosomiasis involves invasion of the CNS. The presence of trypanosomes in perivascular areas is accompanied by intense infiltration of mononuclear cells. Abnormalities in cerebrospinal fluid (CSF) include increased pressure, elevated total protein concentration, and pleocytosis. In addition, trypanosomes are frequently found in CSF.

EPIDEMIOLOGY The trypanosomes that cause sleeping sickness are found only in Africa. Approximately 20,000 new cases are reported each year, but this number is surely an underestimate of the true incidence. Humans are the only reservoir of *T. b. gambiense*, which occurs in widely distributed foci in tropical rain forests of Central and West Africa. Gambiense trypanosomiasis is primarily a problem in rural populations; tourists rarely become infected. Trypano-tolerant antelope species in savanna and woodland areas of Central and East Africa are the principal reservoir of *T. b. rhodesiense*. Cattle also can become infected but generally succumb to the parasite. Since risk results for the most part from contact with tsetse flies that feed on wild animals, humans acquire *T. b. rhodesiense* infection only incidentally, usually while working in areas where infected game and vectors are present. In addition, occasional cases occur among visitors to game parks in East Africa. During the past two decades, 16 cases of imported African trypanosomiasis have been reported to the CDC, most of which were caused by *T. b. rhodesiense*.

CLINICAL COURSE A painful trypanosomal chancre appears in some patients at the site of inoculation of the parasite. Hematogenous and lymphatic dissemination (stage I disease) is marked by the onset of fever. Typically, bouts of high temperatures lasting several days are separated by afebrile periods. Lymphadenopathy is prominent in *T. b. gambiense* trypanosomiasis. The nodes are discrete, movable, rubbery, and nontender. Cervical nodes are often visible, and enlargement of the nodes of the posterior cervical triangle, or Winterbottom's sign, is a classic finding. Pruritus is frequent, and a circinate rash is often present. Inconstant findings include malaise, headache, arthralgias, weight loss, edema, hepatosplenomegaly, and tachycardia.

CNS invasion (stage II disease) is characterized by the insidious development of protean neurologic manifestations that are accompanied by progressive abnormalities in the CSF. A picture of progressive indifference and daytime somnolence develops (hence the designation "sleeping sickness"), sometimes alternating with restlessness and insomnia at night. A listless gaze accompanies a loss of spontaneity, and speech may become halting and indistinct. Extrapyramidal signs may include choreiform movements, tremors, and fasciculations. Ataxia is frequent, and the patient may appear to have Parkinson's

disease, with a shuffling gait, hypertonia, and tremors. In the final phase, progressive neurologic impairment ends in coma and death.

The most striking difference between the West African and East African trypanosomiases is that the latter illness tends to follow a more acute course. Typically, in tourists, systemic signs of infection, such as fever, malaise, and headache, appear before the end of the trip or shortly after the return home. Persistent tachycardia unrelated to fever is common early in the course of *T. b. rhodesiense* trypanosomiasis, and death may result from arrhythmias and congestive heart failure before CNS disease develops. In general, untreated East African trypanosomiasis leads to death in a matter of weeks to months, often without a clear distinction between the hemolymphatic and CNS stages.

DIAGNOSIS A definitive diagnosis of African trypanosomiasis requires detection of the parasite. If a chancre is present, fluid should be expressed and examined directly by light microscopy for the highly motile trypanosomes. The fluid also should be fixed and stained with Giemsa stain. Material obtained by needle aspiration of lymph nodes early in the course of the illness should be examined similarly. Examination of wet preparations and Giemsa-stained thin and thick films of serial blood samples is also useful. If parasites are not found by these methods, the buffy coat from 10 to 15 mL of anticoagulated blood or the pellet obtained by centrifugation of the eluate from 25 to 50 mL of blood passed through a DEAE-cellulose column should be examined. Trypanosomes may be seen in material aspirated from the bone marrow; the aspirate can be inoculated into liquid culture medium, as can blood, buffy coat, lymph node aspirates, and CSF. Finally, *T. b. rhodesiense* infection can be detected by inoculation of these specimens into mice or rats, which results in patent parasitemia in a week or two. Although this method is highly sensitive for the detection of *T. b. rhodesiense*, it unfortunately does not detect *T. b. gambiense* because of host specificity.

It is essential to examine CSF from all patients in whom African trypanosomiasis is suspected. An increase in the CSF cell count is the first abnormality to be detected; increases in opening pressure and in levels of total protein and IgM develop later. Trypanosomes may be seen in the sediment of centrifuged CSF. Any CSF abnormality in a patient in whom trypanosomes have been found at other sites must be viewed as pathognomonic for CNS involvement and thus must prompt specific treatment for CNS disease.

A number of serologic assays are available to aid in the diagnosis of African trypanosomiasis, but their variable sensitivity and specificity mandate that decisions about treatment be based on demonstration of the parasite. These tests are of value for epidemiologic surveys.

℞ TREATMENT

The drugs traditionally used for treatment of African trypanosomiasis are suramin, pentamidine, and organic arsenicals. An addition to this list is eflornithine (difluoromethylornithine), which was approved by the U.S. Food and Drug Administration (FDA) in November 1990 for the treatment of West African trypanosomiasis. In the United States these drugs can be obtained from the CDC. Therapy for African trypanosomiasis must be individualized on the basis of the infecting organism (*T. b. gambiense* or *T. b. rhodesiense*), the presence or absence of CNS disease, adverse reactions, and (occasionally) drug resistance. The choices of drugs for the treatment of African trypanosomiasis are summarized as follows.

Stage I (normal CSF) West African trypanosomiasis (*T. b. gambiense*) should be treated with either suramin or eflornithine. Pentamidine can be used as an alternative drug. Stage II West African trypanosomiasis (abnormal CSF) should be treated with eflornithine.

Stage I East African trypanosomiasis (*T. b. rhodesiense*) should be treated with suramin, and pentamidine can be used as an alternative drug. Since suramin and pentamidine do not penetrate the CNS well and since eflornithine has variable efficacy against *T. b. rhodesiense*, stage II East African trypanosomiasis should be treated with melarsoprol. Patients who cannot tolerate the latter drug should be treated with tryparsamide plus suramin.

Suramin is highly effective against stage I disease. However, it can cause serious adverse effects and must be administered under the close supervision of a physician. A 100- to 200-mg intravenous test dose should be administered to detect hypersensitivity. The dosage for adults is 1 g intravenously on days 1, 3, 7, 14, and 21. The regimen for children is 20 mg/kg (maximum, 1 g) intravenously on days 1, 3, 7, 14, and 21. The drug is given by slow intravenous infusion of a freshly prepared 10% aqueous solution. Approximately 1 patient in 20,000 has an immediate, severe, and potentially fatal reaction to the drug, developing nausea, vomiting, shock, and seizures. Less severe reactions include fever, photophobia, pruritus, arthralgias, and skin eruptions. Renal damage is the most common important adverse effect of suramin. Transient proteinuria often appears during treatment. A urinalysis should be undertaken before each dose, and treatment should be discontinued if proteinuria increases or if casts and red cells appear in the sediment. Suramin should not be given to patients with renal insufficiency.

Eflornithine is highly effective for treatment of both stages of West African trypanosomiasis. In the trials on which the FDA based its approval, this agent cured more than 90 percent of 600 patients with stage II disease. The recommended treatment schedule is 400 mg/kg per day intravenously in four divided doses for 2 weeks followed by 300 mg/kg per day orally for 3 to 4 weeks. Adverse reactions include diarrhea, anemia, thrombocytopenia, seizures, and hearing loss. The efficacy of eflornithine in *T. b. rhodesiense* infection has not been determined. The high dosage and long duration of therapy required are disadvantages that may make widespread use of eflornithine difficult.

Pentamidine is the alternative drug for patients with stage I African trypanosomiasis, although some *T. b. rhodesiense* infections are unresponsive to this agent. The dose for both adults and children is 4 mg/kg per day intramuscularly or intravenously for 10 days. Frequent, immediate adverse reactions include nausea, vomiting, tachycardia, and hypotension. These reactions are usually transient and do not warrant cessation of therapy. Other adverse reactions include nephrotoxicity, abnormal liver function tests, neutropenia, rashes, hypoglycemia, and sterile abscesses.

The arsenical melarsoprol is the drug of choice for the treatment of East African trypanosomiasis with CNS involvement. Melarsoprol cures both stages of the disease and therefore is also indicated for the treatment of stage I disease in patients who fail to respond to or cannot tolerate suramin and/or pentamidine. However, because of its relatively high toxicity, melarsoprol is never the first choice for the treatment of stage I disease. The drug should be given to adults in three courses of 3 days each. The dosage is 2 to 3.6 mg/kg per day intravenously in three divided doses for 3 days followed 1 week later by 3.6 mg/kg per day, also in three divided doses and for 3 days. The latter course is repeated 10 to 21 days later. In debilitated patients, suramin is administered for 2 to 4 days before therapy with melarsoprol is initiated. An 18-mg initial dose of the latter drug, followed by progressive increases to the standard dose, has been recommended. For children, a total of 18 to 25 mg/kg should be given over 1 month. A starting dose of 0.36 mg/kg intravenously should be increased gradually to a maximum of 3.6 mg/kg at 1- to 5-day intervals, for a total of 9 or 10 doses.

Melarsoprol is highly toxic and should be administered with great care. The incidence of reactive encephalopathy has been reported to be as high as 18 percent in some series. Clinical manifestations of reactive encephalopathy include high fever, headache, tremor, impaired speech, seizures, and even coma and death. Treatment with melarsoprol should be discontinued at the first sign of encephalopathy but may be restarted cautiously at small doses a few days after signs have resolved. Extravasation of the drug results in intense

local reactions. Vomiting, abdominal pain, nephrotoxicity, and myocardial damage can occur.

The treatment of patients with stage II East African disease who cannot tolerate melarsoprol is problematic. The combination of the arsenical tryparsamide and suramin is one possible approach, but its efficacy is limited because suramin does not penetrate the CNS well and tryparsamide is much less effective against *T. b. rhodesiense* than it is against *T. b. gambiense*. The schedule for tryparsamide therapy is 30 mg/kg (maximum 2 g) in a single intravenous dose every 5 days for a total of 12 doses; that for suramin treatment is 10 mg/kg intravenously every 5 days, also for a total of 12 injections. Tryparsamide can cause encephalopathy, fever, vomiting, abdominal pain, rash, tinnitus, and a variety of ocular symptoms. Alternatively, eflornithine can be administered as outlined above to patients who cannot tolerate melarsoprol, but, as noted, its effectiveness against *T. b. rhodesiense* is variable.

PREVENTION The trypanosomiases pose complex public-health and epizootic problems in Africa. Considerable progress has been made in some areas through control programs that focus on eradication of vectors and drug treatment of infected humans, but there is no consensus on the best approach to solving the overall problem. Individuals can reduce their risk of acquiring trypanosomiasis by avoiding areas known to harbor infected insects, by wearing protective clothing, and by using insect repellent. Chemoprophylaxis is not recommended, and no vaccine is available to prevent transmission of the parasites.

BIBLIOGRAPHY

CHAGAS' DISEASE

Bocchi EA: Long-term follow-up after heart transplantation in Chagas' disease. Transplant Proc 25:1329, 1993

Hagar JM, Rahimtoola SH: Chagas' heart disease in the United States. N Engl J Med 325:763, 1991

Kirchhoff LV: Is *Trypanosoma cruzi* a new threat to our blood supply? Ann Intern Med 111:773, 1989

————: American trypanosomiasis (Chagas' disease): A persistent problem in Latin America now affects the United States. N Engl J Med 329:639, 1993

———— et al: American trypanosomiasis (Chagas' disease) in Central American immigrants. Am J Med 82:915, 1987

———— et al: Increased specificity of serodiagnosis of Chagas' disease by detection of antibody to the 72- and 90-kilodalton glycoproteins of *Trypanosoma cruzi*. J Infect Dis 155:561, 1987

————: American trypanosomiasis (Chagas' disease). Gastroenterol Clin North Am 25:517, 1996

Ochs DE et al: Postmortem diagnosis of autochthonous acute chagasic myocarditis by PCR amplification of a species-specific DNA sequence of *Trypanosoma cruzi*. Am J Trop Med Hyg 54:526, 1996

Salazar Schettino PM et al: Chagas disease in Mexico. Parasitol Today 4:348, 1988

Schmunis GA: *Trypanosoma cruzi*, the etiologic agent of Chagas' disease: Status in the blood supply in endemic and nonendemic countries. Transfusion 31:547, 1991

SLEEPING SICKNESS

Bryan RT et al: African trypanosomiasis in American travelers: A 20 year review, in *International Travel Medicine*, R Steffen (ed). Berlin, Springer-Verlag, 1990

Jordan AM: *Trypanosomiasis Control and African Rural Development*. London, Longman, 1986

Milord F et al: Efficacy and toxicity of eflornithine for treatment of *Trypanosoma brucei gambiense* sleeping sickness. Trans R Soc Trop Med Hyg 87:652, 1992

Pepin J, Milord F: The treatment of African trypanosomiasis. Adv Parasitol 33:1, 1994

Poltera AA: Pathology of human African trypanosomiasis with reference to experimental African trypanosomiasis and infections of the central nervous system. Br Med Bull 41:169, 1985

Vanhamme L, Pays E: Control of gene expression in trypanosomes. Microbiol Rev 59:223, 1995

Vickerman K: Developmental cycles and biology of pathogenic trypanosomes. Br Med Bull 41:105, 1985

TOXOPLASMA INFECTION

DEFINITION   Toxoplasmosis is the disease caused by infection with the obligate intracellular parasite *Toxoplasma gondii*. Acute infection acquired after birth is asymptomatic but frequently results in the chronic persistence of cysts within the tissues of the host. Both acute and chronic toxoplasmosis are conditions in which the parasite is responsible for the development of clinically evident disease, including lymphadenopathy, encephalitis, myocarditis, and pneumonitis. Congenital toxoplasmosis is an infection of newborns that results from the transplacental passage of parasites from an infected mother to the fetus. These infants usually are asymptomatic at birth but later manifest a wide range of signs and symptoms, including chorioretinitis, strabismus, epilepsy, and psychomotor retardation.

ETIOLOGY   *T. gondii* is an intracellular coccidian that infects both birds and mammals. There are two distinct stages in the life cycle of *T. gondii*: the nonfeline and feline stages. In the nonfeline stage, tissue cysts that contain bradyzoites or sporulated oocysts are ingested by an intermediate host (e.g., a human, mouse, sheep, or pig). The cyst is rapidly digested by the acidic-pH gastric secretions. Bradyzoites or sporozoites are released, enter the small-intestinal epithelium, and transform into rapidly dividing tachyzoites. The tachyzoites are able to infect and replicate in all mammalian cells except red blood cells. Once attached to the host cell, the parasite penetrates the cell and forms a parasitophorous vacuole within which it divides. Parasite replication continues until the number of parasites within the cell approaches a critical mass and the cell ruptures, releasing parasites that infect adjoining cells.

As a result of this process, an infected organ soon shows evidence of cytopathology. Most of the tachyzoites are eliminated by means of humoral and cell-mediated immune responses of the host. Tissue cysts containing many bradyzoites develop 7 to 10 days after the systemic tachyzoite infection. These tissue cysts occur in a variety of host organs but are found principally within the central nervous system (CNS) and muscle, where they may exist for the lifetime of the host. The development of this chronic stage completes the nonfeline portion of the life cycle. Active infection in the immunocompromised host is most likely due to the spontaneous release of encysted parasites that undergo rapid transformation into tachyzoites within the CNS.

The principal stage in the life cycle of the parasite takes place in the cat (the definitive host) and its prey. The parasite's sexual phase is defined by the formation of oocysts within the feline host. This enteroepithelial cycle begins with the ingestion of the bradyzoite tissue cysts and culminates after several intermediate stages in the production of gametes. Gamete fusion produces a zygote, which envelops itself in a rigid wall and is secreted in the feces as an unsporulated oocyst. After 2 to 3 days of exposure to air at ambient temperature, the noninfectious oocyst sporulates to produce eight sporozoite progeny. The sporulated oocyst can be ingested by an intermediate host, such as a person emptying a cat's litter box, a pig rummaging in a barnyard, or perhaps a mouse. It is in the intermediate host that the parasite completes its life cycle.

EPIDEMIOLOGY   *T. gondii* is able to infect a wide range of mammals and birds. Its seroprevalence is dependent on the locale and the age of the population. Generally, hot arid climatic conditions are associated with a low prevalence of infection. In the United States and most European countries, the prevalence of seroconversion increases with age and exposure. For example, in the United States, 5 to 30 percent of individuals 10 to 19 years old and 10 to 67 percent of those over the age of 50 years show serologic evidence of exposure; seroprevalence increases by approximately 1 percent per year. In Central America, France, Turkey, and Brazil, the seroprevalence is much higher, approaching 90 percent by age 40.

ORAL TRANSMISSION   The principal source of human *Toxoplasma* infection remains uncertain. Transmission usually takes place by the oral route and can be attributable to ingestion of either sporulated oocysts from contaminated soil or bradyzoites from undercooked meat. During acute feline infection, a cat may excrete as many as 100 million parasites per day. These very stable sporozoite-containing oocysts are highly infectious and may remain viable for many years in the soil. Humans infected during a well-documented outbreak of oocyst-transmitted infection develop stage-specific antibodies to the oocyst/sporozoite.

Children and adults also can acquire infection from tissue cysts containing bradyzoites. The ingestion of a single cyst is all that is required for human infection. Undercooking or insufficient freezing of meat is an important source of infection in the developed world. In the United States, 10 to 20 percent of lamb products and 25 to 35 percent of pork products show evidence of cysts that contain bradyzoites. The incidence in beef is much lower—perhaps as low as 1 percent. Direct ingestion of bradyzoite cysts in these various meat products leads to acute infection.

In addition to oral transmission, direct transmission of the parasite by blood or organ products during transplantation takes place at a low incidence. Viable parasites can be cultured from refrigerated anticoagulated blood, which may be a source of infection in individuals receiving blood transfusions. *T. gondii* infection also has been reported in kidney and heart transplant recipients who were uninfected before transplantation.

TRANSPLACENTAL TRANSMISSION   About one-third of all women infected with *T. gondii* during pregnancy transmit the parasite to the fetus; the remainder give birth to normal, uninfected babies. Of the various factors that influence fetal outcome, gestational age at the time of infection is the most critical. Few data support a role for recrudescent maternal infection as the source of congenital disease. Thus women who are seropositive before pregnancy usually are protected against acute infection and do not give birth to congenitally infected neonates.

The following general guidelines can be used to evaluate congenital infection. There is essentially no risk if the mother is infected 6 months or more before conception. If infection is acquired less than 6 months before conception, the likelihood of transplacental infection increases as the interval between infection and conception decreases. In pregnancy, if the mother becomes infected during the first trimester, the incidence of transplacental infection is lowest (about 15 percent), but the disease in the neonate is most severe. If maternal infection occurs during the third trimester, the incidence of transplacental infection is greatest (65 percent), but the infant is usually asymptomatic at birth. Recent evidence, however, suggests that infected infants who are normal at birth may have a higher incidence of learning disabilities and chronic neurologic sequelae than uninfected children. Only a small proportion (20 percent) of women infected with *T. gondii* develop clinical signs of infection. Often the diagnosis is first appreciated when routine postconception serologic tests show evidence of specific antibody.

PATHOGENESIS   Upon the ingestion by the host of either tissue cysts containing bradyzoites or oocysts containing sporozoites, the parasites are released from the cysts by a digestive process. Bradyzoites are resistant to the effect of pepsin and quickly invade and multiply within the gastrointestinal tract of the host. Within enterocytes, the parasites undergo morphologic transformation, giving rise to invasive tachyzoites. These tachyzoites are able to induce host secretory immunity, as evidenced by increased levels of parasite-specific IgA. The parasites are disseminated to a variety of organs, particularly lymphatic tissue, skeletal muscle, myocardium, retina, placenta, and (most frequently) the CNS. In these organs, the parasite infects host cells, replicates, and invades the adjoining cells. In this fashion, the hallmarks of the infection develop: cell death and focal necrosis surrounded by an acute inflammatory response.

In the normal immune host, both the humoral and the cellular immune responses are important in controlling infection. Tachyzoites are sequestered by a variety of immune mechanisms, including induction of parasiticidal antibody, activation of macrophages, production of interferon γ (IFNγ), and stimulation of cytotoxic T lymphocytes of the CD8 + phenotype. These antigen-specific lymphocytes are capable of killing both extracellular parasites and target cells infected with parasites. As tachyzoites are cleared from the acutely infected host, tissue cysts containing bradyzoites begin to appear, usually within the CNS and the retina. A number of immune factors, including altered antibody levels within the CNS, IFNγ, and CD4 + and CD8 + T cells, modulate the normal host immune response.

In the immunocompromised or fetal host, the immune factors necessary to control the spread of tachyzoite infection are lacking. This altered immune state gives rise to a progression of focal destruction that results in organ failure (i.e., necrotizing encephalitis, pneumonia, and myocarditis).

Persistence of infection with cysts containing bradyzoites is common in the normal host. This lifelong infection usually remains subclinical. Although bradyzoites are in a slow metabolic phase, cysts do degenerate and rupture within the CNS. This degenerative process, with the development of new bradyzoite-containing cysts, is the most likely stimulus for the persistence of antibody titers in the normal host. Degeneration of these cysts is the most probable source of recrudescent infection in immunocompromised individuals.

PATHOLOGY   Cell death and focal necrosis due to replicating tachyzoites induce an intense mononuclear inflammatory response in any tissue or cell type infected. Tachyzoites rarely can be visualized by routine histopathologic staining of these inflammatory lesions. However, immunofluorescence staining with parasite antigen–specific antibodies can reveal either the organism itself or evidence of antigen. In contrast to this inflammatory process caused by tachyzoites, bradyzoite-containing cysts cause inflammation only at the early stages of development, and even this inflammation may be a response to the presence of tachyzoite antigens. Once the cysts reach maturity, the inflammatory process can no longer be detected, and the cysts remain immunologically quiescent within the brain matrix until they rupture.

Lymph Nodes   During acute infection, lymph node biopsy demonstrates characteristic findings, including follicular hyperplasia and irregular clusters of tissue macrophages with eosinophilic cytoplasm. Granulomas rarely are evident in these specimens. Although tachyzoites are not usually visible, they can be sought either by subinoculation of infected tissue into mice, with resultant disease, or by the polymerase chain reaction (PCR). PCR amplification of DNA fragments representing either p30 (SAG-1) or p22 (SAG-2) antigen has been shown to be an effective and sensitive assay for establishing infection of lymph node tissue by tachyzoites.

Eyes   In the eye, infiltrates of monocytes, lymphocytes, and plasma cells may produce uni- or multifocal lesions. Granulomatous lesions and retinochoroiditis can be observed in the posterior chamber following acute necrotizing retinitis. Other ocular complications of infection include iridocyclitis, cataracts, and glaucoma.

Central Nervous System   During CNS involvement, both focal and diffuse meningoencephalitis can be documented, with evidence of necrosis and microglial nodules. Necrotizing encephalitis in the patient without AIDS is characterized by small diffuse lesions with perivascular cuffing in contiguous areas. In the AIDS population, polymorphonuclear leukocytes may be present in addition to monocytes, lymphocytes, and plasma cells. Cysts containing bradyzoites frequently are found contiguous with the necrotic tissue border. In the mouse model, parasite DNA has been detected by PCR amplification in association with reactivation of CNS toxoplasmosis.

Lungs   Among patients with AIDS who die of toxoplasmosis, 40 to 70 percent have involvement of the heart and lung. Interstitial pneumonitis can develop in the neonate and the immunocompromised patient. Thickened and edematous alveolar septa infiltrated with mononuclear and plasma cells are apparent. This inflammation may extend to the endothelial walls. Tachyzoites and bradyzoite-containing cysts have been observed within the alveolar membrane. Superimposed bronchopneumonia can be caused by other microbial agents.

Heart   Cysts and aggregates of parasites in cardiac muscle tissue are evident in patients with AIDS who die of toxoplasmosis. Focal necrosis surrounded by inflammatory cells is associated with hyaline necrosis and disrupted myocardial cells. Pericarditis is associated with toxoplasmosis in some patients.

Other Sites   Pathologic changes during disseminated infection are similar to those described for the lymph nodes, eyes, and CNS. In patients with AIDS, the skeletal muscle, pancreas, stomach, and kidneys can be involved, with necrosis, invasion by inflammatory cells, and (rarely) the presence of tachyzoites detectable by routine staining. Large necrotic lesions may cause direct tissue destruction. In addition, secondary effects from acute infection of these various organs, including pancreatitis, myositis, and glomerulonephritis, have been reported.

HOST IMMUNE RESPONSE   Acute *Toxoplasma* infection evokes a cascade of protective immune responses in the normal host. *Toxoplasma* enters the host at the gut mucosal level and evokes the production of IgA antibody. This isotype, which constitutes more than 80 percent of all antibody in the mucosa, has now been shown to be a potentially important modulator of protection and indicator of infection. Titers of serum IgA antibody directed at p30 (SAG-1) have been shown to be a useful marker of congenital and acute toxoplasmosis. Milk-whey IgA from acutely infected mothers contains a high titer of antibody to *T. gondii* and is able to block infection of enterocytes in vitro. The predominant parasite antigen recognized by the whey IgA is p30. In mice, IgA intestinal secretions directed at the parasite are abundant and are associated with the induction of mucosal T cells.

If the parasite evades the host mucosal response, both humoral immunity and cellular immunity are evoked. *T. gondii* rapidly induces detectable levels of both IgM and IgG antibodies in serum. Monoclonal gammopathy of the IgG class can occur in congenitally infected infants. IgM levels may be increased in the newborn with congenital infection. The polyclonal IgG antibodies evoked by infection are parasiticidal in vitro in the presence of serum complement and are the basis for the Sabin-Feldman dye test. However, cell-mediated immunity is the major protective response evoked by the parasite during host infection. Macrophages are activated following phagocytosis of antibody-opsonized parasites. This activation can lead to death of the parasite by either an oxygen-dependent or an oxygen-independent process. Recent studies demonstrate that if the parasite is not phagocytosed and enters the macrophage by active penetration, it continues to replicate. In addition, T cells are activated by a variety of parasite antigens. These antigens can be either membrane-associated or cytoplasmic. The CD4 + and CD8 + T cell responses are antigen-specific and further stimulate the production of a variety of important lymphokines that expand the T cell and natural killer cell repertoire. IFNγ is an important factor in eliciting host immune protection against *Toxoplasma* infection. T cells exhibiting both T$_{H1}$ (associated with IFNγ production) and T$_{H2}$ [associated with interleukin (IL) 4 production] have been isolated from seropositive individuals. CD8 + cells appear critical to host immunity. In humans, prolonged alteration in T cell subpopulations is associated with *T. gondii* infection. Both asymptomatic patients and those with active infection may show a depression in the ratio of CD4 + to CD8 + lymphocytes. This shift may be correlated with a disease syndrome but is not necessarily correlated with disease outcome. Human T cell clones of both the CD4 + and the CD8 + phenotypes are cytolytic against parasite-infected macrophages. These T cell clones produce cytokines that are "microbistatic." IL-12 and perhaps IL-7 and IL-15 appear to be important during acute infection, upregulating the production of IFNγ. Recent studies suggest that the effect of IFNγ may be paradoxical, with stimulation of a host downregulatory response as well.

In patients with AIDS, both the humoral response and the cellular response to *T. gondii* are altered. Although infection in the patient with AIDS is believed to be recrudescent, determination of antibody titers is not helpful in establishing reactivation. Because of the severe depletion in CD4 + T cells, quite frequently there is no observed increase in antibody titer during exacerbation of infection. T cells from AIDS patients with reactivation of toxoplasmosis fail to secrete both INFγ and IL-2. This alteration in the production of these critical immune cytokines contributes to the persistence of infection. *Toxoplasma* infection frequently develops late in the course of AIDS, when the loss of T cell–dependent protective mechanisms, particularly CD8+ T cells, becomes most pronounced.

CLINICAL MANIFESTATIONS In the person whose immune system is intact, acute toxoplasmosis is usually asymptomatic and self-limited. This condition can go unrecognized in 80 to 90 percent of adults and children with acquired infection. The asymptomatic nature of this infection makes diagnosis difficult in mothers infected during pregnancy. In contrast, the wide range of clinical manifestations in congenitally infected children includes severe neurologic complications such as hydrocephalus, microcephaly, mental retardation, and retinochoroiditis. If prenatal infection is severe, multiorgan failure and subsequent intrauterine fetal death can occur. In children and adults, chronic infection can persist throughout life, with little consequence to the immunocompetent host.

Toxoplasmosis in the Immunocompetent Person The most common manifestation of acute toxoplasmosis is cervical lymphadenopathy. The nodes may be single or multiple, are usually nontender, are discrete, and vary in firmness. Lymphadenopathy also may be found in suboccipital, supraclavicular, inguinal, and mediastinal areas. Generalized lymphadenopathy occurs in 20 to 30 percent of symptomatic patients. Between 20 and 40 percent of patients with lymphadenopathy also have headache, malaise, fatigue, and fever (usually with a temperature of <40°C). A smaller proportion of symptomatic individuals have myalgia, sore throat, abdominal pain, maculopapular rash, meningoencephalitis, and confusion. Rare complications associated with infection in the normal immune host include pneumonia, myocarditis, encephalopathy, pericarditis, and polymyositis. Symptoms associated with acute infection usually resolve within several weeks, although the lymphadenopathy may persist for some months. In a recent epidemic, toxoplasmosis was diagnosed correctly in only 3 of the 25 patients who consulted physicians. If toxoplasmosis is considered in the differential diagnosis, routine laboratory and serologic screening should be performed before node biopsy.

The results of routine laboratory studies are usually unremarkable except for minimal lymphocytosis, an elevated sedimentation rate, and a nominal increase in liver aminotransferases. Evaluation of cerebrospinal fluid (CSF) in cases with evidence of encephalopathy or meningoencephalitis shows an elevation of intracranial pressure, mononuclear pleocytosis (10 to 50 cells/mL), a slight increase in protein concentration, and (occasionally) an increase in the gamma globulin level. PCR amplification of the *Toxoplasma* DNA target sequence in the CSF may be beneficial. The CSF of chronically infected individuals is normal.

Ocular Infection Infection with *T. gondii* is estimated to cause 35 percent of all cases of chorioretinitis in the United States and Europe. Most ocular involvement is believed to be due to congenital infection, with a very low incidence following acquired infection. Individuals with AIDS also can develop debilitating chorioretinitis. A variety of ocular manifestations are documented, including blurred vision, scotoma, photophobia, and eye pain. Macular involvement occurs with loss of central vision, and nystagmus is secondary to poor fixation. Involvement of the extraocular muscles may lead to disorders of convergence and to strabismus. Ophthalmologic examination should be undertaken in newborns with suspected congenital infection. As the inflammation resolves, vision improves, but episodic flare-ups of chorioretinitis, which progressively destroy retinal tissue and lead to glaucoma, are common.

The ophthalmologic examination reveals yellow-white, cotton-like patches with indistinct margins of hyperemia. As the lesions age, white plaques with distinct borders and black spots within the retinal pigment become more apparent. Lesions usually are located near the posterior pole of the retina; they may be single but are more commonly multiple. Congenital lesions may be unilateral or bilateral and show evidence of massive chorioretinal degeneration with extensive fibrosis. Surrounding these areas of involvement are a normal retina and vasculature. In patients with AIDS, retinal lesions are often large with diffuse necrosis of the retina and include both free tachyzoites and cysts containing bradyzoites.

Infection of the Immunocompromised Person Patients with AIDS and those receiving immunosuppressive therapy for lymphoproliferative disorders are at greatest risk for developing acute toxoplasmosis. This predilection may be due either to reactivation of latent infection or to acquisition of parasites from exogenous sources such as blood or transplanted organs. In individuals with AIDS, more than 95 percent of cases of *Toxoplasma* encephalitis are believed to be due to recrudescent infection. In most of these cases, encephalitis develops when the CD4+ cell count falls below 100 cells/μL. In the immunocompromised individual, the disease may be rapidly fatal if untreated. Thus accurate diagnosis and initiation of appropriate therapy are necessary to prevent fulminant infection.

Toxoplasmosis is a principal opportunistic infection of the CNS in persons with AIDS. Although geographic origin may be related to frequency of infection, it has no correlation with the severity of disease in the immunocompromised host. Individuals with AIDS who are seropositive for *T. gondii* are at a very high risk for developing encephalitis. In the United States, about one-third of the 15 to 40 percent of adult patients with AIDS who are latently infected with the parasite develop *Toxoplasma* encephalitis.

The signs and symptoms of acute toxoplasmosis in the immunocompromised patient are principally within the CNS. More than 50 percent of patients with clinical manifestations have intracerebral involvement. Clinical findings at the time of presentation can range from nonfocal to focal dysfunction. These findings include encephalopathy, meningoencephalitis, and mass lesions. Patients may present with altered mental status (75 percent), fever (10 to 72 percent), seizures (33 percent), headaches (56 percent), and focal neurologic findings (60 percent), including motor deficits, cranial nerve palsies, movement disorders, dysmetria, visual-field loss, and aphasia. Patients who present with evidence of diffuse cortical dysfunction develop evidence of focal neurologic disease as the infection progresses. This altered condition is due not only to the necrotizing encephalitis caused by direct invasion of the parasite but also to secondary effects, including vasculitis, edema, and hemorrhage. The onset of infection can range from an insidious process over several weeks to an acute confusional state with fulminant focal deficits, including hemiparesis, hemiplegia, visual-field defects, localized headache, and focal seizures.

Although lesions can occur anywhere within the CNS, the areas most involved appear to be the brainstem, basal ganglia, pituitary gland, and corticomedullary junction. Brainstem involvement gives rise to a variety of neurologic dysfunctions, including cranial nerve palsy, dysmetria, and ataxia. With basal ganglionic infection, patients may develop hydrocephalus, choreiform movements, and choreoathetosis. Because *Toxoplasma* usually causes encephalitis, meningeal involvement is uncommon, and thus CSF findings may be unremarkable or may include a modest increase in cell count and in protein—but not glucose—concentration.

Cerebral toxoplasmosis needs to be differentiated from other opportunistic infections or tumors within the CNS of those afflicted with AIDS. The differential diagnosis includes herpes simplex encephalitis, cryptococcal meningitis, progressive multifocal leukoencephalopathy, and primary CNS lymphoma. Involvement of the pituitary gland can give rise to panhypopituitarism and hyponatremia from inappropriate secretion of vasopressin (antidiuretic hormone). AIDS-dementia complex may present as cognitive impairment, attention loss, and altered memory. Brain biopsy in those patients who have been treated for *Toxoplasma* encephalitis but who continue to exhibit neurologic dysfunction often fails to identify organisms.

Autopsies of patients infected with *Toxoplasma* have demonstrated multiple organ involvement with or without CNS disease. The organs infected include the lungs, gastrointestinal tract, pancreas, skin, eyes, heart, and liver. *Toxoplasma* pneumonia can occur and can be confused with *Pneumocystis carinii* infection. Respiratory involvement usually presents as dyspnea, fever, and a nonproductive cough and may rapidly progress to acute respiratory failure with hemoptysis, metabolic acidosis, hypotension, and (occasionally) disseminated intravascular coagulation. Histopathologic studies demonstrate necrosis and a mixed cellular infiltrate. The presence of organisms is a helpful diagnostic indicator, but organisms can also be found in healthy tissue. Most commonly, myocardial infection is asymptomatic. However, infection of the heart can be associated with cardiac tamponade or biventricular failure. As discussed previously, ocular involvement can occur without concomitant encephalitis. This infection should be distinguished from chorioretinitis caused by cytomegalovirus, which is usually more hemorrhagic in character. Toxoplasmic retinochoroiditis may be a prodrome to the development of encephalitis.

A presumptive clinical diagnosis of toxoplasmic encephalitis in patients with AIDS is based on clinical presentation, history of exposure as evidenced by positive serology, and radiologic evaluation. When these criteria are used, the predictive value is as high as 80 percent. More than 97 percent of patients with AIDS and toxoplasmosis have IgG antibody to the parasite in their sera. IgM serum antibody is usually not demonstrable. Intrathecal antibody to *T. gondii* may be present. Neuroradiologic evaluation should include double-dose contrast computed tomography (CT) of the head. By this test, single and frequently multiple contrast-enhancing lesions (<2 cm) may be identified. Magnetic resonance imaging (MRI) usually demonstrates multiple lesions and provides a more sensitive evaluation of the efficacy of therapy than does CT. Patients with primary CNS lymphoma are four times more likely than patients with *Toxoplasma* encephalitis to have solitary lesions on an MRI scan. A therapeutic trial of anti-*Toxoplasma* medications frequently is used to assess the diagnosis. Recent studies have shown that treatment of presumptive *Toxoplasma* encephalitis with pyrimethamine/clindamycin results in quantifiable clinical improvement in more than 50 percent of patients by day 3. By day 7, more than 90 percent of treated patients show evidence of improvement. In contrast, if patients fail to respond or have lymphoma, clinical signs and symptoms worsen by day 7. Patients in this category require brain biopsy with or without a change in therapy. This procedure can now be performed by a stereotactic CT-guided method that reduces the potential for complications. Brain biopsy for *T. gondii* identifies organisms in 50 to 75 percent of cases. More recent studies indicate that PCR amplification of target genes significantly increases the sensitivity of detection of parasites.

Congenital Toxoplasmosis   Between 400 and 4000 infants born each year in the United States are affected by congenital toxoplasmosis. Infection of the placenta leads to hematogenous infection of the fetus. As has already been stated, the proportion of fetuses that becomes infected increases but the clinical severity of the infection declines as gestation proceeds. Persistence of the parasite can ultimately result in reactivation and further damage decades later. Factors associated with relatively severe disabilities include delayed diagnosis and initiation of therapy, neonatal hypoxia and hypoglycemia, profound visual impairment, uncorrected hydrocephalus, and increased intracranial pressure. If treated appropriately, upwards of 70 percent of children have normal developmental. neurologic, and ophthalmologic findings at follow-up evaluations. Treatment for 1 year with pyrimethamine and sulfonamide is tolerated with minimal toxicity (see below).

DIAGNOSIS   Tissue and Body Fluid   The diagnosis of acute toxoplasmosis can be made by isolation of the parasite from either blood or other body fluids after subinoculation of the body fluid into the peritoneal cavity of mice. Mice should be tested for organisms in the peritoneal fluid 6 to 10 days after inoculation. If no parasites are found in the mouse's peritoneal fluid, its anti-*Toxoplasma* serum titer can be evaluated 4 to 6 weeks after inoculation. Isolation of *T. gondii* from the patient's body fluids reflects acute infection, whereas isolation from biopsied tissue is an indication only of the presence of tissue cysts and should not be misinterpreted as acute toxoplasmosis. Persistent parasitemia in patients with latent, asymptomatic infection is rare.

Histologic examination of lymph nodes may suggest the characteristic changes described above. Demonstration of tachyzoites in lymph nodes establishes the diagnosis of acute toxoplasmosis. As with subinoculation into mice, demonstration of cysts containing bradyzoites in histologic specimens confirms prior infection with *T. gondii* but is nondiagnostic for acute infection.

Serology   The preceding procedures have great diagnostic value but are limited by difficulties encountered either in the growth of parasites in vivo or in the identification of tachyzoites by histochemical methods. Serologic testing has become the routine method of diagnosis. A wide range of serologic tests that can be used to measure antibody to *T. gondii* are available commercially. The reader is referred to the excellent review of the various tests by Remington and McLeod.

Diagnosis of acute infection with *T. gondii* can be established by detection of the simultaneous presence of IgG and IgM antibody to *Toxoplasma* in serum. The presence of circulating IgA favors the diagnosis of an acute infection. The Sabin-Feldman dye test, the indirect fluorescent antibody test, and the enzyme-linked immunosorbent assay (ELISA) all satisfactorily measure circulating IgG antibody to *Toxoplasma*. Positive IgG titers (>1:10) can be detected as early as 2 to 3 weeks after infection. These titers usually peak at 6 to 8 weeks and decline slowly to a new baseline level that persists for life. It is necessary to measure the serum IgM titer in concert with the IgG titer to better establish the time of infection. The methods currently available for this determination are the double-sandwich IgM-ELISA and the IgM-immunosorbent assay (IgM-ISAGA). Both of these assays are specific and sensitive, and their use precludes the false-positive results associated with rheumatoid factor and antinuclear antibody. The double-sandwich IgA-ELISA is more sensitive than the IgM-ELISA for detecting congenital infection in the fetus and newborn.

The Immunocompetent Adult or Child   For the patient who presents with lymphadenopathy only, a positive IgM titer is an indication of acute infection—and an indication for therapy, if that is clinically warranted (see "Treatment" below). The serum IgM titer should be determined again in 3 weeks. An elevation in the IgG titer without an increase in the IgM titer suggests that infection is present but that it is not acute. If there is a borderline increase in either IgG or IgM, the titers should be assessed again in 3 to 4 weeks.

Ocular Toxoplasmosis   Because of the congenital nature of ocular toxoplasmosis, the serum antibody titer may not correlate with the presence of active lesions in the fundus. In general, a positive IgG titer (measured in undiluted serum if necessary) in conjunction with typical lesions establishes the diagnosis. If lesions are atypical and the titer is in the low-positive range, the diagnosis is presumptive.

The Immunocompromised Host   As discussed above, in patients with AIDS, the presence of IgG and radiologic findings consistent with toxoplasmosis are grounds for a presumptive diagnosis. Attempts to evaluate rising IgG titers or to determine whether IgM is present are not productive. Serologic evidence of infection virtually always precedes the development of *Toxoplasma* encephalitis. It is therefore important to determine the *Toxoplasma* antibody status of all patients infected with human immunodeficiency virus (HIV). Antibody titers may range from negative to 1:1024 in patients with AIDS and *Toxoplasma* encephalitis. Fewer than 3 percent of patients have no demonstrable antibody to *Toxoplasma* at the time of diagnosis. Determination of the intrathecal antibody titer may be useful in identifying prior infection. PCR amplification of genetic material of the parasite found in the CSF may prove diagnostically beneficial in the future.

Patients with toxoplasmic encephalitis have focal or multifocal abnormalities demonstrable by CT or MRI. These findings are not pathognomonic of *Toxoplasma* infection since 40 percent of CNS lymphomas are multifocal and 50 percent are ring-enhancing. Lesions on CT scan are multiple and are located in both hemispheres, with the basal ganglia and corticomedullary junction most commonly involved. A CT scan may underestimate the degree of inflammation during early disease. Double-dose contrast enhancement may increase the sensitivity of diagnosis. For both MRI and CT scans, the rate of false-negative results is approximately 10 percent. The finding of a single lesion on an MRI scan increases the suspicion of primary lymphoma and strengthens the argument for the performance of a brain biopsy. MRI should be performed if the CT scan shows only a single lesion. CT and MRI scans are important for assessment of the response to therapy. As in other conditions, the radiologic response may lag behind the clinical response. Resolution of lesions may take from 3 weeks to 6 months. Some patients show clinical improvement despite worsening radiographic findings.

A presumptive diagnosis of *Toxoplasma* encephalitis should prompt the immediate initiation of therapy. Patients should be monitored for neurologic deterioration during the first 7 days of treatment. After this time, therapy should result in stabilization or improvement in clinical status. After 3 weeks, repeat radiologic studies should detect improvement. If glucocorticoids have been administered, radiologic studies should be repeated at the time of discontinuation to determine whether an exacerbation of disease has occurred. If the patient's clinical condition becomes worse, performance of a biopsy must be strongly considered.

Diagnosis of Congenital Infection The issue of concern when a pregnant woman has evidence of recent *T. gondii* infection is obviously whether the fetus is infected. PCR of the amniotic fluid to detect the B1 gene of the parasite has replaced fetal blood sampling. However, the definitive test for congenital infection is the direct inoculation of placental tissue or of newborn blood or CSF into susceptible mice. Serologic diagnosis is based on the persistence of IgG antibody or a positive IgM titer after the first week of life (a time frame that excludes placental leak). The IgG determination should be repeated every 2 months. An increase in IgM beyond the first week of life is indicative of acute infection. However, up to 25 percent of infected newborns may be seronegative and have normal routine physical examinations. Thus assessment of the eye and the brain, with ophthalmologic testing, CSF evaluation, and radiologic studies, is important in establishing the diagnosis.

℞ TREATMENT

Immunologically competent adults and older children who have only lymphadenopathy do not require specific therapy unless they have persistent and severe symptoms. Patients with ocular toxoplasmosis should be treated for 1 month with pyrimethamine plus either sulfadiazine or clindamycin. A large percentage of patients with chorioretinitis improve clinically with treatment.

Patients with AIDS should be treated for acute toxoplasmosis. Current therapeutic protocols are directed at folate metabolism, protein synthesis, or nucleic acid synthesis of the parasite. Pyrimethamine and trimethoprim inhibit the enzyme dihydrofolate reductase. Inhibitors of protein synthesis, including clindamycin, chlortetracycline, and azithromycin, affect growth of the parasite. Inhibitors of purine synthesis, such as arprinocid, may prove to be important. Atovaquone, which blocks pyrimidine salvage, has demonstrated activity against both *T. gondii* and *P. carinii*.

In the immunocompromised patient, toxoplasmosis is rapidly fatal if untreated. The mainstay of treatment for *Toxoplasma* encephalitis is a combination regimen. Pyrimethamine and sulfadiazine administered together block folic acid metabolism and successfully reduce the parasite burden. Leucovorin (calcium folinate) is given as an adjunct to prevent the bone marrow toxicity associated with pyrimethamine. Both pyrimethamine and sulfadiazine cross the blood-brain barrier. A prominent consequence of dual therapy is the high incidence of associated toxicity (40 percent). Rash may develop during the first 3 weeks in up to 20 percent of patients but does not preclude the use of this combination. Other complications include hematologic effects, crystalluria, hematuria, radiolucent renal stones, and nephrotoxicity. During therapy, serum levels of these drugs may be erratic, but such fluctuations have not been correlated with these complications.

The current regimen consists of pyrimethamine (a 200-mg loading dose followed by 50 to 75 mg/d) plus sulfadiazine (4 to 6 g/d in four divided doses). In addition, the administration of leucovorin (10 to 15 mg/d for 6 weeks) is required. These agents are active only against the tachyzoite stage of the parasite. Thus, after patients complete the initial course (lasting 4 to 6 weeks or until radiologic improvement is documented), they must receive lifelong suppressive therapy with pyramethamine (25 to 50 mg/d) and sulfadiazine (2 to 4 g/d). If sulfadiazine cannot be tolerated, a combination of pyrimethamine (75 mg/d) plus clindamycin (450 mg tid) can be used. It is possible that pyrimethamine (50 to 75 mg/d) is sufficient for chronic suppressive therapy. Congenitally infected neonates are treated with daily oral pyrimethamine (0.5 to 1 mg/kg) and sulfadiazine (100 mg/kg) for 1 year. In addition, therapy with spiramycin (100 mg/kg per day) plus prednisone (1 mg/kg per day) has been shown to be efficacious for congenital infection.

Alternative therapies have been established because of the toxicity associated with the long-term antimicrobial therapy necessary for many individuals infected with *T. gondii*. Dapsone (diaminodiphenyl sulfone), with its longer serum half-life and decreased toxicity, is an effective alternative to sulfadiazine. Spiramycin, which has been used in Europe to treat pregnant women, reduces transplacental transmission. However, spiramycin has been ineffective as primary prophylaxis in patients with AIDS. Clindamycin is well absorbed from the gastrointestinal tract, and serum levels peak 1 to 2 h after administration. The combination of oral pyrimethamine (25 to 75 mg/d) plus intravenous clindamycin (1200 to 4800 mg/d) is effective for patients with AIDS who have *Toxoplasma* encephalitis. Toxic effects of clindamycin include nausea, vomiting, neutropenia, rash, and pseudomembranous colitis. Other macrolides that have been evaluated include roxithromycin, clarithromycin, and azithromycin. A combination of pyrimethamine and clarithromycin appears to be effective. Evidence suggests that the macrolides are not beneficial by themselves. Atovaquone (750 mg tid or qid) is an optional agent for the treatment of individuals who are intolerant of other agents. Glucocorticoids can be used to treat intracerebral edema, but their benefit has not yet been established. It is difficult to assess the benefit of glucocorticoids when they are administered in conjunction with anti-*Toxoplasma* medication. Anticonvulsants are sometimes necessary for the treatment of seizures, but attention should be given to the potential interaction between sulfadiazine and phenytoin. A regimen of trimethoprim-sulfamethoxazole or dapsone plus pyrimethamine with leucovorin may prevent the development of *Toxoplasma* encephalitis in individuals infected with HIV who are seropositive for *T. gondii* after their CD4+ T lymphocyte count falls to 100/μL.

PREVENTION The chances of primary infection with *Toxoplasma* can be reduced by not eating undercooked meat and by avoiding oocyst-contaminated material (i.e., a cat's litter box). Meat should be heated to 60°C or frozen to kill cysts. Hands should be washed thoroughly after work in the garden, and all fruits and vegetables should be washed. Blood intended for transfusion into *Toxoplasma*-seronegative immunocompromised individuals should be screened for antibody to *T. gondii*. Although such serologic screening is not routinely performed, seronegative women should be screened for evidence of infection several times during pregnancy if they are exposed to environmental conditions that put them at risk for infection with *T. gondii*. HIV-positive individuals should closely adhere to these preventive measures.

BIBLIOGRAPHY

Channon JY, Kasper LH: *Toxoplasma gondii*–induced immune suppression by human peripheral blood monocytes: Role of gamma interferon. Infect Immun 64:1181, 1996

Fadul CE et al: Survival of immunoglobulin G–opsonized *Toxoplasma gondii* in nonadherent human monocytes. Infect Immun 63:4290, 1995

Kasper LH, Boothroyd JC: *T. gondii* and toxoplasmosis, in *Immunology and Molecular Biology of Parasitic Infections*, 3d ed, KS Warren, N Agabian (eds). Oxford, Blackwell Scientific, 1993

Luft BJ, Remington JS: Toxoplasmic encephalitis in AIDS. Clin Infect Dis 15:211, 1992

McAuley J et al: Early and longitudinal evaluations of treated infants and children with congenital toxoplasmosis. Clin Infect Dis 18:38, 1994

Podzamczer D et al: Intermittent trimethoprim-sulfamethoxazole compared with dapsone-pyrimethamine for the simultaneous primary prophylaxis of *Pneumocystis* pneumonia and toxoplasmosis in patients infected with HIV. Ann Intern Med 122:755, 1995

Prophylaxis for *Toxoplasma* encephalitis. Infect Dis Alert 11:164, 1992

Remington JS et al: Toxoplasmosis, in *Infectious Diseases of the Fetus and Newborn Infant*, 4th ed, JS Remington, JO Klein (eds). Philadelphia, Saunders, 1994

———, McLeod R: Toxoplasmosis, in *Infectious Diseases in Medicine and Surgery*, J Bartlett et al (eds). Philadelphia, Saunders, 1992

Richards FO Jr et al: Preventing toxoplasmic encephalitis in persons infected with human immunodeficiency virus. Clin Infect Dis 19:S49, 1995

Wong S-Y et al: AIDS-associated toxoplasmosis, in *The Medical Management of AIDS*, 4th ed, MA Sande, PA Volberding (eds). Philadelphia, Saunders, 1994

220

Theodore E. Nash, Peter F. Weller

PROTOZOAL INTESTINAL INFECTIONS AND TRICHOMONIASIS

PROTOZOAL INFECTIONS

GIARDIASIS *Giardia lamblia* is a cosmopolitan protozoal parasite that inhabits the small intestines of humans and other mammals. Giardiasis is one of the most common parasitic diseases worldwide and causes both endemic and epidemic intestinal disease and diarrhea.

Life Cycle and Epidemiology Infection follows the ingestion of the environmentally hardy cysts, which excyst in the small intestine, releasing trophozoites that multiply by binary fission, occasionally to enormous numbers. *Giardia* remains a pathogen of the proximal small bowel and does not disseminate hematogenously. Trophozoites remain free in the lumen or attach to the mucosal epithelium by means of a ventral sucking disk. As a trophozoite encounters altered conditions, it forms a morphologically distinct cyst, which is the stage of the parasite usually found in the feces. Trophozoites may be present and even predominate in loose or watery stools, but it is the resistant cyst that survives outside the body and is responsible for transmission. Cysts do not tolerate heating, desiccation, or continued exposure to feces but do remain viable for months in cold fresh water. The number of cysts excreted varies widely but can approach 10^7 per gram of stool.

Giardia infections are common in both developed and developing countries. Ingestion of as few as 10 cysts is sufficient to cause infection in humans. Because cysts are infectious when excreted or shortly thereafter, person-to-person transmission occurs where fecal hygiene is poor. Giardiasis, as a symptomatic or an asymptomatic infection, is especially prevalent in day-care centers; person-to-person spread also takes place in other institutional settings with poor fecal hygiene and during homosexual contact. If food is contaminated with *Giardia* cysts after cooking or preparation, food-borne transmission can occur. Waterborne transmission accounts for episodic infections (e.g., in campers and other travelers) and for massive epidemics in metropolitan areas. Surface water, ranging from mountain streams to large municipal reservoirs, can become contaminated with fecally derived *Giardia* cysts; outmoded water systems are subject to cross-contamination from leaking sewer lines. The efficacy of water as a means of transmission is enhanced by the small infectious inoculum of *Giardia*, the prolonged survival of cysts in cold water, and the resistance of cysts to killing by routine chlorination methods that are adequate for controlling bacteria. Viable cysts can be eradicated from water by either boiling or filtration. In the United States, *Giardia* is the agent most commonly identified in waterborne epidemics of gastroenteritis, and cross-sectional studies

in selected populations show prevalences from a few tenths of a percent to 50 percent or higher. In developing countries, *Giardia* infections can be extremely common, with cumulative rates close to 100 percent by 2 years of age and prevalences of 20 to 30 percent or higher among adults.

The importance of animal reservoirs as sources of infection for humans is unclear. *Giardia* parasites morphologically similar to those in humans are found in a large number of mammals, including beavers from reservoirs implicated in epidemics, dogs, cats, and ruminants. Although the high degree of isolate heterogeneity noted in humans is consistent with infections originating from different animal sources, animals have not been directly established as sources of human infection.

Giardiasis, like cryptosporidiosis, creates a significant economic burden because of the costs incurred in the installation of water filtration systems required to prevent waterborne epidemics, in the management of epidemics that involve large communities, and in the evaluation and treatment of endemic infections. In the United States, giardiasis results in about the same number of hospitalizations as shigellosis.

Pathophysiology The reasons why some, but not all, infected patients develop clinical manifestations and the mechanisms by which *Giardia* causes alterations in small-bowel function are largely unknown. While trophozoites adhere to the epithelium, they do not cause invasive or locally destructive alterations. The development of lactose intolerance and significant malabsorption in a minority of infected adults and children are clinical signs of the loss of brush border enzyme activities. In most infections the morphology of the bowel is unaltered, but in a few—usually in chronically infected, symptomatic patients—the histopathologic findings (including flattened villi) and the clinical manifestations resemble those of tropical sprue and gluten-sensitive enteropathy. The pathogenesis of diarrhea in giardiasis is not known.

The natural history of *Giardia* infection is not well defined and varies markedly. Infections may be aborted, transient, recurrent, or chronic. Parasite as well as host factors may be important in determining the course of infection and disease. Both cellular and humoral responses develop in human infections, but their precise roles in the control of infection and/or disease are unknown. Because patients with hypogammaglobulinemia commonly suffer from prolonged, severe infections that are poorly responsive to treatment, humoral immune responses appear to be important. The greater susceptibility of the young than of the old and of newly exposed persons than of chronically exposed populations also suggests that at least partial protective immunity may develop. Although no strains of the parasite that are clearly nonpathogenic have been identified, *Giardia* isolates vary biochemically and biologically. The marked biochemical differences among some isolates may help account for the different courses of infection noted in experimentally infected humans and animals. The surface of trophozoites is covered by a family of related cysteine-rich proteins that undergo surface antigenic variation and may contribute to prolonged and/or repeated infections.

Clinical Manifestations Disease manifestations of giardiasis range from asymptomatic carriage to fulminant diarrhea and malabsorption. Most infected persons are asymptomatic, but in epidemics the proportion of symptomatic cases may be higher. Symptoms may develop suddenly or gradually. In persons with acute giardiasis, symptoms develop after an incubation period that lasts at least 5 to 6 days and usually 1 to 3 weeks. Prominent early symptoms include diarrhea, abdominal pain, bloating, belching, flatus, nausea, and vomiting. Although diarrhea is common, upper intestinal manifestations such as nausea, vomiting, bloating, and abdominal pain may predominate. The duration of acute giardiasis is usually in excess of 1 week, although diarrhea often subsides. Individuals with chronic giardiasis may present with or without having experienced an antecedent acute symptomatic episode. Diarrhea is not necessarily prominent, but increased flatus, loose stools, sulfurous burping, and (in some instances) weight loss occur. Symptoms may be continual or episodic and can persist for years. Some persons who have relatively mild symptoms for long periods recognize the extent of their discomfort only in retrospect.

Fever, the presence of blood and/or mucus in the stools, and other signs and symptoms of colitis are uncommon and suggest a different diagnosis or a concomitant illness. Symptoms tend to be intermittent yet recurring and gradually debilitating, in contrast with the acute disabling symptoms associated with many enteric bacterial infections. Because of the less severe illness and the propensity for chronic infections, patients may seek medical advice late in the course of the illness; however, disease can be severe, resulting in malabsorption, weight loss, growth retardation, dehydration, and (in rare cases) death. A number of extraintestinal manifestations have been described, such as urticaria, anterior uveitis, and arthritis; whether these are caused by giardiasis or concomitant processes is unclear.

Giardiasis can be life-threatening in patients with hypogamma-globulinemia and is typically difficult to treat and eradicate. *Giardia* infections can complicate other preexisting intestinal diseases, such as cystic fibrosis. Although *Giardia* can cause enteric illness in patients with AIDS, neither the course of infection nor the response to treatment differs for patients with and without AIDS.

Diagnosis   Giardiasis is diagnosed by the identification of cysts in the feces or of trophozoites in the feces or small intestines. Cysts are oval, measure 8 to 12 μm $\times$ 7 to 10 μm, and characteristically contain four nuclei. Trophozoites are pear-shaped, dorsally convex, flattened parasites with two nuclei and four pairs of flagella. The diagnosis is sometimes difficult to establish. Direct examination of fresh or properly preserved stools as well as concentration methods should be used. Because cyst excretion is variable and may be undetectable at times, repeated examination of stool, sampling of duodenal fluid, and biopsy of the small intestine may be required to detect the parasite. Tests for parasitic antigen in stool, now commercially available, are as sensitive and specific as good microscopic examinations and easier to perform. All of these methods occasionally yield false-negative results.

 TREATMENT
Cure rates with metronidazole (250 mg tid for 5 days) are usually higher than 80 percent; those with furazolidone (100 mg qid for 7 to 10 days) are somewhat lower. The latter agent is frequently used to treat children because it is available as a palatable elixir that is not bitter. Quinacrine, the first effective drug for the treatment of giardiasis, is no longer available.

Patients in whom initial treatment fails can be re-treated with a longer course. Almost all patients respond to therapy and are cured, although some with chronic giardiasis experience delayed resolution of symptoms after eradication of *Giardia*. Those who remain infected after repeated treatments should be evaluated for reinfection through family members, close personal contacts, and environmental sources as well as for hypogammaglobulinemia. In cases refractory to multiple treatment courses, prolonged therapy with metronidazole (750 mg tid for 21 days) has been successful. Tinidazole, not available in the United States, is considered more effective than metronidazole or quinacrine. When children attending day-care centers infect an entire family, treatment of all infected family members, including asymptomatic carriers, may be required to prevent reinfection. Paromomycin, an oral aminoglycoside that is not well absorbed, can be given to symptomatic pregnant women, although the experience accumulated thus far is not a sufficient basis on which to judge how often this agent either eradicates infection or ameliorates symptoms.

Prevention   Although *Giardia* is extremely infectious, disease can be prevented by the exclusive consumption of noncontaminated food and water. Cooking food adequately and boiling or filtering potentially contaminated water prevent infection.

CRYPTOSPORIDIOSIS   The coccidian parasite *Cryptosporidium* is now known to cause diarrheal disease in immunocompetent human hosts and to be especially common among persons with AIDS or other forms of immunodeficiency.

Life Cycle and Epidemiology   Cryptosporidiosis is acquired by the consumption of oocysts, which excyst to liberate sporozoites that in turn enter and infect intestinal epithelial cells. The parasite's further

development involves both asexual and sexual cycles, which produce forms capable of infecting other epithelial cells and of generating oocysts that are passed in the feces. *Cryptosporidium* spp. infect a number of animals and can spread from infected animals to humans. Since oocysts are infectious when passed in feces, person-to-person transmission takes place in day-care centers and among household contacts and medical providers. As with giardiasis, waterborne transmission accounts for infections in travelers and for common-source epidemics. Oocysts are quite hardy and resist killing by routine chlorination.

Pathophysiology   Although intestinal epithelial cells harbor the parasite in an intracellular vacuole, the means by which secretory diarrhea is elicited remain uncertain. No characteristic pathologic changes are found by biopsy. The distribution of infection can be spotty within the principal site of infection, the small bowel. In some cases, cryptosporidia are found in the pharynx, stomach, and large bowel; they have been recovered from the respiratory tract, although the pathogenicity of the infection for human respiratory epithelium has not been determined. Involvement of the biliary tract can cause papillary stenosis, sclerosing cholangitis, or cholecystitis.

Clinical Manifestations   Asymptomatic infections can occur in both immunocompetent and immunocompromised hosts. In immunocompetent persons, symptoms develop after an incubation period of about a week and consist principally of watery nonbloody diarrhea, at times in conjunction with abdominal pain, nausea, anorexia, fever, and/or weight loss. In these hosts, the illness usually subsides after 1 to 2 weeks, whereas in immunocompromised hosts, especially those with AIDS, diarrhea can be chronic, persistent, and remarkably profuse, causing clinically significant fluid and electrolyte depletion. Stool volumes may range from 1 to 25 L/d. Weight loss, wasting, and abdominal pain may be severe. Biliary tract involvement can manifest as midepigastric or right upper quadrant pain.

Diagnosis   Evaluation usually starts with fecal examination for small oocysts, which are 4 to 5 μm in diameter and are smaller than the fecal stages of most other parasites. Detection is enhanced by evaluation of stools (obtained on multiple days) by several techniques, including modified acid-fast and direct immunofluorescent stains and enzyme immunoassays. If low numbers of oocysts are being excreted, Sheather's coverslip flotation method concentrates them for examination. Cryptosporidia also can be identified by light and electron microscopy at the apical surfaces of intestinal epithelium from biopsy specimens of the small bowel and, less frequently, the large bowel.

 TREATMENT
To date, no chemotherapeutic agents effective against *Cryptosporidium* have been identified, although paromomycin (500 to 750 mg qid) may be partially effective for some patients infected with human immunodeficiency virus (HIV). Treatment includes supportive care with replacement of fluids and electrolytes and administration of antidiarrheal agents. Biliary tract obstruction may require papillotomy or T-tube placement. Prevention requires minimizing exposure to infectious oocysts in human or animal feces.

ISOSPORIASIS   The coccidian parasite *Isospora belli* causes human intestinal disease. Infection is acquired by the consumption of oocysts, after which the parasite invades intestinal epithelial cells and undergoes both sexual and asexual cycles of development. Oocysts excreted in stool are not immediately infectious but must undergo further maturation. Although *I. belli* infects many animals, little is known about the epidemiology or prevalence of this parasite in humans. It appears to be more common in tropical and subtropical countries. Acute infections can begin abruptly with fever, abdominal pain, and watery nonbloody diarrhea and may last for weeks or months. In patients who have AIDS or are immunocompromised for other reasons, infections often are not self-limited but rather resemble cryptosporidiosis, with chronic, profuse watery diarrhea. Eosinophilia, which is not found in other enteric protozoan infections, may be detectable. The diagnosis is usually made by detection of the large (~25-μm) oocysts in stool by modified acid-fast staining. Oocyst excretion may be low-level and intermittent; if repeated stool examinations are unrevealing, sampling of duodenal contents by aspiration or a string test (Enterotest) or small-bowel biopsy (often with electron-microscopic examination) may be necessary.

In contrast to cryptosporidiosis, isosporiasis responds to chemotherapy. Trimethoprim-sulfamethoxazole (160/800 mg qid for 10 days and then bid for 3 weeks) has been effective; for patients intolerant of sulfonamides, pyrimethamine (50 to 75 mg/day) can be used. Relapses can occur in persons with AIDS and necessitate maintenance therapy with trimethoprim-sulfamethoxazole (160/800 mg three times a week) or combined sulfadoxine (500 mg) and pyrimethamine (25 mg) once weekly.

CYCLOSPORIASIS Coccidian parasites of the genus *Cyclospora* have been identified as the causative organisms in diarrheal illness formerly ascribed to blue-green algal or *Cyanobacteria*-like forms. This parasite is globally distributed: illness due to *Cyclospora cayetanensis* has been reported in the United States, Asia, Africa, Latin America, and Europe. The epidemiology of this parasite has not yet been fully defined, but waterborne transmission has been recognized as one means of its acquisition. The incubation period may be as brief as a day or two. The full spectrum of illness attributable to *Cyclospora* has not been delineated. Some patients may harbor the infection without symptoms, but many with cyclosporiasis have diarrhea, flulike symptoms, and flatulence and burping. The illness can be self-limited, can wax and wane, or (in many cases) can involve prolonged diarrhea, anorexia, and upper gastrointestinal symptoms, with sustained fatigue and weight loss in some instances. Diarrheal illness may persist for longer than a month. *Cyclospora* can cause enteric illness in patients infected with HIV, albeit at an unknown frequency.

The parasite is detectable in epithelial cells of small-bowel biopsy samples and elicits secretory diarrhea by an unknown means. The absence of fecal blood and leukocytes indicates that disease due to *Cyclospora* is not caused by destruction of the small-bowel mucosa. The diagnosis can be made by detection of spherical 8- to 10-μm oocysts in the stool. These refractile oocysts are variably acid-fast and are fluorescent when viewed with ultraviolet light microscopy. Cyclosporiasis should be considered in the differential diagnosis of prolonged diarrhea, with or without a history of travel by the patient to other countries.

Cyclosporiasis is effectively treated with trimethoprim-sulfamethoxazole (160/800 mg bid for 7 days). Patients infected with HIV, however, may experience relapses after such treatment and thus may require longer-term suppressive maintenance therapy.

MICROSPORIDIOSIS Microsporidia are obligate intracellular spore-forming protozoa that infect many animals and recently have been recognized as causing disease in humans, especially as opportunistic pathogens in AIDS. Microsporidia are members of a distinct phylum, Microspora, which contains dozens of genera and hundreds of species. The various microsporidia are differentiated by their developmental life cycles, by ultrastructural features, and (more recently) by molecular taxonomy based on ribosomal RNA. The organisms' complex life cycles result in the production of infectious spores. Currently, six genera of microsporidia—*Encephalitozoon, Pleistophora, Nosema, Vittaforma, Septata,* and *Enterocytozoon*—are recognized as causes of human disease; a seventh genus—*Microsporidium,* which includes organisms of uncertain taxonomic status—also causes disease in humans. Though some microsporidia are probably prevalent causes of self-limited or asymptomatic infections in immunocompetent patients, little is known of how microsporidiosis is acquired.

Microsporidiosis is most common among patients with AIDS, less common among patients with other types of immunocompromise, and rare among immunocompetent hosts. In patients with AIDS, intestinal infections with *Enterocytozoon bieneusi* and *Encephalitozoon* (formerly *Septata*) *intestinalis* are increasingly recognized to contribute to chronic diarrhea and wasting; these infections are found in 10 to 40 percent of patients with chronic diarrhea. Both organisms have been found in the biliary tracts of patients with cholecystitis. *E. intestinalis* may also disseminate to cause fever, diarrhea, sinusitis, cholangitis, and bronchiolitis. In patients with AIDS, *Encephalitozoon hellem* has caused superficial keratoconjunctivitis as well as sinusitis, respiratory tract disease, and disseminated infection. Myositis due to *Pleistophora* has been documented in two patients. *Nosema, Vittaforma,* and *Microsporidium* have caused stromal keratitis associated with trauma in immunocompetent patients.

Microsporidia are small gram-positive organisms with mature spores measuring 0.5 to 2 μm × 1 to 4 μm. Diagnosis of microsporidial infections in tissue often requires electron microscopy, although intracellular spores can be visualized by light microscopy with hematoxylin and eosin, Giemsa, or tissue Gram's stains. For the diagnosis of intestinal microsporidiosis, chromotrope 2R-based staining and Uvitex 2B or calcofluor fluorescent staining reveal spores in smears of feces or duodenal aspirates. Definitive therapies for microsporidial infections remain to be established. For superficial keratoconjunctivitis due to *E. hellem,* topical therapy with fumagillin suspension has shown promise (see Chap. 213). For enteric infections with *E. bieneusi* and *E. intestinalis* in HIV-infected patients, therapy with albendazole may be efficacious (see Chap. 213).

OTHER INTESTINAL PROTOZOA **Balantidiasis** *Balantidium coli* is a large ciliated protozoal parasite that can produce a spectrum of large-intestinal disease analogous to amebiasis. The parasite is widely distributed in the world. Since it infects pigs, cases in humans are more common where pigs are raised; in Muslim countries, rodents may be important carriers. Infective cysts can be transmitted from person to person and through water, but many cases are due to the ingestion of cysts derived from porcine feces in association with slaughtering, with use of pig feces for fertilizer, or with contamination of water supplies by pig feces.

Ingested cysts liberate trophozoites, which reside and replicate in the large bowel. Many patients remain asymptomatic, but some have persisting intermittent diarrhea, and a few develop more fulminant dysentery. In symptomatic individuals, the pathology in the bowel—both gross and microscopic—is similar to that seen in amebiasis, with varying degrees of mucosal invasion, focal necrosis, and ulceration. Balantidiasis, unlike amebiasis, does not spread hematogenously to other organs. The diagnosis is usually made by detection of the trophozoite stage in stool or sampled colonic tissue. Tetracycline (500 mg qid for 10 days) is an effective therapeutic agent.

***Blastocystis hominis* Infection** *Blastocystis hominis,* long considered a nonpathogenic yeast, is believed by some to be a protozoan capable of causing intestinal disease, although its taxonomy and inherent pathogenicity remain uncertain. Some patients who pass *B. hominis* in their stools are asymptomatic, whereas others have diarrhea and associated intestinal symptoms. Diligent evaluation reveals other potential bacterial, viral, or protozoal causes of diarrhea in some but not all patients with symptoms. Because the pathogenicity of *B. hominis* is uncertain and because therapy for *Blastocystis* infection is neither specific nor uniformly effective, patients with prominent intestinal symptoms should be fully evaluated for other infectious causes of diarrhea. If diarrheal symptoms associated with *Blastocystis* are prominent, either metronidazole (750 mg tid for 10 days) or iodoquinol (650 mg tid for 20 days) can be used.

***Dientamoeba fragilis* Infection** *Dientamoeba fragilis* is unique among intestinal protozoa in that it has a trophozoite stage but not a cyst stage. How trophozoites survive to transmit infection is not known, but the unusually high prevalence of *D. fragilis* infection among persons with pinworm infection raises the possibility that eggs or larvae of *Enterobius* facilitate the transmission of *D. fragilis.* When symptoms develop in *D. fragilis* infection, they are generally mild and include intermittent diarrhea, abdominal pain, and anorexia. The diagnosis is made by the detection of trophozoites in stool, but the lability of these forms accounts for the greater yield when fecal samples are preserved immediately after collection. Since fecal excretion rates vary, examination of several samples obtained on alternate days increases the rate of detection. Iodoquinol (650 mg tid for 20 days), paromomycin (25 to 30 mg/kg per day in three doses for 7 days), or tetracycline (500 mg qid for 10 days) is appropriate for treatment.

Sarcosporidiosis   Various *Sarcocystis* spp. of coccidian parasites are widely distributed agents of infection in numerous animals. These parasites have an obligatory cycle of development involving two hosts. Sexual reproduction occurs in the intestine, with sporocysts passed in the feces; asexual multiplication leads to the development of muscle cysts. Humans can develop intestinal infections—albeit apparently infrequently—by ingesting muscle-stage cysts in undercooked pork or beef. While the full spectrum of the intestinal disease is not defined, a diarrheal illness can ensue, and sporocysts are found in the stool. Alternatively, ingestion of fecally derived sporocysts can lead to the development of cysts in striated or cardiac muscle. Some patients experience muscle pain and swelling, but the frequency and nature of symptoms elicited by muscle involvement are not clear, and these cysts, measuring 100 to 325 μm, also have been found incidentally in muscle specimens. Muscle-stage infections are not followed by further spread in humans. No specific therapy exists for either intestinal or muscle-stage *Sarcocystis* infections in humans.

TRICHOMONIASIS

Various species of trichomonads can be found in the mouth (in association with periodontitis) and occasionally in the gastrointestinal tract. *Trichomonas vaginalis*—one of the most prevalent protozoal parasites in the United States—is a pathogen of the genitourinary tract and a major cause of symptomatic vaginitis.

Life Cycle and Epidemiology   *T. vaginalis* is a pear-shaped, actively motile organism that measures about 10 by 7 μm, replicates by binary fission, and inhabits the lower genital tract of females and the urethra and prostate of males. In the United States, it accounts for about 3 million infections per year in women. While the organism can survive for a few hours in moist environments and could be acquired by direct contact, person-to-person venereal transmission accounts for virtually all cases of trichomoniasis. Its prevalence is greatest among persons with multiple sexual partners and among those with other sexually transmitted diseases.

Clinical Manifestations   Most men infected with *T. vaginalis* are asymptomatic, although some develop urethritis and a few have epididymitis or prostatitis. In contrast, infection in women, which has an incubation period of 5 to 28 days, is usually symptomatic and manifests with malodorous vaginal discharge (often yellow), vulvar erythema and itching, dysuria or urinary frequency (in 30 to 50 percent of cases), and dyspareunia. These manifestations, however, do not clearly distinguish trichomoniasis from other types of infectious vaginitis.

Diagnosis   Detection of motile trichomonads by microscopy of wet mounts of vaginal or prostatic secretions has been the conventional means of diagnosis. Although such microscopy provides an immediate diagnosis, its sensitivity for the detection of *T. vaginalis* is only about 50 to 60 percent in routine evaluations of vaginal secretions. Direct immunofluorescent antibody staining is more sensitive (70 to 90 percent) than wet-mount examinations. *T. vaginalis* can be recovered from the urethra of both males and females and is detectable in males after prostatic massage. Culture of the parasite is the most sensitive means of detection; however, the facilities for culture are not generally available, and detection of the organism takes 3 to 7 days.

℞ TREATMENT

Metronidazole is the mainstay of treatment and may be given either as a single 2-g dose or as 250 mg tid for 7 days. It is important that all sexual partners be treated concurrently to prevent reinfection, especially from asymptomatic males. Alternatives to metronidazole for treatment during pregnancy are not readily available, although use of 100-mg clotrimazole vaginal suppositories nightly for 2 weeks may cure some infections in pregnant women. Reinfection often accounts for apparent treatment failures, but strains of *T. vaginalis* exhibiting high-level resistance to metronidazole have been encountered. Treatment of these resistant infections with higher oral doses, parenteral doses, or concurrent oral and vaginal doses of metronidazole has been successful.

BIBLIOGRAPHY

GENERAL

KAPPUS KD et al: Intestinal parasitism in the United States: Update on a continuing problem. Am J Trop Med Hyg 50:705, 1994

MANNHEIMER SB, SOAVE R: Protozoal infections in patients with AIDS. Cryptosporidiosis, isosporiasis, cyclosporiasis, and microsporidiosis. Infect Dis Clin North Am 8:483, 1994

GIARDIASIS

LENGERICH EJ et al: Severe giardiasis in the United States. Clin Infect Dis 18:760, 1994

OVERTURF GD: Endemic giardiasis in the United States—role of the daycare center. Clin Infect Dis 18:764, 1994

THOMPSON RCA et al: *Giardia: From Molecules to Disease*. Wallingford, UK, CAB International, 1994

CRYPTOSPORIDIOSIS

DUPONT HL et al: The infectivity of *Cryptosporidium parvum* in healthy volunteers. N Engl J Med 332:855, 1995

GOODGAME RW et al: Intestinal function and injury in acquired immunodeficiency syndrome–related cryptosporidiosis. Gastroenterology 108:1075, 1995

WHITE AC JR et al: Paromomycin for cryptosporidiosis in AIDS: A prospective, double-blind trial. J Infect Dis 170:419, 1994

CYCLOSPORIASIS

CENTERS FOR DISEASE CONTROL AND PREVENTION: Outbreaks of *Cyclospora cayetanensis*—United States, 1996. Morb Mort Week Rep 45:549, 1996

HOGE CW et al: Placebo-controlled trial of co-trimoxazole for cyclospora infections among travellers and foreign residents in Nepal. Lancet 345:691, 1995

HUANG P et al: The first reported outbreak of diarrheal illness associated with *Cyclospora* in the United States. Ann Intern Med 123:409, 1995

PAPE JW et al: *Cyclospora* infection in adults infected with HIV. Clinical manifestations, treatment, and prophylaxis. Ann Intern Med 121:654, 1994

MICROSPORIDIOSIS

MOLINA JM et al: Disseminated microsporidiosis due to *Septata intestinalis* in patients with AIDS: Clinical features and response to albendazole therapy. J Infect Dis 171:245, 1995

WEBER R, BRYAN RT: Microsporidial infections in immunodeficient and immunocompetent patients. Clin Infect Dis 19:517, 1994

——— et al: Human microsporidial infections. Clin Microbiol Rev 7:426, 1994

WEISS LM: . . . And now microsporidiosis. Ann Intern Med 123:954, 1995

OTHER INTESTINAL PROTOZOA

PREISS U et al: On the clinical importance of *Dientamoeba fragilis* infections in childhood. J Hyg Epidemiol Microbiol Immunol 35:27, 1991

TRICHOMONIASIS

HEINE P, MCGREGOR JA: *Trichomonas vaginalis:* A reemerging pathogen. Clin Obstet Gynecol 36:137, 1993

KRIEGER JN: Trichomoniasis in men: Old issues and new data. Sex Transm Dis 22:83, 1995

221 *Leo X. Liu, Peter F. Weller*

TRICHINOSIS AND INFECTIONS WITH OTHER TISSUE NEMATODES

Nematodes are elongated, symmetric roundworms and constitute one of the largest phyla in the animal kingdom. Most nematode species are free-living, but some have evolved into parasites of plants and animals, including humans. Parasitic nematodes of medical significance may be broadly classified as intestinal or tissue nematodes, but such a classification system is imprecise. This chapter covers trichinosis, visceral and ocular larva migrans, cutaneous larva migrans, cerebral angiostrongyliasis, and gnathostomiasis. All are zoonotic infections caused by incidental exposure to infectious nematodes. The clinical symptoms of these infections are due largely to invasive larval stages that (except in the case of *Trichinella*) do not reach maturity in humans.

TRICHINOSIS   Trichinosis develops after the ingestion of meat containing cysts of *Trichinella*—for example, pork or meat from a carnivore. While most infections are mild and asymptomatic, heavy infections can cause severe enteritis, periorbital edema, myositis, and (infrequently) death.

Life Cycle and Epidemiology   Five species of *Trichinella* are now recognized as causes of infection in humans. Two species are distributed worldwide: *Trichinella spiralis*, which is found in a great variety of carnivorous and omnivorous animals, and *Trichinella pseudospiralis*, which is found in mammals and birds. *Trichinella nativa* is present in Arctic regions and infects bears; *Trichinella nelsoni* is found in equatorial Africa, where it is common among felid predators and scavengers such as hyenas and bush pigs; and *Trichinella bitovi* is found in temperate areas of Europe and western Asia among carnivores but not among domestic swine.

After the consumption of trichinous meat by the host, encysted larvae are liberated by digestive acid and pepsin. The larvae invade the small-bowel mucosa and mature rapidly into adult worms. After about 1 week, female worms release newborn larvae that migrate via the circulation to striated muscle. The larvae of all species except *T. pseudospiralis* then encyst by inducing a radical transformation in the muscle cell architecture. Although host immune responses may help to expel the adult worms, they have little effect on the muscle-dwelling larvae.

Human trichinosis is most often caused by the ingestion of infected pork products and thus can occur in almost any location where the meat of domestic or wild swine is eaten. Human trichinosis also may be acquired from the meat of other animals, including dogs (in parts of Asia and Africa), horses (in Italy and France), and bears and walruses (in northern regions). Although cattle (being herbivores) are not natural hosts of *Trichinella*, beef has been implicated in outbreaks when contaminated or adulterated with trichinous pork. Laws that prohibit the feeding of uncooked garbage to pigs have greatly reduced the transmission of trichinosis in the United States. About 50 to 100 cases of trichinosis are reported annually in this country, but most mild cases probably remain undiagnosed. Recent U.S. outbreaks have been attributable to undercooked ethnic pork dishes, homemade and commercial sausage, wild boar meat, and walrus meat.

Pathogenesis and Clinical Features   Clinical symptoms of trichinosis arise from the successive phases of parasite enteric invasion, larval migration, and muscle encystment. Most light infections (those with fewer than 10 larvae per gram of muscle) are asymptomatic, whereas heavy infections (which can involve more than 50 larvae per gram of muscle) can be life-threatening. Invasion of the gut by large numbers of parasites occasionally provokes diarrhea during the first week after infection. Abdominal pain, constipation, nausea, or vomiting also may be prominent. The prolonged and fulminant diarrhea noted with Arctic trichinosis probably reflects a response to repeated infection.

Symptoms due to larval migration and muscle invasion begin to appear in the second week after infection. The migrating *Trichinella* larvae provoke a marked local and systemic hypersensitivity reaction, with fever and hypereosinophilia. Periorbital and facial edema is common, as are hemorrhages in the subconjunctivae, retina, and nail beds ("splinter" hemorrhages). A maculopapular rash, headache, cough, dyspnea, or dysphagia sometimes develops. Myocarditis with tachyarrhythmias or heart failure—and, less commonly, encephalitis or pneumonitis—may develop and accounts for most deaths of patients with trichinosis.

Upon onset of larval encystment in muscle 2 to 3 weeks after infection, symptoms of myositis with myalgias, muscle edema, and weakness develop, usually overlapping with the inflammatory reactions to migrating larvae. The most commonly involved muscle groups include the extraocular muscles; the biceps; and the muscles of the jaw, neck, lower back, and diaphragm. Peaking about 3 weeks after infection, symptoms subside only gradually during a prolonged convalescence.

Laboratory Findings and Diagnosis   Blood eosinophilia develops in more than 90 percent of patients with symptomatic trichinosis and may peak at a level of greater than 50 percent between 2 and 4 weeks after infection. Serum levels of IgE and muscle enzymes, including creatine phosphokinase, lactate dehydrogenase, and aspartate aminotransferase, are elevated in most symptomatic patients. Patients should be questioned thoroughly about their consumption of pork or wild-animal meat and about illness in other individuals who ate the same meat. A presumptive clinical diagnosis can be based on fevers, eosinophilia, periorbital edema, and myalgias after a suspect meal. A rise in the titer of parasite-specific antibody (assayed by the bentonite flocculation test), which usually does not occur until after the third week of infection, confirms the diagnosis. Alternatively, a definitive diagnosis requires surgical biopsy of at least 1 g of involved muscle; the yields are highest near tendon insertions. The fresh muscle tissue should be compressed between glass slides and examined microscopically, because larvae may be overlooked by examination of routine histopathologic sections alone.

 TREATMENT

Current anthelmintic drugs are ineffective against *Trichinella* larvae in muscle. Fortunately, most lightly infected patients recover uneventfully with bed rest, antipyretics, and analgesics. Glucocorticoids like prednisone (1 mg/kg daily for 5 days) are beneficial for severe myositis and myocarditis. Mebendazole, like thiabendazole, appears to be active against enteric stages of the parasite, but its efficacy against encysted larvae has not been conclusively demonstrated.

Prevention   Larvae may be killed by cooking pork until it is no longer pink or by freezing it at −15°C for 3 weeks. However, Arctic *T. nativa* larvae in walrus or bear meat are relatively resistant and may remain viable despite freezing.

VISCERAL AND OCULAR LARVA MIGRANS   Visceral larva migrans is a syndrome caused by nematodes that are normally parasitic for nonhuman host species. In humans, the nematode larvae do not typically develop into adult worms but instead migrate through host tissues and elicit eosinophilic inflammation. The most common form of visceral larva migrans is toxocariasis due to larvae of the canine ascarid *Toxocara canis* or, less commonly, the feline ascarid *Toxocara cati*. Rare cases with eosinophilic meningoencephalitis have been caused by the raccoon ascarid *Baylisascaris procyonis*.

Life Cycle and Epidemiology   The canine roundworm *T. canis* is distributed among dogs worldwide. Ingestion of infective eggs by dogs is followed by liberation of *Toxocara* larvae, which penetrate the gut wall and migrate intravascularly into the canine liver, muscle, and other tissues, where most remain in a developmentally arrested state. During pregnancy, some larvae resume migration in bitches and infect puppies prenatally (via transplacental transmission) or after birth (via suckling). Thus, in lactating bitches and puppies, larvae return to the intestinal tract and develop into adult worms, which produce eggs that are released in the feces. Humans acquire toxocariasis mainly by eating soil contaminated by puppy feces containing infective *T. canis* eggs. Visceral larva migrans is most common among children who habitually eat dirt, but most toxocaral infections are subclinical. Reported rates of *Toxocara* seropositivity range from 2 percent in an unselected American population to greater than 20 percent among kindergarten children in the United States and England.

Pathogenesis and Clinical Features   Clinical disease most commonly afflicts preschool children. After humans ingest *Toxocara* eggs, the larvae hatch and penetrate the intestinal mucosa, from which they are carried by the circulation to a wide variety of organs and tissues. The larvae invade the liver, lungs, central nervous system, and other sites, releasing toxic products and provoking intense local eosinophilic granulomatous responses. The degree of clinical illness depends on larval number and tissue distribution, reinfection, and host immune responses. Most light infections are asymptomatic and may be manifest only by blood eosinophilia. Characteristic symptoms of visceral larva migrans include fever, malaise, anorexia and weight loss, cough, wheezing, and rashes. Hepatosplenomegaly is common. These features are often accompanied by extraordinary peripheral eosinophilia, which may approach 90 percent. Uncommonly, seizures or behavioral disorders develop. The rare deaths in this disease are due to severe neurologic, pneumonic, or myocardial involvement.

Diagnosis   In addition to prominent eosinophilia, leukocytosis and hypergammaglobulinemia are usually evident. Transient pulmonary infiltrates are apparent on chest x-rays of about half of patients with symptoms of pneumonitis. The clinical diagnosis can be confirmed by an enzyme-linked immunosorbent assay for toxocaral antibodies. Stool examination, while important in the evaluation of unexplained eosinophilia, is worthless for toxocariasis, since the larvae do not develop into egg-producing adults in humans.

The ocular form of the larva migrans syndrome occurs when *Toxocara* larvae invade the eye. An eosinophilic granulomatous mass, most commonly in the posterior pole of the retina, develops around the entrapped larva. The retinal lesion can mimic retinoblastoma in appearance, and mistaken diagnosis of the latter condition can lead to unnecessary enucleation. The spectrum of eye involvement also includes endophthalmitis, uveitis, and chorioretinitis. Unilateral visual disturbances, strabismus, and eye pain are the most common presenting symptoms. In contrast to visceral larva migrans, ocular toxocariasis usually develops in older children or young adults with no history of pica; these patients seldom have eosinophilia or visceral manifestations.

 TREATMENT
The vast majority of *Toxocara* infections are self-limited and resolve without specific therapy. In patients with severe myocardial, central nervous system, or pulmonary involvement, glucocorticoids may be employed to reduce inflammatory complications. Available anthelmintic drugs, including diethylcarbamazine, mebendazole, and albendazole, have not been shown conclusively to alter the course of larva migrans. Control measures include prohibiting dog excreta in public parks and playgrounds, deworming dogs, and preventing pica in children. Treatment of ocular disease is unsatisfactory, and the role of glucocorticoids or anthelmintic drugs in management is controversial.

CUTANEOUS LARVA MIGRANS   Cutaneous larva migrans ("creeping eruption") is a serpiginous skin eruption caused by burrowing larvae of animal hookworms, usually the dog and cat hookworm *Ancylostoma braziliense*. The larvae hatch from eggs passed in dog and cat feces and mature in the soil. Humans become infected after skin contact with soil in areas frequented by dogs and cats, such as areas underneath house porches or scrub vegetation. Cutaneous larva migrans is especially prevalent among children and in regions with warm humid climates, including the southeastern United States.

After larvae penetrate the skin, erythematous lesions form along the tortuous tracts of their migration through the dermal-epidermal junction; the larvae advance several centimeters in a day. The intensely pruritic lesions may occur anywhere on the body and can be numerous if the patient has lain on the ground. Vesicles and bullae may form later. The animal hookworm larvae do not mature in humans and, without treatment, will die out after several weeks, with resolution of skin lesions. The diagnosis is made readily on clinical grounds, and a skin biopsy only rarely yields diagnostic parasite material. Symptoms can be alleviated by thiabendazole administered orally (25 mg/kg bid) or topically (10% aqueous or petroleum jelly suspension) for 2 to 5 days, by ivermectin (150 to 200 μg/kg one time), or by albendazole (200 mg bid for 2 days).

***ANGIOSTRONGYLUS CANTONENSIS* INFECTION**   *Angiostrongylus cantonensis*, the rat lungworm, is the most common cause of human eosinophilic meningitis.

Life Cycle and Epidemiology   This infection occurs principally in Southeast Asia and the Pacific Basin. *A. cantonensis* larvae produced by adult worms in the rat lung migrate to the gastrointestinal tract and are expelled with the feces. They develop into infective larvae within land snails and slugs. Humans acquire the infection by ingesting raw infected mollusks; vegetables contaminated by mollusk slime; or crabs, freshwater shrimp, and certain marine fish that have themselves eaten infected mollusks. The larvae then migrate to the brain.

Pathogenesis and Clinical Features   The parasites eventually die in the central nervous system, but not before initiating pathologic consequences that, in heavy infections, can result in permanent neurologic sequelae or death. Migrating larvae cause proteolytic damage and marked local eosinophilic inflammation and hemorrhage, with subsequent necrosis and granuloma formation around dying worms. Clinical symptoms develop between 2 and 35 days after the ingestion of larvae. Patients usually present with an insidious or abrupt excruciating frontal, occipital, or bitemporal headache. Neck stiffness, nausea and vomiting, and paresthesias are also common. Fever, cranial and extraocular nerve palsies, seizures, paralysis, and lethargy are uncommon.

Laboratory Findings   Examination of the cerebrospinal fluid is mandatory in suspected cases and usually reveals an elevated opening pressure, a white blood cell count of 150 to 2000/μL, and an eosinophilic pleocytosis of >20 percent. The protein concentration is usually elevated and the glucose level normal. The motile larvae of *A. cantonensis* are only rarely seen in the cerebrospinal fluid. Peripheral-blood eosinophilia may be mild. The diagnosis is generally based on the clinical presentation of eosinophilic meningitis together with a compatible epidemiologic history.

 TREATMENT
Specific chemotherapy has not been shown to be of benefit in angiostrongyliasis; larvicidal agents may actually exacerbate inflammatory brain lesions. Management consists of supportive measures, including the administration of analgesics, sedatives, and—in severe cases—glucocorticoids. In most patients, cerebral angiostrongyliasis has a self-limited course, and recovery is complete. The infection may be prevented by adequately cooking snails, crabs, and prawns and inspecting vegetables for mollusk infestation. Other parasitic causes of eosinophilic meningitis in endemic areas may include gnathostomiasis, paragonimiasis, schistosomiasis, and neurocysticercosis.

GNATHOSTOMIASIS   Infection of human tissues with larvae of *Gnathostoma spinigerum* can cause eosinophilic meningoencephalitis, migratory cutaneous swellings, or invasive masses of the eye and visceral organs.

Life Cycle and Epidemiology Human gnathostomiasis is endemic in Southeast Asia and parts of China and Japan. In nature, the mature adult worms parasitize the gastrointestinal tract of dogs and cats. First-stage larvae hatch from eggs passed into water and are ingested by *Cyclops* species (water fleas). Infective third-stage larvae develop in the flesh of many animal species (including fish, frogs, eels, snakes, chickens, and ducks) that have eaten either infected *Cyclops* or another infected second intermediate host. Humans typically acquire the infection by eating raw or undercooked fish or poultry. The raw fish dishes of *somfak* in Thailand and *sashimi* in Japan account for most cases of human gnathostomiasis. Some cases in Thailand result from the local practice of applying frog or snake flesh as a poultice.

Pathogenesis and Clinical Features Clinical symptoms are due to the aberrant migration of a single larva into cutaneous, visceral, neural, or ocular tissues. After invasion, larval migration may cause local inflammation, with pain, cough, or hematuria accompanied by fever and eosinophilia. Painful, itchy, migratory swellings may develop in the skin, particularly in the distal extremities or periorbital area. Cutaneous swellings usually last about a week but often recur intermittently over many years. Larval invasion of the eye can provoke a sight-threatening inflammatory response. Finally, invasion of the central nervous system results in eosinophilic meningitis with myeloencephalitis, a serious complication due to ascending larval migration along a large nerve track. Patients characteristically present with agonizing radicular pain and paresthesias in the trunk or a limb, which are followed shortly by paraplegia. Cerebral involvement, with focal hemorrhages and tissue destruction, is often fatal.

Diagnosis and Treatment Cutaneous migratory swellings with marked peripheral eosinophilia, supported by an appropriate geographic and dietary history, generally constitute an adequate basis for a clinical diagnosis of gnathostomiasis. However, patients may present with ocular or cerebrospinal involvement without antecedent cutaneous swellings. In the latter case, eosinophilic pleocytosis will be demonstrable (usually along with hemorrhagic or xanthochromic cerebrospinal fluid), but worms will almost never be recovered from the cerebrospinal fluid. Surgical removal of the parasite from subcutaneous or ocular tissue, though rarely feasible, is both diagnostic and therapeutic. Albendazole (400 to 800 mg daily for 21 days) may be helpful. At present, cerebrospinal involvement is managed with supportive measures and generally with a course of glucocorticoids. Gnathostomiasis can be prevented by adequate cooking of fish and poultry in endemic areas.

BIBLIOGRAPHY

ANDREWS JR et al: *Trichinella pseudospiralis* in humans: Description of a case and its treatment. Trans R Soc Trop Med Hyg 88:200, 1994

DAVIES HD et al: Creeping eruption. A review of clinical presentation and management of 60 cases presenting to a tropical disease unit. Arch Dermatol 129:588, 1993

GILLESPIE SH et al: The spectrum of ocular toxocariasis. Eye 7:415, 1993

GLICKMAN LT, MAGNAVAL JF: Zoonotic roundworm infections. Infect Dis Clin North Am 7:717, 1993

HOTEZ PJ: Visceral and ocular larva migrans. Semin Neurol 13:175, 1993

JELINEK T et al: Cutaneous larva migrans in travelers: Synopsis of histories, symptoms, and treatment of 98 patients. Clin Infect Dis 19:1062, 1994

LANDRY SM et al: Trichinosis: Common source outbreak related to commercial pork. South Med J 85:428, 1992

LEWIS JM, MAIZELS RM (eds): *Toxocara and Toxocariasis: Clinical, Epidemiological, and Molecular Perspectives.* London, Institute of Biology, 1993

LIU LX, WELLER PF: Antiparasitic drugs. N Engl J Med 334:1178, 1996

MACLEAN JD et al: Epidemiologic and serologic definition of primary and secondary trichinosis in the Arctic. J Infect Dis 165:908, 1992

MAGNAVAL JF: Comparative efficacy of diethylcarbamazine and mebendazole for the treatment of human toxocariasis. Parasitology 110:529, 1995

MURRELL KD, BRUSCHI F: Clinical trichinellosis. Prog Clin Parasitol 4:117, 1994

WELLER PF, LIU LX: Eosinophilic meningitis. Semin Neurol 13:161, 1993

222 Leo X. Liu, Peter F. Weller

INTESTINAL NEMATODES

More than a billion people worldwide are infected with one or more species of intestinal nematodes. Table 222-1 summarizes biologic and clinical features of infections due to the major intestinal parasitic nematodes. These parasites are most common in regions with poor fecal sanitation, particularly in developing countries in the tropics and subtropics but also in the United States. Although nematode infections are not usually fatal, they contribute to malnutrition and diminished work capacity. Humans may on occasion be infected with nematode parasites that ordinarily infect animals; these zoonotic infections include trichostrongyliasis, anisakiasis, capillariasis, and abdominal angiostrongyliasis.

Intestinal nematodes are roundworms; they range in length from 1 mm to many centimeters when mature (see Table 222-1). Their life cycles are complex and highly varied; some species, including *Strongyloides stercoralis* and *Enterobius vermicularis*, can be transmitted directly from person to person, while others, such as *Ascaris lumbricoides*, *Necator americanus*, and *Ancylostoma duodenale*, require a soil phase for development. Because most helminthic parasites do not self-replicate, the acquisition of a heavy burden of adult worms requires repeated exposure to the parasite in its infectious stage, whether larva or egg. Hence, clinical disease, as opposed to asymptomatic infection, generally develops only with prolonged residence in an endemic area. Eosinophilia and elevated serum IgE levels are features of many helminthic infections and, when unexplained, should always prompt a search for occult helminthiasis. Significant protective immunity to intestinal nematodes appears not to develop in humans, although mechanisms of parasite immune evasion and host immune responses to these infections have not been elucidated in detail.

ASCARIASIS *A. lumbricoides* is the largest intestinal nematode parasite of humans, reaching up to 40 cm in length. An estimated 1 billion people are infected worldwide. Most infected individuals have low worm burdens and are asymptomatic. Clinical disease arises from pulmonary hypersensitivity and intestinal complications.

Life Cycle Adult worms live in the lumen of the small intestine. Mature female *Ascaris* worms are extraordinarily fecund, each producing up to 240,000 eggs a day, which pass with the feces. Ascarid eggs, which are remarkably resistant to environmental stresses, become infective after several weeks of maturation in the soil and can remain infective for years. After infective eggs are swallowed, larvae hatched in the intestine invade the mucosa, migrate via the circulation to the lungs, break into the alveoli, ascend the bronchial tree, and return via swallowing to the small intestine, where they develop into adult worms. Between 2 and 3 months elapse between initial infection and egg production. The adult worms live for approximately 1 to 2 years.

Epidemiology *Ascaris* is widely distributed in tropical and subtropical regions as well as in other humid areas, including the rural southeastern United States. Transmission typically occurs via fecally contaminated soil and is due either to a lack of sanitary facilities or to the use of human manure ("night soil") as fertilizer. With their propensity for hand-to-mouth fecal carriage, younger children in impoverished rural areas are most affected. Infection outside endemic areas, though uncommon, can occur via eggs borne on transported vegetables.

Clinical Features During the lung phase of larval migration, about 9 to 12 days after egg ingestion, patients may develop an irritating nonproductive cough and burning substernal discomfort that is aggravated by coughing or deep inspiration. Dyspnea and blood-tinged sputum are less common. Fever is usually reported, with temperatures sometimes exceeding 38.5°C. Eosinophilia develops during this symptomatic phase and subsides slowly over weeks. Chest x-rays may reveal evidence of eosinophilic pneumonitis (Loeffler's syndrome), with round or oval infiltrates a few millimeters to several centimeters in size. These infiltrates may be transient and intermittent, clearing after several weeks. Where there is seasonal transmission of the parasite, seasonal pneumonitis with eosinophilia may develop in previously infected and sensitized hosts.

In established infections, adult worms in the small intestine usually cause no symptoms. In heavy infections, particularly in children, a large bolus of entangled worms can cause pain and small-bowel obstruction, sometimes complicated by perforation, intussusception, or volvulus. Single worms may cause disease when they migrate into aberrant sites. A large worm can enter and occlude the biliary tree, causing biliary colic, cholecystitis, cholangitis, pancreatitis, and (rarely) intrahepatic abscesses. Migration of an adult worm up the esophagus can provoke coughing and oral expulsion of the worm. In highly endemic areas, intestinal and biliary ascariasis can rival acute appendicitis and gallstones as causes of surgical acute abdomen.

Laboratory Findings Most cases of ascariasis can be diagnosed by the microscopic detection of characteristic mamillated *Ascaris* eggs (65 by 45 μm) in fecal samples. Occasionally, patients present after passing an adult worm—identifiable by its large size and smooth cream-colored surface—in the stool or through the mouth or nose. During the early transpulmonary migratory phase, when eosinophilic pneumonitis occurs, larvae can be found in sputum or gastric aspirates before diagnostic eggs appear in the stool. The eosinophilia that is prominent during this early stage usually decreases to minimal levels in established infection. The large adult worms may be visualized, occasionally serendipitously, on contrast studies of the gastrointestinal tract. A plain abdominal film may reveal masses of worms in gas-filled loops of bowel in patients with intestinal obstruction. Pancreaticobiliary worms can be detected by ultrasound and endoscopic retrograde cholangiopancreatography; the latter method also has been used to extract biliary *Ascaris* worms.

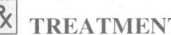 **TREATMENT**
Ascariasis should always be treated to prevent potentially serious complications. Mebendazole or albendazole (which is not yet approved by the Food and Drug Administration) is effective. These benzimidazoles are contraindicated in pregnancy and in heavy infections, in which they may provoke ectopic migration. Pyrantel pamoate and piperazine citrate are safe in pregnancy. Mild diarrhea and abdominal pain are uncommon side effects of these agents. Partial intestinal obstruction should be managed with nasogastric suction, intravenous fluid administration, and instillation of piperazine through the nasogastric tube, but complete obstruction and its severe complications require immediate surgical intervention.

HOOKWORM One-fourth of the world's population is infected with one of the two hookworm species (*A. duodenale* and *N. americanus*). Most infected individuals are asymptomatic. Hookworm disease develops from a combination of factors—a heavy worm burden, a prolonged duration of infection, and an inadequate iron intake—and results in iron-deficiency anemia and, on occasion, hypoproteinemia.

Life Cycle Adult hookworms, which are about 1 cm long, use buccal teeth (*Ancylostoma*) or cutting plates (*Necator*) to attach to the small-bowel mucosa and suck blood (0.2 mL/day per *Ancylostoma* adult) and interstitial fluid. The adult hookworms produce thousands of eggs daily. The eggs are deposited with feces in soil, where rhabditiform larvae hatch and develop over a 1-week period into infectious filariform larvae. Infective larvae penetrate the skin and reach the

Table 222-1

Major Human Intestinal Parasitic Nematodes

Feature	Parasitic Nematode				
	Ascaris lumbricoides (Roundworm)	*Necator americanus, Ancylostoma duodenale* (Hookworm)	*Strongyloides stercoralis*	*Trichuris trichiura* (Whipworm)	*Enterobius vermicularis* (Pinworm)
Global prevalence in humans (millions)	1000	900	50	500	300
Endemic areas	Worldwide	Hot, humid regions	Hot, humid regions	Worldwide	Worldwide
Infective stage	Egg	Filariform larva	Filariform larva	Egg	Egg
Route of infection	Oral	Percutaneous	Percutaneous or autoinfection	Oral	Oral
Gastrointestinal location of worms	Jejunal lumen	Jejunal mucosa	Small-bowel mucosa	Cecum, colonic mucosa	Cecum, appendix
Adult worm size	15–40 cm	7–12 mm	2 mm	30–50 mm	8–13 mm (female)
Pulmonary passage of larvae	Yes	Yes	Yes	No	No
Incubation period* (days)	60–75	40–100	17–28	70–90	35–45
Longevity	1 y	*N. americanus*: 2–5 y *A. duodenale*: 6–8 y	Decades (owing to autoinfection)	5 y	2 months
Fecundity (eggs/day/ worm)	240,000	*N. americanus*: 4000– 10,000 *A. duodenale*: 10,000– 25,000	5000–10,000	3000–7000	2000
Principal symptoms	Rarely gastrointestinal or biliary obstruction	Iron-deficiency anemia in heavy infection	Gastrointestinal symptoms; malabsorption or sepsis in hyperinfection	Gastrointestinal symptoms, anemia	Perianal pruritus
Diagnostic stage	Eggs in stool	Eggs in fresh stool, larvae in old stool	Larvae in stool or duodenal aspirate; sputum in hyperinfection	Eggs in stool	Eggs from perianal skin on cellulose acetate tape
Treatment	Mebendazole Albendazole† Pyrantel pamoate Piperazine citrate	Mebendazole Pyrantel pamoate Albendazole†	Thiabendazole Albendazole† Ivermectin†	Mebendazole Albendazole†	Mebendazole Pyrantel pamoate Albendazole†

* Time from infection to egg production by mature female worm.
† Not approved by the Food and Drug Administration.

lungs by way of the bloodstream. There they invade alveoli and ascend the airways before being swallowed and reaching the small intestine. The prepatent period from skin invasion to appearance of eggs in the feces is about 6 to 8 weeks, but it may be longer with *A. duodenale*. Larvae of *A. duodenale*, if swallowed, can survive and develop directly in the intestinal mucosa. Adult hookworms may survive over a decade but usually live about 6 to 8 years for *A. duodenale* and 2 to 5 years for *N. americanus*.

Epidemiology *A. duodenale* is prevalent in southern Europe, North Africa, and northern Asia, and *N. americanus* is the predominant species in the western hemisphere and equatorial Africa. The two species overlap in many tropical regions, particularly Southeast Asia. In most areas, older children have the greatest incidence and intensity of hookworm infection. In rural areas where fields are fertilized with night soil, older working adults also may be heavily affected.

Clinical Features Most hookworm infections are asymptomatic. Infective larvae may provoke pruritic maculopapular dermatitis ("ground itch") at the site of skin penetration as well as serpiginous tracts of subcutaneous migration (similar to cutaneous larva migrans) in previously sensitized hosts. Larvae migrating through the lungs occasionally cause mild transient pneumonitis, but this condition develops less frequently in hookworm infection than in ascariasis. In the early intestinal phase, infected persons may develop epigastric pain (often with postprandial accentuation), inflammatory diarrhea, or other abdominal symptoms accompanied by eosinophilia. The major consequence of chronic hookworm infection is iron deficiency. Symptoms are minimal if iron intake is adequate, but marginally nourished individuals develop symptoms of progressive iron-deficiency anemia and hypoproteinemia, including weakness, shortness of breath, and skin depigmentation. Intercurrent infections may precipitate frank cardiac failure. Changes in the intestinal mucosa are minimal, and malabsorption is uncommon.

Laboratory Findings The diagnosis is established by the finding of characteristic 40- by 60-μm oval hookworm eggs in the feces. Stool-concentration procedures may be required to detect light infections. Eggs of the two species are indistinguishable. In a stool sample that is not fresh, the eggs may have hatched to release rhabditiform larvae, which need to be differentiated from those of *S. stercoralis*. Hypochromic microcytic anemia, occasionally with eosinophilia or hypoalbuminemia, is characteristic of hookworm disease.

℞ **TREATMENT**

Hookworms can be eradicated with several safe and highly effective anthelmintic drugs, including mebendazole and pyrantel pamoate (see Chap. 214). Mild iron-deficiency anemia often can be treated with oral iron alone. Severe hookworm disease with protein loss and malabsorption necessitates nutritional support and oral iron replacement along with deworming.

Ancylostoma caninum This parasite, the canine hookworm, has been identified as a cause of human eosinophilic enteritis, especially in northeastern Australia. In this zoonotic infection, adult hookworms attach to the small intestine (where they may be visualized by endoscopy) and elicit abdominal pain and intense local eosinophilia. Treatment with mebendazole (100 mg twice daily for 3 days) is effective.

STRONGYLOIDIASIS *S. stercoralis* is distinguished by a capacity, unusual among helminths, to replicate in the human host. This capacity permits ongoing cycles of autoinfection due to internal production of infective larvae. Strongyloidiasis can thus persist for decades without further exposure of the host to exogenous infective larvae. In immunocompromised hosts, large numbers of invasive *Strongyloides* larvae can disseminate widely and can be fatal.

Life Cycle In addition to a parasitic cycle of development, *Strongyloides* can undergo a free-living cycle of development in the soil. This adaptability facilitates the parasite's survival in the absence of mammalian hosts. Rhabditiform larvae passed in feces can transform into infectious filariform larvae either directly or after a free-living phase of development. Humans acquire strongyloidiasis when filariform larvae in fecally contaminated soil penetrate the skin or mucous membranes. The larvae then travel through the bloodstream to the lungs, where they break into the alveolar spaces, ascend the bronchial tree, are swallowed, and thereby reach the small intestine. There the larvae mature into adult worms that penetrate the mucosa of the proximal small bowel. The minute (2-mm-long) parasitic adult female worms reproduce by parthenogenesis; parasitic adult males do not exist. Eggs hatch locally in the intestinal mucosa, releasing rhabditiform larvae that migrate to the lumen and pass with the feces into soil. Alternatively, rhabditiform larvae in the bowel can develop directly into filariform larvae that penetrate the colonic wall or perianal skin and enter the circulation to repeat the migration that establishes ongoing internal reinfection. This autoinfection cycle allows strongyloidiasis to persist for decades after the host has left an endemic area.

Epidemiology *S. stercoralis* is spottily distributed in tropical areas and other hot, humid regions and is particularly common in Southeast Asia, sub-Saharan Africa, and Brazil. In the United States, the parasite is endemic in parts of the South and is found in residents of mental institutions who practice poor hygiene and in immigrants and military veterans who have lived in endemic areas abroad.

Clinical Features In uncomplicated strongyloidiasis, many patients are asymptomatic or have mild cutaneous and/or abdominal symptoms. Recurrent urticaria, often involving the buttocks and wrists, is the most common cutaneous manifestation. Migrating larvae can elicit a pathognomonic serpiginous eruption, *larva currens* ("running larva")—a pruritic, raised, erythematous lesion that advances as rapidly as 10 cm/h along the course of larval migration. Adult parasites burrow into the duodenojejunal mucosa and can cause abdominal (usually midepigastric) pain, which resembles peptic ulcer pain except that it is aggravated by food ingestion. Nausea, diarrhea, gastrointestinal bleeding, mild chronic colitis, and weight loss can occur. Pulmonary symptoms are rare in uncomplicated strongyloidiasis. Eosinophilia is common, with levels fluctuating over time.

The ongoing autoinfection cycle of strongyloidiasis is normally contained by unknown factors of the host's immune system. Abrogation of host immunity after immunosuppressive therapy or with concomitant malignancy or malnutrition leads to hyperinfection, with the generation of large numbers of filariform larvae. Colitis, enteritis, or malabsorption may develop. In disseminated strongyloidiasis, larvae may invade not only gastrointestinal tissues and the lungs but also the central nervous system, peritoneum, liver, and kidney. Moreover, bacteremia may develop due to the entry of enteric flora through disrupted mucosal barriers. Gram-negative sepsis, pneumonia, or meningitis may complicate or dominate the clinical course. Eosinophilia is often absent in severely infected patients. Disseminated strongyloidiasis, particularly in patients with unsuspected infection who are given immunosuppressive drugs, can be fatal. Strongyloidiasis is a frequent complication of infection with human T cell lymphotropic virus type I, but disseminated strongyloidiasis is not common among patients infected with human immunodeficiency virus.

Diagnosis In uncomplicated strongyloidiasis, the finding of rhabditiform larvae in feces is diagnostic. The eggs are almost never detectable because they hatch in the intestine. Rhabditiform larvae are 200 to 250 μm long, with a short buccal cavity that distinguishes them from hookworm rhabditiform larvae. Single stool examinations will detect only about one-third of uncomplicated infections, in which few larvae are passed. Serial examinations or use of the Baermann concentration method improves the sensitivity of stool diagnosis. If the result of stool examination is negative, *Strongyloides* can be assayed by sampling of the duodenojejunal contents by aspiration, biopsy, or the Enterotest string method. An enzyme-linked immunosorbent assay for antibodies to excretory-secretory antigens of *Strongyloides* is a sensitive method of diagnosing uncomplicated infections. In disseminated strongyloidiasis, filariform larvae (550 μm long) should be sought in stool as well as in samples obtained from sites of potential larval migration, including sputum, bronchoalveolar lavage fluid, or surgical drainage fluid.

TREATMENT

Even in the asymptomatic state, strongyloidiasis must be treated because of the potential for fatal hyperinfection. Thiabendazole (25 mg/kg bid) is generally administered for 2 days, but in disseminated strongyloidiasis, treatment should be extended for at least 5 to 7 days or until the parasites are eradicated. Common adverse effects of thiabendazole include nausea, vomiting, diarrhea, dizziness, and neuropsychiatric disturbances. Because thiabendazole is not uniformly effective, stool examinations, eosinophil counts, and monitoring of clinical symptoms should be continued after treatment. Albendazole and ivermectin are newer drugs effective in the treatment of intestinal disease, but, to date, efficacy in disseminated strongyloidiasis has been demonstrated only for thiabendazole.

Strongyloides fülleborni This unusual species, which has been encountered in Africa and Papua, New Guinea, is thought to be transmitted from person to person and via maternal milk. *S. fülleborni* releases membranous sacs filled with eggs into the stool. Most commonly affected are infants and young children, who present with abdominal distention, respiratory distress, vomiting, or diarrhea.

TRICHURIASIS Most infections with the whipworm *Trichuris trichiura* are asymptomatic, but heavy infections may cause gastrointestinal symptoms. Like the other soil-transmitted helminths, whipworm is distributed globally in the tropics and subtropics and is most common among poor children.

Life Cycle A broad posterior section and a thin anterior portion give *Trichuris* its characteristic whiplike shape. The adult worms reside in the colon and cecum, the anterior portions threaded into the superficial mucosa. Thousands of eggs laid daily by adult female worms pass via the feces and mature in the soil. After ingestion, infective eggs hatch in the duodenum, releasing larvae that mature before migrating to the large bowel. The entire cycle takes about 3 months, and adult worms may live for several years.

Clinical Features Tissue reactions to whipworms are mild. Most infected individuals have no symptoms or eosinophilia. Heavy infections may result in abdominal pain, anorexia, and bloody or mucoid diarrhea resembling inflammatory bowel disease. Rectal prolapse can result from massive infections in children, who often suffer from malnourishment and other diarrheal illnesses. Moderately heavy whipworm burdens also contribute to growth retardation.

Diagnosis and Treatment The characteristic 50- by 20-μm lemon-shaped whipworm eggs are readily detected on stool examination. Adult worms, which are 3 to 5 cm long, occasionally can be seen on proctoscopy. Mebendazole is safe and effective for treatment (see Chap. 214).

ENTEROBIASIS (PINWORM) *E. vermicularis* is more common in temperate countries than in the tropics. More than 40 million Americans, particularly schoolchildren, are estimated to be infected with pinworms.

Life Cycle and Epidemiology *Enterobius* adult worms are about 1 cm long and dwell in the bowel lumen. The gravid female worm migrates nocturnally out into the perianal region and releases up to 10,000 immature eggs. The eggs become infective within hours and are transmitted via hand-to-mouth passage. The larvae hatch and mature entirely within the intestine. This life cycle takes about 1 month, and adult worms survive for about 2 months. Self-infection results from perianal scratching and transport of infective eggs on the hands or under the nails to the mouth. Owing to the ease of person-to-person spread, pinworm infections are common among family members and institutionalized populations.

Clinical Features Most pinworm infections are asymptomatic. Perianal pruritus is the cardinal symptom. The itching is often worse at night owing to the nocturnal migration of the female worms, and it may lead to excoriation and bacterial superinfection. Heavy infections have been claimed to cause abdominal pain and weight loss. On rare occasions, pinworms invade the female genital tract, causing vulvovaginitis and pelvic or peritoneal granulomas. Eosinophilia or elevated levels of serum IgE are rare.

Diagnosis Since pinworm eggs are not usually released in the bowel, the diagnosis cannot be made by looking for eggs in the feces. Instead, eggs deposited in the perianal region are detected by the application of clear cellulose acetate tape to the perianal region in the morning. After the tape is transferred to a microscope slide, low-power examination will reveal the characteristic pinworm eggs, which are oval, measure 55 by 25 μm, and are flattened along one side.

 TREATMENT

All affected individuals should be given a dose of mebendazole or pyrantel pamoate, with treatment repeated after 10 to 14 days (see Chap. 214). Treatment of household members is also advocated to eliminate asymptomatic reservoirs of potential reinfection.

TRICHOSTRONGYLIASIS *Trichostrongylus* species that are normally parasites of herbivorous animals occasionally infect humans, particularly in Asia and Africa. This parasite has been termed *pseudohookworm* because of similarities to the hookworms in life cycle and egg morphology. Humans acquire the infection by accidentally ingesting *Trichostrongylus* larvae on contaminated leafy vegetables. The larvae do not migrate in humans but mature directly into adult worms in the small bowel. These worms ingest far less blood than hookworms; most infected people are asymptomatic, but heavy infections may give rise to mild anemia and eosinophilia. *Trichostrongylus* eggs encountered on stool examination resemble those of hookworms but are larger (85 by 115 μm). Appropriate treatment consists of mebendazole (see Chap. 214).

ANISAKIASIS Anisakiasis is a gastrointestinal infection caused by the accidental ingestion in uncooked saltwater fish of nematode larvae belonging to the family Anisakidae. The incidence of anisakiasis in the United States has increased as a result of the growing popularity of raw fish dishes. Most cases occur in Japan, the Netherlands, and Chile, where raw fish—sushi, pickled green herring, and seviche, respectively—are national culinary staples. Anisakid nematodes parasitize large sea mammals such as whales, dolphins, and seals. As part of a complex parasitic life cycle involving marine food chains, infectious larvae migrate to the musculature of a variety of fish. Both *Anisakis simplex* and *Pseudoterranova decipiens* have been implicated in human anisakiasis, but an identical gastric syndrome may be caused by the red larvae of eustrongylid parasites of fish-eating birds. When humans consume infected raw fish, live larvae may be coughed up within 48 h. Alternatively, larvae may immediately penetrate the mucosa of the stomach. Within hours, violent upper abdominal pain accompanied by nausea and occasionally vomiting ensues, mimicking an acute abdomen. The diagnosis can be established by direct visualization on upper endoscopy, outlining of the worm by contrast radiographic studies, or histopathologic examination of extracted tissue. In experienced hands, the first technique is preferable because extraction of the burrowing larvae by endoscopic technique is curative. In addition, larvae may pass to the small bowel, where they penetrate the mucosa and provoke a vigorous eosinophilic granulomatous response. Symptoms may appear 1 or 2 weeks after the infective meal, with intermittent abdominal pain, diarrhea, nausea, and fever resembling the manifestations of Crohn's disease. The diagnosis may be suggested by barium studies and confirmed by curative surgical resection of a granuloma in which the worm is embedded. Anisakid eggs will not be found in the stool, since the larvae do not mature in humans. Anisakid larvae in saltwater fish are killed by cooking to 60°C, freezing at −20°C for 3 days, or commercial blast freezing, but not usually by salting, marinating, or cold smoking.

CAPILLARIASIS Intestinal capillariasis is caused by ingestion of raw fish infected with *Capillaria philippinensis*. Subsequent autoinfection can lead to a severe wasting syndrome. The disease occurs in the Philippines and Thailand and, on occasion, elsewhere in Asia. The natural cycle of *C. philippinensis* involves fish from fresh and brackish water. When humans eat infected raw fish, the larvae mature in the intestine into adult worms, which produce invasive larvae that cause intestinal inflammation and villus loss. Capillariasis has an insidious onset with nonspecific abdominal pain and watery diarrhea. If untreated, progressive autoinfection can lead to protein-losing enteropathy and severe malabsorption and ultimately to death from cachexia, cardiac failure, or superinfection. The diagnosis is established by identification of the characteristic peanut-shaped (20- by 40-μm) eggs on stool examination. Severely ill patients require hospitalization and supportive therapy in addition to prolonged anthelmintic treatment with mebendazole or albendazole (see Chap. 214).

ABDOMINAL ANGIOSTRONGYLIASIS Abdominal angiostrongyliasis is found in Latin America and Africa. The zoonotic parasite *Angiostrongylus costaricensis* causes eosinophilic ileocolitis after the ingestion of contaminated vegetation. *A. costaricensis* normally parasitizes the cotton rat and other rodents, with slugs and snails serving as intermediate hosts. Humans become infected by accidentally ingesting infective larvae in mollusk slime deposited on fruits and vegetables; children are at highest risk. The larvae penetrate the gut wall and migrate to the mesenteric artery, where they develop into adult worms. Eggs deposited in the gut wall provoke an intense eosinophilic granulomatous reaction, and adult worms may cause mesenteric arteritis, thrombosis, or frank bowel infarction. Symptoms may mimic those of appendicitis, including abdominal pain and tenderness, fever, vomiting, and a palpable mass in the right iliac fossa. Leukocytosis and eosinophilia are prominent. A barium enema may reveal ileocecal filling defects, but a definitive diagnosis is usually made surgically with partial bowel resection. Pathologic study reveals a thickened bowel wall with eosinophilic granulomas surrounding the *Angiostrongylus* eggs. In nonsurgical cases, the diagnosis rests solely on clinical grounds because larvae and eggs cannot be detected in the stool. Medical therapy for abdominal angiostrongyliasis is of uncertain efficacy. Careful observation and surgical resection for severe symptoms are the mainstays of treatment.

BIBLIOGRAPHY

ASH LR, ORIHEL TC: *Atlas of Human Parasitology*, 3d ed. Chicago, ASCP Press, 1990

COOPER ES, BUNDY DAP: Trichuris is not trivial. Parasitol Today 4:301, 1988

CROESE J et al: Human enteric infection with canine hookworms. Ann Intern Med 120:369, 1994

CROSS JH: Intestinal capillariasis. Clin Microbiol Rev 5:120, 1992

DUARTE Z et al: Abdominal angiostrongyliasis in Nicaragua: A clinico-pathological study on a series of 12 case reports. Ann Parasitol Hum Comp 66:259, 1991

GENTA RM et al: Strongyloidiasis in US veterans of the Vietnam and other wars. JAMA 258:49, 1987

GYORKOS TW et al: Intestinal parasite infection in the Kampuchean refugee population 6 years after resettlement in Canada. J Infect Dis 166:413, 1992

HAQUE AK et al: Pathogenesis of human strongyloidiasis: Autopsy and quantitative parasitological analysis. Mod Pathol 7:276, 1994

HOTEZ PJ, PRITCHARD DI: Hookworm infection. Sci Am 272:68, 1995

KHUROO MS et al: Hepatobiliary and pancreatic ascariasis in India. Lancet 335:1503, 1990

LIU LX, WELLER PF: Strongyloidiasis and other intestinal nematode infections. Infect Dis Clin North Am 7:655, 1993

OCHOA B: Surgical complications of ascariasis. World J Surg 15:222, 1991

SCHAD GA, WARREN KS (eds): *Hookworm Disease: Current Status and New Directions*. London, Taylor and Francis, 1990

SCHANTZ PM: The dangers of eating raw fish. N Engl J Med 320:1143, 1989 [Editorial]

223 *Thomas B. Nutman, Peter F. Weller*

FILARIASIS AND RELATED INFECTIONS (LOIASIS, ONCHOCERCIASIS, AND DRACUNCULIASIS)

Filarial worms are nematodes that dwell in the subcutaneous tissues and the lymphatics. Eight filarial species infect humans (Table 223-1); of these, four—*Wuchereria bancrofti*, *Brugia malayi*, *Onchocerca volvulus*, and *Loa loa*—are responsible for most serious filarial infections. Filarial parasites, which infect an estimated 140 million persons worldwide, are transmitted by specific species of mosquitoes or other arthropods and have a complex life cycle including infective larval stages that are carried by insects and adult worms that reside in either lymphatic or subcutaneous tissues of humans. The offspring of adults are microfilariae, which, depending on their species, are 200 to 250 μm long and 5 to 7 μm wide, may or may not be enveloped in a loose sheath, and either circulate in the blood or migrate through the skin (see Table 223-1). To complete the life cycle, microfilariae are ingested by the arthropod vector and develop over 1 to 2 weeks into new infective larvae. Adult worms live for many years, whereas microfilariae survive from 3 to 36 months.

Usually, infection is established only with repeated and prolonged exposures to infective larvae. Since the clinical manifestations of filarial diseases develop relatively slowly, these infections should be considered chronic diseases with possible long-term debilitating effects. In terms of the nature, severity, and timing of clinical manifestations, patients with filariasis who are native to endemic areas and undergo lifelong exposure may differ significantly from those who are travelers or who have recently moved to these areas. Characteristically, the disease is more acute and intense in newly exposed individuals than in natives of endemic areas.

LYMPHATIC FILARIASIS

Lymphatic filariasis is caused by *W. bancrofti*, *B. malayi*, or *Brugia timori*. The threadlike adult parasites reside in lymphatic channels or lymph nodes, where they may remain viable for more than two decades.

EPIDEMIOLOGY *W. bancrofti*, the most widely distributed human filarial parasite, affects an estimated 80 million people and is found throughout the tropics and subtropics, including Asia and the Pacific Islands, Africa, areas of South America, and the Caribbean basin. Humans are the only definitive host for the parasite. Generally, the subperiodic form is found only in the Pacific Islands; elsewhere, *W. bancrofti* is nocturnally periodic. (Nocturnally periodic forms of microfilariae are scarce in peripheral blood by day and increase at night, whereas subperiodic forms are present in peripheral blood at all times and reach maximal levels in the afternoon.) Natural vectors for *W. bancrofti* are *Culex fatigans* mosquitoes in urban settings and anopheline or aedean mosquitoes in rural areas.

Brugian filariasis due to *B. malayi* occurs primarily in China, India, Indonesia, Korea, Japan, Malaysia, and the Philippines. *B. malayi* also has two forms distinguished by the periodicity of microfilaremia. The more common nocturnal form is transmitted in areas of coastal rice fields, while the subperiodic form is found in forests. *B. malayi* naturally infects cats as well as humans. *B. timori* exists only on islands of the Indonesian archipelago.

PATHOLOGY The principal pathologic changes result from inflammatory damage to the lymphatics, which is caused by adult worms and not by microfilariae. Adult worms live in afferent lymphatics or sinuses of lymph nodes and cause lymphatic dilatation and thickening of the vessel walls. The infiltration of plasma cells, eosinophils, and macrophages in and around the infected vessels, along with endothelial and connective tissue proliferation, leads to tortuosity of the lymphatics and damaged or incompetent lymph valves. Lymphedema and chronic-stasis changes with hard or brawny edema develop in the overlying skin. These consequences of filariasis are due both to direct effects of the worms and to the immune response of the host to the parasite. These immune responses are believed to cause the granulomatous and proliferative processes that precede total lymphatic obstruction. It is thought that the vessel remains patent as long as the worm remains viable, and that death of the worm leads to enhanced granulomatous reaction and fibrosis. Lymphatic obstruction results, and, despite collateralization of the lymphatics, lymphatic function is compromised.

CLINICAL FEATURES The common manifestations of lymphatic filariasis are asymptomatic microfilaremia, hydrocele, lymphatic inflammation, and lymphatic obstruction. Asymptomatic microfilaremia is found in most infected individuals who are clinically well. Infected males frequently develop disease in the scrotum, primarily because of the presence of adult worms in the lymphatics of the spermatic cord. Hydrocele may develop and, in advanced stages, may evolve into scrotal elephantiasis. Acute lymphangitis and lymphadenitis with high fever ("filarial fevers") are often accompanied by shaking chills and transient local edema. Episodes can recur frequently and usually abate spontaneously after 7 to 10 days. The lymphangitis characteristically develops in a retrograde or descending fashion, extending peripherally from the draining node where the parasite presumably resides. Regional lymph nodes are often enlarged, and the entire lymphatic channel can become indurated and inflamed. Concomitant local thrombophlebitis can develop. In brugian filariasis, a local abscess may form over a lymphatic tract and rupture. Lymphadenitis and lymphangitis involve both the upper and the lower extremities in bancroftian and brugian filariasis, but genital lymphatic involvement develops almost exclusively in relation to *W. bancrofti* infection. Genital involvement can be manifested by funiculitis, epididymitis, and scrotal pain and tenderness.

If lymphatic damage progresses to lymphatic obstruction, the permanent changes associated with elephantiasis may ensue. Brawny edema follows early pitting edema. With thickening of subcutaneous tissues come hyperkeratosis, fissuring of the skin, and hyperplastic changes. Bacterial superinfection of the poorly vascularized tissues is common. In bancroftian filariasis, scrotal lymphedema can develop. If the retroperitoneal lymphatics become obstructed, increased pressure leads to the rupture of renal lymphatics and the development of chyluria, which is usually intermittent and most prominent in the morning.

The clinical manifestations of filarial infections in travelers or transmigrants who have recently entered an endemic region are distinctive. Given a sufficient number of bites by infected vectors, usually over a 3- to 6-month period, recently exposed patients can develop acute lymphatic or scrotal inflammation with or without urticaria and localized angioedema. Lymphadenitis of epitrochlear, axillary, femoral, or inguinal lymph nodes is often followed by retrogradely evolving lymphangitis. Acute attacks are short-lived and, in contrast to filarial fevers in patients native to endemic areas, are usually not accompanied by fever. With prolonged exposure to infected mosquitoes, these attacks, if untreated, become more severe and lead to permanent lymphatic inflammation and obstruction.

DIAGNOSIS A definitive diagnosis can be made only by detection of the parasites and hence can be difficult. Adult worms localized in lymphatic vessels or nodes are largely inaccessible. Microfilariae can be found in blood, in hydrocele fluid, or (occasionally) in other body fluids. Such fluids can be examined microscopically, either directly or—for greater sensitivity—after concentration of the parasites by the passage of fluid through a polycarbonate cylindrical pore filter (pore size, 3 μm) or by the centrifugation of fluid fixed in 2% formalin (Knott's concentration technique). The timing of blood collection is critical and should be based on the periodicity of the microfilariae in the endemic region involved. Many infected individuals do not have microfilaremia, and definitive diagnosis in such cases can be difficult; in some instances, the diagnosis must be made on clinical grounds. In acute episodes, lymphatic filariasis must be distinguished from thrombophlebitis, infection, and trauma. Retrogradely evolving lymphangitis is a characteristic feature that helps distinguish filarial lymphangitis from typically ascending bacterial lymphangitis. Chronic filarial lymphedema must be distinguished from the lymphedema of malignancy, postoperative scarring, trauma, chronic edematous states, and congenital lymphatic-system abnormalities.

Eosinophilia and elevations of serum concentrations of IgE and antifilarial antibody support the diagnosis of lymphatic filariasis. There is, however, extensive cross-reactivity between filarial antigens and antigens of other helminths, including the common intestinal roundworms; thus, interpretations of serologic findings can be difficult. In addition, residents of endemic areas can become sensitized to filarial antigens through exposure to infected mosquitoes without having patent filarial infections.

Assays for circulating antigens of *W. bancrofti* permit the diagnosis of microfilaremic and cryptic (amicrofilaremic) infection. Polymerase

Table 223-1

Characteristics of the Filariae

Organism	Periodicity	Distribution	Vector	Location of Adult	Microfilarial Location	Sheath
Wuchereria bancrofti	Nocturnal	Cosmopolitan areas worldwide, including South America and Africa	*Culex* (mosquitoes)	Lymphatic tissue	Blood	+
		Mainly India	*Anopheles* (mosquitoes)			
		China, Indonesia	*Aedes* (mosquitoes)			
	Subperiodic	Eastern Pacific	*Aedes* (mosquitoes)	Lymphatic tissue	Blood	+
Brugia malayi	Nocturnal	Southeast Asia, Indonesia, India	*Mansonia, Anopheles* (mosquitoes)	Lymphatic tissue	Blood	+
	Subperiodic	Indonesia, Southeast Asia	*Coquilletidia, Mansonia* (mosquitoes)	Lymphatic tissue	Blood	+
Brugia timori	Nocturnal	Indonesia	*Anopheles* (mosquitoes)	Lymphatic tissue	Blood	+
Loa loa	Diurnal	West and Central Africa	*Chrysops* (deerflies)	Subcutaneous tissue	Blood	+
Onchocerca volvulus	None	South and Central America, Africa	*Simulium* (blackflies)	Subcutaneous tissue	Skin, eye	−
Mansonella ozzardi	None	South and Central America	*Culicoides* (midges)	Undetermined site	Blood	−
		Caribbean	*Simulium* (blackflies)			
Mansonella perstans	None	South and Central America, Africa	*Culicoides* (midges)	Body cavities, mesentery, perirenal tissue	Blood	−
Mansonella streptocerca	None	West and Central Africa	*Culicoides* (midges)	Subcutaneous tissue	Skin	−

chain reaction–based assays for DNA of *W. bancrofti* and *B. malayi* in blood have also been developed.

Evaluation of lymphatic function with lymphoscintigraphy can provide useful information in cases of lymphatic filariasis. The procedure involves the intradermal or subcutaneous injection of ^{99}Tc-labeled albumin or ^{99}Tc-labeled dextran [although the latter is not approved by the Food and Drug Administration (FDA)] and subsequent sequential imaging with a gamma camera. In males with suspected lymphatic filariasis, examination of the scrotum by ultrasonography may reveal nodules or lymphatic dilatation. The use of high-frequency (7.5- to 10-MHz) transducers and Doppler techniques may reveal motile worms within the scrotal lymphatics.

℞ TREATMENT

Treatment for lymphatic filariasis is currently limited to diethylcarbamazine (DEC) given at 6 mg/kg per day in either single or divided doses for 2 to 3 weeks. This regimen clears microfilariae from the blood and has a limited but definite effect on adult parasites. If at least some adult parasites survive, as is often the case, microfilaremia along with clinical symptoms can recur within months after therapy. There is some evidence that several courses of DEC or chronic administration of low-dose DEC may effect a cure. Ivermectin, a drug active in onchocerciasis, has been used in trials of therapy for lymphatic filariasis; in a single dose (although not approved by the FDA), it appears to be as effective as DEC at clearing microfilariae. Side effects of treatment with DEC (or ivermectin) include fever, chills, arthralgia, headaches, nausea, and vomiting. Both the development and the severity of these reactions, which may reflect an acute response to the antigens released by dying parasites, are related directly to the number of microfilariae circulating in the blood. These side effects can be avoided either by the initial use of a small dose of DEC, with an increase to a full dose over a few days, or by premedication of the patient with glucocorticoids.

Treatment of chronic lymphatic obstruction is difficult but may be helpful. Elevation of the infected limb, use of elastic stockings, and local foot care eliminate some of the associated symptoms. Surgical decompression with a nodovenous shunt may provide relief for severely affected limbs. Hydroceles can be drained or managed surgically. The management of filarial chyluria is unsatisfactory; neither surgical intervention nor sclerosis of infected lymphatics is effective.

PREVENTION Avoidance of mosquito bites usually is not feasible for residents of endemic areas, but visitors should use insect repellent and mosquito nets. DEC can kill developing filarial larvae and is useful as a prophylactic agent, although the optimal regimen for prophylaxis has not been ascertained. Mass treatment with DEC may reduce community levels of microfilariae so as to interrupt vector-borne transmission among humans.

TROPICAL PULMONARY EOSINOPHILIA

Tropical pulmonary eosinophilia (TPE) is a distinct syndrome that develops in some individuals infected with lymphatic filarial species. This syndrome affects males and females at a ratio of 4:1, often during the third decade of life. The majority of cases have been reported from India, Pakistan, Sri Lanka, Brazil, and Southeast Asia.

CLINICAL FEATURES The main features include a history of residence in filarial endemic regions, paroxysmal cough and wheezing that are usually nocturnal (and probably related to the nocturnal periodicity of microfilariae), weight loss, low-grade fever, adenopathy, and pronounced blood eosinophilia (>3000 eosinophils/μL). Chest x-rays may be normal but generally show increased bronchovascular markings; diffuse miliary lesions or mottled opacities may be present in the middle and lower lung fields. Tests of pulmonary function show restrictive abnormalities in most cases and obstructive defects in half.

Total serum IgE levels (10,000 to 100,000 ng/mL) and antifilarial antibody titers are characteristically elevated.

PATHOLOGY In TPE there is rapid clearance of microfilariae and parasite antigens from the bloodstream by the lungs, and the clinical symptoms result from allergic and inflammatory reactions elicited by the cleared parasites. In some subjects, trapping of microfilariae in other reticuloendothelial organs can cause hepatomegaly, splenomegaly, or lymphadenopathy. A prominent, eosinophil-enriched, intraalveolar infiltrate is often reported. In the absence of successful treatment, interstitial fibrosis can lead to progressive pulmonary damage.

DIFFERENTIAL DIAGNOSIS TPE must be distinguished from asthma, Löffler's syndrome, allergic bronchopulmonary aspergillosis, allergic granulomatosis with angiitis (Churg-Strauss syndrome), the systemic vasculitides (most notably periarteritis nodosa and Wegener's granulomatosis), chronic eosinophilic pneumonia, and the idiopathic hypereosinophilic syndrome. In addition to a geographic history of filarial exposure, useful features for distinguishing TPE include wheezing that is solely nocturnal, very high levels of antifilarial antibodies, and a rapid initial response to treatment with DEC.

℞ TREATMENT

DEC is used at a dosage of 4 to 6 mg/kg of body weight per day for 14 days. Symptoms usually resolve within 3 to 7 days after the initiation of therapy. Relapse, which occurs in approximately 12 to 25 percent of cases (sometimes after an interval of years), requires retreatment.

ONCHOCERCIASIS

Onchocerciasis ("river blindness") is caused by the filarial nematode *O. volvulus*, which infects an estimated 13 million individuals. The majority of individuals infected with *O. volvulus* live in the equatorial region of Africa extending from the Atlantic coast to the Red Sea. About 70,000 persons are infected in Guatemala and Mexico, with smaller foci in Venezuela, Colombia, Brazil, Ecuador, Yemen, and Saudi Arabia. Onchocerciasis is the second leading cause of infectious blindness worldwide.

ETIOLOGY AND EPIDEMIOLOGY Infection in humans begins with the deposition of infective larvae on the skin by the bite of an infected blackfly. The larvae develop into adults, which are typically found in subcutaneous nodules. About 7 months to 3 years after infection, the gravid female releases microfilariae that migrate out of the nodule and throughout the tissues, concentrating in the dermis. Infection is transmitted to other persons when a female fly ingests microfilariae from the host's skin and these microfilariae then develop into infective larvae. Adult *O. volvulus* females and males are about 40 to 60 cm and 3 to 6 cm in length, respectively. The life span of adults can be as long as 18 years, with an average of approximately 9 years. Because the blackfly vector breeds along free-flowing rivers and streams (particularly in rapids) and generally restricts its flight to an area within several kilometers of these breeding sites, both biting and disease transmission are most intense in these locations.

PATHOLOGY Onchocerciasis affects primarily the skin, eyes, and lymph nodes. In contrast to that in lymphatic filariasis, the damage in onchocerciasis is elicited by microfilariae and not by adults. In the skin, there are mild but chronic inflammatory changes that can result in loss of elastic fibers, atrophy, and fibrosis. The subcutaneous nodules, or onchocercomata, consist primarily of fibrous tissues surrounding the adult worm, often with a peripheral ring of inflammatory cells. In the eye, neovascularization and corneal scarring lead to corneal opacities and blindness. Inflammation in the anterior and posterior chambers frequently results in anterior uveitis, chorioretinitis, and optic atrophy. Although punctate opacities are due to an inflammatory reaction surrounding dead or dying microfilariae, the pathogenesis of most manifestations of onchocerciasis is still unclear.

CLINICAL FEATURES **Skin** Pruritus and rash are the most frequent manifestations of onchocerciasis. The pruritus can be incapacitating; the rash is typically a papular eruption that is generalized rather than localized to a particular region of the body. Long-term infection results in exaggerated and premature wrinkling of the skin, loss of elastic fibers, and epidermal atrophy that can lead to loose, redundant skin and hypo- or hyperpigmentation. Localized eczematoid dermatitis can cause hyperkeratosis, scaling, and pigmentary changes. Such lesions are often seen in the lower extremities but can be distributed more extensively.

Onchocercomata These subcutaneous nodules, which can be palpable and/or visible, contain the adult worm. In African patients, they are common over the coccyx and sacrum, the trochanter of the femur, the lateral anterior crest, and other bony prominences; in Latin American patients, they tend to develop preferentially in the upper part of the body, particularly on the head, neck, and shoulders. Nodules vary in size and characteristically are firm and not tender. It has been estimated that, for every palpable nodule, there are four deeper nonpalpable ones.

Ocular Tissue Visual impairment is the most serious complication of onchocerciasis and usually affects only those persons with moderate or heavy infections. Lesions may develop in all parts of the eye. The most common early finding is conjunctivitis with photophobia. In the cornea, punctate keratitis—consisting of acute inflammatory reactions surrounding dying microfilariae manifested as "snowflake" opacities—is frequent in younger patients and resolves without apparent complications. Sclerosing keratitis occurs in approximately 5 percent of persons infected with savannah strains and 1 percent of those infected with forest strains and is the leading cause of onchocercal blindness in Africa. Anterior uveitis and iridocyclitis develop in about 5 percent of infected persons in Africa. In Latin America, complications of the anterior uveal tract (pupillary deformity) may cause secondary glaucoma. Characteristic chorioretinal lesions develop as a result of atrophy and hyperpigmentation of the retinal pigment epithelium and the choriopapillaris. Constriction of the visual field and frank optic atrophy may occur.

Lymph Nodes Mild to moderate lymphadenopathy is frequent, particularly in the inguinal and femoral areas, where the enlarged nodes may hang down in response to gravity ("hanging groin"), sometimes predisposing to inguinal and femoral hernias.

Systemic Manifestations Some heavily infected individuals develop cachexia with loss of adipose tissue and muscle mass. Among adults who become blind, there is a three- to fourfold increase in the mortality rate.

DIAGNOSIS Definitive diagnosis depends on the detection of an adult worm in an excised nodule or, more commonly, of microfilariae in a skin snip. Skin snips are obtained with a corneal-scleral punch, which collects a blood-free skin biopsy sample extending to just below the epidermis, or by lifting of the skin with the tip of a needle and excision of a small (1- to 3-mm) piece with a sterile scalpel blade. The biopsy tissue is incubated in tissue culture medium or in saline on a glass slide or flat-bottomed microtiter plate. After incubation for 2 to 4 h (or occasionally overnight in light infections), microfilariae emergent from the skin can be visualized by low-power microscopy.

℞ TREATMENT

The main goals of therapy are to prevent the development of irreversible lesions and to alleviate symptoms. Surgical excision is recommended when nodules are located on the head, because of the proximity of microfilaria-producing adult worms to the eye, but chemotherapy is the mainstay of management. Ivermectin, a semisynthetic macrocyclic lactone active against microfilariae, is the first-line agent for the treatment of onchocerciasis. It is given orally in a single dose of 150 μg/kg, either yearly or semiannually. After treatment, most individuals have few or no reactions. Pruritus, cutaneous edema, and/or maculopapular rash occurs in approximately 1 to 10 percent of treated individuals. Contraindications to treatment include pregnancy, breast feeding, central nervous system (CNS) disorders that may increase the penetration of ivermectin into the CNS (e.g., meningitis), and an age of less than 5 years. Although ivermectin treatment results in a marked drop in microfilarial density,

its effect may last for only 6 months. Suramin, a potent but potentially toxic macrofilaricidal agent, is recommended only if total cure is necessary. Because of the drug's nephrotoxicity, renal function must be monitored closely during treatment.

PREVENTION Vector control has been beneficial in highly endemic areas in which breeding sites are vulnerable to insecticide spraying, but most areas endemic for onchocerciasis are not suited to this type of control. While persons working in fly-infested areas can minimize the number of bites they sustain by wearing protective garments, this approach is not feasible for the large majority of individuals in endemic foci. No drug has been shown to prevent infection with *O. volvulus*.

LOIASIS

ETIOLOGY AND EPIDEMIOLOGY Loiasis is caused by *L. loa* (the African eye worm), which is present in the rain forests of West and Central Africa. Adult parasites (females, 50 to 70 mm long and 0.5 mm wide; males, 25 to 35 mm long and 0.25 mm wide) live in subcutaneous tissues; microfilariae circulate in the blood with a diurnal periodicity that peaks between 12:00 noon and 2:00 P.M.

CLINICAL FEATURES Manifestations of loiasis in natives of endemic areas may differ from those in temporary residents or visitors. Among the indigenous population, loiasis is often an asymptomatic infection with microfilaremia. Infection may be recognized only after subconjunctival migration of an adult worm or may be manifested by episodic Calabar swellings, evanescent localized areas of angioedema and erythema developing on the extremities and less frequently at other sites. Nephropathy, encephalopathy, and cardiomyopathy are rare. In patients who are not residents of endemic areas, allergic symptoms predominate, episodes of Calabar swelling tend to be more frequent and debilitating, microfilaremia is rare, and eosinophilia and increased levels of antifilarial antibodies are characteristic.

PATHOLOGY The pathogenesis of the manifestations of loiasis is poorly understood. Calabar swellings are thought to result from a hypersensitivity reaction to the adult worm.

DIAGNOSIS Definitive diagnosis of loiasis requires the detection of microfilariae in the peripheral blood or the isolation of the adult worm from the eye or from a subcutaneous biopsy specimen from a site of swelling developing after treatment. In practice, the diagnosis must often be based on a characteristic history and clinical presentation, blood eosinophilia, and elevated levels of antifilarial antibodies, particularly in travelers to the endemic region, who are usually amicrofilaremic. Other clinical findings in the latter individuals include hypergammaglobulinemia, elevated levels of serum IgE, and elevated leukocyte and eosinophil counts.

℞ TREATMENT

DEC (8 to 10 mg/kg per day for 21 days) is effective against both the adult and the microfilarial forms of *L. loa*, but multiple courses are frequently necessary before the disease resolves completely. In cases of heavy microfilaremia, allergic or other inflammatory reactions can take place during treatment, including CNS involvement with coma and encephalitis. Heavy infections are treated initially with low doses of DEC (0.5 mg/kg per day) and glucocorticoids (40 to 60 mg of prednisone per day). If antifilarial treatment has no adverse effects, the prednisone dose can be rapidly tapered and the dose of DEC gradually increased to 8 to 10 mg/kg per day.

Albendazole and ivermectin (although not FDA-approved) have been shown to be effective in reducing microfilarial loads. DEC (300 mg weekly) is an effective prophylactic regimen for loiasis.

STREPTOCERCIASIS

Mansonella streptocerca, found mainly in the tropical forest belt of Africa from Ghana to Zaire, is transmitted by biting midges. The major clinical manifestations involve the skin and include pruritus, papular rashes, and pigmentation changes. Many infected individuals have inguinal adenopathy, although most are asymptomatic. The diagnosis is made by detection of the characteristic microfilariae in skin snips. DEC (6 mg/kg per day in divided doses for 14 to 21 days) is effective in killing both microfilariae and adult worms. As in onchocerciasis, treatment is sometimes accompanied by urticaria, arthralgias, myalgias, headaches, and abdominal discomfort.

MANSONELLA PERSTANS INFECTION

Mansonella perstans, distributed across the center of Africa and in northeastern South America, is transmitted by midges. Adult worms reside in serous cavities—pericardial, pleural, and peritoneal—as well as in the mesentery and the perirenal and retroperitoneal tissues. Microfilariae circulate in the blood without periodicity. The clinical and pathologic features of the infection are poorly defined. Most patients appear to be asymptomatic, but manifestations may include transient angioedema and pruritus of the arms, face, or other parts of the body (analogous to the Calabar swellings of loiasis), fever, headache, arthralgias, and right upper quadrant pain. Occasionally, pericarditis and hepatitis occur. The diagnosis is based on the demonstration of microfilariae in blood or serosal effusions. Perstans filariasis is often associated with peripheral-blood eosinophilia and antifilarial antibody elevations. Although DEC (8 to 10 mg/kg per day for 21 days) is the standard therapeutic agent, there is little evidence that it is effective. Cure is evidenced by the disappearance of symptoms and eosinophilia; multiple courses of therapy are usually required. Mebendazole (100 mg twice daily for 30 days) has been reported to be effective.

MANSONELLA OZZARDI INFECTION

The distribution of *Mansonella ozzardi* is restricted to Central and South America and certain Caribbean islands. Adult worms are rarely recovered from humans. Microfilariae circulate in the blood without periodicity. Although this organism has often been considered nonpathogenic, headache, articular pain, fever, pulmonary symptoms, adenopathy, hepatomegaly, pruritus, and eosinophilia have been ascribed to *M. ozzardi* infection. Diagnosis is made by the detection of microfilariae in peripheral blood. No drug has been proved to be effective for therapy; ivermectin was effective in a single case report.

DRACUNCULIASIS (GUINEA WORM INFECTION)

ETIOLOGY AND EPIDEMIOLOGY Dracunculiasis, caused by *Dracunculus medinensis*, is a parasitic infection whose incidence has declined dramatically because of global eradication efforts. Current estimates suggest that there are only 100,000 cases worldwide, the majority in Sudan and West Africa (particularly Nigeria and Niger). Humans acquire this infection when they ingest water containing infective larvae derived from *Cyclops*, a crustacean that is the intermediate host. Larvae penetrate the stomach or intestinal wall, mate, and mature. The adult male probably dies; the female *Dracunculus* develops over a year and migrates to subcutaneous tissues, usually in the lower extremity. As the thin female *Dracunculus*, ranging in length from 300 cm to 1 m, approaches the skin, a blister forms that, over days, breaks down and forms an ulcer. When the blister opens, large numbers of motile, rhabditiform larvae can be released into stagnant water; ingestion by *Cyclops* completes the life cycle.

CLINICAL FEATURES Few or no clinical manifestations of dracunculiasis are evident until just before the blister forms, when there is an onset of fever and generalized allergic symptoms, including periorbital edema, wheezing, and urticaria. The emergence of the worm is associated with local pain and swelling. When the blister ruptures (usually as a result of immersion in water), the adult worm releases larva-rich fluid, and this release is associated with a relief of symptoms. The shallow ulcer surrounding the emerging adult worm heals over weeks to months. Such ulcers, however, can become secondarily infected, the result being cellulitis, local inflammation, abscess formation, or (uncommonly) tetanus. Occasionally, the adult worm does not emerge but becomes encapsulated and calcified.

DIAGNOSIS The diagnosis is based on the findings developing with the emergence of the adult worm, as described above.

℞ TREATMENT

Gradual extraction of the worm by winding of a few centimeters on a stick each day remains the common and effective practice. Worms may be excised surgically. The administration of thiabendazole (25 mg/kg twice daily for 3 days) or metronidazole (250 mg three times daily for 10 days) may relieve symptoms but has no proven activity against the worm.

PREVENTION Prevention, which remains the only real control measure, depends on the provision of safe drinking water.

ZOONOTIC FILARIAL INFECTIONS

Dirofilariae that affect primarily dogs, cats, and raccoons and *Brugia* parasites that affect small mammals occasionally infect humans incidentally. Because humans are an abnormal host, the parasites never develop fully. Pulmonary dirofilarial infection caused by the canine heartworm *Dirofilaria immitis* generally presents in humans as a solitary pulmonary nodule. Chest pain, hemoptysis, and cough are uncommon. Infections with *Dirofilaria repens* (from dogs) or *Dirofilaria tenuis* (from raccoons) can cause local subcutaneous nodules in humans. Zoonotic *Brugia* infection can produce isolated lymph node enlargement. Eosinophilia levels and antifilarial antibody titers are not commonly elevated. Excisional biopsy is both diagnostic and curative; these infections usually do not respond to chemotherapy.

BIBLIOGRAPHY

ADOLPH PE et al: Diagnosis and treatment of *Acanthocheilonema perstans* filariasis. Am J Trop Med Hyg 11:76, 1962

AMARAL F et al: Live adult worms detected by ultrasonography in human bancroftian filariasis. Am J Trop Med Hyg 50:753, 1994

CENTERS FOR DISEASE CONTROL AND PREVENTION: Progress toward global eradication of dracunculiasis. Morb Mort Week Rep 44:875, 1995

EBERHARD ML, LAMMIE PJ: Laboratory diagnosis of filariasis. Clin Lab Med 11:977, 1991

FREEDMAN DO et al: Lymphoscintigraphic analysis of lymphatic abnormalities in symptomatic and asymptomatic human filariasis. J Infect Dis 170:927, 1994

KLION AD et al: Loiasis in endemic and non-endemic populations: Immunologically mediated differences in clinical presentation. J Infect Dis 163:1318, 1991

MARINKELLE CJ, GERMAN E: Mansonelliasis in the Comisaria del Vaupes of Colombia. Trop Geogr Med 22:101, 1970

MEYERS WM et al: Human streptocerciasis: A clinicopathologic study of 40 Africans (Zairians) including identification of the adult filaria. Am J Trop Med Hyg 21:528, 1972

OTTESEN EA: Filarial infections. Infect Dis Clin North Am 7:619, 1993

———, NUTMAN TB: Tropical pulmonary eosinophilia. Annu Rev Med 43:417, 1992

RO JY et al: Pulmonary dirofilariasis: The great imitator of primary or metastatic lung tumor. A clinicopathologic analysis of seven cases and a review of the literature. Hum Pathol 20:69, 1989

WHO EXPERT COMMITTEE ON FILARIASIS: Lymphatic filariasis: Diagnosis and pathogenesis. Bull WHO 71(2):135, 1993

WHO EXPERT COMMITTEE ON ONCHOCERCIASIS: Onchocerciasis and its control: Fourth report. Technical Report Series No. 852, Geneva, WHO, 1995

SCHISTOSOMIASIS AND OTHER TREMATODE INFECTIONS

The trematodes (flukes) that commonly infect humans live in the intestines, biliary tract, lungs, and venules of the intestines or genitourinary tract. Except in the case of the intestinal schistosomes, which cause a unique type of liver fibrosis, disease is limited primarily to the organs where the parasites reside. The pathophysiology of disease differs among the trematodes. Schistosomiasis is the best understood, and some of the factors important in disease development in this infection appear to apply to infections caused by many of the other trematodes. In endemic areas, large proportions of the population are infected but asymptomatic; the disease is mostly limited to heavily infected persons. Distinct acute and chronic syndromes are recognizable, as are predictable pathologic changes over time. Eosinophilia and fever are common findings in acute disease. Because many of these parasites follow complicated migration routes and/or are poorly adapted to survival in a human host, infections in ectopic locations are an important cause of morbidity.

LIFE CYCLE AND EPIDEMIOLOGY Infections in humans are limited to digenetic trematodes—i.e., those that reproduce sexually and produce eggs in mammalian definitive hosts and reproduce asexually in snails. After eggs reach water, they either hatch immediately or mature before releasing a free-swimming *miracidium*, which seeks out the appropriate intermediate snail host or is ingested by the snail. After a number of cycles of multiplication in the snail, free-swimming *cercariae* are released and, depending on the species, can (1) infect the definitive host; (2) seek out a second intermediate host, such as a fish or crustacean; or (3) encyst on vegetation. The encysted cercaria, or *metacercaria*, is a dormant, relatively resistant form that infects the host following ingestion. With the exception of schistosomes, most trematodes are flat, leaf-shaped parasites that vary in length from 1 mm to 7 cm. They possess two grasping organs called *suckers* and lack a body cavity. The gut usually lacks an anus, and digested food is regurgitated through the oral opening. The surfaces of trematodes are covered by a syncytium of cells, or tegument, through which nutrients are absorbed.

Schistosomes differ in a number of important ways from the other trematodes that infect humans. Most trematodes are hermaphroditic, but the sexes are separate in the schistosomes, and completion of the sexual cycle requires the presence of male and female worms. The adult schistosomes reside in the bloodstream, whereas the other trematodes dwell in the liver, lung, or intestines. In schistosomiasis, humans are infected by free-swimming cercariae that invade the skin; in contrast, in the other trematode infections, humans are infected after ingestion. The eggs of hermaphroditic trematodes possess a characteristic operculum, or caplike structure. The morphology of schistosome ova differs from that of other trematode ova, as described below.

A large number of trematodes can infect humans. With the exception of some species of schistosomes, most trematodes have domestic or wild animals as definitive hosts, and humans are accidentally infected. In highly endemic situations or under particularly advantageous circumstances, humans are able to maintain the life cycle in the absence of the usual definitive host. Some infections are rare or occur in populations in limited geographic areas, while others affect large numbers of persons over extensive areas or produce recognizable syndromes.

DIAGNOSIS A pertinent history is important in the diagnosis of trematode infections. Persons from endemic areas; travelers who are exposed to fresh water or who ingest undercooked fish, crustacea, or potentially contaminated vegetation; and others who ingest locally obtained but potentially contaminated vegetation such as watercress or undercooked, pickled, or smoked fish can be infected. Eosinophilia is common in acute invasive trematode infections. The definitive diagnosis is established by the demonstration of eggs in stool or sputum or by biopsy of the affected tissue. Serologic tests are available for

schistosomiasis, fascioliasis, and paragonimiasis; a positive test is indicative of infection. Serologic tests for other trematode infections may be available in endemic areas or research laboratories.

℞ TREATMENT

Since disease is associated primarily with heavy trematode infection, one of the goals of therapy is to reduce the worm burden to below the level associated with disease. This goal is particularly pertinent in the treatment and prevention of disease in large populations. A number of studies of schistosomiasis and liver fluke infection have demonstrated that treatment does in fact lower the intensity of infection (which is roughly reflected by the number of ova excreted) and result in a marked decrease in disease prevalence. On occasion, a small number of parasites can cause significant disease either by lodging in a strategic location in the tissue that is normally involved (e.g., in the ureter for *Schistosoma haematobium*) or by localizing ectopically [e.g., in the central nervous system (CNS) for *Schistoma* and *Paragonimus*]. Since these complications do not appear to be related to the intensity of infection, elimination of every parasite is a reasonable goal. The pathophysiology of other complications, such as bladder cancer in *S. haematobium* infections and cholangiocarcinoma in liver fluke infections, is unclear; thus, complete elimination of the infection is appropriate. In short, the goals of treatment depend on the person or population involved and the risk of subsequent disease.

Praziquantel is the drug of choice for the treatment of most trematode infections except fascioliasis. Although less costly, other available therapies are inconvenient, have greater side effects, or are experimental. The efficacy of treatment is assessed in most instances by the disappearance of viable ova and/or by the improvement of relevant clinical parameters. Assessment should take place after enough time has passed for ova to have cleared from the tissues or excreta and after damaged worms that were not killed have had a chance to recover, but before reinfection has occurred. Low-level residual infections are not uncommon; patients with such infections can be re-treated if necessary.

SCHISTOSOMIASIS

Three major schistosome species—*Schistosoma mansoni*, *S. haematobium*, and *Schistosoma japonicum*—and a number of less prevalent species infect humans. Both *S. mansoni* and *S. japonicum* adults reside in the venules of the intestine, and the major disease manifestations of these parasites are hepatic. *S. mansoni* is found in parts of South America (Brazil, Venezuela, and Surinam), some Caribbean islands, Africa, and the Middle East, while infections with *S. japonicum* occur in the Far East, mostly in China and the Philippines. *S. haematobium* adults are found mostly in the venules of the urinary tract and cause lesions primarily of the ureters and bladder. Infections with this species occur in Africa and the Middle East. Of lesser importance are *Schistosoma mekongi*, a parasite related to *S. japonicum* that is found along the Mekong River in Indochina, and *Schistosoma intercalatum*, a species found in certain areas of central West Africa. Worldwide, as many as 200 million persons may be infected with schistosomes, and infection of entire communities is common. However, most infected persons experience few or no signs and symptoms, and only a small minority develop significant disease.

LIFE CYCLE The schistosome species infecting humans all share the same basic life cycle but are unique in ways that account for some of the variation in clinical and pathologic findings. Important differences include the length of time before egg laying begins (prepatent period), the location of the adult worms, the number of eggs produced by each pair of worms, the response by the host to the ova, and the eventual fate of retained eggs. The morphology of the parasites and the types of intermediate host snail are also distinct.

Humans become infected after contact with water containing the infective stage of the parasite, which is called a *cercaria*; this microscopic form possesses a forked tail, used for swimming, and a head, which is the anlage of the worm. With the help of secreted enzymes, cercariae penetrate the unbroken skin and transform into *schistosomules*, or developing schistosomes. After 2 to 3 days, the schistosomules migrate to the lungs and then to the portal vein, probably by an intravascular route. In the portal vein, the maturing male and female schistosomes pair. They then migrate to the venules of the mesentery, bladder, or ureters (depending on the species of schistosome), and begin to deposit eggs. The time spent in migration and maturation differs. *S. mansoni* and *S. japonicum* begin depositing eggs around 4 to 5 weeks after infection, while egg deposition begins after 2 to 3 months for *S. haematobium*. Adult worms are about 1 to 2 cm long and migrate in the blood vessels without eliciting a local inflammatory reaction. Adult worms do not multiply in humans, and immunosuppressive therapy does not result in increased numbers of worms.

Once released, eggs are either retained in the tissues at the site of deposition or swept back, mostly to the liver. In the case of the intestinal schistosomes, this transport occurs via the venous portal system. Eggs are deposited mainly in the bladder and ureters by *S. haematobium*. Some of the mature schistosome ova are extruded into the lumen of the intestines, bladder, or ureters. After contact with water they hatch, releasing a miracidium. This free-swimming ciliated stage seeks out the proper intermediate snail vector and burrows into its soft tissues. After 1 to 2 months (depending on the species), the miracidium develops into a primary and then a secondary sporocyst, which, after further development, begins releasing cercariae into the surrounding water. Thousands of cercariae can be released daily from each infected snail. Therefore, one miracidium produces many cercariae, and this arrangement amplifies the number of infective parasites and the risk of infection. Cercariae are most infectious immediately after shedding and are no longer viable 48 h after release, so storage of water for 48 h before contact prevents exposure and infection.

Unlike most other trematodes, schistosomes are of two sexes, but this characteristic is evident only in the adult stage. Ova are laid only when males and females infect the same individual.

PATHOPHYSIOLOGY   A number of factors govern the disease manifestations of schistosomiasis. These include the duration and intensity of infection, the location of egg deposition, host genetics, concurrent infections, and other still undefined factors.

In individuals from endemic areas, initial infection goes unnoticed. There are a number of possible reasons for the lack of symptoms, including age at initial exposure; manner of exposure; and transfer of antigens, antibodies, and anti-idiotypes from the mother to the fetus. In contrast, in visitors to endemic areas, initial infection with schistosomes commonly results in an acute febrile illness (Katayama fever, or acute schistosomiasis), which most likely is a manifestation of the immune response to the developing schistosomes and eggs. These individuals mount a vigorous hypersensitivity response that becomes modulated; they develop elevated levels of eosinophils and immune complexes; and they display a marked reaction to schistosome antigens, which may be measured by lymphocyte blastogenesis. Despite ongoing infection, symptoms subside, as do blastogenic responses to schistosome antigens but not to unrelated antigens such as purified protein derivative of tuberculin. The exudative acute granulomatous response to schistosome eggs is also modulated.

A major factor in the development of disease in humans is the worm burden of the host, which determines the number of eggs produced. The inflammatory and fibrotic response to these eggs accounts for most of the morbidity and mortality associated with schistosomiasis. Factors that limit the survival of the parasite will also limit the development of disease. Immunity exists in experimental animals. In human schistosome infections, protective immunity also is thought to develop, because reinfection rates are reduced in previously treated adults despite continuing water contact. In the first few days after infection, the schistosomule is relatively susceptible to immune attack. A number of systems employing antibody and/or eosinophils, neutrophils, macro-

phages, and complement have been used to kill schistosomules in vitro. However, as the schistosomules mature, they become refractory to these immune responses. In addition, schistosomes coat their tegument with host proteins and evade recognition by the host. Antibodies that block effective killing also may enhance parasite survival. Schistosomule and adult worm antigens have been defined in the hope of developing vaccines; the administration of murine monoclonal antibodies to some of these antigens has reduced worm burdens in challenge infections by about 50 percent, and immunization of rodents with a number of defined antigens has produced similar levels of protection. Successful vaccination with anti-idiotypes also has been reported.

Schistosome eggs elicit a granulomatous response that is best understood in *S. mansoni* infections. The host becomes sensitized to the egg proteins by a T cell–mediated mechanism that induces a larger granuloma. However, with continued infection, the granuloma decreases in size. The mechanisms involved in the induction of granulomas, the immune sensitization that results in an increase in granuloma size, and the immune modulation that leads to a decrease in granuloma size are areas of intense investigation. Studies suggest that granulomatous responses to *S. mansoni* eggs are T_H2-dependent. Administration of interleukin 12—a potent stimulator of the T_H1 response and suppressor of the T_H2 response—at the same time as egg sensitization significantly reduces granuloma formation and subsequent egg-induced fibrosis after challenge infection by replacing the usually predominant T_H2 response to *S. mansoni* eggs with a T_H1 response. This approach offers the promise of controlling disease manifestations by preventing the potentially harmful inflammatory and fibrotic response to eggs. Serum factors, including the anti-idiotypic network, also modulate immune responses. The regulation of granulomas due to *S. japonicum* eggs differs from that of granulomas from *S. mansoni* eggs.

Both eggs and granulomas release factors that induce fibroblast proliferation in vitro. The early cellular response induced by granulomas is followed by fibrosis in vivo; however, liver fibrosis in humans probably involves more than simple fusion of fibrotic granulomas. After years of continued infection, some heavily infected individuals develop end-stage fibrotic lesions, mainly portal fibrosis (Symmers' fibrosis); esophageal varices and splenomegaly often follow in *S. mansoni*, *S. japonicum*, and *S. mekongi* infections, and fibrosis of the ureters and bladder frequently follows in *S. haematobium* infections. After the development of portal fibrosis, eggs are shunted to the lungs via portal-systemic collateral veins, resulting in cor pulmonale in about 15 percent of patients with Symmers' fibrosis. Immune complexes shunted to the systemic circulation cause glomerulonephritis.

Host genetic factors have been found to influence the development of Symmers' fibrosis, although there is no general agreement as to which are important. Moreover, even schistosomes of the same species are genetically diverse, as has been shown by endonuclease restriction analysis, but the effect of this diversity on disease in humans is unknown.

CLINICAL SYNDROMES (See Table 224-1)   **Acute Schistosomiasis**   Acute schistosomiasis, or Katayama fever, follows initial exposure and infection with *S. mansoni* or *S. japonicum*. It rarely follows infection with *S. haematobium*. Acute schistosomiasis is seldom recognized in endemic populations but rather is noted primarily in visitors to endemic areas. Immediately after exposure, patients frequently complain of intense transient itching. From 2 to 6 weeks or longer after exposure, the patient may complain of a variety of symptoms, including fever, chills, headache, hives or angioedema, weakness, weight loss, nonproductive cough, abdominal pain, and diarrhea. Sometimes symptoms abate but return with increased intensity about the time egg laying commences. These symptoms gradually diminish but may last as long as 2 to 3 months. Other newly infected individuals may be asymptomatic or have only minimal symptoms. In these individuals, the diagnosis is established only after further evaluation prompted by suggestive laboratory test results or exposure history. More severe symptoms occur with heavier infections, but light infections may cause severe illness. CNS lesions may develop during acute schistosome infection. The diagnosis of acute schistosomiasis is suggested by the clinical findings and the presence of eosinophilia,

Clinical Manifestations of Disease due to Various *Schistosoma* Species*

Manifestation	S. mansoni	S. japonicum	S. haematobium
Acute toxemic schistosomiasis	+	+	+
Chronic asymptomatic schistosomiasis	+	+	+
Hepatosplenic schistosomiasis	+	+	0
Cor pulmonale	+	+	±
Glomerulonephritis (clinically significant)	+	+	0†
Colonic polyposis	+	+	±
Ectopic lesions			
Brain	±	+	±
Spinal cord	+	±	+
Skin	+	+	+
Chronic cystitis and ureteritis	0	0	+
Mass lesions, bladder and ureters	0	0	+
Bladder cancer	0	0	+
Association with *Salmonella*	+	+	+
Prolonged fever	+	+	+
Urinary carrier state	?	?	+
Swimmers' itch‡	+	+	+

* +, recognized complications of infections by this species; ±, findings much less prominent in individuals infected by this species; 0, complications not present in infections by this species.
† Except with associated *Salmonella* infections.
‡ Usually from schistosomes that do not infect humans.

with values sometimes greater than 50 percent. Leukocytosis, increased levels of immune complexes, and elevated concentrations of IgM, IgG, and IgE are found commonly. Although it has been suggested that immune complexes play a role in the pathophysiology of acute schistosomiasis, glomerulonephritis and vasculitis have not been reported. The specific diagnosis can be established, even before the shedding of ova, by the detection of antibodies to adult schistosome gut antigens or, after egg excretion (5 to 6 weeks after exposure), by appropriate serologic testing and the finding of eggs in the stool or a rectal biopsy sample. Clinically, acute schistosomiasis is frequently misdiagnosed as typhoid fever; in fact, it can be confused with any prolonged febrile illness. Although patients seem to tolerate chemotherapy well, it is unclear whether therapy shortens the course of disease or decreases symptoms. Glucocorticoids may be useful, but their usefulness has not been demonstrated in controlled studies.

Liver Fibrosis   The most important complication of intestinal schistosome infection is the development of periportal or Symmers' fibrosis and portal hypertension (hepatosplenic schistosomiasis). This finding is pathognomonic in *S. mansoni*, *S. japonicum*, and *S. mekongi* infections, but it has been studied best in *S. mansoni* infections, where it normally develops after 10 to 15 years of prolonged exposure and infection. The liver may be enlarged, although in many cases it is small, firm, and nodular, and the left lobe is characteristically prominent. Macroscopic examination shows finger-sized bands of fibrosis ("pipestem" fibrosis) encompassing the large portal tracts. The portal venous tracts are replaced with fibrous tissue; this situation sometimes leads to presinusoidal blockage, portal hypertension, splenomegaly, and esophageal and gastric varices. The intrahepatic pressure is normal. Hepatic function is generally well preserved, and patients commonly present with hematemesis and/or signs and symptoms of splenomegaly. Ascites, hepatic coma, edema, spider angiomas, gynecomastia, and other signs of liver failure occur less frequently than in alcoholic and postnecrotic cirrhosis. Despite repeated episodes of hematemesis, patients may do reasonably well.

In the past, the diagnosis of periportal fibrosis required a wedge biopsy of the liver; needle biopsy specimens are frequently inadequate. Ultrasonograms of the liver show characteristic findings. The fibrotic bands appear as dense echogenic areas surrounding the portal vein and its tributaries. Studies comparing the effectiveness of wedge biopsy of the liver with ultrasonographic examination showed the latter technique to have both a specificity and a sensitivity of 100 percent. Ultrasonography should replace invasive biopsies as the method of choice for the diagnosis of hepatic schistosomiasis.

Ultrasonographic evaluation of *S. mansoni*–infected populations in the Sudan revealed a much higher prevalence of periportal fibrosis than could be identified by physical examination. As many as half the patients studied lacked palpable splenomegaly, and a majority did not give a history of hematemesis. Treatment resulted in regression of periportal fibrosis in some cases.

Patients with periportal fibrosis may not have schistosome eggs in the feces because of previous treatment and/or attrition of adult worms without subsequent reinfection. Since schistosome infections are practically universal in many populations, the mere presence of schistosome eggs in the feces does not establish the diagnosis of schistosomal periportal fibrosis; other liver diseases may be present. It is not clear whether splenectomy or shunting procedures, although used commonly, are beneficial. Mortality among patients with portal fibrosis has not been well studied, but in one group the rate was 8.2 percent after 3.6 years.

Glomerulonephritis and Pulmonary Hypertension   These two complications develop almost exclusively in patients with periportal fibrosis and portal hypertension. Pulmonary hypertension appears to be due to obliteration of pulmonary arterioles by granulomatous inflammation induced by shunted and embolized schistosome eggs. This condition is most frequently recognized with *S. mansoni* and *S. japonicum* infections but is also seen with *S. haematobium*. The association of glomerulonephritis and schistosomiasis has been noted in humans and in experimentally infected animals. This complication is manifested clinically as proteinuria and/or renal failure. Schistosome-specific antibodies and antigens have been detected in the glomeruli of infected patients.

Other Complications   Focal dense deposits of eggs of *S. mansoni* in the large intestine (and less commonly of *S. haematobium* and probably of *S. japonicum*) incite an exudative granulomatous response resulting in the formation of inflammatory polyps. Histologic study reveals that these polyps consist of masses of eggs, inflammatory cells, and fibrotic tissue. The major clinical presentation is bloody diarrhea, sometimes associated with protein-losing enteropathy and anemia. This type of involvement of the bowel is recognized primarily in Egypt and the Sudan. Gastrointestinal symptoms are not greater in most chronically infected patients than in control populations, although blood in the stool has been found more frequently in chronic infection in some studies. Granulomatous masses involving the bowel wall may mimic carcinoma of the bowel. With regard to CNS involvement, *S. mansoni* and *S. haematobium* show a predilection for the spinal cord, while the brain is involved more commonly in *S. japonicum* infections. An increased incidence of brain and/or spinal cord involvement has been noted in foreign visitors infected with *S. haematobium* via contact with water from Lake Malawi in southeastern Africa.

Patients infected with the three major species of schistosomes and subsequently infected with *Salmonella* may develop a prolonged intermittent febrile illness. In *S. haematobium* infections, prolonged excretion of *Salmonella* in the urine is common. In many cases, treatment of the *Salmonella* infection alone is not effective, and specific antischistosomal chemotherapy is also required. *Salmonella* may be protected from host immune responses by residence in the schistosome gut or by adherence to the surface of the schistosome.

SCHISTOSOMA MANSONI   **Epidemiology and Manifestations**   *S. mansoni* is found in South America, in certain Caribbean islands, in Africa, and in the Middle East. The prepatent period is about 4 to 5 weeks. The intermediate hosts are various species in the genus *Biomphalaria*.

Although infection is frequent and sometimes universal in endemic areas, the development of disease is relatively uncommon and depends on a number of factors, including the duration and intensity of infection. In endemic populations, chronic infections are usual, often lasting for decades, and disease manifestations develop in a predictable manner. For the most part, the initial infection of persons living in endemic areas goes unnoticed. Throughout the first decade of life, the intensity of infection—as measured by the number of eggs excreted in the feces—increases in endemic populations, and prevalence rates in this age group often approach 100 percent in highly endemic communities. Few, if any, symptoms are attributable to schistosomiasis during this time. The liver, particularly the left lobe, gradually enlarges and becomes firm. Between 10 and 15 years of age, some heavily infected persons develop splenomegaly, which partly reflects the presence of portal fibrosis and portal hypertension. At about the same time, the number of eggs in the feces decreases; there is evidence to suggest that immune factors as well as decreased water contact are responsible. During the next three decades of life, persons with portal fibrosis and hypertension may experience repeated bouts of hematemesis secondary to esophageal varices or symptoms secondary to a massively enlarged spleen. Because of prior chemotherapy, decreased exposure, or increased host immunity, it is not uncommon for patients with end-stage portal fibrosis to no longer excrete eggs. Adult schistosomes can survive for 20 years or more in the human host but usually live for 5 to 8 years. The prognosis and the potential for reversing complications of infection after appropriate chemotherapy depend on the stage of disease. Ultrasound examination indicates that some regression of periportal fibrosis follows chemotherapy, but in most individuals with advanced periportal fibrosis and clinical manifestations, regression does not occur. Glomerulonephritis and cor pulmonale secondary to schistosomiasis develop exclusively in patients with portal fibrosis. The CNS can become involved at any stage, whatever the intensity of infection.

Diagnosis The diagnosis of *S. mansoni* infection is established by identification of ova in the feces or tissues. The ova are 114 to 175 μm in length and 45 to 68 μm in width and have a prominent lateral spine. In light infections with fewer than 50 eggs per gram of feces, ova may not be detected in the stool without the use of techniques that sample large volumes. Even in light infections, ova can usually be detected in rectal biopsy specimens and are best identified by squashing a small amount of tissue between two glass slides and viewing the tissue microscopically.

Many serologic tests have been employed in the diagnosis of schistosomiasis. These tests are not standardized and differ in sensitivity and specificity. Most current tests have greater than 90 percent sensitivity, and a positive serologic test result is indicative of a present or past infection. An immunofluorescent antibody test employing sections of adult schistosomes to assess the presence of antibodies to schistosome gut antigens has been extremely useful in identifying recently infected persons or those with acute schistosomiasis. Recently, antigen detection assays have been developed that appear to be useful in diagnosing infections and determining treatment response.

℞ TREATMENT

Because drugs used to treat schistosomiasis are relatively safe and effective, most persons with active infections should be treated. These patients carry live eggs that can be identified by microscopy (by an experienced parasitologist), by the presence of flame cells, or by the ability of the eggs to hatch after contact with water. In the past, because of the toxicity of older treatment regimens, chemotherapy was offered only to relatively heavily infected individuals, who were more likely to develop disease than those less intensely infected. However, even in light infections, there is the risk that complications will arise from ectopic location of the schistosome eggs (e.g., in the spinal cord). Relatively few ova may be excreted in schistosomiasis, and their detection therefore may not be easy. Infection may be suggested by a positive result in a serologic test. Because treatment of lightly infected persons with praziquantel is associated with few signs and symptoms, such treatment may be warranted if active infection is likely or cannot be reasonably ruled out. The effectiveness of treatment is evaluated by the cessation of egg excretion after 2 to 3 months. Some types of serologic tests revert to negative after treatment, but these tests are technically difficult to perform and are not generally available. Successful treatment is associated with a reduction of organomegaly and of periportal fibrosis and/or inflammation in some patients. These patients tend to be young people with less severe involvement.

Although a number of drugs are available for the treatment of *S. mansoni* infection, praziquantel and oxamniquine are the drugs of choice (Table 224-2). The two drugs are equally safe and effective in *S. mansoni* infections found in the Caribbean and South America. Because some strains of *S. mansoni* in Africa are relatively resistant to oxamniquine, praziquantel is the better drug. Both drugs can be used in patients with portal fibrosis. The side effects of praziquantel and oxamniquine are frequent but transient and mild. In the author's experience, many of the troublesome side effects associated with praziquantel treatment are the result of the host's response to the injured parasites or ova. Since the worms reside mostly in the intestines, these adverse effects are primarily intestinal and include abdominal pain, lethargy, diarrhea, and fever. In contrast, use of the same drug in the treatment of cysticercosis, in which the worms commonly reside in the CNS, causes symptoms related to the brain. The side effects of oxamniquine include dizziness, tiredness, nausea and vomiting, neuropsychiatric manifestations, and (in rare instances) convulsions.

***SCHISTOSOMA JAPONICUM* Epidemiology and Clinical Manifestations** *S. japonicum* is found in Southeast Asia and is an important health concern in areas of China and the Philippines. The intermediate hosts are amphibious snails of the genus *Oncomelania*. Besides humans, numerous other mammals, such as cattle and water

Table 224-2

Treatment of Schistosomiasis

Species	Drug	Total Dose* (mg/kg of Body Weight)	Regimen
S. haematobium	Praziquantel	40	Single dose or two doses of 20 mg/kg
	Metrifonate†	22.5–30	Single dose of 7.5 to 10 mg/kg given every other week × 3
S. mansoni			
Americas and Caribbean	Oxamniquine	15	Single dose with food
	Praziquantel	40	Single dose or two doses of 20 mg/kg 4 h apart with food
Africa and Middle East	Oxamniquine	60	15 mg/kg twice a day for 2 days with food
	Praziquantel	40	Single dose or two doses of 20 mg/kg 4 h apart with food
S. japonicum or S. mekongi	Praziquantel	60	20 mg/kg every 4 h with food

* All recommended drugs are given orally.
† Available from the Parasitic Diseases Division, Center for Infectious Diseases, Centers for Disease Control and Prevention, Atlanta, GA 30333.

buffalo, are naturally infected and serve as reservoirs of infection. The prepatent period is about 4 weeks.

The course of infection and clinical manifestations for *S. japonicum* are similar to those for *S. mansoni*, but the epidemiology and disease manifestations have been less well studied. Experimental infections with *S. japonicum* are more virulent than those with *S. mansoni*, probably because each *S. japonicum* worm pair produces 10 times as many eggs as each *S. mansoni* worm pair. The granulomas contain clusters of eggs, are larger than those caused by *S. mansoni*, and frequently show central necrosis. As in *S. mansoni* infections, periportal fibrosis is the major clinical manifestation. The other clinical syndromes described in *S. mansoni* infection also occur as complications of *S. japonicum* infection. However, there are some notable differences in disease manifestations, particularly CNS involvement. In acute schistosomiasis associated with *S. japonicum* infections, about 2 to 3 percent of patients experience CNS symptoms and signs that mimic acute encephalitis or a focal neurologic process. Computed tomography shows multiple enhancing lesions. In chronic infections, patients may present with focal lesions of the brain that mimic brain tumors. These lesions contain masses of eggs and granulomas. Uncontrolled studies suggest that treatment with antischistosomal drugs and glucocorticoids is effective.

Diagnosis The principles of diagnosis are similar to those used in *S. mansoni* infection and require the demonstration of the typical ova in the tissues or feces of infected individuals. The eggs are oval in shape, measure 70 to 100 μm by 50 to 65 μm, and have a vestigial spine. Old, calcified, dead eggs are commonly retained in the tissues for long periods and do not indicate active infection. Computed tomography shows a characteristic pattern of calcified eggs in the liver and intestine.

℞ TREATMENT

Most infected persons should be treated. The only safe and effective therapy for *S. japonicum* infections is praziquantel (see Table 224-2).

SCHISTOSOMA MEKONGI *S. mekongi* occurs in the Mekong River in Indochina (Laos, Cambodia, and Thailand). The intermediate host is an aquatic snail, *Tricula aperta*. The eggs are similar to those of *S. japonicum* but are slightly smaller (about 56 by 64 μm) and round. Dogs and human beings frequently are naturally infected. The prepatent period is about 5 weeks. The disease manifestations appear to be similar to those for *S. japonicum* but have not been fully documented. Praziquantel is effective therapy for this infection (see Table 224-2).

SCHISTOSOMA HAEMATOBIUM **Epidemiology and Clinical Manifestations** *S. haematobium* infections occur in extensive areas of Africa and in the Middle East. The intermediate hosts are of the genus *Bulinus*. The prepatent period is 2 to 3 months. Natural infection is primarily limited to human beings.

As in *S. mansoni* infection, the prevalence and intensity of *S. haematobium* infection among persons in endemic areas increase until 10 to 15 years of age. Thereafter, the intensity decreases markedly, while the prevalence rate falls moderately. Owing to the predilection of *S. haematobium* for the veins of the urinary tract, the signs and symptoms caused by the organism result from involvement of the ureters and bladder. In contrast to the asymptomatic period following initial infection with the intestinal schistosomes, dysuria and hematuria are frequently noted 2 to 3 months after *S. haematobium* infection. These findings may continue throughout the course of active infection. Initially, the eggs evoke an intense inflammatory and granulomatous response, which may cause anatomic and/or functional obstruction, hydroureter and hydronephrosis, and masses in the bladder or ureters. Cystoscopic examination may reveal friable masses extending into the bladder, ulceration, petechiae, and granulomas. These early lesions are reversible by antischistosomal chemotherapy. Eggs shed into the urine are usually easily demonstrable. As the infection progresses, the inflammatory component lessens, possibly owing to a modulating effect of the host's immune response, and fibrosis increases, most likely owing to the accumulation of many old and some new lesions. Later, most lesions consist of masses of dead and calcified eggs in fibrous tissue. When the concentration of calcified eggs in the tissues is high enough, radiographic opacification of the affected areas of the urinary tract becomes evident. Fibrotic lesions that cause hydroureter and hydronephrosis are not reversible by antischistosomal chemotherapy. Renal failure occurs in a surprisingly small proportion of infected individuals.

Portal fibrosis and clinically significant glomerulonephritis are not complications of this infection, but passage of eggs into the lungs may result in pulmonary hypertension. Prolonged excretion of *Salmonella* in the urine and intermittent bacteremia are well documented. Urinary tract infections with other bacteria do not appear to be increased in frequency unless there is instrumentation of the urinary tract; however, they may be difficult to eradicate once established. CNS infection most commonly involves the spinal cord, as in *S. mansoni* infections. Although eggs of *S. haematobium* are frequently detected in the feces in low numbers and are often found in rectal biopsy specimens, intestinal polyposis is uncommon. In certain geographic areas, squamous cell cancer of the bladder is thought to be associated with *S. haematobium* infection and is a significant cause of morbidity and mortality.

Diagnosis The diagnosis of *S. haematobium* infection is established by demonstration of the characteristic eggs in the tissues or urine. These eggs measure 112 to 170 μm by 40 to 70 μm, have a prominent terminal spine, and are easily seen in the urine. An increased number of eggs is excreted around midday, and microscopic examination of a centrifuged urine specimen collected at this time usually reveals ova. In light infections, examination of increased volumes of urine is sometimes required. Gross or microscopic hematuria is common in endemic populations, and its presence always suggests the diagnosis in exposed individuals. Antibodies to *S. haematobium* can be detected with *S. mansoni* antigen preparations. Ultrasonographic examinations reveal anatomic alteration of the genitourinary tract.

℞ TREATMENT

Infected persons should be treated. Dead and calcified eggs are common in tissue, are often seen in urine specimens, and should be differentiated from viable eggs. Although a number of drugs have been used to treat *S. haematobium* infection, praziquantel is the treatment of choice (see Table 224-2). Metrifonate—a safe, orally administered agent—is also effective. Its major advantage is low cost, and its major disadvantage is that, to cure infection, it needs to be given in three doses 2 weeks apart.

SCHISTOSOMA INTERCALATUM *S. intercalatum* infection is limited to areas of West Africa. Eggs (140 to 240 μm by 50 to 85 μm) are found in the stool and have a terminal spine. Few symptoms are attributable to this infection, and no cases of portal fibrosis have been reported. Praziquantel is effective for treatment.

SCHISTOSOME DERMATITIS (SWIMMERS' ITCH) When cercariae penetrate the skin, they may provoke a reaction known as *schistosome dermatitis*. Symptoms develop most commonly after penetration by schistosomes that ordinarily infect birds or mammals other than humans. In previously unexposed persons, the initial invasion causes transient itching and occasionally urticaria followed by the development of macules within 24 h and papules after 24 h. Following repeated exposures, the signs and symptoms increase dramatically and occur earlier. Large, pruritic, erythematous papules and (uncommonly) vesicles develop within 24 h. The lesions are most intense 2 to 3 days following exposure and subside after a few days. These lesions represent a delayed hypersensitivity reaction to the invading schistosome. Nonhuman schistosomes do not develop fully in humans, and the signs and symptoms are limited to the skin. A similar dermatitis follows infection with human schistosomes.

Schistosome dermatitis develops after exposure to fresh water in many areas of the world but is particularly common in the north-central and western United States. Dermatitis following seawater exposure (clam diggers' itch) also has been described.

Treatment is based on symptoms. Since cercariae need some time to invade the skin (15 min or less), rapid removal of cercaria-containing droplets after water contact will decrease the intensity of exposure. Limiting the numbers of the intermediate host snail in areas frequented by humans can effectively control exposure.

CONTROL OF SCHISTOSOMIASIS Theoretically, schistosome infections can be controlled by a variety of methods, but the application of these control techniques has generally been only partially successful. Simple and effective health-education measures, such as the elimination of indiscriminate urination and defecation, are difficult to implement in endemic areas. The intermediate molluscan host can be eliminated by the use of molluscicides or the destruction of its habitat. Both methods require dedication of resources and personnel that often are not readily available. Mass chemotherapy of populations has been tried; the need for repeated treatments depends on the degree of reinfection. Some authorities advocate the treatment of persons likely to develop serious disease (e.g., those heavily infected). The methods employed will depend on the nature of the endemic area and the resources available.

OTHER TREMATODES

BILIARY DUCT–DWELLING TREMATODES: *CLONORCHIS SINENSIS, OPISTHORCHIS VIVERRINI, AND OPISTHORCHIS FELINEUS* These closely related trematodes commonly infect the human biliary system, have similar life cycles and routes of infection, appear to have similar pathophysiology and disease manifestations, and produce similar eggs. They are responsible for symptoms and signs related to obstruction of the biliary tract or pancreatic duct and are associated with an increased risk of cholangiocarcinoma. *C. sinensis* is endemic in China, Taiwan, Korea, Japan, and Vietnam; *O. viverrini* is found in Laos and Thailand; and *O. felineus* is found in parts of eastern Europe and the former U.S.S.R.

Life Cycle Humans become infected after ingesting metacercariae in poorly cooked, pickled, or smoked fish. The metacercariae excyst in the small intestine and migrate through the ampulla of Vater into the biliary ducts, where they mature in 3 to 4 weeks. Worms are 7 to 20 mm by 1.5 to 3 mm (depending on the species) and may live for 20 to 25 years (*C. sinensis*).

Pathophysiology Disease manifestations (mostly described for *O. viverrini* and *C. sinensis*) depend on the duration of infection, worm burden, and location of the parasites. Flukes reside mostly in small to medium-sized biliary ducts but at times are also found in the larger biliary ducts as well as the gallbladder. They do not invade the parenchyma of the liver, and most disease manifestations reflect direct or indirect effects of the adult trematodes on the biliary ducts. Their presence leads to adenomatous hyperplasia and varying amounts of periductal inflammation followed by periductal fibrosis. Diffuse and localized dilation of ducts due to obstruction by worms, stones, or strictures is frequently found. Remnants of parasites have been found in biliary stones. The number of persons with disease in a given population increases with the worm burden (thousands of flukes in heavy infections), and manifestations include the findings noted above as well as enlarged gallbladder, cholelithiasis, cholecystitis, and cholangiocarcinoma. The last is found with much greater frequency in *O. viverrini* and *C. sinensis* endemic areas and is an important cause of death. In heavy infections, flukes are also found in the pancreatic duct and may be associated with pancreatitis.

Clinical Manifestations Acute infections are infrequently recognized and are characterized by fever, eosinophilia, and hepatomegaly. In endemic areas, almost the entire population may be infected; however, most are lightly infected and asymptomatic. More heavily infected persons suffer vague constitutional complaints and symptoms associated with cholelithiasis and pancreatitis. The liver may be enlarged and tender. Ascending cholangitis is a serious complication. Cholangiocarcinomas usually are associated with proximal obstruction

and subsequent massive dilation of the biliary ducts. Ultrasonography reveals varying degrees of peripheral dilation of the biliary ducts without proximal obstruction. Biliary stones and flukes also may be noted ultrasonographically. Endoscopic cholangiopancreatography reveals ductal dilation, proliferation, irregularities, and blunting of the terminal branches in a majority of cases. Adult worms are visualized as multiple filling defects.

Diagnosis and Treatment Diagnosis is based on the clinical presentation and the detection of the characteristic ova in the feces or bile. Worms can be visualized by a number of techniques and are frequently noted at surgery. Eggs measure about 30 by 12 μm and are ovoid in shape. At the smaller end, an operculum—a sort of cap—appears to rest on a rim that protrudes slightly from the eggs. The other end is broader and has a median knob. The eggs of *C. sinensis* and *O. viverrini* are difficult to tell apart, but those of *O. felineus* are somewhat longer and thinner. The treatment of choice is praziquantel (25 mg/kg tid for 1 day).

LUNG-DWELLING TREMATODES: *PARAGONIMUS WESTERMANI* AND RELATED SPECIES More than 30 species of *Paragonimus* have been described, and a number of these infect humans. Adult flukes reside mainly in the lungs, but ectopic localization is relatively common. *P. westermani*, found in the Far East, is the most common species causing infection in humans. Others include *Paragonimus skrjabini (szechuanensis)* (China), *Paragonimus heterotrema* (Southeast Asia), *Paragonimus philippinensis* (Philippines), *Paragonimus mexicanus* (Central America and parts of South America), *Paragonimus africanus* (Nigeria and Cameroon), and *Paragonimus uterobilateralis* (Nigeria and other areas of West Africa). *Paragonimus kellicotti* is indigenous to the United States but has rarely been documented in humans.

Life Cycle Humans become infected primarily by ingesting poorly cooked or pickled crabs or crayfish. Metacercariae excyst in the duodenum and within 1 h pass through the intestinal wall into the peritoneal cavity. After 3 to 6 h they migrate into the abdominal wall and then through the diaphragm into the pleura and lung tissue, where they become encapsulated, usually in pairs or triplets. It takes 65 to 90 days for the flukes to develop fully, although symptoms may begin earlier. Eggs are shed around the worm and, with rupture of the contents of the encapsulated cyst into the bronchioles, are excreted in the sputum or swallowed and excreted in the feces. Adults measure 7.5 to 12 mm by 4 to 6 mm by 3.5 to 5 mm and may live for 20 years.

Pathophysiology Disease is caused by the inflammation and fibrosis elicited by the worms in the lungs or in ectopic locations. Manifestations depend on the duration of infection and probably on the intensity of infection, although the latter association is not well documented. Flukes and eggs initially elicit an acute inflammatory response, mostly consisting of eosinophils, which is followed by the formation of a fibrous capsule. In the lung parenchyma, the cysts rupture into the bronchioles, extruding blood, eggs, and inflammatory exudate. Pleura-based lesions cause eosinophilic empyemas that can be confused clinically with tuberculosis. Lesions in long-standing infections exhibit increased fibrosis and decreased inflammatory responses, and some eventually calcify. Not uncommonly, flukes are found in abnormal locations, including the pleura, abdominal wall, viscera, and brain, where they elicit inflammation and fibrosis. Brain involvement is a particularly serious complication. Although frequent and severe bacterial infections may be associated with paragonimiasis, this relationship has not been substantiated. Ectopic lesions of the abdominal wall and liver are hallmarks of *P. skrjabini* infections.

Clinical Manifestations Manifestations can be both acute and chronic. Acute disease is noted infrequently and may include fever, hepatosplenomegaly, cough, eosinophilia, pleural effusions, pulmonary abnormalities, pneumothorax, and signs and symptoms referable to ectopic locations. The findings in chronic infections often include cough, expectoration of rusty or pigmented sputum, and hemoptysis. Dyspnea, chest pain, fever, and constitutional symptoms are found less frequently. Chest x-ray findings are varied, nondiagnostic, and often confused with those of tuberculosis. Localized or multisegmental infiltrates, usually poorly defined, are most common, but nodular, cystic, cavitary, ring shadow patterns are also found. Other findings include pleural effusions, empyemas, pleural thickening, and calcification of lesions. In contrast to the findings in tuberculosis, apical lesions do not predominate, cavities are smooth and regular, and infiltrates are less well defined. Although lung involvement alone appears to cause little mortality, morbidity and mortality are significant with ectopic lesions. In one series, 30.7 and 8.4 percent of hospitalized patients had ectopic lesions and brain involvement, respectively. Both acute and chronic forms of brain involvement are recognized: the former associated with the sudden onset of neurologic symptoms, usually in the presence of pulmonary disease, and the latter most often associated with seizures and long-term deficits. "Soap bubble" calcifications are a characteristic x-ray pattern in chronic neuroparagonimiasis.

Diagnosis and Treatment The diagnosis is established by detection of the characteristic ova in stool or sputum. The golden-brown eggs are unembryonated and measure 80 to 118 μm by 48 to 60 μm. Concentration techniques may be needed for the detection of eggs in lightly infected patients. Serologic tests are available and may be particularly useful in lightly infected individuals or those with suspected ectopic lesions. In acute disease, eggs may not be detected until 2 to 3 months after exposure. Praziquantel is the treatment of choice at 25 mg/kg three times a day for 2 days. Bithionol is also effective but is more toxic.

LIVER-DWELLING TREMATODES: *FASCIOLA HEPATICA* Humans are infected accidentally with this parasite of sheep, cattle, and other ruminants. Acute manifestations consist of a combination of systemic symptoms and signs and manifestations directly referable to invasion of the liver. Chronic disease has many features indistinguishable from those caused by the other liver flukes.

Life Cycle Ruminants become infected after ingestion of metacercariae encysted on aquatic vegetation. Watercress is commonly implicated in human infections. Metacercariae excyst in the duodenum, pass through the intestine into the peritoneum, invade the liver through Glisson's capsule, and eventually reside in the biliary ducts. In humans, the flukes require at least 3 to 4 months to mature, but eggs may not be detected in stool. Adults are relatively large, measuring 30 by 13 mm. Infections occur worldwide in areas where sheep and cattle are raised, including Europe, Australia, and other developed countries. Endogenously acquired infections are rare in the continental United States but occur in Puerto Rico.

Pathophysiology The severity of infection depends on its intensity and duration and the responses of the host. Early manifestations are due to migration of the flukes through the tissues. Punctate hemorrhages, tracts, and nodules are seen on the surface of the liver and constitute points of entry, migration routes, and areas of encapsulated eosinophilic abscesses, respectively. Granulomatous reactions also occur around eggs themselves. In chronic infections, worms reside in the biliary system, and the anatomic changes caused by the worms generally resemble those caused by other liver flukes. However, intermittent obstruction of the biliary passages by worms appears more common in fascioliasis and leads to periods of jaundice.

Clinical Findings Fever, hepatomegaly and/or abdominal pain, and eosinophilia are the hallmarks of acute fascioliasis, which usually begins within 2 to 3 months following ingestion. Nausea, diarrhea, cough, and urticaria are also frequent. Elevation of liver function values is inconstant, anemia is usually evident, and the erythrocyte sedimentation rate is commonly elevated. Untreated, the disease lasts from months to years, but the manifestations change and with time more closely resemble those of other liver fluke infections, including intermittent obstruction, gallbladder and biliary duct thickening, cholecystitis, lithiasis, and the development of strictures. Ectopic localization of flukes is also relatively common and leads to findings related to the invaded tissue. In contrast to the other liver flukes, *F. hepatica* has no apparent association with cholangiocarcinoma. Because exposure is sometimes long-standing, acute and chronic manifestations may occur at the same time. Computed tomography scans show multiple, hypodense, irregular lesions in the liver; ultrasonography sometimes fails to detect these lesions but is helpful in detecting resulting biliary duct pathology.

Diagnosis The presence of fever, eosinophilia, and hepatomegaly or liver pain in the proper clinical setting suggests the diagnosis. Definitive diagnosis is established by the detection of ova in the feces and/or by serologic tests. Ova may not be detected in the feces because the disease becomes manifest before patency, because the ova are unable to pass into the biliary system, or because the worms are in an ectopic location or there is a low level of excretion of ova. Therefore, stool concentration methods should be employed. The ova of *F. hepatica* are immature in the feces, measure 130 to 150 μm by 90 μm, and are indistinguishable from those of *Fasciolopsis buski* (see below).

℞ **TREATMENT**

Although praziquantel is effective for other trematodes, it does not appear to be very effective in *F. hepatica* infection, and bithionol at 30 to 50 mg/kg on alternate days for 10 to 15 doses is the treatment of choice. Infections also have been treated successfully with the experimental drugs triclabendazole and albendazole.

INTESTINE-DWELLING TREMATODES *Fasciolopsis buski* One of the largest parasites infecting humans, *F. buski* measures 20 to 70 mm by 8 to 20 mm by 0.5 to 3 mm and resides in the small intestine and occasionally in the colon or pylorus. Geographically, it is confined to the Far East. The adults attach to the intestinal epithelium, causing ulcerations and localized inflammation. Light infections are generally asymptomatic, but persons heavily infected have diarrhea, fever, and abdominal pain and may develop ascites, anasarca, and intestinal obstruction. The pathophysiology of *F. buski* infection has not been well studied. The diagnosis is established by the detection of ova (indistinguishable from those of *F. hepatica*) in the feces. The treatment of choice is praziquantel (25 mg/kg tid for 1 day).

Heterophyes heterophyes and *Metagonimus yokogawai* The major clinical manifestation of infection with both of these tiny (about 1 mm) intestine-dwelling parasites is diarrhea. Humans acquire infection after the ingestion of undercooked freshwater fish. *H. heterophyes* and *M. yokogawai* are found in the Far East, but the former is also common in the Nile Delta and is present in other areas of the Middle East. The worms attach to and at times burrow into the intestinal mucosa, eliciting inflammatory responses. Ova of *H. heterophyes* have been found in the heart and other organs and have reportedly caused clinically significant myocarditis. The diagnosis is established by the detection of ova in the feces; the ova of the two species are identical and resemble those of *C. sinensis* and related parasites. Praziquantel is the drug of choice (25 mg/kg tid for 1 day).

Nanophyetus salmincola This tiny small-intestine–dwelling trematode has recently infected humans in the Pacific Northwest. It was previously known to infect humans in eastern Siberia. Infections follow the ingestion of undercooked, smoked, or raw fish, usually salmon or trout. Symptoms vary from asymptomatic carriage to watery diarrhea, abdominal pain, bloating, and other gastrointestinal problems. Eosinophilia is found in most cases but is not universal. Unembryonated ova (64 to 97 μm by 34 to 55 μm) appear in the feces after 1 week but are excreted in low numbers so that concentration techniques are needed for detection. The treatment of choice is praziquantel (20 mg/kg tid for 1 day).

BIBLIOGRAPHY

CHEEVER AW: Infection versus disease and hypersensitivity versus immunity. Am J Pathol 142:699, 1993

DRAGANA J, SHER A: Initiation and regulation of CD4+ T-cell function in host-parasite models. Chem Immunol 63:51, 1996

ELKINS DB et al: A high frequency of hepatobiliary disease and suspected cholangiocarcinoma associated with heavy *Opisthorchis viverrini* infection in a small community in northeast Thailand. Trans R Soc Trop Med Hyg 84:715, 1990

FRITSCHE TR et al: Praziquantel for treatment of human *Nanophyetus salmincola (Troglotrema salmincola)* infection. J Infect Dis 160:896, 1989

GUTIERREZ Y: *Diagnostic Pathology of Parasitic Infections with Clinical Correlations.* Philadelphia, Lea & Febiger, 1990

HAGAN P: Reinfection, exposure and immunity in human schistosomiasis. Parasitol Today 8:12, 1992

HOMEIDA M: Diagnosis of pathologically confirmed Symmers' periportal fibrosis by ultrasonography: A prospective blinded study. Am J Trop Med Hyg 39:86, 1988

———— et al: Morbidity associated with *Schistosoma mansoni* infection as determined by ultrasound: A study in Gezira, Sudan. Am J Trop Med Hyg 39:196, 1988

———— et al: Association of the therapeutic activity of praziquantel with the reversal of Symmers' fibrosis induced by *Schistosoma mansoni*. Am J Trop Med Hyg 45:360, 1991

NASH TE et al: Schistosome infections in humans: Perspective and recent findings. Ann Intern Med 97:740, 1982

SAAD AMA et al: Oesophageal varices in region of the Sudan endemic for *Schistosoma mansoni*. Br J Surg 78:1252, 1991

SINGH TS et al: Pulmonary paragonimiasis: Clinical features, diagnosis and treatment of 39 cases in Manipur. Trans R Soc Trop Med Hyg 80:967, 1986

SITHITHAWORN P et al: Quantitative post-mortem study of *Opisthorchis viverrini* in man in northeast Thailand. Trans R Soc Trop Med Hyg 85:765, 1991

TAKEYAMA N et al: Computed tomography findings of hepatic lesions in human fascioliasis: Report of two cases. Am J Gastroenterol 81:1078, 1986

WYNN TA: An IL-12-based vaccination method for preventing fibrosis induced by schistosome infection. Nature 376:594, 1995

YOKOGAWA M: Epidemiology and control of paragonimiasis, in *Parasitic Diseases*, EM Sasa (ed). Tokyo, International Medical Foundation of Japan, 1974, pp 137–149

225 *Thomas B. Nutman, Peter F. Weller*

CESTODES

Cestodes, or tapeworms, are segmented worms. The adults reside in the gastrointestinal tract, but the larvae can be found in almost any organ. Human tapeworm infections can be divided into two major clinical groups. In one group, humans are the definitive hosts, and the adult tapeworms live in the gastrointestinal tract (*Taenia saginata*, *Diphyllobothrium*, *Hymenolepis*, and *Dipylidium caninum*). In the other, humans are intermediate hosts, and larval-stage parasites are present in the tissues. Diseases in this category include echinococcosis, sparganosis, and coenurosis. For *Taenia solium*, the human may be either the definitive or the intermediate host.

The ribbon-shaped tapeworm attaches to the intestinal mucosa by means of sucking cups or grooves located on the head (scolex). Behind the scolex is a short, narrow neck from which proglottids (segments) form. As each proglottid matures, it is displaced further back from the neck by the formation of new, less mature segments. The progressively elongating chain of attached proglottids, called the *strobila*, constitutes the bulk of the tapeworm; it may consist of more than 1000 proglottids and may be several meters long. As each proglottid becomes gravid, eggs are released. Since eggs of the different *Taenia* species are morphologically identical, differences in the morphology of the scolex or proglottids provide the only basis for diagnostic identification to the species level. Most human tapeworms require at least one intermediate host for complete larval development. After ingestion by an intermediate host, an egg develops into a larval oncosphere capable of penetrating the intestinal mucosa. The oncosphere migrates to tissues and develops into an encysted form known as a *cysticercus* (single scolex), a *coenurus* (multiple scolices), or a *hydatid* (cyst with daughter cysts, each containing several scolices). Ingestion by the definitive host of tissues containing a cyst enables a scolex to develop into a tapeworm.

TAENIASIS SAGINATA The beef tapeworm *T. saginata* occurs in all countries where raw or undercooked beef is eaten. It is most prevalent in sub-Saharan African and Middle Eastern countries.

Etiology and Pathogenesis Humans are the only definitive host for the adult stage of *T. saginata*. This tapeworm, which can reach 3 to 8 m in length, inhabits the upper jejunum and has a scolex with four prominent suckers and 1000 to 2000 proglottids. Each gravid segment has 15 to 30 uterine branches (in contrast to 8 to 12 for *T. solium*). The eggs are indistinguishable from those of *T. solium*; each measures 30 to 40 μm and has a thick brown striated shell containing a fully developed embryo. Eggs deposited on vegetation can live for months to years until they are ingested by cattle or other herbivores. The embryo released after ingestion invades the intestinal wall and is carried to striated muscle (predominantly in the hind limbs, diaphragm, and tongue), where it transforms into a cysticercus. When ingested in raw or undercooked beef, this form can infect humans. After the cysticercus is ingested, it takes about 2 months for an adult worm to develop.

Clinical Manifestations Patients become aware of the infection most commonly by noting passage of proglottids in their feces. They may experience perianal discomfort when proglottids are discharged. Although usually minimal or mild, abdominal pain or discomfort, nausea, change in appetite, weakness, and weight loss can occur with *T. saginata* infection.

Diagnosis The diagnosis is made by the detection of eggs or proglottids in the stool as soon as about 3 months after infection. Eggs also may be present in the perianal area; thus, if proglottids or eggs are not found in the stool, the perianal region should be examined with use of a cellophane-tape swab (as in pinworm infection). The distinguishing of *T. saginata* from *T. solium* requires examination of mature proglottids or the scolex. Serologic tests are not helpful diagnostically. Eosinophilia and elevated levels of serum IgE may be detected.

℞ **TREATMENT**
A single dose of praziquantel (5 to 10 mg/kg) is highly effective for therapy.

Prevention The major means of preventing infection is the adequate cooking of beef; exposure to temperatures as low as 56°C for 5 min will destroy cysticerci. Refrigeration or salting for long periods or freezing at −10°C for 9 days also kills cysticerci in beef. General preventive measures include inspection of beef and proper disposal of human feces.

TAENIASIS SOLIUM AND CYSTICERCOSIS The pork tapeworm *T. solium* can cause two distinct forms of infection. The form that develops depends on whether humans are infected with adult tapeworms in the intestine or with larval forms in the tissues (cysticercosis). Humans are the only definitive hosts for *T. solium*; pigs are the usual intermediate hosts, although dogs, cats, and sheep may harbor the larval forms. *T. solium* exists worldwide but is most prevalent in Mexico, Africa, Southeast Asia, eastern Europe, and South America. Cysticercosis occurs in industrialized nations largely as a result of the immigration of infected persons from endemic areas.

Etiology and Pathogenesis The adult tapeworm generally resides in the upper jejunum. Its globular scolex attaches by both sucking disks and two rows of hooklets. Often only one adult worm is present, but that worm may live for up to 25 years. The tapeworm, usually about 3 meters in length, may have as many as 1000 proglottids, each of which produces up to 50,000 eggs. Groups of 3 to 5 proglottids generally are released and excreted into the feces, and the eggs in these proglottids are infective for both humans and animals. The eggs survive in the environment for several months. After ingestion by the intermediate host, eggs embryonate, penetrate the intestinal wall, and are carried to many tissues, with a predilection for striated muscle of the neck, tongue, and trunk. Within 60 to 90 days, the encysted larval stage develops. These cysticerci can survive for long periods. Humans acquire infections that lead to intestinal tapeworms by ingesting undercooked pork containing cysticerci. Infections that cause human cysticercosis follow the ingestion of *T. solium* eggs, usually from fecally contaminated food. Autoinfection may occur if an individual with an egg-producing tapeworm ingests eggs derived from his or her own feces or if eggs pass by reflux from the intestine into the stomach.

Clinical Manifestations Intestinal infections with *T. solium* may be asymptomatic. Epigastric discomfort, nausea, a sensation of hunger, weight loss, and diarrhea are infrequent. Fecal passage of proglottids may be noted by patients.

In cysticercosis, the clinical manifestations are entirely different. Since cysticerci can be found anywhere in the body (most commonly in the brain and the skeletal muscle), their location and size determine the clinical presentation. The manifestations of cysticercosis reflect two distinct processes: the local inflammatory response induced by the parasite and the local effect of the space-occupying lesions. Neurologic manifestations constitute the most common presentation. When inflammation surrounds lesions, seizures and focal neurologic deficits are frequent, and communicating and noncommunicating hydrocephalus and meningitis also can be seen. Generalized, focal, or Jacksonian seizures occur in most cases. Signs of increased intracranial pressure, including headache, nausea, vomiting, changes in vision, dizziness, ataxia, and confusion, often are present. Patients with hydrocephalus may develop papilledema and may experience alterations of mental status. The unusual racemose form of cyticercosis is characterized by grapelike clusters of proliferating larval membranes. This form typically occurs at the base of the brain or in the subarachnoid space and causes chronic meningitis and arachnoiditis. Communicating or noncommunicating hydrocephalus is common. The clinical presentation of neurocysticercosis therefore depends on the number, form, and location of cysticerci, the extent of cyst-associated inflammatory responses, and the duration of disease.

Diagnosis The diagnosis of intestinal *T. solium* infection is made by the detection of eggs or proglottids, as described for *T. saginata*. For cysticercosis, definitive diagnosis requires examination of the cysticercus in an involved tissue, but a diagnosis often can be based on clinical presentation in conjunction with compatible results in radiographic studies—especially computed tomography (CT) and magnetic resonance imaging (MRI)—and serologic tests.

For soft tissue involvement, plain films may reveal multiple calcified "puffed-rice" lesions. For cerebral cysticercosis, CT studies demonstrate parenchymal lesions of varying number and size that are either cystic or solid and may exhibit contrast enhancement. Some or many of the lesions seen by CT may be calcified; thus, multiple punctate calcifications are common findings in neurocysticercosis. Ventricular dilation may be demonstrable, but the CT finding of multiple calcified or noncalcified cystic lesions is strongly suggestive of cerebral cysticercosis. MRI detects cystic structures on T_1- and T_2-weighted images as well as high-intensity rims around cysts, particularly on T_2-weighted images. Use of gadolinium contrast enhances the sensitivity of MRI studies. Because CT is more sensitive in identifying calcified lesions and MRI is better at identifying small cystic lesions, both techniques are useful in evaluating neurocysticercosis.

Most patients with cerebral cysticercosis have cerebrospinal fluid (CSF) pleocytosis with a predominance of mononuclear cells. The glucose level is often decreased and the protein level elevated in CSF. Serologic tests of CSF and sera are helpful in establishing the diagnosis. Of the variety of serologic assays that have been used, many have been complicated by cross-reactivity with other tapeworm, filarial, and echinococcal infections. An immunoblotting technique has improved specificity to 98 percent, with sensitivities reaching 91 percent. Even with this technique, however, patients with single intracranial neurocysticercotic lesions may be seronegative.

℞ **TREATMENT**

Intestinal *T. solium* infection is treated with praziquantel, as specified for *T. saginata* infection. However, praziquantel can evoke an inflammatory response in the central nervous system if concomitant cryptic cysticercosis is present.

The management of cysticercosis can involve chemotherapy, surgery, and supportive medical treatment. Asymptomatic patients with calcified soft tissue or neural lesions generally require no treatment. For symptomatic patients with neurocysticercosis, both praziquantel (50 mg/kg per day in three doses for 15 days) and albendazole (15 mg/kg per day in three doses for 8 to 28 days) are effective. Because both agents provoke inflammatory responses around dying cysticerci, patients receiving either drug should be hospitalized and

given high doses of glucocorticoids during treatment. The efficacy of therapy can be monitored by radiographic imaging. The size of active lesions should decrease within 3 to 6 months. For ocular and spinal lesions, drug-induced inflammation may cause irreversible damage; thus, these lesions as well as those within the ventricles are best managed by surgical resection. Ventricular obstruction may require ventriculostomy or ventriculoperitoneal shunting. Not all neurologic deficits resolve after therapy, and some patients may require continued anticonvulsive treatment.

Prevention Measures for the prevention of intestinal *T. solium* infection consist of the application to pork of precautions similar to those described above for beef with regard to *T. saginata* infection. The prevention of cysticercosis involves minimizing the opportunities for ingestion of fecally derived eggs by means of good personal hygiene, effective fecal disposal, and treatment and prevention of human intestinal infections.

ECHINOCOCCOSIS Echinococcosis is an infection of humans caused by the larval stage of *Echinococcus granulosus*, *Echinococcus multilocularis*, or *Echinococcus vogeli*. *E. granulosus*, which produces unilocular cystic lesions, is prevalent in areas where livestock is raised in association with dogs. This tapeworm species is found in Australia, Argentina, Chile, Africa, eastern Europe, the Middle East, New Zealand, and the Mediterranean region, particularly Lebanon and Greece. *E. multilocularis*, which causes multilocular alveolar lesions that are locally invasive, is found in sub-Arctic or Arctic regions, including Canada, the United States, and northern Europe and Asia. *E. vogeli* causes polycystic hydatid disease and is found only in Central and South America. Like other cestodes, echinococcal species have both intermediate and definitive hosts. The definitive hosts are dogs that pass eggs in their feces. Cysts develop in the intermediate hosts—sheep, cattle, humans, goats, camels, and horses for *E. granulosus* and mice and other rodents for *E. multilocularis*—after the ingestion of eggs. When a dog ingests beef or lamb containing cysts, the life cycle is completed.

Etiology The small (5 mm long) adult *E. granulosus* worm, which lives for 5 to 20 months in the jejunum of dogs, has only three proglottids—one immature, one mature, and one gravid. The gravid segment splits to release eggs that are morphologically indistinguishable from *Taenia* eggs and are extremely hardy. After humans ingest the eggs, embryos escape from the eggs, penetrate the intestinal mucosa, enter the portal circulation, and are carried to various organs, most commonly the liver and lungs. Larvae develop into fluid-filled unilocular hydatid cysts that consist of an external membrane and an inner germinal layer. Daughter cysts develop from the inner aspect of the germinal layer, as do germinating cystic structures called *brood capsules*. New larvae, called *scolices*, develop in large numbers within the brood capsule. The cysts expand slowly over a period of years.

The life cycle of *E. multilocularis* is similar except that small rodents serve as the intermediate hosts. The cyst of *E. multilocularis*, however, is quite different in that the larval form remains in the proliferative phase, the hydatid cyst is always multilocular, and vesicles progressively invade the host tissue by peripheral extension of processes from the germinal layer.

Clinical Manifestations Slowly enlarging echinococcal cysts generally remain asymptomatic until their expanding size or their space-occupying effect in an involved organ elicits symptoms. The liver and the lungs are the most common sites of these cysts. Since a period of 5 to 20 years often elapses before cysts enlarge sufficiently to cause symptoms, they may be discovered incidentally on a routine x-ray or ultrasound study.

Patients with hepatic echinococcosis who are symptomatic most often present with abdominal pain or a palpable mass in the right upper quadrant. Compression of a bile duct or leakage of cyst fluid into the biliary tree may mimic recurrent cholelithiasis, and biliary obstruction can result in jaundice. Rupture of or episodic leakage from a hydatid cyst may produce fever, pruritus, urticaria, eosinophilia, or fatal anaphylaxis. Pulmonary hydatid cysts may rupture into the bronchial tree or peritoneal cavity and produce cough, chest pain, or hemoptysis. By spreading the multitudinous infectious scolices, the rupture of hydatid cysts leads to multifocal dissemination of new cyst-forming elements. Rupture can occur spontaneously or at surgery and in the latter instance is especially likely when a cyst is not recognized to be of echinococcal etiology. Cysts may involve any organ. Other presentations are due to the involvement of bone (invasion of the medullary cavity with slow bone erosion producing pathologic fractures), the central nervous system (space-occupying lesions), and the heart (conduction defects, pericarditis).

The cysts of *E. multilocularis* characteristically present as a slowly growing hepatic tumor, with progressive destruction of the liver and extension into vital structures. Patients commonly complain of upper quadrant and epigastric pain, and obstructive jaundice may be apparent. A minority of patients experience the metastasis of lesions to the lung and brain.

Diagnosis Radiographic and related imaging studies are important in detecting and evaluating echinococcal cysts. Plain films will define pulmonary cysts—usually as rounded irregular masses of uniform density—but may miss other cysts in other organs unless there is cyst wall calcification (as occurs in the liver). MRI, CT, and ultrasound reveal well-defined cysts with thick or thin walls. When older cysts contain a layer of hydatid sand that is rich in accumulated scolices, these imaging methods may detect this fluid layer of different density. However, the most pathognomonic finding, if demonstrable, is that of daughter cysts within the larger cyst. This finding, like eggshell or mural calcification on CT, is indicative of *E. granulosus* infection and helps to distinguish the cyst from carcinomas, bacterial or amebic liver abscesses, or hemangiomas. CT of alveolar hydatid cysts reveals indistinct solid masses with central necrosis and plaquelike calcifications.

A specific diagnosis can be made by the examination of aspirated fluids for scoliceal hooklets, but diagnostic aspiration is not conventionally recommended because of the risk of fluid leakage resulting in either dissemination of infection or anaphylactic reactions. However, CT-guided aspiration of hydatid cysts for diagnosis has been used successfully in some centers. Pretreatment with albendazole (a 1-month course) is believed to minimize biopsy complications. Serodiagnostic assays can be useful, although a negative test does not exclude the diagnosis of echinococcosis. While cysts in the liver are more likely to elicit positive antibody responses than those in the lungs, up to 50 percent of infected individuals may have negative serology. Detection of antibody to specific echinococcal antigens by immunoblotting has the highest degree of specificity, although false-positive findings may be obtained in cysticercosis.

℞ **TREATMENT**

Therapy for echinococcosis is based on considerations of the size, location, and manifestations of cysts and the overall health of the patient. Surgery, when feasible, is the principal definitive method of treatment; *E. granulosus* cysts are excised, or tissue containing *E. multilocularis* cysts is resected. Risks at surgery from leakage of fluid include anaphylaxis and dissemination of infectious scolices. The latter complication has been minimized by the instillation of scolicidal solutions such as hypertonic saline or ethanol, which may cause hypernatremia, intoxication, or sclerosing cholangitis. Albendazole, which has antiechinococcal activity, can be administered adjunctively in the perioperative period and may be useful for medical treatment of echinococcosis. While albendazole has shown efficacy, the exact role of chemotherapy, perhaps combined with percutaneous drainage, remains to be defined. As medical therapy, albendazole, given at a dose of 400 mg twice a day for 12 weeks, is most efficacious against hepatic and pulmonary cysts, although multiple courses may be necessary. Response to treatment is best assessed by repeated evaluation of cysts by CT or MRI, with particular attention to cyst size and consistency.

Prevention In endemic areas, echinococcosis can be prevented by administering praziquantel to infected dogs and by denying dogs access to butchering sites and to the offal of infected animals. Limitation of the number of stray dogs is helpful in reducing the prevalence of infection among humans.

HYMENOLEPIASIS NANA Infection with *Hymenolepis nana*, the dwarf tapeworm, is the most common of all the cestode infections. *H. nana* is endemic in both temperate and tropical regions of the world. Infection is spread by fecal/oral contamination and is common among institutionalized children.

Etiology and Pathogenesis *H. nana* is the only cestode of humans that does not require an intermediate host. Both the larval and adult phases take place in the human. The adult, the smallest tapeworm parasitizing humans, is about 2 cm long and dwells in the proximal ileum. Proglottids, which are quite small and are rarely seen in the stool, release spherical eggs 30 to 44 μm in diameter, each of which contains an oncosphere with six hooklets. The eggs are immediately infective and are unable to survive in the external environment for more than 10 days. *H. nana* also can be acquired by the ingestion of infected insects (especially larval meal-worms and larval fleas). When the egg is ingested by a new host, the oncosphere is freed and penetrates the intestinal villi, becoming a cysticercoid larva. Larvae migrate back into the intestinal lumen, attach to the mucosa, and mature over 10 to 12 days into adult worms. Eggs also may hatch before passing into the stool, causing internal autoinfection with increasing numbers of intestinal worms. Although the life span of adult *H. nana* is only about 4 to 10 weeks, the autoinfection cycle perpetuates the infection.

Clinical Manifestations *H. nana* infection, even with many intestinal worms, is usually asymptomatic. When infection is intense, anorexia, abdominal pain, and diarrhea develop.

Diagnosis Infection is diagnosed by the finding of eggs in the stool.

℞ **TREATMENT**

Praziquantel (25 mg/kg once) is the treatment of choice, since it acts against both the adult worms and the cysticercoids in the intestinal villi.

Prevention Good personal hygiene and improved sanitation can eradicate the disease. Epidemics have been controlled by mass chemotherapy coupled with improved hygiene.

HYMENOLEPIASIS DIMINUTA *Hymenolepis diminuta*, a cestode of rodents, occasionally infects small children, who ingest the adult worm in uncooked cereal foods contaminated by fleas and other insects in which larvae develop. Infection is usually asymptomatic and is diagnosed by the detection of eggs in the stool. Treatment with praziquantel results in cure in most cases.

DIPHYLLOBOTHRIASIS *Diphyllobothrium latum* and other *Diphyllobothrium* species are found in the lakes, rivers, and deltas of the northern hemisphere, Central Africa, and Chile.

Etiology and Pathogenesis The adult worm, the longest tapeworm (up to 25 m), attaches to the ileal and occasionally to the jejunal mucosa by its suckers, which are located on its elongated scolex. The adult worm has 3000 to 4000 proglottids, which release approximately 1 million eggs daily into the feces. If an egg reaches water, it hatches and releases a free-swimming embryo that can be eaten by small freshwater crustaceans (*Cyclops* or *Diaptomus* species). After an infected crustacean containing a developed procercoid is swallowed by a fish, the larva migrates into the fish's flesh and grows into a plerocercoid, or sparganum larva. Humans acquire the infection by ingesting infected raw fish. Within 3 to 5 weeks, the tapeworm matures into an adult in the human intestine.

Clinical Manifestations Most *D. latum* infections are asymptomatic, although manifestations may include transient abdominal discomfort, diarrhea, vomiting, weakness, and weight loss. Occasionally, infection can cause acute abdominal pain and intestinal obstruction; in rare cases cholangitis or cholecystitis may be produced by migrating proglottids. Because the tapeworm absorbs large quantities of vitamin B_{12} and interferes with ileal B_{12} absorption, vitamin B_{12} deficiency can develop. Up to 2 percent of infected patients, especially the elderly, have megaloblastic anemia resembling pernicious anemia and may exhibit neurologic sequelae of B_{12} deficiency.

Diagnosis   The diagnosis is made readily by the detection of the characteristic eggs in the stool. The eggs possess a single shell with an operculum at one end and a knob at the other. Mild to moderate eosinophilia may be detected.

 TREATMENT
Praziquantel (5 to 10 mg/kg once) is highly effective. Parenteral vitamin B_{12} should be given if B_{12} deficiency is manifest.

Prevention   Infection can be prevented by heating fish to 54°C for 5 min or by freezing it at -18°C for 24 h. Placing fish in brine with a high salt concentration for long periods kills the eggs.

DIPYLIDIASIS   *Dipylidium caninum*, a common tapeworm of dogs and cats, may accidentally infect humans. Dogs, cats, and occasionally humans become infected by ingesting fleas harboring cysticercoids. Children are more likely to become infected than adults. Most infections are asymptomatic, but abdominal pain, diarrhea, anal pruritus, urticaria, and eosinophilia can occur. The diagnosis is made by the detection of proglottids in the stool. As in *D. latum* infection, therapy consists of praziquantel. Prevention requires anthelmintic treatment and flea control for pet dogs or cats.

SPARGANOSIS   Humans can be infected by the sparganum, or plerocercoid larva, of a diphyllobothrid tapeworm of the genus *Spirometra*. Infection can be acquired by the consumption of water containing infected *Cyclops*; by the ingestion of infected snakes, birds,

or mammals; or by the application of infected flesh as poultices. The worm migrates slowly in tissues, and infection commonly presents as a subcutaneous swelling. Periorbital tissues can be involved, and ocular sparganosis may destroy the eye. Surgical excision is used to treat localized sparganosis.

COENUROSIS   This rare infection of humans by the larval stage (coenurus) of the dog tapeworm *Taenia multiceps* or *Taenia serialis* results in a space-occupying cystic lesion. As in cysticercosis, involvement of the central nervous system and subcutaneous tissue is most common. Both definitive diagnosis and treatment require surgical excision of the lesion. Chemotherapeutic agents generally are not effective.

BIBLIOGRAPHY

BOTERO D et al: Taeniasis and cysticercosis. Infect Dis Clin North Am 7:683, 1993

FLISSER A: Taeniasis and cysticercosis due to *Taenia solium*. Prog Clin Parasitol 4:77, 1994

GIL-GRANDE LA et al: Randomised controlled trial of efficacy of albendazole in intra-abdominal hydatid disease. Lancet 342:1269, 1993

KAMMERER WS, SCHANTZ PM: Echinococcal disease. Infect Dis Clin North Am 7:605, 1993

SCHAEFER JW, KHAN MY: Echinococcosis (hydatid disease): Lessons from experience with 59 patients. Rev Infect Dis 13:243, 1991

SCHANTZ PM, KRAMER HJ: Larval cestode infections: Cysticercosis and echinococcosis. Curr Opin Infect Dis 8:342, 1995

SCHARF D: Neurocysticercosis: Two hundred thirty eight cases from a California hospital. Arch Neurol 46:77, 1989

PART EIGHT

SECTION 1
DIAGNOSIS

226

Eugene Braunwald

APPROACH TO THE PATIENT WITH HEART DISEASE

The symptoms caused by heart disease result most commonly from myocardial ischemia, from disturbance of the contraction and/or relaxation of the myocardium, from obstruction to blood flow, or from an abnormal cardiac rhythm or rate. Ischemia is manifest most frequently as chest discomfort, while reduction of the pumping ability of the heart commonly leads to weakness and fatigability or, when severe, produces cyanosis, hypotension, syncope, and elevated intravascular pressure behind a failing ventricle; the latter results in abnormal fluid accumulation, which in turn leads to dyspnea, orthopnea, and systemic or pulmonary edema. Obstruction to blood flow, as in valvular stenosis, can cause symptoms resembling those resulting from congestive heart failure. Cardiac arrhythmias often develop suddenly, and the resulting signs and symptoms—palpitation, dyspnea, angina, hypotension, and syncope—generally occur abruptly and may disappear as rapidly as they develop.

A cardinal principle useful in the evaluation of the patient with suspected heart disease is that myocardial or coronary function that may be adequate at rest may be inadequate during exertion. Thus a history of chest discomfort and/or dyspnea that appears only during activity is characteristic of heart disease, while the opposite pattern, i.e., the appearance of these symptoms at rest and their remission during exertion, is rarely observed in patients with organic heart disease.

Patients with cardiocirculatory disease also may be asymptomatic, both at rest and during exertion, but may present an abnormal physical finding, such as a heart murmur, elevated arterial pressure, or an abnormality of the electrocardiogram (ECG) or of the cardiac silhouette on the chest roentgenogram. Patients may exhibit asymptomatic ischemia on an exercise stress test or an ambulatory ECG.

Diseases of the heart and circulation are so common and the laity is so well acquainted with the major symptoms resulting from these disorders that patients, and occasionally physicians, erroneously attribute many noncardiac complaints to cardiovascular disease. The combination of the widespread fear of heart disease with the deep-seated emotional connotations concerning this organ's function results in the frequent development of symptoms that mimic those of organic disease in persons with normal cardiovascular systems. The unraveling of symptoms and signs due to organic heart disease from those not directly related is an important and challenging task in these patients.

Dyspnea, one of the cardinal manifestations of diminished cardiac reserve, is not limited to heart disease but is also characteristic of conditions as diverse as pulmonary disease, marked obesity, and anxiety (Chap. 32). Similarly, chest discomfort may result from a variety of causes other than myocardial ischemia (Chap. 13). Whether heart disease is responsible for these symptoms can frequently be determined by carrying out a careful clinical examination. Noninvasive testing using electrocardiography at rest and during exercise (Chap. 228), echocardiography, roentgenography, and myocardial imaging usually provides important additional information to permit the correct interpretation of symptoms; more specialized invasive examinations (catheterization and angiography; Chap. 229) are occasionally necessary.

DIAGNOSIS As outlined by the New York Heart Association, the elements of a complete cardiac diagnosis include consideration of

1. *The underlying etiology.* Is the disease congenital, infectious, hypertensive, or ischemic in origin?
2. *The anatomic abnormalities.* Which chambers are involved? Which valves are affected? Is there pericardial involvement? Has there been a myocardial infarction?
3. *The physiologic disturbances.* Is an arrhythmia present? Is there evidence of congestive heart failure or of myocardial ischemia?
4. *The extent of functional disability.* How strenuous is the physical activity required to elicit symptoms? The latter should be evaluated in the light of the intensity of therapy.

One example may serve to illustrate the importance of establishing a complete diagnosis. The identification of myocardial ischemia as the etiology of a patient's exertional chest discomfort is of great clinical importance. However, the recognition of ischemia is insufficient to formulate a therapeutic strategy or prognosis until the underlying anatomic abnormalities responsible for the myocardial ischemia, e.g., coronary atherosclerosis or aortic stenosis, are identified and a judgment made as to whether other physiologic disturbances that cause an imbalance between myocardial oxygen supply and demand, such as severe anemia, thyrotoxicosis, or supraventricular tachycardia, play a contributory role. In many instances, the extent of functional disability is a determinant of whether medical or interventional therapy is utilized.

The establishment of a correct and complete cardiac diagnosis often requires the use of six different methods of examination: (1) history, (2) physical examination (Chap. 227), (3) ECG (Chap. 228), (4) chest roentgenogram, (5) noninvasive graphic examinations (echocardiogram, radionuclide and other noninvasive imaging techniques), and occasionally (6) specialized invasive examinations, i.e., cardiac catheterization, angiocardiography, and coronary arteriography (Chap. 229). In order to be most effective, the results obtained from each of these six modalities should be analyzed independently of one another as well as with the information derived from the other methods clearly in mind. Only in this way can one avoid overlooking a subtle, though important, finding. For example, an ECG should be obtained in every patient suspected of having heart disease. It may provide the critical clue in establishing the correct diagnosis, e.g., the finding of a mild atrioventricular conduction disturbance in a patient with unexplained syncope, even when all other methods of examination reveal no abnormal findings, can be the clue that asystole might be the cause. On the other hand, when combined intelligently with the results of other methods of examination, the ECG may provide essential confirmatory data. Thus the knowledge that a patient has an apical diastolic rumbling murmur may direct particular attention to the P waves, and the recognition of left atrial enlargement electrocardiographically supports the suggestion that the murmur is caused by mitral stenosis. The diagnosis can be confirmed by echocardiography, a technique that can also determine the severity of the obstruction and its effects on cardiac function.

Family History In obtaining the history of a patient with known or suspected cardiovascular disease, particular attention should be directed to the family history. Familial clustering is common in many forms of heart disease. Genetic transmission may occur, as in hypertrophic cardiomyopathy (Chap. 239), the Marfan syndrome (Chap. 348), and sudden death associated with a prolonged QT syndrome (Chap. 231). In patients with essential hypertension or coronary atherosclerosis, the genetic component may be less obvious but is also of considerable importance. Familial clustering of cardiovascular diseases may occur not only on a genetic basis but also may be related to familial dietary or behavior patterns, such as excessive ingestion of salt or calories or cigarette smoking.

Assessment of Functional Impairment   When an attempt is made to determine the severity of functional impairment in a patient with heart disease, it is helpful to ascertain with as much precision as possible the level of activity and the rate at which it is performed before symptoms develop. Thus breathlessness that occurs after running up two long flights of stairs denotes far less functional impairment than similar symptoms occurring after taking a few steps on the level. Also, the degree of customary physical activity at work and during recreation should be considered. The development of two-flight dyspnea in a marathon runner may be far more significant than the development of one-flight dyspnea in a previously sedentary person. Similarly, the history must include a detailed consideration of the patient's therapeutic regimen. For example, the persistence or development of edema, breathlessness, and other manifestations of heart failure in a patient whose diet is rigidly restricted in sodium content and who is receiving optimal doses of diuretics is far more grave than the development of similar manifestations of heart failure in the absence of these measures. In an effort to determine the rate of progression of symptoms, and thereby of the severity of the underlying illness, it may be useful to ascertain what, if any, specific tasks the patient could carry out 1 year earlier which he or she cannot carry out now.

Electrocardiogram   Although the ECG is an invaluable aspect of every cardiovascular examination, with the exception of the identification of arrhythmias and of many instances of acute myocardial infarction, it rarely permits establishment of a specific diagnosis. In the absence of other abnormal findings, electrocardiographic changes must not be overinterpreted. The range of normal electrocardiographic findings is wide, and the tracing can be affected significantly by many noncardiac factors, such as age, body habitus, and serum electrolyte concentrations.

Natural History   The natural history of cardiovascular disease must be appreciated. Cardiovascular disorders often present acutely, as in a previously asymptomatic patient with extensive coronary atherosclerosis who develops an acute myocardial infarction or the previously asymptomatic patient with hypertrophic cardiomyopathy whose first clinical manifestation is syncope or even sudden death. However, in both instances, the alert physician may recognize the patient at risk of these complications long before they occur and can often take measures to prevent their occurrence. For example, the patient with acute myocardial infarction may well have had risk factors for atherosclerosis for many years. Had these been recognized, their elimination or reduction might have delayed or even prevented the infarction. Similarly, the patient with hypertrophic cardiomyopathy may have had the familial form of this disorder, and a careful family history might have led to an echocardiographic examination and the recognition of the condition long before the acute manifestations.

PITFALLS IN CARDIOVASCULAR MEDICINE   Increasing subspecialization in internal medicine and the perfection of advanced diagnostic techniques in cardiology can lead to several undesirable consequences, which can be summarized as follows:

1. Failure by the *noncardiologist* to recognize cardiac manifestations of systemic illnesses. Examples of the latter are (a) the Down syndrome (associated with endocardial cushion defect); (b) bony abnormalities of the upper extremities (associated with atrial septal defect in the Holt-Oram syndrome); (c) muscular dystrophies (associated with cardiomyopathy); (d) hemochromatosis and glycogen storage disease (associated with myocardial infiltration and restrictive cardiomyopathy); (e) congenital deafness (associated with prolonged QT interval and serious cardiac arrhythmias); (f) Raynaud's disease (associated with primary pulmonary hyperten-

sion and coronary vasospasm); (g) connective tissue disorders, i.e., the Marfan syndrome, Ehlers-Danlos and Hurler syndromes, and related disorders of mucopolysaccharide metabolism (aortic dilatation, prolapsed mitral valve, a variety of arterial abnormalities); (h) acromegaly (hypertension, accelerated coronary atherosclerosis, conduction defects, cardiomyopathy); (i) hyperthyroidism (heart failure, atrial fibrillation); (j) hypothyroidism (pericardial effusion, coronary artery disease); (k) rheumatoid arthritis (pericarditis, aortic valve disease); (l) scleroderma (cor pulmonale, myocardial fibrosis, pericarditis); (m) systemic lupus erythematosus (valvulitis, myocarditis, pericarditis); (n) sarcoidosis (arrhythmias, cardiomyopathy); and (o) exfoliative dermatitis (high-output heart failure). In patients with these and other systemic disorders a detailed clinical and noninvasive examination of the cardiovascular system should be carried out to identify cardiovascular involvement.

2. Failure by the cardiologist to recognize an underlying systemic illness, such as those listed above, among patients with a cardiac disorder. Patients known or suspected of having heart disease require a detailed general assessment and a search for the frequent *noncardiac* manifestations of systemic disorders with cardiovascular manifestations. For example, infective endocarditis should be considered in patients with known congenital or valvular heart disease with fever, anemia, or albuminuria. A cardiovascular abnormality may provide the clue critical to the recognition of some systemic disorders. For instance, in an elderly person, unexplained atrial fibrillation may provide the first clue to the diagnosis of thyrotoxicosis.

3. Overreliance on and overutilization of laboratory tests, particularly invasive techniques for the examination of the cardiovascular system. Catheterization of the right and left sides of the heart, selective angiography, and coronary arteriography (Chap. 229) provide precise diagnostic information under many circumstances. For example, they aid in establishing a specific anatomic diagnosis and in determining the physiologic consequences of the abnormalities in patients with chest pain of uncertain cause in whom ischemic heart disease is suspected, and in determining the functional significance of valvular abnormalities in patients with rheumatic heart disease being considered for surgical treatment. Although a great deal of attention has been lavished on these specialized examinations, it should be recognized that they serve to *supplement*, not *supplant*, a careful examination carried out by clinical and noninvasive techniques. Sometimes coronary arteriography is carried out in patients with chest pain suspected of having ischemic heart disease instead of taking a careful history; although coronary arteriography may establish whether the coronary arteries are obstructed, the results often do not provide a definite answer to the question of whether a patient's complaint of chest pain is clearly attributable to coronary arteriosclerosis. Catheterization of the left side of the heart is all too frequently employed to determine whether operative treatment of valvular disease is indicated, even before the patient has had a trial of medical therapy.

Despite the enormous value of these invasive tests it must not be overlooked that they entail some small risk to the patient, involve discomfort and substantial cost, and place a strain on existing medical facilities. Therefore, they should be carried out not as part of a "fishing expedition" or as evidence to the patient and the family that "everything is being done," but only if, after detailed clinical examination and assessment by noninvasive tests, the results of the invasive examination can be expected to modify or aid in the patient's management.

℞ **TREATMENT**

After a complete diagnosis has been established, a number of therapeutic options are usually available. Several examples may be used to demonstrate some of the principles of cardiovascular therapeutics:

1. In the absence of evidence of heart disease, a clear, definitive statement to that effect should be made and the patient should *not* be asked to return at intervals for repeated examinations. If

there is no evidence for disease, such continued attention may lead to the patient developing inappropriate anxiety and fixation on the heart.

2. If there is no evidence of cardiovascular disease but the patient has one or more risk factors for the development of ischemic heart disease (Chap. 242), a plan for their reduction should be developed and the patient should be retested at intervals to assess that he or she is complying and that these risk factors are in fact being reduced.

3. Asymptomatic or mildly symptomatic patients with valvular heart disease that is anatomically severe should be evaluated periodically, every 6 to 12 months, by clinical and noninvasive examinations. Early signs of deterioration of ventricular function can be detected in this manner and in appropriate patients may signify the need for cardiac catheterization and surgical treatment before the development of disabling symptoms, irreversible myocardial damage, and an excessive risk of surgical treatment (Chap. 237).

4. It is critical to establish clear criteria for deciding on the form of treatment (medical, angioplasty, or surgical revascularization) in patients with ischemic heart disease (Chap. 244). Mechanical revascularization represents a major therapeutic advance in the treatment of this most common form of heart disease, but operation has probably been employed too widely in the United States; the mere presence of angina pectoris and/or the demonstration of critical coronary arterial narrowing at angiography should not reflexly evoke a decision to treat the patient surgically or by angioplasty. Instead, these forms of treatment should be limited to those patients with ischemic heart disease in whom it has been demonstrated that these treatments are superior to medical treatment.

BIBLIOGRAPHY

BRAUNWALD E (ed): *Heart Disease*, 5th ed. Philadelphia, Saunders, 1997

CHRISTIE LG, CONTI CR: Systematic approach to the evaluation of angina-like chest pain. Am Heart J 102:897, 1981

CONSTANT J: *Bedside Cardiology*, 4th ed. Boston, Little, Brown, 1993

THE CRITERIA COMMITTEE OF THE NEW YORK HEART ASSOCIATION: *Nomenclature and Criteria for Diagnosis*, 9th ed. Boston, Little, Brown, 1994

HURST JW: *Cardiovascular Diagnosis: The Initial Examination.* St. Louis, Mosby, 1993

MARRIOTT HJL: *Bedside Cardiac Diagnosis.* Philadelphia, Lippincott, 1993

SCHMITT BP et al: The diagnostic usefulness of the history of the patient with dyspnea. J Gen Intern Med 1:386, 1986

SUTTON GC: Symptoms of heart disease, in *Diseases of the Heart*, DG Julian (ed). London, Balliere Tindall, 1989, pp 89–99

227

Robert A. O'Rourke, Eugene Braunwald

PHYSICAL EXAMINATION OF THE CARDIOVASCULAR SYSTEM

A meticulous physical examination is a low-cost method for assessing the cardiovascular system and often provides important information for the appropriate selection of additional tests. First, the general physical appearance should be evaluated. The patient may appear tired because of a chronic low cardiac output; the respiratory rate may be rapid in cases of pulmonary venous congestion. Central cyanosis, often associated with clubbing of the fingers and toes, indicates right-to-left cardiac or extracardiac shunting or inadequate oxygenation of blood by the lungs. Cyanosis in the distal extremities, cool skin, and increased sweating result from vasoconstriction in patients with severe heart failure (Chap. 36). Noncardiovascular details can be equally important. For example, the diagnosis of infective endocarditis is highly likely in patients with petechiae, Osler's nodes, and Janeway lesions (Chap. 126).

The blood pressure should be taken in both arms and with the patient supine and upright; the heart rate should be timed for 30 s. Orthostatic hypotension and tachycardia may indicate a reduced blood volume, while resting tachycardia may be due to heart failure.

Careful examination of the optic fundi is essential (Chap. 246), and the retinal vessels may show evidence of systemic hypertension, arteriosclerosis, or embolism. The latter may result from atherosclerosis in larger arteries (e.g., the carotid) or may represent a complication of valvular heart disease (e.g., endocarditis).

Palpation of the peripheral arterial pulses in the upper and lower extremities is necessary to define the adequacy of systemic blood flow and to detect the presence of occlusive arterial lesions. It is also important to examine both legs for evidence of edema, varicose veins, or thrombophlebitis (Chap. 248). The cardiovascular examination includes careful evaluation of both the carotid arterial and the jugular venous pulses, as well as deliberate precordial palpation and attentive cardiac auscultation.

ARTERIAL PRESSURE PULSE The normal central aortic pulse wave is characterized by a fairly rapid rise to a somewhat rounded peak (Fig. 227-1). The anacrotic shoulder, present on the ascending limb, occurs at the time of peak rate of aortic flow just before maximum pressure is reached. The less steep descending limb is interrupted by a sharp downward deflection, synchronous with aortic valve closure, called the *incisura*. As the pulse wave is transmitted peripherally, the initial upstroke becomes steeper, the anacrotic shoulder becomes less apparent, and the incisura is replaced by the smoother dicrotic notch. Accordingly, palpation of a peripheral arterial pulse (e.g., the radial pulse) frequently gives less information than examination of a more central pulse (e.g., the carotid pulse) regarding alterations in left ventricular ejection or aortic valve function. However, certain findings, such as the hyperkinetic pulse of aortic regurgitation or pulsus alternans, are more evident in peripheral arteries (Fig. 227-2). The carotid pulse is best examined with the sternocleidomastoid muscle relaxed and with the head rotated slightly toward the examiner. In palpating the brachial arterial pulse, the examiner can support the subject's relaxed elbow with the right arm while compressing the brachial pulse with the thumb. The usual technique is to compress the artery with the thumb or forefinger until the maximum pulse is sensed. Varying degrees of pressure should then be applied while concentrating on the

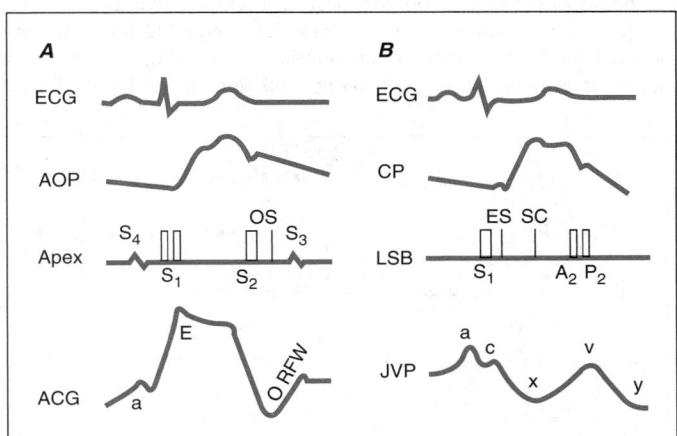

FIGURE 227-1 *A.* Schematic representation of electrocardiogram, aortic pressure pulse (AOP), phonocardiogram recorded at the apex, and apex cardiogram (ACG). On the phonocardiogram, S_1, S_2, S_3, and S_4 represent the first through fourth heart sounds; OS represents the opening snap of the mitral valve, which occurs coincident with the O point of the apex cardiogram. S_3 occurs coincident with the termination of the rapid-filling wave (RFW) of the ACG, while S_4 occurs coincident with the *a* wave of the ACG. *B.* Simultaneous recording of electrocardiogram, indirect carotid pulse (CP), phonocardiogram along the left sternal border (LSB), and indirect jugular venous pulse (JVP). ES, ejection sound; SC, systolic click.

separate phases of the pulse wave. This method, known as *trisection*, is useful for assessing the sharpness of the upstroke, systolic peak, and diastolic slope of the arterial pulse. In most normal persons, a dicrotic wave is not palpable.

A small weak pulse, *pulsus parvus*, is common in conditions with a diminished left ventricular stroke volume, a narrow pulse pressure, and increased peripheral vascular resistance (Fig. 227-2). A *hypokinetic* pulse may be due to hypovolemia, to left ventricular failure, to restrictive pericardial disease, or to mitral valve stenosis. In aortic valve stenosis, the delayed systolic peak, *pulsus tardus*, results from obstruction to left ventricular ejection. In contrast, a large, bounding (*hyperkinetic*) pulse is usually associated with an increased left ventricular stroke volume, a wide pulse pressure, and a decrease in peripheral vascular resistance. This pattern occurs characteristically in patients with an elevated stroke volume, as in complete heart block; with hyperkinetic circulation due to anxiety, anemia, exercise, or fever; or with a rapid runoff of blood from the arterial system (as caused by a patent ductus arteriosus or peripheral arteriovenous fistula). Patients with mitral regurgitation or a ventricular septal defect also may have a bounding pulse, since vigorous left ventricular ejection produces a rapid upstroke in the arterial pulse, even though the duration of systole and the forward stroke volume may be diminished. In aortic regurgitation, the rapidly rising, bounding arterial pulse results from an increased left ventricular stroke volume and an increased rate of ventricular ejection.

The *bisferiens pulse*, which has two systolic peaks, is characteristic of aortic regurgitation (with or without accompanying stenosis) and of hypertrophic cardiomyopathy (Chap. 239). In the latter condition, the pulse wave upstroke rises rapidly and forcefully, producing the first systolic peak ("percussion wave"). A brief decline in pressure follows because of the sudden decrease in the rate of left ventricular ejection during midsystole, when severe obstruction often develops. This pressure trough is followed by a smaller and more slowly rising positive pulse wave ("tidal wave") produced by continued ventricular ejection and by reflected waves from the periphery. The *dicrotic pulse* has two palpable waves, one in systole and one in diastole. It occurs most frequently in patients with a very low stroke volume, particularly in those with dilated cardiomyopathy.

Pulsus alternans is a pattern in which there is regular alteration of the pressure pulse amplitude, despite a regular rhythm (Fig. 227-2). It is due to alternating left ventricular contractile force, usually denotes severe impairment of left ventricular function, and commonly occurs in patients who also have a loud third heart sound. Pulsus

alternans also may occur during or following paroxysmal tachycardia or for several beats following a premature beat in patients without heart disease. In *pulsus bigeminus*, there is also a regular alteration of pressure pulse amplitude, but it is caused by a premature ventricular contraction that follows each regular beat. In *pulsus paradoxus*, the decrease in systolic arterial pressure that normally accompanies the reduction in arterial pulse amplitude during inspiration is accentuated. In patients with pericardial tamponade (Chap. 240), airway obstruction, or superior vena cava obstruction, the decrease in systolic arterial pressure frequently exceeds the normal decrease of 10 mmHg and the peripheral pulse may disappear completely during inspiration.

Simultaneous palpation of the radial and femoral arterial pulses, which normally are virtually coincident, is important to rule out aortic coarctation, in which the latter pulse is weakened and delayed (Chap. 235).

JUGULAR VENOUS PULSE (JVP) The two main objectives of the examination of the neck veins are inspection of their waveform and estimation of the central venous pressure (CVP). In most patients, the right internal jugular vein is best for both purposes. Usually, the pulsation of the internal jugular vein is greatest when the trunk is inclined by less than 30°. In patients with elevated venous pressure, it may be necessary to elevate the trunk further, sometimes to as much as 90°. When the neck muscles are relaxed, shining a beam of light tangentially across the skin overlying the vein exposes the pulsations of the internal jugular vein. Simultaneous palpation of the left carotid artery aids the examiner in deciding which pulsations are venous and in relating the venous pulsations to their timing in the cardiac cycle.

The normal JVP reflects phasic pressure changes in the right atrium and consists of two or sometimes three positive waves and two negative troughs (Fig. 227-1). The positive presystolic *a* wave is produced by venous distention due to right atrial contraction and is the dominant wave in the JVP, particularly during inspiration. Large *a* waves indicate that the right atrium is contracting against an increased resistance (Fig. 227-3), such as occurs with tricuspid stenosis or more commonly with increased resistance to right ventricular filling (pulmonary hypertension or pulmonic stenosis). Large *a* waves also occur during arrhythmias whenever the right atrium contracts while the tricuspid valve is closed by right ventricular systole. Such "cannon" *a* waves may occur regularly (as during junctional rhythm) or irregularly (as in atrioventricular dissociation with ventricular tachycardia or complete heart block). The *a* wave is absent in patients with atrial fibrillation, and there is an increased delay between the *a* wave and the carotid arterial pulse in patients with first-degree atrioventricular block.

The *c* wave, often observed in the JVP, is a positive wave produced by the bulging of the tricuspid valve into the right atrium during right ventricular isovolumetric systole and by the impact of the carotid artery adjacent to the jugular vein. The *x* descent is due both to atrial relaxation and to the downward displacement of the tricuspid valve during ventricular systole. The *x* descent wave during systole is often accentuated in patients with constrictive pericarditis (Fig. 227-3), but this wave is reduced with right ventricular dilation and often is reversed

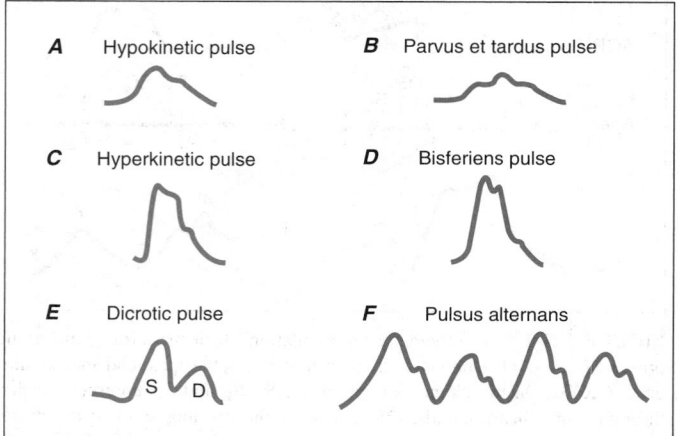

FIGURE 227-2 Schematic representation of arterial pulse waveforms that occur with alterations in cardiac hemodynamics, which may result from normal physiologic responses or may be due to cardiac disease. S, systole; D, diastole. [*Modified from RA O'Rourke, in The Heart, 7th ed, JW Hurst et al (eds). New York, McGraw-Hill, 1990, with permission.*]

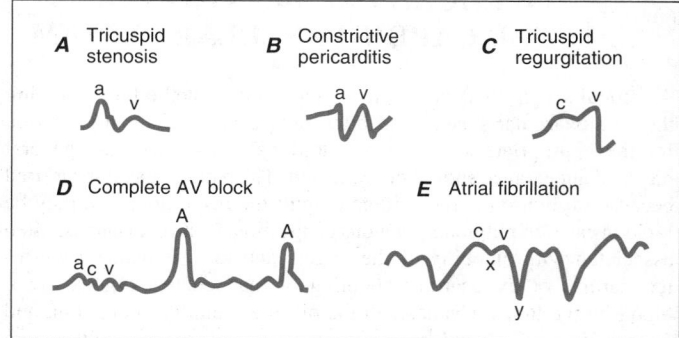

FIGURE 227-3 Abnormal jugular venous pulse waveforms commonly present in patients with cardiac disease and/or arrhythmias. See text. [*Modified from RA O'Rourke, in The Heart, 7th ed, JW Hurst et al (eds). New York, McGraw-Hill, 1990, with permission.*]

in tricuspid regurgitation. The positive, late systolic *v* wave results from the increasing volume of blood in the right atrium during ventricular systole when the tricuspid valve is closed. Tricuspid regurgitation causes the *v* wave to be more prominent; when tricuspid regurgitation becomes severe, the combination of a prominent *v* wave and obliteration of the *x* descent results in a single large positive systolic wave. After the *v* wave peaks, the right atrial pressure falls because of the decreased bulging of the tricuspid valve into the right atrium as right ventricular pressure declines and the tricuspid valve opens (Fig. 227-3).

This negative descending limb—the *y* descent of the JVP—is produced mainly by the opening of the tricuspid valve and the subsequent rapid inflow of blood into the right ventricle. A rapid, deep *y* descent in early diastole occurs with severe tricuspid regurgitation. A venous pulse characterized by a sharp *y* descent, a deep *y* trough, and a rapid ascent to the baseline is seen in patients with constrictive pericarditis or with severe right-sided heart failure and a high venous pressure. A slow *y* descent in the JVP suggests an obstruction to right ventricular filling, as occurs with tricuspid stenosis or right atrial myxoma.

The right internal jugular is the best vein to use for accurate estimation of the central venous pressure. The sternal angle is used as the reference point, because the center of the right atrium lies approximately 5 cm below the sternal angle in the average patient, regardless of body position. The patient is examined at the optimal degree of trunk elevation for visualization of venous pulsations. The vertical distance between the top of the oscillating venous column and the level of the sternal angle is determined; generally it is less than 3 cm (3 cm + 5 cm = 8 cm blood). The most common cause of a high venous pressure is an elevated right ventricular diastolic pressure. In patients suspected of having right ventricular failure who have a normal CVP at rest, the abdominojugular reflux test may be helpful. The palm of the examiner's hand is placed over the abdomen, and firm pressure is applied for 10 s or more. In normal persons, this maneuver does not alter the jugular venous pressure significantly, but when right heart function is impaired, the upper level of venous pulsation usually increases. A positive abdominojugular test is best defined as an increase in JVP during 10 s of firm midabdominal compression followed by a rapid drop in pressure by 4 cm blood on release of the compression. The most common cause of a positive test is right-sided heart failure secondary to elevated left heart filling pressures. Also, abdominal compression may elicit the JVP pattern typical of tricuspid regurgitation when the resting pulse wave is normal. Kussmaul's sign—an increase rather than the normal decrease in the CVP during inspiration—is most often caused by severe right-sided heart failure; it is a frequent finding in patients with constrictive pericarditis or right ventricular infarction.

PRECORDIAL PALPATION The location, amplitude, duration, and direction of the cardiac impulse usually can be best appreciated with the fingertips. The normal left ventricular apex impulse is located at or medial to the left midclavicular line in the fourth or fifth intercostal space and is a tapping, early systolic outward thrust localized to a point not more than 3 cm in diameter. It is due primarily to recoil of the heart as blood is ejected and should be evaluated with the patient supine and in the left lateral position. Left ventricular hypertrophy results in exaggeration of the amplitude, duration, and often size of the normal left ventricular thrust. The impulse may be displaced laterally and downward into the sixth or seventh interspace, particularly in patients with a left ventricular volume load such as occurs in cases of aortic regurgitation or dilated cardiomyopathy.

Additional abnormal features that are detectable at the left ventricular apex include marked presystolic distention of the left ventricle, which is often accompanied by a fourth heart sound in patients with an excessive left ventricular pressure load or myocardial ischemia/infarction, and a prominent early diastolic rapid-filling wave, which is often accompanied by a third heart sound in patients with left ventricular failure or mitral valve regurgitation (Fig. 227-1). A double systolic apical impulse often is palpable in patients with hypertrophic cardiomyopathy.

Right ventricular hypertrophy often results in a sustained systolic lift at the lower left parasternal area, which starts in early systole and is synchronous with the left ventricular apical impulse.

Abnormal precordial pulsations occur during systole in patients with left ventricular dyssynergy due to ischemic heart disease or to diffuse myocardial disease from some other cause. These pulsations often occur in patients with a recent myocardial infarction and may be present in some patients only during episodes of anginal pain. They are most commonly felt in the left midprecordium one or two interspaces above and/or 1 to 2 cm medial to the left ventricular apex. A systolic bulge occurring in the region of the apex is difficult to distinguish from the impulse of left ventricular hypertrophy.

A left parasternal lift is present frequently in patients with severe mitral regurgitation. This pulsation occurs distinctly later than the left ventricular apical impulse, is synchronous with the *v* wave in the left atrial pressure curve, and is due to anterior displacement of the right ventricle by an enlarged, expanding left atrium. A similar impulse occurs to the right of the sternum in some patients with severe tricuspid regurgitation and a giant right atrium. Pulsation of the right sternoclavicular joint may indicate a right-sided aortic arch or aneurysmal dilation of the ascending aorta. Pulmonary artery pulsation is often visible and palpable in the second left intercostal space. While it may be normal in children or thin young adults, in others this pulsation usually denotes pulmonary hypertension, increased pulmonary blood flow, or poststenotic pulmonary artery dilation.

Thrills are palpable, low-frequency vibrations associated with heart murmurs. The systolic murmur of mitral regurgitation may be palpated at the cardiac apex. When the palm of the hand is placed over the precordium, the thrill of aortic stenosis crosses the palm toward the right side of the neck, while the thrill of pulmonic stenosis radiates more often to the left side of the neck. The thrill due to a ventricular septal defect is usually located in the third and fourth intercostal spaces near the left sternal border.

Percussion should be performed in each patient to identify normal or abnormal position of the heart, stomach, and liver. However, in patients with a normal cardiac situs, percussion adds little to careful inspection and palpation in the recognition of cardiac enlargement.

CARDIAC AUSCULTATION

To obtain the most information from cardiac auscultation, the observer should keep in mind several principles: (1) Auscultation should be performed in a quiet room to avoid the distracting noises of normal activity. (2) For optimal auscultation, attention must be focused on the phase of the cardiac cycle during which the auscultatory event is expected to occur. (3) The timing of a heart sound or murmur can be determined accurately from its relation to other observable events in the cardiac cycle—the carotid arterial pulse, the apical impulse, or the JVP. (4) To define the significance of a cardiac sound or murmur, it is often necessary to observe alterations in its timing or intensity during various physiologic and/or pharmacologic interventions (Table 227-1).

HEART SOUNDS The major components of heart sounds are vibrations associated with the abrupt acceleration or deceleration of blood in the cardiovascular system. Studies using simultaneous echocardiographic-phonocardiographic recordings indicate that the first and second heart sounds are produced primarily by the closure of the atrioventricular (AV) and semilunar valves and the events that accompany these closures. The intensity of the *first heart sound* (S_1) is influenced by (1) the position of the mitral leaflets at the onset of ventricular systole, (2) the rate of rise of the left ventricular pressure pulse, (3) the presence or absence of structural disease of the mitral valve, and (4) the amount of tissue, air, or fluid between the heart and the stethoscope. S_1 is louder if diastole is shortened because of tachycardia, if atrioventricular flow is increased because of high cardiac output or prolonged because of mitral stenosis, or if atrial contraction precedes ventricular contraction by an unusually short interval, reflected in a short PR interval. The loud S_1 in mitral stenosis usually signifies that the valve is pliable and that it remains open at the onset of isovolumetric contraction because of the elevated left atrial pressure. A reduction in the intensity of S_1 may be due to poor conduction of sound through the chest wall, a slow rise of the left ventricular pressure pulse, a long PR interval, or imperfect closure due to reduced valve substance, as in mitral regurgitation. S_1 is also soft when the anterior mitral leaflet is immobile because of rigidity and calcification, even in the presence of predominant mitral stenosis.

Splitting of the two high-pitched components of S_1 by 10 to 30 ms is a normal phenomenon (Fig. 227-1). The first component of S_1 is attributed to mitral valve closure, and the second to tricuspid valve closure. Widening of the S_1 is due most often to complete right bundle branch block and the resulting delay in onset of the right ventricular pressure pulse. Reversed splitting of the S_1, in which the mitral component follows the tricuspid component, may be present in patients with severe mitral stenosis, left atrial myxoma, and left bundle branch block.

Splitting of S_2 into audibly distinct aortic (A_2) and pulmonic (P_2) components occurs normally during inspiration, when the augmented inflow into the right ventricle increases its stroke volume and ejection period and thus delays closure of the pulmonic valve. P_2 is coincident with the incisura of the pulmonary artery pressure curve, which is separated from the right ventricular pressure tracing by an interval termed the "hangout time." The absolute value of this interval reflects the resistance to pulmonary blood flow and the impedance characteris-

tics of the pulmonary vascular bed. This interval is prolonged, and physiologic splitting of S_2 is accentuated, in conditions associated with right ventricular volume overload and a distensible pulmonary vascular bed. However, in patients with an increase in pulmonary vascular resistance, the hangout time is markedly reduced, and narrow splitting of S_2 is present. Splitting that persists with expiration (heard best at the pulmonic area or left sternal border) is usually abnormal when the patient is in the upright position. Such splitting may be due to many causes: delayed activation of the right ventricle (right bundle branch block); left ventricular ectopic beats; a left ventricular pacemaker; prolongation of right ventricular contraction with an increased right ventricular pressure load (pulmonary embolism or pulmonic stenosis); or delayed pulmonic valve closure because of right ventricular volume overload associated with right ventricular failure or diminished impedance of the pulmonary vascular bed and a prolonged hangout time (atrial septal defect).

In pulmonary hypertension, P_2 is increased in intensity, and splitting of the second heart sound may be diminished, normal, or accentuated, depending on the cause of the pulmonary hypertension, the pulmonary vascular resistance, and the presence or absence of right ventricular decompensation. Early aortic valve closure, occurring with mitral regurgitation or a ventricular septal defect, also may produce splitting that persists during expiration. It also may occur with constrictive pericarditis. In patients with an atrial septal defect, the proportion of right atrial filling contributed by the left atrium and the venae cavae varies reciprocally during the respiratory cycle, so that right atrial inflow remains relatively constant. Therefore, the volume and duration of right ventricular ejection are not significantly increased by inspiration, and there is little inspiratory exaggeration of the splitting of S_2. This phenomenon, termed *fixed splitting* of the second heart sound, is of considerable diagnostic value.

A delay in aortic valve closure causing P_2 to precede A_2 results in so-called reversed (paradoxic) splitting of S_2. Splitting is then maximal in expiration and decreases during inspiration with the normal delay of pulmonic valve closure. The most common causes of reversed splitting of S_2 are left bundle branch block and delayed excitation of the left ventricle from a right ventricular ectopic beat. Mechanical prolongation of left ventricular systole, resulting in reversed splitting of S_2, also may be caused by severe aortic outflow obstruction, a large aorta-to-pulmonary artery shunt, systolic hypertension, and ischemic heart disease or cardiomyopathy with left ventricular failure. P_2 is normally softer than A_2 in the second left intercostal space; a P_2 that is greater than A_2 in this area suggests pulmonary hypertension, except in patients with atrial septal defect.

The *third heart sound* (S_3) is a low-pitched sound produced in the ventricle 0.14 to 0.16 s after A_2, at the termination of rapid filling. This sound is frequent in normal children and in patients with high cardiac output. However, in patients over 40 years old, an S_3 usually indicates impairment of ventricular function, AV valve regurgitation, or other conditions that increase the rate or volume of ventricular filling. The left-sided S_3 is best heard with the bell piece of the stethoscope at the left ventricular apex during expiration and with the patient in the left lateral position. The right-sided S_3 is best heard at the left sternal border or just beneath the xiphoid and usually is louder with inspiration. Often it is accompanied by the systolic murmur of functional tricuspid regurgitation. Third heart sounds often disappear with treatment of heart failure.

An S_3 that is earlier (0.10 to 0.12 s after A_2) and higher-pitched than normal (a pericardial knock) often occurs in patients with constrictive pericarditis (Chap. 240); its presence depends on the restrictive effect of the adherent pericardium, which halts diastolic filling abruptly.

The *opening snap* (OS) is a brief, high-pitched, early diastolic sound which is usually due to stenosis of an AV valve, most often the mitral valve. It is generally heard best at the lower left sternal border and radiates well to the base of the heart. The A_2-OS interval is inversely related to the height of the mean left atrial pressure and ranges from 0.04 to 0.12 s. In the second intercostal space, an OS is often confused with P_2. However, careful auscultation will reveal both

Table 227-1

Effects of Physiologic and Pharmacologic Interventions on the Intensity of Heart Murmurs and Sounds*

Respiration Systolic murmurs due to TR or pulmonic blood flow through a normal or stenotic valve and diastolic murmurs of TS or PR generally increase with inspiration, as do right-sided S_3 and S_4. Left-sided murmurs and sounds usually are louder during expiration.

Valsalva maneuver Most murmurs decrease in length and intensity. Two exceptions are the systolic murmur of HCM, which usually becomes much louder, and that of MVP, which becomes longer and often louder. Following release of the Valsalva maneuver, right-sided murmurs tend to return to control intensity earlier than left-sided murmurs.

After VPB or AF Murmurs originating at normal or stenotic semilunar valves increase in the cardiac cycle following a VPB or in the cycle after a long cycle length in AF. By contrast, systolic murmurs due to AV valve regurgitation either do not change, diminish (papillary muscle dysfunction), or become shorter (MVP).

Positional changes With *standing,* most murmurs diminish, two exceptions being the murmur of HCM, which becomes louder, and that of MVP, which lengthens and often is intensified. With *squatting,* most murmurs become louder, but those of HCM and MVP usually soften and may disappear. Passive leg raising usually produces the same results.

Exercise Murmurs due to blood flow across normal or obstructed valves (e.g., PS, MS) become louder with both isotonic and submaximal isometric (handgrip) exercise. Murmurs of MR, VSD, and AR also increase with handgrip exercise. However, the murmur of HCM often decreases with near maximum handgrip exercise. Left-sided S_4 and S_3 are often accentuated by exercise, particularly when due to ischemic heart disease.

Pharmacologic interventions During the initial relative hypotension following amyl nitrite inhalation, murmurs of MR, VSD, and AR decrease, while murmurs of aortic stenosis or sclerosis increase. During the later tachycardia phase, murmurs of MS and right-sided lesions also increase. The response in MVP often is biphasic (first softer and then louder than control). The arterial constrictor phenylephrine tends to produce the opposite effects.

Transient arterial occlusion Transient external compression of both arms by bilateral cuff inflation to 20 mmHg over peak systolic pressure augments the murmurs of MR, VSD, and AR, but not murmurs due to other causes.

* TR, tricuspid regurgitation; TS, tricuspid stenosis; PR, pulmonic regurgitation; HCM, hypertrophic cardiomyopathy; MVP, mitral valve prolapse; PS, pulmonic stenosis; MS, mitral stenosis; MR, mitral regurgitation; VSD, ventricular septal defect; AR, aortic regurgitation; VPB, ventricular premature beat; and AF, atrial fibrillation.

components of S_2, followed by the OS. The OS of tricuspid stenosis occurs later in diastole than the mitral OS and is often overlooked in patients with more prominent mitral valve disease.

The *fourth heart sound* (S_4) is a low-pitched, presystolic sound produced in the ventricle during ventricular filling; it is associated with an effective atrial contraction and is heard best with the bell piece of the stethoscope. The sound is absent in patients with atrial fibrillation. The S_4 occurs when diminished ventricular compliance increases the resistance to ventricular filling, and it is present frequently in patients with systemic hypertension, aortic stenosis, hypertrophic cardiomyopathy, ischemic heart disease, and acute mitral regurgitation. Most patients with an acute myocardial infarction and sinus rhythm have an audible S_4. The fourth heart sound is frequently accompanied by visible and palpable presystolic distention of the left ventricle. It peaks in intensity at the left ventricular apex when the patient is in the left lateral position and is accentuated by mild isotonic or isometric exercise in the supine position. The right-sided S_4 is present in patients with right ventricular hypertrophy secondary to either pulmonic stenosis or pulmonary hypertension and frequently accompanies a prominent presystolic *a* wave in the JVP.

An S_4 frequently accompanies delayed AV conduction even in the absence of clinically detectable heart disease. The incidence of an audible S_4 increases with increasing age. Whether an audible S_4 in adults without other evidence of cardiac disease is abnormal remains controversial.

The *ejection sound* is a sharp, high-pitched event occurring in early systole and closely following the first heart sound. Ejection sounds occur in the presence of semilunar valve stenosis and in conditions associated with dilation of the aorta or pulmonary artery. The aortic ejection sound is usually heard best at the left ventricular apex and the second right intercostal space; the pulmonary ejection sound is strongest at the upper left sternal border. The latter, unlike most other right-sided acoustical events, is heard better during expiration.

Nonejection or *midsystolic clicks*, occurring with or without a late systolic murmur, often denote prolapse of one or both leaflets of the mitral valve (Chap. 237). They also may be caused by tricuspid valve prolapse. They probably result from chordae tendineae that are functionally unequal in length on either or both AV valves and are heard best along the lower left sternal border and at the left ventricular apex. Systolic clicks may be single or multiple, and they may occur at any time in systole but usually are later than the systolic ejection sound.

HEART MURMURS Cardiac murmurs result from vibrations set up in the bloodstream and the surrounding heart and great vessels as a result of turbulent blood flow, the formation of eddies, and cavitation (bubble formation as a result of sudden decrease in pressure).

The intensity (loudness) of murmurs may be graded from I to VI. A grade I murmur is so faint that it can be heard only with special effort; a grade IV murmur is commonly accompanied by a thrill; and a grade VI murmur is audible with the stethoscope removed from contact with the chest. The configuration of a murmur may be crescendo, decrescendo, crescendo-decrescendo (diamond-shaped), or plateau. The precise time of onset and time of cessation of a murmur depend on the instant in the cardiac cycle at which an adequate pressure difference between two chambers arises and disappears (Fig. 227-4).

The location on the chest wall where the murmur is best heard and the areas to which it radiates can be helpful in identifying the cardiac structure from which the murmur originates. For example, the murmur of aortic valve stenosis usually is loudest in the second right intercostal space and radiates to the carotid arteries. By contrast, the murmur of mitral regurgitation most often is loudest at the cardiac apex. It may radiate to the left sternal border and base of the heart when the posterior mitral leaflet is predominantly involved or to the axilla and back when the anterior leaflet is more severely affected. In the latter case, the regurgitant blood is directed toward the posterior left atrial wall.

Often it is difficult to classify a cardiac murmur with certainty on the basis of its timing, configuration, location, radiation, pitch, or intensity. However, by noting changes in the characteristics of the murmur during maneuvers that alter cardiac hemodynamics, the aus-

cultator often can identify its correct origin and significance (Table 227-1).

Accentuation of a murmur during inspiration (a maneuver that augments systemic venous return) implies that it originates on the right side of the circulation; expiratory exaggeration has less significance. Prolonged expiratory pressure against a closed glottis (i.e., the Valsalva maneuver) reduces the intensity of most murmurs by diminishing both right and left ventricular filling (i.e., ventricular preload). The systolic murmur associated with *hypertrophic cardiomyopathy* and the late systolic murmur due to *mitral valve prolapse* are exceptions and may be paradoxically accentuated during the Valsalva maneuver. Murmurs due to flow across a normal or obstructed semilunar valve increase in intensity in the cycle following a premature ventricular beat or a long RR interval in atrial fibrillation. In contrast, murmurs due to AV valve regurgitation or a ventricular septal defect do not change appreciably during the beat following a prolonged diastole. Standing, which decreases left ventricular volume, accentuates the murmur of hypertrophic cardiomyopathy and occasionally the murmur due to mitral valve prolapse. Squatting, which increases both venous return and systemic arterial resistance and thus ventricular afterload, increases most murmurs, except those due to hypertrophic cardiomyopathy and mitral regurgitation due to a prolapsed mitral valve, which often decrease. Sustained handgrip exercise, which increases systemic arterial pressure and heart rate, often accentuates the murmurs of mitral regurgitation, aortic regurgitation, and mitral stenosis but usually diminishes those due to aortic stenosis or hypertrophic cardiomyopathy. Pharmacologic interventions include inhalation of amyl nitrite, which reduces systemic arterial pressure and increases blood flow, thereby increasing the intensity of murmurs due to valvular stenosis while diminishing those due to aortic or mitral regurgitation (Table 227-1). Transient external arterial occlusion by the inflation of bilateral arm cuffs to 20 mmHg (2.66 kPa) above systolic blood pressure for 5 s usually intensifies murmurs due to left-sided regurgitant lesions; this method is applicable to almost all patients and does not require administration of any drug.

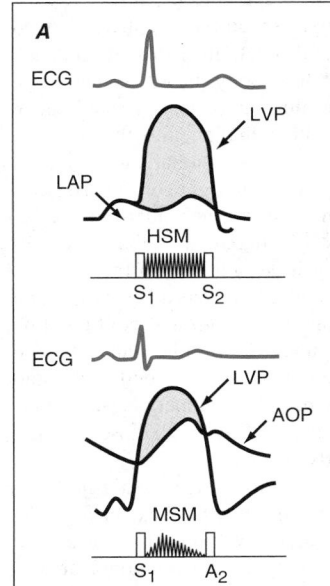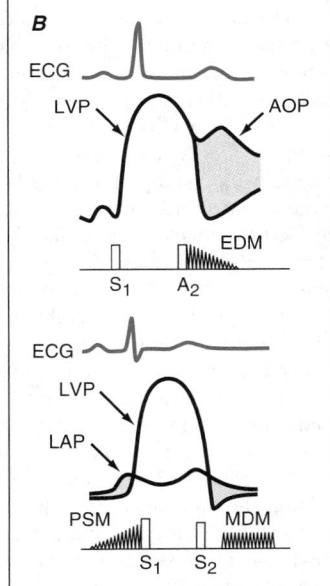

FIGURE 227-4 *A.* Schematic representation of ECG, aortic pressure (AOP), left ventricular pressure (LVP), and left atrial pressure (LAP). The shaded areas indicated a transvalvular pressure difference during systole. HSM, holosystolic murmur; MSM, midsystolic murmur. *B.* Graphic representation of ECG, aortic pressure (AOP), left ventricular pressure (LVP) and left atrial pressure (LAP) with shaded areas indicating transvalvular diastolic pressure difference. EDM, early diastolic murmur; PSM, presystolic murmur; MDM, middiastolic murmur.

Systolic Murmurs *Holosystolic (pansystolic) murmurs* are generated when there is flow between two chambers that have widely different pressures throughout systole, such as the left ventricle and either the left atrium or the right ventricle (Fig. 227-4). The pressure gradient occurs early in contraction and lasts until relaxation is almost complete. Therefore, holosystolic murmurs begin before aortic ejection, and at the area of maximal intensity they begin with S_1 and end after S_2. Holosystolic murmurs accompany mitral or tricuspid regurgitation, ventricular septal defect, and, under certain circumstances, aortopulmonary shunts. Although the typical high-pitched murmur of mitral regurgitation usually continues throughout systole, the shape of the murmur may vary considerably. The holosystolic murmurs of mitral regurgitation and ventricular septal defect are augmented by transient exercise and are diminished by lowering the left ventricular systolic pressure by inhalation of amyl nitrite. The murmur of tricuspid regurgitation associated with pulmonary hypertension is holosystolic and frequently increases during inspiration. Not all patients with mitral or tricuspid regurgitation or ventricular septal defect have holosystolic murmurs (Chap. 237). Often, a mild valvular regurgitant jet, detected by color flow Doppler techniques, is not associated with an audible murmur despite optimal auscultation. Such regurgitant jets usually do not indicate clinical heart disease.

Midsystolic murmurs, also called *systolic ejection murmurs*, which are often crescendo-decrescendo in shape, occur when blood is ejected across the aortic or pulmonic outflow tracts (Fig. 227-4). The murmur starts shortly after S_1, when the ventricular pressure becomes high enough to open the semilunar valve. As the velocity of ejection increases, the murmur gets stronger, and as ejection declines, it diminishes. The murmur ends before the ventricular pressure falls enough to permit closure of the aortic or pulmonic leaflets. When the semilunar valves are normal, an increased flow rate (as occurs in states of elevated cardiac output), ejection into a dilated vessel beyond the valve, or increased transmission of sound through a thin chest wall may be responsible for this murmur. Most benign, functional murmurs are midsystolic and originate from the pulmonary outflow tract. Valvular or subvalvular obstruction of either ventricle also may cause such a midsystolic murmur, the intensity being related to the flow rate.

The murmur of aortic stenosis is the prototype of the left-sided midsystolic murmur. The location and radiation of this murmur are influenced by the direction of the high-velocity jet within the aortic root. In *valvular aortic stenosis*, the murmur is usually maximal in the second right intercostal space, with radiation into the neck. In *supravalvular aortic stenosis*, the murmur is occasionally loudest even higher, with disproportionate radiation into the right carotid artery. In hypertrophic cardiomyopathy, the midsystolic murmur originates in the left ventricular cavity and is usually maximal at the lower left sternal edge and apex, with relatively little radiation to the carotids. When the aortic valve is immobile (calcified), the aortic closure sound (A_2) may be soft and inaudible so that the length and configuration of the murmur are difficult to determine. Midsystolic murmurs also occur in patients with mitral regurgitation or, less frequently, tricuspid regurgitation resulting from papillary muscle dysfunction. Such murmurs due to mitral regurgitation are often confused with those originating in the aorta, particularly in elderly patients.

The patient's age and the area of maximal intensity aid in determining the significance of midsystolic murmurs. Thus, in a young adult with a thin chest and a high velocity of blood flow, a faint or moderate midsystolic murmur heard only in the pulmonic area is usually without clinical significance, while a somewhat louder murmur in the aortic area may indicate congenital aortic stenosis. In elderly patients, pulmonic flow murmurs are rare, while aortic systolic murmurs are common and may be due to aortic dilation, to a significant degree of valvular aortic stenosis, or to nonstenotic deformity (sclerosis) of the aortic valve. Midsystolic aortic and pulmonic murmurs are intensified after amyl nitrite inhalation and during the cardiac cycle following a premature ventricular beat, while those due to mitral

regurgitation are unchanged or softer. Aortic systolic murmurs are diminished by interventions that increase aortic impedance, such as intravenous phenylephrine administration. Echocardiography or cardiac catheterization may be necessary to separate a prominent and exaggerated functional murmur from one due to congenital or acquired semilunar valve stenosis.

Early systolic murmurs begin with the first heart sound and end in midsystole. In *large ventricular septal defects with pulmonary hypertension*, the shunting at the end of systole may be small or absent, resulting in an early systolic murmur. A similar murmur may occur with very *small muscular ventricular septal defects,* the shunt being interrupted in late systole. An early systolic murmur is a feature of *tricuspid regurgitation occurring in the absence of pulmonary hypertension*. This lesion is common in narcotics abusers with infective endocarditis, in whom a tall regurgitant right atrial v wave reaches the level of the normal right ventricular pressure in late systole, confining the murmur to early systole. Patients with acute mitral regurgitation into a noncompliant left atrium and a large v wave often have a loud early systolic murmur that diminishes as the pressure gradient between the left ventricle and left atrium decreases in late systole (Chap. 237).

Late systolic murmurs are faint or moderately loud, high-pitched apical murmurs that start well after ejection and do not mask either heart sound. They are probably related to papillary muscle dysfunction caused by infarction or ischemia of these muscles or to their distortion by left ventricular dilation. They may appear only during angina but are common in patients with myocardial infarction or diffuse myocardial disease. Late systolic murmurs following midsystolic clicks are due to late systolic mitral regurgitation caused by prolapse of the mitral valve into the left atrium (Chap. 237).

Diastolic Murmurs *Early diastolic murmurs* (Fig. 227-4) begin with or shortly after S_2, as soon as the corresponding ventricular pressure falls enough below that in the aorta or pulmonary artery. The high-pitched murmurs of aortic regurgitation or of pulmonic regurgitation due to pulmonary hypertension are generally decrescendo, since there is a progressive decline in the volume or rate of regurgitation during diastole. Faint, high-pitched murmurs of aortic regurgitation are difficult to hear unless they are specifically sought by applying firm pressure with the diaphragm over the left midsternal border while the patient sits leaning forward and holds a breath in full expiration. The diastolic murmur of aortic regurgitation is enhanced by an acute elevation of the arterial pressure, such as occurs with handgrip exercise; it diminishes with a decrease in arterial pressure, as with amyl nitrite inhalation. The diastolic murmur of congenital pulmonic regurgitation without pulmonary hypertension is low- to medium-pitched. The onset of this murmur is delayed because the regurgitant flow is minimal at the onset of pulmonic valve closure when the reverse pressure gradient responsible for the regurgitation is negligible.

Middiastolic murmurs usually arise from the AV valves (Fig. 227-4), occur during early ventricular filling, and are due to disproportion between valve orifice size and flow rate. Such murmurs may be quite loud (grade III), despite only slight AV valve stenosis, when there is normal or increased blood flow. Conversely, the murmurs may be soft or even absent despite severe obstruction if the cardiac output is markedly reduced. When stenosis is marked, the diastolic murmur is prolonged, and the duration of the murmur is more reliable than its intensity as an index of the severity of valve obstruction.

The low-pitched, middiastolic murmur of mitral stenosis characteristically follows the OS. It should be specifically sought by placing the bell of the stethoscope at the site of the left ventricular impulse, which is best localized with the patient on the left side. Frequently, the murmur of mitral stenosis is present only at the left ventricular apex, and it may be increased in intensity by mild supine exercise or by inhalation of amyl nitrite. In tricuspid stenosis, the middiastolic murmur is localized to a relatively limited area along the left sternal edge and may be stronger during inspiration.

Middiastolic murmurs may be generated across the mitral valve in cases of mitral regurgitation, patent ductus arteriosus, or ventricular septal defect, and across the tricuspid valve in cases of tricuspid regurgitation or atrial septal defect. These murmurs are related to the torrential flow across an AV valve, usually follow an S_3, and tend to occur with large left-to-right shunts or severe AV valve regurgitation. A soft middiastolic murmur may sometimes be heard in patients with acute rheumatic fever (Carey-Coombs murmur). It has been attributed to inflammation of the mitral valve cusps or excessive left atrial blood flow as a consequence of mitral regurgitation.

In acute, severe aortic regurgitation, the left ventricular diastolic pressure may exceed the left atrial pressure, resulting in a middiastolic murmur due to "diastolic mitral regurgitation." In severe, chronic aortic regurgitation, a murmur is frequently present that may be either middiastolic or presystolic (Austin-Flint murmur). This murmur appears to originate at the anterior mitral valve leaflet when blood enters the left ventricle simultaneously from both the aortic root and the left atrium.

Presystolic murmurs begin during the period of ventricular filling that follows atrial contraction and therefore occur in sinus rhythm. They are usually due to AV valve stenosis and have the same quality as the middiastolic filling rumble, but they are usually crescendo, reaching peak intensity at the time of a loud S_1. The presystolic murmur corresponds to the AV valve gradient, which may be minimal until the moment of right or left atrial contraction. It is the presystolic murmur that is most characteristic of tricuspid stenosis and sinus rhythm. A right or left *atrial myxoma* may occasionally cause either middiastolic or presystolic murmurs that resemble the murmurs of mitral or tricuspid stenosis.

Continuous Murmurs These begin in systole, peak near S_2, and continue into all or part of diastole. These murmurs result from continuous flow due to a communication between high- and low-pressure areas which persists through the end of systole and the beginning of diastole. A *patent ductus arteriosus* causes a continuous murmur as long as the pressure in the pulmonary artery is much below that in the aorta. The murmur is intensified by elevation of the systemic arterial pressure and is reduced by amyl nitrite inhalation. When pulmonary hypertension is present, the diastolic portion may disappear, leaving the murmur confined to systole. A continuous murmur is uncommon in cases of aortopulmonary septal defect, as that malformation generally is associated with severe pulmonary hypertension. Surgically produced connections and the subclavian–pulmonary artery anastomosis result in murmurs similar to that of a patent ductus.

Continuous murmurs may result from congenital or acquired *systemic arteriovenous fistula*, *coronary arteriovenous fistula*, anomalous origin of the left coronary artery from the pulmonary artery, and communications between the *sinus of Valsalva and the right side of the heart*. Continuous murmurs also may occur in patients with a small atrial septal defect with a high left atrial pressure. Murmurs associated with *pulmonary arteriovenous fistulas* may be continuous but are usually only systolic. Continuous murmurs may also be due to disturbances of flow pattern in constricted systemic (e.g., renal) or pulmonary arteries when marked pressure differences between the two sides of the narrow segment persist; a continuous murmur in the back may be present in *coarctation of the aorta*; *pulmonary embolism* may cause continuous murmurs in partially occluded vessels.

In nonconstricted arteries, continuous murmurs may be due to rapid flow through a tortuous bed. Such murmurs typically occur within the bronchial arterial collateral circulation in cyanotic patients with severe pulmonary outflow obstruction. The "mammary souffle," an innocent murmur heard over the breasts during late pregnancy and in the early postpartum period, may be systolic or continuous. The innocent cervical venous hum is a continuous murmur usually audible over the medial aspect of the right supraclavicular fossa with the patient upright. The hum is usually louder during diastole and can be abolished instantaneously by digital compression of the ipsilateral internal jugular vein. Transmission of a loud venous hum to the area below the clavicles may result in a mistaken diagnosis of patent ductus arteriosus.

Pericardial Friction Rub These adventitious sounds may have presystolic, systolic, and early diastolic scratchy components, may be confused with a murmur or extracardiac sound when heard only in systole. It is best appreciated with the patient upright and leaning forward and may be accentuated during inspiration.

BIBLIOGRAPHY

CRAWFORD MH: *Examination of the Heart*, Part 2: *Inspection and Palpation of Venous and Arterial Pulses*. Chicago, American Heart Association, 1990

EILEN SD et al: Accuracy of precordial palpation for detecting increased left ventricular volume. Ann Intern Med 99:628, 1983

EWY GA: The abdominojugular test: Technique and hemodynamic correlates. Ann Intern Med 109:456, 1988

GREWE K et al: Differentiation of cardiac murmurs by auscultation. Curr Probl Cardiol 13(10):699, 1988

LEMBO NJ et al: Bedside diagnosis of systolic murmurs. N Engl J Med 318:1572, 1988

PERLOFF JK (ed): *Physical Examination of the Heart and Circulation*, 2d ed. Philadelphia, Saunders, 1990

———, BRAUNWALD E: Physical examination of the heart and circulation, in *Heart Disease*, 5th ed, E Braunwald (ed). Philadelphia, Saunders, 1997, pp 15–52

SHAVER JA: Cardiac auscultation: A cost-effective diagnostic skill. Curr Probl Cardiol 20(7):441, 1995

228 *Ary L. Goldberger*

ELECTROCARDIOGRAPHY

The electrocardiogram (ECG or EKG) is a graphic recording of electric potentials generated by the heart. The signals are detected by means of metal electrodes attached to the extremities and chest wall and are then amplified and recorded by the electrocardiograph. ECG *leads* actually display the instantaneous *differences* in potential between these electrodes.

The clinical utility of the ECG derives from its immediate availability as a noninvasive, inexpensive, and highly versatile test. In addition to its use in detecting arrhythmias, conduction disturbances, and myocardial ischemia, electrocardiography may reveal other findings related to life-threatening metabolic disturbances (e.g., hyperkalemia) or increased susceptibility to sudden cardiac death (e.g., QT prolongation syndromes). The advent of coronary thrombolysis or angioplasty in the early therapy of acute myocardial infarction (Chap. 243) has refocused particular attention on the sensitivity and specificity of ECG signs of myocardial ischemia.

ELECTROPHYSIOLOGY (See also Chaps. 230 and 231) Depolarization of the heart is the initiating event for cardiac contraction. The electric currents that spread through the heart are produced by three components: cardiac pacemaker cells, specialized conduction tissue, and the heart muscle itself. The ECG, however, records only the depolarization (stimulation) and repolarization (recovery) potentials generated by the atrial and ventricular myocardium. Under resting conditions, myocardial cells are *polarized*; that is, they carry an electric charge on their surface due to transmembrane ion concentration differences. The charge measured across atrial and ventricular cell membranes is about 90 mV, with the inside negative relative to the outside. When these cells are stimulated above a critical threshold potential, they rapidly depolarize and transiently reverse their membrane polarity. This depolarization process spreads in a wavelike manner through the atria and ventricles. The return of myocardial fibers to their original resting state occurs during repolarization.

The depolarization stimulus for the normal heartbeat originates in the *sinoatrial* (SA) *node* (Fig. 228-1) or *sinus node*, a collection of *pacemaker* cells. These cells fire spontaneously; that is, they exhibit *automaticity*. The first phase of cardiac electrical activation is the spread of the depolarization wave through the right and left atria, followed by atrial contraction. Next, the impulse stimulates pacemaker and specialized conduction tissues in the atrioventricular (AV) nodal and His-bundle areas; together, these two regions constitute the AV junction. The bundle of His bifurcates into two main branches, the right and left bundles, which rapidly transmit depolarization wavefronts to

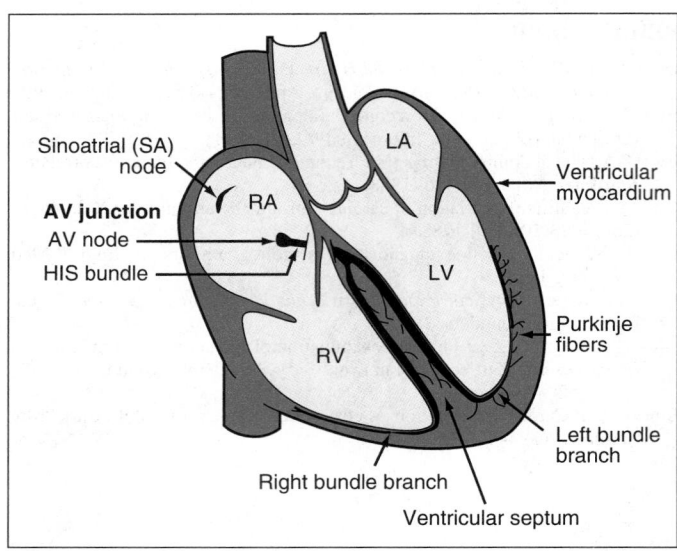

FIGURE 228-1 Schematic of the cardiac conduction system.

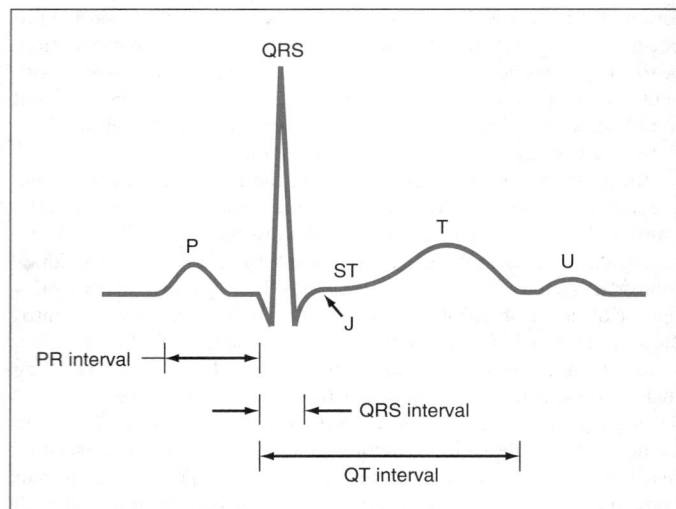

FIGURE 228-2 Basic ECG waveforms and intervals. Not shown is the R-R interval, the time between consecutive QRS complexes.

the right and left ventricular myocardium by way of Purkinje fibers. The main left bundle bifurcates into two primary subdivisions, a left anterior fascicle and a left posterior fascicle. The depolarization wavefronts then spread through the ventricular wall, from endocardium to epicardium, triggering ventricular contraction.

Since the cardiac depolarization and repolarization waves have direction and magnitude, they can be represented by vectors. *Vectorcardiograms* that measure and display these instantaneous potentials are no longer used much in clinical practice. However, the general principles of vector analysis remain fundamental to understanding the genesis of normal and pathologic ECG waveforms. Vector analysis illustrates a central concept of electrocardiography—that the ECG records the complex spatial and temporal summation of electrical potentials from multiple myocardial fibers conducted to the surface of the body. This principle accounts for inherent limitations in both ECG *sensitivity* (activity from certain cardiac regions may be canceled out or may be too weak to be recorded) and *specificity* (the same vectorial sum can result from either a selective gain or a loss of forces in opposite directions).

ECG WAVEFORMS AND INTERVALS The ECG waveforms are labeled alphabetically, beginning with the P wave, which represents atrial depolarization (Fig. 228-2). The QRS complex represents ventricular depolarization, and the ST-T-U complex (ST segment, T wave, and U wave) represents ventricular repolarization. The J point is the junction between the end of the QRS complex and the beginning of the ST segment. Atrial repolarization is usually too low in amplitude to be detected, but it may become apparent in such conditions as acute pericarditis or atrial infarction.

The QRS-T waveforms of the surface (extracellular) ECG correspond in a general way with the different phases of simultaneously obtained ventricular *action potentials*, the intracellular recordings from single myocardial fibers (Fig. 228-3) (see also Chap. 230). The rapid upstroke (phase 0) of the action potential corresponds to the onset of QRS. The plateau (phase 2) corresponds to the isoelectric ST segment, and active repolarization (phase 3) to the inscription of the T wave. Factors that decrease the slope of phase 0 by impairing the influx of Na^+ (e.g., drugs such as quinidine or procainamide, or hyperkalemia) tend to increase QRS duration. Conditions that prolong phase 2 (amiodarone, hypocalcemia) increase the QT interval. In contrast, shortening of ventricular repolarization (phase 3), as by digitalis or hypercalcemia, abbreviates the ST segment.

The electrocardiogram is ordinarily recorded on special graph paper which is divided into 1-mm² gridlike boxes (Fig. 228-4). Since the ECG paper speed is generally 25 mm/s, the smallest (1 mm) horizontal divisions correspond to 0.04 s (40 ms), with heavier lines at intervals of 0.20 s (200 ms). Vertically, the ECG graph measures the amplitude of a given wave or deflection (1 mV = 10 mm with standard calibration; the voltage criteria for hypertrophy mentioned below are given in millimeters). There are four major ECG intervals: R-R, PR, QRS, and QT (Fig. 228-2). The heart rate (beats per minute) can be readily computed from the interbeat (R-R) interval by dividing the number of large (0.20 s) time units between consecutive R waves into 300 or the number of small (0.04 s) units into 1500. The PR interval (normally 120 to 200 ms) measures the time (normally 120 to 200 ms) between atrial and ventricular depolarization, which includes the physiologic delay imposed by stimulation of cells in the AV junction area. The QRS interval (normally 100 ms or less) reflects the duration of ventricular depolarization. The QT interval includes both ventricular depolarization and repolarization times and varies inversely with the heart rate. A rate-related ("corrected") QT interval, QT_c, can be calculated as $QT/\sqrt{R\text{-}R}$ and normally is ≤ 0.44 s.

The QRS complex is subdivided into specific deflections or waves. If the initial QRS deflection in a given lead is negative, it is termed a *Q wave*; the first positive deflection is termed an *R wave*. A negative deflection after an R wave is an *S wave*. Subsequent positive or negative waves are labeled R′ and S′, respectively. Lowercase letters (qrs)

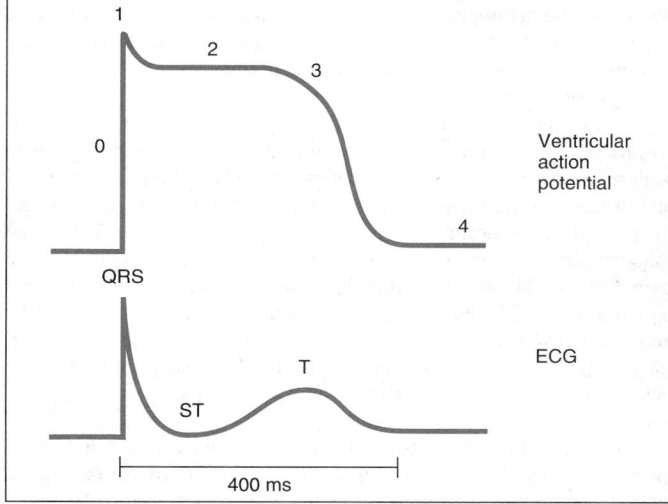

FIGURE 228-3 The QRS-T cycle corresponds to different phases of the ventricular action potential as described in Chap. 230.

are used for waves of relatively small amplitude. An entirely negative QRS complex is termed a *QS wave*.

ECG LEADS The 12 conventional ECG leads record the difference in potential between electrodes placed on the surface of the body. These leads are divided into two groups; six extremity (limb) leads and six chest (precordial) leads. The extremity leads record potentials transmitted onto the *frontal plane* (Fig. 228-5*A*), and the chest leads record potentials transmitted onto the *horizontal plane* (Fig. 228-5*B*). The six extremity leads are further subdivided into three *bipolar* leads (I, II, and III) and three *unipolar* leads (aVR, aVL, and aVF). Each bipolar lead measures the difference in potential between electrodes at two extremities: lead I = left arm − right arm voltages; lead II = left leg − right arm; and lead III = left leg − left arm. The unipolar leads measure the voltage (V) at one locus relative to an electrode (called the *central terminal* or *indifferent electrode*) that has approximately zero potential. Thus, aVR = right arm, aVL = left arm, and aVF = left leg (foot). The lowercase *a* indicates that these unipolar potentials are electrically augmented by 50 percent. The right leg electrode functions as a ground. The spatial orientation and polarity of the six frontal plane leads is represented on the hexaxial diagram (Fig. 228-6).

The six chest leads (Fig. 228-7) are unipolar recordings obtained by electrodes in the following positions: lead V_1, fourth intercostal space, just to the right of the sternum; lead V_2, fourth intercostal space, just to the left of the sternum; lead V_3, midway between V_2 and V_4; lead V_4, midclavicular line, fifth intercostal space; lead V_5, anterior axillary line, same level as V_4; and lead V_6, midaxillary line, same level as V_4 and V_5.

Together, the frontal and horizontal plane electrodes provide a three-dimensional representation of cardiac electrical activity. Each lead can be likened to a different camera angle "looking" at the same events—atrial and ventricular depolarization and repolarization—from different spatial orientations. The conventional 12-lead ECG can be supplemented with additional leads under special circumstances. For example, right precordial leads V_3R, V_4R, etc. are useful in detecting evidence of acute right ventricular ischemia. Esophageal leads may reveal atrial activity not detectable on the surface ECG. Bedside telemetry units and ambulatory ECG (Holter) recordings usually employ only one or two modified leads, respectively. → *Intracardiac electrocardiography and electrophysiologic testing are discussed in Chaps. 230 and 231.*

The ECG leads are configured so that a positive (upright) deflection is recorded in a lead if a wave of depolarization spreads toward the positive pole of that lead, and a negative deflection if the wave spreads toward the negative pole. If the mean orientation of the depolarization vector is at right angles to a given lead axis, a biphasic (equally positive and negative) deflection will be recorded.

GENESIS OF THE NORMAL ECG

P WAVE The normal atrial depolarization vector is oriented downward and toward the subject's left, reflecting the spread of depolarization from the sinus node to the right and then the left atrial myocardium. Since this vector points toward the positive pole of lead II and toward

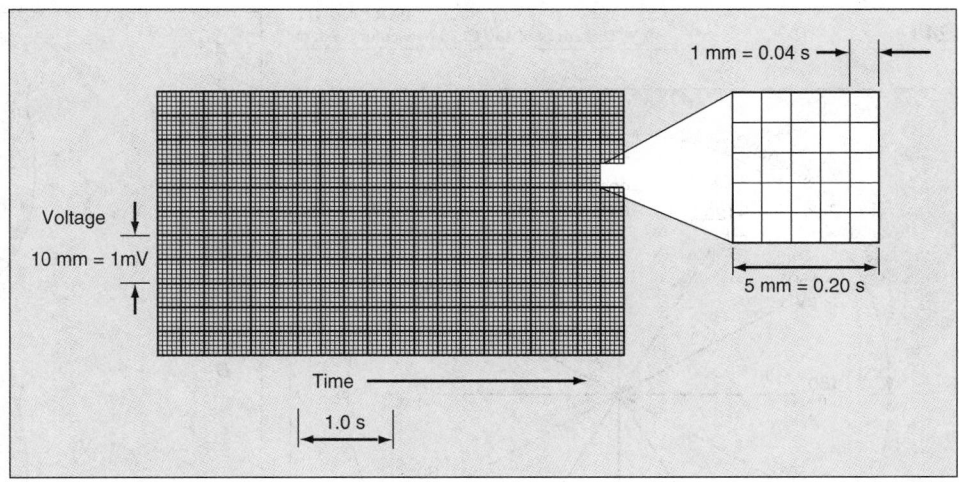

FIGURE 228-4 The ECG graph paper records the time (interval) between cardiac electrical events along the horizontal axis and their amplitude (voltage) along the vertical axis.

the negative pole of lead aVR, the normal P wave will be positive in lead II and negative in lead aVR. By contrast, activation of the atria from an ectopic pacemaker in the lower part of either atrium or in the AV junction region may produce retrograde P waves (negative in lead II, positive in lead aVR).

QRS COMPLEX Normal ventricular depolarization proceeds as a rapid, continuous spread of activation wavefronts. This complex process can be divided into two major, sequential phases, and each phase can be represented by a mean vector (Fig. 228-8). The first phase is depolarization of the interventricular septum from the left to the right (vector 1). The second results from the simultaneous depolarization of the main mass of the right and left ventricles; it is normally dominated by the more massive left ventricle, so that vector 2 points leftward and posteriorly. Therefore, a right precordial lead (V_1) will record this biphasic depolarization process with a small positive deflection (septal r wave) followed by a larger negative deflection (S wave). A left precordial lead, e.g., V_6, will record the same sequence with a small negative deflection (septal q wave) followed by a relatively tall positive deflection (R wave). Intermediate leads show a relative increase in R-wave amplitude (normal R-wave progression) and a decrease in S-wave amplitude progressing across the chest from the right to left. The precordial lead where the R and S waves are of approximately equal amplitude is referred to as the *transition zone* (usually V_3 or V_4) (Fig. 228-9).

The QRS pattern in the extremity leads may vary considerably from one normal subject to another depending on the *electrical axis* of the QRS, which describes the mean orientation of the QRS vector with reference to the six frontal plane leads. Normally, the QRS axis

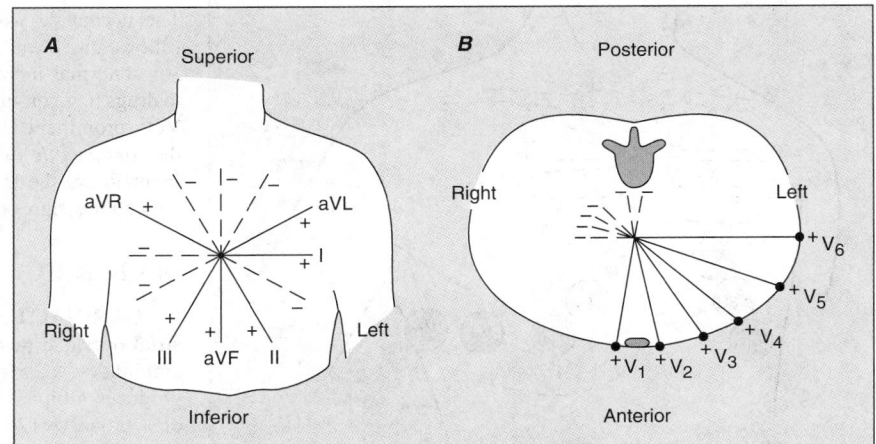

FIGURE 228-5 The six frontal plane (*A*) and six horizontal plane (*B*) leads provide a three-dimensional representation of cardiac electrical activity.

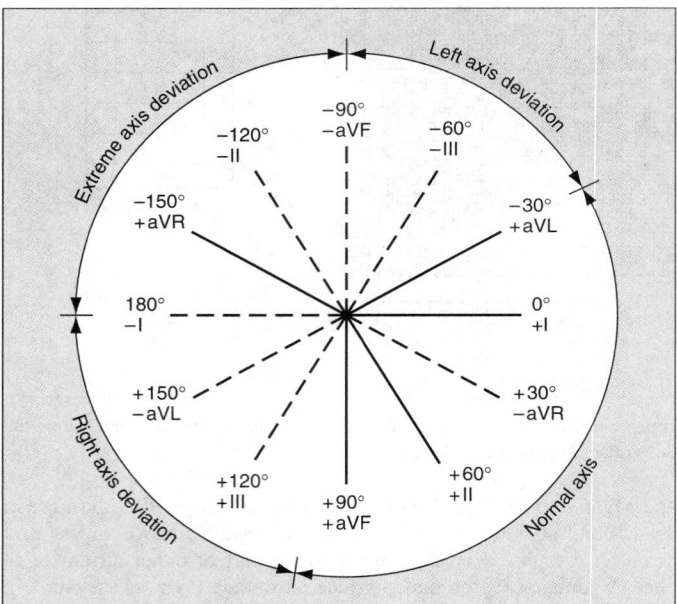

FIGURE 228-6 The frontal plane (extremity or limb) leads are represented on a hexaxial diagram. Each ECG lead has a specific spatial orientation and polarity. The positive pole of each lead axis (*solid line*) and negative pole (*hatched line*) are designated by their angular position relative to the positive pole of lead I (0°). The mean electrical axis of the QRS complex is measured with respect to this display.

ranges from −30° to +100° (Fig. 228-6). An axis more negative than −30° is referred to as *left axis deviation*, while an axis more positive than +100° is referred to as *right axis deviation*. Left axis deviation may occur as a normal variant but is more commonly associated with left ventricular hypertrophy, a block in the anterior fascicle of the left bundle system (left anterior fascicular block or hemiblock), or inferior myocardial infarction. Right axis deviation also may occur as a normal variant (particularly in children and young adults), as a spurious finding due to reversal of the left and right arm electrodes, or in conditions such as right ventricular overload (acute or chronic), infarction of the lateral wall of the left ventricle, dextrocardia, left pneumothorax, or left posterior fascicular block.

T WAVE AND U WAVE Normally, the mean T-wave vector is oriented roughly concordant with the mean QRS vector. Since depolarization and repolarization are electrically opposite processes,

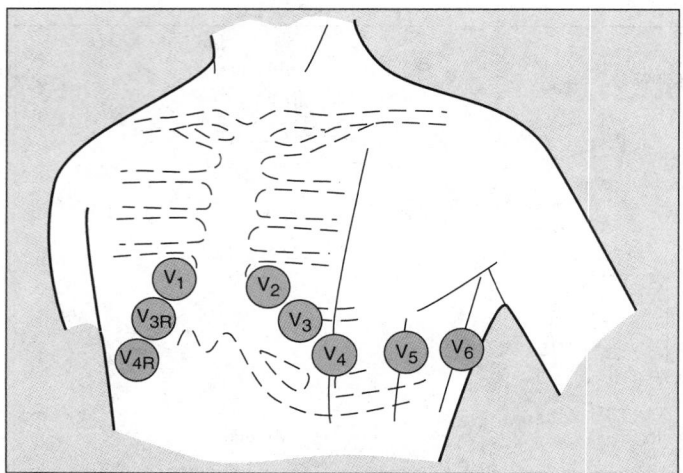

FIGURE 228-7 The horizontal plane (chest or precordial) leads are obtained with electrodes in the locations shown.

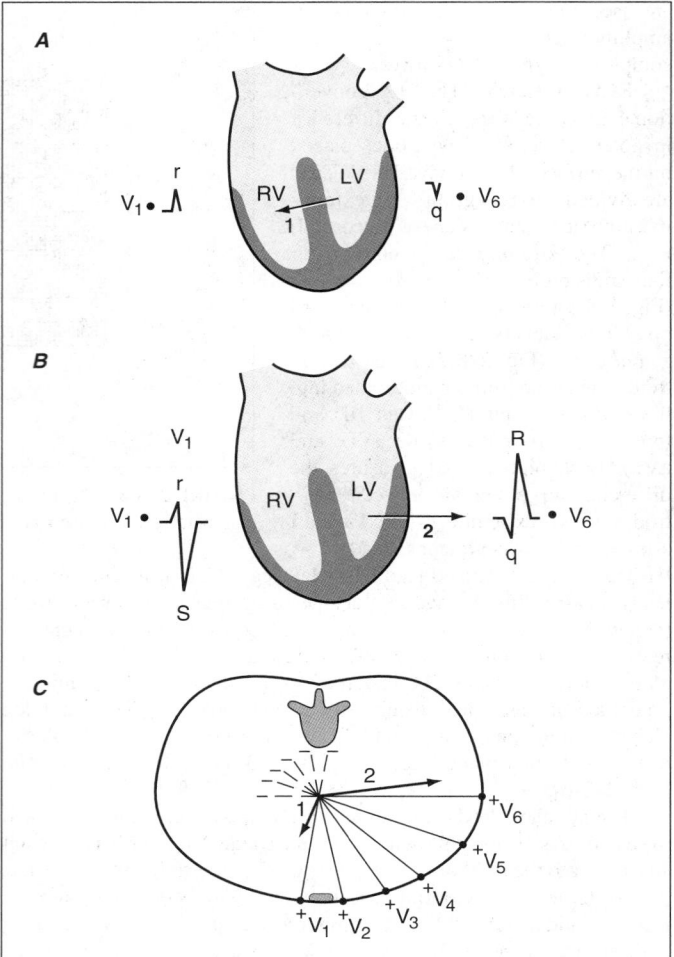

FIGURE 228-8 Ventricular depolarization can be divided into two major phases, each represented by a vector. *A.* The first phase (*arrow 1*) denotes depolarization of the ventricular septum, beginning on the left side and spreading to the right. This process is represented by a small "septal" r wave in lead V_1 and a small septal q wave in lead V_6. *B.* Simultaneous depolarization of the left and right ventricles (LV and RV) constitutes the second phase. Vector 2 is oriented to the left and posteriorly, reflecting the electrical predominance of the LV. *C.* Vectors (*arrows*) representing these two phases are shown in reference to the horizontal plane leads. (*After Goldberger and Goldberger.*)

this normal QRS–T-wave vector concordance indicates that repolarization must normally proceed in the reverse direction from depolarization (i.e., from epicardium to endocardium or from cardiac apex to base). The normal U wave is a small, rounded deflection (≤1 mm) that follows the T wave and usually has the same polarity as the T wave. An abnormal increase in U-wave amplitude is most commonly due to drugs (e.g., quinidine, procainamide, disopyramide) or hypokalemia. Very prominent U waves are a marker of increased susceptibility to the *torsades de pointes* type of ventricular tachycardia (Chap. 231). Inversion of the U wave in the precordial leads is abnormal and may be a subtle sign of ischemia.

MAJOR ECG ABNORMALITIES

CARDIAC ENLARGEMENT AND HYPERTROPHY Right atrial overload (acute or chronic) may lead to an increase in P-wave amplitude (≥2.5 mm) (Fig. 228-10). Left atrial overload typically produces a biphasic P wave in V_1 with a broad negative component or a broad (≥120 ms), often notched P wave in one or more limb leads (Fig. 228-10). This pattern also may occur with left atrial conduction delays in the absence of actual atrial enlargement, leading to the more general designation of *left atrial abnormality*.

Right ventricular hypertrophy due to a pressure load (as from pulmonic valve stenosis or pulmonary artery hypertension) is characterized by a relatively tall R wave in lead V_1 (R ≥ S wave), usually with right axis deviation (Fig. 228-11); alternatively, there may be a qR pattern in V_1 or V_3R. ST depression and T-wave inversion in the right to midprecordial leads are also often present. This so-called ventricular strain pattern is attributed to repolarization abnormalities in hypertrophied muscle. Right ventricular hypertrophy due to ostium secundum–type atrial septal defects, with the accompanying right ventricular volume overload, is commonly associated with an incomplete or complete right bundle branch block pattern with a rightward QRS axis.

Acute cor pulmonale due to pulmonary embolism (Chap. 261) for example, may be associated with a normal ECG or a variety of abnormalities. Sinus tachycardia is the most common arrhythmia, although other tachyarrhythmias, such as atrial fibrillation or flutter, may occur. The QRS axis may shift to the right, sometimes in concert with the so-called $S_1Q_3T_3$ pattern (prominence of the S wave in lead I, Q wave in lead III, with T-wave inversion in lead III). Acute right ventricular dilation also may be associated with poor R-wave progression and T-wave inversions in V_1 to V_4 (right ventricular "strain") simulating acute anterior infarction. A right ventricular conduction disturbance may appear.

Chronic cor pulmonale due to obstructive lung disease (Chap. 238) usually does not produce the classic ECG patterns of right ventricular hypertrophy noted above. Instead of tall right precordial R waves, chronic lung disease more typically is associated with small R waves in right to midprecordial leads (poor R-wave progression) due in part to downward displacement of the diaphragm and the heart. Low-voltage complexes are commonly present, owing to hyperaeration of the lungs.

A number of different voltage criteria for *left ventricular hypertrophy* (Fig. 228-11) have been proposed on the basis of the presence of tall left precordial R waves and deep right precordial S waves [e.g., $SV_1 + (RV_5 \text{ or } RV_6) ≥ 35$ mm; or $(RV_5 \text{ or } RV_6) ≥ 25$ mm]. Repolarization abnormalities (ST depression with T-wave inversions) also may appear (left ventricular "strain" pattern) in leads with prominent R waves. However, prominent precordial voltages may occur as a normal variant, especially in athletic or thin-chested individuals. Left ventricular hypertrophy may increase limb lead voltage (e.g., RaVL ≥ 11 to 13 mm, RaVF ≥ 20 mm; $R_1 + S_{III} ≥ 25$ mm) with or without increased precordial voltage. The presence of left atrial abnormality increases the likelihood of underlying left ventricular hypertrophy in cases with borderline voltage criteria. Left ventricular hypertrophy often progresses to incomplete or complete left bundle branch block. The sensitivity of conventional voltage criteria for left ventricular hypertrophy is decreased in obese persons and in women. ECG evidence for left ventricular hypertrophy is a major noninvasive marker of increased risk of cardiovascular morbidity and mortality, including sudden cardiac death. However, because of false-positive and false-negative diagnoses, the ECG is of limited utility in diagnosing atrial or ventricular enlargement. More definitive information is provided by echocardiography.

BUNDLE BRANCH BLOCKS Intrinsic impairment of conduction in either the right or left bundle system (intraventricular conduction disturbances) leads to prolongation of the QRS interval. With complete bundle branch blocks the QRS interval is ≥ 120 ms in duration; with incomplete blocks the QRS interval is between 100 and 120 ms. The QRS vector is usually oriented in the direction of the myocardial region where depolarization is delayed (Fig. 228-12). Thus,

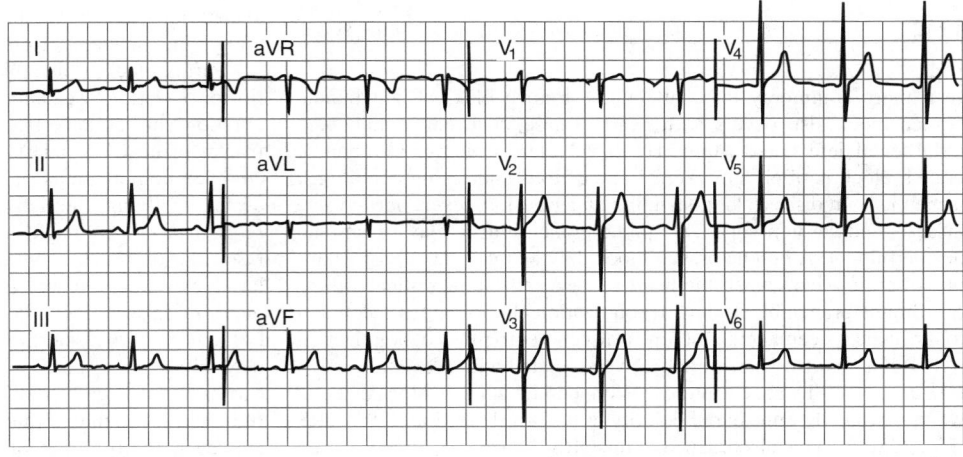

FIGURE 228-9 Normal electrocardiogram from a healthy subject. Sinus rhythm is present with a heart rate of 75 beats per minute. PR interval is 0.16 s; QRS interval (duration) is 0.08 s; QT interval is 0.36 s; the mean QRS axis is about +70°. The precordial leads show normal R-wave progression with the transition zone (R wave = S wave) in lead V_3.

with right bundle branch block, the terminal QRS vector is oriented anteriorly and to the right (rSR′ in V_1 and qRS in V_6, typically). Left bundle branch block alters both early and later phases of ventricular depolarization. The major QRS vector is directed to the left and posteriorly. In addition, the normal early left-to-right pattern of septal activation is disrupted such that septal depolarization proceeds from right to left as well. As a result, left bundle branch block generates wide, predominantly negative (QS) complexes in lead V_1 and entirely positive (R) complexes in lead V_6. A pattern identical to that of left bundle branch block, preceded by a sharp spike, is seen in most cases of electronic right ventricular pacing because of the relative delay in left ventricular activation.

Bundle branch block may occur in a variety of conditions. In subjects without structural heart disease, right bundle branch block is

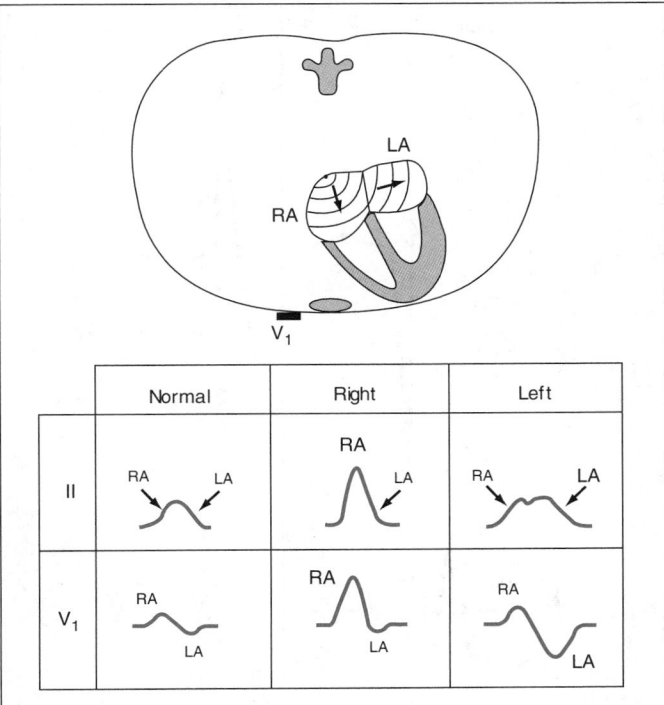

FIGURE 228-10 Right atrial (RA) overload may cause tall, peaked P waves in the limb or precordial leads. Left atrial (LA) abnormality may cause broad, often notched P waves in the limb leads and a biphasic P wave in lead V_1 with a prominent negative component representing delayed depolarization of the LA. *(After MK Park, WG Guntheroth: How to Read Pediatric ECGs, 2d ed. St. Louis, Mosby–Year Book, 1987.)*

seen more commonly than left bundle branch block. Right bundle branch block also occurs with heart disease, both congenital (e.g., atrial septal defect) and acquired (e.g., valvular, ischemic). Left bundle branch block is often a marker of one of four underlying conditions: ischemic heart disease, long-standing hypertension, severe aortic valve disease, and cardiomyopathy. Bundle branch blocks may be chronic or intermittent. A bundle branch block may be rate-related; for example, often it occurs when the heart rate exceeds some critical value.

Bundle branch blocks and depolarization abnormalities secondary to artificial pacemakers not only affect ventricular depolarization (QRS) but are also characteristically associated with *secondary repolarization* (ST-T) abnormalities. With bundle branch blocks, the T wave is typically opposite in polarity to the last deflection of the QRS (Fig. 228-12). This discordance of the QRS–T-wave vectors is caused by the altered sequence of repolarization that occurs secondary to altered depolarization. In contrast, *primary repolarization* abnormalities are independent of QRS changes and are related instead to actual alterations in the electrical properties of the myocardial fibers themselves (for example, in the resting membrane potential or action potential duration), not just to changes in the sequence of repolarization. Ischemia, electrolyte imbalance, and drugs such as digitalis all cause such primary ST–T-wave changes. Primary and secondary T-wave changes may coexist. For example, T-wave inversions in the right precordial leads with left bundle branch block or in the left precordial

leads with right bundle branch block may be important markers of underlying ischemia or other abnormalities.

Partial blocks ("hemiblocks") in the left bundle system (left anterior or posterior fascicular blocks) generally do not prolong the QRS duration substantially but instead are associated with shifts in the frontal plane QRS axis (leftward or rightward, respectively). More complex combinations of fascicular and bundle branch blocks may occur involving the left and right bundle system. Examples of *bifascicular block* include right bundle branch block and left posterior fascicular block, right bundle branch block with left anterior fascicular block, and complete left bundle branch block. Chronic bifascicular block in an asymptomatic individual is associated with a relatively low risk of progression to high-degree AV heart block. In contrast, new bifascicular block with acute anterior myocardial infarction carries a much greater risk of complete heart block. Alternation of right and left bundle branch block is a sign of *trifascicular disease*. However, the presence of a prolonged PR interval and bifascicular block does not necessarily indicate trifascicular involvement, since this combination may arise with AV node disease and bifascicular block. Intraventricular conduction delays also can be caused by extrinsic (toxic) factors that slow ventricular conduction, particularly hyperkalemia or drugs (type 1 antiarrhythmic agents, tricyclic antidepressants, phenothiazines).

Prolongation of QRS duration does not necessarily indicate a conduction delay but may be due to *preexcitation* of the ventricles via a bypass tract, as in the Wolff-Parkinson-White (WPW) syndrome (Fig. 231-10) and related variants. The diagnostic triad of WPW consists of a wide QRS complex associated with a relatively short PR interval and slurring of the initial part of the QRS (delta wave), the latter effect due to aberrant activation of ventricular myocardium. The presence of a bypass tract predisposes to reentrant supraventricular tachyarrhythmias (Chap. 231).

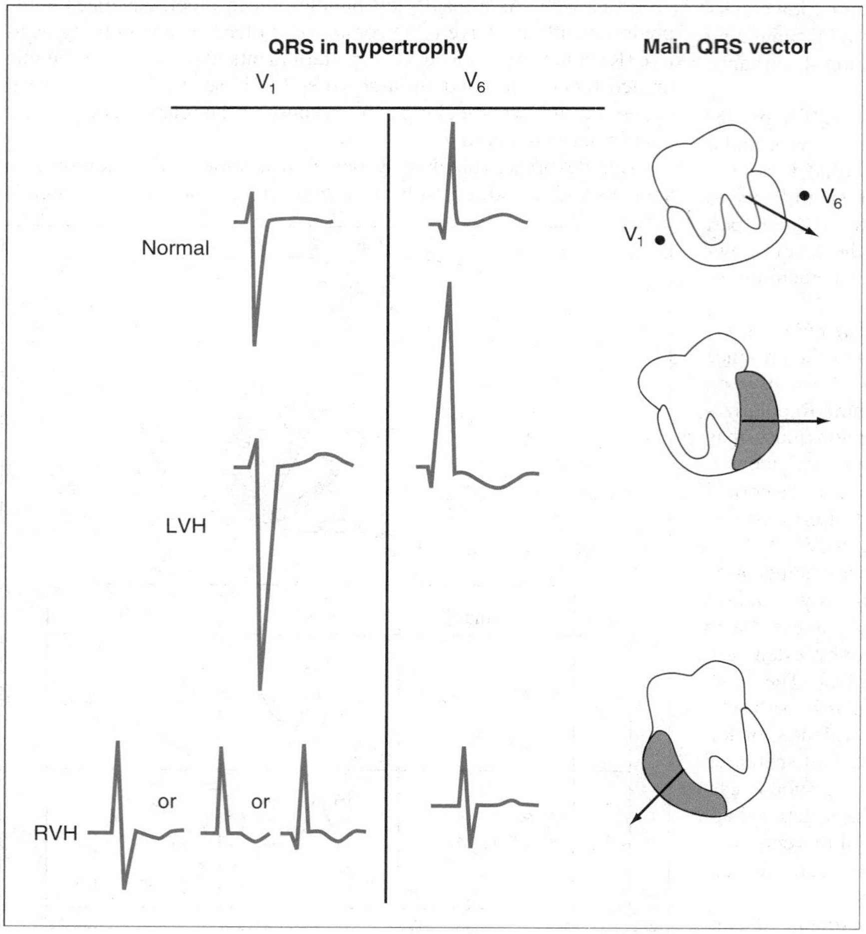

MYOCARDIAL ISCHEMIA AND INFARCTION (See also Chap. 243)   The ECG is a cornerstone in the diagnosis of acute and chronic ischemic heart disease. The findings depend on several key factors: the nature of the process [reversible (i.e., ischemia) versus irreversible (i.e., infarction)], the duration (acute versus chronic), extent (transmural versus subendocardial), and localization (anterior versus inferoposterior), as well as the presence of other underlying abnormalities (ventricular hypertrophy, conduction defects).

Ischemia exerts complex time-dependent effects on the electrical properties of myocardial cells. Severe, acute ischemia lowers the resting membrane potential and shortens the duration of the action potential. Such changes cause a voltage gradient between normal and ischemic zones. As a consequence, current flows between these regions. These so-called currents of injury are represented on the surface ECG by deviation of the ST segment (Fig. 228-13). When the acute ischemia is *transmural*, the ST vector is usually shifted in the direction of the outer (epicardial) layers, producing ST elevations and sometimes, in the earliest stages of ischemia, tall, positive so-called hyperacute T waves over the ischemic zone. With ischemia confined primarily to the *subendocardium*, the ST vector typically shifts toward the subendocardium and ventricular cavity, so that overlying (e.g., anterior precordial) leads show ST-segment depression (with ST elevation in lead aVR). Multiple factors affect the amplitude of acute ischemic ST deviations. Profound ST elevation or depression in multiple leads usually indicates very severe ischemia. Complete

FIGURE 228-11 Left ventricular hypertrophy (LVH) increases the amplitude of electrical forces directed to the left and posteriorly. In addition, repolarization abnormalities may cause ST-segment depression and T-wave inversion in leads with a prominent R wave "strain" pattern. Right ventricular hypertrophy (RVH) may shift the QRS vector to the right; this effect usually is associated with an R, RS, or qR complex in lead V_1. T-wave inversions may be present in right precordial leads ("strain" pattern).

resolution of ST elevation promptly following thrombolytic therapy is a relatively specific, though not sensitive, marker of successful reperfusion.

The ECG leads are more helpful in localizing regions of Q wave than non-Q-wave ischemia. For example, acute anterior wall ischemia leading to Q-wave infarction is reflected by ST elevations or increased T-wave positivity (Fig. 228-14) in one or more of the precordial leads (V_1 to V_6) and leads I and aVL. Anteroseptal ischemia produces these changes in leads V_1 to V_3, apical or lateral ischemia in leads V_4 to V_6. Inferior wall ischemia produces changes in leads II, III, and aVF. Posterior wall ischemia may be indirectly recognized by *reciprocal* ST depressions in leads V_1 to V_3. Prominent reciprocal ST depressions in these leads also occur with certain inferior wall infarcts, particularly those with posterior or lateral wall extension. Right ventricular ischemia usually produces ST elevations in right-sided chest leads (Fig. 228-7). When ischemic ST elevations occur as the earliest sign of acute infarction, they are typically followed within a period ranging from hours to days by evolving T-wave inversions and often by Q waves occurring in the same lead distribution. (T-wave inversions due to evolving or chronic ischemia correlate with prolongation of repolarization and are often associated with QT lengthening.) Reversible transmural ischemia, for example, due to coronary vasospasm (Prinzmetal's variant angina), may cause transient ST-segment elevations without development of Q waves. Depending on the severity and duration of such ischemia, the ST elevations may either resolve completely in minutes or be followed by T-wave inversions that persist for hours or even days. Patients with ischemic chest pain who present with deep T-wave inversions in multiple precordial leads (e.g., V_1 to V_4) with or without cardiac enzyme elevations typically have severe obstruction in the left anterior descending coronary artery system (Fig. 228-15). In contrast, patients whose baseline ECG already shows abnormal T-wave inversions may develop T-wave normalization (pseudonormalization) during episodes of acute transmural ischemia.

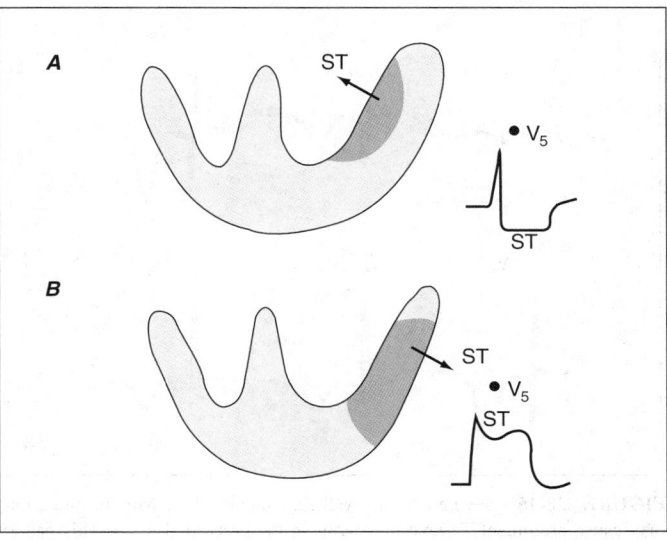

FIGURE 228-13   Acute ischemia causes a current of injury. With predominant subendocardial ischemia (*A*), the resultant ST vector will be directed toward the inner layer of the affected ventricle and the ventricular cavity. Overlying leads therefore will record ST depression. With ischemia involving the outer ventricular layer (*B*) (transmural or epicardial injury), the ST vector will be directed outward. Overlying leads will record ST elevation.

With infarction, depolarization (QRS) changes often accompany repolarization (ST-T) abnormalities. Necrosis of sufficient myocardial tissue may lead to decreased R-wave amplitude or frank abnormal Q waves in the anterior or inferior leads (Fig. 228-16). Previously, abnormal Q waves were considered to be markers of transmural myocardial infarction, while subendocardial infarcts were thought not to produce Q waves. However, careful ECG-pathology correlative studies have indicated that transmural infarcts may occur without Q waves and that subendocardial (nontransmural) infarcts may sometimes be associated with Q waves. Therefore, infarcts are more appropriately classified

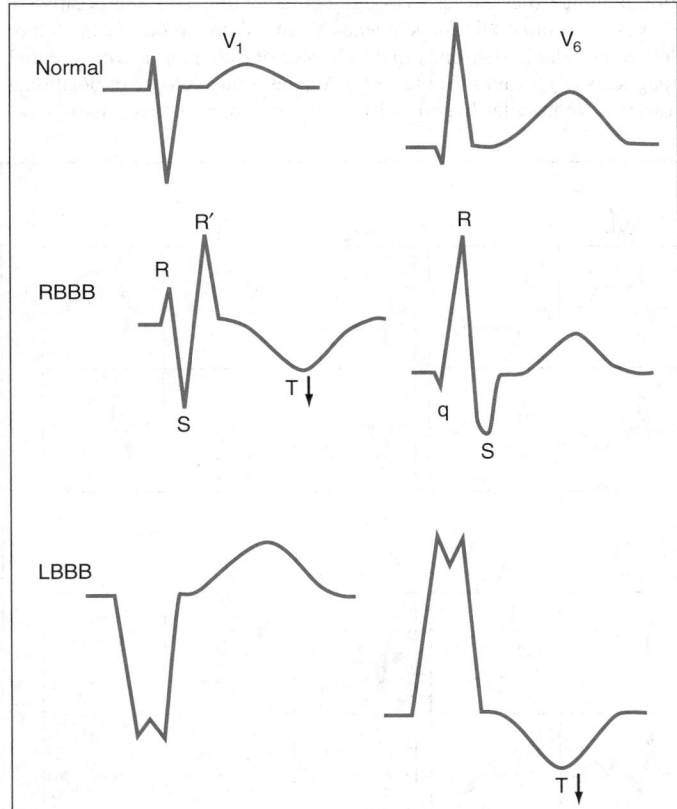

FIGURE 228-12   Comparison of typical QRS-T patterns in right bundle branch block (RBBB) and left bundle branch block (LBBB) with the normal pattern in leads V_1 and V_6. Note the secondary T-wave inversions (*arrows*) in leads with an rSR' complex with RBBB and in leads with a wide R wave with LBBB.

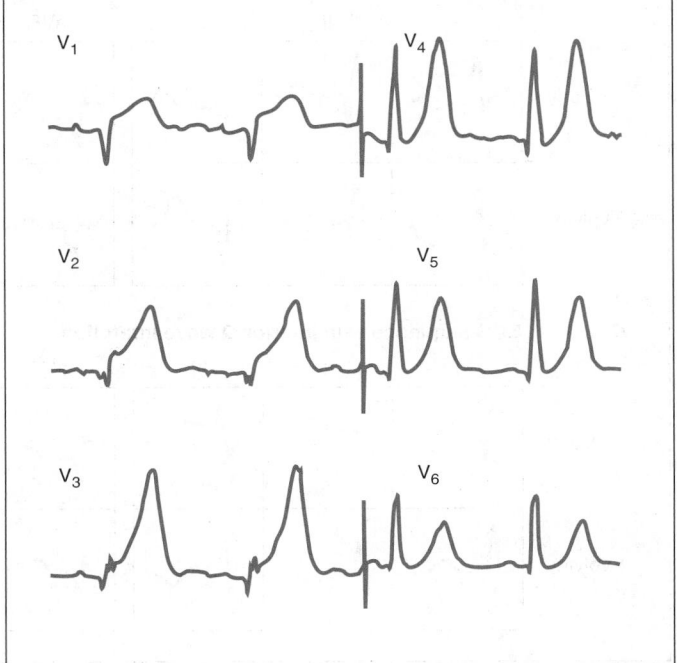

FIGURE 228-14   Hyperacute phase of anteroseptal myocardial infarction (MI). Note the tall positive T waves (V_2 to V_3) along with ST-segment elevations and Q waves (V_1 to V_3).

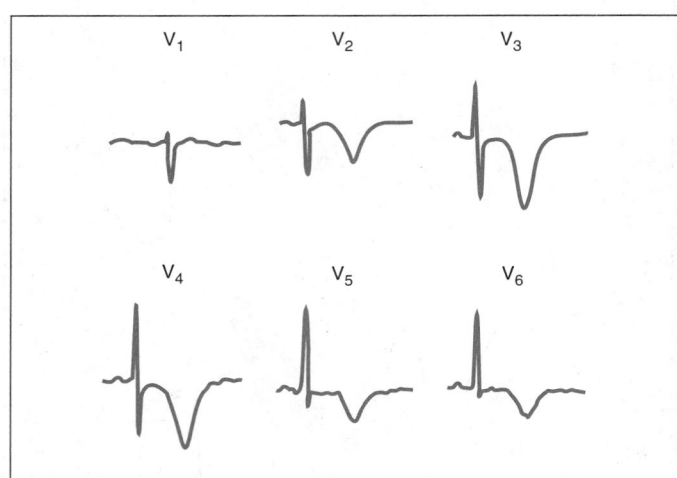

FIGURE 228-15 Severe anterior wall ischemia (with or without infarction) may cause prominent T-wave inversions in the precordial leads. This pattern is usually associated with a high-grade stenosis of the left anterior descending coronary artery.

as "Q-wave" or "non-Q-wave." The major acute ECG changes in syndromes of ischemic heart disease are schematically summarized in Fig. 228-17. Loss of depolarization forces due to posterior or lateral infarction may cause reciprocal increases in R-wave amplitude in leads V_1 and V_2 without diagnostic Q waves in any of the conventional leads. Atrial infarction may be associated with PR-segment deviations due to an atrial current of injury, changes in P-wave morphology, or atrial arrhythmias. In the weeks and months following infarction, these ECG changes may persist or begin to resolve. Complete normalization of the ECG following Q-wave infarction is uncommon but may occur, particularly with smaller infarcts. In contrast, ST-segment elevations that persist for several weeks or more after a Q-wave infarct usually

correlate with a severe underlying wall motion disorder (akinetic or dyskinetic zone), although not necessarily a frank ventricular aneurysm.

ECG changes due to ischemia may occur spontaneously or may be provoked by various exercise protocols (stress electrocardiography) (Chap. 244). In patients with severe ischemic heart disease, exercise testing is most likely to elicit signs of subendocardial ischemia (horizontal or downsloping ST depression in multiple leads). ST-segment elevation during exercise is most often observed after a Q-wave infarct. This repolarization change does not necessarily indicate active ischemia but correlates strongly with the presence of an underlying ventricular wall motion abnormality. However, in patients *without* prior infarction, transient ST-segment elevation with exercise is a reliable sign of transmural ischemia.

The ECG has important limitations in both sensitivity and specificity in the diagnosis of ischemic heart disease. Although a single normal ECG does not exclude ischemia or even acute infarction, a normal ECG *throughout* the course of an acute infarct is distinctly uncommon. Prolonged chest pain without diagnostic ECG changes, therefore, should always prompt a careful search for other noncoronary causes of chest pain (see Chap. 13). Furthermore, the diagnostic changes of acute or evolving ischemia are often masked by the presence of left bundle branch block, electronic ventricular pacemaker patterns, and WPW preexcitation. On the other hand, clinicians may overdiagnose ischemia or infarction based on the presence of ST-segment elevations or depressions, T-wave inversions, tall positive T waves, or Q waves *not* related to ischemic heart disease (pseudoinfarct patterns). For example, ST-segment elevations simulating ischemia may occur with acute pericarditis (Fig. 228-18) or myocarditis or as a normal variant ("early repolarization" pattern). Similarly, tall, positive T waves do not invariably represent hyperacute ischemic changes but also may be caused by normal variants, hyperkalemia, cerebrovascular injury, and left ventricular volume overload due to mitral or aortic regurgitation, among other causes. ST-segment elevations and tall, positive T waves are common findings in leads V_1 and V_2 in left bundle branch or left ventricular hypertrophy in the absence of ischemia. The differential diagnosis of Q waves (Table 228-1) includes physiologic or positional variants, ventricular hypertrophy, acute or chronic noncoronary myo-

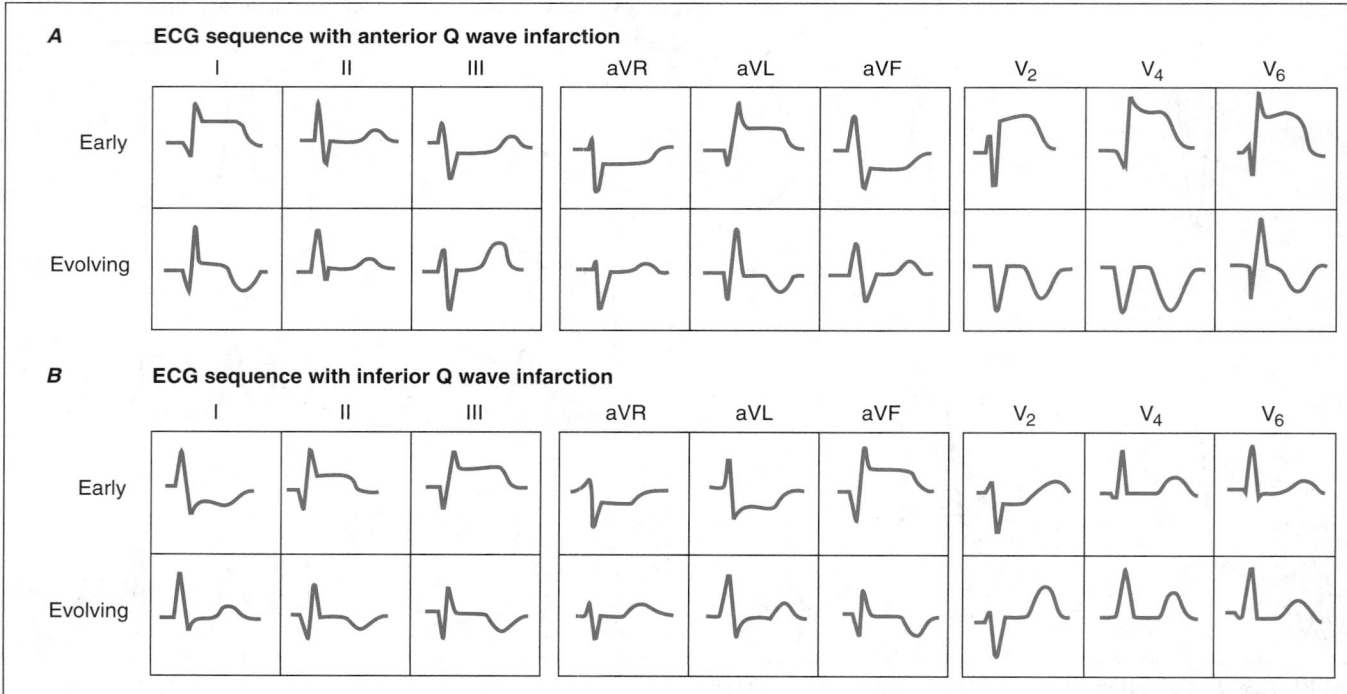

FIGURE 228-16 Sequence of depolarization and repolarization changes with (A) acute anterior and (B) acute inferior wall Q-wave infarctions. With anterior infarcts, ST elevation in leads I, aVL, and the precordial leads may be accom-panied by reciprocal ST depressions in leads II, III, and aVF. Conversely, acute inferior (or posterior) infarcts may be associated with reciprocal ST depressions in leads V_1 to V_3. (*After Goldberger and Goldberger.*)

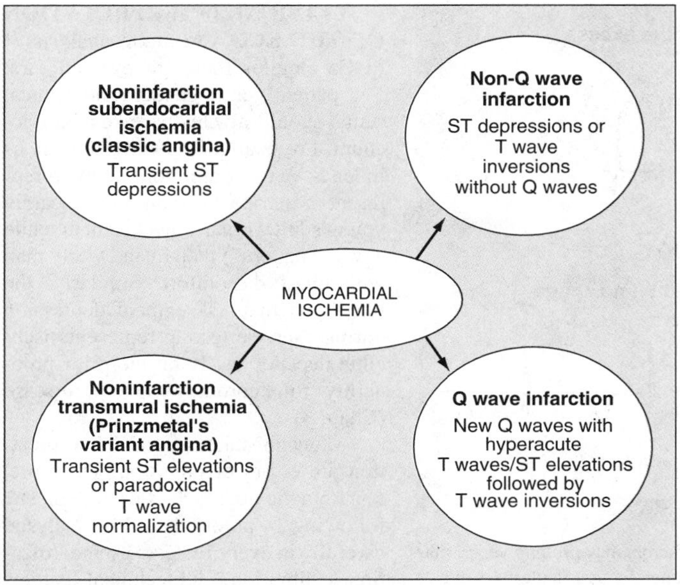

Figure 228-17 Diagram

Noninfarction subendocardial ischemia (classic angina)
Transient ST depressions

Non-Q wave infarction
ST depressions or T wave inversions without Q waves

MYOCARDIAL ISCHEMIA

Noninfarction transmural ischemia (Prinzmetal's variant angina)
Transient ST elevations or paradoxical T wave normalization

Q wave infarction
New Q waves with hyperacute T waves/ST elevations followed by T wave inversions

FIGURE 228-17 Variability of ECG patterns with acute myocardial ischemia. The ECG also may be normal or nonspecifically abnormal. Furthermore, these categorizations are not mutually exclusive. For example, a non-Q-wave infarct may evolve into a Q-wave infarct; ST elevations may be followed by a non-Q-wave infarct; or ST depressions and T-wave inversions may be followed by a Q-wave infarct. *(After Goldberger.)*

Table 228-1

Differential Diagnosis of Q Waves (with Selected Examples)

Physiologic or positional factors
1. Normal variant "septal" q waves
2. Normal variant Q waves in V_1 to V_2, aVL, III, and aVF
3. Left pneumothorax or dextrocardia: loss of lateral R-wave progression

Myocardial injury or infiltration
1. Acute processes: myocardial ischemia or infarction, myocarditis, hyperkalemia
2. Chronic processes: myocardial infarction, idiopathic cardiomyopathy, myocarditis, amyloid, tumor, sarcoid, scleroderma, Chagas' disease, echinococcus cyst

Ventricular hypertrophy/enlargement
1. Left ventricular (poor R-wave progression*)
2. Right ventricular (reversed R-wave progression† or poor R-wave progression, particularly with chronic obstructive lung disease)
3. Hypertrophic cardiomyopathy (may simulate anterior, inferior, posterior, or lateral infarcts)

Conduction abnormalities
1. Left bundle branch block (poor R-wave progression*)
2. Wolff-Parkinson-White patterns

---

* Small or absent R waves in the right to midprecordial leads.
† Progressive decrease in R-wave amplitude from V_1 to the mid- or lateral precordial leads.
SOURCE: After Goldberger

widening of the QRS interval. Severe hyperkalemia eventually causes cardiac arrest with a slow sinusoidal type of mechanism ("sine-wave" pattern) followed by asystole. *Hypokalemia* (Fig. 228-19) prolongs ventricular repolarization, often with prominent U waves. Prolongation of the QT interval (Fig. 228-19) is also seen with drugs that increase the duration of the ventricular action potential—type 1A antiarrhythmic agents and related drugs (e.g., quinidine, disopyramide, procainamide, tricyclic antidepressants, phenothiazines) and type III agents (amiodarone, sotalol). Marked QT prolongation, sometimes with deep, wide T-wave inversions, may occur with intracranial bleeds, particularly subarachnoid hemorrhage ("CVA T-wave" pattern) (Fig. 228-19). Systemic *hypothermia* (Fig. 228-19) also prolongs repolarization, usually with a distinctive convex elevation of the J point (Osborn wave). *Hypocalcemia* typically prolongs the QT interval (ST portion), while *hypercalcemia* shortens it (Fig. 228-20). Digitalis glycosides also shorten the QT interval, often with a characteristic "scooping" of the ST–T-wave complex (*digitalis effect*).

cardial injury, hypertrophic cardiomyopathy, and ventricular conduction disorders. Digitalis, ventricular hypertrophy, hypokalemia, and a variety of other factors may cause ST-segment depression mimicking subendocardial ischemia. Prominent T-wave inversion may occur with ventricular hypertrophy, cardiomyopathy, myocarditis, and cerebrovascular injury (particularly intracranial bleeds; Fig. 228-19), among many other conditions.

METABOLIC FACTORS AND DRUG EFFECTS A variety of metabolic and pharmacologic agents alter the ECG and, in particular, cause changes in repolarization (ST-T-U) and sometimes QRS prolongation. Certain life-threatening electrolyte disturbances may be diagnosed initially and monitored from the ECG. *Hyperkalemia* produces a sequence of changes usually beginning with narrowing and peaking (tenting) of the T waves. Further elevation of extracellular K^+ leads to AV conduction disturbances, diminution in P-wave amplitude, and

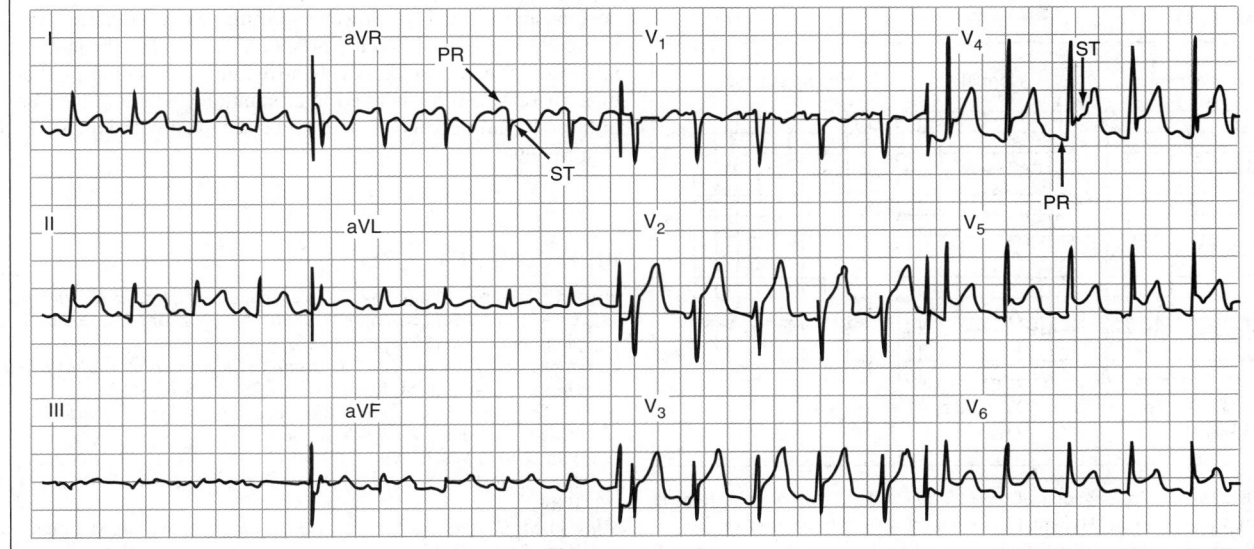

FIGURE 228-18 Acute pericarditis often produces diffuse ST-segment elevations (in this case in leads I, II, aVF, and V_2 to V_6) due to a ventricular current of injury. Note also the characteristic PR-segment deviation (opposite in polarity to the ST segment) due to a concomitant atrial injury current.

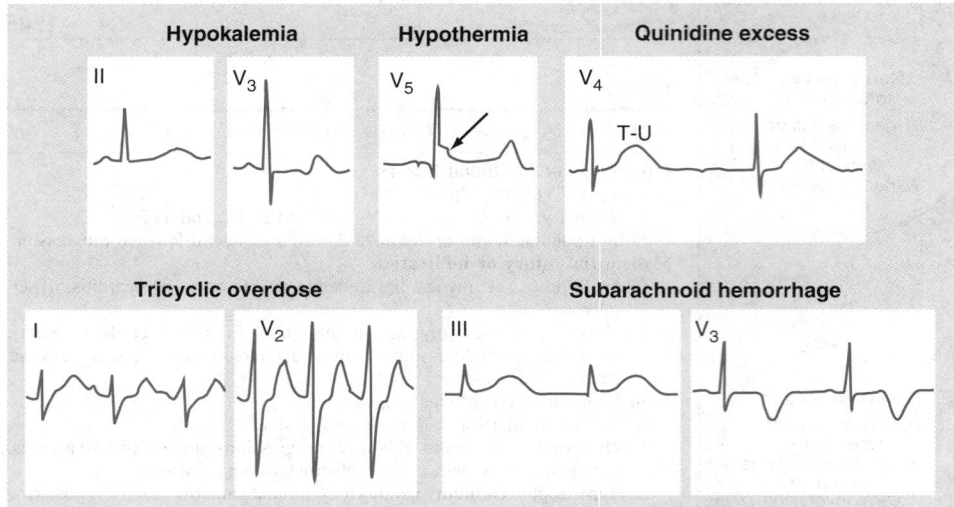

FIGURE 228-19 A variety of metabolic derangements, drug effects, and other factors may prolong ventricular repolarization with QT prolongation or prominent U waves. Repolarization prolongation, particularly if due to hypokalemia or pharmacologic agents, indicates increased susceptibility to torsades de pointes type ventricular tachycardia. Hypothermia is associated with a distinctive convex "hump" at the J point (Osborn wave, *arrow*). Note QRS and QT prolongation along with sinus tachycardia in the case of tricyclic antidepressant overdose.

Many other factors are associated with ECG changes, particularly alterations in ventricular repolarization. T-wave flattening, minimal T-wave inversions or slight ST-segment depression ("nonspecific ST–T-wave changes") may occur with a variety of electrolyte and acid-base disturbances, a variety of infectious processes, central nervous system disorders, endocrine abnormalities, many drugs, ischemia, hypoxia, and virtually any type of cardiopulmonary abnormality. While subtle ST–T-wave changes may be markers of ischemia, transient nonspecific repolarization changes also may occur following a meal or with postural (orthostatic) change, hyperventilation, or exercise in healthy individuals.

ELECTRICAL ALTERNANS Electrical alternans—a beat-to-beat alternation in one or more components of the ECG signal—is a common type of nonlinear cardiovascular response to a variety of perturbations. For example, total electrical alternans (P-QRS-T) with sinus tachycardia is a relatively specific sign of pericardial effusion, often with cardiac tamponade. The mechanism relates to a periodic swinging motion of the heart in the effusion at a frequency exactly one-half the heart rate. ST-T alternans is a sign of electrical instability and may precede ventricular fibrillation.

Accurate analysis of ECGs requires thoroughness and care. The patient's age, gender, and clinical status should always be taken into account. For example, T-wave inversions in leads V_1 to V_3 are more likely to represent a normal variant in a healthy young adult woman ("persistent juvenile T-wave pattern") than in an elderly man with chest discomfort. Similarly, the likelihood that ST-segment depression during exercise testing represents ischemia depends partly on the prior probability of coronary artery disease (Chap. 3).

Many mistakes in ECG interpretation are errors of omission. Therefore, a systematic approach is desirable. The following 14 points should be analyzed carefully in every ECG: (1) standardization (calibration) and technical features (including lead placement and artifacts), (2) heart rate, (3) rhythm, (4) PR interval, (5) QRS interval, (6) QT interval, (7) P waves, (8) QRS voltages, (9) mean QRS electrical axis, (10) precordial R-wave progression, (11) abnormal Q waves, (12) ST segments, (13) T waves, and (14) U waves.

Only after analyzing all these points should the interpretation be formulated. Where appropriate, important clinical correlates or inferences should be mentioned. For example, prolonged ventricular repolarization with prominent U waves should suggest hypokalemia or drug toxicity (e.g., due to quinidine or procainamide) (see Fig. 228-19). The combination of left atrial abnormality (enlargement) and signs of right ventricular hypertrophy suggests mitral stenosis. Low voltage with sinus tachycardia raises the possibility of pericardial tamponade or chronic obstructive lung disease. Sinus tachycardia with QRS and QT (U) prolongation suggests tricyclic antidepressant overdose (Fig. 228-19). Comparison with previous ECGs is essential. → *The diagnosis and management of specific cardiac arrhythmias and conduction disturbances are discussed in Chaps. 230 and 231.*

COMPUTERIZED ELECTROCARDIOGRAPHY Computerized ECG systems are increasingly used. Digital systems provide for convenient storage and immediate retrieval of thousands of ECG records. In recent years, computer programs for ECG analysis have become more reliable. However, despite these advances, computer interpretation of ECGs has important limitations. Incomplete or inaccurate readings are most likely with arrhythmias and complex abnormalities. Therefore, computerized interpretation (including measurements of basic ECG intervals) should not be accepted without careful physician review.

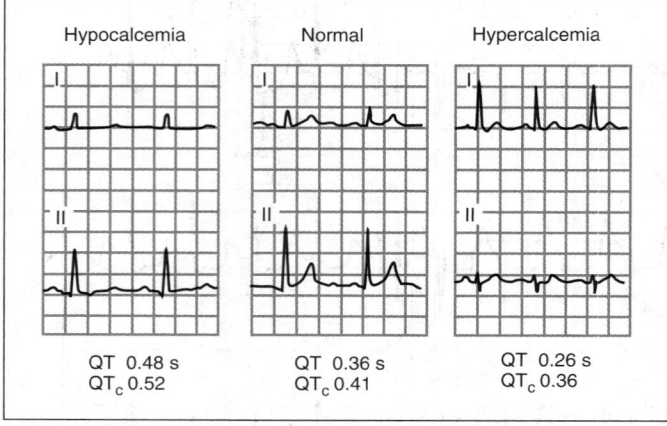

Hypocalcemia	Normal	Hypercalcemia
QT 0.48 s	QT 0.36 s	QT 0.26 s
QT$_c$ 0.52	QT$_c$ 0.41	QT$_c$ 0.36

FIGURE 228-20 Prolongation of the Q-T interval (ST-segment portion) is typical of hypocalcemia. Hypercalcemia may cause abbreviation of the ST segment and shortening of the QT interval.

BIBLIOGRAPHY

FISCH C: Electrocardiography and vectorcardiography, in *Heart Disease: A Textbook of Cardiovascular Medicine*, 5th ed, E Braunwald (ed). Philadelphia, Saunders, 1997, pp 108–152

GOLDBERGER AL: *Myocardial Infarction: Electrocardiographic Differential Diagnosis*, 4th ed. St. Louis, Mosby–Year Book, 1991

————, GOLDBERGER E: *Clinical Electrocardiography: A Simplified Approach*, 5th ed. St. Louis, Mosby–Year Book, 1994

MACFARLAND PW, LAWRIE TDV: *Comprehensive Electrocardiography: Theory and Practice in Health and Disease*. New York, Pergamon Press, 1989

MIRVIS DM: *Electrocardiography: A Physiologic Approach*. St. Louis, Mosby–Year Book, 1993

DIAGNOSTIC CARDIAC CATHETERIZATION AND ANGIOGRAPHY

Cardiac catheterization and angiography remain the gold standard for the assessment of both anatomy and physiology of the heart and vasculature. After initial animal experimentation, cardiac catheterization was first applied to humans in 1929 by Werner Forssmann, who at age 25 performed a right heart catheterization on himself. Although Forssmann's primary goal was to develop a therapeutic technique for the direct delivery of drugs into the heart, the potential for using cardiac catheterization as a diagnostic tool was appreciated by others, especially André Cournand and Dickinson Richards in New York, who shared the Nobel Prize with Forssmann in 1956. Today, more than 1 million cardiac catheterization and angiographic procedures are performed each year for diagnostic purposes, therapeutic intervention, or both. This chapter deals with cardiac catheterization as a diagnostic tool.

INDICATIONS AND CONTRAINDICATIONS Cardiac catheterization is recommended when there is a need to confirm the presence of a clinically suspected condition, define its anatomic and physiologic severity, and determine whether important associated conditions are present. This need most commonly arises when a patient is experiencing significant or increasing symptoms of cardiac dysfunction or when objective measures (such as exercise testing or echocardiography) suggest that the patient is at high risk of rapid deterioration, myocardial infarction, or other adverse events.

While there is debate as to whether cardiac catheterization is necessary in all patients being considered for cardiac surgery, cardiac catheterization and coronary arteriography remain the only techniques capable of defining coronary anatomy with sufficient precision to provide the data for decisions regarding coronary surgery or balloon angioplasty. In patients with other forms of heart disease (e.g., dilated cardiomyopathy, valvular heart disease), cardiac catheterization can provide hemodynamic characterization essential for the design of an appropriate medical regimen as well as for an assessment of prognosis. In some instances, however, decisions regarding cardiac surgery can be made without cardiac catheterization and angiography. Examples of such instances include children with simple congenital heart disease (e.g., patent ductus arteriosus, atrial septal defect), for whom a definitive diagnosis can be established by clinical examination and noninvasive studies, especially echocardiography.

Relative contraindications to cardiac catheterization are listed in Table 229-1.

A history of *allergic reaction* to radiographic contrast agents, which may range from urticaria to frank anaphylactic reaction, is an important relative contraindication to cardiac catheterization; it necessitates appropriate pretreatment with glucocorticoids (prednisone, 20 to 40 mg every 6 h), conventional antihistamines (e.g., diphenhydra-

mine, 25 mg every 6 h), and H$_2$ antagonists (cimetidine, 300 mg every 6 h), starting 18 to 24 h prior to the procedure. Alternatively, one of the newer nonionic contrast agents may be used with less risk of a severe allergic reaction. Despite these precautions, occasional individuals still develop anaphylactic reactions during radiographic contrast angiography, and intravenous epinephrine must be at hand to treat such instances.

COMPLICATIONS OF CARDIAC CATHETERIZATION
Since cardiac catheterization is an invasive technique, it is not surprising that potential complications include death, myocardial infarction, stroke, perforation of the heart or great vessels, and local vascular problems. Table 229-2 lists those characteristics associated with increased risk of death from cardiac catheterization.

TECHNIQUES

Cardiac catheterization is performed with the patient in the fasting state and awake although sedated. Typical sedatives include diazepam (Valium, 5 to 10 mg orally) and diphenhydramine (Benadryl, 25 to 50 mg orally). Prophylactic antibiotics are not necessary. If patients have been anticoagulated chronically with warfarin, this agent must be discontinued at least 48 h prior to the procedure, and the prothrombin time must be less than 18 s if the study is to be done safely. Although cardiac catheterization used to be performed exclusively as an inpatient procedure, current practice is to perform most elective procedures on an outpatient basis.

The technique of cardiac catheterization involves either direct exposure of artery and vein (usually the brachial artery and vein in the antecubital fossa) or catheterization by a percutaneous approach (usually via the femoral artery and vein). Either technique can be used for right and/or left heart catheterization with coronary arteriography, but many procedures (e.g., intraaortic balloon pumping, mitral valve valvuloplasty, coronary atherectomy) require the femoral approach. For a procedure where either approach would be possible, the brachial approach has advantages in the patient with peripheral vascular disease involving the abdominal aorta and iliac or femoral arteries and suspected thrombosis of the femoral or iliac vein or inferior vena cava. Advantages of the percutaneous femoral approach are that arteriotomy and arterial repair are not required; the procedure can be performed repeatedly in the same patient at intervals; infection and thrombophlebitis at the catheterization site are quite rare, and no scar is left. At present, more than 85 percent of cardiac catheterizations are performed by the femoral route.

Table 229-1

Relative Contraindications to Cardiac Catheterization and Angiography

Uncontrolled ventricular irritability: increased risk of ventricular tachycardia and fibrillation during catheterization if ventricular irritability is uncontrolled
Uncorrected hypokalemia or digitalis toxicity
Uncorrected hypertension: predisposes to myocardial ischemia and/or heart failure during angiography
Intercurrent febrile illness
Decompensated heart failure: especially acute pulmonary edema, unless catheterization can be done with patient sitting up
Anticoagulated state: prothrombin time >18 s
Severe allergy to radiographic contrast agent
Severe renal insufficiency and/or anuria: unless dialysis is planned to remove fluid and radiographic contrast load

---

Table 229-2

Patient Characteristics Associated with Increased Mortality from Cardiac Catheterization

Age: Infants (<1 month old) and the elderly (>80 years old) are at increased risk of death during cardiac catheterization. Elderly women appear to be at higher risk than elderly men.
Functional class: Mortality in class IV patients is more than 10 times greater than in class I–II patients.
Severity of coronary obstruction: Mortality for patients with left main coronary artery disease is more than 10 times greater than in patients with one- or two-vessel disease.
Valvular heart disease: Especially when severe and combined with coronary disease, is associated with a higher risk of death at cardiac catheterization than coronary artery disease alone.
Left ventricular dysfunction: Mortality in patients with a left ventricular ejection fraction <30 percent is more than 10 times greater than in patients with an ejection fraction ≥50 percent.
Severe noncardiac disease: Patients with renal insufficiency, insulin-requiring diabetes, advanced cerebrovascular and/or peripheral vascular disease, or severe pulmonary insufficiency have an increased incidence of death and other major complications from cardiac catheterization.

RIGHT HEART CATHETERIZATION This procedure is most commonly performed under fluoroscopic guidance using a balloon flotation catheter, which is advanced from a suitable vein (femoral, brachial, subclavian, or internal jugular) into the superior vena cava, where blood is sampled for oximetry. The catheter is then positioned in the right atrium, where pressure is measured. The balloon is inflated with air or carbon dioxide and advanced sequentially into the right ventricle, pulmonary artery, and pulmonary artery wedge positions. Pressures are recorded in each position. After the wedge pressure is recorded, the balloon is deflated so that pulmonary artery pressure can be monitored and blood samples can be obtained for oximetry. With a thermistor-tipped balloon catheter, cardiac output can be measured using cold saline injection and a small computer (thermodilution technique). Comparison of oxygen saturations in the superior and inferior vena cava, chambers of the right heart, and pulmonary artery permits assessment of the presence of a left-to-right shunt at the atrial, ventricular, or pulmonary artery level, which will be manifested as an increase ("step-up") in oxygen saturation of blood as it traverses these vessels and chambers. As discussed below, measurements of the pulmonary artery and aortic oxygen content and oxygen consumption allow calculation of the cardiac output by the Fick principle as an alternative to use of thermodilution.

The experienced operator will be alert to abnormalities in the course of the catheter during its passage through the right heart chambers, which could indicate the presence of congenital heart disease. For example, the catheter may pass directly from the right to the left atrium through an atrial septal defect, may enter an anomalous pulmonary vein draining into the right atrium, or may pass from the pulmonary artery directly into the aorta through a patent ductus arteriosus.

LEFT HEART CATHETERIZATION When left heart catheterization is done from the *brachial approach*, surgical cut-down is performed in the right (or left) antecubital fossa, with exposure of the brachial artery. An arteriotomy is made, and an appropriate catheter (e.g., a Sones catheter) is advanced under fluoroscopic guidance to the central aorta, where pressure is measured and recorded. Next, the catheter is advanced in retrograde fashion across the aortic valve into the left ventricle, where pressure is measured. If a right heart catheter is in place, this is an appropriate time for simultaneous measurement and recording of left heart, right heart, and peripheral arterial pressures together with a determination of cardiac output by either thermodilution or the Fick principle. These measures allow assessment of possible pressure gradients across the mitral and aortic valves, and catheter pullback on the right side permits assessment of possible gradients across the pulmonic and tricuspid valves. Simultaneous measurement of pressures and cardiac output provides the data for calculation of systemic and pulmonary vascular resistances.

The *percutaneous femoral approach* to left heart catheterization involves puncture of the right (or left) femoral artery with a Seldinger needle, passage of a J-tipped guidewire retrogradely to the abdominal aorta under fluoroscopic guidance, and placement of an intraarterial sheath with a side arm port for flushing. An appropriate catheter (e.g., a pigtail catheter) is then advanced through this sheath and over the guidewire to the descending aorta, at which time the guidewire is removed and the catheter aspirated and flushed vigorously. Under pressure monitoring and fluoroscopic guidance, the catheter is advanced to the ascending aorta, where pressure is recorded simultaneously with peripheral arterial pressure. The subsequent steps in the procedure are identical to those listed for the brachial approach.

An additional method of left heart catheterization is the *transseptal approach*. This approach, which is not commonly employed today except for special diagnostic problems or for purposes of therapeutic intervention (especially mitral valvuloplasty), involves a controlled puncture of the interatrial septum from the right atrial side with a long stainless steel needle. Advancement of a Teflon catheter or sheath over the needle then allows catheterization of the left atrium and catheter passage across the mitral valve into the left ventricle. Rarely, direct catheterization of the left heart through the chest wall is necessary, by *left ventricular puncture* using a needle inserted into the cardiac apex.

CARDIAC ANGIOGRAPHY

Cardiac angiography involves injection of an iodine-based liquid radiopaque contrast agent into a specific cardiac chamber or vessel using either hand injection or power injection through an automated syringe. The contrast agents used today are classified as either high-osmolar or low-osmolar; the low-osmolar contrast agents (including true nonionic contrast agents and the ionic dimer ioxaglate) have a lesser myocardial depressant effect and produce fewer side effects (hypotension, nausea, bradycardia, or a sensation of marked warmth following injection) than earlier high-osmolar agents. They are, however, substantially more expensive than traditional high-osmolar ionic agents, so they are not used routinely in patients who are at low risk for complications with the less expensive high-osmolar contrast agents.

CORONARY ANGIOGRAPHY This common procedure involves the selective injection of a radiographic contrast agent into the coronary arteries. Placement of the catheter tip into the right and left coronary arteries is carried out under fluoroscopic guidance, and contrast agent is injected by hand during recording of the radiographic image. Each coronary artery is usually viewed in several projections to permit assessment of the severity of stenosis and to minimize the overlap of adjacent vessels. In addition to the detection of coronary artery stenoses, coronary angiography is useful for the detection of congenital abnormalities of the coronary circulation, coronary arteriovenous fistulas, and patency of coronary artery bypass grafts. Examples of normal and abnormal coronary anatomy are shown in Figs. 229-1 to 229-3.

LEFT VENTRICULOGRAPHY Injection of radiographic contrast material directly into the left ventricular cavity is an important part of routine left heart catheterization and yields important diagnostic information. A power injector is used to inject 30 to 45 mL of radiographic contrast material into the left ventricular chamber at a rate of 10 to 12 mL/s. Angiographic assessment of the left ventricular silhouette at end-diastole and end-systole permits calculation of the left ventricular chamber volumes and ejection fraction, as well as assessment of regional wall motion abnormalities. The normal left ventricle ejects 50 to 80 percent of its end-diastolic volume with each beat; i.e., its *ejection fraction* is 0.50 to 0.80. In adults, normal values for left ventricular volumes are, for end-diastolic volume, 72 ± 15 mL/m^2 (mean $\pm$ standard deviation) and, for end-systolic volume, 20 ± 8 mL/m^2. Regional abnormalities of wall motion are illustrated in Fig. 229-4 and include diminished inward motion of a myocardial segment (*hypokinesis*), absence of inward movement of a myocardial segment (*akinesis*), and paradoxical systolic expansion of a regional myocardial segment (*dyskinesis*).

Left ventriculography is usually performed in the right anterior oblique projection, which allows assessment of the mitral and aortic valves. Mitral regurgitation is easily visualized as the leakage of radiographic contrast material back into the left atrium during left ventricular systole. Its severity can be estimated qualitatively using a grading system of 1+ (mild; radiographic contrast material clears with each beat and never opacifies the entire left atrium) to 4+ (severe; opacification of the entire left atrium occurs within one beat, and contrast material can be seen refluxing into the pulmonary veins). The *regurgitant fraction* can be calculated by determining the total left ventricular stroke volume (left ventricular end-diastolic volume minus end-systolic volume), subtracting the forward stroke volume (determined by the Fick or indicator-dilution technique), and dividing by the total stroke volume. The cause of mitral regurgitation—for example, myxomatous degeneration of the mitral leaflets and chordal rupture—may sometimes be identified from the left ventricular cineangiogram. Mitral and aortic stenosis can be suspected when the speed and completeness with which the mitral and aortic leaflets open are reduced. Other clues include increased thickness of the mitral and aortic leaflets and the

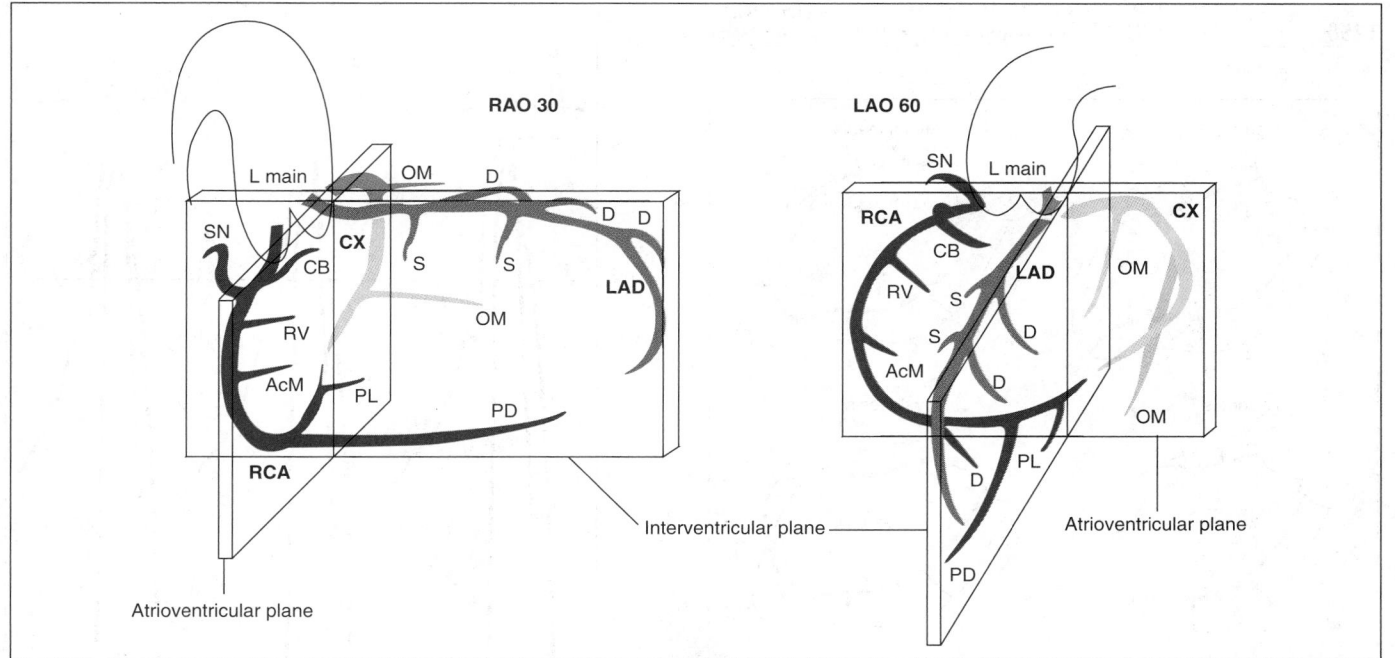

FIGURE 229-1 Representation of coronary anatomy relative to the interventricular and atrioventricular valve planes. Coronary branches are indicated as L Main (left main), LAD (left anterior descending), D (diagonal), S (septal), CX (circumflex), OM (obtuse marginal), RCA (right coronary artery), CB (conus branch), SN (sinus node), AcM (acute marginal), PD (posterior descend-ing, PL (posterolateral left ventricular). RAO, right anterior oblique, LAO, left anterior oblique. [*From DS Baim, W Grossman, in Cardiac Catheterization, Angiography, and Intervention, 5th ed, DS Baim, W Grossman (eds). Baltimore, Williams & Wilkins, 1996.*]

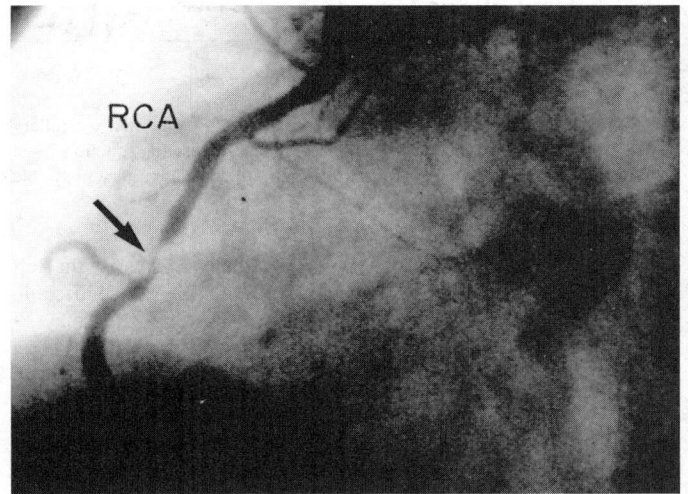

FIGURE 229-2 Coronary angiogram showing a right coronary artery (RCA) with a severe (95 percent) stenosis at its midpoint (*arrow*).

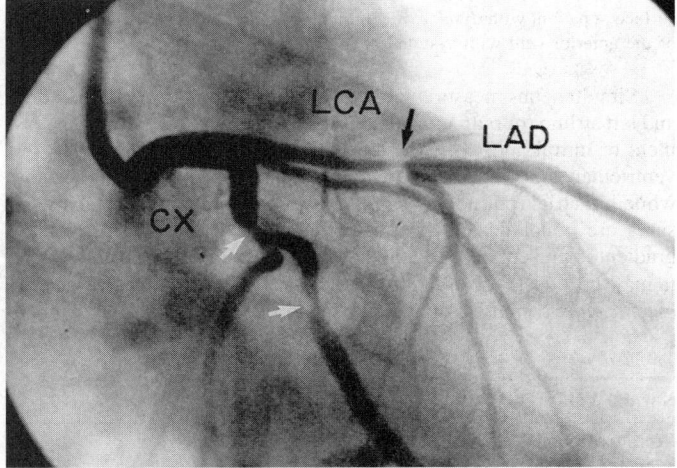

FIGURE 229-3 Coronary angiogram of a left coronary artery (LCA) with a tight stenosis in the proximal left anterior descending (LAD) artery (*black arrow*) immediately prior to the origin of a large septal branch. The circumflex artery (CX) has two moderately severe stenoses (*white arrows*).

presence and extent of leaflet calcification. These findings, however, are usually not useful in estimating the *severity* of physiologic stenosis.

Left ventriculography performed in the left anterior oblique projection permits detection of abnormal communications, such as a ventricular septal defect (Chap. 235). In the most common form of hypertrophic cardiomyopathy (Chap. 239) (idiopathic hypertrophic subaortic stenosis, IHSS), left ventriculography in this projection shows anterior motion of the anterior leaflet of the mitral valve during systole and bulging of the interventricular septum into the left ventricular cavity, especially in the subaortic region. Mural thrombi within the left ventricular chamber may be well visualized during left ventriculography. They occur most commonly in the left ventricular apex.

AORTOGRAPHY Rapid injection of radiographic contrast material into the ascending aorta allows detection of abnormalities involving the aorta and aortic valve. It permits detection and qualitative

assessment of the severity of aortic regurgitation, which is recorded using a 1 + to 4 + scale, as for mitral regurgitation. Abnormal communications between the aorta and right side of the heart, such as a patent ductus arteriosus or ruptured aneurysm of a sinus of Valsalva, may be visualized. Aortography can permit identification of aortic aneurysm and of aortic dissection (Chap. 247) and may visualize an intimal flap within the aortic lumen.

PRESSURE MEASUREMENTS

Pressures within the cardiac chambers and great vessels are recorded routinely during cardiac catheterization and provide important information concerning the function of ventricular myocardium and cardiac valves. Normal values for pressures measured during cardiac catheterization are summarized in Table 229-3.

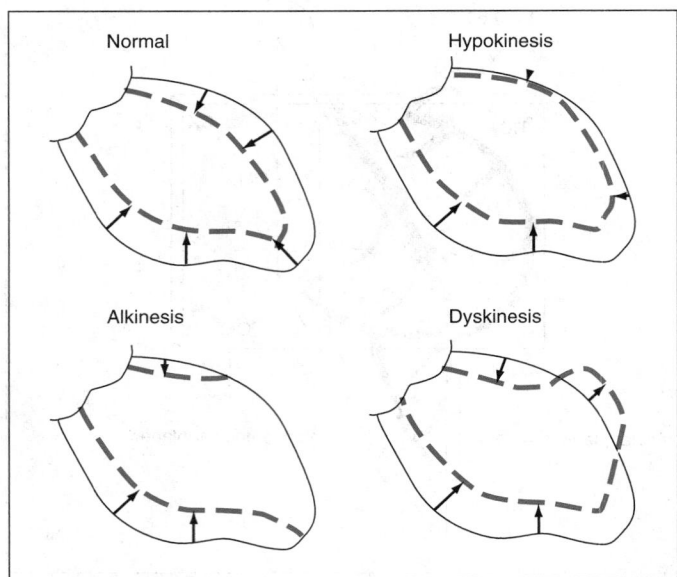

FIGURE 229-4 Diagrammatic representation of end-diastolic (*solid line*) and end-systolic (*dashed line*) silhouettes of left ventricular cineangiograms in various forms of localized wall motion disorder in patients with coronary heart disease. Normal wall motion is symmetric; a patient with *hypokinesis* exhibits reduced contraction, seen here over the anterior and apical surfaces; a patient with *akinesis* exhibits absent wall motion, seen here over the anteroapical surface; a patient with *dyskinesis* exhibits paradoxic bulging of a small portion of the anterior wall with systole.

Simultaneous measurement of pressures in the left ventricle, aorta, and left atrium (or pulmonary capillary wedge position) permits assessment of mitral and aortic valve function. As seen in Fig. 229-5, left ventricular and aortic pressures are essentially equal during systole, while left atrial (pulmonary capillary wedge) and left ventricular pressures are equal during diastole in the normal heart. If a pressure gradient is present between the left ventricle and aorta during systole, it may be due to obstruction at the level of the aortic valve (e.g., *calcific aortic stenosis*) or at the subaortic level (e.g., *hypertrophic*

Table 229-3

Normal Values for Hemodynamic Parameters

Pressures (mmHg)	
Systemic arterial	
Peak systolic/end-diastolic	100–140/60–90
Mean	70–105
Left ventricle	
Peak systolic/end-diastolic	100–140/3–12
Left atrium (or pulmonary capillary wedge)	
Mean	2–10
a wave	3–15
v wave	3–15
Pulmonary artery	
Peak systolic/end-diastolic	15–30/4–12
Mean	9–18
Right ventricle	
Peak systolic/end-diastolic	15–30/2–8
Right atrium	
Mean	2–8
a wave	2–10
v wave	2–10
Resistances [(dyn·s)/cm^5]	
Systemic vascular resistance	700–1600
Pulmonary vascular resistance	20–130
Cardiac index [(L/min)/m^2]	2.6–4.2
Oxygen consumption index [(L/min)/m^2]	110–150
Arteriovenous oxygen difference (mL/L)	30–50

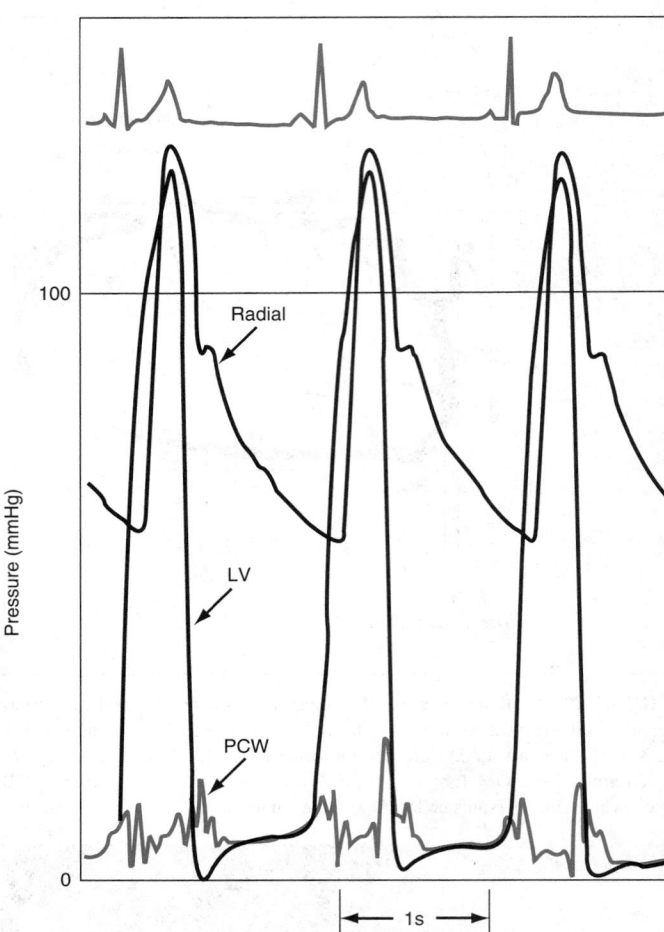

FIGURE 229-5 Left ventricular (LV), radial artery, and pulmonary capillary wedge (PCW) pressures in a patient with normal cardiovascular function. Note the absence of a pressure gradient between the LV and radial artery in systole and between the LV and PCW in diastole.

obstructive cardiomyopathy). A pressure gradient between the left atrium (pulmonary capillary wedge pressure) and the left ventricle in diastole generally indicates *mitral stenosis*, although it also may be seen in rare conditions such as cor triatriatum and left atrial myxoma. An example of a large diastolic pressure gradient in a patient with mitral stenosis is seen in Fig. 229-6. As seen in Fig. 229-7, patients with significant mitral regurgitation may have a prominent *v* wave in the pulmonary capillary wedge pressure, which often increases substantially during modest exercise. Severe *aortic regurgitation* produces a widening of the aortic pulse pressure, with equilibration of aortic and left ventricular pressures in diastole (Fig. 229-8). Right-sided pressures exhibit a characteristic deformity in the presence of valvular heart disease affecting the tricuspid or pulmonic valves. In patients with severe *tricuspid regurgitation*, the right atrial pressure resembles the right ventricular pressure closely in appearance. Mean right atrial pressure and right ventricular end-diastolic pressure are both elevated in tricuspid regurgitation. In *tricuspid stenosis*, there is a pressure gradient between the right atrium and ventricle during diastole.

Characteristic deformities of right and left ventricular diastolic pressures occur in patients with *cardiac tamponade* or *pericardial constriction*. In both conditions there is equalization of left and right ventricular diastolic pressures. However, in constrictive pericarditis, nearly all ventricular filling occurs shortly after mitral and tricuspid valve opening; after this period of rapid filling, ventricular volumes cannot increase further owing to the constricting pericardium. This abnormality produces an abrupt early ventricular diastolic pressure rise with a mid- and late-ventricular pressure plateau, giving the so-called square root sign (Fig. 229-9). In contrast, in tamponade there is equalization of diastolic pressures with a gradual increase throughout diastole.

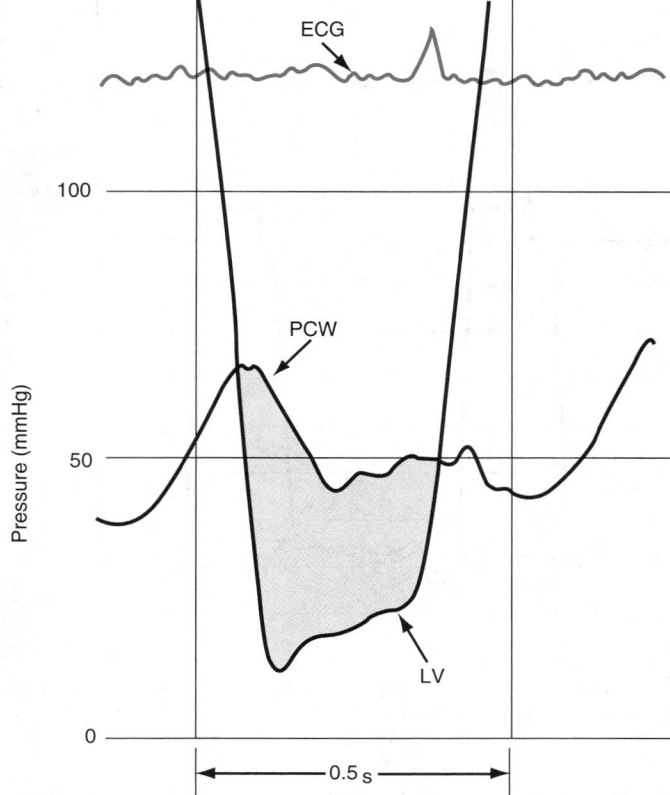

FIGURE 229-6 Pulmonary capillary wedge (PCW) and left ventricular (LV) pressure tracings in a 40-year-old woman with mitral stenosis. This patient also had systemic hypertension and significant elevation of her LV diastolic pressure. [*From BA Carabello, W Grossman, in Cardiac Catheterization, Angiography, and Intervention, 5th ed, DS Baim, W Grossman (eds). Baltimore, Williams & Wilkins, 1996.*]

Congestive heart failure due to myocardial contractile dysfunction is associated with characteristic alterations in the ventricular pressure waveforms seen at cardiac catheterization. Neither the rise nor the decline in isovolumic pressure is as steep as in the normal heart. The reduced slopes of pressure rise and decline are associated with an abbreviated ejection period, giving the left ventricular pressure tracing a triangular appearance (Fig. 229-10). Also, the pressure decline does not continue to zero, so the minimal left ventricular diastolic pressure may be elevated. This hemodynamic finding correlates with an increased ventricular end-systolic volume, which is a sign of depressed contractile function of the left ventricular myocardium.

MEASUREMENT OF FLOW

Systemic and pulmonary blood flows may be measured by either the Fick or the indicator-dilution method. In the normal heart, these flows are equal and constitute the *cardiac output*. Specialized techniques have made it possible to measure coronary artery blood flow (through the use of a catheter- or guidewire-tip-mounted Doppler flowmeter), coronary sinus blood flow (by the thermodilution technique), and renal, cerebral, and femoral blood flows as well.

Cardiac output is most commonly measured by the thermodilution technique, but the standard method, against which this technique and others are calibrated, remains the direct Fick oxygen method. In the direct Fick method, O_2 consumption is measured simultaneously with determination of the arteriovenous oxygen difference across the lungs. Fick's principle states that

$$Q \ (\text{L/min}) = \frac{O_2 \text{ consumption (mL/min)}}{\text{arteriovenous oxygen difference (mL/L)}}$$

In order to compare individuals of different body weights and sizes, O_2 consumption and cardiac output (Q) are commonly divided by

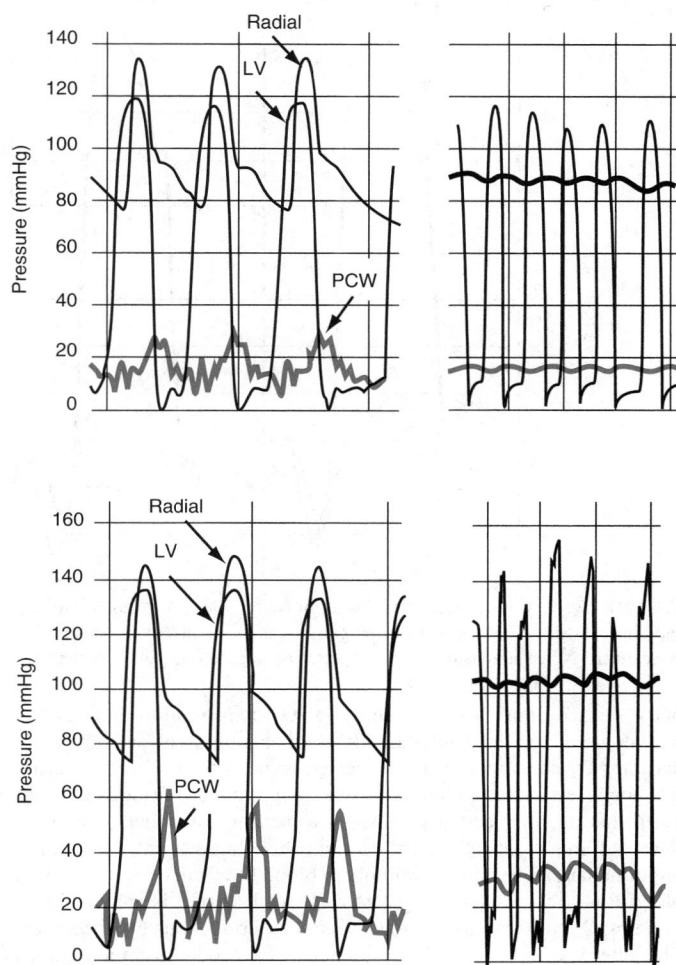

FIGURE 229-7 Hemodynamic findings at rest and during exercise in a patient with mitral regurgitation. Left ventricular (LV), pulmonary capillary wedge (PCW), and radial artery pressure tracings are shown before (*left*) and during (*right*) the sixth minute of supine bicycle exercise. PCW mean pressure and *v* wave increase substantially with exercise. [*From BH Lorell, W Grossman, in Cardiac Catheterization, Angiography, and Intervention, 5th ed, DS Baim, W Grossman (eds). Baltimore, Williams & Wilkins, 1996.*]

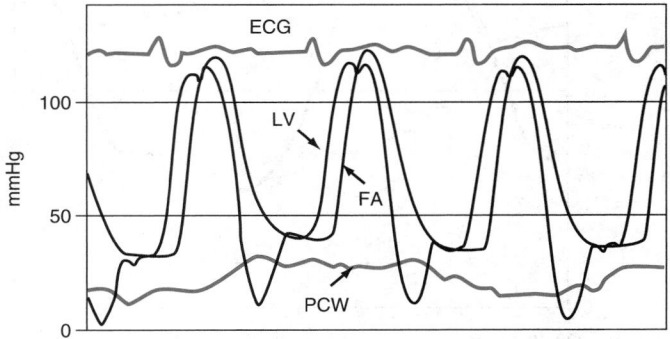

FIGURE 229-8 Severe aortic regurgitation. There is equilibration between the left ventricular (LV) and aortic or femoral artery (FA) pressures in diastole. Also, LV diastolic pressure exceeds pulmonary capillary wedge (PCW) pressure early in diastole, indicating premature closure of the mitral valve (a characteristic feature of severe aortic regurgitation). [*From W Grossman, in Cardiac Catheterization, Angiography, and Intervention, 5th ed, DS Baim, W Grossman (eds). Baltimore, Williams & Wilkins, 1996.*]

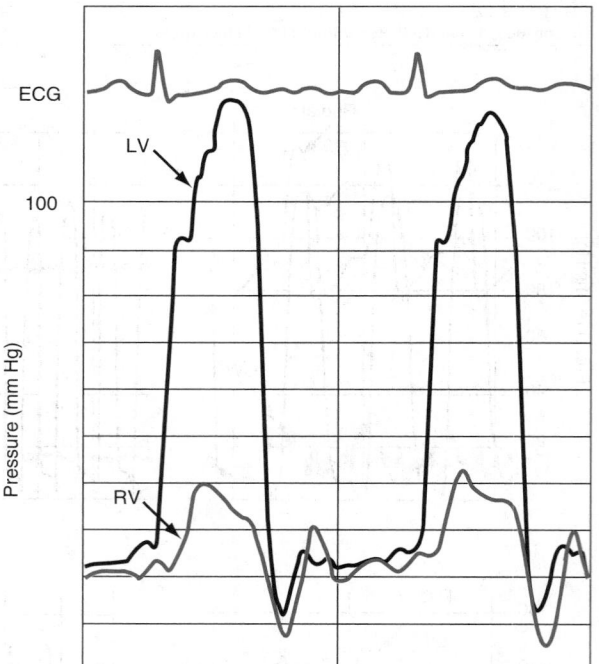

FIGURE 229-9 Left ventricular (LV), right ventricular (RV), and pulmonary capillary wedge (PCW) pressure tracings in a patient with severe constrictive pericarditis. Note the diastolic dip and plateau ("square root sign") pattern for left and right ventricular diastolic pressures (*left*). The wedge pressure (*right*) shows early systolic and early diastolic dips.

body surface area. Normal values for O_2 consumption and cardiac output are given in Table 229-3. Cardiac output is calculated by dividing O_2 consumption by the arteriovenous O_2 difference across the lungs (estimated pulmonary venous–pulmonary arterial O_2 content); this quantity actually provides a measure of *pulmonary blood flow* (Q_p). In patients with a left-to-right shunt at the atrial, ventricular, or pulmonary artery levels, pulmonary blood flow will exceed systemic blood flow. In such cases, systemic blood flow (Q_s) is calculated by dividing O_2 consumption by the systemic arteriovenous O_2 difference. The latter is calculated as the systemic arterial blood O_2 content minus

the mixed venous blood O_2 content as estimated using blood from the chamber immediately proximal to the level of the shunt. The Fick method is most dependable when the cardiac output is low and the arteriovenous oxygen difference is large.

For indicator-dilution measurement of cardiac output using the thermodilution technique, a thermistor is mounted on the tip of a balloon flotation catheter, and the catheter is advanced so that the balloon tip and thermistor are located in the pulmonary artery. Cold dextrose solution or saline is injected via a proximal port on the catheter into the vena cava or right atrium, and the change in temperature monitored at the thermistor is integrated electronically. This integral is inversely proportional to the volume flow rate past the thermistor, and if the temperatures of the injectate and pulmonary artery blood are measured, cardiac output (actually, pulmonary blood flow) can be calculated. In contrast to the Fick method, the indicator-dilution method is least reliable when the cardiac output is low.

Valve Areas and Resistances   Using simultaneous measures of pressure and flow, the resistance to blood flow across the cardiac valves as well as the pulmonary and systemic arteriolar beds may be estimated. Valve areas are calculated using the Gorlin formula:

$$A = \frac{flow}{K\sqrt{\Delta P}}$$

where A = valve orifice area (cm^2), *flow* is the blood flow (mL/s) across the stenotic valve, ΔP is the mean pressure gradient (mmHg) during the period of blood flow, and K is a constant (44.3 for the aortic valve and 37.7 for the mitral valve).

The resistance to blood flow through the systemic vascular bed is

$$SVR = 80(MAP - RA)/SBF$$

where SVR is systemic vascular resistance [(dyn·s)/cm^5], MAP and RA are mean aortic and right atrial pressures (mmHg), 80 is a constant for converting to metric units, and SBF is systemic blood flow (L/min).

Resistance to blood flow through the pulmonary vascular bed is

$$PVR = 80(PA - PCW \text{ or } LA)/PBF$$

where PVR is pulmonary vascular resistance [(dyn·s)/cm^5]; PA, PCW, and LA are pulmonary artery, pulmonary capillary wedge, and left atrial mean pressures, respectively, (mmHg); and PBF is pulmonary blood flow (L/min). Normal values for pulmonary and systemic vascular resistances are given in Table 229-3.

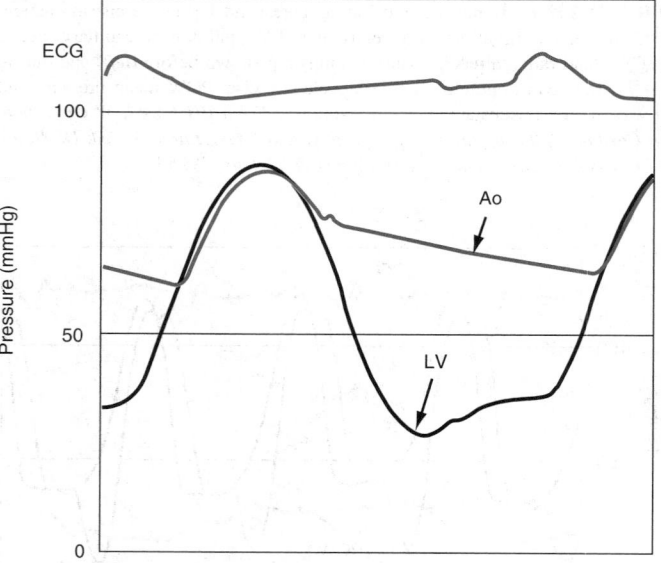

FIGURE 229-10   Left ventricular (LV) and aortic (Ao) pressures in a patient with advanced dilated cardiomyopathy. Marked slowing of the rates of left ventricular pressure rise and fall (impairment of contractility and relaxation) give the LV pressure pulse a triangular appearance. Also, the minimal value for left ventricular diastolic pressure is markedly elevated, suggesting an increased end-systolic volume and a reduced LV ejection fraction. [*From W Grossman, in Cardiac Catheterization, Angiography, and Intervention, 5th ed, DS Baim, W Grossman (eds). Baltimore, Williams & Wilkins, 1996.*]

BIBLIOGRAPHY

Baim DS, Grossman W (eds): *Cardiac Catheterization, Angiography, and Intervention*, 5th ed. Baltimore, Williams & Wilkins, 1996

Davidson CJ et al: Cardiac catheterization, in *Heart Disease*, 5th ed, E Braunwald (ed). Philadelphia, Saunders, 1997, p 177

Godlewski KJ et al: Interpretation of cardiac pathophysiology from pressure waveform analysis: Acute aortic insufficiency. Cathet Cardiovasc Diagn 28:244, 1993

Johnson LW, Krone R: Cardiac catheterization 1991: A report of the Registry

of the Society for Cardiac Angiography and Interventions (SCA&I). Cathet Cardiovasc Diagn 28:219, 1993

Kern MJ et al: Interpretation of cardiac pathophysiology from pressure waveform analysis: Simultaneous left and right ventricular pressure measurements. Cathet Cardiovasc Diagn 28:51, 1993

SECTION 2

DISORDERS OF RHYTHM

Mark E. Josephson, Peter Zimetbaum,
Francis E. Marchlinski, Alfred E. Buxton

| **230** |

THE BRADYARRHYTHMIAS: DISORDERS OF SINUS NODE FUNCTION AND AV CONDUCTION DISTURBANCES

ANATOMY OF THE CONDUCTING SYSTEM Under normal conditions, the pacemaker function of the heart resides in the sinoatrial (SA) node, which lies at the junction of the right atrium and superior vena cava. The SA node is approximately 1.5 cm long and 2 to 3 mm wide and is supplied by the sinus node artery, which arises from either the right coronary artery (60 percent) or the left circumflex coronary artery (40 percent). Once the impulse exits the sinus node and perinodal tissue, it traverses the atrium until it reaches the atrioventricular (AV) node. The blood supply of the AV node is derived from the posterior descending coronary artery (90 percent). The AV node lies at the base of the interatrial septum just above the tricuspid annulus and anterior to the coronary sinus. The electrophysiologic properties of the AV node result in slow conduction, which is responsible for the normal delay in AV conduction, i.e., the PR interval.

The bundle of His emerges from the AV node, enters the fibrous skeleton of the heart, and courses anteriorly across the membranous interventricular septum. It has a dual blood supply from the AV nodal artery and a branch of the anterior descending coronary artery. The branching (distal) portion of the bundle of His gives rise to a broad sheet of fibers that course over the left side of the interventricular septum to form the left bundle branch and a narrow cable-like structure on the right side that forms the right bundle branch. The arborization of both the right and left bundle branches gives rise to the distal His-Purkinje system, which ultimately extends throughout the endocardium of the right and left ventricles.

The sinus node, atrium, and AV node are significantly influenced by autonomic tone. Vagal influences depress automaticity of the sinus node, depress conduction, and prolong refractoriness in the tissue surrounding the sinus node; inhomogeneously decrease atrial refractoriness and slow atrial conduction; and prolong AV nodal conduction and refractoriness. Sympathetic influences exert the opposite effect.

ELECTROPHYSIOLOGIC PRINCIPLES

In the resting state, the interior of most cardiac cells, with the exception of the sinus and AV nodes, is approximately -80 to -90 mV, negative with respect to a reference extracellular electrode. The resting membrane potential is determined primarily by the concentration gradient of potassium across the cell membrane. Activation of cardiac cells results from movement of ions across the cell membrane, causing a transient depolarization known as the *action potential*. The ionic species responsible for the action potential varies among the cardiac

tissues, and the configuration of the action potential is therefore unique to each tissue (Fig. 230-1).

The action potential of the His-Purkinje system and ventricular myocardium has five phases (Fig. 230-2). The rapid depolarizing current (phase 0) is mainly determined by an influx of sodium into myocardial cells followed by a secondary (slower) influx of calcium which produces a slow inward current. The repolarization phases of the action potential (phases 1 to 3) are primarily related to outward flux of potassium. The resting membrane potential is phase 4.

The bradyarrhythmias result from abnormalities either of impulse formation, i.e., automaticity, or of conduction. *Automaticity*, which is normally observed in the sinus node, the specialized fibers of the His-Purkinje system, and some specialized atrial fibers, is the property of a cardiac cell that causes it to depolarize spontaneously during phase 4 of the action potential, leading to the generation of an impulse. To exhibit automaticity, the resting membrane potential must decrease spontaneously until threshold potential is reached and an all-or-none regenerative response occurs. The ionic currents producing spontaneous diastolic depolarization appear to involve the inward current of

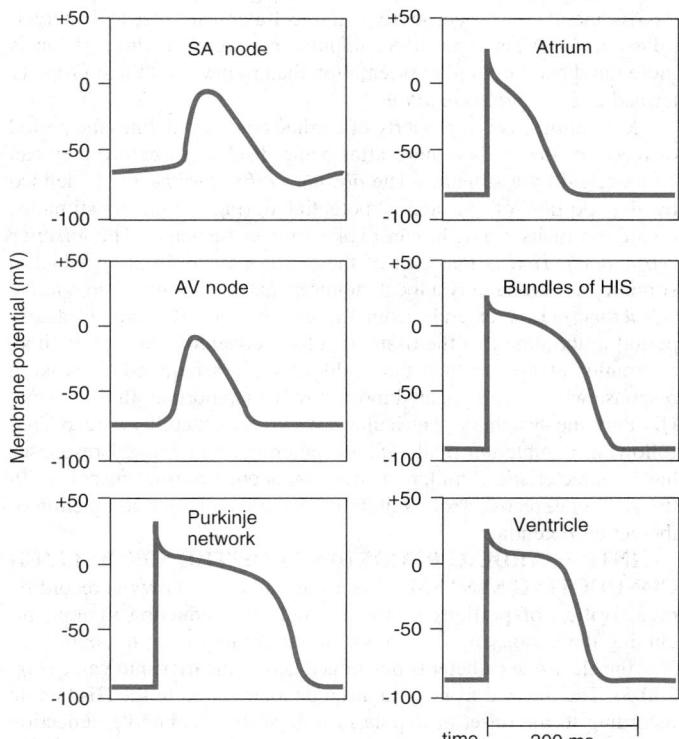

FIGURE 230-1 Action potential configurations in different regions of the mammalian heart. (*From AM Katz, Physiology of the Heart, New York, Raven, 1977.*)

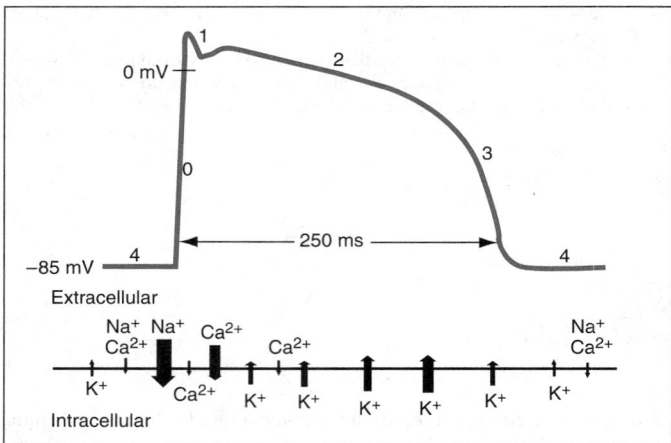

FIGURE 230-2 Schematic representation of the action potential in normal ventricle depicting the direction, strength, and period of flow of the ionic currents underlying the action potential. The arrow's direction and size indicate whether current is inward- or outward-directed and the approximate current strength of the ion identified at the arrow's base. The horizontal position of the arrow corresponds to the same moment in the time course of action potential (see text). The five phases of the action potential are indicated by the numerals placed along the waveform. *(From Ten Eick et al, Prog Cardiovasc Dis 24(2):157, 1981, with permission.)*

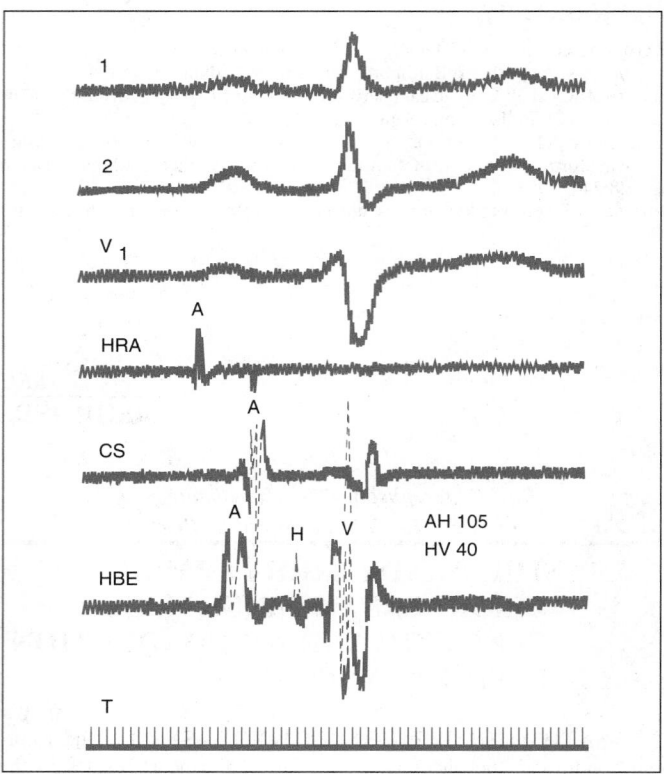

FIGURE 230-3 Normal intracardiac recording. Surface ECG leads I, II, and V_1 are displayed with intracardiac ECGs from the high right atrium (HRA), left atrium from the coronary sinus (CS), and AV junction to obtain a His bundle electrogram (HBE). T, time lines; A, atrial activation; H, His bundle activation; V, ventricular activation. Atrial activation begins in the high right atrium and spreads inferiorly to the low atrial septum, as recorded in the HBE, and the left atrium, as recorded in the CS. The AH and HV intervals represent AV nodal and His-Purkinje conduction times, respectively. Vertical lines = 0.10 s. *(From ME Josephson, SF Seides, Clinical Cardiac Electrophysiology: Techniques and Interpretations. Philadelphia, Lea & Febiger, 1979.)*

either sodium or calcium. The velocity of *conduction*, i.e., impulse propagation through cardiac tissues, depends on the magnitude of inward current, which is directly related to the rate of rise and amplitude of phase 0 of the action potential. The more positive the threshold potential and the slower the rate of depolarization toward threshold, the slower is the rate of rise of phase 0 of the action potential and the slower is the conduction velocity. Disease states or drugs may result in lower rates of rise of phase 0 at any given membrane potential. Passive membrane properties (e.g., intracellular resistance and intercellular coupling) also can affect impulse propagation. Propagation is more rapid parallel to fiber orientation than transverse to it, a property termed *anisotropic conduction*.

Refractoriness is a property of cardiac cells that defines the period of recovery that cells require after being discharged before they can be reexcited by a stimulus. The *absolute refractory period* is defined by that portion of the action potential during which no stimulus, regardless of its strength, can evoke another response. The *effective refractory period* is that part of the action potential during which a stimulus can evoke only a local, nonpropagated response. The *relative refractory period* extends from the end of the effective refractory period to the time that the tissue is fully recovered. During this time, a stimulus of greater than threshold strength is required to evoke a response which is propagated more slowly than normal. In the normal His-Purkinje system or ventricular myocytes, excitability is recovered following completion of the action potential, and evoked responses have characteristics similar to the spontaneous normal response. In the AV node, recovery of excitability occurs well after completion of the action potential.

INTRACARDIAC RECORDINGS OF THE SPECIALIZED CONDUCTING SYSTEM Electrode catheters allow the recording of activation of portions of the specialized conducting system, including the bundle of His. To obtain a recording from the bundle of His, the electrode catheter is positioned across the tricuspid valve (Fig. 230-3). The interval from local atrial depolarization in the His bundle recording to the onset of depolarization of the His bundle deflection is called the *AH interval* (normal = 60 to 125 ms) and represents an indirect method of assessing AV nodal conduction time. The interval from the beginning of the His bundle deflection to the earliest onset of ventricular activation, as measured from any of multiple-surface

electrocardiogram (ECG) leads or the intracardiac ventricular electrogram, is called the *HV interval* (normal = 35 to 55 ms) and represents conduction time through the His-Purkinje system. Electrode catheters can be positioned in the area of the sinus node to record high right atrial activity. Left atrial activity may be recorded directly via a catheter placed across a patent foramen ovale or indirectly using a catheter inserted into the coronary sinus. The atrial activation sequence may be "mapped," and sites of intra- and interatrial conduction abnormalities may be ascertained.

SINUS NODE DYSFUNCTION

The sinus node is normally the dominant cardiac pacemaker because its intrinsic discharge rate is the highest of all potential cardiac pacemakers. Its responsiveness to alterations in autonomic nervous system tone is responsible for the normal acceleration of heart rate during exercise and the slowing that occurs during rest and sleep. Increases in sinus rate normally result from an increase in sympathetic tone acting via beta-adrenergic receptors and/or a decrease in parasympathetic tone acting via muscarinic receptors. Slowing of the heart rate is normally due to opposite alterations. In adults, the normal sinus rate under basal conditions is 60 to 100 beats per minute. Sinus bradycardia is said to exist when the sinus rate is less than 60 beats per minute, and sinus tachycardia when it exceeds 100 beats per minute. However, there is wide variation among individuals, and rates less than 60 beats per minute do not necessarily indicate pathologic states. For example, trained athletes often exhibit resting rates under 50 beats per minute due to increases in vagal tone. Normal elderly individuals also may show marked sinus bradycardia at rest.

ETIOLOGY   Sinus node dysfunction most often is found in the elderly as an isolated phenomenon. Although interruption of the blood supply to the sinus node may produce dysfunction, the correlation between obstruction of the sinus node artery and clinical evidence of sinus node dysfunction is poor. Specific disease states associated with sinus node dysfunction include senile amyloidosis and other conditions associated with infiltration of the atrial myocardium. Sinus bradycardia is associated with hypothyroidism, advanced liver disease, hypothermia, typhoid fever, and brucellosis; it occurs during episodes of hypervagotonia (vasovagal syncope), severe hypoxia, hypercapnia, acidemia, and acute hypertension. However, in most cases of sinus node dysfunction a specific cause cannot be identified.

MANIFESTATIONS   Although marked (≤ 50 beats per minute) sinus bradycardia may cause fatigue and other symptoms due to inadequate cardiac output, more commonly sinus node dysfunction is manifest as paroxysmal dizziness, presyncope, or syncope. These symptoms usually result from abrupt, prolonged sinus pauses caused by failure of sinus impulse formation (sinus arrest) or block of conduction of sinus impulses to the surrounding atrial tissue (sinus exit block). In either case, the ECG manifestation is a prolonged period (>3 s) of atrial asystole. In some patients, sinus node dysfunction is accompanied by abnormalities in AV conduction. In addition to the absence of atrial activity, lower pacemakers fail to emerge during the sinus pauses, resulting in periods of ventricular asystole and syncope. Occasionally, sinus node dysfunction is manifested by an inadequate acceleration in sinus rate in response to a stress such as exercise or fever. In some patients, sinus node dysfunction may become manifest only in the presence of certain cardioactive drugs: cardiac glycosides, beta-adrenergic blocking drugs, verapamil, quinidine, and other antiarrhythmic agents. These agents, which do not cause sinus node dysfunction in normal people, may unmask evidence of sinus node dysfunction in susceptible individuals.

The *sick sinus syndrome* refers to a combination of symptoms (dizziness, confusion, fatigue, syncope, and congestive heart failure) caused by sinus node dysfunction and manifested by marked sinus bradycardia, sinoatrial block, or sinus arrest. Because these symptoms are nonspecific, and because ECG manifestations of sinus node dysfunction are not infrequently intermittent, it may be difficult to prove that such symptoms are actually caused by sinus node dysfunction.

Atrial tachyarrhythmias such as atrial fibrillation, atrial flutter, or atrial tachycardia may be accompanied by sinus node dysfunction. The *bradycardia-tachycardia syndrome* refers to paroxysmal atrial arrhythmia that upon termination is followed by prolonged sinus pauses (Fig. 230-4) or in which there are alternating periods of tachyarrhythmia and bradyarrhythmia. Syncope or presyncope may result from failure of the sinus node to recover function following suppression of automaticity by atrial tachyarrhythmia.

DIAGNOSIS   *First-degree sinoatrial exit block* denotes a prolonged conduction time from the sinus node to the surrounding atrial tissue. It cannot be recognized on a standard (surface) ECG but requires invasive intracardiac recordings (see below). *Second-degree sinoatrial exit block* denotes the intermittent failure of conduction of sinus impulses to the surrounding atrial tissue; it is manifested as the intermittent absence of P waves (Fig. 230-5). *Third-degree*, or *complete, sinoatrial block* is characterized by a lack of atrial activity or by the presence of an ectopic subsidiary atrial pacemaker. On the standard ECG it cannot be distinguished from sinus arrest, but direct intracardiac recordings of sinus node activity permit this distinction. The *bradycardia-tachycardia syndrome* is manifested on the standard ECG as tachyarrhythmias (see Fig. 230-4). Most often these are atrial flutter or fibrillation, although any tachycardia during which the atria are activated may cause overdrive suppression of the sinus node resulting in clinical appearance of this syndrome.

The most important step in the diagnosis is to correlate symptoms with ECG evidence of sinus node dysfunction. While ambulatory ECG (Holter) moni-toring remains a mainstay in evaluating sinus node function, most episodes of syncope are paroxysmal and unpredictable. Single and even multiple 24-h Holter monitor recordings may fail to include a symptomatic episode. Therefore, noting the response to carotid sinus pressure and pharmacologic autonomic "denervation" of the heart is frequently helpful. Carotid sinus pressure is particularly useful in patients in whom paroxysmal dizziness or syncope is compatible with the hypersensitive carotid sinus syndrome (see Chap. 20). In such patients, the response can be dramatic, and sinus pauses in excess of 5 s may occur. Normally, a sinus pause of ≤ 3 s results from 5 s of unilateral carotid sinus massage. However, in elderly patients, pauses >3 s are common and do not necessarily signify a diagnostic response. In all individuals it is important to correlate symptoms with such ECG phenomena. The other noninvasive test of sinus node function involves the use of pharmacologic agents to manipulate the autonomic nervous system and assess the balance of parasympathetic and sympathetic activity on the sinus node. Physiologic or pharmacologic maneuvers that are vagomimetic (Valsalva maneuver or phenylephrine-induced hypertension), vagolytic (atropine), sympathomimetic (isoproterenol or hypotension by nitroprusside), or sympatholytic (beta-adrenergic blocking agents) can be utilized, singly and in combination. These studies are designed to test the response of the sinus node to autonomic stimulation and inhibition and thereby characterize the status of autonomic regulation of the sinus node. Abnormalities of the autonomic control of sinus function are particularly common in patients in whom asymptomatic sinus bradycardia is documented.

Intrinsic Heart Rate   This is a manifestation of the primary activity of the sinus node, and its determination requires chemical autonomic blockade of the heart with a combination of atropine and a beta blocker. Normal values of intrinsic heart rate (in beats per minute) are calculated by the formula $118.1 - (0.57 \times \text{age})$. The use of autonomic blockade can separate patients with asymptomatic sinus bradycardia into a group with primary sinus node dysfunction (slow intrinsic heart rate) and a group with autonomic imbalance (normal intrinsic heart rate). Autonomic blockade is particularly useful when combined with invasive assessment of sinus node function (see Table 230-1). Autonomic blockade may depress conduction in patients with intrinsic disease of the conduction system and should be carried out only in a setting where arrhythmias can be monitored and treated rapidly.

Sinus Node Recovery Time   Sinus node recovery time (SNRT) is evaluated by assessing the response of the sinus node to rapid atrial pacing (Fig. 230-6). When atrial pacing is discontinued, a pause, the *SNRT*, occurs prior to resumption of spontaneous sinus rhythm. When the SNRT is prolonged, the results of this test mimic the prolonged sinus pauses seen following termination of atrial tachyarrhythmias in the bradycardia-tachycardia syndrome (see Fig. 230-4). The SNRT is usually corrected for the spontaneous sinus rate and is normally less than 550 ms. In patients with symptomatic sinus node dysfunction, prolongation of the SNRT is often observed. Patients with abnormally slow intrinsic heart rates usually have an abnormal SNRT, while those with normal intrinsic heart rates have normal recovery times.

Sinoatrial Conduction Time   Determination of the conduction time from the sinus node to the atrium allows for the differentiation of abnormalities of sinoatrial conduction from abnormalities of sinus impulse formation. The conduction time equals one-half the difference

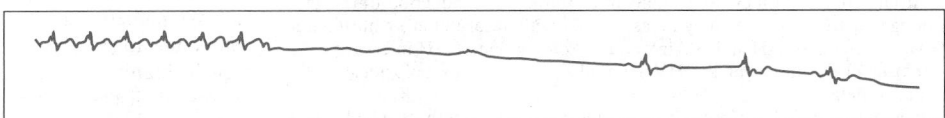

FIGURE 230-4   Tachycardia-bradycardia syndrome. Rhythm strip of ECG lead II showing spontaneous cessation of supraventricular tachycardia followed by a 5.6-s pause prior to resumption of sinus activity. The patient was asymptomatic during supraventricular tachycardia, but the sinus pause caused severe light-headedness.

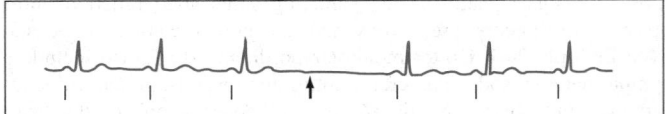

FIGURE 230-5 Second-degree sinoatrial exit block. Surface ECG denoting abrupt absence of P wave during sinus rhythm. Prior to the pause, the sinus rate is regular. The interval of the pause is exactly twice the basal sinus cycle length. The arrow marks the appropriate location for the absent P wave. SA exit block can be 2:1 as above or longer, as shown in Fig. 230-6.

between the pause following termination of brief periods of pacing and the sinus cycle length. Alternatively, the sinus node electrogram can be recorded directly by a catheter electrode placed near the sinoatrial node, and direct measurement of sinoatrial conduction can be obtained.

EVALUATION The electrophysiologic investigation of sinus node dysfunction should be undertaken in patients who have had symptoms compatible with sinus node dysfunction and in whom no documentation of the arrhythmia responsible for these symptoms has been obtained by prolonged Holter monitoring. Asymptomatic patients with sinus bradycardia need *not* be tested, since no therapy is indicated. Similarly, symptomatic patients with ECG documentation of asystole, sinoatrial block or arrest, or the bradycardia-tachycardia syndrome do not require electrophysiologic tests for diagnosis. However, in symptomatic patients without documentation of an arrhythmia, electrophysiologic assessment of sinus node function can yield information that may be used to guide appropriate therapy.

The results of tests of sinus node function must be interpreted with caution. Sinus node dysfunction coexists frequently with other disorders such as AV conduction disturbances, which may cause symptoms such as syncope. Electrophysiologic evaluation of patients with symptoms such as undiagnosed syncope must not stop with the demonstration of abnormalities of sinus node dysfunction or carotid sinus hypersensitivity. Instead, complete evaluation, including His bundle recordings and programmed atrial and ventricular stimulation (see Chap. 231), is necessary to search for additional electrophysiologic abnormalities that could be responsible for symptoms.

Table 230-1

Electrophysiologic Evaluation of the Conduction System

SINUS NODE EVALUATION

1. Sinus node recovery time (SNRT): Amount of time required by the sinus node to recover from overdrive suppression. The SNRT is corrected for the mean sinus rate at baseline. The normal value is <550 ms.
2. Sinoatrial conduction time: Measured from the response of the sinus node to stimulated atrial premature depolarizations or by direct recording from a sinus node electrogram. The normal value is 45–125 ms.
3. Intrinsic heart rate (IHR): Heart rate measured after autonomic blockade with atropine (0.5–2.0 mg IV) and propranolol (1–4 µg/min IV). The normal IHR is calculated by the formula:

$$HR = 118.1 - (0.57 \times age)$$

An abnormally low value suggests sinus node dysfunction.

ATRIOVENTRICULAR CONDUCTION EVALUATION

1. Atrial activation times: Measurement of intraatrial conduction times. Prolonged activation times may be associated with atrial flutter or fibrillation.
2. Measurement of AH and HV intervals: Prolongation of AH interval (>125 ms) or prolongation of the HV interval (>55 ms) may help localize the site of delay.
3. Incremental atrial pacing: To determine the cycle length at which block occurs in the AV node and/or His-Purkinje system. Block below the His bundle at rates of <150 beats per minute portends the development of infra-His block.

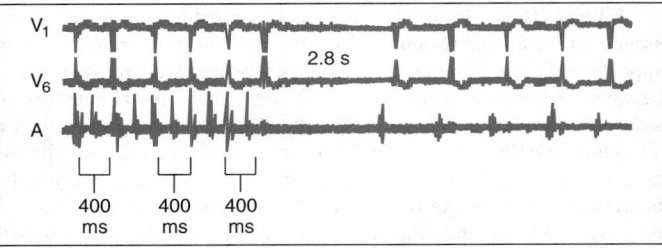

FIGURE 230-6 Example of sinus node recovery time in a patient with symptomatic sinus node dysfunction. Cessation of atrial pacing at 150 beats per minute (cycle length 400 ms) results in a prolonged sinus pause (2.8 s). Surface ECG leads V_1 and V_6 are shown in addition to intracardiac recordings at the high right atrium (A), which demonstrates atrial pacing rate.

℞ TREATMENT

Permanent pacemakers (see p. 1258) are the mainstay of therapy for patients with symptomatic sinus node dysfunction. Patients with intermittent paroxysms of bradycardia or sinus arrest and with the cardioinhibitory form of the hypersensitive carotid sinus syndrome are usually adequately treated by demand ventricular pacemakers. These devices are reliable, relatively inexpensive, and suffice to prevent episodic symptoms due to abrupt bradycardia. Patients with symptomatic chronic sinus bradycardia or frequent prolonged episodes of sinus node dysfunction do better with dual-chamber pacemakers that preserve the normal AV activation sequence. Although theoretically an atrial demand pacemaker should be adequate for patients with sinus node dysfunction, the frequent accompaniment of dysfunction in other portions of the cardiac conduction system usually mandates placement of a pacemaker capable of ventricular pacing. Recent studies suggest that AV sequential pacing also may be useful in preventing atrial fibrillation, an important component of the bradycardia-tachycardia syndrome.

AV CONDUCTION DISTURBANCES

The specialized cardiac conducting system normally ensures synchronous conduction of each sinus impulse from the atria to the ventricles. Abnormalities of conduction of the sinus impulse to the ventricles may portend the development of heart block, which can ultimately lead to syncope or cardiac arrest. In order to evaluate the clinical significance of conduction abnormalities, the physician must assess (1) the site of conduction disturbance, (2) the risk of progression to complete block, and (3) the probability that a subsidiary escape rhythm arising distal to the site of block will be electrophysiologically and hemodynamically stable. This latter point is perhaps the most important, since the rate and stability of the escape pacemaker determine what symptoms result from heart block. The escape pacemaker following AV nodal block is usually in the His bundle, which generally has a stable rate of 40 to 60 beats per minute and is associated with a QRS complex of normal duration (in the absence of a preexisting intraventricular conduction defect). This contrasts with escape rhythms arising in the distal His-Purkinje system, which have lower intrinsic rates (25 to 45 beats per minute), manifest wide QRS complexes with prolonged duration, and are unstable. Although prolonged QRS complexes are invariable when the distal His-Purkinje pacemakers form the escape mechanism, wide QRS complexes also can coexist with AV nodal block and a His bundle rhythm. Therefore, QRS morphology alone may not be adequate to identify the site of block.

ETIOLOGY The AV node is supplied by the parasympathetic and sympathetic nervous systems and is sensitive to variations in autonomic tone. Chronic slowing of AV nodal conduction may be seen in highly trained athletes who have hypervagotonia at rest. A variety of diseases also can influence AV nodal conduction. These include acute processes such as myocardial infarction (particularly inferior), coronary spasm (usually of the right coronary artery), digitalis intoxication, excesses of beta and/or calcium blockers, acute infections such as viral myocarditis, acute rheumatic fever, infectious mononucle-

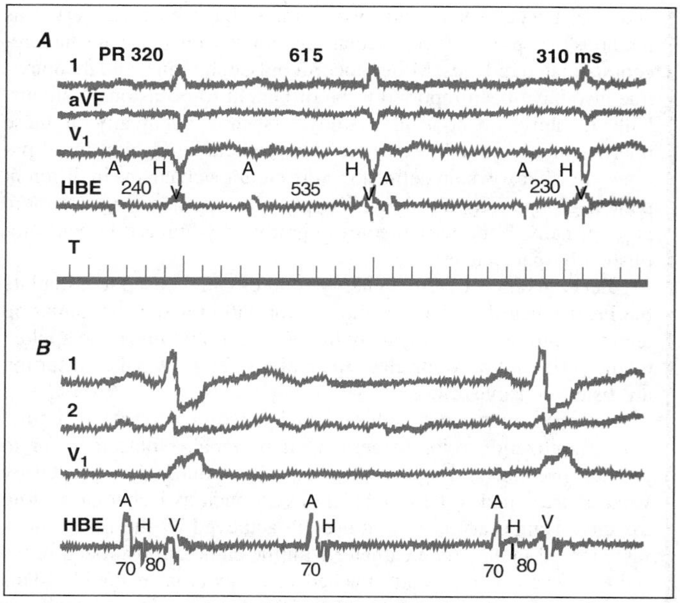

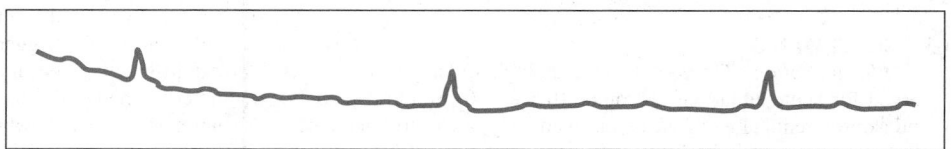

FIGURE 230-7 *A*. Mobitz type I second-degree AV block. Intracardiac recordings demonstrate that the PR prolongation (320, 615 ms) is localized to the AV node (AH 240, 535 ms, respectively). HBE, His bundle electrogram; A, atrium; H, His; V, ventricle. Time lines (T) = 100 ms. *(From ME Josephson, SF Seides, Clinical Cardiac Electrophysiology: Techniques and Interpretations. Philadelphia, Lea & Febiger, 1979.) B*. Mobitz type II second-degree AV block. Intracardiac recordings document block below the His bundle.

osis, and miscellaneous disorders such as Lyme disease, sarcoidosis, amyloidosis, and neoplasms, particularly cardiac mesotheliomas. AV nodal block also may be congenital.

Two degenerative diseases are commonly responsible for damage to the specialized conducting system and produce AV block usually associated with bundle branch block (see Chap. 228). In *Lev's disease*, there is calcification and sclerosis of the fibrous cardiac skeleton, which frequently involves the aortic and mitral valves, the central fibrous body, and the summit of the ventricular septum. *Lenegre's disease* appears to be a primary sclerodegenerative disease within the conducting system itself with no involvement of the myocardium or the fibrous skeleton of the heart. These two diseases are probably the most common causes of isolated chronic heart block in adults. Hypertension and aortic and/or mitral stenosis are specific disorders that either accelerate the degeneration of the conducting system or have a direct effect by calcification and fibrosis involving the conducting system.

First-degree AV block, more properly termed *prolonged AV conduction*, is characterized by a PR interval >0.20 s. Since the PR interval is determined by atrial, AV nodal, and His-Purkinje activation, delay in any one or more of these structures can contribute to a prolonged PR interval. In the presence of a QRS complex of normal duration, a PR interval >0.24 s almost invariably is due to a delay within the AV node. If the QRS is prolonged, delays may be present at any of the levels mentioned above. Delay within the His-Purkinje system is always accompanied by a prolonged QRS duration in addition to a prolonged PR interval. However, as indicated below, it is only with intracardiac recordings that the exact site of delay can be determined.

Second-degree heart block (intermittent AV block) is present when some atrial impulses fail to conduct to the ventricles. Mobitz type I second-degree AV block (AV Wenckebach block) is characterized by progressive PR interval prolongation prior to block of an atrial impulse (Fig. 230-7A). The pause that follows is less than fully compensatory (i.e., is less than two normal sinus intervals), and the PR interval of the first

conducted impulse is shorter than the last conducted atrial impulse prior to the blocked P wave. This type of block is almost always localized to the AV node and associated with a normal QRS duration. It is seen most often as a transient abnormality with inferior wall infarction or with drug intoxication, particularly digitalis, beta blockers, and occasionally calcium channel antagonists. This type of block also can be observed in normal individuals with heightened vagal tone. Although Mobitz type I block can progress to complete heart block, this is uncommon, except in the setting of acute inferior wall myocardial infarction. Even when it does, however, the heart block is usually well tolerated because the escape pacemaker usually arises in the proximal His bundle and provides a stable rhythm. As a result, the presence of Mobitz type I second-degree AV block rarely mandates aggressive therapy. Therapeutic decisions depend on the ventricular response and the symptoms of the patient. If the ventricular rate is adequate and the patient is asymptomatic, observation is sufficient.

In Mobitz type II second-degree AV block, conduction fails suddenly and unexpectedly without a preceding change in PR intervals (Fig. 230-7B). It is generally due to disease of the His-Purkinje system and is most often associated with a prolonged QRS duration. It is important to recognize this type of block because it has a high incidence of progression to complete heart block with an unstable, slow, lower escape pacemaker. Therefore, pacemaker implantation is necessary in this condition. Mobitz type II block may occur in the setting of anteroseptal infarction or in the primary or secondary sclerodegenerative or calcific disorders of the fibrous skeleton of the heart. In so-called high-degree AV block there are periods of two or more consecutively blocked P waves, but intermittent conduction can be demonstrated. Block is usually in the His-Purkinje system, but simultaneous block in the AV node may also be present. Regardless of the site of origin of the escape rhythm, if it is slow and the patient is symptomatic, a cardiac pacemaker is mandatory.

Third-degree AV block is present when no atrial impulse propagates to the ventricles. If the QRS complex of the escape rhythm is of normal duration, occurs at a rate of 40 to 55 beats per minute, and increases with atropine or exercise, AV nodal block is probable. Congenital complete AV block is usually localized to the AV node (Fig. 230-8). If the block is within the His bundle, the escape pacemaker usually is less responsive to these perturbations. If the escape rhythm of the QRS is wide and associated with rates ≤40 beats per minute, block is usually localized in, or distal to, the His bundle and mandates a pacemaker, since the escape rhythm in this setting is unreliable. Some patients with infra-His bundle block are capable of retrograde conduction. In such patients, a "pacemaker syndrome" (see below) may develop if a simple ventricular pacemaker is used. Dual-chambered pacemakers eliminate this potential problem.

AV DISSOCIATION   AV dissociation exists whenever the atria and ventricles are under the control of two separate pacemakers and, while present in complete AV block, can occur in the absence of a primary conduction disturbance. AV dissociation unrelated to heart block may occur under two circumstances: First, it may develop with an AV junctional rhythm in response to severe sinus bradycardia. When the sinus rate and the escape rate are similar and the P waves occur just before, in, or following the QRS complex, *isorhythmic AV dissociation* is said to be present. Treatment usually consists of removal of the offending cause of sinus bradycardia (i.e., discontinuation of digitalis, beta blockers, or calcium antagonists), accelerating the sinus

FIGURE 230-8   Third-degree AV block. Complete heart block with a narrow QRS. In this instance, the block was in the AV node.

node by vagolytic agents, or insertion of a pacemaker if the escape rhythm is slow and results in symptoms. Second, AV dissociation can be caused by an enhanced lower (junctional or ventricular) pacemaker that competes with normal sinus rhythm and frequently exceeds it. This has been called *interference AV dissociation* because the rapid lower pacemaker results in bombardment of the AV node in a retrograde fashion, rendering it refractory to the normal sinus impulses. Thus failure of antegrade conduction is a physiologic response in this circumstance. Interference dissociation commonly occurs during ventricular tachycardia, accelerated junctional or ventricular rhythms seen with digitalis intoxication, myocardial ischemia and/or infarction, or local irritation following cardiac surgery. The accelerated rhythm should be treated with either antiarrhythmic drugs (see Chap. 231), removal of an offending drug, or correction of the metabolic abnormality or ischemia.

INTRACARDIAC ELECTROCARDIOGRAPHIC RECORDINGS IN DIAGNOSIS AND MANAGEMENT The main therapeutic decision in patients with AV conduction disturbance is whether or not a permanent pacemaker is required, and a number of circumstances exist in which His bundle electrocardiography can be a useful diagnostic tool upon which to base this decision. It is unquestionable that patients with *symptomatic* second- or third-degree AV block should be paced, and therefore, these patients do not require electrophysiologic study. However, intracardiac ECG recordings can be useful in at least the following three groups of patients:

1. *Patients with syncope and bundle branch or bifascicular block without documentation of AV block.* In such patients, the demonstration of marked infra-His bundle conduction disturbances, i.e., a prolonged HV interval (>100 ms), may usually be taken as an indication of the need for the insertion of the permanent pacemaker. Complete electrophysiologic evaluation, including atrial and ventricular programmed stimulation, is indicated to help identify other possible cardiac etiologies for the syncope. Since the incidence of significant advanced AV block is low in *asymptomatic* patients who have bifascicular block, electrophysiologic evaluation or permanent pacemakers are not cost-effective. In this group, observation appears most reasonable.

2. *Patients with 2:1 atrioventricular conduction.* Intracardiac recordings are necessary to ascertain the site of the conduction disturbance because the typical ECG features of Mobitz type I or Mobitz type II block cannot be discerned during a 2:1 pattern of AV conduction on the surface ECG. Intracardiac recordings may demonstrate that AV nodal block, intra-His bundle block, infra-His bundle block, or combinations of block may be responsible. A surface ECG finding that suggests an infra-His bundle lesion is the presence of alternating bundle branch block associated with changing PR intervals. Intracardiac recordings in such patients confirm that the block is almost always in the His-Purkinje system. Increasing block with exercise or following atropine suggests intra- or infra-His block. The finding of infra- or intra-His bundle block in patients with asymptomatic second-degree AV block mandates pacemaker therapy because of the high likelihood of the development of symptomatic high-grade AV block and syncope.

3. *Asymptomatic patients with third-degree AV block.* In such patients, electrophysiologic studies may be useful in assessing the stability of the junctional pacemaker. Pacing is indicated when the His bundle escape pacemaker is shown to be unstable by an inadequate response to exercise, atropine, or isoproterenol or by a prolonged junctional recovery time following ventricular pacing.

℞ **TREATMENT**

Pharmacologic Therapy Pharmacologic therapy is usually reserved for acute situations. Atropine (0.5 to 2.0 mg intravenously) and isoproterenol (1 to 4 μg/min intravenously) are useful in increasing heart rate and decreasing symptoms in patients with sinus bradycardia or AV block localized to the AV node. They have an insignificant effect on lower pacemakers. In patients with neurovascular

syncope, beta blockers and disopyramide have been suggested as methods to depress left ventricular function and decrease mechanoreceptor-related reflexes. Mineralocorticoids, ephedrine, and theophylline also have been reported to be of benefit to occasional patients. Unfortunately, no controlled study has shown that any of these pharmacologic modalities works in a predictable fashion in all patients. Further work on delineating different mechanisms in different patient groups may allow us to apply pharmacologic agents more appropriately. Long-term therapy of bradyarrhythmias is best accomplished by pacemakers.

Pacemakers External energy sources can be used to stimulate the heart when disorders in impulse formation and/or transmission lead to symptomatic bradyarrhythmias. Pacer stimuli can be applied to the atria and/or ventricles. Indications for pacemaker insertion are listed in Table 230-2.

TEMPORARY PACING This is usually instituted to provide immediate stabilization prior to permanent pacemaker placement or to provide pacemaker support when a bradycardia is precipitated by what is presumed to be a transient event such as ischemia or drug toxicity. Temporary pacing is usually achieved by the transvenous insertion of an electrode catheter with the catheter positioned in the right ventricular apex and attached to an external generator. This procedure is associated with a small risk of cardiac perforation, infection at the insertion site, and thromboembolism; the risk of the latter two complications increases markedly if the pacing wire is left in place for more than 48 h. The development of an entirely external transthoracic cardiac pacing system may preclude the need for transvenous pacing in selected patients. However, occasional failure of ventricular capture and significant discomfort related to the large current required for effective transthoracic ventricular stimulation preclude the uniform use of this approach.

PERMANENT PACING This mode of pacing is instituted for persistent or intermittent symptomatic bradycardia not related to a self-limiting precipitating factor or for documented infranodal second- or third-degree AV block. Permanent pacing leads are usually inserted transvenously through the subclavian or cephalic vein with the leads positioned in the right atrial appendage for atrial pacing and the right ventricular apex for ventricular pacing. The leads are then attached to the pulse generator, which is inserted into a subcutaneous pocket below the clavicle. Epicardial lead placement is used when (1) transvenous access cannot be obtained, (2) the chest is already open, i.e., in the course of a cardiac operation, and (3) adequate endocardial lead placement cannot be achieved. Most pacemaker generators are powered by lithium batteries. The life expectancy of the generator is related to (1) voltage output required for capture, (2) requirement for incessant or intermittent pacing, and (3) number of cardiac chambers paced. Life expectancy of the simple ventricular demand pacemaker can exceed 10 years.

PACING CODE A code consisting of three to five letters has been developed for describing pacemaker type and function (Table 230-3). The first letter indicates the chamber(s) paced and is designated *V* for ventricular pacing, *A* for atrial pacing, or *D* for dual-chamber (both atrial and ventricular) pacing. The second letter indicates the chamber in which electrical activity is sensed and is also indicated by *A*, *V*, or *D*. An additional designation, *O*, has been used when pacemaker discharge is not dependent on a sensed electrical activity. The third letter refers to the response to a sensed electric signal. The letter *O* represents no response to an underlying electric signal, usually related to the absence of associated sensing function; *I* represents inhibition of pacing function; *T* represents triggering of pacing function; and *D* indicates a dual response, i.e., spontaneous atrial and ventricular activity inhibiting atrial and ventricular pacing and atrial activity triggering a ventricular response. Additional fourth and fifth letters of the pacing code have been recommended to indicate whether the pacemaker is programmable and has rate modulation (fourth) and whether special antitachycardia functions are available (i.e., antitachycardia pacing, *T*, and delivery of high- or low-energy shocks). In the fourth category, *M* represents multiprogrammability and *R* represents rate response ("physiologic") pacing.

Table 230-2

Indications for Permanent Pacing*

ACQUIRED AV BLOCK IN ADULTS

Class I
1. Complete heart block, permanent or intermittent, at any anatomic level, associated with any anatomic level, associated with any one of the following complications:
   a. Symptomatic bradycardia. In the presence of complete heart block, symptoms must be presumed to be due to the heart block unless proved to be otherwise.
   b. Congestive heart failure.
   c. Ectopic rhythms and other medical conditions that require drugs that suppress the automaticity of escape pacemakers and result in symptomatic bradycardia.
   d. Documented periods of asystole ≥ 3.0 s or any escape rate < 40 beats per minute in symptom-free patients.
   e. Confusional states that clear with temporary pacing.
   f. Post-AV junction ablation, myotonic dystrophy.
2. Second-degree AV block, permanent or intermittent, regardless of the type or the site of block, with symptomatic bradycardia.
3. Atrial fibrillation, atrial flutter, or rare cases of supraventricular tachycardia with complete heart block or advanced AV block, bradycardia, and any of the conditions described under a. The bradycardia must be related to digitalis or drugs known to impair AV conduction.

Class II
1. Asymptomatic complete heart block, permanent or intermittent, at any anatomic site, with ventricular rates of 40 beats per minute or faster.
2. Asymptomatic type II second-degree AV block, permanent or intermittent.
3. Asymptomatic type I second-degree AV block at infra-His or intra-His levels.

Class III
1. First-degree AV block.
2. Asymptomatic type I second-degree AV block at the supra-His (AV node) level.

AFTER MYOCARDIAL INFARCTION

Class I
1. Persistent advanced second-degree AV block or complete heart block after acute myocardial infarction with block in the His-Purkinje system (bilateral bundle branch block).
2. Transient advanced AV block and associated bundle branch block.

Class II
1. Persistent advanced block at the AV node.

Class III
1. Transient AV conduction disturbances in the absence of intraventricular conduction defects.
2. Transient AV block in the presence of isolated left anterior hemiblock.
3. Acquired left anterior hemiblock in the absence of AV block.
4. Persistent first-degree AV block in the presence of bundle branch block not demonstrated previously.

BIFASCICULAR AND TRIFASCICULAR BLOCK

Class I
1. Bifascicular block with intermittent complete heart block associated with symptomatic bradycardia.

2. Bifascicular or trifascicular block with intermittent type II second-degree AV block without symptoms attributable to the heart block.

Class II
1. Bifascicular or trifascicular block with syncope that is not proved to be due to complete heart block, but other possible causes for syncope are not identifiable.
2. Markedly prolonged HV (>100 ms).
3. Pacing-induced infra-His block.

Class III
1. Fascicular block without AV block or symptoms.
2. Fascicular block with first-degree AV block without symptoms.

SINUS NODE DYSFUNCTION

Class I
1. Sinus node dysfunction with documented symptomatic bradycardia. In some patients this will occur as a consequence of long-term (essential) drug therapy of a type and dose for which there are no acceptable alternatives.

Class II
1. Sinus node dysfunction, occurring spontaneously or as a result of necessary drug therapy, with heart rates < 40 beats per minute when a clear association between significant symptoms consistent with bradycardia and the actual presence of bradycardia has not been documented.

Class III
1. Sinus node dysfunction in asymptomatic patients, including those in whom substantial sinus bradycardia (heart rate < 40 beats per minute) is a consequence of long-term drug treatment.
2. Sinus node dysfunction in patients in whom symptoms suggestive of bradycardia are clearly documented not to be associated with a slow heart rate.

HYPERSENSITIVE CAROTID SINUS AND NEUROVASCULAR SYNDROMES

Class I
1. Recurrent syncope associated with clear, spontaneous events provoked by carotid sinus stimulation; minimal carotid sinus pressure induces asystole of >3 s duration in the absence of any medication that depresses the sinus node or AV conduction.

Class II
1. Recurrent syncope without clear, provocative events and with a hypersensitive cardioinhibitory response.
2. Syncope with associated bradycardia reproduced by a head-up tilt with or without isoproterenol or other forms of provocative maneuvers and in which a temporary pacemaker and a second provocative test can establish the likely benefits of a permanent pacemaker.

Class III
1. A hyperactive cardioinhibitory response to carotid sinus stimulation in the absence of symptoms.
2. Vague symptoms, such as dizziness, light-headedness, or both, with a hyperactive cardioinhibitory response to carotid sinus stimulation.
3. Recurrent syncope, light-headedness, or dizziness in the absence of a cardioinhibitory response.

* Class I: agreement that permanent pacemaker should be implanted. Class II: divergence of opinion regarding need for implantation. Class III: agreement that pacemaker is unnecessary.
SOURCE: LS Dreifus et al, with permission.

Table 230-3

The NASPE/BPEG Generic Pacemaker Code

Position Category	I Chamber(s) Paced	II Chamber(s) Sensed	III Response to Sensing	IV Programmability, Rate Modulation	V Antitachyarrhythmia Function(s)
	O, None	O, None	O, None	O, None	O, None
	A, Atrium	A, Atrium	T, Triggered	P, Simple programmable	P, pacing (antitachyarrhythmia)
	V, Ventricle	V, Ventricle	I, Inhibited	M, Multiprogrammable	S, Shock
	D, Dual (A + V)	D, Dual (A + V)	D, Dual (T + I)	C, Communicating	D, Dual (P + S)
				R, Rate modulation	
Manufacturer's designation	S, single (A or V)	S, (A or V)			

SOURCE: Zipes, DP: Cardiac pacemakers and antiarrhythmia devices, in *Heart Disease: A Textbook of Cardiovascular Medicine,* 5th ed, E Braunwald (ed). Philadelphia, Saunders, pp 705–741.

It follows from the described code that the standard VVIR (ventricular demand pacemaker) paces the ventricle, senses the ventricle, is inhibited by sensed spontaneous ventricular activity, and has rate modulation, while the DDDR pulse generator is capable of sensing and pacing both the atria and ventricles and has a dual response to the sensed atrial and ventricular activity as described above (Fig. 230-9). Both pacemakers have rate modulation (*R*). "Physiologic" pacemakers use sensors (muscular activity, respiratory rate, temperature, O_2 saturation, QT interval, etc.) as methods to allow the pacemaker to increase the heart rate in response to physiologic demands, i.e., exercise. These pacemakers are essential when chronotropic incompetence is present and an increase in heart rate is required to enhance physiologic performance. Studies have shown that such "physiologic" pacemakers improve exercise tolerance and relieve symptoms to a greater degree than fixed-rate pacemakers.

Selection of the appropriate pacemaker and pacing mode depends on the clinical condition and the type of bradyarrhythmia being treated. The two most common pacing mode selections are DDD and VVI. DDD provides AV sequential pacing, which is ideally suited for the relatively young and active patient who has intact sinus node function or intermittent dysfunction and high-grade persistent or intermittent AV block. The DDD mode will allow for physiologic atrial sensed and ventricular paced rates and improve exercise tolerance. AV synchrony and dual-chamber pacing also may be desirable in patients with borderline hemodynamic reserve who are dependent on atrial contribution to cardiac output and in those patients who develop the pacemaker syndrome (see below) in response to ventricular demand pacing.

Rate-responsive DDD (i.e., DDDR) pacing is indicated when chronotropic incompetence is present in a patient who requires AV synchrony. The DDD pacing mode is contraindicated in chronic atrial fibrillation or flutter, because rapid and irregular ventricular pacing will occur to the upper rate limit. In some cases this will produce a more rapid ventricular rate than the patient's own rate in the absence of a pacemaker. DDD pacemakers must either automatically switch or be reprogrammed to the VVI mode. Almost all such pacemakers are now combined with some form of rate responsiveness so that when the device functions in the VVI mode, it also will respond to physiologic demands (VVIR).

Chronotropic insufficiency (i.e., the inability of the sinus rate to accelerate) is a contraindication for a DDD pacemaker, since such a pacemaker will act as a "fixed-rate" pacemaker at the programmed lower rate. In these situations, a rate-adaptive or "physiologic" pacemaker is indicated (VVIR or DDDR). In patients with impaired sinus node function or chronic atrial fibrillation, a sensor-driven, rate-adaptive pacemaker must be implanted. As mentioned earlier, these pacemakers automatically adjust ventricular pacing rates to a sensed indicator of exertion. The DDD pacing mode also may be contraindicated in patients with intermittent or persistent ventriculoatrial conduction, who may develop pacemaker-mediated tachycardia (see below).

PROGRAMMABILITY OF PACEMAKERS This allows for modification of pacing function after implantation and for adaptation to changes in clinical needs. Pacemaker programming is accomplished by activation of the programming head positioned over the implanted pulse generator after making the desired changes in programmable parameters (see Table 230-3). A radio frequency system is routinely used to communicate the program to the pacemaker. A high degree of sophistication is required to recognize the presence and causes of pacemaker malfunction and their treatment.

COMPLICATIONS Adverse effects of permanent pacing are usually associated with failure or malfunction of the pacing system. These problems are usually secondary to over- or undersensing, output failure, and/or lead fracture or displacement. Two other problems may occur. The *pacemaker syndrome* consists of fatigue, dizziness, syncope, and distressing pulsations in the neck and chest and can be associated with adverse hemodynamic effects. The pathophysiologic contributors to the pacemaker syndrome include (1) loss of atrial contribution to ventricular systole; (2) vasodepressor reflex initiated by cannon *a* waves, which are caused by atrial contractions against a closed tricuspid valve and observed in the jugular venous pulse (Chap. 227); and (3) systemic and pulmonary venous regurgitation due to atrial contraction against a closed AV valve. The symptoms associated with the pacemaker syndrome can be prevented by maintaining AV synchrony by dual-chamber pacing or, in the case of a ventricular demand pacemaker, by programming an escape rate 15 to 20 beats per minute below that of the paced rate (i.e., hysteresis). As a result of this programming, sinus activity and thus atrial contraction will be less likely to occur at the same time as ventricular pacing and ventricular contraction. The second major problem peculiar to dual-chamber pacemakers is the development of *pacemaker-mediated tachycardia*. In this instance, retrograde depolarization of the atria, resulting from a premature ventricular depolarization or a paced ventricular complex, is sensed and leads to subsequent triggering of ventricular pacing. This, in turn, can result in repetition of the phenomenon of ventriculoatrial conduction with the development of an endless-loop, pacemaker-mediated tachycardia. It may be corrected by reprogramming the atrial refractory period.

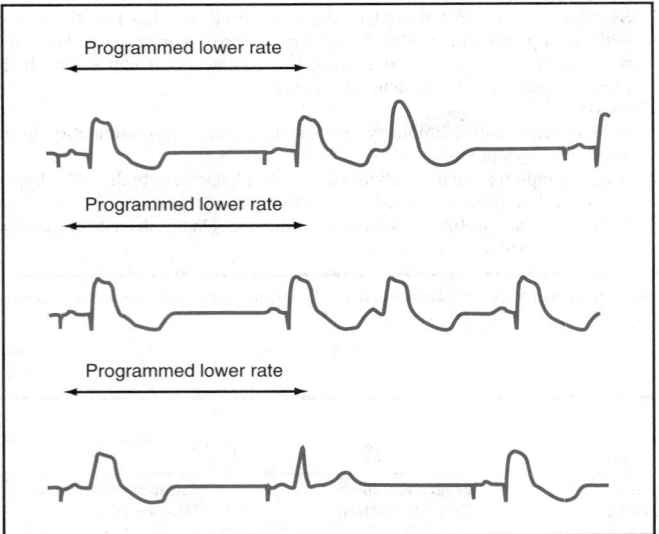

FIGURE 230-9 Normally functioning DDD pacemaker. All three panels show a lead II rhythm strip at 50 mm/s. The programmed lower rate is approximately 55 beats per minute. (*Top*) AV sequential pacing with a paced AV interval of 160 ms is shown for the first two complexes. A VPC occurs and is sensed, resetting the cycle. (*Middle*) The first beat is AV paced, but spontaneous sinus P waves and APC trigger a ventricular paced complex with a sensed P to QRS of 120 ms. (*Bottom*) After the first AV paced complex, a paced atrial complex conducts to the ventricle with a PR of 120 ms, inhibiting the ventricular pacemaker.

BIBLIOGRAPHY

BAROLD SS, ZIPES DP: Cardiac pacemakers and antiarrhythmia devices, in *Heart Disease: A Textbook of Cardiovascular Medicine,* 5th ed, E Braunwald (ed). Philadelphia, Saunders, 1997, p 705

——— et al: Electrocardiography of contemporary DDD pacemakers. Basic concepts: Upper rate response, retrograde ventriculoatrial conduction and differential diagnosis of pacemaker tachycardias, in *Electrical Therapy for Cardiac Arrhythmias: Pacing, Antitachycardia Devices, Catheter Ablation,* S Saksena, N Goldschlager (eds). Philadelphia, Saunders, 1990, p 225

BERNSTEIN AD et al: The NASPE/BPEG generic pacemaker code for antibradyarrhythmias and adaptive-rate pacing and antitachyarrhythmia devices. PACE 10:794, 1987

DREIFUS LS et al: Guidelines for implantation of cardiac pacemakers and antiarrhythmic devices: A report of the American College of Cardiology/ American Heart Association Task Force on Assessment of Diagnostic and Therapeutic Cardiovascular Procedures (Committee on Pacemaker Implantation). J Am Coll Cardiol 18:1, 1991

ELLENBOGEN KA et al: New insights into pacemaker syndrome gained from hemodynamic, humoral and vascular responses during ventriculo-atrial pacing. Am J Cardiol 65(1):53, 1990

HUANG SK et al: Carotid sinus hypersensitivity in patients with unexplained syncope: Clinical, electrophysiologic and long-term follow-up observations. Am Heart J 116:989, 1988

JOSEPHSON ME: Clinical Electrophysiology, 2d ed. Philadelphia, Lea and Febiger, 1993, chaps 4, 5, 6, 13

MENDES LA, DAVIDOFF R: Cardiogenic seizure with bradyarrhythmia: Documentation of the mechanism during asystole. Am Heart J 125:1786, 1993

MICHAËLSON M, JANZON A: Isolated congenital complete atrioventricular block in adult life. A prospective study. Circulation 92:442, 1995

REINOLD SL et al: Risk factors for the development of recurrent atrial fibrillation: Role of pacing and clinical variables. Am Heart J 129:1127, 1995

SRA JS et al: Comparison of cardiac pacing with drug therapy in the treatment of neurocardiogenic (vasovagal) syncope with bradycardia or asystole. N Engl J Med 328:1085, 1993

WALLER BF et al: Anatomy, histology and pathology of the cardiac conduction system: Part II. Clin Cardiol 16:347, 1993

231 | *Mark E. Josephson, Peter Zimetbaum, Alfred E. Buxton, Francis E. Marchlinski*

THE TACHYARRHYTHMIAS

MECHANISMS OF TACHYARRHYTHMIAS

Tachyarrhythmias may be divided into disorders of impulse propagation and disorders of impulse formation. Disorders of impulse propagation (reentry) are generally considered to be the most common mechanism of sustained paroxysmal tachyarrhythmia. The requirements for initiating reentry include (1) electrophysiologic inhomogeneity (i.e., differences in conduction and/or refractoriness) in two or more regions of the heart connected with each other to form a potentially closed loop; (2) unidirectional block in one pathway; (3) slow conduction over an alternative pathway, allowing time for the initially blocked pathway to recover excitability; and (4) reexcitation of the initially blocked pathway to complete a loop of activation (Fig. 231-1). Repetitive circulation of the impulse over this loop can produce a sustained tachyarrhythmia. While anatomic obstacles may underlie reentry and provide an inexcitable center around which the impulse can circulate, they are not essential. Reentrant arrhythmias can be reproducibly initiated and terminated by premature complexes and rapid stimulation. The response of these arrhythmias to stimulation can help distinguish them from arrhythmias caused by triggered activity.

Disorders of impulse formation can be subdivided into tachyarrhythmias caused by enhanced automaticity and those caused by triggered activity. In addition to the sinus node, automatic pacemaker activity can be observed in specialized atrial fibers, fibers of the atrioventricular (AV) junction, and Purkinje fibers (see Chap. 230). Myocardial cells do not normally possess pacemaker activity. Enhancement of normal automaticity in latent pacemaker fibers or the development of abnormal automaticity due to partial depolarization of the resting membrane occurs as a consequence of a variety of pathophysiologic states, which include (1) increased endogenous or exogenous catecholamines, (2) electrolyte disturbances (e.g., hyperkalemia), (3) hypoxia or ischemia, (4) mechanical effects (e.g., stretch), and (5) drugs (e.g., digitalis). Tachycardia caused by automaticity cannot be started or stopped by pacing.

Rhythms due to *triggered activity* are events that do not occur spontaneously but require a change in cardiac frequency as a trigger. Triggered activity may be caused by early afterdepolarizations, which occur during phases 2 and 3 of the action potential, or delayed afterdepolarizations, which occur following completion of phase 3 of the action potential (see Fig. 230-2). Triggered activity has been observed in atrial, ventricular, and His-Purkinje tissue under conditions such as increased local catecholamine concentration, hyperkalemia, hypercal-

cemia, and digitalis intoxication (delayed afterdepolarizations) or during bradycardia, hypokalemia, or other situations prolonging action potential duration (early afterdepolarizations). All of these conditions produce an accumulation of intracellular calcium. With increasing amplitude of the afterdepolarizations, threshold can be reached and repetitive activity produced. The exact role of triggered activity in spontaneous clinical arrhythmias is unknown, but tachyarrhythmias associated with digitalis intoxication, accelerated idioventricular rhythm in acute infarction and/or reperfusion, and exercise-induced ventricular tachycardia (VT) are believed to be caused by triggered activity due to delayed afterdepolarizations. Torsades de pointes (polymorphic VT associated with long QT intervals) may be caused by triggered activity due to early afterdepolarizations.

The use of electrophysiologic studies, i.e., intracardiac recordings and programmed stimulation, has greatly expanded the understanding of the mechanisms of tachyarrhythmias. In addition to helping diagnose arrhythmias, these techniques may be of value in determining the most appropriate types of therapy because they allow the physician to observe the hemodynamic and symptomatic consequences of the arrhythmia in the presence or absence of therapy. Electrophysiologic studies of tachycardias require the positioning of multiple electrode catheters at critical areas within the heart. These electrodes must be capable of both stimulating and recording from multiple sites in the atria and/or ventricles.

PREMATURE COMPLEXES

ATRIAL PREMATURE COMPLEXES (APCs) APCs can be found on 24-h Holter monitoring in over 60 percent of normal adults. APCs are usually asymptomatic and benign, although at times they may be associated with palpitations. In susceptible patients, they can initiate paroxysmal supraventricular tachycardias. APCs may originate from any location in either atrium, and they are recognized on the electrocardiogram (ECG) as early P waves with a morphology that differs from the sinus P wave (Fig. 231-2A). While APCs usually conduct to the ventricles when they occur late in the cardiac cycle, early APCs may reach the AV conduction system while it is still in its relative refractory period, resulting in a conduction delay manifested by prolonged PR interval following the premature P wave (Fig. 231-2A). Very early APCs may even block in the AV node if this structure is encountered during its effective refractory period. APCs, whether conducted or not, are usually followed by a pause before a return to sinus activity. Most commonly, an APC enters and resets the sinus node, so the sum of the pre- and postextrasystolic PP intervals

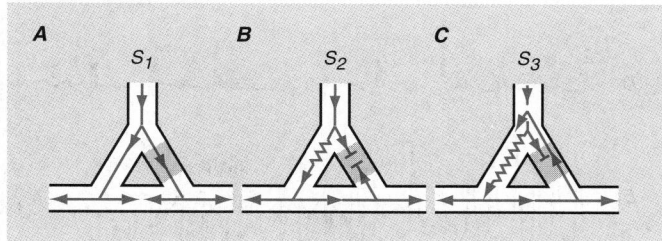

FIGURE 231-1 Schema of reentry. Y branching of the Purkinje system to ventricular muscle is shown in panels *A* through *C*. The right limb (*grey area*) of the Purkinje system has a longer refractory period than the left. *A*. During a slow stimulated rate (S₁), conduction proceeds normally over both Purkinje fibers, resulting in collision in the ventricular muscle. *B*. An early premature stimulus (S₂) results in block in the Purkinje fiber on the right and slow conduction down the left. The impulse conducts through the ventricle and attempts to reenter the initial site of block but fails because this site has not fully recovered excitability. *C*. An earlier stimulus (S₃) again results in block on the left. The resulting slower propagation down the left fiber provides enough time for the initial site of block to recur and allows the impulse to conduct through it to produce a reentrant circuit.

is less than the sum of two sinus PP intervals (Fig. 231-2A). In this case, the pause is said to be less than fully compensatory. The QRS complex following most APCs is normal, although early APCs may be followed by aberrantly conducted QRS complexes due to the premature complex falling within the relative refractory period of the His-Purkinje system.

Since most APCs are asymptomatic, treatment is not required. When they cause palpitations or trigger paroxysmal supraventricular tachycardias (see below), treatment may be useful. Factors that precipitate APCs, such as alcohol, tobacco, or adrenergic stimulants, should be identified and eliminated, and in their absence, mild sedation or the use of a beta blocker may be tried.

AV JUNCTIONAL COMPLEXES The site of origin of these complexes is thought to be in the bundle of His, since the normal AV node in vivo possesses no automaticity. AV junctional complexes are less common than either atrial or ventricular premature complexes and are more often associated with cardiac disease or digitalis intoxication. Junctional premature impulses can conduct both antegradely to the ventricles and retrogradely to the atrium and, on rare occasions, may fail to conduct in either direction. Premature AV junctional complexes can be recognized by normal-appearing QRS complexes that are not preceded by a P wave. Retrograde P waves (inverted in leads II, III, and aVF) may be observed after the QRS complex.

While often asymptomatic, junctional premature complexes may be associated with palpitations and cause cannon *a* waves, which may result in distressing pulsations in the neck. When symptomatic, they should be treated like APCs.

VENTRICULAR PREMATURE COMPLEXES (VPCs) These are among the most common arrhythmias and occur in patients with and without heart disease. Of adult males, ≥60 percent will

exhibit VPCs during a 24-h Holter monitoring. In patients without heart disease, VPCs have not been shown to be associated with any increased incidence in mortality or morbidity. VPCs may occur in up to 80 percent of patients with previous myocardial infarction, and in this setting, if frequent (>10 per hour) and/or complex (occurring in couplets), they have been associated with increased mortality. However, cardiac mortality in such patients usually occurs in association with significantly impaired ventricular function. While frequent and complex ventricular ectopy is an independent risk factor, it is not as strong a risk factor as is impaired ventricular function. Moreover, even though ventricular tachycardia and/or fibrillation may be the basis for the sudden death in these patients, this does not a priori establish a cause-and-effect relation between spontaneous ectopy and life-threatening ventricular tachycardia or fibrillation. Very early cycle (R-on-T) VPCs have been stated by some to increase the risk of sudden death. Although this has been observed during acute ischemia and in the setting of QT prolongation, frequently, VT or fibrillation is precipitated by VPCs that occur after the T wave of the prior beat.

VPCs are recognized by wide (usually >0.14 s), bizarre QRS complexes that are not preceded by P waves (Fig. 231-3A). They may bear a relatively fixed relationship to the preceding sinus complex (i.e., fixed coupled VPCs). When fixed coupling is not present and the interval between VPCs has a common denominator, *ventricular parasystole* is said to be present (Fig. 231-4). Under these circumstances, the VPCs are a manifestation of abnormal automaticity of a protected ventricular focus. Because this focus is not penetrated by sinus impulses, it is not reset by them, and the interectopic intervals remain relatively fixed (≤120 ms variation of mean RR cycle length).

VPCs may occur singly; in patterns of bigeminy, in which every sinus beat is followed by a VPC; in trigeminy, in which two sinus beats are followed by a VPC; in quadrigeminy, etc. Two successive VPCs are termed *pairs* or *couplets*, while three or more consecutive VPCs are termed *ventricular tachycardia* when the rate exceeds 100 beats per minute. VPCs may have similar morphologies (monomorphic, or uniform) or different morphologies (polymorphic, or multiformed) (Fig. 231-3C).

Most commonly, VPCs are not conducted retrogradely to the atrium to reset the sinoatrial node. Thus they produce a fully compensatory pause; i.e., the interval between conducted sinus beats that bracket the VPC equals two basic RR intervals. Ventricular impulses also may manifest retrograde conduction to the atrium and cause inverted P waves in leads II, III, and aVF. This retrograde atrial activation can reset the sinus node, and the pause that results may therefore be less than compensatory. In many instances, the VPC will not be associated with retrograde ventriculoatrial (VA) conduction but may block retrogradely in the AV node. This renders the AV node refractory to the subsequent sinus beat and causes slowed conduction (i.e., prolonged PR interval) or block of the next sinus P wave. This prolonged PR interval is said to be a manifestation of concealed retrograde conduction of the ventricular impulse into the AV node. A VPC that does not produce any manifestation of retrograde concealed conduction and fails to influence the oncoming sinus impulse is termed an *interpolated VPC*.

VPCs can cause palpitations or neck pulsations secondary to either the occurrence of cannon *a* waves or the increased force of contraction due to postextrasystolic potentiation of ventricular contractility. Patients with frequent VPCs or bigeminy may rarely develop syncope or lightheadedness because the VPCs do not result in an adequate stroke volume and the cardiac output is reduced by the "halving" of the heart rate.

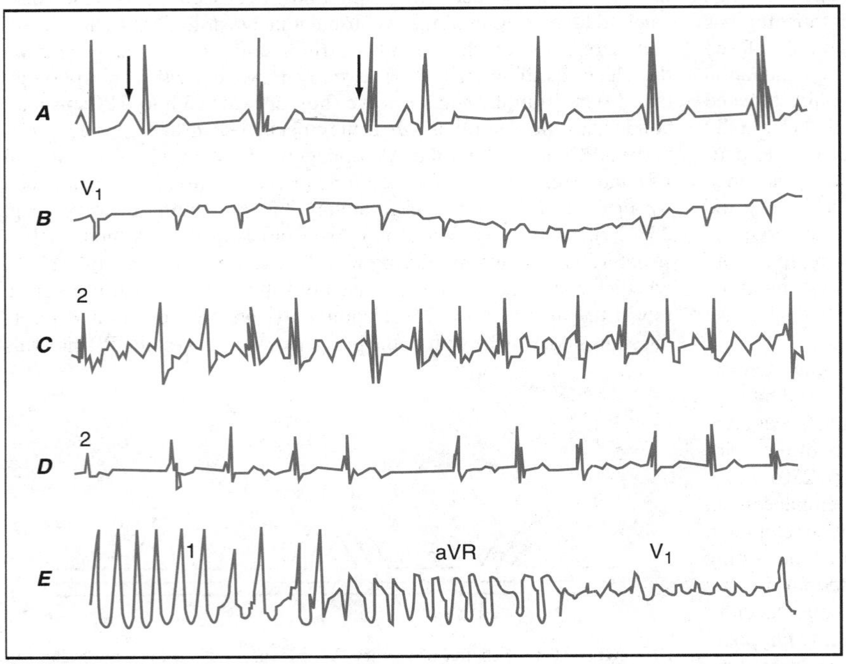

FIGURE 231-2 *A.* ECG lead II. Sinus rhythm with two atrial premature complexes (*arrows*). Note the difference in P-wave configuration between sinus and the premature atrial complexes. In addition, note that the PR interval of the premature complexes is prolonged, due to slowed conduction of the premature impulse through the AV conduction system. *B.* ECG lead V₁. Atrial tachycardia with varying degrees of AV block, typical of digitalis toxicity. *C.* ECG lead II. Atrial flutter. Note the characteristic sawtooth baseline seen in the inferior ECG leads during atrial flutter. Variable degrees of AV conduction block are present. *D.* ECG lead II. Atrial fibrillation. Note the irregular wavy baseline without discrete atrial activity. The ventricular response is irregularly irregular. *E.* ECG leads I, aVR, and V₁. Atrial fibrillation in a patient with Wolff-Parkinson-White syndrome. Note the extremely rapid, grossly irregular ventricular rate with wide, bizarre QRS complexes.

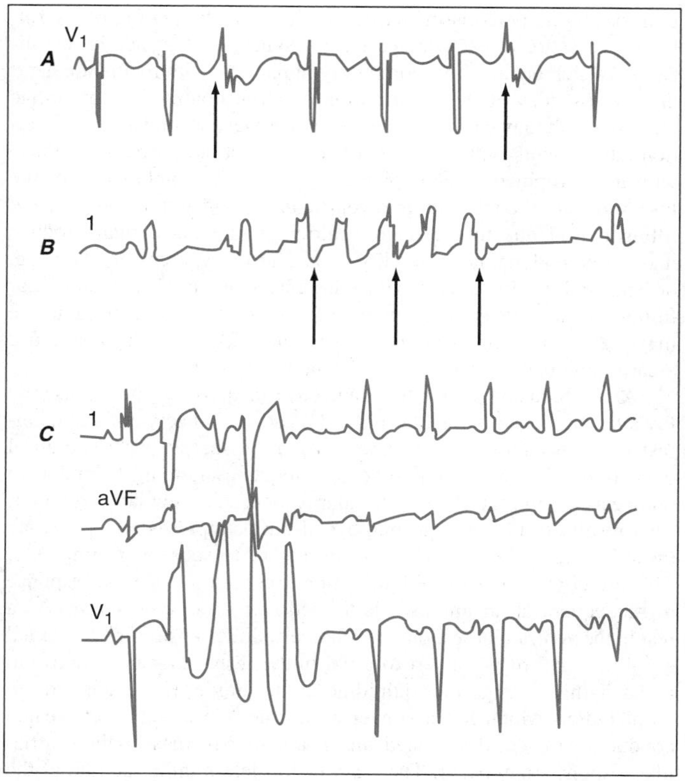

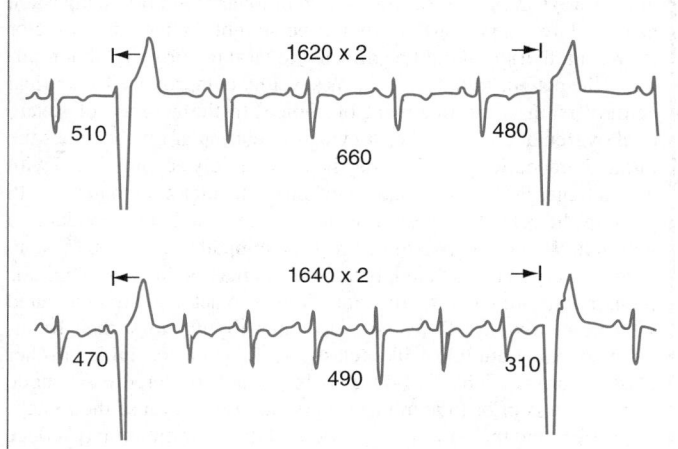

FIGURE 231-3 *A.* Single ventricular ectopy. During sinus rhythm, two premature ventricular complexes (*arrows*) occur. Note that the QRS configuration is bizarre, different from that during sinus rhythm. The premature ventricular complexes are not preceded by P waves. The QRS width of the premature complexes is approximately 160 ms. The pause surrounding the premature complexes is fully compensatory, the sinus beat after the premature complex occurring on time. *B.* A 5-beat run of nonsustained ventricular tachycardia having a uniform morphology. Although intraventricular conduction during sinus rhythm is slightly prolonged, during the run of ventricular tachycardia the QRS duration is further prolonged. Note that 2:1 VA conduction is present during ventricular tachycardia. Retrograde P waves are denoted by the arrows. *C.* Simultaneous recordings of ECG leads I, aVF, and V₁. A 4-beat run of polymorphic nonsustained ventricular tachycardia is demonstrated. No two consecutive QRS complexes are the same. Polymorphic VT is not associated with a prolonged QT interval in this case.

FIGURE 231-4 Ventricular parasystole. At varying sinus cycle lengths during exercise, interectopic intervals remain constant at 1620 to 1640 ms. However, the coupling intervals between sinus and ectopic complexes vary between 510 and 310 ms.

TREATMENT

In the absence of cardiac disease, isolated asymptomatic VPCs, regardless of configuration and frequency, need no treatment. When arrhythmias are symptomatic, the symptoms should first be addressed by either allaying the patient's anxiety or, if this is not successful, reducing the frequency of the VPCs with antiarrhythmic agents. Beta-adrenergic blockers may be successful in managing VPCs that occur primarily in the daytime or under stressful situations and in specific settings such as mitral valve prolapse and thyrotoxicosis. Class I antiarrhythmic agents may be tried should this be unsuccessful. In patients with cardiac disease, frequent VPCs are associated with an increased risk of sudden and nonsudden cardiac death, and many physicians have attempted to eliminate or reduce the frequency of these VPCs in an attempt to reduce this risk. However, the cause-and-effect relationship of the VPCs to fatal events has never been established. The ability of pharmacologic antiarrhythmic therapy guided by continuous ECG monitoring to reduce the risk of sudden death in patients with frequent (≥6 per minute) VPCs was tested by the Cardiac Arrhythmia Suppression Trial (CAST). This study compared mortality in patients whose ectopy was suppressed by one of three agents (encainide, flecainide, or moricizine) and then randomized to treat with either the "effective" drug or placebo. After a mean follow-up of 2 years, the study was discontinued because both the sudden death and overall mortality rate were significantly increased in patients receiving antiarrhythmic agents. This study has shown that in patients having the characteristics of the study population, abolition of ventricular ectopy by pharmacologic therapy cannot be used as a marker to define reduction of the risk of sudden death after myocardial infarction and, in fact, may increase mortality. Ongoing studies are examining the ability of more advanced techniques, such as electrophysiologic testing, to reduce the rate of sudden death in higher-risk patients, i.e., those with left ventricular ejection fractions of ≤40 and nonsustained VT (≥3 consecutive VPCs).

Antiarrhythmic agents also can produce the lethal arrhythmias that they are given to prevent (proarrhythmic effects). Thus therapy directed toward VPCs in the setting of chronic cardiac disease may result in an inappropriate and costly use of agents without proven efficacy and with potential side effects in many patients. The high incidence of side effects and the frequent exacerbation of arrhythmias caused by all antiarrhythmic drugs make it mandatory to monitor patients being treated with such agents.

In acute myocardial infarction, the greatest incidence of primary ventricular fibrillation occurs within the first 24 h (Chap. 243). Temporary prophylactic antiarrhythmic therapy with lidocaine or procainamide was formerly recommended for all patients with acute infarction, regardless of the presence or degree of spontaneous ectopy. However, failure to improve overall survival and drug toxicity have led most physicians to recommend prophylactic antiarrhythmic therapy only to young patients with complicated infarctions, where a favorable risk-benefit ratio may be obtained. Other studies have shown that intravenous beta blockers also may reduce the incidence of primary ventricular fibrillation.

TACHYCARDIAS

Tachycardias refer to arrhythmias with three or more complexes at rates exceeding 100 beats per minute; they occur more often in structurally diseased than in normal hearts. Those paroxysmal tachycardias that are initiated by APCs or VPCs are considered to be due to reentry, except some of the digitalis-induced tachyarrhythmias, which are probably due to triggered activity (see below).

If the patient is hemodynamically stable, an attempt should be made to determine the mechanism and origin of the tachycardia, since this will usually lead to an appropriate therapeutic decision. Information to be obtained from the ECG includes (1) the presence, frequency, morphology, and regularity of P waves and QRS complexes; (2) the relationship between atrial and ventricular activity; (3) a comparison of the QRS morphology during sinus rhythm and during the tachycardia; and (4) the response to carotid sinus massage or other vagal maneuvers. It is useful first to compare a 12-lead ECG during the tachycardia with one recorded during sinus rhythm. One also can utilize the electrodes situated at the end of a flexible pacing catheter inserted into the esophagus behind the left atrium to record atrial activity.

Observation of the jugular venous pulse can provide clues to the presence of atrial activity and its relationship to ventricular ectopy. Intermittent cannon *a* waves suggest AV dissociation, while persistent cannon *a* waves suggest 1:1 VA conduction. Flutter waves may be seen or no atrial activity may be apparent, as in the presence of atrial flutter and fibrillation, respectively. The arterial pulse also may manifest AV dissociation or atrial fibrillation by demonstrating variations in amplitude. A first heart sound of variable intensity during a regular rhythm also suggests AV dissociation or atrial fibrillation.

Carotid sinus pressure should only be applied while the patient is electrocardiographically monitored with resuscitative equipment available to manage the rare episode of asystole and/or ventricular fibrillation associated with this procedure. Carotid sinus massage should not be performed in patients with carotid arterial bruits. The patient should be positioned flat with the neck extended. Massage of one carotid bulb at a time should be performed by applying firm pressure just underneath the angle of the jaw for up to 5 s. Alternative vagomimetic maneuvers include the Valsalva maneuver, immersion of the face in cold water, and administration of 5 to 10 mg edrophonium.

SINUS TACHYCARDIA In the adult, sinus tachycardia is said to be present when the heart rate exceeds 100 beats per minute: sinus tachycardia rarely exceeds 200 beats per minute and is not a primary arrhythmia; instead, it represents a physiologic response to a variety of stresses, such as fever, volume depletion, anxiety, exercise, thyrotoxicosis, hypoxemia, hypotension, or congestive heart failure. Sinus tachycardia has a gradual onset and offset. The ECG demonstrates P waves with sinus contour preceding each QRS complex. Carotid sinus pressure usually produces modest slowing with a gradual return to the previous rate upon cessation. This contrasts with the response of paroxysmal supraventricular tachycardias, which may slow slightly and terminate abruptly.

℞ TREATMENT

Sinus tachycardia should not be treated as a primary arrhythmia, since it is almost always a physiologic response to a demand placed on the heart. As such, the therapy should be directed to the primary disorder. This may involve institution of digitalis and/or diuretics for heart failure and oxygen for hypoxemia, treatment of thyrotoxicosis, volume repletion, aspirin for fever, or tranquilizers for emotional upset.

ATRIAL FIBRILLATION (AF) This common arrhythmia may occur in paroxysmal and persistent forms. It may be seen in normal subjects, particularly during emotional stress or following surgery, exercise, or acute alcoholic intoxication. It also may occur in patients with heart or lung disease who develop acute hypoxia, hypercapnia, or metabolic or hemodynamic derangements. Persistent AF usually occurs in patients with cardiovascular disease, most commonly rheumatic heart disease, nonrheumatic mitral valve disease, hypertensive cardiovascular disease, chronic lung disease, atrial septal defect, and a variety of miscellaneous cardiac abnormalities. AF may be the presenting finding in thyrotoxicosis. So-called lone AF, which occurs in patients without underlying heart disease, is considered to represent the tachycardia phase of the tachycardia-bradycardia syndrome (p. 1255).

The morbidity associated with AF is related to (1) excessive ventricular rate, which in turn may lead to hypotension, pulmonary conges-

tion, or angina pectoris in susceptible individuals; (2) the pause following cessation of AF, which can cause syncope; (3) systemic embolization, which occurs most commonly in patients with rheumatic heart disease; (4) loss of the contribution of atrial contraction to cardiac output, which may cause fatigue; and (5) anxiety secondary to palpitations. In patients with severe cardiac dysfunction, particularly those with hypertrophied, noncompliant ventricles, the combination of the loss of the atrial contribution to ventricular filling and the abbreviated filling period due to the rapid ventricular rate in AF can produce marked hemodynamic instability, resulting in hypotension, syncope, or heart failure. In patients with mitral stenosis, in whom ventricular filling time is critical, development of AF with a rapid ventricular rate may precipitate pulmonary edema (see Chap. 237). AF may also cause a cardiomyopathy related to persistent rapid rates.

AF is characterized by disorganized atrial activity without discrete P waves on the surface ECG (Fig. 231-2*D*). Atrial activation is manifested by an undulating baseline or by more sharply inscribed atrial deflections of varying amplitude and frequency ranging from 350 to 600 beats per minute. The ventricular response is irregularly irregular. This results from the large number of atrial impulses that penetrate the AV node, making it partially refractory to subsequent impulses. This effect of nonconducted atrial impulses to influence the response to subsequent atrial impulses is termed *concealed conduction*. As a result, the ventricular response is relatively slow, considering the actual atrial rate. AF may convert to atrial flutter, especially in response to antiarrhythmic drugs like quinidine or flecainide. If AF converts to atrial flutter, which has a slower atrial rate, the effect of concealed conduction may be diminished, and a paradoxic increase in the ventricular response may occur. The main factor determining the rate of the ventricular response is the functional refractory period of the AV node or the most rapid paced rate at which 1:1 conduction through the AV node can be observed.

If, in the presence of AF, the ventricular rhythm becomes regular and slow (e.g., 30 to 60 beats per minute), complete heart block is suggested, and if the ventricular rhythm is regular and rapid (e.g., ≥100 beats per minute), a tachycardia arising in the AV junction or ventricle should be suspected. Digitalis intoxication is a common cause of both phenomena.

Patients with AF exhibit a loss of *a* waves in the jugular venous pulse and variable pulse pressures in the carotid arterial pulse. The first heart sound usually varies in intensity. On echocardiography, the left atrium is frequently enlarged, and in patients in whom the left atrial diameter exceeds 4.5 cm, it may not be possible to convert AF to sinus rhythm or to maintain the latter, despite therapy.

℞ TREATMENT

In acute AF, a precipitating factor such as fever, pneumonia, alcoholic intoxication, thyrotoxicosis, pulmonary emboli, congestive heart failure, or pericarditis should be sought. When such a factor is present, therapy should be directed toward the primary abnormality. If the patient's clinical status is severely compromised, electrical cardioversion is the treatment of choice. In the absence of severe cardiovascular compromise, slowing of ventricular rate becomes the initial therapeutic goal. This may be most rapidly accomplished with beta-adrenergic blockers and/or calcium channel antagonists. Both prolong the refractory period of the AV node and slow conduction within it. When catecholamine levels or sympathetic nervous system tone is likely to be elevated, beta blockers may be favored. Digitalis preparations are less effective, take longer to act, and are associated with more toxicity. Conversion to sinus rhythm may then be attempted, using quinidine-like (class IA) drugs or flecainide or other class IC drugs (Table 231-1). It is important to increase AV node refractoriness prior to administering such drugs because their vagolytic effect and their ability to convert AF to atrial flutter may reduce the concealed conduction and lead to an excessively rapid ventricular response. Beta-adrenergic blockers are especially useful in this regard. If medical therapy fails to convert AF in 24 h, electrical cardioversion is useful; it generally requires 100 to 200 W·s of energy. In situations where AF has been present for 48 to 72 h or

Table 231-1

Classification of Antiarrhythmic Drugs

Class I Drugs that reduce maximal velocity of phase of depolarization (V_{max}) due to block of inward Na^+ current in tissue with fast response action potentials
   A $\downarrow V_{max}$ at all heart rates and $\uparrow$ action potential duration, e.g., quinidine, procainamide, disopyramide
   B Little effect at slow rates on V_{max} in normal tissue; $\downarrow V_{max}$ in partially depolarized cells with fast response action potentials
     Effects increased at faster rates
     No change or $\downarrow$ in action potential duration, e.g., lidocaine, phenytoin, tocainide, mexiletine
   C $\downarrow V_{max}$ at normal rates in normal tissue
     Minimal effect on action potential duration, e.g., flecainide, propafenone, moricizine
Class II Antisympathetic agents, e.g., propranolol and other beta-adrenergic blockers: $\downarrow$ SA nodal automaticity, $\uparrow$ AV nodal refractoriness, and $\downarrow$ AV nodal conduction velocity
Class III Agents that prolong action potential duration in tissue with fast-response action potentials, e.g., bretylium, amiodarone, sotalol
Class IV Calcium (slow) channel blocking agents: $\downarrow$ conduction velocity and $\uparrow$ refractoriness in tissue with slow-response action potentials, e.g., verapamil, diltiazem

Drugs that cannot be classified by this schema:
   Digitalis
   Adenosine

more, anticoagulation should be started at least 2 weeks prior to and continued for 2 weeks following any attempt at cardioversion, either pharmacologic or electrical. Anticoagulation appears to decrease the incidence of systemic embolization associated with cardioversion. Some advocate the use of transesophageal echocardiography. In the absence of clot, cardioversion can be undertaken and anticoagulation started immediately. It is less likely for chronic AF to convert to or remain in sinus rhythm in the presence of long-standing rheumatic heart disease and/or when the atria are markedly enlarged. It is also unlikely for patients with lone AF to be converted to and maintained in sinus rhythm.

The goal of therapy in patients in whom AF cannot be converted to sinus rhythm is control of the ventricular response. This can usually be accomplished by digitalis, beta blockers, or calcium channel blockers singly or in combination. In occasional patients, the ventricular response cannot be controlled by pharmacologic therapy alone. In such patients, the creation of complete heart block by radiofrequency catheter ablation of the AV junction followed by permanent pacemaker implantation is appropriate. Surgical or direct-current catheter ablation of the AV junction is rarely required to achieve AV block.

If sinus rhythm is restored electrically or pharmacologically, quinidine or related agents as well as the class IC agents (e.g., flecainide) or amiodarone may be used to prevent recurrence. In patients in whom cardioversion is unsuccessful or in whom AF is likely to recur, it is probably wisest to allow the patient to remain in AF and to control the ventricular response with calcium antagonists, beta-adrenergic blockers, or digitalis glycosides. Since such patients are always at risk of systemic embolization, particularly in the presence of organic heart disease, chronic anticoagulation must be considered. Several studies have now demonstrated conclusively that the incidence of embolization in patients with AF not associated with valvular heart disease is reduced by chronic anticoagulation with warfarin-like agents. Aspirin also may be effective for this purpose, but the data supporting its use are less extensive.

ATRIAL FLUTTER This arrhythmia occurs most often in patients with organic heart disease. Flutter may be paroxysmal, in which case there is usually a precipitating factor, such as pericarditis or acute respiratory failure, or it may be persistent. Atrial flutter (as well as AF) is very common during the first week following open-heart surgery. Atrial flutter is usually less long-lived than is AF, although on occasion it may persist for months to years. Most commonly, if it

lasts for more than a week, atrial flutter will convert to AF. Systemic embolization is less common in atrial flutter than in AF.

Atrial flutter is characterized by an atrial rate between 250 and 350 beats per minute. Typically, the ventricular rate is half the atrial rate, i.e., approximately 150 beats per minute. If the atrial rate is slowed to <220 beats per minute by antiarrhythmic agents such as quinidine, which also possess vagolytic properties, the ventricular rate may rise suddenly because of the development of 1:1 AV conduction. Classically, flutter waves are seen as regular sawtooth-like atrial activity, most prominent in the inferior leads (Fig. 231-2C). When the ventricular response is regular and not a simple fraction of the atrial rate, complete AV block is present, which may be a manifestation of digitalis toxicity. Activation mapping suggests that atrial flutter is a form of atrial reentry localized to the right atrium.

℞ **TREATMENT**

The most effective treatment of atrial flutter is direct-current cardioversion, which can be accomplished at low energy (25 to 50 W·s) under mild sedation. Higher energies (100 to 200 W·s) are often used because they are less likely to cause *atrial fibrillation,* which not infrequently occurs following lower energy delivery. In patients who develop atrial flutter following open-heart surgery or recurrent flutter in the setting of acute myocardial infarction, particularly if they are being treated with digitalis, atrial pacing (using temporary pacing wires implanted at the time of operation or a pacing lead inserted into the atrium pervenously) at rates of 115 to 130 percent of the atrial flutter rate can usually convert the atrial flutter to sinus rhythm. Atrial pacing also may result in the conversion of atrial flutter to AF, which allows for easier control of the ventricular response. If immediate conversion of atrial flutter is not mandated by the patient's clinical status, the ventricular response should first be slowed by blocking the AV node with a beta blocker, calcium antagonist, or digitalis. Digitalis is the least effective and occasionally converts atrial flutter into AF. Once AV nodal conduction is slowed with any of these drugs, an attempt to convert flutter to sinus rhythm using a class I (A or C) agent or amiodarone should be made. Increasing doses of the drug selected are administered until the rhythm converts or side effects occur.

Quinidine, quinidine-like drugs, flecainide, propafenone, and amiodarone (Table 231-2) may be useful in preventing recurrences of both atrial flutter and atrial fibrillation.

PAROXYSMAL SUPRAVENTRICULAR TACHYCARDIAS (PSVT) In most cases, functional differences in conduction and refractoriness in the AV node or the presence of an AV bypass tract provide the substrate for the development of PSVT (previously termed *paroxysmal atrial tachycardia*). Electrophysiologic studies have demonstrated that reentry is responsible for the vast majority of cases of PSVT (Fig. 231-5). Reentry has been localized to the sinus node, atrium, AV node, or a macroreentrant circuit involving conduction in the antegrade direction through the AV node and retrograde through an AV bypass tract. Such a bypass tract also may conduct antegradely, in which case the Wolff-Parkinson-White (WPW) syndrome is said to be present. When the bypass tract manifests only retrograde conduction, it is termed a *concealed bypass tract* (Fig. 231-5B). In these cases, the QRS complex during sinus rhythm is normal. In the absence of the WPW syndrome, reentry through the AV node or through a concealed bypass tract makes up more than 90 percent of all PSVTs.

AV NODAL REENTRANT TACHYCARDIA There is no age or disease predisposition for the development of AV nodal reentrant tachycardia, the most common cause of supraventricular tachycardia. It is, however, more commonly observed in women. It usually presents as a regular narrow QRS complex tachycardia at rates of 120 to 250 beats per minute. APCs that initiate the arrhythmia are almost always associated with a prolonged PR interval. Retrograde P waves may be

Table 231-2   Drugs Used to Treat Cardiac Tachyarrhythmias

Drug	Sinus Node	Atrium and Ventricle	AV Node	His-Purkinje System	AV Bypass Tracts
ELECTROPHYSIOLOGIC EFFECTS					
Digoxin and other cardiac glycosides	NC; pts with sinus node disease may develop sinus exit block or arrest	Controversial	↑ ERP, ↓ conduction velocity, due to drug action and vagomimetic effects	NC	NC or ↓ ERP
Adenosine	↓ automaticity	Atrium: ↓ ERP Ventricle: no effect	↓ conduction velocity		
Quinidine (class IA)	NC; may suppress sinus node if node disease exists	↑ ERP; ↓ conduction velocity	↓ or NC in ERP; NC in conduction velocity	↓ automaticity; ↓ conduction velocity; ↑ ERP	↑ ERP may abolish all conduction
Procainamide (class IA)	NC	↑ ERP; ↓ conduction velocity	↓ or NC in ERP; ↓ or NC in conduction velocity	↓ automaticity; ↓ conduction velocity; ↑ ERP	↑ ERP may abolish conduction
Disopyramide (class IA)	NC	↑ ERP; ↓ conduction velocity	↓ or NC in ERP; NC in conduction velocity	↓ automaticity; ↑ ERP; ↓ conduction velocity	↑ ERP may abolish conduction
Lidocaine (class IB)	NC	NC in ERP	NC or ↓ in ERP	NC or ↓ ERP	NC, ↓, or ↑ in ERP
Phenytoin (class IB)	NC	NC in ERP	NC or ↓ in ERP; NC or ↑ in conduction velocity	↓ in ERP; ↓ automaticity	
Tocainide (class IB)	NC	NC	NC	NC; ↓ automaticity	↑ ERP
Mexiletine (class IB)	NC; pts with sinus node disease may develop sinus arrest	NC	Variable and inconsistent effects on conduction and refractoriness	↑ ERP; NC or ↓ conduction velocity	
Flecainide (class IC)	NC; pts with sinus node disease may develop exit block or arrest	↓ conduction velocity; ↑ ERP	↓ conduction velocity; ↑ ERP	↓ conduction velocity	↓ conduction velocity; ↑ ERP; may abolish all conduction
Propafenone (class IC) (also beta blocker)	No significant effect	↓ conduction velocity; ↑ ERP	↓ in conduction velocity; ↑ ERP	↓ conduction velocity; ↑ ERP	↑ ERP
Moricizine (class IC)	No significant effect	Atrium: NC in ERP; ↓ conduction velocity Ventricle: slight increase in ERP; ↓ conduction velocity	↓ conduction velocity	↓ conduction velocity	
Propranolol, atenolol, metoprolol (class II)	↓ sinus rate; ↑ sinus node recovery time	NC	↑ ERP; ↓ conduction velocity	NC	NC
Bretylium (class III)	Initial increase in sinus rate, followed by decrease	↑ ERP	NC	NC	
Amiodarone (class III)	↓ sinus rate	↑ ERP	↑ ERP; ↓ conduction velocity	↑ ERP; ↓ conduction velocity	↑ ERP
Sotalol (class III) (also beta blocker)	↓ sinus rate	↑ ERP	↑ ERP; ↓ conduction velocity	↑ ERP	↑ ERP
Verapamil, diltiazem (class IV)	↓ sinus rate	NC	↑ ERP; ↓ conduction velocity	NC	NC

NOTE: NC, no change; ↑, increase; ↓, decrease; ERP, effective refractory period; AF, atrial fibrillation; VT, ventricular tachycardia; AV, atrioventricular; VF, ventricular fibrillation; SVT, supraventricular tachycardia; VPCs, ventricular premature complexes; CHF, congestive heart failure.

Table 231-2

Indications	Side Effects and Toxicity
CLINICAL EFFECTS	
Slowing of ventricular rate during AF, flutter, and other atrial tachycardias in the absence of preexcitation; slowing, termination and/or prevention of SVT due to AV nodal reentry and AV reentry utilizing bypass tracts; may terminate or prevent intraatrial reentrant tachycardias; ineffective in prevention of automatic atrial tachycardias	Atrial tachycardia, VT, AV nodal block, accelerated junctional rhythms, atrial and ventricular premature depolarizations, VT, VF, anorexia, nausea, vomiting, acceleration of ventricular rate during AF flutter in the presence of preexcitation causing VF
Acute termination of regular reentrant SVT involving the AV node	Transient atrial standstill following termination of SVT; transient hypotension
Atrial and ventricular extrasystoles; atrial and ventricular tachyarrhythmias; all types of SVT; control of ventricular rate in pts with preexcitation and AF and flutter	Anorexia, nausea, vomiting, diarrhea, cinchonism, tinnitus, confusion, hearing and visual changes; thrombocytopenia, hemolytic anemia, rash, drug interactions, elevation of digoxin levels; phenytoin and phenobarbital will decrease quinidine levels; QT prolongation associated with polymorphic VT (torsades de pointes); conversion of nonsustained to sustained acceleration of ventricular response to atrial flutter and fibrillation
Same as quinidine	Anorexia, nausea, confusion, hallucinations, agranulocytosis, and lupus erythematosus–like syndrome; QT prolongation associated with polymorphic VT (torsades de pointes); marked elevations in the primary metabolic rate (NAPA); may be more likely to cause polymorphic VT; conversion of nonsustained to sustained VT; acceleration of ventricular response to atrial flutter and fibrillation
Same as quinidine	Anticholinergic actions, including dry mouth, blurred vision, urinary retention, hesitancy, constipation, narrow-angle glaucoma, congestive heart failure, especially in patients with abnormal ventricular function and QT prolongation associated with polymorphic VT (torsades de pointes)
Same as quinidine	Dizziness, parasthesias, confusion, delirium, seizures, coma; may depress sinus node in pts with underlying sinus node disease; may suppress escape foci in pts with complete heart block; congestive heart failure or liver disease increases risk of side effects
VT and VF, especially during acute ischemia and myocardial infarction	Gingival hypertrophy, rash, blood dyscrasias, nystagmus, ataxia, stupor, coma, lupus erythematosus syndrome, lymph node hyperplasia, peripheral neuropathy, hypocalcemia, hyperglycemia, phlebitis, and hypotension during IV administration
Tachyarrhythmias induced by digitalis; occasionally effective for ventricular tachyarrhythmias not induced by digitalis, alone or in combination with other antiarrhythmic agents; polymorphic VT associated with increased QT	Ataxia, tremor, paresthesias, light-headedness, nausea, rash, lupus erythematosus syndrome, pulmonary fibrosis, bone marrow suppression; may exacerbate heart failure in pts with ventricular dysfunction
VT, VF, frequent VPCs	Nausea, vomiting, ataxia, tremor, gait disturbances, rash
Refractory atrial and ventricular tachyarrhythmias; SVT due to AV node reentry and AV bypass tracts	Refractory polymorphic VT without increased QT if dose is increased too rapidly or in pts with abnormal conduction system; sinus arrest in pts with normal sinus node function; nausea, dizziness, blurred vision; may precipitate heart failure in pts with ventricular dysfunction
Refractory atrial and ventricular tachyarrhythmias; SVT due to AV node reentry and AV bypass tracts	May exacerbate arrhythmias (increase frequency, convert nonsustained to sustained tachycardias); negative inotropic actions may worsen CHF; beta-blocking activity may worsen asthma, AV block, visual blurring, dizziness, paresthesias, taste disturbances
Atrial tachyarrhythmias including AF, SVT (not approved by the FDA for therapy of these arrhythmias), ventricular tachycardias	May exacerbate ventricular tachycardia; dizziness, nausea
Slowing of ventricular rate during AF, atrial flutter, and other atrial tachycardias in the absence of preexcitation; SVT due to AV nodal reentry, reentry utilizing bypass tracts; arrhythmias induced by exercise; arrhythmias occurring in the presence of hyperthyroidism; polymorphic VT associated with congenital long QT syndrome.	Sinus bradycardia, AV node block, congestive heart failure, bronchospasm, masking symptoms of hypoglycemia
Atrial and ventricular tachyarrhythmias (not FDA approved for atrial arrhythmias)	Initially, transient hypertension; subsequent hypotension increased in upright position; the hypotensive effect can be prevented by tricyclic drugs; nausea, vomiting
Refractory VT and VF, especially due to acute ischemia	Marked sinus bradycardia, complete heart block; IV administration may cause hypotension; increased QT associated with polymorphic VT; increased T_4, hypo- and hyperthyroidism; peripheral neuropathy; proximal myopathy, pulmonary fibrosis; increased liver enzymes; hepatitis; blue-gray skin discoloration; corneal microdeposits; elevation of digoxin levels; potential of oral coagulants; exacerbation of CHF, polymorphic VT associated with QT prolongation
Refractory atrial and ventricular tachyarrhythmias; refractory SVT due to AV nodal reentry and AV reentry utilizing bypass tracts; not approved by FDA for atrial arrhythmias; atrial and ventricular extrasystoles and tachyarrhythmias (not yet approved by the FDA)	Sinus bradycardia, AV node block, congestive heart failure, constipation, peripheral edema, drug interactions
Slowing of ventricular rate during atrial fibrillation, atrial flutter, and other atrial tachycardias in the absence of preexcitation: SVT due to AV nodal reentry, reentry utilizing bypass tracts; idiopathic left ventricular tachycardia	Exacerbation of heart failure, sinus bradycardia, AV block, asystole, hemodynamic collapse; all occur more frequently in patients with sinus bradycardia, heart failure, or in patients who are also receiving a beta blocker.

1267

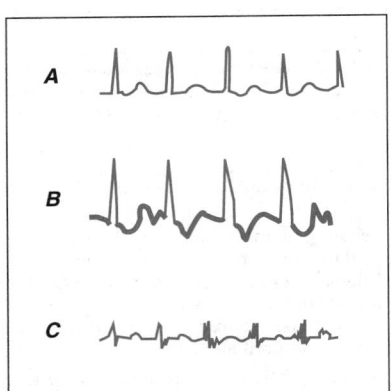

FIGURE 231-5 Examples of reentrant PSVT. *A*. AV nodal reentry. No P waves are visible. *B*. AV reentry using a concealed bypass tract. Inverted retrograde P waves are superimposed on the T wave. *C*. Intraatrial reentry. P waves precede the QRS complex.

absent, buried in the QRS complex, or appear as distortions at the terminal parts of the QRS complex (Fig. 231-5*A*).

AV nodal reentrant PSVT (Fig. 231-6) can be reproducibly initiated and terminated by appropriately timed atrial premature stimuli. The onset of the tachycardia is almost always associated with prolongation of the PR interval due to marked AV nodal conduction delay (prolonged AH interval) following the APC that is critical for the genesis of the arrhythmia. The sudden prolongation of the AH interval is consistent with the concept of dual AV nodal pathways: (1) a beta (fast) pathway, which exhibits rapid conduction and a long refractory period; and (2) an alpha (slow) pathway, which has a short refractory period but conducts slowly. During sinus rhythm, only conduction

over the fast pathway is manifest, resulting in a normal PR interval (see Fig. 231-6). Atrial extrastimuli at a critical coupling interval are blocked in the beta pathway because of its longer refractory period and are conducted slowly through the alpha pathway. If conduction down the alpha pathway is slow enough to allow the previously refractory beta pathway time to recover excitability, a single atrial echo or sustained tachycardia ensues. A critical balance between conduction velocity and refractoriness within the node is required to sustain AV nodal reentry. Retrograde atrial and antegrade ventricular activation occur simultaneously, explaining why P waves may not be apparent on the surface ECG.

Clinical Features AV nodal reentry may produce palpitations, syncope, and heart failure depending on the rate and duration of the arrhythmia and the presence and severity of any underlying heart disease. Hypotension and syncope may occur because of the sudden loss of the atrial contribution to ventricular filling; this also can lead to a marked increase in atrial pressure, acute pulmonary edema, and a reduction in ventricular filling. Simultaneous atrial and ventricular contraction produces cannon *a* waves with each heartbeat.

℞ TREATMENT

In patients without hypotension, vagal maneuvers, particularly carotid sinus massage, can terminate the arrhythmia in 80 percent of cases. If hypotension is present, raising the blood pressure by the cautious use of intravenous phenylephrine in 0.1-mg increments may terminate the arrhythmia alone or in combination with carotid sinus pressure. If these maneuvers are unsuccessful, verapamil (2.5 to 10 mg intravenously) or adenosine (6 to 12 mg intravenously) is the agent of choice. We prefer to use adenosine because of its extremely short half-life, lessening the consequences of any side effects. Beta blockers also may be used to slow or terminate the tachycardia but are agents of second choice. Digitalis glycosides have a slower onset of action and should *not* be used for acute therapy. When these drugs fail to terminate the tachycardia, or when the tachycardia is recurrent, atrial or ventricular pacing via a temporary pacemaker

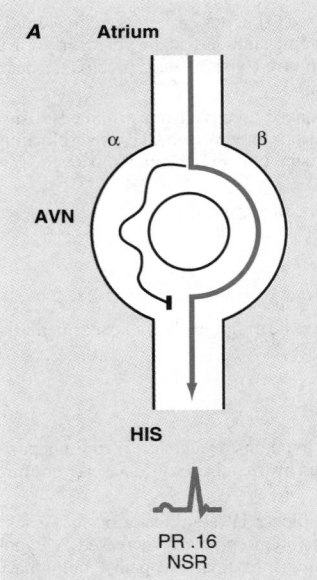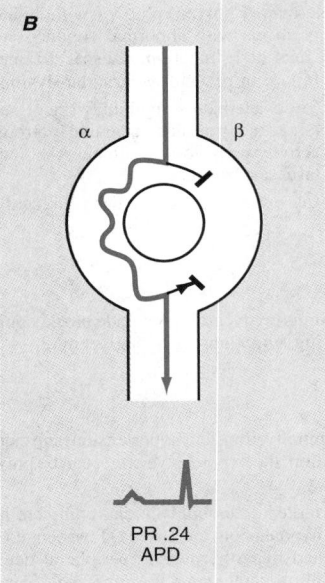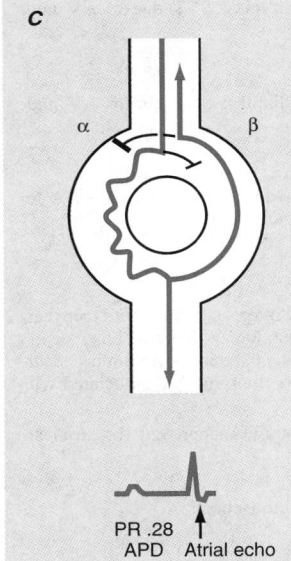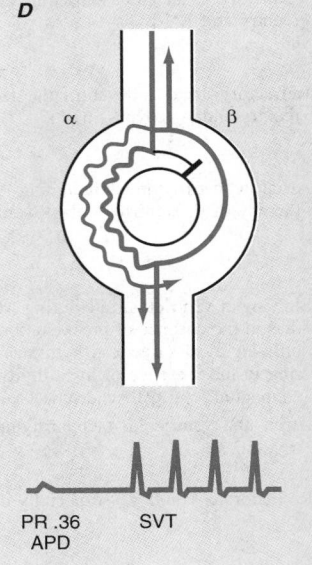

FIGURE 231-6 Mechanism of AV nodal reentry: The atrium, AV node (AVN), and His bundle are shown schematically. The AV node is longitudinally dissociated into two pathways, with different functional properties. The alpha pathway conducts relatively slowly while the beta pathway conducts rapidly (see text). In each panel of this diagram, blue lines denote excitation in the AV node, which is manifest on the surface electrocardiogram, while black lines denote conduction, which is concealed and not apparent on the surface electrocardiogram. *A*. During sinus rhythm (NSR) the impulse from the atrium conducts down both pathways. However, only conduction over the fast (beta) pathway is manifest on the surface ECG, producing a normal PR interval of 0.16 s. *B*. An atrial premature depolarization (APD) blocks in the beta pathway.

The impulse conducts over the alpha pathway to the His bundle and ventricles, producing a PR interval of 0.24 s. Because the impulse is premature, conduction over the alpha pathway occurs more slowly than it would during sinus rhythm. *C*. A more premature atrial impulse blocks in the beta pathway, conducting with increased delay in the alpha pathway, producing a PR interval of 0.28 s. The impulse conducts retrogradely up the beta pathway producing a single atrial echo. Sustained reentry is prevented by subsequent block in the alpha pathway. *D*. A still more premature atrial impulse blocks initially in the beta pathway, conducting over the alpha pathway with increasing delay producing a PR interval of 0.36 s. Retrograde conduction occurs over the beta pathway and reentry occurs, producing a sustained tachycardia (SVT). *(After Josephson.)*

inserted pervenously may be used to terminate the arrhythmia. However, if severe ischemia and/or hypotension is caused by the tachycardia, dc cardioversion should be considered.

AV nodal reentry can usually be prevented by the use of drugs that act primarily on the antegrade slow pathway (such as digitalis, beta blockers, or calcium channel antagonists) or on the fast pathway (class IA or IC; see Table 231-2). We favor as initial therapy digitalis, beta blockers, or calcium channel antagonists because the risk-benefit ratio associated with treatment with these agents is more favorable than that of IA or IC agents. Drugs most likely to avert recurrences prevent induction of the arrhythmias by programmed stimulation. This technique utilizes temporary pacemaker catheters connected to a physiologic stimulator capable of variable rate pacing and stimulation with one or more precisely timed premature impulses. In symptomatic patients who require chronic therapy, radiofrequency catheter modification of the AV node should be considered. This technique can cure AV nodal reentry in >90 percent of cases and has been proven to be safe, although a 1 to 2 percent risk of AV block requiring a permanent pacemaker exists.

AV REENTRANT TACHYCARDIA PSVT due to AV reentry incorporates a concealed AV bypass tract as part of the tachycardia circuit. Thus the impulse passes antegradely from the atria through the AV node and His-Purkinje system to the ventricles and then retrogradely through the (concealed) bypass tract back to the atrium. Patients with this disorder manifest the same type of PSVT as do patients with the WPW syndrome (see below), but the bypass tract cannot conduct in an antegrade direction during sinus rhythm or other atrial tachyarrhythmias.

AV reentrant tachycardia can be initiated and terminated by either APCs or VPCs. Initiation of PSVT by a VPC is virtually diagnostic of AV reentry. Alternation of the QRS complexes occurs in approximately one-third of such tachycardias. Since atrial activation must follow ventricular activation during AV reentry, the P wave usually occurs after the QRS complex (see Fig. 231-5B).

Atrial activation mapping is of major value in evaluating the origin of these tachycardias. Most concealed bypass tracts are left-sided. Thus, during PSVT or during ventricular pacing, the earliest activation sequence is recorded in the left atrium, usually via a catheter in the coronary sinus (Fig. 231-7). This eccentric atrial activation is quite distinct from the normal retrograde activation sequence in which the earliest activation of the atria is in the area of the AV junction. The ability of a ventricular stimulus to conduct to the atrium at a time when the bundle of His is refractory and the termination of the tachycardia by a ventricular stimulus that does not reach the atrium are diagnostic of retrograde conduction over a concealed bypass tract.

Rx **TREATMENT**
This is similar to the treatment for AV nodal reentry tachycardia. Although pharmacologic agents may be used, patients who require chronic therapy should be considered candidates for radiofrequency catheter ablation of the bypass tract. This requires detailed electrophysiologic study to exclude other arrhythmias that may be responsible for patients' symptoms and to determine the location of the bypass tract(s). The efficacy of this procedure exceeds 90 percent, with minimal risks. In the remaining small number of patients failing catheter ablation, surgical ablation or pharmacologic therapy can be used.

SINUS NODE REENTRY AND OTHER ATRIAL TACHYCARDIAS Reentry in the region of the sinus node or within the atria is invariably initiated by APCs. These arrhythmias are less common than AV nodal or AV reentry and are more often associ-

ated with underlying cardiac disease. During sinus node reentry, the P-wave morphology is identical to that occurring in sinus rhythm, but the PR interval is prolonged. This is in contrast to sinus tachycardia, in which the PR interval tends to shorten. With intraatrial reentry, the P-wave configuration differs from that during sinus rhythm, and the PR interval is prolonged (see Fig. 231-5C).

Rx **TREATMENT**
Sinus node and atrial reentrant arrhythmias are managed like other reentrant PSVTs, except that catheter ablation is less successful because multiple foci may be present.

NONREENTRANT ATRIAL TACHYCARDIAS These may be a manifestation of digitalis intoxication or may be associated with severe pulmonary or cardiac disease, with hypokalemia, or with the administration of theophylline or adrenergic drugs. Multifocal atrial tachycardia (MAT) (Fig. 231-8) is particularly common following theophylline administration. By definition, MAT requires three or more consecutive P waves of different morphologies at rates greater than 100 beats per minute. MAT usually has an irregular ventricular rate because of varying AV conduction. There is a high incidence of atrial fibrillation (50 to 70 percent) in patients with MAT. Treatment should be directed at the underlying disorder. The digitalis-induced arrhythmias are caused by triggered activity. In such atrial tachycardias with AV block secondary to digitalis intoxication (see Fig. 231-2B), the atrial rate rarely exceeds 180 beats per minute, and typically 2:1 block is present. Atrial arrhythmias precipitated by digitalis usually can be treated by withdrawal of the drug.

Automatic atrial tachycardias not caused by digitalis are difficult to terminate, and in such cases the main goal of therapy should be to control the ventricular response, either by drugs that affect the AV node, such as digitalis, beta blockers, or calcium channel antagonists, or by ablation techniques. Catheter ablation and surgery have been employed to eradicate the arrhythmia's focus or create heart block for rate control.

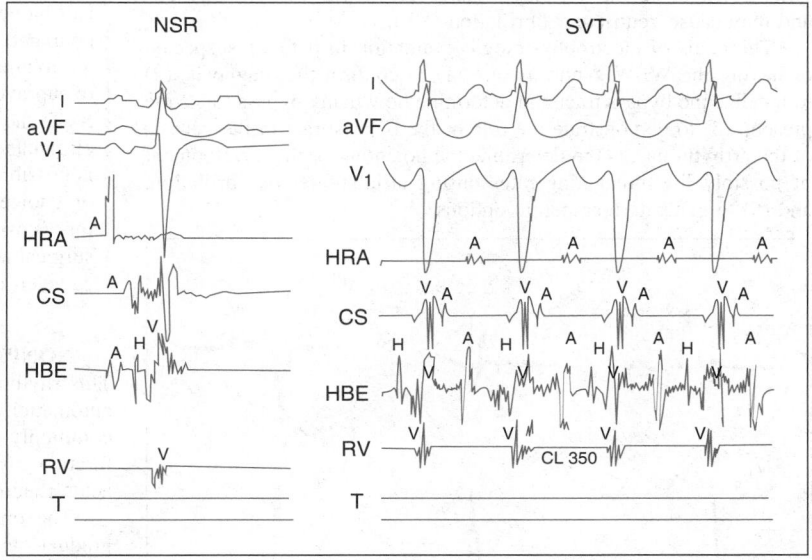

FIGURE 231-7 Intracardiac recordings during supraventricular tachycardia using a left-sided AV bypass tract. Intracardiac recordings during sinus rhythm (NSR) and in supraventricular tachycardia (SVT) are shown. ECG leads I, aVF, and V₁ are displayed with electrograms from the high right atrium (HRA), coronary sinus (CS), His bundle (HBE), and right ventricle (RV). During NSR, the QRS complex and the AH and HV intervals are normal. During SVT the retrograde atrial activation sequence is abnormal. The earliest site of atrial activation is in the CS, which is followed by activation in the HBE and HRA. This activation sequence is diagnostic of a left-sided AV bypass tract conduction retrogradely from ventricle to atrium. *[From ME Josephson, in Update IV, Harrison's Principles of Internal Medicine, KJ Isselbacher et al (eds), New York, McGraw-Hill, 1983; used with permission.]*

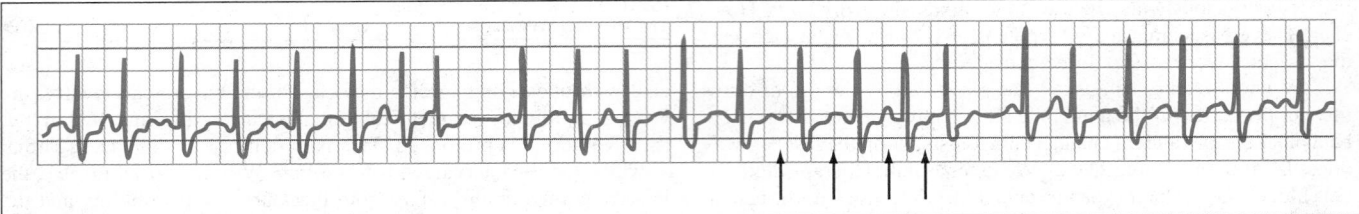

FIGURE 231-8 Multifocal atrial tachycardia. A lead I rhythm strip demonstrates a multifocal atrial tachycardia defined by ≥3 consecutive P waves of variable morphology and rate >100 beats per minute (*arrows*).

PREEXCITATION (WPW) SYNDROME The most frequently encountered type of ventricular preexcitation is that associated with AV bypass tracts. These connections are composed of strands of atrial-like muscle which may occur almost anywhere around the AV rings. The term *Wolff-Parkinson-White syndrome* is applied to patients with both preexcitation on the ECG and paroxysmal tachycardias. AV bypass tracts can be associated with certain congenital abnormalities, the most important of which is Ebstein's anomaly.

AV bypass tracts that conduct in an antegrade direction produce a typical ECG pattern of a short PR interval (<0.12 s), a slurred upstroke of the QRS complex (delta wave), and a wide QRS complex. This pattern results from a fusion of activation of the ventricles over both the bypass tract and the AV nodal His-Purkinje system (Fig. 231-9). The relative contribution of activation over each system determines the amount of preexcitation.

During PSVT in WPW, the impulse is usually conducted antegradely over the normal AV system and retrogradely through the bypass tract. The characteristics are identical to those described on p. 1265. Rarely (approximately 5 percent), tachycardias occurring in patients with WPW will exhibit a reverse pattern with antegrade conduction through the bypass tract and retrograde conduction through the normal AV system. This produces a tachycardia with a wide QRS complex in which the ventricles are totally activated by the bypass tract. Atrial flutter and AF also occur commonly in patients with WPW syndrome. Since the bypass tract does not have the same decremental conducting properties as the AV node, the ventricular responses during atrial flutter or fibrillation may be unusually rapid (see Fig. 231-2E) and may cause ventricular fibrillation (VF).

The goals of electrophysiologic evaluation in patients suspected of having the WPW syndrome are (1) to confirm the diagnosis, (2) to localize the bypass tract and determine how many bypass tracts are present, (3) to demonstrate the role of the bypass tract in the genesis of the arrhythmias, (4) to determine the potential for the development of possibly life-threatening rates during atrial flutter or fibrillation, and (5) to evaluate therapeutic options.

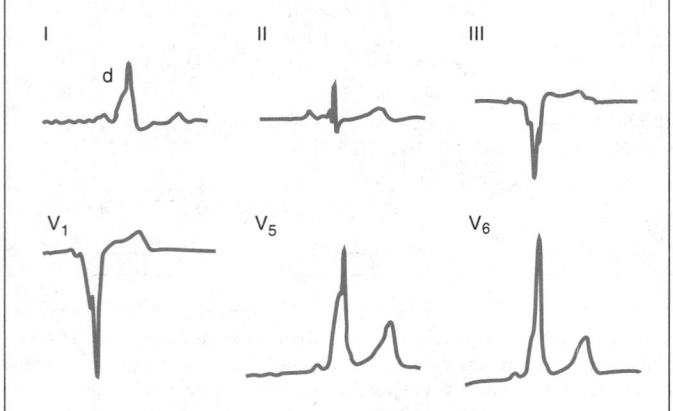

FIGURE 231-9 ECG in WPW syndrome. There is a short PR interval (0.11 s), a wide QRS complex (0.12 s), and slurring on the upstroke of the QRS produced by early ventricular activation over the bypass tract (delta wave, d in lead I). The negative delta waves in V₁ are diagnostic of a right-sided bypass tract. Note the Q wave (negative delta wave) in lead III, mimicking myocardial infarction.

℞ **TREATMENT**

Pharmacologic therapy is aimed at altering the electrophysiologic properties (i.e., refractoriness or conduction velocity) of one or more components of the reentrant circuit. This is most often accomplished by agents such as beta blockers or calcium channel blockers that slow conduction and increase refractoriness of the AV node or by agents such as quinidine or flecainide that slow conduction and increase refractoriness primarily in the bypass tract. Some drugs may affect multiple sites (Fig. 231-10).

Acute management of episodes of PSVT in patients with WPW syndrome is similar to that of PSVT in patients with concealed bypass tracts.

In patients with the WPW syndrome and AF, dc cardioversion should be carried out if there is a life-threatening, rapid ventricular response. Alternatively, lidocaine (3 to 5 mg/kg) or procainamide (15 mg/kg) administered intravenously over 15 to 20 min will usually slow the ventricular response. Caution should be employed when using digitalis or intravenous verapamil in patients with the WPW syndrome and AF, since these drugs can shorten the refractory period of the accessory pathway and can increase the ventricular rate, thereby placing the patient at increased risk for VF. Chronic oral therapy with verapamil is not associated with this risk. In addition to these drugs, beta-blocking agents are of no utility in controlling the ventricular response during AF when conduction proceeds over the bypass tract. Although atrial or ventricular pacing can almost always terminate PSVT in patients with the WPW syndrome, they can induce AF. As such, chronic pacemaker therapy is to be discouraged.

While surgical ablation of bypass tracts offers a permanent cure of supraventricular tachycardia (SVT) and most AFs associated with SVT, the advent of radiofrequency catheter ablation has virtually eliminated the need for surgery. Catheter ablation of bypass tracts is possible in more than 90 percent of patients and is the treatment of choice in patients with symptomatic arrhythmias. It is safer, more cost-effective, and just as successful as surgery. Nevertheless, surgical ablation may be required in the occasional patient in whom catheter ablation fails.

NONPAROXYSMAL JUNCTIONAL TACHYCARDIA
This rhythm usually results from conditions that produce enhanced automaticity or triggered activity in the AV junction and is most commonly due to digitalis intoxication, inferior wall myocardial infarction, myocarditis, endogenous or exogenous catecholamine excess, acute rheumatic fever, or aftereffects of valve surgery.

The onset of nonparoxysmal junctional tachycardia is usually gradual, with a "warm-up" period prior to stabilization of the rate, which can range from 70 to 150 beats per minute, faster rates usually being associated with digitalis intoxication. Nonparoxysmal junctional tachycardia is recognized by a QRS complex identical to that of sinus rhythm. The rate can be influenced by autonomic tone and can be increased by catecholamines, vagolytic agents, or exercise and slowed somewhat by carotid sinus pressure. When this rhythm is due to digitalis intoxication, it usually is associated with AV block and/or dissociation. Soon after cardiac surgery, retrograde conduction is more likely to be present because of the heightened sympathetic state.

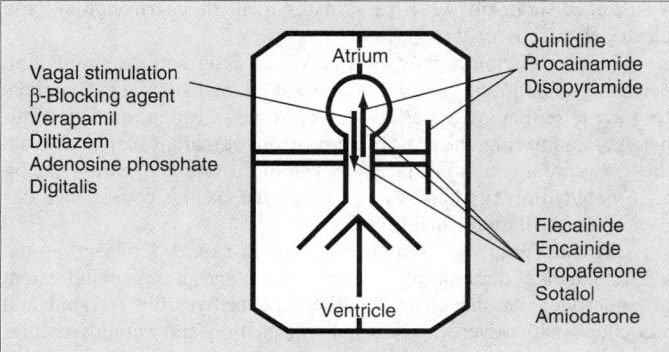

FIGURE 231-10 Site of action of antiarrhythmic agents in the WPW syndrome. The atrium, ventricle, antegrade conduction through the AV node (↓), retrograde conduction through the AV node (↑), and the bypass tract are shown. Drugs on the left affect antegrade AV nodal conduction. Type IA drugs on the upper right affect retrograde conduction over the node and antegrade conduction over the bypass tract. Drugs on the lower right affect conduction in both directions in the AV node and the bypass tract.

℞ TREATMENT

This is directed toward elimination of the underlying etiologic factors. Since digitalis is the most common cause of this rhythm, discontinuation of this drug is indicated. If the rhythm is associated with other serious manifestations of digitalis intoxication, such as ventricular or atrial irritability, active intervention with lidocaine or a beta blocker may be useful, and in some instances, use of digitalis antibodies (Fab fragments) should be considered. Cardioversion of this rhythm should not be attempted, particularly in the setting of digitalis intoxication. When AV conduction is intact, atrial pacing can capture and override the junctional focus and provide the AV synchrony necessary to maximize cardiac output. Nonparoxysmal junctional tachycardia usually is not a chronic, recurrent problem, and attention to the acute precipitating events can often resolve the tachycardia.

VENTRICULAR TACHYCARDIA *Sustained ventricular tachycardia* is defined as VT that persists for more than 30 s or requires termination because of hemodynamic collapse. VT generally accompanies some form of structural heart disease, most commonly chronic ischemic heart disease associated with a prior myocardial infarction. Sustained VT also may be associated with nonischemic cardiomyopathies, metabolic disorders, drug toxicity, or prolonged QT syndrome, and it occurs occasionally in the absence of heart disease or other predisposing factors. Nonsustained VT (three beats to 30 s) is also associated with cardiac disease but occurs in its absence more often than the sustained arrhythmia. While nonsustained VT usually does not produce symptoms, sustained VT is almost always symptomatic and is often associated with marked hemodynamic compromise and/or the development of myocardial

ischemia. A fixed anatomic substrate, not acute ischemia, is responsible for most recurrent episodes of sustained uniform VT. Acute ischemia appears to have little role in the genesis of sustained uniform VT associated with chronic infarction but may play a role in the degeneration of stable VT into VF or initiation of polymorphic VT. Most episodes of VF begin with VT.

The ECG diagnosis of VT is suggested by a wide-complex QRS tachycardia at a rate exceeding 100 beats per minute. The QRS configuration during any episode of VT may be uniform (monomorphic) (Fig. 231-3*B*), or it may vary from beat to beat (polymorphic) (Fig. 231-3*C*). *Bidirectional tachycardia* refers to VT that shows an alternation in QRS amplitude and axis. Typically this appears as a QRS with a right bundle branch block pattern with alternating superior (leftward) and inferior axes (rightward). While the rhythm is usually quite regular, slight irregularity may exist. Atrial activity may be dissociated from ventricular activity, or the atria may be depolarized retrogradely. The onset of the tachycardia is generally abrupt, but in nonparoxysmal tachycardias it can be gradual. Paroxysmal VT is usually initiated by a VPC.

It is important to distinguish supraventricular tachycardia with aberration of intraventricular conduction from VT because the clinical implications and management of these two arrhythmias are totally different. The most important clinical predictor of VT is the presence of structural heart disease. The observation of intermittent cannon *a* waves and varying first heart sounds suggests AV dissociation and is diagnostic of VT. In a majority of cases, the diagnosis can and should be made by close examination of the 12-lead ECG. Pharmacologic maneuvers, such as administration of intravenous verapamil or adenosine, can be hazardous and should be avoided. It is always useful to have a 12-lead ECG recorded during sinus rhythm for comparison with that during tachycardia. When the tracing obtained during sinus rhythm demonstrates the same morphologic features as those during the tachycardia, the diagnosis of PSVT with aberration is favored. An infarction pattern on the sinus rhythm tracing suggests the potential presence of the anatomic substrate necessary for VT. Characteristics of the 12-lead ECG during the tachycardia that suggest a ventricular origin for the arrhythmia are (1) a QRS complex >0.14 s in the absence of antiarrhythmic therapy, (2) AV dissociation (with or without fusion or captured beats) or variable retrograde conduction (Fig. 231-11), (3) a superior QRS axis in the presence of a right bundle branch block pattern, (4) concordance of the QRS pattern in all precordial leads (i.e., all positive or all negative deflections), and (5) other QRS patterns (morphology) with prolonged duration that are inconsistent with typical right or left bundle branch block patterns. (See Table 231-3 for a detailed synopsis of ECG criteria that favor the diagnosis of VT over SVT for wide complex tachycardia.) A wide, complex, bizarre tachycardia that is very irregular suggests AF with conduction over an AV bypass tract (see Fig. 231-2*E*). Similarly, a QRS complex in excess of 0.20 s is uncommon during VT in the absence of drug therapy and is more common with preexcitation. Intravenous verapamil

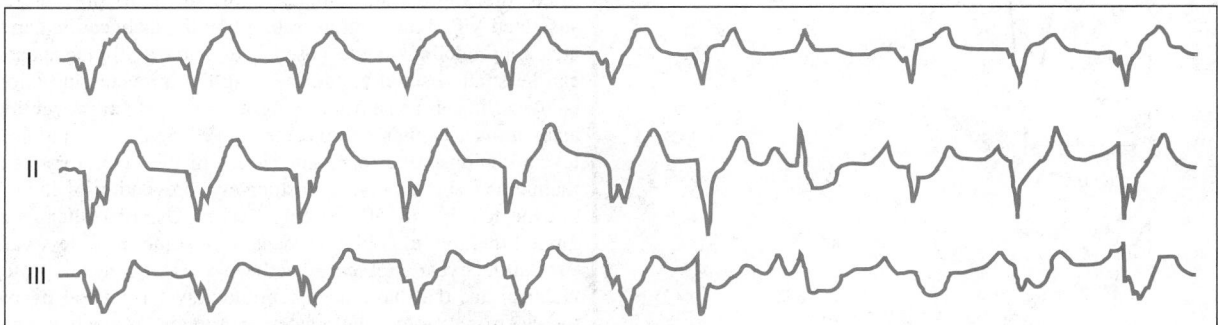

FIGURE 231-11 Ventricular tachycardia with AV dissociation. P waves are dissociated from the underlying wide complex rhythm and result in fusion and capture beats (complexes 7 and 8).

will stop most recalcitrant SVTs involving the AV junction, but it is rarely effective for VT. Because of this property, verapamil has been utilized to attempt to differentiate SVT with aberrant conduction from VT. However, this is extremely hazardous, since intravenous verapamil can precipitate cardiac arrest in patients with VT.

It has been possible to replicate sustained uniform VT in more than 95 percent of patients with this arrhythmia using programmed stimulation. In most patients the tachycardia is initiated with ventricular premature stimuli. A sustained monomorphic VT with a morphology identical to that of the spontaneous arrhythmia is the rule. The clinical significance of polymorphic VT initiated by programmed stimulation is not clear, since more aggressive stimulation (i.e., the use of three or four extrastimuli) can induce polymorphic VT and even VF in some normal subjects and in patients who have never had a clinical arrhythmia.

Sustained uniform VT can be terminated by programmed stimulation or rapid pacing in at least 75 percent of patients; the remainder require cardioversion. The ability to reproducibly initiate and terminate

Table 231-3

Wide Complex Tachycardia

ECG CRITERIA THAT FAVOR VENTRICULAR TACHYCARDIA

1. AV dissociation
2. QRS width: >0.14 s with RBBB configuration
          >0.16 s with LBBB configuration
3. QRS axis: left axis deviation with RBBB morphology
          extreme left axis deviation (northwest axis) with LBBB morphology
4. Concordance of QRS in precordial leads
5. Morphologic patterns of the QRS complex
      RBBB: mono- or biphasic complex in V_1
            RS (*only with left axis deviation*) or QS in V_6

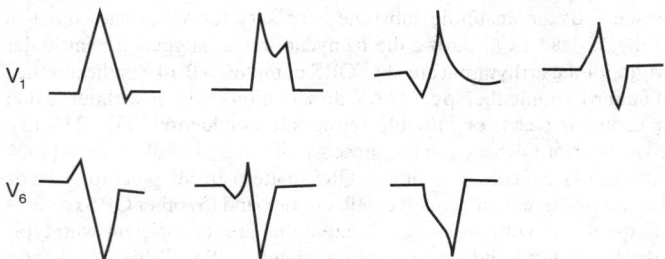

      LBBB: broad R wave in V_1 or $V_2 \geq 0.04$ s
           onset of QRS to nadir of S wave in V_1 or V_2 of ≥ 0.07 s
           notched downslope of S wave in V_1 or V_2
           Q wave in V_6

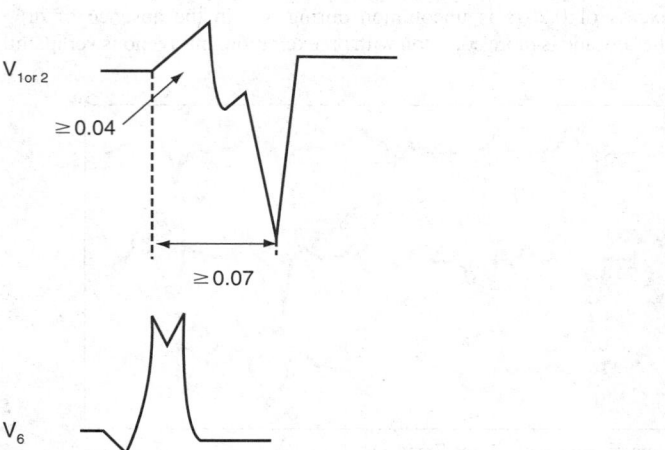

a sustained, uniform VT permits assessment of pharmacologic and electrical therapy of these arrhythmias.

The reproducible termination of VT by programmed stimulation permits evaluation of the effectiveness of antitachycardia pacemakers for long-term therapy of paroxysmal episodes of arrhythmia. Unfortunately, rapid pacing, the most effective form of therapy, can accelerate the tachycardia and/or produce VF. Therefore, antitachycardia pacing is a viable form of therapy only when the pacing device includes backup defibrillation capabilities.

Clinical Features   Symptoms resulting from VT depend on the ventricular rate, duration of the tachycardia, and presence and extent of underlying cardiac disease. When the tachycardia is rapid and associated with severe myocardial dysfunction and cerebrovascular disease, hypotension and syncope are common. However, the presence of hemodynamic stability does not preclude a diagnosis of VT. The rate, loss of the atrial contribution to ventricular filling, and abnormal sequence of ventricular activation are important factors producing a decreased cardiac output during VT.

The *prognosis* of VT depends on the underlying disease state. If sustained VT develops within the first 6 weeks following acute myocardial infarction, the prognosis is poor, with a 75 percent mortality rate at 1 year. Patients with nonsustained VT following myocardial infarction have a threefold greater risk of death than a comparable group of patients without this arrhythmia. However, a cause-and-effect relationship between the nonsustained tachycardia and subsequent sudden death has not been established. Patients without heart disease who have uniform VT have a good prognosis and have an extremely low risk of sudden death.

℞ TREATMENT

The risk-benefit ratio of treating each specific type of VT should be considered before beginning therapy. This is important because antiarrhythmic agents can produce or exacerbate the very arrhythmias that they are given to prevent. In general, patients with VT but without organic heart disease have a benign course; such patients with asymptomatic, nonsustained VT need not be treated because their prognosis will not be affected. An exception is the patient with congenital long QT syndrome. Such patients have recurrent polymorphic VT and a high mortality from sudden death if untreated. Patients with sustained VT in the absence of heart disease usually require therapy because the arrhythmia causes symptoms. These tachycardias may respond to beta blockers, verapamil, or class IA or IC or class III agents. In patients with VT and organic heart disease, if marked hemodynamic compromise is present or if there is evidence of ischemia, congestive heart failure, or central nervous system hypoperfusion, the rhythm should be promptly terminated by dc cardioversion (see below). If the patient with organic heart disease tolerates the VT well, pharmacologic therapy may be tried. Procainamide is probably the most effective agent for acute therapy. It may or may not terminate the tachycardia but almost always slows the rate. In stable patients in whom these drugs do not terminate the arrhythmia, a pacing catheter can be inserted pervenously into the right ventricular apex, and the tachycardia can be terminated by overdrive pacing.

Programmed stimulation is probably the most effective way to select the appropriate antiarrhythmic agent to prevent recurrent, sustained VT. After demonstrating that the tachycardia can be initiated reproducibly in the absence of antiarrhythmic agents, drugs can be studied serially, and the drug that prevents initiation of the tachycardia can be selected; long-term successful prevention of the arrhythmia can then be expected in 90 percent of patients. Drug levels demonstrated to be successful in the laboratory need to be maintained chronically. Unfortunately, prevention of inducible VT is expected in only 50 percent of cases. Use of Holter monitor for guided therapy, although advocated by some, is of less value.

Antitachycardia pacing has been used as a means to terminate tachycardias that have been reproducibly terminated by pacing in the electrophysiology laboratory. Automatic antitachycardia pacing devices are not used alone because pacing during VT may accelerate tachycardia, converting a stable arrhythmia into an unstable one and resulting in severe hemodynamic compromise. However, devices combining antitachycardia pacing with an implantable cardioverter/defibrillator (ICD) (see below) afford a "backup" means of terminating unstable arrhythmias.

The advent of endocardial catheter and intraoperative mapping led to the development of surgical techniques for the management of VT. Activation mapping permits localization of the site of origin of the arrhythmia. In centers in which expertise in mapping is available, operation has been successfully employed to cure tachycardias in the majority of patients in whom it has been undertaken. Even though most patients with VT and ischemic heart disease have markedly impaired left ventricular function and multivessel coronary artery disease, the operative mortality rate has ranged between 8 and 15 percent. Following operation, more than 90 percent of survivors are controlled either off (two-thirds of patients) or on (one-third) antiarrhythmic agents that were previously ineffective in controlling these rhythms.

Specific Types of VT *Torsades de pointes* ("twisting of the points") (Fig. 231-12) refers to VT characterized by polymorphic QRS complexes that change in amplitude and cycle length, giving the appearance of oscillations around the baseline. This rhythm is, by definition, associated with QT prolongation. The latter may result from electrolyte disturbances (particularly hypokalemia and hypomagnesemia), use of a variety of antiarrhythmic drugs (especially quinidine), phenothiazines and tricyclic antidepressants, liquid protein diets, intracranial events, and bradyarrhythmias, particularly third-degree AV block. It also may occur as an isolated idiopathic congenital or acquired anomaly.

The electrocardiographic hallmark is polymorphic VT preceded by marked QT prolongation, often in excess of 0.60 s. These patients often have multiple episodes of nonsustained polymorphic VT associated with recurrent syncope, but they also may develop VF and sudden cardiac death.

Therapy should be directed at removing the precipitating factors, i.e., correcting metabolic abnormalities and removing drugs that have induced the prolonged QT interval. In the setting of drug-induced torsades de pointes, atrial or ventricular overdrive pacing and the administration of magnesium also have been useful in terminating and preventing the arrhythmia. For patients with the congenital prolonged QT interval syndrome, beta-adrenergic blocking agents have been the mainstay of therapy; agents that shorten the QT interval also may be useful (e.g., phenytoin). Cervicothoracic sympathectomy has been proposed as a form of therapy for congenital prolonged QT syndrome, but it is not often effective as the sole therapy. Pacing in combination with beta blockers and sympathectomy is often required.

Polymorphic tachycardias associated with normal QT intervals in patients with ischemic heart disease that are initiated by "R-on-T" VPCs are probably caused by reentry, and their treatment is totally different. This is not true torsades de pointes. In such cases, class I or III agents may be the most effective form of therapy and should be administered in full antiarrhythmic doses. However, these arrhythmias also may result from acute, severe ischemia and will only respond to abolition of the ischemia, usually by revascularization.

Accelerated idioventricular rhythm This arrhythmia, also termed *slow VT*, with a rate that ranges from 60 to 120 beats per minute, usually occurs in acute myocardial infarction, often during reperfusion. It also may be seen following cardiac operations; in patients with cardiomyopathy, rheumatic fever, or digitalis intoxication; as well as in patients with no evidence of heart disease. The rhythm is usually transient and rarely causes significant hemodynamic compromise or symptoms.

Treatment is rarely necessary and should usually be considered only if symptoms arise due to impaired hemodynamics, most commonly due to AV dissociation. In most cases, atropine can accelerate the sinus rate to overdrive the ventricular rhythm.

VENTRICULAR FLUTTER AND VENTRICULAR FIBRILLATION (VF) (See Fig. 231-13; see also Chap. 39) These arrhythmias occur most often in patients with ischemic heart disease. They also occur following administration of antiarrhythmic drugs, particularly those which induce prolonged QT intervals and torsades de pointes (see above), in patients with severe hypoxia or ischemia, and in those with WPW who develop AF with an extremely rapid ventricular response (see p. 1270). Electrical accidents frequently cause cardiac arrest due to the development of VF. The onset of these arrhythmias is rapidly followed by loss of consciousness and, if untreated, death. Episodes of cardiac arrest recorded during Holter monitoring reveal that approximately three-fourths of the sudden deaths are due to VT or VF.

In patients with nonischemic VF, the onset usually begins with a short run of rapid VT, which is initiated by a relatively late coupled VPC. In patients with acute myocardial infarction or ischemia, however, VF is usually precipitated by a single early ventricular complex beat falling on the T wave (the vulnerable period), which produces a rapid VT that degenerates into VF (see Fig. 231-13).

The clinical setting in which VF occurs is important. Most patients who have primary VF within the first 48 h of the onset of acute infarction have a good long-term prognosis, with a very low rate of recurrence or sudden cardiac death. Their short-term mortality may, however, be slightly increased. In contrast, patients who experience VF unassociated with the development of acute myocardial infarction have a recurrence rate of 20 to 30 percent in the year following the event (see Chap. 39).

Ventricular flutter usually appears as a sine wave with a rate between 150 and 300 beats per minute. These oscillations make it impossible to assign a specific morphology to the arrhythmia and in some cases to distinguish it from rapid VT. VF is recognized by grossly irregular undulations of varying amplitudes, contours, and rates (see Fig. 231-13). Electrophysiologic studies have demonstrated that regardless of the apparent gross irregularity on the surface ECG, VF usually starts out with a rapid repetitive sequence of VT that ultimately breaks down into multiple wavelets of reentry.

Electrophysiologic studies have been useful in patients who have been resuscitated from cardiac arrest. Programmed stimulation has demonstrated that in approximately 70 percent of such patients one can reproducibly initiate a sustained VT. Treatment is discussed in Chap. 39.

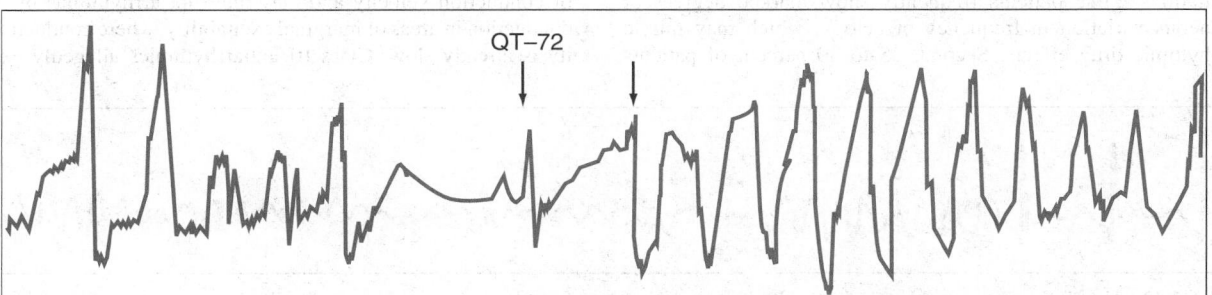

FIGURE 231-12 Torsades de pointes. Polymorphic VT is associated with a pause and QT at 0.72 s.

℞ TREATMENT

Pharmacologic Antiarrhythmic Therapy Prior to initiation of pharmacologic antiarrhythmic therapy, potential aggravating factors such as transient metabolic abnormalities, congestive heart failure, or acute ischemia must be corrected; in some cases this may suffice to control arrhythmias. In addition, the potential role of drugs as a cause or exacerbating factor in the development of the arrhythmia must be considered. It must be recognized that we do not have a good understanding of the effects of antiarrhythmic agents on the spontaneous onset of tachyarrhythmias. In some cases, they may facilitate the onset.

Antiarrhythmic drugs are used in three principal situations: (1) to terminate an acute arrhythmia, (2) to prevent recurrence of an arrhythmia, and (3) to prevent a life-threatening arrhythmia for which the patient is perceived to be at risk but which has never occurred. (The acute pharmacologic therapy of tachyarrhythmias is summarized in Table 231-4.)

Most currently available antiarrhythmic agents have a relatively low toxic/therapeutic ratio; all can exert proarrhythmic effects, and therefore they may exacerbate underlying arrhythmias. Serum levels can be determined for most currently available antiarrhythmic agents. Standards for therapeutic and toxic levels can serve only as a rough guide for selecting the appropriate dose in any individual patient. In the final analysis, the therapeutic level in a given patient is the concentration that achieves the desired antiarrhythmic effect, and the toxic level for each patient is the concentration at which undesirable side effects occur. Since many adverse effects are directly related to drug concentrations, the lowest serum level that achieves an effective antiarrhythmic response should be chosen.

In order to determine the therapeutic level for a patient, one must have a standard to judge drug efficacy. For a patient with an incessant arrhythmia, antiarrhythmic drugs may be administered empirically until the arrhythmia is suppressed. If a reproducible precipitating factor such as exercise can be identified, serial drug testing during such a provocative maneuver may be performed. Unfortunately, most arrhythmias are sporadic and occur unpredictably without identifiable precipitating factors. In these cases, if one waits to observe spontaneous recurrences on each antiarrhythmic drug, assessment of drug efficacy may require months. This type of assessment of efficacy may be adequate for arrhythmias that are not life-threatening. However, this mode of assessment is inadequate for arrhythmias that compromise hemodynamic stability, result in syncope, or cause cardiac arrest. In such cases, two methods for determination of arrhythmic drug efficacy have been utilized. The first, which consists of continuous ECG monitoring in the control state and then in the presence of antiarrhythmic drugs, has been used in order to determine the effect that each drug has on spontaneous atrial or ventricular ectopy. This method presupposes that the mechanism responsible for sustained arrhythmias is the same as that causing isolated premature depolarizations (which may or may not be true) and that therefore eradication of isolated ectopy will correlate with prevention of sustained arrhythmias. This method has a number of limitations. First, patients frequently show marked degrees of spontaneous variation in frequency of ectopy, which may mimic antiarrhythmic drug effects. Second, 25 to 30 percent of patients

Table 231-4

Acute Pharmacologic Therapy of Tachyarrhythmias

Arrhythmia	Drug
Atrial tachyarrhythmias (including AF and atrial flutter) in patients without preexcitation	Initially verapamil, diltiazem, or beta-blocking agent to control ventricular response, then procainamide or quinidine
Atrial tachyarrhythmias (including AF and atrial flutter) in patients with preexcitation	Procainamide
SVT with regular rate and narrow QRS complex	Adenosine
	Verapamil
Sustained monomorphic VT	Procainamide
	Lidocaine

NOTE: AF, atrial fibrillation; SVT, supraventricular tachycardia; VT, ventricular tachycardia.

with sustained ventricular arrhythmias such as VT or VF demonstrate only rare spontaneous ectopy. Finally, many patients demonstrate a dissociation between the effects of antiarrhythmic agents on spontaneous ectopy and the effects of the same agent on sustained arrhythmias.

An alternative method to assess drug efficacy is programmed stimulation. Numerous studies have demonstrated that most clinically occurring supraventricular and ventricular tachyarrhythmias may be reproducibly initiated and terminated safely using this technique. Studies are performed initially in a baseline state in the absence of antiarrhythmic drugs (Fig. 231-14). If the patient's clinical arrhythmia can be reproducibly initiated, then the ability of individual antiarrhythmic drugs to prevent reinduction of the arrhythmia can be assessed either after the drug is administered intravenously or after several days of oral loading in order to achieve a steady-state serum concentration. Use of this method assumes that (1) the induced and spontaneous arrhythmias are identical, and (2) prevention of induction of arrhythmias will correlate with prevention of recurrent spontaneous tachycardias on the same drug regimen. This technique has been validated in patients with a variety of reentrant PSVTs, VT, and VF. The technique is safe when carefully performed, the potential complications being those of any intravascular catheterization. Appropriate interpretation of the results of programmed stimulation is critically dependent on correlating the patient's spontaneous arrhythmias with those induced in the laboratory, with regard to rate and morphology, in order to be certain that the arrhythmia induced in the laboratory represents the same arrhythmia that occurred spontaneously and caused symptoms.

CLASSIFICATION OF ANTIARRHYTHMIC DRUGS A number of classifications of antiarrhythmic drugs have been proposed; the most frequently used is a modification of one proposed by Vaughan-Williams (see Table 231-1). This classification is based in part on the ability of antiarrhythmic drugs to modify the cardiac cellular (1) excitatory currents (Na^+ or Ca^{2+}), (2) action potential duration, and (3) automaticity (phase 4 depolarization). These effects of the drugs on isolated cardiac cells are thought to account for some of the antiarrhythmic properties of the drugs. Thus depression of excitatory currents by class I and class IV antiarrhythmics results in slowing of conduction velocity and may interrupt arrhythmias by blocking conduction in areas of marginal excitability, where conduction velocity is already slow. Class III antiarrhythmics allegedly exert their

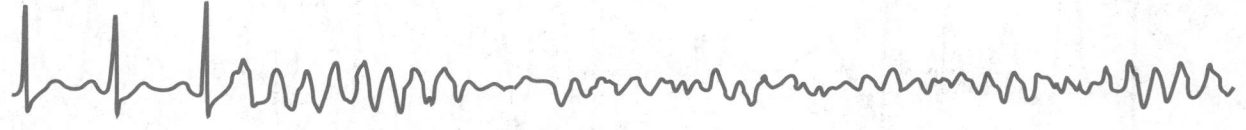

FIGURE 231-13 Ventricular fibrillation. In a patient with coronary disease ventricular fibrillation is initiated by a VPC that produces a rapid polymorphic ventricular tachycardia which rapidly degenerates to ventricular fibrillation (note the undulating baseline with indistinguishable systole and diastole).

Control   230/min

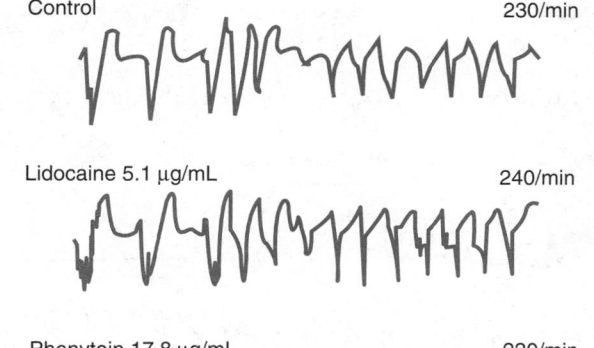

Lidocaine 5.1 µg/mL   240/min

Phenytoin 17.8 µg/mL   230/min

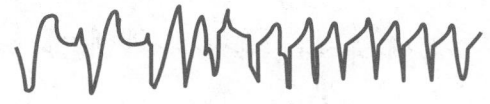

Procainamide 14.8 µg/mL

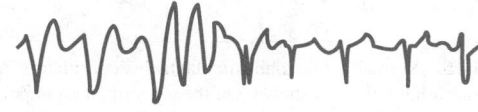

Quinidine 4.8 µg/mL

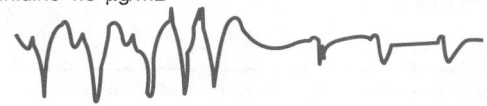

Disopyramide 6.5 µg/mL   190/min

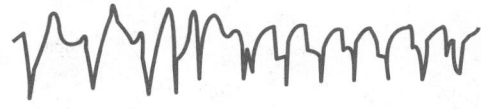

FIGURE 231-14 Selections of an effective antiarrhythmic drug for ventricular tachycardia by programmed stimulation. From top to bottom, the effects of programmed stimulation during the control state and following administration of several antiarrhythmic agents. During the control state two ventricular extrastimuli initiate the ventricular tachycardia at a rate of 230 per minute. Lidocaine, phenytoin, and disopyramide at the plasma levels shown failed to prevent induction of the tachycardia. Both procainamide and quinidine at the plasma levels shown prevented initiation of sustained tachycardia. Chronic oral quinidine therapy effectively prevented recurrences of the arrhythmia. *(From JA Kastor et al, N Engl J Med 304:1004, 1981; reprinted by permission.)*

action by increasing refractoriness through prolongation of the action potential duration. However, this classification has a number of limitations. The electrophysiologic effects of these drugs in vivo may differ from their effects on isolated cells. Also, the effects of heart rate and fiber geometry are not considered. Not all drugs (e.g., adenosine) fit into the classifications. Finally, some drugs (e.g., amiodarone) exhibit properties consistent with multiple classes. The uses and actions of currently available antiarrhythmic drugs are summarized in Tables 231-2 and 231-5.

Electrical Therapy of Tachyarrhythmias PACEMAKERS Cardiac pacing can be used to terminate and in selected cases prevent recurrent supraventricular and ventricular arrhythmias. Because many tachyarrhythmias appear to be due to a reentrant mechanism with the impulse traveling in a circuit, a properly timed paced impulse can penetrate and prematurely depolarize part of the circuit, rendering it refractory to the next circulating wavefront and thereby interrupting

the circus movement. Pacing therapy for arrhythmias is generally reserved for patients whose arrhythmias are refractory to drug therapy and who remain hemodynamically stable during the tachycardia. All forms of pacing therapy require repeated demonstration of their effectiveness and reliability in terminating the arrhythmias during electrophysiologic testing prior to implantation of the pacing device.

The type of pacing device and modality selected for arrhythmia termination depends on (1) the rate of the tachycardia (rates >160 beats per minute are rarely terminated by a single premature stimulus), (2) the type of arrhythmia (atrial flutter and VT are rarely terminated by single extrastimuli), and (3) concomitant drug therapy.

Because many tachycardias cannot be terminated by single premature stimuli, pacemakers have been developed that allow for multiple extrastimuli (burst pacing) to be introduced. In the current era, antitachycardia pacing is almost exclusively for ventricular arrhythmias because of the success of radiofrequency ablative therapy for supraventricular arrhythmias.

Cardiac pacing also has been used to prevent ventricular tachyarrhythmias. Polymorphic VT associated with a long QT interval and bradycardia (torsades de pointes, p. 1273) is most likely to respond. Pacing the atrium and/or ventricle at rates between 90 and 120 beats per minute appears to increase the homogeneity of electrical recovery and markedly reduces the propensity for a recurrence of arrhythmias.

Pacemakers may be self-contained or energized by an external radiofrequency source. The self-contained pacemaker may function automatically [i.e., it incorporates an arrhythmia recognition program (circuit)], or it may be activated by an external magnet. The major advantage of a fully automatic system is that there is no need for the patient to recognize the arrhythmia in order for termination to occur. The advantages of the externally activated system include (1) the decreased risk of unnecessary treatment because of faulty sensing, and (2) the opportunity to initiate monitoring at the time of attempted termination of arrhythmia. This type of monitoring is frequently helpful if pacing techniques are employed to terminate VT, given the risk of acceleration of the arrhythmia by pacing.

The limitations of pacing therapy are primarily related to (1) the changes in the characteristics of the arrhythmia over time such that programmed pacing parameters no longer terminate the tachycardia, (2) the risk of acceleration of the tachycardia with the development of AF when stimulating the atrium and the development of rapid VT and VF when stimulating the ventricles, and (3) inappropriate recognition of supraventricular tachyarrhythmias as ventricular tachycardias, leading to delivery of therapy unnecessarily, which can initiate VT or VF. Future pacing generators that can perform cardioversion and defibrillation will increase the applicability of pacing therapy for the treatment of arrhythmias (see below).

CARDIOVERSION AND DEFIBRILLATION Electrical cardioversion and defibrillation remain the most reliable methods for terminating arrhythmias. By depolarizing all or at least a large portion of excitable myocardium in a near homogeneous fashion, the electrical shock can interrupt reentrant arrhythmias. External cardioversion is routinely performed by placing two paddles 12 cm in diameter in firm contact with the chest wall, with one paddle usually located to the right of the sternum at the level of the second rib and the other in the left anterior axillary line in the fifth intercostal space. If the patient is conscious, a short-acting barbiturate to act as an anesthetic or an amnesic drug such as diazepam or midazolam should be administered to prevent patient discomfort. A person skilled in maintaining an airway should be present.

Energy is delivered synchronously with the QRS complex for all arrhythmias except ventricular flutter and VF, since asynchronous shocks can produce VF. The amount of energy used will vary with the type of tachycardia being treated. With the exception of AF,

SVTs can frequently be terminated with energy levels in the range of 25 to 50 W·s, while AF usually requires ≥100 W·s for termination. For terminating VT, energy levels ≥100 W·s should probably be employed. While energies as low as 25 W·s may be used successfully, they also have a higher incidence of producing VF or AF. At least 200 W·s of energy should be used for initial attempts at terminating VF. If the initial shock fails, all repeated attempts at defibrillation should be with the maximum energy that the defibrillator is capable of delivering (320 to 400 W·s).

Indications for cardioversion depend on the clinical setting and the patient's general condition. Any tachycardia (except sinus tachycardia) that produces hypotension, myocardial ischemia, or heartfailure warrants consideration of prompt termination using external cardioversion. Arrhythmias that fail to terminate with pharmacologic therapy also may be terminated by electrical cardioversion. Transient bradycardias and supraventricular and ventricular irritability following cardioversion are common and usually do not warrant antiarrhythmic intervention.

IMPLANTED CARDIOVERSION/DEFIBRILLATION ICD devices have been developed that will promptly recognize and terminate life-threatening ventricular arrhythmias. These devices can deliver <1 to 40 W·s, the amount of which can be programmed. Current devices have antitachycardia pacing capabilities such that VT can be sensed and terminated without resorting to a painful shock. In such devices, high-energy shocks are reserved for hypotensive VT, acceleration of VT, or failure to terminate VT after a programmed

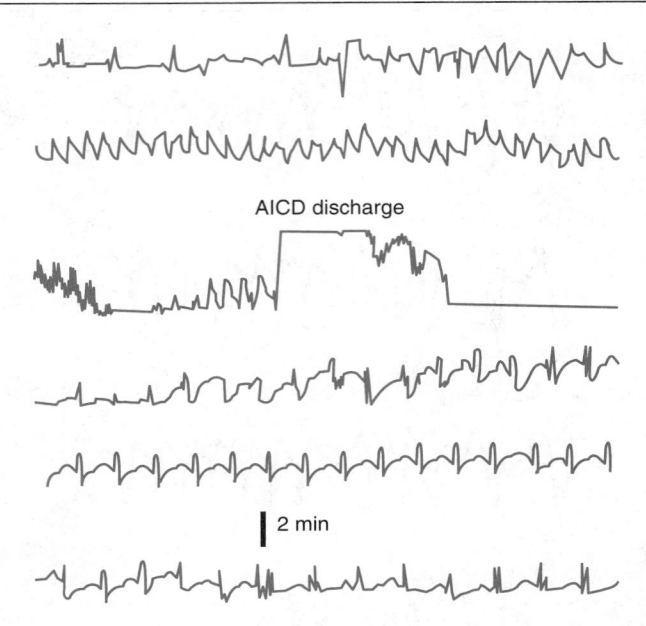

FIGURE 231-15 Normally functioning implantable defibrillators. A continuous Holter monitoring tracing is shown. On the top strip, a rapid polymorphic tachycardia is initiated which beats more uniformly. The automatic implantable cardioverter-defibrillator (AICD) senses the rhythm and delivers a shock which restores sinus rhythm.

Table 231-5

Dose, Serum Half-Life ($t_{1/2}$) Following Oral Administration, and Route of Metabolism of Drugs Used in Treatment of Arrhythmias

Drug	Mode of Administration	$t_{1/2}$ (Oral), h	Route of Metabolism
Digoxin	IV, 0.25–1.5 mg		Renal
	Oral, 0.75–1.5 mg loading dose over 12–24 h	36	
	Maintenance, 0.23–0.50 mg/d		
Propranolol	IV, 0.5–1 mg/min to total dose of 0.15–0.2 mg/kg		Hepatic
	Oral, 10–200 mg q 6 h	3–6	
Esmolol	IV, loading dose of 500 μg/kg/min for 1 min followed by maintenance infusion of 50 μg/kg/min for 4 min; if effect is inadequate, repeat load followed by maintenance of 100 μg/kg/min, up to a maximum maintenance of 200 μg/kg/min. $t_{1/2}$ I.V. = 9 min	NA	
Metoprolol	IV, load with 5–10 mg q 5 min for 3 doses, then 3 mg q 6 h	3–4	
	Oral, 25–100 mg bid		
Verapamil	IV, 2.5–10 mg over 1–2 min to total of 0.15 mg/kg		Hepatic
	Oral, 80–120 mg q 6–8 h	3–8	
Diltiazem	IV, load with 0.25 mg/kg over 2 min; if response is inadequate, repeat after 15 min with 0.35 mg over 2 min	NA	
	Maintenance dose is 10–15 mg/h		
	Oral, 180–360 mg qd or in divided dosages		
Quinidine	IV, 20 mg/min to total of 10–15 mg/kg		Hepatic: 80%
	Oral, 200–400 mg q 6 h	5–9	Renal: 20%
Procainamide	IV, 40–50 mg/min to total of 10–20 mg/kg		Hepatic: 50%
	Oral, 500–1000 mg q 4 h	3–5	Renal: 50%
Disopyramide	Oral, 100–300 mg q 6–8 h	8–9	Renal: 50%
			Hepatic: 50%
Lidocaine	IV, 20–50 mg/min to total of 5-mg/kg loading dose followed by 1–4 mg/kg	1–2	Hepatic: 100%
Phenytoin	IV, 20 mg/min total dose to 1000 mg		Hepatic
	Oral, 1000-mg loading over 24 h	18–36	
	Maintenance, 100–400 mg/d		
Tocainide	Oral, 400–600 mg q 8–12 h	10–17	Hepatic-renal
Bretylium	IV, 1–2 (mg/kg)/min to total of 5–10 mg/kg	8–14	Renal
	Maintenance, 0.5–2 mg/min		
Amiodarone	IV, 5–10 mg/kg		Unknown
	Oral, load 800–1400 mg/d for 1–2 weeks	Unknown	
	Maintenance, 100–600 mg/d		
Moricizine	Oral, 200–400 mg q 8 h	2–6	Hepatic
Propafenone	Oral, 450–900 mg q 8 h	5–8	Hepatic
Sotalol	Oral, 80–160 mg q 12 h for atrial fibrillation; up to 320 mg q 12 h for ventricular arrhythmias. Dose adjusted based on creatinine clearance	10–20	Renal: 90%
Adenosine	IV bolus, 6–12 mg	<10 s	
Mexiletine	Oral, 100–300 mg q 6–8 h	9–12	Hepatic: 100%
Flecainide	Oral, begin at 50–100 mg bid; increase by no more than 50 mg not more often than every 4 days to a maximum of 400 mg daily	7–23	Hepatic: 75%
			Renal: 25%

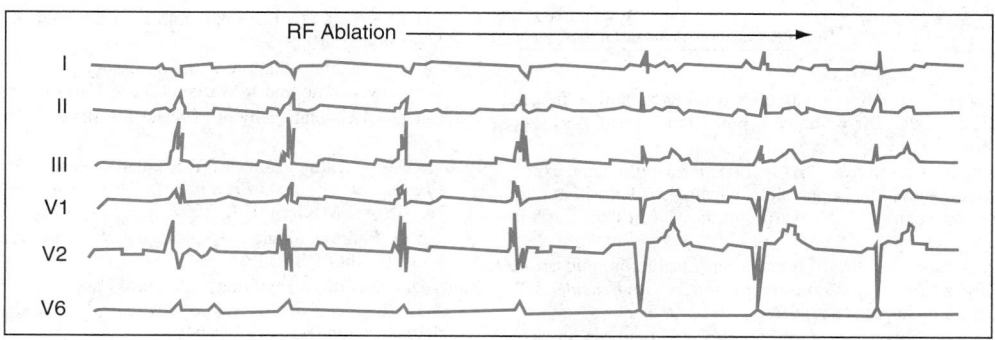

FIGURE 231-16 Radiofrequency ablation in Wolff-Parkinson-White syndrome. Leads I, II, III, V₁, V₂, and V₆ are shown. Preexcitation using a left lateral bypass tract is present in the final four complexes. Following the third complex, radiofrequency energy is applied. By the second beat, preexcitation is lost as the bypass tract is destroyed.

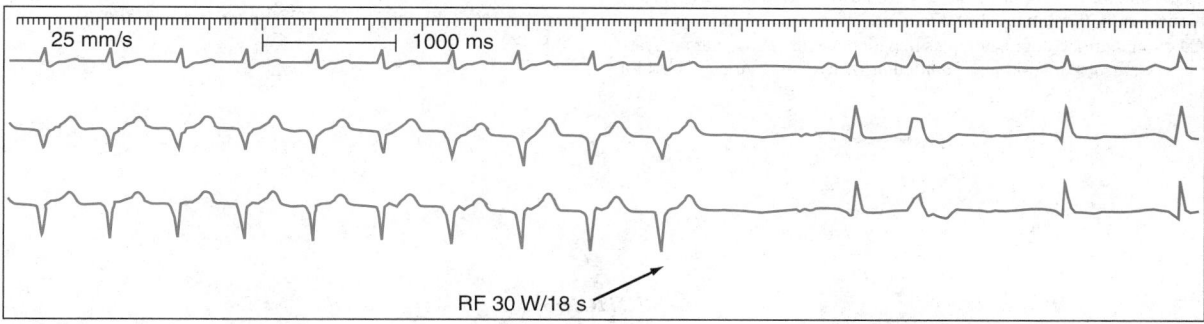

FIGURE 231-17 Radiofrequency ablation of idiopathic ventricular tachycardia in a patient with prior infarction. Leads I, II, and III are shown. Ventricular tachycardia with a right bundle branch block and left axis deviation is shown in a patient with a prior inferior wall infarction. Radiofrequency applied to the site of origin terminates the tachycardia.

duration (see Fig. 231-15). ICDs now can be implanted transvenously, and some are small enough to be implanted in a manner similar to pacemakers. Clinical trials testing the function of these devices in patients with drug-refractory ventricular arrhythmias have demonstrated survival from sudden death at 1 year ranging between 92 and 100 percent. Currently, ICDs should be considered for patients with VT that is not hemodynamically tolerated. They are also indicated for patients with cardiac arrest whose arrhythmias are refractory to drug therapy or in whom there are no good endpoints to assess drug efficacy.

The most frequent problem with the device has been its inappropriate discharge in the absence of sustained ventricular arrhythmias. Additional potential problems include an increase in defibrillation threshold and decrease in tachycardia rates below the rate cut-off of the device in response to many antiarrhythmic drugs. Permanently implanted ventricular pacemakers may interfere with the device's ability to sense VF. This can be avoided by using committed bipolar pacing systems. Diagnostic features of newer, all-in-one devices are able to identify the probable cause of an ICD discharge (e.g., AF, SVT, fractured lead) and to adjust pharmacologic therapy or reprogram the device to avoid such inappropriate shocks. These newer devices have the capability to take a "second look" prior to shock delivery and thus may abort delivery for self-terminating arrhythmias. In addition, the range of candidates suitable for implantation will be expanded because the newer devices have the capability of shock therapy for patients whose arrhythmias do not cause loss of consciousness.

ABLATIVE THERAPY FOR ARRHYTHMIAS Catheter-based mapping techniques have provided a nonoperative approach to the identification and cure of a variety of arrhythmias. In fact, catheter ablation techniques are now the procedures of choice for symptomatic patients with (1) concealed or manifest (WPW) bypass tracts, (2) AV nodal reentrant SVT, (3) typical atrial flutter, and (4) poorly controlled ventricular responses to atrial arrhythmias, most commonly AF. Successful ablation of bypass tracts and modifications of the AV node by radiofrequency energy are extremely successful and cost-effective and are the procedure of choice for patients with recurrent episodes (Fig. 231-16). The creation of AV block with implantation of a pacemaker is the method of choice in managing patients with AF and poorly controlled ventricular response. Idiopathic VTs (Fig. 231-17) that are associated with coronary artery disease are also amenable to ablation but the result is somewhat less successful.

Surgical therapy is now relegated to cases of sustained VT associated with coronary artery disease when operative intervention is needed for coronary bypass surgery and/or aneurysmectomy or VT associated with specific structural abnormalities (e.g., idiopathic left ventricle aneurysm, s/p surgery for tetralogy of Fallot). It also may be undertaken for the unusual instances of failed catheter ablation for SVTs associated with bypass tracts.

BIBLIOGRAPHY

ALMENDRAL J et al: The importance of antitachycardia pacing for patients presenting with ventricular tachycardia. Pacing Clin Electrophysiol 16:535, 1993

BAROLD SS, ZIPES DP: Cardiac pacemakers and antiarrhythmic devices, in *Heart Disease: A Textbook of Cardiovascular Medicine,* 5th ed, E Braunwald (ed). Philadelphia, Saunders, 1997, pp 705–741

BRUGADA J et al: The complexity of mechanisms in ventricular tachycardia. Pacing Clin Electrophysiol 16:680, 1993

CALKINS H et al: Diagnosis and cure of the Wolff-Parkinson-White syndrome or paroxysmal supraventricular tachycardias during a single electrophysiologic test. N Engl J Med 324:1612, 1991

COX JL: Surgical management of cardiac arrhythmias, in *Cardiac Pacing and Electrophysiology,* N El-Sherif, P Samet (eds). Philadelphia, Saunders, 1991, p 436

DREIFUS LS: Guidelines for implantation of cardiac pacemakers and antiarrhythmic devices: A report of the American College of Cardiology/American Heart Association Task Force on Assessment of Diagnostic and Therapeutic Cardiovascular Procedures (Committee on Pacemaker Implantation). J Am Coll Cardiol 18:1, 1991

ECHT DS et al: Mortality and morbidity in patients receiving encainide, flecainide, or placebo: The Cardiac Arrhythmia Suppression Trial (CAST). N Engl J Med 324:781, 1991

GUARDIAN MULTICENTER INVESTIGATORS GROUP: Long term multicenter experience with a second-generation implantable pacemaker-defibrillator in patients with malignant ventricular tachyarrhythmias. J Am Coll Cardiol 19:490, 1992

GUIRAUDON GM et al: Surgery for atrial flutter, atrial fibrillation, and atrial tachycardia, in *Cardiac Electrophysiology: From Cell to Bedside,* DP Zipes, J Jalife (eds). Philadelphia, Saunders, 1990, p 915

JACKMAN WM et al: Catheter ablation of accessory atrioventricular pathways (Wolff-Parkinson-White syndrome) by radiofrequency current. N Engl J Med 324:1605, 1991

JOSEPHSON ME: *Clinical Cardiac Electrophysiology,* 2d ed. Philadelphia, Lea & Febiger, 1993

KADISH A, GOLDBERGER J: Ablative therapy for atrioventricular nodal reentry arrhythmias. Prog Cardiovasc Dis 37:273, 1995

KIM YH et al: Nonpharmacologic therapies in patients with ventricular tachyarrhythmias. Catheter ablation and ventricular tachycardia surgery. Cardiol Clin 11:85, 1993

KUTALEK SP, DREIFUS LS: Implantable cardioverter-defibrillators. Adv Intern Med 38:421, 1993

PLUMB VJ: Catheter ablation of the accessory pathways of Wolff-Parkinson-White syndrome and its variants. Prog Cardiovasc Dis 37:295, 1995

PRITCHETT ELC: Management of atrial fibrillation. N Engl J Med 326:1264, 1991

RODEN DM: Treatment of cardiovascular diseases: Arrhythmias, in *Clinical Pharmacology: Basic Principles in Therapeutics,* KL Melmon et al (eds). New York, McGraw-Hill, 1992, pp 151–185

WYSE DG: Pharmacologic therapy in patients with ventricular tachyarrhythmias. Cardiol Clin 11:65, 1993

ZIPES DP: Specific arrhythmias: Diagnosis and treatment, in *Heart Disease: A Textbook of Cardiovascular Medicine,* 5th ed, E Braunwald (ed). Philadelphia, Saunders, 1997, p 640–704

———: Genesis of cardiac arrhythmias: Electrophysiological considerations, in *Heart Disease: A Textbook of Cardiovascular Medicine,* 5th ed, E Braunwald (ed). Philadelphia, Saunders, 1997, p 548–592

———: Management of cardiac arrhythmias: Pharmacological, electrical, and surgical techniques, in *Heart Disease: A Textbook of Cardiovascular Medicine,* 5th ed, E Braunwald (ed). Philadelphia, Saunders, 1997, p 593–639

SECTION 3

DISORDERS OF THE HEART

| 232 | *Eugene Braunwald* |

NORMAL AND ABNORMAL MYOCARDIAL FUNCTION

CELLULAR BASIS OF CARDIAC CONTRACTION

The *myocardium* is composed of individual striated muscle cells (fibers), normally 10 to 15 μm in diameter and 30 to 60 μm in length (Fig. 232-1*A*). Each fiber contains multiple cross-banded strands (myofibrils) that run the length of the fiber and are, in turn, composed of serially repeating structures, the sarcomeres. The cytoplasm between the myofibrils contains other cell constituents (Fig. 232-1*B*), such as the single centrally located nucleus, numerous mitochondria, and intracellular membrane system, the sarcoplasmic reticulum.

The *sarcomere,* the structural and functional unit of contraction, is delimited by two adjacent dark lines, the Z lines (Fig. 232-1*C*). The distance between Z lines varies with the degree of contraction or stretch of the muscle and ranges between 1.6 and 2.2 μm. Within the confines of the sarcomere are alternating light and dark bands, giving the myocardial fibers their striated appearance under the light microscope. At the center of the sarcomere is a dark band of constant length (1.5 μm), the A band, which is flanked by two lighter bands, the I bands, which are of variable length. The sarcomere of heart muscle, like that of skeletal muscle, is made up of two sets of interdigitating myofilaments (Fig. 232-1*D*). Thicker filaments, composed principally of the protein myosin, traverse and are limited to the A band. They are about 10 nm (100 Å) in diameter, with tapered ends, and measure 1.5 to 1.6 μm in length. Thinner filaments, composed primarily of actin, course from the Z line through the I band into the A band. They are approximately 5 nm (50 Å) in diameter and 1.0 μm in length. Thus there is overlapping of thick and thin filaments only within the A band, while the I band contains only thin filaments (Fig. 232-1*C*). On electron-microscopic examination, bridges may be seen to extend between the thick and thin filaments within the A band.

THE CONTRACTILE PROCESS The sliding model for muscle rests on the fundamental observation that the thick and thin filaments are constant in overall length during both contraction and relaxation. With activation, repeated interactions take place at the bridges between the actin and myosin filaments, and the actin filaments are propelled further into the A band. In the process, the A band remains constant in length, whereas the I band shortens and the Z lines move toward one another.

The *myosin* molecule is a complex, asymmetric fibrous protein with a molecular weight of about 500,000; it has a rodlike portion that is about 150 nm (1500 Å) in length with a globular portion at its end. This globular portion of the myosin is the site of adenosine triphosphatase (ATPase) activity and also forms the bridges between the myosin and actin. In forming the thick myofilament, which is composed of 300 longitudinally stacked myosin molecules, the rodlike segments of the myosin molecules are laid down in an orderly, polarized manner, leaving the globular portions projecting outward so that they can interact with actin to generate force and shortening (Fig. 232-2). *Actin* has a molecular weight of 47,000. The thin filament is composed of a double helix of two chains of actin molecules wound about each other on a larger molecule, tropomyosin, which serves as a "backbone" to the thin filament. A group of these regulatory proteins, troponins C, I, and T, are spaced at regular intervals on this filament (Fig. 232-3). In contrast to myosin, actin has no intrinsic enzymatic activity, but it has the ability to combine reversibly with myosin in the presence of ATP and Mg^{2+}, which activates the myosin ATPase. In relaxed muscle this interaction is inhibited by tropomyosin. *Titin* is a large, flexible, myofibrillar protein that connects myosin to the Z line. Its stretching is believed to contribute to the elasticity of the heart.

During activation of the myocyte, Ca^{2+} becomes attached to troponin C, which results in a conformational change in the regulatory protein tropomyosin, which in turn exposes the actin cross-bridge interaction sites. Repetitive interaction between myosin heads and actin filaments is termed *cross-bridge cycling,* which results in sliding of the actin along the myosin filaments, ultimately causing muscle shortening and/or the development of tension. The splitting of ATP then dissociates the myosin cross-bridge from the actin. In the presence of ATP (Fig. 232-2), linkages between actin and myosin filaments are made and broken cyclically as long as sufficient Ca^{2+} is present; these linkages are broken when Ca^{2+} concentration falls below a critical level, and the troponin-tropomyosin complex once more prevents interactions between the myosin cross-bridges and the actin filaments. Ionic calcium is a principal mediator of the inotropic state of the heart; most positive inotropic drugs, including the digitalis glycosides, beta-adrenergic agonists, and phosphodiesterase inhibitors, act by increasing the concentrations of Ca^{2+} in the vicinity of the myofilaments. Cyclic AMP enhances the phosphorylation of troponin I, a protein that accelerates cardiac relaxation.

The *sarcoplasmic reticulum* (Fig. 232-1*B*) is a complex network of anastomosing intracellular channels that invests the myofibrils. It is less profuse in cardiac than in skeletal muscle. Its longitudinally disposed membrane-lined tubules are closely applied to the surfaces of individual sarcomeres but have no direct continuity with the outside of the cell. However, closely related to the sarcoplasmic reticulum, both structurally and functionally, are the transverse tubules or T system, formed by tubelike invaginations of the sarcolemma that extend into the myocardial fiber along the Z lines, i.e., the ends of the sarcomeres.

CARDIAC ACTIVATION At rest, the cardiac cell is polarized; i.e., the interior has a negative charge relative to the outside of the cell, with a transmembrane potential of -80 to -100 mV (Chap. 230). The sarcolemma, which in the resting state is largely impermeable to Na^+, has a Na^+- and K^+-stimulating pump requiring ATP that extrudes Na^+ from the cell; the pump plays a critical role in establishing this resting potential. Thus, on the inside of the cell $[K^+]$ is relatively high and $[Na^+]$ is far lower, while in the extracellular milieu $[Na^+]$ is high and $[K^+]$ is low. At the same time, in the resting state, the extracellular $[Ca^{2+}]$ greatly exceeds the free intracellular $[Ca^{2+}]$.

During the plateau of the action potential (phase 2) there is a slow inward current that reflects primarily a movement of Ca^{2+} into the cell (Fig. 232-4), although the absolute quantity of Ca^{2+} that crosses the surface membrane is relatively small and itself appears to be incapable of bringing about full activation of the contractile apparatus. The depolarizing current not only extends across the surface of the cell but penetrates deeply into the cell by way of the ramifying T system; this current triggers the release of much larger quantities of Ca^{2+} from the sarcoplasmic reticulum, a process termed *regenerative release* of Ca^{2+}. This rise in intracellular Ca^{2+} is the key step in initiating myocyte contraction.

The Ca^{2+} released from the sarcoplasmic reticulum then diffuses toward the sarcomere and, as already described, combines with troponin C. By repressing this inhibitor of contraction, Ca^{2+} activates the myofilaments to produce contraction. During repolarization the

sarcoplasmic reticulum reaccumulates Ca^{2+} against a concentration gradient. This is an energy-requiring process that lowers the concentration of Ca^{2+} in the vicinity of the myofibrils to a level that inhibits the actin-myosin interaction responsible for contraction and in this manner leads to relaxation. Thus, the cell membrane, transverse tubules, and sarcoplasmic reticulum, with their ability to transmit an action potential, to release, and then to reaccumulate Ca^{2+}, appear to play a fundamental role in the rhythmic contraction and relaxation of heart muscle.

The ATP formed from substrate oxidation is the principal source of energy for almost all of the mechanical work of contraction performed by the myocardial cell. The high-energy phosphate stores in ATP are in equilibrium with those in the form of creatine phosphate.

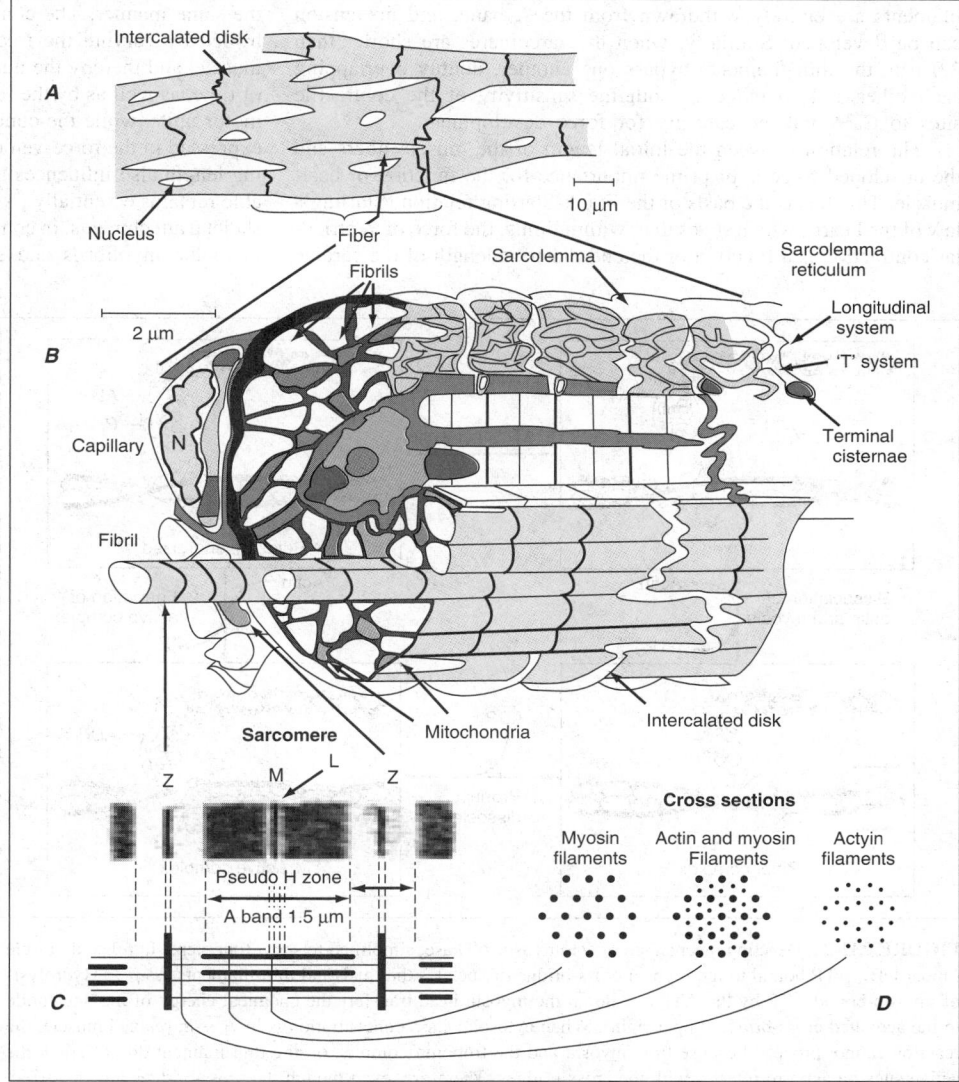

FIGURE 232-1 Microscopic structure of heart muscle. *A.* Myocardium as seen under the light microscope. Branching of fibers is evident. Each fiber, or cell, contains a centrally located nucleus. *B.* Myocardial cell, reconstructed from electron micrographs. Each cell is composed of multiple parallel fibrils. Each fibril is composed of serially connected sarcomeres (N, nucleus). *C.* Sarcomere from a myofibril, with diagrammatic representation of myofilaments. Thick filaments (1.5 μm long, composed of myosin) form the A band, and thin filaments (1 μm long, composed primarily of actin) extend from the Z line through the I band into the A band. The overlapping of thick and thin filaments is seen only in the A band. *D.* Cross sections of the sarcomere indicate the specific lattice arrangements of the myofilaments. In the center of the sarcomere only the thick, or myosin, filaments arranged in a hexagonal array are seen. In the distal portions of the A band, both thick and thin, or actin, filaments are found, with each thick filament surrounded by six thin filaments. In the I band only thin filaments are present. (*From E Braunwald et al, Mechanisms of Contraction of the Normal and Failing Heart, Boston, Little, Brown, 1968.*)

muscle, which in turn is closely related to the ventricular end-diastolic volume.

The activity of myosin ATPase determines the rate of forming and breaking of the actin-myosin cross-bridges and ultimately the velocity of muscle contraction.

THE ROLE OF MUSCLE LENGTH In all striated muscle, including cardiac muscle, the force of contraction depends on initial muscle length. The sarcomere length associated with the most forceful contraction is approximately 2.2 μm. At this length the two sets of myofilaments of the sarcomere are situated so as to provide the greatest area for their interaction. The length of the sarcomere also appears to regulate the extent of activation of the contractile system, i.e., its sensitivity to Ca^{2+}. According to this concept, termed *length-dependent activation*, at the optimal sarcomere length of 2.2 μm the myofilament sensitivity to Ca^{2+} is maximal. When sarcomere length is increased to 3.65 μm, the thin filaments are entirely withdrawn from the A band, and no tension can be developed. Similarly, when the sarcomeres are shorter than 2.0 μm, the thin filaments bypass one another, doubly overlapping each other and so reducing both the sensitivity of the contractile sites to Ca^{2+} and the capacity for force development.

The relation between the initial length of the muscle fibers and the developed force is of prime importance for the function of heart muscle. This forms the basis of the Frank-Starling relation (Starling's law of the heart), which states that, within limits, the force of ventricular contraction is a function of the end-diastolic length of the cardiac

MYOCARDIAL MECHANICS

THE FORCE-VELOCITY CURVE The mechanical activity of all striated muscle may be expressed externally in two ways: shortening and the development of tension. Hill showed in skeletal muscle that the velocity of shortening is inversely related to the tension development, an expression of the so-called force-velocity relation, now recognized to be a fundamental property of muscle. Expressed simply, the greater the load the muscle is called upon to lift, the lower the velocity of shortening and vice versa. The force-velocity relation also applies to cardiac muscle. However, in this respect there is a basic difference between skeletal and cardiac muscle. Skeletal muscle fibers have a single, essentially fixed, force-velocity curve; i.e., at any given muscle length, force and velocity are always related to each other in the same manner. The contractile activity of skeletal muscle is controlled by varying the frequency of nerve impulses stimulating the muscle, and thereby the number of contractions of each fiber per unit of time, as well as by the recruitment of additional muscle fibers, i.e., motor units, while the contractile properties of each individual fiber, expressed in the force-velocity curve, remain constant. Although resting length also influences the characteristics of contraction, this variable remains essentially fixed in vivo because of the skeletal muscles' skeletal attachments. In contrast, the number of cardiac cells and within them the myofibrils and sarcomeres that become activated during each contraction is constant. However, the contractile activity of the myocardium is readily altered under physiologic conditions by changes in resting fiber length and by changes in the inotropic state, i.e., the contractility, both of which shift the myocardial force-velocity curve. Many neurohumoral influences affect contractility, but the most important influence is the adrenergic nervous system operating via its neurotransmitter, norepinephrine.

Cardiac muscle exhibits an inverse relation between the force against which it contracts, i.e., the afterload, and the extent and velocity of shortening. The myocardial force-velocity curve obtained in isolated heart muscle represents this inverse relation and can be used to describe myocardial performance.

VENTRICULAR EJECTION AND FILLING

Analysis of the heart as a pump has classically centered on the relation between the end-diastolic volume of the ventricle (which is related to the length of the muscle fibers) and its stroke volume (the Frank-Starling relation). The end-diastolic or "filling" pressure of the ventricle is sometimes used as a surrogate for the end-diastolic volume. In the heart-lung preparation the stroke volume within limits correlates directly with the diastolic fiber length (preload) and inversely with the arterial resistance (afterload), and the failing heart delivers a smaller-than-normal stroke volume from a normal or elevated end-diastolic volume. The relation between the ven-

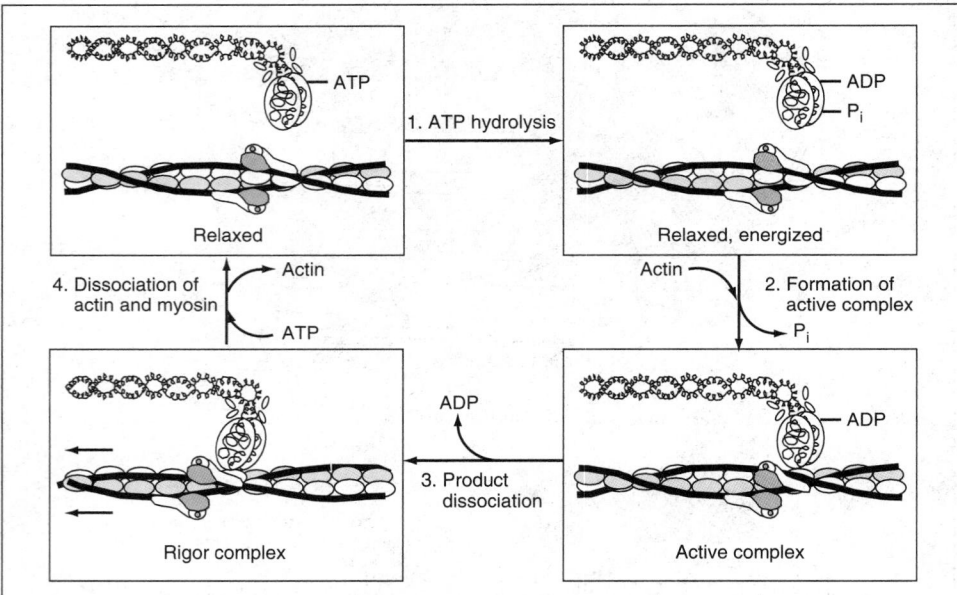

FIGURE 232-2 Reaction mechanism of actomyosin ATPase, simplified to show four steps. In relaxed muscle (upper left), ATP bound to the myosin cross-bridge dissociates the thick and thin filaments. *Step 1:* Hydrolysis of myosin-bound ATP by the ATPase site on the myosin head transfers the chemical energy of the nucleotide to the activated cross-bridge (upper right). When cytosolic Ca^{2+} concentration is low, as in relaxed muscle, the reaction cannot proceed because tropomyosin and the troponin complex on the thin filament do not allow the active sites on actin to interact with the cross-bridges. Therefore, even though the cross-bridges are energized, they cannot interact with actin. *Step 2:* When Ca^{2+} binding to troponin C has exposed active sites on the thin filament, actin interacts with the myosin cross-bridges to form an active complex (lower right) in which the energy derived from ATP is retained in the actin-bound cross-bridge, whose orientation has not yet shifted. *Step 3:* The muscle contracts when ADP dissociates from the cross-bridge; this step leads to the formation of the low-energy rigor complex (lower left), in which the chemical energy derived from ATP hydrolysis has been expended to perform mechanical work (the "rowing" motion of the cross-bridge). *Step 4:* The muscle returns to its resting state, and the cycle ends when a new molecule of ATP binds to the rigor complex and dissociates the cross-bridge from the thin filament. This cycle continues until calcium is dissociated from troponin C in the thin filament, which causes the contractile proteins to return to the resting state with the cross-bridge in the energized state. *[From AM Katz, in WS Colucci (ed), Heart Failure: Cardiac Function and Dysfunction, in Atlas of Heart Diseases, vol 4, E Braunwald (series ed), Philadelphia, Current Medicine, 1995.]*

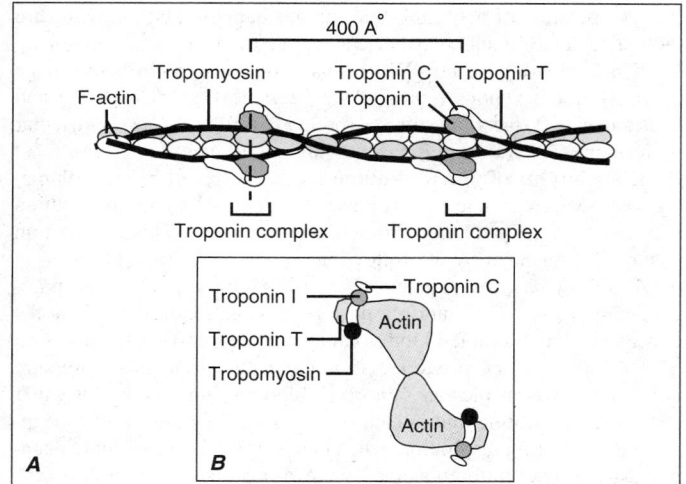

FIGURE 232-3 Structure of the thin filament. *A.* The "backbone" of the thin filament, seen in a longitudinal view, is F-actin, which contains two strands of actin monomers (light blue and white). Troponin complexes, made up of one molecule each of troponin C, troponin I, and troponin T, are distributed at approximately 400-Å intervals along the thin filament. Elongated tropomyosin molecules (solid) lie in the grooves between the two actin strands. *B.* A cross section of the thin filament at the level where the troponin complexes are located shows probable relationships between actin, tropomyosin, and the three components of the troponin complex. The strength of the bond linking troponin I and actin varies, depending on whether Ca^{2+} is bound to troponin C. *[From AM Katz: Molecular and cellular basis of contraction, in WS Colucci (ed): Heart Failure: Cardiac Function and Dysfunction, in E Braunwald (Series ed): Atlas of Heart Diseases, vol 4. Philadelphia, Current Medicine, 1995, p 1.5. Adapted from Katz. With permission of the publisher.]*

tricular end-diastolic pressure and the stroke work of the ventricle (the ventricular function curve) provides a useful definition of the level of the contractile, or inotropic, state of the ventricle. An increase in ventricular contractility is accompanied by a shift of the ventricular function curve upward and to the left [greater stroke work at any level of ventricular end-diastolic pressure (or volume), or lower end-diastolic pressure at any level of stroke work], while depression of contractility is characterized by a shift downward and to the right.

During the adrenergic stimulation of the myocardium accompanying exercise, relatively little change in ventricular end-diastolic volume occurs, while cardiac output, aortic flow velocity, stroke work, and the rate of ventricular pressure development are all augmented, sometimes greatly, reflecting an increase in myocardial contractility.

The important influence of the adrenergic neurotransmitter, norepinephrine (Chap. 70), on the mechanical properties of the myocardium has long been recognized. Direct stimulation of the cardiac adrenergic nerves augments ventricular function as a consequence of the release of norepinephrine from adrenergic nerve endings in the heart. Norepinephrine activates myocardial beta receptors and thereby increases the concentration of cyclic AMP (see Fig. 232-9, p. 1286). The latter, in turn, causes a more rapid, forceful contraction by phosphorylating the Ca^{2+} channel in the myocardial sarcolemma, thereby enhancing the influx of Ca^{2+} into the myocyte which, in turn, acts on the contractile apparatus, as described on p. 1279. The adrenergic effects are evidenced by tachycardia, a reduction in cardiac dimensions, increased velocity of ejection, and an enhanced rate of tension development.

ASSESSMENT OF CARDIAC FUNCTION Several techniques are available for defining impaired cardiac function in patients. With the patient at rest, the cardiac output and stroke volume may be depressed, but not uncommonly these variables are within normal limits, even in the presence of heart failure. A more sensitive index is the ejection fraction, i.e., the ratio of stroke volume to end-diastolic

volume (normal value $= 67 \pm 8$ percent), which may be estimated by radiocontrast or radionuclide angiography or echocardiography and which is frequently depressed in systolic heart failure even when the stroke volume itself is normal. Alternatively, the detection of abnormally elevated ventricular end-diastolic volumes (normal value $= 70 \pm 20$ mL/m^2) in the presence of a normal or presumably normal stroke volume signifies impairment of left ventricular systolic function. A limitation of the measurement of cardiac output, ejection fraction, and ventricular volume in the assessment of cardiac function is that these variables are influenced strongly by ventricular loading conditions. Thus, a depressed ejection fraction and lowered cardiac output may be observed in patients with normal ventricular function but reduced preload, as occurs in hypovolemia, or with increased afterload, as occurs in acutely elevated arterial pressure.

The end-systolic left ventricular pressure-volume relationship is a particularly useful index of ventricular performance since it is independent of both preload and afterload. At any level of myocardial contractility, left ventricular end-systolic volume varies inversely with end-systolic pressure; as contractility declines, end-systolic volume (at any level of end-systolic pressure) rises. Noninvasive techniques, particularly echocardiography and radionuclide angiography, are of great value in the clinical assessment of myocardial function. They provide measurements of end-systolic volume (or end-systolic dimension) that can be related to systolic arterial pressure also determined noninvasively. In addition, they provide convenient measurements of ejection fraction and systolic shortening rate and allow measurement of ventricular filling (see below).

Exercise A useful technique for evaluating ventricular performance involves the measurement of the circulatory changes occurring during exercise. Thus, left ventricular performance may be estimated accurately by measuring the left ventricular end-diastolic pressure, cardiac output, and total-body O_2 consumption at rest and during exercise. In persons with normal cardiac function, the cardiac output rises by more than 500 mL/min for each 100-mL increase in minute O_2 consumption. The left ventricular end-diastolic pressure at rest is less than 12 mmHg and rises slightly, remains unchanged, or decreases slightly during exercise, while stroke volume usually rises, especially when exercise is carried out in the upright position. The failing left ventricle, on the other hand, is characterized by an elevation of end-diastolic pressure during exercise to above 12 mmHg, accompanied by either no change or a fall in stroke volume and a subnormal increase in cardiac output related to the increase in minute O_2 consumption. The overall performance of the cardiopulmonary system in delivering oxygen to the metabolizing tissue can be estimated by measuring the maximal O_2 consumption achieved during escalating treadmill exercise ($\dot{V}max_{O_2}$). Normal values exceed 20 mL/min per kilogram body weight, while values under 10 mL/min per kilogram represent severe impairment of function, usually seen in patients with severe heart failure and a poor prognosis.

The potential value of stressing the left ventricle in assessing its performance is emphasized by the fact that the normal range of left ventricular end-diastolic pressure, cardiac index, and ventricular stroke work in the resting state is wide, with values that frequently overlap those seen in patients with ventricular dysfunction. The response to stress may prove useful not only in the detection of the impairment of myocardial function but also in expressing the severity of such impairment quantitatively.

Diastolic Performance This important variable is best assessed by continuously measuring the flow velocity across the mitral valve using Doppler echocardiography. Normally, the flow velocity is more rapid in early diastole than during atrial systole; with impaired relaxation the rate of early diastolic filling declines, while the rate of presystolic filling rises. With severe impairment of filling the pattern is "pseudo-normalized" and early ventricular filling becomes more rapid as left atrial pressure upstream to the stiff left ventricle rises (Fig. 232-5).

CONTROL OF CARDIAC PERFORMANCE AND OUTPUT

The extent of shortening of mammalian heart muscle and, therefore, the stroke volume of the intact ventricle are determined by three influences: (1) the length of the muscle at the onset of contraction, i.e., the preload; (2) the inotropic state of the muscle, i.e., the position of its force-velocity-length relation; and (3) the tension that the muscle is called upon to develop during contraction, i.e., the afterload. Heart rate determines the cardiac output at any stroke volume as long as the other three influences are maintained. Ventricular filling is influenced by the extent and speed of myocardial relaxation, which in turn is determined by the rate of uptake of Ca^{2+} by the sarcoplasmic reticulum; the latter may be augmented by positive inotropic stimuli and reduced by ischemia. Filling may be impeded by the stiffness of the ventricular wall, which may be increased by ventricular hypertrophy and conditions that infiltrate the myocardium, or by an extrinsic constraint (e.g., pericardial compression).

VENTRICULAR END-DIASTOLIC VOLUME (PRELOAD) At any level of inotropic state and afterload, the performance of the myocardium is influenced profoundly by ventricular end-diastolic fiber length and therefore by diastolic ventricular volume,

i.e., by operation of the Frank-Starling mechanism. The following are the major determinants of ventricular preload in the intact organism:

Total Blood Volume When this is depleted, as in hemorrhage or dehydration, venous return to the heart declines (Chap. 38) and ventricular end-diastolic volume (preload) falls, as does ventricular performance, as reflected in stroke volume and ventricular work.

Distribution of Blood Volume At any given blood volume, the ventricular end-diastolic volume is influenced by its distribution between the intra- and extrathoracic compartments. This distribution in turn is influenced by the following:

1. *Body position.* Gravitational forces tend to pool blood in dependent portions. Thus, upright posture augments extrathoracic at the expense of intrathoracic blood volume and reduces ventricular work.

2. *Intrathoracic pressure.* Normally, mean intrathoracic pressure is negative, which increases thoracic blood volume and ventricular end-diastolic volume and enhances the return of blood to the heart, particularly during inspiration, when this pressure becomes more negative. Elevation of intrathoracic pressure, as occurs during the Valsalva maneuver or prolonged bouts of coughing or with positive-pressure ventilation, tends to impede venous return, diminish intrathoracic blood volume, and ultimately reduce stroke volume and ventricular work.

3. *Intrapericardial pressure.* When this pressure is elevated, as in pericardial tamponade (Chap. 240), there is interference with cardiac filling, and the resultant reduction in ventricular diastolic volume reduces stroke volume and ventricular work.

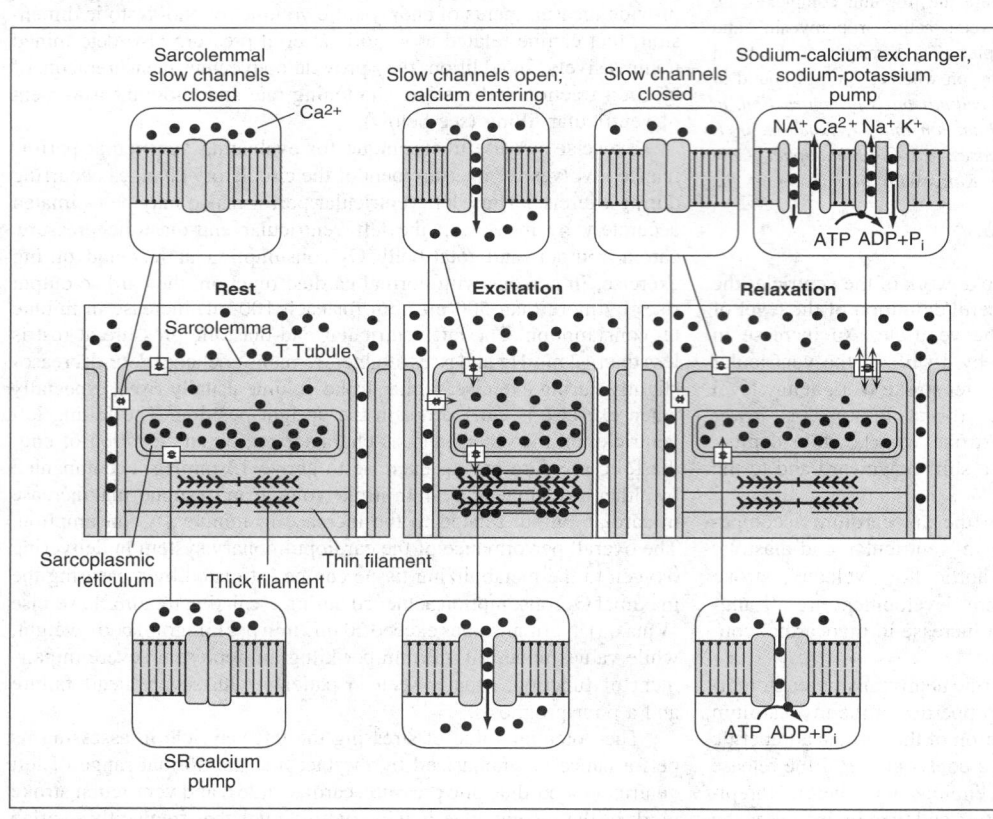

FIGURE 232-4 Calcium fluxes that activate contraction are downhill, and those that cause relaxation are uphill. As depicted in heart muscle at rest, calcium channels in the sarcolemmal membrane are closed; intracellular calcium is stored in the sarcoplasmic reticulum. With excitation and membrane depolarization, voltage-sensitive sodium channels (not shown) and calcium channels in the sarcolemma open to allow rapid entry of extracellular sodium and calcium. Entry of calcium is believed to cause release of calcium from the sarcoplasmic reticulum that initiates contraction. Reuptake of calcium by the sarcoplasmic reticulum by an ATP-dependent calcium pump is essential for the heart to relax. Importantly, contraction is activated mainly by passive calcium fluxes from the sarcoplasmic reticulum. By contrast, during diastole calcium must be pumped out of the cytosol to accomplish relaxation. Energy also must be expended during diastole to restore sodium and calcium gradients across the sarcolemma, which provide for the depolarizing ionic currents that generate the action potential. Sodium transport is accomplished by the sarcolemmal sodium pump (Na^+, K^+-ATPase), which utilizes ATP to pump sodium out of the cell in exchange for potassium. The resultant sodium gradient is largely responsible for active transport of calcium out of the cell during relaxation, via sodium-calcium exchange. [*Reproduced by permission from AM Katz, VE Smith, Hosp Prac, 19(1):69, 1984. Illustration by Bunji Tagawa.*]

4. *Venous tone.* The venous system is not a simple system of passive conduits between the systemic capillary bed and the right atrium. Instead, the smooth muscle in the walls of the venules and veins responds to a variety of neural and humoral stimuli. Venoconstriction occurs during muscular exercise, deep respiration, fright, or marked hypotension, tending to diminish extrathoracic and to augment intrathoracic and intraventricular blood volumes and ventricular performance.

5. *The pumping action of skeletal muscle.* During muscular exercise the contracting skeletal muscles squeeze blood out of the venous bed and, with the aid of the venous valves, displace it centrally, thereby increasing intrathoracic blood volume, ventricular end-diastolic volume, and ventricular work.

Atrial Contraction Vigorous, appropriately timed atrial contraction augments ventricular filling and end-diastolic volume. The atrial contribution to ventricular filling, the so-called atrial kick, is of particular importance in patients with concentric ventricular hypertrophy, in whom the loss of atrial systole (as in atrial fibrillation) tends to reduce ventricular end-diastolic pressure and volume, ultimately lowering myocardial performance. The atrial contribution to ventricular filling may also be reduced by atrioventricular dissociation, prolongation or abbreviation of the P-R interval, and depression of the inotropic state of the atrium.

INOTROPIC STATE (MYOCARDIAL CONTRACTILITY) A number of factors determine

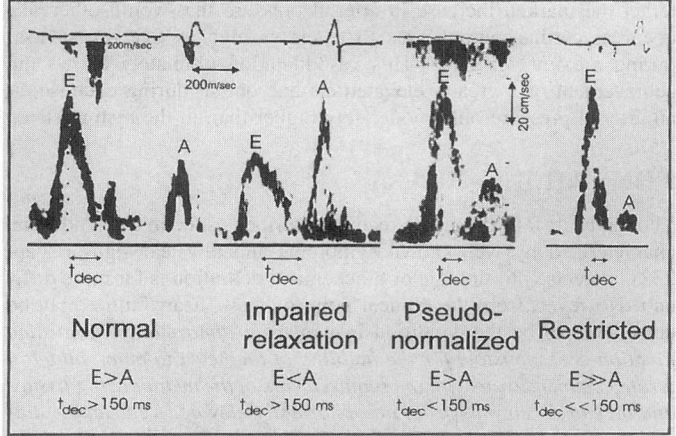

FIGURE 232-5 Patterns of left ventricular filling, as recorded by diastolic Doppler mitral flow velocities. In the normal pattern there is a large E wave and a small A wave. There are three abnormal patterns of mitral filling representing progressively worsening left ventricular diastolic performance. With "impaired relaxation" the E wave is less than the A wave. In the "pseudonormalized" pattern the E wave is larger than the A wave. In the "restricted" filling pattern E is much larger than A with a very short t_{dec}. *(From Little and Braunwald.)*

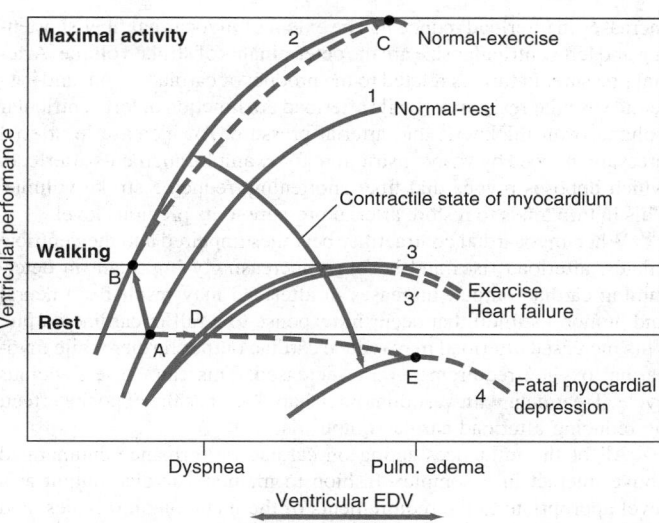

FIGURE 232-6 Diagram showing the interrelations among influences on ventricular end-diastolic volume (EDV) through stretching of the myocardium and the contractile state of the myocardium. Levels of ventricular EDV associated with filling pressures that result in dyspnea and pulmonary edema are shown on the abscissa. Levels of ventricular performance required when the subject is at rest, while walking, and during maximal activity are designated on the ordinate. The broken lines are the descending limbs of the ventricular-performance curves, which are rarely seen during life but which show the level of ventricular performance if end-diastolic volume could be elevated to very high levels. For further explanation see text. *(Modified from E Braunwald et al, Mechanisms of Contraction of the Normal and Failing Heart, Boston, Little, Brown, 1968.)*

the level of ventricular performance at any given ventricular end-diastolic volume, i.e., the position of the ventricular function curve (Fig. 232-6). These influences may be considered to operate by modifying myocardial force-velocity relations. In the final analysis, most of these influences act by altering the concentration of Ca^{2+} in the vicinity of the myofilaments, which in turn trigger cross-bridge cycling (p. 1279).

Adrenergic Nerve Activity (See also Chap. 70) The quantity of norepinephrine released by adrenergic nerve endings in the heart is determined by the adrenergic nerve impulse traffic; alterations in the frequency of these nerve impulses modify the quantity of norepinephrine released and acting on the beta-adrenergic receptors in the myocardium. This mechanism is the most important one that acutely modifies the myocardial contractility under physiologic conditions.

Circulating Catecholamines (See also Chap. 70) When it is stimulated by adrenergic nerve impulse, the adrenal medulla releases catecholamines, which, when they reach the heart, augment the inotropic state and the frequency of contraction.

The Force-Frequency Relation The position of the myocardial force-velocity curve also is influenced by the rate and rhythm of cardiac contraction; e.g., ventricular extrasystoles result in postextrasystolic potentiation, presumably by increasing the Ca^{2+} that enters the cardiac cell. The contractility of the normal (but not of the failing) heart is augmented by an increase in frequency.

Exogenously Administered Inotropic Agents Isoproterenol, dopamine, dobutamine, and other sympathomimetic agents, cardiac glycosides, calcium, amrinone, milrinone, and other phosphodiesterase inhibitors all improve the myocardial force-velocity relation and therefore may be used to stimulate ventricular performance.

Physiologic Depressants Included among these are severe myocardial hypoxia, ischemia, and acidosis. Acting either singly or in combination, these influences depress the myocardial force-velocity curve and left ventricular work at any given ventricular end-diastolic volume.

Pharmacologic Depressants These include procainamide, disopyramide, calcium antagonists such as verapamil, beta blockers, and large doses of barbiturates, alcohol, and general anesthetics as well as many other drugs.

Loss of Myocytes When a sufficiently large portion of ventricular myocardium becomes nonfunctional or necrotic, as occurs transiently during ischemia (Chap. 244) and permanently in myocardial infarction (Chap. 243), total ventricular performance at any given level of end-diastolic volume becomes depressed. Programmed cell death (apoptosis) can cause scattered loss of myocytes and, when

sufficiently widespread, can impair ventricular function and cause heart failure.

Intrinsic Myocardial Depression Although the fundamental mechanisms responsible for depression of myocardial contractility in most cases of chronic congestive heart failure secondary to prolonged ventricular overload or cardiomyopathy remain to be elucidated (p. 1287), it is now apparent that in this condition the inotropic state of individual surviving myocytes is depressed, and as a consequence the ventricular performance at any ventricular preload and afterload is lowered.

VENTRICULAR AFTERLOAD The stroke volume is ultimately a function of the extent of ventricular fiber shortening. In the intact heart, as in isolated cardiac muscle, extent (and velocity) of shortening of ventricular muscle fibers at any level of diastolic fiber length (preload) and myocardial inotropic state are inversely related to the afterload, i.e., the load that opposes shortening. In the intact heart the afterload may be defined as the tension or stress developed in the ventricular wall during ejection. Therefore, the afterload is determined by the aortic pressure as well as the volume and thickness of the ventricular cavity. Laplace's law indicates that the tension of the myocardial fiber is a function of the product of the intracavitary ventricular pressure and ventricular radius divided by the wall thickness. Therefore, at any given level of aortic pressure, the afterload faced by a dilated left ventricle of normal thickness is higher than that encountered by a ventricle of normal size. Conversely, at the same aortic pressure and ventricular diastolic volume, the afterload of a thick-walled ventricle is lower than of a thin-walled chamber. The aortic pressure is determined by the peripheral vascular resistance, the physical characteristics of the arterial tree, and the volume of blood it contains at the onset of ejection.

The critical role played by the ventricular afterload in cardiovascular regulation is shown in Fig. 232-7. As already noted, increases in both preload and contractility increase myocardial fiber shortening, while increases in afterload reduce it. The extent of myocardial fiber shortening and left ventricular size are the determinants of stroke volume. Arterial pressure, in turn, is related to the product of cardiac output and systemic vascular resistance, while afterload is a function of left ventricular volume, wall thickness, and arterial pressure. An increase in arterial pressure induced by vasoconstriction, for example, augments afterload, which opposes myocardial fiber shortening, reducing stroke volume. This in turn tends to restore arterial pressure to its previous level.

When myocardial contractility becomes impaired and the ventricle dilates, afterload rises and becomes increasingly important in determining cardiac output. Increases in afterload may result from neural and humoral stimuli that occur in response to a fall in cardiac output. This increased afterload may reduce cardiac output further while myocardial oxygen requirements are increased. This can cause a vicious cycle. Treatment with vasodilators (Chap. 233) has the opposite effect; by reducing afterload cardiac output rises.

All of the influences acting on cardiac performance enumerated above interact in a complex fashion to maintain cardiac output at a level appropriate to the requirements of the metabolizing tissues, and in a normal person interference with any one of these mechanisms may not influence the cardiac output. For example, a moderate reduction of blood volume *or* the loss of the atrial contribution to ventricular contraction can ordinarily be sustained without a reduction in the cardiac output at rest. Other factors, such as increases in the frequency of adrenergic nerve impulses to the heart and in heart rate, will, in a normal individual, serve as compensatory mechanisms, augment contractility, and sustain cardiac output. In individuals with normal hearts, the preload, which in turn is related to the volume of blood available for filling the heart, rather than the inotropic state of the myocardium or the afterload limits cardiac output. An improvement of myocardial contractility or the reduction of afterload with nitroprusside causes little elevation of the cardiac output in normal individuals. On the other hand, in the presence of congestive heart failure, the cardiac output usually is limited by the depression of myocardial contractility and a positive inotropic drug and/or reduction of afterload raises cardiac output (Chap. 233).

EXERCISE The hemodynamic changes that occur normally during exercise in the upright position are complex (Fig. 232-6). The hyperventilation, the pumping action of the exercising muscles, and the venoconstriction during exercise all tend to augment venous return and hence ventricular filling and preload. Simultaneously, the increase in the adrenergic nerve impulses to the myocardium, the increased concentration of circulating catecholamines, and the tachycardia that all occur during exercise combine to augment the contractile state of the myocardium (Fig. 232-6, curves 1 and 2) and lead to an elevation of stroke work and stroke volume, with no change or even a decrease of end-diastolic pressure and volume (Fig. 232-6, points A and B). Vasodilatation occurs in the exercising muscles, thus tending to counteract the marked increase in arterial pressure that would otherwise occur as cardiac output rises to levels as high as five times basal during maximal exercise. This vasodilatation ultimately allows the achievement of a greatly elevated cardiac output during exercise, at an arterial pressure only moderately higher than in the resting state.

THE FAILING HEART

Though heart failure may be readily described as a clinical syndrome, characterized by well-known symptoms and physical signs (Chap. 233), a precise physiologic or biochemical definition is far more difficult. However, from the clinical point of view, heart failure may be considered to be the condition in which *an abnormality of cardiac function is responsible for the inability of the heart to pump blood at a rate commensurate with the requirements of the metabolizing tissues and/or can do so only from an abnormally elevated ventricular diastolic volume.* Abnormalities during systole and/or diastole may be present in heart failure (Fig. 232-8). In so-called *systolic heart failure* (p. 1288), an impairment of myocardial contractility causes weakened systolic contraction, which leads, ultimately, to a reduction in stroke volume, inadequate ventricular emptying, cardiac dilatation, and often elevation of ventricular diastolic pressure. Idiopathic dilated cardiomyopathy (Chap. 239) is the prototype of systolic heart failure.

In *diastolic heart failure* (p. 1288) the principal abnormality is impaired relaxation and filling of the ventricle and leads to an elevation of ventricular diastolic pressure at any given diastolic volume. Failure of relaxation can be functional and transient, as during ischemia, while impaired ventricular filling can be caused by a stiffened, thickened ventricle (Fig. 232-5). Typical conditions in which diastolic failure occurs are restrictive cardiomyopathy secondary to infiltrative conditions, such as amyloidosis or hemochromatosis, as well as hypertrophic cardiomyopathy (Chap. 239). The concentric hypertrophy associated with chronic hypertension can also impair ventricular filling but rarely causes overt heart failure. In many patients with cardiac hypertrophy and dilatation, systolic and diastolic failure coexist; the ventricle both empties and fills abnormally. There may be cardiac dilatation, but the ventricle's pressure-volume relation is shifted, raising the ventricular diastolic pressure at any given volume.

Though a defect in myocardial contraction is characteristic of systolic heart failure, this defect may result from a primary abnormality in the heart muscle, as in cardiomyopathy, or it may be secondary to a chronic excessive work load as in hypertension or valvular heart disease. In ischemic heart disease systolic heart failure results from a loss in the quantity of normally contracting cells (secondary to myocardial infarction) or from transient loss of function in reversibly impaired myocardium.

It is important to distinguish heart failure from (1) states of circulatory insufficiency in which myocardial function is not primarily impaired, such as cardiac tamponade or hemorrhagic shock; (2) conditions in which there is circulatory congestion because of abnormal salt and water retention but in which there is no serious disturbance of the heart's function, such as in acute glomerulonephritis; and (3) conditions in which a normal myocardium is suddenly presented with a load that exceeds its capacity, such as accelerated hypertension or rupture of a valve cusp secondary to infective endocarditis.

ADAPTIVE MECHANISMS A number of mechanisms aid the heart faced with an increased hemodynamic burden, such as pressure or volume overload, or which has sustained loss of myocardium. These adaptive mechanisms include: (1) the Frank-Starling mechanism operating through an increase in preload (p. 1280); (2) the development of myocardial hypertrophy, which restores elevated ventricular wall stress to normal; (3) redistribution of a subnormal cardiac output away from the skin, skeletal muscle, and kidneys with maintenance of blood flow to vital organs such as the

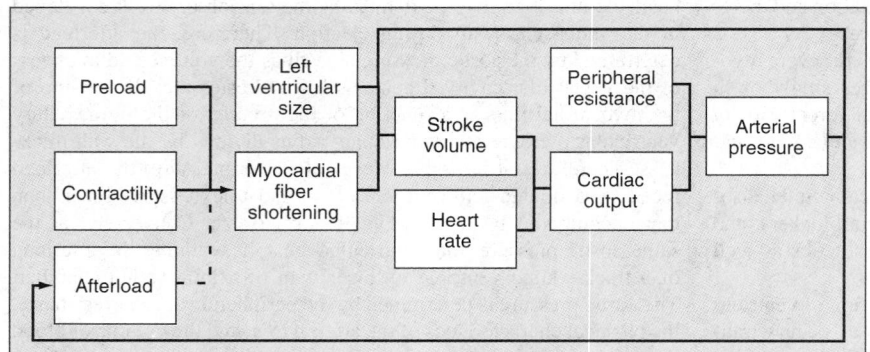

FIGURE 232-7 Scheme of interactions among various components that regulate cardiac activity. Solid lines indicate an augmenting effect; broken line represents an inhibiting effect. (*From E Braunwald, N Engl J Med 290:1124–1129, 1420–1425, 1974.*)

brain and the heart itself; and (4) neurohumoral adjustments, which tend to maintain arterial pressure and are discussed on p. 1283 and in Chap. 70.

The contractility of strips of myocardium removed from failing animal hearts has been shown to be depressed soon after the imposition of a pressure overload. The laying down of additional myofibrils (compensatory hypertrophy) often restores contractility to normal, but when the overload is maintained for prolonged periods, myocardial contractility again declines. Myocytes isolated from the left ventricles of patients with heart failure secondary to dilated cardiomyopathy exhibit reduced shortening.

The failing ventricle may still eject a normal or nearly normal stroke volume despite considerable depression of function through an increase in preload (end-diastolic volume), i.e., through the operation of the Frank-Starling mechanism. As outlined above (p. 1280), an increase in the initial volume of the ventricle is associated with stretching of the sarcomere, which increases the interaction between actin and myosin filaments and their sensitivity to Ca^{2+}.

BIOCHEMICAL ABNORMALITIES IN HEART FAILURE There is no unifying theory providing a biochemical basis for heart failure. The common forms of low-output heart failure, secondary to coronary atherosclerosis, hypertension, cardiomyopathy, and certain valvular and congenital lesions, are characterized by an absolute or a relative reduction in the external work delivered by the heart, although myocardial oxygen consumption remains normal or is only slightly lowered. Therefore, the external efficiency, i.e., the ratio of external work performed to energy consumed, is often depressed.

Alterations in Energy Metabolism When heart failure occurs in the presence of acute or chronic ischemia, it can be attributed to reduced myocardial energy supplies. However, in some forms of experimental and clinical heart failure without ischemia, myocardial energy stores in the form of creatine phosphate are decreased, as is the activity of the enzyme creatine kinase required for the shuttling of high-energy phosphate between creatine phosphate and adenosine diphosphate, suggesting that reductions in myocardial energy reserves may be responsible.

Alterations in Regulatory Proteins There is considerable evidence that changes in the regulatory proteins occur in chronic heart failure. These changes include a reduction of myosin ATPase activity, which could be caused by an alteration in the expression of troponin T and/or of myosin light kinase 2, two proteins that could be responsible for lowering the rate of interaction between myosin and actin myofilaments.

Abnormalities of Excitation-Contraction Coupling Substantial evidence supports the view that in many forms of heart failure the delivery of Ca^{2+} to the contractile sites is reduced, thereby impairing cardiac performance. However, the molecular basis of this abnormality, indeed the subcellular structures involved, i.e., the sarcolemma, T tubules, and/or sarcoplasmic reticulum, have yet to be defined. There is, however, evidence for a reduction in the messenger RNAs of the proteins regulating Ca^{2+} movements, including the sarcolemmal Ca^{2+} channels, as well as the Ca^{2+} release channels and the Ca^{2+} uptake pump, which play critical roles in the movement of Ca^{2+} between the sarcoplasmic reticulum and the cytoplasm and vice versa, respectively. Impaired expression of the genes encoding these proteins can impair both myocardial contraction and relaxation and thereby contribute to the development of diastolic heart failure. In addition, a reduction of Ca^{2+} release by the sarcoplasmic reticulum to the myofilaments can cause systolic heart failure.

NEUROHUMORAL ADJUSTMENTS A reduction in cardiac performance evokes a series of neurohumoral adjustments, which may be considered to be both adaptive and maladaptive. Although they are useful because they maintain arterial perfusion pressure in

the face of a reduction of cardiac output, they increase the hemodynamic burden and oxygen requirements of the failing ventricle.

The Renin-Angiotensin-Aldosterone System When cardiac output declines, the renin-angiotensin-aldosterone system (Chap. 332) is activated. Concentrations of circulating angiotensin II and aldosterone are both increased, the former contributing to excess vasoconstriction and the latter to the retention of salt and water. Patients with heart failure are usually improved by blocking this system with angiotensin-converting enzyme inhibitors, angiotensin II receptor blockers, and aldosterone antagonists (Chap. 233).

The Adrenergic Nervous System In patients with heart failure the levels of circulating norepinephrine may be markedly elevated, reflecting the increased activity of the adrenergic nervous system; indeed the prognosis varies inversely with the concentration. This increased activity of the adrenergic neurons supports ventricular contractility in congestive heart failure. Heart failure is intensified when large doses of beta-adrenergic blocking agents are administered to such patients. However, the chronic adrenergic stimulation in heart failure may also increase afterload by raising vascular resistance and cause arrhythmias and further myocardial damage directly. The latter may be further prevented by the cautious administration of gradually increasing doses of beta blockers (p. 1296).

The density of adrenergic receptors and concentration of cardiac norepinephrine are both reduced in chronic, severe heart failure. These changes are accompanied by a reduction in the activity of adenylate cyclase, which may lower the intracellular concentration of cyclic AMP. The latter in turn reduces the activation of protein kinase, the phosphorylation of Ca^{2+} channels, transarcolemmal Ca^{2+} entry, as well as the phosphorylation of phospholamban, a protein in the sarcoplasmic reticulum, thereby depressing the reuptake of Ca^{2+} by the latter (Fig.

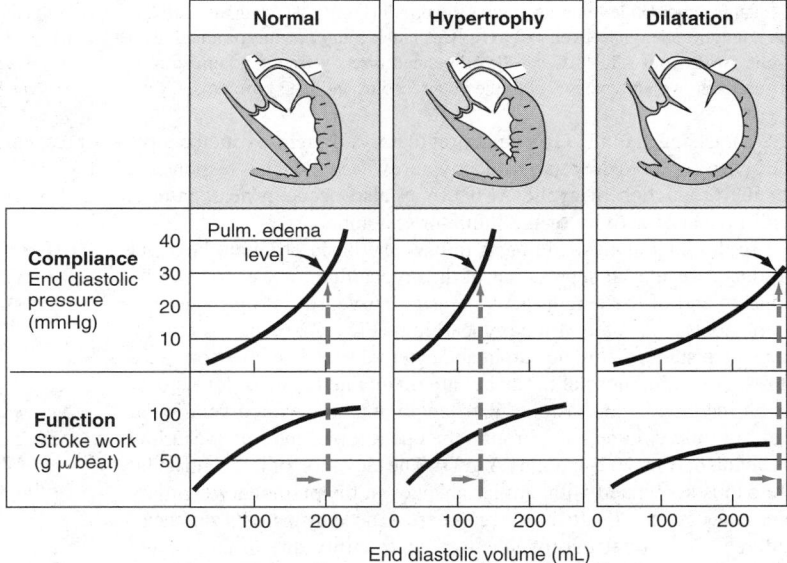

FIGURE 232-8 Relationship between left ventricular end-diastolic volume and (1) end-diastolic pressure (*top*), describing the *compliance* of the left ventricle, i.e., its *diastolic* properties; and (2) left ventricular stroke work (*bottom*), describing the ventricle's *systolic* function curve. The normal left ventricle (*left*) reaches an end-diastolic pressure of 30 mmHg (pulmonary edema level) when its end-diastolic volume is elevated to 200 mL. The concentrically hypertrophied left ventricle (*center*) exhibits normal systolic function since the relation between left ventricular end-diastolic volume and stroke work is unchanged, but there is "diastolic failure" in that end-diastolic pressure reaches pulmonary edema level (i.e., 30 mmHg) at a lower level than normal (i.e., 130 mL). The dilated ventricle (*right*) exhibits "systolic failure" in that the maximal stroke work and the stroke volume at any level of end-diastolic volume are depressed. The left ventricle displays increased diastolic compliance, i.e., distensibility, with a higher than normal end-diastolic volume (280 mL) required to reach the pulmonary edema level. (*Reprinted with permission from R Gorlin, Prim Cardiol 6:84, 1980.*)

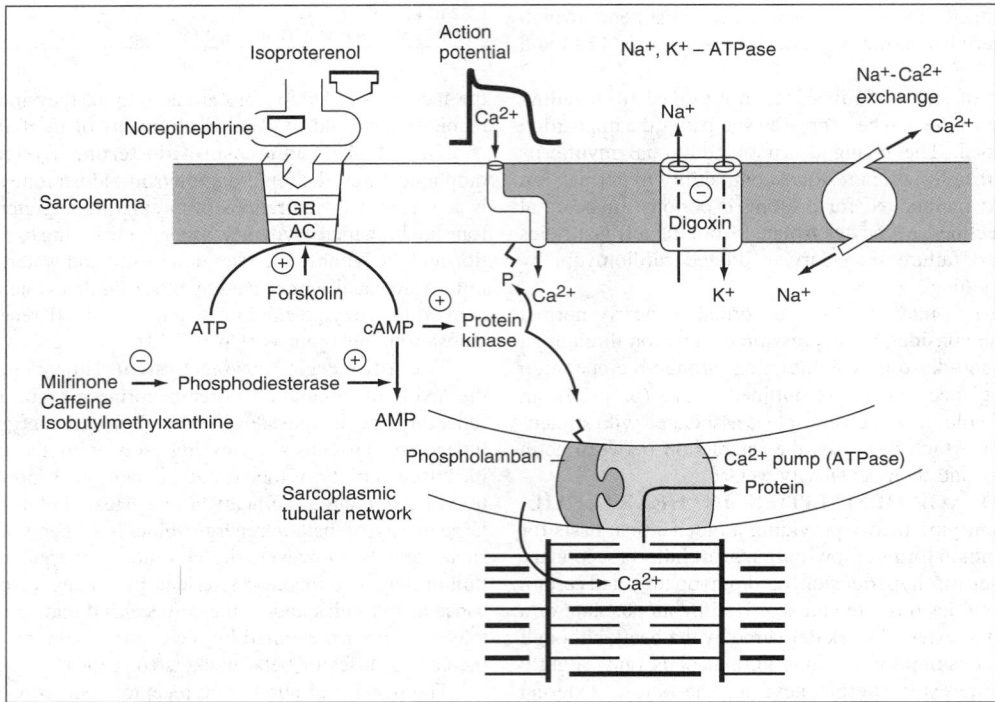

FIGURE 232-9 Schematic representation of influences on intramyocardial Ca²⁺ concentration and excitation-contraction coupling. The action potential is associated with intracellular entry of Na⁺ and the extrusion of K⁺ (not shown) and the entry of Ca²⁺ (shown). The Na⁺-Ca²⁺ exchanger depends on concentration gradients and does not require ATP. Not shown is the energy-dependent sarcolemmal Ca²⁺ pump which extrudes Ca²⁺ from the cell. Isoproterenol and norepinephrine, the latter shown intraneuronally, stimulate the beta-adrenergic receptor in the outer sarcolemma. The beta receptor is coupled to G (guanine nucleotide–binding regulatory) proteins (GR), which in turn activate the catalytic adenylate cyclase (AC). The latter catalyzes the production of cyclic AMP from ATP. AC can be stimulated directly by the administration of forskolin, which bypasses both the beta receptor and the G proteins. Cyclic AMP activates protein kinase, which in turn enhances the phosphorylation of the Ca²⁺ channel, increasing transarcolemmal Ca²⁺ influx. Activated protein kinase also phosphorylates phospholamban, which in its phosphorylated form enhances the uptake of Ca²⁺ by the sarcoplasmic tubular network. Phosphodiesterase catalyzes the breakdown of cyclic AMP to AMP while milrinone, caffeine, and isobutylmethylxanthine inhibit phosphodiesterase, thereby augmenting cyclic AMP concentration. Digoxin inhibits the Na⁺, K⁺-ATPase in the sarcolemma, inhibiting Na⁺ efflux from and K⁺ influx into the cell. As a consequence the intracellular Na⁺ concentration falls and Na⁺-Ca²⁺ exchange is reduced, thereby raising intracellular Ca²⁺. P represents phosphorylation. *(From AMD Feldman et al: Circulation 75:331, 1987, with permission of the American Heart Association, Inc.)*

232-9). Changes in the G (guanine regulatory) proteins, which couple the beta receptor to the catalytic adenylate cyclase (which is responsible for the production of cyclic AMP), may also occur in heart failure, with increased activity of the inhibitory subunit.

In the final analysis, in heart failure, the basic problem, however produced, resides in depressions of the myocardial force-velocity relationship and of the length–active tension curve, reflecting reductions in the contractile state of the myocardium (Fig. 232-6, curves 1 to 3). In many instances, cardiac output and external ventricular performance at rest are within normal limits but are maintained at these levels only by an increased end-diastolic fiber length and an elevated ventricular end-diastolic volume, i.e., through the operation of the Frank-Starling mechanism (Fig. 232-6, points A to D). The elevation of left ventricular preload is associated with similar changes in the pulmonary capillary pressure, contributing to the dyspnea experienced by patients with heart failure. The normal improvement of contractility due to augmented adrenergic activity during exercise is attenuated or even prevented by norepinephrine depletion and downregulation of myocardial beta receptors, which occur in severe heart failure (Fig. 232-6, curves 3 and 3′). The factors that tend to augment ventricular filling during exercise in the normal individual push the failing myocardium along its flattened length–active tension curve, and although the left ventricle may perform somewhat better, this occurs only as a consequence of an inordinate elevation of ventricular end-diastolic volume and pressure and, therefore, of the pulmonary capillary pressure. The latter intensifies dyspnea and therefore plays an important role in limiting the intensity of exercise that the patient can perform. Left ventricular failure becomes fatal when the myocardial length–active tension curve is depressed (Fig. 232-6, curve 4) to the point at which cardiac performance fails to satisfy the requirements of the peripheral tissues even

at rest, and/or the left ventricular end-diastolic and pulmonary capillary pressures are elevated to levels that result in pulmonary edema (Fig. 232-6, point E).

BIBLIOGRAPHY

ANVERSA P et al: Myocyte death in heart failure. Curr Opin Cardiol 11:245, 1996

ARAI M et al: Sarcoplasmic reticulum gene expression in cardiac hypertrophy and heart failure. Circ Res 74:555, 1994

COLUCCI WS (ed): *Heart Failure: Cardiac Function and Dysfunction*, in *Atlas of Heart Diseases*, vol 4, E Braunwald (series ed). Philadelphia, Current Medicine, 1995

———, BRAUNWALD E: Pathophysiology of heart failure, in *Heart Disease*, 5th ed, E Braunwald (ed). Philadelphia, Saunders, 1997, pp 394–420

FORBES MS, SPERELAKIS N: Ultrastructure of mammalian cardiac muscle, in *Physiology and Pathophysiology of the Heart*, 3d ed, N Sperelakis (ed). Boston, Kluwer Academic, 1995, pp 1–35

HEIN S et al: Altered expression of titin and contractile proteins in failing human myocardium. J Mol Cell Biol 26:1291, 1994

KATZ AM: Heart failure, in *Physiology of the Heart*, 2d ed. New York, Raven Press, 1992, pp 638–668

LITTLE WC, BRAUNWALD E: Assessment of cardiac function, in *Heart Disease*, 5th ed, E Braunwald (ed). Philadelphia, Saunders, 1997, pp 421–444

OPIE LH: Mechanisms of cardiac contraction and relaxation, in *Heart Disease*, 5th ed, E Braunwald (ed). Philadelphia, Saunders, 1997, pp 360–393

REEVES JP: Cardiac sodium-calcium exchange system, in *Physiology and Pathophysiology of the Heart*, 3d ed, N Sperelakis (ed). Boston, Kluwer Academic, 1995, pp 309–318

SCHWARTZ K, MERCADIER J-J: Molecular and cellular biology of heart failure. Curr Opin Cardiol 11:227, 1996

SOLARO RJ et al: Regulatory proteins and diastolic relaxation, in *Diastolic Relaxation of the Heart*, BH Lorell, W Grossman (eds). Boston, Kluwer Academic, 1994, pp 43–53

WOLFF MR et al: Rate of tension development in cardiac muscle varies with level of activator calcium. Circ Res 76:154, 1995

HEART FAILURE

Heart failure is the pathophysiologic state in which an abnormality of *cardiac* function is responsible for the failure of the heart to pump blood at a rate commensurate with the requirements of the metabolizing tissues *and/or* can do so only from an abnormally elevated diastolic volume. Heart failure is frequently, but not always, caused by a defect in myocardial contraction, and then the term *myocardial failure* is appropriate. The latter may result from a primary abnormality in heart muscle, as occurs in the cardiomyopathies and in viral myocarditis (Chap. 239). Myocardial failure also may result from extramyocardial abnormalities, such as coronary atherosclerosis which leads to myocardial ischemia and infarction, as well as from abnormalities of the heart valves in which the heart muscle is damaged by the long-standing excessive hemodynamic burden imposed by the valvular abnormality, and/or by the rheumatic process (Chap. 236).

In other patients with heart failure, however, a similar clinical syndrome is present but without any detectable abnormality of *myocardial* function. In some of these patients the normal heart is suddenly presented with a mechanical load that exceeds its capacity, such as an acute hypertensive crisis, rupture of an aortic valve cusp, or massive pulmonary embolism. Heart failure, in the presence of normal myocardial function, also occurs in chronic conditions in which there is impairment of filling of the ventricles due to a mechanical abnormality such as tricuspid and/or mitral stenosis, constrictive pericarditis without myocardial involvement, endocardial fibrosis, and some forms of hypertrophic cardiomyopathy. In many patients with heart failure, particularly those with valvular or congenital heart disease, a combination of impaired myocardial function and mechanical abnormality exists.

Heart failure should be distinguished from (1) conditions in which there is circulatory congestion consequent to abnormal salt and water retention but in which there is no disturbance of cardiac function per se (the latter syndrome, termed the *congested state*, may result from the abnormal salt and water retention of renal failure or from excess parenteral administration of fluids and electrolytes) and (2) noncardiac causes of inadequate cardiac output, including shock due to hypovolemia and redistribution of blood volume (Chap. 38).

The ventricles respond to a chronically increased hemodynamic burden with the development of hypertrophy. With volume overload when the ventricle is called on to deliver an elevated cardiac output for prolonged periods, as in valvular regurgitation, it develops *eccentric hypertrophy*, i.e., cavity dilatation, with an increase in muscle mass so that the ratio between wall thickness and ventricular cavity size remains relatively constant. With chronic pressure overload, as in valvular aortic stenosis or untreated hypertension, it develops *concentric hypertrophy*, in which the ratio between wall thickness and ventricular cavity size increases. In both conditions, a stable hyperfunctioning state may exist for many years, but myocardial function may ultimately deteriorate, leading to heart failure. Heart failure represents a major public health problem in industrialized nations. It appears to be the only common cardiovascular condition that is increasing in prevalence and incidence. In the United States, heart failure is responsible for almost 1 million hospital admissions and 40,000 deaths annually. Since heart failure is more common in the elderly, its prevalence is likely to continue to increase as the population ages.

CAUSES OF HEART FAILURE

In evaluating patients with heart failure, it is important to identify not only the *underlying cause* of the heart disease but also the *precipitating cause* of heart failure. The cardiac abnormality produced by a congenital or acquired lesion such as valvular aortic stenosis may exist for many years and produce no clinical disability. Frequently, however, clinical manifestations of heart failure appear for the first time in the course of some acute disturbance that places an additional load on a myocardium that chronically is excessively burdened. The heart may be compensated but have little additional reserve, and the additional load imposed by a precipitating cause results in further deterioration of cardiac function. Identification of such precipitating causes is of critical importance because their prompt alleviation may be lifesaving. In the absence of underlying heart disease, these acute disturbances do not usually, by themselves, lead to heart failure.

PRECIPITATING CAUSES

1. *Infection.* Patients with pulmonary vascular congestion are also more susceptible to pulmonary infections; any infection may precipitate heart failure. The resulting fever, tachycardia, and hypoxemia and the increased metabolic demands may place a further burden on the overloaded, but compensated myocardium of a patient with chronic heart disease.

2. *Anemia.* In the presence of anemia, the oxygen needs of the metabolizing tissues can be met only by an increase in the cardiac output (Chap. 59). Although such an increase in cardiac output can be sustained by a normal heart, a diseased, overloaded, but otherwise compensated heart may be unable to augment sufficiently the volume of blood that it delivers to the periphery. In this manner, the combination of anemia and previously compensated heart disease can lead to inadequate oxygen delivery to the periphery and precipitate heart failure.

3. *Thyrotoxicosis and pregnancy.* As in anemia and fever, in thyrotoxicosis and pregnancy, adequate tissue perfusion requires an increased cardiac output. The development or intensification of heart failure may actually be one of the first clinical manifestations of hyperthyroidism in a patient with underlying heart disease that was previously compensated (Chap. 331). Similarly, heart failure not infrequently occurs for the first time during pregnancy in women with rheumatic valvular disease, in whom cardiac compensation may return following delivery.

4. *Arrhythmias.* In patients with compensated heart disease, arrhythmias are among the most frequent precipitating causes of heart failure. They exert a deleterious effect for a variety of reasons: (a) Tachyarrhythmias reduce the time period available for ventricular filling. In patients with ischemic heart disease, tachyarrhythmias also may cause ischemic myocardial dysfunction. (b) The dissociation between atrial and ventricular contractions characteristic of many arrhythmias results in the loss of the atrial booster pump mechanism, thereby raising atrial pressures. (c) In any arrhythmia associated with abnormal intraventricular conduction, myocardial performance may become further impaired because of the loss of normal synchronicity of ventricular contraction. (d) Marked bradycardia associated with complete atrioventricular block or other severe bradyarrhythmias reduces cardiac output unless stroke volume rises reciprocally; this compensatory response cannot occur with serious myocardial dysfunction even in the absence of heart failure.

5. *Rheumatic and other forms of myocarditis.* Acute rheumatic fever and a variety of other inflammatory or infectious processes affecting the myocardium may impair myocardial function in patients with or without preexisting heart disease (Chaps. 236 and 239).

6. *Infective endocarditis.* The additional valvular damage, anemia, fever, and myocarditis that often occur as a consequence of infective endocarditis may, singly or in concert, precipitate heart failure (Chap. 126).

7. *Physical, dietary, fluid, environmental, and emotional excesses.* The augmentation of sodium intake, the inappropriate discontinuation of medications to treat heart failure, blood transfusions, physical overexertion, excessive environmental heat or humidity, and emotional crises all may precipitate heart failure in patients with heart disease who were previously compensated.

8. *Systemic hypertension.* Rapid elevation of arterial pressure, as may occur in some instances of hypertension of renal origin or upon discontinuation of antihypertensive medication, may result in cardiac decompensation (Chap. 246).

9. *Myocardial infarction.* In patients with chronic but compensated ischemic heart disease, a fresh infarct, sometimes otherwise silent clinically, may further impair ventricular function and precipitate heart failure (Chap. 243).

10. *Pulmonary embolism.* Physically inactive patients with low cardiac output are at increased risk of developing thrombi in the veins of the lower extremities or the pelvis. Pulmonary emboli may result in further elevation of pulmonary arterial pressure, which in turn may produce or intensify ventricular failure. In the presence of pulmonary vascular congestion, such emboli also may cause pulmonary infarction (Chap. 261).

A systematic search for these precipitating causes should be made in every patient with the new development or recent intensification of heart failure, especially if it is refractory to the usual methods of therapy. If properly recognized, the precipitating cause of heart failure usually can be treated more effectively than the underlying cause. Therefore, the prognosis in patients with heart failure in whom a precipitating cause can be identified, treated, and eliminated is more favorable than it is in patients in whom the underlying disease process has advanced to the point of producing heart failure.

FORMS OF HEART FAILURE

Heart failure may be described as *systolic* or *diastolic*, *high-output* or *low-output*, *acute* or *chronic*, *right-sided* or *left-sided*, and *forward* or *backward*. These descriptors are often useful in a clinical setting, particularly early in the patient's course, but late in the course of chronic heart failure the differences between them often become blurred.

SYSTOLIC VERSUS DIASTOLIC FAILURE The distinction between these two forms of heart failure, described on p. 1284 and in Fig. 232-8, relates to whether the principal abnormality is the inability to contract normally and expel sufficient blood (systolic failure) or to relax and fill normally (diastolic failure). The major clinical manifestations of systolic failure relate to an inadequate cardiac output with weakness, fatigue, reduced exercise tolerance, and other symptoms of hypoperfusion, while in diastolic failure they relate principally to an elevation of filling pressures. In many patients, particularly those who have both ventricular hypertrophy *and* dilatation, abnormalities both of contraction and relaxation coexist.

Diastolic heart failure may be caused by increased resistance to ventricular inflow and reduced ventricular diastolic capacity (constrictive pericarditis and restrictive, hypertensive, and hypertrophic cardiomyopathy), impaired ventricular relaxation (acute myocardial ischemia, hypertrophic cardiomyopathy), and myocardial fibrosis and infiltration (dilated, chronic ischemic, and restrictive cardiomyopathy).

HIGH-OUTPUT VERSUS LOW-OUTPUT HEART FAILURE It is useful to classify patients with heart failure into those with a low cardiac output, i.e., *low-output heart failure*, and those with an elevated cardiac output, i.e., *high-output heart failure*. The former occurs secondary to ischemic heart disease, hypertension, dilated cardiomyopathy, and valvular and pericardial disease, while the latter is seen in patients with heart failure and hyperthyroidism, anemia, pregnancy, arteriovenous fistulas, beriberi, and Paget's disease. In clinical practice, however, low-output and high-output heart failure cannot always be readily distinguished. The normal range of cardiac output is wide [2.2 to 3.5 (L/min)/m²], and in many patients with so-called low-output heart failure the cardiac output may actually be just within the normal range at rest (although it is lower than it had been previously), but it fails to rise normally during exertion. On the other hand, in patients with so-called high-output heart failure the output may not exceed the upper limits of normal (although it would have been elevated had it been measured before heart failure supervened), but rather it may have fallen to the upper limit of normal. Regardless of the *absolute* level of the cardiac output, however, cardiac failure may be said to be present when the characteristic clinical manifestations described below are accompanied

by a depression of the curve relating ventricular end-diastolic volume to cardiac performance (see Fig. 232-6).

An integral physiologic component of *systolic* heart failure (p. 1284) is the delivery of an inadequate quantity of oxygen required by the metabolizing tissues. In the absence of peripheral shunting of blood, this is reflected in an abnormal widening of the normal arterial–mixed venous oxygen difference (35 to 50 mL/L in the basal state). In mild cases, such an abnormality may not be present at rest but becomes evident only during exertion or other hypermetabolic states. In patients with high cardiac output states, such as those associated with arteriovenous fistula or thyrotoxicosis, the arterial–mixed venous oxygen difference is normal or low. The mixed venous oxygen saturation is raised by the admixture of blood that has been diverted from the metabolizing tissues, and it may be presumed that even in these patients the delivery of oxygen to the latter is reduced despite the normal or even elevated mixed venous oxygen saturation. When heart failure occurs in such patients, the arterial–mixed venous oxygen difference, regardless of the absolute value, still exceeds the level that existed prior to the development of heart failure. Therefore, the cardiac output, though normal or even elevated, is lower than before heart failure supervened.

The mechanisms responsible for the development of heart failure in patients whose cardiac outputs are initially high are complex and depend on the underlying disease process. In most of these conditions the heart is called on to pump abnormally large quantities of blood in order to deliver the normal quota of oxygen to the metabolizing tissues. The burden placed on the myocardium by the increased flow load resembles that produced by chronic regurgitant valvular lesions. In addition, thyrotoxicosis and beriberi also may impair myocardial metabolism directly, while severe anemia may interfere with myocardial function by producing myocardial anoxia, especially in the presence of underlying obstructive artery disease.

ACUTE VERSUS CHRONIC HEART FAILURE The prototype of acute heart failure is the patient who is entirely well but who suddenly develops a large myocardial infarction or rupture of a cardiac valve. Chronic heart failure is typically observed in patients with dilated cardiomyopathy or multivalvular heart disease that develops or progresses slowly. Acute heart failure is usually largely systolic, and the sudden reduction in cardiac output often results in systemic hypotension without peripheral edema. In chronic heart failure, arterial pressure tends to be well maintained until very late in the course, but there is often accumulation of edema. Despite these obvious differences in clinical presentation, there is no fundamental distinction between acute and chronic heart failure. For example, intensive efforts to prevent expansion of blood volume by means of dietary sodium restriction and the administration of diuretics will frequently delay the development of exertional dyspnea and edema in patients with chronic valvular heart disease (i.e., it will mask the clinical manifestations of chronic heart failure) until an acute episode, such as an arrhythmia or infection, precipitates acute heart failure. Without intensive efforts to restrict blood volume, the same patients would have been considered to have been suffering from chronic heart failure, even though their underlying myocardial disease was no further advanced.

RIGHT-SIDED VERSUS LEFT-SIDED HEART FAILURE Many of the clinical manifestations of heart failure result from the accumulation of excess fluid behind either one or both ventricles (Chaps. 32 and 37). This fluid usually localizes upstream to (behind) the specific cardiac chamber that is initially affected. For example, patients in whom the left ventricle is mechanically overloaded (e.g., aortic stenosis) or weakened (e.g., postmyocardial infarction) develop dyspnea and orthopnea as a result of pulmonary congestion, a condition referred to as *left-sided heart failure*. In contrast, when the underlying abnormality affects the right ventricle primarily (e.g., valvular pulmonic stenosis or pulmonary hypertension secondary to pulmonary thromboembolism), symptoms resulting from pulmonary congestion such as orthopnea or paroxysmal nocturnal dyspnea are less common, and edema, congestive hepatomegaly, and systemic venous distention, i.e., clinical manifestations of *right-sided heart failure*, are more prominent. However, when heart failure has existed for months or years, such localization of excess fluid behind the failing ventricle may no longer exist. For example, patients with long-standing aortic valve disease or systemic hypertension may have ankle edema, congestive hepatomegaly, and systemic venous distention late in the course of their disease, even though the abnormal hemodynamic burden initially was placed on the left ventricle. This occurs in part because of the secondary pulmonary hypertension and resultant right-sided heart failure but also because of the retention of salt and water characteristic of all forms of heart failure (Chap. 37). The muscle bundles composing both ventricles are continuous, and both ventricles share a common wall, the interventricular septum. Also, biochemical changes that occur in heart failure and that may be involved in the impairment of myocardial function (Chap. 232), such as norepinephrine depletion and alterations in the activity of myosin ATPase, occur in the myocardium of *both* ventricles, regardless of the specific chamber on which the abnormal hemodynamic burden is placed initially.

BACKWARD VERSUS FORWARD HEART FAILURE For many years a controversy has revolved around the question of the mechanism of the clinical manifestations resulting from heart failure. The concept of *backward heart failure* contends that in heart failure, one or the other ventricle fails to discharge its contents or fails to fill normally. As a consequence, the pressures in the atrium and venous system behind the failing ventricle rise, and retention of sodium and water occurs as a consequence of the elevation of systemic venous and capillary pressures and the resultant transudation of fluid into the interstitial space (Chap. 37). In contrast, the proponents of the *forward heart failure* hypothesis maintain that the clinical manifestations of heart failure result directly from an inadequate discharge of blood into the arterial system. According to this concept, salt and water retention is a consequence of diminished renal perfusion and excessive proximal tubular sodium reabsorption and of excessive distal tubular reabsorption through activation of the renin-angiotensin-aldosterone system.

A rigid distinction between *backward* and *forward* heart failure (like a rigid distinction between right and left heart failure) is artificial, since both mechanisms appear to operate to varying extents in most patients with heart failure. However, the rate of onset of heart failure often influences the clinical manifestations. For example, when a large portion of the left ventricle is suddenly destroyed, as in myocardial infarction, although stroke volume and blood pressure are suddenly reduced (both manifestations of forward failure), the patient may succumb to acute pulmonary edema, a manifestation of backward failure. If the patient survives the acute insult, clinical manifestations resulting from a chronically depressed cardiac output, including the abnormal retention of fluid within the systemic vascular bed, may develop. Similarly, in the case of massive pulmonary embolism, the right ventricle may dilate and the systemic venous pressure may rise to high levels (backward failure), or the patient may develop shock secondary to low cardiac output (forward failure), but this low-output state may have to be maintained for some days before sodium and water retention sufficient to produce peripheral edema occurs.

REDISTRIBUTION OF CARDIAC OUTPUT The redistribution of cardiac output serves as an important compensatory mechanism when cardiac output is reduced. This redistribution is most marked when a patient with heart failure exercises, but as heart failure advances, redistribution occurs even in the basal state. Blood flow is redistributed so that the delivery of oxygen to vital organs, such as the brain and myocardium, is maintained at normal or near-normal levels, while flow to less critical areas, such as the cutaneous and muscular beds and viscera, is reduced. Vasoconstriction mediated by the adrenergic nervous system is largely responsible for this redistribution, which in turn may be responsible for many of the clinical manifestations of heart failure, such as fluid accumulation (reduction of renal flow), low-grade fever (reduction of cutaneous flow), and fatigue (reduction of muscle flow).

SALT AND WATER RETENTION (See also Chap. 37)

When the volume of blood pumped by the left ventricle into the systemic vascular bed is reduced, a complex sequence of adjustments occurs that ultimately results in the abnormal accumulation of fluid. On the one hand, many of the troubling clinical manifestations of heart failure are secondary to this excessive retention of fluid; on the other, this abnormal fluid accumulation and the expansion of blood volume that accompanies it also constitute an important compensatory mechanism that tends to maintain cardiac output and therefore perfusion of the vital organs. Except in the terminal stages of heart failure, the ventricle operates on an ascending, albeit depressed and flattened, function curve (Fig. 232-6), and the augmented ventricular end-diastolic volume and pressure characteristic of heart failure must be regarded as helping to maintain the reduced cardiac output, despite causing pulmonary and/or systemic venous congestion.

Congestive heart failure is also characterized by a complex series of neurohumoral adjustments. The activation of the adrenergic nervous system is discussed on p. 1285; there is also activation of the renin-angiotensin-aldosterone system and increased release of antidiuretic hormone. These influences elevate systemic vascular resistance and enhance sodium and water retention and potassium excretion. These actions are, to a minor extent, opposed by the release of atrial natriuretic peptide, which also occurs in congestive heart failure. Patients with severe heart failure may exhibit a reduced capacity to excrete a water load, which may result in dilutional hyponatremia. In the presence of heart failure, effective filling of the systemic arterial bed is reduced, a condition that initiates the renal and hormonal changes mentioned above.

The elevation of systemic venous pressure and the alterations of renal and adrenal function characteristic of heart failure vary in their relative importance in the production of edema in different patients with heart failure. The renin-angiotensin-aldosterone axis is activated most intensely by acute heart failure, and its activity tends to decline as heart failure becomes chronic. In patients with tricuspid valve disease or constrictive pericarditis, the elevated venous pressure and the transudation of fluid from systemic capillaries appear to play the dominant role in edema formation. On the other hand, severe edema may be present in patients with ischemic or hypertensive heart disease, in whom systemic venous pressure is within normal limits or is only minimally elevated. In such patients, the retention of salt and water is probably due primarily to a redistribution of cardiac output and a concomitant reduction in renal perfusion, as well as activation of the renin-angiotensin-aldosterone axis. Regardless of the mechanisms involved in fluid retention, untreated patients with chronic congestive heart failure have elevations of total blood volume, interstitial fluid volume, and body sodium. These abnormalities diminish after clinical compensation has been achieved by treatment.

CLINICAL MANIFESTATIONS OF HEART FAILURE

Dyspnea Respiratory distress that occurs as the result of increased effort in breathing is the most common symptom of heart failure (Chap. 32). In early heart failure, dyspnea is observed only during activity, when it may simply represent an aggravation of the breathlessness that occurs normally under these circumstances. As heart failure advances, however, dyspnea appears with progressively less strenuous activity. Ultimately, breathlessness is present even when the patient is at rest. The principal difference between exertional dyspnea in normal persons and in patients with heart failure is the degree of activity necessary to induce the symptom. Cardiac dyspnea is observed most frequently in patients with elevations of pulmonary venous and capillary pressures. Such patients usually have engorged pulmonary vessels and interstitial pulmonary edema, which may be evident on radiologic examination. This reduces the compliance of the lungs and thereby increases the work of the respiratory muscles required to inflate the lungs. The activation of receptors in the lungs results in the rapid, shallow breathing characteristic of cardiac dyspnea. The oxygen cost of breathing is increased by the excessive work of the respiratory muscles. This is coupled with the diminished delivery of oxygen to these muscles, which occurs as a consequence of the reduced cardiac output and which may contribute to fatigue of the respiratory muscles and the sensation of shortness of breath.

Orthopnea   Dyspnea in the recumbent position is usually a later manifestation of heart failure than exertional dyspnea. Orthopnea occurs because of the redistribution of fluid from the abdomen and lower extremities into the chest causing an increase in the pulmonary capillary hydrostatic pressure, as well as elevation of the diaphragm accompanying supine posture. Patients with orthopnea must elevate their heads on several pillows at night and frequently awaken short of breath or coughing (the so-called nocturnal cough) if their heads slip off the pillows. The sensation of breathlessness usually is relieved by sitting upright, since this position reduces venous return and pulmonary capillary pressure, and many patients report that they find relief from sitting in front of an open window. In far-advanced heart failure, orthopnea may become so severe that patients cannot lie down at all and must spend the entire night in a sitting position. On the other hand, in other patients with long-standing, severe left ventricular failure, symptoms of pulmonary congestion may actually diminish with time as the function of the right ventricle becomes impaired.

Paroxysmal (Nocturnal) Dyspnea   This term refers to attacks of severe shortness of breath and coughing that generally occur at night, usually awaken the patient from sleep, and may be quite frightening. Though simple orthopnea may be relieved by sitting upright at the side of the bed with legs dependent, in the patient with paroxysmal nocturnal dyspnea, coughing and wheezing often persist even in this position. The depression of the respiratory center during sleep may reduce ventilation sufficiently to lower arterial oxygen tension, particularly in patients with interstitial lung edema and reduced pulmonary compliance. Also, ventricular function may be further impaired at night because of reduced adrenergic stimulation of myocardial function. *Cardiac asthma* is closely related to paroxysmal nocturnal dyspnea and nocturnal cough and is characterized by wheezing secondary to bronchospasm—most prominent at night. *Acute pulmonary edema* (Chap. 32) is a severe form of cardiac asthma due to marked elevation of pulmonary capillary pressure leading to alveolar edema, associated with extreme shortness of breath, rales over the lung fields, and the transudation and expectoration of blood-tinged fluid. If not treated promptly, acute pulmonary edema may be fatal.

Cheyne-Stokes Respiration   Also known as *periodic* or *cyclic respiration*, Cheyne-Stokes respiration is characterized by diminished sensitivity of the respiratory center to arterial P_{CO_2}. There is an apneic phase, during which the arterial P_{O_2} falls and the arterial P_{CO_2} rises. These changes in the arterial blood stimulate the depressed respiratory center, resulting in hyperventilation and hypocapnia, followed in turn by recurrence of apnea. Cheyne-Stokes respiration occurs most often in patients with cerebral atherosclerosis and other cerebral lesions, but the prolongation of the circulation time from the lung to the brain that occurs in heart failure, particularly in patients with hypertension and coronary artery disease and associated cerebral vascular disease, also appears to precipitate this form of breathing.

Fatigue, Weakness, and Abdominal Symptoms   These nonspecific but common symptoms of heart failure are related to the reduction of perfusion of skeletal muscle. Exercise capacity is reduced by the limited ability of the failing heart to increase its output and deliver oxygen to the exercising muscle. Anorexia and nausea associated with abdominal pain and fullness are frequent complaints and may be related to the congested liver and portal venous system.

Cerebral Symptoms   In severe heart failure, particularly in elderly patients with accompanying cerebral arteriosclerosis, reduced cerebral perfusion, and arterial hypoxemia, there may be alterations in the mental state characterized by confusion, difficulty in concentration, impairment of memory, headache, insomnia, and anxiety. *Nocturia* is common in heart failure and may contribute to insomnia.

PHYSICAL FINDINGS (See Chap. 227)   In moderate heart failure, the patient appears to be in no distress at rest except that he or she may be uncomfortable when lying flat for more than a few minutes. In more severe heart failure, the pulse pressure may be diminished, reflecting a reduction in stroke volume, and occasionally, the diastolic arterial pressure is elevated as a consequence of generalized vasoconstriction. In acute heart failure, hypotension may be prominent. There may be cyanosis of the lips and nail beds and sinus tachycardia, and the patient may insist on sitting upright. *Systemic venous pressure* is often abnormally elevated in heart failure and may be recognized by observing the extent of distention of the jugular veins. In the early stages of heart failure, the venous pressure may be normal at rest but may become abnormally elevated during and immediately after exertion as well as with sustained pressure on the abdomen (positive abdominojugular reflux).

Third and fourth heart sounds are often audible but are not specific for heart failure, and *pulsus alternans*, i.e., a regular rhythm in which there is alternation of strong and weak cardiac contractions and therefore alternation in the strength of the peripheral pulses, may be present. Pulsus alternans, a sign of severe heart failure, may be detected by sphygmomanometry and in more severe instances by palpation; it frequently follows an extrasystole and is observed most commonly in patients with cardiomyopathy or hypertensive or ischemic heart disease.

Pulmonary Rales   Moist, inspiratory, crepitant rales and dullness to percussion over the lung bases are common in patients with heart failure and elevated pulmonary venous and capillary pressures. In patients with pulmonary edema, rales may be heard widely over both lung fields; they are frequently coarse and sibilant and may be accompanied by expiratory wheezing. Rales may, however, be caused by many conditions other than left ventricular failure. Some patients with long-standing heart failure have no rales because of increased lymphatic drainage of alveolar fluid.

Cardiac Edema (See Chap. 37)   This is usually dependent, occurring in the legs symmetrically, particularly in the pretibial region and ankles in ambulatory patients, in whom it is most prominent in the evening, and in the sacral region of individuals at bed rest. Pitting edema of the arms and face occurs rarely and then only late in the course of heart failure.

Hydrothorax and Ascites   Pleural effusion in congestive heart failure results from the elevation of pleural capillary pressure and transudation of fluid into the pleural cavities. Since the pleural veins drain into *both* the systemic and pulmonary veins, hydrothorax occurs most commonly with marked elevation of pressure in both venous systems but also may be seen with marked elevation of pressure in either venous bed. It is more frequent in the right pleural cavity than in the left. *Ascites* also occurs as a consequence of transudation and results from increased pressure in the hepatic veins and the veins draining the peritoneum (Chap. 46). Marked ascites occurs most frequently in patients with tricuspid valve disease and constrictive pericarditis.

Congestive Hepatomegaly   An enlarged, tender, pulsating liver also accompanies systemic venous hypertension and is observed not only in the same conditions in which ascites occurs but also in milder forms of heart failure from any cause. With prolonged, severe hepatomegaly, as in patients with tricuspid valve disease or chronic constrictive pericarditis, enlargement of the spleen, i.e., congestive splenomegaly, also may occur.

Jaundice   This is a late finding in congestive heart failure and is associated with elevations of both the direct- and indirect-reacting bilirubin; it results from impairment of hepatic function secondary to hepatic congestion and the hepatocellular hypoxia associated with central lobular atrophy. Serum transaminase concentrations are frequently elevated. If hepatic congestion occurs acutely, the jaundice may be severe and the enzymes strikingly elevated.

Cardiac Cachexia   With severe chronic heart failure there may be serious weight loss and cachexia because of (1) elevation of circulating concentrations of tumor necrosis factor; (2) elevation of the metabolic rate, which results in part from the extra work performed by the respiratory muscles, the increased oxygen needs of the hypertrophied heart, and/or the discomfort associated with severe heart failure; (3)

anorexia, nausea, and vomiting due to central causes, to digitalis intoxication, or to congestive hepatomegaly and abdominal fullness; (4) impairment of intestinal absorption due to congestion of the intestinal veins; and (5) rarely, in patients with particularly severe failure of the right side of the heart, protein-losing enteropathy.

Other Manifestations With reduction of blood flow, the extremities may be cold, pale, and diaphoretic. Urine flow is depressed, and the urine contains albumin and has a high specific gravity and a low concentration of sodium. In addition, prerenal azotemia may be present. In patients with long-standing severe heart failure, impotence and depression are common.

ROENTGENOGRAPHIC FINDINGS In addition to the enlargement of the particular chambers characteristic of the lesion responsible for heart failure, distention of pulmonary veins and redistribution to the apices is common in patients with heart failure and elevated pulmonary vascular pressures. Also, pleural effusions may be evident and associated with interlobar effusions.

DIFFERENTIAL DIAGNOSIS The diagnosis of congestive heart failure may be established by observing some combination of the clinical manifestations of heart failure described above, together with the findings characteristic of one of the etiologic forms of heart disease. Table 233-1 shows the Framingham criteria, which are useful in the diagnosis of heart failure. Since chronic heart failure is often associated with cardiac enlargement, the diagnosis should be questioned, but is by no means excluded, when all chambers are normal in size. Two-dimensional echocardiography is particularly useful in assessing the dimensions of each cardiac chamber. Heart failure may be difficult to distinguish from pulmonary disease, and the differential diagnosis is discussed in Chap. 32. Pulmonary embolism also presents many of the manifestations of heart failure, but hemoptysis, pleuritic chest pain, a right ventricular lift, and the characteristic mismatch between ventilation and perfusion on lung scan should point to this diagnosis (see Chap. 261).

Ankle edema may be due to varicose veins, cyclic edema, or gravitational effects (Chap. 37), but in these patients there is no jugular venous hypertension at rest or with pressure over the abdomen. Edema secondary to renal disease can usually be recognized by appropriate renal function tests and urinalysis and is rarely associated with elevation of venous pressure. Enlargement of the liver and ascites occur in patients with hepatic cirrhosis and also may be distinguished from heart failure by normal jugular venous pressure and absence of a positive abdominojugular reflux.

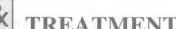 **TREATMENT**

The treatment of heart failure may be divided logically into three components: (1) removal of the precipitating cause, (2) correction of the underlying cause, and (3) control of the congestive heart failure state. The first two are discussed in other chapters together with each specific disease entity or complication. An example is the treatment of pneumococcal pneumonia and acute heart failure (removal of the precipitating cause) followed by mitral valvotomy (correction of the underlying cause) in a patient with mitral stenosis. In many instances, surgical treatment will correct or at least alleviate the underlying cause. The third component of the treatment of heart failure, i.e., control of the congestive heart failure state, may, in turn, be divided into three categories: (1) reduction of cardiac work load, including both the preload and the afterload; (2) control of excessive retention of salt and water; and (3) enhancement of myocardial contractility. The vigor with which each of these measures is pursued in any individual patient should depend on the severity of heart failure. Following effective treatment, recurrence of the clinical manifestations of heart failure can often be prevented by continuing those measures that were originally effective.

While a simple rule for the treatment of all patients with heart failure cannot be formulated because of the varied etiologies, hemodynamic features, clinical manifestations, and severity of heart failure, insofar as the treatment of chronic congestive failure is concerned, the administration of an angiotensin-converting enzyme inhibitor (e.g., lisinopril 10 mg q.d.) has been shown to retard the development of heart failure and should be begun early in patients with cardiac dilatation and/or hypertrophy, even if they are asymptomatic. Then, as symptoms develop, simple measures such as moderate restriction of activity and sodium intake should be tried (Fig. 233-1). If these and the ACE inhibitor are insufficient, therapy with a combination of a diuretic, a vasodilator, and usually a digitalis glycoside is then begun. The next step is more rigorous restriction of salt intake and higher doses of loop diuretics, sometimes accompanied by other diuretics. If heart failure persists, hospitalization with rigid salt restriction, bed rest, intravenous vasodilators, and positive inotropic agents comes next. In some patients, the order in which these measures are applied may be altered.

Table 233-1

Framingham Criteria for Diagnosis of Congestive Heart Failure*

MAJOR CRITERIA

Paroxysmal nocturnal dyspnea
Neck vein distention
Rales
Cardiomegaly
Acute pulmonary edema
S_3 gallop
Increased venous pressure (>16 cmH$_2$O)
Positive hepatojugular reflux

MINOR CRITERIA

Extremity edema
Night cough
Dyspnea on exertion
Hepatomegaly
Pleural effusion
Vital capacity reduced by one-third from normal
Tachycardia ($\geq$120 bpm)

MAJOR OR MINOR

Weight loss $\geq$4.5 kg over 5 days' treatment

* To establish a clinical diagnosis of congestive heart failure by these criteria, at least one major and two minor criteria are required.

SOURCE: KKL Ho et al, Circulation 88:107, 1993.

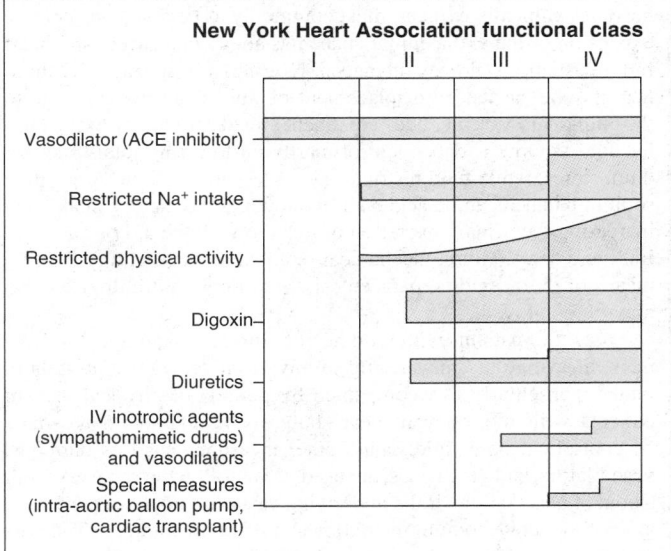

FIGURE 233-1 Overview of the treatment of heart failure. *[From RA Kelly, TW Smith: Treatment of stable heart failure: Digitalis and diuretics, in Heart Failure: Cardiac Function and Dysfunction, in WS Colucci (ed), Atlas of Heart Diseases, vol 4, E Braunwald (series ed), Philadelphia, Current Medicine, 1995.]*

Reduction of Cardiac Work Load This consists of reducing physical activity, instituting emotional rest, and reducing afterload. Modest restriction of physical activity in mild cases and rest in bed or in a chair in severe failure remain cornerstones in the treatment of heart failure. Meals should be small in quantity but perhaps more frequent, and every effort should be made to diminish the patient's anxiety; sometimes drugs such as diazepam (2 to 5 mg tid) for several days are useful. Physical and emotional rest tends to lower arterial pressure and reduce the load on the myocardium by diminishing the requirements for cardiac output. These influences act in concert to diminish the need for redistribution of the cardiac output, and in many patients, particularly those with mild heart failure, simple bed rest and mild sedation often result in an effective diuresis.

Rest should be maintained for 1 to 2 weeks in patients with overt congestive failure and should be continued for several days after the patient's condition has stabilized. The hazards of phlebothrombosis and pulmonary embolism which occur with bed rest may be reduced with anticoagulants, leg exercises, and elastic stockings. *Absolute* bed rest rarely is required or advisable, and the patient should be encouraged to sit in a chair and be given toilet privileges unless heart failure is extreme. Heavy sedation should be avoided, but small doses of tranquilizers may be helpful in calming the emotionally disturbed patient during the first few days of therapy and in permitting much-needed sleep. In patients with chronic, moderately severe heart failure, additional periods of bed rest on weekends frequently allow continuation of gainful employment. Following recovery from heart failure, the patient's activities should be assessed, and often, professional, community, and/or family responsibilities must be curtailed. Intermittent rest during the day (e.g., a scheduled 1-h nap or rest following lunch) and the avoidance of strenuous exertion are often helpful once compensation has been restored. Weight reduction by restriction of caloric intake in obese patients with heart failure also diminishes cardiac work load and is an essential component of the therapeutic program. Vasodilator therapy (p. 1293) may be considered a form of reduction of the cardiac work load. This form of therapy has been shown not only to ameliorate heart failure but also to retard its development in patients with left ventricular dysfunction.

Control of Excessive Fluid Many of the clinical manifestations of heart failure result from hypervolemia and expansion of the interstitial fluid volume. By the time fluid retention due to heart failure becomes clinically evident, most commonly as edema, considerable expansion of the extracellular space has already occurred, and heart failure usually is already advanced. Exertional dyspnea and orthopnea may be caused by displacement of fluid from the systemic to the pulmonary vascular bed. Treatment aimed at reducing extracellular fluid volume is dependent primarily on lowering total-body sodium stores, while fluid restriction is of less importance. A negative sodium balance can be achieved by reducing the dietary intake and increasing the urinary excretion of this ion with the aid of diuretics. In severe heart failure, mechanical removal of extracellular fluid by means of thoracentesis, paracentesis, and, rarely, ultrafiltration also may be employed.

DIET In patients with mild heart failure, considerable improvement in symptoms may result simply from reducing the sodium intake, particularly if accompanied by periods of physical rest. In patients with more severe heart failure, the sodium intake must be controlled more rigidly, and other measures, such as diuretics, vasodilators, and glycosides, are used. Even following recovery from a bout of heart failure, if the underlying cause has not been corrected, at least moderate sodium restriction should be maintained. The normal diet contains approximately 6 to 10 g sodium chloride; this intake can be reduced by half simply by excluding salt-rich foods and salt added at the table. Reduction of the ordinary dietary intake to approximately one-fourth of normal may be achieved if, in addition, all salt is omitted from cooking. In patients with severe heart

failure, in whom the daily sodium chloride intake should be reduced to between 500 and 1000 mg, milk, cheese, bread, cereals, canned vegetables and soups, some salted cuts of meat, and some fresh vegetables, including spinach, celery, and beets, must be eliminated. A variety of fresh fruit, green vegetables, specially processed breads and milk, and salt substitutes are permissible, but it is difficult to keep such diets palatable over the long term. Water intake may be ad libitum in all but the most severe forms of congestive heart failure. Late in the course of heart failure, dilutional hyponatremia may develop in patients who are unable to excrete a water load, sometimes because of excessive secretion of antidiuretic hormone. In such cases, water intake as well as sodium intake must be restricted.

Attention also must be directed to the caloric content of the diet. Calories should be restricted in obese patients with heart failure. On the other hand, in patients with severe heart failure and cardiac cachexia, an attempt must be made to maintain nutritional intake and to avoid caloric and vitamin deficiencies; nutritional supplements may be in order.

DIURETICS A variety of diuretic agents are available (Table 246-4, p. 1387), and in patients with mild heart failure, almost all are effective. However, in the more severe forms of heart failure, the selection of diuretics is more difficult, and abnormalities in serum electrolytes must be taken into account. Overtreatment must be avoided, since the resultant hypovolemia may reduce cardiac output, interfere with renal function, and produce profound weakness and lethargy. The following is a list of the most widely used diuretics:

1. *Thiazide diuretics.* These agents are used widely in clinical practice because of their effectiveness when administered orally. In patients with chronic heart failure of mild or moderate severity, the continued administration of a thiazide diuretic abolishes or diminishes the need for rigid dietary sodium restriction, although salty foods and table salt still should be avoided. Thiazides are well absorbed following oral administration; chlorothiazide and hydrochlorothiazide reach their peak action in 4 h, and diuresis persists for approximately 12 h. Thiazide diuretics reduce the reabsorption of sodium and chloride in the first half of the distal convoluted tubule and a portion of the cortical ascending limb of the loop of Henle, and water follows the unreabsorbed salt. Thiazides fail to increase free water clearance, and in some instances reduce it, supporting the hypothesis that these drugs inhibit selective reabsorption of sodium chloride in the distal cortical diluting segment, at a site where the urine is normally diluted (Chap. 269). This may result in the excretion of a hypertonic urine and may contribute to dilutional hyponatremia. As a consequence of increased delivery of sodium to the distal nephron, sodium-potassium ion exchange is enhanced, and kaliuresis results. In contrast to the loop diuretics, which enhance calcium excretion, the thiazides have the opposite effect. These drugs are effective and useful in the treatment of heart failure as long as the glomerular filtration rate exceeds approximately 50 percent of normal.

Chlorothiazide is administered in doses of up to 500 mg every 6 h. Many derivatives of this compound are available but differ principally in dosage and duration of action and therefore offer few, if any, significant advantages over the parent compound, except for chlorthalidone, which may be administered once daily. Potassium depletion and metabolic alkalosis (the latter due to increased H^+ secretion as a substitute for the depleted intracellular stores of potassium and increased proximal tubular reabsorption of filtered HCO_3^- when there is relative depletion of the extracellular fluid volume) are the chief adverse metabolic effects following prolonged administration of the thiazides, of metolazone, and of the loop diuretics. Hypokalemia may enhance seriously the dangers of digitalis intoxication, induce fatigue and lethargy, and may be prevented by the oral supplementation of potassium chloride. However, the solution is not palatable and may be hazardous in patients with renal failure. Therefore, to prevent potassium depletion in patients receiving thiazide diuretics, intermittent dosage schedules, e.g., omitting the diuretic every third day, and the addition of a potassium-retaining diuretic, such as a spironolactone or triamterene, may be preferable.

Other side effects of thiazides include reduction of the excretion of uric acid, which may lead to hyperuricemia, and a hyperglycemic effect, which rarely may precipitate hyperosmolar coma in the poorly regulated diabetic patient. Skin rashes, thrombocytopenia, and granulocytopenia also have been reported.

2. *Metolazone.* This quinethazone derivative has a site of action and potency similar to those of the thiazides but has been reported to be effective in the presence of moderate renal failure. The usual dose is 5 to 10 mg/d.

3. *Furosemide, bumetanide, ethacrynic acid, piretanide, and torsemide.* These "loop" diuretics are similar physiologically but differ chemically. These extremely powerful diuretics reversibly inhibit the reabsorption of sodium, potassium, and chloride in the thick ascending limb of Henle's loop, apparently by blocking a cotransport system in the luminal membrane. They may induce renal cortical vasodilatation and can produce rates of urine formation that may be as high as one-fourth of the glomerular filtration rate. While other diuretics lose their effectiveness as blood volume is restored to normal levels, the loop diuretics remain effective despite the elimination of excessive extracellular fluid volume. The major side effects of these agents are due to this marked diuretic potency, which on rare occasions may result in contraction of the plasma volume, circulatory collapse, reductions in the renal blood flow and glomerular filtration rate, and the development of prerenal azotemia. Metabolic alkalosis is produced by a large increase in the urinary excretion of chloride, hydrogen, and potassium ions. Hypokalemia (see discussion of thiazides, above) and hyponatremia may occur, and hyperuricemia and hyperglycemia are observed occasionally, as with thiazide diuretics. The reabsorption of free water is decreased.

All five drugs are readily absorbed orally and are excreted in the bile and urine. They are usually effective by mouth and intravenously. Weakness, nausea, and dizziness may complicate the administration of all loop diuretics; ethacrynic acid has been associated with transient or even permanent deafness as well as with skin rash and granulocytopenia.

These extremely effective diuretics are useful in all forms of heart failure, particularly in otherwise refractory heart failure and pulmonary edema. They have been shown to be effective in patients with hypoalbuminemia, hyponatremia, hypochloremia, hypokalemia, and reductions in the glomerular filtration rate and to produce a diuresis in patients in whom thiazide diuretics and aldosterone antagonists, alone and in combination, are ineffective.

In patients with refractory heart failure, the action of loop diuretics may be potentiated by intravenous administration and the addition of other diuretics, i.e., thiazides, carbonic anhydrase inhibitors, osmotic diuretics, and the potassium-sparing diuretics—spironolactone, triamterene, and amiloride. The latter agents act on the cortical collecting ducts, are relatively weak, and therefore are rarely indicated as sole agents. However, their potassium-sparing properties make them particularly useful in conjunction with the more potent kaliuretic agents, the loop diuretics, and thiazides. The potassium-sparing agents fall into two classes, as noted below.

4. *Aldosterone antagonists.* The 17-spironolactones resemble aldosterone structurally and act on the distal half of the convoluted tubule and the cortical portion of the collecting duct by competitive inhibition of aldosterone, thereby blocking the exchange between sodium and both potassium and hydrogen in the distal tubules and collecting ducts. These agents produce a sodium diuresis, and in contrast to the thiazides, ethacrynic acid, and furosemide, they result in potassium retention. Although secondary hyperaldosteronism exists in some patients with congestive heart failure, the spironolactones are effective even in patients in whom the serum aldosterone concentration is within normal limits. Aldactone A may be administered in doses of 25 to 100 mg three to four times daily by mouth. The maximal effect of this regimen is not observed for approximately 4 days. Spironolactones are most effective when administered in combination with thiazide and/or loop diuretics. The opposing action of these drugs on urine and serum potassium makes possible a sodium diuresis without either hyper- or hypokalemia when spirono-

lactone and one of these other agents are administered in combination. Also, since spironolactone, triamterene, and amiloride act on the distal tubule, they are particularly effective when used in combination with one of these other diuretics that act more proximally.

Spironolactone, triamterene, and amiloride should not be administered alone to patients with hyperkalemia, renal failure, or hyponatremia. Reported complications include nausea, epigastric distress, mental confusion, drowsiness, gynecomastia, and erythematous eruptions.

5. *Triamterene and amiloride.* These two drugs exert renal effects similar to those of the spironolactones; i.e., they block sodium reabsorption and secondarily inhibit potassium secretion in the distal tubules. However, their fundamental mechanism of action differs from that of the spironolactones, since they are active in adrenalectomized animals and their action does not depend on the presence of aldosterone. The effective dose of triamterene is 100 mg once or twice daily, and that of amiloride is 5 mg daily. Side effects include nausea, vomiting, diarrhea, headache, granulocytopenia, eosinophilia, and skin rash. Both triamterene and the chemically unrelated diuretic amiloride resemble Aldactone A in that their diuretic potency is not great, but they are effective in preventing the hypokalemia characteristic of the administration of thiazides, furosemide, and ethacrynic acid. A number of diuretic preparations contain a combination of a thiazide and either triamterene or amiloride in a single capsule. They may be useful in patients who develop hypokalemia with a thiazide but should not be used in patients with impaired renal function and/or hyperkalemia.

When making a *choice of diuretics*, orally administered thiazides and metolazone are the agents of choice in the treatment of chronic cardiac edema of mild to moderate degree in patients without hyperglycemia, hyperuricemia, or hypokalemia. Spironolactones, triamterene, and amiloride are not potent diuretics when used alone, but they potentiate other diuretics, particularly the thiazide and loop diuretics. However, in patients with heart failure and severe secondary hyperaldosteronism, spironolactone may be quite effective. Ethacrynic acid, bumetanide, and furosemide, given alone or with spironolactone or triamterene, are the agents of choice in patients with severe heart failure refractory to other diuretics. In very severe heart failure, the combination of a thiazide, a loop diuretic, and a potassium-sparing diuretic is required.

Vasodilator Therapy In many patients with heart failure, left ventricular afterload is increased as a consequence of the several neural and humoral influences that act to constrict the peripheral vascular bed. These include the previously mentioned increased activity of the adrenergic nervous system, elevation of circulating catecholamines, and activation of the renin-angiotensin system, and perhaps increased circulating antidiuretic hormone. In addition to the vasoconstriction, the ventricular end-diastolic and end-systolic volumes rise in systolic heart failure. As a consequence of the operation of Laplace's law, which relates myocardial wall tension to the product of intraventricular pressure and radius (both of which may become elevated in heart failure), the aortic impedance, i.e., the force that opposes left ventricular ejection, or the ventricular afterload, rises. Vasoconstriction is generally considered to be a useful compensatory mechanism that allows blood flow to vital organs to persist in the presence of hypovolemia and many forms of shock associated with reduction of the total cardiac output (Chap. 38). However, in the presence of impaired cardiac function, the increase in afterload may reduce cardiac output further.

As shown in Fig. 232-7 (p. 1284), afterload is a major determinant of cardiac function. When cardiac function is normal, a moderate elevation in afterload does not reduce stroke volume significantly, because the resultant increase in left ventricular end-diastolic volume, i.e., preload, can be tolerated easily. However, when myocardial systolic function is impaired, such an increase in preload evoked by an elevation of afterload may raise ventricular end-diastolic and pulmonary capillary pressures to levels that may produce severe pulmonary congestion or even pulmonary edema. In many patients with heart failure, the ventricle is already operating at the peak, flat portion of its Frank-Starling curve (Fig. 232-6 p. 1283), and any additional increase in aortic impedance (afterload) will reduce stroke volume. Conversely, a modest reduction of afterload has no significant effect on stroke volume in normal individuals, but in patients with heart failure it tends to restore hemodynamics to normal by elevating the stroke volume of the failing ventricle and reducing the elevated ventricular filling pressure.

The pharmacologic reduction of impedance to left ventricular ejection with vasodilator drugs represents an important adjunct in the management of heart failure. This approach may be particularly helpful but is by no means limited to patients with acute systolic heart failure due to myocardial infarction (Chap. 243), valvular regurgitation (Chap. 237), elevated systemic vascular resistance and/or arterial pressure, and marked cardiac dilatation. The reduction of afterload by means of a variety of vasodilators reduces left ventricular end-diastolic pressure, volume, and oxygen consumption while raising stroke volume and cardiac output and causing only modest reduction in aortic pressure. Vasodilators should, of course, not be used in patients with hypotension.

In patients with both acute and chronic heart failure secondary to ischemic heart disease, cardiomyopathy, or valvular regurgitation who are treated with vasodilators, cardiac output rises, the pulmonary wedge pressure falls, the signs and symptoms of heart failure are relieved, and a new steady state is achieved in which cardiac output is higher and afterload lower with no or only mild reduction of arterial pressure (Fig. 233-2). Furthermore, the reduction of an elevated left end-diastolic pressure may improve subendocardial perfusion, further improving myocardial contraction.

Vasodilator therapy is useful in the treatment of all forms of systolic heart failure, ranging from the mild-chronic to the severe-acute forms. Vasodilators are *not* useful in the management of isolated diastolic heart failure.

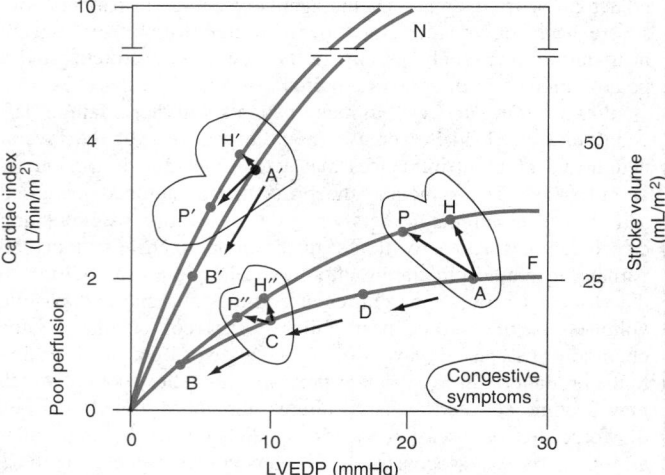

FIGURE 233-2 Effects of various vasodilators on the relationship between left ventricular end-diastolic pressure (LVEDP) and cardiac index or stroke volume in normal (N) and failing (F) hearts. H represents hydralazine or any other pure arterial dilator. It produces only a minimal increase in cardiac index in the normal individual (A′ → H′) or in the patient with heart failure with normal LVEDP (C → H″). In contrast, it elevates output in the patient with heart failure and elevated LVEDP (A → H). P represents a balanced vasodilator, such as sodium nitroprusside or an ACE inhibitor. It reduces filling pressure in all patients, elevates cardiac output in patients with heart failure and elevated LVEDP (A → P), lowers cardiac output in normal individuals (A′ → P′), and has little effect on cardiac output in heart failure patients with normal filling pressures (C → P″). *(From Smith et al, with permission.)*

The several available vasodilators vary in their hemodynamic effects, locus and duration of action, and mode of administration (Table 246-4, p. 1387). Some vasodilators, such as hydralazine, minoxidil, and the alpha-adrenergic blocking agents, such as prazosin, act predominantly on the arterial bed and primarily increase stroke volume; others, such as nitroglycerin and isosorbide dinitrate, act almost entirely on the venous side of the circulation. The latter agents cause pooling of blood in the venous bed and act primarily to reduce ventricular filling pressures. ACE inhibitors, prazosin, and sodium nitroprusside are "balanced vasodilators," i.e., they act on both the arterial and venous beds. Some agents, such as sodium nitroprusside, must be administered by continuous intravenous infusion; nitroglycerin requires administration in ointment patch or intravenous forms when a prolonged effect is desired; and isosorbide dinitrate is most effective when it is administered by the sublingual route.

The ideal vasodilator for the treatment of *acute* heart failure should have a rapid onset and brief duration of action when administered by intravenous infusion; sodium nitroprusside (0.1 to 3.0 μg/kg per minute) qualifies as such a drug, but its use requires careful monitoring of the arterial pressure and, if possible, of the pulmonary artery wedge pressure in an intensive care unit. For the treatment of chronic congestive heart failure, the agent should be effective on oral administration, and its action should persist for at least 6 h. ACE inhibitors (e.g., captopril, 10 to 50 mg tid) satisfy these requirements and have, quite properly, become the most useful and widely used vasodilators. It is advisable to commence therapy with very low doses, particularly in patients receiving diuretics, in order to avoid hypotension and gradually increase the dose.

Vasodilators are potent and effective in acutely improving the deranged hemodynamics of heart failure, and there is evidence in favor of a beneficial chronic effect as well. Studies with ACE inhibitors have demonstrated a favorable long-term reduction of symptoms and enhancement of exercise tolerance. Importantly, these drugs and, to a lesser extent, the combination of hydralazine and isosorbide dinitrate prolong survival of patients with heart failure. The administration of ACE inhibitors has been shown to prevent or retard the development of heart failure in patients with left ventricular dysfunction but without heart failure and to reduce long-term mortality when it is begun in such patients shortly after acute myocardial infarction. Direct acting vasodilators, such as hydralazine or minoxidil, may be useful when added to an ACE inhibitor in patients who have failed ACE inhibitor therapy.

Enhancement of Myocardial Contractility—Digitalis The improvement of myocardial contractility by means of cardiac glycosides is useful in the control of heart failure.

Digoxin, which has a half-life of 1.6 days, is filtered in the glomeruli and secreted by the renal tubules; 85 percent is excreted in the urine. The ratio of digoxin clearance to endogenous creatinine clearance is 0.8, and the percentage of the body's total stores of digoxin lost per day can be calculated as $(14 \pm 0.2) \times$ creatinine clearance in milliliters per minute. Significant reductions of the glomerular filtration rate reduce the elimination of digoxin and, therefore, may prolong digoxin's effect, allowing it to accumulate to toxic levels if it is administered in patients with impaired renal function. The administration of most diuretics does not alter the excretion of digoxin significantly, but spironolactone can inhibit tubular secretion of digoxin, resulting in significant accumulation of the drug. In patients with normal renal function, a plateau concentration in the blood and tissue is reached after 5 days of daily maintenance treatment without a loading dose (see Fig. 68-2).

MECHANISM OF ACTION The most important effect of digitalis on cardiac muscle is to shift its force-velocity relation upward (Chap. 232). This positive inotropic effect is exhibited in normal, nonfailing hypertrophied, and failing hearts. In the absence of heart failure, however, when cardiac output is not limited by cardiac contractility, the drug does not elevate the output.

Excitation-contraction coupling (p. 1279) is the membrane and intracellular process most likely involved in producing the positive inotropic effect of digitalis glycosides. These drugs inhibit transmembrane sodium and potassium movement by inhibition of the monovalent cation transport enzyme–coupled Na^+,K^+-ATPase. The latter, localized to the sarcolemma, appears to be the receptor for cardioactive glycosides, whose action results in an increase in intracellular sodium content; this, in turn, increases intracellular calcium concentration through a Na^+-Ca^{2+} exchange carrier mechanism. The increased myocardial uptake of calcium augments calcium released to the myofilaments during excitation and, therefore, invokes a positive inotropic response.

Cardiac glycosides also produce alterations in the electrical properties of both the contractile cells and the specialized automatic cells, leading to increased automaticity and ectopic impulse activity. The conduction velocity is slowed, which is conducive to the development of reentry. Thus the known electrophysiologic effects of digitalis glycosides are capable of explaining the development of the arrhythmias associated with digitalis intoxication, i.e., ventricular arrhythmias and ventricular fibrillation.

The glycosides also prolong the effective *refractory period* of the atrioventricular node, largely as a result of an enhanced vagal effect. This helps to explain the slowing of ventricular rate produced by digitalis in atrial flutter and fibrillation.

Digitalis slows the sinus rate usually only in the presence of heart failure, in part due to an effect on the central nervous system leading to withdrawal of sympathetic activity and increased vagal action.

In addition, the digitalis glycosides also exert an action on the peripheral vasculature, causing venous and arterial constriction in normal individuals and reflex dilatation resulting from withdrawal of sympathetic constrictor activity in patients with congestive heart failure.

USE IN HEART FAILURE Digitalis is particularly effective in patients with heart failure accompanied by atrial flutter and fibrillation and a rapid ventricular rate, who benefit from both slowing of the ventricular rate and the positive inotropic effect. Although digitalis does not improve survival in patients with sinus rhythm and left ventricular systolic failure, it reduces the need for hospitalization for heart failure in such patients. By stimulating myocardial contractility moderately, digitalis improves ventricular emptying; i.e., it increases cardiac output, augments the ejection fraction, promotes diuresis, and reduces the elevated diastolic pressure and volume and end-systolic volume of the failing ventricle with consequent reduction of symptoms resulting from pulmonary vascular congestion and elevated systemic venous pressure. It is most beneficial in patients in whom ventricular contractility is impaired secondary to chronic ischemic heart disease or when hypertensive, valvular, or congenital heart disease imposes an excessive volume or pressure load. It is of relatively little value in most forms of cardiomyopathy, myocarditis, beriberi with heart failure, mitral stenosis, thyrotoxicosis (all with sinus rhythm), chronic constrictive pericarditis (Chap. 240), and any form of diastolic heart failure (p. 1288).

DIGITALIS INTOXICATION Digitalis intoxication is a serious and potentially fatal complication. The lethal dose of most glycosides is approximately 5 to 10 times the minimal effective dose and only about twice the dose that leads to minor toxic manifestations. Advanced age, acute myocardial infarction or ischemia, hypoxemia, magnesium depletion, renal insufficiency, hypercalcemia, electrical cardioversion, and hypothyroidism all may reduce tolerance to digitalis. The most common precipitating cause of digitalis intoxication, however, is depletion of potassium stores, which occurs often in patients with heart failure as a result of diuretic therapy and secondary hyperaldosteronism. Since it is not necessary for a patient to receive a maximally tolerated dose of digitalis to derive a beneficial effect, even small doses provide some therapeutic action; this point should be considered if these drugs are to be used in patients prone to toxicity, particularly the elderly.

Anorexia, nausea, and vomiting, which are among the earliest signs of digitalis intoxication, are caused by direct stimulation of centers in the medulla. The most frequent disturbance of cardiac rhythm is ventricular premature beats, bigeminy, ventricular tachycardia, and, rarely, ventricular fibrillation. Atrioventricular block of varying degrees of severity may occur. Nonparoxysmal atrial tachycardia with variable atrioventricular block is quite characteristic of digitalis intoxication. Sinus arrhythmia, sinoatrial block, sinus arrest, and atrioventricular junctional and multifocal ventricular tachycardia also may occur. Chronic digitalis intoxication may be insidious in onset and characterized by exacerbations of heart failure, weight loss, cachexia, neuralgias, gynecomastia, yellow vision, and delirium.

The administration of quinidine, verapamil, amiodarone, and propafenone to patients receiving digoxin raises the serum concentration of the latter by reducing both the renal and nonrenal elimination of digoxin and by reducing its volume of distribution. These drugs increase the propensity to digitalis intoxication, and the dose of digitalis should be reduced by half in patients receiving these drugs. Serum digoxin concentrations and electrocardiograms should be followed carefully when these drugs are administered to digitalized patients.

The radioimmunoassay for digoxin makes possible the correlation of serum glycoside levels with the presence of toxicity. In patients receiving standard maintenance doses of digoxin (0.125 to 0.375 mg daily) in whom no sign of intoxication is present, serum concentrations approximate 1 to 1.5 ng/mL. When signs of intoxication are present, serum levels of more than 2 ng/mL are often found. Since many factors other than the serum concentration determine digitalis intoxication, and since there is considerable overlap in serum glycoside concentrations in patients with and without toxicity, these levels cannot be used as a sole guide to digitalis dosage. However, when taken together with findings on the clinical examination and electrocardiogram, they add useful information to the clinical evaluations of digitalis intoxication. In addition, they will indicate whether a patient for whom the history of digitalis intake is in doubt has, in fact, been receiving the drug.

Treatment of digitalis intoxication When tachyarrhythmias result from digitalis intoxication, withdrawal of the drug and treatment with potassium, phenytoin, a beta-adrenoceptor blocker, or lidocaine are indicated. Potassium should be administered cautiously and by the oral route whenever possible if hypokalemia is present. *Potassium must not be employed in the presence of atrioventricular block or hyperkalemia.* Lidocaine is effective in the treatment of digitalis-induced ventricular tachyarrhythmias in the absence of preceding atrioventricular block. A cardiac pacemaker may be required in digitalis-induced atrioventricular block. Electrical conversion may be lifesaving in digitalis-induced ventricular fibrillation but is usually ineffective in other tachyarrhythmias secondary to digitalis intoxication. Quinidine and procainamide are of limited value in the treatment of digitalis intoxication. Fab fragments of purified, intact digitalis antibodies are a potentially lifesaving approach to the treatment of severe intoxication.

Sympathomimetic Amines (See also Chap. 70) Five sympathomimetic amines that act largely on beta-adrenergic receptors—norepinephrine, epinephrine, isoproterenol (isoprenaline), dopamine, and dobutamine—improve myocardial contractility in various forms of heart failure (Table 70-1, p. 437). The latter two agents appear to be most effective in the management of heart failure; they must be administered by constant intravenous infusion and are useful in patients with intractable heart failure, particularly those with a reversible component, such as exists in patients who have undergone cardiac surgery, and in some instances of myocardial infarction and shock or pulmonary edema. While they improve the hemodynamics in these conditions, it is not clear that they improve survival. Their administration should be accompanied by careful and continuous monitoring of the electrocardiogram, arterial pressure, and, if possible, pulmonary artery wedge pressure.

DOPAMINE (p. 1256) This naturally occurring immediate precursor of norepinephrine has a combination of actions that makes it particularly useful in the treatment of a variety of hypotensive states and congestive heart failure. At very low doses, i.e., 1 to 2 (μg/kg)/min, it dilates renal and mesenteric blood vessels through stimulation of specific dopaminergic receptors, thereby augmenting renal and mesenteric blood flow and sodium excretion. In the range of 2 to 10 (μg/kg)/min, dopamine stimulates myocardial beta receptors but induces relatively little tachycardia, while at higher doses it also stimulates alpha-adrenergic receptors and elevates arterial pressure.

DOBUTAMINE This synthetic catecholamine acts on beta$_1$, beta$_2$, and alpha receptors. It exerts a potent inotropic action, has only a modest cardioaccelerating effect, and lowers peripheral vascular resistance, but since it simultaneously raises cardiac output, it has little effect on systemic arterial pressure. Dobutamine, given in continuous infusions of 2.5 to 10 (μg/kg)/min, is useful in the treatment of acute heart failure without hypotension. Like the other sympathomimetic amines, it may be particularly valuable in the management of patients requiring relatively short-term inotropic support—up to 1 week—in conditions that are reversible, such as the cardiac depression that sometimes follows open-heart surgery, or in patients with acute heart failure who are being prepared for operation, including cardiac transplantation. Adverse effects include sinus tachycardia, tachyarrhythmias, and hypertension.

A major problem with all sympathomimetics is the loss of responsiveness, apparently due to "downregulation" of adrenergic receptors, which becomes evident within 8 h of continuous administration. This problem may be managed by intermittent therapy.

AMRINONE AND MILRINONE These bipyridines are noncatecholamine, nonglycoside agents that exert both positive inotropic and vasodilator actions by inhibiting a specific phosphodiesterase. They are suitable for intravenous use only; by simultaneously stimulating cardiac contractility and dilating the systemic vascular bed they reverse the major hemodynamic abnormalities associated with severe heart failure.

ANTICOAGULANTS Patients with advanced heart failure are at increased risk of pulmonary emboli secondary to venous thrombosis and to systemic emboli secondary to intracardiac thrombi. Patients with heart failure and additional risk factors such as atrial fibrillation, previous venous thrombosis, and pulmonary or systemic emboli should receive heparin followed by warfarin.

BETA-ADRENOCEPTOR BLOCKERS While large doses of beta-adrenergic receptor blockers can intensify heart failure, the administration of gradually escalating doses of drugs such as metoprolol, carvedilol, and bucindolol have been reported to improve the symptoms of heart failure and, in some patients, to improve left ventricular function and exercise tolerance and retard the progression of heart failure. In patients with moderately severe heart failure (classes II and III), the administration of 5 mg metoprolol bid, increasing over 6 weeks to a target dose of 50 to 75 mg bid may prove beneficial.[1]

Diastolic Heart Failure The major goal in the treatment of this condition is to eliminate or reduce the causes of diastolic dysfunction, such as ventricular hypertrophy, fibrosis, or ischemia. The second is to reduce pulmonary and/or systemic venous congestion, a major consequence of diastolic dysfunction (Table 233-2).

Management of Arrhythmias Premature ventricular contractions and episodes of asymptomatic ventricular tachycardia are common in advanced heart failure. Sudden death, presumably due to ventricular fibrillation, is responsible for about one-half of all deaths in this condition. (The remainder are due to failure of the cardiac pump.) The management of arrhythmias should commence with correction of electrolyte and acid-base disturbances (Chaps. 49 and 50), especially diuretic-induced hypokalemia, as well as digitalis

---

[1] Beta-adrenoceptor blockers have not been approved for the treatment of heart failure at the time of this writing.

Table 233-2

Management of Diastolic Dysfunction

Reduce the congestive state
   Salt restriction, diuretics, angiotensin-converting enzyme (ACE) inhibitors
   Dialysis or plasmapheresis
Maintain atrial contraction
   Direct-current or pharmacologic cardioversion
   Sequential atrioventricular pacing
Prevent tachycardia and promote bradycardia
   Beta blockers, calcium blockers
   Radiofrequency ablation and pacing
Treat and prevent myocardial ischemia
   Nitrates, beta blockers, calcium blockers
   Bypass surgery, angioplasty
Control hypertension and promote regression of hypertrophy
   Antihypertensive agents
Attenuate neurohormonal activation
   Beta blockers, ACE inhibitors
Prevent fibrosis and promote regression of fibrosis
   ACE inhibitors, spironolactone
   Anti-ischemic agents
Improve ventricular relaxation
   Beta-adrenergic agonists
   Systolic unloading
   Treat ischemia
   Calcium blockers (in hypertrophic cardiomyopathy)

SOURCE: WH Gaasch et al, Management of left ventricular diastolic dysfunction in *Cardiovascular Therapeutics*, TW Smith (ed), Philadelphia, Saunders, 1996

---

intoxication (p. 1295). Treatment with class I antiarrhythmics such as quinidine, procainamide, or flecainide (Chap. 231) is fraught with danger because these drugs are proarrhythmic in patients with heart failure. Amiodarone (p. 1295), on the other hand, is well tolerated and is the drug of choice for patients with atrial fibrillation and symptomatic tachyarrhythmia and perhaps for frequent, prolonged asymptomatic ventricular tachyarrhythmias as well. In patients who have been resuscitated from sudden death, the automatic implantable defibrillator may prevent recurrence and back-up pacing may prevent sudden death due to bradyarrhythmias. It is not yet clear whether these devices alter overall mortality or only the mode of death in patients with advanced heart failure.

Refractory Heart Failure When the response to ordinary treatment is inadequate, heart failure is considered to be refractory. Before assuming that this condition simply reflects advanced, perhaps pre-terminal, myocardial depression, careful consideration must be given to several possibilities: (1) an underlying and overlooked cause of the heart disease that may be amenable to specific surgical or medical therapy, such as silent aortic or mitral stenosis, infective endocarditis, hypertension, or thyrotoxicosis; (2) one or a combination of the precipitating causes of heart failure, such as pulmonary or urinary tract infection, recurrent pulmonary emboli, arterial hypoxemia, anemia, or arrhythmia; and (3) complications of overly vigorous therapy, such as digitalis intoxication, hypovolemia, or electrolyte imbalance.

Recognition and proper treatment of the aforementioned complications are likely to make the patient responsive to therapy again. Perhaps the most common complication results from overzealous treatment with diuretics. When administered too rapidly, these drugs can produce sudden hypovolemia before edema fluid can be mobilized to replace the loss of blood volume, the result being a shocklike state with evidence of systemic hypoperfusion in the presence of edema. The chronically excessively diuresed patient may have exchanged the hazards of pulmonary edema and the inconvenience of systemic edema for a persistently depressed cardiac output with its associated weakness, lethargy, prerenal azotemia, and sometimes cardiac cachexia. Temporarily easing salt restriction and diuretic administration may overcome this difficulty, but as heart failure worsens, this course of action may lead to increased pulmonary congestion, which is equally unacceptable.

Hyponatremia is a late manifestation of refractory heart failure. It, too, may be a complication of overaggressive diuresis leading to reduced glomerular filtration rate and decreased delivery of NaCl to the diluting sites in the distal tubule. Hyponatremia also may result from nonosmotic stimuli for the continued secretion of antidiuretic hormone. Therapy involves improvement of the cardiovascular status, if possible (sometimes requiring the administration of a sympathomimetic amine such as dopamine or dobutamine), as well as temporary cessation of diuretic therapy and restriction of oral water intake. Hypertonic saline is very rarely indicated because total-body sodium is usually elevated, not depressed, in heart failure.

The combination of an intravenously administered vasodilator, such as sodium nitroprusside, along with a potent sympathomimetic amine, such as dopamine or dobutamine, often results in an additive effect, raising cardiac output and lowering filling pressure. Intravenous amrinone or milrinone, sometimes accompanied by the administration of an ACE inhibitor, also may be useful in patients with refractory heart failure.

In hospitalized patients with refractory heart failure, therapy guided by hemodynamic measurements provided by a balloon flotation (Swan-Ganz) catheter may be helpful. The goal of manipulating diuretics, vasodilators, and inotropic agents is to achieve a pulmonary capillary wedge pressure of 15 to 18 mmHg, a right atrial pressure of 5 to 8 mmHg, a cardiac index > 2.2 (L/min)/m^2, and a systemic vascular resistance of 800 to 1200 dynes $\cdot$ s $\cdot$ cm^{-5}. Once these values are achieved, the patient can usually be converted from intravenous to oral therapy.

CARDIAC TRANSPLANTATION When patients with heart failure become unresponsive to a combination of all the aforementioned therapeutic measures, are in New York Heart Association class IV, and are deemed unlikely to survive 1 year, they should be considered for cardiac transplantation (see Chap. 234).

Treatment of Acute Pulmonary Edema Pulmonary edema secondary to left ventricular failure or mitral stenosis is described in Chap. 32. It is life-threatening and must be considered a medical emergency. As is the case for the more chronic forms of heart failure, in the treatment of pulmonary edema, attention must be directed to identifying and removing any precipitating causes of decompensation, such as an arrhythmia or infection. However, because of the acute nature of the problem, a number of additional nonspecific measures are necessary. If it does not delay treatment unduly, recording pulmonary vascular pressures through a Swan-Ganz catheter and intraarterial pressure directly is advisable. The first six measures listed below are ordinarily applied simultaneously or nearly so.

1. Morphine is administered intravenously repetitively, as needed, in doses from 2 to 5 mg. This drug reduces anxiety, reduces adrenergic vasoconstrictor stimuli to the arteriolar and venous beds, and thereby helps to break a vicious cycle. Naloxone should be available in case respiratory depression occurs.

2. Because the alveolar edema interferes with oxygen diffusion, resulting in arterial hypoxemia, 100% oxygen should be administered, preferably under positive pressure. The latter increases intraalveolar pressure and therefore reduces transudation of fluid from the alveolar capillaries and impedes venous return to the thorax, reducing pulmonary capillary pressure.

3. The patient should be maintained in the sitting position, with the legs dangling along the side of the bed, if possible, which also tends to reduce venous return.

4. Intravenous loop diuretics, such as furosemide or ethacrynic acid (40 to 100 mg), or bumetanide (1 mg) will, by rapidly establishing a diuresis, reduce circulating blood volume and thereby hasten the relief of pulmonary edema. In addition, when given intravenously, furosemide also exerts a venodilator action, reduces venous return, and reduces pulmonary edema even before the diuresis commences.

5. Afterload reduction is achieved with intravenous sodium nitroprusside at 20 to 30 μg/min in patients whose systolic arterial pressures exceed 100 mmHg.

6. Inotropic support should be provided by dopamine or dobutamine as described on p. 1296. Patients with systolic heart failure who are not receiving digitalis should receive 1.0 mg digoxin intravenously.

7. Sometimes, aminophylline (theophylline ethylenediamine), 240 to 480 mg intravenously, is effective in diminishing bronchoconstriction, increasing renal blood flow and sodium excretion, and augmenting myocardial contractility.

8. If the above-mentioned measures are not sufficient, rotating tourniquets should be applied to the extremities.

After these emergency therapeutic measures have been instituted and the precipitating factors treated, the diagnosis of the underlying cardiac disorder responsible for the pulmonary edema must be established if it is not already known. After stabilization of the patient's condition, a long-range strategy for prevention of future episodes of pulmonary edema must be established, and this may require surgical treatment.

PROGNOSIS

The prognosis in heart failure depends primarily on the nature of the underlying heart disease and on the presence or absence of a precipitating factor that can be treated. When one of the latter can be identified and removed, the outlook for immediate survival is far better than if heart failure occurs without any obvious precipitating cause. In the latter situation, survival usually ranges between 6 months and 4 years depending on the severity of the heart failure (Fig. 233-3). Also, the long-term prognosis for heart failure is most favorable when the underlying forms of heart disease can be treated. The prognosis also can be estimated by observing the response to treatment. When clinical improvement occurs with only modest dietary sodium restriction and small doses of diuretics, the outlook is far better than if, in addition to these measures, intensive diuretic therapy and vasodilators are necessary. Other factors that have been shown to be associated with a poor prognosis in heart failure include a severely depressed ejection fraction (<25 percent), a reduced maximal O_2 uptake [<15 (mL/kg)/min], the inability to walk on the level and at a normal pace for more than 3 min, reduced (<133 mEq/L) serum sodium concentration, reduced (<3 mEq/L) serum potassium concentration, elevated circulating atrial natriuretic peptide and norepinephrine concentrations, as well as frequent ventricular extrasystoles on Holter monitoring. A large fraction of patients with congestive heart failure die suddenly, presumably of ventricular fibrillation. Unfortunately, there is no evidence that this complication can be prevented by the administration of antiarrhythmic agents.

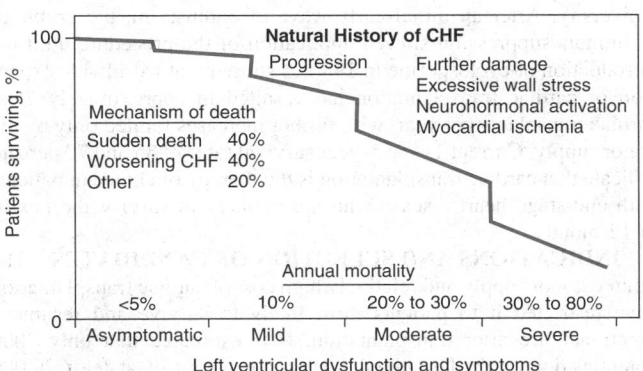

FIGURE 233-3 The natural history of congestive heart failure (CHF). Once left ventricular systolic dysfunction is present, it usually progresses, albeit not predictably. As left ventricular dysfunction progresses and symptoms increase, mortality rate increase and the process becomes inexorable. Myocyte loss and fibrosis become irreversible. An effective preventive measure must be introduced before onset or early in the course of progressive left ventricular dysfunction. *(From BM Massie and NH Shah, with permission.)*

BIBLIOGRAPHY

CODY RJ: Optimising ACE inhibitor therapy of congestive heart failure. Clin Pharmacokinet 24:59, 1993

COLUCCI WS (ed): *Heart Failure: Cardiac Function and Dysfunction*, in *Atlas of Heart Diseases*, vol 4, E Braunwald (series ed). Philadelphia, Current Medicine, 1995

——— et al: Clinical aspects of heart failure, in *Heart Disease*, 5th ed, E Braunwald (ed). Philadelphia, Saunders, 1996, pp 445–470

FRANCIS GS et al: Neurohumoral activation in preclinical heart failure. Remodeling and the potential for intervention. Circulation 87 (Suppl 5):IV90, 1993

GRODEN DL: Vasodilator therapy for congestive heart failure. Lessons from mortality trials. Arch Intern Med 153:445, 1993

KANNEL WB: Epidemiologic aspects of heart failure, in *Heart Failure: Current Concepts and Management*, Cardiology Clinics Series 7/1, KT Weber (ed). Philadelphia, Saunders, 1989

KELLY RA, SMITH TW: Pharmacological treatment of heart failure, in *Goodman and Gilman's The Pharmacological Basis of Therapeutics*, 9th ed. New York, McGraw-Hill, 1996, pp 809–838

KUBO SH, COHN JN: Long-term treatment of the ambulatory patient with heart failure, in *Cardiovascular Therapeutics*, TW Smith (ed). Philadelphia, Saunders, 1996, pp 210–231

MASSIE BM, SHAH NH: The heart failure epidemic: Magnitude of the problem and potential mitigating approaches. Curr Opin Cardiol 11:221, 1996

SLATTON ML, EICHORN EJ: β-blocker therapy for heart failure. Curr Opin Cardiol 11:263, 1996

SMITH TW et al: Management of heart failure, in *Heart Disease*, 5th ed, E Braunwald (ed). Philadelphia, Saunders, 1997, pp 492–514

SOLVD INVESTIGATORS: Effect of enalapril on survival in patients with reduced left ventricular ejection fractions and congestive heart failure. N Engl J Med 325:293, 1991

STEVENSON LW, COLUCCI WS: Management of patients hospitalized with heart failure, in Cardiovascular Therapeutics, TW Smith (ed). Philadelphia, Saunders, 1996, pp 199–209

SWEDBERG K: Reduction in mortality by pharmacological therapy in congestive heart failure. Circulation 87 (Suppl 5):IV126, 1993

WILCOX CS: Diuretics, in *The Kidney*, 5th ed, BM Brenner, FC Rector Jr (eds). Philadelphia, Saunders, 1996, pp 2299–2330

234   *John S. Schroeder*

CARDIAC TRANSPLANTATION

Orthotopic allograft cadaver cardiac transplantation as a treatment for end-stage cardiac disease will achieve its thirtieth anniversary on December 7, 1997. On that day in 1967 Dr. Christiaan Barnard accomplished the first successful cardiac transplant in a human, quickly followed by Dr. Norman Shumway and Dr. Richard Lower at Stanford University. After an initial early wave of enthusiasm, the problems of immunosuppression slowed application of the procedure until the introduction of cyclosporine in 1980. A subsequent worldwide expansion of cardiac transplantation has resulted in approximately 2500 cardiac transplants per year, with further increases limited only by the donor supply. Current 1- and 5-year survival rates of 85 and 70 percent indicate that cardiac transplantation is the therapy of choice in patients with end-stage heart disease who are unlikely to survive the next 6 to 12 months.

INDICATIONS AND SELECTION OF CANDIDATES   The limited donor supply and relatively high cost of cardiac transplantation have restricted it to patients most likely to survive and resume a functional life after transplantation. It is estimated that only 2000 potential donors in the United States, for a pool of at least 20,000 candidates based on current guidelines, become available yearly. Attempts to increase donor awareness in both physicians and the public are being made. Optimal candidates for this procedure are those who would be expected to return to a functional life if their hearts were replaced (Table 234-1). This requires a mentally vigorous, medically compliant person who has not suffered extensive other end-stage organ damage from cardiac failure, does not have other systemic disease

Table 234-1

Indications and Contraindications for Cardiac Transplantation

INDICATIONS

1. End-stage heart disease that limits prognosis for survival over 2 years or severely limits daily quality of life despite optimal medical and other surgical therapy
2. No secondary exclusion criteria
3. Suitable psychosocial profile and social support system
4. Suitable physiologic/chronologic age

EXCLUSION CRITERIA

1. Active infectious process
2. Recent pulmonary infarction
3. Insulin-requiring diabetes with evidence of end-organ damage
4. Irreversible pulmonary hypertension [pulmonary vascular resistance (PVR) poorly responsive to nitroprusside with PVR > 2 or pulmonary systolic pressure > 50 mmHg at peak dose or at mean arterial pressure of 65–70 mmHg]
5. Presence of circulating cytotoxic antibodies
6. Presence of active peptic ulcer disease
7. Active or recent malignancy
8. Presence of severe chronic obstructive pulmonary disease or chronic bronchitis
9. Substance or alcohol abuse
10. Presence of peripheral or cerebrovascular disease
11. Other systemic diseases that would jeopardize rehabilitation posttransplant

such as severe diabetes mellitus or collagen vascular disease, or is not positive for human immunodeficiency virus. Long-standing pulmonary hypertension or recurrent pulmonary emboli and infarction may result in irreversible pulmonary hypertension leading to intraoperative death. Several heart transplant centers have initiated cardiac transplantation for newborns with left ventricular hypoplasia, but long-term survival experience is still very limited.

Timing of the recommendation to undergo cardiac transplantation can be difficult and requires assessment of the patient's current disability, stability of course, and likelihood of surviving the next 6 to 12 months. Generally, left ventricular ejection fractions under 15 to 20 percent and presence of serious ventricular arrhythmias indicate a 1-year survival rate of 50 percent or less. Estimating prognosis remains very challenging. A maximal oxygen uptake during exercise (maximal $\dot{V}_{O_2}$) of <10 mL O_2 per kilogram per minute usually indicates poor likelihood of survival for 1 year and has been a criterion for transplant candidacy in some programs. Maximal $\dot{V}_{O_2}$ values between 10 and 14 mL O_2 per kilogram per minute are in a borderline range, with values >14 usually predicting good 1 to 2 year survival. The increasing acceptance of cardiac transplantation as a treatment modality for heart failure without a corresponding increase in donor availability has led to prolonged waiting times of as much as 2 years or more. This longer waiting time has led to more rigorous medical care of the patient awaiting transplant with meticulous monitoring of electrolytes, fluid status, and overall well-being. Aggressive therapy for congestive heart failure with high-dose angiotensin-converting enzyme inhibitors and beta blockers and meticulous monitoring of serum electrolytes and renal function have led to stabilization and many times some improvement in the functional status of patients awaiting a donor. This has led to as many as 30 to 40 percent of listed patients being placed "on hold" based on their improved status. Whether these patients can maintain their improved state or will subsequently deteriorate remains to be seen. Recurrent hospitalizations may be required. Patients may become dopamine/dobutamine-dependent to maintain adequate cardiac output. This dependency moves the patient to the highest ("status I") priority for a donor heart.

In addition to these pharmacologic bridges to transplantation, mechanical bridges are occasionally used where pharmacologic therapy is no longer effective. Three approaches are currently used. The first is intraaortic balloon pumping, which can increase cardiac output by 15 to 20 percent. The second is a left ventricular assist device (LVAD), which empties blood via a tube placed in the apex of the left ventricle and pumps it with an electrically driven "bellows-type" mechanism into the abdominal aorta. This approach is highly effective and has been used for several months with successful subsequent transplantation. Limitations include right ventricular failure and/or high pulmonary vascular resistance, since the LVAD does not "unload" the right ventricle. Blood clotting in the device remains a problem, in addition to the obvious problems of infection. Finally, total mechanical heart replacement is also applied in some transplant centers. This complete replacement circumvents the problem of right ventricular failure but is limited by the greater complexity of the device, which can lead to clotting and systemic emboli. Patients who underwent mechanical assistance *and* received a donor heart have 1-year survival statistics similar to those who went directly to transplantation.

Tissue cross-matching between donor and recipient has generally not been done because of difficulty in obtaining good matches and lack of correlation between match and outcome. Size, ABO matching, negative lymphocyte cross-match, and avoidance of a transplantation from a cytomegalovirus (CMV)-positive donor to a CMV-negative recipient are more important.

OPERATIVE PROCEDURE The surgeon removes the diseased heart but leaves the posterior wall of the right atrium in place and the superior and inferior venae cavae intact. The posterior wall of the left atrium is also left in situ with pulmonary veins intact. The donor heart is then removed in toto with the posterior wall of the right and left atria incised, which allows suturing of left atrial donor rim to recipient rim and right atrial donor rim to recipient rim, with anastomosis of the aorta and pulmonary artery.

IMMUNOSUPPRESSION AND REJECTION Controlling rejection while avoiding the adverse side effects of immunosuppressive agents is pivotal to successful transplantation. Rejection is characterized by perivascular infiltration of killer T lymphocytes, which migrate into the myocardium and cause cellular necrosis if not checked. Since early rejection can be silent, it is important to detect it before necrosis occurs. Immunologic monitoring of activated T lymphocytes in peripheral blood offers clues to the timing of a rejection process but has not been sufficiently reliable to dictate antirejection therapy. Therefore, repeated percutaneous transvenous right ventricular endomyocardial biopsies via the right internal jugular vein are required for histologic determination of the state of immunosuppression and rejection.

One widely used scheme for grading the stages of rejection is as follows: cannot rule out rejection, mild early rejection, moderate rejection, and severe rejection. Serial biopsies are taken every 1 to 2 weeks early after transplantation, with gradually widening intervals depending on the patient's course and rejection history. Prolongation of isovolumic relaxation time measured by echocardiography also may provide early clues to rejection.

Immunosuppressive therapy regimens vary but usually include triple therapy with cyclosporine, azathioprine, and prednisone. Prophylactic courses of monoclonal antibody OKT3 or antithymocyte globulin also may be given early after transplantation. Careful monitoring of the adverse side effects of these agents is extremely important because they include nephrotoxicity, bone marrow suppression, and opportunistic infections.

EARLY COURSE AND COMPLICATIONS It is rare for a cardiac transplant patient to have a completely uncomplicated postoperative course. In the immediate postoperative period, right-sided heart failure due to pulmonary vascular disease is most life-threatening. During the 2 to 3 weeks after transplantation, the patient is hospitalized with meticulous monitoring for evidence of rejection and infections, repeated percutaneous transvenous endomyocardial biopsies, and adjustment of immunosuppressive drugs. During the ensuing 4 to 6 weeks, infectious complications, including bacterial, viral, and protozoan infections, are common. A successful transplant program requires a highly aggressive and sophisticated approach to diagnosis and therapy of infections in the immunocompromised host. Depending on the degree of cardiac cachexia preoperatively, the patient is usually functional at 1 week and discharged from the hospital at 2 to 3 weeks if no major complication occurs.

The average first-year cost ranges from $100,000 to $150,000, depending on the need for repeated hospitalization and cardiac biopsies, and is occasionally much higher. Yearly costs for immunosuppressive agents range from $5000 to $10,000, in addition to the expense of medical surveillance for rejection or complications.

PHYSIOLOGY AND FUNCTION Since the allografted heart remains denervated, cardiac function differs from that of the innervated heart during both rest and exercise. The electrocardiogram of a recipient shows two P waves; the P wave of the recipient's heart reflects the residual sinus node and posterior walls of the remaining native atria but is dissociated from the QRS, since the depolarization impulse does not cross the suture line. Although it does not control donor heart rate, the recipient's sinus node remains innervated and under the influence of the autonomic nervous system. The donor sinus node controls the rate of the transplanted heart. The donor heart's P wave has a regular PR interval, reflecting conduction to the ventricles. Since the controlling sinus node is denervated, it maintains a heart rate of 100 to 110 beats per minute, and rate increase depends on alterations in chronotropic agents perfusing the sinus node. Partial reinnervation may occur in some patients late after transplantation. This is manifested primarily by the occurrence of angina-like symptoms in patients who have developed accelerated graft atherosclerosis (see below).

Ventricular function in response to isometric and isotonic exercise has been studied extensively. The early response to exercise is more dependent on the Frank-Starling mechanism and change in ventricular volume and filling pressure. As exercise proceeds and catecholamines are released with their positive inotropic and chronotropic effects, cardiac output begins to rise. The cardiac transplant recipient can achieve approximately 70 percent of the maximal cardiac output expected for his or her age, easily sufficient for the stresses of everyday life.

LATE COURSE AND COMPLICATIONS Although the rejection process partially subsides, lifelong administration of immunosuppressive drugs, albeit at lower doses, is still required and remains a hazard. Infectious complications and unsuspected rejection continue to occur, requiring ongoing surveillance and monitoring. Routine cardiac biopsies are performed at 3-month intervals to monitor for unsuspected early rejection. Acute rejection or infection predominates in the first year after transplantation. Chronic rejection (i.e., accelerated coronary vascular disease) becomes the most important cause of death after the first year. The process is a fibrointimal hyperplasia that can go undetected by coronary arteriography at first and then cause diffuse atherosclerotic changes. Risk factors for its development may include repeated rejection episodes and elevated lipid levels. CMV infections also have been associated with higher frequency of this disease. Angina is rare, and patients may present with sudden death or silent myocardial infarction. This diffuse accelerated vascular process affects both proximal and distal coronary vessels so that standard approaches, such as angioplasty or coronary artery bypass grafting, are not generally useful but occasionally are successful.

Uncontrolled trials with anticoagulation, aspirin, and improved immunosuppression with cyclosporine have done little to lower this frequency; 40 to 50 percent of patients show arteriographic evidence of coronary vascular disease 5 years after transplantation. Retransplantation has been employed for some patients with severe graft atherosclerosis, but it is limited by the scarcity of donors and poorer survival expectations after the second transplant. Diltiazem has been reported to reduce the severity and occurrence of this accelerated vascular process when started at the time of transplantation. Recently, pravastatin has been reported not only to lower lipid levels but to have a beneficial effect on rejection, 1-year survival, and incidence of coronary vasculopathy. The mechanism is under investigation.

In addition to the well-known hazards of long-term glucocorticoid usage, the immunosuppressed patient is at increased risk for neoplasia. An unusual form of lymphoma can occur frequently in extranodal locations, which is linked to prior Epstein-Barr viral infection. This lymphoma can be polyclonal or monoclonal, is associated with excessive immunosuppression, and may respond to simply lowering doses of cyclosporine and administration of acyclovir rather than requiring more aggressive chemo- or radiotherapy. Many cases regress fully and do not recur.

HEART-LUNG TRANSPLANTATION

Patients with congenital heart disease with Eisenmenger's complex (Chap. 235) or primary pulmonary hypertension (Chap. 260) are now considered for heart-lung transplantation. The surgical technique is similar to that for heart transplantation, except that the pulmonary venous attachments to the left atrium are left intact, and a tracheal anastomosis is required. The postoperative period is more complex, since the lungs may be rejected separately from the heart, requiring repeated endobronchoscopic biopsies when rejection is suspected. The immunosuppressive regimen is similar to that for heart transplants, except that glucocorticoids are avoided in the first 1 to 2 weeks to allow healing of the tracheal anastamosis. Long-term survival has in the past been limited by obliterative bronchiolitis due to chronic unrecognized rejection; survival rates have been approximately 60 percent at 1 year and 50 percent at 2 years but appear to be improving. Heart-lung transplants also have been applied to primary pulmonary hypertension, but more recent experience with single-lung transplants for these patients has been satisfactory, thus utilizing scarce donors more effectively. Single-lung transplants are also being applied increasingly for patients with advanced emphysema. Double-lung transplants for patients with cystic fibrosis also have become the operation of choice for this group. →*For further discussion, see Chap. 267.*

BIBLIOGRAPHY

CAREY NR: Diagnostic criteria of chronic rejection in transplanted hearts. Transplant Proc 25:2026, 1993

GAO S-Z et al: Progressive coronary luminal narrowing after cardiac transplantation. Circulation 82(Suppl IV):IV-269, 1990

GRATTAN MT et al: Cytomegalovirus infection is associated with cardiac allograft rejection and atherosclerosis. JAMA 261:3561, 1989

HALLE AA 3RD et al: Coronary angioplasty, atherectomy and bypass surgery in cardiac transplant recipients. Int J Cardiol 49:119, 1995

KOBASHIGAWA JA et al: Effect of pravastatin on outcomes after cardiac transplantation. N Engl J Med 333:621, 1995

REEDY JE et al: Bridge to heart transplantation: Importance of patient selection. J Heart Transplant 9:475, 1990

REITZ B: Heart and heart-lung transplantation, in E Braunwald (ed). *Heart Disease*, 5th ed, Philadelphia, Saunders, 1997, p 515

SCHROEDER JS et al: A preliminary study of diltiazem in the prevention of coronary artery disease in heart-transplant recipients. N Engl J Med 328:30, 1993

TANIO JW, EISEN HJ: Medical aspects of cardiac transplantation. Hosp Pract 28:61, 1993

235 | *William F. Friedman, John S. Child*

CONGENITAL HEART DISEASE IN THE ADULT

Congenital heart disease complicates approximately 1 percent of all live births. Substantial numbers of affected infants reach adulthood because of successful medical and/or surgical management, or because the alteration caused in cardiovascular physiology is well tolerated.

ETIOLOGY AND PREVENTION Congenital cardiovascular malformations are generally the result of aberrant embryonic development of a normal structure, or failure of such a structure to progress beyond an early stage of embryonic or fetal development. Malformations are due to complex multifactorial genetic and environmental causes. Recognized chromosomal aberrations and mutations of single genes account for fewer than 10 percent of all cardiac malformations (Table 235-1).

The presence of a cardiac malformation as one component of the multiple system involvement in Down's, Turner's, and the trisomy 13-15(D₁) and 17-18 (E) syndromes may be anticipated in occasional pregnancies by detection of abnormal chromosomes in fetal cells obtained from amniotic fluid or chorionic villus biopsy. Identification in such cells of the enzyme disorders characteristic of Hurler's syndrome, homocystinuria, or type II glycogen storage disease may also allow one to predict cardiac disease.

PATHOPHYSIOLOGY The anatomic and physiologic changes in the heart and circulation due to any specific congenital cardiocirculatory lesion are not static but rather progress from prenatal life to adulthood. Thus, malformations that are benign or escape detection in childhood may become clinically significant in the adult. For example, the functionally normal, congenitally bicuspid aortic valve may thicken and calcify with time, resulting in significant aortic stenosis; or the well-tolerated left-to-right shunt of an atrial septal defect may not result in cardiac decompensation, with or without pulmonary hypertension, until the fourth or fifth decade.

Pulmonary Hypertension This is a common companion of many congenital cardiac lesions, and the status of the pulmonary vascular bed is often the principal determinant of the clinical manifestations, the course, and the feasibility of surgical repair. Increases in pulmonary arterial pressure result from elevation of pulmonary blood flow and/or resistance, the latter due sometimes to an increase in vascular tone but usually the result of obstructive, obliterative structural changes within the pulmonary vascular bed. Because pulmonary vascular obstructive disease can be the determining factor in assessing the advisability of operation, it is important to quantify and compare pulmonary to systemic flows and resistances in patients with severe pulmonary hypertension. The causes of pulmonary vascular obstructive disease are unknown, although increased pulmonary blood flow, increased pulmonary arterial blood pressure, elevated pulmonary venous pressure, polycythemia, systemic hypoxemia, acidosis, and the bronchial circulation have been implicated. The designation *Eisenmenger syndrome* is applied to patients with a large communication between the two circulations at the aortopulmonary, ventricular, or atrial levels and bidirectional or predominantly right-to-left shunts because of high-resistance and obstructive pulmonary hypertension. No specific treatment has proved beneficial for obstructive pulmonary vascular disease, although single lung transplantation and intracardiac defect repair, or total heart-lung transplantation show promise (see Chaps. 234 and 267).

Erythrocytosis The chronic hypoxemia in cyanotic congenital heart disease results in *erythrocytosis* due to increased erythropoietin production (see Chap. 36). The commonly used term *polycythemia* is a misnomer because white cell counts are normal and platelet counts are normal to decreased. Cyanotic patients with erythrocytosis may have compensated or decompensated hematocrits. Compensated erythrocytosis with iron-replete equilibrium hematocrits rarely results in symptoms of hyperviscosity at hematocrits less than 65 percent and occasionally with hematocrits of 70 percent or more. Therapeutic phlebotomy is rarely required in compensated erythrocytosis. In contrast, patients with decompensated erythrocytosis fail to establish equilibrium with unstable, rising hematocrits and recurrent hyperviscosity symptoms. Therapeutic phlebotomy, a two-edged sword, allows temporary relief of symptoms but begets instability of the hematocrit and compounds the problem by iron depletion. Iron-deficiency symptoms are usually indistinguishable from those of hyperviscosity; progressive symptoms after recurrent phlebotomy are usually due to iron depletion with hypochromic microcytosis. Iron depletion results in a larger number of smaller (microcytic) hypochromic red cells that are less capable of carrying oxygen and less deformable in the microcirculation. Because these microcytes are less deformable in the microcirculation and there are more of them relative to the plasma volume, the viscosity is greater than for an equivalent hematocrit with fewer, larger, iron-replete, deformable cells. As such, iron-depleted erythrocytosis results in increasing symptoms due to decreased oxygen delivery to the tissues.

Table 235-1

Syndromes with Associated Cardiovascular Involvement

Syndrome	Major Cardiovascular Manifestations	Major Noncardiac Abnormalities
HERITABLE AND POSSIBLY HERITABLE		
Ellis–van Creveld	Single atrium or atrial septal defect	Chondrodystrophic dwarfism, nail dysplasia, polydactyly
TAR (thrombocytopenia-absent radius)	Atrial septal defect, tetralogy of Fallot	Radial aplasia or hypoplasia, thrombocytopenia
Holt-Oram	Atrial septal defect (other defects common)	Skeletal upper limb defect, hypoplasia of clavicles
Kartagener	Dextrocardia	Situs inversus, sinusitis, bronchiectasis
Laurence-Moon-Biedl	Variable defects	Retinal pigmentation, obesity, polydactyly
Noonan	Pulmonary valve dysplasia, cardiomyopathy (usually hypertrophic)	Webbed neck, pectus excavatum, cryptorchidism
Tuberous sclerosis	Rhabdomyoma, cardiomyopathy	Phakomatosis, bone lesions, hamartomatous skin lesions
Multiple lentigines (leopard) syndrome	Pulmonic stenosis	Basal cell nevi, broad facies, rib anomalies, deafness
Rubenstein-Taybi	Patent ductus arteriosus (others)	Broad thumbs and toes, hypoplastic maxilla, slanted palpebral fissures
Familial deafness	Arrhythmias, sudden death	Sensorineural deafness
Osler-Rendu-Weber	Arteriovenous fistulas (lung, liver, mucous membranes)	Multiple telangiectasia
Apert	Ventricular septal defect	Craniosynostosis, midfacial hypoplasia, syndactyly
Crouzon	Patent ductus arteriosus, aortic coarctation	Ptosis, craniosynostosis, maxillary hypoplasia
Hypertrophic cardiomypathy	Asymmetric septal hypertrophy	Family history of sudden death
Incontinentia pigmenti	Patent ductus arteriosus	Irregular pigmented skin lesions, patchy alopecia, hypodontia
Alagille (arteriohepatic dysplasia)	Peripheral pulmonic stenosis, pulmonic stenosis	Biliary hypoplasia, vertebral anomalies, prominent forehead, deep-set eyes
DiGeorge	Interrupted aortic arch, tetralogy of Fallot, truncus arteriosus	Thymic hypoplasia or aplasia, parathyroid aplasia or hypoplasia, ear anomalies
Friedreich's ataxia	Cardiomyopathy and conduction defects	Ataxia, speech defect, degeneration of spinal cord dorsal columns
Muscular dystrophy	Cardiomyopathy	Pseudohypertrophy of calf muscles, weakness of trunk and proximal limb muscles
Cystic fibrosis	Cor pulmonale	Pancreatic insufficiency, malabsorption, chronic lung disease
Sickle cell anemia	Cardiomyopathy, mitral regurgitation	Hemoglobin SS
Conradi-Hünermann	Ventricular septal defect, patent ductus arteriosus	Asymmetric limb shortness, early punctate mineralization, large skin pores
Cockayne	Accelerated atherosclerosis	Cachectic dwarfism, retinal pigment abnormalities, photosensitivity dermatitis
Progeria	Accelerated atherosclerosis	Premature aging, alopecia, atrophy of subcutaneous fat, skeletal hypoplasia
CONNECTIVE TISSUE DISORDERS		
Cutis laxa	Peripheral pulmonic stenosis	Generalized disruption of elastic fibers, diminished skin resilience, hernias
Ehlers-Danlos	Arterial dilatation and rupture, mitral regurgitation	Hyperextensible joints, hyperelastic and friable skin
Marfan	Aortic dilatation, aortic and mitral incompetence	Gracile habitus, arachnodactyly with hyperextensibility, lens subluxation
Osteogenesis imperfecta	Aortic incompetence	Fragile bones, blue sclera
Pseudoxanthoma elasticum	Peripheral and coronary arterial disease	Degeneration of elastic fibers in skin, retinal angioid streaks
INBORN ERRORS OF METABOLISM		
Pompe's disease	Glycogen storage disease of heart	Acid maltase deficiency, muscular weakness
Homocystinuria	Aortic and pulmonary arterial dilatation, intravascular thrombosis	Cystathionine synthetase deficiency, lens subluxation, osteoporosis
Mucopolysaccharidosis:		
Hurler, Hunter	Multivalvular and coronary and great artery disease, cardiomyopathy	Hurler: Deficiency of α-L-iduronidase, corneal clouding, coarse features, growth and mental retardation
		Hunter: Deficiency of sulfoiduronide sulfatase, coarse facies, clear cornea, growth and mental retardation
Morquio, Scheie, Maroteaux-Lamy	Aortic incompetence	Morquio: Deficiency of N-acetylhexosamine sulfate sulfatase, cloudy cornea, normal intelligence, severe bony changes involving vertebrae and epiphyses
		Scheie: Deficiency of α-L-iduronidase, cloudy cornea, normal intelligence, peculiar facies
		Maroteaux-Lamy: Deficiency of arylsulfatase B, cloudy cornea, osseous changes, normal intelligence

(continued)

Table 235-1

Syndromes with Associated Cardiovascular Involvement *(Continued)*

Syndrome	Major Cardiovascular Manifestations	Major Noncardiac Abnormalities
CHROMOSOMAL ABNORMALITIES		
Trisomy 21 (Down's syndrome)	Endocardial cushion defect, atrial or ventricular septal defect, tetralogy of Fallot	Hypotonia, hyperextensible joints, mongoloid facies, mental retardation
Trisomy 13 (D)	Ventricular septal defect, patent ductus arteriosus, double-outlet right ventricle	Single midline intracerebral ventricle with midfacial defects, polydactyly, nail changes, mental retardation
Trisomy 18 (E)	Congenital polyvalvular dysplasia, ventricular septal defect, patent ductus arteriosus	Clenched hand, short sternum, low-arch dermal-ridge pattern on fingertips, mental retardation
Cri-du-chat (short-arm deletion-5)	Ventricular septal defect	Cat cry, microcephaly, antimongoloid slant of palpebral fissures, mental retardation
XO (Turner)	Coarctation of aorta, bicuspid aortic valve	Short female, broad chest, lymphedema, webbed neck
XXXY and XXXXX	Patent ductus arteriosus	XXXY: hypogenitalism, mental retardation, radial-ulnar synostosis XXXXX: small hands, incurving of fifth fingers, mental retardation
SPORADIC DISORDERS		
VATER association	Ventricular septal defect	Vertebral anomalies, anal atresia, tracheo-esophageal fistula, radial and renal anomalies
CHARGE association	Tetralogy of Fallot (other defects common)	Colobomas, choanal atresia, mental and growth deficiency, genital and ear anomalies
Williams	Supravalvular aortic stenosis, peripheral pulmonic stenosis	Mental deficiency, "elfin" facies, loquacious personality, hoarse voice
Cornelia de Lange	Ventricular septal defect	Micromelia, synophrys, mental and growth deficiency
Shprintzen (velocardiofacial)	Ventricular septal defect, tetralogy of Fallot, right aortic arch	Cleft palate, prominent nose, slender hands, learning disability
Long QT (Jervell and Lange-Nielson, Romano-Ward)	Long QT interval, ventricular arrythmias	Family history of sudden death, congenital deafness (not in Romano-Ward)
TERATOGENIC DISORDERS		
Rubella	Patent ductus arteriosus, pulmonic valvular and/or arterial stenosis, atrial septal defect	Cataracts, deafness, microcephaly
Alcohol-induced	Ventricular septal defect (other defects)	Microcephaly, growth and mental deficiency, short palpebral fissures, smooth philtrum, thin upper lip
Phenytoin-induced	Pulmonic stenosis, aortic stenosis, coarctation, patent ductus arteriosus	Hypertelorism, growth and mental deficiency, short phalanges, bowed upper lip
Thalidomide-induced	Variable	Phocomelia
Lithium-induced	Ebstein's anomaly, tricuspid atresia	None

Hemostasis is abnormal in cyanotic congenital heart disease, due in part to the increased blood volume and engorged capillaries, abnormalities in platelet function and sensitivity to aspirin or nonsteroidal anti-inflammatory agents, and abnormalities of the extrinsic and intrinsic coagulation system. Oral contraceptives are contraindicated for cyanotic women because of the enhanced risk of vascular thrombosis.

The risk of stroke is greatest in children less than 4 years old with cyanotic heart disease and iron deficiency, often with dehydration as an aggravating cause. In contrast, adults with cyanotic congenital heart disease do not appear to be at increased risk for stroke, unless there are excessive, injudicious phlebotomies or inappropriate use of aspirin or anticoagulants.

Symptoms of hyperviscosity can be produced in any cyanotic patient with erythrocytosis if dehydration causes a reduction of plasma volume. Phlebotomy, when required for symptoms of hyperviscosity not due to dehydration or iron deficiency, is a simple outpatient removal of 500 mL of blood over 45 min with isovolumetric replacement with isotonic saline (5% dextrose if congestive heart failure exists). Acute phlebotomy without volume replacement is contraindicated. Iron repletion in decompensated iron-depleted erythrocytosis ameliorates iron-deficiency symptoms but must be done gradually to avoid a sudden excessive rise in hematocrit and resultant hyperviscosity.

PREGNANCY The physiologic alterations during normal gestation (see Chap. 7) can create symptoms and physical findings that may be attributed erroneously to heart disease. Dyspnea due to progesterone and elevated diaphragms in association with peripheral edema and fatigability may be attributed inappropriately to heart failure. The jugular venous pulsations normally become more apparent after the twentieth week. Elevation of the diaphragms can cause basal rales (which disappear with deep breathing). Both ventricles are more easily palpated due to the normal increase in ventricular volumes and elevation of the diaphragm. Third heart sounds, already relatively frequent in normal nongravid young women, increase in frequency and intensity with pregnancy because of increased heart rate and volume of flow across the mitral and tricuspid valves. Midsystolic murmurs across the pulmonary outflow tract and supraclavicular systolic murmurs are caused by increased cardiac output. Venous hums and mammary souffles are usual during pregnancy.

These normal circulatory changes may impinge upon the woman's cardiac reserve. The mother is most at risk if she has a cardiovascular lesion associated with pulmonary vascular disease and pulmonary hypertension (e.g., Eisenmenger's physiology or mitral stenosis) or left ventricular outflow tract obstruction (e.g., aortic stenosis) but also risks death with any malformation that may cause heart failure or a hemodynamically important arrhythmia (Table 235-2). Women with aortic coarctation or Marfan's syndrome are at risk for aortic dissection. Patients with cyanotic heart disease, pulmonary hypertension, or Marfan's syndrome should not become pregnant; those with correctable lesions should be counseled about the risks of pregnancy with an uncorrected malformation versus repair and later pregnancy. The effect of pregnancy in postoperative patients depends upon the outcome of the repair including the presence and severity of residua, sequelae, or complications. Contraception is an important topic with such patients.

Table 235-2

CHAPTER 235
Congenital Heart Disease in the Adult **1303**

Tolerance of Pregnancy by Patients with Various Congenital Cardiac Malformations

Well Tolerated	Intermediate Effect	Poorly Tolerated
NYHA class I	NYHA class II–III	NYHA class IV
Left-right shunts without PHTN	Repaired transposition of the great arteries	Right-left shunt, unrepaired cyanotic heart disease
Aortic or mitral valvular regurgitation (mild-moderate)	Fontan repairs	PHTN and/or pulmonary vascular disease (e.g., Eisenmenger's, "primary PHTN")
Pulmonic or tricuspid regurgitation (if low pressure, even severe)	Aortic or mitral stenosis (moderate)	Aortic or mitral stenosis (severe)
Pulmonic stenosis (mild-moderate)	Ebstein's anomaly	Pulmonic stenosis (severe)
Well-repaired tetralogy of Fallot		Marfan's or aortic coarctation

NOTE: NYHA, New York Heart Association; PHTN, pulmonary hypertension.

Tubal ligation should be considered in those in whom pregnancy is strictly contraindicated.

INFECTIVE ENDOCARDITIS (See also Chap. 126) Routine antimicrobial prophylaxis is recommended for all patients with congenital heart disease and for the majority of patients after operative repair of the lesion, but it should be recognized that antibiotic prophylaxis is not uniformly effective. Nonetheless, it is recommended for all dental procedures, gastrointestinal and genitourinary surgery, and diagnostic procedures such as proctosigmoidoscopy and cystoscopy. The clinical and bacteriologic profile of infective endocarditis in patients with congenital heart disease has changed with the advent of intracardiac surgery and of prosthetic devices. Two major predisposing causes of infective endocarditis are a susceptible cardiovascular substrate and a source of bacteremia. Prophylaxis includes both chemotherapeutic (antimicrobial) and nonchemotherapeutic (hygienic) measures. Meticulous dental and skin care is required.

EXERCISE Advice on athletics and exercise is governed by the nature of the exercise and by the type and severity of the congenital cardiovascular lesion. Patients with lesions characterized by left ventricular outflow tract obstruction, if more than mild to moderate, or pulmonary vascular disease risk syncope or even sudden death. In Fallot's tetralogy, isotonic exercise–induced decrease in systemic vascular resistance relative to the right ventricular outflow obstruction augments the right-to-left shunt, increases hypoxemia, and causes an increase in subjective breathlessness due to the response of the respiratory center to the changes in blood gases and pH.

INSURABILITY AND EMPLOYABILITY Most patients with congenital heart disease must pay significantly more than standard life insurance rates, assuming their anomaly places them in a category that companies have determined is eligible for insurance. There is a paucity of actuarial survival data beyond adolescence for most cardiac lesions that have undergone operative repair. Accordingly, it is often difficult to convince insurance companies to offer insurance at reasonable cost to individual patients whose long-term prognosis is quite good.

Employment is affected by the patient's physical capacity relative to the type of job sought. Job discrimination exists, often because the employer is reluctant to accept health insurance responsibilities. Further, eligibility for some occupations is governed by public safety regulations, e.g., airline pilots, bus drivers.

SPECIFIC CARDIAC DEFECTS

Table 235-3 provides a classification of cardiac anomalies that recognizes the general categories of clinical presentation, functional consequences, and site of origin of congenital defects.

Categorizing the defect(s) in an individual patient requires an answer to a number of basic questions. Is the patient acyanotic or cyanotic? Is pulmonary arterial blood flow increased or not? Does the malformation originate in the left or right side of the heart? Which is the dominant ventricle? Is pulmonary hypertension present or not? With the above information as a foundation, using more refined diagnostic techniques such as transthoracic (precordial) and transesophageal echocardiography and Doppler imaging, magnetic resonance imaging, and/or hemodynamic study and angiocardiography leads to a precise anatomic and functional assessment.

ACYANOTIC CONGENITAL HEART DISEASE WITH A LEFT-TO-RIGHT SHUNT

ATRIAL SEPTAL DEFECT This is a common cardiac anomaly in adults that occurs more frequently in females. The *sinus venosus* type occurs high in the atrial septum near the entry of the superior vena cava and is associated frequently with anomalous connection of pulmonary veins from the right lung to the junction of the superior vena cava and right atrium. *Ostium primum* anomalies are a form of atrioventricular septal defect that lie immediately adjacent to the atrioventricular valves, either of which may be deformed and incompetent. Ostium primum defects occur commonly in patients with Down's syndrome, although the more complex atrioventricular septal defects with a common atrioventricular valve and a posterior defect of the basal portion of the interventricular septum are more characteristic of this chromosomal defect. The most common atrial septal defect involves the fossa ovalis, is midseptal in location, and is of the *ostium secundum* type. This type of defect should not be confused with a *patent foramen ovale*. Anatomic obliteration of the foramen ovale ordinarily follows its functional closure soon after birth, but residual "probe patency" is a normal variant; atrial septal defect denotes a true deficiency of the atrial septum and implies functional and anatomic patency.

The magnitude of the left-to-right shunt through an atrial septal defect depends on the defect size, the diastolic properties of both ventricles, and the relative impedance in the pulmonary and systemic circulations. The left-to-right shunt causes diastolic overloading of the right ventricle and increased pulmonary blood flow.

Patients with atrial septal defect are usually asymptomatic in early life, although there may be some physical underdevelopment and an increased tendency for respiratory infections; cardiorespiratory symptoms occur in many older patients. Beyond the fourth decade, a significant number of patients develop atrial arrhythmias, pulmonary arterial hypertension, bidirectional and then right-to-left shunting of blood, and cardiac failure. Patients exposed to the chronic environmental hypoxia of high altitude tend to develop pulmonary hypertension at younger ages. In some older patients, left-to-right shunting across the defect increases as progressive systemic hypertension and/or coronary artery disease result in reduced compliance of the left ventricle.

Physical Examination Examination usually reveals a prominent right ventricular cardiac impulse and palpable pulmonary artery pulsation. The first heart sound is normal or split, with accentuation of the tricuspid valve closure sound. Increased flow across the pulmonic valve is responsible for a midsystolic pulmonary ejection murmur. The second heart sound is widely split and is relatively fixed in relation to respiration. A middiastolic rumbling murmur, loudest at the fourth intercostal space and along the left sternal border, reflects increased flow across the tricuspid valve. In patients with ostium primum defects, an apical thrill and holosystolic murmur indicate associated mitral or tricuspid incompetence or a ventricular septal defect.

The physical findings are altered when an increase in the pulmonary vascular resistance results in diminution of the left-to-right shunt. Both the pulmonary and tricuspid murmurs decrease in intensity, the pulmonic component of the second heart sound and a systolic ejection sound are accentuated, the two components of the second heart sound may fuse, and a diastolic murmur of pulmonic regurgitation appears. Cyanosis and clubbing accompany the development of a right-to-left shunt.

In adults with an atrial septal defect and atrial fibrillation, the physical findings may be confused with the findings of mitral stenosis with pulmonary hypertension because the tricuspid flow murmur and widely split second heart sound may be mistakenly thought to represent the diastolic murmur of mitral stenosis and the mitral "opening snap," respectively.

Electrocardiogram In patients with an ostium secundum defect, the ECG usually shows right axis deviation and an rSr′ pattern in the right precordial leads representing delayed posterobasal activation of the ventricular septum and enlargement of the right ventricular outflow tract. An ectopic atrial pacemaker or first-degree heart block occurs occasionally in patients with defects of the sinus venosus type. In patients with an ostium primum defect, the right ventricular conduction defect is characteristically accompanied by left axis deviation and by superior orientation and counterclockwise rotation of the QRS loop in the frontal plane. Varying degrees of right ventricular and right atrial hypertrophy may occur with each type of defect, depending on the height of the pulmonary artery pressure. *Chest roentgenograms* reveal enlargement of the right atrium and ventricle, dilatation of the pulmonary artery and its branches, and increased pulmonary vascular marking.

Echocardiogram This shows pulmonary arterial and right ventricular dilatation, and anterior systolic (paradoxical) or flat interventricular septal motion if a significant right ventricular volume overload is present. The defect may be visualized directly from subcostal, right parasternal, or apical echocardiographic windows. In most institutions, two-dimensional echocardiography, supplemented by conventional or color Doppler flow examination, has supplanted cardiac catheterization as the confirmatory test for atrial septal defect. Transesophageal echocardiography is indicated if the transthoracic echocardiogram is ambiguous, which is often the case with sinus venosus defects. Cardiac catheterization is then employed if inconsistencies exist in the clinical data, if significant pulmonary hypertension or associated malformations are suspected, or if coronary artery disease is a possibility.

℞ **TREATMENT**

Operative repair, ideally in children between 3 and 6 years of age, should be advised for all patients with uncomplicated atrial septal defects in whom there is significant left-to-right shunting, i.e., with pulmonary-to-systemic flow ratios exceeding approximately 2.0:1.0. Excellent results may be anticipated, at low risk, even in patients beyond 40 years of age in the absence of pulmonary hypertension. The defect is closed, usually with a patch of pericardium or of prosthetic material, with the patient on cardiopulmonary bypass. In patients with ostium primum defects, cleft, deformed, and incompetent valves often require repair. Intraoperative transesophageal echocardiography is used to monitor the surgical results of mitral valve repair. Operation should not be carried out in patients with small defects and trivial left-to-right shunts, or in those with severe pulmonary vascular disease without a significant left-to-right shunt.

Patients with atrial septal defect of the sinus venosus or ostium secundum types rarely die before the fifth decade. During the fifth and sixth decades the incidence of progressive symptoms, often leading to severe disability, increases substantially. Medical management should include prompt treatment of respiratory tract infections, antiarrhythmic medications for atrial fibrillation or supraventricular tachycardia, and the usual measures for hypertension, coronary disease, or heart failure (see Chap. 233), if these complications occur. The risk of infective endocarditis is quite low unless the defect is complicated by valvular regurgitation or has recently been repaired with a patch (see Chap. 126).

VENTRICULAR SEPTAL DEFECT Defects of the ventricular septum are common as isolated defects and as one component of a combination of anomalies. The opening is usually single and situated in the membranous portion of the septum. The functional disturbance is dependent primarily on its size and on the status of the pulmonary vascular bed, rather than on the location of the defect. Only small or moderate-size defects are usually seen initially in adulthood as the vast majority of patients with isolated large defects come to medical and, often, surgical attention very early in life.

A wide spectrum exists in the natural history of ventricular septal defect, ranging from spontaneous closure to congestive cardiac failure and death in early infancy. Within this spectrum is the possible development of pulmonary vascular obstruction, right ventricular outflow tract obstruction, aortic regurgitation, and infective endocarditis. Spontaneous closure is more common in patients born with a small ventricular septal defect and occurs in early childhood in most patients.

Patients with large ventricular septal defects and pulmonary hypertension are those at greatest risk for developing pulmonary vascular obstruction. Thus, large defects should be corrected surgically early in life when pulmonary vascular disease is still reversible or not yet developed. In patients with severe pulmonary vascular obstruction (Eisenmenger syndrome), symptoms in adult life consist of exertional dyspnea, chest pain, syncope, and hemoptysis. The right-to-left shunt leads to cyanosis, clubbing, and erythrocytosis. In all patients, the degree to which pulmonary vascular resistance is elevated before operation is a critical factor determining prognosis. If the pulmonary vascular resistance is one-third or less of the systemic value, progression of pulmonary vascular disease after operation is unusual. However, if a moderate to severe increase in pulmonary vascular resistance exists preoperatively, either no change or a progression of pulmonary vascular disease is common postoperatively.

Right ventricular outflow tract obstruction develops in approximately 5 to 10 percent of patients who present in infancy with a moderate to large left-to-right shunt. With time, as subvalvular right ventricular outflow tract obstruction progresses, the findings in these patients begin to resemble more closely those of the cyanotic tetralogy of Fallot.

In approximately 5 percent of patients, incompetence of the aortic valve results from insufficient cusp tissue or prolapse of the cusp through the interventricular defect; the aortic regurgitation then complicates and usually dominates the clinical course.

Two-dimensional *echocardiography* with conventional or color Doppler examination can usually define the number and location of defects in the ventricular septum and detect associated anomalies. Hemodynamic and angiographic study may be employed to assess the status of the pulmonary vascular bed and clarify details of the altered anatomy.

℞ **TREATMENT**

Surgery is not recommended for patients with normal pulmonary arterial pressures with small shunts (pulmonary-to-systemic flow ratios of less than 1.5 to 2.0:1.0). Operative correction is indicated when there is a moderate to large left-to-right shunt with a pulmonary-to-systemic flow ratio that exceeds 1.5:1.0 or 2.0:1.0, in the absence of prohibitively high levels of pulmonary vascular resistance.

PATENT DUCTUS ARTERIOSUS The ductus arteriosus is a vessel leading from the bifurcation of the pulmonary artery to the aorta just distal to the left subclavian artery. Normally, the vascular channel is open in the fetus but closes immediately after birth. The flow across the ductus is determined by the pressure and resistance relationships between the systemic and pulmonary circulations and by the cross-sectional area and length of the ductus. In most adults with this anomaly, pulmonary pressures are normal and a gradient and shunt from aorta to pulmonary artery persist throughout the cardiac cycle, resulting in a characteristic thrill and a continuous "machinery" murmur with a late systolic accentuation at the upper left sternal edge. In adults who were born with a large left-to-right shunt through the ductus arteriosus, pulmonary vascular obstruction (Eisenmenger syndrome) with pulmonary hypertension, right-to-left shunting, and cyanosis have usually developed. Severe pulmonary vascular disease results in reversal of flow through the ductus, unoxygenated blood is shunted to the descending aorta, and the toes, but not the fingers, become cyanotic and clubbed, a finding termed *differential cyanosis*. The leading causes of death in adults with patent ductus are cardiac failure and infective endocarditis; occasionally severe pulmonary vascular obstruction may cause aneurysmal dilatation, calcification, and rupture of the ductus.

℞ TREATMENT

In the absence of severe pulmonary vascular disease and predominant left-to-right shunting of blood, the patent ductus should be surgically ligated or divided. Transcatheter closure is experimental, using coils, buttons, plugs, and umbrellas. Operation should be deferred for several months in patients treated successfully for infective endocarditis, because the ductus may remain somewhat edematous and friable.

AORTIC ROOT TO RIGHT HEART SHUNTS The three most common causes of aortic root to right heart shunts are congenital aneurysm of an aortic sinus of Valsalva with fistula, coronary arteriovenous fistula, and anomalous origin of the left coronary artery from the pulmonary trunk. *Aneurysm of an aortic sinus of Valsalva* consists of a separation or lack of fusion between the media of the aorta and the annulus fibrosis of the aortic valve. Rupture usually occurs in the third or fourth decade of life; most often the aorticocardiac fistula is between the right coronary cusp and the right ventricle, but occasionally, when the noncoronary cusp is involved, the fistula drains into the right atrium. Abrupt rupture causes chest pain, bounding pulses, a continuous murmur accentuated in diastole, and volume overload of the heart. Diagnosis is confirmed by two-dimensional and Doppler echocardiographic studies; cardiac catheterization quantifies the left-to-right shunt, and thoracic aortography visualizes the fistula. Medical management is directed at cardiac failure, arrhythmias, or endocarditis. At operation, the aneurysm is closed and amputated, and the aortic wall is reunited with the heart, either by direct suture or with a prosthesis.

Coronary arteriovenous fistula, an unusual anomaly, consists of a communication between a coronary artery and another cardiac chamber, usually the coronary sinus or right atrium or ventricle. The shunt is usually of small magnitude, and myocardial blood flow is not usually compromised. Potential complications include infective endocarditis, thrombus formation with occlusion and distal embolization, rupture of an aneurysmal fistula, and rarely, pulmonary hypertension and congestive failure. A loud, superficial, continuous murmur at the lower or midsternal border usually prompts a further evaluation of asymp-

tomatic patients. Doppler echocardiography demonstrates the site of drainage; if the site of origin is proximal, it may be detectable by two-dimensional echocardiography. Retrograde thoracic aortography

Table 235-3

Classification of Congenital Heart Disease

ACYANOTIC WITH LEFT-TO-RIGHT SHUNT

I. Atrial level shunt
  A. Atrial septal defect
    1. Ostium primum
    2. Ostium secundum
    3. Sinus venosus
  B. Atrial septal defect with mitral stenosis (Lutembacher's syndrome)
  C. Partial anomalous pulmonary venous connection
II. Ventricular level shunt
  A. Ventricular septal defect
    1. Inlet septum
    2. Muscular septum
    3. Perimembranous septum
    4. Infundibular septum
  B. Ventricular septal defect with aortic regurgitation
  C. Ventricular septal defect with left ventricular to right atrial shunt

III. Aortic root to right heart shunt
  A. Ruptured sinus of Valsalva aneurysm
  B. Coronary arteriovenous fistula
  C. Anomalous origin of the left coronary artery from the pulmonary trunk
IV. Aortopulmonary level shunt
  A. Aortopulmonary window
  B. Patent ductus arteriosus
V. Multiple level shunts
  A. Complete common atrioventricular canal
  B. Ventricular septal defect with atrial septal defect
  C. Ventricular septal defect with patent ductus arteriosus

ACYANOTIC WITHOUT A SHUNT

I. Left heart malformations
  A. Congenital obstruction to left atrial inflow
    1. Pulmonary vein stenosis
    2. Mitral stenosis
    3. Cor triatriatum
  B. Mitral regurgitation
    1. Atrioventricular septal (endocardial cushion)
    2. Congenitally corrected transposition of the great arteries
    3. Anomalous origin of the left coronary artery from the pulmonary trunk
    4. Miscellaneous (double-orifice mitral valve, congenital perforations, accessory commissures with anomalous chordal insertion, congenitally short or absent chordae, cleft posterior leaflet, parachute mitral valve, etc.)
  C. Primary dilated endocardial fibroelastosis

  D. Aortic stenosis
    1. Discrete subvalvular
    2. Valvular
    3. Supravalvular
  E. Aortic valve regurgitation
  F. Coarctation of the aorta
II. Right heart malformations
  A. Acyanotic Ebstein's anomaly of the tricuspid valve
  B. Pulmonic stenosis
    1. Subinfundibular
    2. Infundibular
    3. Valvular
    4. Supravalvular (stenosis of pulmonary artery and its branches)
  C. Congenital pulmonary valve regurgitation
  D. Idiopathic dilatation of the pulmonary trunk

CYANOTIC

I. Increased pulmonary blood flow
  A. Complete transposition of the great arteries
  B. Double-outlet right ventricle of the Taussig-Bing type
  C. Truncus arteriosus
  D. Total anomalous pulmonary venous connection
  E. Single ventricle without pulmonic stenosis
  F. Common atrium
  G. Tetralogy of Fallot with pulmonary atresia and increased collateral arterial flow
  H. Tricuspid atresia with large ventricular septal defect and no pulmonic stenosis
  I. Hypoplastic left heart (aortic atresia, mitral atresia)

II. Normal or decreased pulmonary blood flow
  A. Tricuspid atresia
  B. Ebstein's anomaly with right-to-left atrial shunt
  C. Pulmonary atresia with intact ventricular septum
  D. Pulmonic stenosis or atresia with ventricular septal defect (tetralogy of Fallot)
  E. Pulmonic stenosis with right-to-left atrial shunt
  F. Complete transposition of the great arteries with pulmonic stenosis
  G. Double-outlet right ventricle with pulmonic stenosis
  H. Single ventricle with pulmonic stenosis
  I. Pulmonary arteriovenous fistula
  J. Vena caval to left atrial communication

OTHER

I. Congenitally corrected transposition of the great arteries
II. The cardiac malpositions
III. Congenital complete heart block

SOURCE: Modified from JK Perloff, *The Clinical Recognition of Congenital Heart Disease*, Philadelphia, Saunders, 1991.

or coronary arteriography permits identification of the size and anatomic features of the fistulous tract, which may be closed by suture obliteration.

The third anomaly causing a shunt from the aortic root to the right heart is *anomalous origin of the left coronary artery from the pulmonary artery.* Myocardial infarction and fibrosis commonly lead to death within the first year, though up to 20 percent of patients survive to adolescence and beyond without surgical correction. The diagnosis is supported by the electrocardiographic findings of an anterolateral myocardial infarction. Operative management of adults consists of coronary artery bypass with an internal mammary artery graft or saphenous vein–coronary artery graft.

ACYANOTIC CONGENITAL HEART DISEASE WITHOUT A SHUNT

CONGENITAL AORTIC STENOSIS Malformations that cause obstruction to left ventricular outflow include congenital valvular aortic stenosis, discrete subaortic stenosis, supravalvular aortic stenosis, and hypertrophic obstructive cardiomyopathy (Chap. 239).

Valvular Aortic Stenosis This malformation occurs three to four times more often in males than in females. The congenital bicuspid aortic valve, which is not necessarily stenotic, is one of the most common congenital malformations of the heart, although it may go undetected in early life. Because bicuspid valves may become stenotic with time or be the site of infective endocarditis, the lesion may be difficult to distinguish in adults from acquired rheumatic or degenerative calcific aortic stenosis.

The dynamics of blood flow associated with a congenitally deformed, rigid aortic valve commonly lead to thickening of the cusps and, in later life, to calcification. Hemodynamically significant obstruction causes concentric hypertrophy of the left ventricular wall and dilatation of the ascending aorta.

→ *The clinical manifestations and hemodynamic abnormalities are discussed in Chap. 237*

℞ TREATMENT

The medical management of congenital valvular aortic stenosis includes prophylaxis against infective endocarditis and, in patients with diminished cardiac reserve, the administration of digitalis and diuretics and sodium restriction while awaiting operation. If severe aortic stenosis is present, strenuous physical activity should be avoided even when the patient is asymptomatic, and participation in competitive sports should probably be restricted in patients with milder degrees of obstruction. Aortic valve replacement is indicated in adults with critical obstruction, an aortic valve area < 1.0 cm², and symptoms secondary to left ventricular dysfunction or myocardial ischemia or hemodynamic evidence of left ventricular dysfunction. In asymptomatic children or adolescents or young adults with critical aortic stenosis without valvular calcification or these features, aortic balloon valvuloplasty is often useful (Chap. 245). If surgery is contraindicated in older patients because of a complicating medical problem such as malignancy or renal or hepatic failure, balloon valvuloplasty may provide short-term improvement. It may serve as a bridge to aortic valve replacement in patients with severe heart failure.

Subaortic Stenosis The most common form of subaortic stenosis is the *idiopathic hypertrophic* variety, also termed *hypertrophic cardiomyopathy,* which is present at birth in about one-third of the patients and is discussed in Chap. 239. In contrast, both clinically and physiologically, the *discrete* form of subaortic stenosis resembles valvular aortic stenosis. The lesion usually consists of a membranous diaphragm or fibrous ring encircling the left ventricular outflow tract just beneath the base of the aortic valve. Echocardiography demonstrates the subaortic obstruction; Doppler studies show turbulence proximal to the aortic valve and also detect and quantify the pressure gradient and

severity of aortic regurgitation. Treatment consists of excision of the membrane or fibrous ridge.

Supravalvular Aortic Stenosis This anomaly consists of a localized or diffuse narrowing of the ascending aorta originating just above the level of the coronary arteries at the superior margin of the sinuses of Valsalva. In contrast to other forms of aortic stenosis, the coronary arteries are subjected to the elevated pressures that exist within the left ventricle and are often dilated and tortuous.

COARCTATION OF THE AORTA Narrowing or constriction of the lumen of the aorta may occur anywhere along its length but is most common distal to the origin of the left subclavian artery near the insertion of the ligamentum arteriosum. Coarctation occurs in about 7 percent of patients with congenital heart disease, is twice as common in males as in females, and is most frequent in patients with gonadal dysgenesis. Clinical manifestations depend on the site and extent of obstruction and the presence of associated cardiac anomalies, most commonly a bicuspid aortic valve. Aneurysmal arterial dilatation of the circle of Willis produces a high risk of sudden rupture and death.

Most children and young adults with isolated, discrete coarctation are asymptomatic. Headache, epistaxis, cold extremities, and claudication with exercise may occur, and attention is usually directed to the cardiovascular system when a heart murmur or hypertension in the upper extremities and absence, marked diminution, or delayed pulsations in the femoral arteries are detected on physical examination. Enlarged and pulsatile collateral vessels may be palpated in the intercostal spaces anteriorly, in the axillae, or posteriorly in the interscapular area. The upper extremities and thorax may be more developed than the lower extremities. A midsystolic murmur over the anterior part of the chest, back, and spinous processes may become continuous if the lumen is narrowed sufficiently to result in a high-velocity jet across the lesion throughout the cardiac cycle. Additional systolic and continuous murmurs over the lateral thoracic wall may reflect increased flow through dilated and tortuous collateral vessels. The electrocardiogram usually reveals left ventricular hypertrophy. Roentgenograms may show a dilated left subclavian artery high on the left mediastinal border and a dilated ascending aorta. Indentation of the aorta at the site of coarctation and pre- and poststenotic dilatation (the "3" sign) along the left paramediastinal shadow are almost pathognomonic. Notching of the ribs, an important radiographic sign, is due to erosion by dilated collateral vessels. Two-dimensional echocardiography from para- or suprasternal windows identifies the site and length of coarctation, while Doppler studies record and quantify the pressure gradient. Transesophageal echocardiography and magnetic resonance imaging or digital angiography allow visualization of the length and severity of the obstruction and the associated collateral arteries. In adults, cardiac catheterization is indicated primarily to evaluate the coronary arteries.

The chief hazards result from severe hypertension and include the development of cerebral aneurysms and hemorrhage, rupture of the aorta, left ventricular failure, and infective endocarditis.

℞ TREATMENT

This is usually surgical; resection and end-to-end anastomosis or subclavian flap angioplasty are employed commonly, although it may be necessary to use a tubular graft, patch, or bypass conduit if the narrowed segment is long. Systemic hypertension postoperatively, in the absence of residual coarctation, appears to be related to the duration of preoperative hypertension. Postsurgical recoarctation may be successfully treated with percutaneous balloon dilatation.

PULMONARY STENOSIS WITH INTACT VENTRICULAR SEPTUM Obstruction to right ventricular outflow may be localized to the supravalvular, valvular, or subvalvular levels or occur at a combination of these sites. Multiple sites of narrowing of the peripheral pulmonary arteries are a feature of *rubella embryopathy* and may occur with both the familial and sporadic forms of supravalvular aortic stenosis. Valvular pulmonic stenosis is the most common form of isolated right ventricular obstruction.

The severity of the obstructing lesion, rather than the site of narrowing, is the most important determinant of the clinical course.

In the presence of a normal cardiac output, a peak systolic transvalvular pressure gradient between 50 and 80 mmHg is considered to be moderate stenosis; levels below and above that range are classified as mild and severe, respectively. Patients with mild pulmonic stenosis are generally asymptomatic and demonstrate little or no progression in the severity of obstruction with age. In patients with more significant stenosis, the severity may increase with time. Symptoms vary with the degree of obstruction. Fatigue, dyspnea, right ventricular failure, and syncope may limit the activity of older patients, in whom moderate or severe obstruction may prevent an augmentation of cardiac output with exercise. In patients with severe obstruction, the systolic pressure in the right ventricle may exceed that in the left ventricle, since the ventricular septum is intact. Right ventricular ejection is prolonged with moderate or severe stenosis, and the sound of pulmonary valve closure is delayed and soft. Right ventricular hypertrophy reduces the compliance of that chamber, and a forceful right atrial contraction is necessary to augment right ventricular filling. A fourth heart sound, prominent *a* waves in the jugular venous pulse, and, occasionally, presystolic pulsations of the liver reflect vigorous atrial contraction. The clinical diagnosis is supported by a right parasternal lift and harsh systolic ejection murmur and thrill at the upper left sternal border, typically preceded by a systolic ejection sound, if the obstruction is valvular. The holosystolic decrescendo murmur of tricuspid regurgitation may accompany severe pulmonic stenosis, especially in the presence of congestive heart failure. Cyanosis usually reflects right-to-left shunting through a patent foramen ovale or atrial septal defect. In patients with supravalvular or peripheral pulmonary arterial stenosis, the murmur is systolic or continuous and is best heard over the area of narrowing, with radiation to the peripheral lung fields.

The *electrocardiogram* may be helpful in assessing the degree of right ventricular obstruction. In mild cases, the electrocardiogram is often normal, whereas moderate and severe stenoses are associated with right axis deviation and right ventricular hypertrophy. A ventricular strain pattern, as well as high-amplitude P waves in leads II and V_1, indicating right atrial enlargement, is associated with severe stenosis. The chest roentgenogram with mild or moderate pulmonic stenosis often shows a heart of normal size and normal vascularity of the lungs. In the presence of valvular stenosis, poststenotic dilatation of the main and left pulmonary arteries may be evident. With severe obstruction and resultant right ventricular failure, right atrial and ventricular enlargement are generally evident. The pulmonary vascularity may be reduced with severe stenosis, right ventricular failure, and/or a right-to-left shunt at the atrial level. Two-dimensional *echocardiography* visualizes pulmonary valve morphology; the outflow tract pressure gradient can be estimated by Doppler ultrasonography.

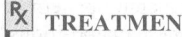**TREATMENT**

The cardiac catheter technique of balloon valvuloplasty (Chap. 229) is usually effective. Direct surgical relief of moderate and severe obstruction may be accomplished at a low risk. Multiple stenoses of the peripheral pulmonary arteries are usually inoperable, but narrowing of a single branch or at the bifurcation of the main pulmonary trunk may be corrected.

CYANOTIC CONGENITAL HEART DISEASE WITH INCREASED PULMONARY BLOOD FLOW

COMPLETE TRANSPOSITION OF THE GREAT ARTERIES In this condition the aorta arises from the right ventricle to the right of and anterior to the pulmonary artery, which emerges from the left ventricle (Fig. 235-1, *left panel*). This results in two separate and parallel circulations, and some communication between them must exist after birth to sustain life. Most patients have an interatrial communication, two-thirds have a patent ductus arteriosus, and about one-third have an associated ventricular septal defect. Transposition is more common in males and accounts for approximately 10 percent of cyanotic heart disease.

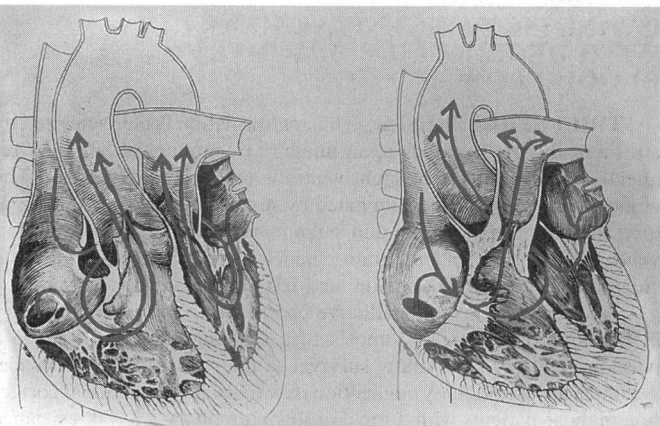

FIGURE 235-1 Complete transposition of the great arteries is depicted in the left panel. The aorta arises from the right ventricle and the pulmonary artery from the left ventricle. The only mixing between the two circulations occurs across a patent foramen ovale. In the right panel, the tetralogy of Fallot cartoon illustrates the two most important anatomic findings, a large ventricular septal defect and right ventricular outflow tract obstruction. A right-to-left shunt is shown across the ventricular septum.

The course is determined by the degree of tissue hypoxia, the ability of each ventricle to sustain an increased work load in the presence of reduced coronary arterial oxygenation, the nature of the associated cardiovascular anomalies, and the status of the pulmonary vascular bed. Pulmonary vascular obstruction develops by 1 to 2 years of age in patients with an associated large ventricular septal defect or large patent ductus arteriosus in the absence of obstruction to left ventricular outflow.

TREATMENT

The balloon or blade catheter or surgical creation or enlargement of an interatrial communication in the neonate is the simplest procedure for providing increased intracardiac mixing of systemic and pulmonary venous blood. Systemic–pulmonary artery anastomosis may be indicated in the patient with severe obstruction to left ventricular outflow and diminished pulmonary blood flow. Intracardiac repair may be accomplished by rearranging the venous returns so that the systemic venous blood is directed to the mitral valve and thence to the left ventricle and pulmonary artery, while the pulmonary venous blood is diverted through the tricuspid valve and right ventricle to the aorta (Mustard or Senning operation). Preferably, this malformation is corrected in infancy by transposing both coronary arteries to the posterior artery and transecting, contraposing, and anastomosing the aorta and pulmonary arteries (arterial switch operation). For those patients with a ventricular septal defect in whom it is necessary to bypass a severely obstructed left ventricular outflow tract, corrective operation employs an intracardiac ventricular baffle and extracardiac prosthetic conduit to replace the pulmonary artery (Rastelli procedure).

SINGLE VENTRICLE This is a family of complex lesions with both atrioventricular valves or a common atrioventricular valve opening to a single ventricular chamber. Associated anomalies include abnormal great artery positional relationships, pulmonic valvular or subvalvular stenosis, and subaortic stenosis.

Survival to adulthood depends upon a relatively normal pulmonary blood flow and good ventricular function. Modifications of the Fontan approach are generally applied to these patients with creation of a pathway(s) from the systemic veins to the pulmonary arteries.

CYANOTIC CONGENITAL HEART DISEASE WITH DECREASED PULMONARY BLOOD FLOW

TRICUSPID ATRESIA   This malformation is characterized by atresia of the tricuspid valve, an interatrial communication, and, frequently, hypoplasia of the right ventricle and pulmonary artery. The clinical picture is usually dominated by severe cyanosis due to obligatory admixture of systemic and pulmonary venous blood in the left ventricle. The electrocardiogram characteristically shows right atrial enlargement, left axis deviation, and left ventricular hypertrophy.

Atrial septostomy and palliative operations to increase pulmonary blood flow, often by anastomosis of a systemic artery or vein to a pulmonary artery, may allow survival to the second or third decade. A Fontan atriopulmonary connection may then allow functional correction in those patients with normal or low pulmonary arterial resistance pressure and good left ventricular function.

EBSTEIN'S ANOMALY   Characterized by a downward displacement of the tricuspid valve into the right ventricle, due to anomalous attachment of the tricuspid leaflets, the Ebstein tricuspid valve tissue is dysplastic and results in tricuspid regurgitation. The abnormally situated tricuspid orifice produces an "atrialized" portion of the right ventricle lying between the atrioventricular ring and the origin of the valve, which is continuous with the right atrial chamber. Often the right ventricle is hypoplastic. Although the clinical manifestations are variable, some patients come to initial attention because of progressive cyanosis from right-to-left atrial shunting, or symptoms due to tricuspid regurgitation and right ventricular dysfunction, or paroxysmal atrial tachyarrhythmias. Diagnostic findings by two-dimensional echocardiography include the abnormal positional relation between the tricuspid and mitral valves with apical displacement of the septal tricuspid leaflet. Tricuspid regurgitation is quantified by Doppler examination. Surgical approaches include prosthetic replacement of the tricuspid valve when the leaflets are tethered or repair of the native valve.

TETRALOGY OF FALLOT   The four components of the tetralogy of Fallot are ventricular septal defect, obstruction to right ventricular outflow, aortic override (straddle) of the ventricular septal defect, and right ventricular hypertrophy (Fig. 235-1, right panel).

The severity of right ventricular outflow obstruction determines the clinical presentation. The severity of hypoplasia of the right ventricular outflow tract varies from mild to complete (pulmonary atresia). Pulmonary valve stenosis and supravalvular and peripheral pulmonary arterial obstruction may coexist; rarely there is unilateral absence of a pulmonary artery (usually the left). A right-sided aortic arch and descending aorta occur in about 25 percent of patients with tetralogy.

The relationship between the resistance to blood flow from the ventricles into the aorta and into the pulmonary vessels plays a major role in determining the hemodynamic and clinical picture. Thus, the severity of obstruction to right ventricular outflow is of fundamental significance. When the obstruction is severe, the pulmonary blood flow is reduced markedly, and a large volume of desaturated systemic venous blood is shunted from right to left across the ventricular septal defect. Severe cyanosis and erythrocytosis occur, and symptoms and sequelae of systemic hypoxemia are prominent. In many infants and children the obstruction is mild but progressive.

The *electrocardiogram* ordinarily shows right ventricular and, less often, right atrial hypertrophy. Radiologic examination characteristically reveals a normal-sized, boot-shaped heart (*coeur en sabot*) with prominence of the right ventricle and a concavity in the region of the pulmonary conus. The pulmonary vascular markings are typically diminished, and the aortic arch and knob may be on the right side. Two-dimensional echocardiography from the parasternal or subcostal windows demonstrates the malalignment of the ventricular septal defect and the subpulmonary stenosis. Selective angiocardiography with right ventricular injection provides architectural details of the right ventricular outflow tract, pulmonary valve and annulus, and caliber of the main branches of the pulmonary artery; coronary arteriography identifies the anatomy and course of the coronary arteries.

℞ **TREATMENT**

Factors that may complicate the treatment of patients with tetralogy of Fallot include infective endocarditis, paradoxic embolism, excessive erythrocytosis, coagulation defects, and cerebral infarction or abscess. Corrective operation is advisable at some point for almost all patients with this anomaly. Successful correction avoids progressive infundibular obstruction, delayed growth, and complications due to hypoxemia and excessive erythrocytosis. The size of the pulmonary arteries rather than the age or size of the infant or child is the most important determinant in establishing candidacy for primary repair. Pronounced hypoplasia of the pulmonary arteries is a relative contraindication for an early corrective surgical procedure. When this problem is present, a palliative operation, such as creation of a systemic arterial–pulmonary arterial shunt, is carried out and is usually followed by complete correction, which can be carried out at a lower risk later in childhood.

OTHER FORMS OF CONGENITAL HEART DISEASES

CONGENITALLY CORRECTED TRANSPOSITION   The two fundamental anatomic abnormalities in this malformation are transposition of the ascending aorta and pulmonary trunk and inversion of the ventricles. This arrangement results in desaturated systemic venous blood passing from the right atrium through the mitral valve to the left ventricle and into the pulmonary trunk, whereas arterialized pulmonary venous blood flows from the left atrium through the tricuspid valve to the right ventricle and into the aorta. Thus, the circulation is corrected functionally. The clinical presentation, course, and prognosis of patients with congenitally corrected transposition vary depending on the nature and severity of any complicating intracardiac anomalies. Ebstein-type anomalies of the left-side tricuspid atrioventricular valve, ventricular septal defect, obstruction to outflow from the venous ventricle, and congenital heart block are often associated with corrected transposition. The diagnosis of the malformation and associated lesions can often be established by two-dimensional echocardiography and Doppler examination.

MALPOSITIONS OF THE HEART   Positional anomalies refer to conditions in which the cardiac apex is in the right side of the chest (dextrocardia), or at the midline (mesocardia), or in which there is a normal location of the heart in the left side of the chest but abnormal position of the viscera (isolated levocardia). Knowledge of the position of the abdominal organs and of the branching pattern of the main stem bronchi is important in categorizing these malpositions. When dextrocardia occurs *without* situs inversus, when the *visceral situs is indeterminate*, or if *isolated levocardia* is present, associated, often complex, multiple cardiac anomalies are usually present. In contrast, mirror-image dextrocardia is usually observed with complete situs inversus, which occurs most frequently in individuals whose hearts are otherwise normal.

SURGICALLY MODIFIED CONGENITAL HEART DISEASE

Because of the enormous strides in cardiovascular surgical techniques that have occurred in the past 20 years, a large number of long-term survivors of corrective operations in infancy and childhood have reached adulthood. These patients are often challenging because of the diversity of anatomic, hemodynamic, and electrophysiologic residua and sequelae of cardiac operations.

The proper care of the survivor of operation for congenital heart disease requires that the clinician understand the details of the malformation prior to operation, pay meticulous attention to the details of the operative procedure, and recognize the postoperative residua (conditions left totally or partially uncorrected), sequelae (conditions

Table 235-4

Potential Late Postoperative Problems

Residual shunts
Residual ventricular outflow obstruction
Residual valvular anomalies
Systemic arterial hypertension
Pulmonary vascular obstruction
Arrhythmias and conduction defects
Myocardial dysfunction
Prosthetic valve malfunction
Prosthetic conduit obstruction
Infective endocarditis

caused by surgery), and the complications that may have resulted from the operation. With the exception of ligation and division of an uncomplicated patent ductus arteriosus, almost every other surgical repair of an anomaly leaves behind or causes some abnormality of the heart and circulation that may range from trivial to serious. Intraoperative transesophageal echocardiography assists in detecting unsuspected lesions, in monitoring the repair, and in verifying a satisfactory result or directing further repair. Thus, even with results that are considered clinically to be good to excellent, continued long-term postoperative follow-up is advisable.

Table 235-4 lists the categories of common late postoperative problems. Cardiac operations importantly involving the atria, such as closure of atrial septal defect, repair of total or partial anomalous pulmonary venous return, or venous switch corrections of complete transposition of the great arteries (the Mustard or Senning operations), may be followed years later by sinus node or atrioventricular node dysfunction or by atrial arrhythmias. Intraventricular surgery may also result in electrophysiologic consequences, including complete heart block necessitating pacemaker insertion to avoid sudden death. In addition, valvular problems may arise late after initial cardiac operation. An example is the progressive stenosis of an initially nonobstructive bicuspid aortic valve in the patient who underwent aortic coarctation repair. Such aortic valves may also be the site of infective endocarditis. After repair of the ostium primum atrial septal defect, the cleft mitral valve may become progressively incompetent. Tricuspid regurgitation may also be progressive in the postoperative patient with tetralogy of Fallot if right ventricular outflow tract obstruction was not relieved adequately at initial surgery. In many patients with surgically modified congenital heart disease, inadequate relief of an obstructive lesion, or a residual regurgitant lesion, or a residual shunt will cause or hasten the onset of clinical signs and symptoms of myocardial dysfunction. Despite a good hemodynamic repair, many patients with a subaortic right ventricle will develop right ventricular decompensation and signs of "left heart failure." In many patients, particularly those who were cyanotic for many years before operation, a preexisting compromise in ventricular performance is due to the original underlying malformation.

A final category of postoperative problems involves the use of prosthetic valves, patches, or conduits in the operative repair. The special risks include infective endocarditis, thrombus formation, and premature degeneration and calcification of the prosthetic materials. There are many patients in whom extracardiac conduits are required to correct the circulation functionally and often to carry blood to the lungs from the right atrium or right ventricle. These conduits may develop intraluminal obstruction and, if they include a prosthetic valve, it may show progressive calcification and thickening.

BIBLIOGRAPHY

CHILD JS: Echo-Doppler and color-flow imaging in congenital heart disease. Cardiol Clin 8:289, 1990
———, MARELLI AJ: The application of transesophageal echocardiography in the adult with congenital heart disease, in *Transesophageal Echocardiography*, G Maurer (ed). New York, McGraw-Hill, 1994, pp159–188
DAJANI AS et al: Prevention of bacterial endocarditis. Recommendations of the American Heart Association. JAMA 264:2919, 1990

FRIEDMAN WF: Congenital heart disease in infancy and childhood, in *Heart Disease*, 5th ed, E Braunwald (ed). Philadelphia, Saunders, 1997, pp 877–962
GRAHAM TP JR et al: Task Force 1: Congenital heart disease. 26th Bethesda Conference: Recommendations for determining eligibility for competition in athletes with cardiovascular abnormalities. J Am Coll Cardiol 24:845, 1994
HIRSCH R et al: Diagnosis in adolescents and adults with congenital heart disease. Prospective assessment of individual and combined roles of magnetic resonance imaging and transesophageal echocardiography. Circulation 90:2937, 1994
KONSTANTINIDES S et al: A comparison of surgical and medical therapy for atrial septal defect in adults. N Engl J Med 333:469, 1995
PERLOFF JK: Congenital heart disease and pregnancy. Clin Cardiol 17:579, 1994
———, CHILD JS: *Congenital Heart Disease in Adults*. Philadelphia, Saunders, 1991

236

Edward L. Kaplan

RHEUMATIC FEVER

Acute rheumatic fever is much less common at the close of the twentieth century than it was 50 years earlier. In the late 1940s, patients with rheumatic fever and rheumatic heart disease accounted for more than half of schoolchildren recognized to have cardiovascular problems in the United States. During the Second World War, there were more than 20,000 cases of acute rheumatic fever in U.S. Navy personnel alone. The incidence of rheumatic fever has declined remarkably in the industrialized countries of the world, where the disease has become rare. However, in many developing countries, which account for almost two-thirds of the world's population, streptococcal infections, rheumatic fever, and rheumatic heart disease remain a very significant public health problem. The magnitude of the problem in these countries today is similar to that in North America 50 years ago.

The decreased incidence of acute rheumatic fever and the low prevalence of rheumatic heart disease in industrialized countries have led many physicians and public health authorities to the incorrect conclusion that these conditions are no longer a problem. However, starting in the 1980s unexpected scattered outbreaks of acute rheumatic fever among both adults and children in North America have confirmed the capacity for this potentially serious illness to reappear and pose significant public health problems. Neither antimicrobial agents nor other public health measures have been totally effective in the control of rheumatic fever.

EPIDEMIOLOGY   The epidemiology of acute rheumatic fever is identical to that of group A streptococcal upper respiratory tract infections (Chap. 143). As is the case for streptococcal sore throat, acute rheumatic fever most often occurs in children; the peak age-related incidence is between 5 and 15 years. Most initial attacks in adults take place at the end of the second and beginning of the third decades of life. Rarely, initial attacks occur as late as the fourth decade and recurrent attacks may be seen even later; attacks have been documented in the fifth and sixth decades.

Epidemiologic risk factors classically associated with individual attacks and especially with outbreaks of acute rheumatic fever include lower standards of living, especially crowding; the disease has been more common among socially and economically disadvantaged populations. However, the outbreaks in the United States in the late 1980s and early 1990s cannot be explained entirely by these factors. The large Utah outbreak of almost 300 cases during 7 years affected patients in primarily middle-class families with ready access to medical care. Therefore, one can conclude that the organism itself as well as the degree of host/herd immunity to the prevalent serotypes in an affected community are equally important risk factors.

Studies have shown that approximately 3 percent of individuals with untreated group A streptococcal pharyngitis will develop rheumatic fever. The epidemiology of rheumatic fever is also influenced by the serotypes of group A streptococci present in a population. The concept of "rheumatogenecity" of specific strains is largely based upon epidemiologic evidence associating certain serotypes with rheumatic fever (serotypes 5, 6, 18, etc.). Mucoid or highly encapsulated strains have been associated with rheumatic fever.

PATHOGENESIS More than half a century ago the pioneering studies of Lancefield differentiated beta-hemolytic streptococci into several serologic groups. This ultimately led to the association of infection by the group A organism of the oropharynx (not of other sites) and the subsequent development of acute rheumatic fever. However, the mechanism(s) responsible for the development of rheumatic fever after an infection remains elusive. Historically, approaches to understanding the pathogenesis of rheumatic fever have been grouped into three major categories: (1) direct infection by the group A streptococcus, (2) a toxic effect of streptococcal extracellular products on the host tissues, and (3) an abnormal or dysfunctional immune response to one or more as yet unidentified somatic or extracellular antigens produced by all (or perhaps only by some) group A streptococci.

There is insufficient evidence to support direct infection of the heart as the inciting event. Additionally, while toxins such as streptolysin O and others have been postulated to be responsible for this sequel, there is relatively little convincing evidence at the present time. Major efforts have focused on an abnormal immune response by the human host to one or more group A streptococcal antigens. The hypothesis of "antigenic mimicry" between human and bacterial antigens has been studied extensively and has concentrated on two interactions. The first is the similarity between the group-specific carbohydrate of the group A streptococcus and the glycoprotein of heart valves; the second involves the molecular similarity between either streptococcal cell membrane or streptococcal M protein and sarcolemma or other moieties of the human myocardial cell. The possibility of a predisposing genetic influence in some individuals is one of the most tantalizing of the incompletely understood factors that might contribute to the susceptibility to rheumatic fever. The precise genetic factors influencing the attack rate have never been adequately defined. Observations have been described that support the concept that this nonsuppurative sequel to a group A streptococcal infection results from an abnormal immune response by the human host. Thus differences in immune responses to streptococcal extracellular antigens have been reported, with a unique surface marker on non-T lymphocytes of rheumatic fever patients.

DIAGNOSIS There is no specific laboratory test that can establish a diagnosis of rheumatic fever. The diagnosis, therefore, is a clinical one but requires supporting evidence from the clinical microbiology and clinical immunology laboratories. Because of the variety of signs and symptoms associated with the rheumatic fever syndrome, in 1944 Jones first proposed criteria to assist the clinician in standardizing the diagnosis of rheumatic fever. The most recent modification of the *Jones criteria* was published in 1992 by a Special Writing Group of the American Heart Association (Table 236-1).

There are five criteria termed *major* because they are most commonly found in patients with rheumatic fever: carditis, migratory polyarthritis, Sydenham's chorea, subcutaneous nodules, and erythema marginatum.

The *carditis* of acute rheumatic fever is a pancarditis involving the pericardium, myocardium, and endocardium. In most published series, between 40 and 60 percent of patients with acute rheumatic fever have evidence of carditis, which is characterized by one or more of the following: sinus tachycardia, the murmur of mitral regurgitation, an S_3 gallop, a pericardial friction rub, and cardiomegaly. The introduction of echocardiography has assisted in the identification of subtle abnormalities of the mitral valve, and these may be present in an additional 20 percent of patients who do not have an audible heart murmur. A prolonged PR interval and evidence of heart failure may be present as well.

Healing of the rheumatic valvulitis may cause fibrous thickening and adhesion, resulting in the most serious complication of rheumatic fever, i.e., valvular stenosis and/or regurgitation (Chap. 237). The mitral valve is involved most frequently, followed by the aortic valve. Even minor degrees of rheumatic valvular involvement can lead to susceptibilities to infective endocarditis (Chap. 126). Although rheumatic pericarditis can cause a serous effusion, fibrin deposits, and even pericardial calcification, it does not lead to constrictive pericarditis.

A *migratory polyarthritis* is present in as many as 75 percent of cases, most often affecting the ankles, wrists, knees, and elbows over a period of days. It usually does not affect the small joints of the hands or feet and seldom involves the hip joints. Since salicylates and other anti-inflammatory drugs usually cause prompt resolution of joint symptoms, it is important that the clinician *not* prescribe these medications until it is determined whether the arthritis is migratory. The arthritis of acute rheumatic fever is extremely painful. Pain can be controlled with codeine or similar analgesics until the diagnosis is established. The difference between arthralgia (joint pain) and arthritis (joint pain and swelling) must be understood. Too often, arthralgia is used (incorrectly) as a major criterion.

Sydenham's chorea occurs in fewer than 10 percent of patients with rheumatic fever. The latent period between the onset of the initiating streptococcal infection and the onset of Sydenham's chorea may be as long as several months. While differing from the other manifestations, this central nervous system disorder is a part of the rheumatic fever complex and should be managed as such. Many patients who appear to have only chorea may present several decades later with evidence of typical rheumatic valvular disease. There is no definitive laboratory test for establishing a diagnosis of Sydenham's chorea, and the diagnosis is one of exclusion. Patients with Sydenham's chorea should be given secondary prophylaxis for prevention of recurrent attacks, even if they do not appear to have rheumatic heart disease.

Subcutaneous nodules and *erythema marginatum* are rare major manifestations, usually present in fewer than 10 percent of cases. Subcutaneous nodules are found over extensor surfaces of joints, are seen most often in patients with long-standing rheumatic heart disease, and are extremely rare in patients experiencing an initial attack. Erythema marginatum is an uncommon manifestation. It is an evanescent macular eruption with rounded borders—usually concentrated on the trunk.

The *minor criteria* (Table 236-1) are nonspecific and may be present in many clinical conditions.

To fulfill the Jones criteria, either two major criteria, or one major criterion and two minor criteria, *plus* evidence of an antecedent streptococcal infection are required. The latter may be provided by recovery of the organism on culture or by evidence of an immune response to one of the commonly measured group A streptococcal antigens (e.g., anti-streptolysin O, anti-deoxyribonuclease B, anti-hyaluronidase). Since the accurate diagnosis of rheumatic fever has future medical

Table 236-1

The Jones Criteria for Rheumatic Fever, Updated 1992

Major Criteria	Minor Criteria
Carditis	Clinical
Migratory polyarthritis	Fever
Sydenham's chorea	Arthralgia
Subcutaneous nodules	Laboratory
Erythema marginatum	Elevated acute phase reactants
	Prolonged PR interval

plus

Supporting evidence of a recent group A streptococcal infection
(e.g., positive throat culture or rapid antigen detection test; and/or elevated or increasing streptococcal antibody test)

SOURCE: Modified from the Special Writing Group of the American Heart Association.

and financial implications, the clinician is obligated to evaluate any patient completely until the suspected diagnosis is either established or excluded. Group A streptococcal pyoderma is *not* thought to predispose to rheumatic fever.

Both the clinical microbiology and the clinical immunology laboratories have important roles in confirming the diagnosis of rheumatic fever. An attempt should be made to recover the organism from a throat culture, although group A streptococci can be recovered from the upper respiratory tract of only 25 to 40 percent of patients. If a rapid antigen detection test is used but is negative, a confirmatory throat culture should be performed. It is helpful to obtain two or three cultures from the throat at the time the diagnosis is suspected but before initiating antibiotic therapy.

At least 80 percent of patients with acute rheumatic fever have an elevated anti-streptolysin O titer at presentation. If one employs two additional streptococcal antibody tests such as the anti-DNAse B or anti-hyaluronidase test, the percentage of patients who show evidence of a preceding group A streptococcal infection will rise to more than 95 percent. While an initially elevated titer is convincing, being able to demonstrate a rise in titer from the acute to the convalescent phase is a more reliable means of documenting the recent infection. If three antibody tests are done and there is no evidence of a preceding infection, the diagnosis must be seriously reconsidered.

℞ TREATMENT

There are two necessary therapeutic approaches to patients with acute rheumatic fever: anti-streptococcal therapy and therapy for the clinical manifestations of the disease. At the time of diagnosis, *all* patients with acute rheumatic fever should be treated as if they have a group A streptococcal infection, whether or not the organism is recovered by culture. In addition to the relatively large percentage of such patients who may have a negative throat culture at the time of diagnosis, others may have only a few organisms present in the throat. Conventional antibiotic treatment should be started immediately: a complete 10-day course in adults of either oral penicillin V (500 mg twice daily), or erythromycin (250 mg four times daily) for those with penicillin allergy. Many choose intramuscular benzathine penicillin G (a single intramuscular injection of 1.2 million units) for the treatment of the presumed streptococcal infection; this will also serve as the first prophylactic treatment for the prevention of recolonization of the upper respiratory tract in the future. Intramuscular benzathine penicillin G has been reported to result in a transient elevation of the sedimentation rate.

Following the initial anti-streptococcal therapy, secondary prophylaxis should be initiated to prevent subsequent colonization of the upper respiratory tract with group A streptococci. Recommendations of the American Heart Association and of the World Health Organization are for intramuscular injection of 1.2 million units of benzathine penicillin G every 4 weeks or for oral penicillin V (250 mg twice daily) or oral sulfadiazine (1.0 g daily). Recent studies have shown that in those individuals who are at high risk for recurrence of rheumatic fever, intramuscular benzathine penicillin G given every 3 weeks is more effective in reducing the risk of recurrence. Secondary prevention should not be discontinued in patients with rheumatic heart disease, those with a history of multiple attacks of rheumatic fever, or those within 10 years of an attack.

Medical therapy for the manifestations of rheumatic fever depends on the clinical status of the patient. For adult patients with the arthritis of rheumatic fever, salicylates in doses escalating to 2 g four times daily are very effective and will result in marked clinical improvement, often within 12 h. When this prompt relief does not occur, one should reexamine the original diagnosis. Salicylates may be given for 4 to 6 weeks and gradually tapered so as to prevent a rebound. The erythrocyte sedimentation rate is one method for determining the rate of taper for salicylates. Usually this requires at least 2 weeks. There are no conclusive data to support using nonsteroidal anti-inflammatory drugs for acute rheumatic fever. There is no indication for the use of glucocorticoids solely for the treatment of the arthritis of rheumatic fever.

Most experienced physicians believe that there is a role for glucocorticoids in patients with severe carditis accompanied by congestive heart failure. However, neither salicylates nor glucocorticoids influence the future development of valvular heart disease. In adults, prednisone can be started in doses as high as 30 mg four times daily in especially severe cases, and, as the patient improves, salicylates can be added during the tapering of the steroid dose; this may require 4 to 6 weeks.

In the presence of congestive heart failure, conventional medical measures (see Chap. 233) are indicated. In the past, patients with acute rheumatic fever were kept at complete bed rest for months. This is inappropriate unless there is a specific reason such as persistent active carditis or severe heart failure. Patients with arthritis will begin to feel better very soon after anti-inflammatory therapy is begun. They may be released from bed rest but should not resume full activity until signs of inflammatory process have abated and the acute-phase reactants have returned to normal.

BIBLIOGRAPHY

BISNO AL et al: Streptococcal infections that fail to cause recurrences of rheumatic fever. J Infect Dis 136:278, 1977

COMMITTEE ON RHEUMATIC FEVER, ENDOCARDITIS AND KAWASAKI DISEASE OF THE COUNCIL ON CARDIOVASCULAR DISEASE IN THE YOUNG OF THE AMERICAN HEART ASSOCIATION: Treatment of acute streptococcal pharyngitis and prevention of rheumatic fever: A statement for health professionals. Pediatrics 96:758, 1995

DAJANI A: Rheumatic fever, in *Heart Disease*, 5th ed, E Braunwald (ed). Philadelphia, Saunders, 1997, pp 1769–1775

KAPLAN EL: Global assessment of rheumatic fever and rheumatic heart disease at the close of the century. The influences and dynamics of population and pathogens: A failure to realize prevention? (The T. Duckett Jones Memorial Lecture.) Circulation 88:1964, 1993

———: The group A streptococcal upper respiratory tract carrier state: An enigma. J Pediatr 97:337, 1980

LUE HC et al: Long-term outcome of patients with rheumatic fever receiving benzathine penicillin G prophylaxis every three weeks versus every four weeks. J Pediatr 125:812, 1994

MARKOWITZ M, GORDIS L: *Rheumatic Fever*. Philadelphia, Saunders, 1972

SPECIAL WRITING GROUP OF THE COMMITTEE ON RHEUMATIC FEVER, ENDOCARDITIS AND KAWASAKI DISEASE OF THE COUNCIL ON CARDIOVASCULAR DISEASE IN THE YOUNG OF THE AMERICAN HEART ASSOCIATION: Guidelines for the diagnosis of rheumatic fever. Jones criteria, 1992 Update. JAMA 268:2069, 1992

VEASY GL et al: Persistence of acute rheumatic fever in the intermountain area of the United States. J Pediatr 24:9, 1994

237 *Eugene Braunwald*

VALVULAR HEART DISEASE

The role of physical examination in the evaluation of patients with valvular disease is also considered in Chap. 227; of electrocardiography in Chap. 228; of cardiac catheterization and angiography in Chap. 229; and of balloon valvuloplasty in Chap. 245.

MITRAL STENOSIS

ETIOLOGY AND PATHOLOGY Two-thirds of all patients with mitral stenosis (MS) are female. MS is generally rheumatic in origin; rarely, it is congenital. Pure or predominant MS occurs in approximately 40 percent of all patients with rheumatic heart disease. The valve leaflets are diffusely thickened by fibrous tissue and/or calcific deposits. The mitral commissures fuse, the chordae tendineae fuse and shorten, the valvular cusps become rigid, and these changes, in turn, lead to narrowing at the apex of the funnel-shaped valve. While the initial insult to the mitral valve is rheumatic, the later changes may be a nonspecific process resulting from trauma to the valve caused by altered flow patterns due to the initial deformity. Calcification of the stenotic mitral valve immobilizes the leaflets and narrows the orifice further. Thrombus formation and arterial embolization may arise from the calcific valve itself.

PATHOPHYSIOLOGY In normal adults the mitral valve orifice is 4 to 6 cm^2. In the presence of significant obstruction, i.e., when the orifice is less than approximately 2 cm^2, blood can flow from the left atrium to the left ventricle only if propelled by an abnormally elevated left atrioventricular pressure gradient (Fig. 229-6), the hemodynamic hallmark of MS. When the mitral valve opening is reduced to 1 cm^2, a left atrial pressure of approximately 25 mmHg is required to maintain a normal cardiac output. The elevated pulmonary venous and capillary pressures reduce pulmonary compliance, causing exertional dyspnea. The first bouts of dyspnea are usually precipitated by clinical events that increase the rate of blood flow across the mitral orifice, resulting in further elevation of the left atrial pressure (see below). In order to assess the severity of obstruction, both the transvalvular pressure gradient and flow rate must be measured (Chap. 229). The latter is dependent not only on the cardiac output but on the heart rate as well. An increase in heart rate shortens diastole proportionately more than systole and diminishes the time available for flow across the mitral valve. Therefore, at any given level of cardiac output, tachycardia augments the transvalvular gradient and elevates further the left atrial pressure. (Similar considerations apply to the tricuspid valve.)

The left ventricular diastolic pressure is normal in isolated MS; coexisting aortic valve disease, systemic hypertension, mitral regurgitation (MR), ischemic heart disease, and perhaps the residua of damage produced by rheumatic myocarditis are sometimes responsible for elevations that reflect impaired left ventricular function and/or reduced left ventricular compliance. Left ventricular dysfunction, as reflected in reduced ejection fraction, occurs in about one-fourth of patients with severe, chronic MS. This may be a consequence of prolonged reduction of preload and extension of the scarring from the valve into the adjacent myocardium. In pure MS and sinus rhythm, the elevated left atrial and pulmonary artery wedge pressures exhibit a prominent atrial contraction (*a* wave) and a gradual pressure decline after mitral valve opening (*y* descent). In severe MS and whenever the pulmonary vascular resistance is significantly increased, the pulmonary arterial pressure is elevated even when the patient is at rest, and in extreme cases it may approach the systemic arterial pressure. Further elevations of left atrial, pulmonary capillary, and pulmonary arterial pressures occur during exercise. When the pulmonary arterial systolic pressure exceeds approximately 50 mmHg in patients with MS, or for that matter with any lesion affecting the left side of the heart, the increased right ventricular afterload impedes the emptying of this chamber, and right ventricular end-diastolic pressure and volume usually rise.

Cardiac Output The hemodynamic response to mitral obstruction ranges from a normal cardiac output at rest and a high left atrioventricular pressure gradient to a reduced cardiac output and low transvalvular pressure gradient. In the majority of patients with moderate MS, the cardiac output is normal or almost so at rest but rises subnormally during exertion. In patients with severe MS, particularly those in whom the pulmonary vascular resistance is strikingly elevated, the cardiac output is subnormal at rest and may fail to rise or may even decline during activity. The depressed cardiac output in patients with MS is related primarily to the obstruction of the mitral orifice but also may be due to the impairment of the function of either ventricle.

Pulmonary Hypertension The clinical and hemodynamic features of MS are influenced importantly by the level of the pulmonary artery pressure. Pulmonary hypertension results from (1) the passive backward transmission of the elevated left atrial pressure; (2) pulmonary arteriolar constriction, which presumably is triggered by left atrial and pulmonary venous hypertension (reactive pulmonary hypertension); (3) interstitial edema in the walls of the small pulmonary vessels; and (4) organic obliterative changes in the pulmonary vascular bed.

Severe pulmonary hypertension results in tricuspid and pulmonary incompetence as well as right-sided heart failure. The changes in the pulmonary vascular bed also may be considered to exert a protective effect; the elevated precapillary resistance reduces the likelihood of symptoms of pulmonary congestion by reducing the surge of blood into the pulmonary capillary bed during activity which then dams up behind the stenotic mitral valve. However, this protection occurs at the expense of a reduced cardiac output.

SYMPTOMS AND COMPLICATIONS In temperate climates the latent period between the initial attack of rheumatic carditis (in the increasingly rare circumstances in which a history of one can be elicited) and the development of symptoms due to MS is generally on the order of two decades; most patients begin to experience disability in the fourth decade. Studies carried out prior to the development of mitral valvuloplasty revealed that once a patient with MS becomes seriously symptomatic, continuous progression of the disease to death usually occurs in 2 to 5 years. In economically deprived areas, particularly on the Indian subcontinent, in Central America, and the Middle East, MS tends to progress more rapidly and frequently causes serious symptoms before the age of 20 years. On the other hand, slowly progressive MS in the elderly is being recognized with increasing frequency in the United States and western Europe.

When valvular obstruction is mild, many of the physical signs of MS may be present in the absence of any symptoms. However, even in patients whose mitral orifices are large enough to accommodate a normal blood flow with only mild elevations of left atrial pressure, elevations of pulmonary capillary pressure leading to dyspnea and cough may be precipitated by extreme exertion, excitement, fever, severe anemia, paroxysmal tachycardia, sexual intercourse, pregnancy, and thyrotoxicosis. As stenosis progresses, lesser stresses precipitate dyspnea, and the patient becomes limited in his or her daily activities. Redistribution of blood from the dependent portions of the body to the lungs, which occurs when the recumbent position is assumed, leads to orthopnea and paroxysmal nocturnal dyspnea. *Pulmonary edema* develops when there is a sudden surge in flow across a markedly narrowed mitral orifice. When moderately severe MS has existed for several years, *atrial arrhythmias*—premature contractions, paroxysmal tachycardia, flutter, and fibrillation—occur with increasing frequency. The rapid ventricular rate associated with untreated or inadequately treated atrial fibrillation is frequently responsible for acute exacerbations of dyspnea. The development of permanent atrial fibrillation often marks a turning point in the patient's course and is generally associated with acceleration of the rate at which symptoms progress.

Hemoptysis (Chap. 33) results from rupture of pulmonary-bronchial venous connections secondary to pulmonary venous hypertension. It occurs most frequently in patients who have elevated left atrial pressures *without* markedly elevated pulmonary vascular resistances and is almost never fatal. True hemoptysis must be distinguished from the bloody sputum that occurs with pulmonary edema, pulmonary infarction, and bronchitis, three conditions that occur with increased frequency in the presence of MS.

As the condition progresses and the pulmonary vascular resistance rises or when tricuspid stenosis (TS) or tricuspid regurgitation (TR) develops, symptoms secondary to pulmonary congestion sometimes diminish, and the episodes of acute pulmonary edema and hemoptysis may become reduced in frequency and severity. Elevation of pulmonary vascular resistance further increases right ventricular systolic pressure, leading to right ventricular failure, fatigue, abdominal discomfort due to hepatic congestion, and edema.

Recurrent pulmonary emboli (Chap. 261), sometimes with infarction, are an important cause of morbidity and mortality late in the course of MS. *Pulmonary infections*, i.e., bronchitis, bronchopneumonia, and lobar pneumonia, commonly complicate untreated MS. *Infective endocarditis* is rare in *pure* MS but is not uncommon in patients with combined stenosis and regurgitation. *Chest pain* occurs in about 10 percent of patients with severe MS; it may be due to pulmonary hypertension or myocardial ischemia secondary to coronary atherosclerosis; often the cause cannot be discovered.

Pulmonary Changes In addition to the aforementioned changes in the pulmonary vascular bed, fibrous thickening of the walls of the alveoli and pulmonary capillaries occurs commonly in MS. The vital capacity, total lung capacity, maximal breathing capacity, and oxygen uptake per unit of ventilation are reduced (Chap. 250), and in patients with severe MS, the latter fails to rise normally during exertion. Pulmonary compliance falls further as pulmonary capillary pressure rises during exercise. In some patients, airway resistance is abnormally increased. These alterations in pulmonary mechanics contribute to an increase in the work of breathing and are responsible for dyspnea. The diffusing capacity may be reduced, particularly during exertion, as a result of structural changes in the diffusing surface and reduction of the pulmonary capillary blood volume. These changes in the lungs are due, in part, to increased transudation of fluid from the pulmonary capillaries into the interstitial and alveolar space. As in other conditions in which left atrial pressure is elevated, pulmonary blood flow in the erect position is displaced from the basal to the apical segments of the lung (Chap. 250). The increased capacity of the pulmonary lymphatic system to drain excess fluid retards the development of alveolar edema.

Thrombi and Emboli *Thrombi* may form in the left atria, particularly in the enlarged atrial appendages of patients with MS. If they *embolize*, they do so most commonly to the brain, kidneys, spleen, and extremities. Embolization occurs much more frequently in patients with atrial fibrillation or unstable rhythms, in older patients, and in those with a reduced cardiac output, and it is seen in patients with relatively mild, as well as in those with severe, obstruction. Thus systemic embolization may be the presenting complaint in otherwise asymptomatic patients with mild MS. At operation, thrombi are *not* found more frequently in the left atria of patients with a past history of embolization than in those without this complication, indicating that it is usually the freshly formed clots that dislodge. Patients who have had one or more systemic emboli have an increased predilection for further embolic episodes. Rarely, a large pedunculated thrombus or a free-floating clot may suddenly obstruct the stenotic mitral orifice. Such "ball valve" thrombi produce syncope, angina, and changing auscultatory signs with alterations in position, findings that resemble those produced by a left atrial myxoma (Chap. 241).

PHYSICAL FINDINGS (See also Chap. 227) **Inspection** In patients with severe MS, there may be a malar flush with pinched and blue facies. In patients with sinus rhythm who have severe pulmonary hypertension or associated TS, the jugular venous pulse reveals prominent *a* waves due to vigorous right atrial systole. When atrial fibrillation is present, the jugular pulse reveals only a single expansion during systole (*c-v* wave). The systemic arterial pressure is usually normal or slightly low.

Palpation A right ventricular tap along the left sternal border signifies an enlarged right ventricle. The first heart sound may be palpable in patients with pliable valve leaflets. In patients with pulmonary hypertension, the impact of pulmonary valve closure can usually be felt in the second and third left intercostal spaces just left of the sternum. A diastolic thrill is frequently present at the cardiac apex, particularly in the left lateral recumbent position.

Auscultation The first heart sound (S_1) is generally accentuated and snapping, and since the mitral valve does not close until the left ventricular pressure reaches the level of the elevated left atrial pressure, this sound is often slightly delayed, causing a prolonged Q-S_1 interval on phonocardiography, particularly in patients with severe stenosis. In patients with pulmonary hypertension, the pulmonary component of the second heart sound (P_2) is often accentuated, and the two components of the second heart sound are closely split. A pulmonary systolic ejection click may be heard in patients with severe pulmonary hypertension and marked dilatation of the pulmonary artery. The opening snap (OS) of the mitral valve is most readily audible in expiration at, or just medial to, the cardiac apex but also may be easily heard along the left sternal edge or at the base of the heart. This sound generally follows the sound of aortic valve closure (A_2) by 0.05 to 0.12 s; that is, it follows P_2. Since the OS occurs when the left ventricular pressure falls below the left atrial pressure, the time interval between A_2 closure and OS varies inversely with the severity of the

MS. The intensities of the OS and S_1 correlate with the mobility of the anterior mitral leaflet.

The OS is followed by a low-pitched, rumbling, diastolic murmur, heard best at the apex with the patient in the left lateral recumbent position. It is accentuated by exercise carried out just before auscultation and reduced during the strain of a Valsalva maneuver. In general, the duration of this murmur correlates with the severity of the stenosis. In patients with sinus rhythm, the murmur often reappears or becomes reaccentuated during atrial systole, as atrial contraction reelevates the rate of blood flow across the narrowed orifice. Soft (grade I or II/VI) systolic murmurs are commonly heard at the apex or along the left sternal border in patients with pure MS and do not necessarily signify the presence of MR. Hepatomegaly, ankle edema, ascites, and pleural effusion, particularly in the right pleural cavity, may occur in patients with right MS and right ventricular failure.

Associated Lesions With severe pulmonary hypertension, a pansystolic murmur produced by functional TR may be audible along the left sternal border. Characteristically, this murmur is accentuated by inspiration, diminishes during forced expiration (Carvallo's sign) or during performance of the Valsalva maneuver, and it should not be confused with the apical pansystolic murmur of MR, since management of the two valvular lesions is quite different.

The recognition of associated MR is of considerable clinical importance in patients with MS. A presystolic murmur and an accentuated S_1 speak against the presence of serious associated MR, but when the S_1 and/or the OS are soft or absent in a patient with mitral valve disease who also has an apical systolic murmur, it is likely that significant MR and/or serious calcification of the deformed mitral valve leaflets are present. A third heart sound at the apex often signifies that the MR is serious; this sound is generally duller, lower pitched, and follows the OS. Occasionally, in patients with pure MS, physical signs may falsely suggest MR. Thus, in the presence of severe pulmonary hypertension and right ventricular failure, a third heart sound may originate from the right ventricle. The enlarged right ventricle may rotate the heart in a clockwise direction and form the cardiac apex, giving the examiner the erroneous impression of left ventricular enlargement. Under these circumstances, the rumbling diastolic murmur and the other auscultatory features of MS become less prominent or may even disappear and be replaced by the systolic murmur of functional TR which is mistaken for MR. When cardiac output is markedly reduced in a patient with MS, the typical auscultatory findings, including the diastolic rumbling murmur, may not be detectable (silent MS), but they may reappear as compensation is restored. Associated TS also tends to obscure many of the physical signs of MS.

The Graham Steell murmur of pulmonary regurgitation, a high-pitched, diastolic, decrescendo blowing murmur along the left sternal border, results from dilatation of the pulmonary valve ring and occurs in patients with mitral valve disease and severe pulmonary hypertension. This murmur may be indistinguishable from the more common murmur produced by aortic regurgitation (AR), except that it is rarely audible at the second right intercostal space and may disappear following successful surgical treatment of the MS.

LABORATORY EXAMINATION **Electrocardiogram** In MS and sinus rhythm, the P wave usually suggests left atrial enlargement (Chap. 228). It may become tall and peaked in lead II and upright in lead V_1 when severe pulmonary hypertension or TS complicates MS and right atrial enlargement occurs. The QRS complex may be normal, even in patients with critical MS. However, with severe pulmonary hypertension, right axis deviation and right ventricular hypertrophy are often present. When the electrocardiogram shows left ventricular hypertrophy, it generally indicates that an additional lesion which places a significant burden on the left ventricle, such as MR, aortic valve disease, or hypertension, is present.

Echocardiogram The echocardiogram is the most sensitive and specific noninvasive method for diagnosing MS. Transthoracic two-dimensional color Doppler flow echocardiographic imaging and Doppler ultrasound provide critical information, including an estimate of the transvalvular gradient and of mitral orifice size, the presence and severity of accompanying MR, the extent of restriction of valve leaflets, their thickness, and the degree of distortion of the subvalvular apparatus. In addition, echocardiography provides an assessment of the size of the cardiac chambers, an estimation of the pulmonary artery pressure, and an indication of the presence and severity of associated TR and pulmonic regurgitation. Transesophageal echocardiography provides superior images and should be employed when transthoracic imaging is inadequate for guiding therapy.

Roentgenogram   The earliest changes are straightening of the left border of the cardiac silhouette, prominence of the main pulmonary arteries, dilatation of the upper lobe pulmonary veins, and backward displacement of the esophagus by an enlarged left atrium. In patients with mild or moderate MS, the heart is not grossly enlarged. In severe MS, however, all chambers and vessels upstream to the narrowed valve are prominent, including the atria, pulmonary arteries and veins, right ventricle, and superior vena cava. Kerley B lines are fine, dense, opaque, horizontal lines that are most prominent in the lower and midlung fields and that result from distention of interlobular septa and lymphatics with edema when the resting mean left atrial pressure exceeds approximately 20 mmHg. In patients who have had multiple hemoptyses, hemosiderin-containing macrophages fill the air spaces, and if they become confluent, they result in a fine, diffuse nodulation most prominent in the lower lung fields (pulmonary hemosiderosis).

DIFFERENTIAL DIAGNOSIS   Significant MR may be associated with a prominent diastolic murmur at the apex, but this murmur commences slightly later than in patients with MS, and there is often clear-cut evidence of left ventricular enlargement. An apical pansystolic murmur of at least grade III/VI intensity as well as a third heart sound should arouse the suspicion of significant associated regurgitation. Similarly, the apical middiastolic murmur associated with AR (Austin Flint murmur) may be mistaken for MS. TS, which occurs rarely in the absence of MS, may mask many of the clinical features of MS. Echocardiography is particularly useful in detecting MS in patients who have or are suspected of having other valve lesions and in defining the severity of the various lesions.

Primary pulmonary hypertension (Chap. 260) results in a number of the clinical and laboratory features observed in MS. It occurs most frequently in young women. The OS and diastolic rumbling murmur are absent, and the pulmonary artery wedge and left atrial pressures are normal, as is the size of the left atrium on echocardiography. *Atrial septal defect* (Chap. 235) also may be mistaken for MS; in both conditions there is often clinical, electrocardiographic, and roentgenographic evidence of right ventricular enlargement and accentuation of the pulmonary vascularity. The widely split S_2 of atrial septal defect may be confused with the mitral OS, and the diastolic flow murmur across the tricuspid valve may be mistaken for the mitral diastolic murmur. However, the absence of left atrial enlargement and of Kerley B lines and the demonstration of fixed splitting of S_2 favor atrial septal defect over MS.

Left atrial myxoma (Chap. 241) may obstruct left atrial emptying, causing dyspnea, a diastolic murmur, and hemodynamic changes resembling those of MS. However, patients with left atrial myxoma often demonstrate findings suggestive of a systemic disease, with weight loss, fever, anemia, systemic emboli, and elevated erythrocyte sedimentation rate and serum IgG concentration. Usually an OS is not audible, and the auscultatory findings frequently change with body position. The diagnosis can be established by demonstrating a characteristic echo-producing mass in the left atrium by two-dimensional echocardiography.

CARDIAC CATHETERIZATION AND ANGIOCARDIOGRAPHY   Left heart catheterization (Chap. 229) is helpful in deciding whether valvulotomy is necessary in the rare patient in whom it is difficult to estimate the severity of obstruction by noninvasive tests. It is helpful in assessing associated lesions such as aortic stenosis

(AS) and AR. Catheterization and coronary arteriography are not usually necessary to aid in the decision regarding surgery in younger patients with typical findings of severe obstruction on clinical examination and echocardiography. In males over 45 years and females over 55 years and younger patients with coronary risk factors, coronary angiography is usually advisable preoperatively, in order to detect patients with critical coronary obstructions that should be bypassed at the time of operation. Catheterization and left ventricular angiography are also indicated in most patients who have undergone previous mitral valve operations and who have redeveloped serious symptoms; in such patients, clinical assessment may be particularly difficult, and the hemodynamic studies allow determination of the severity of the lesion and intelligent planning of the reoperation.

℞ **TREATMENT**

In the asymptomatic adolescent with mitral valve disease, penicillin prophylaxis of beta-hemolytic streptococcal infections (Chap. 236) and prophylaxis for infective endocarditis (Chap. 126) are important. In symptomatic patients, some improvement usually occurs with restriction of sodium intake and maintenance doses of oral diuretics. Digitalis glycosides do not alter the hemodynamics and usually do not benefit patients with pure stenosis and sinus rhythm but are necessary for slowing the ventricular rate of patients with atrial fibrillation. Small doses of beta blockers (e.g., atenolol 25 to 50 mg/d) may be added when cardiac glycosides fail to control ventricular rate in patients with atrial fibrillation or flutter. Hemoptysis is treated by measures designed to diminish pulmonary venous pressure, including bed rest, the sitting position, salt restriction, and diuresis. Anticoagulants should be administered for at least 1 year in patients with MS who have suffered systemic and/or pulmonary embolization and continuously in those with atrial fibrillation.

If atrial fibrillation is of relatively recent origin in a patient whose MS is not severe enough to warrant surgical treatment or balloon valvuloplasty, reversion to sinus rhythm pharmacologically or by means of electrical countershock is indicated. Usually this should be undertaken following 3 weeks of anticoagulant treatment. Conversion to sinus rhythm is rarely helpful in patients with severe MS, particularly those in whom the left atrium is especially enlarged or in whom atrial fibrillation has been present for more than 1 year, since reversion to atrial fibrillation is common.

Mitral Valvulotomy   Unless there is a specific contraindication, mitral valvulotomy is indicated in the symptomatic patient with pure MS whose effective orifice is less than approximately 1.0 cm². Operation usually not only results in striking symptomatic and hemodynamic improvement but also prolongs survival. In uncomplicated cases, the surgical mortality rate should be less than 2 percent. However, there is no evidence that surgical treatment improves the prognosis of patients with slight or no functional impairment. Therefore, unless recurrent systemic embolization has occurred, valvulotomy is *not* recommended for patients who are entirely asymptomatic, regardless of hemodynamic findings. When there is little symptomatic improvement following valvulotomy, it is likely that the procedure was ineffective, that it induced MR, or that associated valvular or myocardial disease was present. The recurrence of symptoms several years after what appeared to be a satisfactory initial result is usually due to an inadequate valvulotomy, but progression of other valvular lesions, restenosis of the mitral valve, or some combination of these conditions also may be responsible. More than half of all patients undergoing mitral valvulotomy require reoperation by 10 years. In the *pregnant patient* with MS, valvulotomy should be carried out if pulmonary congestion occurs despite intensive medical treatment.

An "open" operation using cardiopulmonary bypass is usually preferable to closed commissurotomy. In addition to opening the valve commissures, it is important to loosen any subvalvular fusion of papillary muscles and chordae tendineae and to remove large deposits of calcium, thereby improving valvular function, and to remove atrial thrombi. In patients with significant associated MR, those in whom the valve has been severely distorted by previous operative manipulation, or those in whom the surgeon does not find it possible to improve valve function significantly, the valve may have to be replaced with a prosthesis. Since the operative mortality of replacement of the mitral valve is still approximately 4 percent, and since there are long-term complications of valve replacement, patients in whom preoperative evaluation suggests the possibility that replacement may be required should be operated on only if they have *critical* MS, i.e., an orifice <0.6 cm^2/m^2 body surface area and are in the New York Heart Association class III, i.e., symptomatic with ordinary activity, despite optimal medical therapy. The overall 10-year survival of operative survivors following mitral valve replacement is approximately 65 percent. Long-term prognosis is worse in older patients and those with marked disability and striking depression of the cardiac index preoperatively.

Percutaneous Balloon Valvuloplasty This is an alternative to surgical mitral valvulotomy in patients with pure or predominant rheumatic MS. It is the procedure of choice in young patients without extensive valvular calcification, thickening, subvalvular deformity, or MR; in them the results are similar to those of surgical valvuloplasty. It is particularly useful in pregnant women but also may be used in older patients with severe valvular deformity who are poor operative candidates (Fig. 245-7).

MITRAL REGURGITATION

ETIOLOGY Chronic rheumatic heart disease is the cause of severe MR in about one-third of cases. In contrast to MS, rheumatic MR occurs more frequently in males. The rheumatic process produces rigidity, deformity, and retraction of the valve cusps and commissural fusion, as well as shortening, contraction, and fusion of the chordae tendineae. MR also may occur as a congenital anomaly (Chap. 235), most commonly as a defect of the endocardial cushions. MR may occur with fibrosis of a papillary muscle in patients with healed myocardial infarction as well as in patients with infarction involving the base of a papillary muscle. Transient regurgitation also may occur during periods of ischemia involving a papillary muscle or the adjacent myocardium and may accompany bouts of angina pectoris. MR may occur with marked left ventricular enlargement of any cause in which dilatation of the mitral annulus and lateral displacement of the papillary muscles interfere with coaptation of the valve leaflets. In hypertrophic cardiomyopathy, the anterior leaflet of the mitral valve is displaced anteriorly during systole, leading to regurgitation (Chap. 239). Calcification of the mitral annulus of unknown cause, presumably degenerative, which occurs most commonly in elderly women, also can be responsible for significant MR. The *prolapsing mitral valve leaflet syndrome* (see below) is another important cause of MR. *Acute* MR may occur secondary to infective endocarditis involving the valve or chordae tendineae, in acute myocardial infarction with rupture of a papillary muscle or one of its heads, as a consequence of trauma, or following apparently spontaneous chordal rupture.

Regardless of cause, severe MR is often progressive, since enlargement of the left atrium places tension on the posterior mitral leaflet, pulling it away from the mitral orifice and thereby aggravating the valvular dysfunction. Similarly, the dilatation of the left ventricle increases the regurgitation, which in turn enlarges further the left atrium and ventricle, causing chordal rupture and resulting in a vicious cycle; hence the aphorism, "mitral regurgitation begets mitral regurgitation."

PATHOPHYSIOLOGY The resistance to left ventricular emptying is reduced in patients with MR. As a consequence, the left ventricle is decompressed into the left atrium during ejection, and with the reduction in left ventricular size there is a rapid decline in left ventricular tension, i.e., a progressive reduction in left ventricular afterload. The initial compensation to acute MR consists of more complete systolic emptying of the left ventricle. However, left ventricular volume increases progressively as the severity of the regurgitation increases and the function of the left ventricle deteriorates. This is often accompanied by a depressed forward cardiac output. The regurgitant volume varies directly with the left ventricular systolic pressure and

the size of the regurgitant orifice; the latter, in turn, is influenced profoundly by the degree of left ventricular dilatation.

The *v* wave in the left atrial pressure pulse is usually prominent. During early diastole, as the distended left atrium suddenly empties, there is a particularly rapid *y* descent as long as there is no associated MS (Fig. 229-7). In chronic MR, there is often an increase in left ventricular compliance, so ventricular volume may be increased with little elevation in end-diastolic pressure. The effective (forward) cardiac output is usually reduced in seriously symptomatic patients. A brief, early diastolic atrioventricular pressure gradient may occur in patients with pure regurgitation as a result of the torrential flow of blood across a normal-sized mitral orifice.

The prompt appearance of contrast material in the left atrium following its injection into the left ventricle signifies the presence of MR. The regurgitant volume can be measured by determining the difference between the total left ventricular stroke volume estimated angiocardiographically and the effective forward stroke volume determined by the Fick method (Chap. 229). Qualitative, but clinically useful, estimates of the severity of regurgitation may be made by Doppler echocardiography, color Doppler flow echocardiographic imaging, and observation on cineangiograms of the degree of left atrial opacification following the injection of contrast material into the left ventricle.

The compliance, i.e., the pressure-volume relationship, of the left atrium and pulmonary venous bed affects the clinical picture. Patients with *normal or reduced compliance* usually have *acute* MR, little enlargement of the left atrium, but marked elevation of the left atrial pressure, particularly of the *v* wave. Pulmonary edema is common. Patients with a *marked increase in left atrial compliance* are the opposite end of the spectrum, having severe long-standing severe MR, marked enlargement of the left atrium, and normal or only slightly elevated left atrial and pulmonary artery pressures. These patients usually complain of severe fatigue and exhaustion secondary to a low cardiac output, while symptoms resulting from pulmonary congestion are less prominent; atrial fibrillation is almost invariably present. Most common are patients whose clinical and hemodynamic features are between those in the other two groups, with variable degrees of enlargement of the left atrium and with significant elevation of the left atrial pressure. Symptoms are secondary to both reduced cardiac output and pulmonary congestion.

SYMPTOMS Fatigue, exertional dyspnea, and orthopnea are the most prominent complaints in patients with chronic, severe MR. Hemoptysis and systemic embolism also occur less frequently in MR than in MS. Right-sided heart failure, with painful hepatic congestion, ankle edema, distended neck veins, ascites, and TR, may be observed in patients with MR who have associated pulmonary vascular disease and marked pulmonary hypertension. In patients with *acute*, severe MR, left ventricular failure with acute pulmonary edema and/or cardiovascular collapse is common.

PHYSICAL FINDINGS The arterial pressure is usually normal, and in severe MR the arterial pulse is often characterized by a sharp upstroke. The jugular venous pulse shows abnormally prominent *a* waves in patients with sinus rhythm and marked pulmonary hypertension and prominent *v* waves in those with accompanying severe TR.

Palpation A systolic thrill is often palpable at the cardiac apex, the left ventricle is hyperdynamic with a brisk systolic impulse and a palpable rapid-filling wave, and the apex beat is often displaced laterally. When the left atrium is markedly enlarged, it may extend anteriorly, and its expansion may be palpable along the sternal border late during ventricular systole, resembling a right ventricular lift. The combination of retraction of the left ventricle and expansion of the left atrium during systole may produce a characteristic rocking motion of the chest with each cardiac cycle. A right ventricular tap and the shock of pulmonary valve closure may be palpable in patients with marked pulmonary hypertension.

Auscultation The first heart sound is generally absent, soft, or buried in the systolic murmur; an accentuated mitral closure sound is useful in excluding severe regurgitation. In patients with severe MR, the aortic valve may close prematurely, resulting in wide splitting of the second heart sound. An OS indicates associated MS but does not exclude predominant regurgitation. A low-pitched third heart sound (S_3) occurring 0.12 to 0.17 s after the aortic valve closure sound, i.e. at the completion of the rapid-filling phase of the left ventricle, is believed to be caused by the sudden tensing of the papillary muscles, chordae tendineae, and valve leaflets and is an important auscultatory feature of severe MR. The absence of an S_3 indicates that if MR exists, it may not be severe. The S_3 may be followed, often after a brief interval, by a short, rumbling, diastolic murmur, even in the absence of MS. A fourth heart sound is often audible in patients with acute, severe MR of recent onset who are in sinus rhythm. A presystolic murmur is not ordinarily heard in patients with pure MR and sinus rhythm but is present when there is significant associated MS.

A systolic murmur of at least grade III/VI intensity, is the most characteristic auscultatory finding in severe MR. It is usually holosystolic (Chap. 227), but it may be decrescendo and cease in late systole in patients with acute, severe MR when the tall v wave in the left atrial pressure pulse reduces the late systolic left ventricular–atrial pressure gradient. In MR due to papillary muscle dysfunction or mitral valve prolapse (MVP), the systolic murmur commences in midsystole (see below). The systolic murmur is usually most prominent at the apex and radiates into the axilla. However, in patients with ruptured chordae tendineae or primary involvement of the posterior mitral leaflet, the regurgitant jet strikes the left atrial wall adjacent to the aortic root, and the systolic murmur is transmitted to the base of the heart and therefore may be confused with the murmur of aortic stenosis (AS). In patients with ruptured chordae tendineae the systolic murmur may have a cooing or "sea gull" quality; in patients with a flail leaflet the murmur may have a musical quality. The systolic murmur of MR is intensified by isometric strain but is reduced during the Valsalva maneuver.

LABORATORY EXAMINATION **Electrocardiogram** In patients with sinus rhythm there is evidence of left atrial enlargement, but right atrial enlargement also may be present when pulmonary hypertension is severe. Chronic, severe MR with left atrial enlargement is generally associated with atrial fibrillation. In many patients there is no clear-cut electrocardiographic evidence of enlargement of either ventricle. In others the signs of left ventricular hypertrophy are present.

Echocardiogram Doppler echocardiography and color Doppler flow imaging are the most accurate noninvasive techniques for the detection and estimation of MR. The left atrium is usually enlarged and/or exhibits increased pulsations; the left ventricle may be hyperdynamic. With ruptured chordae tendineae or a flail leaflet, coarse, erratic motion of the involved leaflets may be noted. Findings that help to determine the etiology of MR can often be identified. These include vegetations associated with infective endocarditis, incomplete coaptation of the anterior and posterior mitral leaflets, and annular calcification, as well as left ventricular dilatation, aneurysm, or dyskinesis. The echocardiogram in patients with MVP is described below.

Roentgenogram The left atrium and left ventricle are the dominant chambers; in chronic cases, the former may be massively enlarged and forms the right border of the cardiac silhouette. Pulmonary venous congestion, interstitial edema, and Kerley B lines are sometimes noted. Marked calcification of the mitral leaflets occurs commonly in patients with long-standing combined MR and MS. Calcification of the mitral annulus may be visualized. Contrast left ventriculography is useful in the quantification of MR.

℞ TREATMENT

Medical The nonsurgical management of MR is directed toward restricting those physical activities that regularly produce dyspnea and excessive fatigue, reducing sodium intake, and enhancing sodium excretion with the appropriate use of diuretics (Chap. 233). Vasodilators and digitalis glycosides increase the forward output of the failing left ventricle. Intravenous nitroprusside (Chap. 233) or nitroglycerin to reduce afterload and thereby the volume of regurgitant flow are useful in stabilizing patients with acute and/or severe MR. Angiotensin-converting enzyme (ACE) inhibitors are useful in chronic MR, as is hydralazine. The same considerations as in patients with MS apply to the reversion of atrial fibrillation to sinus rhythm. In the late stages of heart failure anticoagulants and leg binders are used to diminish the likelihood of venous thrombi and pulmonary emboli.

Surgical In the selection of patients for surgical treatment, the chronic, often slowly progressive nature of the disease must be balanced against the immediate risks and long-term uncertainties attendant on valve reconstruction or replacement. Patients with MR who are asymptomatic or who are limited only during strenuous exertion are not considered to be candidates for surgical treatment, since their condition may remain stable for many years. On the other hand, unless there are contraindications, surgical treatment should be offered to patients with severe MR whose limitations do not allow them to work full time or to perform normal household activities despite optimal medical management. Even in patients with mild symptoms, surgical treatment is indicated when left ventricular dysfunction is progressive, with left ventricular end-systolic volume (estimated angiographically) rising above 50 mL/m² and/or endsystolic cavity dimension on echocardiography rising above 45 mm/m². In patients with chronic heart failure, the risk of surgery rises sharply, the recovery of impaired left ventricular function is incomplete, and the long-term survival is reduced. However, conservative management has little to offer these patients, so operative treatment may be indicated even at an advanced stage of the disease, and occasionally, the clinical and hemodynamic improvement following surgical treatment in patients with advanced disease is dramatic. Though most patients who survive operation appear to be greatly improved, some degree of myocardial dysfunction may persist.

When surgical treatment is contemplated, right- and left-sided heart catheterization and left ventricular angiocardiography are generally indicated. These studies are helpful in confirming the presence of severe regurgitation and aid in the identification of patients with primary myocardial disease and relatively mild, functional MR, who usually do not benefit from operation. Hemodynamic studies are also helpful in detecting and assessing the severity of any associated valve lesions, which may have to be dealt with at the time of operation or which may limit the patient's ultimate improvement if they are left untreated. Coronary angiography identifies patients who require concomitant coronary revascularization.

Surgical treatment of MR, especially that caused by valves that are markedly deformed, with shrunken, calcified leaflets secondary to rheumatic fever, requires replacement of the valve with a prosthesis, although in an increasing fraction of patients, particularly those with severe annular dilatation, flail leaflets, MVP, ruptured chordae, or infective endocarditis, reconstruction of the mitral valve apparatus (mitral valvuloplasty) and/or mitral annuloplasty with an annuloplasty ring may be successful. Valve reconstruction should be carried out whenever feasible since the operative risk is about half (1 to 4 percent) of that associated with valve replacement. Also, reconstruction spares the patient the long-term adverse consequences of valve replacement (i.e., thromboembolic and hemorrhagic complications in the case of mechanical prostheses and late valve failure necessitating repeat valve replacement in the case of bioprostheses). In addition, by preserving the integrity of the papillary muscles and subvalvular apparatus, mitral valvuloplasty maintains left ventricular function.

MITRAL VALVE PROLAPSE

MVP, also variously termed the *systolic click-murmur syndrome, Barlow's syndrome, floppy-valve syndrome,* and *billowing mitral leaflet syndrome,* is a common, but highly variable, clinical syndrome resulting from diverse pathogenic mechanisms of the mitral valve apparatus. Among these are excessive or redundant mitral leaflet tissue, which is commonly involved with myxomatous degeneration and greatly increased concentration of acid mucopolysaccharide. It is a frequent finding in patients with heritable disorders of connective tissue, including the Marfan syndrome (Chap. 348), osteogenesis imperfecta, and the Ehler-Danlos syndrome. In most patients with MVP, however, myxomatous degeneration is confined to the mitral valve leaflets without other clinical or pathologic manifestations of disease; the posterior leaflet is usually more affected than the anterior, and the mitral valve annulus is often greatly dilated. In many patients, elongated redundant chordae tendineae cause or contribute to the regurgitation.

In the majority of patients with MVP, the cause is unknown, but in some it appears to be a genetically determined collagen tissue disorder. A reduction in the production of type III collagen has been incriminated, and electron microscopy has revealed fragmentation of collagen fibrils. MVP may be associated with thoracic skeletal deformities similar to but not as severe as those in Marfan's syndrome, including a high arched palate and alterations of the chest and thoracic spine. MVP also may occur as a sequel of acute rheumatic fever, in chronic rheumatic heart disease and following mitral valvulotomy, in ischemic heart disease, and in cardiomyopathies, as well as in 20 percent of patients with ostium secundum atrial septal defect.

MVP may lead to excessive stress on the papillary muscles, which in turn leads to dysfunction and ischemia of the papillary muscles and subjacent ventricular myocardium; rupture of chordae tendineae and progressive annular dilatation and calcification also contribute to valvular regurgitation, which then places more stress on the diseased mitral valve apparatus, thereby creating a vicious cycle. The electrocardiographic changes (see below) and ventricular arrhythmias appear to result from regional ventricular dysfunction related to increased stress placed on the papillary muscles.

CLINICAL FEATURES MVP is more common in females and has been noted in a wide age range but most commonly between the ages of 14 and 30 years. There is an increased familial incidence in some patients, suggesting an autosomal dominant form of inheritance. MVP encompasses a broad spectrum of severities, ranging from patients with only a systolic click and murmur and mild prolapse of the posterior leaflet of the mitral valve to those with severe MR due to chordal rupture and massive prolapse of both leaflets. In many patients, this condition progresses over years or decades.

Most patients are asymptomatic and remain so for their entire lives. Although severe MR is a relatively uncommon complication of MVP, the latter is now the most common cause of isolated *severe* MR in the United States. Arrhythmias, most commonly ventricular premature contractions and paroxysmal supraventricular and ventricular tachycardia, have been reported and may cause palpitations, lightheadedness, and syncope. Sudden death is a very rare complication. Many patients have chest pain that is difficult to evaluate. It is often substernal, prolonged, poorly related to exertion, and rarely resembles typical angina pectoris. Transient cerebral ischemic attacks secondary to emboli from the mitral valve due to endothelial disruption have been reported. Infective endocarditis may occur in patients with MR associated with MVP.

Auscultation The most important finding is the mid- or late (nonejection) systolic click, which occurs 0.14 s or more after the first heart sound and is thought to be generated by the sudden tensing of slack, elongated chordae tendineae or by the prolapsing mitral leaflet when it reaches its maximum excursion. Systolic clicks may be multiple and may be followed by a high-pitched late systolic crescendo-decrescendo murmur, occasionally "whooping" or "honking," which is heard best at the apex. The click and murmur occur earlier with standing, the Valsalva maneuver, or inhalation of amyl nitrate, interventions that decrease left ventricular volume, exaggerating the propensity of mitral leaflet prolapse. Conversely, squatting and isometric exercise, which increase left ventricular end-diastolic volume, diminish mitral prolapse, and the click-murmur complex is delayed and may even disappear. Some patients have a midsystolic click without the murmur; others have the murmur without a click.

LABORATORY EXAMINATION The *electrocardiogram* most commonly is normal but may show biphasic or inverted T waves in leads II, III, and aVF and occasionally supraventricular or ventricular premature contractions. *Two-dimensional echocardiography* is particularly useful in identifying the abnormal position and prolapse of the mitral valve leaflets; a useful echocardiographic definition of MVP is systolic displacement (in the parasternal view) of the mitral valve leaflets into the left atrium with coaptation superior to the plane of the mitral annulus. Thickening of the mitral valve leaflets identifies a subgroup of patients at higher risk of infective endocarditis and the development of severe MR. *Color-imaging* and *Doppler studies* are helpful in revealing and evaluating accompanying MR. *Angiocardiography* generally shows prolapse of the posterior and sometimes of both mitral valve leaflets and, rarely, severe MR.

 TREATMENT

The management of patients with MVP consists of reassurance of the asymptomatic patient without severe MR or arrhythmias, the prevention of infective endocarditis with antibiotic prophylaxis in patients with a systolic murmur and/or thickening of mitral valve leaflets on endocardiography and the relief of the atypical chest pain; beta blockers have been found to be helpful in this regard, although their use is empirical. Antiarrhythmic agents as dictated by electrophysiologic studies should be administered if symptomatic tachyarrhythmias have occurred. If the patient is symptomatic from severe MR, mitral valve repair (or rarely, replacement) is indicated. Antiplatelet aggregation agents such as aspirin should be given to patients with transient ischemic attacks, and if these are not effective, anticoagulants should be employed.

AORTIC STENOSIS

AS occurs in about one-fourth of all patients with chronic valvular heart disease; approximately 80 percent of adult patients with symptomatic valvular AS are male.

ETIOLOGY AS may be congenital in origin, it may be secondary to rheumatic inflammation of the aortic valve, or it may be due to degenerative calcification of the aortic cusps of unknown cause. The *congenitally affected valve* may already be stenotic at birth (see Chap. 235) and may become progressively more fibrotic, calcified, and stenotic. In others the valve may be congenitally deformed, usually bicuspid, without serious narrowing of the aortic orifice during childhood; its abnormal architecture makes its leaflets susceptible to otherwise ordinary hemodynamic stresses, which ultimately lead to valvular thickening, calcification, increased rigidity, and narrowing of the aortic orifice.

Rheumatic endocarditis of the aortic leaflets produces commissural fusion, resulting sometimes in a bicuspid valve. This, in turn, makes the leaflets more susceptible to trauma and ultimately leads to calcification and further narrowing. By the time the obstruction to left ventricular outflow causes serious clinical disability, the valve is usually a rigid calcified mass, and careful examination may make it difficult or even impossible to determine the etiology of the underlying process. Rheumatic AS is almost always associated with rheumatic involvement of the mitral valve. A rheumatic etiology is favored by a history of active rheumatic fever and by associated severe aortic regurgitation.

Idiopathic calcific AS (also known as senile, sclerotic, or sclerocalcific AS) is a common disorder in the elderly, and may be associated with fibrosis and fusion of the valve cusps; the pathologic process is considered to be a degenerative one—a "wear-and-tear" phenomenon. It may produce many of the characteristic systolic murmurs of AS. However, the valvular obstruction is usually relatively mild and of little, if any, hemodynamic significance; it may, on occasion, produce critical obstruction.

OTHER FORMS OF OBSTRUCTION TO LEFT VENTRIC-ULAR OUTFLOW Besides valvular AS, three other lesions may be responsible for obstruction to left ventricular outflow.

1. *Hypertrophic cardiomyopathy.* This condition is characterized by marked hypertrophy of the left ventricle, involving in particular the interventricular septum of the left ventricular outflow tract, and may cause subaortic obstruction, as described in Chap. 239.
2. *Discrete congenital subvalvular AS.* This congenital anomaly is produced by either a membranous diaphragm or a fibrous ridge just below the aortic valve (Chap. 235).
3. *Supravalvular AS.* This uncommon congenital anomaly is produced by narrowing of the ascending aorta or by a fibrous diaphragm with a small opening just above the aortic valve (Chap. 235).

PATHOPHYSIOLOGY The obstruction to left ventricular outflow produces a systolic pressure gradient between the left ventricle and aorta. When severe obstruction is suddenly produced experimentally, the left ventricle responds by dilatation and reduction of stroke volume. However, in patients the obstruction may be present at birth and/or increases gradually over the course of many years, and left ventricular output is maintained by the presence of left ventricular hypertrophy. This serves as a useful compensatory mechanism because it reduces toward normal the systolic stress developed by each segment of myocardium. A large transaortic valvular pressure gradient may exist for many years without a reduction of cardiac output, left ventricular dilatation, or the development of symptoms; ultimately, these changes occur.

A peak systolic pressure gradient exceeding 50 mmHg in the face of a normal cardiac output or an effective aortic orifice less than approximately 0.5 cm^2/m^2 of body surface area, i.e., less than approximately one-third of the normal orifice, is generally considered to represent critical obstruction to left ventricular outflow. The left ventricular pressure pulse exhibits a rounded summit as the contraction of this chamber becomes progressively more isometric. The elevated left ventricular end-diastolic pressure observed in many patients with severe AS does not necessarily signify the presence of left ventricular dilatation or failure but may reflect diminished compliance of the hypertrophied left ventricular wall.

A large *a* wave in the left atrial pressure pulse is usually present in severe AS. Loss of an appropriately timed, vigorous atrial contraction, as occurs in atrial fibrillation or atrioventricular dissociation, may result in a rapid aggravation of symptoms. Although the cardiac output at rest is within normal limits in the majority of patients with severe AS, it may fail to rise normally during exercise. Late in the course the cardiac output and left ventricular–aortic pressure gradient decline, and the mean left atrial, pulmonary artery wedge, pulmonary arterial, and right ventricular pressures rise.

The hypertrophied left ventricular muscle mass elevates myocardial oxygen requirements. In addition, even in the absence of obstructive coronary artery disease, there may be interference with coronary blood flow, because the pressure compressing the coronary arteries exceeds the coronary perfusion pressure. Metabolic evidence of myocardial ischemia can be demonstrated in patients with AS both in the presence and in the absence of coronary arterial narrowing.

A significant fraction of patients with rheumatic AS has associated mitral valve disease. AS intensifies the severity of MR by increasing the pressure driving blood from the left ventricle to the left atrium.

SYMPTOMS AS is rarely of hemodynamic or clinical importance until the valve orifice has narrowed to approximately one-third of normal, i.e., to 0.5 cm^2/m^2 in adults. Even critical AS may exist for many years without producing any symptoms because of the ability of the hypertrophied left ventricle to generate the elevated intraventricular pressures required for a normal stroke volume.

Most patients with pure or predominant AS have gradually increasing obstruction for years but do not become symptomatic until the fifth to seventh decades. Exertional dyspnea, angina pectoris, and syncope are the three cardinal symptoms. Often there is a history of insidious progression of fatigue and dyspnea associated with gradual curtailment of activities. *Dyspnea* results primarily from elevation of the pulmonary capillary pressure; the latter is caused by elevations of left atrial and left ventricular end-diastolic pressures secondary to reduced compliance and/or left ventricular dilatation. *Angina pectoris* usually develops somewhat later and reflects an imbalance between the augmented myocardial oxygen requirements and reduced oxygen availability; the former results from the increased myocardial mass and intraventricular pressure, while the latter may result from accompanying coronary artery disease, which is not uncommon in patients with AS, as well as from compression of the coronary vessels by the hypertrophied myocardium. Therefore, angina may occur in severe AS even without obstructive epicardial coronary artery disease. *Exertional syncope* may result from a decline in arterial pressure caused by vasodilatation in the exercising muscles and inadequate vasoconstriction in nonexercising muscles in the face of a fixed cardiac output or from a sudden fall in cardiac output produced by an arrhythmia.

Since the cardiac output at rest is usually well maintained until late in the course, marked fatigability, weakness, peripheral cyanosis, and other clinical manifestations of a low cardiac output are usually not prominent until this stage is reached. Orthopnea, paroxysmal nocturnal dyspnea, and pulmonary edema, i.e., symptoms of left ventricular failure, also occur only in the advanced stages of the disease. Severe pulmonary hypertension leading to right ventricular failure and systemic venous hypertension, hepatomegaly, atrial fibrillation, and TR are usually preterminal findings.

When AS and MS coexist, the reduction of cardiac output induced by MS lowers the pressure gradient across the aortic valve and thereby masks many of the clinical findings produced by AS. Left heart catheterization is helpful in defining the relative importance of each valvular abnormality.

PHYSICAL FINDINGS The systemic arterial pressure is usually within normal limits. In the late stages, however, when stroke volume declines, the systolic pressure may fall and the pulse pressure narrow. Systemic hypertension is unusual in patients with marked AS, and a basal systolic arterial pressure exceeding 200 mmHg practically excludes severe narrowing of this valve. The peripheral arterial pulse, as palpated in the carotid or brachial arteries, rises slowly to a delayed sustained peak (pulsus parvus et tardus). In the elderly, the stiffening of the arterial wall may mask this important physical sign. A palpable double systolic arterial pulse, the so-called bisferiens pulse, excludes pure or predominant AS and signifies dominant aortic regurgitation. In the late stages of valvular AS, when the pulse pressure is reduced, the pulse amplitude may be so small that the anacrotic nature of the pulse and the delay in its upstroke may become difficult to appreciate. In many patients the *a* wave in the jugular venous pulse is accentuated. This results from the diminished distensibility of the right ventricular cavity caused by the bulging, hypertrophied interventricular septum.

Palpation The apex beat is usually active and displaced laterally, reflecting the presence of left ventricular hypertrophy. A double apical impulse may be appreciated, particularly with the patient in the left lateral recumbent position; the first outward expansion occurs during atrial systole and reflects the important contribution made by atrial contraction to ventricular filling, while the second occurs during ventricular systole and usually is forceful and sustained during ejection. The right ventricle is palpable when pulmonary hypertension develops in the late stages. A systolic thrill is generally present at the base of the heart, in the jugular notch, and along the carotid arteries, but occasionally it is palpable only during expiration and with the patient leaning forward. In patients who do not have marked pulmonary emphysema, a thick chest wall, thoracic deformity, or heart failure, the absence of a systolic thrill suggests that the AS is relatively mild.

Auscultation The rhythm is generally regular until very late in the course; at other times, atrial fibrillation should suggest the possibility of associated mitral valve disease. An early systolic ejection sound, actually the OS of the aortic valve, is frequently audible in children and adolescents with congenital *noncalcific* valvular AS. This sound usually disappears when the valve becomes calcified and rigid. The sound of aortic valve closure also can be identified most frequently in patients with AS who have pliable valves, and calcification diminishes the intensity of this sound as well. As AS increases in severity, left ventricular systole may become prolonged so that the aortic valve closure sound no longer precedes the pulmonic valve closure sound, and the two components may become synchronous, or aortic valve closure may even follow pulmonic valve closure, causing paradoxic splitting of the second heart sound (Chap. 227). Frequently, a fourth heart sound is audible at the apex and reflects the presence of left ventricular hypertrophy and an elevated left ventricular end-diastolic pressure; a third heart sound generally occurs when the left ventricle dilates and fails.

The murmur of AS is characteristically an ejection systolic murmur that commences shortly after the first heart sound, increases in intensity to reach a peak toward the middle of ejection, and ends just before aortic valve closure (Chap. 227). It is usually low-pitched, rough, and rasping in character, loudest at the base of the heart, most commonly in the second right intercostal space. It is transmitted to the jugular notch and upward along the carotid arteries. Occasionally, it is transmitted downward and to the apex and may be confused with the systolic murmur of MR; the latter, however, is usually holosystolic. In almost all patients with severe obstruction, the murmur is at least grade III/VI. In patients with mild degrees of obstruction or in those with severe stenosis with heart failure in whom the stroke volume and therefore the transvalvular flow rate are reduced, the murmur may be relatively soft and brief.

LABORATORY EXAMINATION **Electrocardiogram** This reveals left ventricular hypertrophy in the majority of patients with severe AS (Chap. 228). In advanced cases, ST-segment depression and T-wave inversion (left ventricular "strain") in standard leads I and aVL and in the left precordial leads are evident. However, there is no close correlation between the electrocardiogram and the hemodynamic severity of obstruction, and the absence of electrocardiographic signs of left ventricular hypertrophy does not exclude severe obstruction. The presence of left atrial enlargement should suggest the possibility of associated mitral valve disease.

Echocardiogram The key findings are left ventricular hypertrophy and in patients with valvular calcification, multiple, bright, thick, echoes from within the aortic root. Eccentricity of the aortic valve cusps is characteristic of congenitally bicuspid valves. Transesophageal imaging displays the obstructed orifice. Left ventricular dilatation and reduced systolic shortening reflect impairment of left ventricular function. The transaortic valvular gradient can be estimated by Doppler echocardiography. Echocardiography is particularly useful for identifying valvular abnormalities such as MS and AR, which sometimes accompany AS, and for differentiating valvular from obstructive hypertrophic cardiomyopathy.

Roentgenogram The chest roentgenogram may show no or little overall cardiac enlargement for many years, since the development of concentric left ventricular hypertrophy is the initial response to obstruction to left ventricular outflow. Hypertrophy without dilatation may produce some rounding of the cardiac apex in the frontal projection and slight backward displacement in the lateral view; critical AS is often associated with poststenotic dilatation of the ascending aorta. Aortic calcification is usually readily apparent on fluoroscopic examination with an image intensifier or by echocardiography; *the absence of valvular calcification in an adult suggests that severe valvular AS is not present*. In later stages of the disease as the left ventricle dilates, there is increasing evidence of left ventricular enlargement, roentgenographic signs of pulmonary congestion, as well as enlargement of the left atrium, pulmonary artery, and right side of the heart.

Catheterization and Angiocardiography Catheterization of the left side of the heart and coronary arteriography should generally be carried out in patients suspected of having severe AS, particularly before a final decision concerning operative treatment is made. The goals are to (1) determine the severity of the aortic obstruction, often previously estimated by Doppler echocardiography; (2) assess the status of left ventricular function; and (3) determine the location of the left ventricular outflow obstruction. These investigations are especially indicated in the following:

1. Young, asymptomatic patients with noncalcific congenital AS (Chap. 235), in order to define the severity of obstruction to left ventricular outflow, since operation (which does not usually require aortic valve replacement) or balloon valvuloplasty may be indicated in them if severe AS is present, even in the absence of symptoms.
2. Patients in whom it is suspected that the obstruction to left ventricular outflow may not be at the aortic valve but rather in the sub- or supravalvular regions.
3. Patients with clinical signs of AS and symptoms of myocardial ischemia, in whom associated coronary artery disease is suspected. An effort should be made to determine whether AS or coronary atherosclerosis is primarily responsible for the symptoms, and coronary arteriography should be carried out in addition to catheterization of the left side of the heart.
4. Patients with multivalvular disease, in whom the role played by each valvular deformity should be defined to aid in the planning of definitive operative treatment.

NATURAL HISTORY Death in patients with severe AS occurs most commonly in the seventh and eighth decades. Based on data obtained at postmortem examination in patients *not treated surgically*, the average time to death after the onset of various symptoms was as follows: angina pectoris, 3 years; syncope, 3 years; dyspnea, 2 years; and congestive heart failure, 1.5 to 2 years. Moreover, in more than 80 percent of patients who died with AS, symptoms had existed for less than 4 years. Congestive heart failure was considered to be the cause of death in one-half to two-thirds of patients. Among adults dying with valvular AS, sudden death, which presumably results from an arrhythmia, occurred in 10 to 20 percent and at an average age of 60 years. However, the vast majority of sudden deaths occur in previously symptomatic patients.

℞ **TREATMENT**

All patients with moderate or severe AS require careful periodic follow-up. In patients with *severe* AS, strenuous physical activity should be avoided even in the asymptomatic stage. Digitalis glycosides, sodium restriction, and the cautious administration of diuretics are indicated in the treatment of congestive heart failure, but care must be taken to avoid volume depletion. While nitroglycerin is helpful in relieving angina pectoris, vasodilator therapy for heart failure is usually of little value and may, in fact, be harmful.

Surgical Treatment The most critical decision in the management of AS concerns the advisability of surgical treatment which, in the majority of adults with calcific AS and critical obstruction (aortic orifice <0.5 cm^2/m^2 body surface area), consists of valve replacement. In most instances, it is prudent to postpone operation in patients with severe calcific AS who are asymptomatic, since their future course is difficult to predict and they may continue to do well for many years. However, they should be followed carefully by clinical examination for the development of symptoms and by serial echocardiograms for evidence of deteriorating left ventricular function; operation is generally indicated in patients with severe AS and progressive left ventricular dysfunction, even if they are asymptomatic. In patients without heart failure, the operative risk of aortic valve replacement is approximately 4 percent.

When angina pectoris, syncope, or left ventricular decompensation develops in adults with severe valvular AS, the outlook, despite medical treatment, is very poor and can be improved significantly by replacement of the aortic valve. The operative risk in this group of patients (approximately 7 to 10 percent) is considerably lower than the risk incurred by nonoperative treatment; moreover, the symptomatic improvement in some survivors of operation has been remarkable. There is evidence that regression of left ventricular hypertrophy may occur following relief of obstruction.

Operation should, if possible, be carried out before frank left ventricular failure develops; at this late stage, the operative risk is high (15 to 20 percent), and evidence of myocardial disease may persist even when the operation is technically successful. Furthermore, long-term postoperative survival also correlates inversely with preoperative left ventricular dysfunction. Nonetheless, in view of the very poor prognosis of such patients when they are treated medically, there is usually little choice but to advise immediate surgical treatment. In patients in whom severe AS and coronary artery disease coexist, relief of the AS and revascularization of the myocardium by means of aortocoronary bypass grafting may result in striking clinical and hemodynamic improvement.

Since many patients with calcific AS are elderly, particular attention must be directed to the adequacy of hepatic, renal, and pulmonary function before valve replacement is recommended. The mortality rate depends to a substantial extent on the patient's preoperative clinical and hemodynamic state. The 10-year survival rate of patients with aortic valve replacement is approximately 60 percent. Approximately 15 percent of bioprosthetic valves evidence primary valve failure in 10 years, requiring re-replacement, and an approximately equal percentage of patients with mechanical prostheses develop significant hemorrhagic complications as a consequence of treatment with anticoagulants.

Percutaneous Balloon Aortic Valvuloplasty This procedure, described in Chap. 245, is an alternative to surgery in children and young adults with congenital AS. It is not commonly employed in elderly patients with severe calcific AS because of a high restenosis rate. Nonetheless, this procedure has been employed in patients who are too ill or frail to undergo operation, in patients with life-threatening AS and advanced extracardiac disease, and as a "bridge to surgery" in patients with severe left ventricular dysfunction.

AORTIC REGURGITATION

ETIOLOGY Approximately three-fourths of patients with pure or predominant AR are males; females predominate among patients with AR who have associated mitral valve disease. In approximately two-thirds of patients with AR the disease is rheumatic in origin, resulting in thickening, deformation, and shortening of the individual aortic valve cusps, changes that prevent their proper opening during systole and closure during diastole. A rheumatic origin is less common in patients with isolated AR. Acute AR also may result from infective endocarditis, which can develop on a valve previously affected by rheumatic disease, a congenitally deformed valve, or rarely a normal aortic valve, and perforate or erode one or more of the leaflets. Patients with discrete membranous subaortic stenosis often develop thickening of the aortic valve leaflets, which in turn leads to mild or moderate degrees of AR and makes these valves particularly susceptible to endocarditis. AR also may occur in patients with congenital bicuspid aortic valves. Prolapse of an aortic cusp, resulting in progressive chronic AR, occurs in approximately 15 percent of patients with ventricular septal defect (Chap. 235). Congenital fenestrations of the aortic valve occasionally produce mild AR. Although traumatic rupture of the aortic valve is an uncommon cause of acute AR, it does represent the most frequent serious lesion observed in patients surviving nonpenetrating cardiac injuries. In patients with AR due to primary valvular disease, dilatation of the aortic annulus may occur secondarily and intensify the regurgitation.

AR, both acute and chronic, also may be due entirely to marked aortic dilatation, i.e., aortic root disease, without primary involvement of the valve leaflets; widening of the aortic annulus and separation of the aortic leaflets are responsible for the AR. Syphilis and ankylosing rheumatoid spondylitis may be associated with cellular infiltration and scarring of the media of the thoracic aorta, leading to aortic dilatation,

aneurysm formation, and severe regurgitation. In syphilis of the aorta, the involvement of the intima may narrow the coronary ostia, which in turn may be responsible for myocardial ischemia. Cystic medial necrosis of the ascending aorta, which may or may not be associated with other manifestations of the Marfan syndrome, idiopathic dilatation of the aorta, osteogenesis imperfecta, and severe hypertension all may widen the aortic annulus and lead to progressive AR. Occasionally, AR is caused by retrograde dissection of the aorta involving the aortic annulus.

The coexistence of hemodynamically significant AS with AR usually excludes all the rarer forms of AR because it occurs almost exclusively in patients whose AR is on a rheumatic or congenital basis.

PATHOPHYSIOLOGY The total stroke volume ejected by the left ventricle (i.e., the sum of the effective forward stroke volume and the volume of blood that regurgitates back into the left ventricle) is increased in AR. In patients with wide-open (*free*) AR, the volume of regurgitant flow may equal the effective forward stroke volume. In contrast to MR, in which a fraction of the left ventricular stroke volume is delivered into the low-pressure left atrium, in AR the entire left ventricular stroke volume is ejected into a high-pressure zone, the aorta. An increase in the left ventricular end-diastolic volume (increased preload) constitutes the major hemodynamic compensation for AR. The dilatation of the left ventricle allows this chamber to eject a larger stroke volume without requiring any increase in the relative shortening of each myofibril. Therefore, severe AR may occur with a normal effective forward stroke volume and a normal ejection fraction [total (forward plus regurgitant) stroke volume/end-diastolic volume], together with an elevated left ventricular end-diastolic pressure and volume. However, through the operation of Laplace's law (which indicates that myocardial wall tension is the product of intracavitary pressure and left ventricular radius), left ventricular dilatation increases the left ventricular systolic tension required to develop any given level of systolic pressure. As left ventricular function deteriorates, the end-diastolic volume rises and the ejection fraction and forward stroke volume decline. Deterioration of left ventricular function often precedes the development of symptoms. Considerable thickening of the left ventricular wall also occurs with chronic AR, and at autopsy the hearts of these patients may be among the largest encountered, sometimes exceeding 1000 g in weight.

The reverse pressure gradient from aorta to left ventricle, which is responsible for the aortic regurgitant flow, falls progressively during diastole, accounting for the decrescendo nature of the diastolic murmur. Equilibration between aortic and left ventricular pressures may occur toward the end of diastole in patients with severe AR, particularly when the heart rate is slow, and the left ventricular end-diastolic pressure may be elevated, occasionally to extremely high levels (>40 mmHg). Rarely, in acute, severe AR, the left ventricular pressure exceeds the left atrial pressure toward the end of diastole (Fig. 229-8), and this reversed pressure gradient closes the mitral valve prematurely or causes diastolic MR.

In patients with severe AR, the effective forward cardiac output usually is normal or only slightly reduced at rest, but often it fails to rise normally during exertion. Early signs of left ventricular dysfunction include reductions in the fraction of systolic shortening and in the ejection fraction, determined by echocardiography or radionuclide or contrast angiography. In advanced stages there may be considerable elevation of the left atrial, pulmonary artery wedge, pulmonary arterial, and right ventricular pressures and lowering of the forward cardiac output at rest.

Myocardial ischemia may occur in patients with AR because myocardial oxygen requirements are elevated by both left ventricular dilatation and elevated left ventricular systolic tension. However, the major portion of coronary blood flow occurs during diastole, when arterial pressure is subnormal, thereby reducing coronary perfusion pressure. This combination of increased oxygen demand and reduced supply may cause myocardial ischemia.

HISTORY A family history may frequently be elicited from patients with AR associated with the Marfan syndrome. A history compatible with infective endocarditis may sometimes be elicited from patients with rheumatic or congenital involvement of the aortic valve, and the infection often precipitates or seriously aggravates preexisting symptoms. Ankylosing spondylitis is usually self-evident.

Patients with severe AR may remain asymptomatic for as long as 10 to 15 years.

In chronic, severe AR, uncomfortable awareness of the heartbeat, especially on lying down, may be an early complaint. Sinus tachycardia during exertion or with emotion or premature ventricular contractions may produce particularly uncomfortable palpitations, as well as head pounding. These complaints may persist for many years before the development of exertional dyspnea, usually the first symptom of diminished cardiac reserve. This is followed by orthopnea, paroxysmal nocturnal dyspnea, and excessive diaphoresis. Chest pain occurs frequently, even in younger patients, and it is not necessary to invoke the presence of coronary artery disease to explain this symptom in patients with severe AR. Anginal pain may develop at rest as well as during exertion. Nocturnal angina may be a particularly troublesome symptom, and it may be accompanied by marked diaphoresis. The anginal episodes can be prolonged and often do not respond satisfactorily to sublingual nitroglycerin. Systemic fluid accumulation, including congestive hepatomegaly, ankle edema, and ascites, may develop very late in the course of the disease.

In patients with acute, severe AR, as may occur in infective endocarditis or trauma, the left ventricle cannot dilate sufficiently to maintain stroke volume, and left ventricular diastolic pressure rises rapidly with associated elevations of left atrial and pulmonary capillary pressures. Pulmonary edema and/or cardiogenic shock may develop rapidly.

PHYSICAL FINDINGS Even prior to the examination of the heart of the patient with free AR, the jarring of the entire body and the bobbing motion of the head with each systole can be appreciated, and the abrupt distention and collapse of the larger arteries are easily visible. The examination should be directed toward the detection of conditions predisposing to AR, such as the Marfan syndrome, rheumatoid spondylitis, and ventricular septal defect.

Arterial Pulse A rapidly rising "water-hammer" pulse, which collapses suddenly as arterial pressure falls rapidly during late systole and diastole (Corrigan's pulse), and capillary pulsations, an alternate flushing and paling of the skin at the root of the nail while pressure is applied to the tip of the nail (Quincke's pulse), are characteristic of free AR. A booming, "pistol-shot" sound can be heard over the femoral arteries (Traube's sign), and a to-and-fro murmur (Duroziez's sign) is audible if the femoral artery is lightly compressed with a stethoscope.

The arterial pulse pressure is widened, with an elevation of the systolic pressure, sometimes to as high as 300 mmHg, and a depression of the diastolic pressure. The measurement of arterial diastolic pressure with a sphygmomanometer may be complicated by the fact that systolic sounds are frequently heard with the cuff completely deflated. However, the level of cuff pressure at the time of muffling of the Korotkoff sounds generally corresponds fairly closely to the true intraarterial diastolic pressure. The severity of AR does not always correlate directly with the arterial pulse pressure, and severe regurgitation may exist in patients with arterial pressures in the range of 140/60 mmHg. As the disease progresses and the left ventricular end-diastolic pressure rises markedly, the arterial diastolic pressure may actually rise also, since the aortic diastolic pressure cannot fall below the left ventricular end-diastolic pressure.

Palpation The apex beat is heaving and displaced laterally and inferiorly. The systolic expansion and diastolic retraction of the apex are prominent and contrast sharply with the sustained systolic thrust characteristic of severe AS. A diastolic thrill is often palpable along the left sternal border, and a prominent systolic thrill may be palpable in the jugular notch and transmitted upward along the carotid arteries. This thrill and the accompanying systolic murmur are due to the markedly increased blood flow across the aortic orifice and do not necessarily signify the coexistence of AS. In many patients with pure AR or with combined AS and AR, the carotid arterial pulse is bisferiens, i.e., with two systolic waves separated by a trough.

Auscultation In patients with severe AR, the aortic valve closure sound is usually diminished or absent. A third heart sound and systolic ejection sound are frequently audible, and occasionally, a fourth heart sound also may be heard. The murmur of AR is typically a high-pitched, blowing, decrescendo diastolic murmur, heard best in the third intercostal space along the left sternal border. In patients with mild regurgitation, this murmur is brief, but as the severity increases, the murmur generally becomes louder and longer, and in patients with free AR it is usually holodiastolic. When the murmur is soft, it can be heard best with the diaphragm of the stethoscope and with the patient sitting up, leaning forward, and with the breath held in forced expiration. In patients in whom the AR is caused by primary valvular disease, the diastolic murmur is usually louder along the left than the right sternal border. However, when the murmur is heard best along the right sternal border, it suggests that the AR is caused by aneurysmal dilatation of the aortic root. "Cooing" or musical diastolic murmurs suggest eversion of an aortic cusp vibrating in the regurgitant stream. Unless it is trivial in magnitude, the AR is usually accompanied by peripheral signs such as a widened pulse pressure or a collapsing pulse. On the other hand, with the Graham Steell murmur of pulmonary regurgitation, there usually is clinical evidence of severe pulmonary hypertension, including a loud and palpable pulmonary component of the second heart sound.

A midsystolic ejection murmur is frequently audible in AR. It is generally heard best at the base of the heart and is transmitted along the carotid vessels. This murmur may be quite loud without signifying obstruction; it is often higher pitched, shorter, and less rasping in quality than the ejection systolic murmur heard in patients with predominant AS. A third murmur frequently heard in patients with severe AR is the Austin Flint murmur, a soft, low-pitched, rumbling middiastolic bruit. It is probably produced by the displacement of the anterior leaflet of the mitral valve by the aortic regurgitant stream but does not appear to be associated with hemodynamically significant mitral obstruction. Both the Austin Flint murmur and the rumbling diastolic murmur of MS are loudest at the apex, but the murmur of MS is usually accompanied by a loud first heart sound and immediately follows the OS of the mitral valve, while the Austin Flint murmur is often shorter in duration than the murmur of MS; in patients with sinus rhythm the latter exhibits presystolic accentuation. The auscultatory features of AR are intensified by isometric exercise such as strenuous handgrip, which augments systemic resistance, and reduced by inhalation of amyl nitrite. A blowing holosystolic murmur at the apex, which is transmitted to the axilla, also may be heard in patients with AR who have marked left ventricular dilatation and functional MR.

In *acute*, severe AR, the elevation of left ventricular end-diastolic pressure may lead to early closure of the mitral valve, an associated middiastolic sound, a soft or absent S_1, a pulse pressure that is not particularly wide, and a soft, short diastolic murmur.

LABORATORY EXAMINATION **Electrocardiogram** In patients with mild AR, there may be no electrocardiographic abnormalities, but with severe, chronic AR, the electrocardiographic signs of left ventricular hypertrophy become manifest (Chap. 228). In addition, these patients frequently exhibit ST-segment depression and T-wave inversion in leads I, aVL, V_5, and V_6 ("left ventricular strain"). Left axis deviation and/or QRS prolongation denote diffuse myocardial disease, generally associated with patchy fibrosis, and usually signify a poor prognosis.

Echocardiogram This reveals increased systolic excursion of the posterior left ventricular wall; the extent and velocity of wall motion are normal or even supernormal, until myocardial contractility declines. A rapid, high-frequency fluttering of the anterior mitral leaflet produced by the impact of the aortic regurgitant jet is a characteristic finding. The echocardiogram is also useful in determining the cause of AR, by detecting dilatation of the aortic annulus. Thickening and failure of coaptation of the leaflets also may be noted. Color Doppler flow echocardiographic imaging is very sensitive in the detection of

AR, and Doppler echocardiography is helpful in assessing its severity. Serial two-dimensional echocardiography is valuable in evaluating left ventricular performance and in detecting progressive myocardial dysfunction.

Roentgenogram In severe chronic AR, the apex is displaced downward and to the left in the frontal projection, and frequently the cardiac shadow extends below the left diaphragm. Left ventricular enlargement also may be apparent in the left anterior oblique and lateral projections, in which the left ventricle is displaced posteriorly and encroaches on the spine. In patients in whom primary valvular disease is responsible for the AR, the ascending aorta and aortic knob may be moderately dilated. When AR is caused by primary disease of the aortic wall, aneurysmal dilatation of the aorta may be noted, and the aorta may fill the retrosternal space in the lateral view.

Cardiac Catheterization and Angiography These tests should be carried out to aid in the decision regarding surgical treatment. In addition to providing an accurate measurement of the magnitude of regurgitation and the status of left ventricular function, the condition of the coronary arterial bed may be evaluated.

℞ **TREATMENT**
Although operation constitutes the principal treatment of AR and should be carried out before the development of heart failure, the latter usually does respond initially to treatment with digitalis glycosides, salt restriction, diuretics, and vasodilators, especially ACE inhibitors. Digitalis also may be indicated in patients with severe regurgitation and dilated left ventricles without symptoms of frank left ventricular failure. Cardiac arrhythmias and infections are poorly tolerated in patients with free AR and must be treated promptly and vigorously. Although nitroglycerin and long-acting nitrates are not as helpful in relieving anginal pain as in patients with ischemic heart disease, they are worth a trial. Patients with syphilitic aortitis should receive a full course of penicillin therapy (Chap. 174).

Surgery In deciding on the advisability and proper timing of surgical treatment, two points should be kept in mind: (1) patients with chronic AR usually do not become symptomatic until *after* the development of myocardial dysfunction, and (2) surgical treatment often does not restore normal left ventricular function. Therefore, in patients with severe AR, careful clinical follow-up and noninvasive testing with echocardiography at approximately 6-month intervals are necessary if operation is to be undertaken at the optimal time, i.e., after the onset of left ventricular dysfunction but prior to the development of severe symptoms. Operation can be deferred as long as the patient remains asymptomatic *and* retains normal left ventricular function. In general, operation should be carried out even in asymptomatic patients with progressive left ventricular dysfunction and a left ventricular ejection fraction <50 percent, a left ventricular or end-systolic volume >55 mL/m^2, or end-systolic diameter >55 mm.

Replacement of the aortic valve with a suitable mechanical or tissue prosthesis is generally necessary in patients with rheumatic AR and in many patients with other forms of regurgitation. Rarely, when a leaflet has been perforated during an episode of infective endocarditis or torn from its attachments to the aortic annulus, surgical repair may be possible. When AR is due to aneurysmal dilatation of the annulus and ascending aorta rather than to primary valvular involvement, it may be possible to reduce the regurgitation by narrowing the annulus or by excising a portion of the aortic root without replacing the valve. More frequently, however, regurgitation can be eliminated only by replacing the aortic valve, excising the aneurysm responsible for the regurgitation, and replacing the latter with a graft. This formidable procedure entails a higher risk than aortic valve replacement alone.

As in patients with other valvular abnormalities, both the operative risk of aortic valve replacement and late mortality are largely dependent on the stage of the disease and on myocardial function

at the time of operation; patients with marked cardiac enlargement and prolonged left ventricular dysfunction experience an operative mortality of approximately 10 percent and a late mortality of approximately 5 percent per year despite a technically satisfactory operation. Nonetheless, because of the poor prognosis with medical management, even patients with left ventricular failure should be considered for operation.

ACUTE AORTIC REGURGITATION Infective endocarditis, aortic dissection, and trauma are the most common causes of severe, acute AR. Since the left ventricle has not had time to dilate, stroke volume declines and ventricular diastolic pressure rises markedly; the arterial pulse pressure is often not markedly widened, and the physical signs characteristic of severe chronic AR may be absent. Premature closure of the mitral valve is common and can be recognized by echocardiography. The first heart sound is soft or absent; the aortic diastolic murmur is characteristically brief. Patients present with pulmonary congestion and edema, as well as hypotension secondary to a low cardiac output. Acute, severe regurgitation requires prompt surgical treatment, which may be lifesaving.

TRICUSPID STENOSIS

TS, a relatively uncommon valvular lesion in North America and western Europe, is more common on the Indian subcontinent and in Latin America. It is generally rheumatic in origin and is more common in women than in men. It does not occur as an isolated lesion but is usually observed in association with MS. Hemodynamically significant TS occurs in 5 to 10 percent of patients with severe MS; rheumatic TS is commonly associated with some degree of regurgitation.

PATHOPHYSIOLOGY A diastolic pressure gradient between the right atrium and ventricle can be recorded with a double-lumen cardiac catheter. It is augmented when the transvalvular blood flow increases during inspiration and is reduced during expiration. A *mean* diastolic pressure gradient exceeding 4 mmHg is usually sufficient to elevate the mean right atrial pressure to levels that result in systemic venous congestion and, unless sodium intake has been restricted and diuretics administered, it is associated with ascites and edema. In patients with sinus rhythm, the right atrial *a* wave may be extremely tall and may even approach the level of the right ventricular systolic pressure. The resting cardiac output is usually depressed and fails to rise during exercise. The low cardiac output is responsible for the normal or only slightly elevated left atrial, pulmonary arterial, and right ventricular systolic pressures despite the presence of MS.

SYMPTOMS Since the development of MS generally precedes that of TS, many patients initially have symptoms of pulmonary congestion. Amelioration of the latter should raise the possibility that TS may be developing. Characteristically, patients complain of relatively little dyspnea for the degree of hepatomegaly, ascites, and edema that they present. Fatigue secondary to a low cardiac output and discomfort due to refractory edema, ascites, and marked hepatomegaly are common in patients with TS and/or regurgitation. In some patients, TS may be suspected for the first time when symptoms of right ventricular failure persist after an adequate mitral valvulotomy.

PHYSICAL FINDINGS Since TS usually occurs in the presence of other obvious valvular disease, the diagnosis may be missed unless it is specifically considered and searched for. Severe TS is associated with marked hepatic congestion, often resulting in cirrhosis, jaundice, serious malnutrition, anasarca, and ascites. Congestive hepatomegaly and, in cases of severe tricuspid valve disease, splenomegaly are present. The jugular veins are distended, and in patients with sinus rhythm there may be giant *a* waves. The *v* waves are less conspicuous, and since tricuspid obstruction impedes right atrial emptying during diastole, there is a slow *y* descent. In patients with sinus rhythm there may be prominent presystolic pulsations of the enlarged liver as well.

The right ventricle and the shock of pulmonic valve closure are usually not palpable. Indeed, a giant *a* wave in the jugular venous pulse without palpatory evidence of pulmonary hypertension or right ventricular enlargement should suggest the possibility of TS. On auscultation, the pulmonic closure sound is not accentuated, and occasionally, an OS of the tricuspid valve may be heard approximately 0.06 s after pulmonic valve closure. The diastolic murmur of TS has many of the qualities of the diastolic murmur of MS, and since TS almost always occurs in the presence of MS, the less common valvular lesion may be missed. However, the tricuspid murmur is generally heard best along the left lower sternal margin and over the xiphoid process and is most prominent during presystole in patients with sinus rhythm. The diastolic murmur is reduced in amplitude as the stethoscope is inched laterally, only to intensify or reappear as the mitral murmur at the apex. The murmur is augmented during inspiration, and it is reduced during expiration and particularly during the Valsalva maneuver, when tricuspid blood flow is reduced. This finding is often most easily elicited when the patient is in the erect position.

LABORATORY EXAMINATION The features of right atrial enlargement (Chap. 228) include tall, peaked P waves in lead II, as well as prominent, upright P waves in lead V_1. The *absence* of electrocardiographic evidence of right ventricular hypertrophy in a patient with right-sided heart failure who is believed to have MS should suggest associated tricuspid valve disease. The chest roentgenograms in patients with combined TS and MS show particular prominence of the right atrium and superior vena cava without much enlargement of the pulmonary artery and with less evidence of pulmonary vascular congestion than occurs in patients with isolated MS. On echocardiographic examination, the tricuspid valve is usually thickened; the transvalvular gradient can be estimated by Doppler echocardiography.

℞ **TREATMENT**

Patients with TS generally exhibit marked systemic venous congestion; intensive salt restriction and diuretic therapy are required during the preoperative period. Such a preparatory period may diminish hepatic congestion and thereby improve hepatic function sufficiently so that the risks of operation are diminished. Surgical treatment of the tricuspid valve is not ordinarily indicated at the time of mitral valve surgery in patients with *mild* TS. On the other hand, definitive surgical relief of the TS should be carried out, preferably at the time of mitral valvulotomy, in patients with moderate or severe TS who have mean diastolic pressure gradients exceeding approximately 5 mmHg and tricuspid orifices less than 1.5 to 2.0 cm². TS is almost always accompanied by significant TR. Open-heart operations utilizing cardiopulmonary bypass may permit substantial improvement of tricuspid valve function. If this cannot be accomplished, the tricuspid valve may have to be replaced with a prosthesis, preferably a tissue valve.

TRICUSPID REGURGITATION

Most commonly, TR is functional and secondary to marked dilatation of the right ventricle and the tricuspid annulus. Functional TR may complicate right ventricular enlargement of any cause, including inferior wall infarcts that involve the right ventricle, and it is commonly seen in the late stages of heart failure due to rheumatic or congenital heart disease with severe pulmonary hypertension, as well as in ischemic heart disease, cardiomyopathy, and cor pulmonale. It is in part reversible if pulmonary hypertension is relieved. Rheumatic fever may produce organic TR, often associated with TS. Infarction of right ventricular papillary muscles, tricuspid valve prolapse, carcinoid heart disease, endomyocardial fibrosis, infective endocarditis, and trauma all may produce TR. Less commonly, regurgitation results from congenitally deformed tricuspid valves, and it occurs with defects of the atrioventricular canal as well as with Ebstein's malformation of the tricuspid valve (Chap. 235).

As is the case for TS, the clinical features of TR result primarily from systemic venous congestion and reduction of cardiac output. With the onset of TR in patients with pulmonary hypertension, symptoms of pulmonary congestion diminish, but the clinical manifestations of right-sided heart failure become intensified. The neck veins are distended with prominent *v* waves, and marked hepatomegaly, ascites, pleural effusions, edema, systolic pulsations of the liver, and positive hepatojugular reflux are common. A prominent right ventricular pulsation along the left parasternal region and a blowing holosystolic murmur along the lower left sternal margin, which may be intensified during inspiration and reduced during expiration or the Valsalva maneuver, are characteristic findings; atrial fibrillation is usually present.

The electrocardiogram usually shows changes characteristic of the lesion responsible for the enlargement of the right ventricle that leads to TR. Roentgenographic examination usually reveals enlargement of both the right atrium and ventricle. Echocardiography may be helpful by demonstrating right ventricular dilatation and prolapsing or flail tricuspid leaflets; the diagnosis of TR can be made by color flow echocardiography, and the severity estimated by Doppler examination. The latter is also useful in estimating pulmonary artery pressure.

In patients with severe TR, the cardiac output is usually markedly reduced, and the right atrial pressure pulse may exhibit no *x* descent during early systole but a prominent *c-v* wave with a rapid *y* descent. The mean right atrial and the right ventricular end-diastolic pressures are often elevated.

℞ **TREATMENT**

Isolated TR, without pulmonary hypertension, such as that occurring as a consequence of infective endocarditis or trauma, is usually well tolerated and does not require operation. Indeed, even total excision of an infected tricuspid valve is often well tolerated if the pulmonary artery pressure is normal. Treatment of the underlying cause of heart failure usually reduces the severity of functional TR. In patients with mitral valve disease and TR due to pulmonary hypertension and massive right ventricular enlargement, effective surgical correction of the mitral valvular abnormality results in lowering of the pulmonary vascular pressures and gradual reduction or disappearance of the TR without direct treatment of the tricuspid valve. However, recovery may be much more rapid in patients with severe secondary TR if, at the time of mitral valve replacement, tricuspid annuloplasty (generally with the insertion of a plastic ring) or, in the rare instance of severe organic tricuspid valve disease, tricuspid valve replacement is performed. Surgical treatment of the TR also should be carried out in patients with severe regurgitation secondary to deformity of the tricuspid valve due to rheumatic fever, particularly those *without* severe pulmonary hypertension.

PULMONIC VALVE DISEASE

The pulmonic valve is affected by rheumatic fever far less frequently than are the other valves, and it is uncommonly the seat of infective endocarditis. The most common acquired abnormality affecting the pulmonic valve is regurgitation secondary to dilatation of the pulmonic valve ring as a consequence of severe pulmonary hypertension. This produces the Graham Steell murmur, a high-pitched, decrescendo, diastolic blowing murmur along the left sternal border, which is difficult to differentiate from the far more common murmur produced by AR. It is usually of little hemodynamic significance; indeed, surgical removal or destruction of the pulmonic valve by infective endocarditis does not produce heart failure unless serious pulmonary hypertension is also present. The *carcinoid syndrome* may cause pulmonic stenosis and/or regurgitation. → *Congenital pulmonic stenosis* is discussed in Chap. 235.

VALVE REPLACEMENT

The results of replacement of any valve are dependent primarily on (1) the patient's myocardial function at the time of operation, (2) the technical abilities of the operative team and the quality of the postoperative care, and (3) the durability, hemodynamic characteristics, and thrombogenicity of the prosthesis. Increased operative mortality is associated with the degree of preoperative functional disability and pulmonary hypertension. Late complications of replacement of any valve, which fortunately are declining in incidence, include paravalvular leakage, thromboemboli, bleeding due to anticoagulants, mechanical dysfunction of the prosthesis, and infective endocarditis.

The considerations regarding the choice between a bioprosthetic (tissue) and artificial mechanical valve are similar in the mitral and aortic positions and in the treatment of stenotic, regurgitant, or mixed lesions. All patients who have undergone replacement of any valve with a mechanical prosthesis must be maintained permanently on anticoagulants. The primary advantage of bioprostheses over mechanical prostheses is the reduction of thromboembolic complications, and except for patients with chronic atrial fibrillation, few such instances have been associated with their use. The major disadvantage of bioprosthetic valves is their mechanical deterioration. This results in the need to replace the prosthesis in 30 percent of patients by 10 years and 50 percent by 15 years. Bioprostheses are ordinarily not used in younger patients (<35 years) because of accelerated deterioration but are particularly useful in the elderly (>70 years), in whom there is more concern about chronic anticoagulation than about long-term (>15 years) valve durability. These valves are also indicated in women who expect to become pregnant, as well as others in whom anticoagulation may be contraindicated. Alternative bioprostheses are homograft (allograft) aortic valves obtained from cadavers and cryopreserved, as well as pulmonary autograft transplanted into the aortic position. In patients without the above contraindications, particularly those under 65 years, a mechanical prosthesis may be preferable. Many surgeons now select the St. Jude prosthesis, a double-disk tilting prosthesis, for replacement of both aortic and mitral valves because of somewhat more favorable hemodynamic characteristics and a suggestion of lower thrombogenicity.

BIBLIOGRAPHY

ANTUNES MJ, FRANCO CG: Advances in surgical treatment of acquired valve disease. Curr Opin Cardiol 11:139, 1996
BLOOMFIELD P et al: Twelve year comparison of a Bjork-Shiley mechanical heart valve with porcine bioprostheses. N Engl J Med 324:573, 1991
BRAUNWALD E: Valvular heart disease, in *Heart Disease*, 5th ed, E Braunwald (ed). Philadelphia, Saunders, 1997, pp 1007–1076
DAVID TE: Update on mitral valve repair. Ann Thorac Surg 59:1257, 1995
ENRIQUEZ-SARANO M et al: Valve repair improves the outcome of surgery for mitral regurgitation: Multivariate analysis. Circulation 91:1022, 1995
FELDMAN T: Rheumatic heart disease. Curr Opin Cardiol 11:126, 1996
GAASCH WH, EISENHAUER AC: The management of mitral valve disease. Curr Opin Cardiol 11:114, 1996
——— et al: Managing asymptomatic patients with chronic mitral regurgitation. Chest 108:842, 1995
GRAY RJ, HELFANT RH: Timing of surgery for valvular heart disease. Cardiovasc Clin 23:209, 1993
HESS OM et al: Diastolic dysfunction in aortic stenosis. Circulation 87(Suppl 5):IV73, 1993
KIRKLIN JW, BARRATT-BOYES BG: Part III. Acquired valvular heart disease, in *Cardiac Surgery*, 2d ed, JW Kirklin, BG Barratt-Boyes (eds). New York, Wiley, 1993, p 425
LINDROOS M et al: Factors associated with calcific aortic valve degeneration in the elderly. Eur Heart J 15:865, 1994
RAHIMTOOLA S (ed): *Valvular Heart Disease*, in E Braunwald (series ed), *Atlas of Heart Diseases*, vol 11. Philadelphia, Current Medicine, 1996
REED D et al: Prediction of outcome after mitral valve replacement in patients with symptomatic chronic mitral regurgitation. Circulation 84:23, 1991
REYES VP et al: Percutaneous balloon valvuloplasty compared with open surgical commissurotomy for mitral stenosis. N Engl J Med 331:961, 1994
SLATE J et al: Comparison of cardiac catheterization and Doppler echocardiography in the decision to operate in aortic and mitral valve disease. J Am Coll Cardiol 17:1026, 1991
ZUPPIROLI A et al: Natural history of mitral valve prolapse. Am J Cardiol 75:1028, 1995

238 *Eugene Braunwald*

COR PULMONALE*

DEFINITIONS *Cor pulmonale* is enlargement of the right ventricle secondary to diseases of the lung, thorax, or pulmonary circulation. It is sometimes accompanied by right ventricular failure, with an elevation of transmural right ventricular end-diastolic pressure. Approximately 20 percent of hospital admissions for heart failure are caused by right ventricular failure associated with cor pulmonale. More than half of the patients with chronic obstructive lung diseases (COLD) have cor pulmonale, and this condition constitutes between 5 and 10 percent of all adult heart diseases in the United States. Cor pulmonale constitutes a higher percentage of all forms of heart disease in countries where the incidence of obstructive lung disease is higher, such as the United Kingdom.

NORMAL FUNCTION OF THE PULMONARY CIRCULATION

The pulmonary circulation is interposed between the right and left ventricles for the purpose of gas exchange, the filtering out of particles, and the chemical modification of the blood, such as the conversion of angiotensin I to angiotensin II. Normally, flow through the pulmonary vascular bed depends not only on the pumping action of the right ventricle but also on respiratory movements and the contraction of the left ventricle. Respiratory motion facilitates pulmonary blood flow by aspirating blood into the thorax on inhalation; the blood is then propelled forward by the positive pressure of exhalation acting on a one-way valved system.

The stroke volume of the right ventricle, as of the left, is regulated by its preload, contractility, and afterload (Chap. 232). Since the right ventricle is a relatively thin, compliant reservoir, acute changes in venous return (e.g., an increase with inhalation and decline with exhalation) are accommodated with little change in transmural right ventricular pressure. However, the ability of the right ventricle to increase its systolic pressure is limited. Normally, the right ventricular afterload, which is closely related to the pulmonary artery pressure, is low. The pulmonary artery pressure normally rises slightly when blood is displaced into the chest at the start of exercise; on assuming recumbency; or with cold, anxiety, or pain. A driving pressure of only about 5 cmH$_2$O between the pulmonary artery (15 cmH$_2$O) and the left atrium (10 cmH$_2$O) normally propels the entire cardiac output of approximately 5 L/min at rest through the lungs, and only a modest increase in pressure is necessary to drive a flow of up to 25 L/min through the pulmonary capillary bed during maximal exercise.

The resistance of the pulmonary circulation (R), i.e., the pulmonary vascular resistance (p. 1252), is calculated as the intravascular driving pressure (DP), i.e., pulmonary artery pressure minus pulmonary venous or left atrial pressure, divided by the pulmonary blood flow rate ($\dot{Q}$). The caliber of a distensible vessel depends on its transmural pressure. R increases when vessels collapse, narrow, or lengthen, or when the viscosity of the blood increases.

$$R = Kl\mu/r^4$$

where K = constant; l = length; r = radius; and μ = viscosity. There is no single value of R that describes the pulmonary vascular bed because the relationship between driving pressure and flow is not linear; calculated R decreases with increasing pulmonary blood flow because pulmonary vessels are distended and collapsed vessels are recruited (Fig. 238-1).

PATHOPHYSIOLOGY The severity of right ventricular enlargement in cor pulmonale is a function of the increase in afterload. When the pulmonary vascular resistance is elevated and relatively

---

* This chapter was co-authored by the late Dr. John Butler in the 13th edition.

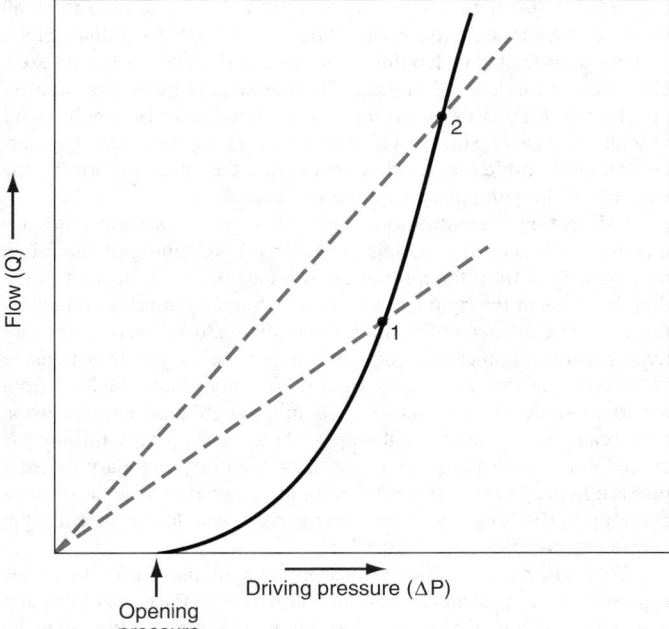

FIGURE 238-1 Relationship between flow and driving pressure ("vascular resistance") in the pulmonary circulation. Note that it does not pass through zero at the origin since an opening pressure must be overcome before flow starts. Thus the calculated vascular resistance (reciprocal of relationship of flow to pressure, dashed lines) falls (1 → 2) as flow increases. *(After R Graham et al, J Appl Physiol 54:1277, 1983, with permission.)*

fixed, as in pulmonary vascular or severe parenchymal lung disease, an elevation in cardiac output as occurs with physical exertion can elevate pulmonary artery pressure markedly. Right ventricular afterload can be augmented when lung volume is enlarged, as in COLD, due to the compression of the alveolar capillaries and the lengthening of the pulmonary vessels. Right ventricular afterload can also increase when lung volume is reduced following extensive pulmonary resection, as well as in restrictive lung diseases in which pulmonary vessels are compressed and distorted. Right ventricular afterload rises with hypoxic pulmonary vasoconstriction caused by hypoxia or acidosis, which are important causes of pulmonary hypertension. Hypoxic vasoconstriction in regions of the lung affected by disease distributes blood flow to normally ventilated regions. Hypoxic vasoconstriction results from alveolar, rather than intravascular, hypoxia and is made worse by hypercarbia, probably because of the associated acidosis. When the hematocrit becomes markedly elevated with chronic hypoxemia, the increase in blood viscosity can aggravate the pulmonary hypertension. Chronic hypoxic pulmonary vasoconstriction may cause pulmonary vascular disease with endothelial swelling and medial hypertrophy (see below).

The elevation of right ventricular afterload responsible for cor pulmonale is caused principally by pulmonary vascular or parenchymal disease. The principal syndromes and their pathophysiologic mechanisms are summarized in Table 238-1.

PULMONARY VASCULAR DISEASES

In these conditions the right ventricular afterload is elevated as a consequence of the restriction to pulmonary blood flow. In cor pulmonale secondary to pulmonary vascular disease, pulmonary hypertension is usually more severe than in pulmonary parenchymal disease. Chronic cor pulmonale secondary to pulmonary vascular disease may result from repeated pulmonary emboli, pulmonary vasculitis, pulmonary vasoconstriction secondary to high altitude, congenital heart disease with left-to-right shunting (e.g., atrial or ventricular septal defect, patent ductus arteriosus; Chap. 235), as well as pulmonary venoocclusive disease. When the cause of elevated pulmonary vascular resistance responsible for cor pulmonale is unknown, the condition is referred to as *primary pulmonary hypertension* (Chap. 260).

COR PULMONALE DUE TO PULMONARY EMBOLI This condition is associated with two distinct syndromes.

Acute Cor Pulmonale It has been estimated that in the United States about 50,000 people die each year from pulmonary emboli (Chap. 261). Probably half die within the first hour from acute right heart failure due to massive or multiple emboli. A large embolic burden causes a sudden, low-output state resulting from the right ventricle's inability to generate the high pressure necessary to drive blood through the acutely compromised pulmonary vascular bed. Depression of cardiac output can also occur with a moderate-sized embolism if the pulmonary circulation has been critically compromised by previous pulmonary vascular or parenchymal disease. The right ventricle begins to fail when systolic pressure is suddenly forced to double, i.e., to exceed approximately 40 to 45 mmHg. Acute right ventricular failure secondary to pulmonary embolism is suggested by the history of the sudden onset of severe dyspnea and cardiovascular collapse in a patient with, or predisposed to, venous thrombosis.

Clinical manifestations The low cardiac output causes pallor, sweating, hypotension, and a rapid pulse of small amplitude. The neck

Table 238-1

Cor Pulmonale

Mechanisms	Responses	Characteristics
PULMONARY VASCULAR DISEASES		
Emboli, large or multiple	Fall in cardiac output due to acute obstruction	Acute cor pulmonale Right ventricular distention Shock
Emboli, small; vasculitis; widespread lung damage (ARDS)	Pulmonary hypertension due to widespread hypoxia and microvascular obstruction	Subacute cor pulmonale Right ventricular distention Breathlessness and fever
Emboli, medium and recurrent; primary pulmonary hypertension; diet or drug vasopathy	Pulmonary hypertension due to vascular obstruction Low or normal cardiac output	Chronic cor pulmonale Right heart hypertrophy Breathlessness
RESPIRATORY DISEASES		
Obstructive Chronic bronchitis and emphysema; chronic asthma	Pulmonary hypertension due to hypoxia, vascular stretching and loss of vessels Heart beat impeded externally by lung hyperinflation Normal or high output	Chronic cor pulmonale "Blue bloater" or "Pink puffer" (see Chap. 258)
Restrictive 1. Intrinsic: interstitial fibrosis, lung resection	Hypertension due to hypoxia, vascular distortion and loss Normal or low output	Chronic cor pulmonale Breathlessness Hyperventilation
2. Extrinsic: obesity, myxedema, muscle weakness, kyphoscoliosis, upper airway obstruction, diminished respiratory drive, high altitude	Hypertension due to alveolar hypoxia Normal or high output	Chronic cor pulmonale Peripheral edema Hypoventilation

NOTE: ARDS, adult respiratory distress syndrome.

veins are distended and often exhibit the prominent *v* waves of tricuspid regurgitation. The liver may be pulsatile, distended, and tender. A systolic murmur of tricuspid regurgitation at the left sternal border may be accompanied by a presystolic (S_4) gallop sound. Arterial blood gas frequently shows hypoxemia due to ventilation/perfusion mismatching and a low Pa_{CO_2} due to hyperventilation.

℞ **TREATMENT**

If the cardiac output remains adequate to sustain the patient during the critical first 2 or 3 h, the natural lytic response usually results in fragmentation of the clot so that the patient survives. Although it has been shown that treatment with thrombolytic agents lyses clots more rapidly than does heparin (Chap. 261), this therapy is probably indicated only when blood flow is critically reduced and not improving. In acute cor pulmonale and in right ventricular failure due to acute right ventricular infarction, expansion of blood volume helps to maintain cardiac output. When hypoxic pulmonary vasoconstriction contributes to pulmonary hypertension, inhalation of 100% O_2 may help to reduce right ventricular afterload.

Chronic Cor Pulmonale Secondary to Pulmonary Vascular Disease In contrast to acute, massive thromboembolism, when the elevation in pulmonary vascular resistance and the development of right ventricular hypertrophy develop gradually, higher pulmonary vascular pressures, sometimes even approaching systemic arterial levels, may be generated. Chronic cor pulmonale can be caused by recurrent, medium-sized emboli that fail to lyse, but organize and recanalize. Particles from intravenous drug abuse, parasites, or tumor tissue that embolizes into the pulmonary vascular bed also may cause persistent pulmonary hypertension. Chronic cor pulmonale also can be caused by *primary pulmonary hypertension* (Chap. 260) or any chronic widespread vasculitis, such as occurs in association with the collagen vascular disorders and that affects the pulmonary vascular bed, particularly the CREST syndrome (Chap. 314).

Clinical Manifestations Breathlessness is a characteristic feature of pulmonary hypertension due to pulmonary vascular disease. It may be distressing during mild exertion or even at rest and is *not* relieved by sitting upright. An unproductive cough is another frequent complaint. Anterior chest pain, due to acute dilation of the root of the pulmonary artery or right ventricular ischemia, can occur. The elevation in systemic venous pressure can cause hepatomegaly and ankle edema.

Patients with pulmonary hypertension and consequent cor pulmonale often have tachypnea that is evident both on mild exertion and at rest and may even persist during sleep. Occasionally there is cyanosis due to arterial hypoxemia and low cardiac output. A right ventricular heave may be palpable along the left sternal border or in the epigastrium, and a high-pitched pulmonary ejection click may be audible to the left of the upper sternum. The second (pulmonary) component of the second heart sound is intensified and may be palpable; fixed splitting of the second heart sound may be present, and a right ventricular protodiastolic gallop (S_3), which increases during inspiration, may be present. A systolic murmur of tricuspid regurgitation, which is augmented by inspiration (p. 1323), is often audible; occasionally, a diastolic murmur of pulmonary regurgitation also is heard. Prominent *a* (and sometimes also *v*) waves in the jugular venous pulse are evident. The onset of right ventricular failure is reflected by an increase of venous pressure, the development of larger *v* waves associated with worse tricuspid regurgitation, a hepatojugular reflux, and a gallop rhythm with both third and fourth heart sounds. These physical findings of right ventricular failure can disappear rapidly when pulmonary artery pressure is suddenly reduced by relief of hypoxemia.

Hypocarbia due to alveolar hyperventilation is an important feature of chronic pulmonary hypertension secondary to pulmonary vascular disease. Usually there are no abnormalities on spirometry, but the ratio of dead space to tidal volume may be high, particularly when large-vessel obstruction is present. The diffusing capacity of the lung is reduced when a capillary vasculitis and/or loss of capillary blood volume is associated with pulmonary vascular disease. Typically, exercise causes a marked fall in Pa_{O_2}. The assessment of exercise capacity may be a useful way of following changes in the severity of pulmonary vascular disease in patients with chronic cor pulmonale, because exercise ability is limited by cardiac output and the latter, in turn, by the severity of the pulmonary vascular obstruction.

Laboratory Examination On *radiologic examination* the pulmonary trunk and hilar vessels are enlarged. Widening of the hilum may be judged from the ratio of the distance between the start of the first divisions of the right and left main pulmonary arteries divided by the transverse diameter of the thorax; a ratio >0.36 suggests pulmonary hypertension. Another radiologic indicator of pulmonary hypertension is widening of the descending right pulmonary artery shadow, from a normal value of <16 mm to >20 mm. Ventilation and perfusion lung scans and systemic venography showing deep vein thrombosis are helpful in confirming the diagnosis of embolic pulmonary vascular disease. In the presence of severe pulmonary hypertension, the electrocardiogram (ECG) shows P pulmonale, right axis deviation, and right ventricular hypertrophy (Chap. 228).

Echocardiography allows measurement of the thickness of the right ventricular wall and can show enlargement of the right ventricular cavity in relation to the left. The interventricular septum may be displaced leftward. Right ventricular systolic pressure can be estimated from measurement of the peak tricuspid regurgitant flow and pulmonic regurgitant flow with Doppler echocardiography.

Magnetic resonance imaging is useful for measuring right ventricular mass, wall thickness, cavity volume, and ejection fraction.

Failure of the right ventricular ejection fraction (measured by radionuclide ventriculography) to increase on exercise appears to be a good indicator of pulmonary hypertension and/or intrinsic right ventricular dysfunction. Myocardial perfusion scintigraphy with thallium 201 or sestamibi is also useful for diagnosing cor pulmonale, since the hypertrophied right ventricle is visualized by these radionuclides. (Normally the right ventricle is not imaged because of the much greater uptake by the left ventricle.)

Cardiac catheterization is necessary for the precise measurement of pulmonary vascular pressures, the determination of pulmonary vascular resistance, and its response to oxygen and vasodilators. Catheterization is sometimes indicated in patients with cor pulmonale to exclude congenital and left heart diseases, and it allows pulmonary angiography to be carried out to confirm the nature of the pulmonary vascular obstruction. Measurements of pulmonary vascular pressures and flow should also be made during exercise to look for abnormal pressure increments or poor responses of cardiac output.

Lung biopsy can be useful in demonstrating vasculitis in some types of pulmonary vascular disease such as the collagen vascular diseases, rheumatoid arthritis, and Wegener's granulomatosis.

PARENCHYMAL PULMONARY DISEASES

Cor pulmonale may be caused by both obstructive and restrictive lung diseases, more frequently the former. In these conditions there are usually only modest elevations of pulmonary artery pressure. The development of cor pulmonale confers a poor prognosis on patients with respiratory disease; in patients with cor pulmonale and right ventricular failure, the 3-year survival is approximately 40 percent. Respiratory diseases causing cor pulmonale are often associated with distortions of the lung that affect the position of the heart, so that cardiac physical signs are altered.

CHRONIC OBSTRUCTIVE LUNG DISEASE (See Chap. 258) This is the most common cause of chronic cor pulmonale. The enlargement of the right ventricle is attributed to the mild-to-moderate pulmonary hypertension that is common in severe obstructive bronchitis and emphysema. Pulmonary artery systolic pressure is typically in the range of 40 to 50 mmHg, far below the systemic levels that appear to be tolerated in patients with congenital heart disease and in those with primary pulmonary hypertension. Patients with cor pulmonale due to COLD usually have an advanced form of the disease with $FEV_1 < 1.0$ L (Chap. 250) and $Pa_{O_2} \leq 60$ mmHg. Right ventricular failure secondary to COLD often occurs when there is "acute-on-chronic" respiratory failure with intensification of hypoxemia.

Pulmonary hypertension in COLD is due to the pulmonary vasoconstriction caused by the alveolar hypoxia, acidemia, and hypercarbia; by the mechanical effects of the high lung volume on the pulmonary vessels; by the loss of small vessels in the vascular bed in regions of emphysema and lung destruction; and sometimes by the increased cardiac output and blood viscosity caused by polycythemia secondary to hypoxia. Of these causes hypoxia is undoubtedly the most important. Pulmonary artery pressure rises further on exercise and often falls acutely on inspiration of 100% O_2. Cardiac output tends to be high in the absence of heart failure if hypoxia and hypercarbia are present. Because of the importance of hypoxic pulmonary vasoconstriction in causing pulmonary hypertension, the hypoventilating "blue bloater" with alveolar hypoxia and hypercarbia more frequently suffers from pulmonary hypertension and consequent cor pulmonale than does the emphysematous "pink puffer" without alveolar hypoxia. Ischemic left ventricular dysfunction is a frequent accompaniment since patients with cor pulmonale secondary to COLD usually have a history of heavy cigarette smoking, a major risk factor for ischemic heart disease. The elevation of pulmonary artery pressure may be secondary, in part, to the increase in left atrial pressure resulting from left-heart dysfunction. Almost half of all patients who die with cor pulmonale due to COLD also have left ventricular hypertrophy on postmortem examination.

Right ventricular failure often complicates cor pulmonale when patients with COLD develop ventilatory failure with hypoxia and hypercarbia. When there is a worsening of the airflow due to increasing airway obstruction, the resulting hypoxia and hypercarbia may increase cardiac output by their vasodilator effect on the systemic arteriolar bed. Hypoxic pulmonary vasoconstriction is intensified, and both supraventricular and ventricular arrhythmias may occur. The liver becomes palpable and tender because it is engorged and displaced downward by the low diaphragm; a hepatojugular reflux may be present.

An exacerbation of airway obstruction elevates intrathoracic pressure, which impedes venous return, raises jugular venous pressure, and may cause peripheral edema, even in the absence of heart failure. This elevation of venous pressure secondary to airway obstruction is *not* necessarily associated with an increase in the transmural right ventricular pressure, the hallmark of right ventricular failure. The venous hypertension due to airflow obstruction declines, sometimes very rapidly, with relief of the obstruction.

Pathology In COLD right ventricular hypertrophy increases progressively. The main pulmonary arteries are enlarged, and the muscular pulmonary arteries show prominent longitudinal muscle, fibrosis, and elastic changes that continue into the arterioles, where the media becomes muscularized. The small vessels and capillaries are distorted or disappear in regions of lung hyperinflation.

Clinical Manifestations A history of a productive cough and dyspnea, perhaps with wheezing, is frequently elicited. Breathlessness limits the patient's ability in the minor stresses of daily living. Frequently there is a history of emergency hospital admissions because of respiratory infection, sometimes necessitating mechanical ventilation. In breathing oxygen, there may be increasing somnolence or other symptoms of hypercarbia such as recurring headaches, confusion, and even vomiting which, when combined with blurred optic discs (also due to cerebral vasodilation), constitutes the "pseudo tumor cerebri" syndrome. Hypoxia due to hypoventilation is usually worse at night, particularly when severe snoring leads to obstructive apnea (Chap. 264).

Physical findings Often there is nicotine staining of the fingers, a tell-tale sign reflecting many years of heavy cigarette smoking. The skin may be warm and the arterial pulse bounding in the high cardiac output state induced by hypoxia and hypercarbia. The distention of the chest due to the airflow obstruction and the rhonchi and wheezes secondary to chronic bronchitis usually make cardiac auscultation

difficult. A right-sided protodiastolic gallop sound (S_3) and a systolic murmur of tricuspid regurgitant may be audible. Signs of right-heart failure are, as discussed above, difficult to separate from those due to severe airflow obstruction. However, a sudden worsening of peripheral edema and rise of systemic venous pressure when atrial fibrillation occurs or when pulmonary infection supervenes are usually considered to be evidence of heart failure. This may be supported by the presence of a positive hepatojugular reflux. The distinction is important since patients can survive for years with the high systemic venous pressure and edema secondary to airflow obstruction but usually have a poor prognosis after right-heart failure develops.

Laboratory Examination *Pulmonary function studies* show marked airflow obstruction with hypoxemia and hypercarbia. Exercise is limited by ventilatory rather than cardiac dysfunction until right ventricular failure develops. The *chest roentgenogram* reveals hyperinflation, which makes the degree of right-heart enlargement difficult to assess. The central pulmonary arteries are large, but the vessels are narrowed and disappear at the periphery, particularly in regions of the lungs that are markedly emphysematous. The ECG is relatively insensitive in demonstrating right-heart enlargement because the enlarged lungs are poor electrical conductors and the inspiratory position of the chest is associated with a vertically positioned heart. Arrhythmias, particularly atrial fibrillation and multifocal atrial tachycardia, are common.

Echocardiographic imaging is often difficult because of the air in the distended lungs, but it usually reveals an increased cross section of the right ventricular cavity and abnormal thickening of the right ventricular wall. Myocardial perfusion scintigraphy shows an abnormally high ratio of right-to-left ventricular uptake.

Right heart catheterization can be carried out at the bedside with a balloon-tipped, flow-directed, multilumen catheter fitted with thermocouples for measuring cardiac output by thermodilution (Chap. 229). The pulmonary artery wedge pressure is usually normal in patients at rest who have uncomplicated cor pulmonale. Cardiac catheterization may be useful in assessing the severity of the pulmonary hypertension and its response to respiring oxygen as well as left ventricular function. Pressure measurements during exercise study may be helpful, particularly in assessing the contribution of left-heart dysfunction to the clinical state.

℞ TREATMENT

First, medical management of the acute and/or chronic lung disease must be optimal (Chaps. 258 and 265). Alveolar hypoxia should be corrected by improving alveolar ventilation through relieving the airflow obstruction and by judiciously increasing the inspired O_2 concentration. Long-term O_2 therapy is helpful in patients with severe COLD and reduces pulmonary artery pressure and pulmonary vascular resistance. When the lung disease improves and pulmonary vasoconstriction secondary to the alveolar hypoxia and hypercarbia are corrected, tachypnea and the signs attributed to right-heart failure are relieved. Bronchodilators and antibiotics lessen the airflow obstruction, and diuretics relieve the edema. Loop diuretics must be used with care since they may cause a metabolic alkalosis and thereby blunt the respiratory drive. Digitalis should be used in the presence of overt right ventricular failure, and slow phlebotomy should be considered when the hematocrit exceeds 55 to 60 percent.

RESTRICTIVE LUNG DISEASES Cor pulmonale in a variety of restrictive disorders affecting the lung (Chap. 259) is often associated with obliteration of the pulmonary vascular bed by lung destruction and fibrosis. Treatment of the underlying disorder and management of right ventricular failure, as described above, are indicated.

DISORDERS OF VENTILATION A variety of disorders of the neuromuscular apparatus, diaphragm, and chest wall cause pulmonary hypertension and cor pulmonale secondary to chronic hypoxia and/or compression of pulmonary vessels. Disorders of ventilatory control, including the sleep apnea syndrome, and upper airways obstruction may be responsible for chronic hypoxia and secondary pulmonary hypertension, cor pulmonale, and, when the latter are severe, eventual right ventricular failure. Management of these patients consists of treating the underlying disorder, as discussed in Chaps. 263 and 264, the inhalation of oxygen, and the management of right ventricular failure with diuretics and digoxin.

BIBLIOGRAPHY

BRADLEY TD, PHILLIPSON EA: Central sleep apnea. Clin Chest Med 13:493, 1992

FERGUSON GT, CHERNIACK RM: Management of chronic obstructive pulmonary disease. N Engl J Med 328:1017, 1993

JAIN D, ZARET BJ: Assessment of right ventricular function. Role of nuclear imaging techniques. Cardiol Clin 10:23, 1992

KLINGER JR, HILL NS: Right ventricular dysfunction in chronic obstructive pulmonary disease: Evaluation and management. Chest 99:715, 1991

LOH E: Cor pulmonale, in *Cardiopulmonary Diseases and Cardiac Tumors*, S Goldhaber (ed), in *Atlas of Heart Diseases*, vol 3, E Braunwald (series ed). Philadelphia, Current Medicine, 1995, pp 1.1–1.24

MACNEE W: Pathophysiology of cor pulmonale in chronic obstructive pulmonary disease. Am J Respir Crit Care Med 150:833, 1994

PATTYNAMA PMT et al: Early diagnosis of cor pulmonale with MR imaging of the right ventricle. Radiology 182:375, 1992

SALVATERRA CG, RUBIN LJ: Investigation and management of pulmonary hypertension in chronic obstructive pulmonary disease. Am Rev Respir Dis 148:1414, 1993

WEITZENBLUM E et al: Benefit from long-term O₂ therapy in chronic obstructive pulmonary disease patients. Respiration 59(Suppl I):14, 1992

——— et al: Pulmonary hemodynamics in patients with chronic obstructive pulmonary disease before and during an episode of peripheral edema. Chest 105:1377, 1994

WIEDEMANN HP, MATTHAY RA: Cor pulmonale, in *Heart Disease*, 5th ed, E Braunwald (ed). Philadelphia, Saunders, 1997, pp 1604–1625

| 239 | *Joshua Wynne, Eugene Braunwald* |

THE CARDIOMYOPATHIES AND MYOCARDITIDES

The cardiomyopathies are diseases that involve the myocardium primarily and are not the result of hypertension or congenital, valvular, coronary, arterial, or pericardial abnormalities.* When the cardiomyopathies are classified on an etiologic basis, two fundamental forms are recognized: (1) a primary type, consisting of heart muscle disease of unknown cause, and (2) a secondary type, consisting of myocardial disease of known cause or associated with a disease involving other organ systems (Table 239-1). (In the World Health Organization classification, *specific cardiomyopathy* is used to describe heart muscle diseases associated with certain systemic or cardiac disorders; examples include hypertensive and metabolic cardiomyopathy. In many

cases it is not possible to arrive at a specific etiologic diagnosis, and thus it is often more desirable to classify the cardiomyopathies on the basis of differences in their pathophysiology and clinical presentation (Tables 239-2 and 239-3).

DILATED CARDIOMYOPATHY

Left and/or right ventricular systolic pump function is impaired, leading to cardiac enlargement and often producing symptoms of congestive heart failure. Mural thrombi are often present, particularly in the left ventricular apex. Histologic examination reveals extensive areas of interstitial and perivascular fibrosis. Myocyte necrosis and cellular infiltration may be present but are not prominent. [The prevalence of this condition appears to be increasing.] Although no cause is apparent in many cases, dilated cardiomyopathy probably is the end result of myocardial damage produced by a variety of toxic, metabolic, or infectious agents. Dilated cardiomyopathy may be the late sequel of acute viral myocarditis, possibly mediated through an immunologic mechanism. Although most commonly a disease of middle-aged men and more common in African-Americans, it may occur in any patient population. A reversible form of dilated cardiomyopathy may be found with alcohol abuse, pregnancy, selenium deficiency, hypophosphatemia, hypocalcemia, thyroid disease, cocaine use, and chronic uncontrolled tachycardia. Approximately 20 percent of patients have familial forms of the disease. The disease is genetically heterogeneous; autosomal dominant, autosomal recessive, and X-linked transmission have been documented. *Right ventricular dysplasia* is a unique cardiomyopathy marked by progressive replacement of the right ventricular wall with adipose tissue. Often associated with ventricular arrhythmias, the clinical course is variable but sudden death is a constant threat.

CLINICAL MANIFESTATIONS   Symptoms of left- and right-sided congestive failure, manifested by dyspnea on exertion, fatigue, orthopnea, paroxysmal nocturnal dyspnea, peripheral edema, and palpitations, develop gradually in most patients. Some patients have left ventricular dilatation for months or even years before becoming symp-

* Diffuse myocardial fibrosis secondary to multiple myocardial scars produced by extensive coronary arterial narrowing and occlusion can impair left ventricular function and is frequently referred to as *ischemic cardiomyopathy*. This is a colloquial use of the term, however, and should be avoided; the term *cardiomyopathy* should be restricted to a condition *primarily* involving heart muscle. In so-called ischemic cardiomyopathy the *primary* involvement is of the coronary vessels.

Table 239-1

Etiologic Classification of Cardiomyopathies

PRIMARY MYOCARDIAL INVOLVEMENT

Idiopathic (D,R,H)
Familial (D,H)
Eosinophilic endomyocardial disease (R)
Endomyocardial fibrosis (R)

SECONDARY MYOCARDIAL INVOLVEMENT

Infective (D)	Connective tissue disorders (D)
Viral myocarditis	Systemic lupus erythematosus
Bacterial myocarditis	Polyarteritis nodosa
Fungal myocarditis	Rheumatoid arthritis
Protozoal myocarditis	Progressive systemic sclerosis
Metazoal myocarditis	Dermatomyositis
Spirochetal	Infiltrations and granulomas (R,D)
Rickettsial	Amyloidosis
Metabolic (D)	Sarcoidosis
Familial storage disease (D,R)	Malignancy
Glycogen storage disease	Neuromuscular (D)
Mucopolysaccharidoses	Muscular dystrophy
Hemochromatosis	Myotonic dystrophy
Fabry's disease	Friedreich's ataxia (H,D)
Deficiency (D)	Sensitivity and toxic reactions (D)
Electrolytes	Alcohol
Nutritional	Radiation
	Drugs
	Peripartum heart disease (D)

NOTE: The principal clinical manifestation(s) of each etiologic grouping is denoted by D (dilated), R (restrictive), or H (hypertrophic) cardiomyopathy.

SOURCE: Adapted from the WHO/ISFC task force report on the definition and classification of cardiomyopathies, 1980.

Table 239-2

CHAPTER 239
The Cardiomyopathies and Myocarditides **1329**

Clinical Classification of Cardiomyopathies

1. Dilated: Left and/or right ventricular enlargement, impaired systolic function, congestive heart failure, arrhythmias, emboli
2. Restrictive: Endomyocardial scarring or myocardial infiltration resulting in restriction to left and/or right ventricular filling
3. Hypertrophic: Disproportionate left ventricular hypertrophy, typically involving septum more than free wall, with or without an intraventricular systolic pressure gradient; usually of a nondilated left ventricular cavity

tomatic. Others develop symptoms after recovery from a viral infection. Although vague chest pain may be present, typical angina pectoris is unusual and suggests the presence of concomitant ischemic heart disease.

PHYSICAL EXAMINATION Variable degrees of cardiac enlargement and findings of congestive heart failure are noted. In patients with advanced disease, the pulse pressure is narrow and the jugular venous pressure is elevated. Third and fourth heart sounds are common, and mitral or tricuspid regurgitation may occur. Diastolic murmurs, valvular calcification, and severe hypertension reduce the likelihood of cardiomyopathy.

LABORATORY EXAMINATIONS The chest roentgenogram demonstrates enlargement of the cardiac silhouette due to left ventricular enlargement, although generalized cardiomegaly often is seen. The lung fields may demonstrate evidence of pulmonary venous hypertension and interstitial or alveolar edema. The electrocardiogram often shows sinus tachycardia or atrial fibrillation, ventricular arrhythmias, left atrial enlargement, diffuse nonspecific ST-T wave abnormalities, and sometimes intraventricular conduction defects. Echocardiography and radionuclide ventriculography show left ventricular dilatation, with normal or minimally thickened or thinned walls, and systolic dysfunction (reduced ejection fraction).

Cardiac catheterization usually is performed only to exclude ischemic heart disease. The left ventricular end-diastolic, left atrial, and pulmonary capillary wedge pressures usually are elevated; when failure of the right side of the heart supervenes, the right ventricular end-diastolic, right atrial, and central venous pressures also rise. Angiography reveals a dilated, diffusely hypokinetic left ventricle, often with some degree of mitral regurgitation; the coronary arteries are normal, thereby excluding so-called ischemic cardiomyopathy. Transvenous endomyocardial biopsy (Chap. 229) usually is not necessary, but may be helpful in excluding certain conditions such as myocardial infiltration by amyloid.

℞ TREATMENT

Most patients pursue an inexorably downhill course, and the majority, particularly those over 55 years of age, die within 5 years of the onset of symptoms. Spontaneous improvement or stabilization occurs in about a quarter of patients. Death is due to either congestive heart failure or ventricular tachy- or bradyarrhythmia; sudden death is a constant threat. Systemic embolization is common, and although the issue is controversial, all patients without contraindications should be considered for chronic anticoagulation. Strenuous exertion should be interdicted. Standard therapy of heart failure with salt restriction, diuretics, digitalis, and vasodilators may produce symptomatic improvement. Mortality

is reduced by angiotensin-converting enzyme inhibitors and the combination of hydralazine and isosorbide dinitrate. Some patients with dilated cardiomyopathy who have biopsy evidence of myocardial inflammation have been treated with immunosuppressive therapy, but long-term evidence of efficacy is lacking. Others have been treated cautiously with gradually increasing doses of beta-adrenergic blockers with apparent clinical benefit. Antiarrhythmic agents are best avoided for fear of proarrhythmic and other side effects, unless they are needed to treat symptomatic or serious arrhythmias. Implantation of an automatic internal defibrillator is useful in patients with malignant arrhythmias. In patients with advanced disease who are refractory to medical therapy, cardiac transplantation should be considered (Chap. 234).

ALCOHOLIC CARDIOMYOPATHY Individuals who consume large quantities of alcohol over many years may develop a clinical picture identical to idiopathic dilated cardiomyopathy; indeed, alcoholic cardiomyopathy is the major form of secondary dilated cardiomyopathy in the western world. Ceasing alcohol consumption before severe heart failure has developed may halt the progression or even reverse the course of this disease, unlike the idiopathic variety, which is marked by progressive deterioration. Alcoholic patients with advanced heart failure have a poor prognosis, particularly if they continue to drink; fewer than one-quarter survive 3 years. The key to the treatment of alcoholic cardiomyopathy is total and permanent abstinence. The toxic effect of alcohol on striated muscle often extends beyond the heart to cause myopathy in skeletal muscles. A second presentation of alcoholic cardiotoxicity may be found in individuals without overt heart failure and consists of recurrent supraventricular or ventricular tachyarrhythmias. Termed the *holiday heart syndrome*, it typically appears after a drinking binge; atrial fibrillation is seen most frequently, followed by atrial flutter and ventricular premature depolarizations. Other patients develop left ventricular hypertrophy, perhaps related to concomitant systemic hypertension; they may present with symptoms of pulmonary congestion due to abnormal diastolic stiffness (diminished compliance) of the left ventricle.

Table 239-3

Laboratory Evaluation of the Cardiomyopathies

	Dilated	Restrictive	Hypertrophic
Chest roentgenogram	Moderate to marked cardiac enlargement Pulmonary venous hypertension	Mild cardiac enlargement	Mild to moderate cardiac enlargement
Electrocardiogram	ST-segment and T-wave abnormalities	Low voltage, conduction defects	ST-segment and T-wave abnormalities Left ventricular hypertrophy Abnormal Q waves
Echocardiogram	Left ventricular dilatation and dysfunction	Increased left ventricular wall thickness Normal or mildly reduced systolic function	Asymmetric septal hypertrophy (ASH) Systolic anterior motion (SAM) of the mitral valve
Radionuclide studies	Left ventricular dilatation and dysfunction (RVG)	Normal or mildly reduced systolic function (RVG)	Vigorous systolic function (RVG) Perfusion defect (^{201}Tl)
Cardiac catheterization	Left ventricular dilatation and dysfunction Elevated left- and often right-sided filling pressures Diminished cardiac output	Normal or mildly reduced systolic function Elevated left- and right-sided filling pressures	Vigorous systolic function Dynamic left ventricular outflow obstruction Elevated left- and right-sided filling pressures

NOTE: RVG, radionuclide ventriculogram; ^{201}Tl, thallium 201.

PERIPARTUM CARDIOMYOPATHY Cardiac dilatation and congestive heart failure of unexplained cause may develop during the last trimester of pregnancy or within 6 months after delivery; most women develop symptoms in the month before or immediately after delivery. The cause of this disorder is unknown, but in some patients endomyocardial biopsy has shown evidence of a myocarditis. Necropsy shows cardiac enlargement, often with mural thrombi, along with histologic evidence of myocardial degeneration and fibrosis. The patient who develops peripartum cardiomyopathy typically is multiparous, African American, and over the age of 30, although the disease may be found in a wide spectrum of patients. The symptoms, signs, and treatment are similar to those in patients with idiopathic dilated cardiomyopathy. The mortality rate is quite variable but may be as high as 25 to 50 percent. The prognosis in these patients appears to be closely related to whether the heart size returns to normal after the first episode of congestive heart failure. If it does, subsequent pregnancies may sometimes be well tolerated; if the heart remains enlarged, however, further pregnancies frequently produce increasing myocardial damage, ultimately leading to refractory congestive heart failure and death. Those who recover should be encouraged to avoid further pregnancies, particularly if cardiomegaly persists.

NEUROMUSCULAR DISEASE (See also Chap. 383) Cardiac involvement is common in many of the muscular dystrophies. In *Duchenne's progressive muscular dystrophy*, myocardial involvement is most frequently indicated by a distinctive and unique electrocardiographic pattern consisting of tall R waves in right precordial leads with an R/S ratio greater than 1.0, often associated with deep Q waves in the limb and lateral precordial leads. These electrocardiographic abnormalities appear to result from selective transmural necrosis of the posterobasal left ventricle and associated papillary muscle. A variety of supraventricular and ventricular arrhythmias are frequently found. Rapidly progressive congestive heart failure may develop despite extended periods of apparent circulatory stability during which the only detectable abnormalities are in the electrocardiogram. *Myotonic dystrophy* is characterized by a variety of electrocardiographic abnormalities, especially disorders of impulse formation and particularly conduction, but other overt clinical evidence of heart disease is uncommon. Because of the abnormalities of impulse generation and conduction, syncope and sudden death are major hazards; in appropriate patients, insertion of a permanent pacemaker may be effective. In *limb-girdle dystrophy* and *fascioscapulohumeral dystrophy*, cardiac involvement is uncommon and seldom severe. Involvement of the heart is very common in *Friedreich's ataxia* (manifested by abnormal electrocardiographic or echocardiographic findings), with as many as half the patients developing cardiac symptoms. The electrocardiogram most commonly demonstrates ST-segment and T-wave abnormalities. The echocardiogram may demonstrate left ventricular hypertrophy, with either symmetric or asymmetric hypertrophy of the left ventricular septum compared with the free wall. Although morphologically similar to some cases of hypertrophic cardiomyopathy, cellular disarray is lacking.

DRUGS A variety of pharmacologic agents may damage the myocardium acutely, producing a pattern of inflammation (myocarditis), or they may lead to chronic damage of the type seen with idiopathic dilated cardiomyopathy. Certain drugs produce only electrocardiographic abnormalities, while others may precipitate fulminant congestive heart failure and death. The anthracycline derivatives, particularly *doxorubicin* (Adriamycin), are powerful antineoplastic agents that, when given in high doses (more than 550 mg/m^2 for doxorubicin), may produce fatal heart failure. The incidence of heart failure is related not only to the dose of the drug but also to the presence or absence of several risk factors (cardiac irradiation, age greater than 70 years, underlying heart disease, hypertension, treatment with cyclophosphamide); at any dose patients with these risk factors have an eight- to tenfold greater frequency of developing heart failure than do patients lacking them. Radionuclide ventriculography and endocardial biopsy may document preclinical deterioration of left ventricular function and allow appropriate dose adjustments; by so monitoring left ventricular function, it is often possible to continue doxorubicin even in patients at high risk for developing heart failure. Recent efforts to modify the dose schedule by giving the drug more slowly have further reduced the risk of cardiotoxicity.

Some patients with congestive heart failure, even those with severe depression of left ventricular function, have demonstrated recovery of cardiac function with aggressive management with digitalis, diuretics, and vasodilators. In others, late asymptomatic contractile dysfunction is common, even in those without initial cardiotoxicity. Children may demonstrate reduced myocardial hypertrophy and mass over time, presumably due to doxorubicin's inhibition of myocardial cell growth. High-dose *cyclophosphamide* may produce congestive heart failure acutely or within 2 weeks of administration; a characteristic histopathologic feature is myocardial edema and hemorrhagic necrosis. Rarely, patients treated with *5-fluorouracil* will develop chest pain and electrocardiographic changes of myocardial ischemia or infarction. Electrocardiographic changes and arrhythmias may result from treatment with tricyclic antidepressants, the phenothiazines, emetine, lithium, and various aerosol propellants. *Cocaine abuse* is associated with a variety of life-threatening cardiac complications, including sudden death, myocarditis, dilated cardiomyopathy, and acute myocardial infarction (resulting from coronary spasm and/or thrombosis with or without underlying coronary artery stenosis). Nitrates and calcium antagonists have been used as well to treat a variety of cocaine-induced cardiotoxicities; beta-adrenergic blockers should be avoided.

HYPERTROPHIC CARDIOMYOPATHY

This disease is characterized by left ventricular hypertrophy, typically of a nondilated chamber, without obvious cause such as hypertension or aortic stenosis. Two features of the disease have attracted the greatest attention: (1) heterogeneous left ventricular (LV) hypertrophy, often with preferential hypertrophy of the interventricular septum resulting in asymmetric septal hypertrophy (ASH); and (2) a dynamic left ventricular outflow tract pressure gradient, related to a narrowing of the subaortic area as a consequence of the midsystolic apposition of the anterior mitral valve leaflet against the hypertrophied septum, i.e., systolic anterior motion (SAM) of the mitral valve. Initial studies of this disease emphasized the dynamic "obstructive" features, and it has been termed *idiopathic hypertrophic subaortic stenosis* (IHSS), *hypertrophic obstructive cardiomyopathy* (HOCM), and *muscular subaortic stenosis*. It has become clear, however, that only about one-quarter of patients with hypertrophic cardiomyopathy demonstrate an outflow tract gradient. The ubiquitous pathophysiologic abnormality is not systolic but rather *diastolic* dysfunction (Chap. 232), characterized by increased stiffness of the hypertrophied muscle that results primarily from an abnormality in calcium handling with attendant intracellular calcium overload. This results in elevated diastolic filling pressures and is present despite a hyperdynamic left ventricle.

The pattern of hypertrophy is distinctive in hypertrophic cardiomyopathy and differs from that seen in secondary hypertrophy (as in hypertension). Most patients have striking regional variations in the extent of hypertrophy in different portions of the left ventricle, and the majority demonstrate a ventricular septum whose thickness is disproportionately increased when compared with the free wall. Other patients may demonstrate disproportionate involvement of the apex or left ventricular free wall; 10 percent or more of patients have concentric involvement of the ventricle. All, however, show a bizarre and disorganized arrangement of cardiac muscle cells in the septum, with disorganization of the myofibrillar architecture, whether or not a systolic intraventricular pressure gradient is present, along with a variable degree of myocardial fibrosis and thickening of the small intramural coronary arteries.

About half of all cases of hypertrophic cardiomyopathy have a positive family history compatible with autosomal-dominant transmission. About 40 percent of these are associated with mutations of the beta cardiac myosin heavy chain gene on chromosome 14, with certain mutations associated with more malignant prognoses. About 15 percent have a mutation of the cardiac troponin T gene, 10 percent a mutation of myosin binding protein L, and about 5 percent a mutation of the α tropomyosin gene. The remainder of familial cases presumably are due to mutations of other genes. Echocardiographic studies have confirmed that about one-third of the first-degree relatives (i.e., parents, siblings, and children) of patients with familial hypertrophic cardiomyopathy have evidence of the disease, although in many of these patients the extent of hypertrophy is mild, no outflow tract pressure gradient is present, and symptoms are not prominent. Since the hypertrophic characteristics may not be apparent in childhood and often appear first in adolescence, a single normal echocardiogram in a child does not entirely exclude the presence of the disease.

In contrast to the obstruction produced by a fixed narrowed orifice, such as valvular aortic stenosis, the pressure gradient in hypertrophic cardiomyopathy, when present, is dynamic and may change between examinations and even from beat to beat. Obstruction appears to result from further narrowing of an already small left ventricular outflow tract by SAM of the mitral valve against the hypertrophied septum. While SAM may be found in a variety of other conditions besides hypertrophic cardiomyopathy, it is *always* found when obstruction is present in hypertrophic cardiomyopathy. Three basic mechanisms are involved in the production of the dynamic pressure gradient: (1) increased left ventricular contractility, (2) decreased ventricular volume (preload), and (3) decreased aortic impedance and pressure (afterload). Interventions that increase myocardial contractility, such as exercise, isoproterenol, and digitalis glycosides, and those that reduce ventricular volume, such as the Valsalva maneuver, sudden standing, nitroglycerin, amyl nitrite, or tachycardia, all may cause an increase in the gradient and the murmur. Conversely, elevation of arterial pressure by phenylephrine, squatting, sustained handgrip, augmentation of venous return by passive leg raising, and expansion of the blood volume all increase ventricular volume and ameliorate the gradient and murmur.

CLINICAL FEATURES Many patients with hypertrophic cardiomyopathy are asymptomatic and may be relatives of patients with known disease. Unfortunately, the first clinical manifestation of the disease may be sudden death, frequently occurring in children and young adults, often during or after physical exertion. In symptomatic patients, the most common complaint is dyspnea, largely due to increased stiffness of the left ventricular walls, which impairs ventricular filling and leads to elevated left ventricular diastolic and left atrial pressures. Other symptoms include angina pectoris, fatigue, syncope, and near-syncope ("graying-out spells"). Symptoms are not related to the presence or severity of an outflow gradient. Most patients with gradients demonstrate a double or triple apical precordial impulse, a rapidly rising carotid arterial pulse, and a fourth heart sound. The hallmark of obstructive hypertrophic cardiomyopathy is a systolic murmur, which is typically harsh, diamond-shaped, and usually begins well after the first heart sound, since ejection is unimpeded early in systole. The murmur is best heard at the lower left sternal border as well as at the apex, where it is often more holosystolic and blowing in quality, no doubt due to the mitral regurgitation that usually accompanies obstructive hypertrophic cardiomyopathy.

LABORATORY EVALUATION The *electrocardiogram* commonly shows left ventricular hypertrophy and widespread, deep, broad Q waves that suggest an old myocardial infarction. Many patients demonstrate arrhythmias, both atrial (supraventricular tachycardia or atrial fibrillation) and ventricular (ventricular tachycardia), during ambulatory (Holter) monitoring. *Chest roentgenography* may be normal, although a mild to moderate increase in the cardiac silhouette is common. The mainstay of the diagnosis of hypertrophic cardiomyopathy is the *echocardiogram*, which demonstrates left ventricular hypertrophy, often with the septum 1.3 or more times the thickness of the high posterior left ventricular free wall. The septum may demonstrate an unusual ground glass appearance, probably related to its abnormal cellular architecture and myocardial fibrosis. SAM of the mitral valve is found in patients with pressure gradients. The left ventricular cavity typically is small in hypertrophic cardiomyopathy, with vigorous pos-

terior wall motion but reduced septal excursion. A rare form of hypertrophic cardiomyopathy, characterized by apical hypertrophy, is often associated with giant negative T waves on the electrocardiogram and a "spade-shaped" left ventricular cavity on angiography; it usually has a benign clinical course. *Radionuclide scintigraphy* with thallium 201 frequently reveals evidence of myocardial perfusion defects even in asymptomatic patients.

Although cardiac catheterization is not required to diagnose hypertrophic cardiomyopathy, the two typical *hemodynamic* features are an elevated left ventricular diastolic pressure due to diminished left ventricular compliance and, when obstruction is present, a systolic pressure gradient between the body of the left ventricle and the subaortic region. When a gradient is not present, it often can be induced by provocative maneuvers such as infusion of isoproterenol, inhalation of amyl nitrite, or the Valsalva maneuver.

℞ **TREATMENT**

Competitive sports and probably strenuous activity should be proscribed. Beta-adrenergic blockers often are used and may ameliorate angina pectoris and syncope in one-third to one-half of patients to some degree. Resting intraventricular pressure gradients usually are unchanged, although these drugs may limit the increase in the gradient that occurs during exercise. It is not known whether beta-adrenergic blockers offer any protection against sudden death. It is not established whether any antiarrhythmic agent, for that matter, is effective in this setting. However, amiodarone appears to be effective in reducing the frequency of supraventricular as well as life-threatening ventricular arrhythmias. Verapamil and diltiazem may reduce the stiffness of the ventricle, reduce the elevated diastolic pressures, increase exercise tolerance, and, in some instances, reduce the severity of outflow tract gradients, although adverse side effects occur in about one-quarter of patients. Disopyramide has been used in some patients to reduce left ventricular contractility and the outflow gradient. Dual-chamber permanent pacing recently has gained favor because it improves symptoms and reduces the outflow gradient in some patients with severe symptoms, presumably by altering the pattern of ventricular contraction. Infarction of the interventricular septum induced by ethanol injections into the septal artery has also been reported to reduce obstruction. The insertion of an implantable automatic defibrillator should be considered in patients surviving cardiac arrest and those with high-risk ventricular tachyarrhythmias. A surgical myotomy/myectomy of the hypertrophied septum may result in lasting symptomatic improvement in about three-quarters of operated patients, but the mortality of 3 to 5 percent limits the operation to severely symptomatic patients with large pressure gradients who are unresponsive to medical management. The effect of any of these therapies on the natural history is not clear. Digitalis, diuretics, nitrates, and beta-adrenergic agonists are best avoided if possible, particularly in patients with known left ventricular outflow tract pressure gradients.

PROGNOSIS The natural history of hypertrophic cardiomyopathy is variable, although many patients demonstrate an improvement or stabilization of symptoms with time. Atrial fibrillation is common late in the course of the disease; its onset may lead to an increase in symptoms, presumably due to loss of the atrial contribution to filling of the thickened ventricle. Infective endocarditis occurs in fewer than 10 percent of patients, and endocarditis prophylaxis is indicated, particularly in patients with resting obstruction and mitral regurgitation. Progression of hypertrophic cardiomyopathy to left ventricular dilatation and dysfunction without an outflow gradient has been reported but is unusual; in about 5 to 10 percent of patients, however, some degree of left ventricular systolic impairment, wall thinning, and chamber enlargement occurs over time. The major cause of mortality in hypertrophic cardiomyopathy is sudden death, which may occur in asymptomatic patients or interrupt an otherwise stable course in symptomatic ones. Predictors of sudden death include age less than 30 years, ventricular tachycardia on ambulatory monitoring, marked ventricular hypertrophy, syncope (especially in children), genetic mutations associated with an increased risk, and a family history of sudden death. There is no correlation between the risk of sudden death and the severity of symptoms or the presence or severity of an outflow tract pressure gradient. Since sudden death often occurs during or just after physical exertion, strenuous exercise should be avoided in all patients, regardless of symptoms. It is likely that most deaths, particularly those that are sudden, are due to ventricular arrhythmias.

RESTRICTIVE CARDIOMYOPATHY

The hallmark of the restrictive cardiomyopathies is abnormal diastolic function (Chap. 232); the ventricular walls are excessively rigid and impede ventricular filling. Myocardial fibrosis, hypertrophy, or infiltration due to a variety of causes is usually responsible. The infiltrative diseases, which represent important causes for secondary restrictive cardiomyopathy, also may show some impairment of systolic function. Myocardial involvement with *amyloid* is a common cause of secondary restrictive cardiomyopathy, although restriction is also seen in hemochromatosis, glycogen deposition, endomyocardial fibrosis, sarcoidosis, Fabry's disease, the eosinophilias, neoplastic infiltration, and myocardial fibrosis of diverse causes. In many of these conditions, particularly those with substantial concomitant endocardial involvement, partial obliteration of the ventricular cavity by fibrous tissue and thrombus contributes to the abnormally increased resistance to ventricular filling.

The inability of the ventricle to fill limits cardiac output and raises filling pressure. Therefore, exercise intolerance and dyspnea are usually the most prominent symptoms. As a result of persistently elevated venous pressure, these patients commonly have dependent edema, ascites, and an enlarged, tender liver. The jugular venous pressure is elevated and does not fall normally, or it may rise with inspiration (Kussmaul's sign). The heart sounds may be distant, and third and fourth heart sounds are common. In contrast to constrictive pericarditis, which the restrictive cardiomyopathies resemble in many respects, the apex impulse is usually easily palpable, and mitral regurgitation is more common. The electrocardiogram shows low-voltage, nonspecific ST-T-wave changes and various arrhythmias. Pericardial calcification on x-ray, which would suggest constrictive pericarditis, is absent. Echocardiography typically reveals symmetrically thickened left ventricular walls and normal or slightly reduced ventricular volumes and systolic function. Doppler recordings demonstrate accentuated early diastolic filling. Cardiac catheterization shows a decreased cardiac output, elevation of the right and left ventricular end-diastolic pressures and a dip-and-plateau configuration of the diastolic portion of the ventricular pressure pulse resembling that seen in constrictive pericarditis. As in the latter condition, the x and y descents of the atrial pressure pulse are prominent, resulting in a "W"-shaped pattern.

Differentiation from constrictive pericarditis may be difficult (Chaps. 229 and 240). This distinction is of importance because the latter condition is potentially curable by operation. Helpful in the differentiation of these two diseases are right ventricular transvenous endomyocardial biopsy (by revealing myocardial infiltration or fibrosis in restrictive cardiomyopathy) and computed tomography or magnetic resonance imaging (by demonstrating a thickened pericardium in constrictive pericarditis). Treatment usually is disappointing, except for hemochromatosis (where desferoxamine has been helpful in reducing myocardial iron content).

ENDOMYOCARDIAL FIBROSIS This is a progressive disease of unknown cause that occurs most commonly in children and young adults residing in tropical and subtropical Africa, particularly Uganda and Nigeria. Endomyocardial fibrosis is a frequent cause of heart failure in Africa, accounting for up to one-quarter of deaths due to heart disease. The condition is characterized by fibrous endocardial

lesions of the inflow portion of the right or left ventricle (or both) and often involves the atrioventricular valves, producing valvular regurgitation. The apex of the ventricles may be obliterated by a mass of thrombus and fibrous tissue. In some ways this disease resembles eosinophilic endomyocardial disease (see below), although they occur in quite different geographic areas and age groups and generally are felt to be different diseases.

The clinical picture depends on which ventricle and atrioventricular valve show predominant involvement; left-sided involvement results in symptoms of pulmonary congestion, while predominant right-sided disease presents features of a restrictive cardiomyopathy. Medical treatment is often disappointing, and surgical excision of the fibrotic endocardium and replacement of the involved atrioventricular valve have led to substantial symptomatic improvement in some patients.

EOSINOPHILIC ENDOMYOCARDIAL DISEASE Also called *Loeffler's endocarditis* and *fibroplastic endocarditis*, this disease appears to be a subcategory of the hypereosinophilic syndrome in which the heart is predominantly involved, with cardiac damage the apparent result of the toxic effects of eosinophilic proteins. Typically, the endocardium of either or both ventricles thickens markedly, with involvement of the underlying myocardium. Large mural thrombi may develop in either ventricle, thereby compromising the size of the ventricular cavity and serving as a source of pulmonary and systemic emboli. Hepatosplenomegaly and localized eosinophilic infiltration of other organs are usually present. Management with diuretics, afterload-reducing agents, and anticoagulation in conjunction with glucocorticoids and cytotoxic drugs (hydroxyurea in particular), appears to have improved survival substantially. Surgical treatment, as for endomyocardial fibrosis, may be helpful.

DIFFERENTIAL DIAGNOSIS Involvement of the heart is the most frequent cause of death in *primary amyloidosis* (Chap. 309), while clinically significant cardiac involvement is uncommon in the secondary form. Focal deposits of amyloid in elderly patients (*senile cardiac amyloidosis*) are common and usually clinically insignificant. Aspiration of abdominal fat or biopsy of the rectal mucosa, gingiva, liver, kidney, or myocardium permits the diagnosis to be made before death in over three-quarters of cases. The heart is firm, rubbery, and noncompliant, and four clinical presentations (alone or in combination) are seen: (1) diastolic dysfunction (restrictive cardiomyopathy), (2) systolic dysfunction, (3) arrhythmias, and (4) orthostatic hypotension. The two-dimensional echocardiogram may be helpful in making the diagnosis of amyloidosis and may show a thickened myocardial wall with a distinctive "speckled" appearance.

Hemochromatosis (Chap. 342) often is the result of multiple transfusions or a hemoglobinopathy; the familial (autosomal recessive) form should be suspected if cardiomyopathy occurs in the setting of diabetes mellitus, hepatic cirrhosis, and increased skin pigmentation. The diagnosis may be confirmed by endocardial biopsy. Phlebotomy may be of some benefit if employed early in the course of the disease. Continuous subcutaneous administration of deferoxamine may reduce body iron stores and result in clinical improvement.

Myocardial *sarcoidosis* (Chap. 320) is generally associated with other manifestations of systemic disease and may cause restrictive as well as congestive features, since cardiac infiltration by sarcoid granulomas results not only in increased stiffness of the myocardium but also in diminished systolic contractile function. A variety of arrhythmias, including atrioventricular block, have been noted. A common cardiac manifestation of systemic sarcoidosis is right heart overload due to pulmonary artery hypertension as a result of parenchymal pulmonary involvement. The *carcinoid syndrome* results in endocardial fibrosis and stenosis and/or regurgitation of the tricuspid and/or pulmonary valve (Chap. 237).

MYOCARDITIDES

Myocarditis, i.e., cardiac inflammation, is most commonly the result of an infectious process. Myocarditis also may result from a hypersensitivity to drugs or may be caused by radiation, chemicals, or physical agents. In an unknown number of cases, acute myocarditis progresses to chronic dilated cardiomyopathy. While almost every infectious agent is capable of producing myocarditis (Table 239-1), clinically significant acute myocarditis in the United States is caused most commonly by viruses, especially coxsackievirus B. The clinical manifestations range from an asymptomatic state, with the presence of myocarditis inferred only by the finding of transient electrocardiographic ST-T-wave abnormalities, to a fulminant condition with arrhythmias, heart failure, and death. In some patients myocarditis simulates acute myocardial infarction, with chest pain, electrocardiographic changes, and elevated serum levels of myocardial enzymes.

Physical examination usually is normal, although more severe cases may show a muffled first heart sound, along with a third heart sound and a murmur of mitral regurgitation. A pericardial friction rub may be audible in patients with associated pericarditis.

Though viral myocarditis is most often self-limited and without sequelae, severe involvement may recur, and it is likely that acute viral myocarditis occasionally progresses to a chronic form and to dilated cardiomyopathy. Patients with viral myocarditis often give a history of a preceding upper respiratory febrile illness, and viral nasopharyngitis or tonsillitis may be evident clinically. The isolation of virus from the stool, pharyngeal washings, or other body fluids and changes in specific antibody titers are helpful clinically.

Experimental studies suggest that exercise may be deleterious in patients with viral myocarditis, and strenuous activity should be proscribed until the electrocardiogram has returned to normal. Patients who develop congestive heart failure respond to the usual measures (digitalis, diuretics, salt restriction), but they appear to be unusually sensitive to digitalis. Arrhythmias are common and are occasionally difficult to manage. Deaths attributed to heart failure, tachyarrhythmias, and heart block have been reported, and it seems prudent to monitor the electrocardiogram of patients with arrhythmias, especially during the acute illness.

HUMAN IMMUNODEFICIENCY VIRUS (HIV) MYOCARDITIS (See also Chap. 308) Many HIV-infected patients have subclinical cardiac involvement, including pericardial effusion, right-sided chamber enlargement, and neoplastic involvement. Overt clinical involvement is seen in 10 percent of HIV patients, and the most common finding is left ventricular dysfunction that in some cases appears to be due to infiltration of the myocardium by the virus itself. In other patients the heart is affected by any of the various opportunistic infections common in AIDS, such as toxoplasmosis, as well as by cardiac metastases in Kaposi's sarcoma. The clinical manifestations of cardiac involvement may be incorrectly attributed to concurrent noncardiac problems such as pneumonia. This is unfortunate, since the dilated cardiomyopathy of HIV infection may respond at least transiently to standard therapy with digitalis, diuretics, and vasodilators.

BACTERIAL MYOCARDITIS Bacterial involvement of the heart is uncommon, but when it does occur, it is usually as a complication of bacterial endocarditis (typically due to *Staphylococcus aureus* and enterococci). Myocardial abscess formation may involve the valve rings and interventricular septum. *Diphtheritic myocarditis* develops in over one-quarter of the patients with diphtheria, is one of the most serious complications, and is the most common cause of death due to diphtheria (Chap. 144). Cardiac damage is due to the liberation of a toxin that inhibits protein synthesis and leads to a dilated, flabby, hypocontractile heart; the conducting system is frequently involved as well. Cardiomegaly and severe congestive heart failure typically appear after the first week of illness. Prompt therapy with antitoxin is crucial; antibiotic therapy is also indicated but is of less urgency.

CHAGAS' DISEASE Chagas' disease, caused by the protozoan *Trypanosoma cruzi* and transmitted by an insect vector (Chap. 218), produces an extensive myocarditis that typically becomes evident years after the initial infection. It is one of the most common causes of heart disease encountered in Central and South America; in rural endemic areas 20 to 75 percent of the population may be affected. An increasing number of cases are found in the United States as patients migrate from endemic areas. Although only about 1 percent of infected individ-

uals have an acute illness, which may include acute myocarditis, upwards of one-third develop chronic myocardial damage many years later. The chronic form is characterized by dilatation of several cardiac chambers, fibrosis and thinning of the ventricular wall, aneurysm formation (especially at the left ventricular apex), and mural thrombi. Chronic progressive heart failure is the rule and is associated with poor survival. The electrocardiogram is abnormal in most patients with cardiac involvement and typically shows right bundle branch block and left anterior hemiblock which may progress to complete atrioventricular block. The *echocardiogram* may reveal a unique pattern of hypokinesis of the posterior left ventricular wall and relatively preserved septal motion. Ventricular arrhythmias are common and are seen especially during and after exertion; oral amiodarone appears to be particularly effective in treating ventricular tachyarrhythmias. The cause of death is either intractable congestive heart failure or an arrhythmia, with a minority of patients dying from embolic phenomena. Therapy is directed toward amelioration of the congestive heart failure and arrhythmias; progressive conduction system disease and heart block may require implantation of a pacemaker. Anticoagulation (if feasible) may reduce the risk of thromboembolism. Medical therapy often is unsatisfactory or unavailable (especially in poor rural areas), however, and a more promising tactic in endemic areas has been the institution of public health measures, particularly the use of insecticides to eliminate the vector.

GIANT CELL MYOCARDITIS This rare myocarditis of unknown cause is characterized by the presence of multinucleated giant cells in the myocardium. It usually causes rapidly fatal congestive heart failure and arrhythmia in young to middle-aged adults. At necropsy, the distinctive features include cardiac enlargement, ventricular thrombi, grossly visible serpiginous areas of myocardial necrosis in both ventricles, and microscopic evidence of giant cells within an extensive inflammatory infiltrate. The cause of giant cell myocarditis remains obscure, although it occurs in association with thymoma, systemic lupus erythematosus, and thyrotoxicosis. Although glucocorticoids usually are tried, no therapy has been shown conclusively to be efficacious.

LYME CARDITIS (See also Chap. 178) Lyme disease is caused by a tick-borne spirochete and is most common in the Northeast, upper Midwest and Pacific Coastal regions of the United States during the summer months. About 10 percent of patients develop symptomatic cardiac involvement, with atrioventricular nodal conduction abnormalities and their consequences, such as syncope. Concomitant myopericarditis is not uncommon, and mild asymptomatic left ventricular dysfunction may occur. Intravenous ceftriaxone or penicillin is used in all but the mildest forms of Lyme carditis, in which case oral amoxicillin or doxycycline is employed. Hospitalization with electrocardiographic monitoring is indicated in patients with second or third degree atrioventricular block. A temporary pacemaker may be needed for symptomatic heart block; the utility of glucocorticoids in reversing heart block is uncertain, but they are usually employed.

BIBLIOGRAPHY

ANAN R et al: Prognostic implications of novel beta cardiac myosin heavy chain gene mutations that cause familial hypertrophic cardiomyopathy. J Clin Invest 93:280, 1994

CANNON RO et al: Results of permanent dual-chamber pacing in symptomatic nonobstructive hypertrophic cardiomyopathy. Am J Cardiol 73:571, 1994

DEC GW, FUSTER V: Medical progress: Idiopathic dilated cardiomyopathy. N Engl J Med 331:1564, 1994

HAGAR JM, RAHIMTOOLA SH: Chagas' heart disease. Curr Probl Cardiol 20:827, 1995

HERSKOWITZ A et al: Myocarditis and cardiotropic viral infection associated with severe left ventricular dysfunction in late-stage infection with human immunodeficiency virus. J Am Coll Cardiol 24:1025, 1994

KASPER EK et al: The causes of dilated cardiomyopathy: A clinicopathologic review of 673 consecutive patients. J Am Coll Cardiol 23:586, 1994

KLONER RA, HALE S: Unraveling the complex effects of cocaine on the heart. Circulation 87:1046, 1993

KYLE RA: Amyloidosis. Circulation 91:1269, 1995

MARON BJ et al: 26th Bethesda conference: Recommendations for determining eligibility for competition in athletes with cardiovascular abnormalities. Task Force 3: Hypertrophic cardiomyopathy, myocarditis and other myopericardial diseases and mitral valve prolapse. J Am Coll Cardiol 24:880, 1994

MASON JW et al: A clinical trial of immunosuppressive therapy for myocarditis. N Engl J Med 333:269, 1995

McKENNA WJ et al: Diagnosis of arrhythmogenic right ventricular dysplasia/cardiomyopathy. Task Force of the Working Group Myocardial and Pericardial Disease of the European Society of Cardiology and of the Scientific Council on Cardiomyopathies of the International Society and Federation of Cardiology. Br Heart J 71:215, 1994

NAKAO S et al: An atypical variant of Fabry's disease in men with left ventricular hypertrophy. N Engl J Med 333:288, 1995

O'CONNELL JB et al: Treatment of end stage dilated cardiomyopathy. Br Heart J 72:S52, 1994

RICHARDSON P et al: Report of the 1995 World Health Organization/International Society and Federation of Cardiology Task Force on the Definition and Classification of Cardiomyopathies. Circulation 93:841, 1996

ROBIOLIO PA et al: Carcinoid heart disease. Correlation of high serotonin levels with valvular abnormalities detected by cardiac catheterization and echocardiography. Circulation 92:790, 1995

SINGH SN et al: Amiodarone in patients with congestive heart failure and asymptomatic ventricular arrhythmia. N Engl J Med 333:77, 1995

STOCKINS BA et al: Prognosis in patients with diphtheric myocarditis and bradyarrhythmias: Assessment of results of ventricular pacing. Br Heart J 72:190, 1994

WATKINS H et al: Mutations in the genes for cardiac troponin T and α-tropomyosin in hypertrophic cardiomyopathy. N Engl J Med 332:1058, 1995

WYNNE J, BRAUNWALD E: The cardiomyopathies and myocarditides, in *Heart Disease*, 5th ed, E. Braunwald (ed). Philadelphia, Saunders, 1997, pp 1404–1463

240 *Eugene Braunwald*

PERICARDIAL DISEASE

NORMAL FUNCTIONS OF THE PERICARDIUM The visceral pericardium is a serous membrane that is separated by a small amount (15 to 50 mL) of fluid, an ultrafiltrate of plasma, from a fibrous sac, the parietal pericardium. The pericardium prevents sudden dilatation of the cardiac chambers during exercise and with hypervolemia. As the result of the development of a negative intrapericardial pressure during ejection, it facilitates atrial filling during ventricular systole. The pericardium also restricts the anatomic position of the heart, minimizes friction between the heart and surrounding structures, prevents displacement of the heart and kinking of the great vessels, and probably retards the spread of infections from the lungs and pleural cavities to the heart. Notwithstanding the foregoing, total absence of the pericardium does not produce obvious clinical disease. In partial left pericardial defects the main pulmonary artery and left atrium may bulge through the defect; very rarely, herniation and subsequent strangulation of the left atrium may cause sudden death.

ACUTE PERICARDITIS

Acute pericarditis, by far the most common pathologic process involving the pericardium, may be classified both clinically and etiologically (Table 240-1). Pain, a pericardial friction rub, electrocardiographic changes, and pericardial effusion with cardiac tamponade and paradoxic pulse are cardinal manifestations of many forms of acute pericarditis and will be considered prior to a discussion of the most common forms of the disorder.

Chest pain is an important but not invariable symptom in various forms of acute pericarditis (Chap. 13); it is usually present in the acute infectious types and in many of the forms presumed to be related to hypersensitivity or autoimmunity. Pain is often absent in a slowly developing tuberculous, postirradiation, neoplastic, or uremic pericarditis. The pain of pericarditis is often severe. It is characteristically retrosternal and left precordial, referred to the back and the trapezius ridge. Often the pain is pleuritic consequent to accompanying pleural inflammation, i.e., sharp and aggravated by inspiration, coughing, and changes in body position, but sometimes it is a steady, constricting pain that radiates into either arm or both arms and resembles that of myocardial ischemia; therefore, confusion with myocardial infarction is common. Characteristically, however, the pericardial pain may be relieved by sitting up and leaning forward and is intensified by lying supine. There is often a pleural component, with aggravation of the pain with coughing and deep inspiration. The differentiation of acute myocardial infarction from acute pericarditis becomes perplexing when, with acute pericarditis, the serum transaminase and creatine kinase levels rise, presumably because of concomitant involvement of the epicardium. However, these enzyme elevations, if they occur,

Table 240-1

Classification of Pericarditis

CLINICAL CLASSIFICATION

I. Acute pericarditis (<6 weeks)
   A. Fibrinous
   B. Effusive (serous or sanguineous)
II. Subacute pericarditis (6 weeks to 6 months)
   A. Effusive-constrictive
   B. Constrictive
III. Chronic pericarditis (>6 months)
   A. Constrictive
   B. Effusive
   C. Adhesive (nonconstrictive)

ETIOLOGIC CLASSIFICATION

I. Infectious pericarditis
   A. Viral (coxsackievirus A and B, echovirus, mumps, adenovirus, hepatitis, HIV)
   B. Pyogenic (pneumococcus, streptococcus, staphylococcus, *Neisseria*, *Legionella*)
   C. Tuberculous
   D. Fungal (histoplasmosis, coccidioidomycosis, *Candida*, blastomycosis)
   E. Other infections (syphilitic, parasitic)
II. Noninfectious pericarditis
   A. Acute myocardial infarction
   B. Uremia
   C. Neoplasia
     1. Primary tumors (benign or malignant)
     2. Tumors metastatic to pericardium (lung and breast cancer, lymphoma, Hodgkin's disease)
   D. Myxedema
   E. Cholesterol
   F. Chylopericardium
   G. Trauma
     1. Penetrating chest wall
     2. Nonpenetrating
   H. Aortic dissection (with leakage into pericardial sac)
   I. Postirradiation
   J. Familial Mediterranean fever
   K. Familial pericarditis
     1. Mulibrey nanism*
   L. Acute idiopathic
III. Pericarditis presumably related to hypersensitivity or autoimmunity
   A. Rheumatic fever
   B. Collagen vascular disease (SLE, rheumatoid arthritis, scleroderma, acute rheumatic fever, Wegener's granulomatosis)
   C. Drug-induced (e.g., procainamide, hydralazine, phenytoin, isoniazide, doxorubicin)
   D. Postcardiac injury
     1. Postmyocardial infarction (Dressler's syndrome)
     2. Postpericardiotomy
     3. Posttraumatic

---

* An autosomal recessive syndrome, characterized by growth failure, muscle hypotonia, hepatomegaly, ocular changes, enlarged cerebral ventricles, mental retardation, and chronic constrictive pericarditis.

are quite modest, given the extensive electrocardiographic ST-segment elevation in pericarditis.

The *pericardial friction rub* is the most important physical sign; it may have up to three components per cardiac cycle and is high-pitched, scratching, and grating, as described in Chap. 227; it can sometimes be elicited only when firm pressure with the diaphragm of the stethoscope is applied to the chest wall at the left lower sternal border. It is heard most frequently during expiration with the patient in the sitting position. The rub is often inconstant and the loud to-and-fro leathery sound may disappear within a few hours, possibly to reappear the following day.

The *electrocardiogram* in acute pericarditis without massive effusion usually displays changes secondary to acute subepicardial inflammation (see Fig. 228-18, p. 1245). There is widespread elevation of the ST segments, involving two or three standard limb leads and V_2 to V_6, with reciprocal depressions only in aVR and sometimes V_1. Usually there are no significant changes in QRS complexes, except for some reduction in voltage in patients with large pericardial effusions. After several days, the ST segments return to normal, and only then do the T waves become inverted. In contrast, in acute myocardial infarction, reciprocal depression of ST segments is usually more prominent; QRS changes occur, particularly the development of Q waves, as well as notching and loss of the amplitude of R waves; and T-wave inversions usually occur within hours *before* the ST segments have become isoelectric. Sequential electrocardiograms are useful in distinguishing acute pericarditis from acute myocardial infarction. In the latter, elevated ST segments return to normal within hours. Early repolarization is a normal variant and also may cause widespread ST-segment elevation, most prominent in left precordial leads. However, in this condition the T waves are usually tall and the ST/T ratio is under 0.25, but it exceeds this number in acute pericarditis. Depression of the PQ segment (below the TP segment) also is common and reflects atrial involvement. With large pericardial effusions, the QRS voltage is reduced; atrial premature beats and atrial fibrillation are sometimes noted.

PERICARDIAL EFFUSION Usually associated with pain and/or the above-mentioned electrocardiographic changes characteristic of pericarditis and an enlargement of the cardiac silhouette, pericardial effusion is especially important clinically when it develops within a relatively short time, since it may lead to cardiac tamponade. Differentiation from cardiac enlargement may be difficult, but heart sounds tend to become faint; the friction rub may disappear or remain clearly audible, and the apex impulse may vanish, but sometimes it remains palpable albeit medial to the left border of cardiac dullness. The base of the left lung may be compressed by pericardial fluid, producing Ewart's sign, a patch of dullness beneath the angle of the left scapula. The chest roentgenogram may show a "water bottle" configuration of the cardiac silhouette, but it also may be normal or almost so. Lucent pericardial fat lines may be seen deep within the cardiopericardial silhouette. Fluoroscopic examination may show the ventricular pulsations to be diminished.

Diagnosis of Pericardial Effusion Echocardiography is the most effective diagnostic laboratory technique available, since it is sensitive, specific, simple, noninvasive, and may be performed at the bedside. The presence of pericardial fluid is recorded by two-dimensional transthoracic echocardiography as a relatively echo-free space between the posterior pericardium and left ventricular epicardium in patients with small effusions and a space between the anterior right ventricle and the parietal pericardium just beneath the anterior chest wall with larger effusions (Fig. 240-1). In patients with large effusions the heart may swing freely within the pericardial sac; when severe, the extent of this motion alternates and may be associated with electrical alternans. Echocardiography also allows localization and estimation of the quantity of pericardial fluid. When pericardial effusion causes tamponade, during inspiration right ventricular diameter increases while left ventricular diameter and mitral valve opening decrease. Often the right ventricular cavity is reduced, and there is late diastolic inward motion (collapse) of the right ventricular free wall and of the right atrium. Doppler ultrasound shows exaggerated

tricuspid and pulmonic flow with reciprocal changes in mitral flow during inspiration. The diagnosis of pericardial fluid or thickening may be confirmed by computed tomography (CT) or magnetic resonance imaging (MRI); these techniques may be superior to echocardiography in detecting loculated pericardial effusions.

When it is deemed desirable to remove pericardial fluid for diagnostic and/or therapeutic purposes, a needle attached to a properly grounded electrocardiographic lead is inserted into the pericardial space, usually through a subxiphoid approach, and, if possible, using echocardiographic control. Intrapericardial pressure should be measured before fluid is withdrawn. Pericardial effusion nearly always has the physical characteristics of an exudate. Bloody fluid is commonly due to tuberculosis or tumor but may also be found in the effusion of rheumatic fever; in post-cardiac injury and post-myocardial

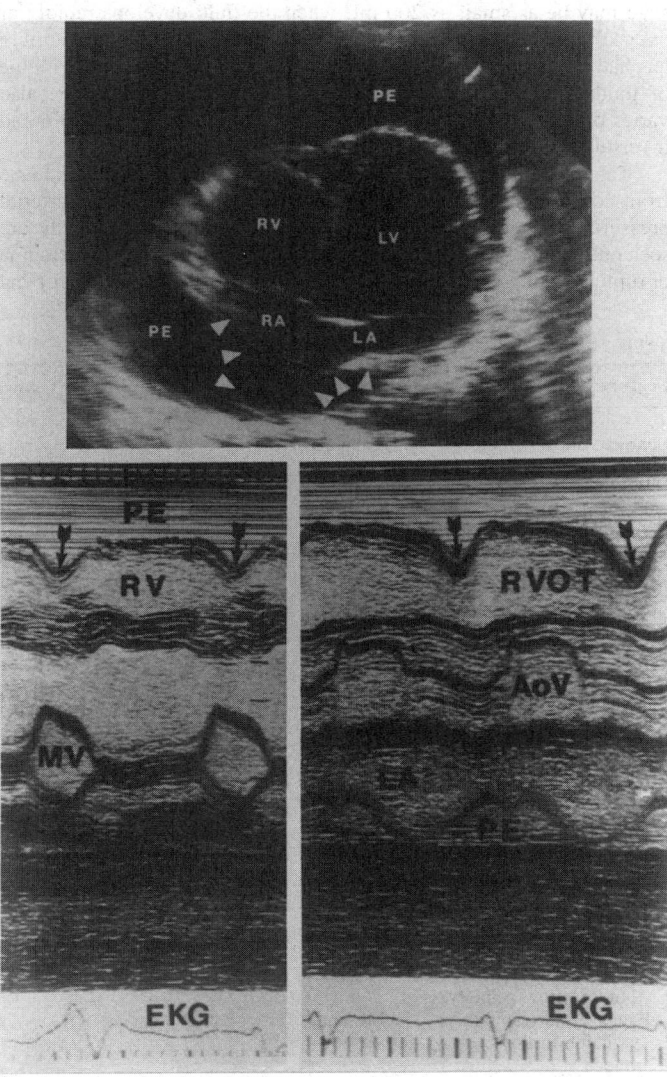

FIGURE 240-1 Two-dimensional (*upper panel*) and M-mode (*lower panels*) echocardiograms of a patient with a malignant pericardial effusion and cardiac tamponade. The two-dimensional image shows a large pericardial effusion (PE) adjacent to the borders of the right ventricle (RV), right atrium (RA), and left ventricle (LV). The effusion is sufficiently large that fluid is also present behind the left atrium (LA). Diastolic compression (white arrowheads) of both the right and left atria is present. The M-mode images also show striking diastolic compression (dark arrows) of the right ventricle during diastole when the mitral valve (MV) is open and compression of the right ventricular outflow tract (RVOT) in early to mid-diastole after aortic valve (AoV) closure. (*From Lorell, with permission.*)

infarction, especially following the administration of anticoagulants; and in uremic pericarditis.

CARDIAC TAMPONADE The accumulation of fluid in the pericardium in an amount sufficient to cause serious obstruction to the inflow of blood to the ventricles results in cardiac tamponade. This grave complication may be fatal if it is not recognized and treated promptly. The three most common causes of tamponade are neoplastic disease, idiopathic pericarditis, and uremia, but it also results from bleeding into the pericardial space either following cardiac operations and trauma (including cardiac perforation during diagnostic procedures) or from tuberculosis and hemopericardium; the latter may result when a patient with any form of acute pericarditis is treated with anticoagulants. The three principal features of tamponade are elevation of intracardiac pressures, limitation of ventricular filling, and reduction of cardiac output. The amount of fluid necessary to produce this critical state may be as small as 200 mL when the fluid develops rapidly or over 2000 mL in slowly developing effusions when the pericardium has had the opportunity to stretch and adapt to the increasing volume of fluid. The volume of fluid required to produce tamponade also varies directly with the thickness of the ventricular myocardium and inversely with the thickness of the parietal pericardium.

Table 240-2 lists the features that distinguish cardiac tamponade from constrictive pericarditis. The classic findings of falling arterial pressure, rising venous pressure, and faint heart sounds usually are seen only with severe, acute tamponade, as occurs with cardiac trauma or rupture. Tamponade may also develop more slowly, and the clinical manifestations resemble those of heart failure, including dyspnea, orthopnea, hepatic engorgement, and jugular venous hypertension. A high index of suspicion for cardiac tamponade is required, since, in many instances, no obvious cause for pericardial disease is apparent, and tamponade should be considered in any patient with hypotension and elevation of jugular venous pressure with a prominent x descent; in contrast to constrictive pericarditis, often the y descent is diminutive or absent. A positive Kussmaul sign (see below) is rare in cardiac tamponade, as is a pericardial knock. Their presence suggests that an organizing process and epicardial constriction are present in addition to effusion. A widening of the area of flatness to percussion across the anterior aspect of the chest wall, a paradoxical pulse (see below), relatively clear lung fields, diminished pulsations of the cardiac silhouette on fluoroscopy, enlargement of the cardiac silhouette (especially in subacute or chronic tamponade), reduction in amplitude of the QRS complexes, and *electrical alternans* of the P, QRS, and T waves should raise the suspicion of cardiac tamponade.

Since immediate treatment of tamponade may be lifesaving, prompt measures to establish the diagnosis by echocardiography should be undertaken. The right atrial pressure is elevated with prominence of the x but not of the y descent (Table 240-2). If measured, the pericardial pressure is also elevated and equal to the right atrial pressure. There is "equalization" of pressures, i.e., the pulmonary artery wedge is equal, or close, to right atrial, right ventricular, and pulmonary artery diastolic pressures. The "square root" sign in the ventricular pressure pulses and the prominent y descent in atrial and jugular venous pressure are characteristic of constrictive pericarditis (see below) and are rarely present in tamponade. In an emergency, pericardiocentesis may be carried out without cardiac catheterization but, whenever possible, after confirmation of the clinical diagnosis by echocardiography.

Paradoxical Pulse This important clue to the presence of cardiac tamponade consists of *a greater than normal (10 mmHg) inspiratory decline in systolic arterial pressure*. When severe, it may be detected by palpating weakness or disappearance of the arterial pulse during inspiration, but usually sphygmomanometric measurement of systolic pressure during slow respiration is required (Fig. 240-2).

Since both ventricles share a tight incompressible covering, i.e., the pericardial sac, in cardiac tamponade the inspiratory enlargement of the right ventricle compresses and reduces left ventricular volume substantially; leftward bulging of the interventricular septum further reduces the left ventricular cavity as the right ventricle enlarges during inspiration. Thus in cardiac tamponade the normal inspiratory augmentation of right ventricular volume causes an exaggerated reciprocal reduction in left ventricular volume. Also, respiratory distress increases the fluctuations in intrathoracic pressure, which exaggerates the mechanism just described. Right ventricular infarction (Chap. 243) may resemble cardiac tamponade with hypotension, ele-

Table 240-2

Features That Distinguish Constrictive Pericarditis From Similar Clinical Disorders

Characteristic	Tamponade	Constrictive Pericarditis	Restrictive Cardiomyopathy	RVMI*
Clinical				
Pulsus paradoxus	Common	Usually absent	Rare	Rare
Jugular veins				
Prominent y descent	Absent	Usually present	Rare	Rare
Prominent x descent	Present	Usually present	Present	Rare
Kussmaul's sign	Absent	Present	Absent	Absent
Third heart sound	Absent	Absent	Rare	May be present
Pericardial knock	Absent	Often present	Absent	Absent
Electrocardiogram				
Low ECG voltage	May be present	May be present	May be present	Absent
Electrical alternans	May be present	Absent	Absent	Absent
Echocardiography				
Thickened pericardium	Absent	Present	Absent	Absent
Pericardial calcification	Absent	Often present	Absent	Absent
Pericardial effusion	Present	Absent	Absent	Absent
RV size	Usually small	Usually normal	Usually normal	Enlarged
Myocardial thickness	Normal	Normal	Usually increased	Normal
Right atrial collapse and RVDC	Present	Absent	Absent	Absent
Increased early filling, ↑ mitral flow velocity	Absent	Present	Present	May be present
Exaggerated respiratory variation in flow velocity	Present	Present	Absent	Absent
CT/MRI				
Thickened/calcific pericardium	Absent	Present	Absent	Absent

mately one-third of patients with constrictive pericarditis. Paradoxical pulse is not pathognomonic of pericardial disease because it may be observed in restrictive cardiomyopathies (Chap. 239) and in some cases of hypovolemic shock, chronic obstructive airways disease, and severe bronchial asthma.

Low-pressure tamponade refers to mild tamponade in which the intrapericardial pressure is increased from its slightly subatmospheric levels to +5 to +10 mmHg; in some instances hypovolemia coexists. As a consequence, the central venous pressure is normal or only slightly elevated while arterial pressure is unaffected. The patients are asymptomatic or complain of mild weakness and dyspnea. The diagnosis is aided by echocardiography, and both hemodynamic and clinical manifestations improve following pericardiocentesis.

℞ TREATMENT

The patient should be observed frequently for the development of an effusion; if a moderate or large effusion is already present, the patient should be hospitalized and watched for signs of tamponade. In the presence of an effusion, arterial and venous pressures and heart rate should be monitored or followed carefully and serial echocardiograms obtained. If manifestations of tamponade appear, pericardiocentesis must be carried out at once, since relief of the intrapericardial pressure may be lifesaving. A small catheter advanced over the needle inserted into the pericardial cavity may be left in place to allow draining of the pericardial space if fluid reaccumulates. When a *diagnostic* pericardiocentesis of a large effusion is carried out, an attempt should be made to remove as much fluid as possible.

VIRAL OR IDIOPATHIC FORM OF ACUTE PERICARDI-TIS

This disorder is frequent and may be confused with other, more serious illnesses. In some cases, an A or B coxsackievirus or the virus of influenza, echovirus type 8, mumps, herpes simplex, chickenpox, or adenovirus has been isolated from pericardial fluid and/or appropriate elevations in viral antibody titers have been noted; in many instances, acute pericarditis has occurred in association with illnesses of known viral origin and, presumably, was caused by the same agent. Commonly, there is an antecedent infection of the respiratory tract, but in many patients such an association is not evident and viral isolation and serologic studies are negative. Acute pericarditis occurs in patients infected with human immunodeficiency virus (HIV). Most frequently, a viral causation cannot be established, nor can it be excluded; the term *acute idiopathic pericarditis* is then appropriate.

Acute pericarditis occurs at all ages but is more frequent in young adults. Regardless of the specific cause, the clinical manifestations are similar. Pericarditis is often associated with pleural effusions and pneumonitis. The appearance of fever and precordial pain at about the same time, often 10 to 12 days after a presumed viral illness, constitutes an important feature in the differentiation of acute pericarditis from myocardial infarction, in which pain precedes fever. The constitutional symptoms are usually mild to moderate, but occasionally the initial symptoms are stormy, the temperature rising to 40°C. The disease ordinarily runs its course in a few days to 4 weeks, but one or more recurrences occur in about one-fourth of patients. Although accumulation of some pericardial fluid is common, tamponade is unusual, and constrictive pericarditis develops rarely. A pericardial friction rub is often audible. The ST-segment alterations in the electrocardiogram are usually transitory, but the abnormal T waves may persist for several years or indefinitely and be a source of confusion in persons without a clear history of pericarditis. Pleuritis and pneumoni-tis frequently accompany pericarditis. The erythrocyte sedimentation rate is elevated; granulocytosis followed by lymphocytosis is common.

Viral or idiopathic pericarditis is usually self-limited and abates within 1 month. One or more episodes of recurrent pericarditis occur in up to one-fourth of patients. Constrictive pericarditis (p. 1339) is a rare complication.

℞ TREATMENT

There is no specific therapy, but bed rest and anti-inflammatory treatment with aspirin, if necessary up to 900 mg qid, may be given. If this is ineffective, one of the nonsteroidal anti-inflammatory agents, such as indomethacin (25 to 75 mg qid) or a glucocorticoid (e.g., prednisone, 20 to 80 mg daily) usually suppresses the clinical manifestations of the acute illness and may be useful in patients in whom the purulent and tuberculous forms of pericarditis have been excluded. Anticoagulants should be avoided. After the patient has been asymptomatic and afebrile for about a week, the dose of the anti-inflammatory agent is gradually tapered. When recurrences are multiple, frequent, disabling, and continue beyond 2 years, pericar-diectomy may be effective in terminating the illness.

POST-CARDIAC INJURY SYNDROME An acute form of pericarditis may appear under a variety of circumstances that have one common feature: previous injury to the myocardium, with blood in the pericardial cavity. The syndrome has been observed when the injury has been induced in the course of a cardiac operation (postperi-cardiotomy syndrome). It may develop after cardiac trauma (Chap. 241), e.g., a stab wound, contusions after a nonpenetrating blow to the chest, or perforation of the heart with a catheter. Rarely, it follows myocardial infarction (Dressler's syndrome; Chap. 243).

The principal symptom is the pain of acute pericarditis, which usually develops 1 to 4 weeks following the cardiac injury but sometimes appears only after a lapse of months. Recurrences are common and may occur up to 2 years or more after the injury. Fever with temperature up to 40°C, pericarditis, pleuritis, and pneumonitis are the outstanding features, and the bout of illness usually subsides in 1 or 2 weeks. The pericarditis may be of the fibrinous variety, or it may be a pericardial effusion, which is often serosanguineous, rarely causes tamponade, and may be accompanied by arthralgias. Leukocytosis, an increased sedimentation rate, and electrocardiographic changes typical of acute pericarditis also may occur.

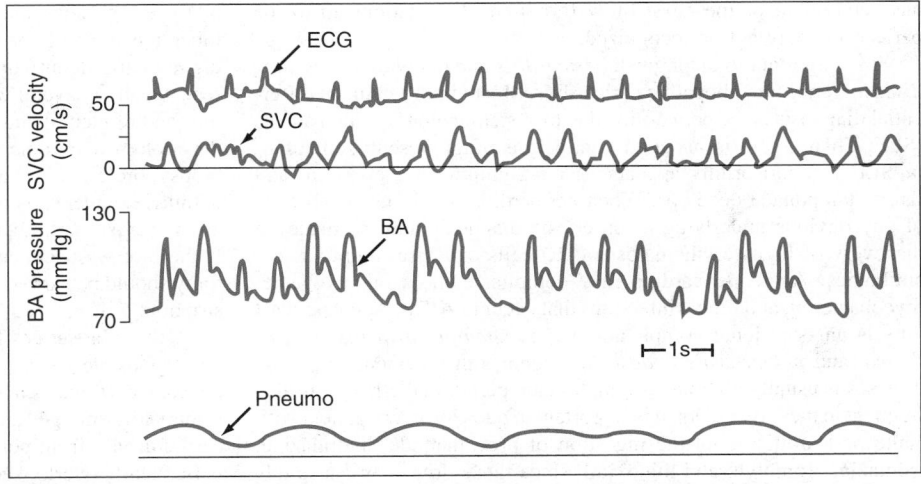

FIGURE 240-2 Simultaneous recording of electrocardiogram (ECG), blood flow velocity in the superior vena cava (SVC), brachial arterial pressure (BA), and the pneumogram (Pneumo) in a patient with cardiac compression and paradoxical pulse. A downward deflection of the pneumogram denotes inspiration, when SVC blood velocity rises and arterial pressure falls (paradoxical pulse). Arterial pressure is maintained during prolonged expiratory pause.

The mechanisms responsible for this syndrome have not been identified, but they are probably the result of a hypersensitivity reaction in which the antigen originates from injured myocardial tissue and/or pericardium; the suggested designation of *post-cardiac injury syndrome* for this group of disorders implies that they may have a common pathogenetic mechanism. Circulating autoantibodies to myocardium occur frequently, but their precise role has not been defined. Viral infection also may play an etiologic role, since antiviral antibodies are often elevated in patients who develop this syndrome following cardiac surgery.

The clinical picture of the post-cardiac injury syndrome mimics acute viral or acute idiopathic pericarditis. Moreover, it is possible that the recurrences that occur so frequently in the latter condition are not always caused by an exacerbation of the original (presumably viral) infection but that the original injury may have initiated the sequence of events that culminates in the post-cardiac injury syndrome.

Often no treatment is necessary aside from aspirin and analgesics. The management of pericardial effusion and tamponade has already been discussed. When the illness is followed by a series of disabling recurrences, therapy with a nonsteroidal anti-inflammatory agent or a glucocorticoid is usually effective.

DIFFERENTIAL DIAGNOSIS Since there is no specific test for *acute idiopathic pericarditis* the diagnosis is one of exclusion. Consequently, all other disorders that may be associated with acute fibrinous pericarditis must be considered. When associated with *acute myocardial infarction*, acute fibrinous pericarditis may be confused with acute viral or idiopathic pericarditis; this complication of infarction, described in Chap. 243, is characterized by the occurrence of fever, pain, and a friction rub in the first 4 days following the development of the infarct (to be distinguished from the pericarditis in Dressler's syndrome, which is a form of post-cardiac injury pericarditis and which occurs a week or two following myocardial infarction). Electrocardiographic abnormalities (such as the appearance of Q waves, brief ST-segment elevations with reciprocal changes, and earlier T-wave changes in myocardial infarction), the extent of the elevations of myocardial enzymes, and the total clinical picture are helpful in differentiating pericarditis from acute myocardial infarction. A common diagnostic error is mistaking acute viral or idiopathic pericarditis for acute myocardial infarction and vice versa.

Pericarditis secondary to post-cardiac injury is differentiated from acute idiopathic pericarditis chiefly by timing. If it occurs within a few weeks of a myocardial infarction or a chest blow, it may be justified to conclude that the two are probably related. If the infarct has been silent or the chest blow forgotten, the relationship to the pericarditis may not be recognized.

It is important to distinguish *pericarditis due to collagen vascular disease* from acute idiopathic pericarditis. Most important in the differential diagnosis is the pericarditis due to systemic lupus erythematosus (SLE; Chap. 312). In this condition, pain is often present; sometimes in SLE the pericarditis appears as an asymptomatic effusion, and rarely, tamponade develops. When pericarditis occurs in the absence of any obvious underlying disorder, the diagnosis may be made on discovery of lupus erythematosus (LE) cells or a rise in antinuclear antibodies. Acute pericarditis may complicate the viral, pyogenic, mycobacterial, and fungal infections that occur in AIDS. Acute pericarditis is an occasional complication of *rheumatoid arthritis*, *scleroderma*, and *polyarteritis nodosa*, but again, other evidence of these diseases is usually obvious. Asymptomatic pericardial effusion is also frequent in these disorders. It is important to question every patient with acute pericarditis about the ingestion of procainamide, hydralazine, isoniazid, cromolyn, and minoxidil, since these drugs can cause this syndrome.

The pericarditis of *acute rheumatic fever* is generally associated with evidence of severe pancarditis and with cardiac murmurs (Chap. 236). *Pyogenic (purulent) pericarditis* is usually secondary to cardiothoracic operations, immunosuppressive therapy, rupture of the esoph-

agus into the pericardial sac, or rupture of a ring abscess in a patient with infective endocarditis and with septicemia complicating aseptic pericarditis. It is accompanied by fever, chills, septicemia, and evidence of infection elsewhere. *Tuberculous pericarditis* (see Chap. 171) may present as an acute pericarditis, associated with fever, weight loss, and other clinical manifestations of active systemic tuberculosis; the diagnosis may be aided by a positive tuberculin test and evidence of pulmonary or mediastinal tuberculosis. Tubercle bacilli can be cultured from the pericardial space only infrequently, and a biopsy of the pericardium with bacteriologic and histologic examination may be required. Alternatively, tuberculous pericarditis may present as a chronic asymptomatic effusion, as subacute effusive-constrictive pericarditis (see below), or as frank chronic constrictive pericarditis (see below).

Uremic pericarditis (Chap. 271) occurs in up to one-third of patients with chronic uremia and is seen most frequently in patients undergoing chronic hemodialysis. It may be fibrinous and is generally associated with an effusion that may be sanguineous. A friction rub is common, but pain is usually absent. Treatment with an anti-inflammatory agent and intensification of hemodialysis is usually adequate. Occasionally, tamponade occurs and pericardiocentesis is required. When uremic pericarditis is recurrent, persistent, or very troubling, it may be necessary to perform pericardiectomy. Pericarditis due to *neoplastic diseases* results from extension or invasion of primary or metastatic tumors (most commonly carcinoma of the lung and breast, malignant melanoma, lymphoma, and leukemia) to the pericardium; pain, atrial arrhythmias, and tamponade are complications that occur occasionally. *Mediastinal irradiation* for neoplasm may cause acute pericarditis and/or chronic constrictive pericarditis after eradication of the tumor. Unusual causes of acute pericarditis include syphilis, fungal infection (histoplasmosis, blastomycosis, aspergillosis, and candidiasis), and parasitic infestation (amebiasis, toxoplasmosis, echinococcosis, trichinosis).

CHRONIC PERICARDIAL EFFUSIONS Chronic pericardial effusions are sometimes encountered in patients without an antecedent history of acute pericarditis. They may cause few symptoms per se, and their presence may be detected by finding an enlarged cardiac silhouette on chest roentgenogram.

Tuberculosis This is a common cause of chronic pericardial effusion, although less so in the United States than in other parts of the world (Chap. 171). The symptoms are often those of a chronic, systemic illness in a patient with pericardial effusion. It is important to bear this condition in mind when a middle-aged or elderly person with fever has enlargement of the cardiac silhouette of undetermined origin, with or without elevation of venous pressure. Weight loss, fever, and fatigability are sometimes observed. Inasmuch as treatment is quite effective, overlooking a tuberculous pericardial effusion may have serious consequences. A chest roentgenogram for pulmonary tuberculosis should be obtained, and a search for tuberculosis in other organs carried out; tuberculin skin tests should be performed and repeated after several weeks; and cultures and smears of gastric washings and of pleural and pericardial fluid should be obtained. Finally, if the etiology of chronic pericardial effusion is still obscure, a pericardial biopsy, preferably by a limited thoracotomy, should be performed. If definitive evidence is then still lacking but the specimen shows caseation necrosis, antituberculous chemotherapy is indicated (Chap. 171). If the biopsy specimen shows a thickened pericardium, pericardiectomy should be carried out in order to prevent the development of constriction.

Other Causes of Chronic Pericardial Effusion *Myxedema* may be responsible for a pericardial effusion that is sometimes massive but rarely, if ever, causes cardiac tamponade. The cardiac silhouette is markedly enlarged and an echocardiogram is necessary to distinguish cardiomegaly from pericardial effusion. The diagnosis of myxedema is frequently overlooked. It is important, therefore, to carry out appropriate tests for thyroid function (Chap. 331) as well as echocardiography in patients with an enlarged cardiac outline of undetermined origin. *Cholesterol pericardial disease* produces large pericardial effusions with a high cholesterol content, which may induce an inflammatory response and constrictive pericarditis.

Neoplasms, SLE, rheumatoid arthritis, mycotic infections, radiation therapy, pyogenic infections, severe chronic anemia, and chylopericardium also may cause chronic pericardial effusion and should be considered and specifically looked for in such patients.

Aspiration and analysis of the pericardial fluid are often helpful in diagnosis. In infections the organism can often be identified by smear or culture. Grossly sanguineous pericardial fluid results most commonly from a neoplasm, tuberculosis, uremia, or slow leakage from an aortic aneurysm.

CHRONIC CONSTRICTIVE PERICARDITIS

This disorder results when the healing of an acute fibrinous or serofibrinous pericarditis or a chronic pericardial effusion is followed by obliteration of the pericardial cavity with the formation of granulation tissue. This gradually contracts and forms a firm scar, encasing the heart and interfering with filling of the ventricles. In some reports, a high percentage of all cases has been of tuberculous origin. In the United States tuberculosis is now an infrequent cause. Chronic constrictive pericarditis also may follow purulent infection, trauma, cardiac operation of any type, mediastinal irradiation, histoplasmosis, neoplastic disease (especially breast cancer and lymphoma), acute viral or idiopathic pericarditis, rheumatoid arthritis, SLE, and chronic renal failure with uremia treated by chronic dialysis. In many patients the cause of the pericardial disease is undetermined, and in them an asymptomatic or forgotten bout of viral pericarditis, acute or idiopathic, may have been the inciting event. The heart also may be constricted and compressed by malignant tumors or organized blood clot in the pericardial cavity.

The basic physiologic abnormality in symptomatic patients with chronic constrictive pericarditis, as in those with cardiac tamponade, is the inability of the ventricles to fill because of the limitations imposed by the rigid, thickened pericardium or the tense pericardial fluid. In constrictive pericarditis, ventricular filling is unimpeded during early diastole but is reduced abruptly when the elastic limit of the pericardium is reached, while in cardiac tamponade, ventricular filling is impeded throughout diastole. In chronic constrictive pericarditis, stroke volume is reduced and the end-diastolic pressures in both ventricles and the mean pressures in the atria, pulmonic veins, and systemic veins are all elevated to about the same levels. Despite these hemodynamic changes, myocardial function may actually be normal or only slightly impaired; instead, the ventricles may be considered to be underloaded.

In constrictive pericarditis, the central venous and right and left atrial pressure pulses display an M-shaped contour, with prominent x and y descents; the y descent (absent or diminished in cardiac tamponade) is the most prominent deflection and is interrupted by a rapid rise in pressure during early diastole, when ventricular filling is impeded by the constricting pericardium. These characteristic changes are transmitted to the jugular veins, where they may be recognized by inspection. In constrictive pericarditis, both ventricular pressure pulses exhibit characteristic "square root" signs during diastole. These hemodynamic changes, although characteristic, are not pathognomonic of constrictive pericarditis but also may be observed in cardiomyopathies characterized by restriction of ventricular filling, as discussed in Chap. 239.

CLINICAL AND LABORATORY FINDINGS (See Table 240-2) Weakness, fatigue, weight loss, and anorexia are common. The patient often appears to be chronically ill with decreased skeletal muscle mass and a protuberant abdomen. Dyspnea, though absent or slight at rest, is usually present on exertion, and orthopnea is common, although not severe. However, attacks of acute left ventricular failure (acute pulmonary edema) practically never occur. The cervical veins are distended and may remain so even after intensive diuretic treatment, and venous pressure may fail to decline during inspiration (Kussmaul's sign). The pulse pressure is normal or reduced. In about one-third of the cases a paradoxical pulse can be detected. Congestive hepatomegaly is pronounced and may impair hepatic function; ascites is common and is usually more prominent than dependent edema. In about half of

patients the heart is normal in size; if it is enlarged, the enlargement is rarely extreme. The apical pulse is reduced in intensity, retracts in systole, and moves outward in diastole. The heart sounds may be distant; an early third heart sound, i.e., a pericardial knock, occurring 0.09 to 0.12 s after aortic valve closure that coincides with a sudden deceleration in ventricular filling, is often conspicuous, and murmurs are usually absent. The apex beat is poorly defined. Because of the high sustained venous pressure, congestive splenomegaly may make the spleen palpable. In the absence of infective endocarditis or tricuspid valve disease, splenomegaly in a patient with congestive heart failure should arouse suspicion of constrictive pericarditis. Protein-losing gastroenteropathy, due to impaired lymphatic drainage from the small intestine, and the nephrotic syndrome, or marked proteinuria or hypoalbuminemia, may complicate chronic constrictive pericarditis.

The *electrocardiogram* frequently displays low voltage of the QRS complex and diffuse flattening or inversion of the T waves. P mitrale may be present in patients with sinus rhythm; atrial fibrillation is present in about one-third of patients.

Systemic and/or pulmonary venous congestion is initially the result of impaired filling of the ventricles caused by the restrictive action of the inelastic pericardium. However, the fibrotic process may extend into the myocardium and cause myocardial scarring, and venous congestion may then be due to the combined effects of the myocardial and pericardial lesions. The interference with filling reduces the work of the heart, and perhaps this leads to myocardial atrophy. The latter probably accounts for the delayed beneficial effects of operative treatment observed in some patients with advanced disease.

Inasmuch as the usual physical signs of cardiac disease (murmurs, cardiac enlargement) may be inconspicuous or absent in chronic constrictive pericarditis, hepatic enlargement and dysfunction associated with intractable ascites may lead to a mistaken diagnosis of cirrhosis of the liver. This error can be avoided if the neck veins are inspected carefully in all patients with ascites and hepatomegaly. *Given a clinical picture resembling hepatic cirrhosis, but with the added feature of distended neck veins, careful search for calcification of the pericardium by chest roentgenography and echocardiography should be carried out and may disclose this curable or remediable form of heart disease.* Calcification occurs in only about one-half of these patients, usually in those with long-standing pericardial constriction. Most patients with chronic constrictive pericarditis show pericardial thickening on echocardiographic examination, and there is a distinctive pattern of transvalvular flow velocity on Doppler echocardiography. There is a reduction in blood flow velocity in the pulmonary veins and across the mitral valve during inspiration, with the opposite occurring during expiration. However, echocardiography cannot definitively exclude the diagnosis. MRI and CT scanning are more accurate than echocardiography in establishing or excluding the presence of a thickened pericardium. Pericardial thickening and even pericardial calcification, however, are not synonymous with constrictive pericarditis since they may occur without seriously impairing ventricular filling.

Prolonged hepatic congestion often leads to hypoalbuminemia, hyperbilirubinemia, and other abnormal tests of hepatocellular function.

DIFFERENTIAL DIAGNOSIS Like cor pulmonale (Chap. 238), chronic constrictive pericarditis may be associated with severe systemic venous hypertension but little pulmonary congestion; the heart usually is not enlarged, and a striking inspiratory fall in arterial pressure may be present. However, in cor pulmonale advanced parenchymal pulmonary disease is usually obvious and venous pressure *falls* during inspiration; i.e., Kussmaul's sign is negative. *Tricuspid stenosis* (p. 1322) also may simulate chronic constrictive pericarditis; congestive hepatomegaly, splenomegaly, ascites, and venous distention may be equally prominent, and the manifestations of left-sided heart failure may be inconspicuous. However, in tricuspid stenosis, the characteristic murmur, the almost universal coexistence of mitral stenosis, the absence of a paradoxical pulse, and the absence, in the jugular venous pulse, of the steep, deep y descent followed by a rapid ascent (manifested by the diastolic shock on palpation and its audible equivalent, the pericardial knock) facilitate the clinical differentiation.

Because constrictive pericarditis can be corrected surgically, it is important, though often difficult, to distinguish chronic constrictive pericarditis from restrictive cardiomyopathy (Chap. 239), which has a similar physiologic abnormality, i.e., restriction of ventricular filling. In many of these patients the ventricular wall is thickened on echocardiographic examination.

The features favoring the diagnosis of restrictive cardiomyopathy are a well-defined apex beat, enlargement of the heart, and pronounced orthopnea with attacks of acute left ventricular failure, left ventricular hypertrophy, gallop sounds (in place of a pericardial knock), bundle branch block, and in some cases abnormal Q waves on the electrocardiogram. At catheterization, patients with chronic constrictive pericarditis usually have left atrial or pulmonary arterial wedge pressure equaling right atrial pressure, the latter often exceeding 15 mmHg despite intensive medical treatment for heart failure. The pulmonary artery systolic pressure is often less than 50 mmHg, and the right ventricular end-diastolic pressure often reaches one-third of the systolic pressure. In contrast, in patients with restrictive cardiomyopathy, the left atrial usually exceeds the right atrial pressure by more than 5 mmHg, the mean right atrial pressure is often below 15 mmHg following intensive treatment with diuretics, the pulmonary artery systolic pressure often exceeds 50 mmHg, and the right ventricular end-diastolic pressure is usually less than one-third of the systolic pressure, while the cardiac output is markedly depressed. The volumes of both ventricles, as determined by angiography or echocardiography, are characteristically reduced or normal in constrictive pericarditis, and the ejection fractions are normal or almost so. The left ventricular end-diastolic volume also may be normal in some cardiomyopathies, but it is frequently elevated in others in which the ejection fraction is markedly reduced; the latter finding militates strongly against the diagnosis of constrictive pericarditis. The echocardiogram in chronic constrictive pericarditis characteristically shows pericardial thickening, i.e., a distinct echo posterior to the left ventricular wall, and paradoxical septal motion. The left ventricular wall moves sharply outward in early diastole and then remains flat. The definitive diagnosis of restrictive cardiomyopathy, when it is due to an infiltrative disease such as amyloidosis, can often be established by endomyocardial biopsy. CT scanning and MRI are very useful in distinguishing between restrictive cardiomyopathy and chronic constrictive pericarditis.

When a patient has progressive, disabling, and unresponsive congestive failure, and if he or she displays any of the features of constrictive heart disease, the most careful and detailed clinical and laboratory studies must be carried out in order to detect or exclude constrictive pericarditis, which is potentially a curable condition. Cardiac catheterization, angiocardiography, endomyocardial biopsy, and MRI may be required.

Occult Constrictive Disease Patients with this condition may have unexplained fatigue, dyspnea, and chest pain. No overt manifestations of pericardial disease are present, but following the rapid intravenous infusion of 1 L of saline solution, diastolic equilibration of intracardiac atrial and ventricular pressures found in overt constrictive pericarditis occur. Although symptomatic improvement may follow pericardiectomy, this procedure should not be carried out in asymptomatic persons.

 TREATMENT
Pericardial resection is the only definitive treatment of constrictive pericarditis, but dietary sodium restriction and diuretics are useful during preoperative preparation. The benefits derived from cardiac decortication are often striking, and the improvement, though slight

at first, usually is progressive over a period of months. The risk of this operation depends on the extent of penetration of the myocardium by the calcific process, by the severity of myocardial atrophy, by the extent of secondary impairment of hepatic and/or renal function, and by the patient's general condition. Operative mortality is in the range of 5 to 15 percent; the patients with the most severe and/or advanced disease are at highest risk. Therefore, surgical treatment should be carried out relatively early in the course.

Many cases of constrictive pericarditis are of tuberculous origin. Antituberculous therapy during the phase of effusion may prevent the development of constriction, and such therapy should be carried out before and after operation if a tuberculous origin is suspected or cannot be excluded in a patient with chronic constrictive pericarditis (Chap. 171).

SUBACUTE EFFUSIVE-CONSTRICTIVE PERICARDITIS This form of pericardial disease is characterized by the combination of a tense effusion in the pericardial space and constriction of the heart by thickened pericardium. It shares a number of features both with chronic pericardial effusion (p. 1338) producing cardiac compression and with pericardial constriction. It may be caused by tuberculosis, multiple attacks of acute idiopathic pericarditis, radiation, traumatic pericarditis, uremia, and scleroderma. The heart is generally enlarged, and a paradoxical pulse and a prominent x descent (without a prominent y descent) are present in the atrial pressure pulse. Following pericardiocentesis, the physiologic findings may change from those of cardiac tamponade to those of pericardial constriction, with a "square root" sign in the ventricular pressure pulse and a prominent y descent in the atrial and jugular venous pressure pulses. Furthermore, the intrapericardial pressure and the central venous pressure may decline, but not to normal. In many patients the condition progresses to the chronic constrictive form of the disease. Wide excision of both the visceral and parietal pericardium is usually effective.

OTHER DISORDERS OF THE PERICARDIUM

Pericardial cysts appear as rounded or lobulated deformities of the cardiac silhouette, most commonly at the right cardiophrenic angle. They do not cause symptoms, and their major clinical significance lies in the possibility of confusion with a tumor, ventricular aneurysm, or massive cardiomegaly. *Tumors* involving the pericardium are most commonly secondary to malignant neoplasms originating in or invading the mediastinum, including carcinoma of the bronchus and breast, lymphoma, and melanoma. The most common *primary* malignant tumor is the mesothelioma. The usual clinical picture of malignant pericardial tumor is an insidiously developing, often bloody, pericardial effusion. Surgical exploration is required to establish a definitive diagnosis and to carry out definitive or, more commonly, palliative treatment.

BIBLIOGRAPHY

CUJER B et al: Echocardiography in pericardial diseases, in *Marcus' Cardiac Imaging: A Companion to Braunwald's Heart Disease*, 2d ed, DJ Skorton et al (eds). Philadelphia, Saunders, 1996, pp 404–419

FOWLER NO: Tuberculous pericarditis. JAMA 266:99, 1991

HANCOCK EW: Subacute effusive-constrictive pericarditis. Circulation 43:183, 1971

KHAN AH: The postcardiac injury syndromes. Clin Cardiol 15:67, 1992

LORELL B: Pericardial diseases, in *Heart Disease*, 5th ed, E Braunwald (ed). Philadelphia, Saunders, 1997, pp 1478–1534

OH JK et al: Diagnostic role of Doppler echocardiography in constrictive pericarditis. J Am Coll Cardiol 23:154, 1994

SAGRISTA SAULEDA J et al: Purulent pericarditis: Review of a 20-year experience in a general hospital. J Am Coll Cardiol 22:1661, 1993

SHABETAI R: Treatment of pericardial disease, in *Cardiovascular Therapeutics: A Companion to Braunwald's Heart Disease*, TW Smith (ed). Philadelphia, Saunders, 1996, pp 742–750

SOLER-SOLER J: Massive chronic idiopathic pericardial effusion, in *Pericardial Disease: New Insights and Old Dilemmas*, J Soler-Soler et al (eds). Dordrecht, The Netherlands, Kluwer Academic, 1990, pp 153–165

STANFORD W, THOMPSON BH: Cardiac masses and pericardial disease: Imaging by electron-beam computed tomography, in *Marcus' Cardiac Imaging: A Companion to Braunwald's Heart Disease*, 2d ed, DJ Skorton et al (eds). Philadelphia, Saunders, 1996, pp 863–870

TIRILOMIS T et al: Pericardiectomy for chronic constrictive pericarditis: Risks and outcome. Eur J Cardiothorac Surg 8:487, 1994

VAITKUS PT, KUSSMAUL WG: Constrictive versus restrictive cardiomyopathy: A reappraisal and update of diagnostic criteria. Am Heart J 122:1431, 1991

——— et al: Treatment of malignant pericardial effusion. JAMA 272:59, 1994

Table 241-1

Relative Incidence of Primary Tumor of the Heart

Type	Percent
BENIGN	
Myxoma	30.5
Lipoma	10.5
Papillary fibroelastoma	9.9
Rhabdomyoma	8.5
Fibroma	4.0
Hemangioma	3.5
Teratoma	3.3
Mesothelioma of the AV node	2.8
Other benign tumors	2.1
Total	75.1
MALIGNANT	
Sarcomas	18.6
Lymphoma	1.6
Other malignant tumors	4.7
Total	24.9

SOURCE: Modified from HA McAllister, JJ Fenoglio, in Atlas of Tumor Pathology, Washington, Armed Forces Institute of Pathology, 1978, fasc 15, 2d series.

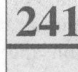

241   *Wilson S. Colucci, Eugene Braunwald*

CARDIAC TUMORS, CARDIAC MANIFESTATIONS OF SYSTEMIC DISEASES, AND TRAUMATIC CARDIAC INJURY

TUMORS OF THE HEART

PRIMARY TUMORS Primary tumors of the heart are rare and are often classified as "benign" histologically (Table 241-1). However, since all cardiac tumors have the potential for causing life-threatening complications, and many are now curable by surgery, it is important that this diagnosis be made whenever possible. Approximately three-quarters are *histologically* benign, and the remainder are malignant, in almost all cases sarcomas.

Clinical Presentation Cardiac tumors may present with a wide array of cardiac and noncardiac manifestations. There may be signs and symptoms of all the more common forms of heart disease, including chest pain, syncope, heart failure, murmurs, arrhythmias, conduction disturbances, and pericardial effusion or tamponade. The specific signs and symptoms produced are most closely related to the location of the tumor.

Myxoma Myxomas are the most common type of primary cardiac tumor for all age groups, accounting for one-third to one-half of all cases at postmortem and for approximately three-quarters of the tumors that are treated surgically. They occur at all ages and show no sex preference. Although the large majority of myxomas are sporadic, some are familial with autosomal dominant transmission or are part of a syndrome that involves a complex of abnormalities including lentigines or pigmented nevi, primary nodular adrenal cortical disease with or without Cushing's syndrome, myxomatous mammary fibroadenomas, testicular tumors, and/or pituitary adenomas with gigantism or acromegaly. Certain constellations of findings have been referred to as the *NAME syndrome* (nevi, atrial myxoma, myxoid neurofibroma, and ephelides) or the *LAMB syndrome* (lentigines, atrial myxoma, and blue nevi). Approximately 7 percent of cardiac myxomas are familial or part of the *syndrome myxoma* with complex abnormalities described above.

Most authorities consider myxoma to be a true neoplasm, while others have suggested that it is formed by organization of an intracardiac thrombus attached to the endocardium. The large majority of sporadic myxomas are solitary and located in the atria, particularly the left, where they arise from the interatrial septum in the vicinity of the fossa ovalis. Sporadic myxomas may also occur in the ventricles or may be found in multiple locations. In contrast to sporadic myxomas, familial or syndrome myxoma tumors tend to occur in younger individuals, are more often multiple in location, and are more likely to have postoperative recurrences, probably reflecting their multicentric nature (Table 241-2). Most are pedunculated on a fibrovascular stalk and average 4 to 8 cm in diameter. The most common clinical presentation resembles that of mitral valve disease, either stenosis as a result of tumor prolapse into the mitral orifice during diastole or regurgitation as a consequence of injury to the valve by tumor-induced trauma. Ventricular myxomas may cause outflow obstruction and may therefore mimic subaortic or subpulmonic stenosis.

The symptoms and signs of atrial myxomas are highly dependent on position, intermittent, and sudden in onset as a result of changes in tumor position with gravity. On auscultation, a characteristic low-pitched sound, termed a "tumor plop," is audible during early or middiastole and is thought to result from the tumor abruptly stopping as it strikes the ventricular wall. Myxomas may also present with peripheral or pulmonary emboli, or any of several noncardiac signs and symptoms including fever, weight loss, cachexia, malaise, arthralgia, rash, clubbing, Raynaud's phenomenon, hypergammaglobulinemia, anemia, polycythemia, leukocytosis, elevated erythrocyte sedimentation rate, thrombocytopenia, or thrombocytosis. Not surprisingly, myxomas are frequently misdiagnosed as endocarditis, collagen vascular disease, or noncardiac tumor.

Two-dimensional echocardiography is useful in the diagnosis of cardiac myxoma and allows determination of the site of tumor attachment and tumor size, important considerations in the planning of surgical excision. Computed tomography and particularly magnetic resonance imaging may provide important information regarding the size, shape, composition, and surface characteristics of the tumor. Because myxomas may be familial, echocardiographic screening of first-degree relatives is appropriate, particularly if the patient is young and has multiple tumors or other evidence of syndrome myxoma. While cardiac catheterization and angiography are often performed

Table 241-2

Comparison of Clinical Features of Sporadic Myxoma and Syndrome Myxoma

Feature	Sporadic	Syndrome
Age (year) (range)	56 (39–82)	25 (10–56)
Female/male ratio	2.7:1	1.8:1
Patients (no.)	70	44
Cardiac myxomas (no.)	72	103
Distributions of myxomas (%):		
Atrial/ventricular	100/0	87/13
Single/multiple	99/1	50/50
Biatrial	0	23
Recurrent	0	18
Freckling (%)	0	68
Noncardiac tumors (%)	0	57
Endocrine neoplasm (%)	0	30
Familial (%)	0	14

SOURCE: HJ Vidaillet et al, Br Heart J 57:247, 1987

prior to surgery, catheterization of the chamber from which the tumor originates is attended by the risk of dislodgment of tumor emboli. In many centers catheterization is no longer considered mandatory when adequate noninvasive information is available and other cardiac diseases (e.g., coronary artery disease) are not considered likely.

 TREATMENT

Surgical excision utilizing cardiopulmonary bypass is indicated and is generally curative. Myxomas recur in approximately 12 to 22 percent of familial cases and in about 1 to 2 percent of sporadic cases; tumor recurrence is most likely due to multifocal lesions in the former and inadequate resection in the latter.

Other Benign Tumors Cardiac *lipomas*, although relatively common, are usually incidental findings at postmortem examination and seldom result in symptoms. However, they may grow as large as 15 cm and present with symptoms due to mechanical interference with cardiac function, arrhythmias, or conduction disturbances, or as an abnormality of the cardiac silhouette on chest x-ray. *Papillary fibroelastomas*, similarly, are relatively common findings on cardiac valves or the adjacent endothelium at postmortem but seldom result in clinical symptoms. Occasionally, these growths may cause mechanical interference with valvular function. *Rhabdomyomas* and *fibromas*, the most frequent tumors in infants and children, most commonly occur in the ventricles, and therefore produce signs and symptoms by mechanical obstruction, which may mimic valvular stenosis, congestive heart failure, restrictive or hypertrophic cardiomyopathy, and pericardial constriction. Rhabdomyomas are probably hamartomatous growths, are multiple in about 90 percent of cases, and may be associated with tuberous sclerosis, adenoma sebaceum, and benign kidney tumors in approximately 30 percent of patients. Calcification of a cardiac tumor strongly suggests that it is a fibroma, although myxomas and sarcomas may also be calcified. *Hemangiomas* and *mesotheliomas* are generally small tumors, most often intramyocardial in location, and may cause atrioventricular conduction disturbances and even sudden death as a result of their propensity for location in the region of the AV node.

Sarcomas Cardiac sarcomas may be of several histologic types, but in general are characterized by a rapidly downhill course leading to the patient's death in weeks to months from the time of presentation as a result of hemodynamic compromise, local invasion, or distant metastases. Sarcomas commonly involve the right side of the heart, and because of their rapid growth, invasion of the pericardial space and obstruction of the cardiac chambers or venae cavae are common. Sarcomas also can occur on the left side of the heart and they may be mistaken for myxomas. At the time of presentation these tumors have often spread too extensively for surgical excision. While there are scattered reports of palliation with surgery, radiotherapy, and/or chemotherapy, the overall experience with cardiac sarcomas is poor. The one exception to this appears to be cardiac lymphosarcomas, which may respond to a combination of chemo- and radiotherapy.

TUMORS METASTATIC TO THE HEART Tumors metastatic to the heart are several times more common than primary tumors, and as the life expectancy of patients with various forms of malignant neoplasms is extended by more effective therapy, the frequency of cardiac metastases will also increase. Although cardiac metastases occur in 1 to 20 percent of all tumor types, the incidence is especially high in malignant melanoma and, to a somewhat lesser extent, in leukemia and lymphoma. In absolute numbers, cardiac metastases are most common in carcinoma of the breast and lung, reflecting the high incidence of these cancers. Cardiac metastases almost always occur in the setting of widespread primary disease, and most often there is either primary or metastatic disease elsewhere in the thoracic cavity. Nevertheless, occasionally a cardiac metastasis may be the initial presentation of a tumor elsewhere in the body.

Cardiac metastases reach the heart via the bloodstream, lymphatics, or direct invasion and generally are small, firm nodules; diffuse infiltrations may also occur, especially with sarcomas or hematologic neoplasms. The pericardium is most often involved, followed by myocardial involvement of any chamber, and, rarely, by involvement of the endocardium or cardiac valves.

Cardiac metastases result in clinical manifestations only about 10 percent of the time, and rarely are they the cause of death. In most patients they are *not* the cause of the presenting clinical features but occur in the setting of a previously recognized malignant neoplasm. While cardiac metastases may present a large number of nonspecific signs and symptoms, the most common are dyspnea, signs of acute pericarditis, cardiac tamponade, a rapid increase in the cardiac silhouette on chest x-ray, the new onset of an ectopic tachyarrhythmia, AV block, and congestive heart failure. As with primary cardiac tumors, the clinical presentation is more closely related to the location and size of the tumor than to its histologic type. Many of these signs and symptoms may also occur with myocarditis, pericarditis, or cardiomyopathy resulting from radiotherapy or chemotherapy.

The electrocardiographic findings are entirely nonspecific and may include ST-T-wave changes, decreased QRS voltage, arrhythmias, and conduction disturbances. On chest roentgenography the cardiac silhouette is most often normal but may reveal a pericardial effusion or bizarre contour. Echocardiography is useful for the diagnosis of pericardial effusion and the visualization of larger metastases. Computed tomography, magnetic resonance imaging, and radionuclide imaging with gallium or thallium may provide useful anatomic information. Angiography may delineate discrete lesions, and pericardiocentesis can allow a specific cytologic diagnosis. Since most patients with cardiac metastases have widespread disease, therapy generally consists of pericardiocentesis when there is hemodynamic compromise and treatment directed at the primary tumor. The removal of a malignant effusion by pericardiocentesis, with or without concomitant instillation of a sclerosing agent (e.g., tetracycline), or placement of a pericardial window for drainage to the pleural space may palliate symptoms and delay or prevent reaccumulation of the effusion.

CARDIAC EFFECTS OF CANCER THERAPY → *See Chap. 239.*

CARDIOVASCULAR MANIFESTATIONS OF SYSTEMIC DISEASES

DIABETES MELLITUS (See Chap. 334) There is an increased incidence of large vessel atherosclerosis and myocardial infarction in patients with insulin- and non-insulin-dependent diabetes mellitus. Coronary artery disease is the most common cause of death in adults with diabetes mellitus. Diabetes mellitus is an independent risk factor for coronary artery disease, and the incidence of coronary artery disease is related to the duration of diabetes. In patients with diabetes mellitus, myocardial infarctions are not only more frequent but also tend to be larger in size and more likely to result in complications such as heart failure, shock, and death. Diabetic patients are more likely to have an abnormal or absent pain response to myocardial ischemia, probably as a result of generalized autonomic nervous system dysfunction. Ambulatory electrocardiographic monitoring has shown that up to 90 percent of the episodes of ischemia are silent in diabetic patients with coronary artery disease; the presentation of ischemia may be exertional or episodic dyspnea, flash pulmonary edema, arrhythmias, heart block, or syncope. Because coronary artery disease is more common in diabetics and often is not associated with typical anginal symptoms, the threshold for the diagnosis should be low, particularly when the duration of disease is long and other risk factors for coronary artery disease (e.g., hypertension, smoking, hyperlipidemia) are present. In such patients, exercise testing should be used to detect ischemia and to determine the need for cardiac catheterization and therapeutic interventions.

Diabetic patients may also have myocardial dysfunction characteristic of a restrictive cardiomyopathy in the absence of large-vessel coronary artery disease, with abnormal relaxation of the myocardium, and evidenced clinically by elevated left ventricular filling pressures. Histologically, these patients have interstitial fibrosis with increased amounts of collagen, glycoprotein, triglycerides, and cholesterol in the myocardial interstitium, and in some cases intimal thickening, hyaline deposition, and inflammatory changes have been observed in small intramural arteries. Diabetic patients have an increased risk of developing clinical heart failure, even after correction for the presence of coronary artery disease, hypertension, and obesity, and it is likely that diabetic cardiomyopathy contributes to excessive cardiovascular morbidity and mortality of these patients. There is some evidence that insulin therapy results in an amelioration of the myocardial dysfunction.

MALNUTRITION AND THIAMINE DEFICIENCY (BERIBERI) Malnutrition (See Chap. 74) In patients whose intake of protein, calories, or both is severely deficient, the heart may become thin, pale, and flabby with myofibrillar atrophy and interstitial edema. The systolic pressure and cardiac output are low and the pulse pressure narrow. Generalized edema is common and is due to a combination of factors, including reduced serum oncotic pressure and myocardial dysfunction. Such profound states of malnutrition, termed *marasmus* in the case of caloric deficiency or *kwashiorkor* in the case of relative protein deficiency, are most common in underdeveloped countries. However, significant nutritional heart disease may also occur in developed nations, particularly in patients with chronic diseases such as AIDS, in the semistarvation that can occur in anorexia nervosa, or in patients with severe cardiac failure in whom gastrointestinal hypoperfusion and venous congestion may cause anorexia and malabsorption. Open-heart surgery poses an increased risk in such patients, who may benefit from preoperative intensive hyperalimentation. Deficient nutrients and minerals should be replaced gradually since rapid expansion of the intravascular space may stress the weakened heart and result in overt congestive heart failure.

Thiamine Deficiency (See Chap. 79) In many cases, malnutrition is accompanied by thiamine deficiency, although this hypovitaminosis may also occur in the presence of an adequate protein and caloric intake, particularly in the Far East, where polished rice deficient in thiamine may be a major dietary component. Because of the widespread use of thiamine-enriched flour in western nations, this disease is seen primarily in alcoholics and food faddists. However, there is evidence that patients with chronic heart failure frequently have thiamine deficiency also, which can be quantified biochemically by the measurement of the erythrocyte thiamine-pyrophosphate effect (TPPE). A high TPPE, which indicates thiamine deficiency, has been found in 20 to 90 percent of patients with chronic heart failure. The basis for thiamine deficiency in these patients appears to be related to both reduced dietary intake and a diuretic-induced increase in the urinary excretion of thiamine. The acute administration of thiamine to such patients increases the left ventricular ejection fraction and the excretion of salt and water.

Clinically, there is usually evidence of generalized malnutrition, peripheral neuropathy, glossitis, and anemia. The characteristic cardiovascular syndrome is that of high-output heart failure with tachycardia, increased cardiac output, and often elevated filling pressures in the left and right sides of the heart. The major cause of the high-output state is vasomotor depression, the precise mechanism of which is not understood but which leads to a reduced systemic vascular resistance. The cardiac examination reveals a wide pulse pressure, tachycardia, a third heart sound, and, frequently, an apical systolic murmur. The electrocardiogram may show decreased voltage, a prolonged QT interval, and T-wave abnormalities; the chest x-ray generally shows a large heart with signs of congestive heart failure. The response to thiamine is often dramatic, with an increase in systemic vascular resistance, decrease in cardiac output, clearing of pulmonary congestion, and a reduction in heart size often occurring in 12 to 48 h. Although the response to digitalis and diuretics may be poor prior to thiamine therapy, these agents may be important *after* thiamine is given, since the left ventricle may not be capable of dealing with the increased workload presented by the return of vascular tone.

OBESITY (See Chap. 75) Although not defined as a disease per se, severe obesity, particularly when it occurs in an upper-body distribution, is associated with an increase in cardiovascular morbidity and mortality, due in part to hypertension, glucose intolerance, and atherosclerotic coronary artery disease, all of which are more prevalent in obese patients. In addition, these patients have a distinct abnormality of the cardiovascular system characterized by increases in total and central blood volumes, cardiac output, and left ventricular filling pressure. It appears that cardiac output is elevated in order to help supply the metabolic needs of the excessive adipose tissue. Left ventricular filling pressure is often at the upper limits of normal and rises excessively with exercise. As a result of chronic volume overload, eccentric cardiac hypertrophy with cardiac dilatation and abnormal ventricular function may develop. Pathologically, there are left and, in some cases, right ventricular hypertrophy and generalized cardiac dilatation, which is not due simply to fatty infiltration of the myocardium. Although these patients may develop pulmonary congestion, peripheral edema, and exercise intolerance, these findings may be difficult to recognize in massively obese patients. Weight reduction is the most effective therapy and results in reduction in blood volume and in the return of cardiac output toward normal. However, rapid weight reduction may cause cardiac arrhythmias and sudden death due to electrolyte imbalance. Digitalis, sodium restriction, and diuretics may also be useful. This form of heart disease should be distinguished from the Pickwickian syndrome (Chap. 263), which may share several of the cardiovascular features but, in addition, frequently has components of central apnea, hypoxemia, pulmonary hypertension, and cor pulmonale.

THYROID DISEASE (See Chap. 331) Thyroid hormone exerts a major influence on the cardiovascular system by a number of direct and indirect mechanisms, and not surprisingly, cardiovascular effects are prominent in both hypo- and hyperthyroidism. Thyroid hormone causes increases in total-body metabolism and oxygen consumption that indirectly place an increased workload on the heart. In addition, although the exact mechanism has not been defined, thyroid hormone exerts direct inotropic, chronotropic, and dromotropic effects that are similar to those seen with adrenergic stimulation (e.g., tachycardia, increased cardiac output). It has been shown that thyroid hormone increases the synthesis of myosin and of Na^+,K^+-ATPase, as well as the density of myocardial beta-adrenergic receptors.

Hyperthyroidism Patients may present with palpitations, systolic hypertension, fatigue, or, in patients with underlying heart disease, angina or heart failure. Sinus tachycardia is found in about 40 percent of patients, and atrial fibrillation in about 15 percent. Other findings include a hyperactive precordium, a widened pulse pressure, an increase in the intensity of the first heart sound and the pulmonic component of the second heart sound, and a third heart sound. An increased incidence of mitral valve prolapse has been associated with hyperthyroidism, and in some cases there may be a midsystolic murmur heard best at the left sternal border with or without a systolic ejection click. A systolic scratchy sound, the *Means-Lerman scratch*, may occasionally be heard at the left second intercostal space during expiration and is thought to result from the rubbing of the hyperdynamic pericardium against the pleura. Elderly patients with hyperthyroidism, so-called apathetic hyperthyroidism, may present with only the cardiovascular manifestations of thyrotoxicosis, such as atrial fibrillation, which may be resistant to therapy until the hyperthyroidism is controlled. Angina pectoris and congestive heart failure are unusual unless there is coexistent underlying heart disease, and in many cases will resolve with therapy of the hyperthyroidism.

Hypothyroidism There is a reduction in cardiac output, stroke volume, heart rate, blood pressure, and pulse pressure. In about one-third of patients there is a pericardial effusion which only rarely results in tamponade. Increased capillary permeability results in pleural and pericardial effusions. Other clinical signs include cardiomegaly, bradycardia, weak arterial pulses, and distant heart sounds. Although the signs and symptoms of myxedema may suggest the diagnosis of congestive heart failure, in the absence of other cardiac disease, myocardial failure is uncommon. The electrocardiogram generally shows sinus bradycardia and low voltage and may show prolongation of the QT interval, decreased P-wave voltage, prolonged AV conduction time, intraventricular conduction disturbances, and nonspecific ST-T-wave abnormalities. Chest x-ray may show cardiomegaly, often with a "water bottle" configuration, pleural effusions, and, in some cases, evidence of congestive heart failure. Pathologically, the heart is pale, dilated, and flabby, often with myofibrillar swelling, loss of striations, and interstitial fibrosis.

Patients with hypothyroidism frequently have elevations of cholesterol and triglycerides and severe atherosclerotic coronary artery disease. Prior to treatment with thyroid hormone, patients with hypothyroidism frequently do not have angina pectoris, presumably because of the low metabolic demands made by their condition. However, such patients, especially when elderly, are prone to angina and myocardial infarction during replacement of thyroid hormone, and this should always be done with care, starting with very low doses which are increased gradually.

MALIGNANT CARCINOID (See Chap. 95) These tumors elaborate a variety of vasoactive amines (e.g., serotonin), kinins, indoles, and other substances believed to be responsible for the diarrhea, flushing, and labile blood pressure seen in these patients. The cardiac lesions due to gastrointestinal carcinoids are almost exclusively in the right side of the heart and occur only when there are hepatic metastases, suggesting that the substance responsible for the cardiac lesions is inactivated by passage through the liver and lungs. Similar lesions occur in the left side of the heart when there is a right-to-left shunt or the tumor is located in the lungs. Fibrous plaques are found on the endothelium of the cardiac chambers, valves, and great vessels. These plaques, which result in distortion of the cardiac valves, consist of smooth-muscle cells embedded in a stroma of acid mucopolysaccharide and collagen and presumably result from healing of endothelial injury. The clinical syndrome is most often that of tricuspid regurgitation, pulmonic stenosis, or both. In some cases a high-output state may occur, presumably as a result of a decrease in systemic vascular resistance due to a vasoactive substance released by the tumor. Progression of the cardiac lesions does not appear to be affected by treatment with serotonin antagonists, and in some severely symptomatic patients valve replacement is indicated. Coronary artery spasm, presumably due to a circulating vasoactive substance, may occur in patients with carcinoid syndrome.

PHEOCHROMOCYTOMA (See Chap. 333) In addition to causing hypertension, which may be labile or sustained, the high circulating levels of catecholamines may also cause direct myocardial injury. Focal myocardial necrosis and inflammatory cell infiltration are seen in about 50 percent of patients who die with pheochromocytoma and may contribute to clinically significant left ventricular failure and pulmonary edema. Left ventricular function and congestive heart failure may resolve after removal of the tumor. In addition, hypertension results in left ventricular hypertrophy.

RHEUMATOID ARTHRITIS AND THE COLLAGEN VASCULAR DISEASES Rheumatoid Arthritis (See Chap. 313) There may be inflammation of any or all parts of the heart in patients with rheumatoid arthritis. *Pericarditis* is the most common cause of clinically apparent disease and may be found by echocardiography in 10 to 50 percent of all patients with rheumatoid arthritis, particularly those with subcutaneous nodules. However, only a small fraction of these patients have clinical evidence of pericarditis, which usually follows a benign course but occasionally may progress to cardiac tamponade or constrictive pericarditis. The pericardial fluid is generally an exudate, with decreased concentrations of complement and glucose and elevated cholesterol. Treatment is directed at the underlying rheumatoid arthritis and may include glucocorticoids. Pericardiectomy is usually required in cases of tamponade or persistent effusion. *Coronary arteritis* with intimal inflammation and edema is present in about 20 percent of cases but only rarely results in angina pectoris or myocardial infarction. The cardiac valves, most often the mitral and aortic, may be involved by inflammation and granuloma

formation that in some cases may cause clinically significant regurgitation due to valve deformity. Myocarditis rarely results in cardiac dysfunction.

Seronegative Arthropathies The seronegative arthropathies (Chaps. 317 and 325), ankylosing spondylitis, Reiter's syndrome, psoriatic arthritis, and the arthritides associated with ulcerative colitis and regional enteritis may be accompanied by a pancarditis and proximal aortitis; the latter may result in aortic regurgitation and may extend into the anterior mitral valve ring and/or AV node. Conduction disturbances are common, occurring in up to one-third of patients; they are more common in patients with aortic valve disease and appear to be associated with the presence of the HLA-B27 antigen. Both aortic regurgitation and AV block are more common in patients with peripheral joint involvement and long-standing disease; treatment with aortic valve replacement and permanent pacemaker placement may be required. Up to one-fifth of patients with peripheral joint involvement and disease for more than 30 years have significant aortic regurgitation. Occasionally, aortic regurgitation precedes the onset of arthritis, and, therefore, the diagnosis of a seronegative arthritis should be considered in young males with isolated aortic regurgitation.

Systemic Lupus Erythematosus (SLE) (See Chap. 312) Pericarditis is common, occurring in about two-thirds of patients, and generally pursues a benign course, although rarely tamponade or constriction may result. The characteristic *endocardial lesions* of SLE, described by Libman and Sacks, consist of wartlike lesions most often located at the angles of the AV valves or on the ventricular surface of the mitral valve. Hemodynamically important valvular regurgitation is rare. Patients with the antiphospholipid syndrome have a higher incidence of cardiovascular abnormalities including valvular disease (particularly regurgitant lesions), a variety of thrombotic disorders (venous and arterial thrombosis, thrombocytopenia, premature stroke), myocardial infarction, pulmonary hypertension, and cardiomyopathy. Myocarditis generally parallels the activity of the disease, and although common histologically, seldom results in clinical heart failure unless associated with hypertension. Although arteritis of large coronary arteries may rarely result in myocardial ischemia, there is also an increased frequency of coronary atherosclerosis that may be related to hypertension or glucocorticoid therapy.

TRAUMATIC HEART DISEASE

Cardiac damage may be due to both penetrating and nonpenetrating injuries. The most frequent cause of a *nonpenetrating injury* is impact of the chest against the steering wheel of an automobile. Serious injury of the heart may ensue even though no external sign of thoracic trauma is evident. Although the commonest injury is myocardial contusion, any structure of the heart may be affected by the trauma. If the valvular apparatus is ruptured, a loud heart murmur produced by valvular regurgitation may appear, followed by the development of rapidly progressive heart failure.

Myocardial contusion may cause arrhythmias, bundle branch block, or electrocardiographic abnormalities resembling those of infarction, and so it is important to bear trauma in mind as a cause of otherwise unexplained electrocardiographic changes. Similarly, myocardial contusion may produce positive radionuclide scans and regional impairment of ventricular function, as occurs in myocardial infarction (Chap. 243). Myocardial contusions are often not immediately appreciated. Increased serum creatine kinase (CK) MB levels may be seen in about 20 percent of patients, but false-positive MB elevations may be seen in the presence of massive injuries associated with large increases in total CK. Pericardial effusion may occur weeks or even months after the accident. In these cases, the pericardial effusion is a manifestation of the postcardiac injury syndrome, which resembles the postpericardiotomy syndrome (Chap. 240). The most serious consequence of nonpenetrating injury is rupture, either of the atria or of the ventricles. Although generally immediately fatal, survival of cardiac rupture has been reported in up to 40 percent of cases of patients who survived long enough to reach a specialized trauma center. Hemopericardium may also follow tearing of a pericardial vessel or coronary artery.

℞ TREATMENT

Acute myocardial failure resulting from rupture of a valve usually requires operative correction. The treatment of an uncomplicated myocardial contusion, with or without myocardial infarction, is similar to that for a myocardial infarction, except that anticoagulation is contraindicated, and should include monitoring for the development of complications such as arrhythmias and cardiac rupture (Chap. 243). Pericardial hemorrhage often leads to constriction, which must be treated by decortication.

Penetrating injuries of the heart, produced by bullets or stab wounds, usually result in immediate or very rapid death because of hemopericardium or massive hemorrhage. However, up to half of such patients may survive if they are resuscitated and/or survive long enough to reach a specialized trauma center. Another common cause of penetrating injuries is the fracture or dislodgment of an intravenous or intracardiac catheter or pacemaker lead. Immediate thoracotomy should be carried out if there is cardiac tamponade and/or shock, whether the trauma was penetrating or nonpenetrating. Pericardiocentesis may be helpful in patients with tamponade, but usually only as a holding maneuver. Patients who suffer penetrating injuries of the heart should be carefully examined several weeks after the event to rule out a ventricular septal defect or mitral regurgitation that may have gone undetected at the time of emergency surgery. Sometimes the patient survives the acute incident and presents with a cardiac murmur and congestive heart failure. A left-to-right shunt due to traumatic ventricular septal defect, aortopulmonary artery fistula, or coronary arteriovenous fistula may be suspected and confirmed by cardiac catheterization and angiocardiography. Operation is indicated if hemodynamically significant abnormalities are present or if a foreign body, e.g., a bullet, is lodged in the heart.

Rupture of the aorta is a common consequence of chest trauma. Indeed, rupture of the aorta at the isthmus or just above the aortic valve is the most common vascular deceleration injury. The clinical presentation is similar to that in aortic dissection (Chap. 247). The arterial pressure and pulse amplitude may be increased in the upper extremities and decreased in the lower extremities, and on chest roentgenogram there may be widening of the mediastinum. Occasionally, the rupture is limited by the aortic adventitia and results in a silent false aneurysm that may be discovered months or years after the injury. When great vessel rupture is due to a penetrating injury, there is usually a hemothorax and, less often, a hemopericardium. Hematoma formation may compress major vessels, and arteriovenous fistulae may be formed, sometimes resulting in high-output congestive heart failure.

BIBLIOGRAPHY

COBLYN JS, WEINBLATT M: Rheumatic diseases and the heart, in *Heart Disease*, 5th ed, E Braunwald (ed). Philadelphia, Saunders, 1997, p 1776

COHN PR, BRAUNWALD E: Traumatic heart disease, in *Heart Disease*, 5th ed, E Braunwald (ed). Philadelphia, Saunders, 1997, p 1535

COLUCCI WS, BRAUNWALD E: Primary tumors of the heart, in *Heart Disease*, 5th ed, E Braunwald (ed). Philadelphia, Saunders, 1997, p 394

DUFLOU J et al: Sudden death as a result of heart disease in morbid obesity. Am Heart J 130:306, 1995

HENDERSON VJ et al: Cardiac injuries: Analysis of an unselected series of 251 cases. J Trauma 36:341, 1994

IMPERATO-MCGINLEY J et al: Reversibility of catecholamine-induced cardiomyopathy in a child with a pheochromocytoma. N Engl J Med 316:793, 1987

KOISTINEN MJ et al: Asymptomatic coronary artery disease in diabetes: Relation to common risk factors, lipoproteins, apoproteins and apo E polymorphism. Acta Diabetol 31:210, 1994

LADENSON PW: Recognition and management of cardiovascular disease related to thyroid dysfunction. Am J Med 88:638, 1990

O'NEILL TW et al: The heart in ankylosing spondylitis. Ann Rheum Dis 51:705, 1992

REYNEN K: Cardiac myxomas. N Engl J Med 333:1610, 1995

ROBIOLIO PA: Carcinoid heart disease. Correlation of high serotonin levels with valvular abnormalities detected by cardiac catheterization and echocardiography. Circulation 92:790, 1995

ROLDAN C et al: Systemic lupus erythematosus valve disease by transesophageal echocardiography and the role of antiphospholipid antibodies. J Am Coll Cardiol 20:1127, 1992

SHAHIAN DM et al: Etiology and management of chronic valve disease in antiphospholipid antibody syndrome and systemic lupus erythematosus. J Card Surg 10:133, 1995

SHIMON I et al: Improved left ventricular function after thiamine supplementation in patients with congestive heart failure receiving long-term furosemide therapy. Am J Med 98:485, 1995

SMITH MK: Transesophageal echocardiography in the diagnosis of rupture of the aorta. N Engl J Med 332:356, 1995

UUSITUPA MI et al: Diabetic heart muscle disease. Ann Med 22:377, 1990

SECTION 4
VASCULAR DISEASE

242	*Peter Libby*

ATHEROSCLEROSIS

Atherosclerosis leads as a cause of death and disability in the developed world. The name, derived from Greek, refers to the thickening of the arterial intima (*sclerosis*, "hardening") and accumulation of lipid (*athere*, "gruel") that characterize the typical lesion. Despite our familiarity with this disease, some of its fundamental characteristics remain poorly recognized and understood. Although many generalized or systemic risk factors predispose to its development, this disease preferentially affects certain regions of the circulation. Atherosclerosis causes distinct clinical manifestations depending on the circulatory ity (Chap. 248). Involvement of the splanchnic circulation can cause mesenteric ischemia and bowel infarction. Atherosclerosis can affect the kidney directly (e.g., causing renal artery stenosis), and, in addition, the kidney is a frequent site of atheroembolic disease. Renal artery atherosclerosis can also contribute to the pathogenesis of hypertension, itself a risk factor for the development of atherosclerosis (Chap. 277).

Even in a given arterial bed, atherosclerosis tends to occur focally, typically in certain predisposed regions, while sparing adjacent segments. For example, in the coronary circulation, the proximal left anterior descending coronary artery has a particular predilection for developing atherosclerotic occlusive disease. Likewise, atherosclerosis preferentially affects the proximal portions of the renal arteries, and, in the cerebrovascular circulation, the carotid bifurcation. Other arteries, such as the internal mammary arteries, seldom harbor atherosclerotic

decades. However, the growth of atherosclerotic plaques probably is discontinuous rather than smoothly linear, with periods of relative quiescence punctuated by episodes of rapid evolution. After a generally prolonged "silent" period, atherosclerosis may become clinically manifest. The clinical expressions of atherosclerosis may be chronic, as in the development of stable effort-induced angina pectoris or predictable and reproducible intermittent claudication. Alternatively, a much more dramatic acute clinical event, such as a myocardial infarction or cerebrovascular accident, may be the first manifestation of atherosclerosis. Other individuals never experience clinical manifestations of arterial disease, even though the presence of widespread atherosclerosis is demonstrated post mortem. Recently, understanding of the reasons why this disease can be stable, unstable, or clinically silent has advanced, as will be discussed below.

The way in which atherosclerosis affects an arterial segment also varies, an additional feature of the heterogeneity and complexity of this disease. Atheromas are usually thought of as stenotic lesions, causing flow limitation or arterial occlusion. However, atherosclerosis can also cause ectasia and development of aneurysmal disease with an increase in lumen caliber. This expression of atherosclerosis frequently occurs in the aorta, creating a predisposition to rupture or dissection rather than to stenosis or occlusion.

The heterogeneity of this disease and the diversity of its causes, natural histories, and clinical manifestations seem difficult to explain. However, contemporary research provides some fundamental pathobiologic principles that provide a basis for understanding this multifaceted process. To furnish a background for a clinical approach to patients with atherosclerotic disease, this chapter will consider the phases in the formation, progression, and complication of lesions. In particular, the chapter will emphasize emerging aspects of the biology of atherosclerosis that provide insight into its pathogenesis, in relation to the prevention or limitation of atherosclerosis and therapies for reducing its manifestations.

INITIATION OF ATHEROSCLEROSIS   Lipoprotein Accumulation and Modification   In normal human adults, the intimal layer of arteries contains some resident smooth muscle cells embedded in extracellular matrix and is covered with a monolayer of vascular endothelial cells (Fig. 242-1A). Taken together, experimental results in animals and studies of human atherosclerosis suggest that the "fatty streak" represents the initial lesion of atherosclerosis. The formation of these early lesions probably results from focal accumulation of lipoproteins in regions of the intimal layer of the artery (Fig. 242-2B). Lipoprotein particles transport lipids such as cholesterol and triglycerides in association with proteins and phospholipids that render the lipids soluble in blood. Low-density lipoprotein (LDL) particles, rich in cholesterol, are an example of an atherogenic lipoprotein (see Chap. 341). The accumulation of lipoprotein particles in the arterial intima during early atherogenesis may not result simply from an increase in the permeability or leakiness of the overlying endothelium. Rather, these lipoproteins may collect in the intima of arteries because they bind to constituents of the extracellular matrix, which increases their residence time in the arterial wall. Lipoproteins that accumulate in the extracellular space of the arterial intima often associate with proteoglycan molecules of the arterial extracellular matrix. At sites of lesion formation, the balance of different matrix constituents may vary in important ways. For example, of the three major classes of proteoglycans, a relative excess of heparan sulfate molecules in relation to keratan sulfate or chondroitin sulfate may promote the retention of lipoprotein particles by binding them and slowing their egress from nascent lesions.

Lipoprotein particles in the extracellular space of the intima, particularly those bound to matrix macromolecules, may undergo chemical modifications. Accumulating evidence supports a potentially pathogenic role for such modifications in atherogenesis. Two types of alterations are of particular interest in relation to how risk factors promote atherogenesis: oxidation and nonenzymatic glycation. Lipoproteins

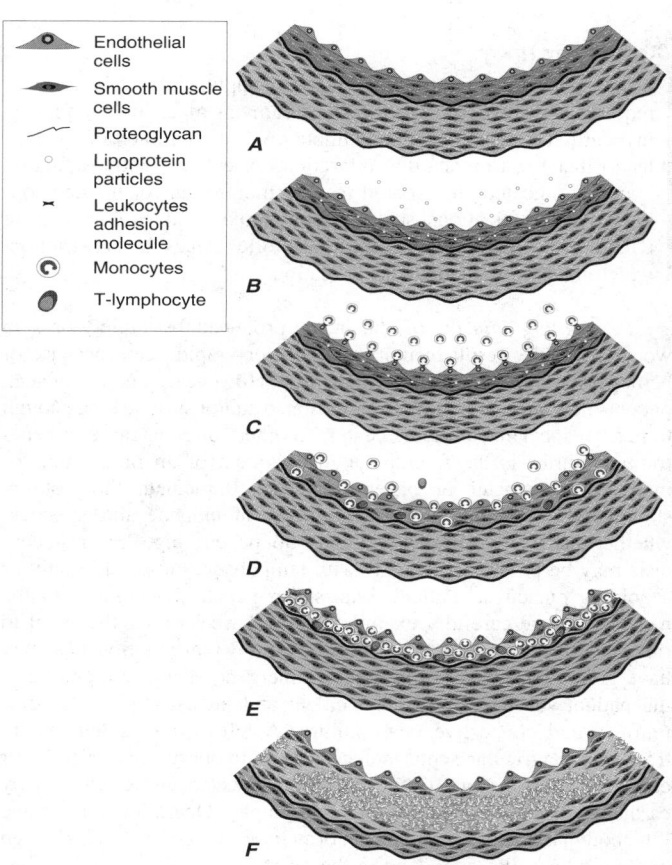

	Endothelial cells
	Smooth muscle cells
	Proteoglycan
	Lipoprotein particles
	Leukocytes adhesion molecule
	Monocytes
	T-lymphocyte

FIGURE 242-1   Fatty Streak Formation. *A.* The normal artery. The normal artery consists of three layers. The intima, lined by a monolayer of endothelial cells in contact with the blood, contains smooth muscle cells embedded in extracellular matrix. The internal elastic lamina forms the border of the intima with the underlying tunica media. The media contains layers of smooth muscle cells invested with a collagen- and elastin-rich extracellular matrix. Elastic arteries such as the aorta contain concentric lamellae of smooth muscle cells sandwiched between dense bands of elastin. Muscular arteries have a looser organization of smooth muscle cells dispersed within the matrix. The external elastic lamina forms the border of the media with the adventitia. The adventitia contains nerves, some mast cells, and is the origin of the vasa vasorum which supply blood to the outer two-thirds of the tunica media. *B.* Accumulation of lipoprotein particles. Lipoprotein particles can accumulate in the intima of arteries, particularly when the ambient concentration is increased by hypercholesterolemic states. The lipoprotein particles often associate with constituents of the extracellular matrix, notably proteoglycans. Sequestration within the intima separates lipoproteins from some plasma antioxidants and can favor oxidative modification. Such modified lipoprotein particles may trigger a local inflammatory response responsible for signaling subsequent steps in lesion formation. *C.* Adhesion of leukocytes. In hypercholesterolemia, adhesion of mononuclear leukocytes to the luminal endothelium occurs early. The augmented expression of various adhesion molecules for leukocytes probably triggers this first step in the recruitment of white blood cells to the site of a nascent arterial lesion. *D.* Penetration of leukocytes. Once adherent, some white blood cells migrate into the intima. The directed migration of leukocytes probably depends on chemoattractant factors, including modified lipoprotein particles themselves and chemoattractant cytokines such as the chemokine macrophage chemoattractant protein 1 (MCP-1) produced by vascular wall cells in response to modified lipoproteins. *E.* Accumulation of leukocytes. Leukocytes resident in the evolving fatty streak can divide and exhibit augmented expression of receptors for modified lipoproteins (scavenger receptors). These mononuclear phagocytes imbibe lipids and transform into foam cells, whose cytoplasm is filled with lipid droplets. *F.* Formation of the fibrous cap and lipid core. As the fatty streak evolves into a more complicated atherosclerotic lesion, smooth muscle cells accumulate in the expanding intima and the amount of extracellular matrix increases. The fibrous cap, formed of extracellular matrix elaborated by the smooth muscle cells in the intima, characteristically overlies a lipid-rich core filled with macrophages. In addition to dividing, these core cells may die, releasing their lipid contents into the extracellular space.

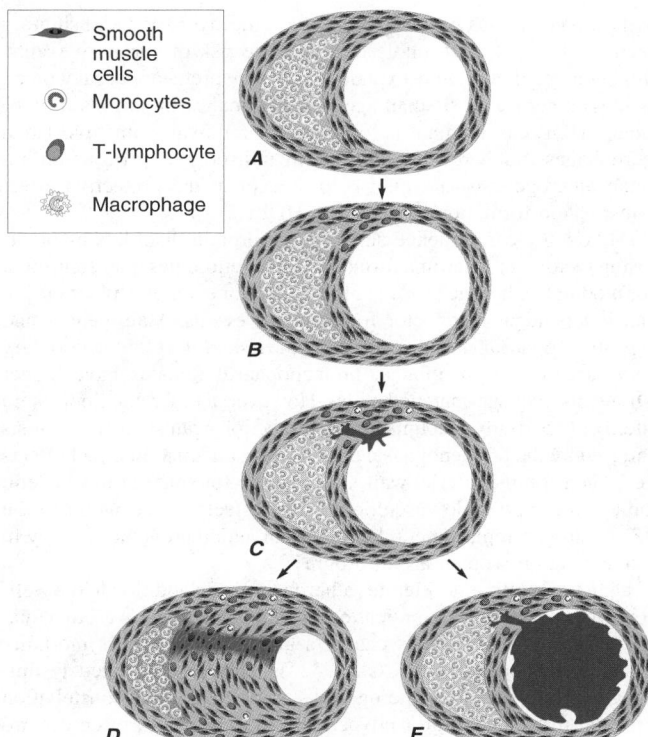

Smooth
muscle
cells

Monocytes

T-lymphocyte

Macrophage

A

B

C

D

E

FIGURE 242-2   Plaque Rupture, Thrombosis, and Healing. *A.* Arterial remodeling during atherogenesis. During the first part of their history, atheromas often grow in an abluminal direction and do not encroach on the lumen. The compensatory enlargement of the artery in this phase accounts in part for the tendency of coronary arteriography to underestimate the degree of atherosclerosis. *B.* Focal inflammation characterizes unstable atherosclerotic plaques. Foci of inflammation often occur in atheromas. Analyses of lesions that have ruptured and caused fatal myocardial infarction characteristically show a prominent infiltration of macrophages and T lymphocytes. Both the leukocytes and the intrinsic vascular cells around points of plaque rupture show markers of inflammatory activation. *C.* Rupture of the plaque's fibrous cap causes thrombosis. A physical disruption of the atherosclerotic plaque (*c*) commonly causes arterial thrombosis by allowing blood coagulant factors to contact the thrombogenic collagen in the arterial extracellular matrix and tissue factors produced by macrophage-derived foam cells in the lipid core of the lesion. A site of plaque rupture thus serves as a nidus for thrombus formation. The normal artery wall has several fibrinolytic and antithrombotic mechanisms that tend to resist thrombosis and lyse clots that begin to form in situ. Such antithrombotic or thrombolytic molecules include thrombomodulin, tissue and urokinase-type plasminogen activators, heparan sulfate proteoglycans, prostacyclin, and nitric oxide. These mechanisms may prevail, or they may be overwhelmed, allowing the clot to propagate (as in *E*). *D.* Healing of a mural thrombus leads to lesion fibrosis and progression and luminal narrowing. Instances of thrombosis in which the thrombus undergoes lysis or is organized into a mural thrombus without occluding the vessel instances may be clinically silent. The subsequent thrombin-induced fibrosis and healing cause a fibroproliferative response that can lead to a more fibrous lesion. Specifically, local thrombin activation can stimulate smooth muscle proliferation. Proteins released from platelets, including platelet-derived growth factors and transforming growth factor β, may also augment collagen production by smooth muscle cells and modulate their growth. Thus, healing may can promote lesion fibrosis and luminal encroachment. Interestingly, such a sequence of events may convert an unstable atheroma with a thin, rupture-prone fibrous cap into a more stable fibrous plaque with a reinforced cap. Angioplasty of unstable coronary lesions may stabilize the lesions by a similar mechanisms. *E.* Plaque rupture with a propagated, occlusive thrombus can cause acute myocardial infarction. When a persistent, occlusive thrombus forms in a coronary artery, the consequences depend on the degree of existing collateral circulation. In a patient with chronic multivessel occlusive coronary artery disease, collateral channels have usually formed. In such circumstances, even a total arterial occlusion may cause no myocardial infarction or may cause an unexpectedly modest or "non-Q-wave" infarct. In the patient with less advanced disease who lacks substantial stenotic lesions, sudden plaque rupture and arterial occlusion commonly produce Q wave infarction.

sequestered from plasma antioxidants in the extracellular space of the intima may be particularly susceptible to oxidative modification. Oxidatively modified LDL, rather than being chemically homogenous, actually comprises a variable and incompletely defined mixture. Both the lipid and the protein moieties of these particles can participate in oxidative processes. Modifications of the lipids may include formation of hydroperoxides, lysophospholipids, oxysterols, and aldehydic breakdown products of fatty acids. Modifications of the apoprotein moieties may include breaks in the peptide backbone as well as derivatization of certain amino acid residues (typically the side chain amino group of lysine) with components of the oxidized lipids (9-hydroxynonenol or malondialdehyde). Considerable evidence supports the presence of such chemical entities in atherosclerotic lesions. In diabetics with sustained hyperglycemia, nonenzymatic glycation of apolipoproteins and other arterial proteins likely occurs and may likewise alter the function of these components and their propensity to accelerate atherogenesis. A good deal of experimental work suggests that both oxidatively modified and glycated lipoproteins or lipoprotein constituents can contribute to many of the subsequent cellular events of lesion development.

Leukocyte Recruitment and Foam-Cell Formation   Recruitment of leukocytes is the second step in formation of the fatty streak (Fig. 242-1*C*). The main white blood cell types typically found in the evolving atheroma are cells of the mononuclear lineage—monocytes and lymphocytes. A number of adhesion molecules or receptors for leukocytes expressed on the surface of arterial endothelial cells likely participate in the recruitment of leukocytes to the nascent fatty streak. Adhesion molecules of particular interest in this regard include vascular cell adhesion molecule 1 (VCAM-1) and intercellular adhesion molecule 1 (ICAM-1) (members of the immunoglobulin superfamily) and P-selectin (a member of a distinct family of leukocyte receptors known as selectins). Lysophosphatidylcholine, a constituent of oxidatively modified LDL, can augment the expression of VCAM-1. This example illustrates how the accumulation of lipoproteins in the arterial intima may be linked to leukocyte recruitment and subsequent events in lesion formation.

Laminar shear forces, such as those present in most regions of normal arteries, can suppress the expression of leukocyte adhesion molecules such as VCAM-1. Sites where atherosclerotic lesions commonly form (e.g., branch points) often have disturbed laminar flow. Also, the laminar shear of normal blood flow augments the production by endothelial cells of nitric oxide (NO). In addition to its well-known vasodilator properties, this molecule, at the low levels constitutively produced by arterial endothelium, can act as a local anti-inflammatory autacoid, for example acting to limit local VCAM-1 expression. Thus, the normal endothelium, by secreting NO at a steady low level, can maintain vasodilation and resist the adhesion of leukocytes. Local disturbances in hemodynamic forces may influence such cellular mechanisms that protect against atherosclerotic lesion initiation and may help explain the focal distribution of atherosclerotic lesions.

Having adhered to the surface of the arterial endothelial cell by interacting with a receptor such as VCAM-1, the monocytes and lymphocytes penetrate the endothelial layer and take up residence in the intima (Fig. 242-1*D*). In addition to constituents of modified lipoproteins, cytokines (a class of protein mediators of inflammation) can regulate the expression of adhesion molecules involved in leukocyte recruitment. For example the cytokines interleukin (IL) 1 and tumor necrosis factor-α (TNFα) induce or augment the expression of VCAM-1 and ICAM-1 on endothelial cells. Since modified lipoproteins can induce cytokine release from vascular wall cells, this pathway may provide an additional link between the accumulation and modification of lipoproteins and leukocyte recruitment. The directed migration of leukocytes into the arterial wall may also result from the actions of modified lipoprotein. For example, in vitro assays suggest that oxidized LDL promotes the chemotaxis of leukocytes. Also, oxidatively modified lipoproteins can elicit the production by vascular wall cells of chemoattractant cytokines such as monocyte chemoattractant protein 1 (MCP-1).

Once resident in the intima, the mononuclear phagocytes differentiate into macrophages, which ultimately become lipid-laden foam cells (Fig. 242-1*E–F*). The transformation of mononuclear phagocytes into foam cells requires the uptake of lipoprotein particles by receptor-mediated endocytosis. One might suppose that the well-recognized LDL receptor would mediate this uptake. However, patients and animals that lack effective LDL receptors for genetic reasons (e.g., familial hypercholesterolemia) have abundant arterial lesions and extraarterial xanthomata rich in macrophage-derived foam cells. Also, exogenous cholesterol suppresses expression of the LDL receptor, so that under conditions of hypercholesterolemia the level of this receptor decreases. Alternative candidates for receptors that mediate the lipid loading of foam cells include the macrophage scavenger receptor that preferentially endocytose modified lipoproteins and other receptors for oxidized LDL or for beta very low density lipoprotein (VLDL), a type of lipoprotein abundant in certain hypercholesterolemic states (see Chap. 341). By imbibing lipids from the extracellular space, the mononuclear phagocytes may participate in clearing the lipoproteins accumulating in the developing lesion. Some lipid-laden macrophages may leave the artery wall, functioning to clear lipid from the artery. Lipid accumulation, and hence a tendency to form an atheroma, occurs if more lipid enters the artery wall than leaves it via mononuclear phagocytes or other pathways. Macrophages thus may play a vital role in the balance of lipid metabolism in the arterial wall during atherogenesis. Some foam cells in the expanding intimal lesion perish, perhaps by apoptosis (programmed cell death) and/or other means. The death of mononuclear phagocytes results in the formation of a lipid-rich *necrotic core* in the lesion, a feature characteristic of more complicated atherosclerotic plaques (Figs. 242-1*F* and 242-2*A*).

Like the vascular wall cells, macrophages taking up modified lipoproteins may produce cytokines and growth factors that elicit some of the further cellular events in lesion complication. A number of growth factors or cytokines elaborated by mononuclear phagocytes can stimulate smooth muscle cell proliferation and the production of extracellular matrix, which accumulates in atherosclerotic plaques. IL-1 and TNF-α are examples of cytokines that can induce local production of growth factors, incuding forms of platelet-derived growth factor and fibroblast growth factor, which may play a role in plaque evolution and complication. Other cytokines, particularly interferon γ derived from activated T cell lesions, can inhibit smooth muscle proliferation and the synthesis of interstitial forms of collagen. These examples illustrate how atherogenesis likely depends on a complex balance between mediators that can promote lesion formation and other pathways that can mitigate it.

Factors That Modulate Atheroma Initiation Elaboration of small molecules by activated mononuclear phagocytes and vascular wall cells in the evolving lesion may also modulate atherogenesis. Phagocytic leukocytes (as well as vascular endothelial and smooth muscle cells) can produce reactive oxygen species when appropriately stimulated. Such reactive oxygen species can modulate the growth of smooth muscle cells, activate inflammatory gene expression via the nuclear factor κB transcriptional control system, and annihilate nitric oxide radicals, decreasing the effect of NO. However, macrophages in the lesion may be activated to express the inducible form of the enzyme that synthesizes NO, known as inducible NO synthase. This high-capacity form of the enzyme can produce relatively large, potentially cytotoxic amounts of nitric oxide radicals. While the low concentrations of NO· produced by the constitutive NO synthase in endothelial cells may have beneficial effects, the higher levels produced by activated phagocytes may be deleterious.

Export by phagocytes may be one response to local lipid overload in the evolving lesion. Another mechanism—reverse cholesterol transport mediated by high-density lipoprotein (HDL)—may provide an independent pathway for removal of lipid from the atheroma. Multiple observational studies have established a tight inverse relationship between the level of HDL cholesterol and the risk of coronary events. A higher level of HDL may explain in part why premenopausal women have less atherosclerosis than age-matched males. In various in vitro models, HDL can mediate net cholesterol removal from lipid-laden macrophages. Such reverse cholesterol transport may occur during human atherogenesis and may help to explain the protective effect against lesion formation provided by HDL.

Although clear evidence supports lipoprotein disorders as predisposing factors for atheroma formation, other etiologies may contribute to or modulate atherogenesis (Table 242-1). For example, hypertension is an independent risk factor for coronary events. Male gender and the postmenopausal state also augment the risk of developing coronary artery disease. As mentioned, premenopausal females have higher HDL levels than age-matched males. However, a favorable lipoprotein pattern only partially accounts for the protection against atherosclerosis conferred by the premenopausal state. Poorly understood direct effects of estrogens on the arterial wall may account for some of this benefit. Studies on the possible vasculoprotective effects of estrogen and the role of estrogen replacement therapy as an antiatherogenic strategy in postmenopausal women are in progress.

Diabetes mellitus accelerates atherogenesis. In addition to the well-known microvascular complications of diabetes, macrovascular disease such as atherosclerosis causes a great deal of excess mortality in the diabetic population (see Chap. 334). Diabetes-associated dyslipidemias strongly promote atherogenesis. In particular, the constellation of insulin resistance, high triglycerides, and low HDL, often accompanied by central adiposity and hypertension, that is common in type II diabetics seems to accelerate atherogenesis potently. As noted above, hyperglycemia may promote the nonenzymatic glycation of LDL. LDL modified in this manner, like oxidatively modified LDL, may signal many of the initial events in atherogenesis. Other lipoproteins, such as triglyceride-rich particles or lipoprotein (a), may also contribute to accelerated atherogenesis in diabetic individuals.

Lipoprotein (a) [Lp(a); it is often called "lipoprotein little a" to distinguish it from apolipoprotein AI] provides a potential link between hemostasis and blood lipids. The Lp(a) particle consists of an apoprotein (a) molecule bound by a sulfhydryl link to the apolipoprotein B moiety of an LDL particle. Apoprotein (a) has homology with plasminogen, and it may inhibit fibrinolysis by competing with plasminogen. Other risk factors for atherosclerosis related to blood clotting include elevated levels of fibrinogen or of plasminogen-activator inhibitor 1 (PAI-1), an inhibitor of fibrinolysis. Multiple studies have established a correlation between plasma fibrinogen levels and coronary risk. Synthesis of fibrinogen, an acute-phase reactant, increases in inflammatory states. Thus, hyperfibrinogenemia in patients with established atherosclerosis may be a secondary phenomenon but nonetheless may contribute to lesion evolution and thrombotic risk. Polymorphisms in the gene encoding PAI-1 may also correlate with manifestations of atherosclerosis. Yet another nonlipid risk factor for coronary events, elevated levels of homocysteine, may act by promoting thrombosis, although the pathophysiology of this association is uncertain.

The relationship between tobacco abuse and atherosclerosis also remains poorly understood. The rapid reduction in the risk of cardiac events that occurs after cessation of cigarette smoking implies that tobacco may promote thrombosis or some other determinant of plaque stability as well as the evolution of the atherosclerotic lesion itself. For example, tobacco smokers have elevated fibrinogen levels, a variable associated with increased atherosclerosis and acute cardiovascular events, as noted above. In other situations, antecedent inflammatory states may predispose to atherosclerosis. For example, the panarteritis caused by Kawasaki disease in childhood may promote development of vascular lesions in the arteries of adults (Chap. 319). Infectious agents continue to be proposed as instigators or potentiators of atherogenesis. Both viral and microbial pathogens have been invoked in this context (e.g., herpesviruses and *Chlamydia*). In some patients, immune or autoimmune reactions may contribute to atherogenesis. In the accelerated form of coronary arteriopathy that plagues heart transplant recipients (Chap. 234), immune factors may be important in pathogenesis. The roles of the immune response and of infectious diseases in usual atherosclerosis remain speculative.

Known genetic defects in lipoprotein metabolism account for only a fraction of the familial risk for coronary artery disease, so other genetic factors must also contribute. Mechanisms of disease susceptibility involving the arterial wall might account for some of the genetic predisposition to atherosclerosis not explained by lipoprotein disorders. Application of molecular genetic techniques should help to identify new polymorphisms linked to coronary risk and may eventually shed light on new pathophysiologic mechanisms.

ATHEROMA EVOLUTION AND COMPLICATION Involvement of Arterial Smooth Muscle Cells Although the fatty streak commonly precedes the development of a more advanced atherosclerotic plaque, not all fatty streaks progress to atheromas. Fatty streaks occur in populations not prone to late lesions (e.g., indigenous Africans). These findings raise several questions. Why do only some fatty streaks progress to fibrous lesions? By what mechanisms do fatty streaks evolve into more complex lesions? While accumulation of lipid-laden macrophages is the hallmark of the fatty streak, accumulation of fibrous tissue typifies the more advanced atherosclerotic lesion. The smooth muscle cell synthesizes most of the extracellular matrix of the complex atherosclerotic lesion. Thus, the arrival of smooth muscle cells and their elaboration of extracellular matrix is probably a critical transition, yielding a fibrofatty lesion in place of a simple accumulation of macrophage-derived foam cells.

Recent research has provided insight into the mechanisms that may trigger the migration and smooth muscle cells into the evolving intimal lesion, the proliferation of these cells in the lesion, and the accumulation of extracellular matrix. Cytokines and growth factors elicited by modified lipoproteins or other agents from both vascular wall cells and infiltrating leukocytes can modulate functions of the smooth muscle cell. For example, platelet-derived growth factors elaborated by activated endothelial cells can stimulate the migration of smooth muscle cells. This mechanism might induce smooth muscle cells resident in the tunica media to migrate into the intima (Fig. 242-1F). Various growth factors produced locally can stimulate the proliferation both of smooth muscle cells resident in the intima and of those that have migrated from the media. Transforming growth factor β, among other mediators, potently stimulates interstitial collagen production by smooth muscle cells. These mediators may arise not only from neighboring vascular cells or leukocytes (a paracrine pathway), but in some instances from the cell that responds to the factor (an autocrine pathway). Together, these alterations in smooth muscle cells, signaled by these local mediators, can hasten transformation of the fatty streak into a lesion richer in fibrous smooth muscle cells and extracellular matrix.

Traditionally atherosclerosis research has focused on the proliferation of smooth muscle cells. However, smooth muscle cells actually replicate rather slowly in complicated atherosclerotic lesions. Estimates of the rate of smooth muscle cell division at a given time in such lesions show a replicative rate below 1 percent. Such observations do not exclude bursts of proliferative activity at certain junctures in the history of an atheroma, perhaps in association with local thrombin generation due to microvascular hemorrhage or formation of a microthrombus at a site of localized endothelial denudation, as discussed below. On the other hand, cell death has been recognized as a component of atherogenesis since the time of Virchow in the mid-nineteenth century. Indeed, complex atheromas often have a primarily fibrous character, lacking the hyper-cellular appearance of less advanced lesions and actually exhibiting a paucity of smooth muscle cells. This relative lack of smooth muscle cells in advanced atheromas may result from the ultimate predominance of cytostatic mediators such as transforming growth factor β or interferon γ, which can inhibit smooth muscle cell proliferation. Also, smooth muscle cells as well as macrophages in advanced atherosclerotic lesions can undergo apoptosis. Some of the same cytokines that activate atherogenic functions of vascular wall cells can also trigger apoptosis in these cells.

Factors That Modulate Atheroma Progression and Complication In addition to locally produced mediators and traditional atherogenic risk factors, signals related to blood coagulation and thrombosis likely contribute to atheroma evolution and complication. Current evidence suggests that fatty streak formation begins without frank denuding endothelial injury or desquamation. However, in advanced fatty streaks, microscopic breaches in the endothelium may occur. Microthrombi rich in platelets can form at such sites of limited endothelial denudation, owing to the exposure of the highly thrombogenic matrix of the underlying basement membrane. Activated platelets release numerous factors that can promote the fibrotic response. In addition to platelet derived growth factor and transforming growth factor β, low-molecular-weight mediators such as serotonin can also alter smooth muscle function. Most of these microthrombi probably resolve without clinical manifestations by a process of local fibrinolysis, resorption, and endothelial repair.

As atherosclerotic lesions advance, abundant plexi of microvessels develop in connection with the artery's vasa vasorum. These new microvascular networks may contribute to lesion complication in several ways. The vessels of these networks provide an abundant surface area for leukocyte trafficking and may serve as the portal by which white blood cells enter and leave the established atheroma. These microvessels may also be foci for intraplaque hemorrhage. Like the neovessels in the diabetic retina, plaque microvessels may be friable and likely to rupture and produce focal hemorrhage. Such a vascular leak would lead to thrombosis in situ and to the generation of thrombin from prothrombin. In addition to its role in blood coagulation, thrombin can modulate many aspects of vascular cell function; among other effects, it can stimulate the proliferation of and the release of cytokines from smooth muscle cells and the production of growth factors such as platelet-derived growth factors by endothelial cells. Atherosclerotic plaques often contain fibrin and hemosiderin, indications that

Table 242-1

Risk Factors for Atherosclerosis

Factor	Evidence for Causality	Modifiable	Comment
Hypercholesterolemia	Strong	Yes	
Low HDL level	Strong	Yes	Varies inversely with plasma triglyceride level
Hypertension	Strong	Yes	
Male gender	Strong	No	
Diabetes mellitus	Strong	Possibly	Effectiveness of stringent glycemic control uncertain
Family history of premature coronary artery disease	Strong	No	Premature onset before age 55 in first-degree relative
High lipoprotein (a) level	Strong	Modestly	Skewed distribution (see text)
Cigarette smoking	Good	Yes	
Post-menopausal state	Good	Possibly	Estrogen replacement therapy being evaluated
Hyperfibrinogenemia	Good	Possibly	Fibric acid derivatives may reduce
Hyperhomocysteinemia	Good	Yes	Some patients respond to folate supplementation
Physical inactivity	Good	Yes	
Obesity	Good	Yes	
Angiotensin converting enzyme polymorphism	Controversial	No	Homozygous deletion mutant associated with myocardial infarctions

episodes of intraplaque hemorrhage are an element in plaque complication.

Established atherosclerotic plaques also frequently accumulate calcium. Proteins specialized for binding calcium and usually associated with bone also occur in atherosclerotic lesions. For example, osteocalcin, osteopontin, and bone morphogenetic proteins localize in atherosclerotic plaques. In fact, complication of the atherosclerotic plaque recapitulates many aspects of bone formation.

Thus, during the evolution of the atherosclerotic plaque, a complex balance between entry and egress of lipoproteins and leukocytes, cell proliferation and cell death, extracellular matrix production and remodeling, as well as calcification and neovascularization contribute to lesion formation. Multiple and often competing signals trigger these various cellular events. There is a growing recognition of the links between atherogenic risk factors and the altered behavior of intrinsic vascular wall cells and infiltrating leukocytes that underlie the complex pathogenesis of these lesions.

CLINICAL SYNDROMES OF ATHEROSCLEROSIS Atherosclerotic lesions are ubiquitous in Western societies. Most atheromas produce no symptoms, and many never cause clinical manifestations. Numerous patients with diffuse atherosclerosis may succumb to unrelated illnesses without ever having experienced a clinically significant manifestation of atherosclerosis. What accounts for this variability in the clinical expression of atherosclerotic disease?

Arterial remodeling during atheroma formation represents a frequently overlooked but clinically important feature of lesion evolution. During the initial phases of atheroma development, the plaque usually grows in the direction away from the lumen (abluminally). Vessels affected by atherogenesis tend to increase in diameter, a type of vascular remodeling known as compensatory enlargement. Not until the plaque covers more than about 40 percent of the circumference of the internal elastic lamina does it begin to encroach on the arterial lumen. Thus, during much of its history, an atheroma will not cause stenosis that can limit blood flow.

Later in the history of the plaque, flow-limiting stenoses commonly form. Many such plaques manifest themselves by stable syndromes such as demand-induced angina pectoris or intermittent claudication in the extremities. In the coronary and other circulations, even occlusion due to atheroma does not invariably lead to infarction. The hypoxic stimulus of repeated bouts of ischemia characteristically induces the formation of collateral vessels in the myocardium, mitigating the consequences of an acute occlusion of an epicardial coronary artery. On the other hand, many lesions that cause acute or unstable atherosclerotic syndromes, particularly in the coronary circulation, may arise from atherosclerotic plaques that do not produce a flow-limiting stenosis. Such lesions may produce only minimal luminal irregularities on traditional angiograms and often do not meet the traditional criteria for "significance" by arteriography. The instability of such nonocclusive stenoses may explain why myocardial infarction is the first manifestation of coronary artery disease in about a third of all cases and why these patients report no prior history of angina pectoris, a syndrome usually caused by flow-limiting stenoses.

Pathologic studies afford considerable insight into the microanatomic reasons for the instability of plaques that are not critically stenotic. The culprit usually is a superficial erosion of the endothelium or a frank plaque rupture or fissure that gives rise to a thrombus. Such a thrombus may cause an episode of unstable angina pectoris or, if occlusive and relatively persistent, an acute myocardial infarction (Fig. 242-2E). In the case of carotid atheroma, a deeper ulceration that provides a nidus for formation of platelet thrombi may underlie the unstable syndromes that cause transient ischemic attacks.

Rupture of the plaque's fibrous cap permits coagulation factors in the blood to contact highly thrombogenic tissue factor, a procoagulant protein, expressed by macrophage foam cells in the plaque's lipid-rich core. If the ensuing thrombus is nonocclusive or transient, the episode of plaque disruption may not cause symptoms or may result

in ischemic symptoms such as rest angina (Fig. 242-2C). Occlusive thrombi that endure will often cause acute myocardial infarction, particularly in the absence of a well-developed collateral circulation supplying the affected territory. Repetitive episodes of plaque disruption and healing are one likely mechanism by which the fatty streak can evolve into a more complex fibrous lesion (Fig. 242-2D). The healing process in arteries, as in skin wounds, involves the laying down of new extracellular matrix and fibrosis.

Not all atheromas have the same propensity to rupture. Studies of the pathology of culprit lesions that have caused acute myocardial infarction show several characteristic features. These plaques tend to have a thin fibrous cap, a relatively large lipid core, and a high content of macrophages (Fig. 242-2A). Morphometric studies show that macrophages and T lymphocytes predominate at the site of plaque rupture (Fig. 242-2B) and that these sites contain relatively few smooth muscle cells. The cells that concentrate at sites of plaque rupture bear markers of inflammatory activation. The presence of the transplantation or histocompatibility antigen HLA-DR provides one convenient gauge of the degree of inflammation in cells in atheromas. Resting cells in normal arteries seldom express this transplantation antigen. However, macrophages and smooth muscle cells at sites of human coronary artery plaque disruption do bear it. Thus, the presence of macrophages and T cells positive for HLA-DR indicates an ongoing inflammatory response at sites of plaque rupture (Fig. 242-2B).

Inflammatory mediators may actually regulate processes that govern the integrity of the plaque's fibrous cap and hence its propensity to rupture. For example, the T cell–derived cytokine interferon γ, found in atherosclerotic plaques and required to induce the HLA-DR present at sites of rupture, can inhibit the growth and collagen synthesis of smooth muscle cells. Cytokines derived from activated macrophages, such as TNFα and IL-1 in addition to T cell–derived interferon γ, can elicit the expression of proteinases that can degrade the extracellular matrix of the plaque's fibrous cap. Thus, inflammatory mediators can both impair the collagen synthesis required for maintenance and repair of the fibrous cap and trigger degradation of extracellular matrix macromolecules, processes that should weaken the cap and enhance its vulnerability to rupture. In contrast, plaques with a dense extracellular matrix and relatively thick fibrous cap and without a substantial lipid core seem generally resistant to rupture and unlikely to provoke thrombosis (Fig. 242-2D).

PREVENTION AND TREATMENT OF ATHEROSCLEROSIS The prevention of atherosclerosis presents a long-term challenge to all health care professionals and to public health policy (Table 242-2). Both individual practitioners and organizations providing health care should strive to help patients to optimize their risk factor profile long before atherosclerotic disease becomes manifest. The care plan for all patients seen by physicians should include measures to assess and minimize cardiovascular risk. Physicians must counsel patients regarding the health risk of tobacco abuse and provide guidance regarding smoking cessation. Likewise, physicians should advise all patients about prudent dietary and exercise habits for maintaining ideal body weight. Obesity, particularly the male pattern of centripetal or visceral fat accumulation, can promote an atherogenic dyslipidemia characterized by elevated plasma triglycerides, low HDL levels, and glucose intolerance. Physicians should encourage their patients to take responsibility for modifiable risk factors. Conscientious counseling and patient education may delay or lessen the need for pharmacologic measures.

As part of an overall strategy for limiting atherosclerosis, hypertension should be controlled, by drug therapy if necessary (see Chap. 246). Most patients with diabetes mellitus die of atherosclerosis and its complications. It remains unproven that "tight" glycemic control can slow atherosclerosis and its complications in insulin-dependent diabetic patients. However, in view of the evidence that such strict euglycemia does favorably alter the development of microvascular complications of diabetes, special attention to glycemic control appears desirable for all such patients.

Lowering of Lipid Levels Current national guidelines recommend cholesterol screening in all adults (Table 242-3). They also recommend obtaining a fasting lipid profile (including total cholesterol, triglycerides, LDL cholesterol and HDL cholesterol) in all patients with known vascular disease and in those with several risk factors or elevated total cholesterol. Dietary measures, including specific consultation by health professionals with training in nutrition, should be offered to all patients with hyperlipidemia as defined by the National Cholesterol Education Project Adult Treatment Panel II. A "normal" total cholesterol level should not be taken as reassurance in an individual whose HDL cholesterol level is below 40 mg/dL or who has additional risk factors for coronary heart disease. Many patients with established atherosclerosis fall into this category.

Pharmacologic Treatment or Prevention of Atherosclerosis—Examples of the Evidence Base

Risk Factor	Treatment	Strength of Evidence for Effectiveness/Limitations of Therapy
High LDL level	Statins	Prevents coronary events, stroke; lowers total mortality in selected populations
High Lp(a) level	Nicotinic acid	May increase noncardiac mortality
High plasma triglyceride level	Fibric acid derivatives	May increase noncardiac mortality
Low HDL level	Nicotinic acid	Effective, but not proven to lower morbidity/mortality
Hypertension	Thiazide diuretics	Meta-analysis indicates reduced coronary events
Hyperglycemia	Insulin	Proven to reduce microvascular complications of diabetes; not yet proven to limit macrovascular disease
Hyperhomocysteinemia	Folic acid	Lowers homocysteine level in some individuals; not shown to influence atherosclerosis or its manifestations
High fibrinogen level	Fibric acid derivatives	May increase noncardiac mortality

They should be particularly encouraged to adopt life-style measures such as diet and exercise programs aimed at increasing their levels of HDL cholesterol. In all patients with HDL cholesterol levels below 40 mg/dL, the physician must carefully weigh the potential adverse effects on HDL cholesterol levels of any medication. In particular, thiazide diuretics and beta-adrenergic blocking agents may adversely affect the lipid profile. Both of these classes of agents can raise triglycerides and lower HDL cholesterol, a point that should be borne in mind when selecting agents for long-term administration or with the goal of primary prevention in patients who have hypertension but no overt atherosclerosis. This concern about beta blockers should not discourage the practitioner from using these agents in appropriately selected survivors of acute myocardial infarction, however. Multiple well-designed clinical trials have established the efficacy of these agents in the prevention of cardiac death following myocardial infarction (Chap. 243).

The role of drug therapy in reducing the manifestations of atherosclerosis in asymptomatic patients with manifest vascular disease is incompletely defined. In asymptomatic patients with heterozygous familial hypercholesterolemia, the use of drugs to lower LDL levels reduces atherosclerosis in both men and women. The West of Scotland Study recently established that the use of pravastatin, a hydroxymethylglutaryl-coenzyme A (HMGCoA) inhibitor, to lower lipid levels reduced cardiac events and total mortality in a cohort of patients who had not had a myocardial infarction but who had cholesterol levels exceeding 250 mg/dL and elevated LDL levels.

Recent information also provides evidence for a benefit of drug therapy in patients with hypercholesterolemia and established coronary artery disease. The Scandinavian Simvastatin Survival Study showed a decrease in total mortality as well as in myocardial infarctions, cardiovascular death, and surgical or angioplastic revascularization procedures in patients with prior myocardial infarction treated with the HMGCoA inhibitor simvastatin. The incidence of cerebrovascular accidents also declined with simvastatin treatment in this cohort. No increase in noncardiac mortality occurred, providing reassurance that the excess noncardiac mortality encountered with some other forms of lipid-lowering therapy does not occur with HMGCoA reductase inhibitors over the period of study. Likewise, a meta-analysis of experience with controlled clinical trials of pravastatin shows a decrease in overall mortality and cardiovascular events. Even survivors of acute myocardial infarction with "average" cholesterol levels have reduced risk of recurrent coronary events when receiving an HMGCoA reductase inhibitor as shown by the recent Cholesterol and Recurrent Events (CARE) trial. Thus, it appears that effective lowering of LDL levels by treatment with an HMGCoA reductase inhibitor reduces cardiovascular morbidity and total mortality in patients with known coronary artery disease.

Curiously, it does not appear that lipid-lowering therapies exert their beneficial effects on cardiovascular events by causing a marked regression of obstructive coronary lesions (Table 242-4). Angiographically monitored studies of lipid lowering have shown at best modest reductions in coronary artery stenoses over the duration of study, even though these studies all showed a resounding decrease in coronary events. These benefits may instead accrue from stabilization of atherosclerotic lesions. For example, the improved cholesterol balance resulting from a reduction in lipid levels may lead to a net egress of lipids from atherosclerotic lesions, resulting in a decrease in the proinflammatory aspects of lipid overloading discussed above. The beneficial effect on cardiovascular events of the lowering of LDL levels produced by HMGCoA reductase treatment seems to require 6 months to up to 2 years of treatment to appear. Improvement of vasomotor responses to endothelium-dependent vasodilators appears to be much more rapid, occurring in 6 months or less. The observations suggest that HMGCoA reductase inhibitors may act on the arteries of hypercholesterolemic individuals by two or more mechanisms. The more rapid effect on endothelium-dependent vasomotor responses could involve an increase in vascular nitric oxide production or a decrease in the production of superoxide anion, a molecule that inactivates nitric oxide, by lesional leukocytes or vascular cells. This effect on the endothelium or on periluminal cells follows the same time course as the reduction in plasma LDL cholesterol (weeks to months). The reduction in cardiovascular events may require removal of lipid and reduced activation of lesional macrophage foam cells from deeper in the lesions, processes that may require many months, perhaps accounting for the slower onset of the stabilizing effect of HMGCoA reductase treatment.

Treatment Decisions Based on LDL Cholesterol Level

Patient Category	LDL Cholesterol Level, mg/dL (mmol/L)	
	Initial	Goal
DIETARY THERAPY		
Without CHD and with fewer than two risk factors	≥160 (4.1)	<160 (4.1)
Without CHD and with two or more risk factors	≥130 (3.4)	<130 (3.4)
With CHD	>100 (2.6)	≤100 (2.6)
DRUG TREATMENT		
Without CHD and with fewer than two risk factors	≥190 (4.9)	<160 (4.1)
Without CHD and with two or more risk factors	≥160 (4.1)	<130 (3.4)
With CHD	≥130 (3.4)	≤100 (2.6)

ABBREVIATION: CHD, coronary heart disease
SOURCE: Summary of the second report of the National Cholesterol Education Program (NCEP) Expert Panel on Detection, Evaluation, and Treatment of High Blood Cholesterol in Adults (Adult Treatment Panel II). JAMA 269:3015, 1993.

Elliott M. Antman, Eugene Braunwald

ACUTE MYOCARDIAL INFARCTION

Table 242-4

Summary of Results of Lipid-Lowering Trials

Study	Treatment Regimen	Regression, %	Reduction, Event, %
NHLBI	Diet + colestipol	7	33
CLAS-1	Diet + colestipol + niacin	16	25
POSCH	Partial ileal bypass + colestipol	14	35
FATS	Lovastatin or niacin + colestipol	39	80
CLAS-II	Diet + colestipol + niacin	18	43
STARS	Diet + colestipol	38	69
SCRIP	Diet + resin/niacin/lovastatin/fibrate	21	50

SOURCE: Adapted from BG Brown et al: Lipid lowering and plaque regression. New insights into prevention of plaque disruption and clinical events in coronary disease. Circulation 87:1781, 1993.

Large-scale clinical studies currently in progress should provide evidence regarding the utility of certain potential new avenues for antiatherosclerotic therapy. The treatments under evaluation include antioxidant vitamin supplementation as well as estrogen replacement therapy for postmenopausal women. Observational studies, small clinical trials, and evaluation of surrogates for disease, as well as current concepts of the biology of atherosclerosis, suggest that such therapies may prove beneficial. However their general use, particularly by lower-risk individuals, should await the results of rigorous prospective studies designed to define doses and appropriate patient groups and to evaluate the possibility of adverse or unwanted effects.

Estrogen Therapy The case of estrogen therapy illustrates some of the complexities encountered in formulating therapeutic strategies. In men, high-dose estrogen treatment causes an increase in mortality, probably owing to an increase in thromboembolic risk. In postmenopausal women, administration of estrogen either alone or combined with a progestin can improve biochemical variables associated with risk for coronary heart disease (lowering LDL levels, raising HDL levels, and lowering fibrinogen levels). Observational studies in women also indicate that estrogen replacement therapy has a beneficial effect in terms of cardiovascular events. However, unopposed estrogen replacement (i.e., without simultaneous progestin treatment) augments endometrial atypia and adenomatous changes. The balance between the possible increased risk of breast or uterine cancer and the cardiovascular benefit from this treatment remains uncertain. The variety of estrogen doses and dosage forms, and the inclusion of progestin cotherapy, complicates the design of controlled clinical trials aimed at monitoring clinical cardiovascular events. Such trials are underway, however, and their results should make it easier to formulate public health policy in this area. In the meantime, the practitioner must decide whether to recommend estrogen replacement therapy on the basis of an assessment of the balance of risks and benefits for individual patients in the light of their profiles of coronary risk factors, breast cancer, and personal preferences.

BIBLIOGRAPHY

BERLINER J et al: Atherosclerosis: Basic mechanisms—oxidation, inflammation, and genetics. Circulation 91:2488–2496, 1995

DAVIES MJ: A macro and micro view of coronary vascular insult in ischemic heart disease. Circulation 82:1138, 1990

FUSTER V: Mechanisms leading to myocardial infaction: Insights from vascular biology. Circulation 90:2126, 1994

LIBBY P: The molecular bases of the acute coronary syndromes. Circulation 91:2844, 1995

ROSS R: The pathogenesis of atherosclerosis: A perspective for the 1990s. Nature 362:801, 1993

STEINBERG D et al: Beyond cholesterol. Modifications of low-density lipoprotein that increase its atherogenicity. N Engl J Med 320:915, 1989

Myocardial infarction is one of the most common diagnoses in hospitalized patients in industrialized countries. In the United States, approximately 1.5 million myocardial infarctions occur each year. The mortality rate with acute infarction is approximately 30 percent, with more than half of these deaths occurring before the stricken individual reaches the hospital. Although the mortality rate after admission for myocardial infarction has declined by about 30 percent over the last two decades, approximately 1 of every 25 patients who survives the initial hospitalization dies in the first year after myocardial infarction. Survival is markedly reduced in elderly patients (over age 65), whose mortality rate is 20 percent at 1 month and 35 percent at 1 year after infarction.

PATHOPHYSIOLOGY: ROLE OF ACUTE PLAQUE RUPTURE

Myocardial infarction generally occurs when there is an abrupt decrease in coronary blood flow following a thrombotic occlusion of a coronary artery previously narrowed by atherosclerosis. Slowly developing, high-grade coronary artery stenoses usually do not precipitate acute infarction because of the development of a rich collateral network over time. Instead, infarction occurs when a coronary artery thrombus develops rapidly at a site of vascular injury. This injury is produced or facilitated by factors such as cigarette smoking, hypertension, and lipid accumulation. In most cases, infarction occurs when an atherosclerotic plaque fissures, ruptures, or ulcerates and when conditions (local or systemic) favor thrombogenesis, so that a mural thrombus forms at the site of rupture and leads to coronary artery occlusion. Histologic studies indicate that the coronary plaques prone to rupture are those with a rich lipid core and a thin fibrous cap. After an initial platelet monolayer forms at the site of the ruptured plaque, a variety of agonists (collagen, ADP, epinephrine, serotonin) promote platelet activation. Following agonist stimulation, there is production and release of thromboxane A_2 (a compound capable of inducing vasoconstriction), further platelet activation, and potential resistance to thrombolysis.

In addition to generation of thromboxane A_2, activation of platelets by agonists promotes a conformational change in the glycoprotein IIbIIIa receptor. Once converted to its functional state, this receptor develops a high affinity for the sequence arginine-glycine-aspartic acid (called the RGD sequence) on the fibrinogen alpha chain and also for a dodecapeptide sequence on the fibrinogen gamma chain. Since fibrinogen is a multivalent molecule, it can bind to two different platelets simultaneously, resulting in platelet cross-linking and aggregation.

The coagulation cascade is activated on exposure of tissue factor in damaged endothelial cells at the site of the ruptured plaque. Factors VII and X are activated, ultimately leading to the conversion of prothrombin to thrombin, which then converts fibrinogen to fibrin. Fluid-phase and clot-bound thrombin participate in an autoamplification reaction leading to further activation of the coagulation cascade. The culprit coronary artery eventually becomes occluded by a thrombus containing platelet aggregates and fibrin strands.

In rare cases, infarction may be due to coronary artery occlusion caused by coronary emboli, congenital abnormalities, coronary spasm, and a wide variety of systemic—particularly inflammatory—diseases. Ultimately, the amount of myocardial damage caused by coronary occlusion depends on the territory supplied by the affected vessel, whether or not the vessel becomes totally occluded, native factors that can produce early spontaneous lysis of the occlusive thrombus, the quantity of blood supplied by collateral vessels to the affected tissue, and the demand for oxygen of the myocardium whose blood supply has been suddenly limited.

Patients at increased risk of developing acute myocardial infarction include those with unstable angina or Prinzmetal's variant angina (Chap. 244) and those with multiple coronary risk factors (Chap. 242). Less common underlying medical conditions predisposing patients to infarction include hypercoagulability, collagen vascular disease, cocaine abuse, and intracardiac thrombi or masses that can produce coronary emboli.

CLINICAL PRESENTATION

In roughly one-half of cases, a precipitating factor appears to be present prior to myocardial infarction, such as vigorous physical exercise, emotional stress, or a medical or surgical illness. Myocardial infarction may commence at any time of the day or night, but the frequency is highest in the morning within a few hours of awakening. This circadian peak may be due to a combination of an increase in sympathetic tone and an increased tendency to thrombosis between 6:00 A.M. and 12 noon. *Pain* is the most common presenting complaint in patients with myocardial infarction. In some instances, the discomfort may be severe enough to be described as the worst pain the patient has ever felt. The pain is deep and visceral; adjectives commonly used to describe it are *heavy*, *squeezing*, and *crushing*, although occasionally it is described as stabbing or burning (Chap. 13). It is similar in character to the discomfort of angina pectoris but usually is more severe and lasts longer. Typically the pain involves the central portion of the chest and/or the epigastrium, and on occasion it radiates to the arms. Less common sites of radiation include the abdomen, back, lower jaw, and neck. The frequent location of the pain beneath the xiphoid and patients' denial that they may be suffering a heart attack are chiefly responsible for the common mistaken impression of indigestion. The pain of myocardial infarction may radiate as high as the occipital area but not below the umbilicus. It is often accompanied by weakness, sweating, nausea, vomiting, anxiety, and a sense of impending doom. The discomfort may commence when the patient is at rest. When the pain begins during a period of exertion, it does not usually subside with cessation of activity, in contrast to angina pectoris.

Although pain is the most common presenting complaint, it is by no means always present. The incidence of painless infarcts is greater in patients with diabetes mellitus, and it increases with age. In the elderly, myocardial infarction may present as sudden-onset breathlessness, which may progress to pulmonary edema. Other less common presentations, with or without pain, include sudden loss of consciousness, a confusional state, a sensation of profound weakness, the appearance of an arrhythmia, evidence of peripheral embolism, or merely an unexplained drop in arterial pressure. The pain of myocardial infarction can simulate pain from acute pericarditis (Chap. 240), pulmonary embolism (Chap. 261), acute aortic dissection (Chap. 247), and costochondritis. These conditions should therefore be considered in the differential diagnosis.

PHYSICAL FINDINGS Most patients are anxious and restless, attempting unsuccessfully to relieve the pain by moving about in bed, altering their position, and stretching. Pallor associated with perspiration and coolness of the extremities occurs commonly. The combination of substernal chest pain persisting for more than 30 min and diaphoresis strongly suggests acute myocardial infarction. Although many patients have a normal pulse rate and blood pressure, within the first hour of infarction, about one-fourth of patients with anterior infarction have manifestations of sympathetic nervous system hyperactivity (tachycardia and/or hypertension), and up to one-half with inferior infarction show evidence of parasympathetic hyperactivity (bradycardia and/or hypotension).

The precordium is usually quiet, and the apical impulse may be difficult to palpate. In patients with anterior wall infarction, an abnormal systolic pulsation caused by dyskinetic bulging of infarcted myocardium may develop in the periapical area within the first days of the illness and then may resolve. Other physical signs of ventricular dysfunction that may be present include, in order of decreasing incidence, fourth (S_4) and third (S_3) heart sounds, decreased intensity of heart sounds, and, in more severe cases, paradoxical splitting of the second heart sound (Chap. 227). A transient apical systolic murmur due to dysfunction of the mitral valve apparatus may be midsystolic or late systolic in timing. A pericardial friction rub is heard in many patients with transmural myocardial infarction at some time in the course of the disease, if they are examined frequently. The carotid pulse is often decreased in volume, reflecting reduced stroke volume. Jugular venous distention with clear lung fields should raise suspicion of right ventricular infarction. Temperature elevations up to 38°C may be observed during the first week after acute myocardial infarction; however, a temperature exceeding 38°C should prompt a search for other causes. The arterial pressure is variable; in most patients with transmural infarction, systolic pressure declines by approximately 10 to 15 mmHg from the preinfarction state.

LABORATORY FINDINGS

The laboratory tests of value in confirming the diagnosis of myocardial infarction may be divided into four groups: (1) the electrocardiogram (ECG), (2) serum cardiac markers, (3) cardiac imaging, and (4) nonspecific indexes of tissue necrosis and inflammation.

ELECTROCARDIOGRAM The *electrocardiographic manifestations* of acute myocardial infarction are described in Chap. 228. Transmural infarction is often present if the ECG demonstrates Q waves or loss of R waves; nontransmural infarction may be present if the electrocardiogram shows only transient ST-segment and T-wave changes. However, electrocardiographic-pathologic correlations are far from perfect and, therefore, a more rational nomenclature for designating electrocardiographic infarction is now commonly in use, with the terms *Q-wave* and *non-Q-wave infarction* replacing the terms *transmural* and *nontransmural infarction*, respectively.

Total occlusion of the infarct artery produces ST-segment elevation, and most such individuals ultimately evolve a Q-wave myocardial infarction. A small proportion may sustain only a non-Q wave myocardial infarction. When the obstructing thrombus is subtotally occlusive, obstruction is transient, or a rich collateral network is present, no ST-segment elevation is seen. Most such patients are diagnosed as having unstable angina, or, if a serum cardiac marker is detected, as having non-Q wave myocardial infarction. A minority of patients who present initially without ST-segment elevation may develop a Q-wave infarction. The presentations that constitute the spectrum ranging from unstable angina through non-Q-wave myocardial infarction to Q-wave myocardial infarction are called the *acute coronary syndromes* (Fig. 243-1).

SERUM CARDIAC MARKERS Certain proteins, called *serum cardiac markers*, are released into the blood in large quantities from necrotic heart muscle after myocardial infarction. The rate of liberation of specific proteins differs depending on their intracellular location and molecular weight, and the local blood and lymphatic flow. The temporal pattern of protein release is of diagnostic importance, but contemporary urgent reperfusion strategies necessitate making a decision (based largely on a combination of clinical and ECG findings) before the results of blood tests have returned from the central laboratory. Rapid whole-blood bedside assays for serum cardiac markers are now available and may facilitate management decisions, particularly in patients with nondiagnostic electrocardiograms.

Creatine phosphokinase (*CK*) rises within 4 to 8 h and generally returns to normal by 48 to 72 h. An important drawback of total CK measurement is its lack of specificity for myocardial infarction, as CK may be elevated with skeletal muscle trauma. A two- to threefold elevation of total CK may follow an intramuscular injection, for example. This ambiguity may lead to the erroneous diagnosis of myocardial infarction in a patient who has been given an intramuscular injection of a narcotic for chest pain of noncardiac origin. Other potential sources of total CK elevation worth noting are (1) muscular diseases, including muscular dystrophy, myopathies, and polymyositis; (2) electric cardioversion; (3) cardiac catheterization; (4) hypothyroidism; (5) stroke;

(6) surgery; and (7) skeletal muscle damage secondary to trauma, convulsions, and prolonged immobilization.

The MB isoenzyme of CK has the advantage total over CK that it is not present in significant concentrations in extracardiac tissue and therefore is considerably more specific. However, cardiac surgery, myocarditis, and electric cardioversion often result in elevated serum levels of the MB isoenzyme. A ratio (relative index) of CKMB mass:CK activity ≥ 2.5 percent suggests but is not diagnostic of a myocardial rather than skeletal muscle source for the CKMB elevation. This ratio is less useful when levels of total CK are high owing to skeletal muscle injury or when the total CK level is within the normal range but CKMB is elevated.

Rather than attempting to make the diagnosis of a myocardial infarction on the basis of a single measurement of CK and CKMB, clinicians should evaluate a series of measurements obtained over the first 24 h. Skeletal muscle release of CKMB typically produces a "plateau" pattern, whereas myocardial infarction produces a CKMB elevation that peaks at approximately 20 h after the onset of coronary occlusion. When released into the circulation, the myocardial form of CKMB (CKMB2) is acted on by the enzyme carboxypeptidase, which cleaves a lysine residue from the carboxy terminus to produce an isoform (CKMB1) with a different electrophoretic mobility. A CKMB2:CKMB1 ratio of >1.5 is highly sensitive for the diagnosis of myocardial infarction, particularly after 4 to 6 h have elapsed since coronary occlusion.

Cardiac-specific troponin T (cTnT) and *cardiac-specific troponin I (cTnI)* have different amino acid sequences than the skeletal muscle forms of these proteins. This difference has permitted the development of quantitative assays for cTnT and cTnI using highly specific monoclonal antibodies. Since cTnT and cTnI are not normally detectable in the blood of healthy individuals but may increase after myocardial infarction to levels over 20 times higher than the cutoff value (usually set only slightly above the noise level of the assay), measurement of cTnT or cTnI is of considerable diagnostic utility. These new serum cardiac markers are particularly valuable when there is clinical suspicion of either skeletal muscle injury or a small myocardial infarction that may be below the detection limit for CK and CKMB measurements. Levels of cTnI may remain elevated for 7 to 10 days after myocardial infarction, and cTnT levels may remain elevated for up to 10 to 14 days. Thus, measurement of cTnT or cTnI is preferable to measurement of lactate dehydrogenase (LDH) and its isoenzymes in patients with suspected myocardial infarction who come to medical attention more than 24 to 48 h after the onset of symptoms.

Myoglobin is released into the blood within only a few hours of the onset of myocardial infarction. Although myoglobin is one of the first serum cardiac markers that rises above the normal range after myocardial infarction, it lacks cardiac specificity, and it is rapidly excreted in the urine, so that blood levels return to the normal range within 24 h of the onset of infarction.

Many clinical centers have begun to use cTnT or cTnI rather than CKMB as the routine serum cardiac marker for diagnosis of myocardial infarction, although any of these analytes remains clinically acceptable. It is not cost-effective to measure both a cardiac-specific troponin and CKMB at all time points in every patient. However, in view of the prolonged elevation of cardiac-specific troponins (>1 week), episodes of recurrent ischemic discomfort and suspected recurrent myocardial infarction are more readily diagnosed with a serum cardiac marker that remains elevated in the blood more briefly, such as CKMB or myoglobin.

While it has long been recognized that the *total* quantity of protein released correlates with the size of the infarct, the *peak* protein concentration correlates only weakly with infarct size. Recanalization of a coronary artery occlusion (either spontaneously or by mechanical or pharmacologic means) in the early hours of myocardial infarction will cause earlier and higher peaking (at about 8 to 12 h after reperfusion) of serum cardiac markers.

Characteristic rises occur in serum cardiac markers in virtually all patients with clinically proven myocardial infarction. CK and CKMB levels generally do not rise in unstable angina. However, approximately one-third of patients who are considered to have unstable angina on the basis of a lack of CK or CKMB elevation have elevations of cTnT or cTnI, probably indicating the presence of microinfarction. The finding of an elevated cardiac-specific troponin level, even in the presence of normal CK and CKMB values, is indicative of an adverse prognosis, and such patients should be considered to have sustained myocardial infarction and managed as described below.

The *nonspecific reaction* to myocardial injury is associated with polymorphonuclear leukocytosis, which appears within a few hours after the onset of pain, persists for 3 to 7 days, and often reaches levels of 12,000 to 15,000 leukocytes per microliter. The erythrocyte sedimentation rate rises more slowly than the white blood cell count, peaking during the first week and sometimes remaining elevated for 1 or 2 weeks.

CARDIAC IMAGING *Two-dimensional echocardiography* is the most frequently employed imaging modality in patients with acute myocardial infarction. Abnormalities of wall motion are almost universally present. Even when no ST-segment elevation is seen, echocardiographically detectable wall motion abnormalities may be observed. Although acute infarction cannot be distinguished from an old myocardial scar or from acute severe ischemia by echocardiography, the ease and safety of the procedure make its use appealing as a screening tool. In the emergency department setting, early detection of the presence or absence of wall motion abnormalities by echocardiography can aid in management decisions, such as whether or not thrombolytic agents should be administered. Echocardiographic estimation of left ventricular function is useful prognostically; detection of reduced function serves as an indication for therapy with an angiotensin converting enzyme inhibitor (see "Angiotensin Converting Enzyme Inhibitors," below). Echocardiography may also identify the presence of right ventricular infarction, ventricular aneurysm, pericardial effusion, and

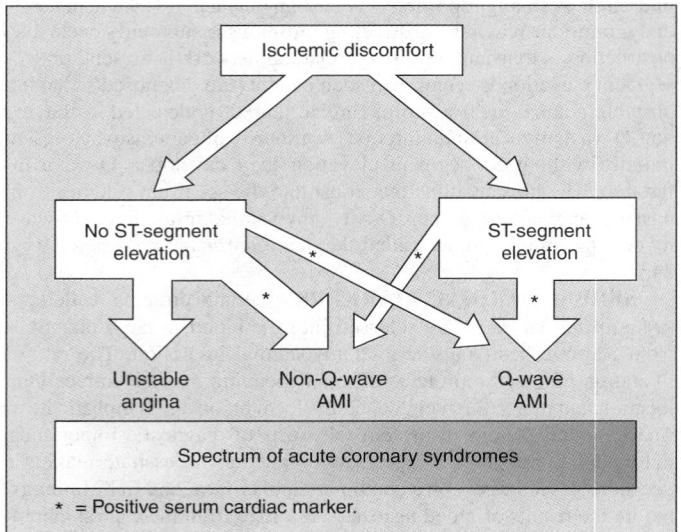

FIGURE 243-1 Acute coronary syndromes. Patients with ischemic discomfort may present with or without ST-segment elevation on the electrocardiogram. Of patients with ST-segment elevation, most (*large arrow*) ultimately develop a Q-wave acute myocardial infarction (AMI), while a minority (*small arrow*) develop a non-Q-wave AMI. Of the patients who present without ST-segment elevation, most (*large arrows*) are ultimately diagnosed as having either unstable angina or non-Q-wave AMI on the basis of the presence or absence of a cardiac marker such as CKMB detected in the serum; a minority of such patients ultimately develop a Q-wave AMI. The clinical conditions in the spectrum ranging from unstable angina through non-Q-wave AMI to Q-wave AMI are referred to as the acute coronary syndromes. [*From EM Antman, E Braunwald: Acute Myocardial Infarction, in Heart Disease, A Textbook of Cardiovascular Medicine, 5th ed, E Braunwald (ed). Philadelphia, Saunders, 1997.*]

left ventricular thrombus. In addition, Doppler echocardiography is useful in the detection and quantitation of a ventricular septal defect and mitral regurgitation, two serious complications of acute myocardial infarction.

Several radionuclide imaging techniques are available for evaluating patients with suspected acute myocardial infarction. However, these imaging modalities are used less often than echocardiography because they are more cumbersome and they a lack sensitivity and specificity in many clinical circumstances. Myocardial perfusion imaging with thallium 201 or technetium 99m sestamibi, which are distributed in proportion to myocardial blood flow and concentrated by viable myocardium, will reveal a defect ("cold spot") in most patients during the first few hours after development of a transmural infarct. However, although perfusion scanning is extremely *sensitive*, it cannot distinguish acute infarcts from chronic scars and thus is not *specific* for the diagnosis of *acute* myocardial infarction. Radionuclide ventriculography, carried out with ^{99m}Tc-labeled red blood cells, frequently demonstrates wall motion disorders and reduction in the ventricular ejection fraction in patients with acute myocardial infarction. While of value in assessing the hemodynamic consequences of infarction, and in aiding in the diagnosis of right ventricular infarction when the right ventricular ejection fraction is depressed, this technique is also quite nonspecific, as many cardiac abnormalities other than myocardial infarction alter the radionuclide ventriculogram.

MANAGEMENT

PREHOSPITAL CARE   The prognosis in acute myocardial infarction is largely related to the occurrence of two general classes of complications: (1) electrical complications (arrhythmias) and (2) mechanical problems ("pump failure"). Most out-of-hospital deaths from myocardial infarction are due to the sudden development of ventricular fibrillation. The vast majority of deaths due to ventricular fibrillation occur within the first 24 h of the onset of symptoms, and, of these, over half occur in the first hour. Therefore, the major elements of prehospital care of patients with suspected acute myocardial infarction include (1) recognition of symptoms by the patient and prompt seeking of medical attention; (2) rapid deployment of an emergency medical team capable of performing resuscitative maneuvers, including defibrillation; and (3) expeditious transportation of the patient to a hospital facility that is continuously staffed by physicians and nurses skilled in managing arrhythmias, providing advanced cardiac life support, and initiating prompt reperfusion therapy. The biggest delay usually occurs not during transportation to the hospital but rather between the onset of pain and the patient's decision to call for help. This delay can best be reduced by education of the public by health care professionals concerning the significance of chest pain and the importance of seeking early medical attention. Increasingly, monitoring and treatment are carried out by trained personnel in the ambulance, further shortening the time between the onset of the infarction and appropriate treatment.

INITIAL MANAGEMENT IN THE EMERGENCY DEPARTMENT   In the emergency department, the goals for the management of patients with suspected acute myocardial infarction include control of cardiac pain, rapid identification of patients who are candidates for urgent reperfusion therapy, triage of lower-risk patients to the appropriate location in the hospital, and avoidance of inappropriate discharge of patients with acute myocardial infarction. Many aspects of the treatment of acute myocardial infarction are initiated in the emergency department and then continued during the in-hospital phase of management.

Aspirin is now considered an essential element in the management of patients with suspected acute myocardial infarction and is effective across the entire spectrum of acute coronary syndromes (Fig. 243-1). Rapid inhibition of cyclooxygenase in platelets followed by a reduction of thromboxane A_2 levels is achieved by buccal absorption of a chewed 160 to 325 mg tablet in the emergency department. This measure should be followed by daily oral administration of aspirin in a dose of 160 to 325 mg.

Since patients with acute myocardial infarction may develop hypoxemia secondary to ventilation-perfusion abnormalities from left ventricular failure and intrinsic pulmonary disease, it has been a common practice to routinely administer *supplemental oxygen*, via the belief that an increase in the oxygen tension of the inspired air will protect the myocardium. In patients whose arterial oxygen saturation is normal as estimated by pulse oximetry or measured by an arterial blood gas specimen, supplemental oxygen is of limited clinical benefit and therefore is not cost-effective. However, when hypoxemia is demonstrated, oxygen should be administered by nasal prongs or face mask (2 to 4 L/min) for the first 6 to 12 h after infarction; the patient should then be reassessed to determine if there is a continued need for such treatment.

CONTROL OF PAIN   *Morphine* is an extremely effective analgesic for the pain associated with myocardial infarction. However, it may reduce sympathetically mediated arteriolar and venous constriction, and the resulting venous pooling may reduce cardiac output and arterial pressure. This complication does not contraindicate morphine use. Hypotension associated with venous pooling usually responds promptly to elevation of the legs, but in some patients volume expansion with intravenous saline is required. The patient may experience diaphoresis and nausea, but these events usually pass and are replaced by a feeling of well-being associated with the relief of pain. Morphine also has a vagotonic effect and may cause bradycardia or advanced degrees of heart block, particularly in patients with posteroinferior infarction. These side effects usually respond to atropine (0.5 mg intravenously). Morphine is routinely administered by repetitive (every 5 min) intravenous injection of small doses (2 to 4 mg) rather than by the subcutaneous administration of a larger quantity, because absorption may be unpredictable by the latter route.

Before morphine is administered, sublingual *nitroglycerin* can be given safely to most patients with myocardial infarction. Up to three 0.4-mg doses should be administered at about 5-min intervals. In addition to diminishing or abolishing chest discomfort, nitroglycerin, once considered contraindicated in the setting of acute myocardial infarction, may be capable of both decreasing myocardial oxygen demand (by lowering preload) and increasing myocardial oxygen supply (by dilating infarct-related coronary vessels or collateral vessels). However, therapy with nitrates should be avoided in patients who present with low systolic arterial pressure (<100 mmHg) or in whom there is clinical suspicion of right ventricular infarction (inferior infarction on electrocardiogram, elevated jugular venous pressure, clear lungs, and hypotension). An idiosyncratic reaction to nitrates, consisting of sudden marked hypotension, sometimes occurs but can usually be reversed promptly by the rapid administration of intravenous atropine. In patients whose initially favorable response to sublingual nitroglycerin is followed by the return of chest pain, particularly if accompanied by other evidence of ongoing ischemia such as further ST-segment or T-wave shifts, the use of intravenous nitroglycerin should be considered.

Intravenous *beta blockers* are also useful in the control of the pain of acute myocardial infarction. These drugs have been shown to control pain effectively in some patients, presumably by diminishing myocardial oxygen demand and hence ischemia. More important, there is evidence that intravenous beta blockers reduce in-hospital mortality, particularly in high-risk patients (see "Beta-Adrenoceptor Blockers," below). A commonly employed regimen is metoprolol, 5 mg every 2 to 5 min for a total of three doses, provided the patient has a pulse greater than 60 beats per minute, systolic pressure greater than 100 mmHg, a PR interval of less than 0.24 sec, and rales that are no higher than 10 cm up from the diaphragm. Fifteen minutes after the last intravenous dose, an oral regimen is initiated of 50 mg every 6 h for 48 h followed by 100 mg every 12 h.

Unlike beta blockers, *calcium antagonists* are of little value in the acute setting, and there is evidence that they may be associated with an increased mortality risk.

MANAGEMENT STRATEGIES (Fig. 243-2) The primary tool for screening patients and making triage decisions is the initial 12-lead electrocardiogram. When ST-segment elevation of at least 1 mm is present in at least two contiguous leads, a patient should be considered a candidate for *reperfusion therapy* (Fig. 243-2A). If no contraindications are present (see "Contraindications and Complications," under "Thombolysis," below), thrombolytic therapy should ideally be initiated within 30 min. The process of selecting patients for thrombolysis versus primary percutaneous transluminal coronary angioplasty is discussed below. If the presenting electrocardiogram shows new or presumably new ST-segment depression and/or T-wave inversion, patients should be treated as though they are suffering from either unstable angina or non-Q-wave myocardial infarction (a distinction to be made on the basis of serial electrocardiograms and serum cardiac marker measurements). In the absence of ST-segment elevation, thrombolysis is not helpful, and evidence exists suggesting that it may be harmful. Pharmacotherapy for patients presenting without ST-segment elevation has not been studied as rigorously as that for patients who present with ST-segment elevation, but contemporary practice typically includes measures to control cardiac pain (as discussed above), aspirin, infusion of nitroglycerin, and either infusion of unfractionated heparin or subcutaneous administration of a low-molecular-weight heparin preparation. Further management recommendations for patients without ST segment elevation are outlined in Fig. 243-2B.

LIMITATION OF INFARCT SIZE The amount of myocardium that becomes necrotic owing to a coronary artery occlusion is determined by factors other than just the site of occlusion (Fig. 243-3). While the central zone of the infarct contains necrotic tissue that is irretrievably lost, the fate of the surrounding ischemic myocardium may be improved by timely restoration of coronary perfusion (Fig. 243-3, line B), reduction of myocardial oxygen demands, prevention of the accumulation of noxious metabolites, and blunting of the impact of mediators of reperfusion injury (e.g., calcium overload and oxygen-derived free radicals). Although up to one-third of patients with acute myocardial infarction may achieve spontaneous reperfusion of the infarct-related coronary artery and experience improved healing of infarcted tissue, it is now possible to minimize the infarct size by accelerating reperfusion either pharmacologically (by thrombolysis) or mechanically (by angioplasty). Protection of the ischemic myocardium by the maintenance of an optimal balance of myocardial oxygen through adequate pain control, treatment of congestive heart failure, and minimization of tachycardia and hypertension extends

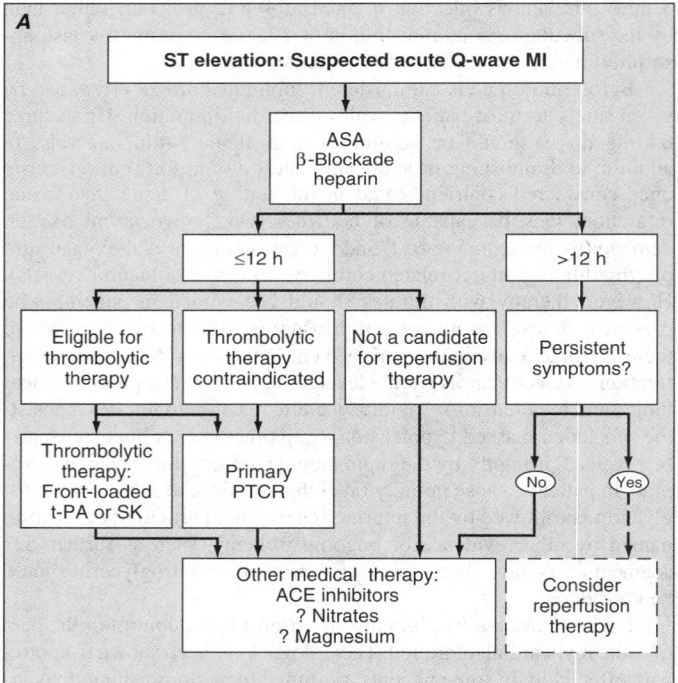

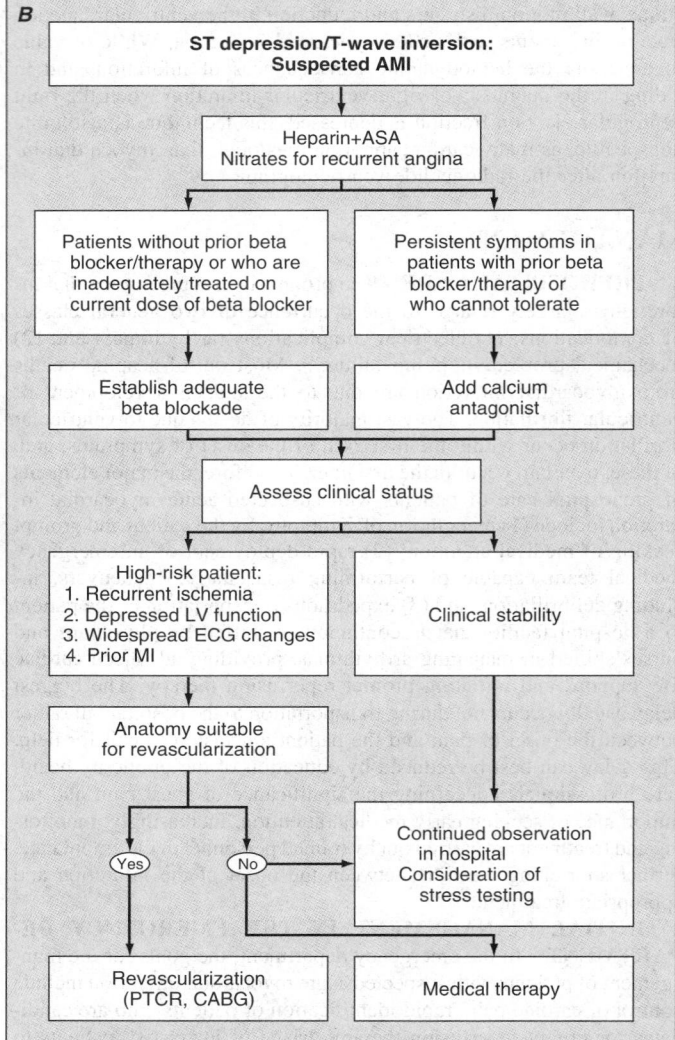

FIGURE 243-2 Management strategies for patients with myocardial infarction. *A.* All patients suspected of having a Q-wave myocardial infarction (MI) (i.e., ST-segment elevation on ECG) should receive aspirin (ASA), beta blockers (in the absence of contraindications), and an antithrombin [particularly if tissue-type plasminogen activator (t-PA) is used for thrombolytic therapy]. Heparin is probably not required in patients receiving streptokinase (SK). Patients treated within 12 h who are eligible for thrombolytic therapy should expeditiously receive either t-PA or SK or be considered for primary percutaneous transluminal coronary revascularization (PTCR). Immediate, primary PTCR is also to be considered when lytic therapy is contraindicated. Patients treated after 12 h should receive the initial medical therapy noted above and, on an individual basis, may be candidates for ACE inhibitors (particularly if left ventricular function is impaired). Further information is required to clarify the role of magnesium. *B.* All patients without ST elevation should be treated with an antithrombin and aspirin. Nitrates should be administered for recurrent episodes of angina. Adequate beta blockade should then be established; when that is not possible or contraindications exist, a calcium antagonist can be considered. Patients at high risk should be triaged to cardiac catheterization with plans for revascularization if clinically suitable, while patients who are clinically stable can be treated more conservatively with continued observation in the hospital and consideration of a stress test to screen for any provocable myocardial ischemia. (CABG, coronary artery bypass grafting; LV, left ventricular.) *[Modified from EM Antman: Overview of medical therapy, in RM Califf (ed): Acute Myocardial Infarction and Other Acute Ischemic Syndromes, in E Braunwald (Series ed): Atlas of Heart Diseases, vol. 8. Philadelphia, Current Medicine 1996.]*

the "window" of time for the salvage of myocardium by reperfusion strategies.

Glucocorticoids and nonsteroidal anti-inflammatory agents, with the exception of aspirin, should be avoided in the setting of acute myocardial infarction. They can impair infarct healing and increase the risk of myocardial rupture, and their use may result in a larger infarct scar. In addition, they can increase coronary vascular resistance, thereby potentially reducing flow to ischemic myocardium.

THROMBOLYSIS The thrombolytic agents tissue plasminogen activator (tPA), streptokinase, and anisoylated plasminogen streptokinase activator complex (APSAC) have been approved by the Food and Drug Administration for intravenous use in the setting of acute myocardial infarction. These drugs all act by promoting the conversion of plasminogen to plasmin, which subsequently lyses fibrin thrombi. Although considerable emphasis used to be placed on a distinction between more fibrin-specific agents, such as tPA, and non-fibrin-specific agents, such as streptokinase, it is now recognized that these differences are only relative, as some degree of systemic fibrinolysis occurs with tPA. The principal goal of thrombolysis is prompt restoration of coronary arterial patency. When assessed angiographically, flow in the culprit coronary artery is described by a simple qualitative scale called the TIMI grading system: grade 0 indicates complete occlusion of the infarct related artery; grade 1 indicates some penetration of the contrast material beyond the point of obstruction but without perfusion of the distal coronary bed; grade 2 indicates perfusion of the entire infarct vessel into the distal bed but with flow that is delayed compared with that of a normal artery; and grade 3 indicates full perfusion of the infarct vessel with normal flow. Early reports frequently lumped TIMI grades 2 and 3 under the general category of *patency*, but it is now recognized that grade 3 flow is the goal of reperfusion therapy, because full perfusion of the infarct-related coronary artery yields far better results in terms of infarct size, maintenance

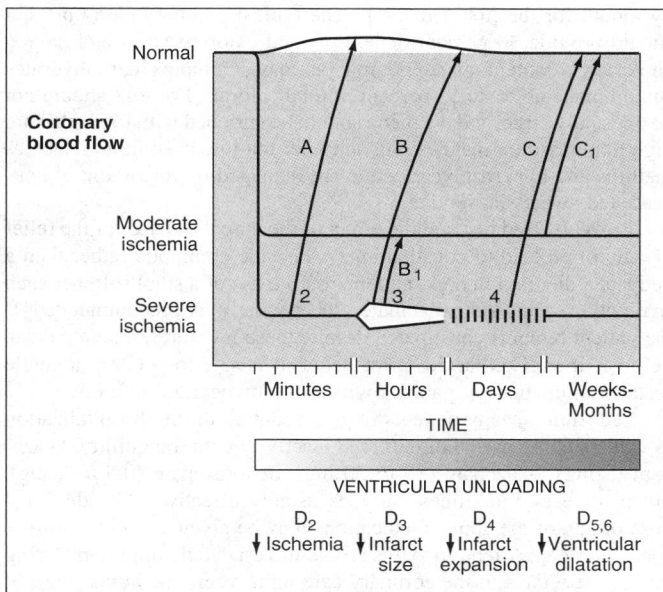

FIGURE 243-3 Therapeutic maneuvers in various stages of ischemia and infarction. Severely ischemic tissue (line 2) may be reperfused quickly with restoration of coronary blood flow to normal, thereby averting myocardial infarction (line A). Tissue undergoing infarction (3) may be reperfused, leading to sparing of myocardial tissue (line B) around a central core of necrotic myocardium. If only a moderate improvement in blood flow is achieved (B_1 = TIMI grade 1 or 2 flow), the myocardium may remain noncontractile although viable, i.e., hibernating. After completion of the infarct (4), late reperfusion (line C) may still be useful. Mechanical reperfusion of moderately ischemic myocardium (C_1) may restore the contractility of hibernating myocardium to normal. Ventricular unloading may be useful throughout the pre-infarct and post-infarct periods. Unloading may reduce ischemia (D_2), infarct size (D_3), infarct expansion (D_4), and ventricular dilation ($D_{5,6}$). *(From E Braunwald, MA Pfeffer, Am J Cardiol 68:4D, 1991.)*

of left ventricular function, and reduction of mortality over the short and long term.

Thrombolytic therapy can reduce the relative risk of in-hospital death by up to 50 percent when administered within the first hour of the onset of symptoms of myocardial infarction, and much of this benefit is maintained for 1 or more years. Appropriately employed thrombolytic therapy appears to reduce infarct size, limit left ventricular dysfunction, and reduce the incidence of serious complications such as septal rupture, cardiogenic shock, and malignant ventricular arrhythmias. Since myocardium can be salvaged only before it has been irreversibly injured, the timing of thrombolytic therapy is of extreme importance in achieving maximum benefit. While the upper time limit depends on specific factors in individual patients, it is clear that "every minute counts" and that patients treated within 1 to 3 h of the onset of symptoms generally benefit most. Although the reduction of mortality is more modest, benefit of therapy remains in many patients seen 3 to 6 h after the onset of infarction, and some benefit appears to be possible up to 12 h, especially if chest discomfort is still present and ST segments remain elevated in electrocardiographic leads that do not yet demonstrate new Q waves. In addition to the possibility of early treatment, clinical factors that favor proceeding with thrombolytic therapy include anterior wall injury, hemodynamically complicated infarction, and widespread ECG evidence of myocardial jeopardy. While younger patients (less than 65 years old) achieve a greater relative reduction in mortality rate than elderly patients, the higher absolute mortality rate (15 to 25 percent) in elderly patients results in similar absolute reductions in mortality rate (about 10 lives saved per 1000 patients treated with thrombolytics).

Intriguing data are accumulating to indicate that improved ventricular function and reduced mortality may also be achieved by *late coronary reperfusion* (Fig. 243-3, line C). The benefits of late reperfusion cannot be attributed to a reduction of infarct size but appear to result from improvement of tissue healing in the infarct zone with prevention of infarct expansion, enhancement of collateral flow, improvement of myocardial contractile performance, and reduction in the tendency to electrical instability. In addition, *hibernating myocardium* (i.e., poorly contractile myocardium in a zone that is supplied by a stenotic infarct-related coronary artery with slow antegrade perfusion, Chap. 244) may show improved contraction following angioplasty to increase coronary blood flow (Fig. 243-3, line C^1).

tPA is more effective than streptokinase at restoring full perfusion—i.e., TIMI grade 3 coronary flow—and has a small edge in improving survival as well. The current recommended regimen of tPA consists of a 15-mg bolus followed by 50 mg intravenously over the first 30 min, followed by 35 mg over the next 60 min. Streptokinase is administered as 1.5 million units intravenously over 1 h.

Contraindications and Complications Clear contraindications to the use of thrombolytic agents include a history of cerebrovascular hemorrhage at any time, a nonhemorrhagic stroke or other cerebrovascular event within the past year, marked hypertension (a reliably determined systolic arterial pressure greater than 180 mmHg and/or a diastolic pressure greater than 110 mmHg) at any time during the acute presentation, suspicion of aortic dissection, and active internal bleeding (excluding menses). While advanced age is associated with an increase in hemorrhagic complications, the benefit of thrombolytic therapy in the elderly appears to justify its use in most cases, particularly if no other contraindications are present and the amount of myocardium in jeopardy appears to be substantial.

Relative contraindications to thrombolytic therapy, which require careful assessment of the risk:benefit ratio, include current use of anticoagulants (international normalized ratio of >2 to 3), a recent (within 2 weeks) invasive or surgical procedure or prolonged (>10 min) cardiopulmonary resuscitation, known bleeding diathesis, pregnancy, a hemorrhagic ophthalmic condition (e.g., hemorrhagic diabetic retinopathy), active peptic ulcer disease, and a history of severe hypertension that is currently adequately controlled. Because of the risk of an allergic reaction, patients should not receive streptokinase if that agent had been received within the preceding 5 days to 2 years.

Allergic reactions to streptokinase occur in approximately 2 percent of cases. While a minor degree of hypotension occurs in 4 to 10 percent of patients given these agents, marked hypotension occurs, though rarely, in association with severe allergic reactions.

Hemorrhage is the most frequent and potentially the most serious complication. Since bleeding episodes that require transfusion are more common when patients require invasive procedures, unnecessary venous or arterial interventions should be avoided in patients receiving thrombolytic agents. Hemorrhagic stroke is the most serious complication and occurs in approximately 0.5 to 0.7 percent of cases. This rate increases with advancing age, with patients older than 70 years experiencing roughly twice the rate of intracranial hemorrhage as those younger than 65 years. Large-scale intervention trials have suggested that the rate of intracranial hemorrhage with tPA is slightly higher than that seen with streptokinase.

Routine angiography after thrombolysis with the intent of performing angioplasty on underlying coronary artery stenoses in the culprit vessel is not recommended owing to higher rates of abrupt closure of the infarct-related coronary artery with a need for urgent coronary artery bypass surgery as well as a trend toward an increase in mortality rate. Instead, after thrombolytic therapy, cardiac catheterization and coronary angiography should be carried out if either (1) there is evidence of failure of reperfusion (persistent chest pain and ST-segment elevation beyond 90 min) in which case a *rescue angioplasty* should be considered, or (2) there is coronary artery reocclusion (reelevation of ST segments and/or recurrent chest pain) or recurrent ischemia develops (such as recurrent angina in the early hospital course or a positive exercise stress test prior to discharge), in which case an *elective angioplasty* should be considered. Coronary artery bypass surgery should be reserved for patients whose coronary anatomy is unsuited to angioplasty but in whom revascularization appears to be advisable because of extensive jeopardized myocardium or recurrent ischemia.

Primary Percutaneous Transluminal Coronary Angioplasty (See also Chap. 245) Primary percutaneous transluminal coronary angioplasty (PTCA) without preceding thrombolysis carried out on an emergency basis in the first few hours of infarction is also effective in restoring perfusion in acute myocardial infarction. It has the advantage of being applicable to patients who have contraindications to thrombolytic therapy but otherwise are considered appropriate candidates for reperfusion. It appears to be more effective than thrombolysis in opening occluded coronary arteries and, when performed by experienced operators in dedicated medical centers, is associated with a better short-term and long-term clinical outcome. Efforts are underway to determine whether the advantages of primary PTCA reported from organized research efforts can be replicated in routine clinical practice. However, this technique is expensive in terms of personnel and facilities, and its applicability is seriously limited by logistic considerations.

Subgroups of patients in whom direct PTCA may provide a special benefit over thrombolytic therapy include patients with cardiogenic shock and others at high risk because of advanced age (>70 years) or hemodynamic compromise (systolic arterial pressure <100 mmHg).

HOSPITAL PHASE MANAGEMENT

CORONARY CARE UNITS These units are routinely equipped with a system that permits continuous monitoring of the cardiac rhythm of *each* patient and hemodynamic monitoring in *selected* patients. Defibrillators, respirators, noninvasive transthoracic pacemakers, and facilities for introducing pacing catheters and flow-directed balloon-tipped catheters are also usually available. Equally important is the organization of a highly trained team of nurses who can recognize arrhythmias, adjust the dosage of antiarrhythmic, vasoactive, and anticoagulant drugs, and perform cardiac resuscitation, including electroshock, when necessary.

Patients should be admitted to a coronary care unit early in their illness when it is expected that they will derive benefit from the sophisticated and expensive care provided (e.g., adjustment of intravenous nitroglycerin infusion rate, hemodynamic monitoring, and initiation of afterload reduction for left ventricular failure). The availability of electrocardiographic monitoring and trained personnel outside the coronary care unit has made it possible to admit lower-risk patients (e.g., those not hemodynamically compromised and without active arrhythmias) to "intermediate care units."

The duration of stay in the coronary care unit is dictated by the ongoing need for intensive care. If a myocardial infarction has been ruled out (ideally within 8 to 12 h) and symptoms are controlled with oral therapy, patients may be transferred out of the coronary care unit. Also, patients who have a confirmed acute myocardial infarction but who are considered to be at low risk (no prior infarction and no persistent chest discomfort, congestive heart failure, hypotension, or cardiac arrhythmias) may be safely transferred out of the coronary care unit in 24 to 36 h.

Activity Factors that increase the work of the heart during the initial hours of infarction may increase the size of the infarct. Therefore, patients with acute infarction should be kept at bed rest for the first 12 h. However, in the absence of complications, patients should be encouraged, under supervision, to resume an upright posture by dangling their feet over the side of the bed and sitting in a chair within the first 24 h. This practice is both psychologically beneficial and usually results in a reduction in the pulmonary capillary wedge pressure. Provided no hypotension occurs, by the third day patients typically are ambulating in their room with increasing duration and frequency, and they may shower or stand at the sink to bathe. By day 4 to 5 after infarction, patients should be increasing their ambulation progressively to a goal of 600 feet at least three times a day.

Diet Because of the risk of emesis and aspiration soon after infarction, patients should receive either nothing or only clear liquids by mouth for the first 4 to 12 h. The typical coronary care unit diet should provide 30 percent or less of total calories as fat and have a cholesterol content of ≤300 mg per day. Complex carbohydrates should make up 50 to 55 percent of total calories. Portions should not be unusually large, and the menu should be enriched with foods that are high in potassium, magnesium, and fiber but low in sodium. Diabetes mellitus and hypertriglyceridemia are managed by restriction of concentrated sweets in the diet.

Bowels Bed rest and the effect of the narcotics used for the relief of pain often lead to constipation. A bedside commode rather than a bedpan, a diet rich in bulk, and the routine use of a stool softener such as dioctyl sodium sulfosuccinate (200 mg daily) are recommended. If the patient remains constipated despite these measures, a laxative can be prescribed. Contrary to prior belief, it is safe to perform a gentle rectal examination on patients with acute myocardial infarction.

Sedation Many patients require sedation during hospitalization to withstand the period of enforced inactivity with tranquillity. Diazepam (5 mg), oxazepam (15 to 30 mg), or lorazepam (0.5 to 2 mg), given three or four times daily, is usually effective. An additional dose of any of the above medications may be given at night to ensure adequate sleep. Attention to this problem is especially important during the first few days in the coronary care unit, where the atmosphere of 24-hour vigilance may interfere with the patient's sleep. However, sedation is no substitute for reassuring, quiet surroundings. It is to be noted that many drugs used in the coronary care unit, such as atropine, H_2 blockers, and narcotics, can produce delirium, particularly in the elderly. This effect should not be confused with agitation, and it is wise to conduct a thorough review of the patient's medications before arbitrarily prescribing additional doses of anxiolytics.

PHARMACOTHERAPY FOR ACUTE INFARCTION

ANTITHROMBOTIC AGENTS The use of antiplatelet and antithrombin therapy during the initial phase of myocardial infarction is based on extensive laboratory and clinical evidence that thrombosis plays an important role in the pathogenesis of acute infarction. The primary goal of treatment with antiplatelet and antithrombin agents is to establish and maintain patency of the infarct-related artery. A secondary goal is to reduce the patient's tendency to thrombosis and thus the likelihood of mural thrombus formation or deep venous thrombosis, either of which could result in pulmonary embolization. The degree to which antiplatelet and antithrombin therapy achieves these goals partly determines how effectively it reduces the risk of mortality from acute myocardial infarction.

As noted previously (see "Initial Management in the Emergency Department," above), the standard antiplatelet agent for patients with acute myocardial infarction is aspirin. The most compelling evidence for the benefits of antiplatelet therapy (mainly with aspirin) in acute myocardial infarction is found in the comprehensive overview by the Antiplatelet Trialists' Collaboration. Data from nearly 20,000 patients with acute myocardial infarction enrolled in nine randomized trials were pooled and revealed a reduction in the mortality rate from 11.7 percent in control patients to 9.3 percent in patients receiving antiplatelet agents. This corresponds to the prevention of 24 deaths for every 1000 patients treated. Similarly, 2 strokes and 12 recurrent infarctions are prevented for every 1000 patients treated with antiplatelet therapy.

The glycoprotein IIb/IIIa receptor is the focus of intense investigation by basic and clinical scientists. Because platelet-rich thrombi are more resistant to thrombolytic agents than platelet-poor thrombi and because platelet aggregates appear to play a role in reocclusion after initially successful thrombolysis, glycoprotein IIb/IIIa inhibition may facilitate thrombolysis and reduce the rate of reocclusion of reperfused vessels. Compounds have been developed that are capable of blocking the glycoprotein IIb/IIIa receptor. These drugs appear promising in the management of myocardial infarction patients undergoing angioplasty and may also prove useful in the medical management of patients both with and without ST segment elevation at presentation.

The standard antithrombin agent used in clinical practice is heparin. Despite numerous clinical trials, the precise role of heparin in patients treated with thrombolytic agents remains uncertain. The available data fail to show any convincing benefit of heparin with respect to either coronary arterial patency or mortality rate when heparin is added to a regimen of aspirin and a non-fibrin-specific thrombolytic agent such as streptokinase. Although not conclusively proven, it appears that the immediate administration of intravenous heparin, in addition to a regimen of aspirin and tPA, helps to facilitate thrombolysis and to establish and maintain patency of the infarct-related artery. This effect is achieved at the cost of an increased risk of bleeding. Most clinicians who use tPA also administer a bolus and infusion of heparin. Commonly employed heparin regimens include a bolus of 5000 units followed by a maintenance infusion of 1000 units per hour or a bolus of 70 units per kilogram followed by a maintenance infusion of 15 units per kilogram per hour. The activated partial thromboplastin time during maintenance therapy should be 1.5 to 2 times the control value.

For patients who do not receive thrombolytic therapy, the minimum antithrombin therapy consists of 7500 units of heparin subcutaneously every 12 h until the patient is ambulatory, to prevent deep venous thrombosis. If the patient is at an increased risk of systemic or pulmonary thromboembolism (i.e., if the patient has an anterior location of the infarction, severe left ventricular dysfunction, congestive heart failure, a history of embolism, two-dimensional echocardiographic evidence of mural thrombus, or atrial fibrillation), full intravenous heparin in the dose noted above should be initiated, followed by at least 3 months of warfarin therapy.

BETA-ADRENOCEPTOR BLOCKERS The benefits of beta blockers in patients with acute myocardial infarction can be divided into those that occur immediately when the drug is given acutely and those that accrue over the long term when the drug is given for secondary prevention following an index infarction. Acute intravenous beta blockade improves the myocardial oxygen supply-demand relationship, decreases pain, reduces infarct size, and decreases the incidence of serious ventricular arrhythmias. An overview of the data from 27,000 patients enrolled in nine randomized trials in the prethrombolytic era indicates that intravenous followed by oral beta blockade

is associated with a 15 percent relative reduction in mortality, nonfatal reinfarction, and nonfatal cardiac arrest. In patients who undergo thrombolysis soon after the onset of chest pain, no incremental mortality reduction is seen with beta blockers, but recurrent ischemia and reinfarction are reduced.

Beta blocker therapy after myocardial infarction thus is useful for most patients except those in whom it is specifically contraindicated (patients with heart failure or severely compromised left ventricular function, heart block, orthostatic hypotension, or a history of asthma) and perhaps those whose excellent long-term prognosis (defined as an expected mortality rate of less than 1 percent per year) markedly diminishes any potential benefit (patients with normal ventricular function, no complex ventricular ectopy, and no angina).

ANGIOTENSIN CONVERTING ENZYME INHIBITORS
These drugs reduce mortality following myocardial infarction; the mortality benefits of angiotensin converting enzyme (ACE) inhibitors are additive to those achieved with aspirin and beta blockers. The maximum benefit is seen in high-risk patients (those who are elderly or have an anterior infarction, a prior infarction, and/or globally depressed left ventricular function) but there is also evidence suggesting that a short-term benefit occurs when ACE inhibitors are prescribed unselectively to all hemodynamically stable patients with infarction (i.e., those with a systolic pressure greater than 100 mmHg). The mechanism involves a reduction in ventricular remodeling after infarction (see "Ventricular Dysfunction," below) with a subsequent reduction in the risk of congestive heart failure. The rate of recurrent infarction also may be lower in patients treated chronically with ACE inhibitors after infarction.

ACE inhibitors should be prescribed within 24 h to all myocardial infarction patients with overt congestive heart failure as well as to hemodynamically stable patients with ST-segment elevation or left bundle branch block. There is little evidence to support the use of ACE inhibitors in myocardial infarction patients who present without ST-segment changes or only with ST-segment depression and without congestive heart failure. Prior to hospital discharge, left ventricular function should be assessed with an imaging study. ACE inhibition should be continued indefinitely in patients who have clinically evident congestive heart failure or in whom an imaging study shows a reduction in global left ventricular function or a large regional wall motion abnormality.

OTHER AGENTS Although the actual impact on mortality is slight (three to four lives saved per 1000 patients treated), *nitrates* (intravenous or oral) may be useful in the relief of pain associated with acute myocardial infarction. Favorable effects on the ischemic process and ventricular remodeling (see below) have led many physicians to routinely use intravenous nitroglycerin (5 to 10 μg/min initial dose and up to 200 μg/min as long as hemodynamic stability is maintained) for the first 24 to 48 h after the onset of infarction.

Results of multiple trials of different *calcium antagonists* have failed to establish a role for these agents in the treatment of most patients with myocardial infarction, in contrast to the more consistent data that exist for other drugs (e.g., beta blockers, aspirin, thrombolytic agents). The routine use of calcium antagonists cannot be recommended.

Intracellular *magnesium* levels are frequently reduced in patients with myocardial infarction, but this deficit is not adequately reflected in serum measurements, as magnesium is predominantly an intracellular ion, and less than 1 percent of the total body stores of magnesium are intravascular. Whether giving routine empirical supplemental infusions of magnesium to high-risk patients with myocardial infarction is beneficial remains an open question. At present, all patients should have a serum magnesium measurement on admission, and any demonstrated deficits should be corrected to minimize the risk of arrhythmias. There does not appear to be any benefit in the routine use of magnesium when it is administered late (greater than 6 h) or to patients with an uncomplicated infarction who have a low mortality risk.

COMPLICATIONS OF MYOCARDIAL INFARCTION AND THEIR TREATMENT

VENTRICULAR DYSFUNCTION Following myocardial infarction, the left ventricle undergoes a series of changes in shape, size, and thickness in both the infarcted and noninfarcted segments. This process is referred to as *ventricular remodeling* and generally precedes the development of clinically evident congestive heart failure in the months to years after infarction. Soon after myocardial infarction, the left ventricle begins to dilate. Acutely, this results from expansion of the infarct (i.e., slippage of muscle bundles, disruption of normal myocardial cells, and tissue loss within the necrotic zone, resulting in disproportionate thinning and elongation of the infarct zone). Later, lengthening of the noninfarcted segments occurs as well. The overall chamber enlargement that occurs is related to the size and location of the infarct, with greater dilation following infarction of the apex of the left ventricle and causing more marked hemodynamic impairment, more frequent heart failure, and a poorer prognosis. Progressive dilation and its clinical consequences may be ameliorated by therapy with ACE inhibitors and other vasodilators (e.g., nitrates) (Fig. 243-2). Thus, in patients with a lowered ejection fraction (less than 40 percent), regardless of whether or not heart failure is present, ACE inhibitors should be prescribed.

HEMODYNAMIC ASSESSMENT Pump failure is now the primary cause of in-hospital death from acute myocardial infarction. The extent of ischemic necrosis correlates well with the degree of pump failure and with mortality, both early (within 10 days of infarction) and later. The most common clinical signs are pulmonary rales and S_3 and S_4 gallop rhythms. Pulmonary congestion is also frequently seen on the chest roentgenogram. Elevation of left ventricular filling pressure and pulmonary artery pressure are the characteristic hemodynamic findings, but it should be appreciated that these findings may result from a reduction of ventricular compliance (diastolic failure) and/or a reduction of stroke volume with secondary cardiac dilation (systolic failure) (Chap. 232).

A classification originally proposed by Killip divides patients into four groups: class I, no signs of pulmonary or venous congestion; class II, moderate heart failure as evidenced by rales at the lung bases, S_3 gallop, tachypnea, or signs of failure of the right side of the heart, including venous and hepatic congestion; class III, severe heart failure, pulmonary edema; and class IV, shock with systolic pressure less than 90 mmHg and evidence of peripheral vasoconstriction, peripheral cyanosis, mental confusion, and oliguria. The expected hospital mortality rate of patients in these clinical classes when this classification was established in 1967 was as follows: class I, 0 to 5 percent; class II, 10 to 20 percent; class III, 35 to 45 percent; and class IV, 85 to 95 percent. With advances in management, the mortality rate has fallen, perhaps by as much as one-third to one-half, in each class.

Hemodynamic evidence of abnormal left ventricular function appears when contraction is seriously impaired in 20 to 25 percent of the left ventricle. Infarction of 40 percent or more of the left ventricle usually results in cardiogenic shock (see below). Positioning of a balloon flotation catheter in the pulmonary artery permits monitoring of left ventricular filling pressure; this technique is useful in patients who exhibit hypotension and/or clinical evidence of heart failure. Cardiac output can also be determined with a pulmonary artery catheter. With the addition of intraarterial pressure monitoring, systemic vascular resistance can be calculated as a guide to adjusting vasopressor and vasodilator therapy. Some patients with acute myocardial infarction have markedly elevated left ventricular filling pressures (>22 mmHg) and normal cardiac indexes [>2.6 and >3.6 L/(min/m²)], while others have relatively low filling pressures (<15 mmHg) and reduced cardiac indexes. The former patients usually benefit from diuresis, while the latter may respond to volume expansion by means of intravenous administration of colloid-containing solutions.

Hypovolemia This is an easily corrected condition that may contribute to the hypotension and vascular collapse associated with myocardial infarction in some patients. Hypovolemia may be secondary to previous diuretic use, to reduced fluid intake during the early stages of the illness, and/or to vomiting associated with pain or medications. Consequently, hypovolemia should be identified and corrected in patients with acute myocardial infarction and hypotension before more vigorous forms of therapy are embarked on. Central venous pressure reflects right rather than left ventricular filling pressure and is an inadequate guide for adjustment of blood volume, since left ventricular function is almost always affected much more adversely than right ventricular function in acute myocardial infarction. The optimal left ventricular filling or pulmonary artery wedge pressure may vary considerably among patients. Each patient's ideal level (generally approximately 20 mmHg) is reached by cautious fluid administration during careful monitoring of oxygenation and cardiac output. Eventually, the cardiac output plateaus and further increases in left ventricular filling pressure only increase congestive symptoms and decrease systemic oxygenation without raising arterial pressure.

℞ TREATMENT

The management of heart failure in association with myocardial infarction is similar to that of acute heart failure secondary to other forms of heart disease (avoidance of hypoxemia, diuresis, afterload reduction, inotropic support) (Chap. 233), except that the benefits of digitalis administration in acute myocardial infarction are unimpressive. On the other hand, diuretic agents are extremely effective, as they diminish pulmonary congestion in the presence of systolic and/or diastolic heart failure. A fall in left ventricular filling pressure and an improvement in orthopnea and dyspnea follow the intravenous administration of furosemide. This drug should be used with caution, however, as it can result in a massive diuresis with associated decrease in plasma volume, cardiac output, systemic blood pressure, and hence coronary perfusion. Nitrates in various forms may be used to decrease preload and congestive symptoms. Oral isosorbide dinitrate, topical nitroglycerin ointment, or intravenous nitroglycerin all have the advantage over a diuretic of lowering preload through venodilation without decreasing the total plasma volume. In addition, nitrates may improve ventricular compliance if ischemia is present, as ischemia causes an elevation of left ventricular filling pressure. The patient with pulmonary edema is treated as described in Chap. 233, but vasodilators must be used with caution to prevent serious hypotension. As noted earlier, ACE inhibitors are an ideal class of drugs for management of ventricular dysfunction following myocardial infarction, especially for the long term.

CARDIOGENIC SHOCK In recent years, efforts to reduce infarct size and prompt treatment of ongoing ischemia and other complications of myocardial infarction appear to have reduced the incidence of cardiogenic shock from 20 percent to about 7 percent. Only 10 percent of patients with this condition present with it on admission, while 90 percent develop it during hospitalization. Typically, patients who develop cardiogenic shock have severe multivessel coronary artery disease with evidence of "piecemeal" necrosis extending outward from the original infarct zone.

It is useful to consider cardiogenic shock as a form of severe left ventricular failure. This syndrome is characterized by marked hypotension with systolic arterial pressure of <80 mmHg and a marked reduction of cardiac index [<1.8 L/(min/m²)] in the face of an elevated left ventricular filling (pulmonary capillary wedge) pressure (>18 mmHg). Hypotension alone is not a basis for the diagnosis of cardiogenic shock, because many patients who make an uneventful recovery will have serious hypotension (systolic pressure of <80 mmHg) for several hours. Such patients often have low left ventricular filling pressures, and their hypotension usually resolves with the administration of intravenous fluids. In contrast to hypovolemic hypotension, cardiogenic shock is generally associated with a mortality rate of >70 percent; however, recent efforts to restore perfusion by coronary angioplasty or surgical revascularization suggest that this high mortality rate can be lowered by as much as one-half.

Risk factors for the in-hospital development of shock include advanced age, a depressed left ventricular ejection fraction on admission, a large infarct, previous myocardial infarction, and a history of diabetes mellitus. Patients with several of these risk factors should be considered for cardiac catheterization and mechanical reperfusion (by angioplasty or surgery) *before* the development of shock.

Pathophysiology of Severe Power Failure A marked reduction in the quantity of contracting myocardium is the cause of cardiogenic shock in myocardial infarction. The initial insult reduces arterial pressure, and the reduction in coronary perfusion pressure and myocardial blood flow initiates a vicious cycle that further impairs myocardial function and may increase the size of the infarct. Arrhythmias and metabolic acidosis also contribute to this deterioration, because they are the result of inadequate perfusion. It is this positive feedback loop that accounts for the high mortality rate associated with the shock syndrome.

Rx **TREATMENT**

The physiology and ominous prognosis of this condition dictate that all patients with shock should, if possible, have continuous monitoring of arterial pressure and of left ventricular filling pressure (as reflected in the pulmonary capillary wedge pressure measured with a pulmonary artery balloon catheter) as well as frequent determinations of cardiac output. When pulmonary edema coexists, endotracheal intubation may be necessary to ensure oxygenation. The relief of pain is important, as some vasodepressor reflex activity may be a response to severe pain. However, narcotics should be used cautiously, in view of their propensity to lower arterial pressure. The primary objective of treatment is to maintain coronary perfusion by raising the arterial blood pressure with vasopressors (see below), intraaortic balloon counterpulsation, and manipulation of blood volume to a level that ensures an optimum left ventricular filling pressure (approximately 20 mmHg). The latter may require either infusion of crystalloid or diuresis.

In patients seen within the first 4 to 8 h of the onset of infarction, early reperfusion by PTCA (see "Primary Percutaneous Transluminal Coronary Angioplasty," above) may improve left ventricular function dramatically, thereby interrupting the cycle of hemodynamic deterioration.

Vasopressors A variety of intravenous drugs may be used to augment arterial pressure and cardiac output in patients with cardiogenic shock. Unfortunately, all have important disadvantages or problems, and none has been shown to change the outcome in patients with established shock. *Isoproterenol* is a sympathomimetic amine that is now rarely used in the treatment of shock due to myocardial infarction. Although this agent increases contractility, it also produces peripheral vasodilation and increases heart rate. The resulting increase in myocardial oxygen consumption and reduction of coronary perfusion pressure may extend the area of ischemic injury. *Norepinephrine* (Chap. 70) is a potent alpha-adrenergic agent with powerful vasoconstrictor properties that also possesses beta-adrenergic activity and therefore enhances contractility. Because the increase in afterload and contractility associated with its use causes a marked increase in myocardial oxygen consumption, it should be reserved for desperate situations or for patients with cardiogenic shock and reduced systemic vascular resistance. It should be started at 2 to 4 μg/min. If pressure cannot be maintained with a dosage of 15 μg/min, it is unlikely that a further increase will be beneficial. *Dopamine* (Chap. 70) is useful in many patients with power failure. At low doses [2 to 10 μg/kg per min], the drug has positive chronotropic and inotropic effects as a consequence of beta receptor stimulation. At higher doses, a vasoconstrictor effect results from alpha receptor stimulation. At lower doses [≤2 μg/kg per min], dopamine also has the unique effect of dilating the renal and splanchnic vascular beds and apparently has little effect on myocardial oxygen consumption. Intravenous dopamine is started at an infusion rate of 2 to 5 μg/kg per min, and the dosage is increased every 2

to 5 min up to a maximum of 20 to 50 μg/kg per min. Systolic arterial blood pressure should be maintained at approximately 90 mmHg. *Dobutamine* is a synthetic sympathomimetic amine with positive inotropic action and minimal positive chronotropic or peripheral vasoconstrictive activity in the usual dosage range of 2.5 to 10 μg/kg per min. It should not be employed when a vasoconstrictor effect is required. However, in patients with less profound degrees of hypotension, dobutamine may be an extremely useful agent, particularly if positive chronotropy is to be avoided.

Amrinone and *milrinone* are positive inotropic agents without catecholamine structure or activity that act by inhibiting phosphodiesterase. These drugs resemble dobutamine in pharmacologic activity, although they have a more potent vasodilating action. For amrinone, an initial loading dose of 0.75 mg/kg is given over 2 to 3 min. If effective, it is followed by an infusion of 5 to 10 μg/kg per min. If necessary, the dose may then be increased up to 15 μg/kg per min for short periods. Milrinone is given as a loading dose of 50 μg/kg over 10 min followed by a maintenance infusion of 0.375 to 0.75 μg/kg per min.

Aortic Counterpulsation In cardiogenic shock, mechanical assistance with an intraaortic balloon pumping system capable of augmenting both diastolic pressure and cardiac output may be helpful. A sausage-shaped balloon at the end of a catheter is introduced percutaneously into the aorta via the femoral artery, and the balloon is automatically inflated during early diastole, thereby augmenting coronary blood flow. The balloon collapses in early systole, thereby reducing the afterload against which left ventricular ejection takes place. Improvement in hemodynamic status has been observed with balloon pumping in a large number of patients. In the absence of early revascularization, however, long-term survival following this mode of therapy in patients with cardiogenic shock is still disappointing. The balloon counterpulsation system may best be reserved for patients whose condition merits mechanical (surgical or angioplastic) intervention (e.g., patients with continuing ischemia, ventricular septal rupture, or mitral regurgitation) and in whom a successful result is likely to reverse the cardiogenic shock. Intraaortic balloon pumping is contraindicated if aortic regurgitation is present or aortic dissection is suspected.

There is reason to believe that results of therapy for the shock syndrome secondary to myocardial infarction, while improving gradually as a result of meticulous attention to the details outlined above, will continue to be disappointing overall because a large fraction of patients with the syndrome have large areas of infarcted myocardium with severe, diffuse coronary atherosclerosis. There is suggestive evidence that dramatic results can be achieved with emergency revascularization surgery, or more commonly, coronary angioplasty. However, only a minority of patients developing cardiogenic shock have prompt access to these expensive techniques, and it is hoped that the widespread and early application of thrombolytic therapy will reduce the amount of myocardium that becomes necrotic and thereby reduce the incidence of this syndrome.

RIGHT VENTRICULAR INFARCTION Approximately one-third of patients with inferoposterior infarction demonstrate at least a minor degree of right ventricular necrosis. An occasional patient with inferoposterior left ventricular infarction also has extensive right ventricular myocardial infarction, and rare patients present with infarction limited primarily to the right ventricle. Clinically significant right ventricular infarction causes signs of severe right ventricular failure (jugular venous distention, Kussmaul's sign, hepatomegaly) with or without hypotension. ST-segment elevations of the right-sided precordial electrocardiographic leads, particularly lead V_4R, are frequently present in the first 24 h in patients with right ventricular infarction. Two-dimensional echocardiography is helpful in determining the degree of right ventricular dysfunction. Catheterization of the right side of the heart often reveals a distinctive hemodynamic pattern resembling cardiac tamponade or constrictive pericarditis (steep right atrial "y" descent and an early diastolic dip and plateau in right ventricular waveforms) (Chap. 240). Therapy consists of volume expansion to maintain adequate right ventricular preload and efforts to improve left ventricular performance with attendant reduction in pulmonary capillary wedge and pulmonary arterial pressures.

MECHANICAL CAUSES OF HEART FAILURE **Free Wall Rupture** Myocardial rupture is a dramatic complication of myocardial infarction that is most likely to occur during the first week after the onset of symptoms; its frequency increases with the age of the patient. First infarction, a history of hypertension, no history of angina pectoris, and a relatively large Q-wave infarct are associated with a higher incidence of cardiac rupture. The clinical presentation typically is a sudden loss of pulse, blood pressure and consciousness while the electrocardiogram continues to show sinus rhythm (*apparent* electromechanical dissociation). The myocardium continues to contract, but forward flow is not maintained as blood escapes into the pericardium. Cardiac tamponade (Chap. 240) ensues, and closed-chest massage is ineffective. This condition is almost universally fatal, although dramatic cases of urgent pericardiotensis followed by successful surgical repair have been reported.

Ventricular Septal Defect The pathogenesis of perforation of the ventricular septum is similar to that of free wall rupture, but the chance of successful therapy is greater. Patients with ventricular septal rupture present with sudden, severe left ventricular failure in association with the appearance of a pansystolic murmur, often accompanied by a parasternal thrill. It is often impossible to differentiate this condition from rupture of a papillary muscle with resulting mitral regurgitation, and the presence in both conditions of a tall "v" wave in the pulmonary capillary wedge pressure further complicates the differentiation. The diagnosis of ventricular septal defect can be established by the demonstration of a left-to-right shunt (i.e., an oxygen step-up at the level of the right ventricle) by means of limited cardiac catheterization performed at the bedside using a flow-directed balloon catheter. Color flow doppler echocardiography can also be extremely useful for making this diagnosis at the bedside. A prolonged period of hemodynamic compromise may produce end-organ damage and other complications that can be avoided by early intervention, including nitroprusside infusion and intraaortic balloon counterpulsation.

The physiology of acute mitral regurgitation is similar to that of acute ventricular septal perforation in that the level of aortic systolic pressure partly determines the regurgitant volume, the principal difference being the chamber into which the regurgitant fraction is ejected. In septal perforation, a fraction of left ventricular output is ejected into the right ventricle. As in mitral regurgitation, lowering of the aortic systolic pressure by mechanical (intraaortic balloon counterpulsation) and/or pharmacologic (nitroglycerin or nitroprusside) means can decrease the hemodynamic compromise caused by perforation.

Mitral Regurgitation (See also Chap. 237) The reported incidence of apical systolic murmurs of mitral regurgitation during the first few days after the onset of a myocardial infarction varies widely (from 10 to 50 percent of patients) depending on the population studied and the acumen of the observers. Whether audible or angiographically demonstrated, mitral regurgitation is of hemodynamic importance in only a minority of these patients.

The most common cause of mitral regurgitation following myocardial infarction is dysfunction of the mitral valve due to ischemia or infarction. Left ventricular dilatation or alteration in the size or shape of the ventricle due to impaired contractility or to aneurysm formation causes disordered contraction of the papillary muscles. A papillary muscle, or, more commonly, the head of a papillary muscle, may rupture. Left ventricular function may deteriorate dramatically, with superimposition of severe mitral regurgitation. The major element in the differential diagnosis is perforation of the ventricular septum as discussed above. Surgical repair or replacement of the mitral valve may lead to dramatic improvement in patients in whom acute heart failure results primarily from severe mitral regurgitation due to papillary muscle rupture or dysfunction and in whom global ventricular function is relatively good.

If aortic systolic pressure is lowered in patients with mitral regurgitation, a greater fraction of the left ventricular output will be ejected antegradely, thus lessening the regurgitant fraction. To this end, both intraaortic balloon counterpulsation, which lowers the aortic systolic pressure mechanically, and the infusion of nitroglycerin or sodium nitroprusside, which reduce systemic vascular resistance, have been used with success in the interim management of patients with severe mitral regurgitation in the setting of acute myocardial infarction. Ideally, definitive operative treatment should be postponed until pulmonary congestion has cleared and the infarct has had time to heal. However, if the patient's hemodynamic and/or clinical condition does not improve or stabilize, surgical treatment should be undertaken, even in the acute stage.

ARRHYTHMIAS (See also Chaps. 230 and 231) The incidence of arrhythmias after myocardial infarction is higher in patients seen early after the onset of symptoms. The mechanisms responsible for infarction-related arrhythmias include autonomic nervous system imbalance, electrolyte disturbances, ischemia, and slowed conduction. An arrhythmia can usually be managed successfully if trained personnel and appropriate equipment are available when it develops. Since mortality from arrhythmia is greatest during the first few hours after infarction, it is obvious that the effectiveness of treatment relates directly to the speed with which patients come under medical observation. The prompt management of arrhythmias constitutes a significant advance in the treatment of myocardial infarction.

Ventricular Premature Beats Infrequent, sporadic ventricular premature depolarizations occur in almost all patients with infarction and do not require therapy. Whereas in the past, frequent, multifocal, or early diastolic ventricular extrasystoles (so-called warning arrhythmias) were routinely treated with antiarrhythmic drugs to reduce the risk of development of ventricular tachycardia and ventricular fibrillation, pharmacologic therapy is now reserved for patients with sustained ventricular arrhythmias. *Prophylactic antiarrhythmic therapy* (either intravenous lidocaine early or oral agents later) is *contraindicated* for ventricular premature beats in the absence of clinically important ventricular tachyarrhythmias, as such therapy may actually increase late mortality. Beta-adrenoceptor blocking agents are effective in abolishing ventricular ectopic activity in infarction patients and in the prevention of ventricular fibrillation. As described above (see "Beta-Adrenoceptor Blockers"), they should be used routinely in patients without contraindications. In addition, hypokalemia and hypomagnesemia are risk factors for ventricular fibrillation in patients with acute myocardial infarction; the serum potassium concentration should be adjusted to approximately 4.5 mmol/L and magnesium to about 2.0 mmol/L.

Ventricular Tachycardia and Fibrillation Within the first 24 h of myocardial infarction, ventricular tachycardia and fibrillation can occur without prior warning arrhythmias. The occurrence of ventricular fibrillation can be reduced by prophylactic administration of intravenous lidocaine. However, prophylactic use of lidocaine has not been shown to reduce overall mortality from acute myocardial infarction. In fact, in addition to causing possible noncardiac complications, lidocaine use may predispose to an excess risk of bradycardia and asystole. For these reasons, and with earlier treatment of active ischemia, more frequent use of beta-blocking agents, and the nearly universal success of electrical cardioversion or defibrillation, routine *prophylactic* antiarrhythmic drug therapy is no longer recommended. It should be reserved for patients who cannot reach a hospital or for those treated in hospitals that lack the constant presence in the coronary care unit of a physician or nurse trained in the recognition and treatment of ventricular fibrillation.

Sustained ventricular tachycardia that is well tolerated hemodynamically should be treated with an intravenous regimen of lidocaine [bolus of 1.0 to 1.5 mg/kg; infusion of 20 to 50 μg/kg per min], procainamide (bolus of 15 mg/kg over 20 to 30 min; infusion of 1 to 4 mg/min), or amiodarone (bolus of 75 to 150 mg over 10 to 15 min followed by infusion of 1.0 mg/min for 6 h and then 0.5 mg/min); if it does not stop promptly, electroversion should be used (Chap. 231). Electroshock (an unsynchronized discharge of 200 to 300 J) is used immediately in patients with ventricular fibrillation or when ventricular tachycardia causes hemodynamic deterioration. Ventricular tachycardia or fibrillation that is refractory to electroshock may be more responsive after treatment with epinephrine (1 mg intravenously or 10 mL of a 1:10,000 solution via the intracardiac route), bretylium (a 5-mg/kg bolus), or amiodarone (a 75 to 150-mg bolus).

Ventricular arrhythmias, including the unusual form of ventricular tachycardia known as *torsade de pointes* (Chap. 231), may occur in infarct patients as a consequence of other concurrent problems (such as hypoxia, hypokalemia, or other electrolyte disturbances) or of the toxic effects of an agent being administered to the patient (such as digoxin or quinidine). A search for such secondary causes should always be undertaken.

Although in-hospital mortality is increased, the long-term survival is good in patients who survive to hospital discharge after *primary* ventricular fibrillation, i.e., ventricular fibrillation that is a primary response to acute ischemia and is not associated with predisposing factors such as congestive heart failure, shock, bundle branch block, or ventricular aneurysm. This result is in sharp contrast to the poor prognosis for patients who develop ventricular fibrillation *secondary* to severe pump failure. In patients who develop ventricular tachycardia or ventricular fibrillation late in their hospital course (i.e., after the first 48 h), the mortality rate is increased both in hospital and during long-term follow-up. Such patients should be considered for electrophysiologic study (Chap. 231).

Accelerated Idioventricular Rhythm   Accelerated idioventricular rhythm (AIVR, "slow ventricular tachycardia"), a ventricular rhythm with a rate of 60 to 100 beats per minute, occurs in 25 percent of patients with myocardial infarction. It often occurs transiently during thrombolytic therapy at the time of reperfusion. The rate of AIVR is usually similar to that of the sinus rhythm that precedes and follows it, and this similarity of rate plus the relatively minor hemodynamic effects make this rhythm more difficult to detect except by electrocardiographic monitoring. For the most part, AIVR is benign and does not presage the development of classic ventricular tachycardia. Most episodes of AIVR do not require treatment if the patient is monitored carefully, as degeneration into a more serious arrhythmia is rare, and, if it occurs, AIVR can generally be readily treated with a drug that increases the sinus rate (atropine).

Supraventricular Arrhythmias   Sinus tachycardia is the most common type of supraventricular arrhythmia. If it occurs secondary to another cause (such as anemia, fever, heart failure, or a metabolic derangement), the primary problem should be treated first. However, if it appears to be due to sympathetic overstimulation, for example as part of a hyperdynamic state, then treatment with a beta blocker is indicated. Other common arrhythmias in this group are atrial flutter and atrial fibrillation, which are often secondary to left ventricular failure. Digoxin administration is usually the treatment of choice for supraventricular arrhythmias if heart failure is present. If heart failure is absent, beta blockers, verapamil, or diltiazem are suitable alternatives for controlling the ventricular rate, as they may also help control ischemia. If the abnormal rhythm persists for more than 2 h with a ventricular rate in excess of 120 beats per minute, or if tachycardia induces heart failure, shock, or ischemia (as manifested by recurrent pain or ECG changes), a synchronized electroshock (100 to 200 J) should be used.

Accelerated junctional rhythms have diverse causes but may be seen in patients with inferoposterior infarction. Digitalis excess must be ruled out as a cause. In some patients with severely compromised left ventricular function, the loss of appropriately timed atrial systole results in a marked decrease in cardiac output. Right atrial or coronary sinus pacing is indicated in such instances.

Sinus Bradycardia   Treatment of sinus bradycardia is indicated if hemodynamic compromise results from the slow heart rate. Atropine is the most useful drug for increasing heart rate and should be given

intravenously in doses of 0.5 mg initially. If the rate remains below 50 to 60 beats per minute, additional doses of 0.2 mg, up to a total of 2.0 mg, may be given. Persistent bradycardia (<40 beats per minute) despite atropine may be treated with electrical pacing. Isoproterenol should be avoided.

Atrioventricular and Intraventricular Conduction Disturbances (See also Chap. 230)   Both the in-hospital mortality rate and the post-discharge mortality rate of patients who have complete atrioventricular (AV) block in association with anterior infarction are markedly higher than those of patients who develop AV block with inferior infarction. This difference is related to the fact that heart block in inferior infarction is commonly a result of increased vagal tone and/or the release of adenosine and therefore is transient. In anterior wall infarction, heart block is usually related to ischemic malfunction of the conduction system, which commonly is associated with extensive myocardial necrosis.

Temporary electrical pacing provides an effective means of increasing the heart rate of patients with bradycardia due to AV block. However, acceleration of the heart rate may have only a limited impact on prognosis in patients with anterior wall infarction and complete heart block in whom the large size of the infarct is the major factor determining outcome. It should be carried out if it improves hemodynamics, however. Pacing does appear to be beneficial in patients with inferoposterior infarction who have complete heart block associated with heart failure, hypotension, marked bradycardia, or significant ventricular ectopic activity. A subgroup of these patients, those with right ventricular infarction, often respond poorly to ventricular pacing because of the loss of the atrial contribution to ventricular filling. In such patients, dual-chamber atrioventricular sequential pacing may be required.

External noninvasive pacing electrodes should be positioned in a "demand" mode for patients with sinus bradycardia (rate < 50 beats per minute) that is unresponsive to drug therapy, Mobitz II second-degree AV block, third-degree heart block, or bilateral bundle branch block (e.g., right bundle branch block plus left anterior fascicular block). Retrospective studies suggest that permanent pacing may reduce the long-term risk of sudden death due to bradyarrhythmias in the rare patient who develops combined persistent bifascicular and transient third-degree heart block during the acute phase of myocardial infarction.

OTHER COMPLICATIONS   Recurrent Chest Discomfort   Recurrent angina develops in approximately 25 percent of patients hospitalized for acute myocardial infarction. This percentage is even higher in patients who undergo successful thrombolysis. Since recurrent or persistent ischemia often heralds *extension* of the original infarct or *reinfarction* in a new myocardial zone and is associated with a doubling of risk following acute myocardial infarction, patients with these symptoms should be considered for repeat thrombolysis or referred for prompt coronary arteriography and mechanical revascularization. Repeat administration of a thrombolytic agent is an alternative to early mechanical revascularization.

Pericarditis (See also Chap. 240)   Pericardial friction rubs and/or pericardial pain are frequently encountered in patients with acute transmural myocardial infarction. This complication can usually be managed with aspirin (650 mg qid). It is important to diagnose the chest pain of pericarditis accurately, since failure to appreciate it may lead to the erroneous diagnosis of recurrent ischemic pain and/or infarct extension, with resulting inappropriate use of anticoagulants, nitrates, beta blockers, or coronary arteriography. Anticoagulants potentially could cause tamponade in the presence of acute pericarditis (as manifested by either pain or persistent rub), and therefore should not be used unless there is a compelling indication.

An infrequently occurring syndrome (post-myocardial infarction syndrome or Dressler's syndrome), characterized by fever and pleuropericardial chest pain, is thought to be due to an autoimmune pericarditis, pleuritis, and/or pneumonitis. It may begin from a few days to 6 weeks after myocardial infarction and usually responds promptly to therapy with salicylates.

Thromboembolism Clinically apparent thromboembolism complicates acute myocardial infarction in approximately 10 percent of cases, but embolic lesions are found in 20 percent of patients in necropsy series, suggesting that thromboembolism is often clinically silent. Thromboembolism is considered to be at least an important contributing cause of death in 25 percent of infarct patients who die following admission to the hospital. Arterial emboli originate from left ventricular mural thrombi, while most pulmonary emboli arise in the leg veins.

Thromboembolism typically occurs in association with large infarcts (especially anterior), heart failure, and a left ventricular thrombus detected by echocardiography. The incidence of arterial embolism from a clot originating in the ventricle at the site of an infarction is small but real. Two-dimensional echocardiography reveals left ventricular thrombi in about one-third of patients with anterior wall infarction but in few patients with inferior or posterior infarction. Arterial embolism often presents as a major complication, such as hemiparesis when the cerebral circulation is involved or hypertension if the renal circulation is compromised. When a thrombus has been clearly demonstrated by echocardiographic or other techniques or when a large area of regional wall motion abnormality is seen even in the absence of a detectable mural thrombus, systemic anticoagulation should be undertaken (in the absence of contraindications), as the incidence of embolic complications appears to be markedly lowered by such therapy. The appropriate duration of therapy is unknown, but 3 to 6 months is probably prudent.

Left Ventricular Aneurysm The term *ventricular aneurysm* is usually used to describe *dyskinesis* or local expansile paradoxical wall motion. Normally functioning myocardial fibers must shorten more if stroke volume and cardiac output are to be maintained in patients with ventricular aneurysm; if they cannot, overall ventricular function is impaired. True aneurysms are composed of scar tissue and neither predispose to nor are associated with cardiac rupture.

The complications of left ventricular aneurysm do not usually occur for weeks to months following myocardial infarction; they include congestive heart failure, arterial embolism, and ventricular arrhythmias. Apical aneurysms are the most common and the most easily detected by clinical examination. The physical finding of greatest value is a double, diffuse, or displaced apical impulse. Ventricular aneurysms are readily detected by two-dimensional echocardiography, which may also reveal a mural thrombus in an aneurysm.

Rarely, myocardial rupture may be contained by a local area of pericardium, along with organizing thrombus and hematoma. Over time, this *pseudoaneurysm* enlarges, maintaining communication with the left ventricular cavity via a narrow neck. Because spontaneous rupture of a pseudoaneurysm often occurs, this defect should be surgically repaired if recognized.

POSTINFARCTION RISK STRATIFICATION AND MANAGEMENT

Many clinical factors have been identified that are associated with an increase in cardiovascular risk following initial recovery from a myocardial infarction. Some of the most important factors include persistent ischemia (spontaneous or provoked), depressed left ventricular ejection fraction (less than 40 percent), rales above the lung bases on physical examination or congestion on chest radiograph, and symptomatic ventricular arrhythmias. Other features associated with increased risk include a history of previous myocardial infarction, age over 70 years, diabetes, prolonged sinus tachycardia, hypotension, the occurrence of ST-segment changes at rest without angina ("silent ischemia"), an abnormal signal-averaged electrocardiogram, nonpatency of the infarct-related coronary artery (if angiography is undertaken), and persistent advanced heart block or a new intraventricular

conduction abnormality on the electrocardiogram. Therapy must be individualized depending on the relative importance of the risk(s) present.

The goal of preventing reinfarction and death following recovery from myocardial infarction has led to strategies to evaluate risk following infarction. Early after infarction, this evaluation generally involves the use of noninvasive testing. In stable patients, submaximal exercise stress testing may be carried out prior to hospital discharge to detect residual ischemia and ventricular ectopy, and to provide the patient with a guideline for exercise in the early recovery period. Alternatively, or in addition, a maximal (symptom-limited) exercise stress test may be carried out 4 to 6 weeks after infarction. Evaluation of left ventricular function at rest and during exercise is usually warranted as well. Recognition of a depressed left ventricular ejection fraction by echocardiography or radionuclide ventriculography identifies patients who should receive ACE inhibitors (see "Angiotensin Converting Enzyme Inhibitors," above). Patients in whom angina is induced at relatively low workloads, those who have a large reversible defect on perfusion imaging or a depressed ejection fraction and demonstrable ischemia, and those in whom exercise provokes symptomatic ventricular arrhythmias should be considered at high risk for recurrent myocardial infarction or death from arrhythmia, and cardiac catheterization with coronary angiography and/or invasive electrophysiologic evaluation is advised.

Exercise tests also aid in formulating an individualized exercise prescription, which can be much more vigorous in patients who tolerate exercise without any of the above-mentioned adverse signs. Additionally, predischarge stress testing may provide an important psychological benefit, building the patient's confidence by demonstrating a reasonable exercise tolerance. Furthermore, particularly when no arrhythmias or signs of ischemia are identified, the patient benefits by the physician's reassurance that objective evidence suggests no immediate jeopardy.

In many hospitals a cardiac rehabilitation program with progressive exercise is initiated in the hospital and continued after discharge. Ideally, such programs should include an educational component that informs patients about their disease and its risk factors.

The usual duration of hospitalization for an uncomplicated myocardial infarction is 5 to 6 days. The remainder of the convalescent phase may be accomplished at home. During the first 2 weeks, the patient should be encouraged to increase activity by walking about the house and outdoors in good weather. Normal sexual activity may be resumed during this period. After 2 weeks, the physician must regulate the patient's activity on the basis of exercise tolerance. It is during this period of increasing activity that the patient may become aware of profound fatigue. Postural hypotension may still be a problem. Most patients will be able to return to work within 2 to 4 weeks.

SECONDARY PREVENTION OF INFARCTION

A variety of secondary preventive measures are at least partly responsible for the improvement in long-term mortality and morbidity following myocardial infarction. Long-term treatment with an antiplatelet agent following a myocardial infarction is associated with a 25 percent reduction in the risk of recurrent infarction, stroke, or cardiovascular mortality (36 fewer events for every 1000 patients treated). In addition, in patients taking aspirin chronically, myocardial infarctions tend to be smaller and are more likely to be non-Q-wave in nature. ACE inhibitors should be used indefinitely by patients with clinically evident heart failure, a moderate decrease in global ejection fraction, or a large regional wall motion abnormality to prevent late ventricular remodeling and recurrent ischemic events.

The chronic routine use of oral beta-adrenoceptor blockers for at least 2 years following acute myocardial infarction is supported by well-conducted placebo-controlled trials that have convincingly demonstrated reductions in the rates of total mortality, sudden death, and, in some instances, reinfarction. In contrast, calcium antagonists are not recommended for routine secondary prevention.

Evidence suggests that warfarin lowers late mortality and the incidence of reinfarction after an acute myocardial infarction. Since studies comparing aspirin and warfarin therapy separately or in combination have not yet been completed, most physicians use aspirin routinely in all patients without contraindications and add warfarin in patients at increased risk of embolism (see "Thromboembolism," above).

Finally, risk factors for *atherosclerosis* (Chap. 242) should be discussed with the patient, and, when possible, favorably modified. In particular, efforts should be made to ensure the cessation of smoking and the control of hypertension and hyperlipidemia (the target low-density lipoprotein level is less than 100 mg/dL). In addition, regular physical exercise and reduction of emotional stress should be encouraged. Hormone replacement therapy should be considered for post-menopausal women recovering from myocardial infarction, although the question of whether to use this modality may be complex given individual patient preferences and the small but finite risk of breast cancer.

BIBLIOGRAPHY

AMERICAN HEART ASSOCIATION: *Heart and Stroke Facts: 1995 Statistical Supplement.* Dallas, American Heart Association, 1995

ANTIPLATELET TRIALISTS' COLLABORATION: Collaborative overview of randomized trials of antiplatelet therapy. I: Prevention of death, myocardial infarction, and stroke by prolonged antiplatelet therapy in various categories of patients. BMJ 308:81, 1994

ANTMAN EM: Magnesium in acute MI. Timing is critical. Circulation 92:2367, 1995

————: Overview of medical therapy. In R Califf (ed): *Acute Myocardial Infarction and Other Acute Ischemic Syndromes,* in E Braunwald (Series ed): *Atlas of Heart Diseases,* vol. 8. Philadelphia, Current Medicine, 1996

———— et al: Evaluation of a rapid bedside assay for detection of serum cardiac troponin T. J Am Med Assoc 273:1279, 1995

CALIFF RM: Acute myocardial infarction. In *Cardiovascular Therapeutics,* TW Smith (ed). Philadelphia, Saunders, 1996, p 127

————, BENGTSON JR: Cardiogenic shock. N Engl J Med. 330:1724, 1994

COMMITTEE ON RADIONUCLIDE IMAGING: ACC/AHA Task Force Report: Guidelines for clinical use of cardiac radionuclide imaging. J Am Coll Cardiol 25:521, 1995

EPSTEIN AE et al: Mortality following ventricular arrhythmia suppression by encainide, flecainide, and moricizine after myocardial infarction. The original design concept of the Cardiac Arrhythmia Suppression Trial (CAST). J Am Med Assoc 270:2451, 1993

FALK E et al: Coronary plaque disruption. Circulation 92:657, 1995

FIBRINOLYTIC THERAPY TRIALISTS (FTT) COLLABORATIVE GROUP: Indications for fibrinolytic therapy in suspected acute myocardial infarction: Collaborative overview of early mortality and major morbidity results from all randomised trials of more than 1000 patients. Lancet 343:311, 1994

FUSTER V et al: The pathophysiology of coronary artery disease and the acute coronary syndromes. N Engl J Med. 326:242, 1992

GOLDMAN, L: Cost and quality of life: Thrombolysis and primary angioplasty. J Am Coll Cardiol 25:38S, 1995

JULIAN D, BRAUNWALD E (eds): *Management of Acute Myocardial Infarction,* London, Saunders, 1994

KINCH JW, RYAN TJ: Right ventricular infarction. N Engl J Med 330:1211, 1994

LIBBY P: Molecular basis of the acute coronary syndromes. Circulation 91:2844, 1995

MAGGIONI AP et al: Age-related increase in mortality among patients with first myocardial infarctions treated with thrombolysis. N Engl J Med 329:1442, 1993

MICHELS KB, YUSUF S: Does PTCA in acute myocardial infarction affect mortality and reinfarction rates? A quantitative verview (meta-analysis) of the randomized clinical trials. Circulation 91:476, 1995

NATIONAL HEART ATTACK ALERT PROGRAM COORDINATING COMMITTEE — 60 MINUTES TO TREATMENT WORKING GROUP: Emergency department: Rapid identification and treatment of patients with acute myocardial infarction. Ann Emerg Med. 23:311, 1994

PATRONO C: Aspirin as an antiplatelet drug. N Engl J Med 330:1287, 1994

PFEFFER JM et al: Angiotensin-converting enzyme inhibition and ventricular remodeling after myocardial infarction. Annu Rev Physiol 57:805, 1995

RAVKILDE J et al: Independent prognostic value of serum creatine kinase isoenzyme MB mass, cardiac troponin T and myosin light chain levels in suspected acute myocardial infarction. Analysis of 28 months of follow-up in 196 patients. J Am Coll Cardiol 25:574, 1995

ROGERS W et al: Treatment of myocardial infarction in the United States (1990 to 1993). Observations from the National Registry of Myocardial Infarction. Circulation 90:2103, 1994

RYAN TJ et al: Guidelines for the management of patients with acute myocardial infarction. A report of the American College of Cardiology/American Heart Association Task Force on Practice Guidelines. J Am Coll Cardiol 28:1328, 1996

THE GUSTO INVESTIGATORS: An international randomized trial comparing four thrombolytic strategies for acute myocardial infarction. N Engl J Med 329:673, 1993

THE TIMI IIIB INVESTIGATORS: Effects of tissue plasminogen activator and a comparison of early invasive and conservative strategies in unstable angina and non-Q-wave myocardial infarction: Results of the TIMI IIIB Trial. Circulation 89:1545, 1994

VAN BERGEN PFMM et al: Costs and effects of long-term oral anticoagulant treatment after myocardial infarction. J Am Med Assoc. 273: 925,1995

WEISMAN HF, HEALY B: Myocardial infarct expansion, infarct extension, and reinfarction: Pathophysiologic concepts. Prog Cardiovasc Dis 30:73, 1987

YUSUF S et al: Beta blockade during and after myocardial infarction: An overview of the randomized trials. Prog Cardiovasc Dis 27:335, 1985

244 *Andrew P. Selwyn, Eugene Braunwald*

ISCHEMIC HEART DISEASE

ETIOLOGY AND PATHOPHYSIOLOGY

Ischemia refers to a lack of oxygen due to inadequate perfusion, which results from an imbalance between oxygen supply and demand. The most common cause of myocardial ischemia is atherosclerotic disease of epicardial coronary arteries. Coronary artery disease (CAD) is the most common, serious, chronic, life-threatening illness in the United States, where more than 11 million persons have CAD. This condition causes more deaths, disability, and economic costs than many other illnesses.

By reducing the lumen of the coronary arteries, atherosclerosis causes an absolute decrease in myocardial perfusion in the basal state or limits appropriate increases in perfusion when the demand for flow is augmented. Coronary blood flow can also be limited by arterial thrombi, spasm, and rarely coronary emboli as well as by ostial narrowing due to luetic aortitis. Congenital abnormalities, such as anomalous origin of the left anterior descending coronary artery from the pulmonary artery, may cause myocardial ischemia and infarction in infancy, but this cause is very rare in adults. Myocardial ischemia can also occur if myocardial oxygen demands are abnormally increased, as in severe ventricular hypertrophy due to hypertension or aortic stenosis. The latter can present with angina that is indistinguishable from that caused by coronary atherosclerosis. A reduction in the oxygen-carrying capacity of the blood, as in extremely severe anemia or in the presence of carboxyhemoglobin, is a rare cause of myocardial ischemia. Not infrequently, two or more causes of ischemia will coexist, such as an increase in oxygen demand due to left ventricular hypertrophy and a reduction in oxygen supply secondary to coronary atherosclerosis. Often such a combination leads to clinical manifestations of ischemia.

Although the large epicardial coronary arteries are capable of constriction and relaxation, in healthy persons they serve largely as conduits and are referred to as *conductance vessels*, while the intramyocardial arterioles normally exhibit striking changes in tone and are therefore referred to as *resistance vessels*. Abnormal constriction or failure of normal dilation of the coronary resistance vessels also can cause ischemia. When it causes angina this condition is sometimes referred to as *microvascular angina*.

The normal coronary circulation is dominated and controlled by the heart's requirements for oxygen. This need is met by the ability of the coronary vascular bed to vary its resistance (and therefore blood flow) considerably while the myocardium extracts a high and relatively fixed percentage of oxygen (Chap. 13). Normally, intramyocardial resistance arterioles demonstrate an immense capacity for dilation. For example, the changing oxygen needs with exercise and emotional stress affect coronary vascular resistance and in this manner regulate the supply of oxygen and substrate (*metabolic regulation*). The coronary resistance vessels also adapt to physiologic alterations in blood pressure in order to maintain coronary blood flow at levels appropriate to myocardial needs (*autoregulation*).

CORONARY ATHEROSCLEROSIS (See also Chap. 242) Epicardial coronary arteries are a major site of atherosclerotic disease. The major risk factors for atherosclerosis [high plasma low-density lipoprotein (LDL), low plasma high-density lipoprotein (HDL), cigarette smoking, hypertension, and diabetes mellitus] are thought to disturb the normal functions of the vascular endothelium. Dysfunction of vascular endothelium and an abnormal interaction with blood monocytes and platelets lead to subintimal collections of abnormal fat, cells, and debris (i.e., atherosclerotic plaques), which develop at irregular rates in different segments of the epicardial coronary tree and lead eventually to segmental reductions in cross-sectional area. The relationship between pulsatile flow and luminal stenosis is complex, but experiments have shown that when a stenosis reduces the cross-sectional area by approximately 75 percent, a full range of increases in flow to meet increased myocardial demand is not possible. When the luminal area is reduced by more than approximately 80 percent, blood flow at rest may be reduced, and further minor decreases in the stenotic orifice can reduce coronary flow dramatically and cause myocardial ischemia.

Segmental atherosclerotic narrowing of epicardial coronary arteries is caused most commonly by the formation of a plaque, which is subject to fissuring, hemorrhage, and thrombosis. Any of these events can temporarily worsen the obstruction, reduce coronary blood flow, and cause clinical manifestations of myocardial ischemia, as described below. The location of the obstruction will influence the quantity of myocardium rendered ischemic and thus determine the severity of the clinical manifestations. Severe coronary narrowing and myocardial ischemia are frequently accompanied by the development of collateral vessels, especially when the narrowing develops gradually. When well developed, such vessels can provide sufficient blood flow to sustain the viability of the myocardium at rest but not during conditions of increased demand.

Once stenosis of a proximal epicardial artery has reduced the cross-sectional area by more than approximately 70 percent, the distal resistance vessels (when they function normally) dilate to reduce vascular resistance and maintain coronary blood flow. A pressure gradient develops across the proximal stenosis, and poststenotic pressure falls. When the resistance vessels are maximally dilated, myocardial blood flow becomes dependent on the pressure in the coronary artery distal to the obstruction. In these circumstances ischemia in the region perfused by the stenotic artery can be precipitated by increases in myocardial oxygen demands caused by physical activity, emotional stress, and/or tachycardia. Changes in the caliber of the stenosed coronary artery due to physiologic vasomotion, pathologic spasm, or small platelet plugs can all upset the critical balance between oxygen supply and demand and thus precipitate myocardial ischemia.

EFFECTS OF ISCHEMIA The inadequate oxygenation induced by coronary atherosclerosis may cause transient disturbances of the mechanical, biochemical, and electrical functions of the myocardium. The abrupt development of severe ischemia, as occurs with total or subtotal occlusion, is associated with almost instantaneous failure of normal muscle contraction and relaxation. The relatively poor perfusion of the subendocardium causes more intense ischemia of this portion of the wall. Ischemia of large portions of the ventricle will cause transient left ventricular failure, and if the papillary muscles are involved, mitral regurgitation can complicate this event. When ischemia is transient, it may be associated with angina pectoris; when

it is prolonged, it can lead to myocardial necrosis and scarring with or without the clinical picture of acute myocardial infarction (see Chap. 243). Coronary atherosclerosis is a focal process that usually causes nonuniform ischemia. Regional disturbances of ventricular contractility cause segmental bulging (dyskinesia), which can greatly reduce myocardial pump function.

Underlying these mechanical disturbances are a wide range of abnormalities in cell metabolism, function, and structure. When oxygenated, the normal myocardium metabolizes fatty acids and glucose to carbon dioxide and water. With severe oxygen deprivation, fatty acids cannot be oxidized, and glucose is broken down to lactate; intracellular pH is reduced, as are the myocardial stores of high-energy phosphates, adenosine triphosphate (ATP), and creatine phosphate. Impaired cell membrane function leads to potassium leakage and the uptake of sodium by myocytes. The severity and duration of the imbalance between myocardial oxygen supply and demand will determine whether the damage is reversible or whether it is permanent, with subsequent myocardial necrosis.

Ischemia also causes characteristic changes in the electrocardiogram (ECG) such as repolarization abnormalities, as evidenced by inversion of the T wave and, when more severe, by displacement of the ST segment (Chap. 228). Transient ST-segment depression often reflects subendocardial ischemia, while transient ST-segment elevation is thought to be caused by more severe transmural ischemia. Another important consequence of myocardial ischemia is electrical instability, which may lead to ventricular tachycardia or ventricular fibrillation (Chap. 231). Most patients who die suddenly from ischemic heart disease do so as a result of ischemia-induced malignant ventricular tachyarrhythmias (Chap. 39).

ASYMPTOMATIC VERSUS SYMPTOMATIC CORONARY ARTERY DISEASE Postmortem studies on accident victims and military casualties in western countries have shown that coronary atherosclerosis often begins to develop prior to age 20 and is widespread even among adults who were asymptomatic during life. When all age groups are considered, ischemic heart disease is the most common cause of death not only in men but also in women (Chap. 6). Exercise stress tests in asymptomatic persons may show evidence of silent myocardial ischemia, i.e., exercise-induced ECG changes not accompanied by angina; coronary angiographic studies of such persons may reveal obstructive CAD (p. 1374). Postmortem examination of patients with obstructive CAD without a history of any clinical manifestations of myocardial ischemia often shows macroscopic scars secondary to myocardial infarction in regions supplied by diseased coronary arteries. According to population studies, approximately 25 percent of patients who survive acute myocardial infarction may not reach medical attention, and these patients carry the same adverse prognosis as those who present with the classic clinical syndrome (Chap. 243). Sudden death may be unheralded and is a common presenting manifestation of ischemic heart disease (Chap. 39). Patients can also present with cardiomegaly and heart failure secondary to ischemic damage of the left ventricular myocardium that caused no symptoms prior to the development of heart failure; this condition is referred to as *ischemic cardiomyopathy*. In contrast to the asymptomatic phase of ischemic heart disease, the symptomatic phase is characterized by chest discomfort due to either angina pectoris or acute myocardial infarction (Chap. 243). Having entered the symptomatic phase, the patient may exhibit a stable or progressive course, revert to the asymptomatic stage, or suddenly die.

STABLE ANGINA PECTORIS

This episodic clinical syndrome is due to transient myocardial ischemia. Various diseases that cause myocardial ischemia as well as the numerous forms of discomfort with which it may be confused are discussed in Chap. 13. Males constitute approximately 70 percent of all patients with angina pectoris and an even greater fraction of those younger than 50 years of age.

HISTORY The typical patient with angina is a 50- to 60-year-old man or 65- to 75-year-old woman who seeks medical help for troublesome or frightening chest discomfort, usually described as heaviness, pressure, squeezing, smothering, or choking and only rarely as frank pain. When the patient is asked to localize the sensation, he or she will typically press on the sternum, sometimes with a clenched fist, to indicate a squeezing, central, substernal discomfort. This symptom is usually crescendo-decrescendo in nature and lasts 1 to 5 min. Angina can radiate to the left shoulder and to both arms and especially to the ulnar surfaces of the forearm and hand. It can also arise in or radiate to the back, neck, jaw, teeth, and epigastrium.

Although episodes of angina are typically caused by exertion (e.g., exercise, hurrying, or sexual activity) or emotion (e.g., stress, anger, fright, or frustration) and are relieved by rest, they may also occur at rest (see "Unstable Angina Pectoris," p. 1373) and at night while the patient is recumbent (angina decubitus). The patient may be awakened at night distressed by typical chest discomfort and dyspnea. The pathophysiology of nocturnal angina is analogous to that of paroxysmal nocturnal dyspnea (Chap. 233), i.e., the expansion of the intrathoracic blood volume that occurs with recumbency causes an increase in cardiac size and myocardial oxygen demand that lead to ischemia and transient left ventricular failure.

The threshold for the development of angina pectoris varies from person to person and may vary by time of day and emotional state. Many patients report a fixed threshold for angina, which occurs predictably at a certain level of activity. In these patients oxygen supply is fixed and ischemia is precipitated by an increase in myocardial oxygen demand. In other patients the threshold for angina may vary considerably within any given day and from day to day. In such patients variations in oxygen supply, most likely due to changes in coronary vascular tone, may play an important role. A patient may report symptoms upon minor exertion in the morning (a short walk or shaving) yet by midday may be capable of much greater effort without symptoms. Angina may be precipitated by unfamiliar tasks, a heavy meal, or exposure to cold.

Sharp, fleeting chest pain or prolonged, dull aches localized to the left submammary area are rarely due to myocardial ischemia. However, angina pectoris may be atypical in location and may not be strictly related to provoking factors. In addition, this symptom may exacerbate and remit over days, weeks, or months, and its occurrence can be seasonal.

Systematic questioning of the patient with suspected ischemic heart disease is important to uncover a positive family history of premature ischemic heart disease (under the age of 45 years in first-degree male relatives and under 55 in female relatives), diabetes, hyperlipidemia, hypertension, cigarette smoking, and other risk factors for coronary atherosclerosis.

PHYSICAL EXAMINATION The physical examination is often normal in the patient with stable angina. The general examination may reveal signs of risk factors associated with coronary atherosclerosis such as xanthelasma, xanthomas (Chap. 242), or diabetic skin lesions. There may also be signs of anemia, thyroid disease, and nicotine stains on the fingertips from cigarette smoking. Palpation can reveal thickened or absent peripheral arteries, signs of cardiac enlargement, and abnormal contraction of the cardiac impulse (left ventricular akinesia or dyskinesia). Examination of the fundi may reveal increased light reflexes and arteriovenous nicking as evidence of hypertension (Table 35-2), while auscultation can uncover arterial bruits, a third and/or fourth heart sound, and, if acute ischemia or previous infarction has impaired papillary muscle function, an apical systolic murmur due to mitral regurgitation. These auscultatory signs are best appreciated with the patient in the left decubitus position. Aortic stenosis, aortic regurgitation (Chap. 237), pulmonary hypertension, and hypertrophic cardiomyopathy (Chap. 239) must be excluded, since these disorders may cause angina even in the absence of coronary artery disease. Examination during an anginal attack is useful, since ischemia can cause transient left ventricular failure with the appearance of a third and/or fourth heart sound, a dyskinetic cardiac apex, mitral regurgitation, and even pulmonary edema.

LABORATORY EXAMINATION Although the diagnosis of ischemic heart disease can be made with confidence from a typical history, a number of simple laboratory tests can be helpful. The urine should be examined for evidence of diabetes mellitus and renal disease, since both these conditions may accelerate atherosclerosis. Similarly, examination of the blood should include measurements of lipids (cholesterol—total, low density, and high density), glucose, creatinine, hematocrit, and, if indicated based on the physical examination, thyroid function. A chest x-ray is important, since it may show the consequences of ischemic heart disease, i.e., cardiac enlargement, ventricular aneurysm, or signs of heart failure. Calcification of the coronary arteries can sometimes be identified on chest fluoroscopy. These signs can support the diagnosis of CAD and are important in assessing the degree of cardiac damage and the effects of treatment for heart failure.

Electrocardiogram A 12-lead ECG recorded at rest is normal in about half the patients with typical angina pectoris, but there may be signs of an old myocardial infarction (Chap. 228). Although repolarization abnormalities, i.e., T-wave and ST-segment changes and intraventricular conduction disturbances at rest, are suggestive of ischemic heart disease, they are nonspecific, since they can also occur in pericardial, myocardial, and valvular heart disease or with anxiety, changes in posture, drugs, or esophageal disease. Typical ST-segment and T-wave changes that accompany episodes of angina pectoris and disappear thereafter are more specific. The most characteristic changes include displacement of the ST segment that is similar in every way to that induced during a stress test (see below). The ST segment is usually depressed during angina but may be elevated—sometimes strikingly so—in Prinzmetal's angina.

Stress Testing The most widely used test in the diagnosis of ischemic heart disease involves recording the 12-lead ECG before, during, and after exercise on a treadmill or using a bicycle ergometer. The test consists of a standardized incremental increase in external workload while the patient's ECG, symptoms, and arm blood pressure are continuously monitored. Performance is usually symptom-limited, and the test is discontinued upon evidence of chest discomfort, severe shortness of breath, dizziness, fatigue, ST-segment depression of greater than 0.2 mV (2 mm), a fall in systolic blood pressure exceeding 10 mmHg, or the development of a ventricular tachyarrhythmia. This test seeks to discover any limitation in exercise performance and establish the relationship between chest discomfort and the typical ECG signs of myocardial ischemia. The ischemic ST-segment response is generally defined as flat depression of the ST segment of more than 0.1 mV below the baseline (i.e., the PR segment) and lasting longer than 0.08 s. This type of depression is designated "square wave" or "plateau" and is flat or downsloping (Fig. 244-1). Upsloping or junctional ST-segment changes are not considered characteristic of ischemia and do not constitute a positive test. Although T-wave abnormalities, conduction disturbances, and ventricular arrhythmias that develop during exercise should be noted, they are also not diagnostic. Negative exercise tests in which the target heart rate (85 percent of maximal heart rate for age and sex) is not achieved are considered to be nondiagnostic. When applying and interpreting ECG stress testing, one must first consider the probability that CAD exists in the patient or population under study (i.e., pretest probability). Overall, false-positive or -negative results can occur in 15 percent of cases. However, a positive result on exercise indicates that the likelihood of CAD is 98 percent in males over 50 years of age with a history of typical angina pectoris who develop chest discomfort during the test. The likelihood decreases progressively and significantly if the patient has atypical or no chest pain. The incidence of false-positive tests is significantly increased in asymptomatic men under the age of 40 or in premenopausal women with no risk factors for premature atherosclerosis (Bayes' theorem—Table 3-3). It is also increased in patients taking cardioactive drugs such as digitalis and quinidine, or in those with intraventricular conduction disturbances, resting abnormalities of the ST segment and the T wave, myocardial hypertrophy, or abnormal serum potassium levels. Obstructive disease limited to the circumflex coronary artery may result in a false-negative stress test since the posterior portion of the heart which this vessel supplies is not well represented on the surface 12-lead ECG. Since the overall sensitivity of exercise stress electrocardiography is only about 75 percent, a negative result does not exclude CAD, although it makes the likelihood of three-vessel or left main CAD extremely unlikely.

The physician should be present throughout the exercise test, and it is important to measure total duration of exercise, the times to the onset of ischemic ST-segment change and chest discomfort, the external work performed (generally expressed as a stage of exercise), and the internal cardiac work performed; the last is represented by the heart rate–blood pressure product. The depth of the ST-segment depression and the time needed for recovery of these ECG changes are also important. Because the risks of exercise testing are small but real—estimated at one fatality and two nonfatal complications per 10,000 tests—equipment for resuscitation should be available. Modified (heart rate–limited rather than symptom–limited) exercise tests can be performed safely in patients as early as 7 days after myocardial infarction.

The normal response to exercise includes a progressive increase in heart rate and blood pressure. Failure of the blood pressure to increase or an actual decrease in blood pressure with signs of ischemia during the test is an important adverse prognostic sign, since it may reflect ischemia-induced global left ventricular dysfunction. The presence of pain or severe (>0.2 mV) ST-segment depression at a low workload and ST-segment depression that persists for more than 5 min after the termination of exercise increases the specificity of the test and suggests severe ischemic heart disease and a high risk of further adverse events.

The information gained from an exercise test can be enhanced by stress myocardial perfusion imaging after the intravenous administration of a radioisotope such as thallium 201 or technetium 99m sestamibi during exercise (or a pharmacologic stress); the imaging is carried out both immediately after cessation of exercise and 4 h later (Fig. 244-2). Technetium 99m can also be used to label the blood pool for gated radioisotope angiography, which provides a measure of ventricular volume and ejection fraction at rest and during exercise. A reduction in ejection fraction during exercise is an important, albeit nonspecific, finding, and when present in CAD suggests the presence of severe ischemia and/or multivessel coronary disease.

An important fraction of patients who need noninvasive stress testing to identify myocardial ischemia and increased risk of coronary events cannot exercise because of peripheral vascular or musculoskeletal disease. In these circumstances intravenous dipyridamole or adenosine can be used in place of exercise. The development of a transient perfusion defect with a tracer such as radioactive thallium or technetium 99m sestamibi is used to detect myocardial ischemia. Ambulatory monitoring of the ECG can assess myocardial ischemia as episodes of ST-segment depression. These techniques are sensitive and capable of identifying patients with ischemia who are at increased risk of coronary events.

Two-dimensional echocardiography of the left ventricle can assess both global and regional wall motion abnormalities due to myocardial infarction or persistent ischemia. Stress (exercise or dobutamine) echocardiography may cause the emergence of regions of akinesis or dyskinesis not present at rest. Stress echocardiography, like stress myocardial perfusion imaging, is more sensitive than exercise electrocardiography in the diagnosis of CAD.

Coronary Arteriography (See Chap. 229) This diagnostic method outlines the coronary anatomy and can be used to detect important evidence of coronary atherosclerosis or to exclude this condition. By this means, one can assess the severity of obstructive lesions and when combined with left ventricular angiocardiography can evaluate both global and regional function of the left ventricle.

Indications Coronary arteriography is indicated in (1) patients with chronic stable or unstable angina pectoris who are severely symptomatic despite medical therapy and who are being considered for revascularization, i.e., percutaneous transluminal coronary angioplasty (PTCA) or coronary artery bypass graft surgery; (2) patients with troublesome symptoms that present diagnostic difficulties in whom there is need to confirm or rule out the diagnosis of CAD; and (3) patients judged to be at high risk of sustaining coronary events based on signs of severe ischemia on noninvasive testing, regardless of presence or severity of symptoms (see below).

Examples of other possible clinical situations include:

1. Patients with chest discomfort suggestive of angina pectoris but a negative exercise test who require a definitive diagnosis for guiding medical management, alleviating psychological stress, career or family planning, or insurance purposes.
2. Patients who have been admitted repeatedly to the hospital for suspected acute myocardial infarction but in whom this diagnosis

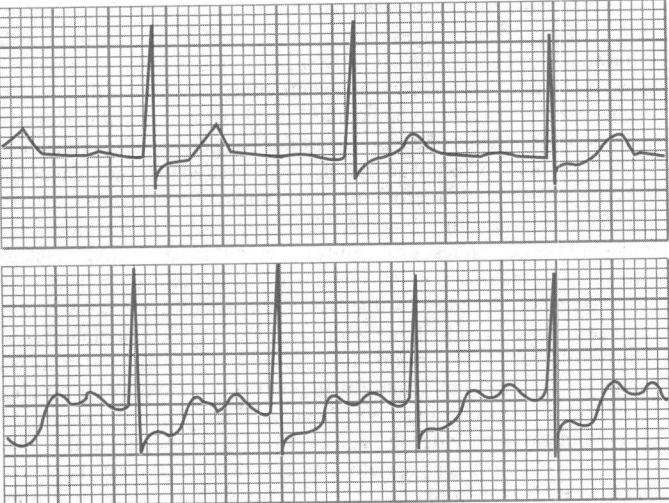

FIGURE 244-1 Lead V$_4$ at rest (*top*) and after 4½ min of exercise (*bottom*). There is 3 mm (0.3 mV) of horizontal ST-segment depression, indicating a positive test for ischemia. [*Modified from BR Chaitman Exercise Stress Testing, in E Braunwald (ed), Heart Disease, 5th ed, Philadelphia, Saunders, 1997, pp 153–176.*]

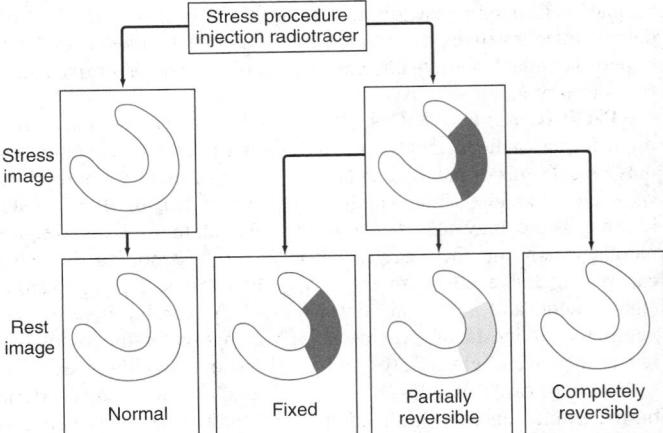

FIGURE 244-2 Interpretation of stress (exercise) and rest myocardial perfusion images. A normal image will show homogeneous accumulation of radiotracer on the exercise and rest (or delayed) image. An area with decreased uptake of the radiotracer (which appears as a darker area on a perfusion image) is referred to as a *defect*. A patient with a fixed perfusion defect will have an abnormal exercise image and an identical rest or delayed redistribution image (scarring). A partially reversible perfusion defect appears as an abnormal exercise image and an improved but still abnormal rest image (ischemia and scarring). A reversible perfusion defect appears as an abnormal exercise image and a normal rest or delayed image (ischemia). [*From FJ Wackers, in GA Beller (ed), Chronic Ischemic Heart Disease, in E Braunwald (series ed), Atlas of Heart Diseases, Philadelphia, Current Medicine, 1994.*]

has not been established and in whom the presence or absence of CAD should be determined.

3. Patients with careers that involve the safety of others (e.g., airline pilots) who have questionable symptoms, suspicious or positive noninvasive tests, and in whom there are reasonable doubts about the state of the coronary arteries.

4. Patients with aortic stenosis or hypertrophic cardiomyopathy and angina in whom the pain could be due to CAD.

5. Male patients aged 45 and females aged 55 years of age or older who will undergo valve replacement and who may or may not have clinical evidence of myocardial ischemia.

6. Patients who are at high risk after myocardial infarction because of the recurrence of angina, heart failure, frequent ventricular premature contractions, or signs of ischemia in the stress test.

7. Patients with angina pectoris, regardless of severity, in whom noninvasive testing reveals signs of severe ischemia.

PROGNOSIS

The principal prognostic indicators in patients with ischemic heart disease are the functional state of the left ventricle, the location and severity of coronary artery narrowing, and the severity or activity of myocardial ischemia. Angina pectoris of recent onset, unstable angina, angina that is unresponsive or poorly responsive to medical therapy or is accompanied by symptoms of congestive heart failure all indicate an increased risk for adverse coronary events. The same is true for the physical signs of heart failure, episodes of pulmonary edema, or for echocardiographic (or roentgenographic) evidence of cardiac enlargement. An abnormal resting ECG or positive evidence of myocardial ischemia during a stress test also indicate increased risk. Most importantly, the following signs during noninvasive testing indicate a high risk for coronary events: a strongly positive exercise test showing onset of myocardial ischemia at low workloads [$\geq$0.1 mV ST-segment depression in stage I (Bruce protocol) of the exercise test; $\geq$0.2 mV ST depression in any stage; ST depression for >5 min following the cessation of exercise; a decline in systolic pressure >10 mmHg during exercise; the development of ventricular tachyarrhythmias during exercise]; the development of large or multiple perfusion defects or increased lung uptake during stress radioisotope perfusion imaging; and a decrease in left ventricular ejection fraction during exercise on radionuclide ventriculography.

On cardiac catheterization, elevations in left ventricular end-diastolic pressure and ventricular volume and a reduced ejection fraction are the most important signs of left ventricular dysfunction and are associated with a poor prognosis. Patients with chest discomfort but normal left ventricular function and normal coronary arteries have an excellent prognosis. In patients with normal left ventricular function and mild angina but with critical stenoses ($\geq$70 percent luminal diameter) of one, two, or three epicardial coronary arteries, the 5-year mortality rates are approximately 2, 8, and 11 percent, respectively. Obstructive lesions of the proximal left anterior descending coronary artery are associated with a greater risk than are lesions of the right or left circumflex coronary artery, since the former vessel usually perfuses a greater quantity of myocardium. Critical stenosis of the left main coronary artery is associated with a mortality of about 15 percent per year.

With any degree of obstructive CAD, mortality is greatly increased when left ventricular function is impaired; conversely, at any level of left ventricular function, the prognosis is influenced importantly by the quantity of myocardium perfused by the critically obstructed vessels. Therefore, it is useful to collect all the evidence substantiating past myocardial damage (ECG and ventriculographic evidence of myocardial infarction), residual left ventricular function (ejection fraction), and risk of future damage from coronary events (extent of coronary disease and severity of ischemia defined by noninvasive stress testing). The larger the amount of established myocardial necrosis, the less the heart is able to withstand additional damage and the poorer the prognosis. All the above signs of past damage plus the risk of future damage should be considered indicators of risk.

The segmental atherosclerotic plaques in epicardial arteries go through phases of inflammatory cellular activity, degeneration, endothelial instability, abnormal vasomotion, platelet aggregation, and fissuring or hemorrhage. These factors can temporarily worsen the stenosis and cause abnormal reactivity of the vessel wall, thus exacerbating the manifestations of ischemia. The recent onset of symptoms, the appearance of severe ischemia during stress testing, and unstable angina pectoris (p. 1373) all reflect episodes of rapid progression in coronary lesions.

℞ TREATMENT

Each patient must be evaluated individually with respect to his or her expectations and goals, control of symptoms, and prevention of adverse clinical outcomes such as myocardial infarction and premature death. The degree of disability as well as the physical and emotional stress that precipitate angina must be carefully recorded in order to set treatment goals. Each management plan should consist of the following: (1) explanation and reassurance, (2) identification and treatment of aggravating conditions, (3) adaptation of activity, (4) treatment of risk factors that will decrease the occurrence of adverse coronary outcomes, (5) drug therapy for angina, and (6) consideration of mechanical revascularization.

Explanation and Reassurance Patients with ischemic heart disease need to understand their condition as best they can and to realize that a long and useful life is possible even though they suffer from angina pectoris or have experienced and recovered from an acute myocardial infarction. Offering case histories of persons in public life who have lived with coronary disease as well as results of national studies showing improved outcomes can be of great value when encouraging patients to resume or maintain activity and return to their occupation. A planned program of rehabilitation can encourage patients to lose weight, improve exercise tolerance, and control risk factors with more confidence.

Identification and Treatment of Aggravating Conditions A number of conditions that are not primarily cardiac in nature may either increase oxygen demand or decrease oxygen supply to the myocardium and may precipitate or exacerbate angina. In the former category, obesity, hypertension, and hyperthyroidism may be treated successfully in order to reduce the frequency of anginal attacks. Decreased myocardial oxygen supply may be due to reduced oxygenation of the blood (e.g., in pulmonary disease or, when carboxyhemoglobin is present, due to cigarette or cigar smoking) or decreased oxygen-carrying capacity (e.g., in anemia). Correction of these abnormalities, if present, may reduce or even eliminate anginal symptoms.

Adaptation of Activity Therapy of angina due to episodes of myocardial ischemia consists of eliminating the discrepancy between the demand of the heart muscle for oxygen and the ability of the coronary circulation to meet this demand. Most patients can be made to understand this fundamental concept and utilize it in the rational programming of activity. Many tasks that ordinarily evoke angina may be accomplished without symptoms simply by reducing the speed at which they are performed. Patients must appreciate the diurnal variation in their tolerance of certain activities and should reduce their energy requirements in the morning and immediately after meals. Sometimes it is helpful to alter the eating pattern, taking small and more frequent meals.

It may be necessary to recommend a change in employment or residence to avoid physical stress; however, with the exception of manual laborers, most patients with ischemic heart disease can usually continue to function merely by allowing more time to complete each task. In some patients, anger and frustration may be the most important factors precipitating myocardial ischemia. If these cannot be avoided, training in stress management may be useful. A treadmill exercise test to determine the approximate heart rate at which ischemic ECG changes or symptoms develop may be helpful in the development of a specific exercise program. Ambulatory recording of the ECG during daily activities may also be helpful in this regard.

Treatment of Risk Factors Although the treatment of risk factors was developed for the primary prevention of coronary atherosclerosis, there is growing evidence that it can reduce the occurrence of myocardial infarction and death both in subjects without clinical disease as well as those with a history of chronic angina or an acute coronary syndrome. A family history of premature coronary disease is an important indicator of increased risk and should trigger a search for treatable risk factors such as hyperlipidemia, hypertension, and diabetes. Obesity impairs the treatment of other risk factors, and when the patient is more than 30 percent above ideal body weight it increases the risk of adverse coronary events. In addition, obesity is often accompanied by two other risk factors—hypertension and hyperlipidemia. The treatment of obesity and these accompanying risk factors is an important component of any management plan.

Cigarette smoking accelerates coronary atherosclerosis in both sexes and at all ages and increases the risk of myocardial infarction and death. By increasing myocardial oxygen needs and reducing oxygen supply it aggravates angina. Smoking cessation studies have demonstrated important benefits with a significant decline in the occurrence of these adverse outcomes. The physician's message must be clear and strong and supported by programs that achieve and monitor abstinence. Hypertension (Chaps. 35 and 246) is associated with increased risk of adverse clinical events from coronary atherosclerosis as well as stroke. In addition, the left ventricular hypertrophy that results from sustained hypertension aggravates ischemia. There is evidence that long-term, effective treatment of hypertension can decrease the occurrence of adverse coronary events. Diabetes mellitus (Chap. 334) accelerates coronary and peripheral atherosclerosis and is frequently associated with dyslipidemias and increases in the risk of angina, myocardial infarction, and sudden coronary death. Strict control of diabetes is helpful in lowering the elevated levels of plasma LDL cholesterol and triglyceride in this condition.

The lowering of lipid levels is a critical aspect of the management of established CAD (see Chaps. 242 and 341). Patients with LDL cholesterol concentrations exceeding 3.2 mmol/L (125 mg/dL) should have these levels reduced. HMG-CoA reductase inhibitors (statins) are especially effective in this regard when they are added to a diet that restricts the intake of saturated fats. Two large clinical trials have shown that effective lowering of LDL cholesterol concentration can reduce the need for coronary revascularization as well as the occurrence of adverse events such as heart attack and death. Hypertriglyceridemia and low levels of HDL should be treated aggressively, as outlined in Chap. 341.

Physical conditioning usually improves the exercise tolerance of patients with angina and exerts substantial psychological benefits. It may also improve the chances of surviving a myocardial infarction. An exercise program within the limits of each patient's threshold for the development of angina pectoris should be encouraged.

RISK REDUCTION IN WOMEN WITH CAD The incidence of clinical CAD in premenopausal women is very low. However, following the menopause, the atherogenic risk factors increase (e.g., increased LDL, reduced HDL) and the rate of clinical coronary events accelerates to the levels observed in men. Women have not given up cigarette smoking as effectively as have men. Diabetes mellitus, which is more common in women, greatly increases the occurrence of clinical CAD and amplifies the deleterious effects of hypertension, hyperlipidemia, and smoking. The postmenopausal use of hormone replacement therapy (estrogen with or without a progestin) reduces adverse coronary outcomes but should not be given to patients at higher than usual risk of breast cancer. Cardiac catheterization and coronary revascularization are often applied more sparingly in women and at a later, and more severe, stage of the disease than in

men. These factors likely explain the modest increase in complications. Although many of the clinical trials to date have not represented women adequately, the evidence is that when cholesterol lowering, beta blockers after myocardial infarction, and coronary artery bypass grafting are applied in the appropriate patient groups, women enjoy the same benefits of improved outcome as do men.

Drug Therapy The commonly used drugs for angina pectoris are summarized in Table 244-1.

NITRATES This valuable class of drugs in the management of angina pectoris acts by causing systemic venodilation, thereby reducing myocardial wall tension and oxygen requirements, as well as by dilating the epicardial coronary vessels and increasing blood flow in collateral vessels. The absorption of these agents is most rapid and complete through the mucous membranes. For this reason, nitroglycerin is administered sublingually in tablets of 0.4 or 0.6 mg. Patients with angina should be instructed to take the medication both to relieve angina and also in anticipation of stress (exercise or emotional) that is likely to induce an episode. The value of this prophylactic use of the drug cannot be overemphasized.

Table 244-1

Drugs Commonly Used for Angina Pectoris

Drug	Usual Dose	Side Effects	Contraindications
NITRATES			
Sublingual NTG	0.3–0.6 mg	Flushing, headache	Intolerance of side effects
Isosorbide dinitrate SR	80–120 mg	Flushing, headache, tolerance after 24 h	As above, worsening ischemia on withdrawal
Transdermal NTG	0.4–1.2 mg/h for 12–14 h	Flushing, headache, tolerance after 24 h	As above, worsening ischemia on withdrawal
Isosorbide-5-monitrate		Flushing, headache, tolerance after 24 h	As above, worsening ischemia on withdrawal
Oral	20–30 mg bid		
Oral SR	60–240 mg once daily		
BETA-ADRENOCEPTOR BLOCKING DRUGS			
Propranolol	20–80 mg qid	Depression, constipation, impotence, bronchospasm, heart failure, bradycardia	Asthma, AV conduction block, heart failure
Metoprolol	25–200 mg bid	As above	As above
Atenolol	50–150 mg once daily	As above	As above
CALCIUM CHANNEL BLOCKING DRUGS			
Nifedipine XL	30–90 mg once daily	Hypotension, flushing, edema, worsening angina	Hypotension, intolerance of side effects
Diltiazem SR	60–120 mg bid	Constipation, AV conduction block, worsening heart failure	AV conduction block, impaired LV function, bradycardia
Verapamil SR	180–240 mg once daily	Constipation, AV conduction block, worsening heart failure	AV conduction delay, impaired LV function, bradycardia
Amlodipine	5–10 mg once daily	Edema	Intolerance of side effects

NOTE: NTG, nitroglycerin; SR, slow release; XL, slow release preparation.

Headache and a pulsating feeling in the head are the most common side effects of nitroglycerin and fortunately only rarely become disturbing at the doses usually required to relieve or prevent angina. Nitroglycerin deteriorates with exposure to air, moisture, and sunlight, so that if the drug neither relieves discomfort or headache nor produces a slight sensation of burning at the sublingual site of absorption, the preparation may be inactive and a fresh supply should be obtained. If relief is not achieved after the first dose of nitroglycerin, a second or third dose may be given at 5-min intervals. If discomfort continues despite treatment, the patient should consult a physician or report promptly to a hospital emergency room for evaluation of possible unstable angina or acute myocardial infarction (Chap. 243).

Asking the patient with recently diagnosed angina pectoris to record the occurrence of pain as well as nitroglycerin consumption is often helpful to the physician attempting to tailor a management program. Such a diary may also be valuable for detecting changes in the frequency or severity of discomfort that may signify the development of unstable angina pectoris and/or herald an impending myocardial infarction.

None of the long-acting nitrates is as effective as sublingual nitroglycerin for the acute relief of angina. These preparations can be swallowed, chewed, or administered as a patch or paste by the transdermal route. They can provide effective plasma levels for up to 24 h, but the therapeutic response is highly variable. Different preparations and/or administration during the daytime should be tried only to prevent discomfort in the individual patient while avoiding side effects such as headache and dizziness. Individual dose titration is important in order to prevent side effects. Useful preparations include isosorbide dinitrate (10 to 60 mg PO bid or tid), nitroglycerin ointment (0.5 to 2.0 in. qid), or sustained-release transdermal patches (5 to 25 mg/d). Long-acting nitrates are relatively safe and can be used together with intermittent sublingual nitroglycerin to relieve discomfort and prevent attacks of angina. The nitrates likely bind to guanylate cyclase in vascular smooth muscle cells, oxidize sulfhydryl groups, and are converted to *S*-nitrosothiols. This leads to an increase in cyclic guanosine monophosphate which causes cell relaxation of vascular smooth muscle. Tolerance with loss of efficacy develops with 12 to 24 h of continuous exposure to all of the long-acting nitrates due to depletion of sulfhydryl groups and to counterregulatory alterations in intravascular fluid balance with fluid retention. In order to minimize the effects of tolerance, the minimum effective dose should be used and a minimum of 8 h each day kept free of the drug so as to restore any useful response(s).

BETA-ADRENOCEPTOR BLOCKADE (See also Chap. 70)   These drugs represent an important component of the pharmacologic treatment of angina pectoris. They reduce myocardial oxygen demand by inhibiting the increases in heart rate and myocardial contractility caused by adrenergic activity. Beta blockade reduces these variables most strikingly during exercise while causing only small reductions in heart rate, cardiac output, and arterial pressure at rest. Propranolol is usually administered in an initial dose of 20 to 40 mg four times a day and is increased as tolerated to 320 mg per day in divided doses. Long-acting beta-blocking drugs (atenolol, 50 to 100 mg/d, and nadolol, 40 to 80 mg/d) offer the advantage of once-a-day dosage (Table 70-1). The therapeutic aims include relief of angina and ischemia. These drugs can also reduce mortality and reinfarction when given to patients after myocardial infarction. Side effects include fatigue, impotence, cold extremities, intermittent claudication, bradycardia, impaired atrioventricular conduction, left ventricular failure, bronchial asthma, and intensification of the hypoglycemia produced by oral hypoglycemic agents and insulin. Reducing the dose or even discontinuation of the drug may be necessary if these side effects develop and persist.

CALCIUM ANTAGONISTS   Slow-release nifedipine (30 to 90 mg once daily), verapamil (80 to 120 mg tid), diltiazem (30 to 90 mg qid), amlodipine (2.5 to 10 mg daily) and other calcium antagonists are all coronary vasodilators that produce variable and dose-depen-

dent reductions in myocardial oxygen demand, contractility, and arterial pressure. These combined pharmacologic effects are advantageous and make these agents quite effective in the treatment of angina pectoris. Verapamil and diltiazem may produce symptomatic disturbances in cardiac conduction and bradyarrhythmias, exert negative inotropic actions, and are more likely to worsen left ventricular failure, particularly when used in combination with beta blockers in patients with left ventricular dysfunction. Although useful effects are usually achieved when calcium antagonists are combined with beta blockers and nitrates, careful individual titration of dose is essential with these potent combinations. Variant (Prinzmetal's) angina responds particularly well to calcium antagonists, supplemented when necessary by nitrates. Nifedipine as well as other calcium antagonists are now formulated as long-acting preparations including diltiazem (60 to 120 mg twice daily) and verapamil (180 to 240 mg once daily). Verapamil should not ordinarily be combined with beta-adrenoreceptor blocking drugs because of the combined effects on heart rate and contractility. Diltiazem can be combined with beta blockers with caution and only in patients with normal ventricular function and no conduction disturbances. Nifedipine or amlodipine and the beta blockers have complementary actions on coronary blood supply and myocardial oxygen demands. While the former decreases blood pressure and dilates coronary arteries, the latter slows heart rate and decreases contractility. Nifedipine and the other second-generation dihydropyridine calcium antagonists (nicardipine, isradipine, amlodipine, and felodipine) are potent vasodilators and useful in the simultaneous treatment of angina and hypertension. Short-acting dihydropyridines should be avoided in patients with acute coronary syndromes because of the risk of precipitating infarction, particularly in the absence of beta blockers.

TREATMENT OF ANGINA AND HEART FAILURE   Transient left ventricular failure with angina can be controlled by the judicious use of nitrates, calcium antagonists, and even beta blockers. For patients with established congestive heart failure the increased left ventricular wall tension raises myocardial oxygen demand. Treatment of congestive heart failure with angiotensin-converting enzyme inhibitors, diuretics, and digitalis (Chap. 233) will decrease heart size, wall tension, and myocardial oxygen demands, which, in turn, will help to control angina and ischemia. Nocturnal angina can often be relieved by the treatment of heart failure; however, there is no benefit—and possibly aggravation of angina—when these drugs are used in patients with angina, a normal heart size and no evidence of heart failure. Nitrates are particularly useful and can simultaneously improve the disturbed hemodynamics of congestive heart failure by vasodilatation, thereby reducing preload, and relieve angina by preventing or reversing myocardial ischemia. There is some evidence that amlodipine is a calcium antagonist that is well tolerated by patients with left ventricular dysfunction and a valuable agent in the treatment of angina in patients with heart failure. The combination of congestive heart failure and angina in patients with CAD usually indicates a poor prognosis and warrants serious consideration of cardiac catheterization and mechanical revascularization, if possible (see p. 1373).

CHOICE BETWEEN BETA-ADRENERGIC RECEPTOR BLOCKADE AND CALCIUM ANTAGONISTS FOR INITIAL THERAPY   Since beta blockers have been shown to improve life expectancy following myocardial infarction (p. 1359), they may be preferable in patients with chronic CAD. However, calcium antagonists are indicated in patients with the following: (1) angina and a history of asthma or chronic obstructive pulmonary disease; (2) sick-sinus syndrome or significant arteriovenous conduction disturbances; (3) Prinzmetal's angina; (4) symptomatic peripheral vascular disease; and (5) adverse reactions to beta blockers—depression, sexual disturbances, fatigue. Many patients with angina do well with a combination of a beta blocker and dihydropiridine calcium antagonist.

ASPIRIN   Aspirin is an irreversible inhibitor of platelet cyclooxygenase activity and thereby interferes with platelet activation.

Chronic administration of 100 to 325 mg orally per day has been shown to reduce coronary events in asymptomatic adult men, patients with asymptomatic ischemia after myocardial infarction, patients with chronic stable angina, and patients who have survived unstable angina and myocardial infarction. Administration of this drug should be considered in all patients with CAD in the absence of side effects such as gastrointestinal bleeding, allergy, or dyspepsia.

CORONARY REVASCULARIZATION

While the basic management of patients with ischemic heart disease, which is a lifelong condition, is medical, as described above, many patients are improved by coronary revascularization procedures, as described below. These interventions should be employed in conjunction with but do not replace the continuing need to modify risk factors.

PERCUTANEOUS TRANSLUMINAL CORONARY ANGIOPLASTY AND RELATED CATHETER-BASED TECHNIQUES (See also Chap. 245) PTCA is a widely used method to achieve revascularization of the myocardium in patients with symptomatic ischemic heart disease and suitable stenoses of epicardial coronary arteries. Whereas patients with stenosis of the left main coronary artery and those with three-vessel CAD (especially with associated impaired left ventricular function) who require revascularization are best treated with coronary artery bypass surgery, PTCA is widely employed in patients with symptoms and evidence of ischemia due to stenoses of one or two vessels, and even selected patients with three-vessel disease, and may offer many advantages over surgery.

After a flexible guidewire is advanced into a coronary artery and across the stenosis to be dilated, a miniature balloon catheter is advanced over the guidewire and into the stenosis followed by repeated inflations until the stenosis is decreased or relieved. The development of a range of steerable guidewires, low-profile balloon catheters, and balloon catheters that also allow coronary flow during inflation have all helped to decrease complications, reach more distal lesions, and dilate more complex stenoses. In suitable stenoses affecting epicardial arteries that are ≥ 3 mm in diameter, a tubular metal stent can be expanded inside the dilated stenosis in order to achieve little or no residual stenosis, and to reduce the incidence of restenosis.

Indications and Patient Selection The most common clinical indication for PTCA is angina pectoris, stable or unstable, accompanied by evidence of ischemia in an exercise test. This symptom should be sufficiently severe to warrant the consideration of bypass graft surgery. PTCA is more effective than medical therapy for the relief of angina. The value of this procedure in reducing the occurrence of coronary death and myocardial infarction has not been established, and therefore it is not generally indicated in asymptomatic or mildly symptomatic patients. PTCA can be used to dilate stenoses in native coronary arteries as well as in bypass grafts in patients who have recurrent angina following coronary artery surgery. This is an important indication when the technical difficulties and the increased mortality that accompanies reoperation are considered. Angioplasty has also been carried out in patients with recent total occlusion (within 3 months) of a coronary artery and severe angina; in this group the primary success rate is decreased to approximately 50 percent.

Risks When coronary stenoses are discrete and symmetric, two and three vessels can be dilated in sequence. However, cautious case selection is essential in order to avoid a prohibitive risk of complications. Female gender, advanced age, stenoses with thrombus, left ventricular dysfunction, stenosis of an artery perfusing a large segment of myocardium without collaterals, long eccentric or irregular stenoses, and calcified plaques all increase the likelihood of complications but are not absolute contraindications, while left main coronary artery stenosis *is* an absolute contraindication. The major complications are usually due to dissection or thrombosis with vessel occlusion, uncontrolled ischemia, and ventricular failure. In experienced hands, the overall mortality rate should be less than 1 percent, the need for emergency coronary surgery less than 3 percent, and the occurrence of clinical myocardial infarction less than 5 percent of cases. Minor complications occur in 5 to 10 percent of patients and include occlusion of a branch of a coronary artery, release of CK-MB into the circulation, and complications of arterial catheterization.

Efficacy Primary success, i.e., adequate dilation (an increase in luminal diameter >20 percent and a residual diameter obstruction <50 percent) with relief of angina, is achieved in approximately 90 percent of cases. Recurrent stenosis of the dilated vessels occurs in 30 to 45 percent of cases within 6 months of the balloon procedure, and angina will recur within 6 to 12 months in 25 percent of cases. This recurrence of symptoms and restenosis is more common in patients with diabetes mellitus, unstable angina, incomplete dilation of the stenosis, dilation of the left anterior descending coronary artery, and stenoses containing thrombi. Dilation of arteries that are totally occluded and of stenotic or occluded vein grafts also exhibit a high incidence of restenosis. It is usual clinical practice to administer aspirin for months after the procedure. Although aspirin may help prevent acute coronary thrombosis during and immediately following PTCA, there are no controlled clinical trials that have demonstrated that these medications or any other can clearly reduce the incidence of restenosis. Successful deployment of a metal stent lowers the restenosis rate to 20 to 30 percent at 6 months but initially requires vigorous antiplatelet therapy (aspirin and Ticlopidine).

If patients do not develop restenosis or angina within the first year after angioplasty, the prognosis for maintaining improvement over the subsequent 4 years is excellent. If restenosis occurs, PTCA can be repeated with the same success and risk, but the likelihood of restenosis increases with the third or subsequent attempt.

Between 30 and 50 percent of patients with symptomatic CAD who require revascularization can be treated by PTCA and need not undergo coronary artery bypass surgery. Successful angioplasty is less invasive and expensive than coronary artery surgery, usually requires only 2 days in the hospital, and permits considerable savings in the initial cost of care; however, this economic benefit is greatly reduced over time because of the greater need for follow-up and for repeat procedures. Successful PTCA also allows earlier return to work and the resumption of an active life.

CORONARY ARTERY BYPASS GRAFTING In this procedure, a section of a vein (usually the saphenous) is used to form a connection between the aorta and the coronary artery distal to the obstructive lesion. Alternatively, anastomosis of one or both of the internal mammary arteries to the coronary artery distal to the obstructive lesion may be employed and is now preferred whenever possible.

Although some indications for coronary artery bypass surgery are controversial, certain areas of agreement exist:

1. The operation is relatively safe, with mortality rates less than 1 percent when the procedure is performed by an experienced surgical team in patients without serious comorbid disease and normal left ventricular function.

2. Intraoperative and postoperative mortality increases with the degree of ventricular dysfunction, comorbidities, age above 80 years, and surgical inexperience. The effectiveness and risk of coronary artery bypass grafting vary widely depending on case selection and the skill and experience of the surgical team, so that the latter must be taken into account when a patient is being considered as a candidate for this procedure.

3. *Occlusion of vein grafts* is observed in 10 to 20 percent during the first postoperative year and in approximately 2 percent per year during 5- to 7-year follow-up and 4 percent per year thereafter. Long-term patency rates are considerably higher for internal mammary artery implantations; in patients with left anterior descending coronary artery obstruction, survival is better when coronary bypass involves the internal mammary artery rather than a saphenous vein.

4. Angina is abolished or greatly reduced in approximately 90 percent of patients following complete revascularization. Although this is usually associated with graft patency and restoration of blood

flow, the pain may also have been alleviated as a result of infarction of the ischemic segment or a placebo effect. Within 3 years, angina recurs in about one-fourth of patients but is rarely severe.

5. Coronary artery bypass grafting does not appear to reduce the incidence of myocardial infarction in patients with chronic ischemic heart disease; perioperative myocardial infarction occurs in 5 to 10 percent of cases, but in most instances these infarcts are small.

6. Mortality is reduced by operation in patients with stenosis of the left main coronary artery as well as in patients with three-vessel CAD and impaired left ventricular function. However, there is no evidence that coronary artery bypass surgery improves survival in patients with one- or two-vessel disease who have chronic stable angina and normal left ventricular function or in patients with one-vessel disease and impaired left ventricular function. Evidence is conflicting concerning the effects of operation on survival in patients with impaired left ventricular function and obstructive disease of two coronary arteries, one of which is the proximal left anterior descending artery.

Indications for coronary artery bypass grafting are usually based on the severity of symptoms, coronary anatomy, and ventricular function. The ideal candidate is male, less than 75 years of age, has no other complicating disease, has troublesome or disabling symptoms that are not adequately controlled by medical therapy or does not tolerate medical therapy and wishes to lead a more active life, and has severe stenoses of several epicardial coronary arteries with objective evidence of myocardial ischemia as a cause of the chest discomfort. Great symptomatic benefit can be anticipated in such patients. When the patient has a disturbance of left ventricular function or critical obstructions in more than one major artery and in whom noninvasive testing shows a high risk of an adverse outcome (p. 1368), coronary artery bypass grafting may, in addition, prolong life.

Congestive heart failure and/or left ventricular dysfunction (ejection fraction <40 percent) are associated with a higher perioperative mortality and were once considered to be contraindications to coronary artery bypass grafting. However, it has now become clear that revascularization of chronically ischemic, noncontractile but viable (so-called hibernating) myocardium can improve left ventricular function and survival. Hibernating myocardium can be detected by positron emission tomographic (PET) scanning, which typically exhibits a mismatch between myocardial perfusion, which is reduced, and metabolism, an indicator of viability, which is sustained. Alternatively, the early or late uptake of thallium 201 in regions of myocardium that fail to contract on echocardiography or the conversion of noncontractile segments to contractile myocardium after low-dose intravenous dobutamine is a more practical approach for detecting hibernating myocardium in which function can be expected to improve by revascularization.

The Choice Between a Catheter-Based Technique and Coronary Bypass Surgery (See Table 244-2) A number of randomized trials have compared PTCA and coronary bypass surgery in patients with multivessel CAD who were suitable technically for both procedures. The occurrence of death or myocardial infarction has been found to be similar between both groups for up to 5 years. In patients with diabetes plus disease of two or more coronary arteries, bypass surgery results in significantly better outcomes and survival and should be the technique of choice. In addition, the recurrence of angina and stenosis and the need for additional revascularization was much higher in the angioplasty group (about 50 percent) than in the surgery group (about 10 percent). Based on these trials and observational studies, we now recommend that patients with an unacceptable level of angina despite optimal medical management should be considered for revascularization. Patients with single- or two-vessel disease with normal global left ventricular function and anatomically suitable lesions are ordinarily advised initially to undergo PTCA, coronary stenting, or other catheter-based procedure (Chap. 245). Patients with two- or three-vessel disease and impaired global left ventricular function (left ventricular ejection fraction <45 percent) or diabetes mellitus or those with lesions unsuitable for catheter-based procedures should

be considered for coronary bypass surgery as the initial method of revascularization.

UNSTABLE ANGINA PECTORIS

The following three patient groups may be said to have unstable angina pectoris: (1) patients with new onset (<2 months) angina that is severe and/or frequent (≥3 episodes per day); (2) patients with accelerating angina, i.e., those with chronic stable angina who develop angina that is distinctly more frequent, severe, prolonged, or precipitated by less exertion than previously; (3) those with angina at rest. Unstable angina may be primary, i.e., occur in the absence of an extracardiac condition that has intensified myocardial ischemia, or it may be precipitated by a condition extrinsic to the coronary vascular bed that has intensified myocardial ischemia, such as anemia, fever, infection, tachyarrhythmias, emotional stress, or hypoxemia. Unstable angina may also develop shortly after myocardial infarction. Unstable angina, particularly when it is characterized by rest pain with ST-segment changes on the ECG or occurs in the postinfarction state, is associated with a relatively high risk of death, myocardial (re)infarction, or intractable angina requiring revascularization. Patients with rest pain frequently develop a third or fourth heart sound during the episode and in some instances exhibit transient left ventricular failure.

When unstable angina is accompanied by objective ECG evidence of transient myocardial ischemia (ST-segment changes and/or T-wave inversions during episodes of chest pain), it is associated with critical stenoses in one or more major epicardial coronary arteries in about 85 percent of cases. The atherosclerotic lesions may have a complicated morphology, with evidence of superimposed thrombosis in approximately 25 to 60 percent of cases. Segmental spasm in the vicinity of atherosclerotic plaques may also play a role in the development of unstable angina. The prognosis is excellent with medical management (see below) in the minority of patients without critical or fixed coronary stenosis.

℞ TREATMENT

The patient with rest pain or severe angina developing after myocardial infarction should be admitted promptly to the hospital for observation, further diagnosis, and treatment. Concomitant conditions that

Table 244-2

Comparison of Revascularization Procedures in Multivessel Disease

Procedure	Advantages	Disadvantages
Percutaneous transluminal coronary angioplasty	Less invasive Shorter hospital stay Lower initial cost Easily repeated Effective in relieving symptoms	Restenosis High incidence of incomplete revascularization Relative inefficiency in patients with severe left ventricular dysfunction Uncertain long-term outcome (>10 years) Limited to specific anatomic subsets Poor outcome in diabetics with 2 plus coronary disease
Coronary artery bypass grafting	Effective in relieving symptoms Improved survival in certain subsets Ability to achieve complete revascularization Wider applicability	Cost Increased risk of a repeat procedure due to late graft closure Morbidity

SOURCE: Modified from DP Faxon, in GA Beller (ed), *Chronic Ischemic Heart Disease*, in E Braunwald (series ed), *Atlas of Heart Diseases*, Philadelphia, Current Medicine, 1994.

can intensify ischemia, such as uncontrolled tachycardia, hypertension and diabetes mellitus, cardiomegaly, heart failure, arrhythmias, thyrotoxicosis, and any acute febrile illness should be sought and treated. Acute myocardial infarction should be ruled out by means of serial ECGs and measurements of plasma cardiac enzyme activity.

Continuous ECG monitoring should be carried out, and the patients should receive reassurance and sedation. Thrombus formation frequently complicates this condition. Therefore, intravenous heparin should be given for 3 to 5 days to maintain the partial thromboplastin time at 2 to 2.5 times control, together with or followed by oral aspirin at a dose of 325 mg/d. A beta-adrenoceptor blocking drug should be administered with a calcium antagonist if necessary, but with caution and an awareness of the possible side effects discussed above. Dosages of these agents should be raised rapidly, but the patient must be observed carefully to avoid bradycardia, heart failure, and hypotension. Nitroglycerin should be given by the sublingual route as needed for symptoms. Intravenous nitroglycerin is quite effective, especially in patients with episodes of ischemia that are particularly severe or prolonged. It is begun at a dosage of 10 µg/min and is raised in 5-µg/min increments to a level at which chest pain is abolished but systolic arterial pressure is maintained or reduced only slightly and other side effects are avoided.

The majority of patients (approximately 80 percent) improve with such treatment over a 48-h period. However, the clinical outcome is highly variable. If angina and/or ECG evidence of ischemia do not diminish within 24 to 48 h of the comprehensive treatment described above in patients with no obvious contraindications for revascularization, then cardiac catheterization and coronary arteriography should be performed. If the anatomy is suitable, PTCA can be performed with surgical standby. PTCA in this condition, particularly in the presence of thrombus, is attended by a slightly increased risk of acute closure and ischemia. If angioplasty cannot be done, coronary artery bypass grafting should be considered to relieve symptoms and myocardial ischemia and as a means of preventing myocardial damage. The factors that influence the choice between catheter-based and surgical revascularization are similar to that in chronic stable angina.

If the patient's symptoms and signs are controlled on medical therapy, a diagnostic exercise ECG should be obtained near the time of hospital discharge. If there is evidence of severe myocardial ischemia and/or evidence of a high risk of coronary events (p. 1368), consideration should be given to catheterization and, depending on the findings, revascularization. It should be recognized that severe CAD is often present in patients with unstable angina who respond to medical therapy. Many patients in whom the unstable state is controlled are left with severe chronic stable angina and ultimately require mechanical revascularization.

PRINZMETAL'S VARIANT ANGINA This relatively uncommon form of unstable angina is characterized by recurrent, prolonged attacks of severe ischemia, caused by episodic focal spasm of an epicardial coronary artery. Approximately three-fourths of patients with Prinzmetal's angina exhibit a fixed obstruction within 1 cm of the site of spasm. Patients with this condition are often in their thirties and forties, i.e., younger than patients with unstable angina secondary to coronary atherosclerosis. Ischemic pain usually occurs at rest or awakens the patient from sleep and is characterized by multilead ST-segment elevation. The diagnosis may be confirmed by detecting transient spasm occurring spontaneously or following a provocative stimulus (intravenous ergonovine, intracoronary acetylcholine, hyperventilation) on coronary arteriography. While long-term survival is excellent, complications include episodes of disabling pain, myocardial infarction, serious ventricular arrhythmias, atrioventricular block, and, rarely, sudden death.

℞ TREATMENT

Management of the acute attack consists of multiple doses of sublingual nitroglycerin and short-acting nifedipine (10 to 30 mg); hypotension should be avoided. In chronic management, long-acting nitrates and calcium antagonists are useful. Beta-adrenergic blockers are of little value, while prazosin, a selective alpha-adrenoceptor blocker, may be useful. Occasionally, mechanical revascularization is helpful in patients with accompanying severe discrete obstructive lesions.

ASYMPTOMATIC (SILENT) ISCHEMIA

Obstructive CAD, acute myocardial infarction, and transient myocardial ischemia are frequently asymptomatic. During continuous ambulatory ECG monitoring, the majority of ambulatory patients with typical chronic stable angina are found to have objective evidence of myocardial ischemia (ST-segment depression) during episodes of chest discomfort while they are active outside the hospital, but many of these patients also appear to have more frequent episodes of asymptomatic ischemia. In addition, there is a large (but as yet unknown) number of totally asymptomatic people with severe coronary atherosclerosis who exhibit ST-segment changes during activity. Evidence of frequent episodes of ischemia (symptomatic and asymptomatic) during daily life appears to indicate an increased likelihood of adverse coronary events such as death and myocardial infarction. The widespread use of exercise ECG during routine examinations has also defined some of these heretofore unrecognized patients with asymptomatic CAD. Longitudinal studies have demonstrated an increased incidence of coronary events (sudden death, myocardial infarction, and angina) in asymptomatic patients with positive exercise tests. In addition, patients with asymptomatic ischemia after suffering a myocardial infarction are at far greater risk for a second coronary event. Patients who seek evaluation and who have asymptomatic ischemia should be subjected to a detailed noninvasive examination utilizing stress ECG and, if necessary, radionuclide scintigraphy.

℞ TREATMENT

The management of patients with asymptomatic ischemia must be individualized. Thus, the physician should consider the following: (1) the degree of positivity of the stress test, particularly the stage of exercise at which ECG signs of ischemia appear, the magnitude and number of the perfusion defect(s) on thallium scintigraphy, and the change in left ventricular ejection fraction which occurs on radionuclide ventriculography or ECG during ischemia and/or during exercise; (2) the ECG leads showing a positive response, with changes in the anterior precordial leads indicating a less favorable prognosis than changes in the inferior leads; and (3) the patient's age, occupation, and general medical condition. Most would agree that an asymptomatic 45-year-old commercial airline pilot with 0.4 mV ST-segment depression in leads V_1 to V_4 during mild exercise should undergo coronary arteriography, whereas the asymptomatic, sedentary 75-year-old retiree with 0.1 mV ST-segment depression in leads II and III during maximal activity need not. However, there is no consensus about the appropriate procedure in the large majority of patients for whom the situation is less extreme. Patients with evidence of severe ischemia on noninvasive testing (as outlined earlier) should undergo coronary arteriography. Asymptomatic patients with silent ischemia, three-vessel CAD, and impaired left ventricular function may be considered appropriate candidates for coronary artery bypass surgery.

The treatment of risk factors, particularly lipid lowering as described above, as well as aspirin and beta blockers have been shown to reduce events and improve outcomes in asymptomatic as well as symptomatic patients with ischemia and coronary disease. While the incidence of asymptomatic ischemia can be reduced by treatment with beta blockers, calcium channel antagonists, and long-acting nitrates, it is not clear whether this is necessary or desirable in patients who have not suffered a myocardial infarction. However, there is evidence that beta-adrenoceptor blockade begun

7 to 35 days after acute myocardial infarction improves survival (Chap. 243).

BIBLIOGRAPHY

THE BARI INVESTIGATORS: Comparison of coronary bypass surgery with angioplasty in patients with multivessel diseases. N Engl J Med 335:217, 1996

BERLINER JA et al: Atherosclerosis: Basic mechanisms, oxidation, inflammations, and genetics. Circulation 91:2488, 1995

BITTL JA: Advances in coronary angioplasty. N Engl J Med 335:1290, 1996

BRAUNWALD E et al: Diagnosing and managing unstable angina. Circulation 90:613, 1994

CALVIN JE et al: Risk stratification in unstable angina. Prospective validation of the Braunwald classification. JAMA 273:136, 1995

DIAMOND GA: Prior restraint: A Bayesian perspective on the optimization of technology utilization for diagnosis of coronary artery disease. Am J Cardiol 76:82, 1995

EAKERS ED: Cardiovascular disease in women. Circulation 88:1999, 1993

FARMER JA, GOTTO AM: Risk factors for coronary artery disease, in *Heart Disease*, 5th ed, E Braunwald (ed). Philadelphia, Saunders, 1997, pp 1126–1160

FISCHMAN DL et al: A randomized comparison of coronary stent placement and balloon angioplasty in the treatment of coronary artery disease. N Engl J Med 331:496, 1994

GERSH BJ et al: Chronic coronary artery disease, in *Heart Disease*, 5th ed, E Braunwald (ed). Philadelphia, Saunders, 1997, pp 1289–1365

HOLDRIGHT D et al: Comparison of the effect of heparin and aspirin versus aspirin alone on transient myocardial ischemia and in-hospital progress in patients with unstable angina. Am J Cardiol 24:39, 1994

KING SB et al: A randomized trial comparing angioplasty with coronary bypass surgery. N Engl J Med 331:1044, 1994

LEVINE GN et al: Cholesterol reduction in cardiovascular disease: Clinical benefits and possible mechanisms. N Engl J Med 332:512, 1995

MASERI A: *Ischemic Heart Disease*. New York, Churchill Livingstone, 1995

NYMAN I et al: Prevention of serious cardiac event by low-dose aspirin in patients with silent myocardial ischemia. Lancet 340:497, 1992

PAFFENBERGER RS JR: The association of changes in physical activity level and other life style characteristics with mortality among men. N Engl J Med 328:538, 1993

PARISI AF et al: A comparison of angioplasty with medical therapy in the treatment of single-vessel coronary artery disease. N Engl J Med 326:10, 1992

PATRONO C: Aspirin as an antiplatelet drug. N Engl J Med 330:1287, 1994

PEPI TRIAL WRITING GROUP: Effects of estrogen or estrogen/progestin regimens on heart disease risk factors in post menopausal women: The Post Menopausal Estrogen/Progestin Interventions (PEPI) Trial. JAMA 273:199, 1995

RYAN TJ et al: Special report: Guidelines for Percutaneous Transluminal Coronary Angioplasty. A report of the American Heart Association/American College of Cardiology Task Force on Assessment of Diagnostic and Therapeutic Cardiovascular Procedures. Circulation 88:2987, 1993

SCANDINAVIAN SIMVASTATIN SURVIVAL STUDY GROUP: Randomized trial of cholesterol lowering in 4444 patients with coronary heart disease: The Scandinavian Simvastatin Survival Study (4S). Lancet 344:1383, 1994

SELWYN AP et al: Pathophysiology of ischemia in patients with coronary artery disease. Prog Cardiovasc Dis 35:1, 1992

Table 245-1

Therapeutic Applications of Cardiac Catheterization

Treatment of coronary stenoses and occlusions
 Percutaneous transluminal coronary angioplasty (PTCA)
 Laser techniques
 Intravascular stents
 Atherectomy
Treatment of valvular stenoses
 Balloon valvuloplasty (aortic, mitral, pulmonic)
Treatment of congenital defects
 Atrial septostomy
 Umbrella closure of patent ductus arteriosus and defects in atrial or ventricular septum
 Coil closure of undesired collateral vessels

TREATMENT OF CORONARY STENOSES AND OCCLUSIONS WITH CORONARY ANGIOPLASTY

Percutaneous transluminal coronary angioplasty (PTCA) is an important form of therapy for coronary artery disease (see Chap. 244). More than 400,000 PTCA procedures are performed each year in the United States, exceeding the number of coronary bypass operations. Since PTCA is performed using local anesthesia, during a short (1- to 3-day) hospitalization, its use in suitable patients can greatly decrease expense and recovery time compared to coronary bypass surgery, although the procedure-related mortality of elective PTCA (0.4 to 1.0 percent), is similar to that of elective coronary bypass surgery.

INDICATIONS The main indication for PTCA is the presence of one or more coronary stenoses that are approachable by balloon catheters and that are thought to be responsible for a clinical syndrome warranting revascularization (Fig. 245-1). Moreover, the risks and benefits of revascularization by PTCA should compare favorably with those of conventional surgery. Significant left main stenosis and multivessel disease in which vessels supplying significant areas of viable myocardium are not approachable by PTCA (owing to chronic total occlusion or other unfavorable anatomic features) constitute relative contraindications to PTCA if surgery is technically possible. Randomized trials comparing PTCA to bypass surgery in patients with multivessel coronary artery disease suggest that, while the two procedures have equivalent in-hospital and 3- to 5-year mortalities, more PTCA patients (40 to 50 percent versus 7 to 10 percent) will require a second revascularization procedure (generally a repeat PTCA to treat restenosis) to maintain an equivalent level of symptom relief.

For most patients, the clinical syndrome being treated is moderately severe, chronic, stable angina that persists despite medical antian-

245

Donald S. Baim, William Grossman

CORONARY ANGIOPLASTY AND OTHER THERAPEUTIC APPLICATIONS OF CARDIAC CATHETERIZATION

The development of catheter-based therapies for the treatment of cardiovascular disease has led to creation of the field known as *interventional cardiology*. In current practice, interventional cardiology provides a safe and effective alternative to conventional surgery for many patients with ischemic, valvular, and congenital heart disease (Table 245-1).

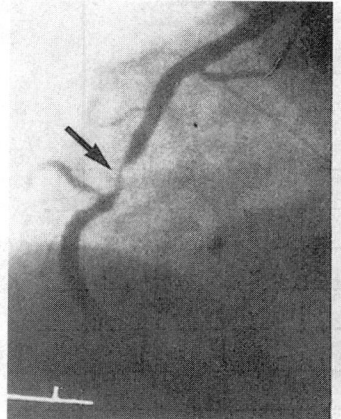
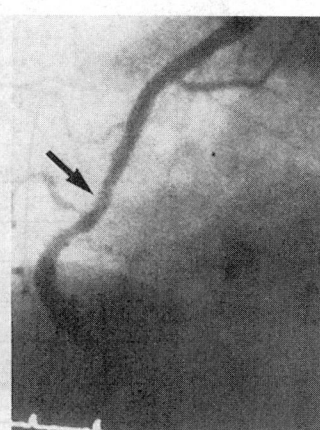

FIGURE 245-1 Right coronary angioplasty in a patient with unstable angina. The lesion is shown before (*left panel*) and after (*right panel*) inflation of the PTCA balloon catheter.

ginal therapy. Approximately 15 percent of current PTCA patients, however, have only mild anginal symptoms despite suitable coronary anatomy and objective evidence of ischemia (i.e., an abnormal exercise test). At the other extreme, many patients have more pressing indications for PTCA, including unstable angina or even acute myocardial infarction (with or without prior thrombolytic therapy).

As the clinical indications for PTCA have broadened, so have its anatomic capabilities. Thus, PTCA no longer is restricted to proximal, discrete, subtotal, concentric, noncalcified lesions, as was the case initially. Angioplasty catheters with smaller deflated profiles, controlled by highly steerable guidewires, can now be advanced successfully across severe stenoses located virtually anywhere in the coronary tree. These balloon catheters tolerate inflation pressures up to 20 atm, adequate to dilate even calcific lesions. Totally occluded coronary arteries (particularly ones that have been occluded for less than 6 months) can be crossed and dilated effectively, although the success rate remains somewhat lower than for subtotal lesions (i.e., 60 percent versus 90 percent for subtotal stenotic lesions). In addition to lesions in the native coronary tree, obstructions in saphenous vein or internal mammary artery bypass grafts also can be dilated successfully to treat postbypass angina. If multiple lesions are responsible for the clinical syndrome, most or all such lesions can generally be dilated during a single procedure.

RESULTS The current PTCA success rate (for dilating a target stenosis by >50 percent of the adjacent normal vessel diameter without producing an associated complication) exceeds 90 percent. About half the failures result from inability to cross the target lesion with the guidewire or balloon catheter, particularly when that target lesion is a chronic total occlusion. The remaining failures are due to excessive local dissection (separation of coronary artery intima from media) resulting from attempted dilatation. While some local dissection is present in virtually all successful PTCA procedures, more extensive dissection (particularly in association with local thrombus formation or vasospasm) can lead to abrupt closure of the dilated segment soon after withdrawal of the balloon catheter. Routine use of vasodilators (nitrates and calcium channel antagonists), anticoagulation (heparin, 10,000 to 15,000 units during the procedure), and antiplatelet therapy (acetylsalicylic acid, 325 mg/day starting at least 24 h prior to PTCA and continued for 3 to 6 months after the procedure) helps to prevent abrupt closure due to spasm and/or thrombus formation. Newer antithrombins (hirudin) or anti-platelet agents (blockers of IIb/IIIa receptors) may further reduce the incidence of ischemic complications within 72 h of PTCA. Closure due to dissection frequently can be reversed by repeat dilatation or, if that is unsuccessful, by the placement of a coronary stent (Fig. 245-2, and see below). When these measures fail, emergency bypass surgery may be necessary to restore blood flow and prevent myocardial infarction. While emergency bypass surgery is needed currently in only 1 to 2 percent of PTCA attempts, this potential difficulty means that angioplasty can be performed only in hospitals where immediate cardiac surgery is available.

FOLLOW-UP After successful PTCA of all "culprit" lesions, marked improvement or complete resolution of the presenting ischemic syndrome should be evident. In approximately 20 to 30 percent of patients, however, evidence of ischemia returns within 6 months, due to so-called restenosis of the dilated segment. This development appears to result from excessive local fibrointimal proliferation and vessel constriction triggered by vessel wall injury and the adhesion of platelets to the freshly dilated surface. To date, despite considerable effort, no pharmacologic strategy has substantially reduced this restenosis rate. When recurrent ischemia develops more than 6 months after PTCA, it usually reflects progression of disease at another site, rather than restenosis. When repeat PTCA is used to treat either restenosis or disease progression, only about 10 percent of patients require bypass surgery during the 5 years following a successful PTCA procedure.

NEWER NONBALLOON TECHNIQUES While conventional balloon angioplasty offers unmatched anatomic versatility, the difficulty of using it for certain anatomic lesion types (e.g., calcified, eccentric, ostial, thrombus-containing, or bifurcation lesions) has fostered the development of a number of newer, nonballoon techniques. These techniques—which include stenting, atherectomy, and ablative laser treatment—moved from clinical investigation to routine clinical practice during the early 1990s and now account for 60 to 70 percent of coronary interventions in many centers. If used appropriately, these new techniques can improve the success, safety, and long-term results (restenosis rate) in lesion types that are difficult to treat using balloon techniques alone. Although most of these procedures cost more in terms of catheter expense, much of this cost can be recouped by the reduction in long-term expenses for the treatment of restenosis.

Stents These are metallic scaffolds that can be positioned in a diseased vessel segment to create a normal vessel lumen by resisting elastic recoil and obliterating any local dissection. By providing a larger acute lumen than does conventional balloon angioplasty, they can also reduce the incidence of subsequent restenosis by nearly one-third. The wire coil design was approved by the Food and Drug

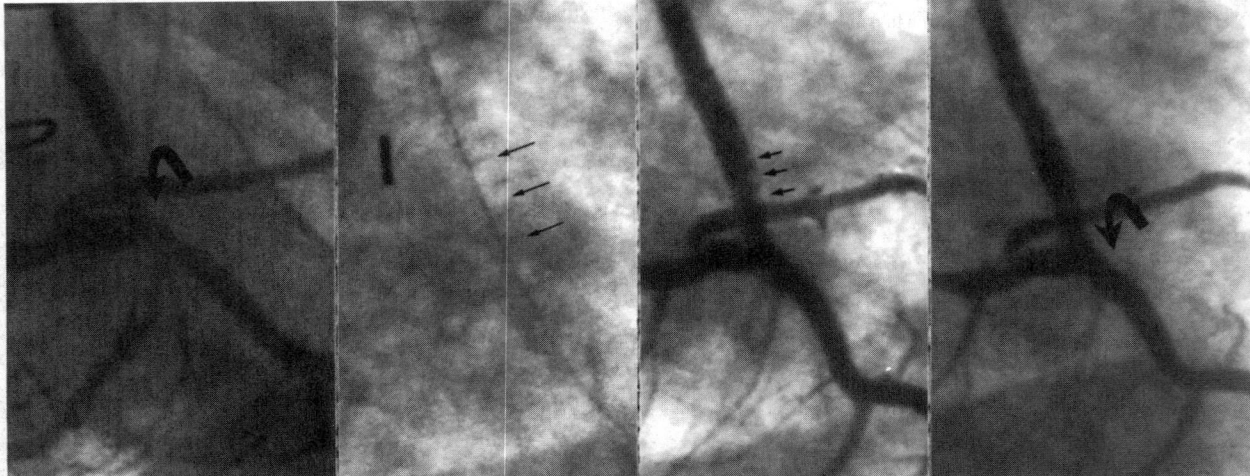

FIGURE 245-2 Placement of coronary stent for dissection after angioplasty. *Left-hand panel*: A prominent filling defect (*curved arrow*) is visible at the site of attempted PTCA in the distal anastomosis of a saphenous vein graft to the circumflex. *Left center panel*: The coils of a Gianturco-Roubin stent are faintly visible (*arrows*). *Right center panel*: Angiogram following stent placement shows small filling defects (*arrows*) representing prolapse of dissected plaque between stent coils. *Right panel*: Following high-pressure postdilation, luminal appearance is near normal (*curved arrow*). The availability of coronary stents to manage actual and threatened abrupt closure has dramatically reduced the need for emergency bypass surgery in current angioplasty practice.

Administration (FDA) in 1993 for use in stabilizing actual or threatened abrupt closure, while the slotted tube design was approved in 1994 for elective treatment of native coronary lesions. In clinical practice, however, both stents have been used widely in other circumstances, including restenotic lesions and saphenous vein grafts (Fig. 245-3). Early experience suggested that these metallic implants were prone to thrombotic occlusion, either acute (<24 h) or subacute (1 to 14 days with a peak at 6 days), and that an aggressive anticoagulation regimen (aspirin, dipyridamole, low-molecular-weight dextran, and warfarin) was needed to prevent such thrombosis. This aggressive anticoagulant regimen led to longer hospitalization and an increased incidence of local vascular complications at the femoral arterial entry site. More recent data, however, suggest that many of these thrombotic complications were the result of incomplete stent expansion, and that more attention to full initial deployment allows the same stents to be used with only antiplatelet drugs (aspirin and ticlopidine), with more acceptable thrombosis and vascular complication rates (each <1 percent). On the basis of the overwhelming clinical success of these two early stents, more than a dozen second-generation designs (including stents that are easier to deliver or are coated with heparin or other bioactive agents) are now emerging from the FDA approval process.

Atherectomy While both balloon angioplasty and stenting enlarge the coronary lumen by displacing plaque, atherectomy catheters provide much of their lumen enlargement by removing plaque mass from the treated lesion. *Directional* atherectomy does so by using a special catheter with a windowed steel cylinder at its tip. Inflation of a low-pressure positioning balloon on the back of the cylinder presses plaque into the window, where it is cut and trapped by a spinning cup-shaped cutter (Fig. 245-4). This device was the first of the nonballoon technologies to reach clinical practice and it is still the treatment of choice for noncalcified lesions at the origin of the left anterior descending artery or at major coronary bifurcations. *Rotational* atherectomy uses burrs of various sizes (diameter 1.25 to 2.38 mm) that are coated

on their leading half with small diamond chips. The burr is spun at 160,000 to 180,000 rpm as it is advanced through a coronary lesion over a leading guidewire. The diamond chips grind through the obstructing plaque, pulverizing it into small (5 to 25 μm) particles, which pass through the distal coronary microcirculation. This device has emerged as an effective treatment for calcified, long (>20 mm), or ostial lesions; frequently it is followed by low-pressure balloon dilation and occasionally by stent placement (Fig. 245-5). *Extraction* atherectomy uses a combination of distal cutting blades rotating at low speed and continuous vacuum aspiration to remove coronary obstructions. The device has limited cutting efficiency, and its use is now confined to softer lesions (e.g., atherosclerotic saphenous vein grafts) or thrombotic lesions. Newer aspiration devices based on the Venturi effect may be able to remove clot more efficiently with less vessel disruption.

Lasers Laser light [at wavelengths from the ultraviolet (308 nm) to the mid-infrared (2000 μm)] can be delivered to obstructing coronary plaques through small optical fibers bundled into flexible catheters whose outer diameter is between 1.2 and 2.0 mm. When these catheters are pulsed with laser energy as they are advanced through a coronary obstruction over a guidewire, they can ablate noncalcified coronary plaque by a combination of photoacoustic (blast), thermal, and photochemical effects. Although lasers have been used to treat ostial as well as diffuse coronary lesions, acceptance of the technique has been limited by the expense of the device and the fact that these lesions can be treated by other techniques, such as rotational atherectomy. Unique applications—such as use of a laser guidewire designed to cross total occlusions—may help entrench the technique. Earlier laser-thermal devices (in which a metal cap or the vessel wall was heated through a transparent angioplasty balloon) were tried but abandoned because of excessive vessel injury and late restenosis.

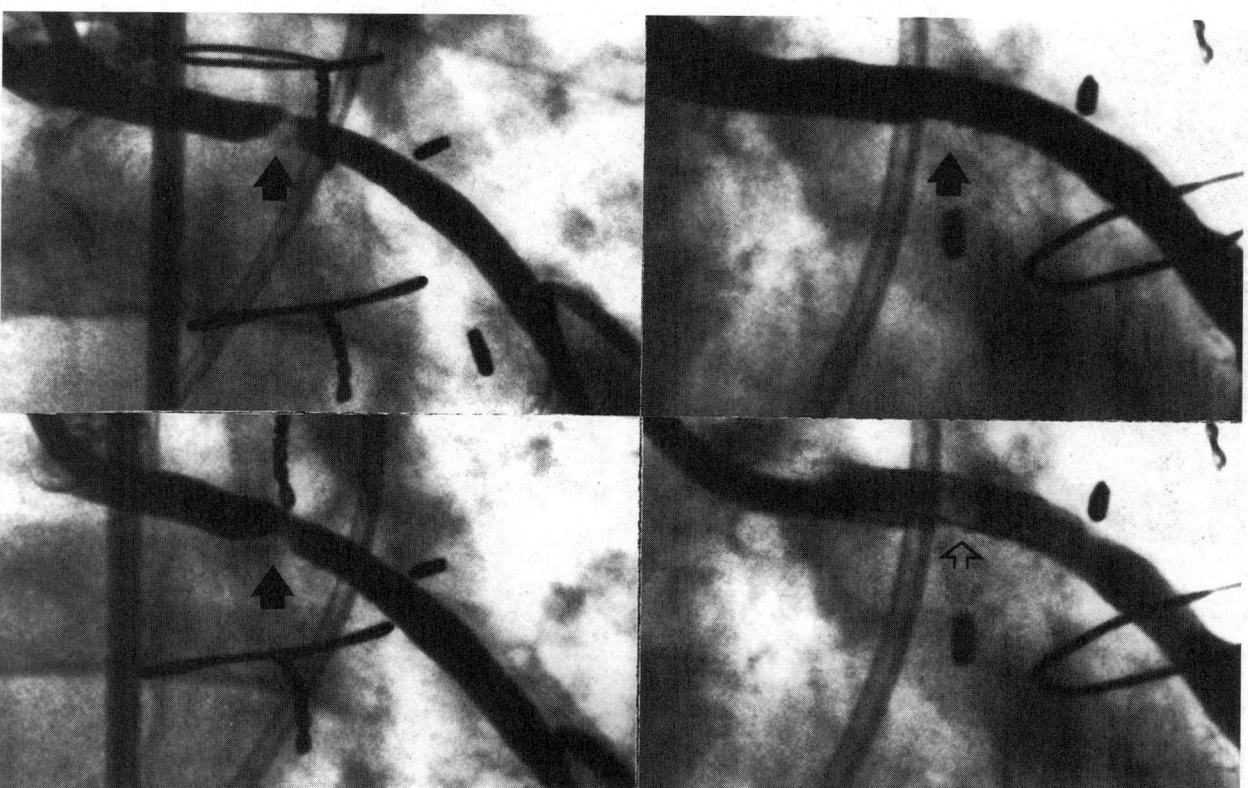

FIGURE 245-3 Stenting of a diseased saphenous vein graft. *Upper left*: Severe eccentric stenosis in an 8-year-old saphenous vein graft to the left anterior descending coronary artery. *Lower left*: Following balloon dilatation, significant stenosis persists owing to elastic recoil of the graft atherosclerotic plaque. *Upper right*: Further lumen enlargement following placement of a slotted-tube stent (*arrow*). *Lower right*: Diamond pattern is visible (*open arrow*) as contrast clears from the graft.

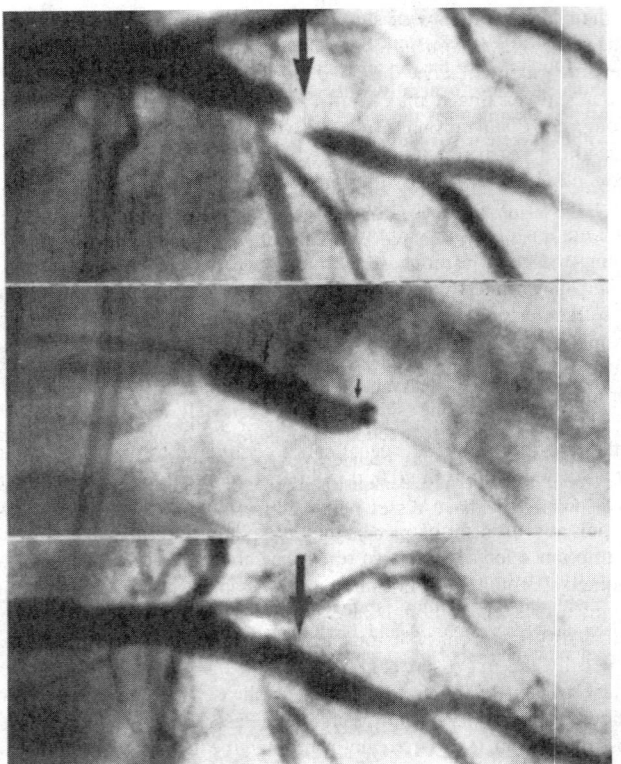

FIGURE 245-4 *Top*: Eccentric, ulcerated lesion in the mid-left anterior descending coronary artery. *Middle*: Lesion being treated by directional atherectomy. *Bottom*: the resulting large, smooth lumen.

TREATMENT OF VALVULAR STENOSIS: BALLOON VALVULOPLASTY

Once the efficacy of balloon dilatation for vascular stenoses was demonstrated, cardiologists treating both pediatric and adult patients applied the technique to the treatment of stenotic cardiac valves. The technique was used first for congenital pulmonic and aortic stenosis but has now been extended to acquired rheumatic and calcific stenoses of the mitral and aortic valves.

PULMONIC VALVULOPLASTY Although congenital pulmonic stenosis is mainly a pediatric disease, it is sometimes encountered in adults (see Chap. 235). Transvalvular pressure gradients of >50 mmHg may produce exertional symptoms or lead to progressive right ventricular hypertrophy or failure. Using a guidewire placed into the pulmonary artery from the femoral vein, one or more valvuloplasty balloons with a combined cross-sectional area as much as 20 percent larger than the pulmonic valve annulus are positioned within the stenotic valve and inflated with liquid contrast medium at pressures of 3 to 5 atm. This typically reduces the transvalvular gradient from 75 to 15 mmHg. Balloon pulmonary valvuloplasty now stands as the preferred therapy for this lesion.

MITRAL VALVULOPLASTY The main application of balloon mitral valvuloplasty is in patients with rheumatic mitral stenosis, in whom stenosis results primarily from commissural fusion with associated leaflet thickening. Such patients—who previously would have undergone open or closed surgical commissurotomy—are now treated almost exclusively by balloon valvuloplasty (Chap. 237). Patients with other kinds of problems (left atrial thrombus, mitral regurgitation, subvalvular disease, or leaflet thickening or rigidity) have less satisfactory results with either surgical commissurotomy or balloon valvuloplasty and are better treated by surgical valve replacement.

The usual approach to balloon mitral valvuloplasty involves transseptal puncture (right atrium to left atrium) followed by passage of a guidewire across the stenotic valve and into the left ventricle. One or more balloon catheters with a dilating area equivalent to a single 23-

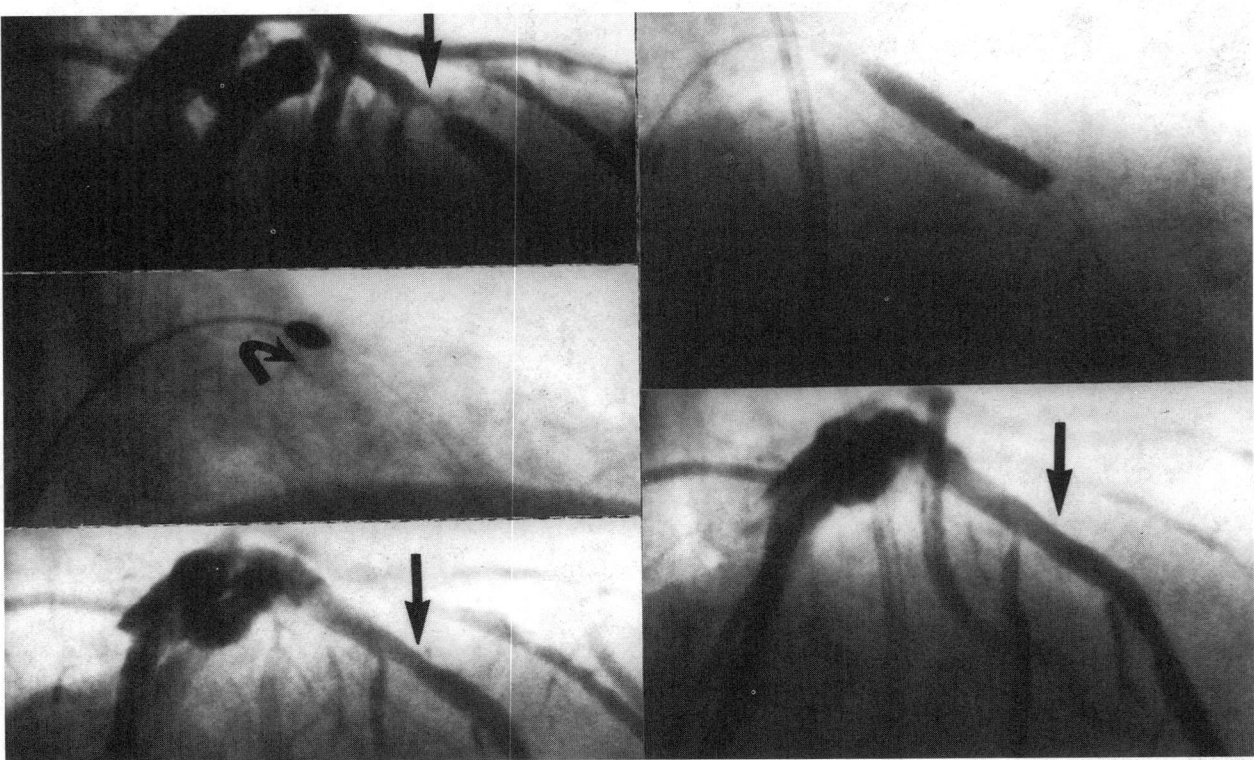

FIGURE 245-5 Rotational atherectomy for a calcified lesion in the mid-left anterior descending coronary artery. *Upper left*: Calcified lesions such as this one (*arrow*) used to be treated by high-pressure balloon inflation, although that commonly resulted in severe local dissection. *Middle left*: In current practice, such lesions are generally treated by rotational atherectomy, shown here using a 2.0-mm diamond-chip–coated burr (*curved arrow*). *Lower left*: Following burr passage, much of the calcified lesion has been ablated (*arrow*). *Upper right*: After rotational atherectomy, inflation of the balloon at low pressure (4 atm) results in full balloon expansion. *Lower right*: Large, smooth lumen present after balloon postdilation.

to 30-mm diameter balloon are advanced over this guidewire and inflated within the stenotic valve. Alternatively, the newer Inoue balloon (Fig. 245-6) can be used to provide faster and more effective dilatation than is achieved with conventional cylindrical balloon designs. Successful dilatation separates fused commissures and enhances leaflet compliance, thus increasing the effective diastolic valve area from 0.9 to 2.0 cm² or more (Fig. 245-7). Although this opening is still restricted compared with the 3.5- to 5-cm² area of a normal mitral valve, it provides excellent symptomatic relief and is equivalent to or approaches the increase in orifice size resulting from surgical mitral commissurotomy or prosthetic mitral valve replacement.

The main complications of balloon mitral valvuloplasty relate to the potential for cardiac perforation during transseptal puncture (approximately 2 percent of patients) and the chance of systemic embolization (approximately 1 percent of patients) despite preprocedure echocardiographic exclusion of patients with left atrial thrombus.

AORTIC VALVULOPLASTY Balloon aortic valvuloplasty may be performed in children with congenital aortic stenosis and in adults with rheumatic or acquired calcific aortic stenosis. Some patients with rheumatic aortic stenosis have leaflet fusion, but the problem in acquired calcific aortic stenosis is due more to rigidity of the valve leaflets themselves. In the latter group of patients, balloon valvuloplasty fractures leaflet calcium (providing new hinge points along which the valve leaflets can open) and temporarily expands the aortic annulus.

The most common approach to balloon aortic valvuloplasty consists of femoral arterial puncture with retrograde passage of a guidewire and balloon (inflated diameter 18 to 23 mm) across the valve. Overdilatation of the valve annulus may cause leaflet avulsion and is generally avoided. Balloon aortic valvuloplasty typically increases the effective systolic valve area from 0.6 to 1.0 cm². The resulting valve area is still small compared with that of a normal aortic valve (3 to 4 cm²) or with the effective area of an inflated 20-mm balloon (3.1 cm²), but it does relieve symptoms at rest or during mild to moderate exertion in most patients with critical aortic stenosis. Unfortunately, the relatively small effective orifice achieved and the high incidence of valvular restenosis (up to 50 percent within 1 year after dilatation) make balloon aortic valvuloplasty most applicable as a temporary palliation for elderly patients who are poor risks for valve replacement or as a "bridge" to valve replacement.

TREATMENT OF CONGENITAL MALFORMATIONS

Pediatric interventional cardiologists have developed a number of innovative techniques to correct or palliate congenital cardiac lesions. Some were described above—balloon dilatation of stenotic pulmonary arteries, surgical stent placement, and balloon valvuloplasty—but others are unique to the pediatric population.

ATRIAL SEPTOSTOMY In certain patients with cyanotic congenital heart disease, such as some with transposition of the great vessels, it is desirable to produce or enlarge an atrial septal defect to facilitate passage of oxygenated blood into the right side of the heart. This can be achieved by passage of a balloon catheter from the right to left atrium across a patent foramen ovale, followed by forceful withdrawal of the inflated balloon. Alternatively, a catheter with a concealed blade can be passed across the septum. The blade can then

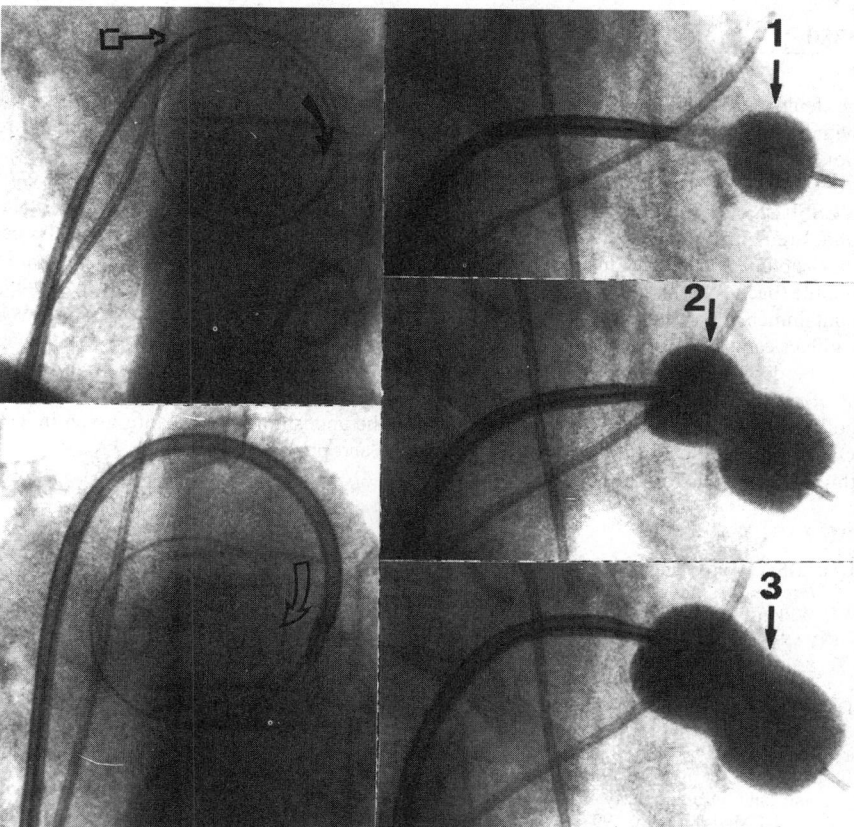

FIGURE 245-6 Inoue balloon for mitral valvuloplasty. Compared to earlier cylindrical balloons, the unique Inoue balloon permits fast and safe dilatation of stenotic mitral valves. *Upper left*: Transseptal puncture has been used to pass a coiled guidewire (*curved arrow*) and tapered dilator (*boxed arrow*) into the left atrium. *Lower left*: The deflated Inoue catheter is advanced into the left atrium over this guidewire (*open curved arrow*). *Upper right*: Partial inflation of the balloon helps it float across the mitral valve and into the left ventricle (1), whereupon it is pulled back against the mitral leaflets. *Middle right*: Further balloon inflation causes expansion of the proximal part of the balloon (2), trapping the mitral orifice between the proximal and distal portions of the balloon. *Lower right*: With the balloon thus anchored, full expansion of its central portion (3) effectively dilates the stenotic valve.

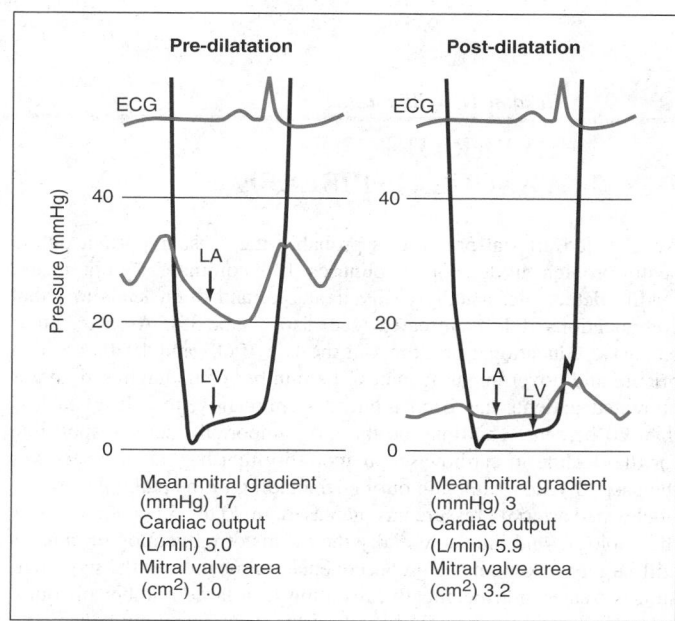

FIGURE 245-7 Hemodynamic results of mitral valvuloplasty in a 38-year-old woman with mitral stenosis. The transmitral gradient [from the left atrium (LA) to the left ventricle (LV)], cardiac output, and calculated mitral valve area are shown before (*left panel*) and after (*right panel*) balloon dilatation.

be deployed in the left atrium to incise the septum as the catheter is withdrawn. The resulting septal incision can be widened by conventional balloon septostomy.

CLOSURE OF UNDESIRED SHUNTS OR COLLATERAL VESSELS   A variety of appliances have been developed to close undesired intracardiac shunts, including defects in the atrial or ventricular septum and patent ductus arteriosus. These devices resemble a double (back-to-back) umbrella, which can be folded into a cylinder for containment in a catheter. Under fluoroscopic guidance, the delivery catheter can be positioned across the target defect so that the umbrella can be deployed to block undesired flow.

Smaller vascular shunts can be closed using special coils. These coils can be placed in a catheter and delivered to the undesired vessel. Once in place, the coil interferes with blood flow and promotes local thrombotic occlusion of the target vessel.

BIBLIOGRAPHY

BAIM DS: Coronary angioplasty, in *Cardiac Catheterization, Angiography and Intervention*, 5th ed, D Baim, W Grossman (eds). Baltimore, Williams & Wilkins, 1996

BERMAN AD et al: Balloon valvuloplasty, in *Cardiac Catheterization, Angiography and Intervention*, 5th ed, D Baim, W Grossman (eds). Baltimore, Williams & Wilkins, 1996

DETRE K et al: Has improvement in PTCA intervention affected long-term prognosis? The NHLBI PTCA Registry experience. Circulation 91:2868, 1995

FISCHMAN DL et al: A randomized comparison of coronary stent placement and balloon angioplasty in the treatment of coronary artery disease. N Engl J Med 331:496, 1994

PERRY SB et al: Pediatric interventions, in *Cardiac Catheterization, Angiography and Intervention*, 5th ed, D Baim, W Grossman (eds). Baltimore, Williams & Wilkins, 1996

POCOCK SJ et al: Metaanalysis of randomized trials comparing coronary angioplasty with bypass surgery. Lancet 346:1184, 1995

RYAN TJ et al: Guidelines for percutaneous transluminal coronary angioplasty—a report of the ACC/AHA task force. J Am Coll Cardiol 22:2033, 1993

THE EPIC INVESTIGATORS: Use of a monoclonal antibody against the platelet glycoprotein IIb/IIIa receptor in high-risk coronary angioplasty. N Engl J Med 330:956, 1994

246   *Gordon H. Williams*

HYPERTENSIVE VASCULAR DISEASE

An elevated arterial pressure is probably the most important public health problem in developed countries. It is common, asymptomatic, readily detectable, usually easily treatable, and often leads to lethal complications if left untreated (see also Chap. 35). As a result of extensive educational programs in the late 1960s and 1970s by both private and government agencies, the number of undiagnosed and/or untreated patients has been reduced significantly, to a level of less than 20 percent. This may be the most important factor responsible for the decline in cardiovascular mortality that has taken place over the past 20 years. Although our understanding of the pathophysiology of elevated arterial pressure has increased, in 90 to 95 percent of cases the etiology (and thus potentially the means of prevention or cure) is still largely unknown. As a consequence, in most cases the hypertension is treated nonspecifically, resulting in a large number of minor side effects and a relatively high (~50 percent) noncompliance rate.

PREVALENCE   The prevalence of hypertension depends on both the racial composition of the population studied and the criteria used to define the condition. In a white suburban population like that in the Framingham Study, nearly one-fifth of individuals have blood pressures greater than 160/95, while almost one-half have pressures greater than 140/90. An even higher prevalence has been documented in the nonwhite population. In females the prevalence is closely related to age, with a substantial increase occurring after age 50. This increase is presumably related to the hormonal changes of menopause. Thus, the ratio of hypertension frequency in women versus men increases from 0.6 to 0.7 at age 30 to 1.1 to 1.2 at age 65.

The prevalence of various forms of secondary hypertension depends on the nature of the population studied and on how extensive the evaluation is. There are no available data to define the frequency of secondary hypertension in the general population, although in middle-aged males it has been reported to be 6 percent. On the other hand, in referral centers where patients undergo an extensive evaluation, it has been reported to be as high as 35 percent. The various forms of hypertension are outlined in Table 246-1, and their relative frequencies are given in Table 246-2.

ESSENTIAL HYPERTENSION

Patients with arterial hypertension and no definable cause are said to have *primary*, *essential*, or *idiopathic hypertension*. Undoubtedly, the primary difficulty in uncovering the mechanism(s) responsible for the

Table 246-1

Classification of Arterial Hypertension

SYSTOLIC HYPERTENSION WITH WIDE PULSE PRESSURE

I. Decreased compliance of aorta (arteriosclerosis)
II. Increased stroke volume
   A. Aortic regurgitation
   B. Thyrotoxicosis
   C. Hyperkinetic heart syndrome
   D. Fever
   E. Arteriovenous fistula
   F. Patent ductus arteriosus

SYSTOLIC AND DIASTOLIC HYPERTENSION (INCREASED PERIPHERAL VASCULAR RESISTANCE)

I. Renal
   A. Chronic pyelonephritis
   B. Acute and chronic glomerulonephritis
   C. Polycystic renal disease
   D. Renovascular stenosis or renal infarction
   E. Most other severe renal diseases (arteriolar nephrosclerosis, diabetic nephropathy, etc.)
   F. Renin-producing tumors
II. Endocrine
   A. Oral contraceptives
   B. Adrenocortical hyperfunction
      1. Cushing's disease and syndrome
      2. Primary hyperaldosteronism
      3. Congenital or hereditary adrenogenital syndromes (17α-hydroxylase and 11β-hydroxylase defects)
   C. Pheochromocytoma
   D. Myxedema
   E. Acromegaly
III. Neurogenic
   A. Psychogenic
   B. Diencephalic syndrome
   C. Familial dysautonomia (Riley-Day)
   D. Polyneuritis (acute porphyria, lead poisoning)
   E. Increased intracranial pressure (acute)
   F. Spinal cord section (acute)
IV. Miscellaneous
   A. Coarctation of aorta
   B. Increased intravascular volume (excessive transfusion, polycythemia vera)
   C. Polyarteritis nodosa
   D. Hypercalcemia
   E. Medications, e.g., glucocorticoids, cyclosporine
V. Unknown etiology
   A. Essential hypertension (>90% of all cases of hypertension)
   B. Toxemia of pregnancy
   C. Acute intermittent porphyria

Table 246-2

CHAPTER 246
Hypertensive Vascular Disease **1381**

Prevalence of Various Forms of Hypertension in the General Population and in Specialized Referral Clinics*

Diagnosis	General Population, %	Specialty Clinic, %
Essential hypertension	92–94	65–85
Renal hypertension:		
Parenchymal	2–3	4–5
Renovascular	1–2	4–16
Endocrine hypertension:		
Primary aldosteronism	0.3	0.5–12
Cushing's syndrome	<0.1	0.2
Pheochromocytoma	<0.1	0.2
Oral contraceptive–induced	0.5–1	1–2
Miscellaneous	0.2	1

* Estimates based on a number of reports in the literature.

hypertension in these patients is attributable to the variety of systems that are involved in the regulation of arterial pressure—peripheral and/or central adrenergic, renal, hormonal, and vascular—and to the complexity of the interrelations of these systems. Several abnormalities have been described in patients with essential hypertension, often with a claim that one or more of them are primarily responsible for the hypertension. While it is still uncertain whether these individual abnormalities are primary or secondary, varying expressions of a single disease process or reflective of separate disease entities, the accumulating data increasingly support the latter hypothesis. Therefore, just as pneumonia is caused by a variety of infectious agents, even though the clinical picture observed may be similar, so essential hypertension likely has a number of distinct causes. Thus, the distinction between primary and secondary hypertension has become blurred, and the approach to both the diagnosis and therapy of hypertensive patients has been modified. For example, when a group of patients with essential hypertension is separated into a distinct subset (e.g., low-renin essential hypertension), the patients have not been reclassified as having a form of secondary hypertension but rather remain in the essential hypertensive group. In this chapter, individuals in whom a specific structural organ or gene defect is responsible for hypertension are defined as having a *secondary* form of hypertension. In contrast, individuals in whom generalized or functional abnormalities may be the cause of hypertension, even if the abnormalities are discrete, are defined as having *essential* hypertension.

HEREDITY Genetic factors have long been assumed to be important in the genesis of hypertension. Data supporting this view can be found in animal studies as well as in population studies in humans. One approach has been to assess the correlation of blood pressure in families (familial aggregation). From these studies, the minimum size of the genetic factor can be expressed by a correlation coefficient of approximately 0.2. However, the variation in the size of the genetic factor in different studies reemphasizes the probably heterogeneous nature of the essential hypertensive population. In addition, most studies support the concept that the inheritance is probably multifactorial or that a number of different genetic defects each have an elevated blood pressure as one of their phenotypic expressions. Finally, both monogenic defects (e.g., glucocorticoid-remediable aldosteronism and Liddle's syndrome) and susceptibility genes (e.g., the angiotensinogen gene) have now been reported which have as one of their consequences an increased arterial pressure (see below and Chap. 332).

ENVIRONMENT A number of environmental factors have been implicated in the development of hypertension, including salt intake, obesity, occupation, alcohol intake, family size, and crowding. These factors have all been assumed to be important in the increase in blood pressure with age in more affluent societies, in contrast to the decline in blood pressure with age in less affluent groups.

SALT SENSITIVITY The environmental factor that has received the greatest attention is salt intake. Even this factor illustrates the heterogeneous nature of the essential hypertensive population, in

that the blood pressure in only approximately 60 percent of hypertensives is particularly responsive to the level of sodium intake. The cause of this special sensitivity to salt varies, with primary aldosteronism, bilateral renal artery stenosis, renal parenchymal disease, and low-renin essential hypertension accounting for about half the patients. In the remainder, the pathophysiology is still uncertain, but postulated contributing factors include chloride intake, calcium intake, a generalized cellular membrane defect, insulin resistance, and "nonmodulation" (see below).

ROLE OF RENIN Renin is an enzyme secreted by the juxtaglomerular cell of the kidney and linked with aldosterone in a negative feedback loop (see Chap. 332). While a variety of factors can modify its rate of secretion, the primary determinant is the volume status of the individual, particularly as related to changes in dietary sodium intake. The end product of the action of renin on its substrate is the generation of the peptide angiotensin II. The response of target tissues to this peptide is uniquely determined by the prior dietary electrolyte intake. For example, sodium intake normally modulates adrenal and renal vascular responses to angiotensin II. With sodium restriction, adrenal responses are enhanced and the renal vascular responses reduced. Sodium loading has the opposite effect. The range of plasma renin activities observed in hypertensive subjects is broader than in normotensive individuals. In consequence, some hypertensive patients have been defined as having *low-renin* and others as having *high-renin* essential hypertension.

Low-Renin Essential Hypertension Approximately 20 percent of patients who by all other criteria have essential hypertension have suppressed plasma renin activity. This situation is more common in African-American than in white patients. Though these patients are not hypokalemic, they have been reported to have expanded extracellular fluid volumes, and it has been suggested but not proved that they have sodium retention and renin suppression due to excessive production of an unidentified mineralocorticoid. On the other hand, some studies have suggested that the adrenal cortex of some of these patients has an increased sensitivity to angiotensin II as the underlying mechanism. Not only does this hypothesis potentially explain their low plasma renin activity, it also suggests the cause of their hypertension. On a diet with a normal or high sodium content, aldosterone production will not be suppressed normally, leading to a mild degree of hyperaldosteronism with its resulting increased sodium retention, volume expansion, and increase in blood pressure. Since this altered sensitivity has been reported even in patients with normal-renin hypertension, it is likely that patients with low-renin hypertension are not a distinct subset but rather form part of a continuum of patients with essential hypertension.

Nonmodulating Essential Hypertension Another subset of hypertensive patients have an adrenal defect opposite to that observed in low-renin patients—a reduced adrenal response to sodium restriction. In these individuals, sodium intake does not modulate either adrenal or renal vascular responses to angiotensin II. Hypertensives in this subset have been termed *nonmodulators* because of the absence of the sodium-mediated modulation of target tissue responses to angiotensin II. These individuals make up 25 to 30 percent of the hypertensive population, have plasma renin activity levels that are normal to high if measured when the patient is on a low-salt diet, and have hypertension that is salt-sensitive because of a defect in the kidney's ability to excrete sodium appropriately. Furthermore, the abnormality appears to be genetically determined (associated with a certain allele of the angiotensinogen gene), and it can be corrected by the administration of a converting-enzyme inhibitor.

High-Renin Essential Hypertension Approximately 15 percent of patients with essential hypertension have plasma renin activity levels above the normal range. It has been suggested that plasma renin plays an important role in the pathogenesis of the elevated arterial pressure in these patients. However, most studies have found that saralasin (a substance that, like losartan, acts as a competitive antagonist of angiotensin II) significantly reduces blood pressure in less than half of these patients. This finding has led some investigators to postulate that the elevated renin levels and blood pressure may both be secondary to an increase in adrenergic system activity. It has been proposed that, in patients with angiotensin-dependent high-renin hypertension whose arterial pressures are lowered by an angiotensin II antagonist, the mechanism responsible for the increase in renin and, therefore, for the hypertension is the nonmodulating defect.

SODIUM ION VERSUS CHLORIDE OR CALCIUM Most studies assessing the role of salt in the hypertensive process have assumed that it is the sodium ion that is important. However, some investigators have suggested that the chloride ion may be equally important. This suggestion is based on the observation that feeding chloride-free sodium salts to salt-sensitive hypertensive animals fails to increase arterial pressure. Calcium also has been implicated in the pathogenesis of some forms of essential hypertension. A low calcium intake has been associated with an increase in blood pressure in epidemiologic studies; an increase in leukocyte cytosolic calcium levels has been reported in some hypertensives. Finally, calcium entry blockers are effective antihypertensive agents. Several studies have reported a potential link between the salt-sensitive forms of hypertension and calcium. It has been postulated that salt loading in combination with a defect in the kidney's ability to excrete salt may lead to a secondary increase in circulating natriuretic factors. One of these factors, the so-called digitalis-like natriuretic factor, inhibits ouabain-sensitive sodium-potassium ATPase and thereby leads to intracellular calcium accumulation and a hyperreactive vascular smooth muscle.

CELL MEMBRANE DEFECT Another postulated explanation for salt-sensitive hypertension is a generalized cell membrane defect. This hypothesis derives most of its data from studies on circulating blood elements, particularly red blood cells, in which abnormalities in the transport of sodium across the cell membrane have been documented. Since both increases and decreases in the activity of different transport systems have been reported, it is likely that some abnormalities are primary and some are secondary. It has been assumed that this abnormality in sodium transport reflects an undefined alteration in the cell membrane and that this defect occurs in many, perhaps all, cells of the body, particularly the vascular smooth muscle cells. The defect leads to an abnormal accumulation of calcium in vascular smooth muscle, resulting in a heightened vascular responsiveness to vasoconstrictor agents. This defect has been proposed to be present in 35 to 50 percent of essential hypertensive persons on the basis of studies using red cells. Other studies suggest that the abnormality in red cell sodium transport is not fixed but can be modified by environmental factors.

The common final pathway in all these hypotheses is an increase in cytosolic calcium resulting in increased vascular reactivity. However, as described above, several mechanisms might produce this calcium accumulation.

INSULIN RESISTANCE Insulin resistance and/or hyperinsulinemia have been suggested as being responsible for the increased arterial pressure in some patients with hypertension. While it is clear that a substantial fraction of the hypertensive population has insulin resistance and hyperinsulinemia, it is less certain that this is more than an association. Insulin resistance is common in patients with non-insulin-dependent diabetes mellitus (NIDDM) or obesity. Both obesity and NIDDM are more common in hypertensive than in normotensive subjects. However, several studies have found that hyperinsulinemia and insulin resistance are present even in lean hypertensive patients without NIDDM, suggesting that this relationship is more than a coincidence.

Hyperinsulinemia can increase arterial pressure by one or more of four mechanisms. An underlying assumption in each case is that some, but not all, of the target tissues of insulin are resistant to its effects. Specifically, tissues involved in glucose homeostasis are resistant (thereby producing the hyperinsulinemia), while tissues in-

volved in the hypertensive process are not. First, hyperinsulinemia produces renal sodium retention (at least acutely) and increases sympathetic activity. Either or both of these effects could lead to an increase in arterial pressure. Another mechanism is vascular smooth-muscle hypertrophy secondary to the mitogenic action of insulin. Finally, insulin also modifies ion transport across the cell membrane, thereby potentially increasing the cytosolic calcium levels of insulin-sensitive vascular or renal tissues. This mechanism would increase arterial pressure for reasons similar to those described above for the membrane-defect hypothesis. It is important to point out, however, that the role of insulin in controlling arterial pressure is only vaguely understood, and, therefore, its potential as a pathogenic factor in hypertension remains unclear.

Few of the features of hypertension discussed above remain constant in a given patient. Some may be a reflection of the current metabolic and hormonal status of the patient rather than a permanent feature of the disease process. For example, at one point a patient might have insulin resistance secondary to obesity, which could lead to sodium retention, intravascular volume expansion, and renin suppression. This patient would be labeled as having "low-renin essential hypertension." If the patient lost weight, however, the salt-retaining tendency would be reversed. If the blood pressure did not normalize, the patient might then have "normal or high-renin essential hypertension." Thus, the features reviewed above should not be considered mutually exclusive or permanent characteristics in a given patient with hypertension.

FACTORS THAT MODIFY THE COURSE OF ESSENTIAL HYPERTENSION Age, race, sex, smoking, alcohol intake, serum cholesterol, glucose intolerance, and weight may all alter the prognosis of this disease. The younger the patient when hypertension is first noted, the greater is the reduction in life expectancy if the hypertension is left untreated. In the United States, urban blacks have about twice the prevalence of hypertension as whites and more than four times the hypertension-induced morbidity rate. At all ages and in both white and nonwhite populations, females with hypertension fare better than males, and the prevalence of hypertension in premenopausal females is substantially less than that in age-matched males or postmenopausal women. Yet, compared with their normotensive counterparts, females with hypertension run the same relative risk of a morbid cardiovascular event as males do. Accelerated atherosclerosis is an invariable companion of hypertension. Thus, it is not surprising that independent risk factors associated with the development of atherosclerosis, such as an elevated serum cholesterol, glucose intolerance, and/or cigarette smoking, significantly enhance the effect of hypertension on mortality rate regardless of age, sex, or race (Chap. 242). There also is no question that a positive correlation exists between obesity and arterial pressure. A gain in weight is associated with an increased frequency of hypertension in subjects with normal blood pressure, and weight loss in obese subjects with hypertension lowers their arterial pressure and, if they are being treated for hypertension, the intensity of therapy required to keep them normotensive. Whether these changes are mediated by changes in insulin resistance is unknown.

NATURAL HISTORY Because essential hypertension is a heterogeneous disorder, variables other than the arterial pressure modify its course. Thus, the probability of developing a morbid cardiovascular event with a given arterial pressure may vary as much as 20-fold depending on whether associated risk factors are present (Table 246-3). Although exceptions have been reported, most untreated adults with hypertension will develop further increases in arterial pressure with time. Furthermore, it has been demonstrated from both actuarial data and experience in the era prior to effective therapy that untreated hypertension is associated with a shortening of life by 10 to 20 years, usually related to an acceleration of the atherosclerotic process, with the rate of acceleration in part related to the severity of the hypertension. Even individuals who have relatively mild disease—i.e., without evidence of end organ damage—that is left untreated for 7 to 10 years have a high risk of developing significant complications. Nearly 30 percent will exhibit atherosclerotic complications, and more than 50 percent will have end organ damage related to the hypertension itself,

Table 246-3

CHAPTER 246
Hypertensive Vascular Disease **1383**

Risk Factors for an Adverse Prognosis in Hypertension

Black race
Youth
Male sex
Persistent diastolic pressure >115 mmHg
Smoking
Diabetes mellitus
Hypercholesterolemia
Obesity
Excess alcohol intake
Evidence of end organ damage
  A. Cardiac
    1. Cardiac enlargement
    2. Electrocardiographic signs of ischemia or left ventricular strain
    3. Myocardial infarction
    4. Congestive heart failure
  B. Eyes
    1. Retinal exudates and hemorrhages
    2. Papilledema
  C. Renal: impaired renal function
  D. Nervous system: cerebrovascular accident

such as cardiomegaly, congestive heart failure, retinopathy, a cerebrovascular accident, and/or renal insufficiency. Thus, even in its mild forms, hypertension is a progressive and lethal disease if left untreated.

SECONDARY HYPERTENSION

As noted earlier, in only a small minority of patients with elevated arterial pressure can a specific cause be identified. Yet these patients should not be ignored for at least two reasons: (1) correction of the cause may cure their hypertension, and (2) these secondary forms of the disease may provide insight into the etiology of essential hypertension. Nearly all the secondary forms of hypertension are related to an alteration in hormone secretion and/or renal function and are discussed in detail in other chapters.

RENAL HYPERTENSION (See also Chap. 277)   Hypertension produced by renal disease is the result of either (1) a derangement in the renal handling of sodium and fluids leading to volume expansion or (2) an alteration in renal secretion of vasoactive materials resulting in a systemic or local change in arteriolar tone. The main subdivisions of renal hypertension are renovascular hypertension, including preeclampsia and eclampsia, and renal parenchymal hypertension. A simple explanation for *renal vascular hypertension* is that decreased perfusion of renal tissue due to stenosis of a main or branch renal artery activates the renin-angiotensin system, described in Chap. 332. Circulating angiotensin II elevates arterial pressure by directly causing vasoconstriction, by stimulating aldosterone secretion with resulting sodium retention, and/or by stimulating the adrenergic nervous system. In practice, only about one-half of patients with renovascular hypertension have an absolute elevation in renin activity in peripheral plasma, although when renin measurements are referenced against an index of sodium balance, a much higher fraction have inappropriately high values.

Activation of the renin-angiotensin system also has been offered as an explanation for the hypertension in both acute and chronic *renal parenchymal disease*. In this formulation, the only difference between renovascular and renal parenchymal hypertension is that the decreased perfusion of renal tissue in the latter case results from inflammatory and fibrotic changes involving multiple small intrarenal vessels. There are enough differences between the two conditions, however, to suggest that other mechanisms are active in renal parenchymal disease. Specifically, (1) peripheral plasma renin activity is elevated far less frequently in renal parenchymal than in renovascular hypertension; (2) cardiac output is said to be normal in renal parenchymal hypertension (unless uremia and anemia are present) but slightly elevated in renovascular hypertension; (3) circulatory responses to tilting and to the Valsalva maneuver are exaggerated in the latter condition; and (4) blood volume tends to be high in patients with severe renal parenchy-

mal disease and low in patients with severe unilateral renovascular hypertension. Alternative explanations for the hypertension in renal parenchymal disease include the possibilities that the damaged kidneys (1) produce an unidentified vasopressor substance other than renin, (2) fail to produce a necessary humoral vasodilator substance (perhaps prostaglandin or bradykinin), (3) fail to inactivate circulating vasopressor substances, and/or (4) are ineffective in disposing of sodium. In the last case, the retained sodium would be responsible for the hypertension as outlined earlier. Although all these explanations, including participation of the renin-angiotensin system, probably have some validity in individual patients, the hypothesis involving sodium retention is particularly attractive. It is supported by the observation that those patients with chronic pyelonephritis or polycystic renal disease who are salt wasters do not develop hypertension and by the observation that removal of salt and water by dialysis or diuretics is effective in controlling arterial pressure in most patients with renal parenchymal disease.

A rare form of renal hypertension results from the excess secretion of renin by juxtaglomerular cell tumors or nephroblastomas. The initial presentation is similar to that of hyperaldosteronism, with hypertension, hypokalemia, and overproduction of aldosterone. However, in contrast to primary aldosteronism, peripheral renin activity is *elevated instead of subnormal*. This disease can be distinguished from other forms of secondary aldosteronism by the presence of normal renal function and unilateral increases in renal vein renin concentration without a renal artery lesion.

ENDOCRINE HYPERTENSION   Adrenal Hypertension Hypertension is a feature of a variety of adrenal cortical abnormalities. In *primary aldosteronism* (Chap. 332), there is a clear relationship between the aldosterone-induced sodium retention and the hypertension. Normal individuals given aldosterone develop hypertension only if they also ingest sodium. Since aldosterone causes sodium retention by stimulating renal tubular exchange of sodium for potassium, hypokalemia is a prominent feature in most patients with primary aldosteronism, and, therefore, the measurement of serum potassium provides a simple screening test. The effect of sodium retention and volume expansion in chronically suppressing plasma renin activity is critical for the definitive diagnosis. In most clinical situations, plasma renin activity and plasma or urinary aldosterone levels parallel each other, but in patients with primary aldosteronism, aldosterone levels are high and relatively fixed because of autonomous aldosterone secretion, whereas plasma renin activity levels are suppressed and respond sluggishly to sodium depletion. Primary aldosteronism may be secondary to either a tumor or bilateral adrenal hyperplasia. It is important to distinguish between these two conditions preoperatively, since usually the hypertension in the latter case is not modified by operation.

The sodium-retaining effect of large amounts of glucocorticoids (perhaps resulting in part from saturation of the 11β-hydroxysteroid hydrogenase enzyme system in the kidney by the increased concentration of cortisol) also offers an explanation for the hypertension in severe cases of Cushing's syndrome (Chap. 332). Moreover, increased production of mineralocorticoids also has been documented in some patients with Cushing's syndrome. However, the hypertension in many cases of Cushing's syndrome does not seem volume-dependent, leading investigators to speculate that it may be secondary to glucocorticoid-induced production of renin substrate (angiotensin-mediated hypertension). In the forms of the adrenogenital syndrome due to C-11 or C-17 hydroxylase deficiency (Chap. 332), deoxycorticosterone accounts for the sodium retention and the resulting hypertension, which is accompanied by suppression of plasma renin activity.

In patients with pheochromocytoma (Chap. 333), increased secretion of epinephrine and norepinephrine by a tumor (most often located in the adrenal medulla) causes excessive stimulation of adrenergic receptors, which results in peripheral vasoconstriction and cardiac stimulation. This diagnosis is confirmed by demonstrating increased urinary excretion of epinephrine and norepinephrine and/or their metabolites.

Acromegaly (See also Chap. 328) Hypertension, coronary atherosclerosis, and cardiac hypertrophy are frequent complications of this condition.

Hypercalcemia (See also Chap. 353) The hypertension which occurs in up to one-third of patients with hyperparathyroidism ordinarily can be attributed to renal parenchymal damage due to nephrolithiasis and nephrocalcinosis. However, increased calcium levels also can have a direct vasoconstrictive effect. In some cases, the hypertension disappears when the hypercalcemia is corrected. Thus, paradoxically, the increased serum calcium level in hyperparathyroidism raises blood pressure, while epidemiologic studies suggest that a high calcium intake lowers blood pressure. To further confuse the issue, calcium entry–blocking agents are effective antihypertensive agents. Additional studies are needed to resolve these seemingly conflicting observations.

Oral Contraceptives Several years ago, a common cause of endocrine hypertension was the use of estrogen-containing oral contraceptives. However, several recent studies suggest that this is no longer true, probably owing to the lower estrogen content of modern oral contraceptives. In patients receiving these agents who do become hypertensive, the mechanism is likely to be activation of the renin-angiotensin-aldosterone system. Thus, both volume (aldosterone) and vasoconstrictor (angiotensin II) factors are important. The estrogen component of oral contraceptive agents stimulates the hepatic synthesis of the renin substrate angiotensinogen, which in turn favors the increased production of angiotensin II and secondary aldosteronism. Some women taking oral contraceptives have increased plasma concentrations of angiotensin II and aldosterone with some increase in arterial pressure. However, only a small number actually have an increase in arterial pressure to a level greater than 140/90, and, in about half of these, the hypertension will remit within 6 months of stopping the drug.

Why some women taking oral contraceptives develop hypertension and others do not is unclear but may be related to (1) increased vascular sensitivity to angiotensin II, (2) the presence of mild renal disease, (3) familial factors (over one-half have a positive family history for hypertension), (4) age (hypertension is significantly more prevalent in women over age 35), (5) the estrogen content of the contraceptive, and/or (6) obesity. Indeed some investigators have suggested that the oral contraceptives are simply unmasking women with essential hypertension.

COARCTATION OF THE AORTA (See also Chap. 235) The hypertension associated with coarctation may be caused by the constriction itself or perhaps by the changes in the renal circulation, which result in an unusual form of renal arterial hypertension. The diagnosis of coarctation usually is evident from physical examination and routine x-ray findings.

EFFECTS OF HYPERTENSION

Patients with hypertension die prematurely; the most common cause of death is heart disease, with stroke and renal failure also frequent, particularly in patients with significant retinopathy.

EFFECTS ON THE HEART Cardiac compensation for the excessive workload imposed by increased systemic pressure is at first sustained by concentric left ventricular hypertrophy, characterized by an increase in wall thickness. Ultimately, the function of this chamber deteriorates, the cavity dilates, and the symptoms and signs of heart failure appear (Chap. 232). Angina pectoris also may occur because of the combination of accelerated coronary arterial disease and increased myocardial oxygen requirements as a consequence of the increased myocardial mass (Chap. 244). On physical examination, the heart is enlarged and has a prominent left ventricular impulse. The sound of

aortic closure is accentuated, and there may be a faint murmur of aortic regurgitation. Presystolic (atrial, fourth) heart sounds appear frequently in hypertensive heart disease, and a protodiastolic (ventricular, third) heart sound or summation gallop rhythm may be present. Electrocardiographic changes of left ventricular hypertrophy (Chap. 228) may occur, but the electrocardiogram substantially underestimates the frequency of cardiac hypertrophy compared with that observed with the echocardiogram. Evidence of ischemia or infarction may be observed late in the disease. Most deaths due to hypertension result from myocardial infarction or congestive heart failure.

NEUROLOGIC EFFECTS The neurologic effects of long-standing hypertension may be divided into retinal and central nervous system changes. Because the retina is the only tissue in which the arteries and arterioles can be examined directly, repeated ophthalmoscopic examination provides the opportunity to observe the progress of the vascular effects of hypertension (Table 35-2). The Keith-Wagener-Barker classification of the *retinal changes* in hypertension has provided a simple and excellent means for serial evaluation of hypertensive patients. Increasing severity of hypertension is associated with focal spasm and progressive general narrowing of the arterioles, as well as the appearance of hemorrhages, exudates, and papilledema. These retinal lesions often produce scotomata, blurred vision, and even blindness, especially when there is papilledema or hemorrhages of the macular area. Hypertensive lesions may develop acutely and, if therapy results in significant reduction of blood pressure, may show rapid resolution. Rarely, these lesions resolve without therapy. In contrast, retinal arteriolosclerosis results from endothelial and muscular proliferation, and it accurately reflects similar changes in other organs. Sclerotic changes do not develop as rapidly as hypertensive lesions, nor do they regress appreciably with therapy. As a consequence of increased wall thickness and rigidity, sclerotic arterioles distort and compress the veins where the two vessel types cross in their common fibrous sheath, and the reflected light streak from the arterioles is changed by the increased opacity of the vessel wall.

Central nervous system dysfunction also occurs frequently in patients with hypertension. Occipital headaches, most often occurring in the morning, are among the most prominent early symptoms of hypertension. Dizziness, light-headedness, vertigo, tinnitus, and dimmed vision or syncope also may be observed, but the more serious manifestations are due to vascular occlusion, hemorrhage, or encephalopathy (Chap. 366). The pathogeneses of the former two disorders are quite different. *Cerebral infarction* is secondary to the increased atherosclerosis observed in hypertensive patients, whereas *cerebral hemorrhage* is the result of both the elevated arterial pressure and the development of cerebral vascular microaneurysms (Charcot-Bouchard aneurysms). Only age and arterial pressure are known to influence the development of the microaneurysms. Thus, it is not surprising that arterial pressure shows a better association with cerebral hemorrhage than with either cerebral or myocardial infarction.

Hypertensive encephalopathy consists of the following symptom complex: severe hypertension, disordered consciousness, increased intracranial pressure, retinopathy with papilledema, and seizures. The pathogenesis is uncertain but probably is not related to arteriolar spasm or cerebral edema. Focal neurologic signs are infrequent and, if present, suggest that infarction, hemorrhage, or transient ischemic attacks are more likely diagnoses. Although some investigators have suggested that prompt lowering of arterial pressure in these patients may adversely affect cerebral blood flow, most studies indicate that this is not the case.

EFFECTS ON THE KIDNEY (See also Chap. 277) Arteriosclerotic lesions of the afferent and efferent arterioles and the glomerular capillary tufts are the most common renal vascular lesions in hypertension and result in a decreased glomerular filtration rate and tubular dysfunction. Proteinuria and microscopic hematuria occur because of glomerular lesions, and approximately 10 percent of the deaths caused by hypertension result from renal failure. Blood loss in hypertension occurs not only from renal lesions; epistaxis, hemoptysis, and metrorrhagia also occur frequently in these patients.

With Hypertension The detailed initial evaluation of the hypertensive patient is outlined in Chap. 35. It includes the critical elements of the history, physical examination, and basic laboratory investigation that aid in arriving at appropriate diagnostic and therapeutic decisions (see Table 35-2).

DIAGNOSIS OF SECONDARY HYPERTENSION Certain clues from the history, physical examination, and basic laboratory studies may suggest an unusual cause for the hypertension and dictate the need for special studies. For example, the abrupt onset of severe hypertension and/or the onset of hypertension of any severity under the age of 25 or after the age of 50 years should lead to laboratory tests to exclude renovascular hypertension and pheochromocytoma. A history of headaches, palpitations, anxiety attacks, unusual sweating, hyperglycemia, and weight loss also should lead to tests to exclude pheochromocytoma. The presence of an abdominal bruit should lead to a workup for renovascular hypertension, and the finding on physical examination of bilateral upper abdominal masses consistent with polycystic renal disease should lead to the performance of an abdominal ultrasound examination or intravenous pyelogram. An elevated creatinine or blood urea nitrogen level, associated with proteinuria and hematuria, should prompt a detailed workup for renal insufficiency (Chap. 269). Special studies for secondary hypertension are also indicated if there is therapeutic failure with the initial drug program. The specific diagnostic measures depend on the most likely causes of secondary hypertension.

Pheochromocytoma (See also Chap. 333) The easiest and best screening procedure for pheochromocytoma is the measurement of catecholamines or their metabolites in a 24-h urine sample collected while the patient is hypertensive. Measurement of plasma catecholamine levels also may be useful. These tests may be indicated even in patients who do not have episodic hypertension, since over half the patients with pheochromocytoma have fixed hypertension. Provocative tests are seldom, if ever, indicated, although occasionally a suppressive test may be useful.

Cushing's Syndrome (See also Chap. 332) A 24-h urine test for cortisol or the administration of 1 mg of dexamethasone at bedtime, followed by the measurement of plasma cortisol at 7 to 10 A.M., is the best test to screen for the presence of Cushing's syndrome. A urine cortisol level of less than 2750 nmol (100 μg) or suppression of the plasma cortisol level to below 140 nmol/L (5 μg/dL) effectively rules out Cushing's syndrome.

Renovascular Hypertension (See also Chap. 277) The standard screening test for renal vascular hypertension has been the rapid-sequence intravenous pyelogram (IVP). Features suggestive of renal ischemia include (1) unilateral delayed appearance and excretion of contrast material, (2) a difference in kidney size of greater than 1.5 cm, (3) an irregular renal silhouette, suggesting partial infarction or atrophy, (4) indentations on the ureter or renal pelvis, possibly due to dilated ureteral arteries (collateral notching), and (5) hyperconcentration of contrast medium in the collecting system of the smaller kidney. When these criteria are used, the false-positive rate is 11 percent and the false-negative rate 12 percent.

In many centers the IVP has been replaced by one or more of the following tests. (1) The digital subtraction angiogram has been received with considerable enthusiasm as a more precise screening test for renal vascular disease. Its ultimate place as a screening test is unclear, however, because of its relatively high cost and the need for an arterial rather than a venous injection. (2) The captopril-induced renogram takes advantage of the dependence of the renal vasculature on angiotensin II. Thus, when individuals with renal artery stenosis are given a converting-enzyme inhibitor (captopril) that reduces angiotensin II levels on the stenotic side, the result will be a renal blood flow pattern demonstrating a reduced uptake and delayed excretion as assessed by the isotope renogram. (3) Renal duplex ultrasound provides both an anatomic assessment (from B-mode imaging) and a functional assessment (from Doppler imaging) of the renal arteries. Thus, in theory, it should provide the most accurate noninvasive assessment. However, its precision is very dependent on the skill and expertise of the radiologist. Thus, in many centers, the converting enzyme inhibitor–induced renogram has displaced the IVP as the screening procedure of choice. The renal duplex ultrasound is favored in a few centers.

The definitive test for surgically correctable renal disease is the combination of a renal angiogram and renal vein renin determinations. The renal arteriogram both establishes the presence of a renal arterial lesion and aids in the determination of whether the lesion is due to atherosclerosis or to one of the fibrous or fibromuscular dysplasias. It does not, however, prove that the lesion is responsible for the hypertension, nor does it permit prediction of the chances of surgical cure. It must be noted (1) that renal artery stenosis is a frequent finding by angiography and at postmortem in normotensive individuals, and (2) that essential hypertension is a common condition and may occur in combination with renal arterial stenosis that is not responsible for the hypertension. Bilateral renal vein catheterization for measurement of plasma renin activity is therefore used to assess the functional significance of any lesion noted on arteriography. When one kidney is ischemic and the other is normal, all the renin released comes from the involved kidney. In the most straightforward situation, the ischemic kidney has a significantly higher venous plasma renin activity than the normal kidney, by a factor of 1.5 or more. Moreover, the renal venous blood draining the uninvolved kidney exhibits levels similar to those in the inferior vena cava below the entrance of the renal veins.

Significant benefit from operative correction may be anticipated in at least 80 percent of patients with the findings described above if care is taken to prepare the patient properly before renal vein blood sampling, i.e., by discontinuing renin-suppressing drugs, such as beta blockers, for at least 10 days; restricting the patient to a low sodium intake for 4 days; and/or giving a converting-enzyme inhibitor for 24 h. When obstructing lesions in the _branches_ of the renal arteries are demonstrated by arteriography, an attempt to obtain blood samples from the main _branches_ of the renal vein should be made in an effort to identify a localized intrarenal arterial lesion responsible for the hypertension.

Primary Aldosteronism (See also Chap. 332) These patients almost always exhibit hypokalemia. Diuretic therapy often complicates the picture when the hypokalemia is first observed and needs to be assessed. Given the presence of hypokalemia, the relation between plasma renin activity and the aldosterone level becomes the key to the diagnosis of primary aldosteronism. The aldosterone concentration or excretion rate is high and plasma renin activity is low in primary aldosteronism, and these levels are relatively unaffected by changes in sodium balance. A critical part of the evaluation after primary aldosteronism has been established is to determine whether disease is unilateral or bilateral, because surgical removal of the lesion usually reduces arterial pressure only in patients with unilateral disease.

Plasma Renin Activity Measurements Some studies have suggested that the plasma renin level should be measured in most hypertensive patients and related to a 24-h urine sodium excretion rate to assess whether high, low, or normal renin levels are present. It has been proposed that this information may be important for both therapeutic and prognostic reasons. However, as noted earlier, it is unclear, on the basis of the available data and treatment programs, that these random measurements are really useful except in patients with findings suggestive of renal vascular disease or mineralocorticoid excess in whom lateralizing renal vein renin levels or suppressed peripheral renin levels may be of diagnostic and/or therapeutic significance.

℞ TREATMENT

Indications for Therapy Virtually every patient with a diastolic arterial pressure that persistently exceeds 90 mmHg, or any patient over 65 years of age with a systolic arterial pressure over

160 mmHg, is a candidate for diagnostic studies and for subsequent treatment. Furthermore, at any given level of blood pressure elevation, the ultimate risk of developing hypertensive vascular complications is greater in men than in women and in younger than in older persons. It may be argued, then, that it is hard to justify producing the uncomfortable side effects of therapy in, for example, an asymptomatic woman over 70 years of age with a diastolic pressure of 90 mmHg. On the other hand, it is easy to justify side effects in a man of 30 with a diastolic pressure exceeding 110 mmHg because such a person may be expected to receive the greatest benefit from therapy. Fortunately, the choice of treatment is such that a satisfactory program to control arterial pressure with minimal side effects can be developed for most patients, particularly as more studies assessing the impact of specific therapeutic agents on the patient's quality of life are reported.

A reasonable guideline would be that all patients with a diastolic pressure repeatedly above 90 mmHg should be treated unless specific contraindications exist. Patients with isolated *systolic* hypertension (levels greater than 160 mmHg) also should be treated if they are over age 65. It is uncertain that individuals under age 65 who have isolated systolic hypertension will benefit from therapy until the results of a well-controlled, prospective study are completed. Patients with labile hypertension or isolated systolic hypertension who are not treated should have regular follow-up examinations at 6-month intervals because of the frequent development of progressive and/or sustained hypertension. Finally, if coronary artery disease or associated cardiovascular risks are present, then treatment of a patient with a lower blood pressure may be warranted. For example, patients with angina pectoris or diabetes mellitus with diastolic blood pressures between 85 and 90 mmHg may be candidates for antihypertensive therapy.

The identification of an operable form of secondary hypertension does not automatically mean that surgical treatment is indicated. The decision depends on the age and general health of the patient, the natural history of the lesion, and the response of the arterial pressure to drug therapy. In patients with renovascular hypertension, the feasibility of renal angioplasty, the advantages of surgical repair versus nephrectomy, and the degree of overall renal functional impairment must be considered. Age and general health are important in patients with renovascular hypertension due to arteriosclerosis, because there is no evidence that repair of the stenosis increases life expectancy in the elderly patient with other evidence of vascular disease. Knowledge of the natural history of the disease is especially important when making a decision in the case of a young patient with renal artery stenosis due to fibrous dysplasia. If the arteriographic appearance suggests that the stenosis is due to intimal or subadventitial fibroplasia, the lesion may be expected to progress, and operation or angioplasty is required. Medial fibroplasia, on the other hand, often remains stable, and operation or angioplasty may not be necessary if pressure can be controlled by drug therapy.

The decision regarding operation also should be considered carefully in patients with primary aldosteronism when neither abdominal computed tomography nor bilateral adrenal venography demonstrates a tumor, because such patients may prove to have multinodular hyperplasia. In that case, bilateral adrenalectomy would be required to eliminate the aldosterone excess, and, even then, hypertension would usually persist. If hypokalemia can be controlled by spironolactone or other drug therapy and arterial pressure lowered with antihypertensive agents, then it is reasonable to withhold operative treatment.

GENERAL MEASURES Nondrug therapeutic intervention is probably indicated in all patients with sustained hypertension and probably in most with labile hypertension. The general measures employed include (1) relief of stress, (2) dietary management, (3) regular aerobic exercise, (4) weight reduction (if needed), and (5) control of

other risk factors contributing to the development of arteriosclerosis. Relief of emotional and environmental stress is one of the reasons for the improvement in hypertension that occurs when a patient is hospitalized. Though it is usually impossible to extricate the hypertensive patient from all internal and external stresses, he or she should be advised to avoid unnecessary tensions. In rare instances, it may be appropriate to recommend a change of job or of life-style. It has been suggested that relaxation techniques also may lower arterial pressure. However, it is uncertain that these techniques alone have much long-term effect.

Dietary management has three aspects:

1. Because of the documented efficacy of sodium restriction and volume contraction in lowering blood pressure, patients previously were instructed to curtail sodium intake drastically. Some investigators have suggested that this is not necessary. They base their conclusion on two observations: (1) In many patients the blood pressure is not sensitive to the level of sodium intake, and (2) diuretics provide another method of decreasing body sodium stores in individuals whose blood pressure is sodium-sensitive. However, meta-analyses of previous diet studies have documented a 5-mmHg reduction in systolic pressure and a 2.6-mmHg reduction in diastolic pressure when sodium intake is reduced by approximately 75 mEq/day. In addition, several reports have documented that, while mild sodium restriction has little if any direct action on blood pressure, it significantly potentiates the efficacy of nearly all antihypertensive agents. Thus, by making it possible to control blood pressure with lower doses of drugs, sodium restriction leads to a reduction in side effects. In addition, it is quite clear that in some hypertensive patients, as noted above, the level of sodium intake does influence the blood pressure. Thus, since there is no apparent risk to mild sodium restriction, the most practical approach now is to advise mild dietary sodium restriction (up to 5 g NaCl per day), which can be achieved by eliminating all additions of salt to food that is prepared normally. Some studies also have reported a lowering of arterial pressure related to an *increase* in potassium and/or calcium intake. For example, in one meta-analysis, dietary potassium supplements of 50 to 120 mEq/day reduced blood pressure by about the same amount as salt restriction (by 6 mmHg systolic and 3.4 mmHg diastolic). While the advisability of these forms of dietary alteration is still controversial, the fact that a moderately high calcium intake (1.5 g elemental calcium daily) probably also reduces the extent of age-related osteoporosis, combined with the results of the potassium supplementation studies, indicate that they are probably useful adjuncts.

2. Caloric restriction should be urged for patients who are overweight. Some obese patients will show a significant reduction in blood pressure simply as a consequence of weight loss. In the Trial of Antihypertensive Interventions and Management (TAIM) study, weight reduction (average 4.4 kg over 6 months) lowered blood pressure by 2.5 mmHg.

3. A restriction in the intake of cholesterol and saturated fats is recommended, as this diet modification may diminish the incidence of arteriosclerotic complications. Reducing or eliminating alcohol intake is also beneficial. Regular exercise is indicated within the limits of the patient's cardiovascular status. Not only is exercise helpful in controlling weight, but also there is evidence that physical conditioning itself may lower arterial pressure. Isotonic exercises (jogging, swimming) are better than isometric exercises (weight lifting) since the latter, if anything, raises arterial pressure. The dietary management outlined above is aimed at the control of other risk factors. Probably the most significant additional step that could be taken in this area would be to convince the smoker to give up cigarettes.

DRUG THERAPY FOR HYPERTENSION (Table 246-4)

To make rational use of antihypertensive drugs, the sites and mechanisms of their action must be understood. In general, there are six classes of drugs: diuretics, antiadrenergic agents, vasodilators, calcium entry blockers, angiotensin-converting enzyme (ACE) inhibitors and angiotensin receptor antagonists.

Table 246-4

Drugs Used in Treatment of Hypertension—Listed According to Site of Action

Site of Action	Drug	Dosage	Indications	Contraindications/Cautions	Frequent or Peculiar Side Effects
DIURETICS					
Renal tubule	Thiazides: e.g., hydrochlorothiazide	Depends on specific drug Oral: 12.5–25 mg daily or twice daily	Mild hypertension; as adjunct in treatment of moderate to severe hypertension	Diabetes mellitus, hyperuricemia, primary aldosteronism	Potassium depletion, hyperglycemia, hyperuricemia, hypercholesterolemia, dermatitis, purpura, depression, hypercalcemia
	Loop-acting: e.g., furosemide	Oral: 20–80 mg 2 or 3 times a day	Mild hypertension; as adjunct in severe or malignant hypertension, particularly with renal failure	Hyperuricemia, primary aldosteronism	Potassium depletion, hyperuricemia, hyperglycemia, hypocalcemia, blood dyscrasias, rash, nausea, vomiting, diarrhea
	Potassium-sparing: Spironolactone	Oral: 25 mg 2 to 4 times daily	Hypertension due to hypermineralocorticoidism; as adjunct to thiazide therapy	Renal failure	Hyperkalemia, diarrhea, gynecomastia, menstrual irregularities
	Triamterene	Oral: 50–100 mg 1 or 2 times daily			Hyperkalemia, nausea, vomiting, leg cramps, nephrolithiasis, GI disturbances
	Amiloride	Oral: 5–10 mg daily			
ANTIADRENERGIC AGENTS					
Central	Clonidine	Oral: 0.05–0.6 mg twice daily	Mild to moderate hypertension, renal disease with hypertension		Postural hypotension, drowsiness, dry mouth, rebound hypertension after abrupt withdrawal, insomnia
	Guanabenz	Oral: 4–16 mg twice daily			
	Guanfacine	Oral: 1–3 mg daily			
	Methyldopa (also acts by blocking sympathetic nerves)	Oral: 250–1000 mg twice daily IV: 250–1000 mg every 4–6 h (tolerance may develop)	Mild to moderate hypertension (oral), malignant hypertension (IV)	Pheochromocytoma, active hepatic disease (IV), during MAO inhibitor administration	Postural hypotension, sedation, fatigue, diarrhea, impaired ejaculation, fever, gynecomastia, lactation, positive Coombs' tests (occasionally associated with hemolysis), chronic hepatitis, acute ulcerative colitis, lupus-like syndrome
Autonomic ganglia	Trimethaphan	IV: 1–6 mg/min	Severe or malignant hypertension	Severe coronary artery disease, cerebrovascular insufficiency, diabetes mellitus (on hypoglycemic therapy), glaucoma, prostatism	Postural hypotension, visual symptoms, dry mouth, constipation, urinary retention, impotence
Nerve endings	Rauwolfia alkaloids: Reserpine	Oral: 0.05–0.25 mg daily	Mild to moderate hypertension in young patient	Pheochromocytoma, peptic ulcer, depression, during MAO inhibitor administration	Depression, nightmares, nasal congestion, dyspepsia, diarrhea, impotence
	Guanethidine	Oral: 10–150 mg daily	Moderate to severe hypertension	Pheochromocytoma, severe coronary artery disease, cerebrovascular insufficiency, during MAO inhibitor administration	Postural hypotension, bradycardia, dry mouth, diarrhea, impaired ejaculation, fluid retention, asthma
	Guanadrel	Oral: 5–50 mg twice daily			
Alpha receptors	Phentolamine	IV: 1–5 mg bolus	Suspected or proved pheochromocytoma	Severe coronary artery disease	Tachycardia, weakness, dizziness, flushing
	Phenoxybenzamine	Oral: 10–50 mg once or twice daily (tolerance may develop)	Proved pheochromocytoma		Postural hypotension, tachycardia, miosis, nasal congestion, dry mouth
	Prazosin	Oral: 1–10 mg twice daily	Mild to moderate hypertension	Use with caution in the elderly	Sudden syncope, headache, sedation, dizziness, tachycardia, anticholinergic effect, fluid retention
	Terazosin	Oral: 1–20 mg daily			
	Doxazosin	Oral: 1–8 mg daily			

(continued)

Table 246-4—*(Continued)*

Drugs Used in Treatment of Hypertension—Listed According to Site of Action

Site of Action	Drug	Dosage	Indications	Contraindications/ Cautions	Frequent or Peculiar Side Effects
Beta receptors	Propranolol	Oral: 10–120 mg 2 to 4 times daily	Mild to moderate hypertension (especially with evidence of hyperdynamic circulation); as adjunct to hydralazine therapy	Congestive heart failure, asthma, diabetes mellitus (on hypoglycemic therapy), during MAO inhibitor administration, COPD, sick sinus syndrome, 2d or 3d degree heart block	Dizziness, depression, bronchospasm, nausea, vomiting, diarrhea, constipation, heart failure, fatigue, Raynaud's phenomenon, hallucinations, hypertriglyceridemia, hypercholesterolemia, psoriasis; sudden withdrawal may precipitate angina or myocardial injury in patients with heart disease
	Metoprolol	Oral: 25–150 mg twice daily			
	Nadolol	Oral: 20–120 mg daily			
	Atenolol	Oral: 25–100 mg daily			
	Timolol	Oral: 5–15 mg twice daily			
	Betaxolol	Oral: 10–20 mg daily			
	Carteolol	Oral: 2.5–10 mg daily			
	Pindolol	Oral: 5–30 mg twice daily			Less resting bradycardia than other beta blockers
	Acebutolol	Oral: 200–600 mg twice daily			
Alpha/Beta receptor	Labetalol	Oral: 100–600 mg twice daily IV: 2 mg/min			Similar to beta blockers with more postural effects

VASODILATORS

Site of Action	Drug	Dosage	Indications	Contraindications/ Cautions	Frequent or Peculiar Side Effects
Vascular smooth muscle	Hydralazine	Oral: 10–75 mg 4 times daily IV or IM: 10–50 mg every 6 h (tolerance may develop)	As adjunct in treatment of moderate to severe hypertension (oral), malignant hypertension (IV or IM), renal disease with hypertension	Lupus erythematosus, severe coronary artery disease	Headache, tachycardia, angina pectoris, anorexia, nausea, vomiting, diarrhea, lupuslike syndrome, rash, fluid retention
	Minoxidil	Oral: 2.5–40 mg twice daily	Severe hypertension	Severe coronary artery disease	Tachycardia, aggravates angina, marked fluid retention, hair growth on face and body, coarsening of facial features, possible pericardial effusions
	Diazoxide	IV: 1–3 mg/kg up to 150 mg rapidly	Severe or malignant hypertension	Diabetes mellitus, hyperuricemia, congestive heart failure	Hyperglycemia, hyperuricemia, sodium retention
	Nitroprusside	IV: 0.5–8 (μg/kg)/min	Malignant hypertension		Apprehension, weakness, diaphoresis, nausea, vomiting, muscle twitching, cyanide toxicity

ANGIOTENSIN CONVERTING ENZYME INHIBITORS

Site of Action	Drug	Dosage	Indications	Contraindications/ Cautions	Frequent or Peculiar Side Effects
Converting enzyme	Captopril	Oral: 12.5–75 mg twice daily	Mild to severe hypertension, renal artery stenosis	Renal failure (reduction of dose), bilateral renal artery stenosis, pregnancy	Leukopenia, pancytopenia, hypotension, cough, angioedema, urticarial rash, fever, loss of taste, acute renal failure in bilateral renal artery stenosis, hyperkalemia
	Benazepril	Oral: 10–40 mg daily			Same as captopril, but little evidence for leukopenia, but perhaps increased frequency of cough and angioedema. All can be given once daily, but side effects are reduced if one-half dose is given twice daily. Fosinopril is excreted more in bile than the others.
	Enalapril	Oral: 2.5–40 mg daily			
	Enalaprilat	IV: 0.625–1.25 mg over 5 minutes every 6–8 h			
	Fosinopril	Oral: 10–40 mg daily			
	Lisinopril	Oral: 5–40 mg daily			
	Quinapril	Oral: 10–80 mg daily			
	Ramipril	Oral: 2.5–20 mg daily			

(continued)

Table 246-4—(*Continued*)

Drugs Used in Treatment of Hypertension—Listed According to Site of Action

Site of Action	Drug	Dosage	Indications	Contraindications/Cautions	Frequent or Peculiar Side Effects
ANGIOTENSIN RECEPTOR ANTAGONISTS					
	Losartan	Oral: 25–50 mg once or twice daily	Mild to severe hypertension, renal artery stenosis	Pregnancy, bilateral renal artery stenosis	Hypotension, acute renal failure in bilateral renal artery stenosis, hyperkalemia
CALCIUM CHANNEL ANTAGONISTS					
Vascular smooth muscle	Nifedipine	Oral: 10–30 mg 4 times daily or as XL form 30–90 mg daily	Mild to moderate hypertension	Heart failure, 2d or 3d degree heart block	Tachycardia, flushing, gastrointestinal disturbances, hyperkalemia, edema, headache
	Amlodipine	Oral: 2.5–10 mg daily			
	Felodipine XL	Oral: 5–10 mg daily			
	Isradipine	Oral: 2.5–10 mg daily			
	Nicardipine	Oral: 20–40 mg 3 times daily			
	Benzothiazepines: Diltiazem	Oral: 30–90 mg 4 times daily or as CD form 180–300 mg daily	Mild to moderate hypertension	Heart failure, 2d or 3d degree heart block	Same as nifidepine, except no tachycardia or edema, but can cause heart block, constipation, and liver dysfunction
	Phenylalkylamine: Verapamil	Oral: 30–120 mg 4 times daily or as SR form 120–480 mg daily	Mild to moderate hypertension	Heart failure, 2d or 3d degree heart block	

DIURETICS (See also Chap. 233)   The thiazides are the most frequently used and most extensively investigated members of this group, and their early effect certainly is related to sodium diuresis and volume depletion. A reduction in peripheral vascular resistance also has been reported by some workers to be important in the long term. Traditionally, thiazide diuretics have formed the cornerstone of most therapeutic programs designed to lower arterial pressure, and they are usually effective within 3 to 4 days. Furthermore, they have been shown to reduce mortality and morbidity in long-term trials. However, in recent years there has been increasing resistance to their routine use, primarily because of their adverse metabolic effects, which include hypokalemia due to renal potassium loss, hyperuricemia due to uric acid retention, carbohydrate intolerance, and hyperlipidemia. The more potent loop-acting diuretics furosemide and bumetanide also have been shown to be antihypertensive, but they have been used less extensively for this indication, primarily because of their shorter duration of action. Spironolactone causes renal sodium loss by blocking the effect of mineralocorticoids, and, therefore, it may be more effective in patients whose mineralocorticoid levels are excessive, such as patients with primary or secondary aldosteronism. Although they do not compete directly with aldosterone, triamterene and amiloride act at the same site as spironolactone to impede sodium reabsorption. They are effective in the same situations as spironolactone, except that triamterene has little intrinsic antihypertensive effect. Their major disadvantage is that they can produce hyperkalemia, particularly in patients with impaired renal function. Any of these three potassium-sparing diuretics also can be given along with thiazide diuretics to minimize renal potassium loss.

ANTIADRENERGIC AGENTS (See also Chap. 70)   These drugs act at one or more sites—centrally on the vasomotor center, in peripheral neurons, where they modify catecholamine release, or in target tissues, where they block adrenergic receptor sites. Drugs that appear to have predominant *central actions* are *clonidine, methyldopa, guanabenz,* and *guanfacine.* These drugs and their metabolites are predominantly alpha-receptor agonists. Stimulation of alpha$_2$ receptors in the vasomotor centers of the brain *reduces* sympathetic outflow, thereby reducing arterial pressure. Usually a fall in cardiac output and heart rate also occurs, more commonly with clonidine and guanabenz, but the baroreceptor reflex is intact. Thus, postural symptoms are absent. However, rebound hypertension may occur rarely when these drugs, particularly clonidine and guanabenz, are stopped. This effect is probably secondary to an increase in norepinephrine release, which is inhibited by these agents owing their agonist effect on presynaptic alpha receptors.

Another class of antiadrenergic agents consists of the *ganglionic blocking drugs,* which are used infrequently now. Because of their side effects, ganglionic blocking agents are now usually reserved for the rapid lowering of arterial pressure by parenteral administration of the short-acting agent *trimethaphan* in patients with severe hypertension.

Various drugs act at *postganglionic adrenergic nerve endings,* but they are rarely used now because of their side effects. *Guanethidine* and its shorter-acting analogue guanadrel block the release of norepinephrine from adrenergic nerve endings. They usually reduce cardiac output and lower systolic more than diastolic blood pressure. They also produce a greater postural effect than the other drugs that act at the nerve endings, and orthostatic hypotension is a frequent side effect.

The last group of drugs affecting the adrenergic system are those that block the *peripheral adrenergic receptors,* alpha, beta, or both (see also Chap. 70).

Alpha-Adrenergic Receptor Blockers   *Phentolamine* and *phenoxybenzamine* block the action of norepinephrine at *alpha*-adrenergic receptor sites. These two compounds block both presynaptic (alpha$_2$) and postsynaptic (alpha$_1$) alpha receptors, and the former action accounts for the tolerance which develops. *Prazosin* is more effective because it selectively blocks only *postsynaptic alpha* receptors, i.e., alpha$_1$ receptors. Thus, presynaptic alpha activity remains, suppressing norepinephrine release, and tolerance occurs only infrequently. Accordingly, prazosin produces less tachycardia but more postural hypotension than direct-acting vasodilators, such as hydralazine, and rarely can produce substantial hypotension following the first dose.

Beta-Adrenergic Receptor Blockers (See also Chap. 244)   A number of effective *beta-adrenergic receptor blocking agents* are available that block sympathetic effects on the heart and should be most effective in reducing cardiac output and in lowering arterial pressure when there is increased cardiac sympathetic nerve activity. In addition, they block the adrenergic nerve–mediated release of renin from the renal juxtaglomerular cells, and this action may be an important component of their blood pressure–lowering action. Beta-adrenergic blockers are particularly useful when employed in conjunction with vascular smooth muscle relaxants, which tend to evoke a reflex increase in heart rate, and with diuretics, the administration of which often results in an elevation of circulating renin activity. In practice, beta blockers appear to be effective even when there is no evidence of increased sympathetic tone, with about one-half or more of all hypertensive patients showing a fall in pressure. Furthermore, like diuretics, they have been shown to reduce morbidity and mortality in long-term clinical trials. However, these agents can precipitate congestive heart failure and asthma in susceptible individuals, and they must be used with caution in diabetics receiving hypoglycemic therapy because they inhibit the usual sympathetic responses to hypoglycemia. Cardioselective beta-blocking agents (so-called beta$_1$ blockers: metoprolol, atenolol) have been developed and may be superior to nonselective beta blockers such as propranolol and timolol in patients with bronchospasm. Nadolol, a nonselective beta blocker, unlike other drugs of this class, is excreted unchanged in the urine and has a half-life of 14 to 20 h; only one dose a day is required. Atenolol also usually only needs to be given once a day. Pindolol and acebutolol are nonselective beta blockers that have partial agonist activity and, therefore, produce less bradycardia. Labetalol exerts both alpha- and beta-adrenergic blocking actions. Thus, it lowers arterial pressure not only by the same complex actions as do beta blockers but also directly by reducing systemic vascular resistance. Usually it has a more rapid onset of action but produces more postural symptoms and chronic sexual dysfunction than the other beta blockers.

VASODILATORS *Hydralazine* is the most versatile of the drugs that cause direct relaxation of vascular smooth muscle; it is effective both orally and parenterally, and acts mainly on arterial resistance rather than on venous capacitance vessels, as evidenced by lack of postural effects. Unfortunately, the effect of hydralazine on peripheral resistance is partly negated by a reflex increase in sympathetic discharge that raises heart rate and cardiac output. This response limits the usefulness of hydralazine, especially in patients with severe coronary artery disease. However, the efficacy of hydralazine can be increased if it is given in conjunction with a beta blocker or a drug such as methyldopa or clonidine, all of which block reflex sympathetic stimulation of the heart. A serious side effect of doses of hydralazine exceeding 300 mg/d has been the production of a lupus erythematosus–like syndrome.

Minoxidil is even more potent than hydralazine but unfortunately produces significant hypertrichosis and fluid retention and, therefore, is mainly limited to patients with severe hypertension and renal insufficiency.

Diazoxide, a thiazide derivative, is restricted in its application to acute situations. It is not a diuretic; in fact, it causes sodium retention. However, like other thiazides, it reduces carbohydrate tolerance. It must be given rapidly intravenously to guarantee an effect. It begins to act immediately to lower blood pressure, and its effects may last for several hours. *Nitroprusside* given intravenously also acts as a direct vasodilator, with onset and offset of actions that are almost immediate. *Nitroglycerin* is a third direct-acting vasodilator useful as an intravenous agent. These latter three drugs are useful only for the treatment of hypertensive emergencies (Table 246-5).

ACE INHIBITORS Drugs from several of the categories discussed above have been shown to possess an additional action resulting in inhibition of renin secretion. These include clonidine, reserpine, methyldopa, and beta blockers. A second group of drugs inhibit the enzyme converting angiotensin I into angiotensin II, the angiotensin converting enzyme (ACE). These agents are useful because they not only inhibit the generation of a potent vasoconstrictor (angiotensin II) but also may retard the degradation of a potent vasodilator (bradykinin), alter prostaglandin production (an effect most notable with captopril), and can modify the activity of the adrenergic nervous system. They are especially useful in renal or renovascular hypertension, as well as in accelerated and malignant hypertension. However, in patients with bilateral renal artery stenosis, rapid deterioration of renal function may occur. They are also as effective in mild, uncomplicated hypertension as beta blockers and thiazides—and probably have fewer side effects, particularly ones that adversely affect the patient's quality of life.

These drugs should be used with caution when the renin system is activated (for example, by severe heart failure, prior diuretic therapy, or substantial salt restriction) to avoid profound hypotension. Usually, diuretics are stopped 2 to 3 days before administration of an ACE inhibitor is begun and are added back later if needed.

ANGIOTENSIN RECEPTOR ANTAGONISTS These drugs have effects similar to those of ACE inhibitors. However, instead of blocking the production of angiotensin II, they competitively inhibit its binding to the angiotensin II AT$_1$ receptor subtype. Their utility and tolerability are similar to those of the ACE inhibitors, but they do not cause cough or angioedema.

CALCIUM CHANNEL ANTAGONISTS There are three subclasses of calcium channel antagonists: the phenylalkylamine derivatives (e.g., verapamil), the benzothiazepines (e.g., diltiazem), and the dihydropyridines (e.g., nifedipine). To date, there is only one therapeutic agent in each of the first two classes but a number of agents in the third class. All three subclasses modify calcium entry into cells by interacting with specific binding sites on the α_1 subunit of the L-type voltage-dependent calcium channel. Thus, since there are other calcium channels (e.g., the T and N types), the actions of these drugs only partially modify total calcium transport into cells. The relative specificity of each agent stems from the fact that each class has a unique binding site on the α_1 subunit, and these sites are variably

Table 246-5

Therapeutic Agents Used to Treat Malignant Hypertension

Drug	Route	Starting Dose	Time Course of Action			Oral Preparation Available
			Onset	Peak	Duration	
IMMEDIATE ONSET						
Nitroprusside	Continuous IV	0.25 μg/kg/min	<1 min	1–2 min	2–5 min	No
Trimethaphan	Continuous IV	0.5 mg/min	<1 min	1–2 min	2–5 min	No
Nitroglycerin	Continuous IV	5 μg/min	1–5 min	2–6 min	3–10 min	No
Diazoxide	IV bolus	50 mg q 5–10 min up to 600 mg	1–5 min	2–4 min	4–12 h	No
DELAYED ONSET						
Enalaprilat	IV	1.25 mg q 6 h	10–15 min	3–4 h	6–24 h	Yes
Hydralazine	IV, IM	5–10 mg q 20 min × 3	10–20 min	20–40 min	4–12 h	Yes
Labetalol	IV	20–80 mg q 10 min up to 300 mg	5 min	20–30 min	3–6 h	Yes
Nifedipine	Sublingual	10–20 mg	5–15 min	30–60 min	3–6 h	Yes

expressed in different tissues. Thus, while agents from all three sub-classes cause vasodilation, usually only dihydropyridines produce reflex tachycardia. Diltiazem and verapamil can both slow atrioventricular conduction—a feature not observed with the dihydropyridines. While calcium channel antagonists are also useful in angina pectoris (see Chap. 244), because of their negative inotropic actions, they should be used with caution in hypertensive patients with heart failure. The short-acting dihydropyridines, such as nifedipine, should be used with caution for long-term therapy in hypertensive patients, since they have been reported to increase the incidence of acute coronary events. Verapamil, diltiazem, or long-acting dihydropyridines should be used instead.

APPROACH TO DRUG THERAPY (Fig. 246-1) The aim of drug therapy is to use the agents just described, alone or in combination, to return arterial pressure to normal levels with minimal side effects. Ideally, one would choose a therapeutic program that specifically corrects the underlying defect resulting in the elevated blood pressure—for example, treatment with spironolactone for patients with primary aldosteronism. As our knowledge of the mechanisms underlying the hypertension in individual patients increases, more specific drug programs will become available. Such programs presumably will result in normalization of blood pressure with fewer side effects. In the absence of this information, an empirical approach is used, which takes into consideration efficacy, safety, impact on the quality of life, compliance, ease of administration, and cost. When used in combination, drugs are chosen for their different sites of action. However, except for those patients with severe hypertension (average diastolic blood pressure >130 mmHg), in whom intensive therapy with several agents simultaneously usually is required, most patients should be treated *initially* with a single agent.

Since many effective antihypertensive agents are available, a number of useful therapeutic regimens have been developed, with the ideal program still unclear. Initial therapy with a diuretic or beta blocker has been the usual first approach, particularly as these are the only agents proven to reduce mortality. However, this practice does not mean that other effective antihypertensives would fail to have the same beneficial effect if used in similar trials. Thus, ACE inhibitors and calcium channel antagonists are also effective as first-line therapy, replacing the old stepped-care approach. The physician is therefore required to choose from four classes of agents for initial therapy, with little evidence that one is more effective than another. It has been suggested, and the author agrees, that an ACE inhibitor or some calcium channel antagonists be used first, because of their lower side effects, with a slight preference for ACE inhibitors because of their longer duration of action, potentially fewer adverse effects, and increased compliance rates. Angiotensin receptor antagonists may also be included, with the caution that their long-term efficacy and side effects are unknown. The choice of one drug over the others is empirical.

The schema outlined in Fig. 246-1 takes into account the presently available data on effectiveness, adverse reactions, compliance, impact on quality of life, and economic impact (including cost, usage of health care resources, and quality and quantity of work performance) in deciding when to use a given agent. This approach is applicable to all patients in whom an indication for a specific form of therapy is lacking. Because of its lower cost, low-dose thiazide therapy, e.g., 25 mg of hydrochlorothiazide (or its equivalent) daily, often has been the first choice. However, three major concerns with widespread thiazide usage have arisen: relatively poor compliance rates (approximately 80 percent), which probably reflect an adverse effect on the patient's quality of life, adverse metabolic effects (hypokalemia, hypomagnesemia, hyperglycemia, and hypercholesterolemia), and potentially an increased frequency of cardiac arrhythmias, including sudden death, probably secondary to the electrolyte disturbances. These concerns, coupled with the eight- to tenfold increase in cost associated with the frequent need for potassium supplementation or a potassium-sparing diuretic, have caused some to suggest that thiazides should play a more restricted role in initial antihypertensive therapy, being limited to individuals who have volume expansion. Thus, ACE inhibitors, beta blockers, and some calcium channel antagonists are probably the preferred agents for first-line therapy for hypertension, with beta blockers being particularly useful in patients with a hyperactive hemodynamic state, as in hypertension with an elevated heart rate.

Under any circumstances, the agent should be started at a low dose, e.g., 25 mg of atenolol, 25 mg of captopril, 5 mg of enalapril, or 120 mg of diltiazem (or their equivalents) in divided doses as needed (Table 246-4). If arterial pressure is lowered to less than 140/90 with any of these agents, no further therapy is indicated (see Fig. 246-1). If arterial pressure has not reached this level after 1 to 3 months, the next step is to double the dose of the primary agent. If hypertension still is not controlled, then 25 mg of hydrochlorothiazide (or its equivalent) per day should be added. Thiazides potentiate the action of ACE inhibitors and probably of beta blockers, and their antihypertensive effect is at least additive to that of calcium channel antagonists. Combining diuretics with ACE inhibitors is particularly appealing because the adverse metabolic effects of the thiazide will in part be ameliorated by the ACE inhibitor. Beta blockers and calcium antagonists do not have this advantage. Indeed, beta blockers and thiazides may actually potentiate each other's adverse effects, insofar as electrolyte alterations (hypokalemia) and metabolic actions (hypercholesterolemia) are concerned.

If therapy with two drugs does not achieve blood pressure control, the primary agent should be increased to full dose, e.g., 100 mg of captopril or atenolol, 20 mg of enalapril, or 360 mg of diltiazem. While doses larger than these can be used, it is probably advisable to switch to another medication rather than increase the dose further.

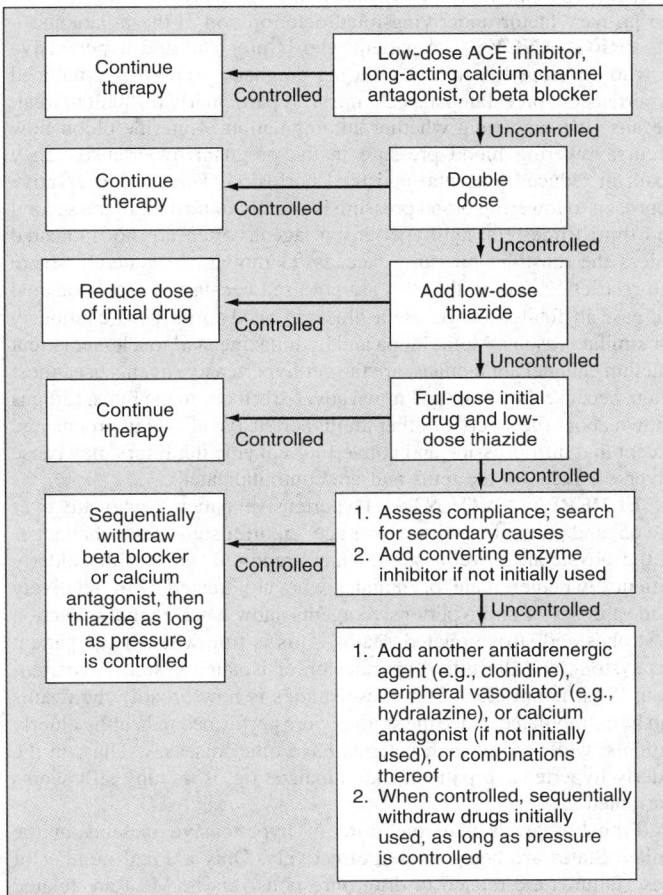

FIGURE 246-1 Schematic approach to the patient with hypertension for whom no specific form of therapy is known or available and who does not have volume expansion.

Occasionally, increasing the thiazide dose to the equivalent of 50 mg of hydrochlorothiazide daily may bring about control of the hypertension; however, thiazide doses higher than this are seldom, if ever, warranted because they almost invariably produce significant side effects. If the blood pressure is still not controlled, then a detailed search for a secondary cause of hypertension, as outlined above, is indicated. If none is found, then a dietary assessment often will reveal a high sodium intake. With reduction in salt intake to 5 g/d or less, blood pressure often is controlled. If the blood pressure is still not controlled, then the primary agent should be switched, maintaining the thiazide. Caution should be used if an ACE inhibitor was not the original agent, as administration of such an agent to a patient who already is taking a diuretic may lead to profound hypotension. If none of these changes produces better control of arterial pressure, then the combination of a calcium channel antagonist and an ACE inhibitor, or triple therapy, usually with a diuretic, ACE inhibitor, and hydralazine, may be effective.

If the blood pressure is controlled, then a stepwise reduction in the dose and/or withdrawal of some of the agents should be done to determine the minimal therapeutic program that will maintain the blood pressure at 140/90 mmHg or less.

Fewer than 5 percent of patients will still be hypertensive at this point. In them, one first should consider the reasons for therapeutic failure, as shown in Table 246-6. If none can be identified, then one of the other agents, such as one of the vasodilators listed in Table 246-4 (e.g., hydralazine) or an antiadrenergic agent (e.g., prazosin or clonidine) should be added. If blood pressure is controlled, previous drugs are withdrawn sequentially to determine the minimal therapeutic program that will maintain a normal blood pressure.

While the recommendations outlined above are satisfactory for a large majority of patients, it is important to use a flexible approach, because individual patients may respond differently to individual drugs and drug combinations. For those patients requiring multiple drugs, once the appropriate combination has been found, the use of a single formulation with the appropriate combination of drugs may simplify the regimen and thereby increase compliance. Every effort should be made to reduce the number of times each day the patients must interrupt their schedules for the medication. Pharmacologic treatment of essential hypertension is usually lifelong, and since most patients are asymptomatic, compliance with a complex regimen may be a serious problem, particularly if the therapeutic regimen has a negative impact on the quality of the patient's life. Finally, it is uncertain what level of arterial pressure should be accepted as representing adequate control. It is clear that reducing diastolic blood pressure to below 90 mmHg is appropriate and reduces morbidity and/or mortality. However, whether a reduction to a level below 85 mmHg is warranted, particularly in elderly patients, remains controversial.

Five groups of patients with hypertension require special consideration because of associated conditions. These groups are considered in the following sections.

RENAL DISEASE Reduction of arterial pressure in hypertensive patients with impaired renal function is often accompanied initially by an increase in serum creatinine. This change does not represent further structural renal damage and should not deter the physician from continuing the therapy, since achievement of blood pressure control may eventually reduce the value toward normal. However, if serum creatinine increases in a patient treated with a converting-enzyme inhibitor, care needs to be exercised, because these patients may have bilateral renal artery disease. Their renal function will continue to deteriorate as long as the converting-enzyme inhibitor is given. Thus, converting-enzyme inhibitors should be used cautiously in patients with impaired renal function, and renal function should be assessed frequently (every 4 to 5 days) for the first 3 weeks. While converting-enzyme inhibitors are contraindicated in patients with bilateral renal artery stenosis, these are the drugs of choice in patients with unilateral renal artery stenosis and a normally functioning contralateral kidney, and probably also in patients with chronic renal failure with or without diabetes mellitus.

CORONARY ARTERY DISEASE In these patients, who also may be taking cardiac glycosides, thiazides should be used judiciously, and a reduction in serum potassium levels should be watched for and, if found, should be corrected rapidly. Beta blockers should be withdrawn carefully, if at all, in these patients. Finally, calcium channel antagonists and converting-enzyme inhibitors may be useful in these patients because they minimize a number of potential adverse reactions that accompany the use of other therapeutic agents, particularly non-specific vasodilators.

DIABETES MELLITUS The diabetic patient with hypertension is particularly challenging to treat because many of the agents used to lower blood pressure can affect glucose metabolism adversely. Converting-enzyme inhibitors may be particularly useful in these individuals. They have no known adverse effects on glucose or lipid metabolism and minimize the development of diabetic nephropathy by reducing renal vascular resistance and renal perfusion pressure—the primary factor underlying renal deterioration in these patients.

PREGNANCY The patient who is pregnant and hypertensive or who develops hypertension during pregnancy (pregnancy-induced hypertension, preeclampsia, eclampsia) is particularly difficult to treat. Because it is uncertain whether autoregulation of uterine blood flow occurs, lowering blood pressure in the pregnant hypertensive may result in reduced placental and fetal perfusion. Thus, a conservative approach to lowering blood pressure is usually indicated. In the second and third trimesters, antihypertensive agents often are not indicated unless the diastolic pressure exceeds 95 mmHg. In general, severe salt restriction and/or diuretics are not used because of the associated increase in fetal wastage. Beta blockers need to be used cautiously for similar reasons. Methyldopa and hydralazine, and to a lesser extent calcium channel antagonists, are the antihypertensive agents used most often, because they have no known adverse effects on the fetus. Little is known about the safety of other antihypertensive agents in pregnancy, except that nitroprusside and converting-enzyme inhibitors may cause adverse effects on the fetus and are contraindicated.

ELDERLY PATIENTS Hypertensive patients who are over age 65, and particularly those over age 75, offer substantial challenges to the physician. Several studies have reported that healthy elderly patients, whether male or female, who are treated with relatively modest doses of antihypertensive agents show a substantial reduction in strokes and stroke-related deaths. This is true whether the patient has systolic and diastolic hypertension or isolated systolic hypertension. What is not clear from these studies is how broadly the results can be extrapolated, since the studies were performed in healthy elderly patients, while many such patients have other diseases. Thus, in the elderly hypertensive patient, individualization of therapy still seems warranted.

Probably fewer than one-third of hypertensive patients in the United States are being treated effectively. Only a small number of these failures are related to drug unresponsiveness. Most are related to (1) failure to detect hypertension, (2) failure to institute effective treatment of an asymptomatic hypertensive patient, and (3) failure of the asymptomatic hypertensive patient to adhere to therapy. To help with the latter problem, patients must be educated to continue treatment

Table 246-6

Reasons for Poor Therapeutic Response in Patients with Hypertension

Inadequate patient compliance
Volume expansion
  Caused by excessive sodium intake
  Caused by nondiuretic antihypertensive agent
Excessive weight gain
Inadequate doses
Drug antagonism
Cold remedies
Sympathomimetics
Oral contraceptives (estrogens)
Adrenal steroids
Secondary forms of hypertension

once an effective regimen has been identified. Side effects and inconveniences of treatment must be minimized or counteracted in order to obtain the patient's continued cooperation.

MALIGNANT HYPERTENSION

In addition to marked blood pressure elevation in association with papilledema and retinal hemorrhages and exudates, the full-blown picture of malignant hypertension may include manifestations of hypertensive encephalopathy, such as severe headache, vomiting, visual disturbances (including transient blindness), transient paralyses, convulsions, stupor, and coma. These manifestations have been attributed to spasm of cerebral vessels and to cerebral edema. In some patients who have died, multiple small thrombi have been found in the cerebral vessels. Cardiac decompensation and rapidly declining renal function are other critical features of malignant hypertension. Oliguria may, in fact, be the presenting feature. The vascular lesion characteristic of malignant hypertension is fibrinoid necrosis of the walls of small arteries and arterioles, and this development can be reversed by effective antihypertensive therapy.

The pathogenesis of malignant hypertension is unknown. However, at least two independent processes—dilation of cerebral arteries and generalized arteriolar fibrinoid necrosis—contribute to the associated signs and symptoms. The cerebral arteries dilate because the normal autoregulation of cerebral blood flow decompensates as a result of the markedly elevated arterial pressure. Cerebral blood flow therefore is excessive, producing the encephalopathy associated with malignant hypertension. Many patients also show evidence of a microangiopathic hemolytic anemia; this secondary phenomenon could contribute to the deterioration of renal function. Most patients also have elevated levels of peripheral plasma renin activity and increased aldosterone production, and these effects may be involved in causing vascular damage.

Perhaps less than 1 percent of hypertensive patients develop the malignant phase, which can occur in the course of both essential and secondary hypertension. Rarely, it is the first recognized manifestation of the blood pressure problem, and it is unusual for it to occur in patients under treatment. The average age at diagnosis is 40, and men are affected more often than women. Prior to the availability of effective therapy, the life expectancy after diagnosis of malignant hypertension was less than 2 years, with most deaths being due to renal failure, cerebral hemorrhage, or congestive heart failure. With the advent of effective antihypertensive therapy, at least half the patients survive for more than 5 years.

℞ TREATMENT

Malignant hypertension is a medical emergency that requires immediate therapy. However, it needs to be distinguished from severe hypertension, since overly aggressive therapy in malignant hypertension could result in a potentially hazardous reduction in myocardial and cerebral perfusion. The initial aims of therapy should be (1) correction of medical complications and (2) reduction of diastolic pressure by one-third, but not to a level below 95 mmHg. The drugs available for treatment of malignant hypertension can be divided into two groups on the basis of time of onset of action (see Table 246-5). Those in the first group act within a few minutes but are not satisfactory for long-term management. If the patient is having convulsions, and if arterial pressure must be reduced rapidly, then one from the immediate-acting group should be used.

The first three agents in this group require continuous infusion and close monitoring. *Nitroprusside* is given by continuous intravenous infusion at a dose of 0.25 to 8.0 μg/kg per min. It is probably the agent of choice in this condition, since it dilates both arterioles and veins. It has the advantage over the ganglionic blockers of not being associated with the development of tachyphylaxis and can be used for days with few side effects. The dosage must be controlled with an infusion pump. *Nitroglycerin* affects veins more than arterioles and is given by continuous infusion at a rate of 5 to 100 μg/min. It is particularly useful in the treatment of hypertension

following coronary bypass surgery, myocardial infarction, left ventricular failure, or unstable angina pectoris. *Diazoxide* is the easiest agent to administer, for no individual titration of dosage is required. However, it is probably less effective than the other agents. It primarily affects arteriolar and not venous tone. A dose of 50 to 150 mg is given rapidly intravenously, and the antihypertensive effect appears in 1 to 5 min. The same dose can be repeated in 5 to 10 min, if necessary, or when the pressure begins to rise, usually after several hours. The total dose should not exceed 600 mg/d. In an occasional patient, pressure may drop below normal levels after diazoxide administration. This drug should not be used in patients in whom aortic dissection or myocardial infarction is suspected. Because it can increase the force of myocardial contraction, often a beta blocker is given concomitantly. *Enalaprilat*, an intravenous form of the ACE inhibitor *enalapril*, also has proven effective, particularly in individuals with left heart failure. Finally, intravenous *labetalol* may be particularly useful in patients with a myocardial infarct or angina because it prevents an increase in heart rate. However, it may be ineffective in patients previously treated with beta blockers and is contraindicated in patients with heart failure, asthma, bradycardia, or heart block. It also may serve as an alternative therapy in patients with eclampsia who are unresponsive to hydralazine. *Trimethaphan*, a ganglionic blocker, is given at a rate of 0.5 to 5 mg/min. Currently, it is seldom used. It also dilates arterioles and veins. The patient should be in the sitting position, and the pressure should be monitored closely, preferably in an intensive care unit. Monitoring may be more complex than with nitroprusside, but trimethaphan may be the better therapy in acute aortic dissection.

Patients given any of these agents also should receive other medications effective for long-term control. Those in the second group in Table 246-5 require 30 min or more to produce their full effect, but they have the advantage of being satisfactory for subsequent oral administration and for long-term management of the patient's hypertension. If such a delay in the achievement of the full effect is acceptable, intravenous *hydralazine* is effective in many patients within 10 min; an effective protocol involves giving 10-mg doses intravenously every 10 to 15 min until the desired effect has been obtained or until a total of 50 mg has been administered. The total amount required for response may then be repeated intramuscularly or intravenously every 6 h. Hydralazine should be used with caution in patients with significant coronary artery disease and should be avoided in patients manifesting myocardial ischemia or aortic dissection. It is effective in preeclampsia. Sublingual *nifedipine* has been reported to be useful, although it may produce tachycardia.

Furosemide is an important adjunct to the therapy just discussed. Given either orally or intravenously, it serves to maintain sodium diuresis in the face of a falling arterial pressure and thus will speed recovery from encephalopathy and congestive heart failure as well as maintain the sensitivity to the primary antihypertensive drug. Digitalis (Chap. 233) also may be indicated if there is evidence of cardiac decompensation.

In patients with malignant hypertension in whom the existence of pheochromocytoma is suspected, urine should be collected for measurement of the products of catecholamine metabolism, and drugs that might release additional catecholamines, such as methyldopa, reserpine, and guanethidine, must be avoided. The parenteral drug of choice in these patients is phentolamine, administered with care to avoid a precipitous reduction in arterial pressure.

There is hope even for patients who fail to respond sufficiently to any of the forms of therapy and who show progressive deterioration in renal function. In some, a period of peritoneal dialysis or hemodialysis to deplete extracellular fluid has resulted in better blood pressure control and eventual improvement in renal function. In other patients with refractory hypertension and renal failure who do not respond to volume depletion or hypotensive therapy, including minoxidil administration—particularly those with marked elevation of plasma renin activity—bilateral nephrectomy has resulted in amelioration of hypertension; subsequently, these patients have been maintained on chronic dialysis or have received renal homografts. However, bilateral nephrectomy should be avoided where possible because (1) the loss of renal erythropoietin will contribute to the associated anemia; (2) vitamin D metabolism may be adversely affected; and (3) all residual renal function will be lost.

BIBLIOGRAPHY

CALHOUN DA et al: Treatment of hypertensive crisis. N Engl J Med 323:1177, 1990

FRIES ED: The efficacy and safety of diuretics in treating hypertension. Ann Intern Med 122:223, 1995

FROHLICH ED et al: The heart in hypertension. N Engl J Med 327:998, 1992

HOLLENBERG NK, WILLIAMS GH: Abnormal renal function, sodium-volume homeostasis, and renin system behavior in normal-renin essential hypertension: The evolution of the non-modular concept, in JH Laragh et al (eds): *Hypertension. Pathophysiology, Diagnosis, and Management*, 2d ed. New York, Raven, 1995, vol 2, p 1837

INSUA JT et al: Drug treatment of hypertension in the elderly: A meta-analysis. Ann Intern Med 121:355, 1994

JAFFE LS, SEELY EW: The heterogeneity of the blood pressure response to hormonal contraceptives. Curr Opin Endo Diab 2:257, 1995

JOINT NATIONAL COMMITTEE ON DETECTION, EVALUATION AND TREATMENT OF HIGH BLOOD PRESSURE: The fifth report. Arch Intern Med 153:154, 1993

LEWIS EJ et al: The effect of angiotensin converting enzyme inhibition on diabetic nephropathy. N Engl J Med 329:1456, 1993

LIEBSON PR et al: Comparison of five antihypertensive monotherapies and placebo for change in left ventricular mass in patients receiving nutritional-hygienic therapy in the Treatment of Mild Hypertension Study (TOMHS). Circulation 91:698, 1995

MORTENSEN RM, WILLIAMS GH: Aldosterone action (physiology), in LJ DeGroot et al (eds): *Endocrinology*, 3d ed. Philadelphia, Saunders, 1994, p 1668

NALLY VJ et al: Diagnostic criteria of renovascular hypertension with captopril renography. A consensus statement. Am J Hypertension 4:749S, 1991

NATIONAL HIGH BLOOD PRESSURE EDUCATION PROGRAM WORKING GROUP: National High Blood Pressure Education Program Working Group report on hypertension in diabetes. Hypertension 23:145, 1994

PSATY BM et al: The risk of incident myocardial infarction associated with antihypertensive drug therapies. Circulation 91:925, 1995

SPEDDING M, PAOLETTI R: Classification of calcium channels and the sites of action of drugs modifying channel function. Pharmacol Rev 44:363, 1992

STERN N, TUCK ML: Mechanisms of hypertension in diabetes mellitus, in JH Laragh et al (eds): *Hypertension: Pathophysiology, Diagnosis and Management*. New York, Raven 1995, p 1698

SYSTOLIC HYPERTENSION IN THE ELDERLY PROGRAM COOPERATIVE RESEARCH GROUP: Implications of the Systolic Hypertension in the Elderly Program. Hypertension 21:335, 1993

WILLIAMS GH: Genetic approaches to understanding the pathophysiology of complex human traits. Kidney Int 46:1550, 1994

WILLIAMS GH: Quality of life considerations in therapeutic decision-making: Antihypertensive therapy as a model, in M Bergener et al (eds): *Aging, Health and Healing*. New York, Springer, 1995, p 257

247

Victor J. Dzau, Mark A. Creager

DISEASES OF THE AORTA

The aorta is the conduit through which the blood ejected from the left ventricle is delivered to the systemic arterial bed. In adults, its diameter is approximately 3 cm at the origin, 2.5 cm in the descending portion in the thorax, and 1.8 to 2 cm in the abdomen. The aortic wall consists of a thin intima composed of endothelium, subendothelial connective tissue, and an internal elastic lamina; a thick tunica media composed of smooth-muscle cells and extracellular matrix; and an adventitia composed primarily of connective tissue and enclosing the vasa vasorum and nervi vascularis. In addition to its conduit function, the viscoelastic and compliant properties of the aorta also subserve a buffering function. The aorta is distended during systole to enable a portion of the stroke volume to be stored, and it recoils during diastole so that blood continues to flow to the periphery during diastole. Because of its continuous exposure to high pulsatile pressure and shear stress, the aorta is particularly prone to injury and disease resulting from mechanical trauma (Table 247-1). The aorta is also more prone to rupture than any other vessel, especially with the development of aneurysmal dilatation, since its wall tension, as governed by Laplace's law (i.e., proportional to the product of pressure and radius), is intrinsically high.

AORTIC ANEURYSM

An *aneurysm* is defined as a pathologic dilatation of a segment of a blood vessel. A *true aneurysm* involves all three layers of the vessel wall and is distinguished from a *pseudoaneurysm*, in which the intimal and medial layers are disrupted and the dilatation is lined by adventitia only and sometimes by perivascular clot. Aneurysms also may be classified according to their gross appearance. A *fusiform aneurysm* affects the entire circumference of a segment of the vessel, resulting in a diffusely dilated lesion. In contrast, a *saccular aneurysm* involves only a portion of the circumference, resulting in an outpouching of the vessel wall.

The most common pathologic condition associated with aortic aneurysm is atherosclerosis. It is controversial whether atherosclerosis itself actually causes aortic aneurysm or develops as a secondary event in the dilated aorta. Causality is implied by studies that have shown that many patients with aortic aneurysms have coexisting risk factors and atherosclerosis in other blood vessels. Familial clusterings of abdominal aortic aneurysms occur in 20 percent of patients, suggesting a hereditary basis of the disease. A mutation of the gene encoding type III procollagen has been implicated. Additional causes of aortic aneurysm include cystic medial necrosis; syphilis, tuberculosis, or other bacterial infections; Takayasu arteritis; giant cell arteritis; seronegative spondyloarthropathies; rheumatoid arthritis; and trauma. Congenital aortic aneurysms may be primary or associated with other anomalies, such as a bicuspid aortic valve or aortic coarctation.

Aortic aneurysms are also classified according to location, i.e., abdominal versus thoracic. Those in the abdominal aorta are almost always associated with atherosclerosis. Aneurysms of the ascending thoracic aorta are caused most often by cystic medial necrosis. Aneurysms of the descending thoracic aorta are *usually* contiguous with infradiaphragmatic aneurysms and, as with the latter, are associated with atherosclerosis.

Aortic aneurysms usually do not produce symptoms. However, as they expand, they may become painful. Compression or erosion of adjacent tissue by aneurysms also may cause symptoms. The formation of mural thrombi within the aneurysm may predispose to peripheral embolization. Occasionally, an aneurysm may leak, leading to extravasation of blood into the vessel wall and the periadventitial area and causing acute pain and local tenderness. This is usually a harbinger of rupture and represents a medical emergency. More often, acute rupture occurs without any prior warning, and this complication is always life-threatening.

Table 247-1

Diseases of the Aorta: Classification and Etiology

Aortic aneurysm	**Aortic occlusion**
Atherosclerosis	Atherosclerosis
Cystic medial necrosis	Thromboembolism
Syphilitic infection	**Aortitis**
Mycotic infection	Syphilitic aortitis
Rheumatic aortitis	Rheumatic aortitis
Trauma	Takayasu's arteritis and aortic arch
Aortic dissection	syndromes
Cystic medial necrosis	Giant cell arteritis
Systemic hypertension	
Atherosclerosis	

ATHEROSCLEROTIC ANEURYSMS Seventy-five percent of atherosclerotic aneurysms are located in the distal abdominal aorta below the renal arteries. An abdominal aneurysm commonly produces no symptoms and is usually detected on routine examination as a palpable, pulsatile, and nontender mass, or it is an incidental finding during an abdominal x-ray or ultrasound performed for other reasons. Some patients may complain of strong pulsations in the abdomen, others of lower back pain. Rarely, there is leakage of the aneurysm with severe pain and tenderness. Acute pain and hypotension occur with rupture of the aneurysm, requiring emergency operation.

Abdominal radiography may demonstrate the calcified outline of the aneurysm. However, about 25 percent of aneurysms are not calcified and cannot be visualized by plain x-ray. An abdominal ultrasound can delineate the transverse and longitudinal dimensions of an abdominal aortic aneurysm and may detect mural thrombus. Abdominal ultrasound is useful for serial documentation of aneurysm size and could be used to screen patients at risk for developing aortic aneurysms, such as those with affected siblings, peripheral atherosclerosis, or peripheral artery aneurysms. Abdominal aortography is used commonly for evaluating patients with aneurysm for surgery, but this procedure carries a small risk of complications, such as bleeding, allergic reactions, and atheroembolism. This technique is useful in documenting the extent of the aneurysm, especially its upper and lower limits, and the extent of associated atherosclerotic vascular disease. However, since the presence of mural clots may reduce the luminal size, aortography may underestimate the diameter of an aneurysm. Computed tomography (CT) with contrast and magnetic resonance imaging (MRI) are accurate noninvasive tests to determine the location and size of thoracic and abdominal aortic aneurysms and are becoming the gold standard for the detection and follow-up of aortic aneurysms.

Prognosis is related to both the size of the aneurysm and the severity of coexistent coronary artery and cerebral vascular diseases. The risk of rupture increases with the size of the aneurysm. The 5-year risk of rupture for aneurysms less than 5 cm in diameter is 1 to 2 percent, whereas it is 20 to 40 percent for aneurysms greater than 5 cm in diameter.

℞ TREATMENT

Operative excision with replacement with a graft is indicated for abdominal aneurysms of any size that are expanding rapidly or that are associated with symptoms. For asymptomatic aneurysms, surgery is indicated if the diameter is greater than 6.5 cm. Operation may be recommended in patients with aneurysm diameters of 4 to 5 cm, except for patients with exceptionally high operative risk. Serial noninvasive follow-up of smaller (<5 cm) aneurysms is an alternative to immediate surgery. In surgical candidates, careful preoperative cardiac and general medical evaluations (followed by appropriate therapy of complicating conditions) are essential. Preexisting coronary artery disease, congestive heart failure, pulmonary disease, diabetes, and advanced age add to the risk of surgery. If clinically indicated, preoperative evaluation should identify high-risk coronary artery disease using an exercise stress test or dipyridamole thallium scanning. Noninvasive tests, such as stress or dobutamine echocardiography or ambulatory electrocardiographic monitoring for silent ischemia, are favored in some institutions. Perioperative management should include the placement of a Swan-Ganz catheter and arterial line to monitor and optimize left ventricular filling pressure, cardiac output, and arterial pressure, especially during clamping and declamping of aorta, as well as during the immediate postoperative period. With careful preoperative cardiac evaluation and postoperative care, which includes Swan-Ganz catheterization, operative mortality approximates 1 to 2 percent. Following acute rupture, the mortality of emergency operation is generally greater than 50 percent.

CYSTIC MEDIAL NECROSIS *Cystic medial necrosis* is the term used to describe the degeneration of collagen and elastic fibers in the tunica media of the aorta, as well as medial cell losses that are replaced by multiple clefts of mucoid material. Cystic medial necrosis

characteristically affects the proximal aorta, results in circumferential weakness and dilatation, and leads to the development of fusiform aneurysms involving the ascending aorta and the sinuses of Valsalva. This condition is particularly prevalent in patients with the Marfan syndrome and Ehlers-Danlos syndrome type IV (Chap. 348) but is also seen in pregnancy, hypertension, valvular heart disease, and sometimes as an isolated condition in patients without any other apparent disease. The clinical manifestations include expanding aneurysms, rupture, and aortic regurgitation.

℞ TREATMENT

Because of this potential complication, the management of patients with Marfan's syndrome includes echocardiography to evaluate aortic root size, aortic valve regurgitation, and mitral and tricuspid prolapse and/or regurgitation. Patients with thoracic aortic aneurysms, and particularly Marfan patients with evidence of aortic root dilatation, should be given long-term beta-blocker therapy. Operative repair is indicated in patients with symptomatic thoracic aortic aneurysms and in those in whom the aortic root diameter exceeds 6 cm. In patients with Marfan's syndrome, thoracic aortic aneurysms >5 cm should be considered for repair. In pregnant Marfan patients with aortic root diameter <4 cm, beta-blockade therapy is indicated throughout pregnancy, with frequent surveillance of the aorta with echocardiography. Transluminal placement of endovascular stent grafts for treatment of descending thoracic aortic aneurysms is undergoing investigation.

MYCOTIC ANEURYSM This rare condition develops as the result of staphylococcal, streptococcal, or salmonella infections of the aorta, usually at an atherosclerotic plaque. Blood cultures are usually positive and reveal the nature of the infecting agent. The aneurysms are usually saccular. Treatment requires parenteral antibiotics and surgical excision.

TRAUMA Aortic rupture may develop following penetrating injury or blunt trauma. Horizontal deceleration injury may tear the aortic isthmus at the site of insertion of the ligamentum arteriosum. Other causes of aortic aneurysm, such as syphilitic infection and rheumatic vasculitides, are discussed below under "Aortitis."

AORTIC DISSECTION

Aortic dissection is caused by a circumferential or, less frequently, transverse tear of the intima. It usually occurs along the right lateral wall of the ascending aorta where the hydraulic shear stress is high. The initiating event is either a medial hemorrhage that dissects into and disrupts the intima or a primary intimal tear with secondary dissection into the media. Another common site is the descending thoracic aorta just below the ligamentum arteriosum. The pulsatile aortic flow then dissects along the elastic lamellar plates of the aorta and creates a false lumen. The dissection usually propagates distally down the descending aorta and into its major branches, but it also may propagate proximally. In some cases, a secondary distal intimal disruption occurs, resulting in the reentry of blood from the false to the true lumen.

There are at least two important pathologic and radiologic variants: intramural hematoma without an intimal flap and penetrating ulcer. The clinical picture and therapeutic management of intramural hematoma are similar to those for classic aortic dissection. On the other hand, penetrating ulcers are usually localized and not associated with extensive propagation. They are primarily found in the distal portion of the descending thoracic aorta and are associated with extensive atherosclerotic disease. The ulcer can erode beyond the intimal border, leading to medial hematoma, and may progress to false aneurysm formation or rupture.

DeBakey and coworkers classified aortic dissections as type I, in which an intimal tear occurs in the ascending aorta but which involves the descending aorta as well; type II, in which the dissection is limited

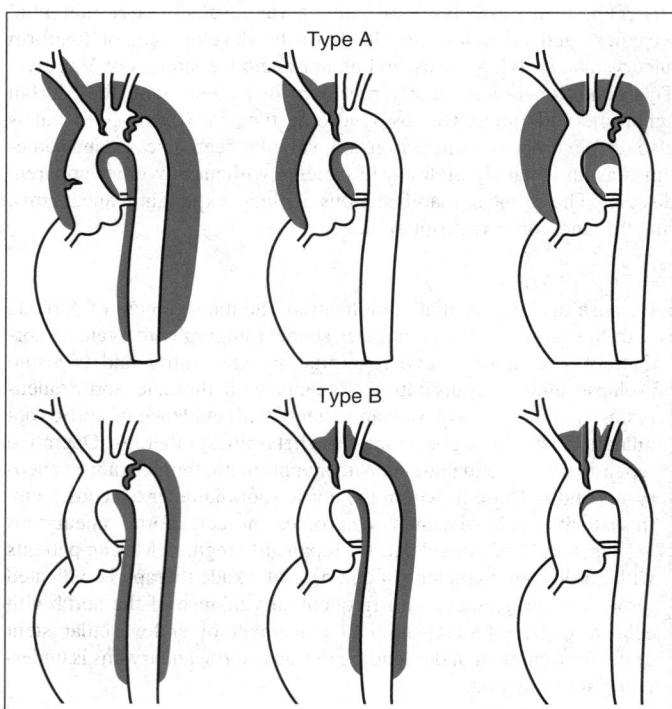

FIGURE 247-1 Classification of aortic dissections. Stanford classification: Top panels illustrate type A dissections that involve the ascending aorta independent of site of tear and distal extension; type B dissections (*bottom panels*) involve transverse and/or descending aorta without involvement of the ascending aorta. DeBakey classification: Type I dissection involves ascending to descending aorta (*top left*); type II dissection is limited to ascending or transverse aorta, without descending aorta (*top center + top right*); type III dissection involves descending aorta only (*bottom left*). [*From DC Miller, in Aortic Dissection, RM Doroghazi, EE Slater (eds), New York, McGraw-Hill, 1983, with permission.*]

to the ascending aorta; and type III, in which the intimal tear is located in the descending area with distal propagation of the dissection (Fig. 247-1). Another classification (Stanford) is that of type A, in which the dissection involves the ascending aorta (proximal dissection), and type B, in which it is limited to the descending aorta (distal dissection). From a management standpoint, classification into type A or B is more practical and useful, since DeBakey types I and II are managed in a similar manner.

The factors that predispose to aortic dissection include systemic hypertension, a coexisting condition in 70 percent of patients, and cystic medial necrosis. Aortic dissection is the major cause of morbidity and mortality in patients with the Marfan syndrome (Chap. 348). The incidence is also increased in patients with congenital aortic valve anomalies (e.g., bicuspid valve), in those with coarctation of the aorta, and in otherwise normal women during the third trimester of pregnancy.

CLINICAL MANIFESTATIONS The peak incidence is in the sixth and seventh decades. Men are more affected than women by a ratio of 2:1. The presentations of aortic dissection and its variants are the consequences of intimal tear, dissecting hematoma, occlusion of involved arteries, and compression of adjacent tissues. Acute aortic dissection presents with the sudden onset of pain (Chap. 13), which is often described as very severe and tearing and is associated with diaphoresis. The pain may be localized to the front or back of the chest, often the interscapular region, and typically migrates with propagation of the dissection. Other symptoms include syncope, dyspnea, and weakness. Physical findings may include hypertension or hypotension, loss of pulses, aortic regurgitation, pulmonary edema, and neuro-

logic findings due to carotid artery obstruction (hemiplegia, hemianesthesia) or spinal cord ischemia (paraplegia). Bowel ischemia, hematuria, and myocardial ischemia have all been observed. These clinical manifestations reflect complications resulting from the dissection occluding the major arteries. Furthermore, clinical manifestations may result from the compression of adjacent structures (e.g., superior cervical ganglia, superior vena cava, bronchus, esophagus) by the expanding dissection aneurysm and include Horner's syndrome, superior vena caval syndrome, hoarseness, dysphagia, and airway compromise. Hemopericardium and cardiac tamponade may complicate a type A lesion with retrograde dissection. Acute aortic regurgitation is an important and common (over 50 percent) complication of proximal dissection. This is the outcome of either a circumferential tear that widens the aortic root or a disruption of the annulus by dissecting hematoma that tears a leaflet(s) or displaces it below the line of closure. Signs of aortic regurgitation include bounding pulses, a wide pulse pressure, a diastolic murmur often radiating to the right sternal border, and evidence of congestive heart failure. The clinical manifestation depends on the severity of the regurgitation.

In dissections involving the ascending aorta, the chest x-ray often reveals a widened superior mediastinum. A pleural effusion (usually left-sided) also may be present. In dissections of the descending thoracic aorta, a widened mediastinum also may be observed on chest x-ray. In addition, the descending aorta may appear to be wider than the ascending portion. An electrocardiogram that shows no evidence of ischemia is helpful in distinguishing aortic dissection from myocardial infarction. Rarely, the dissection involves the right or left coronary ostium and causes acute myocardial infarction. The diagnosis of aortic dissection can be established by aortography or by the use of noninvasive techniques such as two-dimensional echocardiography, CT scan, or MRI. Aortography may be used to document the diagnosis; identify the entry point, the intimal flap, and the false and true lumina; and to establish the extent of dissection into the major arteries. Coronary angiography may be performed concomitantly in high-risk patients in the evaluation and preparation for surgery. The sensitivity of aortography is 70 percent for visualizing internal flap, 56 percent for the site of intimal tear, and 87 percent for false lumen. It is unable to recognize intramural hemorrhage. Transthoracic echocardiography can be performed simply and rapidly and has an overall sensitivity of 60 to 85 percent. For diagnosing proximal ascending aortic dissections, its sensitivity ranges from 80 to 100 percent; it is less useful for detecting dissection of the arch and descending thoracic aorta. Transesophageal echocardiography (Fig. 247-2) requires greater skill and patient cooperation but is very accurate in identifying dissections of the ascending and descending thoracic aorta, but not the arch, achieving 98 percent sensitivity and specificity. CT scan and MRI are each highly accurate in identifying the intimal flap and the extent of the dissection. They are useful in recognizing intramural hemorrhage and penetrating ul-

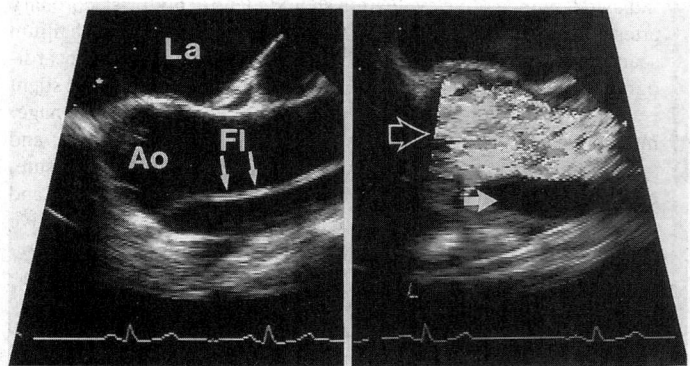

FIGURE 247-2 Aortic dissection. *Left.* Transesophageal echocardiogram of the ascending aorta demonstrating a freely mobile flap within the lumen of the vessel. Ao, aorta; La, left atrium; Fl, flap. *Right.* When color Doppler was superimposed on the image, the true lumen (*open arrow*) was easily separated from the false lumen (*solid arrow*).

cers. MRI also can detect blood flow, which may be useful in characterizing antegrade versus retrograde dissection. These noninvasive tests are now becoming the diagnostic procedures of choice. Their relative utility depends on the availability and expertise in individual institutions as well as on the hemodynamic stability of the patient, with CT and MRI obviously less suitable for more unstable patients.

℞ TREATMENT

Medical therapy should be initiated as soon as the diagnosis is considered. The patient should be admitted to an intensive care unit for monitoring hemodynamics and urine output. Unless hypotension is present, therapy should be aimed at reducing cardiac contractility and systemic arterial pressure, and thereby shear stress. For acute dissection, unless contraindicated, beta-adrenergic blockers should be administered via the parenteral route, using either intravenous propranolol, metoprolol, or the short-acting esmolol to achieve a heart rate of approximately 60 beats per minute. This should be accompanied by sodium nitroprusside infusion to lower systolic blood pressure to 120 mmHg or less. Recently, labetalol (p. 1388), a drug with both beta- and alpha-adrenergic blocking properties, also has been used as a parenteral agent in the acute therapy of dissection.

Trimethaphan, a ganglionic blocker, may be used if nitroprusside or labetalol cannot be employed. Experience with calcium antagonists is limited. Direct vasodilators, such as diazoxide and hydralazine, are contraindicated because these agents can increase hydraulic shear and may propagate dissection.

For ascending aortic dissection (type A), emergent or urgent surgical correction, which includes reconstruction of the aortic wall, is the preferred treatment. The overall in-hospital mortality rate after surgical treatment of patients with aortic dissection is reported to be 15 to 20 percent. The major causes of perioperative mortality and morbidity include myocardial infarction, paraplegia, renal failure, tamponade, hemorrhage, and sepsis. For uncomplicated and stable distal dissection (type B), medical therapy is the preferred treatment unless there is clinical evidence of propagation, compromise of major branches of the aorta, impending rupture, or continued pain. The in-hospital mortality rate of medically treated patients with type B dissection is 15 to 20 percent. Long-term therapy for patients with aortic dissection (with or without surgery) consists of the control of hypertension and reduction of cardiac contractility with the use of beta blockers plus other antihypertensive agents such as angiotensin-converting enzyme inhibitor or calcium antagonist. Patients with chronic type B dissection should be followed on an outpatient basis every 6 to 12 months by CT scan with contrast or MRI to detect propagation. Marfan patients are at high risk for postdissection complications. The long-term prognosis for patients with treated dissections is generally good with careful follow-up; the 10-year survival rate is approximately 60 percent.

AORTIC OCCLUSION

CHRONIC ARTERIOSCLEROTIC OCCLUSIVE DISEASE Chronic occlusive disease usually involves the distal abdominal aorta below the renal arteries. Frequently the disease extends to the common iliac arteries, but it may spare the external iliac arteries. Because of the slowly progressive nature of the atherosclerotic process, the natural history of aortic occlusion is usually chronic and insidious. Claudication characteristically involves the lower back, buttocks, and thighs and may be associated with impotence in males (Leriche syndrome). The severity of the symptoms depends on the adequacy of collaterals. With sufficient collateral blood flow, a complete occlusion of the abdominal aorta may occur without the development of ischemic symptoms. The physical findings include absence of femoral and other distal pulses bilaterally and the detection of an audible bruit over the abdomen (usually at or below the umbilicus) and the common femoral arteries. Atrophic skin, loss of hair, and coolness of the lower extremities are usually observed. In advanced ischemia, rubor on dependency and pallor on elevation can be seen.

The diagnosis is usually established by the physical examination and noninvasive testing, including leg pressure measurements, Doppler velocity analysis, and pulse volume recordings. The anatomy may be defined by abdominal aortography prior to revascularization. Operative treatment is indicated in patients with debilitating symptoms and/or with the development of leg ischemia.

ACUTE OCCLUSION Acute occlusion in the distal abdominal aorta represents a medical emergency because it threatens the viability of the lower extremities. It usually results from an occlusive embolus that almost always originates from the heart. Rarely, acute occlusion may occur as the result of in situ thrombosis in a preexisting severely narrowed segment of the aorta or plaque rupture and hemorrhage into such an area.

The clinical picture is one of acute ischemia of the lower extremities. Severe rest pain, coolness, and pallor of the lower extremities and the absence of distal pulses bilaterally are the usual manifestations. Diagnosis should be established rapidly by aortography. Emergency thrombectomy or revascularization is indicated.

AORTITIS

Aortitis frequently affects the ascending aorta and may result in aneurysmal dilatation and aortic regurgitation; it occasionally obstructs branch vessels of the aorta.

SYPHILITIC AORTITIS This late manifestation of luetic infection (Chap. 174) usually affects the proximal ascending aorta, particularly the aortic root, resulting in aortic dilatation and aneurysm formation. Syphilitic aortitis may occasionally involve the aortic arch or the descending aorta. The aneurysms may be saccular or fusiform and are usually asymptomatic, but compression of and erosion into adjacent structures may result in symptoms; rupture also may occur.

The initial lesion is an obliterative endarteritis of the vasa vasorum, especially in the adventitia. This is an inflammatory response to the invasion of the adventitia by the spirochetes. Destruction of the aortic media occurs as the spirochetes spread into this layer, usually via the lymphatics accompanying the vasa vasorum. Destruction of collagen and elastic tissues leads to dilation of the aorta, scar formation, and calcification. These changes account for the characteristic radiographic appearance of a calcified ascending aortic aneurysm.

The disease typically presents as an incidental radiographic finding 15 to 30 years after initial infection. Symptoms may result from aortic regurgitation, narrowing of coronary ostia due to syphilitic aortitis, compression of adjacent structures (e.g., esophagus), or rupture. Diagnosis is established by a positive serologic test, i.e., VDRL or fluorescent treponemal antibody (see Chap. 174). Treatment includes penicillin and surgical excision and repair.

RHEUMATIC AORTITIS Rheumatoid arthritis (Chap. 313), ankylosing spondylitis (Chap. 317), psoriatic arthritis (Chap. 325), Reiter's syndrome (Chap. 317), Behçet's syndrome (Chap. 318), relapsing polychondritis, and inflammatory bowel disorders may all be associated with aortitis involving the ascending aorta. The inflammatory lesions usually involve the ascending aorta and may extend to the sinuses of Valsalva, the mitral valve leaflets, and adjacent myocardium. The clinical manifestations are aneurysm, aortic regurgitation, and involvement of the cardiac conduction system.

TAKAYASU'S ARTERITIS AND OTHER AORTIC ARCH SYNDROMES Inflammatory diseases of the aortic arch resulting in obstruction of the aorta and its major arteries characterize this major group of diseases. Takayasu's arteritis is also termed *pulseless disease* because of the frequent occlusion of the large arteries originating from the aorta. It also may involve the descending thoracic and abdominal aorta and occlude large branches such as the renal arteries. Aortic aneurysms may also occur. The pathology is a panarteritis with marked intimal hyperplasia, medial and adventitial thickening, and, in chronic form, fibrotic occlusion. The disease is most prevalent in young females of Asian descent. During the acute stage, fever, malaise, weight loss, and other systemic symptoms may be evident. An elevation of the erythrocyte sedimentation rate is common. The chronic stages of the disease present with symptoms related to large artery occlusion, such as upper extremity claudication, cerebral ischemia, and syncope. The chronic disease is intermittently active. Since the process is progressive and there is no definitive therapy, the prognosis is usually poor. Glucocorticoids and immunosuppressive agents have been reported to be effective in some patients during the acute phase. Occasionally, anticoagulation prevents thrombosis and complete occlusion of a large artery. Surgical bypass of a critically stenotic artery may be necessary.

GIANT CELL ARTERITIS (See Chap. 319) Primarily large and medium-sized arteries are affected. The pathology is that of focal granulomatous lesions involving the entire arterial wall. It may be associated with polymyalgia rheumatica (Chap. 22). Obstruction of medium-sized arteries (e.g., temporal and ophthalmic arteries) and of major branches of the aorta and the development of aortitis and aortic regurgitation are some of the complications of the disease. High-dose glucocorticoid therapy may be effective when given early.

BIBLIOGRAPHY

CIGARROA JE et al: Diagnostic imaging in the evaluation of suspected aortic dissection: Old standards and new directions. N Engl J Med 328:35, 1993

CREAGER MA et al: Aneurysmal disease of the aorta and its branches, in *Vascular Medicine*, J Loscalzo et al (eds). Boston, Little, Brown, 1996, pp 907–925

ERNST CB: Abdominal aortic aneurysm. N Engl J Med 328:1167, 1993

EVANS JM et al: Increased incidence of aortic aneurysm and dissection in giant cell (temporal) arteritis. A population based study. Ann Intern Med 122:502, 1995

GUILMET D et al: Aortic dissection: Anatomic types and surgical approaches. J Cardiovasc Surg 34:23, 1993

ISSELBACHER EM et al: Diseases of the aorta, in *Heart Disease*, 5th ed, E Braunwald (ed). Philadelphia, Saunders, 1997, pp 1546–1581

KULVANIEMI H et al: Genetic causes of aortic aneurysms: Unlearning at least part of what the textbooks say. J Clin Invest 88:1441, 1991

NIENABER CA et al: The diagnosis of thoracic aortic dissection by noninvasive imaging procedures. N Engl J Med 328:1, 1993

——— et al: Intramural hemorrhage of the thoracic aorta. Diagnostic and therapeutic implications. Circulation 92:1465, 1995

O'GARA PT, DESANCTIS RN: Aortic dissection in vascular medicine. J Loscalzo et al (eds). Boston, Little, Brown, 1996, pp 927–950

SHORES J et al: Progression of aortic dilatation and the benefit of long-term beta-adrenergic blockade in Marfan's syndrome. N Engl J Med 330:1335, 1994

SPITTELL PC et al: Clinical features and differential diagnosis of aortic dissection: Experience with 236 cases (1980 through 1990). Mayo Clin Proc 68:642, 1993

248 *Mark A. Creager, Victor J. Dzau*

VASCULAR DISEASES OF THE EXTREMITIES

ARTERIAL DISORDERS

ATHEROSCLEROSIS OF THE EXTREMITIES Atherosclerosis (arteriosclerosis obliterans) is the leading cause of occlusive arterial disease of the extremities in patients over 40 years old; the highest incidence occurs in the sixth and seventh decades of life. As in patients with atherosclerosis of the coronary and cerebral vasculature, there is an increased prevalence of peripheral atherosclerotic occlusive disease in individuals with hypertension, hypercholesterolemia, and diabetes mellitus and in cigarette smokers. Atherosclerosis of the extremities is seen most frequently in elderly males.

Pathology (See Chap. 242) Segmental lesions causing stenosis or occlusion are usually localized in large and medium-sized vessels. The pathology of the lesions includes atherosclerotic plaques with calcium deposition, thinning of the media, patchy destruction of muscle and elastic fibers, fragmentation of the internal elastic lamina, and thrombi composed of platelets and fibrin. The primary sites of involvement are the abdominal aorta and iliac arteries (30 percent of symptomatic patients), the femoral and popliteal arteries (80 to 90 percent of patients), and the more distal vessels, including the tibial and peroneal arteries (40 to 50 percent of patients). Atherosclerotic lesions occur preferentially at arterial branch points, sites of increased turbulence, altered shear stress, and intimal injury. Involvement of the distal vasculature is most common in elderly individuals and patients with diabetes mellitus.

Clinical Evaluation The most common *symptom* is intermittent claudication, which is defined as a pain, ache, cramp, numbness, or a sense of fatigue in the muscles; it occurs during exercise and is relieved by rest. The site of claudication is distal to the location of the occlusive lesion. For example, buttock, hip, and thigh discomfort occurs in patients with aortoiliac disease (Leriche syndrome), whereas calf claudication develops in patients with femoral-popliteal disease. Symptoms are far more common in the lower than in the upper extremities because of the higher incidence of obstructive lesions in the former region. In patients with severe arterial occlusive disease, rest pain may develop. Patients will complain of pain or a feeling of cold or numbness in the foot and toes. Frequently, these symptoms occur at night when the legs are in a "neutral" position and improve when the legs are in a dependent position. With severe ischemia, rest pain may be present.

Important *physical findings* of chronic arterial insufficiency include decreased or absent pulses distal to the obstruction, the presence of bruits over the narrowed artery, and muscle atrophy. With more severe disease, hair loss, thickened nails, smooth and shiny skin, reduced skin temperature, and pallor or cyanosis are frequent physical signs. In addition, ulcers or gangrene may occur. Elevation of the legs and repeated flexing of the calf muscles produce pallor of the soles of the feet, whereas rubor, secondary to reactive hyperemia, may develop when the legs are dependent. The time required for rubor to develop or for the veins in the foot to fill when the patient's legs are transferred from an elevated to a dependent position is related to the severity of the ischemia and the presence of collateral vessels. Patients with severe ischemia may develop peripheral edema because they keep their legs in a dependent position much of the time. Ischemic neuritis can result in numbness and hyporeflexia.

Noninvasive Testing The history and physical examination are usually sufficient to establish the diagnosis of peripheral arterial occlusive disease. An objective assessment of the severity of disease is obtained by noninvasive techniques. These include digital pulse volume recordings, Doppler flow velocity waveform analysis, duplex ultrasonography (which combines B-mode imaging and pulse-wave Doppler examination), segmental pressure measurements, transcutaneous oximetry, stress testing (usually using a treadmill), and tests of reactive hyperemia. In the presence of significant arterial occlusive disease, the volume displacement in the leg is decreased with each pulse, and the Doppler velocity contour becomes progressively flatter. Duplex ultrasonography is often useful in detecting stenotic lesions in native arteries and bypass grafts.

Arterial pressure can be recorded noninvasively along the legs by serial placement of sphygmomanometric cuffs and use of a Doppler device to auscultate or record blood flow. Normally, blood pressure in the legs and arms is similar. Indeed, ankle pressure may be slightly higher than arm pressure due to pulse-wave reflection. In the presence of hemodynamically significant stenoses, the arterial pressure in the leg is decreased. Thus, if one were to obtain a ratio of the ankle and brachial artery pressures, it would be >1.0 in normal individuals and <1.0 in patients with occlusive disease. A ratio of <0.5 is consistent with severe ischemia.

Treadmill testing allows the physician to assess functional limitations objectively. Decline of the ankle-brachial systolic pressure ratio immediately after exercise may provide further support for the diagnosis of arterial occlusive disease in patients with equivocal symptoms and findings on examination. Exercise testing also allows simultaneous evaluation for the presence of coronary artery disease.

Contrast angiography should not be used for routine diagnostic testing but is performed prior to potential revascularization. It is useful in defining the anatomy to assist operative planning and is also indicated if nonsurgical interventions are being considered, such as percutaneous transluminal angioplasty or thrombolysis. Recent studies have suggested that magnetic resonance angiography has diagnostic accuracy comparable to that of contrast angiography.

Prognosis The natural history of patients with peripheral arterial occlusive disease is influenced primarily by the extent of coexisting coronary artery and cerebral vascular disease. Studies using coronary angiography have estimated that approximately one-half of patients with symptomatic peripheral arterial occlusive disease also have significant coronary artery disease. Life-table analysis has indicated that patients with claudication have a 70 percent 5-year and a 50 percent 10-year survival rate. Most deaths are either sudden or secondary to myocardial infarction. The likelihood of symptomatic progression of peripheral arterial occlusive disease appears less than the chance of succumbing to coronary artery disease. Approximately 70 percent of nondiabetic patients who present with mild to moderate claudication remain symptomatically stable. Improvement may occur in 10 to 15 percent of patients; deterioration is likely to occur in the remainder, with approximately 5 percent of the group ultimately undergoing amputation. The prognosis is worse in patients who continue to smoke cigarettes or who have diabetes mellitus.

℞ TREATMENT

Therapeutic options include supportive measures, pharmacologic treatment, nonoperative interventions, and surgery. Supportive measures include meticulous care of the feet, which should be kept clean and protected against excessive drying with moisturizing creams. Well-fitting and protective shoes are advised to reduce trauma. Sandals and shoes made of synthetic materials that do not "breathe" should be avoided. Elastic support hose should be avoided, as they reduce blood flow to the skin. In patients with ischemia at rest, shock blocks under the head of the bed together with a canopy over the feet may improve perfusion pressure and ameliorate some of the rest pain.

Treatment of associated factors that contribute to the development of atherosclerosis should be initiated. The importance of discontinuing cigarette smoking cannot be overemphasized. The physician must assume a major role in this life-style modification. It is important to control blood pressure in hypertensive patients but to avoid hypotensive levels. Treatment of hypercholesterolemia is advocated, although reduction in cholesterol levels has not been shown unequivocally to reverse peripheral atherosclerotic lesions. However, it has been shown to prevent or to slow progression of the disease and to improve survival in patients with coronary atherosclerosis. Patients with claudication also should be encouraged to exercise regularly and at progressively more strenuous levels. Supervised exercise training programs may improve muscle efficiency and prolong walking distance. Patients also should be advised to walk for 30 to 45 min daily, stopping at the onset of claudication and resting until the symptoms resolve before resuming ambulation. Other forms of exercise, such as bicycle riding and swimming, provide overall cardiovascular and psychological benefit and often are tolerated better than walking.

Pharmacologic Management This form of treatment of patients with peripheral arterial occlusive disease has not been as successful as the medical treatment of coronary artery disease (Chap. 244). In particular, vasodilators as a class have not proved to be beneficial. During exercise, peripheral vasodilation occurs normally distal to sites of significant arterial stenoses. As a result, perfusion pressure falls, often to levels less than that generated in the interstitial tissue by the exercising muscle. Drugs such as alpha-adrenergic blocking agents, calcium channel antagonists, papaverine, and other vasodilators have not been shown to be effective in patients with occlusive arterial disease. Pentoxifylline, a substituted xanthine derivative, has been reported to decrease blood viscosity and to increase red cell flexibility, thereby increasing blood flow to the microcircula-

tion and enhancing tissue oxygenation. Several placebo-controlled studies have reported that pentoxifylline increased the duration of exercise in patients with claudication, but its efficacy has not been confirmed in all clinical trials. Preliminary studies suggest that long-term parenteral administration of vasodilator prostaglandins decreases pain and facilitates healing of ulcers in patients with severe limb ischemia and improves walking distance in patients with claudication.

Platelet inhibitors, particularly aspirin, have been reported to decrease progression of atherosclerosis in patients with peripheral arterial occlusive disease. Aspirin also reduces the risk of adverse cardiovascular events in patients with peripheral atherosclerosis. Ticlopidine, a drug that inhibits platelet aggregation via its effect on ADP-dependent platelet-fibrinogen binding, also reduces cardiovascular morbidity and mortality in patients with claudication. The anticoagulants heparin and warfarin have not been shown to be effective in patients with chronic arterial occlusive disease but may be useful in acute arterial obstruction secondary to thrombosis or systemic embolism. Similarly, thrombolytic intervention using drugs such as streptokinase, urokinase, or recombinant tissue plasminogen activator may have a role in the treatment of acute thrombotic arterial occlusion but is not effective in patients with chronic arterial occlusion secondary to atherosclerosis.

Revascularization Revascularization procedures, including nonoperative as well as operative interventions, are usually reserved for patients with progressive, severe, or disabling symptoms and ischemia at rest, as well as for individuals who must be symptom-free because of their occupation. Angiography should be performed mainly in patients who are being considered for a revascularization procedure. Nonoperative interventions include percutaneous transluminal angioplasty (PTA), laser angioplasty, atherectomy, and stent placement (Chap. 245). PTA of the iliac artery is associated with a higher success rate than PTA of the femoral and popliteal arteries. Approximately 90 to 95 percent of iliac PTAs are initially successful, and the 3-year patency rate is in excess of 75 percent. Patency rates may be higher if a stent is placed in the iliac artery. The initial success rate for femoral-popliteal PTA is approximately 80 percent, with a 60 percent 3-year patency rate. Patency rates are influenced by the severity of pretreatment stenoses; the prognosis of total occlusive lesions is worse than that of nonocclusive stenotic lesions. Laser angioplasty usually is used in conjunction with PTA and results in similar patency rates. The efficacy of percutaneous atherectomy and stent placement is being addressed in clinical trials.

Several operative procedures are available for treating patients with aortoiliac and femoral-popliteal artery disease. The preferred operative procedure depends on the location and extent of the obstruction(s) and general medical condition of the patient. Operative procedures for aortoiliac disease include aortobifemoral bypass, axillofemoral bypass, femoral-femoral bypass, and aortoiliac endarterectomy. The most frequently used procedure is the aortobifemoral bypass using knitted Dacron grafts. Immediate graft patency approaches 99 percent, and 5- and 10-year graft patency in survivors is in excess of 90 and 80 percent, respectively. Operative complications include myocardial infarction and stroke, infection of the graft, peripheral embolization, and sexual dysfunction from interruption of autonomic nerves in the pelvis. Operative mortality ranges from 1 to 3 percent, mostly due to ischemic heart disease.

Operative therapy for femoral-popliteal artery disease includes in situ and reverse autogenous saphenous vein bypass grafts, placement of polytetrafluoroethylene (PTFE) or other synthetic grafts, and thromboendarterectomy. Operative mortality ranges from 1 to 3 percent. The long-term patency rate depends on the type of graft used, the location of the distal anastomosis, and the patency of runoff vessels beyond the anastomosis. Patency rates of femoral-popliteal saphenous vein bypass grafts at 1 year approach 90 percent and at 5 years, 70 to 80 percent. Five-year patency rates of infrapopliteal saphenous vein bypass grafts are 60 to 70 percent. In contrast, 5-year patency rates of infrapopliteal PTFE grafts are less than 30 percent. Lumbar sympathectomy alone or as an adjunct to aortofemoral reconstruction has fallen into disfavor.

Preoperative cardiac risk assessment may identify individuals especially likely to experience an adverse cardiac event during the perioperative period. Patients with angina, prior myocardial infarction, ventricular ectopy, or heart failure are among those at increased risk. Noninvasive tests, such as treadmill testing (if feasible), dipyridamole thallium or Sesta-MIBI scintigraphy, and ambulatory ischemia monitoring permit further stratification of patient risk. Patients with abnormal test results require close supervision and adjunctive management with antianginal medications. It is not known whether coronary angiography and coronary arterial revascularization reduce overall perioperative mortality in high-risk patients undergoing peripheral vascular surgery, but these procedures should be considered in patients suspected of having left main or three-vessel coronary artery disease.

FIBROMUSCULAR DYSPLASIA   This is a hyperplastic disorder affecting medium-sized and small arteries. It occurs predominantly in females and usually involves renal and carotid arteries but can affect extremity vessels such as the iliac and subclavian arteries. The histologic classification includes intimal, medial, and periadventitial dysplasia. Medial dysplasia is the most common type and is characterized by hyperplasia of the media with or without fibrosis of the elastic membrane. It is identified angiographically by a "string of beads" appearance caused by thickened fibromuscular ridges contiguous with thin, less involved portions of the arterial wall. When limb vessels are involved, clinical manifestations are similar to those for atherosclerosis, including claudication and rest pain. PTA and surgical reconstruction have been beneficial in patients with debilitating symptoms or threatened limbs.

THROMBOANGIITIS OBLITERANS   Thromboangiitis obliterans (Buerger's disease) is an inflammatory occlusive vascular disorder involving small and medium-sized arteries and veins in the distal upper and lower extremities. Cerebral, visceral, and coronary vessels also may be affected. This disorder develops most frequently in men under age 40. The prevalence is higher in Asians and individuals of eastern European descent. While the cause of thromboangiitis obliterans is not known, there is a definite relationship to cigarette smoking and an increased incidence of HLA-B5 and -A9 antigens in patients with this disorder.

In the initial stages of thromboangiitis obliterans, polymorphonuclear leukocytes infiltrate the walls of the small and medium-sized arteries and veins. The internal elastic lamina is preserved, and thrombus may develop in the vascular lumen. As the disease progresses, mononuclear cells, fibroblasts, and giant cells replace the neutrophils. Later stages are characterized by perivascular fibrosis and recanalization.

The clinical features of thromboangiitis obliterans often include a triad of claudication of the affected extremity, Raynaud's phenomenon (p. 1401), and migratory superficial vein thrombophlebitis. Claudication is usually confined to the lower calves and feet or the forearms and hands, because this disorder primarily affects distal vessels. In the presence of severe digital ischemia, trophic nail changes, painful ulcerations, and gangrene may develop at the tips of the fingers. The physical examination shows normal brachial and popliteal pulses but reduced or absent radial, ulnar, and/or tibial pulses. Arteriography is helpful in making the diagnosis. Smooth, tapering segmental lesions in the distal vessels are characteristic, as are collateral vessels at sites of vascular occlusion. Proximal atherosclerotic disease is usually absent. The diagnosis can be confirmed by excisional biopsy and pathologic examination of an involved vessel.

There is no specific treatment except abstention from tobacco. The prognosis is worse in individuals who continue to smoke, but results are discouraging even in those who do stop smoking. Arterial bypass of the larger vessels may be used in selected instances, as well as local debridement, depending on the symptoms and severity of ischemia. Antibiotics may be useful; anticoagulants and glucocorticoids are not helpful. If these measures fail, amputation may be required.

VASCULITIS   Other vasculitides may affect the arteries supplying the upper and lower extremities. Takayasu's arteritis and giant cell (temporal) arteritis are discussed in Chap. 319.

ACUTE ARTERIAL OCCLUSION   This results in the sudden cessation of blood flow to an extremity. The severity of ischemia and the viability of the extremity depend on the location and extent of the occlusion and the presence and subsequent development of collateral blood vessels. There are two principal causes of acute arterial occlusion: embolism and thrombus in situ.

The most common sources of arterial emboli are the heart, aorta, and large arteries. Cardiac disorders that cause thromboembolism include atrial fibrillation, both chronic and paroxysmal; acute myocardial infarction; ventricular aneurysm; cardiomyopathy; infectious and marantic endocarditis; prosthetic heart valves; and atrial myxoma. Emboli to the distal vessels also may originate from proximal sites of atherosclerosis and aneurysms of the aorta and large vessels. Less frequently, an arterial occlusion results paradoxically from a venous thrombus that has entered the systemic circulation via a patent foramen ovale or other septal defect. Arterial emboli tend to lodge at vessel bifurcations because the vessel caliber decreases at these sites; in the lower extremities, emboli lodge most frequently in the femoral artery, followed by the iliac artery, aorta, and popliteal and tibioperoneal arteries.

Acute arterial thrombosis in situ occurs most frequently in atherosclerotic vessels at the site of a stenosis or aneurysm and in arterial bypass grafts. Trauma to an artery also may result in the formation of an acute arterial thrombus. Arterial occlusion may complicate arterial punctures and placement of catheters. Less frequent causes include the thoracic outlet compression syndrome, which causes subclavian artery occlusion, and entrapment of the popliteal artery by abnormal placement of the medial head of the gastrocnemius muscle. Polycythemia and hypercoagulable disorders (Chaps. 111 and 119) are also associated with acute arterial thrombosis.

Clinical Features   The symptoms of an acute arterial occlusion depend on the location, duration, and severity of the obstruction. Often, severe pain, paresthesia, numbness, and coldness develop in the involved extremity within 1 h. Paralysis may occur with severe and persistent ischemia. Physical findings include loss of pulses distal to the occlusion, cyanosis or pallor, mottling, decreased skin temperature, muscle stiffening, loss of sensation, weakness, and/or absent deep tendon reflexes. If acute arterial occlusion occurs in the presence of an adequate collateral circulation, as is often the case in acute graft occlusion, the symptoms and findings may be less impressive. In this situation, the patient complains about an abrupt decrease in the distance walked before claudication occurs or of modest pain and paresthesia. Pallor and coolness are evident, but sensory and motor functions are generally preserved. The diagnosis of acute arterial occlusion is usually apparent from the clinical presentation. Arteriography is useful for confirming the diagnosis and demonstrating the location and extent of occlusion.

℞ **TREATMENT**

Once the diagnosis is made, the patient should be anticoagulated with intravenous heparin to prevent propagation of the clot. In cases of severe ischemia of recent onset, and particularly when limb viability is jeopardized, immediate intervention to ensure reperfusion is indicated. Surgical thromboembolectomy or arterial bypass procedures are used to restore blood flow to the ischemic extremity promptly, particularly when a large proximal vessel is occluded.

Intraarterial thrombolytic therapy is effective when acute arterial occlusion is caused by a thrombus in an atherosclerotic vessel or arterial bypass graft. Thrombolytic therapy also may be indicated when the patient's overall condition contraindicates surgical intervention or when smaller distal vessels are occluded, thus preventing surgical access. Intraarterial streptokinase is administered as a bolus injection of 25,000 to 250,000 IU followed by a continuous infusion of 5000 to 15,000 IU/h. One approach for administering intraarterial urokinase is to give a bolus of 150,000 to 250,000 IU followed by 240,000 IU/h for 2 h, 120,000 IU/h for 2 h, and then 60,000 IU/h. Clinical trials are now in progress to assess the efficacy of intraarterial recombinant tissue plasminogen activator (tPA). Meticulous observation for hemorrhagic complications is required during intraarterial thrombolytic therapy.

If the limb is not in jeopardy, a more conservative approach that includes observation and administration of anticoagulants may be taken. Anticoagulation prevents recurrent embolism and reduces the likelihood of thrombus propagation. It can be initiated with intravenous heparin and followed by oral warfarin. Recommended dosages are the same as those used for deep vein thrombosis (see later). Emboli resulting from infectious endocarditis, the presence of prosthetic heart valves, or atrial myxoma often require surgical intervention to remove the cause.

ATHEROEMBOLISM   Atheroembolism constitutes a subset of acute arterial occlusion. In this condition, multiple small deposits of fibrin, platelet, and cholesterol debris embolize from proximal atherosclerotic lesions or aneurysmal sites. Atheroembolism may occur after intraarterial procedures. Since the emboli tend to lodge in the small vessels of the muscle and skin and may not occlude the large vessels, distal pulses usually remain palpable. Patients complain of acute pain and tenderness at the site of embolization. Digital vascular occlusion may result in ischemia and the "blue toe" syndrome; digital necrosis and gangrene may develop. Localized areas of tenderness, pallor, and livedo reticularis (see below) occur at sites of emboli. Skin or muscle biopsy may demonstrate cholesterol crystals.

Ischemia resulting from atheroemboli is notoriously difficult to treat. Usually neither surgical revascularization procedures nor thrombolytic therapy is helpful because of the multiplicity, composition, and distal location of the emboli. Some evidence suggests that platelet inhibitors prevent atheroembolism. Surgical intervention to remove or bypass the atherosclerotic vessel or aneurysm that causes the recurrent atheroemboli may be necessary.

THORACIC OUTLET COMPRESSION SYNDROME   This is a symptom complex resulting from compression of the neurovascular bundle (artery, vein, or nerves) at the thoracic outlet as it courses through the neck and shoulder. Cervical ribs, abnormalities of the scalenus anticus muscle, proximity of the clavicle to the first rib, or abnormal insertion of the pectoralis minor muscle may compress the subclavian artery and brachial plexus as these structures pass from the thorax to the arm. Patients may develop shoulder and arm pain, weakness, paresthesia, claudication, Raynaud's phenomenon, and even ischemic tissue loss and gangrene. Examination is often normal unless provocative maneuvers are performed. Occasionally, distal pulses are decreased or absent and digital cyanosis and ischemia may be evident. Tenderness may be present in the supraclavicular fossa. Abducting the affected arm by 90° and externally rotating the shoulder may precipitate symptoms. Several additional maneuvers are used to confirm the diagnosis of vascular compression and to suggest the location of the abnormality. These include the scalene maneuver (extension of the neck and rotation of the head to the side of the symptoms), the costoclavicular maneuver (posterior rotation of shoulders), and the hyperabduction maneuver (raising the arm 180°), which may cause subclavian bruits and loss of pulses in the arm. A chest x-ray will indicate the presence of cervical ribs. The electromyogram will be abnormal if the brachial plexus is involved.

℞ TREATMENT
Most patients can be managed conservatively. They should be advised to avoid the positions that cause symptoms. Many patients benefit from shoulder girdle exercises. Surgical procedures such as removal of the first rib or resection of the scalenus anticus muscle are necessary occasionally for relief of symptoms or treatment of ischemia.

ARTERIOVENOUS FISTULA   Abnormal communications between an artery and a vein, bypassing the capillary bed, may be congenital or acquired. Congenital arteriovenous fistulas are the result of persistent embryonic vessels that fail to differentiate into arteries and veins; they may be associated with birthmarks, can be located in almost any organ of the body, and frequently occur in the extremities. Acquired arteriovenous fistulas are either created to provide vascular access for hemodialysis or occur as a result of a penetrating injury such as a gunshot or knife wound or as complications of arterial catheterization or surgical dissection. An infrequent cause of arteriovenous fistula is rupture of an arterial aneurysm into a vein.

The clinical features depend on the location and size of the fistula. Frequently, a pulsatile mass is palpable, and a thrill and bruit lasting throughout systole and diastole are present over the fistula. With long-standing fistulas, clinical manifestations of chronic venous insufficiency, including peripheral edema, large, tortuous varicose veins, and stasis pigmentation become apparent because of the high venous pressure. Evidence of ischemia may occur in the distal portion of the extremity. Skin temperature is higher over the arteriovenous fistula. Large arteriovenous fistulas may result in an increased cardiac output with consequent cardiomegaly and high-output heart failure (Chap. 233).

Diagnosis   The diagnosis is often evident from the physical examination. Compression of a large arteriovenous fistula may cause reflex slowing of the heart rate (Nicoladoni-Branham sign). Arteriography can confirm the diagnosis and is useful in demonstrating the site and size of the arteriovenous fistula.

℞ TREATMENT
Management of arteriovenous fistulas may involve surgery, radiotherapy, or embolization. Congenital arteriovenous fistulas are often difficult to treat because the communications may be numerous and extensive, and new ones frequently develop after ligation of the most obvious ones. Many of these lesions are best treated conservatively using elastic support hose to reduce the consequences of venous hypertension. Occasionally, embolization with autologous material, such as fat or muscle, or with hemostatic agents, such as gelatin sponges or silicon spheres, is used to obliterate the fistula. Acquired arteriovenous fistulas are usually amenable to surgical treatment that involves division or excision of the fistula. Occasionally, autogenous or synthetic grafting is necessary to reestablish continuity of the artery and vein.

RAYNAUD'S PHENOMENON   Raynaud's phenomenon is characterized by episodic digital ischemia, manifested clinically by the sequential development of digital blanching, cyanosis, and rubor of the fingers or toes following cold exposure and subsequent rewarming. Emotional stress also may precipitate Raynaud's phenomenon. The color changes are usually well demarcated and are confined to the fingers or toes. Typically, one or more digits will appear white when the patient is exposed to a cold environment or touches a cold object. The blanching, or pallor, represents the ischemic phase of the phenomenon and results from vasospasm of digital arteries. During the ischemic phase, capillaries and venules dilate, and cyanosis results from the deoxygenated blood that is present in these vessels. A sensation of cold or numbness or paresthesia of the digits often accompanies the phases of pallor and cyanosis.

With rewarming, the digital vasospasm resolves, and blood flow into the dilated arterioles and capillaries increases dramatically. This "reactive hyperemia" imparts a bright red color to the digits. In addition to rubor and warmth, patients often experience a throbbing, painful sensation during the hyperemic phase. Although the triphasic color response is typical of Raynaud's phenomenon, some patients may develop only pallor and cyanosis; others may experience only cyanosis.

Pathophysiology   Raynaud originally proposed that cold-induced episodic digital ischemia was secondary to exaggerated reflex sympathetic vasoconstriction. This theory is supported by the fact that alpha-adrenergic blocking drugs as well as sympathectomy decrease the frequency and severity of Raynaud's phenomenon in some patients. An alternative hypothesis is that the digital vascular responsiveness to cold or to normal sympathetic stimuli is enhanced. It is also possible that normal reflex sympathetic vasoconstriction is superimposed on local digital vascular disease or that there is enhanced adrenergic neuroeffector activity.

Raynaud's phenomenon is broadly separated into two categories: the idiopathic variety, termed *Raynaud's disease*, and the secondary variety, which is associated with other disease states or known causes of vasospasm (Table 248-1).

Raynaud's Disease This appellation is applied when the secondary causes of Raynaud's phenomenon have been excluded. Over 50 percent of patients with Raynaud's phenomenon have Raynaud's disease. Women are affected about five times more often than men, and the age of presentation is usually between 20 and 40 years. The fingers are involved more frequently than the toes. Initial episodes may involve only one or two fingertips, but subsequent attacks may involve the entire finger and may include all the fingers. The toes are affected in 40 percent of patients. Although vasospasm of the toes usually occurs in patients with symptoms in the fingers, it may happen alone. Rarely, the earlobes and the tip of the nose are involved. Raynaud's phenomenon occurs frequently in patients who also have migraine headaches or variant angina. These associations suggest that there may be a common predisposing cause for the vasospasm.

Results of physical examination often are entirely normal; the radial, ulnar, and pedal pulses are normal. The fingers and toes may be cool between attacks and may perspire excessively. Thickening and tightening of the digital subcutaneous tissue (sclerodactyly) develop in 10 percent of patients. Angiography of the digits for diagnostic purposes is not indicated.

In general, patients with Raynaud's disease appear to have the milder forms of Raynaud's phenomenon. Less than 1 percent of these patients lose a part of a digit. After the diagnosis is made, the disease spontaneously improves in approximately 15 percent of patients and progresses in about 30 percent.

Secondary Causes of Raynaud's Phenomenon Raynaud's phenomenon occurs in 80 to 90 percent of patients with systemic sclerosis (scleroderma) and is the presenting symptom in 30 percent (Chap. 314). It may be the only symptom of scleroderma for many years. Abnormalities of the digital vessels may contribute to the development of Raynaud's phenomenon in this disorder. Ischemic fingertip ulcers may develop and progress to gangrene and autoamputation. About 20 percent of patients with systemic lupus erythematosus (SLE) have Raynaud's phenomenon (Chap. 312). Occasionally, persistent digital ischemia develops and may result in ulcers or gangrene. In most severe cases, the small vessels are occluded by a proliferative endarteritis.

Table 248-1

Classification of Raynaud's Phenomenon

Primary or idiopathic Raynaud's phenomenon: Raynaud's disease
Secondary Raynaud's phenomenon
  Collagen vascular diseases: scleroderma, systemic lupus erythematosus, rheumatoid arthritis, dermatomyositis, polymyositis
  Arterial occlusive diseases: atherosclerosis of the extremities, thromboangiitis obliterans, acute arterial occlusion, thoracic outlet syndrome
  Pulmonary hypertension
  Neurologic disorders: intervertebral disk disease, syringomyelia, spinal cord tumors, stroke, poliomyelitis, carpal tunnel syndrome
  Blood dyscrasias: cold agglutinins, cryoglobulinemia, cryofibrinogenemia, myeloproliferative disorders, Waldenström's macroglobulinemia
  Trauma: vibration injury, hammer hand syndrome, electric shock, cold injury, typing, piano playing
  Drugs: ergot derivatives, methysergide, beta-adrenergic receptor blockers, bleomycin, vinblastine, cisplatin

Raynaud's phenomenon occurs in about 30 percent of patients with dermatomyositis or polymyositis (Chap. 315). It frequently develops in patients with rheumatoid arthritis and may be related to the intimal proliferation that occurs in the digital arteries.

Atherosclerosis of the extremities is a frequent cause of Raynaud's phenomenon in men over age 50. Thromboangiitis obliterans is an uncommon cause of Raynaud's phenomenon but should be considered in young men, particularly in those who are cigarette smokers. The development of cold-induced pallor in these disorders may be confined to one or two digits of the involved extremity. Occasionally, Raynaud's phenomenon may follow acute occlusion of large and medium-sized arteries by a thrombus or embolus. Embolization of atheroembolic debris may cause digital ischemia. The latter situation often involves one or two digits and should not be confused with Raynaud's phenomenon. In patients with the thoracic outlet syndrome, Raynaud's phenomenon may result from diminished intravascular pressure, stimulation of sympathetic fibers in the brachial plexus, or a combination of both. Raynaud's phenomenon occurs in patients with primary pulmonary hypertension (Chap. 260); this is more than coincidental and may reflect a neurohumoral abnormality that affects both the pulmonary and digital circulations.

A variety of blood dyscrasias may be associated with Raynaud's phenomenon. Cold-induced precipitation of plasma proteins, hyperviscosity, and aggregation of red cells and platelets may occur in patients with cold agglutinins, cryoglobulinemia, or cryofibrinogenemia. Hyperviscosity syndromes that accompany myeloproliferative disorders and Waldenström's macroglobulinemia also should be considered in the initial evaluation of patients with Raynaud's phenomenon.

Raynaud's phenomenon occurs often in patients whose vocations require the use of vibrating hand tools, such as chain saws or jackhammers. The frequency of Raynaud's phenomenon also seems to be increased in pianists and typists. Electric shock injury to the hands or frostbite may lead to the later development of Raynaud's phenomenon.

Several drugs have been causally implicated in Raynaud's phenomenon. These include ergot preparations, methysergide, beta-adrenergic receptor antagonists, and the chemotherapeutic agents bleomycin, vinblastine, and cisplatin.

TREATMENT

Most patients with Raynaud's phenomenon experience only mild and infrequent episodes. These patients need reassurance and should be instructed to dress warmly and avoid unnecessary cold exposure. In addition to gloves and mittens, patients should protect the trunk, head, and feet with warm clothing to prevent cold-induced reflex vasoconstriction. Tobacco use is contraindicated.

Drug treatment should be reserved for the severe cases. The calcium channel antagonists, especially nifedipine (10 to 30 mg tid) and diltiazem (30 to 90 mg tid), decrease the frequency and severity of Raynaud's phenomenon. Long-acting preparations of these drugs also may be effective. Adrenergic blocking agents, such as reserpine (0.25 to 0.5 mg qid), have been shown to increase nutritional blood flow to the fingers. Some, but not all, patients achieve satisfactory results with long-term reserpine therapy. Moreover, systemic use of this drug is limited by side effects of hypotension, nasal stuffiness, lethargy, and depression. The postsynaptic alpha$_1$-adrenergic antagonist prazosin (1 to 5 mg tid) has been used with favorable responses. Doxazosin and terazosin also may be effective. Other sympatholytic agents, such as methyldopa, guanethidine, and phenoxybenzamine, may be useful in some patients. Treatment with vasodilator prostaglandins is under investigation, and has been reported to improve symptoms in patients with scleroderma. Surgical sympathectomy is helpful in some patients who are unresponsive to medical therapy, but benefit is often transient.

ACROCYANOSIS In this condition, there is arterial vasoconstriction and secondary dilation of the capillaries and venules with resulting persistent cyanosis of the hands and, less frequently, the feet. Cyanosis may be intensified by exposure to a cold environment. Women are affected much more frequently than men, and the age of onset is usually less than 30 years. Generally, patients are asymptomatic but seek medical attention because of the discoloration. Examination reveals normal pulses, peripheral cyanosis, and moist palms. Trophic skin changes and ulcerations do *not* occur. The disorder can be distinguished from Raynaud's phenomenon because it is persistent and not episodic, the discoloration extends proximally from the digits, and blanching does not occur. Ischemia secondary to arterial occlusive disease usually can be excluded by the presence of normal pulses. Central cyanosis and decreased arterial oxygen saturation are not present. Patients should be reassured and advised to dress warmly and avoid cold exposure. Pharmacologic intervention is not indicated.

LIVEDO RETICULARIS In this condition, localized areas of the extremities develop a mottled or netlike appearance of reddish to blue discoloration. The mottled appearance may be more prominent following cold exposure. The idiopathic form of this disorder occurs equally in men and women, and the most common age of onset is in the third decade. Patients with the idiopathic form usually are asymptomatic and seek attention for cosmetic reasons. Livedo reticularis also can occur following atheroembolism (see above). Rarely, skin ulcerations develop. Patients should be reassured and advised to avoid cold environments. No drug treatment is indicated.

PERNIO (CHILBLAINS) This is a vasculitic disorder associated with exposure to cold; acute forms have been described. Raised erythematous lesions develop on the lower part of the legs and feet in cold weather. These are associated with pruritus and a burning sensation, and they may blister and ulcerate. Pathologic examination demonstrates angiitis characterized by intimal proliferation and perivascular infiltration of mononuclear and polymorphonuclear leukocytes. Giant cells may be present in the subcutaneous tissue. Patients should avoid exposure to cold, and ulcers should be kept clean and protected with sterile dressings. Sympatholytic drugs may be effective in some patients.

ERYTHROMELALGIA (ERYTHERMALGIA) This disorder is characterized by burning pain and erythema of the extremities. The feet are involved more frequently than the hands, and males are affected more frequently than females. Erythromelalgia may occur at any age but is most common in middle age. It may be primary or secondary to disorders such as hypertension, polycythemia vera, essential thrombocytosis, or it may occur as an adverse effect of drugs such as nifedipine or bromocriptine. Patients complain of burning in the extremities that is precipitated by exposure to a warm environment and aggravated by a dependent position. The symptoms are relieved by exposing the affected area to cool air or water or by elevation. Erythromelalgia can be distinguished from ischemia secondary to arterial occlusive disorders and peripheral neuropathy because the peripheral pulses are present and the neurologic examination is normal. There is no specific treatment; aspirin may produce relief in patients with erythromelalgia secondary to myeloproliferative disease. Treatment of associated disorders in secondary erythromelalgia may be helpful.

FROSTBITE In this condition, tissue damage results from severe environmental cold exposure or from direct contact with a very cold object. Tissue injury results from both freezing and vasoconstriction. Frostbite usually affects the distal aspects of the extremities or exposed parts of the face, such as the ears, nose, chin, and cheeks. Superficial frostbite involves the skin and subcutaneous tissue. Patients experience pain or paresthesia, and the skin appears white and waxy. After rewarming, there is cyanosis and erythema, wheal and flare formation, edema, and superficial blisters. Deep frostbite involves muscle, nerves, and deeper blood vessels. It may result in edema of the hand or foot, vesicles and bullae, tissue necrosis, and gangrene.

Initial treatment is rewarming, performed in an environment where reexposure to freezing conditions will not occur. Rewarming is accomplished by immersion of the affected part in a water bath at temperatures of 40 to 44°C (104 to 111°F). Massage, application of ice water, and extreme heat are contraindicated. The injured area should be cleansed with soap or antiseptic and sterile dressings applied. Analgesics are often required during rewarming. Antibiotics are used if there is evidence of infection. The efficacy of sympathetic blocking drugs is not established. Following recovery, the affected extremity may exhibit increased sensitivity to cold.

VENOUS DISORDERS

Veins in the extremities can be broadly classified as either superficial or deep. In the lower extremity, the superficial venous system includes the greater and lesser saphenous veins and their tributaries. The deep veins of the leg accompany the major arteries. Perforating veins connect the superficial and deep systems at multiple locations. Bicuspid valves are present throughout the venous system to direct the flow of venous blood centrally.

VENOUS THROMBOSIS The presence of thrombus within a superficial or deep vein and the accompanying inflammatory response in the vessel wall is termed *venous thrombosis* or *thrombophlebitis*. Initially, the thrombus is composed principally of platelets and fibrin. Red cells become interspersed with fibrin, and the thrombus tends to propagate in the direction of blood flow. The inflammatory response in the vessel wall may be minimal or characterized by granulocyte infiltration, loss of endothelium, and edema.

The factors that predispose to venous thrombosis were initially described by Virchow in 1856 and include stasis, vascular damage, and hypercoagulability. Accordingly, a variety of clinical situations are associated with increased risk of venous thrombosis (Table 248-2). Venous thrombosis may occur in more than 50 percent of patients having orthopedic surgical procedures, particularly those involving the hip or knee, and in 10 to 40 percent of patients who undergo abdominal or thoracic operations. The prevalence of venous thrombosis is particularly high in patients with cancer of the pancreas, lungs, genitourinary tract, stomach, and breast. Approximately 10 to 20 percent of patients with idiopathic deep vein thrombosis have or develop clinically overt cancer; there is no consensus on whether these individuals should be subjected to intensive diagnostic workup to search for occult malignancy. Risk of thrombosis is increased following trauma, such as fractures of the spine, pelvis, femur, and tibia. Immobilization, regardless of the underlying disease, is a major predisposing cause of venous thrombosis. This fact may account for the relatively high incidence in patients with acute myocardial infarction or congestive heart failure. The incidence of venous thrombosis is increased during pregnancy, particularly in the third trimester and in the first month postpartum, and in individuals who use estrogens. A variety of clinical disorders that produce systemic hypercoagulability, including resistance to activated protein C (factor V Leiden); antithrombin III, protein C, and protein S deficiencies; antiphospholipid syndrome; systemic lupus erythematosus; myeloproliferative diseases; dysfibrinogenemia; and disseminated intravascular coagulation, may cause venous thrombosis. Venulitis occurring in thromboangiitis obliterans, Behçet's disease, and homocysteinuria also may cause venous thrombosis.

Table 248-2

Conditions Associated with an Increased Risk for Development of Venous Thrombosis

Surgery
  Orthopedic, thoracic, abdominal, and genitourinary procedures
Neoplasms
  Pancreas, lung, ovary, testes, urinary tract, breast, stomach
Trauma
  Fractures of spine, pelvis, femur, or tibia; spinal cord injuries
Immobilization
  Acute myocardial infarction, congestive heart failure, stroke, postoperative convalescence
Pregnancy
Estrogen use (for replacement or contraception)
Hypercoagulable states
  Resistance to activated protein C; deficiencies of antithrombin III, protein C, or protein S; antiphospholipid antibodies; myeloproliferative diseases; dysfibrinogenemia; disseminated intravascular coagulation
Venulitis
  Thromboangiitis obliterans, Behçet's disease, homocysteinuria
Previous deep vein thrombosis

DEEP VENOUS THROMBOSIS   The most important consequences of this disorder are pulmonary embolism (Chap. 261) and the syndrome of chronic venous insufficiency. Deep thrombosis of the iliac, femoral, or popliteal veins is suggested by unilateral leg swelling, warmth, and erythema. Tenderness may be present along the course of the involved veins, and a cord may be palpable. There may be increased tissue turgor, distension of superficial veins, and the appearance of prominent venous collaterals. In some patients, deoxygenated hemoglobin in stagnant veins imparts a cyanotic hue to the limb, a condition called *phlegmasia cerulea dolens*. In markedly edematous legs, the interstitial tissue pressure may exceed the capillary perfusion pressure, causing pallor, a condition designated *phlegmasia alba dolens*.

The diagnosis of deep venous thrombosis of the calf is often difficult to make at the bedside. This is so because only one of multiple veins may be involved, allowing adequate venous return through the remaining patent vessels. The most common complaint is calf pain. Examination may reveal posterior calf tenderness, warmth, increased tissue turgor or modest swelling, and, rarely, a cord. Increased resistance or pain during dorsiflexion of the foot (Homans' sign) is an unreliable diagnostic sign.

Deep venous thrombosis occurs less frequently in the upper extremity than in the lower extremity, but the incidence is increasing because of greater utilization of indwelling central venous catheters. The clinical features and complications are similar to those described for the leg.

Diagnosis   The noninvasive test used most often to diagnose deep venous thrombosis is duplex venous ultrasonography (B-mode, i.e., two-dimensional, imaging and pulse-wave Doppler interrogation). By imaging the deep veins, thrombus can be detected either by direct visualization or by inference when the vein does not collapse on compressive maneuvers. The Doppler ultrasound measures the velocity of blood flow in veins. This velocity is normally affected by respiration and by manual compression of the foot or calf. Flow abnormalities occur when deep venous obstruction is present. The positive predictive value of duplex venous ultrasonography approaches 95 percent for proximal deep vein thrombosis. In the calf, because calf veins are more difficult to visualize than proximal veins, the sensitivity of this technique is only 50 to 75 percent, although its specificity is 95 percent.

Impedance plethysmography measures changes in venous capacitance during physiologic maneuvers. Venous obstruction blunts the normal changes in venous capacitance that occur following inflation and deflation of a thigh cuff. The predictive value of this test for detecting occlusive thrombi in proximal veins is approximately 90 percent. However, it is much less sensitive for diagnosing deep venous thrombosis of the calves.

Magnetic resonance imaging is another noninvasive means to detect deep vein thrombosis. Its diagnostic accuracy for assessing proximal deep vein thrombosis is similar to that of duplex ultrasonography. It is useful in patients with suspected thrombosis of the superior and inferior venae cavae or pelvic veins.

Deep venous thrombosis also can be diagnosed by venography. Contrast medium is injected into a superficial vein of the foot and directed to the deep system by the application of tourniquets. The presence of a filling defect or absence of filling of the deep veins is required to make the diagnosis.

Deep vein thrombosis must be differentiated from a variety of disorders that cause unilateral leg pain or swelling, including muscle rupture, trauma, or hemorrhage; a ruptured popliteal cyst; and lymphedema. It may be difficult to distinguish swelling caused by the postphlebitic syndrome from that due to acute recurrent deep venous thrombosis. Leg pain also may result from nerve compression, arthritis, tendinitis, fractures, and arterial occlusive disorders. A careful history and physical examination can usually determine the cause of these symptoms.

℞ **TREATMENT**

Anticoagulants (See also Chap. 261)   Prevention of pulmonary embolism is the most important reason for treating patients with deep vein thrombosis, since in the early stages the thrombus may be loose and poorly adherent to the vessel wall. Patients should be placed in bed, and the affected extremity should be elevated above the level of the heart until the edema and tenderness subside. Anticoagulants prevent thrombus propagation and allow the endogenous lytic system to operate. Heparin should be administered intravenously as an initial bolus of 7500 to 10,000 IU, followed by a continuous infusion of 1000 to 1500 IU/h. The rate of the heparin infusion should be adjusted so that the activated partial thromboplastin time (aPTT) is approximately twice the control value. Subcutaneous injection of heparin has been used as an alternative form of therapy. In less than 5 percent of patients, heparin therapy may cause thrombocytopenia. Infrequently, these patients develop arterial thrombosis and ischemia. Heparin treatment should be maintained for at least 5 to 7 days. Low-molecular-weight (4000 to 6000 daltons) heparins are reported to be as effective as or better than conventional, unfractionated heparin in preventing extension or recurrence of venous thrombosis. Depending on the specific preparation, low-molecular-weight heparin is administered subcutaneously, in fixed doses, once or twice daily. The incidence of thrombocytopenia is less with low-molecular-weight heparin than with conventional preparations. Warfarin is administered during the first week of treatment with heparin and may be started as early as the first day of heparin treatment if the aPTT is therapeutic. It is important to overlap heparin treatment with oral anticoagulant therapy for at least 4 to 5 days because the full anticoagulant effect of warfarin is delayed. The dose of warfarin should be adjusted to maintain the prothrombin time at an international normalized ratio (INR) of 2.0 to 3.0. The use of anticoagulants for isolated deep vein thrombosis of the calf is controversial. However, approximately 20 to 30 percent of calf thrombi propagate to the thigh, thereby increasing the risk of pulmonary embolism. Also, isolated calf vein thrombosis has been identified as a cause of embolic stroke via a patent foramen ovale.

Anticoagulant treatment is indicated for patients with proximal deep vein thrombosis, since pulmonary embolism may occur in approximately 50 percent of untreated individuals. The incidence of pulmonary embolism in patients presenting with deep calf vein thrombosis is 5 to 20 percent. Therefore, patients with calf vein thrombosis should either receive anticoagulants or be followed with serial noninvasive tests to determine whether proximal propagation has occurred. Anticoagulant treatment should be continued for 3 to 6 months for patients with acute idiopathic deep vein thrombosis and for those with a temporary risk factor for venous thrombosis to decrease the chance of recurrence. The duration of anticoagulant treatment for patients with calf vein thrombosis should be at least 6 weeks. The duration of treatment is indefinite for patients with recurrent deep vein thrombosis and for those in whom associated causes, such as malignancy or hypercoagulability, have not been eliminated. If treatment with anticoagulants is contraindicated because of a bleeding diathesis or risk of hemorrhage, protection from pulmonary embolism can be achieved by mechanically interrupting the flow of blood through the inferior vena cava. Inferior vena cava plication generally has been replaced by percutaneous insertion of a filter.

Thrombolytics   Thrombolytic drugs such as streptokinase, urokinase, and tissue plasminogen activator also may be used, but there is no evidence that thrombolytic therapy is more effective than anticoagulants in preventing pulmonary embolism. However, early administration of thrombolytic drugs may accelerate clot lysis, preserve venous valves, and decrease the potential for developing postphlebitic syndrome.

Prophylaxis   Prophylaxis should be considered in clinical situations where the risk of deep vein thrombosis is high. Low-dose heparin (5000 units 2 h prior to surgery and then 5000 units every 8 to 12 h postoperatively), warfarin, and external pneumatic compression are all useful. Low-dose heparin reduces the risk of deep vein thrombosis associated with thoracic and abdominal surgery and with prolonged bed rest. Low-molecular-weight heparins have been shown to prevent deep vein thrombosis in patients undergoing general or orthopedic surgery. They are said to be more effective than conventional heparin and to cause an equal or lower incidence of bleeding. Warfarin in a dose that yields a prothrombin time equivalent to an INR of 2.0 to 3.0 is effective in preventing deep vein thrombosis associated with bone fractures and orthopedic surgery. Warfarin is started the night before surgery and continued throughout the convalescent period. External pneumatic compression devices applied to the legs are used to prevent deep vein thrombosis when even low doses of heparin or warfarin might cause serious bleeding, as during neurosurgery or transurethral resection of the prostate.

SUPERFICIAL VEIN THROMBOSIS Thrombosis of the greater or lesser saphenous veins or their tributaries—i.e., superficial vein thrombosis—does not result in pulmonary embolism. It is associated with intravenous catheters and infusions, occurs in varicose veins, and may develop in association with deep vein thrombosis. Migrating superficial vein thrombosis is often a marker for a carcinoma and also may occur in patients with vasculitides, such as thromboangiitis obliterans. The clinical features of superficial vein thrombosis are easily distinguished from those of deep vein thrombosis. Patients complain of pain localized to the site of the thrombus. Examination reveals a reddened, warm, and tender cord extending along a superficial vein. The surrounding area may be red and edematous.

℞ TREATMENT

Treatment is primarily supportive. Initially, patients can be placed at bed rest with leg elevation and application of warm compresses. Nonsteroidal antiinflammatory drugs may provide analgesia but also may obscure clinical evidence of thrombus propagation. If a thrombosis of the greater saphenous vein develops in the thigh and extends toward the saphenofemoral vein junction, it is reasonable to consider anticoagulant therapy to prevent extension of the thrombus into the deep system and a possible pulmonary embolism.

VARICOSE VEINS Varicose veins are dilated, tortuous superficial veins that result from defective structure and function of the valves of the saphenous veins, from intrinsic weakness of the vein wall, from high intraluminal pressure, or, rarely, from arteriovenous fistulas. Varicose veins can be categorized as primary or secondary. Primary varicose veins originate in the superficial system and occur two to three times as frequently in women as in men. Approximately half of patients have a family history of varicose veins. Secondary varicose veins result from deep venous insufficiency and incompetent perforating veins or from deep venous occlusion causing enlargement of superficial veins that are serving as collaterals.

Patients with venous varicosities are often concerned about the cosmetic appearance of their legs. Symptoms consist of a dull ache or pressure sensation in the legs after prolonged standing; it is relieved with leg elevation. The legs feel heavy, and mild ankle edema develops occasionally. Extensive venous varicosities may cause skin ulcerations near the ankle. Superficial venous thrombosis may be a recurring problem, and, rarely, a varicosity ruptures and bleeds. Visual inspection of the legs in the dependent position usually confirms the presence of varicose veins.

Varicose veins usually can be treated with conservative measures. Symptoms often decrease when the legs are elevated periodically, when prolonged standing is avoided, and when elastic support hose are worn. External compression stockings provide a counterbalance to the hydrostatic pressure in the veins. Small symptomatic varicose veins can be treated with sclerotherapy, in which a sclerosing solution is injected into the involved varicose vein and a compression bandage is applied. Surgical therapy usually involves extensive ligation and stripping of the greater and lesser saphenous veins and should be reserved for patients who are very symptomatic, suffer recurrent superficial vein thrombosis, and/or develop skin ulceration. Surgical therapy also may be indicated for cosmetic reasons.

CHRONIC VENOUS INSUFFICIENCY Chronic venous insufficiency may result from deep vein thrombosis and/or valvular incompetence. Following deep vein thrombosis, the delicate valve leaflets become thickened and contracted so that they cannot prevent retrograde flow of blood; the vein becomes rigid and thick-walled. Although most veins recanalize after an episode of thrombosis, the large proximal veins may remain occluded. Secondary incompetence develops in distal valves because high pressures distend the vein and separate the leaflets. Primary deep venous valvular dysfunction also may occur without previous thrombosis. Patients with venous insufficiency often complain of a dull ache in the leg that worsens with prolonged standing and resolves with leg elevation. Examination demonstrates increased leg circumference, edema, and superficial varicose veins. Erythema, dermatitis, and hyperpigmentation develop along the distal aspect of the leg, and skin ulceration may occur near the medial and lateral malleoli. Cellulitis may be a recurring problem. Patients should be advised to avoid prolonged standing or sitting; frequent leg elevation is helpful. Graduated compression stockings should be worn during the day. These efforts should be intensified if skin ulcers develop. Ulcers should be treated with applications of wet to dry dressings and, occasionally, dilute topical antibiotic solutions. Commercially available dressings comprising antiseptic solutions and compressive bandages may be applied and should be changed weekly until healing occurs. Recurrent ulceration and severe edema may be treated by surgical interruption of incompetent communicating veins. Rarely, surgical valvuloplasty and bypass of venous occlusions are employed.

LYMPHATIC DISORDERS

Lymphatic capillaries are blind-ended tubes formed by a single layer of endothelial cells. The absent or widely fenestrated basement membrane of lymphatic capillaries allows access to interstitial proteins and particles. Lymphatic capillaries merge to form larger vessels which contain smooth muscle and are capable of vasomotion. Small and medium-sized lymphatic vessels empty into progressively larger channels, most of which drain into the thoracic duct. The lymphatic circulation is involved in the absorption of interstitial fluid and in the response to infection.

LYMPHEDEMA Lymphedema may be categorized as primary or secondary (Table 248-3). The prevalence of primary lymphedema is approximately 1 per 10,000 individuals. Primary lymphedema may be secondary to agenesis, hypoplasia, or obstruction of the lymphatic vessels. It may be associated with the Turner syndrome, the Noonan syndrome, the yellow nail syndrome, the intestinal lymphangiectasia syndrome, and lymphangiomyomatosis. Women are affected more frequently than men. There are three clinical subtypes: congenital lymphedema, which appears shortly after birth; lymphedema praecox, which has its onset at the time of puberty; and lymphedema tarda, which usually begins after age 35. Familial forms of congenital lymphedema (Milroy's disease) and lymphedema praecox (Meige's disease) may be inherited in an autosomal dominant manner with variable penetrance; autosomal or sex-linked recessive forms are less common.

Table 248-3

Causes of Lymphedema

Primary
    Congenital (includes Milroy's disease)
    Lymphedema praecox (includes Meige's disease)
    Lymphedema tarda
Secondary
    Recurrent lymphangitis
    Filariasis
    Tuberculosis
    Neoplasm
    Surgery
    Radiation therapy

Secondary lymphedema is an acquired condition resulting from damage to or obstruction of previously normal lymphatic channels (see Table 248-3). Recurrent episodes of bacterial lymphangitis, usually caused by streptococci, are a very common cause of lymphedema. The most common cause of secondary lymphedema worldwide is filariasis (Chap. 223). Tumors, such as prostate cancer and lymphoma, also can obstruct lymphatic vessels. Both surgery and radiation therapy for breast carcinoma may cause lymphedema of the upper extremity. Less common causes include tuberculosis, contact dermatitis, lymphogranuloma venereum, rheumatoid arthritis, pregnancy, and self-induced or factitious lymphedema following application of tourniquets.

Lymphedema is generally a painless condition, but patients may experience a chronic dull, heavy sensation in the leg, and most often they are concerned about the appearance of the leg. Lymphedema of the lower extremity, initially involving the foot, gradually progresses up the leg so that the entire limb becomes edematous. In the early stages, the edema is soft and pits easily with pressure. In the chronic stages, the limb has a woody texture, and the tissues become indurated and fibrotic. At this point the edema may no longer be pitting. The limb loses its normal contour, and the toes appear square. Lymphedema should be distinguished from other disorders that cause unilateral leg swelling, such as deep vein thrombosis and chronic venous insufficiency. In the latter condition, the edema is softer, and there is often evidence of a stasis dermatitis, hyperpigmentation, and superficial venous varicosities.

The evaluation of patients with lymphedema should include diagnostic studies to clarify the cause. Abdominal and pelvic ultrasound and computed tomography can be used to detect obstructing lesions such as neoplasms. Lymphoscintigraphy and lymphangiography are rarely indicated, but either can be used to confirm the diagnosis or to differentiate primary from secondary lymphedema. Lymphoscintigraphy involves the injection of radioactively labeled technetium-containing colloid into the distal subcutaneous tissue of the affected extremity. In lymphangiography, contrast material is injected into a distal lymphatic vessel that has been isolated and cannulated. In primary lymphedema, lymphatic channels are absent, hypoplastic, or ectatic. In secondary lymphedema, lymphatic channels usually are dilated, and it may be possible to determine the level of obstruction.

 TREATMENT

Patients with lymphedema of the lower extremities must be instructed to take meticulous care of their feet to prevent recurrent lymphangitis. Skin hygiene is important, and emollients can be used to prevent drying. Prophylactic antibiotics are often helpful, and fungal infection should be treated aggressively. Patients should be encouraged to participate in physical activity; frequent leg elevation can reduce the amount of edema. Patients can be fitted with graduated compression hose to reduce the amount of lymphedema that develops with upright posture. Occasionally, intermittent pneumatic compression devices can be applied at home to facilitate reduction of the edema. Diuretics are contraindicated and may cause depletion of intravascular volume and metabolic abnormalities. Recently, microsurgical lymphovenous anastomotic procedures have been performed to rechannel lymph flow from obstructed lymphatic vessels into the venous system.

BIBLIOGRAPHY

BROWSE NL: The diagnosis and management of primary lymphedema. J Vasc Surg 3:181, 1986

COFFMAN JD: *Raynaud's Phenomenon.* New York, Oxford University Press, 1989

CRIQUI MH et al: Mortality over a period of 10 years in patients with peripheral arterial disease. N Engl J Med 326:381, 1992

EUROPEAN WORKING GROUP ON CRITICAL LEG ISCHEMIA: Second European consensus document on chronic critical leg ischemia. Circulation 84:IV1, 1991

GARDNER AW, POEHLMAN ET: Exercise rehabilitation programs for the treatment of claudication pain. A meta-analysis. JAMA 274:975, 1995

GOLDHABER SZ: Thrombolysis in venous thromboembolism. An international perspective. Chest 94:176S, 1990

HIRSH J, HOAK J: Management of deep vein thrombosis and pulmonary embolism. A statement of health care professionals. Circulation 93:2212, 1996

ISNER JM, ROSENFIELD K: Redefining the treatment of peripheral artery disease. Role of percutaneous revascularization. Circulation 88:1534, 1993

LENSING AW et al: Treatments of deep venous thrombosis with low-molecular weight heparins. A meta-analysis. Arch Intern Med 155:601, 1995

LOSCALZO J et al: *Vascular Medicine*, 2d ed. Boston, Little, Brown, 1996

OLIN JW et al: The changing clinical spectrum of thromboangiitis obliterans. Circulation 82:IV3, 1990

PEARSON SD et al: A critical pathway to evaluate suspected deep vein thrombosis. Arch Intern Med 155:1773, 1995

RADACK K, WYDERSKI RJ: Conservative management of intermittent claudication. Ann Intern Med 113:135, 1990

SCHULMAN S et al: A comparison of six weeks with six months of oral anticoagulant therapy after a first episode of venous thromboembolism. N Engl J Med 332:1661, 1995

SMITH GD et al: Intermittent claudication, heart disease risk factor, and mortality: The Whitehall study. Circulation 82:1925, 1990

YOUNG JR et al: *Peripheral Vascular Diseases.* St. Louis, Mosby Year Book, 1996

COLOR ATLAS

COLOR ATLASES

I. Atlas of Dermatology

    A. Common Skin Diseases and Lesions

    B. Cutaneous Neoplasms

    C. Pigmented Lesions—Benign and Malignant

    D. Infectious Disease and the Skin

    E. Immunologically Medicated Skin Disease

    F. Skin Manifestations of Internal Disease

II. Atlas of Endoscopic Findings

III. Atlas of Funduscopic Examination

IV. Atlas of Hematology

I. Atlas of Dermatology

Stephen F. Templeton / Thomas J. Lawley

A. Common Skin Diseases and Lesions

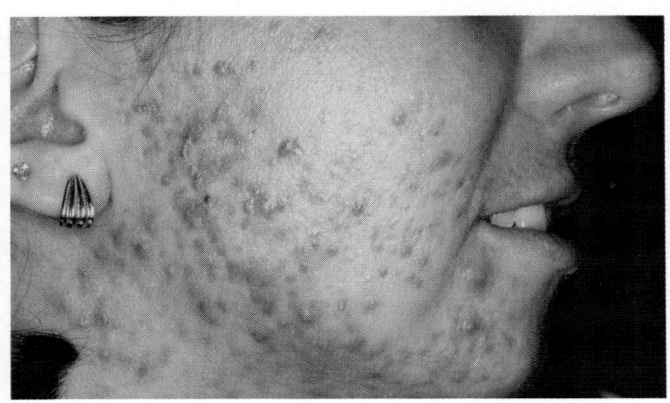

IA-1 **Acne vulgaris** with inflammatory papules, pustules, and comedones

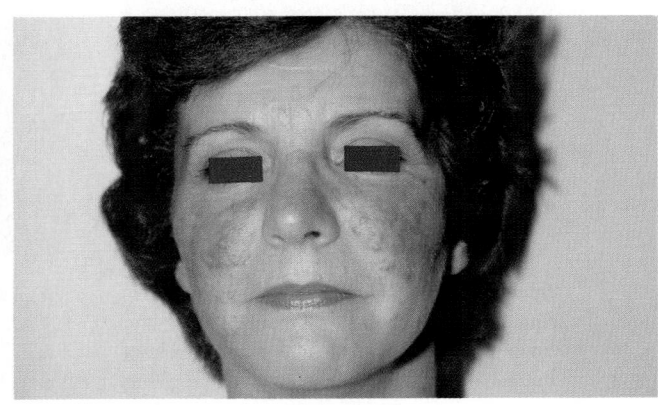

IA-2 **Acne rosacea** with prominent facial erythema, telangiec-tasias, scattered papules, and small pustules

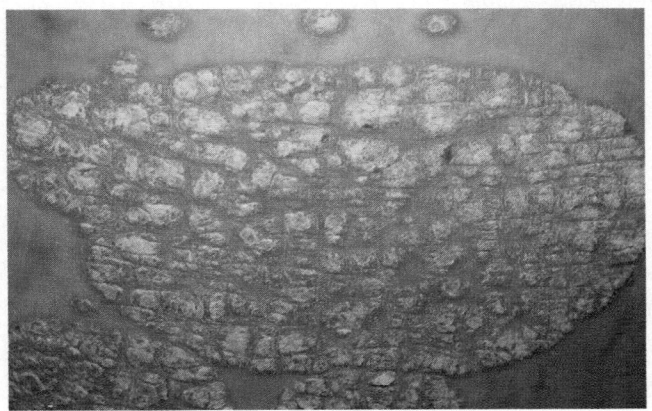

IA-3 **Psoriasis** is characterized by small and large erythematous plaques with adherent silvery scale.

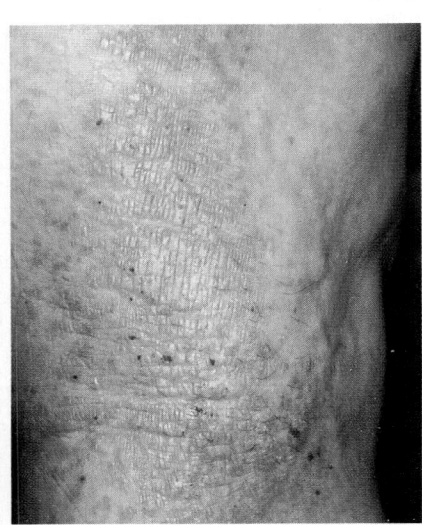

IA-4 **Atopic dermatitis** with excoriated, lichenified plaques in the popliteal fossa

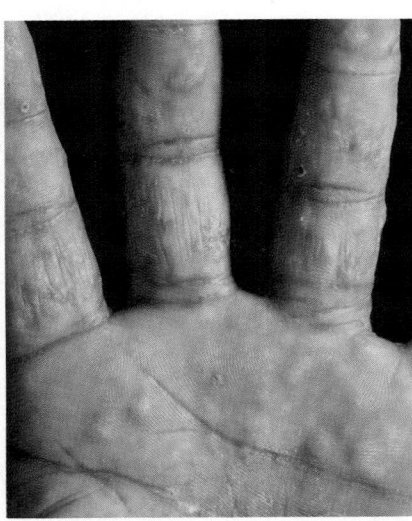

IA-5 **Dyshidrotic eczema,** characterized by deep-seated vesicles and scaling on palms and lateral fingers, is often associated with an atopic diathesis.

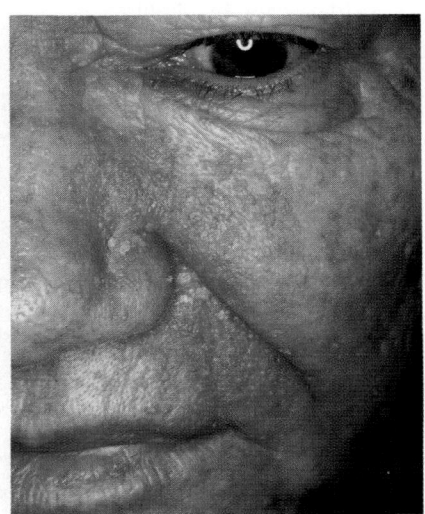

IA-6 **Seborrheic dermatitis** showing central facial erythema with overlying greasy, yellowish scale

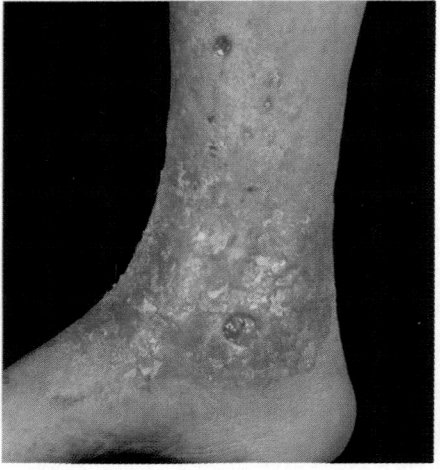
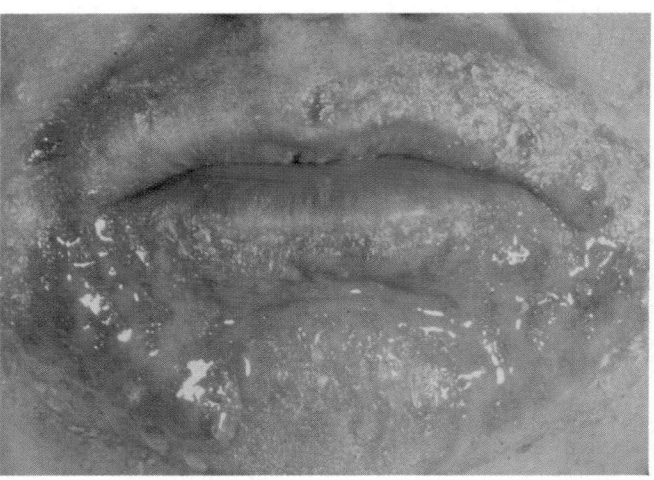

IA-7 **Stasis dermatitis** showing erythematous, scaly, and oozing patches over the lower leg. Several stasis ulcers are also seen in this patient.

IA-8 **Allergic contact dermatitis,** acute phase, with sharply demarcated, weeping, eczematous plaques in a perioral distribution

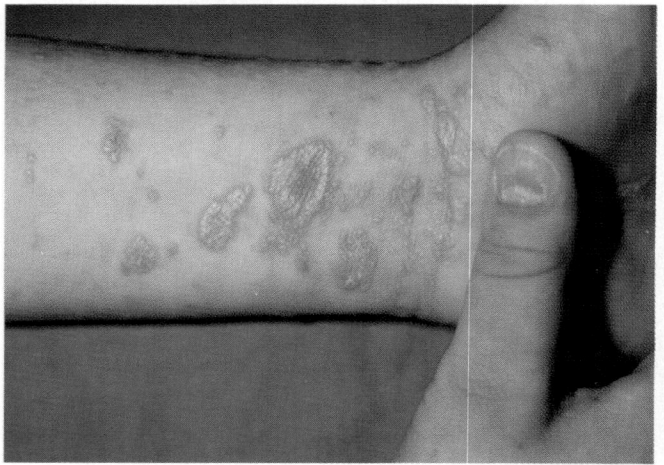
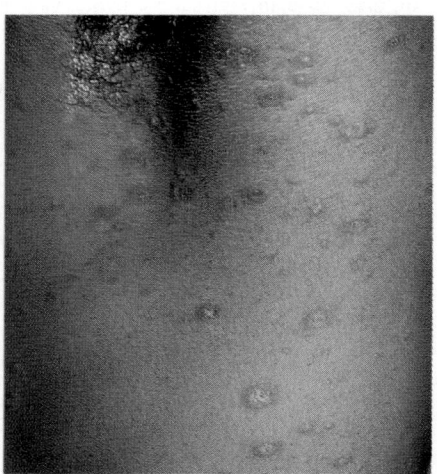

IA-9 **Lichen planus** showing multiple flat-topped, violaceous papules and plaques. Nail dystrophy as seen in this patient's thumbnail may also be a feature.

IA-10 **Pityriasis rosea** Multiple round to oval erythematous patches with fine central scale are distributed along the skin tension lines on the trunk.

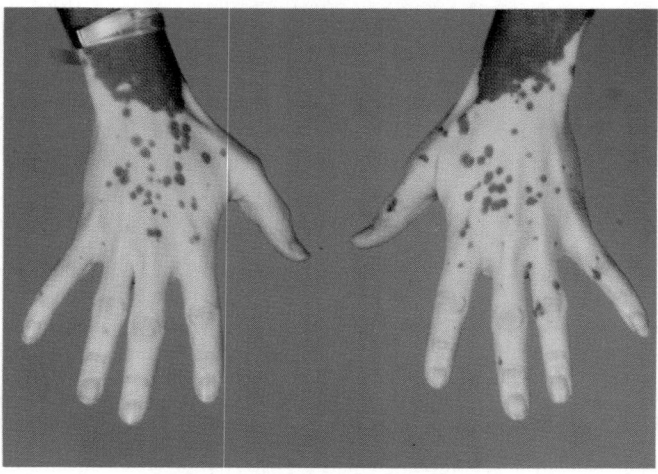

IA-11 **Vitiligo** in a typical acral distribution demonstrating striking cutaneous depigmentation, as a result of loss of melanocytes

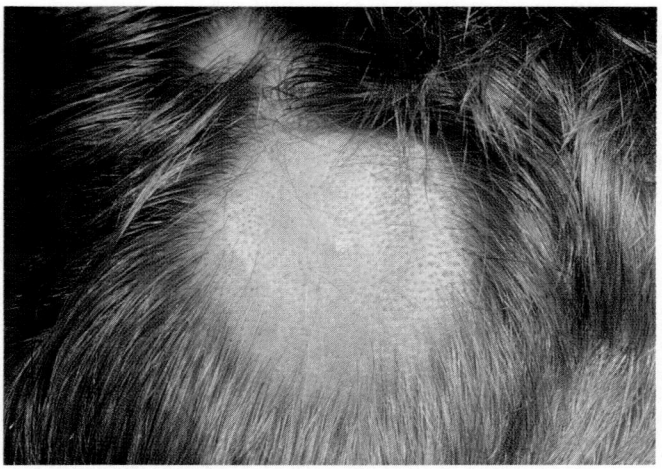

IA-12 **Alopecia areata** characterized by a sharply demarcated circular patch of scalp completely devoid of hairs. Follicular orifices are preserved, indicating a nonscarring alopecia.

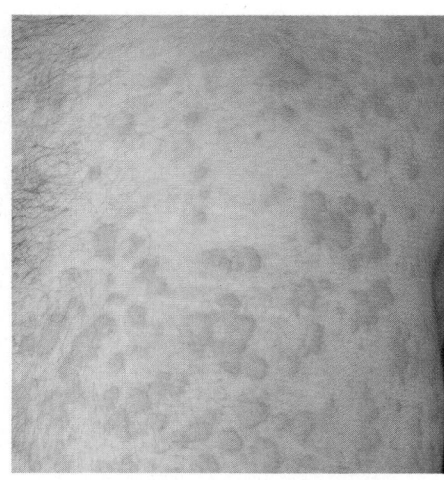

IA-13 **Urticaria** showing characteristic discrete and confluent, edematous, erythematous papules and plaques

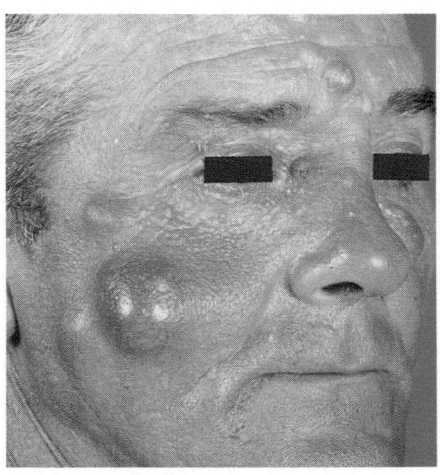

IA-14 **Epidermoid cysts** Several inflamed and noninflamed firm, cystic nodules are seen in this patient. Often a patulous follicular punctum is observed on the overlying epidermal surface.

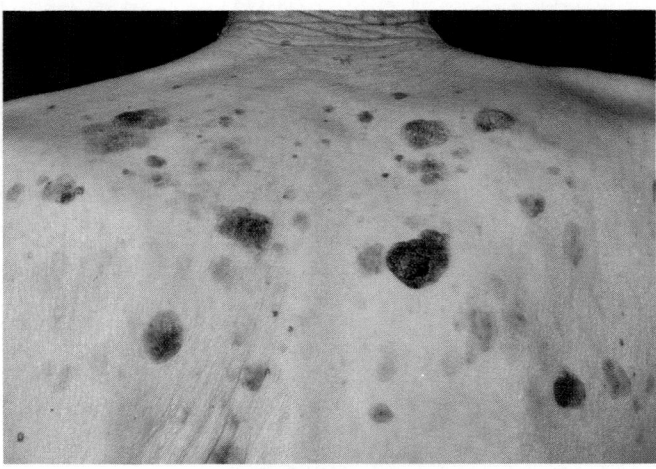

IA-15 **Seborrheic keratoses** are seen as "stuck on," waxy, verrucous papules and plaques with a variety of colors ranging from light tan to black.

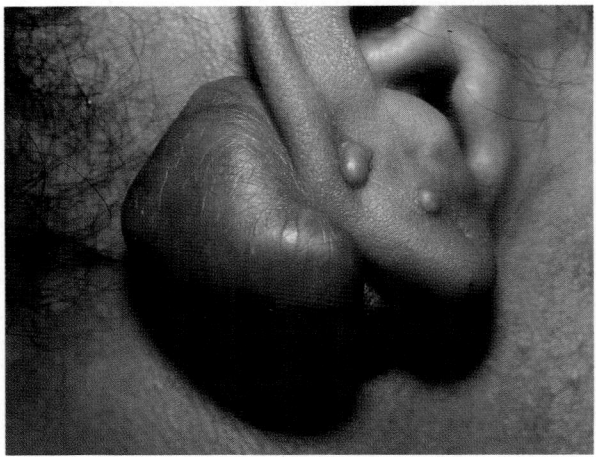

IA-16 **Keloids** resulting from ear piercing, with firm exophytic flesh-colored to erythematous nodules of scar tissue.

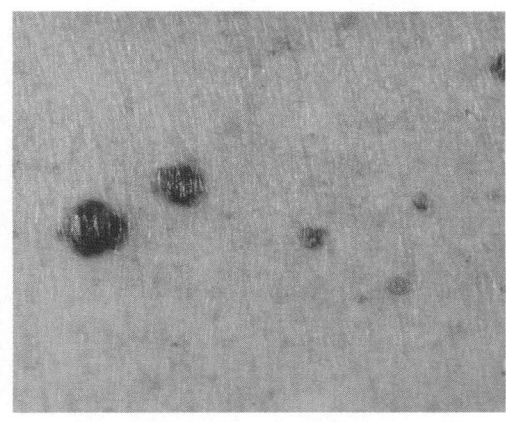

IA-17 **Cherry hemangiomas** are very common and arise in middle-aged to older adults. They are characterized by multiple erythematous to dark-purple papules usually located on the trunk.

B. Cutaneous Neoplasms

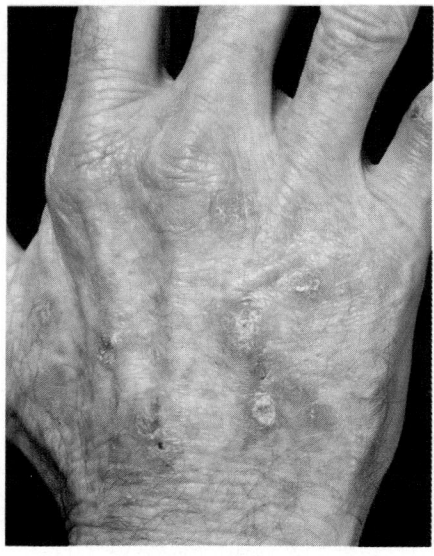

IB-18 **Actinic keratoses** consist of hyperkeratotic erythematous papules and patches on sun-exposed skin. They arise in middle-aged to older adults and have some potential for malignant transformation.

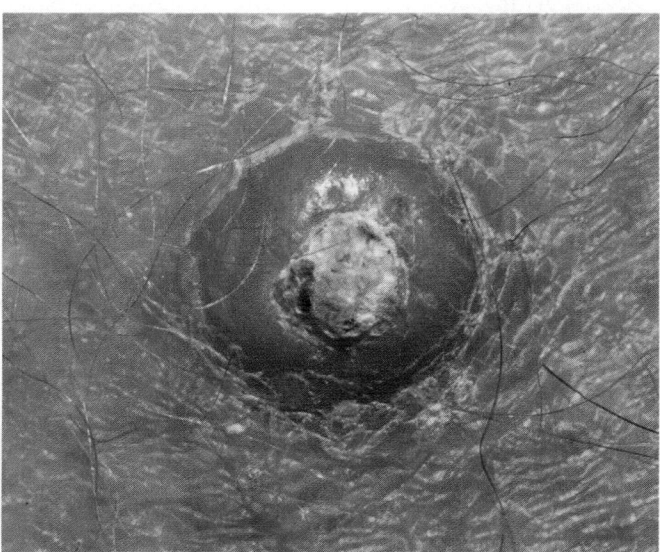

IB-19 **Keratoacanthoma** is a low-grade squamous cell carcinoma that presents as an exophytic nodule with central keratinous debris.

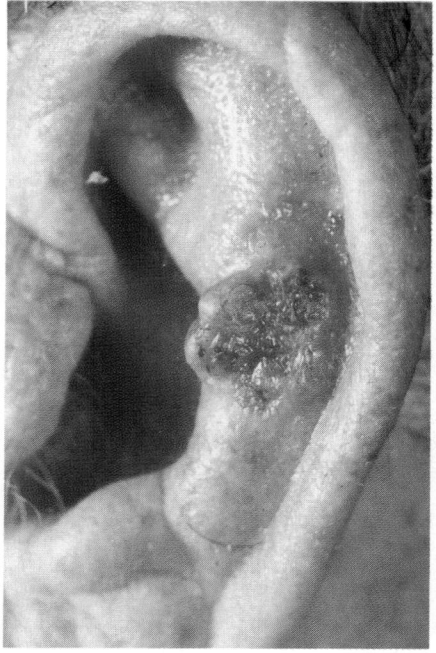

IB-20 **Basal cell carcinoma** showing central ulceration and a pearly, rolled, telangiectatic tumor border

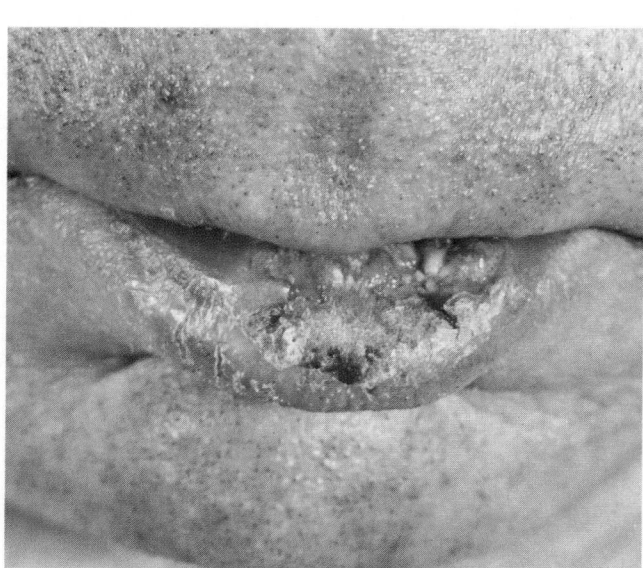

IB-21 **Squamous cell carcinoma** seen here as a hyperkeratotic crusted and somewhat eroded plaque on the lower lip. Sun-exposed skin such as the head, neck, hands, and arms are other typical sites of involvement.

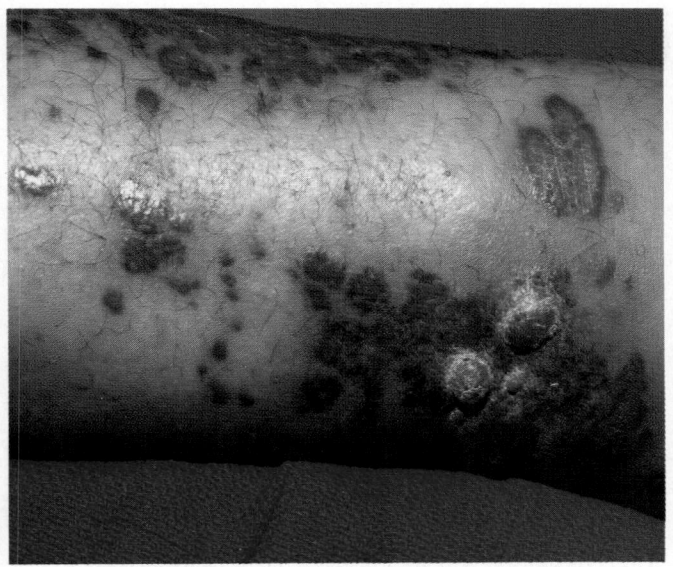

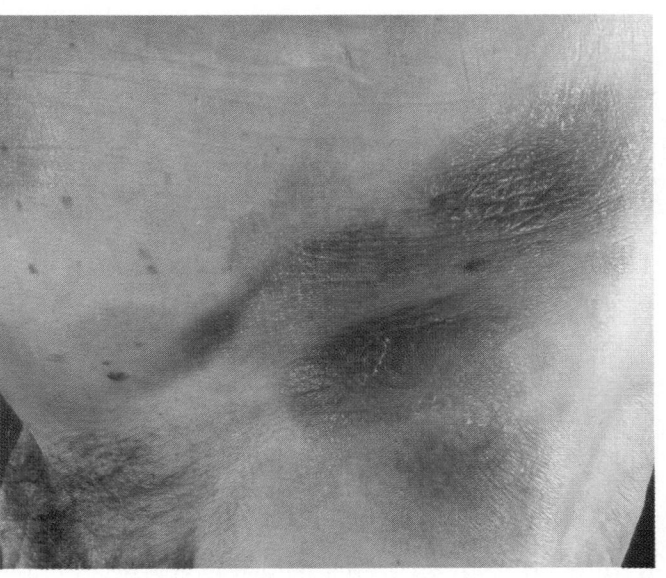

IB-22 **Kaposi's sarcoma** in a patient with AIDS demonstrating patch, plaque, and tumor stages

IB-23 **Mycosis fungoides** is a cutaneous T cell lymphoma, and plaque stage lesions are seen in this patient.

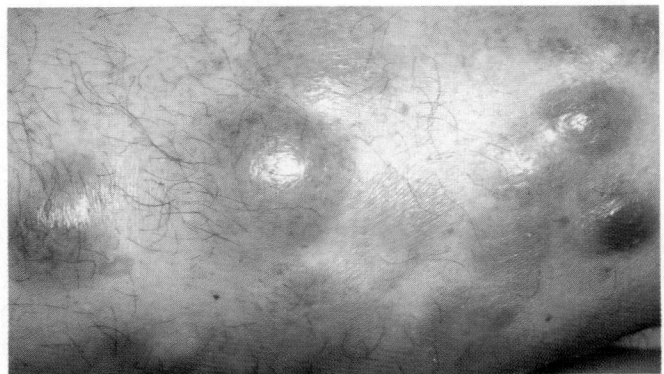

IB-24 **Non-Hodgkin's lymphoma** involving the skin with typical violaceous, "plum-colored" nodules

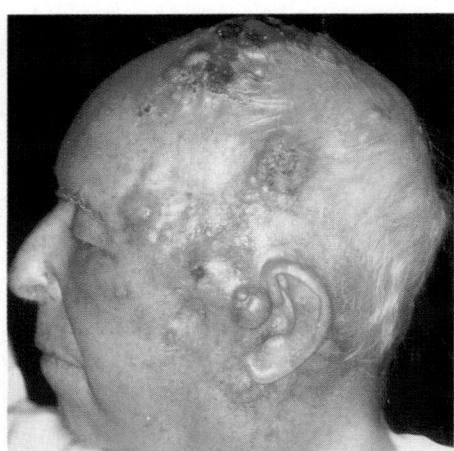

IB-25 **Metastatic carcinoma** to the skin is characterized by inflammatory, often ulcerated dermal nodules.

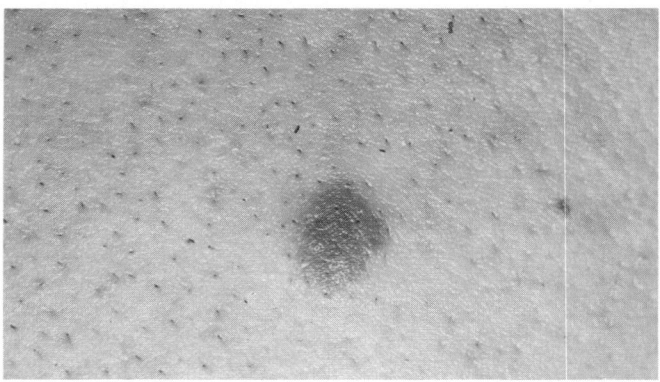

IC-26 **Nevus** Nevi are benign proliferations of nevomelanocytes characterized by regularly shaped hyperpigmented macules or papules of a uniform color.

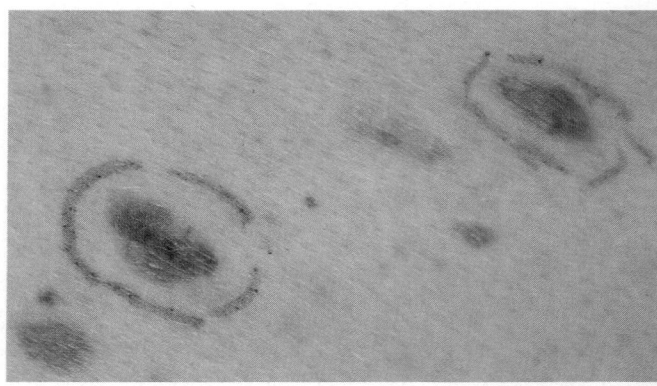

IC-27 **Dysplastic nevi** are irregularly pigmented and shaped nevo-melanocytic lesions that may be associated with familial melanoma.

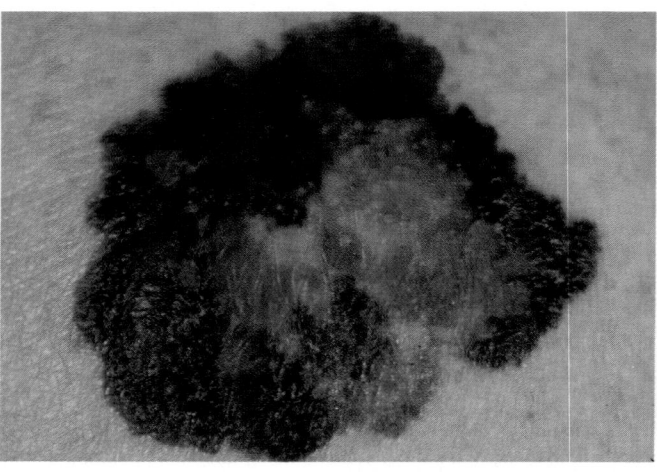

IC-28 **Superficial spreading melanoma** is the most common type of malignant melanoma and demonstrates color variegation (black, blue, brown, pink, and white) and irregular borders.

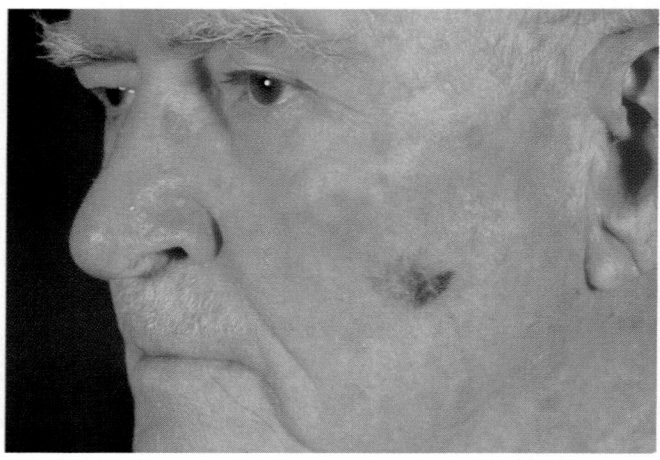

IC-29 **Lentigo maligna melanoma** occurs on sun-exposed skin as a large, hyperpigmented macule or plaque with irregular borders and variable pigmentation.

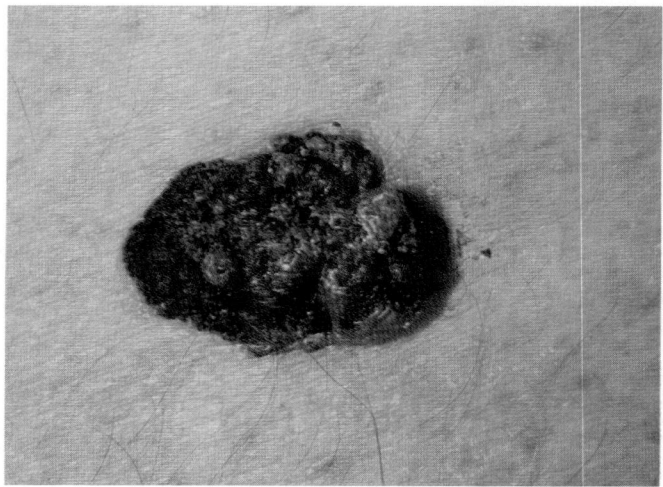

IC-30 **Nodular melanoma** most commonly manifests itself as a rapidly growing, often ulcerated or crusted black nodule.

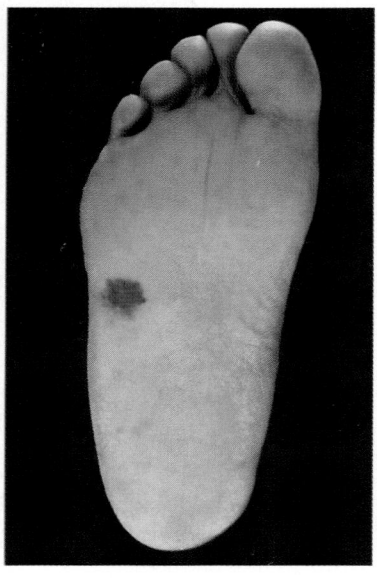

IC-31 **Acral lentiginous melanoma** is more common in blacks, Asians, and Hispanics and occurs as an enlarging hyperpigmented macule or plaque on the palms and soles. Lateral pigment diffusion is present.

D. Infectious Disease and the Skin

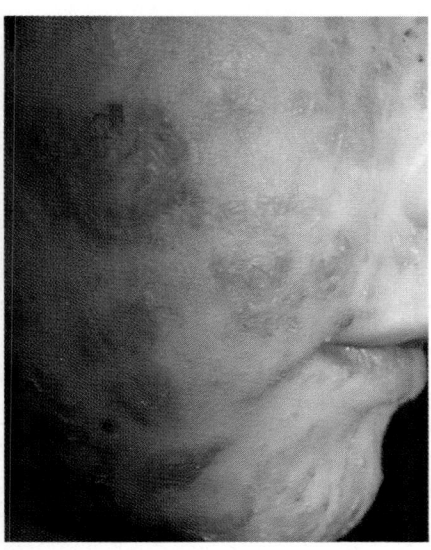

ID-32 **Impetigo contagiosa** is a superficial streptococcal or *S. aureus* infection consisting of honey-colored crusts and erythematous weeping erosions. Occasionally bullous lesions may be seen.

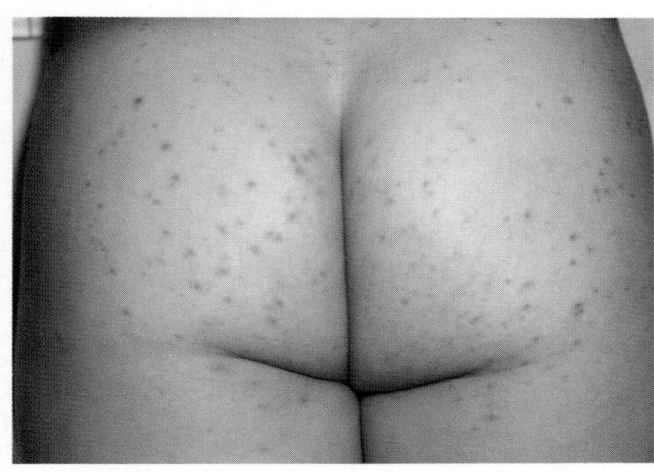

ID-33 **Folliculitis** is a bacterial infection of hair follicles and is seen as erythematous follicular papules and pustules.

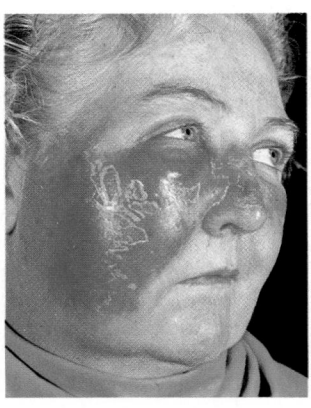

ID-34 **Erysipelas** is a streptococcal infection of the superficial dermis and consists of well-demarcated, erythematous, edematous, warm plaques.

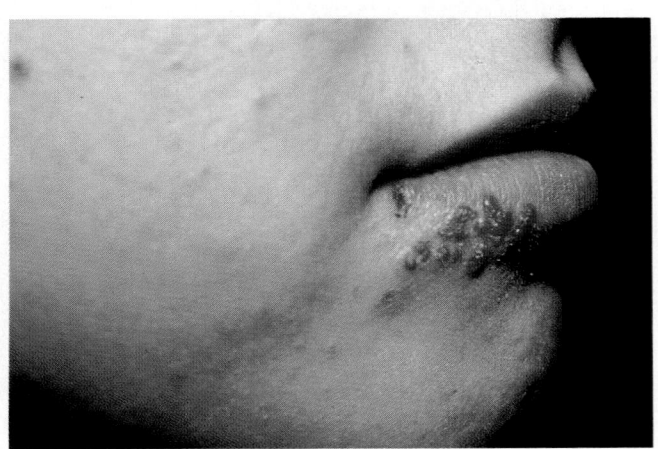

ID-35 **Herpes simplex**   Grouped vesiculopustules on an erythematous base characterize primary HSV infections.

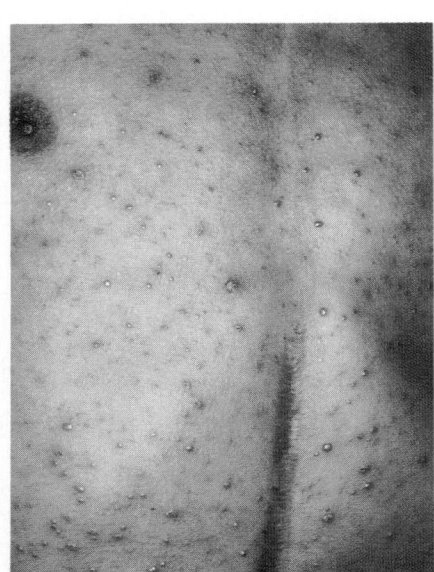

ID-36 **Varicella** showing numerous lesions in various stages of evolution: vesicles on an erythematous base, umbilicated vesicles, and crusts

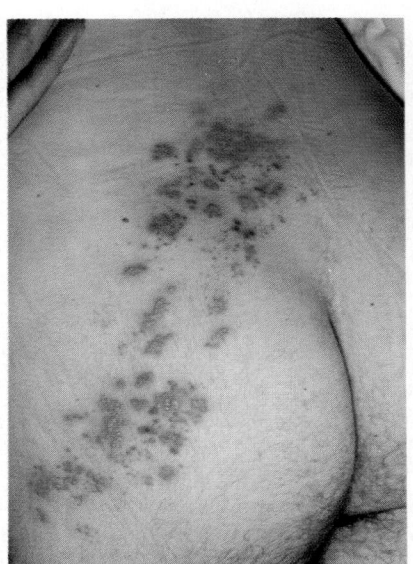

ID-37 **Herpes zoster** is seen in this HIV-infected patient as hemorrhagic vesicles and pustules on an erythematous base grouped in a dermatomal distribution.

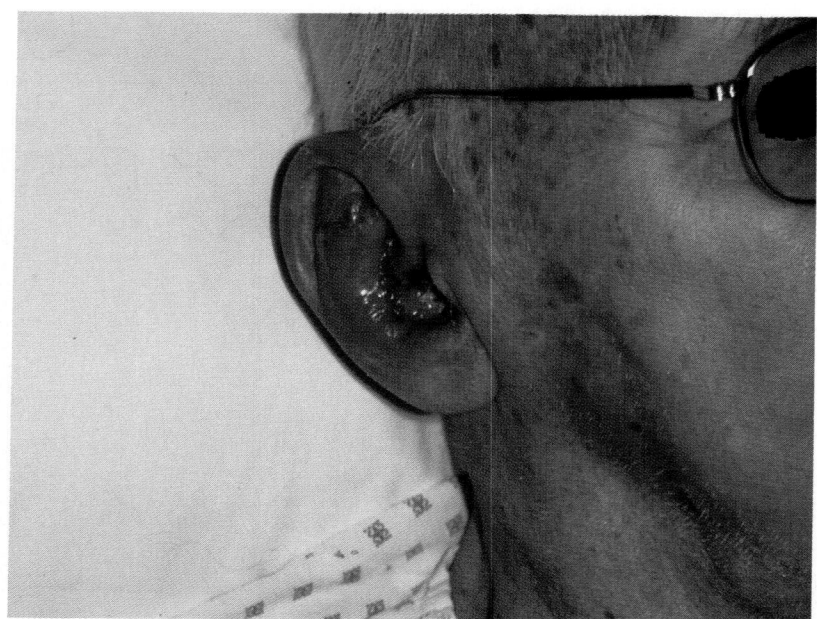

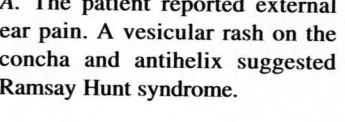

ID-38 **Spread of herpes zoster with chemotherapy**

A. The patient reported external ear pain. A vesicular rash on the concha and antihelix suggested Ramsay Hunt syndrome.

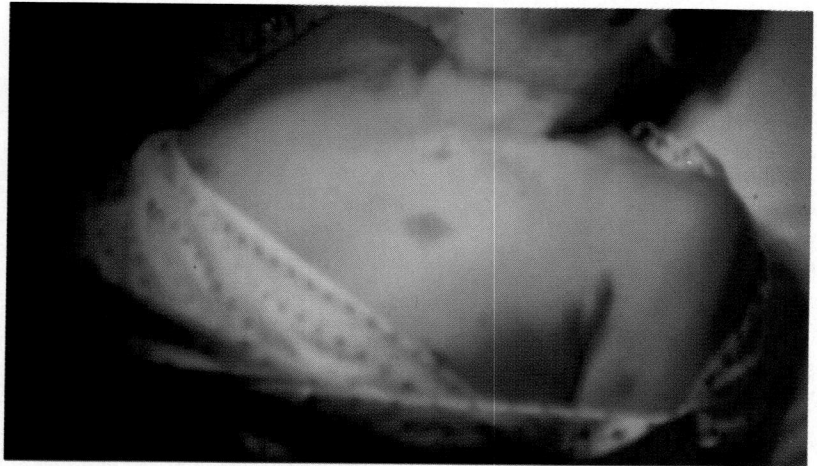

B. After chemotherapy for prostate cancer, the patient developed disseminated zoster, which was eventually controlled with acyclovir.

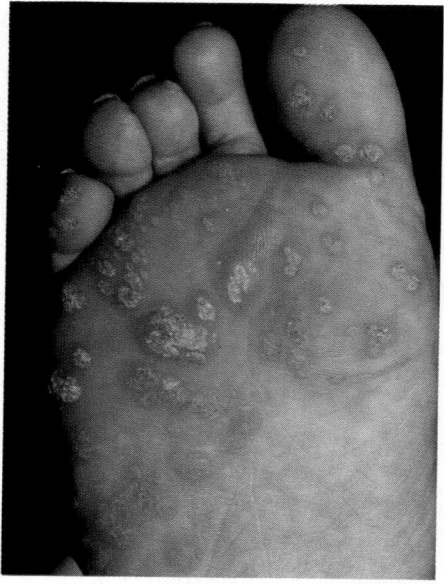

ID-39 **Verrucae** characterized as multiple hyperkeratotic verrucous papules

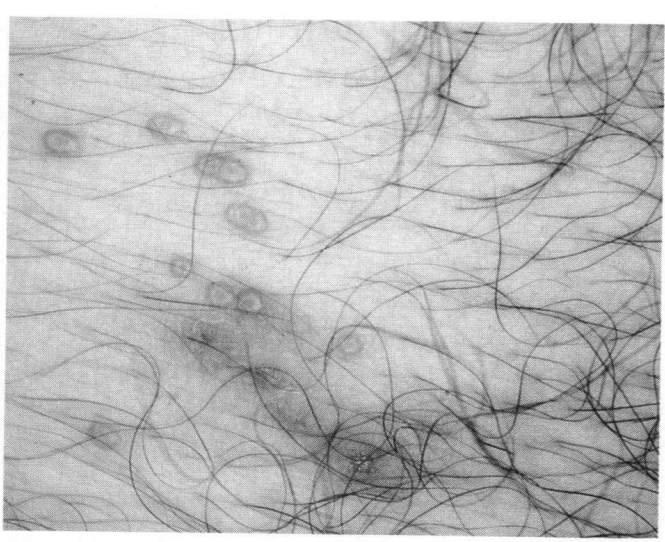

ID-40 **Molluscum contagiosum** is a cutaneous poxvirus infection characterized by multiple umbilicated flesh-colored or hypopigmented papules.

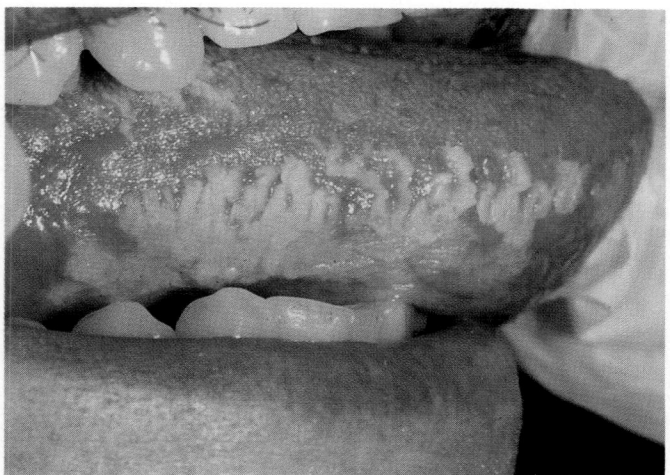

ID-41 **Oral hairy leukoplakia** often presents as white plaques on the lateral tongue and is associated with Epstein-Barr virus infection.

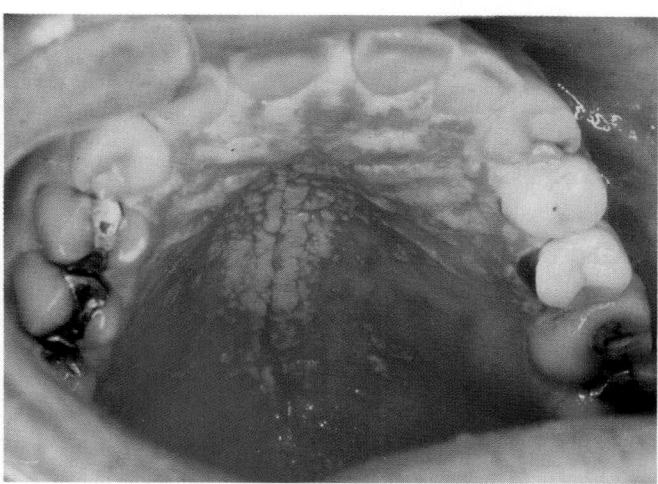

ID-42 **Pseudomembranous oral candidiasis** Adherent white, mucoid plaques with an erythematous halo seen here on the palate often indicate an immunocompromised state.

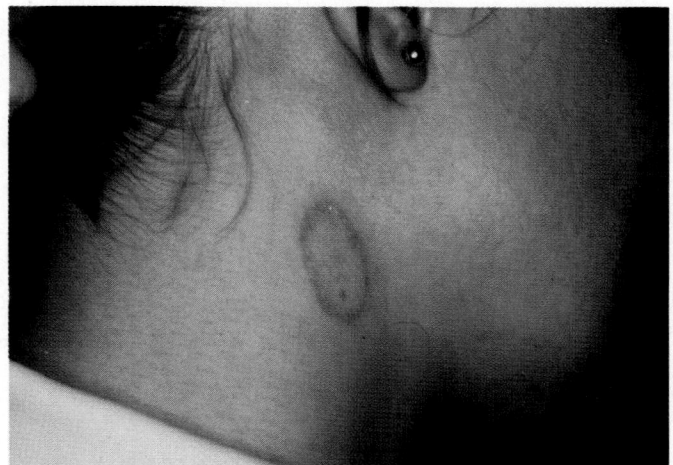

ID-43 **Tinea corporis** is a superficial fungal infection seen here as an erythematous annular scaly plaque with central clearing.

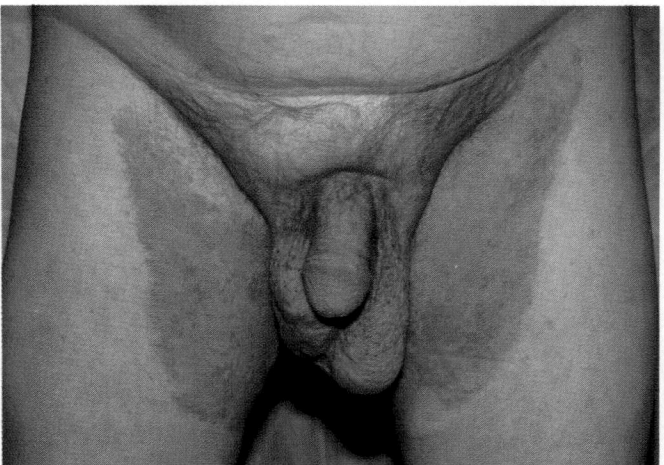

ID-44 **Tinea cruris** is a superficial dermatophyte infection with bilateral scaly, erythematous, annular plaques extending from the inguinal crease to the upper thighs.

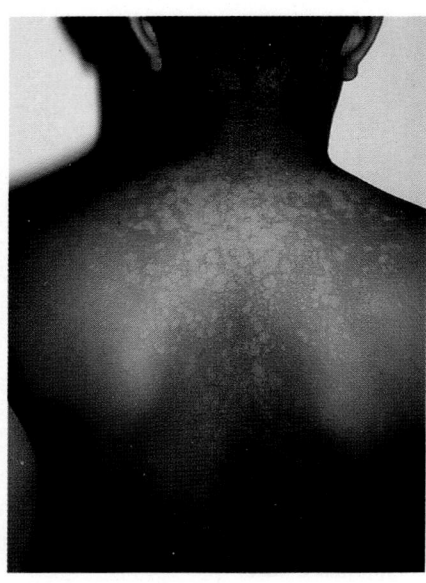

ID-45 **Tinea versicolor** is a superficial cutaneous fungal infection showing a wide variety of lesions. Finely scaling patches may be small or large, hyperpigmented or hypopigmented.

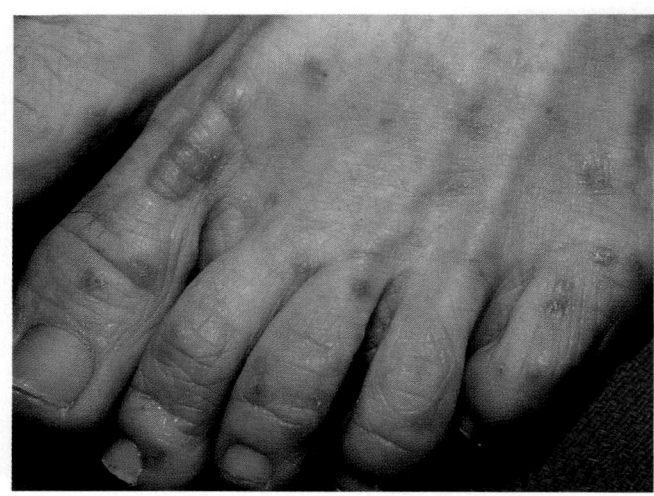

ID-46 **Scabies** showing typical scaling erythematous papules and few linear burrows

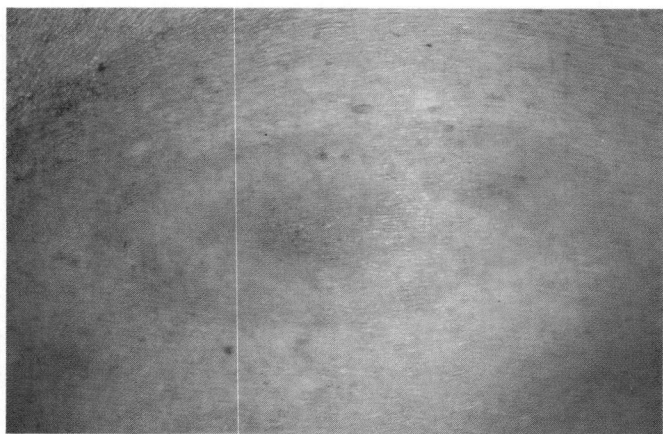

ID-47 **Erythema chronicum migrans** is the early cutaneous manifestation of Lyme disease and is characterized by erythematous annular patches, often with a central erythematous papule at the tick bite site.

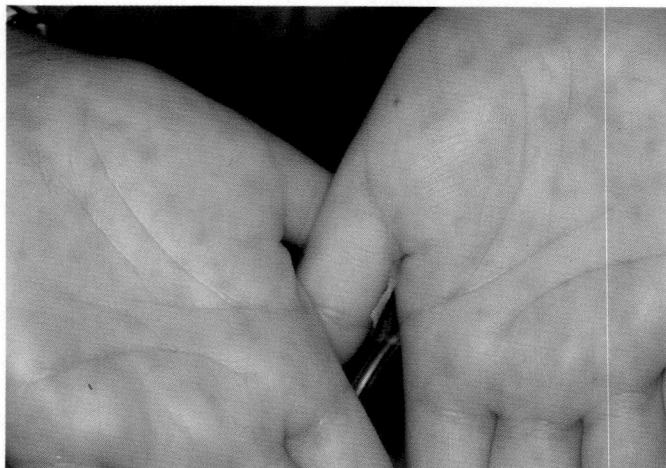

ID-48 **Rocky Mountain spotted fever** demonstrating faint erythematous palmar macules in the early phase of the disease. Lesions may become hemorrhagic (purpuric) as the disease progresses.

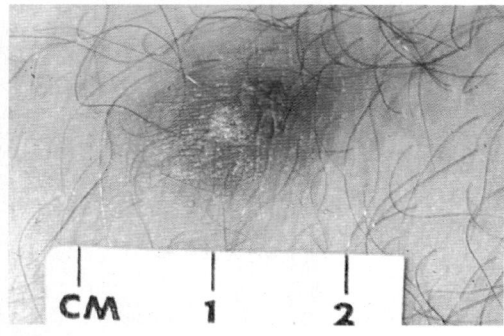

ID-49 **Disseminated gonococcemia** in the skin is seen as hemorrhagic papules and pustules with purpuric centers in an acral distribution.

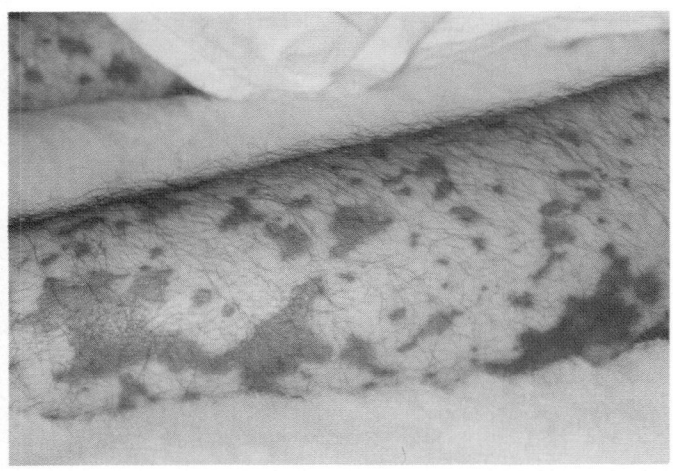

ID-50 **Fulminant meningococcemia** with extensive angular purpuric patches

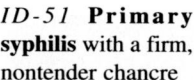

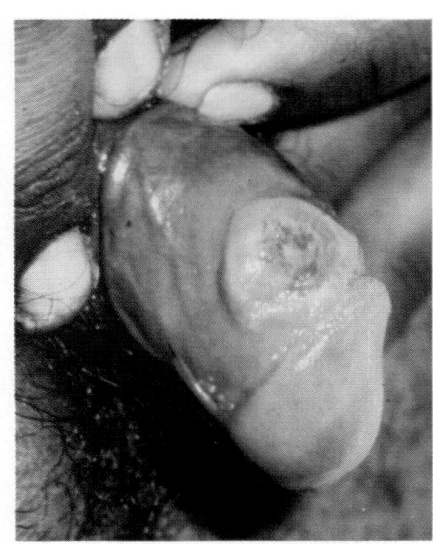

ID-51 **Primary syphilis** with a firm, nontender chancre

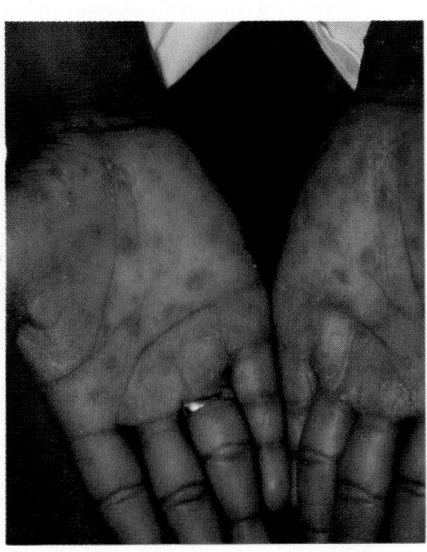

ID-53 **Secondary syphilis** commonly affects the palms and soles with scaling, firm, red-brown papules.

ID-52 **Secondary syphilis** demonstrating the papulosquamous truncal eruption

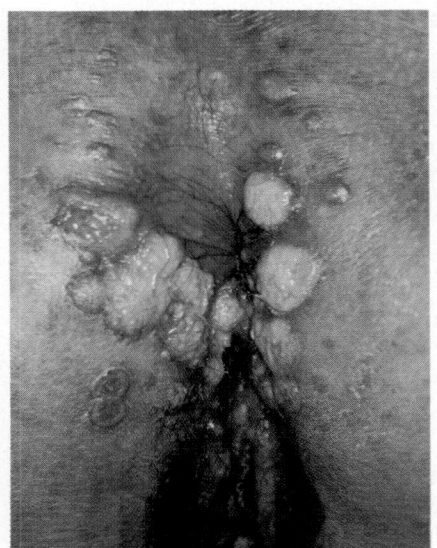

ID-54 **Condylomata lata** are moist, somewhat verrucous intertriginous plaques seen in secondary syphilis.

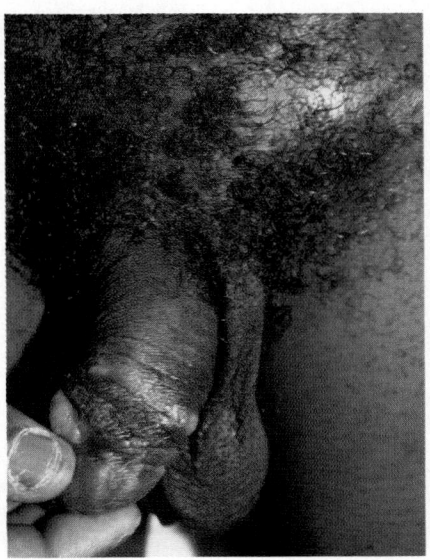

ID-55 **Chancroid** with characteristic penile ulcers and associated left inguinal adenitis (bubo)

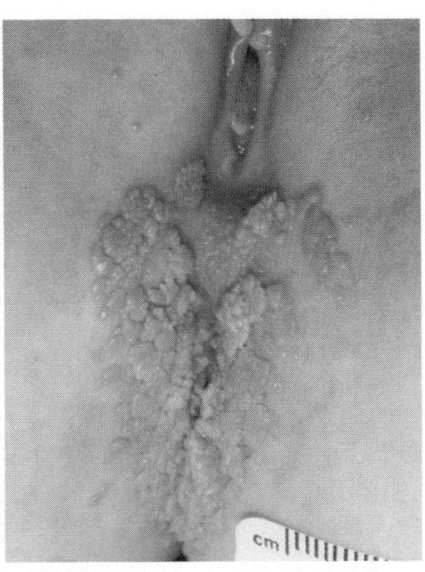

ID-56 **Condylomata acuminata** are lesions induced by human papillomavirus (HPV) and in this patient are seen as multiple verrucous papules coalescing into plaques.

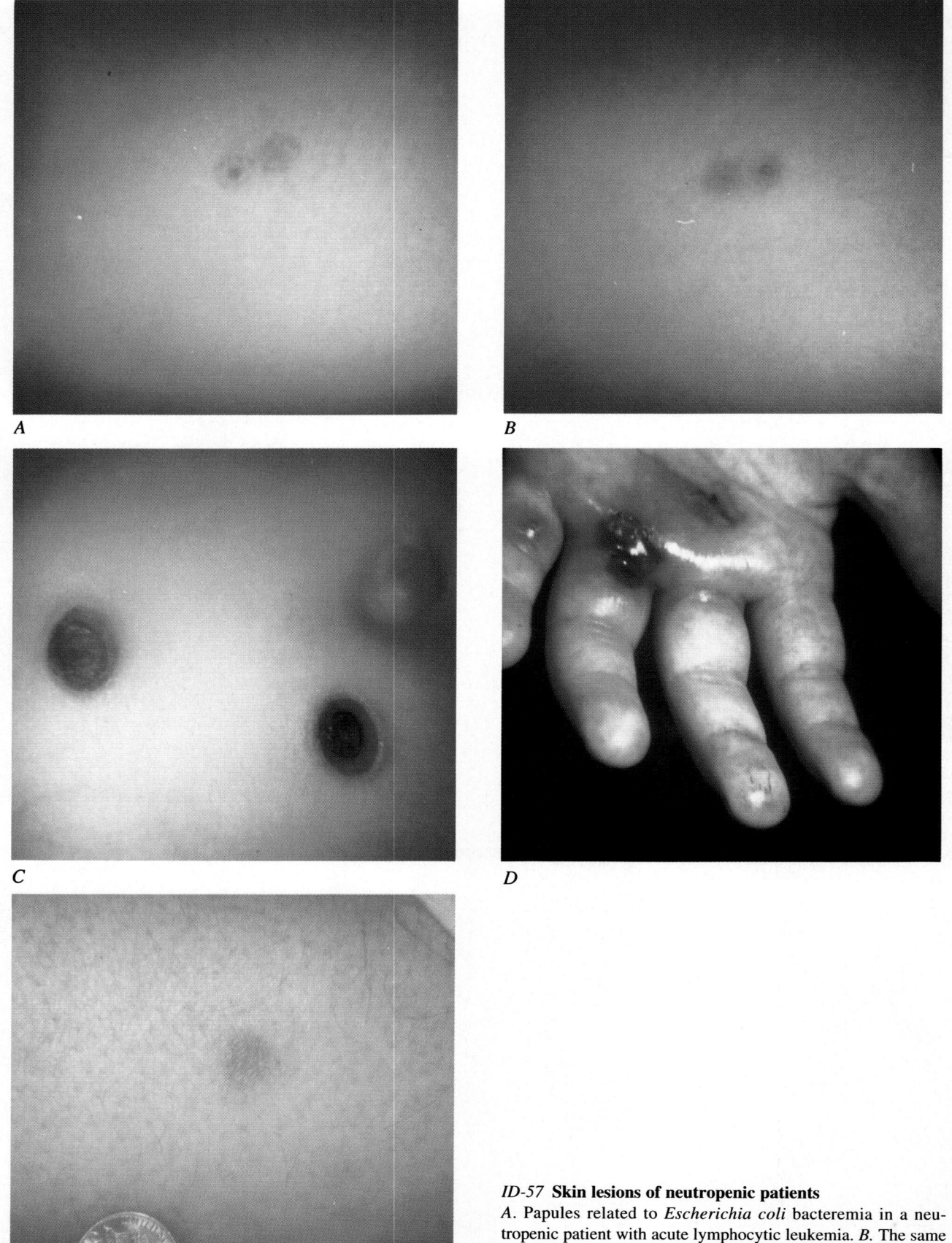

ID-57 **Skin lesions of neutropenic patients**
A. Papules related to *Escherichia coli* bacteremia in a neutropenic patient with acute lymphocytic leukemia. *B.* The same
papule 2 h later. *C.* The same lesion the following day. *D.*
Ecthyma gangrenosum in a neutropenic patient with *Pseudomonas aeruginosa* bacteremia. *E.* Papule in a neutropenic
patient with *Candida tropicalis* fungemia.

E. Immunologically Mediated Skin Disease

IE-58 **Systemic lupus erythematosus** showing prominent, scaly, malar erythema. Involvement of other sun-exposed sites is also common.

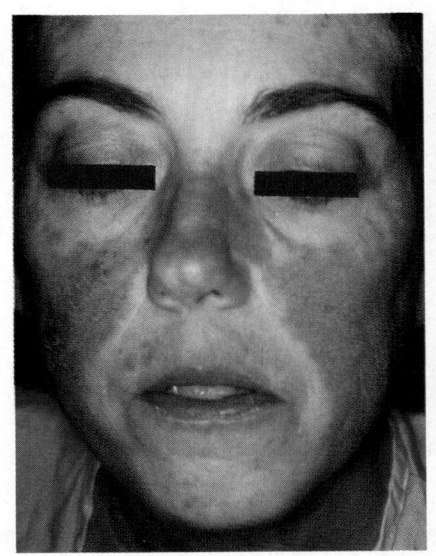

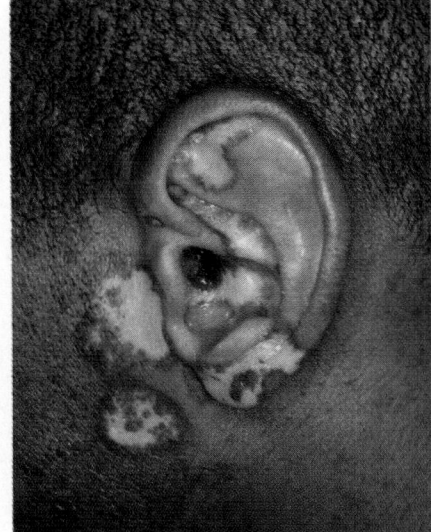

IE-59 **Discoid lupus erythematosus** Violaceous, hyperpigmented, atrophic plaques, often with evidence of follicular plugging, which may result in scarring, are characteristic of this cutaneous form of lupus.

IE-60 **Dermatomyositis** Periorbital violaceous erythema characterizes the classic heliotrope rash.

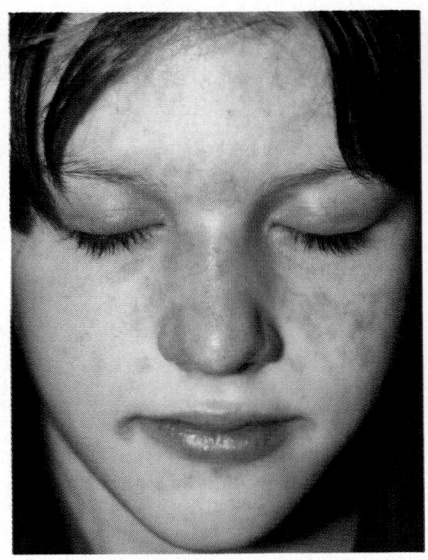

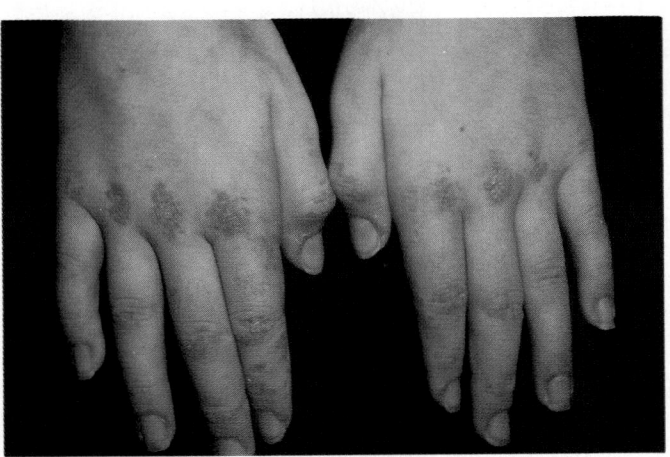

IE-61 **Dermatomyositis** often involves the hands as erythematous flat-topped papules over the knuckles (Gottron's sign) and periungal telangiectasias.

IE-63 **Scleroderma** is characterized by typical expressionless, mask-like facies.

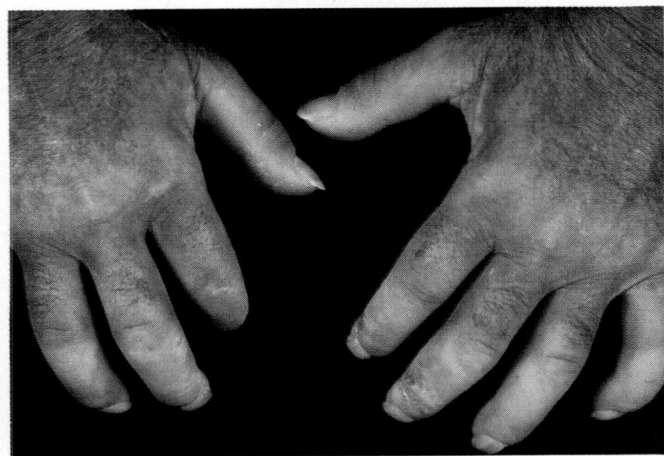

IE-62 **Scleroderma** showing acral sclerosis and focal digital ulcers

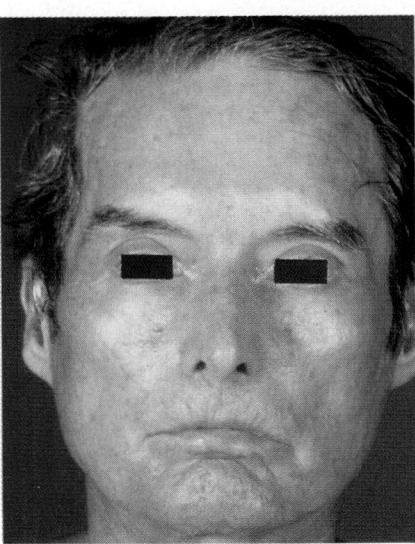

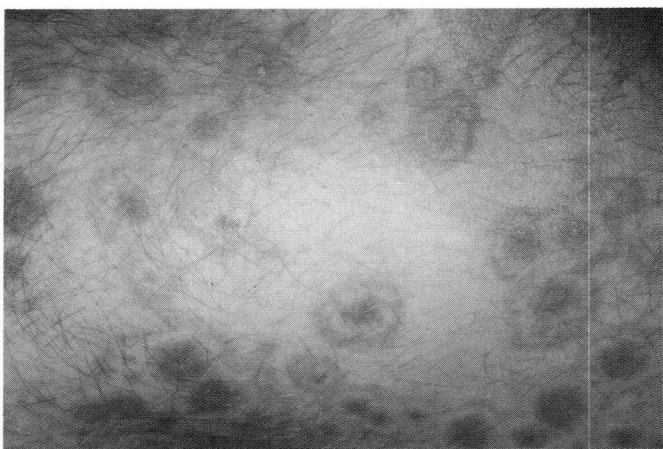

IE-64 **Erythema multiforme** is characterized by multiple erythematous plaques with a target or iris morphology and usually represents a hypersensitivity reaction to drugs or infections (especially herpes simplex virus).

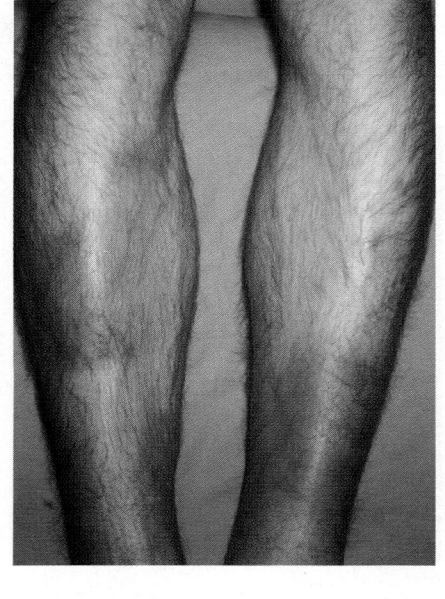

IE-65 **Erythema nodosum** is a panniculitis characterized by tender deep-seated nodules and plaques usually located on the lower extremities.

IE-66 **Vasculitis** Palpable purpuric papules on the lower legs are seen in this patient with cutaneous small vessel vasculitis.

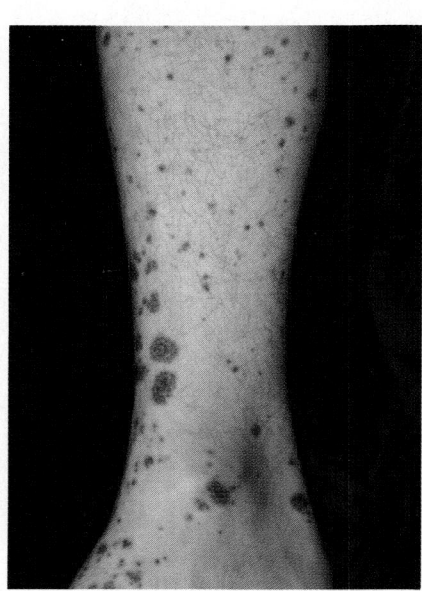

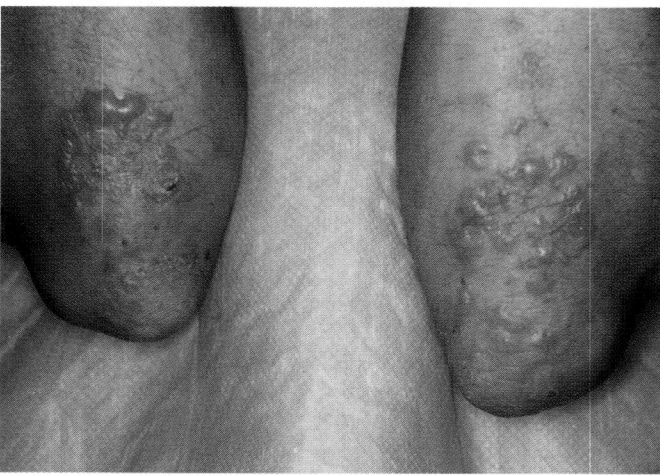

IE-67 **Pemphigus vulgaris** demonstrating flaccid bullae that are easily ruptured, resulting in multiple erosions and crusted plaques

IE-69 **Bullous pemphigoid** with tense vesicles and bullae on an erythematous, urticarial base

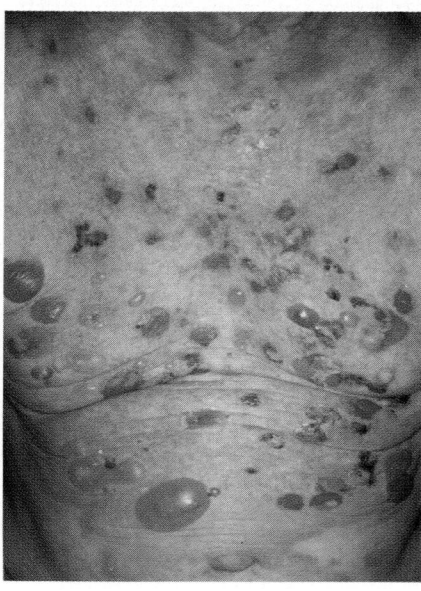

IE-68 **Dermatitis herpetiformis** manifested by pruritic, grouped vesicles in a typical location. The vesicles are often excoriated and may occur on knees, buttocks, and posterior scalp.

F. Skin Manifestations of Internal Disease

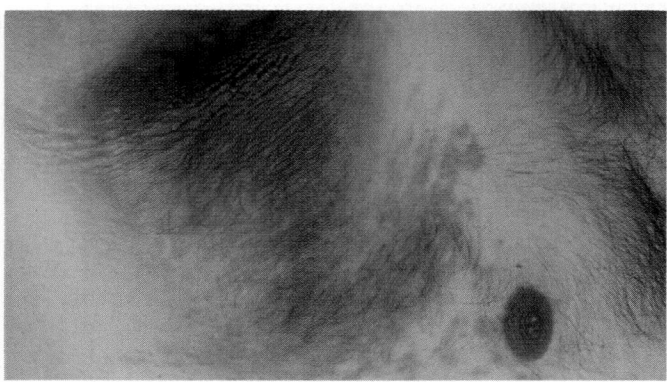

IF-70 **Acanthosis nigricans** demonstrating typical hyperpigmented axillary plaques with a velvet-like, verrucous surface

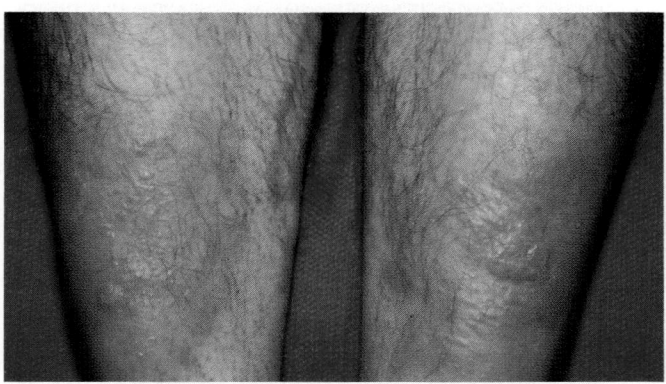

IF-71 **Pretibial myxedema** manifesting as waxy, infiltrated plaques in a patient with Graves' disease

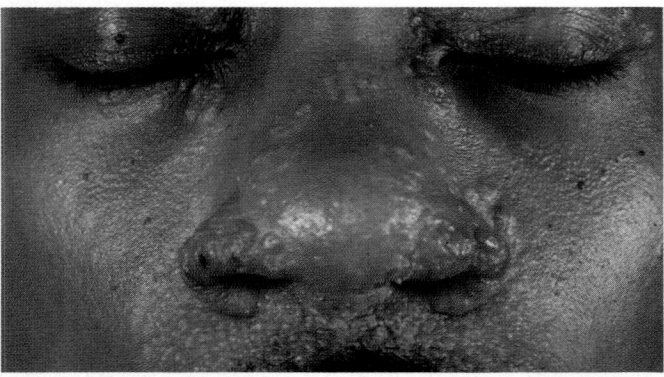

IF-72 **Sarcoid** Infiltrated papules and plaques of variable color are seen in a typical paranasal and periorbital location.

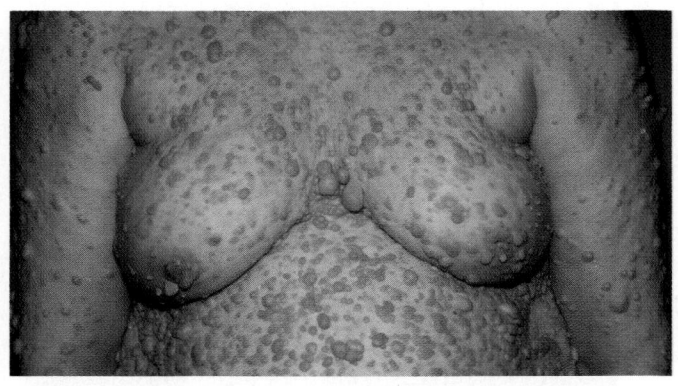

IF-73 **Neurofibromatosis** demonstrating numerous flesh-colored cutaneous neurofibromas

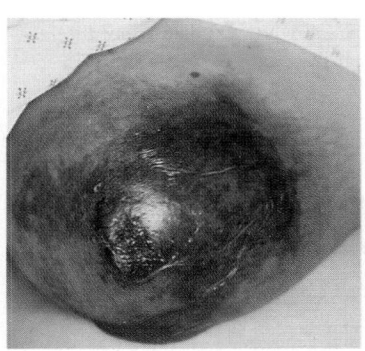

IF-74 **Coumarin necrosis** showing cutaneous and subcutaneous necrosis of a breast. Other fatty areas such as buttocks and thighs are also common sites of involvement.

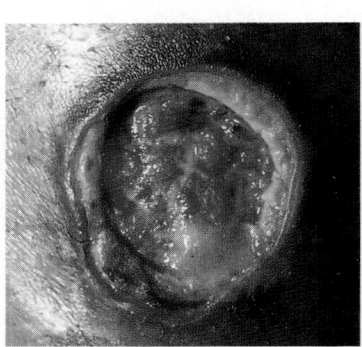

IF-75 **Pyoderma gangrenosum** showing a somewhat purulent ulcer with violaceous and undermined wound edges

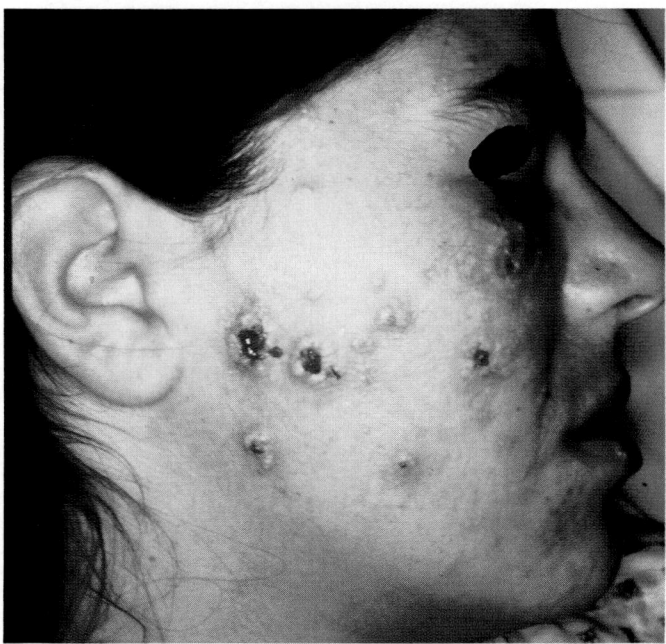

IF-76 **Plaques of Sweet's syndrome** in a patient with acute myelocytic leukemia.

II. Atlas of Endoscopic Findings

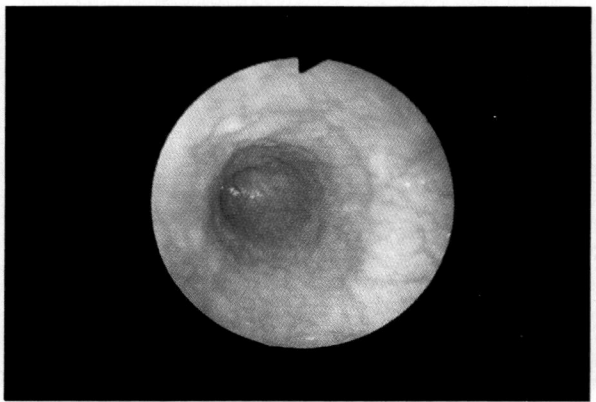

II-1 **Normal esophagus** Fine vasculature can be seen

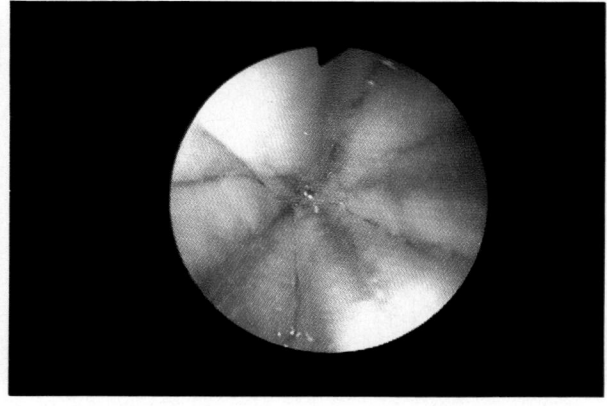

II-2 **Peptic regurgitant esophagitis** Linear red streaks with a central white streak extend up the esophagus

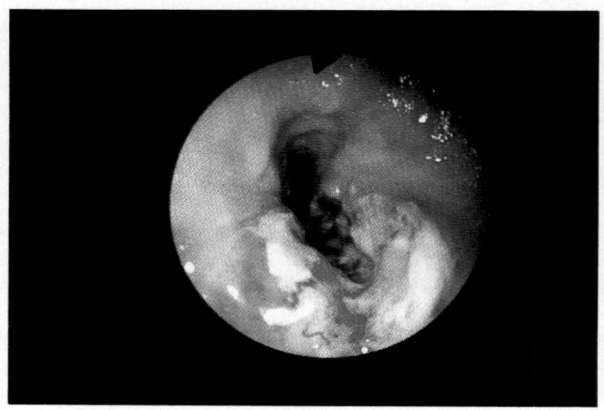

II-3 **Ulcerated squamous cell carcinoma,** with a depressed center, involving one wall of the esophagus

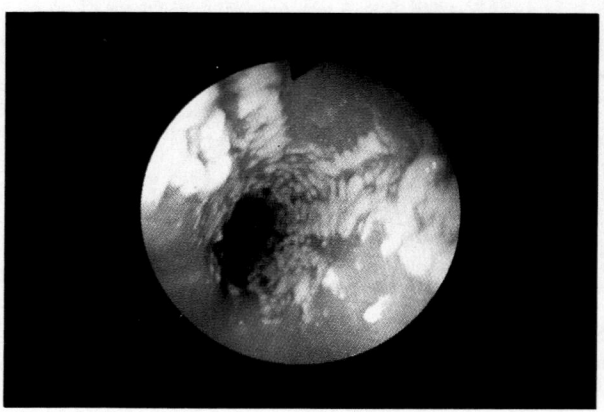

II-4 **Moniliasis of the esophagus** A white exudate is seen with underlying erythematous mucosa

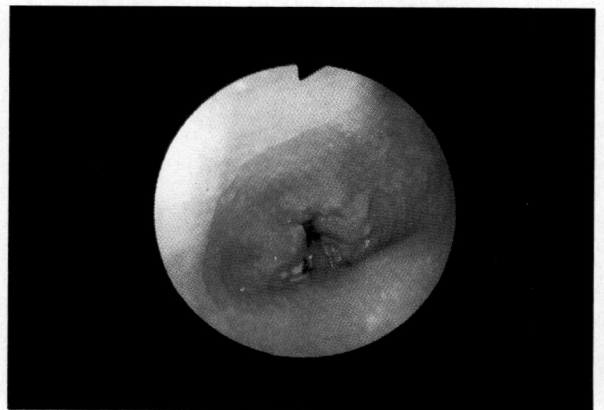

II-5 **Barrett's metaplasia of the esophagus with an adeno-carcinoma** The squamocolumnar junction is noted in the proximal esophagus. A mucosal irregularity in the center of the photograph was an adenocarcinoma.

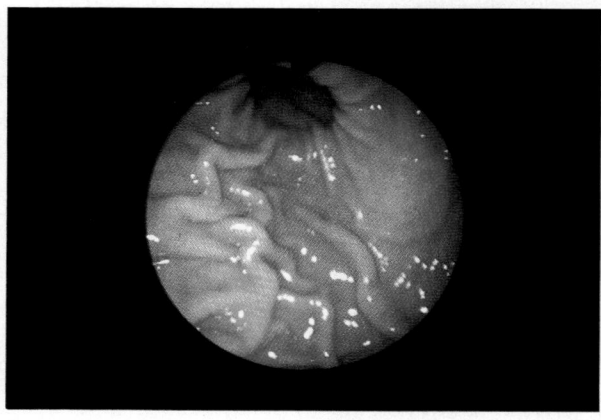

II-6 **Normal body of the stomach with rugal folds**

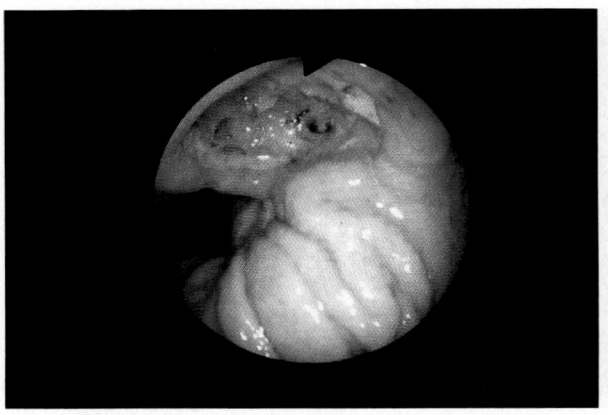

II-7 **Large, benign, lesser curve gastric ulcer**   The folds end at the ulcer margin.

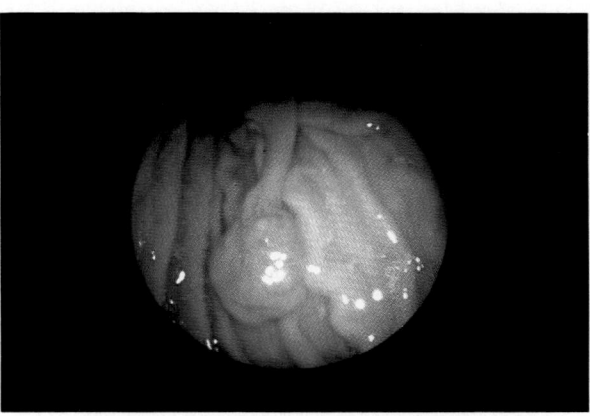

II-8 **Gastric polyp**   The histologic type must be determined by excision and pathologic examination.

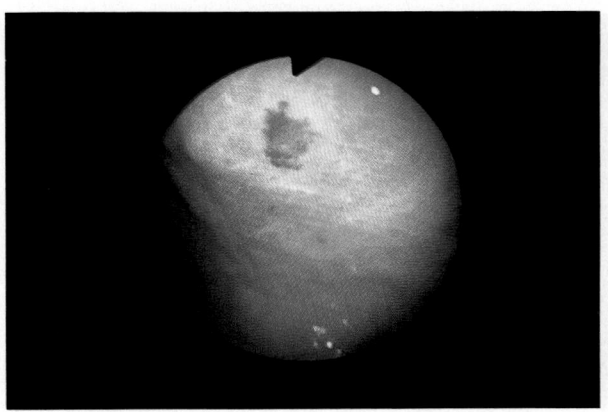

II-9 **Arteriovenous malformation of the gastric mucosa**

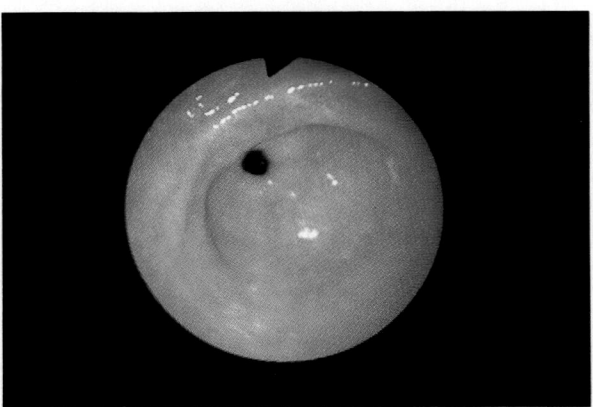

II-10 **Normal pylorus**   Note the absence of gastric rugal folds in the antrum proximal to the pylorus.

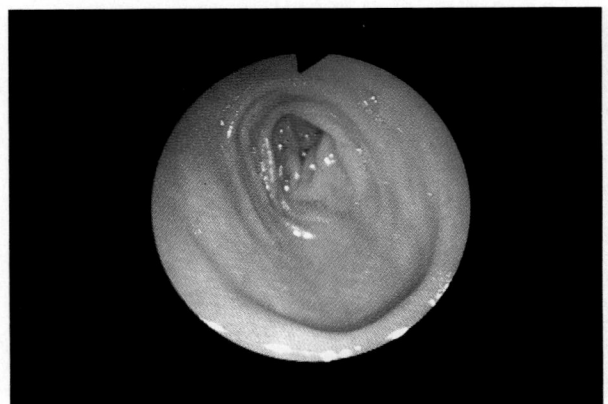

II-11 **Normal duodenal bulb**

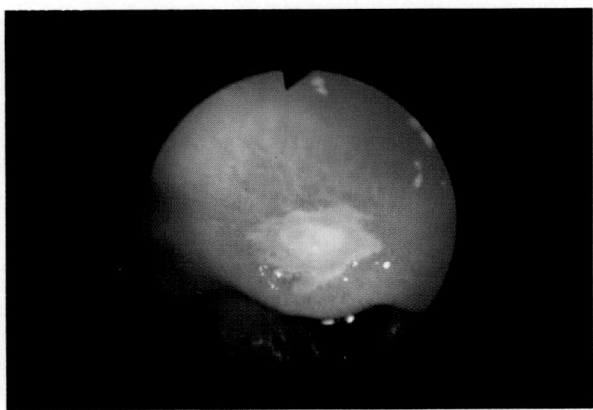

II-12 **Duodenal ulcer**   A typical ulcer with a clean base is seen on the anterior surface of the duodenal bulb.

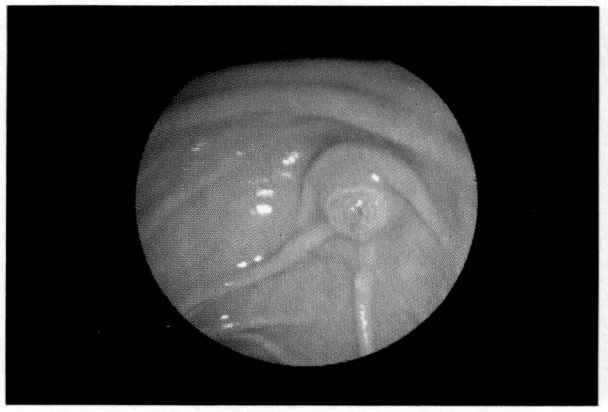

II-13 **Normal papilla of Vater** The fold pattern surrounding the papilla is normal; bile is seen adjacent to the papilla.

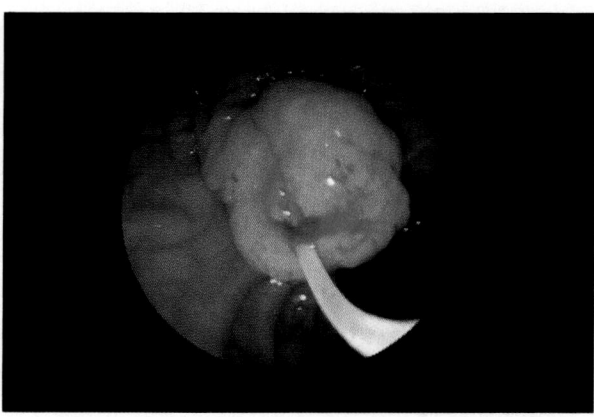

II-14 **Periampullary carcinoma** The mass at the papilla of Vater has been catheterized during ERCP.

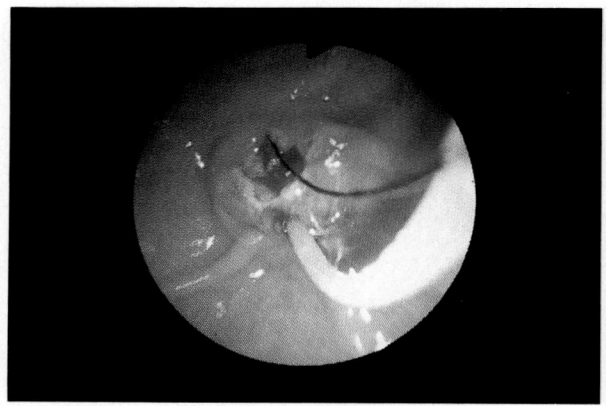

II-15 **Endoscopic papillotomy** A papillotome has been passed into the papilla, the wire bowed, and an incision made, with electrosurgical current, in the superior aspect of the papilla.

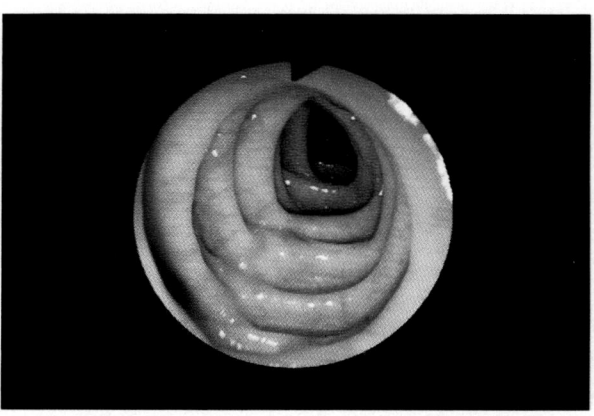

II-16 **Normal colon** Typical folds and vascular pattern can be seen.

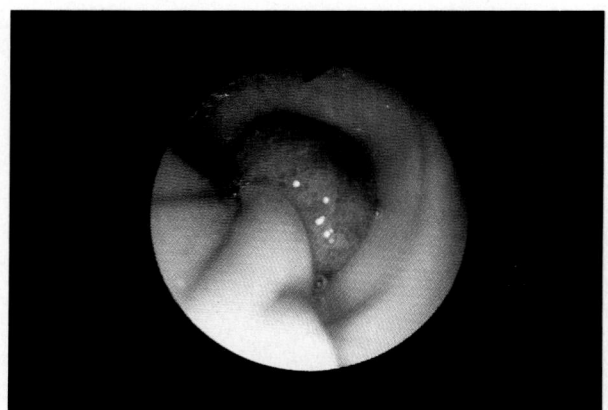

II-17 **Colonic adenomatous polyp** The polyp is erythematous; a stalk is seen covered with normal mucosa.

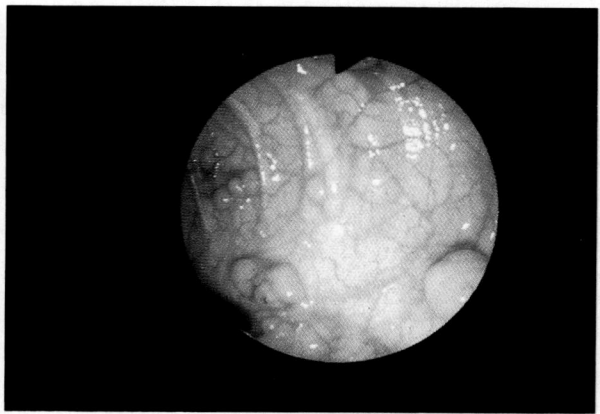

II-18 **Multiple, small, colonic adenomatous polyps** in a case of familial polyposis coli. This colon must be removed to prevent the development of cancer.

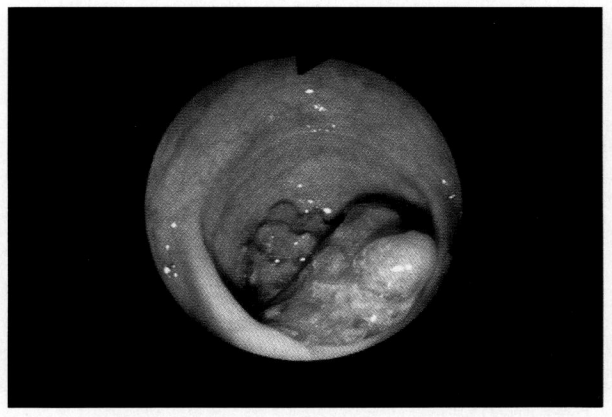

II-19 **Colon adenocarcinoma** The cancer is multilobed and growing into the lumen.

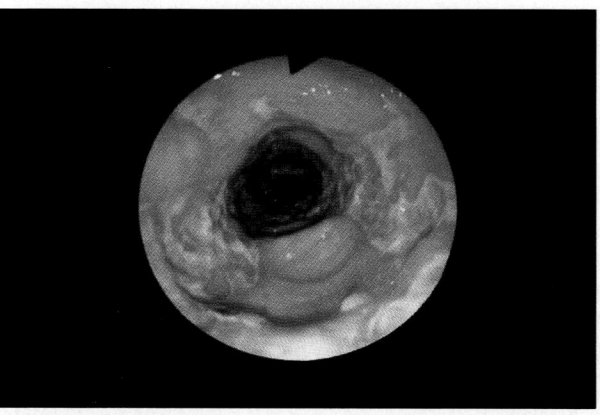

II-20 **Crohn's colitis** with linear, serpiginous, white-based ulcers surrounded by colonic mucosa that is relatively normal

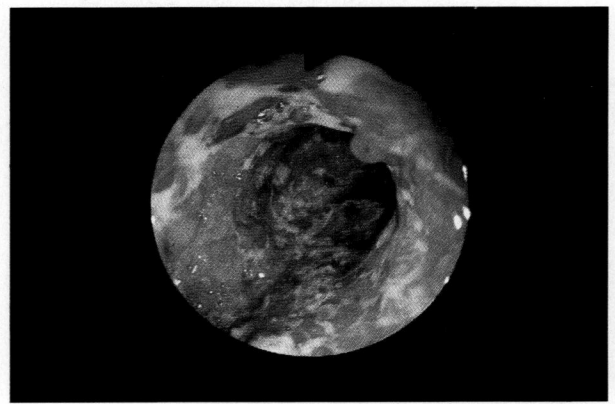

II-21 **Severe ulcerative colitis** with diffuse ulceration, bleeding, and exudation

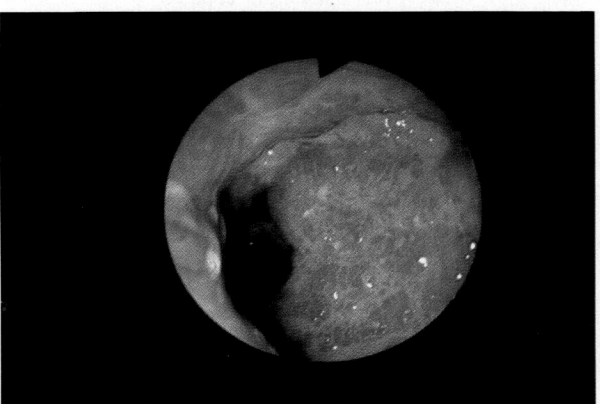

II-22 **Kaposi's sarcoma involving the colon** in a patient with AIDS. The erythematous lesions involve most of the colonic mucosa in the photograph.

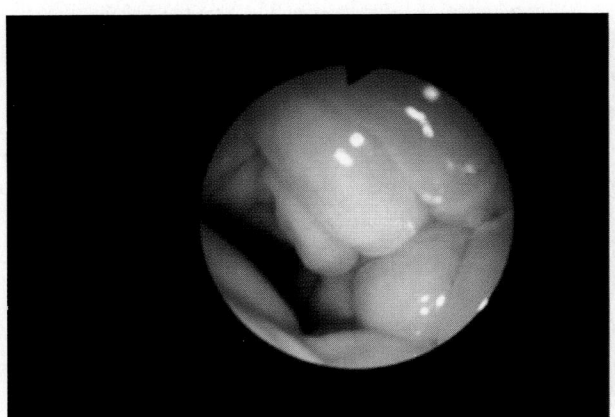

II-23 **Colonic varices** Multiple, serpiginous, subepithelial structures impinge on the colonic lumen.

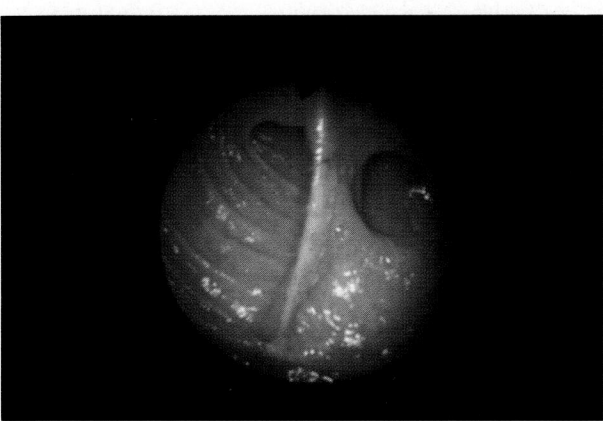

II-24 **Ileal pouch** The mucosa appears normal in this pouch reconstructed from ileum to provide a reservoir after total proctocolectomy and ileoanal anastomosis.

III. Atlas of Funduscopic Examination

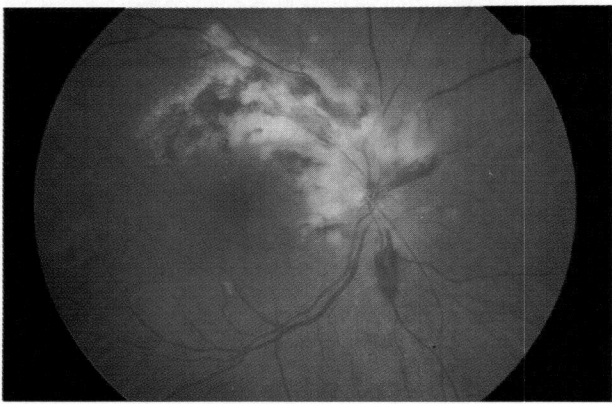

III-1 **Cytomegalovirus** in a patient with AIDS appears as an arcuate zone of retinitis with hemorrhages and optic disc swelling. Often CMV is confined to the retinal periphery, beyond view of the direct ophthalmoscope.

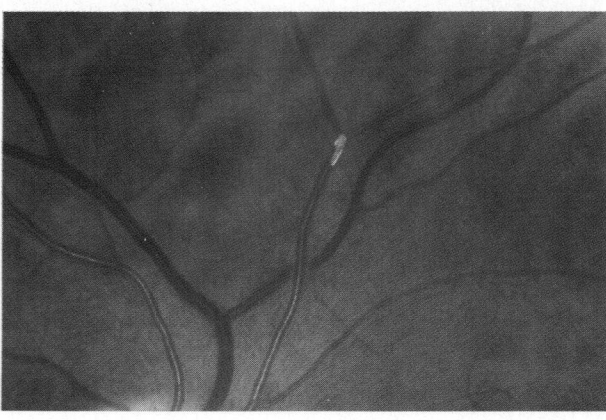

III-2 **Hollenhorst plaque** lodged at the bifurcation of a retinal arteriole proves that a patient is shedding emboli from either the carotid artery, great vessels, or heart.

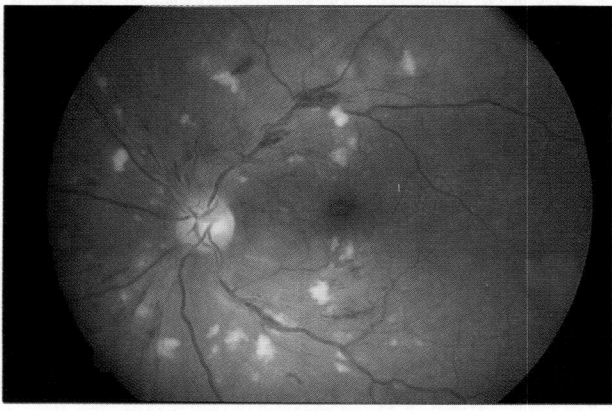

III-3 **Hypertensive retinopathy** with scattered flame (splinter) hemorrhages and cotton wool spots (nerve fiber layer infarcts) in a patient with headache and a blood pressure of 234/120

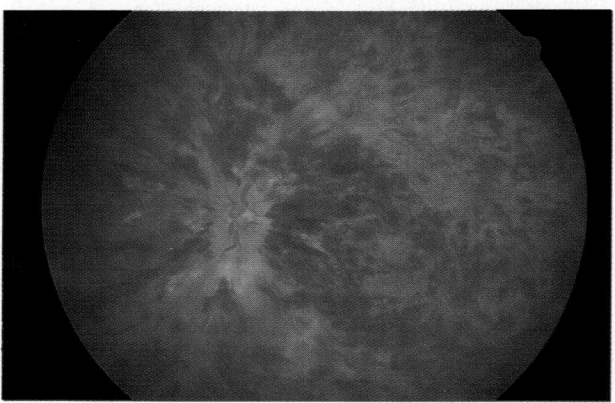

III-4 **Central retinal vein occlusion** can produce massive retinal hemorrhage ("blood and thunder"), ischemia, and vision loss.

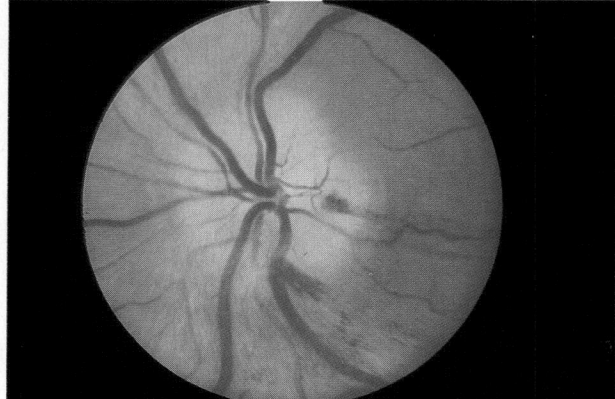

III-5 **Anterior ischemic optic neuropathy** from temporal arteritis in a 78-year old woman with pallid disc swelling, hemorrhage, visual loss, myalgia, and an erythrocyte sedimentation rate of 86 mm/h

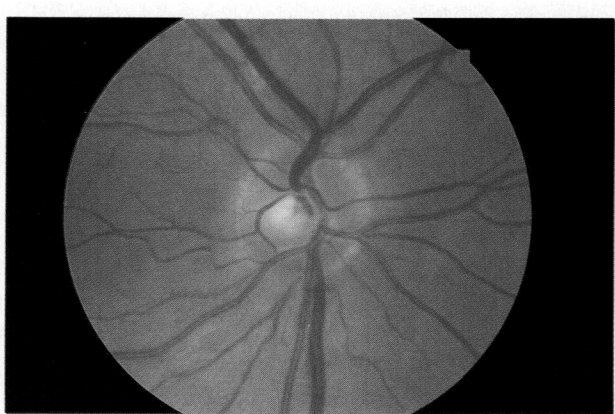

III-6 **Retrobulbar optic neuritis** is characterized by a normal fundus examination initially, hence the rubric, "the doctor sees nothing, and the patient sees nothing." Optic atrophy develops after severe or repeated attacks.

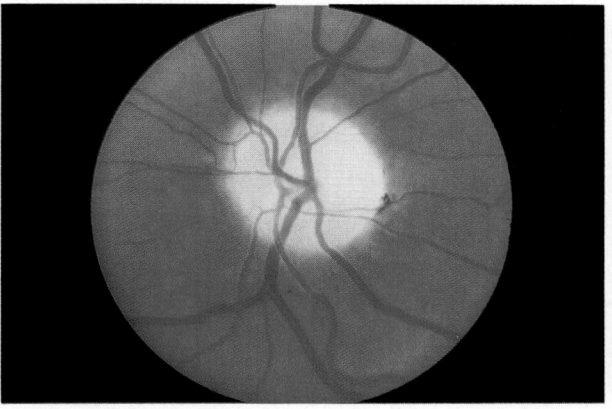

III-7 **Optic atrophy** is not a specific diagnosis but refers to the combination of optic disc pallor, arteriolar narrowing, and nerve fiber layer destruction produced by a host of eye diseases, especially optic neuropathies.

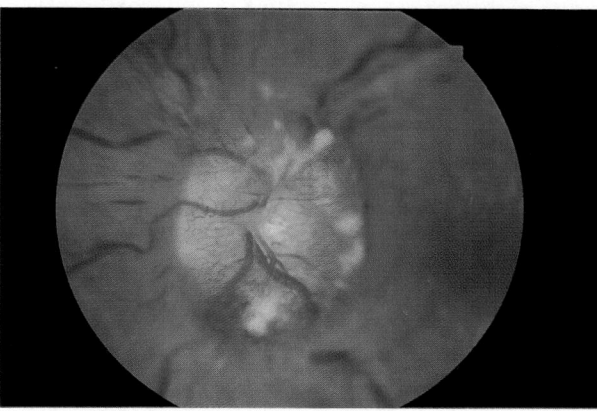

III-8 **Papilledema** means optic disc edema from raised intracranial pressure. This obese young woman with pseudotumor cerebri was misdiagnosed as a migraineur until fundus examination was performed, showing optic disc elevation, hemorrhages, and cotton wool spots.

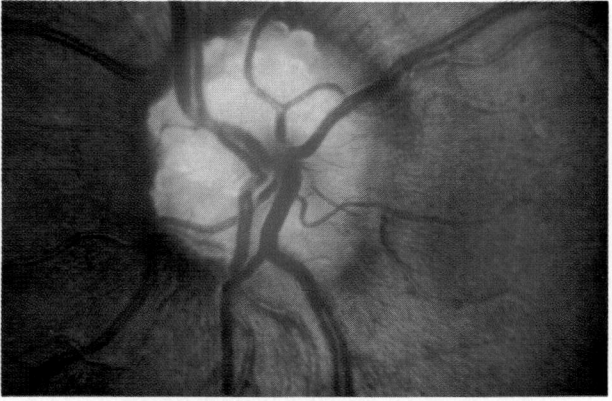

III-9 **Optic disc drusen** are calcified deposits of unknown etiology within the optic disc. They are sometimes confused with papilledema.

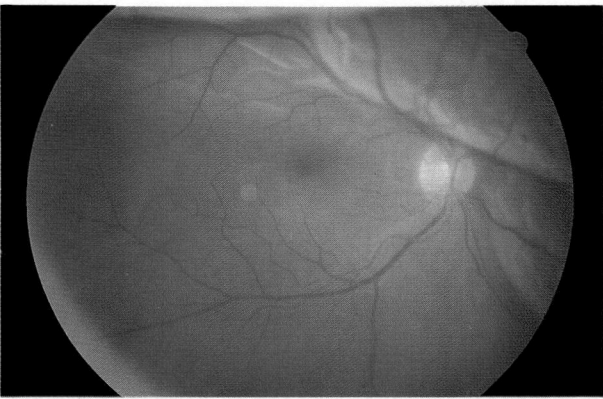

III-10 **Retinal detachment** appears as an elevated sheet of retinal tissue with folds. In this patient the fovea was spared, so acuity was normal, but a superior detachment produced an inferior scotoma.

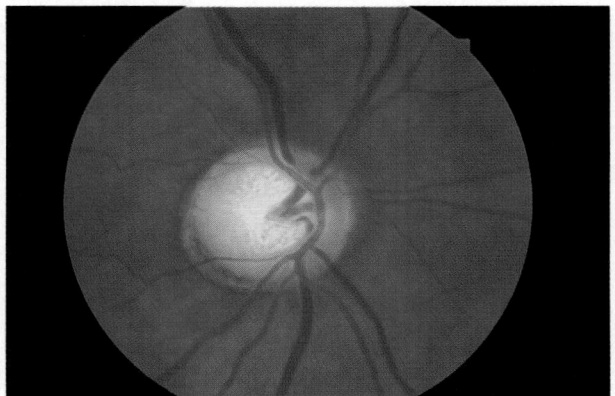

III-11 **Glaucoma** results in "cupping" as the neural rim is destroyed and the central cup becomes enlarged and excavated. The cup-to-disc ratio is about 0.7/1.0 in this patient.

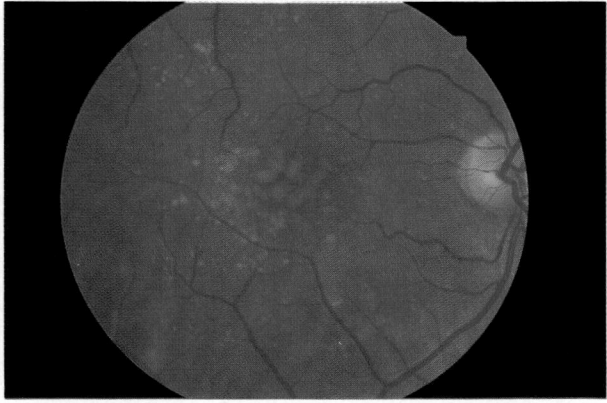

III-12 **Age-related macular degeneration** begins with the accumulation of drusen within the macula. They appear as scattered yellow subretinal deposits.

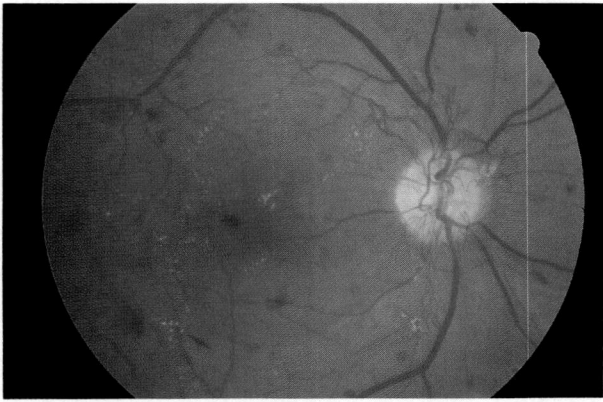

III-13 **Diabetic retinopathy** results in scattered hemorrhages and yellow exudates. This patient has neovascular vessels proliferating from the optic disc, requiring urgent pan retinal laser photocoagulation.

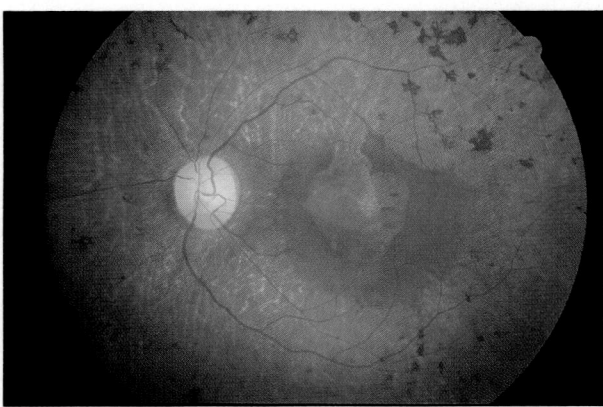

III-14 **Retinitis pigmentosa** with black clumps of pigment in the retinal periphery known as "bone spicules." There is also atrophy of the retinal pigment epithelium, making the vasculature of the choroid easily visible.

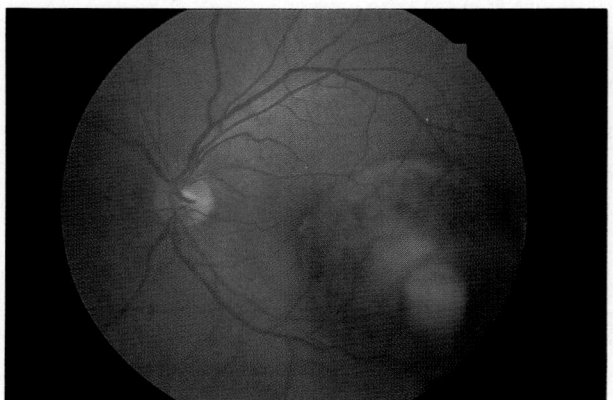

III-15 **Melanoma** of the choroid, appearing as an elevated dark mass in the inferior temporal fundus, just encroaching upon the fovea.

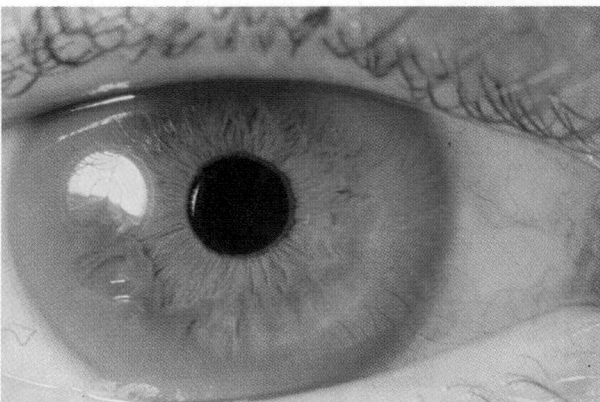

III-16 **Kayser-Fleischer ring** develops in Wilson's disease from copper deposition in Descemet's membrane, producing brownish discoloration of the peripheral cornea. It should not be confused with the yellow-white lipid ring of arcus senilis, which is common in the elderly and occasionally signifies hyperlipidemia, especially when it appears at a young age.

IV. Atlas of Hematology

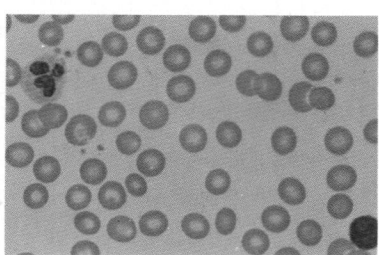

IV-1 **Normal blood smear** Normal red blood cells are round, possess an area of central pallor, appear slightly smaller than the nucleus of a mature lymphocyte, and vary little in size (anisocytosis) or in shape (poikilocytosis).

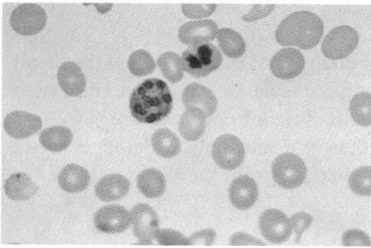

IV-2 **Megaloblastic anemia** Oval macrocytes, well filled with hemoglobin, are admixed with lesser numbers of small teardrop-shaped red blood cells. Note also hypersegmented granulocyte.

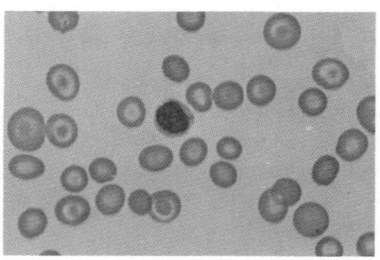

IV-3 **Liver disease** Round macrocytes of rather uniform size are seen. Many of the macrocytes are also target cells.

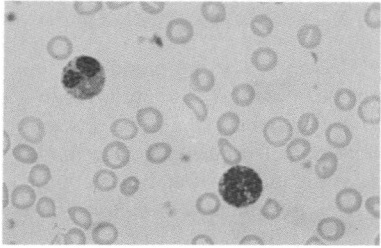

IV-4 **Iron-deficiency anemia** In severe iron deficiency, the red blood cells are smaller than normal (microcytosis), and their central area of pallor is expanded (hypochromia) so that the cells appear to have only a thin rim of hemoglobin.

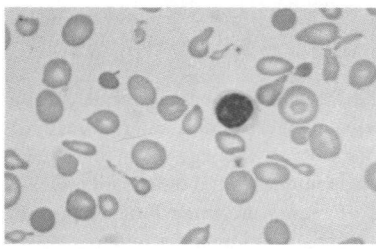

IV-5 **ß Thalassemia intermedia** Microcytic and hypochromic red blood cells are seen that resemble the red blood cells of severe iron deficiency anemia shown in Fig. IV-4. Many elliptical and teardrop-shaped red blood cells are noted.

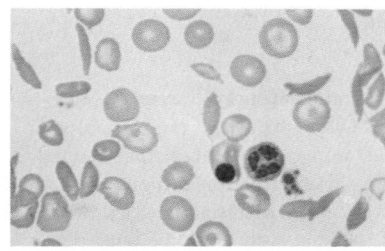

IV-6 **Sickle cell anemia** The elongated and crescent-shaped red blood cells seen on this smear represent circulating irreversibly sickled cells. Target cells and a nucleated red blood cell are also seen.

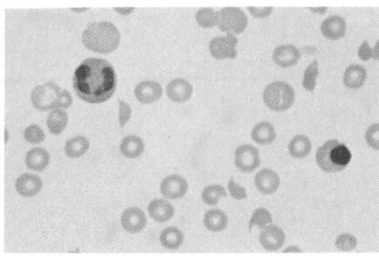

IV-7 **Traumatic hemolysis** The helmet-shaped red blood cell and the small triangular-shaped red blood cells seen on this smear represent morphologic evidence of mechanical damage to red blood cells within the blood vessels.

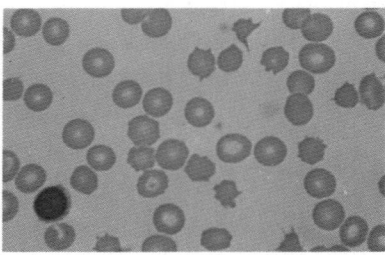

IV-8 **Spur cell anemia** Spur cells are recognized as distorted red blood cells containing several irregularly distributed thornlike projections. Cells with this morphologic abnormality are also called acanthocytes.

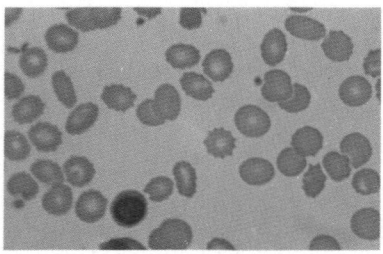

IV-9 **Uremia** The red blood cells in uremia may acquire numerous, regularly spaced, small spiny projections. Such cells, called burr cells or echinocytes, are readily distinguishable from the irregularly spiculated acanthocytes shown in Fig. IV-8.

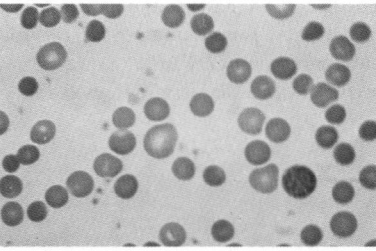

IV-10 **Hereditary spherocytosis** Small, densely staining red blood cells are seen that have lost their central area of pallor (microspherocytes). Microspherocytes may also be found in other hemolytic disorders (Fig. IV-11).

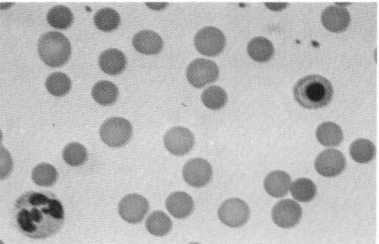

IV-11 **Immunohemolytic anemia** Microspherocytes are seen on this blood smear along with several macrocytes with a slight purple tinge (polychromasia). The latter represent new red blood cells released early from the bone marrow. The microspherocytes seen in immunohemolytic anemia may be indistinguishable from the microspherocytes seen in hereditary spherocytosis (Fig. IV-10).

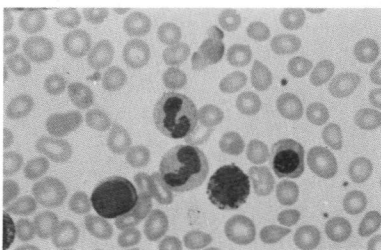

IV-12 **Leukoerythroblastic smear** Teardrop-shaped red blood cells indicative of membrane damage from collagen fibers, a nucleated red blood cell indicative of premature release of erythroid precursors, and immature myeloid cells indicative of extramedullary hematopoiesis are noted. This peripheral blood smear is related to marrow fibrosis, either primary myelofibrosis or secondary myelophthisis.

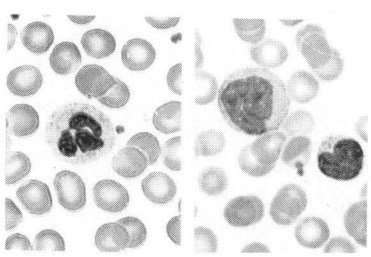

A   *B*

IV-13 A. **Normal granulocyte** The normal granulocyte has a segmented nucleus with heavy, clumped chromatin; fine neutrophilic granules are dispersed throughout its cytoplasm.

B. **Normal monocyte and lymphocyte** The normal monocyte is a large cell with an indented or folded nucleus containing loose, strand-like chromatin; the cytoplasm is a blue-gray color and usually contains fine azurophilic granules. The normal lymphocyte is a smaller cell. Its nucleus is usually round but may be indented, as in the cell shown in this plate. The nuclear chromatin has a smudgy appearance; the cytoplasm is blue.

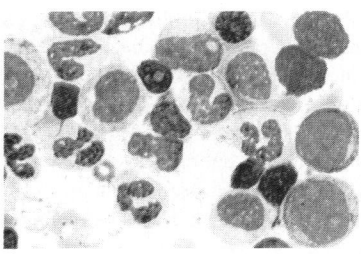

IV-15 **Normal granulocyte precursors in marrow** The earliest granulocytic precursor (myeloblast) possesses a round nucleus with fine, punctate chromatin and one or more nucleoli; the cytoplasm is blue. As nuclear differentiation proceeds, the nucleoli disappear, the chromatin coarsens, and the nucleus becomes increasingly indented and finally segmented. As cytoplasmic differentiation proceeds, azurophilic granules appear and the cytoplasm changes color from blue to the yellow-pink-gray hue of the mature granulocyte, and as this occurs the azurophilic granules become obscured by fine neutrophilic granules.

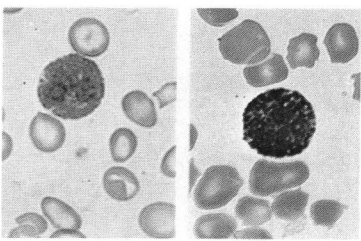

A   *B*

IV-14 A. **Normal eosinophil** The eosinophil contains large, bright-orange granules; the nucleus is bilobed.

B. **Basophil** The basophil contains large purple-black granules that fill the cell and obscure the nucleus.

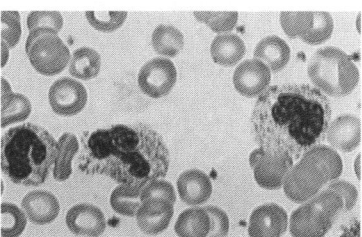

IV-16 **Neutrophils with toxic granulation** In infection and other toxic states, azurophilic granules may become visible in mature granulocytes as coarse, dark-staining cytoplasmic granules.

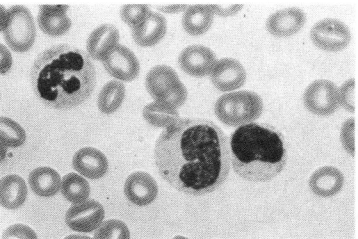

IV-17 **Band with Döhle body** *(center)* Döhle bodies are discrete, blue-staining non-granular areas found in the periphery of the cytoplasm of the neutrophil in infections and other toxic states. They represent aggregates of rough endoplasmic reticulum.

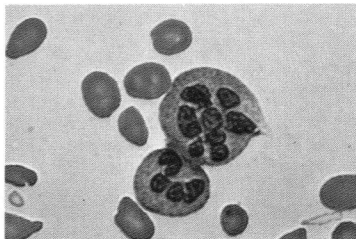

IV-18 **Hypersegmentation** Frequent five-lobed granulocytes on a blood smear or granulocytes with more than five lobes are evidence of hypersegmentation, an important clue to the diagnosis of megaloblastic anemia.

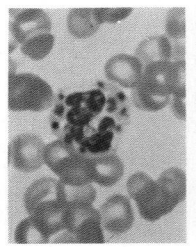 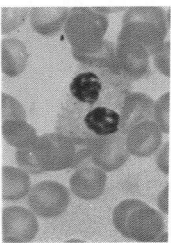

A *B*

IV-19 *A.* **Chédiak-Higashi anomaly** In this ultimately fatal disorder, the granulocytes contain huge cytoplasmic granules, formed from aggregation and fusion of azurophilic and specific granules. Large, abnormal granules are found in other granule-containing cells throughout the body. *B.* **Pelger-Hüet anomaly** In this benign disorder, the majority of granulocytes are bilobed. The nucleus frequently has a spectacle-like or "pince-nez" configuration.

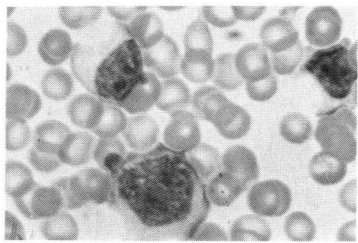

IV-20 **Reactive lymphocytes** (infectious mononucleosis) Reactive lymphocytes are usually large, and contain abundant cytoplasm. The nucleus may be eccentrically placed and may have irregular borders and indentations (not seen on this plate). The cytoplasm contains areas that stain a darker blue due to their increased content of RNA. The cytoplasm may be indented where it abuts against a red blood cell.

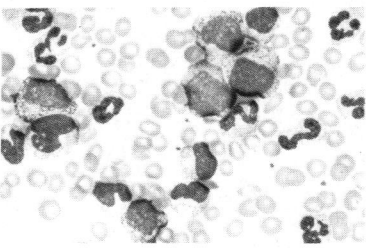

IV-21 **Chronic granulocytic leukemia** The peripheral WBC count is high due to increased numbers of granulocytes and their precursors. The majority of the WBCs are segmented granulocytes or band forms, but myelocytes (as seen on this plate) and promyeloblasts (not seen on this plate) may also be found on review of the blood smear.

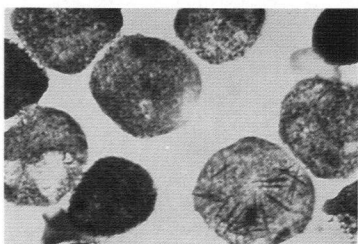

IV-22 **Leukemic cell in acute promyelocytic leukemia** Note multiple Auer rods.

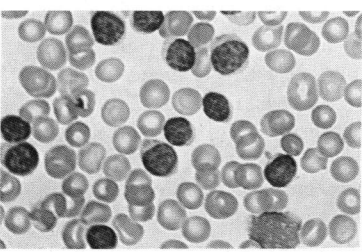

IV-23 **Chronic lymphocytic leukemia** The peripheral WBC count is high due to increased numbers of small, well-differentiated lymphocytes. However, the leukemic lymphocytes are fragile, and substantial numbers of broken, smudged cells are usually also present on the blood smear.

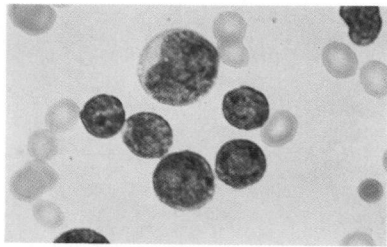

IV-24 **Leukemic cells in acute lymphoblastic leukemia** characterized by round or convoluted nuclei, high nuclear/cytoplasmic ratio and absence of cytoplasmic granules

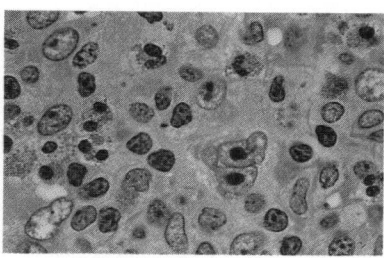

IV-25 **Hodgkin's disease, mixed cellularity**   A Reed-Sternberg cell is present near the center of the field; a large cell with a bilobed nucleus and prominent nucleoli. The majority of the cells are normal lymphocytes, neutrophils, and eosinophils that form a pleiomorphic cellular infiltrate.

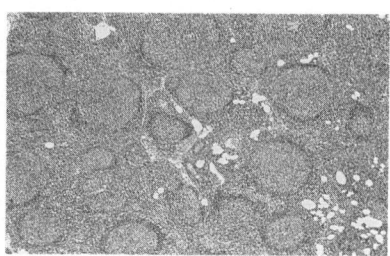

IV-26 **Follicular lymphoma**   The normal nodal architecture is effaced by nodular expansions of tumor cells. Nodules vary in size and mimic normal lymphoid follicles.

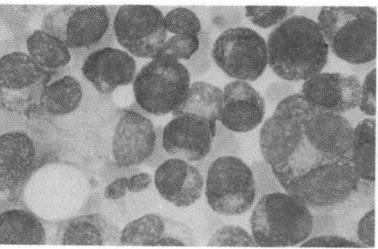

IV-27 **Multiple myeloma** (marrow)   The cells bear the characteristic morphologic features of plasma cells, round or oval cells with an eccentric nucleus composed of coarsely clumped chromatin, a densely basophilic cytoplasm, and a perinuclear clear zone (hof) containing the Golgi apparatus. Binucleate and multinucleate malignant plasma cells also can be seen.

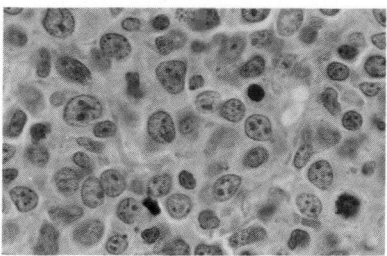

IV-28 **Diffuse large B cell lymphoma** The neoplastic cells are large with vesicular nuclear chromatin and prominent nucleoli.

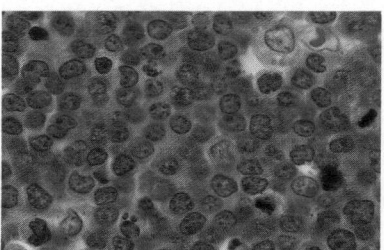

IV-29 **Burkitt's lymphoma**   The neoplastic cells are homogeneous, medium-sized B cells with frequent mitotic figures, a morphologic correlate of high growth fraction. Reactive macrophages are scattered through the tumor and their pale cytoplasm in a background of blue-staining tumor cells gives the tumor a so-called "starry sky" appearance.

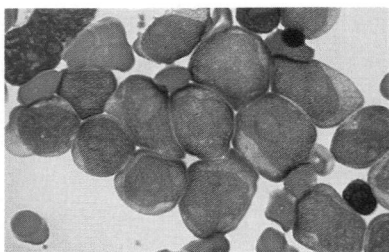

IV-30 **Acute myelocytic leukemia** This marrow section shows sheets of primitive myeloblasts with numerous large nucleoli.

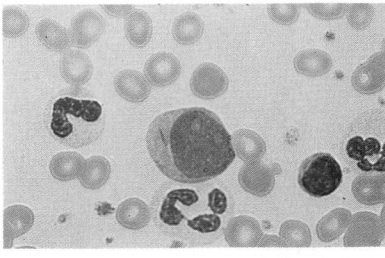

IV-31 **Auer rod** This peripheral blood smear shows a myeloblast with a single Auer rod in the cytoplasm. Auer rods, when present, are usually seen in acute myelocytic leukemia.

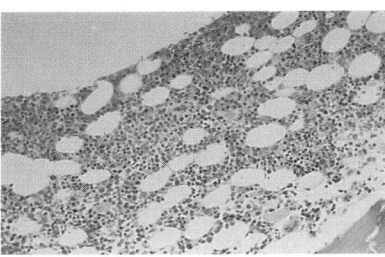

IV-32 **Normal bone marrow biopsy** This is a low power view of an H&E-stained section of normal marrow. Note that the nucleated cellular elements account for about 40 to 50 percent and the fat *(clear areas)* accounts for about 50 to 60 percent of the area.

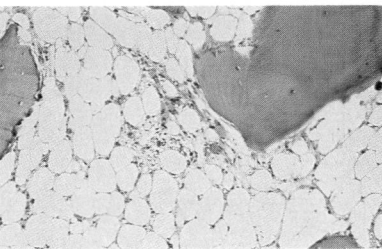

IV-33 **Aplastic anemia** This marrow section shows only fat with nearly complete absence of hematopoietic tissue.

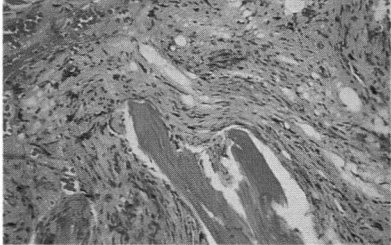

IV-34 **Marrow fibrosis** This marrow section shows the marrow cavity replaced by fibrous tissue composed of reticulin fibers and collagen. When this fibrosis is due to a primary hematologic process, it is called *myelofibrosis.* When the fibrosis is secondary to a tumor or a granulomatous process, it is called *myelophthisis.*

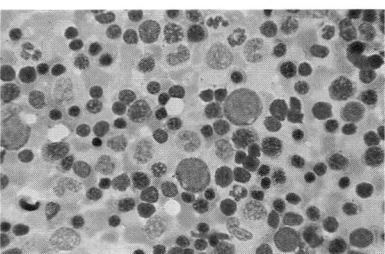

IV-35 **Erythroid hyperplasia** This marrow section shows an increase in the fraction of cells in the erythroid lineage as might be seen in a healthy marrow compensating for acute blood loss or hemolysis. The E/G ratio is greater than 1/1.

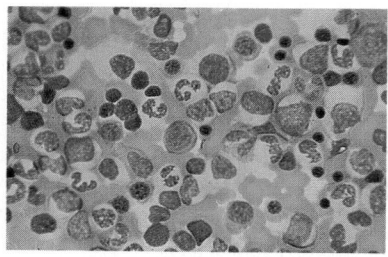

IV-36 **Granulocytic hyperplasia** This marrow section shows an increase in the fraction of cells in the myeloid or granulocytic lineage as might be seen in a healthy marrow responding to infection. The E/G ratio is less than 1/3.

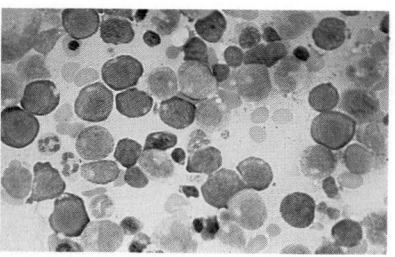

IV-37 **Megaloblastic erythropoiesis** This marrow section demonstrates so-called nuclear-cytoplasmic dissociation; the cytoplasm of erythroblasts is filled with hemoglobin demonstrating nearly complete maturation while the nuclei have loose chromatin characteristic of more immature erythroid cells. The slow nuclear maturation is related to a decrease in DNA synthesis related to an insufficient supply of reduced folate to synthesize thymidylate. DNA synthesis inhibitors can produce this picture, as can folate and B_{12} deficiency.

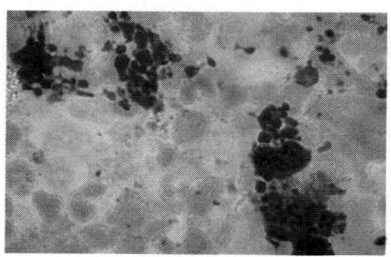

IV-38 **Marrow iron stores** This marrow section is stained with Prussian blue. Iron takes up the stain and is concentrated in reticuloendothelial cells. This picture shows normal iron stores. In iron deficiency states, no stainable iron is detectable. In the anemia of chronic disease, iron is present but cytokines prevent its mobilization and utilization in heme synthesis.

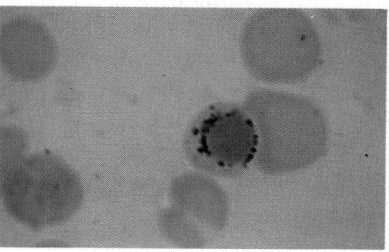

IV-39 **Ringed sideroblast** Refractory anemia with ringed sideroblasts (RARS) is in the spectrum of myelodysplastic syndromes. This marrow Prussian blue stain shows an orthochromatic normoblast with a collar of blue granules surrounding the nucleus. The blue granules represent iron-laden mitochondria.

SOURCES OF PHOTOGRAPHS

I. DERMATOLOGY

Robert Swerlick, M.D.   IA-1 Acne rosacea; IA-9 Lichen planus; IA-12 Alopecia areata; ID-33 Folliculitis; IE-65 Erythema nodosum; IE-66 Vasculitis

S. Wright Caughman, M.D.   IC-30 Nodular melanoma; ID-35 Herpes simplex; ID-50 Fulminant meningococcemia; ID-58 Condylomata acuminatum

Alvin Solomon, M.D.   IC-29 Lentigo maligna melanoma; ID-53 Secondary syphilis of the palms

Mary Spraker, M.D.   ID-32 Impetigo contagiosa

Kim Yancey, M.D.   IF-74 Coumarin necrosis

John Greenspan, Ph.D.   ID-41 Oral hairy leukoplakia; ID-42 Pseudomembranous oral candidiasis

Gregory Cox, M.D.   ID-51 Primary syphilis

Marilynne McKay, M.D.   IE-59 Discoid lupus erythematosus

James Krell, M.D.   IE-60 Dermatomyositis

Yale Resident's Slide Collection   ID-40 Molluscum contagiosum; ID-48 Rocky Mountain spotted fever; ID-69 Bullous pemphigoid; ID-47 Erythema chronicum migrans; ID-54 Condylomata lata; ID-64 Erythema multiforme

Kalman Watsky, M.D.   IA-1 Acne vulgaris

Jean Bolognia, M.D.   IA-6 Seborrheic dermatitis; IB-24 Non-Hodgkin's lymphoma

Robert Hartman, M.D.   ID-36 Varicella

Irwin Braverman, M.D.   IA-4 Atopic dermatitis

II. ENDOSCOPIC FINDINGS

FE Silverstein and **GN Tytgat**   *Atlas of Gastrointestinal Endoscopy,* New York, Gower Medical Publishing, 1987   All photographs except II-12, II-23, II-24

GN Tytgat   II-12, II-23, II-24

III. FUNDUSCOPIC FINDINGS

Jonathan C. Horton, M.D., Ph.D.   All photographs, III-1 to III-16

IV. HEMATOLOGY

Elaine Jaffe, M.D.   IV-25 to IV-29

Robert S. Hillman, M.D., and **Kenneth A. Ault, M.D.**   *Hematology in General Practice,* New York, McGraw-Hill, 1995. Courtesy of the American Society of Hematology Slide Bank. IV-30 to IV-39

APPENDICES

A

LABORATORY VALUES OF CLINICAL IMPORTANCE

INTRODUCTORY COMMENTS

All laboratory appendices should be interpreted with caution since normal values differ widely among clinical laboratories. The values given in this Appendix are meant primarily for use with this text. In preparing the Appendix, the editors have taken into account the fact that the system of international units (SI, système international d'unités) is now used in most countries and in most medical and scientific journals.[1] However, clinical laboratories in many countries continue to report values in traditional units. Therefore, both systems are used in the Appendix. Values in SI units appear first, and traditional units appear in parentheses after the SI units. The dual system is also used in the text except for (1) those instances in which the numbers remain the same but only the terminology is changed (mmol/L for meq/L or IU/L for mIU/mL), when only the SI units are given; and (2) most pressure measurements (e.g., blood and cerebrospinal fluid pressures), when the traditional units (mmHg, mmH₂O) are used. In all other instances in the text the SI unit is followed by the traditional unit in parentheses. The SI base units, SI derived units, other units of measure referred to in Appendix A, and SI prefixes are listed in Tables A-1 to A-3 at the end of Appendix A. Conversions from one system to another can be made as follows:

$$mmol/L = \frac{mg/dL \times 10}{atomic\ weight}$$

$$mg/dL = \frac{mmol/L \times atomic\ weight}{10}$$

ASCITIC FLUID

See Chapter 46

BODY FLUIDS AND OTHER MASS DATA

Body fluid, total volume: 50 percent (in obese) to 70 percent (lean) of body weight
 Intracellular: 0.3–0.4 of body weight
 Extracellular: 0.2–0.3 of body weight
Blood
 Total volume:
  Males: 69 mL per kg body weight
  Females: 65 mL per kg body weight
 Plasma volume:
  Males: 39 mL per kg body weight
  Females: 40 mL per kg body weight
 Red blood cell volume:
  Males: 30 mL per kg body weight (1.15–1.21 L/m² of body surface area)
  Females: 25 mL per kg body weight (0.95–1.00 L/m² of body surface area)

[1] Young DS: Implementation of SI units for clinical laboratory data. Ann Intern Med 106:114, 1987

CEREBROSPINAL FLUID[2]

		Conversion Factor (CF) C × CF = SI
Osmolarity	292–297 mmol/kg water (292–297 mOsm/L)	—
Electrolytes:		
Sodium	137–145 mmol/L (137–145 meq/L)	—
Potassium	2.7–3.9 mmol/L (2.7–3.9 meq/L)	—
Calcium	1.0–1.5 mmol/L (2.1–3.0 meq/L)	0.5
Magnesium	1.0–1.2 mmol/L (2.0–2.5 meq/L)	0.5
Chloride	116–122 mmol/L (116–122 meq/L)	—
CO_2 content	20–24 mmol/L (20–24 meq/L)	—
P_{CO_2}	6–7 kPa (45–49 mmHg)	0.1333
pH	7.31–7.34	
Glucose	2.2–3.9 mmol/L (40–70 mg/dL)	0.05551
Lactate	1–2 mmol/L (10–20 mg/dL)	0.1110
Total protein:	0.2–0.5 g/L (20–50 mg/dL)	0.01
Albumin	0.066–0.442 g/L (6.6–44.2 mg/dL)	0.01
IgG	0.009–0.057 g/L (0.9–5.7 mg/dL)	0.01
IgG index[3]	0.29–0.59	
Oligoclonal bands (OGB)	<2 bands not present in matched serum sample	
Ammonia	15–47 μmol/L (25–80 μg/dL)	0.5872
Creatinine	44–168 μmol/L (0.5–1.9 mg/dL)	88.40
Myelin basic protein	<4 μg/L	—
CSF pressure	50–180 mmH₂O	—
CSF volume (adult)	~150 mL	—
Leukocytes		
Total	<5 per mL	—
Differential:		
Lymphocytes	60–70 percent	—
Monocytes	30–50 percent	—
Neutrophils	None	—

[2] Since cerebrospinal fluid concentrations are equilibrium values, measurements of the same parameters in blood plasma obtained at the same time are recommended. However, there is a time lag in attainment of equilibrium, and cerebrospinal levels of plasma constituents that can fluctuate rapidly (such as plasma glucose) may not achieve stable values until after a significant lag phase.

[3] $IgG\ index = \dfrac{CSF\ IgG(mg/dL) \times serum\ albumin(g/dL)}{Serum\ IgG(g/dL) \times CSF\ albumin(mg/dL)}$

CHEMICAL CONSTITUENTS OF BLOOD

See also function tests, especially "Metabolic and Endocrine Tests."

	Conversion Factor (CF) C × CF = SI
Acetoacetate, plasma: <100 μmol/L (<1 mg/dL)	97.95
Albumin, serum: 35–55 g/L (3.5–5.5 g/dL)	10.00
Aldolase: 0–100 nkat/L (0–6 U/L)	16.67
Alpha₁ antitrypsin, serum: 0.8–2.1 g/L (85–213 mg/dL)	0.01
Alpha fetoprotein (adult), serum: <30 μg/L (<30 ng/mL)	—
Aminotransferases, serum:	
Aspartate (AST, SGOT): 0–0.58 μkat/L (0–35 U/L)	0.01667
Alanine (ALT, SGPT): 0–0.58 μkat/L (0–35 U/L)	0.01667
Ammonia, as NH₃, plasma: 6–47 μmol/L (10–80 μg/dL)	0.5872
Amylase, serum: 0.8–3.2 μkat/L; 60–180 U/L	0.01667
Angiotensin-converting enzyme (ACE): <670 nkat/L (<40 U/L)	16.67
Anticonvulsant drug levels: see Fig. 365-8	
Arterial blood gases:	
[HCO₃⁻]: 21–28 mmol/L (21–30 meq/L)	—
P₍CO₂₎: 4.7–5.9 kPa (35–45 mmHg)	0.1333
pH: 7.38–7.44	—
P₍O₂₎: 11–13 kPa (80–100 mmHg)	0.1333
Ascorbic acid (vitamin C), serum: 23–57 μmol/L (0.4–1.0 mg/dL)	56.78
Barbiturates, serum: normal, nondetectable	
Phenobarbital, "potentially fatal" level: approximately 390 μmol/L (9 mg/dL)	43.06
Most short-acting barbiturates, "potentially fatal" levels: approximately 150 μmol/L (35 mg/L)	4.419
β-Hydroxybutyrate, plasma: <300 μmol/L (<3 mg/dL)	96.05
Bilirubin, total, serum (Malloy-Evelyn): 5.1–17 μmol/L (0.3–1.0 mg/dL)	17.10
Direct, serum: 1.7–5.1 μmol/L (0.1–0.3 mg/dL)	17.10
Indirect, serum: 3.4–12 μmol/L (0.2–0.7 mg/dL)	17.10
Calciferols (vitamin D), plasma:	
1,25-dihydroxyvitamin D [1,25(OH)₂D]: 40–160 pmol/L (16 to 65 pg/mL)	2.4
25-hydroxyvitamin D [25(OH)D]: 20–200 nmol/L (8–80 ng/mL)	2.496
Calcium, ionized: 1.1–1.4 mmol/L (4.5–5.6 mg/dL)	0.2495
Calcium, plasma: 2.2–2.6 mmol/L (9–10.5 mg/dL)	0.2495
Carbon dioxide content, plasma (sea level): 21–30 mmol/L (21–30 meq/L)	—
Carbon dioxide tension (P₍CO₂₎), arterial blood (sea level): 4.7–5.9 kPa (35–45 mmHg)	0.1333
Carbon monoxide content, blood: symptoms with over 20 percent saturation of hemoglobin	
Carotenoids, serum: 0.9–5.6 μmol/L (50–300 μg/dL)	0.01863
Ceruloplasmin, serum: 270–370 mg/L (27–37 mg/dL)	10.00
Chloride, serum (as Cl⁻): 98–106 mmol/L (98–106 meq/L)	—
Cholesterol: see Table A-4	
Complement, serum:	
C3: 0.55–1.20 g/L (55–120 mg/dL)	0.01
C4: 0.20–0.50 g/L (20–50 mg/dL)	0.01
Copper, serum: 11–22 μmol/L (70–140 μg/dL)	0.1574

	Conversion Factor (CF) C × CF = SI
Creatine kinase, serum (total):	
Females: 0.17–1.17 μkat/L (10–70 U/L)	0.01667
Males: 0.42–1.50 μkat/L (25–90 U/L)	0.01667
Creatine kinase-MB: 0–7 μg/L	—
Creatinine, serum: <133 μmol/L (<1.5 mg/dL)	88.40
Digoxin serum:	
Therapeutic level: 0.6–2.8 nmol/L (0.5–2.2 ng/mL)	1.281
Toxic level: >3.1 nmol/L (>2.4 ng/mL)	1.281
Ethanol, blood:	
Behavioral changes: >4.3 mmol/L (>20 mg/dL)	0.2171
Legal intoxication: >17 mmol/L (>80 mg/dL)	0.2171
Coma and death: >65 mmol/L (>300 mg/dL)	0.2171
Fatty acids, free (nonesterified), plasma: 180 mg/L (<18 mg/dL)	10.00
Ferritin, serum:	
Women: 10–200 μg/L (10–200 ng/ml)	
Men: 15–400 μg/L (15–400 ng/ml)	
Fibrinogen, plasma: see "Hematologic Evaluations: Platelets and Coagulation"	—
Fibrinogen split products: see "Hematologic Evaluations: Platelets and Coagulation"	—
Folic acid, red cell: 340–1020 nmol/L cells (150–450 ng/mL cells)	2.266
Folic acid, serum: 7–36 nmol/L cells (3–16 ng/mL cells)	—
Gastrin, serum: 40–200 ng/L (40–200 pg/mL)	—
Glucose (fasting), plasma:	
Normal: 4.2–6.4 mmol/L (75–115 mg/dL)	0.05551
Diabetes mellitus: >7.8 mmol/L [>140 mg/dL (on more than one occasion)]	0.05551
Glucose, 2 h postprandial, plasma:	
Normal: <7.8 mmol/L (<140 mg/dL)	0.05551
Impaired glucose tolerance: 7.8–11.1 mmol/L (140–200 mg/dL)	0.05551
Diabetes mellitus: >11.1 mmol/L on more than one occasion (>200 mg/dL)	0.05551
Hemoglobin, blood (sea level):	
Male: 140–180 g/L (14–18 g/dL)	10.00
Female: 120–160 g/L (12–16 g/dL)	10.00
Hemoglobin A₁c: up to 6 percent of total hemoglobin	—
Immunoglobulins, serum:	
IgA: 0.9–3.2 g/L (90–325 mg/dL)	0.01
IgD: 0–0.08 g/L (0–8 mg/dL)	0.01
IgE: <0.00025 g/L (<0.025 mg/dL)	0.01
IgG: 8.0–15.0 g/L (800–1500 mg/dL)	0.01
IgM: 0.45–1.5 g/L (45–150 mg/dL)	0.01
Iron, serum: 9–27 μmol/L (50–150 μg/dL)	0.1791
Iron-binding capacity, serum: 45–66 μmol/L (250–370 μg/dL)	0.1791
Saturation: 0.2–0.45 (20–45 percent)	
Lactate dehydrogenase, serum: 1.7–3.2 μkat/L (100–190 U/L)	0.01667
Lactate dehydrogenase isoenzymes, serum (agarose):	
Fraction 1 (of total): 0.14–0.25 (14–26 percent)	0.01
Fraction 2: 0.29–0.39 (29–39 percent)	0.01
Fraction 3: 0.20–0.25 (20–26 percent)	0.01
Fraction 4: 0.08–0.16 (8–16 percent)	0.01
Fraction 5: 0.06–0.16 (6–16 percent)	0.01
Lactate, venous plasma: 0.6–1.7 mmol/L (5–15 mg/dL)	0.1110
Lead, serum: <1.0 μmol/L (<20 μg/dL)	0.04826
Lipase, serum: 0–2.66 μkat/L (0–160 U/L)	0.01667
Lipids: see Table A-4	—

	Conversion Factor (CF) C × CF = SI
Lipids, triglyceride, serum: see "Triglycerides"	—
Lipoprotein: see Table A-4	—
Lithium, serum:	
Therapeutic level: 0.6–1.2 mmol/L (0.6–1.2 meq/L)	—
Toxic level: >2 mmol/L (2 meq/L)	—
Magnesium, serum: 0.8–1.2 mmol/L (1.8–3 mg/dL)	0.4114
Osmolality, plasma: 285–295 mmol/kg serum water (285–295 mosmol/kg serum water)	
Oxygen content:	
Arterial blood (sea level): 17–21 volume percent	—
Venous blood, arm (sea level): 10 to 16 volume percent	—
Oxygen percent saturation (sea level):	
Arterial blood: 0.97 mol/mol (97 percent)	0.01
Venous blood, arm: 0.60–0.85 mol/mol (60–85 percent)	0.01
Oxygen tension (P_{O_2}) blood: 11–13 kPa (80–100 mmHg)	0.1333
pH, blood: 7.38–7.44	—
Phenytoin, plasma: See Fig. 365-8	
Phosphatase, acid, serum: 0.90 nkat/L (0–5.5 U/L)	—
Phosphatase, alkaline, serum: 0.5–2.0 nkat/L (30–120 U/L)	—
Phosphorus, inorganic, serum: 1.0–1.4 mmol/L (3–4.5 mg/dL)	0.3229
Potassium, serum: 3.5–5.0 mmol/L (3.5–5.0 meq/L)	
Protein, total, serum: 55–80 g/L (5.5–8.0 g/dL)	10.00
Protein fractions, serum:	
Albumin: 35–55 g/L [3.5–5.5 g/dL (50–60 percent)]	10.00
Globulin: 20–35 g/L [2.0–3.5 g/dL (40–50 percent)]	10.00
Alpha$_1$: 2–4 g/L [0.2–0.4 g/dL (4.2–7.2 percent)]	10.00
Alpha$_2$: 5–9 g/L [0.5–0.9 g/dL (6.8–12 percent)]	10.00
Beta: 6–11 g/L [0.6–1.1 g/dL (9.3–15 percent)]	10.00
Gamma: 7–17 g/L [0.7–1.7 g/dL (13–23 percent)]	10.00
Pyruvate, venous, plasma: 60–170 μmol/L (0.5–1.5 mg/dL)	113.6
Quinidine, serum:	
Therapeutic range: 4.6–9.2 μmol/L (1.5–3 mg/L)	3.082
Toxic range: 15.4–18.5 μmol/L (5–6 mg/L)	3.082
Salicylate, plasma: 0 mmol/L	—
Therapeutic range: 1.4–1.8 mmol/L (20–25 mg/dL)	0.07240
Toxic range: >2.2 mmol/L (>30 mg/dL)	0.07240
Sodium, serum: 136–145 mmol/L (136–145 meq/L)	—
Steroids: see "Metabolic and Endocrine Tests"	—
Transferrin, serum: 2.3–3.9 mg/L (230–390 μg/dL)	10.00
Triglycerides: <1.8 mmol/L (<160 mg/dL)	0.01129
Troponin I, serum: 0–0.4 μg/L (0–0.4 ng/mL)	—
Troponin T, serum: 0–0.1 μg/L (0–0.1 ng/mL)	—
Urea nitrogen, serum: 3.6–7.1 mmol/L (10–20 mg/dL)	0.3570
Uric acid, serum:	
Men: 150–480 μmol/L (2.5–8.0 mg/dL)	59.48
Women: 90–360 μmol/L (1.5–6.0 mg/dL)	59.48
Vitamin A, serum: 0.7–3.5 μmol/L (20–100 μg/dL)	0.03491
Vitamin B$_{12}$, serum: 148–443 pmol/L (200–600 pg/mL)	0.7378
Zinc, serum: 11.5–18.5 μmol/L (75–120 μg/dL)	0.1530

CIRCULATORY FUNCTION TESTS

Arteriovenous oxygen difference: 30–50 mL/L
Cardiac output (Fick): 2.5–3.6 L/m^2 of body surface area per minute
Contractility indexes:
  Maximum left ventricular *dp/dt*: 1650 mmHg/s (range, 1320–1880, mmHg/s)
  (*dp/dt*)/DP when DP = 40 mmHg: 37.6 ±12.2 s^{-1} (DP, diastolic pressure)
  Mean normalized systolic ejection rate (angiography): 3.32 ± 0.84 end-diastolic volumes per second
  Mean velocity of circumferential fiber shortening (angiography) 1.66 ± 0.42 circumferences per second
Ejection fraction, stroke volume/end-diastolic volume (SV/EDV): normal range: 0.55–0.78; average: 0.67
End-diastolic volume: 75 mL/m^2 (range, 60–88 mL/m^2)
End-systolic volume: 25 mL/m^2 (range, 20–33 mL/m^2)
Left ventricular work:
  Stroke work index: 30–110 (g·m)/m^2
  Left ventricular minute work index: 1.8–6.6 [(kg·m)/m^2]/min
  Oxygen consumption index: 110–150 mL
Maximum oxygen uptake: normal range 20–60 mL/min; average: 35 mL/min
Pulmonary vascular resistance: 20–120 (dyn·s)/cm^5 (2–12 kPa·s/L)
Systemic vascular resistance: 770–1500 (dyn·s)/cm^5 (77–150 kPa·s/L)

GASTROINTESTINAL TESTS

See also "Stool Analysis."

Absorption tests:
  D-Xylose absorption test: After an overnight fast, 25 g xylose is given in aqueous solution by mouth. Urine collected for the following 5 h should contain 33–53 mmol (5–8 g) (or >20 percent of ingested dose). Serum xylose should be 1.7–2.7 mmol (25–40 mg/dL) 1 h after the oral dose.
  Vitamin A absorption test: A fasting blood specimen is obtained and 200,000 units of vitamin A in oil is given by mouth. Serum vitamin A levels should rise to twice fasting level in 3–5 h.
Bentiromide test (pancreatic function): 500 mg bentiromide (chymex) orally; *p*-aminobenzoic acid (PABA) measured in plasma and/or urine
  Plasma: >3.6 (±1.1) μg/mL at 90 min
  Urine: >50 percent recovered as PABA in 6 h

Gastric juice:	Conversion Factor (CF) C × CF = SI
Volume:	
24 h: 2–3 L	
Nocturnal: 600–700 mL	
Basal, fasting: 30–70 mL/h	
Reaction:	
pH: 1.6–1.8	
Titratable acidity of fasting juice: 4–9 μmol/s (15–35 meq/h)	0.261
Acid output:	
Basal:	
Females (mean ± 1 SD): 0.6 ± 0.5 μmol/s (2.0 ± 1.8 meq/h)	0.2778
Males (mean ± 1 SD): 0.8 ± 0.6 μmol/s (3.0 ± 2.0 meq/h)	0.2778
Maximal (after subcutaneous histamine acid phosphate 0.004 mg/kg body weight and preceded by 50 mg promethazine or after betazole 1.7 mg/kg body wt or pentagastrin 6 μg/kg body wt):	
Females (mean ± 1 SD): 4.4 ± 1.4 μmol/s (16 ± 5 meq/h)	0.2778
Males (mean ± 1 SD): 6.4 ± 1.4 μmol/s (23 ± 5 meq/h)	0.2778

Conversion
Factor (CF)
C × CF = SI

Basal acid output/maximal acid output ratio: 0.6 or less

Gastrin, serum: 40–200 ng/L (40–200 pg/mL) —

Secretin test (pancreatic exocrine function): 1 unit per kg body wt, intravenously

  Volume (pancreatic juice): >2.0 mL/kg in 80 min —

  Bicarbonate concentration: >80 mmol/L (>80 meq/L) —

  Bicarbonate output: >10 mmol in 30 min (>10 meq in 30 min) —

METABOLIC AND ENDOCRINE TESTS

Conversion
Factor (CF)
C × CF = SI

Adrenocorticotropin (ACTH) plasma, 8 A.M.: 2–11 pmol/L (9–52 pg/mL) — 0.2202

Adrenal cortex function tests: see Chap. 332 —

Adrenal medulla function tests: see Chap. 333 —

Adrenal steroids, plasma:

  Aldosterone, 8 A.M.: <220 pmol/L (patient supine, 100 meq Na and 60–100 meq K intake) (<8 ng/dL) — 27.74

  Cortisol:

    8 A.M.: 140–690 nmol/L (5–25 µg/dL) — 27.59

    4 P.M.: 80–330 nmol/L (3–12 µg/dL) — 27.59

  Dehydroepiandrosterone (DHEA): 7–31 nmol/L (2–9 µg/L) — 3.467

  Dehydroepiandrosterone sulfate (DHEA sulfate): 1.3–6.8 µmol/L (500–2500 µg/L) — 0.002714

  11-Deoxycortisol (compound S): <30 nmol/L (<1 µg/dL) — 28.86

  17-Hydroxyprogesterone:

    Women: follicular phase, 0.6–3 nmol/L (0.20–1 µg/L); luteal phase 1.5–10.6 nmol/L (0.5–3.5 µg/L) — 3.026 / 3.026

    Men: 0.2–9 nmol/L (0.06–3 µg/L) — 3.026

Adrenal steroids, urinary excretion

  Aldosterone: 14–53 nmol/d (5–19 µg/d) — 2.774

  Cortisol, free: 55–275 nmol/d (20–100 µg/d) — 2.759

  17-Hydroxycorticosteroids: 5.5–28 µmol/d (2–10 mg/d) — 2.759

  17-Ketosteroids:

    Men: 20–69 pmol/d (6–20 mg/d) — 3.467

    Women: 20–59 µmol/d (6–17 mg/d) — 3.467

Angiotensin II, plasma, 8 A.M.: 10–30 nmol/L (10–30 pg/mL) —

Arginine vasopressin (AVP), plasma:

  Random fluid intake: 1.5–5.6 pmol/L (1.5–6 ng/L) — 0.92

Calcitonin, plasma: <50 ng/L (<50 pg/mL) —

Catecholamines, urinary excretion:

  Free catecholamines: <590 nmol/d (<100 µg/d) — 5.911

  Epinephrine: <275 nmol/d (<50 µg/d) — 5.458

  Metanephrines: <7 µmol/d (<1.3 mg/d) — 5.458

  Norepinephrine: 89–473 nmol/d (15–80 µg/d) — 5.91

  Vanillylmandelic acid (VMA): <40 µmol/d (<8 mg/d) — 5.046

Glucagon, plasma: 50–100 ng/L (50–100 pg/mL) —

Gonadal function tests: see Chaps. 336 and 337 —

Gonadal steroids, plasma:

  Androstenedione:

    Women: 3.5–7.0 nmol/L (1–2 ng/mL) — 3.492

    Men: 3.0–5.0 nmol/L (0.8–1.3 ng/mL) — 3.492

Conversion
Factor (CF)
C × CF = SI

Estradiol:

  Women: 70–220 pmol/L (20–60 pg/mL), higher at ovulation — 3.671

  Men: <180 pmol/L (<50 pg/mL) — 3.671

Progesterone:

  Men, prepubertal girls, preovulatory women, and postmenopausal women: <6 nmol/L (<2 ng/mL) — 3.180

  Women, luteal, peak: 6–60 nmol/L (2–20 ng/mL) — 3.180

Testosterone:

  Women: <3.5 nmol/L (<1 ng/mL) — 3.467

  Men: 10–35 nmol/L (3–10 ng/mL) — 3.467

  Prepubertal boys and girls: 0.17–0.7 nmol/L (0.05–0.2 ng/mL) — 3.467

Gonadotropins, plasma:

  Women, mature, premenopausal, except at ovulation:

    FSH: 1.4–9.6 IU/L (1.4–9.6 mIU/mL) —

    LH: 0.8–26 IU/L (0.8–26 mIU/mL) —

  Ovulatory surge:

    FSH: 2.3–21 IU/L (2.3–21 mIU/mL) —

    LH: 25–57 IU/L (25–57 mIU/mL) —

  Postmenopausal women:

    FSH: 34–96 IU/L (34–96 mIU/mL) —

    LH: 40–104 IU/L (40–104 mIU/mL) —

  Men, mature:

    FSH: 0.9–15 IU/L (0.9–15 mIU/mL) —

    LH: 1.3–13 IU/L (1.3–13 mIU/mL) —

  Children of both sexes, prepubertal:

    LH: 1.0–5.9 IU/L (1.0–5.9 mIU/mL) —

Growth hormone, after 100 g glucose by mouth: <2 µg/L (<2 ng/ml) —

Human chorionic gonadotropin, β subunit (β-hCG), plasma:

  Men and nonpregnant women: <3 IU/L (<3 mIU/mL) —

Insulin, serum or plasma, fasting: 43–186 pmol/L (6–26 µU/mL) — 7.175

Insulin-like growth factor I (somatomedin C, IGF-1/SM C): see Chap. 329 —

Oxytocin: random 1–4 pmol/L (1.25–5 ng/L) — 0.80

  Ovulatory peak in women 4–8 pmol/L (5–10 ng/L) —

Pancreatic islet function tests: see Chap. 334 —

Parathyroid function tests: see Chap. 354 —

Pituitary function tests: see Chaps. 328 to 330 —

Pregnancy tests: see Chap. 337 —

Prolactin, serum: 2–15 µg/L (2–15 ng/mL) —

Renin-angiotensin function tests: see Chap. 332 —

Semen analysis: see Chap. 336 —

Thyroid function tests:

  Dynamic tests of thyroid function: see Chap. 331 —

  Radioactive iodine uptake, 24 h: 5–30 percent (range varies in different areas due to variations in iodine intake) —

  Resin T_3 uptake: 0.25–0.35 (25–35 percent) (varies among laboratories; for calculation of free T4 estimate, see Chap. 331) — 0.01

  Reverse triiodothyronine (rT_3), plasma: 0.15–0.61 nmol/L (10–40 ng/dL) — 0.01536

  Thyroid-stimulating hormone (TSH): 0.4–5 mU/L (0.4–5 µU/mL) —

  Thyroxine (T_4), serum radioimmunoassay: 64–154 nmol/L (5–12 µg/dL) — 12.86

  Triiodothyronine (T_3), plasma: 1.1–2.9 nmol/L (70–190 ng/dL) — 0.01536

See Table A-9

RENAL FUNCTION TESTS

	Conversion Factor (CF) C × CF = SI
Clearances (corrected to 1.72 m² body surface area):	
Measures of glomerular filtration rate:	
Insulin clearance (C1):	
Males (mean ± 1 SD): 2.1 ± 0.4 mL/s (124 ± 25.8 mL/min)	0.01667
Females (mean ± 1 SD): 2.0 ± 0.2 mL/s (119 ± 12.8 mL/min)	0.01667
Endogenous creatinine clearance: 1.5–2.2 mL/s (91–130 mL/min)	0.01667
Urea: 1.0–1.7 mL/s (60–100 mL/min)	0.01667
Measures of effective renal plasma flow and tubular function:	
p-Aminohippuric acid clearance (C1$_{PAH}$):	
Males (mean ± 1 SD): 10.9 ± 2.7 mL/s (654 ± 163 mL/min)	0.01667
Females (mean ± 1 SD): 9.9 ± 1.7 mL/s (594 ± 102 mL/min)	0.01667
Concentration and dilution test:	
Specific gravity of urine:	
After 12-h fluid restriction: 1.025 or more	—
After 12-h deliberate water intake: 1.003 or less	—
Protein excretion, urine: <0.15 g/d (<150 mg/d)	0.01
Males: 0–0.06 g/d (0–60 mg/d)	0.01
Females: 0–0.09 g/d (0–90 mg/d)	0.01
Specific gravity, maximal range: 1.002–1.028	—
Tubular reabsorption, phosphorus: 79–94 percent of filtered load	—

HEMATOLOGIC EVALUATIONS

See also "Chemical Constituents of Blood."

	Conversion Factor (CF) C × CF = SI
Bone marrow: see Table A-6	—
Carboxyhemoglobin:	
Nonsmoker: 0–0.023 (0–2.3 percent)	0.01
Smoker: 0.021–0.042 (2.1–4.2 percent)	0.01
Erythrocyte:	
Count: 4.15–4.90 × 10¹²/L (4.15–4.90 × 10⁶/mm³)	—
Distribution width: 0.13–0.15 (13–15 percent)	—
Glucose-6-phosphate dehydrogenase: 12.1 ± 2 IU/gHb (WHO)	—
Life span:	
Normal survival: 120 days	—
Chromium-labeled, half-life ($t_{1/2}$): 28 days	—
Mean corpuscular hemoglobin (MCH): 28–33 pg/cell (28–33 pg/cell)	—
Mean corpuscular hemoglobin concentration (MCHC): 320–360 g/L (32–36 g/dL)	10.00
Mean corpuscular volume (MCV): 86–98 fl (86–98 µm³)	—
Ham's test (acid serum): negative	—
Haptoglobin, serum 0.5–2.2 g/L (50–220 mg/dL)	0.01
Hematocrit	
Males: 0.42–0.52 (42–52%)	—
Females: 0.37–0.48 (37–48%)	—

	Conversion Factor (CF) C × CF = SI
Hemoglobin:	
Plasma: 0.01–0.05 g/L (1–5 mg/dL)	0.01
Whole blood:	
Males: 8.1–11.2 mmol/L (13–18 g/dL)	—
Females: 7.4–9.9 mmol/L (12–16 g/dL)	—
Hemoglobin A₂ (HbA₂): 0.015–0.035 (1.5–3.5 percent)	0.01
Hemoglobin, fetal (HbF): <0.02 (<2 percent)	0.01
Leukocytes:	
Alkaline phosphatase (LAP): 0.2–1.6 µkat/L (13–100 µ/L)	—
Count: 4.3–10.8 × 10⁹/L (4.3–10.8 × 10³/mm³)	—
Differential:	
Neutrophils: 0.45–0.74 (45–74 percent)	
Bands: 0–0.04 (0–4 percent)	
Lymphocytes: 0.16–0.45 (16–45 percent)	
Monocytes: 0.04–0.10 (4–10 percent)	
Eosinophils: 0–0.07 (0–7 percent)	
Basophils: 0–0.02 (0–2 percent)	
Methemoglobin: <2 mg/L (<2 µg/mL)	—
Osmotic fragility:	
Slight hemolysis: 0.45–0.39 percent	—
Complete hemolysis: 0.33–0.30 percent	—
Platelets and coagulation parameters:	
Alpha₂ antiplasmin: 70–130 percent	
Antithrombin III: 80–120 percent	
Bleeding time:	
Simplate: <7 min	
Euglobulin lysis time: >2 h	
Factor II: 60–100 percent	
Factor V: 60–100 percent	
Factor VII: 60–100 percent	
Factor IX: 60–100 percent	
Factor X: 60–100 percent	
Factor XI: 60–100 percent	
Factor XII: 60–100 percent	
Factor XIII: 60–100 percent	
Fibrinogen: 200–400 mg/dL	
Plasminogen: 2.4–4.4 CTA U/mL	
Protein C (antigenic assay): 58–148 percent	
Protein S (antigenic assay): 58–148 percent	
Partial thromboplastin time (activated PTT): comparable to control	
Prothrombin time (quick one-stage): control ± 1 s	
Platelets: 130–400 × 10⁹/L (130,000–400,000/mm³)	
Thrombin time: control ± 3 s	
von Willebrand's antigen: 60–150 percent	
Protoporphyrin, free erythrocyte (FEP): 0.28–0.64 µmol/L of red blood cells (16–36 µg/dL of red blood cells)	0.0177
Red cells: (see "Erythrocytes")	
Schilling test: 7–40 percent of orally administered vitamin B₁₂ excreted in urine	
Sedimentation rate:	
Westergren, <50 years of age:	
Males: 0–15 mm/h	
Females: 0–20 mm/h	
Westergren, >50 years of age:	
Males: 0–20 mm/h	
Females: 0–30 mm/h	
Sucrose hemolysis: negative	
Viscosity	
Plasma: 1.7–2.1	
Serum: 1.4–1.8	
White blood cells: (see "Leukocytes")	

STOOL ANALYSIS

	Conversion Factor (CF) C × CF = SI
Bulk:	
Wet weight: <197.5 (115 ± 41) g/d	—
Dry weight: <66.4 (34 ± 15) g/d	—
Alpha₁ antitrypsin: 0.98 (±0.17) mg/g dry weight stool	—
Coproporphyrin: 600–1500 nmol/d (400–1000 µg/d)	1.527
Fat (on diet containing at least 50 g fat): <6.0 (4.0 ± 1.5) g/d when measured on a 3-day (or longer) collection	
Percent of dry weight: 0.30 (<30.4 percent)	0.01
Coefficient of fat absorption: >0.95 (>95 percent)	0.01
Fatty acid:	
Free: 0.01–0.10 (1–10 percent of dry matter)	0.01
Combined as soap: 0.005–0.12 (0.5–12 percent of dry matter)	0.01
Nitrogen: <1.7 (1.4 ± 0.2) g/d	—
Protein content: minimal	—
Urobilinogen: 68–470 µmol/d (40–280 mg/d)	1.693
Water: 0.65 (approximately 65 percent)	0.01

URINE ANALYSIS

See also "Metabolic and Endocrine Tests"

	Conversion Factor (CF) C × CF = SI
Acidity, titratable: 20–40 mmol/d (20–40 meq/d)	—
Ammonia: 30–50 mmol/d (30–50 meq/d)	—
Amylase: 35–260 Somogyi units/h	—
Amylase/creatinine clearance ratio [(Cl$_{am}$/Cl$_{cr}$) × 100]: 1–5	—
Bentiromide (pancreatic function): 50 percent excreted in 6 h as p-amino benzoic acid (PABA) after 500 mg oral bentiromide	—
Calcium (10 meq/d or 200-mg/d calcium diet): <3.8 mmol/d (<7.5 meq/d)	0.5
Catecholamines: see under "Metabolic and Endocrine Tests"	—
Copper: 0–0.4 µmol/d (0–25 µg/d)	0.01574
Coproporphyrins (types I and III): 150–460 nmol/d (100–300 µg/d)	1.527
Creatine, as creatinine:	
Adult males: <380 µmol/d (<50 mg/d)	7.625
Adult females: <760 µmol/d (<100 mg/d)	7.625
Creatinine: 8.8–14 mmol/d (1.0–1.6 g/d)	8.840
Glucose, true (oxidase method): 0.3–1.7 mmol/d (50–300 mg/d)	0.5551
5-Hydroxyindoleacetic acid (5-HIAA): 10–47 µmol/d (2–9 mg/d)	5.230
Lead: <0.4 µmol/d (<80 µg/d)	0.004826
Protein: <0.15 g/d (<150 mg/d)	0.1
Porphobilinogen: none	—
Potassium: 25–100 mmol/d [25–100 meq/d (varies with intake)]	—
Sodium: 100–260 mmol/d [100–260 meq/d (varies with intake)]	—
Urobilinogen: 1.7–5.9 µmol/d (1–3.5 mg/d)	1.693
D-Xylose excretion: 5 to 8 g within 5 h after oral dose of 25 g	—

Table A-1

SI and Other Units

Quantity	Name of Unit	Symbol for Unit	Derivation of Units
SI BASE UNITS			
Length	meter	m	
Mass	kilogram	kg	
Time	second	s	
Thermodynamic temperature	Kelvin	K	
Amount of substance	mole	mol	
SI DERIVED UNITS			
Area	square meter	m²	
Force	newton	N	(m·kg)/s²
Pressure	pascal	Pa	N·m²
Work, energy	joule	J	N·m
Celsius temperature	degree Celsius	°C	K
OTHER UNITS RETAINED FOR USE			
Time	minute	min	
	hour	h	
	day	d	
Volume	liter	L	

Table A-2

Radiation Derived Units

Quantity	Old Unit	SI Unit	Name for SI Unit (and Abbreviation)	Conversion
Activity	curie (Ci)	Disintegrations per second (dps)	becquerel (Bq)	1 Ci = 3.7 × 10¹⁰ Bq 1 mCi = 37 mBq 1 µCi = 0.037 MBq or 37 GBq 1 Bq = 2.703 × 10⁻¹¹ Ci
Absorbed dose	rad	joule per kilogram (J/kg)	gray (Gy)	1 Gy = 100 rad 1 rad = 0.01 Gy 1 mrad = 10⁻³ cGy
Exposure	roentgen (R)	coulomb per kilogram (C/kg)	—	1 C/kg = 3876 R 1 R = 2.58 × 10⁻⁴ C/kg 1 mR = 258 pC/kg
Dose equivalent	rem	joule per kilogram (J/kg)	sievert (Sv)	1 Sv = 100 rem 1 rem = 0.01 Sv 1 mrem = 10 µSv

Table A-3

SI Prefixes and Their Symbols

Factor	Prefix	Symbol for Prefix
10⁹	giga	G
10⁶	mega	M
10³	kilo	k
10²	hecto	h
10¹	deka	da
10⁻¹	deci	d
10⁻²	centi	c
10⁻³	milli	m
10⁻⁶	micro	µ
10⁻⁹	nano	n
10⁻¹²	pico	p
10⁻¹⁵	femto	f
10⁻¹⁸	alto	a

Table A-4

Classification of Total Cholesterol, LDL-Cholesterol, and HDL-Cholesterol Values

	Total Plasma Cholesterol	LDL-Cholesterol	HDL-Cholesterol	Conversion Factor (C to SI)
Desirable	<5.20 mmol/L (<200 mg/dL)	<3.36 mmol/L (<130 mg/dL)	>1.55 mmol/L (>60 mg/dL)	0.02586
Borderline	5.20–6.18 mmol/L (200–239 mg/dL)	3.36–4.11 mmol/L (130–159 mg/dL)	0.9–1.55 mmol/L (35–60 mg/dL)	0.02586
Undesirable	≥6.21 mmol/L (≥240 mg/dL)	≥4.14 mmol/L (≥ 160 mg/dL)	<0.9 mmol/L (<35 mg/dL)	0.02586

SOURCE: Modified from the report of the Expert Panel on Detection, Evaluation, and Treatment of High Blood Cholesterol in Adults: Second Report of the National Cholesterol Education Program (NCEP) expert panel on detection, evaluation, and treatment of high blood cholesterol (Adult Treatment Panel II). Circulation 89:1329, 1994.

Table A-5

Normal Values of Doppler Echocardiographic Measurements in Adults

	Range	Mean
RVD (cm)	0.9 to 2.6	1.7
LVID (cm)	3.5 to 5.7	4.7
Posterior LV wall thickness (cm)	0.6 to 1.1	0.9
IVS wall thickness (cm)	0.6 to 1.1	0.9
Left atrial dimension (cm)	1.9 to 4.0	2.9
Aortic root dimension (cm)	2.0 to 3.7	2.7
Aortic cusps separation (cm)	1.5 to 2.6	1.9
Percentage of fractional shortening	34 to 44%	36%
Mitral flow (m/sec)	0.6 to 1.3	0.9
Tricuspid flow (m/sec)	0.3 to 0.7	0.5
Pulmonary artery (m/sec)	0.6 to 0.9	0.75
Aorta (m/sec)	1.0 to 1.7	1.35

NOTE: RVD, right ventricular dimension; LVID, left ventricular internal dimension; LV, left ventricle; IVS, interventricular septum.
SOURCE: From H Feigenbaum, *Echocardiography,* 5th ed, Philadelphia. Lea & Febiger, 1994

Table A-6

Differential Nucleated Cell Counts of Bone Marrow

	Normal, Mean%*	Range, %†		Normal, Mean%*	Range, %†
Myeloid	56.7		Erythroid	25.6	
Neutrophilic series	53.6		Pronormoblasts	0.6	0.2–1.3
Myeloblast	0.9	0.2–1.5	Basophilic normoblasts	1.4	0.5–2.4
Promyelocyte	3.3	2.1–4.1	Polychromatophilic normoblasts	21.6	17.9–29.2
Myelocyte	12.7	8.2–15.7			
Metamyelocyte	15.9	9.6–24.6	Orthochromatic normoblasts	2.0	0.4–4.6
Band	12.4	9.5–15.3	Megakaryocytes	<0.1	
Segmented			Lymphoreticular	17.8	
Eosinophilic series	3.1	1.2–5.3	Lymphocytes	16.2	11.1–23.2
Basophilic series	<0.1	0–0.2	Plasma cells	2.3	0.4–3.9
			Reticulum cells	0.3	0–0.9

* From MM Wintrobe et al, *Clinical Hematology,* 8th ed. Philadelphia, Lea & Febiger, 1981.
† Range observed in 12 healthy men.

Table A-7

Erythrocytes and Hemoglobin: Normal Values at Various Ages

Age	Red Blood Cell Count,* 10^{12}/L	Hemoglobin,* g/L (g/dL)	Vol. Packed RBCs,* mL/dL	Corpuscular Values MCV, fL	MCH, pg	MCHC, g/L (g/dL)	MCD, μm
Days 1–13	5.1 ± 1.0	195 ± 50 (19.5 ± 5)	54.0 ± 10.0	106–98	38–33	340–360 (36–34)	8.6
Days 14–60	4.7 ± 0.9	140 ± 33 (14 ± 3.3)	42.0 ± 7.0	90	30	330 (33)	8.1
3 months to 10 years	4.5 ± 0.7	122 ± 23 (12.2 ± 2.3)	36.0 ± 5.0	80	27	340 (34)	7.7
11–15 years	4.8	131 (13.14)	39.0	82	28	340 (34)	
Adults:							
Females	4.8 ± 0.6	140 ± 20 (14 ± 2)	42.0 ± 5.0	90 ± 7	29 ± 2	340 ± 20 (34 ± 2)	7.5 ± 0.3
Males	5.4 ± 0.9	160 ± 20 (16 ± 2)	47.0 ± 5.0	90 ± 7	29 ± 2	340 ± 20 (34 ± 2)	7.5 ± 0.3

* The range of values represents almost the extremes of observed variations (93 percent or more) at sea level. The blood values of healthy persons should fall well within these mean ± SD figures.
NOTE: MCV, mean corpuscular volume; MCH, mean corpuscular hemoglobin; MCHC, mean corpuscular hemoglobin concentration; MCD, mean corpuscular diameter.
SOURCE: MM Wintrobe et al, *Clinical Hematology,* 8th ed, Philadelphia, Lea & Febiger, 1981.

Table A-8

Normal Leukocyte Count, Differential Count, and Hemoglobin Concentration at Various Ages

Age	Leukocytes, Total	Neutrophils Total	Band	Segmented	Eosinophils	Basophils	Lymphocytes	Monocytes
12 mo	11.4(6.0–17.5)	3.5(1.5–8.5) *31*	0.35 *3.1*	3.2 *28*	0.3(0.05–0.7) *0.4*	0.05(0–0.20) *0.4*	7.0(4.0–10.5) *61*	0.55(0.05–1.1) *4.8*
4 yr	9.1(5.5–15.5)	3.8(1.5–8.5) *42*	0.27(0–1.0) *3.0*	3.5(1.5–7.5) *39*	0.25(0.02–0.65) *2.8*	0.05(0–0.20) *0.6*	4.5(2.0–8.0) *50*	0.45(0–0.8) *5.0*
6 yr	4.3(1.5–8.0)	0.25(0–1.0) *51*	4.0(1.5–7.0) *3.0*	4.0(1.5–7.0) *48*	0.23(0–0.65) *2.7*	0.05(0–0.20) *0.6*	3.5(1.5–7.0) *42*	0.40(0–0.8) *4.7*
10 yr	8.1(4.5–13.5)	4.4(1.8–8.0) *54*	0.24(0–1.0) *3.0*	4.2(1.8–7.0) *51*	0.20(0–0.60) *2.4*	0.04(0–0.20) *0.5*	3.1(1.5–6.5) *38*	0.35(0–0.8) *4.3*
21 yr	7.4(4.5–11.0)	4.4(1.8–7.7) *59*	0.22(0–0.7) *3.0*	4.2(1.8–7.0) *56*	0.20(0–0.45) *2.7*	0.04(0–0.20) *0.5*	2.5(1.0–4.8) *34*	0.30(0–0.8) *4.0*

NOTE: Values are expressed as "cells $\times 10^9$/L." The numbers in italic are percentages.

SOURCE: E Beutler et al (eds), *Williams Hematology*, 5th ed, New York, McGraw-Hill, 1995. By permission.

Table A-9

Summary of Values Useful in Pulmonary Physiology

	Symbol	Typical Values — Man Aged 40, 75 kg, 175 cm Tall	Woman Aged 40, 60 kg, 160 cm Tall
PULMONARY MECHANICS			
Spirometry—volume-time curves:			
Forced vital capacity	FVC	4.8 L	3.3 L
Forced expiratory volume in 1 s	FEV_1	3.8 L	2.8 L
FEV_1/FVC	FEV_1%	76%	77%
Maximal midexpiratory flow	MMF (FEF 25–27)	4.8 L/s	3.6 L/s
Maximal expiratory flow rate	MEFR (FEF 200–1200)	9.4 L/s	6.1 L/s
Spirometry—flow-volume curves:			
Maximal expiratory flow at 50% of expired vital capacity	V_{max} 50 (FEF 50%)	6.1 L/s	4.6 L/s
Maximal expiratory flow at 75% of expired vital capacity	V_{max} 75 (FEF 75%)	3.1 L/s	2.5 L/s
Resistance to airflow:			
Pulmonary resistance	RL (R_L)	<3.0 (cmH_2O/s)/L	
Airway resistance	Raw	<2.5 (cmH_2O/s)/L	
Specific conductance	SGaw	>0.13 cmH_2O/s	
Pulmonary compliance:			
Static recoil pressure at total lung capacity	Pst TLC	25 ± 5 cmH_2O	
Compliance of lungs (static)	CL	0.2 L cmH_2O	
Compliance of lungs and thorax	C(L + T)	0.1 L cmH_2O	
Dynamic compliance of 20 breaths per minute	C dyn 20	0.25 ± 0.05 L/cmH_2O	
Maximal static respiratory pressures:			
Maximal inspiratory pressure	MIP	>90 cmH_2O	>50 cmH_2O
Maximal expiratory pressure	MEP	>150 cmH_2O	>120 cmH_2O
LUNG VOLUMES			
Total lung capacity	TLC	6.4 L	4.9 L
Functional residual capacity	FRC	2.2 L	2.6 L
Residual volume	RV	1.5 L	1.2 L
Inspiratory capacity	IC	4.8 L	3.7 L
Expiratory reserve volume	ERV	3.2 L	2.3 L
Vital capacity	VC	1.7 L	1.4 L
GAS EXCHANGE (SEA LEVEL)			
Arterial O_2 tension	Pa_{O_2}	12.7 ± 0.7 kPa (95 ± 5 mmHg)	
Arterial CO_2 tension	Pa_{CO_2}	5.3 ± 0.3 kPa (40 ± 2 mmHg)	
Arterial O_2 saturation	Sa_{O_2}	0.97 ± 0.02 (97 ± 2%)	
Arterial blood pH	pH	7.40 ± 0.02	
Arterial bicarbonate	HCO_3^-	24 + 2 meq/L	
Base excess	BE	0 ± 2 meq/L	
Diffusing capacity for carbon monoxide (single breath)	DL_{CO}	0.42 mLCO/s/mmHg (25 mL CO/min/mmHg)	
Dead space volume	V_D	2 ml/kg body wt	
Physiologic dead space; dead space-tidal volume ratio	V_D/V_T		
Rest		≤35% V_T	
Exercise		≤20% V_T	
Alveolar-arterial difference for O_2	$P(A - a)_{O_2}$	≤2.7 kPa ≤20 kPa (≤20 mmHg)	

INSTRUCTIONS FOR COLLECTION AND TRANSPORT OF SPECIMENS FOR CULTURE

It is absolutely essential that the microbiology laboratory be informed of the site of origin of the sample to be cultured and of the infections that are suspected. This information determines the selection of culture media and the length of culture time.

Type of Culture (Synonyms)	Specimen	Minimum Volume	Container	Other Considerations
BLOOD				
Blood, routine (blood culture for aerobes, anaerobes, and yeasts)	Whole blood	10 mL in each of 2 bottles for adults and children; 5 mL, if possible, in each of 2 bottles for infants; less for neonates	See below.[a]	See below.[b]
Blood for fungi/ *Mycobacterium* spp.	Whole blood	10 mL in each of 2 bottles, as for routine blood cultures, or in Isolator tube requested from laboratory	Same as for routine blood culture	Specify "hold for extended incubation," since fungal agents may require 4 weeks or more to grow.
Blood, Isolator (lysis centrifugation)	Whole blood	10 mL	Isolator tubes	Use mainly for isolation of fungi, *Mycobacterium,* or other fastidious aerobes and for elimination of antibiotics from cultured blood in which organisms are concentrated by centrifugation.
RESPIRATORY TRACT				
Nose	Swab from nares	1 swab	Sterile culturette or similar transport system containing holding medium	Swabs made of calcium alginate may be used.
Throat	Swab of posterior pharynx, ulcerations, or areas of suspected purulence	1 swab	Sterile culturette or similar swab specimen collection system containing holding medium	See below.[c]
Sputum	Fresh sputum (not saliva)	2 mL	Commercially available sputum collection system or similar sterile container with screw cap	*Cause for rejection:* Care must be taken to ensure that the specimen is sputum and not saliva. Examination of Gram's stain, with number of epithelial cells and PMNs noted, can be an important part of the evaluation process. Induced sputum specimens should not be rejected.
Bronchial aspirates	Transtracheal aspirate, bronchoscopy specimen, or bronchial aspirate	1 mL of aspirate or brush in transport medium	Sterile aspirate or bronchoscopy tube, bronchoscopy brush in a separate sterile container	Special precautions may be required, depending on diagnostic considerations (e.g., *Pneumocystis*).
STOOL				
Stool for routine culture; stool for *Salmonella, Shigella,* and *Campylobacter*	Rectal swab or (preferably) fresh, randomly collected stool	1 g of stool or 2 rectal swabs	Plastic-coated cardboard cup or plastic cup with tight-fitting lid. Other leak-proof containers are also acceptable.	If *Vibrio* spp. are suspected, the laboratory must be notified, and appropriate collection/transport methods should be used.
Stool for *Yersinia, E. coli* O157	Fresh, randomly collected stool	1 g	Plastic-coated cardboard cup or plastic cup with tight-fitting lid	*Limitations:* Procedure requires enrichment techniques.
Stool for *Aeromonas* and *Plesiomonas*	Fresh, randomly collected stool	1 g	Plastic-coated cardboard cup or plastic cup with tight-fitting lid	*Limitations:* Stool should not be cultured for these organisms unless also cultured for other enteric pathogens.

(continued)

Type of Culture (Synonyms)	Specimen	Minimum Volume	Container	Other Considerations
UROGENITAL TRACT				
Urine	Clean-voided urine specimen or urine collected by catheter	0.5 mL	Sterile, leak-proof container with screw cap or special urine transfer tube	See below.[d]
Urogenital secretions	Vaginal or urethral secretions, cervical swabs, uterine fluid, prostatic fluid, etc.	1 swab or 0.5 mL of fluid	Transwab containing Amies transport medium or similar system containing holding medium for *Neisseria gonorrhoeae*; modified Todd-Hewitt broth for group B *Streptococcus* surveillance cultures	Vaginal swab samples for "routine culture" should be discouraged whenever possible unless a particular pathogen is suspected. For detection of multiple organisms (e.g., group B *Streptococcus, Trichomonas, Chlamydia,* or *Candida* spp.), 1 swab per test should be obtained.
BODY FLUIDS, ASPIRATES, AND TISSUES				
Cerebrospinal fluid (lumbar puncture)	Spinal fluid	1 mL for routine cultures; ≥5 mL for *Mycobacterium*	Sterile tube with tight-fitting cap	Do not refrigerate; transfer to laboratory as soon as possible.
Body fluids	Aseptically aspirated body fluids	1 mL for routine cultures	Sterile tube with tight-fitting cap. Specimen may be left in syringe used for collection if the syringe is capped before transport.	For some body fluids (e.g., peritoneal lavage samples), increased volumes are helpful for isolation of small numbers of bacteria.
Biopsy and aspirated materials	Tissue removed at surgery, bone, anticoagulated bone marrow, biopsy samples, or other specimens from normally sterile areas	1 mL of fluid or a 1-g piece of tissue	Sterile "culturette"-type swab or similar transport system containing holding medium. Sterile bottle or jar should be used for tissue specimens.	Accurate identification of specimen and source is critical. Enough tissue should be collected for both microbiologic and histopathologic evaluations.
Wounds	Purulent material or abscess contents obtained from wound or abscess without contamination by normal microflora	2 swabs or 0.5 mL of aspirated pus	Culturette swab or similar transport system or sterile tube with tight-fitting screw cap. For simultaneous anaerobic cultures, send specimen in anaerobic transport device or closed syringe.	*Collection:* Abscess contents or other fluids should be collected in a syringe (see above) when possible to provide an adequate sample volume and an anaerobic environment.
SPECIAL RECOMMENDATIONS				
Fungi	Specimen types listed above may be used. When urine or sputum is cultured for fungi, a first morning specimen is usually preferred.	1 mL or as specified above for individual listing of specimens. Large volumes may be useful for urinary fungi.	Sterile, leak-proof container with tight-fitting cap	*Collection:* Specimen should be transported to microbiology laboratory within 1 h of collection. Contamination with normal flora from skin, rectum, vaginal tract, or other body surfaces should be avoided.
Mycobacterium (acid-fast bacilli)	Sputum, tissue, urine, body fluids	10 mL of fluid or small piece of tissue. Swabs should not be used.	Sterile container with tight-fitting cap	Detection of *Mycobacterium* spp. is improved by use of concentration techniques. Smears and cultures of pleural, peritoneal, and pericardial fluids often have low yields. Multiple cultures from the same patient are encouraged. Culturing in liquid media shortens the time to detection.
Legionella	Pleural fluid, lung biopsy, bronchoalveolar lavage fluid, bronchial/transbronchial biopsy. Rapid transport to laboratory is critical.	1 mL of fluid; any size tissue sample, although a 0.5-g sample should be obtained when possible	—	—
Anaerobic organisms	Aspirated specimens from abscesses or body fluids	1 mL of aspirated fluid or 2 swabs	An appropriate anaerobic transport device is required.[e]	Specimens cultured for obligate anaerobes should be cultured for facultative bacteria as well.

(continued)

Type of Culture (Synonyms)	Specimen	Minimum Volume	Container	Other Considerations

Type of Culture (Synonyms)	Specimen	Minimum Volume	Container	Other Considerations
Viruses[f]	Respiratory secretions, wash aspirates from respiratory tract, nasal swabs, blood samples (including buffy coats), vaginal and rectal swabs, swab specimens from suspicious skin lesions, stool samples (in some cases)	1 mL of fluid, 1 swab, or 1 g of stool in each appropriate transport medium	Fluid or stool samples in sterile containers or swab samples in viral culturette devices (kept on ice but not frozen) are generally suitable. Plasma samples and buffy coats in sterile collection tubes should be kept at 4 to 8°C. If specimens are to be shipped or kept for a long time, freezing at −80°C is usually adequate.	Most samples for culture are transported in holding medium containing antibiotics to prevent bacterial overgrowth and viral inactivation. Many specimens should be kept cool but not frozen, provided they are transported promptly to the laboratory. Procedures and transport media vary with the agent to be cultured and the duration of transport.

[a] For samples from adults and children, two bottles (smaller for pediatric samples) should be used: one with dextrose phosphate, tryptic soy, or another appropriate broth and the other with thioglycollate or another broth containing reducing agents appropriate for isolation of obligate anaerobes. For special situations (e.g., suspected fungal infection, culture-negative endocarditis, or mycobacteremia), different blood collection systems may be used (Isolator systems; see table).

[b] *Collection:* An appropriate disinfecting technique should be used on both the bottle septum and the patient. Do not allow air bubbles to get into anaerobic broth bottles. *Special considerations:* There is no more important clinical microbiology test than the detection of blood-borne pathogens. The rapid identification of bacterial and fungal agents is a major determinant of patients' survival. Bacteria may be present in blood either continuously (as in endocarditis, overwhelming sepsis, and the early stages of salmonellosis and brucellosis) or intermittently (as in most other bacterial infections, in which bacteria are shed into the blood on a sporadic basis). Most blood culture systems employ two separate bottles containing broth medium: one that is vented in the laboratory for the growth of facultative and aerobic organisms and a second that is maintained under anaerobic conditions. In cases of suspected continuous bacteremia/fungemia, two or three samples should be drawn before the start of therapy, with additional sets obtained if fastidious organisms are thought to be involved. For intermittent bacteremia, two or three samples should be obtained at least 1 h apart during the first 24 h.

[c] Normal microflora includes alpha-hemolytic streptococci, saprophytic *Neisseria* spp., diphtheroids, and *Staphylococcus* spp. Aerobic culture of the throat ("routine") includes screening for and identification of beta-hemolytic *Streptococcus* spp. and other potentially pathogenic organisms. Although considered components of the normal microflora, organisms such as *Staphylococcus aureus, Haemophilus influenzae,* and *Streptococcus pneumoniae* will be identified by most laboratories, if requested. When *Neisseria gonorrhoeae* or *Corynebacterium diphtheriae* is suspected, a special culture request is recommended.

[d] (1) Clean-voided specimens, midvoid specimens, and Foley or indwelling catheter specimens that yield ≥50,000 organisms/mL and from which no more than three species are isolated should have organisms identified. (2) Straight-catheterized, bladder-tap, and similar urine specimens should undergo a complete workup (identification and susceptibility testing) for all potentially pathogenic organisms, regardless of colony count. (3) Certain clinical problems (e.g., acute dysuria in women) may warrant identification and susceptibility testing of isolates present at concentrations of <50,000 organisms/mL.

[e] Aspirated specimens in capped syringes or other transport devices designed to limit oxygen exposure are suitable for the cultivation of obligate anaerobes. A variety of commercially available transport devices may be used. Contamination of specimens with normal microflora from the skin, rectum, vaginal vault, or another body site should be avoided. Collection containers for aerobic culture (such as dry swabs) and inappropriate specimens (such as refrigerated samples; expectorated sputum; stool; gastric aspirates; and vaginal, throat, nose, and rectal swabs) should be rejected as unsuitable.

[f] Laboratories generally use diverse methods to detect viral agents, and the specific requirements for each specimen should be checked before a sample is sent.

INDEX

Bold number indicates the start of the chapter that contains the main discussion of the topic; numbers with "f" and "t" refer to figure and table pages and are listed at the end of the entries.

ISBN 0-07-912013-X

90000

9 780079 120137

SETCODE

ISBN 0-07-020292-3

90000

9 780070 202924

VOL 1

TOPICAL CONTENTS